TEXTBOOK OF CRITICAL CARE

Third Edition

Senior Editor:

Stephen M. Ayres, MD, FCCM

Professor of Medicine
Dean Emeritus, School of Medicine
Director, International Health Programs
Virginia Commonwealth University
Medical College of Virginia
Richmond, Virginia

Editors:

Ake Grenvik, MD, PhD, FCCM

Professor of Anesthesiology, Medicine, and Surgery
Director, Multidisciplinary Critical Care Training Program
University of Pittsburgh Medical Center
Pittsburgh, Pennsylvania

Peter R. Holbrook, MD, FCCM

Professor of Anesthesia and Pediatrics
George Washington University School of Medicine
Chairman, Critical Care Medicine
Director, Intensive Care Units
Children's National Medical Center
Washington, D.C.

William C. Shoemaker, MD, FCCM

Professor of Surgery, UCLA School of Medicine
Chairman, Department of Emergency Medicine
Vice Chairman, Department of Surgery
King-Drew Medical Center
Los Angeles, California

W.B. SAUNDERS COMPANY
A Division of Harcourt Brace & Company
Philadelphia London Toronto Montreal Sydney Tokyo

W.B. SAUNDERS COMPANY
A Division of
Harcourt Brace & Company

The Curtis Center
Independence Square West
Philadelphia, Pennsylvania 19106

Library of Congress Cataloging-in-Publication Data

Textbook of critical care / [edited by] William C. Shoemaker . . . [et al.]— 3rd ed.

p. cm.

Includes bibliographical references and index.

ISBN 0–7216–5422–3

1. Critical care medicine. I. Shoemaker, William C. [DNLM: 1. Critical Care. 2. Intensive Care Units. WX 218 T355 1995]

RC86.7.T453 1995

616′.028—dc20

DNLM/DLC 94-27360

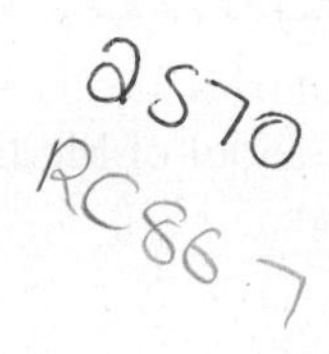

Cover illustration: Molecular model of tumor necrosis factor (cachectin). Courtesy of Stephen R. Sprang, PhD.

Textbook of Critical Care ISBN 0–7216–5422–3

Printed in the United States of America.

Last digit is the print number: 9 8 7 6 5 4 3 2 1

DEDICATED TO

THE FOUNDERS OF THE SOCIETY OF CRITICAL CARE MEDICINE

Who saw so clearly
even though they looked through a darkened glass

and to

Mrs. Norma Shoemaker
Executive Director
Society of Critical Care Medicine

The Society of Critical Care Medicine was founded in 1970 by a group of physicians dedicated to caring for the critically ill and injured. The Society's primary purpose, as envisioned by those founding members, was to improve the quality of critical care multidisciplinary research, education, and patient care.

David Allan, MD*
Henrik Bendixen, MD
Reuben Cherniack, MD
J. Francis Dammann, MD
Louis R.M. Del Guercio, MD, FCCM
John J. Downes, MD
H. Barrie Fairley, MD
Peter L. Frommer, MD
William J. Grace, MD*
Ake Grenvik, MD, PhD, FCCM
John Howard, MD
John M. Kinney, MD
John W. Kirklin, MD
Myron B. Laver, MD*
F. John Lewis, MD
Bernard Lown, MD
Alan Nahum, MD
John J. Osborn, MD
Henning Pontoppidan, MD
Peter Safar, MD, FCCM
William C. Shoemaker, MD, FCCM
Herbert Shubin, MD*
Morely Singer, MD
Paul R. Swyer, MD
Burton A. Waisbren, MD
Max Harry Weil, MD, PhD, FCCM
Robert F. Wilson, MD, FCCM
Peter M. Winter, MD

*Deceased

NOTICE

CONTRIBUTORS

Edward Abraham, MD, FCCM
Section Head, Critical Care Medicine, and Associate Professor, Division of Pulmonary Sciences and Critical Care Medicine, University of Colorado Health Sciences Center; Director, Medical Intensive Care Unit, University Hospital, Denver, Colorado
T and B Cell Function in Critical Illness

Norman S. Abramson, MD
Associate Professor, University of Pittsburgh; Chairman, Department of Emergency Medicine, Cleveland Clinic Foundation, Cleveland, Ohio; Investigator, International Resuscitation Research Center, University of Pittsburgh Medical Center, Pittsburgh, Pennsylvania
Cardiopulmonary-Cerebral Resuscitation

Kareem Abu-Elmagd, MD
Assistant Professor of Surgery, University of Pittsburgh Medical Center; Assistant Professor of Surgery, Pittsburgh Transplant Institute, Pittsburgh, Pennsylvania
Intestinal and Multiple Organ Transplantation

W. Keith Adkins, MD, PhD
Resident Physician, Department of Surgery, University of South Alabama Medical Center, Mobile, Alabama
Regulation of Capillary Exchange of Fluid and Protein

Maurice S. Albin, MD, MSc(Anesth)
Professor of Anesthesiology and Neurological Surgery, University of Texas Health Science Center at San Antonio, San Antonio, Texas
Acute Spinal Cord Trauma

Charles G. Alex, MD
Assistant Professor of Medicine, Loyola University of Chicago, Stritch School of Medicine; Director, Medical and Respiratory Intensive Care Units, Edward Hines, Jr. Veterans Administration Hospital, Hines, Illinois
Assessment of Pulmonary Function in Critically Ill Patients

Harry L. Anderson, III, MD
Assistant Professor of Surgery, University of Pennsylvania School of Medicine; Attending Physician, Division of Trauma and Surgical Critical Care, Department of Surgery, Hospital of the University of Pennsylvania, Philadelphia, Pennsylvania
Extracorporeal and Intravascular Gas Exchange Devices

Derek C. Angus, MB, ChB, MPH, MRCP(UK), FCCP
Assistant Professor of Anesthesiology/Critical Care Medicine, School of Medicine, University of Pittsburgh; Assistant Professor of Anesthesiology/Critical Care Medicine, University of Pittsburgh Medical Center, Presbyterian University Hospital, Pittsburgh, Pennsylvania
Disasters and Critical Care Medicine; Pancreas and Islet Cell Transplantation

John M. Armitage, MD
Mary Washington Hospital, Fredericksburg, Virginia
Intensive Care of the Cardiac Transplant Recipient

Deborah K. Armstrong, PharmD, FCCM
Regional Clinical Manager, Owen Healthcare, Inc., Newport Beach, California
Providing Pharmaceutical Services in Critical Care Areas

Jeffrey S. Augenstein, MD, PhD
Associate Professor of Surgery and Anesthesiology, University of Miami School of Medicine, and Jackson Memorial Hospital, Miami, Florida
Computerization: Solutions to Problems in the Input, Manipulation, and Storage of Intensive Care Unit Data

Raymond F. Austin, Jr., MD
Assistant Professor of Radiology, Medical College of Virginia/Virginia Commonwealth University, Attending Radiologist, Medical College of Virginia Hospital, Richmond, Virginia
Computed Tomography of the Abdomen in the Critical Care Patient

Donald C. Axon, FAIA
Part-time Associate, University of Southern California; Medical Facilities Architect, Los Angeles, California
The Critical Care Unit: Design Recommendations and Standards

Stephen M. Ayres, MD, FCCM
Professor of Medicine, Dean Emeritus, School of Medicine, and Director, International Health Programs, Medical College of Virginia/Virginia Commonwealth University, Richmond, Virginia
The Promise of Critical Care: Effective and Humane Care in an Era of Cost Containment; Infection with HIV, AIDS, and the Intensive Care Unit; The Hyperthermic Syndromes; The Ethics of Resource Allocation in the Intensive Care Unit

Timothy J. Babineau, MD
Instructor in Surgery, Harvard Medical School; Deaconess-Harvard Surgical Service; Instructor, Department of Surgery, Deaconess Hospital, Boston, Massachusetts
Total Parenteral Nutrition: Priorities and Practice

Edward D. Ball, MD
Professor of Medicine, University of Pittsburgh School of Medicine; Chief, Division of Hematology/Bone Marrow Transplant;

Director, Bone Marrow Transplantation Program, University of Pittsburgh Medical Center, Pittsburgh, Pennsylvania
Bone Marrow Transplantation

Nils U. Bang, MD
Professor of Medicine and Pathology, Indiana University School of Medicine; Attending Physician, Indiana University Hospitals; Department of Medicine, Hematology/Oncology Section, Indiana University Medical Center, Indianapolis, Indiana
Thrombolytic Therapy in Acute Myocardial Infarction; Diagnosis and Management of Bleeding Disorders

Steven J. Barker, PhD, MD
Professor and Chairman, University of California at Irvine, Orange, California
Anesthesia in the High-Risk Patient

William H. Barth, Jr., MD
Assistant Professor of Obstetrics and Gynecology, Uniformed Services University of the Health Sciences, F. Edward Hébert School of Medicine, Bethesda, Maryland; Chief of Obstetrics, Wilford Hall Medical Center, San Antonio, Texas
Critical Care Medicine and the Obstetric Patient

Robert H. Bartlett, MD
Professor of Surgery, University of Michigan Medical School; Attending Physician, and Division Chief of Critical Care, Section of General Surgery, and Director, Surgical Intensive Care Unit, University of Michigan Medical Center, Ann Arbor, Michigan
Extracorporeal and Intravascular Gas Exchange Devices

Claudia Bartz, PhD, RN
Chief, Department of Nursing Science, and Colonel, Army Nurse Corps, Army Medical Department Center and School, Fort Sam Houston, Texas
Families in Critical Care: Environment, Needs, and Barriers to Care

Donald P. Becker, MD
Professor and Chief, Division of Neurosurgery, UCLA School of Medicine; Attending Physician at UCLA Medical Center, VA Medical Center, Harbor Medical Center, Los Angeles, California
Intracranial Pressure Monitoring

Paul E. Bellamy, MD
Professor of Medicine, UCLA School of Medicine, Los Angeles, California; Medical Director, Medical Intensive Care Unit, Medical Advisor, Respiratory Therapy Department; and Medical Director, Medical Observation Unit, UCLA Medical Center, Los Angeles, California
Preventing Complications in the Intensive Care Unit

Rinaldo Bellomo, MBBS, MD, FRACP
Full-Time Staff Specialist and Coordinator of Intensive Care Research, Intensive Care Unit, Austin Hospital, Heidelberg, Victoria, Australia
Hemofiltration; Drug-Kidney Interactions

Michael K. Belz, MD
Clinical Instructor, Medical College of Virginia/Virginia Commonwealth University; Attending Physician, McGuire Veterans Affairs Hospital; Private Consultant, Richmond, Virginia
Pacemakers and Implantable Cardioverter Defibrillators in the Intensive Care Unit Setting

Marvin Bergsneider, MD
Assistant Professor, Division of Neurosurgery, UCLA School of Medicine, Los Angeles; Attending Surgeon, UCLA Medical Center, Los Angeles; Attending Surgeon, Harbor-UCLA Medical Center, Torrance, California
Intracranial Pressure Monitoring

Gordon R. Bernard, MD
Professor of Medicine, Vanderbilt University School of Medicine; Director, Medical Intensive Care Unit, Vanderbilt University Medical Center, Nashville, Tennessee
Increased Lung Vascular Permeability: Mediators and Therapies

Bruce Beutler, MD
Associate Investigator, Howard Hughes Medical Institute; Associate Professor of Internal Medicine, University of Texas Southwestern Medical Center at Dallas, Dallas, Texas
Endotoxin-Induced Factors That Provoke Shock and Their Receptors

Morris I. Bierman, MD
Associate Professor of Anesthesia/Critical Care Medicine, University of Pittsburgh School of Medicine; Director, Cardiothoracic Intensive Care Unit, Presbyterian University Hospital, Pittsburgh, Pennsylvania
Transesophageal Echocardiography; Independent Lung Ventilation; Lung Transplantation: Thirty Years of Progress

Nicholas G. Bircher, MD
Assistant Professor, University of Pittsburgh; Associate Director, Surgical Intensive Care Unit; Staff Anesthesiologist, Montefiore University Hospital; Associate Director, International Resuscitation Research Center, University of Pittsburgh Medical Center, Pittsburgh, Pennsylvania
Cardiopulmonary-Cerebral Resuscitation

Carole Birdsall, EdD, RN, CCRN
Associate Professor, Hunter Bellevue School of Nursing, City University; Staff Nurse Per Diem, Critical Care Division, The New York Hospital, Cornell Medical Center, New York, New York
Aspects of Critical Care Nursing Practice: Looking Back to Face the Challenge of the Future

Michael H. Bishop, DO
Assistant Professor of Surgery and Emergency Medicine, Charles R. Drew University of Medicine and Health Sciences Center; Staff Trauma Surgeon and Emergency Physician, King-Drew Medical Center, Los Angeles, California
Clinical Algorithms for Resuscitation in Acute Emergency Conditions

George L. Blackburn, MD, PhD
Associate Professor of Surgery, Harvard Medical School; Director, Nutrition Support Service, Deaconess Hospital, Boston, Massachusetts
Total Parenteral Nutrition: Priorities and Practice

Thomas P. Bleck, MD, FCCM
Associate Professor of Neurology and Neurological Surgery, The John T. and Louise Nerancy Professor in Neurology, University of Virginia; Director, Neuroscience Intensive Care Unit, University of Virginia, Charlottesville, Virginia
Seizures in the Critically Ill; Neuromuscular Disorders in Critical Care

Elana J. Bloom, MD
Assistant Professor of Medicine, University of Pittsburgh School of Medicine; Staff Physician, University of Pittsburgh Medical Center, Pittsburgh, Pennsylvania
Bone Marrow Transplantation

Glenn H. Bock, MD
Associate Professor of Pediatrics, F. Edward Hébert School of Medicine, Uniformed Services University of the Health Sciences, Bethesda, Maryland; Medical Co-Director, Pediatric Kidney Center, Fairfax Hospital for Children, Fairfax, Virginia
Acute Renal Failure in Infants and Children

Philip G. Boysen, MD, FACP, FCCM
Professor and Chairman, Department of Anesthesiology, School of Medicine, University of North Carolina at Chapel Hill, Chapel Hill, North Carolina
Near-Drowning: Adults and Children; Pulmonary Aspiration of Stomach Contents

Pierre G. Braquet, PhD, DSc
General and Research Manager, Institut Henri Beaufour, Robinson, France
Platelet-Activating Factor in Septic Shock

Gordon L. Bray, MD
Director of Clinical Development, Baxter Biotech–Hyland Division, Glendale, California
Bleeding Disorders of Childhood

David Bregman, MD, FACC, FACS
Senior Cardiothoracic Surgeon and Professor of Clinical Surgery, Columbia University College of Physicians and Surgeons; Attending Surgeon, Presbyterian Hospital, New York, New York; Cardiothoracic Surgeon, St. Joseph's Medical Center, Paterson; and Passaic Hospital, Passaic, New Jersey
Intra-Aortic Balloon Counterpulsation

Kenneth L. Brigham, MD
Professor of Medicine, Vanderbilt University School of Medicine; The Joe and Morris Werthan Professor of Investigative Medicine, and Director, Division of Pulmonary and Critical Care Medicine, Vanderbilt University, Nashville, Tennessee
Increased Lung Vascular Permeability: Mediators and Therapies

Timothy J. Broderick, MD
Cardiovascular Research Fellow, Medical College of Virginia/Virginia Commonwealth University, Richmond, Virginia
Ventricular Assist Devices and Artificial Hearts

Brian A. Broznick, CPTC
Executive Director, Center for Organ Recovery and Education, Pittsburgh, Pennsylvania
History and Organization of Organ Transplantation

D. A. Bruce, MB, ChB
Clinical Associate Professor of Neurosurgery, The University of Texas Southwestern Medical School; Attending Neurosurgeon, Department of Neurosurgery, Childrens Medical Center of Dallas, Dallas, Texas
Pediatric Neurosurgical Emergencies

Christopher W. Bryan-Brown, MD, FCCM
Professor of Anesthesiology, Albert Einstein College of Medicine, Yeshiva University; Vice Chairman, Department of Anesthesiology, Montefiore Medical Center, Bronx, New York
Pulmonary Gas Exchange, Transport, and Delivery

Timothy G. Buchman, PhD, MD, FACS, FCCM
Professor of Surgery, Washington University School of Medicine, and Chief, Burns/Trauma/Critical Care, Barnes Hospital, St. Louis, Missouri
Regulation of Gene Expression

Ross Bullock, MD, PhD
Lind Lawrence Associate Professor, Division of Neurosurgery, Medical College of Virginia/Virginia Commonwealth University, Richmond, Virginia
Management of Head Trauma

David J. Burchfield, MD
Associate Professor of Pediatrics, University of Florida College of Medicine, Gainesville, Florida
Pediatric Resuscitation

Mitchell S. Cairo, MD, FAAP
Director of Hematology/Oncology Research and Bone Marrow Transplantation, and Chairman, Pediatric Subspecialty Faculty, Children's Hospital of Orange County, Orange, California
Colony-Stimulating Factors

James E. Calvin, MD, FRCPS, FACC
Associate Professor of Medicine, Rush Medical College; Director, Coronary Care Unit, Rush-Presbyterian-St. Luke's Medical Center, Chicago, Illinois
Applied Cardiovascular Physiology in the Critically Ill

Wayne N. Campbell, MD
Assistant Professor of Medicine, Division of Infectious Diseases, R. Adams Cowley Shock Trauma Center, University of Maryland School of Medicine, Baltimore, Maryland
Prevention and Management of Infections in Critically Ill Trauma Victims and Patients with Hematologic Malignancies

Robert L. Carithers, Jr., MD
Professor of Medicine, and Director, Hepatology Services, University of Washington Medical Center, Seattle, Washington
Severe Liver Disease

Graziano C. Carlon, MD
Professor of Clinical Anesthesiology, Cornell University Medical College; Chief, Critical Care Medicine Service, Department of Anesthesiology and Critical Care Medicine, Memorial-Sloan-Kettering Cancer Center, New York, New York
Intensive Care of the Cancer Patient

Richard W. Carlson, MD, PhD
Department of Medicine, University of Illinois College of Medicine, Peoria, Illinois
Building Bedside Collaborative Practice

Adrian Casavilla, MD
Assistant Professor of Surgery, University of Pittsburgh Medical Center; Assistant Professor of Surgery, Pittsburgh Transplant Institute, Pittsburgh, Pennsylvania
Intestinal and Multiple Organ Transplantation

Ned H. Cassem, MD
Associate Professor of Psychiatry, Harvard Medical School; Chief of Psychiatry, Massachusetts General Hospital, Boston, Massachusetts
Psychiatric Problems of the Critically Ill Patient

Donna A. Castello, DO
Instructor and Assistant Attending Physician, Department of Anesthesiology, Albany Medical Center, Albany, New York
Conventional Airway Access

Leo A. Celi, MD
Fellow, Infectious Disease, Harvard Medical School; Fellowship Combined Harvard Infectious Disease Program, Beth Israel Hospital, Boston, Massachusetts
Toxic Shock Syndrome

John M. Chandler, MD
Assistant Professor, Uniformed Services University of Health Sciences; Director of Critical Care Education, National Naval Medical Center, Bethesda, Maryland
Independent Lung Ventilation

Lakshmipathi Chelluri, MD
Associate Professor of Anesthesiology/Critical Care Medicine and Medicine, School of Medicine, University of Pittsburgh; Director, Surgical Intensive Care Unit, Presbyterian-University Hospital, University of Pittsburgh Medical Center, Pittsburgh, Pennsylvania
Critical Care of Kidney Transplant Recipients

Bart Chernow, MD, FACP
Professor of Medicine, Anesthesia and Critical Care, The Johns Hopkins University School of Medicine; Physician-in-Chief, Department of Medicine, Sinai Hospital of Baltimore, Baltimore, Maryland
Adrenal Dysfunction in the Intensive Care Unit

John William Christman, MD
Associate Professor of Medicine, Vanderbilt University; Director, Medical Intensive Care Unit, Veterans Affairs Medical Center, Nashville, Tennessee
Pulmonary Host Defense and Inflammatory Lung Disease

Michael J. Cinoman, MD
Fellow, Children's Hospital of Pittsburgh, Pittsburgh, Pennsylvania
Neonatal and Pediatric Transport Programs

Cathleen Clancy, MD
Clinical Instructor, Department of Emergency Medicine, National Capital Poison Center, Georgetown University, Washington, District of Columbia; Medical Director, Maryland Poison Center, Maryland University, Baltimore, Maryland
Poisoning

Terry P. Clemmer, MD
Professor of Medicine, University of Utah; Director of Critical Care, LDS Hospital, Salt Lake City, Utah
Computers in the Intensive Care Unit: A Match Meant to Be!

Jacqueline J. Coalson, PhD
Professor of Pathology, University of Texas Health Science Center at San Antonio, San Antonio, Texas
Pathophysiologic Features of Infant and Adult Respiratory Distress Syndromes; Bacterial Pneumonia in Adult Respiratory Distress Syndrome

Patricia E. Cole, PhD, MD
Assistant Professor of Radiology, Medical College of Virginia/Virginia Commonwealth University; Assistant Professor of Radiology, Medical College of Virginia Hospitals, Richmond, Virginia
Interventional Radiology in the Critically Ill

Arthur H. Combs, MD, FCCM
Associate Professor of Medicine, Medical College of Pennsylvania; Director, Medical Intensive Care Unit, Medical College Hospitals, Medical College of Pennsylvania, Philadelphia, Pennsylvania
Critical Care Practice in the Era of Consumerism

Alasdair K. T. Conn, MD, FACS
Assistant Professor of Surgery, Harvard Medical School; Chief of Emergency Services and Visiting Surgeon, Massachusetts General Hospital, Boston, Massachusetts
Transport of the Critically Ill Patient

James A. Cook, PhD
Professor of Physiology, Medical University of South Carolina, Charleston, South Carolina
Prostaglandins, Thromboxanes, Leukotrienes, and Other Products of Arachidonic Acid

Arthur Cooper, MD
Associate Professor of Clinical Surgery, College of Physicians and Surgeons of Columbia University; Chief of Pediatric Surgical Critical Care, Harlem Hospital Center, New York, New York
Pediatric Trauma (Basic Principles)

Lynn Coppage, MD
Assistant Professor of Radiology, Medical University of South Carolina; Attending Physician, Medical University Hospital, Charleston Memorial Hospital, and Ralph H. Johnson Veterans Administration Medical Center, Charleston, South Carolina
Imaging of the Chest in the Intensive Care Setting

Paul Corso, MD, FACS, FACC
Associate Clinical Professor, George Washington University; Senior Attending Physician, Washington Adventist Hospital, Senior Attending Physician, Vice Chairman, Department of Surgery, and Acting Chief, Division of Cardiac Surgery, Washington Hospital Center, Washington, District of Columbia
Postoperative Care of the Adult Cardiac Surgical Patient

Joseph M. Darby, MD
Associate Professor of Anesthesiology/Critical Care Medicine, University of Pittsburgh School of Medicine; Director, Trauma/Neurology Intensive Care Unit, Presbyterian University Hospital, Pittsburgh, Pennsylvania
Controversies in Brain Death Certification; Organ Donor Categories and Management

Lakshmana Das Narla, MD
Associate Professor, Departments of Radiology and Pediatrics, Medical College of Virginia/Virginia Commonwealth University, Richmond, Virginia
Chest Imaging in Pediatric Intensive Care

Joseph F. Dasta, MSc(Pharm), FCCM, FCCP
Associate Professor, The Ohio State University, College of Pharmacy, Columbus, Ohio
Providing Pharmaceutical Services in Critical Care Areas

James Dauber, MD
Professor of Medicine, University of Pittsburgh, Pittsburgh, Pennsylvania
Lung Transplantation: Thirty Years of Progress

Guy de Lisle Dear, MB, FRCA
Assistant Professor of Anesthesiology, Duke University; Attend-

ing Anesthesiologist, Duke University Medical Center, Durham, North Carolina
Hyperbaric Oxygen in Critical Care

R. Phillip Dellinger, MD, MSc
Professor and Director, Pulmonary and Critical Care Medicine, University of Missouri–Columbia; Chief, Pulmonary and Critical Care Medicine, Harry S. Truman Veterans Administration Hospital, Columbia, Missouri
Fiberoptic Bronchoscopy in Critical Care Medicine

Margarida deMagalhaes-Silverman, MD
Assistant Professor of Medicine, University of Pittsburgh School of Medicine; Staff Physician, University of Pittsburgh Medical Center, Pittsburgh, Pennsylvania
Bone Marrow Transplantation

Robert H. Demling, MD
Professor of Surgery, Harvard University, Cambridge; Director, Longwood Area Trauma Center, Brigham and Women's Hospital, Boston, Massachusetts
Management of the Burn Patient; Smoke Inhalation Injury; Hypothermia and Cold-Related Injuries

Michael A. DeVita, MD
Assistant Professor of Anesthesiology/Critical Care Medicine, University of Pittsburgh School of Medicine; Director, Surgical Intensive Care Unit, Montefiore University Hospital and University of Pittsburgh Medical Center, Pittsburgh, Pennsylvania
Foregoing Life-Sustaining Therapy in Intensive Care

Donald J. Deyo, DVM
Assistant Professor, Department of Anesthesiology, University of Texas Medical Branch at Galveston, Galveston, Texas
Brain Function Monitoring

David J. Diehl, MD
Assistant Professor of Psychiatry, University of Pittsburgh School of Medicine, Pittsburgh, Pennsylvania
Positron Emission Tomography: Basic Principles and Potential Applications in the Critically Ill

Bruce Dobkin, MD
Professor of Clinical Neurology, UCLA School of Medicine; Director, Neurological Rehabilitation Program, UCLA Medical Plaza, Los Angeles, California
Cerebral Vascular Emergencies

Forrest Dodson, MD
Assistant Professor of Surgery, Department of Surgery, University of Pittsburgh School of Medicine; Staff Member, Presbyterian University Hospital, Pittsburgh, Pennsylvania
Future of Transplantation (Including Xenografting)

Michael Donahoe, MD
Assistant Professor of Medicine, University of Pittsburgh School of Medicine; Director, Medical Intensive Care Unit, Presbyterian University Hospital, Pittsburgh, Pennsylvania
Acute Respiratory Failure in Chronic Obstructive Pulmonary Disease

Albert D. Donnenberg, PhD
Assistant Professor of Medicine and Research Director, Bone Marrow Transplant Program, University of Pittsburgh School of Medicine, Pittsburgh, Pennsylvania
Bone Marrow Transplantation

John B. Downs, MD
Professor and Chairman, Department of Anesthesiology, University of South Florida College of Medicine; Chief, Department of Anesthesiology, Tampa General Hospital, Tampa, Florida
Airway Pressure Therapy

John J. Downes, MD
Professor of Anesthesia and Pediatrics, University of Pennsylvania School of Medicine; Director, Department of Anesthesiology and Critical Care Medicine, The Children's Hospital of Philadelphia, Philadelphia, Pennsylvania
Distal Airway Disorders in Infants and Children: Bronchiolitis and Asthma

Howard R. Doyle, MD
Assistant Professor of Surgery, University of Pittsburgh School of Medicine; Medical Director, Section of Computational Medicine, Pittsburgh Transplantation Institute, University of Pittsburgh Medical Center, Pittsburgh, Pennsylvania
Multiple Organ Procurement

Jeffrey M. Drazen, MD
Professor of Medicine, Harvard Medical School; Chief, Respiratory Division, Brigham and Women's Hospital, Boston, Massachusetts
Life-Threatening Asthma

Rodney M. Durham, MD
Assistant Professor of Surgery, Department of Surgery, Division of Trauma Service and Surgical Critical Care, St. Louis University, St. Louis, Missouri
Abdominal and Pelvic Trauma

Christopher Eager, MD
Cardiovascular Surgeon, Washington Hospital Center; Cardiovascular and Thoracic Surgeon, Cardiovascular and Thoracic Surgical Associates, Washington, D.C.
Postoperative Care of the Adult Cardiac Surgical Patient

Thomas D. East, PhD
Associate Professor of Anesthesiology, Bioengineering and Medical Informatics, University of Utah; Director of Informatics Research, Pulmonary Division, LDS Hospital, Salt Lake City, Utah
Computerized Management of Mechanical Ventilation

David H. Ebb, MD
Instructor in Pediatrics, Harvard University; Assistant Pediatrician, Massachusetts General Hospital, Boston, Massachusetts
Bleeding Disorders of Childhood

Frederick J. Ehlert, PhD
Associate Professor, College of Medicine, University of California, Irvine, California
Receptor Physiology

Kenneth A. Ellenbogen, MD
Associate Professor of Medicine and Director of Cardiac Electrophysiology, Medical College of Virginia/Virginia Commonwealth University, and McGuire Veterans Administration Medical Center, Richmond, Virginia
Pacemakers and Implantable Cardioverter Defibrillators in the Intensive Care Unit Setting

I. Alan Fein, MD
President, Critical Care Management Consultants, Albany, New York; Intensivist, Baptist Hospital of Miami, Miami, Florida
The Utilization and Allocation of Critical Care Resources

Sandra L. Fein, MA, RN
Doctoral Candidate, Organizational Studies, State University of New York at Albany; Community Psychologist/Management Consultant, Critical Care Management Consultants, Inc., Albany, New York
The Utilization and Allocation of Critical Care Resources

Mitchell P. Fink, MD
Associate Professor of Surgery, Harvard Medical School; Chief, Division of Trauma and Surgical Critical Care, Beth Israel Hospital, Boston, Massachusetts
Failure of the Gastrointestinal Tract Barrier

Charles J. Fisher, Jr., MD, FCCM
Professor of Medicine, Ohio State University School of Medicine; Head, Section of Critical Care Medicine and Director, Critical Care Research Unit, Department of Pulmonary and Critical Care Medicine, The Cleveland Clinic Foundation, Cleveland, Ohio
Toxic Shock Syndrome

Alpha A. Fowler, III, MD
Professor of Medicine and Director of Research, Division of Pulmonary and Critical Care Medicine, Medical College of Virginia/Virginia Commonwealth University, Richmond, Virginia
The Structural Basis of Pulmonary Function

Arthur M. Freedman, MD
Assistant Professor of Radiology, Medical College of Virginia Hospitals; Attending Radiologist, Medical College of Virginia/Virginia Commonwealth University, Richmond, Virginia
Interventional Radiology in the Critically Ill

Bradley P. Fuhrman, MD
Professor of Pediatrics and Anesthesiology and Chief, Division of Pediatric Critical Care, Children's Hospital of Buffalo, Buffalo, New York
Congestive Heart Failure in Infants and Children

John J. Fung, MD, PhD
Chief, Division of Transplant Surgery, and Associate Professor of Surgery, Department of Surgery, University of Pittsburgh; Chief, Division of Transplant Surgery, Presbyterian University Hospital and University of Pittsburgh Medical Center, Pittsburgh, Pennsylvania
Principles of Immunosuppression; Intensive Care of Liver Transplant Recipients; Future of Transplantation (Including Xenografting)

T. James Gallagher, MD, FCCP, FCCM
Professor of Anesthesiology and Surgery, University of Florida College of Medicine; Chief, Division of Critical Care Medicine, Shands Hospital, Gainesville, Florida
Sedatives and Muscle Relaxants in the Intensive Care Unit

Tomas Ganz, PhD, MD
Professor of Medicine, Department of Medicine, UCLA School of Medicine, Los Angeles, California
Macrophage Function

Reed M. Gardner, PhD
Professor of Medical Informatics, University of Utah; Co-Director of Medical Informatics, LDS Hospital, Salt Lake City, Utah
Electrocardiography and Pressure Monitoring: How to Obtain Optimal Results; Computerized Management of Mechanical Ventilation; Computers in the Intensive Care Unit: A Match Meant to Be!

Edward R. Garrity, Jr., MD
Associate Professor of Clinical Medicine, Stritch School of Medicine, Loyola University; Section Chief, Pulmonary and Critical Care Medicine, Foster G. McGraw Hospital; Medical Director, Lung Transplant Program, Pulmonary Function Laboratory, Loyola University Medical Center, Maywood, Illinois
Weaning from Mechanical Ventilation

Raúl J. Gazmuri, MD, PhD
Instructor, Finch University of Health Sciences, The Chicago Medical School; Director of Research, Medical Service and Staff Member of the Critical Care Section, North Chicago Veterans Administration Medical Center, North Chicago, Illinois
Options for Augmenting the Efficacy of Closed-Chest Cardiopulmonary Resuscitation

Todd W. B. Gehr, MD
Associate Professor of Medicine, Division of Nephrology, Department of Internal Medicine, and Director of Acute Dialysis, Medical College of Virginia/Virginia Commonwealth University, Richmond, Virginia
Clinical Assessment of Renal Function; Adult Acute and Chronic Renal Failure

Janet Geisel, MSN, RN
PhD Candidate, Medical University of South Carolina, Charleston, South Carolina
Prostaglandins, Thromboxanes, Leukotrienes, and Other Products of Arachidonic Acid

Jeffrey A. Gelfand, MD
Acting Chairman and Professor of Medicine, Department of Medicine, Tufts University School of Medicine; Associate Physician-in-Chief, New England Medical Center, Boston, Massachusetts
Cytokines

Eileen R. Gillan, MD
Assistant Professor of Pediatrics, University of Connecticut; Attending Physician, Department of Pediatric Hematology and Oncology, John Dempsey Hospital, Farmington, Connecticut
Colony-Stimulating Factors

Salvatore R. Goodwin, MD
Associate Professor of Anesthesiology and Pediatrics, Medical Director, Pediatric Intensive Care, and Program Director, Pediatric Critical Care Medicine, University of Florida, Gainesville, Florida
Near-Drowning: Adults and Children

A. Gerson Greenburg, MD, PhD
Professor of Surgery, Brown University School of Medicine; Surgeon-in-Chief, The Miriam Hospital, Providence, Rhode Island
Intraoperative and Postoperative Transfusion Therapy

George A. Gregory, MD
Professor of Anesthesia and Pediatrics, University of California, San Francisco, California
Resuscitation of the Newborn

Ake Grenvik, MD, PhD, FCCM
Professor of Anesthesiology, Medicine, and Surgery, University of Pittsburgh School of Medicine; Director, Multidisciplinary

Critical Care Training Program, University of Pittsburgh Medical Center, Pittsburgh, Pennsylvania
Air Embolization; Laryngotracheal Injury from Prolonged Tracheal Intubation; Surgical Airway, Cricothyroidotomy, and Tracheotomy: Procedures, Complications, and Outcome; Controversies in Brain Death Certification; History and Organization of Organ Transplantation; Organ Donor Categories and Management; Future of Transplantation (Including Xenografting); Foregoing Life-Sustaining Therapy in Intensive Care

Bartley P. Griffith, MD
Professor of Surgery, University of Pittsburgh School of Medicine; Chief, Division of Cardiothoracic Surgery, University of Pittsburgh Medical Center, Pittsburgh, Pennsylvania
Intensive Care of the Cardiac Transplant Recipient; Lung Transplantation: Thirty Years of Progress

Anthony H. Guarino, MD
Resident in Anesthesia, Department of Anesthesia, Johns Hopkins University School of Medicine, Baltimore, Maryland
Adrenal Dysfunction in the Intensive Care Unit

Philippe Guinot, MD
General and Clinical Manager, Institut Henri Beaufour, Paris, France
Platelet-Activating Factor in Septic Shock

Guillermo Gutiérrez, PhD, MD, FCCM
Professor of Medicine, University of Texas Health Science Center; Division Director, Pulmonary and Critical Care Medicine, Hermann Hospital, Houston, Texas
Tissue Oxygenation and High-Energy Phosphate Metabolism; Pulmonary Gas Exchange, Transport, and Delivery

David W. Haas, MD
Assistant Professor of Medicine, Vanderbilt University School of Medicine; Director of Clinical Infectious Diseases, Vanderbilt University Medical Center, Nashville, Tennessee
Central Nervous System Infections

Steven M. Hall, MD
Attending Radiologist, Sentara Hampton General Hospital, Hampton, Virginia
Computed Tomography of the Abdomen in the Critical Care Patient

Perry V. Halushka, PhD, MD
Professor of Pharmacology and Medicine, Medical University of South Carolina, Charleston, South Carolina
Prostaglandins, Thromboxanes, Leukotrienes, and Other Products of Arachidonic Acid

Jiho Han, MD
Instructor in Medicine, and Fellow in Interventional Cardiology and Critical Care Medicine, Medical College of Virginia/Virginia Commonwealth University, Richmond, Virginia
Echocardiography in Critical Care

Gary D. V. Hankins, MD
Professor, Obstetrics and Gynecology, F. Edward Hébert School of Medicine, Uniformed Services University of the Health Sciences, Bethesda, Maryland; Chairman, Department of Obstetrics and Gynecology, Wilford Hall Medical Center, Lackland Air Force Base, Texas
Critical Care Medicine and the Obstetric Patient

Robert L. Hardesty, MD
Professor of Surgery, Division of Cardiothoracic Surgery, University of Pittsburgh School of Medicine, Pittsburgh, Pennsylvania
Intensive Care of the Cardiac Transplant Recipient; Lung Transplantation: Thirty Years of Progress

John M. Harlan, MD
Professor and Head, Division of Hematology, University of Washington, Seattle, Washington
Neutrophil-Endothelial Cell Interactions

Geoffrey O. Hartzler, MD, FACC
Clinical Professor of Medicine, University of Missouri; Medical Director, Cardiovascular Clinical Research Center, Mid-America Heart Institute of St. Luke's Hospital, Kansas City, Missouri
Interventional Therapies for Cardiogenic Shock

Maurene A. Harvey, RN, MPH, CCRN, FCCM
Consultants in Critical Care, Inc., Glendale, California
The Critical Care Unit: Design Recommendations and Standards; Building Bedside Collaborative Practice

Andrea Hastillo, MD
Associate Professor of Medicine, Medical College of Virginia/Virginia Commonwealth University; Attending Physician, Medical College of Virginia Hospitals, Richmond, Virginia
Diagnosis and Treatment of Cardiac Arrhythmias

Elizabeth A. Henneman, RN, MS, CCRN
Assistant Clinical Professor, UCLA School of Nursing; Clinical Nurse Specialist, Medical Intensive Care Unit, UCLA Medical Center, Los Angeles, California
Preventing Complications in the Intensive Care Unit

Daniel A. Henry, MD
Chairman, Division of Diagnostic Radiology, Department of Radiology, Medical College of Virginia/Virginia Commonwealth University, Richmond, Virginia
Imaging of the Chest in the Intensive Care Setting

Lynn J. Hernan, MD
Assistant Professor of Pediatrics and Anesthesiology; Director, Critical Care Resident Education, and Associate Director, Pediatric Critical Care, Children's Hospital of Buffalo, Buffalo, New York
Congestive Heart Failure in Infants and Children

Carl Anthony Hess, MD
Assistant Clinical Professor and Director, Pain Management Center, Department of Anesthesiology, Irvine Medical Center, University of California, Orange, California
Acute Pain in the Intensive Care Unit

Michael L. Hess, MD
Professor of Medicine, Medical College of Virginia/Virginia Commonwealth University; Attending Physician, Medical College of Virginia Hospitals, Richmond, Virginia
Diagnosis and Treatment of Cardiac Arrhythmias

Rosemary Hickey, MD
Associate Professor of Anesthesiology, University of Texas Health Science Center at San Antonio, San Antonio, Texas
Acute Spinal Cord Trauma

Peter R. Holbrook, MD, FCCM
Professor of Anesthesia and Pediatrics, George Washington University School of Medicine; Chairman, and Critical Care Medicine Director, Intensive Care Units, Children's National Medical Center, Washington, D.C.
Caring for a Child in an Adult Intensive Care Unit; Evaluation of the Child After Resuscitation and Stabilization

Elizabeth Hingsbergen, MD
Assistant Professor, Department of Radiology, Medical College of Virginia/Virginia Commonwealth University, Richmond, Virginia
Chest Imaging in Pediatric Intensive Care

Chester B. Hollinger, Jr., MD
Attending Physician, Department of Critical Care, St. Francis Medical Center, Pittsburgh, Pennsylvania
Capnography and Respiratory Monitoring

Karen W. Hollingsworth, RN, MS, CCRN
Clinical Director of Nursing, Critical Care GENESYS, Regional Medical Center, Flint, Michigan
Electrocardiography and Pressure Monitoring: How to Obtain Optimal Results

David Hosford, PhD
Director of Communications, Beaufour-Ipsen, Robinson, France
Platelet-Activating Factor in Septic Shock

John W. Hoyt, MD, FCCM
Clinical Professor of Anesthesiology and Critical Care, University of Pittsburgh; Chairman, Critical Care Department, St. Francis Medical Center, Pittsburgh, Pennsylvania
The Critical Care Unit: Design Recommendations and Standards; Capnography and Respiratory Monitoring

Eric H. Hubli, MD
Associate Craniomaxillofacial Surgeon, International Craniofacial Institute, Cleft Lip and Palate Treatment Center, Dallas, Texas
Hypothermia and Cold-Related Injuries

Christophe Van Huffel, PhD
Research Associate, Howard Hughes Medical Institute, University of Texas Southwestern Medical Center, Dallas, Texas
Endotoxin-Induced Factors That Provoke Shock and Their Receptors

Russell D. Hull, MBBS, MSc
Professor, University of Calgary; Director, Clinical Trials Unit, Foothills Hospital, Calgary, Alberta, Canada
Treatment of Massive Pulmonary Embolism; Diagnosis and Treatment of Venous Thromboembolism

Thomas K. Hunt, MD
Professor of Surgery and Vice Chairman for Research Affairs, Department of Surgery, University of California, San Francisco, California
Critical Care of Wounds and Wounded Patients

Louis J. Ignarro, PhD
Professor of Pharmacology, UCLA School of Medicine, Los Angeles, California
Physiologic and Pathophysiologic Significance of Nitric Oxide

Robert M. Jackson, MD
Associate Professor of Medicine, Division of Pulmonary and Critical Care Medicine, University of Alabama at Birmingham; Staff Physician, Pulmonary Section/Department of Medicine, Veterans Administration Medical Center, Birmingham, Alabama
Oxygen Therapy and Toxicity

Judith Jacobi, PharmD, FCCM
Affiliate Assistant Professor of Clinical Pharmacy, Purdue University, West Lafayette, Indiana; Adjunct Assistant Professor of Pharmacy Practice, Butler University, Indianapolis, Indiana; Critical Care Pharmacy Specialist, St. Vincent Hospital, Indianapolis, Indiana
Providing Pharmaceutical Services in Critical Care Areas

Michael R. Jacobs, MB, BCh, PhD, MRC Path
Professor, Pathology Department, Case Western Reserve University School of Medicine; Director, Clinical Microbiology Department, University Hospitals of Cleveland, Cleveland, Ohio
Laboratory Diagnosis of Infection

Khursheed N. Jeejeebhoy, MB, BS, PhD, FRCP(C)
Professor of Medicine and Senior Staff Physician, University of Toronto and St. Michael's Hospital, Toronto, Ontario, Canada
Nutrition in Critical Illness

Dennis M. Jensen, MD
Professor of Medicine, Division of Gastroenterology, UCLA Medical Center, Los Angeles, California
Severe Gastrointestinal Hemorrhage

Howard Jolles, MD
Associate Professor, Division of Diagnostic Radiology, Department of Radiology, Medical College of Virginia/Virginia Commonwealth University, Richmond, Virginia
Imaging of the Chest in the Intensive Care Setting

Robert M. Kacmarek, PhD, RRT
Assistant Professor, Department of Anesthesia, Harvard Medical School; Director, Respiratory Care, Massachusetts General Hospital, Boston, Massachusetts
Principles of Respiratory Care

Allen B. Kaiser, MD
Professor of Medicine, Vanderbilt University School of Medicine; Vice Chairman for Clinical Affairs, Department of Medicine, Vanderbilt University Medical Center, Nashville, Tennessee
Central Nervous System Infections

Peter W. Kakavas, MD
Instructor, Rush Medical College; Fellow, Cardiology, Rush-Presbyterian-St. Luke's Medical Center, Chicago, Illinois
Applied Cardiovascular Physiology in the Critically Ill

Yoogoo Kang, MD
Professor of Anesthesiology and Critical Care Medicine, University of Pittsburgh School of Medicine; Director, Hepatic Transplantation Anesthesiology Division, University of Pittsburgh Medical Center, Pittsburgh, Pennsylvania
Multiple Organ Procurement

Jill D. Kaplan, MD
Instructor in Neurology, Harvard Medical School; Assistant in Neurology, Massachusetts General Hospital; Director of Spaulding Rehabilitation Hospital/Massachusetts General Hospital Stroke Program, Spaulding Rehabilitation Hospital, Boston, Massachusetts
Postoperative Confusion

Joan E. Kapusnik-Uner, PharmD
Associate Clinical Professor of Pharmacy, University of California at San Francisco; Clinical Pharmacist in Infectious Diseases, San Francisco General Hospital, San Francisco, California
Antimicrobial Therapy in the Critical Care Setting

Robert Katz, MD
Associate Professor, Pediatrics, University of New Mexico School of Medicine; Director, Pediatric Intensive Care Unit, University Hospital, Albuquerque, New Mexico
Acute Parenchymal Disease in Childhood

Elizabeth S. Kaufman, MD, FACC
Senior Instructor in Medicine, Case Western Reserve University School of Medicine; Director of Cardiac Electrophysiology, MetroHealth Medical Center, Cleveland, Ohio
Electrocardiography

Clifford J. Kavinsky, MD, PhD
Assistant Director, Section of Cardiology, Rush-Presbyterian-St. Luke's Medical Center, Chicago, Illinois
Severe Heart Failure in Cardiomyopathy: Pathogenesis and Treatment

Richard L. Keenan, MD
Professor Emeritus, Department of Anesthesiology, Medical College of Virginia/Virginia Commonwealth University, Richmond, Virginia
The Hyperthermic Syndromes

Stephen Keim, MD
Assistant Professor of Medicine, University of Pittsburgh; Staff Physician, Presbyterian University Hospital-University of Pittsburgh Medical Center, Pittsburgh, Pennsylvania
Conduction Disturbances in the Critically Ill

Dennis L. Kelleher, PhD
Trauma Research Coordinator, Fairfax Regional Trauma Center, Fairfax Hospital, Falls Church, Virginia
Epidemiology of Trauma

John M. Kellum, MD, FACS
Professor, Department of Surgery, Medical College of Virginia/Virginia Commonwealth University; Attending Surgeon, Medical College of Virginia Hospitals, Richmond, Virginia
Intra-Abdominal Sepsis

Andrew S. Kenler, MD
Fellow in Surgery, New England Deaconess Hospital, Harvard Medical School, Boston, Massachusetts
Total Parenteral Nutrition: Priorities and Practice

Gary J. Kerkvliet, MD
Clinical Instructor, The Johns Hopkins University School of Medicine; Chief Medical Resident, Sinai Hospital of Baltimore, Baltimore, Maryland
The Critically Ill Diabetic

Michael B. Kesselbrenner, MD, FACC, FACP
Associate Professor, Seton Hall School of Graduate Medicine; Attending Cardiologist, Valley Hospital, Ridgewood; Director, Critical Care Unit, Barnett Memorial Hospital Center; Attending Cardiologist, St. Joseph's Medical Center, Paterson, New Jersey
Intra-Aortic Balloon Counterpulsation

Pavel L. Khimenko, MD, PhD
Postdoctoral Fellow, University of South Alabama College of Medicine, Mobile, Alabama
Regulation of Capillary Exchange of Fluid and Protein

Anton I. Kidess, MBBS, MD
Fellow, Department of Medicine, Pulmonary and Critical Care Section, The University of Oklahoma Health Sciences Center; Fellow, Department of Medicine, Pulmonary and Critical Care Section, Veterans Administration Medical Center, Oklahoma City, Oklahoma
Pulmonary Edema

Thomas Killip, MD
Professor of Medicine, Albert Einstein College of Medicine; Executive Vice President, Beth Israel Medical Center, New York, New York
Management of Myocardial Infarction

Christina I. Klufas, MD
Clinical Assistant Professor, Departments of Anesthesiology/Critical Care Medicine, University of Pittsburgh School of Medicine; Staff Intensivist, St. Francis Medical Center, Pittsburgh, Pennsylvania
Organ Donor Categories and Management

William A. Knaus, MD
Professor, Department of Anesthesia and Medicine; Director, Intensive Care Research Unit, George Washington University Medical Center, Washington, D.C.
Severity of Illness Indices and Outcome Prediction: Development and Evaluation; Outcome Prediction for Specific Conditions

Matyas Koltai, MD, PhD
Consultant in Pharmacology, Institut Henri Beaufour, Robinson, France
Platelet-Activating Factor in Septic Shock

Robert L. Kormos, MD
Associate Professor of Surgery and Director, Artificial Heart Program, University of Pittsburgh, Pittsburgh, Pennsylvania
Multiple Organ Procurement; Intensive Care of the Cardiac Transplant Recipient

Harry B. Kram, MD, FCCM
Associate Professor of Surgery and Emergency Medicine, Charles R. Drew Postgraduate School of Medicine; Attending Staff, King-Drew Medical Center, Los Angeles, California
Intraoperative Hemostasis

David J. Kramer, MD
Associate Professor of Anesthesiology/Critical Care Medicine and Assistant Professor of Medicine and Surgery, University of Pittsburgh School of Medicine; Co-Director, Liver Transplant Intensive Care Unit Service, University of Pittsburgh Medical Center, Pittsburgh, Pennsylvania
Intensive Care of Liver Transplant Recipients; Pancreas and Islet Cell Transplantation

John W. Kreit, MD
Assistant Professor of Medicine, Division of Pulmonary, Allergy, and Critical Care Medicine, University of Pittsburgh School of Medicine; Director, Medical Intensive Care Unit, Montefiore University Hospital, Pittsburgh, Pennsylvania
The Work of Breathing; Approach to the Patient with Acute Respiratory Failure

Vladimir Kvetan, MD, FCCM, FCCP
Associate Professor of Anesthesiology and Medicine, Albert Einstein College of Medicine; Attending Physician, Montefiore Medical Center, New York, New York
Disasters and Critical Care Medicine

Kenneth K. W. Lee, MD
Assistant Professor, University of Pittsburgh; Attending Surgeon, University of Pittsburgh Medical Center, Presbyterian University Hospital, Montefiore University Hospital, and St. Margaret Memorial Hospital, Pittsburgh, Pennsylvania
Acute Gastrointestinal Disorders; General Surgical Complications in Transplant Patients

Howard Levy, MD
Associate Professor, University of New Mexico; Acting Co-Chairman, Pulmonary and Critical Care Medicine; and Chief of Critical Care Medicine, University Hospital, University of New Mexico Health Sciences Center, Albuquerque, New Mexico
Identification of Previously Undiagnosed Disease: Hantavirus Pulmonary Syndrome

Peter Linden, MD, DMD
Assistant Professor of Anesthesiology and Medicine, Department of Anesthesiology, Division of Critical Care, University of Pittsburgh School of Medicine; Associate Director, Liver Transplant Intensive Care Unit, Presbyterian University Hospital, Pittsburgh, Pennsylvania
Infections After Solid Organ Transplantation

Carl-Eric Lindholm, MD, PhD
Professor of Laryngobronchology, University of Uppsala School of Medicine, Uppsala, Sweden
Laryngotracheal Injury from Prolonged Tracheal Intubation; Surgical Airway, Cricothyroidotomy, and Tracheotomy: Procedures, Complications, and Outcome

Toby L. Litovitz, MD
Director, National Capital Poison Center, Washington, D.C.
Poisoning

Sandra Lookinland, PhD, RN
Professor, Department of Nursing, California State University; Clinical Nurse Researcher, Community Hospitals of Central California, Fresno, California
Stress Management of Staff, Family, and Patients

Thomas G. Luerssen, MD, FACS, FAAP
Associate Professor, Neurological Surgery, Indiana University Medical Center; Chief, Pediatric Neurosurgical Service, James Whitcomb Riley Hospital for Children, Indianapolis, Indiana
The Critical Care of the Neurosurgical Patient

Philip D. Lumb, MBBS, FCCM
Professor of Anesthesiology and Surgery and Chairman, Department of Anesthesiology, Albany Medical College; Anesthesiologist-in-Chief and Co-Director, Surgical Intensive Care Unit, Albany Medical Center Hospital, Albany, New York
Conventional Airway Access; Sedatives and Muscle Relaxants in the Intensive Care Unit

Ignazio Roberto Marino, MD
Assistant Professor of Surgery, University of Pittsburgh; Associate Director, Transplant Division, Veterans Administration Medical Center, Pittsburgh, Pennsylvania; Professor of Surgery, University of Milan, Milan, Italy
Multiple Organ Procurement

Lawrence F. Marshall, MD
Professor, Neurological Surgery, University of California at San Diego; Chief, Neurological Surgery, University of California at San Diego Hospitals, San Diego, California
The Critical Care of the Neurosurgical Patient

G. Daniel Martich, MD, FCCP
Assistant Professor of Critical Care, University of Pittsburgh Medical Center; Attending Physician, Cardiothoracic Intensive Care Unit, Presbyterian University Hospital, Pittsburgh, Pennsylvania
Intensive Care of the Cardiac Transplant Recipient

Tom Masciangelo, MD
Fellow, Pulmonary Transplantation, Baylor College of Medicine, Houston, Texas
Transesophageal Echocardiography

Henry Masur, MD
Clinical Professor of Medicine, George Washington University School of Medicine, Washington, D.C.; Chief, Critical Care Medicine Department, Clinical Center, National Institutes of Health, Bethesda, Maryland
Pneumonia in the Immunosuppressed Patient

John E. Mazuski, MD, PhD
Assistant Professor of Surgery, Department of Surgery, Division of Trauma Service and Surgical Critical Care, St. Louis University, St. Louis, Missouri
Abdominal and Pelvic Trauma

D. Robert McCaffree, MD
Professor of Medicine, University of Oklahoma Health Sciences Center; Chief of Staff, Veterans Administration Medical Center, Oklahoma City, Oklahoma
Pulmonary Edema

Jerry McCauley, MD
Associate Professor, School of Medicine, University of Pittsburgh; Director, Department of Nephrology, University of Pittsburgh Medical Center, Presbyterian University Hospital, Pittsburgh, Pennsylvania
Critical Care of Kidney Transplant Recipients

Joe M. McCord, PhD
Professor of Biochemistry and Medicine, University of Colorado Health Sciences Center, Denver, Colorado
Oxygen-Derived Free Radicals

David J. McConkey, PhD
Assistant Professor, Department of Cell Biology, The University of Texas M. D. Anderson Cancer Center, Houston, Texas
Cellular Signaling and Cell Death

Kristine M. McCulloch, MD
Associate Professor of Pediatrics, University of Illinois College of Medicine; Attending Neonatologist, University of Illinois Hospital, Chicago, Illinois
Surfactant Physiology, Metabolism, Function, and Replacement Therapy

Mary McDonald, MD
Fellowship in Hepatology/Gastroenterology, University of Washington, Seattle, Washington; Private Practice in Gastroenterology, Mercy Medical Center, Oshkosh, Wisconsin
Severe Liver Disease

Richard J. Melker, MD, PhD
Associate Professor of Anesthesiology, Surgery, and Pediatrics, University of Florida College of Medicine, Gainesville, Florida
Pediatric Resuscitation

Mark A. Mintun, MD
Associate Professor of Radiology and Psychiatry, University of Pittsburgh School of Medicine; Medical Director, PET Facility, University of Pittsburgh Medical Center, Pittsburgh, Pennsylvania
Positron Emission Tomography: Basic Principles and Potential Applications in the Critically Ill

Cres B. Miranda, MD, FACC
Cardiologist, Cardiovascular Center of Southern Nevada, Las Vegas, Nevada
Interventional Therapies for Cardiogenic Shock

Jerome H. Modell, MD
Senior Associate Dean for Clinical Affairs; Associate Vice-President for University Health Science Center Affiliations; and Professor, Department of Anesthesiology, University of Florida College of Medicine, Gainesville, Florida; Attending Physician, Shands Hospital, Gainesville Veterans Administration Medical Center, Gainesville, Florida; and University Medical Center, Jacksonville, Florida
Near-Drowning: Adults and Children; Pulmonary Aspiration of Stomach Contents

Richard E. Moon, MD, FACP, FCCP, FRCP(C)
Associate Professor of Anesthesiology and Assistant Professor of Pulmonary Medicine, Duke University; Attending Anesthesiologist and Pulmonologist, Duke University Medical Center, Durham, North Carolina
Hyperbaric Oxygen in Critical Care

Alan H. Morris, MD
Professor of Medicine, Pulmonary Division, University of Utah Medical School; Director of Research, Pulmonary Division, LDS Hospital, Salt Lake City, Utah
Computerized Management of Mechanical Ventilation

William J. Morris, MD
Pediatric Neurosurgeon, Mary Bridge Children's Hospital, Tacoma, Washington
Pediatric Neurosurgical Emergencies

Loren D. Nelson, MD
Associate Professor of Surgery and Anesthesiology, Vanderbilt University; Director, Surgical Intensive Care Unit, Vanderbilt University Medical Center, Nashville, Tennessee
Initial Assessment of the Multiple Trauma Patient

Dane J. Nichols, MD
Assistant Professor of Clinical Medicine, University of Illinois College of Medicine; Director, Medical Intensive Care Unit, St. Francis Medical Center, Peoria, Illinois
Building Bedside Collaborative Practice

Ronald Lee Nichols, MD, MS, FACS
William Henderson Professor of Surgery and Professor of Microbiology and Immunology, Department of Surgery, Tulane University School of Medicine; Attending Surgeon, Tulane University Medical Center Hospital, New Orleans, Louisiana
Infections in the Surgical Critical Care Unit

J. V. Nixon, MD
Professor of Medicine, Medical College of Virginia/Virginia Commonwealth University; Director, Echocardiography Laboratories, Medical College of Virginia Hospitals, Richmond, Virginia
Echocardiography in Critical Care

Scott Norwood, MD, FACS, FCCM
Director of Trauma Services, East Texas Medical Center, Tyler, Texas
Catheter-Related Infections and Associated Bacteremia

Walter J. O'Donnell, MD
Instructor in Medicine, Harvard Medical School; Associate Physician and Medical Director, Pulmonary Function Laboratory, Brigham and Women's Hospital, Boston, Massachusetts
Life-Threatening Asthma

Steven L. Orebaugh, MD
Resident in Anesthesiology, University of Pittsburgh Medical Center, Pittsburgh, Pennsylvania
Air Embolization

Richard A. Orr, MD
Associate Professor, Anesthesiology/Critical Care Medicine and Pediatrics; Associate Director, Pediatric Intensive Care Unit; Medical Director, Pediatric Transport, Children's Hospital of Pittsburgh, Pittsburgh, Pennsylvania
Neonatal and Pediatric Transport Programs

Michele C. Papo, MD
Assistant Professor of Pediatrics and Anesthesiology; Director, Critical Care Fellowship Program; and Associate Director, Pediatric Critical Care, Children's Hospital of Buffalo, Buffalo, New York
Congestive Heart Failure in Infants and Children

Margaret M. Parker, MD
Associate Professor of Pediatrics, SUNY at Stony Brook; Director, Pediatric Intensive Care Unit, University Medical Center at Stony Brook, New York
The Heart in Sepsis

Joseph E. Parrillo, MD
James B. Herrick Professor of Medicine, Rush Medical College; Chief, Sections of Cardiology and Critical Care Medicine; Medical Director, Rush Heart Institute, Rush-Presbyterian-St. Luke's Medical Center, Chicago, Illinois
Severe Heart Failure in Cardiomyopathy: Pathogenesis and Treatment

M. H. Parsa, MD
Associate Clinical Professor of Surgery, Columbia University College of Physicians and Surgeons; Attending Surgeon; Director, Trauma Center; Chief, Vascular Access and Intravenous Hyperalimentation Service, Harlem Hospital Center, New York, New York
Intravascular Access and Long-Term Maintenance; Invasive and Noninvasive Physiologic Monitoring; Enteral Feeding; Nutritional Failure

William T. Peruzzi, MD
Associate Professor and Chief of Critical Care Medicine, Department of Anesthesia, Northwestern University Medical School; Associate Medical Director, Respiratory Care Services, Northwestern Memorial Hospital, Chicago, Illinois
Interpretation of Blood Gases

Sharon L. Pilmer, MD
Assistant Professor of Anesthesia and Pediatrics, University of Pennsylvania School of Medicine; Assistant Anesthesiologist and Director of the Respiratory Rehabilitation Service, The Children's Hospital of Philadelphia, Philadelphia, Pennsylvania
Distal Airway Disorders in Infants and Children: Bronchiolitis and Asthma

Steven M. Pincus, MD, PhD
Assistant Professor of Medicine, University of Pittsburgh School of Medicine; Staff Physician, University of Pittsburgh Medical Center, Pittsburgh, Pennsylvania
Bone Marrow Transplantation

Graham F. Pineo, MD
Professor of Medicine, University of Calgary; Director, Clinical Trials Unit, Calgary General Hospital, Calgary, Alberta, Canada
Treatment of Massive Pulmonary Embolism; Diagnosis and Treatment of Venous Thromboembolism

Michael R. Pinsky, MD
Professor of Anesthesiology, Critical Care Medicine and Medicine, University of Pittsburgh; Director of Research, University of Pittsburgh Medical Center, Pittsburgh, Pennsylvania
Hemodynamic Effects of Artificial Ventilation

Murray M. Pollack, MD
Professor, Anesthesiology and Pediatrics, George Washington University School of Medicine; Associate Director, Pediatric Intensive Care Unit, and Director, Center for Health Services and Clinical Research, Children's Research Institute, Children's National Medical Center, Washington, D.C.
Evaluating Pediatric Intensive Care Units

Fred Plum, MD
Professor and Chairman, Department of Neurology and Neuroscience, New York Hospital–Cornell Medical Center; Neurologist in Chief, New York Hospital, New York, New York
Evaluation of the Comatose Patient

David T. Porembka, DO, FCCM, FCCP
Associate Professor of Anesthesiology and Surgery; Associate Director of Surgical Intensive Care; and Director of Transesophageal Echocardiography, University of Cincinnati, Cincinnati, Ohio
Transesophageal Echocardiography

David J. Powner, MD
Professor, Departments of Anesthesiology/Critical Care Medicine and Medicine, University of Pittsburgh School of Medicine, Pittsburgh, Pennsylvania
Controversies in Brain Death Certification; Organ Donor Categories and Management

Donald S. Prough, MD
Professor and Chairman, Department of Anesthesiology, The University of Texas Medical Branch; Medical Director, Surgical Intensive Care Unit, John Sealy Hospital, Galveston, Texas
Brain Function Monitoring

Eric C. Rackow, MD
Professor and Vice Chairman, Department of Medicine, New York Medical College, New York, New York
Options for Augmenting the Efficacy of Closed-Chest Cardiopulmonary Resuscitation

Louis Rakita, MD, CM, FACP, FRCP(C), FACC
Professor Emeritus of Medicine, Case Western Reserve University School of Medicine; Former Director, Division of Cardiology, MetroHealth Medical Center, Cleveland, Ohio
Electrocardiography

David D. Ralph, MD
Associate Professor, Pulmonary/Critical Care Medicine, University of Washington School of Medicine; Medical Director, Critical Care Unit, University of Washington Medical Center, Seattle, Washington
Severe Liver Disease

Jukka Räsänen, MD
Associate Professor, Department of Anesthesiology, University of South Florida College of Medicine; Staff Anesthesiologist, Tampa General Hospital, Tampa, Florida
Airway Pressure Therapy

Gary E. Raskob, BSc, MSc
Assistant Professor, Department of Biostatistics and Epidemiology, and Department of Medicine, University of Oklahoma Health Sciences Center, Oklahoma City, Oklahoma
Diagnosis and Treatment of Venous Thromboembolism

Keith Reemstma, MD
Emeritus Professor of Surgery and Chief of Surgery, Columbia-Presbyterian Medical Center, New York, New York
Intra-Aortic Balloon Counterpulsation

H. David Reines, MD, FACS, FCCM
Professor of Surgery, Tufts University School of Medicine, Boston, Massachusetts; Chief of Surgery, Newton-Wellesley Hospital, Newton, Massachusetts
Prostaglandins, Thromboxanes, Leukotrienes, and Other Products of Arachidonic Acid; Preoperative Assessment of Critically Ill Patients

Jorge Reyes, MD
Assistant Professor of Surgery, University of Pittsburgh Medical Center; Chief, Pediatric Transplant Surgery, Pittsburgh Transplant Institute, Pittsburgh, Pennsylvania
Intestinal and Multiple Organ Transplantation

Camillo Ricordi, MD
Professor of Surgery, Diabetes Research Institute; Chief, Division of Cellular Transplantation, and Co-Director, Diabetes Research Institute, Miami, Florida
Pancreas and Islet Cell Transplantation

William C. Roberts, MD
Executive Director, Baylor Cardiovascular Institute, Baylor University Medical Center, Dallas, Texas
The Coronary Arteries in Unstable Angina Pectoris, Acute Myocardial Infarction, and Sudden Coronary Death

Dudley F. Rochester, MD
Professor Emeritus, University of Virginia School of Medicine; Attending Physician, University of Virginia Hospital, Charlottesville, Virginia
Respiratory Muscle Failure in Critical Illness

Robert M. Rogers, MD
Professor and Chief, Division of Pulmonary, Allergy, and Critical Care Medicine, University of Pittsburgh School of Medicine; Di-

rector, Comprehensive Lung Center, University of Pittsburgh Medical Center, Pittsburgh, Pennsylvania
The Work of Breathing; Approach to the Patient with Acute Respiratory Failure; Acute Respiratory Failure in Chronic Obstructive Pulmonary Disease

Jonathan D. Root, MD
Assistant Professor of Neurology, Cornell University Medical College; Director, Neurology-Neurosurgery Special Care Unit, New York Hospital-Cornell Medical Center, New York, New York
Evaluation of the Comatose Patient

Allan H. Ropper, MD
Professor of Neurology, Tufts University School of Medicine; Chief, Division of Neurology, St. Elizabeth's Medical Center, Boston, Massachusetts
Critical Care Neurology; Postoperative Confusion

Alan J. Rosenbloom, MD
Assistant Professor, Department of Anesthesiology/Critical Care Medicine, University of Pittsburgh School of Medicine; Assistant Professor, Department of Anesthesiology/Critical Care Medicine, Presbyterian University Hospital, University of Pittsburgh Medical Center, Pittsburgh, Pennsylvania
Principles of Immunosuppression

Lewis J. Rubin, MD
Professor of Medicine and Physiology and Head, Division of Pulmonary and Critical Care Medicine, University of Maryland School of Medicine, Baltimore, Maryland
Pulmonary Hypertension

Edward J. Ruley, MD
Professor of Pediatrics, F. Edward Hébert School of Medicine, Uniformed Services University of the Health Sciences, Bethesda, Maryland; Medical Co-Director, Pediatric Kidney Center, Fairfax Hospital for Children, Falls Church, Virginia
Hypertensive Emergencies in Infants and Children; Acute Renal Failure in Infants and Children

Edmund J. Rutherford, MD
Assistant Professor of Surgery and Associate Chief of Surgical Critical Care, Vanderbilt University Medical Center, Nashville, Tennessee
Initial Assessment of the Multiple Trauma Patient

Witold B. Rybka, MD
Associate Professor of Medicine, University of Pittsburgh School of Medicine; Staff Physician and Clinical Director, Adult Bone Marrow Transplant Program, University of Pittsburgh Medical Center, Pittsburgh, Pennsylvania
Bone Marrow Transplantation

Peter Safar, MD
Distinguished Service Professor, University of Pittsburgh; Director, International Resuscitation Research Center, University of Pittsburgh Medical Center, Pittsburgh, Pennsylvania
Cardiopulmonary-Cerebral Resuscitation

Michael Salem, MD
Assistant Professor of Surgery and Anesthesiology and Director, Surgical Critical Care and Surgical Research, George Washington University School of Medicine, Washington, D.C.
Adrenal Dysfunction in the Intensive Care Unit

Merle A. Sande, MD
Professor and Vice-Chairman, Department of Medicine, University of California at San Francisco; Chief, Medical Service, San Francisco General Hospital, San Francisco, California
Antimicrobial Therapy in the Critical Care Setting

Mark H. Sanders, MD, FCCP
Associate Professor of Medicine and Anesthesiology, University of Pittsburgh School of Medicine; Chief, Pulmonary Sleep Disorders Program, University of Pittsburgh Medical Center, Pittsburgh, Pennsylvania
Positive-Pressure Ventilation Without Tracheal Intubation

Andrew J. Satin, MD
Associate Professor of Obstetrics and Gynecology, F. Edward Hébert School of Medicine, Uniformed Services University of the Health Sciences, Bethesda, Maryland; Assistant Chief of Obstetrics, Wilford Hall Medical Center, Lackland Air Force Base, Texas
Critical Care Medicine and the Obstetric Patient

Thomas J. Savides, MD
Assistant Clinical Professor of Medicine, Division of Gastroenterology, University of California, San Diego Medical Center, San Diego, California
Severe Gastrointestinal Hemorrhage

Joseph M. Scheller, MD
Assistant Professor of Pediatrics, University of Maryland, Baltimore, Maryland
Status Epilepticus in Children

Stephen C. Schimpff, MD
Professor of Medicine, Oncology, and Pharmacology, University of Maryland School of Medicine; Executive Vice President, University of Maryland Medical System, Baltimore, Maryland
Prevention and Management of Infections in Critically Ill Trauma Victims and Patients with Hematologic Malignancies

Christine R. Schneyer, MD
Assistant Professor of Medicine, Division of Endocrinology, Johns Hopkins School of Medicine; Associate Director, Division of Endocrinology, Sinai Hospital of Baltimore, Baltimore, Maryland
The Critically Ill Diabetic

Sidney H. Schnoll, MD, PhD
Professor of Internal Medicine, Psychiatry, and Pharmacology and Toxicology, Medical College of Virginia/Virginia Commonwealth University; Chairman, Division of Substance Abuse Medicine; Medical College of Virginia Hospitals, Richmond, Virginia
Drug Abuse, Overdose, and Withdrawal Syndromes

Luke O. Schoeniger, PhD, MD
Fellow in Surgery, The Johns Hopkins University School of Medicine; Senior Resident in Surgery, The Johns Hopkins Hospital, Baltimore, Maryland
Regulation of Gene Expression

Anton C. Schoolwerth, MD
Professor of Medicine and Physiology and Chairman, Division of Nephrology, Department of Internal Medicine, Medical College of Virginia/Virginia Commonwealth University, Richmond, Virginia
Clinical Assessment of Renal Function; Adult Acute and Chronic Renal Failure

Wolfgang H. Schraut, MD, PhD
Professor of Surgery, University of Pittsburgh; Attending Surgeon, University of Pittsburgh Medical Center Hospitals; Consulting Surgeon, Veterans Administration Hospital; Presbyterian University Hospital, Montefiore University Hospital, Magee Women's Hospital, Veterans Administration Hospital, Pittsburgh, Pennsylvania
Acute Gastrointestinal Disorders

Robert Selby, MD
Associate Professor of Surgery, University of Pittsburgh Medical Center; Associate Professor of Surgery, Pittsburgh Transplant Institute, Pittsburgh, Pennsylvania
Intensive Care of Liver Transplant Recipients; Intestinal and Multiple Organ Transplantation

Michael G. Seneff, MD
Assistant Professor, Anesthesia and Medicine; Director, Intensive Care Unit, George Washington University Medical Center, Washington, D.C.
Severity of Illness Indices and Outcome Prediction: Development and Evaluation; Outcome Prediction for Specific Conditions

Curtis N. Sessler, MD
Associate Professor of Medicine, and Medical Director, Medical Respiratory Intensive Care Unit, Virginia Commonwealth University/Medical College of Virginia, Richmond, Virginia
The Structural Basis of Pulmonary Function

Barry A. Shapiro, MD
Professor and Vice Chairman and Director, Critical Care Medicine, Department of Anesthesia, Northwestern University Medical School; Medical Director, Respiratory Care Services, Northwestern Memorial Hospital, Chicago, Illinois
Interpretation of Blood Gases; Blood Gas Monitoring

Leland Shapiro, MD
Fellow, Division of Geographic Medicine and Infectious Diseases, New England Medical Center, Boston, Massachusetts
Cytokines

Marc J. Shapiro, MD
Associate Professor of Surgery and Anesthesiology and Chief, Division of Trauma Service and Surgical Critical Care, St. Louis University, St. Louis, Missouri
Abdominal and Pelvic Trauma

Ronald Shapiro, MD
Associate Professor, School of Medicine, University of Pittsburgh; Associate Professor of Surgery, University of Pittsburgh Medical Center, Presbyterian-University Hospital, Pittsburgh, Pennsylvania
Critical Care of Kidney Transplant Recipients; Future of Transplantation (Including Xenografting)

William C. Shoemaker, MD, FCCM
Professor of Surgery, UCLA School of Medicine; Chairman, Department of Emergency Medicine, and Vice Chairman, Department of Surgery, King-Drew Medical Center, Los Angeles, California
Diagnosis and Treatment of the Shock Syndromes; Clinical Algorithms for Resuscitation in Acute Emergency Conditions; Intravascular Access and Long-Term Maintenance; Invasive and Noninvasive Physiologic Monitoring; Pericardial Tamponade; Pathophysiology and Management of Adult Respiratory Distress Syndrome; Enteral Feeding; Nutritional Failure

William J. Sibbald, MD, FRCP(C)
Professor, Faculty of Medicine, University of Western Ontario; Coordinator, Critical Care Trauma Centre, Victoria Hospital, London, Ontario, Canada
Applied Cardiovascular Physiology in the Critically Ill

Dean F. Sittig, PhD
Assistant Professor, Biomedical Informatics and Biomedical Engineering, Vanderbilt University, Nashville, Tennessee
Computers in the Intensive Care Unit: A Match Meant to Be!

M. Leon Skolnick, MD
Professor of Radiology, Department of Radiology, University of Pittsburgh School of Medicine; Attending Radiologist, Presbyterian University Hospital, Pittsburgh, Pennsylvania
Critical Care Applications of Sonography

Tod B. Sloan, MD, PhD
Professor of Anesthesiology, University of Texas Health Science Center at San Antonio, San Antonio, Texas
Acute Spinal Cord Trauma

Robert C. Smallridge, MD, FACP
Professor of Medicine, Uniformed Services University of the Health Sciences, Bethesda, Maryland; Director, Division of Medicine, Walter Reed Army Institute of Research, Washington, D.C.
Thyroid Emergencies

Howard S. Smith, MD
Instructor, Department of Anesthesiology, Albany Medical College; Director, Acute and Chronic Pain Management, Stratton Veterans Administration Medical Center, Albany, New York
Conventional Airway Access

Robert A. Smith, MS, RRT, FCCM
Assistant Professor, Department of Anesthesiology, University of South Florida College of Medicine, Tampa, Florida
Principles of Mechanical Ventilation

Stephanie E. Spottswood, MD, MSPH
Assistant Professor, Departments of Radiology and Pediatrics, Medical College of Virginia/Virginia Commonwealth University, Richmond, Virginia
Chest Imaging in Pediatric Intensive Care

Sidney Starkman, MD
Assistant Clinical Professor of Medicine/Emergency Medicine and Neurology, UCLA School of Medicine; Director, Comprehensive Emergency Neurology Program, UCLA Medical Center, Los Angeles, California
Cerebral Vascular Emergencies

Thomas E. Starzl, MD, PhD
Professor of Surgery, Department of Surgery, University of Pittsburgh School of Medicine; Staff Member, Presbyterian University Hospital; Director, Pittsburgh Transplantation Institute, Pittsburgh, Pennsylvania
Multiple Organ Procurement; Intestinal and Multiple Organ Transplantation; Future of Transplantation (Including Xenografting)

David L. Steed, MD
Professor of Surgery, University of Pittsburgh School of Medicine; Vascular Surgeon, University of Pittsburgh Medical Center, Pittsburgh, Pennsylvania
General Surgical Complications in Transplant Patients

Michael L. Steer, MD
Professor of Surgery, Harvard Medical School; Chief of General Surgery and Associate Surgeon-in-Chief, Beth Israel Hospital, Boston, Massachusetts
Acute Pancreatitis

Keith L. Stein, MD, FCCP, FCCM
Associate Professor of Anesthesiology/Critical Care Medicine, Mayo School of Medicine, Rochester, Minnesota; Chief, Critical Care Medicine, Mayo Clinic Jacksonville, Jacksonville, Florida
Transesophageal Echocardiography; High-Frequency Ventilation and Oscillation; Independent Lung Ventilation; Organ Donor Categories and Management; Intensive Care of the Cardiac Transplant Recipient; Lung Transplantation: Thirty Years of Progress

Steven M. Steinberg, MD
Associate Professor, Department of Surgery, Tulane University, New Orleans, Louisiana
Infections in the Surgical Critical Care Unit

David M. Steinhorn, MD
Assistant Professor of Pediatrics and Anesthesiology and Co-Director, Pediatric Critical Care, Children's Hospital of Buffalo, Buffalo, New York
Congestive Heart Failure in Infants and Children

Ronald A. Stiller, MD, PhD, FCCP
Assistant Professor of Medicine and Anesthesiology, University of Pittsburgh School of Medicine; Director, Noninvasive Ventilation Unit, University of Pittsburgh Medical Center, Pittsburgh, Pennsylvania
Positive-Pressure Ventilation Without Tracheal Intubation

James K. Stoller, MD
Associate Professor of Medicine, Ohio State University School of Medicine, Columbus, Ohio; Head, Section of Respiratory Therapy, Department of Pulmonary and Critical Care Medicine, Cleveland Clinic Foundation, Cleveland, Ohio
Principles of Respiratory Care

Bryant W. Stolp, MD, PhD
Associate, Departments of Anesthesiology and Cell Biology, Duke University; Attending Anesthesiologist, Duke University Medical Center, Durham, North Carolina
Hyperbaric Oxygen in Critical Care

Patrick J. Strollo, MD, FCCP
Assistant Professor of Medicine, University of Pittsburgh School of Medicine; Associate Director, Pulmonary Sleep Evaluation Laboratory, University of Pittsburgh Medical Center, Pittsburgh, Pennsylvania
Positive-Pressure Ventilation Without Tracheal Intubation

Susan A. Stuart, RN, BSN, CPTC
Organ Procurement Coordinator, Center for Organ Recovery and Education, Pittsburgh, Pennsylvania
History and Organization of Organ Transplantation

Dale Swift, MD
Clinical Assistant Professor of Neurosurgery, The University of Texas Southwestern Medical School; Attending Neurosurgeon, Department of Neurosurgery, Children's Medical Center of Dallas, Dallas, Texas
Pediatric Neurosurgical Emergencies

Karen N. Swisher, MS, JD
Associate Professor of Health Law, Department of Health Administration, and Department of Legal Medicine; and Associate Director, The Williamson Institute, Medical College of Virginia, Richmond, Virginia
Legal Issues Involved in the Delivery of Critical Care Medicine; The Ethics of Resource Allocation in the Intensive Care Unit

Richard A. Szucs, MD
Assistant Professor of Radiology, Medical College of Virginia/Virginia Commonwealth University; Attending Physician, Medical College of Virginia Hospitals, Richmond, Virginia
Computed Tomography of the Abdomen in the Critical Care Patient

Aubrey E. Taylor, PhD
Professor and Chairman, Department of Physiology, University of South Alabama College of Medicine, Mobile, Alabama
Regulation of Capillary Exchange of Fluid and Protein

Robert W. Taylor, MD
Assistant Clinical Professor, St. Louis University School of Medicine, St. John's Mercy Medical Center/St. Louis University; Director of Critical Care Medicine Fellowship, St. John's Mercy Medical Center/St. Louis University, St. Louis, Missouri
Adult Respiratory Distress Syndrome

Patrick Tchou, MD
Associate Professor of Medicine, University of Pittsburgh; Staff Physician, University of Pittsburgh Medical Center, Pittsburgh, Pennsylvania
Conduction Disturbances in the Critically Ill

Charles Teo, MD
Assistant Professor, Department of Neurosurgery, University of Arkansas for Medical Sciences; Vice-Chief, Division of Pediatric Neurosurgery, Arkansas Children's Hospital, Little Rock, Arkansas
Pediatric Neurosurgical Emergencies

Jaime Tisnado, MD, FACR, FACC
Professor of Radiology, Medical College of Virginia/Virginia Commonwealth University; Attending Radiologist, Cardiovascular and Interventional Radiology, Medical College of Virginia Hospitals; Chairman, Department of Radiology, Hunter Holmes McGuire Veterans Affairs Medical Center, Richmond, Virginia
Interventional Radiology in the Critically Ill

Martin J. Tobin, MD
Professor of Medicine, Loyola University of Chicago Stritch School of Medicine; Program Director, Division of Pulmonary and Critical Care Medicine, Foster G. McGaw Hospital, Maywood; and Edward Hines Jr. Veterans Administration Hospital, Loyola University Medical Center, Hines, Illinois
Assessment of Pulmonary Function in Critically Ill Patients; Weaning from Mechanical Ventilation

Satoru Todo, MD
Professor of Surgery, University of Pittsburgh Medical Center; Professor of Surgery, Pittsburgh Transplant Institute, Pittsburgh, Pennsylvania
Intestinal and Multiple Organ Transplantation

Gail T. Tominaga, MD
Assistant Professor of Surgery, University of California at Irvine, Irvine, California; Surgical Attending Physician, Department of

Surgery, University of California at Irvine Medical Center, Orange, California
Plasma and Blood Substitutes

Tor Inge Tønnessen, MD, PhD
Associate Professor, Department of Anesthesiology and Intensive Care, University of Oslo; Associate Professor, Norwegian National Hospital, Oslo, Norway
Intracellular pH and Electrolyte Regulation

Arthur L. Trask, MD, FACS
Clinical Associate Professor, Department of Surgery, Georgetown University, Washington, District of Columbia; Chief, Trauma Services, Fairfax Hospital, Falls Church, Virginia
Epidemiology of Trauma

Steven J. Trottier, MD
Assistant Clinical Professor, St. Louis University School of Medicine, St. John's Mercy Medical Center/St. Louis University, St. Louis, Missouri
Adult Respiratory Distress Syndrome

Jonathan D. Truwit, MD
Associate Professor of Medicine; Interim Chief, Pulmonary and Critical Care; and Director of Medical Intensive Care Unit, University of Virginia Hospital, Charlottesville, Virginia
Respiratory Muscle Failure in Critical Illness

Andreas G. Tzakis, MD
Professor of Surgery and Chief, Division of Transplantation, University of Miami, Miami, Florida
Pancreas and Islet Cell Transplantation; Intestinal and Multiple Organ Transplantation

Nicholas B. Vedder, MD
Assistant Professor, Department of Surgery, University of Washington, Seattle, Washington
Neutrophil-Endothelial Cell Interactions

Dharmapuri Vidyasagar, MD
Professor of Pediatrics, Department of Pediatrics, University of Illinois at Chicago College of Medicine; Director of Neonatology, Neonatal Unit, University of Illinois Hospital, Chicago, Illinois
Surfactant Physiology, Metabolism, Function, and Replacement Therapy

Sid M. Viner, MD
Clinical Assistant Professor of Medicine, University of Calgary, Calgary, Alberta, Canada
High-Frequency Ventilation and Oscillation

Thomas Vrobel, MD, FACP, FACC
Associate Professor of Medicine, Case Western Reserve University School of Medicine; Staff Physician, MetroHealth Medical Center, Cleveland, Ohio
Electrocardiography

Rade B. Vukmir, MD
Assistant Professor, University of Pittsburgh Department of Anesthesiology/Critical Care Medicine and Emergency Medicine, University of Pittsburgh; Attending Physician, University of Pittsburgh Medical Center, Pittsburgh, Pennsylvania
Laryngotracheal Injury from Prolonged Tracheal Intubation; Surgical Airway, Cricothyroidotomy, and Tracheotomy: Procedures, Complications, and Outcome

Bertil K. J. Wagner, PharmD
Assistant Professor, Department of Pharmacy Practice, Rutgers–The State University of New Jersey College of Pharmacy; Adjunct Assistant Professor, Departments of Surgery and Anesthesia, University of Medicine and Dentistry of New Jersey–Robert Wood Johnson Medical School, Piscataway, New Jersey
Drug Monitoring

John C. Wain, MD
Assistant Professor, Harvard Medical School; Assistant Surgeon, Massachusetts General Hospital, Boston, Massachusetts
Life-Threatening Hemoptysis

John D. Ward, MD, FCCM
Professor, Pediatric Neurological Surgery, Division of Neurological Surgery, Medical College of Virginia/Virginia Commonwealth University; Staff; St. Mary's Hospital, HCA Henrico Doctor's Hospital, and HCA Chippenham Hospital, Richmond, Virginia
Management of Head Trauma

Kenneth Waxman, MD, FACS
Professor, University of California at Irvine; Staff Physician, Director of Trauma Services and Surgical Intensive Care, University of California at Irvine Medical Center, Orange, California
The Acute Abdomen; Plasma and Blood Substitutes; Physiologic Response to Injury

Andrew S. Wechsler, MD
Stuart McGuire Professor, Department of Surgery; Professor of Physiology, Medical College of Virginia; Cardiothoracic Surgeon (Chief) and Chairman of Surgery, Medical College of Virginia Hospitals, Richmond, Virginia
Ventricular Assist Devices and Artificial Hearts

Lawrence R. Wechsler, MD
Clinical Associate Professor of Neurology, University of Pittsburgh Medical School, Pittsburgh, Pennsylvania
Critical Care Neurology

Richard E. Weibley, MD, MPH
Associate Professor of Pediatrics, Section of Critical Care, University of South Florida; Medical Director, Pediatric Intensive Care Unit, Tampa General Hospital, Tampa, Florida
Proximal Airway Disorders in the Pediatric Patient

Max Harry Weil, MD, PhD
Distinguished University Professor, and President of the Institute of Critical Care Medicine; Adjunct Professor of Medicine, UCLA; Adjunct Professor of Medicine, Northwestern University Medical School; Consultant, Desert Hospital, Palm Springs, California; Visiting Physician, Nothwestern Memorial Hospital, Chicago; Consultant, Highland Park Hospital, Highland Park, Illinois; Honorary Physician, Cedars Sinai Medical Center, Los Angeles, California
Options for Augmenting the Efficacy of Closed-Chest Cardiopulmonary Resuscitation

Howard M. Weinberg, DO
Assistant Clinical Professor of Medicine, Department of Medicine, University of Medicine and Dentistry of New Jersey, John F. Kennedy Hospitals, Stratford; Attending Physician, Our Lady of Lourdes Medical Center, Camden, New Jersey
Intra-Aortic Balloon Counterpulsation

Joel Weinthal, MD, FAAP
Physician, Division of Hematology/Oncology and Bone Marrow Transplantation, Children's Hospital of Orange County, Orange, California
Colony-Stimulating Factors

Randall C. Wetzel, MB, BS, FCCM, FAAP
Associate Professor, Departments of Anesthesiology/Critical Care Medicine and Pediatrics, Johns Hopkins University School of Medicine; Chief, Division of Pediatric Anesthesia, and Director, Pediatric Recovery Room, The Johns Hopkins Hospital, Baltimore, Maryland
Pediatric Monitoring

Rodney A. White, MD
Professor of Surgery, UCLA School of Medicine; Chief, Vascular Surgery, and Associate Chairman, Department of Surgery, Harbor-UCLA Medical Center, Torrance, California
Diagnosis and Therapy of Emergent Vascular Diseases

Peter Wilson, MD
Department of Surgery, Vanderbilt University, Nashville, Tennessee
Regulation of Capillary Exchange of Fluid and Protein

Robert F. Wilson, MD, FACS, FCCM
Professor of Surgery, Wayne State University School of Medicine; Chief of Surgery and Director, Trauma Services, Detroit Receiving Hospital, Detroit, Michigan
Thoracic Injuries

Thomas C. Witt, MD
Clinical Instructor, Division of Neurological Surgery, Indiana University Medical Center, Indianapolis, Indiana
The Critical Care of the Neurosurgical Patient

Ginger Schafer Wlody, RN, EdD, FCCM
Assistant Clinical Professor, UCLA School of Nursing; Assistant Chief, Quality Management, Department of Veterans Affairs Medical Center, Los Angeles, California
The Impact of Healthcare and Technology Trends on Critical Care Practice

Mark A. Wood, MD
Assistant Professor of Medicine and Co-Director, Cardiac Electrophysiology Laboratory, Medical College of Virginia and McGuire Veterans Administration Medical Center, Richmond, Virginia
Pacemakers and Implantable Cardioverter Defibrillators in the Intensive Care Unit Setting

David Woods, PharmD
Assistant Clinical Professor of Pharmacy, University of California at San Francisco; Critical Care Pharmacist, San Francisco General Hospital, San Francisco, California
Antimicrobial Therapy in the Critical Care Setting

Stuart J. Youngner, MD
Professor of Medicine, Psychiatry, and Biomedical Ethics, Case Western Reserve University School of Medicine; Director, Clinical Ethics Program, University Hospitals of Cleveland, Cleveland, Ohio
Medical Futility

David D. Zabel, MD
Resident, Department of Surgery, Medical Center of Delaware, Newark, Delaware
Critical Care of Wounds and Wounded Patients

Barbara J. Zarowitz, PharmD, FCCP
Associate Professor of Pharmacy Practice, College of Pharmacy and Allied Health Professions, Wayne State University; Clinical Manager, Department of Pharmacy Services, Henry Ford Hospital, Detroit, Michigan
Pharmacologic Principles

Jack E. Zimmerman, MD
Professor of Anesthesia and Medicine, George Washington University Medical Center, Washington, D.C.
Severity of Illness Indices and Outcome Prediction: Development and Evaluation; Outcome Prediction for Specific Conditions

Janice L. Zimmerman, MD, FACP, FCCP, FCCM
Associate Professor of Clinical Medicine, Baylor College of Medicine; Director, Medicine Emergency Center; Critical Care Attending Physician, Ben Taub General Hospital, Houston, Texas
Hypertensive Crises: Emergencies and Urgencies

PREFACE TO THE THIRD EDITION

The Third Edition of the *Textbook of Critical Care,* like its two preceding editions, is a multiauthor text. The editors have attempted to assemble, under one cover, the views of those authorities who have contributed most to the science and art of caring for critically ill patients. Their studies and practice have fashioned the newest medical discipline—Critical Care Medicine. It seems appropriate that this edition be dedicated to those giants in the field who founded the Society of Critical Care Medicine in 1970 and who had the vision to establish a body of evolving specialized knowledge for the care of individuals hospitalized in the newly developed intensive care units. The development of the discipline is detailed in Chapter 1, which emphasizes the multidisciplinary nature of a specialty that attempts to harness high technology for the service of the individual patient; high touch as blended with high tech!

The growth of scientific knowledge in this and other medical fields has been explosive. Older methods of information diffusion such as books, journals, and conferences are often unable to keep pace with the rapidly advancing front of medical knowledge. This growth is dramatically evidenced by the increased size of the Society's journal, *Critical Care Medicine.* The first volume, published in 1973, contained 292 pages; in contrast, the 1993 volume numbered 2,025 pages and, when bound, was more than four inches thick. Other methods of information diffusion are necessary, and this textbook—and others like it—may soon give way to electronic methods of information storage, retrieval, and transfer.

There is no better evidence of the extraordinary growth of scientific information than that which paralleled the preparation of chapters by the authors of this textbook. When manuscripts for this book were begun more than a year ago, the historical scourge of the elderly, the pneumococcus, was still universally sensitive to the penicillins. By late 1994, resistant strains were commonplace, and vancomycin was recommended by many as the initial treatment for pneumococcal meningitis and other severe infections caused by the ubiquitous organism.* Although other recent developments in concept and practice may not have been as dramatic as the change in the sensitivity of the pneumococcus to penicillin, the authors were asked to add important new information during the publishing process so that the text could be as current as possible.

Transplantation has become the method of choice for treatment of single organ failure. Survival and quality of life after transplantation are far greater than with conventional medical therapy, and thus a full section of this textbook has been devoted to the management of transplantation patients.

Each chapter is meant to stand as a complete essay, and substantial overlap in subject matter has been encouraged in order to give balance to each subject area. Although specific points of fact may not necessarily be in opposition, the clinical experience of different members of the healthcare team is often quite different so that their own practices provide important insight into the care of extremely complex problems. There is some truth to the old observation that surgical patients tend to be overhydrated, whereas those cared for by internists are often volume-depleted. The editors have taken care to adjudicate, whenever possible, differences of opinion over long-standing issues such as the use of colloid solutions and steroids.

We have made this text as comprehensive as possible. Norma Shoemaker, the highly respected and long-serving executive director of the Society of Critical Care Medicine, has pointed out the different "dimensions" of knowledge required of individual physicians and nurses. Medical students graduate with great breadth of knowledge but limited depth. Most residency training frequently requires a progressive narrowing of focus as the individual learns more and more about less and less. The subspecialist, almost by definition, has great depth of knowledge but, sadly, can enjoy but little breadth of knowledge. Intensivists and other primary care practitioners, in contrast, need extensive breadth of information but may have difficulty in maintaining their depth of information. Only comprehensive texts like this, together with access to appropriate medical journals and electronic information sources, can supply the instant depth necessary for clinical decision making.

Many have assisted in the preparation of this book. We would particularly like to thank Mrs. Inger Grenvik, Ms. Sandra Valkhoff, Dr. Gordon Archer, Dr. Michael Hess, and Ms. Anne Flippin for their assistance in the preparation of many sections of this textbook.

W.C.S.
S.M.A.
A.G.
P.R.H.

*Quagliarello VJ, Scheld WM: New perspectives on bacterial meningitis. Clin Infect Dis 1993; 17:603.

CONTENTS

SECTION XIV TRANSPLANTATION 1600

Ake Grenvik

SECTION XV ISSUES IN PATIENT CARE 1717

Joann I. Lamb

SECTION XVI ORGANIZATION AND MANAGEMENT OF CRITICAL CARE 1752

Joann I. Lamb and Stephen M. Ayres

SECTION XVII ETHICAL DECISION MAKING IN CRITICALLY ILL PATIENTS 1793

Joann I. Lamb and Stephen M. Ayres

SECTION I

INTRODUCTION

Stephen M. Ayres, MD

CHAPTER 1

The Promise of Critical Care: Effective and Humane Care in an Era of Cost Containment

Stephen M. Ayres, MD

The evolution of a comprehensive and "standard" textbook of critical care medicine, the third edition of the *Textbook of Critical Care*,[1] parallels the rapid development of the new discipline of critical care medicine itself. It represents the rational application of high-technology medicine to seriously ill and injured people and provides a detailed knowledge base for those practitioners—physicians, nurses, respiratory therapists, physical therapists, and others—who apply this exponentially growing knowledge base at the bedside. The third edition is a direct descendant of the first book on critical care—*Care of the Critically Ill*,[2] first published in 1966; *Critical Care: State of the Art*, first published by the Society of Critical Care Medicine in 1980[3]; and the first edition of the Society's *Textbook of Critical Care*, published in 1984.[4]

The 1966 textbook set the stage for what might be considered the guiding principle of critical care medicine:

It has become "apparent that although certain well-established concepts provided the basis for treatment of such patients, they could not be applied unless continuous quantitative observations were made. We have emphasized circulatory and respiratory derangements because they are usually present in the critically ill. . . . Our goal has been to present a workable framework enabling the physician to reevaluate continually his treatment by constant observation of his own efforts and critical assessment of the growing literature in this area."[1]

The first edition of the *Textbook of Critical Care* echoed the importance of understanding basic pathophysiology and emphasized the interdisciplinary nature of critical care medicine:

"Is critical care more than the sum of the life-threatening parts of traditional medical specialties? To us, the answer is a resounding yes! Justification for critical care is primarily an operational one in which the discipline is committed to objective evaluation of physiologic mechanisms that underlie vital organ failures and the development of therapeutic programs and life-support systems for life-threatening problems that produce maximum effectiveness. The Society of Critical Care Medicine and this book, we hope, address these issues."[3]

This third edition appears as the United States rapidly moves to change dramatically the way its healthcare is financed and delivered. Any health reform plan will certainly require physicians to act as managers of resource allocation as well as diagnosticians and caregivers. The vast amount of new information contained in this third edition is weighty evidence of the need for students and physicians to develop new methods of acquiring and retrieving information. Intensivists have served as resource managers and should be well prepared to take on this important new role in an expanded fashion. They have also led the way in the use of protocols and guidelines as methods for reducing reams of data into useful approaches to diagnosis and treatment.

There is almost universal interest in the principle of *case management*. The concept is usually applied to primary care practitioners. A physician or other health professional such as a nurse practitioner or, in some situations, a medical social worker coordinates the care of an individual in an attempt to provide the best care possible in a cost-effective manner. The medical and nursing directors in the intensive care unit (ICU) are, in effect, case managers who manage resources for each patient in their unit. Their success in bringing order to what many consider the chaotic and willy-nilly use of high technology could provide a model for case managers in primary care.

HEALTHCARE REFORM AND THE DELIVERY OF CRITICAL CARE

The United States, almost alone among the developed countries in its unwillingness to provide health insurance for its people, is at a great crossroads as it once more attempts to develop a program ensuring universal healthcare security. The international flavor of critical care medicine and the growing literature comparing outcomes and costs of other systems will certainly provide a rational pathway to what has worked well in other environments.

At first glance, much of the promise of biomedical science seems to have been fulfilled. Today, 71% of Americans can expect to live to the age of 70 years; only 32% could reach that age in 1900. Much of this improvement in health status can be attributed to the almost exponential growth of scientific knowledge, in general, and the ability to apply that knowledge to the maintenance of health and the treatment of disease. This increase in survivorship has been almost linear and was achieved for much of the century without much increase in cost. The acceleration of healthcare costs began in the late 1960s as total United States health expenditures rose from 27.1 billion dollars in 1960 to 752 billion dollars in 1991. Calculated on a per capita basis, total expenditures rose from $143 per American in 1960 to $2868 in 1991. It is the continuing growth in these costs that staggers the imagination. Per cent yearly increases have ranged from 8.9% to 11.7%, but they have been below 10% during only 1 year—1988. Assuming that expenditures will continue to grow at a rate of 10%, total costs will be 1 trillion dollars in 1994, with per capita expenses averaging $3800. Droll and scholarly economists—some call economics the "dismal science"—often become downright emotional when they watch how healthcare spending reduces other opportunities for individual investment. The percentage of the gross domestic product consumed by healthcare rose from 5.3% in 1960 to 13.2% in 1991. Incredibly, one seventh of the American economy is engaged in delivering healthcare.

The United States leads the way in the cost of healthcare and spends 258% more per capita than Ireland, 182% more than the United Kingdom, 91% more than Germany, 85% more than France, 73% more than Sweden, and 40% more than Canada. Life expectancy is 73.1 years for males in the United States, 74.6 in Ireland, 72.4 in the United Kingdom, 71.8 in Germany, 72.3 in France, 74.2 in Sweden, and 73.0 in Canada. Costs are rising in the other developed countries, however, and shared cross-national experiences may suggest the most efficient ways of delivering high-quality healthcare. United States President William Clinton, in his healthcare reform proposals, has suggested a middle ground between the existing fee-for-service American system and the more rigorously controlled systems found in other countries. Whether "managed competition" is able to control costs and preserve quality remains to be seen, but cost containment will certainly remain an important requirement, even in the United States.

Critical care professionals have been in the forefront of the effort to improve the delivery of healthcare and make it more cost effective. Critics of the healthcare system often point to the excessive use of expensive and poorly evaluated technology in the futile care of hopelessly ill and injured people, even though intensivists led the way in studying their own practice patterns. The cost of caring for such individuals is certainly high, and a study by the Office of Technology Assessment[5] reported that the total hospital costs for patients who spend any time in an ICU during hospitalization ranged from 28% to 34% of total hospital costs. Parno and colleagues[6] carefully studied hospital charges and long-term survival in 558 ICU and 124 non-ICU patients admitted to a large community medical center in Massachusetts. They found that although 9.5% of total hospital admissions to the 950-bed general hospital required intensive care, those patients accounted for 30% of hospital charges. Only 14% of total hospital charges for this 9.5% of patients were related to care within the ICU itself.

Critical care in its various forms has a central role in the access to medical care for millions of Americans who have experienced it, as well as for those who may in their lifetime depend on it for management of life-threatening injury or disease. Because it is a dramatic display of medical intervention at its best, critical care runs the risk of being viewed in terms that would conceptualize it as an end in itself. The truth is that it is part of a medical system that is expected to contribute its share of service for the welfare of the entire society. As part of the fabric of medical care, critical care has all of the strengths and weaknesses and is subject to all of the criticisms and changes that characterize the health and medical effort in this last period of the 20th century. Simply because the stakes and costs for this sort of care are so high, ill-considered changes could seriously damage the American healthcare effort, whereas carefully planned and rational changes in the way such care is delivered could improve the quality and decrease the cost of medical care in general.

THE BEGINNINGS OF CRITICAL CARE MEDICINE

At first, the mission of intensivists was one of salvage. Wartime experience had shown that early replacement of volume deficits with blood plasma and normal saline could save lives, and these techniques were put to peacetime use. Wondrous new technology showed that death could be delayed or actually prevented by the use of iron lungs, dialyzers, defibrillators, and transplanted or mechanical hearts. The diffusion of new information varied widely, and differences in clinical approach soon labeled physicians as "aggressive" or "conservative" depending on whether they chose to err on the side of action or inaction.

The discipline slowly evolved and shifted from an emphasis on life-support measures to an understanding of how to prevent the development of irreversible organ failure and to a better understanding of when to vigorously hold onto life in our patients and when to accept the futility of the struggle and help them pass quietly into eternity. We have made a good deal of progress toward treating life-threatening illness but are still a long way from a fundamental understanding of what determines survival and recovery in many common situations. Perhaps a look back at where we have been and an honest assessment of where we are at this moment can help us advance as rapidly as possible to where we need to be.

Students studying the regulation of the blood volume or cardiac output during critical illness may not realize the debt owed to those great thinkers of the past century who, working with simple and often crude measuring devices, began to understand the complex regulatory capacity of the human body. These scientists set down the fundamental principles of what later became the practice of critical care medicine.

The great French physiologist Claude Bernard pointed out the fallacy of continually attempting to better quantify clinical observations without linking those observations to carefully planned experiments. He argued that "the most useful path for physiology and medicine to follow now is to seek to discover new facts instead of trying to reduce to equations the facts which science already possesses." In a marvelous example that might serve as a warning to those today who prefer statistical analysis of sometimes trivial data to the development of testable hypotheses in the critical care unit, Bernard told the story of a contemporary physiologist who "took urine from a railroad station urinal where people of all nations passed, and who believed he could thus present an analysis of *average* European urine!" Bernard laid out his concepts of experimentation in his 1865 masterpiece, *An Introduction to the Study of Experimental Medicine*.[7] His carefully planned experiments had allowed him to hypothesize and test the concept that

> "*animals have really two environments: a milieu extérieur* in which the organism is situated, and a *milieu intérieur* in which the tissue elements live. The living organism does not really exist in the *milieu extérieur* (the atmosphere if it breathes, salt or fresh water if it is in that element) but in the liquid *milieu intérieur* which surrounds and bathes all the tissue elements. . . . All the vital mechanisms, however varied they may be, have only one object, that of preserving constant the conditions of the *milieu intérieur*."

Seventy years after Bernard's formulation of the milieu intérieur, Walter B. Cannon, Professor of Physiology at Harvard, introduced the term *homeostasis* to describe the "coordinated physiological processes" that maintain a steady state for most systems. His studies into the "ways in which these self-regulatory agencies operate to preserve constancy of the fluid matrix" set the stage for the development of therapeutic methods aimed at promoting that constancy and form the basis of the pathophysiologic approach to serious illness. He could well be called "the father of critical care." His book, *The Wisdom of the Body*,[8] told how he and his colleagues in France in 1917 found that reduced blood pressure led to decreased bicarbonate concentration (the only available test to measure the carbon dioxide combining power). Fifty years before the widespread use of lactate measurements to estimate cellular oxygenation, his studies showed that "the alkali reserve rarely falls below normal . . . until the systolic pressure is less than 80 mm Hg. Furthermore, just as in the experiments performed at Dijon, the greater the reduction of the blood pressure below that critical level, the greater is the fall in the alkali reserve." Sixty years before the concept of supply-dependent oxygen consumption became widely discussed, Cannon's colleague Aub found that in experimental shock, basal metabolism (oxygen consumption) fell 18.5% and 33%, respectively, when the blood pressure was reduced to 70 and 60 mm Hg, respectively.

WERNER FORSSMANN CATHETERIZES HIS OWN HEART

Intracardiac catheterization, one of the bedrock techniques of critical care medicine, was introduced in 1929 by a young German surgeon, who had graduated from the Berlin medical school the previous year. Forssmann, as a medical student, was impressed by the experimental work of the French physiologists Bernard, Chauveau, and Marey. Chauveau and Marey[9] had earlier measured the intracardiac pressures of horses, and although warned by his superiors that human catheterization was not safe, Forssmann, in the summer of 1929, performed the catheterization on himself without prior animal research. He was advised by his superior to write the paper describing his self-catheterization, published in November 1929[10] from a therapeutic rather than a diagnostic perspective in order to deflect some of the expected uproar.

Until Forssmann's discovery, cardiac output could not be measured by the direct Fick principle in humans, even though it had been used by Gréhant and Quinquaud in animals in 1886.[11] Baumann, a German physician, apparently unaware of the new technique of cardiac catheterization, measured cardiac output in humans by direct cardiac puncture in 1930,[12] a method that would hardly have been useful in the modern critical care unit. Klein, an internist in Prague, used Forssmann's cardiac catheterization method to obtain mixed venous blood and studied cardiac output in 30 patients, thus establishing the method that was soon to become the standard in the field.[13]

Not everyone was enchanted with Forssmann's method. Grollman[14] wrote that it was

"not only dangerous to the subject but useless so far as cardiac output determinations are concerned. The formation of thrombi which is very likely with the introduction of a foreign body into the blood stream renders the method too hazardous for its possible future use. The nature of the operation also precludes its use as a means of determining cardiac output for the unavoidable psychic effect accompanying the procedure will elevate the cardiac output considerably and thus vitiate any results obtained. This method must thus be considered merely as a clinical curiosity."

The use of Forssmann's technique to accurately measure intracardiac pressure awaited the development of Wiggers'[15] optical manometer toward the end of the decade. The coupling of Forssmann's technique with Wiggers' manometer was to open a new page in the history of cardiac physiology. The technique lay unused for almost 10 years, probably because of the warnings expressed by authorities like Grollman.[14] It was rediscovered by Andre Cournand and Dickinson Richards in 1940,[16] who used it to study traumatic shock in the emergency wards of New York City's Bellevue Hospital. They used right atrial catheterization to obtain mixed venous blood, and they calculated cardiac output from the arteriovenous oxygen content difference to calculate cardiac output from the Fick equation. They concluded that traumatic shock was a "rapid or precipitate failure of the circulation, usually associated with inadequate return flow of blood to the heart. The chief findings were decreased cardiac output, low pressure in the right auricle, low arterial pressure, and decreased blood volume." They found that oxygen delivery was markedly reduced and that the arteriovenous oxygen difference was increased in an effort to maintain oxygen consumption. In recognition of the important contribution to the diagnosis and treatment of cardiopulmonary disorders made possible by the discovery of cardiac catheterization, Richards, Cournand, and Forssmann were awarded the Nobel Prize for Medicine in 1956.

Renewed interest in hemorrhagic shock came with the Second World War when Carl Wiggers,[15] of Case Western Reserve University in Cleveland, focused on the irreversible shock that followed sustained blood loss. Cannon had demonstrated that adrenosympathetic responses became exhausted after prolonged hemorrhage, but Wiggers believed that factors other than that were necessary to explain irreversibility. The problem, he wrote in 1950, "is not advanced appreciably by the assertions that the metabolic machinery is wrecked or that stagnant anoxia, reflexes or toxic actions are concerned. The agents which induce peripheral vascular failure and myocardial depression must be identified."

CRITICAL CARE BECOMES AN ORGANIZED DISCIPLINE

The newest healthcare specialties, critical care medicine and critical care nursing, were practiced informally for many years and gained form through wartime experiences with hemorrhagic shock, sepsis, and acute renal failure. Improved triage and transportation systems during each of the recent wars led to a progressive decrease in the incidence of acute renal failure and demonstrated the importance of early restoration of blood volume and oxygen delivery, leading to the concept of the so-called *golden hour,* which has become one of the guiding principles of critical care.

The application of advanced technology to life support began with Drinker's development of the whole-body negative-pressure respirator, or "iron lung." These respirators saved many lives in individuals stricken with poliomyelitis and brain stem paralysis. The first acute care units arose in Scandinavia in the early 1950s in order to centralize respirators and health professionals. Those who wish to better understand the incredibly complex burden placed on physicians and nurses by the presence of the extremely contagious and frequently fatal poliovirus in the environment might wish to read the republication of Drinker and McKhann's pioneer article describing the invention of the iron lung.[17] Accompanying the article is a startling photograph showing more than 50 iron lungs in use in a Los Angeles County hospital in the 1950s. As a reminder of the importance of basic research, parallel progress in virology and immunology led to a vaccine that prevented poliomyelitis and, almost overnight, eliminated the need for iron lungs.

In the beginning, anesthesiologists had a leading role in the application of advanced technology to seriously ill patients. Anesthesiologists were in the hospital for much of each day, were skilled at intubation, and were accustomed to dealing with seriously ill patients after surgery. Peter Safar, an anesthesiologist, organized the first special care unit in the United States at the Baltimore City Hospital in 1958 and coined the term *intensive care unit.*[18] The development of the direct current defibrillator[19] and closed-chest cardiac massage[20] made the organization of resources in a coronary care unit inevitable and accelerated the development of ICUs in general.

The discipline gained intellectual structure when 26 individual physicians representing medicine, anesthesiology, pediatrics, and surgery met in 1970 and founded the Society of Critical Care Medicine. The founders agreed that the Society should be interdisciplinary and international in nature. The Society's journal, *Critical Care Medicine,* skillfully edited by William Shoemaker, became a major focus for the exchange of scientific information throughout the world. Recognizing the importance of the dissemination of the basic principles of critical care medicine to all of its practitioners, the Society began to publish an annual review of the discipline in 1980[3] and published the first edition of the *Textbook of Critical Care* in 1984.[4]

Nurses involved in critical care had already developed an organization for coronary care nurses in 1969, The American Association for Cardiovascular Nurses, and broadened its constituency by renaming itself the American Association of Critical Care Nurses (AACN) in 1971. The association's official scientific journal, *Heart and Lung: The Journal of Critical Care,* began publication in 1972 as critical care's first interdisciplinary journal with a nurse-physician editor team at the helm. Twenty years later, the Association's *American Journal of Critical Care* replaced *Heart and Lung* as the official journal. It reaches thousands of nurses and other health professionals, including physicians, and has become a major intellectual resource for the setting of high standards in the field of critical care. The AACN today has almost 80,000 members.

The AACN developed a certification program for experienced nurses in 1973, which became the CCRN. The four medical specialties, after first attempting to develop a joint board certification process, developed separate examinations for each discipline. The anesthesiologists, surgeons, and pediatricians gave their first examination in 1986; the internists gave theirs in the fall of 1987. Today, 6293 physicians hold subspecialty certification in critical care medicine. Critical care medicine has entered the mainstream of American medicine.

INTENSIVE CARE UNITS PROLIFERATE WORLDWIDE

Nearly forty years after the opening of the first ICU at the Baltimore City Hospital in 1958,[18] there are now an estimated 7434 ICUs in the United States and thousands more around the world. An important study conducted by the Society of Critical Care Medicine in partnership with the American Hospital Association, in 1992,[21] described the current topography of critical care. In a mammoth effort that involved the cooperation of critical care physicians and nurses throughout the country, the authors of the study evaluated responses from 2876 separate ICUs, representing 38% of the national total. Figures 4 and 5 in their article reveal information that must make instrument manufacturers giddy. The wide availability of equipment promises patients an excellent chance at surviving events of critical illness if enough trained physicians, nurses, and other health professionals are available to make the most of some incredibly sophisticated hardware. Most units have considerable equipment: 97.8% of ICUs can perform continuous electrocardiographic monitoring, although because the study found that only 18% to 23% of registered nurses are certified by the AACN, it is not clear who is performing the necessary on-line interpretation of complex cardiac arrhythmias. An impressive 97.8% of hospitals are equipped with mechanical ventilators, 96% have pulse oximeters, and 95.8% can perform invasive arterial blood pressure monitoring.

Differences among units begin to emerge when one looks at the ability to monitor cardiovascular hemodynamic function or to support the function of organ systems such as the kidneys or the brain. Only 14.9% of hospitals with less than 100 beds provided mixed venous oximetry, whereas this was available in 54.5% of hospitals with more than 500 beds. Hemodialysis and intracranial monitoring were available in 19.2% and 11.7% of the smallest hospitals and in 76.8% and 61.7% of the largest hospitals. Size and to a lesser extent affiliation with a medical school were associated with a broader range of critical care resources.

THE SCIENTIFIC BASIS OF CRITICAL CARE MEDICINE

The discipline of critical care was initially focused on problems of the heart and lungs and on life-support efforts for individuals whom others had considered to be "hopelessly ill." As many of those deemed by conventional wisdom to be "incurables" left the hospital and returned to useful lives, the aims of the discipline changed. Attention turned to the study of basic pathophysiologic and biochemical mechanisms in an effort to correct individual organ dysfunction before serious stressor forces such as hypovolemia, hypoxemia, and sepsis set the stage for the arrival of multiple organ system dysfunction and failure.

The multi-institutional study organized by the Division of Lung Diseases of the National Institutes of Health (NIH)[22] to study extracorporeal membrane oxygenation for acute respiratory failure found that two thirds of the 490 patients studied had failure of organ systems other than the lungs. The mortality rate was 40% when only the lungs were involved; death rates, however, rose to 85% in the 162 patients with renal failure, to 79% in the patients with central nervous system involvement, and to 77% in the 116 patients with sepsis. The *number* of additional organs involved and not the *nature* of the organ system itself appeared to determine mortality. Involvement of one additional organ increased mortality to 55%, three additional organs to 85%, and four to 100%.

It took many years for modern intensive care science to begin to answer the critical question asked by Cannon and Wiggers and given new importance by the NIH study: Why do cells die? Attention began to shift from the irreversibility of hemorrhagic shock to the incredibly lethal nature of endotoxin. Lewis Thomas summed up evolving research in the field of immunology when he wrote in *The Lives of a Cell,* "It is our response to (bacteria) that makes the disease. Our arsenals for fighting off bacteria are so powerful and involve so many different defense mechanisms, that we are more in danger from them than from the invaders. We live in the midst of explosive devices; we are mined."[23] The demonstration in the 1970s that sepsis could occur without bacteremia and might be the cause of the deadly syndrome of multiple organ failure warned physicians that undiagnosed infection might be more common than previously believed.

Many of the chapters in the third edition of the *Textbook of Critical Care* detail the ways in which scientists began to explore the mediators that might lead to cell death. Leukocytes activated by complement had been suggested as cell killers but did not seem to be toxic enough to explain the syndrome of multiple organ failure. Clowes and colleagues[24] believed that a cleavage fragment of interleukin-1 was the toxic factor, whereas Baracos and associates[25] suggested that interleukin-1 released prostaglandin E_2 and that those two factors interacted to produce the proteolytic effect.

Two years later, Beutler[26] and his group at Rockefeller University isolated a monokine secreted by macrophages stimulated with endotoxin that completely suppressed the synthesis of lipoprotein lipase and had the same activity as tumor necrosis factor activity. Beutler and coworkers[27] then demonstrated that an antibody to cachectin blocked the production of multiple organ failure in mice given endotoxin but could not prevent the development of fever. A collaborative study with the Cornell group[28] demonstrated that recombinant human cachectin produced hypotension, metabolic acidosis, hemoconcentration, diffuse pulmonary inflammation and hemorrhage, ischemic and hemorrhagic lesions of the gastrointestinal tract, hyperglycemia, and hypoglycemia. Although Beutler and his group[26] had earlier and conservatively suggested that cachectin was "clearly only one of the mediators responsible for the numerous pathologic effects of lipopolysaccharide," it was now suggested that "a single protein mediator (cachectin) is capable of inducing many of the deleterious effects of endotoxin."[28] The two research groups, with assistance from Chiron Research Laboratories, then demonstrated conclusively that cachectin was necessary for the development of septic shock. A potent neutralizing monoclonal anticachectin antibody was administered to baboons 1 and 2 hours before they received an LD_{100} dose of live *Escherichia coli.* Unprotected animals developed the classic syndrome of septic shock; animals receiving the monoclonal antibody 2 hours before receiving live bacteria did not develop shock; and animals treated 1 hour before infection failed to develop shock but died of renal and pulmonary failure.[29]

The cachectin story is but one of the many examples of how molecular science has allowed intensivists to look into the cell and determine the causes of its malfunction. Many find the use of the term *cachectin* (the molecule is also called *tumor necrosis factor*) particularly appropriate because so many critically ill and toxic patients are cachectic indeed.

MAKING CRITICAL CARE MORE EFFECTIVE

Critical care, at its very best, matches professional skills and healthcare resources with patient need at a moment when life appears to hang in the balance and the likelihood of death or survival is dependent on the quality and appropriateness of those skills and resources. Unlike many other medical disciplines, critical care is a system of sickness care that begins with transportation to an appropriate hospital, provides urgent care en route to a hospital or in an emergency department, and then initiates an organized approach to comprehensive treatment in a special care unit.

Evaluation of the critical care process has been part of the discipline since its inception and is the purpose of the third edition of the *Textbook of Critical Care.* In 1983, for example, many critical care professionals participated in a systematic assessment by the NIH Office of Medical Applications of Research. That organization has since then been incorporated into a larger and free-standing entity, the Agency for Health Care Policy and Research.

A consensus development conference was held in Washington, D.C., in March of 1983 and concluded that modern therapeutic interventions benefit many patients admitted to critical care units but that the evidence of benefit was equivocal in another large group of patients.[30] The weight of clinical opinion supported the belief that intensive care was useful for this larger population but that the risk of iatrogenic illnesses and complications could outweigh any potential benefit. The panel also concluded that limited resources should not be devoted to patients "without reasonable prospects of recovery when patients who need these services are being turned away due to lack of capacity." Concerns over the ethics of resource allocation and termination of life support echoed the just concluded report of the *President's Commission for the Study of Ethical Problems in Medicine and Biomedical and Behavioral Research: Deciding to Forego Life-Sustaining Treatment.*[31]

EVALUATING THE PRACTICE OF CRITICAL CARE

The rapid introduction of new and expensive technology into critical care and other healthcare disciplines caused many to wonder whether these new technologies were all they were stated to be by their inventors. Paul Ellwood, the pediatrician-healthcare analyst whose home in Jackson Hole, Wyoming, has become a mecca for those involved in healthcare reform, coined the term *outcomes management* in his 1988 Shattuck lecture:

"Outcomes management is a technology of patient experience designed to help patients, payers, and providers make rational medical care-related choices based on better insight into the effects of these choices on the patient's life."[32]

Another pediatrician, William Roper, and his colleagues at the Health Care Financing Administration attempted to operationalize the Ellwood approach by describing an "effectiveness initiative."[33] Traditionally, medical effectiveness measures the efficacy of medical interventions in actual practice whereas medical appropriateness deals with the use of an intervention in a given clinical situation evaluation. Roper chose to collapse both terms and use the word *effectiveness* in a broad manner.

Knaus and colleagues[34] retrospectively measured the severity of illness and mortality rates in 13 American hospitals. Mortality rates varied from 59% to 158% of predicted. The researchers suggested that those ICUs with the lowest death rates had certain important characteristics: They followed standard approaches or protocols and did not permit each physician to develop a completely unique treatment plan for each patient; a medical director with considerable authority for managing admission and discharge policies and for coordinating the care of individual physicians was present; critical care nurses had a high level of educational achievement; and nurses and physicians had a strong collegial relationship. A prospective pilot project organized by the AACN[35] studied an ICU that demonstrated the same elements identified by Knaus and associates.[34] The mortality rate for 192 patients was 51% of predicted, new complications did not occur, and both staff and patient satisfaction was high. The ability of specially trained critical care physicians to lower mortality rates in ICUs was shown by two studies. Reynolds and colleagues[36] reported that the mortality due to septic shock decreased from 74% to 23% when specially trained physicians supervised care. Brown and Sullivan[37] found a 52% decrease in ICU deaths when a full-time critical care specialist was recruited and coordinated the care of the patient's own physician.

PROFESSIONAL AND PUBLIC PARTNERSHIPS FOR BETTER AND MORE AFFORDABLE CRITICAL CARE

On November 13 and 14, 1989, The Foundation for Critical Care sponsored a forum, "Critical Care in the United States: An Agenda for the 1990s." The forum concluded that substantial major improvements in life expectancy and enhanced quality of life for all Americans could be achieved without incurring substantial additional costs if the access to critical care and the management of the critically ill or injured patient were better organized.

The attendees concluded that rapid access to hospital emergency rooms and ICUs is vital because there is firm evidence that the greatest likelihood for survival after critical illness or injury occurs when an individual promptly receives care appropriate for the specific clinical situation. Similar levels of prehospital care should be available to all, and there seems to be no rational explanation for the presence of well-trained paramedics in one geographic location but not in another. Standards exist for paramedic training in some states but not in others.

The forum also concluded that there is strong evidence that the process or manner of providing critical care is an important determinant of survival. The level of collaboration between physicians and nurses and the organization of human resources, rather than the technical capability of individual practitioners, seems to determine outcome. The better the management of human resources, the better the outcome, independent of resources. On-site physician and nurse leaders ensure that patients' needs are matched in the availability of resources by the implementation of sound admission and discharge policies. Effective clinical managers perform triage and attempt to resolve conflict among health practitioners, particularly among physicians. In many units, physician managers are managers in name only and do not perform triage, make decisions, or resolve conflicts. Nurses are forced, in the absence of a working medical director, to make moment-to-moment decisions that determine patients' outcomes. A collaborative nurse-physician relationship usually suggests that physician leadership is present within the units on a reliable and regular basis. The most successful units seem to use nurse resources carefully. Clerical tasks such as seeking laboratory reports, managing patient records, performing certain housekeeping tasks, and making various phone calls are performed by individuals other than nurses.

The third edition of the *Textbook of Critical Care* appears at the beginning of a new phase in American, and indeed worldwide, healthcare delivery. Whether the uniquely American idea of managed competition will work and be adopted by other countries or whether it will prove to be ineffective and be replaced a single-payor system remains to be seen. It is clear, however, that broadly trained healthcare professionals must be at the core of any successful system and should replace the hordes of business and accounting executives who know more about turning profits than caring for the ill. This text aims to prepare new health professionals, physicians and nurses, to take on this leadership responsibility. The continuous accumulation of knowledge aided by computer-assisted informatics, the constant use of deductive and inductive reasoning, respect and affection for individual patients, and the ability to wisely allocate resources for the general population under care will ensure that health professionals of good character and gracious modesty will manage the rational system of tomorrow.

References

1. Shoemaker WC, Ayres SM, Grenvik A, et al: Textbook of Critical Care. 3rd ed. Philadelphia, WB Saunders, 1995.
2. Ayres SM, Giannelli S: The Care of the Critically Ill. New York, Appleton-Century-Crofts, 1966.
3. Shoemaker WC, Thompson WC (eds): Critical Care: State of the Art. Society of Critical Care Medicine, Fullerton, CA, 1980.
4. Shoemaker WC, Thompson WC, Holbrook PR: Textbook of Critical Care. Philadelphia, WB Saunders, 1984.
5. Berenson RA: Intensive Care Units (ICUs): Clinical Outcomes, Costs and Decision-Making. Office of Technology Assessment, Washington, DC, United States Congress, 1984.
6. Parno RP, Teres D, Lemeshow S, et al: Hospital charges and long-term survival of ICU versus non-ICU patients. Crit Care Med 1982; 10:569–574.
7. Bernard C; Greene HC, trans: An Introduction to the Study of Experimental Medicine (1865). New York, Dover Publications, 1927.
8. Cannon W: The Wisdom of the Body. New York, WW Norton & Co, 1932, Chapter 1.
9. Chauveau A, Marey EJ: Appareils et Expériences Cardiographiques. *In*: Mémoires de L'Académie Imperiale de Médicine. Tome XXVI, Paris, 1863.
10. Forssmann W: Die Sondierung des rechten Herzens. Klin Wochenschr 1929; 8:2085–2087; addendum, 1929; 8:2287.
11. Gréhant H, Quinquaud CE: Recherches expérimentales sur la mesure du volume de sang qui traverse les poumons en un temps donné. Comptes Rendus de La Societé de Biologie 1886; 30:159.
12. Baumann H: Über die Verwertbarkeit der verschiedenen Methoden zur Minutenvolumenbestimmung. Z Krebsforsch, 1930; 22:610.
13. Klein O: Zur Bestimmung des zirkulatorischen Minutenvolumens beim Menschen nach dem Fickschen Prinzip mittels Herzsondierung. Munch Med Wochenschr 1930; 77:1311
14. Grollman A: The Cardiac Output in Health and Disease. Springfield, IL, Charles C Thomas, 1932.
15. Wiggers CA: Physiology of Shock. New York, The Commonwealth Fund, 1950, Chapter 51.
16. Cournand A, Ranges HA: Catheterization of the right auricle in man. Proc Soc Exp Biol Med 1941; 46:462.
17. Drinker P, McKhann C: The use of a new apparatus for the prolonged adminstration of artificial respiration. I. A fatal case of poliomyelitis. JAMA 1929; 92:1658; reprinted 1986; 255:1473.
18. Safar P, DeKornfeld T, Pearson J, et al: Intensive care unit. Anesthesia 1961; 16:275–284.
19. Zoll PM, Linenthal AJ, Gibson P, et al: Termination of ventricular fibrillation in man by externally applied countershock. N Engl J Med 1956; 254:727.
20. Kouwenhoven WB, Jude JR, Knickerbocker GG: Closed chest cardiac massage. JAMA 1960; 173:1064.
21. Groeger JS, Strosberg M, Halpern N, et al: Descriptive analysis of critical care units in the United States. Crit Care Med 1992; 20:846–863.
22. Extracorporeal Support for Respiratory Failure: A Collaborative Study in Response to RFP-NHLI-7320. Washington, DC, National Heart, Lung and Blood Institute, 1979.
23. Thomas L: The Lives of a Cell. New York, Bantam Books, 1975, p 92.
24. Clowes GHA, George BC, Ville CA, et al: Muscle proteolysis induced by a circulating peptide in patients with sepsis or trauma. N Engl J Med 1983; 308:515–552.
25. Baracos V, Rodemann HP, Dinarello CA, et al: Stimulation of muscle protein degradation and prostaglandin E_2 release by leukocytic pyrogen (interleukin-1). N Engl J Med 1983; 308:533–558.
26. Beutler J, Mahoney N, LeTrang N, et al: Purification of cachectin, a lipoprotein lipase suppressing hormone secreted by endotoxin-induced RAW 264.7 cells. J Exp Med 1985; 161:984–995.
27. Beutler B, Milsark IW, Cerami AC: Passive immunization against cachectin/tumor necrosis factor protects mice from lethal effect of endotoxin. Science 1985; 229:869–871.
28. Tracey KJ, Beutler B, Lowry SF, et al: Shock and tissue injury induced by recombinant human cachectin. Science 1987; 234:470–474.
29. Tracey KJ, Fong Y, Hesse DG, et al: Anti-cachectin/TNF monoclonal antibodies prevent septic shock during lethal bacteremia. Nature 1987; 330:662–666.
30. Parillo JE, Ayres SM (Eds): Major Issues in Critical Care Medicine Consensus Conference. Baltimore, Williams & Wilkins, 1984.
31. President's Commission for the Study of Ethical Problems in Medicine and Biomedical and Behavioral Research: Deciding to Forgo Life-Sustaining Treatment. Washington, DC, U.S. Government Printing Office Publication No. 83-600503, 1983.
32. Ellwood PM: Shattuck lecture—outcomes management: A technology of patient experience. N Engl J Med 1988; 318:1549–1556.
33. Roper WL, Winkenwerder W, Hackbarth JD, et al: Effectiveness in health care: An initiative to evaluate and improve medical practice. N Engl J Med 1988; 319:1197–1202.
34. Knaus WA, Draper EA, Wagner DP: An evaluation of outcome from intensive care in major medical centers. Ann Intern Med 1986; 104:410.
35. Mitchell PH, Armstrong SA, Simpson TF, et al: American Association of Critical Care Nurses demonstration project: Profile of excellence in critical care nursing. Heart Lung 1989; 18:219–237.

36. Reynolds HN, Haupt MT, Thill-Baharozian MC, et al: Impact of critical care physician staffing on patients with septic shock in a university hospital medical intensive care unit. JAMA 1988; 252:2023–2027.
37. Brown JJ, Sullivan G: Effect on ICU mortality of a full-time critical care specialist. Chest 1989; 96:127–129.

CHAPTER 2

The Critical Care Unit: Design Recommendations and Standards

John W. Hoyt, MD, FCCM
Maurene A. Harvey, RN, MPH, CCRN, FCCM
Donald C. Axon, FAIA

A single phrase, *form follows function,* should be the basis for design recommendations for the critical care unit. It would be impossible to list in this chapter all the individual state rules, regulations, and standards for intensive care unit (ICU) design. Some states require windows for each patient, but others do not. Some states require a toilet in the room for each patient, but others do not. In this chapter, it is much more important to briefly describe the function of an ICU and then to examine in detail the form that facilitates that function. Those readers involved in the process of designing an ICU are referred to their local and state hospital construction and engineering regulations in order to be in compliance with applicable statutes and practices.

It seems appropriate at the beginning of this text on critical care to define the critically ill patient and the role of the ICU. There are two aspects to defining the critically ill patient. First is the issue of monitoring. Critically ill patients are those patients in unstable physiologic situations in whom small changes in organ function may lead to a serious deterioration in overall body function with irreversible organ system damage or death. Intermittent or continuous monitoring is directed at finding these small changes early to provide optimal treatment and restore a more stable physiologic situation and thus prevent organ system damage and death.

The second aspect that defines critically ill patients is the need for special treatment. This treatment may be intermittent, such as portable dialysis, or continuous, such as mechanical ventilation. This treatment may be directed at curing the patient, such as antibiotic therapy, or sustaining the patient, such as life support with an intra-aortic counterpulsation balloon. Critical care is the monitoring of patients with life-threatening illnesses and the provision of therapy to them.[1] For critical care services to function most effectively there must be a harmonious interaction among human, technologic, pharmacologic, and spatial resources.[2]

Critical care encompasses more than monitoring and life support. It comprises a multidisciplinary and multiprofessional team working together in a geographic area of the hospital 24 hours a day, 7 days a week, attempting to guide patients with life-threatening illnesses through their physiologic instabilities to recovery and discharge from the hospital. In the past, critical care services were provided by attending physicians admitting patients to ICUs staffed by nurses. Physicians made rounds once or twice a day and prescribed tests and treatments for nurses to carry out in their absence. This care delivery model requires a smaller and more limited ICU design, which is not discussed in this chapter. Recommendations from the Society of Critical Care on the delivery of level I critical care services require design and space considerations for an integrated team of healthcare workers.[3] This chapter discusses design recommendations and standards for a critical care unit to be staffed by a multidisciplinary and multiprofessional team.

To finish the discussion of critical care unit function, permitting us to go on to an analysis of form, the multidisciplinary and multiprofessional critical care team must be defined. *Multidisciplinary* commonly refers to the physician members of the team who provide the day-to-day bedside medical coverage of the ICU. Critical care physicians include specialists in the disciplines of anesthesiology, internal medicine, pediatrics, and surgery. These primary boards all offer examinations for a certificate of special competence in critical care after completing a 1- to 3-year fellowship, depending on circumstances such as primary specialty. *Multiprofessional* refers to the basic philosophy of critical care that there must be a partnership among physicians, nurses, respiratory therapists, pharmacists, social workers, dieticians, and so forth in the management of critically ill patients.

The multiprofessional team is led by a system of collaborative practice in which a critical care nursing director and a critical care medical director share in the administration and management of the critical care unit. They each have their own areas of responsibility and different lines of reporting within the hospital, but within the ICU they must be partners in providing high-quality monitoring and life support to patients with life-threatening illnesses. The critical care nursing director is responsible for a staff of bedside nurses who provide patient care by working 8- to 12-hour shifts. The critical care medical director is responsible for other critical care attending physicians and possibly house staff composed of critical care fellows and residents. This team is responsible for bedside medical coverage using a "sleep-in" ICU call system.

Thus, when analyzing the form that must follow function in the ICU, needs must be met for patients, families, physicians, nursing care, and respiratory therapy space—to name just a few of the function factors that must be considered. The critical care nursing director must have an office in or near the ICU to be available to the ICU nursing staff. The critical care medical director must have an office in or near the ICU to be available to evaluate patients' problems and to begin corrective therapy. Lounge space, call rooms, conference rooms, and so forth must be available if the form of the ICU is to meet the function of the modern critical care team. Detailed information on all the ancillary spaces needed by a critical care team is presented later in this chapter.

BEDSIDE SPATIAL RELATIONSHIPS

In discussing a critical care unit to be staffed by a multidisciplinary and multiprofessional team, it is necessary to address the issue of unit size and distribution of beds. The Task Force on Guidelines of the Society of Critical Care Medicine has recommended 12 beds as an ideal size for a critical care unit.[2] Because of the close working relationship between nurses, doctors, patients, and family, the ICU is commonly viewed as a family or community.[4] This community has various psychosocial needs if its members are to work in a cooperative relationship. That cooperative relationship is probably most functional in a 12-bed unit. An

ICU of larger size leads to the appearance of chaos. A smaller unit has fewer personnel to work with each other during times of crises.

A frequent controversy in critical care is the issue of unit specialization.[5] On one side of the issue, opposed to specialization, is the inefficiency of multiple small departmental ICUs—for example, a neurology ICU, a neurosurgical ICU, a respiratory ICU, and a medical ICU. Obvious overlaps exist in such a situation, and much of this sort of division usually represents internecine institutional turf struggles with little recognition of the needs of patients or of the ICU staff. On the other side of the issue, in favor of specialization, is the value of a nursing/physician team doing things they are very familiar with in large volume, leading to expertise and high quality. An institution with a large volume of liver transplants, for example, most certainly benefits from a very specialized liver transplantation ICU as long as the average occupancy of the unit can be maintained at 80% to 90%.

It seems that the best recommendation for unit specialization may rest with institutional data on volume of patients. By grouping ICUs of various medical and surgical specialization together, in either a horizontal or vertical manner, these ICUs can share resources such as a *stat* laboratory and a satellite pharmacy. This arrangement leads to substantial cost efficiency by sharing staff such as respiratory therapists, social workers, pharmacists, and others. Physicians and nurses may choose not to cross-cover ICUs of different specialty, but other healthcare workers should be able to work in different specialty units.

The recommended number of beds in a critical care center of multiple ICUs is dependent on the desire of the critical care team for immediate or delayed bed availability. The Canadian Department of National Health and Welfare has suggested a formula for determining the needed number of ICU beds based on past use figures.[6] If a hospital is proposing a critical care center of multiple 12-bed units, it can determine the required number of beds by examining the previous hospital ICU occupancy. For example, a previous occupancy of 30 beds with a desire for a 80% probability of an available bed would require that this hospital build 34 beds. Thus, three 12-bed pods with a total of 36 beds would easily meet the needs of the critical care center.

However, if this critical care center wants a 99% probability that an ICU bed will be available, it must build at least 42 beds and is probably advised to consider four 12-bed pods, or 48 beds. This will certainly require shifting some patients within specialized ICUs to optimize efficiency.[4] This calculation is based on the following formula:

$$\text{Numbers of beds} = \text{average census} + (\text{square root of average census}) \times (Z)$$

Z = a constant dependent on the probability *(P)* of having an ICU bed available

P	Z
99%	2.33
95%	1.65
90%	1.28
85%	1.044
80%	0.804

The decision on the probability of bed availability depends on other hospital resources. For example, if the hospital has a small and poorly monitored emergency medicine department, it should probably pick a 90% or 95% probability that an ICU bed will be available. Likewise, if the hospital has a busy operating room with a small recovery room that must run efficiently with little backlog of patients, then there should be enough ICU beds to have a high probability (90–95%) of immediate admission of a critically ill patient to the ICU from the operating room.

In addition to decisions about the size of an ICU and the total number of hospital ICU beds, decisions must be made about the spatial distribution of ICU beds and their relationship to each other. Three designs are commonly used, each having its advantages and disadvantages. First is the large, open design similar to a recovery room with many beds arranged side by side around the perimeter of a room with the head of the bed against the wall. Second is the private room, related from an evolutionary perspective to early coronary care unit designs, in which rooms surround a central station with a clear view of each patient. Finally, there are groups of two-bed or four-bed pods, commonly with separate nursing stations in each room.

The disadvantage of the open design is a high level of constant activity, leading to the appearance of chaos with excessive amounts of noise. Patients have no privacy, and families have no privacy when visiting at the bedside. The advantage of the open design, particularly if the unit has 12 beds or less, is the sense of community among the staff working together and helping each other at various bedsides. This open type of unit has commonly been criticized from an infectious disease standpoint.[7] However, no evidence exists that an open unit with appropriate infectious disease controls, such as hand washing, has a higher infection rate than an ICU with private rooms.[8]

At the opposite end of the spectrum is the ICU design with only private rooms. This frequently requires a staffing ratio of one nurse per patient and may well leave a patient unattended when a nurse leaves the bedside to obtain supplies or to talk privately with a family. Much can be done with the design of such a unit to improve observation of other patients and improve efficiency. Installation of sliding glass doors as access from the hallway or between rooms and generous stocking of each bedside with equipment and supplies can reduce the risk of patients being left unattended at a critical time.

Still to be considered is a sense of community within the ICU and nurses working cooperatively with each other and other healthcare workers to provide patient care. Many ICU patients do not require one nurse per bedside, yet the private room design mandates a high staffing ratio of one nurse per patient for safety reasons. As an intermediate solution, two-bed or, better yet, four-bed pods of ICU beds solve the chaos issues of the large, open unit and the sense of individual isolation and staff inefficiency of the private rooms. Two or three nurses may commonly be assigned to four patients in a four-bed pod, leading to efficient use of nursing personnel and preservation of the sense of community among nurses helping each other from bedside to bedside.

A 12-bed ICU might have two 4-bed pods, one 2-bed pod, and two isolation rooms for special infectious disease precautions. If the isolation rooms are spatially related to the two-bed pod divided by sliding glass doors, the space can be opened up for efficient staffing when patients do not require isolation. Each nursing pod should have its own nursing station, medication cart, supplies, monitors, and communication equipment. The central station in this design becomes an area for the unit secretary and other individuals not directly involved in hands-on patient care.

The Task Force on Guidelines of the Society of Critical Care Medicine, in its 1988 recommendations on ICU design, did not take a position on an open versus a private room ICU. That was probably appropriate considering the wide range of opinions on the topic and many individual institutional variations that are likely to influence this decision. On the other hand, with the present cost-conscious environment of healthcare, it seems unwise for any institution to prospectively construct an ICU with only private rooms. There is just too much variability in severity of illness among patients and too much fluctuation in healthcare staffing patterns to make this a cost-efficient model.

BEDSIDE DESIGN

Bedside space is key to the delivery of care to ICU patients. It has been recommended that there be 150 to 200 sq ft per bedside in an open design unit and 200 to 250 sq ft per bedside in a private room design. Considering the array of monitoring and life-support devices from mechanical ventilators and intra-aortic counterpulsation balloons to dialysis machines and x-ray equipment, one should always attempt to choose the upper limit of these recommendations.[9] For the two-bed or four-bed pod design, 200 sq ft per bedside seems a reasonable compromise.

There should be an additional 2½ to 3 times this space to support the operations of the critical care unit.[2] For 12 beds in a four-bed pod design, there must be 2400 sq ft of space around the bedsides and an additional 7200 sq ft of support space, for a total space allocation of 9600 sq ft. The distribution of these additional 7200 sq ft of space is discussed later.

The organization and spatial relationships of each individual bedside are key to the efficient delivery of care. Most older ICUs have been designed on the recovery room model, with the head of the bed against the wall. Utilities such as oxygen, compressed air, vacuum, and electricity are also delivered from the wall at the head of the bed and are commonly blocked by the position of the patient. Emergent access to a patient's head for intubation and other airway management can be almost impossible. For that reason, modern ICUs are built like operating rooms, with a patient's bed away from the wall, or in the case of a private cubicle, in the middle of the room.

Utilities can be delivered from a power column that stands at one corner of the head of the bed or from an overhead boom as they frequently are in an operating room (Fig. 2–1). This arrangement permits quick and efficient 360° access to a patient and facilitates management of emergency situations. There have been recommendations for a "life island"[10] or peninsula arrangement to put monitoring, communication, utilities, and equipment immediately at the fingertips of the nurse and yet permit ease of access to a patient.

One of the most significant changes now occurring in critical care is the application of computer equipment to the management of information collected in the ICU. Bedside workstations are connected to the bedside monitor to record vital signs automatically. Intermittent measurements, nursing and physician progress notes, and patient orders are entered in the ICU patient data management system. The bedside workstation is connected to the laboratory to acquire information on all laboratory determinations. Workstations are also connected to each other on a local area

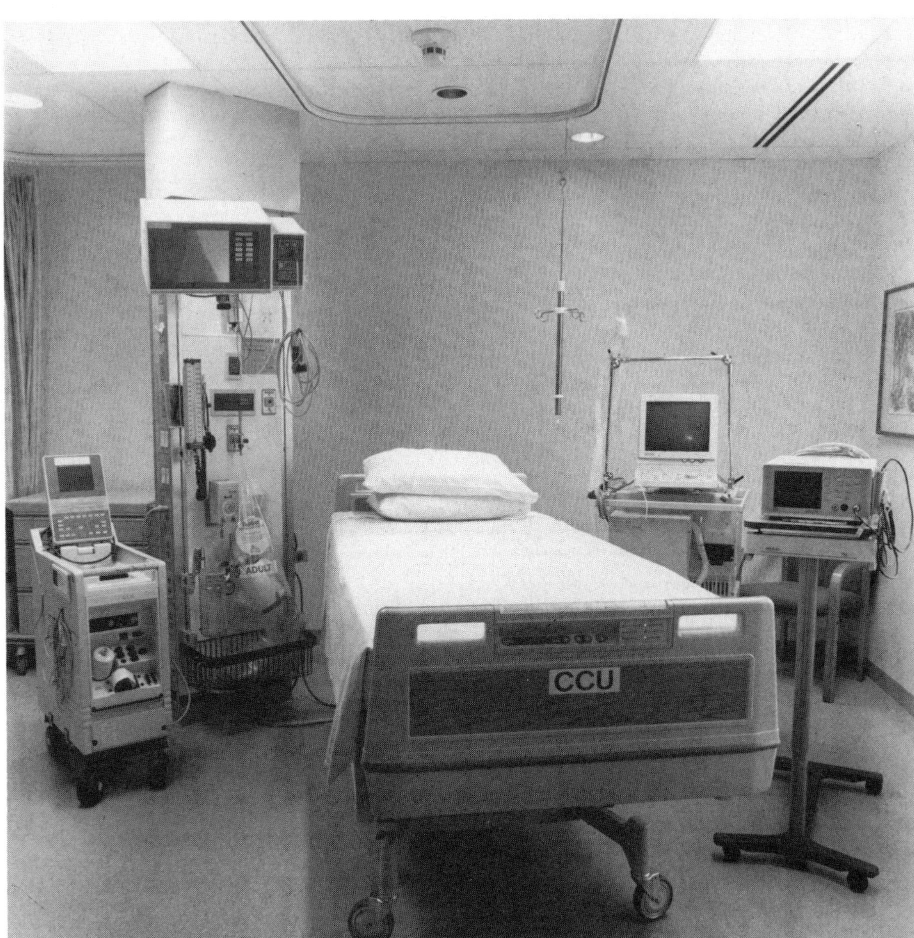

Figure 2–1. The use of 200 to 250 sq ft of space per bedside with placement of the bed in the middle of the room markedly improves access to the patient. This arrangement at Swedish Medical Center (Englewood, CO) won a design award from the Society of Critical Care Medicine. The unit provides adequate room for an intra-aortic counterpulsation balloon, monitor/utility tower, ventilator, and other monitoring equipment without cluttering the bedside.

network for sharing information with a file server. All patient information enters an archival system for long-term patient records.

In 1993, less than 5% of ICUs in the United States were fully computerized as just described. Computerization will most certainly be a growing trend in the future, and ICU bedsides must have space for a computer communication system to be used by all ICU bedside healthcare workers. In addition, phones and intercoms are needed to facilitate verbal communication both inside and outside the ICU. Needless to say, there has to be space and appropriate spatial design for a wide array of bedside monitors, infusion pumps for intravenous administration of medications, and other life-support devices such as mechanical ventilators.

One substantial change in the delivery of critical care services during the past 10 years has been away from the concept of a central station (Fig. 2–2). The original coronary care unit design of a central station with a monitor watcher observing multiple electrocardiogram traces is not relevant to a critical care center. The idea of a quiet, carpeted bedside with a nurse observing at a distance was appropriate only to the previous treatment of cardiac patients when little could be done except prevent fatal cardiac arrhythmias. Modern critical care units operate with nurses, doctors, and respiratory therapists providing constant vigilance at the bedside. Thus, monitoring equipment must be at the bedside, and the monitor-based central station has little value and adds substantial additional capital and personnel cost.

Bedsides need to be fully equipped with disposable supplies, medications, and equipment to preserve the concept of healthcare worker vigilance. Various sorts of mobile storage carts can be exchanged on a daily basis to facilitate restocking of bedside supplies. All efforts must be made to minimize the time that the bedside healthcare team must leave a patient unattended.

The clear and concise recommendations for bedside utilities summarized in Table 2–1 were devised by the Society of Critical Care Medicine Task Force on Guidelines on critical care unit design.

ANCILLARY AND NONBEDSIDE INTENSIVE CARE UNIT AREAS

Flow patterns—the way that staff, visitors, equipment, supplies, and information stream in and out of the ICU—are one of the primary determinants of unit efficiency. The ability for ICU staff to save a few minutes each time on activities that occur frequently is obviously cost effective.

It is probably preferable for visitors and staff to have separate access routes. When a family watches all of the comings and goings in the unit, they often feel excessively anxious because they may assume that any activity relates to their loved one. In most institutions, safety is mandatory, and control over public access is no longer an option.

Experts on time and motion studies can identify design shortcomings. It is important to give patient safety the highest priority. Flow patterns to patients should be the quickest, clearest paths to and from those departments with which the ICU interacts most. To ensure speed, doors should open automatically or by a touchless device and

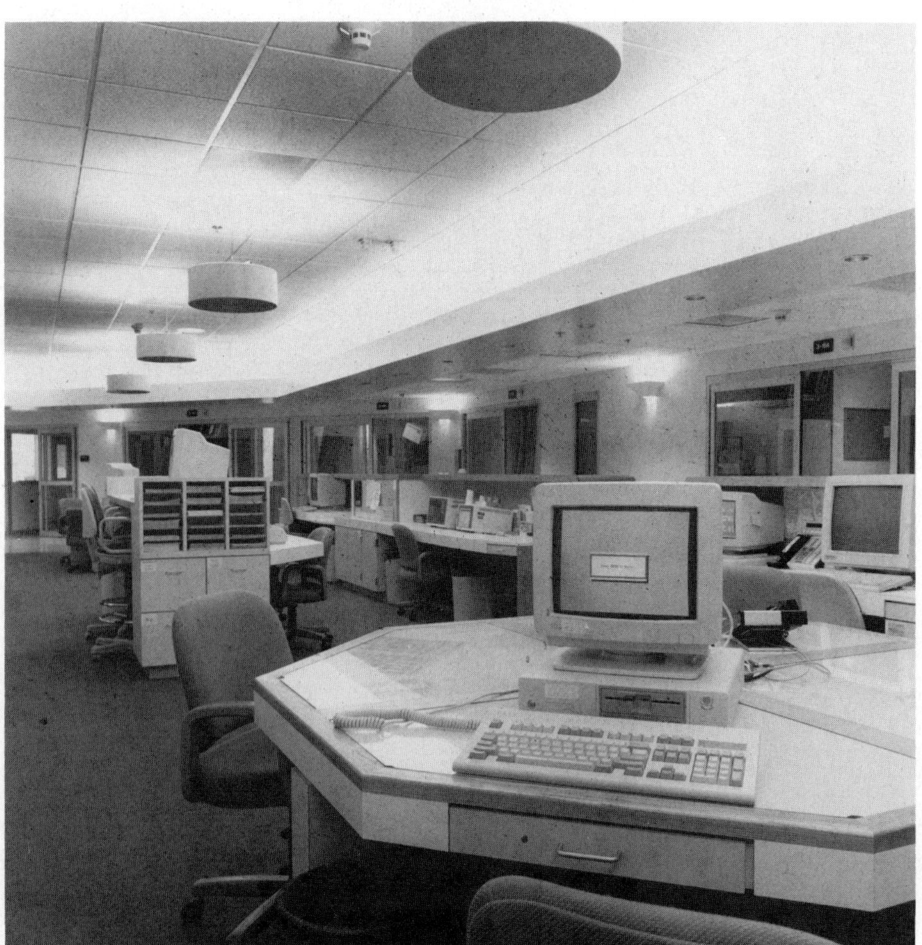

Figure 2–2. The central station with a monitor watcher has been replaced by computerized monitoring equipment that trends abnormal cardiac beats and sounds an alarm when dangerous cardiac rhythm problems occur in a patient or patients. The new equipment allows the central station space (as seen in this photograph) to be used for clerical work and for charting by nurses and physicians. The arrangement provides a spacious and convenient communication center for the ICU staff. This clerical area was designed by Swedish Medical Center (Englewood, CO) and won a design award from the Society of Critical Care Medicine.

TABLE 2–1. Task Force on Guidelines, Society of Critical Care Medicine: Selected Recommendations of Standards for Critical Care Unit Design

Standard	*Required*	*Desirable*	*Optional*
Standard 2: Floor Plan			
Distinct unit	x		
Controlled access	x		
Adjacent to			
Elevator		x	
Emergency room		x	
Operating room		x	
Recovery room		x	
Laboratory			x
Radiology			x
Other critical care units			x
Step-down unit		x	
No through traffic	x		
Unit size			
<12 beds/central station		x	
2½–3 times bed space square footage		x	
Fire/safety features	x		
Services			
Air conditioning/heating	x		
Plumbing, separate service	x		
Grounded electric, separate service	x		
Emergency power source	x		
Circuit breaker access	x		
Lighting	x		
Windows		x	
Ability to be opened		x	
Light control		x	
Color scheme			
Neutral tones		x	
Accent color/design			x
Standard 3: Patient Bed Area			
Minimum space: adult unit-pediatric may elect smaller area/bed if cribs are used			
Open unit: 150–200 sq ft		x	
Room: 225–250 sq ft		x	
Sinks:			
In each room or between beds	x		
Elbow, knee, or foot-operated faucets		x	
Patient lavatory/commode		x	
Patient privacy control		x	
Signals			
Modulated	x		
Musical tones		x	
Staff location system		x	
Sound-absorbing floor covering		x	
Standard 5: Patient Room/Area Services			
Grounded electrical outlets	x		
11 110-V outlets	x		
18 110-V outlets		x	
220-V electrical outlet			x
Oxygen outlets: 2 per bed	x		
Oxygen outlets: 3 or more per bed		x	
Compressed air outlets			
1 per bed	x		
2 or more per bed		x	
Vacuum outlets			
2 per bed	x		
3 per bed		x	
Air conditioning/heating	x		
Humidity 30–60%	x		
Lighting			
Low-level, 35 ft-c night lighting	x		
Overhead 20 to >100 ft-c general	x		
150 ft-c	x		
Standard 8: Isolation Rooms			
250 sq ft	x		
Private bathroom/commode		x	
Anteroom: 20 sq ft	x		
Sink	x		
Storage shelves/cabinets	x		
Reverse/forward airflow		x	
Standard 10: Information and Communication Center			
House telephones	x		
Intercommunications systems	x		
Emergency code alarm system	x		
Glass enclosed		x	
Dictation areas			x
Emergency telephone		x	
Standard 12: Clerical Space			
Shelving		x	
Cabinets (include filing)	x		
Drawers	x		
Separate areas			
Secretarial	x		
Charting		x	
Computer terminal/printer		x	
Hospital information system		x	
Management information system	x		
Nursing information system		x	
Stand-alone system			x
Patient acuity classification system		x	
Standard 13: Readily Accessible Storage			
Crash cart alcoves	x		
Electrical outlet	x		
Medication station	x		
Enclosed area		x	
Glass wall(s)		x	
Refrigerator	x		
Lockable cabinet (narcotics)	x		
Countertop work area	x		
Sink	x		
Storage cabinet/drawers	x		
Standard 20: Equipment Store Room			
Separate room	x		
Peripheral location		x	
Size equal to 100 sq ft per bed		x	
Electrical outlets for battery charging	x		
Standard 21: Staff Lounge			
Separate room (spacious, comfortable, private)	x		
Perimeter location	x		
Controlled access to locker room	x		
Toilet facilities	x		
Environmental control	x		
Telephone	x		
Intercommunications systems		x	
Emergency code alarm signal	x		
Standard 22: Nourishment Preparation Area (if present)			
Distinct area		x	
Countertop work area	x		
Stovetop		x	
Sink	x		
Refrigerator	x		
Microwave		x	
Space for food cart		x	

Table continued on following page

TABLE 2–1. Task Force on Guidelines, Society of Critical Care Medicine: Selected Recommendations of Standards for Critical Care Unit Design *Continued*

Standard	*Required*	*Desirable*	*Optional*
Standard 23: Physician Sleep Room (where required by unit activity)			
Separate room	x		
Adjacent to unit	x		
Toilet/shower facilities	x		
Telephone	x		
Emergency code alarm signal	x		
Intercommunications system			x
Standard 25: Conference Room			
Location			
Peripheral		x	
Exterior to but adjacent to unit			x
Lockable closet		x	
Telephone	x		
Intercommunications systems		x	
Emergency code alarm signal	x		
Separate classroom			x
Adjustable air conditioning/heat		x	
Standard 26: Office Space			
Separate offices			
Physician director	x		
Nurse director		x	
Head nurse	x		
Staff development instructor			x
Clinical specialist			x
Social worker			x
Secretary (between physician director and nurse director or head nurse)		x	
Telephone	x		
Intercommunications systems			x
Standard 27: Public Space			
Separate room		x	
Comfortable space accommodating 1½ to 2 seats per patient bed		x	
Adjacent to			
Unit	x		
Receptionist area	x		
Television		x	
Telephone			
House	x		
Public	x		
Intercommunications systems		x	
Toilet facilities			
Access from facility		x	
Adjacent to facility			x
Shower facilities			x
Private family consultation room			x
Sleep/rest cubicles			x
Environmental control	x		
Windows		x	

(Adapted from Task Force on Guidelines, Society of Critical Care Medicine: Recommendations for critical care unit design. Crit Care Med 1988; 16:796–806.)

elevators should be summoned by an override key mechanism. To facilitate a clear route, corners must be maneuverable by all the potential transport equipment. Floor materials and floor seams must allow unencumbered flow, and elevators must be large enough to carry patients and life-support equipment.

There are many ways to transmit information in the hospital, including telephones, fax machines, computers, and pneumatic tube systems. The latter can also accommodate small supplies and drugs. One step-saving method of delivering supplies and medications kept at the ICU bedside is to use *nurse servers,* which are cupboards that open into the room as well as to the outside hall, often with shelves on turnstiles. If medications are delivered in this fashion, doors must be equipped with locks. Some units have one nurse server for clean supplies and another for dirty or used supplies. Careful thought needs to be given to supply systems and their placement. Saving steps means saving time and money as well as enhancing patient safety by decreasing the amount of time the staff is away from the bedside.

A key issue with supplies is availability at the bedside or near the bedside, in the ICU or outside the ICU. The goal of nursing is to make routinely used supplies conveniently available without unnecessary clutter or cost. Storing too much inventory is costly, but so is wasting time looking for items when supplies are depleted. Some ICUs find it helpful to have several specialized and standardized bedside supply carts—one for neurosurgical patients, one for cardiothoracic surgery patients, one for trauma patients, and so on.

It should be emphasized that proper function of a unit is best achieved when the decision about what to store and where to store it precedes the decision about how to store it. The space in patients' rooms and throughout a unit can then be designed to meet identified needs.

Items can be stored in dedicated rooms, cupboards, closets, open or closed compartments, fixed shelving or movable carts, and drawers or bins made of plastic or metal—all of which work superbly if well planned. Rooms and closets or cupboards hide the equipment from view but make it harder for new personnel to find important supplies. Staff often leave enclosed areas open to save time. Orientation of storage areas to the line of vision of the staff and away from patients and the public may solve the problem of a cluttered appearance.

One strategy for solving space problems is the use of multipurpose rooms with flexible interior design, furniture, and partitions or collapsible walls. One area can serve as a conference room, classroom, report room, lounge, family grieving or counseling room, and library/learning/resource center. A variety of lighting, table, and seating options are necessary to make such a multipurpose room functional.

Important additional needs for the nursing staff include men's and women's lockers with toilets and showers, a staff lounge and space for mailboxes, and a communication center. Physicians need appropriate and private areas to review patients' records, reflect, consult, and dictate. Physician call rooms are required. Respiratory therapists, nurses, and physicians have needs for office space. Flexible office space can be used by other service providers such as social workers, dieticians, and chaplains.

Just as the degree of attention to meeting personnel needs makes a statement about how the institution values employees, the degree of attention to addressing family needs makes a statement about the value of the families. Approximately two seats per patient in the family waiting room are considered adequate. Various seating options (sofas, small groupings of tables and chairs, private areas) and lighting choices make the room more flexible. Phones with privacy, nutrition services, private communication centers, and education or entertainment equipment are important. The appropriate choice of finishes, colors, and decorative design can make the room soothing and humane.

Specific Support Areas

Every unit needs areas for medication preparation, nutrition services, radiology, and equipment storage. An ICU with a multidisciplinary critical care team needs a satellite pharmacy, *stat* laboratory, and possibly a procedure room.

The number of medication preparation areas depends on the size of the unit and whether medications are delivered to the bedside and stored there. Patients should be visible to the nurses working in a medication preparation area. Likewise, nurses at the bedside should be able to see medication preparation areas to guard the security of medications, needles, and syringes from the public. Both the medication and the nutrition areas need sinks and counter space. A microwave oven and refrigerator are essential. Most state and Occupational Safety and Health Administration (OSHA) regulations are clear about keeping these areas separate from laboratory specimens.

Radiographs are often kept in the ICU during a patient's stay. X-ray view boxes can be movable or fixed, embedded in counters or walls, multiple or single. Inconvenient or informal storage methods waste time. Fixed storage cubicles, divided bins, or rotating view boxes with storage capability are useful. Digital technology to retrieve x-ray images from the radiology department on computer screens is available in a few centers and is most practical. A critical care center of multiple 12-bed ICUs may find the need to create a satellite radiology room to store radiographs, house portable machines, and develop films.

Among the support areas most important to a multidisciplinary critical care team is a *stat* laboratory. These facilities are based on analyzing heparinized whole blood samples instead of serum samples as is done in most central laboratories. On 0.5 to 1.0 mL of whole heparinized blood, an ICU *stat* laboratory should be able to perform blood gas analysis; measure hemoglobin oxygen saturation; make electrolyte determinations of sodium, potassium, and chloride values; and measure glucose levels. Because there is no need to centrifuge the sample to obtain serum and because *stat* laboratory equipment is designed to operate quickly, these results can be available to the bedside critical care team within 5 to 10 minutes of acquiring the sample. Other possible *stat* laboratory services can include measurement of hematocrit, lactate, ionized calcium, and ionized magnesium.

Similarly, point-of-care laboratory devices are rapidly developing. They are small, accurate, safe, and user friendly, and they can decrease turnaround times for laboratory results. Although each machine is small, the need for several types of machines may evolve with the need for a sink, counter, and small refrigerator.

Point-of-care single-patient analyzers using sensors such as optodes inserted through arterial catheters may well be a significant future critical care technology. Such analysis is expensive but is faster than the present ICU *stat* laboratory. In the meantime, and even after further evolution of point-of-care equipment, *stat* laboratories improve patient care by providing rapid, accurate blood chemical analysis. Data from *stat* laboratories should be transmitted by computer technology to the bedside nurse for manual entry on the critical care flow sheet or automatic entry on the patient data management system.

In addition, a satellite pharmacy can be of substantial assistance to the critical care team. This might be headed up by a critical care pharmacist who regularly makes rounds with the physicians to determine patients' medication needs. The pharmacy can then prepare continuous-infusion medications such as inotropic therapy with dobutamine, deliver intermittently used medications such as antibiotics, and be involved in the preparation of total parenteral nutrition solutions. The personnel of a satellite pharmacy, working as critical care team members, can improve the quality of patient care and make administration of medication substantially more efficient for patients, bedside nurses, and physicians.

A procedure room may be helpful in the ICU and improve patient safety. Transporting critically ill patients on life support outside the ICU requires a heavy investment in time, equipment, and personnel. Specific procedures such as fluoroscopy may be better performed in a specially equipped ICU procedure room to save patients from a longer wait or a longer trip to radiology.

A common ICU design error is inadequate equipment storage space. It is difficult to appreciate how much space special beds, ventilators, cooling machines, electrocardiography machines, intravenous controllers, balloon pumps, traction/fixation equipment, suction machines, transport equipment, scales, wheelchairs, and carts can require. Many of them must be plugged in to recharge batteries, and banks of electrical outlets are essential. Equipment storage spaces should have sturdy, large shelves and wide room access with touchless door openers. If adequate equipment storage room is not provided, hallways take the equipment overflow, the ICU appears cluttered and obstructed, and the potential arises for violation of fire and safety codes.

Selection of the finishings is important in creating a soothing environment that reduces stress. Soft finishes in soothing color schemes are cost effective and important. The basic colors should be classic rather than trendy. The accent colors are much easier to change over time. Carpets are improving in durability and ease of care but still impede the transport of heavy, rolling equipment such as occupied beds. They should be used as much as practical because they absorb sound, are easier to stand on, and soften the look of the unit. Sheet vinyl is also improving in quality and is probably best used for halls and patient bedside areas.

Ceiling design and materials are important because they are what patients look at most and because they can be part of a noise-abatement system. It is recommended that the noise level not exceed 45 dB during the day, 40 dB in the evening, and 25 dB at night.[11] Devices that monitor the noise level can be purchased to assist in meeting standards. Inclusion of sound barriers, soffits, and offset doors in the unit design can decrease the baseline noise level considerably, as can soft materials on walls, curtains, glass, and carpets.

Many units have dramatically improved their impact by using skylights, gardens, aquariums, plants, artwork, and special lighting. Although some of these seem superfluous and expensive, user satisfaction is a valuable outcome because the critical care team seeks to provide high-quality care and serve patients and families.

INTENSIVE CARE UNIT PLANNING AND DESIGN

Many hospitals have outdated ICUs designed and constructed in the 1970s or earlier. In the 1980s and 1990s, an explosion of technology made old designs and bedside space of 100 to 150 sq ft per bed obsolete. For that reason, ICU remodeling and new construction of critical care centers are commonplace in hospitals, particularly busy tertiary care facilities, where as many as 10% to 15% of total beds can be devoted to monitoring and life support of critically ill patients.

There are two keys to successful ICU construction projects. First is the involvement of as many people from the ICU as possible, and second is spending as much time as possible on preliminary work before beginning the actual design phase. Gathering preliminary information from all the healthcare workers who affect the ICU can allow significant cost and functional decisions to be made early. These decisions have an important impact on the entire life span of the project.

Ultimately, a design team must be chosen after preliminary information has been assembled. Design team members should be chosen based on their experience as caregivers, their healthcare specialty, their ability to share information and think creatively, their willingness to listen and treat other members with respect, and finally their ability to reach consensus. The term *team member* encompasses the many different disciplines that are normally involved in the day-to-day operation of an ICU. This group needs to be heard and to be active participants with the engineers and architects who will establish the final design. It should include nursing staff, respiratory therapists, physicians, and other support staff involved in the day-to-day operation of the ICU.

The first meeting of the design team should be led by a facilitator who can explain the project and sequence of events. Team member assignments and responsibilities should be clarified for each participant. It should be made clear that the success of the project depends on all team members carrying out their parts of the project in a complete and timely fashion. A time line or schedule should be developed for the team and recorded in the programming manual. Future meetings should be scheduled and task forces developed to solve specific problems. The design team and task forces should use questionnaires to gather information and facilitate planning. Finally, a full program of activities is developed, beginning with the design phase and going through the construction phase to the final phase of moving in.

The design team should look at the mission statement of both the institution and the ICU as it begins its work. The mission of a trauma ICU differs from the mission of a medical ICU, and these differences must be addressed in the design process. In the high-technology critical care unit of the 1990s, it is unlikely that a turnkey design package purchased from engineers can meet the diverse needs of medical versus surgical versus pediatric intensive care.

Past experience is important to the design team, recognizing good and bad aspects of previous ICU work experiences. These past experiences may generate design concepts that can be reviewed based on the SWOT theory of strengths, weaknesses, opportunities, and threats. The design team should visit other ICUs and other hospitals to obtain new ideas. The Society of Critical Care Medicine has a file on ICU design as a result of its competition for ICU design awards. This file contains videotape and accompanying portfolio information that may be helpful to the design team. Also helpful are state and federal documents such as the one by Health and Human Services (HHS), *Guidelines for Construction and Equipment of Hospital and Medical Facilities,* which has a chapter on ICU design.[12]

A very important design issue for critical care is the proximity of other hospital facilities. Radiology, emergency medicine, and operating and recovery rooms need to be near to the critical care unit or connected by open and easily navigated hallways and elevators. Critically ill patients never remain stationary in an ICU bed in a critical care unit. They are commonly admitted from the emergency medicine department. They frequently need extensive diagnostic work using nuclear medicine, computed tomography, and magnetic resonance imaging. Surgery is frequently required even for medical patients. The ICU staff must be prepared to move even the sickest patients to distant locations such as the cardiac catheterization laboratory. The more these diagnostic and therapeutic parts of the hospital can be located near the ICU, the greater the safety and efficiency of care to patients with life-threatening illnesses.[12]

Finally, the design team should prepare a list of expectations during the early planning process. Each team member should have a list of expectations that serves as a personal guide during the planning and design process. Expectations should be stated in a clear and objective manner in terms of form, function, economy, and time.[13] These expectations then serve as the criteria for success when the project is completed.

As noted at the beginning of this chapter, *form follows function* is the key to a successful critical care unit design. The critical care team is multiprofessional and multidisciplinary in nature. The remodeling or design of the ICU must also be multiprofessional and multidisciplinary in nature if ICU healthcare workers are going to have ownership in the critical care unit and committment to high-quality patient care. The design team must first determine ICU function in substantial detail, and form will follow automatically within the resources of the institution.

References

1. Cullen DJ: Results and costs of intensive care. Anesthesiology 1977; 47:203.
2. Task Force on Guidelines, Society of Critical Care Medicine: Recommendations for critical care unit design. Crit Care Med 1988; 16:796–806.
3. Task Force on Guidelines, Society of Critical Care Medicine: Guidelines for categorization of services for the critically ill patient. Crit Care Med 1991; 19:279–285.
4. Fein IA: Critical care unit design: Environmental and psychosocial considerations. *In:* Managing the Critical Care Unit. Fein IA, Strosberg MA (Eds). Rockville, MD, Aspen Publishers, 1987, pp 113–126.
5. Meyer C: Visions of tomorrow's ICU. Am J Nurs 1993; 93:27–31.
6. Hudson LD: Design of the intensive care unit from a monitoring point of view. Respir Care 1985; 30:549–559.
7. Du Moulin G: Minimizing the potential for nosocomial pneumonia: Architectural, engineering, and environmental considerations for the intensive care unit. Eur J Clin Microbiol Infect Dis 1989; 8:69–74.
8. Preston GA, Larson El, Stamm WE: The effect of private isolation rooms on patient care practices, colonization and infection in an intensive care unit. Am J Med 1981; 70:641–645.
9. Hoyt JW: Complications of design and construction of the intensive care unit. *In:* Complications in Critical Care Medicine. Lumb PD, Bryan-Brown CW (Eds). Chicago, Year Book Medical Publishers, 1988, pp 312–325.
10. Hoyt JW, Page C, Maffeo C: Considerations for ICU bedside design. Crit Care Med 1983; 11:256.
11. Edwards GB, Schuring LM: Sleep protocol—a research-based practice change. Crit Care Nurse 1993; 13:84–88.
12. AIA Committee on Architecture for Health and US Department of Health Care and Human Services: Guidelines for Construction and Equipment of Hospitals and Medical Facilities. Washington, DC, AIA Press, 1993.
13. Pena W: Problem Seeking. 2nd ed. Boston, Cahners Books International, 1977.

CHAPTER 3

Caring for a Child in an Adult Intensive Care Unit

Peter R. Holbrook, MD

An unknown number of children are cared for in nonpediatric intensive care units (ICUs). Usually, this is because pediatric care must be provided in response to an emergency and transfer to an appropriate pediatric facility is not possible. The elective admission of children to adult ICUs is becoming increasingly less common. The present chapter reviews current issues related to this matter.

All would agree that the overarching principle is the provision of optimal care for children who must be cared for in ICUs. Unfortunately, data indicate that critically ill children cared for in nontertiary care pediatric intensive care facilities fare less well than their severity-matched counterparts in a tertiary setting.[1] Although these data concerned only patients with respiratory failure and head trauma, other data suggest that improved results can be attained at hospitals or units caring for many patients with a given condition.[2–4]

Many observers believe that children should be cared for in dedicated pediatric ICUs.[5] For example, in Australia, a specific recommendation against caring for children in adult ICUs exists.[6]

The Pediatric Section of the Society of Critical Care Medicine and the American Academy of Pediatrics Section on Critical Care as well as its Committee on Hospital Care have defined two levels of ICUs for children.[7] Their guidelines state that pediatric ". . . critical care is provided primarily at one level." However, the guidelines ". . . recognize the need for an additional level of care in geographically isolated regions with a small population base, to allow stabilization of critically ill children prior to transfer to another center and to avoid long-distance transfers for disorders of less complexity or those of low acuity." These latter units, termed level II units, ". . . generally care for fewer severely ill patients." The document goes on to say that patients in level II units ". . . will have less complex and more stable disorders whose course is more predictable . . ." than those patients in level I units.

Although these recommendations currently lack the force of regulation or law, they do represent the opinion of experts, and their respective organizations stand behind them. Similarly, the guidelines represent the minimum requirements. The document states clearly that the ". . . guidelines are not intended as a statement of the ideal or ultimate requirements for pediatric ICUs." Rather, they provide recommendations that are ". . . current, necessary, and attainable in 1993."

The American Academy of Pediatrics/Society of Critical Care Medicine document deals with the characteristics of the patient care unit, not with the care of the individual patient. As previously stated, children are cared for in adult ICUs for a variety of reasons. The adult ICU that cares for children should be aware of these organizations' guidelines. Further elaboration on some of the points may assist those who occasionally encounter children in the adult ICU environment.

The guidelines call for distinct and separate units for children that are ". . . equal in status with all other special care units." The pediatric ICU should have a committee consisting of physicians, nurses, respiratory therapists, and others involved in the unit's activities. Importantly, the pediatric ICU committee should ". . . participate in delineation of privileges of all personnel (both MD and non-MD) within the unit." Careful attention to the delineation of privileges may help to prevent catastrophes that may occur when personnel function outside their areas of expertise.

Appropriate policies should be developed for pediatric ICUs. Safety concerns that must be addressed are obvious (e.g., siderails must be present on cribs); however, a less obvious issue that must also be considered is nosocomial infection. The pediatric patient is at high risk of nosocomial infection. Visitation policies should also be developed. It should be noted that visitation policies in many pediatric ICUs routinely allow for nearly around-the-clock presence of family members at patients' bedsides.

The physical facilities that are required as well as extensive drug and equipment needs (e.g., for pediatric endotracheal intubation equipment, ventilators, and monitors) must be well defined. Policies on maintenance and monitoring are also required.

Personnel requirements include the availability of a medical director and a 24-hour in-house physician staff of at least the second postgraduate year. Consultant personnel who can be available to the pediatric ICU within 30 minutes are listed. Nursing leadership is provided by an experienced nurse manager who has had pediatric critical care training. The particular skills of staff nurses should be highlighted. The availability of respiratory therapy staff members who are familiar with the techniques of ventilating infants and children is also important. In addition, the requirement for social workers and others familiar with the needs of children is clear.

Hospital support services must be able to respond to the needs of pediatric patients and should be able to perform laboratory assays of pediatric microspecimens, have a pharmacy supplied with medications in pediatric dosages, and be able to run cardiovascular and neurologic diagnostic studies on children.

The adult ICU that cares for children is advised to adhere to the American Academy of Pediatrics/Society of Critical Care Medicine recommendations. High-quality care and organizational or equipment requirements may prove to be too costly to maintain. Fortunately, the availability of transport systems (see Chapter 12) can allow for the smooth and safe transport of critically ill children to centers best equipped to address their needs.

References

1. Pollack MM, Alexander SR, Clarke N, et al: Improved outcomes from tertiary center pediatric intensive care: A statewide comparison of tertiary and nontertiary care facilities. Crit Care Med 1991; 19:150–159.
2. Luft HS, Bunker A, Enthoven A: Should operations be regionalized? An empirical study of the relation between surgical volume and mortality. N Engl J Med 1979; 301:1364.
3. Flood AB, Scott WR, Ewy W: Does practice make perfect? I. The relation between hospital volume and outcomes and other hospital characteristics. Med Care 1984; 22:98.
4. Hughes RG, Hunt SS, Luft HS: Effects of surgeon volume and hospital volume on quality of care in hospitals. Med Care 1987; 25:489.
5. Shann F: Australian view of paediatric intensive care in Britain. Lancet 1993; 342:69.
6. National Health and Medical Research Council: Management of seriously ill children in adult intensive care units. Report of the 94th Session of the Council Canberra, Commonwealth of Australia, 1982.
7. Committee on Hospital Care and Pediatric Section of the Society of Critical Care Medicine: Guidelines and Levels of Care for Pediatric Intensive Care Units. Pediatrics 1993; 92:166–175.

SECTION II
RESUSCITATION

William C. Shoemaker • Peter R. Holbrook

CHAPTER 4

Cardiopulmonary-Cerebral Resuscitation

Peter Safar, MD • Norman S. Abramson, MD
Nicholas G. Bircher, MD

Before the 1950s, airway obstruction, apnea, and pulselessness outside the hospital meant certain death.[1] In the hospital but outside the operating room, resuscitation rarely succeeded.[1] In the operating room, open-chest cardiopulmonary resuscitation (CPR) has been practiced since about 1900 with good results.[1] In the late 1950s, modern standard external CPR was initiated by several investigators.[1, 2] Brain-oriented resuscitation was initiated in the 1960s, extending CPR into cardiopulmonary-cerebral resuscitation (CPCR) (Fig. 4–1, and Table 4–1).[2] This chapter summarizes new perspectives and assumes that readers are familiar with CPR guidelines.[2–8]

The goal of CPCR is to save "hearts and brains too good to die"[1, 2] by reversing airway obstruction (usually due to coma), hypoventilation, apnea, sudden cardiac death (usually due to coronary artery disease), exsanguinating hemorrhage (usually due to trauma), and other acute dying processes.[9, 10, 11] The outcome of CPCR attempts should be evaluated in terms of quality of life. For every victim, the emergency medical services delivery team should estimate the duration of cardiac arrest (no blood flow), CPR (low blood flow), and severe hypoxemia and determine the quality of survival in terms of overall and cerebral performance categories (Table 4–2).[2]

The CPCR system, as developed by Safar, consists of three phases—basic life support (BLS), advanced life support (ALS), and prolonged life support (PLS)—and each phase consists of three steps (steps ABC, DEF, and GHI, respectively) (see Fig. 4–1). Historically,[1] in the late 1950s, step A (airway control without devices) (Fig. 4–2) was documented by Safar; step B (exhaled air ventilation) by Elam, Safar, and Gordon; and step C (closed-chest cardiac massage) by Kouwenhoven's group. BLS is merely a stopgap, providing borderline oxygenation until ALS can be instituted. The institution of ALS should begin as rapidly as possible to restore spontaneous circulation. ALS involves a combination of step D (drugs and fluids), step E (electrocardiography [ECG]), and step F (fibrillation treatment, i.e., electric defibrillation). Although originally designed for open-chest CPR, ALS was modified for closed-chest CPR. Once out of immediate danger, a still-comatose patient requires PLS. Hospital intensive care units (ICUs) were initiated for respiratory intensive care in Scandinavia in the early 1950s; their use was expanded to provide life support in multiple organ failure, first at the Baltimore City Hospital in 1958. Mobile ICUs were initiated in Prague and Moscow around 1960.

CPR or CPCR is carried out according to American Heart Association (AHA)[3–7] and international guidelines.[2, 8] The science of modern CPCR, also called *reanimatology*,[11] is based on the pathophysiology of dying[9] (Figs. 4–3 and 4–4). The word *anima*, "the mind," implies that resuscitation should be focused on the brain. Outcome after CPCR attempts depends on the presence of preinsult derangements, the duration and type of the primary insult (cardiac arrest), and the occurrence and mitigation of secondary postreoxygenation derangements, the postresuscitation syndrome.[9, 11] The CPCR system is only as effective as the weakest link in the life-support chain, which extends from the scene via transportation to the hospital emergency room, operating room, and ICU.[2] This "emergency and critical care medicine" delivery system should be multidisciplinary and should provide a continuum of emergency resuscitation (BLS and ALS) and long-term resuscitation (PLS).[2] PLS, in the form of intensive medical care (in the United States called *critical care medicine*) is most often needed for patients who have needed no emergency resuscitation. The authors term the combination of the science, art, and delivery of emergency critical care medicine *resuscitation medicine*.

TABLE 4–1. Standard Brain-Oriented Life Support*

Basic Life Support–Advanced Life Support
Perform according to guidelines.[2–7]
During CPR attempts, cool head if feasible.
During steps A, B, and C, increase perfusion pressure with intravenous or intratracheal epinephrine.
  Use titrated high-dose epinephrine (e.g., 1 mg/70 kg per minute of estimated arrest time over 3 min)
  Earliest possible defibrillation.
For prolonged external CPR steps A, B, C, consider use of a mechanical device.
In ALS-resistant cases, switch to open-chest CPR or cardiopulmonary bypass early.

Prolonged Life Support (Throughout Coma)
After restoration of heartbeat, aim for brief hypertensive bout, then normotension.
Normotension (mean arterial pressure 90–100 mm Hg), titrated with fluids, vasopressor, vasodilator as needed.
Mechanical ventilation for about 12 h.
Normocapnia or mild hypocapnia.
Moderate hyperventilation (Pa_{CO_2} 25–35 mm Hg).
Moderate hyperoxia (Pa_{O_2} >100 mm Hg).
Arterial pH 7.3–7.5. Arterial base deficit <7 mmol/L (with $NaHCO_3$).
Immobilization (partial neuromuscular paralysis) as needed.
Sedation (diazepam, barbiturate, narcotic) as needed.
Anticonvulsants (diazepam, phenytoin) as needed for seizure activity.
Normalization of hematocrit, electrolytes, osmolality, glucose.
Steroid (short-term) optional.
Normothermia. Prevention of hyperthermia.
  If feasible, permit earliest mild hypothermia of 34–36°C to about 12 h postarrest.
  Keep core temperature above 32°C.
Standard intensive care for all vital organ systems.
Position head slightly elevated. Turn trunk periodically from side to side.
See also Table 5 of Safar.[16]

*Recommended by the authors for clinical use.

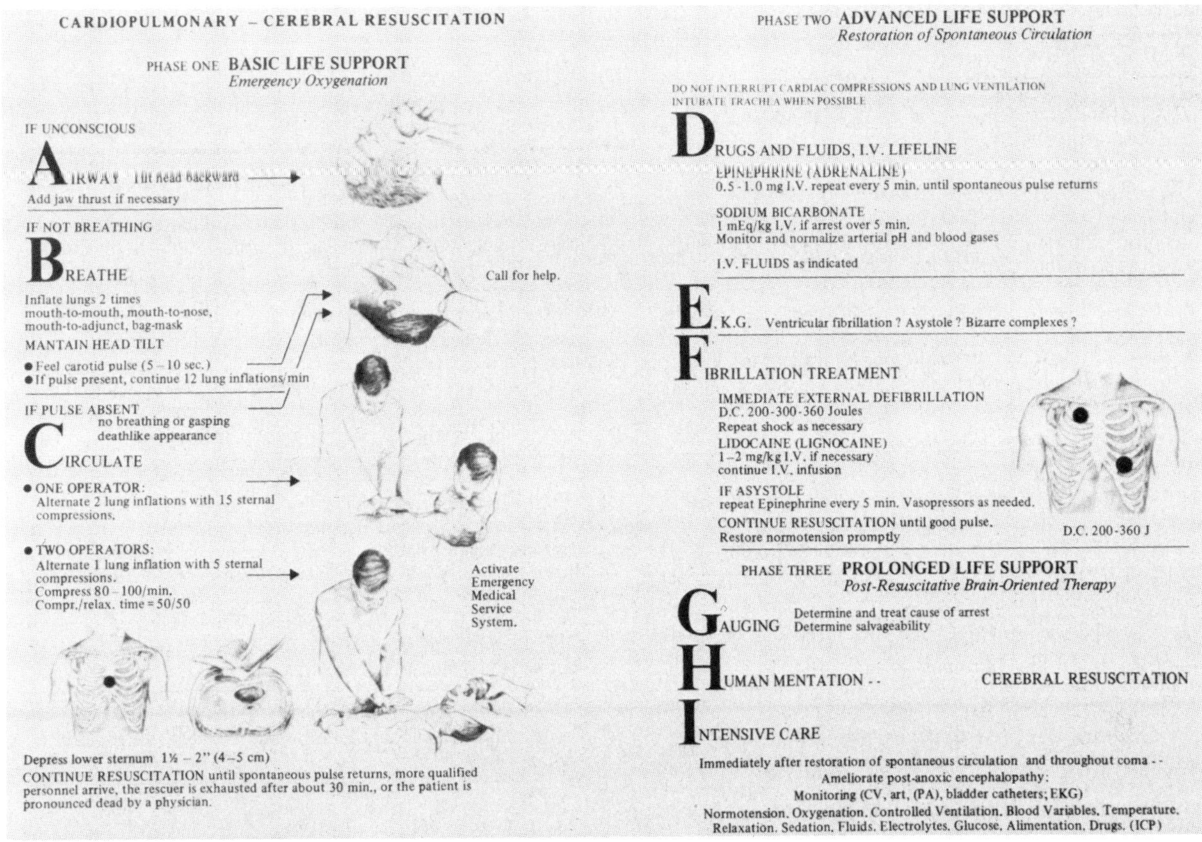

Figure 4–1. Phases and steps of CPCR.
Step A: Airway control includes backward tilt of the head, forward displacement of the mandible, opening of the mouth, and insertion of a pharyngeal or tracheal tube.
Step B: Breathing support is by intermittent positive-pressure ventilation with exhaled air, air, or oxygen.
Step C: Circulation support consists of external or internal cardiac massage.
Steps A, B, and C constitute basic life support (BLS).
Step D: Drugs and fluids.
Step E: Electrocardiography.
Step F: Fibrillation treatment.
Steps D, E, and F constitute advanced life support (ALS), that is, for restoration of spontaneous circulation and other functions.
Steps G–I: Prolonged life support is a combination of Steps G (gauged [i.e., titrated]), H (humanized [i.e., brain-oriented]), and I (intensive) care.
(From Safar P, Bircher N: Cardiopulmonary Cerebral Resuscitation: Guidelines by the World Federation of Societies of Anesthesiologists [WFSA]. 3rd ed. Philadelphia, WB Saunders, 1988.)

The results of CPR attempts so far in industrialized urban communities have been remarkable but less than optimal overall.[2–8, 12] In fewer than 50% of CPR attempts (outside hospitals or in hospitals but outside special care units) has spontaneous circulation been restored. One half of those patients whose circulation was restored died in the hospital, primarily of heart or brain failure. Among the long-term survivors, 10% to 30% have suffered permanent brain damage. Fewer than 10% of CPR attempts overall (outside or in hospitals) have led to discharge from hospitals. However, among those patients in whom CPR was initiated within 4 minutes by bystanders at the scene and restoration of spontaneous circulation was accomplished within 8 minutes (with defibrillation and drug therapy) by an ambulance team trained in ALS, about 40% have been discharged.[12] Initiation and effective performance of CPR by bystanders is associated with improved outcome rates.[12] In general, bystanders seem to perform steps A and B less effectively than they do chest compressions. The needed universal public education in BLS as part of life-supporting first aid, which the authors of this chapter have recommended since the 1960s, is far from implementation. Although in special care units, airway obstruction, apnea, and pulselessness should be and often are reversed with almost 100% success, nevertheless, CPR attempts for secondary arrests occurring in hospital wards have had dismal results because of underlying diseases with multiple organ failure.

In 1992, the American Heart Association Emergency Cardiac Care Committee again updated CPR standards, mainly by changing emphases.[7] The guidelines conference proceedings,[13] however, provide some more forward-looking recommendations, including considerations for ALS pharmacology.[13–15] With these guidelines, the need, challenges, and opportunities to extend CPR to CPCR have finally been acknowledged.[16]

Reperfusion and reoxygenation after normothermic total circulatory arrest lasting more than 5 minutes provoke the postresuscitation syndrome (see Figs. 4–3 and 4–4).[10] Survival depends primarily on the recovery of extracerebral organs. The quality of survival depends primarily on the recovery of human mentation.

Novel therapies may mitigate secondary derangements,

TABLE 4–2. Outcome Evaluation of Patients After Cardiac Arrest or Coma: Overall (Jennett) and Cerebral Performance Categories*

Cerebral Performance Category (CPC)		*Overall Performance Category (OPC)*	
Evaluate *only* cerebral performance capabilities.	Check (√) one	Reflects cerebral *plus* noncerebral status. Evaluate *actual* overall performance.	Check (√) one
CPC 1. Good cerebral performance Conscious, alert, normal cerebral function. May have minor psychologic or neurologic deficits that do not significantly compromise cerebral or physical function.	☐	*OPC 1. Good overall performance* Conscious, alert, capable of normal life. Good cerebral performance (CPC 1) plus slight or no functional disability from noncerebral organ system dysfunction.	☐
CPC 2. Moderate cerebral disability Conscious, alert, sufficient cerebral function for activities of daily life (e.g., dress, travel by public transportation, food preparation). May have hemiplegia, seizures, ataxia, dysarthria, dysphasia, or permanent memory or mental changes.	☐	*OPC 2. Moderate overall disability* Conscious, alert. Moderate cerebral disability alone (CPC 2) *or* moderate disability from noncerebral organ system dysfunction alone, *or both.* Performs independent activities of daily life (dress, travel, food preparation) *or* able to work in part-time sheltered environment. Disabled for competitive work. CPC may be 1 or 2.	☐
CPC 3. Severe cerebral disability Conscious, has at least limited cognition. Dependent on others for daily support (i.e., institutionalized or at home with exceptional family effort) because of impaired brain function. Includes wide range of cerebral abnormalities, from ambulatory patients who have severe memory disturbance or dementia precluding independent existence, to paralyzed patients who can communicate with their eyes only (e.g., the locked-in syndrome).	☐	*OPC 3. Severe overall disability* Conscious. Severe cerebral disability alone (CPC 3) *or* severe disability from noncerebral organ system dysfunction *or both.* Dependent on others for daily support. CPC may be 1, 2 or 3.	☐
CPC 4. Coma/vegetative state Not conscious, unaware of surroundings, *no cognition.* No verbal or psychologic interaction with environment. May *appear* awake because of spontaneous eye opening or sleep–wake cycle. Includes all degrees of unresponsiveness that are neither CPC 3 (conscious) nor CPC 5 (coma that satisfies brain death criteria).	☐	*OPC 4. Coma/vegetative state* Definition same as CPC 4.	☐
CPC 5. Brain death (with beating heart) or death (without beating heart) Apnea, areflexia, "coma," electroencephalographic silence.	☐	*OPC 5. Death (without beating heart)* Apnea, areflexia, "coma," no pulses (see text). Includes CPC 5.	☐
CPC A. Anesthesia (CNS depressants) Uncertain as to above categories because of anesthetic, other CNS depressant drug or relaxant effects.	☐	*OPC A. Anesthesia (CNS depressant)* Uncertain as to above categories because anesthetic, other CNS depressant drug or relaxant effects.	☐
Time achieved: ☐ Hour ☐ Minute		Time achieved: ☐ Hour ☐ Minute	

Compared with baseline status *before* the insult, the patient's *intellectual* function *now* is (check [√] one in each column):

		Patient opinion	Family opinion	Examiner opinion
Unchanged	(1)	☐	☐	☐
Worsened	(2)	☐	☐	☐
Unsure	(3)	☐	☐	☐
Other or unable to determine	(4)	☐	☐	☐

Explain: ______________________________

____

(From Safar P, Bircher N: Cardiopulmonary Cerebral Resuscitation, Guidelines by the World Federation of Societies of Anesthesiologists [WFSA]. 3rd ed. Philadelphia, WB Saunders, 1988.)
*Recommended by the authors for routine clinical use.
Abbreviations: CNS = central nervous system.

thereby improving survival and neurologic recovery.[16] A new, clinically feasible, maximally effective CPCR protocol cannot yet be recommended, although many such approaches are still being investigated in about 10 centers.[16, 17, 17a] Current research is aimed at maximizing cardiovascular resuscitation, circulatory stabilization, and the support of recovery from postischemic-anoxic encephalopathy. These attempts should achieve consistent reversibility and recovery without brain damage from at least 10 minutes of normothermic total circulatory arrest.[16, 17] In the United States, this achievement might save an additional 100,000 lives without brain damage each year,[18] because the present average mobile ICU (ALS) ambulance response times of 8 to 10 minutes cannot be reduced further. Although cardiac arrest in both dogs and humans has been reversed occasionally after up to 20 minutes of normothermic absence of flow, arrest times longer than 5 minutes are still followed in most cases by some permanent neurologic deficit. The heart and

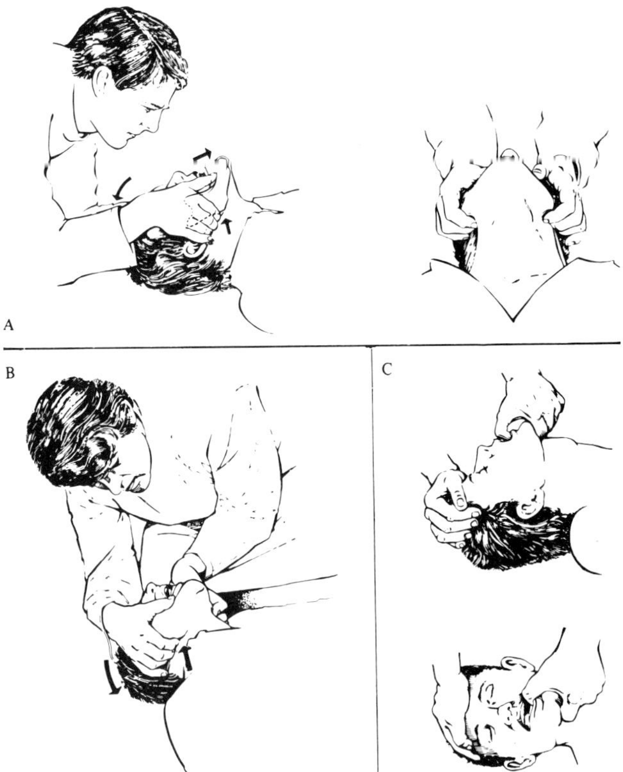

Figure 4–2. Optimal airway control maneuver without use of equipment. The triple airway maneuver consists of tilting the head backward, displacing the mandible forward, and opening the mouth. *A*, Operator at patient's vertex (for spontaneously breathing patient). *B*, Operator at side of patient for direct mouth-to-mouth ventilation. Seal nose with your cheek for mouth-to-mouth breathing. Seal mouth with your other cheek for mouth-to-nose breathing. *C*, Modified triple airway maneuver with thumb-jaw lift method (for relaxed patient only). (From Safar P, Bircher N: Cardiopulmonary Cerebral Resuscitation: Guidelines by the World Federation of Societies of Anesthesiologists [WFSA]. 3rd ed. Philadelphia, WB Saunders, 1988. Illustration © Asmund S. Laerdal, Stavanger, Norway, 1981.)

TABLE 4–3. Novel Brain-Oriented Life Support*

1. In ALS-resistant cases, switch early to open-chest CPR[10, 23] or emergency CPB.[10, 24]
2. Hypertensive reperfusion (optimize steps A, B, and C. After restoration of heartbeat, induce systolic arterial pressure 150–200 mm Hg for 1–5 min).[10, 16, 22] Continue with controlled normotension or mild hypertension throughout coma to 12 h.
3. Calcium entry blocker therapy (e.g., nimodipine, IV 10 μg/kg, as early as possible)[29] perhaps even during CPR steps A, B, and C, followed by 10 $\mu g \cdot kg^{-1} \cdot h^{-1}$ for 12 h. Use optimal mean arterial pressure control.
4. Mild cerebral resuscitative hypothermia:
   Conduct feasibility trials with various rapid brain-cooling methods, for use by paramedics, for use by physicians.
   Monitor and control brain temperature (tympanic membrane or nasopharyngeal) at 34–35°C from immediately after cardiac arrest to about 12 h.[16, 32–35]
   Keep core temperature (esophageal or central venous) above 32°C. Prevent shivering.

*Recommended by the authors for clinical trials.

brain seem to be similarly vulnerable to complete circulatory arrest; however, although necrosis in up to 50% of cardiac myocytes may not obviate restoration of cardiac pumping, necrosis in a few cerebral neurons in critical areas does impair human mentation. The mechanisms of the selective vulnerability of some but not all neurons or myocytes are still poorly understood.

Current laboratory research has revealed increasingly effective CPCR methods.[16] Some of these methods are ready for evaluation on patients, in and outside hospitals (Table 4–3), including modifications of BLS,[19–21] automatic external defibrillation,[7] new drug therapy for ALS,[13–15] reflow promotion by brief hypertension,[22] and improved cardiovascular resuscitability (in ALS-resistant cases) with early use of open-chest CPR[23] or emergency closed-chest cardiopulmonary bypass (CPB).[24] In addition, significantly effective pharmacologic[25–31] and physical cerebral resuscitation measures have been documented.[32–35] The most promising method is mild resuscitative cerebral hypothermia induced immediately after cardiac arrest.[32–35] Other treatments with mechanistic rationale still need documentation by reliable outcome studies in animals (Table 4–4). Fifteen years of experience with the development and use of cardiac arrest and CPCR outcome models in large animals[16] has taught requirements for such models to make cerebral resuscitation results valid (see Table 1 in Safar[16]). Fifteen years of experience with a multicenter clinical study mechanism of sudden cardiac death and CPCR[25, 27, 36] has taught requirements for and limitations of such studies (see Table 2 in Safar[16]) (Fig. 4–5, and Table 4–5). These "brain resuscitation clinical trials" (BRCTs) have influenced the development of international

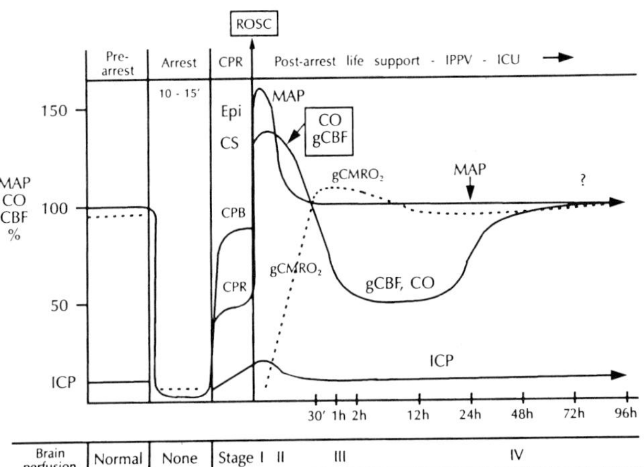

Figure 4–3. Diagram of perfusion failure in the brain and extracerebral organs after cardiac arrest. Reperfusion failure in the brain (proved) and extracerebral organs (suspected) after ventricular fibrillation cardiac arrest, followed by cardiopulmonary resuscitation (CPR) or cardiopulmonary bypass (CPB) for restoration of spontaneous circulation (ROSC). After no blood flow for 10 to 15 minutes, despite control of normal mean arterial pressure (MAP), global cerebral blood flow (gCBF) and cardiac output (CO) go through four postarrest stages: Stage I, multifocal no-reflow (prevented with high reperfusion pressure); Stage II, brief diffuse global hyperemia, with a transient increase in intracranial pressure (ICP); Stage III, delayed protracted global hypoperfusion, with low gCBF and normal ICP, accompanied by normal or supranormal global cerebral oxygen uptake, between about 2 and 12 hours after cardiac arrest (mismatching of oxygen delivery to oxygen uptake); and Stage IV, variable blood flow, accompanied by outcome as either resolution, permanent deficit, or brain death. (From Safar P: Cerebral resuscitation after cardiac arrest: Research initiatives and future directions. Ann Emerg Med 1993; 22[Pt 2]:324.)

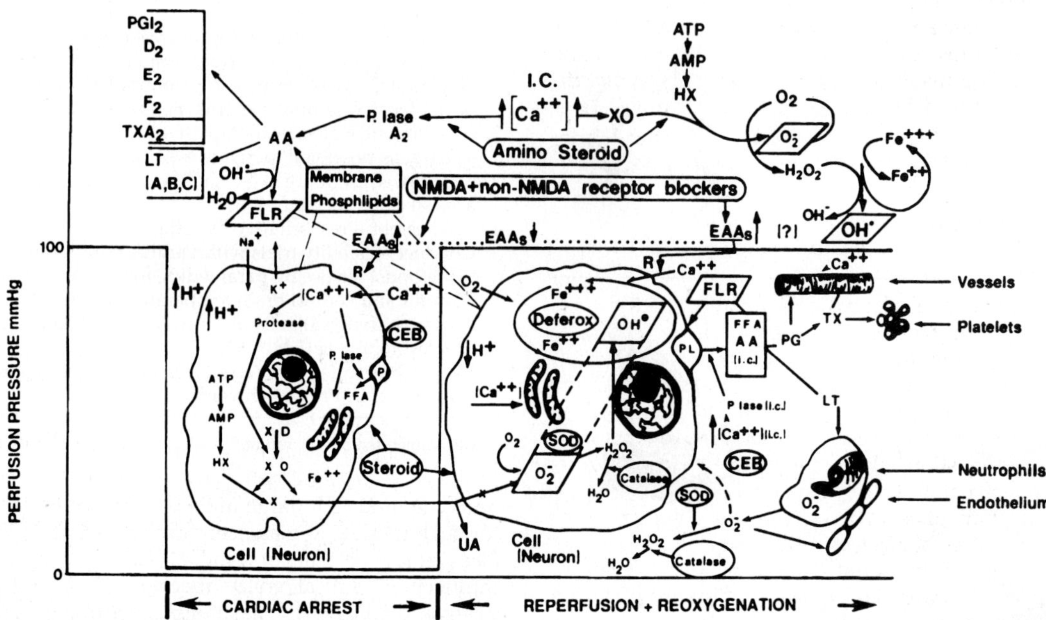

Figure 4–4. Diagram of biochemical cascades in cerebral neurons (hypothesized) or extracerebral organ cells (partially documented) during and after cardiac arrest. (For references, see text.)

Normally, the calcium gradient between the intracellular space ($[Ca^{2+}]i$) and the extracellular space ($[Ca^{2+}]e$) is 1:10,000, that is, 0.1 μmol:1 mmol. Calcium regulators include Ca/Mg adenosine triphosphatase (ATPase), the endoplasmic reticulum (ER), mitochondria, and arachidonic acid (AA). With stimulation, different cell types respond with an increase in $[Ca^{2+}]i$, which results from the release of bound Ca^{2+} in the ER, an influx of $[Ca^{2+}]e$, or both.

During anoxia, the level of adenosine triphosphate (ATP) decreases to near zero in all tissues at different rates, depending on stores of oxygen and substrate. This decrease is fastest in the brain; in the heart, it occurs more slowly. This causes an increase in $[Ca^{2+}]i$, which activates phospholipase (P.lase) A_2, which in turn breaks down membrane phospholipids (PL) into free fatty acids (FFA), particularly AA. It also activates proteolytic enzymes. The hydrolysis of ATP via adenosine monophosphate (AMP) leads to an accumulation of hypoxanthine (HX). Increased $[Ca^{2+}]i$ level enhances the conversion of xanthine dehydrogenase (XD) to xanthine oxidase (XO), priming the neuron for the production of the oxygen free radical (O_2^-). The levels of excitatory amino acid neurotransmitters (EAAs), particularly glutamate and aspartate, increase in the extracellular fluid. Increased [EAA]e level activates NMDA and non-NMDA receptors (R), thereby increasing calcium influx and mobilizing stores of $[Ca^{2+}]i$. Loss of ATP induces intracellular to extracellular potassium leakage. Increased extracellular potassium level also activates EAA receptors by membrane depolarization. In cerebral neurons, these changes occur in the cell body and at the presynaptic level.

During reoxygenation, increased levels of at least three free radical species (in *oblique boxes*) that break down membranes and collagen and worsen microcirculatory failure may be formed: superoxide (O_2^-), hydroxyl radical ($OH^\cdot$), and free lipid radicals (FLR). Hydroxyl radical may or may not be important in the brain. Superoxide may be formed from three sources: (1) from AA directly, (2) from the previously described XO system, and (3) from the activation of neutrophils in the microvasculature (due to the increase in leukotriene [LT] production) or after diapedesis from the microvasculature. Increased O_2^- level leads to increased H_2O_2 production as a result of the intracellular action of superoxide dismutase (SOD). The H_2O_2 is controlled by intracellular catalase. Increased O_2^- level further leads to increased $OH^\cdot$ level as a result of the Fenton reaction ($Fe^{2+} \leftrightarrows Fe^{3+}$), with iron liberated from mitochondria. Also, AA causes increased activity of the cyclooxygenase pathway to produce prostaglandins (PG), including thromboxane (TX) A_2, and of the lipoxygenase pathway to produce LTs. Reoxygenation restores ATP via oxidative phosphorylation, which may result in massive uptake of $[Ca^{2+}]i$ into mitochondria. Thus, mitochondria, loaded with bound Ca^{2+}, may self-destruct; increased $[Ca^{2+}]i$ level by itself and via the triggering of free radical reactions may result in lipid peroxidation, membrane leaks, and cell death. Neuronal damage can be caused (in part) by increased extracellular EAA level (excitotoxicity), resulting in increased $[Ca^{2+}]i$ level. In the brain after cardiac arrest during reoxygenation and thereafter, free radical reactions, increase of $[Ca^{2+}]i$, and increase of extracellular EAAs may be epiphenomena.

Nitric oxide (NO), the endothelium-derived relaxing factor, is ubiquitous. It is formed from L-arginine. Nitric oxide is one of many molecular species involved in the complex adaptive mechanisms of the macro- and microcirculations and in nonspecific immunity as a cytotoxic agent. In the brain, NO is also a neurotransmitter that acts in inhibitory and excitatory neurons and is able to neutralize O_2^-. The exact roles and places for NO in this diagram—some of which might be deleterious, and others beneficial—are still unknown (see the following two reviews: Snyder SH, Bredt DS: Biological roles of nitric oxide. Sci Am 1992; 266:68–77, *and* Nussler AK, Billiard TR: Inflammation, immunoregulation and inducible nitric oxide synthase. J Leukoc Biol 1993; 54:171–178.)

Treatment potentials during or immediately after reperfusion (*in oval boxes*) with the previously presented rationale at this time include: superoxide dismutase and other free radical scavengers; catalase; deferoxamine; calcium entry blockers; XO inhibitors; intracellular buffers; corticosteroids (membrane stabilizers); aminosteroids ("lazaroids," lipid peroxidation inhibitors); and combinations of NMDA and non-NMDA EAA receptor blockers. Mild hypothermia seems to be a nonspecific mitigator of deleterious reoxygenation cascades.[32–35] Single- and combination-treatment protocols deserve evaluation in animal outcome models.

(From Safar P: Cerebral resuscitation after cardiac arrest: Research initiatives and future directions. Ann Emerg Med 1993; 22[Pt 2]:324.)

guidelines for uniform reporting of data to describe the process and outcome of clinical cardiac arrest and CPCR.[37]

When considering novel treatments in acute medicine, one must differentiate among treatments initiated before the insult *(protection)*, those during the insult *(preservation)*, and those to reverse the insult and support recovery *(resuscitation)*. Also, one must differentiate between terminal states (such as shock or asphyxia) and clinical death (potentially reversible cardiac arrest).

BASIC LIFE SUPPORT

Airway Control

The most common site of airway obstruction is the hypopharynx.[1, 2] During coma due to any cause in humans (but not in dogs), when the head is in the flexed or midposition, the relaxed tongue and neck muscles fail to lift the base of the tongue and epiglottis from the posterior pharyngeal wall (see Fig. 4–1). The nasal passage is sometimes obstructed by congestion, blood, mucus, or a valvelike behavior of the soft palate that blocks exhalation, regardless of whether the patient is in the lateral, supine, or prone position. Other causes of airway obstruction include foreign matter, laryngospasm, bronchospasm, bronchial secretions, mucosal edema, aspiration of gastric contents or foreign matter, and inflammatory processes.

Thus, emergency airway control (see Fig. 4–1 step A) should start with stretching the anterior neck structures by tilting the head backward, using chin support, and, if necessary, adding forward displacement of the mandible and opening of the mouth (the triple airway maneuver) (see Fig. 4–2). An unconscious patient should be placed supine and horizontal, with the head tilted backward and aligned with the neck and chest. The legs may be elevated to centralize the blood volume. The prone position makes the face inaccessible. When an unconscious patient is breathing spontaneously and adequately and the rescuer cannot keep holding the head, the stable side position is preferred, with the head maintained tilted backward. The next step should be an attempt at positive-pressure inflation of the lungs.

TABLE 4–4. Novel (Experimental) Cardiopulmonary-Cerebral Resuscitation Methods*

1. Intracarotid/intra-aortic fluids, drugs, cooling
2. Maximizing cerebral oxygen delivery with titrated hemodilution by fluorocarbon or stroma-free hemoglobin plus hypertension, cerebral vasodilation, osmotherapy, control of Pa_{CO_2}, and other measures
3. Titrated cerebral acid-base balance
4. Drug combinations that prevent reoxygenation injury
   - New free radical scavengers and iron chelators
   - New calcium entry blockers
   - New amino steroids
5. Drug combinations that prevent excitotoxicity
   - New NMDA receptor blockers
   - New non-NMDA receptor blockers
   - Phenytoin or other antiepileptics
   - Various anesthetics
6. Anti-inflammatory (anticomplement) treatments
7. Blood detoxification (leukapheresis, plasmapheresis, blood exchange)
8. Metabolic support (pyruvate, fructose)
9. Support of neuronal repair mechanisms

*Recommended by the authors for evaluation in reliable models of outcome in large animals (see Table 1 of Safar[16]).

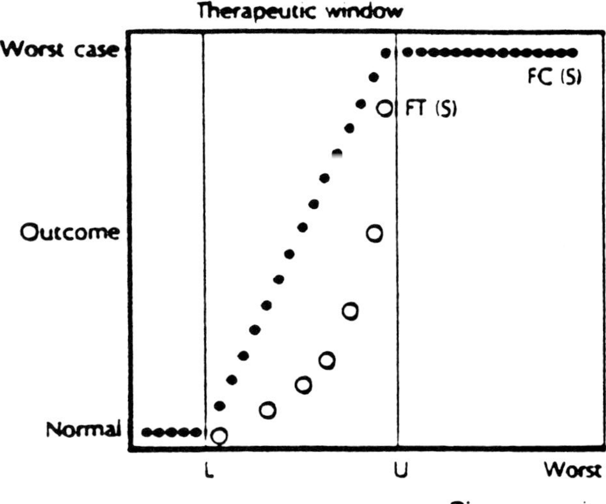

Figure 4–5. Clinical therapeutic window of opportunity. The relationship between disease severity and outcome is shown. • = control group; ○ = treatment group, treatment opportunity outside the therapeutic window is equal to control; FC = function at outcome (predicted or observed) for the control group as a function of disease severity (S); FT = function at outcome (predicted or observed) for the treatment group as a function of S; L = lower limit of therapeutic efficacy; U = upper limit of therapeutic efficacy. (From Bircher NG: CPCR: Brain resuscitation mediators, glucose, and anesthetics. Curr Opin Anesthesiol 1990; 3:259.)

In cases of suspected foreign body obstruction, which method to use for loosening and expelling foreign matter in the upper air passages (back blows, abdominal thrusts, chest thrusts, finger sweep) remains controversial.[8] Abdominal thrusts produce a weak cough effect. Back blows produce higher airway pressures than thrusts when the airway is closed, but they may either loosen the object or further impact it in a standing or sitting victim. Back blows are not recommended by the American Heart Association, but they are recommended abroad.[7, 8]

Devices for airway control may be considered for use in BLS and ALS. Nasopharyngeal and oropharyngeal tubes still require backward tilt of the head. Use of the esophageal obturator and esophageal gastric tube airway has been accompanied by an increased risk of complications.[3–7] The pharyngotracheal lumen airway is inserted blindly into the oropharynx and can result in either esophageal or tracheal placement. The use of the pharyngotracheal lumen airway, the esophageal-tracheal tube, and the laryngeal mask needs further evaluation.[3–7]

Endotracheal intubation with a cuffed tube is preferred to control the airway. Patients who tolerate an intubation attempt need an endotracheal tube. Details of intubation techniques should be studied and practiced,[2] including equipment needed, orotracheal versus nasotracheal intubation, rapid-sequence intubation, intubating the awake patient, difficulties encountered during intubation attempts, tactile orotracheal intubation, transillumination orotracheal intubation, use of the lighted stylet, fiberoptic laryngoscopic intubation, special considerations for the intubation of infants and small children, extubation, and complications. A gastric tube should be inserted as soon as feasible. An alternative to endotracheal intubation is cricothyrotomy, performed by trained personnel.[2] Tracheotomy (below the cricoid cartilage) should be an elective procedure.

TABLE 4–5. Clinical Studies of Pharmacologic Methods of Brain Resuscitation After Cardiac Arrest

	Pittsburgh BRCT I[25]	*Oslo*[31]	*Pittsburgh BRCT II*[27]	*Helsinki*[30]	*Berlin*[42]
Sample size	262	60	520	155	400
International	Yes	No	Yes	No	No
Multicenter	Yes	No	Yes	No	Yes
Randomized	Yes	Yes	Yes	Yes	Yes
Double-blind	No	Yes	Yes	Yes	Yes
Drug tested	Thiopental	Nimodipine (low-dose)	Lidoflazine	Nimodipine (high-dose)	Flunarizine
Overall statistical effect on outcome	No *	No	No *	No *	Not published

(Adapted from Gustafson I, Edgren E, Hulting J: Brain-oriented intensive care after resuscitation from cardiac arrest. Resuscitation 1992; 24:245.)
*Suggestive benefit in subgroups.
Abbreviation: BRCT = Brain Resuscitation Clinical Trial study group.

Clearing the pharyngeal airway and the tracheobronchial tree may require strong suction. In massive aspiration of solid foreign matter, ventilation bronchoscopy, using a large-bore, rigid ventilation bronchoscope rather than the popular flexible, small-bore fiberoptic bronchoscope, can be a life-saving resuscitative measure. Bronchodilation and bronchial clearing are important maneuvers in the management of status asthmaticus, severe bronchitis, near-drowning, and aspiration. Tension pneumothorax can asphyxiate a patient rapidly by lung collapse and bronchial kinking and compression due to mediastinal displacement. In suspected tension pneumothorax, confirmation by needle puncture (in the anterior upper thorax) and insertion of a large-bore chest tube (open or closed technique) should not be delayed until confirmation by radiography.[2]

Breathing Support

Currently recommended methods of artificial ventilation are based on intermittent inflation of the lungs with positive pressure applied to the airway, followed by passive exhalation at atmospheric pressure.[2] If direct mouth-to-mouth ventilation is impossible, one should try mouth-to-nose ventilation.[2] During ventilation via mask, which closes the mouth, nasal obstruction can be overcome with use of the triple airway maneuver (see Fig. 4–2) or insertion of an oropharyngeal or nasopharyngeal tube under the mask. Pressing the cricoid cartilage backward can counteract gastric insufflation and passive regurgitation. When high inflation pressures are needed, endotracheal intubation is preferable.

The chance that a rescuer might become infected during direct mouth-to-mouth ventilation (with hepatitis or the human immunodeficiency virus) is minimal. No such transmission has been documented.[2,7,8] Although transmission of human immunodeficiency virus via blood is a real possibility, such transmission via saliva has not been documented. Laypersons should carry a saliva filter, facemask, or face shield. Health professionals should carry a valved exhaled air ventilation device that directs the victim's exhaled air away from the operator. Adjuncts should include an adapter for optional oxygen enrichment.

The self-refilling bag-valve unit, when attached to an oronasal facemask, is difficult to use, but when it is attached to a tracheal tube it is easy to use and highly effective. For a nonintubated patient, mouth-valve-mask ventilation with oxygen is recommended, because both of the rescuer's hands are free to provide mask fit, head tilt, and jaw thrust.

Devices for ventilation may be considered for use in BLS and ALS. Oxygen-powered, pressure-cycled ventilators and resuscitator-inhalators are obsolete. A manually triggered, oxygen-powered resuscitator should provide 100% oxygen at less than 40 L/min and should have an inflation pressure-relief valve that opens at approximately 60 cm H_2O and, for spontaneously breathing victims, an oxygen demand system that requires no additional breathing effort. Automatic "transport ventilators" may be used effectively in lieu of bag-valve-tracheal tube devices during and after CPR.[2, 7, 8] Expiratory retardation is used to prevent intrapulmonary airway collapse during exhalation in cases of asthma and emphysema. Ventilation-perfusion mismatching calls for an increased inhaled oxygen concentration and positive end-expiratory pressure, which should be titrated according to arterial and mixed venous oxygen values. Spontaneous breathing of oxygen with positive airway pressure, without the use of a mechanical ventilator, can be effective in increasing the partial pressure of arterial oxygen in hypoxemic patients, even without the use of an endotracheal tube.

Circulation Support

Cardiac arrest is "the clinical picture of sudden cessation of circulation in a patient who was not expected to die at the time."[2] Cardiac arrest is recognized when all the following are present: unconsciousness, apnea or gasping, deathlike appearance, and no pulse in the carotid and femoral arteries. Primary cardiac arrest results from either ventricular fibrillation (VF) (which may be preceded by ventricular tachycardia [VT]) or asystole (as, for example, due to heart block or drug overdose). Secondary cardiac arrest results from asphyxia or exsanguination, usually in mechanical asystole (pulselessness) with ECG complexes continuing in the form of pulseless electric activity or electromechanical dissociation. This is relatively easy to reverse. However, defibrillation may change VF to secondary electromechanical dissociation, which may be difficult to reverse. If primary VF remains untreated, it weakens and becomes electric asystole; but with reperfusion, VF resumes.

Pulselessness is determined by palpating the carotid artery (see Fig. 4–1). In cardiac arrest, emergency artificial circulation is most readily produced by intermittent external chest compressions (see Fig. 4–1). The blood flow produced by standard external CPR is unpredictably low—between 0% and 30% of normal.[2–7] Because pressing on the sternum creates right atrial pressure peaks almost as high as arterial pressure peaks, perfusion pressures are low as well. Blood flow can be optimized by a 50:50 compression-relaxation ratio and is little influenced by compression rates between 40 and 120 per minute. In adults, a rate of about 80 compressions per minute (one to two compressions per second) is recommended. The currently recommended rates and ratios of ventilations to sternal compressions (2:15 for nonintubated patients and 1:5 for intubated patients) are a compromise. During CPR, the trachea should be intubated as soon as possible, without interrupting chest compressions for more than 15 seconds at a time. Once the endotracheal tube has been inserted, lung inflations during CPR need not be synchronized with chest compressions. If performed optimally, standard external CPR is sometimes capable of preserving cerebral and myocardial viability in dogs and patients for more than 30 minutes, even after cardiac arrest (no blood flow) times of 5 to 10 minutes.[2, 3–7, 16]

Blood flow seems to be generated by variable combinations of heart-pump and chest-pump mechanisms (see Chapter 5). Coronary and cerebral perfusion pressures generated by external CPR can be augmented by epinephrine. Attempts to augment blood flow with simultaneous ventilation-compression CPR did not lead to improved outcome in dogs[2] or human patients.[19] These techniques to increase airway pressure are not considered to be BLS, because they require an endotracheal tube and mechanical devices. Administration of CPR via an inflatable vest to take advantage of fluctuation in overall intrathoracic pressure does not require an endotracheal tube, but application of the vest device is limited to ambulance personnel.[19a] Improving blood flow during BLS with intermittent abdominal compression CPR[20] or active compression-decompression CPR[21a, 21b] appears promising, but these methods have yet to undergo controlled clinical trials.

Guidelines call for performing steps A, B, and C in this sequence (see Fig. 4–1). In witnessed VF (i.e., VF that occurs in the presence of a trained bystander), coached vigorous coughing, if the patient is still conscious, can maintain consciousness for a few minutes. Performing steps C, A, and B in that sequence is physiologically sound advice[2] in witnessed sudden cardiac arrest, because the aortic blood retains oxygen without ventilation until recirculation begins.[21c] Even sudden cardiac arrest, however, is often preceded by hypoxemia, requiring steps A and B to be performed first. Moreover, laypersons should not be confused with two sequences.

During CPR with steps A, B, and C, the earliest possible attempts at electric defibrillation should be made. Epinephrine should be given intravenously or intratracheally, and CPR should be continued until a strong spontaneous pulse is restored. In asphyxial cardiac arrest (mechanical asystole), a spontaneous pulse may return after a few minutes of effective CPR, without the need for countershock; or CPR can provoke secondary VF.[9]

Precordial thumping by fist cannot be expected to terminate VF, but it can (unpredictably) transform ventricular tachycardia into either sinus rhythm or VF.[6] Repetitive thumping (once per second) and sternal compressions (as for artificial circulation), however, are effective methods of mechanical pacing.[2]

In cases of trauma, circulation support goes beyond external cardiac resuscitation (which in itself has little to offer in an exsanguinated victim). Measures that may be needed in trauma include manual control of external hemorrhage, airway control, artificial ventilation, primary and secondary survey, extrication, positioning for shock, intravenous fluid resuscitation to prevent cardiac arrest from blood loss (not necessarily to restore normotension, which might provoke renewed bleeding), use of a tourniquet, control of internal hemorrhage below the diaphragm with the use of military antishock trousers, and resuscitative surgery.

ADVANCED LIFE SUPPORT

Defibrillation

Electric therapy for life-threatening cardiac dysrhythmias[2] consists mainly of direct-current external electric countershocks for VT or VF, as well as external or transvenous electric pacing for complete heart block (severe bradycardia) or asystole. Additional steps include a simple chest thump for witnessed VT or VF, repetitive chest thumps (fist pacing) for heart block with bradycardia, and synchronized cardioversion for atrial fibrillation or VT with pulse.

Although appropriate drug therapy can often prevent VF, pharmacologic defibrillation has proved unreliable. Electric countershock, the most rapid, effective, and accepted method for terminating VT or VF, has been recognized since the turn of the century, but it was not used in clinical practice until the 1940s. Spontaneous cessation of VF without countershock is rare in humans and large animals, although it is common in small animals. Defibrillating electric shocks produce simultaneous depolarization of all myocardial fibers, after which spontaneous contractions may start if the myocardium is oxygenated and not acidotic.

Low-voltage alternating current (such as that found in the household), which sends less than 2 A through the heart, can induce VF. High-voltage electric shock that sends more than 2 A through the heart (such as defibrillating shocks or lightning) produces a sustained contraction in the normally beating heart and can terminate VF. The energy that defibrillators discharge is measured in watt-seconds or joules (J). Direct-current countershock is produced by a capacitor-discharge–type defibrillator delivering up to 360 J in about 0.01 second. Low resistance between the electrodes and chest wall via the use of saline-soaked or electrode gel pads is important. Transthoracic impedance can be reduced by pressing the electrodes on the chest to lower high-resistance lung volume. The recommended levels of energy are a compromise between the need to consistently deliver shocks sufficient to stop VF and to prevent energy-dose–related myocardial damage. The present recommendation to terminate VF is to deliver a 200-300-360–J sequence of external shocks. Other dysrhythmias require less energy (e.g., 100 J for VT, atrial fibrillation, and paroxysmal supraventricular tachycardia, and 25–50 J for atrial flutter). Myocardial damage can be caused by excessive electric current. However, the importance of promptly restoring spontaneous circulation outweighs the risk of slight myocardial damage resulting from electric shock.

Guidelines for external defibrillation[2, 7] recommend an initial two to three shocks of about 3 J/kg (in adults, 200–300 J). External paddles should be 10 cm in diameter for adults, 8 cm for children, and 4.5 cm for infants. (For open-chest CPR, energies of about 0.5 J/kg are suggested; paddles should be 6 cm in diameter for adults, 4 cm for children, and 2 cm for infants.)

In witnessed cardiac arrest, external countershocks should ideally be applied within 30 to 60 seconds of the onset of VF—that is, before the heart becomes hypoxic or acidotic and before the start of CPR with steps A, B, and C (see Fig. 4–1). If these countershocks are unsuccessful within 60 seconds of collapse, CPR must be started. In unwitnessed cardiac arrest, CPR with steps A, B, and C may be needed for 1 to 2 minutes to reoxygenate the myocardium before an attempt to defibrillate. Good electric contact should be provided without using gel between the electrodes. One paddle should be placed to the right of the upper half of the sternum, below the clavicle, and the other to the left of the cardiac apex, below the left nipple. Polarity influences the ECG reading but not the success of defibrillation. Defibrillation attempts should begin with 200 J (for 70-kg adults) and a quick look at the ECG; if VT or VF continues, immediately apply 300 J and, if unsuccessful, then apply 360 J. These three shocks should be given in rapid succession and followed by CPR steps A, B, and C. Countershocks with 360 J (maximum available) should then be repeated, without interrupting chest compressions more than 10 seconds at a time. If several shocks fail despite optimal chest compressions and intermittent positive-pressure ventilation, then epinephrine, lidocaine, and sodium bicarbonate ($NaHCO_3$) should be given in this sequence. If this fails, bretylium is indicated. Patients have occasionally recovered after several hours of external CPR with multiple defibrillation attempts.[2–7]

Recommendations to improve the success of defibrillation include repositioning the paddle electrodes, because VF may appear as asystole; correcting electrode placement; creating a close interface between the paddles and the chest wall; using heavy pressure on the paddle electrodes; pressing the paddles on the chest to expel air from the lungs; following the recommendations for energy; allowing brief intervals between a series of about three shocks, sufficient only to recharge the defibrillator; checking defibrillators regularly for energy delivery; and monitoring blood gases and pH.

The efficacy of automatic external electric defibrillation is well established.[2, 7, 7a] Portable defibrillators that read the ECG, recognize VF, and discharge countershocks automatically or semi-automatically (giving audio orders to the operator) are among the latest resuscitation technologies for use by emergency medical technicians and trained laypersons. These new devices (such as the Laerdal Heartstart 2000, the Physio-Control LifePak 200, and the Cardiac Resuscitation Corp. Heart Aid) identify VF and automatically deliver external countershocks of 200 to 360 J. They use disposable stick-on chest electrodes and record the ECG for medical review. The Laerdal unit also provides a programmed printout of critical ECG data. In clinical trials, automatic external defibrillators have not shocked a patient inappropriately.[13] Automatic internally implanted defibrillators (with cup electrodes that fit over the apex and base of the heart) have been developed for ambulatory patients at risk of sudden death due to VF. These defibrillators monitor the ECG continuously, recognize VF of more than 20 seconds' duration, and provide 10- to 20-J shocks from a 250-g implanted, biocompatible minidefibrillator.

Adrenergic Agents

Epinephrine (adrenaline) helps to restore spontaneous normotension in cardiac arrest of more than about 1 to 2 minutes' duration, irrespective of the ECG diagnosis.[2, 7] The stimulating effect of epinephrine on α receptors increases systemic peripheral vascular resistance without constricting the coronary and cerebral vessels and thereby improves myocardial (and cerebral) blood flow during CPR with steps A, B, and C. This in turn facilitates the return of spontaneous cardiac contractions.[14] The stimulating effect of epinephrine on β receptors is probably unimportant during cardiac compressions but may be advantageous once spontaneous cardiac action has started. Although epinephrine can produce VF, it can also help convert fine VF into coarse VF, which is more susceptible to termination by electric countershock.

It has been recommended that epinephrine be given in doses of 1 mg/70 kg body weight as an IV bolus or diluted in 10 mL of isotonic sodium chloride intratracheally. Larger doses are more effective in animal models, but clinical results with high-dose epinephrine have so far been confusing (see *Clinical Trials of Cardiopulmonary-Cerebral Resuscitation*, later). One of the authors (Safar) recommends that clinical CPR ALS start with an epinephrine dose of 1 mg/70 kg for each estimated minute of arrest time beyond 3 minutes and to titrate additional doses according to need. Other sympathomimetic amines that primarily stimulate α receptors, such as norepinephrine, metaraminol, phenylephrine, and methoxamine, also help to restore spontaneous circulation.[13] Sympathomimetic amines that stimulate only the β receptors, such as isoproterenol, low-dose dopamine, and dobutamine, do not aid in restoration of spontaneous circulation and are not indicated during CPR.[13, 14]

Buffer Agents

$NaHCO_3$ is the second or third agent of choice in cardiac arrest,[2, 7, 13–15] after epinephrine and lidocaine. The benefit derived from the present routine use of $NaHCO_3$ during CPR with steps A, B, and C is unknown. This agent should be given only after prolonged arrest or CPR time to neutralize the fixed acids coming from ischemic tissues after circulatory arrest. This is particularly needed in order to prevent the arterial pH from decreasing below 7.2 during the early phase after restoration of spontaneous circulation, when acids from previously ischemic tissues are washed out. During cardiac arrest, arterial acidemia poses no problem, because with the low blood flow produced by external CPR and hyperventilation by intermittent positive-pressure ventilation, arterial pH is usually normal or high. During low-flow states in venous blood and tissues, pH is low and partial pressure of carbon dioxide is high.[13–15] As a donor of carbon dioxide, $NaHCO_3$ can transiently worsen hypercarbia, unless its administration is (as it should be) accompanied by transient controlled hyperventilation and administration of epinephrine to improve perfusion. Excessive use of $NaHCO_3$ leads to arterial alkalemia, which may make the heart even less resuscitable and create a "stone heart." Other alleged side effects of $NaHCO_3$ administration[14, 15] might be clinically relevant only if this drug is used in excessive doses. On the other hand, acidemia (pH $<$7.2) can hamper resuscitation by causing vasodilation, myocardial depression, and capillary leakage and by counteracting the effects of catecholamines. In dogs with VF no flow of 10 minutes, $NaHCO_3$ added to epinephrine improved restoration of heartbeat and 24-hour outcome.[15a]

Present recommendations[7] call for epinephrine to be administered first, followed by $NaHCO_3$, 1 mmol/kg IV once during CPR with steps A, B, and C but only when cardiac arrest (no blood flow) of at least 2 to 5 minutes' duration may have occurred. The administration of $NaHCO_3$ should be repeated not more than every 10 minutes during the low-flow state of CPR and should be titrated as soon as possible according to arterial pH, aiming for pHa values of 7.3 to 7.5 or to normalize the calculated base deficit.[14]

Mechanical External Cardiopulmonary Resuscitation

Although mechanical external CPR devices of the past had diverse problems, those currently available offer some advantages during prolonged clinical resuscitation efforts. Carefully operated, they provide consistent chest compressions and higher arterial pressures in humans, and they allow an additional rescuer to attend to other tasks. Nonetheless, the use of mechanical external CPR devices during transportation, although recommended for use on ALS-resistant patients, has not yet been shown to influence outcome.[14]

Open-Chest Cardiopulmonary Resuscitation

Open-chest CPR is physiologically superior but logistically inferior to standard external CPR.[23] Between 1900 and 1960 (when closed-chest CPR became universal), open-chest CPR produced high survival rates with good brain function when practiced in hospitals, usually in operating rooms.[1, 2, 23] Even direct cardiac massage up to 2.5 hours after arrest led to recovery. Open-chest CPR produces higher cerebral and coronary perfusion pressures than external CPR but is limited to use by physicians in hospitals. Mullie and colleagues[39] have performed open-chest CPR outside the hospital, without objection from bystanders.

Direct compression of the heart produces better arteriovenous perfusion pressures and better overall, cerebral, and coronary blood flows than do sternal compressions; the latter increase the overall intrathoracic pressure, which in turn increases venous and arterial pressure simultaneously. Thus, open-chest CPR provides a better chance for sustaining cerebral and myocardial viability and restoring spontaneous circulation. In addition, open-chest CPR permits direct palpation and observation of the heart, which helps guide drug and fluid therapy and electric countershocks in difficult, protracted CPR efforts. Finally, the open-chest method permits direct compression of a bleeding site in intrathoracic exsanguination and, in cases of intra-abdominal hemorrhage, allows temporary compression or clamping of the thoracic aorta above the diaphragm.

Indications for open-chest CPR are: (1) chest already open (in the operating room), (2) suspected intrathoracic hemorrhage, (3) suspected intra-abdominal exsanguination (for clamping the lower thoracic aorta), (4) suspected massive pulmonary embolism, (5) hypothermic cardiac arrest (open-chest CPR permits direct warming of the heart), (6) inability of external CPR to produce a carotid or femoral pulse (as in cases with chest or spine deformities or severe emphysema with barrel chest), and (7) suspected long duration of unwitnessed cardiac arrest and optimal external CPR ALS unable to promptly restore spontaneous normotension within 5 to 10 minutes. Indications 1 to 6 have been part of the national[3–7] and international[2] recommendations, whereas indication 7 has been added by the authors.[2]

The technique of open-chest CPR includes endotracheal intubation and intermittent positive-pressure ventilation with positive end-expiratory pressure provided by a second operator. Mouth-to-mouth ventilation during thoracotomy is feasible but difficult. A skin incision over the fourth or fifth left intercostal space is followed by entering the chest bluntly and cutting the intercostal muscles with Mayo scissors, avoiding the intercostal neurovascular bundle and the internal mammary artery if possible. The intercostal space is pulled open, and a rib spreader is inserted if available. One should start heart compressions without first opening the pericardium, compressing about once per second and adjusting the compression force and rate to the filling of the heart. Sterile equipment is not essential. The operator, standing to the patient's left, faces cephalad and places the thumb of the left hand over the left ventricle posteriorly and the second through fifth fingers over the right ventricle anteriorly. While compressing the ventricles, avoiding the atria, one feels for the wormlike motion of VF. One should compress the descending aorta with the other hand if feasible. Heart compressions may be more effective by compressing the heart against the sternum or using two hands. If uncertain about VF, the pericardium should be opened. Epinephrine may be injected into the cavity of the left ventricle. If needed, $NaHCO_3$ should be given intravenously. Defibrillation is provided using two internal electrodes with saline-soaked gauze pads as previously described, one placed behind the heart over the left ventricle and the other over the right ventricle. Start with 0.5-J/kg shocks. External transthoracic countershock with the chest open is also possible. In massive pulmonary thromboembolism, direct heart massage plus breaking up the clots may be effective. Mechanical open-chest cardiac compression devices, such as the Anstadt cup or other mechanical means of physically pressurizing the pericardium, are convenient and effective but also require special experience to be used effectively. In suspected cardiac tamponade, rapid needle puncture alongside the xiphoid process may obviate the need for thoracotomy.

Emergency Cardiopulmonary Bypass

Wherever clinically feasible, CPB permits control over the flow, pressure, oxygenation, temperature, and composition of blood as rapidly as cannulation can be accomplished. The widespread clinical use of the heart-lung machine for open-heart surgery (by personnel to perform perfusion in the operating room) has not been paralleled by its use for resuscitation outside the operating room, where a portable CPB unit is needed.[24] Some uncontrolled clinical trials of emergency CPB for pulselessness due to pulmonary thromboembolism or hypothermia have been carried out. In 10 studies of dogs with prolonged cardiac arrest, venoarterial pumping without thoracotomy, performed by a portable apparatus with a membrane oxygenator and self-regulating centrifugal pump, primed with plasma substitute, emergency CPB proved superior to external CPR ALS in achieving restoration of spontaneous circulation and cerebral recovery.[24] Clinical trials of closed-chest emergency CPB with femoral cannulation are ongoing. Uses in trauma-related arrests, for inducing and reversing "profound hypothermic suspended animation," and for prolonged assisted circulation (over days) would be enabled by heparin-bonded CPB circuits to avoid systemic heparinization, which can cause cerebral hemorrhage.

Emergency CPB is a competitor for open-chest CPR to treat cases of complicated, prolonged, intractable cardiac arrest. The advantages of CPB over open-chest CPR include full control over reperfusion pressure patterns, arterial oxygen transport, blood composition, and prolonged assisted circulation without thoracotomy. A disadvantage is the longer time required for insertion of the venae cavae drainage catheter and the femoral artery cannula. This is difficult when a patient's body is bounced by the motion of sternal compressions. Cerebral resuscitation is also enhanced by CPB, which permits delivery of brain resuscitation agents that depress the cardiovascular system. With the use of CPB in cardiac arrest, after an initial reperfusion of several minutes, the authors favor early defibrillation to let the left ventricle drain itself by spontaneous beating. Most of the venous return to the right ventricle can be drained through the extracorporeal circuit. More than 50% of prehospital attempts at external CPR ALS fail to restart the heart. Therefore, clinical trials of mechanical CPR or emergency CPB, perhaps even initiated outside the hospital by physician-staffed ambulance teams, are indicated.

BRAIN-ORIENTED LIFE SUPPORT

After prolonged cardiac arrest (no blood flow), the cerebral postresuscitation syndrome seems to consist of eight derangements that can be therapeutically prevented or mitigated[16]: (1) inadequate energy (adenosine triphosphate); (2) impaired ionic pump (intracellular edema); (3) tissue acidosis; (4) perfusion failure, causing inadequate oxygen delivery (see Fig. 4–3); (5) excitotoxicity of neurons; (6) free radical–triggered chemical cascades leading to reoxygenation injury (see Fig. 4–4); (7) inflammatory tissue reaction (unproven after cardiac arrest); and (8) extracerebral derangements, including intoxication from postanoxic viscera (which seems to have only a transiently negative effect on the brain) and blood derangements due to stasis. After brain trauma, one might add three further derangements—(1) direct tissue tearing and destruction; (2) damage to neurons by blood (heme); and (3) brain swelling.

After cardiac arrest, the immediate no-reflow phenomenon seems to be preventable by normotensive or hypertensive reperfusion. Then, after transient hyperemia, delayed protracted cerebral hypoperfusion follows, the cause of which is multifactorial and unclear. Intracranial pressure after cardiac arrest remains normal except for progression to brain death. Low cerebral venous oxygen values reflect a mismatching of oxygen delivery to oxygen need. Mitigation of this condition is possible, at least transiently, with hypertension, hemodilution, and vasodilation, which seem to improve outcome.[22] Novel treatments ready for clinical trials (see Table 4–3) include mild resuscitative cerebral hypothermia,[32–35] promotion of oxygen delivery,[22] and buffer therapy.[15a] Standard brain-oriented life support (see Table 4–1) currently seems to be uncontroversial.

Studies involving drug treatments to prevent reoxygenation injury cascades (see Fig. 4–4) have yielded no convincing evidence of improved cerebral outcome, except for the use of calcium entry blockers.[26–31] Mild hypothermia (34°C) is safe for the cardiovascular system. In contrast, moderate hypothermia (30°C) has serious side effects. Results of four controlled, randomized outcome studies in dogs[32–35] have shown that mild resuscitative hypothermia for 1 to 2 hours after cardiac arrest mitigates brain damage, provided cooling is initiated within 15 minutes after reperfusion. These data have been confirmed by three other groups using a model of incomplete forebrain ischemia in rats.[16] Resuscitative mild hypothermia also seems beneficial after focal brain ischemia and brain trauma, when more time for the induction of cooling is possible.[16]

The therapeutic effect of even mild cooling is probably the result of a synergism of multiple potentially beneficial mechanisms, including the suppression of free radical–triggered cascades that lead to membrane breakdown, tightening of membranes, suppression of excitotoxicity, preservation of adenosine triphosphate and ionic membrane balance, and reduction of oxygen requirements (see the bibliographies of Safar[16] and Leonov and colleagues[32]). Interestingly, moderate hypothermia or deep hypothermia (15°C), which clearly has a greater protective effect than mild hypothermia when induced before and during arrest, when induced with reperfusion from normothermic arrest, resulted in worse outcome for heart and brain.[34]

Mild hypothermia induced immediately after normothermic arrest of 10 or 12 minutes and continued for several hours reduced functional deficit and histologic brain damage[32–35] but did not result in histologically normal brains. This observation suggests that other treatments will have to be added. The effects of combination treatments on outcome are now being evaluated in reliable animal models (see Table 4–4). The best functional and morphologic recovery of the brain in dogs has been recently achieved with a physical combination treatment of mild hypothermia and cerebral blood flow promotion with hypertension, hemodilution, and normocapnia.[45] Because of the difficulty of inducing even mild cerebral hypothermia rapidly after cardiac arrest, clinical feasibility trials of various methods of noninvasive and invasive cooling are urgently needed (see Table 8 of Safar[16]).

WHEN NOT TO START AND WHEN TO STOP CARDIOPULMONARY-CEREBRAL RESUSCITATION

Emergency resuscitation should not be started when a patient is in the terminal stages of an incurable disease, the order "do not attempt resuscitation" (DNAR) has been specified, or another reason to withhold CPR is considered acceptable.[2, 7] For initiation of emergency resuscitation, time should not be wasted on contemplation or consultation. When in doubt, CPR steps A through F (see Fig. 4–1) should be initiated. When contraindicated, PLS should be discontinued. Discontinuance of efforts to provide emergency resuscitation (CPR steps A through F) should be determined on the basis of cardiac death, not brain death. Cardiac death is evident when the heartbeat cannot be restarted despite a maximum effort for at least 30 minutes. Electromechanical dissociation is not proof of irreversibility. As long as VF or VT is present, a chance to restore spontaneous circulation still exists. Emergency CPB during irreversible heart failure might in the future serve as a bridge until emergency implantation of an artificial or donor heart can be performed. After initial partial neurologic recovery, dilated fixed pupils and apnea may develop. Before brain death can be certified, more than 24 hours of extracerebral organ stabilization may be required. Neurologic signs of brain death are frequently associated with vasopressor-resistant hypotension. In protracted coma without brain death, the medical decision to terminate life support for persistent vegetative state (letting the patient die) is part of critical care triage, namely, determining the appropriate level of care. Irreversibility of the vegetative stage should be determined on the basis of published predictive criteria, clinical judgment, and laboratory data. This decision should be made by an experienced physician, who should also seek advice from consultants. Letting a patient die of natural causes should take place in a dignified setting, which can be provided even in the ICU.

CLINICAL TRIALS OF CARDIOPULMONARY-CEREBRAL RESUSCITATION

For resuscitation science to move from laboratory experiments to clinical use, evidence in support of benefit of a new therapy must first be established. This process begins with the development of a reliable, clinically relevant outcome model using animals (see Table 1 of Safar[16]). Such animal experiments are complex, labor intensive, and expensive. With success of the tested therapy, human trials may be performed, which are even more complex, labor intensive, and expensive. Clinical studies must meet certain requirements (see Table 2 of Safar[16]). A favorable benefit-risk profile should be demonstrated before the routine clinical use of a potentially hazardous, labor-intensive, and expensive new treatment is justified.

Clinical trials are not as easily controlled as laboratory trials and often use crude outcome measures with lesser powers of resolution. On the other hand, re-creating human disease (such as coronary atherosclerosis) in animals is often impossible. Clinical trials of cerebral resuscitation after cardiac arrest have not yet confirmed the value of any of the therapies that have been demonstrated to be beneficial in reliable outcome models using animals. Reasons for this may include (1) the background noise of clinical trials (which tends to obscure small treatment differences); (2) the logistic difficulties of conducting clinical research in emergency situations (which, by encouraging deviations in protocol, tend to limit the chance to demonstrate small treatment differences); and (3) the lack of taking advantage of identifying and focusing on appropriate study populations, such as those patients who may actually benefit from the experimental therapy.

Concerning case selection, patients whose severity of disease is minimal all may have good outcomes after standard CPR. Those with severe disease may be beyond the help of any novel intervention. Inclusion of either of these extremes dilutes the observed results. The "therapeutic window of opportunity" includes primarily patients whose disease severity is such that a beneficial experimental therapy may improve outcome (see Fig. 4–5). Timing of a clinical trial is also important. With the publication of positive case reports, clinicians quickly tend to believe that a new therapy for a hopeless disease is of proven value. Once a scientific clinical trial is conducted, the previously accumulated convincing anecdotal evidence of benefit is frequently disproved.

Cardiopulmonary Resuscitation

The current challenge for resuscitation medicine is to advance beyond our ability to restart an arrested heart by maximizing long-term survival with normal neuropsychologic function, within biologic limits. Clinical data confirm the obvious—that the duration of cardiac arrest in part determines post-CPR mortality and neurologic disability; hence, the rationale for rapid-response emergency medical services systems. Similarly, the duration of CPR is associated with poor outcome; hence, the search for increasingly efficient techniques to rapidly restore stable spontaneous circulation.

In VF, the earlier that defibrillation is attempted, the higher is the success rate in restarting the heart. The resulting shorter ischemic insult correlates with improved neurologic recovery. If initial countershocks are unsuccessful or if a patient is in cardiac arrest without VF, adrenergic drug therapy is indicated. Choice and dose of adrenergic agents are controversial. Higher doses of epinephrine (5- to 10-fold greater than "standard doses") have been tested in controlled and uncontrolled clinical studies. A small, randomized trial showed an increased rate of return of spontaneous circulation with 5-mg doses of epinephrine.[40] One large study in Japan noted improved restoration of spontaneous circulation. Three large randomized clinical trials[41–43] did not demonstrate beneficial effect on survival or neurologic recovery. The preliminary results of our BRCT III, a trial of increasing doses of epinephrine (5, 10, and 15 mg), tested in about 3000 patients with cardiac arrest randomized into treatment or control group, suggest enhanced restoration of spontaneous circulation, more post-arrest dysrhythmias, and no overall significant group difference in mortality or cerebral recovery rates after high-dose epinephrine.[43]

Cerebral Resuscitation

The brain benefits from interventions that minimize the duration of the ischemic insult and augment the effectiveness of CPR BLS or ALS. The first prospective controlled clinical study of sudden death and CPCR was the BRCT I (performed during 1979–1984), which randomly tested the efficacy of thiopental loading on survival and neurologic recovery.[25] The BRCT II (1985–1989) tested the efficacy of the calcium entry blocker lidoflazine.[26–28] The BRCT III (1989–1994) tested the efficacy of increasingly high doses of epinephrine. In all three trials, the standard therapy protocol was a simplified version that was suggested by earlier animal experiments (see Table 4–1).

In BRCT I, almost 300 patients were randomized and monitored for up to 12 months (see Table 4–5). Despite various logical but theoretic mechanisms of action, promising animal data, and suggestive evidence of benefit accumulated in clinical feasibility and pilot trials, high-dose barbiturate loading within 30 minutes of restoration of spontaneous circulation from cardiac arrest did not result in a significantly higher incidence of good cerebral recovery compared with standard therapy alone. A subgroup of patients with severe insult, however, showed a numerically better result with thiopental.

In the 1980s, calcium entry blocking drugs were being applied to an ever increasing variety of medical problems. Two such experimental drugs, lidoflazine,[26] and nimodipine,[29] were then of greatest interest for brain resuscitation because both had demonstrated benefit in animal models of global brain ischemia. Early experience with lidoflazine administration in patients undergoing open-heart surgery had shown it to be safe.

In BRCT II, more than 500 comatose survivors of cardiac arrest were randomized into lidoflazine versus standard treatment groups (see Table 4–5).[27, 28] No significant difference was noted between treatment and control groups overall in the proportion of patients who achieved good cerebral outcome. When patients who developed postarrest hypotension or rearrest were excluded from the analysis, the lidoflazine group had a higher proportion of patients with good cerebral outcome.[28] Such subgroup selection after randomization, although unavoidable, is scientifically unacceptable.

From our large data base of more than 800 victims of cardiac arrest in BRCT I and II, other important findings were demonstrated:

1. Clinical confirmation that long durations of arrest and resuscitation efforts are strongly associated with poor neurologic outcome
2. Clinical confirmation that after restoration of heartbeat, high arterial reperfusion pressure correlates with good cerebral recovery, and vice versa
3. Determination that cardiac arrests without CPR of greater than 5 minutes' duration do not always lead to irreversible brain damage
4. Identification of reliable, early (within 72 h) clinical predictors of the persistent vegetative state
5. Determination that advanced age, although associated with increased mortality after CPR, is not associated with worse neurologic outcome
6. Evidence that steroid administration is unassociated with improved neurologic outcome after cardiac arrest

Clinical investigations of other calcium entry blockers have also been conducted (see Table 4–5). A randomized clinical trial in Helsinki of nimodipine loading after cardiac arrest focused on a study population thought to have the best chance of recovery—that is, cases of prehospital VF with BLS started within 10 minutes and ALS within 20 minutes of cardiac arrest, and spontaneous circulation restored within 30 minutes.[30] A total of 155 patients were monitored for up to 1 year. No overall improvement in survival or neurologic recovery was noted. However, improved survival and neurologic recovery at 1 year were found in a subgroup of patients in whom ALS was started 10 minutes or longer after cardiac arrest. Exclusion of patients who had ALS started more than 20 minutes after arrest may have eliminated those least likely to benefit. Subsequently, a clinical trial by the same researchers has been initiated to focus on this patient subgroup.

Another, smaller, study in Oslo of low-dose nimodipine found improved cerebral blood flow after cardiac arrest (the main endpoint of the study) but no improvement in neurologic outcome.[31] Perhaps the dose tested was too low or the sample size too small. Lower intracranial pressure and better cerebral blood flow occurred with nimodipine, but these variables did not correlate with better neurologic outcome.

Finally, a randomized clinical trial tested flunarizine, yet another experimental calcium entry blocker proposed for brain resuscitation of comatose survivors of cardiac arrest (see Table 4–5).[44] The drug was administered early (within 15 min after restoration of spontaneous circulation) by physicians staffing mobile ICU ambulances in order to show whether the experimental treatment was beneficial.

Which methods are currently the most effective for clinical cerebral resuscitation after cardiac arrest? The authors believe that the protocol defined for general life support (see Table 4–1) is beneficial, although its advantage over "usual care" is difficult to prove. Although strong evidence supports many of the components of our recommended combination treatment protocols, such as control of reperfusion pressure and correction of acidemia, some aspects, such as control of blood glucose levels and administration of steroids, are still controversial. For other components such as immediate postarrest mild cerebral hypothermia, the logistic feasibility should be tested.[32–35] For the moment, improved outcome can be expected by simply improving the delivery of established therapies and, as feasible, raising transiently reperfusing pressure and rapidly lowering brain temperature for a few hours.[16]

As the pathophysiology of cardiac arrest continues to unfold and (not surprisingly) become more complex, it seems likely that effective therapeutic protocols will require multifaceted approaches that are titrated according to monitored derangements.[16] Although this approach has already extended the 5-minute arrest reversibility limit to 10 minutes in several series of animal experiments,[16, 17, 22, 32–35, 45] clinical documentation of combination treatments has not yet been attempted.

CONCLUSIONS

Reversibility of terminal states (with pulse) is discussed in other chapters of this book. Reversibility of clinical death (without pulse) has been the focus of this chapter. Outside the hospital, initiation of emergency resuscitation with CPR BLS requires public education in life-supporting first aid. Continuing with effective ALS both outside and in the hospital and effective PLS in the hospital requires skilled team members and experienced team leaders. Guided experience with life support of anesthetized patients in operating rooms and with resuscitation of patients outside the hospital and in emergency departments is the best training. The lifesaving potential of emergency resuscitation efforts outside the ICU, using simple and inexpensive means, exceeds that of long-term resuscitation efforts in the ICU, using complex and expensive means. Cardiac arrest in the hospital ICU usually occurs secondary to other complications and should be either prevented or anticipated. To achieve maximum reversibility of clinical death to survival with good cerebral outcome, response times must be minimized. Researchers should continue to attempt extension of the 5-minute limit of reversibility from cardiac arrest by preventing or mitigating the multifaceted postresuscitation syndrome. The principal challenges are the stunned or permanently failing myocardium and postischemic-anoxic encephalopathy. Both require mechanism-specific, titrated combination treatments. For cerebral resuscitation, laboratory evidence has documented benefit from the immediate postarrest promotion of blood flow, mild hypothermia, and calcium entry blocker therapy. Improved drug cocktails should be designed and evaluated. With coordinated multicenter efforts, socioeconomically important advances using novel methods of CPCR should be possible before the year 2000. As hopes are raised, we must "keep our enthusiasm, but let strict verification be our guide" (Pasteur).

ACKNOWLEDGMENTS

The authors' research was supported in part by the Asmund S. Laerdal Foundation and the National Institutes of Health. Ms. Nancy Arora helped edit, and Ms. Fran Mistrick and Ms. Connie Arelt helped prepare the manuscript.

References

Because of limitation of space we are citing primarily reviews, which list original publications.

1. Safar P: History of cardiopulmonary-cerebral resuscitation. *In*: Cardiopulmonary Resuscitation. Kaye W, Bircher N (Eds). New York, Churchill Livingstone, 1989, pp 1–53.
2. Safar P, Bircher N: Cardiopulmonary Cerebral Resuscitation, Guidelines by the World Federation of Societies of Anesthesiologists (WFSA). 3rd ed. Philadelphia, WB Saunders, 1988.
3. American Heart Association and National Academy of Sciences–National Research Council: Standards for cardiopulmonary resuscitation (CPR) and emergency cardiac care (ECC). JAMA 1966; 198:372.
4. American Heart Association and National Academy of Sciences–National Research Council: Standards for cardiopulmonary resuscitation (CPR) and emergency cardiac care (ECC). JAMA 1974; 277(Suppl):833.
5. American Heart Association: Standards for cardiopulmonary resuscitation (CPR) and emergency cardiac care (ECC). JAMA 1980; 244(Suppl):453.
6. American Heart Association: Standards for cardiopulmonary resuscitation (CPR) and emergency cardiac care (ECC). JAMA 1986; 255(Suppl):2841.
7. American Heart Association: Guidelines for cardiopulmonary resuscitation and emergency cardiac care. JAMA 1992; 268:2171.

7a. Cummins RO, Eisenberg MS, Graves JR, et al: Automatic external defibrillators used by emergency medical technicians: A controlled clinical trial. Crit Care Med 1985; 13:945.

8. European Resuscitation Council, Brighton, England: Guidelines for basic life support. Resuscitation 1992; 24:103.
9. Safar P, Bircher N: The pathophysiology of dying and reanimation. *In*: Principles and Practice of Emergency Medicine. 3rd ed. Vol 1. Schwartz GR, Cayten CG, Mangelsen MA, et al (Eds). Philadelphia, Lea & Febiger, 1992, pp 3–41.
10. Safar P, Bircher N: Cardiopulmonary cerebral resuscitation: Basic and advanced life support. *In*: Principles and Practice of Emergency Medicine. 3rd ed. Vol 1. Schwartz GR, Cayten CG, Mangelsen MA, et al (Eds). Philadelphia, Lea & Febiger, 1992, pp 89–268.
11. Negovsky VA: Postresuscitation disease. Crit Care Med 1988; 16:942.
12. Eisenberg MS, Horwood BT, Cummins RO, et al: Cardiac arrest and resuscitation: A tale of 29 cities. Ann Emerg Med 1990; 19:179.
13. Brown CG, Paraskos JA (Eds): Proceedings of the 1992 National Conference on Cardiopulmonary Resuscitation and Emergency Cardiac Care. Ann Emerg Med 1993; 22:275.
14. Bircher NG: Physiology and pharmacology of standard cardiopulmonary resuscitation. *In*: Cardiopulmonary Resuscitation. Kaye W, Bircher NG (Eds). New York, Churchill Livingstone, 1989, pp 55–86.

15. von Planta M, Bar-Joseph G, Wiklund L, et al: Pathophysiologic and therapeutic implications of acid-base changes during CPR. Ann Emerg Med 1993; 22:404.
15a. Bircher NG, Vukmir RB, Safar P: Arrest interval and sodium bicarbonate influence end-tidal carbon dioxide during CPR in dogs. Anesthesiology 1993; 78:A293.
16. Safar P: Cerebral resuscitation after cardiac arrest. Research initiatives and future directions. Ann Emerg Med 1993; 22:324.
17. Safar P, Grenvik A, Abramson N, et al (Eds): International resuscitation research symposium on the reversibility of clinical death. Crit Care Med 1988; 16:919.
17a. Safar P, et al (eds): International Resuscitation Research Conference, May 1994, Pittsburgh, PA. In preparation for Crit Care Med, 1995.
18. Eisenberg M: Personal communication, 1992.
19. Krischer JP, Fine EG, Weisfeldt ML, et al: Comparison of prehospital conventional and simultaneous compression-ventilation cardiopulmonary resuscitation. Crit Care Med 1989; 17:1263.
19a. Halperin HR, Tsitlik JE, Gelfand M, et al: A preliminary study of cardiopulmonary bypass by circumferential compression of the chest with use of a pneumatic vest. N Engl J Med 1993; 329:762.
20. Sack JB, Kesselbrenner MB, Bregman D: Survival from in-hospital cardiac arrest with interposed abdominal counter pulsation during CPR. JAMA 1992; 267:379.
21. Cohen TJ, Tucker KJ, Lurie KG, et al: Active compression-decompression. A new method of cardiopulmonary resuscitation. JAMA 1992; 267:2916.
21a. Cohen TJ, Goldner BG, Maccaro PC, et al: A comparison of active compression-decompression cardiopulmonary resuscitation with standard cardiopulmonary resuscitation for cardiac arrests occurring in the hospital. N Engl J Med 1993; 329:1918.
21b. Schultz JJ, Coffeen P, Sweeney M, et al: Evaluation of standard and active compression-decompression CPR in an acute human model of ventricular fibrillation. Circulation 1994; 89:684.
21c. Lesser R, Bircher N, Safar P, et al: Sternal compression before ventilation in cardiopulmonary bypass. Prehosp Disaster Med 1985; 1:239.
22. Sterz F, Leonov Y, Safar P, et al: Hypertension with or without hemodilution after cardiac arrest in dogs. Stroke 1990; 21:1178.
23. Bircher N, Safar P: Open-chest CPR: An old method whose time has returned. Am J Emerg Med 1984; 2:568.
24. Safar P, Abramson NS, Angelos M, et al: Emergency cardiopulmonary bypass for resuscitation from prolonged cardiac arrest. Am J Emerg Med 1990; 8:55.
25. Brain Resuscitation Clinical Trial I Study Group, Abramson NS, Safar P, et al: Randomized clinical study of thiopental loading in comatose survivors of cardiac arrest. N Engl J Med 1986; 314:397.
26. Vaagenes P, Cantadore R, Safar P, et al: Amelioration of brain damage by lidoflazine after prolonged ventricular fibrillation cardiac arrest in dogs. Crit Care Med 1984; 12:846.
27. Brain Resuscitation Clinical Trial II Study Group, Abramson NS, Sutton-Tyrrell K, et al: A randomized clinical study of a calcium-entry blocker (lidoflazine) in the treatment of comatose survivors of cardiac arrest. N Engl J Med 1991; 324:1225.
28. Abramson NS, Kelsey SF, Safar P, et al: Simpson's paradox and clinical trials: What you find is not necessarily what you prove. Ann Emerg Med 1992; 21:1480.
29. Steen PA, Gisvold SE, Milde JH, et al: Nimodipine improves outcome when given after complete cerebral ischemia in primates. Anesthesiology 1984; 62:406.
30. Roine RO, Kaste M, Kinnamen A, et al: Nimodipine after resuscitation from out-of-hospital ventricular fibrillation: A placebo-controlled, double-blind randomized trial. JAMA 1990; 264:3171.
31. Forsman M, Aarseth HP, Nordby HK, et al: Effects of nimodipine on cerebral blood flow and cerebrospinal fluid pressure after cardiac arrest. Correlation with neurologic outcome. Anesth Analg 1989; 68:436.
32. Leonov Y, Sterz F, Safar P, et al: Mild cerebral hypothermia during and after cardiac arrest improves neurologic outcome in dogs. J Cereb Blood Flow Metab 1990; 10:57.
33. Sterz F, Safar P, Tisherman S, et al: Mild hypothermic cardiopulmonary resuscitation improves outcome after prolonged cardiac arrest in dogs. Crit Care Med 1991; 19:379.
34. Weinrauch V, Safar P, Tisherman S, et al: Beneficial effect of mild hypothermia and detrimental effect of deep hypothermia after cardiac arrest in dogs. Stroke 1992; 23:1454.
35. Kuboyama K, Safar P, Radovsky A, et al: Delay in cooling negates the beneficial effect of mild resuscitative cerebral hypothermia after cardiac arrest in dogs: A prospective, randomized, controlled study. Crit Care Med 1993; 21:1348.
36. Abramson NS: Resuscitation research: A clinical perspective. *In*: Critical Care. State of the Art. Carlson RW, Reines HD (Eds). Society of Critical Care Medicine, Anaheim, CA, 1992, pp 107–128.
37. Cummins R, Chamberlain D, Abramson NS, et al: Recommended guidelines for uniform reporting of data from out-of-hospital cardiac arrest: The Utstein style. Circulation 1991; 84:960.
38. Criley JM, Blaufuss AJ, Kissel GL, et al: Cough-induced cardiac compression: Self-administered form of cardiopulmonary bypass. JAMA 1976; 236:1246.
39. Mullie, A, Lust P, Pennickx J, et al: Open chest cardiopulmonary resuscitation in the prehospital environment (Abstract). Proceedings 9th World Congress of Anaesthesiologists, Washington, DC, May 1988, Vol 1. p A0317.
40. Lindner KH, Koster R: Vasopressor drugs during cardiopulmonary bypass. Resuscitation 1992; 24:147.
41. Brown CG, Martin D, Pepe P, et al: A comparison of standard-dose and high-dose epinephrine in cardiac arrest outside the hospital. N Engl J Med 1992; 327:1051.
42. Stiell IG, Hebert PC, Weitzman BN, et al: High-dose epinephrine in adult cardiac arrest. N Engl J Med 1992; 327:1045.
43. Callahan M, Madsen CD, Barton CW, et al: A randomized clinical trial of high-dose epinephrine and norepinephrine vs standard-dose epinephrine in prehospital cardiac arrest. JAMA 1992; 268:2667.
44. Schröeder R: Personal communication, 1991.
45. Safar P, Xiao F, Radovsky A, et al: Clinically feasible mild hypothermic combination treatments after cardiac arrest in dogs can improve or worsen neurologic outcome (Abstract). Proceedings of the 2nd CPR Congress of the European Resuscitation Council. Mainz, Germany, October 1994. In preparation for Resuscitation.

CHAPTER 5

Options for Augmenting the Efficacy of Closed-Chest Cardiopulmonary Resuscitation

Raúl J. Gazmuri, MD, PhD • Max Harry Weil, MD, PhD • Eric C. Rackow, MD

HISTORICAL PERSPECTIVE

The development of methods by which ventricular fibrillation could be reversed by external transthoracic countershock, systemic blood flow could be generated by external compression of the chest, and gas exchange could be sustained by mouth-to-mouth ventilation ushered in the era of modern closed-chest cardiopulmonary resuscitation (CPR). In a landmark study more than three decades ago, Jude and coworkers reported on the successful restoration of spontaneous circulation by the closed-chest method in 107 of 138 episodes of in-hospital cardiac arrest.[1] Closed-chest resuscitation became the method of choice for routine cardiac resuscitation in the hospital and confined the once popular open-chest direct cardiac compression to settings in which thoracotomy is readily available during surgical operations or when cardiac arrest occurs following traumatic injury to the chest. The techniques of precordial compression and mouth-to-mouth ventilation were then taught to medical personnel, paraprofessionals, and lay people and were rapidly implemented for the initial management of cardiac arrest. With the nationwide implementation of basic and advanced life support, priorities in the management of cardiac arrest were identified. The importance of early defibrillation was recognized because ventricular fibrillation is the primary cause of cardiac arrest in more than 80% of out-of-hospital victims and because survival with return to productive life is inversely related to the time elapsed between collapse and the beginning of the resuscitation effort.[2, 3]

Approximately 500,000 individuals suffer an episode of sudden cardiac death in the United States each year. It is estimated that fewer than 3% of these victims leave the hospital alive and return to productive lives. However, in selected communities (in the United States and abroad) that have remarkably efficient emergency medical systems, as many as 30% of victims of sudden cardiac death survive. Prompted in part by these encouraging experiences, the American Heart Association has introduced the concept of the "Chain of Survival." It emphasizes that survival is contingent on the rapidity and sequence with which the resuscitation interventions are delivered.[3] The Chain of Survival calls for (1) *early* activation of the emergency medical system; (2) *early* basic CPR, including precordial compression and artificial ventilation; (3) *early* defibrillation, ideally by the first responder; and (4) *early* advanced cardiac care, including tracheal intubation and medications. It is expected that such a tiered response would improve the dismal outcome of out-of-hospital cardiac arrest. The development of automated external defibrillation has facilitated early defibrillation by first responders, emergency medical technicians, and paramedical personnel. Implementation of strategies for early defibrillation in selected communities has strikingly increased the survival success from approximately 5% to 15%.

Despite the universal acceptance and implementation of modern CPR, the science of cardiac resuscitation is in its infancy. Research has developed slowly and has sprouted only within the past 5 to 10 years. New concepts have emerged, and interventions that were once routine, such as administration of alkalizing agents and calcium salts, have now been abandoned because of their unproven benefits and potential risks.[4] One of the most significant research accomplishments within the past decade is the recognition that re-establishment of myocardial blood flow above critical thresholds is crucial for successful resuscitation when initial defibrillation fails.[5–9] As a result, substantial research efforts now focus on options by which the hemodynamic efficacy of CPR may be increased by physical or pharmacologic interventions. Promising new methods have emerged. These include interposed abdominal compression,[10, 11] active compression-decompression,[12–14] circumferential chest compression,[15] and extracorporeal circulation utilizing peripheral vascular access.[16–20] Although no persuasive evidence yet exists to support that these new methods improve the long-term outcome after cardiac arrest, it is hoped that hemodynamically more effective techniques may expand the time window for successful cardiac and cerebral resuscitation.

MECHANISM OF BLOOD FLOW DURING PRECORDIAL COMPRESSION

The mechanism by which blood flow is generated during precordial compression is the subject of continuous debate. The pioneers of modern day CPR postulated in the early 1960s that blood flow resulted from direct compression of the heart between the sternum and the spine.[21] However, subsequent observations in dogs and in human patients challenged this concept.[22, 23] With each precordial compression, comparable increases in the pressures in the left and right sides of the heart occurred. It therefore seemed unlikely that direct compression of the heart was responsible for the flows generated. These observations were complemented by clinical observations made by Criley and coworkers in the mid-1970s on what they termed "cough-CPR."[24] When human patients developed ventricular fibrillation during cardiac catheterization, vigorous coughing promoted systemic blood flows that maintained mental alertness until restoration of spontaneous circulation by external defibrillation could be accomplished. The mechanism of cough-CPR was then investigated in dogs by Rosborough and associates.[25] Cough was emulated by rhythmic stimulations of the cervical vagosympathetic trunks synchronously with intermittent closure of the airway. Prominent increases in intrathoracic pressure were coincident with each cough. The mitral and aortic valves opened, and blood flowed from the pulmonary vasculature into the left ventricle and from the left ventricle into the aorta. These observations supported the theory that a generalized increase in intrathoracic pressure rather than selective compression of the heart is the mechanism of blood flow generation during precordial compression. The theory behind this mechanism, also referred to as the "thoracic pump" mechanism, postulates that chest compression generates global increases in intrathoracic pressure that are transmitted to intrathoracic vascular structures. The pulmonary vascular bed is then compressed and its blood ejected through the left side of the heart into the thoracic aorta and large arteries. The heart therefore acts as a passive conduit, and both mitral and aortic valves open during chest compression (Fig. 5–1). During chest relaxation, the thoracic reservoir is refilled with blood from extrathoracic veins. Retrograde flow into the systemic veins is largely prevented by the closure of venous valves located at the superior thoracic outlet and by dynamic compression of

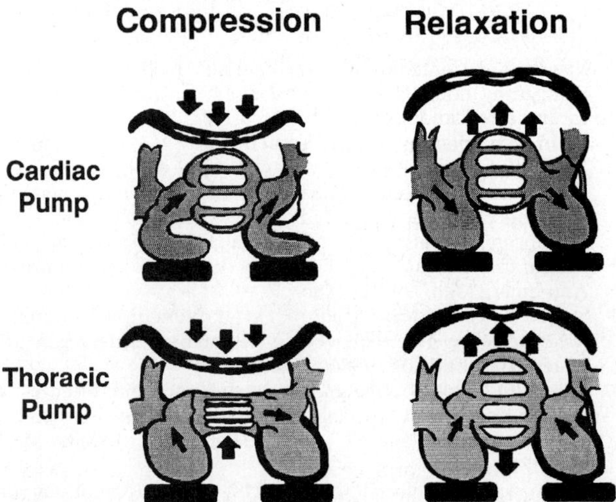

Figure 5–1. Proposed mechanisms of blood flow generation during precordial compression. According to the cardiac pump mechanisms, blood is ejected from the right ventricle into the pulmonary circuit and from the left ventricle into the systemic circuit by direct compression of the heart. Back flow is prevented by the closure of atrioventricular valves. The thoracic pump theory holds that a global increase in intrathoracic pressure propels blood from the pulmonary to the systemic circuit.

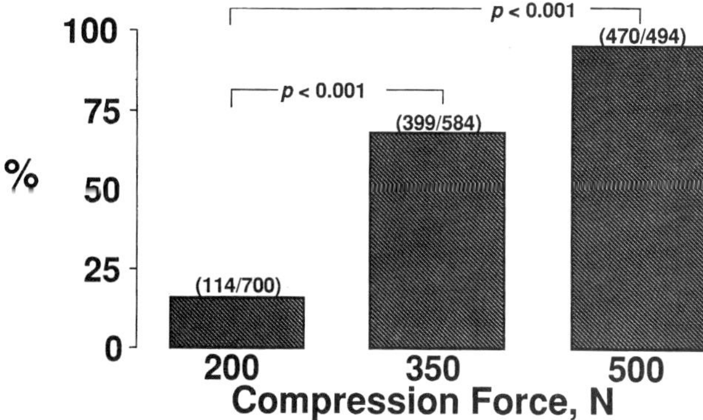

Figure 5–2. Echocardiographic assessment of mitral valve closure at increasing compression force (measured in newtons [N]) during closed-chest resuscitation in pigs (n = 7). Depth of compression was correspondingly increased to 15%, 20%, and 25% of the anteroposterior chest diameter. (Adapted from Hackl W, Simon P, Mauritz W, et al: Echocardiographic assessment of mitral valve function during mechanical cardiopulmonary resuscitation in pigs. Anesth Analg 1990; 70:350–356.)

the inferior vena cava at the inferior thoracic outlet.[26, 27] Early studies in human patients in whom transthoracic echocardiograms were obtained after prolonged unsuccessful closed-chest resuscitation failed to demonstrate changes in ventricular dimensions and closure of the mitral valve during precordial compression.[28, 29] These studies provided additional support to the notion that the heart was passive.

It is noteworthy, however, that the venous valve at the superior thoracic outlet operates not only when the intrathoracic pressure is globally increased but also when such is prevented by excision of the diaphragmatic domes so that the thoracic cavity is vented to the atmosphere during compression. The venous valve also operates when the heart is directly (manually) compressed.[30] Accordingly, valve function at the superior thoracic outlet does not secure that a thoracic pump mechanism operates. The thoracic pump mechanism has also been disputed on the basis of animal and human echocardiographic observations obtained after much shorter intervals of untreated cardiac arrest. In a porcine model of cardiac arrest, precordial compression was associated with decreases in left and right ventricular chamber dimensions, closure of the mitral valve, and opening of the aortic valve.[31] Injection of agitated saline solution containing microbubbles into the right and left ventricular cavities demonstrated forward blood flow across the pulmonic and aortic valves during precordial compression. In a subset of animals, however, in which precordial compression failed to restore spontaneous circulation, chamber deformation and valve function disappeared typically 5 minutes after start of precordial compression. This was attributed to progressive myocardial stiffness associated with myocardial ischemia.[32] Accordingly, it is likely that failure to observe decreased chamber dimensions and valve function in the early human reports represented "irreversible" failure of myocardial function. More recent echocardiographic studies in human patients also support the cardiac pump mechanism as the prevailing factor accounting for forward blood flow.[33–35] Redberg and coworkers[35] reported on successful transesophageal echocardiographic recordings in 18 patients obtained within 7 minutes after the start of precordial compression. In each instance, chest compression was associated with mitral valve closure and chest relaxation with mitral valve opening. Mitral valve closure was accompanied by reduction in left ventricular dimensions as previously demonstrated in animals. In a similar echocardiographic study in human patients, Porter and associates[34] reported mitral valve closure in 12 of 17 patients during precordial compression. Patients in whom the mitral valve remained opened during compression had more prolonged downtimes and were less likely to be resuscitated.

Closure of the mitral valve during compression requires that the ventricular pressure exceed the atrial pressure.[36] Such a ventriculoatrial pressure gradient is more likely to occur when the force of compression is directly transmitted to the heart; this gradient is likely to be attained at high force and velocity of compression[37] (Fig. 5–2). High-impulse compression favors closure of the mitral valve and, therefore, a cardiac pump mechanism. This contrasts with low-impulse compression, which typically favors a thoracic pump mechanisms.[36] Accordingly, the original concept proposed by Kouwenhoven and colleagues[1, 21] that forward blood flow is produced by direct cardiac compression has not been discarded. During clinical resuscitation, when the chest is compressed between 80 and 100 times per minute and force of approximately 500 N is applied, direct cardiac compression is the likely mechanism of blood flow.

DISTRIBUTION OF BLOOD FLOW DURING PRECORDIAL COMPRESSION

Precordial compression generates systemic blood flows that rarely exceed one fourth of normal flows. However, cardiac arrest and the low flow states that are produced by precordial compression trigger an intense and generalized neuroendocrine response that serves to redistribute the scant flow generated by external means toward the more vital coronary and cerebral circuits. Prominent increases occur in the levels of circulating catecholamines, cortisol, vasopressin, angiotensin II, and other stress response hormones.[38–40] Epinephrine and norepinephrine released into the systemic circulation activate vascular α_1-, α_2-, and β_2-adrenergic receptors. The α-vasoconstrictor actions of epinephrine and norepinephrine predominate. These actions, in conjunction with those of vasopressin and angiotensin II, promote peripheral vasoconstriction, which accounts for reduction of blood flow to the skin, skeletal muscle, splanchnic circulation, and kidneys.[41] The blood flow to the adrenal glands is remarkably preserved, especially in successfully resuscitated animals (Fig. 5–3). This may contribute to the increased levels of circulating catecholamines and cortisol that

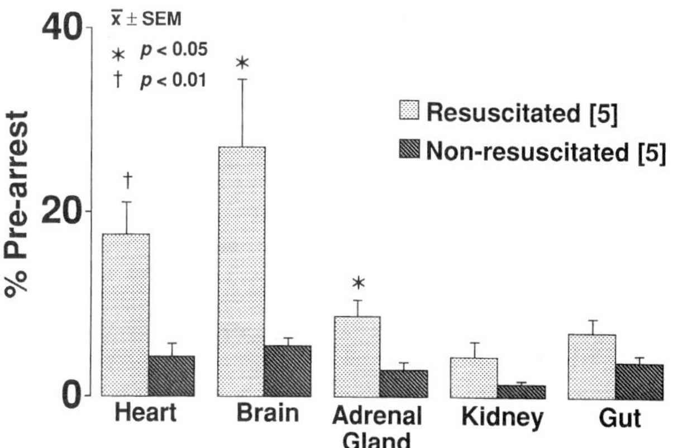

Figure 5–3. Organ blood flow measurements utilizing radioactive microspheres in a rodent model of cardiac arrest. Precordial compression was initiated 4 minutes after induction of ventricular fibrillation. Spontaneous circulation was successfully restored by external transthoracic countershock in 5 of 10 animals after 9 minutes of ventricular fibrillation. (Adapted from Duggal C, Weil MH, Gazmuri RJ, et al: Regional blood flow during closed-chest cardiac resuscitation in rats. J Appl Physiol 1993; 74:147–152.)

are characteristic of cardiac arrest. Peripheral vasoconstriction raises aortic pressure and favors perfusion to the more vital coronary and cerebral circuits.

Notwithstanding this prominent neuroendocrine response, the coronary blood flows generated by precordial compression rarely exceed 40% of normal.[42] This is insufficient to meet the oxygen requirements of the fibrillating heart, which are comparable to those of the normally beating heart. Consequently, myocardial ischemia with striking increases in myocardial tissue partial pressure of carbon dioxide (P_{CO_2}), lactate level, and hydrogen ion concentration invariably develops during cardiac arrest.[43]

Much greater cerebral blood flows are generated by precordial compression. It typically exceeds 50% but may exceed 90% when the resuscitation effort is initiated immediately after onset of cardiac arrest.[42, 44] Such levels exceed the critical threshold flow (16–18 mL $\cdot$ min^{-1} $\cdot$ 100 g^{-1}) required for neuronal function and cerebral viability.[45] The differences in flows between the heart and the brain are largely explained by the function of the venous valves at the superior thoracic inlet. The valves impede backflow into the cerebral circuit such that a pressure gradient across the cerebral circuit is maintained during both the compression and the relaxation phase. In contrast, the pressure gradient across the coronary circuit is restricted to the interval of chest relaxation, when the aortic pressure exceeds the pressures in the left ventricular cavity and in the right atrium. During chest compression, concurrent increases in the aortic, right atrial, and intramyocardial pressures preclude blood flow across the coronary circuit.[46]

IMPORTANCE OF MYOCARDIAL BLOOD FLOW

During cardiac arrest, myocardial ischemia prompts maximum coronary vasodilation such that myocardial blood flow becomes essentially pressure dependent. Even though the resistance across the coronary circuit may be increased by the mechanical effects of ventricular fibrillation and by the myocardial stiffness produced by ischemia, myocardial blood flow is remarkably well correlated with the pressure gradient between the aorta and the right atrium during the relaxation phase of precordial compression[47, 48] (Fig. 5–4). This pressure gradient across the coronary circuit is termed *coronary perfusion pressure* and has been identified as the single most important hemodynamic determinant of successful cardiac resuscitation. Coronary perfusion pressure thresholds highly predictive of successful restoration of spontaneous circulation have been identified both in animal models and in human victims of cardiac arrest. In a porcine model of ventricular fibrillation, increases in coronary perfusion pressure above 10 mm Hg by precordial compression prior to attempts at defibrillation were predictive of return of spontaneous circulation in more than 80% of the instances.[8] Coronary perfusion pressure thresholds of 20 mm Hg have been documented in rodent and canine models of cardiac arrest.[5, 7] These threshold levels specifically apply to settings in which CPR is initiated within less than 4 minutes of untreated cardiac arrest. After more prolonged intervals, substantially greater perfusion pressures are required for successful cardiac resuscitation.[49] In human patients, a coronary perfusion pressure of 15 mm Hg seems to be the minimum threshold for successful resuscitation.[6] Increases in coronary perfusion pressure above this critical threshold is associated with proportionate increases in the rate of return of spontaneous circulation. Resuscitation rates of greater than 70% when the coronary perfusion pressure generated by precordial compression exceeded 20 mm Hg were reported by Paradis and coworkers[6] (Fig. 5–5). Nevertheless, none of the successfully resuscitated patients survived long enough to be discharged alive from the hospital. Accordingly, the coronary perfusion pressure is not predictive of ultimate outcome. Multiple factors have been implicated, including the time interval between arrest and attempted resuscitation, the duration of the resuscitation effort, the underlying disease state, and the immediate precipitating event.

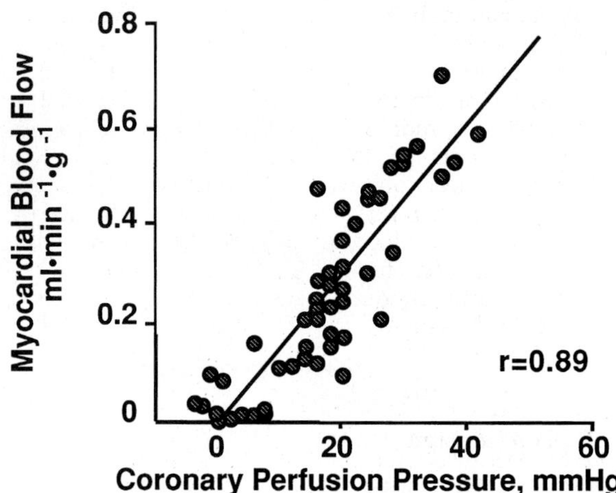

Figure 5–4. Myocardial blood flow, measured using radioactive microspheres, increases in linear relation to the coronary perfusion pressure in dogs. Coronary perfusion pressure corresponds to the pressure gradient between the aorta and the right atrium measured at mid-diastole. (Adapted from Ralston SH, Voorhees WD, Babbs CF: Intrapulmonary epinephrine during prolonged cardiopulmonary resuscitation: Improved regional blood flow and resuscitation in dogs. Ann Emerg Med 1984; 13:79–86.)

EFFICACY OF CONVENTIONAL CARDIOPULMONARY RESUSCITATION

Because the pressures and flows generated by precordial compression characteristically fail to fully meet the metabolic requirements of tissues, organ viability during precordial compression is maintained only for a brief interval. Close attention should therefore be paid to options that may

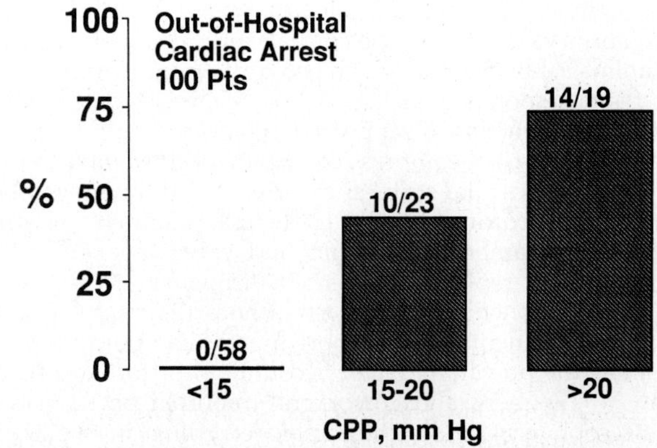

Figure 5–5. Coronary perfusion pressure (CPP) during closed-chest resuscitation in out-of-hospital victims of cardiac arrest. (Adapted from Paradis NA, Martin GB, Rivers EP, et al: Coronary perfusion pressure and the return of spontaneous circulation in human cardiopulmonary resuscitation. JAMA 1990; 263:1106–1113. Copyright 1990, American Medical Association.)

provide maximum hemodynamic effects. During chest compression, the site, depth (and force), rate, and duration of compression are the main determinants of the flows generated. Venous return to the thorax and preload of the arrested heart have more recently been recognized as important determinants of the forward blood flow that is generated by chest compression. In addition, the anatomic and physical characteristics of the chest wall, the adequacy of the intravascular blood volume, the state of the vascular capacitance and the changes in arterial resistance and venous compliance, although incompletely understood, also moderate the flows and pressures generated.

CHEST COMPRESSION

Site of Compression

In earlier American Heart Association Guidelines and Standards of CPR,[50] midsternal compression was recommended for infants and newborns based on studies in cadavers that indicated a more cephalic location of the heart within an infant's thorax. However, more recent radiographic studies in infants and young children have confirmed that the heart consistently lies under the lower third of the sternum.[51] This has practical implications for CPR. When midsternal compression was compared with compression of the lower third of the sternum in pediatric patients during cardiac arrest, the lower compression site yielded higher systolic and mean aortic pressures.[52] In adults, the site of compression initially proposed by Kouwenhoven and coworkers in 1960 is still deemed appropriate.[53] It is in the lower half of the sternum and conforms to the anatomic relationships between the ventricles and the thoracic structures.

Depth and Force of Compression

A minimum compression depth of approximately 2.5 cm must be exceeded before blood flow is generated. Thereafter, blood flow increases in direct proportion to the compression depth[54] (Fig. 5–6). In small dogs, Sanders and associates[55] observed increases in coronary perfusion pressure and end-tidal carbon dioxide pressure when the compression force was increased from 40 to 80 lb. In human patients, the coronary perfusion pressure correlates with the force of compression; however, substantial variability among individual patients does exist.[56] When excessive force is applied, the risk of injury to the rib cage and sternum is increased, with potential laceration of intrathoracic and intra-abdominal viscera. Disruption of the thoracic cage also limits elastic recoil which compromises re-expansion of the thoracic cavity and venous return of blood to the heart.

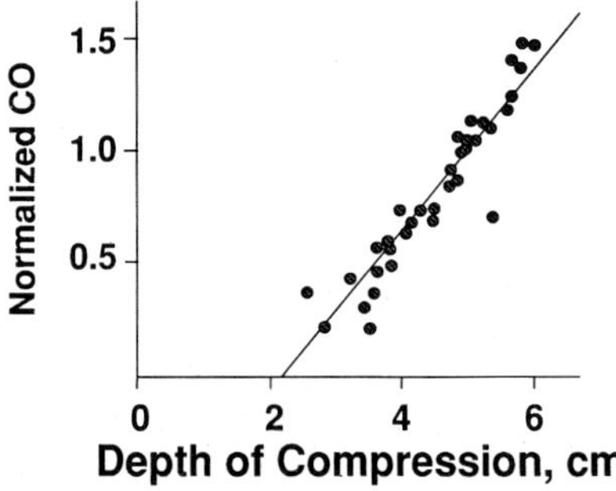

Figure 5–6. Blood flow generated as a function of depth of compression during closed-chest resuscitation in 8 dogs. Cardiac output (CO) is represented as a fraction of the cardiac output generated at a compression depth of 5 cm. (Adapted from Babbs CF, Voorhees WD, Fitzgerald KR, et al: Relation of blood pressure and flow during CPR to chest compression amplitude: Evidence for an effective compression threshold. Ann Emerg Med 1983; 12:527–532.)

Rate of Compression

When the compression rate is increased from 60 to 120 compressions per minute under experimental conditions, systemic and myocardial blood flow increase by approximately twofold.[47, 57, 58] The increases in compression rate do not appear to increase the risk of traumatic injuries to the chest. Experimentally, initial resuscitability, 24-hour survival, and neurologic recovery are increased by higher compression rates that do not exceed 150 compressions per minute. Excessively high compression rates shorten the diastolic interval and compromise both venous return and myocardial perfusion. In human patients, increases in the compression rate from 60 to 120 compressions per minute were associated with greater than 50% increases in coronary perfusion pressure.[56]

Duration of Compression

The optimal duration of compression appears to range from 40% to 50% of the compression-relaxation cycle. This is typically attained in patients during manual compression of the heart at a rate of 80 to 100 compressions per minute.

Traumatic Complications

The risk of potentially serious traumatic injuries to thoracic and abdominal structures during cardiac resuscitation ranges from 10% to 40%. At autopsy, approximately 30% of victims have rib fractures, and almost 20% have sternal fractures.[59, 60] In a minority, these account for mediastinal and pericardial hemorrhages or cardiac contusion, or both. Less frequent but potentially lethal complications include laceration of the atria, ventricles, or large vessels, lacerations of the liver and spleen, and gastroesophageal tears. These risks are increased when less experienced operators assume unconventional positions, compress at unconventional sites, or apply excessive force. The incidence of complications increases as the duration of the resuscitation procedure is increased, especially in elderly individuals.[60] Pulmonary edema has been reported in as many as 40% of successfully resuscitated patients; however, its mechanism is not well understood.[61]

LIMITATIONS OF CONVENTIONAL CARDIOPULMONARY RESUSCITATION

Notwithstanding its optimal deployment, the closed-chest method rarely secures more than one third of the normal systemic and myocardial blood flows. Moreover, the efficacy of precordial compression progressively diminishes as the duration of the resuscitation effort increases such that myocardial and cerebral blood flow are progressively lessened.[42] Previously cited was the role of ischemia in reducing myocardial compliance and, therefore, compressibility. Decreases in the hemodynamic efficacy of precordial compression has also been addressed; these decreases are explained, at least in part, by chest wall deformation and corresponding loss of elastic recoil. Impairment in venous return to the intrathoracic vascular structures is a consequence. The efficacy of precordial compression also decreases when intravascular volume is decreased or when vascular capacitance is increased. However, these are not likely to be of consequence in out-of-hospital cardiac arrest settings except after traumatic injuries. Finally, operator fatigue is also an important limitation of protracted precordial compression.[62] These issues are of practical importance if the time window of successful resuscitation and subsequent long-term survival are to be increased. Conventional closed-chest resuscitation has limited hemodynamic efficacy, and it is likely to be effective only in settings in which CPR is initiated after a brief interval of untreated cardiac arrest. After 30 minutes of unsuccessful resuscitation, no conventional CPR interventions are likely to be redeeming, except when cardiac arrest occurs in the unique setting of hypothermia.

ALTERNATIVE CLOSED-CHEST RESUSCITATION METHODS

During the past 20 years, investigators have searched for alternative methods that would enhance the myocardial and cerebral blood flows generated by external means. Early efforts were directed at options for augmenting the intrathoracic pressures generated during compression with the assumption that such would augment forward blood flow. These methods included compression against an occluded airway,[63, 64] simultaneous compression and ventilation,[65] continuous abdominal binding,[66] and a combination of these methods. Attempts to increase venous return were also made by the use of lower body pneumatic compressive garments,[67] and expansion of the intravascular volume by rapid fluid administration.[68] These techniques, however, failed to provide consistent increases in myocardial and cerebral flows. Disproportionate increases in central venous (and intracranial) pressures reduced the pressure gradient across the cerebral and coronary circuits. Currently, no survival advantage from these methods has been proven on the basis of experimental studies. Nonetheless, continuous research efforts, including refinement of these early techniques and introduction of new approaches, culminated with the development of more promising resuscitation methods. Encouraging clinical studies comparing these new methods with conventional CPR have appeared in the literature.

Interposed Abdominal Compression

Described in the early 1980s by Ralston and coworkers,[10] the interposed abdominal compression method involves midline compression of the abdomen at a site equidistant from the xiphoid process and the umbilicus. The abdomen is compressed at a pressure of 150 to 200 mm Hg during the relaxation phase of precordial compression.[11, 69] Implementation of interposed abdominal compression requires an additional rescuer who compresses the abdomen during the relaxation phase of precordial compression (Fig. 5–7). Interposed abdominal compression transfers venous blood from the vena cava and splanchnic circulation into the thorax. Compression of the aorta decreases the infradiaphragmatic aortic runoff. Accordingly, venous return to the heart and redistribution of arterial flow to structures above the diaphragm are improved. In dogs, interposed abdominal compression increased cardiac output and coronary perfusion pressure twofold, but without added risk of aspiration of gastric contents or major injury to intra-abdominal viscera.[70] In a randomized study involving 103 adult victims of in-hospital cardiac arrest, interposed abdominal compression significantly increased the rate of return of spontaneous circulation and the rate of survival to hospital discharge.[11] The results of this study, however, contrasted with the experience in victims of out-of-hospital cardiac arrest in whom interposed abdominal compression failed to improve the success of CPR.[69]

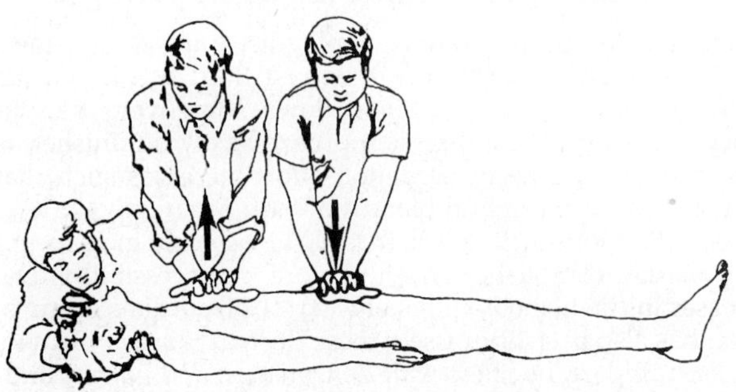

Figure 5–7. Artist's rendition of rescuers performing interposed abdominal compression. (Adapted from Ralston SH, Babbs CF, Niebauer MJ: Cardiopulmonary resuscitation with interposed abdominal compression in dogs. Anesth Analg 1982; 61:645–651.)

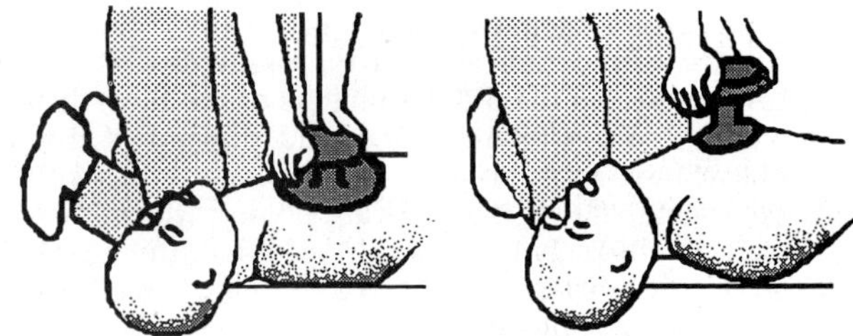

Figure 5–8. Active compression-decompression CPR.

Active Compression-Decompression

Re-expansion of the thoracic cavity during conventional closed-chest CPR is a passive event that relies on the elastic recoil of the chest. In 1992, Cohen and coworkers reported on the hemodynamic effects of active re-expansion of the thoracic cavity.[12, 71] Utilizing a hand-held suction device, the anterior chest wall was manually lifted during the relaxation phase of chest compression (Fig. 5–8). The technique was suggested by an anecdotal report of a successful cardiac resuscitation when a household drain plunger applied to the anterior chest wall was utilized. In preliminary studies in dogs, active compression-decompression significantly augmented cardiac output, systolic arterial pressure, and the coronary perfusion pressure when it was compared with conventional precordial compression and "passive decompression." Comparable observations of active compression-decompression in 10 adults demonstrated increases in forward blood flow, systolic arterial pressure, and diastolic filling time.[12] Based on echocardiographic observation of patients, significant increases in the left ventricular volume were observed at the end of active decompression without change in the ventricular volume at the end of compression.[72] Accordingly, active compression-decompression favors augmented venous return to the heart. Microsphere measurements demonstrate increases in cerebral and myocardial blood flows.[14] In randomized studies of 62 victims of in-hospital cardiac arrest, active compression-decompression significantly increased the success rate of initial resuscitation (62% vs. 30%) and 24-hour survival (45% vs. 9%). However, only 2 of 62 patients survived and were discharged alive from the hospital.[13] Both had undergone active compression-decompression. Additional studies in the setting of out-of-hospital cardiac arrest are anticipated.

Circumferential Chest Compression

Cyclic increases in intrathoracic pressure may generate forward blood flow during cardiac arrest. Early studies in dogs with simultaneous ventilation and compression had demonstrated improved carotid blood flow.[65] This, in part, provided the incentive for randomized studies on more than 900 patients with either conventional CPR or simultaneous ventilation and compression. The results were disappointing because both initial resuscitation and ultimate survival were not improved.[73] A vest device was then developed for circumferential compression of the chest (Fig. 5–9). In human patients, circumferential chest compression significantly increased the maximum aortic pressure and the coronary perfusion pressure.[15] A statistically insignificant increase in the success of initial resuscitation efforts (47% vs. 8%) and 24-hour survival (18% vs. 6%) was subsequently reported. Nevertheless, no patients survived hospitalization. Circumferential chest compression may still prove to be equally or more effective than precordial compression with less risk of injury to the rib cage and intrathoracic organs.

Extracorporeal Circulation

Although technically more demanding, extracorporeal circulation that utilizes peripheral vascular access is presently the hemodynamically most effective intervention for cardiac resuscitation.[16, 18, 20, 74] Normal systemic and organ blood flows may be sustained for prolonged intervals without the physical trauma and the progressive hemodynamic deterioration associated with conventional closed-chest methods. With the development of portable systems, preprimed circuits, and heparin-coated vascular interfaces, along with advances in procedures for rapid peripheral vascular catheterization, the method has become an attractive and increasingly popular option for emergent support of the failing or arrested heart. Experimentally, extracorporeal circulation is a strikingly effective option for restoration of spontaneous circulation.[16, 20, 74, 75] More than 90% of animals are typically resuscitated by extracorporeal circulation even after untreated intervals of cardiac arrest prolonged to 10 to 15 minutes. The experience in human patients is largely confined to the in-hospital setting and especially to the catheterization laboratory, coronary care units, and emergency departments.[17, 18] The cumulative experience with emergent extracorporeal support at 17 institutions in the United States was recently reported by the National Cardiopulmonary Support Registry.[20] Between 1984 and 1991, extracorporeal circulation was utilized for the management of cardiac arrest in 125 patients in whom conventional CPR had failed. Adequate hemodynamic support with a mean aortic pressure equal or greater than 60 mm Hg and a systemic blood flow equal or greater than 2 L/m² was achieved in more than 75% of the instances. Restoration of spontaneous circulation was accomplished in 25 patients (20%); 17 of these (14%) were alive after 30 days. Accordingly, a significant proportion of patients in whom conventional CPR had failed were successfully resuscitated by extracorporeal support. Approximately 75% of the survivors had undergone major diagnostic or therapeutic cardiopulmonary interventions during cardiopulmonary support. These included pulmonary and arterial angiography, angioplasty, and pulmonary embolectomy. Extracorporeal circulation therefore emerges as a highly effective clinical option for initial cardiac resuscitation for patients who do not respond to a brief trial of conventional resuscitation maneuvers. It also provides hemodynamic support for potentially lifesaving diagnostic and therapeutic procedures.

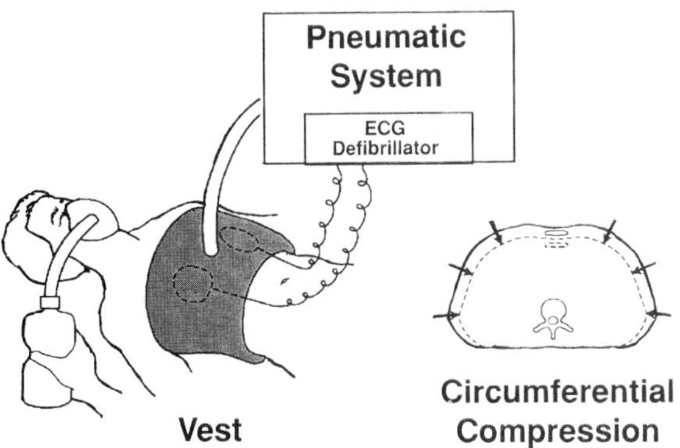

Figure 5–9. The pneumatic system directs compressed air into the vest. The vest is cyclically inflated 60 times per minute at a pressure of between 180 and 250 mm Hg. Inflation is maintained for 40% to 50% of each compression-decompression cycle. (Adapted from Halperin HR, Tsitlik JE, Gelfand M, et al: A preliminary study of cardiopulmonary resuscitation by circumferential compression of the chest with use of a pneumatic vest. N Engl J Med 1993; 329:762–768. Adapted, by permission, from the New England Journal of Medicine.)

The role of extracorporeal circulation for the routine management of cardiac arrest and especially for the victim of out-of-hospital sudden cardiac death remains to be defined. The widespread application of extracorporeal support is constrained by the availability of trained personnel, the cost of instrumentation, and the insecure proof of ultimate clinical benefit. However, it is likely that the use of hemodynamically more potent methods early in the course of the resuscitation effort will not only favor initial resuscitation but also favorably impact on long-term outcomes after successful resuscitation from cardiac arrest.

Pharmacologic Adjuncts

With respect to the vast resuscitation polypharmacy, only agents that prompt peripheral vasoconstriction and thereby enhance myocardial blood flow are of proved benefit for successful resuscitation.[14, 76, 77] Epinephrine has been the preferred agent for routine management. However, there is increasing evidence that its β-adrenergic action may be detrimental. The beta$_1$-agonist action increases myocardial oxygen demands during ventricular fibrillation such that it may exacerbate ischemic injury.[78] Its beta$_2$-agonist action has unfavorable effects on the distribution of pulmonary blood flow such that pulmonary exchange of carbon dioxide and oxygen is impared.[79] The beta$_2$-agonist action also competes with the peripheral vasoconstrictor actions of alpha$_1$- and alpha$_2$-agonists. These issues are likely to be of practical importance.

A controversy in which "low"-dose epinephrine is contrasted with "high"-dose epinephrine has emerged. Since three well-controlled clinical trials have recently failed to demonstrate improved resuscitation outcome when high-dose epinephrine was compared with conventional low-dose use, the routine use of doses that exceed 1 mg in the adult have been discouraged.[80–82]

Although more selective alpha agonists or nonadrenergic peripheral vasoconstrictor agents may emerge as more appropriate alternatives, their ultimate benefit remains to be proved in controlled clinical trials. Following successful cardiac resuscitation when systemic and myocardial blood flow has been restored, inotropic beta$_1$ stimulation may be appropriate for the management of postresuscitation myocardial dysfunction.

MONITORING THE RESUSCITATION EFFORT

Although significant advances in resuscitation research have been made, the clinical implementation of new concepts and techniques has been hampered by the lack of objective hemodynamic measurements with which the resuscitation procedure can be guided. Palpation of peripheral pulses lacks specificity and sensitivity with respect to the forward blood flow, the coronary perfusion pressure, and the likelihood of restoring spontaneous circulation. However, with the recent recognition that elimination of carbon dioxide is flow limited, the measurement of end-expiratory P_{CO_2} (P_{ETCO_2}) has emerged as a practical option for continuous hemodynamic monitoring during cardiac resuscitation.[9, 41, 55, 62, 83–87] P_{ETCO_2} correlates with the cardiac output and the coronary perfusion pressure generated by precordial compression. The vigor of manual chest compression may vary widely among rescuers and may progressively diminish as the rescuer becomes more fatigued. Rescuer fatigue has been anecdotally documented by Kalenda[62] with capnographic recordings of expired carbon dioxide tension during CPR in human patients. However, the greater problem of operator fatigue has not been extensively investigated. With new options for augmenting forward blood flow by interposed abdominal compression, active compression-decompression, and circumferential chest compression, P_{ETCO_2} may serve as a monitor and quantitative indicator for the assessment and titration of the hemodynamic effects of these new interventions.

P_{ETCO_2} also serves to prognosticate the likelihood that ongoing resuscitation maneuvers may restore spontaneous circulation.[85] Figure 5–10 demonstrates the relation between P_{ETCO_2} and the resuscitation outcome in human patients. When their P_{ETCO_2} exceeds 10 mm Hg, more than 50% of cardiac arrest victims are likely to be successfully resuscitated. To the contrary, when resuscitation efforts fail to produce increases in P_{ETCO_2} to levels exceeding 10 mm Hg, there is little likelihood that spontaneous circulation may be restored. Failure of conventional cardiac resuscitation methods may then call for more elaborate interventions and, in selected cases, invasive open-chest direct cardiac compression and extracorporeal circulation.

The return of spontaneous circulation is readily identified by an abrupt increase in P_{ETCO_2} to levels that transiently exceed normal values. Accordingly, the resuscitation procedure does not need to be interrupted for verification of the return of organized electrical activity and spontaneous pulsation.

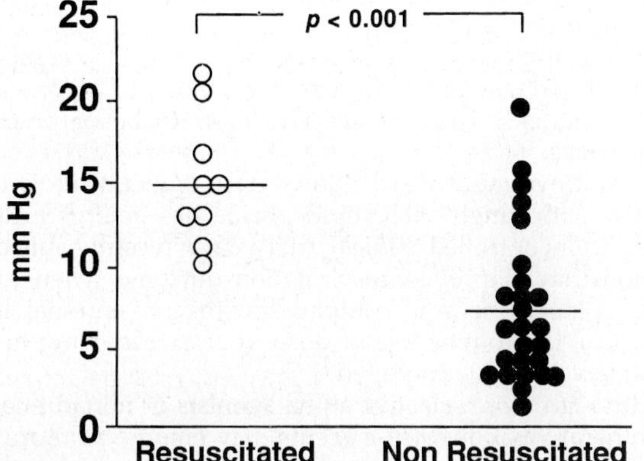

Figure 5–10. Mean P_{ETCO_2} during closed-chest resuscitation in 35 human victims of cardiac arrest. (Adapted from Sanders AB, Kern KB, Otto CW, et al: End-tidal carbon dioxide monitoring during cardiopulmonary resuscitation. JAMA 1989; 262:1347–1351. Copyright 1989, American Medical Association.)

References

1. Jude JR, Kouwenhoven WB, Knickerbocker GG: Cardiac arrest: Report of application of external cardiac massage on 118 patients. JAMA 1961; 178:1063–1070.
2. Weaver WD, Cobb LA, Hallstrom AP, et al: Factors influencing survival after out-of-hospital cardiac arrest. J Am Coll Cardiol 1986; 7:752–757.
3. Improving survival from sudden cardiac arrest: The "Chain of Survival" concept. Circulation 1991; 83:1832–1847.
4. Emergency Cardiac Care Committee and Subcommittees, American Heart Association: Guidelines for cardiopulmonary resuscitation and emergency cardiac care: Part III. Adult advanced cardiac life support. Cummins RO, Ornato JP, Thies WH (Writing group). JAMA 1992; 268:2199–2241.
5. Niemann JT, Criley JM, Rosborough JP, et al: Predictive indices of successful cardiac resuscitation after prolonged arrest and experimental cardiopulmonary resuscitation. Ann Emerg Med 1985; 14:521–528.
6. Paradis NA, Martin GB, Rivers EP, et al: Coronary perfusion pressure and the return of spontaneous circulation in human cardiopulmonary resuscitation. JAMA 1990; 263:1106–1113.
7. von Planta I, Weil MH, von Planta M, et al: Cardiopulmonary resuscitation in the rat. J Appl Physiol 1988; 65:2641–2647.
8. Gazmuri RJ, von Planta M, Weil MH, et al: Cardiac effects of carbon dioxide–consuming and carbon dioxide–generating buffers during cardiopulmonary resuscitation. J Am Coll Cardiol 1990; 15:482–490.
9. Gudipati CV, Weil MH, Bisera J, et al: Expired carbon dioxide: A noninvasive monitor of cardiopulmonary resuscitation. Circulation 1988; 77:234–239.
10. Ralston SH, Babbs CF, Niebauer MJ: Cardiopulmonary resuscitation with interposed abdominal compression in dogs. Anesth Analg 1982; 61:645–651.
11. Sack JB, Kesselbrenner MB, Bregman D: Survival from in-hospital cardiac arrest with interposed abdominal counterpulsation during cardiopulmonary resuscitation. JAMA 1992; 267:379–385.
12. Cohen TJ, Tucker KJ, Lurie KG, et al: Active compression-decompression: A new method of cardiopulmonary resuscitation. Cardiopulmonary Resuscitation Working Group. JAMA 1992; 267:2916–2923.
13. Cohen TJ, Goldner BG, Maccaro PC, et al: A comparison of active compression-decompression cardiopulmonary resuscitation with standard cardiopulmonary resuscitation for cardiac arrest occurring in the hospital. N Engl J Med 1993; 329:1918–1921.
14. Lindner KH, Pfenninger EG, Lurie KG, et al: Effects of active compression-decompression resuscitation on myocardial and cerebral blood flow in pigs. Circulation 1993; 88:1254–1263.
15. Halperin HR, Tsitlik JE, Gelfand M, et al: A preliminary study of cardiopulmonary resuscitation by circumferential compression of the chest with use of a pneumatic vest. N Engl J Med 1993; 329:762–768.
16. Levine LR, Gorayeb M, Safar P, et al: Cardiopulmonary bypass after cardiac arrest and prolonged closed-chest CPR in dogs. Ann Emerg Med 1987; 16:620–627.
17. Moore CH, Rubin JM, Schnitzler RN, et al: Experience and directions using cardiopulmonary support in fifty-three consecutive cases. ASAIO Trans 1991; 37:M340–M342.
18. Dembitsky WP, Moreno-Cabral RJ, Adamson RM, et al: Emergency resuscitation using portable extracorporeal membrane oxygenation. Ann Thorac Surg 1993; 55:304–309.
19. Sugimoto JT, Baird E, Bruner C: Percutaneous cardiopulmonary support in cardiac arrest. ASAIO Trans 1991; 37:M282–M283.
20. Hill JG, Bruhn PS, Cohen SE, et al: Emergent applications of cardiopulmonary support: A multiinstitutional experience. Ann Thorac Surg 1992; 54:699–704.
21. Kouwenhoven WB, Jude JR, Knickerbocker GG: Closed-chest cardiac massage. JAMA 1960; 173:1064–1067.
22. Weale FE, Rothwell-Jackson RL: The efficiency of cardiac massage. Lancet 1962; 1:990–992.

23. MacKenzie GJ, Taylor SH, McDonald AH, et al: Haemodynamic effects of external cardiac compression. Lancet 1964; i:1342–1345.
24. Criley JM, Blaufuss AH, Kissel GL: Cough-induced cardiac compression: Self-administered form of cardiopulmonary resuscitation. JAMA 1976; 236:1246–1250.
25. Rosborough JP, Hausknecht M, Niemann JT, et al: Cough supported circulation. Crit Care Med 1981; 9:371–372.
26. Niemann JT, Rosborough JP, Hausknecht M, et al: Pressure-synchronized cineangiography during experimental cardiopulmonary resuscitation. Circulation 1981; 64:985–991.
27. Fisher J, Vaghaiwalla F, Tsitlik JE, et al: Determinants and clinical significance of jugular venous valve competence. Circulation 1982; 65:188–196.
28. Rich S, Wix HL, Shapiro EP: Clinical assessment of heart chamber size and valve motion during cardiopulmonary resuscitation by two-dimensional echocardiography. Am Heart J 1981; 102:368–373.
29. Werner JA, Green HL, Janko CL, et al: Visualization of cardiac valve motion in man during external chest compression using two-dimensional echocardiography: Implications regarding the mechanism of blood flow. Circulation 1981; 63:1417–1421.
30. Gazmuri RJ, Weil MH, Tang WC, et al: Simultaneous aortic, jugular bulb, and right atrial pressures during cardiopulmonary resuscitation in humans (Letter). Circulation 1990; 81:1158–1159.
31. Deshmukh HG, Weil MH, Gudipati CV, et al: Mechanism of blood flow generated by precordial compression during CPR: I. Studies on closed chest precordial compression. Chest 1989; 95:1092–1099.
32. Hearse DJ, Garlick PB, Humphrey SM: Ischemic contraction of the myocardium: Mechanisms and prevention. Am J Cardiol 1977; 39:986–993.
33. Kühn C, Juchems R, Frese W: Evidence for the 'cardiac pump theory' in cardiopulmonary resuscitation in man by transesophageal echocardiography. Resuscitation 1991; 22:275–282.
34. Porter TR, Ornato JP, Guard CS, et al: Transesophageal echocardiography to assess mitral valve function and flow during cardiopulmonary resuscitation. Am J Cardiol 1992; 70:1056–1060.
35. Redberg RF, Tucker KJ, Cohen TJ, et al: Physiology of blood flow during cardiopulmonary resuscitation: A transesophageal echocardiographic study. Circulation 1993; 88:534–542.
36. Feneley MP, Maier GW, Gaynor JW, et al: Sequence of mitral valve motion and transmitral blood flow during manual cardiopulmonary resuscitation in dogs. Circulation 1987; 76:363–375.
37. Hackl W, Simon P, Mauritz W, et al: Echocardiographic assessment of mitral valve function during mechanical cardiopulmonary resuscitation in pigs. Anesth Analg 1990; 70:350–356.
38. Lindner KH, Strohmenger HU, Ensinger H, et al: Stress hormone response during and after cardiopulmonary resuscitation. Anesthesiology 1992; 77:662–668.
39. Prengel AW, Lindner KH, Ensinger H, et al: Plasma catecholamine concentrations after successful resuscitation in patients. Crit Care Med 1992; 20:609–614.
40. Woodhouse SP, Lewis-Driver D, Eller H: Catecholamines during cardiopulmonary resuscitation for cardiac arrest. Resuscitation 1992; 24:263–272.
41. Duggal C, Weil MH, Gazmuri RJ, et al: Regional blood flow during closed-chest cardiac resuscitation in rats. J Appl Physiol 1993; 74:147–152.
42. Schleien CL, Dean JM, Koehler RC, et al: Effect of epinephrine on cerebral and myocardial perfusion in an infant animal preparation of cardiopulmonary resuscitation. Circulation 1986; 73:809–817.
43. Kette F, Weil MH, Gazmuri RJ, et al: Intramyocardial hypercarbic acidosis during cardiac arrest and resuscitation. Crit Care Med 1993; 21:901–906.
44. Voorhees WD, Babbs CF, Tacker WAJ: Regional blood flow during cardiopulmonary resuscitation in dogs. Crit Care Med 1980; 8:134–136.
45. Sharbrough FW, Mersick JM, Sundt TM: Correlation of continuous electroencephalograms with cerebral blood flow measurements during carotid endarterectomy. Stroke 1973; 4:674–683.
46. Bellamy RF, DeGuzman LR, Pedersen DC: Coronary blood flow during cardiopulmonary resuscitation in swine. Circulation 1984; 69:174–180.
47. Wolfe JA, Maier GW, Newton JRJ, et al: Physiologic determinants of coronary blood flow during external cardiac massage. J Thorac Cardiovasc Surg 1988; 95:523–532.
48. Ralston SH, Voorhees WD, Babbs CF: Intrapulmonary epinephrine during prolonged cardiopulmonary resuscitation: Improved regional blood flow and resuscitation in dogs. Ann Emerg Med 1984; 13:79–86.
49. Gazmuri RJ, Weil MH, Terwilliger K, et al: Extracorporeal circulation as an alternative to open-chest cardiac compression for cardiac resuscitation. Chest 1992; 102:1846–1852.
50. Standards and guidelines for cardiopulmonary resuscitation (CPR) and emergency cardiac care (ECC). JAMA 1980; 244:453–509.
51. Phillips GWL, Zideman DA: Relation of infant heart to sternum: Its significance in cardiopulmonary resuscitation. Lancet 1986; i:1024–1025.
52. Orlowski JP: Optimum position for external cardiac compression in infants and young children. Ann Emerg Med 1986; 15:667–673.
53. Emergency Cardiac Care Committee and Subcommittees, American Heart Association: Guidelines for cardiopulmonary resuscitation and emergency cardiac care: Part II. Adult basic life support. JAMA 1992; 268:2184–2198.
54. Babbs CF, Voorhees WD, Fitzgerald KR, et al: Relation of blood pressure and flow during CPR to chest compression amplitude: Evidence for an effective compression threshold. Ann Emerg Med 1983; 12:527–532.
55. Sanders AB, Atlas M, Ewy GA, et al: Expired P_{CO_2} as an index of coronary perfusion pressure. Am J Emerg Med 1985; 3:147–149.
56. Swenson RD, Weaver WD, Niskanen RA, et al: Hemodynamics in humans during conventional and experimental methods of cardiopulmonary resuscitation. Circulation 1988; 78:630–639.
57. Maier GW, Tyson GS, Olsen CO, et al: The physiology of external cardiac massage: High impulse cardiopulmonary resuscitation. Circulation 1984; 70:86–101.
58. Feneley MP, Maier GW, Kern KB, et al: Influence of compression rate on initial success of resuscitation and 24-hour survival after prolonged manual cardiopulmonary resuscitation in dogs. Circulation 1988; 77:240–250.
59. Powner DJ, Holcombe PA, Mello LA: Cardiopulmonary resuscitation related injuries. Crit Care Med 1984; 12:54–55.
60. Krischer JP, Fine EG, Davis JH, et al: Complications of cardiac resuscitation. Chest 1987; 92:287–291.
61. Dohi S: Postcardiopulmonary resuscitation pulmonary edema. Crit Care Med 1983; 11:434–437.
62. Kalenda Z: The capnogram as a guide to the efficacy of cardiac massage. Resuscitation 1978; 6:259–263.
63. Rudikoff MT, Maughan WL, Effron M, et al: Mechanism of blood flow during cardiopulmonary resuscitation. Circulation 1980; 61:345–352.
64. Redding JS, Haynes RR, Thomas JD: "Old" and "new" CPR manually performed in dogs. Crit Care Med 1981; 9:386–387.
65. Chandra N, Weisfeldt ML, Tsitlik JE, et al: Augmentation of carotid flow during cardiopulmonary resuscitation by ventilation at high airway pressure simultaneous with chest compression. Am J Cardiol 1981; 48:1053–1063.
66. Niemann JT, Rosborough JP, Ung S, et al: Hemodynamic effects of continuous abdominal binding during cardiac arrest and resuscitation. Am J Cardiol 1984; 53:269–274.
67. Lee HR, Wilder RJ, Downs P, et al: MAST augmentation of external cardiac compression: Role of changing intrapleural pressure. Ann Emerg Med 1981; 10:560–565.
68. Ditchey RV, Lindenfeld J: Potential adverse effects of volume loading on perfusion of vital organs during closed-chest resuscitation. Circulation 1984; 69:181–189.
69. Mateer JR, Stueven HA, Thompson BM, et al: Interposed abdominal compression CPR versus standard CPR in prehospital cardiopulmonary arrest: Preliminary results. Ann Emerg Med 1984; 13:764–766.
70. Voorhees WD, Niebauer MJ, Babbs CF: Improved oxygen delivery during cardiopulmonary resuscitation with interposed abdominal compressions. Ann Emerg Med 1983; 12:128–135.
71. Cohen TJ, Tucker KJ, Redberg RF, et al: Active compression-decompression resuscitation: A novel method of cardiopulmonary resuscitation. Am Heart J 1992; 124:1145–1150.

72. Redberg RF, Tucker K, Schiller NB: Transesophageal echocardiography during cardiopulmonary resuscitation. Cardiol Clin 1993; 11:529–535.
73. Krischer JP, Fine EG, Weisfeldt ML, et al: Comparison of prehospital conventional and simultaneous compression-ventilation cardiopulmonary resuscitation. Crit Care Med 1989; 17:1263–1269.
74. Gazmuri RJ, Weil MH, von Planta M, et al: Cardiac resuscitation by extracorporeal circulation after failure of conventional CPR. J Lab Clin Med 1991; 118:65–73.
75. Safar P, Abramson NS, Angelos M, et al: Emergency cardiopulmonary bypass for resuscitation from prolonged cardiac arrest. Am J Emerg Med 1990; 8:55–67.
76. Brown CG, Birinyi F, Werman HA, et al: The comparative effects of epinephrine versus phenylephrine on regional cerebral blood flow during cardiopulmonary resuscitation. Resuscitation 1986; 14:171–183.
77. Little CM, Hobson JL, Brown CG: Angiotensin II effects in a swine model of cardiac arrest. Ann Emerg Med 1993; 22:244–247.
78. Ditchey RV, Lindenfeld J: Failure of epinephrine to improve the balance between myocardial oxygen supply and demand during closed-chest resuscitation in dogs. Circulation 1988; 78:382–389.
79. Tang W, Weil MH, Gazmuri RJ, et al: Pulmonary ventilation/perfusion defects induced by epinephrine during cardiopulmonary resuscitation. Circulation 1991; 84:2101–2107.
80. Callaham M, Madsen CD, Barton CW, et al: A randomized clinical trial of high-dose epinephrine and norepinephrine vs standard-dose epinephrine in prehospital cardiac arrest. JAMA 1992; 268:2667–2672.
81. Stiell IG, Herbert PC, Weitzman BN, et al: High-dose epinephrine in adult cardiac arrest. N Engl J Med 1992; 327:1045–1050.
82. Brown CG, Martin DR, Pepe PE, et al: A comparison of standard-dose and high-dose epinephrine in cardiac arrest outside the hospital. N Engl J Med 1992; 327:1051–1055.
83. Gazmuri RJ, Weil MH, Bisera J, et al: End-tidal carbon dioxide tension as a monitor of native blood flow during resuscitation by extracorporeal circulation. J Thorac Cardiovasc Surg 1991; 101:984–988.
84. Lewis LM, Stothert J, Standeven J, et al: Correlation of end-tidal CO_2 to cerebral perfusion during CPR. Ann Emerg Med 1992; 21:1131–1134.
85. Callaham M, Barton C: Prediction of outcome of cardiopulmonary resuscitation from end-tidal carbon dioxide concentration. Crit Care Med 1990; 18:358–362.
86. Sanders AB, Kern KB, Otto CW, et al: End-tidal carbon dioxide monitoring during cardiopulmonary resuscitation. JAMA 1989; 262:1347–1351.
87. Falk JL, Rackow EC, Weil MH: End-tidal carbon dioxide concentration during cardiopulmonary resuscitation. N Engl J Med 1988; 318:607–611.

CHAPTER 6

Resuscitation of the Newborn

George A. Gregory, MD

Birth is a time of marked physiologic transformation, as evidenced by the profound changes in the cardiovascular and respiratory systems. If these developments fail to occur, either death or survival with central nervous system (CNS) injury frequently ensues. This chapter describes the causes and effects of cardiorespiratory insufficiency at birth and discusses methods by which they can be corrected. It includes the recommendations of the American Heart Association where possible.

CARDIORESPIRATORY PHYSIOLOGY

The lungs evolve from the foregut of the fetus by the 14th day of gestation. By the 20th week, the airways are lined with cuboidal epithelium and the pulmonary capillaries are present. By 26 to 28 weeks, the capillaries are in contact with the developing terminal airways, and extrauterine life is possible for the first time in significant numbers of infants. By 30 to 32 weeks' gestation, the cuboidal epithelium is flattened and thinned, making gas transfer easier.

At 20 weeks' gestation, large quantities of surface active material are present within the alveolar lining (type II) cells.[1] By 28 to 32 weeks' gestation, some of this material is found on the surface lining of the distal airways. Surface active material is present in terminal airways after 34 to 38 weeks' gestation. Thyroxin, steroids, and catecholamines[1–4] release surface active material from type II cells in the fetus; at birth, breathing stimulates its release.[5]

Fetal airways contain approximately 30 mL/kg of plasma ultrafiltrate, which is continuously produced in the lungs and discharged into the mouth. Some of this fluid is swallowed; the remainder is expelled into the amniotic fluid.[6, 7] About 300 mL of lung fluid is produced each day.[8] Normally no amniotic fluid is present in lung fluid. With fetal gasping, however, 30 to 60 mL of amniotic fluid is drawn into the lungs, thereby contaminating the fetal lung fluid. Removal of lung fluid is initiated during labor,[9] continued during delivery, and completed after birth[10] (Fig. 6–1). Preterm and term neonates born by cesarean section, without a trial of labor, have more lung water and more difficulty adapting to extrauterine life than do term babies born vaginally.

Infants normally breathe within 30 seconds after birth and sustain respiration by 90 seconds afterward. The initial outward recoil of the chest at birth helps fill the lungs with air. Mild acidosis, hypercarbia, hypoxia, pain, cold, touch, noise, and umbilical cord clamping all stimulate breathing and sustain rhythmic respiration.[11, 12] Severe acidosis, hypoxia, CNS injury, and maternal use of drugs (such as narcotics, barbiturates, local anesthesia, magnesium, and alcohol) depress respiration.

The fetal circulation is in parallel; that of adults is in series[13, 14] (Fig. 6–2). The fetal right ventricle ejects two thirds of the combined ventricular output, and the left ventricle ejects one third.[15] This imbalance occurs because of intracardiac and extracardiac shunts (foramen ovale and ductus arteriosus). The foramen ovale allows oxygenated blood from the placenta to enter the left atrium. From there it enters the left ventricle and aorta. Poorly oxygenated blood from the superior vena cava enters the right atrium and right ventricle and is ejected into the pulmonary artery. Ninety per cent of pulmonary artery blood bypasses the lungs and joins descending aorta blood (via the ductus arteriosus).[15] The remaining 10% of the right ventricular output perfuses the fetal lungs.

Lung expansion, breathing, increased pH, and raised alveolar oxygen tensions decrease pulmonary vascular resistance (PVR) and increase pulmonary blood flow at birth.[6, 16] Hypoxia, acidosis, hypovolemia, hypoventilation, atelectasis, and a cold environment increase the PVR.[17, 18] Combined hypoxia and acidosis increase PVR more than either of these stimuli alone.

The decrease in PVR at birth reduces pulmonary arterial pressure and increases pulmonary blood flow. At the same time, systemic vascular resistance (SVR), arterial pressure, and cardiac output increase. The combination of reduced PVR and increased SVR reduces right-to-left shunting of blood through the ductus arteriosus. The increased pulmo-

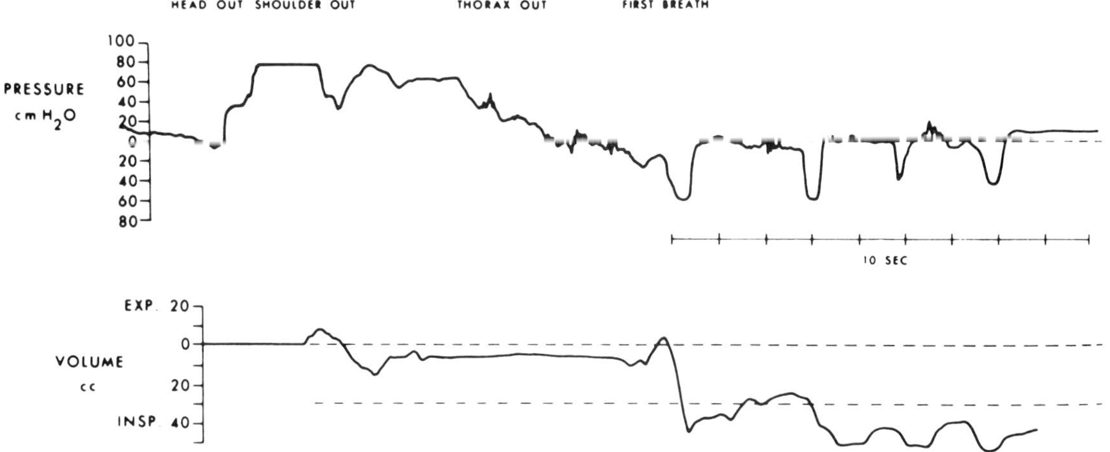

Figure 6–1. Intrathoracic pressures of the infant during delivery. Note the increased intrathoracic pressure when the mouth and head have been delivered. (Reproduced with permission from Gregory GA: Resuscitation of the newborn. Anesthesiology 1975; 43:225.)

nary blood flow augments blood return to the left atrium, thus raising left atrial pressure above right atrial pressure and closing the foramen ovale. Anatomic closure of the foramen ovale may not occur for months, if ever.

In full-term infants, the ductus arteriosus is closed by oxygen, acetylcholine, parasympathetic nerve stimulation, and prostaglandins.[19–21] A partial pressure of arterial oxygen (PaO_2) of 55 to 85 mm Hg (the PaO_2 of healthy, term infants) closes the ductus arteriosus of term lambs, whereas a PaO_2 of 300 to 500 mm Hg causes insignificant constriction of the ductus arteriosus in preterm lambs.[22] Complete closure of the ductus arteriosus may not occur for 10 to 14 days in term infants or for several months in preterm infants. Hypothermia, hypoxia, and acidosis may re-establish right-to-left shunting of blood through the ductus arteriosus during the first few weeks of life.

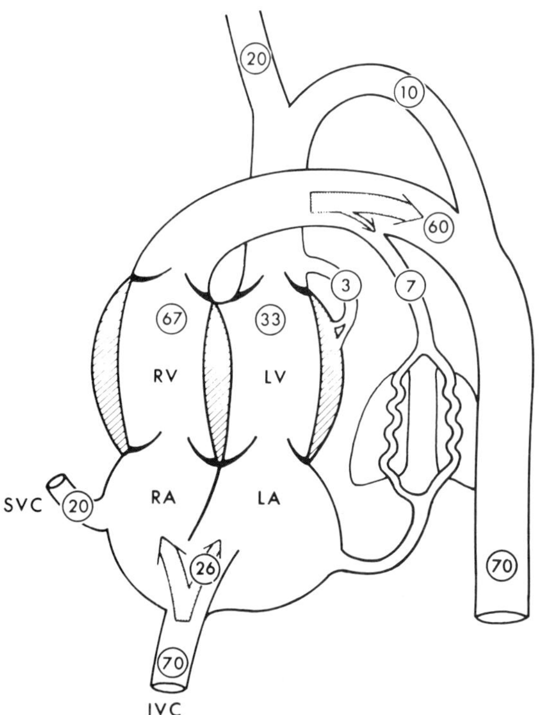

Figure 6–2. Diagram of the fetal circulation. The numbers within the circles are percentages of the combined ventricular output. (Reproduced with permission from Gregory GA: Resuscitation of the newborn. Anesthesiology 1975; 43:225.)

Asphyxia is common in fetuses and neonates. In fetuses, it is caused by maternal hypoxia (e.g., cyanotic congenital heart disease, congestive heart failure, or respiratory failure), reduced placental-umbilical blood flow (e.g., maternal hypotension, catecholamine secretion, or abruptio placentae), or placental diseases (e.g., calcification, infarction, or infection). In fetal asphyxia, the PaO_2 decreases from a normal of 25 to 40 mm Hg to less than 5 mm Hg in 2 minutes (Fig. 6–3) because the fetus's only oxygen store is in blood. The partial pressure of arterial carbon dioxide ($PaCO_2$) rises rapidly because carbon dioxide (CO_2) cannot be removed. In less than 5 minutes, combined metabolic and respiratory acidosis reduce the pH to 7.0 or less.[23]

In early asphyxia, cardiac output is normal but its distribution is altered.[24] Blood flow to the liver, kidneys, gut, muscle, and skin is reduced; flow to the heart, brain, adrenal glands, and placenta is maintained at prehypoxic levels or is increased.[25] This redistribution of blood flow helps maintain the oxygenation and nutrition of these vital organs. The heart rates of hypoxemic fetuses depend on stored energy reserves (glycogen) to sustain their function; when these stores are consumed, the myocardium fails and arterial pressure and cardiac output decrease. The pH is usually less than 7.0 at this point. Bradycardia (less than 100 beats per minute) severely reduces cardiac output. Central venous pressure increases as a result of both venous constriction and myocardial failure.

Intrapartum asphyxia may increase or decrease a neonate's blood volume,[26] but hypovolemia is more frequent and occurs in the presence of (1) partial occlusion of the umbilical vessels (such as the umbilical cord around the neck or umbilical cord compression); (2) hemorrhage from the fetoplacental unit (such as abruptio placentae or transection of the placenta during cesarean section); (3) maternal hypotension (such as shock, trauma, or anesthesia); or (4) asphyxia.

ASSESSMENT OF THE FETUS AT BIRTH

The Apgar score is still a useful guide to neonatal well-being and resuscitation.[27, 28] This system evaluates five variables (Table 6–1) at 1 and 5 minutes of age. If the Apgar score is 7 or less at 5 minutes of age, the score should be

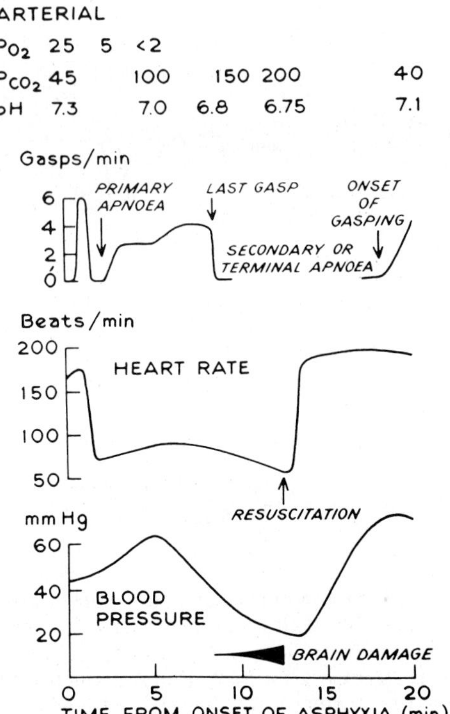

Figure 6–3. The response of newborn monkeys to asphyxia. (Reproduced with permission from Dawes GS: Foetal and Neonatal Physiology, Chicago, Year Book Medical Publishers, 1968.)

redetermined every 5 minutes for a total of 20 minutes. Each variable is given a score from 0 to 2, and the Apgar score at each time is the sum of these scores. The score at 1 minute was previously shown to correlate with both acidosis and survival,[29] but with better resuscitation, this no longer appears to be true. The 5-minute score may predict neurologic outcome.[30, 30a] To be of value, each Apgar variable must be evaluated at both 1 and 5 minutes of age. Resuscitation should start immediately if indicated by inadequate heart rate or respiration. It should not be delayed until the 1-minute Apgar score is obtained.

HEART RATE. The heart rate of healthy neonates is usually 120 to 160 beats per minute. A heart rate of less than 120 beats per minute reduces the cardiac output and tissue perfusion. A heart rate less than 100 beats per minute severely reduces cardiac output and requires treatment.

RESPIRATORY EFFORT. Healthy neonates breathe 30 to 60 times per minute and usually have no pause between inspiration and expiration, thus helping to maintain their functional residual capacity. Apnea occurs with severe acidosis, asphyxia, maternal use of drugs, infections (such as meningitis or septicemia), and CNS injury. Tachypnea (more than 60 breaths per minute) occurs with hypoxemia, hypovolemia, acidosis (metabolic and respiratory), CNS hemorrhage, pulmonary gas leaks, and pulmonary disease (e.g., hyaline membrane disease, aspiration syndromes, or infections).

MUSCLE TONE. Most infants are active at birth and respond to stimuli by moving their extremities. Asphyxia, maternal drugs, CNS injury, amyotonia congenita, and myasthenia gravis decrease a neonate's muscle tone. Flexion contractures, absent joint creases, or both suggest a lack of movement in utero and probable CNS injury.

REFLEX IRRITABILITY. Infants respond to having an extremity flicked by withdrawing the extremity and to insertion of a nasal catheter by grimacing or crying. Lack of response to these stimuli suggests the presence of hypoxia, acidosis, sedation by maternal drug use, CNS injury, or congenital muscle disease.

COLOR. All infants have a blue-tinged cast to their skin at birth. Sixty seconds later, most infants are entirely pink, except for their hands and feet. If central cyanosis is still present at 90 seconds of age, low cardiac output, methemoglobinemia, polycythemia, congenital heart disease, and pulmonary disorders (such as respiratory distress syndrome, airway obstruction, hypoplastic lungs, or diaphragmatic hernia) should be suspected—particularly if the neonate remains blue despite ventilation with oxygen.

Infants who are pale at birth are often asphyxiated, hypovolemic, acidotic, or anemic, or they have congenital heart disease; if heart disease is present, it is usually a left-sided obstructive lesion such as mitral atresia, aortic atresia, or coarctation or hypoplasia of the aorta. Infants who are entirely pink at birth may be intoxicated with alcohol or magnesium, or they may be alkalotic ($pH > 7.5$). Those who are ruborus are usually polycythemic.

RESUSCITATION EQUIPMENT

If neonatal resuscitation is to proceed smoothly, all delivery room personnel must know the location of the resuscitation equipment and be skilled in its use. The proper function and correct calibration of this equipment should be determined daily and just before each birth.

The resuscitation bed should allow positioning of an infant's head below the body, both to aid in the removal of lung fluid and to decrease aspiration of gastric contents. A servo-controlled infrared heater maintains a neonate's temperature between 36°C and 37°C. Two suction devices are needed, one to clear secretions from the mouth and airway of the neonate and the other to evacuate a pneumothorax should this become necessary.

TABLE 6–1. The Apgar Scoring System*

	Apgar Score		
Variable	*0*	*1*	*2*
Heart rate	Absent	Less than 100 bpm	More than 100 bpm
Respiratory effort	Absent	Slow, irregular	Good, crying
Color	Blue, pale	Body pink, extremities blue (acrocyanosis)	Completely pink
Reflex irritability (response to insertion of a nasal catheter)	Absent	Grimace	Cough, sneeze
Muscle tone	Limp	Some flexion of extremities	Active motion

*Each variable is evaluated individually and scored from 0 to 2 at both 1 and 5 minutes of age. The score at each time period is the sum of the scores of the individual variables. A score of 10 is perfect.

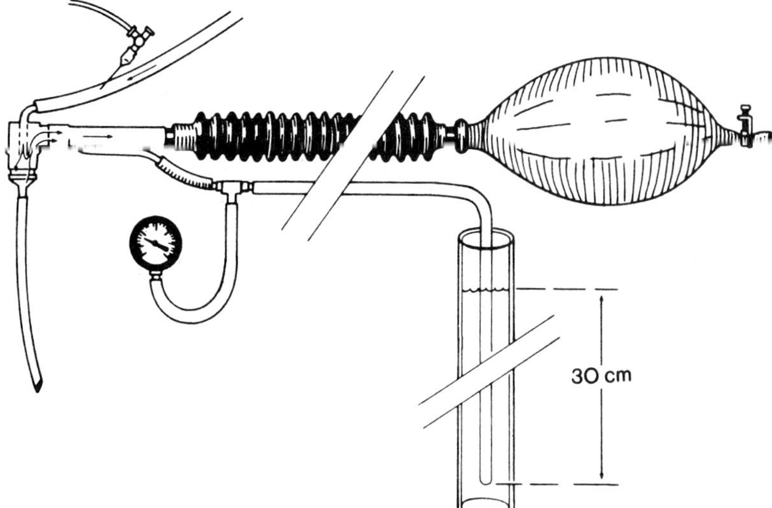

Figure 6–4. A modified Ayres T piece, which allows positive end-expiratory pressure and has a "pop-off" valve to reduce the likelihood of a pneumothorax. (From Gregory GA, Kitterman JA, Phibbs RH, et al: Treatment of the idiopathic respiratory-distress syndrome with continuous positive airway pressure. N Engl J Med 1971; 284:1333. Reproduced with permission from The New England Journal of Medicine.)

The equipment for tracheal intubation should include sizes 0 and 00 straight laryngoscope blades; a small laryngoscope handle; 2.5-, 3.0-, and 3.5-mm endotracheal tubes; and 5-, 6-, and 8-French suction catheters that easily pass through the endotracheal tubes. An extra light bulb and batteries for the laryngoscope should be stored in the delivery room.

The ventilation system should permit maintenance of positive end-expiratory pressure and allow ventilatory rates of 1 to 150 breaths per minute. This is most easily done with a modified Ayres T piece (Fig. 6–4). The ventilation system should not have one-way valves because they often stick, especially at high gas flows and high respiratory rates. If the valve sticks, it may not be possible for the neonate to exhale, in which case hypercarbia and a pneumothorax may develop.

Blood gas and pH determinations are required during resuscitation. Blood for these determinations is most easily obtained from an umbilical artery catheter. However, while the umbilical artery catheter is being inserted, a pulse oximeter should be applied to a finger or toe to guide oxygen therapy until the catheter is in place (Fig. 6–5).

The heart rate and electrocardiogram (needle electrodes) should be monitored continuously in sick neonates during resuscitation. Arterial and central venous pressures should also be monitored continuously when appropriate.

INITIAL EVALUATION

The inverted triangle published by the American Heart Association is a good guide to care needed in the delivery room (Fig. 6–6). Proceeding from top to bottom is a logical way to ensure that patients obtain the care needed. Someone besides the obstetrician (e.g., an anesthesiologist, pediatrician, or neonatologist) should evaluate and resuscitate the neonate at birth. If intrauterine asphyxia is diagnosed or strongly suspected (Table 6–2), at least two assistants are needed, one to aid ventilation and the other to insert an umbilical artery catheter and correct acid-base and blood volume abnormalities. A resuscitation plan should be developed before the infant's birth, if possible.

As an infant's head is delivered, the mouth and nose should be suctioned with a bulb syringe. Once delivered, the neonate should be held at the level of the introitus and dried with a towel to stimulate crying and reduce evaporative heat loss. If the neonate is held below the level of the introitus while the umbilical arteries are still pulsating, the blood volume is increased and he or she may develop polycythemia.[31–35] Polycythemia increases the incidence of high PVR, hypoxia, acidosis, and CNS injury. Raising the neonate above the level of the introitus, especially placing him or her on the mother's abdomen, may cause hypovolemia.

Once breathing is established and the umbilical cord stops pulsating, the cord should be clamped and cut and the neonate handed to the person responsible for resuscitation. Stripping blood from the umbilical cord to the neonate may increase blood volume,[36] respiratory rate,[37] lung water,[38] pulmonary artery pressure, and $Paco_2$,[39] whereas lung compliance, functional residual capacity, and Pao_2 may decrease.[37] Early cord clamping, on the other hand, may de-

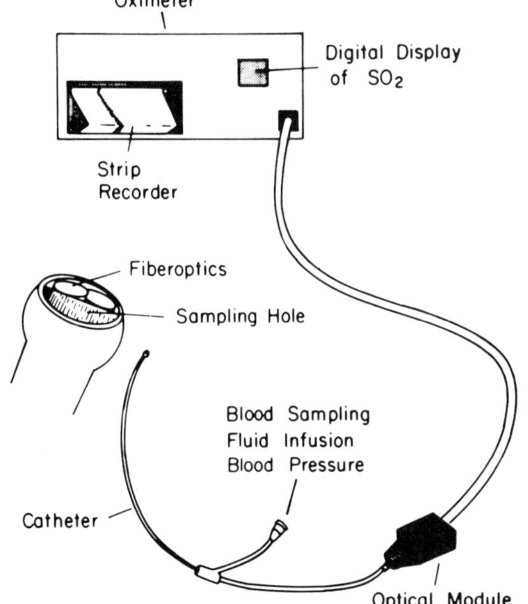

Figure 6–5. The oximetric system for measuring arterial oxygen saturation continuously. The catheter contains fiberoptics that transmit light to and from blood passing the catheter tip. (Reproduced with permission from Wilkinson AR, Phibbs RH, Gregory GA: Continuous measurement of oxygen saturation in sick newborn infants. J Pediatr 1978; 93:1016.)

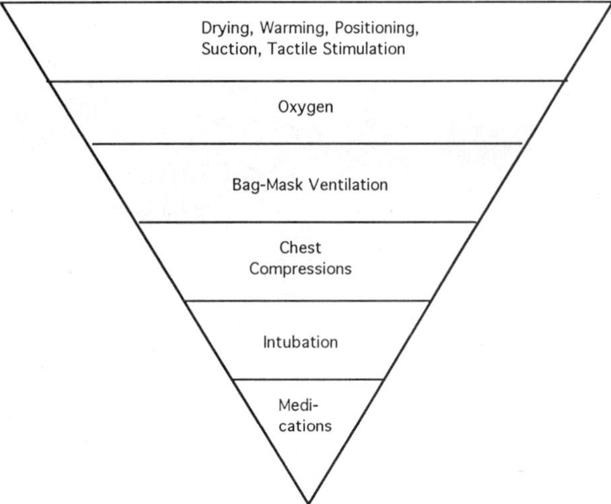

Figure 6–6. Inverted pyramid reflecting the approximate relative frequencies of neonatal resuscitative efforts. Note that a majority of infants respond to simple measures. (Reproduced with permission. Textbook of Pediatric Advanced Life Support, 1988, 1990. Copyright American Heart Association.)

prive the neonate of as much as 30 mL/kg of blood[40] (Fig. 6–7). However, if the neonate is asphyxiated (flaccid, pale, limp, or cyanotic), the umbilical cord should be clamped as soon as possible and the neonate handed to the resuscitator. *Remember that early cord clamping almost always causes hypovolemia.*

After the umbilical cord is cut, the neonate should be placed in a radiantly heated resuscitation bed. The airway should be cleared by gently suctioning the mouth and nose with a bulb syringe. Prolonged suctioning must be avoided because it can induce vomiting, hypoxia, and dysrhythmias (usually bradycardia).

If the respiratory pattern and color are normal at 1 minute of age (top level of triangle, Fig. 6–6), the only requirement is to dry the neonate, keep her or him warm, administer blow-by oxygen until the neonate is pink, and pass a suction catheter into the posterior pharynx through each nostril to rule out choanal atresia. The latter should be done early,

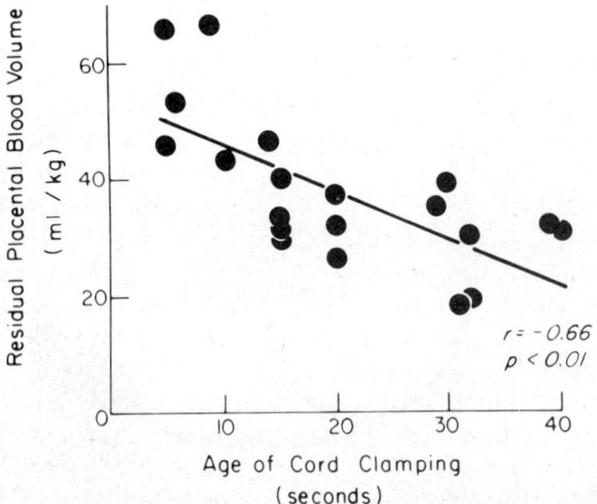

Figure 6–7. The effects of early and late cord clamping on placental blood volume. (Reproduced with permission from Ogata ES, Kitterman JA, Phibbs RH: The effect of time of cord clamping and maternal blood pressure on placental transfusion with cesarean section. Am J Obstet Gynecol 1977; 128:197.)

TABLE 6–2. Disorders Frequently Associated with Asphyxia at Birth

Maternal conditions
1. Older primigravida (older than 35 y)
2. Diabetes
3. Hypertension
4. Toxemia
5. Maternal treatment with any of the following:
   a. Glucocorticoids
   b. Diuretics
   c. Antimetabolites
   d. Reserpine, lithium
   e. Magnesium
   f. Ethyl alcohol
   g. β-Adrenergic drugs (to stop premature labor)
6. Abnormal estriol levels
7. Anemia (hemoglobin <10 g/dL)
8. Blood type or group isoimmunization
9. Previous birth of child with a hereditary disease
10. Current maternal infection or infection during pregnancy with rubella, herpes simplex, syphilis
11. Abruptio placentae
12. Placenta previa
13. Antepartum hemorrhage
14. History of birth of previous infant with jaundice, thrombocytopenia, cardiorespiratory distress, congenital anomalies
15. Narcotic, barbiturate, tranquilizer, or psychedelic drug use
16. Ethyl alcohol intoxication
17. History of previous neonatal death
18. Prolonged rupture of membranes

Conditions of labor and delivery
1. Forceps delivery other than low elective
2. Vacuum extraction delivery
3. Breech presentation and delivery or other abnormal presentation
4. Cesarean section
5. Prolonged labor
6. Prolapsed umbilical cord
7. Cephalopelvic disproportion
8. Maternal hypotension
9. Sedative or analgesic drugs given intravenously within 1 hour of delivery or intramuscularly within 2 hours of delivery

Fetal conditions
1. Multiple births
2. Polyhydramnios
3. Meconium-stained amniotic fluid
4. Abnormal heart rate or rhythm
5. Acidosis (fetal scalp capillary blood)
6. Decreased rate of growth (uterine size)
7. Premature delivery
8. Amniotic fluid surfactant test negative or intermediate within 24 hours of delivery

Neonatal conditions
1. Birth asphyxia
2. Birth weight (inappropriate for gestational age)
3. Meconium staining of the skin, nails, or umbilical cord
4. Signs of cardiorespiratory distress

because choanal atresia can be lethal. Once patency of the nares is ensured, the catheter should be passed through the mouth and advanced into the stomach. Failure of the catheter to enter the stomach suggests that the patient has esophageal atresia. If the catheter enters the stomach and more than 25 mL of fluid is removed, the patient may have a small bowel obstruction.

The 1-minute Apgar score reflects a neonate's condition at birth and may indicate the need for resuscitation. However, it is also important to carefully re-evaluate the Apgar score at 5 minutes of age; some infants who look well at 1 minute are sick by 5 minutes of age.

Most infants (90%) have a 1-minute Apgar score of 8 to 10 and require only nasal and oral suctioning, drying of the skin, and maintenance of a normal body temperature (top level of triangle). When stable, these infants can be wrapped in a warm blanket and handed to the parents.

Infants with 1-minute Apgar scores of 5 to 7 have suffered mild asphyxia just before birth (level 2 of triangle). They usually respond to vigorous stimulation during drying and to having oxygen blown over their face. If they respond slowly, a bag and mask can be used to ventilate their lungs with 80% to 100% oxygen. With appropriate care, such infants are usually well by 5 minutes of age. Blood gases measured at 2 minutes of age usually show a PaO_2 of 50 to 70 mm Hg; a $PaCO_2$ of 40 to 50 mm Hg; a pH of 7.15 to 7.25, and a base deficit of approximately 10 mEq/L. By 10 minutes of age, the pH and base deficit of these patients usually are normal and the $PaCO_2$ is less than 40 mm Hg.

Infants with Apgar scores of 3 to 4 at 1 minute of age are moderately depressed (level 3 of triangle). They are usually cyanotic and have poor respiratory efforts at birth. With bag-and-mask ventilation, their cardiac output improves and their skin becomes pink. If they have never breathed, it may be difficult to ventilate their lungs by bag and mask because their airway resistance exceeds that of the esophagus. In that case, gas preferentially enters the esophagus, stomach, and gut during bag-and-mask ventilation, further interfering with ventilation. Therefore, if a neonate has not breathed spontaneously, it is usually preferable to insert an endotracheal tube before assisting ventilation. Blood gas and pH measurements should be obtained from a doubly clamped segment of umbilical cord as soon as possible. If the pH is less than 7.2, blood gas and pH values should be obtained from a warmed heel or preferably from a radial or temporal artery. If the patient has a base deficit greater than 10, it may be necessary to administer sodium bicarbonate ($NaHCO_3$).

PULMONARY RESUSCITATION

Infants with an Apgar score of 2 or less are severely asphyxiated and require *immediate* resuscitation (levels 4–6 of triangle).

The trachea should be intubated immediately, and the lungs should be ventilated 30 to 60 times per minute with 80% to 100% oxygen and positive pressure. Every fifth breath should be held for 2 to 3 seconds to expand atelectatic lungs and remove lung fluid. Maintaining a positive end-expiratory pressure of 2 to 4 cm H_2O often improves oxygenation.

Tracheal Intubation

An infant's larynx is located more anteriorly than that of an adult. Extending the head displaces the infant's larynx even more anteriorly, making tracheal intubation more difficult. If the head is placed in a neutral or "sniffing" position (Fig. 6–8), the trachea is most easily visualized. The laryngoscope should be held with the thumb and index finger of the left hand while the chin is grasped with the ring and middle fingers. This fixes the head, hand, and laryngoscope into a single unit and reduces the incidence of pharyngeal trauma if the patient's head moves. The handle of the laryngoscope blade should be pulled up and out at 45°, and pressure should be applied over the hyoid bone with the small finger of the left hand. The latter moves the larynx posteriorly and improves one's view of the larynx. The endotracheal tube should then be inserted 1 to 2 cm below the vocal cords, depending on the infant's size. A small gas leak should be present between the tube and the trachea when 15 to 30 cm H_2O of pressure is generated. The appropriate size of endotracheal tube is usually 2.5 mm internal diameter for infants weighing less than 1.5 kg, 3.0 mm for 1.5- to 2.5-kg infants, and 3.5 mm for infants over 2.5 kg. If the endotracheal tube is the same width as the widest portion of the fingernail of the small finger, it fits the trachea appropriately more than 90% of the time.

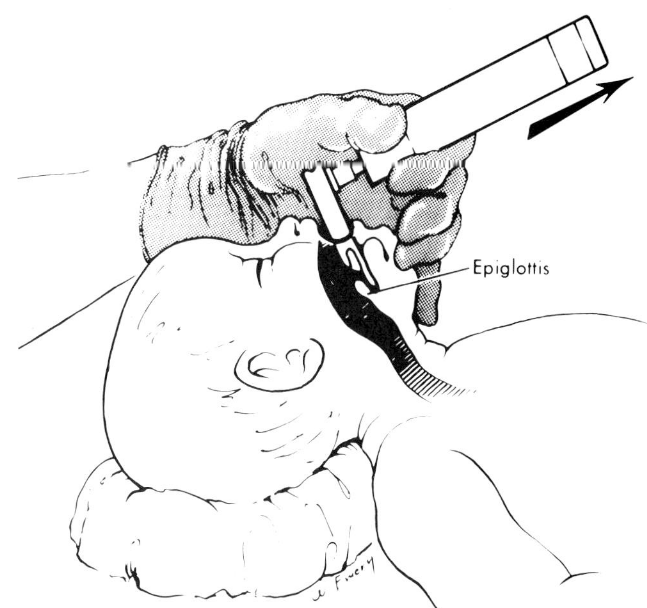

Figure 6–8. Laryngoscopy of the newborn infant. (Reproduced with permission from Gregory GA: Cardiopulmonary resuscitation of the newborn. *In* The Anesthesiologist, the Mother, and the Newborn. Baltimore, Williams & Wilkins, 1974, pp 200–209.)

The lungs should be expanded with an anesthesia bag, and the effects of ventilation should be closely monitored. If the PaO_2 rises above 80 mm Hg or the oxygen saturation exceeds 95%, the inspired oxygen concentration should be reduced in 5% to 10% decrements until the PaO_2 is 50 to 70 mm Hg or the oxygen saturation is 87% to 95%. This is especially important for preterm neonates, who may develop retrolental fibroplasia when the PaO_2 is 100 to 150 mm Hg for a few hours. An infant's heart rate should be monitored continuously during endotracheal intubation to detect dysrhythmias or bradycardia.

Adequacy of Ventilation

The adequacy of ventilation is best assessed by physical examination and blood gas determination. Both sides of the chest should rise equally and simultaneously with inspiration. If one side rises before the other, endobronchial intubation may have occurred or the neonate may have a pneumothorax or a congenital lung anomaly. Breath sounds are well transmitted in these small chests and may be normal despite the presence of atelectasis or a pneumothorax. The breath sounds should be heard over the stomach, but they should not be as loud as those heard over the chest. If they are as loud, determine whether esophageal intubation has occurred or whether the patient has a tracheoesophageal fistula. With adequate ventilation, cyanosis should disappear, the heart rate should rise to normal, and the patient should establish rhythmic breathing. Most asphyxiated infants have normal lungs; therefore, it is uncommon to require more than 25 cm H_2O of pressure to expand their lungs. *Excessive airway pressure is the major cause of pulmonary gas leaks during resuscitation.* Infants with stiff lungs (as found in erythroblastosis fetalis, congenital anomalies of the lung, or pulmonary edema) require high ventilation pressures and are prone to pulmonary gas leaks. If inadequate pressures are used to ventilate the lungs, however, hypoxia, acidosis, CNS injury, and death may occur. Therefore, sufficient pressure should be applied during inspiration to move the chest a normal amount. If pulmonary gas leaks occur, they should be drained with a thoracostomy tube.

Routine Tracheal Suctioning

Ten to 15% of women have meconium staining of their amniotic fluid. Sixty per cent of the infants born to these women have meconium in their trachea at birth.[41] After birth, breathing moves meconium into the periphery of the lungs, unless the meconium is removed before or immediately after the onset of breathing. Sixteen per cent of meconium-stained infants have some respiratory difficulties during the first few days of life. Ten per cent have a pneumothorax or pneumomediastinum on chest radiographs, but only one third of these have respiratory distress.

Because of the seriousness of the complications associated with meconium aspiration, thick particulate or "pea soup" meconium should be removed from the trachea as soon as possible after birth. Thin, watery meconium does not need to be removed. Meconium is most effectively removed by applying a suction device to the end of the endotracheal tube and applying negative pressure as the tube is withdrawn from the trachea. If the laryngoscope is kept in place as the endotracheal tube is removed, the endotracheal tube can be reinserted immediately if meconium is suctioned from the trachea. After suctioning twice, gently ventilate the lungs with oxygen. Absence of meconium in the mouth and posterior pharynx does not preclude its presence in the trachea.[41] Oxygen should be blown over the infant's face, and the heart rate should be monitored continuously during laryngoscopy and tracheal suctioning. Suctioning the stomach reduces the likelihood of regurgitation and aspiration of meconium at a later time. Meconium aspiration has been reviewed elsewhere.[42] Routine tracheal suctioning is also appropriate after severe vaginal bleeding.

VASCULAR RESUSCITATION

Vascular resuscitation is the least understood and least practiced area of neonate resuscitation. It is seldom mentioned in textbooks, despite the fact that hypovolemia is common in asphyxiated neonates at birth.

If the response to ventilation and tactile stimulation is not immediate, an umbilical artery catheter should be inserted to determine blood gas and pH values, measure arterial pressure, expand blood volume, and administer drugs. An umbilical venous catheter (with its tip is above the diaphragm) allows central venous pressure to be determined and to be used as an index of adequate volume replacement. The normal central venous pressure of neonates is 4 to 12 cm H_2O (discussed later).

CORRECTION OF ACIDOSIS

Respiratory acidosis is corrected by assisting ventilation. Metabolic acidosis is improved by correcting blood volume deficits and infusing $NaHCO_3$. However, $NaHCO_3$ administration is associated with several potentially serious problems: (1) $NaHCO_3$ is very hypertonic. Therefore, the likelihood of intracranial hemorrhage occurring in preterm neonates increases when $NaHCO_3$ is given rapidly and in large volumes. (2) The complete reaction of $NaHCO_3$ with hydrogen ions produces approximately 1250 mL of CO_2/50 mEq of $NaHCO_3$; some of this CO_2 is buffered. If ventilation is adequate, most of the CO_2 is immediately exhaled and the Pa_{CO_2} rises less than 4 mm Hg. On the other hand, if ventilation is inadequate (as it usually is in asphyxiated infants), the Pa_{CO_2} rises markedly and death may ensue. Hypercarbia dilates the cerebral vessels and increases cerebral blood flow, further increasing the likelihood of intracranial hemorrhage. To avoid these complications, $NaHCO_3$ should be given slowly (not faster than 1 $mEq \cdot kg^{-1} \cdot min^{-1}$) while the patient is artificially ventilated. (3) Administering $NaHCO_3$ also may induce hypotension (Fig. 6–9). (4) $NaHCO_3$ administration does not increase the intracellular acidosis of the neonatal brain.[43]

If the Apgar score is 2 or less at 2 minutes of age or 5 or less at 5 minutes, despite adequate ventilation and stimulation, a blood gas sample should be sent to the laboratory, and 2 to 3 mEq/kg of $NaHCO_3$ should be given while artificially ventilating the lungs. $NaHCO_3$ should not be infused into an umbilical venous catheter if the tip of the catheter is in the liver because doing so may cause hepatic necrosis. Blood gases and pH should be monitored after giving the drug. If the pH is 7.1 or less and the Pa_{CO_2} is less than 45 mm Hg, one fourth of the base deficit can be corrected with $NaHCO_3$. If the pH is greater than 7.1, ventilation of the

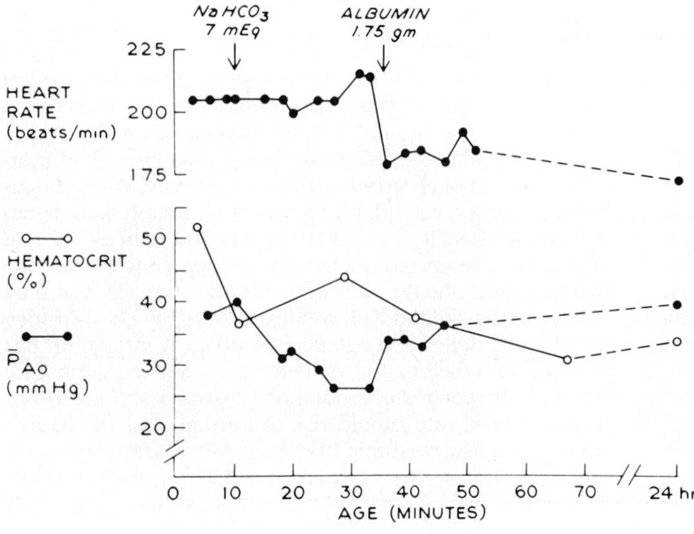

Figure 6–9. The effects of sodium bicarbonate on arterial blood pressure (PAO), heart rate and hematocrit (Hct). Note that hypotension occurred following the administration of $NaHCO_3$. The Hct decreased as fluid was pulled into the intravascular space to compensate for the hypovolemia that was present since birth. Raising pH decreased the peripheral vasoconstriction produced by the preexisting acidosis. Giving albumin increased the arterial pressure to normal. Based on the final Hct, the infant's initial blood volume was approximately 30% less than predicted. (Used with permission of Ross Products Division, Abbott Laboratories, Columbus, OH, from Report of the 59th Ross Conference on Pediatric Research, © 1969 Ross Products Division, Abbott Laboratories.)

neonate's lungs should be continued and another blood gas measurement should be obtained in 5 minutes. If the repeat blood gas determination does not show an increased pH, one fourth of the base deficit should be corrected with $NaHCO_3$ while continuing to ventilate the lungs.

Metabolic acidosis occurs when heart failure or hypovolemia reduces tissue perfusion. Raising the pH to 7.25 or greater usually improves cardiac output, increases liver perfusion, and decreases metabolic acid production (Fig. 6–10). If hypoglycemia is the cause of heart failure, the serum glucose level should be raised to 45 to 90 mg/dL by infusing 5 mL/kg of 10% dextrose solution over 3 to 5 minutes. This glucose bolus should be followed with continuous infusion of 10% glucose. Hyperglycemia should be avoided because it worsens neurologic outcome.[44–46] If the heart failure is due to congenital cardiac anomalies or hypoxic myocardial depression, the cardiac output should be increased by infusing isoproterenol (start with 0.05 $\mu g \cdot kg^{-1} \cdot min^{-1}$ and increase the dose as necessary). Isoproterenol usually raises the cardiac output, but the heart rate must be increased to 160 to 190 beats per minute. In rare instances (e.g., congenital heart block), it may be necessary to treat congenital bradycardia with a transvenous pacemaker immediately after birth. Dopamine may also improve cardiac output, but much larger doses may be required (5 to 100 $\mu g \cdot kg^{-1} \cdot min^{-1}$) to achieve normal blood pressure and normal perfusion for infants.[47] If the acidosis is due to hypovolemia, as it usually is, the blood volume should be increased.

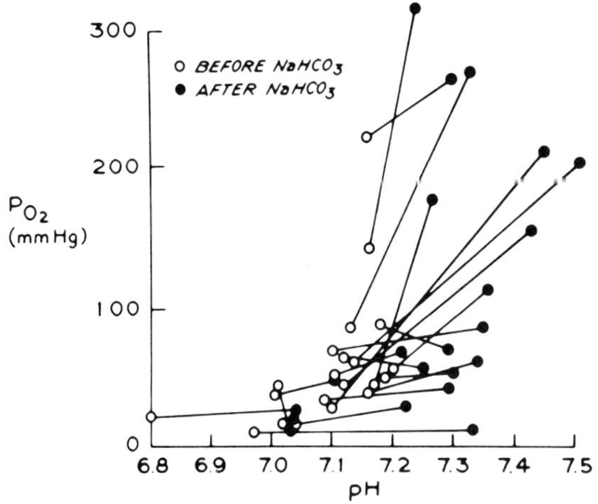

Figure 6–10. The effects of sodium bicarbonate infusion on Pa_{O_2} and pH when ventilation was held constant in asphyxiated infants. The Pa_{O_2} rose when the pH rose above 7.10 to 7.20. (Reproduced with permission from Gregory GA: Resuscitation of the newborn. Anesthesiology 1975; 43:225.)

CORRECTION OF HYPOVOLEMIA

Hypovolemia is detected by measuring arterial pressure and by physical examination. Approximately 60% of asphyxiated preterm infants are hypovolemic at birth, partly because of the appropriate early clamping of their umbilical cords (see Fig. 6–7).[40] Infants who have partial umbilical cord occlusion, abruptio placentae, or accidental placental transection during a cesarean section are usually hypovolemic.

Arterial blood pressure can be measured with a Doppler system or an indwelling arterial catheter and strain gauge.[48] During resuscitation, the latter is advantageous because arterial pressure is measured continuously. In the author's experience, the mean arterial pressure, which increases with increasing gestational age (Table 6–3), is more representative of a patient's condition than the systolic or diastolic pressure; if the systolic pressure decreases more than 5 mm Hg with each inspiration, the neonate may be hypovolemic.

Central venous pressure is also helpful in deciding whether a neonate is hypovolemic. This pressure is normally 4 to 12 cm H_2O at end-expiration. If it is less than 4 cm H_2O, hypovolemia should be suspected.

Hypovolemic infants are usually pale and have poor capillary filling and poor peripheral perfusion (Table 6–4). Their extremities are cold, and their pulses (especially the radial and posterior tibial) are weak or absent. Infants intoxicated with alcohol or magnesium are usually pink, peripherally dilated, hypotensive, and often acidotic.

The key to treating hypovolemia is intravascular volume expansion with blood, plasma, or crystalloid. If it is suspected that a neonate may be hypovolemic at birth, O-negative, low-titer blood should be crossmatched against the mother before birth; one unit of packed cells and one unit

TABLE 6–3. Average Systolic, Diastolic, and Mean Arterial Blood Pressures (mm Hg) During the First 12 Hours of Life in Normal Infants

	Hours											
	1	*2*	*3*	*4*	*5*	*6*	*7*	*8*	*9*	*10*	*11*	*12*
Body weight 1001–2000 g												
Systolic	49	49	51	52	53	52	52	52	51	51	49	50
Diastolic	26	27	28	29	31	31	31	31	31	30	29	30
Mean	35	36	37	39	40	40	39	39	38	37	37	38
Birth weight 2001–3000 g												
Systolic	59	57	60	60	61	58	64	60	63	61	60	59
Diastolic	32	32	32	32	33	34	37	34	38	35	35	35
Mean	43	41	43	43	44	43	45	43	44	44	43	42
Birth weight >3000 g												
Systolic	70	67	65	65	66	66	67	67	68	70	66	66
Diastolic	44	41	39	41	40	41	41	41	44	43	41	41
Mean	53	51	50	50	51	50	50	51	53	54	51	50

TABLE 6–4. Relationship of Skin Color, Capillary Refill Time, Pulse Volume, and Extremity Temperature to Hypovolemia

Amount of Volume Depletion	*Skin Color*	*Capillary Refill Time (s)*	*Posterior Tibial Pulse Volume*	*Skin Temperature*
None	Pink	<2	+ + + +	Warm
5%	Pale	3–4	+ +	Cold from midcalf and midforearm out
10%	Gray	4–5	0	Cold midthigh and upper arm out
15%	Mottled	>5	0	Entire extremity cold

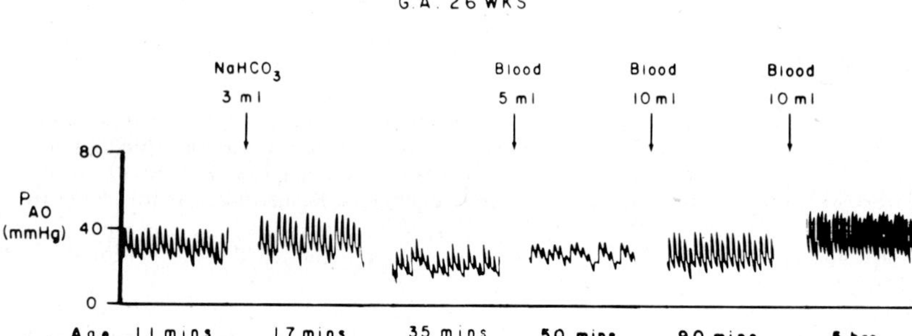

Figure 6–11. The effect of hypovolemia in a preterm infant. PAO equals mean arterial pressure. (Reproduced with permission from Gregory GA: Resuscitation of the newborn. Anesthesiology 1975; 43:225.)

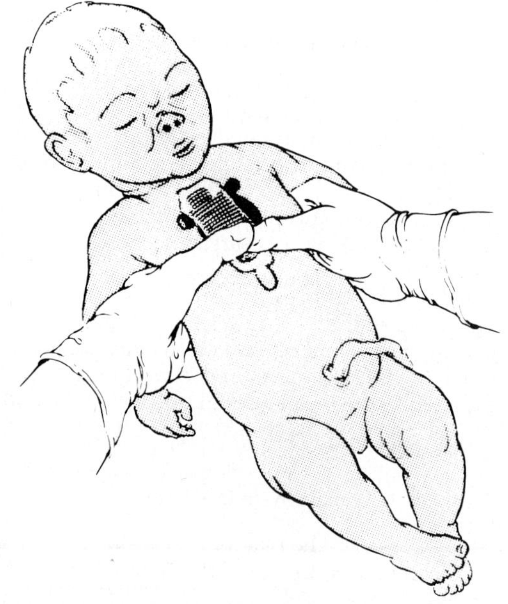

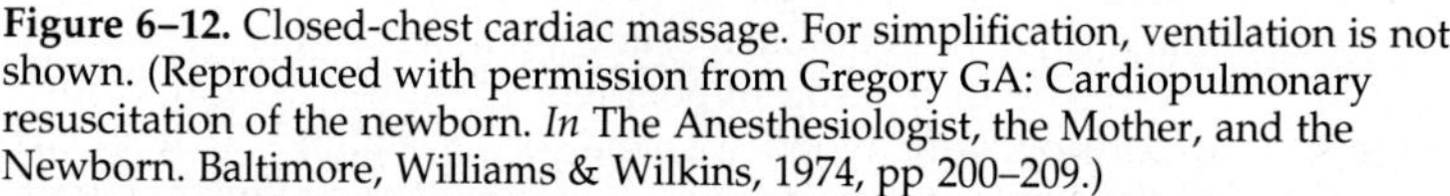

Figure 6–12. Closed-chest cardiac massage. For simplification, ventilation is not shown. (Reproduced with permission from Gregory GA: Cardiopulmonary resuscitation of the newborn. *In* The Anesthesiologist, the Mother, and the Newborn. Baltimore, Williams & Wilkins, 1974, pp 200–209.)

TABLE 6–5. Drugs Used During Resuscitation

Drug	*Indication*	*Dose**	*Route*	*Response*	*Complication*
Atropine	Bradycardia	0.03 mg/kg	IV	Increased heart rate	Marked tachycardia, diminished cardiac output
Calcium gluconate	Low cardiac output	100 mg/kg over 5–10 min (ECG monitoring)	IV	Improved cardiac output	Bradycardia, dysrhythmias
Epinephrine	"Flat line" ECG	0.1 mL/kg of a 1:10,000 solution	IV	"Flat line" ECG converted to some rhythmic response	Hypertension, ventricular fibrillation
Isoproterenol	Bradycardia, hypotension, low cardiac output	4 mg/250 mL 5% dextrose in water, until heart rate increases	IV	Increased heart rate, improved cardiac output	Dysrhythmias, low cardiac output if heart rate >180–200 bpm

*Doses given are starting doses and may have to be increased. Most drugs tend to be more effective when pH >7.15.
Abbreviations: ECG = electrocardiogram.

of whole blood should be brought to the delivery room in separate sealed plastic ice chests. If the blood is not used within 4 hours, it can be returned to the blood bank.

If crossmatched blood is unavailable, blood can be withdrawn sterilely from the umbilical placental arteries and veins into a syringe containing 1 to 2 units of heparin per milliliter of blood. After the blood is filtered, it can be given to the neonate. Placental blood vessels of asphyxiated babies frequently contain large amounts of blood.[40] Blood group incompatibility is not a concern because blood in the placental vessels belongs to the neonate; giving placental blood poses a small risk of infection, and it takes several minutes to obtain the blood. If blood is not available, give 1 to 2 g of 25% albumin per kilogram or 10 mL/kg of plasma or lactated Ringer's solution. The volume of fluid required to raise the blood pressure to normal may be enormous; at times it exceeds 50% of the blood volume (85 mL/kg) (Fig. 6–11), particularly if the placenta is abrupted or if it is transected during a cesarean section.

Overexpansion of the intravascular volume and hypertension should be avoided because asphyxiated infants are unable to autoregulate their cerebral circulation.[49–50a] Thus, overexpansion of the blood volume and hypertension increase the likelihood of an intracranial hemorrhage, especially in premature neonates.[51]

Pulmonary gas leaks or high airway pressures cause hypotension because they interfere with the venous return to the heart. Hypoglycemia, hypocalcemia, and hypomagnesemia also cause hypotension. Alcohol- and magnesium-induced hypotension usually respond to blood volume expansion. Hypermagnesemic neonates also may respond to an infusion of 100 to 200 mg of calcium gluconate.

Polycythemia (a hematocrit > 65%) occurs with delayed cord clamping, with holding the neonate below the introitus after birth, and with stripping the umbilical cord of blood. The hyperviscosity that accompanies polycythemia can reduce the pulmonary blood flow and increase the right-to-left shunting of blood through the ductus arteriosus and foramen ovale. When polycythemia is present, the hematocrit should be reduced to 50% to 55% by an exchange transfusion with plasma or albuminated saline (4 g albumin per 100 mL saline). The sequelae of polycythemia include cardiac and renal failure, as well as cerebral, intestinal, and renal vascular thrombosis.

CARDIAC MASSAGE

If the heart rate is less than 100 beats per minute and fails to increase when the patient is ventilated with 100% oxygen by bag and mask, the trachea should be intubated, the lungs ventilated with oxygen, and closed-chest massage begun. Both thumbs should be placed at the junction of the lower and middle third of the body of the sternum, with the fingers encircling the chest to support the back (Fig. 6–12). The sternum is compressed 1 to 2 cm or 0.5 to 0.75 in (approximately one third of the distance to the anterior vertebral column) at a rate of 100 to 150 times per minute. Ventilation of the lungs occurs 40 to 60 times per minute and is continuous during cardiac massage. The effectiveness of cardiac massage is best monitored by measuring the arterial pressure. If this is not available, the pupil size should be monitored. The pupils should be in the midposition or constricted. If they are dilated (and atropine has not been given), cerebral blood flow and oxygenation are inadequate.

Ideally, each chest compression should generate a systolic pressure of 80 mm Hg. This pressure, in conjunction with compression of about 120 times per minute, maintains diastolic pressure greater than 25 mm Hg, which is probably adequate for coronary perfusion.

All resuscitation drugs should be infused in the smallest volume possible to reduce the risk of hypervolemia (Table 6–5).[52] This means filling the dead space of the catheter and tubing with high drug concentrations, which may cause serious dysrhythmias or cardiac arrest if the drugs are flushed in rapidly. To avoid these complications, three times the volume of the catheter and stopcock should be withdrawn before injecting anything into the catheter. It is preferable to infuse vasoactive drugs into a separate intravenous line. Because acidosis decreases the effectiveness of resuscitation drugs, the pH should be raised above 7.2 as soon as possible.

References

1. Platzker ACG, Kitterman JA, Mescher EJ, et al: Surfactant in the lung and tracheal fluid of the fetal lamb and acceleration of its appearance by dexamethasone. Pediatrics 1971; 56:554.
2. Ballard PL: Hormones and lung maturation: Thyroid hormone effects and binding. *In*: Monographs on Endocrinology. Gross F, Grumbach MM, Labhart A (Eds). Heidelberg, Springer-Verlag, 1986, pp 197–230.
3. Platzker ACG, Kitterman JA, Clements JA, et al: Surfactant appearance and secretion in the fetal lamb lung in response to dexamethasone. Pediatr Res 1972; 6:406.
4. Lawson EW, Brown EB, et al: Influence of epinephrine on fetal pulmonary fluid release and surfactant production. Am Rev Respir Dis 1978; 118:1023.
5. Lawson EW, Birdwell RL, Huang PS, et al: Augmentation of pulmonary surfactant secretion by lung expansion at birth. Pediatr Res 1979; 13:611.
6. Adams FH, Moss AJ, Fagan L: The tracheal fluid of the foetal lamb. Biol Neonate 1963; 5:151.
7. Ross FB: Comparison of foetal pulmonary fluid with foetal plasma and amniotic fluid. Nature 1963; 199:1100.
8. Mescher EJ, Platzker ACG, Ballard PL, et al: Ontogenicity of tracheal fluid pulmonary surfactant and plasma corticoids in the fetal lamb. J Appl Physiol 1975; 39:1017.
9. Bland RD, McMillan DD, Bressack MA, et al: Clearance of liquid from lungs of newborn rabbits. J Appl Physiol 1980; 49:171.
10. Karlberg P: The adaptive changes in the immediate postnatal period, with particular reference to respiration. J Pediatr 1960; 56:585.
11. Chernick V, Fariday EE, Pagatakhan RD: Role of the peripheral and central chemoreceptors in the initiation of fetal respiration. J Appl Physiol 1975; 38:407.
12. Jansen AH, Chernick V: Site of chemosensitivity in fetal sheep. J Appl Physiol 1975; 39:1.
13. Dawes GS: Foetal and Neonatal Physiology. Chicago, Year Book Medical Publishers, 1968.
14. Rudolph AM, Heymann MA: Fetal and neonatal circulation and respiration. Annu Rev Physiol 1974; 36:187.
15. Rudolph AM: Congenital Diseases of the Heart. Chicago, Year Book Medical Publishers, 1974.
16. Rudolph AM, Yuen S: Response of the pulmonary vasculature to hypoxia and H+ ion concentration changes. J Clin Invest 1966; 45:399.
17. Cassen S, Dawes GS, Mott JC, et al: The vascular resistance of the foetal and newly ventilated lung of the lamb. J Physiol 1964; 171:61.
18. Brady JP, Rigatto H: Pulmonary capillary flow in infants. Circulation 1969; (Suppl III):50.
19. Asali NS, Morris JA, Smith RW, et al: Studies on ductus arteriosus circulation. Circ Res 1963; 13:478.
20. Heymann HS, Rudolph AM: Constriction of the ductus arteriosus by acetylcholine in premature infants. Circulation 1971; 43:11.
21. Evans N: Diagnosis of patent ductus arteriosus in the preterm newborn. Arch Dis Child 1993; 68:58.
22. McMurphy DM, Heymann HA, Rudolph AM, et al: Develop-

mental changes in constriction of the ductus arteriosus. Responses of oxygen to vasoactive agents in the isolated ductus arteriosus of the fetal lamb. Pediatr Res 1972; 6:231.
23. Dawes GS: Foetal and Neonatal Physiology. Chicago, Year Book Medical Publishers, 1968.
24. Behrman RE, Lees MH, Peterson EN, et al: Distribution of circulation in the normal and asphyxiated fetal primate. Am J Obstet Gynecol 1970; 108:956.
25. Biehl DR, Coté J, Wade JG, et al: Uptake of halothane by the foetal lamb *in utero*. Can Anaesth Soc J 1983; 30:24.
26. Yao AC, Lind J: Blood volume in the asphyxiated term neonate. Biol Neonate 1972; 21:199.
27. Apgar V: A proposal for a new method of evaluation of the newborn infant. Curr Res Anesth 1953; 32:260.
28. Apgar V, James LS: Further observations on the newborn scoring system. Am J Dis Child 1962; 104:419.
29. James LS, Weisbrot IM, Prince CE, et al: The acid-base status of human infants in relation to birth asphyxia and onset of respiration. J Pediatr 1958; 52:379.
30. Drage JS, Berendes H: Apgar scores and outcome of the newborn. Pediatr Clin North Am 1966; 13:635.
30a. Lam BC, Yeung CY: Perinatal features of birth asphyxia and neurologic outcome. Acta Paediatr Jpn 1992; 34:17.
31. Yao AC, Moinain H, Lind J: Distribution of blood between infant and placenta after birth. Lancet 1969; ii:871.
32. Black VD, Lubchenco LO, Koops BL, et al: Neonatal hyperviscosity: Randomized study of effect of partial plasma exchange transfusion on long-term outcome. Pediatrics 1985; 75:1048.
33. Van der Elst CW, Molteno CD, Molan AF, et al: The management of polycythemia in the newborn infant. Early Hum Dev 1980; 4:393.
34. Hart A, Ulrich M: Late prognosis in untreated neonatal polycythemia with minor or no symptoms. Acta Pediatr Scand 1982; 71:629.
35. Black VD, Lubchenco LO, Luckey DW, et al: Developmental and neurologic sequelae of neonatal hyperviscosity syndrome. Pediatrics 1982; 69:426.
36. Gunther H: The transfer of blood between baby and placenta in the minutes after birth. Lancet 1957; i:1277.
37. Oh W, Lind J, Gessner IH: The circulatory and respiratory adaptation to early and late cord clamping in newborn infants. Acta Pediatr Scand 1966; 55:17.
38. Cassidy G: Effect of caesarean section on neonatal body water spaces. N Engl J Med 1971; 285:887.
39. Oh W, Arcilla RA, Lind J, et al: Arterial blood gases and acid balance in the newborn infant. Effects of cord clamping at birth. Acta Pediatr Scand 1966; 55:593.
40. Ogata ES, Kitterman JA, Phibbs RH: The effect of time of cord clamping and maternal blood pressure on placental transfusion with cesarean section. Am J Obstet Gynecol 1977; 128:197.
41. Gregory GA, Gooding C, Phibbs RH, et al: Meconium aspiration in infants, a prospective study. J Pediatr 1974; 85:848.
42. Katz VL, Bowes WA Jr: Meconium aspiration syndrome: Reflections on a murky subject. Am J Obstet Gynecol 1992; 166:171.
43. Sessler D, Mills P, Gregory GA, et al: Effects of bicarbonate on arterial and brain intracellular pH in neonatal rabbits recovering from hypoxic lactic acidosis. J Pediatr 1987; 111:817–823.
44. Welsh FA, Sims RE, McKee AE: Effect of glucose on recovery of energy metabolism following hypoxia-oligemia in mouse brain: Dose-dependence and carbohydrate specificity. J Cereb Blood Flow Metab 1983; 3:486.
45. Gardiner M, Smith ML, Kagstrom E, et al: Influence of blood glucose concentration on brain lactate accumulation during severe hypoxia and subsequent recovery of brain energy metabolism. J Cereb Blood Flow Metab 1982; 2:429.
46. Ginsberg MD, Welsh FA, Budd WA: Deleterious effect of glucose pretreatment on recovery from diffuse cerebral ischemia in the cat. Stroke 1980; 11:347.
47. Perez CA, Reimer JM, Schreiber MD, et al: Effect of high dose dopamine on urine output in newborn infants. Crit Care Med 1986; 14:1045.
48. Versmold HT, Kitterman JA, Phibbs RH, et al: Aortic blood pressure during the last 12 hours of life in infants with birth weight 610–4,200 grams. Pediatrics 1981; 67:607.
49. Lou HC, Lassen NA, Friis-Hansen B: Impaired autoregulation of cerebral blood flow in the distressed newborn infant. J Pediatr 1979; 94:118.
50. Lou HC, Lassen NA, Friis-Hansen B: Is arterial hypertension crucial for the development of cerebral hemorrhage in premature infants? Lancet 1979; i:1215.
50a. Del TJ, Louis PT, Goddard FJ: Cerebrovascular regulation and neonatal brain injury. Pediatr Neurol 1991; 7:3.
51. Lou HC, Lassen NAS, Tweed WA, et al: Pressure passive cerebral blood flow and breakdown of the blood-brain barrier in experimental fetal asphyxia. Acta Pediatr Scand 1979; 68:57.
52. Burchfield DJ, Berkowitz ID, Berg RA, et al: Medications in neonatal resuscitation. Ann Emerg Med 1993; 22:435.

CHAPTER 7

Pediatric Resuscitation

Richard J. Melker, MD, PhD • David J. Burchfield, MD

Cardiopulmonary resuscitation (CPR) is most frequently performed on very old and very young patients. After the first 6 weeks of life and especially after the first year, CPR is rarely necessary in children because of the low incidence of critical illness in this age group. Pediatric CPR is primarily used either outside the hospital, in the emergency department after accidents, or in the intensive care unit on children with a wide variety of medical and surgical illnesses.

For adults, CPR is usually used in the setting of cardiac arrest. Circulatory arrest is rare in children; respiratory arrest is far more common. If assisted ventilation and external chest compression are used as temporizing measures while the underlying cause of the arrest is corrected, the outcome is more likely to be successful. Prolonged CPR is an ominous sign, especially when the cause of the arrest is either unrecognized or uncorrectable. This chapter briefly reviews the recently revised American Heart Association's (AHA) recommendations for performing CPR on children[1] and stresses areas of controversy in these recommendations. It also emphasizes recent studies that have elucidated differences between adults and children in the blood flow mechanism during CPR.

RECOMMENDATIONS FOR BASIC LIFE SUPPORT

A detailed description of the CPR technique in children has recently been updated.[1] In infants younger than 1 year, external chest compression is performed at a rate of at least 100 compressions per minute. Downward compression should last for 50% of each cycle; mouth-to-mouth ventilation with a tidal volume of 12 mL/kg is performed during a 1.0- to 1.5-second pause after every fifth compression. This results in approximately 15 breaths per minute and 80 compressions per minute. These recommendations were adopted in 1986 to reduce the likelihood of gastric insufflation during ventilation in a patient with an unprotected airway. By increasing inspiratory time, lower flow rates occur, resulting in lower intraoral pressure; if this pressure remains lower than the lower esophageal sphincter opening pressure, lung inflation rather than gastric insufflation is likely. The recommendation is the same for either one or two rescuers.

For children 1 to 8 years of age, external chest compression is performed at a rate of 100 compressions per minute, compression being maintained for 50% of each cycle. Ventilation with an inspiratory time of 1.0 to 1.5 second is given after every fifth compression, resulting in a rate of 15 breaths per minute; the technique is the same for one or two rescuers. For children older than 8 years, adult CPR techniques are recommended. For two rescuers, the compression rate has been increased to 80 to 100 per minute, with a 1.5- to 2.0-second pause for ventilation after every fifth compression.[2]

The AHA's 1986 standards for pediatric resuscitation[3] simplified the 1980 recommendations[4] in order to improve the lay public's retention of pediatric CPR skills. There have been only minor revisions from the 1986 guidelines in both pediatric and adult CPR recommendations and only where scientific evidence warranted. Particular emphasis is placed on the use of rescue breathing for respiratory arrest, because this is the most frequent and reversible cause of cardiac arrest in children.

CARDIOPULMONARY RESUSCITATION IN THE PEDIATRIC INTENSIVE CARE UNIT

The pediatric intensive care unit provides the most sophisticated environment available to care for critically ill children. Properly trained personnel and readily available equipment should optimize the performance and outcome of CPR. The most recent edition of the *Textbook of Advanced Cardiac Life Support* includes chapters dealing specifically with the resuscitation of infants and children; topics include airway control and ventilation, drug therapy, intravenous and intra-arterial techniques, and defibrillation.[5] In addition, the *Textbook of Pediatric Advanced Life Support*,[6] first published in 1988, provides detailed descriptions of all aspects of infant and child resuscitation. Clearly, the use of advanced life-support techniques by the pediatric critical care specialist should improve arrest outcome when compared with the use of basic life-support procedures alone.

Respiratory or cardiac arrest can result from myriad causes. Although CPR cannot completely restore perfusion to the brain and heart, it should allow additional time to correct any causes of reversible arrest.

Ventilatory failure per se is not difficult to treat; death due to uncomplicated reversible causes is now rare. Continuous positive airway pressure or positive pressure breathing with positive end-expiratory pressure can sustain oxygenation and ventilation for prolonged periods. In complicated cases, treatment of the underlying cause of respiratory failure determines the outcome. Maintenance of adequate perfusion during cardiac arrest is far more difficult than maintenance of ventilation after respiratory arrest. Further studies must be performed to define the ventilation and external chest compression variables and the sequencing of these procedures for children of different ages in order to understand how CPR can be optimized.

Data published since the previous edition of the *Textbook of Advanced Cardiac Life Support* provide further support for a different mechanism for blood flow in infants—and possibly small children—than in adults. Until quite recently, alternative techniques for optimizing blood flow have been based on experimental models that simulate adult human physiology. These CPR techniques are designed to maximize phasic changes in intrathoracic pressure and thus increase the extrathoracic pressure gradient between the carotid artery and the internal jugular vein.

Blood flow in adults is rarely the result of direct cardiac compression. Studies have shown that blood flow during CPR in a piglet model of blood flow in infants is most likely the result of direct cardiac compression and is thus similar to open-chest cardiac massage.[7, 8] Using standard CPR, cerebral and myocardial blood flows were 50% and 17% of prearrest levels, respectively, after 5 minutes, compared with less than 10% of prearrest levels in adult animals. Of equal importance, there was only a slight increase in intrathoracic vascular pressures when switching from conventional CPR to simultaneous compression-ventilation CPR (SCV-CPR). Although SCV-CPR improves cerebral blood flow when compared with conventional CPR in adult animal models,[9] piglet studies suggest that vascular pressures generated with conventional CPR are high, and changing to SCV-CPR provides little increase. Another study compared prolonged (50 min) conventional and SCV-CPR in a piglet model to test the hypothesis that SCV-CPR may be preferable by counteracting the progressive chest deformity seen in neonatal pigs.[10] The increasing deformity is accompanied by a sharp fall in aortic pressure and in cerebral and myocardial blood flow. This study found comparable myocardial and cerebral flows both initially and after prolonged CPR with either method. Thus, SCV-CPR appears to offer no advantages over conventional CPR in a neonatal model. As a child grows older and larger and the chest wall becomes less compliant, manipulating intrathoracic pressure should become more important. An intriguing new method of CPR has been described: active compression-decompression CPR (ACD-CPR). With this method, the chest is actively decompressed with a hand-held suction device after each compression. In a preliminary study using a model of endotracheally intubated but nonventilated adult dogs, ACD-CPR improved coronary perfusion pressure, systolic arterial pressure, cardiac output, and minute ventilation.[11] Additionally, in preliminary data in humans, ACD-CPR provided improved hemodynamic parameters when compared with conventional and mechanical "thumper" CPR.[12] Although no studies have yet been performed in children or in a pediatric animal model, the concept of re-expanding the chest wall with active decompression is compelling. Clearly, further study is warranted.

Although changes in CPR technique offer one strategy for improving blood flow during cardiac arrest, pharmacologic intervention also appears to have additive value. Studies have shown that epinephrine, through its α-adrenergic effects, improves cerebral and myocardial blood flow during both conventional and SCV-CPR in adult animal models.[13] Previous studies found the same salutary epinephrine effects in a piglet model.[7, 8] After epinephrine infusion, cerebral blood flow approximated prearrest blood flow, whereas myocardial blood flow increased to 37% of prearrest blood flow after 5 minutes of CPR. Both cerebral and myocardial blood flows remained elevated with epinephrine during prolonged CPR.

Epinephrine appears to exert its beneficial effects by preventing or reversing arterial collapse and by vasoconstricting peripheral vascular beds. Cerebral blood flow is increased by the selective redistribution of common carotid artery blood flow to the internal carotid artery, rather than by an increase in total carotid arterial blood flow. Myocardial blood flow is improved because epinephrine increases aortic diastolic pressure but does not alter right atrial diastolic pressure and, thus, increases coronary perfusion pressure.

In 1992, the AHA recommended an initial epinephrine dose of 0.02 mg/kg.[14] This dose is based on extrapolation of the adult-recommended dose of 0.5 to 1.0 mg, or 0.007 to 0.014 mg/kg in a 70-kg person. However, studies in animals have found that doses up to 10 times higher than that currently recommended appear to improve cerebral blood flow,[15] left ventricular output, and coronary pressure[16] and hasten return of spontaneous circulation[17] during ventricular fibrillation. Adults receiving CPR during ventricular fibrillation also show improved hemodynamics with higher than recommended doses of epinephrine.[18, 19] In recent reports, return of spontaneous circulation was induced in 8 of 20 pediatric patients with epinephrine doses of 0.2 mg/kg after standard doses failed, whereas none of the control group, who received 0.01 mg/kg epinephrine, had return of spontaneous circulation.[20, 21]

At present, SCV-CPR and other alternative CPR techniques must be viewed as experimental; they require further research before they can be used routinely in pediatric patients. The AHA has noted that CPR guidelines lag behind the most recent advances and therefore suggests that the ventilation and chest compression rates, as well as their sequencing, should be used at the discretion of the physician who is most aware of the patient's underlying conditions and cardiac arrest. In the pediatric ICU setting, the physician may elect to use alternative ventilation and compression sequences rather than those routinely recommended for use in advanced life-support settings outside the hospital.

The AHA has reaffirmed its 1986 indications for other drugs used during advanced life support for adults.[22] The pediatric standards for advanced life support reflect these recommendations. Specifically, it is recognized that sodium bicarbonate is overused during cardiac arrest, especially in brief episodes. Sodium bicarbonate use should be accompanied by blood gas measurements or the physician's knowledge of the patient's prearrest condition. The recommended initial dose is 1.0 mEq/kg, with subsequent doses of 0.5 mEq/kg every 10 minutes. The indications for calcium chloride remain unchanged, largely owing to mounting data that this agent is not of value during asystole or electromechanical dissociation. Additionally, calcium accumulates in the brain and myocardium and may have negative effects on outcome. Therefore, calcium chloride is only indicated in patients who are documented or suspected as being hypocalcemic but should be considered in the treatment of hyperkalemia, hypermagnesemia, and calcium channel blocker overdose. Isoproterenol is no longer considered an option.

References

1. American Heart Association: Guidelines for cardiopulmonary resuscitation and emergency cardiac care. Part V. Pediatric basic life support. JAMA 1992; 268:2251.
2. American Heart Association: Guidelines for cardiopulmonary resuscitation and emergency cardiac care. Part II. Adult basic life support. JAMA 1992; 268:2184.
3. American Heart Association: Guidelines for cardiopulmonary resuscitation and emergency cardiac care. Part IV. Pediatric basic life support. JAMA 1986; 255:2954.
4. American Heart Association: Guidelines for cardiopulmonary resuscitation and emergency cardiac care. Part III. Basic life support in infants and children. JAMA 1980; 244:468.
5. American Heart Association: Resuscitation of infants and children. *In:* Textbook of Advanced Cardiac Life Support. 2nd ed. Dallas, American Heart Association, 1990, p 257.
6. American Heart Association and American Academy of Pediatrics: Textbook of Pediatric Advanced Life Support. Dallas, American Heart Association, 1988.
7. Koehler RC, Michael JR, Guerci AD, et al: Beneficial effect of epinephrine infusion on cerebral and myocardial blood flows during CPR. Ann Emerg Med 1985; 14:8.
8. Schleien C, Dean J, Koehler R, et al: Effects of epinephrine on cerebral and myocardial perfusion in an infant preparation of cardiopulmonary resuscitation. Circulation 1986; 73:809.
9. Koehler RC, Chandra N, Guerci AD, et al: Augmentation of cerebral perfusion by simultaneous chest compression and lung inflation with abdominal binding after cardiac arrest in dogs. Circulation 1983; 67:266.
10. Berkowitz ID, Chantarojanasiri T, Koehler RC, et al: Blood flow during cardiopulmonary resuscitation with simultaneous compression and ventilation in infant pigs. Pediatr Res 1989; 26:558.
11. Cohen TJ, Tucker KJ, Redberg RF, et al: Active compression-decompression resuscitation: A novel method of cardiopulmonary resuscitation. Am Heart J 1992; 124:1145.
12. Cohen TJ, Tucker KJ, Lurie KG, et al: Active compression-decompression: A new method of cardiopulmonary resuscitation. JAMA 1992; 267:2916.
13. Michael JR, Guerci AD, Koehler RC, et al: Mechanisms by which epinephrine augments cerebral and myocardial perfusion during cardiopulmonary resuscitation in dogs. Circulation 1984; 69:822.
14. American Heart Association: Guidelines for cardiopulmonary resuscitation and emergency cardiac care. Part VI. Pediatric advanced life support. JAMA 1992; 268:2262.
15. Brown CG, Werman HA, Davis EA, et al: Comparative effect of graded doses of epinephrine on regional brain blood flow during CPR in a swine model. Ann Emerg Med 1986; 15:1138.
16. Linder KH, Ahnefeld RW, Bowdler IM: Comparison of different doses of epinephrine on myocardial perfusion and resuscitation success during cardiopulmonary resuscitation in a pig model. Am J Emerg Med 1991; 9:27.
17. Brunette DD, Jameson SJ: Comparison of standard versus high-dose epinephrine in the resuscitation of cardiac arrest in dogs. Ann Emerg Med 1990; 19:8.
18. Gonzalez ER, Ornato JP, Garnett AR, et al: Dose-dependent vasopressor response to epinephrine during CPR in human beings. Ann Emerg Med 1989; 18:920.
19. Paradis NA, Martin GB, Rosenberg J, et al: The effect of standard and high-dose epinephrine on coronary perfusion pressure during prolonged cardiopulmonary resuscitation. JAMA 1991; 265:1139.
20. Goetting MG, Paradis NA: High-dose epinephrine in refractory pediatric cardiac arrest. Crit Care Med 1989; 17:1258.
21. Goetting MG, Paradis NA: High-dose epinephrine improves outcome from pediatric cardiac arrest. Ann Emerg Med 1991; 20:22.
22. American Heart Association: Standards and guidelines for cardiopulmonary resuscitation and emergency cardiac care. Part V. Pediatric advanced life support. JAMA 1986; 255:2961.

CHAPTER 8

Critical Care Medicine and the Obstetric Patient

Gary D. V. Hankins, MD • William H. Barth, Jr., MD • Andrew J. Satin, MD

Women who are pregnant or who have recently been delivered are increasingly being admitted to intensive care units. Pregnant patients are unique for a number of reasons and represent a substantial challenge to the healthcare team because of these differences. First, in a continuing or ongoing pregnancy, at least two patients must be considered, the mother and the fetus. With multifetal gestations, the number of patients is correspondingly higher. Second, pregnant women have many physiologic adaptations as a consequence of the pregnancy, and these alter the definition of normal for the diverse variables that are routinely monitored in intensive care units. Additionally, some of these changes such as a reduction in the colloid oncotic pressure or the functional residual capacity (FRC) of the lungs may uniquely predispose pregnant women to more significant injury, given any relative degree of insult, than would occur in their nonpregnant counterparts. Finally, pregnancy presents the opportunity for a host of disease processes that are unique to pregnancy itself and that never occur outside of pregnancy, such as amniotic fluid embolus (AFE) syndrome.

The purpose of this chapter is multiple. The physiologic changes of pregnancy are reviewed, with an emphasis on those areas where the physiology renders pregnant patients uniquely susceptible to injury. The principal areas accounting for maternal mortality, hypertensive diseases of pregnancy, obstetric hemorrhage, and trauma are also reviewed. When treating a pregnant woman and her fetus, it is important to realize that one must meet the usual standards established for patients in intensive care units as well as those established for a pregnant woman and her fetus.

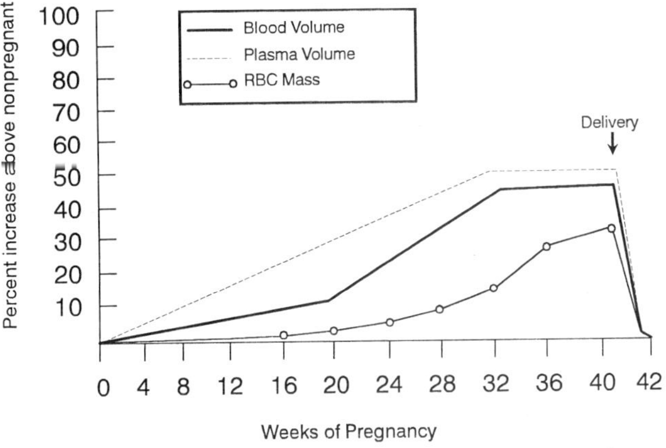

Figure 8–1. Blood volume changes during pregnancy. (From Scott DE: Anemia during pregnancy. Obstet Gynecol Annu 1972; 1:219.)

CARDIORESPIRATORY CHANGES DURING PREGNANCY

By the late first trimester, significant changes in plasma volume have occurred. The increase in plasma volume plateaus at approximately a 45% to 50% increase above nonpregnant levels at 32 weeks, remaining stable thereafter until delivery.[1] The red blood cell mass also increases progressively; however, the increase first occurs at a later point in pregnancy, persists until term, and is approximately 33% above nonpregnant levels. As demonstrated in Figure 8–1, the relatively greater increase in plasma volume than red blood cell mass results in a physiologic anemia of pregnancy, with the greatest divergence between red blood cell mass and plasma volume occurring at approximately 28 weeks of gestation. The magnitude of pregnancy hypervolemia shows considerable variation among different women despite a tendency for the same plasma volume pattern to be repeated in successive pregnancies for any given individual.[2, 3] The absolute increase in blood volume is positively correlated with the number of fetuses. The overall increase in blood volume for singleton pregnancies is approximately 1600 mL, compared with approximately 2000 mL for twin pregnancies. Teleologically, this is perhaps a very important compensatory physiologic change of pregnancy inasmuch as a pregnant woman is basically her own ambulatory blood bank. Indeed, with the usual blood loss of 1000 mL at the time of cesarean delivery, a pregnant woman will be expected to increase her hematocrit in the postpartum period relative to that immediately before surgery. In pregnant women with preeclampsia or eclampsia, the vascular space is not expanded to the extent that it would be in the absence of hypertensive disease and in fact is closer to the volume of a nonpregnant patient than a pregnant patient. Accordingly, preeclamptic patients tolerate blood loss poorly compared with their counterparts without hypertensive diseases of pregnancy. In contrast, volume expansion is normal in women with chronic hypertension.

Blood Pressure

Systolic and diastolic blood pressures decrease during pregnancy, and the lowest readings are usually obtained in the late second trimester at around 28 weeks of gestation. Thereafter follows a gradual recovery toward nonpregnant values as the 40th week of pregnancy is reached.[4, 5] In pregnancy, blood pressure measured in the lateral decubitus position usually is lowest whereas that in the supine position is highest (Fig. 8–2). It is generally accepted that after the 20th week of gestation and certainly after the 28th week of gestation, blood pressure should be measured in positions other than supine because the possibility of relative to complete obstruction of the inferior vena cava by the gravid uterus may yield inaccurate measurements. In women at bed rest, blood pressures are obtained from the superior arm with the patient either in the left or right lateral recumbent position.

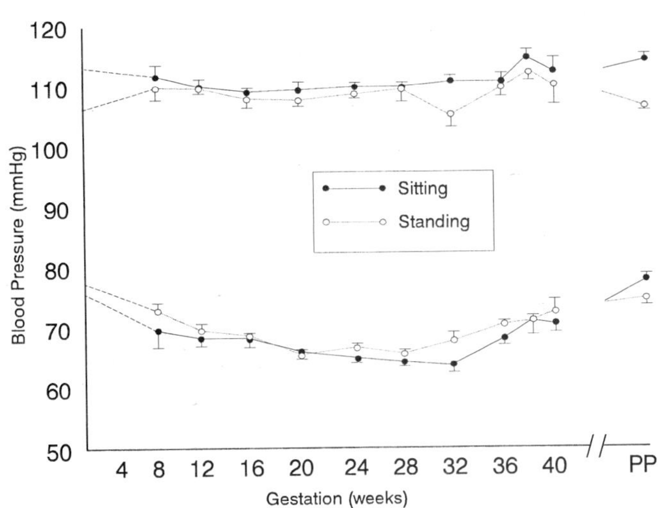

Figure 8–2. Sequential changes in average systolic and diastolic blood pressures, with subjects sitting and standing throughout pregnancy (n = 69 patients with standard errors of the mean). Postpartum values drawn on the ordinate are used as a baseline, and *dotted lines* represent the presumed changes during the first 8 weeks. (From Wilson M, Morganti AA, Zervodakis I, et al: Blood pressure, the renin-aldosterone system, and sex steroids throughout normal pregnancy. Am J Med 1980; 68:97.)

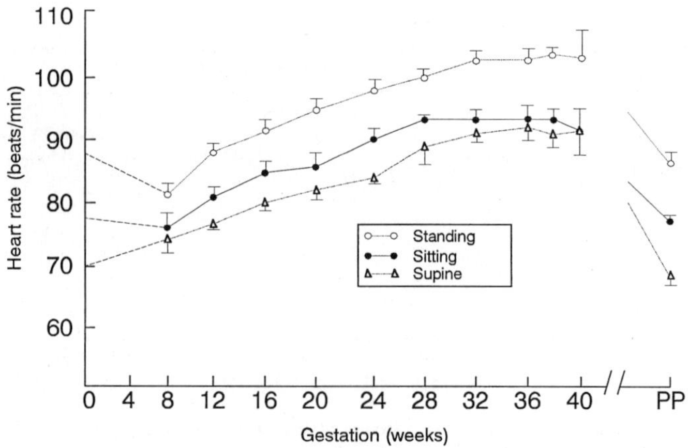

Figure 8–3. Sequential changes in mean heart rate in three positions throughout pregnancy (n = 69 patients with standard errors of the mean). (From Wilson M, Morganti AA, Zervodakis I, et al: Blood pressure, the renin-aldosterone system, and sex steroids throughout normal pregnancy. Am J Med 1980; 68:97.)

Heart Rate

Maternal heart rate increases occur as early as the seventh week of pregnancy, and by late pregnancy maternal heart rate averages approximately 20% over postpartum values (Fig. 8–3).[5]

Cardiac Output

Maternal cardiac output increases as early as 10 weeks' gestation and peaks at 30% to 50% over control values by the late second trimester. This rise, from approximately 4.5 to 6.0 L/min, is sustained for the remainder of pregnancy if cardiac output is measured in the lateral decubitus position.[6,7] As shown in Figure 8–4, highest cardiac outputs when measured in women in the late third trimester are obtained in the knee-chest, right lateral, and left lateral positions. A significant fall in cardiac output occurs in the supine position, with an even further reduction in the standing position.

The increase in cardiac output results from increases in both heart rate and stroke volume. Several theories have been set forth in an effort to explain the mechanism responsible for the stroke volume increases that contribute to higher cardiac output during early pregnancy. The increased stroke volume cannot be explained on the basis of increased left ventricular filling pressures because pulmonary artery diastolic and capillary wedge pressures do not significantly change.[6,8] It has been proposed that the increased plasma volume, cardiac output, and heart rate during pregnancy are similar to the hemodynamic changes following the development of an arteriovenous fistula, much as is occurring in the uteroplacental circulation. Others have suggested that left ventricular dilatation is related to hormonal factors and is analogous to the decreased venous tone observed with normal pregnancy or after administration of oral contraceptives.

Systemic and Pulmonary Vascular Resistance

Vascular resistance changes during pregnancy are related to both mechanical and hormonal factors. Development of the uteroplacental circulation leads to a major low-resistance circuit that reduces cardiac afterload. Other possible causes of the peripheral vasodilatation of pregnancy include the extraordinarily high levels of estrogen and progesterone as well as local production and effects of prostaglandins.[9–11] The decrease in systemic vascular resistance (SVR) during pregnancy reflects the combination of decreased mean arterial pressure and increased cardiac output. Bader and associates[8] used cardiac catheterization to document the lowest values for SVR (980 dyne · s/cm^5 · m^2) during the 14th to the 24th week of pregnancy. According to their observations, this parameter rose progressively toward a nonpregnant value of 1240 dyne · s/cm^5 · m^2 by term. These observations are consistent with those of Clark and colleagues[6] who found the mean SVR during the late third trimester to be 1210 ± 266 dyne · s/cm^5 · m^2.

Pulmonary Vascular Resistance

Pulmonary vascular resistance had not been measured directly in healthy pregnant women before the investigation by Clark and associates.[6] It was widely held that it did not differ from the values obtained when not pregnant. However, when determined using a pulmonary artery catheter, the resistance at 36 to 38 weeks of gestation was 78 ± 22 dyne · s/cm^5 · m^2. This is a value lower than prior estimates obtained by noninvasive techniques.

Labor Hemodynamics

Baseline hemodynamic values in nonlaboring healthy pregnant, postpartum, and nonpregnant women are shown in Table 8–1.[6,7,12] Superimposed on these background changes are the physiologic events such as labor or the pathologic

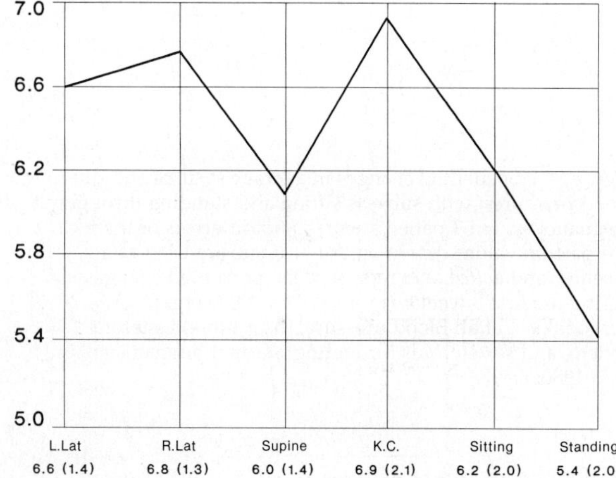

Figure 8–4. Hemodynamics of normal pregnancy—position change and cardiac output.

TABLE 8–1. Hemodynamic Values in Healthy Nonpregnant, Pregnant, and Postpartum Women

	*Hemodynamic Values in Subjects**		
Parameter (Units)	*Nonpregnant Gestation*	*36–38 Weeks*	*Postpartum*
Heart rate (bpm)	60–100	83 ± 10	71 ± 10
Central venous pressure (mm Hg)	5–10	3.6 ± 2.5	3.7 ± 2.6
Mean pulmonary artery pressure (mm Hg)	15–20	†	†
Pulmonary capillary wedge pressure (mm Hg)	6–12	7.5 ± 1.8	6.3 ± 2.1
Mean arterial pressure (mm Hg)	90–110	90.3 ± 5.8	86.4 ± 7.5
Cardiac output (L/min)	4.3–6.0	6.2 ± 1.0	4.3 ± 0.9
Stroke volume (mL/beat)	57–71	74.7	60.6
Systemic vascular resistance (dyne · s/cm^5 · m^2)	900–1400	1210 ± 266	1530 ± 520
Pulmonary vascular resistance (dyne · s/cm^5 · m^2)	<250	78 ± 22	119 ± 47

(Adapted from Rosenthal MH: Intrapartum intensive care management of the cardiac patient. Clin Obstet Gynecol 1981; 24:789–807, and Clark SL, Cotton DB, Lee W, et al: Central hemodynamic assessment of normal term pregnancy. Am J Obstet Gynecol 1989; 161:1439–1442.)

*Where available, data are given as mean ± SD. Pregnancy values determined with patient in left lateral decubitus position.

†Not reported.

events such as severe preeclampsia. One example of the cumulative effects of pregnancy and various pregnancy complications, such as premature labor treated with a β-sympathomimetic tocolytic drug, on the cardiovascular system is demonstrated in Figure 8–5.

With the onset of labor, healthy women have a 40% increase in cardiac output above their basal third-trimester level. The demands are further increased by factors such as twins, anemia, infection, or hyperthyroidism. Indeed, during labor, it is not unusual to have cardiac outputs of 10 to 16 L/min. The magnitude of increase in cardiac output in laboring women is related to the degree of pain control afforded them. The increase in cardiac output during the first and second stages of labor is not as pronounced when a patient is given conduction anesthesia as when given only local anesthesia.[13–15]

The repetitive and forceful uterine contractions of labor may have significant implications for a woman's central hemodynamic stability if she is compromised for some reason (e.g., valvular heart disease, cardiomyopathy, or ischemic heart disease). With each uterine contraction, approximately 300 to 500 mL of blood reenters the central circulation. This blood is expelled from both the uterine and placental circulations and from the lower extremities as the uterus rises off the inferior vena cava during the contraction.[16, 17] These changes are analogous to giving a woman a full unit of whole blood over 30 to 60 seconds. The usual response of a healthy parturient is a very transient increase in right atrial pressure and a transient increase in maternal heart rate, but the filling pressures at all times remain within the realm of physiologic normalcy. In patients who have cardiac compromise, as alluded to earlier, pathologic elevations of central venous and wedge pressures have been noted to accompany the uterine contractions (Fig. 8–6).[18] Undoubtedly, the compromised cardiovascular system is at risk of decompensation and overt failure when challenged repetitively by these sudden and dramatic volume boluses that occur with every uterine contraction.

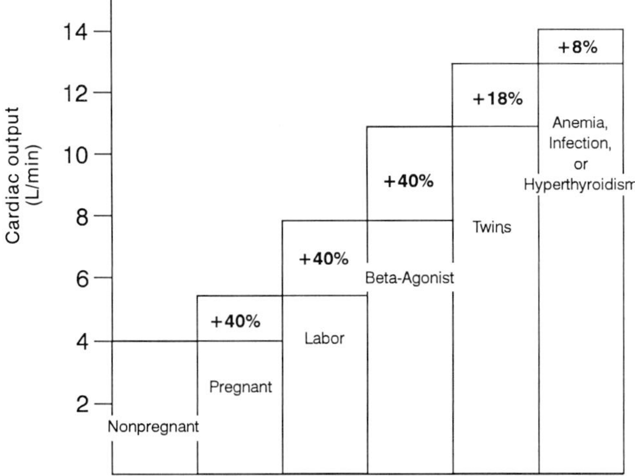

Figure 8–5. Cumulative effects of pregnancy and of various pregnancy complications on cardiac output.

Postpartum Hemodynamics

Significant hemodynamic fluctuations, reflecting the net effect of blood loss at delivery and the body's physiologic compensation to peripartum hemorrhage, occur in the immediate postpartum period. The puerperium has also been characterized by changes in cardiac output, stroke volume, and heart rate. Ueland and Hansen[14] measured these parameters in 13 patients who received caudal anesthesia and found a 59% increase in cardiac output and a 71% increase in stroke volume by 10 minutes postpartum. One hour postpartum, the cardiac output was elevated 49% and stroke volume 67% above baseline. Measured as late as 4 to 5 days postpartum, cardiac output has been elevated to approximately 18% to 29% above prelabor values. The return of cardiac output to nonpregnant values has been variably reported to range from 2 to 4 weeks postpartum.[19, 20]

During the first week after delivery, Chesley and colleagues reported a 2-L decrease in the sodium space compartment associated with 3 kg of weight loss.[21] This well-known postpartum diuresis usually occurs between the second and fifth day and provides a physiologic mechanism by which increased extracellular fluid accumulated during pregnancy can be dissipated. The potential clinical significance of this phenomenon is illustrated by Hankins and coworkers,[22] who reported significant and pathologic elevations in pulmonary capillary wedge pressures (PCWPs) in a select group of preeclamptic women who manifested these events 48 to 72 hours postpartum. These investigators suggested that this phenomenon was due to mobilization of extracellular or extravascular fluid before diuresis. In this regard, postpartum pulmonary edema may develop in

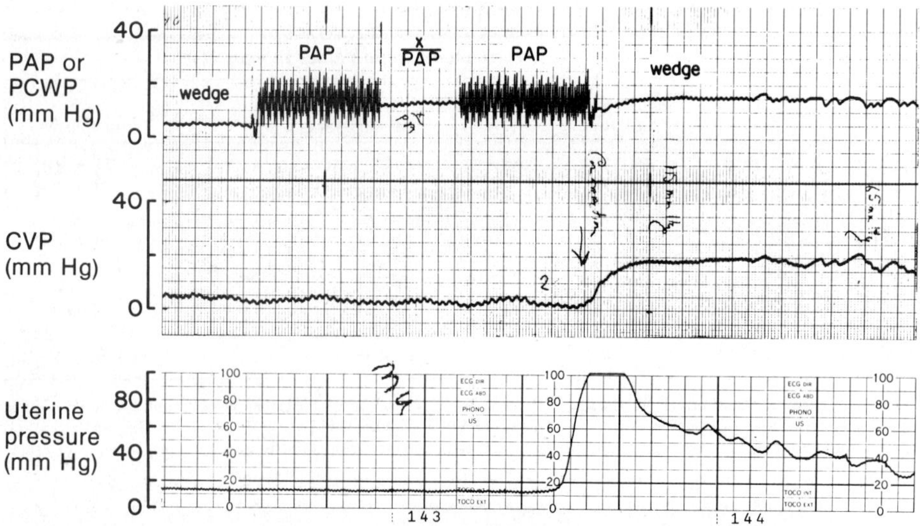

Figure 8–6. Effect of a uterine contraction (change in uterine pressure) on maternal pulmonary capillary wedge and central venous pressures in case reports. (*Abbreviations*: PAP = pulmonary artery pressure; PCWP and wedge = pulmonary capillary wedge pressure; X/PAP = mean pulmonary artery pressure; CVP = central venous pressure.)

high-risk patients who fail to diurese before mobilization of extravascular fluid. Indeed, pulmonary edema in pregnancy most commonly occurs in the postpartum period.

RESPIRATORY SYSTEM

Pulmonary Physiology

Four lung volumes and four lung capacities are used to describe pulmonary physiology. These are shown in Figure 8–7 along with the expected effects of pregnancy. Except for residual volume and lung capacities derived therefrom, these can be measured using direct spirometric techniques (discussed later). According to de Swiet,[23] physiologic changes induced by pregnancy can be summarized as follows:

1. Vital capacity may be increased by 100 to 200 mL in some women.
2. Inspiratory capacity increases by about 300 mL by late pregnancy.
3. Expiratory reserve volume decreases from 1300 mL to 1100 mL.
4. Residual volume decreases from 1500 mL to 1200 mL.
5. FRC, a sum of expiratory reserve and residual volumes, is reduced considerably by 500 mL.
6. Tidal volume increases considerably from about 500 to 700 mL.
7. Minute ventilation increases 40%, from 7.5 to 10.5 L/min, and because the respiratory rate is unchanged, this is primarily due to increased tidal volume.

The sum of these changes substantively increases ventilation due to deeper but not more frequent breathing. These changes presumably are induced to help supply increased basal oxygen consumption, which increases by 20 to 40 mL/min in the second half of pregnancy.

Among the physiologic changes that apparently predispose pregnant women to an amplification of any effect of a pulmonary insult is the effect of loss of lung volume indicated by low critical closing volume (CCV). In a normal healthy person, all regions of the lung are open at the end of a full inspiration. Normally, the FRC exceeds the CCV. With a lung injury and loss of volume, however, FRC may no longer exceed the CCV; and when breathing with low tidal volumes, segments of lung may collapse and result in reduced compliance and increased intrapulmonary shunt. During pregnancy, the CCV does not change but the FRC declines. Indeed, the FRC, as noted earlier, reduces considerably, and by the third trimester of pregnancy, tidal volume and CCV may overlap even in the absence of a lung injury. This may explain why the morbidity and mortality of virtually all pneumonic processes are significantly higher in pregnant than in nonpregnant women.[24, 25]

Just as many of the parameters involved in lung volume change in pregnancy, so do blood gas values by virtue of changes in ventilation. The normal maternal partial pressure of arterial oxygen (Pao_2) varies from 101 to 108 mm Hg early in pregnancy and falls to 90 to 100 mm Hg near term. The increased CCV, as previously discussed,[26, 27] is responsible for the widened alveolar-arterial oxygen gradient, which averages 20 mm Hg in the third trimester.[28] The nor-

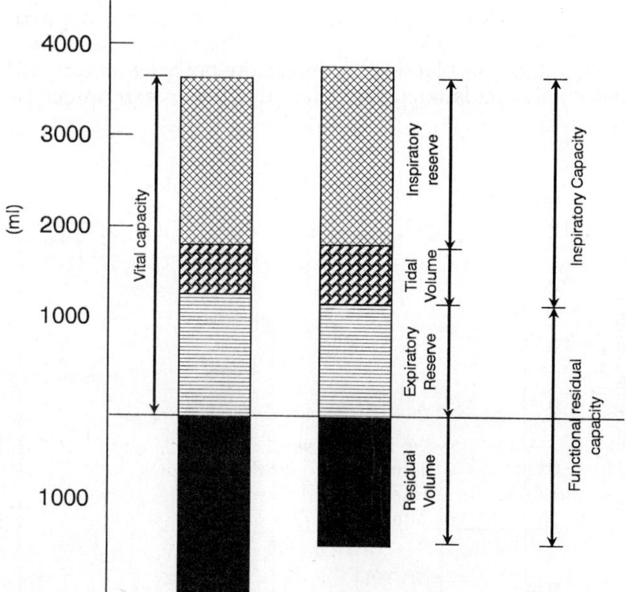

Figure 8–7. Lung volumes and capacities in nonpregnant patients compared with those in late pregnancy. (From de Swiet M: The respiratory system. *In*: Clinical Physiology in Obstetrics. 2nd ed. London, Blackwell Scientific, 1991, pp 83–100. Reprinted by permission of Blackwell Scientific Publications, Inc.)

mal physiologic increase in minute ventilation during pregnancy is reflected by a partial pressure of arterial carbon dioxide ($Paco_2$) of 27 to 32 mm Hg and an increase in pH from 7.40 to 7.45.[27]

COLLOID OSMOTIC PRESSURE

Oian and coworkers measured Starling forces in 10 normal patients in the first trimester of pregnancy and in 10 additional normal women in the third trimester.[29, 30] Values for plasma colloid oncotic pressure (COP_p) in early pregnancy (23.2 ± 0.8 mm Hg) were statistically higher than values obtained in the third trimester (21.1 ± 1.2 mm Hg). Using subcutaneous wicks placed at the level of the thorax and ankle of pregnant volunteers, these same investigators collected interstitial fluid and were able to quantitate its colloid oncotic pressure (COP_i). Values obtained in the ankle were found to be lower than those in the thorax. In addition, a marked reduction in COP_i was noted when comparing first- and third-trimester values, a decline that exceeded the fall of COP_p with advancing gestation. The COP_i values in the thorax were 13.1 ± 1.2 mm Hg in the first trimester and 8.4 ± 0.8 mm Hg in the third trimester, whereas corresponding values for the ankle were 9.6 ± 1.8 and 5.5 ± 1.4 mm Hg, respectively. It was hypothesized that as pregnancy progressed, an increase in capillary filtration secondary to elevated capillary hydrostatic pressure initially would lead to a fall in COP_i by simple dilution. To account for the greater decline in COP_i as compared with COP_p with advancing gestation, proteins would have to be removed from the interstitium at increased rates. It was proposed that an increase in lymphatic flow would effect such a reduction in the protein concentration of the interstitium. The same investigators measured interstitial fluid hydrostatic pressure (P_i) by inserting specialized steel cannulas into the subcutaneous tissue of pregnant patients. The P_i was noted to be subatmospheric and to increase with advancing gestational age. The P_i of the thorax was recorded at −1.6 ± 0.7 mm Hg in the first trimester, increasing to −1.2 ± 0.9 mm Hg in the third trimester of pregnancy. Likewise, the P_i at the level of the ankle increased from −0.9 ± 0.5 to −0.1 ± 0.4 mm Hg when first- and third-trimester measurements were compared.

Having measured three of the four Starling forces in pregnant patients, these investigators then calculated capillary hydrostatic pressure (P_c) from the Starling equation. Their calculations were based on the assumption that flow across the capillary membrane was zero. Because this would dictate that the lymphatic flow was zero, the investigators admitted that their calculated capillary hydrostatic pressures were an underestimate of the true values. Second, they assumed that the capillary reflection coefficient was 1.0, denoting that capillaries are impermeable to proteins. A significant increase in P_c with advancing gestational age was noted at the level of both the thorax and ankle. Thoracic P_c was noted to increase from 8.3 ± 1.9 mm Hg in the first trimester to 11.5 ± 2.3 mm Hg in the third trimester. Similarly, ankle P_c increased from 12.7 ± 2.2 to 15.5 ± 2.3 mm Hg.

In summary, pregnancy is associated with a moderate fall in COP_p and a rise in P_c. Such alterations of these Starling forces would tend to increase fluid filtration from the intravascular compartment to the interstitium. A progressive fall in COP_i exerts a protective effect. Despite this mechanism, increasing P_c in late gestation probably overwhelms this mechanism, allowing increased fluid egress from the capillaries.

Weil and associates[31a] reported that the mean COP_p in healthy nonpregnant ambulatory adult volunteers was 25.4 ± 2.3 mm Hg. A slightly lower COP_p has been noted in female patients when compared with their male counterparts. A downward trend is also noted with advancing age. Maternal COP_p values in normal pregnancy decrease and reach a nadir at approximately 34 to 36 weeks of gestation (Fig. 8–8). This trend closely parallels the decrease in maternal serum albumin concentrations. A mean value at term is reported to be 22.4 ± 0.54 mm Hg. This change is consistent with simple dilution of plasma proteins secondary to a rise in plasma volume. Because albumin is thought to be the major protein responsible for plasma oncotic pressure, Robertson and Cheyne[31] proposed that the fall in albumin concentration that occurs in pregnancy is the probable explanation for declining COP_p in the gravid state.

Measurements of COP_p at term in patients with pregnancy-induced hypertension have revealed values that are lower than those from a similar group of normotensive patients (17.9 ± 0.68 mm Hg versus 22.0 ± 0.48 mm Hg).[32, 33] The degree of hypertension, however, does not seem to correlate with the magnitude of reduction in the COP_p. When compared with intrapartum values, values of COP_p measured in the first 24 hours postpartum have revealed a significant reduction. Cotton and coworkers[34] reported a

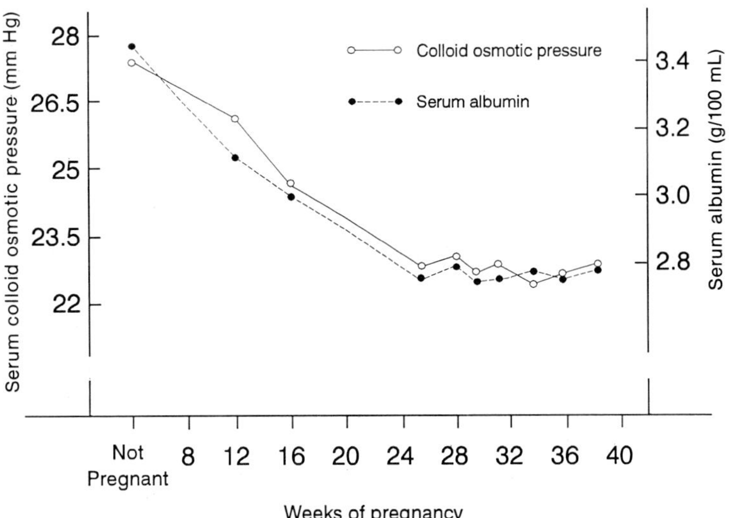

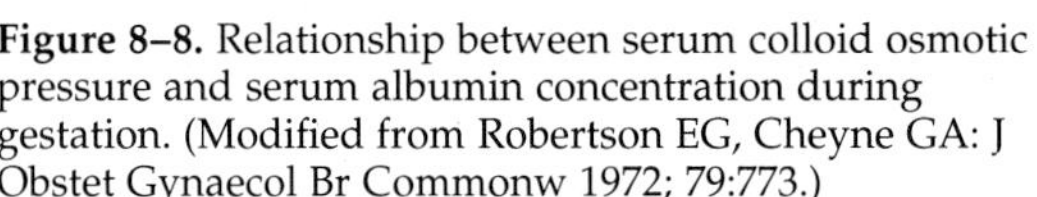
Figure 8–8. Relationship between serum colloid osmotic pressure and serum albumin concentration during gestation. (Modified from Robertson EG, Cheyne GA: J Obstet Gynaecol Br Commonw 1972; 79:773.)

COP_p value of 15.4 ± 2.1 mm Hg postpartum compared with a value of 21.0 ± 2.1 mm Hg in the intrapartum period. The nadir of the COP_p appears to occur from 6 to 16 hours after delivery and is consistent with effects secondary to mobilization of interstitial fluid. The corresponding postpartum fall in preeclamptic patients is even greater, falling to as low as 13 to 14 mm Hg in the postpartum period.[33] Similar to the alteration in lung volumes, these alterations in the colloid oncotic pressures and their impact on Starling forces may well predispose pregnant women to greater risk of pulmonary edema given any absolute degree of insult, without regard to whether the primary genesis is hydrostatic pressure or increased pulmonary capillary permeability.

TRAUMA DURING PREGNANCY

Physical trauma complicates approximately 1 in every 12 pregnancies,[35, 36] and trauma and various forms of violence are leading causes of death in women of reproductive age. It is therefore not surprising that trauma is a leading cause of nonobstetric maternal death.

Blunt Abdominal Trauma

Motor vehicle accidents are the leading cause of trauma during pregnancy, followed by falls and direct assaults on the abdomen.[37–39] Battering occurs frequently during pregnancy, and rates of recurrence are high. It has been reported that 1 of every 12 women in an inner-city population was battered at some time during her pregnancy.[40]

Intra-abdominal injuries are of particular concern after blunt abdominal trauma. Serious retroperitoneal hemorrhage following lower abdominal and pelvic trauma occurs more frequently in pregnant women than in their nonpregnant counterparts.[41] The increased size of the pelvic organs, particularly the uterus, and the greatly increased blood flow into this area are predisposing factors. Conversely, bowel injuries occur less frequently during pregnancy because the bowel is protected by the enlarged uterus. In the upper abdomen, splenic rupture is the most common cause of intraperitoneal hemorrhage after trauma. Liver and renal injuries account for most of the remaining serious abdominal injuries.

Because the uterus and its contents are subject to serious and even catastrophic injury, trauma during pregnancy is a unique event. Abruptio placentae complicates 1% to 5% of minor injuries and 40% to 50% of major life-threatening injuries.[37–39, 41, 42] Placental separation results from deformation of the elastic myometrium around the relatively inelastic placenta.[43] Shearing of the placental edge from the underlying decidua basalis results, with this separation further propagated by increased intrauterine pressure resulting from impact. Frequent findings include vaginal bleeding, uterine tenderness, uterine contractions, fetal tachycardia, late decelerations, fetal acidosis, fetal bradycardia, and fetal death.[38, 42]

Differentiation of labor from early abruptio placentae is difficult after trauma. In a trauma victim who is beyond 20 weeks of gestation, electronic monitoring appears to be particularly sensitive in identifying patients with uterine contractile activity or abruptio placentae. The presence of vaginal bleeding and tetanic or hypertonic contractions is presumptive evidence of abruptio placentae. The effectiveness of tocolytics in abating preterm uterine contractions in this setting is uncertain. If used, tocolytics, particularly β-mimetic agents, can also produce fetal or maternal tachycardia, which may confuse or delay the diagnosis of abruptio placentae.

Uterine rupture is an infrequent but life-threatening complication of trauma. It accounts for less than 1% of all injuries during pregnancy and usually tends to occur when direct abdominal impact is associated with substantial force. Uterine rupture ranges clinically from only subtle findings such as uterine tenderness or a nonreassuring fetal heart rate pattern without changes in maternal vital signs to the alternate extreme of rapid onset of maternal hypovolemia with possible fetal and maternal death.

Direct fetal injury is an infrequent complication of trauma during pregnancy. Numerous cases of direct fetal injury have been reported, but because it is such an uncommon event, the incidence remains uncertain. Direct fetal injury from blunt abdominal trauma most often involves the fetal skull and brain. Figure 8–9 shows a massive and lethal intracranial bleed in a fetus of 26 weeks' gestation whose mother was involved in a head-on motor vehicle collision at approximately 10 miles per hour at impact. Although the accident was lethal to the fetus, which succumbed 48 hours after hospital admission of the mother, the mother sustained no injuries. The most commonly described mechanism of fetal head injury involves simultaneous fracture of the maternal pelvis in late gestation when the fetal head is engaged. If the force is sufficient to result in pelvic fracture, the fetus in vertex presentation often sustains a skull fracture. Even a nonvertex fetus has been reported to sustain significant intracranial trauma, presumably from the accel-

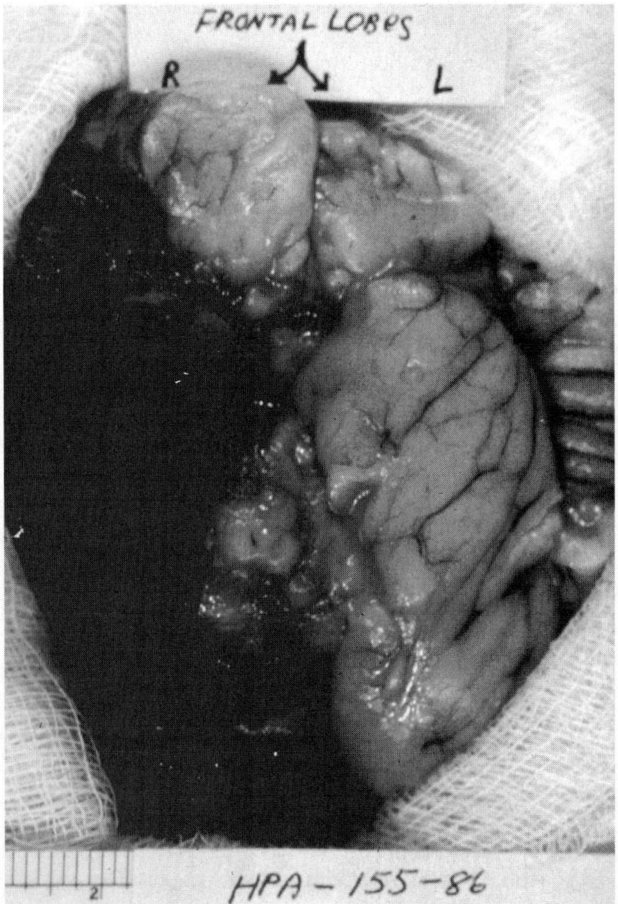

Figure 8–9. A massive and lethal intracranial bleed in a fetus of 26 weeks' gestation whose mother was involved in a head-on motor vehicle collision (approximately 10 miles per hour at impact). Although the fetus died 48 hours after hospital admission of the mother, the mother sustained no injuries.

eration-deceleration forces, and at times with minimal maternal trauma.

Penetrating Trauma

Gunshot and stab wounds make up most types of penetrating abdominal trauma. A number of reports have described self-inflicted penetrating wounds, in most cases as an effort by the woman to abort the pregnancy. Penetrating abdominal trauma during pregnancy has remarkably disparate prognoses for the fetus and the woman. Visceral injuries to the mother complicate only 19% of gunshot wounds to the uterus, whereas the fetus is injured nearly two thirds of the time.[44] Isolated injuries to the umbilical cord, fetal membranes, and placenta have been reported. Subsequent perinatal mortality varies from 41% to 71%. In contrast, maternal mortality occurs in less than 5% of cases of penetrating trauma. The extent and severity of maternal and fetal injury due to gunshot wounds depend on a number of factors, including the size and velocity of the bullet; the anatomic region penetrated; the angle of entry; deflection of the bullet's trajectory by muscle, bone, or viscera; the gestational age of the fetus; and the distance from which the missile was shot. Bullets tend to tumble once they have entered the body, and much more damage frequently occurs than suggested by the entrance wound. Accordingly, any abdominal gunshot wound requires exploration. Conversely, the extent of stab wound injuries is limited by the length and width of the penetrating object. As opposed to gunshot wounds, with stab wounds, observation may be warranted in selected cases if both the mother and fetus are stable and the index of suspicion for significant intra-abdominal bleeding is low.

Evaluation and Treatment

Treatment priorities are the primary consideration in the early management of injured pregnant women. These priorities are identical to those in nonpregnant patients, and pregnancy should not result in any restriction of the usual diagnostic, pharmacologic, or resuscitative procedures or maneuvers. It is important to follow a methodic evaluation that ensures complete assessment and stabilization of the mother. If attention is drawn to the fetus before the woman is stabilized, serious or life-threatening maternal injuries may be overlooked, or circumstances that can compromise fetal oxygenation (e.g., maternal hypoxemia, hypovolemia, or supine hypotension) may be ignored, with resultant lessening of the likelihood of both maternal and fetal survival.

EVALUATION AND TREATMENT OF THE MOTHER

Uterine Displacement

Pregnant women require certain considerations that need not be addressed in their nonpregnant counterparts. Included is deflection of the uterus off the inferior vena cava and abdominal aorta when a patient is in a supine position and beyond midpregnancy. This can be effected by having the patient lie in the lateral decubitus position. If a patient must remain supine, as in cases of suspected spinal injury or when cardiopulmonary resuscitation is being administered, manual deflection of the uterus to the left with a hand and placement of a wedge under the patient's hip or backboard assist in accomplishing uterine displacement.

Peritoneal Lavage

Pregnancy is not a contraindication to peritoneal lavage; however, if a patient is known to be pregnant, then open peritoneal lavage is preferred over blind needle insertion to lessen the likelihood of injury to the uterus or to other displaced intra-abdominal organs. Open peritoneal lavage has been shown to be safe, sensitive, and specific during pregnancy.[45] The indications for peritoneal lavage after trauma during pregnancy are identical to those in nonpregnant counterparts. Peritoneal lavage is unnecessary if clinically obvious intraperitoneal bleeding is present.

EVALUATION AND TREATMENT OF FETUS

The use of electronic fetal monitoring in pregnant trauma victims beyond 20 weeks of gestation may assist in the early diagnosis of abruptio placentae. In one study, no case of placental abruption occurred in trauma patients who did not have uterine contractions or who had contractions at a frequency of less than one every 10 minutes after 4 hours of fetal monitoring. Conversely, of those women who had uterine contractions with greater frequency, almost 20% had placental abruption. Importantly, abnormal fetal heart rate tracings, including tachycardia and late decelerations, were frequently noted in cases of abruptio placentae. Because abruptio placentae usually becomes apparent shortly after injury, monitoring should be initiated after the woman is stabilized. Monitoring should be continued and further evaluation carried out if uterine contractions, a nonreassuring fetal heart rate pattern, vaginal bleeding, significant uterine tenderness or irritability, serious maternal injury, or rupture of the amniotic membranes is present. If these findings are not present, the patient may be discharged or transferred.[46] Other studies[47] have concluded that monitoring periods of 2 to 6 hours are adequate if no uterine contractions, uterine tenderness, or bleeding is observed. On discharge, the patient should be instructed to return if she develops vaginal bleeding, leakage of fluid, decreased fetal movement, or severe abdominal pain.

The incidence of fetal-maternal hemorrhage is four- to fivefold higher in pregnant women who have experienced trauma than in uninjured controls.[36, 37, 48] The mean volume of fetal-maternal hemorrhage is also significantly higher in women experiencing trauma than in uninjured controls. Among women who exhibit evidence of fetal-maternal hemorrhage due to trauma, the mean estimated blood volume is usually less than 15 mL and more than 90% of the hemorrhages are less than 30 mL. Therefore, administration of 300 μg of immunoglobulin D would protect nearly all D-negative trauma victims from D isoimmunization. The routine use of the Kleihauer-Betke assay or other similar quantitative assays of fetal-maternal hemorrhage may be useful in identifying those few unsensitized, D-negative trauma victims who exhibit a greater than 30-mL transfusion. Additional immunoglobulin D may be administered to patients so identified. Complications of fetal-maternal hemorrhage other than isoimmunization have been described in a limited number of patients. Fetal and neonatal anemia, fetal cardiac arrhythmia, and fetal death all have been reported. It is unclear whether the information gained from routine use of Kleihauer-Betke assay or similar testing designed to demonstrate fetal-maternal hemorrhage can prevent adverse outcomes from these complications.

The use of ultrasonography after trauma during pregnancy does not appear to be as sensitive as electronic fetal and uterine monitoring for diagnosing abruptio placentae. Sonography may be useful for pregnant trauma victims for establishment of gestational age, placental localization, determination of fetal well-being or demise, and estimation of amniotic fluid volume. Ultrasonography may also reveal the presence of intra-abdominal fluid and may increase the index of suspicion for intraperitoneal hemorrhage.

When exploratory laparotomy is required, the fetus usually tolerates surgery and anesthesia well if maternal oxygenation and uterine perfusion can be maintained. When the uterus has been penetrated by an object or projectile, the fetus has probably been injured. If the fetus is alive, the decision to perform cesarean delivery should be weighed against the likelihood of fetal survival. Factors involved in this decision include gestational age at the time of injury, the condition of the fetus based on antenatal testing that may have been performed, the extent of injury to the uterus (i.e., cesarean hysterectomy may be necessary with extensive injuries), and whether the gravid uterus allows adequate exploration of the peritoneal cavity. The need to perform a laparotomy in and of itself is not an indication to proceed with cesarean delivery. If the uterus has been penetrated and delivery is to be effected, a pediatric surgeon and a neonatologist should be available if possible.

AMNIOTIC FLUID EMBOLISM

Pathophysiology

AFE was first described by Meyer in 1926.[49] The dramatic presentation as cardiopulmonary collapse, pulmonary edema, or profuse hemorrhage, either alone or in combination,[49–51] along with the maternal mortality of up to 80%,[52] has made AFE a topic of intense interest. Precise definition of the pathophysiology of AFE has been thwarted by our inability to predict its occurrence and by its relatively low incidence, complicating between 1 in 15,000 and 1 in 20,000 pregnancies. Although more than 300 cases of purported AFE have been described in the literature, observations on central hemodynamics have to date been limited in number (Table 8–2).[53] Currently, observations have been obtained only after acute cardiopulmonary decompensation, and by virtue of the catastrophic nature of the presentation, central hemodynamic measurements have first been possible several hours after the acute event and frequently under clinical conditions requiring use of potent vasoactive agents in support of the cardiac system and mechanical ventilation to support the pulmonary system.

In animal studies, which have been relied on to evaluate the acute phase of AFE, the most reproducible occurrence has been acute elevations in the pulmonary artery pressure. Indeed, this has been the dominant effect reported in those models; however, it persisted for only a very short time, with a peak at approximately 10 minutes after the amniotic fluid was infused and return to baseline values by 30 minutes after the infusion.[54] One study demonstrated an acute elevation in not only pulmonary pressures and resistances but in systemic pressures and resistances as well. Although these effects were seen with all types of amniotic fluid, the fluids containing meconium had by far the most pronounced effects. Of note, neither filtration nor boiling of the amniotic fluid blocked the pressor effect, implying that it is both heat stable and soluble.[53]

As noted in Table 8–2, 12 of the 14 women in whom measurements were taken had mean pulmonary artery pressures at or greater than 1 SD above the mean, with 5 of 14 being greater than 2 SD above the mean values obtained in pregnancy. Similarly, in 10 of the 12 women who had a pulmonary vascular resistance calculated, the values were greater than 2 SD above the mean. Thus, although previous interpretations had concluded that the pulmonary vascular resistance and the mean pulmonary artery pressures were not elevated in pregnant women with AFE, that conclusion was based on comparison with nonpregnant values, and indeed there is an elevation when compared with normative data for pregnancy.

Accepting then that abnormalities of pulmonary pressures and resistances are present in women who have sustained an AFE, they are nonetheless minimal relative to the degree of left ventricular dysfunction that is manifested in those fortunate enough to survive the acute event. The PCWP has exceeded 3 SD above the mean in 86% of the cases. The absolute value was greater than or equal to 18 mm Hg in 50%, a level that would be universally accepted as abnormally elevated.

Thus, the pathophysiology of AFE would appear to involve transient but marked elevations in pulmonary and systemic vascular resistances with resultant hypertension, peaking approximately 10 minutes after the embolus occurs and returning toward a baseline value within 30 minutes. With the pulmonary hypertension and pulmonary arterial spasm, a significant shunt occurs, resulting in arterial hypoxemia (Fig. 8–10).

Women seem particularly predisposed to arrhythmias and cardiopulmonary collapse during the acute event. Those women who can be successfully resuscitated or stabilized during the initial phase then enter a second phase of the disease characterized by left ventricular failure and pulmonary capillary injury. The left ventricular failure likely results from a combination of hypoxic insult, acidemia, and perhaps coronary arterial spasm, thereby magnifying the already significant systemic injury by further insult at the local level of myocardium.[55] At this stage, attention to correcting and stabilizing oxygenation and cardiac performance is the dominant clinical problem.

TABLE 8–2. Hemodynamic Indices in Patients with Amniotic Fluid Embolism

Case	*MPAP (mm Hg)*	*PCWP (mm Hg)*	*PVR (dyne · s/cm⁵ · m²)*	*LVSWI (g · m/m²)*
1	20	14	83	Clinical LVF
2	31	26	206	Clinical LVF
3	27	21	86	33
4	23	14	277	Nuclear scan LV
5	27*	18	—	Clinical LVF
6	29	19	138	19
7	18	16	133	3
8	42	31	215	12
9	21	16	137	31
10	25	14	135	40
11	—	9	—	—
12	19	27	250	15
13	48	32	200	5.0 CI MR
14	16	12	134	1.4 CI

*Pulmonary artery diastolic pressure (PADP).

Abbreviations: MPAP = mean pulmonary artery pressure; nl = normal (nl 13 ± 5 mm Hg, mean ± SD)[38]; PCWP = pulmonary capillary wedge pressure (nl 7.5 ± 1.8 mm Hg, mean ± SD)[38]; PVR = pulmonary vascular resistance (nl 78 ± 22 dyne · s/cm^5 · m^2, mean ± SD)[38]; LVSWI = left ventricular stroke work index (nl 48 ± 6 g · m/m^2, mean ± SD)[38]; LVF = left ventricular failure; CI = cardiac index; MR = mitral regurgitant murmur.

Coagulopathy

In addition to hemodynamic collapse and pulmonary injury, 40% of patients surviving the initial hemodynamic insult may develop a coagulopathy, ranging from disseminated intravascular coagulation to minor disturbances in platelet count or other aberrations of coagulation.[54, 56] Although the nature of the coagulopathy demonstrated in humans with AFE syndrome has not been satisfactorily explained, the potent thromboplastin-like effects of trophoblasts are well established, and these effects may have a greater role in the

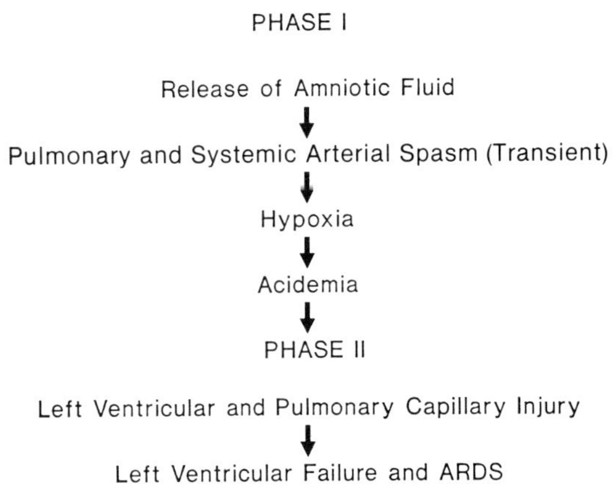

PHASE I

Release of Amniotic Fluid

↓

Pulmonary and Systemic Arterial Spasm (Transient)

↓

Hypoxia

↓

Acidemia

↓

PHASE II

Left Ventricular and Pulmonary Capillary Injury

↓

Left Ventricular Failure and ARDS

Figure 8–10. Hemodynamic alterations in human amniotic fluid embolism. Phase I is resolved within 30 minutes of the acute event, whereas phase II has been documented an hour or more following presumed embolization.

coagulopathy of AFE than has previously been appreciated. Clinical observation generally supports a more pronounced coagulopathy in those instances of meconium particulate contamination of the amniotic fluid, cases with overt chorioamnionitis at the time of the embolism, and cases with intrauterine fetal demise. In all of these settings, the fluid is apparently laden with materials capable of activating the extrinsic coagulation cascade.

Clinical Presentation

As previously outlined, AFE syndrome appears to be a biphasic process (see Fig. 8–10). The initial disturbances involve profound alterations in hemodynamics and oxygenation. In about 20% of cases, a clinically evident seizure occurs as one of the first observations. Similarly, some degree of consumptive coagulopathy can be demonstrated in up to 40% of cases, a bleeding diathesis alone being the presenting manifestation in 10% to 15% of cases.[54, 57, 58] The classic presentation, however, remains that of sudden dyspnea and variable degrees of hypotension. If a woman is still pregnant and fetal monitoring is being used, then the tracing may well show evidence of alterations in fetal heart rate patterns suggestive of compromise even before the woman experiences symptoms. Survivors of the initial hemodynamic collapse are at high risk for evolution of acute respiratory failure, occurring in up to 70% of patients. The respiratory failure appears to be secondary to a combination of depressed left ventricular function with elevated pressures; however, the degree of injury is disproportionate to the pressures and suggestive of a simultaneous permeability defect. Patients who develop a significant coagulopathy often have the hemorrhage compounded by concurrent uterine atony attributable to a myometrial depressant effect of amniotic fluid.[59] Coagulopathy is also frequently manifested by persistent bleeding from venipuncture sites and surgical wounds. Decreased fibrinogen, elevated levels of fibrin split products, prolonged partial thromboplastin and prothrombin times, and thrombocytopenia are common. Women who have required a cesarean delivery very often have obvious bleeding into the abdominal cavity. Caution is advised in reoperating on these women before correcting the coagulopathy with blood and blood products.

Diagnosis

The diagnosis of AFE can be made and classically has been made at autopsy via demonstration of squamous cells or debris in the pulmonary artery vasculature. In this setting, routine hematoxylin-eosin stain may be insufficient to demonstrate fetal elements and special stains such as acid mucopolysaccharide or Alcian blue may be required. The diagnosis of AFE syndrome is primarily based on the presentation and clinical history. Specimens of blood from the pulmonary artery have been touted for diagnosis, because squamous cells and other debris of presumed fetal origin have been aspirated from the central venous or pulmonary artery circulation of living patients with AFE syndrome. Unfortunately, similar debris has been recovered from healthy nonpregnant volunteers, as well as from specimens from men who had pulmonary artery catheters inserted for a host of indications.[52, 60]

When considering the AFE syndrome, it is important to evaluate alternative diagnoses, such as septic shock, aspiration pneumonia, acute myocardial infarction, pulmonary thromboembolism, and, when coagulopathy is a dominant feature, placental abruption. Finally, bupivacaine anesthetic toxicity presents a clinical picture that is virtually indistinguishable from AFE syndrome.

Treatment

Treatment is directed toward three goals: (1) oxygenation, (2) maintenance of both cardiac output and blood pressure, and (3) combating what is usually a self-limited coagulopathy. Generally accepted goals of therapy include maintenance of systolic blood pressure of greater than 90 mm Hg, urinary output of greater than 25 mL/h, and PaO_2 of greater than 60 mm Hg or hemoglobin saturation of greater than or equal to 90%. If a patient is in full cardiac arrest, cardiopulmonary resuscitation is instituted in much the same fashion as in a nonpregnant patient. Alterations in cardiopulmonary resuscitation are discussed subsequently. Oxygen should be administered in the highest concentrations that are readily available. If a patient is unconscious, she should be intubated and ventilated with 100% oxygen when feasible. Because maternal hypotension is usually secondary to cardiac shock, treatment includes optimization of cardiac preload by rapid volume infusion as well as early inotropic support with dopamine if the patient remains hypotensive. Because pulmonary injury is likely to occur from both ventricular dysfunction and alterations in pulmonary capillary permeability, institution of pulmonary artery catheterization is usually helpful in guiding hemodynamic management. After initial resuscitation and correction of hypotension, fluid therapy should be restricted to maintenance levels to minimize pulmonary edema. Abnormalities in clotting functions or clinical bleeding should be treated aggressively with specific components, and the clinician should avoid the temptation to re-explore the patient, even in the setting of intra-abdominal bleeding, until the coagulation defect has been corrected. In AFE syndrome, the liberal use of consultants is encouraged.

HYPERTENSION

Hypertensive disorders remain the second most common cause of maternal mortality in the United States. Pregnancy may induce hypertension in a previously normotensive gravida or exacerbate pressures in a chronically hypertensive patient (Table 8–3). How or why chorionic villi incite vasospasm, hypertension, and multiorgan dysfunction or failure is uncertain. However, there is no doubt that without skillful management, severe hypertensive disease may kill the mother and fetus. The goals of therapy for severe preeclampsia or eclampsia are simple: (1) prevent convulsions, (2) control extreme blood pressure elevations, and (3) effect

TABLE 8–3. Hypertensive Disease in Pregnancy

I. Pregnancy-induced hypertension
   A. Preeclampsia
      1. Mild
      2. Severe
   B. Eclampsia
II. Chronic hypertension
III. Chronic hypertension with superimposed pregnancy-induced hypertension
   A. Superimposed preeclampsia
   B. Superimposed eclampsia

TABLE 8–4. Signs and Symptoms of Severe Preeclampsia

Blood pressure	> 160/110 mm Hg
Proteinuria	> 5 g/24 h
Oliguria	< 400–500 mL/24 h
Central nervous system	Cerebral or visual disturbances
Pulmonary	Pulmonary edema or cyanosis
Gastrointestinal	Epigastric or right upper quadrant pain
	Impaired liver function
Hematologic	Thrombocytopenia

delivery. We review the definitions and pathophysiology of preeclampsia, severe preeclampsia and eclampsia superimposed on chronic hypertension, and controversies in management and outline a simple and time-proven management scheme. Severe preeclampsia and eclampsia should be considered obstetric emergencies because they may lead to long-term maternal multiple end-organ damage and even maternal and fetal death.

Hypertensive disease of pregnancy has been referred to by many names through the years, including *toxemia, gestosis, pregnancy-associated hypertension, pregnancy-induced hypertension, preeclampsia, eclampsia, preeclampsia superimposed on chronic hypertension,* and *transient hypertension.* In 1986, the American College of Obstetricians and Gynecologists proposed the following definitions and classifications of hypertensive disorders in pregnancy or puerperium.[61] Hypertension is defined as a diastolic blood pressure of 90 mm Hg or greater or a systolic blood pressure of 140 mm Hg or greater or a rise in diastolic blood pressure of at least 15 mm Hg or systolic blood pressure of 30 mm Hg above prepregnancy baseline. It is important to note that blood pressure normally drops 10 mm Hg in the first and second trimesters, and therefore, relative increases must be based on prepregnancy values. Preeclampsia is the development of hypertension with proteinuria, nondependent edema (usually visible in the face and hands and associated with a 5-lb weight gain per week) or both after 20 weeks' gestation. Proteinuria is defined as 300 mg or more in 24 hours or 100 mg/dL in at least two random urine specimens collected 6 hours apart. A preeclamptic woman who has no history of a seizure disorder and who develops convulsions is said to have eclampsia. Chronic hypertension implies hypertensive disease that either antedates pregnancy, is not associated with hydatidiform mole, or persists 6 weeks postpartum.

The pathophysiology of preeclampsia is incompletely understood and somewhat controversial. Various inciting causes have been suggested, including abnormal placentation, as well as immunologic, endocrine, and genetic responses to pregnancy. Regardless of the initial mechanism, preeclampsia is characterized by generalized vasospasm. Women with preeclampsia or eclampsia exhibit an increased vascular reactivity to vasoactive agents. Gant and colleagues observed that normotensive gravidas were refractory to the effect of infused angiotensin II, whereas women destined to become preeclamptic failed to develop pregnancy-induced refractoriness to angiotensin II.[62] Vasospasm or sensitivity to vasoactive agents in gravidas with preeclampsia may be due to a relative prostaglandin imbalance with an increase in thromboxane A_2 and prostaglandin F_2 (vasoconstrictive prostaglandins) as compared with prostaglandin I_2 and prostaglandin E (vasodilating prostaglandins).[63] The National Institute of Child Health and Disease Maternal-Fetal Medicine Network conducted a double-blind placebo-controlled trial of low-dose aspirin in an attempt to reduce hypertensive disease in pregnancy.[64] No differences in gestational hypertension or perinatal outcomes were noted between the aspirin and placebo group. Importantly, use of aspirin was associated with a higher incidence of abruptio placentae. Thus, to date, no known method exists to predict which gravidas will develop preeclampsia, and no proven therapy can prevent its onset. We now focus our attention on the diagnosis and management of severe hypertensive disease.

Severe preeclampsia is diagnosed when blood pressure exceeds 160/110 mm Hg or when maternal end-organ disease or placental abruption, fetal growth retardation, fetal distress, or fetal death is evident. Signs and symptoms of severe preeclampsia are listed in Table 8–4. Importantly, preeclampsia of any severity can rapidly evolve to eclampsia or severe preeclampsia. Convulsions are usually but not always preceded by any of the following: scotomata, right upper quadrant pain, hyperreflexia, thrombocytopenia, or hemoconcentration. In the authors' experience, epigastric or right upper quadrant pain, believed secondary to hepatocellular necrosis and stretching of Glisson's capsule due to edema, is a most ominous sign. Laboratory abnormalities consistent with preeclampsia (Table 8–5) may include hemoconcentration, thrombocytopenia, and renal and hepatic insufficiency. In the United States, the medication most commonly used to control and prevent eclamptic seizures is magnesium sulfate ($MgSO_4 \cdot 7H_2O$ USP). The mechanism of action of $MgSO_4$ is controversial, but evidence suggests it acts centrally on the cerebral cortex.[65] Plasma magnesium levels between 4 and 7 mEq/L (4.8–8.4 mg/dL) are reported to be therapeutic for seizure prophylaxis. Pritchard and associates[65] reported a combined regimen of intravenous and intramuscular $MgSO_4$ in which 4 g of 20% $MgSO_4 \cdot 7H_2O$ was given IV over 2 to 4 minutes and 10 g was given IM (5 g in each buttock) as a loading dose, followed by 5 g IM every 4 hours.[66] Because intramuscular administration is painful, we prefer to load $MgSO_4$ with 4 g IV over 2 to 6 minutes, followed by a continuous intravenous infusion of 2 g/h. Careful attention is paid to signs of magnesium toxicity (Table 8–6) and to serum magnesium levels, and the dosage adjusted accordingly. Importantly, magnesium is secreted in the urine, and women with severe preeclampsia may indeed have or develop renal insufficiency. We therefore advocate placing a Foley catheter and monitoring serum creatinine values, and we strictly record and monitor intravenous fluid input and urine output. In an eclamptic

TABLE 8–5. Laboratory Abnormalities That May Be Consistent with Preeclampsia

Hematocrit	Increased
Platelet count	Decreased
Serum glutamic-oxaloacetic transaminase	Increased
Prothrombin time/partial thromboplastin time	Increased
Serum creatinine level	Increased

TABLE 8–6. Signs and Symptoms of Progressive Hypermagnesemia

Hot flushes	Respiratory arrest
Loss of reflexes	Cardiac arrest
Respiratory depression	

woman who has a seizure before initiation of $MgSO_4$ seizure prophylaxis, care must be taken during the seizure to prevent injury and protect her airway from aspiration. The initial 4 g IV infusion is administered. Most seizures end during $MgSO_4$ administration. If seizure activity continues, another 2 g IV of $MgSO_4$ may be given. If seizures continue, various treatments including amobarbital, diazepam, pentobarbital, and thiopental (Table 8–7) have been successful. Once seizures are arrested, serum magnesium levels may be measured and $MgSO_4$ infusion adjusted accordingly.

Phenytoin, which is commonly used to treat epilepsy, has been advocated for use for seizure prophylaxis and treatment in preeclampsia and eclampsia. The small studies in which it has been given to prevent seizures in eclamptic women are unconvincing. Dommisse, in a randomized study of $MgSO_4$ versus phenytoin, noted a 36% failure rate in women given phenytoin despite therapeutic serum levels.[67] In a report of nearly 5000 preeclamptic women given $MgSO_4$ for seizure prophylaxis, Cunningham and Leveno reported a failure rate of 1 in 700.[68] Thus, in America, $MgSO_4$ remains the treatment of choice for seizure prophylaxis and treatment of women with preeclampsia or eclampsia.

The degree to which blood pressure should be lowered remains controversial, because a profound decrease in blood pressure may result in uteroplacental insufficiency and subsequent fetal distress. Thus, the goal of antihypertensive therapy in severe preeclampsia is not normotension but prevention of extremes of blood pressure. We recommend maintaining diastolic levels between 90 and 110 mm Hg. Many agents have been administered to women with severe hypertension to control blood pressure (Table 8–8). Lindheimer and Katz and the report of the National High Blood Pressure Education Program Working Groups suggested guidelines for treating severe hypertension during labor; intravenous hydralazine remains the most widely studied and the drug of choice.[69, 70] Fetal distress presumably due to decreased placental blood flow rarely occurs when small intravenous doses of hydralazine are used to maintain diastolic blood pressure between 90 and 110 mm Hg.[4] We recommend an initial 5-mg IV bolus and then administration of 5 to 10 mg every 20 minutes. Labetalol, an α- and β-adrenergic blocker, has had more widespread use. Patients may receive an initial dose of 20 mg IV with escalating doses of 20, 40, 80, 80, and 80 mg every 10 minutes to a maximum cumulative dose of 300 mg or until the desired diastolic blood pressure is obtained.[71] A constant labetalol infusion of 0.5 mg · kg^{-1} · h^{-1} with an increase in dose every 30 minutes by 0.5 mg · kg^{-1} · h^{-1} to a maximum of 3 mg · kg^{-1} · h^{-1} has also been described.[72]

TABLE 8–7. Secondary Agents for Treatment of Eclamptic Seizures

Initial Agent	*Intravenous Dose (mg)*
Amobarbital	250
Diazepam	1–10
Thiopental	100
Pentobarbital	100

TABLE 8–8. Therapies for Treating Severe Hypertension in Pregnancy

Agent	*Dosage*
Hydralazine	5 mg IV bolus, followed by 5–10 mg every 20–30 min
Labetalol	20 mg IV, followed by escalating doses every 10 min to a maximum cumulative dose of 300 mg
Diazoxide	30-mg miniboluses
Sodium nitroprusside	0.25 μg · kg^{-1} · min^{-1}, increasing by 0.25 μg · kg^{-1} · min^{-1} every 5 min titrated to effect
Nifedipine	10 mg PO, repeated in 30 min if necessary

There should be little doubt that severe preeclampsia near or at term warrants delivery of the fetus. Remote from term, attempts to temporize may be taken; however, we strongly believe that delivery should be accomplished regardless of fetal age if severe hypertension or evidence of progressive end-organ damage persists after a period of observation.

The route of delivery (i.e., vaginal or cesarean) is based on an evaluation of maternal and fetal risks. Vaginal delivery, if accomplishable and tolerated by the fetus, is nearly always safer for the mother. Induction of labor with intravenous oxytocin and continuous electronic fetal monitoring may be used by various regimens.[73, 74]

The use of lumbar epidural analgesia in severely preeclamptic women in active labor must be performed with caution by individuals with special training and familiarity with this disease. Specifically, hypotension with resultant decreased uteroplacental insufficiency must be averted while avoiding central volume overload in women with possible pulmonary capillary leak. Epidural analgesia for labor and vaginal delivery may reduce pain, anxiety, and catecholamines and may lead to less extremes of hypertension. However, the use of epidural analgesia may be contraindicated in women with evidence of a fulminant coagulopathy. Unfortunately, to date, a randomized study of the efficacy and safety of epidural analgesia versus general anesthesia for women with severe preeclampsia is nonexistent.

General anesthesia may be accomplished rapidly and should be the anesthetic choice in cases of acute fetal distress. Furthermore, general anesthesia is rarely associated with hypertension, and the amount of intervention with volume expansion is less than with epidural anesthetics. Concern had been raised that severe hypertension after tracheal intubation may increase maternal intracranial pressure and result in significant neurologic and circulatory morbidity.[75] Despite this concern, to date, not a single case of a preeclamptic woman sustaining central nervous system hemorrhage during tracheal intubation has been reported.[76]

Administration of large volumes of fluid to severely preeclamptic women, whether to avoid or treat hypotension resulting from medical therapy or epidural-induced sympathetic blockade, is problematic.[77, 78] Although women who have severe preeclampsia and eclampsia often manifest oliguria and may have intravascular contraction, aggressive fluid infusion may lead to pulmonary and cerebral edema.[79] This phenomenon probably results from internal damage to the vessels and inappropriately distributed fluid between intravascular and extravascular spaces. The risk of pulmonary edema increases postpartum because some women mobilize their extravascular volume before the initiation of diuresis.[22]

For women with severe preeclampsia with oliguria before delivery, some have advocated use of invasive central hemodynamic monitoring. The American College of Obstetricians and Gynecologists has concluded that the majority of severely preeclamptic women can and should be cared for without invasive monitoring.[7]

Clark and associates described three hemodynamic subsets of preeclampsia with oliguria based on Swan-Ganz measurements (Table 8–9).[80] They advocated volume replacement for those with a low PCWP, low-dose dopamine for those with a normal PCWP, and fluid restriction for those with an increased PCWP. Although invasive hemodynamic monitoring has been an excellent research tool, the fact that most women with preeclampsia have decreased or contracted plasma volume[80] suggests that most patients would fall into Clark's first subset, Clark's second subset would be rare, and the third subset may result from overly aggressive fluid management (see Table 8–9).

Fluid management of severe preeclampsia during labor and before delivery requires strict monitoring of fluid intake and output. The authors place a Foley catheter and a pulse co-oximeter and attempt to infuse no more than 125 mL of fluid per hour, including the fluid incorporated in the oxytocin and $MgSO_4$ infusions. If urine output becomes less than 100 to 120 mL in a 4-hour period, a single fluid challenge of 500 to 1000 mL of normal saline is administered. If no response occurs, no further fluid challenges are performed. If pulmonary edema develops secondary to ventricular failure or fluid overload, most of these women respond quickly to intravenous furosemide. Oliguria associated with preeclampsia, unless also associated with blood loss, reverses after delivery; thus, vigorous hydration with colloids, crystalloid, or volume expanders appears to be unnecessary and potentially dangerous.[79] Invasive monitoring should be considered when multiple compounding conditions are present along with preeclampsia, as in sepsis or underlying maternal cardiopulmonary disease. Importantly, if central invasive hemodynamic monitoring is needed, then a pulmonary artery catheter is needed. Central venous pressure when low normal does not correlate with PCWP in women with preeclampsia.[81] Management decisions (i.e., volume expansion) based on central venous pressure readings may be dangerous. Labor should be closely monitored with continuous fetal heart rate monitoring and uterine tocodynamometry because uteroplacental insufficiency with concomitant fetal distress and placental abruption may occur. Furthermore, pediatric specialists should be advised of the maternal condition and should be available at the time of delivery.

In summary, the time-proven antepartum therapy for severe preeclampsia or eclampsia includes $MgSO_4$ for seizure prophylaxis, intravenous hydralazine for extremes of hypertension, meticulous fluid therapy, and delivery.

After delivery, a woman with severe preeclampsia may be less tolerant of blood loss because she does not possess the usual "hypervolemia" of pregnancy. With an average blood loss of approximately 500 mL at vaginal delivery and 1500 mL with cesarean, a preeclamptic woman may lose approximately one third of her blood volume at delivery.

TABLE 8–9. Clark's Hemodynamic Subsets in PIH Complicated by Oliguria

Subset	*Pulmonary Capillary Wedge Pressure*	*Systemic Vascular Resistance*	*Ventricular Function*
1	Low	Increased	Hyperdynamic
2	Normal or slight increase	Normal	Normal
3	High	High	Depressed

This loss, combined with the possibility of capillary endothelial leak secondary to vasospasm in preeclampsia, suggests that when oliguria follows delivery, hematocrit should be checked and excessive blood loss should be treated with blood transfusion. Importantly, hypertensive women who become "cured" and are normotensive may really be exhibiting intravascular volume depletion. Maintenance of hematocrit greater than 25% to 30% and urine output greater than 30 mL/h with aggressive use of blood transfusion is time proven and still an effective therapeutic goal. $MgSO_4$ should be continued for a minimum of 24 hours postpartum and sometimes longer if elevations of blood pressure do not resolve.

SUMMARY

The most practical, efficient, and economical means of caring for critically ill obstetric patients who require invasive monitoring and ventilatory support or both depend on the number of pregnant women cared for at a particular facility, including women referred to that facility. Although some obstetric services have a sufficient volume and acuity of such women, the majority encounter fewer than 20 such patients per year. Accordingly, arrangements are needed either to care for these women in surgical or medical intensive care units or to have specialized rooms designated in the labor and delivery suite where necessary equipment quickly can be assembled to provide appropriate care. For a woman who is undelivered, ideal care is provided best by specially trained obstetricians and obstetric nurses with extensive knowledge and experience in critical care medicine. In the absence of such key individuals, a team of physicians and nurses is assembled to include those with special expertise sufficient to deal with all problem areas. Physician members of the team should include an obstetrician, assisted by other providers who may include anesthesiologists, pulmonologists, cardiologists, nephrologists, and intensivists. With an ongoing pregnancy, both obstetric and intensive care nurses may be required.

The medical record of women needing such care is very likely to come under subsequent review. Accordingly, documentation and clarity of the record not only assist with the ongoing day-to-day care but also stand one well in any subsequent reviews. In taking care of such women, it is important to recognize that with the crossover of multiple specialties, many professional standards and guidelines may need to be met simultaneously. Included would be those promulgated by organizations such as the Society of Critical Care Medicine, the American College of Obstetricians and Gynecologists, and the Association of Women's Health Obstetrics and Neonatal Nursing. As regards care of obstetric patients, familiarity with Standards for Obstetric-Gynecologic Services and Guidelines for Perinatal Care is recommended.[82, 83]

References

1. Scott DE: Anesthesia during pregnancy. Obstet Gynecol Annu 1972; 1:219.
2. Lund CJ, Donovan JC: Blood volume during pregnancy. Am J Obstet Gynecol 1967; 98:393.
3. Pritchard JA: Changes in the blood volume during pregnancy and delivery. Anesthesiology 1965; 26:393.
4. Pritchard JA, Cunningham FG, Pritchard SA: The Parkland Memorial Hospital protocol for treatment of eclampsia: Evaluation of 245 cases. Am J Obstet Gynecol 1984; 148:951.
5. Wilson M, Morganti AA, Zervodakis I, et al: Blood pressure, the renin-aldosterone system, and sex steroids throughout normal pregnancy. Am J Med 1980; 68:97.

6. Clark SL, Cotton DB, Lee W, et al: Central hemodynamic assessment of normal term pregnancy. Am J Obstet Gynecol 1989; 161:1439.
7. American College of Obstetricians and Gynecologists: Invasive Hemodynamic Monitoring in Obstetrics and Gynecology. ACOG Technical Bulletin 175. Washington, DC, ACOG, 1992.
8. Bader RA, Bader MG, Rose DJ, et al: Hemodynamics at rest and during exercise in normal pregnancy as studied by cardiac catheterization. J Clin Invest 1955; 34:1524.
9. Walters WAW, Lim YL: Cardiovascular dynamics in women receiving oral contraceptive therapy. Lancet 1969; 2:879.
10. Greiss FC, Anderson SG: Effect of ovarian hormones on the uterine vascular bed. Am J Obstet Gynecol 1970; 107:829.
11. Gerber JG, Payne NA, Murphy RC, et al: Prostacyclin produced by the pregnant uterus in the dog may act as a circulating vasodepressor substance. J Clin Invest 1981; 67:632.
12. Rosenthal MH: Intrapartum intensive care management of the cardiac patient. Clin Obstet Gynecol 1981; 24:789.
13. Ueland K, Hansen JM: Maternal cardiovascular dynamics. II. Posture and uterine contractions. Am J Obstet Gynecol 1969; 103:1.
14. Ueland K, Hansen JM: Maternal cardiovascular dynamics. III. Labor and delivery under local and caudal anesthesia. Am J Obstet Gynecol 1969; 103:8.
15. Ueland K, Metcalfe J: Circulatory changes in pregnancy. Clin Obstet Gynecol 1975; 18:41.
16. Adams JQ, Alexander AM: Alterations in cardiovascular physiology during labor. Obstet Gynecol 1958; 12:542.
17. Hendricks CH, Quilligan EJ: Cardiac output during labor. Am J Obstet Gynecol 1958; 76:969.
18. Hankins GDV, Wendel GD, Leveno KJ, et al: Myocardial infarction during pregnancy. A review. Obstet Gynecol 1985; 65:139.
19. Adams JQ: Cardiovascular physiology in normal pregnancy: Studies with the dye-dilution technique. Am J Obstet Gynecol 1964; 67:741.
20. Metcalfe J: Oxygen supply and fetal growth. J Reprod Med 1985; 30:301.
21. Chesley LC, Valenti C, Uichano L: Alterations in body fluid compartments and exchangeable sodium in early puerperium. Am J Obstet Gynecol 1959; 77:1054.
22. Hankins GDV, Wendel GD Jr, Cunningham FG, et al: Longitudinal evaluation of hemodynamic changes in eclampsia. Am J Obstet Gynecol 1984; 150:506.
23. de Swiet M: The respiratory system. *In*: Clinical Physiology in Obstetrics. 2nd ed. Hytten F, Chamberlain G (Eds). London, Blackwell Scientific Publications, 1991, pp 83–100.
24. Bevan DR, Holcroft A, Loh L, et al: Closing volume and pregnancy. Br Med J 1974; 1:13.
25. Holcroft A, Bevan DR, O'Sullivan JC, et al: Airway closure and pregnancy. Anaesthesia 1977; 32:517.
26. Weinberger SE, Weiss ST, Cohen WR, et al: Pregnancy and the lung. Am Rev Respir Dis 1980; 121:559.
27. Noble PW, Lavee AE, Jacobs MM: Respiratory diseases in pregnancy. Obstet Gynecol Clin North Am 1988; 15:391–428.
28. Awe RJ, Nicotra MB, Newsom TD, et al: Arterial oxygenation and alveolar-arterial gradients in term pregnancy. Obstet Gynecol 1979; 53:182.
29. Oian P, Maltau JM, Noddeland H, et al: Oedema-preventing mechanisms in subcutaneous tissue of normal pregnant women. Br J Obstet Gynaecol 1985; 92:1113.
30. Oian P, Maltau JM: Calculated capillary hydrostatic pressure in normal pregnancy and preeclampsia. Am J Obstet Gynecol 1987; 157:102.
31. Robertson EG, Cheyne GA: Plasma biochemistry in relation to oedema of pregnancy. J Obstet Gynaecol Br Commonw 1972; 79:769.
31a. Weil MH, Morissette S, Michaels S, et al: Routine plasma colloid osmotic pressure measurements. Crit Care Med 1974; 2:229.
32. Nguyen HN, Clark SL, Greenspoon J, et al: Peripartum colloid osmotic pressures: Correlation with serum proteins. Obstet Gynecol 1986; 68:807.
33. Benedetti TJ, Carlson RW: Studies of colloid osmotic pressure in pregnancy-induced hypertension. Am J Obstet Gynecol 1979; 135:308.
34. Cotton DB, Gonik B, Spillman T, et al: Intrapartum to postpartum changes in colloid osmotic pressure. Am J Obstet Gynecol 1984; 149:174.
35. Peckham CH, King RW: A study of intercurrent conditions observed during pregnancy. Am J Obstet Gynecol 1963; 87:609.
36. Pearlman MD, Tintinalli JE, Lorenz RP: A prospective controlled study of outcome after trauma during pregnancy. Am J Obstet Gynecol 1990; 162:1502.
37. Goodwin TM, Breen MT: Pregnancy outcome and fetomaternal hemorrhage after noncatastrophic trauma. Am J Obstet Gynecol 1990; 162:665.
38. Pearlman MD, Tintinalli JE, Lorenz RP: Blunt trauma during pregnancy. N Engl J Med 1990; 323:1609.
39. Rothenberger D, Quattlebaum FW, Perry JF Jr, et al: Blunt maternal trauma: A review of 103 cases. J Trauma 1978; 18:173.
40. Helton AS, McFarlane J, Anderson ET: Battered and pregnant: a prevalence study. Am J Public Health 1987; 77:1337.
41. Elliott M: Vehicular accidents and pregnancy. Aust N Z J Obstet Gynaecol 1966; 6:279.
42. Crosby WM, Costiloe JP: Safety of lap-belt restraint for pregnant victims of automobile collisions. N Engl J Med 1971; 284:632.
43. Crosby WM, Snyder RG, Snow CC, et al: Impact injuries in pregnancy. I. Experimental studies. Am J Obstet Gynecol 1968; 101:100.
44. Buchsbaum HJ: Penetrating injury of the abdomen. *In*: Trauma in Pregnancy. Buchsbaum HJ (Ed). Philadelphia, WB Saunders, 1979, pp 82–100.
45. Esposito TJ, Gens DR, Smith LG, et al: Evaluation of blunt abdominal trauma occurring during pregnancy. J Trauma 1989; 29:1628.
46. Williams JK, McClain L, Rosemurgy AS, et al: Evaluation of blunt abdominal trauma in the third trimester of pregnancy: maternal and fetal considerations. Obstet Gynecol 1990; 75:33.
47. Mostello DJ, Jacobson RL, Siddiqui TA: Surveillance after noncatastrophic trauma in the pregnant patient: How much is enough? Abstract No. 97. Presented at the Tenth Annual Meeting of the Society of Perinatal Obstetricians; January 23–27, 1990.
48. Rose PG, Strohm PL, Zuspan FP: Fetomaternal hemorrhage following trauma. Am J Obstet Gynecol 1985; 153:844–847.
49. Meyer JR: Brasil-medico 1926; 2:301.
50. Steiner PE, Luschbaugh CC: Maternal pulmonary embolism by amniotic fluid. JAMA 1941; 117:1245.
51. Liban E, Raz S: A clinicopathologic study of fourteen cases of amniotic fluid embolism. Am J Clin Pathol 1969; 51:477.
52. Clark SL, Greenspoon JS, Aldahl D, et al: Severe preeclampsia with persistent oliguria: Management of hemodynamic subsets. Am J Obstet Gynecol 1986; 154:490.
53. Hankins GDV, Snyder RR, Clark SL, et al: Acute hemodynamic and respiratory effects of amniotic fluid embolism in the pregnant goat model. Am J Obstet Gynecol 1993; 168:1113.
54. Clark SL: Amniotic fluid embolism. Clin Perinatol 1986; 13:801.
55. Richards DS, Carter LS, Corke B, et al: The effect of human amniotic fluid on the isolated perfused rat heart. Am J Obstet Gynecol 1988; 158:210.
56. Cron RS, Kilkenny GS, Wirthwein C, et al: Amniotic fluid embolism. Am J Obstet Gynecol 1952; 64:1360.
57. Courtney LD, Allington LM: Effect of amniotic fluid on blood coagulation. Br J Haematol 1972; 113:911.
58. Morgan M: Amniotic fluid embolism. Anaesthesia 1979; 34:29.
59. Courtney LD: Amniotic fluid embolism. Obstet Gynecol Surv 1974; 29:169.
60. Lee W, Ginsburg KA, Cotton DB, et al: Squamous and trophoblastic cells in the maternal pulmonary circulation identified by invasive hemodynamic monitoring during the peripartum period. Am J Obstet Gynecol 1986; 155:999.
61. American College of Obstetricians and Gynecologists: Management of Preeclampsia. ACOG Technical Bulletin 91. Washington, DC, ACOG, 1986.
62. Gant NF, Daley GL, Chand S, et al: A study of angiotensin II pressor response throughout primigravid pregnancy. J Clin Invest 1973; 52:2682.
63. Romero R, Lockwood C, Oyarzun E, et al: Toxemia: New concepts in an old disease. Semin Perinatol 1988; 12:302.
64. Sibai B, Caritis S, Phillips E, et al: Prevention of preeclampsia: Low-dose aspirin in nulliparous women: A double-blind placebo controlled trial. Am J Obstet Gynecol 1993; 168:286.

65. Pritchard JA: The use of magnesium sulfate in preeclampsia-eclampsia. J Reprod Med 1979; 23:107.
66. Borges LF, Guler G: Effect of magnesium on epileptic foci. Epilepsia 1978; 19:81.
67. Dommisse J: Phenytoin sodium and magnesium sulphate in the management of eclampsia. Br J Obstet Gynaecol 1990; 97:104.
68. Cunningham FG, Leveno KJ: Management of Pregnancy-Induced Hypertension. Handbook of Hypertension. New York, Elsevier, 1988.
69. Lindheimer MD, Katz AI: Hypertension in pregnancy. N Engl J Med 1985; 313:675.
70. National High Blood Pressure Education Program Working Group report on high blood pressure during pregnancy. Am J Obstet Gynecol 1990; 163:1689.
71. Mabie WC, Gonzales AR, Sibai BM, et al: A comparative trial of labetalol and hydralazine in the acute management of severe hypertension complicating pregnancy. Obstet Gynecol 1987; 70:328.
72. Michael CA: Intravenous labetalol and intravenous diazoxide in severe hypertension complications in pregnancy. Aust N Z J Obstet Gynecol 1986; 26:26.
73. American College of Obstetricians and Gynecologists: Induction and augmentation of labor. ACOG Technical Bulletin 157. Washington, DC, ACOG, 1991.
74. Satin AJ, Leveno KJ, Sherman ML, et al: High- versus low-dose oxytocin for labor stimulation. Obstet Gynecol 1992; 80:111.
75. Fox EJ, Sklar GS, Hill CH, et al: Complications related to the pressor response to endotracheal intubation. Anesthesiology 1977; 47:524.
76. Hankins GDV, Cunningham FG: Severe preeclampsia and eclampsia: Controversies in management. Williams Obstetrics. 18th ed. Suppl 12. Norwalk, CT, Appleton & Lange, 1991.
77. Benedetti TJ, Kales, Williams V: Hemodynamic observations in severe preeclamptic complicated by pulmonary edema. Am J Obstet Gynecol 1985; 152:330.
78. Kirshon B, Moise KJ, Cotton DB, et al: Role of volume expansion in severe preeclampsia. Surg Obstet Gynecol 1988; 167:367.
79. Cunningham FG, MacDonald PC, Gant NF: Williams Obstetrics. 18th ed. Norwalk, CT, Appleton & Lange, 1989.
80. Clark SL, Pavlova A, Horenstein J, et al: Squamous cells in the maternal pulmonoembolism. Am J Obstet Gynecol 1986; 154:104.
81. Clark SL, Cotton DB: Clinical indications for pulmonary artery catheterization in the patient with severe preeclampsia. Am J Obstet Gynecol 1988; 158:453.
82. American College of Obstetricians and Gynecologists: Standards for Obstetric-Gynecologic Services. 7th ed. Washington, DC, ACOG, 1989.
83. American Academy of Pediatrics and the American College of Obstetricians and Gynecologists: Guidelines for Perinatal Care. 3rd ed. Washington, DC, ACOG, 1992.

CHAPTER 9

Evaluation of the Child After Resuscitation and Stabilization

Peter R. Holbrook, MD

Diagnostic evaluation of the child after resuscitation and stabilization occasionally occurs in the adult intensive care unit. It should be emphasized that the variety of diagnostic possibilities and the relative rarity of life-threatening events in childhood should lead the careful physician to consult a qualified pediatric specialist. While such consultation is actively being sought—or, in the rare case, when it is difficult to obtain—some diagnostic guidelines may be helpful.

TRAUMA

Children rarely survive cardiac arrest that is caused by trauma. In those few who do, the diagnosis and therapy will have occurred at the time of the initial evaluation. More commonly seen is the child who has been resuscitated from hypovolemic shock. The source of the blood loss that has led to hypovolemic shock may not be immediately apparent. In children, blood can "hide" around pelvic or femoral fractures or in the retroperitoneal space. Bleeding in the latter region may be associated with blunt abdominal trauma but with minimal physical findings. It is understood that bleeding inside the skull that is sufficient to cause hypovolemic symptoms in a child does not occur without dominant neurologic findings; however, profuse bleeding from a scalp wound may be sufficient to cause shock in a child (see Chapter 159).

The cause of a traumatic incident may not be clear. In any child, especially in one under the age of 3 years, the possibility of child abuse or neglect should be carefully considered. An implausible explanation for a child's injuries or parental inconsistency on questioning should trigger concern. If abuse or neglect is suspected, the physician is obligated by law to report the event to the appropriate authorities and is generally excluded from civil or criminal liability.

CARDIORESPIRATORY ARREST

Successful resuscitation from cardiac arrest in a child is rare (see also Chapter 7). Primarily, this is a result of the paucity of primary, reversible rhythm disturbances in childhood. Similarly, if restoration of spontaneous circulation has occurred, the child should be assessed for primary rhythm disturbances. Arrhythmias in children are not due to coronary artery disease except in certain families with a history of hyperlipidemia. Rather, they are primary in nature, such as prolonged QT syndrome or Wolff-Parkinson-White syndrome. Ventricular dysrhythmias are commonly found in adolescents and are rarely problematic.

Cardiac infections may cause sudden death. Myocarditis may escape clinical detection prior to the onset of lethal dysrhythmia or overwhelming congestive heart failure. Pericarditis with effusion may cause tamponade symptomatology.

Idiopathic hypertrophic subaortic stenosis develops in adolescence and may cause sudden death on exertion. An additional cause of death on exertion is congenital coronary abnormality (most commonly, the presence of an aberrant left coronary artery).

RESPIRATORY ARREST

Successful resuscitation of a child from respiratory arrest is substantially more likely. Causes of respiratory collapse include airway obstruction, which usually (but not invariably) occurs in a child under the age of 2 years. Obstruction may be at the supraglottic (as in diphtheria, supraglottitis, or related syndromes), glottic (ingestion of foreign bodies or the presence of congenital malformations at or near the vocal cords), or subglottic (as with croup and bacterial tracheitis) areas. Chronic airway obstruction may result in apnea. In both acute and chronic situations, stridor is usually elicited on the taking of the patient's history. An exception to this is the child whose obstruction is due to a foreign body (see Chapter 81).

The number of pediatric deaths due to asthma has been increasing. Although the majority of fatalities continue to be caused by progressive respiratory failure that develops over a period of hours or days, death due to asthma of sudden onset and short duration is being increasingly recognized. In the latter case, children may have symptoms of less than 1 hour's duration and may present to the medical care system with cardiac arrest. The occurrence of sudden onset asthma is not confined to patients with historically severe asthma,[1] and biologic differences among such children (increased neutrophil counts compared with eosinophil counts in the airway submucosa) have been reported.[2] Additional information on asthma may be found in Chapter 82.

CENTRAL NERVOUS SYSTEM COLLAPSE

Catastrophic intracranial events may occur without warning in children. Most frequently, they result from increased intracranial pressure. Inapparent asphyxia, unwitnessed trauma to the head or higher cervical cord, or intracranial bleeding may be underlying causes. A patient may complain of a severe headache before collapsing with intracranial bleeding (aneurysm, arteriovenous malformation, or bleeding into a tumor), or he or she may have no symptoms before collapse. Patients may experience unwitnessed status epilepticus, which renders them unconscious. Electroencephalography is indicated in these cases (see Chapter 172).

VASCULAR COLLAPSE

Overwhelming sepsis is a risk for a child of any age, but it is particularly common in newborns and immunosuppressed children. It may be confused with coarctation of the aorta in the newborn (which is distinguished by weak or absent femoral pulses) or with ingestions (see Chapter 130). Carbon monoxide poisoning is a risk if the child's history reveals exposure to fuel combustion. Similarly, the classic triad of polydipsia, polyuria, and polyphagia may go unnoticed in the active child until diabetic ketoacidosis becomes manifest. Dehydration due to fluid loss is usually evident clinically. Aggressive efforts to restore fluid balance are essential.

For additional information on sudden death in children, the reader is referred to a recent review.[3]

It should be noted that it is not always possible to determine a precise cause of death in children. Sudden infant death syndrome is, by definition, due to uncertain cause and accounts for over 50% of deaths in children between the ages of 1 month and 1 year. Even in older children, complete autopsy findings may fail to reveal a cause in as many as 10% of patients.

References

1. Robertson CF, Rubinfeld AR, Bowes G: Pediatric asthma deaths in Victoria: The mild are at risk. Pediatr Pulmonol 1992; 13:95–100.
2. Sur S, Crotty TB, Kephart GM, et al: Sudden onset fatal asthma: A distinct entity with few eosinophils and relatively more neutrophils in airway submucosa. Am Rev Respir Dis 1993; 148:713–719.
3. Holbrook PR: Sudden unexpected death. *In*: Textbook of Pediatric Critical Care. Holbrook PR (Ed). Philadelphia, WB Saunders, 1993, pp 94–97.

CHAPTER 10

Near-Drowning: Adults and Children

Salvatore R. Goodwin, MD • Philip G. Boysen, MD, FACP, FCCM • Jerome H. Modell, MD

Drowning has been defined in numerous ways. Modell defined *drowning without aspiration* as death secondary to respiratory obstruction and asphyxia while submerged in water. He defined *drowning with aspiration* as death secondary to changes from aspiration of water while submerged. *Near-drowning without aspiration* is survival, at least initially, after asphyxia from submersion in water. *Near-drowning with aspiration* describes survival, at least initially, after aspiration of and submersion in water. Modell later revised these definitions as follows: *To drown, with or without aspiration,* is to die while submerged in water. *To near-drown, with or without aspiration,* is to suffocate by submersion in water and to survive at least temporarily. *Delayed death* may occur secondary to near-drowning after an apparently successful initial resuscitation.

In 1980 Levin suggested the following definitions[1]: *Drowning* is a submersion injury that causes death within 24 hours of the incident. *Near-drowning* is a submersion injury after which the patient survives for at least 24 hours. Many of these patients eventually die from organ damage caused by the initial injury or from complications resulting from that injury. The latter set of definitions is frequently used among clinicians caring for children.[2]

Over the past five decades, the emphasis on the pathophysiologic changes that occur during drowning and near-drowning has shifted. During the 1940s and 1950s, the emphasis was primarily on the changes in serum electrolyte concentrations, blood volume, and blood density that occurred under experimental conditions of drowning by total immersion. During the 1960s and 1970s, pulmonary insufficiency, acid-base changes, and changes in cardiovascular performance that occurred after near-drowning were emphasized. In the 1980s, techniques reputed to minimize neurologic damage were highlighted, and early reports appeared promising. Although the latter issue remains an important concern, to date no intervention has been shown conclusively to alter recovery from neurologic injury that occurs secondary to near-drowning.[3–5] Until such time as effective cerebral resuscitation interventions are discovered, it seems that the most significant impact on this important public health problem will likely be in the areas of prevention and rescuer care. In this chapter, we address the issues of epidemiology, pathophysiology, treatment, and prevention of near-drowning as well as issues of outcome prediction.

EPIDEMIOLOGY

Drowning is responsible for the loss of more than 9000 lives annually in the United States.[6] It ranks as the fourth most common cause of injury-related death in all age groups, the third in toddlers, and the second in unintentional injury among adolescents (Table 10–1). Although these data are from a national data base, individual regions may vary considerably with respect to the prevalence of drowning. In Milwaukee County, Wisconsin, drowning ranks third be-

TABLE 10–1. Fatal Injuries to Children (<19 Years), 1986

Cause	*Number*
Motor vehicle accidents	10,535
Homicide	2877
Suicide	2151
Drowning	2062
Fire/burns	1619

(Adapted with permission from Fatal injuries to children—United States, 1986. MMWR 1990; 39:442–551.)

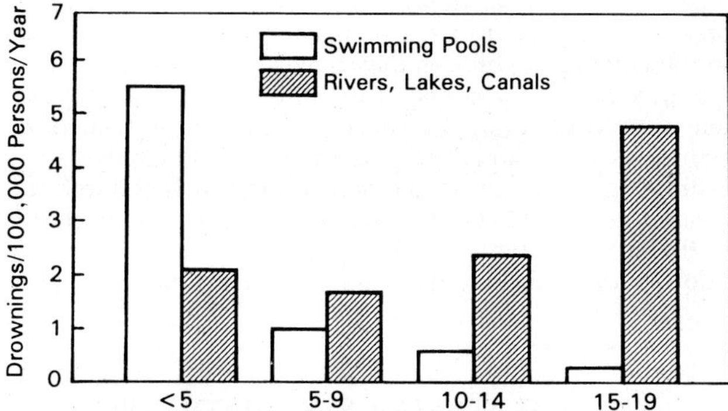

Figure 10–2. Drowning rates by age at selected sites in Sacramento County, CA, among children aged 0 to 19 years from 1974 to 1984. (From Wintemute GJ, Kraus JF, Teret SP, et al: Drowning in childhood and adolescence: A population based study. Am J Public Health 1987; 77:830. Copyright 1987, American Public Health Association.)

hind house fires and firearms as a cause of fatal injury. Surprisingly, motor vehicle accidents rank fourth and account for only 7% of fatal injuries.[6a] It is estimated that for every drowning there are three to five near-drownings severe enough to require hospitalization.[7] Wintemute reported that approximately 25% of near-drowning patients who are seen in the emergency room require hospitalization.[7] Severe neurologic impairment may result in as many as 20% of those survivors who require hospitalization. Thus, the magnitude of submersion accidents as a public health issue is enormous.

Male victims demonstrate bimodal frequency peaks at age 1 to 2 years and as adolescents between 15 and 19 years. Their death rates level off but are always considerably higher than those of females (Fig. 10–1). Older children and adults drown primarily in rivers, lakes, and canals, whereas toddlers drown primarily in private swimming pools and account for 75% of all pool drownings[7] (Fig. 10–2). It is important to recognize that any container of water into which a toddler can fit is a potential drowning site (Table 10–2). Persons with seizure and syncopal disorders are at increased risk of drowning. Improper judgment, overestimation of swimming ability, hyperventilation before underwater swimming, boating and diving accidents, and alcohol use are other contributing factors in drowning among older children and adults.

PATHOPHYSIOLOGY

Ten to 12% of drowning victims may not actually aspirate water.[8] Instead, they die from acute asphyxia while submerged, possibly resulting from laryngospasm or breath holding. The remaining victims aspirate freshwater, seawater, brackish water, or any of a variety of other liquids. The pathophysiologic changes caused by drowning depend on the quantity and quality of liquid aspirated and on the duration of hypoxemia that has occurred.

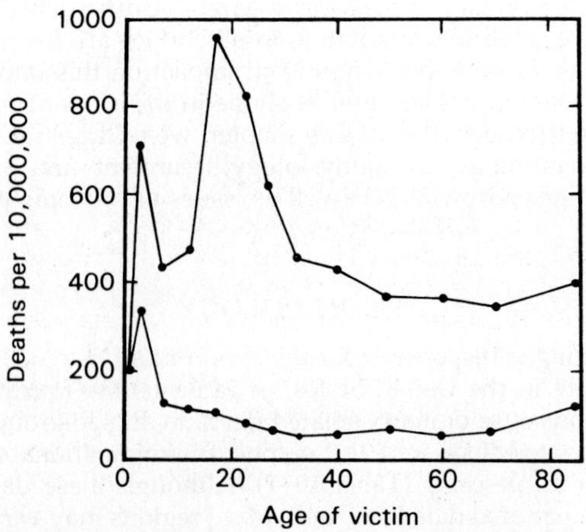

Figure 10–1. Drowning rate in the United States from 1977 to 1979 for males (*top line*) and females (*bottom line*). (From Spyker DA: Submersion injury. Pediatr Clin North Am 1985; 32:113–125.)

No two near-drowned victims are exactly alike: the state of health of each individual may have been different immediately before the accident, various quantities of water may have been aspirated, and the patient may have been submerged after maximal inhalation or exhalation. Furthermore, one patient may have succumbed from physical exhaustion, whereas another may have suffered a myocardial infarction or loss of consciousness.

Some investigators have placed considerable emphasis on water temperature. Immersing one's face in cold water (below 20°C) during breath holding evokes the diving reflex, which imposes a severe bradycardia and intense peripheral vasoconstriction and shunts blood to the heart and brain. This reflex is much less well developed in humans than in some other animals, and its relevance in cold-water drowning has been questioned.[9] Extremely cold water rapidly causes total-body hypothermia, decreasing oxygen consumption and therefore prolonging the time that hypoxia can be tolerated. This is especially true for infants, who cool rapidly because of their large body surface area: weight ratio. However, excessive cooling (below 30°C) alters cardiac function, sometimes causing fatal arrhythmias such as ventricular fibrillation. Whereas some persons cannot be re-

TABLE 10–2. Relative Contribution of Various Submersion Media to Drowning Accidents

Media	%
Seawater	1–2
Freshwater	98
Swimming pools	
Private	50
Public	3
Lakes, rivers, streams	20
Bathtubs	15
Buckets of water	4
Fish tanks or ponds	4
Toilets	1
Washing machines	1

(From Orlowski JP: Drowning, near-drowning and ice-water submersions. Pediatr Clin North Am 1987; 34:77.)

suscitated to a normal state even after brief submersion, others have regained normal cerebral function after submersion for as long as 10 minutes in warm water and 40 minutes in extremely cold water.[10] Thus, because of the complexity of factors involved in near-drowning accidents, each patient must be evaluated individually.

Pulmonary Changes

Aspiration of either freshwater or seawater decreases pulmonary compliance. Seawater is hypertonic; therefore, fluid is drawn from the plasma into the alveoli. These fluid-filled but perfused alveoli produce a large intrapulmonary shunt (Fig. 10–3). In contrast, aspirated freshwater is rapidly absorbed into the circulation and redistributed. Freshwater alters the surface tension properties of pulmonary surfactant so that alveoli become unstable. This results in unventilated or poorly ventilated alveoli that continue to be perfused, thus causing intrapulmonary shunt and an increased degree of hypoxia. Aspiration of either freshwater or seawater causes pulmonary edema, which also contributes to the intrapulmonary shunt. Many near-drowned patients suffer severe cerebral hypoxia, which, in addition, can precipitate neurogenic pulmonary edema.

Cardiovascular Changes

Near-drowned victims sometimes exhibit profound bradycardia or intense peripheral vasoconstriction, so that it is difficult to ascertain at the scene of the accident whether mechanical cardiac activity is present. Bradycardia may be secondary to a physiologic diving reflex in cold water or to profound hypoxia. Intense peripheral vasoconstriction could also be secondary to hypothermia or to a sharp increase in the level of circulating catecholamine. Other patients may be in a state of asystole.

The changes in cardiovascular function that occur in victims of near-drowning are predominantly secondary to changes in the partial pressure of arterial oxygen tension (PaO_2) and acid-base balance. Variations in blood volume and serum electrolyte concentrations also contribute to cardiovascular changes. However, less than 15% of drowning victims aspirate sufficient water to cause changes of this magnitude.

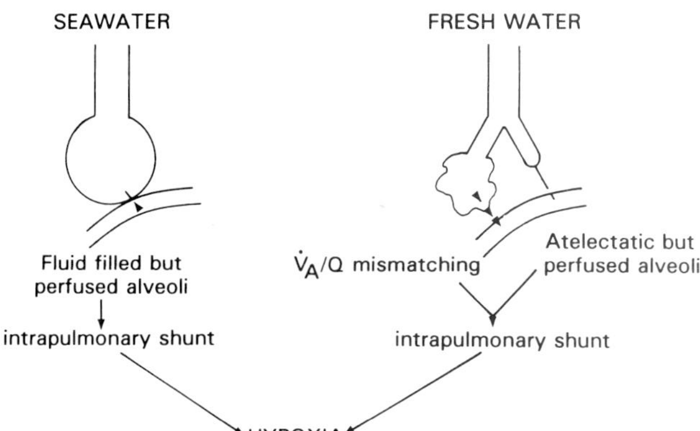

Figure 10–3. Effects of aspiration. After seawater aspiration, fluid fills the alveoli, producing intrapulmonary shunt. After freshwater aspiration, alteration of surfactant causes the partial collapse and complete atelectasis of alveoli, which produces intrapulmonary shunt. Aspiration of either type of water causes hypoxia.

Arterial blood pressure after near-drowning varies. Central venous pressure (CVP) increases immediately after aspiration of small quantities of freshwater or seawater and then rapidly returns to normal. After aspiration of larger quantities of freshwater, increased CVP usually returns to normal within approximately 1 hour and may even drop below normal as absorbed fluid is redistributed and pulmonary edema occurs. Aspiration of large quantities of seawater causes an initial but transient increase in CVP, followed by a rapid decrease in CVP—secondary to pulmonary edema—which causes a decrease in the effective circulating blood volume.

Central Nervous System Changes

Although the global ischemia from drowning or near-drowning affects all organs, the primary morbidity and mortality frequently are due to brain ischemia. The primary injury is from hypoxemia and ischemia, which occur at the time of submersion and continue until adequate ventilation, oxygenation, and perfusion are restored. Continuing ischemia with resultant secondary injury may occur even after effective cardiopulmonary resuscitation (CPR) as a result of reperfusion injury, hypotension, hypoxia, and increased intracranial pressure (ICP) from cerebral edema.

Consciousness is lost after varying lengths of time, usually after 2 to 3 minutes of the onset of apnea and hypoxia. Irreversible brain damage begins to occur after 4 to 10 minutes of anoxia. This presumes that hypoxia begins within seconds of submersion and is followed by absent perfusion within 2 to 6 minutes. The normothermic brain is very unlikely to recover after 8 to 10 minutes of anoxia. Although other organs can survive as long as 45 minutes of anoxia and be resuscitated, the brain cannot. If these patients survive, it is often in a chronic vegetative state. The rapid onset of cerebral hypothermia will markedly reduce metabolic activity and thereby prolong the time before irreversible brain damage occurs in victims of submersion.

The prognosis for normal survival of persons who arrive at the hospital either awake or with a blunted level of consciousness is excellent with intensive pulmonary and cardiovascular care. Forty to 50% of children who are comatose on admission survive normally. In data culled from several studies, 21% of children who presented with a Glasgow Coma Scale (GCS) score of 3 survived normally (Table 10–3).[4, 5, 11–14]

Patients who remain comatose for a period of time but awaken within 24 hours are likely to recover completely but may be at risk for delayed postanoxic demyelination. This is a very rare sequela of anoxic injury reported most often in carbon monoxide intoxication but which may occur in various other types of anoxia. The syndrome is described as follows: after awaking within 24 hours, the patient resumes normal activity in 4 to 5 days, which lasts for 2 to 10 days. The patient then abruptly becomes irritable and confused, clumsy, and subsequently spastic. Deterioration may progress to coma and death, or complete recovery may occur. Pathologic changes observed in most cases involve extensive cerebral hemispheric demyelination, the cause of which is unknown. The authors have never witnessed this complication after near-drowning, but its remote possibility should be considered. Patients and their families should be cautioned to return for medical care if central nervous system (CNS) symptoms return after discharge.

Cerebral Edema

Diffuse cerebral edema frequently occurs as a result of cytotoxic injury caused by severe global CNS anoxia and is-

TABLE 10–3. Glasgow Coma Scale (GCS) Score in Near-Drowned Children on Arrival to the Pediatric Intensive Care Unit (PICU)

Study	*No. in Series*	*No. with GCS Score 3 in the PICU*	*No. with GCS Score 3 Who Had Normal Survival*
Hildebrand et al[11]	26	6	0
Nussbaum and Maggi[5]	31	31	12
Allman et al[4]	66	37	0
Frewen et al[13]	13	6	2
Conn and Barker[14]	205	46	14
Dean and McComb[12]	101	20	3
Total	442	146	31

chemia. This anoxic and ischemic injury is considered the primary CNS injury. Toxic metabolites and further ischemia from elevated ICP and compromised cerebral perfusion are believed to contribute to further or secondary CNS injury. Cerebral edema can occur rapidly but often takes as long as 3 days to reach maximum swelling. Some patients with profound CNS injury and even brain death never show signs of cerebral edema on examination or computed tomographic scan.[15]

Blood Volume and Electrolyte Changes

Volume overload and hyponatremia can occur after aspiration of large volumes of freshwater, and hypovolemia and hypernatremia can occur after aspiration of large volumes of seawater. Although studies that subjected animals to total immersion until death confirm these theories, humans who survive long enough to receive hospital care rarely exhibit these disturbances. Thus, it is unlikely that these surviving patients have aspirated a sufficient volume of water to cause significant fluid and electrolyte changes. Even though a transient hypervolemia may follow near-drowning in freshwater, fluid rapidly redistributes, and a sufficient amount may leak from the intravascular space into the lung to render the patient hypovolemic within 1 hour.[16] Significant elevations of plasma hemoglobin concentrations are rare.

Although much attention has been given to the sequelae of aspirated water, it is also important to remember that sometimes large quantities of water can be ingested into the gastrointestinal tract before loss of consciousness. This has been reported to result in electrolyte and fluid disturbances after near-drowning in the Dead Sea[17] and also in infants during swimming lessons.[18] Also, it may increase the likelihood of vomiting during resuscitation, with resultant gastric aspiration injury.

Almost all near-drowning victims have normal or near-normal serum electrolyte concentrations when they are measured at the hospital. Serum potassium concentration, which is usually normal in humans who near-drown in freshwater or seawater, may be lower than normal when measured at the hospital. Hyperkalemia can result from tissue damage from global hypoxia.

Renal Changes

Renal function of patients who are resuscitated after near-drowning usually remains intact. However, albuminuria, hemoglobinuria, oliguria, and anuria can all occur. Renal damage may progress to acute tubular necrosis, which is likely secondary to severe hypoxia, although lactic acidosis and changes in renal blood flow may also contribute.

TREATMENT

Rescuer Management

Cardiopulmonary Resuscitation

The primary objective of emergency therapy for the near-drowned victim is to restore ventilation, perfusion, arterial blood gas tensions, and acid-base status to normal as rapidly as possible. The victim must be removed from the water immediately, and basic CPR must be applied. Because hypoxia increases rapidly with each second of apnea, it is imperative that emergency measures be taken immediately to initiate artificial respiration. If it is not feasible to remove the victim from the water immediately, then mouth-to-mouth ventilation should begin as soon as the rescuer reaches the victim. Some victims who are apneic still have effective cardiac activity; therefore, restoration of ventilation improves myocardial oxygenation and cardiac output. In others, a persistent, marked decrease in cardiac output or even asystole may be present. In these situations, closed-chest cardiac massage must be initiated as soon as possible. The single most important consequence of near-drowning that may prevent a normal recovery is irreversible CNS hypoxia. Therefore, the ability of the first responder to institute proper CPR and restore spontaneous ventilation and heartbeat frequently determines the quality of long-term survival. If the victim has not aspirated water, and if effective ventilation and circulation are established before permanent circulatory and neurologic changes occur, the prognosis is excellent. These patients frequently regain consciousness at the scene. Although they may be described as sleepy, lethargic, or foggy, these symptoms clear rapidly, and the patient usually does not require further therapy.

If water has been aspirated, however, alterations of pulmonary function persist. Initiating effective artificial ventilation promptly is more important than draining fluid from the lungs, particularly because the quantity of water aspirated frequently is not large and freshwater is absorbed from the lungs within minutes. Occasionally, victims of drowning and near-drowning swallow large quantities of water before completely losing consciousness. Therefore, it is important to ensure a clear airway so that the stomach is not overdistended during resuscitation, which may cause the patient to regurgitate and aspirate gastric contents. Because few near-drowned victims aspirate large quantities of water that remain in the lungs and many vomit and may aspirate stomach contents, a subdiaphragmatic thrust maneuver as described by Heimlich should be considered only when the airway cannot be cleared by other means—such as a jaw thrust—and mechanical obstruction is suspected. It should be remembered, however, that an abdominal thrust may cause an expulsion of the gastric contents, thereby increasing the risk of aspiration.[19]

Supplemental Oxygen

Even if the patient breathes spontaneously after rescue or initial resuscitation, the rescuer should not be lulled into a false sense of security. A patient may be able to converse with the rescuer and still have an extremely low PaO_2 or pH. Supplemental oxygen should be given until an actual measurement of arterial oxygen saturation or tension confirms it to be unnecessary. All near-drowned victims should be taken to the hospital for further evaluation and therapy. During transport, ventilatory and circulatory assistance should be provided, as indicated.

Hospital Management

All patients who required resuscitation should be admitted to the hospital (Fig. 10–4). Patients who are alert, were known to have been submersed less than 1 minute, required no CPR of any type, and were never symptomatic can be considered near-miss accidents and sent home. Those who have regained consciousness by the time they arrive at the emergency room and who require no further intervention should be observed at least overnight. Patients with altered mental status or respiratory dysfunction should be admitted to an intensive care unit (ICU) with the physical and human resources necessary to care for multisystem injuries. Initial therapy emphasizes cardiopulmonary support and prevention of secondary CNS injury.[20]

Pulmonary Support

The degree of intrapulmonary shunting that occurs after near-drowning is variable but has been observed to exceed 70% of the cardiac output in both animals and humans. The application of mechanical ventilation with positive end-expiratory pressure (PEEP) to the airway can dramatically improve ventilation-perfusion ratios. In many patients who are capable of sufficient minute ventilation to clear carbon dioxide adequately, this can be accomplished by permitting the patient to breathe spontaneously with continuous positive airway pressure (CPAP). The exact amount of CPAP should be determined on an individual basis, and its effects on intrapulmonary shunt, arterial oxygen tension, and cardiovascular function should be assessed. The optimal level is the lowest venous admixture achieved without adversely affecting cardiac output.

Many patients have minimal intrapulmonary shunting as a result of aspiration or resolve the lesion rapidly with appropriate therapy. These patients can usually be monitored with pulse oximetry with or without a few arterial blood samples for blood gas and pH determination. Those with persistent hypoxia will require frequent blood gas and pH measurements and are best managed with arterial catheter placement.

If the patient is sufficiently alert to maintain airway patency, CPAP can be applied with a specially designed, tight-fitting mask at levels up to 10 to 12 mm Hg. Obtunded patients will need endotracheal intubation. If the patient cannot easily maintain a normal partial pressure of arterial CO_2 ($PaCO_2$) with spontaneous ventilation, mechanical ventilation should be added to the regimen. Although both mechanical ventilation and PEEP can decrease cardiac output, frequently this decrease is secondary to hypovolemia. If a normal effective circulating blood volume is maintained by supplemental fluid administration, cardiac output may actually increase as PEEP or CPAP increases and PaO_2 improves.

Occasional bronchospasm after near-drowning can be treated with an aerosol of bronchodilating agent. The pulmonary edema that accompanies near-drowning is best controlled by titrating PEEP or CPAP to an optimal level. Once this level is reached, the amount of PEEP or CPAP should not be decreased rapidly or discontinued abruptly (e.g., to suction the patient's trachea) because even very short interruptions can cause an afflux of pulmonary edema fluid, a profound increase in intrapulmonary shunt, and a decrease in PaO_2.

Corticosteroid and prophylactic antibiotic therapy is not recommended for the pulmonary lesion caused by near-drowning. Experiments with animal models indicate that corticosteroids can interfere with normal pulmonary healing.[21] Empiric use of broad-spectrum antibiotics may impose the risk of infection with resistant organisms. It is better to withhold antibiotics unless there are definite clinical signs of infection or the fluid in which the drowning occurred is highly contaminated.

Adult respiratory distress syndrome (ARDS) occasionally results from aspiration in near-drowned patients. Although the surfactant washout and destruction that occur in seawater and freshwater, respectively, seem to predispose these patients to ARDS, surprisingly few patients experience this complication. Those patients in whom ARDS does develop are susceptible to all of the associated complications, which are discussed elsewhere in this text. Severe ARDS can develop with any type of near-drowning but may be more common with contaminated or unusual types of fluids. In the authors' experience, a child who near-drowned in detergent water in a washing machine and who experienced severe ARDS with barotrauma ultimately had a good recovery (Fig. 10–5).

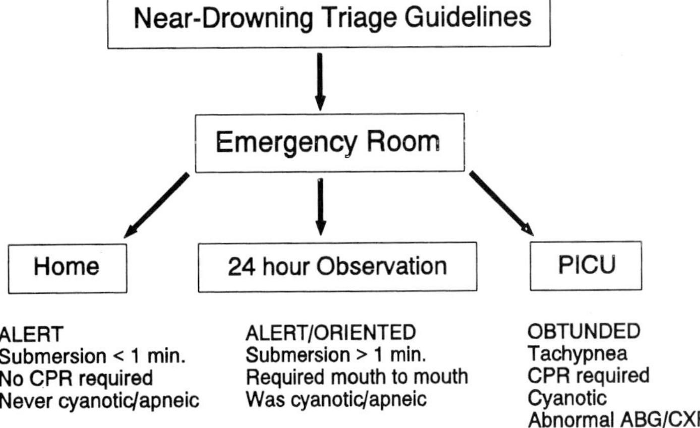

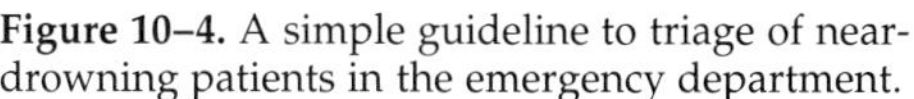
Figure 10–4. A simple guideline to triage of near-drowning patients in the emergency department.

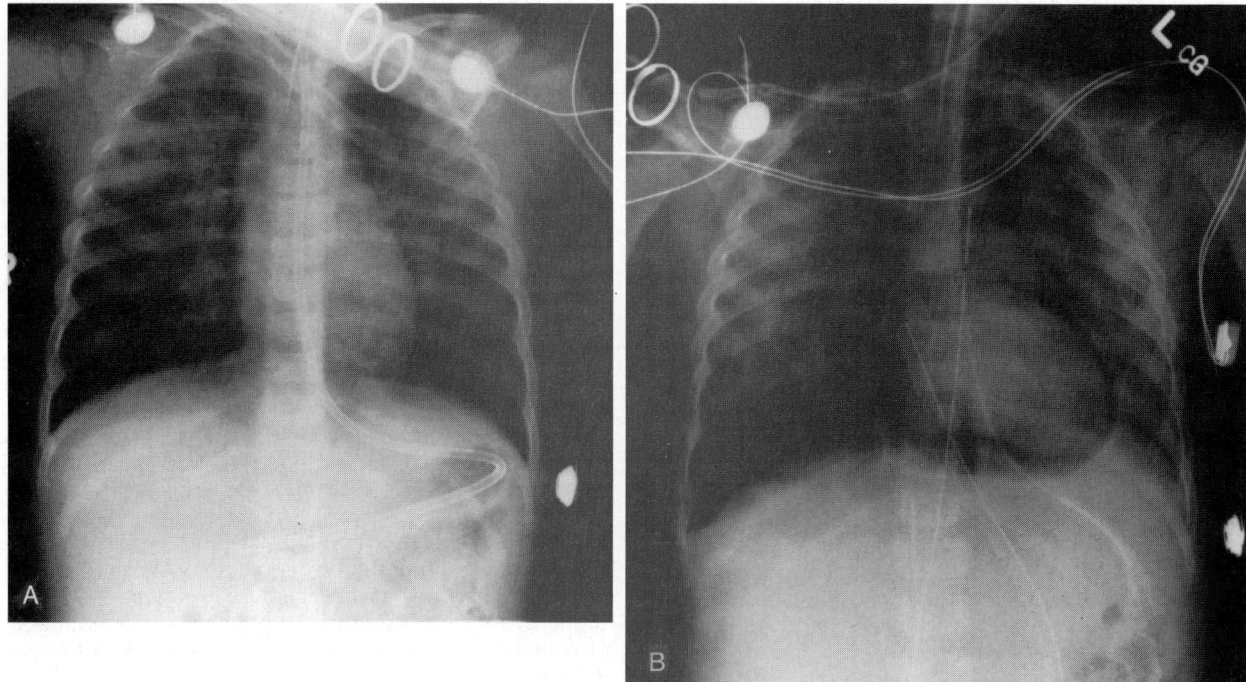

Figure 10–5. Radiographs of an 18-month-old girl who nearly drowned in detergent water in a washing machine. *A*, Radiograph taken on the day of admission showing the presence of diffuse bilateral infiltrates. *B*, Radiograph taken on the 4th hospital day after the development of a pneumothorax, pneumomediastinum, and pneumopericardium. Appropriate drainage tubes have been placed. The child survived and recovered normally.

Many strategies of mechanical ventilation have been advocated for the treatment of ARDS. Our current practice is to use the technique that can provide adequate oxygenation with the lowest inspiratory pressures and oxygen concentrations possible. We allow $PaCO_2$ to rise above normal if a pH of 7.2 or greater is maintained in deference to using high peak airway pressures. This "gentilation," also known as "controlled hypoventilation" or "permissive hypercapnia," may decrease overdistension of alveoli and barotrauma in patients with a variety of types of respiratory failure.[22–24a] In spontaneously breathing patients, we use pressure support ventilation to help decrease the work of breathing imposed by the decreased lung compliance and by the breathing circuit and endotracheal tube. In selected cases, pressure control–inverse ratio ventilation is helpful in reducing shunt and peak airway pressure (Table 10–4).[25–28] This technique may allow collapsed or fluid-filled alveoli to participate in gas exchange with less chance of overdistending the more normal alveoli. Familiarity with this technique and the potential complications is essential before its use.

The potential efficacy of exogenous surfactant in ARDS is currently being investigated in several multicenter trials. There is some evidence that this will be beneficial.[29] Artificial surfactant has been shown to be effective and safe in treating respiratory distress syndrome in newborns. One clinical study has reported encouraging results using surfactant in patients with ARDS secondary to sepsis.[30] In this study, mortality at 14 days after 5 days of therapy was decreased from 50% in the placebo group to 25% and 35% in the two groups receiving high and low concentrations, respectively, of nebulized artificial surfactant. There was also a significant improvement in alveolar-arterial oxygen gradient in both treatment groups compared with controls. Artificial surfactant (Exosurf) is administered at a dose of 5.0 ml/kg in both newborns and older patients. In newborns, direct instillation is used, whereas in older patients it is nebulized continuously over the treatment period.

Extracorporeal life support for respiratory failure in one of several forms has also come back into use in the pediatric population. Although its use has gained widespread acceptance in newborns with meconium aspiration syndrome and congenital diaphragmatic hernia, it has not yet been proven

TABLE 10–4. Several Reports Comparing Pressure Control–Inverse Ratio Ventilation to Conventional Ventilation in Terms of Changes in Peak Inspiratory Pressures and Some Index of Oxygenation*

		PIP (cm H_2O)		*PaO_2 (mm Hg)*		*FIO_2*	
Study	*N*	*Pre*	*Post*	*Pre*	*Post*	*Pre*	*Post*
Lain et al[25]	19	48	32	66	89		
Anderson[26]	67	70	44			1.0	.45
Abraham and Yoshihara[27]	9	44	39	63	76		
Tharatt et al[28]	89	66	46	69	80		

*Values are given pre- and postinstitution of pressure control–inverse ratio ventilation.
Abbreviations: PIP = peak inspiratory pressure; PaO_2 = partial pressure of arterial oxygen; FIO_2 = fraction of inspired oxygen.

to be beneficial in older children with respiratory failure. Its efficacy in this setting is unknown and should be considered experimental.

Cardiovascular Support

Near-drowned adults and children will present with any of the entire gamut of cardiovascular disturbances. Those who have suffered profound hypoxemia may have serious damage to any or all end-organs. Myocardial ischemia may be a cause of cardiogenic shock; fluid translocation from gut ischemia may cause hypovolemic shock; and associated head injuries can cause neurogenic shock. Patients may be temporarily hypervolemic from swallowed or aspirated water, or they may be euvolemic or hypovolemic. Renal ischemia and diuretic therapy may cause urine output to be unreliable as an indicator of adequacy of intravascular volume. Thus, complex fluid and hemodynamic changes may necessitate the use of invasive hemodynamic monitoring.

At the minimum, every patient should have vital signs (pulse, respiration, blood pressure, and temperature) monitored, and serial determinations of arterial blood gas tensions and pH should be made as indicated. Also, the electrocardiogram and the urinary output of patients who require any type of prolonged support should be monitored closely. Those patients requiring CPAP and in whom it is helpful to quantitate intrapulmonary shunt may require pulmonary artery catheter placement. Titration of CPAP in patients who are hypovolemic may result in a decrease in venous return, which may decrease cardiac output. This problem can usually be avoided by appropriate volume loading guided by the measurement of central pressures and cardiac output.

Central Nervous System Support

Therapy for CNS injury associated with near-drowning should be directed at preventing further secondary injury. Therapy can be viewed in three separate areas: general management, ICP control, and brain resuscitation. As stated previously, although the latter two issues have been areas of intense interest over the last decade, they have not altered outcome in those patients with anoxic/ischemic CNS injury.

General Management

Adequate perfusion must be ensured, along with support of oxygenation and ventilation as needed and cardiovascular support. In general, fluid restriction is used to limit cerebral edema and in anticipation of inappropriate antidiuretic hormone secretion. However, it is essential to provide adequate fluid to support the circulation as needed. Hypo-osmotic states and high or low blood glucose concentrations may also adversely affect outcome. Fever should be controlled because hyperthermia increases cerebral metabolic rate and oxygen consumption with increases in ICP. Seizures also increase ICP by the same mechanism and should be aggressively controlled.

Intracranial Pressure Control

That ICP can be controlled in ischemic injury by the various known interventions has been reasonably well documented. However, that outcome is improved by these interventions has not been documented.[3-5] This has slowly changed the practice of ICP control and monitoring in the last 5 years. Although ICP monitoring, hyperventilation, pentobarbital coma, and diuretic therapy were all part of an aggressive ICP control regimen in near-drowning patients a short time ago, the more invasive and potentially dangerous interventions have for the most part been abandoned.[3-5] We have surveyed all of the pediatric intensive care medicine fellowship programs in the United States and have determined that ICP monitoring and pentobarbital coma are rarely used and that the noninvasive practices of hyperventilation, head elevation, and diuretics are used frequently, but not universally, throughout the United States. Steroids are of no benefit in this type of cytotoxic edema and may worsen outcome. Hypothermia was also used in the past but has not proven to alter outcome and may impair immune responses.

For patients with suspected elevations in ICP, we use head elevation, hyperventilation, fluid restriction if indicated, and diuretic therapy. Our survey supports this continued practice. We may institute more aggressive therapy in the obtunded but not flaccid patient (a Glasgow Coma Scale [GCS] score of 5 to 8) (Table 10–5) who later becomes flaccid or decerebrate and has evidence of cerebral edema. Twenty per cent of our survey participants would use ICP

TABLE 10–5. Glasgow Coma Scale Score for Adults and Children and Infants

Response Score	*Adults and Children*	*Infants*
Eye Opening		
4	Spontaneous	Spontaneous
3	To verbal stimuli	To speech
2	To pain	To pain
1	None	None
Verbal		
5	Oriented	Coos, babbles
4	Confused	Irritable
3	Inappropriate words	Cries to pain
2	Nonspecific sounds	Moans to pain
1	None	None
Motor		
6	Follows commands	Normal spontaneous movements
5	Localizes pain	Withdraws to touch
4	Withdraws to pain	Withdraws to pain
3	Decorticates to pain	Decorticates to pain
2	Decerebrates to pain	Decerebrates to pain
1	Flaccid	Flaccid

(Modified from James HE, Trauner DA: The Glasgow Coma Scale. *In*: Brain Insults in Infants and Children. James HE (Ed). Orlando, Grune & Stratton, 1985, p 181.)

monitoring and only 9% would use pentobarbital coma in this setting.

Brain Resuscitation

All of the modalities of brain resuscitation remain investigational at this point. The effect of free radical scavengers, calcium channel blockers, dimethyl sulfoxide, opiate receptor antagonists, prostaglandin blockers, and anesthetics in reducing secondary injury remains to be elucidated.

Outcome Prediction

Perhaps the most frustrating aspect of caring for near-drowning patients is providing aggressive care to those whose outcome is suspected to be dismal. However, because of many "miraculous recovery" reports, the clinician feels obligated to provide this care, all the while knowing that if the patient survives it will be almost certainly in a persistent vegetative state. For this reason, many predictive methods have been tested. Factors such as submersion time longer than 5 minutes, initial pH of less than 7.1, requirement for continued CPR once the patient reaches the hospital, persistence of coma in the emergency room and the ICU, fixed and dilated pupils, elevated ICP, and young age are all associated with a bad outcome. However, all of these predictors suffer from the same shortcoming: the presence of the unacceptable error of false pessimism.

Any predictive tool has the possibility of yielding two types of error: false pessimism and false optimism. The latter, predicting a good outcome when a bad outcome occurs, causes disappointment but is an acceptable type of error. False pessimism, predicting a bad outcome when in fact a good outcome is possible, may result in limiting care when it may be helpful. Any predictive tool that permits this error to occur, even to a degree as low as 1% to 5%, has limited usefulness. None of us would withhold therapy on a near-drowned victim if the predictive tool told us that as many as 5 of 100 patients in that condition could survive without severe handicap. Each predictive tool should be viewed in the context of the potential for these types of errors.

Cardiac Arrest

Several reports have documented that the chance of intact survival is extremely low for a near-drowned victim who requires CPR in the emergency room.[31, 32] One clear exception to this involves ice-water injuries, in which normal outcomes have been reported in asystolic patients.[33]

Level of Consciousness

Many authors attempted to correlate outcome with some measurement of consciousness. Modell and Conn suggested a classification system primarily for the purpose of comparing results of clinical studies.[34] This system is analogous to the GCS, which has been used extensively to predict outcome from coma of various causes.[35] Patients who arrive in the ICU with a GCS of 3 (flaccid coma) (see Table 10–5) are believed to have a universally poor prognosis. However, many clinical reports document the potential for intact survival in this situation. It is again clear that false pessimism is unacceptably present (see Table 10–3).[4, 5, 11–14]

Clinical Scoring System

Orlowski attempted to combine several prognostic indicators into a scoring system (Table 10–6).[36] Here again, in 5 of 100 accidents, a falsely pessimistic prediction was made.

Evoked Potentials

We have found, as have others, that multimodality evoked potential recordings are very helpful in predicting outcome in coma from all causes.[37] We have identified 1023 comatose patients in 20 studies who had evoked potential recordings performed (Table 10–7). In this group, false pessimism was essentially nonexistent. Of the five cases of false pessimism, only one was a valid prediction. This case involved a child who was struck by lightning and was flaccid with absent evoked potentials, who regained consciousness and evoked potentials and recovered normally. The remaining four were reporting errors or involved neonates, in whom this technology is known to be unreliable. This information, combined with the clinical information derived from both the Orlowski score and the GCS, can be used to help determine who should receive aggressive therapy. The technology does require skilled technical support and professionals with experience in performing and interpreting these signals.

TABLE 10–6. Orlowski Criteria for Predicting Prognosis After Drowning*

1. Age ≤3 years
2. Estimated maximum submersion ≥5 minutes
3. No attempts at CPR within 10 minutes of rescue
4. Coma on admission to emergency room
5. Arterial pH <7.11.

(From Orlowski JP: Prognostic factors in pediatric cases of drowning and near-drowning. Ann Emerg Med 1979; 8:176.)

*The presence of any of the five unfavorable prognostic factors is given a value of 1. A score of 2 or less is associated with a 90% chance of recovery. A score of 3 or more is associated with a 5% chance of recovery.

Abbreviation: CPR = cardiopulmonary resuscitation.

Prevention

To address prevention of drowning and near-drowning accidents, it is essential to understand the circumstances most commonly associated with accident victims in different age groups. The profile of a toddler playing in the yard and wandering into the pool area when the mother, who has not been trained in basic life support, goes inside to answer the telephone characterizes a large number of submersion injuries.

Location

Toddlers drown primarily in residential pools and account for 75% of all pool drownings. The older age group drowns primarily in rivers, lakes, and canals. It is important to recognize that any container of water into which a toddler can fit is a potential drowning site. Drownings in hot tubs, spas, and whirlpools have increased as much as 10-fold in some states over the last two decades.[38] Again, access and poor supervision are the main contributors to this trend, but some are related to entrapment by the suction. Solar pool covers represent another water hazard to children.[39]

Poor Judgment

Many drownings are a result of poor judgment on the part of either the caregiver or the victim. Brief lapses of supervision for various reasons are responsible for a large number of toddler drownings. Overestimation of swimming ability, disregard for safety rules, and alcohol use are responsible for many adolescent and adult drownings. Unfamiliarity with the effect of hyperventilation, which causes a loss of consciousness and subsequent drowning, before underwater swimming is also a significant factor.

Swimming Ability

Thirty-five per cent of drowned victims can swim. This is not surprising in the adolescent group. Whether swimming

TABLE 10–7. Use of Multimodality Evoked Potential (MEP) Recordings to Predict Outcome in Comatose Children and Adults*

Year	*Author*	*n*	*Patient Age*	*Modality of EPs*	*False Pessimism*	*False Optimism*
1978	de la Torre	17	A,C	SEPs	0	0
1980	Tsubokawa	64	A,C	BAEPs	0	3
1981	Narayan	133	A,C	MEPs	0	12
	Goldie	88	A	MEPs	0	5
	Lindsay	32	A	MEPs	0	5
1984	Anderson	39	A	MEPs	0	2
	Rosenberg	25	A,C	BAEPs	0	7
	Jain	15	A,C	BAEPs	1	6
1985	Karnaze	45	A	BAEPs	0	5
	Dear	30	N	BAEPs	2	—
	Steinhart	23	C	BAEPs	0	2
	Frank	5	C	MEPs	0	0
1986	Walser	63	A	SEPs	0	17
	Cant	35	A	MEPs	0	3
1987	De Meirleir	73	C	SEPs	1	0
1988	Elwany	68	A	BAEPs	0	13
	Ahmed	60	A	SEPs	0	—
	Nataloni	30	C	BAEPs	0	7
1989	Taylor	37	C	SEPs/VEPs	1	0
1990	Judson	100	A,C	SEPs	0	12
1991	Goodwin	41	C	MEPs	0	2
	Total	1023			5	101

(Modified with permission from Goodwin SR, Friedman WA, Bellefleur M: Is it time to use evoked potentials to predict outcome in comatose children and adults? Crit Care Med 1991; 19:518.)

*Of 1023 cases, there were only 5 cases of false pessimism reported; when assessed carefully only 1 was valid. The 101 cases of false optimism are an expected and acceptable type of error. See text for discussion.

Abbreviations: A = adults; C = children; SEPs = somatosensory evoked potentials; BAEPs = brainstem auditory evoked potentials; VEPs = visual evoked potentials.

ability in the toddler age group increases or decreases the risk of drowning is a subject of considerable debate.[40] Even though children younger than 3 years can be taught to float, keep their heads above water, and propel themselves, they cannot be expected to react appropriately in an emergency. Some investigators also believe that these children may lose their fear of the water and be at increased risk. None of these concerns have been proven.

Seizure Disorder

Patients with a known seizure disorder have a four to five times higher risk of drowning.[7] Although restriction of swimming is not practical, it is essential for these patients to be observed closely by trained personnel while swimming.

Barriers

In 80% of all residential pool drownings, the child gains access to the pool from the house or play area.[41] Many states require fences around yards with pools; however, none requires the pool to be isolated from the play area or house (Fig. 10–6). It is estimated that 80% of pediatric drowning can be prevented by effective barriers.[42, 43] In New Zealand, the 1987 Fencing of Swimming Pools Act mandates that the fence must enclose the pool, not the property, and that self-closing and self-latching gates be used. An 80% reduction in drownings is predicted with this legislation as opposed to only 8% if boundary fencing requirements are used.[43]

CPR

The drowning victim frequently receives either no CPR or CPR from an untrained provider. Even if the victim has been submerged only for a few minutes, anoxia will continue until effective CPR is performed. Thus, universal training in CPR should significantly improve outcome statistics after drowning and near-drowning.

ABCs of Prevention

In children, the elementary components, or the ABCs, of prevention consist of *A*dult supervision, *B*arriers that are effective, and *C*PR training for parents and pool owners. Although supervision and CPR training are educational issues, barrier legislation is a public health issue. Healthcare providers can be the prime force in initiating efforts to change local and state ordinances to require effective barriers. Using isolation fencing and self-closing, self-latching gates will save more lives than all of the heroic efforts that have been attempted in cerebral resuscitation.

Drowning prevention in adults will continue to be a matter of education on safety issues involving breath-hold div-

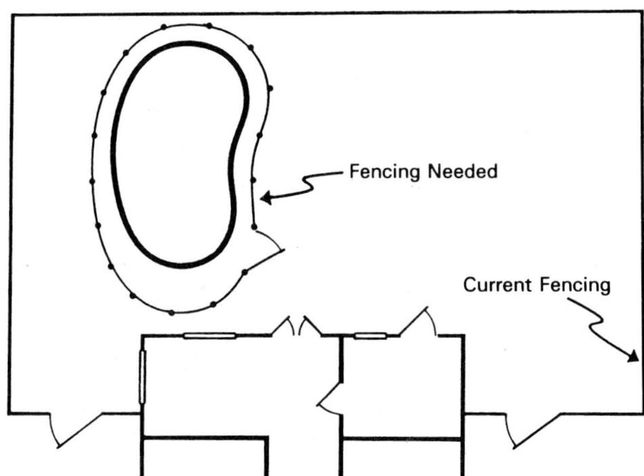

Figure 10–6. Current yard and pool fencing as recommended by Wintemute (From Wintemute GJ: Childhood drowning and near-drowning in the United States. Am J Dis Child 1990; 144:663. Copyright 1990, American Medical Association.)

ing, diving into shallow water, alcohol use, and seizure complications. Legislation on alcohol use and boating will undoubtedly have some favorable impact on boating-related drownings.

ACKNOWLEDGMENT

The authors thank Suzanne M. White for her editorial assistance.

References

1. Levin DL: Near-drowning. Crit Care Med 1980; 8:590.
2. Fields AI: Near-drowning in the pediatric population. Crit Care Clin 1992; 8:113.
3. Bohn DJ, Biggar WD, Smith CR, et al: Influence of hypothermia, barbiturate therapy, and intracranial pressure monitoring on morbidity and mortality after near-drowning. Crit Care Med 1986; 14:529.
4. Allman FD, Nelson WB, Pacentine GA, et al: Outcome following cardiopulmonary resuscitation in severe pediatric near-drowning. Am J Dis Child 1986; 140:571.
5. Nussbaum E, Maggi JC: Pentobarbital therapy does not improve neurologic outcome in nearly-drowned, flaccid-comatose children. Pediatrics 1988; 81:630.
6. Baker SP, O'Neill B, Karpf RD: The Injury Fact Book. Lexington, MA: DC Heath, 1984, p 155.

6a. Weesner CL, Hargarten SW, Aprahamian C, et al: Fatal childhood injury patterns in an urban setting. Ann Emerg Med 1994; 23:231–236.

7. Wintemute GJ: Childhood drowning and near-drowning in the United States. Am J Dis Child 1990; 144:663.
8. Cot C: Les asphyxies accidentelles (submersion, electrocution, intoxication oxycarbonique). *In*: Etude Clinique, Therapeutique et Preventive. Paris, Editions Medicales N. Maloine, 1931.
9. Hayward JS, Hay C, Matthews BR: Temperature effect on the human dive response in relation to cold water near-drowning. J Appl Physiol 1984; 56:202–206.
10. Siebke H, Breivek H, Rod T, et al: Survival after 40 min submersion without cerebral sequelae. Lancet 1975; i:1275.
11. Hildebrand CA, Hartmann AG, Arcinue EL, et al: Cardiac performance in pediatric near-drowning. Crit Care Med 1988; 16:331.
12. Dean JM, McComb JG: Intracranial pressure monitoring in severe pediatric near-drowning. Neurosurgery 1981; 9:627.
13. Frewen TC, Sumabat WO, Han VK, et al: Cerebral resuscitation therapy in pediatric near-drowning. J Pediatr 1985; 106:615.
14. Conn AW, Barker GA: Fresh water drowning and near-drowning: An update. Can Anaesth Soc J 1984; 31:538.
15. Taylor T, Quencer RM, Holzman BH, et al: Central nervous system ischemic insult in children due to near-drowning. Radiology 1985; 156:641.
16. Tabeling BB, Modell JH: Fluid administration increases oxygen delivery during continuous positive airway pressure ventilation after freshwater near-drowning. Crit Care Med 1983; 11:693.
17. Modell JH: Serum electrolyte changes in near-drowning victims (Editorial). JAMA 1985; 253:557.
18. Goldberg GN, Lightner ES, Morgan W, et al: Infantile water intoxication after a swimming lesson. Pediatrics 1982; 70:599.
19. Modell JH: Is the Heimlich maneuver appropriate as first treatment for drowning? (Editorial). Emerg Med Serv 1981; 10:63.
20. Modell JH: Drowning. *In*: Edema. Staub NC, Taylor AE (Eds). New York, Raven Press, 1984, pp 679–694.
21. Wynne JW, Reynolds JC, Hood CI, et al: Steroid therapy for pneumonitis induced in rabbits by aspiration of foodstuff. Anesthesiology 1979; 51:11.
22. Kolobow T, Moretti MP, Fumagalli R, et al: Severe impairment in lung function induced by high peak airway pressure during mechanical ventilation. Am Rev Respir Dis 1987; 135:312.
23. Darioli R, Perret C: Mechanical controlled hypoventilation in status asthmaticus. Am Rev Respir Dis 1984; 129:385.
24. Hicking KG, Henderson SJ, Jackson R: Low mortality associated with permissive hypocapnea in severe adult respiratory distress syndrome. Intensive Care Med 1990; 16:372.

24a. Slutsky AS: American College of Chest Physicians Consensus Conference: Mechanical ventilation. Chest 1993; 104:1833–1859.

25. Lain DC, DiBenedetto R, Morris SL, et al: Pressure control inverse ratio ventilation as a method to reduce peak inspiratory pressure and provide adequate ventilation and oxygenation. Chest 1989; 95:1081.
26. Anderson JB: Ventilatory strategy in catastrophic lung disease: Inverse ratio ventilation (IRV) and combined high frequency ventilation (CHFV). Acta Anaesthesiol Scand 1989; 33:145.
27. Abraham E, Yoshihara G: Cardiorespiratory effects of pressure controlled inverse ratio ventilation in severe respiratory failure. Chest 1989; 96:1356.
28. Tharatt RS, Allen RP, Albertson TE: Pressure controlled inverse ratio ventilation in severe adult respiratory failure. Chest 1988; 94:755.
29. Lewis JF, Jobe AH: Surfactant and the adult respiratory distress syndrome. Am Rev Respir Dis 1993; 147:218–233.
30. Reins HD, Silverman H, Hurst J, et al: Effects of two concentrations of nebulized surfactant (Exosurf) in sepsis-induced adult respiratory distress syndrome (ARDS). Crit Care Med 1992; 20:S61.
31. Nichter MA, Everett PB: Childhood near-drowning: Is cardiopulmonary resuscitation always indicated? Crit Care Med 1989; 17:993.
32. O'Rourke P: Outcome of children who are apneic and pulseless in the emergency room. Crit Care Med 1986; 14:466.
33. Biggart MJ, Bohn D: Effect of hypothermia and cardiac arrest on outcome of near drowning accidents in children. J Pediatr 1990; 117:179.
34. Modell JH, Conn AW: Current neurological considerations in near-drowning. Can Anaesth Soc J 1980; 27:197.
35. Dean M, Kaufman ND: Prognostic indicators in pediatric near-drowning: The Glasgow Coma Scale. Crit Care Med 1981; 9:536.
36. Orlowski JP: Drowning, near-drowning, and ice-water submersions. Pediatr Clin North Am 1987; 34:77.
37. Goodwin SR, Friedman WA, Bellefleur M: Is it time to use evoked potentials to predict outcome in comatose children and adults? Crit Care Med 1991; 19:518.
38. Shinaberger CS, Anderson CL, Fraus JF: Young children who drown in hot tubs, spas, and whirlpools in California: A 26-year survey. Am J Public Health 1990; 80:613.
39. Sulkes SB, van der Jagt EW: Solar pool blankets: Another water hazard. Pediatrics 1990; 85:1114.
40. Flynn TG: Committee on pediatric aspects of physical fitness, recreation, and sports: Position statement on swimming instruction for infants. Pediatrics 1980; 65:847.
41. Wintemute FJ, Kraus JF, Teret SP, Wright M: Drowning in childhood and adolescence: A population-based study. Am J Public Health 1987; 77:830.
42. Ferfusson BA, Horwood LJ: Risks of drowning in fenced and unfenced domestic swimming pools. N Z Med J 1984; 97:777.
43. Hassal IB: Thirty-six consecutive under 5 year old domestic swimming pool drownings. Aust Paediatr J 1989; 25:143.

CHAPTER 11

Transport of the Critically Ill Patient

Alasdair K. T. Conn, MD, FACS

Within the last quarter century, there has been a dramatic increase in the number and types of intensive care units (ICUs) both in the United States and abroad. These ICUs may be serving a discreet subset of a hospital's population—the critically ill—or may function as a regional resource, such as burn units, level III neonatal units, or shock trauma units. When appropriately used, this capability has been demonstrated to improve survival in critically ill patients; but this has meant that patients may need to be transported over relatively large distances to obtain access to these ICUs. Even within an institution, patients may need to be transferred from one ICU to another or from the ICU to the operating room or radiologic suite.

In this chapter, the role of prehospital and interhospital transport of the adult critically ill is discussed, although many of the techniques and equipment that are used on interfacility transport can also be of benefit for intrafacility transport. As political forces gather to control healthcare costs within the United States, an increased regionalization of critical care is likely; and so the interfacility transport of these patients becomes essential for health system viability. The hypothesis that transport of the critically ill to the hospital best capable of managing that acute illness or injury will be encouraged in the hope that this will allow the efficiencies of high volume and yet achieve optimal patient outcomes.

Interfacility transports are not recorded in any national data base; however, an indication of the rapid growth of critical transfer may be gained from the aeromedical experience.[1]

The hospital-based helicopter programs have increased from 101 programs in July 1985 to 178 in July 1991, a 76% increase. These figures are for hospital-based rotor-craft programs and do not include transports performed by public service helicopter systems or those provided by the military. Many of these hospital-based helicopter programs have now developed both ground and fixed-wing transport services; many hospitals also have independently developed specialized transport teams, particularly in the neonatal and pediatric arenas.

ISSUES

Transport Team Composition

The decision to transfer a patient is a medical one and must be made by the referring physician. Once the receiving facility has ascertained that they have the capability of acceptance, the next decision concerns the mode of transport and the composition of the transporting crew. At this time, there are no national guidelines as to which patients may be transferred solely by paramedics, which will require a nurse in attendance, and which mandate that a physician be in attendance. Paramedics are certified on a state-by-state basis, and either state or local jurisdictional regulations may limit the capability of paramedics in providing an extended scope of practice to manage the more critical interfacility transfer patients. Paramedics should, for example, not be managing unfamiliar equipment such as ventilators; and there is a legal liability should adverse patient outcomes be experienced. Certain states will allow an extended scope of practice but only with close monitoring by a responsible physician and the ability to obtain verbal orders either by radio or cellular telephone (on-line medical direction).

A registered nurse with additional intensive care training and experience is frequently used during the more complex transfers; however, there is a continued debate as to whether a physician is an essential component of the transferring team. One survey[2] compiled from 126 hospital-based aeromedical programs shows that 97% use at least two attendants. Of the 3% that only use one medical attendant, 75% use registered nurses and 25% use paramedics. Among programs that use two attendants, the most common mix was a flight nurse/flight medic (53%), followed by a nurse/other medical attendant (usually a respiratory therapist) (20%), a nurse/physician (11%), and a nurse/nurse (11%). Other combinations make up the remaining 5%. Several attempts have been made to determine whether a physician is a required component of these transport teams or whether the need for a physician can be predetermined.[3–5] Unfortunately, many of these studies are retrospective, subjective, contain no patient outcome data, and are mostly questionnaires to the existing crew as to whether having a physician would be of assistance. One prospective study[6] of two helicopters served by the same facility—one staffed with a physician/nurse crew and the other with a nurse/paramedic crew—did show a difference in outcome. However, the number of patients in each group was relatively small.

In addition, although there was a statistically significant difference in survival, the authors themselves noted that placing a physician on board a helicopter to achieve improved patient outcome on 1 flight in 50 must be given "critical consideration." The qualifications of the physicians have received relatively little investigation; many programs are using resident physicians in training, and there is little information as to whether the level of training of the physicians is a determining factor in patient outcome. Several of these studies also suffer from using mortality as the sole end measure rather than cost, length of hospital stay, or morbidity; and it may be that death is not the correct outcome measurement to gauge transport effectiveness. Several programs ascribe considerable value to the presence of a physician even though only 11% of patients fly with physicians on board.[1] It has been previously demonstrated that tube thoracostomy, cricothyrotomy, initiation of pharmacologic paralysis, and endotracheal intubation can be performed safely by nonphysicians.[7, 8] Furthermore, on more specialized flights, an experienced nurse or respiratory therapist may be more familiar with a ventilator than a physician; and a pump technician may be more familiar with a malfunctioning intra-aortic balloon pump than either an attending or a resident physician.

The controversy as to whether the physician is an essential component of all interfacility critical transport teams for air and, by implication, for ground transports is still unresolved. Further studies should address whether patients can be identified pretransport who might benefit from the presence of a physician; in addition, such studies should attempt to identify pertinent skills and level of training of such physicians. Some of the skills might be acquired by alternative flight personnel.

Transport Mode

After selection of the composition of the transport team, the next decision concerns the mode of transport.[9] The current options are ground transport (usually in a specially equipped or modified ground ambulance) and either rotor-wing aircraft (helicopter) or fixed-wing aircraft (airplane). In many areas of the United States and Canada, all three options are available, and under extremely rural locations such as Alaska, the use of fixed-wing aircraft becomes imperative. Factors that influence the mode of transport include the distance and duration of transport, the techniques that the transport personnel might need to provide to the patient, the urgency for the patient to obtain access to tertiary care, the diagnosis and complications that the patient might incur during air versus ground transport, local weather conditions, geography, vehicle availability, and the requirement and availability of a proceed-out team. Sometimes the patient is sufficiently unstable that transport should be effected as soon as possible.

Ground Ambulance

Ground ambulance vehicles are usually widely available, can be used in all types of weather, and should be used for most short-distance transfers. Ground ambulances fall under two main types: basic life support and advanced life support (ALS). ALS ambulances have as part of their standard equipment monitor defibrillators, endotracheal tubes, and several medications and are staffed by paramedics. Although ALS vehicles are primarily used for emergency medical services (EMS) response, they can be called on to provide interfacility transfers. If the ambulance, however, has as its primary mission the response to the local jurisdiction, they may not wish to take the vehicle out of service for a long transport to a tertiary facility.

Ground ambulances can be limited by surface traffic conditions such as construction or inclement weather. If ground ambulances are used, one should ensure that they have the necessary outlets and supporting generators for managing ventilators or balloon pumps. Appropriate back-up supplies (electrical, extra oxygen tanks) should be available in case of vehicle or electrical failure. Most ambulances have radio communication capability. During long-distance transports, it is wise to ensure that the receiving facility has the ability to communicate directly. Cellular telephones can be used in urban areas.

Ground ambulance is the most widely used and the cheapest type of interfacility transport mode, and strong consideration should be made if the transport distance is 30 miles or shorter.

Helicopter

Helicopters should be considered (if available) for transfers of intermediate range (i.e., 30–150 miles). Although the speed depends on the model and power plant of the helicopter design, ground speeds of between 120 and 180 mph can be achieved. Helicopters are dispatched from tertiary facilities or from urban airports. Helicopters may be multipurpose, serving as police or search and rescue rotor-craft as well as a medical function, or dedicated, providing only medical transports. On notification of an impending flight, helicopters usually require a 2- to 4-minute warm-up time before liftoff. Thus, allowing for system activation, they can be airborne within 5 to 6 minutes of flight request.

Most aircraft are configured to be immediately available for scene or emergency department response. Reconfiguration for specialized flights such as neonatal transfers, balloon pumps, or high-risk maternity may require additional time for aircraft preparedness. Helicopters usually fly under Federal Aviation Administration visual flight rules (VFRs), but many programs have chosen to equip their aircraft so they can fly by instrument flight rules (IFRs). It should be indicated that scene responses and responses to hospitals require VFR because IFRs mandate filing a flight plan and landing at an airport with appropriate instrumentation. The liftoff capability depends on the type of helicopter used, but most used for medical response can manage two patients of up to 250 pounds each. The internal configuration will depend on aircraft selection, although several standard interior designs are available.

Helicopters are expensive: The capital cost is between $1 million and $5 million depending on whether one is using a single-engine or a dual-engine aircraft and whether the system will require a larger aircraft with IFR capability. Many programs lease the helicopter from a vendor. Usually included in such a lease is the cost of dedicated pilots, mechanics, and back-up aircraft. Typically, there is an additional charge per flight hour to cover the cost of aircraft maintenance. The fuel burn is normally between 50 and 100 gallons per flight hour and is usually borne by the hospital. In programs that are not hospital based, relationships usually exist allowing specialized equipment and personnel to fly on more critical transfers.

Helicopters cannot fly in freezing rain or in dense fog. Because of the high degree of sophistication, helicopter transport should be used only for those patients who have been shown to benefit from this expensive technology. An approximate annual budget for one dual-engine, EMS-configured aircraft is between $1 million and $3 million, depending on how the medical crew is accounted for. These programs attempt to obtain reimbursement from third-party payers but may require continued subsidy by tertiary institutions.

Fixed-Wing Aircraft

Fixed-wing aircraft should be considered for longer flights (more than 150 miles). A fixed-wing aircraft usually has IFR capability and will fly from airport to airport; the ground transportation is required at air-transfer initiation and completion. Most aircraft performing medical transports have the capability of being pressurized, although under certain clinical circumstances, it may be advisable to pressurize to ground level. Aircraft cabins on commercial airliners are pressurized between 6000 and 8000 feet depending on the altitude reached; medical transport over long distances may need similar pressurization. Air pressure at these levels affects not only the patient's condition but also the calibration of the monitors or ventilators that are being used for clinical support. Those being transferred to hyperbaric facilities for the bends, for example, may require pressurization at ground level; and for other patients who are ventilator dependent or when oxygen delivery and cardiac output may be critical, anticipation of the effects of pressurization on patient condition is essential. Fixed-wing aircraft vary considerably in price and complexity but are cheaper than rotor-craft on an hour-to-hour basis. Transcontinental or intercontinental flights of ventilated patients can now be performed.

Liability and Legal Issues

Interfacility transport has come under increasing legal scrutiny within the last few years. All physicians involved in interfacility transport should be aware of the passage of the (Consolidated Omnibus Budget Reconciliation Act in 1986 (Section 9121, Amendments to the Social Security Law in 1985; and Section 1867, Special Responsibilities for Hospital and Emergency Cases in 1985). These rules have been subsequently amended by the Omnibus Reconciliation Act of 1989, which was enacted in 1990. These laws refer to emergency transfers of unstable patients and were originally drafted to address transfers of uninsured patients; however, these two acts provide a framework of legal responsibility, and this has been accepted in interfacility transfers. Physicians should be familiar with these acts;[10–12] briefly, the sending facility is responsible for initiating the transfer and for selecting the mode of transportation. When one selects the mode of transportation, one is also selecting the level of expertise of the transferring personnel and indirectly the equipment in the transporting vehicle. The sending physician is responsible for determining the risks of transfer and, for emergency transfers, has to attest in writing that the benefits to the patient after successful transfer outweigh the risks of the transfer itself. The receiving facility is responsible for ensuring that there is available space and personnel. The amended 1989 act further noted that receiving facilities that have specialized units—noted as burn units, shock trauma units, and neonatal ICUs—cannot refuse transfers if space is available. This was designed as a nondiscrimination clause and is an attempt to prevent receiving facilities from selecting nonindigent transfers for acceptance while denying access to those without the ability to pay. ICUs that may be closed because of high census should have a mechanism of monitoring their refusal of patient transfers if they are to be compliant with these regulations.

For institutions that provide transfer programs, there are other liability concerns such as workmen's compensation and disability insurance for the transporting personnel and regular audiometry (important for helicopter crews). In addition, directors' and officers' insurance may be required of governing and administrative personnel. Flight programs may also require hull insurance to cover aircraft loss and insurance to cover property damage in the case of a crash over a densely populated area.

Flight programs should comply with the U.S. Occupational Safety and Health Administration regulations for their crew members; exposure and risk are different than those for in-hospital personnel and must be addressed in relation to program configuration.

Outcome Data

Many attempts have been made in the literature to support the concept of regionalization of care using transport technology; efforts have followed one of four themes:

1. Outcomes of the critically ill in tertiary centers matched for severity are better than outcomes in community hospitals
2. Critical patients can be transferred over long distances without an adverse outcome and, hence, by implication achieve the benefit of tertiary care (vide supra)
3. Subsets of critically ill transferred patients have improved outcomes compared with national norms
4. An established healthcare system that incorporates critical transfer as an integral part of system function provides better societal outcomes than compatible communities without an integrated system

Pollack and colleagues,[13] in studying the outcome of critically injured children with head trauma and respiratory failure in Oregon, compared mortality in three tertiary facilities with 71 nontertiary hospitals. Using a risk of mortality score developed for the pediatric population, they demonstrated that outcomes in nontertiary facilities were poorer than those in tertiary facilities. Furthermore, they found that the difference in outcome was more pronounced the higher the expected mortality. In their most critical group, which is defined as a mortality risk of greater than 30%, the odds of dying in a nontertiary versus a tertiary facility was a factor of 8 ($P < .05$). Pollack and colleagues suggested that pediatric survival from a broader range of disorders could potentially be improved by regionalization of pediatric care. A similar study[14] examining the outcome of the multiply-traumatized patient was published by Kilberg and associates in 1988. These authors examined patients with a CRAMS (*C*irculation, *R*espiration, *A*bdomen, *M*otor, *S*peech) score[15] of 4 or less and compared the outcome of patients transferred to a level I trauma center with that of patients in community hospitals; they concluded that there was a significant difference. They also commented that there were no patient deaths as a result of delay at the accident scene awaiting helicopter arrival or during the longer transport times when by-passing a local facility by ground.

Management of the critically ill has been related to the volume of patients for both coronary artery bypass surgery[16] and trauma,[17] offering further support for regionalization. In other studies, transport of the critically ill has been shown not to increase mortality in patients with respiratory distress,[18] in cardiac patients,[19] and in pediatric patients.[20] In a study of emergency aeromedical transport of 104 patients with acute myocardial infarction,[21] transfer by helicopter was not detrimental to patient outcome.

The TRISS (*TR*auma score *I*njury *S*everity *S*core) methodology[22] has been used to demonstrate improved outcomes in trauma patients transferred by helicopter compared with national norms.[23] An expanded study with more than 1200 patients from seven aeromedical programs demonstrated similar improvement.[24]

Systems of care have been shown to benefit the multiply-traumatized patient and the head-injury patient.[25–27] However, analysis of such systems has not defined the specific contribution made by appropriate triage, transport, or improvement in definitive care at the receiving institution.

Studies of this nature provide support for regionalization of critical care, of which transport is an essential component.

EQUIPMENT AND MONITORING

Interfacility critical care transport requires interfacility critical care management. The patient should be monitored, and the transporting vehicle should have the ability to transfer necessary equipment. Back-up battery supply in case of electrical failure should be available, and additional oxygen should be carried to supply patient needs in case of vehicle breakdown. In colder climates, maintenance of a warm environment in case of vehicle failure is also important. It should be emphasized that the transport environment is different from the ICU, and compromises may be necessary to ensure that equipment is small, light, and rugged and can function under adverse circumstances.

Medications

Lists of appropriate medications to be used on critical transport have been published for pediatric patients,[28, 29] obstetric patients,[30] neonates,[31] and adult patients.[32] All transferring personnel managing these patient subsets should be aware of the use and complications of all of these medications and ensure that the expiratory dates on medications are acceptable. Guidelines should be in place for the involvement of the sending physician, the transferring personnel, and the receiving physician as well as for the use of on-line medical direction, either by radio or cellular telephone.

Ventilators

Several ventilators have been designed that may be used for the transport environment. The exact choice will depend on mission profile, choice of the medical director, and usually compatibility with the receiving ICU staff. Most programs now monitor the patients continuously, both by electrocardiogram monitor and pulse oximetry; continuous oximetry can identify clinically unrecognized hypoxia.[33, 34] Small, robust monitors can be used to measure intra-arterial pressure, pulmonary artery pressure, and intracranial pressure should the patient require it.

Some programs now provide the capability of transferring patients on left ventricular assist devices or intra-aortic balloon pumps; these have been configured to fit inside helicopters and fixed-wing aircraft. For further information, readers are referred to specific transport programs performing these difficult transfers.

EDUCATION AND TRAINING

Physicians

Physicians involved in critical care transport may function as off-line medical control (i.e., supervising training, developing medical protocols, standing orders and quality assurance); as on-line medical control by providing consultation to transferring personnel either by radio or cellular telephone; or as integral members of the transport team. A survey of medical directors of critical care air-transport services showed that only 15% were members of the Society of Critical Care Medicine despite the fact that 70% of patients being transferred by these services were critically ill interfacility transfers.[35] The majority of online medical control is provided by emergency physicians who are familiar with providing medical direction to EMS paramedics. Most physicians who provide such consultation have obtained training and are familiar with the radio equipment and the rules and regulations governing their use.

Crew Qualifications

Paramedic

Paramedics have completed a curriculum outlined by the Department of Transportation and need to be certified by a state licensing examination. They have knowledge of all emergency situations and can usually perform defibrillation, endotracheal intubation, and cricothyrotomy, although use of these skills may be modified at either the state or local level. The paramedic corresponds to the aeromedical crew level II in the American College of Surgeons document.[32]

Critical Care Transport Nurse

There are no national guidelines at this time for critical care transport nurses and no requirement for state or national licensure other than being a registered nurse. Many flight programs have developed flight nurse curriculums, but training depends on the program profile. Critical care transport registered nurses should have knowledge of the management of obstetric, neonate, pediatric, burn, cardiac, and psychiatric patients. In addition, those teams that are involved with aviation should have knowledge of altitude physiology, aircraft safety, aviation communication, and crash and survival. Facilities and crew should be subjected to ongoing curriculum development and quality assurance by a medical director. The medical director should perform regular audits and be responsible for continuing education.

REIMBURSEMENT AND COST

In hospital-based transport teams involving ground ambulances, often the sponsoring facility supports the medical crew and assumes the liability for the patient. The sponsoring institution enters into a contract with an ambulance company, which provides the ambulance, a driver, and in some cases paramedical personnel. Clear delineation of authority and responsibility should be outlined by contract, together with a clear understanding of the financial support of the program. Ground ambulance services are often covered by third-party payers, but a medical necessity form may be required justifying transfer before payment is made.

Helicopter programs usually lease the helicopter as well as support mechanics, pilots, and back-up aircraft for both scheduled and unscheduled maintenance. Medical crew salaries are handled by the hospital, and the hospital providing medical direction assumes legal responsibility for the medical management. Most programs attempt to bill third-party payers, but recovery is not usually sufficient to maintain financial viability. Charges and reimbursement are quite variable nationally;[36, 37] and the charge structure may vary depending on whether crew costs and equipment costs are placed in the hospital cost base or within the flight program. Some third-party payers only recognize transport to the closest medical facility that is capable of managing the care of that individual even though this may be in contrast to the EMS plan for the state or region or those of traditional referral lines.

THE FUTURE

Pressure to control healthcare costs while providing improved patient outcome will mandate regionalization of all critical illness. Transport technology already exists with the ability to transfer extremely critical patients over long distances with minimal detrimental effects. As integrated healthcare-delivery networks are established, moving critical patients expeditiously within a system will gradually emerge as a subspecialty of both critical care and emergency medicine.

References

1. Collett H: Transport survey. J Air Med Transport 1992; 11:25–28.
2. Collett H: 1988 program survey. Hospital Aviation 1989; 8:19–21.
3. Carraway RP, Bremer ME, Lewis BR, et al: Why a physician? Aeromedical transport of the trauma victim (Abstract). J Trauma 1984; 24:650.
4. Rhee KJ, Strozeski M, Burney RE, et al: Is a flight physician needed for helicopter emergency services? Ann Emerg Med 1986; 15:174–177.
5. Snow N, Hull C, Stevens J: Physician staffing on a helicopter emergency service. Emerg Care Q 1986; 2:40–45.
6. Baxt WG, Moody P: The impact of physicians as part of the aeromedical prehospital team in patients with blunt trauma. JAMA 1987; 257:3246–3250.
7. Gervin AS: Cricothyrotomy by flight paramedics. Aeromed J 1988; 3:22.
8. Boyle M, Sheets C: Surgical cricothyrotomy performed by air ambulance flight nurses: A five-year experience. J Air Med Transport 1989; 8:60.
9. Schneider C, Gomez M, Lee R: Evaluation of ground ambulance, rotor-wing and fixed-wing aircraft services. Crit Care Clin 1992; 8:533–564.
10. Beckman P: COBRA can bite. J Emerg Med Service 1989; 8:11–12.
11. Frew SA: Emergency medical services legal issues for the emergency physician. Emerg Med Clin North Am 1990; 8:41–55.
12. Dunn JD: Legal aspects of transfers. *In*: Problems in Critical Care. Philadelphia, JB Lippincott, 1990, pp 447–448.
13. Pollack MM, Alexander SR, Clarke N, et al: Improved outcomes from tertiary center pediatric intensive care: A statewide comparison of tertiary and non-tertiary care facilities. Crit Care Med 1991; 19:150–159.
14. Kilberg L, Clemmer TP, Clawson J, et al: Effectiveness of implementing a trauma triage system or outcome: A prospective evaluation. J Trauma 1988; 28:1493–1498.
15. Gornican SP: CRAMS scale: Field range of trauma victims. Ann Emerg Med 1982; 11:132–135.
16. Hannan EL, O'Donnel JF, Kilburn H, et al: Investigation of the relationship between volume and mortality for surgical procedures performed in New York hospitals. JAMA 1989; 262:503–510.
17. Smith RF, Frateschi L, Sloan EP, et al: The impact of volume of outcome in seriously injured trauma patients: Two years' experience of the Chicago trauma system. J Trauma 1990; 30:1066–1076.
18. Harless KW, Morris AH, Cengiz M, et al: Civilian ground and air transport of adults with acute respiratory failure. JAMA 1978; 240:361–365.

19. Rubinstein D, Treister NW, Kapoor AS, et al: Transfer of acutely ill cardiac patients for definitive care. JAMA 1988; 259:1695–1698.
20. Usher R: Changing mortality rates with perinatal intensive care and regionalization. Perinatol 1977; 3:309–314.
21. Kaplan L, Walsh D, Burney RE: Emergency aeromedical transport of patients with acute myocardial infarction. Ann Emerg Med 1987; 16:55–57.
22. Boyd CR, Tolson MA, Copes WS: Evaluating trauma care: The TRISS method. J Trauma 1987; 27:370–378.
23. Baxt WG, Moody P: The impact of a rotorcraft aeromedical emergency care science on trauma mortality. JAMA 1983; 249:3047–3051.
24. Baxt WG, Moody P, Cleveland HC, et al: Hospital based rotorcraft aeromedical emergency care services and trauma mortality: A multicenter study. Ann Emerg Med 1985; 14:859–864.
25. Shackford SR, Hollingsworth-Findlund P, Cooper GF: The effect of regionalization upon the quality of trauma care as assessed by concurrent audit before and after institution of a trauma system: A preliminary report. J Trauma 1986; 26:812–818.
26. Cales RH: Trauma mortality in Orange County: The effect of implementation of a regional trauma system. Ann Emerg Med 1984; 13:1–10.
27. Shackford SR: Cause of decline in head injury mortality in San Diego, California. J Neurosurg 1985; 62:528–531.
28. Hackel A, Simon JE, Wingert WA, et al: Committee on hospital care guidelines for air and ground transportation of pediatric patients. Pediatrics 1986; 78:943–950.
29. Day S, McCloskey K, et al: Pediatric interhospital critical care transport: Consensus of national leadership conference. Pediatrics 1991; 88:696–704.
30. Giles HR: Maternal transport. Clin Obstet Gynecol 1979; 6:203.
31. MacDonald MG: Infant transport equipment checklist. *In*: Emergency Transport of the Perinatal Patient. MacDonald MG, Miller MK (Eds). Boston, Little, Brown and Co, 1989, p 410.
32. Committee on Trauma, American College of Surgeons: Resources for Optimal Care of the Injured Patient. Chicago, IL, American College of Surgeons, 1990.
33. Gudgell S, Vukov LF, Farrell MB: Pulse oximetry in rotorwing transport. Aeromed J 1987; 2:81.
34. Short L, Hecker RB, Middaugh RE, et al: A comparison of pulse oximeters during helicopter flight. J Emerg Med 1989; 7:639–643.
35. Poulton TJ, Kisicki PA: Medical directors of critical care air transport services. Crit Care Med 1987; 15:784–785.
36. Collett H: 1992 transport charge survey. J Air Med Transport 1992; 11:25.
37. Schneider C: Counting the cost. Emergency 1989; 7:39–43.

CHAPTER 12

Neonatal and Pediatric Transport Programs

Michael I. Cinoman, MD • Richard A. Orr, MD

Injured or sick children must be moved from one site to another for numerous reasons. A *scene run* refers to the transfer of a patient by local emergency medical service (EMS) personnel to the nearest available emergency department or designated hospital from either the patient's home or the scene of an accident. The personnel attending these transports often provide the first line of emergency care to critically ill patients. *Interhospital transport* refers to the transfer of a patient from a hospital where initial stabilization is provided to one where definitive treatment is provided. *Intrahospital transport* refers to the transfer of a patient between locations within a hospital and typically involves moving a patient from the emergency department or operating room to a patient ward or taking a patient for a diagnostic study.

The goal of all transports should be to provide the same quality of care that the patient received before transport without increased morbidity or mortality. However, limitations of monitoring capability, diminished resources, and general hazards associated with a moving environment all increase the risk of morbidity to these patients during transport. Although decisions are made daily regarding the mode of travel and the staffing of pediatric transports, little research supports the validity of the decision-making process. One prospective study found the morbidity during the first 2 hours to be twice as high in critically ill pediatric patients transported by nonspecialized teams compared with patients admitted directly to the pediatric intensive care unit (PICU) from within the hospital.[1] Because most transport systems were designed for adult patients, pediatric transports are particularly fraught with problems. A prospective survey of 100 pediatric emergency transports found 340 problems with these transports. Of these problems, 24% were believed to be preventable by improved education of referring physicians (including, e.g., the unrecognized need for ventilatory support and difficulties with airway selection) and 28% were deemed preventable by better organization of the pediatric emergency transport system. Difficulties associated with the transport environment itself (such as vibration, noise, air turbulence) were uncommon.[2] According to one source, "Perhaps there is no element in the continuum of critical care services that is less understood and laced with monocular biases than the transport of patients to and between hospitals."[3] Children appear to be at higher risk for morbidity during interhospital transport than at other times during their overall care.

INDICATIONS FOR INTERHOSPITAL TRANSPORT

Patients are transported from one hospital to another to obtain a better level of care than is provided by the referring institution. In most cases, transport from a community hospital to a tertiary care center involves a child whose medical requirements exceed the capability of the primary institution. Nonpediatric centers may not be optimally prepared to handle pediatric emergencies because of limited resources or lack of proper training of the caregivers.[3a] In some cases, children may require subspecialty consultation for unusual diseases or those confined to the pediatric population. In other cases, patients may be referred for surgical care or advanced life support to units dedicated to the care of critically ill children.

RESPONSIBILITY FOR THE PATIENT DURING TRANSPORT

The responsibility for the patient's care during a transport may depend on who makes the decision for transport and the composition of the transport team. When the receiving hospital will not be transporting the patient, it must be notified of the impending transfer before it occurs. Otherwise, the referring hospital has been considered to have "abandoned" the patient, which is defined as the "unilateral termination of a physician-patient relationship by the physician, without the patient's consent and without giving the patient sufficient opportunity to secure the services of another competent physician."[3b] Under a new law, the Consolidated Omnibus Budget Reconciliation Act, legal liability has been expanded beyond previous standards. This act requires the transferring hospital to assume responsibility not only for the safe transfer of a patient until arrival at the receiving hospital but also for the medical integrity of the receiving hospital and for the appropriateness of the patient's transfer.[4]

When the receiving hospital provides a transport team, it should assume full responsibility for the patient when its team arrives at the referring hospital. However, if the receiving institution only provides advice over the telephone and asks the referring hospital to arrange transport, responsibility is jointly shared between the referring and receiving hospitals.[4a] In either case, the decision regarding the composition of the transport team, made by both the transferring and receiving institutions, will ultimately determine who is responsible for the patient during the transport.

COMPOSITION OF THE TRANSPORT TEAM

Perhaps the greatest controversy in pediatric transport medicine involves the question of who should be directly caring for the patient during the transport.

No Team

One option is simply to have the parents of the patient transport their child in their own vehicle. Because no trained medical caregiver is present in this situation and the responsibility for the patient rests with the referring physician, this method should be undertaken only for a patient whose condition will not deteriorate during transport. This form of transport also suffers from unpredictable delays because parents have no control over traffic and weather conditions and may not take their child directly to the receiving center.

Local Emergency Medical Services

Many interhospital transfers do not involve critically ill children and can be accomplished safely using local EMS. The advantages of this form of transport are the relatively low cost, availability of trained medical personnel should some intervention be necessary, and decreased time spent in city traffic.

Some problems are associated with using EMS, particularly in the transport of children. The focus of EMS training is primarily on the adult population, and some systems fail to meet the needs of children.[4a–d] In evaluating the ability of paramedics to assess children, one study found that paramedics' assessments agreed with those of the physicians only 50% of the time and that paramedics were more likely to underestimate the severity of a pediatric patient's problem.[5] A retrospective review of pediatric transports involving EMS personnel who had training in pediatric intubation revealed an intubation success rate during transport of only 64%, with the rate decreasing to only 50% in children younger than 1 year.[6] This rate differs markedly from the success rate in adults in other EMS systems (85–95%).[7] Another retrospective study examined paramedics' success with intravenous access in children and found that access was attempted in 80% of patients who met the criteria for placement of intravenous catheters in the field, with a success rate of 84%. The success rate decreased to 49% in patients younger than 6 years.[8] One study proposed a computer model for overall "time to intubation" in children with impending respiratory failure. The model takes into account success rates for the intubation of children by paramedics and travel time from the scene to the emergency department. In this model in areas in which the success rates for paramedics were poor, police transports demonstrated shorter times to intubation for short runs from the scene to the emergency department, whereas paramedic transports demonstrated shorter times to intubation for longer runs. The authors concluded that police care transport of ill children should be considered in the development of an urban pediatric EMS.[9] These studies do not suggest that EMS is inappropriate in the transport of children but rather that, particularly where intubation or intravenous access may be necessary, transport by other means or those more experienced with these procedures should be considered. Improved paramedic training in pediatric advanced life support might also be helpful in areas in which the failure rates for intubation and intravenous catheter insertion are unacceptably high.

Additional Personnel from the Referring Hospital

Ambulance transport with added personnel and equipment from the referring hospital can provide an additional level of care. This option is less costly and possibly faster than the use of a critical care transport team. A disadvantage is that it results in the loss of personnel from the referring hospital. This form of transport is usually indicated in cases in which a dedicated transport team is unavailable or when arrival at the receiving hospital is deemed "time dependent."[9a] A physician is often included on these transports because the patient is critically ill. It must be remembered that if the members of the hospital staff are uncomfortable managing the patient in the emergency department, they will likely be even more so in an ambulance, where access to anesthesia, radiology, and some types of monitoring are not available.

Dedicated Transport Teams

These teams vary in composition and may include any combination of a physician, nurse, paramedic, or respiratory therapist. A dedicated pediatric transport team should be able to deliver care to a child during transport equivalent to that found in a PICU. Transport should occur without deterioration in the child's clinical status. Any medications or interventions necessary to maintain stability should be delivered by those caregivers who have experience in their use and performance. In most cases, a physician, particularly one who is trained in critical care or emergency medicine, has the most experience in making decisions and performing interventions on critically ill children. Therefore, ideally, a physician should be present during the transport of a child who requires intensive care. However, most emergency or critical care physicians are limited resources and have other clinical responsibilities. The difficulty comes in trying to determine which patients will require the skills of specialized personnel before the transport itself.

The ability to predict the need for and composition of a suitable, dedicated pediatric transport team based on a patient's pretransport severity of illness is one of the most active and controversial areas of research in the field of pediatric transport. For adults and neonatal patients, data suggest that physicians are not always needed as part of the transport team.[9b] Neonates in particular tend to have a limited number of problems that are common, and transport teams using dedicated neonatal transport nurses have been shown to have success rates similar to using physician-based teams.[10] However, older infants and children can have numerous problems causing them to be critically ill. One study of a system using physicians on all pediatric transports found that physicians subjectively believed they were necessary during transport only 46% of the time.[11] In a follow-up study by the same principal investigator, physicians were prospectively asked to decide subjectively whether they would be necessary during the transport based on information available before transport. They were then asked the same question again after the transport was completed. Physicians underestimated their need during transport in only 2% of all transports, whereas 25% overestimated their need during transport.[12]

Rather than relying on a physician's subjective opinion for the composition of the transport team, current research has sought methods to predict the need for specialized skills during transports. These skills usually involve interventions (intubation) or the administration of various medications (epinephrine or diazepam). Such studies attempted to stratify patients according to their pretransport severity of illness, which could be assessed using combinations of data derived from vital signs, clinical status, diagnosis, previously performed interventions, or numerous laboratory tests available before transport. In one study, the criteria of intubation and age of less than 1 year with unstable vital signs most accurately predicted the need for major interventions and the presence of a physician during transport.[13]

Other work has sought to use previously validated severity of illness scores for children to predict the need for critical care during transport. The pediatric risk of mortality (PRISM) score has been validated to predict mortality for patients admitted to PICUs on the basis of vital signs, laboratory data, and clinical status obtained on the first day of hospitalization (see Chapter 199). One study showed that deterioration during transport rarely occurred (4%) in patients with a PRISM score less than 10; the authors concluded that referring hospital personnel are capable of safely transporting such patients.[14] However, 25% of the patients in this study who experienced physiologic deterioration during transport had a PRISM score of less than 10. Other studies found that the PRISM score did not predict the need for a physician's presence during transport,[15, 15a] whereas another showed that the PRISM score underestimates the requirement for major interventions during transport.[16] These findings are not surprising because the PRISM score was validated for the purpose of determining in-hospital mortality in critically ill patients, and many patients with a low risk of mortality may still require interventions and medications during transport (as in patients with asthma or seizures), whereas others with a high risk of mortality actually require little care during transport (as in patients with chronic liver failure who are being referred for evaluation for transplantation).

Newer work must focus on developing severity of illness scores based on data that are readily available on patients before their transport. These scores must be predictive for outcome variables such as the need for critical interventions or administration of medications, which would indicate the need for specialized personnel during the transport. Because paramedic-based teams have a higher than acceptable rate of failure to diagnose and treat ill children adequately, and because currently available severity of illness scores do not allow stratification of children to predict their needs during transport adequately, decisions regarding the composition of the transport team should be made cautiously.

MODES OF TRANSPORT

Patients may be transported by ground or air depending on their needs. Factors to be considered include space, speed of transport, cost, distance, and severity of illness.

Ground-Based Vehicle

The ambulance is the most frequently used vehicle for ground transport. The advantages for pediatric transport include a relatively large work area, minimal cost when compared with other modes of transport, the availability of assistance from paramedics, and general availability of these vehicles. However, the greatest advantage over air transport is in the ability to stop quickly during the transport, which immediately removes the interference of noise and vibration and allows attending personnel to perform patient intervention when necessary. The disadvantages of ground transport are the time required to transport patients great distances and the need to contend with heavy traffic.

Aeromedical Transport Services

Civilian, hospital-based aeromedical transport services were developed in the 1970s initially to transport trauma victims to a trauma center. The greatest advantage of aeromedical transport for children is the speed of the transport. When the transport is needed in densely populated areas or over a long distance, a helicopter can perform this task more quickly than a ground-based transport. The disadvantages of aeromedical transport are noise and a cramped work area, which make clinical assessment and the performance of procedures difficult in any patient. Accurate assessment of breath sounds is impossible in a helicopter.[16a] Costs are high compared with ground transport. The national average charge for a 100-mile round-trip helicopter transport is approximately $2400.[16b]

Fixed-wing aircraft can also be used but generally only for distances greater than 150 miles when ground transport and helicopter transport are unfeasible. Fixed-wing aircraft may be used for shorter distances, but they lose the advantage of cost and time saved. Additional advantages include a larger work area and quieter conditions than are found in a helicopter. When an increase in altitude could potentially worsen a patient's condition (as with pneumothorax or pneumopericardium), cabin pressure can be controlled within limits. The disadvantages include the cost of transport and need for airports in the vicinity of both the referring and receiving hospitals. Probably the greatest disadvantage is the total time required to transport the patient. Most fixed-wing aircraft operators require some time for flight planning and crew preparation, sometimes taking up to an hour before departing to the pickup site. The patient must be transported from the referring hospital by ambulance to the aircraft and then back to an ambulance for transfer to the receiving hospital. In our experience, fixed-wing aircraft transport generally takes a minimum of 4 to 5 hours once the request is made regardless of the transport distance and even under the best of circumstances.

More than 180 aeromedical transport services operate in the United States, and many transport children as well as adults.[16c] With most of these services, team composition varies for the transport of children; the most common is a flight nurse and paramedic. In 1986, the American Academy of Pediatrics (AAP) published guidelines for the transport of children.[17] Nevertheless, one survey of aeromedical transport services showed poor compliance with these guidelines.[18] In particular, all aeromedical transport services surveyed agreed to transport children; however, only 20% had personnel with pediatric training, and only 9% had medical directors or transport coordinators who were pediatric specialists. Only 30% varied transport team composition based on the patient's condition, as has been recommended by the AAP and many researchers.

BASIC PRINCIPLES OF PEDIATRIC TRANSPORT

Although a great deal of research has been published regarding the transport of both adults and neonates, no rigid criteria have been established for the transport of children. The AAP guidelines provide only the most general principles for the transport of children. Much of what has been published to date suggests that many problems exist in pediatric transport as it is presently practiced in many areas, and only recently has an effort been made to study solutions to these problems.

Administration

In its 1986 guidelines for transport of children, the AAP stated that "the most important component of a pediatric transport system is medical control by a qualified pediatric specialist."[17] The director should be trained in either pediatric critical care or emergency medicine. This person is responsible for the design and daily management of the program, including selecting the transport team, defining transport protocols, and acting as liaison with both the hospital administration and other physicians in the community. The director has the ultimate responsibility for patient care and quality control during transport. Questions and complaints from the referring hospitals should be handled by the medical director. The director may also have to handle financial issues such as contracts with ambulance services, protocols for the transport of uninsured patients, and possibly even the salaries of employees.

Protocol

The specifics of the transport process are defined by protocols that are individualized for specific programs and specific areas of the country. A dedicated pediatric transport team must be able to mobilize quickly to respond to the needs of the referring community. This can occur only if predetermined lines of communication are in place, equipment is prepared, and dedicated team members are available at all times. Simple computer programs can calculate and print pediatric drug doses for patients according to their age and weight. Finally, a transport team must have agreements with both ambulance and aeromedical transport companies to have priority when their services are needed.[18]

Communication

Because each transport begins with communication between the referring and receiving hospitals, all transport systems should have a protocol for patient referrals. The referring hospital should make contact and initiate the transport process with the receiving hospital as soon as the patient has been initially stabilized. A list of commonly used referral centers should be posted by the telephone. The initial telephone contact is an extremely important time during the transport process because the receiving center will decide on team composition and make recommendations to the referring center according to information obtained at this time.

One study has shown that data obtained during the initial telephone call significantly underestimate the patient's severity of illness (as measured by a PRISM score) compared with data obtained by the transport team once it has actually arrived to care for the patient.[19] This finding is probably due to both miscommunication between the referring and receiving hospitals and clinical deterioration of the patient from the time of the initial telephone referral. Such data emphasize the need for expedient yet thorough telephone communication. An organized approach to the initial telephone referral will allow complete patient information to be communicated in just minutes. Many referring hospitals prefer having a critically ill child transferred as rapidly as possible because of the lack of equipment and medications specifically designed for children as well as their limited experience in treating children. However, it is in the patient's best interest to have information carefully and completely provided over the telephone to assist the receiving hospital.

The receiving hospital, particularly if it is a tertiary care pediatric facility, should have a dedicated system in place to service referrals from the surrounding community. A telephone number other than the hospital operator or emergency department should be dedicated for transport referrals. The number should be publicized and well known at community hospitals in the area. A designated physician should be available at all times to receive transport calls as a priority. A log should be kept both as a permanent record of the telephone referral and as a guide to prompt the physician to obtain complete information before transport. The telephone log should record pertinent information, including the patient's weight, vital signs, neurologic status, brief history of illness, and relevant laboratory and x-ray film results. The receiving hospital should conclude the call by making recommendations for additional patient care that are easily within the means of the referring hospital. They should also be advised to prepare the patient for transport and prevent delays once the transport team has arrived.

Communication must not end with the initial telephone referral. The referring hospital should be encouraged to relate updates to the receiving hospital if the patient's condition changes, and the receiving hospital should notify the referring hospital of their mode of transport and estimated time of arrival as soon as these are known. The receiving hospital should provide the referring physician with follow-up information at least on arrival of the patient and 1 week later.

General Preparation at the Referring Hospital

In general, a referring hospital that agrees to accept children must be prepared to care for them until transport is available. They should follow standard resuscitation guidelines for children. Dosages for pediatric resuscitation drugs should be posted. Equipment that is designed for children, including all sizes of endotracheal tubes, intravenous catheters, and ventilation bags and masks, should be available in all hospitals. Healthcare workers (paramedics, nurses, and physicians) in community hospitals that care for children should be trained in pediatric advanced life support and recertified every 2 years to stay current with life-support recommendations and skills.

In the short term, before the arrival of the transport team, the referring hospital can prepare the patient for transport to reduce the time the team will need to spend at the referring hospital. Informed consent to transport should be discussed with the patient's family. IV catheters and endotracheal tubes must be secured before transport. Kanter and colleagues[1] found that endotracheal tubes plugged or dislodged and IV access was lost in 15% of children during transport compared with a 3.6% incidence of the same mishaps occurring in PICU patients with the same severity of illness during the first 2 hours after admission to the intensive care unit (ICU). The patient's records and x-ray films should be copied in advance. Any blood products that may be necessary during transport should be ordered as soon as possible. Telephone numbers of the laboratories performing the tests should be included in the patient's records to allow the receiving hospital to follow culture results.

Equipment

The equipment used in pediatric transport must be as compact as possible and have some ability to operate by battery power for 4 to 6 hours. Any team dedicated to transporting infants must have a transport isolette to provide a warm environment because these patients are at risk for hypothermia as a result of their small size and relatively large body surface area. Often these isolettes include built-in monitors and ventilators. A transport ventilator should be simple to use; for example, it should be flow generated, time cycled, pressure limited, and able to conserve gas consumption. Positive end-expiratory pressure must be provided either directly through the ventilator or through valves in the expiratory limb of the circuit. The oxygen requirements for each patient must be estimated before transport, and approximately twice that amount should be available in the event of delays. Transport ventilators can deplete gas supplies rapidly and should be used only by an experienced respiratory therapist or nurse.

A pediatric transport team should always carry enough supplies to ensure the provision of a level of care equivalent to that found in a PICU because many community emergency departments are limited in their ability to care for children. These supplies include ventilation masks, intravenous catheters, nasal cannulas, chest tubes, blood pressure cuffs, oral and nasal airways, laryngoscopes, and endotracheal tubes of all sizes (Table 12–1). A suggested list of medications is shown in Table 12–2.

Scoop and Run?

Undue pressure is often placed on transport teams, both paramedic based and specialized, to get the patient out of the referring hospital as rapidly as possible. This pressure to "scoop and run" comes from several sources. Some teams try to apply the golden hour of trauma to all pediatric transports and attempt to deliver patients to the receiving center as rapidly as possible because they believe that this improves patient outcome. The staff of the emergency department in the referring hospital may hope to have the patient out quickly because of their discomfort in caring for sick children and to make room for other patients who may be waiting for their services. Because air medical services are an industry as well as a profession, flight crews may operate under a directive to capture as many flights as possible to maximize revenue and compete with other services.

The optimal time that a team should spend at the referring hospital is not clearly defined[19a]; however, it logically varies depending on the severity and type of illness, duration of transport, amount of care already being provided at the referring hospital, and level of expertise of the transport team. The concept of the golden hour was created 20 years ago for trauma victims whose chances for survival at that time improved considerably if transferred to a tertiary care center within 1 hour of sustaining their injuries.[19b] This principle, which was found to be true for severely injured trauma patients, has been extrapolated to many areas of the field of transport, including pediatrics. The golden hour principle may indeed hold true for patients whose most urgent need is surgical and when little can be done until the patient arrives in the operating room. However, as previously discussed, most morbidity that occurs during pediatric transport relates to inadequate airway management or the inability to obtain vascular access when necessary. Experienced individuals need relatively little time to stabilize the airway and circulation of a child even if intubation and vascular access are required. This care is much more difficult to deliver in the noisy, moving transport environment if the patient deteriorates and requires it emergently. Although currently unproved, adequate attention to a child's "ABCs" (*a*irway, *b*reathing, and *c*irculation) at the referring hospital by those experienced in pediatric care may more effectively reduce the mortality and morbidity seen in the transport of critically ill children than rapid transfer to a tertiary care center.

TABLE 12–1. Equipment and Supplies for Transport

Respiratory Equipment
Oxygen tanks
Oxygen hood
Bag, valve, masks (all sizes)
Pressure manometer
Intubation equipment
  Endotracheal tubes
    Uncuffed, 2.0–6.5
    Cuffed, 5.0–8.0
  Oral airways
  Laryngoscopes
  Magill forceps
Ventilator
Nebulizer for aerosols
Suction equipment

Monitors
Electrocardiograph
Respiratory
Temperature
Pressure
Defibrillator (pediatric paddles)
Pulse oximeter
Stethoscope
Blood pressure cuffs

Procedure Packs
Cutdown kit
Thoracostomy kit
Venous catheterization kits

Fluids, Infusion Devices
5% dextrose in water
0.9% saline
5% albumin
Lactated Ringer's solution
Infusion pumps
Intravenous catheters

Miscellaneous
Skin-preparation solutions
Tape
Electrodes

TABLE 12–2. Medications for Transport

Resuscitation
Epinephrine
Sodium bicarbonate
Atropine
Glucose
Naloxone
Lidocaine
Isoproterenol

Cardiovascular
Adenosine
Digoxin
Dopamine/dobutamine
Prostaglandin E_1
Furosemide
Hydralazine
Phenylephrine

Central Nervous System
Phenobarbital
Phenytoin
Lorazepam
Thiopental
Dexamethasone

Pulmonary
Aminophylline
Albuterol
Racemic epinephrine
Methylprednisolone

Sedation/Analgesia
Morphine
Midazolam
Fentanyl

Antibiotics
Ampicillin/nafcillin
Cefotaxime/ceftriaxone
Aminoglycoside
Clindamycin

Muscle Relaxants
Pancuronium/vecuronium

Miscellaneous
Potassium chloride
Calcium chloride
Heparin
Charcoal
Insulin

INTRAHOSPITAL TRANSPORT

In recent years, technologic radiographic advances, such as magnetic resonance imaging, computed tomography, and angiography, have given the medical field many additional tools to aid in the diagnosis and treatment of critically ill patients. However, because most of this equipment is not portable, patients must be moved from the ICU or emergency room to another location in the hospital. Patients are transported throughout the hospital for other reasons, including transfer from unit to unit, transfer to and from the operating room, and transfer to the cardiac catheterization laboratory. In some cases, patients may be moved from their primary site of care for extended periods to areas of the hospital that have limited monitoring equipment and personnel with little experience in caring for the critically ill. Intrahospital transports occur as frequently as, if not more than, out-of-hospital transports, and in some instances the risk may be greater.[19c]

Although research efforts have been limited, much of the work on intrahospital transport has shown that critically ill patients are at risk for numerous problems during transport. The adverse events that occur are equipment related as well as physiologic. Sixty-eight per cent of critically ill adult patients transported for diagnostic studies, with an average transport time of 81 minutes, experienced serious physiologic changes in blood pressure, heart rate, respiratory rate, or oxygen saturation that required an adjustment in support.[20] In a study of patients with severe head injury, adverse events (hypertension, increased intracranial pressure) occurred in 50% of transports.[21] Even relatively brief adult transports from the operating room to the ICU were found to have a surprisingly high incidence (13%) of adverse events.[22] In a study of critically ill pediatric patients from our institution, major adverse events (blood gas deterioration, endotracheal tube mishaps, less than 5% decrease in oxygen saturation, 20% change in vital signs, or medication error) occurred in 36% of patients transported from the operating room to the ICU and in 64% of patients transported for other reasons.[22a]

The goal of intrahospital transport of critically ill children is the same as that of all transports: It should occur with care equivalent to that delivered in the ICU and without an increase in mortality or morbidity. Although certainly unproved, it has been suggested that a critical care physician should be present during the intrahospital transport of any patient who is intubated or hemodynamically or neurologically unstable.[22b] Another suggestion is that a respiratory therapist should accompany the team if the patient is intubated or unstable from a respiratory standpoint.[22c] Advance preparation with adequate resuscitation is always important. In the study of head-injured patients, treatment of increased intracranial pressure in the 2 hours before transfer prevented associated complications during transfer of these patients.[21] Thorough monitoring and the use of equipment specifically designed for intrahospital transport may also help reduce adverse events. Link and colleagues[23] showed a significant decrease in problems during intrahospital transport of adults after the institution of a transport unit equipped with the following: independent power supply; respirator; capnometer; monitor with electrocardiograph; intracranial, intra-arterial blood pressure measuring capability; and two syringe pumps.

The optimal mode of ventilation for intubated critically ill patients during intrahospital transport is uncertain. Braman and associates[24] demonstrated that patients who were being manually ventilated had a greater incidence of clinically significant changes in hemodynamic status and blood gas values during transport (75%) than did those being ventilated with portable volume ventilation. However, Weg and Haas,[25] in a single-blind prospective study, found that patients who were being manually ventilated had no greater incidence of significant changes in hemodynamic status or blood gas values than did those being mechanically ventilated. These authors concluded that manual ventilation was safe for intrahospital transport; however, as they pointed out, less than 25% of their patients required any positive end-expiratory pressure. In patients with greater ventilatory demands, portable transport ventilators may be of value. The issue has not been examined in infants and children. However, children often require higher respiratory rates and smaller tidal volumes than adults, and duplicating mechanical ventilatory settings with manual ventilation may be more difficult than in adults, particularly in pediatric patients requiring a significant amount of ventilatory support.

References

1. Kanter RK, Boeing NM, Hannan WP, et al: Excess morbidity associated with interhospital transport. Pediatrics 1992; 90:893.
2. Henning R, McNamara V: Difficulties encountered in transport of the critically ill child. Pediatr Emerg Care 1991; 7:133.
3. American Academy of Pediatrics, American College of Obstetricians and Gynecologists: Guidelines for Perinatal Care. Elk Grove Village, IL, American Academy of Pediatrics, 1988, pp 209–222.

3a. Ludwig S, Fleisher G, Henretig F, et al: Pediatric training in emergency medicine residency programs. Ann Emerg Med 1982; 11:170.

3b. George JE: General legal principles. *In*: Law and Emergency Care. George JE (Ed). St Louis, CV Mosby, 1980, 1–18.

4. Frew SA, Roush WR, LaGreeca K: COBRA: Implications for emergency medicine. Ann Emerg Med 1988; 17:835.

4a. Venkataraman ST, Rubenstein JS, Orr RA: Interhospital transport: A pediatric perspective. Crit Care Clin 1992; 8:515.

4b. Graham CJ, Stuemky J, Lera TA: Emergency medical services preparedness for pediatric emergencies. Pediatr Emerg Care 1993; 9:329.

4c. Seidel JS, Hornbein M, Yoshiyama K, et al: Emergency medical services and the pediatric patient: Are the needs being met? Pediatrics 1984; 73:769.

4d. Seidel JS: Emergency medical services and the pediatric patient: Are the needs being met? II. Training and equipping emergency medical services providers for pediatric emergencies. Pediatrics 1986; 78:808.

5. Schonfield NA, Park K, Lev R, et al: Paramedic physical assessment and intervention in children (SAEM abstract). Ann Emerg Med 1989; 18:437.
6. Aijian P, Tsai A, Knopp R, et al: Endotracheal intubation of pediatric patients by paramedics. Ann Emerg Med 1989; 18:489.
7. Stewart R, Pris P, Winter P, et al: Field endotracheal intubation by paramedical personnel, success rates and complications. Chest 1984; 85:341.
8. Lillis KA, Jaffe DM: Prehospital intravenous access in children. Ann Emerg Med 1992; 21:1430.
9. Sacchetti A, Carraccio C, Feder M: Pediatric EMS transport: Are we treating children in a system designed for adults only? Pediatr Emerg Care 1992; 8:4.

9a. McCloskey K, Orr R: Pediatric transport issues in emergency medicine. Emerg Med Clin North Am 1991; 9:475.

9b. Baxt WG, Moody P: The impact of a physician as part of the aeromedical prehospital team in patients with blunt trauma. JAMA 1987; 257:3246.

10. Thompson TR: Neonatal transport nurses: An analysis of their role in the transport of newborn infants. Pediatrics 1980; 65:887.
11. McCloskey KA, King WD, Byron L: Pediatric critical care transport: Is a physician always needed on the team? Ann Emerg Med 1989; 18:247.
12. McCloskey KA, Johnston C: Critical care interhospital transports: Predictability of the need for a pediatrician. Pediatr Emerg Care 1990; 6:89.
13. McCloskey KA, Faries G, King WD, et al: Variables predicting the need for a pediatric critical care transport team. Pediatr Emerg Care 1992; 8:1.

14. Kanter RK, Tompkins JM: Adverse events during interhospital transport: Physiologic deterioration associated with pretransport severity of illness. Pediatrics 1989; 84:43.
15. Rubenstein JS, Gomez MA, Rybicki L: Can the need for a physician as part of the pediatric transport team be predicted? A prospective study. Crit Care Med 1992; 20:1657.
15a. Strauss RH, Rooney B: Critical care pediatrician-led transports: Physician interventions and predictiveness of outcome. Pediatr Emerg Care 1993; 9:270.
16. Orr RA, Venkataraman ST, Cinoman MI: Pretransport pediatric risk of mortality score (PRISM) underestimates the requirement for intensive care or major interventions during interhospital transport. Crit Care Med 1994; 22:101–107.
16a. Hunt RC, Bryan DM, Brinkley VS, et al: Inability to assess breath sounds during air medical transport by helicopter. JAMA 1991; 265:1982.
16b. 1992 Transport Charge Survey. J Air Med Transport 1992; 11:25.
16c. Aeromedical service directory. Hosp Aviat 1987; 6:3.
17. American Academy of Pediatrics, Committee on Hospital Care: Guidelines for air and ground transportation of pediatric patients. Pediatrics 1986; 78:943.
18. Strauss RH: Aeromedical transport services accepting pediatric patients and their abidance by published guidelines. Pediatr Emerg Care 1992; 8:318.
19. Whitfield JM, Costello ST, Young-Lashley S, et al: The telephone evaluation of severity of illness of the neonatal/pediatric patient prior to interhospital transfer. J Air Med Transport 1991; 10:82.
19a. Whitfield JM, Buser MK: Transport stabilization times for neonatal and pediatric patients prior to interfacility transfer. Pediatr Emerg Care 1993; 9:69.
19b. Cowley RS, Hudson F, Scanlan E, et al: An economical and proved helicopter program for transporting the emergency critically ill and injured patient in Maryland. J Trauma 1973; 13:1029.
19c. Venkataraman ST, Orr RA: Intrahospital transport of critically ill patients. Crit Care Clin 1992; 8:525.
20. Indeck M, Peterson S, Smith J, et al: Risk, cost, and benefit of transporting ICU patients for special studies. J Trauma 1988; 28:1020.
21. Andrews PJD, Piper IR, Dearden NM, et al: Secondary insults during intrahospital transport of head-injured patients. Lancet 1990; 335:327.
22. Insel J, Weissman C, Kemper M, et al: Cardiovascular changes during transport of critically ill and postoperative patients. Crit Care Med 1986; 14:539.
22a. Wallen EA, Venkataraman ST, Orr RA, et al: Adverse events during intrahospital transport of critically ill children. Crit Care Med 1991; 19:S79.
22b. Orr RA, McCloskey DA: Mobilizing critical care for interhospital and intrahospital transport. *In*: Lumb PD, Shoemaker WC (Eds): Critical Care: State of the Art. Vol. 11. Fullerton, CA, Society of Critical Care Medicine, 1990, pp 303–320.
22c. Ramsey CB, Holbrook PR: Pediatric Critical Care Transport. *In*: Textbook of Pediatric Critical Care. Holbrook PR (Ed): Philadelphia, WB Saunders, 1993, pp 1108–1116.
23. Link J, Krause H, Wagner W, et al: Intrahospital transport of critically ill patients. Crit Care Med 1990; 18:1427.
24. Braman SS, Dunn SM, Amico CA, et al: Complications of intrahospital transport in critically ill patients. Ann Intern Med 1987; 107:469.
25. Weg J, Haas C: Safe intrahospital transport of critically ill ventilator-dependent patients. Chest 1989; 96:631.

CHAPTER 13

Diagnosis and Treatment of the Shock Syndromes

William C. Shoemaker, MD

This chapter reviews the pathophysiology, outcome prediction, and therapy of postoperative, hemorrhagic, traumatic, and septic shock. A mechanistic model was generated from the sequential pattern of hemodynamic and oxygen transport parameters of survivors and nonsurvivors. Methods for outcome prediction were described and tested. Decision rules and a branch chain decision tree (clinical algorithm) for therapy were developed and tested prospectively.

RECOGNITION AND DIAGNOSIS OF SHOCK

Shock is a syndrome or symptom complex that is recognized clinically by subjective symptoms and signs such as cold clammy skin, pallor, altered mental status, weak thready pulse, and unstable vital signs. Routine standard therapeutic management in many instances is also directed toward correction of these subjective and very imprecise findings.

Traditionally, shock is classified by etiology as hemorrhagic, postoperative, cardiogenic, traumatic, neurogenic, or septic.[1–16] These etiologic categories are described by clinical signs and symptoms, laboratory findings, and the presumed primary pathophysiology; rather simplistic therapy based on these descriptions was developed for each etiology (Table 13–1). This approach is simple, easily understood, and generally accepted, but it is also seriously misleading.

The essential problem of this one-dimensional approach is that it proposes simplistic one-dimensional therapy for complex physiologic problems. Moreover, in actual clinical practice, each primary etiologic event does not begin and end with a single pathophysiologic defect that, when therapeutically corrected, leads to survival. Rather, the primary precipitating event of each etiologic type of shock sets in motion neural and neurohormonal compensations as well as numerous cascades that activate various biochemical mediators and inflammatory responses that are an integral part of the shock syndromes.

THE NATURE OF SHOCK

Essentially, the primary initiating event of shock syndromes is poor tissue perfusion from either low blood flow or unevenly distributed flow. This occurs early in the course of shock and stimulates physiologic mechanisms and biochemical mediators that lead to organ dysfunction. Death from shock usually results from multiple organ failure.

Irrespective of the initiating events of shock syndromes, concomitant interacting circulatory changes occur in blood pressure, flow, and volume and in oxygen transport patterns; these changes lead to local tissue hypoxia, organ dysfunction, multiple organ failure, and death. In this context, it may be helpful to use the sequential pattern of changes to separate early primary events from subsequent secondary and tertiary responses and their subsequent sequelae.[7, 9–25]

TABLE 13–1. Approach to Various Etiologic Types of Shock

Hemorrhagic	*Cardiogenic*	*Traumatic*	*Septic*
Signs and Symptoms			
Pallor, fainting	Pallor, fainting	History of injury	Fever, chills
Skin clammy, cold	Skin clammy, cold	Physical evidence of injury, fractures	Skin warm
Tachycardia	Arrhythmias	Oliguria	Tachycardia
Oliguria	Oliguria	Tachycardia	Oliguria
Collapse	Collapse	Collapse	Altered mental status
			Collapse
Laboratory			
↓ Hct, Hgb	↑ Cardiac enzymes	Radiography, CT	Positive smears and cultures
	ECG	Angiograms for organ and vascular injury	
Pathophysiology			
↓ Blood volume	↓ Cardiac output	Direct injury to organs and tissue	↓ Peripheral resistance
Therapy			
1. Fluids	1. Antiarrhythmics	1. Repair injuries	1. Antibiotics
2. Blood	2. Vasopressors	2. Fluids	2. Fluids
3. Control bleeding	3. Vasodilators	3. Blood	3. Drain abscesses

(Modified from Shoemaker WC: Circulatory mechanisms of shock and their mediators. Crit Care Med 1987; 15:787–794. Copyright Williams & Wilkins.)
Abbreviations: ECG = electrocardiography; CT = computed tomography.

CONVENTIONAL APPROACH TO THE DEVELOPMENT OF A THERAPEUTIC PLAN

The conventional approach to therapy consists of a one-at-a-time search for specific defects, their documentation, and then their correction. This approach to each specific defect followed by its normalization leads to fragmented, episodic patient care.[10] Therapy based on this approach unfortunately is not maximally effective.

Since shock is recognized clinically by the presence of hypotension, tachycardia, and oliguria, these superficial manifestations are often treated with vasopressors and diuretics as if they were the primary defects and as though the return of the circulatory values to their normal ranges is the goal of therapy. However, the underlying physiologic problem may continue unabated, even if the secondary manifestations of the syndrome are "cosmetically" corrected. Although most patients eventually get the therapeutic interventions that they need, these interventions are not necessarily administered at the right time, in the right amount, or in the right order.[16] Most importantly, therapy of shock, irrespective of the precipitating event, ideally should address the problems and interactions of the major circulatory components: the heart and the lungs, and tissue perfusion.

CRITIQUE OF THE CONVENTIONAL APPROACH TO THERAPY

The real danger is that the conventional approach focuses on the restoration of the superficial manifestations of shock with crystalloid solutions (crystalloids), diuretics, and vasopressors may leave the underlying tissue perfusion alteration uncorrected. The danger of maintaining normal values for central venous pressure (CVP) and vital signs is that compensatory increases in cardiac function and tissue perfusion may be limited by suboptimal preload.

Diuretics may restore urine output at the expense of blood volume, which may be deficient. Crystalloids rapidly distribute into the interstitium and only slightly increase blood volume and the cardiac index (CI). When tissue oxygenation is not evaluated by determination of oxygen delivery ($\dot{D}O_2$) and oxygen consumption ($\dot{V}O_2$) early in the course of acute critical illness, perfusion abnormalities may not be recognized until the appearance of adult respiratory distress syndrome (ARDS) or other organ failure.[18]

PATHOPHYSIOLOGY OF SHOCK SYNDROMES

It is crucial to develop a mechanistic physiologic model of shock and from this to develop coherent, organized therapeutic plans. Therapy intuitively based on simplistic notions, anecdotal information, or inadequate monitoring is likely to be suboptimal. Moreover, if the pathophysiology is not understood or if monitoring is not appropriate, death may be attributed to a patient's disease rather than to the inappropriateness and ineffectiveness of therapy.

The natural histories of various types of clinical shock produced by hemorrhage, accidental injury, surgery, sepsis, and cardiac problems and various combinations of these were described from the temporal viewpoint beginning with the time of the precipitating etiologic event. These descriptions were based on serial measurements obtained during periods remote from therapy; that is, before therapy was begun or after the immediate direct effects of therapy were over. The distinctive hemodynamic and oxygen transport patterns of survivors and nonsurvivors of the various clinical etiologies were described and the pathophysiology characterized.[7, 9–25]

Physiologic mechanisms may be elucidated by comparison of survivor and nonsurvivor patterns. The patterns of survivors represent the effects of the precipitating etiologic events and the patients' own compensations augmented by therapy. The patterns of nonsurvivors represent the overwhelming effects of the shock syndrome or inadequate compensations or both. Therapeutic strategies should be based on circulatory mechanisms that have demonstrated survival value; that is, the goals of therapy are to attain the hemodynamic and oxygen patterns of the survivors of each clinical and etiologic group.

Physiologic Methods

Monitoring with systemic arterial and pulmonary arterial catheters provides frequent measurements of arterial and venous pressures in the systemic (mean arterial pressure [MAP] and CVP) and pulmonary (MAP and pulmonary artery occlusion pressure [PAOP]) circulations, cardiac output, arterial and mixed venous gases, hemoglobin (Hbg), and Hgb saturations are measured simultaneously with cardiac output; they also are used to calculate $\dot{D}O_2$, $\dot{V}O_2$, oxygen extraction, pulmonary venous admixture or shunting ($\dot{Q}sp/\dot{Q}t$), the ratio of the arterial partial pressure of oxygen to the inspired oxygen fraction ($Pa O_2/FI O_2$), and alveolar-arterial oxygen gradient ($PA O_2 - Pa O_2$). All flow-related and volume-related variables in this chapter are indexed to body surface area. The variables, abbreviations, units, formulas, normal values, and optimal values defined by high-risk survivors of postoperative shock are shown in Table 13–2.[9–11, 19]

Time: A Crucial Factor for Pathophysiologic Description

In order to evaluate the possible causal mechanisms of shock, it is necessary to describe the time-course and sequence of events and to differentiate primary events from secondary or tertiary events. An early event may or may not be causally related to a subsequent event, but a late event can be excluded as the cause of an earlier event.

Most reports have described hemodynamic and oxygen transport variables in various etiologic types of shock in terms of their mean values and standard deviation (SD) or standard error of the mean (SEM) as if only a single time line were to exist[1–6]; that is, the data were expressed in terms unrelated to the time of onset of the syndrome, the temporal sequence, the progression of the syndrome, or the time of death or recovery. Occasionally, reference is made to values obtained in the early or late stages, but only rarely are complete temporal patterns of the monitored variables presented for survivors and nonsurvivors so that evaluations could be made at comparable time periods.

A major part of this problem is the difficulty encountered in identifying the time of onset of shock (e.g., shock from sepsis, occult hemorrhage, and anaphylaxis syndromes) as well as the time-course of the shock syndromes. Even if the time of onset of shock (or the time of the precipitating event) could be identified and if this time were used as a "zero" time, then the subsequent time-course would not necessarily be in phase with the progression of the syndrome because shock may develop rapidly or slowly owing to the severity of the etiologic event, the associated clinical problems, and the vigorousness of therapeutic efforts. Alternatively, the initial low point (nadir) of MAP or CI values has been used to identify an early time point of the syndrome.[9] Similarly, the restoration of normal MAP or the highest compensatory changes, such as CI, $\dot{D}O_2$, or $\dot{V}O_2$ values, after resuscitation represents another identifiable point. The initial low and the subsequent highest CI or $\dot{V}O_2$ value define two points that partially describe a time frame for the syndrome. This is roughly similar to the concept of the "peak and trough" levels for antibiotics.

Hemodynamic and Oxygen Transport Patterns of Survivors and Nonsurvivors of Surgical Operations

The surgical operation represents a controlled form of trauma and provides a unique opportunity to describe and analyze the temporal patterns of shock because the exact

TABLE 13–2. Cardiorespiratory Variables: Abbreviations, Units, Calculations, Normal Values, Optimal Values, and Predictive Capacity

	Abbreviations	*Units*	*Measurements or Calculations*	*Normal Values*	*Optimal Values*	*Per cent Correct*
Volume-Related Variables						
Mean arterial pressure	MAP	mm Hg	Direct measurement	82–102	>84	76
Central venous pressure	CVP	cm H_2O	Direct measurement	1–9	<5	62
Central blood volume	CBV	ml/m²	CBV = MTT × CI × 16.7	660–1000	>925	61
Stroke index	SI	ml/m²	SI = CI ÷ HR	30–50	>48	67
Hemoglobin	Hgb	g/dL	Direct measurement	12–16	>12	66
Mean pulmonary artery pressure	MPAP	mm Hg	Direct measurement	11–15	<19	68
Wedge pressure	WP	mm Hg	Direct measurement	0–12	>9.5	70
Blood volume	BV	mL/m²	BV = PV ÷ (1−Hct)* × surface area	Men, 2.74 Women, 2.37	>3.0 >2.7	76
Red blood cell mass	RCM	mL/m²	RCM = BV − PV	Men, 1.1 Women, 0.95	>1.1 >0.95	85
Flow-Related Variables						
Cardiac index	CI	L/min · m²	Direct measurement	2.8–3.6	>4.5	70
Left ventricular stroke work	LVSW	g · m/m²	LVSW = SI × MAP × 0.0144	44–68	>55	74
Left cardiac work	LCW	kg · m/m²	LCW = CI × MAP × 0.0144	3–4.6	>5	76
Right ventricular stroke work	RVSW	g · m/m²	RVSW = SI × MPAP × 0.0144	4–8	>13	70
Right cardiac work	RCW	kg · m/m²	RCW = CI × MPAP × 0.0144	0.4–0.6	>1.1	69
Stress-Related Variables						
Systemic vascular resistance	SVR	dyne · s/cm⁵ · m²	SVR = 79.92 (MAP−CVP)† ÷ CI	1760–2600	<1450	62
Pulmonary vascular resistance	PVR	dyne · s/cm⁵ · m²	PVR = 79.92 (MPAP−WP)† ÷ CI	45–225	<226	77
Heart rate	HR	beat/min	Direct measurement	72–88	<100	60
Rectal temperature	temp	°F	Direct measurement	97.8–98.6	>100.4	64
Oxygen-Related Variables						
Hgb saturation	SaO_2	%	Direct measurement	95–99	>95	67
Arterial carbon dioxide tension	$PaCO_2$	mm Hg	Direct measurement	36–44	>30	69
Arterial pH	pH		Direct measurement	7.36–7.44	>7.47	74
Mixed venous oxygen tension	$P\bar{v}O_2$	mm Hg	Direct measurement	33–53	>36	68
Arterial-mixed venous oxygen content difference	$C(a-\bar{v})O_2$	mL/dL	$C(a-\bar{v})O_2 = CaO_2 - C\bar{v}O_2$	4–5.5	<3.5	68
Oxygen delivery	$\dot{D}O_2$	mL/min · m²	$\dot{D}O_2 = CaO_2 \times CI \times 10$	520–720	>550	76
Oxygen consumption	$\dot{V}O_2$	mL/min · m²	$\dot{V}O_2 = C(a-\bar{v})O_2 \times CI \times 10$	100–180	>167	69
Oxygen extraction rate	O_2 ext	%	$O_2\ ext = (CaO_2 - C\bar{v}O_2) \div CaO_2$	22–30	<31	69

(Modified from Shoemaker WC, Appel P, Bland R: Use of physiologic monitoring to predict outcome and to assist in clinical decisions in critically ill postoperative patients. Am J Surg 1983; 146:43–50.)

*Hematocrit corrected for packing fraction and large ratio of vessel hematocrit to total body hematocrit.

†Venous pressures expressed in mm Hg.

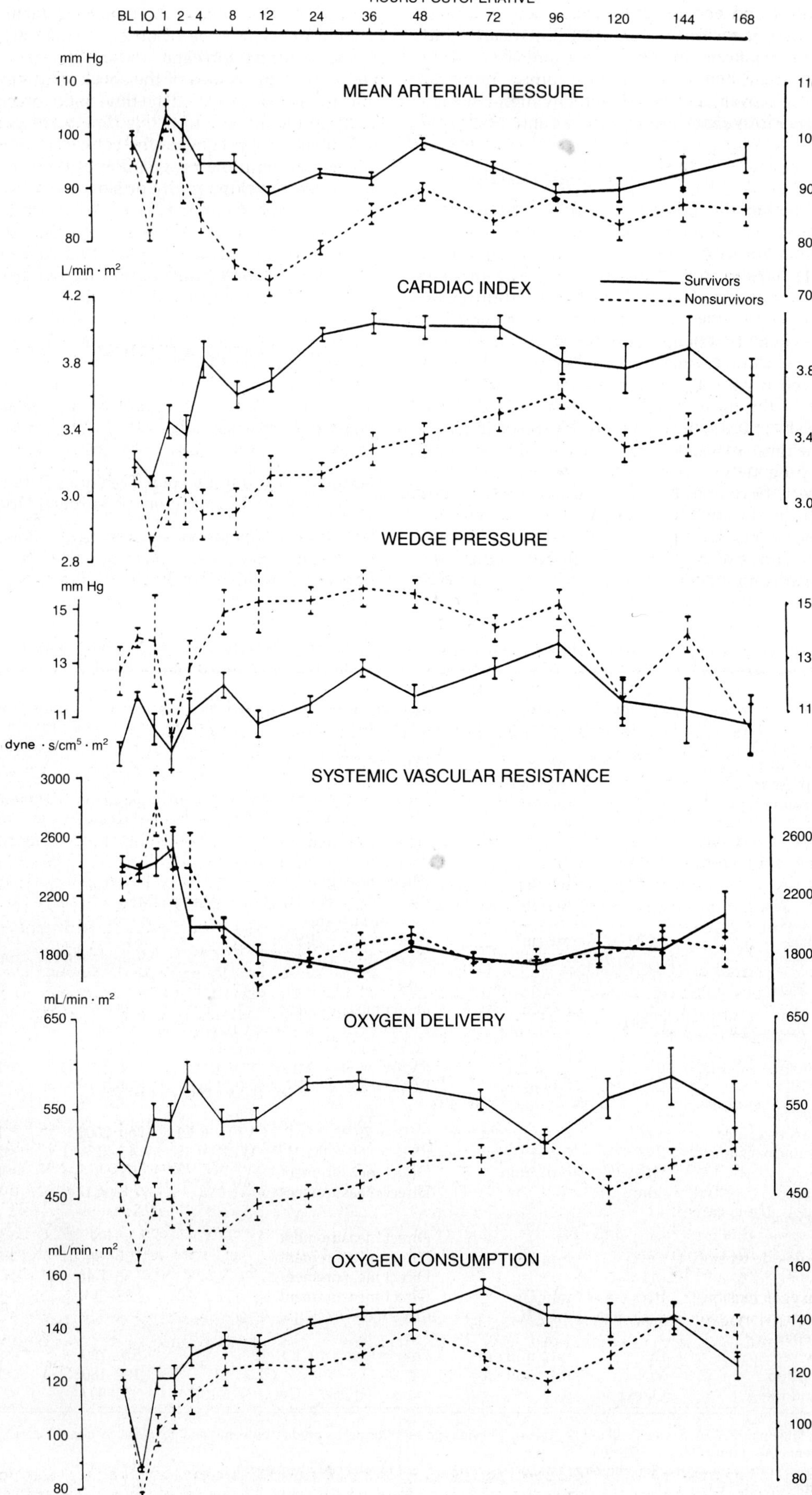

Figure 13–1 *See legend on opposite page*

times of the start and end of an operation are well documented. Physiologic measurements may be obtained in a preillness baseline control period, during and after the operation or the initial hemodynamic crisis, and throughout the subsequent recovery periods of survivors and nonsurvivors. This descriptive approach to physiologic events provides the basic data for a mechanistic model of the reperfusion injury of postoperative shock. It may also serve as a model for other etiologic types of shock.

Circulatory patterns in several large series of critically ill surgical patients were observed over their temporal course in the perioperative periods in order to characterize hemodynamic and oxygen transport patterns after surgical trauma in a temporal context (i.e., the actual time elapsed from the beginning or the end of the surgical operation).[11, 16–19] Many associated preoperative conditions, including age, sepsis, accidental trauma, stress, hypovolemia, cirrhosis, hypertension, prior myocardial infarction, stroke, and chronic congestive cardiac failure, may greatly affect these patterns.[12] More important, the vigorousness and effectiveness of therapy may also affect these patterns.

The physiologic pattern of postoperative survivors compared with the pattern of those who died provides the basis for evaluating the nature and biologic importance of circulatory compensations. Changes from the normal range in survivors described the effects of surgical trauma and successful compensatory responses that have survival value, whereas abnormal findings of nonsurvivors may reflect the effects of overwhelming trauma, inadequate compensations, or both.

The circulatory effects of operative trauma per se may be characterized by the hemodynamic and oxygen transport patterns of patients who preoperatively had normal cardiac output and no evidence of associated circulatory conditions (Fig. 13–1). Intraoperatively, the mean CI, $\dot{D}O_2$, and $\dot{V}O_2$ decreased from normal preoperative values in both survivors and nonsurvivors, but the decrease in CI, $\dot{D}O_2$, and $\dot{V}O_2$ was greater in the nonsurvivors.

Postoperative variations in the routinely recorded vital signs of both groups were minimal. In survivors, however, the mean CI, $\dot{D}O_2$, and $\dot{V}O_2$ increased during the first 12 postoperative hours. The postoperative values reached at their peaks were as follows: CI > 4.5 L/min · m^2; $\dot{D}O_2 > 600$ mL/min · m^2; and $\dot{V}O_2 > 170$ mL/min · m^2. The nonsurvivors maintained normal or near normal values for CI, $\dot{D}O_2$, and $\dot{V}O_2$; these values, although usually within the normal range, were significantly less than those of the survivors. Nonsurvivors' oxygen extraction ratios increased in partial compensation for inadequate tissue oxygenation. Despite normal blood gases, the nonsurvivors' $\dot{Q}sp/\dot{Q}t$ and $PAO_2 - PaO_2$ values increased intraoperatively and postoperatively.[9, 11]

Preoperative patients with low cardiac output included elderly patients, those with cardiac failure, and those with hypovolemia from dehydration or hemorrhagic shock. Postoperatively, they developed compensatory increases in CI, $\dot{D}O_2$, and $\dot{V}O_2$ that were similar to but less intense than those of patients with normal preoperative values. That is, the survivors' CI, $\dot{D}O_2$, and $\dot{V}O_2$ values increased in the postoperative period from their low preoperative baseline values, whereas the nonsurvivors maintained lower postoperative CI, $\dot{D}O_2$, and $\dot{V}O_2$ values and high PAOP. The nonsurvivors also had significantly greater increases in the pulmonary vascular resistance index (PVRI) and $\dot{Q}sp/\dot{Q}t$.[13]

High preoperative CI values in patients with sepsis, trauma, stress, and advanced cirrhosis suggest preoperative compensatory circulatory responses. Postoperatively, the mean CI, $\dot{D}O_2$, and $\dot{V}O_2$ values of these patients increased above their high preoperative baseline values; the temporal pattern of these increases also was greater in the survivors at comparable time periods than in the nonsurvivors. The PAOP, PVRI, and $\dot{Q}sp/\dot{Q}t$ were higher in the nonsurvivors than in the survivors. Both groups maintained their mean intravascular pressures and other non–flow-related variables in their preoperative ranges, which were relatively normal.[13, 19]

Sequential Patterns of Survivors and Nonsurvivors in Hemorrhagic Shock

With rapid blood loss, which is defined as major hemorrhage that occurs in less than 4 hours, the pattern of hemorrhagic shock was characterized by reduced blood pressure, CI, CVP, PAOP, mixed venous oxygen saturation ($S\bar{v}O_2$), pH, hematocrit, $\dot{D}O_2$, and $\dot{V}O_2$ concomitant with an increased systemic vascular resistance index (SVRI) and oxygen extraction ratio. With moderate degrees of hypovolemia, the initial PaO_2 values were usually normal, but in the presence of severe hypovolemia, hyperpnea and tachypnea occurred usually with near-normal PaO_2 and pH values but low arterial partial pressure of carbon dioxide ($PaCO_2$) values, indicating respiratory alkalosis. When shock was prolonged, poor tissue perfusion and inadequate tissue oxygenation led to acidosis, increased lactate levels, and base deficits. The initial compensatory responses included increased heart rate, which increased CI by neural and neurohormonal mechanisms; increased SVRI, which tended to maintain arterial pressures in the face of decreasing flow; and increased oxygen extraction ratios, which improved tissue oxygenation when blood flow was reduced.[20]

When blood loss was slow, defined as hemorrhage that occurs for longer than 4 hours, the hemorrhagic shock pattern showed greater reductions in hematocrit and lesser reductions in MAP, CI, $\dot{D}O_2$, and $\dot{V}O_2$. Moreover, the reduced rate of $\dot{V}O_2$ was lower quantitatively but more prolonged than that occurring after rapid losses of comparable quantities of blood. After the hemorrhage was stopped and blood volume was restored with appropriate fluids, the recovery period of survivors was characterized by supranormal values for CI, $\dot{D}O_2$, and $\dot{V}O_2$.[10]

Shock After Accidental Trauma

The hemodynamic and oxygen transport patterns after accidental trauma were similar to those described after surgery except that after accidental injuries wider variations in the patterns occurred because of marked differences in the amount and location of injuries, associated blood loss, organ injury, and the time delays to complete resuscitation.[7, 21, 22] Nonsurvivors were shown to have greater initial reductions in MAP, CI, $\dot{D}O_2$, and $\dot{V}O_2$ and lesser elevations in these parameters in the early postresuscitation period (i.e., the first 24 hours after the time of injury).[21, 22] However, after 3 or 5 days, septic complications and organ failures led to

Figure 13–1. Temporal patterns of MAP, CI, pulmonary artery wedge pressure, systemic vascular resistance, $\dot{D}O_2$ index, and $\dot{V}O_2$ index for survivors and nonsurvivors in the preoperative control period and intraoperative period as well as at various time intervals in the postoperative period. The *dots* represent mean values; the *vertical bars* represent SEM.

higher $\dot{V}O_2$ values for nonsurvivors that were associated with increased body metabolism, particularly in the preterminal stage.[21, 22]

In 65 trauma patients with severe shock from blood loss of greater than 3000 mL and injury severity scores of greater than 20, Bishop and coworkers[21, 22] observed a mortality rate of 12% when the accumulated delays were less than 24 hours from the time of injury to the time postoperatively when optimal supranormal values were achieved. By contrast, when these accumulated delays were greater than 24 hours, or when supranormal optimal values were not achieved, the mortality rate was 40%.

Hemodynamic and Oxygen Transport Patterns in Septic Shock

Time relationships necessary to define circulatory patterns in postoperative patients are marked by the time of onset or the end of the surgical operation; the subsequent temporal circulatory patterns can be related to either of these times. Sepsis, by contrast, is often a more subtle disorder with an insidious onset. Time relationships are obscure, and progression from localized infection to generalized infection with systemic manifestations, to the septic syndrome, to the septic shock, and to death may be gradual and not readily apparent. This progression may not be recognized until advanced stages. On the other hand, fulminating sepsis may lead to rapid cataclysmic deterioration and demise.

Septic shock is also difficult to understand because of the heterogenous groups of patients who are affected; that is, widely different clinical manifestations occur in postoperative, post-traumatic, urologic, respiratory failure, and general internal medicine patients. Sepsis may be the primary disorder, or it may be a complication. Sepsis also may be the expected consequence in patients with obstruction to the normal flow of biologic fluids (urine, bile, or gastrointestinal fluids), immunodeficiencies, and late-stage malignancies.

Sequential hemodynamic and oxygen transport patterns of survivors and nonsurvivors were described in a series of 378 consecutive internal medicine and surgical septic shock patients to differentiate primary from secondary and tertiary events and to evaluate possible underlying mechanisms and their therapeutic implications.[23, 24] Owing to the gradual transitions between the stages of shock but also to the wide variation in the duration of each stage, we used specific criteria to define the following stages: (1) an early period that began with the first recorded increase in cardiac output; (2) a middle period, which was the time 48 hours before and after the maximum metabolic activity, defined as the period characterized by the highest recorded rate of oxygen consumption; and (3) a late period, which was the time 48 hours before death or recovery; the last of these was defined as the time when the patient had recovered sufficiently to allow discontinuation of measurements and the removal of the catheters (Fig. 13–2).

The earliest hemodynamic changes were increased heart rate, CI, and $\dot{D}O_2$. Early transient reductions in $\dot{V}O_2$ that preceded the temperature elevations and hypotension were

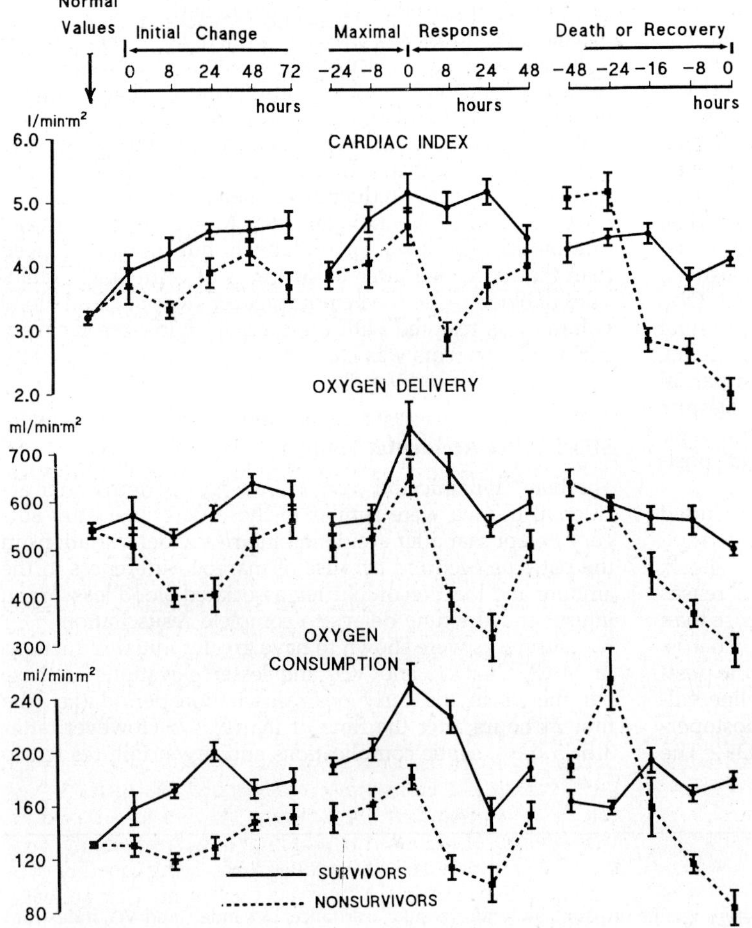

Figure 13–2. Temporal patterns of CI, $\dot{D}O_2$, and $\dot{V}O_2$ values in early *(left)*, middle *(center)*, and late *(right)* stages of septic shock compared with normal values *(extreme left column)*. See text for definitions of the stages. (From Shoemaker WC, Appel PL, Kram HB, et al: Sequence of physiologic patterns in surgical septic shock. Crit Care Med 1993; 21:1876.)

observed in both survivors and nonsurvivors. Subsequently, in the early and middle periods, progressive increases in CI, $\dot{D}O_2$, and $\dot{V}O_2$ were noted. These increases were greater in the survivors than in the nonsurvivors at comparable time periods.[23–24]

Although 84% of the patients with sepsis were consistently hyperdynamic, transient hypodynamic episodes, defined as CI < 2.5 L/min · m² in approximately 10% of the measurements, were seen. Also, in 8% of the nonsurvivors, transient preterminal hypermetabolic periods, defined as $\dot{V}O_2$ > 200 mL/min · m², were also observed; these usually occurred 18 to 72 hours prior to death and were followed by a progressive downhill course. In the nonsurvivors' terminal period, MAP, CI, $\dot{D}O_2$, and $\dot{V}O_2$ fell abruptly. Thus, increases in CI and $\dot{D}O_2$ represent physiologic compensations for circulatory deficiencies that limit body metabolism and compromise survival.[23, 24]

Hankeln and associates[25] reported that postoperative and cardiac patients with ARDS who did survive had supranormal CI and $\dot{D}O_2$; in their series, nonsurvivors had lower values than did survivors. Others also observed increased CI, $\dot{D}O_2$, and $\dot{V}O_2$ in septic shock patients.[26–29] Abraham and colleagues[26] demonstrated additional increases in $\dot{D}O_2$ and $\dot{V}O_2$ after fluid loading with colloids in septic shock patients with peritonitis. Others have corroborated the increased CI, $\dot{D}O_2$, and $\dot{V}O_2$ in septic shock patients given fluids or inotropes.[30–33] Edwards and colleagues[34, 35] took the concept one step further by driving $\dot{D}O_2$ and $\dot{V}O_2$ to optimal supranormal values with the administration of fluids and dobutamine; using this approach, they demonstrated improved survival rates in severely ill septic shock patients. In prospective randomized studies on medical patients with septic shock, Tuchschmidt and coworkers[36] showed reduced mortality when CI was driven to 6 L/min · m² with fluids and dobutamine.

Cardiogenic Shock

Traditionally, the Starling myocardial performance curve, defined by a CI of 2.5 L/min · m² and an arbitrary PAOP of 18 or 20 mm Hg, is used to evaluate clinical subsets of cardiogenic shock. Four quadrants described by the Starling curve and PAOP identify the physiologic impairments of these four subsets and suggest therapies appropriate to these conditions.[37]

Chronic congestive cardiac failure and acute circulatory failure in chronic cardiac patients have been extensively studied; reduced CI and MAP with high PAOP and SVRI were commonly found. Although numerous studies have documented these CI–venous pressure relationships, only two studies of cardiogenic shock after acute myocardial infarction have reported the relationships of CI, $\dot{D}O_2$, and $\dot{V}O_2$. DaLuz and associates[38] reported oxygen transport data in seven patients, all of whom had received adrenergic drugs before the measurements were made. Creamer and coworkers[39] reported on 19 postinfarction patients in cardiogenic shock. Fourteen patients had a CI of 1.3 ± 0.5 L/min · m² before therapy; in response to therapy, they developed a CI of 2.5 ± 0.4 L/min · m² associated with marked increases in $\dot{D}O_2$ from 230 ± 69 mL/min · m² to 397 ± 60 mL/min · m² and $\dot{V}O_2$ from 103 ± 31 mL/min · m² to 124 ± 22 mL/min · m²; 13 of these 14 patients survived. Two other patients with a mean CI of 0.9 ± 0.4 L/min · m² died before therapy could be given, and three other patients spontaneously recovered. The authors concluded that in cardiogenic shock, supply-dependent $\dot{V}O_2$, although not as elevated as in septic shock, was nevertheless an important component of both pathophysiology and therapy.[39] Other goals of therapy included an increase in $\dot{D}O_2$ from 300 to 400 mL/min · m², a decrease in oxygen extraction ratio to about 30%, and an increase in $S\bar{v}O_2$ to approximately 70%.[40]

EVALUATION OF PATHOPHYSIOLOGY

Functional Circulatory Assessment

Circulatory function may be assessed by oxygen transport and oxygen metabolism values because oxygen consumption is (1) essential to life, (2) impaired in shock states, (3) considerably different in survivors and nonsurvivors, (4) measures overall body metabolism, and (5) is a sensitive monitored variable for outcome from acute circulatory failure.[6–36] Technically, $\dot{D}O_2$ and $\dot{V}O_2$ are convenient to measure because oxygen has the highest extraction ratio of any blood constituent. $\dot{V}O_2$ measurements reflect the state of body metabolism reasonably well, since oxygen cannot be stored and sizable oxygen debts cannot be accumulated for appreciable periods of time without significant adverse consequences. Therefore, at a given point of time, the $\dot{V}O_2$ measures the overall rate of oxidative metabolism—that is, the amount of oxygen burned per minute, which is not necessarily the optimal $\dot{V}O_2$ nor what the patient actually needs, but rather the amount of oxygen actually consumed per minute at the time of the measurement.

Rationale and Experimental Basis for Monitoring

The hypothesis was that outcome would be improved if the hemodynamic and oxygen transport values of survivors were rapidly achieved by aggressive therapy within 8 to 12 hours of the onset. This was tested in a randomized series of high-risk surgical patients with the median CI, $\dot{D}O_2$, and $\dot{V}O_2$ values of survivors as the goals of therapy. The optimal goals for patients with preoperative hyperdynamic states from sepsis, trauma, and cirrhosis are somewhat higher, whereas the goals for patients with preoperative hypodynamic states, the elderly, hypovolemic, and cardiac patients are somewhat lower than those for patients with normal preoperative values.

The major premise of these clinical studies has been that death in critical illness follows physiologic patterns that are independent of the clinical diagnosis and independent of the surgical operation. Although many clinicians feel that there are too many clinical differences among individual patients to develop a therapeutic plan based on common physiologic patterns, we found that the similarities of patients' sequential hemodynamic and oxygen transport patterns outweighed individual patients' clinical differences. This suggested that basic underlying physiologic mechanisms are reflected by their common hemodynamic and oxygen transport patterns.

The second premise is that the supranormal values empirically seen in survivors reflect the effects of surgical operations, trauma, hypovolemia, sepsis, and other types of stress as well as the effects of circulatory compensations, whereas the relatively normal or subnormal values of the nonsurvivors reflect the overwhelming effects of the surgery and trauma or infection or inadequate circulatory compensations, or both.

The important assumption is that physiologic criteria for the management of the life-threatening illness or for sepsis can be developed from the patterns of survivors. Based on extensive observations, it was assumed that physiologic patterns of patients who survived life-threatening illnesses provide objective criteria that may be used as the first approximation to goals of therapy.

Definition of Optimal Goals: Normal Versus Supranormal Values As Criteria for Therapy

The median values for a non–septic shock surgical patient without associated preoperative cardiovascular problems were shown to be a CI ≥ 4.5 L/min · m^2 (normal: 3.2 ± 0.2 L/min · m^2), $\dot{D}O_2$ ≥ 600 (usually 800–1000) mL/min · m^2 (normal: 520 ± 57 mL/min · m^2), and $\dot{V}O_2$ of 167 ± 18 mL/min · m^2 (normal: 130 ± 17 mL/min · m^2).[9, 11–19] In the septic shock patient, these values are CI ≥ 5.5 L/min · m^2, $\dot{D}O_2$ ≥ 1000 mL/min · m^2, and $\dot{V}O_2$ ≥ 190 mL/min · m^2.[23, 24] In the trauma patient, these values are CI ≥ 5.0 L/min · m^2, $\dot{D}O_2$ ≥ 800 mL/min · m^2, and $\dot{V}O_2$ ≥ 180 mL/min · m^2.[21, 22] The empirically determined "supranormal" values were used as a guide of first approximation to "optimal" goals for physiologic therapy, whereas the values of the nonsurvivors' patterns served as an early warning of potentially lethal patterns.

Hemodynamic and Oxygen Transport Patterns in Relation to Oxygen Debt in Critically Ill Postoperative Patients

Since $\dot{V}O_2$ reflects the rate at which oxygen is utilized, and not the rate that is required, it is necessary to estimate oxygen need independently to evaluate the potential oxygen debt in high-risk surgical patients. The $\dot{V}O_2$ need may be estimated from the patient's own preoperative values under normal, steady-state conditions with correction terms used to estimate the $\dot{V}O_2$ need when he or she is under general anesthesia and at various body temperatures. This value was extrapolated into the intraoperative period and the early postoperative period. Lowe and Ernst[41] reported $\dot{V}O_2$ under anesthesia in healthy elective patients, $\dot{V}O_2$ (anesth) = 10 × kg$^{0.72}$. This "$\dot{V}O_2$ (anesth)" value was also corrected for temperature and was used to estimate the $\dot{V}O_2$ need during the time that the patient underwent general anesthesia. This value was usually about 100 mL/min · m^2. The temperature correction assumed that metabolic activity increased or decreased at the rate of 7% per degree Fahrenheit.[18] After the anesthetic was reversed in the immediate postoperative period, the $\dot{V}O_2$ need was estimated from the patient's own preoperative baseline $\dot{V}O_2$ corrected for the effects of temperature. The temperature-corrected baseline preoperative $\dot{V}O_2$ was extrapolated as the estimated "$\dot{V}O_2$-need" in the immediate postoperative period. Thus, the net cumulative amount of intraoperative and postoperative oxygen deficit was calculated from the measured $\dot{V}O_2$ minus the $\dot{V}O_2$ need estimated from the patient's own resting preoperative control values corrected for both temperature and anesthesia conditions and integrated over time.

Figure 13–3 shows the patterns of selected hemodynamic and oxygen transport variables in a series of 253 consecutively monitored, surviving and nonsurviving, high-risk surgical patients in the preoperative, intraoperative, and immediate postoperative period.[18] CI, $\dot{D}O_2$, and $\dot{V}O_2$ of survivors without organ failure were highest and those who survived with organ failure were intermediate, whereas the values of those who subsequently died were lowest. The mean nonsurvivor values, however, were usually within the normal range. The magnitude and duration of the calculated $\dot{V}O_2$ deficit was greatest for nonsurvivors, somewhat less for survivors with organ failure, and least for survivors without organ failure.

The oxygen debt was also calculated in the prospective randomized study of high-risk surgical patients (Fig. 13–4). This study evaluated the effects of the empirically observed supranormal values of critically ill postoperative survivors.[18] Significantly smaller oxygen debts were not observed in protocol patients who had supranormal oxygen transport values as therapeutic goals compared with control group patients who had normal values as therapeutic goals.

Capillary Leak and Water Distribution Changes in Shock

Unquestionably, capillary leaks sometimes occur in the late stage of shock syndromes, particularly in those patients with sepsis. The major unanswered questions are: When does this leak occur? What is the magnitude of the leak? and, How can it be measured under clinical conditions? At the present time, we do not have direct evidence to answer these questions. The finding of pink, frothy fluid in pulmonary edema indicates leakage of red blood cells across the alveolocapillary membrane. A capillary leak is suggested by widespread peripheral edema, pulmonary edema, hypotension, oliguria, and multiple organ failures, especially in the terminal state. Intravenous administration of tracer doses of labeled albumin or high-molecular-weight dextrans may be

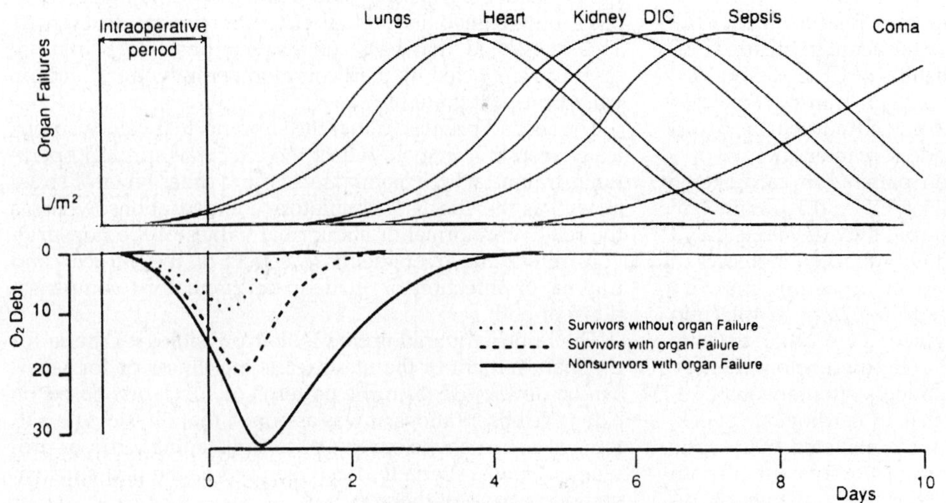

Figure 13–3. Postoperative appearance of various organ failures (above the horizontal lines). Net cumulative oxygen deficit for nonsurvivors *(solid line)*, survivors without organ failure *(dotted line)*, and survivors with organ failure *(dashed line)* calculated for intraoperative periods and successive time periods after operation (below the horizontal lines). (From Shoemaker WC, Appel P, Kram HB: Role of oxygen debt in the development of organ failure, sepsis and death in high-risk surgical patients. Chest 1992; 102:208–215.)

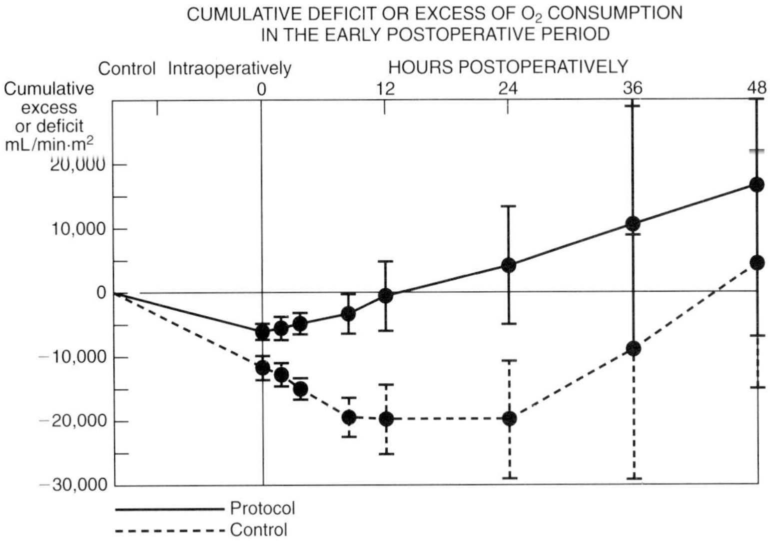

Figure 13–4. Net cumulative $\dot{V}O_2$ debt for protocol and control patients in a prospective randomized trial of supranormal values of survivors as therapeutic goals. (Data from Shoemaker WC, Appel PL, Kram HB, et al: Prospective trial of supranormal values of survivors as therapeutic goals in high-risk surgical patients. Chest 1988; 94:1176.)

recovered in bronchial secretions, indicating the presence of alveolocapillary leaks. In terminal and preterminal patients, evidence of capillary leak is suggested by the failure of transfusions and intravenous fluid infusions to maintain vascular pressures, flow, and circulatory function. However, no direct quantitative measurements of the amount of capillary leak are available in the clinical setting.

Water distribution changes may be attributed to Starling forces, cardiac failure, fluid overload, massive crystalloid infusions, hypoalbuminemia, nutritional failure, capillary leak, or the terminal stage of most diseases. In practice, however, it is not possible to know when the capillary leak begins or how much of a leak is present at any given time.

Operationally, it is likely that there is little or no leak in the early stages of shock states, particularly when significant increases in CI, $\dot{D}O_2$, and $\dot{V}O_2$ occur in response to colloid administration. In the middle stage of shock, when there are satisfactory $\dot{D}O_2$ and $\dot{V}O_2$ responses, some leak may occur, but not enough to deter satisfactory circulatory responses to fluid therapy. From the practical vantage point, fluids—including colloids—may be given as long as they are effective in improving CI, $\dot{D}O_2$, and $\dot{V}O_2$. When they cease to be effective, resort may be made to transfusions and the use of inotropic agents and vasopressors.

Body Composition Changes in Shock

Body compositional measurements in the late stage of shock reveal expanded total-body water and interstitial water with contracted plasma volume and intracellular fluid.[42–44] These body composition abnormalities are also produced by massive crystalloid infusions that predominantly expand the interstitial fluid compartment and only minimally correct blood volume.[45–48] The presence of overexpanded interstitial water and excessive total-body water does not mean that blood volume deficits have been corrected, since hypovolemia often occurs in the presence of massive peripheral edema. The increased interstitium does not contribute to circulatory function but may actually aggrevate the problems of oxygen transport by increasing the diffusion pathway and the diffusion time of oxygen as it travels from the intravascular space to the cell membrane.

A Physiologic Mechanistic Model of Shock

We have developed a physiologic mechanistic model of shock based on descriptions of the temporal patterns of hemodynamic and oxygen transport variables of survivors and nonsurvivors in shock states due to various events. These descriptions suggest that tissue hypoxia from poor tissue perfusion is the basic underlying physiologic defect of all shock syndromes. Tissue hypoxia may be initiated by inadequate or maldistributed blood flow, hypovolemia, vascular occlusion, cardiac insufficiency or failure, anesthetic-induced cardiodepression, and hypoxemia. Increased metabolic demands may be caused by inflammatory responses, fever, wound healing after accidental or surgical trauma, and sepsis. Inadequate flow or increased demands may, when extensive, produce tissue hypoxia, organ dysfunction, organ failure, and death.

In this physiologic model of shock, reduced tissue oxygenation is the primary event, and increases in CI and $\dot{D}O_2$ are compensations that may, if sufficient and timely, alleviate the antecedent tissue hypoxia. In shock, there is a similar pattern of reduced blood flow and tissue hypoxia followed by increased flow and oxygenation.

The extent and duration of the antecedent tissue hypoxic event as well as the extent and duration of the optimal CI and $\dot{D}O_2$ responses must be studied, and the effects of standardized therapeutic regimens must be tested prospectively so that more explicit guidelines for the management of high-risk critically ill patients can be developed.

In shock syndromes, local tissue hypoxia stimulates the release of neuroendocrine peptides, hormones, and stress ("heat shock") proteins that alter T cell and B cell function as well as immunosuppressive factors. Activated T cells and other hematopoietic cells produce various cytokines, including tumor necrosis factor and interleukins (IL-1, IL-2, IL-6, and IL-8). The activated lymphocytes and monocytes have receptors for hormones and are able simultaneously to synthesize and secrete the same hormones and messengers. Activation of leukocytes by these and other biochemical mechanisms produces oxygen free radicals that, although extremely short lived, produce major tissue damage.[49–51]

Relation of Physiologic Patterns to Biochemical Mediators

Many cascades have been shown to produce biologically active mediators of shock and multiple organ failures. These include the compliment system; leukotrienes, thromboxane, prostaglandins, and other eicosanoids from the breakdown of arachidonic acid; the bradykinin-renin system; the T and B lymphocyte functional responses; cytokines; and the production of bacterial antigens. These and other influences are reviewed in detail in Chapters 21, 22, and 23.

Major unanswered questions concern the interactions of these mediators with patterns of hemodynamic changes. Key to understanding these interactions are the time relationships of activation of each of these mediators to the temporal hemodynamic and oxygen transport patterns of the evolving shock syndromes. This information is needed to clarify whether circulatory events stimulate mediators, or whether mediator activations produce the hemodynamic and oxygen transport patterns that lead to organ failure and death.

The serum levels of IL-1, IL-6, and IL-8 and tumor necrosis factor have been demonstrated to rise within hours of the induction of experimental endotoxemia and the intravenous infusion of bacteria.[52] We[53] and others[54–56] have demonstrated experimentally and clinically the activation of IL-6, IL-8, and tumor necrosis factor when sepsis or ARDS occurs after trauma. Increased release of each of these cytokines is associated with an acute-phase reaction and the hypermetabolic state.

The sequence of physiologic changes in relation to activation of cytokines, compliment factors, and other chemical mediators needs to be elucidated. It is likely that these cytokines, the compliment system, and oxygen free radicals play major roles in modulating the alterations in oxygen metabolism and hemodynamic parameters associated with shock and sepsis in affecting the metabolic responses that determine outcome in various clinical settings. The elevations of plasma IL-6 and IL-8 levels reach their maxima after post-traumatic ARDS becomes manifest, but hemodynamic and oxygen transport variables occur before ARDS.[53] It is also likely that monoclonal antibody therapy and anti–tumor necrosis factor therapy as well as free radical scavenger promotion may become useful approaches to the management of septic and other types of shock.

Physiologic Compensations and Their Therapeutic Implications

Physiologic compensatory responses maintain overall circulatory function at a higher than normal level after surgery, accidental trauma, sepsis, and other types of shock. Organ failure occurs when these responses fail to compensate adequately.[18, 19] Increased cardiac output may compensate for reduced hematocrit, low Pa_{O_2}, or uneven blood flow, all of which produce inadequate tissue oxygenation.[14] Since this compensatory increase in flow has survival value, therapy should augment cardiac output; the use of β-blockers to reduce high cardiac output values or tachycardia in patients with traumatic or septic shock may lead to circulatory and metabolic deterioration and arrest. An understanding of physiologic responses to stress in mechanistic terms is essential to identify and then to augment compensatory responses that are needed for survival. If the physiology is misunderstood and the therapy is inappropriate, death may be attributed to the patient's disease rather than to the inappropriate therapy.

Systemic Vascular Resistance and the Distribution of Blood Flow

A commonly stated concept is that shock syndromes, particularly septic shock, primarily result from the interacting influences of vasodilation, reduced peripheral vascular resistance index (SVRI), low blood pressure, and low blood flow. If a reduced SVRI were the pathogenic cause of shock, it would be logical to increase SVRI with vasopressors. However, a low SVRI is not well correlated with death, nor is a normal or high SVRI correlated with survival.[12–17] Moreover, correction of a low SVRI with vasopressors does not improve outcome. On the contrary, vasopressors tend to intensify microcirculatory maldistribution of flow by their α-adrenergic action, which produces even more uneven vasoconstriction and worsens the flow maldistributions.

A low SVRI is not a good measure of "distributive shock" because SVRI represents only the ratio of pressure to flow and not the distribution of flow. According to Ohm's law—R = e/i—resistance (R) is the ratio of pressure (i) to flow (e) in direct current circuits; it is not applicable to alternating currents or periodic functions. A high SVRI occurs when the CI is low (e.g., after hemorrhage), and a low SVRI occurs when flow is high and pressure is normal or low (e.g., after trauma, surgery, or sepsis). Because the SVRI is directly related to the CI, the total body blood flow, it does not reflect microcirculatory flow maldistributions. Furthermore, organ vascular circuits are in parallel, and the resistance of the whole system is largely determined by the circuit with the lowest resistance. Thus, if one organ's resistance decreases while all other organ resistances increase, the calculated total resistance is decreased. Thus, the SVRI is not a good measure of microcirculatory flow distributions, nor is it an appropriate criterion for therapy.

Distributive Shock

The term "distributive shock" has been used as a designation for a type of high-flow shock under the assumption that flow is not normally distributed. Used in this context, it is a theoretic designation that is not defined by criteria that can be quantitatively measured at the bedside. Unevenly distributed flow has been directly observed with in vivo microscopy in experimental animals. Maldistributed blood flow also has been well documented clinically by incident light microscopy in selected accessible microscopic fields such as the scleral conjunctiva, nail bed, and the surface of parenchymal organs (e.g., the liver during surgical operations).

Direct observations document the phenomenon, but they are not necessarily representative of all microscopic fields and do not quantitatively measure the extent of this problem throughout the body. Thus, flow maldistribution is a physiologic concept and a pathogenic mechanism that may be relevant in most, if not all, shock states. More explicit quantitative criteria that are clinically measurable are needed for distributive shock to qualify as a diagnostic classifier of a specific type of clinical shock.

Tissue Oxygenation As a Physiologic Cause of Organ Failure and Death

The development of therapeutic plans and priorities depends on an accurate evaluation of the pathophysiology. Inadequate cardiac and respiratory functions are directly measurable; in contrast, inadequate tissue perfusion and oxygenation are more difficult to measure and more subtle in appearance but of greater consequence in terms of outcome. Inadequate tissue perfusion with either low or high flow leads to tissue hypoxia, which when extensive in degree and protracted in time produces organ dysfunction, multiple organ failures, and death. Most instances of death after surgery, trauma, sepsis, and other acute cardiorespiratory disorders are preceded by multiple organ failures. In fact, organ failures are the most common proximate causes of intensive care unit (ICU) deaths.

When the early manifestations of shock are alleviated by

therapy that is insufficient to correct poor tissue oxygenation, the resultant oxygen debt may not be recognized until the appearance of organ failures, including sepsis in the uncontaminated patient, acute cardiac failure or arrest, renal failure, shock lung, disseminated intravascular coagulation, hepatic failure, and coma.[18]

Colloids produced greater CI, $\dot{D}O_2$, $\dot{V}O_2$, and blood volume effects than did crystalloids in our series of critically ill patients. Colloids also produced greater CI effects than did packed red blood cells, but the latter often produced greater $\dot{V}O_2$ increases, particularly in patients with low hematocrits.

Cardiac Depression As a Physiologic Mechanism

In septic shock, terminal states, and cardiogenic problems as well as during inhalation anesthesia, moderate degrees of cardiodepression occur. However, this cardiodepression may be counteracted by compensatory adrenomedullary stress responses that stimulate cardiac contractility. The balance between the cardiodepression and the adrenal medullary stress response results in a wide range of cardiac function from hypodynamic to hyperdynamic states. This balance is also affected by the degree of shock, the presence of associated medical conditions, the capacity of the heart to compensate, blood volume status, and the temporal stage of the shock state.[23]

The predominant physiologic effects of inotropic and fluid therapy (principally colloid therapy) are to stimulate cardiac function and increase CI. In septic shock and the late stage of postoperative and post-traumatic shock, the therapeutic action of fluids may be less effective and shorter in duration than in early nonseptic shock. Irrespective of these limitations, it is important to obtain the optimal effectiveness with fluids and inotropic agents to maximize outcome despite the cardiodepressant aspects of septic or late-stage nonseptic shock.

PREDICTION OF OUTCOME

Relative Importance of Circulatory Variables in Outcome Prediction

Frequently recorded hemodynamic and oxygen transport measurements describe the temporal patterns of survivors and nonsurvivors and provide essential information needed to elucidate underlying physiologic mechanisms and their relevance to outcome. Each variable's biologic importance may be independently evaluated by its ability to predict outcome, which is also a criterion of its usefulness for clinical decision-making. If a variable is not related to outcome, it should not be relevant to therapy. However, if it does predict outcome, it may reflect important pathophysiologic mechanisms and, therefore, provide a useful criterion for therapeutic decisions.

The percentages of correctly predicted outcomes for each monitored variable were calculated at each stage and for all stages in a series of postoperative patients.[15, 16, 19] The commonly measured variables were the poorest predictors. By contrast, oxygen transport–related variables were excellent outcome predictors and, therefore, were clinically important. This concept has been corroborated by studies of both surgical and medical shock.[25–36]

Outcome Prediction from Survivors' and Nonsurvivors' Patterns

Multivariate nonparametric statistical analyses were developed empirically to evaluate each variable and to incorporate all variables into an overall outcome assessment. The average score for each variable's prediction was computed, and the average of all scores was calculated to give an overall predictive index for a patient at various postoperative time periods.[13, 15, 16] This predictive analysis also provided an objective, physiologic, and heuristic basis for therapeutic decisions. The sole criterion of this empiric physiologic analysis was survival. More importantly, predictors objectively reflect severity of illness and express prediction and severity in quantitative statistical terms.

Figure 13–5 shows a significant separation between survivors and nonsurvivors in the prospective series beginning 2 to 4 hours postoperatively.[16] The predictors objectively analyze the complex physiologic problems with no preconceptions and a minimum number of assumptions. The criteria are determined solely by the observed values of critically ill surgical patients who survived as compared with the values of those who subsequently died.

Outcome prediction for each hemodynamic and oxygen transport variable varies from stage to stage as patients' shock syndromes evolve; that is, predictors are stage-specific; $\dot{D}O_2$ and the pulmonary vascular resistance index (PVRI) are good predictors in the early stage, but not in the late stage; and MAP is a poor early predictor, but a good

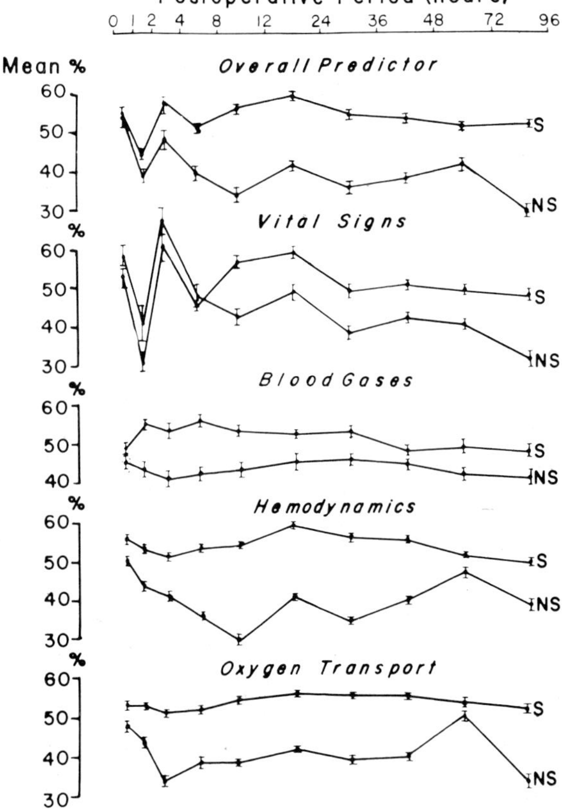

Figure 13–5. *Uppermost section,* Overall predictor for survivors (S) and nonsurvivors (NS) at each time interval postoperatively. *Second section,* Predictions calculated from the vital sign variables for S and NS. *Third section,* Predictions calculated from the blood gas variables for S and NS. *Fourth section,* Predictions calculated from the hemodynamic variables for S and NS. *Lowermost section,* Predictions calculated from the oxygen transport variables for S and NS. The *dots* represent mean values; the *vertical bars* represent SEM. (From Bland RD, Shoemaker WC: Probability of survival as a prognostic and severity of illness score in critically ill surgical patients. Crit Care Med 1985; 13:91.)

late predictor. Most variables predict outcome well in the late stage, but by this time, clinical judgment is also excellent, and the usefulness of predictors is minimal.[11-16]

THERAPY

Therapeutic Goals

Optimal therapeutic goals for high-risk postoperative patients may be defined empirically by outcome predictors and by the values of survivors of life-threatening critical illnesses. Criteria from two large retrospective series and several prospective series[11-16, 19] include the following: (1) CI, 4.5 L/min · m^2, 50% greater than normal; (2) $\dot{D}O_2$, 600 to 1000 mL/min · m^2, greater than normal; (3) $\dot{V}O_2$, 170 mL/min · m^2, 30% greater than normal; and (4) blood volume that is 500 mL in excess of the norm (i.e., 3.2 L/m^2 for men, and 2.8 L/m^2 for women).[11] These increased values are needed to overcome poorly distributed blood volume and blood flow as well as to supply the increased metabolic need associated with wound healing, fever, and the accumulated oxygen debt. Severely traumatized, stressed, septic shock, cirrhotic, and burn patients may require even higher values whereas cardiac patients have lower values (Table 13–3).[11-12]

The standard approach to therapy often results in a fragmented, uncoordinated plan that leads to episodic and sometimes contradictory therapy. An alternative approach is to base therapy on survivors' patterns confirmed by outcome predictions. The hypothesis is that the survivors' patterns represent the effects of the etiologic event plus the patients' compensatory responses. The patterns of survivors provide information needed to define therapeutic goals, whereas the patterns of nonsurvivors represent overwhelming effects of shock and inadequate compensations. This hypothesis was tested in prospective clinical trials.[18, 19]

Prospective Clinical Trials of Supranormal Oxygen Transport

In the initial prospective studies, the hypothesis was tested that if patients' CI, $\dot{D}O_2$, and $\dot{V}O_2$ are promptly brought up to the optimal values, survival would be increased and morbidity reduced. A therapeutic plan that used the empirically defined median values of survivors as therapeutic goals was prospectively tested in clinical trials against a control group for which normal values were used as the therapeutic goals.[19] Both protocol and control groups had the same availability of radiography and laboratory tests, monitoring, nursing care, ancillary facilities, and therapy. In the first study, patients whose critical illnesses were specified by prearranged criteria were prospectively allocated to control or protocol services. Comparison of the clinical data, clinical diagnoses, operations, and associated medical conditions demonstrated that the patients in the protocol group were at least as ill as and probably more ill than those in the control group. However, about one third of these patients entered the trial at various times postoperatively; these patients had much less improvement in outcome with the protocol compared with those who were studied immediately postoperatively.[19] Subsequently, this hypothesis was more rigorously tested by identifying high-risk patients preoperatively with predetermined criteria and by randomizing them to one of three therapeutic regimens: (1) CVP catheter, with the observed values made available by this catheter brought to their normal range; (2) pulmonary artery catheter, with the hemodynamic and oxygen transport values made available by this catheter brought to their normal range as goals; and (3) pulmonary artery catheter, with the supranormal optimal values of CI, $\dot{D}O_2$, and $\dot{V}O_2$ as goals of therapy. All eligible high-risk patients were randomized preoperatively; the trial was strictly randomized with the use of sealed opaque envelopes that contained cards identifying one of the three monitoring/therapeutic approaches. The results showed no statistically significant difference between the mortality of patients managed with a CVP catheter (23%) and those with a pulmonary artery catheter with normal values as therapeutic goals (33%). However, use of optimal goals with the pulmonary artery catheter led to a significant reduction (4%) in mortality. Moreover, the number of complications, hospital days, ICU days, and ventilator days as well as hospital costs were reduced (Table 13–4). The survivors' oxygen transport values were achieved promptly in 68% of protocol patients with only rapid, vigorous fluid therapy and in the remainder with the addition of dobutamine; 7% of patients also required vasodilators.[19]

The results of these prospective clinical trials suggest that most postoperative deaths are due to physiologic problems that can be identified, described, predicted, and prevented. Therapy for various categories of critically ill patients should be defined by physiologic criteria of the survivors of each group. Therapy should be monitored to obtain the optimal physiologic goals within the first 8 to 12 hours after surgery.[19]

A Therapeutic Plan Using a Branch Chain Decision Tree

Strategies for achieving therapeutic goals were determined empirically by evaluating the relative effectiveness of each therapy to produce the desired goals. Decision rules were generated from the patterns of survivors and nonsurvivors and from these patients' responses to specific therapeutic interventions. A branch chain decision tree was developed from these decision rules, and priorities were determined based on the effects of the various therapies (Fig. 13–6). A branch chain decision tree helps to achieve these therapeutic goals expeditiously by providing a coherent, organized patient management plan. The plan is prophylactic in that it aims to maintain the patient in the optimal hemodynamic state and to prevent the development of tissue hypoxia, organ failure, and death from deficits in blood volume and circulatory function as determined by hemodynamic and oxygen transport patterns. It should not be necessary to wait

TABLE 13–3. Maximum Cardiac Index, Oxygen Delivery, and Oxygen Consumption Values in Various Types of Shock*

Etiologic Type	*CI (L/min · m^2)*	*$\dot{D}O_2$ (mL/min · m^2)*	*$\dot{V}O_2$ (mL/min · m^2)*
High-risk surgery	4.5 ± 0.2	600 ± 1	167 ± 18
Trauma	5.0 ± 0.3	800 ± 46	180 ± 24
Sepsis	5.5 ± 0.3	1000 ± 52	190 ± 26
Acute myocardial infarction	2.5 ± 0.4	400 ± 60	124 ± 22

*Values are Mean ± SEM

TABLE 13–4. Clinic Data of a Prospective Randomized Clinical Trial

	CVP	*PA–Control*	*PA–Protocol*
Age in years	55.2 ± 30	5.34 ± 2.5	56.4 ± 3.1
Hospital days	22.2 ± 2.8	25.2 ± 3.4	19.3 ± 2.4
ICU days	11.5 ± 1.7	15.8 ± 3.1	10.2 ± 1.6*
Ventilator days	4.6 ± 1.4	9.4 ± 3.4	2.3 ± 0.5*
Intraoperative deaths	0	1	0
Postoperative deaths, No (%)	7 (23%)	10 (33%)	1 (4%)*
Organ failures	22	31	1
Other complications	9	8	10
Average costs	$30,748	$37,335	$27,665
Average cost per survivor	$40,106	$58,950	$28,690

*Significantly different from the PA–control group, $P < .05$.
(Modified from Shoemaker WC, Appel PL, Krom HB, et al: Prospective trial of supranormal values of survivors as therapeutic goals in high-risk surgical patients. Chest 1988; 94:1176.)

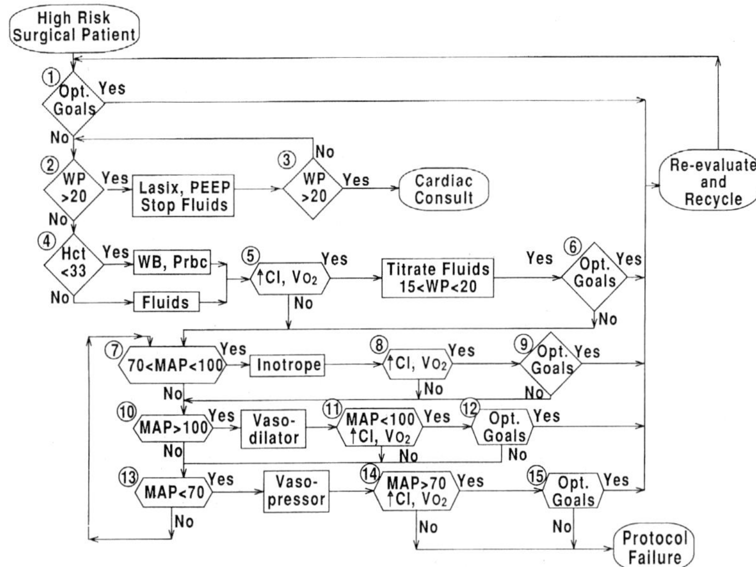

Figure 13–6. Branch chain decision tree for postoperative ICU patients. Preliminary evaluation of high-risk critically ill patients by routine ICU work-up that includes arterial blood gas analysis, chest radiography, routine blood chemistry studies, electrocardiography, and coagulation studies. These tests should either have been performed or be in process, and the observed defects corrected.
Step 1: Measure CI, $\dot{D}O_2$, $\dot{V}O_2$, and blood volume (BV) to determine whether the patient has reached the optimal goals. If CI < 4.5 L · min^{-1} · m^2, $\dot{D}O_2$ < 600 mL · min^{-1} · m^2, $\dot{V}O_2$ < 170 mL · min^{-1} · m^2, or BV < 3 L/m^2 (for men) or < 2.7 L/m^2 (for women), proceed to Step 2, but if the goals are reached, the objective of the algorithm has been achieved; re-evaluate and repeat at intervals to maintain these goals.
Step 2: Measure pulmonary artery wedge pressure (WP). If WP > 20 mm Hg, proceed to Step 3; if WP < 20 mm Hg proceed to Step 4.
Step 3: If WP > 20 mm Hg give furosemide at increasing dose levels (20, 40, 80, 160 mg IV) if there is clinical or x-ray evidence of salt and water overload or if there are clinical findings of pulmonary congestion. If not, consider administering vasodilators, nitroprusside, or nitroglycerin if MAP > 80 mm Hg and systolic pressure > 120 mm Hg. Repeat to titrate the dose as needed to reduce WP to < 15 mm Hg but to maintain MAP at > 80 mm Hg. If unsuccessful, place patient on a cardiac protocol.
Step 4: If hematocrit (Hct) < 33%, give 1 unit of whole blood (WB) or 2 units of packed red blood cells (Prbc). If Hct > 33%, give a fluid load (volume challenge) consisting of one of the following (depending on clinical indications of plasma volume deficit or hydration state): 500 mL of 5% plasma protein fraction; 500 mL of 5% albumin; 100 mL of 25% albumin (25 g); 500 mL of 6% hydroxyethyl starch; 500 mL of 6% dextran-60; or 1000 mL of lactated Ringer's solution or normal saline.
Step 5: If the blood or fluid load improved any of the optimal therapeutic goals defined in Step 1, proceed to Step 6; if none of them was improved, proceed to Step 7.
Step 6: If goals are not reached, repeat Steps 2 through 6 until these goals are met or until WP > 20 mm Hg.
Step 7: If MAP is between 70 and 100 mm Hg, give dobutamine by constant intravenous infusion in doses to increase CI, $\dot{D}O_2$, and $\dot{V}O_2$.
Step 8: Titrate dobutamine, beginning with 2 μg · kg^{-1} · min^{-1} and gradually increasing the dosing to a rate of up to 20 μg · kg^{-1} · min^{-1} or greater provided that CI, $\dot{D}O_2$, or $\dot{V}O_2$ improve or until the goals are met.
Step 9: If the goals are reached, re-evaluate and recycle. If goals are not reached or if it becomes evident that higher doses of the drug are not more effective or that they produce hypotension and tachycardia, continue dobutamine administration at its most effective dosing range.
Step 10: If MAP > 100 mm Hg, give a vasodilator (e.g., sodium nitroprusside, nitroglycerin, labetalol, or prostaglandin E_1) in gradually increasing doses provided improvement in CI, $\dot{D}O_2$, or $\dot{V}O_2$ occurs.
Step 11: Titrate vasodilators to decrease MAP and to increase CI, $\dot{D}O_2$, and $\dot{V}O_2$. If no improvement in CI, $\dot{D}O_2$, or $\dot{V}O_2$ occurs with vasodilator use or if hypotension (MAP < 70 mm Hg, SAP < 110 mm Hg) ensues, discontinue vasodilator use. If improvement occurs in CI, $\dot{D}O_2$, or $\dot{V}O_2$, titrate the vasodilator to maximum effect consistent with satisfactory arterial pressures.
Step 12: If the optimal goals are reached, re-evaluate and recycle at intervals.
Step 13: If these goals are not reached and if MAP < 80 mm Hg and SAP < 110 mm Hg, give dopamine or other vasopressor.
Step 14: Titrate the vasopressor in the lowest possible doses to maintain arterial pressures, MAP > 80 mm Hg, SAP > 110 mm Hg and to optimize CI, $\dot{D}O_2$, and $\dot{V}O_2$. If the goals and the pressures cannot be maintained, the patient is considered to be a protocol failure.
Step 15: If the goals are reached, re-evaluate and recycle. Consider additional therapy to further increase CI, $\dot{D}O_2$, and $\dot{V}O_2$, assuming greater than expected tissue hypoxia from poor tissue perfusion. (Modified from Shoemaker WC, Appel PL, Bland RD: Use of physiologic monitoring to predict outcome and to assist in clinical decisions in critically ill postoperative patients. Am J Surg 1983; 164:43.)

for patients to develop deficits before therapy is initiated. To be optimally effective, therapy should be started as soon as possible in order to achieve the maximally compensated physiologic status before the microcirculatory defects become irreversible or before the capillary leak becomes widespread and resistant to therapy.

Blood Volume and Fluid Status

The first and most important therapeutic goal for hemorrhagic, traumatic, neurogenic, and septic shock is to restore blood volume; however, criteria for demonstrating this goal's achievement are not well defined. The use of tachycardia and reduced MAP, CVP, PAOP, urine output, and hematocrit values was based on experimental and clinical observations made immediately after sudden acute hemorrhage and the subsequent resuscitation. Although useful during acute hypovolemia, these values, including PAOP, unfortunately do not reflect the blood volume status during a patient's subsequent ICU course. Moreover, in critically ill postoperative patients, these commonly used clinical criteria were unreliable when compared with careful measurements of blood volume.[57]

Contrary to the approach of many internists, surgeons are often accused of overly aggressive fluid administration in the presence of minimal clinical indications, especially in patients with surgical or accidental trauma. Medical patients, especially those with chronic cardiac, renal, pulmonary, and hepatic disorders, often have excessive amounts of salt and water and thus require diuretics and fluid restriction.

Fluid therapy controversies often arise from a common misconception: the failure to diagnose deficient plasma volume clinically in the presence of excessive interstitial (extracellular) water. As an example, the patient with peripheral edema obviously has too much interstitial water, but may also have hypovolemia. Frequently, postoperative shock patients have maldistributed flow with contracted plasma volume but increased interstitial water.[42–45] This is also commonly seen in the inadequately resuscitated trauma patient and in the patient resuscitated with massive crystalloid infusion regimens. Therapy should be aimed at improving circulatory function by restoring plasma volume, not by overloading an already expanded interstitial space.

Restoration of blood volume is the most important correctable therapeutic problem in acute circulatory shock. It is, therefore, essential to have a reliable means to assess this volume. Measurement of plasma volume with iodine 125–labeled albumin or of red blood cell mass with chromium 55–labeled red blood cells is time-consuming, expensive, and usually performed only in research centers. The CVP and PAOP, which can be repeated at frequent intervals or monitored continuously, were thought to have the needed accuracy and have largely replaced blood volume measurement methods for patients with most clinical conditions. CVP and PAOP rapidly decrease with acute hemorrhage and increase immediately after fluid therapy. High venous pressures are associated with both acute blood volume overload and cardiac failure. However, after a variable period of time in the ICU, venous pressures are notably unreliable indicators of blood volume status because of compliance changes of the walls of veins. In the postoperative ICU period, venous pressures accommodate to either high or low blood volumes with PAOP values that usually remain in the range of about 8 to 12 mm Hg. Figure 13–7 illustrates the values of over 1700 carefully measured blood volumes relative to the commonly monitored variables thought to reflect blood volume.[57] The latter fail to reflect blood volume changes over a wide range of values.

Figure 13–8 illustrates the scatter of blood volume values relative to their corresponding CVP values. Although CVP and PAOP may accurately measure venous pressures, they do not accurately reflect blood volume in most ICU patients. However, they are useful to determine the capacity of the vascular system to accept more volume without the production of pulmonary edema and to prevent acute blood volume overload during rapid fluid restoration. Furthermore, peripheral edema as well as pulmonary edema may result from massive crystalloid infusions that expand the interstitial space without exceeding "safe" venous pressures or fully restoring plasma volume.[45]

Daily weight assessments and fluid balance measurements are used to monitor fluid management, but both of these reflect total body water or changes in body water, not blood volume. The distribution of body water between the plasma, interstitium, and intracellular compartments can be definitively measured only by isotopic body composition studies.[42–44]

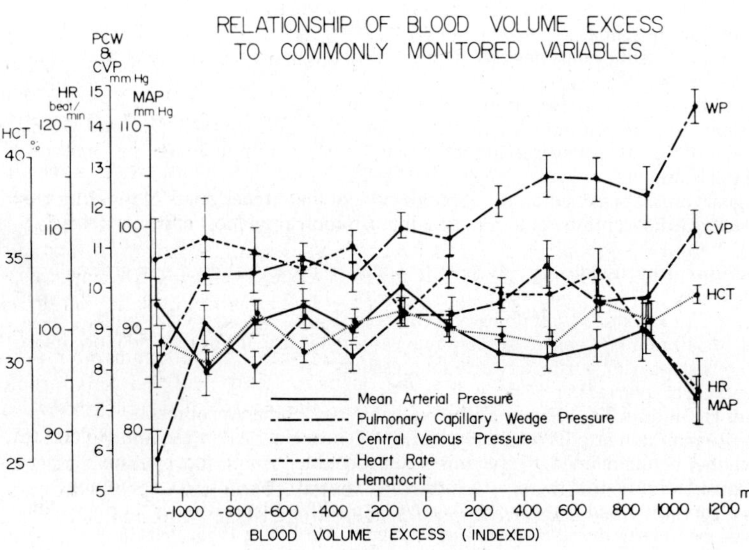

Figure 13–7. BV index values plotted against Hct, heart rate (HR), CVP, WP, and MAP on the *y*-axis. Blood volume values are expressed as milliliters of excess (+) or deficit (−) from the patient's predicted norm indexed to body surface area. Note the very poor correlation of the commonly monitored variables. (From Shippy CR, Appel PL, Shoemaker WC: Reliablity of clinical monitoring to assess blood volume in critically ill patients. Crit Care Med 1984; 12:107.)

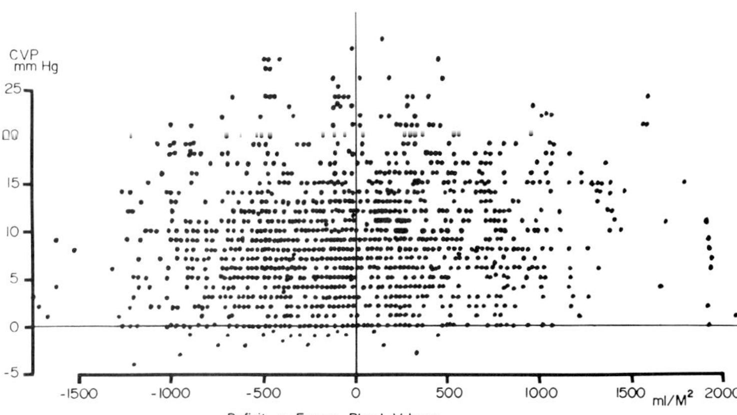

Figure 13–8. BV index values plotted against their simultaneously measured CVP values. (From Shippy CR, Appel PL, Shoemaker WC: Reliability of clinical monitoring to assess blood volume in critically ill patients. Crit Care Med 1984; 12:107.)

Volume Therapy

Vigorous and rapid volume loading that does not exceed PAOP values greater than 18 or 20 mm Hg is the first and most important therapy. It is easier to achieve the therapeutic goals with colloids, which expand the plasma volume without overexpansion of the interstitial water, than with crystalloids, which primarily are distributed in the interstitial water.[19, 45–48, 58] Plasma volume restoration cannot be assumed in the presence of pitting edema in patients who have received large volumes of crystalloids because hypovolemia frequently occurs together with expansion of interstitial water. Moreover, it can not be assumed that one third of the extracellular water will remain in the intravascular space while two thirds is distributed in the interstitium because these often quoted conclusions were based on radiosulfate measurements made under normal conditions.[45] In critically ill patients, only 20% of 1000 mL of crystalloids remained in the circulation by the end of a 1-hour infusion, and 40 minutes later almost all of that had gone into the interstitial space.[45] In conditions of peripheral edema, we prefer to give concentrated (25%) albumin, which increases colloidal osmotic pressure and expands plasma volume by shifting interstitial water back into the plasma volume.[45, 46] Subsequently, diuretics may be used to reduce plasma volume, if this becomes a problem.

In control studies of critically ill patients, 500 mL of 5% albumin persisted for 3.5 to 4.5 hours, whereas 500 mL of hydroxyethyl starch lasted 5 to 6 hours, and dextran 40 and gelatin about 1.5 to 2 hours; crystalloids lasted 40 minutes.[46, 48]

Inotropic Agents

After the maximum effect of fluids has been obtained, administration of an inotropic agent such as dobutamine may be started at about 5 $\mu g \cdot kg^{-1} \cdot min^{-1}$; the appropriate dose is obtained by titration to achieve the optimal goals in terms of CI, $\dot{D}O_2$, and $\dot{V}O_2$. Dobutamine produced marked and significant increases in CI and stroke index, cardiac and stroke work, and $\dot{D}O_2$, and $\dot{V}O_2$ as well as decreases in systemic and pulmonary vascular resistances and venous inflow pressures (CVP and PAOP); blood gases, pH, and $\dot{Q}sp/\dot{Q}t$ were not significantly changed.[58–60]

The effects of dobutamine at various doses are summarized in Figure 13–9. The data show pronounced changes beginning at the 2.5-$\mu g \cdot kg^{-1} \cdot min^{-1}$ dose, with greater flow effects occurring at greater doses. CI, $\dot{D}O_2$, and $\dot{V}O_2$ significantly increased after dobutamine was administered in septic shock patients, but these changes were less in the septic shock patients compared with the nonseptic shock patients. Vasopressors produced greater increases in blood pressure than did dobutamine but less improvement in $\dot{D}O_2$ and $\dot{V}O_2$, particularly in large doses.[59]

The effects of dobutamine were observed in a small group of patients before and after a fluid load consisting of 500 or 1000 mL of 5% albumin was given. Greater flow effects with little or no hypotension and tachycardia were observed when blood volume was adequately restored before infusion. The hypovolemic patient is extremely sensitive to vasodilators and may rapidly deteriorate if blood volume is not restored prior to vasodilation. Additional fluids must be given if hypotension occurs following administration of dobutamine or other vasodilators. Stimulation of the empty heart with an inotropic vasodilator may produce severe hypotension and dysrhythmias. When dobutamine produces sudden severe hypotension, this reaction may be reversed with rapid administration of fluids.[60]

Vasodilator Therapy

If a patient has normal or high MAP with a high SVRI, vasodilation with nitroglycerin, nitroprusside, labetalol, hydralazine, or prostaglandin (alprostadil [PGE_1]) may be considered; the optimal dose is obtained by titration to achieve improved CI without production of hypotension (i.e., MAP > 80 mm Hg; systolic arterial pressure (SAP) > 100 mm Hg).

Vasopressor Therapy

Vasopressors are indicated for hypotension after volume therapy has been given. Hypotension, defined as MAP less than 70 mm Hg and diastolic pressures less than 50 mm Hg, should be prevented because blood flow to the heart and brain is largely driven by pressure. However, the α-adrenergic effects of vasopressors also intensify the uneven vasoconstriction produced by neural mechanisms. This uneven metarteriolar constriction raises blood pressure but at the expense of uneven microcirculatory flow. Since dopamine, norepinephrine, and epinephrine, in contrast to methoxamine, have inotropic action that increases CI, the net effect on tissue perfusion and oxygenation is the balance between the favorable increase of blood flow and the unfavorable maldistribution of flow from uneven vasoconstriction. For this reason, the smallest doses of vasopressors needed to maintain the minimum satisfactory blood pressure are recommended because no administered amount of vasopressors will make up for inadequate blood volume.

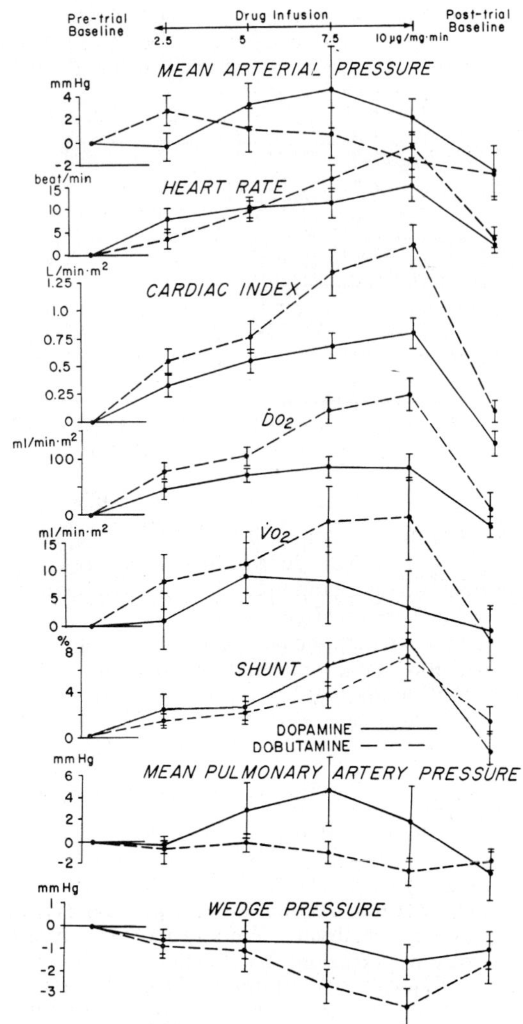

Figure 13–9. Hemodynamic and oxygen transport effects of dobutamine *(dashed line)* and dopamine *(solid line)* in 25 high-risk postoperative patients in a prospective, random-ordered crossover trial. (Modified from Shoemaker WC, Appel PL, Kram HB: Comparison of dobutamine and dopamine in prospective crossover clinical trials in critically ill postoperative patients. Chest 1988; 96:120.)

Strategy for Treatment of Shock

Similar underlying physiologic alterations occur in patients with severe accidental trauma, stress, and sepsis, but the optimal goals are not quantitatively the same as those for postoperative patients—that is, the underlying physiologic defects may be qualitatively similar and the metabolic requirements may be greater, but more aggressive therapy may be needed to achieve the optimal goals. The increased $\dot{V}O_2$ in patients with severe trauma, stress, sepsis, and hypercatabolic states indicates increased metabolic requirements. However, greater than normal metabolism should not be interpreted to mean that all metabolic needs have been met; even greater rates of $\dot{V}O_2$ may be needed. The strategy in each case is to try to open up unevenly vasoconstricted arteriolar-capillary networks by vigorous volume loading and then to increase blood flow with the use of inotropic agents and, subsequently, vasodilators to overcome vasoconstricted metarteriolar circuits.

Optimal goals can be calculated as the mean for a given etiologic type of shock or for a given type of patient population. However, the optimal goals cannot be precisely defined for individual patients because of interpatient variations in baseline $\dot{V}O_2$ requirements, prior associated medical conditions, the amount and duration of oxygen debt, compensatory capacities, and many other factors. The optimal values after trauma and sepsis are more widely variable than are those after elective surgery because the widely varying extent of injury and the virulence of the infectious agent produce wide variations in the increases of metabolic demands. A broad range of circulatory function is required to supply these increased metabolic needs.

The answer to this dilemma is an operational definition of goals; to resolve the issue of whether the patient with high $\dot{V}O_2$ has enough $\dot{V}O_2$, the $\dot{D}O_2$ is increased until no further increase in $\dot{V}O_2$ occurs (unless limited by PAOP in instances of fluid loading or by tachycardia $>$130 beats per minute with inotropic agents, and hypotension $<$80 mm Hg MAP or $<$110 mm Hg systolic arterial pressure with vasodilators). Thus, tissue oxygen demand is inferred indirectly by an empirical trial of therapy. If therapy increases CI, $\dot{D}O_2$, and $\dot{V}O_2$, it may be assumed that it opened up additional microcirculatory channels that perfused relatively hypoxic tissues, which then extracted more oxygen. Since tissues cannot take up more oxygen than they use, the increased $\dot{V}O_2$ after therapy indicates that an oxygen debt exists and that this debt has been at least partially satisfied. In this approach, PAOP is not used as a measure of blood volume because it clearly does not reflect blood volume.[57] Rather, PAOP is used as an upper limit for volume therapy or for the rate of volume infusion so that pulmonary edema can be avoided.

Vasopressors are used as a last resort to maintain sufficient MAP to provide for coronary and cerebral perfusion after the maximum effects of fluids, inotropes and vasodilators have been achieved. The hemodynamic effectiveness of each agent given separately should be established before agents are combined.

Elderly and cardiac patients have considerably different physiologic problems and different compensatory mechanisms than do patients with normal hearts but multiple organ dysfunction. The heart may be the weak link in the former, but circulatory transport functions are likely to limit survival in the latter. An appropriate strategy in cardiac patients may be to stimulate cardiac function with inotropic agents and to reduce cardiac work by afterload reduction with vasodilators; preload should be augmented, but overdilation should be avoided.

The most important principles in these complex clinical conditions are (1) documentation of baseline hemodynamic and oxygen transport variables, (2) measurement of changes with each appropriate agent to determine the relative effectiveness of alternative therapies, and (3) titration of the dose to achieve optimal or near-optimal values.

Potential Use of Monoclonal Antibodies and Free Radical Scavengers

Clinical trials of two types of monoclonal endotoxin and anti–tumor necrosis factor antibodies have not provided the anticipated good results and Food and Drug Administration approval at the time of this writing. Additional clinical trials are being undertaken. It is doubtful that any single agent will be sufficient to reverse the complex multifactorial shock state. It is likely that these and other ancillary agents, such as steroids, prostaglandins, and cyclooxygenase inhibitors, will have a role after a patient's major circulatory variables are corrected with fluids and inotropic agents.

Antioxidant vitamins and antioxidant enzymes, including

superoxide dismutase, catalase, and glutathione peroxidase, although not commercially available, may eventually be helpful in restoring and maintaining an appropriate balance between oxidants and antioxidants.

References

1. Wiggers CJ: Physiology of Shock. New York, Commonwealth Fund, 1940.
2. Cournand A, Riley RL, Bradley SE, et al: Studies of the circulation in clinical shock. Surgery 1943; 13:964.
3. Clowes GHA Jr, Del Guercio LRM: Circulatory response to trauma of surgical operations. Metabolism 1960; 9:67.
4. Wilson RF, Thal AP, Kinding PH, et al: Hemodynamic measurements in shock. Arch Surg 1965; 91:124.
5. Heilbrunn A, Allbritten FF: Cardiac output during and following surgical operation. Ann Surg 1960; 152:197.
6. Del Guercio LRM, Commarswamy RF, Feins NR, et al: Pulmonary arteriovenous admixture and the hyperdynamic state in surgery for portal hypertension. Surgery 1964; 56:57.
7. Shoemaker WC, Printen KJ, Amato JJ, et al: Hemodynamic patterns after acute anesthetized and unanesthetized trauma. Arch Surg 1967; 95:492.
8. Siegel J, Goldwyn PM, Friedman HP: Pattern and process in the evolution of human septic shock. Surgery 1971; 70:232.
9. Shoemaker WC, Montgomery ES, Kaplan E, et al: Physiologic patterns in surviving and nonsurviving shock patients. Arch Surg 1973; 106:630.
10. Shoemaker WC: Shock states: Pathophysiology, monitoring, outcome prediction, and therapy. *In:* Textbook of Critical Care. 2nd ed. Shoemaker WC, Ayres SM, Grenvik A, et al (Eds). Philadelphia, WB Saunders, 1989, pp 977–993.
11. Bland RD, Shoemaker WC, Abraham E, et al: Hemodynamic and oxygen transport patterns in surviving and nonsurviving postoperative patients. Crit Care Med 1985; 13:85.
12. Bland RD, Shoemaker WC: Common physiologic patterns in general surgical patients: Hemodynamic and oxygen transport changes during and after operation in patients with and without associated medical problems. Surg Clin North Am 1985; 65:793.
13. Shoemaker WC, Bland RD, Appel PL: Therapy of critically ill postoperative patients based on outcome prediction and prospective clinical trials. Surg Clin North Am 1985; 65:811.
14. Shoemaker WC: Circulatory mechanisms of shock and their mediators. Crit Care Med 1987; 15:787.
15. Shoemaker WC, Czer L, Chang P, et al: Cardiorespiratory monitoring in postoperative patients: I. Prediction of outcome and severity of illness. Crit Care Med 1979; 7:237.
16. Bland RD, Shoemaker WC: Probability of survival as a prognostic and severity of illness score in critically ill surgical patients. Crit Care Med 1985; 13:91.
17. Shoemaker WC, Appel PL, Bland RD: Use of physiologic monitoring to predict outcome and to assist in clinical decisions in critically ill postoperative patients. Am J Surg 1983; 164:43.
18. Shoemaker WC, Appel P, Kram HB: Role of oxygen debt in the development of organ failure, sepsis and death in high-risk surgical patients. Chest 1992; 102:208–215.
19. Shoemaker WC, Appel PL, Kram HB, et al: Prospective trial of supranormal values of survivors as therapeutic goals in high-risk surgical patients. Chest 1988; 94:1176.
20. Bassin R, Vladick B, Kim SI, et al: Comparison of hemodynamic responses of two experimental shock models with clinical hemorrhage. Surgery 1971; 69:722.
21. Bishop MH, Shoemaker WC, Appel PL, et al: Influence of time and optimal circulatory resuscitation in high-risk trauma. Crit Care Med 1993; 21:56.
22. Bishop MH, Shoemaker WC, Fleming AW, et al: Relationship between ARDS, hemodynamics, fluid balance and pulmonary infiltration in critically ill surgical patients. Am Surg 1991; 57:785.
23. Shoemaker WC, Appel PL, Kram HB, et al: Temporal hemodynamic and oxygen transport patterns in medical patients with sepsis and septic shock. Chest 1993; 104:1529.
24. Shoemaker WC, Appel PL, Kram HB, et al: Sequence of physiologic patterns in surgical septic shock. Crit Care Med 1993; 21:1876.
25. Hankeln K, Senker R, Schwarten JM, et al: Evaluation of prognostic indices based on hemodynamic and oxygen transport variables in shock patients with adult respiratory distress syndrome. Crit Care Med 1987; 15:1.
26. Abraham E, Bland RD, Cobo JC, et al: Sequential cardiorespiratory patterns associated with outcome in septic shock. Chest 1984; 85:75.
27. Haupt MT, Gilbert EM, Carlson RW: Fluid loading increases oxygen delivery and consumption in septic patients with lactic acidosis. Am Rev Respir Dis 1985; 131:912.
28. Russell JA, Lockhat D, Belzberg M, et al: Oxygen delivery and consumption and ventricular preload are greater in survivors than nonsurvivors of ARDS. Chest 1988; 94:755.
29. Gilbert EM, Haupt MT, Mandanas RT, et al: The effect of fluid loading blood transfusion, and catecholamine infusion on oxygen delivery and consumption in patients with sepsis. Am Rev Respir Dis 1986; 134:873.
30. Rackow EC, Kaufman BS, Falk JL, et al: Hemodynamic response to fluid repletion in patients with septic shock. Circ Shock 1987; 22:11.
31. Packman MI, Rackow EC: Optimal left heart filling pressure during fluid resuscitation of patients with hypovolemia and septic shock. Crit Care Med 1983; 11:165.
32. Astiz ME, Rackow EC, Falk JL, et al: Oxygen delivery and consumption in patients with hyperdynamic septic shock. Crit Care Med 1987; 15:26.
33. Tuchschmidt J, Fried J, Swinney R, et al: Early hemodynamic correlates of survival in patients with septic shock. Crit Care Med 1989; 17:719.
34. Edwards JD, Redmond AD, Nightingale P, et al: Oxygen consumption following trauma. Br J Surg 1988; 75:690.
35. Edwards JD, Brown GCS, Nightingale P, et al: Use of survivors' cardiorespiratory values as therapeutic goals in septic shock. Crit Care Med 1989; 17:1098.
36. Tuchschmidt J, Fried J, Astiz M, et al: Supranormal oxygen delivery improves mortality in septic shock patients. Chest 1992; 102:216–220.
37. Forrester JS, Diamond GA, Swan HJC: Correlation classification of clinical and hemodynamic function after acute myocardial infarction. Am J Cardiol 1977; 39:137.
38. DaLuz P, Cavanilles JM, Michael S: Oxygen delivery, anoxic metabolism and hemoglobin P50 in patients with acute myocardial infarction and shock. Am J Cardiol 1975; 36:148.
39. Creamer J, Edwards JD, Nightingale P: Hemodynamic and oxygen transport variables in cardiogenic shock following acute myocardial infarction and their response to treatment. Am J Cardiol 1990; 65:1297.
40. Edwards JD: Oxygen transport in cardiogenic and septic shock. Crit Care Med 1991; 19:658.
41. Lowe JG, Ernst EA: The Quantitative Practice of Anesthesia: Use of the Closed Circuit. Baltimore, Williams & Wilkins, 1981, pp 146–147.
42. Moore FD, Olesen KH, McMurrey JD, et al: Body Cell Mass and its Supporting Environment: Body Cell Mass in Health and Disease. Philadelphia, WB Saunders, 1963.
43. Davidson I, Haglind E, Gelin LE: Plasma volume, intravascular protein content, hemodynamic and oxygen transport changes during intestinal shock in dogs. Crit Care Med 1980; 8:73.
44. Davidson I, Ottosson J, Reich J: Infusion volumes of Ringer's lactate and 3% albumin solution as they relate to survival after resuscitation of a lethal intestinal ischemic shock. Circ Shock 1986; 18:277.
45. Shoemaker WC, Kram HB: Comparison of the effects of crystalloids and colloids on hemodynamic oxygen transport, mortality and morbidity. *In:* Debates in General Surgery. Simmon RS, Udeko AJ (Eds). Chicago, Year Book Medical Publishers, 1991.
46. Hauser CJ, Shoemaker WC, Turpin I, et al: Hemodynamic and oxygen transport responses to body water shifts produced by colloids and crystalloids in critically ill patients. Surg Gynecol Obstet 1980; 150:811.
47. Shoemaker WC, Matsuda T, State D: Relative hemodynamic effectiveness of whole blood and plasma expanders in burned patients. Surg Gynecol Obstet 1977; 144:909.
48. Appel PL, Shoemaker WC: Fluid therapy in adult respiratory failure. Crit Care Med 1981; 9:862.

49. Abraham E: Physiologic stress and cellular ischemia. Crit Care Med 1991; 19:613–618.
50. Bentler B: Endotoxin, tremor necrosis factor and related mediators. New Horiz 1993; 1:3.
51. McCord JM: Oxygen-derived free radicals. New Horiz 1993; 1:70.
52. Suffredini AF, Fromm RE, Parker MM, et al: The cardiovascular response of normal humans to the administration of endotoxins. N Engl J Med 1989; 321:280–287.
53. Hoch RC, Rodriguez R, Manning T, et al: Effects of accidental trauma on cytokine and endotoxin production. Crit Care Med 1993; 21:839.
54. Pullicino EA, Carli F, Poole S, et al: The relationship between circulating concentrations of interleukin-6, tumor necrosis factor, and the acute phase response to elective surgery and accidental injury. Lymphokine Res 1990; 9:231–238.
55. Van Zee KJ, DeForge LE, Fischer E, et al: IL-8 in septic shock, endotoxemia, and after IL-1 administration. J Immunol 1991; 146:3478–3482.
56. Di Padova F, Pozzi C, Tondre MJ, et al: Selective and early increase of IL-1 inhibitors, IL-6 and cortisol after elective surgery. Clin Exp Immunol 1991; 85:137–142.
57. Shippy CR, Appel PL, Shoemaker WC: Reliablity of clinical monitoring to assess blood volume in critically ill patients. Crit Care Med 1984; 12:107.
58. Shoemaker WC, Appel PL, Kram HB: Oxygen transport measurements to evaluate tissue perfusion and titrate therapy: Dobutamine and dopamine effects. Crit Care Med 1991; 19:672.
59. Shoemaker WC, Appel PL, Kram HB: Hemodynamic and oxygen transport effects of dobutamine in critically ill general surgical patients. Crit Care Med 1986; 14:1032.
60. Shoemaker WC, Appel PL, Kram HB: Comparison of dobutamine and dopamine in prospective crossover clinical trials in critically ill postoperative patients. Chest 1988; 96:120.
61. Luce JM: Introduction of new technology into critical care practice: A history of HA-1A human monoclonal antibiotics against endotoxin. Crit Care Med 1993; 21:1233.

CHAPTER 14

Clinical Algorithms for Resuscitation in Acute Emergency Conditions

William C. Shoemaker, MD • Michael H. Bishop, DO

CLINICAL DECISIONS IN RESUSCITATION

The sudden appearance of an acute emergency may become the prelude to confusion and sometimes disaster. In contrast to elective conditions, time is of the essence. High-risk emergency victims concomitantly require rapid diagnostic, monitoring, and therapeutic decisions that then must be translated expeditiously into action. In patients with multiple life-threatening problems or severe associated preexisting medical conditions, there are minimal margins for error in their resuscitation. For example, hypotensive shock patients have a high risk of death if the right things do not get done in time: Fluid therapy must be initiated quickly and titrated appropriately in the initial resuscitation and continued in the subsequent postshock period to achieve optimal outcome.

The resuscitation and immediate management of high-risk, life-threatening emergencies require expeditious diagnostic work-up, physiologic monitoring, and fluid therapy of shock as well as definitive therapy of the specific injury or disease state. The three major activities—diagnosis, monitoring, and therapy—must be rapidly planned and expeditiously coordinated as the patient moves from the emergency department (ED), to the operating room, or to the intensive care unit (ICU). The challenge is to provide a well-organized, coherent approach prioritized according to the life-threatening aspects of each problem. These crucial decisions involving priorities and therapeutic goals are best defined by branch chain decision trees or clinical algorithms.

TRADITIONAL APPROACH TO CLINICAL DECISION MAKING

In the traditional approach, well-established clinical concepts are usually stated in narrative form and by lists for diagnostic work-up and therapy. These concepts are often supplemented by anecdotal observations, by reviews of the results of specific types of accidents, and by information from experimental shock in anesthetized animals. Traditional approaches focus on general principles distilled from the wealth of clinical experience but leave detailed applications to the bedside clinician. By contrast, clinical algorithms focus on the detailed application of concepts in a systematic organized fashion. The traditional approaches apply generalized rules for all patients of a given diagnostic category. Alternatively, clinical algorithms progressively stratify the patient series by successive clinical criteria defined for each decision node; then they define specific criteria for initiation of therapy as well as titration of therapy to endpoints. The aim of our algorithms is to titrate each therapy to criteria that characterize survival patterns.

Conventional clinical approaches provide lists of diagnostic and laboratory tests that may be appropriate to some therapeutic activities but inappropriate to others; for example, Table 14–1 lists activities and principles for trauma admissions[1] developed more than 25 years ago. The difficulty with these lists of needed clinical and laboratory data are that they leave the impression that perhaps all this information might be needed before making the important initial decisions. By the time one gets halfway down the list, however, there are conflicting historic information, changing clinical signs, and questionable laboratory tests that delay decision making. Conventional approaches to emergency care attempt to be meticulously complete but may be difficult to apply and easily lead to diagnostic tangents. The problem is compounded because formal presentations of diseases in medical texts are organized according to diagnostic categories: The dilemma is that this requires the diagnosis to have been established before therapeutic decisions are made.

By contrast, the algorithmic approach enfolds the diagnostic and monitoring processes into therapeutic management to expedite continuing decision making of all these processes. Each decision may be made as soon as the criterion within the diamond (or hexagon) of each decision node is met without having to wait until all other information needed for subsequent decisions is available.

Common Problems in Resuscitation

Our review of emergency fatalities revealed that most preventable errors occurred not so much because of ignorance but because of the failure to act expeditiously at a crucial moment. Delays in resuscitation may result from disorganized activity, from failure to recognize priorities, and from failure to appreciate the complexities of emergency care. Although usually the correct therapeutic measures eventually are done, they are frequently not done at the right time,

TABLE 14–1. Evaluation, Diagnosis, and Therapy of Trauma Patients

1. Withdraw blood sample for hematocrit, typing, crossmatch, electrolytes, and routine chemistries.
2. Start intravenous fluids.
3. Insert central venous pressure catheter.
4. Examine lungs; tap chest if pneumothorax or hemothorax is suspected.
5. Examine heart.
6. Insert Foley catheter and measure urine output.
7. Measure arterial blood gases.
8. Obtain electrocardiogram.
9. Measure blood volume or hemoglobin/hematocrit.
10. If cardiac tamponade suspected from rising central venous pressure, obtain echocardiogram, computed tomographic scan, or pericardiocentesis.
11. Examine abdomen; if blunt trauma with organ damage is suspected, perform diagnostic peritoneal lavage.
12. Examine the patient thoroughly for evidence of fractures, wounds, and other injuries.
13. Search for sources of obscure bleeding.
14. Search for sources of infection; perform a culture of available body fluids.
15. Hematologic evaluation: prothrombin time, partial thromboplastin time, platelet count, fibrinogen, bleeding and clotting times.

in the right amount, and in the right order. A major difficulty in organizing priorities for emergency care is that the exigencies of emergency situations preclude carefully controlled scientific studies. Moreover, in most clinicians' minds, the urgent demand for therapy focuses on one or more key issues to the exclusion of other important considerations.

The successful resuscitation of acute emergency victims may depend on the nature and extent of the primary illness or injury, the amount of blood and fluid losses, the patient's age and previous state of health, the number and extent of associated medical conditions, the time delay in instituting therapy, the volume and rate of fluids administered, and the choice of fluids given. Although experienced physicians manage emergency victims with excellent outcomes, it is difficult to describe their approaches objectively so that students, residents, and younger clinicians could emulate them. Less experienced physicians in the community hospital who see limited numbers of major emergency victims may need help to organize priorities and applications of a wide variety of generally accepted principles. The branch chain decision tree provides the vehicle to transfer information and approaches of high-volume experience to a wider array of clinical applications.

From both the organizational and scientific viewpoints, it is difficult to evaluate the wide range of associated medical conditions and preexisting illnesses during emergency resuscitation. Although the general principles of resuscitation and emergency care are well known, the major difficulty operationally is providing the optimal emergency care on the spot, without delay, and without missing important steps. This involves evaluating the process of emergency care by specifically defined criteria and priorities to achieve the best outcome.

Evaluations of these clinical problems from detailed reviews of many clinical series over several decades suggest that delays in decision making and therapy would be prevented and care would be improved if the clinical management was organized in the context of a decision tree. Most medical activity, according to McDonald,[2] consists of simple recognition-response arcs that can be defined by decision rules to deal expeditiously with emergency problems.

USE OF BRANCH CHAIN LOGIC: THE DECISION TREE

Algorithmic Approach

The algorithmic approach to resuscitation is based on the premise that the important clinical problems may be described by clinical criteria and that decision rules can be defined by clinical and physiologic criteria. These decision rules, together with their therapeutic choices, may then be expressed in the format of a branch chain decision tree. This framework provides the skeleton for commonly encountered major clinical problems; it does not preclude other additional care not specified by the decision tree, but it simply provides the organizational outline for expeditious care.

Initially, clinical algorithms were designed for resuscitation of trauma victims in the ED,[3, 4] for paramedical personnel performing triage,[5, 6] and for nurse clinicians and physicians' assistants.[7, 8] More than two decades ago, decision trees were designed to guide physicians in treating acute illness and trauma.[3, 4, 9–20] The branch chain logic is ideally suited to resuscitation and fluid management in patients with shock. Prospective clinical trials have demonstrated improved outcome with a resuscitation algorithm.[12, 13]

Branch chain logic is probably the process clinicians subconsciously use to reason, and algorithms generated by careful analysis may represent formal conceptualizations of thought processes. An algorithm, therefore, uses branch chain logic as a set of formalized procedure rules that may be applied to a specific recurring set of conditions. Usually it is applied to very specific conditions that lend themselves to definitive resolution by breaking down complex problems into a series of components, each having been characterized by specific criteria. In essence, an algorithm is a formalized set of step-by-step instructions with detailed specifications for each aspect of the algorithm. It is essentially a closed system that is designed to accomplish a given task by precisely defined criteria for entry, for each step, for the sequence of steps, and for a specific endpoint at which to stop.

Clinical Algorithm

Clinical algorithms are less rigorously defined than mathematical equations or algorithms used in computer software. Branch chain decision trees or clinical algorithms represent sets of guidelines for clinical care that are less precisely and less quantitatively defined. On the other hand, the term *algorithm* is often misapplied to flow charts that merely describe percentages of clinical groups or outcomes of groups managed by various procedures. The essential features of an algorithm are well-defined sets of criteria that serially specify each sequential decision node.

Each node on the decision tree stratifies the subjects by explicit prearranged criteria and specifies the next action to be taken. This provides a plan that shows at a glance the specific criteria for each decision node, the sequence of this sorting operation, and the tasks to be performed at each decision node. This facilitates more expeditious, consistent, and complete therapy than management hastily arranged by those who happen to be present or on call at the time. It does not readily allow important parts of the process to be neglected.

The branch chain logic approach specifies the minimum information needed to make the first decision; as soon as that information is available, the decision can be made and therapy instituted. In the meantime, information is gathered for the next decision. Thus, the acquisition of the relevant data and the administration of each type of therapy are sequenced to address the most important and urgent decisions first. This approach preselects patients of specifically defined groups in order of their life-threatening probabilities: Each successive selection is based on the prior tests and therapies, so that urgent problems are resolved and the residual population then becomes more homogeneous. This stepwise process provides the organizational framework for accomplishing prioritized objectives of resuscitation without limiting the clinical actions to these activities.

Algorithmic Conventions and Notations

By conventional notations, decision nodes are indicated by diamonds or hexagons; the criteria needed for each decision are indicated by the values shown inside the hexagons. The ovals or balloons give criteria for entrance or exit from the algorithm, whereas the rectangles indicate diagnostic procedures or therapeutic interventions. The decision sequences are shown by arrows indicating the temporal order of the numbered decision nodes.

Common clinical problems that lend themselves to this approach must have very specific and well-defined criteria for each decision. Questions that require interpretation such as, "How sick is the patient?", do not make good decision nodes because they are not answered by a simple "yes" or "no" based on objective data. By contrast, straightforward, routinely managed problems whose answers have been well worked out and clinically tested are easily expressed in the algorithmic format. With these essential tasks addressed, clinicians are then free to concentrate on problems that cannot be easily defined and that require considered judgment and interpretation.

This chapter describes three clinical algorithms for (1) initial fluid resuscitation of emergency hypotensive patients in the ED, (2) subsequent fluid management of the critically ill patient being monitored with a central venous pressure (CVP) catheter, and (3) management of blunt and penetrating wounds of the chest and abdomen. The third decision tree extends the algorithmic approach from the relatively simple fluid management problem to a more comprehensive organization of diagnosis, monitoring, and therapy of trauma. A fourth algorithm for high-risk surgical patients using a pulmonary artery catheter is described in Chapter 13. A fifth algorithm for diagnosis and management of acute pericardial tamponade is described in Chapter 62.

ALGORITHM FOR INITIAL FLUID RESUSCITATION OF HYPOTENSIVE EMERGENCY PATIENTS

Usually the most crucial problem in the hypotensive emergency trauma victim is unrecognized hypovolemia and delay or inadequate fluid resuscitation that leads to increased mortality and morbidity. Upper airway obstruction may be more urgent, but it is less common and usually readily correctable with intubation and mechanical ventilation.

Description and Strategy Conveyed by the Algorithm

An algorithm was designed for fluid therapy in the first 30 to 60 minutes of resuscitation of hypotensive patients entering the ED (Fig. 14–1). It is based on the premise that hypovolemia causes most of the mortality and morbidity of trauma and other acute emergency conditions. The longer the patient is hypovolemic, the more likely there will be shock and its sequela: shock-related organ failure.

The emergency algorithm may be used to illustrate the therapeutic strategy for fluid resuscitation of hypotensive emergencies. In the first decision point, the criterion for initiation of fluid therapy is mean arterial blood pressure (MAP) less than 60 mm Hg or systolic pressure less than 90 mm Hg. The MAP is defined as the diastolic pressure plus one third of the pulse pressure, which is the difference between systolic and diastolic pressures. Thus, in emergency patients, hypotension is all that is needed to start the first liter of saline or lactated Ringer's solution (RL). The second decision point involves the choice of fluids and indicates that patients who are younger than 45 years and who have no cardiac history may be able to tolerate more salt and water; therefore, they are given an additional liter of RL plus 500 mL of colloids. The third decision point is a CVP greater than 15 mm Hg, which defines criteria to slow or stop fluid administration. The fourth decision point, hematocrit (Hct) less than 25%, defines the criteria for use of O-negative or uncrossmatched (type-specific) blood in patients with rapid exsanguinating hemorrhage. Finally, the MAP response to therapy is used as the decision criterion to recycle or to proceed to the next section.

In essence, hypotension is the criterion for starting fluids; age, cardiac history, and Hct define the type and amount of fluids. The young, previously healthy gunshot victim may tolerate large volumes of crystalloids, whereas the elderly cardiac patient on a 1-g salt diet may not. The MAP response is a guide to the effectiveness of the fluids, and the CVP defines the upper limits for volume restoration. The initial MAP is roughly analogous to the accelerator in an automobile, and the CVP and MAP response are analogous to the brakes.

Evaluation of the Effectiveness of the Resuscitation Algorithm

The algorithm was tested prospectively in all hypotensive emergency patients entering a surgical ED over a 2½ year period; half the patients were managed with the algorithm and half by the standard of care of a university-run county hospital; compliance with the algorithm was carefully documented in each patient.[12, 13] Of 6833 emergency admissions, 603 patients (9%) had hypotension either on admission to or during the stay in the ED. In addition, another 135 patients (2%) of all patients, or 22% of the hypotensive patients, normally maintained low MAP (mean ± SD = 75 ± 3 mm Hg) but did not have medical conditions that could account for this hypotension; this was more common in, but not confined to, young females.

Of the 603 hypotensive patients, 6% were admitted in full arrest, 18% in severe shock (MAP = 0–60 mm Hg), and 52% in moderate shock (MAP = 60–80 mm Hg); 24% were initially normotensive but subsequently became hypotensive during initial management in the ED; the average lowest MAP value ± SD was 53 ± 25 mm Hg. There were 114 (19%) deaths and 169 (28%) patients with complications.[12, 13] Eight per cent of all in-hospital complications were shock related; these organ failures and complications included shock lung, acute renal failure, circulatory failure, sepsis in the uncontaminated patient, and possible fluid overload; 25 (52%) of the patients with shock-related organ failures died (Figs. 14–2 and 14–3).

Patients whose management was in compliance with the algorithm had the most rapid resuscitations; as the number of deviations from the algorithm increased, resuscitation times were more prolonged.[12, 13] There was an 85% survival rate in those with satisfactory compliance compared with a 64% survival rate in patients having deviations from the algorithm ($P < .01$). Most of the delays and a majority of the shock-related complications could have been prevented. In essence, there were significantly reduced resuscitation

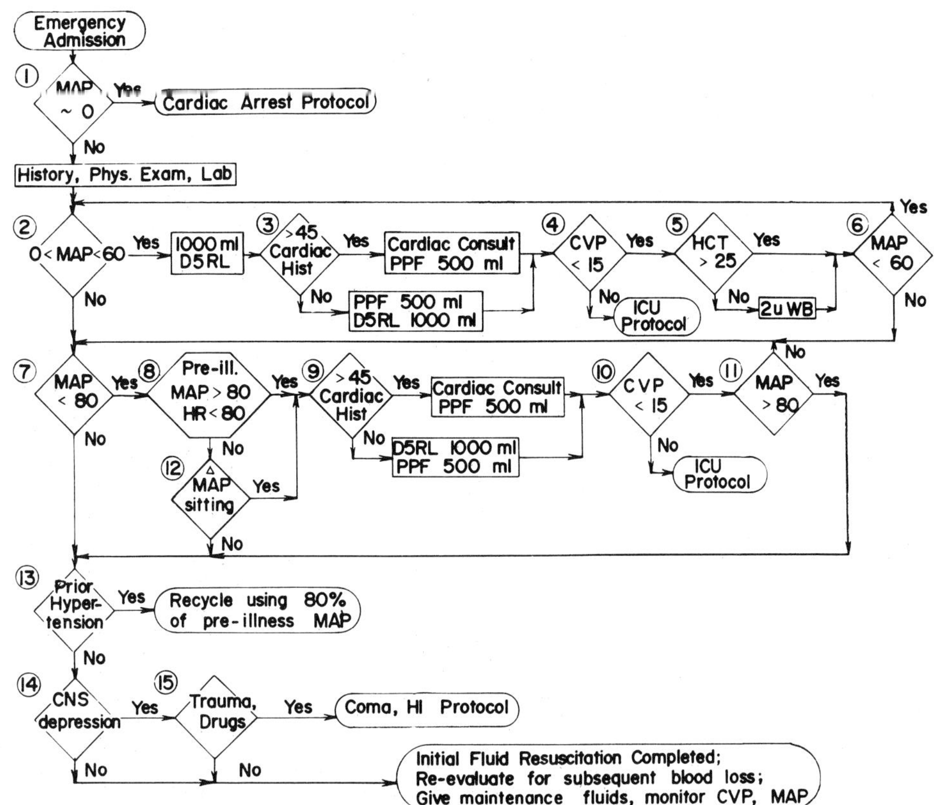

Figure 14–1. Clinical algorithm for the initial (1st hour) resuscitation of emergency admissions. This algorithm was designed for resuscitation of the acute emergency patient to restore circulatory integrity as rapidly as possible without producing fluid overload. *Abbreviations*: MAP = mean arterial blood pressure; RL = lactated Ringer's solution; CVP = central venous pressure; CNS = central nervous system.

Step 1: If the MAP is zero or nearly zero, determine whether cardiac arrest has occurred and begin cardiopulmonary resuscitation immediately. If the patient has an MAP <20 mm Hg, alert personnel for a possible cardiac arrest.

Step 2: If the MAP is <60 mm Hg, immediately start administration of RL or D5RL (dextrose 5% in RL), 1000 mL, and run as rapidly as possible, especially if the MAP is <50 mm Hg.

Step 3: If the patient is <45 years old and does not have a history of cardiac disease, place a CVP line and start another infusion of D5RL, 1000 mL, plus 500 mL of plasma protein fraction (PPF) or artificial colloid through a third intravenous line.

Step 4: Monitor the CVP at frequent intervals during the rapid infusion of these three solutions so as not to exceed values >15 cm H_2O. If the CVP is >15 cm H_2O, go directly to the ICU protocol.

Step 5: If the Hct is <25%, give 2 U of O-negative or type-specific blood. When crossmatched blood becomes available, transfusions of whole blood or packed red cells should be given to maintain Hct at >33%.

Step 6: Rapid restoration of the MAP to 60 mm Hg is the titration endpoint for fluids in this section. If the MAP is <60 mm Hg, recycle from Step 2 through Step 6. If a MAP >60 mm Hg has been achieved, proceed to Step 7.

Step 7: If the MAP is <80 mm Hg, go to Step 8; if not, proceed to Step 13.

Step 8: If the MAP is <80 mm Hg, inquire from the patient or the patient's family or consult a previous hospital record to evaluate the patient's "normal" pre-illness control MAP. If the MAP is <80 mm Hg and the heart rate (HR) is >80 beat/min, measure orthostatic blood pressure (Step 12).

Step 9: As in Step 3, the cardiac patient requires less salt and water but more colloid. If the age of the patient is >45 years or if he or she has a history of cardiac disease, give 500 mL of colloid; if the patient's age is <45 years and he or she has no history of cardiac disease, give 1000 mL of D5RL plus 500 mL of colloid.

Step 10: Fluids may be given safely if the CVP is <15 cm H_2O; if this is exceeded, go to the ICU protocol and continue to give fluids as needed to restore circulatory integrity, provided wedge pressures of 18 mm Hg are not exceeded.

Step 11: If the MAP is >80 mm Hg without exceeding a CVP of >15 cm H_2O, the objective of this cycle has been achieved. If the MAP is <80 mm Hg, recycle Steps 7 through 11.

Step 12: Orthostatic blood pressure is measured. If a 10-mm Hg change in the MAP occurs on sitting or standing, this is presumptive evidence of at least 1000 mL of blood volume deficit.

Step 13: After the MAP has been restored to the normal value (>80 mm Hg), it is still necessary to be sure that the pre-illness blood pressure was normal. If a prior hypertension was observed, the patient should be recycled from Step 7 through Step 13 using 80% of the pre-illness value as the criterion for the adequacy of resuscitation.

Step 14: Examine the patient for evidence of CNS depression, drug poisoning, or drug abuse.

Step 15: Examine the patient for evidence of head injury or other trauma. If trauma is present, the patient should be treated in accordance with a coma–head injury protocol. (Reproduced with permission from Hopkins JA, Shoemaker WC, Chang PC, et al: Results of a clinical trial on the use of an emergency resuscitation algorithm. Crit Care Med 1983, 11: 621.)

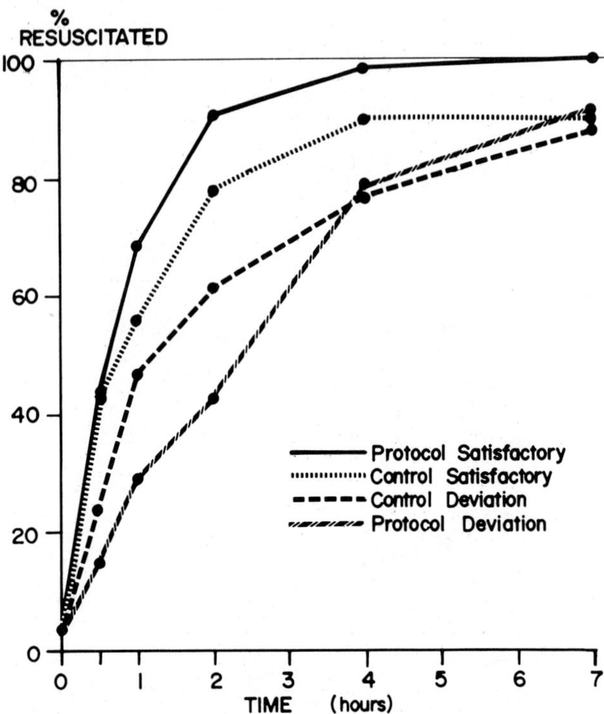

Figure 14–2. Cumulative percentage of patients resuscitated plotted against the time taken for resuscitation in control and protocol patients who had deviations from the algorithm and satisfactory compliance. (Reproduced with permission from Hopkins JA, Shoemaker WC, Chang PC, et al: Results of a clinical trial on the use of an emergency resuscitation algorithm. Crit Care Med 1983; 11:621.)

times and fewer shock-related organ failures, complications, and deaths when patients were resuscitated according to the algorithm.[12, 13]

There were 265 (44%) hypotensive patients who had severe associated medical illnesses; they were more vulnerable to complications and death. The algorithm is most useful in these emergency patients with severe associated illnesses in whom delay or unorganized therapy was more likely to lead to unsatisfactory outcomes. When the algorithm was followed in patients with severe associated illnesses, there were more rapid resuscitation times, shorter ICU stays, shorter hospitalizations, and less mortality.[12]

Fluid restoration by the algorithm in patients with trauma, hemorrhage, or sepsis led to better outcome. However, patients with head injuries did not have significantly improved outcomes, probably because the degree of neurologic damage at the time of injury primarily determined outcome; hypovolemia was usually not the major problem.[12] The data were also stratified according to various clinical criteria, including (1) lowest recorded MAP, (2) age, (3) sex, (4) severity of illness, (5) comorbid conditions, (6) estimated blood loss, and (7) volume of fluids given. In each stratification, the resuscitation times were shorter and the shock-related complications were fewer in patients satisfactorily managed by the algorithm; most of these reduced resuscitation times were statistically significant.[12] The data of this series show that hypovolemia is the most common life-threatening problem and that fluid resuscitation by branch chain logic leads to more rapid and effective resuscitation.

It was also observed that prolonged resuscitation may be tolerated in young patients with only mild hypotension and no other medical problems. By contrast, relatively short delays or small technical problems may be lethal in patients with severe associated medical problems. With limited physiologic reserves, small problems at any stage may be life threatening. Most patients fall somewhere between these two extremes, where moderate degrees of inadequately treated hypovolemia may limit circulatory function and outcome.

ALGORITHM FOR FLUID MANAGEMENT OF PATIENTS WITH CVP CATHETERS

The resuscitation algorithm covers initial intravenous fluid management for the first hour. A branch chain decision tree has been developed for the subsequent management of critically ill or hemodynamically unstable patients who are suspected of having hypovolemia but have only CVP catheters (Fig. 14–4). In this algorithm, MAP, heart rate (HR), urine output, Hct, and CVP were used as criteria. The basic premise under these conditions is that increments of volume expanders may be used to titrate therapy to optimal responses without exceeding safe CVP pressures (less than 18 mm Hg) to obviate fluid overload. This algorithm is useful in managing fluid therapy after the initial resuscitation and in administering fluid challenge to those patients who are suspected of being hypovolemic.

COMPREHENSIVE BRANCH CHAIN DECISION TREE FOR TRAUMA RESUSCITATION

The two algorithms described previously here are addressed to the specific problem of fluid resuscitation based on the assumption that hypovolemia is the most urgent problem in shock. Decision rules for fluid resuscitation are rather straightforward and the decision trees are relatively

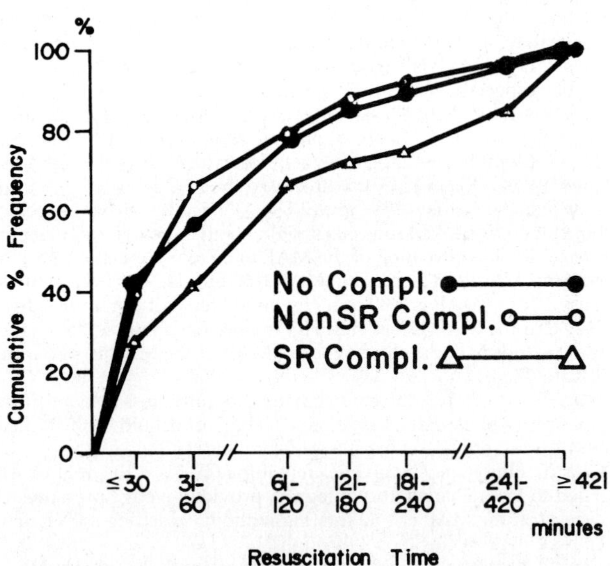

Figure 14–3. Cumulative frequency of resuscitation plotted against the time taken for resuscitation in three groups of patients: those with no complications (No Compl.) indicated by the *solid dots*, those with non–shock-related complications (Non SR Compl.) indicated by the *open dots*, and those with shock-related complications (SR Compl.) indicated by the *triangles*. Note the last group has delayed resuscitation compared with the other two groups. (Reproduced with permission from Hopkins JA, Shoemaker WC, Chang, DC, et al. Results of a clinical trial on the use of an emergency resuscitation algorithm. Crit Care Med 1983; 11:621.)

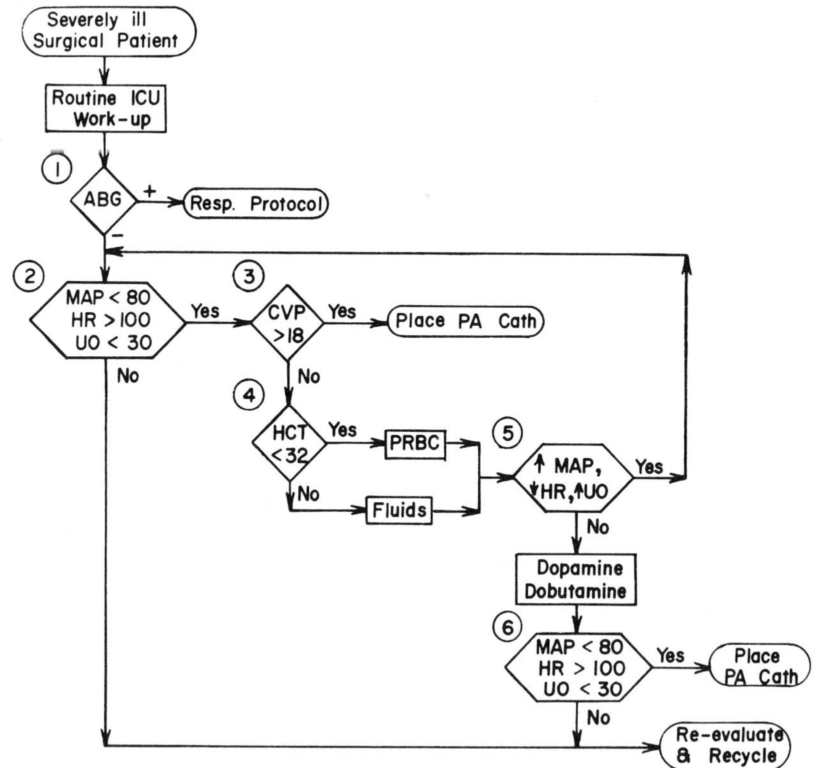

Figure 14–4. Algorithm for subsequent continuing fluid management in patients with CVP catheters. If the routine work-up has not been completed, the following should be ordered: chest radiography, complete blood count and differential, routine electrolytes and blood chemistries (M300), 12-lead electrocardiography, and urinalysis, Hct, prothrombin time, partial thromboplastin time, and platelets if significant blood loss or bleeding tendency is present, as well as other indicated radiographic and laboratory studies. If evidence of sepsis is present, culture blood, urine, or sputum, drain site, and cerebrospinal fluid if appropriate.

Step 1: Assess arterial blood gases (ABG); if abnormal, proceed with respiratory protocol.

Step 2: If MAP is <80 mm Hg, HR is >100 beats/min, or urine output (UO) is <30 mL/h, measure CVP and proceed to Step 3, as inadequate hydration is a likely possibility. If MAP is >80 mm Hg, HR is <100 beats/min, and UO is >30 mL/h, re-evaluate at frequent intervals.

Step 3: If CVP is >18 mm Hg, place a pulmonary artery (PA) catheter; if CVP is <18 mm Hg, measure Hct.

Step 4: If Hct is <32%, give 2 U packed red cells (PRBC) or 1 U whole blood. If Hct is >32%, give 1 L RL or 500 mL plasma protein fraction.

Step 5: If the fluid load given above improves MAP, HR, or UO, this is evidence of hypovolemia or dehydration; proceed to Step 2 to test adequacy of fluid load. If the criteria of Step 2 (MAP >80 mm Hg, HR <100 beats/min, UO >30 mL/h) are met, re-evaluate at intervals; if not, recycle from Step 3 to 5. This fluid cycle may be repeated as long as (1) there is continued improvement and (2) CVP does not exceed 18 mm Hg. However, it is also necessary to search for continued fluid losses. If the fluid load given as described does not improve MAP, HR, or UO, dehydration and hypovolemia are unlikely; start administration of an inotropic agent such as dobutamine or vasopressors in low doses and titrate gradually to achieve the optimal result.

Step 6: If MAP is >80 mm Hg, HR is <100 beat/min, and UO is >30 mL/h, re-evaluate at frequent intervals, but if these goals are not reached, place a PA catheter.

simple, but algorithms that attempt to address the total immediate care of the trauma victim are an order of magnitude more complex than the fluid resuscitation algorithms. Nevertheless, comprehensive decision trees for expeditious resuscitation, including monitoring, diagnosis, and therapy of penetrating and blunt trauma of the chest and abdomen, were designed and tested.[14–20]

The algorithms for trauma are based on the assumption that it is imperative to restore circulatory integrity, to establish a diagnosis, and to begin definitive therapy as rapidly as possible. All three of these activities need to be carried out simultaneously on separate parallel tracts. Cardiopulmonary resuscitation (CPR) for cardiac arrest and fluid therapy for shock are early subroutines.

General Principles and Concepts

1. If the patient is hypotensive or in shock, immediate resuscitation and surgical exploration are mandatory.

2. If the MAP does not immediately respond to adequate volumes of fluids (5–10 L), urgent surgical exploration is mandatory to control the bleeding source. Fluid resuscitation is continued vigorously during the surgical attempts to control bleeding.

3. Gunshot wounds (GSW), except tangential or grazing wounds, should be explored.

4. Stab wounds (SW) without abdominal findings, except for localized tenderness at the wound site, may be considered for conservative (nonoperative) management to avoid negative explorations and shorten the hospital stay.

5. Cardiac tamponade must be considered in SW and GSW of the chest as well as the upper abdomen, flank, and back; about 2% of penetrating chest wounds have tamponade. Elevated CVP is usually the first monitored sign of tamponade.

6. Patients with blunt abdominal trauma and peritoneal signs should be surgically explored urgently with or with-

out diagnostic peritoneal lavage to repair lacerated solid or perforated gastrointestinal injuries.

7. Computed tomographic (CT) scans may be done in hemodynamically stable patients with questionable abdominal signs and in patients with head injuries, coma, or ethanol intoxication.

8. Thoracoabdominal injuries require special consideration and should be explored with less rigorous indication including hypotension, abdominal tenderness, guarding and rebound tenderness, or CT findings.

9. Repeated physical examinations provide important information in questionable cases.

10. Penetrating abdominal wounds are often overdiagnosed and unnecessarily explored, whereas blunt trauma is more frequently underdiagnosed and explored too late.

Algorithm for Blunt and Penetrating Injuries of the Thorax and Abdomen

Figure 14–5 describes a clinical algorithm for the management of blunt and penetrating thoracic and abdominal injuries. It describes the major decision points and suggests criteria for each decision. Table 14–2 lists common problems for blunt and penetrating wounds of the thorax and abdomen; Table 14–3 lists the most common diagnostic procedures, monitoring systems, and therapeutic interventions in the management of trauma patients. These three activities should proceed concurrently along three parallel tracks according to the priorities described by the algorithm. This algorithm describes the clinical conditions and circumstances for the most important management decisions in blunt and penetrating trauma.

The entrance criteria include all patients with either blunt or penetrating injuries from thoracic or abdominal trauma. The general work-up includes rapid physical assessment; this may be pre-empted by emergency situations such as cardiac arrest and severe shock. In the latter circumstances, the work-up should proceed in parallel with resuscitation; the therapy of shock, similar to CPR in cardiac arrest, takes precedence over diagnostic tests and other therapy. The routine minimal work-up should include blood type and crossmatch, spun Hct, complete blood count, portable chest radiograph, prothrombin time, partial thromboplastin time, serum electrolytes (sodium, potassium, chloride, bicarbonate), glucose, blood urea nitrogen, creatinine, and urinalysis. Abdominal radiography, arterial blood gas measurement, additional blood chemistries (such as calcium and amylase), and other tests may be performed if indicated.

Initial feasibility studies of this algorithm were carried out prospectively in a county hospital setting,[15, 16, 18] and, subsequently, a more definitive series of 434 and finally a series of 1000 patients were prospectively evaluated by Bishop and associates.[19, 20] The series of 1000 patients with possible truncal injury was collected over a 13-month period, during which time 2843 trauma patients were evaluated in the ED, 1457 were admitted to the hospital, and 326 were admitted to the surgical ICU (SICU). Of the 1000 patients in the study group, 338 (34%) had blunt trauma (292 accidents involving motor vehicles, 35 assaults, and 11 falls) and 662 (66%) had penetrating injuries (502 truncal GSW, 138 truncal stab wounds, and 22 truncal shotgun wounds). Sixty (6%) patients (37 with penetrating injuries and 23 with blunt trauma) arrived at the ED with no signs of life and no cardiac electrical activity; these patients were pronounced

TABLE 14–2. Common Problems in Blunt and Penetrating Trauma to the Thorax and Abdomen

1. Cardiac or respiratory arrest or both
2. Respiratory distress
3. Circulatory shock
4. Laceration of the heart with or without cardiac tamponade
5. Cardiac contusion
6. Pneumothorax, tension pneumothorax, hemothorax
7. Lacerations of the trachea, bronchus with air leak
8. Sucking chest wound
9. Fractures of ribs with or without flail chest
10. Pulmonary contusion
11. Injury to great vessels
12. Laceration or rupture of esophagus, stomach, small bowel, colon, or bladder
13. Laceration of diaphragm
14. Laceration or rupture of liver, spleen, kidney, or pancreas
15. Vascular injuries
16. Fractures of pelvis, spine, and long bones
17. Retroperitoneal, mesenteric, or omental hematomas

TABLE 14–3. Diagnostic Procedures, Monitoring Systems, and Therapy in Blunt and Penetrating Trauma of the Thorax and Abdomen

Diagnostic Procedure	*Monitoring*	*Therapy*
1. C-spine	1. MAP	1. CPR
2. Chest radiograph, AP and lat	2. Heart rate	2. Fluids, blood
3. Chest tap, chest tube	3. CVP	3. Oxygen by mask
4. Abdominal radiograph: upright, decubitus	4. Urine output	4. Needle thoracentesis
5. An IV urogram	5. ECG	5. Chest tube
6. Echocardiography	6. Hct	6. Tracheal intubation
7. Angiography	7. ABGs	7. Mechanical ventilation
a. Aortic arch		
b. Celiac axis		
c. Internal and external iliac arteries		
d. Peripheral vessels		
8. Bronchoscopy	8. NG tube: output, volume and Hct	8. Thoracotomy, repair of injuries
9. Pericardiocentesis	9. Chest tube: output, volume, and Hct	9. Laparotomy, repair of injuries
10. CT scan		
11. Liver, lung scan		
12. MUGA scan		
13. Endoscopy		
14. Minilap		

Abbreviations: MAP = mean arterial pressure; CPR = cardiopulmonary resuscitation; AP = anteroposterior; lat = lateral; CVP = central venous pressure; IV = intravenous; ECG = electrocardiogram; Hct = hematocrit; ABGs = arterial blood gases; NG = nasogastric; CT = computed tomographic; MUGA = multiple gated acquisition.

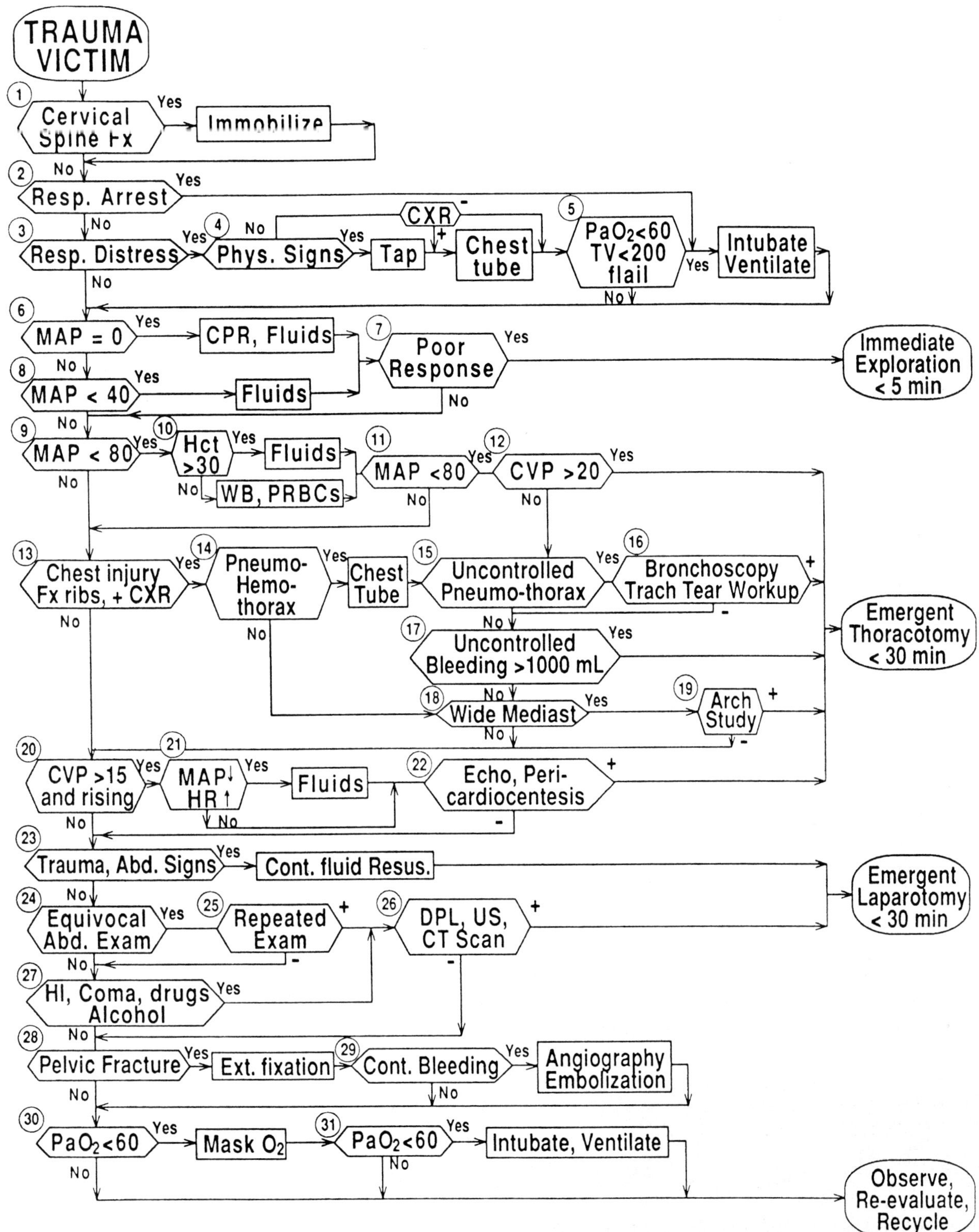

Figure 14–5. Algorithm for the clinical management of blunt and penetrating thoracic and abdominal injuries.

Step 1: If patient has any physical signs (penetrating wounds, contusions, swelling, extremity weakness, or sensory loss) of blunt or penetrating neck injury or has any neck pain, maintain external cervical immobilization, obtain lateral cervical spine radiographs to screen for major cervical injury, and continue resuscitation.

Step 2: If respiratory arrest occurs, intubate and begin mechanical ventilation.

Step 3: If respiratory distress or depressed level of consciousness is present as defined by one or more of the following criteria, proceed to Steps 4 through 8: tachypnea (respiratory rate ≥30 breaths/min), bradypnea (respiratory rate ≤8 breaths/min), sternal retraction, use of accessory breathing muscles, flaring of nasal alae during respiration, cyanosis of the lips or skin, or Glasgow Coma Score (GCS) ≤9.

Step 4: If physical signs of pneumothorax are present, such as hyperresonance, distant or decreased breath sounds, or open chest wounds, perform an immediate needle thoracostomy in the midclavicular line of the second intercostal space (ICS) of the affected side.

Then, place a No. 36 or No. 40 chest tube into the affected hemithorax at ICS 4–5 in the midaxillary line and proceed to Step 5. If no physical signs of tension pneumothorax are observed, obtain a portable chest radiograph (CXR). If the CXR is negative, proceed to Step 5. If the CXR shows a hemothorax or pneumothorax, perform tube thoracostomy and go to Step 5. However, if 1000 mL of blood is immediately obtained from the tube, clamp the tube and obtain a CXR. If after the drainage of 1000 mL of blood the CXR shows an estimated 500 mL or more of blood still in the hemithorax (massive hemothorax), transport the patient to the operating room (OR) for further chest drainage and possible thoracotomy. (Letting chest drainage continue in the emergency department [ED] may precipitate a hypovolemic cardiac arrest.) Colloids (5% albumin or hydroxyethyl starch) should be infused rapidly while the patient is prepared for the OR.

Step 5: Intubate and start mechanical ventilation if one or more of the following conditions exists: $Pa O_2$ is <60 mm Hg on 40% facemask O_2, $Pa CO_2$ is >45 mm Hg, spontaneous tidal volume (VT) is <200 mL, respiratory rate is >30 breaths/min or <8 breaths/min, flail segment exists, or GCS is <9. Adjust ventilator settings to maintain arterial oxygen saturation at ≥93% or $Pa O_2 \geq 60$ mm Hg and $Pa CO_2$ at ≤45 mm Hg. Proceed to Step 6.

Step 6: If the patient has a detectable pulse and blood pressure (BP), proceed to Step 8. If the patient has no detectable BP (MAP = 0), rapidly administer 3 to 5 L of fluids and 2 to 4 U of O-negative blood or packed cells while simultaneously initiating the Advanced Cardiac Life Support (ACLS) protocol. With large-bore intravenous (IV) lines, 1 L of fluid may be given in 2 to 5 minutes. Inserting IV tubing via cut downs into the greater saphenous, antecubital, or basilic vein establishes very effective resuscitation lines. Proceed to Step 7.

Step 7: If, with fluid resuscitation and ACLS, a detectable pulse returns and the MAP rises to ≥40 mm Hg, proceed to Step 9. If a response is obtained but the MAP remains <40 mm Hg, transport the patient to the OR for immediate exploration. If no detectable pulse or BP is obtained with resuscitation, proceed as follows:

1. *For penetrating truncal wounds*: If the patient had signs of life at some time in the field or the ED, perform a left anterior thoracotomy. This is done to relieve pericardial tamponade, to perform direct cardiac massage, to cross-clamp the descending thoracic aorta and increase blood flow to the coronary arteries and brain, and to stop other intrathoracic bleeding. The incision may be easily extended to a trans-sternal thoracotomy (if necessary) to control hemorrhage from the right hemithorax. If the penetrating injury is on the right thorax, a right anterior thoracotomy may be done first to control bleeding from the wound.
2. *For blunt injuries*: Continue maximum volume infusion; perform bilateral needle thoracostomy immediately followed by bilateral tube thoracostomy (midaxillary line, ICSs 4) to relieve tension pneumothorax; and perform pericardiocentesis to diagnose cardiac tamponade. If cardiac tamponade is present, perform left anterior thoracotomy; if either tube thoracostomy drains 1000 mL of blood and flow continues, clamp the tube, continue transfusions, and transport the patient to the OR for thoracotomy. Allowing the tube output to continue may increase intrathoracic hemorrhage and lead to rapid cardiac arrest from hypovolemia.

Step 8: If MAP is >40 mm Hg, proceed to Step 9. If the MAP is <40 mm Hg or systolic arterial pressure (SAP) is <60 mm Hg, insert two large-bore IV (≥16-gauge) catheters (either percutaneously or by cut down) and rapidly infuse 3 to 5 L of fluid. If inferior vena caval injury is suspected, use at least one upper extremity vein for volume infusion. If the MAP remains ≤40 mm Hg for >5 minutes, the patient should be transported to the OR for exploration. If the MAP rises to >40 mm Hg, continue expectant volume loading and proceed to Step 9.

Step 9: If the MAP is >80 mm Hg, proceed to Step 13. If the MAP is <80 mm Hg or SAP is <100 mm Hg, administer IV fluids and proceed to Step 10.

Step 10: Measure hemoglobin (Hgb) or Hct or both. If the Hct is >30%, continue infusing IV fluids. If Hct is <30%, administer 2 U PRBC or 2 U whole blood. Proceed to Step 11.

Step 11: If, after resuscitation, the MAP rises to >80 mm Hg, proceed to Step 13. If the MAP remains <80 mm Hg, insert a CVP catheter and go to Step 12.

Step 12: If the patient's CVP is <20 mm Hg, proceed to step 13. If the CVP is ≥20 mm Hg, continue resuscitation and repeat both MAP and CVP measurements at 5-minute intervals. If, over three consecutive measurements the CVP remains >20 mm Hg with the MAP remaining <80 mm Hg, presume cardiac tamponade is present and transport patient to the OR for exploratory thoracotomy. If the CVP is ≥20 mm Hg and the MAP has risen >80 mm Hg, reduce rate of fluid infusion by 50% and recheck both CVP and MAP at 5-minute intervals. If the CVP subsequently rises to >24 mm Hg, presume cardiac tamponade is present and transport patient to the OR for exploratory thoracotomy. Otherwise, proceed to Step 13.

Step 13: Obtain a portable CXR; if a hemothorax or pneumothorax is present, proceed to Step 14. If a "sucking" chest wound is present, cover injury with petroleum-impregnated gauze and place a chest tube on the affected side. If the CXR is normal and no other clinical signs of thoracic injury are present, proceed to Step 23.

Step 14: If a hemothorax or pneumothorax is present, place a chest tube (>36 French) in midaxillary line at ICS 4 or 5. Replace lost blood using an autotransfusion device if the tube output is >200 mL. Proceed to Step 15. If the patient has no hemothorax or pneumothorax, proceed to Step 18.

Step 15: If a pneumothorax persists despite the proper performance of tube thoracostomy or if an air leak persists, place a second chest tube and go to Step 16.

Step 16: If the pneumothorax/air leak persists after a second tube thoracostomy has been performed on the affected side, proceed with bronchoscopy to evaluate for major tracheobronchial injury. If injury is diagnosed, proceed with thoracotomy and repair. If the second tube thoracostomy controls the air leak, or if the bronchoscopy reveals no tracheobronchial injury, proceed to Step 17.

Step 17: If, after the initial hemothorax is drained, the chest tube accumulates >100 mL of blood per hour for 3 or more hours, proceed with exploratory thoracotomy. If bleeding is controlled, proceed to Step 18.

Step 18: If the mediastinum appears to be of normal width on the CXR and no other signs of a thoracic great vessel injury exist (pleural cap, indistinct aortic arch, obliteration of aortopulmonary window, displacement of nasogastric tube or mainstem bronchus), proceed to Step 20. If the mediastinum appears widened on CXR or if one or more of the other signs of great vessel injury are present, proceed to Step 19.

Step 19: Obtain an aortic and great vessel angiogram. If the angiogram demonstrates great vessel injury, proceed with emergent thoracotomy and repair. For blunt injuries and penetrating thoracoabdominal wounds, a peritoneal tap and lavage should be performed in the OR prior to thoracotomy to rule out intra-abdominal hemorrhage. For patients needing thoracotomy who are also suspected of having intracranial lesions that require operative intervention, a rapid computed tomography (CT) head scan may be obtained before thoracotomy, or diagnostic burr holes may be performed simultaneously with thoracotomy. If the great vessel angiogram has a negative result, go to Step 20.

Step 20: If the patient has clinical signs of cardiac tamponade, such as distended neck veins or distant heart sounds, or both, or has a penetrating injury in proximity to the precordial region, insert a CVP catheter in a subclavian or internal jugular vein. Perform three simultaneous CVP and MAP measurements over a 15-minute period. If the CVP is persistently <15 mm Hg, go to Step 23. If the patient's CVP is >20 mm Hg for three consecutive readings or is >15 mm Hg and rises over three successive measurements, proceed to Step 21.

Step 21: If, after the three readings in Step 20 have been performed, the MAP is <80 mm Hg or the HR is >110 beats/min, give 500 mL of 5% albumin or hetastarch (Hespan) over 10 minutes. After infusion is initiated, proceed to Step 22. If the MAP remains >80 mm Hg and the HR is <110 beats/min, proceed to Step 22 without giving an additional fluid bolus.

Step 22: Obtain echocardiogram or perform pericardiocentesis or subxyphoid window creation. If blood is present in the pericardial sac, assume cardiac tamponade is present and proceed with exploratory thoracotomy or median sternotomy. Also, if at any time the patient's MAP falls >15 mm Hg over a 5-minute period, assume cardiac tamponade is present and proceed with exploratory thoracotomy or median sternotomy. If no blood is found in the pericardial sac, based on the results of echocardiography, pericardiocentesis, or subxyphoid window creation, proceed to Step 23.

Step 23: If the patient has an abdominal or thoracoabdominal gunshot wound (except one with a tangential "grazing" trajectory that could not possibly penetrate the abdominal cavity) or a stab wound with hypotension (MAP <80 mm Hg), diffuse tenderness, rebound tenderness, decreased bowel sounds, or other abdominal findings, exploratory laparotomy should be performed within 30 minutes. Patients with blunt injury and diffuse peritoneal irritation should undergo exploration. If the patient does not have diffuse peritoneal signs, proceed to Step 24.

Step 24: If the patient has a blunt injury or stab wound and has equivocal abdominal examination findings, proceed to Step 25.

Step 25: Perform at least three sequential abdominal examinations over a 15-minute period. If the patient's abdomen becomes nontender, proceed to Step 27. If equivocal examination results persist, proceed to Step 26.

Step 26: Proceed as follows:

1. If the patient has blunt injury, perform peritoneal tap and lavage or triple-contrast abdominal and pelvic CT; if either test has positive results, perform exploratory laparotomy within 30 minutes. If results are negative, proceed to Step 27.
2. If the patient has a stab wound over the rectus sheath, perform local wound exploration; if the wound extends through the anterior rectus sheath, perform either peritoneal tap and lavage or triple-contrast abdominal and pelvic CT. If either test yields positive results, perform exploratory laparotomy within 30 minutes. If the anterior rectus sheath has not been penetrated or if diagnostic test results are negative, proceed to Step 27.
3. If the patient has a stab wound between the lateral rectus sheath and the midaxillary line, either peritoneal tap and lavage or triple-contrast abdominal and pelvic CT should be performed. If either test yields a positive result, perform exploratory laparotomy within 30 minutes. If the patient has a stab wound posterior to the midaxillary line, perform triple-contrast abdominal and pelvic CT. If either test has a positive result, perform exploratory laparotomy within 30 minutes. If diagnostic test results are negative, proceed to Step 27.

Step 27: If the patient has evidence of head injury, drug ingestion, or ethanol intoxication, a normal abdominal examination may be inaccurate, and, therefore, the patient should undergo either peritoneal tap and lavage or triple-contrast abdominal and pelvic CT. If either has a positive result, proceed with exploratory laparotomy within 30 minutes; if results are negative, proceed to Step 28.

Step 28: If no pelvic fracture is present, proceed to Step 30. If the patient has a pelvic fracture, evaluate its stability. If the fracture is stable, proceed to Step 29. If the fracture is unstable, immediately place either Military Anti-Shock Trousers or emergently consult an orthopedist for external fixation.

Step 29: Perform serial Hgb/Hct measurements every 30 minutes. If the patient's Hgb/Hct drops and the patient needs >6 U PRBCs within 6 hours postadmission to maintain Hgb >10 g/dL or Hct >30%, perform pelvic vessel angiography for possible embolization. Proceed to Step 30. If Hgb/Hct remains stable, proceed to Step 30.

Step 30: Obtain measurements of arterial blood gases (ABGs). If the patient's PaO_2 is <60 mm Hg on room air, administer 40% O_2 by facemask and proceed to Step 31. If, on room air, the patient's PaO_2 is >60 mm Hg, observe the patient for subsequent signs of respiratory distress, hypotension, and new symptoms of thoracic or abdominal injury.

Step 31: After 40% O_2 has been administered for 10 minutes, obtain a repeat set of ABG measurements. If the PaO_2 is still <60 mm Hg, intubate, ventilate, and re-evaluate for thoracic or abdominal injury. If the PaO_2 is >60 mm Hg, observe the patient and re-evaluate him or her periodically.

dead on arrival. They were excluded from analysis, leaving 940 patients in the study group. The outcomes of these study patients were evaluated in terms of type of trauma and deviations from the algorithm.[20]

There were 135 deaths (14% mortality) in the study group of the 940 patients. One hundred (16%) of 625 patients with penetrating injuries died, and 35 (11%) of the 315 blunt trauma patients died. There were deviations from the algorithm in 58 (43%) of the 135 fatal cases as opposed to only 69 (9%) of the 805 survivors who were managed in compliance with the algorithm.

There were deviations in the management of 127 (14%) of the 940 study group patients; 58 (46%) of these 127 patients died, whereas only 77 (9%) of 813 patients whose management complied with the algorithm died ($P < .001$). The most common deviations were delayed operation (56 occurrences, 25 deaths, 45% mortality), transport of unstable patients to the CT scan or radiology area (12 occurrences, 6 deaths, 50% mortality), and inappropriate observation instead of operation (12 occurrences, 3 deaths, 25% mortality).

One hundred five (11%) of the 940 patients had injury severity scores (ISSs) greater than 50; 28 of 43 (65%) with deviations from the algorithm died, whereas 48 of 62 (77%) whose management complied with the algorithm died (not significant). Of the 264 patients with ISSs greater than or equal to 20 and less than or equal to 50, 25 of 60 (42%) managed with deviations died, whereas only 23 of 193 (12%) whose management followed the algorithm died ($P < .001$). The remaining 571 patients had ISSs less than 20; 5 of 24 (21%) with deviations died, whereas only 6 of 547 (1%) who complied with the algorithm died ($P < .001$).

The data from this series suggest that the majority of preventable trauma deaths that occur in the periadmission period stem not from misunderstandings of the proper procedural management of trauma but from delays in intended therapy (such as delayed transport to the operating room) and from misassessment of the patients' physiologic status (such as inappropriate transport to the radiology area or inappropriate observation). This is likely due to conventional approaches that focus on the diagnosis and treatment of specific injuries and do not focus on the rapid diagnosis and correction of circulatory derangements that cause early patient mortality.[20]

These data support the hypotheses that branch chain decision trees facilitate expeditious therapy and that therapeutic decisions based on specific, objective criteria rather than subjective clinical assessment will improve outcome when rapid executions of multiple diagnostic and interventional maneuvers are necessary for patient survival. We conclude that patients with serious injuries are salvageable when appropriately and expediently managed and that those with ISSs between 20 and 50 will show the greatest improvement in survival when managed by the algorithm.

PHYSIOLOGIC AND THERAPEUTIC PROBLEMS IN TRAUMA RESUSCITATION

Initial Monitoring

In emergency admissions and in the early phase of shock, the circulation is initially monitored by blood pressure, HR, respiratory rate, temperature, Hct, CVP, electrocardiogram (ECG), hourly urinary output with specific gravity or osmolality, and blood gas-pH measurements. Blood pressure, HR, respiratory rate, and temperature (the so-called vital signs) are used for the initial screening. The Hct is used to diagnose and assess initial blood loss, provided there is time for extracellular water (ECW) to cross the capillary membrane into the plasma volume. Usually it takes 3 to 4 hours for blood losses to change the Hct significantly. CVP is important as an endpoint during initial resuscitation to indicate plasma volume overload. CVP values of 20 mm Hg or more suggest (1) congestive cardiac failure, (2) overtransfusion or overadministration of fluids, or (3) too rapid administration of blood or fluids. The ECG is frequently used to diagnose and monitor suspected arrhythmias. Although it is appropriate for assessment of cardiac rhythm and electrical activity, the ECG is rarely useful in patients with hemorrhage, trauma, or sepsis, except to rule out associated cardiac problems. Urinary output below 30 mL/h may reflect inadequate blood volume, decreased renal blood flow, or impaired renal parenchymal function. If there is no preexisting renal damage, and if urinary specific gravity is greater than 1.018 or urine osmolality is more than 500 mOsm/L, urine output may reflect renal tissue perfusion. However, patients resuscitated with large volumes of sodium-rich fluids may have adequate urine output despite low blood volume. The blood volume measurement, if done properly and accurately, is the most reliable means to evaluate blood volume status, particularly during unstable hemodynamic conditions.[21]

Serial measurements of vital signs, Hct, CVP, hourly urinary output, blood volume, and blood gases provide the necessary information on which decisions for management can be based. However, when blood pressures fall precipitously after hemorrhage, fluid therapy must be started immediately and given vigorously. Subsequently, physiologic monitoring should be started as soon as possible to indicate when conservative therapy should give way to surgical intervention. A systematic record of monitored data provides a continuous evaluation of the circulatory status during initial resuscitation, subsequent therapy, operative intervention, and postoperative management.

Clinical Criteria for Fluid Therapy

The first and most important goal of the treatment of shock and its sequelae is to restore blood volume. However, criteria for achieving this goal have been poorly defined. Clinical studies in this area are often incompletely controlled with poor documentation for the degree of hypovolemia, for the extent of the blood volume correction, and for the time factors involved. The clinical criteria most often used for adequate blood volume restoration are arterial pressure, HR, Hct, urine output, CVP, and pulmonary arterial wedge pressures. In the initial hypotensive period, changes in these clinically monitored variables reflect physiologic compensations and decompensations for hypovolemia. In subsequent periods after the initial resuscitation, when patients become critically ill, most of these variables have been shown to be unreliable for evaluation of hypovolemia when compared with careful blood volume measurements.[21] Although the commonly monitored variables roughly correlate with hypovolemia in the initial hypotensive crisis, this is clearly not the case in the ICU patient in whom venous wall compliance changes compensate for blood volume alterations.[22]

Frequently, the initial resuscitation with sodium-rich solutions restores MAP and urine output without properly correcting unrecognized hypovolemia.[17–23] With massive crystalloid infusions, patients may still have suboptimal blood volume despite marked expansion of the interstitial fluid compartment and restoration of blood pressure. Furthermore, critically ill post-traumatic and postoperative patients, as well as those with malnutrition and chronic wasting diseases, often have hypovolemia with expanded ECW and reduced plasma protein concentrations.[24, 25] This salt and water alteration is intensified by antidiuretic hormone and aldosterone. These fluid maldistributions are frequently unsuspected when vital signs, CVP, and urine output are the only criteria used for the assessment of volume status.

Management of the Trauma Patient Immediately After ED Admission

Severe hypovolemia, severe hypoxia, and upper airway obstruction are the most important and urgent problems of the emergency trauma victim, accounting for the majority of preventable trauma deaths in the early management period. These problems, although frequently life threatening, are usually easily recognized clinically and often readily correctable with appropriate therapy. Severe hypovolemia manifests as pallor, tachycardia, hypotension, altered mental status, oliguria, and cold, clammy skin. Hypoxia may present with cyanosis, ash-gray color, tachypnea, dilated nasal alae, suprasternal and intercostal retraction, and agitation. Upper airway obstruction presents with a wide range of symptoms; partial obstruction produces agitation, tachypnea, stridor, wheezing, and use of accessory breathing muscles, and total obstruction produces apnea, cyanosis, and altered mental status ranging from severe agitation to lethargy and collapse. In extreme cases of these three common problems, rapid fluid administration, endotracheal intubation with mechanical ventilation, and CPR may be needed and take precedence over diagnostic and therapeutic maneuvers. After these catastrophic conditions are addressed and corrected, the other therapeutic goals should be defined and treatment prioritized according to the life-threatening capacity of each condition.

Resuscitation of the Trauma Patient Using Prospectively Tested Physiologic Goals

Approximately 50% of all trauma fatalities occur at the time of or shortly after injury. Lethal hypoxia or exsanguination occurring within 12 to 24 hours after emergency admission is responsible for another 20% of trauma deaths; a small percentage of these patients die in the operating room. However, in most trauma fatalities, patients die either in the early postinjury period or weeks later in the SICU of multiple vital organ failures. These organ failures have their origins in earlier unrecognized tissue hypoxia from hypovolemia. Therapy, therefore, should be directed to the major underlying pathophysiology of shock (i.e., inadequate oxygen transport from low or maldistributed flow at the organ and microcirculatory levels). The low oxygen consumption ($\dot{V}O_2$) in the early period and the normal or high $\dot{V}O_2$ in the middle or late period are often less than needed to meet increased metabolic requirements. In general, therapy should be titrated to attain the optimal goals rather than given as a standardized prescribed dose. Moreover, treatment of one vital organ failure can jeopardize the function of another vital organ. In multiple vital organ failure, therapy of each impaired organ should be titrated to appropriate physiologic goals to avoid compromising the other vital organs. The major objective is to correct the life-threatening physiologic as well as physical problems. At the very least, it is necessary to institute early therapy for potentially lethal circulatory problems before they become irreversible. The longer shock or perfusion deficiencies persist, the more likely are unfavorable outcomes.

Prospective Trial of Supranormal Cardiac Index, Oxygen Delivery, and $\dot{V}O_2$ Values as Therapeutic Goals in Severe Trauma

In an empiric study of a series of 90 severely traumatized patients, 60 of whom survived their initial management period but had significant (>2000 mL) blood loss, Bishop and colleagues[26] observed that the 60 survivors had significantly higher values of cardiac index (CI), oxygen delivery, ($\dot{D}O_2$), and $\dot{V}O_2$ than did the 30 nonsurvivors and that these differences were most pronounced in the first 24 hours postinjury. These empirically observed survivor values were then tested as resuscitation goals in a prospective double-arm formal clinical trial[27] and showed a significant improvement in mortality (18% vs. 34%, $P < .05$) and reduction in shock-related organ failures (mean $\pm$ SD $=$ 0.74 $\pm$ 0.28 per patient vs. 1.62 $\pm$ 0.45 per patient, $P < .05$) compared with conventional treatment. These data support the hypotheses that post-traumatic increases in CI, $\dot{D}O_2$, and $\dot{V}O_2$ are primary physiologic compensations that if inadequate, may result in organ failure and death and that timely therapy to augment these compensations will result in improved survival.

Evaluation of Therapeutic Efficacy

If hemodynamic and oxygen transport variables are measured before, during, and after the administration of a therapeutic agent with a known physiologic action, important information is often revealed about the nature of that disturbed circulation. That is, responsiveness to the action of an agent suggests that a circulatory deficiency was present and that there was also some reserve capacity that could be stimulated to improve function. Failure of response suggests that either the therapy was ineffective, the patient had limited physiologic reserve capacity, or the disorder was irreversible. A trial of therapy with agents of specific actions (e.g., plasma expanders) and agents with inotropic actions (alpha and beta agonists) such as dobutamine, dopamine, isoproterenol, and norepinephrine may thus provide physiologic data that have diagnostic, therapeutic, and prognostic value.

Because bulk transport of oxygen is the important circulatory function, $\dot{V}O_2$ may be used to evaluate the effectiveness of a given therapeutic agent. Short-term changes in $\dot{V}O_2$ during and immediately after administration of a therapeutic agent to patients in shock may reflect changes in tissue perfusion. An immediate increase in $\dot{V}O_2$ after the administration of a specific agent suggests that therapy may have improved tissue perfusion and tissue oxygenation.

Fluid Therapy of Acute Circulatory Problems

The following fluid therapy recommendations for resuscitation of acute hypotensive and hypovolemic problems are proposed: Red blood cell losses should be replaced with red blood cells, water loss from dehydration should be replaced with crystalloids, and plasma volume losses should be replaced with plasma or its colloidal equivalent (i.e., plasma protein fraction, 5% or 25% albumin, hydroxyethyl starch, or other artificial colloids).

Saline, glucose, and RL solution in various combinations are commonly used for initial resuscitation in mild degrees of shock and subsequent replacement of daily fluid losses. In general, 3 to 5 L of fluid usually replace acute losses in mild to moderately ill patients who do not have extrarenal fluid losses and who tolerate nothing by mouth. However, patients with enteric fistulas, diarrhea, vomiting, large volumes of nasogastric suction, and other extrarenal fluid losses may require several times this volume to replace the estimated fluid losses and maintain blood pressure, HR, urine output, CVP, and Hct. After the estimated extrarenal fluid losses are replaced, the optimal volume is best determined by fluid-balance studies that collect, measure, and record urinary, nasogastric suction, fecal, and enteric fistula losses; the estimated insensible losses are added to this. The intraoperative insensible losses occurring when the peritoneal or pleural cavities are opened may be 400 to 700 mL/h (6–9 $mL \cdot kg^{-1} \cdot h^{-1}$) depending on ambient temperature and humidity.

In severe shock, the initial resuscitation should be at least one-third colloids to maintain the administered fluids in the blood volume compartment.[27] However, the ICU patient usually has already been given excessive crystalloids; in these circumstances, fluid challenge with 25 g of concentrated (25%) albumin, 500 mL of plasma protein fraction (5% albumin), or other colloids is recommended. Whole blood or packed red blood cells should be given in sufficient quantities to maintain Hct at about 34%. The therapeutic goals of the critically ill shock and trauma patient are empirically determined by survivors' mean values for CI (5.0 L/min per m^2), $\dot{D}O_2$ (800 mL/min per m^2), and $\dot{V}O_2$ (170 mL/min per m^2).[23, 26, 27]

SUMMARY: THE ALGORITHMIC APPROACH TO DECISION MAKING

The algorithmic approach does not attempt to automate or take away decisions from the physician or to take the art out of medicine. In a sense, algorithms resemble postoperative standing orders that specify the volume and rates for vasopressor or vasodilator infusions at various blood pressures. The resuscitation algorithms are more than just guidelines to organize the care by serial steps; they represent an approach that applies clinically tested principles in a prioritized manner.

Clinical algorithms attempt to find a middle ground between the extreme that all patients are different and must be handled individually and the other extreme that all patient care can be diagrammed and computerized. All patients are certainly different, but for the majority of clinical problems, no matter how complicated, there is a common set of decisions on which diagnosis and therapy are based, and these decisions can be expressed in a logical format. In practice, algorithms are not necessarily meant to be followed slavishly; minor deviations will occur in the work-up by a perceptive, conscientious physician depending on extraneous circumstances not covered by the algorithm. However, carefully thought-out, peer-reviewed protocols that are the result of well-established , literature-supported strategies can be followed in major clinical decisions. Moreover, they have been found to be useful and effective when applied and tested prospectively in real clinical problems.[3–13]

The algorithmic approach places the most common problems in a prioritized order, thereby preselecting the patients coming to each node, and then provides criteria based on decision rules for expeditious diagnostic, monitoring, and therapeutic decisions. Thus, patients in cardiac arrest are immediately given CPR. For those not in arrest, the clinician reads down the decision tree; problems are addressed in the order of their life-threatening capability. Algorithms are particularly useful in crisis situations when time is of great importance, such as the resuscitation of emergency shock and trauma patients. Because of its objectivity and usefulness as a teaching tool, the algorithmic approach is of practical benefit in the training of residents and students in teaching hospitals but is also useful in community hospitals where physicians manage emergency patients less frequently.

Inadequate fluids and delays in resuscitation were clearly related to an increased incidence of shock-related complications: shock lung, acute renal failure, cardiopulmonary arrest, sepsis, cardiac failure, and fluid overload. When the algorithm was followed satisfactorily, faster resuscitation and fewer shock-related complications occurred, particularly in patients with severe associated illnesses in which the margin for error was small. The shorter SICU stay, shorter hospitalization, and reduced mortality in these patients indicate cost effectiveness in this approach. Algorithms provide a potentially useful approach to complex clinical situations fraught with emotionally held opinions, anecdotal descriptions, and judgmatic pronouncements repeated in the manner of a party line.

References

1. Shoemaker WC, Bryan-Brown CW: Resuscitation and immediate care of the critically ill and injured patient. Semin Drug Treat 1973; 3:249.
2. McDonald CJ: Use of a computer to detect and respond to clinical events: Its effect on clinical behavior. Ann Intern Med 1976; 84:162.
3. Shoemaker WC: Algorithm for resuscitation: A systematic plan for immediate care of the injured or postoperative patient. Crit Care Med 1975; 3:127.
4. Shoemaker WC: Algorithm for early recognition and management of cardiac tamponade. Crit Care Med 1975; 3:59.
5. Larsen KT, Vickery MD, Collis PB, et al: A logical algorithmic alternative to a non-system. JACEP 1973; 2:183.
6. Slay LE, Riskin WG: Algorithm-directed triage in an emergency department. JACEP 1976; 5:869.
7. Greenfield S, Anderson H, Winickoff RM, et al: Nurse-protocol management of low back pain: Outcomes, patient satisfaction, and efficiency of primary care. West J Med 1975; 123:350.
8. Sox HC, Sox CH, Tompkins RK: Training of physicians' assistants by a clinical algorithm system. N Engl J Med 1973; 258:818.
9. Ellis BW: Use of logic based flow patterns in the investigation and management of surgical disorders. Br J Surg 1975; 62: 800.
10. Shoemaker WC, Hopkins JA, Greenfield S, et al: Resuscitation algorithm for management of acute emergencies. JACEP 1978; 7:361.
11. Eiseman B, Watkyns R: Surgical Decision Making. Philadelphia, WB Saunders, 1978.
12. Hopkins JA, Shoemaker WC, Chang PC, et al: Results of a clinical trial on the use of an emergency resuscitation algorithm. Crit Care Med 1983; 11:621.
13. Shoemaker WC, Hopkins JA: Clinical aspects of resuscitation with and without an algorithm: Relative importance of various decisions. Crit Care Med 1983; 11:630.
14. Shoemaker WC: Resuscitation of the critically ill patient: Use of branch chain decision trees to improve outcome. Emerg Med Clin North Am 1986; 4:655.
15. Shoemaker WC, Corley RD, Liu M, Harrier HD, et al: Development and testing of a decision tree for blunt trauma. Crit Care Med 1988; 16:1199.
16. Liu M, Shoemaker WC, Kram HB, Harrier HD: Design and prospective evaluation of an algorithm for penetrating truncal injuries. Crit Care Med 1988; 16:1191.
17. Shoemaker WC, Kvetan V, Fyodora V, et al: Clinical algorithm for initial resuscitation in disasters. Crit Care Clin 1991; 7:363.
18. Bishop MH, Shoemaker WC, Jackson G, et al: An algorithm for blunt and penetrating truncal trauma. Crit Care Clin 1991; 7:383.
19. Bishop MH, Shoemaker WC, Jackson G, et al: Evaluation of a single comprehensive algorithm for the management of blunt and penetrating thoracic and abdominal trauma. Am Surgeon 1991; 57:712.
20. Bishop MH, Shoemaker WC, Shori S, et al: Evaluation of a comprehensive algorithm for the management of blunt and penetrating truncal trauma—Report of 1000 cases. J Trauma (in press).
21. Shippy CR, Appel PL, Shoemaker WC: Reliability of clinical monitoring to assess blood volume in critically ill patients. Crit Care Med 1984; 12:107.
22. Wo CJ, Shoemaker WC, Appel PL, Bishop MH: Unreliability of blood pressure and heart rate for evaluation of circulatory stability in emergency resuscitation and critical illness. Crit Care Med 1992; 21:95.
23. Shoemaker WC, Bland RD, Appel PL: Therapy of critically ill postoperative patients based on outcome prediction and prospective clinical trials. Surg Clin North Am 1985; 65:811.
24. Elwyn DH, Bryan-Brown CW, Shoemaker WC: Nutritional aspects of body water dislocations in postoperative and depleted patients. Ann Surg 1975; 182:76.
25. Shoemaker WC, Bryan-Brown CW, Quigley L, et al: Body fluid shifts in depletion and post-stress states and their correction with adequate nutrition. Surg Gynecol Obstet 1973; 136:371.
26. Bishop MH, Wo CJ, Appel PL, et al: Relationship between supranormal circulatory values, time delays, and outcome in severely traumatized patients. Crit Care Med 1993; 21:56.
27. Bishop MH, Shoemaker WC, Kram HB, et al: Prospective trial of survivor values of cardiac index, oxygen delivery, and oxygen consumption as resuscitation endpoints in severe trauma. J Trauma (in press).
28. Shoemaker WC, Schluchter M, Hopkins JA, et al: Comparison of the relative effectiveness of colloids and crystalloids in emergency resuscitation. Am J Surg 1981; 142:73.

CHAPTER 15

Critical Care Medicine in Disasters

Derek C. Angus, MB, ChB, MPH, MRCP(UK), FCCP
Vladimir Kvetan, MD, FCCM, FCCP

Until recently, the role of critical care medicine in response to disaster has been poorly explored, even though many modern principles of medical management for victims of disasters were proposed by leading intensivists during the early years of critical care, when it was seen in practical terms as a continuum from the prehospital arena to the intensive care unit (ICU) setting. Today, the American intensivist devotes the great majority of his or her time to the care of individual patients in a geographically defined, high-technology environment. Critical care training programs do not traditionally provide instruction or experience in disaster management, yet many of the skills of the well-trained intensivist are indispensable for a high-quality response to disaster situations. The critical care physician should be capable of delivering care in a mass casualty situation even in a low-technology or mobile environment. This requires knowledge not only of specific medical conditions but also of field resuscitation, triage, and resource allocation. The intensivist must be prepared to think beyond individual patient care to his or her obligations to the community, which can extend to the regional, national, or even international level.

Since the early 1970s, natural disasters alone (e.g., earthquakes, hurricanes, floods, fires, and tornadoes) have killed about 3 million people and adversely affected at least 800 million people worldwide. In the 1990s, which have been declared by the United Nations as the International Decade of Disaster Reduction, we have already seen terrible man-made disasters superimposed on a background of major geopolitical realignment. Significant activism has been demonstrated by American civilian and military medical professionals in responding to disasters overseas. The experience and its efficacy in improving the outcomes of disaster victims remain to be fully analyzed. As in all undertakings, the best approach is awareness of disaster risks through proper analysis of political, industrial, seismic, and other hazards and through reduction of their impact by training. This chapter briefly reviews the history, classification, and organizational aspects of disaster response with which an intensivist should be acquainted. For a more detailed approach to medical management, the reader is referred to other available texts.[1, 2]

TERMINOLOGY AND HISTORY

Variation in the definitions of disaster is widespread. Clearly, physicians and other healthcare professionals concerned with the analysis of the medical response to disasters must decide on a common nomenclature and classification.[4] *Emergency management,* which encompasses the overall approach to disaster management at a systems level, is rapidly evolving into a sophisticated specialty. For medical systems to develop effective disaster response capability, they must be closely integrated into this overall management system. Consideration of emergency management nomenclature is, therefore, of value.

Hazards are events that have potential to cause catastrophic damage. They include natural phenomena such as earthquakes, hurricanes, and droughts as well as man-made events such as war, transportation mishaps, and hazardous materials spills. *Disasters* are hazards that have impacted on human lives and human activities, causing adverse physical, psychologic, social, economic, or even political effects.[5] The scope of this impact exceeds the affected community's ability to manage the resultant damage. *Medical disasters* constitute a disaster subset; they are characterized by physical or psychological injury or illness, or both, that exceed the medical response capabilities of the communities affected.

Safar delineated three types of medical disasters.[6] The first is an event that, irrespective of its size, is containable by the local Emergency Medical Services (EMSs). This is termed a *multicasualty incident.* The second is an event that overwhelms local response capability and is termed a *mass disaster* (sometimes used interchangeably with *mass casualty incident* [MASSCAL]). The third is termed an *endemic disaster*—for example, the recurrent famines of Ethiopia and Somalia. Medical disasters may also be classified by the speed of impact and the requisite response phase. For example, earthquakes and tornadoes are of *sudden onset* and require an effective response to be very rapid, whereas famine and malnutrition are characteristically *slow-onset* disasters. Birnbaum has suggested further classifying mass disasters and multicasualty incidents by *type* and *scope.*[4] The type reflects the incident's cause (e.g., a train wreck, an earthquake, or a flood), whereas the scope defines the extent of the event in terms of fatalities, injuries, response, and the like.

From an operational perspective, an event becomes a multicasualty incident when its impact exceeds the day-to-day response routine of the local systems and significant local adjustments must occur. This is often called a *Level I response.* A *Level II response* is when this enhanced local response is overwhelmed, and neighboring or regional resources are activated for assistance. A *Level III response* involves state, interstate, and federal resources in the rescue and recovery process.[7] Depending on the human impact and the degree of deviation from normal response capability, MASSCALs and medical disasters may require Level II or Level III responses.

Factors other than overwhelmingly large numbers of casualties may generate a disaster situation. For instance, a compromised medical system or disruption of the usual rapid transport to the hospital may be the affected variable that causes deviation from day-to-day operational activities. The factor that defines an event as a medical disaster may also be only a moderate increase in the number of patients, all of whom are in a narrow diagnostic category that overwhelms the ability to supply the required specialty care (e.g., confined-space medical care to entrapped victims, pulmonary critical care, renal dialysis, and burn care).[7] Both the threshold where an event or hazard becomes a medical disaster and the level of care provided in the disaster very much depend on preceding medical research, planning, coordination, and training. With the onset of a medical disaster, operational priorities change from providing the best care possible for each individual involved to providing the best care possible for the greatest number of victims (i.e., "rationing" of healthcare).

For many years, the only organized medical involvement in disasters was the public health response. This tended to be focused on delayed support for mass disasters and on ongoing support for endemic disasters. Since the formation of the Club of Mainz in 1968 (to later become the World Association for Disaster and Emergency Medicine [WADEM]), physicians concerned with mitigating the immediate loss of life and injury through resuscitation have generated interest and research in a new area of disaster medicine—disaster resuscitology (or reanimatology). This field is concerned primarily with the logistics of applying the principles of emergency medicine, trauma care, and critical care medicine to the much larger scale of multicasualty incidents and mass disasters.[8] Meanwhile, considerable experience was being gained in military medicine from the application of modern resuscitation techniques in combat situations. The Vietnam War demonstrated that effective medical care practiced outside the traditional hospital setting (e.g., field medics, rapid transport, field hospitals) could dramatically reduce morbidity and mortality.[9, 10] The subsequent development of the EMSs throughout the United States, the development of the fields of emergency medicine and trauma and critical care, and the dissemination of first aid concepts have provided the foundation for immediate and effective prehospital and emergency medical response for disaster victims. Practical experience of physicians interested in acute care in unconventional settings such as wilderness medicine and urban search and rescue, developing in parallel with more didactic approaches of professional societies such as the WADEM and the International Trauma Anesthesia and Critical Care Society (ITACCS) with its regular disaster response exercises, have laid groundwork for rational civilian response.

In recent years, the concept of sophisticated disaster medical response in the forms of mobile ICU and renal dialysis teams (the 1988 Armenian earthquake and the 1989 pipeline explosion in Ufa, Russia), military and civilian burn teams (Ufa, Russia, 1989), Disaster Medical Assistance Teams (DMATs) (in St. Croix, U.S. Virgin Islands, 1989, after Hurricane Hugo; and in Florida, 1992, after Hurricane Andrew), and emergency medical teams (the 1988 Armenian earthquake and the 1990 Philippine earthquake) has further expanded the evolving field of disaster medicine.[3, 11–16]

The Society of Critical Care Medicine developed their Task Force on Disasters, later renamed the Critical Care Preparedness Committee, to provide a didactic and clinical forum for intensive care specialists interested in delivery of services in unconventional situations such as disasters, adverse environments, and armed conflict. The Task Force has a clinical response capability; its members have worked on civilian and military medicine disaster response teams[13] and national committees concerned with high-quality, specialized response. The need for high-quality, multidisciplinary critical care response was noted during one of the largest potential man-made disasters: Operation Desert Storm in the Persian Gulf. In collaboration with the Office of the Army Surgeon General, the Task Force recruited approximately 2000 intensive care personnel for 42 large, multidisciplinary teams from 22 states to augment military medicine resources at U.S. military hospitals in Germany.[17]

These efforts have demonstrated that it is possible to rapidly deploy fully equipped specialty ICU teams at remote locations and to create a nationwide system of advanced ICU response without governmental support on short notice.

DISASTER TYPES

Natural Disasters

An *earthquake* is the oscillatory movement of the Earth's surface that follows a release of energy in the Earth's crust.[18] Dislocations of the Earth's crust probably occur secondary to the underlying movement of tectonic plates. When a sudden tectonic plate movement occurs, the crust may first bend and then "snap" to a new position. The vast majority of the world's earthquakes occur around the Pacific rim where they overlie the edge of the Pacific plate. Over 1 million earthquake deaths and serious injuries due to earthquakes have occurred worldwide since the early 1970s; some 1600 deaths caused by earthquakes have been recorded in the United States since colonial times.[19] In addition to the primary movement of the Earth's crust, secondary effects also occur, including tsunamis (tidal waves), landslides, fires, and flooding.

The primary cause of injury following an earthquake is structural collapse and falling debris.[20–24] Consequently, building type is a major determinant with regard to the number of persons injured. Nonreinforced masonry and mud-brick or adobe construction are often the most dangerous because of their high sensitivity to shaking forces. This is reflected by the large casualty tolls following earthquakes in the developing world.[3, 20, 22, 24–26] Further injury can result from flooding, fire, and landslides, and those injured may deteriorate secondary to the effects of the earthquake elsewhere (e.g., delayed access as a result of road damage).[27–32] The most common severe injuries are secondary to major trauma and include fractures, blunt and penetrating trauma, open and closed head injuries, and crush injuries.[3, 19, 26] Airway problems present a particular dilemma because of the need for immediate intervention. Asphyxiation of mildly injured but concussed victims serves as a typical but tragic example of preventable death. The spread of dust is inevitable following building collapse and further complicates airway management.[29] Burn and smoke inhalation injuries often occur as a result of the frequent occurrence of fires following earthquakes. The most famous example of fire devastation and injury following an earthquake was the 1906 earthquake in San Francisco, in which the majority of the 1900 deaths were due to fire.

Late complications include hypothermia, wound infections, sepsis, and gangrene. They are a manifestation of the timing and degree of disaster response. Outbreaks of infectious and communicable diseases and the consequences of starvation and dehydration can also occur if response capacity is inadequate. Such complications are common in many disaster situations and are not specific to earthquakes.

A *volcano* is a hill or mountain built around a vent that is connected to reservoirs of molten rock below the Earth's surface.[31] Buoyancy and gas pressure can cause the molten rock to be driven up through these vents and to break through weaknesses in the surface of the volcano. The ensuing eruption is variable. Molten rock can pour over the edge of the volcano as nonexplosive, slowly moving lava flows, or a violent explosion can propel lava fragments and hot gases into the air. The fragments may fall back to the volcano and slip down the mountain as ash flows. The finer ash particles can be carried in the atmosphere and spread as clouds of hot ash. The heat generated from these flows of gas, ash, and molten rock can melt snow caps and liquefy soils, causing landslides, rapidly moving mud flows (lahars), and floods.[32] Owing to their speed, the most lethal consequences are pyroclastic flows. These are flows of lava fragments and ash in hot gases that accelerate down the side of a volcano at a speed of hundreds of miles per hour and that can spread for several miles.[33, 34]

Volcanic eruptions have claimed more than 266,000 lives in the past 400 years, with the most catastrophic being that on the island of Krakatoa, which resulted in 36,000 deaths. Injury patterns vary, depending on the characteristics of the eruption. One recurring feature, however, is the high proportion of lethal injuries. Contrary to popular belief, lava flows are not the main danger because they proceed slowly and, although they destroy virtually everything in their paths, are easily avoided. The major causes of death and injury are lahars, ashfalls, and pyroclastic flows. The relatively small eruption of snow-capped Nevada del Ruiz in Colombia in 1986 caused the formation of considerable lahars after melting of the icecap. Some 23,000 people died from engulfment in these lahars, including 21,105 of the 29,170 inhabitants of Armero.[35] The proportion of dead to injured was 5:1. The eruption of Mt. Vesuvius in 79 AD buried the towns of Pompeii and Herculaneum with falling ash in only a few hours. They were inundated so completely that their ruins were not discovered for 1700 years. A striking example of a pyroclastic flow was the 1902 eruption of Mt. Pelee in Martinique, when one surge left only a handful of the 28,000 inhabitants of St. Pierre alive.

Death is usually the result of immediate suffocation and, to a lesser degree, burns or blunt trauma. Of those who survive volcanic eruptions, the most common injuries are inhalation lung damage, burns, or blunt trauma.

Cyclones are large, rotating weather systems that form seasonally over tropical oceans.[19] They consist of a calm inner portion of low pressure, known as the "eye," that is surrounded by a wall of rain and high-velocity winds. The wind circles most quickly at the inner edge of the eye and can travel up to 150 miles per hour. They are called *hurricanes* in the Caribbean Ocean and Western Atlantic and *typhoons* in the Western Pacific and South China Sea.[20] The most devastating hurricane in the United States hit Galveston, Texas, in 1900 and killed 6000 people. This remains the most catastrophic disaster in North American history.

The major cause of death and destruction is not the high winds but "storm surges."[36, 37] These are caused by a rise in sea level in response to the profound barometric depression at the center of the cyclone. Consequently, up to 90% of fatalities are from drowning. The Bangladesh cyclones of 1970 and 1991 caused 300,000 and 100,000 deaths, respectively, predominantly secondary to flooding.[38] Other early causes of injury include trauma from building collapse and floating debris.[39] Late morbidity is due to postdisaster cleanup accidents (including electrocution), starvation and dehydration, outbreaks of communicable diseases, and wound contamination.[40] The United States' experience with hurricanes Hugo and Andrew points to the vulnerability of even a highly developed and industrialized society.

A *tornado* is a funnel-shaped cloud that extends toward the ground from the base of a thundercloud, and it is the most lethal and the most violent of all natural atmospheric phenomena. The funnel is composed of extremely high-velocity winds encircling a low-pressure, hollow cavity.[41] Circular wind speeds can exceed 300 miles per hour and are strong enough to propel objects as heavy as automobiles.[42] Tornadoes occur worldwide but are particularly common and severe in the Midwest and Southern regions of the United States. Although hundreds occur every year, most burn out over remotely populated regions, and only 3% cause casualties.[43] Of the 14,600 tornadoes recorded from 1952 until 1973, only 497 caused fatalities, and 26 alone caused more than 50% of the deaths.

Since the early 1940s, 9000 people have died in tornadoes; the most common causes of death were craniocerebral trauma and crush injuries to the trunk. Other causes of injury and death include fractures, spinal cord injuries, lacerations, and contusions.[44–46]

Floods can be divided into three types: flash floods (secondary to heavy rains or dam failures); coastal floods (including storm surges and tsunamis); and river floods.[47] Together, they are the most common type of disaster and account for about half of all disaster-related deaths.[48] The most lethal in recorded history was the 1887 flood of the Hwang Ho (Yellow) River in China, which killed 900,000 people and rendered 2 million others homeless; the worst flood in the United States was the flash flood in Johnstown, Pennsylvania, which killed 2200 people[49]; the massive 1993 floods in the Midwest serve as a reminder that the United States is not immune to this catastrophe. The primary cause of death is drowning.[49] Other causes are principally related to trauma from floating debris and hypothermia.[50] Of those who survive, fewer than 2% require significant medical intervention. Later "complications" include public health concerns, such as contamination of water supplies, overcrowding of refugee shelters, and outbreaks of communicable diseases.[51] Wound infection is common because of contamination; wounds should not be closed in this setting. A notable concern is the displacement of wildlife. In 1973, Ussher reported the occurrence of numerous snakebites, including 6 snakebite-related deaths, after a flood in the Philippines. The snakes were cobras that were driven to higher ground near towns and villages.[52]

The main types of injury seen in natural disasters are summarized in Table 15–1.

Man-Made Disasters

The most destructive and preventable man-made disaster is armed conflict. Escalation of civil strife throughout the globe in places such as Somalia, former Yugoslavia, and Rwanda points to the tremendous destructive potential of the disintegration of civilian authority on the well-being of citizens. Table 15–1 also lists important causes of nonmilitary, man-made disasters and their likely injury patterns. Transport accidents, structural collapses, burn disasters, and acts of terrorism produce many injuries similar to those seen in natural disasters and in day-to-day urban violence. Other types of man-made disasters, such as the release of chemical or radioactive materials, may produce syndromes rarely seen by practicing intensivists.

Although *motor vehicle accidents* cause many deaths each year, rarely do single incidents constitute medical disasters. On the occasion when there is a large number of casualties, a complicating factor, such as the spillage of chemicals from trucks, is often present. In 1982, more than 1000 deaths occurred following a motor vehicle accident involving a gasoline tanker in the Salang Tunnel in Afghanistan. The majority of deaths occurred secondary to inhalation of carbon monoxide released from the combustion of gasoline.[53] Normally, however, the usual pattern of injury is of multiple trauma and fractures. The management of these injuries is well documented throughout the medical literature, and

TABLE 15–1. Common Injury Patterns in Disasters

	Injury Type										
Disaster	*Trauma*	*Crush*	*Head Injury*	*Spinal Injury*	*Fracture*	*Laceration*	*Burns*	*Hypothermia*	*Inhalation*	*Drowning*	*Late Complications**
Natural											
Earthquake	x	x	x	x	x	x	x	x	x		x
Volcano	x						x		x		
Cyclone	x									x	x
Tornado	x	x	x	x	x						
Flood								x		x	x
Man-Made											
Motor vehicle accident	x	x	x	x	x	x					
Rail accident	x	x	x	x	x	x	x				
Aircraft accident	x	x	x	x	x	x	x		x		
Sea accident								x	x	x	x
Hazardous material spill							x		x		
Terrorism	x	x	x	x	x	x					

*Includes starvation, dehydration, wound infection, and communicable diseases.

trauma medicine is now a recognized subspecialty of surgery, anesthesia, and critical care medicine in the United States. In addition, much information regarding extrication, prehospital care, and emergency scene management has been derived from research in this area.

Rail transport is considered one of the safest modes of transportation, with an estimated 0.05 deaths per million hours of travel (private car travel and airline flight are more than 10-fold more lethal).[54] However, serious disasters do occasionally occur. More than 800 perished in June 1981 when a train crashed into the Bagmati river in India. Certain aspects of rail crashes are particularly important. First of all, access is often difficult. For example, trains may crash in narrow cuttings or in tunnels, the result of which can be delayed or inefficient rescue. Second, significant hazards are often present. The line may be electrified, runaway stock may be present, or hazardous materials may be on board. This last problem can be particularly important. Unlike with road transport, a train may be carrying several different chemicals in different cars. When a train crashes, these chemicals may mix and release new and unexpected toxic chemicals that further hamper the rescue response.

Injury patterns are dependent on the circumstances of the crash. The most common injuries are multiple trauma and fractures. However, burns and chemical injuries can be common, depending on the cargo of the train and the secondary effects of the crash. Furthermore, exposure, hypothermia, and drowning are obviously likely if the train crashes into water.

Approximately 60 fatal *air transport* crashes occur each year, and more than half of these are nonsurvivable.[55] On closer study of these crashes, certain patterns emerge. In general, most crashes occur at an airport; survival is more likely if an aircraft has a wide rather than a narrow body and if the crash occurs at an airport.[56–58] Moreover, if there are survivors, the dead usually outnumber those who remain alive. Injury patterns are multiple trauma and crush injuries, burns, fractures, and asphyxiation secondary to combustion of plastic construction products lining the cabin. An autopsy analysis of injuries incurred in the Avianca flight 52 crash in 1990 in New York demonstrated that in a situation when fuel is exhausted and no fire results, primary causes of death are severe head and upper body injuries.[59] Of those who survive, one third will have long-term disability.

The most important feature of aircraft disaster management is airport planning. Therefore, guidelines have been published by the International Civil Aviation Organization, and implementation of all aspects regarding personnel, equipment, training, and drilling is mandatory if effective response is to be achieved.[58]

Sea transport wrecks have caused disasters for centuries. The 1912 sinking of the ocean liner *Titanic* is one of the most infamous disasters of modern times. More recently, the March 1987 sinking of the *Herald of Free Enterprise,* a British cross-channel ferry, less than 5 minutes after its departure from the Belgian port of Zeebrugge caused just under 200 deaths and stirred the United Kingdom into national mourning. Unfortunately, despite vast improvements in ship design over the last hundred years, shipwrecks continue to occur. The principal reasons are classified as vessel unseaworthiness; environmental (predominantly storm) damage; collision; fire; explosion; chemical leakage; and war.[60]

The main causes of death and injury are due to the effects of abandonment. They can be subdivided into immersion (which leads to drowning, hypothermia, and oil contamination), starvation, dehydration, and exposure.

Thermal injuries are seen in nearly all military operations and in many natural disasters. Causes of injury include flames, hot water, and steam, combustible gases and liquids, molten liquids, boiling liquid–expanding vapor explosions, chemical burns, and burns due to explosions.[61] One of the most devastating of such disasters was the accident in June 1989 near Ufa in Russia that involved two trains and a massive hydrocarbon mixture explosion, resulting in 805 traumatized burn victims who were transported to regional and national medical centers. The United States' response included an Army Burn Team and a civilian burn ICU team from New York. This event demonstrated significant progress in both local response capabilities developed in the aftermath of the earthquake in Armenia as well as rapid response by syndrome-specific foreign teams. Another important advance was confirmation of the feasibility of Telemedicine Spacebridge,[62] a satellite-mediated and audio-video-fax link between American and Russian medical centers that permits American consultants to assist their Russian colleagues in the management of medical issues from vastly remote locations.

Hazardous material disasters can produce a variety of diverse injury patterns such as chemical burns, toxic inhalations, and systemic injuries that are often unfamiliar to ICU physicians. Furthermore, although the risk of such spills is rising with the ever increasing volume of chemical production and transport (more than 60,000 different chemicals and radioactive isotopes are produced in the United States), accidents are relatively rare. Historically, the term "hazardous material" was coined by fire departments to describe chemicals or materials that were toxic, flammable, corrosive, explosive, or radioactive. The term is used by the U.S. Department of Transportation to refer to "a substance or material which has been determined by the Secretary of Transportation to be capable of posing an unreasonable risk to health, safety, and property when transported in commerce."

Shipments consist of a few 1-gallon containers, multi-ton loads, or 10,000-gallon tanks that contain hazardous materials. These materials may be released by accident at any point between the manufacturer's shipping dock and the receiving facility. Rail shipments often involve multiple rail cars carrying many different hazardous commodities. These released chemicals may ignite or react with one another and ignite or release newly formed toxic chemicals, producing a plethora of undefined products. This problem is of such a magnitude and is so pervasive throughout the United States that in 1986 Congress passed the Superfund Amendment and Reauthorization Act, and the attached Title III mandates that all communities have detailed plans for dealing with hazardous materials accidents.[63]

An important aspect of field management is that victims whose skin or clothes, or both, are contaminated with chemicals must have their clothing removed at the scene and be decontaminated by washing.[64] However, in the event that there are many contaminated patients or that the EMS personnel dealing with the patients are not properly trained, one may well find such patients arriving at the hospital still contaminated and essentially untreated. In addition, some patients may arrive at the hospital by means other than the EMS ambulances. It is important that medical personnel avoid contact with the patient's skin or clothes. For the most part, ordinary eye protection (goggles) and surgical mask, gown, and gloves are sufficient. Although the potential toxicity of each chemical compound to the treating medical personnel must be evaluated, certain hazardous materials pose a higher than normal risk to the treating medical personnel until the patient has been decontaminated.[65]

Accidents involving *radioactive materials* may occur in a variety of settings, such as laboratory or nuclear medicine facilities, isotope production facilities, and nuclear reactor sites as well as during transport.[66] The most likely irradiation accident that would involve the community is a transportation accident. Community involvement in nuclear reactor accidents is extremely rare, with the Three Mile Island[67] and Chernobyl[68] incidents being the best known; however, the threat of radiation exposure is probably more frightening to the general population than is the threat of injury from all other hazardous materials combined.[69]

It is important to determine the type of radioactive emission (α, β, or γ) and the degree of a patient's exposure (external irradiation, contamination, or incorporation). Alpha particles are the least penetrating of all ionizing radiations and are not an external hazard. However, materials emitting α particles are extremely dangerous when ingested or inhaled. Beta particles are able to penetrate skin or several millimeters of aluminum and are therefore both internal and external hazards. Gamma particles are the most penetrating and, consequently, the most hazardous, passing easily through the human body.

External irradiation, sometimes called an *irradiation accident,* occurs when all or part of the body is exposed to penetrating radiation from an external source. The person having sustained external radiation is not radioactive and can be handled without danger to the EMSs and medical personnel. Contamination with radioactive materials means that radioactive materials in the form of gases, liquids, or solids are deposited on a person's clothes or skin (external contamination) or in his body via an open wound, ingestion, or inhalation (internal contamination). Such persons are potentially hazardous to EMSs and medical personnel who must exercise caution until the patient has been decontaminated. Incorporation means that radioactive atoms are taken up within the body cells or structures. In general, such incorporation depends on the atoms and the chemical properties of the radioactive materials (e.g., radium and strontium incorporate in bone, and iodine in the thyroid gland).

External irradiation of the whole body or a part thereof does not constitute a medical emergency, even if the level of exposure was high. The medical effects are usually not evident for days or weeks, so one can ignore this aspect and treat whatever other medical problems might have developed during the initial accident. When contamination has occurred, however, the victim must be handled with great care because one does not want to cause internal contamination in either the victim or the rescuer; this may lead to incorporation and result in adverse health effects appearing years after the accident. Life-threatening medical problems of victims of radiation accidents always have priority over radiation monitoring, contamination control, and decontamination of the site itself. Once those are taken care of, however, the goals of the rescue personnel are to avoid contaminating the victim further, to avoid contaminating their own skin or becoming internally contaminated, and to prevent the spread of any radioactive materials.[70, 71]

Widespread deposition of radioactive material involving many people is most likely to occur in a nuclear power reactor accident such as that at Three Mile Island or Chernobyl. Chernobyl-type accidents are unlikely to occur in the United States because the plant and reactor designs are reasonably safe. Patients injured by such accidents generally suffer from external contamination and need to be decontaminated carefully. The larger problem is environmental contamination, which introduces radioactivity into the food chain, leading to incorporation.

Accidents causing widespread irradiation, contamination, and incorporation can occur, such as those in Goiânia, Brazil[72], and in Juárez, Mexico.[73] Those accidents occurred when the citizens found abandoned cobalt 60 cancer therapy units and broke them open. The small (1-mm diameter) pellets subsequently were spread over a wide area, contaminating people, homes, streets, and oil. Resolution required massive government mitigation. The Goiânia incident initially manifested itself by a large number of patients with nausea, vomiting, and diarrhea that could not be connected to a microbial source.

The most common act of *terrorism* is the detonation of an explosive device in a large group of people. Analysis of 220 bombings showed that while 89.5% of victims requiring surgery suffer from bone and soft tissue injury, head injury resulted in 71.4% of immediate deaths and 52% of late deaths. Pulmonary blast injury, the most common thoracic trauma syndrome, accounted for 11% of overall mortality.[74]

MANAGEMENT WITHIN THE HOSPITAL DURING AN EMERGENCY

Hospitals are required by the Joint Commission on Accreditation of Healthcare Organizations (JCAHO) to have both internal disaster plans (for mishaps within the hospital system) and external disaster plans (for events removed from the hospital system).[75] These must be updated periodically and practiced in semiannual drills. Despite this specific requirement, the quality and detail of hospital disaster planning are highly variable. Complacency is unwarranted as even a large, busy trauma center can be easily overwhelmed by a moderate number of casualties.[76] Although serious internal disasters are rare, responses to external disasters have been widely reported. Over 4 years, the staff at the Parkland Memorial Hospital in Dallas, Texas, were exposed to three separate aircraft crashes that resulted in large influxes of casualties. These experiences gave the hospital and its staff opportunities to test and improve their disaster planning.[76] This ability to improve planning has also been reported by medical centers situated in regions at high risk for hurricanes.[77] Some logistic issues that should be considered in designing a hospital plan are outlined in the following sections.

Local Conditions

It is important to link the external hospital plan with the emergency plans of surrounding municipalities and airports and to recognize differences between plans in terms of activation, lines of authority, communication channels, and triage principles. Clearly, the hospital must be prepared to respond appropriately to whatever plan is activated. Links should also be forged with other emergency agencies, including the fire fighters, police, and local EMSs.[78]

The hospital should also prepare for realistic disaster situations. If located near a chemical plant, for example, the hospital should be prepared for hazardous material spills and have stocks of appropriate antidotes and treatments. The most commonly anticipated external disasters are those that generate a heavy trauma toll, such as transportation mishaps. These are usually large multicasualty incidents.[79]

Command

The mobilization of personnel, equipment, and supplies is an expensive venture, and false alarms are not relished by hospital administrators. Thus, it is important to establish who has the authority to declare a disaster. It is also crucial to delineate beforehand the line of command responsible for triage of patients and allocation of personnel and resources.

If specific personnel are expected to assume key roles, then the plan must incorporate a method to ensure that these personnel can be reached outside the hospital. Locating personnel may require the deployment of a helicopter, a resource that might otherwise have been used for the transfer of critically ill patients, or the personnel may have sustained serious injury themselves. It is wise, therefore, to plan for alternative personnel to fulfill key roles.

To facilitate administration of the disaster plan, a command post should be set up at a predesignated position in the hospital. This post would be responsible for directing resources and personnel throughout the hospital on the basis of information it receives from outside the hospital regarding the predicted casualty load. In addition, information regarding bed occupancy in the hospital as well as in surrounding hospitals is necessary to aid the post in triage decisions. This center is also responsible for liaison with the media and local, regional, and state emergency management agencies. For these functions to be performed effectively, the disaster plan should outline the different tasks and designate specific roles or personnel.

Communication

A frequent problem in disaster response is the difficulty of obtaining accurate or reliable information from the scene. After the aircraft disaster in northern England in 1989, in which an airliner crashed onto the M1 highway, victims were transferred to three regional trauma centers.[80] However, the transfers occurred in waves, one to each hospital. Thus, all three hospitals had periods of acute overload, since gradual transfer and dispersal of casualties between all hospitals throughout the night did not occur. Furthermore, little warning of the number or nature of the injuries of incoming casualties was given, leaving the hospitals unsure of how to prepare. A similar problem with scene-to-hospital communication occurred in Dallas in 1985. Initial reports of an airline crash stimulated the senior medical staff to activate the disaster plan. However, a rumor of no survival led the hospital administrators to cancel the plan, only to reactivate it as the wounded began to arrive at the emergency department. Both groups, in critiquing their response, suggested the need for a rapid deployment of a physician-led team from the hospital to the scene, not to treat the injured but rather to assess the needs, direct triage, and provide the receiving hospitals with an estimate of the numbers of injured, the types of injury, and the likely time of arrival.

Communication is also needed outside the hospital to recruit off-duty hospital personnel. After the M1 crash, the telephone callout failed completely. Ferguson and coworkers have recommended a cascade system in which each person called is responsible for telephoning five others.[78] Although this system may reduce the burden on the hospital switchboard, to our knowledge it has not been tested in an actual disaster. The high effectiveness of cellular phone systems during the Loma Prieta, California, earthquake has been demonstrated in a situation of damaged or saturated telephone and radio communication networks. The Dallas group stressed the importance of good liaison with the media to secure wide broadcast of the need for hospital personnel to return to the hospital.[76] However, the spread of such information must be exercised with care.

It is also important to be able to communicate with other emergency services and surrounding hospitals. In a disaster, the hospital switchboard often becomes overloaded by the volume of calls from media and the public inquiring about the fate of the injured. One of the hospitals responding to the M1 crash had a direct line to its anesthesia department that bypassed the hospital switchboard.[80] This was perceived as vital to the effective coordination and planning of operating room and ICU resources. Unfortunately, there is no guarantee that all areas vital to a disaster plan will have direct telephone access. Furthermore, the telephone number may be widely accessible and, hence, susceptible to jamming. Therefore, careful planning should probably include the installation of protected telephone lines in critical areas with their numbers listed only in disaster manuals issued to specific personnel.

Telephone lines within the hospital may still become overloaded. Thus, communication of pertinent patient information may break down. In response to the M1 airliner crash, physicians found the only reliable way to obtain laboratory results was on foot. Accompanied by enough personnel, they were able to maintain effective communication for patient care by having people carry samples to the laboratory and wait for the result. Although effective, this approach is a rather inefficient and inadvisable deployment of personnel. Laboratory information may best be transferred on a hospital's mainframe computer, if one exists. However, other information may not be so easily transferred. Previous experience has shown that emergency rooms often function rather autonomously. Patients are rapidly assessed and resuscitated to a variable degree only to be dispatched to different parts of the hospital without clear details regarding their care plans, the presumptive diagnoses, or a record of tests ordered or performed. In response to internal communication problems during their first disaster response, the staff at Parkland Memorial Hospital in Dallas decided to use walkie-talkie units. These were placed in key areas of the hospital to be used in the event of disaster. When a subsequent disaster occurred, the walkie-talkies were found to be very effective in communicating information regarding patient movement, bed status, and so on.

Personnel

Personnel management is crucial. On activation of the disaster plan, it is usual to request that all staff currently on-duty to remain in the hospital beyond the end of their shifts until the situation has stabilized. In addition, off-duty staff may have to be recruited. Hospitals can be overwhelmed by the response of staff coming in from home on hearing about a disaster from the media. An overload of personnel may be followed later by staff exhaustion and no personnel relief. Thus, it is important to devise a scheduling plan that specifically requires willing helpers to return home and await their turn. This will increase efficiency and reduce postincident stress. It is also important to consider that the staff working in the hospital at the time of the disaster are understandably anxious to determine whether their relatives and homes have been affected by the event. It is not uncommon for hospital personnel to depart for their homes as soon as an earthquake strikes, leaving the hospital even less well equipped for the impending casualty load.

The stress of responding to a disaster can exert a significant psychologic toll on hospital staff. Evidence suggests that early counseling by peer groups not involved in the response can help reduce the psychologic impact. This technique, first used among emergency agency personnel, is known as *critical incident stress debriefing.* Provision for such debriefing should be regarded as essential to the disaster plan and should be targeted at all hospital staff, including the hospital administrators and senior medical staff.

Triage

Triage is considered a crucial aspect of disaster management[81]; unfortunately, a form of "reverse triage" frequently occurs when a large volume of ambulatory victims appear in the emergency ward before the medical center is aware of a disaster in progress. It is important to consider the potential of the hospitals to receive certain types of casualties and to decide on-scene which victims should be dispatched to which hospitals. In addition, pooling of victims in one transport vehicle bound for one destination increases the efficiency of the response. Therefore, a triage team should be dispatched to the scene. Depending on the local disaster plan, this team may be dispatched from the principal local hospital and should probably be led by a senior physician such as an emergency medicine physician, intensivist, or trauma surgeon from the local hospital. The team should not be involved in patient transport or individual patient care but devoted simply to quick patient assessment and precise determination of the severity of injury and the subsequent priority for staging and dispatch of patients.

This prioritization is done rapidly to facilitate the timely application of lifesaving procedures to those who are deemed salvageable. Although multiple triage systems have been developed, most follow a basic categorization. Category 1 includes patients who require immediate intervention to save life. Category 2 patients require second priority intervention to avoid significant deterioration and possible death. Even though they also are significantly ill, these patients are well enough to withstand stabilization before definitive intervention and thus can wait while those in category 1 are managed definitively. Patients in category 3 can wait for delayed intervention without undue compromise. These patients have only minor injury for which no initial medical treatment is necessary. Category 4 includes those who are either dead or have sustained injuries thought incompatible with life. Once categorized, the patient may be tagged at the triage center according to a casualty triage color code. An alternative to tagging is to keep patients in color-designated areas. This has the advantage of saving time if large numbers of casualties are arriving simultaneously.

Within the hospital, it is important to apply the principles of triage to existing patients, preferably before a large influx of casualties occurs. Patients should be transferred out of the ICU if at all possible. Prearranged agreement to suspend restrictive policies, such as forbidding the use of intravenous drips outside the ICU, could effectively generate more ICU beds by allowing the transfer of patients out of the ICU during the unconventional situation of a disaster response. Likewise, patients in non-ICU beds might be fit for discharge. To avoid using scarce ambulance services, however, they could be moved to a holding area in the hospital, thus freeing beds for patients being transferred from the ICU. It is important that the guidelines for exercising these triage rules be clarified in the disaster plan beforehand and that the decisions of the triage team be final. Laboratory blood work and radiologic procedures should also be triaged on a priority basis in a manner similar to the mechanism used for field triage of patients.

The casualty reception point should be larger than the average emergency department. The hospital anteroom often is a good choice, especially if it is close to elevators (if operable), the emergency department, and the operating suites. This area should be considered more as a staging area (or secondary triage center) than a treatment area. The physician in charge should be responsible primarily for making triage decisions regarding the need for emergency surgery or intensive care and should have absolute authority. Accurate communication of the number and severity of casualties must be relayed continually to the central command post in the hospital to facilitate preparation of the operating suites, ICUs, hospital wards, and support departments.

The Media, Relatives, and General Public

All disasters are considered prime news events, and hospital disaster plans should include plans to deal with the media. It is wise to designate a media officer whose sole responsibility is to communicate with the media. This allows other personnel critical to the management of the response to work unhindered by the burden of inquisitive reporters. Press releases should be made at regular intervals beginning as soon after the disaster as possible to reduce media curiosity, even if no new information is available.[82] Careful thought should be given to messages that might be disseminated by the media. In the absence of clear direction from the hospital, for example, the media suggested that blood would probably be required in response to the 1985 airliner crash in Dallas. This led to a deluge of volunteers arriving at the Parkland Memorial Hospital's emergency room, impairing access for ambulance crews transporting casualties from the scene.[76] Accordingly, the disaster plan should include guidelines for the communication of clear, early messages to the general public concerning information such as what help might (and might not) be needed, who the contact members are for those inquiring into the status of casualties, and what the role of off-duty personnel should be.

If possible, a specific holding area for the media should be set up. Provision of telephones, facsimile equipment, coffee, and seating is likely to promote good relations between the hospital and the media. This area should be as close to the main clinical areas as possible to allow senior clinical personnel to give short interviews without having to stray far from their duties.[82]

Relatives should be held in a waiting area similar to that recommended for the media. It should, however, be distant from the media. Each family should be asked to designate one representative to facilitate communication, and efforts should be made to provide frequent updates, as in usual clinical practice.

Natural inquisitiveness drives members of the public and the media to extraordinary lengths, especially in the wake of a disaster. Emergency management agencies are well aware of the need to secure the scene of an incident and can quickly cordon off a disaster scene, allowing in only authorized personnel. However, the receiving hospital will also become a site of interest for those seeking information and, without similar levels of security, the ability of the hospital to function effectively can be severely hampered. In their early experiences, Klein and Weigelt reported no security control at either the scene or the hospital, with the resultant meandering of unauthorized personnel throughout both areas.[76] Others have reported the smuggling of media representatives into operating rooms. Thus, the hospital disaster plan should consider who is to enforce security and by what means. Security should be enforced in critical areas such as the operating suite, the ICUs, and the emergency department. The media, family relatives, and other nonhospital personnel should be directed to their respective waiting areas, and authorized personnel should carry identification badges to gain access to restricted areas. If the hospital intends to deploy a triage team to the scene, the plan must also include prior determination of identification procedures to ensure that the team is allowed access.

Documentation

Documentation is often poor in disasters. The lack of documentation not only impedes the ability to critique the response after an event but may hamper the response itself. Different groups have come up with different solutions.[76, 81] Some suggest that routine hospital forms should be used because they are familiar to the staff and, accordingly, efficient to use, whereas forms to be used only in disasters are less familiar and engender inefficiency. Conversely, others have complained that routine forms often require too much information for the time available and suggest the use of special forms that are both brief and feature tearoff tags to facilitate labeling and tracking of patients as they are moved through the hospital. The best solution, although not necessarily the cheapest, is probably to modify existing forms such that they are both familiar through routine use and easily adaptable to an emergency situation.

Internal Disaster Plan

The internal disaster plan usually assumes that the hospital is incapacitated in some way, for instance, following a power failure, but that it has intact outside help. The Armenian earthquake of 1988 destroyed several hospitals entirely. In such an event, the likelihood of receiving timely help from the outside is extremely low, since the entire area is probably devastated, and any help must arrive from distant areas.[83] However, the most likely internal disaster would be one that affects only a particular area of the hospital (e.g., a power failure in one wing). Thus, hospitals should have unit-specific disaster plans. For example, an ICU disaster plan should include alternative sites for the emergency transfer of patients and strategies for the maintenance of life-supporting therapy in the absence of power. These plans should be developed by a multidisciplinary group and should be tested with mock drills, just as is necessary for the larger external disaster plans.

STATE AND REGIONAL CONSIDERATIONS

States are mandated to have, within their government structure, an emergency management capability. Commonly, the responsibility falls on state emergency management agencies or emergency services sectors. The make-up and capabilities of these entities vary markedly among the 50 states. Some, such as California's Office of Emergency Services, are very organized operational and educational entities. They have grouped the state's counties into regions to provide an intermediate response level between the local and state levels.

Each state's medical disaster response is typically coordinated by the state's emergency management agency and the state's department of health. Historically, the primary organized medical response to disasters has consisted of EMS responders that provide triage and very austere medical care and then the transport of involved victims. Meanwhile, management within the hospitals has remained somewhat autonomous of state control and has been characterized by the peculiarities of individual institutions.

NATIONAL CONSIDERATIONS

In the event of a truly catastrophic occurrence, the state's governor may appeal to the President of the United States to declare a disaster in the affected area. A presidential disaster declaration allows activation of considerable federal resources. It is the intent of these resources to supplement and assist, but not to supplant, the affected local and state authorities. The federal resources are catalogued, coordinated, and mobilized in accordance with a detailed and complex Federal Natural Disaster Plan. Within the plan, federal agencies, the Department of Defense, the American Red Cross, and other resources are organized to provide a multitude of Emergency Support Functions (ESFs), which are listed in Table 15–2.

TABLE 15–2. Federal Natural Disaster Plan: Emergency Support Functions (ESFs)

ESF 1	Transportation
ESF 2	Communications
ESF 3	Public works and engineering
ESF 4	Firefighting
ESF 5	Information and planning
ESF 6	Mass care
ESF 7	Resource support
ESF 8	Health and medical services
ESF 9	Urban search and rescue
ESF 10	Hazardous materials
ESF 11	Food
ESF 12	Energy

The support function of primary medical importance is ESF 8, health and medical services. Mass care (ESF 6) has provision for only a first-aid level medical component. The primary federal agency in charge of ESF 8 is the U.S. Public Health Service, and both its own medical personnel and military medical units can be accessed and deployed in addition to the civilian response. The potential scope of this support is extensive (Table 15–3). Within ESF 8, the organization given the task of providing the majority of the prehospital medical care, patient transport (evacuation), and definitive medical care (including intensive care) is the National Disaster Medical System (NDMS). It consists of elements from the Department of Health and Human Services, the Department of Veteran Affairs, the Department of Defense, and the Federal Emergency Management Agency.

The predecessor of NDMS, the Civilian Military Contingency Hospital System, was conceived in the early 1980s as a back-up to the military medical system for casualties of a non-nuclear military conflict. This system evolved into the NDMS as an organized, national "mutual aid" system to be activated in the event of an overwhelming disaster. The system's concept is to provide medical care resources at the disaster site, air evacuation for patients unable to be cared for by local resources, and a commitment of hospital beds nationwide to be made available for these evacuated patients.

The plan also incorporates DMATs to staff the casualty collection points and the receiving airport's reception areas.

TABLE 15–3. Health and Medical Services

Assessment of health/medical needs
Health surveillance
Medical care personnel
Health/medical equipment and supplies
Patient evacuation
In-hospital care
Food/drug/medical device safety
Worker health/safety
Radiation health issues
Chemical (hazardous materials [HAZMAT])
Biologic health issues
Mental health
Public health information
Disease vector control
Water safety/wastewater and solid waste disposal
Victim identification/mortuary service

The original DMAT concept was based on the military model with a specified personnel composition. A command and support unit was also devised, and when combined with three DMATs, was designated as the "clearing staging unit."

The original NDMS concept was to provide medical care from receiving areas near disaster sites and to continue the care through the evacuation stage to definitive care at fixed medical facilities recruited through the system. This has since been developed into highly organized DMAT units that can set up field hospital units and provide hospital care in the prehospital environment. The United States currently has a number of these teams, and many have been shown to be operational through successful response drills. In addition, the concept of specialized DMATs is evolving (Table 15–4). The recent effort of the NDMS National Medical Response Steering Committee includes organized provision for intensive care services within this scope. The concept of a rapidly deployed resuscitation/critical care group by rotary or fixed-wing aircraft was recommended for inclusion within NDMS some years ago.[6] This was not implemented on a clinical level, to our knowledge, until the critical care team was airlifted to Armenia in 1988 in the early phase of the earthquake response. The function, in addition to life support of severely ill postoperative and medical patients, may appropriately extend into difficult triage decisions, critical care transport, and consultation with other groups in the field. This group also is the local medical authority on respiratory care and metabolic support.

Bringing all of the medical entities into NDMS provides multiple benefits. This strategy markedly improves the federal government's ability to respond expeditiously to very realistic disaster medical problems, and it provides an avenue for developed medical teams to obtain the necessary logistic support to respond to a disaster site (transportation, housing, food, communications). Through the legal powers of the U.S. Public Health Service, the NDMS provides licensure and assumes liability for medical teams that cross state lines to provide care. As the NDMS continues to evolve, it appears to be taking on the valuable role of acting as an umbrella organization to catalogue, coordinate, and integrate the varied medical groups that are seriously developing a disaster response capability.

In a national disaster situation, military medicine facilities and other resources can be accessed after a state has requested assistance from the Federal Emergency Management Administration and presidential approval for declaration of a disaster has been received. Some of the specialized resources of military medicine are ideally configured for disaster response. The U.S. Air Force has developed FAST teams (the Flying Ambulance Surgical Trauma teams) after the 1983 bombing of U.S. Marine barracks in Beirut. The teams consist of 20 individuals who can be en route within 2 hours, are self-sufficient for up to 48 hours, and can provide trauma surgical care for up to 50 casualties. An example of their deployment was in the aftermath of the crash in Ethiopia of an aircraft carrying Congressman Leland of Texas. The U.S. Army maintains similar FAST teams (the Forward Army Surgical Teams). The Army teams have advanced critical care capabilities, including hemodynamic monitoring, mechanical ventilation, and other technologies in addition to major trauma surgical capabilities. The U.S. Navy supports MMARTs (Mobile Medical Augmentation Response Teams) with similar capabilities. The U.S. military also has a number of mobile hospital facilities, ranging from the Air Force ATH (Air Transportable Hospital), which is a self-sufficient 50-bed hospital, to the Navy hospital ships that have up to 1000 ward beds and 80 ICU beds with full diagnostic capabilities, including computed tomography scanners. The U.S. military has been increasing its participation in providing disaster relief worldwide, from victims of the cyclones in Bangladesh to the starving population of Somalia.

TABLE 15–4. Specialized Teams

Urban Search and Rescue Team	Dialysis Team
Trauma Team	Critical Care Medicine Team
Pediatric Team	Mortuary Team
Burn Team	Critical Incident Debriefing Team
Hazardous Materials Team	

PEDIATRIC CONSIDERATIONS

Children are among the victims in most disasters.[84] However, few hospitals or community systems are prepared to meet the needs of children in a disaster situation. In January 1990, an Avianca airliner carrying 160 people, including 25 children, crashed in Nassau County, a suburban area of Long Island, New York. An analysis of the pediatric aspects of the disaster response concluded that pediatric survivors "were neither adequately triaged nor transported to appropriate facilities which could optimize their care."[85] Only four of the seven critically injured survivors were treated in available tertiary care trauma centers or pediatric centers. Only one patient was transported directly to one of the higher level centers. This episode is typical of the responses to children in a disaster situation.

Preparation for children is essential for both in-hospital and community disaster planners. In addition to the considerations already noted, in-hospital plans must identify a pediatric triage officer, arrange for a pediatric call-down system, identify areas in the hospital that are prepared to receive children, arrange for specialized medical, nursing, and support services, plan for media management for children, and communicate with other healthcare facilities that may be involved in a disaster response.

The community disaster response should anticipate possible pediatric disasters, arrange for triage officers trained in pediatric management (e.g., pediatric intensivists, pediatric emergency specialists, and pediatric surgeons), and train for pediatric emergencies. Equipment lists for pediatric disasters have been developed.[86]

Several problems are worthy of special mention: assessment and reassessment of patients, documentation, and the effects of psychologic stress. As noted in the Avianca disaster, prehospital pediatric training is often insufficient. Thus, initial assessments may be faulty. An injured child needs to be reassessed as he or she moves through the triage/transport system until his or her condition is finally assessed appropriately. Triage levels may be altered significantly. Coupled with these alterations is the need for careful documentation. Therapy based on one assessment may be inappropriate given a different triage category. There is often little room for error. Administration of resuscitation fluids at the site of an accident serves as a good example.

The handling of injured or dead children can also exact a psychologic toll on bystanders, families, and healthcare workers. The response to this pain may require an extra effort as a part of the disaster response.

SUMMARY

Critical care physicians are important in a quality response to a disaster on a regional, national, and international level.

In this chapter, an overview of disaster medicine from the perspective of an intensivist has been provided.

ACKNOWLEDGMENT

The authors would like to acknowledge the help and contributions of Peter Holbrook, MD.

References

1. Baskett P, Weller R (Eds): Medicine for Disasters. Littleton, MA, PSG Publishing, 1988.
2. Kvetan V: Disaster management. Crit Care Clin 1991; 7:257–484.
3. Klain M, Ricci E, Safar P, et al: Disaster reanimatology potentials: A structured interview study in Armenia: Methodology and preliminary results. Prehosp Disaster Med 1989; 4:135.
4. Birnbaum M: Disaster medicine: Fact or fiction? Prehosp Disaster Med 1989; 4:107.
5. Petroni IJ: Systems affecting the disaster rescue and EMS response. Presented at EMS Today, San Diego, CA, March 8, 1989.
6. Safar P: Resuscitation potentials in mass disasters. J World Assoc Emerg Disaster Med 1986; 2:34.
7. Mulhoney LE, Lasek RW, Paris PM: Natural disaster management. *In:* Management of Wilderness and Environmental Emergencies. Auerbach PS, Geehr EC (Eds). St. Louis, CV Mosby, 1989, p 453.
8. Bissell R, Young K, Abbott L, et al: Management of the Medical Response to Mass Casualties in a Catastrophic Disaster: A Planning Guidance Document. US Public Health Service (in press).
9. Safar P: Introduction to "disaster resuscitology." J World Assoc Emerg Disaster Med 1985; 1(Suppl 1):11.
10. Elseman B: Combat casualty management in Vietnam. J Trauma 1967; 7:3.
11. Heaton LD: Army medical services activities in Vietnam. Mil Med 1966; 131:646.
12. Peel S: Army aeromedical evacuation procedures in Vietnam: Implications for rural America. JAMA 1968; 4:99.
13. Pesola G, Bayshtok V, Kvetan V: American critical care team at a foreign disaster site: The Armenian experience. Crit Care Med 1989; 17:582.
14. Collins AJ: Kidney dialysis treatment for victims of the Armenian earthquake. N Engl J Med 1989; 10:1291.
15. Collins AJ, Burnstein S: Renal failure in disasters. Crit Care Clin 1991; 7:421.
16. Barbera J: Report of Special Medical Response Team response to earthquake in Baguio City, Philippines. Washington, DC, Office of Foreign Disaster Assistance, 1990.
17. Kvetan V: Operation Desert Storm: Task force on disasters and critical care. Crit Care Med 1991; 19:854.
18. San Francisco: Earthquake Planning Scenario for a Magnitude 7.5 Earthquake in the Hayward Fault in the San Francisco Bay Area. California Department of Conservation, Division of Mines and Geology. Washington DC, US Government Printing Office, 1989, Special Publication 78.
19. Office of US Foreign Disaster Assistance: Disaster History: Significant Data on Major Disasters Worldwide, 1900 to Present. Washington, DC, Agency for International Development, 1990, p 1.
20. Noji EK: Natural disasters in disaster management. Crit Care Clin 1991; 7:271.
21. Leonard RB, Teitelman U: Manmade disasters in disaster management. Crit Care Clin 1991; 7:293.
22. American Association for World Health: Should disaster strike—Be prepared. World Health Day Bull, April 7, 1991.
23. US Geological Survey: The Severity of an Earthquake. Washington, DC, US Department of the Interior, Division of Geological Survey, 1990, General Interest Publication 0273494.
24. Glass RI, Urrutia JJ, Sibony S, et al: Earthquake injuries related to housing in a Guatemalan village. Science 1977; 197:638.
25. De Ville de Govet C, Del Cid E, Romero E, et al: Earthquake in Guatemala: Epidemiologic evaluation of the relief effort. Bull Pan Am Health Organ 1976; 10:95.
26. Berberian M: Tabase Golshan (Iran) catastrophic earthquake of 16 September, 1978: A preliminary field report. Disasters 1979; 2:207.
27. Philippines earthquake. Earthquake Eng, September 3, 1990.
28. Barbera JA, Cadoux CG: Search, rescue, and evacuation. Crit Care Clin 1991; 7:321.
29. Kunkle RF: Medical care of entrapped patients in confined spaces. International Workshop on Earthquake Injury. Epidemiology for mitigation and response. In: Johns Hopkins University Proceedings, p. 339, July 10, 1989.
30. Sheng CY: Medical support in the Tangshan earthquake: A review of the management of mass casualties and certain major injuries. J Trauma 1987; 27:1130.
31. Tilling RL: Volcanoes. Washington, DC, US Department of the Interior, Division of Geological Survey, General Interest Publication.
32. Heliker C: Volcanic and Seismic Hazards on the Island of Hawaii. Washington, DC, US Department of the Interior, Division of Geological Survey, 1990, General Interest Publication 259799.
33. Baxter PJ: Volcanoes. *In:* The Public Health Consequences of Disasters. Gregg MB (Ed). Atlanta, Centers for Disease Control, 1989, p 25.
34. Sigurdsson H, Carey S: Volcanic disasters in Latin America and the 13 November 1985 eruption of Nevada del Ruiz volcano in Colombia. Disasters 1986; 10:205.
35. Gueri M, Perez LJ: Medical aspects of the "El Ruiz" avalanche disaster, Colombia. Disasters 1986; 10:150.
36. French JG: Hurricanes. *In:* The Public Health Consequences of Disasters. Gregg MB (Ed). Atlanta, Centers for Disease Control, 1989, p 33.
37. Orlowskii J: Floods, hurricanes and tsunamis. *In:* Medicine for Disasters. Baskett P, Weller R (Eds). Littleton, MA, PSG Publishing, 1988, p 291.
38. Sommer A, Mosley WH: East Bengal cyclone of November, 1970. Lancet 1972; i:1029.
39. Centers for Disease Control: Medical examiner/coroner reports of deaths associated with Hurricane Hugo—South Carolina. MMWR 1989; 38:754.
40. Centers for Disease Control: Update: Work-related electrocutions associated with Hurricane Hugo. MMWR 1989; 38:718.
41. Sanderson LN: Tornadoes. *In:* The Public Health Consequences of Disasters. Gregg MB (Ed). Atlanta, Centers for Disease Control, 1989, p 39.
42. Frazier K: The Violent Face of Nature: Severe Phenomena and Natural Disasters. New York, William Morrow, 1979.
43. Galway G: Relationship of tornado death to severe weather watch areas. Mon Weather Rep 1975; 103:737.
44. Glass RL, Craven RB, Bregman DG, et al: Injuries from the Witchita Falls tornado: Implications for prevention. Science 1980; 207:734.
45. Bakst HJ, Berg RL, Foster FD, et al: The Worchester County Tornado: Medical Study of the Disaster. Washington, DC, National Research Council, Committee on Disaster Studies, 1954, p 1.
46. Mandelbaum I, Nahrwold D, Boyer DW: Management of tornado casualties. J Trauma 1966; 6:353.
47. French JG, Holt KW: Floods. *In:* The Public Health Consequences of Disaster. Gregg MB (Ed). Atlanta, Centers for Disease Control, 1989.
48. Beinin L: Medical Consequence of Natural Disasters. New York, Springer Verlag, 1985, p 1.
49. French J, Ing R, Von Allmen S, et al: Mortality from flash flood: A review of national weather reports, 1969–1981. Public Health Rep 1983; 98:584.
50. Pan American Health Organization: Assessing Needs in the Health Sector after Floods and Hurricanes. Technical Paper 11. Washington, DC, Pan American Health Organization, 1987, p 1.
51. Centers for Disease Control: Medical examiner/coroner reports of deaths associated with Hurricane Hugo—South Carolina. MMWR 1989; 38:754.
52. Ussher JH: Philippine flood disaster. J R Nav Med Serv 1973; 59:81.
53. Fisher J: Road traffic accidents. *In:* Medicine for Disasters. Baskett P, Weller R (Eds). Littleton, MA, PSG Publishing, 1988, p 318.
54. Robertson B: Railway accidents. *In:* Medicine for Disasters. Bas-

kett P, Weller R (Eds). Littleton, MA, PSG Publishing, 1988, p 340.

55. Fahey M: Airport and aircraft accidents. *In:* Medicine for Disasters. Baskett P, Weller R (Eds). Littleton, MA, PSG Publishing, 1988, p 34.
56. Auffret R: Airport disasters. *In:* Proceedings of the 7th World Congress on Emergency and Disaster Medicine, Montreal (in press).
57. Bergot GP: Medical equipment for disaster at airports. J World Assoc Emerg Disaster Med 1985; 1:124.
58. Airport Emergency Planning—Part 7 (Document 9137AN/898). Montreal, Quebec, Canada, International Civil Aviation Organization, 1980.
59. Dulchavsky SA, Geller ER, Iorio DA: Analysis of injuries following the crash of Avianca flight 52. J Trauma 1993; 34:282.
60. Golden F: Shipwreck and exposure. *In:* Medicine for Disasters. Baskett P, Weller R (Eds). Littleton, MA, PSG Publishing, 1988, p 363.
61. Anantharam V: Burn mass disasters: Aetiology, predisposing situations and initial management. Ann Acad Med Singapore 1992; 21:635.
62. Houtchens BA, Clemmer TP, Holloway HC: Telemedicine and international disaster response. Prehosp Dis Med 1993; 8:57.
63. Leonard RB, Calabro JJ, Noji EK, et al: SARA (Superfund Amendments and Reauthorization Act), Title III: Implications for emergency physicians. Ann Emerg Med 1989; 18:1212.
64. Leonard RB: Community planning for hazardous materials disasters. Top Emerg Med 1986; 7:55.
65. Hazardous Materials: Medical Management Protocols. California Emergency Medical Services Authority and the Toxics Epidemiology Program, Los Angeles County, Department of Health Services, March 13, 1989.
66. Rieus RC: Prehospital Management of Radiation Accidents. Oak Ridge, TN, Oak Ridge Associated Universities (prepared for the Federal Emergency Management Agency), February 1984.
67. Smith JS Jr, Fisher JH: Three Mile Island: The silent disaster. JAMA 1981; 245:1656.
68. Geiger HJ: The accident at Chernobyl and the medical response. JAMA 1986; 256:609.
69. Saenger EL: Radiation accidents. Ann Emerg Med 1986; 15:1061.
70. Leonard RB, Ricks RC: Emergency department radiation accident protocol. Ann Emerg Med 1980; 9:462.
71. National Council on Radiation Protection and Measurements: Management of Persons Accidentally Contaminated with Radionuclides. Washington, DC, National Council on Radiation Protection and Measurements, 1980, NCRP Report No 65.
72. International Atomic Energy Agency: The Radiological Accident in Coiana. Vienna, International Atomic Energy Agency, 1988.
73. Marshall E: Juarez: An unprecedented radiation accident. Science 1984; 223:1152.
74. Frykberg ER, Tepas JJ: Terrorist bombings. Ann Surg 1988; 208:569.
75. Joint Commission on Accreditation of Health Care Organizations: Accreditation Manual for Hospitals, 1991. Standard PL 17. Chicago, Joint Commission on Accreditation of Healthcare Organizations, 1990, p 201.
76. Klein JS, Weigelt JA: Disaster management: Lessons learned. Surg Clin North Am 1991; 71:257.
77. Norcross ED, Elliott BM, Adams DB: Impact of a major hurricane on surgical services in a university hospital. Am Surg 1993; 59:28.
78. Ferguson KL, Walleck C, Jastremski M: Disaster management. *In:* Principles of Critical Care. Hall JB, Schmidt GA, Wood LDH (Eds). New York, McGraw-Hill, 1992, p 580.
79. Bissell R, Young K, Abbott L, et al: Management of the medical response to mass casualties in a catastrophic disaster: A planning guidance document. US Public Health Service (in press).
80. Coad NR, Jones MJ, Byrne A, et al: The M1 air crash: The demand placed on anaesthetic and intensive care services at two hospitals. Anaesthesia 1989; 44:851–854.
81. Chion HR, Moreau MM, Gainer PS: Assessment and triage. *In:* Medicine for Disasters. Baskett P, Weller R (Eds). Littleton, MA, PSG Publishing, 1988.
82. Partington AJ, Savage PE: Disaster planning: Managing the media. Br Med J 1985; 291:590.
83. Klain M, Ricci E, Safar P, et al: Disaster reanimatology potentials: A structured interview study in Armenia: I. Methodology and preliminary results. Prehosp Disaster Med 1989; 4:135.
84. Holbrook PR: Pediatric disaster medicine. Crit Care Clin 1991; 7:463–470.
85. van Amerongen RH, Fine JS, Tunik MG, et al: The Avianca plane crash: An emergency medical system's response to pediatric survivors of the disaster. Pediatrics 1993; 92:105–110.
86. Leonard RB: Role of pediatricians in disasters and mass casualty incidents. Pediatr Emerg Care 1988; 4:41.

SECTION III
CELL INJURY AND CELL DEATH

Edward Abraham

CHAPTER 16

Regulation of Gene Expression

Timothy G. Buchman, PhD, MD, FACS, FCCM
Luke O. Schoeniger, PhD, MD

GENES[1]

Genes were originally defined in the context of the science of genetics as loci of developmental information associated with heritable characteristics. A relationship between genetic defects and metabolic abnormalities was first proposed by Garrod in 1909 after he realized that alkaptonuria (subsequently proved to be an error in tyrosine metabolism resulting in the excretion of homogentisic acid) was inherited by mendelian rules. The nature of the relationship between genes and metabolism remained obscure until the 1940s, when Beadle and Tatum demonstrated that each gene was responsible for one enzyme. Enzymes were already recognized to be catalytic proteins, but the genetic material had yet to be identified. In 1944, Avery, MacLeod, and McCarty showed that a newly purified enzyme, deoxyribonuclease, selectively destroyed developmental information otherwise transferable between bacteria, implying that the enzyme's substrate, deoxyribonucleic acid (DNA), was in fact the bacterial "transforming principle." In 1952, Hershey and Chase reported that only the DNA portion of a bacterial virus—and not its protein coat—entered a (bacterial) cell, and this DNA was both necessary and sufficient to program viral replication. In 1953, Watson and Crick proposed a biophysical structure, the double helix, which not only accounted for the characteristic composition of DNA but also suggested a basis for semi-conservative replication using each parental strand of the double helix as template from which a daughter strand was synthesized.

Gene Expression

Although ribonucleic acid (RNA) had been recognized as the link between DNA and protein by the 1950s, it remained for Nirenberg and colleagues to confirm the nature of that link. They prepared cell-free extracts containing ribosomes, transfer RNA molecules, adenosine triphosphate (ATP), and guanosine triphosphate (GTP)—everything except the RNA molecules that would later be termed messenger RNA (mRNA) molecules. When synthetic mRNA molecules (consisting of polymers of a single nucleotide) were added to these extracts, polypeptides consisting of a single amino acid were formed. Using these RNA homopolymers and simple heteropolymers, these investigators proved that RNA was the intermediate between DNA and protein and "cracked the second genetic code" by showing that addition of amino acid residues to a nascent polypeptide was programmed for by particular RNA triplets. If gene expression reflects the number and activation state of protein molecules corresponding to a specific gene, then Nirenberg's work and that of his predecessors unequivocally separated gene expression into distinct and potentially regulatable steps. These include transcription of RNA from a DNA template by a DNA-dependent RNA polymerase; post-transcriptional modification of RNA into messenger form capable of being translated into polypeptide; translation of mRNA into polypeptide by ribosomes; and post-translational modification of the polypeptide chain into active protein.

Gene Expression in the Intensive Care Unit

The spectrum of processes and interventions managed in the intensive care unit ranges from those mechanical problems and solutions that are clearly unrelated to gene expression (e.g., pneumothorax and tube thoracostomy) to those that have an unequivocal genetic basis and therapy (e.g., sickle cell crisis and exchange transfusion). Rather than classify all possible patient presentations and therapies according to the extent to which gene expression might play a part, it is more convenient to classify abnormalities in gene expression and discuss familiar examples.

Congenital Errors

Congenital errors are primarily inherited but may not become clinically significant until childhood or even adulthood; thus, pediatric and adult intensivists confront congenital errors. One common series of error affects the β-globin gene, including sickle cell anemia and β-thalassemia (Cooley's anemia). Although sickle cell anemia had long been recognized as an inherited disease, identification of the molecular error dates only to 1956, when Ingram isolated globin from the blood of patients with sickle cell, cleaved the protein with sequence-specific proteases, and separated the peptide fragments by a combination of electrophoresis and chromatography to create a two-dimensional fingerprint. Ingram showed that a single amino acid substitution in a single gene was sufficient to account for the entire pathologic presentation of sickle cell anemia; subsequent investigators would prove that this substitution was caused by a point mutation in the DNA coding for β-globin. The electrophoretic techniques used by Ingram were subsequently applied to β-thalassemia. The amino acids all were correct, but the amount of β-globin protein produced was insufficient. The fact that β-thalassemia also followed a recessive pattern of mendelian inheritance was proof that genes had two functional domains: a structural domain and a regulatory domain. In other words, the gene encoded not only the amino acid sequence of its protein product but also regulatory information that controlled the rate at which that protein was produced. Subsequent work has established that the most important region regulating expression of a gene (the promoter) is contiguous with the site at which expression of that gene begins, the transcription start site.*

Congenital errors include inherited errors as well as sporadic mutations affecting germline DNA. Treatment has primarily focused on inherited errors and particularly on recessively inherited errors. The reason for this treatment focus is that correction of recessive errors can be accomplished in three distinctly different ways: by replacement of a defective gene by a gene; by replacement of a cell carrying the "correct" gene and its product (such as exchange transfusions for sickle cell anemia); or by replacement of the correct gene product itself (such as the administration of Factor VIII for hemophilia). Another feature of correction of recessive errors is that replacement typically need not be complete: Restoration of a gene product to 1% to 10% of normal levels is often sufficient to correct the biochemical defect. Dominant heritable errors typically cause minimal physiologic disturbances. This is both understandable and fortunate—understandable in that a severe physiologic disturbance mitigates against reproductive success and the mutation would therefore be expected to die out, and fortunate in that correction of a dominant error theoretically requires interventions aimed at every cell with faulty gene expression. Such intervention is now confined to animal research strategies aimed at the fertilized ovum and is beyond the current scope of clinical care.

Acquired Errors in Genes

Acquired errors in genes are very common but almost always silent for two reasons. First, effective immune surveillance identifies and eradicates affected cells. One familiar example of acquired error is the acquisition of new viral genes associated with acute infection. That human viruses commonly produce thousands of progeny per infected cell stands as mute testimony to the efficiency of a normal immune system in eradicating cells that are recognized as having acquired such errors. The second reason that acquired errors in genes and their expression generally are clinically insignificant is that most errors are either insignificant or adversely affect the cell that has acquired the error. It is the uncommon but clinically significant error acquired by a single cell that affects a regulatory protein and either enhances cell replication or prolongs cell survival. Either way, the result is a malignancy. Although a detailed review of the affected genes is more appropriately the province of molecular oncology, these genes are also of interest to intensivists precisely because their products regulate expression of many other genes. They fall into two classes. Tumor suppressor genes (also known as antioncogenes) are genes expressed in normal cells whose products typically regulate key steps in cell replication. Oncogenes are abnormal homologues of normal cellular genes whose products have key roles in the regulation of signal transduction or gene expression.

Abnormal Expression of Normal Genes

Abnormal expression of normal genes is perhaps the error most commonly encountered by intensivists. Examples include the hypoadrenalism and hypothyroidism associated with pituitary ablation; the disseminated inflammatory process that precedes development of the multiple organ dysfunction syndrome, and the rejection of a transplanted allograft. The common theme is that the regulatory failure is due to neither the regulatory nor the structural domain of the affected gene but rather the insufficiency or excess of regulatory signals such as hormones and cytokines. From the standpoint of an individual cell, gene expression is regulated by an affector arm (signals and their transduction) and an effector arm (transcription, translation, and intermediate steps).

Gene Expression in Cell Injury

Injury provides a convenient framework for review of the molecular mechanisms regulating gene expression. For review purposes, a significant injury is operationally defined as a change in the external (to each cell's membrane) environment sufficient to trigger changes in gene expression. This operational definition suggests several areas of interest.

- How are injury signals transduced to alter gene expression?
- What mechanisms regulate transcription of DNA after injury?
- What mechanisms regulate processing of transcripts into mRNA after injury?
- What mechanisms regulate stability of mRNA after injury?
- What mechanisms regulate initiation of translation after injury?
- How does a particular injury signal affect gene expression in diverse cell types?
- How do diverse injury signals affect gene expression in a particular cell type?
- Are there common patterns of gene expression among diverse cell types subjected to diverse injuries?

The definition of a signal is also an operational one: Any environmental change leading to change in gene expression is a signal. The environmental change is typically a change in the local (extracellular) concentration of a particular molecule. Although signal molecules have traditionally been classified according to the distance between site of synthesis and site of action (i.e., endocrine, paracrine, and autocrine), a more useful classification divides signals according to their ability to penetrate the cytoplasmic membrane. Lipophilic thyroid and steroid hormones readily penetrate the cytoplasmic membrane. Receptors for these hormones are intracellular and therefore can have direct roles in the regulation of gene expression. Ligand binding causes these particular receptors to undergo a conformational change, thereby exposing a hidden portion of the receptor that binds promoter regions of DNA in a sequence-specific fashion.

*Familiarity with a couple of conventions relating nomenclature with adjacency and directionality of macromolecules may be helpful. In the nucleus, DNA consist of two strands of polymerized deoxynucleic acid that are in antiparallel orientation. In other words, each strand is directional. Messenger RNA is likewise directional but consists of a single strand homologous to one of the DNA strands and complementary to the other, that latter having served as the template from which the RNA was synthesized. By convention, the DNA strand homologous to the RNA is known as the *coding strand* or *coding sequence.*

Nucleic acid synthesis is likewise directional and occurs when the hydroxyl residue of the 3′ position of the sugar ring (deoxyribose for DNA, ribose for RNA) of the last residue in the polymer is enzymatically joined to a phosphate located at the 5′ position of the sugar ring of the incoming monomer. For any given nucleic acid strand at any given time, there can be one (and only one) free 5′ end and one (and only one) free 3′ end. Because nucleic acid synthesis proceeds by attaching monomers to the free 3′ end of the polymer, it is said to proceed "5′ to 3′." Both DNA synthesis and RNA synthesis (transcription) proceed 5′ to 3′.

The conventions are as follows: Molecular biologists tend to refer to regions of DNA lying 5′ or 3′ with reference to the transcribed region of gene. The promoter region—the most important region regulating transcription—is located immediately 5′ to ("upstream" from) the transcription start site. This location is also described as being immediately upstream from the transcription start site. These RNA transcripts include regions that are never translated into protein but rather serve regulatory purposes. These regions, either upstream or downstream from the coding sequence, are referred to as 5′-UTRs or 3′-UTRs (untranslated regions), respectively. Translation also proceeds 5′ to 3′ with respect to the mRNA, with the 5′-most part of the sequence encoding the N-terminal of the polypeptide.

The two points here are first that the receptor itself is capable of regulating gene expression according to occupancy of its binding site, and second that such regulation occurs as a DNA sequence–specific interaction between the receptor protein and a portion of the promoter. Because these receptors can bind both ligands and particular DNA sequences, transduction of the lipophilic hormone signals requires only this single messenger.

Other signals that are either large (e.g., proteins) or hydrophilic cannot penetrate the cytoplasmic membrane and therefore must be transduced through a receptor molecule extracellularly displayed at the cytoplasmic membrane. Such receptors are typically large, specialized protein molecules that are tightly anchored in (and therefore unable to leave easily) the cytoplasmic membrane. Although signal transduction begins by binding of the signal to this receptor at the cell surface, additional (second) messengers are required to transmit information from the inner aspect of the cytoplasmic membrane through the cell to points where gene expression is regulated. Although some cells (such as antigen-recognition cells) likely have thousands of unique receptors, receptors and their second messengers are amenable to mechanistic classification.

SEVEN-PASS TRANSMEMBRANE RECEPTORS AND G PROTEINS[2]

The largest family of cell surface receptors are functionally linked to a specific class of intracellular molecules called G proteins. The cell surface receptors are members of the seven-pass transmembrane protein family, so called because their amino acid sequence codes include a distinctive pattern of alternating hydrophobic and hydrophilic regions that serve to anchor the protein in the cell membrane: when inserted into the cell membrane, the protein snakes back and forth across the membrane seven times, creating extracellular and intracytoplasmic loops. The variable extracellular segments that determine their unique interactions respond to particular signals such as peptide hormones. The third intracytoplasmic loop is the most variable and appears to select for the particular G protein that will ultimately generate a second messenger.

G Protein Structure and Mechanism

G proteins are heterotrimers consisting of α, β, and γ subunits. The β and γ subunits appear to be common to all G proteins, and thus it is the specific α subunit that defines precisely the activity of a G protein. Alpha subunits also characteristically bind guanylyl nucleotides and hydrolyze GTP into guanosine diphosphate (GDP). Quiescent G proteins are heterotrimers in which the α subunit has GDP in its binding site. Binding of a ligand to a seven-pass transmembrane receptor stimulates the G protein to partially liberate the α subunit from the β/γ complex, which in turn allows replacement of the resident GDP by GTP. Such replacement facilitates full dissociation of the α subunit, freeing it to activate other effector molecules, commonly adenylyl cyclase. The degree of signal amplification (e.g., how much cyclic adenosine monophosphate [cAMP] is generated) is variable and dependent at least in part on the half-life of the GTP residue on the particular α subunit. Hydrolysis of this GTP to GDP causes the α subunit to dissociate from the effector molecule and reassociate with the β/γ complex. Some α subunits ($G\alpha_s$) stimulate their effector, and others ($G\alpha_i$) inhibit it. Intensivists practicing in developing nations are especially familiar with a regulatory error involving this second-messenger system because it is a leading cause of death among children: cholera. Cholera toxin attacks $G\alpha_s$ after GTP binding and prevents hydrolysis to GDP. This particular G protein stimulates adenyl cyclase. The massive diarrhea associated with cholera infection is directly attributable to the consequent sustained high levels of cAMP in intestinal epithelium. Receptor-linked G proteins also regulate the activity of phospholipase Cβ. The second messengers most closely associated with the latter enzyme are diacylglycerol (DAG), which activates protein kinase C, and inositol triphosphate (IP_3), which binds to intracellular receptors on the endoplasmic reticulum, which in turn release calcium ions into the cytosol.

TYROSINE KINASES

The second important family of cell surface receptors includes those hormone receptors that phosphorylate the aromatic hydroxyl group of tyrosine residues embedded in polypeptides. These are called *tyrosine kinases,* and they transduce various polypeptide growth factors, including insulin and platelet-derived growth factors. These receptors are more varied in their structure than the seven-pass transmembrane receptors, yet all highly conserve the domain within the cytoplasmic region that catalyzes the phosphorylation of intracellular proteins. Generally, these receptors are activated by a conformational change induced by ligand binding; the conformational change causes dimerization between like or similar receptor subunits. This dimerization results in cross-phosphorylation between these two tyrosine kinase molecules, a characteristic feature of this receptor family. The intracellular substrates for these tyrosine kinase are numerous, and it has been difficult to prove which ones are most physiologically important. Several tyrosine kinase receptors have been shown to activate phospholipase Cγ, which (like phospholipase Cβ) generates DAG and IP_3.

OTHER RECEPTORS

A large class of injury-relevant membrane receptors are neither coupled to G proteins nor appear to possess intrinsic tyrosine kinase activity. These include receptors for growth hormone, prolactin, and many lymphokines and cytokines. For example, the interleukin-2 receptor has no intrinsic tyrosine kinase activity but interacts with an independent protein kinase when activated by interleukin-2. The binding of the activated interleukin-2 receptor to this protein kinase ($p56^{ick}$) results in changes in gene expression due to subsequent kinase reactions.

Many second messengers appear to converge through messenger-specific protein kinases toward protein phosphorylation as a final common regulatory mechanism.

Cyclic Adenosine Monophosphate

Historically, the first and most well-described second messenger is cAMP. Cyclic AMP acts as an allosteric regulator via activation of the cAMP-dependent protein kinase A (PKA). Cyclic AMP binds to a regulatory subunit of PKA, causing dissociation of another active catalytic subunit. This catalytic subunit then phosphorylates target proteins on serine-threonine residues using ATP as a cosubstrate. PKA activation is well known to regulate metabolic pathways acutely by phosphorylating target enzymes such as those that catalyze glycolysis. In addition to these metabolic and biochemical effects, however, PKA regulates gene expression by phosphorylation of DNA binding proteins that act as transcription factors. By this pathway, cAMP acts as a mediator between cell surface events and transcriptional activity.

Inositol Triphosphate–Calcium

The IP_3 mechanism that augments intracellular calcium concentration has already been suggested. Endotoxin is a familiar activator of this system. This newly released calcium then binds to calmodulin, a highly conserved cytoplasmic protein that can accommodate at least four calcium ions. This activated calmodulin has two primary effects. First, activated calmodulin regulates cAMP levels through activation of cyclic nucleotide phosphodiesterase, which degrades cAMP. Second, activated calmodulin itself activates a multifunctional protein kinase, calmodulin kinase.

Diacyglycerol

DAG, formed by the phospholipase C–catalyzed cleavage of phosphatidylinositol bis-phosphate (PIP_2), mediates an effect on gene expression by activation of protein kinase C, a calcium-dependent protein kinase.

MECHANISMS REGULATING GENE EXPRESSION

Initiation of Transcription

The expression of many genes is transcriptionally controlled through mechanisms that regulate the initiation of transcription. Although some nontranslated genes (e.g., genes coding for ribosomal RNA) are transcribed by RNA polymerases I and III, genes that code for proteins are transcribed by RNA polymerase II. Initiation of RNA synthesis by this enzyme requires several steps that involve binding of both regulatory and synthetic proteins to DNA sequences in the promoter and enhancer regions of genes.

Nucleosomes[3]

Access to DNA is not trivial, because within the nucleus, DNA is ordinarily compacted into nucleosomes. These globular structures are complexes of DNA and histone proteins. Histone proteins surround and charge-neutralize the DNA in a sequence-independent fashion. Each nucleosome includes about 180 base pairs of DNA and forms a structure that resembles beads (histone proteins) on a string (DNA). Although this arrangement is very efficient for close packing of DNA, transcription cannot begin until the nucleosomes are displaced to reveal the DNA sequences.

At least two distinct strategies exist for eukaryotic cells to displace nucleosomes and thereby allow RNA polymerase II to effect gene transcription: persistent displacement and induced displacement. A very few persistent nucleosome-free regions are sustained through the tight, sequence-specific binding of nonhistone proteins to the DNA. This arrangement is crucial to heat shock gene expression, which is the archetypal intracellular stress gene response (discussed later and in Chapter 23). In the more common induced displacement mechanism, histones are initially displaced by the actions of nonspecific activator proteins. The displacement zones, which must include the promoter, are then occupied by sequence-specific DNA binding proteins (e.g., the activated thyroid hormone receptor). These sequence-specific binding proteins that regulate transcription are collectively called *nuclear factors*.

The promoter has at least two functional regions where the nucleosomes have to be displaced promptly. The first region is the core promoter region, which serves as the scaffolding on which RNA polymerase II and general initiation factors will bind to form the so-called transcription complex. The second functional region includes DNA sequences that are the target site of specific nuclear factors that are not required for initiation of transcription per se but regulate the rate at which RNA polymerase II initiates additional rounds of transcription at the core promoter region.

Transcription Complex[4]

Initiation of transcription from the core promoter is a multistage process requiring the action of at least five initiation factor proteins and an ATP cofactor. The first stage of the process is site selection, which culminates in RNA polymerase II locating and binding selectively to the core promoter. First, an initiation protein called the TATA factor (also known as TFIID) locates a highly conserved DNA sequence called the TATA box. This TATA box, a TA-rich region of DNA, is absolutely required for transcription by RNA polymerase II. Binding of TATA factor to the TATA box forms an initial complex. Additional factors (α, TFIIB) and finally RNA polymerase II bind productively to complete the site selection process. However, the complex is not yet stable. Additional factors, ϵ and δ, bind to stabilize protein-DNA contacts and anchor the proteins firmly to the DNA. Only then is the preinitiation complex complete. Subsequent activation of this complex appears to require hydrolysis of a molecule of ATP, which is not incorporated into the nascent RNA chain.

Regulatory Factors

The rate at which initiation of transcription occurs is modulated by the other promoter-enhancer DNA sequences or more precisely by the binding of "factors" (regulatory proteins) to those sequences.[5] The target sequences, also known as regulatory elements, typically are stretches of DNA that are 6 to 20 base pairs in length and that often have dyadic symmetry. The proteins that bind to those elements have highly conserved DNA-binding domains that can be recognized on the basis of the secondary structures predicted by their amino acid sequences. These conserved DNA-binding domains have colorful names reflecting conserved structural features: the *zinc finger*, the *helix-turn-helix*, the *leucine zipper*, and the *basic helix-loop-helix*. It is the minor changes in protein structure adjacent to these regions that account for each factor's specificity with respect to its target element. The interaction of a regulatory element with its nuclear factor can be envisioned as turning on a switch. The rate of initiation of transcription of a particular gene is regulated by the state of several such switches (i.e., a set of regulatory elements that bind specific nuclear factors). This combinatorial approach allows for tissue specificity in gene expression. It also allows for the alteration in the expression of multiple genes on transduction of a single signal.

Clearly, the activation of nuclear factors to initiate binding to regulatory elements must be very fast and tightly controlled. Three general mechanisms are operative.[5,6] The first is compartmentalization—the factor can be sequestered in the cytoplasm and maintained inactive through lack of access to the regulatory elements. Second, the factor can be covalently modified to affect the DNA-binding site. Third, the factor can be covalently modified distant from the DNA-binding site in the region where it interacts with the initiation complex, the so-called transactivation domain. Interestingly, all of these mechanisms have been observed in nuclear factors relevant to injury/critical care. Perhaps more importantly, all rely on protein phosphorylation. Three examples follow.

NF-κB. The nuclear factor NF-κB is a heterodimeric protein. Although it was originally identified in association with B cell–specific transcription factors, it is now recognized to regulate gene expression in response to phorbol esters, antigens, cytokines, ultraviolet irradiation, and virus infection. This heterodimer consists of two subunits, p50 and p65, which themselves are ordinarily bound in the cytoplasm by a third protein molecule, IκB. This IκB is a direct target for protein kinases A and C and, when phosphorylated, dissociates from p50 and p65. It may also be an indirect target for these kinases because the latter augment production of reactive oxygen intermediates and such intermediates also can dissociate IκB from the heterodimer. The free p50/p65 heterodimer easily translocates to the nucleus, where it binds to its response elements.

AP-1. The nuclear factor AP-1 is actually a collection of homodimeric and heterodimeric complexes of the products of two genes called *fos* and *jun*. AP-1 binding is critical to the expression of many genes, including those of the acute-phase response, which results in hepatic synthesis of procoagulants and antiproteases. The jun protein is ordinarily phosphorylated in its DNA-binding domain, where the phosphate residues interfere with DNA binding. In a cascade arrangement, activation of protein kinase C secondarily activates a specific phosphatase that removes the phosphates from the jun protein's DNA-binding domain and thereby allows DNA binding to occur. Interestingly, another kinase can phosphorylate jun in its transactivation domain, further potentiating the initiation of transcription.

CREB. The nuclear factor CREB is a 43-kd protein that activates genes in response to increasing cAMP levels by binding to the cAMP response element (CRE). Here, binding of cAMP to the regulatory subunit of PKA releases the catalytic subunit of that kinase, which itself translocates to the nucleus and phosphorylates CREB in its transactivation domain. CREB's target is apparently promiscuous, because elevated intracellular Ca^{2+} also results in CREB phosphorylation by non-PKA mechanisms.

Enhancers and Locus Control Regions[7]

All genes have promoters. Initiation of transcription of some genes is further regulated by enhancers and by locus control regions. Enhancers differ from promoters by virtue of the great distance (up to 40,000 nucleotides) over which they can influence a particular gene. Enhancers escape not only the adjacency requirement but also the directionality requirement of promoters—that is, they can be flipped end over end and reinserted into the DNA sequence, and work perfectly well. Enhancers typically contain several regulatory elements than can bind activating (or suppressing) factors. Many such factors are cell type specific. Multimerization of enhancers characteristically potentiates transcription. Locus control regions are similar to enhancers but typically regulate the expression of multiple gene loci during normal growth and development. They are functionally distinguished from enhancers in that multimerization does not potentiate transcription. The β-globin locus is an example of a locus regulated by such a control region. Promoters, enhancers, and locus control regions all have regulatory elements, and all appear to regulate initiation of transcription by element-specific binding of regulatory proteins.

Transcript Elongation

Conspicuous by its absence from this discussion is any mention of the rate of elongation of transcripts after initiation. With one notable exception (heat shock, discussed later), this potential regulatory mechanism appears to be unrealized or at least unrecognized. RNA polymerase II adds about 50 nucleotides per second to nascent transcripts, retarded nonspecifically by the requirement to free DNA from nucleosomes.

Transcript Processing: Appearance of Messenger Ribonucleic Acid

Soon after transcription begins, the free 5′ end of the transcript undergoes the first of three modifications required for the transcript to function as mRNA. This first modification is the addition of a methylated cap structure that requires the catalyzed formation of a unique 5′-5′ guanylyl-nucleotidyl phosphodiester bond followed by methylation of guanylyl residue at nitrogen-7. This capping event, although catalyzed, is not considered an important control point in the regulation of gene expression. The second modification to the transcript is the addition of a characteristic polyadenylylate (polyA) tail to the 3′ end of the just completed transcript. This modification is also a two-step process requiring site-directed cleavage of the primary transcript to expose a 3′-hydroxyl group to which polyA is promptly added. Interestingly, the only eukaryotic transcripts that escape this tailing requirement are those that code for histone proteins. The third modification is splicing of the RNA molecule. Splicing is required for many but not all eukaryotic RNAs (heat shock RNA is an important exception) and involves site-specific excision of RNA sequences with resealing of the parent molecule. The process often occurs in defined organelles (spliceosomes). The time required for splicing reactions varies from seconds to a half hour. This splicing time is probably transcript specific but appears to be not subject to acute regulation. Only after all three of these modifications are completed can the transcript be properly identified as mRNA and be transported to the cytoplasm.

Stability of Messenger Ribonucleic Acid[8]

None of modifications catalogued in the preceding paragraph appear to be acutely regulated by external signals. These modifications do, however, strongly affect the stability of the newly synthesized mRNA molecule. Degradation of mRNAs is a highly regulated process that can determine the level of expression of a gene, and the mere existence of highly unstable mRNAs allows for tight titration against transcription rates to precisely fix specific transcript levels. At least seven different destabilizing elements have been found in mRNAs. No structure has yet been identified as conferring special stability on mRNAs: They are intrinsically stable molecules within the cell cytoplasm and remain stable until translated unless one or more of the destabilizing elements is present. Some of the destabilizing elements are nonspecific. For example, as mRNAs age, their polyA tail is progressively shortened. When the polyA tail length falls below a critical level of about 10 residues, degradation of the message occurs quickly. Other destabilizing elements are message and sequence specific. At least one of these now appears crucial to injury and critical care: the uracil-adenine (UA)–rich sequence.

Instability of Cytokine Messenger Ribonucleic Acids[9]

This UA-rich motif (also called the *AU-rich element* [ARE] was initially identified as a repeating octamer in the 3′ untranslated region of mRNA molecules encoding many cytokines, including interferon-β and tumor necrosis factor-α. It was shown to accelerate degradation of these cytokine mRNAs by creating chimeric genes in which the UA-rich sequences were coded into other RNA molecules. These chimeric transcripts became unstable. At least some ARE-containing mRNAs are stabilized in response to discrete changes in external signals or cell metabolism. ARE-binding proteins may influence not only message stability but also translation rates, at least in the case of tumor necrosis factor-α.

TRANSLATION: OVERVIEW[10, 11]

Translation of mRNA into protein is a complex process that consists of three stages: initiation of translation, elongation of the nascent polypeptide chain, and termination/release of the protein from the ribosome. The rate-limiting step in the process, in nearly all cases, occurs during the initiation stage. This stage comprises two steps: An mRNA among many available mRNAs is selected for translation, and then the ribosome identifies the initiator codon in the message and begins translation. Elongation is a cyclic process in which transfer RNA molecules add additional amino acid residues to the C-terminal end of the nascent polypeptide chain. Termination is the release of the completed polypeptide from the ribosome. Initiation involves at least 10 polypeptide cofactors (eIFs), elongation requires at least 4 polypeptide cofactors, and termination requires polypeptide release factor.

Global Regulation of Translation

Global regulation of translation is well characterized and occurs primarily through changes in the phosphorylation state of initiation factors, particularly eIF-2. Cofactor eIF-2 is a cytoplasmic G protein (discussed earlier) that ordinarily cycles through GTP hydrolysis and GDP binding. When eIF-2 is bound to GDP, it becomes accessible to a particular kinase and, if phosphorylated, becomes inactive. Moreover, this inactive form traps another factor (G elongation factor, GEF) crucial for initiation. This trapping mechanism is so powerful that phosphorylation of only 25% of the eIF-2 pool essentially abolishes protein synthesis. It is unclear whether a global decline in translation actually constitutes a specific regulatory mechanism.

Regulation of Specific Messenger Ribonucleic Acid Translation

Very few examples of mRNA-specific proteins regulating translation in eukaryotic cells can be cited. The example that most closely affects injury and critical care concerns the repression of translation of the mRNA coding for the iron-sequestering protein ferritin.[11, 12] Iron concentrations are tightly regulated, owing in part to iron's role in the nonenzymatic production of reactive oxygen species via the Fenton and Haber-Weiss reactions. At the 5′ end of the ferritin mRNA molecule is an iron-responsive element. The (single-stranded) RNA molecule self-hybridizes in this region to form a three-dimensional stem-and-loop structure. The protein that binds to this response element (IRE-BP) is of particular interest because it has aconitase activity (aconitase metabolizes citrate in the tricarboxylic acid cycle). Because aconitase is known to contain a labile iron-sulfur bond, regulation of IRE-BP binding to ferritin RNA could well be based on reversible oxidation of a sulfhydryl group. If iron levels fall, the sulfhydryl group is maintained in the reduced state and IRE-BP remains bound to mRNA. If iron levels rise, the sulfhydryl group oxidizes and the IRE-BP separates, thereby derepressing the translation of the mRNA. Even more intriguing, this same IRE-BP regulates the stability of the transferrin receptor mRNA. Proteins binding specifically to mRNAs coding for the antioxidant enzymes catalase[13] and superoxide dismutase[14] have been described. It is uncertain whether these proteins regulate expression of these gene products. Activation of translation by a specific mRNA-binding protein is rare in bacteria and has not been demonstrated with certainty in any eukaryotic system.

Reinitiation of Translation as a Regulatory Mechanism[11]

Reinitiation of translation in a different reading frame is a complex mechanism that has been observed so far only in yeast. It is of particular interest to intensivists because this regulatory mechanism is triggered by starvation. The mechanism involves the biosynthesis of a yeast-specific transcription factor, GCN4. Although transcripts of GCN4 are made constitutively and ribosomes bind to the message, no protein is made. Apparently, the ribosomes start to scan the message, looking for open reading frames (translation start sites), and get stuck in two small open reading frames upstream from the real coding portion of the message. When the yeasts are starved, the ribosomes scan past through the upstream regions and translate the GCN4 protein. This GCN4 protein is intrinsically active, functioning as a nuclear factor to promote transcription of 30 to 40 genes coding for enzymes required for amino acid biosynthesis.

Termination of Protein Synthesis[15]

Termination of protein synthesis, formerly considered a general and fundamental event culminating in release of the protein product, is increasingly regarded as a pause signal regulating gene expression. The regulatory mechanisms affecting bacterial stop signals have only begun to be recognized; the role of this mechanism in eukaryotic cells must be considered indeterminate at present.

AUTHOR'S PERSPECTIVE. *Whereas management of congenital or acquired errors in gene structure or expression can be directed at a single gene, abnormal expression, particularly that due to signal excess, rarely affects individual genes. No "shock" or "injury" gene has been identified; rather, hundreds of them exist. Although the tools of molecular biology provide unique insight into the mechanisms regulating expression of these genes, it may well be insufficient to explain (much less suggest therapeutic approaches to) critical illnesses such as multiple organ dysfunction syndrome. Basic and clinical investigators have therefore focused on identifying signals transduced at the cell membrane, predicated on the view that neutralization of categorically harmful signals is sufficient to alter adverse gene expression and improve outcome. Unfortunately, individual signals and the genes they ultimately regulate cannot be so easily categorized or manipulated. More sophisticated approaches certainly are required to affect outcome in a predictable and salutary way.*

A more intricate view of signaling and regulation of gene expression in critical illness—one that explicitly accounts for the interactions among multiple genes and multiple programs of gene expression—may ultimately prove even more useful to clinicians. This view predicts that gene expression is a self-organizing process.[16] *In particular, not all combinations of gene expression are possible, and cells are afforded surprisingly few stable metabolic states. This view predicts that signals and their intracellular second messengers converge not merely to regulate changes in gene expression but rather to facilitate transitions among metabolic states characterized according to expression of representative genes. By extension, these regulatory mechanisms would establish an implicit priority among metabolic states, and the collection of signals impinging on each cell would determine the probability of transitions between particular states.*

ACKNOWLEDGMENTS

Supported in part by awards GM 00581, GM 39756, and GM 48095 from the National Institutes of Health.

References

Because of the scope of this chapter and limitations of format, secondary (review) articles and monographs have been listed to facilitate breadth of coverage. Statements with specific references can be found primarily within the review articles cited.

1. Darnell J, Lodish H, Baltimore D: Molecular Cell Biology, 2nd ed. New York, Scientific American, 1990.
2. Karin M: Signal transduction from cell surface to nucleus in development and disease. FASEB J 1992; 6:2581–2590.
3. Workman JL, Buchman AR: Multiple functions of nucleosomes and regulatory factors in transcription. Trends Biochem Sci 1993; 18:90–95.
4. Weliky-Conaway J, Conaway RC: Initiation of eukaryotic messenger RNA synthesis. J Biol Chem 1991; 266:17721–17724.
5. Hunter T, Karin M: The regulation of transcription by phosphorylation. Cell 1992; 70:375–387.
6. Whiteside ST, Goodbourn S: Signal transduction and nuclear targeting: Regulation of transcription factor activity by subcellular localisation. J Cell Sci 1993; 104:949–955.
7. Dillon N, Grosveld F: Transcriptional regulation of multigene loci: Multilevel control. Trends Genet 1993; 9:134–137.
8. Sachs AB: Messenger RNA degradation in eukaryotes. Cell 1993; 74:413–421.
9. Beutler B: Application of transcriptional and posttranscriptional reporter constructs to the analysis of tumor necrosis factor gene regulation. Am J Med Sci 1992; 303:129–133.
10. Hershey JWB: Translational control in mammalian cells. Am Rev Biochem 1991; 60:717–755.
11. Kozak M: Regulation of translation in eukaryotic systems. Annu Rev Cell Biol 1992; 8:197–225.
12. Munro H: The ferritin genes: Their response to iron status. Nutr Rev 1993; 51:65–73.
13. Clerch LB, Massaro D: Oxidation-reduction sensitive binding of lung protein to rat catalase mRNA. J Biol Chem 1992; 267:2853–2855.
14. Fazzone H, Wangner A, Clerch LB: Rat lung contains a developmentally regulated MnSOD binding protein. J Clin Invest 1993; 92:1278–1281.
15. Tate WP, Brown CM: Translational termination: "Stop" for protein synthesis or "pause" for regulation of gene expression. Biochemistry 1992; 31:2443–2449.
16. Kauffman SA: The origins of order: Self-organization and selection in evolution. New York, Oxford University Press, 1993.

CHAPTER 17

Macrophage Function

Tomas Ganz, PhD, MD

Macrophages and their secretory products have a central role in host defense against pathogenic microbes, in the development of protective immunity, in the pathogenesis of septic shock and of acute and chronic infections, and in the pathophysiology of wound healing, tissue remodeling, and fibrosis.[1] In their role as scavenger cells, macrophages sequester and degrade particulates that enter the body by inhalation, trauma, or parenteral injection; they break down accumulated deposits of metabolites and dispose of senescent cells.

MORPHOLOGY AND DEVELOPMENT

Macrophages are mononuclear phagocytes—that is, cells with a single nonsegmented nucleus and the ability to ingest particles into cytoplasmic membrane-lined vacuoles. Some macrophages are freely motile (e.g., alveolar macrophages, peritoneal macrophages); others are fixed in tissues (e.g., liver and colon macrophages). The characteristic ultrastructural features of free macrophages include a ruffled membrane, sometimes with a prominent trailing extension (pseudopod), and a cytoplasm with abundant vacuoles. Some of these vacuoles (pinosomes) contain ingested fluid, others (phagosomes) contain ingested particles, yet others (lysosomes) are acidic vacuoles with digestive enzymes (hydrolases) capable of degrading proteins, complex carbohydrates, nucleic acids, and lipids. Of necessity, most of what we know about macrophages was learned from cells washed free from the pulmonary alveoli or body cavities or released from disaggregated tissues. Critical readers of the literature should be aware that crucial aspects of macrophage behavior may depend on the animal species and strain, the organ from which the macrophages were harvested, and the time and conditions ex vivo.

Most macrophages originate from bone marrow precursors that develop into blood monocytes, which, after a few days in the circulation, enter tissues and mature into macrophages.[2] Macrophages can divide, and this process contributes substantially to maintaining resident macrophage populations. The number of monocytes and macrophages is controlled by hematopoietic hormones,[3] especially interleukin-3 (IL-3, multi-colony-stimulating factor [CSF]), granulocyte-macrophage CSF (GM-CSF), and macrophage CSF (M-CSF, CSF-1). IL-3 is produced by lymphocytes, and GM-CSF by macrophages, lymphocytes, endothelial cells, and fibroblasts. Inflammatory or immune stimuli, acting in part by increasing the levels of IL-1 and tumor necrosis factor-α (TNF-α), increase the production of all three CSFs, ultimately generating more monocytes and macrophages.

Morphologic and biochemical studies of macrophages have described many tissue-specific adaptations that resulted in a confusing nomenclature—for example, *Kupffer's cells* for liver macrophages and *microglia* for brain macrophages. Studies of macrophage-specific marker antigens in mice[4] revealed that all tissues contain macrophages, with particularly high concentrations in bone marrow and lymph nodes. However, when the weight of the organs is taken into account, the largest total numbers of macrophages are found in the liver, small bowel, and colon. The factors that control the differentiation of macrophages into tissue-specific subtypes are not yet understood.

MACROPHAGE RECEPTORS

Macrophages sense their environment by various membrane-associated receptor molecules. Some receptors are exposed to the extracellular fluid, span the macrophage cell membrane, and immerse their intracellular end into the cytoplasm of the macrophage. For other receptors, the functional equivalent of the cytoplasmic tail is generated by transducer and adapter proteins that are associated with the receptor. Occupancy of receptors by their agonists results in transmission of a signal into the cytoplasm and activation of a cascade of biochemical reactions that constitutes the specific response of the cell to each agonist. The responses include cellular movement toward the source of a substance (chemotaxis), localized movement of the membrane in the area of receptor contact (adhesion, spreading, phagocytosis), rearrangement of internal organelles (e.g., fusion of phagocytic vacuoles with lysosomes), synthesis and assembly of systems required for antimicrobial activity (macrophage activation), alteration in the amount or nature of substances released into the extracellular milieu (regulated secretion), or initiation of cell division or cellular remodeling (mitogenesis, differentiation).

MICROBICIDAL FUNCTION AND CYTOTOXICITY

Unlike other phagocytes (i.e., neutrophils, eosinophils, monocytes), macrophages are resident in noninflamed tissues and thus are likely to interact with microbes during the earliest stages (first few hours) of infection. The response of motile macrophages to microbial invasion consists of movement toward the microbes (chemotaxis), recognition and ingestion of microbes (phagocytosis), killing and digestion of the microbes, and recruitment of additional effector cells to the site of infection.

Chemotaxis

Macrophages initiate movement toward microbes when their chemotactic receptors are occupied by (1) substances emitted by the invader (e.g., formylated peptides characteristic of prokaryotic organisms), (2) reaction products resulting from the encounter of microbes with extracellular fluids (e.g., complement fragment C5a), or (3) products released by other cells, including other macrophages, engaged in host defense activity (e.g., leukotriene B_4 [LTB_4]). Each chemotactic substance interacts with its own specialized receptor. Movement of macrophages to the site of invasion is induced by a gradient of concentration of the chemotactic substance that results in higher occupancy of the receptors on the leading edge of the macrophage as compared with its trailing end. Clearly, fixed macrophages cannot actively reach their targets and must instead entrap them. In the liver, lymph nodes, or spleen, macrophages are located near fluid channels that carry lymph or blood, and there they may contribute to removing microbes from these fluids.

Phagocytosis

Once a macrophage reaches its target, it recognizes friend from foe by another set of receptors[5–8] that detect (1) specific antibody covering the invader (recognized by Fc receptors), (2) complement fragments covalently bound to the surface of the invader (recognized by C3b or C3bi receptors), or (3) oligosaccharide moieties not present in the host (recognized by lipopolysaccharide [LPS] receptors, and oligosaccharide receptors also known as *lectins*). The contact of these receptors with ligands on the surface of the target triggers a local rearrangement of the cytoskeleton. The resulting movement of the membrane causes additional receptors to come in contact with ligands on the target, until the whole target is invaginated into the cell (the "zipper" mechanism). The connection to the outside of the cell is then pinched off to form a closed vacuole (phagosome).

Killing

Engagement of phagocytic receptors (especially Fc receptors) activates the microbicidal and digestive machinery of the macrophage, so that reactive oxygen intermediates, microbicidal and cytotoxic proteins, and hydrolytic enzymes are released into the phagocytic vacuole. In addition to these toxins, the microbe sequestered in the vacuole is also exposed to low pH and nutrient deprivation. This arrangement creates a highly biotoxic environment for the microbe while limiting the exposure of surrounding host cells to these potentially injurious influences.

The microbicidal mechanisms activated by phagocytosis include an enzyme system in the phagosomal membrane, the reduced form of nicotinamide-adenine dinucleotide phosphate, which reduces molecular oxygen to superoxide, which is then converted to microbicidal hydrogen peroxide.[9] Another enzyme system, characterized in murine macrophages, generates nitric oxide and related metabolites, some of which are microbicidal or cytotoxic. The role of this system in human macrophages, if any, is not yet clear. Vesicles containing lysozyme, other digestive enzymes, and microbicidal and cytotoxic proteins fuse to the phagosome and deliver their contents. The pH of the vacuole, initially neutral, becomes acidic and may reach less than 5. The concentration of iron and perhaps other nutrients essential for microbes may decrease to a point at which the metabolic function of the microbe is compromised. The combined damage from these changes usually results in the death and digestion of the microbial invader.

Tissue Injury

Several proposed mechanisms would expose host tissues ("innocent bystander cells") to macrophage-derived cytotoxins. These include extracellular leakage of phagosomal contents, secretion of macrophage products in response to stimulation of macrophage plasma membrane in the absence of phagosome formation, and release of preformed cytotoxins by injured or dying macrophages. In cell culture and certain animal models, macrophages can also exert selective cytotoxicity toward tumor cells by both antibody-dependent and antibody-independent mechanisms.[10] The extent to which these mechanisms contribute to tissue injury during infections or to host defense against human neoplasia is not known.

Microbial Countermeasures

Some microbes have evolved mechanisms that allow them to avoid destruction by macrophages. Certain fungi and bacteria are coated with materials that inhibit phagocytosis, others have cell walls or enzyme systems that help resist the macrophage toxins, and others somehow prevent the delivery of microbicidal and digestive proteins to the phagosome. A few species of bacteria can lyse the phagosomal membrane and escape into the cytoplasm (e.g., *Listeria*) and eventually leave the cell to infect its neighbor. Some bacteria (and perhaps all pathogenic ones), after entering the host, begin to synthesize new proteins that appear to be essential to their survival inside the macrophage and other host tissues. Certain pathogens have perfected all these survival mechanisms to the point that the macrophage is the predominant site of their multiplication (e.g., *Legionella, Histoplasma capsulatum*, some mycobacteria). The ability of macrophages to resist these intracellular pathogens is enhanced when they are exposed to various macrophage activating factors, substances that include interferon-γ and TNF-α.

Recruitment of Additional Effector Cells

When stimulated by phagocytosis or certain soluble substances, macrophages release products that attract neutrophils (LTB_4, IL-8) and lymphocytes (IL-8) to the site of infection or inflammation.

SCAVENGING FUNCTION

The ability of macrophages to break down senescent or necrotic cells and foreign particulate matter was appreciated even before their microbicidal role was known. Macrophages remove or degrade dust in the lungs, necrotic cells in wounds, injected particulates impacted in the pulmonary vasculature, and devolving structures during embryonic development. Specialized macrophages (osteoclasts) remodel bones, and other macrophages, in the spleen, recognize and destroy aging erythrocytes. Macrophages in atherosclerotic plaques ingest lipids and cholesterol, forming foam cells. Other macrophages participate in the lysis and degradation of blood clots and hematomas. Foreign body giant cells seen in areas of chronic antigenic or particulate stimulation are terminally differentiated forms of macrophages.

SECRETORY FUNCTION

Macrophages secrete various substances[11] that serve signaling or effector functions (Table 17–1). Some of these substances contribute to the acute response to microbial invasion by recruiting neutrophils to the site (LTB_4, IL-8), generating a systemic febrile response and stimulating the synthesis of acute-phase proteins by the liver (IL-1, IL-6, TNF-α). Other secreted substances can kill microbes (lysozyme), tumor cells (TNF-α), or both (hydrogen peroxide, nitric oxide). Yet other proteins may initiate or promote wound healing by stimulating fibroblast proliferation[12] and the formation of new capillaries[13] (transforming growth factors, basic fibroblast growth factor, platelet-derived growth factor). In animals selectively depleted of monocyte-macrophages, wound healing is impaired. The macrophages also secrete substances that act on other host defense cells: They increase macrophage microbicidal activity (TNF-α) or decrease it (TGF-β), activate T lymphocytes (IL-1), or increase the production of neutrophils in the bone marrow (G-CSF, GM-CSF). The list of active substances secreted by macrophages is continually expanding, and only selected examples are listed in Table 17–1.

ANTIGEN-PRESENTING FUNCTION

Although macrophages are prominent effector cells, they also have an important initiating role in immune responses.[14, 15] When hosts immune to a pathogenic microbe are rechallenged with it, T lymphocytes that recognize the antigens respond by undergoing "activation": They (1) multiply and (2) release various lymphokines. Lymphokines are substances that regulate the function of other host defense cells, including macrophages and T and B lymphocytes. When the activation response was studied in vitro with purified populations of lymphocytes, it was found to be dependent on the presence of nonlymphocyte cells, termed *antigen-presenting cells* (APCs). Although several other cell types (including dendritic cells and endothelial cells) can also fulfill this role, macrophages are efficient APCs.

After phagocytosis by macrophages, microbes are killed and undergo proteolytic digestion. From the microbial proteins, small peptide fragments are generated. Some of these peptide fragments associate with newly synthesized carrier molecules, termed *major histocompatibility complex* (MHC) class II. The MHC class II and its associated peptide are transported to the macrophage membrane and displayed. When the macrophage makes contact with a T lymphocyte possessing receptors that recognize the peptide–MHC II combination, the T cell receptor binds to the peptide–MHC II combination and the T lymphocyte becomes activated. It has been suggested that this mode of antigen presentation prevents T cell receptors from being flooded by excess antigen because most antigens do not bind to the T cell receptor without prior processing and interaction with MHC molecules.

MACROPHAGE ACTIVATION

Previous exposure of the host to certain microbial pathogens (e.g., mycobacteria) subsequently produces an enhanced microbicidal response by macrophages. This response extends not only to the original microbial species but also, at least in part, to other microbes. The morphologic and biochemical changes that accompany the enhanced microbicidal response are defined as *activation*. Activated macrophages display increased plasma membrane ruffling, increased content of hydrolytic enzymes, enhanced production of reactive oxygen intermediates, and increased numbers of MHC class II molecules. The activation response can be reproduced by incubating macrophages with the secretory products of lymphocytes (T and NK cells) that have been challenged with certain microbes or microbial products.[16, 17] Interferon-γ and TNF-α are the most important of the several activating factors purified from lymphocyte secretions. Genetically altered mice that lack interferon-γ or its receptor show poor macrophage activation in response to infection and are highly susceptible to intracellular parasites. Macrophage activation is temporary, and specific factors that can deactivate macrophages have been identified (e.g., TGF-β and macrophage-deactivating factor).

TABLE 17–1. Substances Secreted by Macrophages

Activity	*Substances (Examples)*
Chemotactic for neutrophils	LTB_4, IL-8
Growth factors (wound healing)	TGF-β, platelet-derived growth factor
Angiogenic factors	basic fibroblast growth factor, TGF-α
Growth factors (hematopoietic)	GM-CSF, G-CSF
Acute-phase response, fever, signs of sepsis	TNF-α, IL-1, IL-6
Microbicidal substances	Lysozyme, hydrogen peroxide
Cytotoxic substances	TNF-α, hydrogen peroxide, nitric oxide
Macrophage regulatory factors	TNF-α, TGF-β
Lymphocyte regulatory factors	IL-1, IL-6
Lytic enzymes	Plasminogen activator, collagenase, elastase
Enzyme inhibitors	α_2-Macroglobulin, α_1-antitrypsin

TABLE 17–2. Comparison of Macrophages and Granulocytes

Property	*Macrophages*	*Granulocytes*
Differ by organs and tissues	Yes	No
Mature cells can divide	Yes	No
Life span in tissues	Days to weeks	About 1 d
Phagocytosis	Yes	Yes
Generate reactive oxygen intermediates	Yes	Yes
Contain microbicidal proteins	Few known	Yes
Preformed cytoplasmic granules	Unusual	Abundant
Constitutive secretion	Yes	No
Secretion by degranulation	Limited	Prominent
Protein synthesis	Very active	Minimal
Deoxyribonucleic acid synthesis	Moderate	Inactive
Present antigen to T lymphocytes	Yes	Unknown

MACROPHAGES AND ENDOTOXIN

Entry of gram-negative bacteria into the bloodstream elicits a well-known sequence of responses ranging from rigors and fever to hypoxemia and hypotension. Many if not most of these responses are generated by secretory products released by macrophages that interact with an LPS component of bacteria (LPS, endotoxin). Specifically, exposure of macrophages to LPS induces secretion of IL-1β, TNF-α, and IL-6, factors that can reproduce nearly all of the manifestations of endotoxemia.

Macrophages possess at least three sets of receptors for endotoxin.[16] One set of receptors, CD14, recognizes LPS bound to a serum factor, LPS-binding protein (LBP). CD14 receptor activates the secretion of macrophage mediators. Another class of LPS receptors, CD18, includes multifunctional receptors such as the C3bi (CD11a/CD18) receptor, LFA-1 (CD11b/CD18) receptor, and p150,95 (CD11c/CD18) receptor. These receptors interact with various surfaces, fibrinogen, adhesion molecules on other cells, and complement fragments. In relation to LPS, CD18 receptors may be important for nonopsonic (complement and antibody-free) phagocytosis of gram-negative bacteria and for removal and degradation of LPS from the bloodstream and tissues. The third receptor type that may be important in the metabolism of LPS is the scavenger receptor, best known as the receptor that internalizes acetylated low-density lipoprotein. This receptor takes up various anionic ligands and transports them to lysosomes for degradation. The liver macrophages are particularly rich in scavenger receptors, where they may function to remove endotoxin from portal blood.[17]

MACROPHAGES AND "MICROPHAGES"

The ability of macrophages to ingest and kill microbes was first described at the end of the 19th century by Ilya Mechnikoff, who distinguished them from the smaller "microphages," phagocytic cells today known as *granulocytes*. Although the cells overlap in some of their activities, they differ in many other respects (Table 17–2).

What is the evolutionary advantage of having two sets of phagocytes? It appears that the numerous granulocytes kept ready in several reserve compartments are rapid-deployment, "disposable" phagocytes, particularly well suited for time-limited and massive response to microbial invasion. The short life span and limited synthetic repertoire of granulocytes may make them inhospitable to intracellular parasites that would readily survive and multiply in macrophages. In contrast, the longer-lived and adaptive macrophages are better suited for tissue-specific patrol duties and prolonged response to chronic low-level infections.

CONCLUSION

Macrophages, ubiquitous phagocytic and secretory cells, have a central role in host defense, inflammation, systemic response to infections, scavenging, and wound repair.

References

1. Johnston RB Jr: Monocytes and macrophages. N Engl J Med 1988; 318:747–752.
2. van Furth R: Development and distribution of mononuclear phagocytes. *In*: Inflammation: Basic Principles and Clinical Correlates. 2nd ed. Gallin JI, Goldstein IM, Snyderman R (Eds). New York, Raven Press, 1992, pp 325–339.
3. Golde DW, Baldwin GC: Myeloid growth factors. *In*: Inflammation: Basic Principles and Clinical Correlates. 2nd ed. Gallin JI, Goldstein IM, Snyderman R (Eds). New York, Raven Press, 1992, pp 291–301.
4. Lee SH, Starkey PM, Gordon S: Quantitative analysis of total macrophage content in adult mouse tissues. J Exp Med 1985; 161:475–489.
5. Fridman WH, Bonnerot C, Daeron M, et al: Structural bases of Fc gamma receptor functions. Immunol Rev 1992; 125:49–76.
6. Brown EJ: Complement receptors and phagocytosis. Curr Opin Immunol 1991; 3:76–82.
7. Stahl PD: The mannose receptor and other macrophage lectins. Curr Opin Immunol 1992; 4:49–52.
8. Wright SD: Multiple receptors for endotoxin. Curr Opin Immunol 1991; 3:83–90.
9. Klebanoff SJ: Oxygen metabolites from phagocytes. *In*: Inflammation: Basic Principles and Clinical Correlates. 2nd ed. Gallin JI, Goldstein IM, Snyderman R (Eds). New York, Raven Press, 1992, pp 541–588.
10. Adams DO, Hamilton TA: Macrophages as destructive cells in host defense. *In*: Inflammation: Basic Principles and Clinical Correlates. Gallin JI, Goldstein IM, Snyderman R (Eds). New York, Raven Press, 1992, pp 637–662.
11. Nathan CF: Secretory products of macrophages. J Clin Invest 1987; 79:319–326.
12. Cromack DT, Porras-Reyes B, Mustoe TA: Current concepts in wound healing: Growth factor and macrophage interaction. J Trauma 1990; 30:S129–S133.
13. Sunderkötter C, Goebeler M, Schulze-Osthoff K, et al: Macrophage-derived angiogenesis factors. Pharmacol Ther 1991; 51:195–216.
14. Harding CV: Pathways of antigen processing. Curr Opin Immunol 1991; 3:3–9.
15. Unanue ER: Cellular studies on antigen presentation by class II MHC molecules. Curr Opin Immunol 1992; 4:63–69.
16. Bancroft GJ, Schreiber RD, Unanue ER: Natural immunity: A T-cell–independent pathway of macrophage activation, defined in the scid mouse. Immunol Rev 1991; 124:5–24.
17. Nacy CA, Meltzer MS: T-cell–mediated activation of macrophages. Curr Opin Immunol 1991; 3:330–335.

CHAPTER 18

Oxygen-Derived Free Radicals

Joe M. McCord, PhD

The discovery in 1969 of the enzyme superoxide dismutase (SOD)[1] caused a certain amount of bewilderment in biologic circles. The enzyme catalyzed the seemingly unlikely radical-radical annihilation (or disproportionation) reaction of the superoxide radical ($O_2^{\cdot}$):

$$O_2^{\cdot -} + O_2^{\cdot -} + 2\,H^+ \rightarrow H_2O_2 + O_2$$

Did organisms really possess an enzyme for the purpose of getting rid of free radicals, or was this activity incidental—some sort of curious test-tube artifact? Free radicals had previously been in the domains of radiation chemists, polymer chemists, and plasma physicists, but not biologists. The existence of a free radical–scavenging enzyme implied, of course, the existence of significant biologic sources of free radical production (at least of the superoxide radical). Because the superoxide radical results from the one-electron reduction of molecular oxygen, one obvious possibility was that this radical was a common and unavoidable consequence of using oxygen as a terminal electron acceptor. If this were true, then all aerobic organisms might be expected to need this protective enzyme; strict anaerobes, on the other hand, which *die* in the presence of oxygen, might not be expected to have SOD. A quick survey of "who has SOD and who doesn't" supported this view and led to the further speculation that SOD might be an absolute necessity for oxygen-metabolizing organisms.[2] Studies have confirmed that if *Escherichia coli* is deprived of its two genes encoding SODs, the organism cannot live in oxygen on minimal medium (conditions in which all metabolic pathways are forced into operation), although it survives well anaerobically.[3]

WHAT ARE FREE RADICALS AND ACTIVE OXYGEN SPECIES?

Chemically, a free radical is any molecule containing a single, unpaired electron. Because a covalent bond is formed when a pair of electrons occupies a single molecular orbital, free radicals may be viewed as molecular fragments formed by homolytic cleavage of a bond. (Transition metal ions usually are not considered to be free radicals, although by technical definition they are.) The unpaired electron imparts paramagnetic character to the radical, which displays a characteristic absorption spectrum when placed in a magnetic field, detectable by electron paramagnetic resonance spectroscopy. Molecular oxygen is somewhat of an electronic oddity in that its ground state is a diradical, with *two* unpaired electrons of like spin. This unconventional distribution of electrons makes it impossible for oxygen to accept a spin-matched pair of electrons, as badly as it may want them, until one of its unpaired electrons undergoes a spontaneous spin reversal to make pairing possible. At ordinary collisional frequency, the period of contact is too brief, imposing a kinetic barrier to most oxidative reactions. It is this kinetic barrier that saves us from reacting explosively with an atmosphere of huge thermodynamic potential. It is the same kinetic restriction that renders oxygen an ideal terminal electron acceptor for biologic systems. Enzymes with a binding site for oxygen can keep it in contact with its reductant considerably longer than would occur by simple collision, overcoming the kinetic reluctance to react and rendering available the huge amounts of energy to be derived from giving electrons to molecular oxygen.

Our relationship with oxygen is still an uneasy one. Oxygen has great affinity for four more electrons. (The process of taking away electrons is called *oxidation* because oxygen does it so well. The substance receiving electrons becomes *reduced*.) This complete reduction of oxygen breaks the bonds holding the two nuclei together and, after picking up protons from the solvent, results in the formation of two molecules of water. Occasionally, under normal biologic conditions, oxygen does manage to steal away electrons from other molecules by nonenzymatic autoxidations. Because it cannot accommodate a spin-matched pair, it must settle for stealing electrons one at a time. This breaking up of electron pairs results in free radical formation. The one-electron reduction product of oxygen is the superoxide radical. If two electrons are transferred the product is hydrogen peroxide (H_2O_2), which is not a radical. It is nonetheless still hungry for two more electrons, causing H_2O_2 to be a cytotoxic oxidant. Ferrous iron is capable of transferring a third electron to H_2O_2, causing lysis of the oxygen-oxygen bond. One fragment is reduced to the state of water; the other fragment is the hydroxyl free radical, a highly potent oxidant. It can initiate lipid peroxidation, cause DNA strand breaks, and indiscriminately oxidize virtually any organic molecule. The fact that it is so indiscriminate actually works in our favor; most of the targets it strikes are expendable. *Reactivity* and *toxicity* are not synonymous.[4]

The family of reactive intermediates resulting from incomplete reduction of oxygen includes superoxide radical, H_2O_2, and hydroxyl radical. It is not correct to refer to this group as *oxygen-derived free radicals*, because one member is not a radical. Accordingly, several terms are now in use to refer to this family. *Reactive oxygen metabolites* or *active oxygen* or variations of these are the most common. Occasionally, the terms are intended to include electronically excited oxygen (singlet oxygen) and even hypochlorous acid, produced from H_2O_2 by neutrophil myeloperoxidase.

SUPEROXIDE AND BACTERICIDAL ACTION BY PHAGOCYTES

Nature has a knack for putting things to constructive uses. As free radical biologists were acknowledging the unavoidable production of superoxide and the protective roles of SODs, an insightful observation was made by Bernard Babior. It had long been known that neutrophils display a burst of cyanide-insensitive (i.e., nonmitochondrial) oxygen consumption when they encounter and kill microorganisms. It was further known that this resulted in H_2O_2 production,[5] which is able to kill microorganisms. Babior thought superoxide radical might be a likely candidate to participate in bactericidal action and showed that neutrophils stimulated to engulf latex particles did indeed produce this free radical.[6] The bactericidal roles of the free radical and its metabolites, H_2O_2 and hypochlorous acid, are now well understood.[7] Much subsequent work has characterized a multicomponent NADPH oxidase located in the plasma membrane of the neutrophil.[8] This enzyme may be the only enzyme in the body that produces superoxide by design rather than by accident. The genetic inability to produce superoxide in this instance causes the life-threatening condition known as chronic granulomatous disease. Neutrophils from such individuals have seriously impaired ability to kill microorganisms that have been ingested, leading to multiple recurrent local infections and often to septicemia and death at an early age.[9]

ACTIVE OXYGEN AND TISSUE INJURY

True symbiosis is relatively rare; most life forms do not tolerate being invaded by other life forms. Such a challenge usually precipitates a fight to the death of one party or the other. In higher organisms, the neutrophil is the foot soldier of this war for self preservation. It is programmed in the philosophy of the Old West: "Shoot first and ask questions later." So much is at risk that failure to carry out its mission is unacceptable. It has to be prepared to blast away at *any* antigen it does not recognize, assuming dire consequences if it allows the foreigner to survive. Hence, it is programmed for overkill, not for caution. We pay a substantial price for this ultraconservative policy. The "antibiotics" in the neutrophil's arsenal (superoxide radical, H_2O_2, and hypochlorous acid) are of the broadest possible spectrum. They are not the selective silver bullets of our modern day pharmacopoeia. Therefore, the battlefield becomes littered with casualties. Host tissues are caught in the cross-fire and succumb to the oxidant attack, along with the neutrophils themselves.[10] Infected tissues display the cardinal signs of inflammation (redness, heat, swelling, pain, and loss of function) not necessarily as a result of the invading microbe but largely because of the war waged by the attacking neutrophils and the unavoidable damage to host tissues.

SEPTIC INFLAMMATORY INJURY AND ADULT RESPIRATORY DISTRESS SYNDROME

Adult respiratory distress syndrome (ARDS) is an acute inflammatory process altering the structure and function of the lungs. The disease is a poorly understood response to diverse insults, including traumatic injury and sepsis.[11] ARDS afflicts roughly 150,000 patients annually in the United States.[12] The mortality rate is approximately 60% and has not changed since the disease was described in 1967.[13, 14]

Early descriptions of ARDS revealed neutrophils in interstitial and alveolar spaces as prominent findings.[15–17] Leukopenia associated with respiratory insufficiency has been noted in septic patients.[16] It has been hypothesized that various events known to incite ARDS cause an abnormal accumulation of adherent neutrophils in the vasculature of the lungs, possibly via complement-mediated mechanisms, and that the tissue injury resulting from neutrophil stimulation and release of oxidants contributes to the development of ARDS.[18] Because all neutrophils must pass through the lungs on every roundtrip through the circulation, because the lungs are structurally rather delicate and easily injured, and because loss of pulmonary function for even brief periods results in death, the lungs are a very vulnerable target for neutrophils, whether activated systemically or locally.

ASEPTIC INFLAMMATORY INJURY DUE TO IMMUNE COMPLEX FORMATION

If a pathogenic infection is squelched, the cost of the warfare may be justified. Often, however, the war is waged at a perceived but nonexistent or nonthreatening enemy. This is the case in autoimmune diseases and allergies. When antibody is produced against any antigen, that component is "marked" by the formation of immune complex and is now a designated target for the neutrophil. If the antigen is a soluble component, then circulating immune complex is formed. This may activate neutrophils as described earlier, or the immune complex may localize in the lungs or other tissues, attracting and activating the neutrophils and instigating tissue injury.[19] This mechanism is thought to be active in systemic lupus erythematosus[20] and the associated nephritis,[21] in Crohn's disease (ulcerative colitis or inflammatory bowel disease),[22–24] and in asthma.[25–27] Multiple sclerosis is now being viewed as a possible autoimmune disease,[28–29c] with evidence of active oxygen-mediated injury, as is rheumatoid arthritis.[30, 31] In other types of arthritis, neutrophil activation may result from physical trauma to the joint tissues (osteoarthritis or degenerative joint disease)[31, 32] or from attempts to phagocytose urate crystals (gout).[33–35]

ISCHEMIA-REPERFUSION INJURY AND FREE RADICAL PRODUCTION

A very important family of diseases affecting millions of Americans results from transient circulatory insufficiency to the heart, brain, and other organs. When tissues are injured by ischemia or anoxia, their ability to control the metabolism of oxygen is compromised.[36] Accordingly, reperfusion or reoxygenation causes enhanced free radical production and associated tissue injury and functional impairment. Injured tissues may produce the superoxide radical by several mechanisms, quite apart from neutrophils. These mechanisms have been studied in buffer-perfused isolated organ preparations in which no neutrophils are present.

In tissues containing abundant xanthine dehydrogenase, this enzyme becomes an important source of superoxide on tissue reoxygenation. During ischemia, massive catabolism of the adenine nucleotide pool occurs as a result of the low energy status of the tissue. Adenosine is broken down to inosine and then to hypoxanthine, which accumulates in abundance.[37] Although about 10% of any tissue's xanthine dehydrogenase exists as an oxygen-utilizing superoxide-producing xanthine oxidase, ischemia-induced proteolytic conversion appears to result in even more of the radical-producing form of the enzyme.[36] Hence, a period of ischemia is followed by production of xanthine oxidase (preexisting or newly converted) and an abundance of its purine substrate hypoxanthine. At reperfusion, the remaining substrate, molecular oxygen, reenters the tissue and a burst of superoxide production ensues. Reperfused organs are dramatically protected by inhibitors of xanthine oxidase or by SOD.[38–40] Great tissue and species variability is noted in terms of the content of xanthine dehydrogenase/oxidase. Both rats and dogs contain at least several orders of magnitude higher amounts of xanthine oxidase in their hearts than do rabbits, pigs, and humans.[41–43] The author and others have used the rabbit heart as a model of the xanthine oxidase–deficient human heart. Enzyme-inhibiting doses of allopurinol do not protect the rabbit heart, although protection is still afforded by SOD.[44, 45] This finding implies the existence of xanthine oxidase–independent mechanisms of superoxide production, most likely resulting from ischemic injury to the mitochondria.[46]

In vivo, ischemia-reperfusion injury invariably involves subsequent inflammatory injury.[47] In fact, antineutrophil measures such as administration of an antiadherence monoclonal antibody provide nearly complete suppression of injury to the postischemic feline intestine.[48] If protection in this model may be provided by inhibitors of xanthine oxidase,[40] by SOD,[39] or by antineutrophil measures,[48] how can all these studies be reconciled? The answer seems to lie in the temporal sequence of the events. Relatively small amounts of superoxide radical may be produced in the reperfused tissue by xanthine oxidase, immediately on reperfusion. This superoxide may be insufficient in amount to cause massive tissue injury by itself, but it can initiate an infiltration of neutrophils by activation of a superoxide-dependent chemoattractant.[49] This chemoattractant is activated in even greater amount with the arrival of the first wave of neutrophils, which on stimulation by components leaking from the damaged tissue generate still more superoxide. The factor thus serves to amplify and maintain the process of chemotaxis. Most of the tissue injury results from the oxidants generated by huge numbers of neutrophils invading the tissue. Xanthine oxidase inhibitors, then, block the initial influx of neutrophils. SOD inhibits the initial chemotaxis as well as the amplified and maintenance phases of chemotaxis. Antiadhesion antibodies prevent diapedesis of neutrophils, and thus no infiltration occurs.

IRON EXACERBATES FREE RADICAL INJURY—AND MOST OF US ARE IRON OVERLOADED

From the time it was first realized that iron is a necessary trace element, essential for life itself, the natural tendency was to assume that more must be better. Physicians and scientists were no more immune from this line of reasoning than the rest of society. Accordingly, for several decades we have been sold on the idea of iron-fortified foods, in many cases to our eventual detriment.

When it was realized that biologic systems can produce free radicals and other potent oxidants, the natural tendency of conventional wisdom was to label the oxidants as "bad" and the antioxidants as "good." Things are rarely so simple. Now, after two decades of contemplation and experimentation, there is a growing recognition that a *balance* between oxidants and antioxidants is a more realistic depiction of the relationship. There were many early clues, most of which were ignored or dismissed because of their circumstantial nature or possibly just because they flew in the face of conventional wisdom. With the recognition that life must carefully juggle oxidants against antioxidants has come the recognition that iron, as the most common redox-active transition element present in biologic systems, is an active participant in this precarious balancing act. From a physiologic or clinical perspective, the important point to appreciate is that iron may seriously exacerbate any oxidative stress.

Soon after the discovery that biologic systems can produce superoxide, evidence suggested that in some cases superoxide radical was not acting alone. It appeared to be collaborating with H_2O_2 (the product of its dismutation) to produce a species with much greater oxidizing potential than either of the coconspirators.[50] This new species was presumed to be the hydroxyl radical ($HO^{\cdot}$), one of the most potent oxidants known. It was thought to be generated via a reaction first proposed in 1934 by Haber and Weiss[51]:

$$O_2^{\cdot -} + H_2O_2 \rightarrow O_2 + HO^{\cdot}_2 OH^- \quad \text{[Reaction 1]}$$

Weinstein and Bielski reported the rate constant for this reaction to be so slow that it precluded biologic relevance.[52] Iron, however, was found to catalyze the reaction[53, 54]:

$$O_2^{\cdot -} + Fe^{3+} \rightarrow O_2 + Fe^{2+} \quad \text{[Reaction 2]}$$

$$Fe^{2+} + H_2O_2 \rightarrow Fe^{3+} + HO^{\cdot} + OH^- \quad \text{[Reaction 3]}$$

$$O_2^{\cdot -} + H_2O_2 \rightarrow O_2 + HO^{\cdot} + OH^- \quad \text{[Reaction 1]}$$

This combination of reactions is now commonly referred to as the *iron-catalyzed Haber-Weiss reaction* or as *superoxide-driven Fenton chemistry*, because Reaction 3 had been proposed much earlier by Fenton.[55] It seems proper as well to refer to it simply as Haber-Weiss chemistry, because these researchers postulated all three reactions.[51]

Higher organisms are particularly fastidious about the handling of iron. "Free" or loosely chelated iron is never present in the healthy state. It is transported in the ferric state, bound to transferrin, in a complex that is especially difficult to reduce. Likewise, it is stored in the ferric state by ferritin, a protein found in virtually all tissues and in plasma. Importantly, the superoxide radical is capable of reducing ferritin-bound iron to the ferrous state, whereupon it is released[56, 57]:

$$O_2^{\cdot -} + \text{ferritin-}Fe^{3+} \rightarrow O_2 + \text{ferritin} + Fe^{2+} \quad \text{[Reaction 4]}$$

It is this iron, liberated by the pathologic production of superoxide, that is now free to catalyze Haber-Weiss chemistry. The hydroxyl radical so produced can initiate lipid peroxidation, a free radical chain reaction leading to loss of membrane structure and function. The hydroxyl radical can also attack structural macromolecules[58] and cause deoxyribonucleic acid breaks.[59] The liberated iron can also cause the reductive lysis of the oxygen-oxygen bond in a preexisting lipid hydroperoxide molecule, giving rise to a lipid alkoxyl radical ($LO^{\cdot}$), which may then serve as an initiating radical for lipid peroxidation:

Initiation: $Fe^{2+} + LOOH \rightarrow Fe^{3+} + LO^{\cdot} + OH^-$ [Reaction 5]

$LO^{\cdot} + LH \rightarrow LOH + L^{\cdot}$ [Reaction 6]

Propagation: $L^{\cdot} + O_2 \rightarrow LOO^{\cdot}$ [Reaction 7]

$LOO^{\cdot} + LH \rightarrow LOOH + L^{\cdot}$ [Reaction 8]

If "liberated" iron can seriously exacerbate the component of tissue injury as a result of free radical production, the question arises about whether iron status from a nutritional standpoint might be a predisposing factor in all of the disease states discussed earlier. American males accumulate total body iron stores almost linearly after puberty, commonly reaching iron stores of 2 g or more.[60] Women are protected until the age of menopause, after which time their iron accumulation parallels that of men. The body absorbs dietary iron with an efficiency of about 10%, but it has no mechanism to get rid of excess iron. A study by van der Kraaij and colleagues[61] experimentally addressed the question of whether iron status may affect the extent of reperfusion injury by comparing hearts from normal versus iron-supplemented rats. Langendorff hearts were subjected to 45 minutes of anoxic perfusion, followed by reoxygenation. Under normoxia, the groups behaved identically. After a period of anoxia, however, the iron-loaded hearts displayed ventricular fibrillation and significantly lower recovery of contractility, both of which were returned to control values by perfusion with deferoxamine, a chelator that prevents iron from redox cycling. An ongoing prospective human study has concluded that iron *sufficiency* is associated with hypertension and excess risk of heart attack.[62, 62a] In a study of patients with small cell carcinoma of the lung, Milman and associates[63] found that those patients with the lowest serum ferritin levels at the time of diagnosis had significantly longer survival times.

THE OXIDANT-ANTIOXIDANT BALANCE

In healthy organisms, a relatively delicate balance is maintained among oxidants (such as active oxygen species and transition metals) and antioxidants (such as SOD, catalase, and vitamins E, C, and A). Under pathologic conditions, the balance may be tilted toward the oxidative side as outlined earlier, with the end result being uncontrolled and potentially lethal lipid peroxidation. The antioxidant vitamins E (lipid soluble) and C (water soluble) collaborate to terminate lipid peroxidation chain reactions. A summary of a number of European population studies underscores the protective role of the antioxidant vitamins in heart disease.[64] This study correlated mortality due to ischemic heart disease with two factors considered to be major risk factors, hypertension and serum cholesterol value, as well as with serum vitamin E levels. The correlation was stronger versus vitamin E than with either of the other two factors: The higher the plasma vitamin E level, the lower the mortality rate from heart disease.[64a, 64b]

CONCLUSION

A number of factors contribute to a nearly ubiquitous role for oxygen radical generation under pathologic circumstances. Oxygen is prone to radical generation because of a quirk in its electronic structure. Virtually all cells must deal with the chemically tricky reduction of oxygen in order to generate energy. The fact that neutrophils have learned to put cytotoxic active oxygen to a constructive, bactericidal use is a mixed blessing. Although it saves us from infection, it has enormous potential for host tissue destruction when generated inappropriately, as in autoimmunity.

References

1. McCord JM, Fridovich I: Superoxide dismutase: An enzymic function for erythrocuprein (Hemocuprein). J Biol Chem 1969; 244:6049–6055.
2. McCord JM, Keele BB Jr, Fridovich I: An enzyme-based theory of obligate anaerobiosis: The physiological function of superoxide dismutase. Proc Natl Acad Sci U S A 1971; 68:1024–1027.
3. Natvig DO, Imlay K, Touati D, et al: Human copper-zinc superoxide dismutase complements superoxide dismutase–deficient *Escherichia coli* mutants. J Biol Chem 1987; 262:14697–14701.
4. McCord JM: Superoxide production and human disease. *In*: Molecular Basis of Oxidative Damage by Leukocytes. Jesaitis A, Dratz E (Eds). Boca Raton, CRC Press, 1992, p 225.
5. Iyer GYN, Islam MF, Quastel JH: Biochemical aspects of phagocytosis. Nature 1961; 192:535–541.
6. Babior BM, Kipnes RS, Curnutte JT: Biological defense mechanisms. The production by leukocytes of superoxide, a potential bactericidal agent. J Clin Invest 1973; 52:741–744.
7. Babior BM: Oxygen-dependent microbial killing by phagocytes. N Engl J Med 1978; 298:659–668, 721–725.
8. Babior BM: The respiratory burst oxidase. Trends Biochem Sci 1987; 12:241–243.
9. Babior BM: The respiratory burst oxidase and the molecular basis of chronic granulomatous disease. Am J Hematol 1991; 37:263–266.
10. Salin ML, McCord JM: Free radicals and inflammation: Protection of phagocytosing leukocytes by superoxide dismutase. J Clin Invest 1975; 56:1319–1323.
11. Fowler AA, Hamman RF, Good JT, et al: Adult respiratory distress syndrome: Risk with common predispositions. Ann Intern Med 1983; 98:593–597.
12. Repine JE: Scientific perspectives on adult respiratory distress syndrome. Lancet 1992; 339:466–469.
13. Ashbaugh DG, Bigelow DB, Petty TL, et al: Acute respiratory distress in adults. Lancet 1967; 2:319–323.
14. Bernard GR, Luce JM, Sprung CL, et al: High-dose corticosteroids in patients with the adult respiratory distress syndrome. N Engl J Med 1987; 317:1565–1570.
15. Ratliff NB, Wilson JW, Mikat E, et al: The lung in hemorrhagic shock. IV. The role of the polymorphonuclear leukocyte. Am J Pathol 1971; 65:325–334.
16. Bachofen M, Weibel ER: Alterations of the gas exchange apparatus in adult respiratory insufficiency associated with septicemia. Am Rev Respir Dis 1977; 116:589–615.
17. Pratt PC: Pathology of adult respiratory distress syndrome. *In*: The Lung: Structure, Function and Disease. Thurlbeck WM, Abell MR (Eds). Baltimore, Williams & Wilkins, 1978, p 43.
18. Tate RM, Repine JE: Neutrophils and the adult respiratory distress syndrome. Am Rev Respir Dis 1983; 128:552–559.
19. Strauss AL, Coe FL, Deutsch L, et al: Factors that predict relapse of calcium nephrolithiasis during treatment: A prospective study. Am J Med 1982; 72:17–24.
20. Jiang XX, Chen FW: The effect of lipid peroxides and superoxide dismutase on systemic lupus erythematosus—a preliminary study. Clin Immunol Immunopathol 1992; 63:39–44.
21. Sato T, Nishikawa M, Higuchi C, et al: Effect of SOD on lupus nephritis. *In*: Medical, Biochemical and Chemical Aspects of Free Radicals. Hayaishi O, Niki E, Kondo M, Yoshikawa T (Eds). Amsterdam, Elsevier Science, 1989, p 735.
22. Emerit J, Pelletier S, Tosoni-Verlignue D, et al: Phase II trial of copper zinc superoxide dismutase (CuZnSOD) in treatment of Crohn's disease. Free Radic Biol Med 1989; 7:145–149.
23. Curran FT, Allan RN, Keighley MRB: Superoxide production by Crohn's disease neutrophils. Gut 1991; 32:399–402.
24. Simmonds NJ, Allen RE, Stevens TRJ, et al: Chemiluminescence assay of mucosal reactive oxygen metabolites in inflammatory bowel disease. Gastroenterology 1992; 103:186–196.
25. Owen S, Pearson D, Suarezmendez V, et al: Evidence of free-radical activity in asthma. N Engl J Med 1991; 325:586–587.
26. Novak Z, Nemeth I, Gyurkovits K, et al: Examination of the role of oxygen free radicals in bronchial asthma in childhood. Clin Chim Acta 1991; 201:247–251.
27. Barnes PJ: Reactive oxygen species and airway inflammation. Free Radic Biol Med 1990; 9:235–243.
28. Hammann KP, Hopf HC: The significance of the inflammatory reactions for the development of clinical signs in multiple sclerosis and acute experimental autoimmune encephalomyelitis as assessed by means of the spontaneous chemiluminescence activity of peripheral blood monocytes. J Neuroimmunol 1988; 20:239–241.
29. Fisher M, Levine PH, Weiner BH, et al: Monocyte and polymorphonuclear leukocyte toxic oxygen metabolite production in multiple sclerosis. Inflammation 1988; 12:123–131.

29a. Fisher M, Plante GM, Doyle EM: Inhibition of inflammatory cell-mediated myelin oxidation and interleukin-1 beta generation by a 21-aminosteroid, U74500A. J Neurol Sci 1993; 119:189–194.

29b. Antel JP, Williams K, Blain M, et al: Oligodendrocyte lysis by CD4(+) t cells independent of tumor necrosis factor. Ann Neurol 1994; 35:341–348.

29c. Lehmann D, Karussis D, Misrachikoll R, et al: Oral administration of the oxidant-scavenger N-acetyl-L-cysteine inhibits acute experimental autoimmune encephalomyelitis. J Neuroimmunol 1994; 50:35–42.

30. Todoroki T, Shingu M, Ezaki I, et al: Superoxide generation by synovial fluid neutrophils enhanced by immune complexes and suppressed by rheumatoid factor in synovial fluid. Rheumatol Int 1986; 6:133–137.
31. Biemond P, Swaak AJ, Penders JM, et al: Superoxide production by polymorphonuclear leucocytes in rheumatoid arthritis and osteoarthritis: In vivo inhibition by the antirheumatic drug piroxicam due to interference with the activation of the NADPH-oxidase. Ann Rheum Dis 1986; 45:249–255.
32. Chen BX, Francis MJ, Duthie RB, et al: Oxygen free radical in human osteoarthritis. Chin Med J (Engl) 1989; 102:931–933.
33. Higson FK, Jones OT: Oxygen radical production by horse and pig neutrophils induced by a range of crystals. J Rheumatol 1984; 11:735–740.
34. Rosen MS, Baker DG, Schumacher HR Jr, et al: Products of polymorphonuclear cell injury inhibit IgG enhancement of monosodium urate–induced superoxide production. Arthritis Rheum 1986; 29:1473–1479.
35. Marcolongo R, Calabria AA, Mazzullo G, et al: The "switch-off" mechanism of spontaneous resolution of acute gout attack. Adv Exp Med Biol 1986; 195 (Pt A):371–379.
36. McCord JM: Oxygen-derived free radicals in post-ischemic tissue injury. N Engl J Med 1985; 312:159–163.
37. Saugstad OD, Schrader H, Aasen AO: Alteration of the hypoxanthine level in cerebrospinal fluid as an indicator of tissue hypoxia. Brain Res 1976; 112:188–189.
38. Granger DN, Rutili G, McCord JM: Superoxide radicals in feline intestinal ischemia. Gastroenterology 1981; 81:22–29.
39. Parks DA, Bulkley GB, Granger DN, et al: Ischemic injury in the cat small intestine: Role of superoxide radicals. Gastroenterology 1982; 82:9–15.

40. Granger DN, McCord JM, Parks DA, et al: Xanthine oxidase inhibitors attenuate ischemia-induced vascular permeability changes in the cat intestine. Gastroenterology 1986; 90:80–84.
41. Grum CM, Ragsdale RA, Ketai LH, et al: Absence of xanthine oxidase or xanthine dehydrogenase in the rabbit myocardium. Biochem Biophys Res Commun 1986; 141:1104–1108.
42. Parks DA, Granger DN: Xanthine oxidase: Biochemistry, distribution and physiology. Acta Physiol Scand 1986; 126(Suppl 548):87–99.
43. Eddy LJ, Stewart JR, Jones HP, et al: Free radical–producing enzyme, xanthine oxidase, is undetectable in human hearts. Am J Physiol 1987; 253(Heart 22):H709–H711.
44. McCord JM, Omar BA, Russell WJ: Sources of oxygen-derived radicals in ischemia-reperfusion. *In*: Medical, Biochemical, and Chemical Aspects of Free Radicals. Hayaishi O, Niki E, Kondo M, et al (Eds). Amsterdam, Elsevier Science, 1989, p 1113.
45. Downey J, Chambers D, Miura T, et al: Allopurinol fails to limit infarct size in a xanthine oxidase–deficient species. Circulation 1986; 74(Suppl II):372.
46. Turrens JF, Beconi M, Barilla J, et al: Mitochondrial generation of oxygen radicals during reoxygenation of ischemic tissues. Free Radic Res Commun 1991; 12–13:681–689.
47. McCord JM: Oxygen-derived radicals: A link between reperfusion injury and inflammation. Fed Proc 1987; 46:2402–2406.
48. Hernandez LA, Grisham MB, Twohig B, et al: Role of neutrophils in ischemia-reperfusion–induced microvascular injury. Am J Physiol 1987; 253(HCP 22):H699–H703.
49. Petrone WF, English DK, Wong K, et al: Free radicals and inflammation: Superoxide-dependent activation of a neutrophil chemotactic factor in plasma. Proc Natl Acad Sci U S A 1980; 77: 1159–1163.
50. Beauchamp C, Fridovich I: A mechanism for the production of ethylene from methional. The generation of the hydroxyl radical by xanthine oxidase. J Biol Chem 1970; 245:4641–4646.
51. Haber F, Weiss J: The catalytic decomposition of hydrogen peroxide by iron salts. Proc R Soc Lond [Biol] Ser A 1934; 147:332–351.
52. Weinstein J, Bielski BHJ: Kinetics of the interaction of HO_2 and O_2^- radicals with hydrogen peroxide. The Haber-Weiss reaction. J Am Chem Soc 1979; 101:58–62.
53. McCord JM, Day ED Jr: Superoxide-dependent production of hydroxyl radical catalyzed by iron-EDTA complex. FEBS Lett 1978; 86:139–142.
54. Halliwell B: Superoxide-dependent formation of hydroxyl radicals in the presence of iron chelates. FEBS Lett 1978; 92:321–326.
55. Fenton HJH: Oxidation of tartaric acid in the presence of iron. J Chem Soc 1894; 65:899–903.
56. Biemond P, van Eijk HG, Swaak AJG, et al: Iron mobilization from ferritin by superoxide derived from stimulated polymorphonuclear leukocytes. Possible mechanism in inflammation diseases. J Clin Invest 1984; 73:1576–1579.
57. Biemond P, Swaak AJ, Beindorff CM, et al: Superoxide-dependent and -independent mechanisms of iron mobilization from ferritin by xanthine oxidase. Implications for oxygen-free-radical–induced tissue destruction during ischaemia and inflammation. Biochem J 1986; 239:169–173.
58. McCord JM: Free radicals and inflammation: Protection of synovial fluid by superoxide dismutase. Science 1974; 185:529–531.
59. Imlay JA, Linn S: DNA damage and oxygen radical toxicity. Science 1988; 240:1302–1309.
60. Cook JD, Finch CA, Smith NJ: Evaluation of the iron status of a population. Blood 1976; 48:449–455.
61. Van der Kraaij AMM, Mostert LJ, van Eijk HG, et al: Iron-load increases the susceptibility of rat hearts to oxygen reperfusion damage: Protection by the antioxidant (+)-cyanidanol-3 and deferoxamine. Circulation 1988; 78:442–449.
62. Salonen JT, Salonen R, Nyyssonen K, et al: Iron sufficiency is associated with hypertension and excess risk of myocardial infarction: The Kuopio Ischaemic Heart Disease Risk Factor Study (KIHD). Circulation 1992; 85:864.
62a. Salonen JT, Nyyssonen K, Korpela H, et al: High stored iron levels are associated with excess risk of myocardial infarction in eastern Finnish men. Circulation 1992; 86:803–811.
63. Milman N, Sengelov H, Dombernowsky P: Iron status markers in patients with small cell carcinoma of the lung—relation to survival. Br J Cancer 1991; 64:895–898.
64. Gey KF, Puska P, Jordan P, et al: Inverse correlation between plasma vitamin E and mortality from ischemic heart disease in cross-cultural epidemiology. Am J Clin Nutr 1991; 53(Suppl): 326S–334S.
64a. Stampfer MJ, Hennekens CH, Manson JE, et al: Vitamin E consumption and the risk of coronary disease in women. N Engl J Med 1993; 328:1444–1449.
64b. Rimm EB, Stampfer MJ, Ascherio A, et al: Vitamin E consumption and the risk of coronary heart disease in men. N Engl J Med 1993; 328:1450–1456.

CHAPTER 19

Prostaglandins, Thromboxanes, Leukotrienes, and Other Products of Arachidonic Acid

Perry V. Halushka, PhD, MD • Janet Geisel, MSN, RN • H. David Reines, MD, FACS, FCCM • James A. Cook, PhD

The first report of the biologic activity of what was subsequently identified as prostaglandins was in 1930,[1] when it was found that extracts of seminal fluid contracted uterine tissue. von Euler[2] attributed the activity of the extract to lipid substances, and because he thought that they came from the prostate named them *prostaglandins.* The structures of two of the prostaglandins (PGE_2 and $PGF_{1\alpha}$) were subsequently elucidated using gas chromatography–mass spectrometry, and with this discovery, research in the field rapidly grew.[3] Thromboxane B_2 (TXB_2) was isolated by Samuelsson and colleagues[4] in 1978 from human platelets. It was the stable metabolite of TXA_2, whose structure was deduced at the time and subsequently was proved to be correct. The name *thromboxane* was chosen because it caused platelet aggregation (thrombosis) and has an oxetane ring system. It was ultimately shown that rabbit aorta–contracting substance was TXA_2.[5] Prostacyclin (PGI_2) was discovered in 1976.[6]

The next major group of arachidonic acid metabolites to be discovered and characterized were the leukotrienes. They derived their name from the observations that they were made by leukocytes and had triene structures.[7] The sulfidopeptide leukotrienes were shown to be the active principles of slow-reacting substance of anaphylaxis (SRS), released from mast cells and neutrophils.[7] Arachidonic acid, dihomo-γ-linolenic acid, and eicosapentaenoic acid are precursors of prostaglandins, thromboxanes, and leukotrienes. The former two are also known as *eicosatetraenoic acid* and *eicosatrienoic acid*, respectively; thus, the name *eicosanoids* is used generically to name the products of these fatty acids.

NOMENCLATURE

The products of fatty acid cyclooxygenase and lipoxygenase pathways are all named with a letter and a number. The letters in the cyclooxygenase pathway metabolites refer to the substitutions on the cyclopentane ring, and in the leukotriene pathway the letters refer to the amino acids coupled to the fatty acid.[7] The numbers refer to the number of double bonds present on the side chains.

SITES OF SYNTHESIS AND PHARMACOLOGIC ACTIVITY OF THE EICOSANOIDS

Fatty Acid Cyclooxygenase Products

The pathway for the metabolism of arachidonic acid is shown in Figure 19–1. PGA, PGB, and PGC are nonenzymatic dehydration products of PGE_2 and are considered artifacts of the extraction procedures. However, PGA is a vasodilator. PGD_2 is synthesized in large quantities by mast cells, being the major cyclooxygenase metabolite in this cell. It and its major metabolite $9\alpha,11\beta,PGF_2$ are potent bronchoconstrictors and are overproduced in mastocytosis.[8] Depending on the vascular bed, it may be either a vasoconstrictor or vasodilator. Vasodilation usually occurs at the lower doses; however, it constricts only the pulmonary artery. It is also synthesized by platelets and inhibits platelet aggregation via increasing intraplatelet cyclic adenosine monophosphate (cAMP) levels. It has yet to be determined if its synthesis is increased in shock.

PGE_2 is synthesized mainly by the kidneys, platelets, and blood vessels but is also synthesized by many other tissues in smaller amounts. It is a vasodilator, natriuretic, and diuretic; it inhibits gastric acid secretion and contracts uterine tissue. Three subtypes of receptors have been identified for PGE_2. They are associated with either stimulation or inhibition of adenylate cyclase and stimulation of phospholipase C.[8] PGE_2 synthesis is significantly increased in shock syndromes (discussed later).

$PGF_{2\alpha}$ is synthesized in many tissues in variable amounts. It is an effective bronchoconstrictor and venoconstrictor, and it contracts uterine smooth muscle. Its synthesis is also increased in sepsis.

PGI_2 is made in large quantities by endothelial cells, macrophages, the lungs, and the kidneys. It is a vasodilator and antiaggregatory substance. It is unstable and has a half-life of about 10 minutes and spontaneously hydrolyzes to form 6-keto-$PGF_{1\alpha}$. The major urinary metabolite of 6-keto-$PGF_{1\alpha}$ is 2,3-dinor-6-keto-$PGF_{1\alpha}$. PGI_2 is a potent stimulator of adenylate cyclase. To date, only one class of receptors has been identified for it.

TXA_2 is synthesized in large quantities by platelets, macrophages, monocytes, and the lungs. It is unstable and has a half-life of only 30 seconds and spontaneously hydrolyzes to form the stable but inactive TXB_2. The major plasma metabolite of TXB_2 is 11-dehydro-TXB_2. The major urinary metabolites are 11-dehydro-TXB_2 and 2,3-dinor-TXB_2. TXA_2 is a very potent vasoconstrictor, bronchoconstrictor, and proaggregatory substance. At least two subtypes of receptors have been identified for TXA_2, the platelet and the vascular smooth muscle cell receptors.[8] Its synthesis is markedly increased in shock syndromes.

Leukotriene B_4 (LTB_4) is synthesized by white blood cells, macrophages, and synovial cells. It is a very potent chemotactic substance for white blood cells.

LTC_4 is synthesized by white blood cells, lung parenchymal tissue, and macrophages. It is converted to LTD_4, the active metabolite of LTC_4. It is a vasoconstrictor and bronchoconstrictor, and it increases capillary permeability and bronchial mucus secretion. Its synthesis is increased during sepsis and adult respiratory distress syndrome (ARDS).[9] The urinary excretion of *N*-acetyl LTE_4, a metabolite of LTD_4, is increased in ARDS and shock.[10]

Arachidonic Acid Release

Release of arachidonic acid from membrane phospholipids is the rate-limiting step in the formation of eicosanoids in nonpathologic states.[11] Stimulation of cells by hormonal and nonhormonal agonists results in activation of phospholipases A_2 and C. Activation of phospholipase A_2 results in the

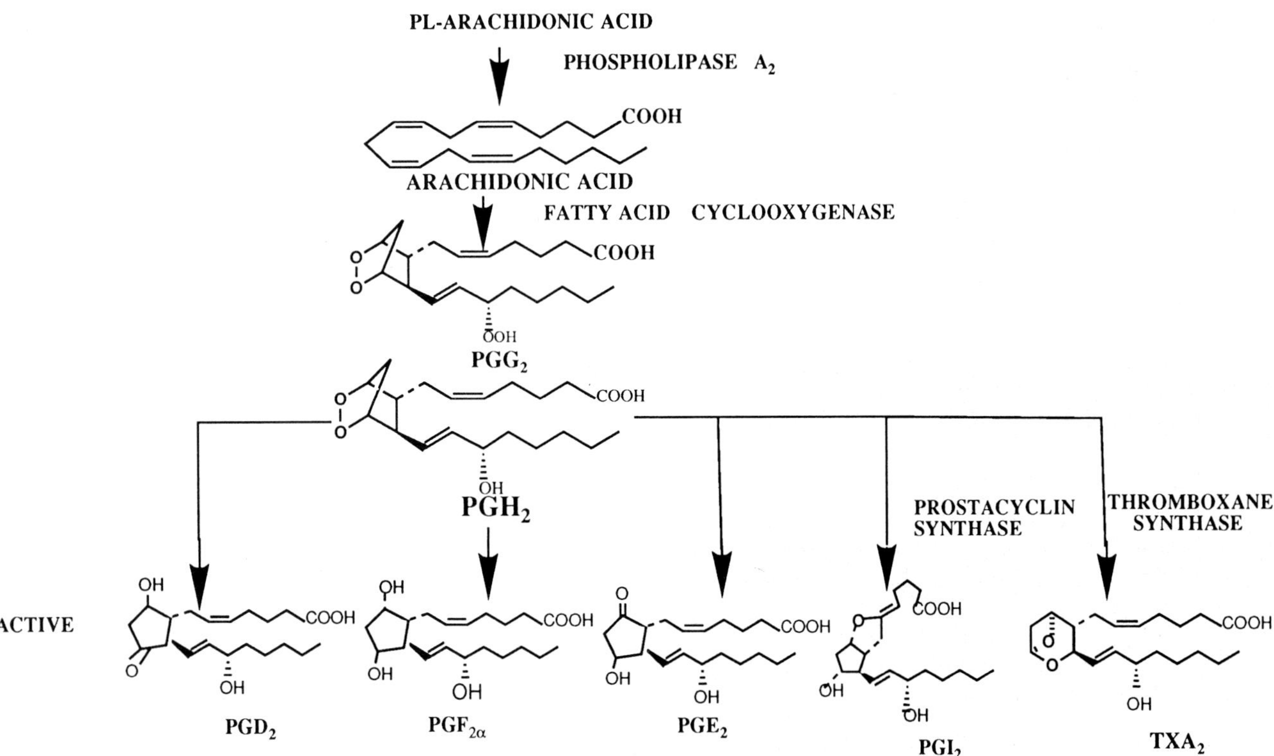

Figure 19–1. Metabolism of arachidonic acid. (From Wagner TR, Halushka PV, Cook JA: Cyclooxygenase products in septic and endotoxic shock. *In*: Handbook of Mediators in Septic Shock. Neugebauer EA, Holaday JW [Eds]. Boca Raton, CRC Press, 1993, pp 395–418. Used with permission.)

release of arachidonic acid from the Sn2 position of phosphatidylcholine, and phosphatidylethanolamine.[12] Isozymes of phospholipase A_2 have been demonstrated to have specificity for catalyzing the release of arachidonic acid preferentially from either phosphatidylcholine or phosphatidylethanolamine.[13] In the other pathway, phospholipase C cleaves phosphatidylinositol 4,5-bisphosphate, resulting in inositol 1,4,5-trisphosphate and 1,2-diacylglycerol, both of which function as intracellular second messengers.[14–17] Diglyceride lipase then releases the arachidonic acid from the diacylglycerol.[18, 19]

The particular phospholipid substrate providing arachidonic acid in response to a specific stimulus may influence whether lipoxygenase or fatty acid cyclooxygenase products are formed. Resident murine macrophages in response to stimuli that activate the lipoxygenase pathway demonstrate dependence on the phospholipase C–diglyceride lipase pathway,[20] whereas endotoxin or phorbol myristate acetate–induced prostaglandin formation is independent of the phospholipase C–diglyceride lipase pathway.

Prostaglandin H Synthase (Fatty Acid Cyclooxygenase)

PGH synthase catalyzes the committed step in the conversion of arachidonic acid to the prostaglandin endoperoxides PGG_2 and PGH_2.[21] PGH_2 is the direct precursor for primary prostaglandins and TXA_2. PGH synthase has been found in most of the organs of all mammalian species but not in all cell types.[22] Subcellular studies demonstrate that PGH synthase is an integral membrane protein concentrated in the endoplasmic reticulum, as well as in the nuclear envelope and the plasma membrane.[22, 23] PGH synthase is approximately 68,000 daltons with species variations attributed to different amounts of *N*-glycosylation and mannose carbohydrate side chains.[24] Two sites of enzymatic activity have been proposed,[25] and heme binding sites are conserved.[26]

PGH synthase possesses two enzymatic activities.[27] The first activity cyclizes an oxygen molecule in a bis-dioxygenase configuration at carbon-9 (C-9) and C-11, converting arachidonic acid to PGG_2. PGH synthase then uses another oxygen molecule to peroxidize this unstable metabolite at C-15, converting PGG_2 into PGH_2. The bound heme of PGH synthase is believed to act as the electron transfer site in these reactions. PGH_2 is the substrate for the enzymes responsible for the synthesis of prostaglandins D_2, E_2, $F_{2\alpha}$, and I_2 and TXA_2, the final product profile being dependent on the specific cell type.

Many fatty acids are substrates for PGH synthase, but arachidonic acid is the most common in vivo.[21] PGH synthase is inhibited by aspirin and all the nonsteroidal anti-inflammatory agents (NSAIDs). Aspirin irreversibly inhibits the enzyme by covalently acetylating a serine residue. In platelets, the inhibition lasts for the life of the platelet (7–10 d) because platelets are not capable of synthesizing new enzyme.

Induction of Prostaglandin Synthase

In response to many agents, the production of eicosanoids appears to be regulated by a combination of arachidonic acid release and induction of additional PGH synthase enzyme protein. Tsai and colleagues[28] have suggested that PGH synthase may reside in two distinct pools—a "constitutive pool" with a long half-life that is inaccessible to released arachidonic acid and a phorbol "stimulated pool" that is an active enzyme with a short half-life. Various mitogens, hormones, and biologic agents that have been reported to induce PGH synthase are epidermal growth factor, platelet-derived growth factor, phorbol myristate acetate, interleukin-1, interleukin-2, and cAMP.[29, 29a–29c] Evidence has been shown that early response genes of the Swiss 3T3 and the chicken embryo fibroblasts code for a unique PGH synthase protein. Two distinct messenger ribonucleic acids (mRNAs) for PGH synthase have also been identified in sheep tracheal mucosa epithelial cells and in cultured rat mesangial cells. The evidence is that a second gene for PGH synthase exists and is transcribed into an mRNA for a PGH synthase isozyme. The latter isoenzyme, designated *PGH synthase-2,* has been cloned from chicken and mouse cells as an early response gene to biologic activators.[29]

Bacterial endotoxin can also induce the synthesis of PGH synthase-2. De novo induction of PGH synthase-2 in murine peritoneal macrophages[30] and human monocytes[31] is blocked by pretreatment with dexamethasone. Also, intravenous endotoxin injection in adrenalectomized mice results in a two- to three-fold induction of PGH synthase-2.[32] Masferrer and colleagues[32] proposed that PGH synthase-1 is a constitutive enzyme present in most cells and tissues and is unaffected by steroids, whereas PGH synthase-2, whose induction is blocked by exogenous steroids in response to endotoxin and interleukin-1 in proinflammatory cells (e.g., macrophages), is under tonic control of endogenous steroids as well. Lee and associates[33] demonstrated that newly synthetized PGH synthase-2 has a role in endotoxin priming of rat alveolar macrophages to synthesize TXB_2 by zymosan. Northern blot analysis using cloned deoxyribonucleic acid probes to the mitogen-inducible PGH synthase demonstrated induction of mRNA specific for the synthase. Thus, induction of the rabbit homologue of PGH synthase-2 may play a part in endotoxin priming for eicosanoid production. These results further corroborate an important role of endotoxin-induced de novo PGH synthase-2 and eicosanoid production. This PGH isozyme has been described as the predominant PGH synthase in inflammatory reactions because of its responsiveness to stimuli and inhibition by dexamethasone.[32, 33a]

Lipoxygenase

The lipoxygenase pathways of arachidonic acid metabolism involve three species of lipoxygenases-5-lipoxygenase, 12-lipoxygenase, and 15-lipoxygenase.[34–36] These enzymes insert a molecule of oxygen into arachidonic acid, respectively, at C-5, C-12, and C-15, forming the 5-, 12-, and 15-hydroxyeicostatetraenoic acids (HETEs). 5-Lipoxygenase demonstrates several unique characteristics compared with the other human lipoxygenases. It is dependent on adenosine triphosphate and Ca^{2+} for activation as well as three additional components.[37, 38] One of these components is an 18-kd protein that is required for both the translocation and activation of 5-lipoxygenase.[37, 39] This protein has been named *5-lipoxygenase–activating protein.* The 5-lipoxygenase metabolizes arachidonic acid to 5-hydroperoxy-eicosatetraenoic acid (5-HPETE). 5-HPETE is further metabolized to 5-HETE and LTA_4. LTA_4 is an unstable intermediate that is rapidly metabolized to LTB_4 by LTA_4 hydrolase, to LTC_4 by LTC_4 synthase, and to other metabolites by nonenzymatic reactions. LTC_4 consists of glutathione covalently bound to arachidonic acid at the C-6 position (a sulfidopeptide leukotriene). The glutamic acid moiety of glutathione is cleaved by a γ-glutamyltranspeptidase to produce LTD_4. LTD_4 is further metabolized by a peptidase or a cysteinylglycinase to form LTE_4. LTE_4 can be *N*-acetylated and subsequently excreted in the urine.

The 12-lipoxygenase metabolizes arachidonic acid to 12-

HPETE and the subsequent metabolites, di-HETE and tri-HETE. 12-Lipoxygenase is found in platelets and is the predominant lipoxygenase in brain tissue. 15-Lipoxygenase is approximately 70 kilodaltons.[40] Its activity is preferentially expressed only in certain cells,[41] but the biologic role of 15-lipoxygenase in these cell types is not fully understood.[42]

Cytochrome P_{450} Metabolism

The newest discovered pathways for the metabolism of arachidonic acid are the cytochrome P_{450} enzymes.[43] They are present in several tissues including the liver, the vascular endothelium, and the thick ascending limb of the loops of Henle. P_{450} metabolites are formed via the epoxidation of arachidonic acid to form 5, 6, 8, 9, 11, 12, 14, and 15 epoxides. These metabolites are made in large quantities in the kidneys and liver. They are in turn metabolized to the corresponding vicinal diols via epoxide hydrolase. Some of these compounds can be further metabolized via cyclooxygenase to active metabolites. Omega and omega-1 metabolism may also occur, resulting in the formation of 20- and 19-HETE, respectively. Whether their synthesis is increased in sepsis or other forms of shock remains to be determined.

INCREASED SYNTHESIS OF EICOSANOIDS IN ENDOTOXEMIA AND SEPSIS

The seminal observation that eicosanoids may be involved in the pathogenesis of endotoxic shock was made by Northover and Subramanian in 1962.[44] They demonstrated that dogs treated with aspirin before exposure to endotoxin had an improved survival compared with controls. At that time, it was not known that aspirin inhibited prostaglandin synthesis. In 1976, Herman and Vane[45] then demonstrated increased levels of PGE-like material in the renal vein of dogs given endotoxin. Taken together, these two observations suggested the possibility that eicosanoids were important in the pathogenesis of septic shock.

Increased synthesis of eicosanoids in response to endotoxemia and sepsis occurs in several animal species and in humans. Increases in plasma levels of TXB_2 and 6-keto-$PGF_{1\alpha}$ can be demonstrated in rats with experimental endotoxemia and sepsis.[34, 46–48] Similar profiles of TXB_2 and 6-keto-$PGF_{1\alpha}$ in plasma are observed in endotoxemic or septic sheep,[49, 50] pigs,[46, 51–55] and baboons.[56, 57] The relative amounts of TXB_2 and 6-keto-$PGF_{1\alpha}$ are influenced by the experimental route of endotoxin administration[58] and the frequency of endotoxin administration.[59] Increases in plasma levels of TXB_2 and 6-keto-$PGF_{1\alpha}$ also parallel shock severity in patients dying of septic shock.[60–62]

5-Lipoxygenase products also are increased in endotoxemic animals and patients with sepsis and ARDS.[63] In endotoxemic rats, Hagmann and colleagues[64] reported increases in biliary *N*-acetyl LTE_4, a stable metabolite of sulfidopeptide leukotrienes. LTC_4 levels are increased in the lungs of rats with experimental endotoxemia.[65] Increased LTB_4 levels are found in bronchoalveolar lavage fluid of endotoxemic pigs[66] and in lung lymph in endotoxemic sheep.[67] Increases in sulfidopeptide leukotrienes and LTB_4 have been demonstrated in the bronchoalveolar lavage fluid of patients with ARDS, a complication associated with sepsis.[10, 68–72]

EFFECT OF EICOSANOID SYNTHESIS INHIBITORS AND RECEPTOR ANTAGONISTS

More direct evidence that eicosanoids mediate endotoxin-induced sequelae is provided by observations that inhibition of eicosanoid synthesis or blockade of specific receptors protects animals from endotoxic shock sequelae. Numerous NSAIDs have been evaluated for potential therapeutic benefit in endotoxemia and sepsis in animal models.[34] These compounds, when used in experimental sepsis or endotoxemia, have generally been found to improve survival or survival time and to reduce cardiopulmonary dysfunction and indices of tissue injury.[34, 46–48] Among the most extensively studied prototype NSAID is ibuprofen. In various species with endotoxemia and sepsis, ibuprofen has been shown to improve systemic hypotension, pulmonary hypertension, protein and fluid extravasation, lung water flux, airway resistance, and oxygen delivery.[34, 48, 53, 58, 73–75] In some studies, however, ibuprofen did not improve shock sequelae.[75] Ibuprofen also alters neutrophil function, including inhibition of neutrophil aggregation responses, organ influx, and adherence.[73, 75] As with other NSAIDs, it is likely that some of these salutary actions are the result of pharmacologic actions of ibuprofen other than inhibition of fatty acid cyclooxygenase. The latter include potential inhibition of LTB_4 production,[75] superoxide anion production,[75] hydroxyl radicals,[76] and burn-induced inhibition of fibrinolysis.[77]

Pretreatment with TXA_2 synthase inhibitors or TXA_2 receptor antagonists improves survival time or attenuates certain shock sequelae in endotoxemic animals. The pathophysiologic events ameliorated by these pharmacologic agents include pulmonary hypertension,[78, 79] reduction in cardiac output, hypotension,[80, 81] decreased renal blood flow, decreased glomerular filtration rate,[79, 81, 82] thrombocytopenia,[78, 81–83] renal glomerular fibrin deposition,[84] and renal glomerular microthrombi.[81] Most studies have shown that the beneficial effect of these drugs was not obtained if they were given after endotoxin. Other studies have failed to demonstrate improved outcome in sepsis and endotoxic shock.[85] Presumably, in these experiments, mediators other than TXA_2 dominate to produce pathophysiologic sequelae contributing to the development of shock and mortality. Use of TXA_2 receptor antagonists in endotoxemia may have several advantages over use of TXA_2 synthase inhibitors. TXA_2 receptor antagonists block the effects of both PGH_2 and TXA_2 to activate TXA_2 receptors but do not produce shunting of PGH_2 to PGI_2 synthesis.

The 5-lipoxygenase inhibitor diethylcarbamazine improved survival of mice in endotoxic shock,[64] and CGS8515 attenuated endotoxin-induced hemoconcentration and hypotension in rats.[86] AA-861, a 5-lipoxygenase inhibitor, attenuated endotoxin-induced neutropenia and concomitant oxygen radical synthesis in rats[87] and improved survival in endotoxemic mice.[88] L651,392, another 5-lipoxygenase inhibitor, blocked endotoxin-induced pulmonary hypertension and bronchoconstriction and increased arterioalveolar oxygen difference and lung microvascular permeability in sheep.[67]

Further evidence for the role of lipoxygenase products in endotoxin-induced shock sequelae is provided by studies using specific leukotriene receptor antagonists in experimental endotoxemia. The sulfidopeptide leukotriene receptor antagonist FPL57231 attenuated endotoxin-induced bronchoconstriction and pulmonary hypertension in sheep and cats.[89, 90] The LTD_4 receptor antagonist SKF104353 prevented endotoxin-induced hemoconcentration and thrombocytopenia and improved survival time in rats.[91] The LTD_4/E_4 receptor antagonist LY171883 improved endotoxin-induced hypotension, hemoconcentration, and leukopenia in rats. Both compounds were shown to prevent acute splanchnic permeability changes induced by endotoxin in rats[92] and mesenteric ischemia in pigs.[46] The LTB_4 receptor antagonist LY233978 has been shown to attenuate endotoxin-induced leukopenia, hemoconcentration, and hypotension in rats.[93] Another LTB_4 receptor antagonist, LY255283, however, only transiently attenuated endotoxin-induced hypotension and hemoconcentration.

Some studies have used combination therapy with cyclooxygenase inhibitors and leukotriene receptor antagonists or lipoxygenase inhibitors. Young and Passmore[94] examined the effect of combined therapy with ibuprofen and LY171883 in canine endotoxic shock. Combined blockade was more effective in maintaining blood pressure and cardiac output but provided no greater protection of renal blood flow or glomerular filtration rate. Turner and colleagues[95] demonstrated good protection with a combined cyclooxygenase and lipoxygenase inhibitor (SKF86002) in a rat model of endotoxin-induced ARDS. The inhibitor blocked the increase in lung wet-dry ratio, total bronchoalveolar lavage protein, hemoconcentration, and thrombocytopenia. Other combination therapies have been shown to be successful. Byrne and associates[96] demonstrated increased survival after delayed cyclooxygenase and histamine blockade in a porcine model of severe sepsis-induced lung injury.

THERAPEUTIC APPROACHES IN PATIENTS

The NSAIDs may have beneficial effects in the treatment of patients with trauma or sepsis. Faist and coworkers[97] studied the effect of indomethacin in a randomized prospective study in 43 patients undergoing major surgical trauma. The cellular immune status was evaluated preoperatively and up to a week after surgery. In contrast to untreated patients, patients receiving indomethacin exhibited improved delayed-type hypersensitivity responses, mitogen-induced lymphocyte transformation, and a lower rate of opportunistic infections. The results suggest that NSAIDs, by preventing impairment of cell-mediated immunity, may reduce susceptibility to sepsis after surgery.

A short course of ibuprofen therapy versus placebo in 30 patients with severe sepsis has been investigated in a randomized two-center study.[9] Ibuprofen (800 mg) or placebo (saline) was given as a retention enema at the time of entry into the study and twice more at 4-hour intervals. Vital signs and number of patients in shock at the time of entry into the study were similar. Urinary levels of 2,3-dinor TXB_2 and 2,3-dinor 6-keto-$PGF_{1\alpha}$ were significantly reduced, along with febrile response, heart rate, and peak airway pressure responses. Importantly, ibuprofen did not produce any signs of worsening renal function. The time to reversal of shock was shortened in the ibuprofen group. Similar beneficial actions of ibuprofen have been reported in human volunteers injected with endotoxin.[98] Ibuprofen pretreatment in these individuals reduced endotoxin-induced mylagia, tachycardia, fever, and plasma stress hormone responses.[98]

These studies provide the impetus for more extensive studies of NSAIDs in trauma, sepsis, and ARDS. Combination therapy approaches with NSAIDs may also prove to be beneficial. Experimentally, combinations of drugs with NSAIDs have been more effective than single-drug treatments.[99–104] Of particular interest, in view of the demonstrated increases of lipoxygenase products in patients with ARDS, is the potential application of lipoxygenase inhibitors or leukotriene receptor antagonists.

ACKNOWLEDGMENTS

This work was supported in part by NIH GM27673. The secretarial assistance of Ms. Janie Nelson is gratefully acknowledged.

References

1. Kurzok R, Lieb CC: Biochemical studies of human semen: The action of semen on the human uterus. Proc Soc Exp Biol Med 1930; 28:268–272.
2. von Euler US: Zur kenntnis der pharmakologischen wirkungen von nativsekre ten und extrakten mannlicher accessorischer geschlechtsdrusen. Naunyn Schmeidebergs Arch Exp Pathol Pharmacol 1934; 175:78–84.
3. Bergstrom S, Sjovall J: The isolation of prostaglandin E from sheep prostate glands. Acta Chem Scand 1960; 14:1701–1705.
4. Samuelsson B, Goldyne M, Granstrom E: Prostaglandins and thromboxanes. Annu Rev Biochem 1978; 47:997–1029.
5. Piper PJ, Vane JR: Release of additional factors in anaphylaxis and its antagonism by anti-inflammatory drugs. Nature 1969; 223:29–33.
6. Moncada S, Gryglewski R, Bunting S: An enzyme isolated from arteries transforms prostaglandin endoperoxides to an unstable substance that inhibits platelet aggregation. Nature 1976; 263:663–665.
7. Samuelsson B, Borgeat P, Hammarstrom S: Introduction of a nomenclature: Leukotrienes. Prostaglandins 1979; 17:785–787.
8. Halushka PV, Mais DE, Mayeux PR, et al: Thromboxane, prostaglandin and leukotriene receptors. Annu Rev Pharmacol Toxicol 1989; 29:213–239.
9. Bernard GR, Reines HD, Halushka PV, et al: Prostacyclin and thromboxane A2 formation is increased in human sepsis syndrome. Effects of cyclooxygenase inhibition. Am Rev Respir Dis 1991; 144:1095–1101.
10. Bernard GR, Korley V, Chee P, et al: Persistent generation of peptido leukotrienes in patients with the adult respiratory distress syndrome. Am Rev Respir Dis 1991; 144:263–267.
11. Irvine RF: How is the level of free arachidonic acid controlled in mammalian cells? Biochem J 1982; 204:3–16.
12. Lapetina EG: Regulation of arachidonic acid production: Role of phospholipases C and A_2. Trends Pharmacol 1982; 3:115–118.
13. Tanaka Y, Amano F, Kishi H, et al: Degradation of arachidonyl phospholipids catalyzed by two phospholipases A_2 and phospholipase C in a lipopolysaccharide-treated macrophage cell line, RAW264.7. Arch Biochem Biophys 1989; 272:210–218.
14. Berridge MJ, Irvine RF: Inositol trisphosphate, a novel second messenger in cellular signal transduction. Nature 1984; 312:315–321.
15. Berridge MJ: Inositol trisphosphate and diacylglycerol as second messengers. Biochem J 1984; 220:345–360.
16. Majerus PW, Connolly TM, Deckmyn H, et al: The metabolism of phosphoinositide-derived messenger molecules. Science 1986; 234:1519–1526.
17. Prpic V, Weiel JE, Somers SD, et al: Effects of bacterial lipopolysaccharide on the hydrolysis of phosphatidylinositol-4,5-bisphosphate in murine peritoneal macrophages. J Immunol 1987; 139:526–533.
18. Bell RL, Kennerly DA, Stanford N, et al: Diglyceride lipase: A pathway for arachidonate release from human platelets. Proc Natl Acac Sci U S A 1979; 76:3238–3241.
19. Moscat J, Herrero C, Garcia BP, et al: Phospholipase C–diglyceride lipase is a major pathway for arachidonic acid release in macrophages. Biochem Biophys Res Commun 1986; 141:367–373.
20. Wightman PD, Dallob A: Regulation of phosphatidylinositol breakdown and leukotriene synthesis by endogenous prostaglandins in resident mouse peritoneal macrophages. J Biol Chem 1990; 265:9176–9180.
21. Smith WL, Marnett LJ: Prostaglandin endoperoxide synthase: Structure and catalysis. Biochim Biophys Acta 1991; 1083:1–17.
22. Smith WL: Prostaglandin synthesis and its compartmentation in vascular smooth muscle and endothelial cells. Annu Rev Physiol 1986; 48:251–262.
23. Smith WL, DeWitt DL, Allen MA: Bimodal distribution of the prostaglandin I_2 antigen in smooth muscle cells. J Biol Chem 1983; 258: 59222–5926.
24. Mutsaers KJGM, van Halbeek H, Kamerling JP, et al: Determination of the structure of the carbohydrate chains of prostaglandin endoperoxine synthase from sheep. Eur J Biochem 1985; 147:569–574.
25. Smith WL, DeWitt DL, Kraemer SA, et al: Structure-function

relationships in sheep, mouse, and human prostaglandin endoperoxide G/H synthases. Adv Prostaglandin Thromboxane Leukot Res 1990; 20:14–21.

26. Lambier AM, Markey CM, Dunford HB, et al: Spectral properties of the higher oxidation states of prostaglandin H synthase. J Biol Chem 1985; 260:14894–14896.
27. Marnett LJ, Chen YN, Maddipati KR, et al: Localization of the peroxidase active site of PGH synthase. Adv Prostaglandin Thromboxane Leukot Res 1989; 19:458–461.
28. Tsai AL, Sanduja R, Wu KK: Evidence for two pools of prostaglandin H synthase in human endothelial cells. Adv Prostaglandin Thromboxane Leukot Res 1991; 21A:141–144.
29. Xie W, Robertson DL, Simmons DL: Mitogen-inducible prostaglandin G/H synthase: A new target for nonsteroidal anti-inflammatory drugs. Drug Dev Res 1992; 25:249–265.

29a. Maier JA, Ragnotti G: An oligomer targeted against protein kinase C alpha prevents interleukin-1 alpha induction of cyclooxygenase expression in human endothelial cells. Exp Cell Res 1993; 205:52–58.

29b. Lyons-Giordano B, Pratta MA, Galbraith W, et al: Interleukin-1 differentially modulates chondrocyte expression of cyclooxygenase-2 and phospholipase A2. Exp Cell Res 1993; 206:58–62.

29c. Zyglewska T, Wu LC, Xu XM, et al: Quantitative analysis of vascular prostaglandin H synthase mRNA levels by competitive polymerase chain reaction. J Lab Clin Med 1993; 122:542–548.

30. Masferrer JL, Zweifel BS, Seibert K, et al: Selective regulation of cellular cyclooxygenase by dexamethasone and endotoxin in mice. J Clin Invest 1990; 86:1375–1379.
31. Fu JY, Masferrer JL, Seibert K, et al: The induction and suppression of prostaglandin H_2 synthase (cyclooxygenase) in human monocytes. J Biol Chem 1990; 265:16737–16740.
32. Masferrer JL, Seibert K, Zweifel B, et al: Endogenous glucocorticoids regulate an inducible cyclooxygenase enzyme. Proc Natl Acad Sci U S A 1992; 89:3917–3921.
33. Lee SH, Soyoola E, Chanmugam P, et al: Selective expression of mitogen-inducible cyclooxygenase in macrophages stimulated with lipopolysaccharide. J Biol Chem 1992; 267:25934–25938.

33a. O'Sullivan MG, Huggins EM Jr, McCall CE: Lipopolysaccharide-induced expression of prostaglandin H synthase-2 in alveolar macrophages is inhibited by dexamethasone but not by aspirin. Biochem Biophys Res Commun 1993; 191:1294–1300.

33b. Phillips TA, Kujubu DA, MacKay RJ, et al: The mouse macrophage activation–associated marker protein, p71/73, is an inducible prostaglandin endoperoxide synthase (cyclooxygenase). J Leukoc Biol 1993; 53:411–419.

34. Cook JA, Halushka PV: Arachidonic acid metabolites in septic Shock. *In*: Multiple Organ Failure. Bihari DJ, Cerra F (Eds). Fullerton, CA, Society of Critical Care Medicine, 1989, pp 101–124.
35. Handerson W Jr: Products of 12- and 15-lipoxygenase. *In*: Mediators of the Inflammatory Process. Henson PM, Murphy RC (Eds). New York, Elsevier, 1989, pp 45–75.
36. Shimizu T, Wolfe LS: Arachidonic acid cascade and signal transduction. J Neurochem 1990; 55:1–15.
37. Rouzer CA, Shimizu T, Samuelsson B: On the nature of the 5-lipoxygenase reaction in human leukocytes: Characterization of a membrane-associated stimulatory factor. Proc Natl Acad Sci U S A 1985; 82:7505–7509.
38. Rouzer CA, Thornberry NA, Bull HG: Kinetic effects of ATP and two cellular stimulatory components on human leukocyte 5-lipoxygenase. Ann N Y Acad Sci 1988; 524:1–11.
39. Rouzer CA, Ford HA, Morton HE, et al: MK886, a potent and specific leukotriene biosynthesis inhibitor blocks and reverses the membrane association of 5-lipoxygenase in ionophore-challenged leukocytes. J Biol Chem 1990; 265:1436–1442.
40. Sigal E, Craik CS, Dixon RA, et al: Cloning and expression of human arachidonate 15-lipoxygenase. Trans Assoc Am Physicians 1989; 102:176–184.
41. Nadel JA, Conrad DJ, Ueki IF, et al: Immunocytochemical localization of arachidonate 15-lipoxygenase in erythrocytes, leukocytes, and airway cells. J Clin Invest 1991; 87:1139–1145.
42. Ford HA: Arachidonate 15-lipoxygenase; characteristics and potential biological significance. Eicosanoids 1991; 4:65–74.
43. McGiff JC: Cytochrome P-450 metabolism of arachidonic acid. Annu Rev Pharmacol Toxicol 1991; 31:339–369.
44. Northover BJ, Subramanian G: Analgesic-antipyretic drugs as antagonists of endotoxin shock in dogs. J Pathol Bacteriol 1962; 83:463–468.
45. Herman AG, Vane JR: Release of renal prostaglandins during endotoxin induced hypotension. Eur J Pharmacol 1976; 39:79–90.
46. Fink MP, Rothschild HR, Deniz YF, et al: Systemic and mesenteric O_2 metabolism in endotoxic pigs: Effect of ibuprofen and meclofenamate. J Appl Physiol 1989; 67:1950–1957.
47. Petrak RA, Balk RA, Bone RC: Prostaglandins, cyclo-oxygenase inhibitors, and thromboxane synthetase inhibitors in the pathogenesis of multiple systems organ failure. Crit Care Clin 1989; 5:303–314.
48. Bone RC: Phospholipids and their inhibitors: A critical evaluation of their role in the treatment of sepsis. Crit Care Med 1992; 20:884–890.
49. Morel DR, Huttemeier PC, Skoskiewicz MJ, et al: Dose-dependent effects of a pyridoquinazoline thromboxane synthetase inhibitor on arachidonic acid metabolites and hemodynamics during *E. coli* endotoxemia in anesthetized sheep. Prostaglandins 1987; 33:879–902.
50. Demling RH, Smith M, Gunther R, et al: Pulmonary injury and prostaglandin production during endotoxemia in conscious sheep. Am J Physiol 1981; 240:H348–H353.
51. Hardie EM, Olson NC: Prostaglandin and thromboxane levels during endotoxin-induced respiratory failure in pigs. Prostaglandins Leukot Med 1987; 28:255–265.
52. Schrauwen E, Vandeplassche G, Laekman G, et al: Endotoxin shock in the pig: Release of prostaglandins and beneficial effects of flubiprofen. Arch Int Pharmacodyn Ther 1983; 262:332–334.
53. Nishijima MK, Breslow MJ, Miller CF, et al: Effect of naloxone and ibuprofen on organ blood flow during endotoxic shock in pig. Am J Physiol 1988; 255:H177–H184.
54. Zellner JL, Cook JA, Reines DH, et al: Hemodynamic effects of leukotriene (LT) D_4 and LTD_4 receptor antagonist in the pig. Eicosanoids 1990; 3:219–224.
55. Zellner JL, Cook JA, Reines HD, et al: Effect of a LTD_4 receptor antagonist in porcine septic shock. Eicosanoids 1991; 4:169–175.
56. Harris RH, Zmudka M, Maddox Y, et al: Relationships of TXB_2 and 6-keto-$PGF_{1\alpha}$ to the hemodynamic changes during baboon endotoxic shock. *In*: Advances in Prostaglandins and Thromboxane Research. Samuelsson B, Ramwell RW, Paoletti R (Eds). New York, Raven Press, 1980, pp 843–850.
57. Casey LC, Fletcher JR, Zmudka MI, et al: Prevention of endotoxin-induced pulmonary hypertension in primates by the use of a selective thromboxane synthetase inhibitor, OKY 1581. J Pharmacol Exp Ther 1982; 222:441–446.
58. Demling RH, Wenber H, Hechtman H, et al: Role of subcutaneous tissue endotoxin in the production of prostanoid-induced lung injury: Comparison with intravenous endotoxin response. Circ Shock 1985; 17:147–161.
59. Klosterhalfen B, Hörstmann-Jungemann K, Vogel P, et al: Time course of various inflammatory mediators during recurrent endotoxemia. Biochem Pharmacol 1992; 43:2103–2109.
60. Reines HD, Halushka PV, Cook JA, et al: Plasma thromboxane concentrations are raised in patients dying with septic shock. Lancet 1982; 24:174–175.
61. Oettinger W, Berger D, Beger HG: The clinical significance of prostaglandins and thromboxane as mediators of septic shock. Klin Wochenschr 1987; 65:61–68.
62. Halushka PV, Reines HD, Barrow SE, et al: Elevated plasma 6-keto-prostaglandin $F_{1\alpha}$ in patients in septic shock. Crit Care Med 1985; 13:451–453.
63. Keppler D, Guhlmann A, Huber M, et al: Leukotrienes in shock syndromes: Metabolism and detection in vivo. Adv Prostaglandin Thromboxane Leukot Res 1990; 20:179–186.
64. Hagmann W, Denzlinger C, Keppler D: Production of peptide leukotrienes in endotoxin shock. FEBS Lett 1985; 180:309–313.
65. Chang SW, Westcott JY, Pickett WC, et al: Endotoxin-induced lung injury in rats: Role of eicosanoids. J Appl Physiol 1989; 66:2407–2418.

66. Olson NC, Salzer WL, McCall CE: Biochemical, physiological and clinical aspects of endotoxemia. Mol Aspects Med 1988; 10:511–629.
67. Coggeshall JW, Christman BW, Lefferts PL, et al: Effect of inhibition of 5-lipoxygenase metabolism of arachidonic acid on response to endotoxemia in sheep. J Appl Physiol 1988; 65:1351–1359.
68. Matthay MA, Eschenbacher WL, Goetzl EJ: Elevated concentrations of leukotriene D_4 in pulmonary edema fluid of patients with adult respiratory distress syndrome. J Clin Immunol 1984; 4:479–483.
69. Stephenson AH, Lonigro AJ, Hyers TM, et al: Increased concentrations of leukotrienes in bronchoalveolar lavage fluid of patients with ARDS or at risk for ARDS. Am Rev Respir Dis 1988; 138:714–719.
70. Antonelli A, Bufi M, De Blasi RA, et al: Detection of leukotriene B_4, C_4 and their isomers in arterial, mixed venous blood and bronchoalveolar lavage fluid from ARDS patients. Intensive Care Med 1989; 15:296–301.
71. Davis JM, Meyer JD, Barie PS, et al: Elevated production of neutrophil leukotriene B_4 precedes pulmonary failure in critically ill surgical patients. Surg Gynecol Obstet 1990; 170:495–500.
72. Seeger W, Grimminger F, Barden M, et al: Omega-oxidized leukotriene B_4 detected in the broncho-alveolar lavage fluid of patients with non-cardiogenic pulmonary edema, but not in those with cardiogenic edema. Intensive Care Med 1991; 17: 1–6.
73. Rinaldo JE, Pennock B: Effects of ibuprofen on endotoxin-induced alveolitis: Biphasic dose response and dissociation between inflammation and hypoxia. Am J Med Sci 1986; 29: 29–38.
74. Ward PH, Maldonado M, Moreno M, et al: Oxygen-derived free radicals mediate the cutaneous necrotizing vasculitis induced by epinephrine in endotoxin-primed rabbits. J Infect Dis 1990; 161:1020–1022.
75. Wagner TR, Halushka PV, Cook JA: Cyclooxygenase products in septic and endotoxic shock. *In*: Handbook of Mediators in Septic Shock. Neugebauer EA, Holaday JW (Eds). Boca Raton, CRC Press, 1993, pp 395–418.
76. Hamburger SA, McCay PB: Spin trapping of ibuprofen radicals: Evidence that ibuprofen is a hydroxyl radical scavenger. Free Radic Res Commun 1990; 9:337–342.
77. Rockwell WB, Ehrlich HP: Ibuprofen in acute-care therapy. Ann Surg 1990; 211:78–83.
78. Taneyama C, Sasao J, Senna S, et al: Protective effects of ONO 3708, a new thromboxane A_2 receptor antagonist, during experimental endotoxin shock. Circ Shock 1989; 28:69–77.
79. Cirino M, Morton H, MacDonald C, et al: Thromboxane A_2 and prostaglandin endoperoxide analogue effects on porcine renal blood flow. Am J Physiol 1990; 258:F109–F114.
80. Svartholm E, Bergqvist D, Hedner U, et al: Thromboxane A_2–receptor blockade and prostacyclin in porcine *Escherichia coli* shock. Arch Surg 1989; 124:669–672.
81. Fukumoto S, Tanaka K: Protective effects of thromboxane A_2 synthetase inhibitors on endotoxin shock. Prostaglandins Leukot Med 1983; 11:179–188.
82. Badr KF, Kelley VE, Rennke HG, et al: Roles for thromboxane A_2 and leukotrienes in endotoxin-induced acute renal failure. Kidney Int 1986; 30:474–480.
83. Olanoff L, Cook JA, Eller T, et al: Protective effects of trans-13-APT, a thromboxane receptor antagonist, in endotoxemia. J Cardiovasc Pharmacol 1985; 7:117–120.
84. Westwick J, Fletcher MS, Kakkar VV: Inhibition of thromboxane formation prevents endotoxin-induced renal fibrin deposition in jaundiced rats. *In*: Advances in Prostaglandin and Thromboxane Research. Samuelsson B, Paoletti R, Ramwell P (Eds). New York, Raven Press, 1983, pp 83–91.
85. Furman BL, McKechnie K, Paratt JR: Failure of drugs that selectively inhibit thromboxane synthesis to modify endotoxin shock in conscious rats. Br J Pharmacol 1984; 82:289–294.
86. Matera G, Cook JA, Hennigar RA, et al: Beneficial effects of a 5-lipoxygenase inhibitor in endotoxic shock in the rat. J Pharmacol Exp Ther 1988; 247:363–371.
87. Suematsu M, Miura S, Suzuki M, et al: 5-lipoxygenase inhibitor (AA-861) attenuates neutrophil-mediated oxidative stress on the venular endothelium in endotoxemia. J Clin Lab Immunol 1988; 25:41–45.
88. Ogata M, Matsumoto T, Kamochi M, et al: Protective effects of a leukotriene inhibitor and a leukotriene antagonist on endotoxin-induced mortality in carrageenan-pretreated mice. Infect Immun 1992; 60:2432–2437.
89. Ahmed T, Wasserman MA, Muccitell R, et al: Endotoxin-induced changes in pulmonary hemodynamic and respiratory mechanics. Am Rev Respir Dis 1986; 134:1149–1159.
90. Pacitti N, Bryson SE, McKechnie K, et al: Leukotriene antagonist FPL 57231 prevents the acute pulmonary effects of *Escherichia coli* endotoxin in cats. Circ Shock 1987; 21:155–168.
91. Smith EF III, Kinter LB, Jugus M, et al: Beneficial effects of the peptidoleukotriene receptor antagonist, SK&F 104353, on the responses to experimental endotoxemia in the conscious rat. Circ Shock 1988; 25:21–31.
92. Cook JA, Li EJ, Spicer KM, et al: Effect of leukotriene receptor antagonists on vascular permeability during endotoxic shock. Circ Shock 1990; 32:209–218.
93. Li EJ, Cook JA, Wise WC, et al: Effect of LTB_4 receptor antagonists in endotoxic shock in the rat. Circ Shock 1991; 34:385–392.
94. Young JS, Passmore JC: Hemodynamic and renal advantages of dual cyclooxygenase and leukotriene blockade during canine endotoxic shock. Circ Shock 1990; 32:243–255.
95. Turner CR, Quinlan MF, Schwartz LW, et al: Therapeutic intervention in a rat model of ARDS: I. Dual inhibition of arachidonic acid metabolism. Circ Shock 1990; 32:231–242.
96. Byrne K, Sielaff TD, Michna B, et al: Increased survival time after delayed histamine and prostaglandin blockade in a porcine model of severe sepsis-induced lung injury. Crit Care Med 1990; 18:303–308.
97. Faist E, Ertel W, Cohnert T, et al: Immunoprotective effects of cyclooxygenase inhibition in patients with major surgical trauma. J Trauma 1990; 30:8–17.
98. Revhaug A, Michie HR, Manson JM, et al: Inhibition of cyclooxygenase attenuates the metabolic response to endotoxin in humans. Arch Surg 1988; 123:162–170.
99. Ogletree ML, Begley CJ, King GA, et al: Influence of steroidal and nonsteroidal anti-inflammatory agents on the accumulation of arachidonic acid metabolites in plasma and lung lymph after endotoxemia in awake sheep. Measurements of prostacyclin and thromboxane metabolites and 12-HETE. Am Rev Respir Dis 1986; 133:55–61.
100. Olson NC, Brown TT Jr, Anderson DL: Dexamethasone and indomethacin modify endotoxin-induced respiratory failure in pigs. J Appl Physiol 1985; 58:274–284.
101. Sielaff TD, Sugerman HJ, Tatum JL, et al: Treatment of porcine *Pseudomonas* ARDS with combination drug therapy. J Trauma 1987; 27:1313–1322.
102. Wise WC, Halushka PV, Knapp DR, et al: Ibuprofen, methylprednisolone, gentamicin as conjoint therapy in septic shock. Circ Shock 1985; 17:59–71.
103. Goto M, Zeller WP, Hurley RM: Dexamethasone and indomethacin treatment during endotoxicosis in the suckling rat. Circ Shock 1990; 32:113–122.
104. Butler RR Jr, Wise WC, Halushka PV, et al: Gentamicin and indomethacin in the treatment of septic shock: Effects on prostacyclin and thromboxane A_2 production. J Pharmacol Exp Ther 1983; 225:94–101.

CHAPTER 20

Cellular Signaling and Cell Death

David J. McConkey, PhD

Apoptosis is a process of regulated cell deletion that mediates many important physiologic and pathologic phenomena. Although apoptosis was originally defined by the stereotyped morphologic alterations that accompany the process, studies have revealed the involvement of several biochemical and molecular pathways that are better known for their roles in regulating cell proliferation and differentiation. Intracellular signaling pathways—including Ca^{2+} mobilization, cyclic adenosine monophosphate (cAMP) production, and protein kinase C (PKC) activation—figure prominently in this regulation, as presented later in this chapter.

OCCURRENCE OF APOPTOSIS

A number of critical physiologic processes are mediated by apoptosis. Perhaps the most basic of these is normal cell turnover and cell loss due to aging.[1] In addition, hormone-induced tissue atrophy invariably occurs via apoptosis. Examples include both direct effects of hormones, such as in steroid-induced atrophy of the adrenal cortex and the thymus,[1] as well as hormone withdrawal, as in atrophy of the prostate after androgen ablation,[2, 3] regression of the lactating breast,[4] sloughing of the endometrial lining,[5] and withdrawal of interleukin-2 (IL-2) at the termination of a T cell–mediated immune response.[6] Cell death is common during development,[7] when it mediates fitness-based cell selection processes in the central nervous system[8, 9] and primary lymphoid organs,[10] fusion of the secondary palate,[11] formation of digits,[7, 12] and tadpole tail regression.[13]

Apoptosis is also widespread in cases of "accidental" or pathologic cell death. Toxic chemicals,[14, 15] irradiation,[16, 17] hyperthermia,[15, 18] and hypothermia (cold shock)[19, 20] all apparently induce physical damage that triggers a secondary apoptotic response. Programmed cell death probably also mediates T cell depletion in acquired immunodeficiency syndrome,[21, 22] neural degeneration in Huntington's, Parkinson's, and Alzheimer's diseases[23, 24]; islet cell depletion in diabetes[25]; and tissue injury due to inflammation. Together, these observations indicate that apoptosis is the most important cell death pathway of clinical relevance.

MORPHOLOGIC, BIOCHEMICAL, AND MOLECULAR MECHANISMS IN APOPTOSIS

A critical component of the original conceptual defense of apoptosis as a unique cell death mechanism was that a series of morphologic changes occur within apoptotic cells that can be readily distinguished from those observed in cells undergoing accidental or necrotic cell death.[1] Apoptosis is characterized by plasma and nuclear membrane blebbing and a consequent loss of volume (cell shrinkage). Organelle relocalization and compaction and chromatin condensation follow. Cells give rise to numerous membrane-enclosed fragments (termed *apoptotic bodies*) that are found dispersed within areas of tissues with high rates of apoptotic cell turnover. Apoptotic cells and bodies are subsequently specifically recognized and cleared by neighboring cells and phagocytic cells (tissue macrophages) before loss of membrane integrity. In this manner, cell deletion occurs without consequent inflammation. Organelle function remains grossly intact, although adenosine triphosphate (ATP) levels and rates of messenger ribonucleic acid (mRNA) and protein synthesis may fall precipitously. Some of these features of apoptosis contrast sharply with the changes observed during necrosis, which include cell swelling, obvious plasma membrane disruption, organelle dilation, and inflammation.

Apoptosis is a suicidal cellular response that can involve gene expression, and a common (but not invariant) feature of the process is that it can be blocked by inhibitors of protein (cycloheximide, puromycin) or mRNA (actinomycin D) synthesis.[8, 9, 24] Several groups have identified "lysis genes" whose expression appears to be selectively induced by apoptotic stimuli.[26–31] In addition, genes previously implicated in oncogenesis have important roles in regulating apoptosis. However, it is clear that the minimal components of the apoptotic machinery are constitutively present in most cell types, such that apoptosis can be triggered by cytotoxic T lymphocytes, heat shock, gliotoxin, and diphtheria toxin while mRNA and protein synthesis are totally blocked.[10, 32–34] Indeed, specific macromolecular synthesis inhibitors themselves can directly induce apoptosis.[35] Moreover, inhibition of apoptosis by macromolecular synthesis inhibitors may be due at least in part to depletion of components of the apoptotic machinery possessing rapid turnover rates.[36] Thus, induction of new gene expression is not mandatory for apoptosis, and protein synthesis may be more important to pathway-specific control mechanisms than to production of suicide factors within cells.

The most characteristic biochemical feature of apoptosis is activation of an endogenous nuclear endonuclease, resulting in cleavage of host chromatin at internucleosomal "linker" regions.[37] The result is formation of fragments that appear as a "ladder" after electrophoresis on agarose gels. Notably, endonuclease activation occurs well before plasma membrane integrity is compromised, and deoxyribonucleic acid (DNA) ladders are not observed in necrotic cells.[1] When DNA fragmentation does occur in necrosis, it is typically a postmortem event mediated by release of lysosomal enzymes that generates random DNA cleavage patterns ("smears"). Studies with isolated nuclei have demonstrated the constitutive presence of an endonuclease capable of producing characteristic DNA ladders in most cell types.[38–42] The activity is strictly dependent on Ca^{2+} and Mg^{2+} and can be inhibited by the divalent cation Zn^{2+},[40] calmodulin antagonists,[41] or calcium chelators.[41] Several independent laboratories have reported the isolation and biochemical characterization of candidate Ca^{2+}-dependent apoptosis endonucleases,[43–45] and ongoing experimentation is aimed at precisely defining their role(s) in DNA fragmentation during apoptosis.

Characteristic DNA fragmentation can be induced in some cells that do not appear to constitutively express the Ca^{2+}-dependent enzyme activity, and endonuclease activation in these systems appears to be Ca^{2+} independent. Eastman and colleagues have isolated a candidate endonuclease (DNAse II) from Chinese hamster ovary cells that is active at low pH and that may mediate DNA fragmentation in intact cells.[46] It is conceivable that several independent DNA fragmentation pathways exist within cells and that rapidly dividing or transformed (factor-independent) cells lose expression of or the ability to activate the Ca^{2+} endonuclease. This idea is supported by the observation that sensitivity to induction of Ca^{2+}-dependent endonuclease activation is lost in exponentially growing cell lines[19, 20] and that cytokines and chemical tumor promoters can deplete nuclei of Ca^{2+}-stimulated endonuclease activity in vitro.[47]

The actual function served by endonuclease activation in apoptotic cell death remains the subject of debate. Data from Wyllie's laboratory suggests that endonuclease activation directly causes chromatin condensation in apoptotic cells.[44] Studies with inhibitors have shown that agents that inhibit endonuclease activation often prevent cell death,[32, 40, 48] suggesting that DNA fragmentation may contribute to the mechanism of cell inactivation or killing. However, DNA fragmentation is dispensible for apoptotic cell death in other model systems. For example, cytotoxic T lymphocytes can lyse cells independently of chromatin cleavage.[49] Moreover, although programmed cell death in the nematode *Caenorhabditis elegans* involves endonuclease activation, it is a late event that occurs after phagocytosis.[50] Coupled with the observation that viruses have evolved specific mechanisms to inhibit endonuclease activation in their hosts,[51, 52] these findings support the idea originally advanced by Martz and Howell[53] that the main purpose of DNA fragmentation is to destroy potentially transforming viral or mutant host genetic material before it can be passed on to progeny or neighboring cells. It is certainly possible that endonuclease activation serves multiple functions. In particular, because cytotoxic T cells can kill their targets by necrosis,[10, 54] it would appear that redundant physiologic cell death mechanisms that have evolved do not rely on biochemical events within the potentially apoptosis-resistant target.

Exciting new information on the role of oncogenes and tumor suppressor genes in regulating apoptosis is emerging. Because apoptosis has a central role in regulating cell number in normal tissue homeostasis, it has been widely assumed that malregulation of apoptosis could contribute to neoplasia.[55, 56] Direct support for this model has come from work on *bcl*-2, in that several groups have demonstrated that cells that overexpress *bcl*-2 are resistant to induction of apoptosis.[57–62] The tyrosine kinase encoded by v-*abl*[63] and activated *ras*[64, 64a] also appear to inhibit the process. In contrast, expression of *myc*[65–67] or *fos*[68] appears to facilitate apoptosis, indicating that some oncogenes may actually predispose cells to suicide. Likewise, the tumor suppressor protein p53 also promotes apoptosis, as originally shown by Yonish-Rouach and coworkers in myeloid leukemic cells transfected with a temperature-sensitive p53 construct.[69] This observation has since been confirmed in a human colon tumor line.[70] Lane postulated that p53 may have a general role in preventing replicative amplification of mutant DNA sequences by mediating cell cycle arrest or apoptosis in response to DNA damage.[71] Supporting this notion, results from Lowe and colleagues'[72] and Clarke and associates'[73] laboratories indicate that DNA damage-stimulated apoptosis in response to gamma irradiation or etoposide treatment is blocked in mice lacking p53, although other pathways of apoptosis remain intact. Identification of the mechanisms by which DNA damage and p53 expression elicit apoptosis awaits further experimentation.

CELL SIGNALING IN PROGRAMMED CELL DEATH

Based on its occurrence in development and other physiologic contexts, apoptosis was thought from its inception to be a tightly regulated process involving a network of biologic and molecular pathways triggered specifically by the host. Apoptosis in vivo usually involves the actions of hormones or growth factors and their receptors, strongly suggesting the involvement of cellular signaling mechanisms. Several concrete examples of how particular signal transduction pathways regulate apoptosis in various tissues are discussed next.

Role of Calcium

The strict Ca^{2+} dependence of the endonuclease is strong supportive evidence for a role for Ca^{2+} in the regulation of apoptosis.[38–42] Further support has come from work by Kaiser and Edelman, who showed that glucocorticoid-induced thymocyte apoptosis is associated with enhanced Ca^{2+} influx[74] and can be mimicked by calcium ionophores.[75] Calcium ionophores induce the morphologic changes and endonuclease activation that characterize apoptosis in thymocytes[76] and mimic the effects of testosterone withdrawal in prostatic cells.[77] The author demonstrated a strong direct correlation between the effects of ionophore on the cytosolic Ca^{2+} concentration and DNA fragmentation.[48] Sustained Ca^{2+} elevations have also been observed in response to other stimuli in apoptotic cells,[20, 25, 78–82] and inhibition of these increases with intracellular Ca^{2+} buffering agents, extracellular Ca^{2+} chelators, or Ca^{2+} channel blockers abrogates both endonuclease activation and cell death.[20, 25, 77–81, 83–85] Calmodulin antagonists can also block endonuclease activation.[20, 41, 79–81] The author and his coworkers presented evidence that the calmodulin requirement is linked to the function of a novel ATP-dependent nuclear Ca^{2+} pump that facilitates endonuclease activation by raising intranuclear Ca^{2+} concentrations.[41, 86] These Ca^{2+} signaling mechanisms are summarized in Figure 20–1. In other cell types, however, sustained Ca^{2+} elevations are either not involved in apoptosis[87, 88] or they even inhibit the process. For example, Ca^{2+} ionophores inhibit apoptosis in hematopoietic precursors deprived of IL-3 via a mechanism that involves produc-

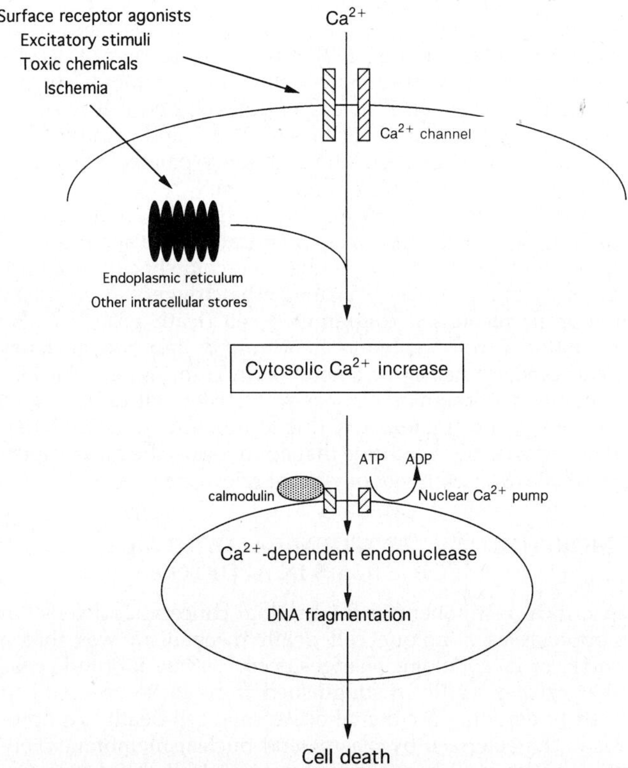

Figure 20–1. Role of Ca^{2+} in apoptosis. Various physiologic and pathologic stimuli induce DNA fragmentation and cell death by triggering sustained increases in the cytosolic Ca^{2+} concentration. These increases in Ca^{2+} are mediated both by release from intracellular stores (including those of the endoplasmic reticulum) and by the opening of plasma membrane Ca^{2+} channels. An adenosine triphosphate (ATP)– and calmodulin-dependent nuclear Ca^{2+} uptake system also appears to be involved.

tion of IL-4.[89,90] In addition, membrane depolarization inhibits apoptosis in neurons deprived of nerve growth factor via a mechanism that involves a Ca^{2+} increase.[91,92] Interestingly, these cells may lack the Ca^{2+}-dependent nuclear endonuclease responsible for apoptotic DNA fragmentation in other systems[88,90] (personal observation), although the nature of the endonuclease involved is not known.

Role of cAMP Cyclic Adenosine Monophosphate

Several years ago Pratt, Martin, and Hassell showed that programmed cell death during fusion of the secondary palatal epithelium involves elevations of cAMP,[11,93] and the cytolytic effects of cAMP on lymphoid cell lines are well known.[28,94,95] Interest in the potential involvement of cAMP in the control of apoptosis is now re-emerging (Fig. 20–2). Studies have demonstrated that series E prostaglandins and pharmacologic agents that elevate cAMP induce endogenous endonuclease activation in lymphocytes.[96,97] The response involves the Ca^{2+}-dependent endonuclease and activation of cAMP-dependent protein kinase (PKA),[96] suggesting that changes in specific target substrate(s) phosphorylation are involved. Because cAMP often exerts its effects via changes in gene transcription and the effects of cAMP on thymocytes are blocked by inhibitors of mRNA or protein synthesis, it is possible that alterations in gene expression are ultimately responsible for triggering apoptosis in the cells. Supporting this notion, Harrigan and colleagues have found evidence that treatment of lymphoid cell lines with cAMP-raising agents or glucocorticoids to induce apoptosis results in overlapping patterns of mRNA expression in the dying cells,[28] and Dowd and Miesfeld have shown that the pathways share overlapping distal elements in their cytolytic mechanisms.[98] Glucocorticoids and cAMP can also act synergistically to promote apoptosis[99,100] (see Fig. 20–2), and we have presented evidence that the cAMP pathway of apoptosis in thymocytes requires glucocorticoid receptor function.[100] Ongoing efforts are aimed at defining more precisely the nature of the relationship between cAMP and the glucocorticoid receptor in lymphoid cells and other cell types.

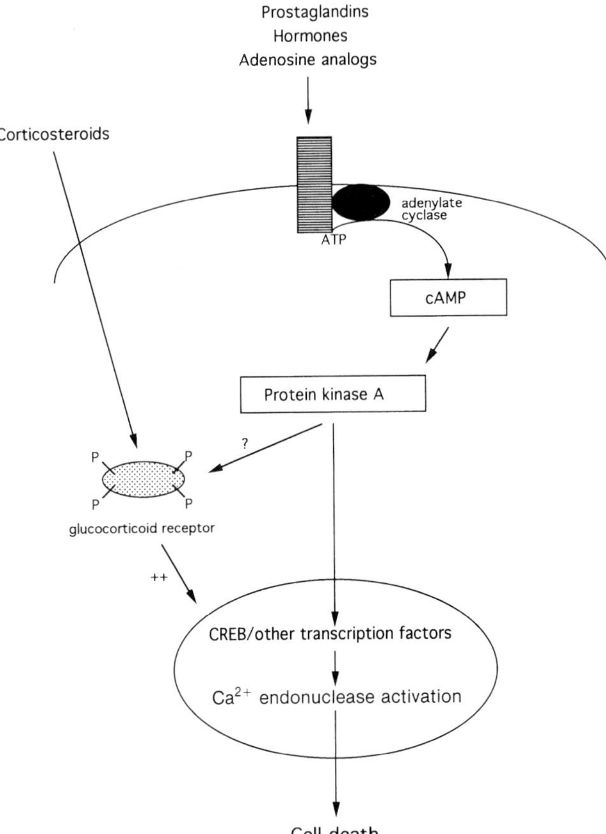

Figure 20–2. Role of the cAMP/PKA signaling pathway in apoptosis. Receptor-mediated activation of adenylate cyclase results in the production of cAMP, which in turn activates the protein serine/threonine kinase, protein kinase A (PKA). Subsequent changes in target substrate phosphorylation (potentially including the glucocorticoid receptor) mediate Ca^{2+}-dependent endonuclease activation via an unknown mechanism that may involve the glucocorticoid receptor or other transcription factors (e.g., *c*AMP *R*esponse *E*lement *B*inding protein, or CREB).

Role of Protein Kinase C

Many physiologic responses to surface receptor engagement involve the early activation of polyphosphoinositide-specific phospholipases C, resulting in production of two important second messengers, inositol triphosphate and diacylglycerol (DAG).[101,102] The primary action of inositol triphosphate appears to involve Ca^{2+} mobilization,[102] whereas DAG exerts its effects via binding to and activating the serine/threonine protein kinase, PKC.[101] Activation of PKC appears to be an important prerequisite for initiation of the events that lead to cell proliferation, including stimulation of $p21^{ras}$ function.[103] PKC has also been implicated in tumor promotion and differentiation.[101]

Most of the evidence for a role for PKC in apoptosis comes from work with phorbol esters, a class of tumor-promoting agents that mimic the effects of DAG to activate the enzyme. Chronic treatment of thymocytes with phorbol esters results in apoptosis.[61,104] The response can be abrogated by PKC inhibitors, suggesting that kinase activation is involved in the response.[104] Curiously, endonuclease activation does not occur immediately but involves a lag period of several hours, during which the phorbol ester can be removed and cells recover. This delay is not observed in thymocytes induced to undergo apoptosis in response to treatment with various other agents. Although the biochemical basis for the lag is not known, it may be related to special transcriptional and translational requirements or, perhaps more likely, to the known ability of phorbol esters to down-regulate PKC protein expression after prolonged exposure of cells to the agents in culture. These possibilities are being investigated.

Physiologic or pharmacologic activators of PKC can also block apoptosis in thymocytes and other cell types[20,47,85,96,104–108] (Fig. 20–3). The protective effects are abrogated with protein kinase antagonists, and possible targets of the kinase include the Na^+/H^+ antiporter,[106] the endonuclease itself,[47] or the *ras* pathway of signal transduction.[64,103] We have proposed that apoptosis may represent a cellular response to imbalanced signal transduction[78] and that activation of PKC in these systems restores balance and possibly promotes alternative cellular responses (proliferation, differentiation). The potential involvement of particular PKC substrates and PKC-responsive transcription factors (see Fig. 20–3) requires further investigation.

Other Second Messengers

Sphingolipids and their metabolites are bioactive molecules with diverse functions.[109] Sphingomyelin is converted into two compounds of particular interest, sphingosine and ceramide. The former is a potent inhibitor of PKC,[109] and the latter is a second messenger that may be involved in the

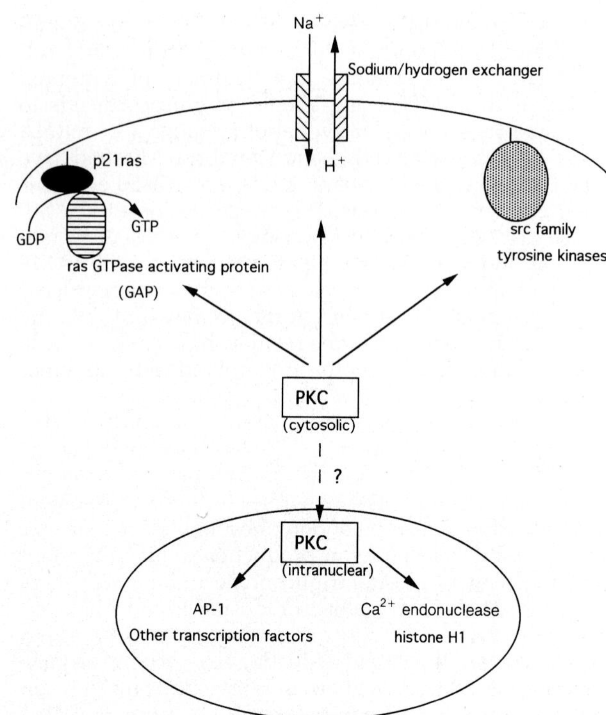

Figure 20–3. Potential mechanisms underlying the inhibition of apoptosis by PKC. Production of DAG or the action of chemical tumor promoters can inhibit endogenous endonuclease activation and cell death via activation of PKC. Possible cytosolic targets of PKC action include inhibition of *ras* GTPase activating protein (GAP), which leads to an inhibition of GTP hydrolysis and promotes *ras* function, stimulation of the Na^+/H^+ exchanger (which in turn leads to an increase in cytosolic pH), and phosphorylation of members of the *src* family of protein tyrosine kinases, which are PKC substrates. Possible nuclear targets include the *fos/jun* heterodimeric transcription factor AP-1, histone H1, and the Ca^{2+}-dependent endonuclease itself.

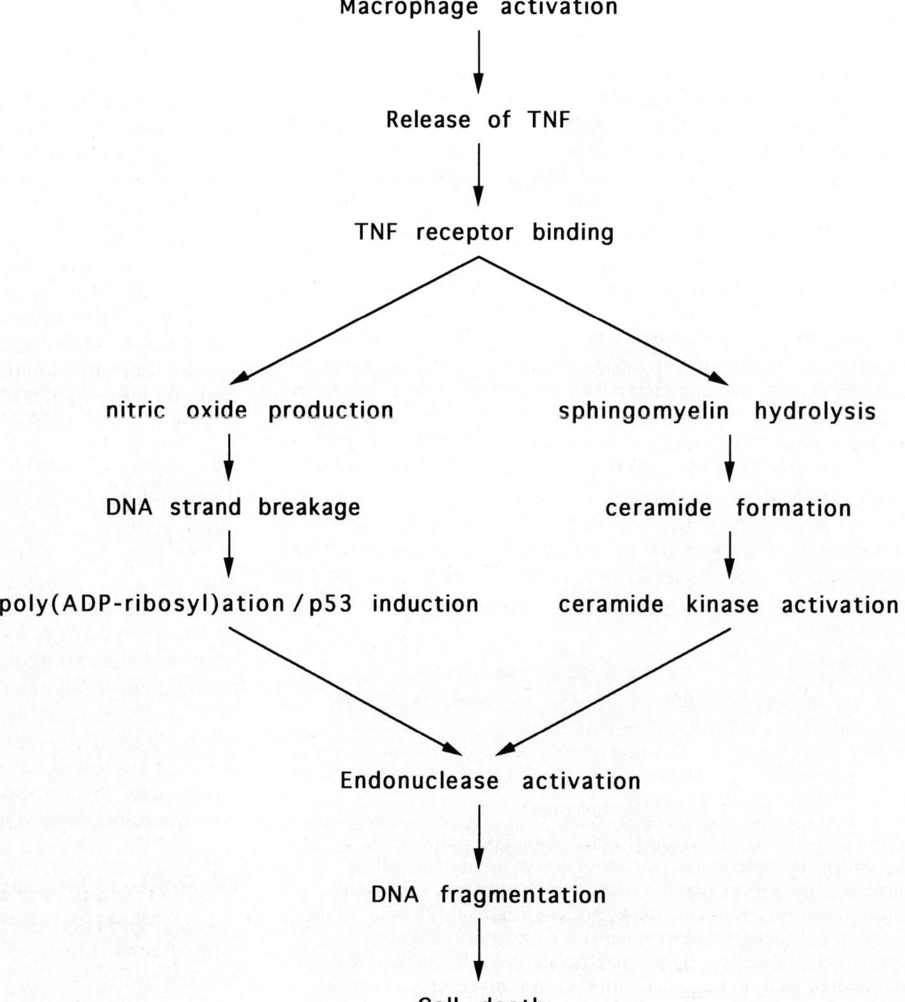

Figure 20–4. Inflammation-directed cell death mediated by TNF. Upon binding of its plasma membrane receptor, TNF triggers a complex signal transduction cascade that involves both sphingomyelin hydrolysis and nitric oxide production, both of which have been implicated in TNF-stimulated apoptosis. The sphingomyelin product ceramide may activate a lipid-sensitive protein kinase, whereas nitric oxide may elicit the DNA damage response by inducing oxidative damage to DNA, p53 induction, and poly(ADP-ribose) polymerase activation. Whether these pathways synergistically promote apoptosis is not known.

effects of steroid hormones, interferon, and tumor necrosis factor (TNF)[110, 111] (Fig. 20–4). TNF stimulates apoptosis in sensitive target cells,[112] and studies by Obeid and coworkers have linked production of ceramide to the response[108] (see Fig. 20–4). Other possible mediators of inflammatory cytokine-mediated tumor cell apoptosis include reactive oxygen species and nitric oxide[113, 114] (see Fig. 20–4), and the relative contribution of each to TNF-induced apoptosis is not yet clear.

Damage to DNA elicits a response involving activation of the nuclear enzyme polyadenosinediphosphate (ADP-ribose) polymerase, which catalyzes the transfer of the ADP-ribose moiety of nicotine adenine dinucleotide (NAD^+) to target proteins.[115] Extensive DNA damage can result in use of the entire cellular NAD^+ pool, leading to ATP depletion due to an inhibition of oxidative phosphorylation; this scenario has been advanced as a form of cellular suicide.[116, 117] The enzyme is directly activated by single- or double-strand breaks in chromatin. Early work suggested that the Ca^{2+}-dependent endonuclease is a target for the enzyme,[118] and we have shown that NAD^+ promotes its activity in vitro.[41] Studies using inhibitors of the enzyme have suggested that poly(ADP-ribose) polymerase activation is involved in apoptosis in response to irradiation.[119] Direct implication of poly(ADP-ribose) polymerase activation in the DNA damage-mediated pathway of apoptosis requires additional investigation.

CELL SIGNALING IN CYTOTOXICITY

The biochemical and molecular mechanisms regulating pathologic apoptosis appear largely similar to those operating under physiologic circumstances. Many cytotoxic chemicals and other pathologic stimuli induce cell killing by disrupting intracellular Ca^{2+} homeostasis,[120–122] and it appears that apoptosis induction commonly underlies their cytotoxicity. Damage to DNA mediated by direct chemical effects or to the production of reactive oxygen species (oxidative stress) also plays an important part, because it elicits the p53-dependent cellular response mechanism that initiates the process. Importantly, apoptosis in these systems is often accompanied by necrosis, and the overall contribution of the two processes to tissue injury probably depends on the degree of insult and the damaging stimulus in question. Expression of oncogenes such as *bcl*-2 also dictates the magnitude of the response.[123, 124] This observation may in part explain the development of tumor resistance to cancer treatment protocols, although the complexity of the response indicates that several factors are involved. Ultimately, it is hoped that knowledge of the underlying biochemistry of the process will allow for the design of protocols to promote apoptosis in tumors and to prevent its induction during tissue injury.

References

1. Wyllie AH, Kerr JFR, Currie AR: Cell death: The significance of apoptosis. Int Rev Cytol 1980; 68:251.
2. Kerr JFR, Searle J: Deletion of cells by apoptosis during castration-induced involution of the rat prostate. Virchows Arch Abt B Zellpathol 1973; 13:87.
3. Kyprianou N, Isaacs JT: Activation of programmed cell death in the rat ventral prostate after castration. Endocrinology 1988; 122:552.
4. Walker NI, Bennett RE, Kerr JFR: Cell death by apoptosis during involution of the lactating breast in mice and rats. Am J Anat 1989; 185:19.
5. Hopwood D, Levison DA: Atrophy and apoptosis in the cyclical human endometrium. J Pathol 1976; 119:159.
6. Duke RC, Cohen JJ: IL-2 addiction: Withdrawal of growth factor activates a suicide program in dependent T cells. Lymphokine Res 1986; 5:289.
7. Saunders JW Jr: Death in embryonic systems. Science 1966; 154:604.
8. Oppenheim RW: Cell death during development of the nervous system. Annu Rev Neurosci 1991; 14:453.
9. Raff MC: Social controls on cell survival and cell death. Nature 1992; 356:397.
10. Cohen JJ, Duke RC, Fadok VA, Sellins KS: Apoptosis and programmed cell death in immunity. Annu Rev Immunol 1992; 10:267.
11. Pratt RM, Martin GR: Epithelial cell death and cyclic AMP increase during palatal development. Proc Natl Acad Sci U S A 1975; 72:874.
12. Ballard KJ, Holt SJ: Cytological and cytochemical studies on cell death and digestion in the foetal rat foot: The role of macrophages and hydrolytic enzymes. J Cell Sci 1968; 3:245.
13. Kerr JFR, Harmon B, Searle J: An electron microscope study of cell deletion in the anuran tadpole tail during spontaneous metamorphosis with special reference to apoptosis of striated muscle fibres. J Cell Sci 1974; 14:571.
14. Searle J, Lawson TA, Abbot PJ, et al: An electron microscope study of the mode of cell death induced by cancer chemotherapeutic agents in populations of proliferating normal and neoplastic cells. J Pathol 1975; 116:129.
15. Barry MA, Behnke CA, Eastman A: Activation of programmed cell death (apoptosis) by cisplatin, other anticancer drugs, toxins, and hyperthermia. Biochem Pharmacol 1990; 40:2353.
16. Umansky SR, Korol BA, Nelipovich PA: In vivo DNA degradation in thymocytes of gamma irradiation and hydrocortisone treated rats. Biochim Biophys Acta 1981; 655:9.
17. Sellins KS, Cohen JJ: Gene induction by gamma irradiation leads to DNA fragmentation in lymphocytes. J Immunol 1987; 139:3199.
18. Harmon BV, Corder AM, Collins RJ, et al: Cell death induced in a murine mastocytoma by 42–47° C heating in vitro: Evidence that the form of death changes from apoptosis to necrosis above a critical heat load. Int J Radiat Biol 1990; 58:845.
19. Soloff BL, Nagle WA, Moss AJ Jr, et al: Apoptosis induced by cold shock in vitro is dependent on cell growth phase. Biochem Biophys Res Commun 1987; 145:876.
20. Perotti M, Toddei F, Mirabelli F, et al: Calcium-dependent DNA fragmentation in human synovial cells exposed to cold shock. FEBS Lett 1990; 259:331.
21. Meyaard L, Otto SA, Jonker RR, et al: Programmed death of T cells in HIV-1 infection. Science 1992; 257:217.
22. Gougeon ML, Montagnier L: Apoptosis in AIDS. Science 1993; 260:1269.
23. Martin JB: Huntington's disease: Genetically programmed cell death in the human central nervous system. Nature 1982; 299:205.
24. Vaux DL: Toward an understanding of the molecular mechanisms of physiological cell death. Proc Natl Acad Sci U S A 1993; 90:786.
25. Juntti-Berggren L, Larsson O, Rorsman P, et al: Increased activity of L-type Ca^{2+} channels exposed to serum from patients with type I diabetes. Science 1993; 261:86.
26. Ellis HM, Horvitz HR: Genetic control of programmed cell death in the nematode *C. elegans*. Cell 1986; 44:817.
27. Buttyan R, Olsson CA, Pintar J, et al: Induction of the TRPM-2 gene in cells undergoing programmed cell death. Mol Cell Biol 1989; 9:3473.
28. Harrigan MT, Baughman G, Campbell NF, et al: Isolation and characterization of glucocorticoid- and cyclic AMP-induced genes in T lymphocytes. Mol Cell Biol 1989; 9:3438.
29. Owens GP, Hahn WE, Cohen JJ: Identification of mRNAs associated with programmed cell death in immature thymocytes. Mol Cell Biol 1991; 11:4177.
30. Ishida Y, Agata Y, Shibahara K, et al: Induced expression of PD-1, a novel member of the immunoglobulin gene superfamily, upon programmed cell death. EMBO J 1992; 11:3887.
31. Baughman G, Lesley J, Trotter J, et al: Tcl-30, a new T cell-specific gene expressed in immature glucocorticoid-sensitive thymocytes. J Immunol 1992; 149:1488.

32. Duke RC, Chervenak R, Cohen JJ: Endogenous endonuclease-induced DNA fragmentation: An early event in cell-mediated cytolysis. Proc Natl Acad Sci U S A 1983; 80:6361.
33. Waring P: DNA fragmentation induced in macrophages by gliotoxin does not require protein synthesis and is preceded by raised inositol triphosphate levels. J Biol Chem 1990; 265:14476.
34. Chang MP, Bramhall J, Graves S, et al: Internucleosmal DNA cleavage precedes diphtheria toxin-induced cytolysis. J Biol Chem 1989; 264:15261.
35. Martin SJ, Lennon SV, Bonham AM, et al: Induction of apoptosis (programmed cell death) in human leukemic HL-60 cells by inhibition of RNA or protein synthesis. J Immunol 1990; 145:1859.
36. McConkey DJ, Hartzell P, Orrenius S: Rapid turnover of endogenous endonuclease activity in thymocytes: Effects of inhibitors of macromolecular synthesis. Arch Biochem Biophys 1990; 278:284.
37. Wyllie AH: Glucocorticoid-induced thymocyte apoptosis is associated with endogenous endonuclease activation. Nature 1980; 284:555.
38. Hewish DR, Burgoyne LA: Chromatin sub-structure. The digestion of DNA at regularly spaced sites by a nuclear deoxyribonuclease. Biochem Biophys Res Comm 1973; 52:504.
39. Vanderbilt JN, Bloom KS, Anderson JN: Endogenous nuclease: Properties and effects on transcribed genes in chromatin. J Biol Chem 1982; 257:13009.
40. Cohen JJ, Duke RC: Glucocorticoid activation of a calcium-dependent endonuclease in thymocyte nuclei leads to cell death. J Immunol 1984; 132:38.
41. Jones DP, McConkey DJ, Nicotera P, et al: Calcium-activated DNA fragmentation in rat liver nuclei. J Biol Chem 1989; 264:6398.
42. Kyprianou N, English HF, Isaacs JT: Activation of a Ca^{2+}-Mg^{2+}-dependent endonuclease as an early event in castration-induced prostatic cell death. Prostate 1988; 13:103.
43. Gaido ML, Cidlowski JA: Identification, purification, and characterization of a calcium-dependent endonuclease (NUC-18) from apoptotic rat thymocytes. J Biol Chem 1990; 266:18580.
44. Arends MJ, Morris RG, Wyllie AH: Apoptosis: The role of the endonuclease. Am J Pathol 1990; 136:593.
45. Peitsch MC, Polzar B, Stephan H, et al: Characterization of the endogenous deoxyribonuclease involved in nuclear DNA degradation during apoptosis (programmed cell death). EMBO J 1993; 12:371.
46. Barry MA, Eastman A: Identification of deoxyribonuclease II as an endonuclease involved in apoptosis. Arch Biochem Biophys 1993; 300:440.
47. McConkey DJ, Hartzell P, Jondal M, et al: Inhibition of DNA fragmentation in thymocytes and isolated thymocyte nuclei by agents that stimulate protein kinase C. J Biol Chem 1989; 264:13399.
48. McConkey DJ, Hartzell P, Nicotera P, et al: Calcium-activated DNA fragmentation kills immature thymocytes. FASEB J 1989; 3:1843.
49. Ucker DS, Obermiller PS, Eckhart W, et al: Genome digestion is a dispensible consequence of physiological cell death mediated by cytotoxic T lymphocytes. Mol Cell Biol 1992; 12:3060.
50. Hedgecock EM, Sulston JE, Thomson JN: Mutations affecting programmed cell deaths in the nematode *Caenorhabditis elegans*. Science 1983; 220:1277.
51. White E, Sabbatini P, Debbas M, et al: The 19-kilodalton adenovirus E1B transforming protein inhibits programmed cell death and prevents cytolysis by tumor necrosis factor alpha. Mol Cell Biol 1992; 12:2570.
52. Henderson S, Rowe M, Gregory C, et al: Induction of *bcl*-2 expression by Epstein-Barr virus latent membrane protein 1 protects infected cells from programmed cell death. Cell 1991; 65:1107.
53. Martz E, Howell DM: CTL: Virus control cells first and cytolytic cells second? Immunol Today 1989; 10:79.
54. Zychlinsky A, Zheng LM, Liu CC, et al: Cytolytic lymphocytes induce both apoptosis and necrosis in target cells. J Immunol 1991; 146:393.
55. Wyllie AH: The biology of cell death in tumors. Anticancer Res 1985; 5:131.
56. Williams GT: Programmed cell death: Apoptosis and oncogenesis. Cell 1991; 65:1097.
57. Hockenberry DM: The *bcl*-2 oncogene and apoptosis. Semin Immunol 1992; 4:413.
58. Hockenbery D, Nunez G, Milliman C, et al: *Bcl*-2 is an inner mitochondrial membrane protein that blocks programmed cell death. Nature 1990; 348:334.
59. Nunez G, London L, Hockenbery D, et al: Deregulated *bcl*-2 gene expression selectively prolongs survival of growth factor-deprived hemopoietic cell lines. J Immunol 1990; 144:3602.
60. Sentman CL, Shutter JR, Hockenbery D, et al: *Bcl*-2 inhibits multiple forms of apoptosis but not negative selection in thymocytes. Cell 1991; 67:879.
61. Strasser A, Harris AW, Cory S: *Bcl*-2 transgene inhibits T cell death and perturbs thymic self-censorship. Cell 1991; 67:889.
62. Siegel RM, Katsumata M, Miyashita T, et al: Inhibition of thymocyte apoptosis and negative antigenic selection in *bcl*-2 transgenic mice. Proc Natl Acad Sci U S A 1992; 89:7003.
63. Evans CA, Owen-Lynch PJ, Whetton AD, et al: Activation of the Abelson tyrosine kinase activity is associated with suppression of apoptosis in hemopoietic cells. Cancer Res 1993; 53:1735.
64. Wyllie AH, Rose KA, Morris RG, et al: Rodent fibroblast tumours expressing *myc* and *ras* genes. Growth, metastasis, and endogenous oncogene expression. Br J Cancer 1987; 56:251.
65. Askew DS, Ashmun RA, Simmons BC, et al: Constitutive *c-myc* expression in an IL-3-dependent myeloid cell line suppresses cell cycle arrest and accelerates apoptosis. Oncogene 1991; 12:1915.
66. Evan GI, Wyllie AH, Gilbert CS, et al: Induction of apoptosis in fibroblasts by *c-myc* protein. Cell 1992; 69:119.
67. Shi Y, Glynn JM, Guilbert LJ, et al: Role for *c-myc* in activation-induced apoptotic cell death in T cell hybridomas. Science 1992; 257:212.
68. Smeyne RJ, Bendrell M, Hayward M, et al: Continuous *c-fos* expression precedes programmed cell death in vivo. Nature 1993; 363:166.
69. Yonish-Rouach E, Resnitzky D, Lotem J, et al: Wild-type p53 induces apoptosis of myeloid leukaemic cells that is inhibited by interleukin-6. Nature 1991; 352:345.
70. Shaw P, Bovey R, Tardy S, et al: Induction of apoptosis by wild-type p53 in a human colon tumor-derived cell line. Proc Natl Acad Sci U S A 1992; 89:4495.
71. Lane DP: p53, guardian of the genome. Nature 1992; 358:15.
72. Lowe SW, Schmitt EM, Smith SW, et al: p53 is required for radiation-induced apoptosis in mouse thymocytes. Nature 1993; 362:847.
73. Clarke AR, Purdie CA, Harrison DJ, et al: Thymocyte apoptosis induced by p53-dependent and independent pathways. Nature 1993; 362:849.
74. Kaiser N, Edelman IS: Calcium dependence of glucocorticoid-induced lymphocytolysis. Proc Natl Acad Sci U S A 1977; 74:638.
75. Kaiser N, Edelman IS: Further studies on the role of calcium in glucocorticoid-induced lymphocytolysis. Endocrinology 1978; 103:936.
76. Wyllie AH, Morris RG, Smith AL, et al: Chromatin cleavage in apoptosis: Association with condensed chromatin morphology and dependence on macromolecular synthesis. J Pathol 1984; 142:67.
77. Martikainen P, Isaacs J: Role of calcium in the programmed death of rat prostatic glandular cells. Prostate 1990; 17:175.
78. McConkey DJ, Orrenius S, Jondal M: Cellular signaling in programmed cell death (apoptosis). Immunol Today 1990; 11:120.
79. McConkey DJ, Hartzell P, Duddy SK, et al: 2,3,7,8-Tetrachlorodibenzo-*p*-dioxin kills immature thymocytes by Ca^{2+}-mediated endonuclease activation. Science 1988; 242:256.
80. McConkey DJ, Nicotera P, Hartzell P, et al: Glucocorticoids activate a suicide process in thymocytes through an elevation of cytosolic Ca^{2+} concentration. Arch Biochem Biophys 1989; 269:365.
81. Zheng LM, Zychlinsky A, Liu CC, et al: Extracellular ATP as a trigger for apoptosis or programmed cell death. J Cell Biol 1991; 112:279.
82. Allbritton NL, Verret CR, Wolley RE, et al: Calcium ion concentrations and DNA fragmentation in target cell destruction

by murine cloned cytotoxic T lymphocytes. J Exp Med 1988; 167:514.
83. McConkey DJ, Chow SC, Orrenius S, et al: NK cell cytotoxicity is dependent on a Ca^{2+} increase in the target. FASEB J 1990; 4:2661.
84. Story MD, Stephens LC, Tomasovic SP, et al: A role for calcium in regulating apoptosis in rat thymocytes irradiated in vitro. Int J Radiat Biol 1992; 61:243.
85. Robertson LE, Chubb S, Meyn RE, et al: Induction of apoptotic cell death in chronic lymphocytic leukemia by 2-chloro-2′-deoxyadenosine and 9-beta-arabinosyl-2-fluoroadenine. Blood 1993; 81:143.
86. Nicotera P, McConkey DJ, Jones DP, et al: ATP stimulates Ca^{2+} uptake and increases the free Ca^{2+} concentration in isolated rat liver nuclei. Proc Natl Acad Sci U S A 1989; 86:453.
87. Bansal N, Houle AG, Melnykovych G: Dexamethasone-induced killing of neoplastic cells of lymphoid derivation: Lack of early calcium involvement. J Cell Physiol 1989; 143:105.
88. Alnemri ES, Litwack G: Activation of internucleosomal DNA cleavage in human CEM lymphocytes by glucocorticoid and novobiocin. Evidence for a non-Ca^{2+}-requiring mechanism(s). J Biol Chem 1990; 265:17323.
89. Rodriguez-Tarduchy G, Collins M, Lopez-Rivas A: Regulation of apoptosis in interleukin-3-dependent hemopoietic cells by interleukin-3 and calcium ionophores. EMBO J 1990; 9:2997.
90. Rodriguez-Tarduchy G, Malde P, Lopez-Rivas A, et al: Inhibition of apoptosis by calcium ionophores in IL-3-dependent bone marrow cells is dependent upon production of IL-4. J Immunol 1992; 148:1416.
91. Martin DP, Johnson EM Jr: Programmed cell death in the peripheral nervous system. *In*: Apoptosis: The Molecular Basis of Cell Death. Vol I. Tomei LD, Cope FO (Eds). Cold Spring Harbor, NY, Cold Spring Harbor Press, 1990, p 247.
92. Edwards SN, Buckmaster AE, Tolkovsky AM: The death programme in cultured sympathetic neurones can be suppressed at the posttranslational level by nerve growth factor, cyclic AMP, and depolarization. J Neurochem 1991; 57:2140.
93. Hassell JR, Pratt RM: Elevated levels of cAMP alters the effect of epidermal growth factor in vitro on programmed cell death in the secondary palatal epithelium. Exp Cell Res 1977; 106:55.
94. Daniel V, Litwack G, Tomkins GM: Induction of cytolysis of cultured lymphoma cells by adenosine 3′:5′-cyclic monophosphate and the isolation of resistant variants. Proc Natl Acad Sci U S A 1973; 70:76.
95. Basile DV, Wood HN, Braun AC: Programming of cells for death under defined experimental conditions: Relevance to the tumor problem. Proc Natl Acad Sci U S A 1973; 70:3055.
96. McConkey DJ, Orrenius S, Jondal M: Agents that elevate cAMP stimulate DNA fragmentation in thymocytes. J Immunol 1990; 145:1227.
97. Kizaki H, Suzuki K, Tadakuma T, et al: Adenosine receptor-mediated accumulation of cyclic AMP-induced T-lymphocyte death through internucleosomal DNA cleavage. J Biol Chem 1990; 265:5280.
98. Dowd DR, Miesfeld RL: Evidence that glucocorticoid- and cyclic AMP-induced apoptotic pathways in lymphocytes share distal events. Mol Cell Biol 1992; 12:3600.
99. Gruol DJ, Campbell NF, Bourgeois S: Cyclic AMP-dependent protein kinase promotes glucocorticoid receptor function. J Biol Chem 1986; 261:4909.
100. McConkey DJ, Orrenius S, Okret S, et al: Cyclic AMP potentiates glucocorticoid-induced endogenous endonuclease activation in thymocytes. FASEB J 1993; 7:580.
101. Nishizuka Y: The role of protein kinase C in cell surface signal transduction and tumour promotion. Nature 1984; 308:693.
102. Berridge MJ: Inositol trisphosphate and calcium signalling. Nature 1993; 361:315.
103. Downward J, Graves JD, Warne PH, et al: Stimulation of p21*ras* upon T-cell activation. Nature 1990; 346:719.
104. Kizaki H, Tadakuma T, Odaka C, et al: Activation of a suicide process of thymocytes through DNA fragmentation by calcium ionophores and phorbol esters. J Immunol 1989; 143:1790.
105. McConkey DJ, Aguilar-Santelises M, Hartzell P, et al: Induction of DNA fragmentation in chronic B-lymphocytic leukemia cells. J Immunol 1991; 146:1072.
106. Rajotte D, Haddad P, Haman A, et al: Role of protein kinase C and the Na^{+}/H^{+} antiporter in suppressing apoptosis by granulocyte macrophage colony-stimulating factor and interleukin 3. J Biol Chem 1992; 267:9980.
107. Forbes IJ, Zalewski PD, Giannakis C, et al: Induction of apoptosis in chronic lymphocytic leukemia cells and its prevention by phorbol ester. Exp Cell Res 1992; 198:367.
108. Obeid LM, Linardic CM, Karolak LA, et al: Programmed cell death induced by ceramide. Science 1993; 259:1769.
109. Hannun YA, Bell RM: Functions of sphingolipids and sphingolipid breakdown products in cellular regulation. Science 1989; 243:500.
110. Kim MY, Linardic C, Obeid L, et al: Identification of sphingomyelin turnover as an effector mechanism for the action of tumor necrosis factor alpha and gamma interferon. J Biol Chem 1991; 266:484.
111. Okazaki T, Bell RM, Hannun YA: Sphingomyelin turnover induced by vitamin D3 in HL-60 cells: Role in cell differentiation. J Biol Chem 1989; 264:19076.
112. Laster SM, Wood JG, Gooding LR: Tumor necrosis factor can induce both apoptotic and necrotic forms of cell lysis. J Immunol 1988; 141:2629.
113. Zimmerman RJ, Marafino BJ Jr, Chan A, et al: The role of oxidant injury in tumor cell sensitivity to recombinant human tumor necrosis factor in vivo. J Immunol 1989; 142:1405.
114. Duerksen-Hughes PJ, Day DB, Laster SM, et al: Both tumor necrosis factor and nitric oxide participate in lysis of simian virus 40-transformed cells by activated macrophages. J Immunol 1992; 149:2114.
115. Lunee J: Introductory review: Involvement of ADP-ribosylation in cellular recovery from some forms of DNA damage. Br J Cancer 1984; 49(Suppl VI):13.
116. Schraufstatter IU, Hinshaw DB, Hyslop PA, et al: Oxidant injury of cells: DNA strand breaks activate polyadenosine diphosphate-ribose polymerase and lead to depletion of nicotinamide adenine dinucleotide. J Clin Invest 1986; 77:1312.
117. Gaal JL, Smith KR, Pearson CK: Cellular euthanasia mediated by a nuclear enzyme: A central role for nuclear ADP-ribosylation in cellular metabolism. Trends Biochem Sci 1987; 12:129.
118. Yoshihara K, Tanigawa Y, Burzio L, et al: Evidence for adenosine diphosphate ribosylation of Ca^{2+}, Mg^{2+}-dependent endonuclease. Proc Natl Acad Sci U S A 1975; 72:289.
119. Nelipovich PA, Nikonova LV, Umansky SR: Inhibition of poly(ADP-ribose) polymerase as a possible reason for activation of Ca^{2+}/Mg^{2+}-dependent endonuclease in thymocytes of irradiated rats. Int J Radiat Biol 1988; 53:749.
120. Kerr JFR: Shrinkage necrosis: A distinct mode of cellular death. J Pathol 1971; 105:13.
121. Orrenius S, McConkey DJ, Bellomo G, et al: Role of Ca^{2+} in toxic cell killing. Trends Pharmacol Sci 1989; 10:281.
122. Trump BF, Berezesky IK: The role of cytosolic Ca^{2+} in cell injury, necrosis, and apoptosis. Curr Opin Cell Biol 1992; 4:227.
123. Tsujimoto Y: Stress-resistance conferred by high level of *bcl*-2 alpha protein in human B lymphoblastoid cell. Oncogene 1989; 4:1331.
124. Miyashita T, Reed JC: *Bcl*-2 oncoprotein blocks chemotherapy-induced apoptosis in a human leukemia cell line. Blood 1993; 81:151.

CHAPTER 21

Cytokines

Leland Shapiro, MD • Jeffrey A. Gelfand, MD

Cytokines are intercellular messenger polypeptides that modulate many biologic responses. They are small, with molecular mass between 8 and 30 kd, and are biologically active at low concentrations (picomolar or less). They differ from classic endocrine hormones in that they are produced by many cell types rather than by discrete organs, are primarily produced de novo in response to stimuli, have little significant role in normal homeostasis, are often induced in response to exogenous (not endogenous) stimuli, and frequently have autocrine and paracrine effects. It is clear from these qualities that the distinctions among cytokines, neurotransmitters, and hormones are mainly functional. The nomenclature of cytokines is confusing. They are variously subdivided into interleukins, interferons, growth factors, stimulating factors, proinflammatory factors, inhibitory factors, activating factors, and so forth. These terms were usually generated descriptively on the basis of physiologic function, target cell type, or order of discovery. Examples include the interleukins (ILs, which currently number 15), macrophage-activating factor, macrophage migration inhibitory factor, tumor necrosis factor (TNF), granulocyte/macrophage colony-stimulating factor, granulocyte colony-stimulating factor, erythropoietin, cardiac depressant factor, platelet-derived growth factor, platelet-activating factor (PAF), leukemia inhibitory factor, ciliary neurotrophic factor, and others. Binding proteins and soluble cytokine receptors have also been identified.

It is clear that cytokines are involved directly or indirectly in the pathogenesis of many diseases, especially those associated with inflammation or cell proliferation. Some of these are systemic inflammatory response syndrome (SIRS)/sepsis, adult respiratory distress syndrome, carcinomatous cachexia, bacterial meningitis, atherosclerotic coronary artery disease, congestive heart failure syndrome, hepatic fibrosis, pulmonary fibrosis, Kawasaki syndrome, solid and hematologic malignancies, hypercalcemia of malignancy, malaria, alcoholic hepatitis, glomerulonephritis, graft rejection, many collagen vascular diseases, and granulomatous diseases. A partial list of conditions associated with increased cytokine production is presented in Table 21–1.

It is often difficult to determine whether cytokines associated with a particular disease represent an epiphenomenon or whether they are causally linked to disease pathophysiology. The best case for a causal role for cytokines in disease is found for IL-1 and TNF in sepsis or, more generally, SIRS. Three lines of evidence support a functional role for cytokines in disease pathophysiology. Proceeding from weakest to strongest, these are

1. Studies demonstrating a correlation between clinical status and cytokine concentrations in body fluids or biopsy specimens[1–6]
2. Administration of cytokines to animals, replicating many, if not all findings of certain diseases or syndromes[7, 8]
3. Selective blockade of specific cytokines, ameliorating or abrogating disease phenomena in animals or humans[7, 9, 10]

In addition to their direct causal role in disease pathophysiology, cytokines can serve as markers of disease activity. This has been shown in clinical studies involving many diseases and various body fluids and secretions. In general, IL-6, the anti-inflammatory cytokine IL-1 receptor antagonist (IL-1ra), and the inhibitory soluble TNF receptors correlate better with disease activity than do the concentrations of circulating proinflammatory cytokines (discussed later).

Exciting developments include the demonstration of complex interactions between host and microorganism involving cytokines. For example, several viruses produce soluble receptors to proinflammatory cytokines. They have immunomodulatory activity and serve as virulence factors in in vivo animal models of inflammatory diseases.[11–15] Certain strains of virulent bacteria have been found to use cytokines directly as growth factors or to bind cytokines at their surface to enhance phagocytic cell entry and virulence.[16, 17] It has also been demonstrated that *Schistosoma mansoni* uses host TNF to facilitate egg laying in a murine model, and plasmodia parasites, which cause malaria, gain access to red blood cells by binding to IL-8 receptors present on the red blood cells' surface.[18, 18a]

CYTOKINES AND SEPSIS (SYSTEMIC INFLAMMATORY RESPONSE SYNDROME)

Sepsis is currently listed as the 13th leading cause of death in the United States, and it is on the rise. Factors thought to account for this increase include an aging population, increased use of invasive therapies and devices, improved survival of individuals with debilitating illnesses, and nosocomial infections persuant to increased hospitalization of chronically ill patients. All of these contribute to the opportunity for infection.

The prevalence of community-acquired bacteremia increased from 7 to 13 cases per 1000 hospital admissions between the mid-1960s and the mid-1970s, with increased risk associated with extremes of age. Some important predisposing factors in the development of bacteremia or sepsis include advanced age, use of intravenous lines and invasive devices, granulocytopenia, prior antibiotic therapy, severe burn injury, functional asplenia, and human immunodeficiency virus infection.

TABLE 21–1. Selected Conditions Associated with Increased Cytokine Production

Condition	*Example(s)*
Infectious disease	Infection due to gram-positive or gram-negative bacteria, fungi, protozoa, viruses, and mycobacteria
Trauma	Burn injury
Autoimmunity	Rheumatoid arthritis, systemic lupus erythematosus, vasculitides
Neoplasia	Many solid and hematologic malignancies
Circulating drugs/medications	Amphotericin B
Cryptogenic inflammatory disease	Sarcoidosis, Kawasaki syndrome, inflammatory bowel disease
Cardiac disease	Acute myocardial infarction, congestive heart failure syndrome
Production of endogenous substances	Cytokines, activated complement components, immune complexes

A plethora of terms associated with "sepsis" abound and need definition.[19] *Bacteremia* is the presence of bacteria in the blood, confirmed by culture. *Septicemia* implies bacteremia with significant clinical manifestations. *Sepsis* is now taken to mean evidence of infection with a systemic response. The *sepsis syndrome* refers to clinical evidence of infection with a systemic response sufficient to produce adverse organ function such as respiratory insufficiency, renal dysfunction, acidosis, or altered mental function. *Septic shock* refers to the sepsis syndrome with documented hypotension (systolic blood pressure <90 mm Hg, or a decrease in mean arterial blood pressure of >40 mm Hg from the baseline). *Refractory septic shock* is defined as septic shock lasting longer than 1 hour with no response to intervention with intravenous fluids or pharmacologic agents. It has been proposed that the more general term *systemic inflammatory response syndrome* be used to describe clinical manifestations of systemic inflammation.[20] The gradations of SIRS correspond to the severity of sepsis beyond and including sepsis syndrome, but SIRS does not imply only the presence or suspicion of infection. It therefore describes the clinical consequences of inflammatory endothelial activation regardless of cause.[21]

At the turn of the century, the focus of physicians was entirely on the microorganisms responsible for producing overwhelming infections, and the prevailing hypothesis was that either "pyogenic" or toxin-producing organisms were required. By the late 1920s, the description of the Shwartzman reaction focused the attention of investigators on the state of the host for the first time. By the 1950s, the endotoxin component of gram-negative bacteria was thought to be a major pathogenic factor in sepsis. By the 1970s complement activation and the activated neutrophil were thought to have major roles in the pathogenesis of sepsis. The importance of the host response was further suggested by the observed consistency of the stereotyped septic response to many different kinds of inciting factors and many types of infecting organisms. In the 1980s, a number of critical endogenous pathogenic mediators, notably the cytokines and arachidonic acid–derived metabolites, were elucidated. It was found that sepsis could be replicated by exogenous cytokine administration in the absence of bacteremia, and septic pathophysiology could be ameliorated by cytokine blockade. An illuminating series of experiments was performed with the C3H/Hej mouse, which has a mutation rendering its mononuclear leukocytes incapable of producing TNF in response to lipopolysaccharide (LPS). Such mice were found to be nearly refractory to LPS toxicity, indicating the primacy of the cytokine response in producing the septic state.[22]

An interesting fact concerning mortality associated with septic shock is that it has not changed significantly during the past 30 years, although the types of patients developing this syndrome probably have. It is remarkable that modern technology has contributed minimally to the survival statistics in this condition. Technologic advances have included invasive monitoring equipment, better diagnostic modalities, more effective vasopressors and inotropes, more powerful antibiotics, and combination antibiotic therapy. Another factor of import is the rapidly rising cost per life saved (or lost) in the face of little added benefit in ultimate outcome. A safe conclusion is that improved antibiotics are not the answer to significant improvement in therapy for this condition.

Although microorganisms can secrete exotoxins, these do not appear to be directly responsible for the majority of damage produced during bacterial sepsis (although diseases such as tetanus, toxic shock syndrome, staphylococcal scalded skin syndrome, and others are toxin mediated).

The sequence of events leading to sepsis presumedly begins with bacteremia. In the outer membrane of all gram-negative bacteria is LPS, or endotoxin, which interacts with the reticuloendothelial system in a way that produces the septic state. Lipid A appears to be the key conserved piece of the endotoxin molecule involved in this interaction.[23, 24] Although not everything is known about the details of events leading to sepsis, a model is emerging, as follows (Fig. 21–1):

1. Endotoxin binds to receptors found on mononuclear leukocytes (monocytes and macrophages).
2. This interaction results in secretion of several cytokines. When produced in excess, the primary cytokines initiating adverse effects are IL-1 and TNF.[2, 25–28]
3. IL-1 and TNF orchestrate the physiology of the septic state by their effects on the temperature set-point (fever induction, possibly hypothermia), vascular resistance and permeability, cardiac function/inotropic state, bone marrow effects (e.g., increased leukocytes), and effects on many enzymes such as lactate dehydrogenase and lipoprotein lipase, which alter energy use by many tissues. At some point, cardiac depressant factor appears to be elaborated, although the identity of this molecule is unclear.[29] All of this morbid physiology can proceed in the absence of inciting endotoxin, as occurs in gram-positive septic shock or after clearance of endotoxin from the circulation. This observation further supports the notion that cytokines, and not the endotoxins themselves, are essential mediators of the multiple effects of sepsis.
4. Many of the effects of cytokines are mediated at the target tissues by nitric oxide, arachidonic acid metabolites (prostaglandins, eicosanoids, PAF), or lipoxygenase derivatives.
5. IL-1 and TNF stimulate the elaboration of other cytokines, producing a cascade effect with the multiple functions of amplification and modulation (both up- and down-regulation) as cytokines beget cytokines.[30, 31] Of special import may be the local production of IL-8 by cells at various organs, which has the function of recruiting and activating polymorphonuclear leukocytes, which can then cause tissue damage and organ dysfunction. In vitro data have documented significant IL-8 production in response to minute concentrations of IL-1 or TNF, suggesting an amplification role for IL-8 of IL-1 or TNF produced at sites of inflammation.
6. The complement, coagulation, and kinin cascades are also activated and have important roles in the septic state.[32–35]
7. Specific and nonspecific anticytokine substances are concomitantly produced, including glucocorticoids, IL-1ra, and soluble cytokine and endotoxin receptors (discussed earlier). Also, some liberated cytokines (IL-4, IL-6, IL-10, transforming growth factor-β [TGF-β]) have anti-inflammatory effects such as decreasing mononuclear cell synthesis of IL-1 and TNF in response to endotoxin.[36–39]

Of clinical relevance, antibiotics may exacerbate the inflammatory response to microorganisms by lysing them, releasing increased quantities of free endotoxin. This may result in increased contact of endotoxin with cytokine-producing cells, subsequently augmenting production of IL-1, TNF, and IL-8.

INTERLEUKIN-1 AND TUMOR NECROSIS FACTOR AS A SYNERGISTIC SEPTIC COMBINATION

The foregoing findings have stimulated some controversy about which cytokine constitutes *the* shock molecule. The seminal work of Beutler and Cerami has made a strong case

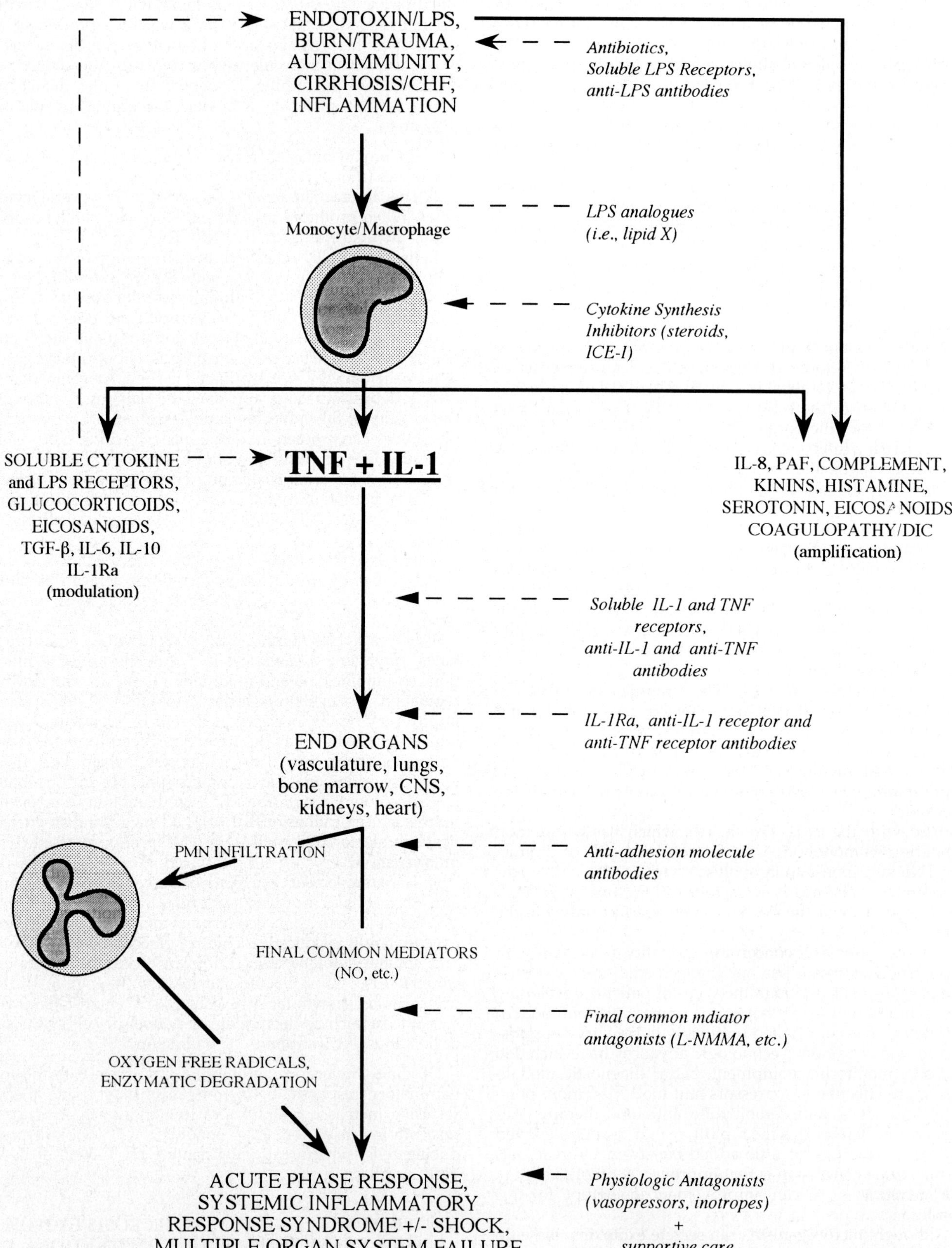

Figure 21–1 *See legend on opposite page*

for TNF being *the* shock cytokine. It has been shown that intravenous endotoxin infusion can produce septic shock while increasing circulating levels of TNF, TNF infusions can replicate all of the physiologic effects of septic shock, TNF serum levels correlate with degree of sepsis in humans (quantitated by APACHE II [Acute Physiology and Chronic Health Evaluation] score), and anti-TNF antibodies can prevent mortality as well as abrogate septic physiology after endotoxin infusion in animals. However, much in vivo and in vitro evidence supports a crucial role for IL-1 as a comediator of the sepsis syndrome. IL-1 has been shown to have nearly identical effects as TNF when administered to animals or humans.

Specifically, TNF or IL-1 infusion into animals results in fever (endogenous pyrogen), anorexia, sleep (hypnotoxin), hypotension, metabolic acidosis, neutrophilia or neutropenia (depending on dose), increased serum levels of adrenocorticotropic hormone, IL-6 and granulocyte/macrophage colony-stimulating factor, decreased serum iron, zinc, hepatic cytochrome P_{450} (hence decreased metabolism of many drugs), thyroxin (possible origin of nonthyroid illness) and albumin levels, increased hepatic synthesis of acute-phase proteins (i.e., serum amyloid A protein), capillary leak (possible origin of adult respiratory distress syndrome), and death. The current consensus includes little doubt about the importance of TNF and IL-1 as comediators of sepsis.[8, 22, 25, 26, 28, 40–42]

The kinetics of IL-1 may be relevant regarding the possibility of therapeutic cytokine modulation in sepsis. In animal models of bacteremia or endotoxemia, circulating TNF levels rise rapidly and peak at 60 to 90 minutes, followed by a delayed increase in circulating IL-1 levels that peak at 180 minutes; similar observations have been made in humans. Experiments have shown that TNF induces IL-1 in vivo.[30, 43, 44] These observations are important because any attempt to treat sepsis by modulating TNF may have to occur very early in the septic state. However, if IL-1 modulation is the target, intervention may be possible later in the disease process.

Evidence of the importance of IL-1 in septic shock is highlighted by experiments showing that blocking IL-1 using IL-1ra in animal models of septic shock decreases morbidity and mortality.[9, 41]

Thus, IL-1 or TNF given intravenously can reproduce the elements of the septic syndrome, and blocking the activities of either experimentally can abrogate the septic state. From a clinical standpoint, the arguments about which cytokine is most important in sepsis are secondary to the fact that IL-1 and TNF appear to act synergistically in producing septic physiology. In animal models of SIRS, injection of TNF or IL-1, which individually produce no significant hemodynamic disarray, can produce hemodynamic shock when infused together.[7] Similar experiments have documented synergistic TNF and IL-1 effects on increasing plasma lactate, glucose, and triglycerides in animals.[45] The teleology of this cytokine redundancy is uncertain, but the clinical implications are not. We may need not block all of the proinflammatory elements of the cytokine cascade; blocking only one or a few of them is likely to produce significant clinical benefit. As alluded to previously, many other mediators of sepsis exist (i.e., complement components, PAF, kinins, prostaglandins), but the extant data implicate IL-1 and TNF as crucial triggers in the initiation of sepsis.

PAF is a phospholipid produced by platelets, endothelium, and mononuclear and polymorphonuclear leukocytes; it has been implicated in the pathophysiology of sepsis. The evidence supporting such a role for PAF is similar to that described earlier for IL-1 and TNF. In fact, some PAF effects are probably mediated by IL-1 and TNF production, whereas some TNF effects are mediated through PAF.[46] The relative contribution of PAF to the septic state is uncertain, but data are accumulating rapidly.[47, 47a]

ROLE OF CYTOKINES IN PROTECTING THE HOST

It appears that some (yet undefined) levels of some cytokines are beneficial but excessive levels are detrimental. One experiment evaluated the role of exogenous IL-1ra in a neonatal rat model of lethal bacteremic sepsis.[48] Compared with control rats, blocking IL-1 activity with the receptor antagonist decreased lethality in this model, whereas very high doses of IL-1ra promoted lethality. The adverse outcome with more complete IL-1 suppression suggests that some quantity of IL-1 is beneficial. Other murine models have demonstrated exacerbation of infection after blockade of IL-1 activity, and pretreatment with low doses of IL-1 or TNF conferred protection from the effects of subsequent infection.[49, 50] Until we know more, the answer to the question of what critical levels of cytokines in disease traverse the boundary of helpful to harmful will have to remain "enough, but not too much."

Using anticytokine strategies to combat infectious/inflammatory conditions is not unprecedented, because this strategy occurs naturally in the course of disease in vivo. The natural control of inflammation has been shown to involve increased production of down-regulating or negative-feedback substances. These include soluble receptors to LPS, TNF, and (possibly) IL-1. Also produced are IL-6, IL-10, and TGF-β, which have anti-inflammatory functions, and IL-1ra is produced. In the course of overwhelming inflammation or infection, however, these natural anticytokine mediators are thought to be produced in insufficient quantities to contain such insults. Hence, one proposed therapeutic strategy is to administer large parenteral doses of these agents (produced by recombinant deoxyribonucleic acid technology) and to use pharmacologic blockade of multiple stages of the proinflammatory cascade simultaneously.

Figure 21–1. Any of a number of initiating factors can interact with mononuclear leukocytes and other cells to stimulate secretion of the key proinflammatory cytokines TNF and IL-1. In sufficiently high circulating concentrations, these two cytokines synergistically orchestrate all the phenomena of the systemic inflammatory response syndrome by proceeding to various end-organs and inducing specific final common mediators of organ dysfunction. Additionally, adhesion molecules are induced with subsequent recruitment and activation of polymorphonuclear leukocytes (aided by the chemotactic cytokine IL-8), which contribute to tissue damage. Amplification and diminution of the inflammatory responses proceed concomitantly with TNF and IL-1 production as shown. Also shown are possible targets for therapeutic intervention. *Abbreviations*: CHF = congestive heart failure; CNS = central nervous system; ICE-I = interleukin-1–converting enzyme inhibitor; IL-1Ra = interleukin-1 receptor antagonist; L-NMMA = L-N-monomethylarginine; NO = nitric oxide; PAF = platelet activating factor; PMN = polymorphonuclear leukocyte; TGF-β = transforming growth factor beta; *solid arrow* = proinflammatory response induction; *dashed arrow with notched head* = naturally occuring down-regulatory responses; *dashed arrow with flat head* = possible areas of therapeutic intervention *(italics)*.

INFLAMMATORY VERSUS ANTI-INFLAMMATORY CYTOKINES

Although more than 30 cytokines have been described, they may be characterized by broad functional categories. Cytokines may have growth-promoting, proinflammatory, or anti-inflammatory activities (Table 21–2). The primary proinflammatory cytokines are IL-1, TNF, and IL-8. IL-1 and TNF have nearly identical effects when injected intravenously in animal models of sepsis. As previously discussed, TNF or IL-1 infusion into animals results in fever, anorexia, sleep, hypotension, metabolic acidosis, and so forth.

IL-8 is a small cytokine with a molecular mass of about 8 kd, with the functions of neutrophilic chemotaxis and activation, as well as angiogenesis.[51, 52] Studies imply an important role for this cytokine in neutrophilic recruitment and activation at sites of inflammation, resulting in amplification of the local inflammatory response as well as tissue damage. IL-8 is secreted by many cell types, including fibroblasts, endothelium, and peripheral blood mononuclear cells. IL-8 secretagogues include endotoxin, IL-1, and TNF. In vitro, significant amounts of this cytokine are produced in response to minute concentrations of these stimulants; 1 to 10 pg/mL IL-1 or TNF can induce significant IL-8 production in human endothelial or fibroblast cell lines.

IL-6 is a cytokine that is also produced by many different cell types in response to various stimuli, including endotoxin, IL-1, and TNF.[53] It circulates in plasma at concentrations higher than those of most other cytokines and is one of the best cytokine markers of inflammatory disease activity in humans. It has both anti-inflammatory and proinflammatory activities owing to its function as a suppressor of proinflammatory cytokine induction, its role as an endogenous pyrogen, and its initiation of the acute-phase response (a property shared by IL-1 and TNF but not IL-8). Unlike IL-1 or TNF, IL-6 in animals does not appear to be causally related to SIRS.[36, 54] IL-1ra is also a marker of disease activity. It has been found clinically that levels of the anti-inflammatory cytokines are more reliable markers of inflammatory disease activity than levels of the proinflammatory cytokines, probably because of the greater magnitude of production or prolonged half-life of the former.

The cytokines IL-6, IL-10, TGF-β, and IL-1ra have activities that can be construed as anti-inflammatory. All can decrease the endotoxin-induced production of IL-1 and TNF in several in vitro and in vivo systems.

SELECTED ANTICYTOKINE STRATEGIES

Anticytokine approaches to infectious/inflammatory diseases have many potential advantages:

- Applicability to many such diseases, because therapy is directed at the final common pathway of inflammation and not at its specific proximate cause. Thus, in the case of SIRS due to infection, these approaches should be equally applicable to gram-positive or fungal conditions as well as to gram-negative ones.
- The margin of safety is likely to be great and the risk of immunogenicity small for many contemplated anticytokine agents, because they are naturally occurring substances, such as IL-1ra and soluble cytokine receptors.
- Specificity of some possible anticytokine agents. For instance, soluble cytokine receptors typically demonstrate a 100- to 1000-fold greater affinity for their respective cytokines than do monoclonal antibodies raised against these same cytokines.

Intracellular production of proinflammatory cytokines can be targeted. Signal transduction following cellular contact with proinflammatory substances leading to elaboration

TABLE 21–2. Proinflammatory Cytokines, Anti-inflammatory Cytokines, and Soluble Tumor Necrosis Factor Receptors

Cytokine (Mass in kd)		*Major Sources*	*Principal Activities*
Proinflammatory	IL-1 (17.5)	Monocyte/macrophage, lymphocyte, neutrophil, endothelium, fibroblast, keratinocyte	Activation of T cells, B cells, natural killer cells, neutrophils, osteoblasts, and endothelium. Induces fever, sleep, anorexia, adrenocorticotropic hormone release, and hepatic acute-phase protein synthesis. Leads to myocardial depression, hypercoagulability, hypotension/shock, and death. Stimulates production of TNF, IL-8, and IL-6. Supression of cytochrome P_{450}, thyroglobulin, and lipoprotein synthesis.
	TNF (17.5)	Monocyte/macrophage, lymphocyte, neutrophil, endothelium, fibroblast, keratinocyte	Activation of T cells, B cells, natural killer cells, neutrophils, osteoblasts, and endothelium. Tumoricidal activity. Induces fever, sleep, anorexia, catabolism, adrenocorticotropic hormone release, hepatic acute-phase protein synthesis. Leads to myocardial depression, hypercoagulability, hypotension/shock, and death. Stimulates production of IL-1, IL-8, and IL-6. Suppression of cytochrome P_{450}, thyroglobulin, and lipoprotein lipase.
	IL-8 (8)	Monocyte/macrophage, lymphocyte, endothelium, fibroblast, keratinocyte	Recruitment and activation of neutrophils, chemotactic for lymphocytes, angiogenesis.
Anti-inflammatory	IL-10, TGF-β (35, 12.5)	T cell, fibroblast	Suppression of B cell and T cell proliferation. Inhibition of LPS-induced monocyte IL-1 and TNF production. Induction of IL-1 Ra.
	IL-6 (21–28)	Monocyte/macrophage, T cell, endothelium, fibroblast, keratinocyte	Induction of fever and the hepatic acute-phase response. Stimulates cortisol production. Decreases IL-1 and TNF production. Participates in activation and proliferation of B and T cells, facilitates immunoglobulin production by B cells.
	IL-1ra (17.5)	Monocyte/macrophage, fibroblast	Specifically inhibits IL-1 effects, including SIRS due to endotoxin or *Escherichia coli* in animal models.
Soluble TNF receptors—derived from TNF receptors p55 and p75 (30 and 40, respectively)		Unknown, but monocyte/macrophage and neutrophil are likely	Specifically inhibits TNF effects, including SIRS due to endotoxin or *Escherichia coli* in animal models.

of TNF and IL-1 can be blocked pharmacologically. Corticosteroids decrease TNF and IL-1 production and have so far demonstrated some therapeutic efficacy, especially in patients with bacterial meningitis. Both thalidomide and pentoxifylline can decrease TNF production, and administration of TGF-β, IL-6, or IL-10 has been shown to decrease induction of TNF and IL-1.[37, 38, 53, 55, 56] A new molecular target is the IL-1–converting enzyme, which converts the biologically inactive pro-IL-1 within cells into the mature, bioactive IL-1 molecule. An IL-1–converting enzyme inhibitor has been found to down-regulate the inflammatory response; these substances are now under investigation as potential therapeutic agents.[57–59]

After IL-1 or TNF production, interventions designed to neutralize them or block interaction with cell surface receptors are possible. Anti-TNF antibodies have been shown to decrease mortality significantly and to ameliorate adverse physiologic changes in animal models of sepsis.[10, 60] This passive immunization treatment for adverse TNF effects has proved effective when administered either before the septic challenge or as late as 30 minutes afterward. A monoclonal murine IgG anti-TNF antibody preparation has been safely administered to humans, and phase-three clinical trials are under way.

IL-1ra is a natural product of monocytes and fibroblasts. It has been found to bind to and block IL-1 receptors, preventing IL-1 activity.[61] This is a unique substance in that it is the only natural competitive antagonist of a cytokine/hormone/neurotransmitter described to date. IL-1ra has reduced mortality by as much as 70% in rabbit, mouse, and primate models of septic shock.[9, 43, 44] An initial prospective, open-label, placebo-controlled phase two trial of IL-1ra in humans with sepsis syndrome documented a 64% reduction in mortality in patients given IL-1ra (133 mg/h) with standard care compared with those in the group given standard care without IL-1ra.[44a] An important finding of these studies was that IL-1ra was noted to be effective even when administered after the onset of septic shock. This finding has clear clinical implications, because it extends the window of opportunity for treating sepsis. A phase-three double-blind trial in 893 patients with SIRS given IL-1ra has been completed. Overall mortality was 34% in patients given placebo (standard care) and 29% in patients administered high-dose IL-1ra by continuous intravenous infusion (2 mg · kg^{-1} · h^{-1} for 72 h) in addition to standard care. Although the overall mortality difference was not statistically significant ($P = .22$), retrospective analysis demonstrated a statistically significant reduction in mortality in those patients with higher predicted mortality based on clinical predictive indices. In 595 enrolled patients with a predicted mortality of 24% or greater, a 22% reduction in mortality was obtained in those patients given IL-1ra compared with controls ($P = .03$).

One of the most potent stimuli for IL-1ra production by mononuclear cells is immunoglobulin. Many provocative questions are thus raised about the mechanism of therapeutic efficacy of immunoglobulin preparations in clinical practice. For example, do immunoglobulin infusions in patients with immune thrombocytopenic purpura work in part by inducing the production of IL-1ra, which subsequently down-regulates the actions of phagocytic cells and acts as an immunosuppressant? This is an important issue, because immunoglobulin preparations are used in many diseases such as immune thrombocytopenic purpura, Kawasaki syndrome, certain immunoglobulin deficiencies, infections (i.e., parvovirus B-19), aplastic anemia, and others.[62–65]

Soluble receptors to TNF (also called TNF-binding proteins [TBPs]) have been found naturally in the circulation. In 1989 and 1990, several groups of researchers isolated two proteins from human urine that specifically bound and inactivated TNF biologic activity.[66–70] They have also been isolated from the supernatants of cultured peripheral blood mononuclear cells, polymorphonuclear neutrophils, and fibroblasts. Subsequent experiments demonstrated that the two TBPs are the extracellular portions of the two types of TNF receptors, probably generated by proteolysis. Current nomenclature designates that the extracellular soluble portion of the type 1 (55–60 kd, 455 residue) TNF receptor be called TBP-1 and that the extracellular soluble portion of the type 2 (75–80 kd, 461 residue) TNF receptor be called TBP-2. TBP-1 and TBP-2 are each about half the mass of their respective receptors, with mass of about 30 kd and 40 kd, respectively. TNF receptors are found on almost all cell types except red blood cells. In the most comprehensive experimental clinical study of TBPs to date, human volunteers were given LPS, 20 units/kg, IV, resulting in an increase in TNF at about 1 hour after infusion (returning to baseline in about 4 h) and was followed in 1 to 2 hours by elevation of plasma levels of TBP-1 (3.7 ng/mL) and TBP-2 (1.4 ng/mL).[71] Soluble receptor levels remained elevated for up to 24 hours after LPS infusion. In a separate study of 12 critically ill patients in a surgical intensive care unit, TNF was elevated in plasma of 37% of patients by enzyme immunoassay and in 20% of those same patients by WEHI-cell cytotoxicity bioassay. However, TBP-1 and TBP-2 were elevated in 94% and 89%, respectively, suggesting that they are more sensitive indicators of disease activity. TBP-1 and TBP-2 concentrations were correlated. These investigators also conducted a follow-up study to evaluate a potential therapeutic role for exogenous administration of TBP-1 in an animal model of septic shock. Six baboons were administered an LD_{100} of live *Escherichia coli*. Three received *E. coli* after a 3-hour intravenous infusion of TBP-1 at a dose expected to produce a 500-fold molar excess of TBP-1 to TNF. The other three baboons received placebo infusions along with *E. coli*. Average circulating steady-state level of TBP-1 was 29 μg/mL. The results were unexpected in that only one death occurred in the placebo group. However, a beneficial effect due to TBP-1 infusion was reflected in greater blood pressure stability and in decreased volume of fluids required to maintain hemodynamic status. Another notable result was that TNF immunoactivity was undetectable, presumedly because of binding to TBP-1, which blocked antibody recognition of TNF epitopes.

In a murine model of lethal endotoxemia, infusion of a TBP-1-immunoglobulin chimera significantly decreased mortality.[72] Therapeutic trials of recombinant TBP-1 in patients with SIRS are pending.

Two IL-1 receptors have been identified—the type 1 receptor (80 kd) present on T cells and fibroblasts and type 2 receptor (65 kd) present on B cells and mononuclear cells. Soluble IL-1 receptor type 1 (sIL-1R1) has been genetically engineered by transfecting cells with a truncated form of the full IL-1 receptor type 1 deoxyribonucleic acid coding only for the extracellular portion of this receptor. There are no reports of a naturally occurring sIL-1R1.

The experimental in vivo activities of sIL-1R1 include

1. Prolongation of survival of allogeneic heart transplants in mice (intraperitoneal or subcutaneous murine sIL-1R1 given on days 0–6 or 0–2 with respect to transplantation)
2. Decreased ipsilateral lymph node enlargement in mice administered irradiated allogeneic splenocytes in the footpad (sIL-1R1 started on day [−1] and given for 3–4 days)
3. Decreased IL-1-assisted B cell proliferation at a 200-fold molar excess of sIL-1R1 to IL-1 (50% decrease in proliferation)

4. Decreased experimental allergic encephalomyelitis in rats

5. Decreased joint inflammatory response in a rat antigen-induced arthritis model (synergy of anti-inflammatory effects with TBP-1 noted)

Some current evidence supports the existence of a natural soluble IL-1 receptor type 2 in human plasma, serum, synovial inflammatory fluid, activated peripheral blood mononuclear cell (PBMC) supernatant, and stimulated Raji cell supernatant (human B cell Burkitt's lymphoma cell line).

A functional role has not yet been demonstrated in vivo for any of these soluble receptors.

The final common mediators of cytokine-induced damage at the multiple end-organs may be antagonized. For example, it has been established that nitric oxide is a major mediator of peripheral vasodilation and decreased vascular resistance during inflammation. Early data show that *N*-monomethyl arginine (an inactive substrate for the enzyme nitric oxide synthase, the enzyme that synthesizes nitric oxide) can reverse some elements of sepsis physiology.[73]

In conclusion, the past decades have seen the discovery of potent new antimicrobial agents and more sophisticated supportive care without substantial improvement in the outcome of septic shock. Mortality from septic shock has remained disappointingly high. New efforts have focused on the host's responses to inflammatory stimuli such as endotoxin, with the hypothesis that the generation of endogenous mediators that provoke this response gives us a point of therapeutic attack in sepsis as well as many other disease states. Despite much promise, interventions specifically designed to modulate cytokine activity in sepsis have yet to produce definitive clinical benefit in humans. There is no more eloquent description of the septic response to infection than that by Lewis Thomas, who wrote in *The Lives of a Cell*[74]:

> *We are likely to turn on every defense at our disposal; we will bomb, defoliate, blockade, seal off, and destroy all the tissues in the area. Leukocytes become more actively phagocytic, release lysosomal enzymes, turn sticky, and aggregate together in dense masses, occluding capillaries and shutting off the blood supply. . . . Pyrogen is released from leukocytes, adding fever to hemorrhage, necrosis, and shock. It is a shambles.*

Attempts will eventually be made to evaluate the efficacy of therapies designed to simultaneously inhibit multiple elements of the proinflammatory cytokine cascade. Therapeutic interventions currently focus on the synergistic toxicity of the cytokines and other mediators, paradoxically giving us the opportunity to gain a therapeutic effect by disarming even one major component of this catastrophic response. Current therapies focusing on the inhibition or antagonism of TNF and IL-1 do just that.

ACKNOWLEDGMENTS

Supported by NIH grants GM21700, AI15614, AI07329, and the Alfond Family Fund.

References

1. Levine B, Kalman J, Mayer L, et al: Elevated circulating levels of tumor necrosis factor in severe heart failure. N Engl J Med 1990; 323:236.
2. Cannon JG, Tompkins RG, Gelfand JA, et al: Circulating interleukin-1 and tumor necrosis factor in septic shock and experimental endotoxin fever. J Infect Dis 1990; 161:79.
3. Chavanet P, Bonnotte B, Guiguet M, et al: High concentrations of intrathecal interleukin-6 in human bacterial and nonbacterial meningitis. J Infect Dis 1992; 166:428.
4. Heney D, Lewis IJ, Evans SW, et al: Interleukin-6 and its relationship to C-reactive protein and fever in children with febrile neutropenia. J Infect Dis 1992; 165:886.
5. Tilg H, Wilmer A, Vogel W, et al: Serum levels of cytokines in chronic liver diseases. Gastroenterology 1992; 103:264.
6. Donnelly SC, Strieter RM, Kunkel SL, et al: Interleukin-8 and development of adult respiratiory distress syndrome in at-risk patient groups. Lancet 1993; 341:643.
7. Okusawa S, Gelfand JA, Ikejima T, et al: Interleukin-1 induces a shock-like state in rabbits. Synergism with tumor necrosis factor and the effect of cyclooxygenase inhibition. J Clin Invest 1988; 81:1162.
8. Tracey KJ, Beutler B, Lowry SF, et al: Shock and tissue injury induced by recombinant human cachectin. Science 1986; 234:470.
9. Ohlsson K, Bjork P, Bergenfeldt M, et al: Interleukin-1 receptor antagonist reduces mortality from endotoxic shock. Nature 1990; 348:550.
10. Tracey K, Fong Y, Hesse DG, et al: Anti-cachectin/TNF monoclonal antibodies prevent septic shock during lethal bacteremia. Nature 1987; 330:662.
11. Spriggs MK, Hruby DE, Maliszewski CR, et al: Vaccinia and cowpox viruses encode a novel secreted interleukin-1-binding protein. Cell 1992; 71:145.
12. Gooding LR: Virus proteins that counteract host immune defenses. Cell 1992; 71:5.
13. Smith CA, Davis T, Anderson D, et al: A receptor for tumor necrosis factor defines an unusual family of cellular and viral proteins. Science 1990; 248:1019.
14. Smith GL, Chang YS: Two vaccinia virus proteins structurally related to the interleukin-1 receptor and the immunoglobulin superfamily. J Gen Virol 1991; 72:511.
15. Upton C, Mossman K, McFadden G: Encoding of a homolog of the IFN-γ receptor by myxoma virus. Science 1992; 258:1369.
16. Luo G, Niesel DW, Shaban RA, et al: Tumor necrosis factor alpha binding to bacteria; evidence for a high-affinity receptor and alteration of bacterial virulence properties. Infect Immun 1993; 61:830.
17. Porat R, Clark BD, Wolff SM, et al: Enhancement of growth of virulent strains of *Escherichia coli* by interleukin-1. Science 1991; 254:852.
18. Amiri P, Locksley RM, Parslow TG, et al: Tumor necrosis factor α restores granulomas and egg-laying in schistosome-infected SCID mice. Nature 1992; 356:604.

18a. Horuk R, Chitnis CE, Darbonne WC, et al: A receptor for the malarial parasite plasmodium vivax: The erythrocyte chemokine receptor. Science 1993; 261:1182.

19. Bone RC: Sepsis, the sepsis syndrome, multi-organ failure: A plea for comparable definitions. Ann Intern Med 1991; 114:332.
20. Bone RC: Toward an epidemiologic and natural history of SIRS (systemic inflammatory response syndrome). JAMA 1992; 268:3452.
21. Dinarello CA, Gelfand JA, Wolff SM: Anticytokine strategies in the treatment of the systemic inflammatory response syndrome. JAMA 1993; 269:1829.
22. Michalek SM, Morre RN, McGhee JR, et al: The primary role of lymphoreticular cells in the mediation of host responses to bacterial endotoxin. J Infect Dis 1980; 141:55.
23. Proctor RA, Will JA, Burhop KE, et al: Protection of mice against lethal endotoxemia by a lipid A precursor. Infect Immun 1986; 52:905.
24. Golenbock DT, Will JA, Raetz CR, et al: Lipid X ameliorates pulmonary hypertension and protects sheep from death due to endotoxin. Infect Immun 1987; 55:2471.
25. Beutler B, Cerami A: Cachectin and tumor necrosis factor as two sides of the same biologic coin. Nature 1986; 320:584.
26. Beutler B, Cerami A: Cachectin: More than a tumor necrosis factor. N Engl J Med 1987; 316:279.
27. Dinarello CA, Wolff SM: The role of interleukin-1 in disease. N Engl J Med 1993; 328:106.
28. Mathison JC, Wolfson E, Ulevitch RJ: Participation of tumor necrosis factor in the mediation of gram-negative bacterial lipopolysaccharide-induced injury in rabbits. J Clin Invest 1988; 1:1925.
29. Parillo JE: Pathogenetic mechanisms of septic shock. N Engl J Med 1993; 328:1471.
30. Dinarello CA, Cannon JG, Wolff SM, et al: Tumor necrosis

factor (cachectin) is an endogenous pyrogen and induces production of interleukin-1. J Exp Med 1986; 163:1433.
31. Schindler R, Mancilla J, Endres S, et al: Correlations and interactions in the production of interleukin-6 (IL-6), IL-1, and tumor necrosis factor (TNF) in human blood mononuclear cells: IL-6 suppresses IL-1 and TNF. Blood 1990; 75:40.
32. Groopman JE, Molina J-M, Scadden DT: Hematopoietic growth factors. N Engl J Med 1989; 321:1449.
33. McCabe WR: Serum complement levels in bacteremia due to gram-negative organisms. N Engl J Med 1973; 288:21.
34. van der Poll T, Buller HR, ten Cate HT, et al: Activation of coagulation after administration of tumor necrosis factor to normal subjects. N Engl J Med 1990; 322:1622.
35. Suffredini AF, Harpel PC, Parrillo JE: Promotion and subsequent inhibition of plasminogen activation after administration of intravenous endotoxin to normal subjects. N Engl J Med 1989; 320:1165.
36. Barton BE, Jackson JV: Protective role of interleukin-6 in the lipopolysaccharide-galactosamine septic shock model. Infect Immun 1993; 61:1496.
37. McCartney FN, Mizel D, Wong H, et al: TGF-beta regulates production of growth factors and TGF-beta by human peripheral blood monocytes. Growth Factors 1990; 4:27.
38. Howard M, O'Garra A, Ishida H, et al: Biological properties of interleukin-10. J Clin Immunol 1992; 12:239.
39. Vannier E, Miller LC, Dinarello CA: Coordinated anti-inflammatory effects of interleukin 4: Interleukin 4 suppresses interleukin 1 production but up-regulates gene expression and synthesis of interleukin 1 receptor antagonist. Proc Natl Acad Sci U S A 1992; 89:4076.
40. Beutler B, Milsark IW, Cerami A: Passive immunization against cachectin/tumor necrosis factor protects mice from lethal effects of endotoxin. Science 1985; 229:869.
41. Wakabayashi G, Gelfand JA, Burke JF, et al: A specific receptor antagonist for interleukin-1 prevents *Escherichia coli*-induced shock. FASEB J 1991; 5:338.
42. Michie HR, Manogue KR, Spriggs DR, et al: Detection of circulating tumor necrosis factor after endotoxin administration. N Engl J Med 1988; 318:1481.
43. Alexander HR, Doherty GM, Buresh CM, et al: A recombinant human receptor antagonist to interleukin-1 improves survival after lethal endotoxemia in mice. J Exp Med 1991; 173:1029.
44. Fischer E, Marano MA, van Zee KJ, et al: Interleukin-1 receptor blockade improves survival and hemodynamic performance in *Escherichia coli* septic shock, but fails to alter host responses to sublethal endotoxemia. J Clin Invest 1992; 89:1551.
44a. Fisher CJ, Slotman GJ, Opal SM, et al: Initial evaluation of human recombinant interleukin-1 receptor antagonist in the treatment of sepsis syndrome: A randomized, open-label, placebo-controlled multicenter trial. Crit Care Med 1994; 22:12.
45. Tredget EE, Yu YM, Zhong S, et al: Role of interleukin 1 and tumor necrosis factor on energy metabolism in rabbits. Am Physiol Soc 1988; 88:E760.
46. Sun X, Hsueh W: Bowel necrosis induced by tumor necrosis factor in rats is mediated by platelet-activating factor. J Clin Invest 1988; 81:1328.
47. Anderson BO, Bensard DD, Harkin AH: The role of platelet activating factor and its antagonists in shock, sepsis and multiple organ failure. Surgery 1991; 172:415.
47a. DeJay SQ, Jeyaseelan R, Torley LW, et al: Effect of CL 184,005, a platelet-activating factor antagonist in a murine model of *Staphylococcus aureus*–induced gram-positive sepsis. J Infect Dis 1994; 169:150.
48. Mancilla J, Garcia P, Dinarello CA: The interleukin-1 receptor antagonist can either reduce or enhance the lethality of *Klebsiella pneumoniae* sepsis in newborn rats. Infect Immun 1993; 61:926.
49. Havell EA, Moldawer LL, Helfgott D, et al: Type 1 IL-1 receptor blockade exacerbates murine listeriosis. J Immunol 1992; 92:1486.
50. van der Meer JWM: The effects of recombinant interleukin-1 and recombinant tumor necrosis factor on non-specific resistance to infection. Biotherapy 1988; 1:19.
51. Baggiolini M, Walz A, Kunkel SL: Neutrophil-activating peptide-1/interleukin 8, a novel cytokine that activates neutrophils. J Clin Invest 1989; 84:1045.
52. Koch AE, Polverini PJ, Kunkel SL, et al: Interleukin-8 as a macrophage-derived mediator of angiogenesis. Science 1992; 258:1798.
53. Kishimoto T: The biology of interleukin 6. Blood 1989; 74:1.
54. Libert C, Vink A, Coulie P, et al: Limited involvement of interleukin-6 in the pathogenesis of lethal septic shock as revealed by the effect of monoclonal antibodies against interleukin-6 or its receptor in various murine models. Eur J Immunol 1992; 22:2625.
55. Moreira AL, Sampaio EP, Zmuidzinas A, et al: Thalidomide exerts its inhibitory action on tumor necrosis factor α by enhancing mRNA degradation. J Exp Med 1993; 177:1675.
56. Strieter RM, Remick DG, Ward PA, et al: Cellular and molecular regulation of tumor necrosis factor alpha production by pentoxiphylline. Biochem Biophys Res Commun 1988; 155:1230.
57. Cerretti DP, Kozlosky CJ, Mosley B, et al: Molecular cloning of the interleukin-1β converting enzyme. Science 1992; 256:97.
58. Ray CA, Black RA, Kronheim SR, et al: Viral inhibition of inflammation: Cowpox virus encodes an inhibitor of the interleukin-1β converting enzyme. Cell 1992; 69:597.
59. Thornberry NA, Bull HG, Calaycay JR, et al: A novel heterodimeric cysteine protease is required for interleukin-1 beta processing in monocytes. Nature 1992; 356:768.
60. Hinshaw LB, Emerson TE, Taylor FB, et al: Lethal *Staphylococcus aureus*–induced shock in primates: Prevention of death with anti-TNF antibody. J Trauma 1992; 33:568.
61. Seckinger P, Lowenthal JW, Williamson K, et al: A urine inhibitor of interleukin-1 activity that blocks ligand binding. J Immunol 1987; 139:1546.
62. Frickhofen N, Abkowitz LL, Safford M, et al: Persistent B19 parvovirus infection in patients infected with human immunodeficiency virus type-1 (HIV-1): A treatable cause of anemia in AIDS. Ann Intern Med 1990; 113:926.
63. Gernsheimer T, Stratton J, Ballem PJ, et al: Mechanisms of response to treatment in autoimmune thrombocytopenic purpura. N Engl J Med 1989; 320:874.
64. Hunter RF, Huang AT: A realistic approach to therapy for severe aplastic anemia. South Med J 1986; 79:1121.
65. Leong YM, Cotran RS, Kurt-Jones E, et al: Endothelial cell activation and high interleukin-1 secretion in the pathogenesis of acute Kawasaki disease. Lancet 1989; 2:1298.
66. Engelmann H, Aderka D, Rubenstein M, et al: A tumor necrosis factor–binding protein purified to homogeneity from human urine protects cells from tumor necrosis factor toxicity. J Biol Chem 1989; 264:11974.
67. Lantz M, Gullberg U, Nilsson E: Characterization in vitro of a human tumor necrosis factor binding protein. A soluble form of a tumor necrosis factor receptor. J Clin Invest 1990; 86:1396.
68. Novick D, Engelmann H, Wallach D: Soluble cytokine receptors are present in normal human urine. J Exp Med 1989; 170:1409.
69. Seckinger P, Isaaz S, Dayer J-M: Purification and biologic characterization of a specific tumor necrosis factor α inhibitor. J Biol Chem 1989; 264:11966.
70. Olsson I, Lantz M, Nilsson E, et al: Isolation and characterization of a tumor necrosis factor binding protein from urine. Eur J Haematol 1989; 42:270.
71. van Zee KJ, Kohno T, Fischer E: Tumor necrosis soluble receptors circulate during experimental and clinical inflammation and can protect against excessive tumor necrosis factor α in vitro and in vivo. Proc Natl Acad Sci U S A 1992; 89:4845.
72. Peppel K, Crawford D, Beutler B: A tumor necrosis factor (TNF) receptor-IgG heavy chain chimeric protein as a bivalent antagonist of TNF activity. J Exp Med 1991; 174:1483.
73. Petros A, Bennett D, Vallance P: Effect of nitric oxide synthase inhibitors on hypotension in patients with septic shock. Lancet 1991; 338:1557.
74. Lewis T: The Lives of a Cell. New York, Viking Press, 1974, p 92.

CHAPTER 22

Endotoxin-Induced Factors That Provoke Shock and Their Receptors

Bruce Beutler, MD • Christophe Van Huffel, PhD

Endotoxic shock could not occur in the absence of cells or factors of hematopoietic origin. So much is evident from studies of the C3H/HeJ mouse and its response to lipopolysaccharide (LPS).[1] These animals, which bear a single-gene mutation that renders them insensitive to LPS,[2, 3] survive challenge with immense quantities of LPS. In itself, this is a remarkable finding. It indicates that all of the biologic actions of LPS, however broad, must traverse a biologic "bottleneck" (i.e., the action of a single protein is required for LPS to cause shock and tissue injury.) No less remarkable, C3H/HeJ mice are restored to a normal level of sensitivity to LPS when transplanted with bone marrow derived from endotoxin-sensitive mice. Additional studies involving the adoptive transfer of macrophages indicate that macrophages are the principal cellular mediator of endotoxic shock.[4] Presumably, these cells produce factors that elicit shock and death.

However, which factors purvey the lethal effect? Over what time interval do these agents act? What beneficial functions do they serve? What signaling mechanisms do they use? In fashioning an effective treatment for endotoxic shock, it is surely necessary to know the answers to these questions.

As in other areas of biomedical research, molecular cloning has powerfully influenced our concept of shock and its origins. Recent work has drawn attention to several protein mediators of endotoxin action as the likely proximal cause of septic shock. The distinction between cell-bound and soluble mediators (cytokines) has been blurred with the discovery that several such proteins exist in both forms. In this review, the regulation and biologic actions of tumor necrosis factor (TNF) and its homologues are discussed because members of this cytokine family have been more clearly linked to the pathogenesis of endotoxic shock than any other proteins.

TUMOR NECROSIS FACTOR LIGAND FAMILY

Abundant evidence points to the involvement of TNF in the mediation of shock. TNF itself fulfills many of the conditions required of a shock mediator. It is principally produced by cells of hematopoietic origin in response to agents that induce shock. Its production is temporally related to the development of shock. Administration of TNF to experimental animals causes shock, and passive immunization against TNF prevents shock. For these reasons, it has long been suspected that TNF mediates the shock state induced by bacterial endotoxin and the wasting diathesis produced by many types of chronic disease.

It has, however, become clear that TNF is but one member of a family of cytokines with varying degrees of structural homology. This cytokine family, in turn, engages a set of receptors that are homologous to one another, activating them by a common mechanism (aggregation) and in some cases transducing similar effects. The TNF family and the TNF receptor family provide an interesting example of coevolution, wherein gene duplication, mutation, and exon shuffling allowed the development of a richly varied set of signaling pathways, whereas only one such pathway may have existed ab initio. Although no TNF-like molecules have been identified in subvertebrate species, indirect data suggest that the TNF and TNF receptor families may have served defensive functions even before the separation of plant and animal kingdoms.[5] Thus, it seems possible that TNF is but one avenue by which a state of shock may be provoked and that parallel pathways, embodied by the structural homologues of TNF, also exist.

TNF-α (a protein originally known as TNF[6] or cachectin[7]) and TNF-β (a protein also known as lymphotoxin) are encoded by tightly linked genes that lie within the major histocompatibility complex.[8, 9] A new member of the family, known as lymphotoxin-β, is encoded by a third, tightly linked member of the family.[10] Sequencing studies may yet reveal other homologues. Although TNF-α and TNF-β are largely secreted, the former can also exist in a membrane-associated form. Lymphotoxin-β is entirely membrane associated and may act to maintain TNF-β in close proximity with the cell membrane. The TNFs, like many other members of this cytokine family, are trimeric proteins. Each TNF has three sites capable of engaging the TNF receptor. These sites are formed by the interface between adjacent subunits.[11–13] In binding to the TNF receptor, the TNF causes receptor aggregation or changes receptor conformation in such a way that a signal is generated; hence, antibodies against the TNF receptor may have agonist activity.[14] The majority of the effects elicited by TNF-α and TNF-β are identical, although certain discrepancies have been reported.[15] The major difference between these cytokines, at a functional level, is to be seen at the level of their production; the two proteins are produced in response to an entirely different stimuli and often by different types of cells.[16] TNF-α is produced largely by macrophages as well as by certain extrahematopoietic cell types. TNF-β is expressed almost exclusively by lymphocytes and their derivatives. Thus, it seems that a common biologic activity may be produced at different sites in response to different inducing agents.

The closest structural relatives of the TNF proteins include the CD40 ligand,[17] the CD27 ligand,[18] and the CD30 ligand.[19] Modeling studies suggest that at least the CD40 ligand is trimeric,* although none has been crystallized to date. They are expressed as integral membrane proteins on the surface of T lymphocytes. Like the TNF molecules, they appear to trigger a biologic response by causing the aggregation of receptors that remain on neighboring cells (either a T lymphocyte or a B cell in the case of CD40 ligand). None of the molecules interact with the receptors for TNF. Ligands for some members of the family remain to be discovered. These include the ligands for the 4-1BB and OX-40 proteins and the Fas antigen (discussed later). Although its receptor is homologous to the TNF family of receptors, nerve growth factor (NGF) is not sufficiently similar to TNF to be classified as a member of the TNF gene family. It might, therefore, be said that a single family of receptors coopted two gene families encoding ligands and directed their development as regulated "triggers" of a biologic response.

The separate members of the TNF gene family have been diverging for a long time. The tree shown in Figure 22–1 *(top)* gives some indication of the evolutionary relationship that defines this protein family. Even the TNF proteins themselves (TNF and lymphotoxin) must be separated by several hundred million years of evolution.

*Jongeneel V: Personal communication, 1994.

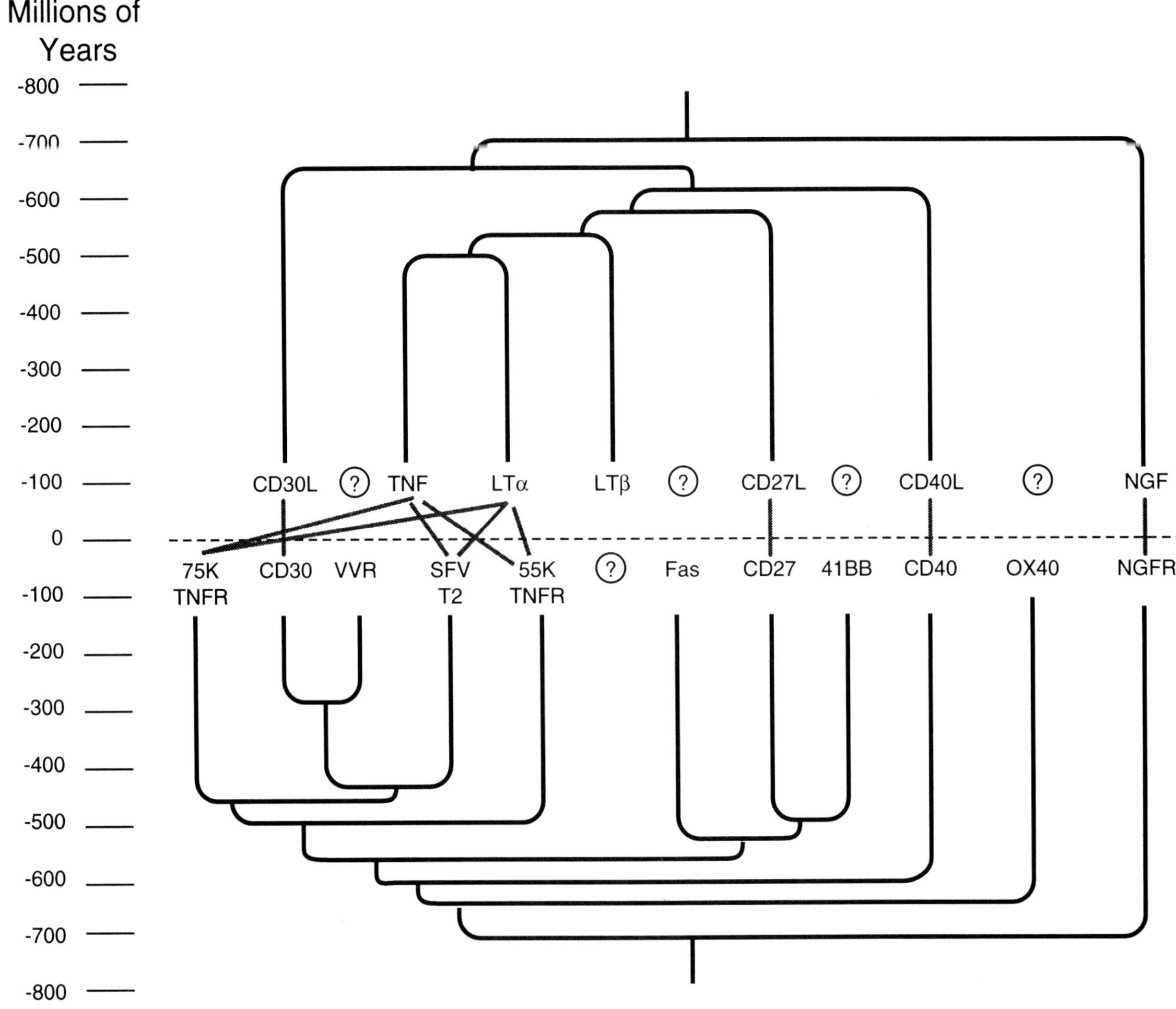

Figure 22–1. The phylogenetic origins of the TNF/NGF ligand and receptor families. Two phylogenetic "trees" were generated by computer-based comparison of the sequence of processed ligands (lacking transmembrane and secretion signal domains) and the extracellular domains of the receptor family members. The connections drawn between ligand and receptor family members indicate direct physical interaction between the molecules. A question mark (?) implies that the sequence of the respective ligand or receptor is not available at present. The time scale is approximate and should be taken only to indicate that, with the exception of some very closely related proteins, the point of phylogenetic divergence is very ancient.

TUMOR NECROSIS FACTOR/NERVE GROWTH FACTOR FAMILY OF RECEPTORS

The TNF/NGF family of receptors is defined by a cysteine-rich motif, present in four copies (the TNF receptors, the NGF receptor, the 4-1BB molecule and the soluble receptors for TNF encoded by viral genomes[20]), three copies (the OX-40 protein, the Fas antigen, and the CD27 molecule), or six copies (the CD30 molecules). All of these molecules are type I integral membrane proteins (N-terminal in the extracellular space), and all are glycosylated. It is probable that none of the molecules exist in a truly monomeric form on the plasma membrane. At a minimum, it appears that they are present as dimers, which undergo conformational change after interaction with their respective ligands.* CD27 is known from biochemical analyses to be a disulfide-linked dimer.[21]

One of the most striking effects of TNF is its ability to trigger programmed cell death (apoptosis) in certain cells that bear the 55 kDa TNF receptor.[22, 23] Indeed, several groups initially purified TNF to homogeneity based on its ability to cause lysis of certain transformed cells in vitro.[24–29] Other members of the TNF receptor family are also involved in apoptotic events; for example, the Fas antigen, CD40, and the 75 kDa NGF receptor seem capable of triggering a cytotoxic response either when engaged by their respective ligand (in the case of the Fas antigen)[30] or when unengaged (in the case of CD40 and NGF receptor).[31–35]

The signals imparted by each of these receptors remain quite mysterious. Although some progress has been made in defining the domains of the TNF receptor and Fas antigen that convey an apoptotic signal,[36] there is as yet little insight into the identity of the next molecule in the pathway. Activation of mitogen-activated protein (MAP) kinases[37] and of sphingomyelinase[38, 39] are each purportedly involved in transduction. Regardless of the signaling events that are involved, the broad consequences of cytokine or receptor deletion have come into very sharp focus as the genes encoding them have been deleted.

*Sprang S: Personal communication, 1994.

The cytoplasmic portion of the TNF/NGF receptor molecules is highly variable. However, a common motif (perhaps related to the production of an apoptotic effect) is observed in the cytoplasmic domain of the 55 kDa TNF receptor, the Fas antigen, and the CD40 protein. Mutations within this domain are known to abolish the transduction of a cytolytic effect by the Fas antigen and by the TNF 55 kDA receptor. The phylogenetic relationship among the genes encoding these proteins, as reconstructed from the nucleotide sequence of the extracellular domains, is illustrated in Figure 22–1 *(bottom).*

Soluble forms of the TNF receptors are known to exist and are presumed to be generated by proteolysis. These monomeric forms of the receptors have a relatively low affinity for TNF, illustrating the importance of dimerization in the achievement of tight binding.[40]

FUNCTION REVEALED BY MUTATION AND "GENE KNOCKOUT"

The interleukins, TNF, and colony-stimulating factors have all been known as important components of a signaling system whereby cells of the immune system communicate with one another, and the induction of certain individual cytokines by other cytokines has given rise to a rather vague notion of the existence of a cytokine network.[41–43] "Cascades" of cytokines are believed to regulate inflammation, hematopoiesis, certain aspects of development, and many other vital processes. Yet an awareness of the general importance of cytokine mediators is not entirely satisfying in the absence of specific details.

Because an understanding of function is usually best advanced by an analysis of the failure of normal function, a great deal of effort has been concentrated on the identification of defects of the cytokine production or activity. Certain diseases can now be attributed to discrete mutations of cytokines[44, 45] or their receptors,[46] and where nature has not provided such mutations, attempts have been made to introduce them artificially.[47–52]

One of the first mutations to be shown to involve a cytokine receptor was the *lpr* mutation of mice,[53, 54] *lpr* (for *l*ymphoproliferation) was shown to be caused by retroposon-mediated interruption of the gene coding for Fas antigen.[53] A second nonfunctional allele of *lpr* (*lpr*[CG]) was shown to result from a point mutation within a conserved region specifying the Fas antigen cytoplasmic domain, a fact that explained certain phenotypic characteristics of this allele.[54] In the absence of Fas expression or activity, the accumulation of an unusual class of T cell (CD4−, CD8−, B220+) was observed, suggesting that these cells, which might normally be removed through an apoptotic mechanism involving the action of the Fas antigen, were retained with resultant lymphoproliferation syndrome. Characteristically, mice with lymphoproliferation acquire a lupus-like syndrome, suggesting a link between apoptosis and the normal control of immune response.

The ligand for Fas antigen has not yet been identified. However, a second mutation, *gld* (for *g*eneralized *l*ymphoproliferative *d*isease), yields a phenotype identical to that caused by *lpr.* On theoretical grounds, it has been argued that the *gld* locus may code for the Fas ligand.[55, 56]

The similarity of the Fas antigen and the 55 kDa TNF receptor made it seem likely that mutations of the latter would also give rise to a syndrome in which faulty apoptosis would produce undesirable accumulation of one or another cell types and perhaps also cells of a lymphoid lineage. However, knockout of the 55 kDa receptor, achieved in two separate laboratories, produced no such phenotype.[51, 52] On the contrary, mice lacking a functional 55 kDa receptor appeared to develop and grow normally. As predicted from passive immunization studies, they showed a marked resistance to the lethal effect of LPS as well as a high level of sensitivity to infection by *Listeria monocytogenes,* which multiplied without restriction in the liver and spleen of the mutant animals, duplicating the earlier noted effect of passive immunization against TNF.[57]

Knockout of the 75 kDa TNF receptor, known for its ability to promote T cell growth, produced no discernible phenotype,* although ongoing investigation may ultimately reveal a defect of some sort. The combination of these two knockouts has yet to be achieved. However, as noted later, other approaches have made it seem likely that a double knockout would yield no more than the sum of its parts.

CD40 ligand mutation causes a failure of normal B cell activation, so that T cells, which normally bear the ligand, cannot trigger the switch between production of immunoglobulin (Ig) M and IgG, IgA, or IgD. In humans, mutation of the CD40 ligand presents itself as an X-linked immunodeficiency characterized by low or absent levels of IgG and normal or high levels of IgM in the plasma.[44, 45, 58] It has been suggested that CD40 ligand prevents apoptosis of B cells, which otherwise occurs as a consequence of antigen presentation and is mediated by the CD40 molecule. This interesting hypothesis suggests that some members of the TNF/NGF receptor family may trigger apoptosis when engaged by their ligands (e.g., the 55 kDa TNF receptor or the Fas antigen), whereas others trigger apoptosis only when not engaged (e.g., CD40 and the NGF receptor).[32–35, 59]

INVOLVEMENT OF TUMOR NECROSIS FACTOR FAMILY MEMBERS IN SHOCK

The pathogenetic role of TNF-α in shock is beyond question. The role played by TNF-β is inferential and less well documented because lymphotoxin is not known to be produced in vivo in response to LPS. Together with TNF-α, however, it may be secreted as a result of exposure to certain bacterial exotoxins (superantigens[60–63]). The involvement of other members of the TNF family in shock is likely but unproven. Because the shock-producing effect of TNF is mediated by the 55 kDa receptor, which causes apoptosis, suspicion must fall on the Fas antigen, the closest structural relative of this protein, in a search for additional shock-producing ligand/receptor couples. Although a simple test of the hypothesis that Fas transduces a part of the endotoxin signal would consist of the administration of LPS to *lpr* (−/−) and (+/+) animals, this approach might easily be confounded by phenotypic effects of the *lpr* mutation (e.g., altered sensitivity to LPS caused by lymphoproliferation, renal disease, and so on), and so far has not been attempted.

The ligand for the Fas antigen has yet to be cloned, and it is unclear whether this molecule is cell bound or soluble. It is highly probable that the Fas ligand is a member of the TNF gene superfamily and that it resides on mouse chromosome 1, because this is the location of the *gld* locus. As noted previously, mutations of the *gld* locus give rise to a lymphoproliferation syndrome indistinguishable from than caused by mutations of the Fas antigen, and it has been widely assumed that *gld* encodes a ligand for Fas.[55, 56] It is known that *gld* is expressed chiefly or entirely by cells of hematopoietic origin[56] as would befit an important mediator of endotoxic shock.[1]

In the absence of other information concerning the ligand

*Goeddel D: Personal communication, 1993.

for Fas, it is not possible to determine whether this cytokine is induced by LPS or whether it becomes widely distributed. However, because agonist antibodies against the Fas antigen can be expected to duplicate the activity (if not necessarily the distribution) of the Fas ligand, it seems reasonable to examine the effects of this antibody in vivo as a first approximation of the activities of Fas ligand.

Precisely, this experiment was recently performed by Ogasawara and coworkers, who noted that intraperitoneal injection of Fas antibody had a rapid lethal effect in mice. Particularly striking was the finding of hepatic necrosis, which these authors attributed to apoptosis occurring in the liver.[64] Although it was suggested that Fas and its ligand might normally cooperate in the programmed lysis of hepatocytes, it must be conceded that mice bearing the *lpr* or *gld* mutations in homozygous form do not suffer from any abnormality of hepatic function or morphogenesis.

The injection of TNF does not trigger hepatic necrosis; notably, the liver is spared in animals that receive a lethal dose of this cytokine (although hepatic injury is a prominent feature of endotoxic shock). Moreover, the toxic effects of TNF are known to be greatly potentiated by agents that injure the liver (e.g., D-galactosamine).[65, 66] It is appealing to consider that the Fas ligand may operate in concert with TNF to produce the full syndrome of septic shock.

No animal model of CD40 or CD40 ligand mutations has been devised, and it is therefore unclear whether CD40 plays any role in the pathogenesis of shock, alongside its clear function in the switch between IgM and IgG synthesis. Moreover, none of the other members of the receptor family (CD27, CD30, 4-1BB, and OX-40) or their respective ligands have been deleted or mutationally altered to date. Therefore, the composite influence exerted by these molecules remains undetermined.

INVOLVEMENT OF OTHER CYTOKINES IN SHOCK

The development of shock is partly a "parallel" process in which several cytokines can, independently, provoke multiple organ failure. It is also partly a cooperative process, or cascade, in which one cytokine induces another and the second induces yet a third, each contributing to the release of more distal toxic products. These aspects of shock are not easily quantitated. However, it is apparent that the more parallel shock proves to be in its development, the more benefit is to be expected from the conjoint administration of several cytokine inhibitors. Alternatively, a single inhibitor of the first agent in the cascade would be as effective as the conjoint administration of inhibitors that act at all subsequent levels of induction if the development of shock is massively cooperative (Fig. 22–2).

Experience to date suggests that both parallel and cooperative features characterize the response to LPS. Hence, endotoxicity traverses a "bottleneck" at the level of the LPS gene product. An inhibitor active at this level might, like the LPS^r mutation, abrogate all effects of LPS, shifting the dose-lethality curve 100- to 1000-fold. The antagonism of specific cytokines is only partially effective. A threefold shift in toxicity is witnessed with the administration of TNF inhibitors.[67–71] A similar attenuation of response is observed with inhibitors of interleukin-1 (IL-1), such as the IL-1 receptor antagonist.[72]

Interferon-γ potentiates many of the effects of TNF, including its toxicity.[73–75] Inhibitors of interferon-γ diminish the toxicity of LPS[76–79] and might, therefore, be expected to play a role in the treatment of shock. Certain other cytokines that participate in the development of shock may, as yet, be undiscovered. Still others, such as IL-10, clearly oppose shock.[80]

DOMINANT-NEGATIVE GENES TO DECIPHER THE FUNCTION OF TUMOR NECROSIS FACTOR–LIKE CYTOKINES

Gene knockout is a definitive technique for determining gene function. When the functional importance is not revealed by knockout as a result of overlap with other genes, however, gene knockout may leave many questions unanswered. Furthermore, to the extent that development may be impaired by deletion of a particular gene, it is often difficult to gauge the function of that gene in animals that have completed development normally. For example, mutation of the IL-2 receptor gamma chain creates a severe combined immunodeficiency disorder syndrome in humans[46]; yet this does not provide insight into the function of IL-2 in humans who possess an intact repertoire of T and B lymphocytes. A more conditional approach to the analysis of gene function is certainly desirable.

Practical considerations limit the application of gene knockout to the analysis of cooperation among cytokines. To study the effect of more than one mutant gene at a time, it is necessary to combine knockout mutations by genetic crossing schemes. This approach may be exceptionally difficult or impossible if the genes are tightly linked. Moreover, the study of cytokine deficiencies in specialized strains of mice (such as NOD or NZW/NZB F1 hybrids) is not easily achieved without extensive backcrossing of the mutation. The analysis of cytokine function in species other than mice is not possible without the creation of a new knockout mutation.

For all of these reasons, a dominant-negative mutational approach to cytokine analysis is often desirable. Soluble receptors for cytokines are capable of abolishing cytokine function if expressed at high enough concentrations in vivo. This is particularly true of receptors that have been artificially dimerized; such molecules can engage their targets with extremely high affinity by virtue of the fact that they combine with two epitopes on the cytokine surface.

High-level expression of cytokine inhibitors may be achieved through the use of adenoviral vectors, which efficiently infect hepatocytes, causing abundant secretion of proteins that they encode.[81] A chimeric protein, consisting of the human 55 kDa TNF receptor fused to a mouse IgG heavy chain, has been expressed at concentrations exceeding 1 mg/mL of plasma in mice transduced with such a replication-defective adenovirus.[82] In the presence of such a high concentration of inhibitor, any TNF-α or TNF-β that might be produced would presumably be ineffective. Indeed, expression of the inhibitor construct produces a phenocopy of 55 kDa TNF receptor knockout.[82]

Because adenoviruses encoding chimeric versions of all members of the TNF receptor family can be produced with relative ease, it may soon be possible to determine the cooperative effects of members of this cytokine family in shock. Other transduction methods, including lipofection, promise to make such studies still simpler by offering a quicker means to the attainment of high-level expression in vivo[83, 84] and by circumventing some of the problems inherent in the adenovirus approach (e.g., antigenicity of the virus).

REGULATION OF THE BIOSYNTHESIS

By blocking cytokine synthesis, it should be possible to abolish most or all untoward reactions to bacterial endotoxin. A great deal of effort has been directed toward this goal, and specific antagonists of the signaling pathway that triggers cytokine release are being studied intensively. The activation of TNF biosynthesis is a paradigm for the study of

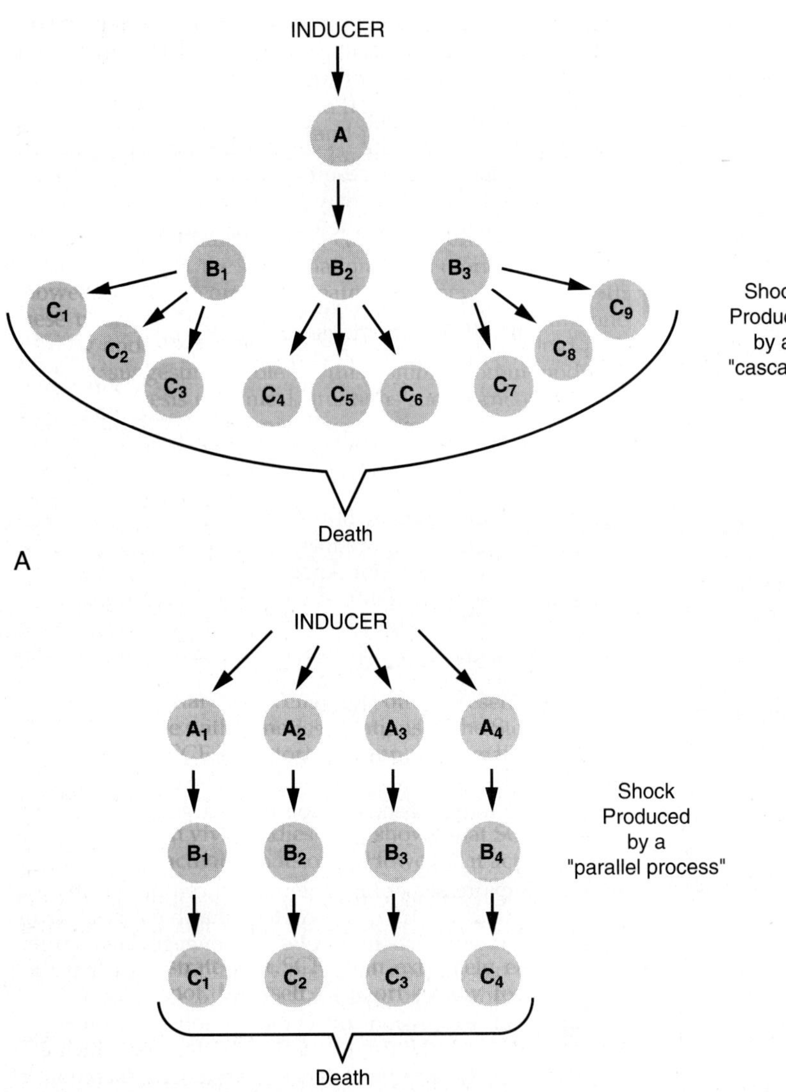

Figure 22–2. The hierarchy of factors that mediate shock. On the one hand, shock may be produced by an inducer that activates a single protein, which, in turn, causes the release of many toxic factors through a cascade mechanism. Alternatively, the inducer may trigger several independent pathways, initiating shock by a parallel sequence of events. The true mechanism of shock pathogenesis undoubtedly involves a combination of cascading and parallel mechanisms.

pathways activated by LPS. The most important features of the LPS signaling pathway, as it applies to TNF, are outlined next.

Host Sensing Mechanism

LPSs are of variable structure but feature a disaccharide backbone containing two phosphate groups and a number of acyl chains, which are attached to still other acyl chains by acyloxyacyl linkages. A polysaccharide moiety of variable size confers antigenicity to the LPS molecule but does not seem to mediate toxicity. Rather, toxicity is a function of the lipid moiety, which engages specific receptors on cells.

The best characterized receptor for LPS is that molecule known as CD14.[85] CD14 resides on a number of cell types including macrophages. It is a glycerolphosphoinositol-linked component of the plasma membrane and may also exist in a secreted form.[86–90] By directly engaging LPS, or LPS linked to LPS-binding protein (LBP), CD14 effectively concentrates the agonist and allows the sensing of minute concentrations of LPS in plasma or in tissues. Transgenic mice that express high levels of CD14 exhibit a modest enhancement in sensitivity to LPS.

However, CD14 is not the product of the LPS gene, which is required for biologic responses to endotoxin. CD14 does not transmit a signal to the cytoplasm and indeed may be bypassed by the application of high concentrations of LPS to cells. Hence, 70Z/3 cells, which lack CD14, are LPS responsive provided that high concentrations of LPS are added to the culture. Likewise, macrophages respond to LPS in the absence of serum (a source of LBP).

Certain monoclonal antibodies against CD14 do not impair LPS binding, yet block further transduction of the LPS signal.[91] Such studies suggest the direct interaction between CD14 and more distal components of the LPS signaling pathway. Interestingly, modified forms of LPS, such as lipid IVa (a form that lacks acyloxyacyl side groups), are capable of directly activating mouse cells but antagonize the response of human cells to LPS.[92–94] Because there appears to be no difference in the binding of lipid IVa to human and mouse CD14,* a direct interaction between LPS and later components of the signaling pathway may reasonably be suspected.

In many ways, the identification of the product of the LPS gene represents a breakthrough in understanding of LPS signal transduction. This protein is, in fact, the gateway to LPS response. It is to be hoped that novel approaches to the cloning of this gene may soon shed light on its function.

*Tobias P: Personal communication, 1992.

Of course, other components of eubacteria, as well as other microorganisms, are capable of activating macrophages to produce cytokines. For example, lipopeptides derived from *Treponema pallidum* and *Borrelia bergdorferi* stimulate macrophages to secrete TNF[95] apparently through a pathway distinct from that used by LPS. The TNF gene is also activated by gram-positive organisms, perhaps through interaction with lipoteichoic acid.* Lipoarabinomannan, as well as other products of mycobacteria, also may act as an inducer of TNF synthesis.[96–98] *Plasmodium* species[99–102] and trypanosomes[103–105] also are capable of activating TNF synthesis, presumably through the action of lipid-bearing inducing molecules.

The molecular targets of these toxins are obscure. Aside from CD14, no biologically relevant receptors for these nonprotein toxins have been identified. It is noteworthy that many of the inducing agents are lipids; however, this observation does not, in itself, provide much information as to the nature of the receptors.

Certain proteins of microbial origin also activate TNF or IL-1 synthesis. Bacterial exotoxins, including Shiga toxin (SLT-I),[106, 107] toxic shock toxin,[108–110] and staphylococcal enterotoxin B[16] have been reported to stimulate TNF production by cultured monocytes or macrophages or in vivo. In mice, SLT-I appears to induce TNF reporter gene expression specifically in renal tissue.[107] This is of interest because the kidney is the principal target of SLT-I action when this exotoxin induces the hemolytic uremic syndrome. It is possible that site-specific expression of the TNF gene, determined by exotoxin receptor specificity, may lead to many different clinical presentations wrought by a single cytokine.

More Distal Signaling Events in the Production of Tumor Necrosis Factor and Related Cytokines

Endotoxin-induced expression of the TNF gene has been thoroughly studied, and at least some of the mechanisms that control TNF biosynthesis apply in the regulation of other cytokines. In studying expression of cytokine genes, the nature of the signaling pathway that activates these genes is examined de facto. It has become apparent, for example, that most cytokine genes are dependent on NF-kB for activation.[111–114] NF-kB is a positively acting transcription factor that, in quiescent cells, exists as a cytoplasmic complex with a second protein that functions as an inhibitor of NF-kB action (IkB). IkB is modified, perhaps by phosphorylation, so as to release NF-kB after cell activation. The NF-kB then translocates to the nucleus, binding to a recognition motif within the promoter of diverse cytokines, and facilitates initiation of transcription.

Other transcription factors, such as AP1 (often consisting of a dimer composed of fos and jun) and NF-AT,[115] may also contribute to activation of many cytokine genes at a transcriptional level. Still other factors may act to influence expression negatively. Thus, the transcriptional response to LPS induction is in at least some cases short lived; this accounts for the decline in TNF biosynthesis after bolus administration of LPS and perhaps for the refractory state that follows challenge.[116]

Transcriptional activation may be blocked by certain drugs, such as dexamethasone,[117–121] pentoxifylline,[117, 122–124] and 2-aminopurine,[117, 125] each of which acts through a distinct mechanism to interfere with signal transduction. Although the precise mechanism of action by which each of these agents acts remains obscure, dexamethasone (like other glucocorticoid hormones) appears to act at a very early stage in the signaling pathway because its application to cells blocks translational activation (see later discussion) as well as transcriptional activation of TNF synthesis within macrophages. Pentoxifylline exerts a specific effect on TNF synthesis (to the exclusion of effects on IL-1 synthesis, for example). It is known to inhibit phosphodiesterase, thereby increasing cytoplasmic cyclic adenosine monophosphate (cAMP) levels and may conceivably exert its action through other effects as well. Elevation of cAMP, whether by inhibition of phosphodiesterase or other mechanisms, strongly inhibits TNF gene transcription.[117] Finally, 2-aminopurine acts as a protein kinase inhibitor and, as such, appears capable of abrogating signals that initiate transcription as well.[117, 125]

Transcriptional activation is but one process by which cytokine release is effected. At least some cytokines, and perhaps most of them, are also translationally repressed by virtue of their content of a (U + A)-rich element within the 3′-untranslated region of their respective messenger ribonucleic acids (mRNAs).[126] Translational repression is overcome by cell activation in the case of the TNF mRNA, which is more efficiently translated after stimulation by LPS,[127] or by ultraviolet light.[128] The molecular events that cause translational repression or favor its release remain to be deciphered, although certain RNA binding proteins may very well be involved.

Clearly, within a common cellular environment, some cytokine genes respond to a given activating signal more strongly than others.[129–131] Moreover, temporal differences in response exist, suggesting that the state of cell activation evolves over time, favoring the activation of one set of genes, then another, and then still others.[132] Commitment to activation also occurs[121] so that some agents (notably glucocorticoids) become ineffectual, and it is necessary to halt the activation process by a different approach at later and later stages.

Post-Translational Processing and Secretion of Cytokines

Most cytokines are expressed as prohormones, bearing a classic signal sequence that dictates their efficient secretion. There are exceptions, however, and with time, the distinction between cytokines and cell-surface proteins has become blurred because many bioactive proteins, capable of engaging specific cell-surface receptors, can exist in both soluble and cell-bound forms.

TNF, for example, has a hydrophobic signal peptide sequence and is, for the most part, efficiently secreted after proteolytic cleavage of the prohormone to yield a mature product through the action of an elastase-like enzyme that has two potential cleavage sites within the murine protein sequence.[133] However, a fraction of the TNF that is synthesized fails to undergo cleavage and, therefore, is diverted to the plasma membrane, where it may retain weak biologic activity.[134, 135] The function of this membrane-associated TNF remains to be determined. It has been observed on both macrophages and on lymphocytes, and certain noncleavable mutants have been produced so as to ensure membrane localization.[135] The physical state of the membrane-associated TNF has yet to be determined. Specifically, given that secreted TNF is a trimeric protein,[136–138] it is not clear whether the major form of membrane-associated TNF is a homotrimer consisting of three prohormone subunits or whether a single prohormone anchors two processed subunits to the membrane.

Some cytokines, such as the IL-1 molecules, are secreted through a different and poorly understood mechanism,

*Beutler B: Unpublished observation.

which may in fact be lysis of the cell.[139, 140] The IL-1 molecules are also produced as prohormones, which undergo cleavage by IL-1 converting enzyme (ICE), the complementary deoxyribonucleic acid for which has now been cloned.[141, 142] ICE is the object of considerable interest because specific ICE antagonists may effectively prevent the formation of biologically active IL-1.

Many cytokines are glycosylated; however, aside from influencing the stability of the protein in circulation, it is unclear that glycosylation functionally alters any of the cytokines, which can effectively engage their receptors whether or not a glycosyl moiety is present.

METHODS FOR BLOCKADE OF TUMOR NECROSIS FACTOR BIOSYNTHESIS

Ultimately, it may be possible to block endotoxin signaling at its root (i.e., at the level of the LPS gene product). This will likely depend on the identification of this protein by one of several cloning strategies. There is sound reason to believe, then, that a state of endotoxin resistance as profound as that witnessed in the C3H/HeJ mouse might be elicited. However, until this goal is achieved, other approaches will undoubtedly be pursued.

The antagonism of LPS by nontoxic analogs[143] and its inhibition by antibodies[144–150] remain viable strategies in principle, although efficacy remains highly controversial.[151] Glucocorticoid hormones, which effectively block endotoxic shock in animals if administered before LPS or bacterial pathogens, are quite ineffective in human clinical trials[152–155] probably because their effect is strictly pre-emptive.[121] Pentoxifylline, amrinone, and other phosphodiesterase inhibitors block TNF gene transcription and can, in animals, prevent endotoxic shock.[122, 156–159] However, the therapeutic index of these agents is extremely small, and their use is not widely contemplated in humans with septic shock. Conceivably, newer, less toxic agents of the same type might find a clinical use.

A number of agents that block specific cytokine mediators are under study in septic shock. These include inhibitors of TNF[160, 161] and IL-1 activity.* There is reason for confidence that combinations of these agents, as noted previously here, might be even more effective than individual inhibitors.

CONCLUSIONS

Although the clinical picture that septic shock presents may be dauntingly complex, the process is, at its origins, strikingly simple. The structure of LPS, the chief initiator of shock produced by gram-negative organisms, is well defined, and it is known that LPS action is entirely dependent on the function of a single gene. Presumably, only a handful of toxic mediators are responsible for the further transmission of toxicity. We may well be optimistic, therefore, that our attempts to block the untoward reactions to bacteria will ultimately succeed. This optimism must be tempered by an awareness of two facts. First, damage that has occurred before initiation of therapy may prove partially or entirely irreversible. We cannot expect cytokine blockade to restore lost function or to repair dead and dying tissues. Second, the blockade of cytokine activity is an immunosuppressive maneuver. Effective antibiotic therapy is therefore absolutely critical to a successful outcome. In the context of the often-stated belief that we are capable of dealing with infection but not with its effects, the goal of blocking cytokine synthesis seems a realistic one.

*Beutler B: Unpublished data.

References

1. Michalek SM, Moore RN, McGhee JR, et al: The primary role of lymphoreticular cells in the mediation of host responses to bacterial endotoxin. J Infect Dis 1980; 141:55.
2. Watson J, Kelly K, Largen M, et al: The genetic mapping of a defective LPS response gene in C3H/HeJ mice. J Immunol 1978; 120:422.
3. Watson J, Riblet R, Taylor BA: The response of recombinant inbred strains of mice to bacterial lipopolysaccharides. J Immunol 1977; 118:2088.
4. Freudenberg MA, Keppler D, Galanos C: Requirement for lipopolysaccharide-responsive macrophages in galactosamine-induced sensitization to endotoxin. Infect Immun 1986; 51:891.
5. Van Den Ackerveken GF, Van Kan JA, Joosten MH, et al: Characterization of two putative pathogenicity genes of the fungal tomato pathogen *Cladosporium fulvum.* Mol Plant-Microb Interac 1993; 6:210.
6. Pennica D, Nedwin GE, Hayflick JS, et al: Human tumor necrosis factor: Precursor structure, expression and homology to lymphotoxin. Nature 1984; 312:724.
7. Beutler B, Greenwald D, Hulmes JD, et al: Identity of tumour necrosis factor and the macrophage-secreted factor cachectin. Nature 1985; 316:552.
8. Nedwin GE, Naylor SL, Sakaguchi AY, et al: Human lymphotoxin and tumor necrosis factor genes: Structure homology and chromosomal localization. Nucleic Acids Res 1985; 13:6361.
9. Muller U, Jongeneel CV, Nedospasov SA, et al: Tumor necrosis factor and lymphotoxin genes map close to H-2D in the mouse major histocompatibility complex. Nature 1987; 325:265.
10. Browning JL, Ngam-ek A, Lawton P, et al: Lymphotoxin β, a novel member of the TNF family that forms a heteromeric complex with lymphotoxin on the cell surface. Cell 1993; 72:847.
11. Sprang SR, Eck MJ: The 3-D structure of TNF. *In*: Tumor Necrosis Factors: The Molecules and Their Emerging Role in Medicine. Beutler B (Ed). New York, Raven Press, 1992, pp 11–32.
12. Banner DW, D'Arcy A, Janes W, et al: Crystal structure of the soluble human 55 kd TNF receptor-human TNFβ complex: Implications for TNF receptor activation. Cell 1993; 73:431.
13. D'Arcy A, Banner DW, Janes W, et al: Crystallization and preliminary crystallographic analysis of a TNF-β-55 kDa TNF receptor complex. J Mol Biol 1993; 229:555.
14. Engelmann H, Holtmann H, Brakebusch C, et al: Antibodies to a soluble form of a tumor necrosis factor (TNF) receptor have TNF-like activity. J Biol Chem 1990; 265:14497.
15. Desch CE, Dobrina A, Aggarwal BB, et al: Tumor necrosis factor-alpha exhibits greater proinflammatory activity than lymphotoxin in vitro. Blood 1990; 75:2030.
16. Nedwin GE, Svedersky LP, Bringman TS, et al: Effect of interleukin 2, interferon-gamma, and mitogens on the production of tumor necrosis factors alpha and beta. J Immunol 1985; 135:2492.
17. Armitage RJ, Fanslow WC, Strockbine L, et al: Molecular and biological characterization of a murine ligand for CD40. Nature 1992; 357:80.
18. Goodwin RG, Alderson MR, Smith CA, et al: Molecular and biological characterization of a ligand for CD27 defines a new family of cytokines with homology to tumor necrosis factor. Cell 1993; 73:447.
19. Smith CA, Gruss H-J, Davis T, et al: CD30 antigen, a marker for Hodgkin's lymphoma, is a receptor whose ligand defines an emerging family of cytokines with homology to TNF. Cell 1993; 73:1349.
20. Smith CA, Davis T, Wignall JM, et al: T2 open reading frame from the Shope fibroma virus encodes a soluble form of the TNF receptor. Biochem Biophys Res Commun 1991; 176:335.
21. Sugita K, Hirose T, Rothstein DM, et al: CD27, a member of the nerve growth factor receptor family, is preferentially expressed on CD45RA + CD4 T cell clones and involved in distinct immunoregulatory functions. J Immunol 1992; 149:3208.
22. Helson L, Green S, Carswell E, et al: Effect of tumour necrosis factor on cultured human melanoma cells. Nature 1975; 258:731.

23. Tartaglia LA, Rothe M, Hu Y-F, et al: Tumor necrosis factor's cytotoxic activity is signaled by the p55 TNF receptor. Cell 1993; 73:213.
24. Matthews N, Ryley HC, Neale ML: Tumour necrosis factor from the rabbit: IV. Purification and chemical characterization. Br J Cancer 1980; 42:416.
25. Ruff MR, Gifford GE: Purification and physico-chemical characterization of rabbit tumor necrosis factor. J Immunol 1980; 125:1671.
26. Abe S, Gatanaga T, Yamazaki M, et al: Purification of rabbit tumor necrosis factor. FEBS Lett 1985; 180:203.
27. Aggarwal BB, Kohr WJ, Hass PE, et al: Human tumor necrosis factor. Production, purification, and characterization. J Biol Chem 1985; 260:2345.
28. Haranaka K, Satomi N, Sakurai A, et al: Purification and partial amino acid sequence of rabbit tumor necrosis factor. Int J Cancer 1985; 36:395.
29. Haranaka K, Carswell EA, Williamson BD, et al: Purification, characterization, and antitumor activity of nonrecombinant mouse tumor necrosis factor. Proc Natl Acad Sci 1986; 83:3949.
30. Trauth BC, Klas C, Peters AMJ, et al: Monoclonal antibody-mediated tumor regression by induction of apoptosis. Science 1989; 245:301.
31. Allsopp TE, Wyatt S, Paterson HF, et al: The proto-oncogene *bcl*-2 can selectively rescue neurotrophic factor-dependent neurons from apoptosis. Cell 1993; 73:295.
32. Rabizadeh S, Oh J, Zhong L, et al: Induction of apoptosis by the low-affinity NGF receptor. Science 1993; 261:345.
33. Tsubata T, Wu J, Honjo T: B-cell apoptosis induced by antigen receptor crosslinking is blocked by a T-cell signal through CD40. Nature 1993; 364:645.
34. Kannan Y, Usami K, Okada M, et al: Nerve growth factor suppresses apoptosis of murine neutrophils. Biochem Biophys Res Commun 1992; 186:1050.
35. Edwards SN, Buckmaster AE, Tolkovsky AM: The death programme in cultured sympathetic neurones can be suppressed at the posttranslational level by nerve growth factor, cyclic AMP, and depolarization. J Neurochem 1991; 57:2140.
36. Tartaglia LA, Ayres TM, Wong GHW, et al: A novel domain within the 55 kd TNF receptor signals cell death. Cell 1993; 74:845.
37. Vietor I, Schwenger P, Li W, et al: Tumor necrosis factor-induced activation and increased tyrosine phosphorylation of mitogen-activated protein (MAP) kinase in human fibroblasts. J Biol Chem 1993; 268:18994.
38. Dbaibo GS, Obeid LM, Hannun YA: Tumor necrosis factor-α (TNF-α) signal transduction through ceramide. Dissociation of growth inhibitory effects of TNF-α from activation of nuclear factor-kappaB. J Biol Chem 1993; 268:17762.
39. Yang Z, Costanzo M, Golde DW, et al: Tumor necrosis factor activation of the sphingomyelin pathway signals nuclear factor kappaB translocation in intact HL-60 cells. J Biol Chem 1993; 268:20520.
40. Peppel K, Beutler B: Biological properties of a recombinant TNF inhibitor. *In*: Bacterial Endotoxin: Recognition and Effector Mechanisms. Levin J, Alving CR, Munford RS, Stütz PL (Eds). New York: Elsevier Science, 1993, pp 447–454.
41. Old LJ: Polypeptide mediator network. Nature 1987; 326:330.
42. Harrison LC, Campbell IL: Cytokines: An expanding network of immuno-inflammatory hormones. Mol Endocrinol 1988; 2:1151.
43. Chatenoud L: Allograft rejection: The role of the cytokine network. Eur Cytokine Netw 1992; 3:509.
44. Korthäuer U, Graf D, Mages HW, et al: Defective expression of T-cell CD40 ligand causes X-linked immunodeficiency with hyper-IgM. Nature 1993; 361:539.
45. Allen RC, Armitage RJ, Conley ME, et al: CD40 ligand gene defects responsible for X-linked hyper-IgM syndrome. Science 1993; 259:990.
46. Noguchi M, Yi H, Rosenblatt HM, et al: Interleukin-2 receptor gamma chain mutation results in X-linked severe combined immunodeficiency in humans. Cell 1993; 73:147.
47. Dalton DK, Pitts-Meek S, Keshav S, et al: Multiple defects of immune cell function in mice with disrupted interferon-gamma genes. Science 1993; 259:1739.
48. Huang S, Hendriks W, Althage A, et al: Immune response in mice that lack the interferon-gamma receptor. Science 1993; 259:1742.
49. Schorle H, Holtschke T, Hünig T, et al: Development and function of T cells in mice rendered interleukin-2 deficient by gene targeting. Nature 1991; 352:621.
50. Kuhn R, Rajewsky K, Muller W: Generation and analysis of interleukin 4 deficient mice. Science 1991; 254:707.
51. Pfeffer K, Matsuyama T, Kündig TM, et al: Mice deficient for the 55 kd tumor necrosis factor receptor are resistant to endotoxic shock, yet succumb to *L. monocytogenes* infection. Cell 1993; 73:457.
52. Rothe J, Lesslauer W, Lötscher H, et al: Mice lacking the tumour necrosis factor receptor 1 are resistant to TNF-mediated toxicity but highly susceptible to infection by *Listeria monocytogenes*. Nature 1993; 364:798.
53. Adachi M, Watanabe-Fukunaga R, Nagata S: Aberrant transcription caused by the insertion of an early transposable element in an intron of the Fas antigen gene of *lpr* mice. Proc Natl Acad Sci U S A 1993; 90:1756.
54. Watanabe-Fukunaga R, Brannan CI, Copeland NG, et al: Lymphoproliferation disorder in mice explained by defects in Fas antigen that mediates apoptosis. Nature 1992; 356:314.
55. Roths JB, Murphy ED, Eicher EM: A new mutation, gld, that produces lymphoproliferation and autoimmunity in C3H/HeJ mice. J Exp Med 1984; 159:1.
56. Allen RD, Marshall JD, Roths JB, et al: Differences defined by bone marrow transplantation suggest that lpr and gld are mutations of genes encoding an interacting pair of molecules. J Exp Med 1990; 172:1367.
57. Havell EA: Evidence that tumor necrosis factor has an important role in antibacterial resistance. J Immunol 1989; 143:2894.
58. DiSanto JP, Bonnefoy JY, Gauchat JF, et al: CD40 ligand mutations in x-linked immunodeficiency with hyper-IgM. Nature 1993; 361:541.
59. Jensen LM, Zhang Y, Shooter EM: Steady-state polypeptide modulations associated with nerve growth factor (NGF)-induced terminal differentiation and NGF deprivation-induced apoptosis in human neuroblastoma cells. J Biol Chem 1992; 267:19325.
60. Kappler J, Kotzin B, Herron L, et al: V-beta specific stimulation of human T cells by staphylococcal toxins. Science 1989; 244:811.
61. Hackett SP, Stevens DL: Superantigens associated with staphylococcal and streptococcal toxic shock syndrome are potent inducers of tumor necrosis factor-β synthesis. J Infect Dis 1993; 168:232.
62. Miethke T, Wahl C, Heeg K, et al: T-cell-mediated lethal shock triggered in mice by the superantigen staphylococcal enterotoxin-B. Critical role of tumor necrosis factor. J Exp Med 1992; 175:91.
63. Miethke T, Gaus H, Wahl C, et al: T-cell dependent shock induced by a bacterial superantigen. Chem Immunol 1992; 55:172.
64. Ogasawara J, Watanabe-Fukunaga R, Adachi M, et al: Lethal effect of the anti-Fas antibody in mice. Nature 1993; 364:806.
65. Galanos C, Freudenberg MA, Reutter W: Galactosamine-induced sensitization to the lethal effects of endotoxin. Proc Natl Acad Sci 1979; 76:5939.
66. Lehmann V, Freudenberg MA, Galanos C: Lethal toxicity of lipopolysaccharide and tumor necrosis factor in normal and d-galactosamine-treated-mice. J Exp Med 1987; 165:657.
67. Opal SM, Cross AS, Kelly NM, et al: Efficacy of a monoclonal antibody directed against tumor necrosis factor in protecting neutropenic rats from lethal infection with *Pseudomonas aeruginosa*. J Infect Dis 1990; 161:1148.
68. Sheehan KCF, Ruddle NH, Schreiber RD: Generation and characterization of hamster monoclonal antibodies that neutralize murine tumor necrosis factors. J Immunol 1989; 142:3884.
69. Mathison JC, Wolfson E, Ulevitch RJ: Participation of tumor necrosis factor in the mediation of gram negative bacterial lipopolysaccharide-induced injury in rabbits. J Clin Invest 1988; 81:1925.
70. Tracey KJ, Fong Y, Hesse DG, et al: Anti-cachectin/TNF monoclonal antibodies prevent septic shock during lethal bacteraemia. Nature 1987; 330:662.

71. Beutler B, Milsark IW, Cerami A: Passive immunization against cachectin/tumor necrosis factor (TNF) protects mice from the lethal effect of endotoxin. Science 1985; 229:869.
72. Ohlsson K, Bjork P, Bergenfeldt M, et al: Interleukin-1 receptor antagonist reduces mortality from endotoxin shock. Nature 1990; 348:550.
73. Chokri M, Freudenberg M, Galanos C, et al: Antitumoral effects of lipopolysaccharides, tumor necrosis factor, interferon and activated macrophages: Synergism and tissue distribution. Anticancer Res 1989; 9:1185.
74. Galanos C, Freudenberg MA: Mechanisms of endotoxin shock and endotoxin hypersensitivity. Immunobiology 1993; 187:346.
75. Tribble H, Schneider M, Bowersox O, et al: Combination immunotherapy with RH TNF and RM IFN G: Increased therapy and toxicity. Fed Proc 1987; 46:561.
76. Heremans H, Van Damme J, Dillen C, et al: Interferon gamma, a mediator of lethal lipopolysaccharide-induced Shwartzman-like shock reactions in mice. J Exp Med 1990; 171:1853.
77. Doherty GM, Lange JR, Langstein HN, et al: Evidence for IFN-gamma as a mediator of the lethality of endotoxin and tumor necrosis factor-alpha. J Immunol 1992; 149:1666.
78. Heinzel FP: The role of IFN-gamma in the pathology of experimental endotoxemia. J Immunol 1990; 145:2920.
79. Silva AT, Cohen J: Role of interferon-gamma in experimental gram-negative sepsis. J Infect Dis 1992; 166:331.
80. Gerard C, Bruyns C, Marchant A, et al: Interleukin 10 reduces the release of tumor necrosis factor and prevents lethality in experimental endotoxemia. J Exp Med 1993; 177:547.
81. Graham FL, Prevec L: Manipulation of adenovirus vectors. *In*: Methods in Molecular Biology. Murray EJ (Ed). Clifton, NJ: Humana Press, 1991, pp 109–128.
82. Kolls J, Peppel K, Silva M, et al: Prolonged and effective blockade of TNF activity through adenovirus-mediated gene transfer. Proc Natl Acad Sci 1994; 91:215.
83. Philip R, Liggitt D, Philip M, et al: In vivo gene delivery. Efficient transfection of T lymphocytes in adult mice. J Biol Chem 1993; 268:16087.
84. Zhu N, Liggitt D, Liu Y, et al: Systemic gene expression after intravenous DNA delivery into adult mice. Science 1993; 261:209.
85. Beck G, Benach JL, Habicht GS: Isolation of interleukin 1 from joint fluids of patients with lyme disease. J Rheumatol 1989; 16:800.
86. Wright SD, Jong MTC: Adhesion-promoting receptors on human macrophages recognize *Escherichia coli* by binding to lipopolysaccharide. J Exp Med 1986; 164:1876.
87. Wright SD, Tobias PS, Ulevitch RJ, et al: Lipopolysaccharide (LPS) binding protein opsonizes LPS-bearing particle for recognition by a novel receptor on macrophages. J Exp Med 1989; 170:1231.
88. Schumann RR, Leong SR, Flaggs GW, et al: Structure and function of lipopolysaccharide binding protein. Science 1990; 249:1429.
89. Wright SD, Ramos RA, Tobias PS, et al: CD14, a receptor for complexes of lipopolysaccharide (LPS) and LPS binding protein. Science 1990; 249:1431.
90. Ferrero E, Goyert SM: Nucleotide sequence of the gene encoding the monocyte differentiation antigen, CD14. Nucleic Acids Res 1988; 16:4173.
91. Lee JD, Kravchenko V, Kirkland TN, et al: Glycosylphosphatidylinositol anchored or integral membrane forms of CD14 mediate identical cellular responses to endotoxin. Proc Natl Acad Sci U S A 1993; 90:9930.
92. Birkland TP, Cornwell RD, Golenbock DT, et al: Comparative study of lipopolysaccharide-, lipid IVa-, and lipid X-induced tumor necrosis factor production in murine macrophage-like cell lines. Adv Exp Med Biol 1990; 256:399.
93. Riedo FX, Munford RS, Campbell WB, et al: Deacylated lipopolysaccharide inhibits plasminogen activator inhibitor-1, prostacyclin, and prostaglandin E_2 induction by lipopolysaccharide but not by tumor necrosis factor-α. J Immunol 1990; 144:3506.
94. Munford RS, Hall CL: Detoxification of bacterial lipopolysaccharides (endotoxins) by a human neutrophil enzyme. Science 1986; 234:203.
95. Radolf JD, Norgard MV, Brandt ME, et al: Lipoproteins of *Borrelia burgdorferi* and *Treponema pallidum* activate cachectin/TNF synthesis: analysis using a CAT reporter construct. J Immunol 1991; 147:1968.
96. Wallis RS, Amir-Tahmasseb M, Ellner JJ: Induction of interleukin 1 and tumor necrosis factor by mycobacterial proteins: The monocyte Western blot. Proc Natl Acad Sci U S A 1990; 87:3348.
97. Valone SE, Rich EA, Wallis RS, et al: Expression of tumor necrosis factor in vitro by human mononuclear phagocytes stimulated with whole *Mycobacterium bovis* BCG and mycobacterial antigens. Infect Immun 1988; 56:3313.
98. Grau GE, Parida SK, Pointaire P, et al: TNF and mycobacteria. *In*: Tumor Necrosis Factors: The Molecules and Their Emerging Role in Medicine. Beutler B (Ed). New York, Raven Press, 1992, pp 329–340.
99. Taverne J, Bate CAW, Sarkar DA, et al: Human and murine macrophages produce TNF in response to soluble antigens of *Plasmodium falciparum*. Parasite Immunol 1990; 12:33.
100. Kwiatkowski D, Cannon JG, Manogue KR, et al: Tumour necrosis factor production in *Falciparum* malaria and its association with schizont rupture. Clin Exp Immunol 1989; 77:361.
101. Taverne J, Bate CAW, Playfair JHL: Induction of TNF in vitro as a model for the identification of toxic malaria antigens. Lymphokine Res 1989; 8:317.
102. Bate CAW, Taverne J, Playfair JHL: Malarial parasites induce TNF production by macrophages. Immunology 1988; 64:227.
103. Hotez PJ, Le Trang N, Fairlamb AH, et al: Lipoprotein lipase suppression in 3T3-L1 cells by a haematoprotozoan-induced mediator from peritoneal exudate cells. Parasite Immunol 1984; 6:203.
104. Goldberg SS, Cordeiro MN, Silva Pereira AA, et al: Release of lipopolysaccharide (LPS) from cell surface of *Trypanosoma cruzi* by EDTA. Int J Parasitol 1983; 13:11.
105. Ketteridge DS: Lipopolysaccharide from *Trypanosoma cruzi*. Trans R Soc Trop Med Hyg 1978; 72:101.
106. Barrett TJ, Potter ME, Strockbine NA: Evidence for participation of the macrophage in Shigalike toxin II-induced lethality in mice. Microb Pathog 1990; 9:95.
107. Harel Y, Weinberg A, Silva M, et al: A reporter transgene indicates renal-specific induction of TNF by shiga-like toxin: Possible involvement of TNF in hemolytic-uremic syndrome (Abstract). J Clin Invest 1993; 92:2110.
108. Fast DJ, Schlievert PM, Nelson RD: Toxic shock syndrome-associated staphylococcal and streptococcal pyrogenic toxins are potent inducers of tumor necrosis factor production. Infect Immun 1989; 57:291.
109. Ikejima T, Dinarello CA, Gill DM, et al: Induction of human interleukin-1 by a product of *Staphylococcus aureus* associated with toxic shock syndrome. J Clin Invest 1984; 73:1312.
110. Ikejima T, Minami M, Gill DM, et al: Human, rabbit and murine interleukin-1 production in response to toxic shock syndrome toxin-1. Unpublished manuscript, 1985.
111. Baeurle PA, Baltimore D: The physiology of the NF-kB transcription factor. *In*: Hormonal control regulation of gene expression. Cohen P, Foulkes JG (Eds). Elsevier, Amsterdam, Biomedical Press, 1991, pp 409–432.
112. Zhang Y, Lin J-X, Vilcek J: Interleukin-6 induction by tumor necrosis factor and interleukin-1 in human fibroblasts involves activation of a nuclear factor binding to a kappaB-like sequence. Mol Cell Biol 1990; 10:3818.
113. Lenardo MJ, Baltimore D: NF-kB: A pleiotropic mediator of inducible and tissue-specific gene control. Cell 1989; 58:227.
114. Lenardo MJ, Fan C-M, Maniatis T, et al: The involvement of NF-kB in beta-interferon gene regulation reveals its role as widely inducible mediator of signal transduction. Cell 1989; 57:287.
115. Castigli E, Pahwa R, Good RA, et al: Molecular basis of a multiple lymphokine deficiency in a patient with severe combined immunodeficiency. Proc Natl Acad Sci U S A 1993; 90:4728.
116. Mathison JC, Virca GD, Wolfson E, et al: Adaptation to bacterial lipopolysaccharide controls lipopolysaccharide-induced tumor necrosis factor production in rabbit macrophages. J Clin Invest 1990; 85:1108.
117. Han J, Huez G, Beutler B: Interactive effects of the TNF promoter and 3′-untranslated regions. J Immunol 1991; 146:1843.

118. Narumi S, Hamilton TA: Dexamethasone selectively regulates LPS-inducible gene expression in murine peritoneal macrophages. Immunopharmacology 1990; 19:93.
119. Ghezzi P, Sipe JD: Dexamethasone modulation of LPS, IL-1, and TNF stimulated serum amyloid A synthesis in mice. Lymphokine Res 1988; 7:157.
120. Han J, Thompson P, Beutler B: Dexamethasone and pentoxifylline inhibit endotoxin-induced cachectin/TNF synthesis at separate points in the signalling pathway. J Exp Med 1990; 172:391.
121. Beutler B, Krochin N, Milsark IW, et al: Control of cachectin (tumor necrosis factor) synthesis: Mechanisms of endotoxin resistance. Science 1986; 232:977.
122. Zabel P, Schade FU, Schlaak M: Inhibition of endogenous TNF formation by pentoxifylline. Immunobiology 1993; 187:447.
123. Waage A, Sorensen M, Stordal B: Differential effect of oxpentifylline on tumour necrosis factor and interleukin-6 production. Lancet 1990; 335:543.
124. Strieter RM, Remick DG, Ward PA, et al: Cellular and molecular regulation of tumor necrosis factor-alpha production by pentoxifylline. Biochem Biophys Res Commun 1988; 155:1230.
125. Goldfeld AE, Maniatis T: Coordinate viral induction of tumor necrosis factor alpha and interferon β in human B cells and monocytes. Proc Natl Acad Sci U S A 1989; 86:1490.
126. Caput D, Beutler B, Hartog K, et al: Identification of a common nucleotide sequence in the 3′-untranslated region of mRNA molecules specifying inflammatory mediators. Proc Natl Acad Sci U S A 1986; 83:1670.
127. Han J, Brown T, Beutler B: Endotoxin-responsive sequences control cachectin/TNF biosynthesis at the translational level. J Exp Med 1990; 171:465.
128. Bazzoni F, Kruys V, Shakhov A, et al: Analysis of TNF promoter responses to ultraviolet light. J Clin Invest 1994; 93:56.
129. Osipovich OA, Fegeding KV, Misuno NI, et al: Differential action of cycloheximide and activation stimuli on transcription of tumor necrosis factor-α, IL-1β, IL-8, and P53 genes in human monocytes. J Immunol 1993; 150:4958.
130. Sillaber C, Bevec D, Butterfield JH, et al: Tumor necrosis factor α and interleukin-1β mRNA expression in HMC-1 cells: Differential regulation of gene product expression by recombinant interleukin-4. Exp Hematol 1993; 21:1271.
131. Hallet M-M, Peyrat M-A, Soulillou J-P, et al: Simultaneous transcription of eleven cytokines in human alloreactive T lymphocyte clones after stimulation by phorbol ester and A23187. Eur Cytokine Netw 1992; 3:477.
132. Fong Y, Tracey KJ, Moldawer LL, et al: Antibodies to cachectin/tumor necrosis factor reduce interleukin 1β and interleukin 6 appearance during lethal bacteremia. J Exp Med 1989; 170:1627.
133. Cseh K, Beutler B: Alternative cleavage of the cachectin/TNF propeptide results in a larger, inactive form of secreted protein. J Biol Chem 1989; 264:16256.
134. Kriegler M, Perez C, DeFay K, et al: A novel form of TNF/cachectin is a cell surface cytotoxic transmembrane protein: Ramifications for the complex physiology of TNF. Cell 1988; 53:45.
135. Perez C, Albert I, DeFay K, et al: A non-secretable cell surface mutant of tumor necrosis factor (TNF) kills by cell to cell contact. Cell 1990; 63:251.
136. Eck MJ, Beutler B, Kuo G, et al: Crystallization of trimeric recombinant human tumor necrosis factor (cachectin). J Biol Chem 1988; 263:12816.
137. Eck MJ, Sprang SR: The structure of tumor necrosis factor-alpha at 2.6A resolution: Implications for receptor binding. J Biol Chem 1989; 264:17595.
138. Jones EY, Stuart DI, Walker NPC: Structure of tumour necrosis factor. Nature 1989; 338:225.
139. Hogquist KA, Nett MA, Unanue ER, et al: Interleukin 1 is processed and released during apoptosis. Proc Nat Acad Sci U S A 1991; 88:8485.
140. Chaplin DD, Hogquist KA: Interactions between TNF and interleukin-1. *In*: Tumor Necrosis Factors: The Molecules and Their Emerging Role in Medicine. Beutler B (Ed). New York, Raven Press, 1992, pp 197–220.
141. Molineaux SM, Casano FJ, Rolando AM, et al: Interleukin 1 beta (IL-1 beta) processing in murine macrophages requires a structurally conserved homologue of human IL-1 beta converting enzyme. Proc Nat Acad Sci U S A 1993; 90:1809.
142. Thornberry NA, Bull HG, Calaycay JR, et al: A novel heterodimeric cysteine protease is required for interleukin-1 beta processing in monocytes. Nature 1992; 356:768.
143. Takayama K, Qureshi N, Beutler B, et al: Diphosphoryl lipid A from *Rhodopseudomonas spaeroides* ATCC 17023 blocks induction of cachectin in macrophages by lipopolysaccharide. Infect Immun 1989; 57:1336.
144. Baumgartner JD, Heumann D, Gerain J, et al: Association between protective efficacy of anti-lipopolysaccharide (LPS) antibodies and suppression of LPS-induced tumor necrosis factor α and interleukin 6. Comparison of O side chain-specific antibodies with core LPS antibodies. J Exp Med 1990; 171:889.
145. Vogel SN, Havell EA: Differential inhibition of lipopolysaccharide-induced phenomena by anti-tumor necrosis factor alpha antibody. Infect Immun 1990; 58:2397.
146. Ziegler E, Fisher C, Sprung C, et al: Prevention of death from gram negative bacteremia and sepsis by HA-1A—a human monoclonal antibody specific for lipid A of endotoxin: Results of phase III trial. Clin Res 1990; 38:304A.
147. Calandra T, Glauser MP, Schellekens J, et al: Treatment of gram-negative septic shock with human IgG antibody to *Escherichia coli* J5: A prospective, double-blind, randomized trial. J Infect Dis 1988; 158:312.
148. Ward DC, Michalek SM, McGhee JR: Monoclonal antibodies to salmonella lipopolysaccharide: Functional analysis of anti-lipid A antibodies. Clin Exp Immunol 1988; 72:157.
149. Braude AI, Douglas H, Davis CE: Treatment and prevention of intravascular coagulation with antiserum to endotoxin. J Infect Dis 1973; 128:S157.
150. Braude AI, Douglas H: Passive immunization against the local Shwartzman reaction. J Immunol 1972; 108:505.
151. Warren HS, Danner RL, Munford RS: Anti-endotoxin monoclonal antibodies (see comments). N Engl J Med 1992; 326:1153.
152. Sheagren JN: Septic shock and corticosteroids. N Engl J Med 1981; 305:456.
153. Pitcairn M, Schuler J, Erve PR, et al: Glucocorticoid and antibiotic effect on experimental gram-negative bacteremic shock. Arch Surg 1975; 110:1012.
154. Luce JM, Montgomery AB, Marks JD, et al: Ineffectiveness of high-dose methylprednisolone in preventing parenchymal lung injury and improving mortality in patients with septic shock. Am Rev Respir Dis 1988; 138:62.
155. Marks JD, Marks CB, Luce JM, et al: Plasma tumor necrosis factor in patients with septic shock: Mortality rate, incidence of adult respiratory distress syndrome, and effects of methylprednisolone administration. Am Rev Respir Dis 1990; 141:94.
156. Semmler J, Wachtel H, Endres S: The specific type IV phosphodiesterase inhibitor rolipram suppresses tumor necrosis factor-α production by human mononuclear cells. Int J Immunopharmacol 1993; 15:409.
157. Sigurdsson GH, Youssef H: Effects of pentoxifylline on hemodynamics, gas exchange and multiple organ platelet sequestration in experimental endotoxic shock. Acta Anaesthesiol Scand 1993; 37:396.
158. Waxman K, Clark L, Soliman MH, et al: Pentoxifylline in resuscitation of experimental hemorrhagic shock. Crit Care Med 1991; 19:728.
159. Schade UF, Bosch JVD, Schonharting MM: Increase of survival rate by pentoxifylline in endotoxic shock. *In*: Pentoxifylline and leukocyte function. Mandell G, Novick W, Jr (Eds). Wiesbaden, Germany, Hoechst, 1988, pp 175–183.
160. Ashkenazi A, Marsters SA, Capon DJ, et al: Protection against endotoxic shock by a tumor necrosis factor receptor immunoadhesin. Proc Natl Acad Sci U S A 1991; 88:10535.
161. Peppel K, Crawford D, Beutler B: A tumor necrosis factor (TNF) receptor-IgG heavy chain chimeric protein as a bivalent antagonist of TNF activity. J Exp Med 1991; 174:1483.

CHAPTER 23

Intracellular pH and Electrolyte Regulation

Tor Inge Tønnessen, MD, PhD

In clinical practice, the most commonly ordered laboratory tests are electrolytes and pH. This is due to the major importance of these parameters for the function of the body. Unfortunately, they largely reflect the extracellular milieu, and what happens intracellularly is not known to clinicians. There is, however, a huge body of knowledge on the regulation of intracellular pH and electrolytes. Yet most of the studies have been carried out in vitro, and the function of these mechanisms in vivo has not been fully elucidated. Fortunately, with the increasing utilization of magnetic resonance imaging (MRI) and positron emission tomographic scanning for real-time measurements of intracellular parameters in vivo, much of this basic knowledge is applied to the understanding of whole-body physiology and pathophysiology. In order for the knowledge to expand further, however, clinicians and clinical scientists need to have knowledge of these basic processes. It is the intent of this chapter to give the clinician some insight into this topic.

Because of the widespread writing on pH and electrolyte disturbances in the clinical literature, certain assumptions have become established, such as:

- Bicarbonate is an extracellular buffer and is not effective to treat intracellular pH disturbances.
- Administration of bicarbonate will give rise to intracellular acidification.
- Acidosis will increase oxygen (O_2) delivery to tissues.
- Under ischemic conditions, lactic acid is the main acid to acidify the cytosol.

In this chapter, these assumptions, among others, are addressed on the basis of recent knowledge that clearly disputes the validity of several of these statements. Also, future treatment of acid-base disorders in the form of drugs to specifically inhibit or stimulate intracellular regulatory mechanisms to normalize the disturbances is discussed. Thus, exciting new treatment for diverse disorders such as cerebral edema, myocardial stunning after cardioplegia, ischemia, inflammation, and cancer might be available by application of the current basic knowledge on how cells regulate their cytosolic pH and electrolytes.

MECHANISMS INVOLVED IN THE REGULATION OF CYTOSOLIC pH

As a result of metabolism, approximately 20,000 mmol of carbon dioxide (CO_2), approximately 1500 to 4500 mmol of lactic acid, and approximately 100 to 200 mmol of other nonvolatile acids are formed each day. Also alkaline compounds, although to a lesser extent, are end products of catabolism. Because of the large acid load, effective regulation of pH in the body is of vital importance because a number of cellular processes are highly pH sensitive.

Intracellular pH is not uniform throughout the cells. The pH of the cytosol (pH_i) is in most cells somewhat lower (0.02–0.3 pH units) than extracellular pH (pH_o). pH_i is not a static value but changes depending on the activation of the cell. pH of cell organelles is markedly different from the cytosolic pH. Thus, lysosomes are very acidic (pH 4.5–5.5), endosomes and Golgi apparatus are somewhat more alkaline (pH 5.5–6.5), and the nucleus is only slightly more acidic than the cytosol.

To achieve a precise regulation of pH in the body despite a very heavy acid load because of cellular metabolism, the four main defense mechanisms are as follows:

1. Physiochemical buffers both in the extracellular fluid and intracellular fluid
2. Transport of acid and base across the cell membrane via specific mechanisms
3. Removal of volatile acid by respiration
4. Removal of nonvolatile acid and absorption of base by the kidneys

Physiochemical Buffering

Extracellular Buffering

The main buffers in the blood and interstitial fluid are proteins, phosphate, and bicarbonate (i.e., weak acids and their conjugate base). Despite the fact that the bicarbonate buffer system has a pK value of 6.1, it is quantitatively the most important extracellular physiologic buffer because of its high concentration (approximately 25 mmol) and the fact that the "weak acid" CO_2 is effectively removed by respiration. The extracellular phosphate concentration is 1 to 2 mmol, and this buffer is therefore much less important. The total extracellular protein concentration is 2 to 4 mmol, but each protein has many buffering residues that make them important buffers.

The extracellular buffering of nonvolatile acids (hydrogen ion [H^+]) is very effective. However, because the bicarbonate/CO_2 complex is the dominating system, buffering of excess CO_2/carbonic acid (H_2CO_3) is rather ineffective extracellularly, and relatively small variations of CO_2 by alteration of respiration may markedly influence pH of the blood plasma. Thus, the main buffering of CO_2/H_2CO_3 takes place intracellularly in red blood cells and tissue cells.

Intracellular Buffering

The main intracellular buffers are proteins, organic phosphates, and bicarbonate. At physiologic concentration of bicarbonate ion (HCO_3^-), it constitutes approximately half of the buffering capacity. In red blood cells, hemoglobin is a particularly effective buffer because of its high concentration and its many histidine residues, the only amino acid with significant buffering power near neutral pH. Importantly, deoxygenated hemoglobin has a higher affinity for protons than its oxygenated counterpart (Haldane effect).

The bicarbonate buffer system is particularly effective because the components of the system (i.e., CO_2 and HCO_3^-) can be independently regulated by the body to maintain a physiologic pH. Because the plasma membranes of all cells are highly permeable to CO_2, intracellular CO_2 concentration is under most circumstances equal to the extracellular concentration. Because of the removal of CO_2 by respiration, the intracellular H_2CO_3 concentration is effectively regulated. Because of this, every HCO_3^- ion can buffer two to four times better than any other physiologic buffer. Not only does CO_2 effectively diffuse across the cell membrane, but there are also specific transporters for HCO_3^-. The intracellular concentration of HCO_3^- can therefore be regulated independently of CO_2, making this buffering system remarkably effective both for intracellular and extracellular buffering.

Transmembrane Transport of Acid and Base

Importance of Transmembrane Transport for Cellular Function

Because of its hydrophobic interior, the lipid bilayer of the plasma membrane is highly impermeable to most polar molecules. This prevents most of the water-soluble content from escaping. To transport these molecules in a controlled manner, cells have evolved very specialized membrane transport proteins. These are large proteins that span the entire membrane by having their α-helixes cross the plasma membrane several times. This arrangement creates an interior of the protein that shields the transported molecules from the hydrophobic lipid membrane. There are two major classes of membrane transport proteins: carrier proteins and channel proteins. *Carrier proteins* (also called *carriers* or *transporters*) bind the specific solute to be transported and undergo a conformational change to transfer the solute across the membrane. *Channel proteins* form water-filled "pores" that extend across the lipid bilayer. These channels can be closed or open; once they are open, electrolytes traverse the channels according to the specificity of the channel and to the transmembrane gradient of the solute. All channel proteins and many carrier proteins allow only *passive transport* (facilitated diffusion) (i.e., the direction of transport is determined by the electrochemical gradient). Transport of a solute against its electrochemical gradient occurs only with carrier proteins and is either *primary active* (i.e., requires metabolic energy most often by the hydrolysis of adenosine triphosphate [ATP]) or *secondary active transport,* which means that the transport of the solute is coupled to the simultaneous or sequential transfer of another solute with a more favorable electrochemical gradient. The latter can be achieved either as a *symport,* in which both solutes are transported in the same direction, or as an *antiport,* in which the solutes are exchanged in the opposite direction (Fig. 23–1). Antiport is often called *exchanger* or *exchange mechanism* in the literature.

All these mechanisms are dependent on the sodium ion (Na^+)/potassium ion (K^+) "pump" for their proper function. This pump is a transmembrane carrier protein with an ATPase function (i.e., it hydrolyzes ATP as a part of the transport mechanisms to harness energy. This enables an active transport of electrolytes against their electrochemical gradient. Because three Na^+ are transported out of the cell in exchange for two K^+, the mechanism is electrogenic and a transmembrane potential is built up. The direct effect of the pump, however, seldom contributes more than 20% of the membrane potential. The rest of the membrane potential emanates from an indirect effect of the pump by building up an outward-directed K^+ gradient, which, because of its membrane permeability, builds up the membrane potential. This permeability is achieved by a K^+ leak channel protein. Most channel proteins have the ability to close and open in response to stimuli. If they are regulated by the electrical status of the cell, they are called *voltage-gated* channels. If their activity is determined by humoral mediators, they are *ligand gated.*

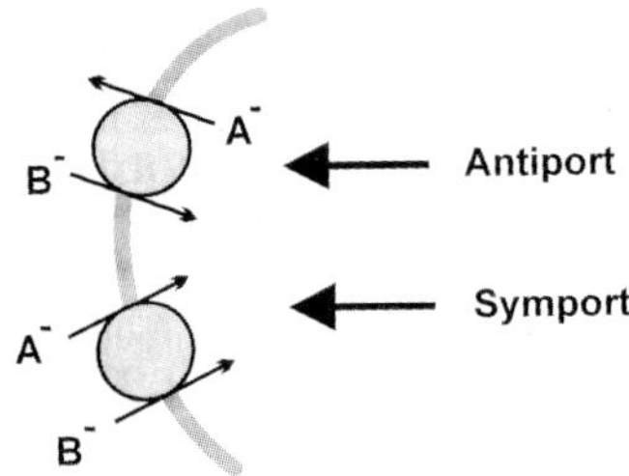

Figure 23–1. Difference in the direction of transport for antiport and symport.

TABLE 23–1. Electroneutral and Electrogenic Processes

Electroneutral Processes	*Electrogenic Processes*
1. Na^+/H^+ antiport	1. Na^+-HCO_3^- symport
2. Na^+-coupled Cl^-/HCO_3^- antiport	2. Proton translocating ATPase
3. Na^+-independent Cl^-/HCO_3^- antiport	
4. H^+/K^+ ATPase	
5. H^+/lactate$^-$ symport	

Abbreviations: ATPase = adenosine triphosphatase; Na^+ = sodium ion; H^+ = hydrogen ion; Cl^- = chlorine ion; HCO_3^- = bicarbonate ion; K^+ = potassium ion.

Mechanisms of Transmembrane Acid and Base Transport

Charged molecules like H^+, hydroxide ion, and HCO_3^- cannot readily cross lipid membranes. To be transported across the cell membrane, they need specific carrier proteins (Table 23–1). Apart from the primary active processes H^+/K^+-ATPase in gastric parietal cells and H^+-translocating ATPase (which directly uses ATP), all the other processes are secondary active (i.e., dependent on the ion gradients [provided by the NA^+/K^+-ATPase] to carry out their transport of acid and base equivalents).

Figure 23–2 depicts the different mechanisms for regulation of pH_i. Mechanisms for elevation of pH_i are found on the left side, whereas mechanisms that decrease pH_i are on the right. As is evident from the figure, electrolyte transport is an integrated part of pH regulation. Consequently, these mechanisms regulate not only pH_i but also intracellular ion concentrations, cell volume, and transcellular transport of electrolytes. Thus, the cells use a small set of transmembrane transport mechanisms to carry out several different tasks. Needless to say, these mechanisms must be precisely regulated for this to occur in a controlled manner.

Na^+/H^+ ANTIPORT. This system catalyzes the entry of extracellular Na^+ in exchange for intracellular H^+, eliciting a rise in pH_i (Fig. 23–3). The exchange process is secondary active driven by the chemical gradients of Na^+ and H^+ and is therefore dependent on the operation of the $Na^+/K^+/$ ATPase.

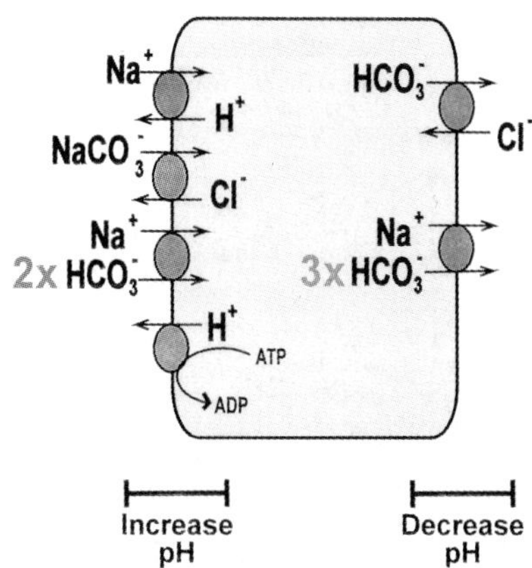

Figure 23–2. The most common mechanisms for transmembrane transport of acid and base.

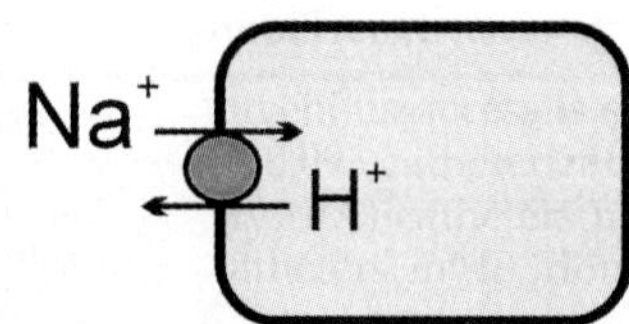

Figure 23–3. The Na^+/H^+ antiport.

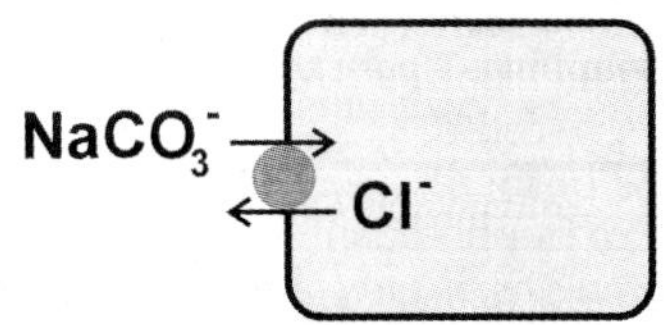

Figure 23–5. Na^+-Coupled Cl^-/HCO_3^- antiport.

The Na^+/H^+ antiport has an internal "pH sensor" (i.e., the activity of the antiport is regulated by the intracellular pH).[1] Thus, the antiport is activated by decreasing pH_i (Fig. 23–4).[2] Cells with steeply regulated antiports (with so-called high Hill coefficient) are thus very sensitive to relatively small changes in pH_i.[3]

The pH sensor on the cytosolic side of the antiport is also important to shut off the activity of the antiport at normal pH_i. This protects the cell from undue alkalinization. Because of the $Na^+_{outside}/Na^+_{inside}$ ratio of greater than 10, pH_i would become greater than 8.0 if the Na^+/H^+ antiport was active at a pH_i higher than the resting pH_i.[4]

The extracellular pH (pH_o) may also greatly influence the transport activity of the antiport. In most cells, extracellular protons may severely reduce the rate of Na^+/H^+ exchange, indicating that this antiport also has an external pH sensor.[5] Thus, when the cells produce acids that acidify the cytosol and the extracellular milieu is neutral because of an effective perfusion, the removal of H^+ from the cell is very effective. If, in contrast, perfusion is marginal, reducing the removal of extracellular acid, the transport of acid via the Na^+/H^+ antiport is markedly inhibited. Also a systemic low pH will decrease the effectiveness of Na^+/H^+ antiport in cells throughout the body, and correction of extracellular pH, which can be achieved clinically, is therefore important for pH_i.

Na^+/H^+ antiport has been detected in the plasma membrane of almost all cells studied.[2, 4] The dynamics of this antiport in different cells vary strongly, and a 30-fold difference in its activity between various cells has been found.[6]

It is beyond doubt that Na^+/H^+ exchange is of major importance in the normalization of pH_i after extensive acidification of the cytosol. Evidence indicates that this antiport in various cells does not contribute to the maintenance of steady-state cytosolic pH at neutral pH_o.[7] In other cell types, however, the Na^+/H^+ antiport is active at a more alkaline pH, and the antiport appears to be important for the maintenance of steady-state pH_i.

Na^+-COUPLED Cl^-/HCO_3^- ANTIPORT. The Na^+-coupled chlorine ion/HCO_3^- antiport most likely exchanges extracellular $NaCO_3^-$ with intracellular Cl^- (Fig. 23–5). $NaCO_3^-$ is formed by one Na^+ and two bicarbonate molecules. This antiport transports two base equivalents for every Na^+ (i.e., $CO_3^- + 2H^+ \leftrightarrow H_2CO_3 \leftrightarrow CO_2$ + water [H_2O]) and thus neutralizes two protons.

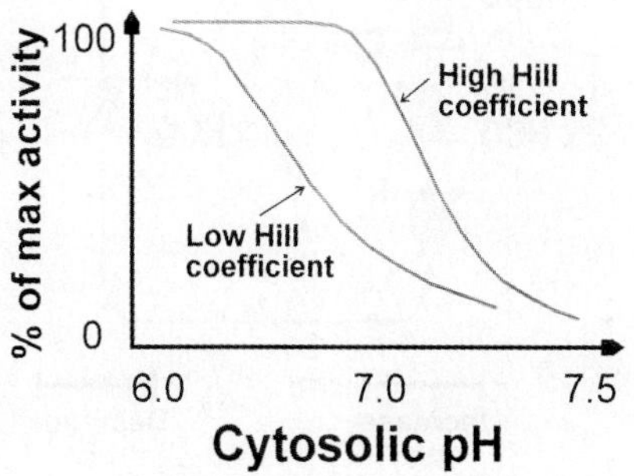

Figure 23–4. Activity of Na^+/H^+ antiport as a function of cytosolic pH.

The role of the Na^+-coupled Cl^-/HCO_3^- antiport in the regulation of pH_i varies between cells. Unlike the Na^+/H^+ antiport, it does not appear to be an omnipresent transport mechanism, although it is found in many of the cells in which pH_i regulation has been studied in the presence of HCO_3^-.[6, 8]

Like the Na^+/H^+ antiport, the activity of the Na^+-coupled Cl^-/HCO_3^- antiport increases as pH_i is decreased, suggesting a cytosolic pH_i-sensitive site on the transport protein.[7–10] Also pH_o appears to regulate the activity of the antiport. Some studies showed a marked inhibition of its activity when pH_o was decreased.[11] In some cells studied, the system is quiescent around neutral pH_i and is activated only when pH_i is lowered.[12] This contrasts with findings in other cells in which the antiport is active also at higher pH_i values. Moreover, in some cells, the antiport appears to be constitutively active (i.e., not fully down-regulated even at high pH_i).[7] The activity of the Na^+-coupled Cl^-/HCO_3^- antiport is often higher than Na^+/H^+ antiport at pH_i near neutrality but not at lower pH_i values.[7] Thus, in many cells, it is the most important mechanism to keep pH_i at a physiologic level.

Na^+/HCO_3^- SYMPORT. This mechanism transports Na^+ and HCO_3^- unidirectionally apparently without exchange of other ions. The transport is electrogenic because of transport of more than one HCO_3^- per Na^+. The Na^+ and HCO_3^- gradient will direct transport of these ions into the cells if the interior is acidic compared with the extracellular space (Fig. 23–6). Thus, under such conditions, this symport will function as an alkalinizing mechanism.[13]

A similar symport has been identified in the basolateral (serosal) membrane of proximal tubular cells in the kidneys, and its function appears to be the main mechanism for HCO_3^- exit across the basolateral membrane in this nephron segment and probably also in the thick ascending loop of Henle (see Fig. 23–6).[14] A coupling ratio of HCO_3^- to Na^+ of 3:1 is sufficient to transport HCO_3^- outward. The transport is energized by the negative membrane potential and the outward gradient of HCO_3^-, thus overcoming the opposing inward gradient for Na^+.

HYDROGEN ION/LACTATE SYMPORT. Lactic acid is noncharged and will therefore to some extent penetrate membranes by nonionic diffusion. The need for a specific transporter for lactic acid is therefore not obvious. Yet, in cardiac muscle cells, skeletal muscle cells, and the placenta, an H^+/

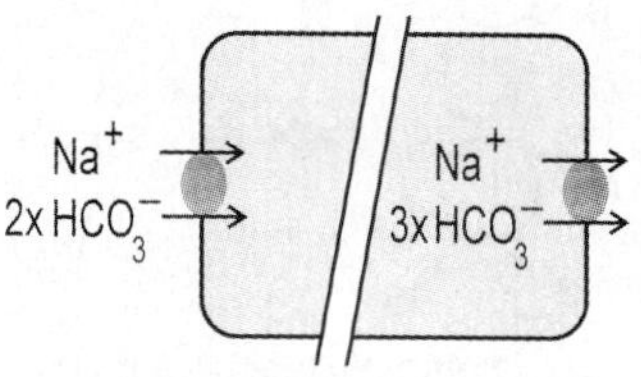

Figure 23–6. The two types of Na^+/HCO_3^- symport.

lactate symport has been identified.[15] These cells produce large amounts of lactic acid, which needs to be transported rapidly out of the cells. The H^+/lactate$^-$ symport is extremely effective in increasing pH_i in these cells during a lactic acid load. It is several times more effective than the Na^+/H^+ antiport, which is also found in these cells. The driving force for export of lactate from the cells is the concentration gradient. Thus, accumulation of lactic acid extracellularly caused by insufficient blood flow to transport lactic acid away will severely decrease the ability of the cells to counteract intracellular acidification.

PROTON TRANSLOCATING ADENOSINE TRIPHOSPHATASES. These "proton pumps" use ATP directly as an energy source to pump protons either into intracellular vesicles (endosomes, lysosomes) (so-called V-type ATPase) or across the plasma membrane (P-type ATPase). These processes will increase the cytosolic pH by pumping protons out of the cells or into these vesicles (Fig. 23–7). Subsequently, many of the vesicles fuse with the plasma membrane by exocytosis and the protons are expelled. It may appear illogical to hydrolyze ATP to get rid of protons inasmuch as hydrolysis of one ATP molecule liberates approximately 0.8 H^+ equivalents into the cytoplasm. However, for the proton ATPases studied, the stoichiometry is two or three H^+ transported per ATP molecule hydrolyzed,[16] making it a cost-effective process. Because the transport of H^+ is electrogenic, it is accompanied by transport of Cl^- through a separate channel to preserve electroneutrality.

Plasma membrane proton pumps have been identified in mammalian renal cells, pancreatic and biliary duct cells, human macrophages and neutrophils, type II pneumocytes, and osteoclasts. In many other cells studied, no evidence for plasma membrane H^+ pumps has been found.

The proton pump possessed by type II pneumocytes and alveolar epithelial cells might explain the low pH in epithelial lining fluid. Osteoclasts secrete protons by this mechanism to produce an acidic environment that resorbs bone.

Na^+-*INDEPENDENT* Cl^-/HCO_3^- ANTIPORT. Under physiologic conditions, the Na^+-independent Cl^-/HCO_3^- antiport exchanges external Cl^- for internal HCO_3^-. This elicits a decrease in pH_i (Fig. 23–8). Thus, this antiport decreases pH_i by extruding base (HCO_3^-), which in turn elevates pH_o. This increase in pH_o may be important in the regulation of extracellular acidosis (see discussion of metabolic acidosis). Also, the regulation of cytosolic Cl^- and cell volume appears to be markedly influenced by the activity of the Na^+-independent Cl^-/HCO_3^- antiport. Furthermore, the antiport is of great importance for the transcellular transport of Cl^- and HCO_3^- in epithelial cells.

This transport system has been most extensively studied in erythrocytes in which the Cl^-/HCO_3^- exchange (often called the Hamburger shift) is mediated by the so-called band 3, one of the most abundant proteins in the red cell membrane. Subsequently, similar anion exchangers have been found in a number of nucleated cells,[6–9, 17–19] and they appear to be nearly ubiquitous proteins in the plasma membrane. Thus, in a study of more than 20 different cell lines,

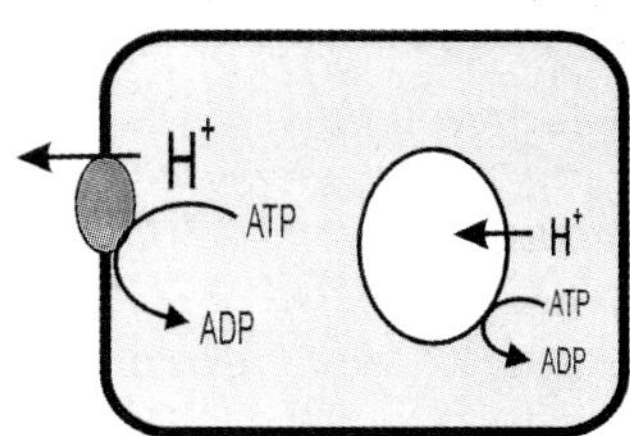

Figure 23–7. H^+-Translocating ATPases.

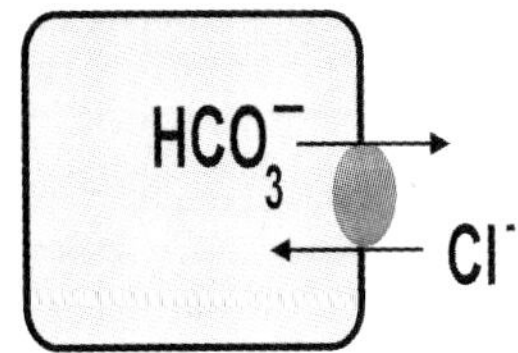

Figure 23–8. Na^+-*In*dependent Cl^-/HCO_3^- antiport.

a Na^+-independent Cl^-/HCO_3^- antiport was found in all but one.[6]

An important property of the Na^+-independent Cl^-/HCO_3^- antiport is its ability to respond to alterations in cytosolic pH (Fig. 23–9).[17] Thus, at higher pH_i, the activity of the antiport increases. The pH_i dependence is present in most cells, although in some cell lines it is presumably absent.[6] The antiport seems to have an internal pH sensor that is sensitive to small alterations in proton/base concentrations, allowing a precise regulation of pH_i by the Na^+-independent Cl^-/HCO_3^- antiport. The pH_i value for transition from low to high activity is different in different cells,[6, 17, 18] and it is regulated by both physiologic ligands and drugs.[9, 20, 21]

Equally as important as the activation of the Na^+-independent Cl^-/HCO_3^- antiport at high pH_i is its deactivation at lower pH_i values. If its activity was not severely decreased at pH_i less than 7.1, it would acidify the cytosol to nonphysiologic values.[19] Thus, the regulation of the antiport to a low-activity state prevents an acidification that would otherwise occur if the antiport continued to work at a high rate.

Physiologic Control of pH_i-Regulating Mechanisms

In recent years, a large number of reports have appeared on the regulation of the activity of ion transport mechanisms by growth factors, hormones, and other physiologic ligands and several drugs. It is beyond the scope of this chapter to discuss in detail different receptors and second-messenger mechanisms involved in these regulations. However, it is noteworthy that all known second-messenger systems have been found to participate. More than one system may take part in the same cell.

The common short-term effect of physiologic ligands is a modification of the pH_i dependence of involved antiports. Thus, most factors activating the Na^+/H^+ antiport or the Na^+-coupled Cl^-/HCO_3^- antiport shift the pH_i value for activation to a more alkaline level (for review see Grinstein et al.[4]) (Fig. 23–10). This means that, at physiologic pH_i, the antiports become active, eliciting a rise in pH_i. Activation of the Na^+-independent Cl^-/HCO_3^- antiport makes it active at a pH_i value lower than normal (Fig. 23–11). This tends to

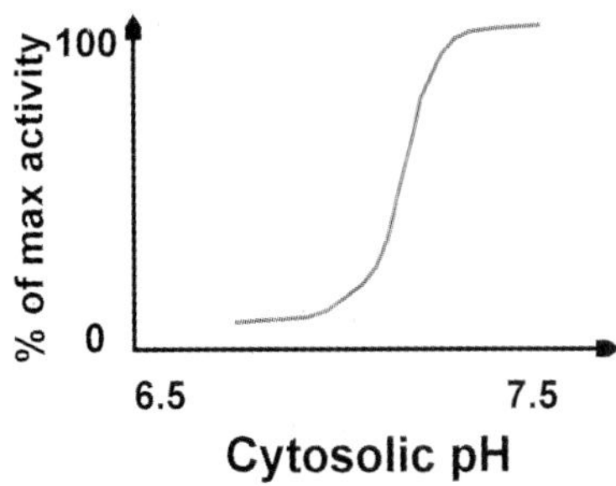

Figure 23–9. Activity of antiport as a function of cytosolic pH.

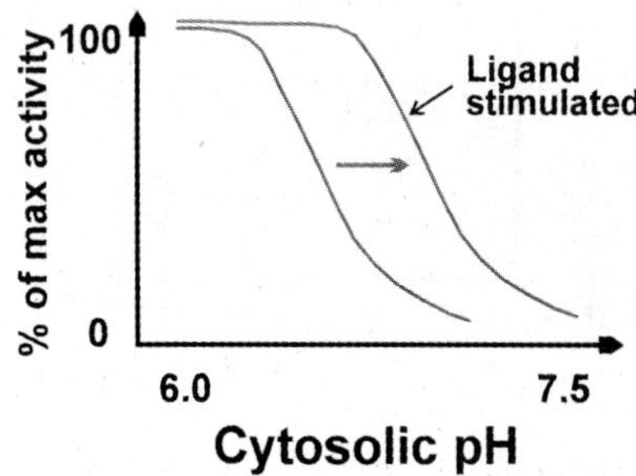

Figure 23–10. Modification of the activity of Na^+/H^+ antiport by ligands.

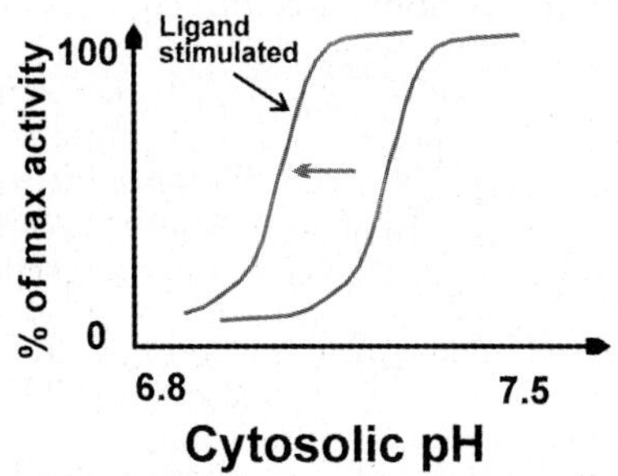

Figure 23–11. Modification of the activity of Na^+-*in*dependent Cl^-/HCO_3^- antiport by ligands.

decrease the pH_i. Thus, depending on which antiport is stimulated, stimulation by a ligand may either increase or decrease pH_i. In many cases, more than one antiport is stimulated by the same ligand. Vasopressin, for instance, was found to stimulate the Na^+/H^+ antiport, the Na^+-coupled Cl^-/HCO_3^- antiport, and the Na^+-independent Cl^-/HCO_3^- antiport in mesangial cells.[9] The resting pH_i did not change, but the cells were more able to withstand acid and base challenges. There are literally hundreds of articles describing different effects of physiologic ligands and drugs on these antiports. A few of these effects are listed in Table 23–2.

Several pathologic conditions and numerous ligands appear to alter the activity of antiports on a long-term basis (i.e., several hours to days). In many cases, the activation of the Na^+/H^+ antiport appears not to be a modification of its pH_i sensitivity but rather an alteration in the maximal transport velocity (V_{max}).[22]

Drug Effects on pH_i-Regulating Mechanisms

The diuretic drug amiloride will, at concentrations obtained in vivo, inhibit Na^+-conducting channels in kidney cells. In higher concentration, however, it is a strong inhibitor of the Na^+/H^+ antiport. It is being used extensively as a research tool to inhibit the Na^+/H^+ antiport in cell experiments. Newer derivatives of amiloride have a more specific inhibitory effect on the Na^+/H^+ antiport without interfering with the Na^+ conducting channel and may be used in vivo to inhibit the Na^+/H^+ antiport.

Diuretic drugs like bumetanide and furosemide exert their action by inhibiting the $Na^+/K^+/2\ Cl^-$ symport in the ascending part of Henle's loop. In higher concentration, they also inhibit the Na^+-independent Cl^-/HCO_3^- antiport, but it is unknown whether this has a clinical consequence. Drugs for relatively specific inhibition of Cl^-/HCO_3^- antiports are also available (DIDS, SITS).

Nonsteroidal anti-inflammatory drugs (NSAIDs) have strong effects on the Na^+-coupled Cl^-/HCO_3^- antiport and the Na^+-independent Cl^-/HCO_3^- antiport. At presumably pharmacologic concentrations, the drugs stimulate the activity of the Na^+-independent Cl^-/HCO_3^- antiport, whereas the Na^+-coupled Cl^-/HCO_3^- antiport is inhibited in several cell lines.[20] The net effect of this is a decrease in pH_i. At higher concentrations, which are found in the gastrointestinal tract after oral intake and systemically in cases of overdoses, the drugs inhibit both Cl^-/HCO_3^- antiports by competitive inhibition probably through interaction with the transport site for the anions.[21] This may be part of the local erosive effect of these drugs, as discussed later in this chapter, and may also be related to acid-base disturbances in case of salicylic acid intoxication. Also, drugs like catecholamines, dopamine, vasopressin, and so on will modify the action of these mechanisms (see Table 23–2).

TABLE 23–2. Effects of Physiologic Ligands and Drugs on Antiports

Compound	*Na^+/H^+ Antiport*	*Na^+-Coupled Cl^-/HCO_3^- Antiport*	*Na^+-Independent Cl^-/HCO_3^- Antiport*
Epinephrine	↑		
Isoproterenol			↑
Vasopressin	↑		↑
Angiotensin II	↑		
Dopamine	↓		↓
Serotonin	↑		↑
Endothelin	↑		
Interleukin-1, 2, 3	↑		
Interferon	↑		
Prolactin	↑		
Parathyroid hormone	↓		
Thyroid hormone	↑		
NSAIDs	↓	↓	↑
Pathway			
cAMP	↓ ↑	↑	↑ ↓
Ca^{2+}	↑		
Protein kinase C	↑		↑ ↓

Abbreviations: NSAIDs = nonsteroidal anti-inflammatory drugs; cAMP = cyclic adenosine monophosphate; Ca^{2+} = calcium ion.

Cooperation Between pH_i-Regulating Mechanisms

All cells possess more than one pH_i-regulating mechanism. pH_i will, therefore, be determined by the relative activity of these mechanisms.[7] Figure 23–12 shows the quantitatively most important mechanisms. Each cell type differs, and no known cell possesses all the depicted mechanisms.

The Na^+/H^+ antiport is present in all cells. In many cell types, it is the main pH-regulating antiport to increase pH_i after an acid load, whereas in other cell types the bicarbonate-dependent antiports are the most important. Thus, in certain cells, the Na^+/H^+ antiport is decisive for steady-state pH, whereas in other cells its activity is not required to keep pH_i normal under resting conditions but only to normalize pH_i after an acid load.

There are two bicarbonate-dependent mechanisms that are able to increase pH_i: namely, the Na^+-coupled Cl^-/HCO_3^- antiport and Na^+/HCO_3^- symport. These two mechanisms appear to be mutually exclusive because they have not been found to appear in the same cell. One or the other of these mechanisms is present in the majority of cells, although in a number of cells examined neither of them is found. The Na^+-coupled Cl^-/HCO_3^- antiport seems to consist of $NaCO_3^-$ exchanged with Cl^-. This mechanism carries one Na^+ and two bicarbonate equivalents into the cells. The carbonate may bind two protons and thereby increase the pH_i in an efficient way with less osmotic load on the cell (i.e., less Na^+ influx per buffering equivalent) than the Na^+/H^+ antiport. The Na^+/HCO_3^- symport will increase pH_i in certain cells when pH_i is lower than pH_o (as mentioned previously, in kidney cells a basolateral Na^+/HCO_3^- symport is the major mechanism for extrusion of HCO_3^- and carries a stoichiometry of 1 Na^+:3 HCO_3^-). All these mechanisms increase their activity as pH_i is lowered and will increase pH_i. However, at low extracellular pH, the effectiveness of these mechanisms is decreased to a different extent in different organs, underlining the necessity of regulating pH_o in clinical situations to increase pH_i. This does not imply that pH_i is merely a passive consequence of pH_o because these mechanisms still have a certain activity even at low pH_o.

Certain cells like macrophages, neutrophils, kidney cells, and pneumocytes, among others, have a proton pump (H^+ translocating ATPase) that extrudes H^+. These cells also possess a Na^+/H^+ antiport and in many cases also a Na^+-coupled Cl^-/HCO_3^- antiport. Why do they need two or three mechanisms to fight acidosis? The reason appears to be that, because Na^+/H^+ antiport and Na^+-coupled Cl^-/HCO_3^- antiport decrease their activity severely at low extracellular pH (even if they are stimulated by low pH_i), these mechanisms do not suffice under extremes of acidity, whereas the proton pumps maintain a high activity even in very acidic environments by overcoming an enormous transmembrane gradient of protons (1:1000, approximately pH_o 4.5). Thus, macrophages and neutrophils in the acidic milieu in an abscess are probably dependent on a proton pump to function satisfactorily.

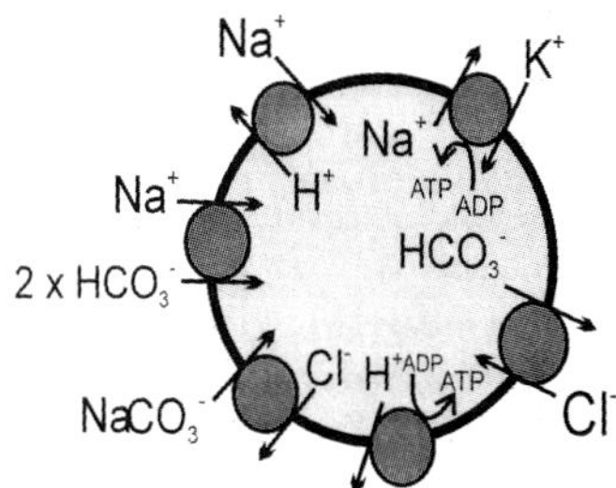

Figure 23–12. Cooperation between the most common mechanisms for regulation of cytosolic pH.

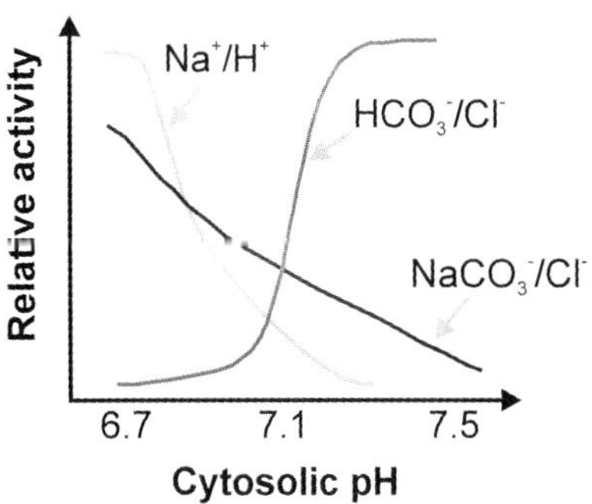

Figure 23–13. Relative activity of different antiports as a function of cytosolic pH.

These mechanisms just mentioned will all increase pH_i. When a critical pH_i level is reached, the Na^+-independent Cl^-/HCO_3^- antiport is activated. At pH_i above neutrality, intracellular HCO_3^- is exchanged for extracellular Cl^-. As a result, the pH_i is reduced. A prerequisite for this to occur in a controlled manner is the striking pH_i dependence for the activation of this antiport. Thus, in most cells, the antiport is idle at pH_i below 7.1 and is then sharply activated at pH 7.2 to 7.4. It should be noted, however, that this transition value is different in various cells and is also dependent on the activation of the cells by various physiologic ligands.

Figure 23–13 shows an example of the activity of the Na^+/H^+ antiport, the Na^+-coupled Cl^-/HCO_3^- antiport, and the Na^+-independent Cl^-/HCO_3^- antiport at different pH values, demonstrating how these mechanisms vary in significance depending on the acid load of the cell. Also, the activity of these mechanisms is significantly changed by many growth factors, other physiologic ligands, and certain drugs (see Table 23–2). Thus, pH_i (or at least the ability to withstand an acid or base load) varies with the activity state of the cell.

To elucidate the effect of bicarbonate-dependent mechanisms on intracellular pH, experiments in vitro can be carried out in the presence or absence of HCO_3^-. From these experiments, the following can be concluded:

1. The intracellular buffering power is approximately doubled in the presence of HCO_3^-.
2. The resting pH is in most cells higher in the presence of bicarbonate.[23] This is due to both the higher buffering power and the activity of the Na^+-coupled Cl^-/HCO_3^- antiport or Na^+/HCO_3^- symport, which will increase pH_i. In a number of cells, however, pH_i has been found to be lower in the presence of HCO_3^- because of a high activity in the Na^+-independent Cl^-/HCO_3^- antiport, which acidifies the cytosol.[7]
3. The recovery from both an acid and an alkali load is faster in the presence of bicarbonate than in its absence. This is due to buffering power plus the activity of HCO_3^--dependent mechanisms.
4. Bicarbonate is, therefore, of major importance for the regulation of intracellular pH and is readily transported across the plasma membrane by specific carrier mechanisms. Thus, it is incorrectly stated in many textbooks that HCO_3^- is not important for regulation of cytosolic pH.

Should metabolic acidosis be treated with bicarbonate? With administration of bicarbonate, an immediate increase in extracellular HCO_3^-, partial pressure of CO_2 (P_{CO_2}) (dependent on the ability of the respiratory system to ventilate), and pH is found. Because CO_2 is freely membrane permeable, an immediate intracellular acidification takes place if extracellular P_{CO_2} is increased. This acidification is very short lived because the bicarbonate treatment has increased the extracellular pH, making the conditions very favorable for a high activity of the Na^+/H^+ antiport and the Na^+-coupled Cl^-/HCO_3^- antiport. Thus, within minutes, the cytosolic pH is higher than before treatment with bicarbonate. Therefore, despite a short-lived acidification, bicarbonate treatment is effective to increase pH_i in cases of metabolic acidosis.

Role of pH_i-Regulating Mechanisms for Excretion of Acid by Respiration

A prerequisite for the functioning of the bicarbonate buffer system is the excretion of CO_2 by the lungs. Some 13,000 to 20,000 mmol of CO_2 are produced daily as the result of oxidative metabolism. This generates H^+ that must be eliminated to prevent acidosis. Because of the high intracellular content of carbonic anhydrase, CO_2 is processed much more rapidly to H^+ and HCO_3^- inside the erythrocytes than in the blood plasma. Simultaneously with CO_2 entering the cells, O_2 leaves and hemoglobin is deoxygenated. Deoxygenated hemoglobin has a higher pK than its oxygenated counterpart, which means that it can buffer more acid (Haldane effect). This provides an effective buffering of protons. Also counteracting acidification is the formation of carbaminohemoglobin from CO_2 and hemoglobin (Fig. 23–14). Hence, relatively large amounts of CO_2 can be added to the blood (1.3 mmol of CO_2/pL) without eliciting a decrease in pH of more than 0.05 pH units. The Haldane effect enables the body to double the amount of CO_2 transported.

The majority (approximately 80%) of CO_2 is transformed to HCO_3^-, which is exported from the erythrocytes into the blood plasma. Bicarbonate must be transported across the erythrocyte membrane very rapidly to ensure an effective transport of CO_2 by the blood. A Na^+-independent Cl^-/HCO_3^- antiport (band 3) is capable of handling this. The antiport protein is abundant in erythrocytes, where it constitutes about 25% to 30% of the total membrane protein[24] with about 10^6 molecules per cell.

Several lines of evidence indicate that the transport of bicarbonate across the red cell membrane is a rate-limiting step in the elimination of CO_2 by the lungs during physical exercise and in other situations of hyperdynamic circulation but not at rest. At rest, about 1.9 mmol of CO_2/min yielding 1.5 mmol of HCO_3^- are transported by the blood. The capillary passage time in the lungs is about 0.7 seconds under these conditions. This is sufficient time for Cl^-/HCO_3^- exchange to reach 99% equilibrium.[25, 26] However, on strenuous exercise, about 6 mmol of CO_2 are transported, and the capillary passage time is decreased to 0.3 seconds because of the increased cardiac output. During this short passage time, Cl^-/HCO_3^- exchange attains only 90% of equilibrium and will therefore limit the elimination of CO_2 by the lungs. Severe anemia and severe salicylate intoxication (which inhibits Cl^-/HCO_3^- exchange) might limit the elimination of CO_2 by the lungs because there is simply not enough antiport activity to carry out this increased transport.[27, 28] In the peripheral tissues, this would be rate limiting, decreasing the ability of the tissues to get rid of CO_2. There would be an increased CO_2 tension in the interstitial fluid, but the amount transported by the blood would be limited because of decreased capacity of the Cl^-/HCO_3^- antiport. An arterial blood gas would not reveal any abnormalities despite a tissue "respiratory" acidosis.

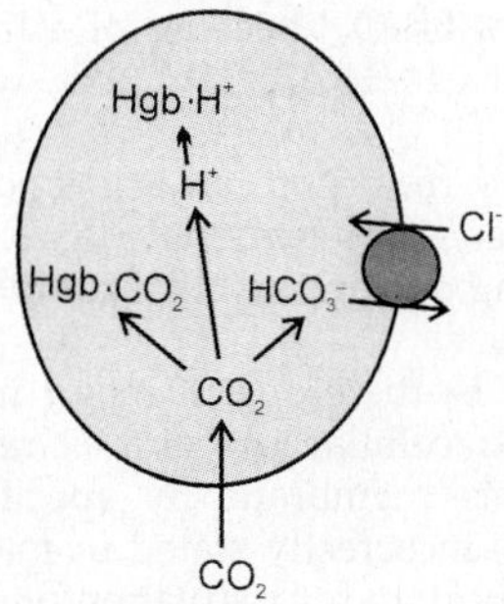

Figure 23–14. Mechanisms of CO_2 transport by red blood cells.

pH disturbances can influence the O_2-hemoglobin dissociation curve. Thus, acidosis shifts the curve to the right, increasing the unloading of O_2, whereas alkalosis has the opposite effect. Of importance is the fact that erythrocytes have a considerable ability to keep their intracellular pH near normal despite systemic alkalosis or acidosis. It is incorrect to assume that hemoglobin is surrounded by the pH value we measure in arterial blood. The effect of pH on the oxygen dissociation curve is therefore clearly less than expected.

Handling of Acid-Base Balance by Renal pH_i-Regulating Mechanisms

In addition to the production of 13,000 to 20,000 mmol of the volatile acid CO_2, there is a daily production of 40 to 200 mmol of nonvolatile acids, mainly from the metabolism of food. During muscular exercise, a substantial amount of lactic acid is also produced (up to 4500 mmol/day). This lactic acid is, to a large extent, metabolized and does not need to be excreted, whereas the other nonvolatile acids are excreted by the kidneys. From this standpoint the function of the kidneys is to excrete H^+ and absorb HCO_3^-.

Preservation of bicarbonate involves two renal processes: (1) the reabsorption of virtually all bicarbonate filtered through the glomeruli, and (2) the reclamation of bicarbonate consumed in the buffering of fixed acids in the blood. The latter process is accomplished through the excretion of equivalent amounts of protons as "titratable acid" in the urine. Approximately 4500 mmol of HCO_3^- are filtered each day, and more than 99.9% are reabsorbed. Of this, 80% to 90% are reabsorbed in the proximal tubules, approximately 5% in the loop of Henle, approximately 3% in the distal tubules, and roughly 1% to 2% in the collecting ducts.

The mechanism of reabsorption of bicarbonate appears to vary in the different nephron segments. The Na^+/H^+ antiport appears to be the major mechanism for export of H^+ across the luminal membrane in the proximal tubule, but at least in the S_3 segment of the proximal tubule and in the distal tubule a proton translocating ATPase is capable of transporting a major part of the H^+ (Fig. 23–15).[29] The exported H^+ reacts with the filtered HCO_3^- to form CO_2 and H_2O. Carbon dioxide diffuses readily across the luminal membrane to form H^+ and HCO_3^- inside the cells. The protons are again exported via the Na^+/H^+ antiport or H^+ ATPase and then reused.

The basolateral exit of bicarbonate can be mediated by a Na^+-3 HCO_3^- symport or a Na^+-independent Cl^-/HCO_3^- antiport.[14, 30] The former mechanism is dominant in the proximal tubule and appears to account for 70% to 80% of the

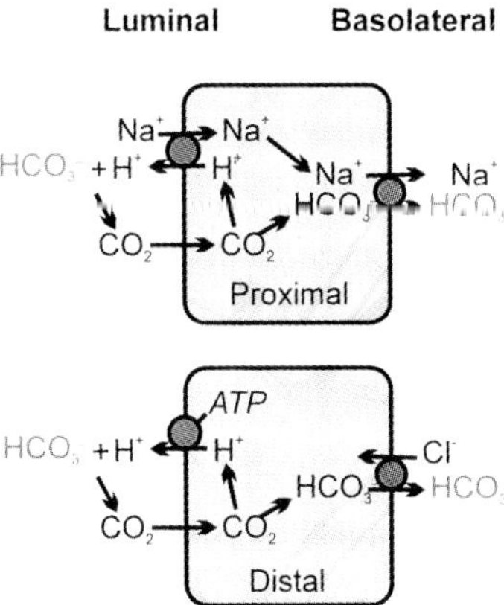

Figure 23–15. Mechanisms for the reabsorption of bicarbonate in the proximal and distal tubule.

HCO_3^- exit, whereas the latter seems to be the dominant mechanism in the more distal part of the nephron. There is a correlation between increased activity of the Na^+-HCO_3^- symport and Na^+-independent Cl^-/HCO_3^- antiport versus increased systemic acid load. The Na^+/H^+ antiport on the luminal side and the Na^+-HCO_3^- symport on the basal side are both stimulated by angiotensin II, which thereby increases bicarbonate absorption.[31] Parathyroid hormone inhibits the reabsorption and reclamation of HCO_3^-. This is achieved by inhibition of Na^+/H^+ antiport by increasing cyclic adenosine monophosphate (cAMP).[32]

It has been demonstrated that the activity of the Na^+/H^+ antiport inhibits renin release.[33] Angiotensin II has been found to stimulate the Na^+/H^+ antiport in renal tubular membranes via a phospholipase A_2-mediated mechanism.[34] Consequently, the inhibitory effect of angiotensin II on renin release appears to be mediated by stimulation of the Na^+/H^+ antiport because an amiloride analog has been demonstrated to inhibit this effect.[33] Hyperosmolarity also inhibits the secretion of renin. This effect is dependent on the Na^+-independent Cl^-/HCO_3^- antiport.

REGULATION OF CELL VOLUME AND ELECTROLYTE CONCENTRATION

The cellular volume is strictly regulated. The plasma membrane of most cells is highly permeable to water, and the cell volume is therefore determined by the content of osmotically active solutes intra- and extracellularly. The cells contain impermeable macromolecules (mainly proteins) that will induce a colloidosmotic swelling as a result of the entry of diffusible ions and water because of the Gibbs-Donnan equilibrium. This swelling is counteracted by ion extruding pumps (mainly the Na^+/K^+ ATPase) and other ion transport mechanisms.

In addition to the effort involved in maintaining a constant volume under resting conditions, many cells are challenged by anisotonic conditions under physiologic and pathophysiologic conditions. Thus, renal cells are exposed both to hyper- and hypotonic urine, blood cells traversing the kidney face areas with high osmolarity, intestinal cells are exposed to anisotonic solutions, and so on. In absorbing and secreting epithelia, the large transcellular transport of ions and water requires effective mechanisms to maintain a normal cell volume. For instance, in kidney proximal tubule cells, the transcellular transport of water each minute is four times the cell volume. In pathophysiologic conditions such as dehydration, hyperglycemic acidosis, edema, and so on, the cells are exposed to conditions that may severely change the cell volume. To counteract the shrinking or swelling in anisotonic media, cells have volume regulatory processes. Swollen cells tend to reduce their volume by loss of potassium chloride (KCl) and accompanying water (regulatory volume decrease [RVD]). Shrunken cells increase their volume by net uptake of sodium chloride (NaCl). Na^+ is then exchanged with K^+ by Na^+/K^+-ATPase, eliciting a net gain of KCl, which results in a concomitant uptake of water (regulatory volume increase [RVI]). The ability to recover the initial volume varies between different cells. Both RVD and RVI are due to activation of ion transport systems, some of which are also involved in the regulation of pH_i.

Regulatory Volume Decrease

Three transport mechanisms have been found to mediate regulatory volume decrease after swelling of the cells: (1) separate conductive K^+ and Cl^- transport pathways (Fig. 23–16); (2) an electroneutral K^+-Cl^- symport; and (3) an electroneutral functionally coupled exchange K^+/H^+ and Cl^-/HCO_3^- antiports. The first-mentioned process appears to be the main mechanism operating in human cells.

Because volume regulatory decrease is elicited in situations in which the hypotonicity is due to hyponatremia, there is often a decrease in pH_i because both the Na^+/H^+ antiport and Na^+-coupled Cl^-/HCO_3^- antiport have less favorable gradients under these conditions.[35]

Regulatory Volume Increase

The transport systems involved in increasing cell volume are as follows: (1) Na^+-K^+-2 Cl^- symport (Fig. 23–17); (2) Na^+-Cl^- symport; and (3) electroneutral Na^+/H^+ antiport functionally coupled to Cl^-/HCO_3^- antiport (Fig. 23–18). A sizable number of cells use both Na^+-K^+-2 Cl^- symport and Na^+/H^+ exchange functionally coupled to Cl^-/HCO_3^- exchange. Cells also increase their volume before cell division. Growth factor–induced stimulation of Na^+-K^+-2 Cl^- symport, Na^+/H^+ exchange, and Na^+-independent Cl^-/HCO_3^- antiport have been reported to elicit these changes.[36, 37]

REGULATION OF INTRACELLULAR ION CONCENTRATION

The regulation of ion concentration is closely related to the regulation of cell volume. The dominant intracellular cation is K^+, and its concentration appears to be mainly controlled by the activity of the Na^+-K^+-ATPase. Thus, even if the

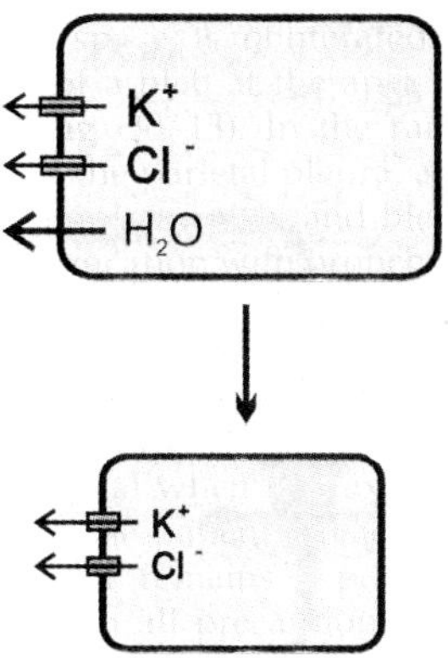

Figure 23–16. Regulatory volume decrease.

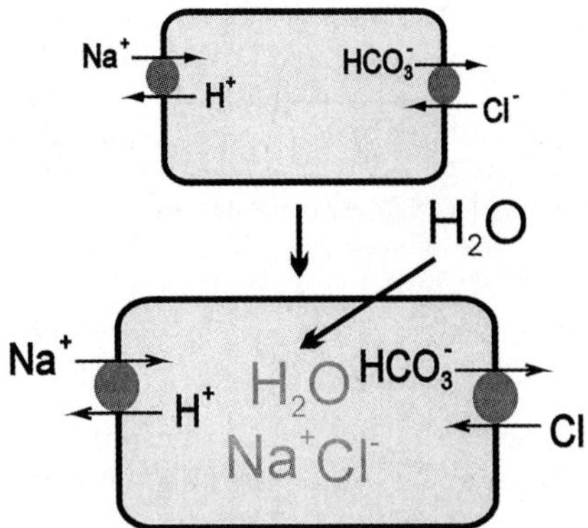

Figure 23–17. Regulatory volume increase.

concentration of Na^+ is increased by activation of Na^+/H^+ exchange, Na^+ is pumped out of the cells again in exchange with K^+. Therefore, in most if not all human cells, K^+ is the predominant intracellular cation, and its concentration does not vary much from one cell type to another.

As far as anions are concerned, the cytosolic concentration varies greatly in different cells. This fact is not well recognized because it is repeatedly stated in textbooks that the transmembrane distribution of Cl^- and therefore the cytosolic concentration of Cl^- are determined by the membrane potential. However, the concentration of $[Cl^-]_i$ varies from approximately 4 mmol in excitable cells (neurons and muscle) to more than 100 mmol in nucleated blood cells.[38] Other cell types contain intermediate concentrations of 40 to 60 mmol. Even in cells with high Cl^- concentration, the membrane potential is 30 to 60 mV. Thus, the internal Cl^- concentration is far above its electrochemical equilibrium. This is due to activity of the Na^+-K^+-2 Cl^- symport, which, because of the ion gradients, will transport considerable amounts of Cl^- into the cells.

The internal concentration of HCO_3^- is dependent on pH_i because CO_2 is highly membrane permeable. Conversely, altering the concentration of HCO_3^- will change pH_i. Because this is achieved by a Cl^-/HCO_3^- exchange, the internal Cl^- concentration is also influenced by pH.

Many cells possess Na^+-independent Cl^-/HCO_3^- antiports, Na^+-coupled Cl^-/HCO_3^- antiports, Na^+-K^+-2 Cl^- symport, and Na^+/H^+ antiports. As discussed previously, all these processes are involved in the regulation of intracellular ion concentrations. Therefore, the dynamic interaction between them will determine the concentration of cations and anions.

TRANSCELLULAR TRANSPORT

Transcellular transport is a property of polarized epithelial cells. Such cells (e.g., renal tubular cells and intestinal epithelial cells) have a different milieu at the apical (luminal) membrane compared with the basolateral (serosal) membrane and therefore transport some solutes in one direction and others in the opposite direction. To accomplish this, the types of transmembrane transport molecules (antiports, symports) have to be different on the luminal and serosal sides.

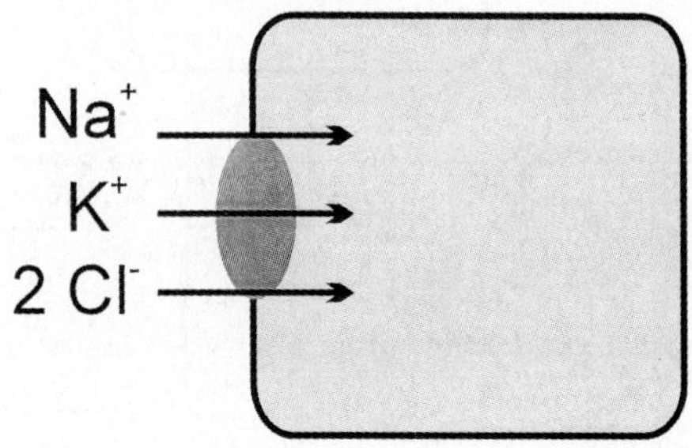

Figure 23–18. The $Na^+/K^+/2\ Cl^-$ symport.

Gastric Cells

In gastric parietal (oxyntic) cells, K^+/H^+-ATPase pumps protons out of the cells at the apical membrane into the gastric lumen in exchange for extracellular K^+ (Fig. 23–19). Protons are accompanied by Cl^-, which leaves the cells through Cl^- conductive channels. A Na^+-independent Cl^-/HCO_3^- antiport is found in the basolateral membrane. This antiport is highly pH_i-dependent as its activity increases with increasing pH_i.[39] The Na^+-independent Cl^-/HCO_3^- antiport fulfills two purposes: influx of Cl^- to substitute for the apical Cl^- efflux; and export of HCO_3^- basolaterally to decrease pH_i, which is markedly increased because of export of H^+ via the apical K^+/H^+-ATPase. Also, Na^+/K^+-ATPase and Na^+/H^+ antiports are found in the basolateral membrane. The Na^+/H^+ antiport is stimulated by secretagogues (histamine and related compounds), thus elevating pH_i to a value at which the Na^+-independent Cl^-/HCO_3^- antiport is active.[39] The mechanism of action for the antiulcer drug omeprazole is to specifically inhibit the H^+/K^+ ATPase.

In mucosal cells of the stomach and duodenum, export of HCO_3^- takes place at the apical membrane to protect the cells against the gastric acid. Bicarbonate reacts with H^+ to form water and CO_2, the latter of which escapes through the mucous barrier secreted by the mucosal cells (Fig. 23–20). By this mechanism, the pH at the luminal surface of the mucosa is near neutrality. A Na^+-independent Cl^-/HCO_3^- antiport is situated in the apical membrane and is partly responsible for the HCO_3^- secretion. In the basolateral membrane, a Na^+-dependent HCO_3^- influx takes place. This transport may occur by a Na^+-coupled Cl^-/HCO_3^- antiport, and the transcellular transport of HCO_3^- would therefore be dependent on the operation of two different Cl^-/HCO_3^- antiports. Interestingly, mucosal cells are protected against luminal acid by supplying HCO_3^- on the serosal side in accordance with the previously mentioned notion of transcellular transport of HCO_3^-. A Na^+/H^+ antiport is located in the basolateral (serosal) membrane. If pH_i decreases because of an influx of H^+ at the luminal membrane, this antiport is activated to increase pH_i. The activity of this antiport increases also by a high pH of the blood on the

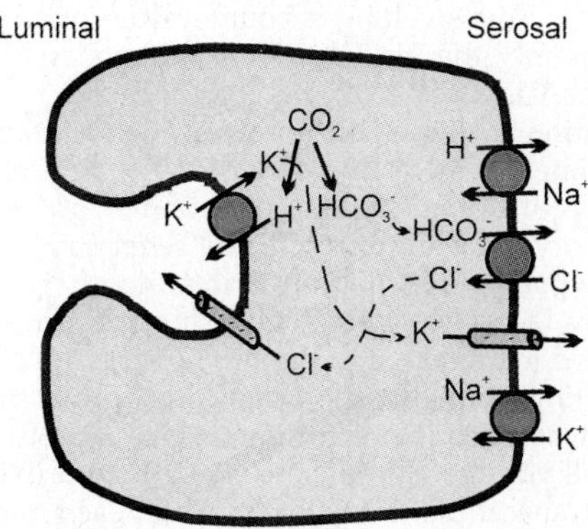

Figure 23–19. Mechanisms for transmembrane transport of electrolytes and acid and base in the parietal cell.

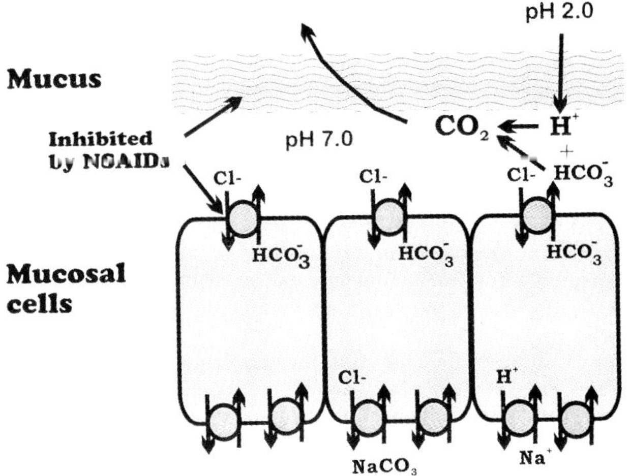

Figure 23–20. Secretion of bicarbonate by gastric mucosal cells.

serosal side. Interestingly, it has been found that a high systemic bicarbonate and pH result in a lower incidence of stress ulcers.

The NSAIDs often give rise to peptic ulcer. This is partly due to a local erosive effect and partly to a systemic effect, but the precise mechanisms of action are not established. High concentrations of NSAIDs strongly inhibited both the Na^+-coupled and the Na^+-independent Cl^-/HCO_3^- antiport.[21] This inhibition of bicarbonate transport will reduce the concentration of bicarbonate to neutralize the gastric acid at the apical surface of the cells and thereby impose an acid load on the cells. This increased acidification of cells exposed to NSAIDs may be toxic and cause peptic ulcer. Also, when the transport of bicarbonate to the external surface of the cells is reduced by NSAIDs, extracellular pH decreases and the NSAID picks up protons to be deionized. Under these conditions, the drug easily penetrates the cell membrane by nonionic diffusion, accumulates inside the cells, and may therefore be toxic to the cells.

Kidney

The transcellular transport of bicarbonate is described earlier in this chapter. In salt-absorbing tubular cells, both the Na^+/H^+ antiport and the Na^+-independent Cl^-/HCO_3^- antiport have been identified on the apical side. Evidence has been presented that a part (30–50%) of the NaCl absorption is mediated by a parallel activity of these two antiports (Fig. 23–21).[40] In this case, H^+ and HCO_3^- are transported out of the cells by these two antiports and immediately enter the cells again as CO_2, thus taking part in a catalytic cycle. Also, in other organs (intestines, gallbladder, salivary glands), such parallel exchange is an important part of the transcellular transport of salt.

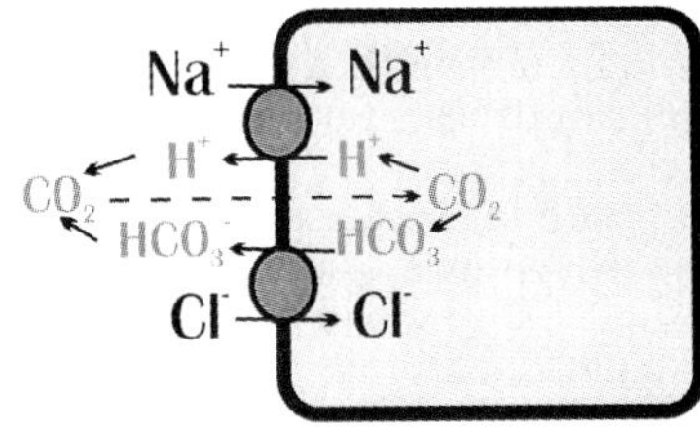

Figure 23–21. Absorption of salt in the renal tubule.

Low dietary NaCl intake increases the activity of Na^+/H^+ antiport to effectively absorb Na^+ and prevent hyponatremia. In contrast, high intake of NaCl down-regulates this antiport. Dopamine working via DA_1 receptors increases the concentration of cAMP and thereby inhibits the Na^+/H^+ antiport, leading to natriuresis. Also, atrial natriuretic peptide appears to have a similar effect.

ROLE OF pH_i-REGULATING MECHANISMS IN PATHOPHYSIOLOGIC CONDITIONS

Acid-Base Disturbances

It should be noted that the definitions of these disturbances are based on measurements of pH and CO_2 and calculation of HCO_3^- and base excess in blood plasma. This does not necessarily reflect the intracellular conditions. Also, most blood gases are measured arterially, which reflects tissue conditions to a lesser extent than venous measurements. The body is remarkably tolerant to changes in acidity. Because we use the logarithmic pH scale to measure acidity, we often forget that, at pH 7.1 compared with 7.4, the amount of free protons is doubled (Table 23–3). Imagine what would happen if the Na^+ or K^+ concentration were doubled!

Metabolic Acidosis

Metabolic acidosis is caused by several disorders. In many cases, there are nonvolatile acids, either endogenous (lactic acid, ketoacids in diabetes mellitus, and so on) or exogenous (salicylate and other intoxications), that bring about the pH disturbance. Lactic acid production under normal conditions is approximately 15 to 30 mmol/kg per day. The maximum capacity of the liver to convert this to glucose via gluconeogenesis or to CO_2 via the citric acid cycle is 3.5 mol per day. If this capacity is exceeded, a lactic acidosis will ensue. In the setting of severe liver failure, lactic acidosis will occur with normal production of lactic acid.

Under conditions of aerobic metabolism, the glycolytic pathway goes via pyruvate to Krebs' cycle and then to oxidative phosphorylation. Under anaerobic conditions, however, the reduced form of nicotinamide-adenine dinucleotide (NAD [NADH]) formed from the glycolytic pathway builds up because it is not used in Krebs' cycle. This depletes the cells of NAD^+, and the glycolytic pathway is halted. To regain NAD^+ to be able to produce ATP, lactic acid is formed according to the following reaction: Pyruvate + NADH + H^+ ↔ lactic acid + NAD^+. This anaerobic pathway generates 2 mol of H^+ per mole of glucose. Thus, a considerable amount of acid is produced. The enzyme catalyzing the formation of lactate, lactate dehydrogenase, is regulated by the pH_i such that an acidosis tends to decrease its activity, whereas an alkalosis increases it. Respiratory alkalosis decreases the elimination of lactate by decreasing its clearance by 40% and thereby increasing its half-life from approximately 15 to 45 minutes. Thus, eliciting alkalosis by treatment under these conditions may increase the lactic acid content.

TABLE 23–3. pH and H^+ Concentrations

pH	*H^+ Concentration (nmol/L)*
7.70	20
7.40	40
7.10	80
7.00	100

Abbreviation: H^+ = hydrogen ion.

It should be noted that lactate production may markedly increase also under conditions in which the cell apparently is not hypoxic. Convincing data show this to be the case in some septic models. Conversely, under anaerobic conditions, many cells do not produce large amounts of lactic acid. Thus, the link between lactate production and anaerobiosis is not straightforward.

Lactic acid and ketoacids are synthesized intracellularly and cause an increased intracellular acid load. The cytosolic buffering power (proteins, phosphate, bicarbonate) attenuates the fall in pH_i. The acids are membrane permeable in their protonated form and to some extent leave the cells by nonionic diffusion. There is, however, evidence that an H^+/lactate$^+$ symport markedly increases the transmembrane transport of protons and lactate in heart and muscle cells. Also, Na^+/H^+ antiport and probably the Na^+-coupled Cl^-/HCO_3^- antiport elevate pH_i in cases of intracellular lactic acidosis, but H^+/lactate symport appears to be the most efficient mechanism when lactic acid is effectively removed extracellularly. If extracellular lactic acid is not removed by a sufficient blood circulation, an extracellular acidosis ensues. This inhibits further removal of lactic acid from the cells, and also the Na^+/H^+ antiport and the Na^+-coupled Cl^-/HCO_3^- antiport are inhibited. Thus, in cases of systemic acidosis, the removal of lactic acid from the cells is strikingly inhibited. Also, in cases of local lactic acidosis caused by hypoperfusion, a severe intracellular acidosis develops because of the dissipation of the inside:outside gradient of lactic acid. Bicarbonate reacts with H^+ to form CO_2, which is not removed, and can give rise to intracellular P_{CO_2} greater than 300 mm Hg.

Interestingly, a disease has been detected in which the patients lack the lactate transporter in their skeletal muscle cells. After muscle exercise, lactate is therefore removed slowly from the intracellular space, and these patients experience muscle pain and fatigue.

In cases of systemic metabolic acidosis, HCO_3 in the blood and interstitial fluid buffers the acids by forming CO_2, which is eliminated by respiration. Hence, the concentration of HCO_3^- decreases considerably. This decrease in HCO_3^- strongly affects the HCO_3 gradient across the cell membrane. Bicarbonate ion therefore tends to leave the cells because of a reversed inside:outside gradient, predominantly by the Na^+-independent Cl^-/HCO_3^- antiport. This lowers pH_i and elevates pH_o. This is functionally equivalent to a net transport of H^+ into the cells. Thus, even though the cell membranes are poorly permeable to H^+ per se, an effective intracellular buffering of extracellular acidosis may be accomplished by the operation of Na^+-independent Cl^-/HCO_3^- antiport.[41] The intracellular space of the body is more than twice the extracellular space, and the intracellular buffering power per volume unit is much higher than extracellularly. Therefore, the indirect import of H^+ by exporting HCO_3^- via the Na^+-independent Cl^-/HCO_3^- antiport is probably an important defense mechanism in systemic acidosis. Thus, compensation for metabolic acidosis is not only hyperventilation and slow compensation by the kidneys but also transport of acid equivalents across the cell membranes to buffer the acid intracellularly. The Na^+/H^+ and the Na^+-coupled Cl^-/HCO_3^- antiport will counteract this increased cytosolic acid load. Because of the decreased extracellular HCO_3^- and low extracellular pH in metabolic acidosis, pH_i is not fully normalized.

Respiratory Acidosis

In cases of respiratory acidosis, P_{CO_2} is increased, resulting in a decreased pH. This acid load cannot be buffered effectively extracellularly by bicarbonate, which is usually the main buffer system. Buffering, albeit insufficient, is achieved by extracellular proteins and phosphate. Because of the high membrane permeability of CO_2, it quickly enters the cells and yields H^+ and HCO_3^-. H^+ is buffered by proteins and phosphate to some extent, but nevertheless an intracellular acidosis ensues. This activates Na^+/H^+ antiport and, depending on the cell type, also Na^+-coupled Cl^-/HCO_3^- antiport. Thus, pH_i will increase but attain a lower value than in situations of lower P_{CO_2} tension. This means that a part of the protons formed by the increased P_{CO_2} are quickly buffered intracellularly. Because the extracellular buffering is slight and H^+ is exported out of the cells by Na^+/H^+ antiport and HCO_3^- is imported into the cells via the Na^+-coupled Cl^-/HCO_3^- antiport, the extracellular pH is not effectively normalized. Thus, the decrease in pH_o is more pronounced than the fall in pH_i.

Slower defense mechanisms against respiratory acidosis than those discussed previously are the elimination of acids and the reabsorption of HCO_3^- by the kidneys. Particularly important in this context is that long-standing acidosis itself may interfere with the response of pH_i-regulating mechanisms. Thus, the Na^+-H^+ antiport, the Na^+-HCO_3^- symport, and the Na^+-independent Cl^-/HCO_3^- antiport, which all are important for reabsorption of HCO_3^- by the kidneys, increase their maximal velocity in response to the increased acid load, enabling them to eliminate acid and absorb HCO_3^- more efficiently. The mechanisms involved in this regulation are not well characterized, but at least in the case of the Na^+-independent Cl^-/HCO_3^- antiport, an increased synthesis of antiports is involved.

Metabolic Alkalosis

Metabolic alkalosis is clinically separated into chloride-responsive and chloride-unresponsive types. The former is due to excess loss of chloride (vomiting, nasogastric suctioning, diuretic therapy), whereas the latter may be due to excess alkali load or excess mineralocorticoid effect. The chloride-responsive type illustrates the close coupling between $[Cl^-]$ and $[HCO_3^-]$.

The generation of metabolic alkalosis in cases of Cl^- loss from the stomach may be partly explained by the action of the Na^+-independent Cl^-/HCO_3^- antiport in the parietal cells. In short, for the parietal cells to secrete large amounts of HCl, Cl^- must be imported across the basolateral membrane, and the HCO_3^-, which is generated when H^+ is formed, must be exported across the basolateral membrane. This is accomplished by a pH_i-regulated Na^+-independent Cl^-/HCO_3^- antiport (see Fig. 23–19). For each H^+ and Cl^- lost by vomiting or nasogastric suction, one HCO_3^- is exported from the parietal cell and elicits an alkalosis. Usually the kidneys are able to excrete HCO_3^- rapidly, but in case of dehydration, which often occurs as a result of the gastrointestinal fluid loss, the kidneys reabsorb almost all Na^+ and water to compensate for the fluid loss. An anion must accompany the reabsorption of Na^+. Because $[Cl^-]$ is low, bicarbonate instead is reabsorbed and the alkalosis persists. Some of the reabsorbed Na^+ is electrically balanced by the excretion of H^+ or K^+. Because H^+ is reduced in metabolic alkalosis, K^+ is excreted. This induces a hypokalemia, which is often found in metabolic alkalosis.

The cells will compensate for an intracellular alkalosis by exporting HCO_3^- in exchange for Cl^- via the Na^+-independent Cl^-/HCO_3^- antiport. This antiport is activated at alkaline pH and is driven by the anion gradients. Thus, if the inwardly directed Cl^- gradient is greater than the HCO_3^- gradient, pH_i will decrease. With increasing systemic alkalosis, the gradient for HCO_3^- and Cl^- will be more unfavorable and the regulation of pH_i less effective. Thus, the intracellular compartment will buffer an extracellular alkalosis. Because of a higher buffering capacity intracellularly than extracellularly, pH_i will remain lower than pH_o.

Respiratory Alkalosis

Because of the high membrane permeability for CO_2, the cytosolic pH is rapidly elevated in respiratory alkalosis. The cells will to some extent counteract this by activating the Na^+-independent Cl^-/HCO_3^- antiport as outlined previously. Because of the higher buffering power inside the cells, the intracellular pH deviation is less than the extracellular change.

In chronic respiratory alkalosis, the $[HCO_3^-]$ will be lowered because of the increased excretion of bicarbonate by the kidneys. The Na^+-HCO_3^- symport, which is one of the main mechanisms to reabsorb HCO_3^- in the proximal tubule, has a decreased transport capacity in cases of chronic alkalosis.

Cardiovascular Function

Effect of pH on Cardiac Function

Studies carried out on the effect of acidification on muscle contractility have shown that a relatively small acidification of heart muscle (approximately 0.2 pH units) has a severe negative inotropic effect, reducing the contractility by 40% to 50%. This is due to a decreased sensitivity of troponin C for Ca^{2+}, to interference of H^+ with cross linking of actin and myosin, and possibly to inhibition of Na^+/Ca^{2+} exchange in the plasma membrane.[42] These studies were done in isolated hearts or myocardial cells (i.e., devoid of sympathetic innervation). In vivo the activation of the sympathetic nervous system by acidosis will compensate for the direct negative inotropic effect of the acid and the cardiovascular effect of a moderate acidosis is minor in normal hearts. This is accomplished by the inotropic effect of the sympathetic transmitters, but also stimulation of the Na^+/H^+ antiport via an alpha receptor plays a role.[42] However, even relatively mild acidosis (pH 7.25) has been found to decrease the stimulatory effect of norepinephrine,[43] and at pH_o 7.00 virtually no stimulatory effect of epinephrine is found. Beta blockers decrease the activity of the Na^+/H^+ antiport. The negative inotropic effect of Ca^{2+} channel blockers is markedly increased by acidosis. In situations in which the sympathetic nervous system is activated to keep the cardiac output sufficient when pH is normal (i.e., congestive heart failure), an acidosis might severely decrease cardiac function. Thus, the arbitrary pH value of 7.2, which is often cited in textbooks as a cutoff value to start treating an acidosis, might be satisfactory for a patient with a normal heart but devastating for a patient with cardiac failure. Furthermore, with low pH, the effect of catecholamines is more tachycardia and peripheral vasoconstriction than increased inotropy. This can jeopardize myocardial oxygenation and increase intramyocardial acidosis. Therefore, the decision for treatment should be based on the cardiovascular parameters of the patient in question and not on a fixed pH value.

During rapid contractions of the heart, lactic acid accumulates. The lactic acid is transported out from the cardiac muscle fibers to a large extent by the H^+/lactate symport. To transport lactic acid out of the cells effectively, the extracellular acid must be rapidly removed by perfusion in diastole. In cases of cardiac ischemia caused by hypoperfusion, lactic acid rapidly accumulates intracellularly and causes a myocardial acidosis (see section on ischemia).

Apart from the lactic acid transporter, the Na^+/H^+ antiport appears to provide the main mechanism for export of protons from cardiac cells. The Na^+/H^+ antiport is regulated by the Ca^{2+}/calmodulin system, ATP, and alpha and probably beta receptors. There is little evidence for the existence of a Na^+-coupled Cl^-/HCO_3^- antiport in adult hearts, but it is found to be important for pH_i regulation in infant hearts.[44] The Na^+-independent Cl^-/HCO_3^- antiport appears to be the main mechanism to extrude base. Recently, evidence has been presented that this antiport is highly pH_i-sensitive and increases its activity with increasing pH_i in a manner similar to other cells. In accordance with this at pH_o of 7.4, pH_i is lower in the presence of bicarbonate than in its absence in vitro. However, the presence of HCO_3^- strongly increases the intracellular buffering power, enabling the cells to resist acid load better.[45]

Vascular Function

In vascular smooth-muscle cells, a Na^+/H^+ antiport, a Na^+-coupled Cl^-/HCO_3^- antiport (or possibly an Na^+-HCO_3^- symport in some preparations), and a Na^+-independent Cl^-/HCO_3^- antiport have been found to participate in pH_i regulation. In several studies, the bicarbonate-dependent mechanisms appear to be quantitatively more important than Na^+/H^+ antiport. Thus, in the presence of bicarbonate, pH_i was found to be higher than in its absence.[46]

Also in vascular smooth muscle, there seems to be a link between contractility and pH_i. Vascular smooth muscle is regulated by several ligands with vasoconstrictory or vasodilatory effects. Many of the vasoconstrictor agents (norepinephrine, epinephrine, serotonin, endothelin, vasopressin, and others) stimulate the Na^+/H^+ antiport and increase pH_i in the absence of HCO_3^-. In the presence of physiologic concentrations of bicarbonate, no changes in pH_i by these ligands were found, ruling out the proposed second-messenger role of pH_i. The reason for the lack of change in pH_i despite the activation of the Na^+/H^+ antiport is that at least serotonin and vasopressin also activate the Na^+-independent Cl^-/HCO_3^- antiport, which counteracts the alkalinization. Also the Na^+-coupled Cl^-/HCO_3^- antiport is stimulated by vasopressin. The result of these actions is that the cells are more able to withstand acid or base loads. Despite this, significant acidosis or alkalosis might interfere with the actions of these physiologic ligands. Thus, alkalosis (pH 7.6) can increase the vasoconstrictory action of norepinephrine, serotonin, and prostaglandin $F_{2\alpha}$. Conversely, acidosis inhibits their action, particularly the effect of norepinephrine. Consequently, the most common effect of in vivo acidosis is dilation of vessels in the systemic circulation, whereas alkalosis is associated with vasoconstriction. It is, however, important to realize that these effects are dependent on the ligands present. The reactivity of pulmonary vessels to acidosis might be vasoconstriction. Thus, acidosis may give rise to pulmonary hypertension. This is particularly evident in the newborn in whom acidosis that elicits pulmonary hypertension can convert the circulatory system to a fetal pattern (persistent fetal circulation). There are, however, contradictory findings in the literature concerning the effect of pH disturbances on the reactivity of pulmonary vessels. Interestingly, alkalosis was found to inhibit hypoxic vasoconstriction of pulmonary vessels by stimulating the production of vasodilatory prostacyclin.

Central Nervous System

In cases of diabetic ketoacidosis, cerebral edema may develop after the extracellular acidosis is corrected.[47] Thus, when the systemic pH is normalized, the mental condition of the patient may be severely disturbed. It has been found that cerebral edema is mainly an intracellular swelling. Ketoacidosis elicits a decrease in pH_i, which should activate the Na^+/H^+ antiport. However, when the extracellular pH is low, the Na^+/H^+ antiport is inhibited.[47] When pH_o is normalized because of treatment, Na^+/H^+ antiport functions at maximal speed to increase cytosolic pH, and the cells gain Na^+ in considerable amounts. It has been found in vitro that this results in intracellular swelling. The concomitant action of the Na^+-independent Cl^-/HCO_3^- antiport increases the intracellular salt and water gain. It therefore appears that the action of these pH_i-regulating antiports may give rise to intracellular edema. In most cells of the body, this may not have serious negative effects, but intracranially a moderate swelling may be life threatening. The combined action of Na^+/H^+ and Na^+-independent Cl^-/HCO_3^- antiports may also increase cell volume in other cases of cerebral edema (i.e., after ischemia and trauma). In vitro inhibition of these antiports abolishes intracellular edema. Effective inhibitors of antiports to be used in vivo will soon be tested for their efficacy in cases of cerebral edema.

Ischemia

In cases of ischemia, not only is the supply of oxygen jeopardized but also the removal of products of metabolism such as lactic acid, CO_2, and protons is severely inhibited. With the decreased supply of O_2, the cells revert to anaerobic metabolism, which they may sustain for different periods of time without damage depending on the cell type. In cells where phosphocreatine is abundant, such as muscle cells, ATP will still be present for 1 to 2 hours of complete ischemia if the muscle is resting. Myocardial cells also contain phosphocreatine, but because of constant activity they cannot tolerate more than 10 to 20 minutes of complete ischemia without severe energy failure. The brain cells contain less phosphocreatine and can be irreversibly damaged by 5 minutes of severe ischemia.

With the lack of oxygen supply, the cells exhaust their ATP stores rapidly. In 5 to 10 minutes, the amount of ATP is less than 10% of normal in most cells providing that no new ATP is formed from phosphocreatine. The breakdown (hydrolysis) of ATP yields protons, which acidify the cells ($ATP + H_2O \rightarrow ADP + P_i + H^+$). How important this is for the immediate cell acidification depends on the cell type. Thus, in cells with little phosphocreatine, the hydrolysis of ATP is unreversed, and a considerable amount of protons are liberated, whereas in cells with a sizable amount of phosphocreatine, protons will be picked up with the transfer of phosphate from phosphocreatine to ATP. Consequently, only when phosphocreatine stores are empty will the cells be acidified.

As soon as ATP stores decrease in the absence of oxygen, the cells can only produce ATP via glycolysis. Under these conditions, NADH is accumulated because it cannot be converted to NAD^+ via oxidative phosphorylation. The only way to convert NADH to NAD^+ under anaerobic metabolism is to produce lactic acid. The accumulation of lactic acid is slower than the unreversed ATP hydrolysis. Studies of ischemic cells indicate that the first acidification of the cells appears to be due to the protons liberated as a result of the breakdown of ATP, whereas lactic acid accumulation may be the major acidification source after 15 to 30 minutes of ischemia.[48] If lactic acid is the major source of acidification, then administration of dichloroacetate and measurement of plasma lactate are relevant clinical actions. If, however, other acids produced as a result of ATP hydrolysis are more important, then neither the administration of dichloroacetate or measurement of plasma lactate would be of benefit.

During ischemia, the acidosis starts intracellularly. Despite this, pH_i has been found to be higher than pH_o, indicating that the cells are able to export H^+ also under ischemic conditions.[49] This is not surprising because Na^+/H^+ antiport, Na^+-coupled Cl^-/HCO_3^- antiport, and Na^+/HCO_3^- symport are not primary active ATP-dependent mechanisms. Thus, for a limited period of time, the cells are able to withstand severe acidification. With continued export of protons and lactic acid, these metabolites accumulate extracellularly. They will be buffered by HCO_3^- in the tissue, giving rise to a high P_{CO_2} (100–400 mm Hg). Because CO_2 is highly membrane permeable, this results in a secondary intracellular acidification. Adding to this acidification is the decreasing effectiveness of pH_i-regulating mechanisms because of their inhibition by low extracellular pH and the dissipation of the Na^+ gradient across the plasma membrane resulting from energy failure and therefore loss of Na^+/K^+ ATPase activity. The cytosolic pH is therefore highly dependent on the removal of extracellular acids and CO_2 to regulate pH_i. Therefore, with zero-flow ischemia, the decrease in pH_i is much more pronounced than, for instance, with hypoxia and normal flow.

Low pH_i per se, as found in ischemic tissue, can lethally damage cells.[50] Interestingly, there has been a reproducible finding of more severe injury after ischemia in brain cells if the research animals or patients are hyperglycemic at the time of ischemia and thereby experience an increased lactic acidosis.[51] However, many cell types can sustain extended periods of low pH_i and still survive. More likely than the acidosis being the major cause of injury is that acidosis facilitates the effects of, for instance, free oxygen radicals, calcium, and so on. Complicating this concept are recent in vitro experiments that, surprisingly, indicate that acidosis in certain instances may protect the cells against hypoxic/ischemic injury.[52] Acidosis slows down the activity of most intracellular enzymes and possibly also enzymes involved in the generation of harmful substances, such as, for instance, free radicals. As long as the cell is not too acidotic, this slowdown of activity might be beneficial under ischemic conditions. It is, however, applicable only to cell types in which low activity during acidosis can be tolerated by the body, such as liver and kidney, but in most cases not myocardial cells. During reperfusion, the extracellular protons and CO_2 are rapidly removed. This leaves the cells with a low pH_i and high pH_o (i.e., the most favorable situation for a rapid regulation of pH_i back to normal). In fact, the regulation of pH_i is so rapid that only 5 to 10 minutes are required for normalization. This suddenly changes the whole metabolism of the cells to high activity including generation of free radicals and other potentially harmful substances. The cells swell because of the rapid influx of Na^+ via the Na^+/H^+ antiport, which might be detrimental intracranially. Thus, it might theoretically be beneficial to inhibit the rapid regulation of pH_i back to normal on reperfusion. Indeed, several articles support this view by showing increased function and cell survival when Na^+/H^+ antiport is inhibited by amiloride or its derivatives.[52, 53] This approach is also feasible clinically and might be an important way to influence cell survival in ischemic conditions.

Inflammation

Polymorphonuclear neutrophils and lymphocytes possess a Na^+/H^+ antiport, a H^+ translocating ATPase, and Na^+-independent Cl^-/HCO_3^- antiport.[54] The activity of the Na^+-independent Cl^-/HCO_3^- antiport in lymphocytes is strongly pH_i dependent.[37] Basophilic cells possess an Na^+/H^+ antiport and a Na^+-coupled Cl^-/HCO_3^-.[54]

The extracellular pH (interstitial pH) is often markedly acidic in inflammatory exudates. This is partly due to the increased production of acid by polymorphonuclear neutrophils and, in some instances, to the production of acid by bacteria. To function properly, the inflammatory cells must withstand this external acid load. Under these circumstances, the Na^+/H^+ antiport is inhibited by the low pH_o, whereas the H^+-translocating ATPase still works very effectively and is able to counteract the acidification to a large extent. *Bacteroides* produce large amounts of succinic acid.[55] This acid is excreted from the bacteria and, because of the high membrane permeability at acidic pH_o, it gains access to the cytosol of the polymorphonuclear neutrophils and causes a strong cytosolic acidification. This inactivates the polymorphonuclear neutrophils. Thus, the excretion of organic acid by bacteria may be a defense mechanism against the immunologic system to considerably increase the virulence of the bacteria.

Almost all NSAIDs are weak acids. They bind strongly to serum albumin, but at low pH a considerable part of the drug is released from the protein. Thus, in acidic inflammatory exudates, these drugs are accumulated and therefore exert a strong action on the inflammatory cells. It has been found that NSAIDs decrease pH_i in certain kidney cells by stimulating the Na^+-independent Cl^-/HCO_3^- antiport and inhibiting the Na^+-coupled Cl^-/HCO_3^- antiport.[20] It is not known whether the same action is present in leukocytes.

Cancer

Cancer cells have a metabolism that in several ways deviates from that of normal cells. Among these is the increased production of lactic acid resulting from anaerobic metabolism. This is caused by both the preferential use of this pathway by cancer cells and the hypoxic conditions that often develop inside tumors. Numerous measurements of tumor pH have been published, and the results show considerable variation. The average tumor pH appears to be 0.5 to 1.5 units lower than in normal tissues, although in some studies a higher pH than normal has been found.[56, 57] The low pH is caused by both increased lactic acid and protons released in the hydrolysis of ATP.

In accordance with the idea that an increased pH_i is necessary or at least permissive for proliferation, some transformed cell lines have been found to have a higher pH_i in vitro than their nontransformed parental cells measured at neutral pH_o.[58] Significantly, in vivo mutant malignant cells lacking the Na^+/H^+ antiport fail to form tumors or these tumors grow at a considerably slower rate than the corresponding cells possessing the antiport.[56, 59] This implies a key role for Na^+/H^+ antiport for tumor growth in vivo. It is tempting to speculate that, because of the lactic acidosis in the tumor, $[HCO_3^-]$ is very low and the cells therefore depend on Na^+/H^+ antiport to keep their pH_i at a value permissive for growth. Thus, the increased activity of the Na^+/H^+ antiport, which is found in some malignant cells, may not be necessary to increase pH_i to a value higher than what is found in normal cells but may be necessary to withstand the increased acid load found in tumors.

From a therapeutic point of view, the idea of exploiting a low pH to kill cells has attracted much attention.[59, 60] Thus, acidic cytostatic drugs gain increased access to cells at low pH_o, whereas alkaline drugs are excluded from the cells. The knowledge of tumor pH measured by ^{31}P MRI spectroscopy could therefore influence the choice of cytostatic drugs. The cells in the acidic interior of the tumor are probably in a nonproliferative state. Because most cytostatics interfere with cell division, these cells may be able to survive and start proliferating later when the majority of the other cells have been killed by the treatment. Therefore, drugs that could further decrease pH_i in these nonproliferating cells to a value incompatible with survival are greatly needed.

SUMMARY

During the last decade, we have witnessed a revolution in our understanding of intracellular regulation of pH and electrolytes. A short summary of our current understanding is as follows:

1. All cells have several transmembrane transport mechanisms (most notably Na^+/H^+ antiport, Na^+-coupled Cl^-/HCO_3^- antiport, Na^+/HCO_3^- symport, H^+-ATPases, and Na^+-independent Cl^-/HCO_3^- antiport) to keep pH_i near normal levels despite heavy acid or base load.
2. These transmembrane transport mechanisms are highly regulated in their activity by both intra- and extracellular pH, natural ligands (paracrine and endocrine hormones, growth factors, vasoactive substances, and so on), and many drugs.
3. The bicarbonate system is the most important buffer system both extra- and intracellularly. The other major buffer system is protein. Prerequisites for the efficacy of the bicarbonate system are the removal of CO_2 by respiration and the transmembrane transport of HCO_3^- via Na^+-coupled Cl^-/HCO_3^- antiport, Na^+/HCO_3^- symport, or Na^+-independent Cl^-/HCO_3^- antiport.
4. The previously mentioned mechanisms are also involved in the regulation of intracellular electrolytes, cell volume, transcellular transport, and membrane potential. Like a network, disturbances in one of the processes markedly influence the others.
5. These processes are obviously involved in acid-base disturbances and are important to correct pH deviations. Equally important, these processes appear to be involved in the pathophysiology of ischemia/reperfusion, cerebral edema, kidney failure, peptic ulcer, heart failure, hypovolemic and septic shock, inflammation, cancer, and so on.
6. With the recent detailed knowledge of the molecular biology of these processes, new drugs that interfere with their activity will be discovered. In fact, several drugs in current use such as amiloride, furosemide, NSAIDs, dopamine, and epinephrine, have been shown to alter the activity of these mechanisms in vitro. Thus, in the future, drug treatment of these disorders will be available, providing a rational approach to their management instead of our current guessing on the beneficial or detrimental effect of bicarbonate administration.

References

1. Aronson PS, Nee J, Suhm MA: Modifier role of internal H^+ in activating Na^+/H^+ exchanger in renal microvillus membrane vesicles. Nature 1982; 299:161–163.
2. Frelin C, Vigne P, Ladoux A, et al: The regulation of the intracellular pH in cells from vertebrates. Eur J Biochem 1988; 174:3–14.
3. Lazdunski M, Frelin C, Vigne P: The sodium/hydrogen exchange system in cardiac cells: Its biochemical and pharmacological properties and its role in regulating internal concentrations of sodium and internal pH. J Mol Cell Cardiol 1985; 17:1029–1042.
4. Grinstein S, Rotin D, Mason MJ: Na^+/H^+ exchange and growth factor-induced cytosolic pH changes: Role in cellular proliferation. Biochim Biophys Acta 1989; 988:73–97.
5. Hoffmann EK, Simonsen LO: Membrane mechanisms in volume and pH regulation in vertebrate cells. Physiol Rev 1993; 69:315–382.
6. Reinertsen KV, Tønnessen TI, Jacobsen J, et al: Role of chloride/bicarbonate antiport in the control of cytosolic pH: Cell-line

differences in activity and regulation of antiport. J Biol Chem 1988; 263:11117–11125.

7. Tønnessen TI, Sandvig K, Olsnes S: Role of $Na(^+)$-H^+ and $Cl(^-)$-HCO_3^- antiports in the regulation of cytosolic pH near neutrality. Am J Physiol 1990; 258:C1117–C1126.
8. Tønnessen TI, Ludt J, Sandvig K, et al: Bicarbonate/chloride antiport in Vero cells: I. Evidence for both sodium-linked and sodium-independent exchange. J Cell Physiol 1987; 132:183–191.
9. Tønnessen TI, Aas AT, Ludt J, et al: Regulation of Na^+/H^+ and Cl^-/HCO_3^- antiports in Vero cells. J Cell Physiol 1990; 143:178–187.
10. Chen LK, Boron WF: Intracellular pH regulation in epithelial cells. Kidney Int [Suppl] 1991; 33:S11–S17.
11. Boron WF, Knakal RC: $Na(^+)$-dependent Cl-HCO_3 exchange in the squid axon: Dependence on extracellular pH. J Gen Physiol 1992; 99:817–837.
12. Ladoux A, Krawice I, Cragoe EJ Jr, et al: Properties of the Na^+-dependent Cl^-/HCO_3^- exchange system in U937 human leukemic cells. Eur J Biochem 1987; 170:43–49.
13. Jentsch TJ, Janicke I, Sorgenfrei D, et al: The regulation of intracellular pH in monkey kidney epithelial cells (BSC-1): Roles of Na^+/H^+ antiport, Na^+-$HCO_3(^-)$-$(NaCO_3^-)$ symport, and Cl^-/HCO_3^- exchange. J Biol Chem 1986; 261:12120–12127.
14. Boron WF, Boulpaep EL: The electrogenic Na/HCO_3 cotransporter. Kidney Int 1989; 36:392–402.
15. Balkovetz DF, Leibach FH, Mahesh VB, et al: A proton gradient is the driving force for uphill transport of lactate in human placental brush-border membrane vesicles. J Biol Chem 1988; 263:13823–13830.
16. Swallow CJ, Grinstein S, Rotstein OD: Cytoplasmic pH regulation in macrophages by an ATP-dependent and N,N'-dicyclohexylcarbodiimide-sensitive mechanism: Possible involvement of a plasma membrane proton pump. J Biol Chem 1988; 263:19558–19563.
17. Olsnes S, Tønnessen TI, Sandvig K: pH-regulated anion antiport in nucleated mammalian cells. J Cell Biol 1986; 102:967–971.
18. Olsnes S, Tønnessen TI, Ludt J, et al: Effect of intracellular pH on the rate of chloride uptake and efflux in different mammalian cell lines. Biochemistry 1987; 26:2778–2785.
19. Olsnes S, Ludt J, Tønnessen TI, et al: Bicarbonate/chloride antiport in Vero cells: II. Mechanisms for bicarbonate-dependent regulation of intracellular pH. J Cell Physiol 1987; 132:192–202.
20. Tønnessen TI, Aas AT, Sandvig K, et al: Effect of anti-inflammatory analgesic drugs on the regulation of cytosolic pH by anion antiport. J Pharmacol Exp Ther 1989; 248:1197–1206.
21. Tønnessen TI, Aas AT, Sandvig K, et al: Inhibition of chloride/bicarbonate antiports in monkey kidney cells (Vero) by nonsteroidal anti-inflammatory drugs. Biochem Pharmacol 1989; 38:3583–3591.
22. Preisig PA, Alpern RJ: Chronic metabolic acidosis causes an adaptation in the apical membrane Na/H antiporter and basolateral membrane $Na(HCO_3)_3$ symporter in the rat proximal convoluted tubule. J Clin Invest 1988; 82:1445–1453.
23. Bierman AJ, Cragoe EJ Jr, de Laat SW, et al: Bicarbonate determines cytoplasmic pH and suppresses mitogen-induced alkalinization in fibroblastic cells. J Biol Chem 1988; 263:15253–15256.
24. Passow H: Molecular aspects of band 3 protein-mediated anion transport across the red blood cell membrane. Rev Physiol Biochem Pharmacol 1986; 103:61–203.
25. Crandall ED, Bidani A: Effects of red blood cell $HCO_3(^-)/Cl^-$ exchange kinetics on lung CO_2 transfer: Theory. J Appl Physiol: Respir, Environ Exercise Physiol 1981; 50:265–271.
26. Wieth JO, Andersen OS, Brahm J, et al: Chloride–bicarbonate exchange in red blood cells: Physiology of transport and chemical modification of binding sites. Philos Trans R Soc Lond: (Biol) 1982; 299:383–399.
27. Crandall ED, Winter HI, Schaeffer JD, et al: Effects of salicylate on HCO_3^-/Cl^- exchange across the human erythrocyte membrane. J Memb Biol 1982; 65:139–145.
28. Wieth JO, Brahm J: Inhibitory effect of salicylate on chloride and bicarbonate transport in human red cells: A possible explanation for the stimulatory effect of salicylate on respiration. Ugesk Laeger 1978; 140:1859–1865.
29. Kurtz I: Apical Na^+/H^+ antiporter and glycolysis-dependent H^+-ATPase regulate intracellular pH in the rabbit S_3 proximal tubule. J Clin Invest 1987; 80:928–935.
30. Nakhoul NL, Chen LK, Boron WF: Intracellular pH regulation in rabbit S_3 proximal tubule: Basolateral Cl-HCO_3 exchange and Na-HCO_3 cotransport. A J Physiol 1990; 258:F371–F381.
31. Geibel J, Giebisch G, Boron WF: Angiotensin II stimulates both $Na(^+)$-H^+ exchange and Na^+/HCO_3^- cotransport in the rabbit proximal tubule. Proc Nat Acad Sci USA 1990; 87:7917–7920.
32. Hensley CB, Bradley ME, Mircheff AK: Parathyroid hormone-induced translocation of Na-H antiporters in rat proximal tubules. Am J Physiol 1989; 257:C637–C645.
33. Kurtz A, Della Bruna R, Scholz H, et al: Amiloride enhances the secretion but not the synthesis of renin in renal juxtaglomerular cells. Pflugers Arch 1991; 419:32–37.
34. Morduchowicz GA, Sheikh-Hamad D, Dwyer BE, et al: Angiotensin II directly increases rabbit renal brush-border membrane sodium transport: Presence of local signal transduction system. J Memb Biol 1991; 122:43–53.
35. Madshus IH, Tønnessen TI, Olsnes S, et al: Effect of potassium depletion of Hep 2 cells on intracellular pH and on chloride uptake by anion antiport. J Cell Physiol 1987; 131:6–13.
36. Paris S, Pouyssegur J: Growth factors activate the bumetanide-sensitive $Na^+/K^+/Cl$-cotransport in hamster fibroblasts. J Biol Chem 1986; 261:6177–6183.
37. Mason MJ, Smith JD, Garcia-Soto JJ, et al: Internal pH-sensitive site couples Cl-$(^-)HCO_3^-$ exchange to Na^+-H^+ antiport in lymphocytes. Am J Physiol 1989; 256:C428–C433.
38. Grinstein S: Intracellular chloride concentration: Determinants and consequences. Prog Clin Biol Res 1987; 254:31–43.
39. Muallem S, Blissard D, Cragoe EJ Jr, et al: Activation of the Na^+/H^+ and Cl^-/HCO_3^- exchange by stimulation of acid secretion in the parietal cell. J Biol Chem 1988; 263:14703–14711.
40. Preisig PA, Rector FC Jr: Role of Na^+-H^+ antiport in rat proximal tubule NaCl absorption. Am J Physiol 1988; 255:F461–F465.
41. Tønnessen TI: Regulation of cytosolic pH in mammalian cells. Oslo, The Norwegian Cancer Society, 1990.
42. Gambassi G, Spurgeon HA, Lakatta EG, et al: Different effects of alpha- and beta-adrenergic stimulation on cytosolic pH and myofilament responsiveness to Ca^{2+} in cardiac myocytes. Circ Res 1992; 71:870–882.
43. Archike FI, Dai S: Influence of pH changes on the actions of verapamil on cardiac excitation-contraction coupling. Eur J Pharmacol 1991; 196:77–83.
44. Nakanishi T, Gu H, Seguchi M, et al: $HCO_3(^-)$-dependent intracellular pH regulation in the premature myocardium. Circ Res 1992; 71:1314–1323.
45. Weissberg PL, Little PJ, Cragoe EJ Jr, et al: The pH of spontaneously beating cultured rat heart cells is regulated by an ATP-calmodulin-dependent Na^+/H^+ antiport. Circ Res 1989; 64:676–685.
46. Putnam RW: pH regulatory transport systems in a smooth muscle-like cell line. Am J Physiol 1990; 258:C470–C479.
47. Van der Meulen JA, Klip A, Grinstein S: Possible mechanism for cerebral oedema in diabetic ketoacidosis. Lancet 1987; 2:306–308.
48. Terrier F, Lazeyras F, Posse S, et al: Study of acute renal ischemia in the rat using magnetic resonance imaging and spectroscopy. Magn Reson Med 1989; 12:114–136.
49. Yan GX, Kleber AG: Changes in extracellular and intracellular pH in ischemic rabbit papillary muscle. Circ Res 1992; 71:460–470.
50. Kraig RP, Petito CK, Plum F, et al: Hydrogen ions kill brain at concentrations reached in ischemia. J Cereb Blood Flow Metab 1987; 7:379–386.
51. Siesjo BK: Pathophysiology and treatment of focal cerebral ischemia: Part I. Pathophysiology. J Neurosurg 1992; 77:169–184.
52. Currin RT, Gores GJ, Thurman RG, et al: Protection by acidotic pH against anoxic cell killing in perfused rat liver: Evidence for a pH paradox. FASEB J 1991; 5:207–210.
53. Meng HP, Lonsberry BB, Pierce GN: Influence of perfusate pH on the postischemic recovery of cardiac contractile function: Involvement of sodium-hydrogen exchange. J Pharmacol Exp Ther 1991; 258:772–777.
54. Swallow CJ, Grinstein S, Sudsbury RA, et al: Cytoplasmic pH regulation in monocytes and macrophages: Mechanisms and functional implications. Clin Invest Med 1991; 14:367–378.

55. Rotstein OD, Nasmith PE, Grinstein S: The bacteroides by-product succinic acid inhibits neutrophil respiratory burst by reducing intracellular pH. Infect Immun 1987; 55:864–870.
56. Tannock IF, Rotin D: Acid pH in tumors and its potential for therapeutic exploitation. Cancer Res 1989; 49:4373–4384.
57. Newell KJ, Tannock IF: Reduction of intracellular pH as a possible mechanism for killing cells in acidic regions of solid tumors: Effects of carbonylcyanide-3-chlorophenylhydrazone. Cancer Res 1989; 49:4477–4482.
58. Gillies RJ, Martinez-Zaguilan R, Martinez GM, et al: Tumorigenic 3T3 cells maintain an alkaline intracellular pH under physiological conditions. Proc Nat Acad Sci USA 1990; 87:7414–7418.
59. Lagarde AE, Franchi AJ, Paris S, et al: Effect of mutations affecting Na^+: H^+ antiport activity on tumorigenic potential of hamster lung fibroblasts. J Cell Biochem 1988; 36:249–260.
60. Rotin D, Wan P, Grinstein S, et al: Cytotoxicity of compounds that interfere with the regulation of intracellular pH: A potential new class of anticancer drugs. Cancer Res 1987; 47:1497–1504.

CHAPTER 24

T and B Cell Function in Critical Illness

Edward Abraham, MD

Important alterations in T and B cell function are associated with critical illness, producing a relatively immunocompromised state in which infection is more likely to occur and, when it does occur, is less able to be controlled.[1, 2] Severe injury, sepsis, blood loss, as well as pharmacologic agents used in critically ill patients, such as aminoglycoside antibiotics and anesthetic agents, produce significant alterations in T and B cell function associated with decreased resistance to infectious insults.[1]

T CELL ACTIVATION AND PROLIFERATION

T cells can be divided into two subsets, $CD4^+$ and $CD8^+$, on the basis of the presence of these T cell receptor (TCR) adjacent-surface molecules. Subpopulations of $CD4^+$ T cells have "helper" functions in augmenting T and B cell proliferation and activation. "Suppressor" $CD8^+$ T cells have been identified and can down-regulate T and B cell activation. $CD8^+$ cells also have cytotoxic functions and can kill tumor cells as well as cells infected intracellularly with virus, bacteria, and fungi. Viral, fungal, bacterial, and nonbacterial antigens, required for cellular activation, are presented to T cells in an appropriately recognizable configuration bound to the major histocompatibility complex (MHC) on the surface of antigen-presenting cells.[3, 4] Many cell types can function as antigen-presenting cells, the most important being tissue dendritic cells, B cells, and macrophages.[5, 6] In general, protein antigens require intracellular processing before being presented to T cells, a role usually undertaken by dendritic cells and macrophages. Polysaccharide antigens, which are common on the membrane of bacteria, can be recognized by immunoglobulin residing on the B cell surface and then directly presented to T cells.

T cell activation is a multistep process (Fig. 24–1) involving (1) antigen being presented in the proper configuration by efficient antigen-presenting cells, (2) T cells with appropriate TCR to recognize the antigen, (3) the presence of T cells that are capable of responding to and becoming activated by antigen (i.e., nonanergic T cells), (4) appropriate interactions by adhesion molecules and other cell-surface molecules permitting presentation of the antigen in the proper stereotaxic format, (5) coregulatory interactions between T and B cells modulated by such surface molecules as CD28 and B7/BB1, and (6) adequate cytokine and other signals between antigen-presenting cells and T cells. Evidence indicates that many of these required steps in T cell activation may be affected by critical illness, resulting in less efficient T cell help in augmenting immune responses and a greater predominance of suppressive T cell effects.

Antigen-presenting ability of macrophages, as well as the expression of MHC class II molecules on the surface of macrophages, is decreased by hemorrhage and severe injury.[2, 7–9] Because $CD4^+$ T cell activation is dependent on the proper configuration of antigen and MHC class II, diminished expression of MHC class II molecules on the macrophage surface may result in inadequate activation of this T cell subpopulation and lack of sufficient "help" to achieve an optimal host response against infection.

Although macrophages probably are not the most important antigen-presenting cells for antigens associated with gram-negative and gram-positive extracellular bacteria, they play a more important role in presenting antigens derived from intracellular bacteria as well as viruses and fungi. Depression of macrophage antigen-presenting capacity, therefore, would be expected primarily to affect resistance to intracellular organisms, normally killed by $CD8^+$ T cells and natural killer cells.[10] Suppression of macrophage antigen-presenting capacity, associated with models of critical illness and likely to occur in patients, may contribute to the emergence of opportunistic intracellular infections, such as those caused by fungi, which are an important clinical problem in the intensive care unit (ICU). Dendritic cells, present in the follicles of lymph nodes as well as in other lymphoid sites, and B cells appear to be much more important antigen-presenting cells than are macrophages. Unfortunately, few studies have investigated the effects of critical illness on the antigen-presenting ability of dendritic or B cells.

The ability of both $CD4^+$ and $CD8^+$ T cells to be activated in an antigen-specific or nonspecific manner appears to be diminished after hemorrhage, burns, and accidental and experimental trauma.[11–15] Hemorrhage and injury are associated with decreased production of T cell–derived cytokines. There also is evidence that messenger ribonucleic acid (mRNA) transcripts and presumably protein production of cytokines, such as transforming growth factor (TGF)-β, capable of inhibiting T and B cell function are increased in models of critical illness. The result of these alterations is a reduction in the ability of T cells to participate efficiently in cellular interactions required to provide optimal host defense against microbial invasion.

Both burns and blood loss are associated with activation of a population of $CD8^+$ cells, capable of inhibiting the activation and proliferation of other T cells.[16–18] Transfer of $CD8^+$ cells from hemorrhaged mice to normal mice results in decreased T cell–mediated cytotoxicity.[12] Such alterations in T cell function may have important clinical implications because they often are associated with a decreased ability to kill cells infected with intracellular organisms, such as fungi. In addition, hemorrhage-activated $CD8^+$ T cells decrease numbers and frequencies of bacterial antigen-specific B cells when transferred to normal mice.[19] Therefore, even though overall T cell, $CD4^+$, and $CD8^+$ proliferation and activation appear to be diminished in models of critical illness, increased activity of a subset of $CD8^+$ cells, able to affect other

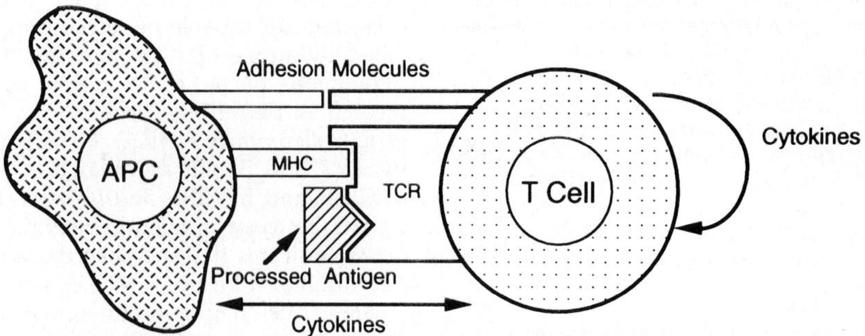

Figure 24–1. T cell activation involves presentation of antigen in a major histocompatibility complex (MHC)–specific manner to engage an antigen-specific T cell receptor (TCR) on the T cell surface. Interaction between the antigen-presenting cell (APC) and the T cell is promoted by adhesion molecules on the surfaces of both cells. Cytokines produced by the T cell and antigen-presenting cell (e.g., interleukin 1, interleukin 2, and others) can modulate the activation state of both cells. In particular, T cell–produced cytokines, such as interleukin 2, can promote further activation of T cells by up-regulating receptor numbers on the surfaces of T cells as well as receptor affinity.

T cells and B cells, also may contribute to the relatively immunocompromised state, characterized most importantly by increased susceptibility to infection, found in critically ill patients.

CYTOKINES

Macrophages, T cells, B cells, as well as many other cell types throughout the body produce relatively small proteins, called *cytokines,* that are capable of affecting the function of cells involved in the immune response (Table 24–1). Cytokines generally have molecular weights between 10,000 and 30,000 d and interact with specific receptors on responding cell surfaces. Soluble receptors also have been identified for several cytokines and may be an important regulatory mechanism modulating cytokine actions. Cytokines often have other actions distinct from their effects on immune response. For example, interleukin (IL)-1 can produce hypotension and fever and appears to have an important role in mediating organ system dysfunction in sepsis.[20–22]

A large number of cytokines are predominantly produced by T cells and are capable of affecting macrophage, T, and B cell function. Recent evidence indicates that $CD4^+$ T cells can be divided into two populations on the basis of their cytokine profiles.[23] Th1 cells are involved in inflammatory functions and produce tumor necrosis factor (TNF)-α, IL-2, and interferon (IFN)-γ, and Th2 cells provide B cell help and produce IL-4, IL-5, and IL-10. IL-10 appears to have an important role in regulating the balance between Th1 and Th2 cell activity because it can down-regulate the production of Th1 cytokines through its actions on macrophages.[24–26]

Studies in injured patients and in animals after trauma and blood loss demonstrate a decrease in Th1-associated cytokines, with increases in at least some cytokines produced by the Th2 population.[27, 28] In particular, production of IL-2 and IFN-γ decreases after hemorrhage and injury, whereas IL-10 is markedly increased and IL-4 slightly increased in this setting.[29] These injury-induced alterations in cytokine production may have important roles in affecting antimicrobial host defenses. IL-2 enhances both T and B cell activation as well as progression to antibody production by B cells.[30, 31] A relative decrease in IL-2 production, therefore, might be expected to result in depressed resistance to infection. In burned mice, treatment with IL-2 restores resistance to bacterial infection associated with fecal peritonitis.[32] Although addition of IL-2 to T cell cultures from injured patients and hemorrhaged mice did not restore T cell proliferation,[33, 34] in vivo treatment with IL-2 was able to increase bacterial antigen-specific plasma cell numbers back to normal levels.[35]

IL-10 has potent down-regulatory effects on cytokine production by Th1 cells and macrophages.[24–26] In particular, IL-10 suppresses cytokine production as well as antigen-specific and nonspecific proliferation of Th1 cells.[24, 25, 36] IL-10 also has been shown to strongly down-regulate the constitutive and inducible expression of MHC class II molecules on macrophages and monocytes.[37] Similarly, the production by macrophages and monocytes of inflammatory mediators, such as IL-1α, IL-6, IL-8, and TNF-α, is inhibited by IL-10.[24, 26, 37] Blood loss and injury have been reported to have profound suppressive effects on the production of IL-1 and IL-6 as well as MHC class II expression and antigen presentation by macrophages.[2, 7–9] These generally suppressive effects of hemorrhage on macrophage functions and on the generation of Th1 cytokines could be mediated through the actions of IL-10, which is produced by $CD4^+$ Th2 cells in increased amounts in models of critical illness and blood loss.[29]

The addition of IFN-γ to macrophage populations causes increased antigen presentation and increased surface expression of MHC class II (Ia). Experiments have shown that therapy with IFN-γ improved macrophage Ia expression after blood loss as well as survival from bacterial infection.[38–41] In contrast, in experimental endotoxemia, the addition of IFN-γ had deleterious effects, presumably through augmenting the toxicity of TNF released in this model.[42] Similarly, IFN-γ is suppressive for immunoglobulin secretion by B cells and because of this, therapy with IFN-γ may be associated with diminished resistance to extracellular organisms, for which circulating and secretory immunoglobulins are of major importance.

Therapies with other cytokines, able to enhance T cell function, also can increase resistance to infection. This has been shown most clearly with IL-1, which improves outcome when provided in various animal models of chronic infection.[43–45] In contrast, in acute septicemia, blocking the actions of IL-1 through the use of an IL-1 receptor antagonist appears to be highly effective in improving outcome.[22] These contrasting results highlight some of the future potential difficulties in using immunomodulatory therapy in infected, critically ill patients.

Mucosal surfaces, such as the lung and intestine, appear to be particularly vulnerable to bacterial colonization and infection in critically ill patients. In models of critical illness,

TABLE 24–1. Major Cytokines and Their Primary Activities

Cytokine	*Actions*
Interleukin-1	Induces fever, acute phase proteins; activates endothelial cells; stimulates T cell proliferation
Interleukin-2	Activates macrophages, stimulates natural killer cell activity, stimulates B cell proliferation and differentiation, activates T cells, stimulates T cell proliferation and differentiation
Interleukin-3	Stimulates eosinophil activity, B cell differentiation, in vivo hematopoiesis
Interleukin-4	Activates macrophages, T and B cells; stimulates B cell proliferation and differentiation; induces IgE receptors on B cells; stimulates T cell proliferation
Interleukin-5	Stimulates eosinophil activity, activates B cells, stimulates IgA isotype selection
Interleukin-6	Induces acute phase proteins; activates T cells; stimulates T cell proliferation and differentiation, B cell differentiation, and antibody production
Interleukin-7	Stimulates T and B cell proliferation
Interleukin-8	Chemotactic for neutrophils, induces neutrophil activation, inhibits neutrophil adhesion to endothelium
Interleukin-10	Suppresses cytokine production by Th1 cells and macrophages/monocytes, diminishes delayed hypersensitivity, suppresses monocyte/macrophage antigen-presenting cell function, down-regulates expression of MHC class II molecules on monocytes/macrophages, suppresses production of reactive nitrogen oxides by macrophages/monocytes, up-regulates MHC class II expression on B cells, augments proliferation and differentiation of B cells
Tumor necrosis factor-α	Activates macrophages; stimulates granulocyte activity, T cell proliferation; induces expression of intracellular adhesion molecules (e.g., ICAM-1); activates endothelial cells; induces fever and acute phase proteins
Transforming growth factor-β	Inhibits proliferation of hematopoietic precursors, inhibits activation and proliferation of T and B cells, stimulates growth of fibroblasts and osteoblasts, produces isotypes switching to IgA
Interferon-α	Induces a cellular antiviral state; stimulates natural killer cell activity, B cell proliferation and differentiation; inhibits T cell proliferation; induces fever
Interferon-β	Induces a cellular antiviral state, stimulates natural killer cell activity, enhances MHC class I expression, induces fever, stimulates B cell proliferation
Interferon-γ	Induces acute-phase protein production, stimulates isotype selection (IgG2a), inhibits B cell activation, activates macrophages
Granulocyte-macrophage colony-stimulating factor	Activates macrophages; stimulates granulocyte activity, eosinophil activity, T cell proliferation, in vivo hematopoiesis
Granulocyte colony-stimulating factor	Stimulates granulopoiesis and granulocyte activity

Abbreviations: IgE = immunoglobulin E; IgA = immunoglobulin A; MHC = major histocompatibility complex.

increases in the transcription of proinflammatory (e.g., IL-1β, TNF-α) and immunoregulatory (e.g., TGF-β, IFN-γ) cytokine genes are found as rapidly as 1 hour after physiologic insults similar to those in critically ill patients.[46] These alterations in cytokine mRNA levels are most prominent in mucosal sites, such as the lung and Peyer's patches, and are not found systemically, such as in the spleen or peripheral blood. Increased mRNA expression at mucosal surfaces and subsequent enhanced production of cytokines, such as TGF-β, capable of inhibiting T and B cell functions may be important factors contributing to the vulnerability of these anatomic sites to infection in critically ill patients.

B CELLS

B cells, through the production of antibodies, have a central role in resistance to extracellular organisms. Secretory antibodies, primarily immunoglobulin (Ig)A, are present at mucosal surfaces, such as the intestines and lung. By binding to bacteria, fungi, and viruses present at mucosal sites, secretory IgA is able to protect the host from systemic invasion. Secretory antibodies do not appear to be capable of fixing complement but do enhance antibody-mediated cellular killing, which may be a primary mechanism contributing to their efficacy in protection against infection at mucosal surfaces. Circulating antibodies are mostly of the IgG and IgM classes and participate in antibacterial resistance by coating bacteria, thereby facilitating complement-mediated killing as well as phagocytosis by neutrophils and macrophages. Both neutrophils and macrophages have receptors on their surfaces (Fc receptors) able to recognize antibody, therefore allowing them to bind to and ingest antibody-coated bacteria.

Achievement of an adequate and appropriate antibody response is dependent on factors relating to B cell populations and dynamics as well as interactions between B cells and other cell types that can affect the state of B cell activation. The factors affecting progression of a resting B cell to become an activated antibody-producing plasma cell are diagrammed in Figure 24–2. In particular, crucial steps affecting the adequacy of an antimicrobial antibody response relate to (1) sufficient numbers of resting B cells committed to producing antibody against the appropriate bacterial antigens, (2) adequate help, primarily provided by $CD4^+$ cells, to achieve activation of resting B cells, (3) absence of inappropriate suppression, primarily by $CD8^+$ T cells, which might inhibit activation of resting B cells to become antibody-producing plasma cells, (4) an appropriate cytokine milieu encouraging B cell progression to antibody production, and (5) sufficient numbers of plasma cells actually producing antibody against the appropriate bacterial antigens.

As B cells leave the bone marrow, they are already committed to producing antibody specific for a single antigen. Most B cells never are activated to produce antibody against

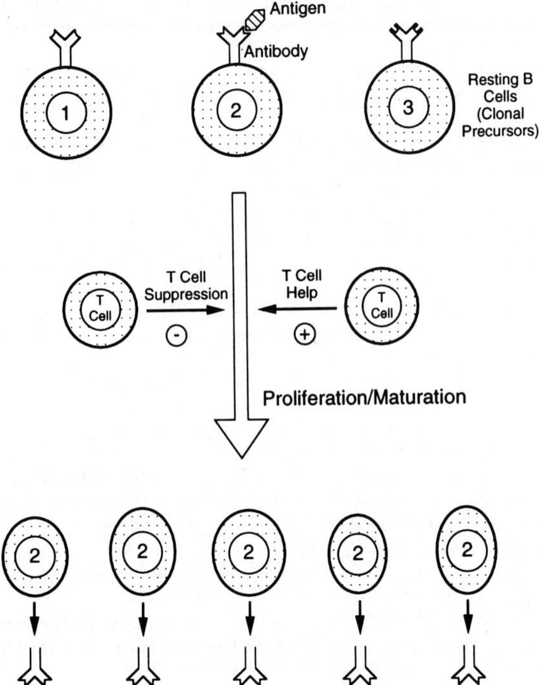

Figure 24–2. Resting B cells become activated after interaction of antigens with antigen-specific antibody on their surface. Each B cell is committed to producing antibody of a single specificity, and small amounts of antibody specific for that antibody are present on the surface of resting B cells. Proliferation and maturation of activated B cells that lead to their becoming antibody-secreting plasma cells are modulated by helper and suppressor influences provided by T cells.

their specifically preprogrammed antigen, and they die within several days of leaving the bone marrow. In the relatively rare case in which a B cell actually does come into contact with its specific antigen, activation, proliferation, and progression to antibody secretion occur. Some of these activated B cells remain in the body, either in systemic or mucosal sites, for periods as long as several years and constitute the "memory" component of the B cell population.

Because B cells are unable to change the specificity of the antibody that they are destined to produce, an adequate antibody response to an infectious episode depends on the numbers of antigen-specific resting B cells (B cell clonal precursors) that are present at the time of infection and that can then be activated and recruited into the antibody-secreting plasma cell pool. Activation of B cell clonal precursors is affected by many factors, including help provided by $CD4^+$ T cells and suppression by $CD8^+$ T cells, and these factors can result in skewing of the actual repertoire so that there are relatively more or less antigen-specific plasma cells than the percentage found among resting B cells. Cytokines can enhance (i.e., IL-2, IL-4, IL-5) or inhibit (i.e., TGF-β, IFN-γ) B cell activation and antibody secretion.

Several studies[47–49] using models for critical illness have shown profound and long-lasting decreases in the numbers of bacterial antigen-specific resting B cells. These alterations are most striking among B cells present at mucosal sites such as the lung and intestine and programmed to produce antibodies to bacterial antigens.[48, 49] Decreased numbers of bacterial antigen-specific resting B cells will translate into an inadequate antibacterial antibody response unless these bacterial antigen-specific B cell clonal precursors are able to be recruited into the plasma cell pool with increased efficiency. Unfortunately, data do not suggest that increased activation of resting B cells occurs in the setting of critical illness.

One could imagine that even if the number of antigen-specific plasma cells is decreased, the smaller number of plasma cells still present could maintain antibody levels by increasing the amount of antibody produced by each cell. This does not appear to occur in models of critical illness. Bacterial antigen-specific secretory antibody titers in the lung have been measured at varying times after experimental hemorrhage and resuscitation, and they showed patterns of decrease that paralleled those found among bacterial antigen-specific pulmonary plasma cell numbers.[50]

CONCLUSIONS

Nosocomial infections occur frequently in critically ill patients, contributing to the high incidence of sepsis and multiple organ system failure in these patients.[51, 52] The widespread abnormalities in T and B cell function associated with critical illness clearly play an important role in the increased susceptibility to infection found in this setting. A major future challenge is to identify which of the multiple alterations in T and B cell function are central in producing the immunocompromised state associated with critical illness. Therapies then can be designed that will appropriately address that immunologic abnormality without affecting other components of the immune system. This concern is far from trivial because almost all of the immunomodulatory agents that we have, such as monoclonal antibodies, cytokines, and cytokine blockers, have multiple immunologic effects.

Nosocomial infections often originate at mucosal surfaces, primarily the lungs.[51–53] Critical illness appears to be associated with marked decreases in the numbers and percentages of resting B cells able to be activated to produce antibodies to bacterial antigens; these findings are most prominent at pulmonary and intestinal sites.[48, 49] These alterations in B cell repertoires result in inadequate levels of secretory antibody at mucosal sites, which may contribute to the increased incidence of bacterial colonization at these surfaces. Similarly, decreased numbers of systemic bacterial antigen-specific B cells are expected to translate into a less efficient antibacterial antibody response should bacteria cross mucosal barriers to invade the bloodstream.

Given the decreased numbers of resting bacterial antigen-specific B cells that accompany critical illness, interventions to enhance the antibody response must be aimed at mechanisms that result in increased antibody production from the remaining B cells. At least three possible interventions could be postulated to be of benefit in this situation. First, vaccination against organisms likely to produce secondary infections if administered early in the hospital course, before numbers of bacterial antigen-specific resting B cells had become severely depleted, could result in enhanced antibody titers and protection against infection.[54] Second, enhanced antibody production by plasma cells may be achieved through the use of cytokines, such as IL-2, IL-4, and IL-6.[55] Third, recruitment of resting bacterial antigen-specific B cells into the antibody-secreting plasma cell pool has been shown to be diminished in models of critical illness because of relatively increased suppressive effects of $CD8^+$ T cells.[19] Therapies, primarily using cytokines or cytotoxic monoclonal antibodies able to recognize and eliminate this $CD8^+$ population, may result in an improved antibacterial antibody response. Most important, determination of the causes in critical illness for the disappearance of bacterial antigen-specific B cell clonal precursors from the peripheral and mucosal B cell pool will permit the development of methodologies able to preserve numbers of these B cells, thereby allowing maintenance of normal antibody responses in the critically ill patient.

Intracellular infections, with organisms such as fungi and *Pneumocystis carinii,* are becoming more common in critically ill patients. T cells are an important component in host defense to intracellular infection, but, as discussed in this chapter, often function inadequately in the setting of critical illness. Future interventions, most likely involving the use of cytokine combinations able to restore T cell activities may have an important role in enhancing resistance to infection. The efficacy of such therapies is suggested by models showing that IL-1, IL-2, and IFN-γ can improve outcome in experimental infection.[32, 38–41, 45] Restoring T cell–T cell interactions, through modulating the effects of activated suppressor $CD8^+$ subpopulations on cytotoxic T cells required for resistance to intracellular infection or through enhancing cytotoxic T cell function directly, may be important in preventing superinfections in the ICU. T cell–T cell interactions also may be modified through cytokine manipulation, such as using IL-10, which will affect Th1–Th2 balance and host defense.

Intact functioning of T and B cell response, as well as maintenance of T cell–B cell interactions, is of central importance in resisting infection. Although critical illness produces multiple alterations in many of these components of immune response, therapies are becoming available that promise to restore immunocompetence in this setting. Such therapies, by preventing nosocomial infections and superinfections in the ICU, should result in significant improvement in patient outcome.

References

1. Abraham E: Host defense abnormalities after hemorrhage, trauma and burns. Crit Care Med 1989; 17:934–939.
2. Chaudry IH, Ayala A, Ertel W, et al: Hemorrhage and resuscitation: Immunological aspects. Am J Physiol 1990; 259:R663–R678.
3. Matis LA: The molecular basis of T cell specificity. Annu Rev Immunol 1990; 8:65–82.
4. Braciale TJ, Braciale VL: Antigen presentation: Structural themes and functional variations. Immunol Today 1991; 12:124–129.
5. Steinman RM: The dendritic cell system and its role in immunogenicity. Annu Rev Immunol 1991; 9:271–296.
6. Brodsky FM, Guagliardi L: The cell biology of antigen processing and presentation. Annu Rev Immunol 1991; 9:707–744.
7. Meldrum DR, Ayala A, Perrin MM, et al: Diltiazem restores IL-2, IL-3, IL-6 and IFN-γ synthesis and decreases host susceptibility to sepsis following hemorrhage. J Surg Res 1991; 51:158–164.
8. Ayala A, Perrin MM, Chaudry IH: Defective macrophage antigen presentation following hemorrhage is associated with the loss of MHC class II (Ia) antigens. Immunology 1990; 70:33–39.
9. Ayala AA, Perrin MM, Wagner MA, et al: Enhanced susceptibility to sepsis following simple hemorrhage: Depression of Fc and C3b receptor mediated phagocytosis. Arch Surg 1990; 125:70–75.
10. Kaufmann SHE: $CD8^+$ T lymphocytes in intracellular microbial infections. Immunol Today 1988; 9:168–173.
11. Stephan RN, Kupper TS, Geha AS, et al: Hemorrhage without tissue trauma produces immunosuppression and enhances susceptibility to sepsis. Arch Surg 1987; 122:62–68.
12. Chang Y-H, Jagels M, Abraham E: Hemorrhage produces depressions in alloantigen specific immune responses in the mouse through activation of suppressor T cells. Clin Exp Immunol 1990; 80:478–483.
13. O'Mahony JB, Palder SB, Wood JJ, et al: Depression of cellular immunity after multiple trauma in the absence of sepsis. J Trauma 1984; 24:869–874.
14. Grbic JT, Mannick JA, Gough DB, et al: The role of prostaglandin E_2 in immune suppression following injury. Surgery 1991; 214:253–262.
15. Abraham E, Freitas AA: Hemorrhage produces abnormalities in lymphocyte function and lymphokine generation. J Immunol 1989; 142:899–906.
16. Abraham E, Chang Y-H: Generation of functionally active suppressor cells by hemorrhage and hemorrhagic serum. Clin Exp Immunol 1988; 72:238–242.
17. Kupper TS, Green DR: Immunoregulation after thermal injury: Sequential appearance of $I\text{-}J^+$, Ly-1 T suppressor inducer and Ly-2 T suppressor effector cells following thermal trauma in mice. J Immunol 1984; 135:3047–3053.
18. Kupper TS, Baker CC, Ferguson TA, et al: A burn induced Ly-2 suppressor T cell lowers resistance to bacterial infection. J Surg Res 1985; 38:606–612.
19. Abraham E, Freitas AA, Jagels M, et al: Transfer of T or $CD8^+$ cells from hemorrhaged mice produces alterations in bacterial antigen specific B cell repertoire in normal syngeneic recipients. Immunobiology 1990; 181:379–387.
20. Durum SK, Schmidt JA, Oppenheim JJ: Interleukin-1: An immunological perspective. Annu Rev Immunol 1985; 3:263–287.
21. Okusawa S, Gelfand JA, Ikejima T, et al: Interleukin-1 induces a shock-like state in rabbits: Synergism with tumor necrosis factor and the effect of cyclooxygenase inhibition. J Clin Invest 1988; 81:1162–1172.
22. Ohlsson K, Bjork P, Bergenfeldt M, et al: An interleukin-1 receptor antagonist reduces mortality from endotoxin shock. Nature 1190; 348:550–552.
23. Mosmann TR, Coffman RL: Th1 and Th2 cells: Different patterns of lymphokine secretion lead to different functional properties. Annu Rev Immunol 1989; 7:145–173.
24. MacNeil IA, Suda T, Moore KW, et al: IL-10, a novel growth cofactor for mature and immature T cells. J Immunol 1990; 145:4167–4173.
25. Fiorentino DF, Zlotnick A, Mosmann TR, et al: IL-10 inhibits cytokine production by activated macrophages. J Immunol 1991; 147:3815–3822.
26. Howard M, O'Garra A: Biological properties of interleukin 10. Immunol Today 1992; 13:198–200.
27. Abraham E, Regan RF: The effects of hemorrhage and trauma on interleukin-2 production. Arch Surg 1985; 120:1341–1345.
28. Wood JJ, Rodrick ML, O'Mahony JB, et al: Inadequate interleukin 2 production: A fundamental immunological deficiency in patients with major burns. Ann Surg 1984; 200:311–320.
29. Abraham E, Chang Y-H: Hemorrhage-induced alterations in function and cytokine production of T cells and T cell subpopulations. Clin Exp Immunol 1992; 90:497–502.
30. Croft M, Swain SL: B cell response to fresh and effector T helper cells: Role of cognate T-B interaction and the cytokines IL-2, IL-4, and IL-6. J Immunol 1991; 146:4055–4064.
31. Owens T: Requirement for noncognate interaction with T cells for the activation of B cell immunoglobulin secretion by IL-2. Cell Immunol 1991; 133:352–361.
32. Gough DB, Moss NM, Jordan A, et al: Recombinant interleukin-2 improves immune response and host resistance to septic challenge in thermally injured mice. Surgery 1988; 104:292–300.
33. Abraham E, Lee RJ, Chang Y-H: The role of interleukin 2 in hemorrhage-induced abnormalities of lymphocyte proliferation. Circ Shock 1986; 18:205–214.
34. Abraham E, Regan RF, Chang Y-H: The lack of effect of recombinant interleukin 2 on trauma-induced abnormalities in lymphocyte proliferation. Crit Care Med 1986; 14:847–851.
35. Abraham E, Chang Y-H: Modulation of the post hemorrhage bacterial polysaccharide antigen specific antibody response by interleukins 2 and 4. Lymphokine Cytokine Res 1992; 4:241–246.
36. Fiorentino DF, Zlotnick A, Viera P, et al: IL-10 acts on the antigen-presenting cell to inhibit cytokine production by Th1 cells. J Immunol 1991; 146:3444–3451.
37. de Waal Malefyt R, Abrams J, Bennett B, et al: Interleukin 10 inhibits cytokine synthesis by human monocytes: An autoregulatory role of IL-10 produced by monocytes. J Exp Med 1991; 174:1209–1220.
38. Ertel W, Morrison MH, Ayala A, et al: Interferon-γ attenuates hemorrhage-induced suppression of macrophage and spleno-

cyte functions and decreases susceptibility to sepsis. Surgery 1992; 111:177–187.
39. Livingston DH, Malangoni MA: Interferon-γ restores immune competence after hemorrhagic shock. J Surg Res 1988; 45:37–43.
40. Malangoni MA, Livingston DH, Sonnenfeld G, et al: Interferon gamma and tumor necrosis factor alpha. Arch Surg 1990; 125:444–446.
41. Hershman MJ, Polk HC, Pietsch JD, et al: Modulation of infection by gamma interferon treatment following trauma. Infect Immun 1988; 56:2412–2418.
42. Heinzel FP: The role of IFN-γ in the pathology of experimental endotoxemia. J Immunol 1990; 145:2920–2924.
43. Dinarello CA: Interleukin-1 and its biologically related cytokines. Adv Immunol 1989; 44:153–167.
44. O'Riordain MG, Collins KH, Pilz M, et al: Modulation of macrophage hyperactivity improves survival in a burn-sepsis model. Arch Surg 1992; 127:152–157.
45. Silver GM, Gamelli RL, O'Reilly M, et al: The effect of interleukin 1 alpha on survival in a murine model of burn wound sepsis. Arch Surg 1990; 125:922–925.
46. Shenkar R, Abraham E: Effects of hemorrhage on cytokine gene transcription. Lymphokine Cytokine Res 1993; 12:237–247.
47. Abraham E, Freitas AA, Coutinho AA: Hemorrhage in mice produces alterations in B cell repertoires. Cell Immunol 1989; 122:208–217.
48. Abraham E, Chang Y-H: Hemorrhage in mice produces alterations in intestinal B cell repertoires. Cell Immunol 1990; 128:165–174.
49. Robinson AS, Abraham E: Hemorrhage in mice produces alterations in pulmonary B cell repertoires. J Immunol 1990; 145:3734–3739.
50. Robinson A, Abraham E: Effects of hemorrhage and resuscitation on bacterial antigen specific pulmonary plasma cell function. Crit Care Med 1991; 19:1285–1293.
51. Reidy JJ, Ramsay G: Clinical trials of selective decontamination of the digestive tract: Review. Crit Care Med 1990; 18:1449–1456.
52. Hammond JMJ, Potgieter PD, Saunders GL, et al: Double-blind study of selective decontamination of the digestive tract in intensive care. Lancet 1992; 340:5–9.
53. Stountenbeek CP, van Saene HKF, Miranda DR, et al: The effect of selective decontamination of the digestive tract on colonization and infection in multiple trauma patients. Intensive Care Med 1984; 10:185–192.
54. Abraham E, Shah S: Intranasal immunization with liposomes containing IL-2 enhances bacterial polysaccharide antigen-specific pulmonary secretory antibody response. J Immunol 1992; 149:3719–3726.
55. Valle A, Aubry JP, Durand I, et al: Il-4 and IL-2 upregulate the expression of antigen B7, the B cell counterstructure to T cell CD28: An amplification mechanism for T-B cell interactions. Int Immunol 1991; 3:229–236.

CHAPTER 25

Neutrophil-Endothelial Cell Interactions

Nicholas B. Vedder, MD • John M. Harlan, MD

The adherence of neutrophils to endothelium is a critical early event in host defense against microorganisms and in the repair of injured tissue. Under certain circumstances, however, the same mechanisms that mediate these normal processes can contribute to vascular and tissue injury. Neutrophil-mediated endothelial injury has been implicated as central to the pathogenesis of disorders produced by tissue ischemia and reperfusion as well as acute inflammatory diseases. Elucidation of the molecular basis of neutrophil-endothelial interactions, therefore, not only is important for understanding the acute inflammatory response but may also suggest new approaches to therapy of a wide range of human disease processes.[1–3]

NEUTROPHIL-MEDIATED INJURY

To carry out their normal functions in host defense and repair, neutrophils are armed with a diverse array of potent effector mechanisms.[2] In response to a spectrum of inflammatory stimuli such as cytokines, activated complement components, platelet-activating factor (PAF), bacterial peptides, or endotoxin, neutrophils are capable of generating and releasing a plethora of inflammatory mediators. These include reactive oxygen species, proteases, peptides, lipid mediators, and vasoactive substances.[3] When activation and release are appropriately controlled and regulated, the toxic substances act on bacteria or other material brought into the neutrophil by phagocytosis, resulting in efficient clearance of pathogens or diseased tissue. Over a century ago, Metchnikoff alluded to a process whereby phagocytic leukocytes could cause tissue injury as a result of uncontrolled release of toxic substances.[4] Neutrophil-mediated vascular and tissue injury with damage to otherwise viable host tissues and organs may result if regulatory mechanisms fail or if activation is initiated in response to diffuse or systemic inflammatory stimuli. The body, of course, has an abundance of endogenous tissue- and plasma-based anti-inflammatory mechanisms to protect itself against such processes.[5] It is abundantly clear, however, that these endogenous mechanisms can become overwhelmed and that neutrophil-mediated vascular and tissue injury can contribute to the pathogenesis of a wide variety of clinical disorders.

Neutrophil adherence to endothelium plays a pivotal role in both neutrophil-mediated defense and repair as well as neutrophil-mediated vascular injury (Fig. 25–1). Observations of the microcirculation using intravital microscopy have elucidated a sequence of events involved in neutrophil-endothelial adhesive interactions at the site of inflammation.[1, 6, 7] In response to inflammatory stimuli, signals are generated that act on both the neutrophil and the endothelial cell to initiate a sequence of events, an early step of which is increased neutrophil and endothelial cell adhesiveness. Neutrophils are first seen leaving the laminar flow stream and rolling along the endothelial wall of postcapillary venules at the site of inflammation. This is then followed by firm adherence to the endothelium, which arrests the neutrophil, followed subsequently by diapedesis and emigration. Once firmly adherent to the endothelium, a protected microenvironment develops beneath the adherent neutrophil in which its proteases, oxidants, or other toxic products can cause injury to the endothelium, inaccessible to circulating anti-inflammatory agents.[5, 8] This direct endothelial injury by activated neutrophils can result in loss of microvascular integrity with edema, hemorrhage, or thrombosis and ultimately organ dysfunction. Increased neutrophil adhesiveness can also cause tissue injury through homotypic adhesion or aggregation. Aggregates of neutrophils adherent to each other can occlude the microcirculation, resulting in tissue hypoperfusion and further ischemic damage.[9] Finally, once emigrated, neutrophils can continue to release toxic products that directly injure tissue and provoke organ damage. It is apparent, therefore, that understanding the cellular and molecular mechanisms that mediate neutrophil adherence to endothelium is central to understanding and potentially modulating neutrophil-mediated injury.

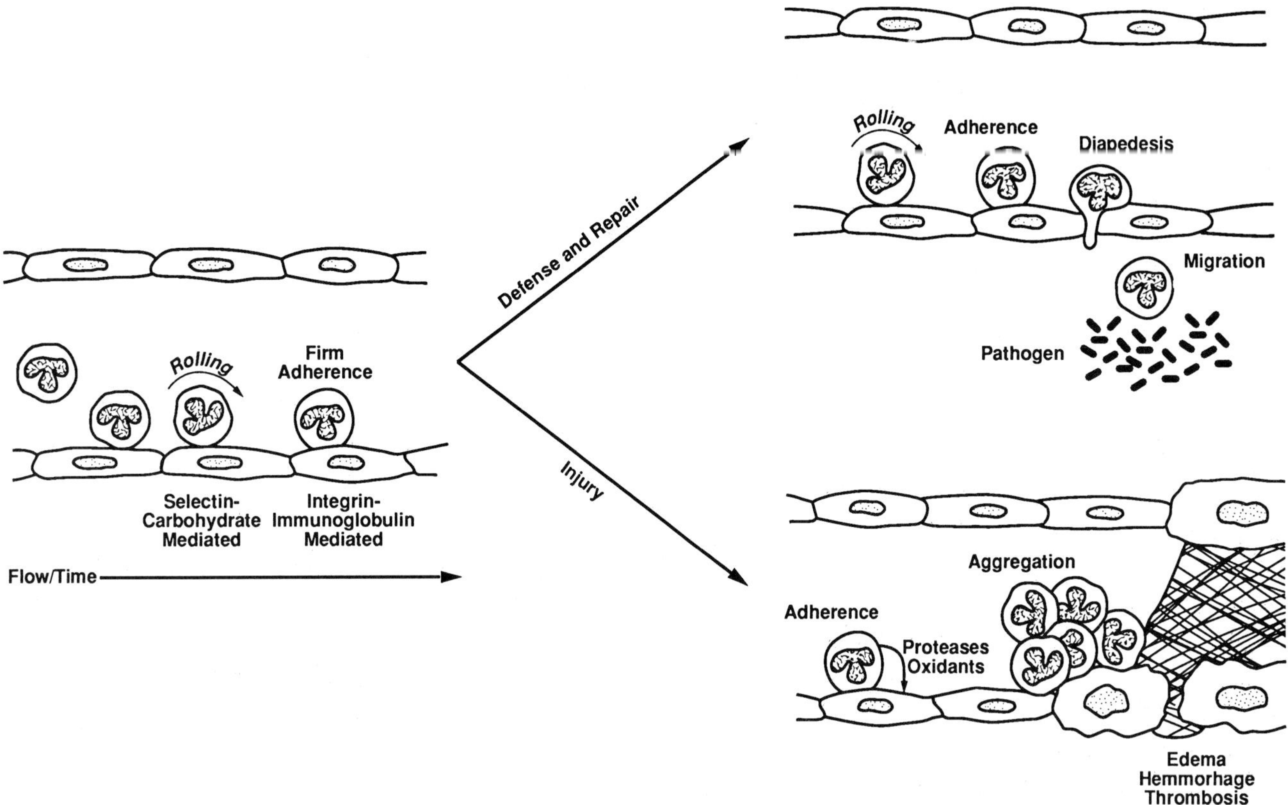

Figure 25–1. Diagrammatic representation of the sequential events that occur at a site of inflammation as neutrophils leave the laminar flow stream of a postcapillary venule. Initial selectin/carbohydrate-mediated rolling along the surface of the endothelium is followed by integrin/immunoglobulin-mediated firm adherence. These two events are required either for neutrophil emigration in the setting of defense and repair or for neutrophil-mediated endothelial injury in pathologic conditions.

MECHANISMS OF ADHESION

Since the time of Cohnheim[10] and Metchnikoff,[4] it was a matter of debate whether alterations in the neutrophil or in the endothelial cell were responsible for the critical adhesive interaction. Not surprisingly, it is now clear that both cell types are involved. In just the past decade, more than a dozen proteins involved in this interaction have been immunologically identified and molecularly cloned and their functions defined in vivo as well as in vitro.[11–13] These adherence molecules are currently classified into two major categories (Fig. 25–2). The first category includes the leukocyte integrin receptors, which interact with ligands on the endothelial cell that are members of the immunoglobulin superfamily.[14] The integrin-immunoglobulin interaction mediates firm adhesion of neutrophils to endothelium at sites of inflammation as well as subsequent diapedesis and emigration. The second category is the selectin receptors, which are lectin-containing proteins that recognize specific carbohydrate counterstructures.[15] Selectin-mediated adhesion is generally a weaker interaction than integrin-immunoglobulin adhesion. However, selectin-mediated adhesion is observed under conditions of flow, whereas integrin-dependent adhesion is sensitive to shear and is optimal under static conditions.[16] Thus, selectin receptors appear to be responsible for the initial transient adhesion of neutrophils that occurs at sites of inflammation, manifested as "rolling." Once slowed by selectin-carbohydrate interactions, local inflammatory stimuli subsequently activate the neutrophils to produce firm integrin-immunoglobulin adhesion.

Integrin/Immunoglobulin-Mediated Adhesion

The recent explosion of knowledge in the field of neutrophil-endothelial cell adhesion originated from studies of a genetic deficiency syndrome known as leukocyte adhesion deficiency (LAD) in which patients manifest recurrent bacterial infections and an inability to suppurate.[17] These patients' neutrophils demonstrate defective adherence functions both in vitro and in vivo as a result of a deficiency of the leukocyte adhesion receptor complex, CD11/CD18.

The CD11/CD18 complex consists of three heterodimeric glycoprotein subunits. Each subunit consists of a light or β-chain polypeptide common to all three subunits, designated CD18, and a distinct heavy or α-chain polypeptide, designated CD11a, CD11b, or CD11c. These subunits are commonly known as LFA-1 (CD11a/CD18); Mac-1, Mo1, or CR3 (CD11b/CD18); and p150,95 (CD11c/CD18). LFA-1 is found on all leukocytes, whereas Mac-1 and p150,95 are found on phagocytes and natural killer cells but not on most lymphocytes. The three CD11 α-chains as well as the CD18 β-chain have been cloned and shown to be members of the integrin superfamily of adhesion receptors, comprising the β_2 subclass, which is unique to leukocytes.[12, 14]

The molecular basis of the CD11/CD18 deficiency syndrome has been demonstrated to be heterogeneous mutations in the common β chain, resulting in a deficient or abnormal β chain that fails to associate with the normal α chain into heterodimers.[17] Without heterodimer formation, neither α- nor β-chain polypeptides are inserted into the plasma membrane. This leads to a severe defect in neutrophil emigration at sites of inflammation because, without functional CD11/CD18, the critical steps of adherence to and diapedesis across endothelium cannot occur.[18] The defect in adhesion-dependent functions of these neutrophils can be reproduced in normal neutrophils by the addition of monoclonal antibodies directed to function-related epitopes of the CD11/CD18 glycoprotein complex.

Studies with cultured human umbilical vein endothelial

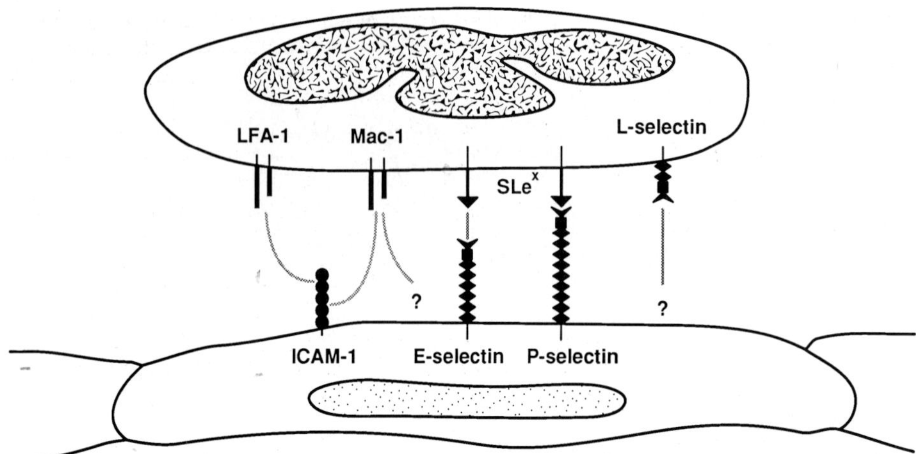

Figure 25–2. Diagrammatic representation of the known neutrophil-endothelial adhesion receptors. The β_2 integrin receptors on neutrophils, LFA-1 (CD11a/CD18) and Mac-1 (CD11b/CD18; both represented as α/β dimers) bind to intercellular adhesion molecule-1 (ICAM-1 [CD54], represented with its five immunoglobulin domains) and another (other) as yet unidentified ligand (ligands) on the endothelial cell. Endothelial E-selectin (CD62E) and P-selectin (CD62P; represented with their N-terminal lectin domain, epidermal growth factor domain, multiple complement regulatory repeat sequences, transmembrane domain, and cytoplasmic domain) bind to carbohydrate ligands, particularly Sialyl Lewis X antigen (SLe^x; CD15s), expressed on glycoproteins or glycolipids of neutrophils. L-selectin (CD62L) on neutrophils binds to (an) as yet unidentified carbohydrate ligands (ligand) on endothelium in the systemic vasculature.

cells (HUVEC) demonstrate that normal neutrophils exhibit a very low level of basal adherence to HUVEC. With stimulation of neutrophils using tumor necrosis factor (TNF)-α, C5a, interleukin(IL)-8, PAF, endotoxin, or bacterial chemotactic peptide, there is a dramatic increase in neutrophil adhesiveness to endothelium (and with many of these substances, an increase in homotypic neutrophil adhesion, i.e., aggregation, as well). Addition of monoclonal antibodies directed to functional epitopes of CD11b or CD18 essentially eliminates this increased adhesiveness and, in so doing, effectively blocks neutrophil-mediated endothelial injury in vitro.[8] Inhibition of tight adherence prevents formation of a closed interface between the adherent neutrophil and the endothelium in which proteases and oxidants released by the activated neutrophil can cause injury to the endothelium.[5] This approach to inhibiting neutrophil-mediated injury, therefore, has a potential significant advantage over antiproteases or antioxidants, which are ineffective once adherence has created a protected microenvironment.

For neutrophils, CD11b/CD18 (Mac-1, Mo1, CR3) appears to be the heterodimer most responsible for firm adhesion, although CD11a/CD18 (LFA-1) is also involved.[19] The mechanism by which CD11b/CD18 augments neutrophil adhesiveness in response to stimulation is not entirely clear. In unstimulated neutrophils, the CD11b/CD18 heterodimer exists on the cell surface and in greater quantities within the secondary or tertiary granules. After stimulation, the contents of these granules are translocated to the cell surface, resulting in a 3- to 10-fold increase in surface-associated CD11b/CD18. This increase in surface expression, however, is neither necessary nor sufficient to cause increased adhesiveness.[20] Instead, the primary mechanism appears to be an activation of surface receptors that produces a conformational change, resulting in a high-avidity binding to ligand. The molecular basis for avidity modulation of the β_2-integrin receptor has not been defined, although allosteric changes induced by intracellular lipids have been suggested.[21] This activation process and avidity modulation are logical targets for manipulating neutrophil adhesion and neutrophil-mediated injury in inflammation.

The endothelial counterstructures for the CD11/CD18 complex include intercellular adhesion molecule (ICAM)-1 and ICAM-2, two members of the immunoglobulin superfamily.[12,14] ICAM-1 is recognized by CD11b/CD18, although there appear to be other as yet unidentified endothelial ligands for CD11b/CD18. ICAM-1 is expressed at low levels on resting endothelial ligands for CD11b/CD18. ICAM-1 is expressed at low levels on resting endothelium in vitro and in vivo, and it is up-regulated over a period of hours in response to inflammatory stimuli, such as lipopolysaccharide (LPS), IL-1β and TNF. Monoclonal antibodies to ICAM-1 inhibit neutrophil adherence to endothelium after inflammatory stimulation in vitro, although to a lesser extend than monoclonal antibodies to CD11b or CD18.

The importance of integrin-immunoglobulin–mediated adhesion to the process of neutrophil-mediated inflammation and injury in vivo is illustrated by animal models of acute inflammation that have used monoclonal antibodies to CD11b, CD18, or ICAM-1. The first such study used intravital microscopy to examine neutrophil-endothelial adhesion and neutrophil-mediated injury in response to superfusion of a chemoattractant.[22] It was shown that a blocking CD18 monoclonal antibody effectively abolished neutrophil adherence to endothelium at the site of inflammation. With blockade of adherence, neutrophil emigration and endothelial injury, as evidenced by plasma leakage, were also effectively inhibited. Similar findings have also been noted with monoclonal antibodies to CD11b and ICAM-1, further demonstrating the central role of the CD11/CD18-ICAM-1 interactions in neutrophil-mediated inflammation and injury.

Another member of the immunoglobulin superfamily, platelet-endothelial cell adhesion molecule-1 (PECAM-1 [CD31]) has been identified and cloned.[22a] It is found on the surface of platelets, at endothelial intercellular junctions, and on cells of myelomonocytic lineage, and it has been shown to play an important role in neutrophil-endothelial adhesion and, particularly, in transendothelial migration of phagocytes.[22b, 22c]

Selectin/Carbohydrate-Mediated Adhesion

Selectin receptors and their carbohydrate counterstructures are the other major category of adhesion molecules involved in neutrophil-endothelial cell adhesion.[15] Recent in vitro and in vivo evidence suggests that selectin-mediated adhesion is relatively resistant to shear forces and plays an important role in the initial rolling of neutrophils along the endothelium at sites of inflammation. The three selectin receptors are L-selectin (CD62L; previously also known as LAM-1, Leu-8, or LECAM-1), E-selectin (CD62E; previously known as ELAM-1), and P-selectin (CD62P; previously known as GMP-140, PADGEM, or CD62). E-selectin is localized to endothelial cells, P-selectin is found on platelets as well as endothelial cells, and L-selectin is expressed only on leukocytes. The selectin molecules consist of an amino-terminal lectin domain, an epidermal growth factor domain, a variable number of complement regulatory repeat sequences, a transmembrane domain, and a carboxy-terminal cytoplasmic domain. Binding occurs between the lectin domain and the specific carbohydrate counterstructure on either the neutrophil (in the case of E- and P-selectin) or the endothelial cell (in the case of L-selectin). For E- and P-selectin receptors, the Sialyl Lewis X (SLe^x; CD15s) antigen is a major counterstructure.[23] Sialyl Lewis X is expressed on a number of glycolipids and glycoproteins, including P-selectin glycoprotein ligand, a mucin-like molecule that may present SLe^x to P- and E-selectin.[24] Sulfation of the carbohydrate ligand may also enhance binding. From studies of two patients with a second form of leukocyte adhesion deficiency (designated LAD type 2), it is clear that the ligand for E- and P-selectin must by fucosylated. The LAD type 2 patients have a general defect in fucose metabolism and are unable to form SLe^x or any other fucosylated structure. They exhibit a defect in neutrophil emigration in vivo, and neutrophils from these patients are unable to bind to E-selectin expressed on HUVEC in vitro.[25]

In cultured HUVEC, P-selectin is not expressed and is minimally expressed on the surface of unstimulated endothelium in vivo but is rapidly inducible within minutes of stimulation with thrombin, histamine, phorbol ester, or hydrogen peroxide.[15] This increased surface expression does not require de novo synthesis because P-selectin is stored within the Weibel-Palade bodies and is quickly translocated to the cell surface in response to stimulation.[26]

In vitro experiments have demonstrated that purified P-selectin bound to platelets is capable of mediating neutrophil rolling at physiologic shear stress rates without causing firm adhesion even with cessation of flow.[16] In contrast, an isolated integrin–ICAM-1 system does not support rolling or adherence at physiologic flow rates but can produce firm adherence once rolling is first induced by P-selectin. P-selectin–mediated adhesion, then, provides an ideal mechanism for initially slowing neutrophils at sites of inflammation so that stimulation can occur, leading to firm, integrin-mediated adhesion and subsequent diapedesis or, under some conditions, to direct endothelial injury.

Unlike P-selectin, L-selectin is constitutively expressed on the neutrophil in the basal state and is rapidly shed from the surface in response to stimulation.[13] L-selectin binds to a cytokine-induced ligand on HUVEC in vitro[27] as well as to high endothelial venules of lymph nodes. Although Gly-CAM-1 and CD34 have been identified as ligands for L-selectin on high endothelial venules in the mouse,[28, 28a] the ligand for L-selectin on systemic endothelium is unknown. Like E- and P-selectin, L-selectin may recognize SLe^x, although this structure has not been identified on the surface of basal or stimulated HUVEC. The importance of L-selectin to neutrophil recruitment at sites of inflammation in vivo is supported by intravital microscopy studies that have demonstrated that monoclonal antibodies to or blocking forms of L-selectin can effectively inhibit neutrophil rolling and subsequent adhesion at sites of early inflammation.[27, 29] Neutrophil emigration and accumulation can be similarly inhibited in models of inflammation by either selectin antibodies or SLe^x oligosaccharide.[29a]

Although E-selectin shares the same binding properties as the other selectins, its time course of induction in vitro is notably different. In contrast to P-selectin, which is rapidly translocated from preformed stores to the endothelial surface within minutes of stimulation, E-selectin requires de novo protein synthesis and, therefore, does not reach peak surface expression for 4 to 6 hours.[15] The agents responsible for inducing E-selectin expression are also different, being primarily the cytokines, IL-1β, TNF-α, and LPS. Although the duration of expression of E-selectin is much longer than P-selectin on HUVEC in vitro, it declines rapidly in comparison to ICAM-1, with much reduced but detectable levels observed 24 hours after stimulation. In vitro studies suggest that the rapid decline results from both a decrease in transcription and rapid internalization. In cultured HUVEC, interferon-γ augments and prolongs E-selectin expression induced by TNF-α,[30] suggesting additional mechanisms of regulation. In contrast to the relatively transient expression of E-selectin observed in vitro, E-selectin has been found to persist at inflammatory sites in vivo. The identification of markedly increased expression of E-selectin in sepsis[31] and at sites of chronic inflammation such as rheumatoid joints[32] and delayed-type hypersensitivity reactions[33] supports this role for E-selectin and suggests that E-selectin may be involved in subacute and chronic inflammatory or immune reactions as well as more acute processes.

Coordination of Neutrophil-Endothelial Cell Interactions

It is evident that the mechanisms involved in neutrophil adherence to endothelium and subsequent neutrophil-mediated endothelial injury are complex and likely quite varied, depending on the vascular bed, the degree and nature of the inflammatory stimulus, and the time course involved. In the healthy state, there is minimal interaction between circulating neutrophils and the vascular endothelium. In response to an extravascular inflammatory stimulus, there is an initial rapidly induced, selectin-mediated rolling at the site of inflammation, likely involving either P- or L-selectin or later through the induction and synthesis of E-selectin. Factors released as part of the early inflammatory process such as thrombin, histamine, and oxidants can initiate P-selectin expression and thereby induce leukocyte rolling, whereas cytokines generated later, such as IL-1 and TNF-α can induce the L-selectin ligand or E-selectin. Rolling allows the neutrophils to come in contact with the endothelium of the inflamed vessels where subsequent activation of the integrin receptors by various agonists produces firm adherence.[13, 16]

PAF or chemotactic peptides such as IL-8 may play important roles in initiating integrin/ICAM-1-mediated adhesion. In vitro, PAF is expressed on the endothelial surface along with P-selectin in response to thrombin, histamine, and oxidizing agents, and PAF can, in turn, result in up-regulation and activation of neutrophil integrins, leading to the second step of firm adhesion. This effect can be blocked by either inhibiting P-selectin or the PAF receptor, suggesting that a coordinated or "juxtacrine" process is involved.[34] IL-8 is a potent neutrophil chemoattractant that is a member of the cys-cys subfamily of chemokinetic proteins. It is produced by endothelial cells and diverse other cell types in response to TNF-α, IL-1, or LPS. Endothelial-derived IL-8 in subendothelial tissue may promote integrin-dependent adherence and diapedesis,[35] although intravascular IL-8 has paradoxically been noted to inhibit emigration.[36]

Additional mechanisms are also involved in the regulation of neutrophil adherence to endothelium. Other cytokines (e.g., TNF-α), infectious agents (N-formyl-methionyl-leucyl-phenylalanine, LPS), and chemotaxins (leukotriene B_4 [LTB_4], C5a) can all increase the surface expression of β_2-integrin (CD11/CD18) receptors, which may be an important factor in augmenting adhesion. As mentioned previously, however, increased surface expression of integrin receptors of itself is insufficient to cause adhesion, and receptor "activation" is required, resulting in a conformational change that increases adhesiveness. Phosphorylation of the amino acids in the cytoplasmic domain of the receptor subunits and binding of a lipid mediator to the intracellular region of the integrin receptor have been suggested potential mechanisms of effecting allosteric changes.[21] However, the precise biochemical basis of this "inside-out" signaling remains to be elucidated.[37]

Similar to the regulation noted in CD11b/CD18, L-selectin has also been observed to transiently bind ligand more avidly with activation.[38] Notably, with continued exposure, many of the stimuli that cause up-regulated surface expression and increased avidity of CD11b/CD18 also produce shedding of L-selectin (i.e., the integrin and selectin receptors are inversely regulated).[13] Loss of L-selectin with activation of neutrophils in the vascular lumen may serve as a mechanism to limit neutrophil recruitment at sites of inflammation.

Although an increase in the avidity of integrin receptors is important for firm adherence, neutrophil migration requires that there also be mechanisms to decrease avidity (i.e., "turn off" the receptor). Indeed, avidity regulation by sequential activation-deactivation of the receptor is essential for movement. "Freezing" integrin receptors in the high-avidity state has been shown to enhance adherence but markedly inhibit transendothelial migration in vitro.[39] The mechanisms involved in "deactivation" of integrin receptors in neutrophils are not yet defined.

There are, therefore, numerous factors involved in the regulation of neutrophil-endothelial adhesive interactions. As our knowledge and understanding of the molecular basis of neutrophil adherence to endothelium increases, the tools for manipulating these processes will continue to expand, allowing more detailed analysis of neutrophil-mediated injury processes and their role in human disease.

IN VIVO MODELS OF NEUTROPHIL-MEDIATED INJURY

Although no human clinical trials using specific agents to inhibit neutrophil-endothelial cell adhesion have been completed to date, there have been multiple studies using monoclonal antibodies to various adhesion receptors to examine the role of neutrophil-mediated injury in a wide variety of animal models (Table 25–1). These studies fall into two major groups: processes involving ischemia-reperfusion and those of an inflammatory or immune origin.[1]

Ischemia-Reperfusion Injury

Ischemia-related cellular, tissue, and organ injuries form the basis of many important clinical disorders including myocardial infarction, stroke, peripheral vascular disease, and circulatory shock. Although much progress has been made in the area of early restoration of perfusion, there is evidence that, in some settings, a significant proportion of the tissue damage triggered by ischemia may be a consequence of events associated with reperfusion of ischemia tissues (i.e., "reperfusion injury"). Oxygen-derived free radicals generated at the time of reperfusion have been identified as potentially important mediators of this reperfusion injury.[40, 41] Another important source of free radicals is the neutrophil, which can also cause injury through the release of proteases and phospholipase products. An important role for neutrophils in ischemia-reperfusion injury is suggested by studies that have shown a close association between neutrophil accumulation and tissue injury in this setting and by studies that have demonstrated injury reduction by depletion of circulating neutrophils.[42]

TABLE 25–1. Antiadhesion Therapy in Experimental Models of Vascular and Tissue Injury*

Ischemia/Reperfusion	*Inflammatory/Immune*
Intestinal ischemia[47]	Inflammatory skin lesions[22, 56]
Tissue reperfusion injury[43, 43a]	Edema in meningitis[57, 57a]
Shock/resuscitation[53, 54]	Endotoxic shock[58, 59]
Myocardial ischemia[48, 49, 49a–c]	Allergic asthma[60]
Skeletal muscle ischemia[51]	Autoimmune diabetes[61]
Central nervous system ischemia[50]	Pulmonary oxygen toxicity[62]
	NSAID-induced gastric injury[63]
	Burns[64, 65]
	Graft rejection[66, 67]
	Inflammatory lung injury[29b, 67a–c]

*Experimental models in which monoclonal antibodies that block neutrophil-endothelial adhesion molecules have been shown to be effective at attenuating injury. These studies fall into two major groups: processes of an inflammatory or immune origin, and those involving ischemia-reperfusion.

Abbreviation: NSAID = nonsteroidal anti-inflammatory drug.

Adherent, activated neutrophils can cause direct endothelial injury, resulting in loss of vascular integrity and producing edema, hemorrhage, and thrombosis (see Fig. 25–1). Another possible mechanism of injury involves adherence of neutrophils to the endothelium of the microvasculature and aggregation of neutrophils within the vessel lumen, leading to occlusion and further ischemia.[9] Thus, a progressive downward spiral may result in which reperfusion induces neutrophil activation and adherence, leading to leukocyte accumulation and endothelial injury, which then results in further ischemia and eventually complete cessation of flow. This may be the basis of what has in the past been called the *no-reflow phenomenon,* which more precisely might be called a *diminishing reflow phenomenon.*[43]

The mechanisms by which neutrophil adherence and injury are initiated in the setting of ischemia-reperfusion are not entirely clear. However, there is good evidence that oxygen-derived free radicals are generated at the time of reperfusion.[40, 41] These can initiate the process of selectin-mediated adhesion, release of PAF, and subsequent integrin-mediated adhesion.[44] The important role of oxygen free radicals in initiating this process has been further demonstrated both in vitro and in vivo.[45, 46]

The use of monoclonal antibodies directed against specific adhesion proteins has been shown to be extremely effective at inhibiting neutrophil accumulation and neutrophil-mediated reperfusion injury in a number of animal models. The first such study examined the role of neutrophils in reperfusion injury of feline gut.[47] A CD18 monoclonal antibody effectively attenuated the increase in plasma leakage that normally occurs after intestinal ischemia and reperfusion.

Studies using the isolated rabbit ear, based on its vascular pedicle, also showed that blocking neutrophil adherence functions with CD18[43] or P-selectin[43a] monoclonal antibody markedly reduced reperfusion-associated edema formation as well as tissue necrosis.[43] In these particular studies, the degree of protection was the same whether antibody was administered before ischemia or after ischemia but immediately before reperfusion. This result provided strong evidence that neutrophil-mediated injury in the setting of ischemia and reperfusion occurs at the time of reperfusion as activated neutrophils flood the vascular bed, causing diffuse endothelial and tissue injury. In this sense, the injury is in fact a true "reperfusion injury."

Inhibition of CD18/ICAM-mediated or selectin/carbohydrate-mediated adherence has also been shown to be effective at attenuating reperfusion injury in myocardium,[48, 49] the central nervous system,[50] and permeability edema in skeletal muscle.[51] Even remote effects of neutrophil-mediated reperfusion injury can be potentially inhibited in this way, as has been shown with the reduction of remote lung injury after hind-limb ischemia-reperfusion.[52]

Hemorrhagic shock followed by resuscitation is another important form of ischemia-reperfusion injury, representing a global or generalized ischemia-reperfusion injury. In this regard, inhibition of CD18-mediated neutrophil adherence and injury has been shown to reduce organ injury, attenuate the generalized microvascular injury, and improve survival in both small animal and subhuman primate models of hypovolemic shock.[53, 54] Once again, this approach is just as effective if treatment is administered after shock but before reperfusion, suggesting that the significant injury that occurs after profound shock and resuscitation is also a reperfusion injury.[55] In these studies, control animals experienced severe hemorrhagic gastritis and a diffuse capillary leak, requiring large volumes of resuscitation fluid to maintain cardiac output. Treatment with a single dose of CD18 monoclonal antibody at the time of resuscitation almost completely prevented both of these events and led to significant reductions in mortality in rabbit survival studies. These findings also suggest that neutrophil-mediated injury may play an important role in the development of multiple organ injury and multiple organ failure syndrome, which is a frequent and devastating consequence of severe traumatic shock.

Inflammatory/Immune Origin

Monoclonal antibodies to adherence molecules have also been used in a variety of models of inflammatory or immune disease processes.[1] A number of studies have shown that CD18 monoclonal antibodies effectively inhibit neutrophil accumulation and permeability edema in inflammatory skin lesions.[22, 56] In addition, both CD18 and anti-ICAM-1 antibodies, as well as saccharides, have been shown to be effective at attenuating injury associated with bacterial meningitis,[57] endotoxic shock,[58, 59] allergic asthma,[60] autoimmune diabetes,[61] pulmonary oxygen toxicity,[62] nonsteroidal-induced gastric mucosal injury,[63] and thermal burns,[64, 65] and attenuating cardiac and renal allograft rejection.[66, 67] Blockade of selectin-carbohydrate interactions has also been demonstrated to reduce vascular and tissue damage in several models of acute inflammatory lung injury.[29b, 67a–67c]

There is evidence to suggest that inhibiting neutrophil adherence in the setting of overt sepsis may actually improve outcome under certain circumstances. CD18 blockade has been shown to improve hemodynamics, reduce fluid requirements, and improve survival in rabbit models of both gram-negative and endotoxic shock.[58] Treatment with a CD11b monoclonal antibody increased survival in endotoxic shock in mice.[59] These studies seem to challenge the evidence from the LAD type 1 syndrome that neutrophil adherence and emigration are necessary for host defense because severely deficient patients often die from sepsis. However, they support the concept that uncontrolled inflammation can be equally deleterious.

THERAPEUTIC POTENTIAL

Given the diverse array of important disease processes in which antiadhesion therapy has shown such striking protective effects in animal models, it is exciting to speculate about the clinical therapeutic potential of such an approach. At this time, there are a number of clinical trials that are either ongoing or planned that will examine the efficacy and safety of antiadhesion therapy. These studies will use either murine or humanized monoclonal antibodies directed to CD11/CD18, ICAM-1, or the selectins or will use small molecules to inhibit either integrin–ICAM-1 or selectin-mediated adhesion.

In contemplating such an approach, however, one must keep in mind that, by inhibiting neutrophil adherence functions, one essentially recreates the LAD syndromes. The risk of infection must be carefully weighed against any potential benefit of this form of therapy. Studies have shown that blocking CD18 does not increase mortality or infectious complications in models of bacterial peritonitis[68] and can actually improve outcome in certain septic models such as bacterial meningitis[57] and gram-negative sepsis,[58] as described previously. It has also been shown, however, that, with extremely high inocula of subcutaneous bacteria, there can be an increase in infectious complications and mortality even after a single dose of CD18 monoclonal antibody, although this effect is not seen with lower, clinically relevant inocula of bacteria,[69] nor is it seen with P-selectin blockade.[69a]

Although these studies suggest that it may be safe to inhibit neutrophil adherence functions for a limited period of time in a carefully defined setting, they also must raise a significant note of caution about completely inhibiting such a basic physiologic process. It stands to reason that the more acute disease processes such as those related to ischemia-reperfusion may be more amenable to and, perhaps, more appropriate for controlled, transient inhibition of adherence.

CONCLUSION

The adhesive interaction between neutrophils and the endothelium is a fundamental event in the acute inflammatory response. Recent in vitro and in vivo studies have yielded important new insights into the basic cellular and molecular mechanisms that mediate these interactions and have provided tools to manipulate them. The result is an increased understanding of the contribution of neutrophils to vascular and tissue injury in acute inflammation and a potential new approach to the treatment of human disease processes.

References

1. Harlan JM, Winn RK, Vedder NB, et al: In vivo models of leukocyte adherence to endothelium. *In*: Adhesion: Its Role in Inflammatory Disease. Harlan JM, Lui D (Eds). New York, WH Freeman, 1992, pp 117–150.
2. Malech HL, Gallin JI: Current concepts: Immunology: Neutrophils in human diseases. N Engl J Med 1987; 317:687–694.
3. Weiss SJ: Tissue destruction by neutrophils. N Engl J Med 1989; 320:365–376.
4. Metchnikoff E: Sur lallutte des cellules de l'organisme contre l'invasion des microbes. Ann Inst Pasteur 1887; 1:321.
5. Harlan JM: Neutrophil-mediated vascular injury. Acta Med Scand Suppl 1987; 715:123–129.
6. Grant L: The sticking and emigration of white blood cells in inflammation. *In*: The Inflammatory Process. Zweifach BL, McCluskey L (Eds). Orlando, FL, Academic Press, 1973, pp 205–249.
7. Movat HZ: The role of endothelium in leukocytes emigration: The views of Cohnheim, Metchnikoff and their contemporaries. Pathol Immunopathol Res 1989; 8:35–41.
8. Diener AM, Beatty PG, Ochs HD, et al: The role of neutrophil membrane glycoprotein 150 (GP-150) in neutrophil-mediated endothelial cell injury in vitro. J Immunol 1985; 135:537–543.
9. Schmid-Schönbein GW: Capillary plugging by granulocytes and the no-reflow phenomenon in the microcirculation. Fed Proc 1987; 46:2397–2401.
10. Cohnheim J: Lectures in General Pathology. London, New Sydenham Society, 1889, pp 242–382.
11. Carlos TM, Harlan JM: Membrane proteins involved in phagocyte adherence to endothelium. Immunol Rev 1990; 114:5–28.
12. Springer TA: Adhesion receptors of the immune system. Nature 1990; 346:425–434.
13. Butcher EC: Leukocyte-endothelial cell recognition: Three (or more) steps to specificity and diversity. Cell 1991; 67:1033–1036.
14. Lobb RR: Integrin-immunoglobulin superfamily interactions in endothelial-leukocyte adhesion. *In*: Adhesion: Its Role in Inflammatory Disease. Harlan JM, Liu DY (Eds). New York, WH Freeman, 1992, pp 1–18.
15. Bevilacqua MP, Nelson RM: Selectins. J Clin Invest 1993; 91:379–387.

16. Lawrence MB, Springer TA: Leukocytes roll on a selectin at physiologic flow rates: Distinction from and prerequisite for adhesion through integrins. Cell 1991; 65:859–873.
17. Anderson DC, Springer TA: Leukocyte adhesion deficiency: An inherited defect in the Mac-1, LFA-1, and p150,95 glycoproteins. Annu Rev Med 1987; 38:175–194.
18. Harlan JM, Killen PD, Senecal FM, et al: The role of neutrophil membrane glycoprotein GP-150 in neutrophil adherence to endothelium in vitro. Blood 1985; 66:167–178.
19. Smith CW, Marlin SD, Rothlein R, et al: Cooperative interactions of LFA-1 and Mac-1 with intercellular adhesion molecule-1 in facilitating adherence and transendothelial migration of human neutrophils in vitro. J Clin Invest 1989; 83:2008–2017.
20. Vedder NB, Harlan JM: Increased surface expression of CD11b/CD18 (Mac-1) is not required for stimulated neutrophil adherence to cultured endothelium. J Clin Invest 1988; 81:676–682.
21. Hermanowski-Vosatka A, Van-Strijp JA, Swiggard WJ, et al: Integrin modulating factor-1: A lipid that alters the function of leukocyte integrins. Cell 1992; 68:341–352.
22. Arfors K-E, Lundberg C, Lindbom L, et al: A monoclonal antibody to the membrane glycoprotein complex CDw18 (LFA) inhibits PMN accumulation and plasma leakage in vivo. Blood 1987; 69:338–340.
22a. Newman PJ, Berndt MC, Gorski J, et al: PECAM-1 (CD31) cloning and relation to adhesion molecules of the immunoglobulin gene superfamily. Science 1990; 247:1219–1222.
22b. Muller WA, Weigl SA, Deng X, et al: PECAM-1 is required for transendothelial migration of leukocytes. J Exp Med 1993; 178:449–460.
22c. Vaporciyan AA, DeLisser HM, Yan HC, et al: Involvement of platelet-endothelial cell adhesion molecule-1 in neutrophil recruitment in vivo. Science 1993; 262:1580–1582.
23. Polley MJ, Phillips ML, Wayner E, et al: CD62 and endothelial cell-leukocyte adhesion molecule 1 (ELAM-1) recognize the same carbohydrate ligand, sialyl-Lewis x. Proc Natl Acad Sci USA 1991; 88:6224–6228.
24. Sako D, Chang XJ, Barone KM, et al: Expression cloning of a functional glycoprotein ligand for P-selectin. Cell 1993; 75:1179–1186
25. Etzioni A, Frydman M, Pollack S, et al: Brief report: Recurrent severe infections caused by a novel leukocyte adhesion deficiency. N Engl J Med 1992; 327:1789–1792.
25a. von-Andrian UH, Berger EM, Ramezani L, et al: In vivo behavior of neutrophils from two patients with distinct inherited leukocyte adhesion deficiency syndromes. J Clin Invest 1993; 91:2893–2897.
26. McEver RP, Beckstead JH, Moore KL, et al: GMP-140, a platelet alpha-granule membrane protein, is also synthesized by vascular endothelial cells and is localized in Weibel-Palade bodies. J Clin Invest 1989; 84:92–99.
27. Ley K, Gaehtgens P, Fennie C, et al: Lectin-like cell adhesion molecule 1 mediates leukocyte rolling in mesenteric venules in vivo. Blood 1991; 77:2553–2555.
28. Lasky LA, Singer MS, Dowbenko D, et al: An endothelial ligand for L-selectin is a novel mucin-like molecule. Cell 1992; 69:927–938.
28a. Baumheter S, Singer MS, Henzel W, et al: Binding of L-selectin to the vascular sialomucin CD34. Science 1993; 262:436–438.
29. von Andrian UH, Chambers JD, McEvoy LM, et al: Two-step model of leukocyte-endothelial cell interaction in inflammation: Distinct roles for LECAM-1 and the leukocyte beta 2 integrins in vivo. Proc Natl Acad Sci USA 1991; 88:7538–7542.
29a. Mulligan MS, Paulson JC, De-Frees S, et al: Protective effects of oligosaccharides in P-selectin–dependent lung injury. Nature 1993; 364:149–151.
30. Leeuwenberg JF, von-Asmuth EJ, Jeunhomme TM, et al: IFN-gamma regulates the expression of the adhesion molecule ELAM-1 and IL-6 production by human endothelial cells in vitro. J Immunol 1990; 145:2110–2114.
31. Redl H, Dinges HP, Buurman WA, et al: Expression of endothelial leukocyte adhesion molecule-1 in septic but not traumatic/hypovolemic shock in the baboon. Am J Pathol 1991; 139:461–466.
31a. Gearing AJ, Newman W: Circulating adhesion molecules in disease. Immunol Today 1993; 14:506–512.
32. Koch AE, Burrows JC, Haines GK, et al: Immunolocalization of endothelial and leukocyte adhesion molecules in human rheumatoid and osteoarthritic synovial tissues. Lab Invest 1991; 64:313–320.
33. Waldorf HA, Walsh LJ, Schechter NM, et al: Early cellular events in evolving cutaneous delayed hypersensitivity in humans. Am J Pathol 1991; 138:477–486.
34. Lorant DE, Topham MK, Whatley RE, et al: Inflammatory roles of P-selectin. J Clin Invest 1993; 92:559–570.
35. Huber AR, Kunkel SL, Todd RF III, et al: Regulation of transendothelial neutrophil migration by endogenous interleukin-8 Science 1991; 254:99–102.
36. Hechtman DH, Cybulsky MI, Fuchs HJ, et al: Intravascular IL-8: Inhibitor of polymorphonuclear leukocyte accumulation at sites of acute inflammation. J Immunol 1991; 147:883–892.
37. O'Toole TE, Katagiri Y, Faull RJ, et al: Integrin cytoplasmic domains mediate inside-out signal transduction. J Cell Biol 1994; 124:1047–1059.
38. Spertini O, Kansas GS, Munro JM, et al: Regulation of leukocyte migration by activation of the leukocyte adhesion molecule-1 (LAM-1) selectin. Nature 1991; 349:691–694.
39. Kuijpers TW, Mul EPJ, Blom M, et al: Freezing adhesion molecules in a state of high-avidity binding blocks eosinophil migration. J Exp Med 1994; 178:279–284.
40. Granger DN, Hollwarth ME, Parks DA: Ischemia-reperfusion injury: Role of oxygen-derived free radicals. Acta Physiol Scand 1986; 548(Suppl):47–63.
41. McCord JM: Oxygen-derived radicals: A link between reperfusion injury and inflammation. Fed Proc 1987; 46:2402–2406.
42. Romson JL, Hook BG, Kunkel SL, et al: Reduction of the extent of ischemic myocardial injury by neutrophil depletion in the dog. Circulation 1983; 67:1016–1023.
43. Vedder NB, Winn RK, Rice CL, et al: Inhibition of leukocyte adherence by anti-CD18 monoclonal antibody attenuates reperfusion injury in the rabbit ear. Proc Natl Acad Sci USA 1990; 87:2643–2646.
43a. Winn RK, Liggitt D, Vedder NB, et al: Anti-P-selectin monoclonal antibody attenuates reperfusion injury to the rabbit ear. J Clin Invest 1993; 92:2042–2047.
44. Patel KD, Zimmerman GA, Prescott SM, et al: Oxygen radicals induce human endothelial cells to express GMP-140 and bind neutrophils. J Cell Biol 1991; 112:749–759.
45. Kubes P, Ibbotson G, Russell J, et al: Role of platelet-activating factor in ischemia/reperfusion-induced leukocyte adherence. Am J Physiol 1990; 259:G300–G305.
46. Suzuki M, Inauen W, Kvietys PR, et al: Superoxide mediates reperfusion-induced leukocyte-endothelial cell interactions. Am J Physiol 1989; 257:H1740–H1745.
47. Hernandez LA, Grisham MB, Twohig B, et al: Role of neutrophils in ischemia-reperfusion-induced microvascular injury. Am J Physiol 1987; 253:H699–H703.
48. Simpson PJ, Todd RF III, Fantone JC, et al: Reduction of experimental canine myocardial reperfusion injury by a monoclonal antibody (Anti-Mo1, Anti-CD11b) that inhibits leukocyte adhesion. J Clin Invest 1988; 81:624–629.
49. Ma XL, Tsao PS, Lefer AM: Antibody to CD-18 exerts endothelial and cardiac protective effects in myocardial ischemia and reperfusion. J Clin Invest 1991; 88:1237–1243.
49a. Ma XL, Weyrich AS, Lefer DJ, et al: Monoclonal antibody to L-selectin attenuates neutrophil accumulation and protects ischemic reperfused cat myocardium. Circulation 1993; 88:649–658.
49b. Weyrich AS, Ma XY, Lefer DJ, et al: In vivo neutralization of P-selectin protects feline heart and endothelium in myocardial ischemia and reperfusion injury. J Clin Invest 1993; 91:2620–2629.
49c. Buerke M, Weyrich AS, Zheng Z, et al: Sialyl Lewis x-containing oligosaccharide attenuates myocardial reperfusion injury in cats. J Clin Invest 1994; 93:1140–1148.
50. Clark WM, Madden KP, Rothlein R, et al: Reduction of central nervous system ischemic injury in rabbits using leukocyte adhesion antibody treatment. Stroke 1991; 22:877–883.
51. Carden DL, Smith JK, Korthuis RJ: Neutrophil-mediated microvascular dysfunction in postischemic canine skeletal muscle: Role of granulocyte adherence. Circ Res 1990; 66:1436–1444.
52. Welbourn CR, Goldman G, Paterson IS, et al: Pathophysiology of ischaemia reperfusion injury: Central role of the neutrophil. Br J Surg 1991; 78:651–655.
52a. Seekamp A, Till GO, Mulligan MS, et al: Role of selectins in

local and remote tissue injury following ischemia and reperfusion. Am J Pathol 1994; 144:592–598.
52b. Seekamp A, Mulligan MS, Till GO, et al: Role of beta 2 integrins and ICAM-1 in lung injury following ischemia-reperfusion of rat hind limbs. Am J Pathol 1993; 143:464–472.
53. Vedder NB, Winn RK, Rice CL, et al: A monoclonal antibody to the adherence-promoting leukocyte glycoprotein, CD18, reduces organ injury and improves survival from hemorrhagic shock in rabbits. J Clin Invest 1988; 81:939–944.
54. Mileski WJ, Winn RK, Vedder NB, et al: Inhibition of CD18-dependent neutrophil adherence reduces organ injury after hemorrhagic shock in primates. Surgery 1990; 108:206–212.
55. Vedder NB, Fouty BW, Winn RK, et al: Role of neutrophils in generalized reperfusion injury associated with resuscitation from shock. Surgery 1989; 106:509–516.
56. Nourshargh S, Rampart M, Hellewell PG, et al: Accumulation of 111In-neutrophils in rabbit skin in allergic and non-allergic inflammatory reactions in vivo: Inhibition by neutrophil pretreatment in vitro with a monoclonal antibody recognizing the CD18 antigen. J Immunol 1989; 142:3193–3198.
57. Tuomanen EI, Saukkonen K, Sande S, et al: Reduction of inflammation, tissue damage, and mortality in bacterial meningitis in rabbits treated with monoclonal antibodies against adhesion-promoting receptors of leukocytes. J Exp Med 1989; 170:959–969.
57a. Granert C, Raud J, Xie X, et al: Inhibition of leukocyte rolling with polysaccharide fucoidin prevents pleocytosis in experimental meningitis in the rabbit. J Clin Invest 1994; 93:929–936.
58. Thomas JR, Harlan JM, Rice CL, et al: Role of leukocyte CD11/CD18 complex in endotoxic and septic shock in rabbits. J Appl Physiol 1992; 73:1510–1516.
59. Burch RM, Noronha-Blob L, Bator JM, et al: Mice treated with a leumedin or antibody to Mac-1 to inhibit leukocyte sequestration survive endotoxin challenge. J Immunol 1993; 150:3397–3403.
60. Wegner CD, Gundel RH, Reilly P, et al: Intercellular adhesion molecule-1 (ICAM-1) in the pathogenesis of asthma. Science 1990; 247:456–459.
61. Hutchings P, Rosen H, O'Reilly L, et al: Transfer of diabetes in mice prevented by blockade of adhesion-promoting receptor on macrophages. Nature 1990; 348:639–642.
62. Wegner CD, Wolyniec WW, LaPlante AM, et al: Intercellular adhesion molecule-1 contributes to pulmonary oxygen toxicity in mice: Role of leukocytes revised. Lung 1992; 170:267–279.
63. Wallace JL, Arfors KE, McKnight GW: A monoclonal antibody against the CD18 leukocyte adhesion molecule prevents indomethacin-induced gastric damage in the rabbit. Gastroenterology 1991; 100:878–883.
64. Bucky LP, Vedder NV, Hong HZ, et al: Reduction of burn injury by inhibiting CD18-mediated leukocyte adherence in rabbits. Plast Reconstr Surg 1994; 19:1473–1480.
65. Mileski W, Borgstrom D, Lightfoot E, et al: Inhibition of leukocyte-endothelial adherence following thermal injury. J Surg Res 1992; 52:334–339.
66. Cosimi AB, Conti D, Delmonico FL, et al: In vivo effects of monoclonal antibody to ICAM-1 (CD54) in nonhuman primates with renal allografts. J Immunol 1990; 144:4604–4612.
67. Flavin T, Ivens K, Rothlein R, et al: Monoclonal antibodies against intercellular adhesion molecule 1 prolong cardiac allograft survival in cynomolgus monkeys. Transplant Proc 1991; 23:533–534.
67a. Mulligan MS, Polley MJ, Bayer RJ, et al: Neutrophil-dependent acute lung injury. Requirement for P-selectin (GMP-140). J Clin Invest 1992; 90:1600–1607.
67b. Mulligan MS, Lowe JB, Larsen RD, et al: Protective effects of sialylated oligosaccharides in immune complex-induced acute lung injury. J Exp Med 1993; 178:623–631.
67c. Mulligan MS, Miyasaka M, Tamatani T, et al: Requirements for L-selectin in neutrophil-mediated lung injury in rats. J Immunol 1994; 152:832–840.
68. Mileski WJ, Winn RK, Harlan JM, et al: Transient inhibition of neutrophil adherence with the anti-CD18 monoclonal antibody 60.3 does not increase mortality rates in abdominal sepsis. Surgery 1991; 109:497–501.
69. Sharar SR, Winn RK, Murry CE, et al: A CD18 monoclonal antibody increases the incidence and severity of subcutaneous abscess formation after high-dose *Staphylococcus aureus* injection in rabbits. Surgery 1991; 110:213–219.
69a. Sharar SR, Sasaki SS, Flaherty LC, et al: P-selectin blockade does not impair leukocyte host defense against bacterial peritonitis and soft tissue infection in rabbits. J Immunol 1993; 151:4982–4988.

CHAPTER 26

Receptor Physiology

Frederick J. Ehlert, PhD

The idea of a "receptor" was first introduced by Ehrlich and Langley around the turn of the century in an attempt to explain the remarkably selective and potent effects that some natural and synthetic chemicals had on biologic tissues. They argued that pharmacologic agents must interact specifically with macromolecular components in tissue to produce physiologic effects. This idea, of course, is now a readily demonstrable fact. Researchers have identified hundreds of receptors and determined the primary sequence of many of these proteins through gene cloning. The precision with which we now think about a receptor is perhaps most spectacularly illustrated with the nicotinic acetylcholine receptor. Electron micrographic analysis of crystallized nicotinic acetylcholine receptors from Torpedo has produced high-resolution pictures showing a channel-like structure with a central pore, presumably representing the microscopic tunnel through which positive cations flow when the receptor binds its neurotransmitter, acetylcholine.[1]

The identification of receptors as the target for many drugs has an important corollary. It implies that drugs do not create new responses in tissues; but rather, they start, stop, or modulate natural physiologic functions. For example, synthetic muscarinic agonists are able to elicit contractions of intestinal smooth muscle because they bind with muscarinic receptors and trigger a signaling cascade that results in the mobilization of calcium and an activation of contractile proteins in the muscle. Obviously, this signaling pathway evolved to respond to neuronally released acetylcholine and not to synthetic drugs. The idea that drugs use physiologic mechanisms applies not only to readily quantifiable responses in peripheral tissues but also to responses that are somewhat more complex. The sensation of euphoria and well-being produced by opiate drugs, like morphine and heroin, implies the existence of reward pathways in the brain whose natural function is to provide positive reinforcement to the organism under appropriate conditions.[2]

Within this general context, one can define many classes or types of receptors. There are the so-called physiologic receptors, which mediate the effects of a variety of neurotransmitters, peptide and steroid hormones, biogenic amines, and eicosanoids. In addition, enzymes, transport proteins, and ion channels are also important receptors for a variety of drugs that usually, but not always, block the function of these proteins. Finally, the cytoskeleton and deoxyribonucleic acid (DNA) itself may constitute the "receptor" for some agents.

The aims of this chapter are to review some of the quantitative aspects of drug receptor interactions and to provide a brief survey of the major families of the physiologic receptors and their signaling mechanisms.

RELATIONSHIP BETWEEN RECEPTOR OCCUPANCY AND RESPONSE

The binding of a reversible drug to a receptor usually obeys the following scheme:

$$D + R \leftrightarrow DR \qquad \text{[Equation 1]}$$

in which D denotes the drug concentration, R denotes the receptor concentration, and DR denotes the drug-receptor complex. At equilibrium, the relationship between the drug-receptor complex and the drug concentration is as follows:

$$[DR] = \frac{[D]R_T}{[D] + K_d} \qquad \text{[Equation 2]}$$

in which R_T denotes that total concentration of receptors and K_d denotes the equilibrium dissociation constant of the drug-receptor complex. The K_d has units of concentration (e.g., molar) and is equivalent to the concentration of drug required for half-maximal receptor occupancy. The K_d is a measure of the affinity of a drug for a receptor. The lower the K_d, the higher the affinity. Scheme 1 is usually called the law of mass action. Its consequences adequately reflect the manner in which a variety of drugs bind with receptors under physiologic conditions.

The size of the response elicited by a drug depends on its intrinsic efficacy and the percentage of receptors that it occupies. It is easier to understand the property of intrinsic efficacy if we consider how the drug-receptor complex behaves in the absence of other ligands or endogenous neurotransmitters. In the absence of drugs, most native receptors are silent. An agonist is a drug that binds to the receptor, turns it on, and triggers a response. The property that enables the agonist to turn on the receptor is called *intrinsic efficacy*. An antagonist is a drug that lacks intrinsic efficacy but is capable of binding to the receptor. Such agents have no effects by themselves but are capable of antagonizing the action of an agonist, whether it be an exogenous drug or an endogenous neurotransmitter. The amount of intrinsic efficacy can vary widely among different drugs, and drugs having a small or intermediate level of intrinsic efficacy are called *partial agonists*.

This general framework may not be entirely sufficient to account for the behavior of all receptor systems. For example, the guanosine triphosphatase (GTPase) activity elicited by opiate receptors is already active in the absence of agonists when this function is measured in brain homogenate in a hypotonic buffer.[3] Under these conditions, the addition of agonists causes a further increase in the GTPase activity, whereas antagonists either have no effect or they inhibit the ongoing basal GTPase activity. In other words, if the receptor is already turned on in the absence of agonists, some antagonists will actually turn off the receptor. To what extent partially turned-on receptors exist in vivo is unknown. To date, the only few receptors that behave in this fashion have been shown to do so under nonphysiologic conditions.

Figure 26–1 shows the relationship between occupancy and response for a highly efficacious agonist (see Fig. 26–1*A*), a less efficacious agonist (see Fig. 26–1*B*), and a partial agonist (see Fig. 26–1*C*). In Figure 1*A*, the dose-response curve for the agonist lies to the left of the occupancy curve, indicating that it only requires a low level of receptor occupancy to produce a maximum response. This behavior is typical for a highly efficacious agonist. In Figure 1*B*, there is closer agreement between the two curves, so that the response is proportional to receptor occupancy. Although this less efficacious agonist is capable of eliciting a maximum response, it can only do so at a much higher level of receptor occupancy compared with the more efficacious agonist shown in Figure 1*A*. In Figure 1*C*, the agonist has little intrinsic efficacy so that it is incapable of eliciting a maximum response even when the receptors are fully occupied. Consequently, the agonist is designated as a partial agonist.

When an agonist is capable of eliciting a maximum response at a submaximal level of receptor occupancy (e.g., see Fig. 1*A*), the situation is referred to as *spare receptors*. Unfortunately, this term has created considerable confusion in the pharmacologic literature. The term does not imply that some of the receptors are extra or unnecessary; rather, it simply means that only a small fraction of the total functional receptor population needs to be occupied by the agonist to elicit a maximum response. The presence of spare receptors enhances the potency of the agonist because lower concentrations of the agonist can produce effective responses. The functional activity of the total receptor population can be appreciated by considering what happens when some of the receptors are inactivated. After partial receptor inactivation, the dose-response curve of a highly efficacious agonist shifts to the right without a decrease in

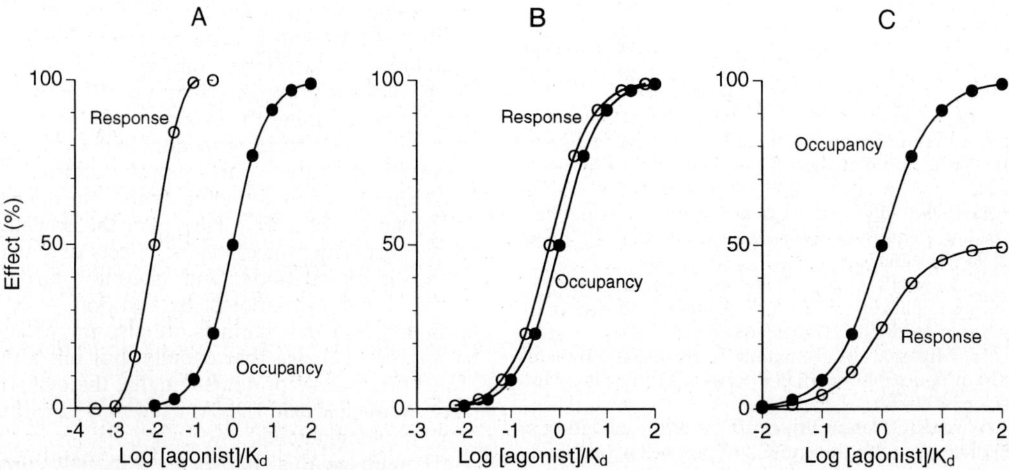

Figure 26–1. Relationship between receptor occupancy (●) and response (○) for a highly efficacious agonist (*A*), a less efficacious agonist (*B*), and a partial agonist (*C*). Both occupancy and response are expressed as percentages of their maximum values and are plotted on the ordinate scale. The concentration of the agonist is expressed on the abscissa as a log of the ratio of the agonist concentration divided by its K_d.

the maximum response. The loss in potency associated with inactivation of some of the receptors illustrates that spare receptors are functional and maintain the sensitivity of the receptor system. Another important point is that the presence of spare receptors does not imply that there is an excess of receptors to effectors. In fact, the converse is usually the case. In many signaling cascades, there is divergence along every step in the pathway. That is, one receptor may interact with several effector molecules, and each effector will generate several second-messenger molecules and so forth. This divergence leads to amplification and thereby enables a relatively small number of agonist-receptor complexes to generate a significant physiologic response.

Because antagonists lack intrinsic efficacy, all that is necessary to describe their interaction with a receptor at equilibrium is the K_d. This parameter can be estimated by measuring an agonist dose-response curve in the absence and presence of the competitive antagonist. A competitive antagonist will shift the log dose-response curve of an agonist to the right in a parallel fashion without causing a decrease in the maximum response. The K_d of the antagonist can be estimated from the shift in the dose-response curve using the following equation:

$$DR - 1 = [A]K_A \qquad \text{[Equation 3]}$$

in which DR (dose ratio) denotes the concentration of agonist causing a half-maximal response in the presence of the antagonist divided by that measured in its absence and [A] denotes the concentration of the antagonist.

The relationships described previously are adequate to account for the interactions of agonists and antagonists with the primary recognition site of a receptor. Some receptors have secondary allosteric sites where drugs can also bind and modify the ability of primary ligands to activate the receptor. One such example is the gamma-aminobutyric acid-A ($GABA_A$) receptor.[4] This receptor is a chloride channel that is regulated by the neurotransmitter GABA. When GABA binds to its site on the $GABA_A$ receptor, it causes the chloride channel to open. In addition to the GABA recognition site, there are other allosteric sites, including one for benzodiazepine-like drugs. A tranquilizing benzodiazepine, like diazepam, binds to the allosteric site and increases the affinity of GABA for its site on the channel, thereby enhancing the effects of GABA. This allosteric effect can account for the pharmacologic properties of benzodiazepines, which include relief from anxiety, sedation, and protection against seizures. In contrast, some β-carboline derivatives bind to the allosteric site and inhibit the binding of GABA. These compounds have been called *inverse agonists* because they elicit responses that are opposite to those of benzodiazepines (i.e., anxiety, convulsions). However, they are more appropriately referred to as allosteric GABA antagonists because they produce their effects by antagonizing GABA. In addition, there are some compounds that bind to the allosteric site and have no effect on the binding of GABA. These compounds (e.g., Ro 151788) are called benzodiazepine antagonists, and, although they have no effects by themselves, they antagonize both the tranquilizing effects of benzodiazepines and the convulsant effects of β-carbolines.

RECEPTOR FAMILIES

Physiologic receptors can be divided into four families on the basis of structural and functional properties. These four families are the ligand-regulated transcription factors, the ligand-regulated enzymes, the ligand-gated ion channels, and the G protein–linked receptors.[5] Each family has a distinct overall structure and general function that is shared by all members of the same family. Within each family, there is usually, but not always, a considerable amount of sequence homology. Regions of high homology within a given family have enabled molecular biologists to use low-stringency hybridization techniques to identify additional members of the same family. In some instances, the endogenous ligands for the cloned receptor protein have not been identified, which has led to their designation as "orphan receptors." A cursory survey of these four receptor families is given next.

Ligand-Regulated Transcription Factors

The ligand-regulated transcription factor superfamily comprises a large group of soluble receptors that bind to DNA and regulate the activity of specific genes in a ligand-dependent manner.[6] This family includes receptors for thyroid hormone, retinoids, vitamin D, and the various steroid hormones including glucocorticoids, mineralocorticoids, androgens, progesterone, and estrogen. Most of these receptors are located in the nucleus. Not surprisingly, the ligands for these receptors can readily penetrate the plasma membrane, and their access to the receptor is controlled by hormone-binding proteins and by enzymatic processing of the ligand itself.

Receptors belonging to the steroid superfamily all share a similar structure having three major domains.[6] Near the center of the sequence is a highly conserved domain of 66 to 68 amino acids that constitutes the DNA-binding region of the receptor. In this domain, the sequence forms two loops that are held in place by a zinc atom that interacts with cysteine residues on opposite sides of the loop. Each of the two loops is called a "zinc finger," and many proteins that bind with DNA have a zinc fingerlike structure. The second major domain of this family of receptors is the carboxy-terminal region, which functions as the ligand-binding domain. This region of the receptor also shows considerable sequence homology, particularly among the androgen, glucocorticoid, mineralocorticoid, and progesterone receptors, which have structurally similar ligands (i.e., steroids). The third major domain is the amino-terminal region, which shows the greatest variation in size and the least conservation in sequence. This domain of the receptor is thought to mediate transcriptional activation.

A variety of evidence supports the existence of these distinct functional domains on steroid receptors. Perhaps the most dramatic evidence of this sort comes from studies on chimeric receptors in which a domain from one receptor is replaced with the corresponding domain from another. For example, when the 66-amino-acid DNA-binding region of the estrogen receptor is replaced with that of the glucocorticoid receptor, a chimeric receptor is formed that turns on a glucocorticoid-inducible gene in the presence of estradiol.[7] Truncated receptors have also yielded clues about functional domains as well as the mechanism of ligand-induced activation. For example, glucocorticoid receptor mutants lacking most of the ligand-binding domain demonstrate constitutive activity.[8] That is, the truncated receptor binds to DNA and causes transcriptional activation in the absence of hormone. Apparently, the ligand-binding domain of the glucocorticoid receptor normally prevents DNA binding and transcriptional activation, whereas the binding of the hormone relieves this tonic inhibition. Finally, several cases of hormonal resistance have been attributed to point mutations in the ligand-binding domain, resulting in diminished hormone binding.[6]

Although the details are unclear, the binding of hormone to its receptor triggers the formation of receptor dimers that subsequently bind to DNA.[6] The site on DNA where binding occurs is called the *hormone response element* (HRE). These sites are located in the regulatory regions of steroid-induced genes, and several have been identified. The consensus sequences of HREs exhibit dyad symmetry, which is consistent with the idea that a receptor dimer interacts with the HRE.

Ligand-Regulated Enzymes

The ligand-regulated enzymes represent a huge superfamily of receptors that can be divided into different families. The unifying structural feature of these receptors is the presence of an extracellular ligand-binding domain that regulates the activity of an intracellular catalytic domain. In most instances, the two domains of the receptor are connected by a single transmembrane-spanning region. This large superfamily includes receptors for a variety of growth factors, cytokines, and peptides.

One of the major groups within the ligand-regulated enzyme superfamily is the receptor tyrosine kinase (RTK) family, which includes receptors for insulin, fibroblast growth factor (FGF), epidermal growth factor (EGF), and platelet-derived growth factor. The structural and functional properties of these receptors have been reviewed,[9, 10] and a brief description of these receptors is given here. As mentioned previously, members of this family have an extracellular ligand-binding domain, an intracellular tyrosine kinase domain, and a transmembrane-spanning domain (Fig. 26–2). Most RTKs are formed from a single polypeptide chain; however, the class II RTKs, which include receptors for insulin and insulin-like growth factor, are heterotetrameric, consisting of two α and two β subunits connected by disulfide bonds (see Fig. 26–2). The two α subunits contribute to the ligand-binding domain, whereas the two β subunits traverse the membrane and possess the tyrosine kinase activity. The class I and II RTKs, which include the EGF receptor and the insulin receptor, have cysteine-rich regions in their extracellular ligand-binding domains. Another class, which includes the FGF receptor, has three immunoglobulin-like domains in the extracellular ligand-binding portion of the receptor. The tyrosine kinase domain is the most highly conserved domain among the different classes of RTKs. This domain contains an adenosine triphosphate–binding site and a tyrosine acceptor site. In the class III RTKs, these two functional regions of the kinase domain are separated by a hydrophilic, proline-rich sequence of 77 to 107 amino acids. The results of studies on chimeric receptors constructed from heterologous ligand binding and kinase domains provide further support for the existence of autonomous functional domains. In each case, the hybrid receptors have displayed the appropriate ligand specificity and kinase activity.

Ligand binding to monomeric RTKs results in dimerization, which is a prerequisite for growth factor–dependent kinase activation. Interestingly, the kinase activity of the tetrameric insulin receptor, which is analogous to an EGF receptor dimer, is much greater than that of the dimeric αβ form of the insulin receptor. The results of ligand-binding studies have demonstrated that growth factors bind to dimeric receptors with higher affinity compared with monomers, suggesting that the tighter binding of the agonist to the dimer provides the drive for receptor aggregation. Once made active by their respective ligands, all RTKs autophosphorylate on several tyrosine residues. Apparently, this autophosphorylation is a requirement for tyrosine kinase activity against heterologous proteins. There are many target proteins for phosphorylation within the cell, and these include a phospholipase C-γ1 (PLC-γ1), a GTPase-activating protein, and the putative regulatory subunit of phosphatidylinositol 3′-kinase.[11] Activation of PLC-γ1 results in the formation of two second messengers, inositol-1,4,5-trisphosphate (IP_3) and diacylglycerol (DAG), which have important roles in calcium mobilization and protein kinase C activation as described later under Signaling Mechanisms of G protein–Linked Receptors. Although many of the details are unclear, activation of RTKs causes a variety of cellular events including DNA synthesis, cellular replication, increased synthesis of protein, stimulation of ion and glucose transport, pinocytosis, and other cytoskeletal and morphologic changes.

Another member of the ligand-regulated enzyme superfamily is the receptor for atrial natriuretic peptide (ANP).[12, 13] This receptor contains an extracellular ligand-binding domain for ANP, a single transmembrane-spanning domain, and an intracellular domain that has guanylate cyclase activity (see Fig. 26–2). The binding of ANP to this receptor causes an increase in the concentration of cyclic guanosine monophosphate (GMP) inside the cell. This second messenger activates a cyclic GMP-dependent protein kinase (protein kinase B), which ultimately triggers a variety of responses including diuresis, natriuresis, and vasorelaxation. Interestingly, the extracellular domain of the ANP re-

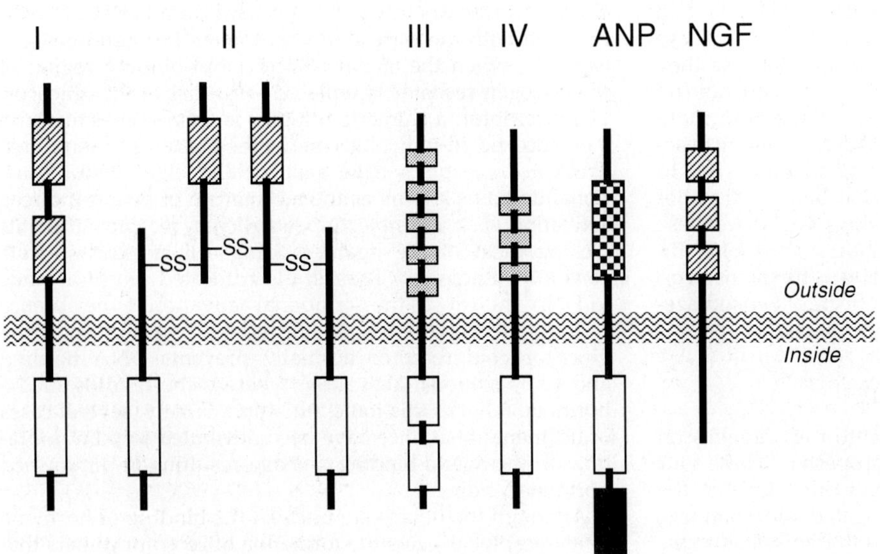

Figure 26–2. Structure of different members of the ligand regulated enzyme superfamily of receptors. The figure shows the transmembrane topography of the primary sequences of the receptor tyrosine kinases (I, II, III, and IV), the receptor for atrial natriuretic peptide (ANP), and the receptor for nerve growth factor (NGF). The *boxes* indicate the various functional domains of the receptor and are shaded according to the following scheme: *diagonal lines* = cysteine-rich domain; *shaded* = immunoglobulin domain; *checkered* = ANP binding domain; *open* = tyrosine kinase domain; and *solid* = guanylate cyclase domain.

ceptor is homologous with an ANP-binding protein that is thought to have a role in the clearance of ANP from the circulation. The proximal portion of the intracellular domain is homologous to the kinase domain of RTKs, although no ANP-induced kinase activity has been detected. The most distal portion of the intracellular domain represents the catalytic domain, and it is homologous to the soluble form of guanylate cyclase.

The last group within the ligand-regulated enzyme superfamily is a family that includes the receptors for nerve growth factor (NGF) and tumor necrosis factor (TNF).[14] These receptors contain three or four cysteine-rich domains in their extracellular ligand-binding domains, a single transmembrane-spanning domain, and an intracellular domain varying in length from 36 to 221 amino acids (see Fig. 26–2). The intracellular domain has an unknown function, and it lacks sequence identity with any other known proteins. It has been suggested that a transmembrane tyrosine kinase can interact with the intracellular domain of the NGF receptor to elicit a biologic signal. Once occupied by their respective ligands, the NGF receptor causes neuronal differentiation and survival, whereas the TNF receptor causes inflammation and tumor cell death.

Ligand-Gated Ion Channels

The ligand-gated ion channels represent a large superfamily that includes receptors for acetylcholine (nicotinic acetylcholine receptor), γ GABA ($GABA_A$ receptor), glycine, and various excitatory amino acids (e.g., glutamate and aspartate).[5] As their name implies, members of this superfamily are ion channels that open up and conduct an ionic current when an agonist ligand binds on them. In the case of the nicotinic acetylcholine receptor of the neuromuscular junction and the Torpedo electric organ, the ionic current is carried by positive monovalent cations, primarily sodium. Evidence suggests that neuronal nicotinic receptors may carry a rapidly desensitizing calcium current.[15] In the case of excitatory amino acid receptors, the ionic current is carried by both sodium and calcium, whereas inhibitory amino acid receptors (i.e., GABA and glycine receptor) carry a chloride current. The ligand-regulated ion channels have a characteristic oligomeric structure. The nicotinic acetylcholine receptor of the neuromuscular junction has a pentameric structure, consisting of two α subunits and one each of β, γ, and δ subunits. These subunits are arranged like the staves in a barrel-like structure having a central pore that is thought to be the channel of the receptor.[1] Although the precise subunit structure of neuronal nicotinic receptors and the other ligand-gated ion channels is unknown, they are thought to be analogous, but not necessarily identical, to that of the neuromuscular nicotinic acetylcholine receptor. For example, it is possible that some ligand-gated ion channels are tetramers, composed of only two α and two β subunits.[16] Moreover, recombinant homomeric $GABA_A$ receptors have been formed by injecting only messenger ribonucleic acid (RNA) for the α subunit into *Xenopus* oocytes, indicating that functional, GABA-regulated ion channels can be formed only from α subunits.[17] However, these homomeric channels do not retain all of the complex allosteric interactions characteristic of native $GABA_A$ receptors, and it is entirely possible that homomeric channels do not occur naturally. Several different subtypes of the individual subunits have been cloned for both the nicotinic and $GABA_A$ receptors, which raises the possibility of a staggering number of channel subtypes based on combinations of different types of subunits. These different subtypes of channels could have different pharmacologic and functional properties and unique developmental profiles. Although this potential diversity represents a colossal task to sort out, it does increase the likelihood of attaining more selective drugs.

The overall structure of the ligand-gated ion channels shows homology with many of the voltage-regulated ion channels, like the sodium channel and the L-type calcium channel.[5] Although the ligand-regulated channels are primarily chemosensitive, their gating characteristics are modified by the potential of the membrane. Conversely, although the voltage-gated ion channels are primarily potential sensitive, they are also modified by a variety of agonistic and antagonistic ligands that bind at different sites on the channel that are often allosterically linked to one another. When considered from this viewpoint, the ligand- and voltage-regulated ion channels form a large superfamily of receptors.

The overall three-dimensional structure and transmembrane topography of the various types of ligand-gated cation and anion channels show considerable homologies, and a description of their general features is given here.[5] Although far from conclusive, the ligand-binding domain of the nicotinic and glycine receptor appears to be on an extracellular domain of the α subunit. In the case of the neuromuscular nicotinic receptor, two molecules of acetylcholine bind to the channel and cause it to open. This scheme is consistent with the subunit structure of the channel (i.e., $\alpha_2\beta\gamma\delta$) and with the positive cooperativity that is characteristic of the binding of acetylcholine to the channel.[5] The different subunits of the channel show considerable homology with each other and contain four transmembrane-spanning domains. Ion selectivity has been occasionally attributed to a putative transmembrane-spanning, amphipathic helix; however, this sequence is only found in the nicotinic acetylcholine receptor. Consequently, both the ionic selectivity role and transmembrane location of the amphipathic helix seem untenable, which limits the transmembrane-spanning domains to four and puts both the amino- and carboxy-terminal ends of the receptor on the same side of the membrane. Clusters of residues having a charge opposite to that of the permiant ion are located at the channel opening in both the nicotinic and $GABA_A$ receptors, and perhaps these amino acids determine the ion selectivity of the channel.

Ligand-gated ion channels are widespread throughout the central and peripheral nervous systems and are responsible for rapid synaptic neurotransmission, characterized by synaptic delays of less than half a millisecond. The nicotinic acetylcholine receptor is present at the neuromuscular junction, where it is responsible for eliciting skeletal muscle contraction in response to impulse flow from α motor neurons. These receptors are the targets for the neuromuscular blocking agents used as adjuncts to general anesthesia.[18] The $GABA_A$ receptor represents the major inhibitory neurotransmitter receptor in the brain, and it is an important target for a variety of drugs used to treat anxiety, convulsions, and insomnia.[19] Excitatory amino acid receptors are also abundant in brain, and inhibitors of these ion channels may have use in preventing the neuronal damage associated with brain ischemia after stroke.

G Protein–Linked Receptors

The G protein–linked family of receptors is perhaps the largest, and it includes receptors for a variety of endogenous neurotransmitters including acetylcholine (muscarinic acetylcholine receptor), catecholamines, histamine, serotonin, eicosanoids, and some peptides.[5] These receptors trigger responses by binding with heterotrimeric G proteins, which in turn activate various effectors, including ion channels and enzymes that generate second messengers (see later discussion). Not only are these receptors involved in neurotransmission at a variety of synapses and junctions throughout the brain and peripheral autonomic nervous system, but members of this family are also involved in the special sensory functions of vision, taste, and olfaction.[20] The light receptor in the retina, rhodopsin, consists of a tightly bound complex between a protein called opsin and a photoactive ligand, 11-*cis* retinal.[21, 22] When light shines on 11-*cis* retinal, it isomerizes to the *trans* isomer, which induces a conformational change in rhodopsin, causing it to activate a G protein called *transducin* (G_T). Ultimately, transducin initiates a cascade of events leading to a hyperpolarizing response in the retinal ganglion cell. This signaling pathway is so highly amplified that a single photon of light has a 50% probability of triggering a response in the retinal ganglion cell. G protein–linked receptors are also involved in olfaction to a remarkable extent. The results of cloning studies on genomic and complementary DNA libraries prepared from the olfactory epithelium indicate that there may be more than 100 different types of odorant receptors in the nose, each of which may be receptive to a different spectrum of odorants.[23]

Receptors belonging to the G protein–linked class all share a similar structure consisting of seven highly conserved, transmembrane-spanning domains of α-helix that are connected to the less conserved amino terminal, carboxy terminal, and intra- and extracellular loops. It is generally assumed that the three-dimensional structure of G protein–linked receptors conforms to that of bacteriorhodopsin, which has been determined by x-ray diffraction.[24] In bacteriorhodopsin, the transmembrane domains run perpendicular to the plane of the membrane and circumscribe a central pore. Retinal and the neurotransmitters for muscarinic and catecholamine receptors are thought to bind at a site within the pore. Accordingly, point mutations in a highly conserved aspartic acid residue in the third transmembrane segment cause a loss in agonist binding at muscarinic[25] and β-adrenergic[26] receptors. Not surprisingly, the part of the receptor involved in G protein coupling is a relatively large, hydrophilic domain that projects into the cytoplasm; namely, the third cytoplasmic (i3) loop. The strongest evidence for the coupling role of the i3 loop comes from studies on chimeric receptors in which the i3 loop of one receptor is replaced with that from another. For example, when the i3 loop of the muscarinic receptor was switched with that of the β-adrenergic receptor, the chimeric receptor triggered β-adrenergic effects in response to muscarinic agonists.[27] Analogous results have been observed in studies on chimers constructed from a variety of other G protein–linked receptors. Interestingly, the i3 loops of several receptors are constitutively active by themselves.[28] Thus, the ligand-binding domain (seven transmembrane segments) of G protein–linked receptors probably exerts a tonic inhibitory effect on the i3 loop, and the binding of neurotransmitter relieves this inhibition.

The G proteins involved in receptor signaling are heterotrimeric, consisting of α, β, and γ subunits.[29, 30] The βγ subunits form a tightly bound complex that functions as a unit. The α subunits of heterotrimeric G protein are close relatives of many other low-molecular-weight G proteins that lack βγ subunits. These small G proteins participate in numerous metabolic processes within the cell that have little to do with transmembrane signaling at the cell surface. The basic function that G proteins accomplish at the expense of GTP hydrolysis is one of transportation between two destinations. In the case of the low-molecular-weight G protein, elongation factor Tu, there is a transport of transfer RNA complexes on the ribosome, whereas in the case of heterotrimeric G proteins, the G protein shuttles between the receptor and its effector. Thus, nature uses G proteins for a variety of roles, and the involvement of heterotrimeric G proteins in receptor signaling at the cell membrane probably represents a highly specialized function.

The α subunit of heterotrimeric G proteins shows the greatest diversity, and more than 20 different types of α subunits have been cloned.[20] By contrast, the βγ subunits seem to be fewer in subtypes, and it appears that more than one type of α subunit can associate with the same dimer of βγ subunits. The α subunits confer selectivity for different receptors as well as effectors; however, the degree of selectivity is not absolute (see later discussion). For example, the M_2 subtype of the muscarinic receptor can interact with more than one type of G protein (e.g., G_o, G_i, and G_{i2}[31]), and a single G protein, like G_i, can interact with more than one type of receptor (e.g., M_2 muscarinic and D_2 dopamine). However, receptors that interact with G_i and G_o are usually ineffective at interacting with G_s and vice versa.[20] There is also selectivity at the level of the G protein–effector interaction. For example, more than one type of G protein can mediate an inhibition of adenylate cyclase activity; however, these G proteins are ineffective at coupling receptors to the phosphoinositide-specific phospholipase C. The α subunit of G proteins binds GTP, resulting in activation and a dissociation of the GTP-α complex from the βγ subunits. In addition, the α subunit has GTPase activity that hydrolyzes GTP to GDP, causing the inactive GDP-α complex to coalesce with the βγ subunits. The α subunits of some G proteins are also substrates for bacterial toxins that catalyze the adenosine diphosphate (ADP) ribosylation of the α subunit. For example, cholera toxin causes an ADP ribosylation of the α subunit of G_s, the G protein that stimulates adenylate cyclase activity. This ADP ribosylation causes an inhibition of the GTPase activity, resulting in an irreversible activation of G_s and, consequently, adenylate cyclase. In contrast, pertussis toxin causes the ADP ribosylation of G_i and G_o, which prevents receptor-mediated activation of G_i and G_o. G_T is a substrate for both cholera toxin and pertussis toxin.

Figure 26–3 shows what happens inside the cell when an agonist activates a G protein–linked receptor. Initially, the G protein is in its trimeric form with GDP tightly bound to it. This inactive form of the G protein is a prerequisite for receptor interaction because the agonist-receptor complex cannot interact with free α or βγ subunits, only the trimeric complex. Although the cell contains high concentrations (approximately 0.1 mmol) of GTP, this nucleotide cannot compete GDP off the G protein because the dissociation rate of GDP from the α subunit is negligible. The binding of agonist to its receptor causes a conformational change so that the i3 loop can interact with the G protein. This interaction allows the agonist to increase the rate of dissociation of GDP so that GTP can now bind to the G protein. The binding of GTP causes a dissociation of the GTP-α subunit from both the βγ subunit and the receptor, resulting in activation. The GTP-α subunit complex is then free to turn on its effector and ultimately trigger the cell's response to the agonist. In some instances, it appears that the βγ subunits elicit the response. The turn-off mechanism is the GTPase activity of the α subunit, which hydrolyzes GTP. The resulting GDP-α subunit then coalesces with the βγ subunits to form the trimeric complex, which is inactive. The cycle can then repeat itself provided that agonist is occupying the receptor.

Several experimental observations support the scheme just described, and a few of these are mentioned here. Muscarinic agonists cause the M_2 receptor to form a stable complex with G_i that can be identified on Western blots with antibodies to G_i or the M_2 receptor.[31] In contrast, antagonists do not promote the formation of a receptor–G protein com-

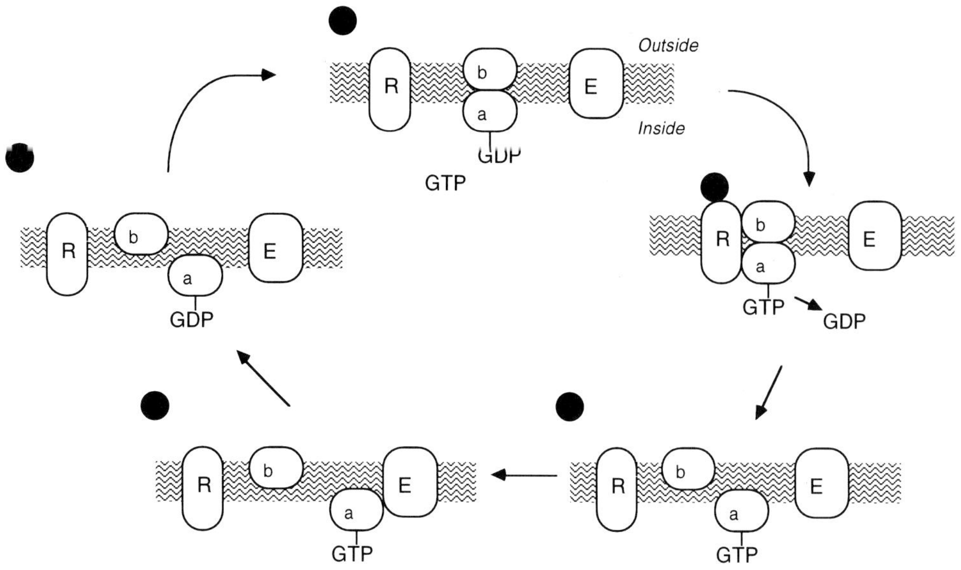

Figure 26–3. Receptor-activated GTPase cycle. The figure shows a schematic diagram of the interaction of an agonist (*solid circle*) with its receptor (R) and the α (a) and βγ (b) subunits of a G protein. The effector is denoted by "E." Further details are given in the text.

plex. Moreover, the ability of the ligand to promote the ternary complex (agonist–receptor–G protein complex) is proportional to the intrinsic efficacy of the agonist.[32] This relationship is shown in Figure 26–4 for M_2 muscarinic receptors in the heart. The propensity of the agonist to generate the ternary complex can be measured in a binding assay, and this parameter is denoted by "receptor-G_i cooperativity" in Figure 26–4*A*. It can be seen that the cooperativity is proportional to intrinsic efficacy for a number of agonists. Another conspicuous feature of most G protein–linked receptors is that the binding of ligands to the receptor is modified by GTP in a manner that is proportional to the intrinsic efficacy of the ligand. Both GTP and GDP cause a reduction in agonist-binding affinity but not antagonist affinity. The relationship between intrinsic efficacy and the inhibitory effect of GTP (GTP shift) on ligand binding to M_2 muscarinic receptors in the heart is shown in Figure 26–4*B* for a number of ligands. The proportional relationship between the negatively cooperative effects of GTP on agonist binding and the intrinsic efficacy of the agonist is readily apparent from the plot.

The relationships shown in Figure 26–4 provide insight into the mechanism of how the receptor works. In considering Figure 26–4, it is important to note that GDP as well as GTP inhibit agonist, but not antagonist, affinity. This effect is allosteric because the agonist and the guanine nucleotide act at different sites. Therefore, the nature of the interaction between the two types of ligands is called *negative heterotropic cooperativity*. One of the properties of allosteric interactions is that they are reciprocal; that is, if GDP or GTP reduces the affinity of the agonist, then the agonist must reduce the affinity of the guanine nucleotide to precisely the same extent.[33] This agonist-mediated reduction in the affinity of GDP causes it to dissociate from the G protein more rapidly, allowing GTP to compete it off the G protein. Although this increase in the dissociation kinetics of GDP is achieved at the cost of reducing the affinity of GTP, it does not result in a decrease in the binding of GTP because GTP is maintained at saturating concentrations inside the cell. For example, K_d of GTP analogs for the G protein is in the nanomolar (10^{-9} mol) range, whereas the concentration of GTP inside the cell is in the millimolar (10^{-3} mol) range. Thus, it can be seen that the agonist-receptor complex works by increasing the dissociation kinetics of GDP from the G protein and that this effect is mediated by negative heterotropic cooperativity.

SIGNALING MECHANISMS OF G PROTEIN–LINKED RECEPTORS

G protein–linked receptors mediate myriad responses at the level of the whole tissue; however, at the subcellular level, these responses seem to be triggered by a relatively small number of transduction mechanisms. This situation illustrates that diversity is achieved through divergence in the signaling pathway and that the factors that determine the

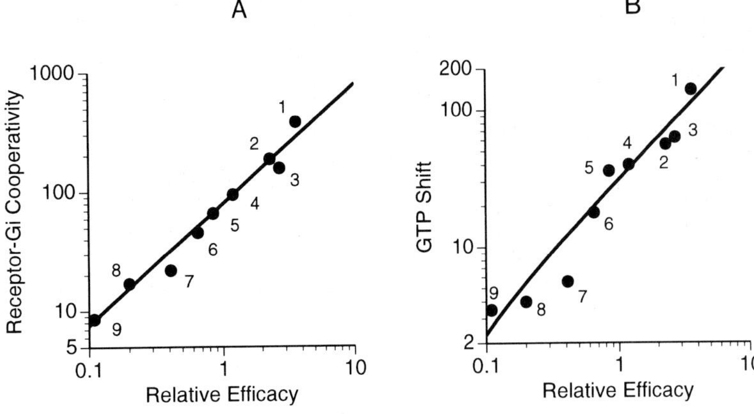

Figure 26–4. Correlation between relative efficacy and agonist-binding properties at M_2 muscarinic receptors. *A,* The positive heterotropic cooperativity between the binding of the agonist and G_i is plotted against the relative efficacy of the agonist as determined by inhibition of adenylate cyclase activity. *B,* The ratio of the concentration of the agonist in the presence and in the absence of GTP is plotted against the relative efficacy of the agonist. *Key:* 1 = oxotremorine-M; 2 = carbachol; 3 = *cis*-dioxolane; 4 = oxotremorine; 5 = (+)-aceclidine; 6 = (−)-aceclidine; 7 = *N*-methylaceclidine; 8 = BM5; 9 = BOK1. (Data from Ehlert FJ: The relationship between muscarinic receptor occupancy and adenylate cyclase inhibition in the rabbit myocardium. Mol Pharmacol 1985; 28:410.)

TABLE 26–1. Signaling Mechanisms of G Protein–Linked Receptors*

Representative receptors	*G protein family*	*Effector*
β_1- and β_2 adrenergic D_1 dopamine H_2 histamine	G_s	Stimulate adenylate cyclase, open calcium channels
M_2 and M_4 muscarinic D_2 dopamine α_2 adrenergic	G_i and G_o	Open potassium channels, close calcium channels, inhibit adenylate cyclase, stimulate PIP_2-PLC, stimulate PLA_2
M_1, M_3, and M_5 muscarinic α_1 adrenergic Angiotensin II	G_q	Stimulate PIP_2-PLC
Rhodopsin	G_T	Stimulate cGMP phosphodiesterase

*Data are taken from Hepler and Gilman.[20]
Abbreviations: phosphatidylinositol-4,5-bisphosphate-PLC = phosphatidylinositol-4,5-bisphosphate-specific phospholipase C; PLA_2 = phospholipase A_2; cGMP = cyclic guanosine monophosphate.

intermediate and distal parts of the signaling mechanism are tissue specific. Thus, calcium mobilization resulting from activation of a phospholipase C-linked receptor in smooth muscle may cause contraction[34]; however, in an exocrine gland, the same transduction mechanism may cause secretion. Some of the major transduction mechanisms of G protein–linked receptors are summarized next and listed in Table 26–1.

Perhaps the most universal mechanism for triggering a response is to increase the concentration of calcium within the cell.[35] Not surprisingly, several different signaling mechanisms ultimately affect the levels of calcium within the cytoplasm. One common mechanism for elevating calcium is through activation of phosphatidylinositol-4,5-bisphosphate-specific phospholipase C (PIP_2-PLC), an enzyme that hydrolyzes the phospholipid PIP_2 into IP_3 and DAG.[36] This membrane-bound enzyme is activated by numerous receptors through G_q and G_o (see Table 26–1). The two hydrolysis products, IP_3 and DAG, act as second messengers within the cell.[37] IP_3 causes a release of calcium from the endoplasmic reticulum and DAG activates protein kinase C. IP_3 is phosphorylated in some cells to inositol-1,3,4,5-tetrakisphosphate (IP_4), which appears to have a role in assisting IP_3 in mobilizing calcium.[38] Both IP_3 and IP_4 are unstable and are sequentially hydrolyzed by phosphatases back to inositol, which is then recycled for synthesis of new PIP_2. The final phosphatase in the sequence, *myo*-inositol-1-phosphatase, is inhibited by lithium. Ultimately, this inhibition leads to an accumulation of inositol-1-phosphate (IP_1) and a depletion in inositol and inositol containing phospholipids (e.g., PIP_2) within the brain. This depletion can lead to a dampening in receptor signaling through the PIP_2-PLC pathway, and it has been suggested that this dampening is the mechanism by which lithium attenuates the symptoms of manic-depressive psychosis.[39] Once calcium is elevated in the cell, it can mediate a variety of effects by binding to calmodulin and activating a variety of kinases and phosphatases. The protein kinase C that is activated by DAG also mediates numerous effects, and it is the target for some tumor-promoting phorbol ester derivatives.

Another important signaling mechanism within the cell is the adenylate cyclase system. G protein–linked receptors that affect adenylate cyclase can be divided into two categories depending on whether they stimulate or inhibit the enzyme.[20] G_s mediates the stimulation, whereas G_i mediates inhibition through a distinct group of receptors. Several different types of adenylate cyclases have been identified, and all of these are activated by the α subunit of G_s (i.e., α_s).[40] The mechanism for inhibition of the enzyme is not entirely clear; it appears that both α_i and the $\beta\gamma$ subunits may be involved, depending on the type of adenylate cyclase. Once cyclic adenosine monophosphate (AMP) rises within the cell, it can mediate a variety of effects through activation of cyclic AMP–dependent protein kinase (protein kinase A). The turn-off mechanism for cyclic AMP is phosphodiesterase, which rapidly hydrolyzes cyclic AMP into AMP.

There are several possibilities for crosstalk between receptors that stimulate adenylate cyclase and those that activate PIP_2-PLC. For example, the type I adenylate cyclase, which is abundant in brain, is activated by calcium.[40] Also, calcium stimulates phosphodiesterase in some tissues. Moreover, the stimulation of adenylate cyclase caused by G_s-linked receptors is enhanced by activation of protein kinase C in some tissues. Finally, α_s-mediated stimulation of the type II and IV adenylate cyclases has been shown to be greatly potentiated by the $\beta\gamma$ subunits, which provides yet another mechanism for receptor crosstalk.

In addition to the second-messenger systems described previously, G protein–linked receptors can also affect a variety of ionic conductances.[41] In several instances, these effects are mediated indirectly by second messengers, whereas in other cases there is direct coupling of G proteins to ion channels. One such example is in the heart, where muscarinic receptors and β-adrenergic receptors cause reciprocal changes in the conductivity of inwardly rectified potassium channels. These effects are mediated by G_i and G_s, respectively, and represent the mechanisms by which the vagus nerve slows heart rate and the cardiac sympathetic nerves increase heart rate.

CELLULAR SIGNALING AND CANCER

Most cancer cells contain mutations in their DNA that presumably cause tumorigenesis.[42] These mutations are of two general forms: (1) recessive, which results in a loss of function of tumor suppressor genes and (2) dominant, which results in a gain in function. The genes that contain these dominant mutations are designated as oncogenes, and their normal counterparts are referred to as proto-oncogenes. Invariably, proto-oncogenes code for proteins that are part of normal receptor signaling cascades within the body. For example, truncated forms of the EGF receptor lacking the ligand-binding domain are constitutively active and cause tumorigenesis.[9] Relatively small changes in signaling proteins are oncogenic in numerous instances. For example, point mutations in G_i have been implicated in carcinoma of the ovary and adrenal gland, whereas point mutations in G_s are present in adenomas of the pituitary gland and carcinoma of the thyroid.[43] Interestingly, these point mutations result in a loss in the GTPase activity of these G proteins, causing them to become constitutively active. There are numerous other examples of oncogene products that are mutated signaling proteins, including ligand regulated transcription factors, RTKs, and low-molecular-weight G proteins. Thus, in numerous instances, tumorigenesis is caused by overactive, unregulated, receptor signaling.

CONCLUSIONS

In considering the diverse mechanisms by which information is transmitted throughout the body by way of receptor signaling, one is struck by two seemingly opposite principals of nature: diversity and redundancy.[44] Nature is redundant in the sense that only four different types of mechanisms can account for the function of what may turn out to be more than 1000 different types of physiologic and sensory receptors. Also, the same general GTPase cycle is harnessed for innumerable functions within the cell, ranging from protein synthesis, secretion, neurotransmission, taste, olfaction, and vision. To accomplish these diverse tasks, nature modifies a given mechanism in an extraordinary number of ways. An appreciation of the diversity and redundancy of nature will aid in the future unraveling of biologic mechanisms and in the development of therapeutic agents to treat disease.

ACKNOWLEDGMENTS

Portions of the author's work cited in this chapter were supported by National Institutes of Health Grants NS30882 and NS26511. Frederick J. Ehlert is a recipient of U.S. Public Service Research Cancer Development Award NS01396 from the National Institute of Neurological Disorders and Stroke.

References

1. Unwin N, Toyoshima C, Kubalek E: Arrangement of the acetylcholine receptor subunits in the resting and desensitized states determined by cryelector microscopy of crystallized Torpedo postsynaptic membranes. J Cell Biol 1988; 107:1123.
2. Stein L, Belluzzi JD: Reinforcement, neurochemical substrates. *In*: Encyclopedia of Neuroscience, Volume II. Adelman G (Ed). Boston, Birkhauser, 1987, pp 1043–1045.
3. Costa T, Herz A: Antagonists with negative intrinsic activity at delta opioid receptors coupled to GTP-binding proteins. Proc Natl Acad Sci U S A 1989; 86:7321.
4. Ehlert FJ: "Inverse agonists," cooperativity and drug action at benzodiazepine receptors. Trends Pharmacol Sci 1986; 7:28.
5. Taylor P, Insel PA: Molecular basis of drug action. *In* Principles of Drug Action. 3rd ed. Pratt WB, Taylor P (Eds). New York, Churchill Livingstone, 1990, pp 103–200.
6. Fuller PJ: The steroid receptor superfamily: Mechanisms of diversity. FASEB J 1991; 5:3092.
7. Green S, Chambon P: Oestradiol induction of a glucocorticoid-responsive gene by a chimaeric receptor. Nature 1987; 325:75.
8. Godowski PJ, Rusconi S, Miesfeld R, et al: Glucocorticoid receptor mutants that are constitutive activators of transcriptional enhancement. Nature 1987; 325:365.
9. Yarden Y, Ullrich A: Growth factor receptor tyrosine kinases. Ann Rev Biochem 1988; 57:443.
10. Jaye M, Schlessinger J, Dionne CA: Fibroblast growth factor receptor tyrosine kinases: Molecular analysis and signal transduction. Biochim Biophys Acta 1992; 1135:185.
11. Cantley LC, Auger KR, Carpenter C, et al: Oncogenes and signal transduction. Cell 1991; 64:281.
12. Chinkers M, Garbers DL, Chang M-S, et al: A membrane form of guanylate cyclase is an atrial natriuretic peptide receptor. Nature 1989; 338:76.
13. Garbers DL: Guanylate cyclase receptor family. Rec Prog Horm Res 1990; 46:85.
14. Mallet S, Barclay AN: A new superfamily of cell surface proteins related to the nerve growth factor receptor. Immunol Today 1991; 12:220.
15. Clarke PB: The fall and rise of neuronal alpha-bungarotoxin binding proteins. Trends Pharmacol Sci 1991; 13:407.
16. Schofield PR, Darlison MG, Fujita N, et al: The brain $GABA_A$ receptor: Cloning and functional expression of the cDNAs encoding its subunits. Nature 1987; 328:221.
17. Verdoorn TA, Draguhn A, Ymer S, et al: Functional properties of recombinant rat $GABA_A$ receptors depend upon subunit composition. Neuron 1990; 4:919.
18. Taylor P: Agents acting at the neuromuscular junction and autonomic ganglia. *In*: The Pharmacological Basis of Therapeutics. 8th ed. Gilman GG, Rall TW, Nies AS, Taylor P (Eds). New York, Pergamon Press, 1990, pp 166–186.
19. Rall TW, Scheifer LS: Drugs effective in the therapy of the epilepsies. *In*: The Pharmacological Basis of Therapeutics. 8th ed. Gilman GG, Rall TW, Nies AS, Taylor P (Eds). New York, Pergamon Press, 1990, pp 436–462.
20. Hepler JR, Gilman AG: G proteins. Trends Biochem Sci 1992; 17:383.
21. Stryer L: The molecules of visual excitation. Sci American 1987; 256:42.
22. Schnapf JL, Baylor DA: How photoreceptor cells respond to light: Sci American 1987; 256:40.
23. Birdsall NJ: Wheel on the sweet smell of success. Trends Pharmacol Sci 1991; 12:283.
24. Findlay JBC, Pappin DJC: The opsin family of proteins. Biochem J 1986; 238:625.
25. Fraser CM, Wang CD, Robinson DA, et al: Site-directed mutagenesis of m1 muscarinic acetylcholine receptors: Conserved aspartic acids play important roles in receptor function. Mol Pharmacol 1989; 36:840.
26. Strader CD, Sigal IS, Candelore MR, et al: Conserved aspartic acid residues 79 and 113 of the beta-adrenergic receptor have different roles in receptor function. J Biol Chem 1988; 263:10267.
27. Wong SK, Parker EM, Ross EM: Chimeric muscarinic cholinergic: Beta-adrenergic receptors that activate G_s in response to muscarinic agonists. J Biol Chem 1990; 265:6219.
28. Lefkowitz RJ, Cotecchia S, Samamama P, et al: Constitutive activity of receptors coupled to guanine nucleotide regulatory proteins. Trends Pharmacol Sci 1993; 14:303.
29. Bourne HR, Sanders DA, McCormick F: The GTPase superfamily: Conserved structure and molecular mechanism. Nature 1991; 349:117.
30. Bourne HR, Sanders DA, McCormick F: The GTPase superfamily: A conserved switch for diverse cell functions. Nature 1990; 348:125.
31. Matesic DF, Manning DR, Luthin GR: Tissue-dependent association of muscarinic acetylcholine receptors with guanine nucleotide-binding regulatory proteins. Mol Pharmacol 1991; 40:347.
32. Ehlert FJ: The relationship between muscarinic receptor occupancy and adenylate cyclase inhibition in the rabbit myocardium. Mol Pharmacol 1985; 28:410.
33. Weber G: Energetics of ligand biding to proteins. Adv Prot Chem 1975; 29:1.
34. Thomas EA, Baker SA, Ehlert FJ: Functional role for the M2 muscarinic receptor in smooth muscle of the guinea pig ileum. Mol Pharmacol 1993; 44:102.
35. Rasmussen H: The cycling of calcium as an intracellular messenger. Sci American 1989; 261:66.
36. Cockcroft S, Thomas GM: Inositol-lipid-specific phospholipase C isoenzymes and their differential regulation by receptors. Biochem J 1992; 288:1.
37. Berridge MJ: The molecular basis of communication within the cell. Sci American 1985; 255:142.
38. Irvine RF: How do inositol 1,4,5-triphosphate and inositol 1,3,4,5-tetrakisphosphate regulate intracellular Ca2+? Biochem Soc Trans 1989; 17:6.
39. Berridge MJ, Downes CP, Hanley MR: Neural and developmental actions of lithium: A unifying hypothesis. Cell 1989; 59:411.
40. Tang WJ, Gilman AG: Adenylyl cyclases. Cell 1992; 70:869.
41. Brown AM: Regulation of heartbeat by G protein-coupled ion channels. Am J Physiol 1990; 259:H1621.
42. Bishop MJ: Molecular themes in oncogenesis. Cell 1991; 64:235.
43. Lyons J, Landis CA, Harsh G, et al: Two G protein oncogenes in human endocrine tumors. Science 1990; 249:655.
44. Koshland DE: The two-component pathway comes to eukaryotes. Science 1993; 262:532.

CHAPTER 27

Physiologic and Pathophysiologic Significance of Nitric Oxide

Louis J. Ignarro, PhD

The field of nitric oxide (NO) research has virtually exploded into numerous and diverse areas of physiology and pathophysiology since the 1987 discovery that mammalian cells synthesize and release NO.[1-3] Before this discovery, most biologists and chemists viewed NO as one of several prominent pollutant gases, especially of the internal combustion engine, that contributes to the formation of smog and acid rain. Nitric oxide, however, had been shown in the mid- to late 1970s to elicit marked biologic actions. Nitric oxide gas, either generated in the laboratory by adding sodium nitrite to hydrochloric acid or purchasing a small gas cylinder commercially, was shown to activate guanylate cyclase, the enzyme that catalyzes the conversion of guanosine triphosphate (GTP) to cyclic guanosine monophosphate (GMP), and to stimulate cyclic GMP formation in mammalian tissues.[4,5] At that time, the biologic significance of cyclic GMP was unknown, although studies from this laboratory indicated that cyclic GMP formation was associated temporally with stimulation of human neutrophil function, including lysosomal enzyme secretion and phagocytosis.[6]

Following the observations that NO and certain nitro compounds such as sodium nitroprusside and nitroglycerin stimulated tissue cyclic GMP formation, we reasoned that NO and cyclic GMP might cause vascular smooth-muscle relaxation. Subsequent experiments in 1979 to 1981 revealed that (1) NO is a potent vasorelaxant; (2) cyclic GMP is the second messenger mediating this important action of NO; and (3) the mechanism of vasodilator action of sodium nitroprusside, nitroglycerin, and isoamyl nitrite is attributed to the chemical conversion of these nitrovasodilators to NO in vascular smooth muscle.[5] Moreover, NO was found to be a potent inhibitor of human platelet aggregation, and this effect was also mediated by cyclic GMP. Thus, the first two biologic actions of NO discovered were vascular smooth-muscle relaxation and inhibition of platelet aggregation, and both initial observations were made before the discovery of endothelium-derived relaxing factor (EDRF) in 1980.

Nitric oxide is 1 of the 10 smallest molecules found in nature, composed of a single atom of nitrogen and a single atom of oxygen (O_2). Yet research during the past 5 years has revealed the multifaceted and complex physiologic and pathophysiologic roles played by NO in at least a dozen different mammalian cell types in various tissues ranging from the brain to the penis. The objective of this chapter is to provide a brief review of the essential chemical and pharmacologic properties of NO and to highlight its principal biologic actions in mammalian cells.

CHEMISTRY OF NITRIC OXIDE

The NO molecule contains an odd number of electrons (five electrons from nitrogen plus six electrons from oxygen). This means that one electron is unpaired (paramagnetism) and renders NO a reactive molecule, a free radical often written as •NO. Free radicals tend to react with other molecules containing unpaired electrons, such as molecular O_2, superoxide anion (O_2^-), and various metals including iron. This chemistry underlies the basis for the physiologic and pathophysiologic actions as well as the biologic inactivation of NO.

Nitric oxide is a gas that is soluble in water to the extent of about 1 to 3 mmol (30–90 mg/L). Biologically active concentrations of NO range from 1 to 100 nmol. Nitric oxide is a very lipophilic molecule that readily permeates lipoprotein membrane barriers, but NO has a limited half-life of less than 3 to 5 seconds because of its spontaneous reactivity with molecular O_2 to yield nitrite (NO_2^-) and, under certain conditions, nitrate (NO_3^-), both of which are relatively inactive biologically at low concentrations. The oxidation of NO is often represented as follows:

$$2{\bullet}NO + O_2 \rightarrow 2\,NO_2$$
$$2NO_2 \rightarrow N_2O_4$$
$$N_2O_4 + H_2O \rightarrow NO_2^- + NO_3^- + 2H^+$$

Various oxidizing agents in the intracellular and extracellular environment can catalyze the more rpaid oxidative inactivation of NO primarily to NO_3^-. One such prominent molecule is oxyhemoglobin (HbO_2) and the reaction is represented next:

$$\underset{(Fe^{2+})}{HbO_2} + {\bullet}NO \rightarrow \underset{(Fe^{3+})}{\text{methemoglobin (metHb)}} + NO_3^-$$

In view of its short half-life, NO must elicit its biologic actions at sites that are very close to its sites of biosynthesis. Thus, the NO molecules synthesized by a given cell generally act on closely adjacent cells. An example is the action of endothelium-derived NO on adjacent vascular smooth-muscle cells (Fig. 27–1). This paracrine action is very different from the endocrine action of chemically stable hormonal substances that act on cells at distant sites. Nitric oxide also elicits autocrine effects (within its cells of origin), the principal effect being a negative feedback modulation of its own synthesis.

Nitric oxide reacts readily with the reduced iron (ferrous; Fe^{2+}) of the heme prosthetic group in cytosolic guanylate cyclase to cause prompt and marked enzyme activation, resulting in stimulation of cyclic GMP biosynthesis. This reaction forms the basis for the biochemical mechanism by which NO relaxes vascular smooth muscle and inhibits platelet function. Cyclic GMP is the second-messenger molecule that expresses the cellular actions of NO. At very high concentrations, NO not only binds to and reacts with the iron in proteins but knocks the iron out of the protein, thereby disrupting the function of the protein and also the cell containing that protein. This constitutes one of the pathophysiologic mechanisms by which NO elicits cytotoxicity on certain target cells and micro-organisms. Another pathophysiologic mechanism involves the reactivity of NO with O_2^- to yield peroxynitrite anion ($ONOO^-$) and related radicals that promote lipid peroxidation and cell damage. The reaction is usually written as follows:

$${\bullet}NO + O_2^- \rightarrow ONOO^-$$
$$ONOO^- + H^+ \rightleftarrows ONOOH$$
$$ONOOH \rightarrow {\bullet}OH + {\bullet}NO_2 \rightarrow NO_3^- + H^+$$

Hemoglobin has a very high binding affinity for NO, even higher than that for carbon monoxide, and inactivates NO by sequestration. Oxyhemoglobin interacts similarly with NO and, in addition, catalyzes the oxidation of NO to NO_3^- as described previously. These properties of HbO_2 ensure a highly localized or restricted biologic action of NO on nearby cells.

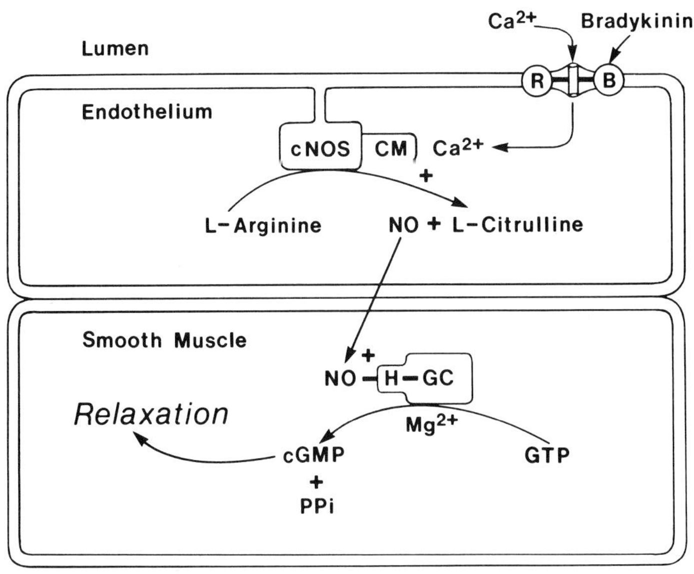

Figure 27–1. Schematic illustration of the interaction between endothelium-derived NO and vascular smooth muscle. In this example of endothelium-dependent vascular smooth muscle relaxation, bradykinin in the blood interacts with selective receptors (B) on the luminal surface of endothelial cells to trigger calcium ion (Ca^{2+}) influx. Other chemical agents in the blood may also interact with their own selective receptors (R) to trigger Ca^{2+} influx. Intracellular Ca^{2+} forms a complex with calmodulin (CM) that is bound to the constitutive isoform of NO synthase (cNOS), thereby causing enzyme activation (+). cNOS catalyzes the conversion of L-arginine to NO plus L-citrulline. The NO generated diffuses readily across membrane barriers into adjacent smooth muscle cells and forms a complex with heme (H) that is bound to the cytosolic guanylate cyclase (GC), thereby causing enzyme activation (+). GC catalyzes the conversion of GTP to cyclic GMP (cGMP) plus inorganic pyrophosphate (PPi) in the presence of magnesium ion (Mg^{2+}). cGMP acts as an intracellular second messenger to effect smooth muscle relaxation.

PHARMACOLOGY OF NITRIC OXIDE

The first two pharmacologic effects discovered for NO more than a dozen years ago turned out to be the most important and relevant for the subsequent studies that led to the identification of EDRF as NO.[7] Nitric oxide is a potent vascular smooth-muscle relaxant, affecting veins as well as arteries. In fact, NO is a more potent venodilator than arteriodilator. The mechanism of action of NO is fairly well established. Nitric oxide binds to the heme prosthetic group of the cytosolic isoform of guanylate cyclase and activates the enzyme, thereby catalyzing the conversion of GTP to cyclic GMP. Cyclic GMP acts as an intracellular amplifier and messenger to cause a rapid decrease in the levels of intracellular free calcium and to inactivate myosin light-chain kinase. By these two mechanisms, the contractile activity of vascular smooth muscle is paralyzed and the muscle relaxes. Clinically useful nitrovasodilators including nitroglycerin, sodium nitroprusside, isoamyl nitrite, and related analogs all work by the same mechanism of action, namely, by being metabolized to NO and thereby stimulating cyclic GMP formation.[8] These nitrovasodilators interact with vascular smooth-muscle cells and undergo chemical biotransformation with the liberation of NO.

Nitric oxide is a potent inhibitor of platelet aggregation induced by adenosine diphosphate, thrombin, arachidonic acid, and related proaggregatory agents.[7] Again, the action of NO is cyclic GMP dependent. Nitric oxide activates cytosolic guanylate cyclase in platelets by heme-dependent mechanisms, and cyclic GMP turns off key calcium-dependent platelet functions by lowering intracellular free calcium levels in platelets. Sodium nitroprusside also inhibits platelet function but nitroglycerin does not. The reason for this apparent dichotomy is that, whereas the nitroprusside anion readily liberates NO on contact with platelets and other cells, nitroglycerin is not metabolized to NO in platelets. In addition to inhibiting platelet aggregation, NO inhibits platelet adhesion to endothelial cell surfaces again by cyclic GMP–dependent mechanisms.

In addition to relaxing vascular smooth muscle, NO also relaxes nonvascular smooth muscle, including that in airways, gastrointestinal tissue, uterus, and the retractor penis muscle of the bull. These observations led to the important discovery of the mechanism by which certain uncharacterized neurons, termed *nonadrenergic-noncholinergic* (NANC), cause inhibitory influences (relaxation) on nonvascular smooth muscle. Electrical stimulation of NANC neurons innervating various nonvascular smooth-muscle preparations caused relaxant responses that were highly characteristic of the relaxant responses elicited by authentic NO. These observations led to the discovery that NO is the NANC neurotransmitter in numerous tissues.[9] Interestingly, vascular smooth muscle in certain arteries, such as cerebral arteries and arteries in the erectile tissue of the penis, is also innervated by inhibitory NANC neurons that release NO on electrical stimulation.[10] Thus, NO is the principal mediator of penile erection in the mammal, and the process is regulated by NANC neurotransmission (Fig. 27–2).

Nitric oxide appears to play a neurotransmitter role in the central nervous system, although its precise function or effects are presently unclear. In the rat, NO is synthesized primarily in the cerebellum, but this may not be the case for other species, including humans. For example, in the bovine species, the cerebellum contains only little NO synthase activity, whereas the cerebrum has the highest NO-forming activity. It is conceivable that NO could function to modulate efferent motor activity. Nitric oxide may play a modulatory role in neuronal plasticity such as long-term potentiation in memory function.

Recent evidence has accumulated that NO may act to inhibit cell proliferation. For example, the induction of large amounts of NO-forming activity in cultured vascular smooth-muscle cells is associated with a reduction in cell proliferation. Thus, it is possible that vascular endothelium-derived NO could regulate the mass of the underlying vascular smooth muscle by regulating cell proliferation. These observations have profound implications in vascular disorders in which the endothelial cell layer is damaged, such as in arteriosclerosis and immune arteritis, both of which are characterized by vascular smooth-muscle hyperplasia. Moreover, balloon angioplasty causes endothelial cell damage, which is often associated with the development of vascular smooth-muscle hyperplasia.

BIOSYNTHESIS OF ENDOGENOUS NITRIC OXIDE

The discovery that EDRF is NO in 1987 was immediately followed by the question, "How is NO synthesized in vascular endothelial cells?" The answer came from an important clue that was provided 2 years earlier from a study on activated macrophages.[11] Murine macrophages incubated in

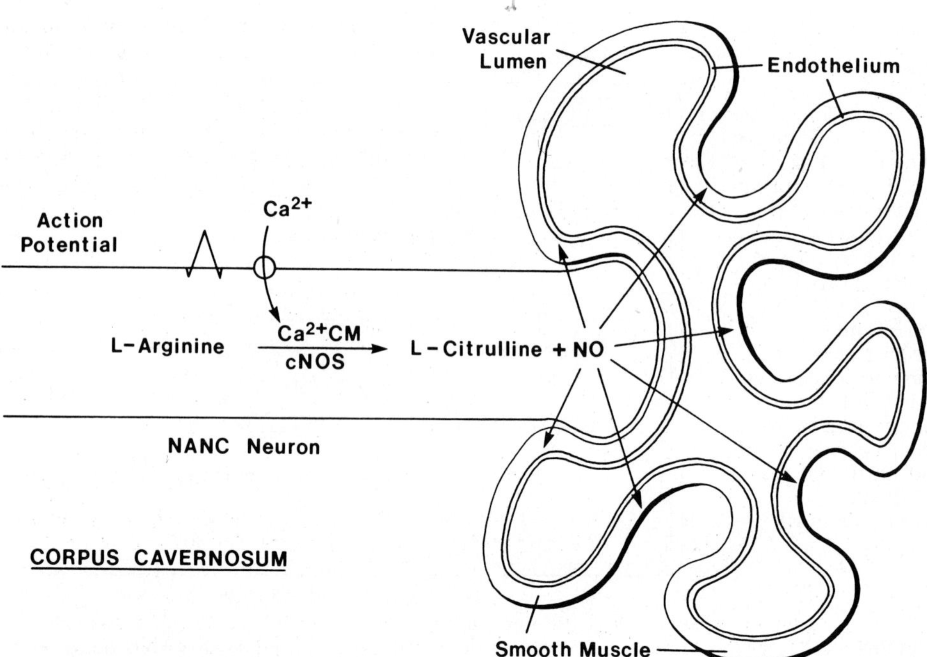

Figure 27–2. Schematic illustration of the role of NO as a neuronal mediator of penile erection. The sinusoidal vascular network of the corpus cavernosum, the erectile tissue of the penis, is innervated by nonadrenergic-noncholinergic (NANC) neurons that travel in the parasympathetic division of the autonomic nervous system. The propagated action potential opens voltage-dependent Ca^{2+} channels to cause Ca^{2+} influx. Intraneuronal Ca^{2+} forms a complex with calmodulin (CM) that is bound to the constitutive isoform of NO synthase (cNOS), and this causes enzyme activation. cNOS catalyzes the conversion of L-arginine to NO plus L-citrulline. The NO generated diffuses out of the NANC neuron in all directions and into the surrounding corpus cavernosum. NO interacts with the corpus cavernosum to cause relaxation by cGMP-dependent mechanisms, as discussed in Figure 27–1. In the corpus cavernosum, the vascular endothelium does not appear to play a role in NANC transmission–related relaxation of vascular smooth muscle.

the presence of *Escherichia coli* lipopolysaccharide were shown to synthesize relatively large quantities of NO_2^- and NO_3^-, the two major oxidation products of NO in aqueous solution. However, the authors did not recognize at the time that NO was an intermediate in the formation of NO_2^- and NO_3^-. Subsequent studies by the same laboratory revealed that the presence of L-arginine in the incubation medium was required for NO_2^- and NO_3^- formation. Concomitant studies by another laboratory also showed that, in addition to NO_2^-, citrulline was a second product generated by activated macrophages.[12] These investigators showed also that NO_2^- and citrulline formation was L-arginine dependent and inhibited by addition of N^G-methyl-L-arginine to the macrophage incubation medium. These earlier observations with macrophages paved the way for the later finding with arterial endothelial cells that NO and citrulline were formed from L-arginine.[13]

Studies from various laboratories soon revealed that, in addition to vascular endothelial cells and macrophages, many other cell types were also capable of synthesizing NO from L-arginine. These additional cell types or tissues include activated neutrophils, platelets, hepatic Kupffer cells, vascular smooth muscle, nonvascular smooth muscle, NANC neurons, and a variety of cell types in the brain. Mammalian cells use an enzyme whose apparent sole important function is to produce NO. This enzyme, NO synthase, catalyzes the conversion of L-arginine to NO, the second product of the reaction being L-citrulline (Fig. 27–3).

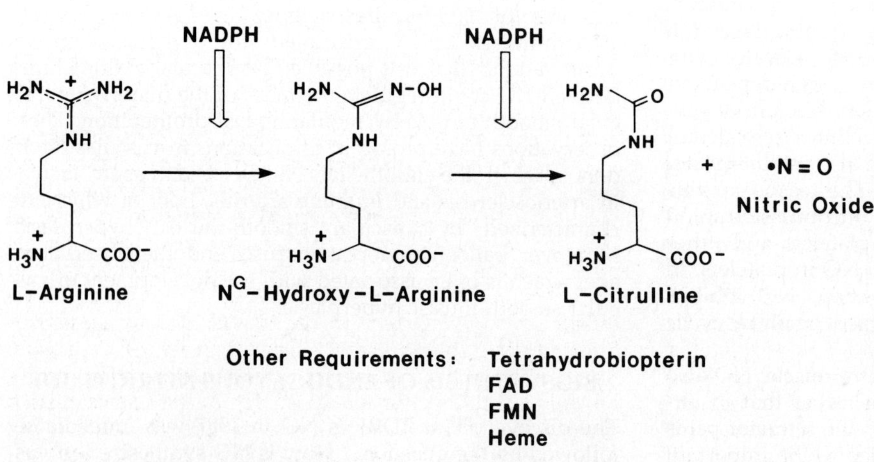

Figure 27–3. Characteristics of the biosynthesis of NO from L-arginine catalyzed by NO synthase. L-Arginine is a basic amino acid in which one of the two equivalent amino nitrogen atoms is oxidized and cleaved to yield NO (•N = O) plus L-citrulline. One of the reaction intermediates is known to be N^G-hydroxy-L-arginine. Nicotinamide-adenine dinucleotide phosphate (reduced form) (NADPH) is a required cofactor for the reaction as illustrated. Additional cofactors required for catalysis include tetrahydrobiopterin, flavin adenine dinucleotide (FAD), flavin mononucleotide (FMN), and heme, all of which function in electron transfer to accommodate the complicated five-electron oxidation of L-arginine to yield NO plus L-citrulline. Molecular oxygen is incorporated into both the NO and L-citrulline reaction products. Both the constitutive and inducible isoforms of NO synthase possess similar cofactor requirements. In addition, cNOS requires Ca^{2+} and calmodulin for enzyme activation.

L-Arginine is a basic amino acid, possessing the basic guanidinium group. One of the two equivalent basic amino nitrogen atoms is oxidized to yield an intermediate, N^G-hydroxy-L-arginine. Then, in a complex series of oxidative steps, the nitrogen is cleaved to yield NO while the remaining carbon takes on an O_2 atom to form a carbonyl, yielding L citrulline. The O_2 atoms incorporated into NO and L-citrulline derive from molecular O_2. This complex oxidative pathway requires the transfer of five electrons from L-arginine, and catalysis is achieved by a single enzyme protein: NO synthase.[14] The reduced form of nicotinamide-adenine dinucleotide phosphate (NADPH) is one cofactor that is required, even for a trace of enzymatic activity. Other reducing cofactors that speed up the reaction and may also be required as well include tetrahydrobiopterin, flavin adenine dinucleotide, and flavin mononucleotide. Nitric oxide synthase also contains bound heme (ferroprotoporphyrin IX). The function of the heme (Fe^{2+} state) is to bind and activate oxygen for subsequent incorporation into NO and citrulline. Thus, heme likely plays a key role in electron transfer and therefore NO biosynthesis. Another function of heme may be to bind NO once NO is formed. The binding of NO to heme on NO synthase causes reversible inhibition of NO synthase activity. This effect may represent a negative feedback regulatory action of NO on its own biosynthesis. We have observed this effect with both the constitutive and inducible isoforms of NO synthase. Such an autocrine effect of NO may represent one key mechanism by which NO regulates its own synthesis.

There are two important forms of NO synthase in mammalian cells.[15] One is constitutive (always present), and the other is inducible (appears only after enzyme synthesis). The constitutive isoform (isoenzyme), in addition to requiring the reducing cofactors discussed previously, is regulated by calcium and calmodulin. That is, the calcium-calmodulin complex binds to and activates the NO synthase. An increase in intracellular free calcium levels results in the formation of enzyme-bound calcium-calmodulin complex, which activates NO synthase and turns on NO production. The apparent affinity of NO synthase for free calcium is about 1 μmol or less. This means that physiologic stimuli that increase intracellular calcium levels from 0.1 to 1 μmol will stimulate NO production in those cells. The second major isoform of NO synthase is inducible. That is, NO synthase activity is undetectable until several hours after enzyme protein synthesis has been initiated by an appropriate cell activator. The inducible isoform is not regulated by calcium or calmodulin. When the enzyme protein is present, it is in the fully activated state.

The inducible isoform of NO synthase is important in tissue macrophages, neutrophils, and hepatic Kupffer cells. In macrophages, for example, appropriate cytokines such as interferon-γ or lipopolysaccharide activate the macrophages and induce the synthesis of NO synthase protein. Four to 6 hours later, detectable quantities of NO and L-citrulline are formed, reaching a maximum after about 24 hours. The function of the NO generated by macrophages in this manner is cytotoxicity to target cells. In a similar manner and for similar purposes, NO can be generated by activated neutrophils and hepatic Kupffer cells. Nitric oxide formation can be induced to occur also in vascular smooth-muscle cells under special pathophysiologic conditions such as septic shock, endotoxin shock, and related disorders. In these conditions, lipopolysaccharide, related bacterial toxins, and cytokines such as interleukin-1 and tumor necrosis factor induce the synthesis of NO synthase in vascular smooth muscle. The result is profound vascular smooth-muscle relaxation, vasodilation, and a decrease in peripheral vascular resistance (hypotension) that is quite difficult to reverse.

The constitutive isoform of NO synthase is important in mediating normal physiologic processes, whereas the inducible isoform appears to be involved in cytotoxicity. Many different cell types possess constitutive NO synthase activity. When studied, the constitutive enzyme exists either in the cytosolic fraction or membrane-bound fraction, but the catalytic properties are indistinguishable with current techniques. The intracellular calcium concentration decides whether NO formation increases in any cell type. Thus, pharmacologic selectivity lies with the extracellular membrane-bound receptors that respond to agonists by promoting calcium influx or promoting the intracellular liberation of bound calcium. For example, acetylcholine, bradykinin, and histamine each interact with selective endothelial cell receptors to trigger calcium influx, NO synthase activation, and NO formation.

METABOLISM OF ENDOGENOUS NITRIC OXIDE

One of the most intriguing properties of NO is its extreme chemical lability at low concentrations in O_2-containing aqueous solution. The biologic half-life of NO in aqueous solution is 3 to 5 seconds and less than 1 second in biologic tissues containing oxyhemoproteins and other biologic oxidants. This means that there is no need for complex enzymatic systems or reuptake mechanisms to promote the termination of action of NO. The biologic activity of NO is terminated rapidly by its oxidation in the presence of O_2 to NO_2^- and NO_3^-. Nitrite is much less active biologically than is NO, and NO_3^- is essentially inactive. Other biochemical processes participate under special conditions to accelerate the oxidative inactivation of NO. Superoxide anion is generated by numerous cell types, including activated macrophages and neutrophils, and vascular endothelial cells during increases in O_2 tension after periods of low O_2 tension. Nitric oxide reacts very rapidly with O_2^- to form a new chemical species, thereby resulting in the inactivation of NO.

The very short half-life of NO requires that any biologic effects be elicited close to its site of biosynthesis. Most of the studies conducted indicate clearly that NO elicits its effects not in its cells of origin but rather in adjacent target cells. Thus, NO must have enough time to exit its cells of origin, permeate its target cells, and elicit a biologic response. The physicochemical properties of NO endow this tiny molecule with the capacity to fulfill its paracrine role as a messenger molecule. Nitric oxide is a small lipophilic molecule that easily and rapidly penetrates lipoidal membrane barriers.

PHYSIOLOGIC ROLES FOR NITRIC OXIDE

The two most widely appreciated biologic roles for NO are vascular smooth-muscle relaxation and inhibition of platelet-induced thrombosis. Both of these effects appear to occur throughout the vascular system within a species and across all species examined thus far. A variety of substances and conditions can stimulate NO formation in vascular endothelial cells. The first substance found to stimulate endothelial NO production was acetylcholine. Acetylcholine interacts with muscarinic receptors on the extracellular surface of endothelial cells to trigger an increase in the concentration of intracellular free calcium, thereby leading to the activation of constitutive NO synthase and increasing NO production. Although the mechanism of vasodilator action of acetylcholine is fairly clear, the physiologic significance of such observations is less clear because cholinergic neurons are not known to innervate vascular endothelial cells, acetylcholine is a quaternary ammonium compound that cannot permeate cell membranes, and any acetylcholine in the blood will be readily hydrolyzed by cholinesterase.

Autacoids, or local tissue hormones such as bradykinin, histamine, serotonin, and other small amines, peptides, and other chemical agents possess selective receptors on vascular endothelial cells in certain blood vessels of some species. Interaction of agonists with these receptors results in a calcium ionophore action, wherby the elevated intracellular free calcium interacts with calmodulin to activate NO synthase and stimulate NO production. Thus, the mechanism of local vasodilator action of these autacoids appears to be attributed to the stimulation of formation and subsequent local action of NO. Such a mechanism involving NO is consistent with the understanding that autacoids elicit local and transient vasodilator responses. Most of the autacoids function in acute inflammatory episodes to increase local blood flow to inflamed regions. Another desirable action of NO is the prevention of local thrombosis or blood clot formation. The chemical properties of NO ensure that the autacoid-mediated response will be localized.

In addition to the endothelium-dependent vasodilator actions of autacoids, nonchemical factors also elicit endothelium-dependent vasodilation by mechanisms that are attributed to NO. Flow-dependent dilation, which has long been recognized but unexplained, is now believed to occur as a result of the shear forces imposed on the vascular endothelial cells by the flowing blood. This tangential force is applied directly to the surface of the endothelial cells and represents a signal for enhanced production of NO. Shear force–induced generation of NO is calcium dependent, L-arginine dependent, and prostaglandin independent and appears to be attributed entirely to NO.[16] Shear force–induced generation of NO may be a major mechanism of antithrombosis because blood flow in any vessel should stimulate NO formation and thereby prevent platelet adhesion and aggregation. The precise mechanisms by which shear force is translated into a chemical signal for NO synthase activation are unknown. It is conceivable that shear force activates a mechanoreceptor that is coupled to a calcium channel, resulting in opening of the latter and consequent elevated intracellular levels of calcium. The mechanoreceptor could be a shear force–sensitive transmembrane potassium channel that is gated to an inward calcium channel. This could constitute the mechanochemical coupling mechanism that translates shear force into NO production. The mediation of flow-dependent dilation by NO is consistent with many past observations that the vasodilator response to shear force is a highly localized and transient phenomenon.

Electrical field stimulation of isolated vascular preparations often causes smooth-muscle relaxation that is mediated by NO. Pulmonary artery from various species responds to electrical field stimulation with smooth-muscle relaxation that is endothelium dependent and mediated by NO.[17] Relaxation is dependent on extracellular calcium and intracellular calmodulin, is accompanied by cyclic GMP accumulation, and is abolished by NO synthase inhibitors. Interestingly, the electrically induced and NO-mediated relaxation does not appear to involve neuronal structures because the sodium channel blocker, tetrodotoxin, does not inhibit the response. Thus, the question remains as to the mechanism by which the electric current is gated to the L-arginine–NO pathway. One possibility is that an electric current near the endothelial cell membrane initially mobilizes intracellular calcium, thereby opening calcium-activated potassium channels, which leads to hyperpolarization. Endothelial cell hyperpolarization would augment the driving force for potential-dependent transmembrane calcium influx and thereby provide the signal for NO synthase activation. Figure 27–4 illustrates some of the players involved in promoting the biosynthesis of NO in vascular endothelial cells.

Other blood vessels relax in response to electrical field stimulation by mechanisms that are endothelium independent and neuron dependent. These relaxant responses appear to involve adrenergic, cholinergic, and NANC transmission. The vasodilator responses to NANC transmission appear to be mediated by NO. Moreover, there are several different nonvascular smooth-muscle tissues that are innervated by NANC neurons and that relax in response to NANC neuronal stimulation. Again, the relaxation responses are mediated by NO. These NANC neurons have been known for what they are not (nonadrenergic and noncholinergic), and they have been referred to as inhibitory NANC neurons because the smooth-muscle response is relaxation rather than contraction.[9] All of the previous observations can easily be explained by the more recent findings that NANC neurons synthesize and release NO, which is responsible for the smooth-muscle relaxation. The blood vessels that are known to undergo NANC-mediated vasodilation are cerebral arteries and penile arteries in the corpus cavernosum, but there are likely to be more. The identification of NO as the physiologic mediator of penile erection has opened the way for reinvestigation of the cause and pharmacologic treatment of impotence.[10] Nonvascular smooth-muscle relaxation that occurs in response to NANC neuronal stimulation includes gastrointestinal, anococcygeal, and airway smooth muscle.

These observations, together with the immunocytochemical evidence for the presence of NO synthase in NANC neurons, indicate that the NANC neurons should be renamed for what they are rather than for what they are not. We propose the terms *nitrosergic neurons* and *nitrosergic transmission* to replace the older and outdated terminology. The *nitros* part of nitrosergic signifies the nitroso functionality of NO and would be compatible with other evidence that S-nitrosothiols are also generated by mammalian cells.

Another potentially important physiologic role for NO may be in regulating cell proliferation, at least in the vascular system. Nitric oxide is believed to retard or inhibit the proliferation of vascular smooth-muscle cells. Activation of cytosolic guanylate cyclase by exogenous NO results in the inhibition of thymidine incorporation into deoxyribonucleic acid by vascular smooth-muscle cells in culture. This observation may explain how endothelial cells retard or regulate proliferation of the underlying smooth-muscle cells. In turn, endothelium-derived NO could account for the knowledge that vascular smooth-muscle cells do not readily proliferate in the presence of a normal functional endothelial cell layer, whereas smooth-muscle hyperplasia often occurs at sites of endothelial cell damage.

Nitric oxide has turned out to be a novel neurotransmitter.[18] Its novelty stems from its extraordinary chemical simplicity, and in this way it differs from the more complex large peptides and other chemicals that serve as neurotransmitters. Nitric oxide synthase has been localized only in discrete populations of neurons. In the pituitary gland, the enzyme is present in neurons originating in the hypothalamus and extending into the posterior lobe of the pituitary gland. Thus, NO may play a role in modulating the release of oxytocin and vasopressin. Nitric oxide synthase is present in the anterior pituitary as well and may function in the regulation of release of corticotropin, growth hormone, thyroid-stimulating hormone, and other hormones. In the adrenal gland, NO synthase is localized in a neuronal plexus that stimulates epinephrine release. In the intestine, NO synthase is localized in the NANC neurons making up the myenteric and Auerbach's plexus. Thus, NO may modulate

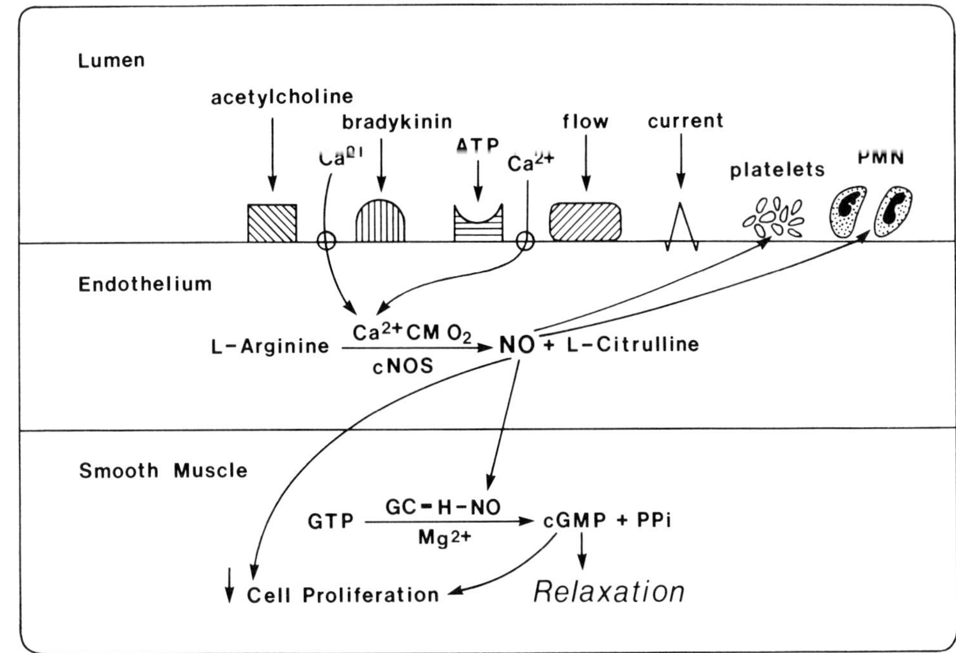

Figure 27–4. Schematic illustration of multiple factors that stimulate formation of endothelium-derived NO and multiple vascular functions of endothelium-derived NO. Various chemical agents in the blood (acetylcholine, bradykinin, adenosine triphosphate [ATP]) as well as mechanical (flow) and electrical (current) forces can interact with selective membrane surface receptors to trigger the influx of Ca^{2+} into endothelial cells. Intracellular Ca^{2+} forms a complex with CM that is bound to cNOS. Oxygen is one of several requirements for catalysis. The NO generated diffuses in all directions. In the underlying smooth muscle, NO causes relaxation by cGMP-dependent mechanisms. NO forms a complex with heme (H) that is bound to GC, thereby causing enzyme activation and formation of cGMP plus PPi. NO also causes inhibition of smooth muscle cell proliferation, but the role of cGMP in this action of NO is unclear. At the luminal surface, NO interacts with platelets and polymorphonuclear leukocytes (PMN) to prevent both adhesion to the endothelial surface and cellular aggregation. These functions of NO are likely mediated by cGMP formed in the platelet and PMN.

peristalsis. In the brain, NO synthase is localized in a variety of structures that also display the presence of NADPH diaphorase, an oxidative enzyme that requires NADPH as an electron donor but whose function is unknown. Evidence is accumulating that NADPH diaphorase and NO synthase are closely related enzymes.

The exact role of NO in the brain remains unknown, but several interesting observations have been made. Nitric oxide synthase and NADPH diaphorase neurons make up about 2% of the cerebral cortex. These neurons clearly survive or resist a variety of neurotoxic insults associated with Huntington's disease, Alzheimer's disease, and stroke. In a laboratory model of stroke, in which N-methyl-D-aspartate (NMDA) causes calcium-dependent, glutamate receptor–mediated neurotoxicity, the toxic action of NMDA was found to be mediated by NO and prevented by NO synthase inhibitors. Also of interest is that the NO synthase–containing neurons were resistant to damage. Only the nearby target cells were adversely affected by NMDA. Thus, in the brain, glutamate-induced neuronal toxicity appears to occur as a result of stimulation of the local production of relatively large quantities of NO. Nitric oxide synthase inhibitors may be useful in the treatment of neurologic disorders mediated by glutamate and NO.

If NO is a neurotransmitter, the characteristics of neurotransmission involving NO would have to differ significantly from that for other classic neurotransmitters. For example, NO is not localized in synaptic vesicles and is synthesized on demand in response to a rise in intracellular calcium triggered by the nerve action potential. The neuronal release of NO occurs as a simple diffusion process rather than by energy-requiring exocytosis. The small lipophilic molecule diffuses rapidly into the broad extraneuronal milieu rather than only into the synaptic cleft. Thus, several different cells adjacent to the neuron can be influenced by the NO released. Nitric oxide diffuses into these target cells and activates cytosolic guanylate cyclase to cause cyclic GMP accumulation, thereby triggering the target cell response. This represents a completely novel signal-transduction mechanism for a novel chemical neurotransmitter. Much research is in progress to elucidate the possible neurotransmitter role of NO in the brain. According to evidence accumulating from models of long-term potentiation and long-term depression in the hypothalamus, NO may be involved in learning and memory. The high specific activity of NO synthase in the cerebellum of rodents suggests that, among other potential functions, NO may play a role in regulating motor movement or coordination.

PATHOPHYSIOLOGIC ROLES FOR NITRIC OXIDE

The first clue that endogenous NO could play a pathophysiologic role in mammalian systems evolved from studies on activated rodent macrophages, which were shown to synthesize relatively large quantities of NO from L-arginine, as discussed previously. The common knowledge that NO becomes a very reactive nitrosating species at acidic pH led to the hypothesis that macrophage-derived NO causes damage to target cells within an acidic pH environment. In addition, the knowledge that NO reacts with other atoms or molecules that also contain unpaired electrons such as iron and related metals suggested that NO reacts with iron-containing proteins to alter their structure and function. As discussed earlier, NO reacts with the iron of the heme prosthetic group of guanylate cyclase in a physiologic manner to activate the enzyme and promote intracellular cyclic GMP formation. Guanylate cyclase activation by NO is a reversible process and represents the only known example of enzyme activation by NO. At higher concentrations, NO can react with heme iron-containing proteins, including guanylate cyclase, or nonheme iron-containing proteins to disrupt their normal physiologic function.

Macrophages are activated by various endotoxins and cytokines, such as interleukin-1 and tumor necrosis factor, derived from cytotoxic T lymphocytes. Lipopolysaccharide plus interferon-γ are often used experimentally to activate macrophages. Activated macrophages rapidly synthesize, or induce the appearance of, NO synthase. Nitric oxide synthase induction can be assessed by monitoring the formation or accumulation of L-citrulline and NO. The quantity of NO generated by activated macrophages is much greater than that generated by vascular endothelial cells under physiologic conditions. Macrophage-derived NO damages target-invading tumor cells, other cells, and a variety of microorganisms including bacteria and parasites. Nitric oxide typically exerts a cytostatic action (inhibits cell division and other cellular functions) rather than a cytocidal action (kills the target cells), but the latter can occur under appropriate conditions. Nitric oxide damages cells by binding to certain enzymes involved in cellular respiration, thereby interfering with their function. Some iron-containing proteins altered by NO include the mitochondrial enzyme aconitase and NADPH oxidoreductase enzymes.

In addition to tissue macrophages derived from the blood, other macrophage-like cells and neutrophils respond to activating substances with the induction of NO synthase and the production of cytotoxic quantities of NO. The hepatic Kupffer cell can be induced by endotoxin and cytokines to generate sufficient quantities of NO that are cytotoxic to adjacent hepatocytes. Under certain conditions, the hepatocytes alone can generate enough NO to be self-destructive. Brain astrocytes and microglial cells are macrophage-like cells that can be activated by certain cytokines to produce enough NO to cause cytotoxicity to nearby cells. Articular chondrocytes have been shown to respond to endotoxin and cytokines with a marked increase in NO production. The implications of these observations in disease are addressed later.

Vascular smooth-muscle cells can also be induced to synthesize large amounts of NO. Endotoxin in combination with cytokines such as interferon-γ, interleukin-1, or tumor necrosis factor induces the appearance of NO synthase in vascular smooth-muscle tissue and cultured cells. These observations offer a plausible explanation of the cause of septic shock or endotoxin shock.

We have observed that the constitutive isoform of NO synthase, under appropriate conditions in vivo, can be rapidly activated to generate large enough quantities of NO to cause marked cellular damage to ventricular muscle.[19] Young piglets, first made hypoxic by allowing them to breathe air with low O_2 tension and then exposed to cardioplegia solution with high O_2 tension during cardiopulmonary bypass, consistently experience the rapid development of conditions favorable for the formation of O_2-derived radicals and accompanying myocardial failure as a result of ventricular muscle damage. At the onset of myocardial reoxygenation, a marked surge in the formation of O_2-derived radicals and NO occurs, and this is accompanied by marked lipid peroxidative damage associated with a decrease in myocardial contractility. Myocardial reoxygenation injury is nearly completely prevented by administration of NO synthase inhibitors to the animals at the time of reoxygenation on cardiopulmonary bypass. These observations reveal that, under appropriate conditions in the intact animal, the constitutive isoform, rather than the inducible isoform, of NO synthase can produce sufficient quantities of NO to be immediately destructive to mammalian ventricular muscle cells. This study suggests also that NO can react with O_2-derived radicals, perhaps O_2^-, in tissues to generate products that are rapidly and markedly cytotoxic.

NITRIC OXIDE AND DISEASE

Nitric oxide undoubtedly plays key supportive roles in the normal function of various cell types, as discussed previously. Thus, a deficiency of NO caused by any mechanism is expected to lead to the development of abnormal cellular or organ function. One such mechanism could be interference with the biosynthesis of NO from L-arginine. Inhibitors of NO synthesis have been tested on intact cells and in intact animals to develop a better understanding of what the physiologic roles of NO might be. Such studies suggested that deficient NO production by vascular endothelial cells could lead to vasoconstriction and perhaps chronic hypertension. Deficient endothelial NO production may also promote platelet adhesion, aggregation, and thrombosis. Likewise, deficient endothelial NO production may promote the local adhesion of neutrophils, especially to areas where the endothelial cell layer is damaged. Local adhesion of neutrophils to blood vessels such as the epicardial coronary arteries could cause vascular damage, coronary vasoconstriction, and myocardial ischemic injury. Because NO causes vasodilation also in the corpus cavernosum, a deficiency in NO production could represent one important cause of erectile dysfunction or impotence. As far as brain function is concerned, any lesions associated with inhibition of NO production could lead to brain dysfunction, such as loss of memory or impaired learning and uncoordinated motor movements. Finally, because NO produced by activated macrophages and related cell types is believed to play a key pathophysiologic role in cytostasis and cytotoxicity, deficient NO production could promote inflammation, infection or superinfection, and tumor growth.

Nitric oxide itself is a chemically unstable gas and is difficult to administer in most situations. Although the administration of NO may be helpful in correcting deficiencies of NO in certain disease states, drugs that incorporate the NO (nitroso) group would be more useful than pure NO gas. Some of the S-nitrosothiols used experimentally, such as S-nitroso-N-acetylpenicillamine, may be appropriate for clinical use as NO donor drugs. Related NO donor drugs are under development by several laboratories for possible clinical use to treat disease states that may be caused by a deficiency in NO. Organic NO_3^- esters (nitroglycerin, isosorbide dinitrate), organic NO_2^- esters (isoamyl nitrite), and inorganic nitroso compounds (nitroprusside) have already been proven to be useful clinically. Nitric oxide gas itself has recently been proven to be of great interest and utility in the potential treatment of hypoxic pulmonary vasoconstriction and possible severe acute pulmonary hypertension (high-altitude pulmonary edema). In very small amounts, the inhalation of NO in an air mixture causes localized pulmonary vasodilation without any significant systemic effects.[20] This has distinct advantages over the systemic administration of NO donor drugs, which would cause marked systemic effects including reflex cardiovascular effects. Recent studies indicate that NO gas may also be effective as a bronchodilator in the treatment of acute respiratory distress syndrome in infants.

In addition to the development of tissue and organ dysfunction resulting from a deficiency of NO, problems can also develop with too much of a good thing. That is, excessive production of NO can cause local and global pathophysiologic responses, and there are numerous examples of this. Excitatory neurotransmission in the brain is closely linked to the stimulation of NO formation by certain neurons in the cerebellum and hippocampus. Excessive excitatory neurotransmission, which occurs in certain cases of head injury and disease, can be mimicked by administration of glutamate and results in excessive NO formation and consequent neurotoxicity, sometimes termed *excitotoxicity*. This cytotoxicity can be prevented by the administration of NO synthase inhibitors. Excessive NO production by other brain cell types that resemble macrophages, such as astrocytes and microglial cells, can provoke local damage to the oligodendrocytes, which normally function to bring about neuronal myelinization. The result could be multiple sclerosis. Outside the brain, the production of excessive amounts of NO can cause serious problems. Excessive local NO production by articular chondrocytes could play a prominent role in mediating local inflammation and cartilage destruction in rheumatoid arthritis and other chronic inflammatory disorders. Another good example is septic shock, which is caused by bacterial toxins that enter the systemic circulation. The marked hypotension that is characteristic of septic shock is often fatal and is attributed to excessive NO production by NO synthase that is induced in the vascular smooth-muscle cells by one or more cytokines. The induction of excessive NO production in hepatic Kupffer cells during septic shock also results in cytotoxicity to the nearby hepatocytes, which stop synthesizing proteins. As discussed previously, excessive NO production that occurs during reoxygenation of hypoxic tissues often causes serious tissue and organ damage that is attributed to a chemical reaction between NO and O_2^- to generate cytotoxic free radicals.

A proper balance of NO production and inactivation in mammalian cells appears to be what is important to preserve the physiologic and pathophysiologic functions of NO without bringing about any detrimental effects attributed to too little or too much NO. Thus, a finite minimal quantity of NO is required for normal physiologic function. Quantities of NO that fall outside this critical range can cause cellular and organ toxicity. Nitric oxide is a unique and fascinating molecule that appears to serve more diverse key roles in mammalian cell function than any other biologic molecule in recent memory.

ACKNOWLEDGMENTS

This work was supported in part by U.S. Public Health Service grants HL35014 and HL40922, a grant from the Laubisch Fund for Cardiovascular Research, and a grant from the Tobacco-Related Disease Research Program. The author thanks Diane Rome Peebles for preparation of the illustrations and Russ Byrns for preparation of the photographs.

References

1. Ignarro LJ, Buga GM, Wood KS, et al: Endothelium-derived relaxing factor produced and released from artery and vein is nitric oxide. Proc Natl Acad Sci USA 1987; 84:9265–9269.
2. Ignarro LJ, Byrns RE, Buga GM, Wood KS: Endothelium-derived relaxing factor from pulmonary artery and vein possesses pharmacological and chemical properties identical to those of nitric oxide radical. Circ Res 1987; 61:866–879.
3. Palmer RMJ, Ferrige AG, Moncada S: Nitric oxide release accounts for the biological activity of endothelium-derived relaxing factor. Nature 1987; 327:524–526.
4. Waldman SA, Murad F: Cyclic GMP synthesis and function. Pharmacol Rev 1987; 39:163–196.
5. Ignarro LJ, Kadowitz PJ: The pharmacological and physiological role of cyclic GMP in vascular smooth muscle relaxation. Ann Rev Pharmacol Toxicol 1985; 25:171–191.
6. Ignarro LJ: Regulation of polymorphonuclear leukocyte, macrophage, and platelet function. *In*: Immunopharmacology. Hadden JW, Coffey RG, Spreafico F (Eds). Plenum Press, 1977, pp 61–86.
7. Ignarro LJ: Biological actions and properties of endothelium-derived nitric oxide formed and released from artery and vein. Circ Res 1989; 65:1–21.
8. Ignarro LJ, Lippton H, Edwards JC, et al: Mechanism of vascular smooth muscle relaxation by organic nitrates, nitrites, nitroprusside and nitric oxide: Evidence for the involvement of S-nitrosothiols as active intermediates. J Pharmacol Exp Ther 1981; 218:739–749.
9. Sanders KM, Ward SM: Nitric oxide as a mediator of nonadrenergic noncholinergic neurotransmission. Am J Physiol 1992; 262:G379–G392.
10. Rajfer J, Aronson WJ, Bush PA, et al: Nitric oxide as a mediator of relaxation of the corpus cavernosum in response to nonadrenergic, noncholinergic neurotransmission. N Engl J Med 1992; 326:90–94.
11. Stuehr DJ, Marletta MA: Mammalian nitrite biosynthesis: Mouse macrophages produce nitrite and nitrate in response to *Escherichia coli* lipopolysaccharide. Proc Natl Acad Sci U S A 1985; 82:7738–7742.
12. Hibbs JB, Taintor RR, Vavrin Z: Macrophage cytotoxicity: Role for L-arginine deiminase activity and imino nitrogen oxidation to nitrite. Science 1987; 235:473–476.
13. Moncada S, Palmer RMJ, Higgs AE: Nitric oxide: Physiology, pathophysiology and pharmacology. Pharmacol Rev 1991; 43:109–142.
14. Tayeh MA, Marletta MA: Macrophage oxidation of L-arginine to nitric oxide, nitrite, and nitrate: Tetrahydrobiopterin is required as a cofactor. J Biol Chem 1989; 264:19654–19658.
15. Forstermann U, Schmidt HHHW, Pollock JS, et al: Isoforms of nitric oxide synthase: Characterization and purification from different cell types. Biochem Pharmacol 1991; 42:1849–1857.
16. Buga GM, Gold ME, Fukuto JM, Ignarro LJ: Shear stress-induced release of nitric oxide from endothelial cells grown on beads. Hypertension 1991; 17:187–193.
17. Buga GM, Ignarro LJ: Electrical field stimulation causes endothelium-dependent and nitric oxide-mediated relaxation of pulmonary artery. Am J Physiol 1992; 262:H973–H979.
18. Snyder SH, Bredt DS: Biological roles of nitric oxide. Sci Am 1992; 266:68–77.
19. Matheis G, Sherman MP, Buckberg GD, et al: Role of L-arginine-nitric oxide pathway in myocardial reoxygenation injury. Am J Physiol 1992; 262:H616–H620.
20. Frostell C, Fratacci M-D, Wain JC, et al: Inhaled nitric oxide: A selective pulmonary vasodilator reversing hypoxic pulmonary vasoconstriction. Circulation 1991; 83:2038–2047.

CHAPTER 28

Platelet-Activating Factor in Septic Shock

Matyas Koltai, MD, PhD • Philippe Guinot, MD
David Hosford, PhD • Pierre G. Braquet, PhD, DSc

Despite considerable advances in the intensive clinical care in the past decade, septic shock still remains the most common cause of death in noncoronary intensive care units.[1–4] The relative lack of effective pharmacologic interventions highlights the complex pathophysiologic events involved in sepsis.[5] To develop a more uniform set of definitions, the American College of Chest Physicians and the Society for Critical Care Medicine recently held a consensus conference that proposed that sepsis and similar disorders be called *systemic inflammatory response syndrome* (SIRS).[6] SIRS frequently leads to the development of acute lung injury, renal failure, and other end-organ dysfunctions; therefore, the consensus conference also proposed the term *multiple organ dysfunction syndrome*.[6] Although not completely understood, septic shock is believed to result from widespread endothelial damage caused by persistent inflammation.[7] Inflammation is a natural defense mechanism; however, when the release of inflammatory mediators exceeds a certain level, the symptoms of SIRS become apparent. The consensus conference made another key decision to restrict the use of the word *sepsis* to cases in which infection is documented, because SIRS can be caused not only by bacterial, viral, fungal, or other infections but also by multiple trauma and tissue injuries, severe burns, hemorrhagic shock, pancreatitis, and other life-threatening conditions. Among the various infections, gram-negative bacteria producing lipopolysaccharide (LPS) are known as a major causative factor in SIRS. Therefore, attenuating the effect of endotoxin is a major problem in the treatment of septic shock.[8] There is much evidence to suggest that, beyond various cytokines and eicosanoids, platelet-activating factor (PAF) also plays an important role in this general, exaggerated inflammatory response.

PAF, characterized structurally as 1–0-alkyl-2(R)-acetyl-glycero-3-phosphocholine, is a potent phospholipid autacoid implicated in inflammation, ischemic disorders and shock. PAF is produced by a variety of cells, including endothelial cells, polymorphonuclear leukocytes (PMNs), platelets, monocytes, basophils, eosinophils, mast cells, and lymphocytes[9–11] and is an important trigger for cell-to-cell interaction,[12, 13] which leads to the release of inflammatory mediators other than PAF. The contribution of PAF to microvascular circulatory failure has recently been reviewed.[14] Studies on the pathophysiologic role of PAF have been facilitated by a variety of compounds that can specifically inhibit the binding of PAF to its receptors in various cells and tissues. PAF antagonists can be broadly divided into two groups: natural compounds and synthetic inhibitors. The latter group consists of compounds having a PAF-related framework or compounds that have a chemical structure unrelated to PAF. With regard to their medicinal chemistry and patent status, readers are referred to a recent overview.[15] In this review, interest is focused on BN 52021, a natural compound isolated from *Ginkgo biloba* leaves,[16] and BN 50739, a synthetic PAF receptor antagonist with a hetrazepine framework.[17] This review summarizes recent knowledge on PAF as potential mediator in animal models of septic shock and examines the potential therapeutic efficacy of specific PAF receptor antagonists.

SYSTEMIC INFLAMMATORY RESPONSE SYNDROME INDUCED BY LIPOPOLYSACCHARIDE

The most important cellular target of endotoxin is the vascular endothelium.[7] As reviewed recently by Ward,[18] injury of endothelial cells is a frequent outcome of the acute inflammatory response and is caused predominantly by toxic oxygen products of activated neutrophils. Killing of endothelial cells by neutrophils includes increased adhesive interactions[19] induced by cytokines, such as tumor necrosis factor (TNF) and interleukin (IL)-1β followed by superoxide production. In acute lung injury, both macrophages and neutrophils are stimulated by immune complexes and complement, and cytokines and PAF are involved in the inflammatory response.[20] Activated macrophages release TNF and up-regulate the formation of leukocyte adhesion molecules in endothelial cells; thus, adherence of PMN to vascular endothelial cells increases. The final step here is also an augmented production of toxic oxygen species.

Cardiovascular Effects of Cytokines in Septic Shock

Peripheral circulation and cardiac function are profoundly altered by cytokines,[21] particularly TNF and IL-1. It is well documented that LPS releases inflammatory mediators, including TNF and ILs, from inflammatory cells.[22]

The principal causes of decreased myocardial contractility related to sepsis are down-regulation of adrenergic receptors, altered calcium ion (Ca^{2+}) handling, myocardial edema, rearrangement of the lipid components in the cellular membrane,[23] and direct or indirect coronary vasoconstriction with consecutive hypoperfusion. Endotoxin itself does not influence the function of isolated heart;[24] therefore, the sepsis-induced myocardial depression is probably due to secondary release of TNF, which causes negative inotropic effect in guinea pigs.[25] TNF and PAF have been suggested to be involved in the formation of myocardial depressant factor[26] in splanchnic artery occlusion-induced shock in anesthetized rats.[27] However, these alterations may not be specific for septic shock because hypoxia itself has been shown to induce IL-1 and TNF release from cultured human mononuclear cells,[28] and circulating TNF levels have been reported to increase in patients with severe chronic heart failure.[29]

Since 1986, when the shock-inducing effect of recombinant TNF was first described,[30] the effects of cytokines on the peripheral circulation have been extensively studied. The principal effects of cytokines are diffuse microvascular plugging,[31] loss of vascular autoregulation, and increased permeability.[32] These symptoms appeared to show oxygen supply dependency phenomenon associated with increased blood lactate levels.[33]

The pathomechanism through which cytokines aggravate septic shock and the therapeutic relevance of this process have been reviewed.[34] In clinical patients, plasma cytokine levels have been shown to be higher in sepsis than in non-septic shock;[35] furthermore, the persistence of elevated plasma concentrations rather than peak levels predicts a poor outcome of the shock state.

Role of Platelet-Activating Factor in the Pathophysiology of Shock States

Although the role of phospholipid mediators and their antagonists has been questioned in sepsis,[36] the role of PAF in various shock conditions has been well established and extensively reviewed.[37, 38] PAF, released from membrane phospholipids by activation of phospholipase A_2 (PLA_2), mimics the shock state by producing hypotension, pulmonary hypertension, thrombocytopenia, myocardial depression, microvascular and multiple organ failure, and death in different animal species.[9–11]

It has been reported that, in correlation with the severity of circulatory collapse, serum PLA_2 activity is markedly elevated in patients with septic shock.[39] In parallel experiments, purified native PLA_2 produced hypotension in experimental animals. In a prospective study of septic shock patients, the relationship of PLA_2 activity to PLA_2 immunoreactivity using radiolabeled *Escherichia coli* phospholipid substrate and an enzyme-linked immunosorbent assay specific for group II human nonpancreatic PLA_2 was apparent. The 554-fold increase in nonpancreatic type II PLA_2 activity observed in this study suggests the involvement of the enzyme and consecutive PAF release in endotoxin shock.

When released, PAF, but not its deacetylated and biologically inactive metabolite lyso-PAF, interacts with its primary target, the vascular endothelial cells.[40, 41] In association with the release of intracellular Ca^{2+} through activation of the phosphatidylinositol pathways,[42, 43] cultured human endothelial cells grown on fibronectin-coated polycarbonate filter retract and lose reciprocal contact and promote iodine 125-albumin diffusion into the cells. It is, therefore, evident that PAF triggers the release of inositol triphosphate (ITP_3), which is a second messenger of many intracellular processes through internal Ca^{2+} signals. The molecular and physiologic properties of these receptors closely resemble the Ca^{2+} mobilizing ryanodine receptors of the muscle. The family of intracellular channels displays the regenerative process of Ca^{2+}-induced Ca^{2+} release responsible for the complex temporospatial patterns of Ca^{2+} waves and oscillations.[44] Such a dynamic signaling pathway controls many cellular processes, including smooth-muscle contraction, cell growth, secretion, and PAF-induced inflammatory responses. Similar mechanisms exist not only in endothelial cells but also in PMNs and platelets.[45, 46] Congenital platelet dysfunction and impaired agonist-induced Ca^{2+} mobilization has been found to be unrelated to a defect in ITP_3 or eicosanoid response, but they are rather due to a lack of phospholipase C activation,[47] suggesting that Ca^{2+} signaling is a highly conserved intracellular process.

Nakamura and colleagues[48] showed that the LPS-induced increase in intracellular Ca^{2+} in platelets and platelet aggregation is blocked by selective PAF receptor antagonists. This finding was also confirmed using the cloned PAF receptors expressed in *Xenopus* oocytes and Chinese hamster ovary cells. In both systems, cells responded to LPS only when PAF receptors were expressed, and specific PAF binding was successfully displaced and reversibly dissociated by LPS. This suggests that PAF receptor activation by LPS may represent a novel and important pathway in the pathogenesis of circulatory collapse and systemic thrombosis caused by endotoxin.

Release of Platelet-Activating Factor Lipopolysaccharide and Bacterial Porins

There is substantial evidence that LPS derived from gram-negative bacteria releases PAF in a great variety of in vitro and in vivo animal models.[49–52] The effect of LPS on the regulation of the surface expression of the PAF in peritoneal macrophages has been studied.[53] Preincubation of IC-21 cultured peritoneal macrophages with LPS increased PAF receptor expression without apparent change in the affinity of the receptor for the ligand. This effect was abolished by actinomycin D and cycloheximide, suggesting that enhanced receptor protein synthesis is involved. Moreover, LPS increased the capability of the IC-21 cells to respond to PAF addition by elevating intracellular free Ca^{2+} without causing an increase in the basal level of intracellular Ca^{2+}.

More recently, another pathway was also demonstrated through which gram-negative bacteria may interact with cellular release of PAF. Porins, a family of hydrophobic proteins located in the outer membrane of the cell wall of gram-negative bacteria, were shown to stimulate the synthesis and release of PAF by mesangial cells in the kidney[54] and PMNs.[55] The increased PAF synthesis was independent from contamination by LPS and generation of TNF. In contrast, PAF synthesis and release induced by LPS showed a biphasic pattern with an early transient peak at 10 minutes followed by a second and sustained peak requiring protein synthesis. The LPS-induced PAF synthesis was prevented by anti-TNF antibodies. Experiments with labeled precursors demonstrated that PAF was synthesized by bacterial porins via the remodeling pathway, which involves acetylation of PAF generated from lyso-PAF by PLA_2 activation. Accordingly, porins induced a sustained mobilization of ^{14}C-arachidonic acid that was inhibited by p-bromodiphenyl bromide, an inhibitor of PLA_2. The activation by porins of PAF synthesis and release depended on the extracellular Ca^{2+} and formation of transmembrane channels determined by a sustained influx of $^{45}Ca^{2+}$ into the cytosol, a process blocked by inhibitors of Ca^{2+}-calmodulin complexes, suggesting the calmodulin mediation of porin-induced increase in PAF synthesis. These experiments explored a new aspect of the interaction of gram-negative bacteria with the PAF-synthesizing machinery of various inflammatory cells. This may contribute to septic shock; however, the role of porin-induced PAF release in sepsis needs further careful experimental analysis.

Similarities Between the Effect of Platelet-Activating Factor and Lipopolysaccharide

The effects of LPS and PAF are qualitatively similar, but the concentration of PAF that induces shock is usually about 500- to 1000-fold less than that of the LPS. This difference in the effective concentrations may be an important indication that endotoxins cause deleterious effects mainly through releasing PAF. Interestingly, in one study, 50 μg/kg IV, LPS or 25 μg/kg IP PAF induced approximately the same degree of intestinal motor disturbances in conscious rats.[56] This relatively small difference between the effective concentrations strongly suggests that the intestinal wall may be the primary site of action of PAF and endotoxin.

The potential role of bacterial translocation across the intestinal wall in the development of septic shock in female Swiss Webster mice has been studied.[57] Animals purchased from different suppliers exhibited different morbidity and mortality after parenteral LPS administration. Increased LPS sensitivity was associated with intestinal disease, gram-negative bacterial overgrowth, and increased bacterial translocation. If there was no LPS-induced increased bacterial translocation, the density of cecal gram-negative flora was lower. Parenteral injection of LPS induced morbidity and mortality without increased bacterial translocation. When PAF was parenterally used instead of LPS, the same findings were observed.

MEDIATORS OF ENDOTOXIN SHOCK

LPS is a potent inflammatory stimulus for the host and triggers the release of endogenous mediators, including TNF, IL-1, PAF, eicosanoids, complement, contact activation system, and opioids.[4] The mediator role of cytokines, PAF, and eicosanoids, with special regard to the sequence of their release in response to LPS as well as the effect of some PAF antagonists on the release process is discussed.

Activated macrophages produce a cytokine, TNF-α, which is one of the principle candidates as mediator of septic shock.[30] Intramesenteric infusion of endotoxin in domestic pigs has been shown to result in early death in 50%,[58, 59] and those animals that die within one-half hour, termed *nonsurvivors*, respond with a rapid, excess TNF-α production but do not release other mediators, suggesting a primary role for TNF-α as mediator of lethal septic shock. However, one may argue that, in these shock-prone pigs, such drastic changes occur after LPS infusion because the release of PAF and thromboxane B_2 (TXB_2) cannot be detected as a result of the fulminant circulatory collapse. Consequently, the extremely high concentration of TNF-α in the blood may not be the cause but rather may be the consequence of a dramatically rapid cell death. The PAF receptor antagonist BN 52021 was ineffective against death in this critical early phase.[59–61] In survivor pigs, sequential release of other meditors, such as PAF and TXB_2, occurs. This later phase of shock was, in turn, effectively alleviated by BN 52021.[59–61]

The time course of TXB_2, 6-keto-prostaglandin (PG) $F_1\alpha$ (6-keto-$PGF_1\alpha$), TNF-α, PAF, and IL-6 release was studied in domestic pigs.[62] In the 18-hour experiment, 0.5 μg/kg of *E. coli* endotoxin was infused intravenously for 30 minutes three times at 0 hour, 5 hours, and 10 hours, and concentrations of various mediators were determined at 0, 15, 30, 45, 60, 120, and 180 minutes after each infusion; pulmonary arterial pressure and cardiac output were controlled as functional parameters. PAF and TXB_2 showed peak plasma levels between 30 and 45 minutes, TNF-α and 6-keto-$PGF_1\alpha$ between 30 and 60 minutes, and IL-6 between 120 and 180 minutes after each LPS infusion. The repeated infusion of LPS-induced characteristic changes in the blood levels of various inflammatory meditors. This study shows that pigs are highly susceptible to LPS even when it is not given intramesenterically close to the intestine. Furthermore, when endotoxin is injected at a sublethal dose, the sequence of mediator release is different from that observed in nonsurvivor pigs after intramesenteric infusion of LPS.[58–61] Another very important finding of this study is that repeated LPS injections induce a different release profile of inflammatory mediators. The release of PAF was sustained after the first and second injections and moderately declined after the third administration. A gradual decrease in plasma concentrations of TNF and TXB_2 was also apparent. In contrast, the release of 6-keto-$PGF_1\alpha$ was continuously increased after repeated challenge with LPS, whereas the maximum level of IL-6 was achieved by the second injection. These results are in favor of the concept that PAF is first released in response to LPS. This is followed by thromboxane A_2 (TXA_2) production. Tumor necrosis factor, PGI_2, and IL-6 are obviously released in the later phase of endotoxin shock.

In rats, Rabinovici and co-workers[63] found that TNF-α reaches peak concentration in plasma at 2 hours after intravenous administration of endotoxin and remains unchanged by BN 50739. These results suggest that those species (e.g., rats in this study) or individuals not prone to the fatal complications of septic shock relatively slowly release TNF-α, the level of which in the blood does not reach excess concentration seen in nonsurvivor pigs.[58–61] This finding may explain why some patients are resistant to intensive clinical care and has put forward the possible therapeutic relevance of an early administration of anti-TNF-α antibodies.[64] In fact, Tracey and colleagues[64] demonstrated that anesthetized baboons infused with a lethal dose of live *E. coli* were protected against fatal circulatory collapse and pulmonary and renal failure when neutralizing anti-TNF antibody fragments were administered 1 hour before bacterial challenge. Another study demonstrated that monoclonal antibodies raised against recombinant human TNF afforded not only prophylaxis but also effective treatment of endotoxic shock in cynomolgus monkeys.[65] CB0006, the monoclonal antibody to human TNF-α, was tried in a phase I study for evaluation of its safety and pharmacokinetics in septic shock patients.[66] After early rise of blood pressure and alleviation of other parameters measured, the protection declined; thus, it was concluded that the beneficial effect of CB0006 conferred by prophylaxis might also extend to treatment, although the "therapeutic window" might be narrow. In contrast, the PAF antagonist TCV-309 has been shown to suppress LPS-induced TNF generation and mortality in mice in which treatment with carrageenan, a sulfated polygalactose, aggravated endotoxin shock.[67] This finding confirms the important role for PAF in LPS-induced TNF release.

Like TNF, IL-1 also plays a central role in the host inflammatory response. IL-1 is produced in large quantity in SIRS; however, most of it binds peripheral receptor sites and remains undetectable. IL-1 affects vascular cells in numerous ways to trigger and amplify the network of events during sepsis that causes vascular congestion, capillary leak, altered coagulation, cellular infiltration, and stimulation of endothelial cells to produce PGI_2 and PGE_2.[68, 69] It appears likely that ILs are mediators of the late phase of SIRS.[62] A naturally occurring human protein anakinra (Antril), inhibits the action of IL-1.[70] Anakinra has been developed for the treatment of septic shock; however, the results of phase III clinical trial have been disappointing.

PAF is released in response to LPS in the pig[58–62] and rat.[63, 67] This parallelism between the severity of LPS-induced shock and the sequential release of PAF and TNF, as well as the experience with repeated infusions of nonlethal dose of endotoxin, suggests that PAF plays a central role in the mediation of septic shock. When the animals survived the most critical half hour of LPS infusion or received a nonlethal dose of LPS, PAF release always preceded the peak of TNF production.[58–62]

The sequence of eicosanoid release also shows characteristic features. In survivor pigs, PAF release was associated with the release of TXB_2, 6-keto-$PGF_1\alpha$, and leukotriene B_4 (LTB_4). The earliest rise of TXB_2 concentration was seen in pigs,[58–62] rabbits,[71] dogs,[72] and rats[63, 73, 74] followed by the elevation of plasma 6-keto-$PGF_1\alpha$, whereas LTB_4 production was the latest. Indomethacin blocked the release of all eicosanoids produced through the cyclooxygenase pathway and augmented the release of lipoxygenase products. An interesting aspect of this inhibitory effect is that the release of 6-keto-$PGF_1\alpha$ was more resistant to indomethacin than that of TXB_2. In accord, PAF receptor antagonists can effectively block TXB_2 production and only moderately decrease the release of 6-keto-$PGF_1\alpha$.

Human Monoclonal Immunoglobulin M Antibody Against Lipopolysaccharide

Research on antibodies that bind the lipid A domain of endotoxin goes back to the early 1980s. Protection against gram-negative bacteremia and endotoxemia with human monoclonal immunoglobulin (Ig) M antibodies in animals was described.[75] HA-1A, a human monoclonal IgM antibody, and E5, a murine monoclonal IgM antibody, both raised against endotoxin, have been developed[76] and have undergone clinical trials. The first randomized, double-blind, placebo-controlled clinical trials[76–78] have indicated that HA-1A and E5 are safe and effective for the treatment of patients with sepsis and gram-negative bacteremia, whereas the second trial produced dubious results that could not confirm the beneficial effect.[79]

POSSIBLE MECHANISMS OF PLATELET-ACTIVATING FACTOR–INDUCED EFFECTS IN SEPTIC SHOCK

Amplification by Platelet-Activating Factor of Mediator Release

As reviewed,[12, 13] there is circumstantial evidence that growth factors and cytokines interact with PAF. Under pathophysiologic conditions like septic shock, cells "primed" by LPS, PAF, or cytokines produce excess amounts of inflammatory mediators, including PAF, cyclooxygenase and 5′-lipoxygenase products, and toxic oxygen species that may result in profound microvascular failure. This concept has been confirmed by recent results. For example, granulocyte monocyte colony-stimulating factor which regulates the growth of hemopoietic progenitor cells, was found to prime mature human phagocytes to PAF, which led to respiratory burst and increased LTB_4 synthesis.[80] When activated by inflammatory stimuli, macrophages produce TNF-α and IL-1, which then induce PAF synthesis in endothelial cells, neutrophils, and macrophages, and an increased respiratory burst occurs.[81–83] Not only can growth factors and cytokines induce PAF release, but also treatment with PAF has been shown to increase cytokine production. In Sprague-Dawley rats, long-term parenteral treatment with PAF dose dependently stimulated IL-1 and IL-2 production in isolated spleen mononuclear cells.[84] Mediator production declined after large doses of PAF and BN 52021 inhibited either the stimulatory or the inhibitory effect of PAF. After stimulation with muraminyl dipeptide, human monocytes produced TNF and IL-1, and PAF significantly enhanced production of both cytokines at two concentration ranges. A major enhancement blocked by BN 52021 was seen between 10^{-8} and 10^{-6} mol, whereas a second increase was observed at 10^{-15} to 10^{-14} mol of PAF, which remained unaltered by the PAF antagonist.[85] In isolated monocytes, PAF augmented the production of both bioactive TNF and IL-1, whereas lyso-PAF, the inactivated phospholipid mediator, had no such effect. After fractionation on a discontinuous Percoll gradient, a denser subpopulation of monocytes responded preferentially to higher PAF concentrations; in contrast, the less dense subpopulation responded to both concentrations. Some of these effects were blocked by BN 52021, indicating an interaction with specific PAF receptors, whereas others, being unaffected by BN 52021, appear to occur through different pathways.

A PAF/cytokine interaction ordinarily results in bell-shaped concentration-effect curves; for example, after stimulatory agonist concentrations that usually produce a concentration-dependent increase of mediator release, a high agonist concentration suppresses mediator release.[85] This might explain why an overall dominance of a single inflammatory mediator may be associated with the lack of the release of other mediators, as demonstrated in nonsurvivor pigs after intramesenteric infusion of LPS.[58–61]

Down-Regulation by Platelet-Activating Factor of Mediator Release

In activated cells, mediator release can be regulated not only by priming or amplification but also through down-regulation. The balance between these processes is fundamental for protecting cells from overstimulation and death. Down-regulatory processes are particularly important in septic shock, during which excess amplification of inflammatory mediator release frequently occurs and leads to death.

Deactivation and receptor down-regulation are independent of pertussis toxin-sensitive G proteins and protein kinase C and appear to depend on the sequential release of various mediators.[86] For example, eicosanoids, particularly PGI_2, have been shown to elevate intracellular cyclic adenosine monophosphate (cAMP) levels, which, in turn, can effectively decrease eicosanoid production in platelets[87, 88] and vascular endothelial cells.[89] PAF is known to induce eicosanoid release, and then increased PGI_2 production can reduce PAF release through a feedback activation of adenylate cyclase.[90, 91] This suggests that PAF plays a central role not only in amplification but also in down-regulation of inflammatory mediator release. Alternatively, TNFs known to stimulate macrophages, PMNs, and endothelial cells to synthesize and release PAF[92] may facilitate PGI_2 production, which then down-regulates the release of TNF. Similarly, IL-1 released at a later phase of septic shock also may trigger down-regulation through PGI_2 and PGE_2 production.[68] The conditions that favor feedback down-regulation of LPS-induced TNF release have not yet been fully understood.

SECOND MESSENGERS AND NITRIC OXIDE IN SEPTIC SHOCK

The L-arginine (NO) synthase–NO system, producing endothelium-dependent vasorelaxation, maintains a constant vasodilator tone.[93] Nitric oxide synthase exists in two forms. A constitutive, Ca^{2+}-dependent enzyme located predominantly in endothelial cells is active under normal conditions inducing transient vasodilation, whereas an inducible, apparently Ca^{2+}-independent enzyme, which was, however, recently shown to involve calmodulin as a subunit,[94] is synthesized de novo by a variety of inflammatory cells in septic shock. These enzymes exhibit similar properties, among which the ability to synthesize NO and activate guanylate cyclase[95] are prevailing, and they show different characteristics, among which the NO-generating capacity is the most significant. The constitutive enzyme produces NO at only picomolar concentrations that can induce transient vasodilation, whereas the inducible enzyme synthesizes nanomolar concentrations of NO; thus, its activation produces a powerful and sustained decrease of blood pressure, leading to a complete paralysis of the vascular wall to vasoconstrictor agents. The inducible enzyme is synthesized in macrophages, PMNs,[96] and freshly isolated human hepatocytes[97] in response to IL-1, TNF, and interferon-γ (IFN) and during endotoxemia.

The LPS-induced, cytokine-related de novo synthesis of this NO synthase has been shown to cause the loss of contractile force of both intact and denuded isolated arterial rings and profoundly decreases vascular resistance in vivo.[98] The induction of NO synthase is inhibited by dexamethasone,[99] providing explanation for the beneficial effect of glucocorticoids in septic shock. Inhibitors of NO synthase, such as N^G-monomethyl-L-arginine (L-NAME), are able to restore vascular reactivity impaired by endotoxin and cytokines.[100]

In one study, [101] a 10-mg/kg bolus of LPS caused a rapid and sustained decrease in blood pressure in male anesthetized Wistar rats, and 60 minutes thereafter the pressor response to norepinephrine (NE) was markedly reduced. The decreased NE response was restored, but control responses remained unchanged by L-NAME. Dexamethasone, a potent inhibitor of the induction of NO synthase, did not alter initial impairment of NE response but significantly attenuated an early blood pressure decrease induced by LPS. The NE response decreased by LPS was prevented 180 minutes after dexamethasone treatment. At 60 minutes after LPS, inducible NO synthase was detected only in the aorta; however, at 180 minutes the enzyme level was increased in a variety of tissues evidently because of the induction of enzyme synthesis, which was prevented by dexamethasone. The conclusion was drawn that the immediate vascular hyporeactivity to NE in endotoxin shock is caused by enhanced formation of NO resulting from the activation of the constitutive enzyme, whereas the delayed impairment of vascular tone and reactivity is due to enhanced NO formation by the LPS-induced enzyme.

The regulation of NO synthase activity with NO has been recognized in a murine macrophage cell line, J774, which expresses NO synthase activity in response to IFN-γ plus LPS from 6 hours up to 48 hours after exposure, with peak level at 12 hours.[102] The decline in NO synthase activity was slowed when cells were cultured in a low L-arginine medium or with added hemoglobin, suggesting that NO itself may be involved in the feedback inhibition. Nitric oxide generators, like S-nitroso-acetyl-penicillamine (SNAP), markedly and concentration dependently inhibited NO synthase activity, whereas the inhibition of protein synthesis had no effect. SNAP directly inhibited the inducible NO synthase extracted from activated J774 cells as well as the constitutive NO synthase extracted from the rat brain. When SNAP was removed from the medium by gel filtration, NO synthase activity was not restored, indicating a NO-induced irreversible inhibition. The generation of NO by the inducible NO synthase is tightly regulated. Cytokines, such as transforming growth factor-β,[103] IL-4,[104] and IL-10[105] are involved in this control mechanism. One may assume that disturbances in the well-controlled regulatory process may lead to the constitutive enzyme to switch to the inducible enzyme. The better understanding of this process may shed more light on the pathomechanism of LPS-induced vascular paralysis.

To determine the in vitro regional vascular reactivity in septic shock, New Zealand white rabbits were injected intravenously with a priming dose of 15 μg/kg of *E. coli* LPS 18 hours before a challenge dose of 200 to 2000 μg/kg was given under pentobarbital anesthesia.[106] LPS markedly lowered blood pressure, and 1 hour later the central ear arteries and kidneys were isolated to monitor perfusion pressure under constant flow conditions. Individual dose-response curves for NE and histamine were performed to assess contractile function and for methacholine (MCh) and sodium nitroprusside (SNP) to control relaxant activity. Contractile dose-response curves were shifted to the right by 2- and 2.7-fold, respectively, in the ear artery isolated from LPS-treated versus vehicle-treated animals, whereas no such difference was seen with the perfused kidney. Relaxation to MCh was similar in the ear artery, whereas in the kidney it was significantly reduced. SNP response was not different in the two tissues. LPS is, therefore, suggested to impair vasoconstriction in the ear artery but cause damage to the endothelium of the renal vascular bed. Intrinsic contraction-relaxation properties of coronary artery rings isolated from LPS-treated dogs that have systemic hypotension and cardiovascular depression induced by LPS were also evaluated.[107] Isolated vassels were stretched to the apex of the length-contractile tension curve; no differences were observed in length-active and length-passive tension (vessel compliance) relationships between controls and LPS. Contractile and relaxant responses were unchanged by LPS treatment except for agents that induce endothelium-dependent vasorelaxation. The impaired response to acetylcholine remained unaltered by the combination of antioxidant therapy with allopurinol, superoxide dismutase, and catalase. This suggests that neither depolarization nor cyclic guanosine monophosphate (cGMP)–dependent vasodilation changes in acute endotoxemia. The effect of free radicals in the impairment of endothelium-dependent vasodilation can also be excluded.

The role of PAF in the vascular paralysis induced by LPS has not been completely understood. In one study performed in anesthesized dogs,[108] small doses of PAF induced coronary dilation, which disappeared after de-endothelization by saponin infusion, suggesting that PAF, presumably though activation of intracellular Ca^{2+} signaling and increased Ca^{2+} release,[43, 44] may induce endothelium-dependent vasodilation. As is well documented (see, for a review, Braquet et al[9]), large doses of PAF produced coronary artery contraction. BN 52021 and WEB 2086 abolished either PAF-induced coronary dilation or constriction. Thrombin-induced PAF release from cultured human umbilical vein endothelial cells has been found to be sensitive to nitrovasodilators.[109] SNP, activating soluble guanylate cyclase with a consecutive increase in cGMP generation, inhibits platelet aggregation. SNP decreases, in a concentration-dependent manner, thrombin-induced PAF synthesis as well. 8-bromo-cGMP, a penetrable nonhydrolyzable analog of cGMP, mimicks the effect of SNP. PAF synthesis requires PLA_2-mediated hydrolysis of a membrane precursor to lyso-PAF, which is, in turn, converted into PAF by an acetyltransferase. Both enzymes are inhibited by SNP, suggesting a new mechanism; thus, endogenous NO may affect vascular tone and endothelium-dependent cellular adhesion. Further research needs to clarify the critical steps at which LPS becomes able to express messenger ribonucleic acid for induction of NO synthase and the role of PAF in the inducible NO synthase–NO system.

Endotoxin, applied at a dose that did not modify blood pressure, has been shown to abolish the acid secretory response induced by pentagastrin in the perfused stomach of the anesthetized rat;[110] L-NAME and indomethacin substantially restored secretory response to pentagastrin. The effect of L-NAME was suspended by pretreatment with L-arginine but not by D-arginine, indicating the involvement of NO in the LPS-induced inhibition of pentagastrin. WEB 2086 partially reversed, whereas a combination of WEB 2086 with L-NAME completely restored, the degree of hydrogen ion output induced by pentagastrin. These results show that NO and PAF may have additive effects against LPS response not only in the vascular wall but also in other tissues; the mechanism through which this interaction is working, however, remains to be elucidated.

In conclusion, septic shock is characterized by an overstimulation of guanylate cyclase, resulting in elevated cGMP levels in the vascular wall and several organs, including the heart, where it may induce cardiac depression.[111] The overall prevalence of cGMP may suppress cAMP-mediated down-regulation of inflammatory mediator release and promote amplification of PAF/cytokine inflammatory feedback network.

EFFECT OF BN 52021 AND BN 50739 IN ENDOTOXIN SHOCK

BN 52021, a natural specific PAF receptor antagonist, is effective in different animal models of endotoxin shock. In the rat, it significantly reduces the late blood pressure–lowering effect of LPS, improves survival rate, alleviates hemodynamic changes,[72, 74] and decreases intestinal motor disturbances.[56] Endotoxin-induced pulmonary platelet recruitment in the guinea pig is also attenuated by BN 52021.[112] In an ovine model, BN 52021 prevented endotoxin-induced pulmonary hypertension and lung edema.[113] Improvement by BN 52021 of LPS-induced hemodynamic changes are associated with decreased TXB_2 release and an almost unaffected 6-keto-$PGF_1\alpha$ release in survivor pigs[59–62] and rats;[72, 74] however, BN 52021 does not change early excessive release of TNF in nonsurvivor pigs.[59]

BN 50739, a novel synthetic PAF receptor antagonist, has been found to markedly attenuate endotoxin-induced alterations in animal models. In rabbits given 50 μg/kg of intravenous LPS, pretreatment with BN 50739 prevented early thrombocytopenia and TXB_2 release and reduced the 24-hour mortality rate from 75% to 22%.[71] Post-treatment with BN 50739 increased the 10-hour survival from 33% to 87%; however, it had no effect on 24-hour lethality. BN 50739 did not affect LPS-induced leukopenia or elevation of plasma TNF-α concentration. In Sprague-Dawley rats injected with 14.4 mg/kg of intravenous LPS, BN 50739 prevented hemoconcentration, reduced 24-hour mortality from 100% to 60%, and attenuated hypotension and TXB_2 release, but leukopenia and thrombocytopenia remained unchanged.[62] Pretreatment with BN 50739 decreased recombinant TNF-induced 24-hour mortality by 65% but did not alter hemoconcentration and thrombocytopenia. The priming effect of PAF on LPS-induced lung injury and cardiovascular collapse was also prevented by BN 50739.[114]

These results clearly indicate that both BN 52021 and BN 50739 are effective protective agents in animal models of endotoxin-induced alterations. The protective effect is marked in the later phase of shock and obviously associated with a significant improvement of hemodynamic changes as well as a profound decrease of PAF-induced TXB_2 release triggered by LPS. The immediate phase of shock, presumably mediated by excess TNF release, which frequently causes early death, cannot be prevented by these agents.

CONCLUSIONS

Considerable evidence has been accumulated to support the concept that a PAF/cytokine autogenerated feedback network is responsible for priming and amplification of inflammatory mediator release in septic shock. Growth factors and cytokines, such as TNF-α, IL-1, and other interleukins, mutually interact with PAF, and the phospholipid mediator amplifies cytokine production; therefore, PAF may be the principal mediator in endotoxin shock. A single factor identified as TNF is suggested to play a pivotal role in the fatal phase of septic shock. Presumably, excess TNF is released as a result of an amplification process primarily triggered by PAF. One may assume that the high TNF concentration in the blood of "nonsurvivors" is the consequence rather than the cause of cell death. The dubious results of clinical trials with anti-TNF antibodies and IL-1Ra, a naturally occurring IL-1 antagonist protein, have increased the debate of the exceptional role of these cytokines in the pathomechanism of septic shock or SIRS induced by gram-negative micro-organisms. There are similar problems with the interpretation of the results obtained in clinical trials of monoclonal IgM antibodies against *E. coli* endotoxin, HA-1A and E5. Future studies need to answer the question regarding the effectivity or inefficiency of this treatment. Perhaps when the plasma concentrations of LPS and cytokines exceed a critical level, treatment fails to save patients' lives. Similarly to individual animals, some patients may be prone to SIRS induced by LPS. With regard the causal role of LPS in septic shock, the putative role of bacterial porins may have to be taken into consideration. The marked release of PAF induced by endotoxin leading to excess TXA_2 production may be responsible for the microvascular failure and death in septic shock. Antagonists of PAF markedly protect against the release of TXA_2 and may interrupt the vicious circle of the amplification process. Alternatively, PAF antagonists may promote the beneficial feedback loop, termed *down*-regulation, because they have relatively little effect on PGI_2 release, being responsible for cAMP generation, an important factor in the down-regulation of inflammatory mediator release. Nitric oxide produced by the inducible NO synthase plays a pivotal role in causing vascular paralysis in LPS-induced SIRS. An exploration of the relationship of PAF to NO synthesis will provide a better understanding of the pathomechanism of septic shock. Several PAF antagonists, including BN 52021, have undergone phase II and phase III clinical trials. The results of these clinical studies may prove the efficacy of these drugs in the clinical management of septic shock induced by gram-negative bacteremia. The strategy in the treatment of SIRS, however, remains multifactorial because little is known about the SIRS caused by micro-organisms other than gram-negative bacteria.

References

1. Dal Nogare AR: Southwestern internal medicine conference: Septic shock. Am J Med Sci 1991; 302:50.
2. Bone RC: A critical evaluation of new agents for the treatment of sepsis. JAMA 1991; 266:1686.
3. Glauser MP, Zanetti G, Baumgartner JD, et al: Septic shock: Pathogenesis. Lancet 1991; 338:732.
4. Zimmerman JJ, Ringer TV: Inflammatory host responses in sepsis. Prog Pediatr Crit Care 1992; 8:163.
5. Bone RC: Towards an epidemiology and natural history of SIRS (systemic inflammatory response syndrome). JAMA 1992; 268:3452.
6. American College of Chest Physicians, Society for Critical Care Medicine Consensus Conference: Definitions for sepsis and organ failure and guidelines for the use of innovative therapies in sepsis. Chest 1992; 101:1644.
7. Bone RC: The pathogenesis of sepsis. Ann Intern Med 1991; 115:457.
8. Bone RC: Attenuating the effects of endotoxin. J Lab Clin Med 1992; 119:323.
9. Braquet P, Touqui L, Shen TS, et al: Perspectives in platelet-activating factor research. Pharmacol Rev 1987; 39:97.
10. Koltai M, Hosford D, Guinot P, et al: Platelet-activating factor (PAF): A review of its effects, antagonists and possible future clinical applications. Drugs 1991; 42:9.
11. Koltai M, Hosford D, Guinot P, et al: Platelet-activating factor (PAF): A review of its effects, antagonists and possible future clinical applications. Drugs 1991; 42:174.
12. Braquet P, Paubert-Braquet M, Bourgain R, et al: PAF/cytokine autogenerated feedback networks in microvascular immune injury: Consequences in shock, ischemia and graft rejection. J Lipid Med 1989; 1:75.
13. Braquet P, Paubert-Braquet M, Koltai M, et al: Is there a case for PAF antagonists in the treatment of ischemic states? Trends Pharmacol Sci 1989; 10:23.
14. Koltai M, Hosford D, Braquet P: The role of PAF and cytokines in microvascular tissue injury. J Lab Clin Med 1992; 19:461.
15. Whittaker M: PAF receptor antagonists: Recent advances. Curr Opin Ther Patent, 1992; 2:583–623.
16. Braquet P, Esanu A, Buisine E, et al: Recent progress in ginkgolide research. Med Res Rev 1991; 11:295.
17. Koltai M, Spinnewyn B, Duverger D, et al: BN 50739. Drugs Future 1991; 16:413.
18. Ward PA: Mechanism of endothelial cell injury. J Lab Clin Med 1991; 118:421.
19. Garrod DR: Cell to cell and cell to matrix adhesion. Br Med J 1993; 306:703.
20. Chang SW: Endotoxin-induced lung vascular injury: Role of platelet activating factor, tumor necrosis factor and neutrophils. Clin Res 1992; 40:528.
21. Berlot G, Vincent JL: Cardiovascular effects of cytokines. Clin Intens Care 1992; 3:199.
22. Ertel W, Morrison MH, Wang P, et al: The complex pattern of cytokines in sepsis: Association between prostaglandins, cachectin and interleukin. Ann Surg 1991; 214:141.
23. Salmond GP, Reeves PJ: Membrane traffics and protein secretion in gram-negative bacteria. Trends Biochem Sci 1993; 18:7.
24. Abel FL: Myocardial function in sepsis and endotoxic shock. Am J Physiol 1989; 257:R1265.
25. Heard SO, Perkins MW, Fink MP: Tumour necrosis factor-alpha causes myocardial depression in guinea pigs. Crit Care Med 1992; 20:523.
26. Lefer AM: Interaction between myocardial depressant factor and vasoactive mediators with ishchemia and shock. Am J Physiol 1987; 252:R193.
27. Zingarelli B, Squadrito, Ioculano M, et al: Platelet activating factor interaction with tumor necrosis factor and myocardial depressant factor in splanchnic artery occlusion shock. Eur J Pharmac 1992; 222:13.
28. Ghezzi P, Dinarello CA, Bianchi M, et al: Hypoxia increases IL-1 and TNF production by human mononuclear cells. Cytokine 1991; 3:189.
29. Levine B, Kalman J, Mayer L, et al: Elevated circulating tumor necrosis factor in severe chronic heart failure. N Eng J Med 1990; 323:236.
30. Tracey KJ, Beutler B, Lowry SF, et al: Shock and tissue injury induced by recombinant human cachectin. Science 1986; 234:470.
31. Van der Poll T, Buller H, ten Cate H, et al: Activation of

coagulation after administration of tumor necrosis factor. N Eng J Med 1990; 322:1622.
32. Vane JR, Anggard EE, Botting RM: Regulatory functions of vascular endothelium. N Eng J Med 1990; 323:27.
33. Bakker J, Vincent JL: The oxygen supply dependency phenomenon is associated with increased blood lactate levels. J Crit Care 1991; 6:152.
34. Christman JW, Wheeler AP, Bernard GR: Cytokines and sepsis: What are the therapeutic implications? J Crit Care 1991; 6:172.
35. Pinsky MR, Vincent JL, Deviere J, et al: Serum cytokine levels in human septic shock: Relation to multiple-system organ failure and mortality. Chest 1993; 103:565.
36. Bone RC: Phospholipids and their inhibitors: A critical evaluation of their role in the treatment of sepsis. Crit Care Med 1992; 20:884.
37. Hosford D, Braquet P: The potential role of platelet activating factor in shock and ischemia. J Crit Care 1990; 5:115.
38. Hosford D, Braquet P: Interaction between platelet-activating factor and lipopolysachharide: Consequences in endotoxemia and sepsis. *In*: Bacterial Endotoxic Lipopolysaccharides: Vol 2. Immunopharmacology and Pathophysiology. Ryan JL, Morrison DC (Eds). Boca Raton, FL, CRC Press, 1992, pp 57–74.
39. Vadas P, Scott K, Smith G, et al: Serum phospholipase A_2 enzyme activity and immunoreactivity in a prospective analysis of patients with septic shock. Life Sci 1992; 50:807.
40. Bussolino F, Camussi G, Aglietta M, et al: Human endothelial cells are a target for platelet-activating factor. J Immunol 1987; 139:2439.
41. Bourgain RH, Maes L, Braquet P, et al: The effect of 1-0-alkyl-2-acetyl-sn-glycero-3-phosphocholine (PAF-acether) on the arterial wall. Prostaglandins 1985; 30:185.
42. Bussolino F, Aglietta M, Sanavio F, et al: Alkyl-ether phosphoglycerides influence calcium fluxes into human endothelial cells. J Immunol 1985; 135:2748.
43. Marquis O, Robaut C, Cavero I: Evidence for the existence and ionic modulation of platelet-activating factor receptors mediating degranulatory responses in human polymorphonuclear leukocytes. J Pharmacol Exp Ther 1989; 250:293.
44. Berridge MJ: Inositol triphosphate and calcium signalling. Nature 1993; 361:315.
45. Gomez-Cambronero J, Durstin M, Molski TF, et al: Calcium is necessary for the platelet-activating factor release in human neutrophils stimulated by physiological stimuli: Role of G-proteins. J Biol Chem 1989; 264:12699.
46. Rink TJ, Sage SO: Calcium signaling in human platelets. Ann Rev Physiol 1990; 52:431.
47. Rao AK, Disa J, Yang X: Concomitant defect in internal release and influx of calcium in patients with congenital platelet dysfunction and impaired agonist-induced calcium mobilization: Thromboxane production is not required for internal release of calcium. J Lab Clin Med 1993; 121:52.
48. Nakamura M, Honda Z, Waga T, et al: Endotoxin transduces Ca^{2+} signalling via platelet-activating factor receptor. FEBS Lett 1992; 314:125.
49. Inarrea P, Gomez-Cambronero J, Pascual J, et al: Synthesis of PAF-acether and blood volume changes in gram-negative sepsis. Immunopharmacology 1985; 9:45.
50. Hsueh W, Gonzalez-Crussi F, Arroyave J: Platelet-activating factor an endogenous mediator for bowel necrosis in endotoxemia. FASEB J 1987; 1:403.
51. Bussolino F, Porcellinin MG, Varese L, et al: Intravascular release of platelet-activating factor in children with sepsis. Thromb Res 1987; 48:619.
52. Lopez-Diez F, Nieto ML, Fernandez-Gallardo S, et al: Occupancy of platelet receptors for platelet-activating factor in patients with septicemia. J Clin Invest 1989; 83:1733.
53. Liu H, Chao W, Olson MS: Regulation of the surface expression of the platelet-activating factor receptor in IC-21 peritoneal macrophages: Effects of lipopolysaccharide. J Biol Chem 1992; 267:20811.
54. Camussi G, Biancone L, Iorio EL, et al: Porins and lipopolysaccharide stimulate platelet activating factor synthesis by human mesangial cells. Kidney Int 1992; 42:1309.
55. Tufano MA, Tetta C, Biancone L, et al: Salmonella typhi murium porins stimulated platelet-activating factor synthesis by human polymorphonuclear neutrophils. J Immunol 1992; 149:1023.
56. Pons L, Droy-Lefaix MT, Braquet P, et al: Role of free radicals and platelet-activating factor in the genesis of intestinal motor disturbances induced by *Escherichia coli* endotoxins in rats. Gastroenterology 1991; 100:946.
57. Wells CL, Barton RG, Wavatne CS, et al: Intestinal bacterial flora, intestinal pathology, and lipopolysaccharide-induced translocation of intestinal bacteria. Circ Shock 1992; 37:117.
58. Mozes T, Zijlstra FJ, Heiligers JPC, et al: Sequential release of tumour necrosis factor, platelet activating factor and eicosanoids during endotoxic shock in anaesthetized pigs: Protective effects of indomethacin. Br J Pharmacol 1991; 104:691.
59. Mozes T, Heiligers JPC, Tak CJAM, et al: Platelet activating factor is one of the mediators involved in endotoxic shock in pigs. J Lipid Med 1991; 4:309.
60. Mozes T, Zijlstra FJ, Heiligers JPC: Interactions between platelet activating factor and eicosanoids during endotoxic shock in anesthetized pigs. Mediat Inflammation 1992; 1:183.
61. Mozes T, Ben Efraim S, Bonta IL: Lethal and non-lethal course of endotoxic shock is determined by interactions between tumor necrosis factor, platelet activating factor and eicosanoids. Pathol Biol 1992; 40:807.
62. Klosterhalfen B, Hörstmann-Jungemann K, Vogel P, et al: Time course of various inflammatory mediators during recurrent endotoxemia. Biochem Pharmacol 1992; 43:2103.
63. Rabinovici R, Yue TL, Farhat M, et al: Platelet activating factor (PAF) and tumor necrosis factor-α (TNF-α) interactions in endotoxemic shock: Studies with BN 50739, a novel PAF antagonist. J Pharmacol Exp Ther 1990; 255:256.
64. Tracey KJ, Fong Y, Hesse DG, et al: Anti-cachectin/TNF monoclonal antibodies prevent septic shock during lethal bacteriaemia. Nature 1987; 330:662.
65. Exley AR, Buurman W, Bodmer M, et al: Monoclonal antibody to recombinant human tumour necrosis factor in the prophylaxis and treatment of endotoxic shock in cynomolgus monkeys. Clin Sci 1989; 76:50.
66. Exley AR, Cohen J, Buurman W, et al: Monoclonal antibody to TNF in severe septic shock. Lancet 1990; 335:1275.
67. Ogata M, Matsumoto T, Koga K, et al: An antagonist of platelet-activating factor suppresses endotoxin-induced tumor necrosis factor and mortality in mice pretreated with carrageenan. Infect Immun 1993; 61:699.
68. Dinarello CA: The proinflammatory cytokines interleukin-1 and tumor necrosis factor and treatment of the septic shock syndrome. J Infect Dis 1991; 163:1177.
69. Dinarello CA: Interleukin-1 and interleukin antagonism. Blood 1987; 77:1627.
70. Conti P, Panara MR, Barbacane M, et al: Human recombinant IL-1 receptor antagonist (ILRa) inhibits leukotriene B_4 generation from human monocyte suspensions stimulated by lipopolysaccharide (LPS). Clin Exp Immunol 1993; 91:526.
71. Yue TL, Farhat M, Rabinovici R, et al: Protective effect of BN 50739, a new platelet-activating factor antagonist, in endotoxin-treated rabbits. J Pharmacol Exp Ther 1990; 254:976.
72. Moore JM, Ernest MA, DiSimone AG, et al: A PAF receptor antagonist, BN 52021, attenuates thromboxane release and improves survival in lethal canine endotoxemia. Circ Shock 1991; 36:53.
73. Gray GA, Furman BL, Parratt JR: Endotoxin-induced impairment of vascular reactivity in the pithed rat: Role of arachidonic acid metabolites. Circ Shock 1990; 31:395.
74. Fletcher JR, DiSimone AG, Earnest M: Platelet activating factor antagonist improves survival and attenuates eicosanoid release in severe endotoxemia. Ann Surg 1990; 211:312.
75. Teng NNH, Kaplan HS, Herbert JM, et al: Protection against gram-negative bacteriemia and endotoxemia with human monoclonal antibodies. Proc Natl Acad Sci USA 1985; 82:1790.
76. Hopkins SJ: HA-1A: Human monoclonal IgM antibody. Drugs Today 1992; 28:13.
77. Ziegler EJ, Fisher CJ, Sprung CL, et al: Treatment of gram-negative bacteremia and septic shock with HA-1A human monoclonal antibody against endotoxin: A randomized, double-blind, placebo-controlled trial. N Engl J Med 1991; 324:429.
78. Greenman RL, Schein RMH, Martin MA, et al: A controlled clinical trial of E5 murine monoclonal IgM antibody to endo-

toxin in the treatment of gram-negative sepsis. JAMA 1991; 266:1097.
79. Warren HS, Danner RL, Munford RS: Anti-endotoxin monoclonal antibodies. N Engl J Med 1992; 326:1153.
80. McColl SR, Krump E, Naccache PH, et al: Granulocyte-macrophage colony-stimulating factor increases the synthesis of leukotriene B_4 by human neutrophils in response to platelet-activating factor: Enhancement of both arachidonic acid availability and 5-lipoxygenase activation. J Immunol 1991; 146:1204.
81. Paubert-Braquet M, Hosford D, Koltz P, et al: Tumor necrosis factor primes PAF-induced superoxide production by human neutrophils: Possible involvement of G proteins. J Lipid Med 1990; 2:S1.
82. Braquet P, Hosford D, Koltz P, et al: Effect of platelet-activating factor on tumor necrosis factor-induced superoxide generation from human neutrophils: Possible involvement of G proteins. Lipids 1991; 26:1071.
83. Pignol B, Hénane S, Sorlin B, et al: Effect of long-term treatment with platelet-activating factor on IL-1 and IL-2 production by rat spleen cells. J Immunol 1990; 145:980.
84. Gatti S, Faggioni R, Echtenacher B, et al: Role of tumour necrosis factor and reactive oxygen intermediates in lipopolysaccharide-induced pulmonary oedema and lethality. Clin Exp Immunol 1993; 91:456.
85. Poubelle PE, Gingras D, Demers C, et al: Platelet-activating factor (PAF-acether) enhances the recombinant production of tumour necrosis factor-alpha and interleukin-1 by subsets of human monocytes. Immunology 1991; 72:181.
86. Schleiffenbaum B, Fehr J: The tumor necrosis factor receptor and human neutrophil function: Deactivation and cross-deactivation of tumor necrosis factor-induced neutrophil responses by receptor down-regulation. J Clin Invest 1990; 86:184.
87. Gorman RR, Bunting S, Miller OV: Modulation of human platelet adenylate cyclase by prostacyclin (PGX). Prostaglandins 1977; 13:377.
88. Tateson JE, Moncada S, Vane JR: Effects of prostacyclin (PGX) on cyclic AMP concentrations in human platelets. Prostaglandins 1977; 13:389.
89. Abigail F, Brotherton A, Hoack JC: Role of Ca^{2+} and cyclic AMP in the regulation of the production of prostacyclin by the vascular endothelium. Proc Natl Acad Sci U S A 1982; 79:495.
90. Zimmerman GA, McIntyre TM, Prescott SM: Production of platelet-activating factor by human vascular endothelial cells: Evidence for a requirement for specific agonists and modulation by prostacyclin. Circulation 1985; 72:718.
91. Heller R, Bussolino F, Ghido D, et al: Protein kinase C and cyclic AMP modulate thrombin-induced platelet-activating factor synthesis in human endothelial cells. Biochim Biophys Acta 1991; 1093:55.
92. Camussi G, Bussolino F, Salvidio G, et al: Tumor necrosis factor/cachectin stimulates peritoneal macrophages, polymorphonuclear neutrophils, and vasular endothelial cells to synthesize and release platelet-activating factor. J Exp Med 1987; 186:1390.
93. Moncada S, Palmer RMJ, Higgs EA: Nitric oxide: Physiology, pathophysiology, and pharmacology. Pharmacol Rev 1991; 43:109.
94. Forstermann U, Pollock JS, Schmidt HH, et al: Calmodulin-dependent endothelium-derived relaxing factor/nitric oxide synthase activity is present in the particulate and cytosolic fractions of bovine aortic endothelial cells. Proc Natl Acad Sci U S A 1991; 88:1788.
95. McCall TB, Felisch M, Palmer RMJ, et al: Identification of N-iminoethyl-L-ornithine as an irreversible inhibitor of nitric oxide synthase in phagocytic cells. Br J Pharmacol 1991; 102:234.
96. Nussler AK, Di Silvio M, Billiar TR, et al: Stimulation of nitric oxide synthase pathway in human hepatocytes by cytokines and endotoxin. J Exp Med 1992; 176:261.
97. Rees DD, Palmer RMJ, Schulz R, et al: Characterization of three inhibitors of endothelial nitric oxide synthase in vitro and in vivo. Br J Pharmacol 1990; 101:746.
98. McKenna TM: Prolonged exposure of rat aorta to low levels of endotoxin in vitro results in impaired contractility: Association with vascular cytokine release. J Clin Invest 1990; 86:160.
99. Radomski MW, Palmer RJM, Moncada S: Glucocorticoids inhibit the expression of inducible, but not the constitutive nitric oxide synthase in vascular endothelial cells. Proc Natl Acad Sci USA 1990; 87:10043.
100. Rees DD, Palmer RMJ, Hodson HF, et al: A specific inhibitor of nitric oxide formation from L-arginine attenuates endothelium-dependent relaxation. Br J Pharmacol 1989; 96:418.
101. Szabo C, Mitchel JA, Thiemermann C, et al: Nitric oxide-mediated hyporeactivity to noradrenaline precedes the induction of nitric oxide synthase in endotoxic shock. Br J Pharmacol 1993; 108:786.
102. Assreuy J, Cunha FQ, Liew FY, et al: Feedback inhibition of nitric oxide synthase activity by nitric oxide. Br J Pharmacol 1993; 108:833.
103. Ding A, Nathan CF, Graycar J, et al: Macrophage deactivating factor and growth factor-β1, β2 and β3 induction of macrophage nitric oxide synthesis by IFN-γ. J Immunol 1990; 145:940.
104. Liew FY, Li Y, Severn A, et al: A possible novel pathway of regulation by murine T helper type-2 (Th_2) cell of activity via modulation of the induction of nitric oxide synthase on macrophages. Eur J Immunol 1991; 21:2489.
105. Cunha FQ, Moncada S, Liew FY: Interleukin-10 (IL-10) inhibits the nitric oxide synthase by IFN-γ in murine macrophages. Biochem Biophys Res Commun 1992; 186:1155.
106. Li T, Croce K, Windquist RJ: Regional differences in the effects of septic shock on vascular reactivity in the rabbits. J Pharmacol Exp Ther 1992; 261:959.
107. Parker JL, Keller RS, DeFily DV, et al: Coronary vascular smooth muscle function in *E. coli* endotoxemia. Am J Physiol 1992; 260:H832.
108. Sagash VF, Zhukova AV, Braquet P: Endothelium-dependent effects of platelet-activating factor in the coronary circulation. J Cardiovasc Pharmacol 1992; 20:S85.
109. Heller R, Bussolino F, Ghigo D, et al: Nitrovasodilators inhibit thrombin-induced platelet-activating factor synthesis in human endothelial cells. Biochem Pharmacol 1992; 44:223.
110. Martinez-Cuesta MA, Barrachina MD, Pique JM, et al: Role of nitric oxide and platelet-activating factor in the inhibition by endotoxin of pentagastrin-stimulated gastric acid secretion. Eur J Pharmacol 1992; 218:351.
111. Opie LH: Role of cyclic nucleotides in the heart metabolism. Cardiovasc Res 1982; 16:483–507.
112. Beijer L, Botting J, Crook P, et al: The involvement of platelet-activating factor in endotoxin-induced pulmonary platelet recruitment in the guinea-pig. Br J Pharmacol 1987; 92:803.
113. Redl H, Vogl C, Schiesser A, et al: Effect of PAF antagonist BN 52021 in an ovine endotoxin shock. J Lipid Med 1990; 2:S195.
114. Rabinovici R, Esser KM, Lysko PG, et al: Priming by platelet-activating factor of endotoxin-induced lung injury and cardiovascular shock. Circ Res 1991; 69:12.

CHAPTER 29

Colony-Stimulating Factors

Joel Weinthal, MD, FAAP • Eileen R. Gillan, MD
Mitchell S. Cairo, MD, FAAP

Colony-stimulating factors (CSFs) are a family of glycoprotein hormones that regulate production and differentiation of hematopoietic cells.[1, 2] Many individual CSFs have now been identified, cloned, and characterized. The CSFs comprise a complex family of cytokines, which are often referred to as hematopoietic growth factors. The term *CSF* was coined because these factors stimulated the formation of clonal colonies in in vitro culture systems. The study of hematopoietic growth factors has now evolved from the laboratory into an expanding number of clinical applications. The clinical utility of these CSFs is based on their extremely potent biologic activity in stimulating primitive and mature hematopoietic cells.

Specific erythroid, myeloid, and lymphoid hematopoietic growth factors have now been cloned and used in experimental systems to help elucidate our understanding of normal hematopoiesis as well as hematopoietic diseases. We are presently using several hematopoietic growth factors in the treatment of patients with hematopoietic and immunologic diseases. CSFs have also been used as adjuvant therapy with intensive chemotherapy to ameliorate the myelosuppressive toxicity. Clinical trials using the commercially available CSFs, granulocyte CSF (G-CSF), granulocyte-macrophage CSF (GM-CSF), and erythropoietin (EPO) as well as some newer CSFs are now underway in an attempt to expand the number of conditions for which they can be used. Recently, CSFs have been used as adjuvant therapy in the treatment of sepsis. This review focuses on the biology of these CSF as well as their current and potential clinical applications in the treatment of hematologic and other disorders.

BIOLOGY OF HEMATOPOIESIS

Hematopoiesis is a complex process that begins with an uncommitted pluripotent hematopoietic stem cell (PPSC), which has the ability to self-renew, proliferate, and differentiate into all of the hematopoietic lineages. Figure 29–1 illustrates our current understanding of the complex interaction of the hematopoietic growth factors at many different stages in hematopoiesis. The ultimate result of this hematopoietic process is a mature, lineage-restricted effector cell that circulates in the bloodstream. The less mature forms of blood cells, known as progenitor cells, can differentiate into different lineages depending on their exposure to individual and combinations of hematopoietic growth factors. Primitive progenitor cells maintain their multipotent potential, whereas more mature progenitor cells become committed as they differentiate into specific lineages. The schematic figure of hematopoiesis is derived from in vitro culture systems in which progenitor cells have been identified and induced with specific growth factors, resulting in differentiated progeny in various culture systems. Early progenitors are called colony-forming units (CFUs) and are named for the lineages that are derived from a specific colony. Thus, a CFU-GM is capable of giving rise to granulocytes and macrophages, whereas a CFU-Meg can give rise only to megakaryocytes. The most primitive CFU studied in colony assays is the CFU-GEMM (granulocyte, erythrocyte, macrophage, and megakaryocyte), which does not contain lymphoid cells or their progenitors and has only limited capability for self-renewal. The in vivo process of hematopoiesis is far more complex, with many other local microenvironmental factors influencing blood cell development. These include many nonhematopoietic cells such as fibroblasts and endothelial cells, which come into contact with hematopoietic progenitors during their maturation and circulation in the bone marrow and blood. Additionally, the true PPSC has yet to be identified, although very small populations of progenitor cells can be isolated that contain stem cells, as demonstrated by their ability to successfully engraft lethally irradiated animals after bone marrow transplantation (BMT).[3]

Each individual hematopoietic growth factor is coded for

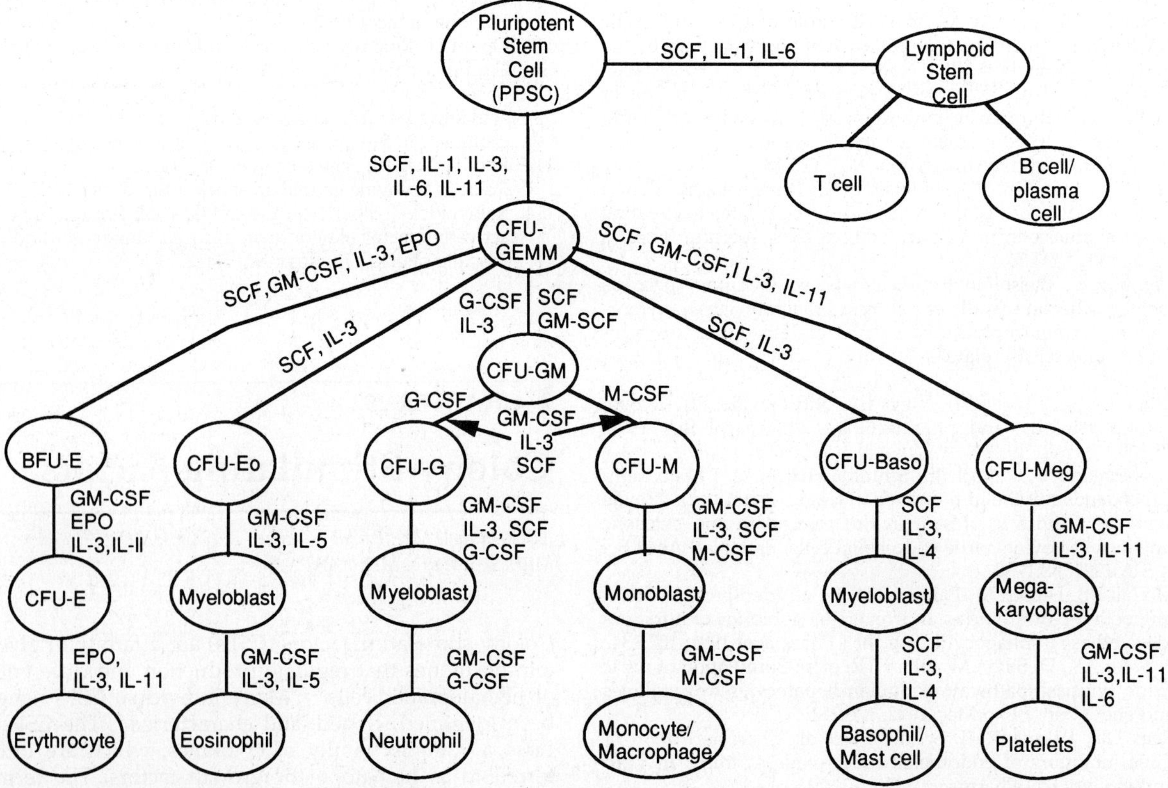

Figure 29–1. Colony-stimulating factors in hematopoiesis. *Abbreviations:* SCF = stem cell factor; IL = interleukin; CSF = colony-stimulating factor; CFU = colony-forming unit; GEMM = granulocyte, erythrocyte, macrophage, and megakaryocyte; GM = granulocyte-macrophage; G = granulocyte; M = macrophage; Eo = eosinophil; Baso = basophil; Meg = megakaryocyte; BFU-E = burst-forming unit-erythroid; EPO = erythropoietin.

by a unique gene, as described in Table 29–1. Many of these genes are located on chromosome 5, which has also been shown to be involved in various hematopoietic disorders such as myeloid leukemia and myelodysplastic syndromes. Each growth factor is produced by a variety of cells and has specific target cells, which are also described in Table 29–1. Regulation of the production of hematopoietic growth factors is a complex process that is not completely understood at this time. As illustrated in Figure 29–1, growth factors exert their influence at multiple stages of differentiation in multiple lineages. Regulation of specific CSF receptors, either through positive or negative cellular and microenvironmental influences, also plays a part in the regulation of normal hematopoiesis. In vitro culture systems have confirmed the important role of the microenvironment as well as exogenous and endogenously produced growth factors in maintaining the hematopoietic process. Abnormal conditions and disease processes such as severe anemia and sepsis result in production of multiple cytokines and growth factors that participate in biologic cascade processes, which serve to up- and down-regulate the production of growth factors and their receptors in a process known as transmodulation. The important role of cytokines in sepsis is discussed in the individual sections on specific CSFs. It is clear that the CSFs play a major role both in the disease and the body's response to disease.

GENERAL PROPERTIES OF THE COLONY-STIMULATING FACTORS

All of the CSF are glycoproteins in the 14,000- to 90,000-kd range. They are monomeric proteins with the exception of M-CSF and IL-5, which exist as homodimers. They are all heavily glycosylated; however, production of recombinant forms of the growth factors in *Escherichia coli* and yeast systems produces nonglycosylated proteins that retain the biologic activity of the specific factor being produced. This group of hormones has an extremely high biologic activity, with concentrations in the picomolar range. Low to nonexistent activity is usually measurable in the blood or marrow; however, increases in the levels of specific growth factors can be measured in response to stimuli such as other growth factors, infection, and severe cytopenia. Table 29–1 shows that the CSF are produced by a variety of cell types including fibroblasts, lymphocytes, endothelial cells, stromal cells, and macrophages. The nomenclature for the CSFs is arrived at by the generic CSF preceded by a prefix that indicates the main cell type stimulated by the specific CSF. For example, G-CSF exerts its primary actions on the granulocyte lineage. There is significant CSF amino acid sequence homology between mammalian species, although some of the CSFs such as multi-CSF or interleukin (IL)-3 have activity that is species specific. Each individual CSF has a specific receptor, although the entire group of CSF receptors is now categorized as a family because of the striking structural subunit homology.[4]

GRANULOCYTE-MACROPHAGE COLONY STIMULATING FACTOR

GM-CSF is a cytokine produced by activated T lymphocytes, macrophages, mast cells, fibroblasts, and other mesenchyma-derived cells that stimulate the production, differentiation, and maturation of myeloid hematopoietic precursors. GM-CSF also enhances the function of mature myeloid cells including neutrophils, monocytes, and eosinophils.[5] The gene encoding GM-CSF is located on chromosome 5q21.32, and it encodes a protein that contains 127

TABLE 29–1. Colony-Stimulating Factors

Cytokine	*Chromosome Location*	*Protein (kd)*	*Cellular Source*	*Progenitor Cell Target*	*Mature Effector Cell Target*
G-CSF	17qll.22	18–22	Monocytes, fibroblasts, endothelial cells	CFU-GEMM, CFU-GM, CFU-G	Neutrophil
GM-CSF	5q21.32	14–35	T lymphocytes, monocytes, fibroblasts, endothelial cells, osteoblasts, smooth-muscle cells, mast cells	CFU-GEMM, CFU-GM, CFU-G, BFU-E, BFU-Eo	Neutrophil, eosinophil, monocyte
M-CSF (CSF-1)	1	47–90	Fibroblasts, monocytes, endothelial cells, placenta	CFU-GM, CFU-M	Monocyte, neutrophil, eosinophil, basophil
(MGF, SCF SLF, KL)	12q14.3	26	Fibroblasts, endothelial cells	PPSC, CFU-GEMM	No known effects
IL-1-α IL-1β	2q13 2q14	17 17	Monocytes, lymphocytes, neutrophils	PPSC, lymphoid stem cell	Monocytes, lymphocytes, neutrophils, osteoclasts, endothelial cells, hepatocytes
IL-3 (multi-CSF)	5q23.31	28	T lymphocytes, monocyte	PPSC, CFU-GEMM, CFU-GM, CFU-M, CFU-G, CFU-Baso, CFU-Meg, CFU-Eo, BFU-E, CFU-E	Eosinophil, neutrophil, basophil, monocyte
IL-6 (INF-β2) BSF-2)	7p15	19–26	T lymphocytes, B cells, monocytes, fibroblasts, endothelial cells	PPSC, CFU-GEMM, CFU-GM, BFU-E	B cell, T cell
IL-11		20	Fibroblasts, endothelial cells	CFU-GEMM, BFU-E, CFU-G, CFU-Meg, CFU-E	Platelet
EPO	7	14–39	Renal tubular cells, hepatocytes	CFU-GEMM, BFU-E, CFU-E	

Abbreviations: CSF = colony-stimulating factor; SCF = stem-cell factor; G = granulocyte; M = macrophage; MGF = mast-cell growth factor; SLF = steel factor; KL = *Kit* ligand; IL = interleukin; EPO = erythropoietin; CFU = colony-forming unit; GEMM = granulocyte, erythrocyte, macrophage, megakaryocyte; PPSC = plurepotent hematopoietic stem cell; Baso = basophilic; Meg = megakaryocyte; E = erythrocyte; Eo = eosinophil; BSF = B cell–stimulating factor.

amino acids with a molecular weight of 14 to 35 kd depending on the degree of glycosylation.[6] GM-CSF acts on relatively early hematopoietic progenitors (see Fig. 29–1) of multiple cell lineages and can act in concert with other CSFs to influence the proliferation of these cells. Low concentrations of GM-CSF are required for viability of neutrophils and monocytes (and their progenitors).[2] Two classes of GM-CSF receptors have been identified, and they are distinguished by their high and low affinity for the cytokine. The receptors are found on hematopoietic cells as well as on endothelial cells and some solid tumor cells.[5]

GM-CSF has been shown to enhance the effector function of mature neutrophils, eosinophils, and macrophage/monocytes. These effects, which have been shown in in vitro and in vivo studies, include augmentation of neutrophil oxidative metabolism, chemotaxis, phagocytosis, leukotriene release, degranulation, and antibody-dependent cellular cytotoxicity (ADCC).[7] Similar effects are found in monocyte/macrophages as well as enhanced intracellular killing, potentiation of antigen processing, and increased production of tumor necrosis factor (TNF), IL-1, and M-CSF. Eosinophils show analogous increases in function as well as an increase in viability and protozoal killing.

Human studies have demonstrated that there is a transient leukopenia with a decrease in circulating neutrophils, eosinophils, and monocytes as well as pulmonary neutrophil sequestration after GM-CSF administration.[8] This is followed by a leukocytosis secondary to neutrophil demargination, increased marrow production, and increased half-life of circulating neutrophils. Phase I studies have shown that GM-CSF is generally well tolerated, although toxicities have included bone pain, myalgias, fever, elevation in transaminases, rash, and facial flushing. Dose-limiting toxicities (16–32 μg/kg) have included a capillary leak syndrome with generalized edema and pleural and pericardial effusions.[1] Biologically active doses have minimal side effects and have allowed GM-CSF to be studied in many clinical settings ranging from bone marrow failure syndromes to infectious diseases.[1]

GM-CSF has been used to treat refractory aplastic anemia in children and adults. The clinical responses have been variable, but most patients have shown an increase in bone marrow cellularity and neutrophil counts while on GM-CSF, with a subsequent return to their baseline state on discontinuation of the cytokine. The responses were best in patients who had higher initial neutrophil counts, although the reticulocyte and platelet responses were inconsistent.[1]

Many studies have evaluated the use of GM-CSF to ameliorate the myelotoxicity of chemotherapy by enhancing neutrophil recovery after cytotoxic therapy. These studies were largely uncontrolled but nonetheless demonstrated the efficacy of GM-CSF in this clinical situation. The propensity of GM-CSF to induce fever in patients in this setting may limit the clinical utility of the drug for postchemotherapy myelosuppression.

GM-CSF has been studied postablative chemotherapy to augment hematopoietic engraftment after BMT. In a randomized, placebo-controlled study in patients undergoing autologous BMT for hematologic malignancies, GM-CSF shortened the duration of neutropenia, antibiotic therapy, and hospitalization.[9] This study led to GM-CSF's U.S. Food and Drug Administration approval in this clinical (auto-BMT) setting. Other studies have examined the use of GM-CSF after allogeneic BMT and have had mixed results. Additionally, the use of GM-CSF to augment the collection of peripheral blood stem cell (PBSC) has been demonstrated,[10] although optimal doses and schedules for this application are still being studied. The goal of PBSC collection is to use these cells to assist or replace harvested bone marrow in autologous transplantation in an effort to decrease the morbidity of this procedure.

GM-CSF has also been used in the therapy of myeloid malignancies including myelodysplastic syndrome (MDS) and acute myeloid leukemia (AML). Malignant myeloid cells express GM-CSF receptors, making GM-CSF administration attractive in an attempt to either stimulate differentiation or proliferation to increase the sensitivity of these cells to cytotoxic therapy. However, the possibility of providing exogenous leukemic growth factor in the form of GM-CSF in this setting is also being examined. GM-CSF has been given to many patients with MDS in several clinical trials. A majority of patients have shown an increase in their neutrophil count, with a minority showing erythrocyte and platelet responses. Infection rates decreased with the increase in neutrophil counts; however, patients still progressed and leukemia developed. Cytogenetic abnormalities were unaffected by treatment with GM-CSF. Several groups have shown that GM-CSF does not increase relapse rates in AML when used after chemotherapy to accelerate marrow recovery[11] or when used in an effort to augment chemotherapy by increasing the cycling or proliferation of malignant leukemic cells.[12] In an analogous fashion, GM-CSF may be used in future clinical trials in the treatment of solid tumors, which express the GM-CSF receptor such as small-cell lung carcinoma and osteosarcoma. Additionally, there are data to suggest that GM-CSF can increase the tumoricidal activity of tissue macrophages.

The use of GM-CSF in nonhematologic diseases has been focused on infectious diseases because GM-CSF can augment effector function of mature blood elements involved in host defense. Additionally, overwhelming bacterial or viral sepsis is often accompanied by granulocytopenia. In combination with antibiotics, GM-CSF may play a role in the therapy of this condition. Several groups have demonstrated a protective effect of GM-CSF in combination with antibiotics in septic, neutropenic mice.[13, 14] Clinical trials using GM-CSF in septic patients are now underway.

GM-CSF has also been studied in patients with acquired immunodeficiency syndrome (AIDS) in an attempt to circumvent the myelosuppression that results from the retroviral infection as well as the myelotoxicity of antiviral chemotherapy. GM-CSF increases peripheral myeloid blood cell counts when used in patients with human immunodeficiency virus (HIV) infection.[1, 15] Patients who were neutropenic from azidothymidine (AZT) or interferon therapy were subsequently able to receive these medications once they began taking simultaneous GM-CSF.[16] In vitro studies have demonstrated that GM-CSF can potentiate antiviral therpy by stimulating HIV replication in monocytes,[17] but clinical correlation in vivo has not yet been reported.

GRANULOCYTE COLONY-STIMULATING FACTOR

G-CSF is a hematopoietic growth factor that exerts its effect on cells of the neutrophil lineage by stimulating proliferation and differentiation of granulocytes and their committed precursors (see Fig. 29–1). G-CSF is considered a late-acting CSF because of its relative lineage specificity. G-CSF also enhances mature neutrophil function. Human G-CSF was first identified after the purification of murine G-CSF by Nicola and associates in 1983.[18] In 1985, Welte and colleagues purified human G-CSF from the bladder carcinoma cell line 5637.[19] The gene for G-CSF was subsequently cloned in 1986[20] and was mapped to chromosome 17q11.22.[21] G-CSF is a single polypeptide chain consisting of 207 amino acids, with 177 making up the mature molecule and 30 of leader sequence. The protein can be heavily glycosylated and therefore has a variable molecular weight of 18 to 22 kd. Recombinant G-CSF has been produced in *E. coli* and has been shown to have a similar activity to the native protein.[22] Endogenous G-CSF is produced primarily by mature macrophages but has also been shown to be produced by endothelial cells, fibroblasts, and mesothelial cells. G-CSF production can be stimulated in these cells by TNF, lipopolyaceharide, IL-1, GM-CSF, IL-3, IL-4, and interferon-γ.[23] In vitro culture and colony assays have demonstrated significant synergistic actions of G-CSF with other CSFs in stimulating hematopoietic progenitors, particularly IL-1, IL-3, IL-6, and stem-cell factor (SCF). (see Fig. 29–1).[23] A specific receptor for G-CSF has been identified[24] and is found on cells in the granulocyte lineage as well as on leukemic cells, placental cells, and endothelial cells.[22] The significance of G-CSF receptors in nonhematopoietic cells is unknown.

The role of G-CSF in steady-state hematopoiesis is unclear; however, in the stressed conditions of sepsis and congenital neutropenia and after cytotoxic chemotherapy, endogenous G-CSF levels increase markedly.[22, 23] Cairo and associates[25] demonstrated that endogenous G-CSF production correlates with myeloid engraftment after autologous and allogeneic BMT. Experimental data have shown that G-CSF can produce a rapid release of bone marrow neutrophils into the circulation and reduce granulocyte maturation time. Multiple animal studies have documented that G-CSF can cause a neutrophilia with little toxicity.[26] Furthermore, G-CSF can enhance the effector function of mature neutrophils by priming oxidative metabolism, promoting chemotaxis and phagocytosis, and augmenting antibody-dependent cellular cytotoxicity.[22, 27] These studies have led to many clinical trials using G-CSF in a variety of conditions and are summarized in the following section. Of note, toxicity from G-CSF has been minimal, with the most common side effect being bone pain, which subsides on discontinuation of the drug.

Bodey and coauthors first demonstrated that the risk of infection in cancer patients receiving myelosuppressive chemotherapy correlates with depth and duration of neutropenia.[28] Several phase II G-CSF studies after chemotherapy have demonstrated clinical efficacy in ameliorating the hematologic and infectious toxicity of intensive treatment regimens. Crawford and colleagues[29] published the results of a double-blind phase III study in small-cell lung cancer patients who were randomized to receive prophylactic G-CSF after chemotherapy cycles. The G-CSF group had a reduced duration and severity of neutropenia as well as a lower incidence of febrile neutropenia, infections, hospitalizations, and antibiotic use.[29] We reported similar findings in children with solid tumors who received intensive myelosuppressive chemotherapy followed by G-CSF compared with historic controls who received the same treatment without G-CSF.[30] However, the optimal G-CSF dose and administration schedule is still to be determined in the postchemotherapy setting and is the focus of many ongoing clinical trials in pediatric and medical oncology.

G-CSF has also been used and studied after myeloablative therapy for BMT in an effort to decrease the neutropenia before engraftment. G-CSF recipients have been shown to have a shorter period of neutropenia, decreased hospital stay, parenteral nutrition, and less mucositis[1, 22] compared with historic controls. Allogeneic BMT results have been similar, although no prospective studies have been done.[22] The use of G-CSF to augment PBSC collection has also been reported.[31] Patients who received G-CSF treatment before PBSC collection had accelerated neutrophil and platelet recovery after auto-BMT and PBSC compared with those who did not receive G-CSF before PBSC collection.

Congenital neutropenia (Kostman's syndrome) is characterized by severe neutropenia and recurrent bacterial infections despite high endogenous levels of G-CSF.[32] This condition was previously treatable only by allogeneic BMT. Two groups have reported a significant increase in neutrophil count as well as a clinical response, as demonstrated by decreased infections, antibiotic use, and hospital stay after G-CSF therapy. Interestingly, this response was not seen with GM-CSF.[33]

Cyclic neutropenia is characterized by a 14- to 28-day periodic fluctuation in blood counts of all lineages. Clinical symptoms usually manifest themselves as infections and mouth ulcers during periods of the neutrophil nadir. Although the underlying problem is believed to be a defect within a multilineage progenitor, G-CSF administration decreased clinical symptoms by reducing the cycling time and increasing the neutrophil nadir.[34]

G-CSF has also been used to treat patients with aplastic anemia. Neutrophil increases have been seen in several studies, but G-CSF has not had any effect on increasing red blood cell or platelet populations.[35] Furthermore, the neutrophil responses have disappeared after cessation of G-CSF. Combination CSF therapy or earlier acting agents may produce better and longer lasting multilineage responses in this disease.

G-CSF has been studied in MDS and myeloid leukemias in an effort to differentiate neoplastic cells and increase normal neutrophils.[36] Interestingly, some MDS patients have shown a reticulocyte response to G-CSF. Although neutrophil recovery is enhanced after chemotherapy for AML, no data for overall clinical response have been reported. G-CSF administration does appear to be safe in this clinical setting despite the presence of G-CSF receptors on the leukemic cells with no increase in relapse rate reported.[23]

G-CSF administration has been used in patients with AIDS to treat the neutropenia that accompanies HIV infection as well as the myelosuppressive side effects of antiretroviral therapy with AZT.[37] Preliminary data do not seem to indicate that G-CSF accelerates the progression of HIV infection, and clinical and laboratory deterioration has not been seen in the reported patients.

Using the neutrophilic and effector enhancement properties of this cytokine, several investigators have studied the use of G-CSF to modulate sepsis in experimental animal models. Yasuda and colleagues demonstrated an increased survival in mice treated with antibiotics and G-CSF after *Pseudomonas aeruginosa* infection.[38] Herbert and co-workers[39] demonstrated improved survival in splenectomized mice challenged with pneumococci that were treated with G-CSF. Pretreatment of neutropenic mice with G-CSF protected them from experimental infection with *Pseudomonas, Staphylococcus aureus, Candida albicans,* and *Serratia marcescens* compared with control animals that died after infection without G-CSF pretreatment.[39] Cairo and others[40] studied the survival of neonatal rats after experimental group B streptococci infection and demonstrated enhanced survival in animals that were pretreated with G-CSF and received antibiotics compared with those that received antibiotics or G-CSF alone. These preclinical data are now being used in designing human clinical trials of G-CSF adjuvant therapy in bacterial sepsis.

ERYTHROPOIETIN

EPO is a sialoglycoprotein hormone that has been identified as the CSF that regulates red blood cell production (erythropoiesis). During the 1950s, investigators were able to demonstrate the transfer of an erythropoietic stimulus from hypoxic rats[41] and anemic rabbits.[42] EPO was first isolated and purified in 1977 by Miyake,[43] and the gene was cloned in 1985 by two groups.[44, 45] The gene has been mapped to chromosome 7.[46] The protein has a molecular weight of 14 to 39 kd depending on the degree of glycosylation. Although it has been known for some time that EPO was produced by the kidney, it has now been shown that 90% of EPO is produced in the kidney and 10% is produced in the liver.[47] EPO is produced in response to anemia or hypoxia by proximal peritubular cells within the kidney.[48] These cells have the ability to detect subtle changes in oxygen tension and regulate EPO production accordingly. EPO levels are measurable in the plasma, and levels increase in states of hypoxia and anemia.[49] A specific EPO receptor has been cloned[50] and is present on the appropriate erythroid progenitors (see Fig. 29–1).

EPO interacts with several other CSFs in stimulating erythroid progenitors known as burst-forming unit erythroid and the CFU-erythroid. GM-CSF, IL-3, IL-1, and the recently described SCF have all been shown to synergize with EPO in promoting erythropoiesis.[51, 52] Additionally, it has been shown that EPO can act in concert with other CSFs to stimulate other nonerythroid lineages including myeloid, monocyte, and megakaryocytic in vivo and in vitro.

The clinical applications of EPO were first studied after the production of recombinant human EPO in 1985. Recombinant EPO was first used in patients with chronic renal failure undergoing dialysis who had the expected deficiency in endogenous EPO secondary to their underlying renal disease. Winearls and colleagues reported on the efficacy of EPO administration three times per week after dialysis in maintaining hematocrits in the 35% range.[53] Subsequent studies have confirmed and expanded these exciting results to further demonstrate that renal failure patients have experienced improvements in appetite, activity level, sense of well-being, uremic coagulopathy, and pruritus as a result of EPO treatment.[54, 55]

Other clinical conditions have been studied with regard to the use of EPO. In a placebo-controlled study, patients with anemia secondary to rheumatoid arthritis have shown a significant improvement in their hematocrit.[56] Patients with AIDS in whom anemia develops secondary to AZT antiviral therapy showed a reticulocyte response if they did not have elevated serum EPO levels before EPO treatment.[1] Miller and coauthors reported that the anemia of cancer was characterized by inappropriately low levels of EPO,[57] leading to several clinical studies that demonstrated the efficacy of EPO administration in cancer patients. Goodnough and colleagues reported another potential clinical application of EPO: augmenting the presurgical collection of autologous blood used for elective operative procedures.[58] They performed a double-blind, placebo-controlled study that demonstrated that patients who received EPO were able to donate more units of blood and these units had a significantly higher hematocrit. A final area of investigation into the use of exogenous EPO is in anemia of premature infants who also have a relative deficiency of EPO. Clinical trials are now underway to assess the efficacy of EPO therapy in the anemia of prematurity.

The toxicity of EPO has been minimal, hypertension has been the most significant side effect seen in renal failure patients. It is believed that the hypertension is exacerbated by a rapid rise in hematocrit[1] and can usually be prevented by careful monitoring of blood counts with appropriate EPO dose modification. Iron deficiency can often accompany anemias secondary to chronic inflammation, cancer, and renal failure. A poor response to EPO therapy in patients may be improved by pretreatment with supplemental iron, and all patients treated with EPO should have their iron stores evaluated by routine laboratory assessment.

MACROPHAGE-COLONY STIMULATING FACTOR

M-CSF was the first myeloid CSF to be defined and was originally called CSF-1. It is now known that M-CSF is produced by fibroblasts, endothelial cells, macrophages, and placental tissue.[59] Of note, T lymphocytes do not produce M-CSF, unlike the other myeloid CSFs. Initial clinical trials were performed with M-CSF that was purified from human urine.[60] Subsequently, the M-CSF gene was cloned,[61] and a recombinant M-CSF has been produced, enabling clinical trials to proceed in larger numbers. The M-CSF gene has been mapped to chromosome 1p13.21[62] and encodes a protein with a molecular weight of 14.5 kd. However, the biologically active protein exists as a homodimer that is variably glycosylated and has a molecular weight of 47 to 90 kd.

M-CSF induces the proliferation and differentiation of committed monocyte/macrophage progenitor cells. M-CSF also enhances the function of mature monocyte/macrophages, which continue to express receptors for this relatively lineage-specific cytokine. The M-CSF receptor is the product of the *fms* proto-oncogene.[63] Mutations in this receptor can lead to dysregulated growth of cells and oncogenesis.

The effects of M-CSF on mature monocytes have been well studied. M-CSF enhances intracellular killing of *Mycobacterium avium–intracellulare* and *C. albicans* as well as ADCC and tumoricidal activity of macrophages.[64] M-CSF also stimulates the production and release of IL-1, TNF, G-CSF, interferon, ferritin, plasminogen activator, thromboplastin, prostaglandins, and superoxide dismutase.[65]

Clinical trials with M-CSF are lagging behind these with G-CSF and GM-CSF, although the previously mentioned enhancement of monocyte and macrophage function make this an attractive cytokine for augmenting host defense and immunotherapy against neoplastic diseases. Komiyama and colleagues[66] reported an increase in leukocyte and neutrophil counts in neutropenic children treated for 7 days with purified urinary M-CSF. Motoyoshi and colleagues treated 24 patients with urinary M-CSF after chemotherapy and demonstrated a decrease in the duration of neutrophil nadir compared with albumin treatment, although fever was a significant side effect in the M-CSF group.[67] Nemunaitis and associates[68] reported the results of a phase 1 trial of recombinant human M-CSF in BMT patients with invasive fungal infections. Dose-related thrombocytopenia was observed in this patient population, although no changes in neutrophil, monocyte, and lymphocyte counts were seen. Overall, 39% of patients with documented infection and 50% with presumed infection survived 100 days after initiation of M-CSF and antifungal therapy compared with a historic control population who had a survival rate of less than 20%. This phase I trial had a mixed population of underlying diseases and variable date of initiation of therapy after BMT, making the hematologic data questionable. However, this study does provide pilot data for a randomized, controlled study to test the efficacy of M-CSF in invasive fungal disease. Furthermore, in vitro studies demonstrate that M-CSF has significant synergy with other CSFs in stimulating marrow progenitor cells.[69] This suggests that the optimal way to achieve the maximal biologic effect of M-CSF in the clinical setting may be to use it in combination with other CSFs. This approach may enter clinical trials in the near future.

MULTICOLONY STIMULATING FACTOR

Multi-CSF, or IL-3, was the last of the initial group of human CSFs to be cloned. It was first purified from the WEHI-3B cell line[70] and is a monomeric glycoprotein with a weight of 28 kd.[71] The gene was cloned in 1986[72] and maps to chromosome 5q23.31 near the GM-CSF gene.[73] Unlike other CSFs, the murine and human IL-3 genes have only minimal homology (29%), explaining the protein's relative species specificity despite the similarity of biologic properties. IL-3 has an extremely broad range of target cells including neutrophil, eosinophil, basophil, monocyte, megakaryocyte, and erythrocyte precursors (see Fig. 29–1). IL-3 is produced by activated T cells, monocytes, and natural killer cells. The IL-3 receptor is part of the cytokine receptor family. Overexpression of IL-3 in an experimental murine gene transfer model led to a myeloproliferative disorder, raising questions about the importance of IL-3 gene regulation in normal hematopoiesis.

IL-3 acts on a broad range of target cells and their progenitors (see Fig. 29–1), and synergism with other growth factors is well documented in murine and human models of hematopoiesis. The combination of IL-3 and GM-CSF has been shown to stimulate megakaryocyte progenitors.[74] Other IL-3 combinations can stimulate T and B lymphocyte growth as well as mast-cell and eosinophil function.[65] IL-3 can affect mature cell function in a manner similar to other CSFs. IL-3 has been shown to increase monocyte tumoricidal activity via increased TNF production, IL-1 activity, ADCC, and antigen expression.[59]

Phase I and II studies of IL-3 are now underway after several reports of IL-3 activity in animals in ameliorating myelosuppressive toxicity of chemotherapy, increasing progenitor cells in peripheral blood, and augmenting multiple hematopoietic lineages after prolonged IL-3 treatment.[75] The combination of IL-3 and IL-6 has been shown to stimulate stem-cell cycling in the mouse[76] as well as in human in vitro assays.[77] Thrombopoiesis in primates was increased with administration of IL-3 followed by IL-6 when compared with IL-3 treatment alone.[78] Sequential IL-3 followed by GM-CSF led to a doubling of leukocyte concentration in treated monkeys compared with control animals. These experiments support the concept that IL-3 can act by priming multipotential progenitors for later acting CSFs.

Recombinant IL-3 has been studied in human trials and has produced significant multilineage increases in hematopoiesis. Neutrophil, lymphocyte, reticulocyte, and platelet counts all increased in a dose-dependent manner.[79] Interestingly, there was a 1-week delay in the increase in leukocyte counts in contrast to the almost immediate leukocytosis seen after G-CSF or GM-CSF administration. This supports the hypothesis that IL-3 acts on an earlier progenitor than the other CSFs. Transient increases in neutrophil counts were seen in patients with aplastic anemia treated with IL-3 without significant reticulocyte or platelet responses.[80] IL-3 is currently being studied in myelodysplastic syndrome. Finally, a clinical trial based on the animal and in vitro data using sequential IL-3 and GM-CSF demonstrated an enhanced neutrophil response and an equivalent platelet response compared with IL-3 treatment alone.[81]

The toxicity data in IL-3 trials to date report side effects similar to those of other CSFs, including headache, fever, bone pain, and myalgia. Combination CSF trials using IL-3 in the future need to better define the role of this unique cytokine in hematopoietic diseases as well as its toxicity when used in this fashion. Concerns about the potential stimulation of neoplastic cells that contain IL-3 receptors are being prospectively studied. Additionally, the role of IL-3 in stimulating other cytokines is being investigated to better understand the mechanism by which IL-3 exerts its actions. However, the ability of IL-3 to increase megakaryopoiesis gives it a unique niche in the design of clinical CSF trials.

The remaining CSFs that have been identified have accumulated few clinical data. Few CSFs have entered formal clinical trials, although they have all been studied in in vitro or animal model systems. Each of these CSFs has unique properties that may give them a role in future clinical applications.

INTERLEUKIN-1

IL-1 activity has now been demonstrated to be elaborated by two individual proteins: IL-1α and IL-1β.[82] IL-1α is located on chromosome 2q13 and is a 31-kd protein, whereas IL-1β maps to chromosome 2q14 and has a weight of 17 kd.[59] IL-1 is produced by monocytes and tissue macrophages as well as lymphocytes and neutrophils.[59] Production of IL-1 is stimulated by immune complexes, endotoxin, viruses, bacteria, and yeast.[59] IL-1 is thought to be involved in the initiation of the acute-phase response to microbial invasion, including fever, increased neutrophil counts, and increased expression of adhesion molecules by endothelial cells.[65] Elevated circulating IL-1 levels have been shown in adults with sepsis[83, 84] and have correlated with mortality rates. A specific IL-1 receptor antagonist (IL-1RA) is naturally produced[85] in response to sepsis, and increased IL-1RA production may play an important role the body's response to septic shock.

The role of IL-1 in hematopoiesis is as an early-acting stimulator of progenitors and stromal cells to produce other CSFs, thereby enabling IL-1 to act in a synergistic fashion with other cytokines. IL-1 induces G-CSF, GM-CSF, and M-CSF production by stromal cells, fibroblasts, and endothelial cells.[59, 65] IL-1 acts synergistically with these CSFs to enhance production of early and late progenitors.[86] IL-1 can up-regulate its own receptors on hematopoietic progenitors, thereby increasing the cell's sensitivity to IL-1 and providing a molecular mechanism for the initiation and autoregulation of the cytokine cascade.[87] IL-1 treatment in animal models has been shown to increase peripheral blood progenitors.[88] In combination with other CSFs, IL-1 enhances recovery after chemotherapy and radiation.[59, 89] These preclinical studies have led to the initiation of IL-1 clinical trials in a variety of settings.[89a]

INTERLEUKIN-6

IL-6 is a 184-amino acid, 26-kd glycoprotein that was originally cloned from a T lymphocyte complementary deoxyribonucleic acid (cDNA) library as a molecule that induced immunoglobulin production by B lymphocytes.[90] It was previously called by many names including interferon-β2, B cell stimulating factor-2, hybridoma/plasmacytoma growth factor, hepatocyte-stimulating factor, and B cell differentiation factor. It is produced by T cells, B cells, monocytes, fibroblasts, endothelial cells, stromal cells, and several tumor cell lines and has a broad range of action on many cell types, as its previous names reflect. IL-6 gene expression is stimulated by LPS, interferon-γ, TNF, plalelet-derived growth factor, IL-1, and various viruses including HIV.[59]

IL-6 is a potent mitogen for B cells[91] and can induce resting T cells and up-regulate IL-2 production.[59] Patients with autoimmune and inflammatory diseases show increased serum levels of IL-6, and overproduction of IL-6 has been shown to cause Castleman's disease in animal models.[92] Serum levels of IL-6 have been shown to be elevated in bacterial sepsis[93] and to correlate with survival, demonstrating the important role of IL-6 in the endogenous cytokine cascade that mediates the host reaction to overwhelming sepsis.

Although we and others have shown that IL-6 has thrombopoietic activity when given for long periods of time,[94] IL-6 has relatively little hematopoietic activity on its own.[95] However, IL-6 has significant multilineage activity in combination with other CSFs. Ikebuchi and co-workers[96] demonstrated that IL-6 and IL-3, when combined, act synergistically to support multilineage progenitor cells. Several investigators demonstrated that this combination can induce quiescent stem cells to cycle and proliferate in in vitro culture systems in murine[97] and human[98] models. These data suggest a clinical role for this CSF combination in augmenting the proliferation of early progenitors in such settings as BMT and peripheral stem-cell collection. Cairo and associates also studied the combination of IL-6 and G-CSF and showed that the sequential treatment of newborn rats with these two cytokines induced a significant increase in bone marrow and extramedullary storage pools of myeloid progenitors, suggesting a role for this combination in modulating myelopoiesis in clinical situations such as neonatal sepsis or sepsis in neutropenic cancer patients.[99]

STEM-CELL FACTOR

SCF is a recently described CSF that is the ligand for the *c-kit* proto-oncogene.[100] It has several other names including mast-cell growth factor, *kit* ligand, and steel factor because this CSF has been shown to be the product of the Steel locus in the mouse.[101] It is a 26-kd protein that maps to chromosome 12q14.3. SCF is produced by fibroblasts, marrow stromal cells, fetal liver cells, and other mesenchymal-derived cells. Mice with genetic mutations in the Steel locus or *c-kit* gene (the SCF receptor) have an abnormal phenotype with a macrocytic anemia, mast-cell deficiency, and defects in melanocytosis and gametogenesis.

In vitro and in vivo studies have shown that SCF has little hematopoietic activity on its own. However, it acts synergistically with many cytokines including G-CSF, GM-CSF, EPO, IL-3, IL-6, IL-1, and M-CSF to enhance proliferation of early progenitors as well as committed cells.[102, 103] These studies demonstrate that SCF is an extremely early acting CSF but does not, by itself, support colony formation or stem-cell proliferation. The best combination of CSFs in supporting and stimulating stem-cell populations is now believed to be SCF, IL-1, IL-3, and IL-6.[104]

Clinical trials will begin to use these CSF combinations in various disease states over the next several years.[104a] Cairo and colleagues demonstrated that the combination of SCF and G-CSF can significantly reduce the mortality of experimental group B streptococci sepsis in a newborn rat model.[105] Several other investigators demonstrated that SCF in combination with other CSFs can produce an in vitro response among progenitor cells from some patients with Diamond-Blackfan anemia, a congenital hypoplastic anemia unresponsive to other CSFs.[106] These preclinical studies suggest that SCF will be used to modulate sepsis as well as treat hematopoietic disease in the future in a manner analogous to other CSFs.

INTERLEUKIN-11

IL-11 is a newly described CSF that is 199 amino acids in length.[107] IL-11 was originally cloned from a primate stromal cell line, PU34, and the human MRC 5 cell line. It has been shown to enhance B cell and plasmacytoma proliferation and synergize with other early acting CSFs, including SCF and IL-3, to enhance multilineage hematopoiesis.[108] IL-11 can stimulate erythroid progenitors in vitro in combination with IL-3, even in the absence of EPO.[109] A unique property of IL-11 may be its thrombopoietic activity. Du and associates[110] demonstrated that administration of IL-11 after BMT in lethally irradiated mice significantly enhanced platelet recovery and reduced the bleeding time compared with control-treated animals. Cairo and coauthors[110a] also showed that administration of IL-11 to newborn rats with experimental sepsis results in a significant increase in the circulating platelet count without affecting red or white blood cell counts. This study also demonstrated that the combination of IL-11 and G-CSF acts synergistically in increasing the circulating neutrophil count while maintaining the IL-11–induced platelet increase, which is not seen with G-CSF alone. Further evaluation of IL-11 alone and in combination with other cytokines in patients with both congenital and acquired platelet disorders will define the role of IL-11 in clinical practice.

PIXY-321

PIXY-321 is a new "fusion" CSF that was synthesized by fusing the cDNA coding regions of GM-CSF and IL-3.[111] The PIXY-321 is produced in a recombinant yeast expression system, and the protein is immunoreactive with both GM-CSF and IL-3 antibodies. A higher binding affinity for the specific receptors on cell lines has been shown, as has an increase in specific activity in stimulating cells compared with individual cytokines or the combination of IL-3 and GM-CSF. Cairo and colleagues showed that PIXY-321 in combination with SCF can significantly enhance colony formation from purified umbilical cord blood progenitor cells.[112] These data may be applied in future studies designed to optimize in vitro expansion of cord blood progenitor cells for BMT and modulation of neonatal hematopoiesis and host defense. Others investigations showed that this novel CSF can stimulate colony formation from chemotherapy-purged bone marrow to a greater extent than can the individual cytokines.

Early animal studies using PIXY-321 demonstrate that this cytokine is able to promote neutrophil and platelet recovery after administration of experimental doses of sublethal irradiation. This bilineage effect may prove to be quite clinically useful after near-ablative chemotherapy or after the intensive preparative regimens used before BMT. In vivo animal studies using PIXY-321 alone and in combination with other CSFs are underway in an effort to augment multilineage hematopoiesis. Human phase I and II trials using PIXY-321 after BMT and intensive chemotherapy are also underway to determine the clinical utility of this novel CSF.[112a]

SUMMARY

Many different CSFs have now been identified, cloned, and studied in vitro and in vivo. ILs now number 1 to 11, and we have chosen to highlight the more clinically promising and relevant ones in this chapter. It is clear that each CSF and their specific combinations will have distinct clinical applications in augmenting hematopoiesis and enhancing the immune system to fight disease and infection. Monoclonal antibodies raised against specific CSF receptors may provide specific clinical bullets to reverse the pathologic effects of dysregulated CSF production seen in sepsis and hematopoietic malignancies. New CSFs are being described and synthesized at a breathtaking pace. The study of CSFs will continue to foster the collaboration of basic science and clinical medicine in finding useful applications for these important new molecules.

References

1. Groopman JE, Molina J-M, Scadden DT: Hematopoietic growth factors biology and clinical applications. N Engl J Med 1989; 321:1449.
2. Metcalf D: Haemopoietic growth factors 1. Lancer 1989; i:825.

3. Spangrude GJ, Heimfeld S, Weissman IL: Purification and characterization of mouse hematopoietic stem cells. Science 1988; 241:58.
4. Park LS, Gillis S: Characterization of hematopoietic growth factor receptors. Prog Clin Biol Res 1990; 352:189.
5. Gasson JC: The molecular physiology of GM-CSF. Blood 1991; 77:1131.
6. Furman WL, Crist WM: Potential uses of recombinant human granulocyte-macrophage colony-stimulating factor in children. Am J Pediatr Hematol Oncol 1991; 13:388.
7. Weisbart RH, Golde DW: Physiology of granulocyte and macrophage colony-stimulating factors in host defense. Hematol Oncol Clin North Am 1989; 3:401.
8. Devereux S, Linch DC, Campos Costa D, et al: Transient leukopenia induced by granulocyte-macrophage colony stimulating factor. Lancet 1987; 1:1523.
9. Nemunaitis J, Rabinowe SN, Singer JW, et al: Recombinant granulocyte-macrophage colony-stimulating factor after autologous bone marrow transplantation for lymphoid cancer. N Engl J Med 1991; 324:1773.
10. Gianni AM, Siena S, Bregni M, et al: Granulocyte-macrophage colony-stimulating factor to harvest circulating haemopoietic stem cells for auto-transplantation. Lancet 1989; 2:580.
11. Ohno R, Tomonaga M, Kobayashi T, et al: Effect of granulocyte colony-stimulating factor after intensive induction therapy in relapsed or refractory acute leukemia. N Engl J Med 1990; 323:871.
12. Cannistra SA, DiCarlo J, Groshek P, et al: Simultaneous administration of granulocyte-macrophage colony-stimulating factor and cytosine arabinoside for the treatment of relapsed acute myeloid leukemia. Leukemia 1991; 5:230.
13. Bermudez LE, Martinelli JC, Gascon R, et al: Protection against gram-negative bacteremia in neutropenic mice with recombinant granulocyte-macrophage colony-stimulating factor. Cytokine 1990; 2:287.
14. Tanaka T, Okamura S, Okada K, et al: Protective effect of recombinant murine granulocyte-macrophage colony-stimulating factor against *Pseudomonas aeruginosa* infection in leukocytopenic mice. Infect Immun 1984; 57:1792.
15. Groopman JE, Mitsuyasu RT, DeLeo MJ, et al: Effect of recombinant human granulocyte-macrophage colony-stimulating factor on myelopoiesis in the acquired immunodeficiency syndrome. N Engl J Med 1987; 317:593.
16. James DL, Allan JD, Tessitore JH, et al: Recombinant human granulocyte-macrophage colony-stimulating factor ameliorates zidovudine-induced neutropenia in patients with acquired immunodeficiency syndrome (AIDS)/AIDS-related complex. Blood 1991; 78:3148.
17. Perno CF, Yarchoan R, Cooney DA, et al: Replication of human immunodeficiency virus in monocytes: Granulocyte/macrophage colony-stimulating factor (GM-CSF) potentiates viral production yet enhances the antiviral effect mediated by 3′-azido-2′3′-dideoxythymidine (AZT) and other dideoxynucleoside congeners of thymidine. J Exp Med 1989; 169:933.
18. Nicola NA, Metcalf D, Matsumoto M, et al: Purification of a factor inducing differentiation in murine myelomonocytic leukemia cells: Identification as granulocyte colony-stimulating factor. J Biol Chem 1983; 258:9017.
19. Welte K, Platzer E, Lu L, et al: Purification and biochemical characterization of human pluripotent hematopoietic colony-stimulating factor. Proc Natl Acad Sci USA 1987; 82:1526.
20. Nagata S, Tsuchiya M, Asano S, et al: Molecular cloning and expression of cDNA for human granulocyte colony-stimulating factor. Nature 1986; 319:415.
21. Simmers RN, Webber LM, Shannon MF, et al: Localization of the G-CSF gene on chromosome 17 proximal to the breakpoint in the t(15;17) in acute promyelocytic leukemia. Blood 1987; 70:330.
22. Lieschke GJ, Burgess AW: Granulocyte colony-stimulating factor and granulocyte-macrophage colony stimulating factor. N Engl J Med 1992; 327:28–35.
23. Demetri GD, Griffin JD: Granulocyte colony-stimulating factor and its receptor. Blood 1991; 78:2791.
24. Nicola NA, Metcalf D: Binding of ^{125}I-labeled granulocyte colony-stimulating factor to normal murine hemopoietic cells. J Cell Physiol 1985; 124:313.
25. Cairo M, Suen Y, Sender L, et al: Circulating granulocyte colony-stimulating factor (G-CSF) levels after allogeneic and autologous bone marrow transplantation: Endogenous G-CSF production correlates with myeloid engraftment. Blood 1992; 79:1869.
26. Welte K, Bonilla MA, Gillio AP, et al: Recombinant human granulocyte colony-stimulating factor: Effects on hematopoiesis in normal and cyclophosphamide-treated primates. J Exp Med 1987; 165:941.
27. Lopez A, Nicola N, Burgess A, et al: Activation of granulocyte cytotoxic function by purified mouse colony-stimulating factors. J Immunol 1983; 131:2983.
28. Bodey G, Buckley M, Sathe Y, et al: Quantitative relationship between circulating leukocytes and infection in patients with acute leukemia. Ann Intern Med 1966; 64:328.
29. Crawford J, Ozer H, Stoller R, et al: Reduction by granulocyte colony-stimulating factor of fever and neutropenia induced by chemotherapy in patients with small-cell lung cancer. N Engl J Med 1991; 325:164.
30. Weinthal J, Gillan E, Hodder F, Cairo M: G-CSF significantly reduces the nadir of neutropenia, hospitalizations, and costs during intensive chemotherapy in children with solid tumors. ASCO Proceedings 1992; 11:362A.
31. Sheridan WP, Begley CG, Juttner CA, et al: Effect of peripheral-blood progenitor cells mobilized by filgrastim (G-CSF) on platelet recovery after high-dose chemotherapy. Lancet 1992; 339:640.
32. Mempel K, Pietsch T, Menzel T, et al: Increased serum levels of granulocyte colony-stimulating factor in patients with severe congenital neutropenia. Blood 1991; 77:1919.
33. Welte K, Zeidler C, Reiter A, et al: Differential effects of granulocyte-macrophage colony-stimulating factor and granulocyte colony-stimulating factor in children with severe congenital neutropenia. Blood 1990; 75:1056.
34. Hammond WP IV, Price TH, Souza LM, et al: Treatment of cyclic neutropenia with granulocyte colony-stimulating factor. N Engl J Med 1989; 320:1306.
35. Kojim S, Fukuda M, Miyajima Y, et al: Treatment of aplastic anemia in children with recombinant human granulocyte colony-stimulating factor. Blood 1991; 77:937.
35a. Kojima S, Matsuyama T: Stimulation of granulopoiesis by high-dose recombinant human granulocyte colony-stimulating factor in children with aplastic anemia and very severe neutropenia. Blood 1994; 83:1474.
36. Negrin RS, Haeuber DH, Nagler A, et al: Treatment of myelodysplastic syndromes with recombinant human granulocyte colony-stimulating factor: A phase I-II trial. Ann Intern Med 1989; 110:976.
37. Miles SA, Mitsuyasu RT, Moreno J, et al: Combined therapy with recombinant granulocyte colony-stimulating factor and erythropoietin decreases hematologic toxicity from zidovudine. Blood 1991; 77:2109.
38. Yasuda H, Ajiki Y, Shimozato T, et al: Therapeutic efficacy of G-CSF alone and in combination with antibiotics against *Pseudomonas aeruginosa* infections in mice. Infect Immun 1990; 58:2502.
39. Matsumoto M, Tamura M, Matsubara S, et al: Mechanism of protective effect of recombinant human granulocyte colony-stimulating factor (rG-CSF) on *Pseudomonas* infection. Microbiol Immunol 1991; 35:461–475.
40. Cairo MS, Plunkett JM, Mauss D, et al: Seven-day administration of recombinant human granulocyte colony-stimulating factor to newborn rats: Modulation of neonatal neutrophilia, myelopoiesis, and group B *Streptococcus* sepsis. Blood 1990; 76:1788–1794.
41. Reissmann KR: Studies of the mechanism of erythropoietic stimulation in parabiotic rats during hypoxia. Blood 1950; 5:372.
42. Erslev A: Humoral regulation of red cell production. Blood 1953; 8:349.
43. Miyake T, Kung CK-H, Goldwasser E: Purification of human erythropoietin. J Biol Chem 1977; 252:5558.
44. Jacobs K, Shoemaker C, Rudersdorf R, et al: Isolation and

characterization of genomic and cDNA clones of human erythropoietin. Nature 1985; 313:806.

45. Lin FK, Suggs S, Lin CH, et al: Cloning and expression of the human erythropoietin gene. Proc Natl Acad Sci USA 1985; 82:7580.
46. Law ML, Cai G-Y, Lin F-K: Chromosomal assignment of the human erythropoietin gene and its DNA polymorphism. Proc Natl Acad Sci USA 1986; 83:6920.
47. Eschbach JW, Egrie JC, Downing MR, et al: Correction of the anemia of end-stage renal disease with recombinant human erythropoietin: Results of a combined phase I and II clinical trial. N Engl J Med 1987; 316:73.
48. Lacombe C, Da Silva J-L, Bruneval P, et al: Peritubular cells are the site of erythropoietin synthesis in the murine hypoxic kidney. J Clin Invest 1988; 81:620.
49. Garcia JF, Ebbe SN, Hollander L, et al: Radioimmunoassay of erythropoietin: Circulating levels in normal and polycythemic human beings. J Lab Clin Med 1982; 99:624.
50. D'Andrea AD, Lodish HF, Wong GG: Expression cloning of the murine erythropoietin receptor. Cell 1989; 57:277–285.
51. Migliaccio G, Migliaccio AR, Adamson JW: In vitro differentiation of human granulocyte/macrophage and erythroid progenitors: Comparative analysis of the influence of recombinant human erythropoietin, G-CSF, GM-CSF and IL-3 in serum depleted and serum deprived cultures. Blood 1989; 72:1452.
52. McNiece IK, Langley KE, Zsebo KM: Recombinant human stem cell factor synergizes with GM-CSF, G-CSF, IL-3 and Epo to stimulate human progenitor cells in the myeloid and erythroid lineages. Exp Hematol 1991; 19:226.
53. Winearls CG, Oliver DO, Pippard MJ, et al: Effects of human erythropoietin derived from recombinant DNA on the anemia of patients maintained by chronic haemodialysis. Lancet 1986; ii:1175.
54. Eschbach JW, Egrie JC, Downing MR, et al: Correction of the anemia of end-stage renal disease with recombinant human erythropoietin: Results of a combined phase I and II clinical trial. N Engl J Med 1987; 316:73.
55. Evans RW, Rader B, Manninen DL: Cooperative multicenter EPO clinical trial group: The quality of life of hemodialysis recipients treated with recombinant human erythropoietin. JAMA 1990; 263:825.
56. Pincus T, Olsen NJ, Russell J, et al: Multicenter study of recombinant human erythropoietin in correction of anemia of rheumatoid arthritis. Am J Med 1990; 89:161.
57. Miller CB, Jones RJ, Piantadosi S, et al: Decreased erythropoietin response in patients with the anemia of cancer. N Engl J Med 1990; 322:1689.
58. Goodnough LT, Rudnik S, Price TH, et al: Increased preoperative collection of autologous blood with recombinant human erythropoietin therapy. N Engl J Med 1989; 321:1163.
59. Holbrook ST, Christensen RD: Hematopoietic growth factors. Adv Pediatr 1991; 38:23–49.
60. Komiyama A, Ishiguro A, Kubo T, et al: Increases in neutrophil counts by purified human urinary colony-stimulating factor in chronic neutropenia of childhood. Blood 1988; 71:41.
61. Kawasaki ES, Ladner M, Wang AM, et al: Molecular cloning of a complementary DNA encoding human macrophage specific factor (CSF-1). Science 1985; 230:291.
62. Morris S, Valentine M, Shapiro D, et al: Reassignment of the human CSF-1 gene to chromosome 1p13-p21. Blood 1991; 78:2013.
63. Sherr CF, Rettenmier CW, Sacca R, et al: The *c-fms* protooncogene product is related to the receptor for the mononuclear phagocyte growth factor, CSF-1. Cell 1985;41:665.
64. Ralph P, Nakoinz I: Stimulation of macrophage tumoricidal activity by the growth and differentiation factor CSF-1. Cell Immunol 1987; 105:270.
65. Robinson B, Quesenberry P: Hematopoietic growth factors: Overview and clinical applications, Part II. Am J Med Sci 1990; 300:237.
66. Komiyama A, Ishiguro A, Kubo T, et al: Increases in neutrophil counts by purified human urinary colony-stimulating factor in chronic neutropenia of childhood. Blood 1988; 71:41.
67. Motoyoshi K, Takaka F, Kusumoto K, et al: Phase I and early phase II studies on human urinary colony-stimulating factor. Jpn J Med 1982; 21:187.
68. Nemunaitis J, Meyers J, Buckner C, et al: Phase I trial of recombinant human macrophage colony-stimulating factor in patients with invasive fungal infections. Blood 1991; 78:907.
69. Caracciolo D, Shirsat N, Wong GG, et al: Recombinant human macrophage colony stimulating factor (M-CSF) requires subliminal concentrations of granulocyte/macrophage (GM)-CSF for optimal stimulation of human macrophage colony formation in vitro. J Exp Med 1987; 166:1851.
70. Ihle JN, Keller T, Henderson L, et al: Procedure for the purification of interleukin-3 to homogeneity. J Immunol 1982; 129:2431.
71. Ihle JN, Keller J, Oroszlan S, et al: Biologic properties of interleukin-3. J Immunol 1983; 131:282–287.
72. Yang Y-C, Ciarletta AB, Temple PA, et al: Human IL-3 (multi-CSF): Identification by expression cloning of a novel hematopoietic growth factor related to murine IL-3. Cell 1986; 47:3.
73. Yang Y-C, Kovacic S, Kriz R, et al: The human genes for GM-CSF and IL 3 are closely linked in tandem on chromosome 5. Blood 1988; 71:958.
74. Bruno E, Miller ME, Hoffman R: Interacting cytokines regulate in vitro human megakaryocytopoiesis. Blood 1989; 73:671.
75. Donahue RE, Seehra J, Metzer M, et al: Human IL-3 and GM-CSF act synergistically in stimulating hematopoiesis in primates. Science 1988; 241:1820.
76. Bodine D, Karlsson S, Nienhuis A: Combination of interleukins 3 and 6 preserves stem cell function in culture and enhances retrovirum-mediated gene transfer into hematopoietic stem cells. Proc Natl Acad Sci USA 1989; 86:8897.
77. Nolta J, Kohn D: Comparison of the effects of growth factors on retroviral vector-mediated gene transfer and the proliferative status of human hematopoietic progenitor cells. Hum Gene Ther 1990; 1:257.
78. Geissler K, Valent Peter, Bettelheim P, et al: In vivo synergism of recombinant human interleukin-3 and recombinant human interleukin-6 on thrombopoiesis in primates. Blood 1992; 79:1155.
79. Ganser A, Lindemann A, Seipelt G, et al: Effects of recombinant human interleukin-3 in patients with normal hematopoiesis and in patients with bone marrow failure. Blood 1990; 76:666.
79a. D'Hondt V, Weynants P, Humblet Y, et al: Dose-dependent interleukin-3 stimulation of thrombopoiesis and neutropoiesis in patients with small-cell lung carcinoma before and following chemotherapy: A placebo-controlled randomized phase Ib study. J Clin Oncol 1993; 11:2063.
80. Ganser A, Lindemann A, Seipelt G, et al: Effects of recombinant human interleukin-3 in aplastic anemia. Blood 1990; 76:1287.
81. Ganser A, Lindemann A, Ottmann OG, et al: Sequential in vivo treatment with two recombinant human hematopoietic growth factors (interleukin-3 and granulocyte-macrophage colony-stimulating factor) as a new therapeutic modality to stimulate hematopoiesis: Results of a phase I study. Blood 1992; 79:2583.
82. March CJ, Mosley B, Larsen A, et al: Cloning sequence and expression of two distinct human interleukin-1 complementary DNAs. Nature 1985; 315:641.
83. Cannon JG, Tompkins RG, Gelfand JA, et al: Circulating interleukin-1 and tumor necrosis factor in septic shock and experimental endotoxin fever. J Infect Dis 1990; 161:79.
84. Calandra T, Baumgartner JD, Grau GE, et al: Prognostic values of tumor necrosis factor/cachectin, interleukin-1, interferon-α and interferon-γ in the serum of patients with septic shock. J Infect Dis 1990; 161:982.
85. Granowitz EV, Santos AA, Poutsiaka DD, et al: Production of interleukin-1-receptor antagonist during experimental endotoxaemia. Lancet 1991; 338:1423.
86. Bartelmez SH, Stanley ER: Synergism between hemopoietic growth factors (HGFs) detected by their effects on cells bearing receptors for a lineage specific HGF: Assay of hemopoietin-1. J Cell Physiol 1985; 122:370.
87. Moore MAS: Clinical implications of positive and negative hematopoietic stem cell regulators. Review Stratton lecture. Blood 1991; 78:1.
88. Fibbe WE, Hamilton MS, Laterveer LL, et al: Sustained en-

graftment of mice transplanted with IL-1-primed blood-derived stem cells. J Immunol 1992; 148:417.
89. Moore MAS, Warren DJ: Synergy of interleukin 1 and granulocyte colony-stimulating factor: In vivo stimulation of stem-cell recovery and hematopoietic regeneration following 5-fluorouracil treatment of mice. Proc Natl Acad Sci USA 1987; 84:7134.
89a. Vadhan-Raj S, Kudelka A, Garrison L, et al: Effects of interleukin-1α on carboplatin-induced thrombocytopenia in patients with recurrent ovarian cancer. J Clin Oncol 1994; 12:707.
90. Wong GG, Clark SC: Multiple actions of interleukin 6 within a cytokine network. Immunol Today 1988; 9:137.
91. Muraguchi A, Hirano T, Tang B, et al: The essential role of B-cell stimulatory factor 2 (BSF-2/IL-6) for the terminal differentiation of B cells. J Exp Med 1988; 167:332.
92. Brandt SJ, Bodine DM, Dunbar CE, et al: Dysregulated interleukin-6 expression produces a syndrome resembling Castleman's disease in mice (Abstract). Blood 1989; 74:48a.
93. Sullivan JS, Kilpatrick L, Costarino AT Jr, et al: Correlation of plasma cytokine elevations with mortality rate in children with sepsis. J Pediatr 1992; 120:510.
94. Cairo M, Plunkett J, Nguyen A, et al: Sequential administration of interleukin-6 and granulocyte-colony-stimulating factor in newborn rats: Modulation of newborn granulopoiesis and thrombopoiesis. Pediatr Res 1991; 30:554.
95. Cairo MS, Plunkett JM, Clark S, et al: In vivo hematological effects of seven days of rhIL-6 in neonatal rats. Am J Pediatr Hematol Oncol 1992; 14:44.
96. Ikebuchi K, Ihle JN, Hirai Y, et al: Synergistic factors for stem cell proliferation: Further studies of the target stem cells and the mechanism of stimulation by interleukin-1, interleukin-6, and granulocyte colony-stimulating factor. Blood 1988; 72:2007.
97. Bodine D, Karlsson S, Nienhuis A: Combination of interleukins 3 and 6 preserves stem cell function in culture and enhances retrovirum-mediated gene transfer into hematopoietic stem cells. Proc Natl Acad Sci USA USA 1989; 86:8897.
98. Nolta J, Kohn D: Comparison of the effects of growth factors on retroviral vector-mediated gene transfer and the proliferative status of human hematopoietic progenitor cells. Hum Gene Ther 1990; 1:257.
99. Cairo M, Plunkett JM, Clark S, et al: In vivo hematological effects of seven days of rhIL-6 in neonatal rats. Am J Pediatr Hematol Oncol 1992; 14:44.
100. Zsebo K, Wypych J, McNiece I, et al: Identification, purification, and biological characterization of hematopoietic stem cell factor from buffalo rat liver-conditioned medium. Cell 1990; 63:195.
101. Zsebo K, Williams D, Geissler E, et al: Stem cell factor is encoded at the S1 locus of the mouse and is the ligand for the c-kit tyrosine kinase receptor. Cell 1990; 63:213.
102. Bernstein I, Andrews R, Zsebo K: Recombinant human stem cell factor enhances the formation of colonies by CD34+ and CD34+lin- cells, and the generation of colony-forming cell progeny from CD34+lin- cells cultured with interleukin-3, granulocyte colony-stimulating factor, or granulocyte-macrophage colony-stimulating factor. Blood 1991; 77:2316.
103. McNiece I, Langley K, Zsebo K: Recombinant human stem cell factor synergizes with GM-CSF, G-CSF, IL-3 and EPO to stimulate human progenitor cells of the myeloid and erythroid lineages. Exp Hematol 1991; 19:226.
104. Moore MAS: Clinical implications of positive and negative hematopoietic stem cell regulators: Review Stratton lecture. Blood 1991; 78:1.
104a. Crawford J, Lau D, Erwin R, et al: A phase I trial of recombinant methionyl human stem cell factor (SCF) in patients (PTS) with advanced non–small cell lung carcinoma (NSCLC). ASCO Proc 1993; 12:135.
105. Cairo M, Plunkett J, Nguyen A, et al: Effect of stem cell factor with and without granulocyte colony-stimulating factor on neonatal hematopoiesis: In vivo induction of newborn myelopoiesis and reduction of mortality during experimental group B streptococcal sepsis. Blood 1992; 80(1):96.
106. Olivieri NF, Grunberger T, Ben-David Y, et al: Diamond-Blackfan anemia: Heterogenous response of hematopoietic progenitor cells in vitro to the protein produce of the steel locus. Blood 1991; 78(9):2211.
107. Paul SR, Bennett F, Calvetti JA, et al: Molecular cloning of a cDNA encoding interleukin 11, a stomal cell-derived lymphopoietic and hematopoietic cytokine. Proc Natl Acad Sci USA 1990; 87:7512.
108. Tsuji K, Lyman SD, Sudo T, et al: Enhancement of murine hematopoiesis by synergistic interactions between steel factor (ligand for *c-kit*), interleukin-11, and other early acting factors in culture. Blood 1992; 79(11):2855.
109. Quesniaux VFJ, Clark SC, Turner K, et al: Interleukin-11 stimulates multiple phases of erythropoiesis in vitro. Blood 1992; 80:1218.
110. Du X, Keller D, Goldman S, et al: Functional effects of interleukin-11 treatment in vivo following bone marrow transplantation and combined modality therapy in mice (Abstract). Exp Hematol 1992; 20:768.
110a. Cairo M, Plunkett J, et al: The combined effects of interleukin-11 (IL-11), stem cell factor (SCF), and granulocyte colony-stimulating factor (G-CSF) on newborn rat hematopoiesis: Significant enhancement of the absolute neutrophil count. Exp Hematol (in press).
110b. Gordon M, Hoffman R, Battiato L, et al: Recombinant human interleukin eleven (Neumega rhIL-11 growth factor; rhIL-11) prevents severe thrombocytopenia in breast cancer patients receiving multiple cycles of cyclophosphamide (C) and doxorubicin (A) chemotherapy. ASCO Proc 1994; 13:133.
111. Curtis B, Williams D, Broxmeyer H, et al: Enhanced hematopoietic activity of a human granulocyte/macrophage colony-stimulating factor: Interleukin 3 fusion protein. Proc Natl Acad Sci USA 1991; 88:5809.
112. Cairo MS, Law P, van de Ven C, et al: The in vitro effects of stem cell factor and PIXY321 on myeloid progenitor formation (CFU-GM) from immunomagnetic separated CD34+ cord blood. Pediatr Res 1992; 32:277.
112a. Vadhan-Raj S, Papadopoulos N, Burgess M, et al: Effects of PIXY321, a granulocyte-macrophage colony-stimulating factor/interleukin-3 fusion protein, on chemotherapy-induced multilineage myelosuppression in patients with sarcoma. J Clin Oncol 1994; 12:715.

SECTION IV
MONITORING

William C. Shoemaker

CHAPTER 30

Intravascular Access and Long-Term Catheter Maintenance

M. H. Parsa, MD • William C. Shoemaker, MD

Established access to the circulation via needles and catheters is essential for monitoring and treating critically ill patients. On the basis of our experience with 20,093 intravascular accesses, from May 1968 to August 1993,[1–7] a variety of techniques for establishing intravascular access are described, and the principles of long-term catheter maintenance as well as the prevention, recognition, and management of complications are reported.

INTRAVENOUS ACCESS

Insertion of Peripheral Vein Conduits

The veins that are visible or palpable through the skin can be further dilated by appropriate application of a tourniquet proximal to the planned site of vein puncture. The skin area of the planned vein-puncture site should be shaved if hair is present and prepared with an iodine antiseptic solution–impregnated gauze; the skin should be rubbed firmly in different directions until all skin debris are removed. Time should be allowed for the antiseptic to take effect before the vein puncture is made. The prepared area should be surrounded by a sterile drape. The venipuncture is then attempted by a steel needle or by a catheter over needle with sterile precautions. After catheter insertion, the skin site should be covered by a topical antimicrobial agent that is effective as long as it is physically present and not rendered ineffective by time and temperature.

We consider 1% silver sulfadiazine cream the most effective topical antimicrobial agent for this purpose and have used it since 1980.[8] A peripheral intravenous access site usually becomes thrombosed as a result of venous cannulas and intravenous infusions within 4 days. We believe that patients who are in need of intravenous access for 10 days or longer should have a subclavian or internal jugular superior vena cava catheter placed initially to avoid multiple peripheral vein punctures and consequent thromboses. Indications for intravenous catheters with central location of the tip are listed in Table 30–1.

Insertion of Nonperipheral Venous Catheters with Central Location of the Tip

The distances of subclavian, internal jugular, and femoral veins on the right side from the venae cavae are shorter and straighter than those of the left-sided veins. Therefore, we prefer accesses via the right-sided veins if conditions permit. Our order of preference based on clinical practicality is as follows:

1. Right supraclavicular approach to the subclavian vein
2. Right infraclavicular approach to the subclavian vein
3. Right internal jugular approach

These three approaches can be exercised in one preparation setting. This order also applies to veins on the left side as the second choice. When these veins are inaccessible bilaterally, the right and then the left femoral veins may be cannulated. In patients with difficult intravenous access, brachial veins may be used for percutaneous cannulation.

Supraclavicular Approach to the Subclavian Vein

The technique is illustrated in Figure 30–1. The subclavian vein consists of a lateral segment over the first rib and a medial segment over the pleural dome. We refer to the medial segment as the junctional segment because it joins the internal jugular vein. Attempts for venipuncture in the medial segment have a high rate of success, but there is a risk that the needle may traverse the vein and puncture the pleural dome and the lung apex (Fig. 30–2).

Infraclavicular Approach to the Subclavian Vein

Again, the needle is advanced toward the vein in the segment over the first rib (Fig. 30–3). When the needle is advanced toward the medial segment, there is the possibility of puncturing the pleural dome alone as well as the apex of the lung (Fig. 30–4). Depending on individual anatomic structures in some patients, the vein is more accessible from below or above the clavicle (Fig. 30–5). In practice, when attempts for supraclavicular approach fail, the infraclavicular approach is usually successful. Conversely, when the infraclavicular approach fails in a primary attempt, the supraclavicular approach is usually successful as a secondary attempt. Puncture of the vein in the second segment is attempted only if attempts to puncture the vein in over-the-rib segment have failed supra- and infraclavicularly.

Approach to the Internal Jugular Vein

When both of the above approaches to the subclavian vein fail, the internal jugular vein is approached from the posterior border of the sternocleidomastoid muscle in the same

TABLE 30–1. Indications for Intravenous Catheters with Centrally Located Tips

1. Central venous pressure monitoring
2. Long-term infusion of hypotonic, hypertonic, potassium-containing, and other irritating solutions/medications
3. Need for long-term (10 days or longer) intravenous catheters
4. Venous hemodialysis
5. No accessible peripheral superficial veins
6. As an access for pulmonary artery catheterization

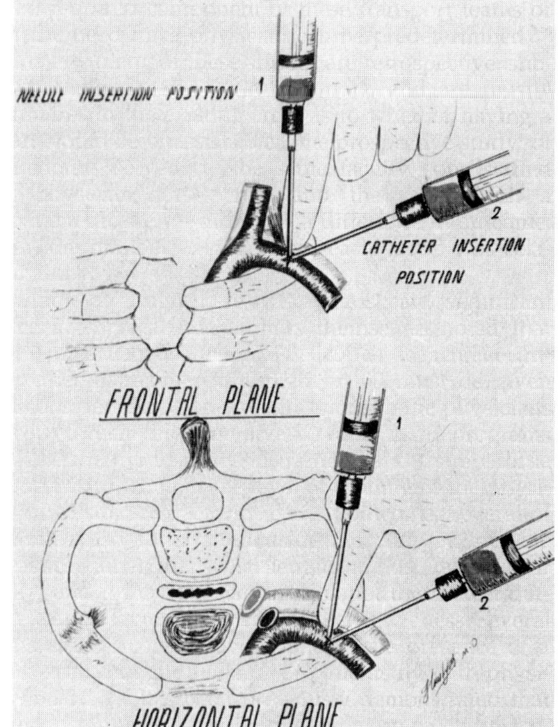

Figure 30–1. Left subclavian vein puncture in the lateral segment over the first rib illustrated in the frontal and horizontal anatomic planes at the level of C-7. The needle is advanced toward the vein perpendicular to the course of the vein. After entry into the vein, the needle is moved to position 2 for alignment with the axis of the vein to pass the catheter. Position 1 facilitates vein puncture. Position 2 facilitates catheterization.

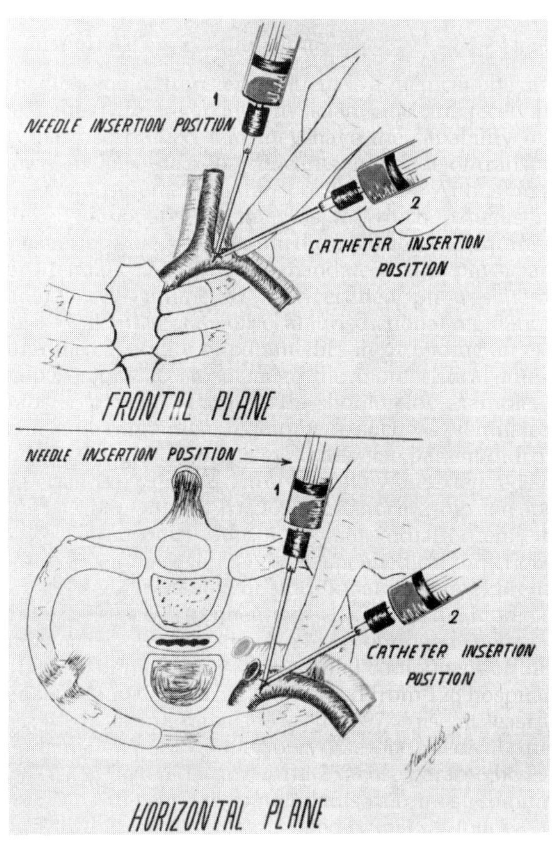

Figure 30–2. Left supraclavicular subclavian vein puncture in the medial segment, over the pleural dome. Should the vein walls coapt in this segment owing to the pressure exerted by the needle, the tip may penetrate the pleural dome and lung apex. Position 1 indicates the appropriate direction for vein puncture. Position 2 indicates the redirection of the needle for vein cannulation.

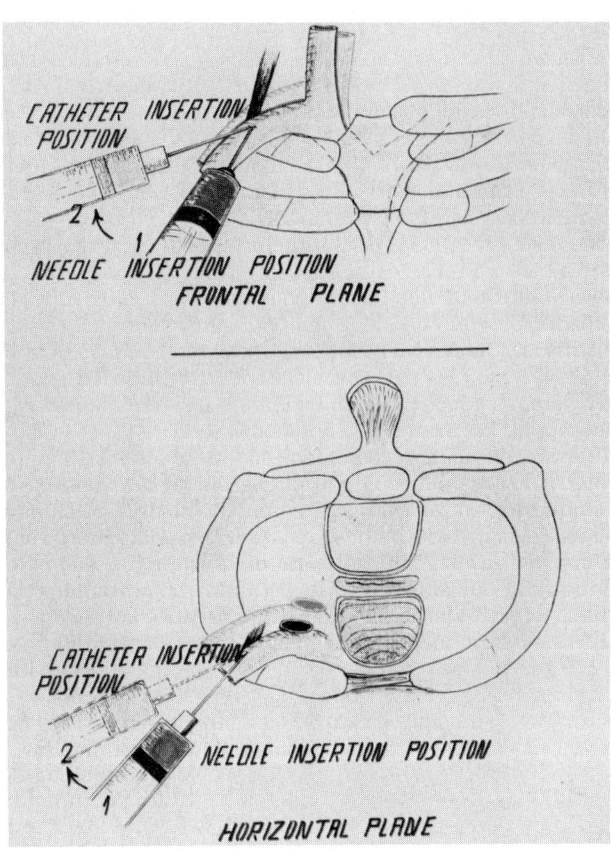

Figure 30–3. Right subclavian vein puncture for cannulation infraclavicularly is illustrated in the frontal and horizontal planes at the level of C-7 in the lateral segment over the first rib. After obtaining a free flow of blood in the syringe in position 1, the needle is moved to position 2 for alignment with the axis of the vein and cannulation.

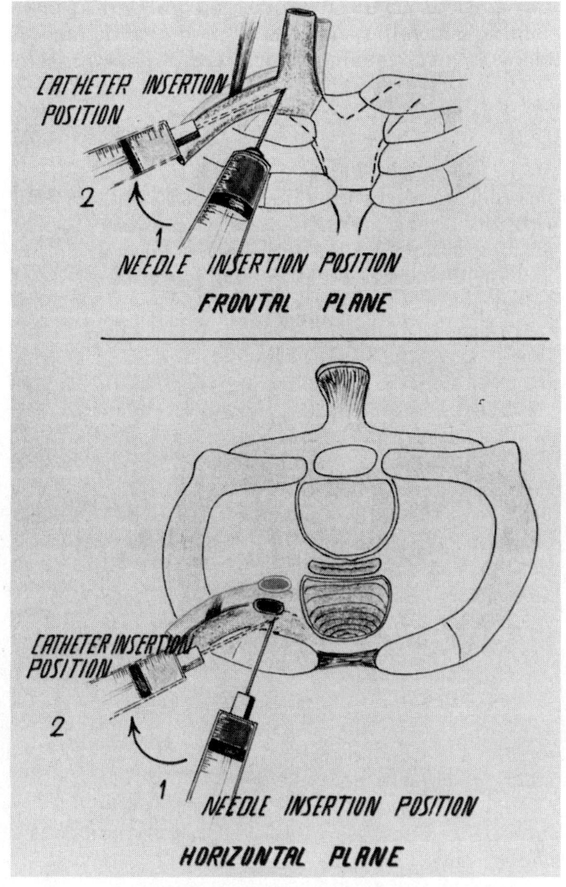

Figure 30–4. Right subclavian vein puncture infraclavicularly in the medial segment of the vein. When the wall of the vein collapses owing to pressure exerted by the needle tip, the needle may puncture the pleural dome and apex of the lung.

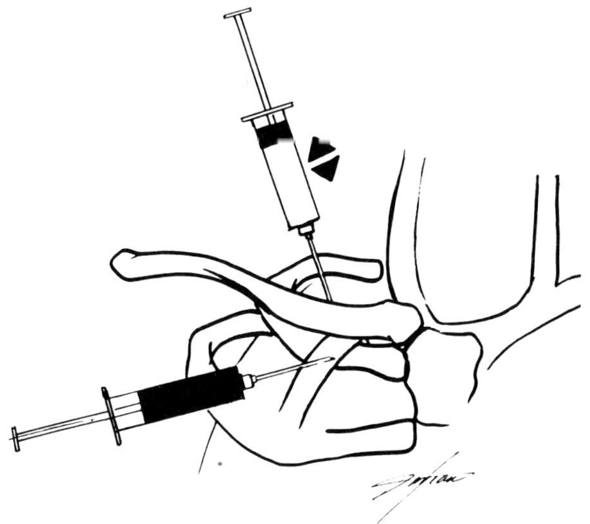

Figure 30–5. When the clavicle is positioned more cephalad, it may obscure the vein sought with a supraclavicular approach, whereas the vein may be easily reached with an infraclavicular approach. The reverse is also true: when the clavicle is positioned more caudad, it does not override the first rib, and the vein is accessed more easily with a supraclavicular approach.

setting (Fig. 30–6). Frequently, when this approach fails, those from the anterior border of the sternocleidomastoid muscle and from the apex of the angle between the sternal and clavicular shafts of the muscle fail also. Therefore, we seldom use the latter two approaches.

Double and Triple Catheters

The main catheter that we have used is polymer resin, 20 cm long and 16 or 19 gauge (IntraCath, Deseret). This catheter is soft, pliable, and nonirritating to the tissues. Consequently, the number of complications resulting from use of this catheter have consistently been low; it is also the least costly. In patients who need more than one (two or three and occasionally four) catheter, the necessary number of catheters have been inserted in one vein or two adjacent veins side by side. We have kept these catheters in place for as long as 2 months and an average of 16 days. Indications for the use of double and triple catheters include the following:

1. Administration of large volumes of fluids
2. Preoperative patients with difficult venous access
3. Administration of highly incompatible medications
4. In difficult cutdowns, when the exposed vein admits two catheters

Unlike double- and triple-lumen catheters, when one of these catheters is inadvertently removed, the other (or others) may remain in place. Each catheter can be used separately as a means of exchange with a Swan-Ganz or hemodialysis catheter. Each catheter can be removed individually when it is no longer functional or when it is not needed. This technique of catheter insertion is simple and important for a beginner to learn. A potential complication is the possibility of transection of the catheter (or catheters) already in place during the second or third needle puncture catheterization attempts[9]; this complication has been avoided in our series by not advancing the needle against undue resistance.

Femoral Vein Approach

The right femoral vein has a shorter distance to the inferior vena cava and the path is straight; therefore, it is the preferred route for cannulation over the left femoral vein. However, femoral inferior vena cava catheters should be inserted only when there is no alternative.[9a, 9b] The catheter tip should reach the inferior vena cava preferably close to the diaphragm. Femoral inferior vena cava catheters should be replaced once a week and removed as soon as possible.

Venous Cannulation by Cutdown

When percutaneous vein cannulation is not safe or the procedure fails, the veins can be surgically exposed and catheterized through a direct needle puncture or a small venotomy.[9a–9c] Techniques of cutdown have been previously reported.[3, 7, 10] Establishing rapid intravenous access by cutdowns, performed under emergency conditions, takes precedence over observing sterile technique. Therefore, catheters inserted under unsterile emergency conditions should be replaced after the emergency condition has been corrected. Cutdowns performed as elective operations should be done in a clean procedure room or the operating room depending on the magnitude of the procedure and the patient's susceptibility to infection.

In spite of exercising rules of sterility, catheters inserted by cutdowns do not last too long. When the size of the vein permits, two catheters should be inserted; if one malfunctions, the other serves the purpose. When large veins are exposed surgically, cannulation should be carried out by using the Seldinger technique rather than by inserting the catheter through the needle to prevent bleeding at the catheter–vein entry site.

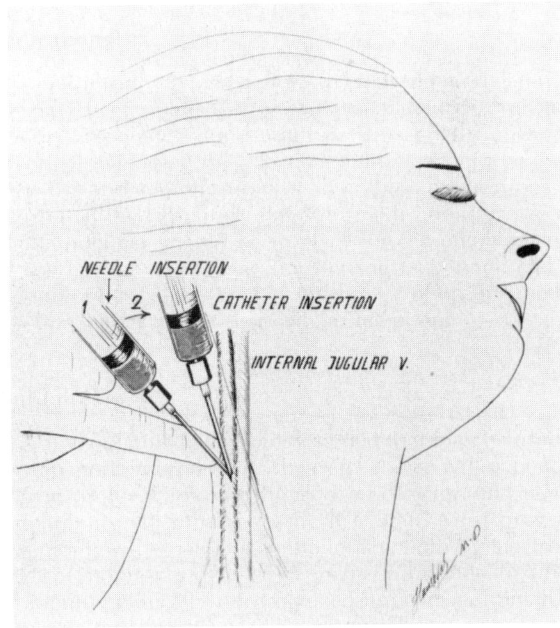

Figure 30–6. Internal jugular puncture from the posterior border of the sternocleidomastoid muscle. The needle is advanced in position 1 at a 45° angle to the muscle and at a 45° angle to the frontal plane anteriorly. After advancing the needle tip behind the muscle, it is positioned in such a manner that it penetrates the vein from the anterior wall rather than from the lateral wall. Once a free flow of blood is obtained in the syringe, the needle is moved to position 2 for alignment with the axis of the vein. The syringe is then detached, and the catheter is inserted.

Summary of Technical Experience

Our experience with intravenous access is shown in Tables 30–2 to 30–4. Among the 20,093 catheterizations performed, we used pulmonary artery (PA) catheters in 63, subcutaneously tunneled Silastic catheters in 48, double- and triple-lumen catheters in 22, venous hemodialysis catheters in 8, and totally implanted Silastic catheters in 30.

Special Venous Catheters

Subcutaneously Tunneled and Totally Implanted Catheters

These catheters can be inserted percutaneously or by cutdown. The outside end of the subcutaneously tunneled catheter is exited through a subcutaneous tunnel in an area conveniently reachable by patients so that they can provide catheter site care.[10a]

The totally implantable catheters with subcutaneous ports were devised to reduce infection.[10b] However, multiple percutaneous punctures into the port can introduce contamination into the catheter. Also, microorganisms may gain access to these catheters, like any other catheter, and produce serious infections[11]; these catheters should not be inserted in patients who are already septic and in infection-prone patients. Before removing tunneled or implanted catheters, a radiograph should be obtained to detect the integrity of the catheter as well as potential problems that may cause the catheter to break off during removal.[12]

Double- and Triple-Lumen Catheters

Insertion of these catheters is more involved technically than that of needle puncture and catheter insertion through the needle. The lumens of these catheters should always have flow of intravenous fluids. Stagnation and lack of flow enhance the growth of microorganisms that may have gained access to the catheter lumen. Therefore, when a lumen is no longer needed, the triple-lumen catheter should be replaced by a double-lumen catheter, and the double-lumen catheter should be replaced by a single-lumen catheter to avoid having a stagnant lumen. When double- and triple-lumen catheters or two to three catheters are used to deliver larger volumes of intravenous fluids, an infusion pump should be used instead to speed up fluid infusions to the desired rate via a single-lumen catheter.

TABLE 30–2. Summary of Experience with Conventional Percutaneous Venous Catheterization Techniques (May 1968–August 1993)

Catheterization by Percutaneous Venipuncture	*Number*
1. Supraclavicular subclavian or junctional*	6208
2. Infraclavicular subclavian	2297
3. Internal jugular from posterior and anterior border of sternocleidomastoid muscle	467
4. External jugular	50
5. Cephalic	50
6. Basilic	50
7. Femoral	352
8. Right brachial	3
9. Left brachial	1
Total catheterizations	9478

*Supraclavicular subclavian vein puncture at the junctional zone of the subclavian and internal jugular veins.

TABLE 30–3. Summary of Experience in Insertion of Intravenous Catheters by Special Techniques (May 1968–June 1985)

Technique	*Access Site/Vein*	*Number*
Double catheter by percutaneous puncture		
Two punctures in one vein	Subclavian	185
	Internal jugular	13
	Femoral	10
Two punctures in adjacent veins	Internal jugular and subclavian	40
One puncture (two guide wires via Swan-Ganz catheter sheath, two catheters over guide wires)	Subclavian	17
	Femoral	2
Double catheters in one vein by cutdown	Internal jugular	1
	External jugular	4
	Cephalic subclavian	6
	External iliac	1
	Common iliac	1
	Inferior vena cava	2
	Gonadal	1
	Axillary	2
Single catheter by cutdown	Subclavian	24
	Internal jugular	20
	Inferior epigastric	7
	Lateral thoracic	6
	Cephalic	60
	Basilic	15
	Brachial	15
	External jugular	25
	Saphenous	100
Intraoperative, abdominal	Gonadal	7
	Portal	22
Thoracotomy	Greater azygos	1
	Right atrium	2
Intracostal	Anterolateral	4
Intrasternal	Body of sternum	1
Intra-arterial	Left subclavian artery	1
Total cases		595
Total catheters		880

TABLE 30–4. Variety and Number of Double and Triple Central Venous Catheters Inserted (in Order of Preference for Safety Based on Clinical Applicability) from July 1985 to August 1993

Approach	*Vein*	*Double Catheters*	*Triple Catheters*
Right supraclavicular	Subclavian	1778	18
Left supraclavicular	Subclavian	1513	20
Right infraclavicular	Subclavian	467	17
Left infraclavicular	Subclavian	482	12
Right posterior sternomastoid border	Internal jugular	119	0
Left posterior sternomastoid border	Internal jugular	104	0
Right supraclavicular and right posterior border	Subclavian and internal jugular	43	4
Left supraclavicular and left posterior border	Subclavian and internal jugular	32	4
Right supraclavicular and right infraclavicular	Subclavian	55	7
Left supraclavicular and left infraclavicular	Subclavian	68	4
Right infraclavicular and right posterior border	Subclavian and internal jugular	15	0
Left infraclavicular and left posterior border	Subclavian and internal jugular	14	0
Right groin	Femoral	41	1
Left groin	Femoral	2	0
Total cases		4822*	
Total catheters		9735	

*Includes two cases each with four catheters (not listed in this table).

Hemodialysis Catheters

The most suitable vein for hemodialysis catheters is the right internal jugular vein because of its straight path to the superior vena cava.[13, 14] Prolonged use of these catheters is associated with clot formation and stenosis of the veins that they pass through, including venae cavae.[15, 16]

Before each dialysis session, the outflow port of these catheters should be vigorously flushed with a 10- to 20-ml syringe filled with sterile solution when the outflow of blood is hindered. Venous hemodialysis catheters should be used for short terms in acute renal failure but not for long term because of their inherent danger of clot formation, infection, vascular erosion, and venous stenosis.

Complications of Intravenous Access

Some of the complications are preventable, and some are not. Complications can increase in number and severity by the susceptibility of the patients (high risk) and limited experience of the team providing care for the patient. Table 30–5 outlines risk factors for complications. We documented all technical complications with 350 catheters inserted in 180 consecutive patients in a 3-month period as a cross-sectional sample of our patient population; the results are shown in Table 30–6. In 9 patients, there were 16 catheter malpositions; in 14 of the malpositions, the catheter was inserted via the subclavian vein and detoured into the homolateral internal jugular vein. In two cases, the catheters coiled in the superior vena cava because of existing mural clots. All but one of the malpositioned catheters were clinically detected and corrected. Routine chest radiograph located and reviewed in 142 of 180 cases corroborated the correct placement that had been predetermined clinically except for the one undetected catheter mentioned previously. Therefore, our clinical accuracy in detecting the position of the catheter without the need for a radiographic study is about 99.3%. Considering other indications for radiographic study for the detection of pneumothorax, phrenic nerve injury, catheter tip erosion, and all otherwise questionable situations, we estimate that 80% of the cases do not require routine radiographic studies after cannulation or during long-term maintenance.

Table 30–7 lists the complications due to specific techniques as well as those common to all techniques when used in the presence of contraindications. The absolute and relative contraindications for subclavian/internal jugular superior vena cava catheterization are listed in Table 30–8.

Inadvertent Arterial Puncture

This is one of the most common complications and occurs in about 5% of cases. Yet in many cases arterial puncture occurs more than once during attempts for a vein puncture/catheterization procedure; thus, in 47 consecutive such cases with arterial puncture, we counted a total of 78 arterial punctures. All arteries adjacent to the veins are at risk for inadvertent puncture (Fig. 30–7).

Lymphatic Trunk Puncture

Lymphatic duct puncture in the thoracic outlet is the second most common complication of subclavian/internal jugular puncture. The incidence increases significantly when subclavian venipuncture is attempted on the left side supraclavicularly in patients with portal hypertension. Lymphatic duct puncture is recognizable by the aspiration of clear or milky fluid in the syringe attached to the puncture needle. When the needle injury to the duct is missed or ignored and the vein is cannulated, especially in patients with high thoracic duct pressure, lymph will continue to ooze from the catheter site. A characteristic of lymph fluid is that it forms clots. When there is lymphorrhagia from around the catheter, the catheter should be removed; unlike the persistent oozing of blood from around the catheter, which usually stops by the placement of a circular stitch (Fig. 30–8), the lymph leakage can be definitively halted only by removing the catheter and applying pressure to the site. Causes of oozing from the catheter site are listed in Table 30–9. Causes of bleeding inside or chylothorax are indicated in Table 30–10. The circular hemostatic suture inserted under the catheter and tied over a cuff of skin should be removed within 48 hours to

TABLE 30–5. Risk Factors in Central Venous Catheterization and Long-Term Maintenance

Inadvertent Arterial Puncture
Hypertension
Coagulopathy
Long and large-bore needles
Lack of experience of the operator*
Tortuous or aneurysmal arteries

Inadvertent Puncture of Lymphatic Ducts
Portal hypertension
Intravenous drug abuse (venous thrombosis increasing lymphatic flow)

Inadvertent Puncture of Lung Apex
Apical blebs
Emaciation
Lung diseases (COPD, PCP, and TB)
Old age
Long needles (relative to the thickness of soft tissue between the skin and lung apex)
History of iatrogenic pneumothorax consequent to central venous catheterization attempts
Mechanical ventilation with a high PEEP and large tidal volume

Air Embolus
Hypovolemia and low venous blood pressure
Labored inspiratory efforts and tachypnea
Inappropriate position of the patient (head elevated) during subclavian/internal jugular vein puncture/cannulation
Accidental disconnection of the catheter from the intravenous tubing (patient in upright position)
Via subclavian or internal jugular catheter tract just removed and skin site not covered by sterile bandage

Intravenous Catheter-Related Infection
Contaminated technique of insertion and/or maintenance
Immunocompromised state
Terminal cancer state
Long-term indwelling intravenous catheter(s)/therapy

Clot Formation
Catheter malposition and retraction/regression
Hypercoagulability states
Catheter infection
Chemically and physically irritative catheters and infusion fluids
Long-term indwelling catheters

Clogging/Obstruction of Catheter/Intravenous Tubing
Sharp kinking of catheter/intravenous tubing
Blood reflux into the catheter after intravenous fluids run dry
Placement of intravenous fluids bags/bottles below the heart level with the intravenous tubings open to allow blood reflux

Accidental Removal of Catheter
Restless and uncooperative patients†
Inexperienced patient care and patient transport team members in protection of central venous catheters‡
Inadequate catheter maintenance by nurses/physicians

Severity of Sequelae of Complications
Delayed recognition
Inappropriate and/or inadequate treatment

*Lack of experience of the operator is a risk factor for all technical complications.
†Lack of patient cooperation is a risk factor for many of the technical and long-term maintenance complications. Restless patients should be deeply sedated and hand restrained at least during the procedure.
‡Lack of experience of long-term maintenance team members is a risk factor for all long-term maintenance complications.
Abbreviations: COPD = chronic obstructive pulmonary disease; PCP = *Pneumocystis carinii* pneumonia; TB = tuberculosis.

TABLE 30–6. Technical Complications* Recorded in 350 Consecutive Catheterizations in 180 Cases During a 3-Month Period

Complications	*Number*	*Percentage of Complications/Cases*	*Percentage of Complications/Catheters*
Catheter detour/malposition	16	8.8	4.5
Oozing/venous blood from catheter site†	13	7.2	3.7
Thoracic duct puncture	11	6.1	3.1
Arterial puncture, inadvertent	9	5.0	2.5
Pneumothorax‡	0	0	0
Total	49	27.1	13.8

*All complications were recognized immediately and resolved without sequelae.
†This is considered a complication when the venous bleeding does not stop by elevating the head of the bed and applying local pressure; a circular hemostatic stitch is then required.
‡Our overall incidence of puncture of lung apex among all cases is 0.99%; among catheters, it is 0.50%. Our overall incidence of puncture of lung apex among all cases resulting in pneumothorax is 0.41%; among all catheters, it is 0.21%.

TABLE 30–7. Potential Complications of Central Venous Catheters in Percutaneous Insertion and Long-Term Maintenance

Subclavian and Internal Jugular Veins
Puncture of the pleural dome alone
Puncture of the pleural dome and lung apex
Clinically/radiologically detectable pneumothorax*
Hemothorax and/or soft tissue and mediastinal hematoma
Needle injury to the adjacent arteries
Puncture of lymphatic ducts, lymphorrhagia, chylomediastinum, and chylothorax
Catheter misplacement in pleural cavity and consequent deposition of fluids and blood infusates in the pleural space
Venous air embolus
Injury to vertebral vessels with consequent brain stem ischemic damage
Subclavian Veins
Injury to brachial plexus directly by the needle or indirectly by the pressure of a tense arterial hematoma
Injury to the clavicle or first-rib periosteums, cartilages, or ligaments and consequent osteitis/chondritis and calcific reactions
Internal Jugular
Needle injury to the vagus nerve, phrenic nerve, cervical sympathetic chain, stellate ganglion, and cervical plexus
Brain infarction caused by injury or clot and air embolism via the carotid artery
Needle injury to the trachea and esophagus
Injury to transverse processes of the cervical vertebrae with consequent reactions and infections of periosteum and bone
Brain infarct caused by venous thrombosis extending to intracranial venous sinuses
All Venipuncture/Cannulation Techniques and Long-Term Catheters
Inadvertent arterial puncture and consequent soft-tissue hematoma, intracavitary and external bleeding, false aneurysm, and arteriovenous fistulas
Detour of the catheter tip into a branch
Catheter tip in apposition to the vein wall and consequent wall perforation/erosion
Catheter tip advanced too far (longer catheters)
Catheter shorter than the desirable length or retraction/regression of catheter tip back into smaller veins
Catheter tip positioned against the blood flow
Clot and fibrinous sleeve formation
Thrombosis of the vein and thromboembolism
Catheter-related infections
Catheter shredding and catheter embolus
Guidewire embolus
External bleeding from catheter skin site (venous or arterial)
Accidental removal of catheters
Clogging of catheters

*A chest x-ray film taken at the end of the forced expiratory phase with the patient in an upright or opposite lateral decubitus position is most sensitive to show a minimal pneumothorax. We do not know the necessary minimal amount of free air in the pleural space that will show as pneumothorax radiologically. Computed tomograph of the chest is more sensitive to show small amounts of pneumothorax. Clinically, 10% to 15% pneumothorax is necessary to sense diminished breath sounds by auscultation while the patient is breathing with normal tidal volume.

prevent skin necrosis and consequent infection. While removing this suture, the sharp edge of the cutting instrument should be directed away from the catheter (Fig. 30–9).

Once the catheter is in place, if hair is to be shaved close to the catheter skin site, the blade strokes should always move away from the catheter to avoid cutting it and resulting in catheter embolism (Fig. 30–10).

Inadvertent Puncture of Air-Containing Structures

Puncture of the pleural dome without puncture of the lung apex has a higher incidence than can be recognized clinically. Puncture of the pleural dome without puncture of the

TABLE 30–8. Contraindications for Subclavian and Internal Jugular Central Venous Catheterization

Absolute and General
Conditions of severe bleeding tendency and coagulopathy states
Persistent shock
Obstruction of the superior and inferior venae cavae, innominate, subclavian, and internal jugular veins and recently failed attempts at cannulation by an experienced operator
Respiratory distress, tachypnea, and labored inspirations
Traumatic injury to the superior vena cava, innominate, internal jugular or subclavian veins
Patient's refusal or retraction of previously given consent
Relative and Specific
In process of cardiopulmonary resuscitation (extrathoracic cardiac compressions)
In restless and uncooperative patients
Infection, burns, or presence of cancerous lymph nodes in the area of planned vein puncture
Tracheostomy with copious secretions close to planned vein puncture site
Left supraclavicular subclavian or internal jugular vein puncture attempt, low in the neck, in cirrhotics
Infraclavicular vein puncture attempt when costoclavicular space is very narrow
Supraclavicular vein puncture attempt when the outer end of clavicle is going steeply cephalad and the position cannot be corrected
Severe hypertension, tortuosity of the arteries, and proximity of an aneurysm to the vein
When attempt in one side has resulted in a severe complication at the time or even previously
When sterile technique cannot be observed in nonemergency intravenous access establishment
Lack of experience of the operator without direct expert supervision

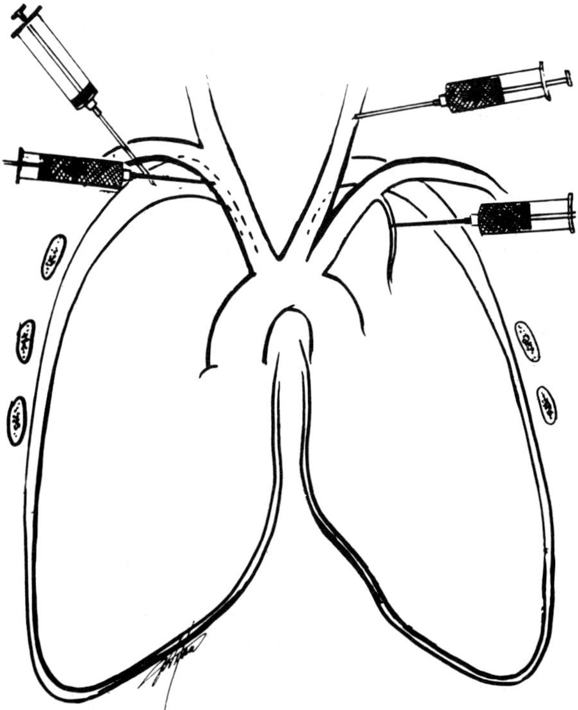

Figure 30–7. Illustration depicting arterial branches that may be inadvertently punctured during attempts for subclavian/internal jugular vein puncture. The top needle on the left has traversed the subclavian artery and has entered the pleural dome simultaneously.

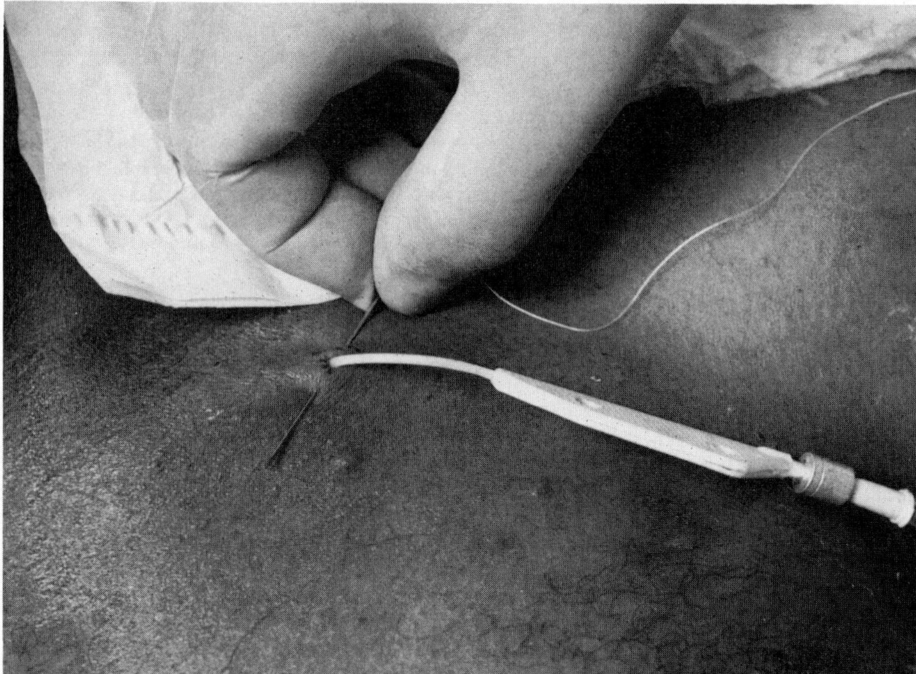

Figure 30–8. A 3–0 polyglycolic acid suture is inserted under the catheter at the skin site. The suture is then tied over a cuff of skin around the catheter to stop the oozing of blood or lymph.

lung apex is clinically recognizable only when pleural fluid, blood, or air from a pre-existing pneumothorax is aspirated. Puncture of air-containing structures is recognized when air is aspirated in the syringe, which is attached to the needle with an airtight connection (Fig. 30–11). When air is aspirated in the syringe, the needle should be kept in place to pass the catheter into the pleural space for removal of pleural free air (Fig. 30–12). Frequently, when the lung does not have apical blebs with major air leaks through the puncture site, this may be the only treatment needed. When air leakage into the pleural space continues, we insert a thoracic vent* with a one-way valve for spontaneous escape of pleural air. This small set is attached to the chest wall by a

*Tru-Close (Davis and Geck).

TABLE 30–9. Causes of External Fluid Leakage and Hemolymphorrhagia at the Catheter Site After Vein Puncture/Catheterization Attempts

Venous Blood
Subclavian vein catheter traversing the external jugular vein at the supraclavicular region
Markedly elevated venous pressure systemically or from segmental venous blockage
Forceful coughing or straining
Sitting or standing up immediately after femoral vein catheterization
Severe coagulopathy
During cardiopulmonary resuscitation (from chest compressions and/or coagulopathy)
Arterial Blood
Needle injury to subcutaneous or deep arteries
Lymph Fluid
Needle injury to the thoracic duct, especially in cirrhotics, and subclavian or jugular lymphatic trunks in supraclavicular, subclavian or internal jugular puncture low in the neck in patients with thrombosis of innominate veins*
Edema Fluid
Pleural Effusion Fluid
When pleural dome has been punctured during venipuncture attempts with the patient in supine position
Intravenous Fluid†
Backing out via the fibrinous sleeve tract
Caused by a puncture in the extravascular soft-tissue portion of the catheter

*Puncture of a tortuous lymphatic trunk during infraclavicular subclavian vein puncture attempts is rare but possible, especially in the left side.
†Intravenous fluid leakage stops by shutting off the intravenous fluid flow.

TABLE 30–10. Causes of Internal Fluid Leakage or Hemolymphorrhagia as the Result of Subclavian or Internal Jugular Vein Puncture/Catheterization Attempts

Subcutaneous, Interstitial, or Mediastinal Collection
Seldom from venous origin unless the venous pressure is too high and the vein has sustained a major injury/tear
Frequently from inadvertent puncture of the following arteries:
- Common carotid
- Transverse cervical artery
- Suprascapular artery
- Subclavian artery
- Innominate artery
- Internal mammary artery
- Vertebral artery
- Small subcutaneous or other unnamed arteries

Lymphorrhagia from the injured thoracic duct or other lymphatic branches/trunks (jugular and subclavian trunks) with high pressure
Pleural Space as Hemo-, Hydro-, or Chylothorax
In patients with coagulopathy and shock, as a result of pleural dome puncture(s)
Puncture of the subclavian or internal jugular vein into the pleural space or catheters traversing these veins into the pleural space
Puncture of the arteries into the pleural space (subclavian, common carotid, innominate, and internal thoracic)
Rupture/decompression of a mediastinal hematoma into the pleural space
Infusion of fluid and/or blood via a catheter misplaced in the pleural space
Chylothorax as a result of simultaneous needle puncture of a lymphatic duct, with high pressure, into the pleural dome space*

*Chylothorax has not been observed in this series.

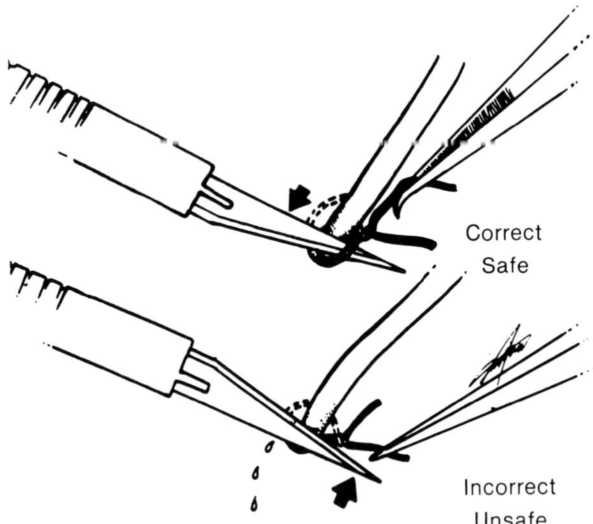

Figure 30–9. When removing the circular hemostatic suture, the cutting edge of the blade cuts away from *(top)*, and not toward, the catheter to avoid catheter transsection and embolus *(bottom)*.

self-adhesive back. The thoracic cannula is inserted in the second or third intercostal space at the midclavicular line. The thoracic vent is inserted at the bedside. After preparation of the skin and infiltration of a local anesthetic, a 0.5-cm incision is made in the skin, and the vent cannula is inserted using an inner trocar. The thoracic vent can be connected to suction if the lung does not expand completely without suction. The vent is removed when air leakage stops, as evidenced by cessation of fluctuation of the red

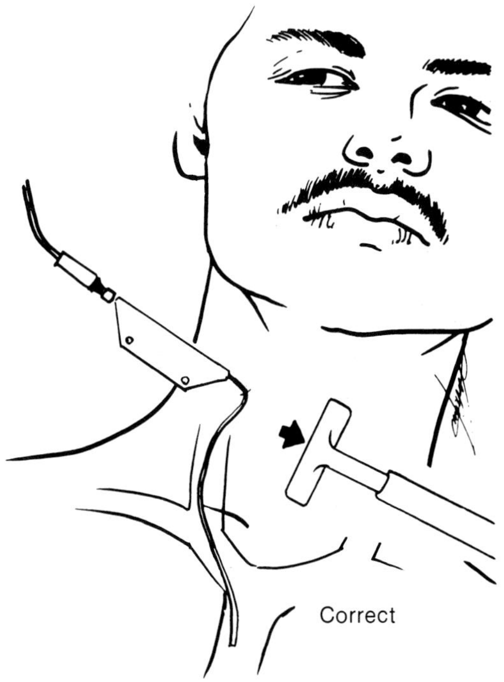

Figure 30–10. When the skin area surrounding the catheter site needs to be shaved and the catheter is already in place, the strokes of the razor are carefully started close to and directed away from the catheter to avoid cutting the catheter and consequent catheter embolus.

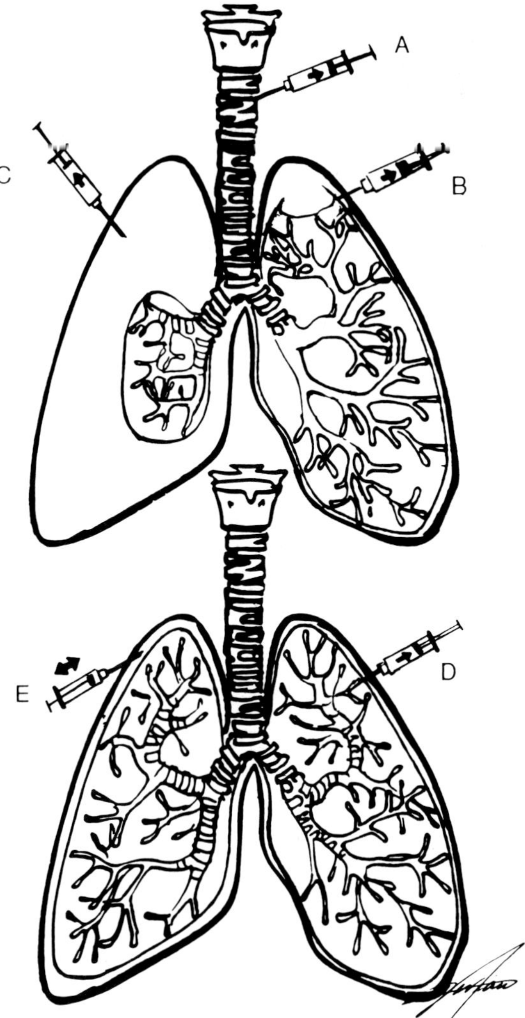

Figure 30–11. The puncture needle intended for the internal jugular or subclavian vein may enter air-containing structures that yield air in the syringe. Needle A has entered the trachea, needle B has entered an apical bleb, and needle C has entered the pleural dome space with pre-existing pneumothorax. Needle D has entered the lung apex, and needle E has entered the pleural dome space only; entry in the pleural dome space yields no air (unless a preexisting pneumothorax is present), whereas all other needle entries shown yield air.

diaphragm. The thoracic vent eliminates the need for a chest tube and pleural drainage sets for these patients with iatrogenic pneumothorax.

When the pleural space is obliterated by pre-existing adhesions, puncture of a bleb at the apex may create soft-tissue emphysema (Fig. 30–13). In the rare case when an apical bleb adheres to the parietal pleura, an adjacent artery may be punctured simultaneously and bleed into the bleb. If the bleb has communication with bronchioles, hemoptysis may occur. Hemoptysis has occurred in two recent cases after this series.

Air Embolus

Air embolus can be lethal when it is excessive[17, 18] or when it is not excessive but the patient already has a severe respiratory compromise; it remains a potentially dangerous complication even when all precautions are taken because air embolus is not always preventable. Most air emboli occur during vein puncture/catheterization. Yet air embolus

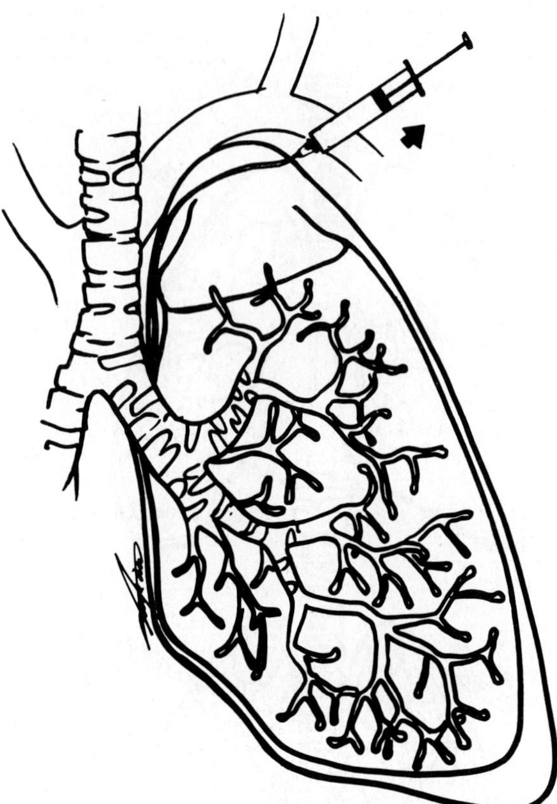

Figure 30–12. When air is aspirated into the syringe from the pleural space, the intravenous catheter should be inserted via the needle into the pleural cavity. The pleural free air can be evacuated with a 20- to 50-mL syringe connected to the catheter interposing a three-way stopcock. In patients who do not have a major air leak, this air aspiration may be all that is needed to clear the free air out of the pleural space. If air leak continues, placement of a chest catheter/tube may be needed.

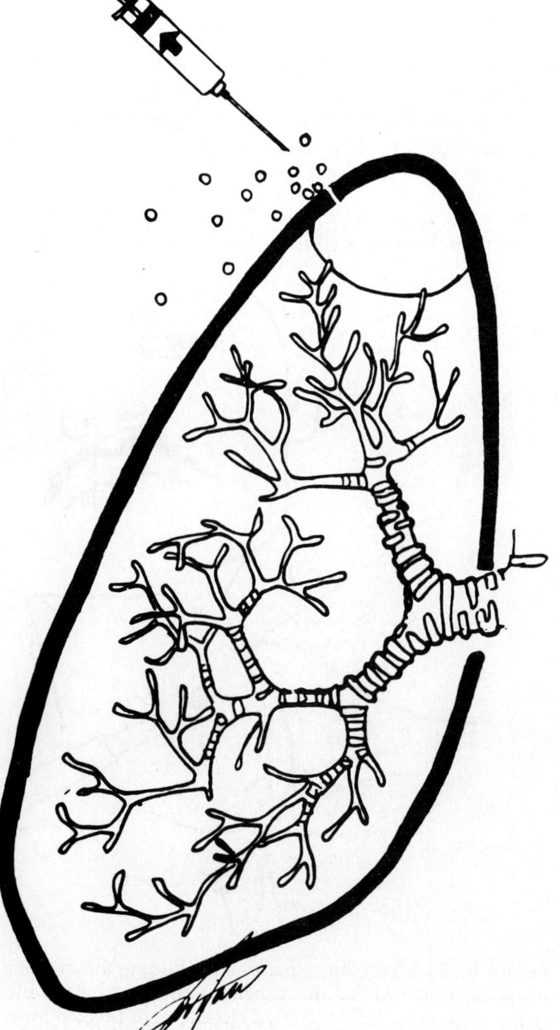

Figure 30–13. Patients with solid pleural adhesions, no pleural space, and an apical bleb that is punctured may develop subcutaneous emphysema.

can occur by disconnecting the central venous catheter from the intravenous tubing or after removing the catheter.[18] Most air emboli that occur as a result of the patient's position are preventable.

Malposition of Catheters

The catheter tip can detour into an unintended vein going in the wrong direction.[19] Malposition can enhance clot formation, catheter-related infections, and catheter erosion. Correct position or malposition of the catheter tip can be assessed clinically (Table 30–11); when necessary, it can be clarified radiologically (Table 30–12). Possible detours and malpositions of central venous catheters are shown in Table 30–13.

Guide wires can be used to rectify malpositioned catheters. Indications for the use of guide wires are listed in Table 30–14. Because of the spring movements of the guide wire, contamination is likely, especially with operators who are not adept in sterile technique.

We have replaced catheters directly via the tract immediately after removal of the existing catheter. The replacement is usually achieved after 7 days of the catheter being in place, especially when the tract is not fibrosed, infected, or zigzagged. The results of catheter exchange without the use of guide wire in 103 cases are listed in Table 30–15. Preexisting larger sized catheters could be replaced by two or more smaller catheters.

Extravascular Catheter-Tip Malpositions

Catheter malpositions could be extravascular in the soft tissues, pleural space, and peritoneal cavity.[20] Such extravascular malpositions occurring during cannulation are due to perforation of the vessels during insertion. Perforations can occur later by erosion when the tip is against the wall, especially by catheters inserted from the left side.[21–27] Catheter erosion can occur within the cardiovascular system without overt clinical evidence. When the tip of the catheter is placed against the atrial septum, it can erode into the left atrium. The tip also may erode through the tricuspid valve cusps.

Clot Formation

An inevitable complication of intravascular catheters is clot formation,[27a] the extent of which depends on the individual patient's state of blood coagulability. The first site to form a clot immediately after insertion is the puncture site into the vein. Within 48 hours, another clot may form close to the tip, and the entire catheter length may become ensheathed in a fibrin sleeve within 4 days. The longer and larger the catheter and the more rigid and irritating the catheter and infusion fluids, the more clots will form (Figs. 30–14 and 30–15). In long terms (4–10 months), all accessible veins may become thrombosed to the extent that venous cannulation becomes impossible. In patients with hypercoagulability states, anticoagulation therapy may prolong the duration of venous patency.[28] Some patients with catheter-related venous thrombosis may have embolization[29–31] perhaps as a result of rapid clot formation before the clots become adherent to the wall of the vein. Others can form potentially life-threatening thrombi.[32–36] Spontaneous closure of existing arteriovenous fistula has occurred because of venous thrombosis.[37]

Patients with blood hypocoagulability states and coagulopathy may be less at risk for venous thrombosis. Venous catheterization in such patients also appears to be reasona-

TABLE 30–11. Clinical Assessment of the Position of Intended Central Venous Catheters

Group	*Criteria*
1. Correctly placed, tip in the center of the vein or parallel to the wall	Catheter length appropriate (not short and not long) Catheter advanced, meeting no resistance Catheter stylet is straight when pulled out, and it can be reintroduced without undue resistance Catheter can be moved back partially and advanced into the vein without resistance Catheter yields blood freely, aspirating it by a syringe even when the catheter is partially withdrawn and readvanced; rapid injection of the blood aspirated in the syringe that produces no pain or sense of awareness in the patient indicates central location* Venous pressure fluctuates with respirations and central venous pressure is as expected.
2. Correctly placed, but the tip is against a vein wall, needing repositioning by manipulation until blood can be aspirated freely	Blood cannot be aspirated freely by a syringe, but there is a blood reflux in the intravenous tubing when the intravenous bottle/bag is lowered below bed level
3. Questionable; these are the catheters that detour into the internal jugular, homolateral subclavian, opposite innominate, homolateral internal thoracic, vertebral, or azygos veins	There was undue resistance to catheter advancement at some point, which was overcome by force If all other criteria in group 1 are present, catheter is correctly placed but the position still needs to be verified by x-ray film If some or all criteria in group 1 do not exist, catheter is misplaced and must be repositioned/replaced before or after x-ray confirmation
4. Definitely misplaced	Advancement met with undue resistance, which is overcome by force; catheter does not yield blood; once it is partially withdrawn, it cannot be readvanced

*This is the only test indicating that the tip of the catheter is not close to and not in apposition to the wall, provided the catheter has no side openings.

TABLE 30–12. Clinical and Radiologic Evidence of Malpositioned Catheters

Location and Position of Tip	*Signs and Symptoms*
Internal jugular, catheter lumen facing cephalad	No respiratory fluctuations of venous pressure Pain on that side of the neck created by rapid injection of fluids via the catheter; intravenous fluid stops running by pressing on the vein cephalad to the tip of catheter; pain and swelling on that side of the neck caused by thrombosis of the vein later on should the malpositioned catheter be left in place No blood return via the catheter after a few days with confirming x-ray evidence of malposition
Left internal mammary	X-ray film shows the catheter to the left of mediastinum and anterior in lateral projection Vague discomfort and pain, anterior chest No fluctuations of venous pressure by respirations No blood return from the catheter after a few days as a result of vein thrombosis Leakage of intravenous fluid from around the catheter skin site after a few days
Vertebral vein	X-ray film shows the catheter tip going cephalad and posteriorly Vague discomfort and patient's awareness of the presence of catheter in the back of the neck; leakage of intravenous fluids from around the skin site of catheter entry and no blood return via catheter after a few days
Greater azygos vein	X-ray film shows the catheter detouring from the superior vena cava course medially and posteriorly Vague discomfort/pain in the back of the chest Leakage of intravenous fluid from around the catheter as a result of venous thrombosis and formation of a fibrinous sleeve along/around the catheter leading the intravenous fluid to outside
Right atrium	Venous pressure 2 to 5 cm of water higher than that of the superior vena cava; x-ray evidence confirms the position
Tip of catheter against tricuspid valve leaklets	Blood can be aspirated by a syringe in diastole, whereas no blood can be aspirated in systole (intermittently)
Tip of catheter against flow of venous blood	Venous pressure 2 to 5 cm of water higher than that when the tip of catheter is in the direction of blood flow Smaller veins become thrombosed and intravenous fluid may leak out via the fibrinous sleeve around catheter
Right ventricle	Venous pressure weakly pulsatile and much higher than central venous pressure Premature ventricular contractions may appear initially or when manipulating catheter; conscious patient can feel irregular contractions associated with anxiety
Tip of catheter against wall of the vein or heart chambers	No blood return by aspiration with a syringe but present by lowering the intravenous bottle/bag below the bed level with the intravenous tubing open
Opposite innominate and subclavian vein (crossing over)	X-ray evidence; swelling of the opposite arm caused by vein thrombosis when the catheter is left in place for a few days
Homolateral axillary vein	Edema and swelling of the arm; pain and tenderness in the axilla; palpable cordlike and tender axillary vein

TABLE 30–13. Possible Detours and Malpositions of Central Venous Catheters in Order of Frequency

Vein and Site of Origin or Course of Catheter	*Possible Malpositions of the Catheter Tip*
Subclavian, infraclavicular	In homolateral internal jugular, axillary, and vertebral veins
Subclavian, supraclavicular	In homolateral internal mammary, opposite innominate, and axillary veins
Internal jugular (left)	In homolateral internal mammary and subclavian veins
Innominate (right)	In left innominate
Superior vena cava	In greater azygos, right atrium, coronary sinus, inferior vena cava, right ventricle, pulmonary artery
Femoral (left)	In ascending lumbar and homolateral internal iliac veins
Femoral (right)	In homolateral internal iliac vein
Inferior vena cava	In right atrium, superior vena cava, right innominate, right internal jugular, right ventricle, pulmonary artery
Internal jugular (left)	Against inferior wall of left innominate, right wall of superior vena cava
Subclavian (left)	Against right wall of superior vena cava
Subclavian (right)	Against left wall of right innominate, inferior wall of left innominate
Femoral (left)	Against superior wall of left common iliac, right wall of inferior vena cava
Femoral (right)	Against left wall of inferior vena cava

bly safe.[38] However, when an inadvertent arterial puncture occurs with simultaneous puncture of the pleural dome, a state of uncontrollable intrapleural bleeding may be encountered, especially in patients with hypertension. Undoubtedly, intravascular catheters in patients with states of blood hypocoagulability are associated with less clot formation and a longer duration of intravascular accessibility. However, these patients are more at risk for bleeding after venous catheterization attempts than those with normal blood coagulability.

TABLE 30–14. Indications for the Use of Guidewire in Insertion of Central Venous Catheter

1. Correction of malpositioned/misdirected catheters
2. Replacement of defective catheters
3. Periodic exchange of central venous catheters in septic patients
4. Elimination of the needle otherwise retained over the catheter
5. Insertion of venous hemodialysis catheters
6. Insertion of double- and triple-lumen catheters
7. Insertion of Swan-Ganz catheter introducer and sheath
8. Insertion of catheters by cutdown (exposure of vessels) and direct needle puncture (to prevent bleeding from puncture site)
9. When a catheter cannot be advanced into a central position of the tip via the puncture needle, a guide wire may first be passed over which the catheter may be advanced

Neurologic Complications

All peripheral nerves and ganglia in proximity of the veins can be injured directly[39, 40] or indirectly by the pressure of a tense hematoma resulting from an inadvertent arterial puncture. Central nervous system complications can result from venous thrombosis originating from internal jugular catheters[41] and from injury to the arteries supplying circulation to the brain.[5, 42, 43]

Catheter and Guidewire Embolism

We consider this complication preventable[44, 45] provided the following two principles are observed:

1. Do not force a catheter or guide wire through a needle when undue resistance has been encountered during advancement.

TABLE 30–15. Summary of Experience with Exchange of Central Venous Catheters Without the Use of Guidewire

Vein(s)/Site(s)	*No. of Catheters/ No. of Cases*	*Catheter(s), Size(s)*	*Range (d)*	*Results*
Right subclavian Supraclavicular	53/35	16-gauge, 19-gauge 8.5-French, 7-French	6–42	Replaced: 50 Failed: 10
Left subclavian Supraclavicular	46/33	16-gauge, 19-gauge 7-French, 8.5-French	5–39	Replaced: 37 Failed: 14
Right subclavian Infraclavicular	12/11	16-gauge, 19-gauge 8.5-French	7–40	Replaced: 16 Failed: 0
Left subclavian Infraclavicular	17/16	16-gauge 8.5-French, 11.5-French	9–37	Replaced: 20 Failed: 1
Right internal jugular	3/3	16-gauge 8.5-French	5–14	Replaced: 5 Failed: 0
Left internal jugular	1/1	16-gauge	45	Replaced: 1 Failed: 0
Right supra- and infraclavicular	8/3	16-gauge	8–21	Replaced: 3 Failed: 5
Left supra- and infraclavicular	3/1	16-gauge	14	Replaced: 3 Failed: 0

Total:
Replaced, each catheter by another catheter or more: 82 cases
Replaced one, failed replacing another of two catheters: 4 cases
Failed replacing catheters: 17 cases
Number of initial catheters: 143
Number of replacement catheters: 135
Number of catheters failed to replace: 30

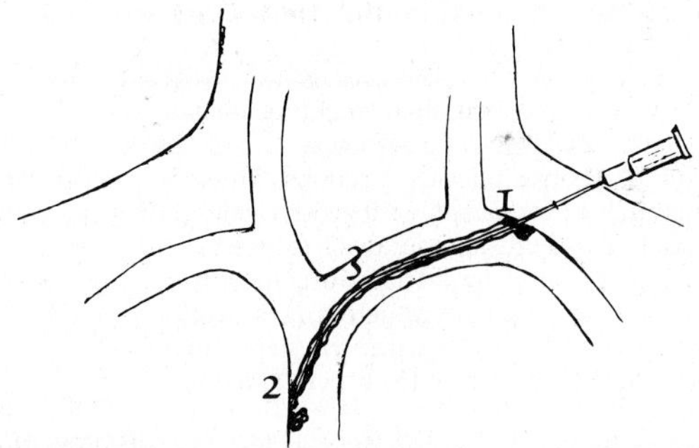

Figure 30–14. Three foci of clot formation exist around a catheter: at the site of vein puncture to seal off the site (1); at the tip of the catheter owing to the irritation of the catheter or intravenous fluids (2); and around the catheter to ensheath it (3).

2. Do not pull out the catheter or guide wire that has been forced in and that does not come out easily.

In the second situation, the needle is first pulled back. Then, if the catheter or guide wire does not come out easily, operative removal by exposure of the resistant site should be attempted.[44, 45] The embolized guide wire or catheter should be retrieved immediately nonoperatively by snare. Operative removal of the embolized catheter or guide wire should be reserved for those that manifest infectious complications that can be cured only by removal.

Arterial Puncture/Cannulation

By taking advantage of pulsation, arteries with percutaneously detectable pulse can be punctured for arterial blood sampling as well as cannulation. The development of noninvasive monitoring of the partial pressure of oxygen and carbon dioxide has diminished the need for invasive intra-arterial monitoring.[46, 47] Accessible arteries include the radial, dorsalis pedis, femoral, brachial, and axillary arteries and the umbilical artery in the newborn.

The radial artery is used more frequently because the cannulation and maintenance of the cannula in place are easy to achieve. Before cannulation of radial artery, however, the adequacy of palmar circulation should be assessed by manual compression and blockage of the radial artery. Preferably, the wrist of the left hand in the right-handed patient or the right hand in the left-handed patient is splinted with as much dorsal flexion as tolerated without interfering with palpation of the pulse. The area is then prepared with an iodine solution and surrounded by sterile drape. A local anesthetic is infiltrated into the skin over the planned arterial puncture site, followed by insertion of a short catheter over the needle or by Seldinger technique. Arterial puncture is recognized by the backing up of bright red, pulsatile blood that has a high pressure in the syringe attached to the cannula. The intra-arterial catheter is affixed to the underlying skin and locked by heparin solution or connected to a pressure monitor. The presence of radial artery cannula may affect the accuracy of pulse oximetry in the same hand.[48] In patients with weak or nonpalpable pulse, the radial or dorsalis pedis artery can be cannulated by cutdown.

The brachial artery at the medial aspect of the upper midarm can be readily cannulated and the cannula effectively maintained in place. The axillary artery may be accessed in adults, children, and neonates. While attempting brachial or axillary artery cannulation, the brachial and axillary veins may be entered inadvertently. When the vein is unintentionally entered with a short arterial catheter, it should not be used for long-term intravenous access[49] because the arterial catheter is not long enough to reach the superior vena cava.[50] In neonates, the umbilical artery cannulation can be used but with due vigilance for the potential complications.[51]

Complications of Intra-Arterial Access

Ischemia from clot formation and infection remains the major potential unpreventable complication of arterial cannulas. Hand ischemia in the newborn is rare.[52] Early complications of arterial indwelling catheters are due to hematoma, infection, thrombosis, and false aneurysms.[53–56] The ischemic sequela can continue as a long-term complication with various clinical manifestations.[57–59] Because of inherent complications, arterial catheters should be placed as atraumatically as possible while maintaining sterile technique. Arterial catheters should be used with definite needs and for as short a time as possible.

Pulmonary Artery Catheter

The PA balloon-tipped (Swan-Ganz) catheter[60] has provided many hemodynamic measurements in understanding and management of pathophysiology in critically ill patients.[61–65] Even though PA catheterization is frequently performed at the bedside, strict rules of operating room sterility must be exercised.

Insertion of Catheter

After preparation, the skin area is widely surrounded by sterile drapes. The operator should wear a cap and a mask. After hand scrub, sterile gown and gloves are worn. We prefer to introduce a 16-gauge catheter in the superior vena cava first; a guide wire is then advanced to only 20 to 25 cm to avoid disturbance in cardiac rhythm.[66, 67] The catheter is then removed. A small incision is made into the skin site using a sharp-tipped scalpel blade, with the back of the blade toward the guide wire, incising the skin away from the guide wire. The introducer is first advanced over the guide wire to ensure smooth insertion free of undue resistance. Inadequate skin incision can interfere with insertion of the introducer and sheath by bending or deforming the sheath, which then may interfere with catheter insertion.

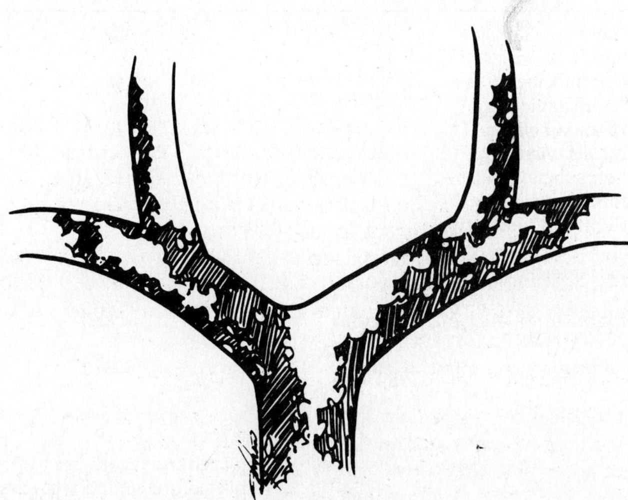

Figure 30–15. The presence of consecutive multiple and long-term central venous catheters eventually results in thrombosis of all of the veins harboring the catheters. The veins become inaccessible to catheterization, even though blood flow is not completely blocked.

TABLE 30–16. Precautions that May Reduce Catheter Infection

Catheterize by the first or second puncture attempt(s).
Remove needle, ordinarily retained over the catheter, by a guide wire to avoid trapping blood and microorganisms between the needle and catheter or between needle and the needle guard.
Keep intravenous fluid flow uninterrupted to prevent blood reflux into the catheter and intravenous tubings.
Flush catheter free from debris by running the intravenous fluid freely several minutes once or twice a day.
Avoid suturing the catheter to the skin; use tape instead.
Prevent pressure sore or soreness of the skin at the site of the catheter hub and intravenous tubing connection by placing a gauze pad underneath.
Provide antiseptic preparation and apply silver sulfadiazine cream at the catheter skin site at least daily, preferably three times daily in infection-prone patients.
Use chemically inert catheters with as short a length, as small a diameter, and as soft a substance as possible.
Remove catheters as soon as possible.
Change site once a week in septic patients, if possible; otherwise, exchange catheter twice a week in septic patients.
Avoid creation of hematoma at the site and fluid, blood, and lymph leakage from around the catheter site.
Leave catheter sites exposed in patients with marked perspiration or burns at the skin site.
Apply waterproof dressings over the catheter site when the patient is showering or when there is a nearby contamination source, and change at least daily.*
Create a subcutaneous tunnel to place the catheter skin exit/entry site away from the nearby source of contamination.
Apply dry gauze dressing over the catheter site, permitting air circulation to keep it dry.

*We only use waterproof transparent adhesive dressing for this purpose and when the patient is showering/bathing.

Intravascular Catheter-Related Infections

Although the risk of catheter infection can be reduced, infection cannot be prevented. Many critically ill patients are infection prone, and it is only a matter of time before they manifest catheter-related infections, unless intravascular catheters are used only intermittently for short periods. Factors that may enhance or prevent the development of catheter infections are listed in Tables 30–16 and 30–17. All intravascular catheters should remain closed to the outside environment. Because central venous manometers can violate the principle of closure and the intravenous fluids remain stagnant in the manometer, we recommend that the pressure be measured without the manometer.[2, 73]

Gauze dressing, which permits air to remain under it, is more advantageous than the semipermeable, transparent dressing.[74] Antibiotic bonding seems promising,[75] but it remains to be proven effective in long-term indwelling catheters, especially for contaminations occurring from within the catheter lumen.

A catheter without the flow of intravenous fluids is particularly vulnerable to the growth of contaminant microorganisms that may exist within the lumen. Antibiotic lock can be effective in the prevention of microbial growth in catheters without intravenous fluid flow.[76] We believe there is a correlation between the amount of clot formation and catheter infection. Anticoagulation and particularly short-term use of intravascular catheters diminish clot formation and may help reduce catheter infection. Currently, catheter-related infection remains a major problem for patients and clinicians.[77–82]

Septic embolization and metastatic infections can occur when there are infected clots or when septicemia develops.[83]

When the subcutaneous tissue is scarred, as in intravenous drug abusers, the skin incision must be carried deep into the scarred tissue. In this situation, the introducer cannot be advanced at once. The introducer is advanced partially and then placed on traction to expose the subcutaneous scar tissue. The tissue is incised with the tip of the scalpel blade, which is introduced between the introducer and the scar tissue; the sharp edge cuts the scar tissue away from the introducer. This process is repeated until only mild resistance is felt against introducer advancement. The introducer and the sheath are then fully advanced. The introducer is then removed, and the PA catheter is inserted and advanced through the sheath with an uninflated balloon to 20 cm in adults; the balloon is then inflated with 1.5 mL of air. If the balloon is inflated after advancement of the catheter to 25 to 30 cm, the tip may have already entered the inferior vena cava. Advancement of the catheter through the heart must be slow and gentle. The pressure tracings indicate the location of the tip of the catheter until it has reached a wedge position. The balloon is deflated soon after reaching wedge position. When replacing a PA catheter, the existing one should be removed before the new one is introduced because of the potential danger of knotting and entanglement of one catheter with the other.

Complications of Pulmonary Artery Catheters

Technical complications specific to PA catheters include failure to pass the catheter, especially in the patient in shock and low-flow state, knotting of the catheter, cardiac arrhythmia, rupture of pulmonary artery and consequent pulmonary hematoma, hemoptysis, and pulmonary artery pseudoaneurysm.[68–70] A catheter should not be kept in place for longer than 3 days; otherwise, the rates of infection and other complications may increase.[71, 72]

TABLE 30–17. Factors that May Lead to Intravenous Catheter-Related Infection

Multiple puncture attempts at one site at one or repeated setting
Hematoma around the catheter soft-tissue tract
Blood clots or stains allowed to remain under the dressing
Fibrin or blood clots retained within the catheter and intravenous tubing
Leakage of lymph, interstitial edema fluid, intravenous fluids, or blood and accumulation of perspirations under the dressing, which keep the catheter site moist
Blood trapped between the catheter inside the needle segment and between the needle and the needle guard
Sutures at the catheter site, especially hemostatic sutures, tied tightly
Catheters with no blood return, ball valve clot at the tip
Catheters with fibrinous sleeve
Catheters inserted close to infection or contamination sources
Short distance between the skin puncture and vein puncture sites
Catheters inserted through skin burns
Misdirected, coiled, and partially withdrawn catheters
Catheters in patients with preexisting sepsis; sepsis is perpetuated
Catheters in patients with long-term intravenous therapy (>4 months)
Long, large-bore, rigid, and/or multiple long-term catheters
Immune deficiency states
Catheters inserted under emergency conditions, during cardiopulmonary resuscitation, and during operative interventions*
Persistent shock
Advanced cancer, renal, and/or hepatic failure
Catheters and intravenous tubings handled by unsterile technique
Unsterile intravenous fluids preparation and administration techniques
Constant moisture at the catheter skin site

*We replace all catheters considered or suspected of being contaminated after the emergency situation is averted.

The most effective and safest way to abort catheter-related infections is to remove the catheter[84] rather than replace it. To overcome the infection, the cause should be eliminated, even if only for a short time.

Avoiding and Managing Other Potentially Dangerous or Lethal Complications

Critically and terminally ill patients may have no vital reserve to tolerate central venous/PA cannulation procedures. Small air emboli in severely respiratory compromised patients can be lethal. Therefore, subclavian and internal jugular vein puncture/cannulation in these patients should be managed with extreme care or avoided altogether. Air embolus can occur via the established central venous catheters in the event of inadvertent disconnection of the intravenous tubing and the catheter.[85] Safe maintenance of the intravascular catheters calls for the necessary education of the patient care personnel as well as the patient.[86, 87]

Catheter-tip erosion may be prevented by using soft and pliable catheters. We have not had catheter erosions in this series. When using semirigid or rigid catheters, the operator must make certain that the tip is not positioned against the vessel wall. The only positive test for proper tip position is to aspirate blood with free flow via the catheter with the opening at the tip only.

At the confluence of major veins, there is a turbulent flow. This turbulence can act as a drill force, driving the tip of the catheter through the wall when it is positioned against the wall in the turbulent area.[86–88] A major turbulent venous blood flow area is at the junction of the innominate veins. When the tip of the catheter enters the heart chambers abutting against the wall, in time cardiac contractions can drive the catheter tip through the wall.

Insertion of central venous and PA catheters is contraindicated in patients with severe coagulation defects. In the event of massive hemothorax after catheter insertion, a chest tube should be inserted and an emergency thoracotomy considered if immediate administration of sufficient coagulation factors fails to stop the bleeding. In the event of massive hemoptysis, the patient should be intubated with a double-lumen endotracheal tube, which can prevent the blood from going into the opposite bronchus; this is a temporary life-saving measure until the source of bleeding is controlled.

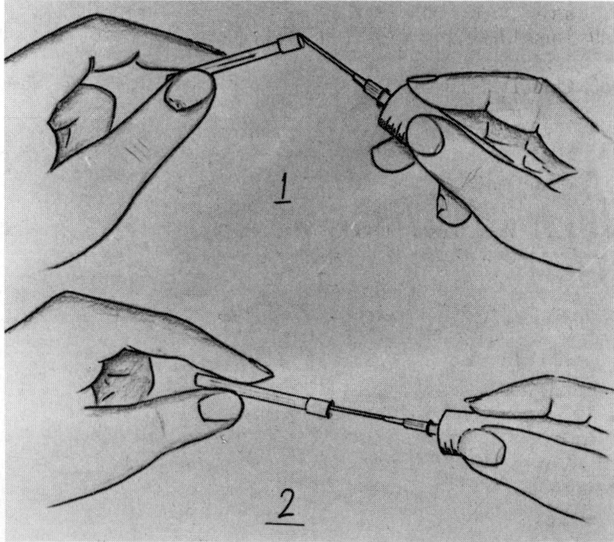

Figure 30–16. The used needle can be safely capped by first advancing the needle tip into the plastic casing at an angle and then by straightening out the angle and advancing the needle fully inside the cap. The second step of capping should *never* be interchanged with the first.

If the guidewire or catheter enters the right ventricle with the possibility of generating ventricular tachycardia or fibrillation, a defibrillator as well as antiarrhythmic medications should be kept available at the bedside.

During injection of fluids or blood, the operator should hold the syringe firmly against the hub of the needle or catheter to prevent spray of fluids or blood.

The local anesthetic bottle should not be held by the assistant but rather placed down on a firm surface until needle entry and then picked up by the assistant to aid in withdrawal of the fluid into the syringe.

While establishing piggybacked infusion or giving intravenous push medications, the main intravenous tubing should be held safely behind the needle being inserted, not unsafely with the hand in front of the needle.

To cap the needle, it should be introduced into the cap at an angle first and then advanced straight forward to avoid needle puncture (Fig. 30–16).

Intravascular access catheters established and maintained with safe and sterile technique by an experienced team and used for the shortest time possible can prove life saving; otherwise, they can prove life threatening. The sicker the patient, the more experienced the operator should be providing the care personally.

ACKNOWLEDGMENT

The authors thank Fernando Tabora, MD, for data collection for Table 30–6 and Cyrus Parsa for typing of the manuscript.

References

1. Parsa MH, Ferrer JM, Habif DV, et al: Intravenous hyperalimentation: Indications, technique and complications. Bull NY Acad Med 1972; 48:920.
2. Parsa MH, Ferrer JM, Habif DV: Safe Central Venous Nutrition: Guidelines for Prevention and Management of Complications. Springfield, IL, Charles C Thomas, 1974.
3. Parsa MH, Tabora F: Establishment of intravenous lines for long-term intravenous therapy and monitoring. Surg Clin North Am 1985; 65:835.
4. Parsa MH, Shoemaker WC: Nutritional failure. *In*: Textbook of Critical Care. Shoemaker WC, Thompson WL, Holbrook PR, et al (Eds). Philadelphia, WB Saunders, 1984, p 664.
5. Parsa MH, Tabora F: Central venous access in critically ill patients in the emergency department. Emerg Med Clin North Am 1986; 4:709.
6. Parsa MH, Tabora F, Freeman HP: Techniques of insertion of double or triple IV catheters in one vein or two adjacent veins. Surg Rounds 1987; 10:43.
7. Parsa MH, Tabora F, Freeman HP: Vascular cannulation techniques in intravenous drug addicts and patients with limited or difficult intravenous access. Contemp Surg 1987; 31:31.
8. Parsa MH, Lau K, Jampayas I, et al: Intravenous catheter-related infection. Infect Surg 1985; 4:789.
9. Smith MB: Another complication of intravenous catheterization: A case report. J Okla State Med Assoc 1990; 83:18.

9a. Treiman GS, Silberman H: Chronic venous access in patients with cancer: Selective use of the saphenous vein. Cancer 1993; 72:760.

9b. Westfall MD, Price KR, Lambert M, et al: Intravenous access in the critically ill trauma patient: A multicentered, prospective, randomized trial of saphenous cutdown and percutaneous femoral access. Ann Emerg Med 1994; 23:541.

9c. Raaf JH, Heil D: Open insertion of right atrial catheters through the jugular veins. Surg Gynecol Obstet 1993; 177:295.

10. Parsa MH, Tabora F, Al-Sawwaf M: Vascular access techniques. *In*: Textbook of Critical Care. 2nd Edition. Shoemaker WC, Ayres S, Grenvik A, et al (Eds). Philadelphia, WB Saunders, 1989, p 122.
10a. Freedman SE, Bosserman G: Tunneled catheters: Technologic advances and nursing care issues. Nurs Clin North Am 1993; 28:851.
10b. Gullo SM: Implanted ports: Technologic advances and nursing care issues. Nurs Clin North Am 1993; 28:859.
11. Heinemann M, Frank G, Oldhafer KJ, et al: Infected intravenous port device causing tricuspid valve regurgitation. Ann Thorac Surg 1991; 51:827.
12. Hinke DH, Zandt-Stastny DA, Goodman LR, et al: Pinch-off syndrome: A complication of implantable subclavian venous access devices. Radiology 1990; 177:353.
13. Cimochowski GE, Worley E, Rutherford WE, et al: Superiority of the internal jugular over the subclavian access for temporary dialysis. Nephron 1990; 54:154.
14. Schillinger F, Schillinger D, Montagnac R, et al: Post catheterisation vein stenosis in haemodialysis: Comparative angiographic study of 50 subclavian and 50 internal jugular accesses. Nephrol Dial Transplant 1991; 6:722.
15. Khanna S, Sniderman K, Simons M, et al: Superior vena cava stenosis associated with hemodialysis catheters. Am J Kidney Dis 1993; 21:278.
16. Surratt RS, Picus D, Hicks ME, et al: The importance of preoperative evaluation of the subclavian vein in dialysis access planning. Am J Roentgenol 1991; 156:623.
17. Rouse DA, Hargrove R: An unusual case of gas embolism. Am J Forensic Med Pathol 1992; 13:268.
18. Phifer TJ, Bridges M, Conrad SA: The residual central venous catheter track: An occult source of lethal air embolism: Case report. J Trauma 1991; 31:1558.
19. Rosa UW, Foreman M, Willsie-Ediger S: Intermittent back pain after central venous catheter placement. JPEN J Parenter Enteral Nutr 1993; 17:91.
20. Eanniello VC II, Jacobs LM, Sahdev P: Intraperitoneal femoral venous catheter insertion with free blood return in presence of tense hemoperitoneum. Am J Emerg Med 1991; 9:157.
21. Beauregard JF, Matsumoto AH, Paul MG, et al: Venobronchial fistula: A complication associated with central venous catheterization for chemotherapy. Cathet Cardiovasc Diagn 1990; 19:49.
22. Winkler TR, Hanlin RJ, Hinke TD, et al: Unusual cause of hemoptysis: Hickman-induced cava-bronchial fistula. Chest 1992; 102:1285.
23. Krasna IH, Krause T: Life-threatening fluid extravasation of central venous catheters. J Pediatr Surg 1991; 26:1346.
24. Mukau L, Talamini MA, Sitzmann JV: Risk factors for central venous catheter-related vascular erosions. JPEN J Parenter Enteral Nutr 1991; 15:513.
25. Rogers BB, Berns SD, Maynard EC, et al: Pericardial tamponade secondary to central venous catheterization and hyperalimentation in a very low birthweight infant. Pediatr Pathol 1990; 10:819.
26. Byard RW, Bourne AJ, Moore L, et al: Sudden death in early infancy due to delayed cardiac tamponade complicating central venous line insertion and cardiac catheterization. Arch Pathol Lab Med 1992; 116:654.
27. Duntley P, Siever J, Korwes ML, et al: Vascular erosion by central venous catheters: Clinical features and outcome. Chest 1992; 101:1633.
27a. Longley DG, Finlay DE, Letourneau JG: Sonography of the upper extremity and jugular veins. AJR Am J Roentgenol 1993; 160:957.
28. Bern MM, Lokich JJ, Wallach SR, et al: Very low doses of warfarin can prevent thrombosis in central venous catheters: A randomized prospective trial. Ann Intern Med 1990; 112:423.
29. Cervia JS, Caputo TA, Davis SD, et al: Septic pulmonary embolism complicating a central venous catheter. Chest 1990; 98:1526.
30. Johnson CW, Miller DL, Ognibene FP: Acute pulmonary emboli associated with guidewire change of a central venous catheter. Intensive Care Med 1991; 17:115.
31. Kreher SK, Ulstad VK, Dick CD, et al: Frequent occurrence of occult pulmonary embolism from venous sheaths during endomyocardial biopsy. J Am Coll Cardiol 1992; 19:581.
32. Kaye GC, Smith DR, Johnston D: Fatal right ventricular thrombus secondary to Hickman catheterisation. Br J Clin Pract 1990; 44:780.
33. Storper IS, Calcaterra TC: Laryngeal edema induced by neck dissection and catheter thrombosis. Am J Otolaryngol 1992; 13:101.
34. Cohen GI, Klein AL, Chan KL, et al: Transesophageal echocardiographic diagnosis of right-sided cardiac masses in patients with central lines. Am J Cardiol 1992; 70:925.
35. Karnik R, Valentin A, Winkler WB, et al: Duplex sonographic detection of internal jugular venous thrombosis after removal of central venous catheters. Clin Cardiol 1993; 16:26.
36. Figuerola M, Tomás MT, Armengol J, et al: Pericardial tamponade and coronary sinus thrombosis associated with central venous catheterization. Chest 1992; 101:1154.
37. Zullo MA, Wallerson DC, Lang S: Formation and spontaneous closure of an arteriovenous fistula after transvenous pacemaker placement. Chest 1991; 100:572.
38. Foster PF, Moore LR, Sankary HN, et al: Central venous catheterization in patients with coagulopathy. Arch Surg 1992; 127:273.
39. Pleasure JR, Shashikumar VL: Phrenic nerve damage in the tiny infant during vein cannulation for parenteral nutrition. Am J Perinatol 1990; 7:136.
40. Zeligowsky A, Szold A, Seror D, et al: Horner syndrome: A rare complication of internal jugular vein cannulation. JPEN J Parenter Enteral Nutr 1991; 15:199.
41. Stephens PH, Lennox G, Hirsch N, et al: Superior sagittal sinus thrombosis after internal jugular vein cannulation. Br J Anaesth 1991; 67:476.
42. Amaral JF, Grigoriev VE, Dorfman GS, et al: Vertebral artery pseudoaneurysm: A rare complication of subclavian artery catheterization. Arch Surg 1990; 125:546.
43. Sloan MA, Mueller JD, Adelman LS, et al: Fatal brainstem stroke following internal jugular vein catheterization. Neurology 1991; 41:1092.
44. Parsa MH: Catheter insertion through steel needle. Crit Care Med 1985; 13:249.
45. Parsa MH: Complications of central venous catheter insertion. Crit Care Med 1992; 20:443.
46. Tremper KK, Shoemaker WC: Continuous CPR monitoring with transcutaneous oxygen and carbon dioxide sensors. Crit Care Med 1981; 9:417.
47. Abraham E, Markle DR, Pinholster G, et al: Noninvasive measurement of conjunctival PCO_2 with a fiberoptic sensor. Crit Care Med 1986; 14:138.
48. Morris RW, Nairn M, Beaudoin M: Does the radial arterial line degrade the performance of a pulse oximeter? Anaesth Intensive Care 1990; 18:107.
49. Parsa MH: Axillary vein cannulation in neonates. Crit Care Med 1993; 21:476.
50. Oriot D, Defawe G: Percutaneous catheterization of the axillary vein in neonates. Crit Care Med 1988; 16:285.
51. Seibert JJ, Northington FJ, Miers JF, et al: Aortic thrombosis after umbilical artery catheterization in neonates: Prevalence of complications on long-term follow-up. Am J Roentgenol 1991; 156:567.
52. Hack WW, Vos A, Okken A: Incidence of forearm and hand ischaemia related to radial artery cannulation in newborn infants. Intensive Care Med 1990; 16:50.
53. Furfaro S, Gauthier M, Lacroix J, et al: Arterial catheter-related infections in children: A 1-year cohort analysis. Am J Dis Child 1991; 145:1037.
54. Swanson E, Freiberg A, Salter DR: Radial artery infections and aneurysms after catheterization. J Hand Surg (Am) 1990; 15:166.
55. McEllistrem RF, O'Toole DP, Keane P: Post-cannulation radial artery aneurysm: A rare complication. Can J Anaesth 1990; 37:907.
56. Falk PS, Scuderi PE, Sherertz RJ, et al: Infected radial artery pseudoaneurysms occurring after percutaneous cannulation. Chest 1992; 101:490.
57. Hack WW, Vos A, van der Lei J, et al: Incidence and duration of total occlusion of the radial artery in newborn infants after catheter removal. Eur J Pediatr 1990; 149:275.
58. Guy RL, Holland JP, Shaw DG, et al: Limb shortening secondary to complications of vascular cannulae in the neonatal period. Skeletal Radiol 1990; 19:423.

59. Taylor LM Jr, Troutman R, Feliciano P, et al: Late complications after femoral artery catheterization in children less than five years of age. J Vasc Surg 1990; 11:297.
60. Swan HJC, Ganz W, Forrester J, et al: Catheterization of the heart in man with use of a flow-directed balloon-tipped catheter. N Engl J Med 1970; 283:447.
61. Shoemaker WC, Printer KJ, Amato JJ, et al: Hemodynamic patterns after acute anesthetized and unanesthetized trauma. Ann Surg 1967; 95:492.
62. Shoemaker WC, Appel PL, Kram HB, et al: Prospective trial of supranormal values of survivors as therapeutic goals in high-risk surgical patients. Chest 1988; 94:1176.
63. Shoemaker WC, Appel P, Bland R: Use of physiologic monitoring to predict outcome and to assist in clinical decisions in critically ill postoperative patients. Am J Surg 1983; 146:43.
64. Shoemaker WC, Appel PL, Kram HB, et al: Sequence of physiologic patterns in surgical septic shock. Crit Care Med 1993; 21:1876.
65. Parsa MH, Al-Sawwaf M, Shoemaker WC: Complications of pulmonary artery catheterization: Cost benefit analysis. Probl Gen Surg 1985; 2:133.
66. Eissa NT, Kvetan V: Guide wire as a cause of complete heart block in patients with pre-existing left bundle branch block. Anesthesiology 1990; 73:772.
67. Stuart RK, Baxter JK, Shikora SA, et al: Reducing arrhythmias associated with central venous catheter insertion or exchange. Nutrition 1992; 8:19.
68. Feng WC, Singh AK, Drew T, et al: Swan-Ganz catheter-induced massive hemoptysis and pulmonary artery false aneurysm. Ann Thorac Surg 1990; 50:644.
69. Cooper JP, Jackson J, Walker JM: False aneurysm of the pulmonary artery associated with cardiac catheterisation. Br Heart J 1993; 69:188.
70. Jondeau G, Lacombe P, Rocha P, et al: Swan-Ganz catheter-induced rupture of the pulmonary artery: Successful early management by transcatheter embolization. Cathet Cardiovasc Diagn 1990; 19:202.
71. Mermel LA, McCormick RD, Springman SR, et al: The pathogenesis and epidemiology of catheter-related infection with pulmonary artery Swan-Ganz catheters: A prospective study utilizing molecular subtyping. Am J Med 1991; 91:197S.
72. Rello J, Coll P, Net A, et al: Infection of pulmonary artery catheters: Epidemiologic characteristics and multivariate analysis of risk factors. Chest 1993; 103:132.
73. Parsa MH, Ferrer JM, Habif DV: A new closed technique for measuring CVP. Res Staff Phys 1971; 17:37.
74. Fitchie C: Central venous catheter-related infection and dressing type. Intensive Crit Care Nurs 1992; 8:199.
75. Kamal GD, Pfaller MA, Rempe LE, et al: Reduced intravascular catheter infection by antibiotic bonding: A prospective, randomized, controlled trial. JAMA 1991; 265:2364.
76. Cowan CE: Antibiotic lock technique. J Intravenous Nurs 1992; 15:283.
77. Kiehn TE, Gorey E, Brown AE, et al: Sepsis due to Rhodotorula related to use of indwelling central venous catheters. Clin Infect Dis 1992; 14:841.
78. Kaye GC, Rodgers H, Smith DR, et al: Bacterial endocarditis of the tricuspid valve after insertion of a central venous catheter. Br J Clin Pract 1990; 44:762.
79. Paut O, Kreitmann B, Silicani MA, et al: Successful treatment of fungal right atrial thrombosis complicating central venous catheterization in a critically ill child. Intensive Care Med 1992; 18:375.
80. Joshi P, Bullingham A, Soni N: Septic atrial thrombus: A complication of central venous catheterization. Anaesthesia 1991; 46:1030.
81. Ullman RF, Gurevich I, Schoch PE, et al: Colonization and bacteremia related to duration of triple-lumen intravascular catheter placement. Am J Infect Control 1990; 18:201.
82. Early TF, Gregory RT, Wheeler JR, et al: Increased infection rate in double-lumen versus single-lumen Hickman catheters in cancer patients. South Med J 1990; 83:34.
83. Kwok T, Coles J: Psoas abscess as a complication of subclavian venous catheterization. Postgrad Med J 1990; 66:771.
84. Raad I, Davis S, Khan A, et al: Impact of central venous catheter removal on the recurrence of catheter-related coagulase-negative staphylococcal bacteremia. Infect Control Hosp Epidemiol 1992; 13:215.
85. Ferrer JM, Parsa MH: Fatal air embolism via subclavian vein. N Engl J Med 1970; 282:688.
86. Parsa MH, Freeman HP: Precautions for long-term maintenance of central venous catheters: The need for patient and personnel education. Part I. Surg Rounds 1992; 15:967.
87. Parsa MH, Freeman HP: Precautions for long-term maintenance of central venous catheters: The need for patient and personnel education: Part II. Surg Rounds 1992; 15:1013.
88. Parsa MH: Fatal cardiac tamponade. JAMA 1983; 249:1707.

CHAPTER 31

Invasive and Noninvasive Physiologic Monitoring

William C. Shoemaker, MD • M.H. Parsa, MD

"All science is measurement."

HELMHOLTZ

Conventionally, readily accessible variables are used for screening, for early warning, and for early correction of circulatory problems. Physiologic monitoring differs from diagnostic methods, which are most often chemical or radiologic tests that are performed infrequently to document data needed for specific diagnoses. However, the distinction between monitoring and diagnostic procedures becomes blurred when chest radiographs, arterial blood gases assessments, serum electrolytes analyses, and coagulation profiles are carried out daily.

No single physiologic measurement or group of measurements can convey all aspects of a patient's condition. Clinical judgment, on the other hand, is subjective, hard to quantify, and cannot be quantitatively applied as a "yardstick." Physiologic data, laboratory and radiographic studies supplement rather than supplant clinical judgment. Physiologic measurements often reinforce clinical opinions and provide baseline values and the subsequent quantitative basis for management. More importantly, these measurements provide objective criteria for the evaluation of physiologic deficiencies separate from the diagnostic evaluation. Making this distinction is particularly important, as most people die not from their diagnosis but from physiologic deficiencies that lead to the failure of vital organs.

Routinely monitored variables are evaluated one-at-a-time, and the abnormalities detected are also corrected one-at-a-time. Recent technical developments in monitoring systems have provided a wide range of physiologic variables that allow extensive assessment of complex interacting circulatory functions. Ideally, however, the interactions of multiple physiologic measurements should be used to analyze early initiating events as an approach to the development of therapeutic plans.

First, the purpose of circulatory monitoring is to obtain frequent, repetitive measurements of circulatory variables so as to allow prompt recognition of circulatory problems. Second, monitoring is done to evaluate physiologic conditions. Third, monitoring is done to institute early corrective therapy. Fourth, monitored circulatory values of survivors are used as criteria to titrate therapy so as to achieve optimal therapeutic goals.

Hemodynamic and oxygen transport variables are available on a routine basis for invasive intensive care unit (ICU) monitoring. Available systems directly measure and calculate 30 or more variables with each cardiac output measurement and with measurements of associated arterial and mixed venous blood gases; serial measurements can provide the temporal pattern of acute circulatory problems as well as the responses to therapeutic interventions.

The uncomplicated elective surgical patient is often monitored postoperatively based on his or her vital signs, electrocardiogram (ECG), urine output, arterial blood gases, and central venous pressure (CVP). More extensive invasive hemodynamic and oxygen transport monitoring may be used preoperatively for evaluation of high-risk surgical patients, during and after surgery; in patients with suspected acute circulatory problems; in patients with myocardial infarction, sepsis, or blood loss; in patients with major trauma, head injury, or blunt injury to the chest or abdomen; and in patients with shock syndromes and other life-threatening conditions.

Invasive hemodynamic and oxygen transport monitoring in ICU patients identifies correctable physiologic deficiencies in their early stages. It supplements clinical guesswork with more objective physiologic criteria and provides the basis for titrating therapy. The ideal rate of invasive monitoring should be about four- or fivefold the expected mortality rate to include all potentially fatal deficiencies that are correctable. Table 31–1 lists high-risk conditions of surgical patients (with an expected mortality rate of about 30%) that are appropriate for invasive monitoring.[1] Hemodynamic monitoring also may be indicated when vital signs and CVP suggest the presence of more extensive circulatory problems.

This chapter summarizes the various circulatory parameters, from routine noninvasive surveillence and screening techniques to invasive hemodynamic and oxygen transport monitoring methods. The monitoring of fetus and child, the ECG, the electroencephalogram, ventilation studies, arterial blood gases analysis, radiology, digital imaging, and cerebral pressure measurement are discussed in subsequent chapters.

TABLE 31–1. High-Risk Criteria for Surgical Patients

Preoperative Patients

1. Previous severe cardiorespiratory illness (e.g., acute MI, COPD, stroke)
2. Extensive ablative surgery planned for carcinoma (e.g., esophagectomy and total gastrectomy, or prolonged surgery [>6 h])
3. Severe multiple trauma (e.g., involving more than three organs or more than two systems; opening of two body cavities [left side of chest and abdomen]; multiple long-bone and pelvic fractures)
4. Massive blood loss (>8 units): BV >1.5 L/m^2 and Hct >20 mL/dL within 48 h before admission
5. Age over 70 y and evidence of limited physiologic reserve of one or more vital organs
6. Shock: MAP <60 mm Hg; CVP <5 mm Hg; UO <20 mL/h; cold, clammy skin
7. Septicemia: positive blood culture, WBC count >12,000/mm^3, spiking fever > 101° F for 48 h, chills
8. Evidence of septic shock (temperature >101° F, WBC count >12,000/mm^3) plus hypotension (MAP <70 mm Hg)
9. Severe nutritional problems associated with a surgical illness: weight loss >20 lb, albumin concentration <3 g/dL, osmolarity <280 mOsm/L
10. Respiratory failure (e.g., Pa_{O_2}, <60 mm Hg or F_{IO_2} >0.4, Qsp/Qt >30%, patient on mechanical ventilation)
11. Acute abdominal catastrophe (e.g., pancreatitis, gangrenous bowel, peritonitis, perforated viscus, and internal gastrointestinal bleeding)
12. CVP >15 mm Hg after fluid resuscitation
13. Acute renal failure: blood urea nitrogen >50 mg/dL, creatinine >3 mg/dL, C_{H_2O} >10 mL/h
14. Acute hepatic failure (bilirubin >3 mg/dL, albumin concentration <3 g/dL, LDH >200U/mL, alkaline phosphatase >100 U/mL, ammonia >120 μg/mL
15. Acute agitation, depressed nervous system, semicoma, or coma

Postoperative Patients

1. Acute catastrophic change, suggesting fresh MI, pulmonary embolus, or postoperative bleeding
2. Hypotension: MAP <70 mm Hg or unstable vital signs
3. Operative misadventure: (e.g., use of <8 units of WB or PRBCs for estimated 4000-mL blood loss in the operating room)
4. Severe sepsis, perforated viscus, gangrenous bowel, peritonitis, pneumonia, positive blood culture, aspiration pneumonia, temperature elevation >101° F for >2 d
5. Any vital organ failure—that is, the same as 9 to 15 of the above list of preoperative conditions
6. Postoperative fluid-electrolyte problem requiring more than 5000 mL of fluids per day
7. Failure to respond to adequate volume therapy, which is replacement of blood losses estimated from sponge and lap counts and as judged by clinical criteria, such as arterial pressure, UO, Hct, level of consciousness, and motor responses

Abbreviations: MI = myocardial infarction; COPD = chronic obstructive pulmonary disease; BV = blood volume; Hct = hematocrit; MAP = mean arterial pressure, UO = urinary output; WBC = white blood cells; LDH = lactate dehydrogenase; WB = whole blood; PRBCs = packed red blood cells.

COMMONLY MONITORED PHYSIOLOGIC VARIABLES

Approximately 25 monitored variables are commonly used for evaluating critically ill and shock patients (Table 31–2). They vary from the vital sign measurements routinely used in all hospital admission departments to the invasive assessment of hemodynamic and oxygen transport variables. Normal values for commonly monitored variables are listed in Table 31–3.

TABLE 31–2. Monitored Physiologic Variables

1. Arterial blood pressure (systolic, diastolic, and mean)
2. Heart rate
3. Temperature
4. Hct and hemoglobin concentration
5. UO rate
6. ECG (see Chapter 32)
7. Serum electrolytes and blood chemistries
8. CVP
9. Arterial blood gases and pH (see Chapters 33 and 34)
10. Pulse oximetry
11. Transcutaneous oxygen and carbon dioxide tensions
12. Blood volume, plasma volume
13. Plasma colloidal osmotic pressure
14. Plasma and urine osmolality, osmolar and free-water clearances
15. Electroencephalogram (see Chapter 38)
16. Intracranial pressure (see Chapter 37)
17. Pulmonary arterial and precapillary wedge pressures
18. Cardiac output and hemodynamic variables
19. Oxygen transport variables
20. Continuous cardiac output and oxygen consumption measurements
21. Ventilatory monitoring (see Chapter 36)
22. Noninvasive cardiac output by ultrasound method
23. Noninvasive cardiac output by thoracic electrical bioimpedance
24. Multicomponent circulatory monitoring

TABLE 31–3. Normal Values for the Most Commonly Monitored Variables

Variable	*Normal Value*	*Units*
Arterial blood pressure	120/80	mm Hg
MAP	80–95	mm Hg
Heart rate	60–80	Beats/min^{1}
Temperature	36–37	degrees Celsius
Hct	42–45	%
Hemoglobin concentration	13–15	g/dL
CVP	−2 to + 6	mm Hg
UO	40–60	mL/h
BV		
Men	2.74	L/m^3
Women	2.37	L/m^2

Vital Signs

Arterial pressures, heart rate, temperature, and respiratory rate—the so-called "vital signs"—are the simplest, most easily measured and most commonly monitored noninvasive circulatory variables. They are useful for screening and are monitored during routine hospital and ICU admissions; physical examinations; daily nursing routines; and in preoperative, intraoperative, and postoperative patients. Vital signs are recorded more frequently during periods of circulatory instability to provide a running graphic record of a patient's condition and may alert attendants to unexpected circulatory problems.

Arterial Pressures

Arterial pressure reflects overall circulatory status but lacks diagnostic specificity. Arterial pressure falls after hypovolemia from blood or fluid loss; during cardiac failure, acute trauma, sepsis, anaphylactoid reactions, and vasovagal attacks; in the presence of neural (spinal cord) lesions; and in the late or terminal stage of most diseases. Decreased blood pressure indicates circulatory decompensation or the failure of a specific therapy; increased pressure may indicate improved circulatory function, adrenal stress response, or excessive vasopressor therapy.

Arterial pressure measurements do not directly reflect reductions of blood flow and volume but rather the failure of circulatory compensations such as the adrenal stress response to hypovolemia. The interactions of blood pressure, flow, and volume are extremely complex, and only the grossest aspects of circulatory status are reflected by serial blood pressure measurements. Arterial pressure measurements are useful for screening and for rapid assessment of trends in emergency conditions—especially trauma and gastrointestinal bleeding—but in and of themselves are of limited physiologic importance.

Normal arterial blood pressure measured with a sphygmomanometer cuff is approximately 120/80 mm Hg for healthy, young adults; this value increases gradually with age. As a rough estimate, the upper limit of normal for systolic pressures is 100 mm Hg plus the patient's age; systolic pressures greater than 160 mm Hg and diastolic pressures greater than 90 mm Hg suggest hypertension. Young adults (especially teenage girls) may normally have blood pressures as low as 90/60 mm Hg. It is important to know the patients' baseline, pre-illness pressures if those individuals whose normal pressures are not within the standard range are to be treated properly.

The pulse pressure is the difference between the systolic pressure and the diastolic pressure. A decreased pulse pressure may precede a decrease in diastolic pressure in a patient developing hypovolemic shock and is a clinical sign of hypovolemia.

Mean arterial pressure (MAP) is defined as the sum of the diastolic pressure and one third of the pulse pressure; alternatively, it may be expressed as one third of the sum of the systolic pressure and twice the diastolic pressure. MAP is also measured directly in various invasive and noninvasive recording systems as a dampened "electrical mean" of the systolic and diastolic pressures. MAP is frequently used in the calculation of derived hemodynamic variables, such as the systemic vascular (peripheral) resistance index, left ventricular stroke work index, and left cardiac work index.

Intra-Arterial Blood Pressure

Apparatuses for the invasive monitoring of blood pressure via the axillary, radial, ulnar, or femoral artery provide continuous display of the waveform along with measurements of systolic and diastolic pressures and of MAP. (The technique of catheter insertion, associated precautions, and its complications are discussed in Chapter 30; and calibration and zeroing and their problems and complications are presented in Chapter 32.)

Intra-arterial pressure measurement with a system consisting of intra-arterial catheters, pressure transducers, and a continuous recording apparatus that has been zeroed and calibrated is more accurate than cuff measurement of pressure. Under normal conditions, pressures obtained from intra-arterial catheters are about 2 to 8 mm Hg greater than cuff-measured pressures. In critically ill patients, intra-arterial pressures may be 10 to 30 mm Hg greater than cuff-measured pressures. Furthermore, cuff-measured pressures are often inaccurate in patients with severe vasoconstriction and low stroke volume. Differences of 50 to 60 mm Hg between intra-arterial catheter–measured and cuff-measured pressures have been reported. The indications for continuous invasive pressure recording are shock, critical illness, marked peripheral vasoconstriction; intraoperative and postoperative monitoring in patients undergoing extensive or life-threatening operations and in patients with other high-risk conditions is also indicated. In these cases, accurate continuous arterial pressure display is needed to observe trends and to titrate therapy. Moreover, arterial catheters allow frequent arterial blood gas measurements.[3]

Pressures should be measured in both arms early in a patient's hospital course because specific unilateral arteriosclerotic or traumatic vascular lesions may produce 10- to 20-mm Hg differences between the left- and right-sided values. Similarly, in trauma to the aorta or femoral artery, differences in cuff pressures between one leg or arm or the other may occur. Normally, the femoral arterial pressures are 5 to 10 mm Hg greater than brachial pressures.

Arterial pressure decreases occur during shock and trauma states; however, these decreases may be delayed and are nonspecific and poorly reflect deficits in blood volume or cardiac function. Pressures may be misleading in the face of falling blood volume and flow because compensatory adrenomedullary and other neurohormonal stress reactions tend to maintain blood pressure, at least transiently, in the face of declining blood flow. Arterial pressure decreases after the compensatory mechanisms are exhausted, but this may occur long after the precipitating event. Severely reduced cardiac output for periods of from 40 minutes to 2 hours before a significant reduction in arterial pressure has been demonstrated.[3, 4] On the other hand, arterial pressure may be restored by saline and other crystalloid solutions well before cardiac output and oxygen transport are corrected.[5]

Noninvasive Blood Pressure Monitoring

Manometric blood pressure measurements obtained with sphygmomanometry using the Korotkoff blood pressure sounds are routinely used to assess systolic and diastolic pressures. Initially, Dinamap (Critikon, Tampa, FL) measured only MAP, but current models display systolic, mean, and diastolic pressures. The instrument is sensitive to motion artifact, particularly muscular activity in the arm. This was the only available noninvasive method until 1970, when crystal microphones and piezoelectric crystals that employed the Doppler principle were developed. Subsequently, microprocessor-based devices such as Infrasonde (Puritan-Bennett, Carlsbad, CA) and Accutorr (Datascope, Paramus, NJ), which use an oscillometric method that automatically inflates and deflates the cuff, were developed. These systems improved sensitivity, particularly in patients with low pressures and low blood flow. The Infrasonde device is an auscultatory method for determining systolic and diastolic pressures. With its use, two crystal microphones are positioned over the bronchial artery; these microphones identify the Korotkoff blood pressure sounds. The cuff deflation rate can be selected by the operator.

The Finapres (Omeda, Denver, CO) has a small cuff that is placed over a finger. The cuff is connected to a very rapidly responding solenoid that inflates and deflates the cuff to keep the finger volume constant while the blood flow pulses increase and decrease the blood volume. In effect, the device tracks the MAP in the digital artery by nulling the pressure changes occurring under the finger cuff. The device displays a waveform that is based on the counterpressure needed to null the digital artery pressure.

Heart Rate

The indications for measuring heart rate are the same as those for determining arterial pressure. Arterial pressure and heart rate are routinely measured at the same time and graphically recorded daily or twice daily on the vital signs sheet of every hospitalized patient's chart or at more frequent intervals intraoperatively, for patients in the ICU, those receiving emergency services, and those in special care units. Heart rate is usually determined by manual palpation of the radial artery just above the wrist for at least 30 seconds. Tachycardia is defined as a heart rate greater than 100 beats per minute. When premature ventricular contractions or other irregularities are present, the heart rate may be determined by auscultation at the apex; the difference between apical and radial rates represents the number of dropped beats. Heart rates may also be measured automatically from either the ECG wave or the arterial pulse wave. In invasive hemodynamic monitoring, the heart rate is used to calculate stroke volume from cardiac output as well as other derived variables.

Heart rate is a nonspecific hemodynamic variable. Increased heart rate is part of an early neurohormonal stress response that also tends to increase flow in the presence of falling pressure. Its increase suggests blood flow and blood volume deficits; the faster the heart rate, the greater the hypovolemia or cardiac impairment. However, heart rate also increases with infection, anxiety, fear, fever, exercise, pain and discomfiture, and other nonspecific stresses.

Bradycardia, defined as a slow heart rate (<50 beats per minute) may occur with inferior myocardial infarction when right coronary artery occlusion produces ischemia that blocks the sinoatrial node; it also may occur with other types of arteriosclerotic heart disease. Bradycardia during low cardiac output is an ominous sign suggesting markedly reduced and inadequate coronary blood flow that compromises myocardial performance. Dysrhythmias associated with cardiac problems require that ECG and other methods be applied for specific diagnosis.

Temperature

Body temperature is measured routinely with the determination of blood pressure, pulse, and respirations. Usually, it is measured either orally (when significant elevations are not expected) or rectally (in ill patients). The central core temperature may be measured at the tympanic membrane or midesophagus for greater accuracy. Pulmonary arterial temperature, which also reflects core temperature, is routinely provided on a continuous basis by the pulmonary artery thermodilution catheter.

Temperature elevations are most often associated with infection, tissue necrosis, late-stage carcinomatosis, Hodgkin's disease, leukemia, hyperthyroidism, malignant hyperthermia, and other hypermetabolic states. Low-grade fever is also present after accidental or surgical trauma and particularly when hematomas, foreign bodies, fistulas, urinary extravasation, or stasis of urinary excretion or of bronchial secretions is present. Hypothermia may occur in some patients with septic shock, reduced metabolism associated with hypothyroidism, malnutrition, severe anemia, and cold exposure. Like arterial pressure and heart rate determination, temperature measurement is a useful but nonspecific screening test.

Hematocrit

The hematocrit, which is a measure of the percentage of red blood cells in a sample of venous blood, has been widely used to assess blood loss after trauma and surgery. In general, hematocrit values are decreased by hemorrhage and increased by dehydration and hypovolemia. The hematocrit is measured on the routine admission of patients as well as in patients with emergency conditions, including trauma and hemorrhage or suspected hemorrhage; fever, dehydration, or other water losses; suspected overtransfusion or overhydration; hemolysis, cell aggregation (sludging) and microthrombi; destruction of red blood cells subsequent to freshwater drowning, envenomation, consumption coagulopathies, and disseminated intravascular coagulation; in patients in postoperative states, especially when intraperitoneal bleeding is suspected; and in patients with acute illnesses, circulatory shock, and sepsis.

To measure hematocrit, blood samples are drawn from a peripheral vein or artery, immediately injected into four or more heparinized capillary tubes, and promptly spun for 4 minutes in a microcentrifuge. The results of replicate samples should agree to within 1%. Alternatively, 4 mL of blood is drawn into a syringe containing 0.1 mL heparin (1000 U/mL) and is immediately placed into a Wintrobe tube; the latter is centrifuged at 2000 *g* for 30 minutes. When blood is drawn for hematocrit measurement and allowed to stand for even brief periods, the red blood cells begin to settle, leaving the top half of the syringe with considerably fewer cells than the bottom half; shaking the sample does not completely eliminate this problem. However, errors of less than 1% can be obtained when the hematocrit tubes are filled immediately after the blood is drawn.

A decreased percentage of red blood cells is an indirect effect of blood loss produced by compensatory transcapillary refilling of plasma volume by interstitial water. This compensation takes a considerable amount of time to occur. If a patient rapidly exsanguinates within a few minutes, the first and the last drops of blood have nearly the same hematocrit.[6] However, a 500-mL blood loss in human volunteers is replaced by interstitial water over an 18-hour period.[6, 7] Replacement occurs at a rate of about 1 mL/min for the first few hours and thereafter at successively decreasing rates. In the severely bled anesthetized dog, replacement occurs at maximum rates of 2.5 mL/min.[8] For these reasons, serial hematocrits at 2- to 4-hour intervals are recorded in the early period of traumatic or postoperative shock when covert blood loss is suspected.

Decreases in serial hematocrits of postoperative and posttraumatic patients can signal the possibility of intra-abdominal hemorrhage, but such measurements are not specific and have severe limitations. Since the hematocrit represents a static measurement of red blood cell concentration in a sample of venous blood, it is affected by a gain or loss of plasma water as well as by a gain or loss of red blood cells. However, it cannot distinguish among the effects of fluids administered intravenously, of fluids leaking from the plasma into the interstitial space, of red blood cells being transfused, of red blood cells dropping out of the circulation via the formation of cell aggregates or microthrombi, and of newly synthesized red blood cells. Therefore, after a patient has been given large volumes of crystalloid and colloid solutions and transfusions, changes in hematocrit are often misleading and are difficult to interpret. Hematocrit determination may be a reasonably good screening test for assessing gross changes in the early stages of hemorrhage, but it does not reliably estimate the subsequent blood volume status.[9]

Urine Output Rate

The rate of urine output is easily measured after bladder catheterization, preferably with a Foley catheter. The urine may be collected in a closed sterile system, and the output is usually recorded hourly. The catheter must be flushed with aseptic solution at regular intervals, since the most common cause of low urine output or anuria in the hospitalized patient is a plugged catheter.

The hourly rate of urine output obtained with the use of an indwelling urethral catheter is a rough approximation of the perfusion to this one vital organ, provided that the patient has an adequate blood volume and no preexisting renal disease. In resuscitation from acute injury, decreased urine flow may reflect low blood volume, poor perfusion of the kidney, or the onset of acute renal failure. However, urine output is not an adequate reflection of tissue perfusion in shock states; we have documented good urine output up to the hour of death in patients with severe septic shock. Other, more precise measures of renal function, such as creatinine, osmolar, and free water clearances, are discussed later in this chapter.

Electrocardiographic Monitoring

The ECG measures voltages at the body surface and is used to assess the electromechanical events of cardiac contraction. Early studies assumed the body to be a homogenous volume conductor with uniform geometry similar to a tank of saline to accommodate the complexities of the three-dimensional character of the body and the varying distances of the heart from the recording electrodes. This assumption has led to a large body of information on the electrophysiology of the heart. In one model, the heart is represented by two charged electrodes: a dipole with one positive pole and one negative pole. The Dutch physiologist Einthoven surrounded this dipole with a hypothetic equilateral triangle. The electrical activity of the heart, represented by the equivalent dipole, changes its magnitude and orientation during the cardiac cycle. The sides of the triangle, which represent the axes of the three standard limb leads, provide a triaxial frame of reference for presenting spatial orientation of the magnitude and the direction of cardiac electrical activity. When combined with the chest (V lead) readings, the model can be further refined to have frontal, sagittal, and horizontal components (see Chapters 32 and 54).

The standard three-lead ECG is recorded from the right arm (RA), left arm (LA), and left leg (LL). The standard limb leads are defined as lead I (LA-RA), lead II (LL-RA), and lead III (LL-LA), where differences in electrical potential produced by the heart are measured across the designated limbs. Small electrodes corresponding to each lead are attached to the chest after application of a conductive salt paste to the skin. These electrodes pick up ECG waveforms, which are continuously displayed and, when desired, recorded on a permanent record at the patient's bedside and at a central monitor station. A 12-lead ECG is essential in the cardiac patient and is useful to rule out cardiac complications in the acutely injured patient, the postoperative patient, and the patient with sepsis. Frequently, lead II or other individual leads may be continuously monitored for arrhythmias.

The 12-lead ECG pattern is specific for diagnosis of cardiac conditions, and continuous ECG display of lead II waveform provides the earliest indication of electrical changes associated with disorders of the cardiac muscle. Continuous ECG monitoring is essential for the patient with acute myocardial infarction because arrhythmias are the most common life-threatening complications. Although done routinely, continuous ECG monitoring of the postoperative general surgical patient is rarely useful, since the incidence of significant arrhythmias is rather low; the authors have found three acute myocardial infarctions after 8000 operations in a county hospital setting. The ECG is probably overused and overemphasized in patients with noncardiac general surgical conditions.[10] Nevertheless, in hypovolemic and traumatic shock, arrhythmias, signs of subendocardial ischemias, and bradycardia occur with inadequate oxygen delivery to the myocardium and may suggest a precardiac arrest state (see Chapter 54).

Assessment of Serum Electrolytes and Blood Chemistries

In acute illness, accidents, and other emergencies, serum sodium, potassium, and chlorine ions, blood glucose, lactate, blood urea nitrogen, and creatinine measurements are routinely taken. Testing of these biochemical indicators confirms or rules out various diagnoses, monitors the progress of various disease states, and assesses the efficacy of therapy in acute, rapidly progressive illnesses. Measurement of serum electrolyte levels are particularly important in patients with arrhythmias from hypokalemia associated with alkalosis from gastric outlet obstruction and other gastrointestinal conditions that produce severe vomiting; hyperkalemia associated with acidosis; hyperglycemia associated with diabetes, stress, trauma and head injury; hypoglycemia associated with insulin reactions, insulinoma, or nutritional deficiency; lactacidemia associated with low cardiac output, hypovolemia for cardiogenic shock; and increasing levels of blood urea nitrogen and creatinine associated with renal failure.

Acidosis characterized by pH <7.2, anion gap of >8 mEq/L, gastric mucosal pH <7.2, measurement of blood lactate levels, and determination of ratios of lactate to pyruvate confirm the presence of anaerobic metabolism, which is usually caused by reduced tissue P_{O_2} due to low flow states and inadequate tissue perfusion as well as metabolic and nutritional disorders. However, in patients in most postoperative and post-traumatic states with predominantly high blood flows, death is more often due to respiratory failure, sepsis, renal failure, disseminated intravascular coagulation, and hepatic failure than to a reduction in blood flow. Under these conditions, lactate values are not as helpful in relating the severity of illness to morbidity and mortality.

Prothrombin time, partial thromboplastin time, fibrinogen determination, fibrin split product, and platelet counts are used to monitor acute bleeding and clotting problems associated with shock, sepsis, trauma, and hemorrhage.

Central Venous Pressure

Following the classic and definitive work on venous pressures by Landis and Hortenstine,[11] Hughes and Magovern[12] used right atrial pressure monitoring to guide blood volume replacement in patients who had undergone thoracotomy. Wilson and coworkers[13] developed the CVP catheters that were eventually widely used for both medical and general surgical patients. Because of its simplicity and availability, CVP monitoring is routinely used to guide fluid therapy after hemorrhage and accidental and surgical trauma, in sepsis, and in emergency conditions associated with blood volume deficits. The catheters are simple to place, and the pressures are easy to read. The most important problem in accurately measuring CVP is the establishment of a consistent "zero" point that can permit meaningful changes to be measured by different individuals on different shifts. The point selected may be marked on the patient's side with a felt-tip pen. A point located 10 cm above the lowest surface of the back or 10 cm below the sternum in the sixth interspace in the supine position represents the point of entrance of the vena cava into the right atrium. The pressure transducer should be moved up or down to this level as the bed is raised or lowered or corrected electronically.

The average CPV values during normal inspiration and expiration in healthy persons are −2 and +6 mm Hg, respectively. A healthy, ambulatory person who is lying down may have CVP values that average about 6 to 8 mm Hg; as the vascular tree accommodates, the CVP values gradually decrease. Eight to 10 mm Hg is commonly used as the upper limit of normal for acutely ill patients. However, critically ill patients receiving mechanical ventilation and positive end-expiratory pressure, who require fluid volume to maintain arterial pressure, may develop CVP values of 20 mm Hg or greater. When CVP values exceed 15 to 18 mm Hg, a pulmonary arterial balloon flotation catheter may be used to measure the pulmonary artery wedge pressure for more precise titration of fluid administration.

Central venous pressure is affected by blood volume, venous wall compliance, right cardiac function, and intrathoracic pressure. Large fluid infusions may produce only small transient CVP changes in hypovolemic patients, but increased blood volume elevates CVP in the overtransfused or stressed patient. Fluid administration may rapidly increase CVP in patients with chronic congestive cardiac failure. Although CVP is low during and immediately after acute hemorrhage, after a patient has remained a day or so in the ICU, his or her blood volume and CVP correlate poorly because of changes in venous wall compliance, despite the presence of major deficits or excesses in blood volume (Figs. 31–1 and 31–2). It is incorrect to assess blood volume status from CVP because the correlation between CVP and blood volume according to conventional thinking is overly simplistic. Many factors influence the CVP values,

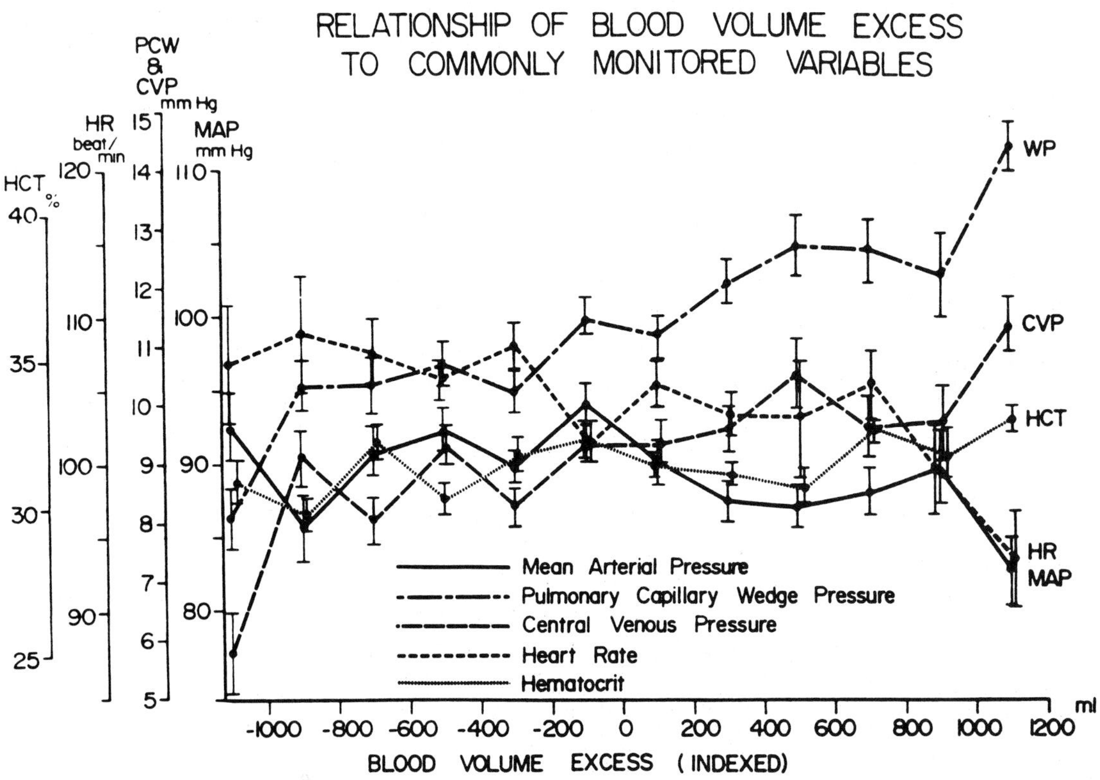

Figure 31–1. Mean ± SEM of the commonly monitored variables on the *y*-axis plotted against their corresponding blood volume excess (+) or deficit (−) indexed. Note the poor capacity of the monitored variables to predict blood volume. (From Shippy CR, Appel PL, Shoemaker WC: Reliability of clinical monitoring to assess blood volume in critically ill patients. Crit Care Med 1984; 12:107.)

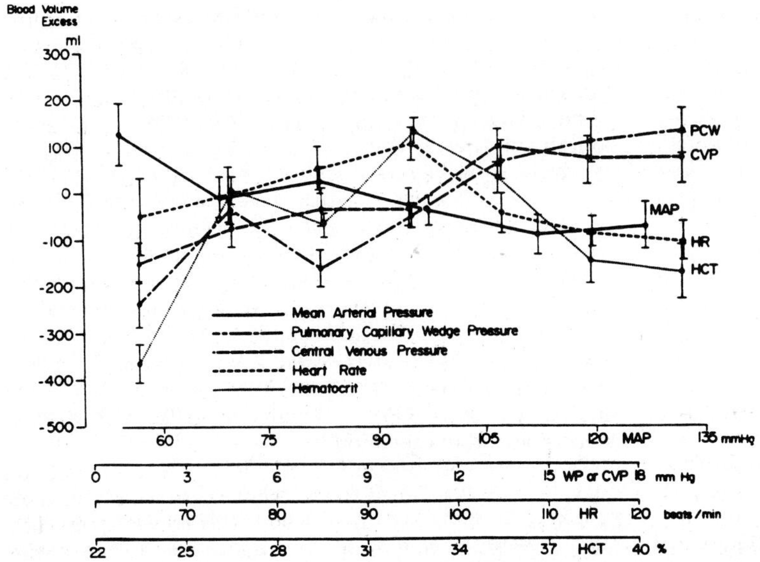

Figure 31–2. Mean ± SEM values of blood volume excess (+) or deficit (−) index on the *y*-axis plotted against their corresponding monitored variables. Note the poor capacity of the blood volume values to predict monitored variables. (From Shippy CR, Appel PL, Shoemaker WC: Reliability of clinical monitoring to assess blood volume in critically ill patients. Crit Care Med 1984; 12:107.)

not the least of which are cardiac performance, blood volume, vascular tone, intrinsic venous tone, increased intra-abdominal or intrathoracic pressures, and vasopressor therapy. Artifacts can be caused by catheter obstruction, motion, and elevation or by lowering of the bed without the making of corresponding changes to the transducer. Obvious errors can be made in establishing a constant baseline in the patient who must be frequently repositioned and whose bed must be lowered or elevated. Methods for placing CVP lines and other vascular access problems are covered in Chapter 30.

Patients with right-sided heart failure classically have distention of the neck veins that reflects increased CVP. In many instances, right-sided heart failure is secondary to left-sided heart failure; in such cases, left atrial, end-diastolic, and, subsequently, pulmonary artery (PA) pressures rise; PA pressure elevations increase the work of the right side of the heart. If the PA systolic pressure is less than 40 mm Hg in chronic conditions, the right ventricle usually maintains normal flow. However, with prolonged elevation of PA pressure, the right ventricle may fail, and CVP can increase. Less commonly, right-sided heart failure occurs with right myocardial infarction and without left-sided heart failure, particularly in patients with pulmonary hypertension. Also, right-sided heart failure may occur in the presence of high pulmonary vascular resistance caused by pulmonary emboli, chronic obstructive lung disease, adult respiratory distress syndrome, and other types of respiratory failure. Wide variation in the CVP may occur (1) if the central line slips into the right ventricle, (2) in severe right-sided heart failure and dilation of the atrioventricular ring, and (3) in cases of tricuspid insufficiency.

CVP measurements are most useful during early resuscitation from acute injury with hypotension; initially, hypovolemia occurs with low CVP. A CVP in excess of 20 to 25 mm Hg usually indicates that too much fluid has been given, that fluids were given too rapidly, or that an exaggerated stress response has occurred. Knowledge of CVP is most helpful when failure of only one organ system has occurred (such as in cardiac failure or uncomplicated blood loss). Increases in CVP or wedge pressures in response to administration of a standardized volume load over a prescribed time period can serve as valuable information; tolerance of a volume load or fluid challenge indicates that the heart and vascular tree have an adequate reserve capacity.

Peripheral venous pressures usually reflect CVP when they are in the high ranges, but measurements of these pressures diverge in the low ranges. The central venous system, including the right atrium, the vena cava, and its major branches act as a unicameral system with nearly equal pressures. In hypovolemia, the extent of the unicameral behavior of the system is limited, and the peripheral venous pressures largely reflect local influences upstream from their site of measurement. By contrast, in the hypervolemic state and in right-sided heart failure, the venous tree is distended by the accumulation of blood behind the right ventricle; as this venous engorgement increases, the dimensions of the unicameral venous tree with respect to pressure measurements also increase. Under such conditions, high peripheral venous pressure values closely correlate with high CVP values.

Arterial Blood Gases and pH

Measurements of arterial blood gases and pH are useful for screening pulmonary function in critically ill patients (Table 31–4). They are essential in patients with respiratory illness and are indicated in the initial evaluation and work-up of patients who have a variety of conditions,[14] including tachypnea, dyspnea, chronic obstructive pulmonary disease, and adult respiratory distress syndrome; of those who have experienced accidental trauma, acute emergency conditions,

TABLE 31–4. Blood Gas Variables, Abbreviations, and Normal Values on Room Air (FIO_2-0.21)

Arterial oxygen tension (PaO_2), 80–95 mm Hg
Mixed venous oxygen tension ($P\bar{v}O_2$), 35–50 mm Hg
Arterial oxygen saturation (SaO_2), 96–99%
Arterial oxygen concentration (CaO_2), 17–20 mL/dL
Mixed venous oxygen concentration ($C\bar{v}O_2$), 12–15 mL/dL
Arteriovenous oxygen difference ($C(a - v)O_2$), 4–5 mL/dL
Arterial carbon dioxide tension ($PaCO_2$), 35–45 mm Hg
Arterial carbon dioxide concentration ($CaCO_2$), 23–27 mmol/L
Mixed venous carbon dioxide tension ($P\bar{v}CO_2$), 40–45 mm Hg
pH, 7.36–7.44
Bicarbonate (HCO_3), 22–28 mEq/L
Base excess or deficit, +3 to −3 mEq/L

extensive surgery, burns and smoke inhalation, and other catastrophic conditions; of patients receiving controlled or assisted ventilation or oxygen therapy; of critically ill patients suspected of having respiratory complications; in preoperative evaluation and postanesthesia surveillance; of patients with fluid and electrolyte problems; of those with restlessness, anxiety or mental confusion; of those who have drug overdose; and of patients with altered mental status or who fail to respond after anesthesia (see Chapter 33).

The first laboratory signs of early lung problems are usually arterial blood gas abnormalities, such as arterial partial pressure of oxygen (PaO_2) values less than 70 mm Hg (arterial hemoglobin saturation [SaO_2] <90%) in the patient breathing room air (fraction of inspired oxygen = [FIO_2] 0.2), arterial partial pressure of carbon dioxide ($PaCO_2$) values greater than 45 mm Hg, and pH values less than 7.3 or greater than 7.5. Respiratory failure is suggested by PaO_2 values less than 50 mm Hg in the patient breathing room air or a PaO_2/FIO_2 less than 250. Usually, the acutely ill patient is given supplementary oxygen by mask or nasal prongs as well as chest therapy. If these measures do not improve the blood gas values, endotracheal intubation and mechanical ventilation should be considered before PaO_2 drops to less than 60 mm Hg. However, patients with chronic respiratory insufficiency may tolerate very low blood gas values and not require mechanical ventilation (see Chapter 33).

Pulse Oximetry

The development of microprocessors and light-emitting diodes has made continuous noninvasive monitoring of arterial oxygenation a routine monitoring method. In this technique, a red diode and an infrared diode are rapidly pulsed in sequence, and the amounts of light transmitted by each during successive heart beats are compared to calculate SaO_2. Continuously measured SaO_2 values are then used to calculate a running average that is then displayed continuously on a monitoring screen.

The oximeter is designed to measure differences in the SaO_2 pulse waveform; thus, without a good waveform, the instrument cannot function accurately. Moreover, it does not distinguish oxyhemoglobin level from the level of carboxyhemoglobin or that of methemoglobin; knowledge of the latter is needed in patients who have been exposed to carbon monoxide.

Pulse oximeters have been shown to be useful during initial resuscitation of trauma patients and of those who have experienced other acute emergencies, during anesthesia, and in critically ill patients with unstable hemodynamics or suspected respiratory problems. These instruments are particularly useful for titration of FIO_2 during mechanical ventilation and during weaning of patients from mechanical ventilation. The frequency of arterial blood gas measurement may be reduced with the use of pulse oximetry. This is important in children and in those with acute, rapidly changing critical illnesses. Disposable probes are used in patients with infectious conditions.

Transcutaneous Oxygen and Carbon Dioxide Monitoring

Clark[15] developed the first practical polarographic electrode in 1956 using a semipermeable polyethylene membrane-covered platinum cathode. This rapidly became the standard for blood gas analysis. Subsequently, Hüch and associates[16] and Eberhard and colleagues[17] described the use of heated Clark electrodes for continuous noninvasive transcutaneous oxygen tension ($PtcO_2$) measurement. Initially, this technique was used as a substitute for PaO_2 determination in neonates to reduce the need for arterial blood sampling, and it was based on the assumption that PaO_2 and $PtcO_2$ were identical or nearly identical to their arterial blood measurements. When differences between the two measurements occurred, they were usually attributed to failure of the $PtcO_2$-measuring instrument. Although $PtcO_2$ usually reflected PaO_2 when the neonate was hemodynamically stable, it was appreciably lower than PaO_2 in the seriously ill neonate with circulatory problems.

In adults, $PtcO_2$ is usually about 80% of the value for PaO_2 during stable or normal hemodynamic conditions[18]; however, when blood flow rate limits body metabolism, $PtcO_2$ tracks flow. In both normal and low-flow states, $PtcO_2$ was used to track oxygen delivery ($\dot{D}O_2$). In essence, $PtcO_2$ is only indirectly related to PaO_2; it is directly related to local tissue perfusion and oxygenation.[19]

The heating of the skin by the transcutaneous electrode changes the structure of the lipoproteins in the stratum corneum from the gel to the sol state. This allows rapid diffusion of oxygen from subcutaneous tissues to the surface electrode. However, the heating affects tissue and blood by decreasing oxygen solubility, shifting the oxyhemoglobin dissociation curve to the right and dilating the local metarterioles. An electrode temperature of 44°C to 45°C allows the $PtcO_2$ to approach PaO_2 in hemodynamically stable patients.[19]

Since $PtcO_2$ values are dependent on both PaO_2 and local blood flow (or local $\dot{D}O_2$), $PtcO_2$ is used to track PaO_2 when flow is adequate and to track flow or $\dot{D}O_2$ when PaO_2 is adequate. In either case, $PtcO_2$ reflects local $\dot{D}O_2$. For example, when the normovolemic patient develops respiratory failure, changes in $PtcO_2$ correspond to those in PaO_2; however, when low-flow circulatory problems develop, $PtcO_2$ values fall markedly below PaO_2 values. From a practical clinical viewpoint, the patterns of the two variables reliably reflect tissue perfusion and tissue oxygenation when used for screening.[19] $PtcO_2$ values greater than 65 mm Hg suggest satisfactory perfusion; values from 40 to 65 mm Hg suggest marginal perfusion; values from 25 to 40 mm Hg suggest impaired tissue perfusion; and values less than 25 mm Hg indicate severe shock.[20]

Measurement of $PtcO_2$ is useful in the management of trauma and other emergency conditions immediately after hospital admission, in the perioperative and postanesthesia period, and in the ICU. Since it measures tissue perfusion, it is an important part of multicomponent noninvasive monitoring systems.[20]

Transcutaneous carbon dioxide tension ($PtcCO_2$) measurement based on the use of the Stowe-Severinghaus carbon dioxide electrode[21] was initially used in neonates to approximate $PaCO_2$. However, the $PtcCO_2$ values parallel but consistently overestimate by 10 to 30 mm Hg the $PaCO_2$ values in both hemodynamically stable neonates and adults.[21]

In shock, $PtcCO_2$ may be greatly elevated to values as high as 100 mm Hg; it is inversely related to cardiac output.[21] Differences between the value of $PaCO_2$ and $PtcCO_2$ reflect accumulation of carbon dioxide in the tissues due to inadequate perfusion and indirectly reflect peripheral perfusion in shock states.

Blood Volume Measurement

Commonly, blood volume is inferred indirectly from measurements of arterial pressure, heart rate, CVP, pulmonary artery occlusion pressure (PAOP), urinary output, and hematocrit. These may be useful during resuscitation of patients who are not very ill; however, they are notably unreliable indicators of blood volume in the critically ill shock patient (see Figs. 31–1 and 31–2). Blood volume measurements that provide definitive answers to the problem of hypovolemia and hypervolemia have largely been replaced by PAOP (wedge pressure) measurements because of the hazards of radioactivity, the time required for measurement, and the cost associated with the measurement of blood volume.

Blood volume measurement is based on a very simple concept: a known amount of a marker or indicator that mixes uniformly with the plasma or blood is injected intravenously, and its concentration or radioactivity is measured in blood samples obtained at timed intervals after injection of the indicator.[9, 22, 23] The concentration of the indicator is inversely proportional to its volume of dilution; the latter is calculated by the standard dilution formula, $C_1V_1 = C_2V_2$, where C_1 and V_2 are the concentration and volume, respectively (i.e., mass of the injected indicator), and C_2 and V_2 are the concentration and volume of the indicator in its volume of distribution at the time of sampling.

Plasma volume was first measured with photometric assay of dyes, such as Evans blue (T1824), that are initially distributed in the plasma volume. This technique has been replaced by radioassay of isotopic iodine–labeled human serum albumin and, to a much lesser extent, by ^{55}Cr-labeled or ^{32}P-labeled erythrocyte assay. The ^{125}I-tagged or ^{131}I-tagged albumin is available and convenient, but red blood cell labels are usually reserved for various research studies.[26] For labeled albumin studies, serum or plasma samples are radioassayed in duplicate for two or more preinjection control samples and for three to six timed postinjection samples; 4% corrections are made for the packing fraction of plasma in the hematocrit measurements, and 6% corrections are made for the difference between venous hematocrit and total body hematocrit.[24–26]

Normal blood volume is 2.74 L/m^2 or 7.5 mL/kg for males, and 2.37 L/m^2 or 7 mL/kg for females. The patient in shock due to hemorrhage, trauma, and sepsis has been found empirically to do better with about 500 mL in excess of the expected norm (i.e., 3.2 L/m^2 for males and 2.9 L/m^2 for females). The extra volume compensates for maldistributions of blood volume, pooling of blood in the splanchnic area, red blood cell aggregation in the microcirculation, and red blood cell microthrombi. Accurate measurements require meticulous isotope dilution to obtain reproducible measurements with an acceptable error of from 8% to 10%.

Blood volume, cardiac functional capacity, and colloidal osmotic pressure (COP) are of major importance in fluid therapy.[5–9, 22, 23] Hypovolemic patients with normal cardiac reserve can readily tolerate volume load (fluid challenge); those with low colloidal osmotic pressure, cardiac problems, and chronic respiratory conditions are less able to tolerate infusion of large volumes of crystalloid solutions without developing pulmonary edema and other complications.

Colloidal Osmotic Pressure

The plasma and interstitial fluids are two aqueous bodies separated by the capillary basement membrane. The latter is a semipermeable membrane that is freely permeable to water and electrolytes but barely permeable to high-molecular-weight compounds such as plasma proteins. Similarly, the cell membrane separates the intracellular water and extracellular water. Water migrates through each membrane to equalize the concentrations of the solutions on either side by a process called *osmosis.* The colloidal osmotic pressure, or oncotic pressure, is the osmotic force exerted on a membrane by macromolecules. It is a measure of the hydrostatic pressure applied to a solution of greater concentration that is just able to prevent the net movement of water across the membrane. Colloidal osmotic pressure, like osmotic pressure, is determined solely by the number of molecules in solution on each side of the membrane.

Normally, plasma water escapes from the vascular space at the arterial end of the capillary, where hydrostatic pressure is greatest. Water returns at the venous end because venous colloid osmotic pressure is greater than that of the interstitial water. It is estimated that the equivalent of the plasma volume (i.e., 3000 mL in the healthy 70-kg man) leaves and returns to the vascular space each minute. By contrast, about 1% of the plasma proteins, mainly albumin, also leave the vascular space per minute, but most of these proteins are returned by way of the lymphatics. About one third of the plasma water may be outside the anatomic confines of the vasculature at any given time. After hemorrhage, capillary refilling of the plasma volume occurs primarily as a result of these osmotic forces.[26]

The distribution of water between the intravascular and interstitial compartments of the systemic circulation depends on the balance of forces described by Starling.[27] The hydrostatic pressures at the arterial end of the capillary are approximately 25 to 35 mm Hg, the tissue pressure—from −2 to +2 mm Hg, the capillary venous pressures—from 10 to 15 mm Hg, the venous oncotic pressures—from 24 to 28 mm Hg, and the interstitial oncotic pressure—about 15 to 20 mm Hg. Normally, the forces that determine net water movement across a capillary are close to zero or slightly negative; excess water driven into the tissues by this low net pressure is returned to the vascular space by the lymphatics. Two to four liters of lymph are returned to the circulation via the thoracic duct each day.

Measurement of Plasma and Urine Osmolality and of Osmolar and Free-Water Clearances

The ability of the kidney to concentrate urine is its most sensitive and important function. This capacity, which conventionally has been inferred from urine output rates and specific gravity, is best evaluated by measurements of the ratio of the osmolalities of urine and plasma (Uosm:Posm) or by determinations of osmolar and free-water clearances. Although Uosm:Posm greater than 1.7 suggests good concentrative ability, in the presence of oliguria, this ratio may be normal even when osmolar clearance is low. Renal function is better evaluated by determination of osmolar clearances, which express the rate of solute removal from the plasma; normally, the osmolar clearance is 120 mL/h, but it is markedly decreased in acute renal failure.

Free-water clearance, which more explicitly considers osmotic clearance with respect to the rate of urinary output, is a more sensitive indicator that may be used to predict the early onset of postoperative acute renal failure. Normally, it is strongly negative, ranging from −25 to −100 mL/h. Transient positive values followed by values close to zero precede the development of acute renal failure. For example, a patient with urine osmolality of 330 mOsm/L, plasma osmolality of 300 mOsm/L, and urine output of 100 mL/h has a relatively normal osmolar clearance (110 mL/h); however, the high free-water clearance (10 mL/h) indicates high-output renal failure.

Osmolality of both plasma and urine is easily measured by using the freezing point depression method (with a Fiske osmometer) or the vapor pressure method. Uosm:Posm is readily calculated from these two measurements. If the rate of urinary output (V) is also measured with the same specimen, the osmolar clearance (Cosm) is

$$\text{Cosm} = \frac{\text{Uosm}}{\text{Posm}} \times \text{V},$$

and the free-water clearance is C_{H_2O} = V − Cosm.

Electroencephalography

Electroencephalography may be used to diagnose and evaluate noninvasive neural function intraoperatively and in critically ill patients with possible central nervous system deficits. It may be used to evaluate and localize cerebral lesions in patients with craniocerebral injuries or other acute neurologic problems. Continuous electroencephalographic monitoring is occasionally used to evaluate cerebral perfusion during the administration of anesthetics as well as during open heart surgery, carotid endarterectomy, cerebrovascular surgery, epilepsy surgery, and induced hypotension for various surgical procedures (see Chapter 38).

Intracranial Pressure Measurement

Cerebral edema rapidly increases intracranial pressures because the brain, unlike other organs, is rigidly confined within the skull. Even small amounts of swelling may displace part of the 120 to 150 mL of cerebrospinal fluid and can result in high tissue pressures, headache, loss of consciousness, coma, and brain death. Increased intracerebral pressures are most frequently seen after closed head injury, intracranial operations, subarachnoid hemorrhage or other vascular accidents as well as in patients with Reye's syndrome, brain tumor, meningitis, and encephalitis.

Continuous intracranial pressure measurement and recording can be obtained with hollow, fluid-filled Richmond screw placed in the subdural space or with a cannula placed in the lateral ventricle. Both the screw and the cannula are inserted through small burr holes made in the parietal region of the calvarium after local anesthesia with 1% or 2% lidocaine has been induced; the nondominant hemisphere usually is selected. The Richmond screw may be placed just beneath the dura; the screw or cannula sensor is attached to a conventional pressure transducer and recording system for measurement, graphic display, and recording of intracranial pressures. The intraventricular cannula is more accurate and less likely to become dampened than is the screw. Cerebrospinal fluid may be withdrawn for culture and chemical analyses or drained during periods of intracranial hypertension (see Chapter 37).

Pulmonary Artery and Precapillary Wedge Pressure Measurement

The balloon-tipped, flow-directed PA (Swan-Ganz) catheter is commonly used to measure PA pressures and PAOP as a means to assess left ventricular filling pressures; this is analogous to the use of CVP values to assess right ventricular filling pressure.[28, 29] The PA catheter is frequently used to differentiate acute cardiac failure from fluid volume problems.[30] It is also used with cardiac output and oxygen transport measurements to monitor the progress of therapy in patients with acute myocardial infarction or other types of cardiac problems, shock, trauma, or other critical illnesses in which the fluid and circulatory status is uncertain. For example, in acute myocardial infarction, the expected hemodynamic pattern is hypotension, low cardiac output, and increased ventricular filling pressure (i.e., PAOP), usually in combination with decreased ventricular contractility and compliance. Monitoring PA pressure and PAOP is indicated to observe the progress of the disease and to titrate various therapeutic interventions.

In normal conditions, left atrial pressure is within 2 or 3 mm Hg of right atrial pressure; but in the higher ranges or in patients with valvular lesions, the mean left atrial pressure or PAOP may be higher than the right atrial pressure or CVP. Marked disparities occur between venous inflow pressures when ventricular disease is predominantly on one side of the heart and when pulmonary vascular resistance is elevated during acute postoperative respiratory failure. Otherwise, PAOP is affected by most of the factors that influence CVP—that is, blood volume, ventricular function, intrathoracic pressures, abdominal distention, and vasopressors—as well as by conditions that may increase afterload.

PA hypotension is frequently seen in hypovolemic shock, but PA hypertension may occur in patients after rapid fluid resuscitation for hypovolemic and traumatic shock as well as in those with congenital intra-atrial and intraventricular defects, chronic obstructive lung disease, and primary pulmonary hypertension. Relatively transient increases in PA pressure usually accompany fluid and transfusion therapy in various shock syndromes.

The PAOP closely parallels left atrial and left ventricular end-diastolic pressures unless significant mitral valve stenosis or pulmonary venous resistance exists (as may be seen in chronic obstructive pulmonary disease patients). In mitral stenosis, high PAOP cannot be taken to mean that left ventricular filling is adequate because of increased pressure gradients across the mitral valve. During and after mitral and aortic valve replacement, left ventricular filling pressures may be measured by using left atrial pressures obtained via a left atrial catheter placed intraoperatively.

PAOP is not a reliable measure of blood volume (see Figs. 31–1 and 31–2).[9] Commonly, in ICU conditions the tone of the pulmonary venous wall accommodates to blood volume deficits or excesses; the CVP and PAOP usually settle to around 8 to 12 mm Hg in patients with either hypovolemia or hypervolemia. Sudden increases in the PAOP to greater than 20 mm Hg may be due to infusion of too much intravenous fluid too rapidly, to inadequate left ventricular contractility, and to high positive end-expiratory pressure or intrathoracic pressure.

Insertion of Pulmonary Artery Balloon Flotation Catheters

The PA balloon flotation catheter is a 100-cm double-, triple-, or quadruple-lumen catheter. In its simplest form, it consists of an inflatable balloon connected to the tip of the catheter's smaller (minor) lumen. The balloon may be inflated with 0.5 to 0.8 mL of air (not water), introduced with a 1- or 2-mL syringe attached to the minor lumen that is suitably marked by a red-handled, on-off valve. The bursting volume of the balloon is less than 3 mL. The major or distal lumen, which terminates at the tip, should be filled with saline before insertion to avoid the small air embolus produced by infusion of fluid into an "empty" catheter.

The quadruple-lumen PA cardiac output catheter has a yellow distal port that is used to withdraw blood samples and to record PA and PAOP measurements; the proximal blue port is for injection of iced glucose solution for cardiac output measurements.[28–30] The quadruple-lumen catheter includes a thermodilution system for cardiac output measurements and pacing electrodes.

The catheter is introduced into the subclavian, jugular, brachial, or femoral vein by percutaneous puncture or; if this is not possible, it can be introduced by cutdown on a suitably sized vein in the antecubital fossa, saphenous system or in another accessible site (see Chapter 30). If the subclavian vein is used, the catheter is advanced centrally about 40 cm (indicated by the markings on the side of the catheter); the hub of the catheter is connected to a suitable pressure transducer and recording device. At this point, the patient is asked to take a deep breath or to cough; sizeable pressure oscillations indicate that the tip of the catheter is in the vena cava. Next, 0.05 to 0.8 mL of air is introduced into the minor lumen, and the catheter is further advanced gently while the attending physician views the pressure waveform. The bloodstream usually carries the catheter into the right atrium, where the atrial A and V waves may be seen (Fig. 31–3). As the catheter is cautiously advanced, the characteristic right ventricular pulse waves become visible. The systolic pressure usually ranges from 20 to 30 mm Hg; the diastolic pressure reading is very close to the CVP or right atrial pressure. As the catheter is advanced further, high-frequency oscillations ("ringing") indicate passage of the catheter's tip through the pulmonary valve and into the PA. At this point, the pulmonary systolic pressure is the same as that of the right ventricle, but the pulmonary diastolic pressure is considerably greater than the right ventricular diastolic pressure.

The inflated balloon is advanced until it reaches a PA branch. The balloon is deflated by removing the syringe; the barrel of the syringe is *not* withdrawn because the thin balloon might be sucked into one of the ports and rupture. When the balloon is gradually reinflated, the pressure at the catheter's tip falls, and the pulse wave dampens; this plateau is called the *wedge pressure* because of its similarity to the pressure obtained when an ordinary cardiac catheter is "wedged" into a small PA branch. The assumption is that a static, nonflowing column of blood that extends from the catheter's lumen to the pulmonary arterioles, capillaries, and veins of the lung segment provides a measure of the pressure downstream from the catheter tip and approximates the pulmonary venous and left atrial pressures.[28–30] For a detailed description of catheter insertion and its complications, see Chapter 30).

Complications of cardiac catheterization include pulmonary infarction, small pulmonary embolus formation, rupture of a branch of the PA, pneumothorax, arteriovenous fistula formation, kinking or looping of the catheter in the right ventricle, knotting of the catheter, arrhythmias, infection, bacterial colonization on the catheter wall, and bleeding from the site of insertion.

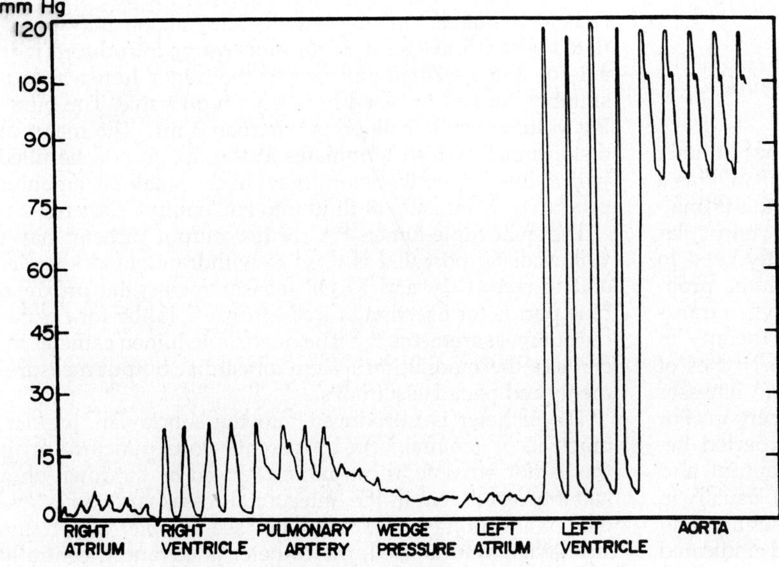

Figure 31–3. Intravascular pressure measurements at various segments of the vascular system, showing the general pattern of the various pressure waveforms from the right atrium, right ventricle, pulmonary artery and, with the inflation of the balloon, wedge pressures; left atrial, left ventricular, and aortic pressure waveforms are then shown.

Cardiac Output and Hemodynamic Variables

The most important aspects of the hemodynamic system are blood pressure, blood volume, and blood flow. Their measurements are easy to make, readily automated, simple in concept, relatively straightforward as a technique, and may be performed by nurses and medical technologists. The rate of blood flow pumped by the heart is measured as cardiac output and is usually expressed as the *cardiac index.* All volume and flow measurements should be indexed by dividing them by the patient's body surface area or weight; this normalization allows comparison of the hemodynamic values of patients with widely varying size and body habitus. The various hemodynamic variables may be calculated from pressure and flow data, using standard formulas (Table 31–5).

In 1887, Fick postulated that if the oxygen content of arterial (Ca_{O_2}) and of mixed venous ($C\bar{v}_{O_2}$) blood were known in addition to the oxygen consumption ($\dot{V}_{O_2}$), then blood flow could be calculated using the following equation:

$$\text{Cardiac output} = \frac{\dot{V}_{O_2}}{Ca_{O_2} - C\bar{v}_{O_2}}$$

The direct Fick method for estimation of cardiac output has become the gold standard against which other methods are evaluated. In clinical situations, the direct Fick method classically required measurement of $\dot{V}_{O_2}$ by spirometry or by timed collection of expired gas in a Douglas bag and simultaneous anaerobic sampling of blood from a systemic artery and the right ventricle or PA at the time of the $\dot{V}_{O_2}$ measurements. Oxygen concentrations were classically measured directly by manometry but now are calculated from hemoglobin concentrations and saturations measured by co-oximetry (Co-Oximeter, Radiometer, Westlake, OH; and Instrument Laboratories, Lexington, MA). Alternatively, $\dot{V}_{O_2}$ may be calculated by metabolic carts that measure inspired and expired oxygen concentrations and tidal volume. This requires meticulous standardization and calibration (see *Continuous Cardiac Output and Oxygen Consumption Measurements*).

The indicator dilution technique for measurement of cardiac output was described by Hamilton and coworkers and is based on a concept originally proposed by Stewart. A measured amount of indicator (e.g., 2–4 mg of indocyanine

TABLE 31–5. Hemodynamic Variables

Variable	*Formula*	*Normal Value*	*Units**
Cardiac index	CI = cardiac output/BSA	3.2 ± 0.2	$L \cdot min^{-1} \cdot m^2$
Systemic vascular resistance index	SVRI = 79.92* (MAP − CVP)/CI	2180 ± 210	$dyne \cdot s/cm^5 \cdot m^2$
Pulmonary vascular resistance index	PVRI = 79.92* (MPAP − WP)/CI	270 ± 15	$dyne \cdot s/cm^5 \cdot m^2$
Mean transit time	Direct measurement	15 ± 1.4	s
Central blood volume	CBV = MTT × CI × 16.7	830 ± 86	mL/m^2
Stroke index	SI = CI/HR	46 ± 5	mL/m^2
Left ventricular stroke work	LVSW = SI × MAP × 0.144*	56 ± 6	$g \cdot m/m^2$
Right ventricular stroke work	RVSW = SI × MPAP × .0144*	8.8 ± 0.9	$g \cdot m/m^2$
Left cardiac work	LCW = CI × MAP × .0144	3.8 ± 0.4	$kg \cdot m/m^2$
Right cardiac work	RCW = CI × MPAP × .0144	0.6 ± 0.06	$kg \cdot m/m^2$

*.0144 and 79.92 are conversion terms.

Abbreviations: BSA = body surface area; MPAP = mean pulmonary artery pressure; WP (or PAOP) = pulmonary artery occlusion pressure (or wedge pressure); MTT = mean transit time; HR = heart rate.

green dye) is injected rapidly into a CVP catheter, and arterial blood is continuously sampled through a constant withdrawal syringe and assayed by a photodensitometer. The cardiac output (CO) is obtained by using the formula

$$CO = \frac{\text{Amount of dye injected,}}{\int_0^\infty c(t)dt}$$

and the mean transit time (MTT) is expressed by the formula

$$MTT = \frac{tc(t)dt}{\int_0^\infty c(t)dt},$$

where t is time and c is concentration of the dye in the arterial blood.

The thermal dilution method is an application of the indicator dilution principle. In this case, the indicator is a measured quantity of iced saline or 5% glucose solution; dilution of the cold solution in the bloodstream is measured by a calibrated thermocouple positioned about 10 cm upstream from the point of injection. Unlike indocyanine green dye or other indicators, the measurable amounts of the thermal indicator do not recirculate; the small amount of cold solution injected into the PA does not affect the temperature of venous blood returning to the right side of the heart. This simplifies calculations of cardiac output. Furthermore, thermodilution may be repeated more frequently than the dye technique, it does not require removal of blood for photometric analysis, and it may be used in conjunction with the PA balloon flotation catheter to obtain simultaneous PAOP.

A low cardiac index is characteristic of hemorrhage, myocardial infarction, and other forms of central pump failure. However, most patients with septic and traumatic shock are characterized by normal or high blood flow (unless they are also hypovolemic). The optimal cardiac index for the critically ill patient who has sustained life-threatening surgical trauma is greater than 4.5 $L \cdot min^{-1} \cdot m^2$, about 50% greater than the values for an unstressed, healthy volunteer. Patients with severe sepsis or burn shock may require more than twice the normal cardiac index. Similarly, stroke index, both left and right ventricular stroke work indexes, and left cardiac work index (LCWI) and right cardiac work index (RCWI) are reduced in hypovolemic and cardiogenic shock but are often increased in septic and traumatic shock. The increased cardiac index, stroke work, and myocardial performance in the latter conditions are part of the body's response to increased circulatory and metabolic requirements and prior oxygen debt from inadequate tissue perfusion associated with severe stress, wound healing, tissue repair, and restoration of body metabolism. Thus, normal values for the unstressed, normal volunteer subject are not appropriate as goals for the critically ill or shock patient.

Increased vascular resistance, a result of neural and neurohumoral (epinephrine and norepinephrine) influences, is a very early transient response to the low cardiac output of hypovolemia and cardiogenic shock. This response maintains arterial pressures in the face of decreasing blood flow, at least for a limited period of time. Hypotension occurs when compensatory responses that increase blood pressure and systemic vascular resistance index values are overwhelmed, exhausted, or attenuated by acidosis and metabolic vasodilatory mechanisms. Pulmonary vascular resistance may increase with trauma, hemorrhage, lung hypoxia, high altitude sickness, adult respiratory distress syndrome, and other forms of stress. An increased pulmonary vascular resistance index, which also is initiated by neural and other mechanisms, precedes the increased pulmonary venous admixture or shunting that occurs with postoperative and post-traumatic adult respiratory distress syndrome.

Oxygen Transport Variables and Other Circulatory Functions

Although cardiac output and PAOP are important hemodynamic variables that reflect cardiac function, the essential overall function of the circulation is to maintain body metabolism by tissue perfusion. This is reflected by the bulk transport of oxygen, carbon dioxide, nutrients, end-products of metabolism destined for excretion, and metabolites such as lactate and pyruvate that will be recycled through distant intracellular metabolic pathways. Of all blood components, oxygen has the highest percentage of extraction. It is therefore the most flow-dependent blood constituent, the most crucial in circulatory failure, and the variable whose arteriovenous gradient is easiest to measure. Hypoxic brain death or permanent neurologic deficit occurs when cardiac arrest persists for more than 4 or 5 minutes.

At the present time, it is not possible to measure tissue perfusion directly. However, the functional circulatory status is best evaluated by observing changes in the temporal patterns of $\dot{V}O_2$ in relation to the patterns of the cardiac index and $\dot{D}O_2$ (Table 31–6).[39,40] A decrease in $\dot{V}O_2$ indicates reduction of the overall rate of oxidative processes. This usually suggests (1) inadequate oxygen transport across the lungs; (2) poor tissue perfusion from maldistribution of systemic blood flow; or (3) decreased metabolic rates resulting from specific disease states (e.g., hypothyroidism, malnutrition, vitamin deficiencies), cancericidal drug therapy and or other metabolic poisoning, hypothermia, and terminal states. An increased in $\dot{V}O_2$ indicates an increase in tissue metabolism from (1) a prior oxygen debt due to low blood flow or maldistributed flow; (2) increased metabolic de-

TABLE 31–6. Oxygen Transport Variables

Variable	*Formula*	*Normal Value*	*Unit*
Arterial Hgb* saturation	Direct measurement	96 ± 1	%
Mixed venous Hgb* saturation	Direct measurement	75 ± 1	%
Arterial oxygen content	$Cao_2 = Sao_2 \times 1.36 \times Hgb + (.0031 \times Pao_2)$	19 ± 1	mL/dL
Mixed venous oxygen content	$C\bar{v}o_2 = S\bar{v}o_2 \times 1.36\ Hgb + (.0031 \times P\bar{v}o_2)$	14 ± 1	mL/dL
Oxygen delivery	$\dot{D}o_2 = CI \times Cao_2$	520 ± 16	$mL \cdot min^{-1} \cdot m^2$
Oxygen consumption	$\dot{V}o_2 = CI\ (Cao_2 - C\bar{v}o_2)$	131 ± 2	$mL \cdot min^{-1} \cdot m^2$
Oxygen extraction	$O_2\ ext = Do_2/Vo_2$	26 ± 1	%

*Hgb = hemoglobin.

mand from tissue hypoxia, sepsis, hyperthermia, post-traumatic states, burns, and hyperthyroidism; and (3) the use of various drugs, anesthetics, adrenergic agonists, such as epinephrine, that stimulate metabolism or poisons, like dinitrophenol, that dissociate oxidative phosphorylation. Infrequent or random measurements of $\dot{V}o_2$ give only a snapshot view of the situation and are usually not useful. By contrast, when therapeutic agents are given one at a time, and when $\dot{V}o_2$ is monitored before, during, and after each therapeutic intervention as well as throughout the course of a critical illness, changes in $\dot{V}o_2$ may reflect changes in tissue perfusion from the improvement in $\dot{D}o_2$ produced by the therapeutic intervention.[31, 32]

A $\dot{V}o_2$ that is greater than normal does not mean that the circulation is adequate, as increased metabolic requirements associated with tissue repair and prior oxygen debt as well as the requirements for restoration of normal function may be considerably greater than normal. Patients with major trauma, sepsis, and burns require appreciable increases in $\dot{V}o_2$—sometimes more than double the normal value. If $\dot{V}o_2$ is greater than normal before therapy but does not increase after therapy, then either tissue perfusion is already adequate or the $\dot{V}o_2$ is inadequate for these circumstances and the therapy ineffective or the circulatory defect is irreversible (as in the late stage of shock). A low or normal $\dot{V}o_2$ before and after therapy suggests that the therapy is ineffective or that the defect is irreversible. When $\dot{V}o_2$ is low before therapy and increases afterward, then either the patient's condition has spontaneously improved or the administered agent has effectively improved tissue perfusion.[31, 32]

Continuous Cardiac Output and Oxygen Consumption Measurements

Historically, continuous $\dot{V}o_2$ was directly measured by external spirometry since before the turn of the century. Because of the considerable errors and artifacts produced by the spirometers, these systems were replaced by collection of expired gas in the Douglas bag for later gas analysis. Subsequently, Guyton[33] measured $\dot{V}o_2$ continuously in animals confined to an airtight box. Westenskow and associates[34] developed a metabolic gas monitor with which gas from the inspiratory and expiratory limbs were sampled and analyzed for oxygen concentrations with a zirconium oxide sensor and for carbon dioxide with an infrared sensor. Hankeln and colleagues[35, 36] developed a microcomputer-assisted monitoring system for the continuous, on-line, real-time calculations of cardiac output and of hemodynamic and oxygen transport variables. This system continuously displays $\dot{V}o_2$, $\dot{V}co_2$, cardiac index, and an array of 20 or more hemodynamic variables calculated from inspired and expired oxygen and carbon dioxide concentrations, minute ventilation, temperature, ECG, heart rate, and intravascular pressures. The data are converted to digital form, processed, displayed on a monitoring screen, and stored for subsequent evaluation. Similar systems are available on metabolic monitoring carts and in newer ventilator models manufactured by Puritan-Bennett (Carlsbad, CA) and Siemans (Cupertino, CA). A method for continuous measurement of cardiac output using frequent thermal impulses has been reported.[37]

When an oximetric PA catheter was used, continuous $S\bar{v}o_2$ and periodic Sao_2 measurements allowed calculation of continuous cardiac output.[36] Generally, this system has reasonably good agreement with the thermodilution cardiac output[38] and was used prospectively to evaluate predictors of outcome in a wide range of clinical conditions.[39] Davies and coworkers[38] have continuously monitored cardiac output using the Westenskow oxiconsumeter system for continuous $\dot{V}o_2$ measurement compared with PA catheter oximetry and pulse oximetry. They reported good agreement with the thermodilution cardiac output method under ideal clinical conditions.

Noninvasive Cardiac Output by Impedance Measurement

Thoracic electric bioimpedance measures the apparent resistance to the flow of a small-amplitude (0.2–4.0 mA) alternating current at 40 to 100 kHz that is applied to the chest.[40–48] Thoracic electric bioimpedance was initiated by Nyboer[40] and developed as a medical instrument by Kubicek and colleagues.[41] In the 1970s, the original system was "bench-tested," tried on astronauts, and developed as the Minnesota Impedance Cardiograph (Surcom, Inc, Minneapolis, MN). Although it seemed to function well in normal patients, the instrument was generally unreliable for sick patients, particularly those with obesity, abnormal body habitus, and severe illnesses. It has been withdrawn from the market.

Subsequently, Sramek made several improvements to the technique, including diastolic clamping of the electrical signal, and Bernstein[42] developed a better mathematical representation of the thorax and corrected for changes in body habitus. Their instrument did work satisfactorily in about two thirds of sick patients when the waveform could be visualized and validated. When the waveform was not routinely examined and validated, comparisons with the standard thermodilution method revealed unacceptable correlation ($r < 0.50$).

Sorba Medical Systems, Inc. (Milwaukee WI), has developed a modification of the Minnesota instrument that has been shown to function well in normal adults and in patients with some illnesses, but to date it has not been shown to be generally reliable in monitoring critically ill patients.

A new impedance system for noninvasive measurement of cardiac output has been developed by Wang and coworkers[43] at Renaissance Technologies, Inc. (Newtown, PA), in association with Drexel University in Philadelphia. The new technology is based on major improvements in the electrode system for data acquisition and on a completely redesigned software system for data analysis, data processing, and data management. Initial clinical evaluations under real clinical conditions have shown improved stability of the signal and satisfactory agreement with simultaneous thermodilution measurement of cardiac output.[44, 45] The Renaissance Technologies system is based on time-frequency distribution technology and uses a digital signal processing technique that provides high signal-to-noise ratios for measurement of mechanical functions of the heart. The system is capable of rapid signal processing with minimal computations because of its all–integer–coefficient filtering technology. This noninvasive estimation of blood flow, when it has been extensively tested, will be a major contribution to the field of managing acute illness of circulatory origin.

Ultrasound Method for Noninvasive Cardiac Output Estimation

The Doppler ultrasound uses frequency shifts of an ultrasound wave reflected from a moving substance to measure cardiac output. In blood flow estimations, sound is reflected from a moving column of red blood cells leaving the heart. Continuous-wave Doppler ultrasound and pulsed Doppler ultrasound systems are commercially available. The transducer of such a system is placed in the suprasternal notch or esophagus and aligned with the ascending aorta. The transducer is directed to find the greatest frequency shift, which indicates the highest blood flow velocity. Integration of a velocity-time curve gives an estimate of the mean velocity. The mean velocity multiplied by the cross-sectional area multiplied by the cosine of the angle of the beam with the axis of the aorta yields stroke volume.[46, 47]

The continuous-wave system uses A-mode or M-mode Doppler estimation of aortic root cross-sectional area, which is usually performed prior to velocity measurement. Bernstein's critique describes the theoretic aspects of and practical problems associated with these methods.[47] Doppler methodology has been greatly enhanced by fast Fourier transform analysis of the Doppler frequencies. A wide variety of transducer designs have made possible greater application of this methodology at the bedside.

Ventilatory Monitoring

Ventilation, the movement of gas in and out of the lungs, is commonly assessed by determination of the tidal volume (V_T), which is the average volume of gas inspired with each breath; the minute volume (MV), which is the mean volume of inspired gas per minute; and the respiratory rate (f), which is the mean number of breaths taken per minute. Less commonly, the respiratory quotient may be measured by spirometry or calculated from the rate of carbon dioxide production (V_{CO_2}) based on end-tidal carbon dioxide tensions (P_{ETCO_2}) measured by mass spectrometry. The dead space (V_{DS}/V_T) is also calculated from the P_{ETCO_2} by using the Bohr equation (see Chapter 36).

INDICATIONS FOR INVASIVE AND NONINVASIVE MULTICOMPONENT MONITORING

The patient who has undergone elective surgery without complications may be easily monitored with routine screening that includes assessment of vital signs, ECG, and CVP. More comprehensive hemodynamic and oxygen transport monitoring is needed in high-risk surgical patients during and after major surgery (see Table 31–1). The mortality rates after major surgical procedures are usually in the range of 1% to 2%, but the mortality rates of many high-risk patients seen in the surgical ICU may be as high as 30%. To reduce these mortality rates, it is advisable to monitor all potentially fatal cases—that is, preoperative patients with risk factors as well as critically ill, medical, septic, and postoperative patients. It may be necessary to monitor at least four or five times the actual number of deaths to be sure that the optimal therapy is given to fatal patients. Invasive hemodynamic monitoring also may be useful when routine screening with monitoring of vital signs, CVP, hematocrit, and blood gases suggests more extensive hemodynamic problems.

Invasive and noninvasive hemodynamic and oxygen transport monitoring can identify correctable physiologic alterations at the earliest possible moment before they become life-threatening or irreversible.[48] Furthermore, such monitoring provides objective circulatory measurements and criteria for therapeutic decision-making. In essence, such monitoring replaces clinical suspicion and guesswork with objectively determined physiologic criteria.

DEVELOPMENT OF PLANS FOR MONITORING IN THE INTENSIVE CARE UNIT

The monitoring functions of an ICU must meet patient needs, the Joint Commission for Accreditation of Hospitals (JCAH) standards, and the expectations of referring physicians. The choice of systems used depends on the clinical load of the hospital, referral patterns, and available expertise in critical care. The single most important factor is the committment of the administration, medical staff, and nursing service. Deficiencies in the physical plant are correctable; human resources and expertise may be recruited, but administration or staff reluctance is the common deterrent to the development of advanced ICU monitoring.

The monitoring functions of an ICU vary from simple electrocardiographic surveillance to comprehensive physiologic monitoring of hemodynamic and oxygen transport functions. The type, extent, and complexity of monitoring functions reflect the overall purpose and function of the ICU. For example, the cardiac ICU and postanesthesia recovery room may only require continuous display of the ECG, heart rate, arterial pressure, pulse oximetry values, and venous pressure at the bedside. In addition to this, the surgical and multidisciplinary ICU may require facilities for comprehensive hemodynamic monitoring that include pulmonary arterial thermodilution cardiac output measurement, arterial and mixed venous blood gas analysis, and serum electrolyte and osmolarity determination. The respiratory ICU may have a sophisticated mass spectrometer for continuous monitoring of expired gases, end-tidal carbon dioxide, dead space, $\dot{V}_{O_2}$, and V_{CO_2}.

Listing the functions that are important to monitor is the first step in the development of a monitoring system for critically ill patients. The second and more difficult step is the development of a system for data reduction and analysis that can objectively assess the course of the patient's circulatory status and that also can be applied to clinical decision-making at the bedside of the critically ill patient. Therapeutic systems and treatment algorithms are discussed in the chapters 13 and 14.

References

1. Shoemaker WC, Kram HB, Appel PL, et al: The efficacy of central venous and pulmonary artery catheters and therapy based upon them in reducing mortality and morbidity. Arch Surg 1990; 125:1332–1338.
2. Adler DC, Bryan-Brown CW: Use of the axillary artery for intravascular monitoring. Crit Care Med 1973; 1:148–150.

3. Wo CJ, Shoemaker WC, Appel PL, et al: Unreliability of blood pressure and heart rate to evaluate cardiac output in emergency resuscitation and critical illness. Crit Care Med 1993; 21:218–223.
4. Monson DO, Shoemaker WC: Sequence of hemodynamic events after various types of hemorrhage. Surgery 1968; 63:738–749.
5. Shoemaker WC, Kram HB: Effects of crystalloids and colloids on hemodynamics, oxygen transport, and outcome in high-risk patients. *In*: Debates in Clinical Surgery. Simmons RC, Udehuo AS (Eds). Chicago, Year Book Medical Publishers, 1990, pp 263–316.
6. Skillman JJ, Awwad HK, Moore FD: Plasma kinetics of the early transcapillary refill after hemorrhage in man. Surg Gynecol Obstet 1967; 123:983–996.
7. Moore FD: Effects of hemorrhage on body composition. N Engl J Med 1965; 273:567–577.
8. Wiggers CJ: Physiology of Shock. New York, Commonwealth Fund, 1950.
9. Shippy CR, Appel PL, Shoemaker WC: Reliability of clinical monitoring to assess blood volume in critically ill patients. Crit Care Med 1984; 12:107.
10. Lewis FJ, Quinn ML: Continuous electrocardiogram monitoring in a surgical intensive care unit. Crit Care Med 1977; 4:73.
11. Landis EM, Hortenstine JC: Functional significance of venous blood pressure. Physiol Rev 1950; 30:1.
12. Hughes RE, Magovern GJ: The relationship between right atrial pressure and blood volume. Arch Surg 1959; 79:238.
13. Wilson JN, Grow JB, Demong CV, et al: Central venous pressure in optimal blood volume maintenance. Arch Surg 1962; 83:563.
14. Clinical Application of Blood Gases. 4th ed. Vol 3. Shapiro BA, Harrison RA, Walton JR (Eds). Chicago, Year Book Medical Publishers, 1990.
15. Clark LC Jr: Monitor and control of blood and tissue oxygen tensions. Trans Am Soc Artif Intern Organs 1956; 2:41.
16. Hüch A, Hüch R, Meinzer K, et al: Eine schnelle behizte Proberflach-electrode zur kontinuierlichen Uberwachung des Po_2 beim Menschen. *In*: Electrodenaufbau und Eigenschaften. Stuttgart, Proc Medizin-Technik, May 16, 1972.
17. Eberhard P, Mindt W, Hammacher K: Perkutane Messung des Sauerstoff-partialdruckes. *In*: Methodik und Anwendungen. Stuttgart, Proc Medizin-Technik, May 16, 1972.
18. Tremper KK, Shoemaker WC: Transcutaneous oxygen monitoring of critically ill adults with and without low flow shock. Crit Care Med 1981; 9:706.
19. Tremper KK, Waxman K, Shoemaker WC: Effects of hypoxia and shock in transcutaneous Po_2 values on dogs. Crit Care Med 1979; 7:526.
20. Shoemaker WC, Appel PL, Kram HB, et al: Multicomponent noninvasive physiologic monitoring of circulatory function. Crit Care Med, 1988; 16:482–490.
21. Tremper KK, Shoemaker WC, Shippy CR, et al: Transcutaneous CO_2 monitoring in adult patients in the ICU and operating room. Crit Care Med 1981; 9:752.
22. Shoemaker WC, Bryan-Brown CW, Quigley L, et al: Body fluid shifts in depletion and poststress states and their correction with adequate nutrition. Surg Gynecol Obstet 1973; 136:371.
23. Shoemaker WC, Monson DO: Effect of whole blood and plasma expanders on volume-flow relationships in critically ill patients. Surg Gynecol Obstet 1973; 137:453.
24. Davis HA: Blood Volume Dynamics. Springfield, Charles C Thomas, 1962.
25. Albert SN: Blood Volume. Springfield, Charles C Thomas, 1963.
26. Moore FD: The body cell mass and its supporting environment: Body composition in health and disease. Philadelphia, WB Saunders, 1963.
27. Starling EH: On the absorption of fluids from the connective tissue spaces. J Physiol 1896; 19:312.
28. Swan HJC, Ganz W, Forrester JS, et al: Catheterization of the heart in man with use of a flow-directed balloon-tipped catheter. N Engl J Med 1970; 283:447.
29. Swan HJC: Role of hemodynamic monitoring in the management of the critically Ill. Crit Care Med 1975; 3:83.
30. Forrester JS, Diamond G, Chatterjee J, et al: Medical therapy of acute myocardial infarction by application of hemodynamic subsets. N Engl J Med 1976; 295:1356–1404.
31. Shoemaker WC, Appel PL, Kram HB: Oxygen transport measurements to evaluate tissue perfusion and titrate therapy. Crit Care Med 1991; 19:672–688.
32. Shoemaker WC, Appel PL, Kram HB, et al: Hemodynamic and oxygen transport monitoring to titrate therapy in septic shock. New Horizons 1993; 1:145–159.
33. Guyton AC: A continuous cardiac output recorder employing the Fick principle. Circ Res 1959; 7:661.
34. Westenskow DR, Culter CA, Wallace WD: Instrumentation for monitoring gas exchange and metabolic rate in critically ill patients. Crit Care Med 1984; 12:183.
35. Hankeln KB, Michelson H, Schipalle M, et al: Microcomputer-assisted monitoring system for measuring and processing cardiorespiratory variables. Crit Care Med 1985; 13:426.
36. Hankeln KB, Michelson H, Kubiak V, et al: Continuous on-line, real-time measurement of cardiac output and derived cardiorespiratory variables in the critically ill. Crit Care Med 1985; 13:1071.
37. Yelderman MD: Continuous measurement of cardiac output with the use of stochastic system identification technique. J Clin Monit 1990; 6:323–332.
38. Davies GG, Jebsen PJR, Glasgow BM, et al: Continuous Fick cardiac output compared to thermodilution cardiac output. Crit Care Med 1986; 14:881.
39. Hankeln KB, Sanker R, Schwarten JW, et al: Evaluation of prognostic indices based on hemodynamic and oxygen transport variables in shock patients with adult respiratory distress syndrome. Crit Care Med 1987; 15:1.
40. Nyboer J: Impedance Plethysmography. Springfield, Charles C Thomas, 1959.
41. Kubicek WG, Karnegis JN, Patterson RP, et al: Development and evaluation of an impedance cardiac output system. Aerospace Med 1966; 37:1208.
42. Bernstein DP: A new stroke volume equation for thoracic electrical bioimpedance: Theory and rationale. Crit Care Med 1986; 14:904.
43. Wang XA, Sun HH, Adamson D, et al: Impedance cardiograph system: A new design. Ann Biomed Eng 1989; 17:535.
44. Wo CJ, Shoemaker WC, Bishop MH: Evaluation of a new thoracic electric impedance device for estimation of cardiac output in critically ill patients. J Clin Monit (in press).
45. Shoemaker WC, Wo CJ, Appel PL, et al: Multi-institution trial of a new impedance system for noninvasive cardiac output measurements. Crit Care Med (in press).
46. Mehta N, Iyane VI, Cummin ARC, et al: Validation of a Doppler technique for beat to beat measurement of cardiac output. Clin Sci 1985; 69:377.
47. Bernstein DP: Noninvasive cardiac output measurement. *In*: Textbook of Critical Care. 2nd ed. Shoemaker WC, Ayres S, Grenvik A (Eds). Philadelphia, WB Saunders, 1989, p 159.
48. Shoemaker WC, Appel PL, Kram HB: Incidence, physiologic description, compensatory mechanisms, and therapeutic implications of monitored events. Crit Care Med 1989; 17:1277.

CHAPTER 32

Electrocardiography and Pressure Monitoring: How to Obtain Optimal Results

Reed M. Gardner, PhD • Karen W. Hollingsworth, RN, MS, CCRN

Electrocardiographic (ECG) monitoring and the direct measurement of blood pressure have become common practices in the modern surgical suite and in intensive care units (ICUs). These monitoring techniques provide current and important data for patient management. However, neither of these physiologic measurement procedures is infallible, and care must be taken to optimize the acquisition of meaningful data. Modern, microcomputer-based bedside ECG monitors not only detect changes in heart rate (HR) and sound an alarm during life-threatening situations but also detect dangerous cardiac arrhythmias. However, if improperly set up or calibrated, this sophisticated monitoring equipment is useless. Optimization of the use of monitoring equipment is crucial for the reliable assessment of physiologic signals and for the minimization of the need for trouble-shooting.[1a, 1b] This chapter reviews methods for optimizing ECG, arterial pressure, and pulmonary artery pressure (PAP) monitoring. Such monitoring is particularly challenging during surgery, when interference from high-frequency electrosurgical equipment is present. High-quality monitoring may also be difficult to perform in a busy ICU and when patients move in their beds.

OPTIMIZING ELECTROCARDIOGRAPHIC MONITORING

ECG monitoring has become a standard practice in the measurement of HR and rhythm. ECG monitoring is used to detect arrhythmias and myocardial ischemia and to assess pacemaker function[1c]; consequently, signal quality must be excellent. The aphorism "garbage in, garbage out" is especially relevant to ECG monitoring, as poor signal quality or the complete lack of an ECG signal is a major frustration. A critical medical strategy is "when in doubt, check the patient first"; in other words, an important reason why no ECG signal is displayed on a monitor might be that the patient does not have one!

The major goal of ECG recording is to faithfully reproduce and display the ECG signal and to eliminate undesired signals known as "noise" or "artifacts." Signals from 60-Hz power lines (50-Hz in Europe) and electrosurgery equipment commonly interfere with ECG signal monitoring as do distortion caused by amplifier nonlinearity, noise, and inadequate frequency response. Poor ECG monitoring quality is a very common clinical problem. However, most of the problems encountered clinically are correctable through the application of technical knowledge and the optimization of technique. Figure 32–1 shows the potential sources of artifact, interference, and distortion, and Table 32–1 lists in outline form the documented ECG monitoring problem areas.

Patient

The electrical signal that is emitted from the heart and that is measured at the skin surface is very small, having an amplitude of only 0.5 to 2 mV. It is measured best when the skin has been properly prepared and when the electrodes have been placed in the best possible positions. Wet or oily skin should be cleansed for about 10 seconds with alcohol and dried to allow maximum electrode adhesion. Hairy skin should be trimmed to optimize adhesion and to make electrode removal less painful to the patient. In surgery, electrodes should be covered with a sterile drape to prevent surgical scrub solution from seeping under the electrodes and loosening the adhesive that holds them in place. Dead cells should be removed from the skin surface to permit the ECG signals to travel more efficiently to the electrodes (Fig. 32–2).[2–9]

The granular layer of the epidermis has a resistance of about 50 kΩ/cm^2.[3] Proper skin preparation reduces electrode resistance from as high as 200 kΩ to as low as 10 kΩ in 90% of patients.[2, 3, 9] Also, a skin potential of approximately 30 mV exists between the inside and the outside of this layer. Stretching the skin decreases this potential to about 25 mV. The 5-mV change is sensed as motion artifact. Abrading this layer by vigorous rubbing of the skin with cotton gauze reduces the potential difference to nearly zero. After the granular layer has been scratched, the conductive gel placed on an electrode can penetrate and disrupt the epidermis and reduce contact resistance. Fifteen to 30 minutes are required for gel penetration. Because the protective skin layer is disrupted during such abrading, mild gels should be used if skin irritation is to be avoided.[3, 9] Figure 32–3 shows how ECG signal level can be improved by proper skin preparation.

Proper placement allows electrodes to receive the maximum ECG signal with a minimum of noise. QRS amplitude is greatest when the thoracic equivalent of lead II configuration occurs.[3] Placement of electrodes over bone prominences such as the sternum or clavicles—and not over areas of loose skin—reduces muscle and motion artifact. In the operating room and ICU, such optimal electrode placement may be impossible because of the location of the operative or wound site.

Other factors that may interfere with ECG monitoring include muscle artifact,[2, 3] skin movement, and respiration. Electromyography has frequency and voltage characteristics similar to those of ECG monitoring. Shivering caused by

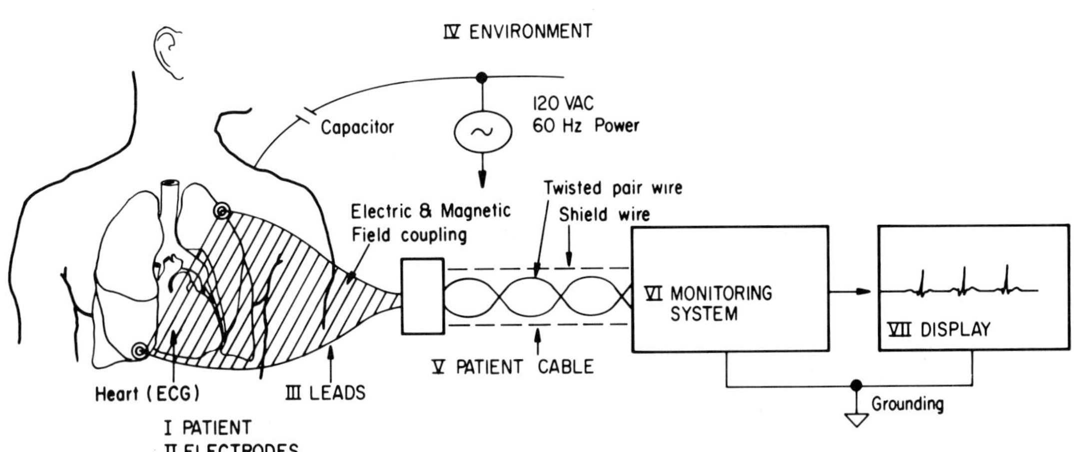

Figure 32–1. Sources of artifact, interference, and distortion during ECG monitoring. Roman numerals I to VII indicate elements involved in signal degeneration.

TABLE 32–1. Electrocardiographic Documented Problem Areas

I. Patient	***V. Patient Cables***
Electrode placement	Loose connections
Skin preparation	Unshielded wire
Wet or oily skin	Untwisted wire
Hairy surface	Cable movement (triboelectric)
Skin irritation	***VI. Monitoring Systems***
Muscle artifact (electromyelography)	Internal noise (thermal/shot)
Motion—bumping, pulling	Input resistance
Chest wall (respiration)	Common mode rejection
II. Electrodes	Gain
Type of electrode	Double trigger (T wave and pacer)
Dissimilar types	Single lead
Dry electrode gel	Frequency response
Electrode motion	Pacemaker signal
Unstable half-cell potential	Defibrillator recovery
Too cold to attach	Electrosurgery nonlinearity
Poor adhesive	Lead continuity detection
Long defibrillator recovery	AC power surges (e.g., brown-outs, spikes)
Skin irritation	***VII. Display***
III. Leads	Improper connections (grounding)
Loose or corroded clips	Frequency response
Poor connections	Loss of pacer spikes
Intermittent wire breaks	Heart rate counting
Cable movement (triboelectric)	Stairstep/resolution (time and amplitude distort)
Unshielded wire	Frozen display
Untwisted wire	
Draped over motors, lights, and transformers	
IV. Environment	
60-Hz power lines	
Electrosurgery	
Motors and transformers	
Bypass pumps	
Intravenous pumps	
Static charge sources	
Fluorescent lights	

Refer to Figure 32–1 for sources of artifact, interference, and distortion, and to the text for preventive measures.

hypothermia or Parkinson tremor may cause electromyographic artifact. Any electromyographic signal occurring between the two electrodes shown in Figure 32–1 adds to the ECG signal and thus reduces signal quality. Motion artifact that is caused by electrode movement (Fig. 32–4) can be minimized not only by proper skin preparation but also by taping the lead wires to prevent any artifact caused by their movement. Electrode artifact that is caused by chest or abdominal wall movement produced during respiration can be minimized by repositioning of the electrodes.

Electrodes

Most electrodes for ECG monitoring are designed for a single use only. To minimize electrode problems, the proper type of electrodes should be used—that is, those that have been designed for clinical monitoring (e.g., not an exercise ECG electrode).[10, 11] Furthermore, the use of electrodes of dissimilar type (e.g., those produced by different manufacturers) can cause large half-cell (battery-like) potentials that may disable the ECG amplifier. Electrodes should be consistently obtained from the same supplier and should conform to the specifications of the American National Standards Institute (ANSI) and the Association for the Advancement of Medical Instrumentation (AAMI).[10] The use of electrode gel that has dried owing to improper storage or the failure to use electrode gel results in high-resistance skin contact, which causes the unstable tracings and 60-Hz interference signal pickup. Electrode gel may become dry because of improper electrode storage or exposure to heat, or if they

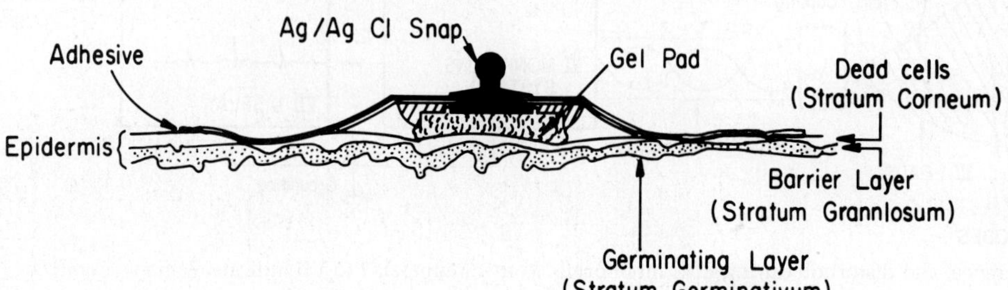

Figure 32–2. Schematic drawing of an ECG electrode attached to the skin.

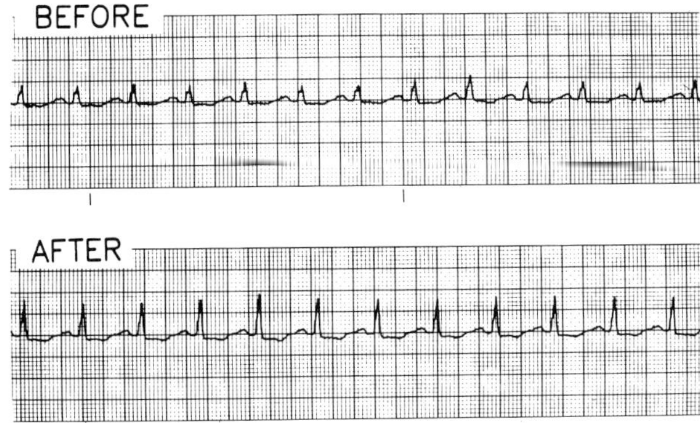

Figure 32–3. An ECG waveform before and after proper skin preparation.

have been removed from the foil-wrapped packages that are designed to prevent gel evaporation.

Unstable half-cell potentials can be minimized by coating the electrode "snap" with silver chloride (Ag/AgCl).[12] ECG electrodes should be of the Ag/AgCl variety, as the half-cell voltage for stainless steel needle electrodes is large and unstable[11, 12, 12a] and, as a result, can produce unacceptably long defibrillator recovery times.[13] The use of needle electrodes, which has been suggested as a solution to the problems of electrode placement during surgery, is not recommended because of the potential hazard of thermal injury that can result from the high current densities associated with electrosurgery.[3, 14] Cold electrodes may not adhere to skin properly and can prematurely detach; thus, cold electrodes should be hand-warmed before they are applied.

Leads

Loosening or corrosion of clips can result in poor contact between the lead wires and the electrode snaps. Increased resistance at these connections can increase the interference from 60-Hz power lines. Poor connections between the lead wires and the patient cable going to the monitor may sometimes be improved by their mere disconnection and reconnection. Suspected intermittent breaks in the lead wires can cause sporadic ECG transmission. When this occurs, these wires should be changed or carefully checked. Cable movement, which causes motion artifact or triboelectric noise, is generated by friction and deformation of the insulation surrounding the wires.[3] It can be minimized by repositioning of the leads.

Shielded lead wires minimize the pickup of alternating-current electrical fields from 60-Hz power lines, electrosurgery machines, and other sources such as radio transmitters (e.g., paging systems and citizen-band radios).[15] Magnetic fields can also cause the induction of signals into lead wires. The two leads that connect the patient to the monitor form a loop (see Fig. 32–1) through which magnetic fields can pass and induce unwanted voltages. There are two ways to minimize the effect of the magnetic fields on ECG monitoring: (1) by not draping the lead wires over power cords, motors, lights, or other electrically powered instruments; and (2) by decreasing the loop area by keeping the lead wires close together (e.g., through the use of twisted pair wires).[15]

Environment

ECG recording is frequently impeded by interference originating from nearby power sources. Electromagnetic sources can cause interference in three ways (see Fig. 32–1): (1) by inducing a voltage in the loop formed by the electrode leads; (2) by inducing an electrical current into the leads, thus creating an interfering voltage drop across the combined skin and electrode resistance; (3) by inducing a voltage between the two recording electrodes and the amplifier grounding point. Figure 32–5 shows an ECG signal that has been affected by 60-Hz interference.

A patient is always coupled to the 60-Hz power line by a very small (but finite) capacitor, the size of which is determined by how close the patient is to the power source (see Fig. 32–1). Voltage introduced to the patient from the power line is known as *common-mode voltage;* this voltage can be as small as a few millivolts if the patient is touching a grounded object or as great as 20 V if the patient grasps an insulated power cord. The common-mode voltage for most patients is typically 1 V (1000 times as great as the ECG signal).[16] The common-mode voltage caused by a 60-Hz power line can be reduced through (1) the use of lead wires that are shielded, which minimize electrical field pickup, and of twisted pair wires that minimize magnetic coupling; (2) the proper placement of cables and equipment; (3) proper preparation of the skin and careful placement of the electrodes, which minimize skin contact resistance; (4) the use of an amplifier system that has excellent common-mode voltage rejection characteristics[3, 15, 17]; and (5) the use of an adaptive computer subtraction method within the bedside monitoring system (as shown in Figure 32–6).

Electrosurgical units that are used by surgeons to cut and coagulate tissue radiate large radio-frequency fields. The interference created by such electrosurgical equipment is a combination of radio-frequency current (800–2000 kHz) and alternating-current AC line frequency (60 Hz).[14] Many ECG monitoring systems are disabled by this interference, particularly when it is caused by spark-gap electrosurgical units. Several passive electrical filters and electronic methods have been implemented in bedside monitors to minimize this interference.[3] Another way to reduce the artifact of an electrosurgical unit is to place the indifferent (right-leg) electrode close to the electrosurgical grounding pad. Also, the ECG bedside monitor should be plugged into a power outlet separate from that of the electrosurgical unit.

Because defibrillator discharge can destroy ECG monitors or force the amplifier into a nonlinear region, the AAMI suggests that an ECG monitor should be able to withstand defibrillator discharges and to recover from them within 5 seconds.[13, 18]

Motors and electrical transformers emit magnetic fields; therefore, it is important to keep the patient, leads, and

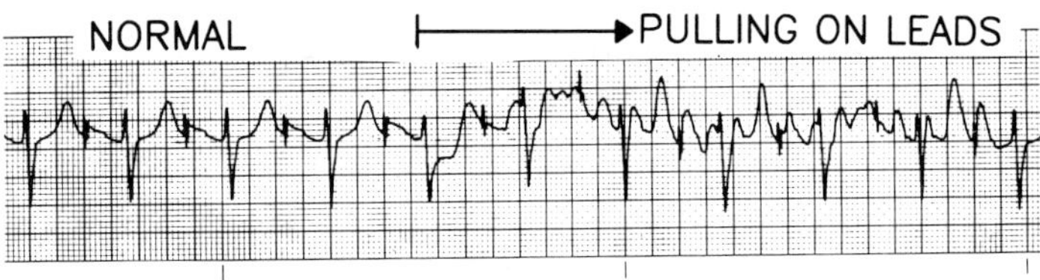

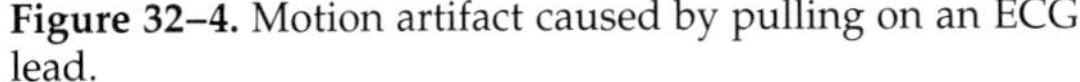

Figure 32–4. Motion artifact caused by pulling on an ECG lead.

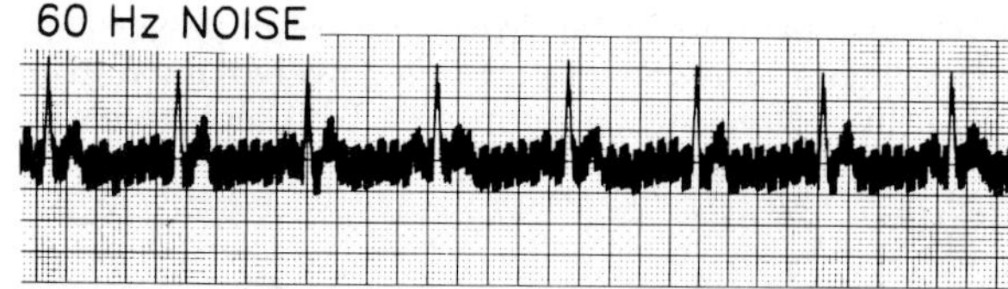

Figure 32–5. An ECG when 60-Hz interference is superimposed.

cables away from these known 60-Hz power sources (which include bypass pumps [which contain motors], infusion pumps,[3, 19] sources of static charge [such as a nurse who has walked across a carpeted floor],[19] and fluorescent lights).[16]

Patient Cables

Since patient cables are susceptible to problems similar to those of ECG leads, patient cables should have good connectors; an intact, shielded wire (to minimize electrical field pickup); and twisted internal wires (to minimize magnetic field pickup). Cable movements can cause triboelectric pickup; therefore, the same precautions that apply to the placement of patient's leads apply to the positioning of the patient's cables. Cables that lead from different pieces of equipment should be individually coiled and not draped over each other.[15]

Monitor

All monitoring systems have monitors and displays that contain amplifiers and processors. The ECG amplifier and processing sections of bedside monitors have benefitted greatly from the advances in solid-state integrated circuit technology. Stable, low-cost, and linear amplifiers with a low level of internal noise, high-input resistance, and high common-mode rejection, were once unavailable; however, the properly designed, modern ECG amplifier seldom causes signal distortion.[20] Low-amplitude ECG signals may be due to the low gain of the ECG amplifier. Therefore, an amplifier gain control is a necessary component of an ECG monitoring system. However, if not carefully executed, a gain change may affect the ischemia detection (ST-segment analysis) available with newer systems.[1] The problem of low QRS amplitude (usually <0.5 mV) can often be solved by better skin preparation or by the changing or moving of electrodes (see Fig. 32–3).

The HR detector, which is intended to detect the QRS complex, sometimes improperly double-triggers on T waves or pacing spikes. Changing the ECG electrode position or switching to a different monitoring lead may circumvent the problem. More modern monitoring systems have the capability to simultaneously monitor and display calibrated signals from multiple ECG leads[20]; as a result, continuous ECG monitoring is not affected by the loss of one lead. Thus, single-lead ECG recording is becoming a thing of the past.

An alternative to determining a possibly false HR from the ECG signal is to derive the HR from the arterial blood pressure signal.

The American Heart Association (AHA) has specified two different ECG monitoring frequency-response ranges: (1) from 0.5 to 50 Hz for monitoring use; and (2) from 0.05 to 100 Hz for diagnostic use.[21] The diagnostic frequency response must be available when monitoring for ischemic changes.[1] The frequency response of the monitoring mode may improve the quality of the ECG tracing by decreasing baseline wander; however, it may falsely depress or elevate the ST segment or even shift an abnormal ST segment toward the isoelectric line.[4] Thus, the diagnostic mode is required for monitoring ischemic changes in the ST segment. Bringing a conventional, 12-lead ECG system to the bedside or the surgery suite to detect ST-segment changes is no longer necessary with the use of new bedside monitoring technology. Indeed, ECG signs of ischemia are now monitored intraoperatively.

Because pacing spikes may be as short as 0.1 ms in duration and have amplitudes of from 50 to 700 mV, they are especially difficult to detect, display, and count.[20] Special analog circuits must detect pacer spikes and "condition" them to be "visible" to the digital sampling system[20]; otherwise, pacing spikes might appear to "come and go," and thus the pacemaker would appear to be working improperly.

A recent advancement in ECG monitoring systems is the introduction of the lead continuity detector. By injecting small, high-frequency, alternating currents into each of the leads, the monitoring system is able to detect whether any given lead has too great a resistance and can give a warning before the lead is completely disconnected or before the electrode gel dries out.

Display

Displays are typically either oscilloscopes or strip-chart recorders. Most oscilloscopes display digitally stored waveforms either in a scrolling mode or "frozen" on the screen. Problems can occur because of improper connections or improper grounding, frequency response limitations (especially when pacemaker spikes are displayed), imperfections in computer algorithms (which can prevent proper HR determinations as a result of artifact on the ECG signal), and distortions (caused by limited display resolution). For example, stair-step changes in the ECG signal on some computer-driven displays can be distracting and prevent proper waveform interpretation.

Summary

A satisfactory waveform should be displayed if the electrodes and cables have been properly placed and if the skin has been properly prepared. If no ECG signal appears, check the patient first; if this does not reveal the source of error, a few quick equipment inspections may demonstrate

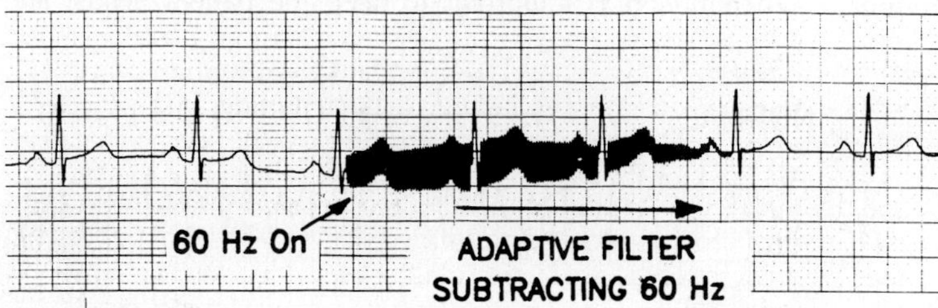

Figure 32–6. An ECG waveform with 60-Hz interference that is quickly detected and eliminated (in about 2 seconds) by an adaptive computer filter algorithm.

the problem. If no tracing is seen at all, ascertain whether the monitor is turned on and plugged into the wall outlet (or has sufficient battery charge) and whether the patient leads are connected. Both cleansing of the skin with mild abrasives and application of good electrodes are essential to good signal quality.

Several devices that simulate a patient's ECG and blood pressure signals are available. These devices should be used at frequent intervals to verify that the monitoring system is operating properly. Inspection, performance validation, and certification of the monitoring equipment by the bioinstrumentation department should be performed at regular intervals. In addition, the bioinstrumentation group should become a part of the trouble-shooting team any time monitoring problems develop.

OPTIMIZING BLOOD PRESSURE MONITORING

In the critically ill patient, PAP, systemic arterial pressure, central venous pressure, and pulmonary capillary wedge pressure are measured frequently. Systemic arterial pressure can be measured with either direct or indirect methods. However, PAP, central venous pressure, and wedge pressure are currently measured only with direct methods. Although the indirect measurement of arterial pressure is imprecise when compared with the direct method,[22] errors in direct pressure measurement are, unfortunately, still very common.

Indirect Blood Pressure Measurement

The Korotkoff auscultatory method for indirect arterial blood pressure measurement has been widely used since it was first described in 1905. The AHA has made recommendations about how indirect arterial pressure should be measured.[22] The auscultatory measurement of arterial pressure usually underestimates the systolic pressure. Cohn showed the serious limitations of both the auscultatory and palpatory methods for measuring blood pressure in hypotensive patients in shock.[23] Since most indirect pressure measurement techniques require cuff inflation, measurements can only be made at intervals. Only recently have prototype devices that allow continuous, noninvasive pressure waveform monitoring been tested clinically.[24, 25]

Contemporary medical technology has produced a variety of devices for the measurement of arterial pressure automatically with oscillometric, stopped-flow, and auscultatory techniques.[26–29] Despite these automated techniques, problems with their application and questions about their accuracy do exist.[27, 30–50, 50a–50d] The popular automated oscillometric devices "under-read" systolic and mean pressures at high arterial pressures and "over-read" them at low arterial pressures.[31, 32] Finnie and coworkers[34] recommended that the oscillometric method be used for measuring systolic and mean blood pressures and that the Korotkoff sound method be used for determining diastolic blood pressure indirectly in critically ill patients.[35–37]

Johnson and Kerr[32] found that five automated noninvasive devices gave unreliable readings for patients with low blood pressure (radial artery systolic pressure > 80 mm Hg). For situations in which they did obtain a pressure, it tended to be an optimistic result. They also reported that invasive techniques were clearly preferable in the critically ill patient with shock.

Despite the well-established safety and convenience of the automatic oscillometric blood pressure systems, a few clinically important problems (e.g., ulnar neuropathy[51] and venostasis[52]) that occur when the cuff is inflated too frequently have been reported. Some recommendations[53] for automated oscillometric blood pressure measurements are as follows:

1. Always verify the HR and pulse rate by using a second method.
2. If the blood pressure as measured with an oscillometric device seems low, immediately compare the oscillometrically determined pulse rate with that on the ECG monitor (for patients without bigeminy); if the pulse rates agree, hypotension exists. If the oscillometric rate is considerably lower then the ECG rate, the blood pressure instrument may have a malfunction.
3. Observe the patient's cuffed extremity for signs of impeded blood flow, especially when cycling quickly (every 1 to 2 minutes).
4. Use the cuffs and connections provided by the manufacturer. The most important factor in determining the accuracy of the indirect blood pressure measurement is the selection of the proper cuff size[54] as recommended by the AHA (cuff sizes are based on limb circumference).

As a general rule, if there is a change in blood pressure as measured by any indirect method, no precipitous clinical action should be taken until a repeat measurement has been made.[31] Any indirect methods for determining pressures in patients with arrhythmias may give inaccurate results. When a rapidly acting drug such as nitroprusside is given, indirect pressure measurements may not be available frequently enough.

Direct Blood Pressure Measurement

Two major purposes for inserting an arterial or pulmonary artery catheter are to measure intravascular pressure and to withdraw blood samples. The direct measurement of blood pressure requires a "plumbing system" that includes a catheter, a stopcock (or stopcocks), connecting tubing, a continuous flush device, a pressure transducer, and a pressure monitor with display (Fig. 32–7). The major problems of blood pressure measurement with a catheter system are (1) improper system zeroing, (2) inadequate dynamic response, and (3) the improper determination of derived data from the available pressure signals.[38–41, 55–61] It would seem that the proper specification and selection of plumbing systems would completely resolve problems (2) and (3), but such is not the case. Since each clinical situation is different, careful setup and testing of the complete monitoring system is essential to the acquisition of accurate data.

Zeroing

The zeroing of the pressure monitoring system is the single most important step in setting up a pressure measuring system. Zeroing errors can make a substantial difference in the recording of all pressures, particularly of those on the right side of the circulatory system, such as PAP, central venous pressure, and wedge pressure. Pressure monitoring systems should be zeroed frequently and always prior to initiation of treatment changes based on the pressure data. Proper zeroing is done by opening an appropriate stopcock to the atmosphere and aligning the resulting fluid-air interface point at the midaxillary line (Fig. 32–8). "Zero" changes can be caused by many factors, including (1) a change in patient position in relation to the pressure transducer (hydrostatic effect); (2) a transducer electrical zero change; (3) pressure amplifier drift; and (4) a transducer that is sensitive to light.[62]

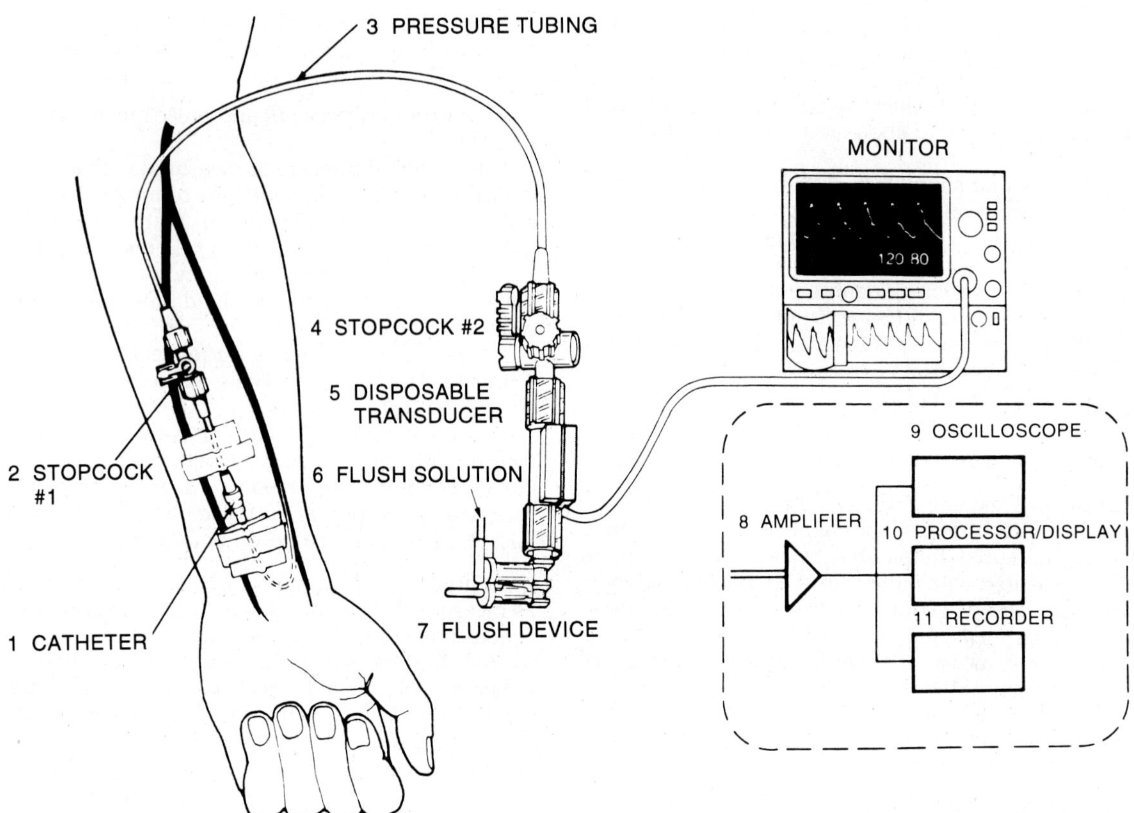

Figure 32–7. The 11 components used to directly monitor blood pressure. The monitoring components are nearly the same independent of whether the catheter is in a radial, brachial, or femoral artery (or in the pulmonary artery). *Note:* The transducer size and plumbing components were enlarged for illustrative purposes.

Calibration

Many of the transducer-associated calibration problems that are caused by improper transducer setups[38, 63, 64] have been eliminated by the use of disposable pressure transducers that meet the ANSI transducer interchangeability standards.[65] Disposable pressure transducers are much more rugged and reliable than the previously used expensive, reusable transducers.[66–68] Disposable transducers are already cost-effective for clinical use. Since the semiconductor manufacturing techniques that are used to make computer components are used to make disposable pressure transducers, the prices of these transducers are also likely to continue to fall.

Most pressure transducers are standardized to a fixed sensitivity of 5 mV per volt of excitation for each millimeter of mercury of pressure applied. If standardized pressure transducers are used, sensitivity adjustment on the monitor is not needed. Pressure calibration checking is not recommended in the clinical setting because of the risk of air embolism or microbiologic contamination of the patient.[69, 70] If calibration errors are suspected, fixed sensitivity monitors can be quickly checked with a transducer simulator. If problems are still suspected, the disposable transducer should be replaced with a new one and the "suspect" transducer tested in the laboratory.

Dynamic Response Testing

The catheter, tubing, continuous flush device, and transducer (plumbing) system used for pressure monitoring can distort the pressure signal.[38, 56–64, 71] A "fast-flush" test ensures that the recorded waveforms and derived parameters are adequate.[55–57] Two methods are used to characterize the "dynamic response" of the catheter, tubing, and transducer systems. The first specifies that the system's frequency response be unvarying up to a specified cutoff frequency; this frequency is determined by the number of harmonics in the original pulse wave (usually 10 harmonics are specified) (Fig. 32–9). The second method uses the specification of the natural frequency (Fn) and damping coefficient (ζ). However, the Fn and damping coefficient parameters are more convenient to use because they can be measured in the actual pressure monitoring system and have been used to define catheter–transducer system dynamics.[55]

Figure 32–10 shows a plot of the Fn and damping coefficient for a pressure monitoring plumbing system. Five areas are defined; only two of these areas produce adequate or optimal reproduction of a patient's pressure waveforms, whereas the other three areas result in distortion. Most catheter, tubing, and transducer plumbing systems are underdamped, and a few have unacceptably low Fn values. If the Fn is less than 7.5 Hz, the pressure waveform will be distorted no matter what the value of the damping coefficient (see Fig. 32–10). However, if the Fn can be increased to 24 Hz, the damping coefficient can range from about 0.15 to 1.1 without distorting the dynamic response of any pressure monitoring system. The Fn should be as high as possible. Theoretically, a high Fn can be obtained in systems with short tubing and in those having catheters with large internal diameters, as well as by using transducers and other components that are noncompliant.

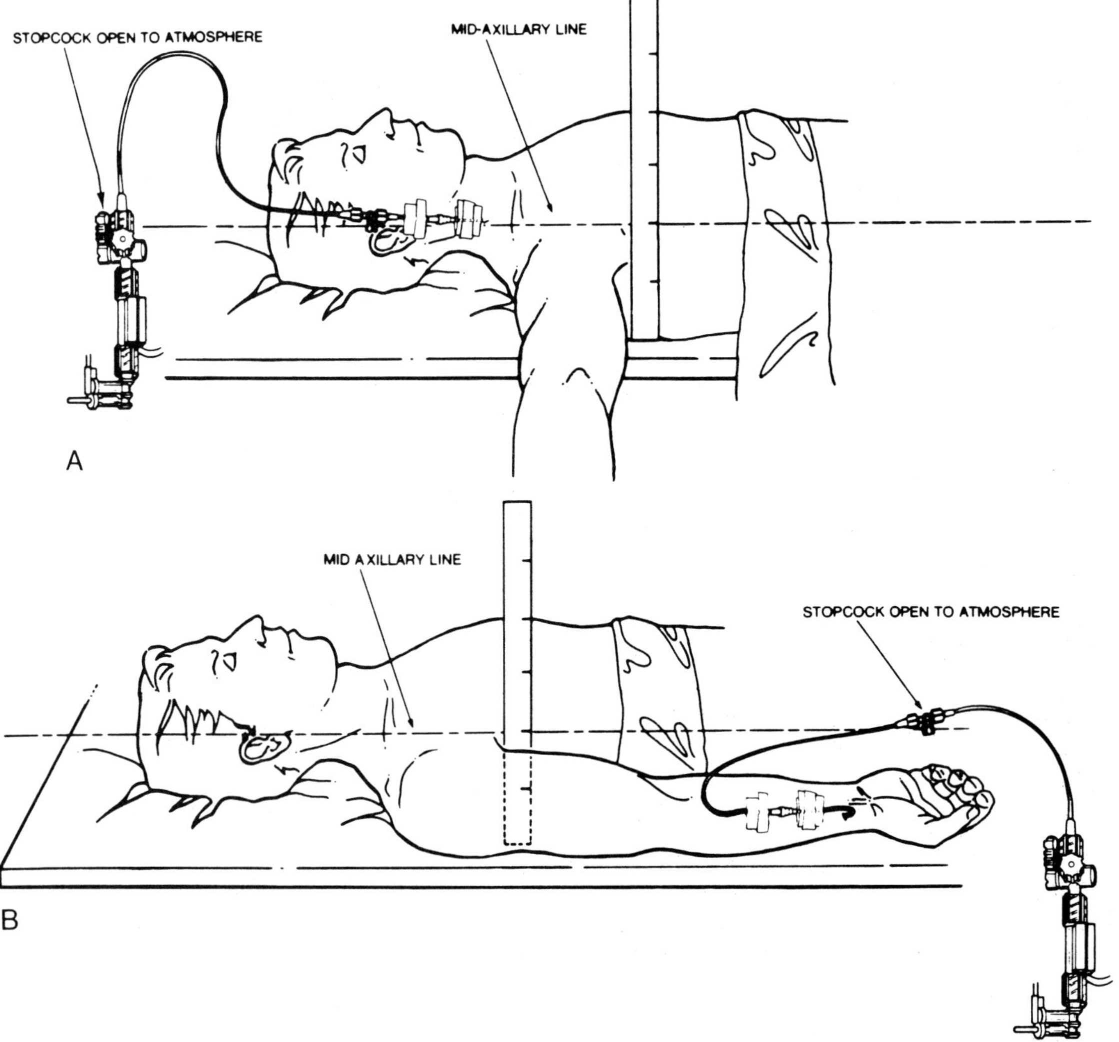

Figure 32–8. Two methods of zeroing a pressure transducer. Note that the location at which the water-air interface occurs should always be at the midaxillary line during zeroing. *A,* The stopcock is placed near the transducer at the midaxillary line. *B,* The stopcock is placed nearer to the catheter at the midaxillary line.

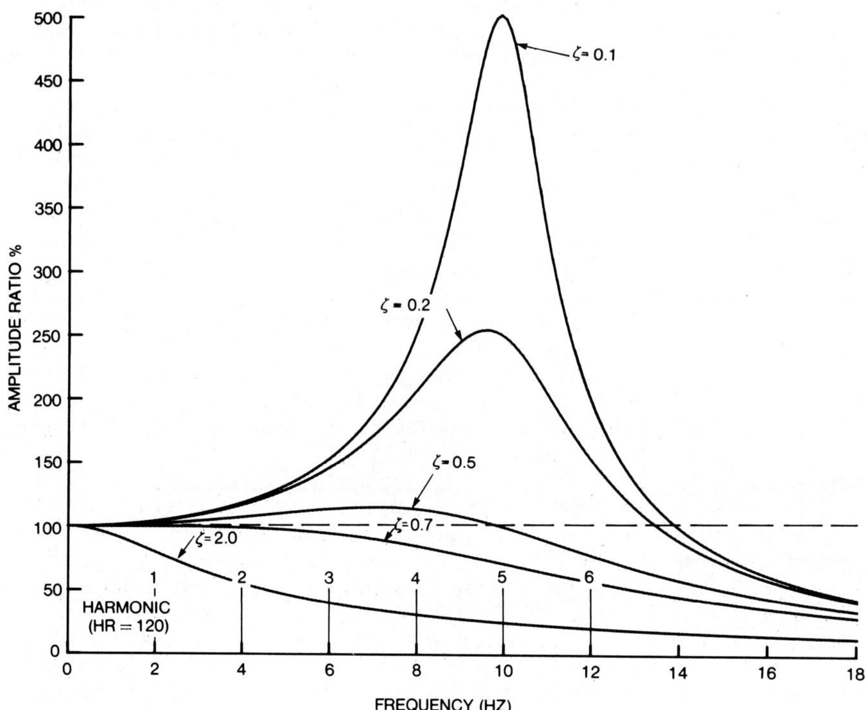

Figure 32–9. Family of frequency versus amplitude ratio plots for five different damping coefficients (ζ). The frequency of the plot shown is 10 Hz. A ζ of 0.1 occurs when a system is very underdamped; a ζ of 2.0 occurs when a system is overdamped. The *dashed line* shows the frequency versus amplitude characteristic that would occur if the system had a "flat" frequency response. Along the frequency axis are plotted the harmonics of the pressure wave if the HR were 120 beats per minute (2/s). Note that by the fifth harmonic (10 Hz), if the ζ were 0.1, the true signal would be amplified fivefold. If the ζ were 2.0, an attenuation to about one fourth of the amplitude would occur. In both cases, gross waveform distortion would occur because neither situation reflects a "high-fidelity" system dynamic response. Fidelity of the system can be improved by (a) increasing the frequency or (b) adjusting the ζ to within a range of 0.5 to 0.7.

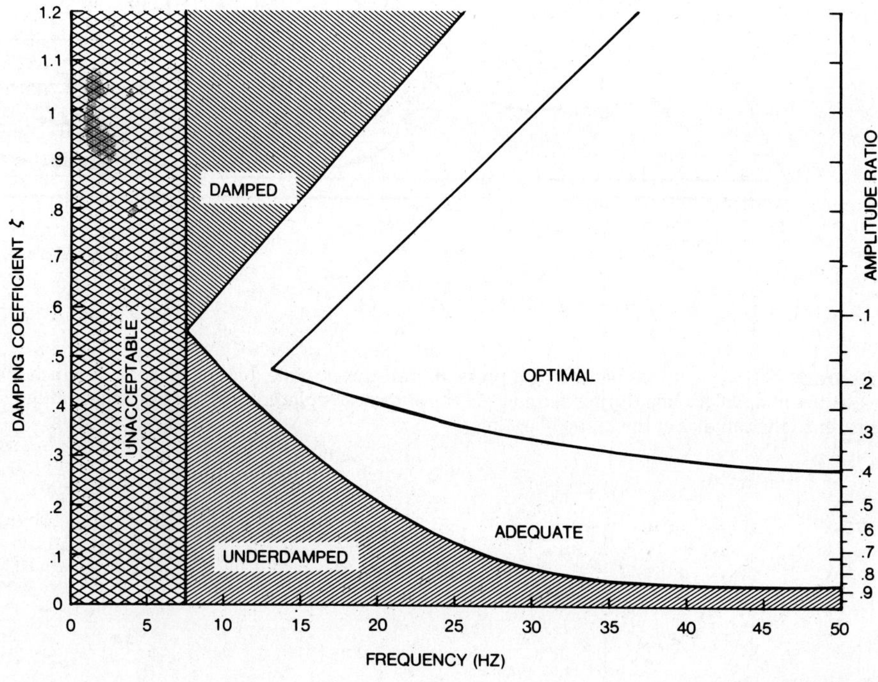

Figure 32–10. A frequency versus damping coefficient ζ plot that illustrates the five areas into which catheter-tubing/transducer systems fall. Systems that are in the optimal area reproduce even the most demanding (fast HR and rapid systolic upstroke) arterial or pulmonary artery waveforms without distortion. Systems that are in the adequate area reproduce most "typical" patient waveforms with little or no distortion. Systems in all other areas cause serious and clinically important waveform distortion. Note that the scale on the right can be used to estimate the ζ from the amplitude ratio determined during fast-flushing.[43] See Figure 32–11 for examples of waveforms.

Fast-flush dynamic response testing should be performed at regular intervals; such testing should always follow a manipulation of the plumbing system—for example, after drawing a blood sample. A fast-flush test is performed by opening the fast-flush valve of the continuous-flush system (e.g., by pulling the pigtail on an Intraflo (Abbott Critical Care, Salt Lake City, UT) or other continuous flush device and by allowing the fast-flush valve to snap closed; see Fig. 32–7). The rapid valve closure generates a square wave that permits a measurement of the plumbing system's Fn and damping coefficient.[55, 56] The fast-flush method is superior to other techniques for ascertaining the plumbing system's dynamic response because it is applied quickly, safely, and easily in the clinical setting (Fig. 32–11). This method tests the entire pressure monitoring system from the catheter tip to the display device.[56] As shown in Figure 32–11, the systolic pressure is the first pressure to be affected by poor dynamic response; the next is the diastolic pressure, which can tolerate much poorer dynamic response characteristics. Finally, note that the mean pressure is hardly affected at all by dynamic response limitation.

Several factors lead to poor dynamic response[57]: (1) the presence of air bubbles in the system; (2) the use of pressure tubing that is too long; (3) the use of pressure tubing that is too compliant; (4) the use of kinked tubing, particularly tubing with T connections; (5) the use of pressure transducers or continuous-flush devices that are too compliant; and (6) clot formation in the catheter.

Although air bubbles may be intentionally added to the plumbing system to "damp" the pressure waveforms, they also decrease the Fn and increase the damping coefficient. Adding air to pressure systems can thus create waveform distortion; it also increases the likelihood of blood clotting at the catheter tip because with added air more blood enters the catheter tip with each pressure pulsation. Clinically, the best method for improving a plumbing system's dynamic response is to improve the Fn. Techniques for increasing the system's Fn include the following:

1. The elimination of air bubbles by using transparent tubing and fluid pathways; air can then be seen and removed. Even a tiny air bubble (e.g., only 1 mm in diameter) in the transducer can result in serious waveform distortion. Since it is likely that air is dissolved in the flush solution, care should be taken to prevent air trapping at any point in the pressure monitoring system.[63]
2. The plumbing system should be simplified by using the fewest components possible. Preassembled pressure monitoring plumbing kits are recommended.[57]
3. Compliant elements should be eliminated; only short lengths of high-quality, low-compliance pressure tubing should be used. Injection-site or compliant stopcocks should not be used.
4. The use of the continuous-flush systems with dilute heparin prevents clot formation by keeping the catheter patent and by preventing "toilet seat" or flap-valve clots.[55, 72–75]

In the majority of situations, application of these techniques results in a system with acceptable frequency response (Fn > 20 Hz). If the plumbing system still does not preform adequately, an adjustable damping device[55, 76] might be used. Although pressure monitoring systems are tested in the laboratory to determine their dynamic characteristics,[55–59] fast-flush tests of each system's dynamic re-

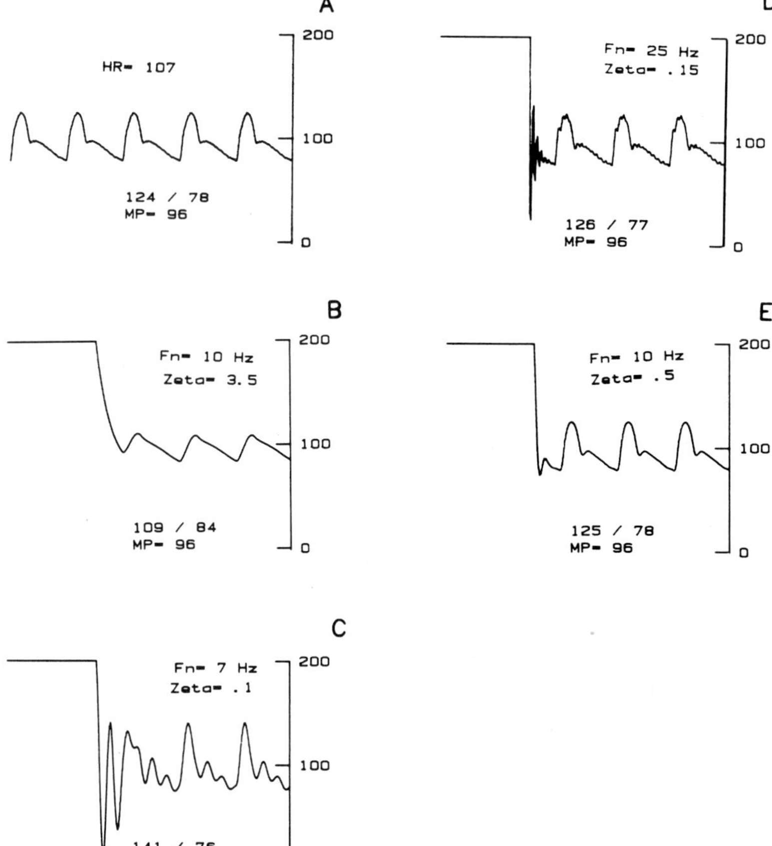

Figure 32–11. Arterial pressure waveforms obtained from the same patient. *A,* The patient's actual arterial pressure waveform is shown as if it were recorded with a catheter-tipped transducer. The systolic pressure is 124 mm Hg, the diastolic pressure is 78 mm Hg, and the mean pressure is 96 mm Hg. *B,* The same patient's arterial waveform when recorded with an "overdamped" system is depicted. Note that the "fast-flush" signal *(upper left)* returns slowly to the patient's waveform. Systolic pressure is underestimated (109 mm Hg), diastolic pressure is overestimated (84 mm Hg), and mean pressure is unchanged. *C,* An "underdamped" condition with low frequency (8 Hz) is shown. After the "fast-flush," the pressure signal oscillates rapidly *(rings).* Systolic pressure is overestimated (141 mm Hg), and mean pressure is correct. *D,* This panel shows an "underdamped" condition but one with a high frequency (25 Hz). Note that the waveform is only slightly distorted and that the systolic (128 mm Hg), diastolic (77 mm Hg), and mean pressures are close to the real pressures. *E,* An ideally damped pressure-monitoring system is shown. The undershoot after the "fast-flush" is small, and the patient's original waveform is adequately reproduced.

sponse in the clinical setting are essential because of individual setup variability.[56,57]

Pressure Monitor

Various electronic filters and processing algorithms that are built into pressure monitors may improperly extract data from the pressure waveform.[76–79] Pressure amplifiers should have a frequency response that extends from 0 (DC) to 50 Hz so that the patient's pressure is not distorted. A calibrated oscilloscope or a strip recorder provides the best view of blood pressure waveforms. These display devices allow the visualization of each pressure waveform in realtime so that respiratory variations, arrhythmias, and artifact can be seen.

Respiratory variations affect the arterial pressure; PAP is especially affected.[78,80–82] Digitally displayed results are available on most monitors and include systolic, diastolic, and mean pressures; some monitors determine HR from the pressure waveform. Systolic pressure is not the same for each heart beat and, as a result, the digital readout appears unstable; this is a problem that faces the monitor's manufacturer. Most manufacturers filter or average the beat-to-beat variability to get a representative systolic pressure. Although filters stabilize the display readings, most monitoring systems do not properly reject artifact.[79–86] Therefore, it is important to compare pressures displayed on a calibrated oscilloscope or recorder with values displayed on the digital readout.[79]

A performance review of three bedside monitors with pressure monitoring capability showed that none of the monitors recognized and rejected the following artifact conditions: (1) zeroing the transducer, (2) fast-flushing the system; and (3) drawing blood from the patient.[79] These conditions occur several times a day during normal patient care and result in the triggering of false alarms and in erroneous data logging. To help eliminate these problems, new pressure monitoring algorithms have been developed for bedside pressure monitors.[87]

Direct Versus Indirect Pressure Comparisons

There are several reasons why the directly measured and indirectly measured pressures do not agree. Even if the mechanics are properly evaluated, differences in pressure measurements can still occur. In addition to the variability caused by respiration, arrhythmias, and artifact, physiologic differences are known.[33–37,43–48] Real differences exist among arterial pressures that are measured in different locations in the arterial system. For example, an amplification of systolic pressure usually occurs as one moves to peripheral vessels; this amplification is similar to that seen in the underdamped system (see Fig. 32–11, Panel C). When measuring arterial pressure, it is desirable to advance the catheter tip to a central location such as the thoracic aorta or subclavian artery. Pressures measured at peripheral sites may not accurately reflect pressures at the central arterial location.[42–48] Often, femoral arterial catheters are inserted and advanced to measure abdominal or thoracic aortic pressures.[86] Central pressures are those that supply the driving force and cause flow to the vital organs, heart, kidney, and brain, and they are thus the most important. If an invasive arterial catheter is placed, great care should be taken to ensure that accurate pressure monitoring data are obtained.[41] Any invasive procedure increases the risk of infection and other complications, whereas inserting a catheter increases the risk of thrombosis.[60] Invasive catheters should be removed promptly when their use is no longer needed.

CONCLUSIONS

Monitoring equipment that is properly set up and used provides nursing and medical staff with an ever-increasing amount of valuable, up-to-date patient information. However, each measuring device can also produce false information. Care must be taken with all instruments to ensure that the useful data are maximized and that the "garbage" is minimized. In most cases, the devotion of care and attention to the details of measuring instrument setup contributes greatly to the achievement of accurate monitoring data.

GLOSSARY*

Artifact A medical term used to describe electrical noise; errors in a test result, graph, or written record.

Common-mode rejection Interference that appears between both signal leads and a common reference plane (ground). *For ECG amplifiers:* the ability to reject the signal common to both ECG leads (usually the high-level signal coupled from the electrical power source [60 Hz]).

Damping coefficient zeta (ζ) A characteristic of a second-order linear system that relates to how quickly it comes to rest after being disturbed.

Distortion An undesired change in waveform.

Frequency response The frequency-dependent relation in both gain and phase difference, between steady-state sinusoidal input and output.

Gain A general term used to denote the ratio of output voltage or power of an amplifier to its input voltage or power.

Half-cell An electrode immersed in a suitable electrolyte that generates a battery voltage. Half-cells are formed with the electrode-electrolyte interface in ECG electrodes.

Input resistance The passive resistance of the input terminal or terminals of an amplifier.

Interference In a data transmission path, either the extraneous power that tends to interfere with the reception of the desired signals or the disturbance of the signal that results.

Internal noise The undesirable electrical noise generated internally in an amplifier system.

Linear amplifier An amplifier in which the output quantity is essentially proportional to the input quantity.

Natural frequency (Fn) For a second-order linear system without damping, the frequency of free oscillations in Hertz (cycles per second).

Noise Unwanted disturbances superimposed upon a useful signal that tend to obscure its information content.

Nonlinear distortion Distortion caused by a deviation from a desired linear relationship between specified output and input measurements of a system.

Shielded wires Wires that are wrapped with foil or a wire screen covering to prevent the pickup of unwanted electric field signals.

Shot noise Noise caused by current fluctuations due to the discrete nature of charge carriers in amplifiers.

Static charge A charge developed on a surface; it usually results from friction.

Thermal noise Noise occurring in electric conductors and resistors as a result of random free electron movement.

Triboelectricity Electricity generated by friction.

Twisted-pair wires Cables composed of two small insulated conductors twisted together in a common covering. Used to prevent the pickup of unwanted magnetic signals.

---

*Definitions adapted from the IEEE Standard Dictionary of Electrical and Electronic Terms. 3rd ed. Frank Jay (Ed). New York, Institute of Electrical and Electronic Engineers, Inc., 1984.

References

1a. Webster JG (Ed): Medical Instrumentation: Applications and Design. 2nd ed. Boston, Houghton-Miffin, 1992.

1b. Gardner RM, Hujcs M: Fundamentals of physiologic monitoring. *In*: Concepts of Physiologic Monitoring/Hemodynamic Pressure Monitoring Systems. AACN Clin Issues Crit Care Nurs 1993; 4:11–24.

1c. Kotrly KJ, Kotter GS, Mortara D, et al: Intraoperative detection of myocardial ischemia with a ST segment trend monitoring system. Anesth Analg 1984; 63:343.

2. Smith M: Rx for ECG monitoring artifacts. Crit Care Nurs 1984; 4:64.
3. Webster JG: Reducing motion artifacts and interference in biopotential recording. IEEE Trans Biomed Eng 1984; 31:823.
4. Kaplan JA: Electrocardiographic monitoring. *In:* Cardiac Anesthesia. Kaplan JA (Ed). New York, Grune & Stratton, 1979, pp 117–166.
5. Kaplan JA: The electrocardiogram and anesthesia. *In:* Anesthesia. Miller RD (Ed). New York, Churchill Livingstone, 1981, pp 203–232.
6. Klinger DR, Schoenberg AA, Worth NP, et al: A comparison of gel-to-gel skin measurements of electrode impedance. Med Instrum 1979; 13:266.
7. Olson WH, Schmincke DR, Henley BL: Time and frequency dependence of disposable ECG electrode–skin impedance. Med Instrum 1979; 13:269.
8. Thakor NV, Webster JG: Electrode studies for the long-term ambulatory ECG. Med Biol Eng Comput 1982; 20:159.
9. Odman S, Oberg P: Movement-induced potentials in surface electrodes. Med Biol Eng Comput 1982; 29:159.
10. American National Standards Institute (ANSI) and Association for the Advancement of Medical Instrumentation (AAMI): American National Standard for Pregelled ECG Disposable Electrodes. Arlington, VA, 1984.
11. Patterson RP: The electrical characteristics of some commercial ECG electrodes. J Electrocardiol 1978; 11:23.
12. Klingler DR, Booth HE, Schoenberg AA: Effects of DC bias currents on ECG electrodes. Med Instrum 1979; 13:257.

12a. Gardner RM: Offset potential of commercial ECG Electrodes (Letter). Heart Lung 1994; 23:267–268.

13. Schoenberg AA, Booth HE, Lyon PC: Development of standard test methods for evaluating defibrillation recovery characteristics of disposable ECG electrodes. Med Instrum 1979; 13:259.
14. DeRose JF, Gadsby PD: Radio-frequency heating under ECG electrodes. Med Instrument 1979; 13:273.
15. Huhta JC, Webster JG: 60-Hz interference in electrocardiography. IEEE Trans Biomed Eng 1973; 20:91.
16. Winter BB, Webster JG: Reduction of interference due to common-mode voltage in biopotential amplifiers. IEEE Trans Biomed Eng 1983; 30:85.
17. Winter BB, Webster JG: Driven-right-leg circuit design. IEEE Trans Biomed Eng 1983; 30:62.
18. Association for the Advancement of Medical Instrumentation (AAMI): Standard for Cardiac Monitors, Heart Rate, and Alarms. Arlington, VA, 1984.
19. Gordon DH: Triboelectric interference in the ECG. IEEE Trans Biomed Eng 1975; 22:252.
20. Evaluation: Patient monitoring system. Health Devices 1985; 14:143.
21. American Heart Association: AHA committee report: Recommendations for standardizing of lead and of specifications for instruments in electrocardiography and vectorcardiography. Circulation 1975; 52:11.
22. Kirkendall WM, Feinleib M, Freis ED, et al: Recommendations for human blood pressure determination by sphygmomanometers. Subcommittee of the AHA Postgraduate Education Committee. Circulation 1980; 62:1146A.
23. Cohn JN: Blood pressure measurement in shock: Mechanisms of inaccuracy in auscultation and palpatory methods. JAMA 1967; 19:972.
24. Smith NT, Wesseling KH, de Wit B: Evaluation of two prototype devices producing noninvasive, pulsatile, calibrated blood pressure measurement from a finger. J Clin Monit 1985; 1:17.
25. Jones RDM, Brown AG, Roulson CJ, et al: The upgraded Finapres 2300e: A clinical evaluation of a continuous noninvasive blood pressure monitor. Anaesthesia 1992; 47:701.
26. Ramsey M: Noninvasive automatic determination of mean arterial pressure. Med Biol Eng Comput 1979; 17:11.
27. Paulus DA: Noninvasive blood pressure measurement. Med Instrum 1981; 15:91.
28. Geddes LA, Voelz M, Combs C, et al. Characterization of the oscillometric method of measurement of indirect blood pressure. Ann Biomed Eng 1982; 10:271.
29. Sheppard LC, Johnson TS, Kirkland JW: Controlled study of brachial artery blood pressure measurement by a new indirect method: J Assoc Adv Med Instrum 1971; 5:297.
30. Davis RF: Clinical comparison of automated auscultatory and oscillometric and catheter-transducer measurement of arterial pressure. J Clin Monit 1985; 1:114.
31. Hutton P, Dye J, Prys-Roberts C: An assessment of the Dinamap 845. Anaesthesia 1984; 39:261.
32. Johnson CJH, Kerr JH: Automatic blood pressure monitors: A clinical evaluation of five models in adults. Anesthesia 1985; 30:471.
33. Nystrom E, Reid KH, Bennett R, et al: A comparison of two automated indirect arterial blood pressure meters: With recordings from a radial artery catheter in anesthetized surgical patients. Anesthesiology 1985; 62:526.
34. Finnie KJC, Watts DG, Armstrong PW: Biases in the measurement of arterial pressure. Crit Care Med 1984; 12:965.
35. Automated sphygmomanometers. Health Devices 1986; 15:187.
36. Physiologic patient monitors. Health Devices 1991; 20:81.
37. Evaluation criteria, test methods, and results for ECG monitors, invasive and noninvasive blood pressure monitors. Health Devices 1991; 20:100.
38. Runciman WB, Rutten AJ, Ilsley AH: An evaluation of blood pressure measurement. Anaesth Intensive Care 1981; 9:314.
39. Runciman WB, Ilsley AH, Rutten AJ: Systemic arterial pressure. Anaesth Intensive Care 1988; 16:54.
40. O'Rourke MF: Wave reflection and the arterial pulse. Arch Intern Med 1984; 144:366.
41. O'Rourke MF: What is blood pressure? Am J Hypertens 1990; 3:803.
42. Stern DH, Gerson JL, Allen FB, et al: Can we trust the direct radial artery pressure immediately following cardiopulmonary bypass? Anesthesiology 1985; 62:557.
43. Gallagher JD, Morre RA, McNicolas KW, et al: Comparisons of radial and femoral arterial blood pressure in children after cardiopulmonary bypass. J Clin Monit 1985; 1:168.
44. Rulf ENR, Mitchell MM, Prakash O, et al: Measurement of arterial pressure after cardiopulmonary bypass with long radial artery catheters. J Cardiothorac Anesth 1990; 4:19.
45. Pauca AL, Wallenhaupt SL, Kon ND, et al: Does radial artery pressure accurately reflect aortic pressure? Chest 1992; 102:1193–1198.
46. Gravlee GP, Brauer SD, O'Rourke MF, et al: A comparison of brachial, femoral, and aortic intra-arterial pressures before and after cardiopulmonary bypass. Anaesth Intensive Care 1989; 17:305.
47. Bazaral MG, Welch M, Golding LAR, et al: Comparison of brachial and radial artery pressure monitoring in patients undergoing arterial bypass surgery. Anesthesiology 1990; 73:38–45.
48. Maruyama K, Horiguchi R, Hashimoto H, et al: Effect of combined infusion of nitroglycerin and nicardipine on femoral–to–radial artery pressure gradient after cardiopulmonary bypass. Anesth Analg 1990; 70:428.
49. Bruner JMR, Krensi LJ, Kunsman JM, et al: Comparison of direct and indirect methods of measuring arterial blood pressure. Parts I to III. Med Instrum 1981; 15:11, 97, and 182.
50. Bruner JMR: Handbook of Measuring Arterial Blood Pressure. Littleton, MA, PSG Publishing, 1978, p 83.

50a. Iyriboz Y, Heraon CM: A proposal for scientific validation of instruments for indirect blood pressure measurement at rest, during exercise, and in critical care. J Clin Monit 1994; 10:163–177.

50b. Bruner JMR: On the calibration of artifacts (Editorial). J Clin Monit 1994; 10:143–146.

50c. Yong P, Geddes LA: A surrogate arm for evaluating the accu-

racy of instruments for indirect measurement of blood pressure. Biomed Instrum Technol 1990; 24:130–135.
50d. Drzewiecki G, Bansal V, Karam E, et al: Mechanics of the occlusive arm cuff and its application as a volume sensor. IEEE Trans Biomed Eng 1993; 40:704–708.
51. Sy WP: Ulnar nerve palsy possibly related to use of automatically cycled blood pressure cuff. Anesth Analg 1981; 60:687.
52. Showman A, Betts EK: Hazard of automatic noninvasive blood pressure monitors. Anesthesiology 1981; 55:717.
53. Roy RC, Morgan L, Beamer D: Factitiously low blood pressure from the Dinamap. Anesthesiology 1983; 55:717.
54. Manning DM, Kuchirka C, Kaminski J: Miscuffing: Inappropriate blood pressure cuff application. Circulation 1983; 68:763.
55. Gardner RM: Direct blood pressure measurement: Dynamic response requirements. Anesthesiology 1981; 54:227.
56. Kleinman B, Powell S, Kumar P, et al: The fast flush does measure the dynamic response of the entire blood pressure monitoring system. Anesthesiology 1992; 77:1215.
57. Heimann PA, Murray WB: Construction and use of catheter-manometer systems. J Clin Monit 1993; 9:45.
58. Shinozaki T, Deane RS, Mazuzan JE: The dynamic responses of liquid-filled catheter systems for direct measurements of blood pressure. Anesthesiology 1980; 53:498.
59. Boutros A, Albert S: Effect of the dynamic response of transducer–tubing system on accuracy of direct pressure measurement in patients. Crit Care Med 1983; 11:124.
60. Toll MO: Direct blood-pressure measurements: Risks, technology evolution and some current problems. Med Biol Eng Comput 1984; 22:2.
61. O'Quin R, Marini JJ: Pulmonary artery occlusion pressure: Clinical physiology, measurement, and interpretation. Am Rev Respir Dis 1983; 128:319.
62. Garrett JS, Vernon DD, Xanos N, et al: Spurious hemodynamic alterations resulting from light sensitive pressure transducers. Crit Care Med 1993; 21:1401–1402.
63. Soule DT, Powner DJ: Air entrapment in pressure monitoring lines. Crit Care Med 1984; 12:520.
64. Barbieri LT, Kaplan JA: Artifactual hypotension secondary to intraoperative transducer failure. Anesth Analg 1983; 62:112.
65. Gardner RM, Kutik M: American National Standard for Interchangeability and Performance of Resistive Bridge-Type Blood Pressure Transducers. New York, American National Standards Institute, 1986.
66. Disposable pressure transducers. Health Devices 1984; 13:268.
67. Gordon VL, Welch JP, Carley D, et al: Zero stability of disposable and reusable pressure transducers. Med Instrum 1987; 21:81.
68. Disposable pressure transducers (evaluation). Health Devices 1988; 17:75.
69. Air embolism during calibration of invasive blood pressure monitoring systems. Health Devices 1982; 11:22.
70. Hazards: Disposable blood pressure transducers: Calibration methods. Health Devices 1993; 22:97.
71. Hunziker P: Accuracy and dynamic response of disposable pressure transducer–tubing systems. Can J Anaesth 1987; 34:409–414.
72. Gardner RM, Bond EL, Clark JS: Safety and efficacy of continuous flush systems for arterial and pulmonary artery catheters. Ann Thorac Surg 1977; 23:534.
73. Clifton GD, Branson P, Kelly HJ, et al: Comparison of normal saline and heparin solutions for maintenance of arterial catheter patency. Heart Lung 1991; 20:115.
74. Hook ML, Reuling J, Luettgen ML, et al: Comparison of the patency of arterial lines maintained with heparinized and nonheparinized infusions. Heart Lung 1987; 16:693.
75. Peterson FY, Kirchoff KT: Analysis of the research about heparinized versus nonheparinized intravascular lines. Heart Lung 1991; 20:631.
76. Abrams JH, Olson ML, Marino JA, et al: Use of a needle valve variable resistor to improve invasive blood pressure monitoring. Crit Care Med 1984; 12:978.
77. Ream AK: Mean blood pressure algorithms. J Clin Monit 1985; 1:138.
78. Ellis DM: Interpretation of beat-to-beat blood pressure values in the presence of ventilator change. J Clin Monit 1985; 1:65.
79. Maloy L, Gardner RM: Monitoring systemic arterial blood pressure: Strip recording versus digital display. Heart Lung 1986; 15:627.
80. Berryhill RE, Benumof JL, Rauscher LA: Pulmonary vascular pressure reading at end of exhalation. Anesthesiology 1978; 49:365.
81. Cengiz M, Crapo RO, Gardner RM: The effect of ventilation on the accuracy of pulmonary artery and wedge pressure measurement. Crit Care Med 1983; 11:502.
82. McGregor M: Pulsus paradoxes. N Engl J Med 1979; 301:480.
83. Morris AH, Chapman RH, Gardner RM: Frequency of technical problems encountered in the measurement of pulmonary artery wedge pressure. Crit Care Med 1984; 12:164.
84. Morris AH, Chapman RH, Gardner RM: Frequency of wedge pressure errors in the ICU. Crit Care Med 1985; 13:705.
85. Bridges EJ, Woods SL: Pulmonary artery pressure measurement: State of the art. Heart Lung 1993; 22:99.
86. Thomas F, Burke JP, Parker J, et al: The risk of infection related to radial vs. femoral sites of arterial catheterization. Crit Care Med 1983; 11:807.
87. Gardner RM, Monis SM, Oehler P: Monitoring direct blood pressure: Algorithm enhancements. IEEE Comput Cardiol 1986; 13:607.

CHAPTER 33

Interpretation of Blood Gases

Barry A. Shapiro, MD • William T. Peruzzi, MD

Respiration is the diffusion of oxygen (O_2) and carbon dioxide (CO_2) molecules across permeable membranes. Respiratory homeostasis encompasses all physiologic mechanisms acting to balance O_2 and CO_2 exchange at the lung and cellular levels. Critically ill patients often require therapeutic interventions to maintain respiratory homeostasis, a clinical demand that depends to a major degree on the availability and interpretation of arterial blood gas values (pH, partial pressure of carbon dioxide [$P{CO_2}$] and oxygen [$P{O_2}$]) and related measurements.

METABOLIC ACID-BASE IMBALANCE

When the arterial pH and $P{CO_2}$ are known, the clinical form of the Henderson-Hasselbalch equation (where the pK = 6.1, the solubility coefficient [s] = 0.0301, and HCO_3^- is the bicarbonate ion)

$$pH = pK + \log \frac{[HCO_3^-]}{s \times P{CO_2}}$$

allows for the calculation of plasma bicarbonate concentration. The normal ranges for these parameters are listed in Table 33–1. The terms *acidosis* and *alkalosis* refer to conditions of abnormal acid-base balance in which the pH need not be abnormal while either the acids or bases are dominant. Essentially, metabolic acidosis and alkalosis are determined by the calculation of the HCO_3^-, whereas blood pH measurement determines *acidemia* and *alkalemia* (an excess or deficit of free hydrogen ion [H^+] activity). Table 33–2 lists the traditional nomenclature in regard to metabolic acid-base imbalance.

Evaluation of Metabolic Acid-Base Abnormalities

Human blood contains an enormous buffering capacity that allows notable changes in acid content to occur with incon-

TABLE 33–1. The Henderson-Hasselbalch Parameters and Their Laboratory Normal Ranges

Variable	*pH*	*P_{CO_2} (mm Hg)*	*$[HCO_3^-]p$ (mmol/L)*
Normal	7.35–7.45	35–45	22–26
Acidotic	<7.35	>45	<22
Alkalotic	>7.45	<35	>26

Abbreviations: HCO_3^- = bicarbonate ion; P_{CO_2} = partial pressure of carbon dioxide.

sequential changes in free H^+ concentration (pH). As diminution of the normal buffering capacity develops, the pH change for any given change in acid content increases. This crucial buffering capacity depends not only on the HCO_3^- concentration but also on the red blood cell mass and other factors.

The concept of base excess/deficit is founded on the premise that the degree of deviation from the normal buffering availability can be calculated independently of compensatory partial pressure of carbon dioxide (P_{CO_2}) changes. A negative base excess is referred to as a base deficit. A base excess within ±3 mmol/L denotes a normal metabolic acid-base status. A base excess within ±5 mmol/L denotes a relatively balanced metabolic acid-base status. An abnormal pH with a base excess outside ±10 mmol/L denotes a clinically significant metabolic acid-base imbalance that may be life threatening; and a base excess of ±5 to 10 mmol/L should be investigated and corrective intervention considered.

Estimating Base Excess

The Pa_{CO_2}–pH relationship is predictable and can be approximated as shown in Table 33–3 if a baseline Pa_{CO_2} of 40 mm Hg and a baseline pH of 7.40 are assumed. An acute increase of 10 mm Hg in the Pa_{CO_2} results in a pH decrease of approximately 0.05; an acute decrease in Pa_{CO_2} of 10 mm Hg results in a pH increase of 0.10. Under normal circumstances, a variance of 10 mmol/L from the normal buffer baseline represents a metabolic pH change of approximately 0.15. Moving the pH decimal point two places to the right results in a two:three relationship (10 ± 15). The steps for estimating the base excess are outlined in Table 33–4.

Mixed Acid-Base Abnormalities

The term *mixed acid-base abnormality* refers to conditions in which respiratory and metabolic imbalances coexist. Most commonly, one imbalance is a consequence of homeostatic mechanisms compensating for the original imbalance. Proper clinical assessment of such blood gas values demands that the respiratory and metabolic components be separately identified and quantified because each will be treated quite differently. Simply stated, when an estimation of the pH at a P_{CO_2} of 40 mm Hg is made, the metabolic component of the acid-base abnormality has been accomplished. The appropriate process for making such an estimation has produced significant debate and controversy for decades[1]; however, these historic concerns should not confuse our clinical ability to interpret arterial blood gas values properly.[2]

There are three generally accepted approaches for estimating the degree of nonrespiratory acid-base imbalance (Table 33–5): (1) calculation of plasma bicarbonate concentration from the measured pH and P_{CO_2}; (2) calculation of the base excess/deficit from the measured pH and P_{CO_2}; and (3) determination of the calculated pH difference from the measured pH and P_{CO_2}. All three methods are clinically appropriate and result in clinically acceptable accuracy.

TABLE 33–2. Traditional Metabolic Acid-Base Nomenclature

Nomenclature	*pH*	*P_{CO_2}*	*$[HCO_3^-]p$*	*BE*
Metabolic Acidosis				
Uncompensated (acute)	↓	N	↓	↓ (−)
Partly compensated (subacute)	↓	↓	↓	↓ (−)
Completely compensated (chronic)	N	↓	↓	↓ (−)
Metabolic Alkalosis				
Uncompensated (acute)	↑	N	↑	↑ (+)
Partly compensated (subacute)	↑	↑	↑	↑ (+)
Completely compensated (chronic)	N	↑	↑	↑ (+)

Abbreviations: P_{CO_2} = partial pressure of carbon dioxide; HCO_3^- = bicarbonate ion; ↑ = increased; ↓ = decreased; N = normal; BE = base excess.

TABLE 33–3. Approximate Pa_{CO_2}–pH Relationship*

Pa_{CO_2} (mm Hg)	*pH*	*$[HCO_3^-]p$ (mmol/L)*
80	7.20	28
60	7.30	26
40	7.40	24
30	7.50	22
20	7.60	20

*Boxed data represent assumed baseline.
Abbreviations: Pa_{CO_2} = partial pressure of arterial carbon dioxide; HCO_3^- = bicarbonate ion.

Anion Gap Concept

Clinical reality requires that metabolic acid-base imbalances be detectable from routine clinical chemistry studies when the arterial pH and P_{CO_2} are not available. The confines of electrical neutrality dictate that significant differences in plasma cation and anion concentrations cannot exist. The *anion gap* is an artificial disparity between the major plasma cations and anions routinely measured,* namely, sodium ion (Na^+, chloride ion (Cl^-), and HCO_3^-. Minor plasma cations include potassium ion, calcium ion, and magnesium ion, and minor plasma anions include phosphates, sulfates,

*Some include potassium because it is commonly measured. However, most do not include potassium because it is not a major plasma cation.

TABLE 33–4. Three Steps for Determining Base Excess* / Deficit†

1. Determine P_{CO_2} variance (difference between measured P_{CO_2} and 40 mm Hg); move decimal point two places to the left.
2. Determine predicted pH: If P_{CO_2} >40 mm Hg, subtract half P_{CO_2} variance from 7.40. If P_{CO_2} <40 mm Hg, add P_{CO_2} variance to 7.40.
3. Estimate base excess/deficit: Determine difference between measured and predicted pH. Move decimal point two places to the right. Multiply by two thirds.

*Base excess: measured pH greater than predicted pH.
†Base deficit (often referred to as a "minus base excess").
Abbreviation: P_{CO_2} = partial pressure of carbon dioxide.

TABLE 33–5. Three Generally Accepted Approaches for Estimating Degree of Nonrespiratory Acid-Base Imbalance

Case Study	*HCO_3^- (mmol/L)*	*Base Excess/Deficit (mmol/L)*	*pH Difference*
Normal	22–26	±3	±.06
Acceptable	20–28	±5	±.10

Abbreviation: HCO_3^- = bicarbonation.

and organic anions such as proteins. The anion gap is calculated as follows:

$$\text{Major plasma cations} - \text{major plasma anions}$$
$$[Na^+] - ([Cl^-] + [HCO_3^-])$$

The anion gap is normally 8 to 16 mmol/L* (12 ± 4 being two SDs from the mean). Plasma albumin normally accounts for approximately 11 mmol/L of the anion gap[3]; therefore, a decreased anion gap is commonly due to either hypoalbuminemia or severe hemodilution. Less commonly, a decreased anion gap is due to an increase in the cations that are not major, such as encountered with lithium toxicity, hypercalcemia, hypermagnesemia, and bromide toxicity.

Anion Gap Acidosis

Any process that increases minor anions should create a metabolic acidosis with an anion gap. This occurs with hyperlactatemia, hyperketonemia, renal failure (increased sulfates, phosphates), excessive organic salt therapy (Ringer's lactate solution, sodium acetate, carbenicillin, high-dose penicillin), and dehydration. Ingestion of salicylates, methanol, ethylene glycol, and others causes accumulation of nonvolatile organic acids, including acetic acid. Rarely, an anion gap may result from decreased minor cations, such as calcium and magnesium, which causes an increase in sodium.

Nonanion Gap Acidosis

A metabolic acidosis without an increased anion gap is typically associated with an increased plasma Cl^- that has replaced depleted plasma HCO_3^-. Such hyperchloremic acidosis is most commonly due to gastrointestinal loss of bicarbonate (diarrhea) or renal wasting of HCO_3^- (renal tubular acidosis).[4]

Hyperlactatemia

Metabolic acidosis attributable to accumulation of organic metabolites, such as lactic acid, should be accompanied by an increased anion gap. It has been traditionally assumed that a nonanion gap metabolic acidosis reliably rules out hyperlactatemia in critically ill patients.[3, 5] However, some studies suggested that more than half of intensive care unit (ICU) patients with hyperlactatemia manifest nonanion gap metabolic acidosis.[6, 7] This is most likely due to the notable incidence of preexisting hypoalbuminemia, hyperchloremia, and mixed acid-base disorders in the ICU population.[8–11]

Because lactate is the end product of anaerobic glucose metabolism, hyperlactatemia is a credible clinical indicator of tissue hypoxia because it reflects anaerobic metabolism in excess of the hepatic/renal uptake. Correlations of hyperlactatemia with mortality in the critically ill patient are well established.[12–14] In view of these factors, lactate levels should be measured when the clinical suspicion of hyperlactatemia exists. Clinical ranges for arterial lactate levels (whole blood) are shown in Table 33–6.

*12–20 mmol/L when the serum potassium is included as a major cation.

TABLE 33–6. Clinical Ranges for Arterial Lactate Levels

Lactate (mmol/L)	*Clinical Terminology*	*Associated Mortality (%)*
<2.5	Normal	—
2.5–4.9	Mild	25–35
5.0–9.9	Moderate	60–75
>10.0	Severe	>95

Sodium Bicarbonate Administration

When sodium bicarbonate is administered intravenously to correct severe metabolic acidemia, it is imperative to quantify the abnormality as a guide to therapy. Table 33–7 demonstrates a procedure for quantifying extracellular bicarbonate deficit. It is generally prudent to administer one half to one third of the calculated deficit and then obtain another blood gas sample in 5 minutes and re-evaluate.

Intravenous sodium bicarbonate solution is an appropriate therapy for reversing metabolic acidemia as long as lung function is adequate and the cardiac output is not significantly low. As illustrated in Figure 33–1, sodium bicarbonate solution adds HCO_3^- to the blood only after the CO_2 load inherent in the sodium bicarbonate solution is eliminated by the lungs. As illustrated in Figure 33–2, when sodium bicarbonate solution is administered to a patient with acute respiratory acidosis, the $Pa{CO_2}$ usually increases and arterial pH decreases because the CO_2 load cannot be eliminated. As illustrated in Figure 33–3, low cardiac output may be a limiting factor in CO_2 excretion. When sodium bicarbonate solution is administered to a patient with very poor cardiac output or ventilatory function, the venous blood demonstrates a paradoxic respiratory acidosis.

ASSESSMENT OF RESPIRATORY ACID-BASE IMBALANCE

Ventilation is gas movement in and out of the pulmonary system and is most readily measured in critically ill patients as the gas volume exhaled in 1 minute (VE). The portion of the VE that respires (removes CO_2 from the blood and transfers O_2 to the blood) is referred to as *alveolar ventilation* (VA); the portion of the VE that does not respire is designated as dead space ventilation (VDS).

Alveolar Ventilation and the Arterial Partial Pressure of Carbon Dioxide

Respiratory acid-base balance depends on the ability of homeostatic systems to maintain a balance between CO_2 production and excretion. The metabolic rate essentially determines the quantity of CO_2 that enters the blood; lung function essentially determines the quantity of CO_2 excreted from the blood. The major determinant of CO_2 excretion is

TABLE 33–7. Quantifying Extracellular Bicarbonate Deficit

1. Base deficit is the millimoles of bicarbonate that is deficient per liter of extracellular water.
2. Approximately 25% of an adult's total body weight in kilograms is equivalent to the number of liters of extracellular water.

$$\frac{\text{Base deficit} \times \text{weight (kg)}}{4} = \text{deficient millimoles of bicarbonate}$$

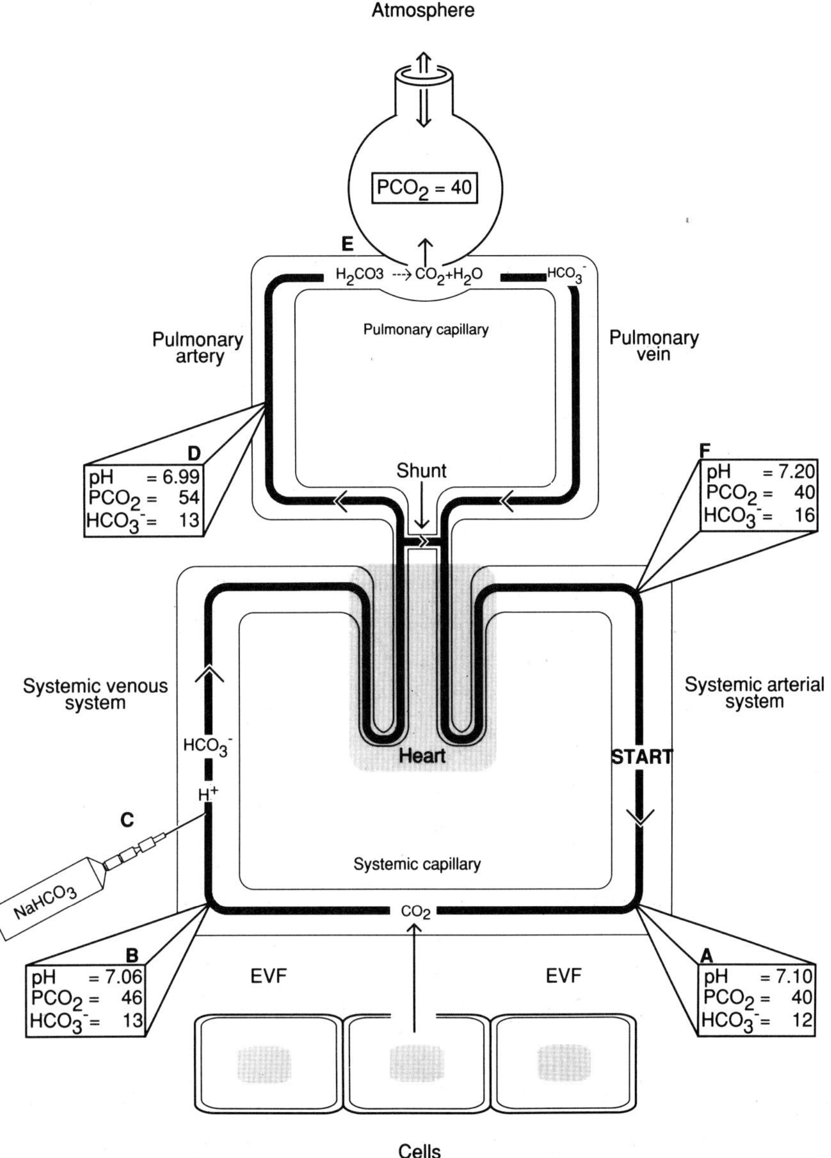

Figure 33–1. Schematic illustration of a single circulation time demonstrating the effect of intravenous sodium bicarbonate ($NaHCO_3$) administration in the presence of metabolic acidemia when the cardiac output and pulmonary reserves are adequate. The schema begins in the systemic arterial system (START), with *box A* representing the original arterial blood pH as 7.10, P_{CO_2} as 40 mm Hg, and HCO_3^- as 12 mmol/L; *box B* represents the systemic venous system blood pH as 7.06, P_{CO_2} as 46 mm Hg, and HCO_3^- as 13 mmol/L prior to intravenous $NaHCO_3$ administration; C represents the site of intravenous $NaHCO_3$ injection, which adds carbonic acid to the blood (essentially a hydrogen ion [H^+] and a bicarbonate ion [HCO_3^-]); *box D* represents the mixed venous blood pH as 6.99, P_{CO_2} as 54 mm Hg, and HCO_3^- as 13 mmol/L after $NaHCO_3$ administration; E represents the process of alveolar CO_2 excretion, which essentially eliminates a hydrogen ion while the bicarbonate ion remains in the blood; *box F* represents the resultant arterial blood pH of 7.20, P_{CO_2} of 40 mm Hg, and HCO_3^- of 16 mmol/L. Note the net HCO_3^- gain from *box A* to *box F*. EVF = extravascular fluid. (From Shapiro BA, Peruzzi WT, Templin R: Clinical Application of Blood Gases. 5th ed. Chicago, Mosby-Yearbook, 1994.)

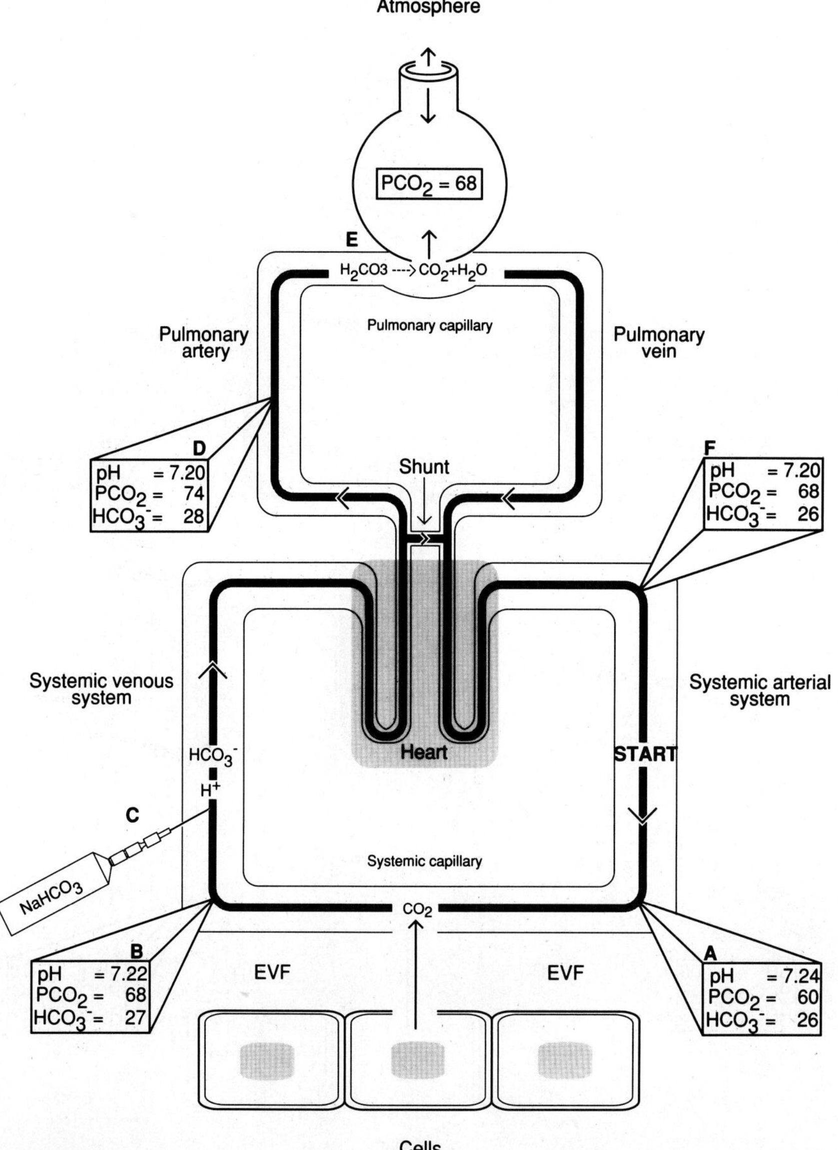

Figure 33–2. Schematic illustration of a single circulation time demonstrating the effect of intravenous $NaHCO_3$ administration when a mixed metabolic and respiratory acidemia is present secondary to an inability of the pulmonary system to adequately excrete CO_2. The schema begins in the systemic arterial system (START), with *box A* representing the original arterial blood pH as 7.24, P_{CO_2} as 60 mm Hg, and HCO_3^- as 26 mmol/L; *box B* represents the systemic venous system blood pH as 7.22, P_{CO_2} as 68 mm Hg, and HCO_3^- as 27 mmol/L prior to intravenous $NaHCO_3$ administration; C represents the site of intravenous $NaHCO_3$ injection, which adds carbonic acid to the blood (essentially a hydrogen ion [H^+] and a bicarbonate ion [HCO_3^-]); *box D* represents the mixed venous blood pH as 7.20, P_{CO_2} as 74 mm Hg, and HCO_3^- as 28 mmol/L after $NaHCO_3$ administration; E represents inadequate alveolar CO_2 excretion and, therefore, essentially no addition of HCO_3^- to the blood; *box F* represents the resultant arterial blood pH of 7.20, P_{CO_2} of 68 mm Hg, and HCO_3^- of 26 mmol/L. Note the increase in P_{CO_2}, decrease in pH, and absence of change in HCO_3^- from *box A* to *box F*. (From Shapiro BA, Peruzzi WT, Templin R: Clinical Application of Blood Gases. 5th ed. Chicago, Mosby-Yearbook, 1994.)

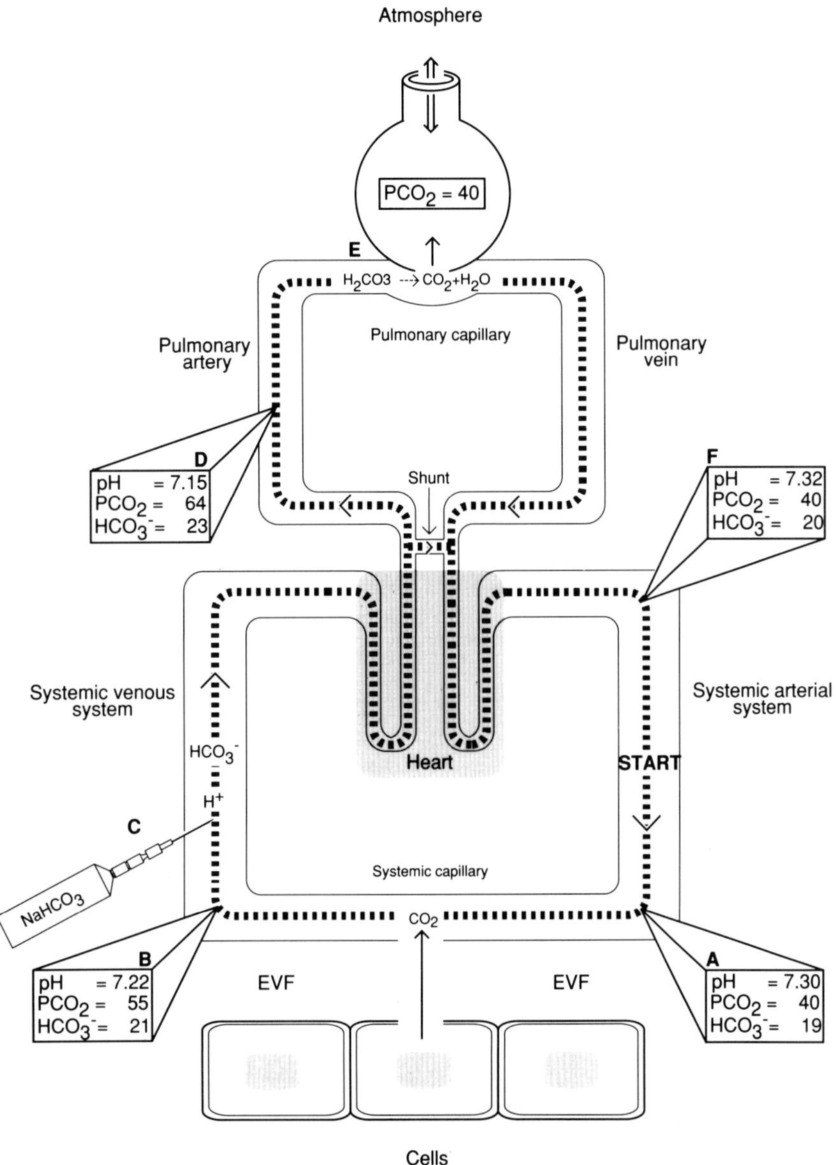

Figure 33–3. Schematic illustration of a single circulation time that demonstrates the effect of intravenous $NaHCO_3$ administration when a metabolic acidemia is present secondary to a low cardiac output (hypoperfusion and lactic acidemia). The diminished cardiac output is represented by the *broken circulation line.* The schema begins in the systemic arterial system (START), with *box A* representing the original arterial blood pH of 7.30, P_{CO_2} of 40 mm Hg, and HCO_3^- of 19 mmol/L; *box B* represents the systemic venous system blood pH as 7.22, P_{CO_2} as 55 mm Hg, and HCO_3^- as 21 mmol/L prior to intravenous $NaHCO_3$ administration; C represents the site of intravenous $NaHCO_3$ injection, which adds carbonic acid to the blood (essentially a hydrogen ion [H^+] and a bicarbonate ion [HCO_3^-]); *box D* represents the mixed venous blood pH as 7.15, P_{CO_2} as 64 mm Hg, and HCO_3^- as 23 mmol/L after $NaHCO_3$ administration; E represents adequate alveolar CO_2 excretion from the diminished blood flow per unit time; *box F* represents the resultant arterial blood pH of 7.32, P_{CO_2} of 40 mm Hg, and HCO_3^- of 20 mmol/L. Note the relatively unchanged values between *box A* and *box F*, while the venous blood is significantly hypercapnic and acidemic as a result of the $NaHCO_3$ administration. (From Shapiro BA, Peruzzi WT, Templin R: Clinical Application of Blood Gases. 5th ed. Chicago, Mosby-Yearbook, 1994.)

the alveolar CO_2 tension (P_{ACO_2}), which varies to some degree among the millions of individual alveoli; however, the Pa_{CO_2} reflects the mean P_{ACO_2} and is the clinical measurement used to reflect the functional status of CO_2 excretion.

It is crucial that significantly abnormal CO_2 production be identified when interpreting the Pa_{CO_2} because the rate of CO_2 production affects the intracellular P_{CO_2}, which in turn influences the rate of CO_2 diffusion into the venous blood. Common circumstances of abnormal CO_2 production are (1) temperature deviation that alters CO_2 production approximately 10%/°C change; (2) excessive muscular activity (shivering, rigor, seizure), which can increase CO_2 production three- to five-fold; (3) "physiologic stress" responses, which are known to increase CO_2 production; (4) sepsis, which is known to alter CO_2 production; and (5) parenteral nutrition with glucose providing more than 50% of the non-protein calories, which can increase CO_2 production two- to eight-fold. We assume a reasonably normal CO_2 production unless specifically stated otherwise.

Dead Space Ventilation

Ventilation is the sum of alveolar and dead space components: $V_E = V_A + V_{DS}$. Increases in V_{DS} will require an increase in V_E to maintain a consistent V_A. Common circumstances that increase V_{DS} are (1) acutely diminished cardiac output, which creates a greater portion of lung that is poorly perfused (high ventilation-perfusion [$\dot{V}/\dot{Q}$] ratio); (2) acute pulmonary emboli, which create ventilated/unperfused alveoli (infinite $\dot{V}/\dot{Q}$); (3) acute pulmonary hypertension, which creates less perfusion of non–gravity-dependent lung (high $\dot{V}/\dot{Q}$); (4) severe acute lung injury (adult respiratory distress syndrome [ARDS]), which creates both zero $\dot{V}/\dot{Q}$ and high $\dot{V}/\dot{Q}$ disease, causing both significant intrapulmonary shunting and V_{DS}; and (5) positive-pressure ventilation (PPV), which favors distribution of ventilation to non–gravity-dependent lung.

Disparity Between Gas Volume Exhaled in 1 Minute and Arterial Partial Pressure of Carbon Dioxide

In normal exercising humans, the minute ventilation increases in proportion to the metabolic rate and cardiac output[15]; therefore, the Pa_{CO_2} remains the same or decreases to a small degree.[16] In contrast, a normal subject undergoing PPV requires a greater than normal minute volume to maintain a normal Pa_{CO_2}; an observation generally attributed to an increase in dead space ventilation.[17, 18]

Clinical observation that minute ventilation (V_E) is increased without an appropriate decrease in Pa_{CO_2} raises the possibility of increased V_{DS}. Table 33–8 assumes a CO_2 production of 200 mL/min and shows the ideal relationship among minute ventilation, alveolar ventilation, and Pa_{CO_2} when the minute ventilation is doubled, redoubled, and halved. The following guidelines are recommended in acutely ill patients: (1) when the measured V_E is associated with a Pa_{CO_2} significantly greater than predicted in Table 33–8 and an increased CO_2 production can be reasonably ruled out, increased V_{DS} is the most likely explanation; (2) when the V_E is associated with a Pa_{CO_2} significantly less than predicted in Table 33–8, diminished CO_2 production or depleted CO_2 stores should be suspected.

TABLE 33–8. Ideal Minute Ventilation (MV), Alveolar Ventilation (VA), and Arterial Carbon Dioxide Tension (Pa_{CO_2}) Relationships*

MV (L)	*VA (L)*	*Pa_{CO_2} (mm Hg)*
3	2	80
6	4	40
12	8	30
24	16	20

*Boxed data represent assumed baseline values.

Traditional Respiratory Acid-Base Balance

Table 33–9 lists the criteria for the traditional nomenclature of respiratory acidosis and respiratory alkalosis.[19, 20] As the Pa_{CO_2} acutely rises, the plasma carbonic acid concentration correspondingly increases, resulting in an increased free H^+ concentration (decreased pH) in the plasma. For example, an acute increase in Pa_{CO_2} from 40 to 80 mm Hg will cause the pH to decrease from 7.40 to nearly 7.20. An increased Pa_{CO_2} in conjunction with the predicted low pH signifies the respiratory acidosis is acute and uncompensated. The kidneys respond to a decreased arterial pH by excreting more H^+ and adding HCO_3^- to the blood. Given time, this renal mechanism will correct the pH to near normal. For example, a Pa_{CO_2} of 80 mm Hg in conjunction with an arterial pH of 7.35 signifies that the respiratory acidosis is chronic or compensated. These inter-relationships of pulmonary and renal responses to acid-base imbalances are predictable and determine the criteria for the traditional approach to respiratory acid-base interpretation.

Concept of Ventilatory Failure

Traditional physiology considers the need to excrete CO_2 in terms of respiratory acid-base balance, inferring that the biologic insult of CO_2 accumulation is the chemically associated accumulation of free H^+. From a clinical viewpoint, the accumulation of CO_2 represents a failure of the pulmonary system to excrete the waste product of metabolism adequately. The concern of the clinician is to specifically determine the ventilatory abnormality, identify interventions that can correct the imbalance, and document the affects of the interventions. Even though the disease process causing CO_2 accumulation may exist outside of the lungs, the inability of the pulmonary system to meet the metabolic demands for CO_2 excretion remains the primary clinical concern. Simply stated, the clinical relevance of respiratory acid-base imbalance is the need to support the processes involved in the elimination of CO_2.

Laboratory normal ranges for blood gas values are listed in Table 33–10. Table 33–11 lists the ventilatory and acid-base nomenclature used in this chapter as well as the criteria for using each term. Experience in critical care medicine has

TABLE 33–9. Traditional Respiratory Acid-Base Nomenclature

Nomenclature	*pH*	*P_{CO_2}*	*[HCO_3^-]*	*BE*
Respiratory Acidosis				
Uncompensated (acute)	↓	↑	N	N
Partly compensated (subacute)	↓	↑	↑	↑
Compensated (chronic)	N	↑	↑	↑
Respiratory Alkalosis				
Uncompensated (acute)	↑	↓	N	N
Partly compensated (subacute)	↑	↓	↓	↓
Compensated (chronic)	N	↓	↓	↓

Abbreviations: P_{CO_2} = partial pressure of carbon dioxide; HCO_3^- = bicarbonate ion; ↓ = depressed; ↑ = elevated; N = normal; BE = base excess.

TABLE 33–10. Laboratory Normal Ranges

Variable	*M*	*1 SD*	*2 SD*
Pa_{CO_2} (mm Hg)	40	38–42	35–45
pH	7.40	7.38–7.42	7.35–7.45

Abbreviation: Pa_{CO_2} = partial pressure of arterial carbon dioxide.

revealed that clinical judgments are rarely influenced by minor variations from the normal ranges of arterial CO_2 and/or pH measurements. Thus, broader arbitrary "acceptable ranges" for arterial pH and P_{CO_2} emerged that are not intended to replace or diminish the importance of normal ranges. Rather, they recognize that minor variations from normal in the seriously ill patient are seldom clinically significant. However, in keeping with tradition and acceptance throughout medical science, we use the normal ranges, hoping readers realize that the acceptable ranges should be kept in mind when considering cardiopulmonary supportive therapy.

Ventilatory failure (respiratory acidosis) is a blood gas diagnosis that refers only to failure of the pulmonary system to provide adequate CO_2 excretion. When clinically significant acute ventilatory failure is present, the following factors must be immediately considered: (1) the need for ventilatory assistance; (2) the adequacy of ventilatory assistance if the patient is receiving mechanical ventilatory support, especially in the presence of significant dead space ventilation; (3) tissue hypoxia should be assumed if concurrent severe hypoxemia is present; and (4) concomitant acute metabolic acidosis is most likely secondary to inadequate perfusion or detrimental work of breathing (WOB).

Impending Ventilatory Failure

Breathing is the process by which the ventilatory pump creates ventilation by cyclic muscle contractions. In essence, we breathe to ventilate, and we ventilate to respire. WOB provided within the limits of cardiopulmonary reserves improves matching of ventilation to perfusion and augments venous return to the heart, factors that can be considered beneficial to the maintenance of respiratory homeostasis. However, if WOB places demands on the cardiopulmonary system that exceed functional reserves, the result is often detrimental to the maintenance of respiratory homeostasis.[21]

Extreme degrees of detrimental WOB are clinically recognized as acute respiratory distress (progressive tachypnea, tachycardia, dyspnea, hypertension, intercostal retraction, use of accessory muscles of ventilation, diaphoresis, and mental status changes); the patient is often described as appearing "fatigued" or "tiring out." Lesser degrees of detrimental WOB are manifested by progressive increases in respiratory rate, heart rate, and systolic blood pressure, onset of diaphoresis and mental confusion, delirium, and even obtundation. Patients able to communicate will invariably complain of dyspnea. The progression of clinical signs is an important element in the diagnosis of detrimental WOB.

The clinical suspicion of detrimental WOB in a patient with an acceptable Pa_{CO_2} suggests that, if no therapeutic interventions to reduce WOB are instituted, acute ventilatory failure (rising Pa_{CO_2} and falling pH) will eventually ensue. This clinical circumstance is referred to as *impending ventilatory failure* and is a clinical diagnosis. Metabolic acidemia and hypoxemia are common in patients with impending ventilatory failure and are rapidly reversed when appropriate ventilatory assistance is instituted.

Acute Respiratory Alkalosis

Clinically significant acute respiratory alkalosis (Pa_{CO_2} <30 mm Hg; pH >7.50) represents an *acute alveolar hyperventilation* and usually indicates an increased WOB. There are three common causes of acute alveolar hyperventilation in the critically ill patient: (1) a homeostatic response to arterial hypoxemia; (2) a homeostatic response to metabolic acidosis; and (3) central nervous system dysfunction. The latter two are seldom concomitant with arterial hypoxemia; in fact, acute respiratory alkalosis without hypoxemia is most commonly secondary to intracranial disease, anxiety, or pain. However, severe anemia, carbon monoxide poisoning, and methemoglobinemia should be ruled out.

Acute Respiratory Alkalosis with Hypoxemia

This blood gas interpretation is almost always attributable to cardiopulmonary disease. When the hypoxemia is due to a pulmonary process that is responsive to oxygen therapy (asthma, bronchitis, noncardiogenic edema, retained secretions, early pneumonia), administering O_2 should decrease the WOB, increase the Pa_{CO_2} toward normal, and decrease the heart rate and blood pressure toward normal. The Pa_{CO_2} will readily approach 70 mm Hg but seldom exceed that tension until the cardiopulmonary work has been significantly reduced. When the hypoxemia is due to a pulmonary process that is refractory to oxygen therapy (consolidated pneumonia, lobar atelectasis, ARDS), the blood gas values and WOB will not significantly change with O_2 administration.

Acute reductions in cardiac output result in decreased mixed venous oxygenation because the tissues must extract O_2 from less blood per unit time. Therefore, any magnitude of preexisting intrapulmonary shunting will have greater hypoxemic effects on the arterial blood because the "shunted" blood is relatively less oxygenated than the nonshunted blood. In response to the hypoxemia, minute ventilation may increase to increase the alveolar partial pressure of O_2 (P_{AO_2}), thus resulting in an acute alveolar hyperventilation with hypoxemia. The hypoxemia attributable to acute myocardial infarction, acute heart failure, and interstitial pulmonary edema is low $\dot{V}/\dot{Q}$ and should respond to O_2 therapy with an increased Pa_{O_2} and signifi-

TABLE 33–11. Nomenclature and Criteria for Clinical Interpretation

Clinical Terminology	*Criteria*
Ventilatory failure (respiratory acidosis)	Pa_{CO_2} >45 mm Hg
Alveolar hyperventilation (respiratory alkalosis)	Pa_{CO_2} <35 mm Hg
Acute ventilatory failure (respiratory acidosis)	Pa_{CO_2} >45 mm Hg, pH <7.35
Chronic ventilatory failure (respiratory acidosis)	Pa_{CO_2} >45 mm Hg, pH 7.36–7.44
Acute alveolar hyperventilation (respiratory alkalosis)	Pa_{CO_2} <35 mm Hg, pH >7.45
Chronic alveolar hyperventilation (respiratory alkalosis)	Pa_{CO_2} <35 mm Hg, pH 7.36–7.44
Acidemia	pH <7.35
Alkalemia	pH >7.45
Acidosis	HCO_3^- <20 mmol/L, BD >5 mmol/L
Alkalosis	HCO_3^- >28 mmol/L, BE >5 mmol/L

Abbreviations: Pa_{CO_2} = partial pressure of arterial carbon dioxide; HCO_3^- = bicarbonate ion; BD = base deficit; BE = base excess.

cantly decreased cardiopulmonary work. Pulmonary edema involving alveolar fluid is usually relatively refractory to oxygen therapy.

Abnormal Peripheral Carbon Dioxide Stores

Intracellular water must have partial pressures of nitrogen, O_2, and CO_2, which are referred to as *gas tissue stores*. Nitrogen is inert and exists in equilibrium throughout all water compartments in the body. When increased O_2 concentrations are administered, the nitrogen stores change relatively rapidly because the inspired fraction of nitrogen is altered. Because O_2 is consumed by the cells, intracellular O_2 tensions are so low that steady-state conditions are almost always present within the confines of biologic viability.[22] However, CO_2 is constantly produced in the cells, dictating that peripheral CO_2 stores are large and change at a relatively slow pace. This makes consideration of CO_2 stores significant in the clinical application of blood gas values.

The CO_2 content of blood constitutes the "central" CO_2 stores. When the P_{ACO_2} changes, the central CO_2 stores are immediately and rapidly affected; however, the extravascular ("peripheral") CO_2 stores are essentially unaffected over several hours. Thus, changes in V_A are rapidly reflected in the central stores (the arterial and mixed venous P_{CO_2}) but not in the peripheral CO_2 stores. Peripheral CO_2 stores are estimated to be approximately 110 L in a 70-kg individual. The vast majority (up to 100 L) is stored in bone and fat, which have relatively poor perfusion so that significant changes would be expected to take days; skeletal muscle represents the next largest component (approximately 5 L) in which significant changes can occur in hours; visceral tissue stores account for the remainder in which significant changes can occur within minutes.

Assuming a normal CO_2 production and minute ventilation, Table 33–12 demonstrates the relationships among changes in peripheral CO_2 stores, mixed venous blood, alveolar gas, and arterial blood. It should be noted that depleted peripheral CO_2 stores allow a normal minute ventilation to result in an unexpectedly low Pa_{CO_2}; conversely, elevated peripheral CO_2 stores allow a normal minute ventilation to result in a greater Pa_{CO_2} than expected.

Depletion of Peripheral Carbon Dioxide Stores

Depletion of peripheral stores occurs when CO_2 excretion exceeds production for significant periods of time. Skeletal muscle depletion of CO_2 stores occurs in a few hours,[23] whereas bone depletion takes several days.[24] Figure 33–4 illustrates that the decreased P_{ACO_2} is secondary to diminished tissue P_{CO_2} rather than to an increased V_A. Therefore, a normal minute ventilation and normal V_{DS} are present in conjunction with a diminished P_{ACO_2}. The key to identifying such a patient is the low Pa_{CO_2} in conjunction with a normal or decreased minute ventilation when a decreased CO_2 production has been clinically excluded. The common occurrence of depleted peripheral CO_2 stores in patients with central nervous system dysfunction underscores the advisability of measuring minute ventilation in conjunction with arterial blood gas measurements in critically ill patients.

TABLE 33–12. Theoretic Relationship of P_{CO_2} Changes When Peripheral CO_2 Stores Are Altered*

CO_2 Stores	*Tissue P_{CO_2}*	*$P\bar{v}_{CO_2}$*	*Alveolar P_{CO_2}*	*Pa_{CO_2}*
Normal	50	46	40	40
Decreased	40	36	30	30
Increased	60	56	50	50

*Carbon dioxide production and minute ventilation are assumed normal.
Abbreviations: CO_2 = carbon dioxide; P_{CO_2} = partial pressure of CO_2; $P\bar{v}_{CO_2}$ = partial pressure of carbon dioxide, mixed venous blood; Pa_{CO_2} = partial pressure of arterial carbon dioxide.

Patients tend to replenish peripheral CO_2 stores within several days after resolution of the precipitating disease. The repletion process can be clinically important when the restoration of peripheral CO_2 stores impacts on the underlying pathophysiologic factors. For example, a patient with a head injury has been hyperventilated on a ventilator for several days and is able to assume spontaneous ventilation because the depleted CO_2 stores allow for the low Pa_{CO_2} to be maintained with a normal minute ventilation. If the patient still has a diminished intracranial compliance, repletion of peripheral CO_2 stores will require an increased minute ventilation to maintain hypocapnia. If the patient is unable to increase minute ventilation without exceeding cardiopulmonary reserves, the repletion of peripheral CO_2 stores may precipitate respiratory distress and increased intracranial pressure. The essential factor is that, as peripheral CO_2 stores are replenished over time, the onset of respiratory distress may be wrongfully attributed to worsening of the intracranial disease. Appropriate interpretation of the blood gas values can alert the clinician to such occurrences.

Increased Peripheral Carbon Dioxide Stores: The "Carbon Dioxide Retainer"

Chronic hypercapnia (Pa_{CO_2} >45 mm Hg; arterial pH >7.35) is most commonly seen in patients with chronic obstructive pulmonary disease. However, it is also seen with chronic restrictive pulmonary disease, morbid obesity (pickwickian syndrome), and rare central nervous system disorders. The increased peripheral CO_2 stores allow for the maintenance of CO_2 homeostasis (lung excretion equal to cellular production) while maintaining an increased P_{ACO_2}. Because inspired gas is essentially void of CO_2, in any steady-state circumstance, a smaller minute ventilation is required to maintain an increased P_{ACO_2} than to maintain a normal P_{ACO_2}.

Chronic hypercapnia (chronic respiratory acidosis, chronic ventilatory failure) involves intracellular adaptation to an increased cellular P_{CO_2}. It appears that such adaptation involves maintenance of mitochondrial function despite intracellular acidosis and significantly diminished O_2 delivery. Extracellular acid-base balance is maintained by accumulating an increased HCO_3^- concentration in concert with a Cl^- deficiency. Available data suggest that shifts in water molecules and Cl^- between the intracellular and extracellular spaces result in a slightly greater extracellular pH than in the normal population.[25] Although these patients are usually on tubular diuretics that waste potassium, it is also true that most of them take potassium supplements. There is ample evidence that this metabolic alkalosis "overcompensation" for the respiratory acidosis is primarily due to these water and Cl^- shifts between the intracellular and extracellular spaces.[25, 26]

Chronically hypercapnic patients have a limited capability to increase cardiopulmonary work in response to stress. Although the majority of these patients will not further hypoventilate when administered O_2, such therapy must be carefully administered because some will become significantly more hypercapnic in response to excessive O_2 administration.[27] Proper interpretation of the arterial blood gas values depends on recognition and differentiation of acute factors from chronic factors.

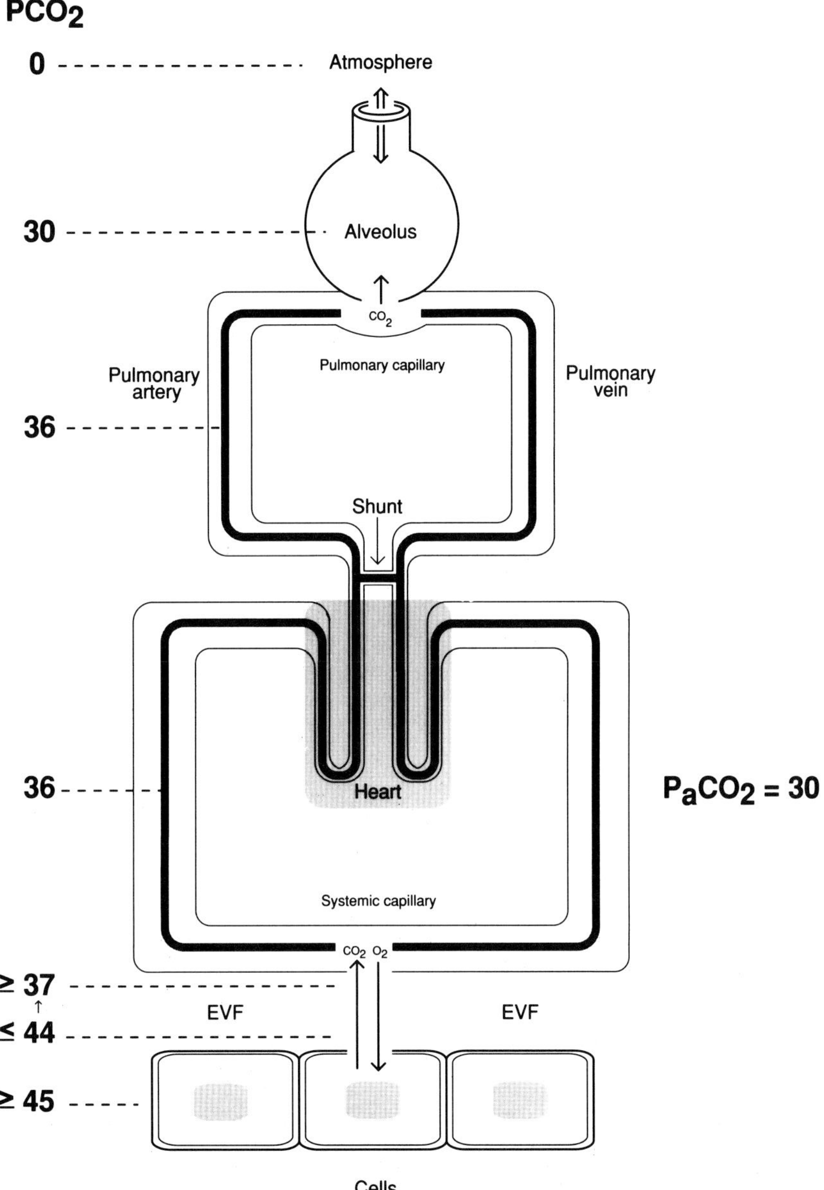

Figure 33–4. Tissue $P\text{CO}_2$ is normally ≥55 mm Hg, which results in a $P\bar{v}\text{CO}_2$ of 46 mm Hg. Normally, a ventilated alveolus presented with a $P\bar{v}\text{CO}_2$ of 46 mm Hg results in a $Pa\text{CO}_2$ of 40 mm Hg. This figure is an illustration of how depleted CO_2 peripheral stores affect the $P_A\text{CO}_2$ and $Pa\text{CO}_2$. The *double-sided arrow* represents normal alveolar ventilation. $P\text{CO}_2$ is expressed in millimeters of mercury. (kPa = mm Hg × 0.133.) (From Shapiro BA, Peruzzi WT, Templin R: Clinical Application of Blood Gases. 5th ed. Chicago, Mosby-Yearbook, 1994.)

Chronic Hypercapnia and Acute Ventilatory Failure
Typical room-air blood gas is as follows: pH <7.35; Pco_2 >60 mm Hg; Po_2 <45 mm Hg. The severity of this condition must be judged by the degree of acute acidemia. Regardless of the Pco_2 level, a pH above 7.30 usually denotes a tolerable change from baseline. If the pH falls below 7.20, evaluation for ventilatory assistance is mandatory. Although lactic acidosis is common in these patients, sodium bicarbonate administration is contraindicated before supporting ventilation because of the added CO_2 load.

Chronic Hypercapnia and Acute Hyperventilation
Typical room-air blood gas is as follows: pH >7.45; Pco_2 >40 mm Hg; Po_2 <50 mm Hg. These blood gas values should be initially interpreted as a "partly compensated metabolic alkalosis with significant hypoxemia." However, diseases causing metabolic alkalemia rarely cause significant hypoxemia! When one is presented with these blood gas values, consideration should be given to the probability that a patient with chronic hypercapnia may transiently respond to an acute stress by hyperventilating, thus "unmasking" the preexisting base excess.

Assessment of Oxygenation

The tissue oxygenation status is a global concept that cannot be directly measured. Further, no available combination of measurements can reliably reflect the oxygenation status of vital tissues in critically ill patients. Therefore, all clinical assessments of the oxygenation status must be based on an evaluation of the arterial blood.

Arterial Oxygenation

The milliliters of oxygen contained in 100 mL of blood are defined as *oxygen content* (mL/dL). The traditional calculation ($1.34 \times \%HbO_2$) + ($Po_2 \times 0.003$), where HbO_2 is oxyhemoglobin, requires measurement of the Po_2(mm Hg), $\%HbO_2$, and the total hemoglobin (Hb) (g/dL). The vast majority of O_2 in the blood exists in chemical combination with Hb, whereas less than 5% is dissolved in the plasma. The quantity of O_2 that moves into (or out of) the blood depends on three factors: (1) the amount of dissolved O_2 (Po_2); (2) the amount of O_2 combined to the Hb ($\%HbO_2$); and (3) the degree to which the Hb binds the O_2 (Hb–O_2 affinity).

The $\%HbO_2$ must be measured by multiwavelength oximetry that measures HbO_2, reduced Hb, carboxyhemoglobin, and methemoglobin. When the HbO_2 is measured by dual-wavelength oximetry (pulse oximetry) or calculated from the arterial pH and Po_2, the assumption is made that only HbO_2 and reduced Hb exist. A decreased Hb–O_2 affinity (shift to the right, increased P_{50} [the Po_2 at which the hemoglobin is 50% saturated when Pco_2, pH, and temperature are normal]) results in a diminished O_2 content that may further limit O_2 delivery; an increased Hb–O_2 affinity will increase the O_2 content but potentially inhibit O_2 unloading to the tissues. Because numerous factors in critically ill patients modify the Hb–O_2 affinity, the presence of hypoxemia demands that both Po_2 and $\%HbO_2$ be assessed.

Defining Arterial Hypoxemia

Oxygen delivery ($\dot{D}o_2$) is the volume of O_2 presented to the tissues in 1 minute ($Cao_2 \times$ cardiac output $\times 10$), where Cao_2 is arterial O_2 concentration. Oxygen consumption ($\dot{V}o_2$) is defined as the volume of oxygen consumed in 1 minute. It is generally agreed that when $\dot{D}o_2$ is three to four times greater than $\dot{V}o_2$, tissue O_2 needs are reasonably satisfied in nonseptic patients.[28]

Deficiencies in arterial O_2 content that demand increased cardiac work to ensure adequate $\dot{D}o_2$ are considered significant arterial oxygenation deficits. Significant arterial hypoxemia is defined as a Pao_2 less than 60 mm Hg or a $\%HbO_2$ less than 90%. When the Pao_2 is greater than 60 mm Hg (>90%HbO_2), the blood O_2 content is close to the maximum for that Hb content and O_2 delivery will depend on cardiac output and capillary perfusion (i.e., there will be little to gain by further increasing the Po_2).

Pao_2 less than 40 mm Hg (most often associated with a $\%HbO_2$ below 75%) reflects not only significantly decreased O_2 content but also Hb molecules less able to release O_2 to tissues. Such severe hypoxemia is a direct threat to tissue oxygenation despite increases in cardiac output. A Pao_2 from 40 to 60 mm Hg may threaten tissue oxygenation if other functions such as cardiac output or total Hb cannot sufficiently compensate for the diminished O_2 content.

Oxygenation Deficits

Correction of arterial hypoxemia greatly depends on delineation of the degree to which each of three essential functions is contributing to the hypoxemia: (1) O_2 transfer across the lungs; (2) cardiac output; and (3) O_2 consumption. Specific identification and quantification of these factors require blood gas analysis of both arterial and pulmonary arterial blood plus cardiac output measurement. Obtaining these values allows calculation of $\dot{D}o_2$, O_2 extraction (O_2 content difference between arterial and mixed venous blood [$Cao_2 - C\bar{v}o_2$]) and the intrapulmonary shunt fraction ($\dot{Q}sp/\dot{Q}t$).

Oxygen Extraction

Oxygen extraction represents the O_2 transferred to the tissues from 100 mL (1 dL) of blood. This relationship can be quantified on a global scale as $Cao_2 - C\bar{v}o_2$. When the $\dot{V}o_2$ is constant, the $Cao_2 - C\bar{v}o_2$ will vary inversely to the cardiac output. As shown in Table 33–13, critically ill patients with adequate cardiac reserves have a $Cao_2 - C\bar{v}o_2$ in the range of 3 to 4 mL/dL.[29] In the absence of anemia and sepsis in a patient with clinically adequate peripheral perfusion, a $Cao_2 - C\bar{v}o$ of 3 to 4 mL/dL suggests there are adequate cardiac reserves to meet further stress if required, whereas a $Cao_2 - C\bar{v}o_2$ of greater than or equal to 5 mL/dL suggests an inadequate cardiac response to the stress.

The relationship between the O_2 supply and O_2 demand can also be reflected in the mixed venous oxygen saturation ($S\bar{v}o_2$) when the Hb content is greater than 10 g%.[30] The availability of technology to continuously measure $S\bar{v}o_2$ lends clinical practicality to this concept.

Lung As an Oxygenator

Blood that goes from the right side to the left side of the heart without contacting alveolar gas (zero $\dot{V}/\dot{Q}$, true shunt) will create hypoxemia by mixing in the left ventricle with blood that has been well oxygenated in the lung. The resultant degree of hypoxemia will be determined by both the amount of blood that shunts and the $\%HbO_2$ saturation of the shunted blood. Alveoli that are poorly ventilated in relation to perfusion (low $\dot{V}/\dot{Q}$) will have a P_{AO_2} that is less than ideal, and blood that respires with these alveoli will be oxygenated to a lesser degree than if exposed to perfect alveoli, causing arterial hypoxemia.

Intrapulmonary Shunt Nomenclature
This subject is controversial, confused, and arbitrary. The sum of anatomic and capillary shunts is most commonly termed *zero $\dot{V}/\dot{Q}$* or *true shunt*, often simply referred to as

TABLE 33–13. Predicted Oxygenation Values in Health and Disease for Pulmonary Artery Blood

	$P\bar{v}O_2$ *(mm Hg)*		$S\bar{v}O_2$ *(mm Hg)*		$CaO_2 - C\bar{v}O_2$ *(mm Hg)*	
Condition	*Range*	*Average*	*Range*	*Average*	*Range*	*Average*
Healthy resting human volunteer	37–33	40	70–76	75	4.5–6.0	5.0
Critically ill patient, cardiovascular reserves excellent	35–40	37	68–75	70	2.5–4.5	3.5
Critically ill patient, cardiovascular stable, limited cardiovascular reserves	30–35	32	56–68	60	4.5–6.0	5.0
Critically ill patient, cardiovascular decompensation	<30	<30	<56	<56	>6.0	>6.0

Abbreviations: $P\bar{v}O_2$ = partial pressure of oxygen, mixed venous blood; $S\bar{v}O_2$ = saturation of oxygen, mixed venous blood; $CaO_2 - C\bar{v}O_2$ = oxygen content difference between arterial and mixed venous blood.

"shunt." Venous admixture is often referred to as "low $\dot{V}/\dot{Q}$," "$\dot{V}/\dot{Q}$ inequity," or "shunt effect."

- $\dot{Q}s/\dot{Q}t$: Classic shunt concept (calculation of the intrapulmonary shunt while breathing 100% inspired O_2 concentrations). Most commonly referred to as "the shunt" because this was originally believed to represent only the zero $\dot{V}/\dot{Q}$ and not venous admixture.
- $\dot{Q}sp/\dot{Q}t$: Physiologic shunt (calculation of the intrapulmonary shunt at less than 100% inspired O_2 concentrations). In a normal person breathing room air, this is a measurement of the normal intrapulmonary shunt; when applied to patients with diseased lungs, it represents the degree of impairment of the lung as an oxygenator; some authors dislike the term *physiologic* applied to a pathologic circumstance.
- $\dot{Q}va/\dot{Q}t$: Venous admixture (calculation of the intrapulmonary shunt at less than 100% inspired O_2 concentrations). Exactly the same as the physiologic shunt; preferred by some to avoid the term *physiologic* in a pathologic circumstance.

The shunt equation is:

$$\frac{\dot{Q}sp}{\dot{Q}t} = \frac{C\acute{c}O_2 - CaO_2}{C\acute{c}O_2 - C\bar{v}O_2}$$

$C\acute{c}O_2$ is the ideal end pulmonary capillary O_2 content that is calculated using the ideal alveolar gas equation to determine the ideal PO_2. The shunt equation calculates that portion of the cardiac output that traverses from the right side to the left side of the heart without increasing O_2 content. The mathematics assumes that the nonshunting blood perfectly oxygenates by exchanging with perfect alveolar gas. Although the intrapulmonary shunt concept does not reflect regional relationships as does the $\dot{V}A/\dot{Q}$ concept, it does reflect the degree to which the lung deviates from ideal as an oxygenator of pulmonary blood. It is this quantitative ability to look at the lung as an oxygenator that makes this measurement unique and valuable in the clinical setting. We use the term $\dot{Q}sp/\dot{Q}t$ in reference to the intrapulmonary shunt calculated with the patient breathing less than 100% oxygen.

INTERPRETIVE GUIDELINES

1. A calculated shunt less than 10% is clinically compatible with normal lungs.
2. A calculated shunt of 10% to 19% denotes a degree of disease that seldom requires significant support.
3. A calculated shunt of 20% to 29% may be life threatening in a patient with limited cardiovascular or nervous system function.
4. A calculated shunt of greater than 30% is potentially life threatening and usually requires significant cardiopulmonary supportive therapy.
5. When significantly low $\dot{V}/\dot{Q}$ mechanisms are present, the shunt calculation will significantly increase as the fraction of inspired O_2 (FIO_2) is decreased from 0.5.

ALTERNATIVES TO THE SHUNT CALCULATION

Shunt calculations require analysis of pulmonary artery blood. Oxygen tension–based indexes (alveolar-arterial difference in partial pressure of O_2, or $PAO_2 - PaO_2$, PAO_2/PaO_2, PaO_2/FIO_2, and so on) do not require mixed venous O_2 analysis but have significant limitations in reliably reflecting shunt fractions in critically ill patients.[31] It appears that the popularity of these indexes is not based on their accuracy or reliability but rather on the fact that they are easily obtained because mixed venous O_2 measurements are not required.

When pulmonary artery blood gases are not available, it makes both physiologic and clinical sense to use an O_2 content index rather than an O_2 tension index. The most widely used O_2 content index, the estimated shunt, is derived by mathematical manipulation of the shunt equation that places the $CaO_2 - C\bar{v}O_2$ in the denominator.[32]

$$\text{Est. } \dot{Q}sp/\dot{Q}t = \frac{C\acute{c}O_2 - CaO_2}{[C\acute{c}O_2 - CaO_2] + [CaO_2 - C\bar{v}O_2]}$$

As shown in Table 33–14, the estimated shunt has been demonstrated to be far superior to all O_2 tension–based indexes in reflecting changes in the $\dot{Q}sp/\dot{Q}t$.[33] The estimated shunt is not an adequate substitute for $\dot{Q}sp/\dot{Q}t$ measurement in critically ill patients, but it is a far more reliable alternative than O_2 tension indexes when pulmonary artery blood is not available.

Hypoxemia and Oxygen Therapy

The PAO_2 results from the dynamic equilibrium between the O_2 molecules delivered to the alveolus (ventilation and FIO_2) and the O_2 molecules diffusing into the pulmonary capillary blood. All other factors remaining constant, increasing the FIO_2 will increase the delivery of O_2 molecules to the alveolus and thereby increase the PAO_2.

The hypoxemia caused by true intrapulmonary shunting (zero $\dot{V}/\dot{Q}$) will be relatively refractory to increases in FIO_2 because the nonshunting blood is well oxygenated; therefore, increasing PAO_2 will add insignificant quantities of O_2 to the pulmonary capillary blood. Hypoxemia secondary to low $\dot{V}/\dot{Q}$ mechanisms is due to a diminished PAO_2; therefore, the arterial hypoxemia is responsive to an increasing FIO_2.

TABLE 33–14. Comparison of Gas Exchange Index

Parameter	M ± SD	Range (Min–Max)	R Value
$\dot{Q}sp/\dot{Q}t$	22.3 ± 11.2	3.0–53.0	—
Estimated shunt	27.6 ± 11.3	2.7–62.3	+0.94
RI*	3.1 ± 2.6	0.3–14.0	+0.74
Pa_{O_2}/PA_{CO_2}	0.3 ± 0.2	0.06–0.77	−0.72
Pa_{O_2}/FI_{O_2}	1.8 ± 0.9	0.1–4.3	−0.71
$PA_{O_2} - Pa_{O_2}$	222.8 ± 141.7	32–611	+0.62

$$*RI = \frac{PA_{O_2} - Pa_{O_2}}{Pa_{O_2}}.$$

Abbreviations: $\dot{Q}sp/\dot{Q}t$ = intrapulmonary shunt fraction; RI = respiratory index; Pa_{O_2} = partial pressure of arterial oxygen; PA_{CO_2} = partial pressure of alveolar carbon dioxide; FI_{O_2} = fraction of inspired oxygen; $PA_{O_2} - Pa_{O_2}$ = alveolar-arterial difference in partial pressure of oxygen.

Aberrant Intracellular Metabolism

Alterations in metabolic rate predictably accompany temperature variation, thyroid dysfunction, and physical activity. Such changes in metabolic rate do not alter the relationship of CO_2 production to O_2 consumption; therefore, the general rules applied to interpretation of arterial pH, Pa_{CO_2}, and Pa_{O_2} remain valid. However, arterial blood gas interpretation requires additional considerations when aberrant metabolism is present, particularly with sepsis, lactic acidosis, and parenteral hyperalimentation.

Sepsis

The hyperdynamic response to sepsis ("warm shock") involves a decreased O_2 extraction ($Ca_{O_2} - C\bar{v}_{O_2}$) which is most likely secondary to decreased oxidative metabolism,[34] resulting in an increased $S\bar{v}_{O_2}$ and, consequently, an improved arterial oxygenation status. A Pa_{CO_2} below normal is most commonly seen with the hyperdynamic phase of septic shock probably because of a decreased CO_2 production[34] and an increased minute ventilation. Blood lactate levels are seldom significantly increased so that a significant component of metabolic acidosis is uncommon. Most of the guidelines for assessing oxygenation are not applicable with sepsis because intracellular O_2 utilization is abnormal. "Cold septic shock" involves tissue hypoperfusion and manifests blood gases similar to all hypoperfusion states.

Lactic Acidosis

Anaerobic metabolism produces lactic acid, a nonvolatile metabolite. The most common cause of anaerobic metabolism is tissue hypoperfusion. Severe hypoxemia or anemia may produce anaerobic metabolism, but most commonly there is a concurrent element of tissue hypoperfusion. The cellular production of lactic acid is unreliably reflected in arterial or central venous blood because specific organ system perfusion and hepatic function are variable. An adequately oxygenated and perfused liver is remarkably capable of rapidly metabolizing lactic acid to carbonic acid. Thus, although certain organ systems (e.g., skeletal muscle, gastrointestinal tract, skin) may produce lactic acid, normal hepatic function can prevent significant accumulation of lactic acid in the core circulation.

The presence of increased blood lactate levels documents the presence of anaerobic metabolism; however, the absence of blood lactate does not imply the absence of anaerobic metabolism. Metabolic acidosis in a patient with severe hypoxemia and/or poor perfusion status must be assumed to be lactic acidosis until proven otherwise. The presence of metabolic acidemia secondary to lactic acid in a patient with shock, seizures, or shivering is a dire circumstance. The absence of metabolic acidemia implies that vital organs may still be reasonably oxygenated, but by no means is that a certainty.

ARTERIAL BLOOD GASES DURING CARDIOPULMONARY RESUSCITATION

Lung function normally determines CO_2 excretion and maintains a venous-to-arterial PCO_2 gradient ($P\bar{v}_{CO_2} - Pa_{CO_2}$) of approximately 8 mm Hg. However, pulmonary blood flow becomes the limiting factor determining CO_2 excretion with cardiopulmonary resuscitation (CPR). The resultant acid-base abnormalities coincident with CPR are unique and demand separate consideration when interpreting arterial blood gases.

Acid-Base Balance During Cardiopulmonary Resuscitation

In spontaneously breathing patients with poor cardiac output the $P\bar{v}_{CO_2} - Pa_{CO_2}$ has been observed to increase 50% to 100%; a 3- to 10-fold increase has been observed in patients receiving CPR.[35] As depicted in Figure 33–5, assuming CPR with normal lungs and increased minute ventilation, a venous "respiratory acidosis" occurs in conjunction with an arterial "respiratory alkalosis."[36] An acute increase in venous P_{CO_2} results in a decreased venous pH with little change in plasma bicarbonate concentration. Because systemic capillary blood is similar to the venous blood, it is inferred that tissue P_{CO_2} and pH will be similar to the venous values.

Inadequate tissue perfusion inevitably leads to anaerobic metabolism and the production of lactic acid. This lactate production has traditionally been considered the primary cause of acidosis during CPR; however, it is now clear that a significant plasma bicarbonate depletion as a result of lactic acid accumulation is seldom present in the first 10 to 15 minutes of CPR.[37] The best explanation for this observation is that hepatic function metabolizes lactate to CO_2 as long as liver oxygenation is adequate; as liver oxygenation gradually diminishes, the lactic acid gradually accumulates. Early lactate production probably increases CO_2 production by the liver and thereby contributes to the venous respiratory acidosis.

The plasma bicarbonate deficit attributable to metabolic acidosis is essentially equal in both the venous and arterial blood. This means that the differences in venous and arterial pH seen in early CPR are due to differences in the respective P_{CO_2} levels. The degree of metabolic acidosis in arterial blood is reflective of total body metabolic acidosis.

Arterial Blood Gases During Cardiopulmonary Resuscitation

Arterial Partial Pressure of Oxygen

All CPR efforts include increasing FI_{O_2} so that it approaches 1.0; therefore, arterial hypoxemia should be attributable to

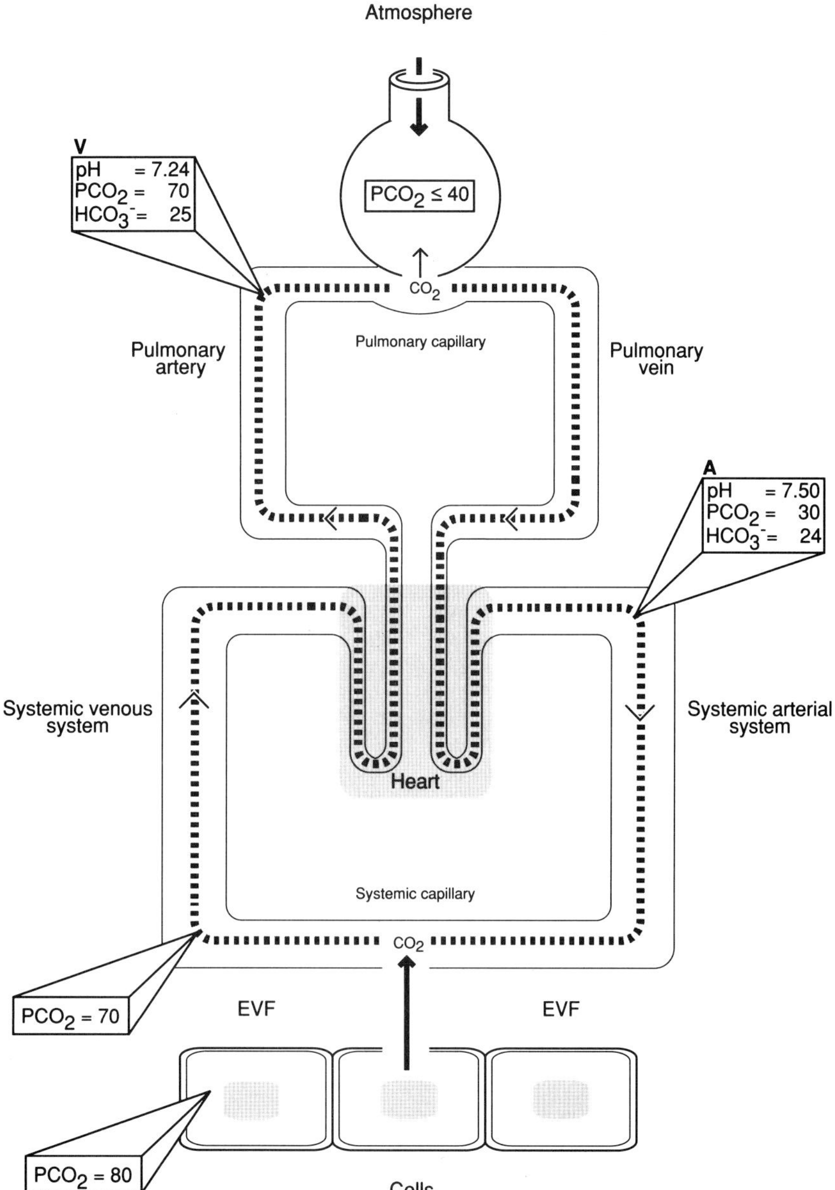

Figure 33–5. The *broken circulation line* represents low cardiac output during cardiopulmonary resuscitation and low cardiac output states. Relatively small volumes of blood perfuse the lungs; this limits CO_2 excretion despite adequate lung function and increased minute volume. This circumstance results in the excretion of less CO_2 in the lungs each minute than is produced in the cells. The systemic arterial blood (*box A*: pH = 7.50; P_{CO_2} = 30 mm Hg; HCO_3^- = 24 mmol/L) shows an acute respiratory alkalemia because of the diminished Pa_{CO_2}. The mixed venous blood (*box V*: pH = 7.24; P_{CO_2} = 70 mm Hg; HCO_3^- = 25 mmol/L) represents an acute respiratory acidosis. Widening of the $P(v-a)_{CO_2}$ gradient correlates with diminishing cardiac output. (From Shapiro BA, Peruzzi WT, Templin R: Clinical Application of Blood Gases. 5th ed. Chicago, Mosby-Yearbook, 1994.)

zero $\dot{V}/\dot{Q}$ mechanisms in the lungs. A $\dot{Q}sp/\dot{Q}t$ in excess of 25% will be associated with hypoxemia during CPR despite a high F_{IO_2}. Careful attention to proper endotracheal tube placement and lung collapse secondary to pneumothorax is essential.

Arterial Partial Pressure of Carbon Dioxide

In CPR dog models with normal lungs, it is possible to avoid arterial acidemia for up to 18 minutes by providing an increase in minute ventilation necessary to maintain the Pa_{CO_2} between 25 and 30 mm Hg.[37] As the $P\bar{v}_{CO_2} - Pa_{CO_2}$ increases during CPR, blood going from the right side to the left side of the heart without exchanging with alveolar gas (true shunt or zero $\dot{V}/\dot{Q}$) will enter the left side of the heart with a P_{CO_2} significantly greater than the blood that has exchanged with alveolar gas. If the lungs have shunting in excess of 20%, the Pa_{CO_2} may be greatly increased despite adequate minute ventilation. The Pa_{CO_2} during CPR cannot be considered to be a reflection of total body CO_2 homeostasis. No particular comfort can be validly derived from a Pa_{CO_2} of less than 40 mm Hg; whereas a Pa_{CO_2} greater than 40 mm Hg reflects either inadequate minute ventilation or significant intrapulmonary shunting.

Arterial pH

Mixed venous pH is always less than the arterial pH. During CPR an arterial pH of less than 7.2 reflects severe tissue acidosis and is a poor prognostic sign.[38] An alkalemic arterial pH during CPR is almost always due to a low Pa_{CO_2} and does not reflect the tissue acid-base state.[39]

A bicarbonate deficiency (metabolic acidosis) will not have a significant disparity between the arterial and venous blood despite differing levels of P_{CO_2}. Therefore, the degree of metabolic acidosis in arterial blood can be considered reflective of total body metabolic acidosis.

TEMPERATURE CORRECTION

Transport of CO_2 and O_2 involves gases in solution that are affected by temperature variation. Simply stated, a blood sample of given O_2 and CO_2 contents will manifest different gas tensions when analyzed at various temperatures. An open system allows for gas exchange with the adjacent environment (e.g., capillary blood or a blood sample exposed to the air). A closed system does not allow mass exchange of gas content (e.g., arterial blood or a gas-tight syringe). Blood samples are in a closed system in which changes in temperature induce alteration of gas tensions. In vivo gas tension alterations resulting from temperature variation occur in an open system in which gas contents can, and do, change.

To obtain true in vivo blood gas values, the temperature of the measuring electrode would have to be adjusted to that of the patient, a process that would add at least 30 minutes to each analysis as well as complicate quality assurance. To avoid these undesirable factors, the pH, P_{CO_2}, and P_{O_2} electrodes are encased in a constant 37°C environment to which the blood sample chamber is also exposed. Thus, independently of the patient's temperature, the pH, P_{CO_2}, and P_{O_2} are analyzed in a closed system at 37°C.

The term *temperature correction* refers to applying mathematical adjustments to the measured 37°C values for the purpose of obtaining a truer reflection of the in vivo gas tensions. Although the derivation of temperature correction formulas is quite empiric in reference to in vitro changes in a closed system, it is generally agreed that they are reasonably accurate within the clinically relevant ranges.[40]

Clinical Relevance of Temperature Correction

The popularity of temperature correcting pH, P_{CO_2}, and P_{O_2} values is based on the observation that large differences in the blood gas values are present when the patient is profoundly hypo- or hyperthermic. This observation leads many to conclude that the 37°C values are "wrong." The danger in this logic is the unfounded conclusion that temperature-corrected values are "right." The scientific truth is that, with significant changes in patient temperature, we do not fully understand the complexity of effects on metabolism, vascular function, and respiration. Therefore, both corrected and uncorrected blood gas values are of uncertain usefulness in patients with significant deviations in body temperature. There is no logical or scientific basis for assuming that temperature-corrected values are better than the 37°C values. In fact, the available technical and biologic data lead to the conclusion that there is no clinical advantage to using values other than those at 37°C.[41]

Although temperature correction of blood gases cannot be considered wrong, several realities lead to the conclusion that blood gas values should be temperature corrected only when specifically requested by the clinician. First, acid-base balance is always best judged by the 37°C values because available data suggest that the "normal" pH is not constant with temperature variation but varies in a predictable fashion that allows the 37°C values to reliably reflect in vivo imbalances.[42] Second, oxygenation is best evaluated with the 37°C values; for example, a temperature-corrected Pa_{O_2} of 42 mm Hg in a 30°C patient does not mean severe hypoxemia exists because the 37°C value is 65 mm Hg, which is acceptable for a normal $\dot{V}_{O_2}$ and is probably acceptable for a $\dot{V}_{O_2}$ diminished by 50%. Third, the assumption that the laboratory has received the patient's true temperature at the time of sampling is not borne out in our experience. Fourth, temperature-corrected values can be confused with uncorrected values and vice versa.

Interpretation of End-Tidal Partial Pressure of Carbon Dioxide

Exhaled gas measurements will reflect the in vivo (temperature-corrected) Pa_{CO_2}. With normal alveolar ventilation and a body temperature of 30°C, the end-tidal P_{CO_2} would be 28 mm Hg and the uncorrected arterial P_{CO_2} would be 40 mm Hg. The clinician must be aware of this circumstance so that the end-tidal P_{CO_2} will not be inappropriately interpreted. The Pa_{CO_2} must be temperature corrected to ensure that the two values are being considered at the same temperature.

Oxygen Tension Indexes

When O_2 tension indexes are used, the Pa_{O_2} must be temperature corrected to reflect the true difference with the calculated alveolar tension.

PERMISSIVE HYPERCAPNIA

Patients with severe lung disease often present the difficulty of deciding the level of hypoxemia that one is willing to accept. Most experts agree that a Pa_{O_2} of 60 mm Hg is adequate for O_2 delivery in the critically ill patient, and few argue with permitting a Pa_{O_2} in the 50s to avoid a deleterious F_{IO_2} or positive end-expiratory pressure levels, provided that cardiovascular function and Hb content are adequate. Therefore, "permissive hypoxemia" is determined by each clinician's convictions and judgments concerning the

TABLE 33–15. General Concepts Guiding Application of Permissive Hypoxemia and Hypercapnia

Permissive Hypoxemia	*Permissive Hypercapnia*
PaO_2 ≥60 mm Hg: acceptable	$PaCO_2$ ≤50 mm Hg: acceptable
PaO_2 50–60 mm Hg if (1) CV function adequate, (2) advancing FIO_2 or PEEP risks lung injury	$PaCO_2$ >50 mm Hg if (1) arterial pH ≥7.25, (2) CV function adequate, (3) advancing pressure limit risks lung injury
PaO_2 <50 mm Hg if increased lung injury deemed a greater risk to survival than the risks of inducing tissue hypoxia	Arterial pH <7.25 if increased lung injury deemed a greater risk to survival than the risks of inducing tissue acidosis

Abbreviations: PaO_2 = partial pressure of oxygen; CV = cardiovascular; FIO_2 = fraction of inspired oxygen; PEEP = positive end-expiratory pressure; $PaCO_2$ = partial pressure of arterial carbon dioxide.

deleterious effects of advancing therapy versus the deleterious effects on cellular oxygenation.

Sufficient animal data and some inferential human data have been published that support the concept that overdistention of alveoli leads to lung injury.[43–45] The concept of permissive hypercapnia is based on the assumption that microprocessor-controlled volume variable ventilators allow for application of airway pressures and tidal volumes that avoid alveolar overdistention. When this limitation of airway pressure results in an increased $PaCO_2$, the hypercapnia is permitted provided that the hazards of alveolar overdistention are judged more deleterious to survival than the potential hazards of allowing the arterial pH to decrease. Most agree that an arterial pH of greater than or equal to 7.25 is usually well tolerated by patients free of preexisting cardiac disease. Table 33–15 compares the general concepts guiding the application of permissive hypoxemia and hypercapnia.

References

1. Severinghaus JW: Acid-base balance controversy (Editorial). J Clin Monit 1991; 7:274–275.
2. Fagan T: Base excess and inappropriate bicarbonate (Letter to the Editor and Reply). J Clin Monit 1993; 9:67–68.
3. Emmett M, Narins RG: Clinical use of the anion gap. Medicine 1977; 56:38–54.
4. Koch SM, Taylor RW: Chloride ion in intensive care medicine. Crit Care Med 1992; 20:227–240.
5. Oh MS, Carroll HJ: The anion gap. N Engl J Med 1977; 297:814–817.
6. Iberti TJ, Leibowitz AB, Papadakos PJ, et al: Low sensitivity of the anion gap as a screen to detect hyperlactatemia in critically ill patients. Crit Care Med 1990; 18:275–277.
7. Mehta K, Kruse JA, Carlson RW: The relationship between anion gap and elevated lactate (Abstract). Crit Care Med 1986; 14:405.
8. Mizock BA: Controversies in lactic acidosis: Implications in critically ill patients. JAMA 1987; 258:497–501.
9. Madias NE, Cohen JJ, Adrogue HJ: Influence of acute and chronic respiratory alkalosis on preexisting chronic metabolic alkalosis. Am J Physiol 1990; 258:479–485.
10. Neary RH, Edwards JD: Metabolic alkalosis and hyperlactatemia. Br Med J 1987; 294:1462.
11. Kruse JA, Carlson RW: Lactate metabolism. Crit Care Clin 1987; 3:725–746.
12. Broder G, Weil MH: Excess lactate: An index of reversibility of shock in human patients. Science 1964; 143:1457–1459.
13. Peretz DI, Scott HM, Duff J, et al: The significance of lactic acidemia in the shock syndrome. Ann NY Acad Sci 1965; 119:1133–1141.
14. Luft D, Deichel G, Schmulling RM, et al: Definition of clinically relevant lactic acidosis in patients with internal diseases. Am J Clin Pathol 1983; 80:484–489.
15. Higgs BE, Clode M, McHardy GJR, et al: Changes in ventilation, gas exchange and circulation during exercise in normal subjects. Clin Sci 1967; 32:329–337.
16. Jones NL, McHardy GJR, Naimark A: Physiologic deadspace and alveolar-arterial gas pressure differences during exercise. Clin Sci 1966; 31:19–29.
17. Bergman NA: Effect of varying respiratory wave forms on distribution of inspired gas during artificial ventilation. Am Rev Respir Dis 1969; 100:518–525.
18. Hedenstierna G, McCarthy G: Mechanics of breathing, gas distribution and functional residual capacity at different frequencies of respiration during spontaneous and artificial ventilation. Br J Anaesth 1975; 47:706–712.
19. Winters RW: Terminology of acid-base disorders. Ann Intern Med 1965; 63:873–884.
20. Bartels H, DeJours P, Kellogg RH, et al: Glossary on respiration and gas exchange. J Appl Physiol 1973; 34:549–558.
21. Shapiro BA, Kacmarek RM, Cane RD, et al: Clinical Application of Respiratory Care. 4th ed. St. Louis, Mosby-Year Book, 1991, pp 252–260.
22. Farhi LE, Rahn H: Gas stores of body and unsteady states. J Appl Physiol 1955; 7:472.
23. Ward SA, Whipp BJ, Koyal S, et al: Influence of body CO_2 stores on ventilatory dynamics during exercise. J Appl Physiol 1983; 55:742–749.
24. Bolot JR, Berstein S, Guerin MA, et al: Iliac crest bone CO_2 and CO_2/C_a ratio in man during respiratory failure. Bull Eur Physiopathol Respir 1976; 12:39–47.
25. Robin ED: Abnormalities of acid-base regulation in chronic pulmonary disease, with special reference to hypercapnia and extracellular alkalosis. N Engl J Med 1963; 268:917–922.
26. Boddy K, Davies DL, Howie AD, et al: Total body and exchangeable potassium in chronic airways obstruction: A controversial area? Thorax 1978; 33:62–66.
27. Milic-Emili J, Aubier M: Some recent advances in the study of the control of breathing in patients with chronic obstructive lung disease. Anesth Analg 1980; 59:865.
28. Shoemaker WC, Appel PL, Waxman K, et al: Clinical trial of survivors' cardiorespiratory patterns as therapeutic goals in critically ill postoperative patients. Crit Care Med 1982; 10:398.
29. Harrison RA, Davison R, Shapiro BA, et al: Reassessment of the assumed A-V oxygen content difference in the shunt calculation. Anesth Analg 1975; 54:198.
30. Stock MC, Shapiro BA, Cane RD: Reliability of $S_{\bar{v}}O_2$ in predicting the A-VDO_2 and the effect of anemia. Crit Care Med 1986; 14:402.
31. Shapiro BA: Assessment of oxygenation: Today and tomorrow. Scand J Clin Lab Invest 1990; 50 (Suppl 203):197–202.
32. Bendixen HH, Egbert LD, Hedley-Whyte J, et al: Respiratory Care. St. Louis, CV Mosby, 1965.
33. Cane RD, Shapiro BA, Templin R, et al: The unreliability of oxygen tension based indices in reflecting intrapulmonary shunting in critically ill patients. Crit Care Med 1988; 16:12–43.
34. Nishijima H, Weil MH, Shubin H, et al: Hemodynamic and metabolic studies on shock associated with gram negative bacteremia. Medicine 1973; 52:287–294.
35. Benjamin E, Paluch TA, Berger SR, et al: Venous hypercarbia in canine hemorrhagic shock. Crit Care Med 1987; 15:516–518.
36. Weil MH, Rackow EC, Trevino R, et al: Difference in acid-base state between venous and arterial blood during cardiopulmonary resuscitation. N Engl J Med 1986; 315:153–156.
37. Sanders AB, Ewy GA, Taft TV: Resuscitation and arterial blood gas abnormalities during prolonged cardiopulmonary resuscitation. Ann Emerg Med 1984; 13:676–679.
38. Suljaga-Pechtel K, Goldberg E, Strickon P, et al: Cardiopulmonary resuscitation in a hospitalized population: Prospective study of factors associated with outcome. Resuscitation 1984; 12:77–95.
39. Ornato JP, Gonzalez ER, Coyne MR, et al: Arterial pH in out of hospital cardiac arrest: Response time as a determinant of acidosis. Am J Emerg Med 1985; 3:498–502.
40. Ashwood ER, Kost G, Kenny M: Temperature correction of blood gas and pH measurement. Clin Chem 1983; 29:1977–1985.

41. Shapiro BA, Harrison RA, Cane RD, et al: Clinical Application of Blood Gases. 4th ed. Chicago, Year Book Medical Publishers, 1989, pp 176–184.
42. Rahn H, Reeves RB, Howell BJ: Hydrogen ion regulation, temperature and evaluation. Am Rev Respir Dis 1975; 112:165–172.
43. Tsuno K, Miura K, Takeya M, et al: Histopathologic pulmonary changes from mechanical ventilation at high peak airway pressures. Am Rev Respir Dis 1991; 143:1115–1120.
44. Parker JC, Hernandez LA, Peevy KJ: Mechanics of ventilator-induced lung injury. Crit Care Med 1993; 21:131–143.
45. Hickling KG: Low volume ventilation with permissive hypercapnia in the adult respiratory distress syndrome. Clin Intens Care 1992; 3:67–68.

CHAPTER 34

Blood Gas Monitoring

Barry A. Shapiro, MD

The scientific origins of electrochemical methods for analysis of blood gases were first described in the 1890s.[1] Those cumbersome and time-consuming techniques were relegated to the research laboratory until 1956, when Leland Clark introduced an electrochemical methodology that allowed clinical laboratory technologists to make accurate measurements consistently within several minutes.[2] However, two decades passed before 24-hour availability of blood gases was a reality in most hospitals.[3]

An *analyzer* is a device that measures fluids, excrement, or tissue permanently removed from the body.[4] Modern blood gas analyzers are highly automated, self-diagnostic, minimal-maintenance instruments. They use microprocessors to calibrate before analysis of every sample and essentially eliminate moment-to-moment technical surveillance. Recently introduced blood gas analyzers can function reliably outside the traditional laboratory setting, even at the bedside; thus, the delay between obtaining the sample and receiving results is significantly reduced.

The major clinical disadvantages of blood gas analyzers are that (1) they provide intermittent data with significant delay secondary to transporting the sample and transmitting the results; (2) the frequency of measurement is limited because blood samples must be permanently removed from the patient; and (3) the blood sample is subject to preanalytic errors.[5] This "gold standard" technology proffers such an unsuitable milieu for obtaining clinically vital information that numerous alternatives have been developed to provide noninvasive and continuous reflections of partial pressures of arterial oxygen (Pa_{O_2}) and carbon dioxide (Pa_{O_2}), a testament, rather than a refutation, for the central importance of arterial blood gas measurements in critical care. In fact, arterial blood gases are presently the most frequently ordered laboratory examination in the operating room and intensive care unit (ICU).[6]

CONTINUOUS VERSUS INTERMITTENT MONITORS

A clinical *monitor* is generically defined as a patient-dedicated apparatus used to observe or record physiologic phenomena without permanently removing body fluids, excrement, or tissue.[4] The verb "monitor" pertains to an individual's act of constant surveillance; the noun "monitor" refers to devices that provide timely information to assist an individual's surveillance. A monitor is noninvasive when application does not require disruption of skin or mucous membrane integrity. Theoretically, a noninvasive monitor should be complication free when appropriately applied and used. An invasive monitor is inevitably associated with some risk of complications despite perfect application and maintenance.

Continuous monitors, like the electrocardiogram, are preferred because they potentially can provide information that may lead to therapeutic intervention before significant physiologic disruption. This proactive capability is enhanced by alarm limits that can be set to alert the bedside practitioner of deviations from the norm and thereby improve the ability to detect problems as early as possible. *Intermittent* monitors, like the sphygmomanometer, are common and useful but are reactive because there must be a reason to initiate the measurement. Of course, intermittent monitors can be automatically cycled very frequently to approach a proactive condition.

Table 34–1 classifies clinical monitors in a descending sequence in terms of desirability. Unfortunately, blood gas analyzers provide the least desirable form of information to aid clinical monitoring: invasive and intermittent with delay. It is no wonder that continuous and noninvasive methods of reflecting blood gases (capnography and oximetry) have gained in popularity. Indeed, it is fair to state that much of the enthusiasm and acceptance for these technologies is due to the undesirability of blood gas analyzers rather than to the accuracy and reliability of the noninvasive devices.

TABLE 34–1. Classification of Clinical Monitors

Classification	*Example*
Noninvasive, continuous	Electrocardiogram monitor
Noninvasive, intermittent	Blood pressure cuff
Invasive, continuous	Transduced blood pressure
Invasive, intermittent	Thermal dilution cardiac output

OPTODE MICROSENSING

In contradistinction to an analyzer, a blood gas *monitor* is a patient-dedicated device that measures arterial pH, Pa_{CO_2}, and Pa_{O_2} without permanently removing blood.[4, 7, 8] Because electrochemical techniques are poorly adaptable to an in vivo environment, an alternative technology is required for the development of blood gas monitors.[9, 10] Advances in fiberoptic and microprocessor technology, combined with optical techniques that alter light without consuming reagents, have led to development of miniaturized sensors that detect change in light (optodes[11]) and have great potential for biomedical applications.[12]

A sensor that operates via electrochemical properties is an electrode; a sensor that operates via optical detection of altered light is an optode.[11] Either transmission-based or fluorescence-based chemistries can be used as indicators for optode microsensing.

Transmission Optodes

As illustrated in Figure 34–1, a transmission optode requires two optic paths. A primary optic path carries a light of known intensity to an indicator where changes in the concentration of an analyte within the indicator cause attenuation of the light by absorption, scattering, reflection outside the fiber, or reflection at the fiber surface. A secondary optic path then carries the attenuated light back to a device that

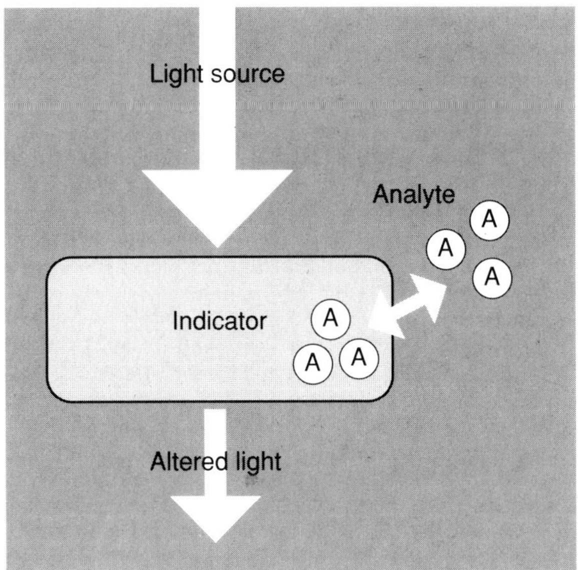

Figure 34–1. The basic principles governing a transmission optode are illustrated. The indicator chamber contains a substance that alters light in a predictably linear manner, depending on the concentration of a specific analyte (A) within the substance. The indicator chamber is in intimate contact with the blood and is separated from it by a membrane freely permeable to the analyte being measured. One optic path (the light source) carries a light of known intensity to the indicator chamber; a second optic path carries the altered light back to a measuring device. (From Shapiro BA, Peruzzi WT, Templin R: Clinical Application of Blood Gases. 5th ed. Chicago, Mosby-Yearbook, 1994.)

quantifies the light. An absorbance-based optode has been described for in vivo pH measurement.[13]

Fluorescent Optodes

A fluorescent dye contains a chemical whose electrons are activated when exposed to an appropriate light intensity. When the light exposure ends, the electrons return to a lower ground state and, in that process, emit a light (fluorescence) of lower frequency or intensity than that of the excitation light source. As illustrated in Figure 34–2, a fluorescent optode is essentially an optic fiber with a fluorescent dye at one end. A light source of known intensity is momentarily turned on, and the light is transmitted down the optic fiber to the fluorescent dye chamber, activating the electrons in the dye. When the light exposure ends, the electrons return to basal activity, and the lower frequency emitted light (fluorescence) will be altered as the concentration of the analyte changes. Fluorescence is augmented as the concentration of hydrogen ion or carbon dioxide (CO_2) increases and is quenched as the concentration of oxygen (O_2) increases. The fluorescent light will be carried by the single optic fiber to a device that quantifies the light. Thus, analyte concentration is determined by measurement of the fluorescence change. These fluorescence-based optodes require only one optic path and have been described for patient-dedicated measurement of pH and partial pressure of CO_2 (P_{CO_2}) and O_2 (P_{O_2})[14–16]

A limitation of fluorescent optodes is the relatively small number of substances that fluoresce. Energy-transfer optodes combine a colorimetric reagent with a fluorescent indicator, greatly increasing the range of substances that can be measured with fluorescent optodes. Optic probes that measure sodium ion, potassium ion, and pH using energy-transfer techniques have been described.[17]

DEMONSTRATION OF CLINICAL FEASIBILITY

To justify routine clinical use in the ICU, a patient-dedicated blood gas monitor must fulfill at least the nine requirements listed in Table 34–2. In 1989, we reported the evaluation of a fluorescent optode intravascular blood gas system intended to measure arterial pH, Pa_{CO_2}, and Pa_{O_2} continuously (CDI 1000 Blood Gas Monitoring System, CDI-3M Healthcare, Tustin, CA).[18] The clinical study was designed to evaluate the performance of the optode system in the operating room and ICU when all patient-interface conditions known to alter function were absent. This resulted in 12 of 23 carefully selected patients meeting the criteria for more than 24 hours. The highly selective patient data confirmed the clinical performance of this device to be within 95% confidence limits that imply the system could have replaced conventional blood gas analysis in these patients. However, only the first three requirements in Table 34–2 were met because of the major patient-interface problems that were subsequently described.[19]

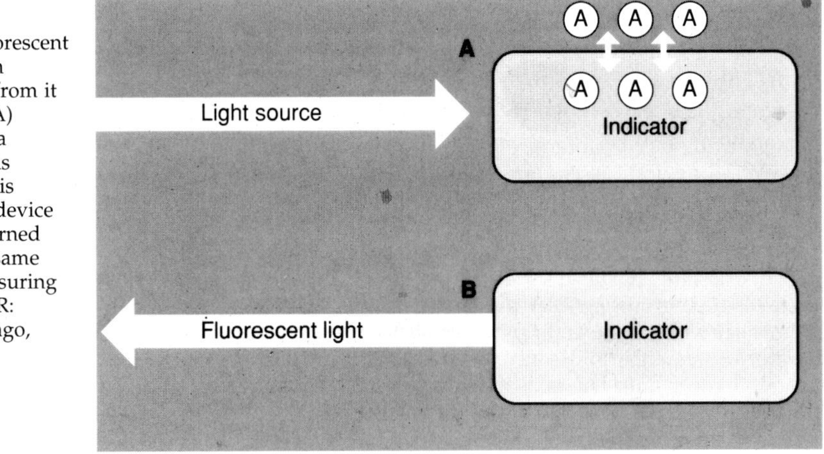

Figure 34–2. The basic principles governing a fluorescent optode are illustrated. The indicator chamber is in intimate contact with the blood and is separated from it by a membrane freely permeable to the analyte (A) being measured. The indicator chamber contains a fluorescent dye (see text). *A*, The fluorescent dye is exposed to a light source of known intensity that is carried down the optic path from the measuring device to the indicator chamber. *B*, The light source is turned off, and the fluorescent light is carried along the same optic path from the indicator chamber to the measuring device. (From Shapiro BA, Peruzzi WT, Templin R: Clinical Application of Blood Gases. 5th ed. Chicago, Mosby-Yearbook, 1994.)

TABLE 34–2. Minimal Requirements for a Blood Gas Monitor in Conjunction with Arterial Catheters

1. Must accurately measure pH, partial pressure of carbon dioxide and oxygen, and temperature with rapid response time
2. Must be operable with a 20-gauge arterial catheter and not negatively affect continuous pressure measurement, obtaining of blood samples, or routine function of the arterial catheter system
3. Must be biocompatible and nonthrombogenic so that the arterial catheter's longevity, reliability, and rate of complications are not negatively affected
4. Must be simple to operate and maintain
5. Must be able to withstand the abuse and rigors of clinical conditions common to the operating room and intensive care unit
6. Must be stable and consistent for at least 72 hours
7. Must not be adversely affected by the reduction in local blood flow or temperature
8. Must not be adversely affected by the hemodynamic changes often encountered in critically ill patients
9. Must be cost effective

CONTINUOUS INTRA-ARTERIAL BLOOD GAS MONITORS

After demonstration of the clinical feasibility of optode microsensing and the description of the patient-interface problems, several companies produced improved intravascular prototypes that rapidly developed to clinically tested devices.

In 1992, the PB 3300 Intra-Arterial Blood Gas Monitor (Puritan-Bennett Corporation, Carlsbad, CA) became available. This device has three fluorescent optodes with significant design improvements that appear to lend accuracy, stability, and dependability for at least 72 hours. Another important feature is that the microsensors are transportable between instruments, allowing for easy patient transfer from the operating room (OR) to the ICU. The Optex BioSentry Optode System (Optex Biomedical, Inc, The Woodlands, TX) incorporates both transmission and fluorescent optodes with a unique side-window sample-chamber configuration that appears to lend stability and precision.[20] The Paratrend of Intravascular Blood Gas Monitoring System (Biomedical Sensors, Malvern, PA) became commercially available in 1993. These continuous blood gas monitors have sophisticated microprocessor systems that provide trend data and alarms. Preliminary data from clinical trials suggest these products meet at least the first six requirements in Table 34–2; how well they meet the final three requirements has yet to be determined, but there is ample justification for optimism.

INTERMITTENT EXTRA-ARTERIAL BLOOD GAS MONITORS

To avoid the patient-interface problems described with intra-arterial devices, an extra-arterial fluorescent optode system has been developed (CDI 2000 Blood Gas Monitoring System; CDI-3M Healthcare, Tustin, CA). This device locates the pH, P_{CO_2}, and P_{O_2} fluorescent optodes within a sensor cassette that is inserted in series with the arterial catheter tubing system near the patient's wrist (Fig. 34–3). To measure pH, P_{CO_2}, and P_{O_2}, a stopcock closes the system to the intravenous fluid source, which then allows arterial blood to flow into the sensor cassette when a subatmospheric pressure is created in an "upstream" reservoir. The placement of the reservoir is such that only intravenous fluid enters the reservoir. The stopcock is then returned to its original position so that the reservoir is isolated and fluid flow from the pressurized bag is restored, allowing blood pressure monitoring to continue. The minimal blood flow occurring in the sensor cassette does not interfere with optode function, and results are displayed within 2 minutes. When the measurement is complete, the blood in the cassette and tubing is returned to the patient by first emptying the intravenous fluid from the reservoir and then flushing the catheter in the routine manner.

In 1993, we reported the clinical performance of this extra-arterial blood gas monitoring system in a prospective, multicenter study.[21] A total of 1341 arterial blood gas measurements were obtained from 117 patients over a 1- to 4-day period. The range of values were 7.14 to 7.64 for pH, 19 to 98 mm Hg (2.5–13.0 kPa) for P_{CO_2}, and 38 to 413 mm Hg (5.1–54.9 kPa) for P_{O_2}. Performance bias (difference between analyzer and monitor mean values) and performance precision (standard deviation of the mean difference between analyzer and monitor) are listed in Table 34–3. Insertion of the sensor cassette into the arterial catheter tubing system did not alter the fidelity of blood pressure readings when there was no preexisting harmonic augmentation of systolic pressure. When harmonic augmentation of systolic pressure was apparent, insertion of the sensor chamber resulted in a "dampening" of systolic pressure of less than 10%. No clinically or statistically significant differences in systolic, diastolic, or mean arterial pressures were evident before, during, or after blood gas measurements attributable to the blood gas monitoring system.

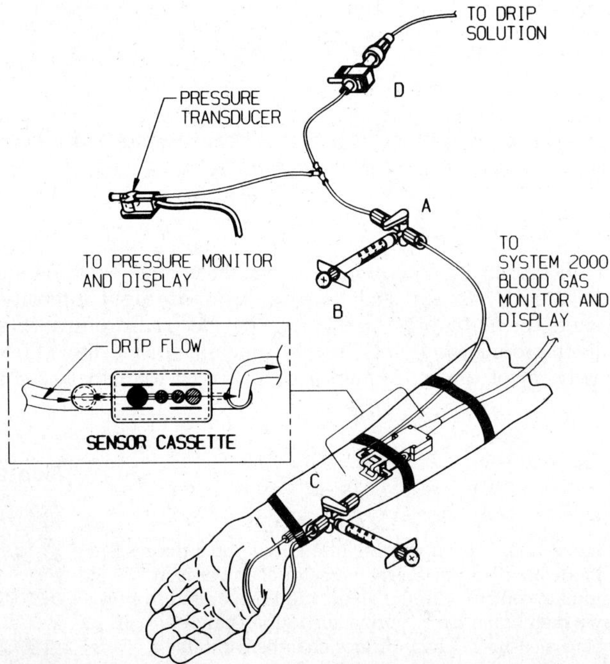

Figure 34–3. A schematic representation of an arterial catheter tubing system with the CDI 2000 Blood Gas Monitoring System in place. The inset depicts a longitudinal section through the sensor cassette that shows the three optodes (pH, P_{CO_2}, P_{O_2}) and the thermistor. *Point A* represents an "upstream" stopcock that allows the aspirating reservoir to function. *Point B* shows a syringe that represents the aspirating reservoir; other devices may also be used. *Point C* represents a stopcock that is available for obtaining blood samples. *Point D* represents a fast-flush mechanism; often, it is in series or parallel with the pressure transducer. (From Shapiro BA, Mahutte CK, Cane RD, et al: Clinical performance of a blood gas monitor: A prospective, multicenter trial. Crit Care Med 1993; 21: 487.)

TABLE 34–3. Bias and Precision of the Blood Gas Monitoring System Values Compared with the Blood Gas Analyzer Values at Four Medical Centers (n = 1341)

Medical Center	*pH*		*P_{CO_2} (mm Hg)*		*P_{O_2} (mm Hg)*	
	Bias	*Precision*	*Bias*	*Precision*	*Bias*	*Precision*
Long Beach	−.005	±.023	−0.5	±2.1	−2.6	±6.5
Northwestern	−.003	±.026	−0.9	±2.2	−2.7	±10.3
Tampa	−.002	±.024	−1.6	±3.0	−3.7	±8.6
Minnesota	−.010	±.039	−1.0	±3.1	1.0	±8.9
Total	−.004	±.027	−0.8	±2.4	−2.2	±8.7

kPa = mm Hg × 0.133.
Abbreviations: P_{CO_2} = partial pressure of carbon dioxide; P_{O_2} = partial pressure of oxygen.

EVALUATION OF BLOOD GAS MONITORS

The clinical availability of blood gas monitors will inevitably result in significant changes in our approach and ability to support cardiopulmonary function in critically ill patients. Such fundamental and pervasive clinical impact demands that a careful and thorough evaluation of such measurement devices be undertaken by the clinician. This requires establishing clear definitions of several terms commonly applied to the study of measuring devices: (1) *accuracy* is the nearness of a measurement to the actual value of the variable being measured; (2) *bias* is a consistent difference in the measured value of a known variable; and (3) *precision* is the closeness to each other of repeated measurements of the same quantity.[22]

Accuracy, bias, and precision can be specifically determined for a given blood gas analyzer in the laboratory because known variables and controlled conditions are available. Unfortunately, consensus of clinical performance standards for modern blood gas machines has not been established[23] because accuracy, bias, and precision vary among commercially available machines[24] and clinical blood gas values are so variable in stable ICU patients.[25] Therefore, the clinical comparison of the performance of an optode-based blood gas monitor with modern blood gas machines must be relatively arbitrary and subjective. To assist the clinician in the interpretation of clinical data, we suggest comparison of stability, consistency, and accuracy of the optode-based blood gas monitor performance in relation to the performance of the electrode-based blood gas machine.

Laboratory Precision

Electrode precision is determined by multiple measurements of a stable sample of known value in a short time frame. For modern blood gas analyzers, electrode precision is generally stated as ±0.01 for pH (the Sanz electrode), ±2% (approximately ±1 mm Hg at 40 mm Hg) for P_{CO_2} (the Severinghaus electrode), and ±3% (approximately ±2.5 mm Hg at 80 mm Hg) for P_{O_2} (the Clark electrode).[23] Using a bovine tonometered blood loop, studies of fluorescent optodes demonstrated optode precision as good as, or better than, the modern blood gas electrodes.[26] Therefore, it is reasonable to compare the clinical performance of these optodes with electrodes because their laboratory precision is comparable.

Performance Stability

It is well known that electrochemical sensors like the Clark (P_{O_2}), Severinghaus (P_{CO_2}), and Sanz (pH) electrodes demonstrate significant "drift" over time, which requires frequent calibration with known standards. Electrode drift is no longer a significant consideration because modern blood gas machines automatically accomplish a one-point calibration with known gas mixtures at intervals that maintain consistent electrode performance. Fluorescent-based optode sensors demonstrate minimal drift in 24 hours (pH <0.005, P_{CO_2} of 0.9 mm Hg [0.12 kPa], and P_{O_2} of 2.1 mm Hg [0.28 kPa]).[18]

Considering the blood gas analyzer values as the standard, the performance stability of an optode-based monitoring system should be reflected in the bias (the difference in the means between the analyzer and monitor).[27] Table 34–3 lists the performance bias of the CDI 2000 Blood Gas Monitoring System, demonstrating that, on average, the monitor values were slightly higher than the analyzer values and were essentially within the ranges considered acceptable for electrode imprecision. This should be interpreted as strong evidence that the performance stability of the blood gas monitor is comparable to that of the modern blood gas machine.

Performance Consistency

To ensure performance consistency of blood gas electrodes over the common range of clinically relevant values, a two-point calibration with known gases and buffers is recommended every 4 to 8 hours. When comparing electrode with optode consistency, linear regression analysis determines multiple correlation coefficients that can suggest how consistently the optode performed using the electrode as the standard. It is appropriate to evaluate more specifically the performance consistency of a blood gas monitoring system by considering each set of measurements as the average of the two measurements compared with the difference between the two measurements as shown in Figure 34–4.[27]

Performance Accuracy

To ensure electrode accuracy, accepted laboratory procedure requires a daily correlation with control solutions. It is relatively easy to produce control solutions for most analytes of clinical interest because they are measured in serum or plasma where essentially no change in analyte concentration occurs with time. Because whole blood is living tissue that continuously alters the concentrations of O_2, CO_2, and hydrogen ion, a control solution that realistically reflects the patient-analytic system would not be stable over time.[28] This means that commercially available stable control solutions for blood gas electrodes do not predictably reflect the patient-analytic system and therefore pose significant difficulties in establishment of target values.[29, 30] These technical factors complicate the quality-control process and play a role in the documented bias and imprecision of modern blood gas electrodes.[15, 31, 32]

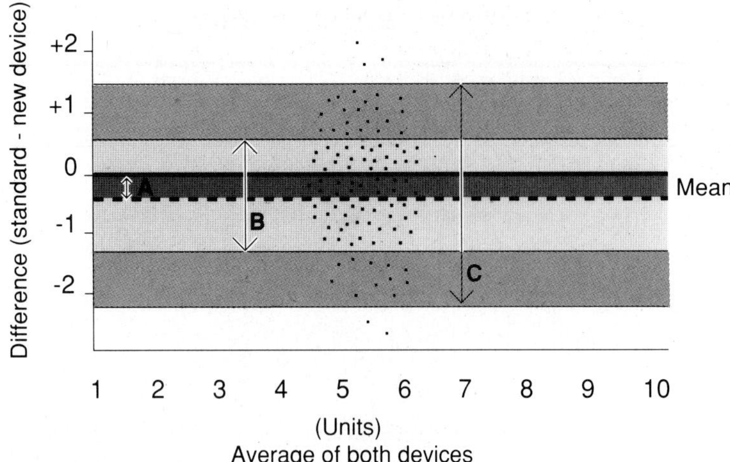

Figure 34–4. A representation of the Bland-Altman method of determining agreement between two measuring devices (see text). A data set contains a measurement made by the standard device and one made by the new device. Each dot on the graph represents a data set determined by the *difference* between the standard device and the new device on the vertical axis; the *average* of the two measurements is on the horizontal axis. *A*, The mean difference between the two devices, which represents the *performance bias*. *B*, Plus or minus one standard deviation of the mean difference, which represents *performance precision*. *C*, Plus or minus two standard deviations of the mean difference, which represents the 95% confidence range for agreement. (From Shapiro BA, Peruzzi WT, Templin R: Clinical Application of Blood Gases. 5th ed. Chicago, Mosby-Yearbook, 1994.)

To demonstrate the accuracy of internal laboratory controls, periodic comparison with a "peer group" of extralaboratory analyzers is recommended. This process is known as *proficiency testing*. The College of American Pathologists provides proficiency testing for blood gas analyzers and promulgates medical usefulness evaluation criteria composed of fixed limits around target values (Table 34–4).[33] Target values are established by calculating the mean value from a peer group of similar machines analyzing a common sample. It must be emphasized that these proficiency criteria are applied to peer groups of the same manufacturers and models of blood gas analyzers because variation between these devices is well known.[15, 23, 24] In fact, recognition of significant bias and imprecision among commercially available blood gas analyzers resulted in the Health Care Finance Administration adopting 1993 proficiency evaluation criteria[8] with even more generous fixed limits than the 1992 College of American Pathologists limits (see Table 34–4). Although we recognize that such proficiency criteria for blood gas electrodes specifically apply to only a group of equivalent analyzers, it seems reasonable to examine the performance of blood gas monitors in relation to these established performance criteria for analyzers.

Recognizing the numerous factors complicating accuracy determinations for blood gas machines, it has been suggested that clinically acceptable accuracy specifications be based on the electrode bias being less than the imprecision and drift.[23, 24] On the basis of this concept, Table 34–5 shows the recommended "acceptable bias" for a newly calibrated sensor.

ADVANTAGES OF A BLOOD GAS MONITOR

Arterial catheters are commonly placed in ICU patients for continuous monitoring of blood pressure and/or frequent diagnostic blood testing. The suitability of a blood gas monitor (Table 34–6) for such patients is obvious providing there is no requirement to alter the size, location, and placement of the arterial catheter, and the routine use and maintenance of the arterial catheter system are unaffected.

Blood gas monitors should significantly reduce therapeutic decision time (the interval from ordering the test to initiating a therapeutic action based on the test results[35]), enabling rapid and dependable titration of common therapeutic modalities such as O_2 administration, positive-pressure ventilation, positive end-expiratory pressure, and alkali therapy. Blood gas monitors do not require the removal of blood from the patient, thereby resulting in a significant conservation of blood loss in critically ill patients.[36, 37] The risk of nosocomial infection from contaminated arterial catheters should be reduced because the integrity of the arterial catheter tubing is not interrupted to obtain blood gas values. The frequency of personnel exposure to the patient's blood would be markedly diminished. Finally, it has been suggested that combining a blood gas monitor with capnography may allow observation of trend changes in both cardiac output and intrapulmonary shunting.[7, 38]

POTENTIAL IMPACT OF BLOOD GAS MONITORS

Assuming an acceptable cost for patient-dedicated blood gas monitors, the advantages listed in Table 34–6 would be reason enough for enthusiasm. We believe these factors represent the tip of the iceberg regarding the impact blood gas monitors will have on patient care in the ICU. We submit that capnography in conjunction with blood gas monitors has the potential to reliably monitor trends in cardiac output and quantify the shunt fraction in the majority of ICU patients. To date, no direct data confirming this concept have yet been published because blood gas monitors have not been available for prolonged study. However, the inferential information referenced next suggests that these concepts will prove clinically useful.

Monitoring Trends of Acute Change in Cardiac Output

Dead space ventilation is defined as that portion of total ventilation that does not respire, dictating that dead space gas does not undergo an increase in P_{CO_2}. It is agreed that the difference between the Pa_{CO_2} and the end-tidal (ET) CO_2

TABLE 34–4. College of American Pathologists (CAP) and Health Care Finance Administration (HCFA) Proficiency Testing Criteria Compared with Precision Performance of the Blood Gas Monitoring System

Parameter	*CAP Limits*	*HCFA Limits*	*Monitor Precision*
Arterial pH	±0.03	±0.04	±0.03
Pa_{CO_2}	±3 mm Hg	±5 mm Hg	±2.4 mm Hg
Pa_{O_2}	±7.5%	±3 SD of PT group	±8.3%

Abbreviations: Pa_{CO_2} = partial pressure of arterial carbon dioxide; Pa_{O_2} = partial pressure of arterial oxygen.
PT = proficiency testing group.
kPa = mm Hg × 0.133.

TABLE 34–5. Acceptable Bias for Blood Gas Electrodes Compared with Bias Performance of the Blood Gas Monitoring System

Parameter	*Acceptable Electrode Bias*	*Monitor Bias*
Arterial pH	0.05	0.004
$Paco_2$ (mm Hg)	3.0	0.8
Pao_2 (mm Hg)	5.0	2.2

kPa = mm Hg × 0.133.
Abbreviations: $Paco_2$ = partial pressure of arterial carbon dioxide; Pao_2 = partial pressure of arterial oxygen.

($Paco_2$ − $PETCO_2$) gradient must be a function of the dead space ventilation and, therefore, changes in the $Paco_2$ − $PETCO_2$ that are not due to technical problems should be attributed to changes in dead space ventilation. The most common clinical causes of alterations in dead space ventilation are (1) lung disease; (2) pulmonary embolic phenomena; and (3) changes in cardiac output. Acute lung disease, including embolic phenomenon, alters ventilation-perfusion ratio ($\dot{V}/\dot{Q}$) in a nonuniform manner and thereby changes the shape of the capnogram. As illustrated in Figure 34–5, when the $Paco_2$ − $PETCO_2$ changes in conjunction with the changes in capnographic configuration, it is reasonable to assume that dead space changes are attributable to changes in lung disease.

The interrelation of cardiac function, pulmonary blood flow, and CO_2 excretion suggests that capnography may be a useful indicator of changes in cardiac function. Animal studies confirm that a controlled decrease in cardiac output results in an acute decrease in $PETCO_2$.[39] Such preliminary data, in conjunction with universally accepted respiratory pathophysiology, suggest that an acute change in the $Paco_2$ − $PETCO_2$ gradient without simultaneous change in capnographic configuration (see Fig. 34–5) should indicate an acute change in cardiac output.[40] The clinical reality of blood gas monitors provides the technologic advance that promises to allow the capnograph to reliably monitor cardiac output changes in response to interventions such as intravenous fluid therapy, inotropic therapy, and diuretic therapy.

Estimating the Intrapulmonary Shunt Fraction

Although far from perfect, calculation of the intrapulmonary shunt fraction is the most reliable clinical means of quantifying disruption of pulmonary O_2 transfer. Because calculation of the shunt fraction requires determination of both arterial and mixed venous O_2 contents, the value is available only in patients with pulmonary artery catheters in place.

TABLE 34–6. Advantages of Blood Gas Monitors in Conjunction with Arterial Catheters

1. They provide a proactive monitor with alarms for early warning of significant changes, perhaps leading to therapeutic intervention before significant physiologic disruption.
2. They furnish immediate and continuing blood gas trends, allowing for more rapid and precise changes in respiratory supportive therapy such as supportive ventilation, positive end-expiratory pressure, and oxygen.
3. They reduce blood loss incident to obtaining data.
4. They reduce the risks of nosocomial infection.
5. They reduce the exposure of personnel to patients' blood.

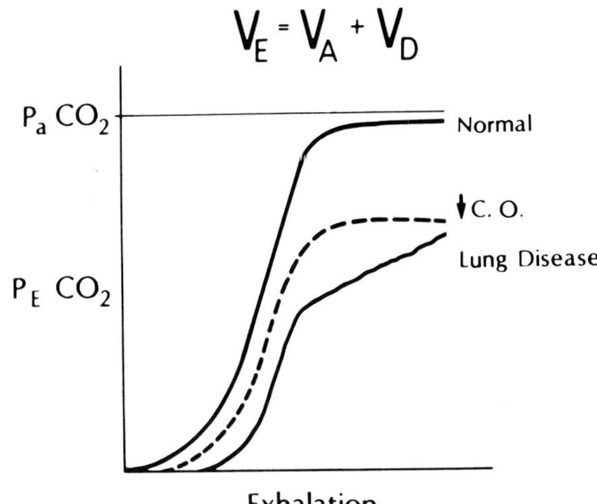

Figure 34–5. Total ventilation ($\dot{V}$E) is composed of both alveolar ventilation ($\dot{V}$A) and dead space ventilation ($\dot{V}$DS). The $Paco_2$ is considered the best reflection of alveolar ventilation. The end tidal Pco_2 is the expired Pco_2 ($PECO_2$) at the end of the plateau. An increase in $\dot{V}$E is manifest as an increase in P(a − ET) CO_2 gradient. The two most common causes of increased DS are decreased cardiac output (C.O.) and lung disease. A decreased pulmonary perfusion (*dashed curve*) results in more alveoli having lower Pco_2; the net result is a decrease in $PECO_2$ but no change in lung emptying pattern. Lung disease involves a change in emptying patterns and, therefore, a change in the shape of the curve. (From Shapiro BA, Peruzzi WT, Templin R: Clinical Application of Blood Gases. 5th ed. Chicago, Mosby-Yearbook, 1994.)

When mixed venous blood is not available, numerous O_2 tension indexes—including alveolar-arterial difference in partial pressure of O_2 (PAO_2 − Pao_2), partial pressure of arterial oxygen (Pao_2) divided by partial pressure of alveolar oxygen, Pao_2 divided by fraction of inspired oxygen (Fio_2), PAO_2 − Pao_2/PAO_2—have been proposed to reflect pulmonary O_2-transfer deficits. The nonlinear relationship between O_2 content and O_2 tension predicts a poor correlation between O_2 tension indexes and shunt fractions, especially in critically ill patients in whom Fio_2 and cardiac output may frequently change. However, these indexes are relatively easy to calculate and continue to enjoy popularity despite their documented unreliability.[41]

Oxygen-content indexes should predictably reflect changes in shunt fractions because O_2 content and hemoglobin saturation have relatively linear relationships. The estimated shunt is the clinical shunt equation with an assumed arterial-mixed venous blood difference in O_2 content of 3.5 mL/dL and has been demonstrated to be superior to tension-based indexes in reflecting the intrapulmonary shunt fraction.[39] A stable cardiac output, indicated by a stable $Paco_2$ − $PETCO_2$ gradient, should validate the assumption that changes in the estimated shunt would reliably quantify changes in the shunt fraction.

CONCLUSION

The clinical availability of blood gas monitors will have as great an effect on ICU and OR care as the introduction of blood gas analyzers had 30 years ago. Although they will not completely replace the need for blood gas analyzers and noninvasive monitors, they will have profound effects on our practices of monitoring and supporting critically ill patients.

References

1. Severinghaus JW, Astrup PB: History of blood gas analysis. Int Anesthesiol Clin 1987; 25:12.
2. Clark LC Jr: Measurement of oxygen tension: An historical perspective. Crit Care Med 1981; 9:960.
3. Hall JR, Shapiro BA: Acute care/blood gas laboratories: Profile of current operations. Crit Care Med 1984; 12:530–533.
4. Shapiro BA: Quality improvement standards for intensive care unit monitors: We must be informed and involved. Crit Care Med 1992; 20:1629–1630.
5. Walton JR, Shapiro BA, Wine C: Pre-analytic error in arterial blood gas measurement (Abstract). Respir Care 1981; 21:1136.
6. Maukkassa FF, Rutledge R, Fakhry SM, et al: ABGs and arterial lines: The relationship to unnecessarily drawn arterial blood gas samples. J Trauma 1991; 30:1087.
7. Shapiro BA: In-vivo monitoring of arterial blood gases and pH. Respir Care 1992; 37:165–169.
8. Medicare, Medicaid and CLIA Programs; Regulations Implementing the Clinical Laboratory Improvement Amendments of 1988 (CLIA '88). Federal Register, February 28, 1992, p 7008.
9. Mahutte CK: On line blood gas monitoring. *In*: Contemporary Management in Critical Care: Respiratory Monitoring. Vol 4. Tobin MJ (Ed). New York, Churchill Livingstone, 1991.
10. Greene GE, Hassell KT, Mahutte CK: Comparison of arterial blood gas with continuous intra-arterial and transcutaneous PO_2 sensors in adult critically ill patients. Crit Care Med 1987; 15:491–494.
11. Optiz N, Lubbers DW: Theory and development of fluorescence-based optochemical oxygen sensors: Oxygen optodes. Int Anesthesiol Clin 1987; 25:177–197.
12. Peterson JL, Vurek GG: Fiber-optic sensors for biomedical applications. Science 1984; 224:123–126.

12a. Wahr JA, Tremper KK: Continuous intravascular blood gas monitoring. J Cardiothorac Vasc Anesth 1994; 8:342–353.

13. Saari LA, Seitz WR: pH sensor based on immobilized fluoresceinamine. Anna Chem 1982; 54:821–825.
14. West JB, Dollery CT, Naimark A: Distribution of blood flow in isolated lung: Relation to vascular and alveolar pressure. J Appl Physiol 1964; 19:713–724.
15. Gehrich JL, Lubbers DW, Optiz N, et al: Optical fluorescence and its application to an intravascular blood gas monitoring system. IEEE Trans Biomed Eng 1986; 33:117–132.
16. Miller WW, Gehrich JL, Hansmann DR, et al: Continuous in vivo monitoring of blood gases. Lab Med 1988; 19:629–635.
17. Angel SM: Optodes: Chemically selective fiber-optic sensors. Spectroscopy 1987; 2:38–46.
18. Shapiro BA, Cane RD, Chomka CM, et al: Preliminary evaluation of an intra-arterial blood gas system in dogs and humans. Crit Care Med 1989; 17:455–460.
19. Mahutte CK, Sassoon CSH, Muro JR, et al: Progress in the development of a fluorescent intravascular blood gas system in man. J Clin Monit 1990; 6:147–157.
20. Zimmerman JL, Dellinger RP: Initial evaluation of a new intra-arterial blood gas system in humans. Crit Care Med 1993; 21:495–500.
21. Shapiro BA, Mahutte CK, Cane RD, et al: Clinical performance of a blood gas monitor: A prospective, multicenter trial. Crit Care Med 1993; 21:487–494.
22. Zar JH: Biostatistical Analysis. 2nd ed. Englewood Cliffs, NJ, Prentice-Hall, 1984.
23. Clausen JL, Murray KM: Clinical applications of arterial blood gases: How much accuracy do we need? J Med Tech 1985; 2:19–32.
24. Wickers EK, Teunissen AJ, Van den Camp RA, et al: A comparative study of the electrode systems of three pH and blood gas apparatus. J Clin Chem Biochem 1978; 16:175–185.
25. Thorson SH, Marini JJ, Pierson DJ, et al: Variability of arterial blood gas values in stable patients in the ICU. Chest 1983; 84:14–18.
26. Miller WW, Yafuso M, Yan CF, et al: Performance of an in-vivo, continuous blood-gas monitor with disposable probe. Clin Chem 1987; 33:1538–1542.
27. Bland JM, Altman DG: Statistical methods for assessing agreement between two methods of clinical measurement. Lancet 1986; i:307–310.
28. Steiner MC, Shapiro BA, Kavanaugh J, et al: A stable blood product for pH-blood gas quality control. Clin Chem 1978; 24:793–795.
29. Leary ET, Graham G, Kenney MA: Commercially available blood gas controls compared with tonometered blood. Clin Chem 1980; 26:1309–1316.
30. Moran RF, Grenier RE: A simple method of setting reliable target values and limits for blood gas quality control materials. Can J Med Tech 1988; 50:95–98.
31. Moran RF: Assessment of quality control of blood gas/pH analyzer performance. Respir Care 1981; 26:538–546.
32. National Committee for Clinical Laboratory Standards: Devices for measuring PO_2 and PCO_2 in blood samples. NCCLS Publication C-21 1983; 3:136–160.
33. Interlaboratory Comparison Program Surveys Manual, Section III: Clinical Chemistry. Northfield, IL, College of American Pathologists, 1992, pp 28–29.
34. Ehrmeyer SS, Laessig RH: 1990 Medicare/CLIA final rules for proficiency testing: Minimum intra-laboratory performance characteristics (CV and bias) needed to pass. Clin Chem 1990; 36:1736–1740.
35. Zaloga GP: Evaluation of bedside testing options for the critical care unit. Chest 1990; 97(Suppl):185S–190S.
36. Salem B, Chernow B, Burke R: Bedside diagnostic testing: Its accuracy, rapidity, and utility in blood conservation. JAMA 1991; 266:382–389.
37. Chernow B, Salem M, Stacey J: Blood conservation: A critical imperative. Crit Care Med 1991; 19:313–314.
38. Shapiro BA, Cane RD: Blood gas monitoring: Yesterday, today and tomorrow. Crit Care Med 1989; 17:573–581.
39. Isserles SA, Breen PH: Can changes in end-tidal PCO_2 measure changes in cardiac output? Anesth Analg 1991; 73:808–814.
40. Smallhout B, Kalenda Z: An Atlas of Capnography. Zeist, The Netherlands, Kerckebosch, 1975.
41. Hess D, Maxwell C, Shefet D: Determination of intrapulmonary shunt: Comparison of an estimated shunt equation and a modified shunt equation with the classic equation. Respir Care 1987; 32:268–273.
42. Shapiro BA: Blood gas monitors: Justifiable enthusiasm with a note of caution. Am J Respir Crit Care Med 1994; 149:850–851.
43. Shapiro BA: Evaluation of blood gas monitors: Performance criteria, clinical impact, and cost-benefit. Crit Care Med 1994; 22:546–548.

CHAPTER 35

Tissue Oxygenation and High-Energy Phosphate Metabolism

Guillermo Gutiérrez, PhD, MD

CELLULAR ENERGY METABOLISM

Cells require a continuous supply of energy to perform their function within an organ and to maintain adequate control over membrane permeability. A failure of cellular energy metabolism results in organ dysfunction and cell death as control is lost over solute and metabolite exchange across the membrane.[1] Cellular energy production is the end result of the metabolism of various foodstuffs, glucose, fat, and protein. Consumption of these substrates results in phosphorylation of adenosine diphosphate (ADP) to adenosine triphosphate (ATP). Energy is stored in a high-energy phosphate bond of ATP, to be released when required by the synthetic or locomotive functions of the cell.[2]

Aerobic Energy Production

Generation of ATP occurs in both the presence and absence of oxygen. Aerobic metabolism is the preferred method of energy generation. Significantly more energy is produced by the cells when substrate consumption is coupled to the consumption of oxygen. After their entry into the cell, glucose and free fatty acids undergo conversion to acetylcoenzyme A (acetyl-CoA), which is completely metabolized in the tricarboxylic acid cycle, also called the Krebs cycle, to water, carbon dioxide, and four electron pairs (Fig. 35–1). Nicotinamide dinucleotide (NAD^+) and flavin adenine dinucleotide (FAD^+) transport the electron pairs to the cytochrome system as NADH and $FADH_2$. The cytochromes are located in the inner mitochondrial membrane. The electrons move down the cytochromes in a chain of oxidation-reduction reactions in which each reaction is associated with progressively lower energy levels, until the final cytochrome reduces molecular oxygen (O_2). This process is called *oxidative phosphorylation*, and it produces three ATP molecules per NADH and two per $FADH_2$.[3]

ATP diffuses to the sites of energy use in the cytosol, such as the myofibrils and the membrane-associated ionic pumps, where a large amount of chemical energy is released from the hydrolysis of one of ATP's high-energy phosphate bond. The ATPases are the enzymes that control the hydrolysis of ATP resulting in the formation of ADP, inorganic phosphate (Pi), and hydrogen ion (H^+):

$$ATP \rightarrow ADP + Pi + H^+$$

ADP, Pi, and H^+ return to the mitochondria, where they serve as substrates for the formation of other ATP molecules. In this manner, the cytosolic concentration of these metabolites is maintained low.

The control of ATP production appears to be a function of the concentrations of ATP, ADP, and Pi, expressed as the phosphate potential[4]:

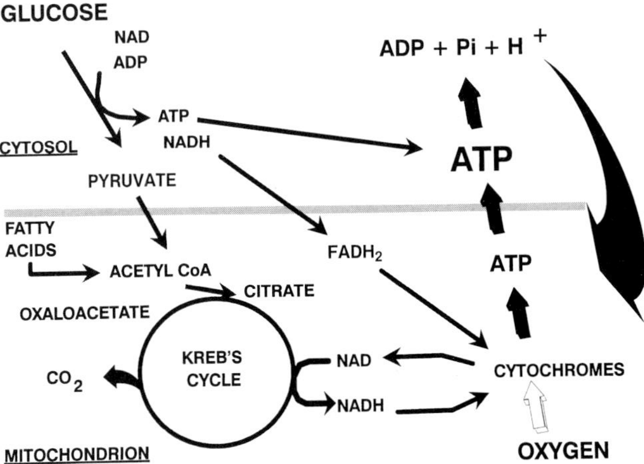

Figure 35–1. The aerobic metabolism of glucose, glycogen, and free fatty acids results in the generation of ATP by oxidative phosphorylation. ATP diffuses directly out of the mitochondria to the sites of energy utilization, or its high energy phosphate bond is carried by the creatine phosphate shuttle. The hydrolysis of ATP releases energy and produces ADP, inorganic phosphate (Pi), and hydrogen ion (H^+). These byproducts of energy metabolism return to the mitochondria to help in the formation of another ATP molecule. *Abbreviations*: NAD = nicotinamide-adenine dinucleotide; NADH = nicotinamide-adenine dinucleotide (reduced form); $FADH_2$ = flavin adenine dinucleotide (reduced form).

$$\text{Phosphate potential} = \frac{[ATP]}{[ADP][Pi]}$$

When the rate of mitochondrial ATP production lags behind the rate of cellular use, ADP and Pi accumulate in the cytosol and the phosphate potential declines. A signal is thus sent to the mitochondria to produce more ATP, and O_2 consumption increases. On the other hand, when cellular energy demand decreases, the rate of ATP hydrolysis and the concentrations of ADP and Pi also decrease. The net result is an increase in phosphate potential and diminished mitochondrial ATP production. This aerobic feedback system permits the cell to adjust ATP production in response to imbalances between energy supply and demand.

The situation is different during strenuous exercise, when aerobic ATP production is limited by the cellular availability of O_2. Under those conditions, the phosphate potential declines rapidly because the rate of ATP hydrolysis is significantly greater than the rate of ATP formation and the tissues must either lower their level of energy use, resulting in muscle fatigue, or turn to anaerobic sources of energy to supplement aerobic ATP production. Hypoxia also results in an imbalance between energy demands and aerobic ATP production, because mitochondrial O_2 delivery is limited by decreases in tissue oxygenation.

Anaerobic Energy Production

The three sources of anaerobic ATP production are glycolysis, the adenylate kinase reaction, and in some tissues that require a ready source of energy supply, the creatine kinase reaction. The adequacy of tissue oxygenation in critically ill patients may be assessed by measuring the metabolic byproducts of these reactions.[5]

The imbalance between the rate of ATP supply to the cell and the demands for energy result in intracellular accumulation of ADP, Pi, and H^+. Changes in concentration of these metabolites serve as feedback signals to modulate the pattern of substrate use by the cells and to promote anaerobic synthesis of ATP. The Pasteur effect, defined as the preferential use of glucose as a metabolic substrate, is an early response to hypoxia.[6] Cells turn preferentially to glycolysis during hypoxia because the number of ATP molecules produced per molecule of O_2 consumed, also called the phosphate-O_2 (P-O) ratio, is greater for glucose than for fat or protein. By increasing glucose metabolism, the hypoxic cell becomes a more efficient consumer of O_2. This metabolic pattern has been observed in the heart during hypoxia[7,8] as the myocytes switch from the consumption of lactate and free fatty acids to the almost exclusive use of glucose.

Hypoxia also depresses protein synthesis by inhibiting peptide chain elongation, resulting in the intracellular accumulation of most amino acids, with the exception of aspartate and glutamate.[9] The concentrations of aspartate and glutamate decrease as they are transaminated with pyruvate to form alanine. Increases in alanine synthesis from pyruvate serve to moderate the formation of lactate during hypoxia.

Anaerobic Sources of Energy

Glycolysis

Glycolysis is a universal cellular reaction to hypoxia, in which glucose or glycogen is metabolized to lactate with the production of ATP. The overall reaction of glycolysis is

$$\text{Glucose} + 2\ ADP + 2\ Pi \rightarrow 2\ \text{lactate} + 2\ ATP$$

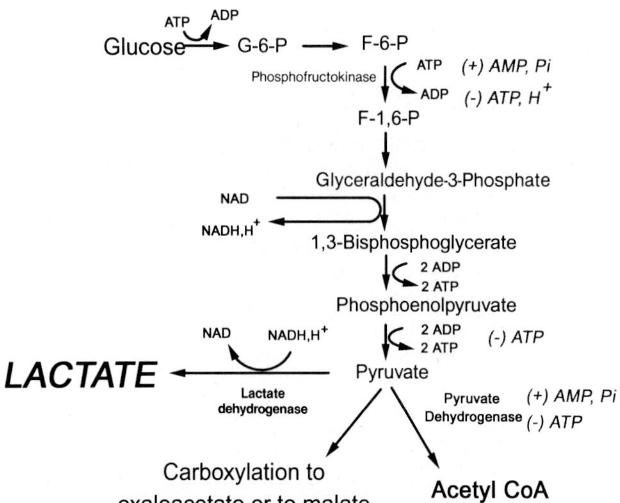

Figure 35–2. Metabolic control of glycolysis. The formation of pyruvate from glucose is a carefully controlled process that accelerates when energy needs are high, as reflected by the cytosolic concentrations of AMP and Pi. Increases in ATP concentration have a negative effect on glycolysis. *Abbreviations*: G-6-P = glucose-6-phosphate; F-6-P = fructose-6-phosphate; F-1,6-P = fructose-1,6-bisphosphate.

The rate of glycolysis is regulated by several key reactions, perhaps the most important being the phosphofructokinase (PFK) reaction,[10] in which fructose-6-phosphate is converted to fructose-1,6-bisphosphate (Fig. 35–2). PFK is strongly inhibited by ATP and H^+ and activated by metabolites whose concentration increases with hypoxia, adenine monophosphate (AMP), and Pi. Consequently, glycolysis is stimulated when the rate of cellular energy use outpaces the rate of ATP production by the mitochondria.

Glycolysis has some disadvantages. The production of ATP by glycolysis is an inefficient process, from the perspective of substrate used to ATP generated. Only 2 mol of ATP are produced per mole of glucose consumed, compared with 38 ATP when glycolysis is coupled to oxidative phosphorylation. Glycolysis also results in cellular acidosis. The source of H^+ generation in glycolysis is controversial, because glycolysis does not generate H^+ when cellular pH is at the physiologic level of 7.2.[11] However, at low intracellular pH values (pH ~ 6.2), the protonation of ADP increases and one H^+ is formed per molecule of lactate generated. Hydrolysis of ATP is the major source of intracellular H^+ during hypoxia. When mitochondrial function is limited by O_2 supply, the recycling of protons by oxidative phosphorylation declines and cytosolic H^+ concentration rises.[12]

Cellular acidosis may inhibit mitochondrial ATP transport, promoting the loss of adenine nucleotides from the mitochondria.[13] The balance between the total adenine nucleotide content (ATP + ADP + AMP) in the mitochondria in relation to that in the cytosol is thus disrupted. Under normoxic conditions, the respective sizes of the adenine nucleotide pools in the cytosol and in mitochondria are balanced.

$$\underbrace{[ATP] + [ADP] + [AMP]}_{\text{cytosol}} \leftrightarrow \underbrace{[ATP] + [ADP] + [AMP]}_{\text{mitochondria}}$$

Hypoxia shifts the distribution of the adenine nucleotides, resulting in an increase in the cytosolic pool. This process may be hastened by decreases in pH, because it favors the net loss of ATP from the mitochondria with increasing acidity of the cytosol. As the adenine nucleotide pool of the mitochondria diminishes, so does the rate of oxidative phosphorylation. The mitochondrial adenylate pool eventually becomes so small that ATP production ceases. After a net loss of adenine nucleotides from the cell, the mitochondria may not be capable of renewing aerobic ATP production when O_2 supply returns to normal.

The Creatine Kinase Reaction

Organs with high metabolic demands, such as the brain, the heart, and skeletal muscle, use the creatine kinase reaction as a ready, anaerobic source of ATP in addition to glycolysis. In this reaction, phosphocreatine (PCr) is metabolized to creatine, transferring its high-energy phosphate bond to ATP. This reaction also helps buffer intracellular acidosis by using H^+,

$$PCr + ADP + H^+ \leftrightarrow ATP + creatine$$

Under physiologic conditions, the creatine kinase reaction is in equilibrium. Increases in ADP and H^+ during hypoxia promote the formation of ATP and creatine, whereas the opposite occurs when the supplies of ATP rise. These changes can be measured in vivo with phosphorus 31 magnetic resonance spectroscopy (^{31}P-MRS).[14]

The creatine kinase reaction also appears to have a significant role in the transport of high-energy phosphates from the mitochondria to the sites of energy use. It has been proposed[15] that high-energy phosphates are transferred from ATP to PCr in the outer mitochondrial wall. PCr is a small molecule that diffuses easily in the cytosol until it reaches the sites of energy use, where it transfers the high-energy phosphate bond to local ADP to form ATP and creatine.

The Adenylate Kinase Reaction

The third anaerobic source of energy is the adenylate kinase reaction, which is present in all cells. The adenylate kinase reaction converts two ADP molecules into one ATP and one AMP:

$$ADP + ADP \rightarrow ATP + AMP$$

This reaction results in the accumulation of AMP, which in turn is dephosphorylated to adenosine by 5′-nucleotidase (Fig. 35–3). The production of AMP leads to the formation of adenosine by the 5′-nucleotidase reaction. Because adenosine is a potent vasodilator,[16] the tissues are thus provided with a metabolic feedback loop capable of promoting local increases in blood flow in response to hypoxia.[17–19] Hester[20] micropipetted adenosine into the venules of the hamster's cremaster muscle and showed that the diffusion of a vasoactive metabolite, such as adenosine, may provide a mechanism by which the tissue can send a signal to cause dilation of the more proximal arterioles. AMP also can be deaminated to inosine monophosphate (IMP) by the AMP deaminase reaction,[17] with the concurrent production of ammonia (NH_3). This metabolic step also helps buffer cytosolic pH:

$$AMP \rightarrow IMP + NH_3$$
$$NH_3 + H^+ \rightarrow NH_4^+$$

Deamination of AMP to IMP is an important metabolic step that attenuates the loss of adenine nucleotides from the cell; otherwise, AMP would be lost in the form of adenosine. The formation of IMP conserves adenine nucleotides and allows resynthesis of AMP by the enzyme succinyl AMP

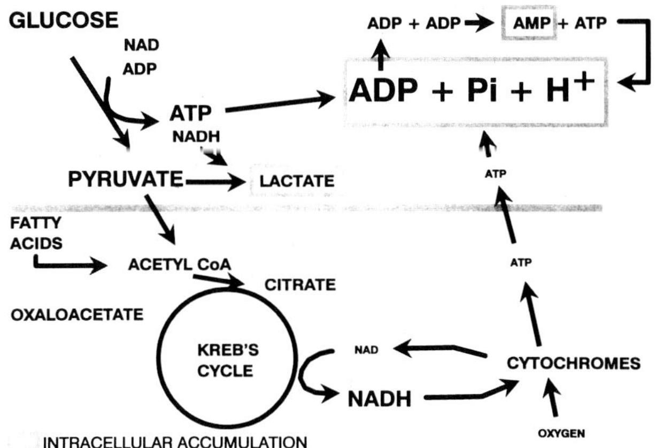

Figure 35–3. During hypoxia, insufficient oxygen is present to maintain the usual turnover rate of the Kreb's cycle, and thus pyruvate accumulates. This results in the formation of lactate and in the accumulation of ADP, Pi, and H^+ in the cytosol. Some ATP is formed anaerobically by the adenylate kinase reaction, which produces increases in AMP concentration.

synthetase during recovery from exercise or hypoxia. Otherwise, adenine nucleotides must be created de novo from small molecule precursors,[21] a relatively slow metabolic process.

METABOLIC INDICES OF TISSUE ENERGY STATE

Lactate Production

Arterial lactate has been proposed as a marker of inadequate tissue oxygenation in critically ill patients[22, 23] (Fig. 35–4). Although an elevated blood lactate level usually signifies generalized tissue hypoxia, a normal value should not be taken as evidence of adequate oxygenation in all organs. Arterial or mixed venous lactate concentrations reflect the pooling of blood from several tissue beds, and elevations in venous lactate flowing from underperfused organs may be dampened or even lost after mixing with venous blood derived from adequately perfused tissues. Therefore, it is not surprising that a clear relationship between lactate levels and the energy status of a patient may be difficult to establish, except in obvious cases of systemic hypoperfusion.[24]

Lactate production for individual organs is a more reliable index of anaerobic metabolism. It can be calculated from measurements of the organ blood flow and the arteriovenous lactate difference. However, measurement of whole-body lactate production may misrepresent the true state of anoxic tissues, because this parameter is influenced by changes in tissue lactate accumulation and washout.[25] Moreover, the kinetics of lactate accumulation in blood are difficult to predict, because lactate is released by the liver in response to circulating catecholamines while simultaneously being metabolized by various organs. Furthermore, results of experimental studies suggest that the relationship between tissue lactate release and regional tissue hypoxia in sepsis may be more complicated than was previously appreciated.[26–28]

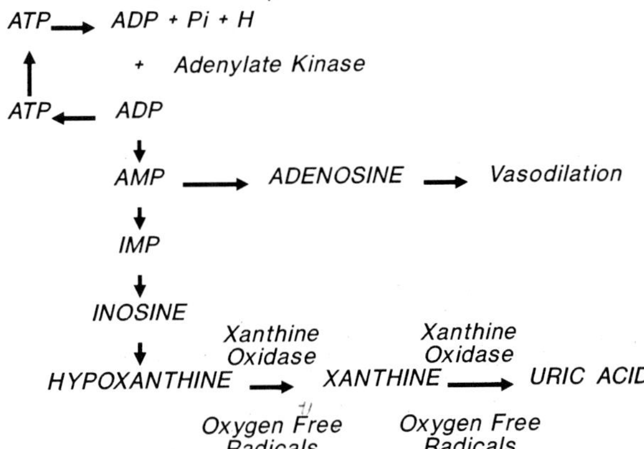

Figure 35–4. The degradation of adenine nucleotides in cellular hypoxia. Increases in ADP concentration resulting from the hydrolysis of ATP leads to the formation of AMP by the adenylate kinase reaction. AMP is either converted to adenosine, a powerful vasodilator, or it is deaminated to inosine monophosphate and eventually it is metabolized to uric acid, resulting in the production of O_2 free radicals by the xanthine oxidase reaction.

Magnetic Resonance Spectroscopy

The use of ^{31}P-MRS offers an unparalleled advantage over other techniques to monitor the adequacy of tissue oxygenation because it measures in a noninvasive manner the levels of high-energy phosphate in skeletal muscle, the brain, and the heart.[29, 30] Furthermore, the use of another isotope, proton MRS, may allow for precise localization and measurement of many biologically active compounds.

High levels of exercise or hypoxia result in accumulation of ADP, Pi, and lactate, as well as decreases in PCr and intracellular pH. The decrease in PCr and the concomitant increase in Pi provide a convenient index of cellular energy state, the PCr:Pi ratio. This index has been used to characterize the state of cell bioenergetics in skeletal muscle, heart, and brain.[31] It appears that the PCr:Pi ratio may be equivalent to the parameter most closely associated with the control of mitochondrial respiration, the phosphate potential.[32]

In the past, the phosphate potential or the PCr:Pi ratio could be measured only by destructive tissue biopsy. This has changed with the introduction of ^{31}P-MRS, a technique that makes it possible to sequentially monitor changes in PCr, Pi, and ATP during hypoxia in an accurate and noninvasive manner. A magnetic resonance spectrometer consists of a radio transmitter capable of directing high-frequency radio waves into a tissue sample placed inside a strong, homogeneous magnetic field. The energy from these radiofrequency waves is absorbed by certain atomic nuclei, and as the radio pulse fades, these nuclei generate electric signals that are used to develop a frequency spectrum.

The MRS spectrum contains several peaks, each corresponding to a different molecule containing the isotope nuclei. Because the peak area is the sum of the resonating nuclei, this area can be used to quantify the concentration of the compound under investigation. Proton, or H^+, an abundant isotope present in fat and water, has been used to obtain tomographic images (magnetic resonance imaging). Given the close association of phosphorus with the various bioenergetic phenomena, ^{31}P-MRS has been very useful to characterize metabolic changes.

Figure 35–5 shows a ^{31}P-MRS spectrum obtained from skeletal muscle. ^{31}P is a naturally occurring isotope that forms part of several important molecules that participate in the transfer of energy within the cell. These peaks correspond to the resonance of Pi, PCr, and the three phosphate bonds of ATP, gamma, alpha, and beta. Because the resonance of ADP also contributes to the gamma and alpha peaks, the concentration of ATP is determined from the area

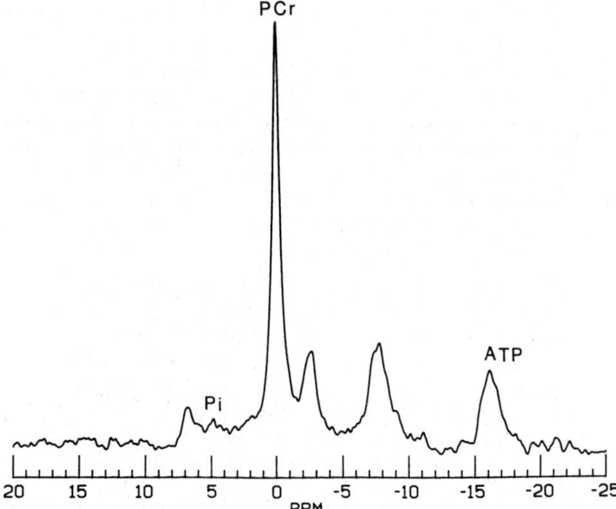

Figure 35–5. A skeletal muscle ^{31}P spectrum obtained with magnetic resonance spectroscopy.

under the beta peak. Intracellular pH can be accurately measured from the separation between the Pi and PCr peaks, the chemical shift.[33] Changes in the peak areas and in the chemical shift can be used as noninvasive measures of changes in cellular energy metabolism. For example, Figure 35–6 illustrates changes in skeletal muscle ^{31}P spectrum of a rabbit subjected to progressive decreases in inspired oxygen fraction. As the animal becomes hypoxic, the Pi peak of the spectrum increases in height and width, whereas the PCr peak becomes smaller.

MRS has several limitations. The signals derived from an MRS experiment represent a spatial and temporal average, and therefore, the technique is inherently poor in spatial localization.[34] The sensitivity of the MRS measurement is strongly dependent on the concentration of the nuclei under study and the length of time during which the spectra are accumulated. MRS can detect metabolites found in concentrations of approximately 1 mmol/L, but it cannot measure

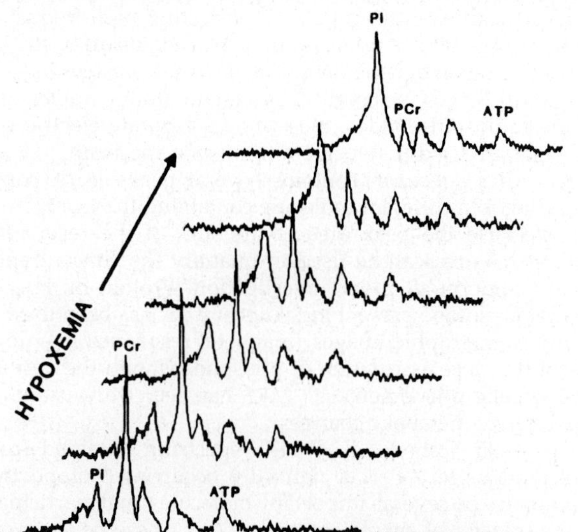

Figure 35–6. Changes in the ^{31}P spectrum from rabbit muscle during periods of progressive hypoxia. PCr decreases, and Pi increases. (From Gutierrez G, Marini C: Cellular response to hypoxia. Update Intens Care Emerg Med 1989; 8:191.)

those present in smaller or trace amounts. The latter include many biologically important molecules, including hormones and drugs.

Individual Organ Perfusion and Metabolism

Hypoxia and sepsis result in major alterations in the distribution of cardiac output. These changes appear to be mediated by local factors, such as the products of metabolism, producing vasodilation. Therefore, local metabolic regulation of blood flow results in its redistribution according to metabolic need, because those organs requiring the greatest levels of energy receive the greatest flow. On the other hand, some organs are better prepared to regulate tissue perfusion than others. An example is skeletal muscle, whose capillary density can increase 20- to 30-fold during exercise. Therefore, even a small metabolic signal during tissue hypoxia may be amplified into a large number of opened capillaries, perhaps explaining why blood flow to resting skeletal muscle increases during hypoxemia. This type of regulation is not available to other organs, such as the intestines, that depend heavily on autonomic reflex regulation.

A technique that appears capable of monitoring metabolic events in critically ill patients is tonometric measurement of intestinal or gastric mucosal pH (pH_i). This parameter provides noninvasive metabolic information from an organ that is at great risk during periods of hypoxia. Measurements of gastric pH_i are highly predictive of morbidity and mortality.[35–38]

Another promising metabolic marker is provided by measurement of the metabolites resulting from the degradation of adenine nucleotides, inosine, hypoxanthine, xanthine, and uric acid. Grum and colleagues[39] noted an increase of these metabolites in the blood of critically ill patients. However, this technique also suffers from the same drawbacks as measurement of blood lactate, because it is a global measurement with low sensitivity. Other biochemicals markers of inadequate tissue oxygenation are the [NAD]-[NADH] ratio and [ATP]-[ADP][P_i]. The other two variables mentioned earlier are technically difficult to obtain and are not in clinical use.

CONCLUSIONS

Alterations in the rate of formation and use of high-energy phosphates determine the well-being of the cells and their ability to survive periods of O_2 deprivation. The past decade has been a time of great advances in our understanding of the interaction between tissue oxygenation, high-energy phosphate concentration, P_i accumulation, and changes in lactate and H^+ production. The future of clinical monitoring in the intensive care unit appears to be in organ-specific measures of cellular metabolism as the earliest warning of impending irreversible cellular damage.

ACKNOWLEDGMENTS

Supported in part by an American Lung Association Cancer Investigator Award.

References

1. Hochachka PW, Guppy M: Metabolic arrest and the control of biological time. Cambridge, MA, Harvard University Press, 1987, pp 10–35.
2. Harold FM: The Vital Force: A Study of Bioenergetics. New York, Freeman, 1986, pp 28–56.
3. Balaban RS: Regulation of oxidative phosphorylation in the mammalian cell. Am J Physiol 1990; 258:C377.

4. Chance B, Nioka S, Leigh JS: Metabolic control principles. *In*: Oxygen Transport and Utilization. Bryan-Brown CW, Ayres SM (Eds). Fullerton, CA, Society for Critical Care Medicine, 1987, pp 215–224.
5. Gutierrez G: Cellular energy metabolism during hypoxia. Crit Care Med 1991; 19:619.
6. Hochachka PW: Defense strategies against hypoxia and hypothermia. Science 1986; 231:234.
7. Myears DW, Sobel BE, Bergmann SR: Substrate use in ischemic and reperfused canine myocardium: Quantitative considerations. Am J Physiol 1987; 253:H1557.
8. Neely JR: Metabolic disturbances after coronary occlusion. Hosp Pract 1989; 24:81.
9. Kao R, Rannels DE, Morgan EH: Effect of anoxia and ischemia on protein synthesis in perfused rat hearts. Circ Res 1976; 38(Suppl):124.
10. Newsholme E: The regulation of phosphofructokinase in muscle. Cardiology 1971; 56:22.
11. Gevers W: Generation of protons by metabolic processes in heart cells. J Mol Cell Cardiol 1977; 9:864.
12. Mainwood GW, Renaud JM: The effect of acid base balance on fatigue of skeletal muscle. Cancer J Physiol Pharmacol 1985; 63:403.
13. Aprille JR: Regulation of the mitochondrial adenine nucleotide pool size in liver: Mechanism and metabolic role. FASEB J 1988; 2:2547.
14. Gadian DG: Nuclear magnetic resonance and its application to living systems. New York, Oxford University Press, 1982, pp 1–20.
15. Bessman SP: The creatine-creatine phosphate energy shuttle. Annu Rev Biochem 1985; 54:831.
16. Berne RM: Adenosine: an important physiological regulator. News Physiol Sci 1986; 1:163–167.
17. Bontemps F, Berghe GVD, Hers HG: Pathways of adenine nucleotide catabolism in erythrocytes. J Clin Invest 1986; 77:824.
18. Wei HM, Kang YH, Merrill GF: Coronary vasodilation during global myocardial hypoxia: Effects of adenosine deaminase. Am J Physiol 1988; 254:H1004.
19. Van Belle H, Goossens F, Wynants J: Formation and release of purine catabolites during hypoperfusion, anoxia, and ischemia. Am J Physiol 1987; 252:H886.
20. Hester RL: Venular-arteriolar diffusion of adenosine in hamster cremaster circulation. Am J Physiol 1990; 258:H1918.
21. Dudley GA, Terjung RL: Influence of aerobic metabolism on IMP accumulation in fast-twitch muscle. Am J Physiol 1985; 248:C37.
22. Kruse J, Haupt M, Puri V, et al: Lactate levels as predictors of the relationship between oxygen delivery and consumption in ARDS. Chest 1990; 98:959–962.
23. Rashkin MC, Bosken C, Baughman RP: Oxygen delivery in critically ill patients. Relationship to blood lactate and survival. Chest 1985; 87:580.
24. Weil MH, Afifi AA: Experimental and clinical studies on lactate and pyruvate as indicators of the severity of acute circulatory failure (shock). Circulation 1970; 41:989.
25. Connett RJ, Gayeski TE, Honig CR: Lactate accumulation in fully aerobic working dog gracilis muscle. Am J Physiol 1984; 246:H120.
26. Hurtado FJ, Gutierrez AM, Silva N, et al: Role of tissue hypoxia as the mechanism of lactic acidosis during *E. coli* endotoxemia. J Appl Physiol 1992; 72:1895.
27. Curtis SE, Cain SM: Regional and systemic oxygen delivery/uptake relations and lactate flux in hyperdynamic, endotoxin-treated dogs. Am Rev Respir Dis 1992; 145:348.
28. Hotchkiss RS, Karl IE: Reevaluation of the role of cellular hypoxia and bioenergetic failure in sepsis. JAMA 1992; 267:1503.
29. Gutierrez G, Pohil JP, Narayana P: Skeletal muscle O_2 consumption and energy metabolism during hypoxemia. J Appl Physiol 1989; 66:2117.
30. Gutierrez G, Andry JM: Nuclear magnetic resonance measurements—clinical applications. Crit Care Med 1989; 17:73.
31. Chance B, Eleff S, Leigh JS: Noninvasive, nondestructive approaches to cell bioenergetics. Proc Nat Acad Sci U S A 1980; 77:7430.
32. Gyulai L, Roth Z, Leigh J, et al: Bioenergetic studies of mitochondrial oxidative phosphorylation using 31-phosphorus NMR. J Biol Chem 1985; 260:3947.
33. Moon R, Richards J: Determination of intracellular pH by ^{31}P magnetic resonance. J Biol Chem 1973; 48:7276.
34. Chance B, Leigh JS, Nioka S: Micro-heterogeneity—the Achilles heel of NMR spectroscopy and imaging: Some calculations for brain ischemia and muscle exercise. New Metabol Res 1985; 2:26.
35. Gutierrez G, Bismar H, Dantzker DR, et al: Comparison of gastric intramucosal pH with measures of oxygen transport and consumption in critically ill patients. Crit Care Med 1992; 20:451.
36. Marik PE: Gastric intramucosal pH. A better predictor of multiorgan dysfunction syndrome and death than oxygen-derived variables in patients with sepsis. Chest 1993; 104:225.
37. Maynard N, Bihari D, Beale R, et al: Assessment of splanchnic oxygenation by gastric tonometry in patients with acute circulatory failure. JAMA 1993; 270:1203.
38. Gutierrez G, Palizas F, Doglio G, et al: Gastric intramucosal pH as a therapeutic index of tissue oxygenation in critically ill patients. Lancet 1992; 339:195.
39. Grum CM, Simon RH, Dantzker DR, et al: Evidence for adenosine tri-phosphate degradation in critically ill patients. Chest 1985; 88:763–767.

CHAPTER 36

Capnography and Respiratory Monitoring

Chester B. Hollinger, Jr., MD • John W. Hoyt, MD, FCCM

Confirming the adequacy of oxygenation and ventilation is an important part of monitoring that is required in the management of critically ill patients. Analysis of arterial blood gases has been the traditional gold standard in the intensive care unit for detection of arterial hypoxemia and hypercarbia. Unfortunately, arterial blood gas analysis is invasive, has potential for inaccurate sampling due to technical error, provides information on an intermittent basis, and frequently imposes a substantial delay between sampling and the availability of results.

Pulse oximeters and capnometers are examples of noninvasive respiratory monitors that have become the standard of care in anesthesia and some intensive care units. Both provide accurate and valuable information when used in the proper context. This chapter explores capnography as a new and evolving monitoring technology in the intensive care unit.

Capnography is the technique of displaying carbon dioxide (CO_2) concentration changes during the respiratory cycle.[1] A capnogram is a continuous record of CO_2 partial pressure or percentage in expired air. It is derived from the Greek words *kapnos*, meaning "smoke," and *gramma*, meaning "something written." A capnogram is typically a graphic display plotting CO_2 on the ordinate and time on the abscissa. A capnometer is a device that measures CO_2 concentrations of inspired and expired gases.[1, 2] The instrument used to record the CO_2 partial pressure in expired air is called a *capnograph*.

Capnography provides a noninvasive means of rapidly identifying problems such as esophageal intubation, inadvertent bronchial intubation, and apnea. It can help prevent potentially disastrous complications due to inadequate alveolar ventilation, as well as unrecognized malfunctions of the breathing circuit or ventilator. Overall, it provides a means to evaluate the integrity of the airway and the quality of a patient's cardiopulmonary function.

When applying the information obtained by capnography to a patient, it is important to remember that capnography is a qualitative rather than a quantitative technique. It can detect abnormal events, but it does not measure the degree of physiologic derangement.[3-5]

CAPNOGRAPHIC ANALYZERS

Two primary methods are available to monitor CO_2 gas—a mass spectrometer and an infrared detector. Infrared capnographs are used to monitor individual patients and function as stand-alone systems. A mass spectrometer is usually a centralized monitoring system serving more than one patient, possibly as many as 20.

Infrared capnographs work on the principle that molecules containing more than one element absorb infrared light in a unique and characteristic manner. In addition, every substance absorbs light at a characteristic wavelength. CO_2 absorbs infrared light at 2600-nm and 4300-nm wavelengths.[6]

Infrared capnographs use a hot wire to emit infrared light and a filter to obtain the desired wavelength. Variable filters can be used so that light with diverse wavelengths measures the concentrations of several different gases. When measuring CO_2, a wavelength of 4300 nm is used. The infrared light is beamed through a calibrated CO_2-filled chamber serving as a control and through the chamber with the gas to be analyzed. Infrared-sensitive photocells receive light from both chambers and calculate the concentrations of CO_2 in the sample gas by comparing it with the known concentrations of CO_2 in the control.[7] The amount of light absorbed is dependent on the concentration of CO_2 molecules in the sample. A semi-conductor, called the *detector*, is used to create an electrical signal that can be processed to display continuous CO_2 concentration. A higher concentration of CO_2 in the gas mixture causes more light to be absorbed and less to arrive at the detector. Infrared CO_2 analyzers provide breath-by-breath measurement of CO_2 concentration. The response time is approximately 100 msec.

Infrared devices can be subdivided into two categories: mainstream, or in-line analyzers, and sidestream, or sampling analyzers. Both types measure CO_2 in gas close to a patient's mouth.

The sidestream analyzer uses suction to withdraw a continuous sample of inspired and expired gas through a capillary tube, which is connected to an adapter, from the patient's airway to the monitor. A water trap is used to remove particles of water before measurement takes place. The advantages of this system include reduction in dead space, simple attachment to the endotracheal tube, less need for miniaturization, and small expense.[8] Sidestream analyzers also allow for the use of zero-CO_2 reference cells or absolute zero-CO_2 gas reference measurements, producing dependable, drift-free performance. A disadvantage is the narrow lumen of the sampling tube, which may become obstructed by pulmonary secretions or condensate. In addition, response time of most sidestream analyzers is not as rapid as that of mainstream analyzers.[7]

The mainstream analyzer has a special flow-through adapter, called the *cuvette*, that is mounted directly in line with the endotracheal tube and ventilator circuit (Fig. 36–1). The cuvette contains an infrared light source and photodetector. It is heated to prevent condensation. The advantages of the mainstream analyzer include a quick response time and absence of delay and interference due to long sampling catheters.[6] Disadvantages include added dead space, the size and weight of the cuvette in the patient's airway, and its cost.[7] The major technical problem is the inability to provide reliable, drift-free, zero-CO_2 reference signals. Rebreathing may be impossible to detect.[8]

Difficulties are involved in applying these principles to infrared analyzers. First, water vapor can interfere with the accuracy of CO_2 analysis in both mainstream and sidestream analyzers. It can condense on the cell windows of the mainstream analyzer, leading to inaccurate analysis of CO_2 concentration. Water vapor can block the sampling capillary of the sidestream analyzer. Calibration can also be affected by water vapor. A second problem is nonlinear absorption of infrared light by CO_2. Manufacturers adjust for this in the design of instruments. Third, background gases, such as nitrogen and nitrous oxide, can cause infrared absorption by accepting kinetic energy from CO_2 molecules. This effect is referred to as *pressure broadening*. Most CO_2 monitors compensate for this either manually or automatically.

The general principle governing the use of mass spectrometry is the release of characteristic ions when a gaseous substance is bombarded with an electron beam.[9] Quadruple filtering and magnetic sector analysis are the two methods of performing mass spectrometry.

All clinical mass spectrometers are sidestream analyzers. The continuously aspirated sample of a patient's respired gases travels through a tube to the mass spectrometer, usually at a site distant from the patient. An electron beam bombards the sample in an ionization chamber. Some of the gas molecules become charged ions of the original substance, and some become ion fragments of the original substance. A detector plate is positioned so that ions unique to that substance strike it. Fragments hitting the detector produce an electric current proportional to the fractional concentration of the gas in the original sample. The electric current is processed by a computer that can digitalize and transform the information to display waveforms, trends, or numeric values.

A mass spectrometer can service as many as 20 patients. It is the only method currently available for clinical breath-by-breath measurement of all respiratory gases. The major drawback is that it must be shared by patients because of the size and expense of the system. Additionally, the response time can be as long as 80 seconds.

PHYSIOLOGY OF CARBON DIOXIDE MEASUREMENT

In a normal lung, CO_2 rapidly diffuses across the capillary-alveolar membrane when ventilation and perfusion are well matched. End-tidal CO_2 (P_{ETCO_2}), defined as the partial pressure equivalent of airway CO_2 concentration at the end of a tidal breath, closely approximates the arterial P_{CO_2} (Pa_{CO_2}) in normal lungs.[8] The assumptions inherent in equating P_{ETCO_2} and Pa_{CO_2} are (1) that P_{ETCO_2} is equal to the P_{CO_2} within ventilated alveoli; (2) that Pa_{CO_2} equals P_{CO_2} within perfused alveoli; and (3) that P_{CO_2} within ventilated alveoli equals the P_{CO_2} within perfused alveoli.[9] The Pa_{CO_2} nearly always equals the P_{CO_2} of perfused alveoli. The disparity between P_{ETCO_2} and Pa_{CO_2} usually occurs because perfused alveolar P_{CO_2} does not equal P_{ETCO_2}. The Pa_{CO_2} closely approximates the mean alveolar P_{CO_2} (PA_{CO_2}) of perfused alveoli, and P_{ETCO_2} approximates the mean PA_{CO_2} of all ventilated alveoli, whether or not they are perfused.

West's three-compartment lung model[10] was used to demonstrate that the end-tidal to arterial P_{CO_2} gradient ($D_{ET\text{-}aCO_2}$) in normal persons is extremely small. The $D_{ET\text{-}aCO_2}$ is

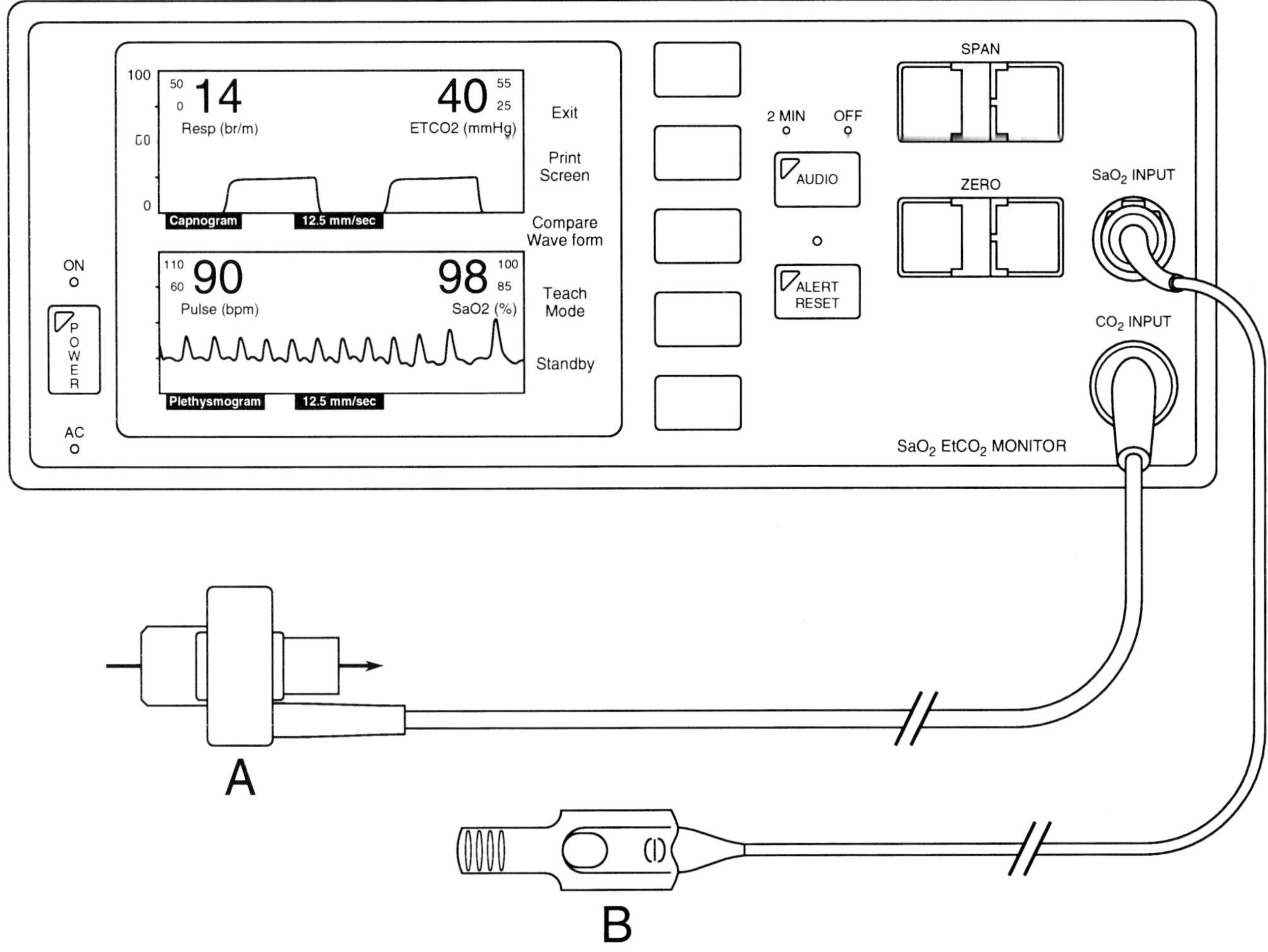

Figure 36–1. A mainstream analyzer. This represents one of the various capnograph models commercially available for use at the bedside. The cuvette *(A)* is attached to the endotracheal tube via a small piece of ventilator tubing and is directly in-line with the ventilator circuit. It also provides a finger probe *(B)* so that simultaneous pulse oximetry readings can be obtained.

approximately 0.6 mm Hg in healthy individuals with a very small dead space ventilation and physiologic shunt (<2%).[11]

The physiologic shunt and dead space ventilation can be increased to approximately 10% when a healthy supine patient is given anesthetic agents or heavy sedation.[11] The PCO_2 of perfused alveolar gas closely approximates $PaCO_2$. However, in end-expiratory gas, which includes gas from both perfused and nonperfused alveoli, the difference between $PETCO_2$ and $PaCO_2$ is significant. This theoretic DET-aCO_2 was confirmed in clinical practice by a number of investigators.[12–15]

The DET-aCO_2 in awake, healthy individuals is negligible, and $PETCO_2$ accurately reflects $PaCO_2$. As dead space ventilation increases, $PETCO_2$ underestimates $PaCO_2$. Various clinical conditions may cause a large difference between $PETCO_2$ and $PaCO_2$; pulmonary parenchymal disease with widely differing ventilation-perfusion ratios and emptying times, hypovolemia with decreased pulmonary artery pressure, excessive positive end-expiratory pressure with increased alveolar pressure, pulmonary vascular occlusive disease, and venous air embolism may cause an increased DET-aCO_2.

Ventilation-perfusion maldistributions[16, 17] and poor sampling of a patient's gas have been cited as the most common reasons for an abnormally wide alveolar-to-arterial difference of CO_2 ($PACO_2$–$PaCO_2$). Dilution with CO_2-free fresh gas can occur in virtually any breathing circuit and is a function of the rate of fresh gas flow into the breathing circuit, the sample aspiration rate, and the expiratory flow rate of the patient's tidal breathing.[18] The $PETCO_2$ value can be falsely lowered if the sample flow rate exceeds the expiratory flow rate, causing some CO_2-free fresh gas to be aspirated by the patient's sampled gas. As exhaled volume decreases, the dilution effect increases. The dilution effect is more prominent in patients with small tidal volumes, such as infants and small children, and does not appear to be a factor in adults with large tidal volumes.

Sampling errors may occur with leaks at the connection between the patient and the airway equipment. This occurs during anesthesia with a poor mask fit and with a loose-fitting endotracheal tube commonly used in infants and small children. The end-tidal value is falsely low.

Incomplete exhalation before the next mechanical or assisted breath, which may occur with small airway obstruction, can falsely lower the end-tidal value. Alveolar gas may not have sufficient time to enter the patient's airway, producing a lower end-tidal reading.

NORMAL CAPNOGRAM

A capnogram is the graphic presentation of the CO_2 concentration at the patient's airway over time. Information about the integrity of the breathing circuit and the patient's cardiopulmonary status can be inferred by the shape of the capnogram.[19]

At the end of normal inhalation, the concentration of CO_2 is highest in the alveoli, where there is an equilibrium with the CO_2 tension and the end-capillary blood. The concentration gradually decreases proximally in the respiratory tree until at some point it reaches zero. At the patient's airway, the concentration of CO_2 is zero.

At the beginning of exhalation, the first gas sampled is the CO_2-free tracheal dead space (Fig. 36–2). Normally, the capnogram should display a segment corresponding to zero CO_2 concentration (segment A–B).

As exhalation continues, CO_2-containing gas from the patient's respiratory tree begins to enter the trachea and eventually arrives at the patient's airway. It appears on the capnograph at point B. As the CO_2 concentration begins to rise, it should produce a sharp, smooth upstroke in the capnogram (segment B–C).

Slowly changing CO_2 concentration over time produces a nearly horizontal alveolar plateau (segment C–D).

Near the end of the exhalation, the CO_2 concentration approaches a value that is the ventilation-weighted average of ventilated lung units, or P_{ETCO_2}. The highest value on the CO_2 plateau is taken as the best approximation of the alveolar CO_2 concentration, estimating arterial P_{CO_2} (point D).

P_{ETCO_2} closely approximates the mean alveolar concentration when the alveolar plateau is achieved. At this point, the difference between the P_{ETCO_2} and the Pa_{CO_2} is minimal, and the P_{ETCO_2} reflects the Pa_{CO_2}. In a patient with normal respiratory function, the P_{ETCO_2} is an underestimate of the Pa_{CO_2} by less than 4 mm Hg, and a slightly positive Pa_{CO_2}–P_{ETCO_2} gradient is produced.[20]

With inhalation, CO_2-free fresh gas is entrained into the patient's airway and the airway CO_2 concentration returns to the baseline (Fig. 36–3). CO_2 concentration should remain at zero until the next exhalation. If CO_2 is rebreathed, the CO_2 concentration at the airway either does not fall to zero or rises above zero as CO_2 is inhaled.[22]

The capnogram may be displayed at normal or slow speed. The normal speed represents a real-time display and provides current information for each breath. In a slow-speed display, fine details are obscured but trends are more easily identified. Alterations in either the normal-speed or slow-speed display can help define abnormalities in the patient or malfunctions in the gas delivery system.

A study of inhaled and exhaled flow and airway pressure using a mechanical lung ventilated with CO_2 noted changes in pressure and flow slightly preceded the deflection in the mainstream capnogram. The sidestream analyzer was out of phase by approximately 3 seconds, an effect attributed to the delay caused by transport of the gas sample through the capillary to the analyzer.[22]

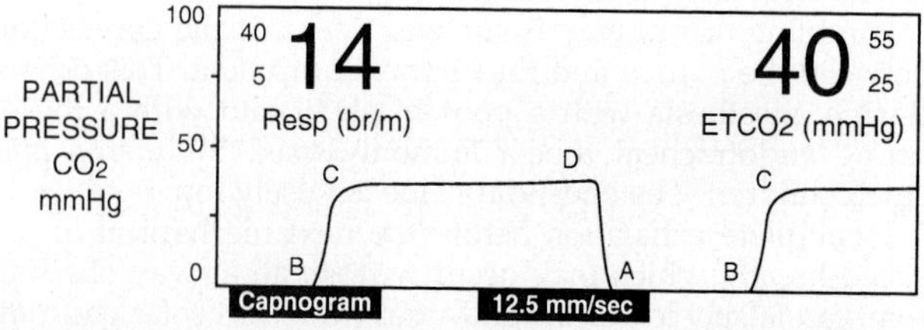

Figure 36–2. A normal capnogram. *Segment A–B* represents the beginning of exhalation, which is free of CO_2 because of the tracheal dead space. *Segment B–C* denotes the detection of CO_2 as exhalation continues. *Segment C–D* is the result of slowly changing CO_2 concentration over time. *Point D* represents end-tidal CO_2, which is the best approximation of arterial P_{CO_2}. Inhalation, which is normally free of CO_2 gas, causes the tracing to return to the zero baseline.

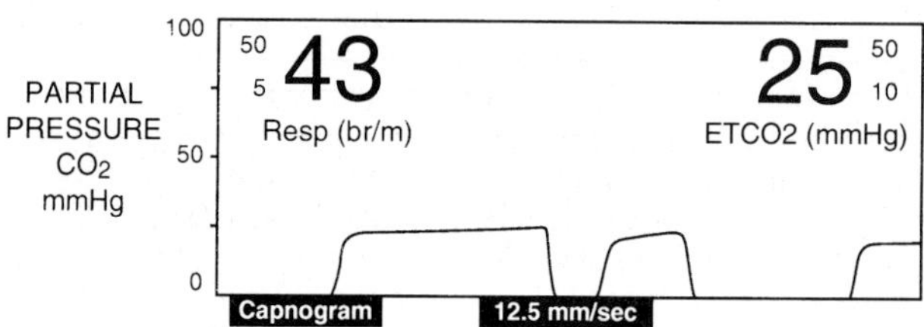

Figure 36–3. Normal capnograms. These tracings represent normal capnograms. The first waveform represents a mechanical breath. The second waveform represents a spontaneous breath with a shorter alveolar plateau. The capnogram only displays CO_2 versus time and is independent of flow rate. Therefore, a capnogram does not reflect the volume of gas exchanged with each breath.

CHANGES IN END-TIDAL CARBON DIOXIDE PRESSURE

Changes in P_{ETCO_2} must be interpreted with close clinical correlation of the patient's condition.[23] The integrity and function of both the patient's cardiopulmonary system and the breathing circuit are reflected by the capnogram,[24] and malfunctions can often be detected by changes in the capnogram.[25]

A sudden drop of P_{ETCO_2} to a zero or near-zero value usually foretells an impending disaster. Critical events that may present this way include esophageal intubation,[26] complete airway disconnection, complete ventilator malfunction, and a totally obstructed endotracheal tube.[27] All of these events are potentially fatal airway disasters and require immediate examination of the patient and the ventilatory circuit. Capnography would greatly enhance detection of such a catastrophic event.

A fall in P_{ETCO_2} values approaching zero and loss of the alveolar plateau denote an absence of full exhalation (Fig. 36–4). This pattern may be caused by a loosely fitting endotracheal tube, a leaking or defective endotracheal tube cuff, partial obstruction of the endotracheal tube, or partial ventilator disconnection.

A progressive drop in P_{ETCO_2} occurring over time almost always signals a potentially serious event involving the cardiopulmonary system. An increase in physiologic dead space ventilation produces this picture. Clinical events that may account for this include sudden hypotension due to massive blood loss, circulatory arrest, and pulmonary embolism due to thrombus or air.

The capnogram may show sustained low P_{ETCO_2} values without a good alveolar plateau with no apparent malfunc-

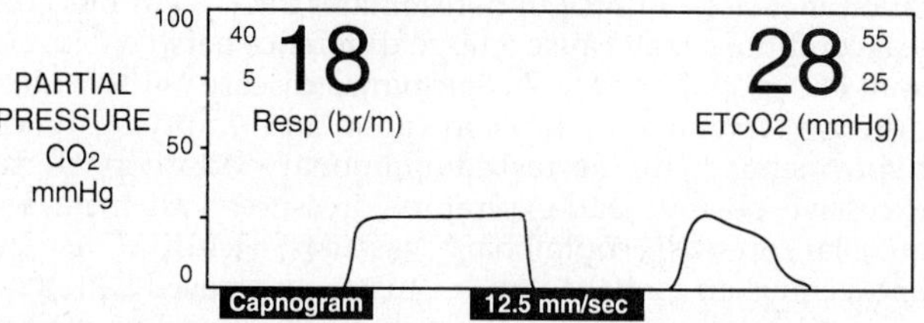

Figure 36–4. Loss of the normal alveolar plateau, as seen in the second tracing, may be caused by a loosely fitting endotracheal tube, a leaking or partially obstructed endotracheal tube cuff, or a partial ventilator disconnection.

tion of the breathing circuit or in the patient's cardiopulmonary status. In this situation, P_{ETCO_2} is not a reliable estimate of alveolar P_{CO_2} and therefore is not an estimate of Pa_{CO_2}. Lack of complete exhalation before the beginning of the next breath, could explain this picture, as could dilution of the patient's tidal volume with fresh gas due to a small tidal volume, high aspiration sample rate, or high fresh gas dilution from the circuit.

Incomplete emptying of the lungs may be produced by bronchospasm or secretions compromising small airway patency. An endotracheal tube that is partially kinked or partially obstructed by cuff herniation may prevent full exhalation of the tidal volume (Fig. 36–5). In small children and other patients who have small tidal volumes, the aspirating sample rate may exceed the expiratory flow rate near the end of exhalation, producing an inadequate alveolar plateau. When this occurs, the aspiration sample is diluted with fresh gas from the breathing circuit. A lower sampling rate may correct the situation; otherwise, the P_{ETCO_2} cannot be used to estimate alveolar ventilation.

In some circumstances, the capnogram displays a low P_{ETCO_2} with a widened P_{ACO_2}–Pa_{CO_2} with preservation of a good plateau. This may represent a malfunction of the capnograph or miscalibration. A sample of a normal person's exhaled gas should be 5% to 6% CO_2 (equivalent to approximately 38–46 mm Hg).

A wide P_{ACO_2}–Pa_{CO_2} noted with a properly functioning capnometer represents excessive dead space ventilation. Chronic obstructive pulmonary disease, pneumonia, bronchopulmonary dysplasia in children, and other pathologic states are commonly associated with large physiologic dead space (Fig. 36–6). Mild pulmonary artery hypoperfusion due to high airway pressures and hypovolemia, noted with dehydration, the use of vasodilators, and hyperventilation, commonly results in a wide P_{ACO_2}–Pa_{CO_2}.

A progressive drop in P_{ETCO_2} with a normal plateau pattern could be due to a falling body temperature, slowly decreasing systemic or pulmonary perfusion, hyperventilation, or reduced CO_2 production.

A steady rise in P_{ETCO_2} with an unchanging morphology may be associated with partial airway obstruction, rising body temperature, a leak in the ventilator circuit with hypoventilation,[28] or absorption of exogenous CO_2.[29]

A partial airway obstruction that reduces effective ventilation without significant interference with exhalation produces an increase in P_{ETCO_2}.

Increasing body temperature results in increased CO_2 production and increased P_{ETCO_2} if ventilation and dead space ventilation remain constant. A rapid rise in P_{ETCO_2} may be noted in malignant hyperthermia.[30, 31]

Acute, transient increases in P_{ETCO_2} may be caused by any factor that suddenly increases the amount of CO_2 reaching the pulmonary circulation. The most common causes are injections of bicarbonate and release of a limb tourniquet. Both of these events should be recognized as benign and expected. In addition, an acute increase in cardiac output may cause an increase in P_{ETCO_2}.

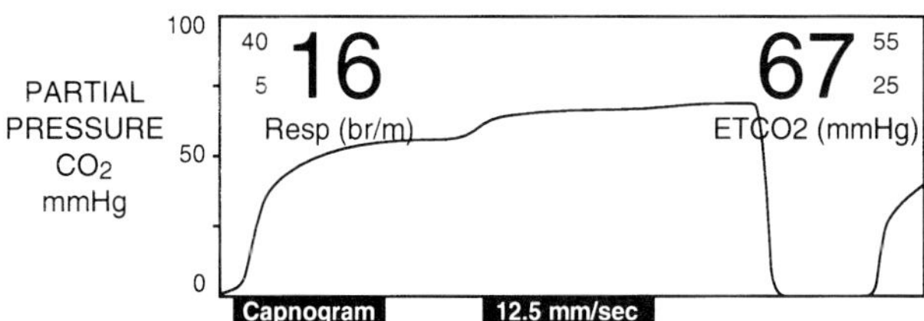

Figure 36–6. A prolonged and upsloping alveolar plateau is typical in a patient with chronic obstructive pulmonary disease. A biphasic aspect of the plateau is caused by alveoli that empty with different time constants owing to varying compliance.

A sudden rise in the baseline of the capnogram with an equal rise in the P_{ETCO_2} value usually signifies some contamination in the sample cell. Cleaning the cell usually corrects the abnormality.

A gradual rise in both baseline and P_{ETCO_2} values suggests that previously exhaled CO_2 is being rebreathed from the circuit (Fig. 36–7). The inspiratory portion of the capnogram fails to reach the zero baseline, and a slanted upstroke may be associated with exhalation. This can be seen in some anesthesia partial rebreathing circuits commonly used in pediatric anesthesia.[32] Malfunctions of a circle system that cause rebreathing would include faulty check valves that allow bidirectional flow instead of unidirectional flow, the presence of a CO_2 absorber bypass circuit, or the presence of exhausted CO_2 absorber.

CLINICAL APPLICATIONS

The concentration of CO_2 measured during exhalation is greatly influenced by various physiologic components, including ventilation-perfusion ratios within the lungs, total CO_2 production, and total alveolar ventilation. In critically ill patients, these variables may not be stable. Therefore, monitoring P_{ETCO_2} alone may not provide adequate warning of changes in the Pa_{CO_2} and is not a reliable substitute for arterial blood gas analysis during weaning or adjustments of mechanical ventilation (Fig. 36–8).

A constant P_{ETCO_2} does not ensure a constant Pa_{CO_2}. Trends in the P_{ETCO_2} in critically ill patients can be misleading because of the wide variability in the Pa_{CO_2}–P_{ETCO_2} gradient that may occur during ventilator changes.[33]

A capnometer can be used to confirm esophageal intubation, to document a changing ventilation-perfusion ratio through a changing Pa_{CO_2}–P_{ETCO_2} gradient, or to demon-

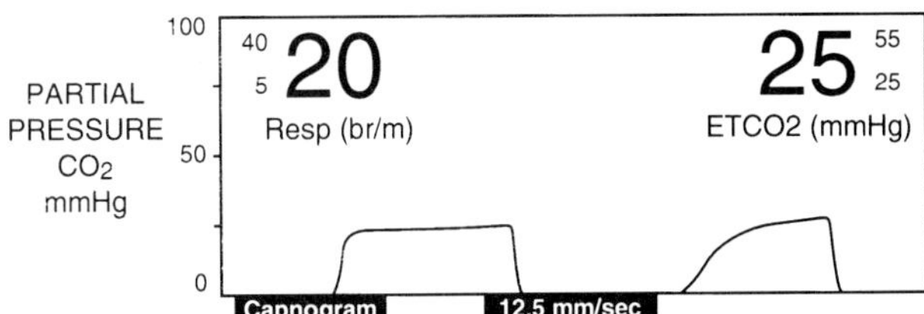

Figure 36–5. The second tracing represents incomplete emptying of the lungs. It may be caused by kinking of an endotracheal tube or by partial obstruction of an endotracheal tube due to cuff herniation. Bronchospasm or secretions that compromise small airway patency could produce the same picture.

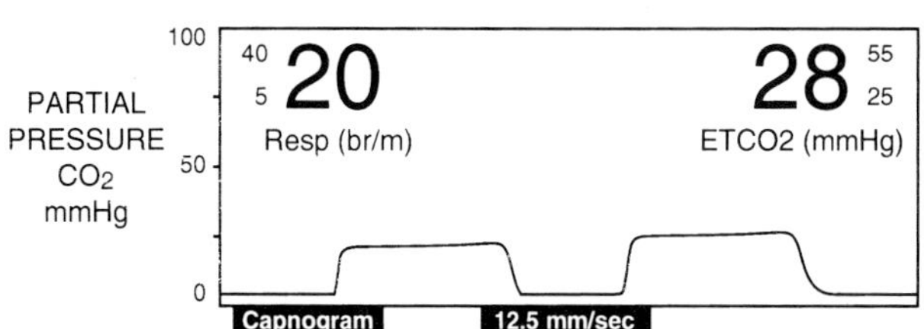

Figure 36–7. The second capnogram is seen during rebreathing of CO_2. The inspiratory portion of the tracing fails to reach the zero baseline, and a slanted upstroke associated with exhalation may be present. Ventilator function should be evaluated in such a case.

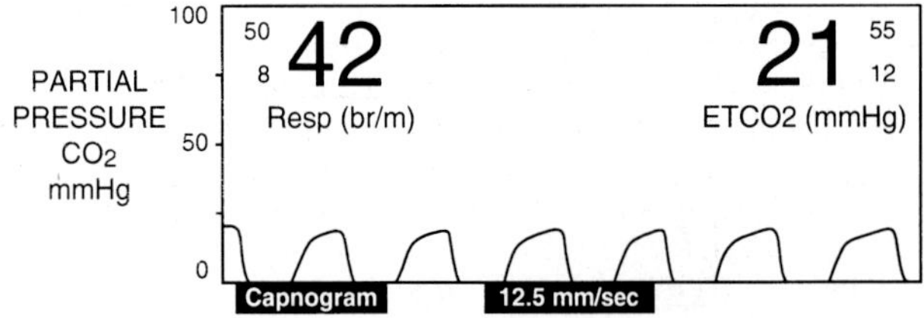

Figure 36–8. The patterns of capnogram may be helped during the weaning process. Tachypnea is readily recognized when a patient fails to be weaned from mechanical support. A chaotic pattern of respirations would also be typical of weaning failure.

strate restoration of the circulation after cardiopulmonary arrest and resuscitation.[34]

CO_2 concentrations of gastric gas and inspired gas are negligible. CO_2 is eliminated in large quantities only through the lungs. Capnography can be used to ensure ventilation of the lungs, as opposed to gastric or esophageal ventilation, by detecting a consistently high CO_2 concentration in the exhaled gas. Expired gas containing CO_2 frequently can be introduced into the stomach when ventilating the lungs with a mask. In this situation, esophageal intubation may result in CO_2 detection in the "exhaled" gas.[26] The P_{ETCO_2} returning from the stomach is considerably less (3–7 mm Hg) than gas exhaled from the lungs (usually 20–45 mm Hg) and rapidly returns to zero after four to five breaths. Keeping this in mind, P_{ETCO_2} measurement can distinguish between tracheal and esophageal intubation and provides evidence that a mask or tube is ventilating the lungs.

CO_2 consistently present in exhaled gases does not necessarily mean that a tracheal tube is in the trachea. A tube placed in the pharynx might ventilate the lungs well, producing a normal P_{ETCO_2}. A tracheal tube that has been dislodged into the pharynx occasionally results in an abnormal exhaled CO_2 waveform. Analyzing expired gases for CO_2 not only helps with the recognition of esophageal intubation but aids in recognition of disconnection from ventilating systems, airway obstruction, and accidental removal of a tracheal tube.[27]

Continuous capnography used during blind nasotracheal intubation in spontaneously breathing patients provides valuable information about the position of the tracheal tube during the entire procedure.[35] Passage of the tip of the tube posterior to the larynx results in immediate disappearance of the CO_2 tracing. Entrance of the tube into the trachea results in a typical plateau waveform in the capnogram.

SUMMARY

Monitoring the exhaled CO_2 concentration waveform and quantitation of P_{ETCO_2} are used clinically in four primary ways: (1) to ensure that an endotracheal tube or mask ventilates the lungs; (2) as an estimate of Pa_{CO_2} in stable patients with normal systemic and pulmonary perfusion; (3) as a reflection of a change in pulmonary blood flow or dead space ventilation; and (4) to detect the addition of excess CO_2 to the systemic circulation.

The P_{ETCO_2} is always less than or equal to Pa_{CO_2} because of the exhaled gas contributed from ventilated but poorly perfused alveoli. A large dead space ventilation causes a wide gradient between P_{ETCO_2} and Pa_{CO_2}.

According to one survey, substantial interest has been expressed about capnography for intensive care medicine. Intensivists have no clear preference for sidestream or mainstream techniques. The survey suggested that the most important reason for the uncommon use of CO_2 monitoring in intensive care when compared with anesthesia is the inability of manufacturers to solve the problem of routinely integrating capnography into the bedside cardiovascular monitor or the ventilator.[36] Capnography is a valuable monitor of cardiopulmonary function in critically ill patients and should achieve growing popularity.

References

1. Carlon GC, Ray CJ, Miodownik S, et al: Capnography in mechanically ventilated patients. Crit Care Med 1988; 16:550–556.
2. Mogue LR, Rantala B: Capnometers. J Clin Monit 1988; 4:115–121.
3. McAslan TC: Automated respiratory gas monitoring of critically injured patients. Crit Care Med 1976; 4:255.
4. Whitesell R, Asiddas C, Gollman D, et al: Relationship between arterial and peak expired carbon dioxide pressure during anesthesia and factors influencing the difference. Anesth Analg 1981; 60:508.
5. Racmer DB, Francis D, Phillip JH, et al: Variation in P_{CO_2} between arterial blood and peak expired gas during anesthesia. Anesth Analg 1983; 62:1065.
6. Gravenstein JS, Paulus DA: Monitoring ventilation and gases. *In*: Clinical Monitoring Practice, 2nd ed. Philadelphia, JB Lippincott, 1987, pp 184–196.
7. Technology Subcommittee of the Working Group on Critical Care, Ontario Ministry of Health: Noninvasive blood gas monitoring: A review for use in the adult critical care unit. Can Med Assoc J 1992; 146:703–712.
8. Blitt CD: Monitoring and patient safety. *In*: Monitoring in Anesthesia and Critical Care Medicine. 2nd ed. Blitt CD (Ed). New York, Churchill Livingstone, 1990, pp 48–63.
9. Stock MC: Noninvasive carbon dioxide monitoring. Crit Care Clin 1988; 4:511–526.
10. West JB: Ventilation: Blood Flow and Gas Exchange. 2nd ed. Oxford, Blackwell Scientific Publications, 1970.
11. Nunn JF: Carbon dioxide. *In*: Applied Respiratory Physiology. 2nd ed. Nunn JF (Ed). Boston, Butterworths, 1977, pp 334–374.
12. Nunn JF, Hill DW: Respiratory deadspace and arterial to end tidal CO_2 difference in anesthetized man. J Appl Physiol 1960; 5:383.
13. Hedenstierna G, McCarthy G: The effect of anesthesia and intermittent positive pressure ventilation with different frequencies on the anatomical deadspace. Br J Anaesthiol 1975; 47:847.
14. Shankar KB, Mosely H, Kumar Y, et al: Arterial to end-tidal carbon dioxide tension difference during caesarean section anaesthesia. Anaesthesia 1986; 41:698.
15. Valentin N, Lomholt B, Thorup M: Arterial to end-tidal carbon dioxide tension difference in children under halothane anaesthesia. Can Anaesth Soc J 1982; 29:12.
16. Comroe JH: Physiology of Respiration: An Introductory Text. Chicago, Year Book Medical Publishers, 1974, p 168.
17. Comroe JH, Forster RE, Dubois AB, et al: The pulmonary circulation and ventilation/blood flow ratios. *In*: The Lung, Clinical Physiology and Pulmonary Function Tests. 2nd ed. Comroe JH (ed). Chicago, Year Book Medical Publishers, 1962, p 77.
18. Schieber RA, Namnoum A, Sugden A, et al: Accuracy of expiratory carbon dioxide measurements using the coaxial and circle breathing circuits in small subjects. J Clin Monit 1985; 1:149.
19. Swedlow DB: Capnometry and capnography: An anesthesia disaster warning system. Semin Anesth 1986; 5:194.
20. Synder JV, Elliot FL, Grenvik A: Capnography. *In*: Respiratory Monitoring in Intensive Care. Spence A (Ed). New York, Churchill Livingstone, 1982, pp 100–121.
21. Nightingale DA, Richards CG, Glars A: An evaluation of rebreathing in modified t-piece system during controlled ventilation in anaesthetized children. Br J Anaesth 1975; 37:762.
22. Gravenstein JS, Paulus D, Hayes T: The capnogram. *In*: Capnography in Clinical Practice. Gravenstein JS, Paulus D (Eds). Boston, Butterworths, 1988, pp 11–30.
23. May WJ: Respiratory monitoring. Int Anesthesiol Clin 1986; 24:159–169.

24. Smalhout B, Kalenda Z: An Atlas of Capnography. Vol I. The Netherlands, Kerckebosch-Zeist, 1975.
25. Smalhout B: A Quick Guide to Capnography and Its Use in Differential Diagnosis. Hewlett-Packard Application Note 78345–9001, Federal Republic of Germany, 1983.
26. Linko K, Paloheimo M, Tammisto T: Capnography for detection of accidental oesophageal intubation. Acta Anaesthesiol Scand 1983; 27:199.
27. Murray IP, Modell JH: Early detection of endotracheal tube accidents by monitoring carbon dioxide concentration in respiratory gas. Anesthesiology 1983; 59:344.
28. Osborn JJ, Raison JC, Beaumont JO, et al: Respiratory causes of "sudden unexplained arrhythmia" in postthoracotomy patients. Surgery 1971; 69:24.
29. Shulman D, Aronson HB: Capnography in the early diagnosis of carbon dioxide embolism during laparoscopy. Can Anaesth Soc J 1984; 31:455.
30. Baudendistel L, Goudsouzian N, Cote C, et al: End-tidal CO_2 monitoring. Its use in the diagnosis and management of malignant hyperthermia. Anaesthesia 1984; 39:1000.
31. Triner L, Sherman J: Potential value of expiratory carbon dioxide measurement in patients considered to be susceptible to malignant hyperthermia. Anesthesiology 1981; 55:482.
32. Fisher DM: Anesthesia Equipment for Pediatrics. *In*: Pediatric Anesthesia. Gregory GA (Ed). New York, Churchill Livingstone, 1983, p 347.
33. Hoffman RA, Krieger BP, Kramer MR, et al: End-tidal carbon dioxide in critically ill patients during changes in mechanical ventilation. Am Rev Respir Dis 1988; 140:1265–1268.
34. Falk JL, Rackow EC, Weil MH: End-tidal carbon dioxide concentration during cardiopulmonary resuscitation. N Engl J Med 1988; 318:607–611.
35. Linko K, Paloheimo M, Tammisto T: Capnography facilitates blind nasotracheal intubation. Acta Anaesthesiol Belg 1983; 43:117.
36. Survey of CO_2 monitors in intensive care. Intensive Care World 1993; 10:20.

CHAPTER 37

Intracranial Pressure Monitoring

Marvin Bergsneider, MD • *Donald P. Becker, MD*

The association of elevated intracranial pressure (ICP) with neurologic dysfunction was postulated in ancient times. At the turn of the century, the measurement of ICP began by lumbar puncture; since that time, monitoring of ICP has undergone extensive evolution. Current technology offers safe, accurate, and reliable techniques of continuously monitoring ICP. The intent of this chapter is to familiarize readers with the basic concepts important to interpretation of ICP measurements, as well as to detail many of the practical aspects necessary for clinical use of this tool.

THE RATIONALE OF INTRACRANIAL PRESSURE MONITORING

Neurologic examination remains the best clinical assessment of patients with intracranial pathology, although its usefulness diminishes as unconsciousness ensues. In comatose patients with elevated ICP, neurologic examination yields too little information on which to base all clinical decisions. The use of other diagnostic tests (such as ICP monitoring, cerebral blood flow [CBF] and metabolism determination) may be necessary to assess the pathophysiologic dynamics occurring at both the cellular and global level.

Elevated ICP, which is always a manifestation of a primary intracranial pathologic process (such as head injury or hydrocephalus), may in turn cause secondary injury as well. This may occur as a physical deformation of the brain stem due to shift of the intracranial contents[1] or due to impaired cerebral perfusion. Clinically, the latter can be assessed by what is termed the *cerebral perfusion pressure* (CPP), defined as the difference between the systemic mean arterial blood pressure (MAP) and the ICP (CPP = MAP − ICP). In the normal brain, adequate CBF is maintained for CPP values greater than 50 mm Hg (pressure autoregulation).[2] The association of CBF and ICP at CPP values greater than 50 mm Hg is complex and not completely understood.[3] CBF is governed by multiple autoregulatory mechanisms: metabolic, carbon dioxide, blood viscosity, and perfusion pressure. Depending on the extent of the brain injury, one or more of these autoregulatory functions may become impaired.[3] In certain clinical situations, ICP may have a significant role in the determination of CBF, because neurologic impairment secondary to reduced CBF has been noted for ICP values greater than 25 mm Hg (normal ICP for adults: 0–10 mm Hg).[4]

The rationale of ICP monitoring is based on the following premises: (1) Identification of subthreshold CPP values can be accomplished only if CPP is continuously determined; (2) elevated ICP may be causally related to reduced CBF in many clinical circumstances, despite "adequate" CPP values; (3) treatment of elevated ICP is not without risks, and therefore, precise, accurate determination of ICP is important; and (4) changes in ICP dynamics may signify the presence of a previously unexpected mass lesion. An ICP greater than 20 mm Hg has been statistically associated with a worsened neurologic outcome in severely head-injured patients.[4–6] In general, most neurosurgeons emphasize measures aimed at lowering ICP and avoiding systemic hypotension, although some institutions regard the absolute CPP as the more important index.[7] In either case, accurate determination and continuous monitoring of ICP are an integral component in the pathophysiology-based approach to the management of these complex cases.

REGULATION OF INTRACRANIAL PRESSURE

ICP assumes importance because the cranium is a rigid enclosure. The intracranial contents, which can be grouped into four components—brain tissue, cerebrospinal fluid (CSF), intravascular blood, and mass lesions (if present)—obey the physical laws governing pressure-volume relationships. An increase in the volume of one of these components must be accompanied by a decrease in volume of another if pressure is to remain constant, because none is compressible. This concept is known as the Monro-Kellie hypothesis.[8, 9] In reality, the cranium is not entirely enclosed, and mechanisms are present to accommodate physiologic and pathologic alterations in intracranial volume. For example, translocation of CSF through the foramen magnum to the distensible spinal subarachnoid space represents an initial, acute-stage buffering mechanism. Thereafter, increased absorption of CSF can further decrease the total CSF volume, which in an average adult is approximately 150 mL.

Inherent ICP buffering mechanisms maintain a relatively constant ICP in response to slow and limited fluctuations in volume of one of the Monro-Kellie components. Once the physical and dynamic limitations of the buffering mechanisms are exhausted, ICP may increase dramatically. The physical limitation is illustrated by the classic cerebral pres-

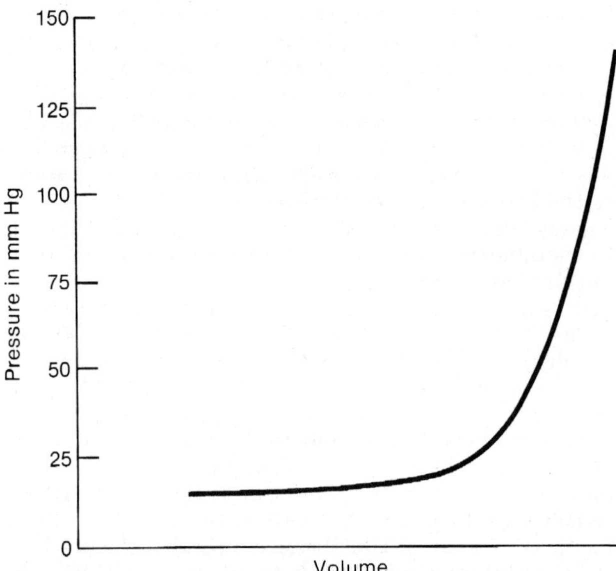

Figure 37–1. Schematic representation of the intracranial pressure-volume relationship, originally proposed by Langfitt.[10] Volume (the abscissa) represents an incremental addition of a space-occupying lesion within the intracranial compartment; it is dimensionless, since the curve shifts across the horizontal plane, depending on the rate of change of volume. ICP is maintained at a normal level until buffering mechanisms are overwhelmed, which results in the exponential increase in pressure.

sure-volume curve[10] (Fig. 37–1). *Cerebral compliance*, defined as the change in volume per unit pressure (analogous to pulmonary compliance), is the inverse of the slope at any given point along the curve. A low-compliance state is represented by the steep portion of the curve, where a small increase in volume results in a large elevation in ICP.

Buffering mechanisms have dynamic limitations as well. The rate of change of volume can have a significant influence on the resultant pressure change, reflecting a finite response time of the buffering mechanisms. For example, in a normal adult, a cough may increase ICP to 60 mm Hg, whereas a slowly growing tumor such as meningioma may reach an enormous size (7 cm in diameter) without elevating ICP. In terms of cerebral capacitance, ICP is a function of a first-degree differential equation in which the rate of change in volume as well as the initial volume state must be known.

ICP measurements cannot be interpreted in isolation, because CPP and cerebral capacitance may have a profound clinical impact. Attempts to quantify the latter have focused on obtaining a measure of compliance only. One such technique, the volume-pressure response (VPR), measured the change in intraventricular pressure after injection or withdrawal of 1 mL of CSF over 1 second.[11] The combination of a normal ICP and an elevated VPR (> 5 mm Hg/mL) was found to have a high positive predictive value for a previously unexpected intracranial mass lesion.[4] Enthusiasm for the technique was blunted by the fact that a large number of patients (17%) died secondary to elevated ICP despite normal VPR measurements. Because of the invasive nature of VPR measurements (and related methods, such as the pressure-volume index), as well as the limited clinical usefulness, this procedure is not routine at most institutions. A bedside gross estimate of cerebral compliance can be obtained by performing a modified Queckenstedt's test, noting the rate and magnitude of the change in ICP with compression of the jugular veins. Prolonged elevations in ICP (5–20 min), known as *plateau waves* or *Lundberg's type A waves*, are another indicator of a low compliance state and have been associated with neurologic deterioration and death.[12]

PATHOPHYSIOLOGY OF ELEVATED INTRACRANIAL PRESSURE

A pathologic process causing intracranial hypertension usually does so as a consequence of one or more etiologic mechanisms. These mechanisms are generally grouped in terms of the Monro-Kellie components and have significance in regard to treatment options.

An increase in brain tissue volume, per se, occurs as one of several forms of cerebral edema.[13] Cytotoxic edema is the product of cellular membrane disruption, usually secondary to ischemia or trauma. Vasogenic edema arises from a breakdown in the blood-brain barrier, normally occurring in the presence of neoplasms and cerebral abscesses. Cerebral edema often has multiple or unclear causes, such as in certain metabolic (fulminant hepatitis), immunologic (Reye's syndrome), and idiopathic (pseudotumor cerebri) processes.

Blockage of the CSF pathways generates elevated pressures because CSF production is independent of pressure, occurring at a constant rate of 20 mL/min. Obstruction of CSF flow occurring within the ventricular system (noncommunicating hydrocephalus) is often caused by discrete masses within or abutting the ventricular space. Focal (lobar) elevations in ICP may result from "trapping" of an isolated part of the ventricular system with the contained choroid plexus (most commonly the temporal horn). Inadequate CSF absorption normally results in a globally elevated ICP, termed *communicating hydrocephalus*, which is usually due to infectious, hemorrhagic, or degenerative injury of the arachnoid granulations.

Excessive intracranial arterial blood volume is not a primary cause of elevated ICP, although loss of cerebrovascular autoregulation may have a significant impact on ICP dynamics (by Poiseuille's law, CBF is proportional to the fourth power of the vessel radius). Excessive CBF (hyperemia) is thought to underlie elevated ICP in some patients.[3, 14] A significant obstruction of venous outflow can cause both acute and chronic elevations in ICP as well.

The most common cerebral mass lesions associated with elevated ICP are hematomas, neoplasms, and infections. Mass lesions can elevate ICP by more than one mechanism. For example, a glioblastoma multiforme tumor arising within a temporal lobe exhibits mass effect based on the tumor bulk itself, the surrounding vasogenic edema, and entrapment of the ventricular horn.

INDICATIONS FOR INTRACRANIAL PRESSURE MONITORING

ICP monitoring is indicated in the treatment of patients in whom intracranial hypertension is suspected and in whom treatment decisions will be influenced by the results. The most common use of ICP monitors is for treatment of head-injured patients. Approximately two thirds of comatose (Glasgow Coma Scale score 8 or less) head-injured patients develop elevated ICP, and therefore, ICP monitors are routinely placed in these patients.[15] Exceptions are occasionally made, such as in the case of an obviously intoxicated patient with a normal head seen on computed tomography.[16] Less common indications for ICP monitoring include illnesses associated with severe brain swelling, such as Reye's syndrome and fulminant hepatitis. ICP monitoring may help diagnostically in certain cases of pseudotumor cerebri and hydrocephalus.

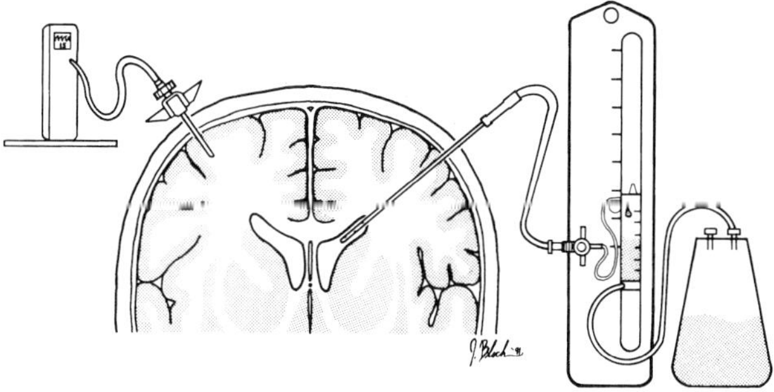

Figure 37–2. On the right, a ventriculostomy is shown to connect to a CSF collection system. The pressure transducer is normally situated in a plane even with the external auditory meatus. The three-way valve allows either pressure monitoring or drainage of CSF. On the left, a distal transducer monitor is shown to insert into the brain parenchyma. The monitor is anchored to the skull by a bolt mechanism.

INTRACRANIAL PRESSURE MONITORING DEVICES

Two fundamental types of ICP monitoring devices are used: those that have a fluid-coupled transducer communicating with the ventricular system and those that incorporate a distal transducer (Fig. 37–2). The decision about which type to use is normally based on ease of ventricular access and the need for CSF drainage. With either method, measured ICP values are computed mean values, analogous to the MAP.

The ventriculostomy (ventricular catheter) is a fluid-coupled system. Under local anesthesia, a twist drill craniostomy is made just anterior to the coronal suture along the midpupillary line (normally on the right, nondominant side) and a Silastic catheter is directed orthogonal to the skull to a depth of 5 cm. The catheter is tunneled beneath the scalp for some distance to lessen the risk of infection. CSF return and a triphasic waveform usually indicate patency and proper catheter placement within the frontal ventricular horn. The transducer is zeroed to the level of the external auditory meatus, which serves as the external landmark even with the foramen of Monro. Ventriculostomies are managed by either continuously monitoring ICP and intermittently draining CSF only when the pressure exceeds 20 mm Hg, or by continuous drainage of CSF, adjusting the level of the collection system to grossly regulate the ICP (by the principle of a hydrostatic fluid column).

Distal pressure-transducer devices (such as the Camino Laboratories monitor) incorporate a counterpressure membrane system, which can be used to measure either tissue or fluid pressure.[17] The transducer is zeroed to atmospheric pressure just before placement, and once inserted, no readjustment is possible. These devices are typically placed in the brain tissue (intraparenchymal) of the frontal lobe and serve diagnostic purposes only. Subdural and hybrid-intraventricular catheter systems are available as well.

RISKS AND PITFALLS IN INTRACRANIAL PRESSURE MONITORING

Rare complications of ICP monitor placement are subdural or intracerebral hematomas, as well as seizures. Infection is the most common morbidity, occurring in 3% to 12% of ventriculostomies.[18–20] Mayhall and colleagues[18] demonstrated the rate of ventriculostomy infection to increase significantly 5 days after placement, and therefore, some centers place a new ventriculostomy every 5 to 7 days, theorizing that colonization and the incidence of infections are reduced. Antibiotic prophylaxis has not been shown to reduce the incidence of ventriculostomy infection.[19]

Inaccurate or misleading measurements are the most common pitfalls encountered in ICP monitoring. A partially obstructed ventricular catheter produces a dampened waveform that underestimates the true pressure. Distal pressure transducers may undergo mechanical or electronic drift of the zero point after several days of use, leading to a bias error of up to 6 mm Hg.[17] Misleading ICP values result from undetected pressure gradients arising from compartmentalization of intracranial contents. Mass lesions in the posterior or middle fossa may produce elevations in ICP, within that compartment, due to dural and bony anatomic constraints. Clinically, this occurs most frequently with cerebellar or anterior temporal lobe hematomas, which can compress the brain stem *without* the elevation of ICP measured from the frontal lobe.[21]

Neuroimaging studies may help to corroborate ICP measurements by demonstrating either focal or global evidence of elevated ICP. The presence of uncal or subfalcian herniation signifies a nonuniform ICP distribution, whereas diffusely elevated ICP is suggested by obliteration of the basal cisterns and cerebral sulci. Hydrocephalus, edema, and mass lesions are usually readily apparent. The identification of a temporal lobe or posterior fossa mass lesion is best made by magnetic resonance imaging, although computed tomography usually reveals clinically significant lesions. When indicated, these neuroimaging studies must be repeated as often as necessary to ensure the validity of the ICP measurements.

TREATMENT OF ELEVATED INTRACRANIAL PRESSURE

The treatment of elevated ICP must be tailored to each individual patient, depending on the cause, severity, and age group. No universally accepted treatment protocol exists; therefore, the following is given as a general overview and reflects preferences at our institution. Regardless of the cause, management of intracranial hypertension should include general measures aimed predominantly at not exacerbating the existing conditions. In addition, high priority is given to identification and removal of surgical lesions. Further, specific measures are typically initiated if the ICP exceeds 20 mm Hg for longer than 5 minutes. These are discussed next in the usual order in which they are instituted, although much variation exists among institutions.

General Measures

Management of elevated ICP requires attention to multiple facets of patient care. In head-injured patients, fluid management must be carefully addressed. Excessive hydration in the acute period (24–72 h) may exacerbate cerebral edema; therefore, mild (75%) fluid restriction is often instituted during this period. Thereafter, a normovolemic state is desired. The maintenance fluid is usually a 5% dextrose solution, which is either isotonic or 0.4% sodium choride. If fluid boluses are necessary, a colloid such as 5% albumin is preferred. Deleterious increases in CBF should be avoided by maintaining an adequate arterial oxygen partial pressure, aggressively treating fevers, and preventing seizures. Cerebral venous drainage can be enhanced by elevating the head of the bed to 30° and administering moderate sedation with narcotics or benzodiazepines (as well as intravenous lidocaine before bronchial suctioning). Hypotension must be avoided.

Specific Measures

Glucocorticoids (such as dexamethasone) are effective in reducing vasogenic edema surrounding tumors and abscesses. Steroids have no effect on cytotoxic edema and have shown no statistical benefit in the treatment of head-injured patients.[22, 23] Significant side effects of steroids include immunosuppression, superinfections, gastric ulcers, poor wound healing, and hyperglycemia.

Ventricular CSF drainage is highly effective in reducing ICP but is often limited by collapse of the ventricular cavity. In the presence of an intracranial mass lesion, ventriculostomy is the method of choice. In other cases, such as pseudotumor cerebri, repeated lumbar puncture may be used for therapeutic purposes.

Hyperventilation reduces ICP by causing vasoconstriction of cerebral arterioles in response to lowered partial pressure of carbon dioxide (P_{CO_2}).[24] An arterial P_{CO_2} of 30 to 35 mm Hg is optimal; lower values may result in focal ischemia due to excessive vasoconstriction. Studies[25, 26] have shown a statistically significant worsened outcome in head-injured patients (Glascow Coma Scale score 4–5) who received prophylactic hyperventilation, as compared with those who did not. It was suggested that prolonged hyperventilation results in the loss of CSF buffering capacity, leading to a hypersensitivity to the normalization of P_{CO_2}, which occurs intermittently during care (such as during tracheal suctioning), and a net increase in the time ICP exceeds 20 mm Hg. Trimethamine, a CSF buffering agent, appeared to counteract this ICP instability and improve outcome. Although not clearly settled, it is generally recommended that hyperventilation be used as a short-term measure (not prophylactically), that the P_{CO_2} be carefully controlled, and that administration of trimethamine be considered if prolonged hyperventilation is required. Once begun, hyperventilation therapy must be slowly tapered off to avoid rebound intracranial hypertension.

Although referred to as an "osmotic agent," mannitol (and related urea) appears to reduce ICP predominantly by improving the rheologic characteristics of blood, thus inducing an autoregulatory vasoconstriction in response to improved perfusion.[27] Early in therapy, the osmotic gradient created across the blood-brain barrier may draw interstitial fluid into the vascular space, although this effect may be minor. The initial dose of mannitol is 1 g/kg body weight given by rapid intravenous infusion, followed by doses of 0.25 to 0.5 g/kg every 6 hours, as dictated by the ICP. Overaggressive treatment may result in a lethal hyperosmolar, nonketotic state. Some physicians alternate mannitol doses with furosemide, 1 mg/kg, to avoid a hyperosmotic state. Serum Na^+ and osmolality levels should be monitored every 6 hours, and treatment adjusted accordingly to achieve but not exceed a serum osmolality of 305 to 310. Mannitol therapy must be gradually reduced in order to leach out the interstitial accumulation of mannitol. Rebound increases in ICP can occur with abrupt cessation of mannitol therapy as a result of reversal of the serum-interstitial osmolality gradient. The diuretic effect of these agents is generally not desired, and fluid management should be adjusted to maintain a normovolemic status. Patients who do not respond to hyperventilation and mannitol generally carry a worse prognosis, presumably reflecting the loss of cerebrovascular autoregulation associated with a severe brain injury.[3]

Neuromuscular paralysis (with vecuronium or a similar agent) in combination with sedation may be helpful in cases in which excessive abnormal motor posturing is problematic. The neurologic examination is no longer obtainable, leaving the ICP monitor as the only measure of treatment effectiveness. Seizure activity remains undetected unless continuous electroencephalographic monitoring is used.

High-dose barbiturates reduce ICP by inducing a coupled decrease in CBF and metabolism.[28] Although these drugs are frequently effective in lowering ICP, clinical studies have not demonstrated a statistical improvement in outcome.[29] Significant myocardial depression and pulmonary complications occur frequently, requiring intense medical management. Despite the risks and unproven efficacy, barbiturate coma is still used by many institutions, including ours, as a measure of last resort.

Decompressive surgery is based on the concept of relieving pressure on critical brain structures by removing either portions of the cranium or nonessential cerebral tissue. Subtemporal decompressions (removal of the squamous part of the temporal bone and opening of the underlying dura) allow lateral herniation of the temporal lobe into the temporalis muscle rather than medially into the midbrain. In extreme cases, an anterior temporal or frontal lobe can be removed unilaterally, usually with minimal deficit (assuming intact contralateral function).

PEDIATRIC CONSIDERATIONS

The physiology of ICP in neonates and infants is altered by a pliable, expandable skull. The anterior fontanelle can serve as a semi-quantitative ICP indicator. In many situations, placement of an ICP monitor is not possible owing to the thin skull and scalp. Dosages of medications are different from those listed earlier and should be tailored accordingly.

References

1. Ropper AH: A preliminary study of the geometry of brain displacement and level of consciousness in patients with acute intracranial masses. Neurology 1989; 39:622–627.
2. Graham DI, Adams JH, Doyle D: Ischemic brain damage in fatal non-missile head injury. J Neurol Sci 1978; 39:213–234.
3. Muizelaar JP: Cerebral circulation after severe head injury: *In*: Textbook of Head Injury. Becker DP, Gudeman SK (Eds). Philadelphia, WB Saunders, 1989, pp 221–240.
4. Miller JD, Becker DP, Ward JD, et al: Significance of intracranial hypertension in severe head injury. J Neurosurg 1977; 47:503–516.
5. Becker DP, Miller JD, Ward JD, et al: The outcome from severe head injury with early diagnosis and intensive management. J Neurosurg 1977; 47:491–502.
6. Marshall LF, Smith RW, Shapiro HM: The outcome with aggressive treatment in severe head injury. Part I. The significance of intracranial pressure monitoring. J Neurosurg 1979; 50:2025.
7. Rosner MJ, Daughton S: Cerebral perfusion pressure management in head injury. J Trauma 1990; 30:933–941.
8. Burrows G: Disorders of the cerebral circulation. Philadelphia, Len & Blanchards, 1848.
9. Lundberg N: The saga of the Monro-Kellie doctrine. *In*: Intracranial Pressure V. Ishii S, Nagai H, Brock M (Eds). Berlin, Springer-Verlag, 1983, pp 66–78.
10. Langfitt TW: Increased intracranial pressure. Clin Neurosurg 1969; 16:436–471.
11. Miller JD: Intracranial volume pressure relationships in pathological conditions. J Neurosurg Sci 1976; 20:203–209.
12. Lundberg N: Continuous recording and control of ventricular fluid pressure in neurosurgical practice. Acta Psychiatr Neurol Scand 1960; 36:1–193.
13. Fishman RA: Brain edema. N Engl J Med 1975; 293:706–711.
14. Bruce DA, Schut L, Bruno LA, et al: Outcome following severe head injuries in children. J Neurosurg 1978; 48:679–688.
15. Becker DP: Common themes in head injury: *In*: Textbook of Head Injury. Becker DP, Gudeman SK (Eds). Philadelphia, WB Saunders, 1989, p 13.
16. Fleischer AS, Payne NS, Tindall GT: Continuous monitoring of intracranial pressure in severe closed head injury without mass lesions. Surg Neurol 1976; 6:31–34.

17. Crutchfield JS, Narayan RK, Robertson CS, et al: Evaluation of a fiberoptic intracranial pressure monitor. J Neurosurg 1990; 72:482–487.
18. Mayhall GC, Archer NH, Lamb VA, et al: Ventriculostomy related infections, a prospective epidemiologic study. N Engl J Med 1984; 310:553–559.
19. Rosner MJ, Becker DP: ICP monitoring, complications, and associated factors. Clin Neurosurg 1976; 23:494–519.
20. Smith RW, Alksne JF: Infections complicating the use of external ventriculostomy. J Neurosurg 1976; 44:567.
21. Piek J, Bock WJ: Continuous monitoring of cerebral tissue pressure in neurosurgical practice—experience with 100 patients. Intensive Care Med 1990; 16:184–188.
22. Braakman R, Schouten HJ, Blaauw van Dishoeck M, et al: Megadose steroids in severe head injury. Results of a prospective double-blind study. J Neurosurg 1983; 58:326–330.
23. Gudeman SK, Miller DJ, Becker DP: Failure of high-dose steroid therapy to influence ICP in patients with severe head injury. J Neurosurg 1979; 51:301–306.
24. Crockard HA, Coppel DL, Morrow WFK: Evaluation of hyperventilation in treatment of head injuries. Br Med J 1973; 4:634–640.
25. Muizelaar JP, Marmarou A, Ward JD, et al: Adverse effects of prolonged hyperventilation in patients with severe head injury: A randomized clinical trial. J Neurosurg 1991; 75:731–739.
26. Ward JD, Choi S, Marmarou A, et al: Effect of prophylactic hyperventilation on outcome in patients with severe head injury. *In*: ICP VII. Hoff JT (Ed). Berlin, Springer-Verlag, 1989.
27. Muizelaar JP, Lutz HA, Becker DP: Effect of mannitol on ICP and CBF and correlation with pressure autoregulation in severely head-injured patients. J Neurosurg 1984; 61:700–706.
28. Michenfelder JD: The interdependency of cerebral function metabolic effects following massive doses of thiopental in the dog. Anesthesia 1974; 41:231–236.
29. Ward JD, Becker DP, Miller JD, et al: Failure of prophylactic barbiturate coma in the treatment of severe head injury. J Neurosurg 1985; 62:383.

CHAPTER 38

Brain Function Monitoring

Donald J. Deyo, DVM • Donald S. Prough, MD

Despite the frequency in intensive care units (ICUs) of patients with acute traumatic and ischemic brain diseases, clinical neurologic monitoring remains rudimentary. Often, only systemic hemodynamics and gas exchange are monitored, an approach that is adequate for many patients in whom cerebral oxygen delivery is dependent primarily on blood pressure and systemic oxygenation. Although clinical experience suggests that morbidity and mortality might be altered by therapeutic alteration of cerebral blood flow (CBF) and cerebral metabolism in some neurologically injured patients, no data confirm the general clinical utility of neurologic monitoring.

This chapter reviews the techniques currently available for cerebral function monitoring and summarizes information about the use of those techniques in common neurologic and neurosurgical diseases. Throughout the chapter, three questions should be constantly kept in mind:

1. In what diseases is the proportion of patients who will develop avoidable injury sufficiently large to justify extensive (and potentially expensive) application of neurologic monitoring devices?
2. Under what circumstances do blood pressure, partial pressures of arterial carbon dioxide and oxygen ($Paco_2$ and Pao_2), and body temperature provide insufficient information about the adequacy of cerebral oxygen delivery (CDo_2 = [CBF] × Cao_2)?
3. Under what circumstances does more precise information about the adequacy of CDo_2 permit therapeutic interventions that improve outcome?

GOALS OF BRAIN MONITORING

Monitoring devices potentially contribute to decreased morbidity and mortality by providing physiologic data that can be integrated into a more effective therapeutic plan. Neurologic monitoring falls into two distinct categories: The first category, which includes electroencephalography (EEG) and evoked potential (EP) monitoring, defines a qualitative threshold of neurologic ischemia. The second category, which includes monitors of intracranial pressure (ICP), CBF, and cerebral metabolism, provides quantitative physiologic information that can potentially define a threshold for changing treatment. Nevertheless, few data quantify the relationship between monitored variables and the risk of preventable neurologic injury. Changes in monitored variables that correlate with various levels of cerebral perfusion are summarized in Table 38–1.

CEREBRAL ISCHEMIA

Virtually all neurologic monitors detect actual or possible cerebral ischemia, defined as CDo_2 insufficient to meet metabolic needs. Cerebral ischemia is traditionally characterized as global or focal and complete or incomplete. Most global cerebral insults, such as hypotension, hypoxemia, and cardiac arrest, are readily detected by systemic monitors. Therefore, brain-specific monitors can provide additional information primarily in situations such as stroke, subarachnoid hemorrhage (SAH) with vasospasm, and cerebral trauma, in which focal cerebral oxygenation may be impaired despite adequate systemic oxygenation and perfusion.

TABLE 38–1. Clinical, Pathophysiologic, and Monitoring Thresholds in Cerebral Ischemia

CBF *(mL·100 g^{-1}·min^{-1})*	*Clinical Changes*	*Pathophysiologic Changes*	*Monitored*
50	Normal		
23	Reversible paralysis		EEG slowing, EP change
20		Na^+-K^+ pump dysfunction	
18	Infarction		EEG flat
15			EP absent
10		K^+ efflux, Ca^{2+} influx	

(From Prough DS: Brain monitoring. *In*: Critical Care: State of the Art. Vol 12. Shoemaker W, Taylor R (Eds). Fullerton, CA, Society of Critical Care Medicine, 1991, p 165.)

The severity of ischemic brain damage is proportional to the magnitude and duration of CDO_2. In monkeys, potentially reversible paralysis develops if regional CBF declines below about 23 mL · 100 g^{-1} · min^{-1}.[1] Infarction of brain tissue, however, requires that CBF remain below 18 mL · 100 g^{-1} · min^{-1}.[1] The tolerable duration of more profound ischemia is inversely proportional to the severity of CBF reduction.

TABLE 38–2. Brain Function Monitors

Cerebral Perfusion	*Cerebral Oxygen Extraction*	*Cerebral Function*
Cerebral blood flow	Jugular bulb saturation	Electroencephalogram
		Processed
		Raw
Cerebral blood flow velocity	Near-infrared spectroscopy	Evoked potentials
Intracranial pressure		

TECHNIQUES OF NEUROLOGIC MONITORING

Brain monitors directly or indirectly assess cerebral perfusion, cerebral oxygen extraction, or cerebral function (Table 38–2). Brain monitors can be classified in terms of the validity of the measurements performed and in terms of the ease with which monitored information can be incorporated into the clinical reasoning process (Table 38–3). The design and use of monitoring devices necessitate tradeoffs among various performance characteristics. For instance, a monitor with high positive predictive value (i.e., that falls outside threshold values only when cerebral ischemia is unequivocally present) is unlikely to sensitively detect less profound ischemia. A monitor that is highly sensitive to changes in cerebral oxygenation frequently warns of small changes that are unlikely to produce brain injury.

If a monitor of brain function detects cerebral ischemia, all that is known is that cerebral oxygenation in a region of brain that contributes to that function has fallen below a critical threshold. Because more severe ischemia produces neurologic injury in less time, it is impossible to predict with certainty if changes in function will be followed by cerebral infarction. In addition, if regional ischemia involves structures that do not participate in the monitored function, infarction could develop without warning.

Cardiorespiratory Monitoring

Blood pressure monitoring and pulse oximetry provide important data about the adequacy of global brain oxygenation. CBF is controlled in normal persons by metabolic demand, pressure autoregulation, $PaCO_2$, and arterial oxygen content (CaO_2). Figure 38–1*A* depicts the normal "coupled" relationship in which CBF is dependent on the cerebral metabolic rate of oxygen ($CMRO_2$), which varies directly with body temperature and with the level of brain activation. Because of the phenomenon of pressure autoregulation, changes in cerebral perfusion pressure do not alter CBF over a range of pressures of approximately 50 to 130 mm Hg (see Fig. 38–1*B*).[2] If $PaCO_2$ is halved, CBF is acutely halved; if $PaCO_2$ doubles, CBF doubles (see Fig. 38–1*C*). In response to decreasing CaO_2, CBF increases, whether the reduction is secondary to a decrease in hemoglobin or in arterial blood oxygen saturation (SaO_2) (see Fig. 38–1*D*).[3,4]

Neurologic Examination

Neurologic examination quantifies changes in consciousness and focal brain dysfunction. The Glasgow Coma Scale has become popular as a brief, reproducible estimate of level of consciousness in critically ill patients. The score should be supplemented by recording pupillary size and reactivity and the status of focal neurologic findings. Impaired consciousness is nonspecific; however, recognition of changing consciousness may warn of various treatable conditions, including progression of intracranial hypertension, developing vasospasm in patients after SAH, delayed post-traumatic intracranial hematomas, or systemic complications of intracranial pathology such as hyponatremia, hypoxemia, or hypercarbia.

Neuroimaging

Cerebral computed tomographic scans, magnetic resonance imaging scans, and radionuclide scans do not function as monitors per se. Rather, they are indicated in response to suspicion of a new or progressive anatomic lesion, such as a subdural or intracerebral hematoma, that will require altered treatment. Computed tomography scanning provides static, discontinuous data, supplies no information about

TABLE 38–3. Glossary of Neurologic Monitor Characteristics

Term	*Definition*
Bias	Average difference (positive or negative) between monitored values and "gold standard" values
Precision	Standard deviation of the differences (bias) between the measurements
Sensitivity	Probability that the monitor will demonstrate cerebral ischemia when cerebral ischemia is present
Positive predictive value	Probability that cerebral ischemia is present when the monitor suggests cerebral ischemia
Specificity	Probability that the monitor will not demonstrate cerebral ischemia when cerebral ischemia is not present
Negative predictive value	Probability that cerebral ischemia is not present when the monitor reflects no cerebral ischemia
Threshold value	The value used to separate acceptable (i.e., no ischemia present) from unacceptable (i.e., ischemia present)
Speed	The time elapsed from the onset of actual ischemia or the risk of ischemia until the monitor provides evidence

(From Prough DS: Brain monitoring. *In:* Critical Care: State of the Art. Vol 12. Shoemaker W, Taylor R (Eds). Fullerton, CA, Society of Critical Care Medicine, 1991, pp 164–165.)

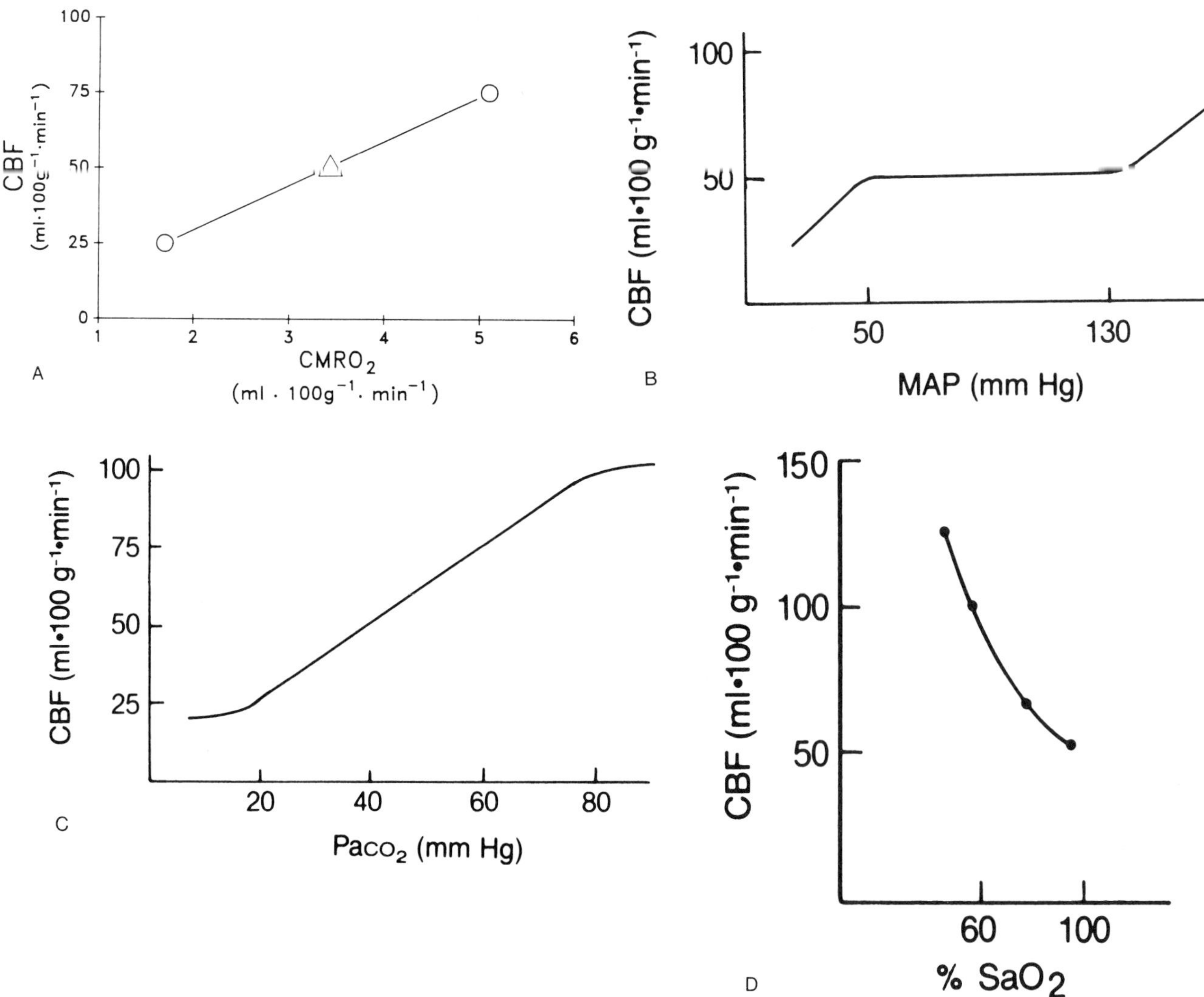

Figure 38–1. *A,* The normal relationship between the cerebral metabolic rate of oxygen consumption ($CMRO_2$) and cerebral blood flow (CBF) is characterized by closely coupled changes in both variables. Normally, CBF is 50 mL · 100 g^{-1} · min^{-1} at a $CMRO_2$ of 3.4 mL · 100 g^{-1} · min^{-1} in adults *(triangle).* As $CMRO_2$ increases or decreases, CBF changes in a parallel fashion *(solid line).* (From Butterworth JF IV, Prough DS: Head trauma. *In:* Intensive Care Medicine. 2nd ed. Rippe JR, Irwin RS, Alpert JS, et al (Eds). Boston, Little, Brown & Co, 1991, with permission from the publisher.) *B,* Effect of mean arterial pressure (MAP) on CBF. Note that changes in MAP produce little change in CBF over a broad range of pressures. If ICP exceeds normal limits, substitute cerebral perfusion pressure (CPP) on the horizontal axis. *C,* Effect of $Paco_2$ on CBF. Changes in $Paco_2$ exert powerful effects on cerebral vascular resistance across the entire clinically applicable range of values. *D,* Effect of arterial oxygen saturation (Sao_2) on CBF. Extreme changes in Sao_2 cause reciprocal changes in CBF.

brain function, and requires moving a critically ill patient out of the ICU. Magnetic resonance imaging scans, which often provide better resolution than computed tomography scans, are incompatible with ferrous metals, a ubiquitous component of life-support equipment. In patients with clinical evidence of brain death, cerebral flow studies (the initial component of radionuclide brain scans) can document cessation of CBF and have generally replaced repeated EEG for confirmation of brain death.[5]

Cerebral Blood Flow Monitoring

The first quantitative clinical method of measurement of CBF, the Kety-Schmidt technique,[6] calculated global CBF from the difference between the arterial and jugular bulb saturation curves of an inhaled, inert gas. Later techniques used extracranial gamma detectors to measure regional cortical CBF from washout curves after intracarotid injection of a radioisotope such as Xenon[133] (^{133}Xe).[7] Carotid puncture was avoided by techniques that measured cortical CBF after inhaled[8] or intravenous administration of ^{133}Xe, using gamma counting of exhaled gas to correct clearance curves for recirculation of ^{133}Xe. Among the obstacles to wider use of ^{133}Xe clearance are technical complexity, cumbersome regulations governing radionuclides, and the sustained stable conditions (5–15 min) required to perform a single measurement.

In most patients, arterial flow velocity can be readily measured in intracranial vessels, especially the middle cerebral artery, using transcranial Doppler ultrasonography. Doppler flow velocity uses the frequency shift, proportional to velocity, observed when sound waves are reflected by moving red blood cells. Blood moving toward the transducer shifts the transmitted frequency to higher frequencies, and blood moving away, to lower frequencies. Velocity is a function of both blood flow rate and vessel diameter. If diameter remains constant, changes in velocity are proportional to changes in CBF; however, intersubject differences in flow velocity correlate poorly with intersubject differences in CBF.[9] Entirely noninvasive, transcranial Doppler ultrasonography can be repeated at frequent intervals or even applied continuously. However, further clinical research is necessary to define those situations in which the excellent capacity for rapid trend monitoring can be exploited.

Intracranial Pressure Monitoring

ICP functions as the outflow pressure for the cerebral circulation, according to the following equation:

$$CPP = MAP - ICP$$

where CPP stands for cerebral perfusion pressure, MAP represents mean arterial pressure, and ICP exceeds jugular venous pressure. Because the skull is not distensible, the brain, cerebrospinal fluid (CSF), and cerebral blood volume have little room to expand without increasing ICP. Although CBF cannot be directly inferred from knowledge of mean arterial pressure and ICP, severe increases in ICP reduce both cerebral perfusion pressure and CBF.

The symptoms and signs of raised ICP are neither sensitive nor specific. The physical findings associated with increasing ICP usually become apparent only when intracranial hypertension has become sufficiently severe to injure the brain. Because ICP cannot otherwise be adequately assessed, direct measurement and monitoring of ICP have become a common intervention. One of three sites—one of the lateral ventricles, the subdural space, or the brain parenchyma—is usually used. Because pressure gradients may exist among various sites, it may be advantageous to monitor in or adjacent to the most severely damaged hemisphere. The problems associated with ICP monitoring fall generally into three categories: risks to patients (i.e., intracranial hemorrhage, cortical damage, and infection), inaccurate data, and inappropriate use or misinterpretation of data.

Ventricular catheterization, performed under strict aseptic technique, is the method of choice for monitoring and CSF drainage in patients with acute intracranial hypertension and excess CSF. However, intraventricular catheters may be difficult to place if cerebral edema or brain swelling has compressed the ventricular system. Intraventricular monitoring can be performed with hollow catheters that are fluid coupled to external pressure transducers or with catheters that are transducer tipped (Camino Laboratories, San Diego, CA). Fiberoptic catheters are less susceptible to short-term malfunction than conventional, fluid-filled catheters.[10] All fluid-coupled systems that passively connect to external transducers must be "zeroed" at the level of the external auditory meatus.

ICP monitoring from the subdural space is usually carried out with fluid-coupled bolts, fluid-coupled subdural catheters, or fiberoptic transducer-tipped catheters. Because subdural bolts are open tubes facing end-on against the brain surface, brain tissue may herniate into the system, obstructing the system and potentially damaging the brain cortex. The fiberoptic system, when inserted subdurally, cannot be calibrated after insertion but demonstrates acceptably low drift.[10] In a series of 46 patients monitored with fiberoptic catheters in the intraparenchymal ($n = 43$) or intraventricular ($n = 3$) positions, 12% developed broken components, 8.6% required repositioning for erroneous readings, and epidural hematomas complicated 3.4%.[11]

In addition to frankly increased ICP, monitoring can also reveal pathologic waveforms and decreased intracranial compliance. B waves, cycling at a rate of two to four per second with an amplitude of 10 mm Hg or greater, warn of possible decompensation of reserve. Plateau, or A waves, which have long been recognized as a sign of impending catastrophe, consist of cyclic increases in ICP, often 50 mm Hg or greater and lasting as long as 15 to 30 minutes.[12]

Brain compliance can be assessed by calculating the pressure-volume index (PVI). This requires the addition of volume to CSF or withdrawal of CSF through a ventricular cannula, then substituting measured values in the following equation:

$$PVI = \frac{V}{\log P_0/P_{m \text{ or } p}}$$

where V is the volume withdrawn or injected; P_0 equals the pressure before withdrawing or injecting fluid; P_m represents the minimum pressure following fluid withdrawal and P_p stands for the peak pressure after volume addition.[13]

Cerebral Oxygen Extraction

Measurements of jugular venous bulb oxygenation reflect the adequacy of CBF as systemic "mixed venous" oxygenation reflects the adequacy of cardiac output. CBF, $CMRo_2$, Cao_2, and jugular venous oxygen content ($Cjvo_2$) are related according to the following equation:

$$CMRo_2 = CBF(Cao_2 - Cjvo_2)$$

Mixed cerebral venous blood, like mixed systemic blood, is a global average and may not reflect marked regional hypoperfusion. Therefore, abnormally low jugular venous saturation suggests the possibility of cerebral ischemia, but normal or elevated jugular venous saturation does not indicate adequate cerebral perfusion. The internal jugular vein can be located by external anatomic landmarks and a "seeker" needle as it is for antegrade passage of central venous catheters or pulmonary artery catheters; however, the catheter is directed toward the mastoid process, below which lies the jugular venous bulb. A skull radiograph can confirm the position (Fig. 38–2). In clinical use, jugular venous blood gas sampling or continuous monitoring has detected unexpected cerebral desaturation.

Near-infrared spectroscopy may eventually offer the opportunity to assess the adequacy of brain oxygenation continuously. Near-infrared light penetrates the skull and, during transmission through or reflection from brain tissue, undergoes changes in wavelength that are proportional to the relative concentrations of oxygenated and deoxygenated hemoglobin in the tissue beneath the field.[14] The absorption (A) of light by a chromophore (i.e., hemoglobin) is defined by Beer's law:

$$A = abc$$

where a stands for the absorption constant, b equals path length of the light, and c is concentration of the chromophore.

Extensive preclinical and clinical data demonstrate the sensitivity of the technique for detecting qualitative changes in brain oxygenation[14–16] (Fig. 38–3). Technical challenges to quantification of the signal include difficulty in determining the path lengths of reflected lights of different wavelengths and estimating the relative proportions of arterial, venous, and capillary blood in the field. Proof that this promising, noninvasive technique is useful awaits clinical validation.

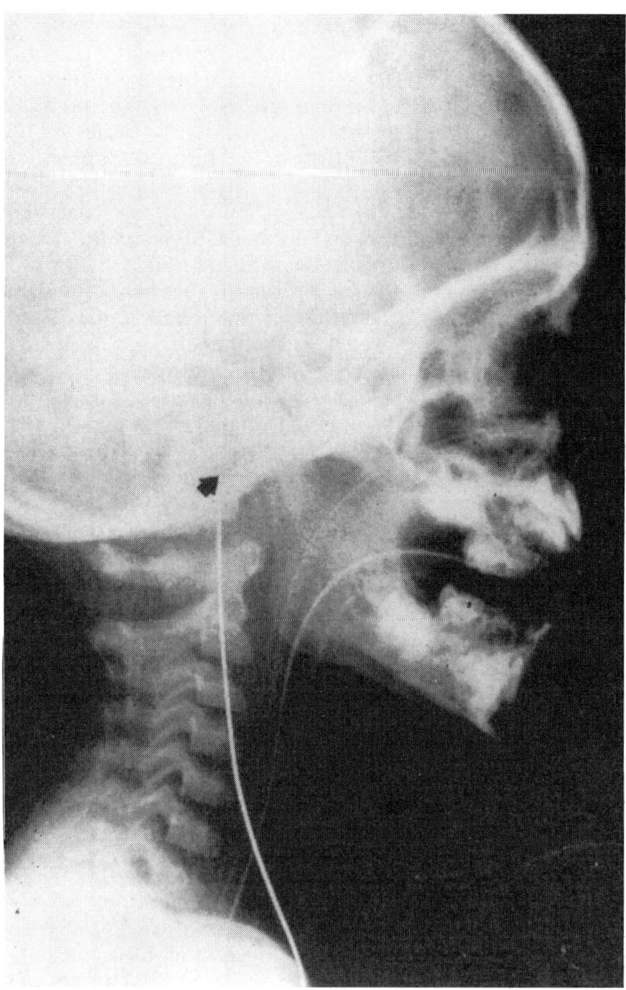

Figure 38–2. Radiograph demonstrating proper position of a jugular bulb catheter tip. The *arrow* indicates the location of the jugular bulb. (From Goetting MG, Preston G: Jugular bulb catheterization: Experience with 123 patients. Crit Care Med 1990; 18:1221.

Electrophysiologic Monitoring

The cortical EEG, altered by mild cerebral ischemia and abolished by profound cerebral ischemia, can be used to indicate potentially damaging hypoperfusion. Although the EEG has not been used extensively in critically ill patients, it may be useful in patients suspected of having isolated seizures or status epilepticus, in defining the depth or the type of coma, and in documenting focal or lateral intracranial abnormalities.

In an ICU, electrical noise from electronic equipment such as monitors and nearby computers may interfere with technically adequate tracings. Continuous EEG recording is cumbersome because of the sheer volume of data (300 pages per hour of hard copy on as many as 16 channels). Therefore, various software has been designed to compress the data. If the complex waveform, consisting of four frequency ranges, delta (<4 Hz), theta (4–8 Hz), alpha (8–13 Hz), and beta (>13 Hz), is filtered and digitized, rapid Fourier analysis of the digitized data can determine the relative amplitude present in each frequency band. Data can then be displayed as a compressed spectral array or a density spectral array, which permits detection of small peaks that might be hidden in the peaks of the density spectral array.[17]

Sensory EPs, which include somatosensory evoked potentials (SSEPs), brain stem auditory evoked potentials (BAEPs), and visual EPs, can be used as qualitative threshold monitors to detect severe neural ischemia. The EEG records the continuous, spontaneous activity of the brain, and EPs evaluate the responses of the brain to specific stimuli. To record SSEPs, a stimulus is applied to a peripheral nerve, usually the median nerve at the wrist, by a low-amplitude current of approximately 20 msec in duration. The resultant sensory (afferent) nerve stimulation is sufficient to provoke a slight thumb twitch. Repeated identical stimuli are applied, and signal averaging is used to visualize the reproducible evoked responses while removing the highly variable background EEG. EPs are described in terms of the amplitude of individual peaks and the delay (latency) from stimulus administration until the appearance of specific portions of the waveform. Because peripheral nerve stimulation can be uncomfortable, SSEPs are usually obtained on comatose patients. SSEPs are unaffected by neuromuscular blocking agents.

The sensitivity of EP monitoring is similar to that of EEG monitoring. EPs, especially BAEPs, are relatively robust, although they are modified by sedatives, narcotics, and anesthetics, as well as by trauma, hypoxia, or ischemia. Because obliteration of EPs occurs only under conditions of profound cerebral ischemia or mechanical trauma, EP monitoring is one of the most specific ways in which to assess neurologic integrity.

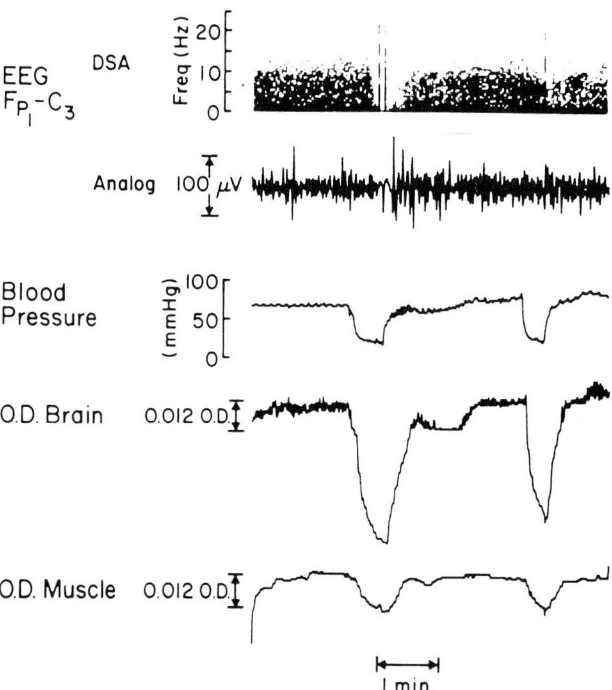

Figure 38–3. Electroencephalogram (EEG, DSA display), analog EEG, blood pressure, and near-infrared spectroscopic estimation of hemoglobin saturation in brain and muscle (O.D. = optical density in brain and muscle) during an episode of ventricular fibrillation in a patient undergoing implantation of an automatic implantable defibrillator. With abrupt cessation of cerebral circulation, O.D. in brain and muscle declined abruptly. After an interval of absent circulation, defibrillation resulted in restoration of perfusion. The postdefibrillation increase in O.D. in the brain may represent transient postischemic hyperemia. (From Smith DS, Levy W, Maris M, et al: Reperfusion hyperoxia in brain after circulatory arrest in humans. Anesthesiology 1990; 73:12.

Extensive use of electrophysiologic techniques in the ICU has been limited by three factors: expensive equipment, the requirement for highly trained technicians, and the need for clinical sophistication in the art of pattern recognition.

SPECIFIC NEUROLOGIC AND NEUROSURGICAL DISEASES

Monitoring in Traumatic Brain Injury

Human acute head injury, sufficiently severe to produce coma (Glasgow Coma Scale score ≤ 8), is associated with substantial cerebrovascular changes. In most patients, CBF is less than the normal value of 50 mL/100 g/min and $CMRO_2$ is well below the normal value of 3.5 mL · 100 g^{-1} · min^{-1}.[18] In some patients with head injury, $CMRO_2$ and CBF are proportionately reduced (i.e., coupling is preserved); in others, CBF substantially exceeds that necessary to meet $CMRO_2$.[18] Patients who demonstrate appropriate coupling with $CMRO_2$ and low CBF may develop a wide cerebral arteriovenous oxygen content difference during hyperventilation, suggesting that hyperventilation therapy should be accompanied by an estimate of the adequacy of cerebral perfusion.[18] Lower CBF correlates with poorer outcome, after adjustment for confounding variables, in head-injured patients.[19]

CBF after head trauma is pressure dependent in approximately one third of patients; two thirds demonstrate intact pressure autoregulation. Neither ICP, neurologic status, nor baseline CBF predicts the status of autoregulation. However, most patients with mass lesions demonstrate defective autoregulation, whereas autoregulation remains intact in many patients without intracranial mass lesions.[20] Transcranial Doppler flow velocity measurements have been used to identify moderate and severe cerebral vasospasm after head injury[21, 21a]; all patients with severe vasospasm (5 of 8 patients with vasospasm in a total group of 30 head-injured patients) had traumatic SAH.[21]

If CBF measurements are unavailable, calculation of the cerebral oxygen extraction or lactate extraction may provide clinically useful information about the adequacy of cerebral perfusion.[21b, 22] Excessive regional vasoconstriction represents a possible mechanism for the reported worsening of outcome[23] in patients hyperventilated after head trauma in comparison with those maintained at a higher level of $PaCO_2$.

Robertson and colleagues reported extensive experience in head-injured patients with monitoring of the cerebral arteriovenous oxygen content difference.[22] In a series of 100 patients, measurements of the cerebral arteriovenous differences of lactate and oxygen content could be used to predict CBF and to differentiate patients with patterns consistent with ischemia or infarction, normal CBF, cerebral hyperemia, and compensated hypoperfusion (Fig. 38–4).[22] Although controversial,[22a] near-infrared spectroscopy offers promise for the noninvasive determination of brain oxygenation.[14, 16, 22b] Near-infrared spectroscopy also has been used to localize post-traumatic intracranial hematomas.[24]

Conceptually, much of the management of acute head injury is intended to maintain adequate CBF; however, CBF is not routinely measured. Most cerebral circulatory information is inferred from knowledge of mean arterial pressure, $PaCO_2$, and measurement of ICP. ICP monitoring is usually considered to be a fundamental part of the care of patients with severe closed head injury (i.e., Glasgow Coma Scale score ≤ 8).[25] Severe intracranial hypertension is the primary cause of death in more than 10% of severely injured patients, and ICP exceeding 20 mm Hg increases morbidity in those who survive.[26] Although many neurosurgeons consider that aggressive monitoring and control of ICP improve outcome in severe head injury,[27] others question whether concurrent improvements in management, rather than ICP monitoring, explain the improvement.

In head-injured patients, clinicians have applied systematic but institutionally specific protocols for avoidance of intracranial hypertension and for reduction of increased ICP when a threshold of 15 or 20 mm Hg is exceeded. In particular, decisions about diuretics, hyperventilation, position changes, and additional diagnostic procedures may be determined by ICP information. The information is considered necessary in patients in whom neuromuscular blocking agents are administered as part of treatment to reduce ICP, because of the inability to perform a comprehensive neurologic examination. If intracranial hypertension is refractory to conventional therapy, ICP monitoring is one of the alternative techniques used to titrate barbiturate coma.[28] In head-injured patients, EP monitoring has been used as a diagnostic and prognostic aid. BAEPs correlate less well with clini-

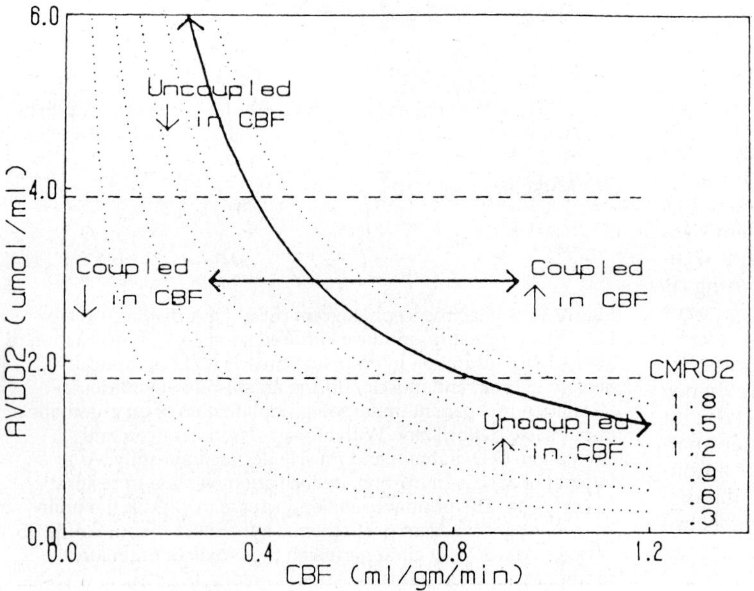

Figure 38–4. Conceptual model of the relationship between CBF and cerebral metabolism in comatose, head-injured patients. In nonischemic brain, the arteriovenous oxygen difference ($AVDO_2$) and CBF vary reciprocally, as illustrated by the *solid curve*, which represents a $CMRO_2$ averaging 0.9 μmol · g^{-1} · min^{-1} (note that this is substantially less than the $CMRO_2$ in normal individuals of 1.5 μmol · g^{-1} · min^{-1}; 15 μmol · g^{-1} · min^{-1} = 3.4 mL of O_2 · 100g^{-1} · min^{-1}). In the presence of cerebral ischemia/infarction *(open arrows)*, $AVDO_2$, and CBF have an unpredictable relationship. (From Robertson CS, Narayan RK, Gokaslan ZL, et al: Cerebral arteriovenous oxygen difference as an estimate of cerebral blood flow in comatose patients. J Neurosurg 1989; 70:222.)

cal outcome than cortical SSEPs,[29] the disappearance of which is a particularly ominous prognostic sign.[29] Multimodality EPs improve the prognostic accuracy of the clinical examination and measurement of ICP.[30]

Monitoring in Ischemic Neurologic Disease

Neurologic monitoring in patients with nontraumatic, ischemic neurologic and neurosurgical conditions has been less extensive than in patients with traumatic coma. After cardiac arrest, some patients develop postischemic hypoperfusion,[31] but $CMRO_2$ tends to be proportionately reduced.[31] Because the cerebral vasodilator nimodipine increased CBF and improved neurologic outcome in animals after complete cerebral ischemia, immediate postresuscitation administration of nimodipine was investigated in patients.[32] However, neurologic outcome was not improved. In some patients, CBF actually increases markedly within 24 to 48 hours after cardiac arrest and is associated with poor prognosis.[33]

Neurologic deterioration after SAH often represents cerebral vasospasm. Although CBF decreases, vasospasm reduces blood vessel diameter, thereby increasing flow velocity in the middle cerebral artery.[34] As vasospasm resolves (and CBF increases), velocity decreases. In patients randomized to receive nicardipine (a calcium entry blocker) or placebo after SAH, the incidence of vasospasm, as reflected in mean middle cerebral artery flow velocities exceeding 120 cm/s, was 23% in the nicardipine versus 49% in the placebo group.[35] Elevated middle cerebral artery velocity has also been used to determine the success of angioplasty to treat intracranial vasospasm.[36] Nevertheless, some investigators find transcranial Doppler ultrasonography to be of questionable value, failing to predict delayed ischemic deficits,[37] even if more sophisticated pulsatility indices are used.[38]

ICP monitoring has been applied in diverse acute ischemic and nonischemic neurologic conditions, including SAH and anoxic cerebral insults.[39] In nontraumatic brain disease, data defining the impact of ICP monitoring on outcome are more fragmentary and less convincing than those available for traumatized patients.

Using a compressed spectral array display of EEG data, Cant and Shaw monitored 51 patients[40] and reported that persistence or return of a peak of activity in the theta or alpha frequency bands within 10 days of the onset of coma was associated with a favorable recovery. In contrast, patients in whom such a peak was lost were likely to die or suffer residual neurologic damage. In patients comatose

TABLE 38–4. Techniques for Assessing Cerebral Circulation

Characteristic	*Evoked Potentials*	*EEG*	*CBF (^{133}Xe Clearance)*	*CBF (Transcranial Doppler Flow Velocity)*	*ICP Monitoring*	*Brain Metabolic Monitoring (Jugular Venous Saturation)*	*Brain Metabolic Monitoring (Near-Infrared Spectroscopy)*
Bias	NA	NA	± 5%	NA	Excellent	Gold standard	Not established
Precision	NA	NA	± 5%	NA	Excellent	Gold standard	Not established
Sensitivity	High for ischemia	Good for ischemia; sensitive to drug effects	Good for 5% change	Good for CBF change (relative)	Good for ICP change; poor for ischemia	Good for global; poor for regional	Good for severe global desaturation
Positive predictive value	Good for ischemia	Poor for ischemia	Good for CBF decrease	Good for CBF change	Good for ICP change; poor for ischemia	Good for global; poor for regional	Not established
Specificity	High for ischemia	Poor for ischemia	Poor for ischemia; good for CBF decrease	Good for CBF change	Good for ICP change; poor for ischemia	Good	Not established
Negative predictive value	Good for ischemia	Fair for ischemia	Poor for ischemia	Poor for ischemia; good for vasospasm	Good for ICP change; poor for ischemia	Good	Not established
Threshold definition	Ischemia (CBF 15–23 mL/100 g/min)	Ischemia (CBF 18–23 mL/100 g/min)	Can be set at desired level	Interpatient variability	15–20 mm Hg or <50 mm Hg cerebral perfusion pressure	Saturation <50	Probably similar to jugular saturation
Speed	Good	Good	Poor	Poor	Good (once inserted)	Fair (good if continuous)	Excellent
Utility in clinical:							
Diagnosis	Good	Good	Poor	Good	Poor	Poor	Untested
Surveillance	Poor	Fair	Poor	Fair in SAH	Good (CHI)	Poor (good if continuous)	Should be excellent
Prognosis	Good	Fair	Fair	Fair in SAH	Good (CHI)	Fair	Untested
Goal-directed therapy	Poor	Poor	Poor	Untested	Fair (CHI); Reye's syndrome	Untested	Potentially valuable but untested

from a mixture of traumatic and ischemic injuries, an alternating pattern of compressed spectral array activity was associated with a more favorable outcome.[41] Alpha coma, unconsciousness associated with an EEG pattern resembling normal wakefulness occurring after brain stem stroke or hypoxic-anoxic cerebral injury, suggests a poor prognosis. Serial EEGs have been used to improve prognostication in children with nontraumatic coma; the worst prognostic findings were low-amplitude activity or electrocerebral silence.[42] Quantitative EEG monitoring has been used to identify delayed ischemic deficits after SAH, occasionally before clinical deterioration.[43] Because of the sensitivity of the EEG to drug effects, either unprocessed or processed EEG monitoring can be used to assess sedation in critically ill patients. It can also be used to provide early evidence of seizure activity or cerebral ischemia.

When used for brain and spinal cord monitoring, EPs are intended to detect deterioration in neurologic function at a time when corrective action may still reverse changes. To a limited extent, EPs have been used to facilitate diagnosis and prognostication in ischemic and hypoxic brain injury. Central conduction time is prolonged in humans who have ischemic complications of SAH.[44] With impending brain death, cortical SSEPs disappear first; BAEPs disappear only when brain death is imminent.[45] Persistence of the medullary components of the SSEP, at a time when the cortical components are no longer present, confirms brain death. In children, absence of the cortical components of SSEPs with preserved brain stem function suggests the likelihood of a chronic vegetative state.[46]

SSEPs persist, although in altered form, during barbiturate administration; BAEPs are resistant to the effects of barbiturates.[47] Central conduction time, a measure of the time required to transmit the response to a stimulus from the periphery to the cortex, appears to be unaffected even by high levels of barbiturates.[48] Therefore, EPs assist in assessing neurologic status even in patients in barbiturate coma.

SUMMARY

Various powerful techniques, all of which can be performed at the bedside of critically ill patients, are available for assessing the cerebral circulation (Table 38–4). The next step in the evolution of neurologic monitoring necessitates the development of physiologically and pharmacologically sound protocols for goal-directed therapy. These must then be carefully tested to determine whether they can reduce morbidity and mortality in patients with critical neurologic illness.

References

1. Jones TH, Morawetz RB, Crowell RM, et al: Thresholds of focal cerebral ischemia in awake monkeys. J Neurosurg 1981; 54:773.
2. Strandgaard S, Paulson OB: Cerebral autoregulation. Stroke 1984; 15:413.
3. Tommasino C, Moore S, Todd MM: Cerebral effects of isovolemic hemodilution with crystalloid or colloid solutions. Crit Care Med 1988; 16:862.
4. Phillis JW, Preston G, DeLong RE: Effects of anoxia on cerebral blood flow in the rat brain: Evidence for a role of adenosine in autoregulation. J Cereb Blood Flow Metab 1984; 4:586.
5. Korein J, Braunstein P, Kercheff I, et al: Radioisotope bolus technique as a test to detect circulatory deficit associated with cerebral death. Circulation 1975; 51:924.
6. Kety SS, Schmidt CF: The determination of cerebral blood flow in man by the use of nitrous oxide in low concentrations. Am J Physiol 1945; 143:53.
7. Olesen J, Paulson OB, Lassen NA: Regional cerebral blood flow in man determined by the initial slope of the clearance of intra-arterially injected ^{133}Xe. Stroke 1971; 2:519.
8. Obrist WD, Thompson HK Jr, Wang HS, et al: Regional cerebral blood flow estimated by ^{133}Xenon inhalation. Stroke 1975; 6:245.
9. Bishop CCR, Powell S, Rutt D, et al: Transcranial Doppler measurement of middle cerebral artery blood flow velocity: A validation study. Stroke 1986; 17:913.
10. Crutchfield JS, Narayan RK, Robertson CS, et al: Evaluation of a fiberoptic intracranial pressure monitor. J Neurosurg 1990; 72:482–487.
11. Yablon JS, Lantner HJ, McCormack TM, et al: Clinical experience with a fiberoptic intracranial pressure monitor. J Clin Monit 1993; 9:171–175.
12. Lundberg N, Troupp H, Lorin H: Continuous recording of the ventricular-fluid pressure in patients with severe acute traumatic brain injury. J Neurosurg 1965; 22:581–590.
13. Maset AL, Marmarou A, Ward JD, et al: Pressure-volume index in head injury. J Neurosurg 1987; 67:832–840.
14. Edwards AC, Richardson C, van der Zee P, et al: Measurement of hemoglobin flow and blood flow by near-infrared spectroscopy. J Appl Physiol 1993; 75:1884.
15. Smith DS, Levy W, Maris M, et al: Reperfusion hyperoxia in brain after circulatory arrest in humans. Anethesiology 1990; 73:12.
16. Kurth CD, Steven JM, Benaron D, et al: Near-infrared monitoring of the cerebral circulation. J Clin Monit 1993; 9:163.
17. Levy WJ, Shapiro HM, Maruchak G, et al: Automated EEG processing for intraoperative monitoring: A comparison of techniques. Anesthesiology 1980; 53:223.
18. Obrist WD, Langfitt TW, Jaggi JL, et al: Cerebral blood flow and metabolism in comatose patients with acute head injury. Relationship to intracranial hypertension. J Neurosurg 1984; 61:241.
19. Robertson CS, Contant CF, Gokaslan ZL, et al: Cerebral blood flow, arteriovenous oxygen difference, and outcome in head injured patients. J Neurol Neurosurg Psychiatry 1992; 55:594–603.
20. Bruce DA, Langfitt TW, Miller JD, et al: Regional cerebral blood flow, intracranial pressure, and brain metabolism in comatose patients. J Neurosurg 1973; 38:131.
21. Martin NA, Doberstein C, Zane C, et al: Posttraumatic cerebral arterial spasm: Transcranial Doppler ultrasound, cerebral blood flow, and angiographic findings. J Neurosurg 1992; 77:575–583.

21a. Steiger HJ, Aaslid R, Stooss R, et al: Transcranial Doppler monitoring in head injury: Relations between type of injury, flow velocities, vasoreactivity, and outcome. Neurosurgery 1994; 34:79.

21b. Chan K-H, Dearden NM, Miller JD, et al: Multimodality monitoring as a guide to treatment of intracranial hypertension after severe brain injury. Neurosurgery 1993; 32:547.

22. Robertson CS, Narayan RK, Gokaslan ZL: Cerebral arteriovenous oxygen difference as an estimate of cerebral blood flow in comatose patients. J Neurosurg 1989; 70:222.

22a. Hirtz DG: Report of the National Institute of Neurological Disorders and Stroke workshop on near infrared spectroscopy. Pediatrics 1993; 91:414.

22b. Villringer A, Planck J, Hock C, et al: Near infrared spectroscopy (NIRS): A new tool to study hemodynamic changes during activation of brain function in human adults. Neurosci Lett 1993; 154:101.

23. Muizelaar JP, Marmarou A, Ward JD, et al: Adverse effects of prolonged hyperventilation in patients with severe head injury: A randomized clinical trial. J Neurosurg 1991; 75:731.
24. Gopinath SP, Robertson CS, Grossman RG, et al: Near-infrared spectroscopic localization of intracranial hematomas. J Neurosurg 1993; 79:43–47.
25. Ward JD: Intracranial pressure monitoring. *In:* Critical Care: State of the Art. Fuhrman BP, Shoemaker WC (Eds). Fullerton, CA, Society of Critical Care Medicine, 1989, pp 173–185.
26. Miller JD, Becker DP, Ward JD, et al: Significance of intracranial hypertension in severe head injury. J Neurosurg 1977; 47:503–516.
27. Saul TG, Ducker TB: Effect of intracranial pressure monitoring and aggressive treatment on mortality in severe head injury. J Neurosurg 1982; 56:498–503.
28. Eisenberg HM, Frankowski RF, Contant CF, et al: High-dose

barbiturate control of elevated intracranial pressure in patients with severe head injury. J Neurosurg 1988; 69:15.
29. Ganes T, Lundar T: EEG and evoked potentials in comatose patients with severe brain damage. Electroencephalogr Clin Neurophysiol 1988; 69:6.
30. Anderson DC, Bundlie S, Rockswold GL: Multimodality evoked potentials in closed head trauma. Arch Neurol 1984; 41:369.
31. Beckstead JE, Tweed WA, Lee J, et al: Cerebral blood flow and metabolism in man following cardiac arrest. Stroke 1978; 9:569.
32. Roine RO, Kaste M, Kinnunen A, et al: Nimodipine after resuscitation from out-of-hospital ventricular fibrillation. A placebo-controlled, double-blind, randomized trial. JAMA 1990; 264:3171.
33. Cohan SL, Mun SK, Petite J, et al: Cerebral blood flow in humans following resuscitation from cardiac arrest. Stroke 1989; 20:761.
34. Aaslid R, Huber P, Nornes H: Evaluation of cerebrovascular spasm with transcranial Doppler ultrasound. J Neurosurg 1984; 60:37.
35. Haley EC Jr, Kassell NF, Torner JC: A randomized trial of nicardipine in subarachnoid hemorrhage: Angiographic and transcranial Doppler ultrasound results. J Neurosurg 1993; 78:548–553.
36. Hurst RW, Schnee C, Raps EC, et al: Role of transcranial Doppler in neuroradiological treatment of intracranial vasospasm. Stroke 1993; 24:299–303.
37. Laumer R, Steinmeier R, Gönner F, et al: Cerebral hemodynamics in subarachnoid hemorrhage evaluated by transcranial Doppler sonography. Part 1. Reliability of flow velocities in clinical management. Neurosurgery 1993; 33:1–9.
38. Steinmeier R, Laumer R, Bondár I, et al: Cerebral hemodynamics in subarachnoid hemorrhage evaluated by transcranial Doppler sonography. Part 2. Pulsatility indices: Normal reference values and characteristics in subarachnoid hemorrhage. Neurosurgery 1993; 33:10–19.
39. Tasker RC, Matthew DJ, Helms P, et al: Monitoring in non-traumatic coma. Part I: invasive intracranial measurements. Arch Dis Child 1988; 63:888.
40. Cant BR, Shaw NA: Monitoring by compressed spectral array in prolonged coma. Neurology 1984; 34:35.
41. Karnaze DS, Marshall LF, Bickford RG: EEG monitoring of clinical coma: The compressed spectral array. Neurology 1982; 32:289.
42. Tasker RC, Boyd S, Harden A, et al: Monitoring in non-traumatic coma. Part II. electroencephalography. Arch Dis Child 1988; 63:895.
43. Labar DR, Fisch BJ, Pedley TA, et al: Quantitative EEG monitoring for patients with subarachnoid hemorrhage. Electroencephalogr Clin Neurophysiol 1991; 78:325–332.
44. Symon L, Hargadine J, Zawirski M, et al: Central conduction time as an index of ischaemia in subarachnoid hemorrhage. J Neurol Sci 1979; 44:95.
45. Garcia-Larrea L, Bertrand O, Artru F, et al: Brain-stem monitoring. II. Preterminal BAEP changes observed until brain death in deeply comatose patients. Electroencephalogr Clin Neurophysiol 1987; 68:446.
46. Frank LM, Furgiuele TL, Etheridge JE Jr: Prediction of chronic vegetative state in children using evoked potentials. Neurology 1985; 35:931.
47. de Weerd AW, Groeneveld C: The use of evoked potentials in the management of patients with severe cerebral trauma. Acta Neurol Scand 1985; 72:489.
48. Hume AL, Cant BR, Shaw NA: Central somatosensory conduction time in comatose patients. Ann Neurol 1979; 5:379.

CHAPTER 39

Pediatric Monitoring

Randall C. Wetzel, MB, BS, FCCM, FAAP

Because of the wide variations in patients' size and age, pediatric intensive care units (ICUs) tend to deal with more diverse normal physiology and a greater host of pathologic problems than do other critical care units. Furthermore, pediatric ICUs routinely treat children suffering from a wide variety of medical and surgical emergencies, as well as postoperative, traumatic, and neurosurgical problems. Each child's underlying disease process and general status must be monitored according to his or her size, age, and disease. All critically ill children routinely require continual surveillance of their vital signs, electrocardiogram (ECG), and respirations. More sophisticated hemodynamic monitoring depends on the nature and complexity of a child's problems. In all cases, the purpose of monitoring is to detect changes and trends in physiologic parameters rather than to measure absolute values.

NONINVASIVE MONITORING TECHNIQUES

Electrocardiography

Continuous ECG display, including a system to record the tracing, is routinely indicated in the pediatric ICU. This is essential to allow rapid identification of arrhythmias, electromechanical dissociation, electrical paradox, bradycardias, and electrical standstill. Appropriate placement of ECG leads is as necessary in children as it is in adults. Accurate interpretation of ST-T changes, electric axis, and arrhythmias requires attention to lead placement. Abnormalities detected during monitoring require further investigation with a 12-lead ECG.

An infant's ECG normally shows right-sided predominance. At birth, the normal frontal QRS vector is about 135°; by 3 months of age, it has decreased to around 75°. By 6 years of age, a child's ECG is similar to an adult's. Abnormal ECGs with bizarre vectors may represent abnormal situs. The determination of ventricular hypertrophy in children requires reference to tables of standard voltage criteria in pediatric cardiology texts.

Ventricular tachycardia and fibrillation are rare in a pediatric ICU. The most common pediatric arrhythmias are sinus arrhythmia, bradyarrhythmia, and supraventricular tachyarrhythmias.[1] Arrhythmias in children generally occur postoperatively or in those children with a history of palpitations or hypotension. Syncopal attacks, seizures mimicking epilepsy, near miss sudden infant death syndrome, and attacks of pallor and vomiting are also associated with the sudden onset of pediatric arrhythmias. ECG monitoring in the pediatric ICU may offer the first clue to the cardiac origin of these symptoms.

Pronounced sinus arrhythmias are occasionally confused with arrhythmias caused by premature atrial contractions or dropped beats. Bradycardia (defined as heart rates of less than 100, 80, and 70 beats per minute in neonates, infants, and older children, respectively) is frequently encountered in critically ill children and may signal hypoxia in a neonate. In older children, bradyarrhythmias are generally postoperative conditions associated with the sick sinus syndrome, especially after a Mustard procedure; heart block, especially Mobitz type II; and bundle branch block, particularly after right ventriculostomy or surgery undoing the system. After complex surgery for congenital heart disease, pacing leads should always be placed.

Supraventricular arrhythmias are common.[2] A child's atrioventricular node and His bundle are less refractory to sinus stimulation than those of an adult; children with sinus tachycardias of 240 to 300 beats per minute show a 1:1 ventricular response. These high rates may be due to a primary conduction disorder. For example, a supraventricular tachycardia exceeding 300 beats per minute in neonates and infants is frequently associated with the Wolff-Parkinson-White syndrome. A shortened PR interval and a slurred upstroke during ventricular depolarization (delta wave) differentiate this condition from the Lown-Ganong-Levine syndrome, which is also due to abnormal conduction pathways but which displays a normal ventricular depolarization sequence.

Other causes of syncopal arrhythmias, seizures, or sudden death include various congenital ventricular depolarization abnormalities. For example, familial prolongation of the QT segment (Romano-Ward syndrome), sometimes associated with deafness (Jervell and Lange-Nielsen syndrome), and the presence of a prominent U wave are associated with episodes of sudden ventricular fibrillation. Ventricular dysrhythmias are generally related to structural anomalies or postoperative cardiac injury.[3] The diagnosis may first become apparent during ECG monitoring in the pediatric ICU.

Echocardiography (see also Chapters 52 and 53)

Echocardiography (Echo) is continuing to replace more invasive monitoring techniques in extremely ill neonates and children, particularly for those children in whom catheter insertion may be difficult, time consuming, or undesirable. Improved ultrasonographic technology and understanding and the advent of transesophageal ultrasound probes have led to increased reliance in this technology, not only for anatomic diagnosis, but also to monitor cardiac function intraoperatively and in the pediatric ICU.[4, 5] Common congenital defects such as an aortoseptal override in the tetralogy of Fallot can be diagnosed directly from an Echo cardiac structure display. In critically ill neonates, Echo can rapidly differentiate the low-output state caused by a hypoplastic left ventricle from sepsis or remediable heart disease: A small, poorly contractile left ventricle with a poorly visualized mitral valve, small aortic root, and large right ventricle is hypoplastic. Echo monitoring can detect right and left atrial myxomas, as well as other malignant intracavitary lesions. Furthermore, Echo is helpful when positioning pulmonary arterial catheters in the right ventricular (RV) outflow tract and in the pulmonary artery (PA).

Cardiac anomalies may also be inferred from abnormal Echos. Patent ductus arteriosus (PDA) and other causes of large left-to-right shunts may overload the left atrium and cause increased left atrial dimensions. By comparing the relatively inflexible aortic root dimension with the hyperexpanded left atrial dimension, it is possible to approximate the degree of volume overload. The normal ratio is about 1:1 in newborns and increases to greater than 1:3 in patients with a left-to-right shunt. Medical closure of the PDA with indomethacin can be monitored by serial Echos, as can the response of an infant's heart to digoxin or surgical ductus ligation. In addition, transesophageal Echo direction of nonoperative correction of congenital heart disease is becoming more frequent.[6]

Contrast Echo monitoring uses a rapid bolus injection of liquid into the circulation, producing highly echogenic "flurries" in the heart chambers and great vessels. The flurries are caused by dissolution of air microbubbles in the injectate, referred to as *microcavitation*. Because these bubbles are usually cleared by the pulmonary circulation, a venous injection should not create echoes on the left side of the heart except in patients with a right-to-left intracardiac shunt. Right-to-left shunting associated with a reopened foramen ovale and elevated PA pressure may follow cardiac surgery or occur during septic shock. It is also associated with persistent transitional circulation. A PDA may be diagnosed by injection through an umbilical artery catheter (UAC) in the aortic arch; suprasternal placement of the transducer demonstrates left-to-right shunting across the PDA from the aorta to the PA. After the placement of a shunt prosthesis, contrast Echo can confirm prosthetic shunt function and patency.

Echo monitoring is the most sensitive means of detecting fluid in the pericardial sac and estimating its volume. It can rapidly establish the presence, extent, and degree of hemodynamic deterioration caused by a pericardial effusion from cardiothoracic surgery, chemotherapy, or sepsis. Echo is also useful to monitor the effects of surgical or medical intervention.

Pediatric Echo monitoring requires rigid standardization. Experience with real-time, two-dimensional Echo has enabled a much clearer understanding of how a child's heart functions in critical situations. The introduction of transesophageal Echo for continuous cardiac function monitoring in children of an appropriate size has expanded the clinical critical care application of Echo.[4–6] Echo observation of heart action in critically ill children routinely provides critical information for diagnosis and to guide therapy. The specific application of Echo technology to the hemodynamics of head injury, postoperative monitoring, pulmonary vascular hemodynamics, and weaning from extracorporeal life support should receive further attention, as should attempts to correlate Echo-derived hemodynamic determinations with invasive methods.

Quantitative Echocardiography for Evaluating Myocardial Performance

Echo monitoring enables clinicians to monitor cardiac contractions, watch the aortic and pulmonary valves open and close, and determine the relative sizes of cardiac chambers. Left ventricular (LV) dimensions are determined from ventricular volumes and standardized by measurement at end-expiration just below the mitral valve ring (Fig. 39–1). The most useful quantitative parameters of myocardial contractility that can be determined by Echo monitoring are the shortening fraction (SF), the mean velocity of circumferential fiber shortening, and the ejection fraction (EF). SF is the most readily useful index of myocardial contractility for serial monitoring of patients in an ICU. SF is the LV end-diastolic dimension (LVED) minus the left ventricular end-systolic dimension (LVES), normalized for end-diastole:

$$SF = \frac{LVED - LVES}{LVED}$$

SF is independent of heart rate; however, decreased myocardial contractility decreases SF. SF values less than 30% denote impaired myocardial contractility. SF is increased when more demand is placed on the myocardium with increased afterload, such as in aortic stenosis and PDA.

The ventricular EF is the ratio of the cubed ventricular dimensions:

$$EF = \frac{LVED^3 - LVES^3}{LVED^3}$$

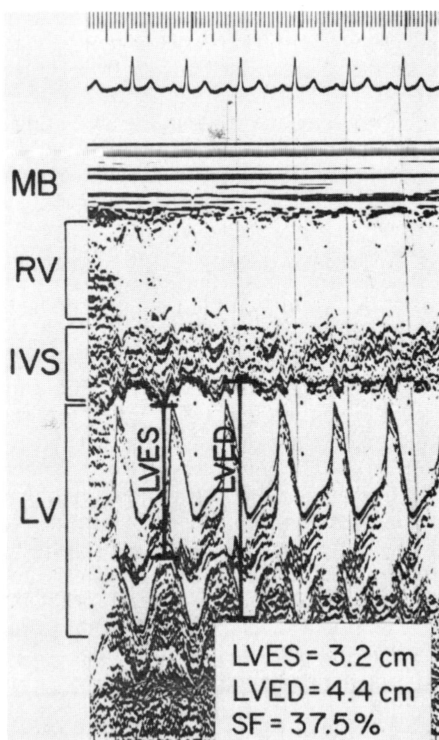

Figure 39–1. Echocardiographic measurement of left ventricular dimensions. The left ventricular end-diastolic (LVED) dimension is the distance from the septal endocardium to the left ventricular free wall endocardium at the end of diastole (electrical). The left ventricular end-systolic (LVES) dimension is the minimal dimension during systole. (From Wetzel RC, Rogers MC: Pediatric Hemodynamic Monitoring. *In*: Critical Care: State of the Art. Vol 2. Fullerton, CA, Society of Critical Care Medicine, 1981, p II [L]:29.)

The lower limit of normal for EF is 55%. This parameter obviously makes great assumptions about ventricular geometry and is only a coarse approximation of ventricular volume ratios. The mean velocity of circumferential fiber shortening (VCF) considers chronotropic influences on myocardial performance and normalizes SF with respect to ventricular ejection time (ET):

$$VCF = (LVED - LVES) / LVED \times ET = SF/ET$$

ET is the duration of blood ejection from the ventricle during each systole (i.e., the time the semilunar valve is open). This corresponds to the isotonic contraction period and is readily determined from the aortic valve echo. ET can be used to differentiate the depressed myocardial function of myopathy from the increased myocardial function associated with left-to-right shunts. The availability of two-dimensional Echo allows bedside assessment of global heart function in an ICU.

The systolic time intervals (STI) are also useful indicators of cardiovascular performance. These include the pre-ejection period (PEP) and the ET. PEP is the time from the onset of electric systole to the opening of the semilunar valve, including depolarization of the ventricular myocardium, closure of atrioventricular valves, and isometric ventricular contraction before valve opening. Although LVSTI values can be determined noninvasively by a combination of ECG, carotid pulsation tracings, and phonocardiography, noninvasive determination of RVSTI values requires Echo monitoring. The PEP-ET ratio often accentuates subtle abnormalities in both or either parameter. An increase in ventricular filling decreases PEP and increases the ET and stroke volume. An increase in the afterload prolongs PEP, shortens ET, and decreases stroke volume. Neither age nor heart rate alters PEP-ET ratio, although both PEP and ET increase with age and decrease with increasing heart rate.

Because STI values are affected by so many variables, their value in determining hemodynamic status is limited. Obviously, a child in septic shock with decreased myocardial contractility and increased systemic vascular resistance (SVR) has a prolonged LVPEP-LVET ratio (Fig. 39–2); however, this value is not helpful in determining whether decreased contractility or increased afterload is primarily responsible. When considered in conjunction with other clinical findings, however, serial STI values may be extremely useful to assess progress and responses to therapy. LVPEP-LVET ratio (normal range 0.30–0.39) is proportional to cardiac index and stroke volume and correlates very well with EF as determined by angiography. LVPEP-LVET ratio decreases with improving clinical status.

RVPEP-RVET ratio (normal range 0.16–0.30) correlates with pulmonary vascular resistance (PVR), mean PA pressure, and PA diastolic pressure. If RVPEP-RVET ratio is less than 0.30, there is a 90% chance that mean PA pressure is less than 35 mm Hg, PA diastolic pressure is less than 25 mm Hg, and the PVR index (PVRI) is less than 240 dyne · cm · 5^{-5}, or 3 R units. If the RVPEP-RVET ratio is greater than 0.40, there is a 90% chance that mean PA pressure is greater than 45 mm Hg, PA diastolic pressure is greater than 25 mm Hg, and PVRI is greater than 5 R units. In the postnatal period, the RVSTI values decrease within days after birth. Normal values for RVPEP-RVET ratio are 0.39

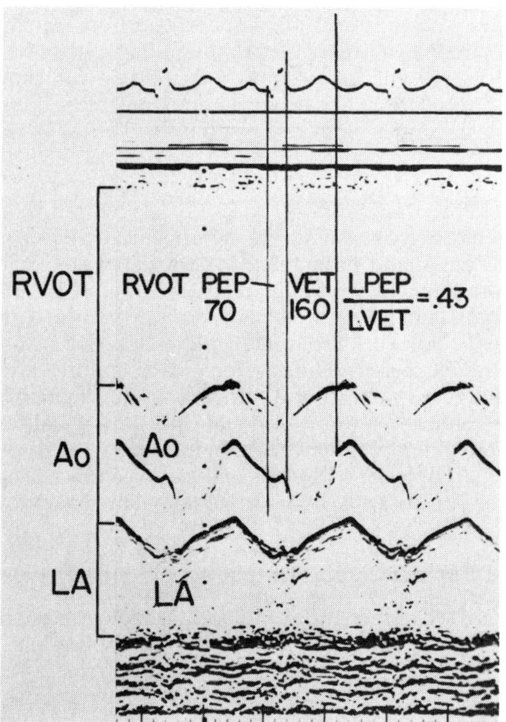

Figure 39–2. Elevated LVPEP-LVET ratio. Note that the PEP is from onset of electrical systole to valve opening and that the ejection time is from opening to closure. In this example, the RVOT is dilated. This patient has severe acute respiratory distress syndrome. All times are in milliseconds.

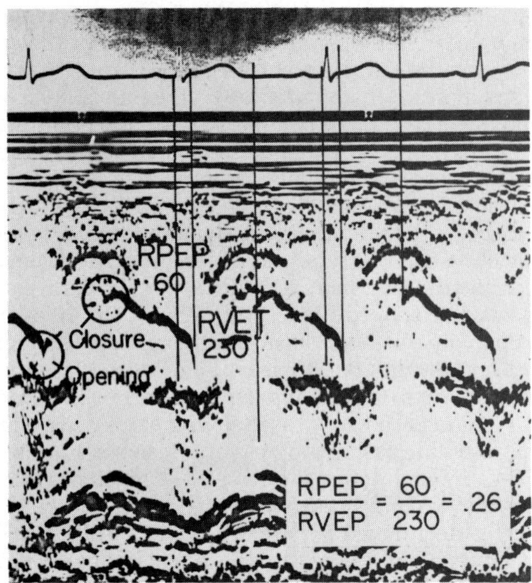

Figure 39–3. Echocardiogram of a neonatal pulmonary valve. Note opening and closure. An RVPEP-RVET ratio of 0.26 is normal for neonates. (From Wetzel RC, Rogers MC: Pediatric Hemodynamic Monitoring. *In*: Critical Care: State of the Art. Vol 2. Fullerton, CA, Society of Critical Care Medicine, 1981, p II [L]:239.)

± 0.05 from 0 to 12 hours, 0.32 ± 0.03 from 12 to 24 hours, 0.31 ± 0.05 from 24 to 48 hours, and 0.28 ± 0.03 after 48 hours (Fig. 39–3). These parameters correlate well with the physiologic PVR decrease during the first few days of life and presumably reflect decreasing RV afterload. Determining RVPEP-RVET ratio has become part of routine diagnostic management and is a method by which to monitor the therapy of newborns in whom persistent transitional circulation prolongs a high PVR. Although mean values are not useful in determining prognosis, decreasing values in survivors correlate with clinical improvement. Conversely, studies in infants with the respiratory distress syndrome show that increased RVPEP-RVET ratios correlate with a poor outcome.

In children, early rises in RVPEP-RVET ratios, before other evidence consistent with neurogenically induced vascular changes and pulmonary hypertension, are prolonged and correlate with intrapulmonary shunting and frank pulmonary edema. Return toward normal values correlates well with recovery from the pulmonary implications of head trauma. Serial STI measurements in children after cardiac surgery yield useful prognostic information; Echo stroke volume determinations and thus cardiac index correlate well with measurements from traditional invasive monitoring. Well-designed studies will lead to an increase in the number of ECG applications in hemodynamic monitoring.

Pulsed Doppler Cardiac Output

Further development of ultrasound technology has enabled determination of cardiac output by the application of the Doppler principle:

$$V = \frac{\Delta f_c}{2f_o \mathrm{Cos}\Theta}$$

which states that the velocity of a moving object (V, e.g., red blood cells) is equal to the ultrasound frequency shift (Δf_c) divided by twice the speed of sound (f_o) times the cosine of the angle of incidence of the ultrasound beam on the directional axis of movement (Θ).[7] CosΘ is generally assumed to be 1, because the angle of incidence is 0 to 15° for a suprasternal approach to the ascending aorta. This technique assumes a uniform velocity profile in the ascending aorta and thus readily measures the mean aortic velocity. Standard Echo monitoring can be used to measure the aortic root diameter, calculate its area (A), and thus determine flow (cardiac output = VA). This technique has been validated in children by Alverson and colleagues,[8] who compared it with Fick's cardiac output determinations (r^2 = 0.96). It has subsequently been used to study infants of diabetic mothers and neonates with transient myocardial dysfunction.[9, 10] Not all studies have been supportive. Notterman and associates reported that compared with thermodilution, pulsed Doppler technology was inadequate to guide therapy in critically ill children.[11]

The Doppler equipment necessary to determine cardiac output is readily available and provides a noninvasive, reliable technique for determining cardiac output, especially in neonates. It is, however, expensive. Newer applications of this technology include placing Doppler crystals endotracheally or esophageally, with at least preliminary good results.[12, 13] Placement of Doppler ultrasound probes intraoperatively may provide direct continuous measurement of aortic output postoperatively.[14]

Nuclear Cardiology

Radionuclide imaging techniques can be used to evaluate both structural and functional aspects of cardiac performance safely and noninvasively in critically ill children. These techniques have proved useful in diagnosing congenital heart disease, demonstrating and quantifying intracardiac shunts, monitoring for myocardial ischemia in neonates, and determining ventricular function indices. By determining radionuclide counts in systole and diastole, EF can be accurately determined by either first-pass or equilibrium methods.[15] By applying the dye-dilution principle and extrapolating the decay curve of LV activity, cardiac output can be determined. Although this approach has been well correlated with invasive techniques in adults, this correlation is not available for children. Several studies have documented the effectiveness of radionuclide imaging in serially assessing myocardial performance in children. For example, in cystic fibrosis, gated blood pool analysis was used to monitor both LV and RV function.[16] Gated blood pool techniques have also proved useful in quantitating both aortic and mitral regurgitation in children. Radionuclide ventriculography has been demonstrated to determine EF reliably, even in complex congenital heart diseases such as the single ventricle.[15] The use of radionuclide techniques in the ICU could potentially provide a noninvasive and effective method to serially monitor cardiac function in critically ill children.

Impedance Cardiography

The concept of thoracic electrical impedance plethysmography as a noninvasive measure of cardiac output holds great fascination for pediatric intensivists.[17] It is noninvasive, easy to apply, and virtually risk free. Unfortunately, this promise has not been fulfilled. The accuracy of impedance cardiography in the electrically charged atmosphere of an ICU is not sufficient to permit monitoring of an individual child's status. This technology may be useful in large populations of stable patients to determine hemodynamic responses to specific interventions.[18] It is inaccurate in the presence of shunts, mechanical ventilation, and low-output states.[19]

Transcutaneous Oxygen Sensors

Providing oxygen at the cellular level is the function of hemodynamic support. Although determining the partial pressure of oxygen is not generally considered to be part of hemodynamic monitoring, the use of transcutaneous oxygen sensors in the pediatric ICU to monitor critically ill children is discussed in Chapter 31.

Pulse Oximetry

The most useful monitor of overall cardiorespiratory function is pulse oximetry.[20] The light-emitting diodes emit light at 660 nm (red) and 925 nm (infrared). The light passes through soft tissues and is detected by a sensor placed 180° from the diode. Because the arterial bed is pulsatile, a cyclic change in the light path length occurs, generating a plethysmographic waveform. The pulse oximeter measures light absorption from this pulsatile waveform only and thus eliminates interference from nonpulsable absorption such as venous blood, soft tissues, and bone. By applying Beer's law (relating the concentration of saturated and unsaturated hemoglobin to absorptivity, path length, and percentage of light transmission), a beat-to-beat measurement of oxyhemoglobin and deoxyhemoglobin is made. This technique is tremendously reliable in children. Apart from providing respiratory function monitoring, it can also detect changes in hemodynamic shunts. For example, in persistence of the fetal circulation, preductal saturation may be 95% to 100% and postductally may be less, thus reflecting the degree of right-to-left transductal shunting. An increase in PVR increases the amount of shunting and decreases the postductal saturation. The author has found this technique to be very valuable in monitoring the extremely stormy hemodynamic course of these children. Pulse oximetry can also be used to assess perfusion distal to arterial catheters, overall perfusion status, and blood pressure.

A further potential application of oximetry is the combination of peripheral pulse oximetry to determine arterial saturation, mixed venous oximetry via an indwelling catheter, and oxygen consumption measurement. The availability of these parameters should allow continuous measurement of cardiac output by applying the Fick principle. Oximetric catheters are available for pediatric use and are routinely placed in the PA to determine mixed venous saturations and in the jugular bulb as a monitor of cerebral perfusion.[21]

INVASIVE MONITORING TECHNIQUES

Peripheral Artery Catheterization

The indications for invasive arterial monitoring in the pediatric ICU are similar to those in the adult ICU.[22] Peripheral artery lines are used to monitor the pulse, blood pressure, and arterial blood gases, as well as to provide ready access for serial blood sampling. Although useful for hemodynamically stable children, noninvasive blood pressure monitoring by either oscillometric or ultrasound techniques frequently overestimates blood pressure in children in shock.[23, 24]

The method for placing peripheral arterial catheters in larger children does not differ significantly from that for adults. Infants and small children require a modified technique. The first step is a modified Allen test, performed to assess the patency of the collateral circulation. The radial and ulnar arteries are compressed so that blood drains from the hand. This may be aided by passive flexion and extension in small children. The ulnar artery is then released, and the entire hand, especially the distal part of the forefinger and thumb, is carefully observed for flushing. Refill should be complete within 10 seconds. A similar procedure can be carried out in the foot by compressing the dorsalis pedis and posterior tibial arteries.[22]

Although palpation usually identifies the vessel and its anatomy in larger patients, it is often inadequate in small infants whose arterial lumen is only a few millimeters wide. In these cases, a Doppler flow detection probe identifies arterial pulsations. Alternatively, a transilluminator focuses intense light on the tissues of a small infant to illuminate the artery as a dark, pulsatile line, allowing cannulation under direct visualization. The tip of the transilluminator may generate enough heat to burn an infant's skin, so a heat filter should be used and contact time should be minimized. After the vessel is identified, the skin over the artery is cleaned and draped using the aseptic technique. The skin is punctured with an 18-gauge needle so that the subsequently inserted small Teflon cannula is not snagged on the skin and thus distorted during its entry into the arterial lumen. In small children, it is useful to tape the hand gently but securely before inserting the cannula. The digits should be left in clear view to monitor blanching or discoloration. After the stylet has transfixed (passed through) the artery, it is withdrawn. The cannula is then slowly withdrawn until blood return is brisk. It is then advanced along the arterial lumen. If percutaneous catheterization fails, an arterial cutdown may be necessary; however, working with a dissected, free artery in a hemorrhagic field is generally less successful than transfixing an immobilized, closed vessel.

A small cannula in a large artery is less likely to produce thromboembolism than a large cannula in a small artery. Although the risk of thromboembolism may be decreased by using the brachial artery in children, this site is avoided because of the potential for limb loss. Increasingly, when smaller arteries cannot be cannulated, the axillary or femoral arteries may be considered. Axillary cannulation is permissible owing to the rich anastomosis around the shoulder and lack of long-term sequelae.[25] The femoral artery has been avoided in the past in children for fear of invading the underlying hip joint capsule and causing osteoarthritis. Its proximity to the perineum, a source of infection, further contraindicates the use of the femoral artery; however, careful aseptic technique should reduce the risk of both complications. A prospective study of femoral artery cannulation in 74 children 1 to 10 years of age revealed a high rate of success (73 of 74 attempts). Transient blanching occurred in 11% of the children. One episode of infection was reported.[26] The use of both femoral vessels on the same side is strongly discouraged because of the likelihood of compromised limb perfusion.[22] Use of the superficial temporal artery is contraindicated because of the risk of temporal lobe infarction due to retrograde perfusion during flushing. For these reasons, radial artery lines are most common; however, the dorsalis pedis and posterior tibial arteries may be similarly cannulated.[22]

Maintenance of arterial lines requires compulsive care and attention. Nothing should be infused through an arterial line other than heparinized saline at a slow rate (2 mL/h). Blood samples that are withdrawn through the catheter should either be discarded or, if the infant is too small to tolerate this blood loss, reinfused through a venous line. A 1-kg infant has approximately 80 mL of blood; hence, 10 2-mL samples contain 25% of his or her blood volume. For this reason, an accurate record of the blood amount withdrawn and the amount of solution flushed or infused through the line should be maintained. Circulation in the limb should be constantly monitored by assessing the patient's color, capillary refill, presence of pulses, and temperature. A pulse oximeter probe distal to the insertion site may serve as an early warning perfusion monitor.

Removal of the peripheral artery lines using an aseptic technique should be followed by continuous occlusive pressure on the arterial site for 10 minutes. Because blood flow is necessary to supply clotting factors to the wound, clamping pressure should not be used. Any duration of bleeding longer than 10 minutes suggests a coagulopathy, and pressure should be continued for another 10 minutes. Pressure dressings are contraindicated because they may compromise the collateral circulation and impair the blood supply to the distal limb.

Complications

Catheter disconnection and bleeding from the catheter and tubing are probably the most frequent catheter-associated complications.[22] Other complications include distal ischemia and infection. Prevention of these complications includes careful monitoring of the perfusion distal to the catheter (pulse oximetry), appropriate site selection, strict aseptic technique, and dressing changes as used for hyperalimentation lines. Connections in the line (e.g., stopcocks) and extension should be minimized. Retrograde perfusion and embolization can occur from any site; thus, careful flushing techniques and avoidance of the temporal arteries are required. This precaution is also important for axillary lines in order to avoid retrograde cerebral embolization.[27] Acute ischemic injury should be constantly monitored for and promptly treated. Long-term sequelae may include nerve injury and carpal tunnel syndrome. Every physician responsible for children with arterial catheters must be aware of how to treat complications.

Interpretation

Attaining normal blood pressure may not be sufficient in treating critically ill children. What is normal for a well child is not normal or necessarily even desirable for a critically ill child. Attention to other parameters of tissue perfusion, such as skin temperature, capillary refill, blood pH, and serum lactate levels, are just as important, because blood pressure is the last parameter to decline in decreased perfusion states. This is particularly true of children, who have less rigid, more responsive vascular beds than adults and who tend to compensate extremely well for a decreased cardiac output.

In children, the frequent presence of a vascular left-to-right shunt may alter the pressure tracing. Children with PDA or aortic incompetence show a widened pulse pressure, rapid diastolic pressure drop, and reduced diastolic pressure. Diastolic pressure analysis can relate left-to-right shunting in these patients to diastolic half-time; arterial pressure decay curves have thus been used to diagnose and monitor the response to therapy.

Central Catheterization

Central catheter insertion is indicated in any child, regardless of size, when the benefit of accurate hemodynamic monitoring outweighs the risks involved. These conditions include: (1) low-output states that are not rapidly responsive to volume loading (i.e., sepsis, hemorrhagic shock, and severe head trauma); (2) uncertain hemodynamic states after cardiothoracic surgery; and (3) situations requiring advanced mechanical ventilatory support.

Central venous catheters can be inserted into the superior vena cava or right atrium via the antecubital, subclavian, jugular, or femoral veins, using meticulous aseptic technique. Although the femoral vein is the preferred site for cardiac angiography studies, prolonged catheterization at this site risks thromboembolism of the iliac veins and inferior vena cava as well as possible sepsis from the perineum. In particular, the proximity of the child's hip capsule to the vein increases the risk of septic arthritis, which can rapidly lead to permanent destruction of the growing hip joint. This pediatric dogma has been challenged. Reports prospectively documenting the safety of femoral venous cannulation have demonstrated that this relatively simple approach has no greater incidence of complications than other central approaches.[28, 29] Central pressures monitored through femoral lines must be cautiously interpreted in children. Abdominal pressure does not accurately reflect right atrial pressure, and when knowing the right atrial pressure is important, care must be taken to ensure right atrial, intrathoracic placement of the distal end of the femoral catheter. The possibility of paradoxical air embolism across either a patent foramen ovale, intraventricular defect (e.g., tetralogy of Fallot), or great vessel shunt must be rigorously avoided by meticulous nursing care.

Left atrial catheters can be directly inserted into the left atrial appendage of the right superior pulmonary vein during surgery to monitor LV filling pressures.[30] These catheters are a potential embolic source downstream from vital cerebral, myocardial, and renal blood supplies; therefore, nothing other than a slow, heparinized continuous flush should be administered through these lines except in the direst of emergencies. If blood cannot be freely aspirated, the catheter should be removed rather than flushed. All connections, transducers, and lines that are connected to the left atrial line should be clearly and obviously marked to avoid inadvertent use. The risk of cerebral embolization and its subsequent permanent neurologic deficit should be made known to all personnel caring for the child. With these precautions, left atrial catheterization is a useful substitute or adjunct for PA catheterization in patients with complex congenital heart disease, those requiring intricate operative repair, or those with abnormal pulmonary vasculature.

PA catheters[22, 31, 32, 32a] can be inserted either operatively in children undergoing cardiothoracic surgery for congenital heart disease or subcutaneously. Operatively, catheters are placed directly in the PA or inserted through the RV outflow tract in the RV infundibulum and from there into the PA. Percutaneously, the vascular entry site selection depends on the patient's size and status, as well as the operator's familiarity with the technique. In children older than about 5 years, selection is no different from that in adults. In smaller children, the choice lies between an internal or external femoral or jugular approach. Internal jugular entry is less desirable in patients at risk for intracranial hypertension, because venous drainage may theoretically be impaired.

Preparation of the PA catheter before its insertion is no different from that described in the adult literature; however, the presence of a right-to-left intracardiac shunt, at either the atrial or ventricular level (as in tetralogy of Fallot), requires added care and full aseptic technique to avoid systemic and subsequent cerebral embolism. Generally, the distance from the insertion site to the second left intercostal space determines how far to insert the catheter. If this distance is exceeded by more than 10 cm, the catheter should be withdrawn and reinserted.

Once vascular access has been obtained, insertion of the catheter into the PA is essentially the same as for adults. A nurse or physician who is not involved in the catheterization should monitor the child during the procedure. Heart tone must be continuously audible so that the operator can listen for ectopic beats. The continuous pressure tracing from a cathode-ray oscilloscope should be used to guide insertion. Manipulating the catheter through the small heart requires patience and a gentle technique but is almost always successful.

Complications

The most common complication during the insertion and positioning of central catheters in children is induction of either atrial or ventricular premature contractions. However, constant vigilance and prompt withdrawal of the catheter prevent these from becoming serious; further treatment is almost never necessary. A second type of complication occurs if the cross-sectional area of the inflated balloon significantly obstructs or occludes the RV outflow tract at the pulmonary valve for more than a few seconds. The result is hypoxemia, bradycardia, hypotension, and rapid decompensation. Third, balloon distention of the pulmonary valve ring and PA can significantly increase the PA systolic and diastolic pressures, especially in neonates recovering from persistent transitional circulation. In children with hyperactive PAs, this sudden PVR increase may be detrimental. Catheter knotting, pulmonary and tricuspid valve damage, catastrophic PA rupture, and even papillary muscle avulsion are also potential hazards.

Thromboembolic complications after catheter insertion are caused by the presence of a foreign body in the circulation. Emboli from the catheter tip or in the introducer sheath can cause pulmonary infarction. Leaving the introducer sheath in situ may allow clot formation between the catheter and the sheath wall, with serious potential for venous embolism. In the presence of a right-to-left intracardiac shunt, this may lead to systemic embolism. The risk of emboli can be reduced by using an introducer with a side-arm attachment, thus allowing continuous flushing of the introducer sheath with a heparinized solution, and by decreasing the length of time the sheath is inserted.

The risk of infection requires meticulous technique, similar to that used for hyperalimentation lines. Changing sites every 72 hours may not be practical in children with limited venous access; however, central catheters should be removed as soon as their monitoring functions are no longer essential. It is not advisable to leave these catheters in position merely to provide venous access.

Blood loss from the entry wound during or after catheter insertion requires careful monitoring and, if necessary, blood replacement. The absence of a preexisting bleeding diathesis should be confirmed before catheter insertion. Platelet consumption coagulopathy may be related to prolonged PA catheterization; daily platelet monitoring is advisable when these lines remain in place for more than a few days.

Measurements

If a child is invasively monitored, pressures and blood samples from all chambers should be studied for abnormal pressure gradients and oxygen saturation variations.[22, 31, 32] Right atrial pressures; RV end-diastolic and systolic pressures; PA systolic, diastolic, and mean pressures; and PA occlusion pressure are required for a complete study. Blood samples from the right atrium, RV, and PA demonstrate any significant left-to-right shunts. Continual monitoring of the PA pressures after catheterization and serial determinations of the cardiac output, PVR, and SVR are indications for leaving the catheter in situ.

The techniques for determining cardiac output by dye dilution, the Fick principle, and thermodilution are essentially the same in children as in adults. Small (2–5 French) thermodilution catheters have been developed for children. Cardiac output is usually expressed as cardiac index, which is the cardiac output per square meter. This value, generally 3.0 to 5.0 $L \cdot min^{-1}$ per square meter, is age independent, although normative data in children have not been determined. Because a child's body surface area is usually less than 1 m^2, the cardiac index is usually greater than the cardiac output, in contrast to these measurements in adults.

Unfortunately, there is no accurate way to assess cardiac output in the presence of valvular regurgitation or intracardiac shunting. Trends may even be misleading. Clearly, the degree of shunting and amount of valvular regurgitation vary with cardiovascular status; for example, increased systemic resistance may increase left-to-right shunting, whereas hypoxia and induced pulmonary vasospasm may enhance a right-to-left shunt. However, it is not possible to predict the degree at which these changes affect cardiac output. An analysis of the complex dynamic relationship between the pulmonary and systemic circulations in the presence of intracardiac shunting requires experience and skill.

SVR and PVR may be used to assess the response to cardiovascular therapy. Resistance is the reciprocal of conductance; it equals the pressure reduction divided by the flow. The pressure reduction across the systemic circulation is the difference between the mean arterial blood pressure (MAP) and the central venous pressure (CVP); therefore, SVR may be indexed as SVRI = (MAP − CVP)/flow. In pediatrics, the flow used is the cardiac index; SVRI is therefore expressed in R units. The normal SVRI in children is 15 to 20 R units. PVRI is similarly described as MPAP − LAP/flow, where MPAP is mean PA pressure and LAP is the left atrial pressure (also called the PA occlusion pressure). PVRI is generally $\frac{1}{20}$ of the SVRI; normal PVRI is 1 to 3 R units.

The determination and relevance of ventricular stroke work indices and other derived parameters of ventricular function are similar in adults and children. Although these calculations are only approximations, they are frequently useful in guiding therapeutic interventions and in monitoring trends in preload, afterload, and contractility. Congenital heart disease and atrial or ventricular intercommunication may equalize right-sided and left-sided pressures, making individual ventricular performance impossible to determine.

Neonatal Catheterization

Catheterization of one of the two umbilical arteries in a neonate is routine for intensive care. In neonates as old as 8 days, UACs can be inserted directly into the cut vessel lumen or by cutdown on the umbilical vessels as they pass caudally from the cord in the abdominal wall. The catheters may be placed either above the diaphragm or below the third lumbar vertebra.[33] The complication rate appears to be high with either position; however, placement below the fourth lumbar vertebra avoids the celiac and mesenteric blood supplies as well as the renal arteries, thereby decreasing the risk of thromboembolism from the vessel intima and catheter tip. Patency is maintained by a slow, continuous infusion of heparinized saline. The standard rate of 2 mL heparin per milliliter of normal saline for infants may provide more sodium than a small premature infant (lighter than 1500 g) can tolerate. No other drugs or solutions are ever infused through these lines. No boluses of blood or blood products should be infused. As with other forms of invasive arterial monitoring, the line must be removed at the slightest sign of complications.

Complications associated with UACs are increasingly recognized, thus narrowing the risk-benefit ratio for these readily sited catheters. Septicemia occurs in up to 8% of these infants, compared with one to three cases per thousand liveborn infants, and is in part attributable to the enforced absence of sterile technique during catheter insertion. Seeding of infection to other sites is particularly hazardous if the hip joint becomes involved. Moreover, prophylactic antibiotics do not appear to be useful and risk superinfection with resistant organisms. Daily cultures of the catheter may identify early infection or dangerous colonization. The duration of catheterization should be minimized.

Vascular occlusion caused by thrombosis, embolism, or vasospasm has been identified postmortem in 3.5% to 48% of neonates with UACs and has also been demonstrated in 24% to 95% of infants with UACs undergoing angiography. Vascular occlusion is generally clinically evident by the blanching of the limbs, absence of arterial pulses, and dark discoloration of the toes. More severe manifestations may include renal artery thromboembolism with hematuria and proteinuria, acute vasomotor nephropathy, renal failure, and hypertension. Embolization of spinal arteries causing paraplegia, embolization of the mesenteric blood supply causing gut infarction, and large areas of tissue gangrene have also been reported. The cause of frequent thromboembolism has been attributed to catheter material (particularly polyvinylchloride), catheter fabrication and design, and clotting abnormalities inherent to the sick neonate (high Factor VIII and low antithrombin III). No long-term defects in leg growth or blood pressure are clearly discernible after these transient vaso-occlusive episodes; however, areas of necrosis and gangrene may necessitate plastic repair or even limb amputation.

Other UAC complications include internal hemorrhage and bleeding from the catheter apparatus due to disconnection. Massive hemorrhage has been reported intraperitoneally as well as into the bladder; an infant can suffer a fatal intravesicular hemorrhage within hours of catheterization. Finally, hypoglycemia may follow an infusion of dextrose-containing solutions into the blood supply of the pancreas, leading to islet cell stimulation and consequent hyperinsulinemia and hypoglycemia. It should be noted that the current trend is away from UACs toward noninvasive monitoring of peripheral sites.

Measurements

Catheters in the descending and abdominal aorta are distal to the ductus arteriosus. If the ductus is patent, blood gas levels measured from UAC samples are lower than actual gas saturations in the carotid artery. Such a situation may lead to inadvertent administration of high inspired oxygen levels and the untoward development of retrolental fibroplasia or pulmonary oxygen toxicity. In the presence of right-to-left ductal shunting, right radial artery blood gases or preductal pulse oximetry reflects saturations in the carotid circulation.

FUTURE TRENDS

The trend toward less invasive monitoring as exemplified by pulse oximetry, Echo monitoring, and nuclear cardiography can be expected to continue. The development and application of other noninvasive techniques for monitoring critically ill children is necessary, not only for clinical application but also to help us understand the pathophysiology of critical illness in children. Additional refinement of Echo and Doppler techniques can be expected. Combination of Echo with Doppler-determined flows may allow real-time continuous evaluation of cardiac dynamic function and output.[34] Smaller, more sophisticated ultrasound crystals will allow more accurate measurement of cardiac output[35] and may be more widely applied intraoperatively. The use of duplex Doppler has been shown to be useful in determining RV outputs in infants.[36]

New applications of noninvasive imaging techniques such as positron emission tomography and nuclear magnetic resonance imaging are being increasingly reported. For example, magnetic resonance imaging can yield accurate structural information in congenital heart disease and assess the function of systemic-to-pulmonary shunts. Positron emission tomography offers the exciting ability not only to determine dynamic functional changes but also to monitor myocardial metabolic activity. Although still remote, the potential for these techniques to allow noninvasive monitoring in critically ill children is being explored.

Probably the single greatest problem in pediatric monitoring is reliable determination of cardiac function indices in postoperative cardiac patients with anatomically abnormal hearts. The assumptions inherent in the classic methods of determining cardiac index make these methods unsuitable for precise monitoring. Understanding the hemodynamic status of these children requires synthesis of data from many monitoring modalities. These may include clinical examination findings, Echo anatomic and functional data, invasive pressure analysis, mixed venous oxygen saturations, and Doppler flow studies to understand the entire hemodynamic status. Combining these with sound clinical judgment is necessary to ensure reliable monitoring of critically ill children.

References

1. Strasburger JF: Cardiac arrhythmias in childhood: Diagnostic considerations and treatment. Drugs 1991; 42:974–983.
2. Gillette PC: Supraventricular arrhythmias in children. J Am Coll Cardiol 1985; 5:122B–129B.
3. Vetter VL: Ventricular arrhythmias in patients with congenital heart disease. Cardiovasc Clin 1992; 22:255–273.
4. Seward JB, Khandheria BK, Oh JK, et al: Transesophageal echocardiography: Technique, anatomic correlations, implementation, and clinical application. Mayo Clin Proc 1988; 63:649–680.
5. Muhiudeen I, Roberson D, Silverman NH, et al: Intraoperative echocardiography in infants and children with congenital cardiac shunt lesions; transesophageal versus epicardial echocardiography. J Am Coll Cardiol 1990; 16:687–695.
6. Stumper O, Witsenburg M, Sutherland GR, et al: Transesophageal echocardiographic monitoring of interventional cardiac catheterization in children. J Am Coll Cardiol 1991; 18:1506–1514.
7. Lees MH: Cardiac output determination in the neonate. J Pediatr 1983; 102:709.
8. Alverson DC, Eldridge M, Dillon T, et al: Noninvasive pulsed Doppler determination of cardiac output in neonates and children. J Pediatr 1982; 101:46.
9. Walther FJ, Siassi B, King J, et al: Cardiac output in infants of insulin-dependent diabetic mothers. J Pediatr 1985; 107:109.
10. Walther FJ, Siassi B, Ramadan N, et al: Cardiac output in newborn infants with transient myocardial dysfunction. J Pediatr 1985; 107:781.
11. Notterman DA, Castello FV, Steinberg C, et al: A comparison of thermodilution and pulsed Doppler cardiac output measurement in critically ill children. J Pediatr 1989; 115:554–560.
12. Singer M, Clarke J, Bennett ED: Continuous hemodynamic monitoring by esophageal Doppler. Crit Care Med 1989; 17:447–452.
13. Jaimovich DG, Shabino CL, Nelson CB: Continuous cardiac output measurement by transtracheal Doppler technique in a pediatric patient with septic shock. Crit Care Med 1992; 20:707–710.
14. Keagy BA, Wilcox BR, Lucas CL, et al: Constant postoperative monitoring of cardiac output after correction of congenital heart defects. J Thorac Cardiovasc Surg 1987; 93:658–664.
15. Beller G: Nuclear cardiology: Current indications and clinical usefulness. *In*: Current Problems in Cardiology. Vol 10. O'Rourke RA (Ed). Chicago, Year Book Medical Publishers, 1985, pp 4–76.
16. Chipps BE, Alderson PO, Roland JMA, et al: Non-invasive evaluation of ventricular function in cystic fibrosis. J Pediatr 1979; 95:379.

17. Tibballs J: A comparative study of cardiac output in neonates supported by mechanical ventilation: Measurement with thoracic electrical bioimpedance and pulsed Doppler ultrasound. J Pediatr 1989; 114:632–635.
18. Michell JJ, Lucking SE, Chaten FC, et al: Trending of impedance-monitored cardiac variables: Method and statistical power analysis of 100 control studies in a pediatric intensive care unit. Crit Care Med 1990; 18:645–650.
19. Miles DS, Gotshall RW, Golden JC, et al: Accuracy of electrical impedance cardiography for measuring cardiac output in children with congenital heart defects. Am J Cardiol 1988; 61:612–616.
20. Fait CD, Wetzel RC, Dean JM, et al: Pulse oximetry in critically ill children. J Clin Monit 1985; 1:232.
21. Gayle MO, Frewen TC, Armstrong RF, et al: Jugular venous bulb catheterization in infants and children. Crit Care Med 1989; 17:385–388.
22. Miller CL, Burrows FA: Invasive monitoring in the pediatric patient. Int Anesthesiol Clin 1992; 30:91–108.
23. Stopfkuchen H: Hemodynamic monitoring in childhood. Intensive Care Med 1989; 15:S27–S31.
24. Weindling AM: Blood pressure monitoring in the newborn. Arch Dis Child 1989; 64:444–447.
25. Lawless S, Orr R: Axillary arterial monitoring of pediatric patients. Pediatrics 1989; 84:273–275.
26. Graves PW, Davis AL, Maggi JC, et al: Femoral artery cannulation for monitoring in critically ill children: Prospective study. Crit Care Med 1990; 18:1363–1366.
27. Butt WW, Gow R, Whyte H, et al: Complications resulting from use of arterial catheters: Retrograde flow and rapid elevation in blood pressure. Pediatrics 1985; 76:250–254.
28. Kanter RK, Zimmerman JJ, Strauss RH, et al: Central venous catheter insertion by femoral vein: Safety and effectiveness for the pediatric patient. Pediatrics 1986; 77:842–847.
29. Stenzel JP, Green TP, Fuhrman BP, et al: Percutaneous femoral venous catheterizations: A prospective study of complications. J Pediatr 1989; 114:411–415.
30. Satur CMR, Stubington SR, Crew AD, et al: Operative insertion of a transvenous left atrial pressure monitoring line. Ann Thorac Surg 1990; 50:1004–1005.
31. Damen J, Wever JEAT: The use of balloon-tipped pulmonary artery catheters in children undergoing cardiac surgery. Intensive Care Med 1987; 13:266–272.
32. Introna RPS, Martin DC, Pruett JK, et al: Percutaneous pulmonary artery catheterization in pediatric cardiovascular anesthesia: Insertion techniques and use. Anesth Analg 1990; 70:562–566.
32a. Abou-Khalil B, Scalea TM, Trooskin SZ, et al: Hemodynamic responses to shock in young trauma patients: Need for invasive monitoring. Crit Care Med 1994; 22:633–639.
33. Squire SJ, Homung TL, Kirchhoff KT: Comparing two methods of umbilical artery catheter placement. Am J Perinatol 1990; 7:8–12.
34. Caidahl K, Mellander M, Sabel K-G, et al: Estimation of stroke volume using Doppler echocardiography and left ventricular echocardiographic dimensions in infants and children. Acta Pediatr Scand Suppl 1986; 329:114–119.
35. Niclou R, Teague SM, Lee R: Clinical evaluation of a diameter sensing Doppler cardiac output meter. Crit Care Med 1990; 18:428–432.
36. Walther FJ, Van Bel F, Ebrahimi M: Duplex versus unguided pulsed Doppler measurements of right ventricular output in newborn infants. Acta Pediatr Scand 1990; 79:41–46.

SECTION V
IMAGING

Stephen M. Ayres

CHAPTER 40
Imaging of the Chest in the Intensive Care Setting

Lynn Coppage, MD • Howard Jolles, MD • Daniel A. Henry, MD

The portable chest radiograph (PCXR) remains the initial and most frequently ordered imaging study in the intensive care unit (ICU) patient population. Efficacy studies have shown that a significant percentage (31–65%) of these portable films have documented an unexpected finding, many of which require a change in catheter or tube position or in patient management.[1–4] It is, therefore, essential that the radiographs be of consistently high quality and that they be obtained and interpreted in a timely fashion. To facilitate this process, we have developed a priority system for ordering portable chest radiographs based on the acuity of patient need, following strict clinical indicators. Our ICU teams have found it useful to conduct daily morning rounds with a radiologist to discuss issues of patient management as they relate to radiologic examinations performed in the intervening time period. This has improved patient care through prompt detection and communication of unsuspected abnormalities in this most critically ill patient population.

Although plain radiographs are the mainstay in radiologic diagnosis of chest disease, imaging has expanded to include bedside sonography, nuclear medicine studies, and computed tomography in the appropriate clinical setting.

TECHNICAL CONSIDERATIONS

Conventional Radiography

Portable radiography of the chest is generally obtained with 75 to 80 kV (peak), the exposure adjusted by varying mA. A wide-latitude film–screen combination may be helpful to minimize errors in exposure. The radiographs are obtained in the anteroposterior projection with the patient upright whenever possible. Because of space limitations in the ICU, a minimum film-tube distance of 40 inches is used rather than the 72 inches preferred in the radiology department.

By its very nature, portable chest radiography suffers from several disadvantages, some technical and others related to the patient. The kilovoltage and milliamperage are limited, so that exposures are relatively long, and image contrast may be excessive.[5] Antiscatter grids are not practical because they result in higher radiation dose and create technical problems of grid cutoff and mandatory film-tube distances. Automatic exposure devices are not commonly available, leading to technical variations that cause difficulty in comparing serial films on the same patient. The illness of the patient, together with multiple associated life-support devices and an inability to control for respiratory and body motion, is an added obstacle to good image quality. Considering that portable chest examinations make up about 50% of all chest films in large institutions,[6] the importance of dedicated, competent, portable radiograph technologists and an effective quality-assurance program cannot be overemphasized.

Digital Radiography

To address these technical and patient-related problems encountered in portable chest radiography, digital image technology has shown promising results. Digital, or computed radiography, uses a phosphor plate rather than film to store the radiographic image and has the advantages of consistent film density, flexible image processing, and lower radiation dose. The diagnostic accuracy and confidence level of these systems are similar to those obtained with conventional screen–film radiography.[7]

Digital image processing identifies the portion of the dynamic range containing the diagnostic information and then adjusts the final output for display at a consistent, optimized contrast and density. It is this compensatory control that obviates repeat examinations because of errors in exposure or the necessity to interpret films of marginal diagnostic quality. These advantages, however, do not obviate the need for accurate patient positioning and alignment of the beam, and there is no time savings for each portable examination. Also, there may be a slight delay in waiting for image processing. Spontaneous downtime can jeopardize the efficiency of the entire portable operation if only one image-processing unit is available. Last, enthusiasm for purchasing a digital radiography system must be tempered by the cost of the unit and associated service fees. Widespread utilization of this technology will likely hinge on the development of hospital-wide computer networks with the capability to both store these images and transmit them locally or to distant sites.[7]

LIFE-SUPPORT CATHETERS AND TUBES

A significant percentage of clinically unsuspected findings on PCXR in the ICU setting relate to malposition or complications of life-support catheters and tubes.[1,2] Bekemeyer and colleagues found that 27% of newly placed catheters or tubes were improperly positioned and that 6% resulted in a radiographically visible complication of the intervention.[2] Although many such abnormalities are not immediately life threatening, some require rapid correction to avoid clinical deterioration in patients with marginal cardiopulmonary reserve.

Endotracheal Tubes

Improper position of endotracheal tubes (ETT) has been demonstrated in 12% to 15% of chest radiographs obtained in intubated patients.[4,8] An analysis of the position of the tube tip as it relates to the carina and the degree of neck

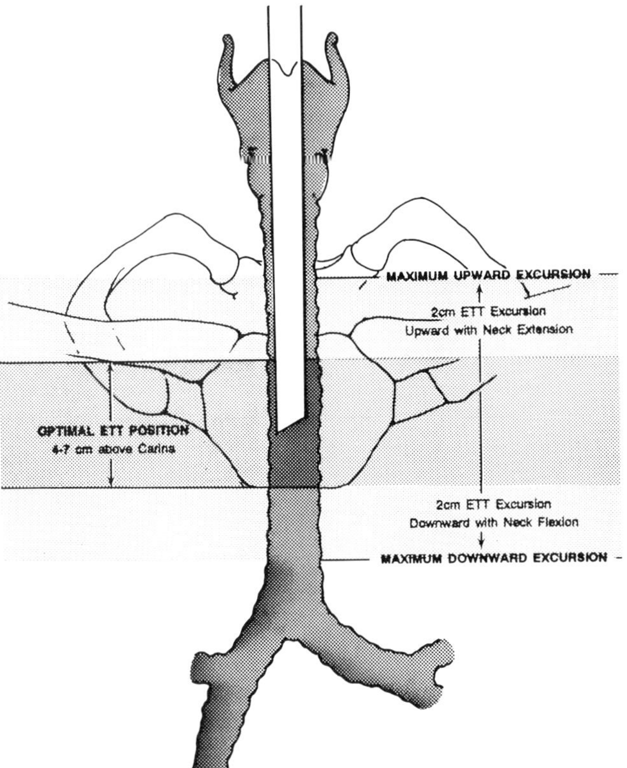

Figure 40–1. Illustration demonstrating the zone of optimal ETT position and maximum safe excursion *(shaded areas)* from the zone boundaries with neck movement. ETT excursion outside these areas may be problematic.

flexion or extension should be routinely performed on each radiograph. Most ETTs have a dense radiopaque strip and a somewhat less dense, but still visible, opposite wall. Optimally, in an adult patient, the tube tip should rest 4 to 7 cm above the carina with the patient's head in a neutral position (i.e., with the mandible, if visible, projecting over the fifth or sixth cervical vertebral body). The location of the carina can be established in most cases by following the inferior wall of the left mainstem bronchus proximally. Because the tube is secured at the nose or mouth, there is up to 2 cm of excursion of the tube tip, downward with neck flexion or upward with extension (Fig. 40–1).[9] In addition, rotation of the head will augment this excursion. Attention should also be paid to the inflated cuff, which should not bulge the tracheal walls, because this may produce ischemia, predisposing to tracheostenosis, tracheomalacia, or tracheoesophageal fistula (Fig. 40–2).

The most common complication detected on the first postintubation PCXR is ETT malposition. Because of the less acute carinal angle on the right, right mainstem intubation occurs more frequently (Fig. 40–3).[8] If this malposition goes undetected, there may be subsequent atelectasis of the left lung accompanied by an increased incidence of contralateral hyperinflation and pneumothorax.[10] Esophageal intubation, although most often apparent clinically, may be first suggested on the chest radiograph by visualization of the ETT lateral to the tracheal wall, gaseous distention of the stomach or esophagus, and displacement of the trachea by the inflated cuff. The optimal radiographic examination to distinguish between tracheal versus esophageal intubation is the 25° right posterior oblique projection with a nasogastric tube in place and the patient's head turned to the right.[11] In 96% of patients, this view is diagnostic.

Mechanical ventilation may alter the appearance of the PCXR considerably.[12] The institution of positive pressure, particularly positive end-expiratory pressure (PEEP), will improve lung volumes and may result in an apparent radiographic improvement. Serial radiographs should, therefore, be interpreted, whenever possible, with knowledge of current ventilatory settings.

Tracheostomy Tubes

Patients requiring long-term assisted ventilation may require placement of a tracheostomy tube (TT). Postplacement radiographs, including a lateral film when feasible, should be assessed for proper TT alignment and position (i.e., the tube should overlay the air column and run parallel to the

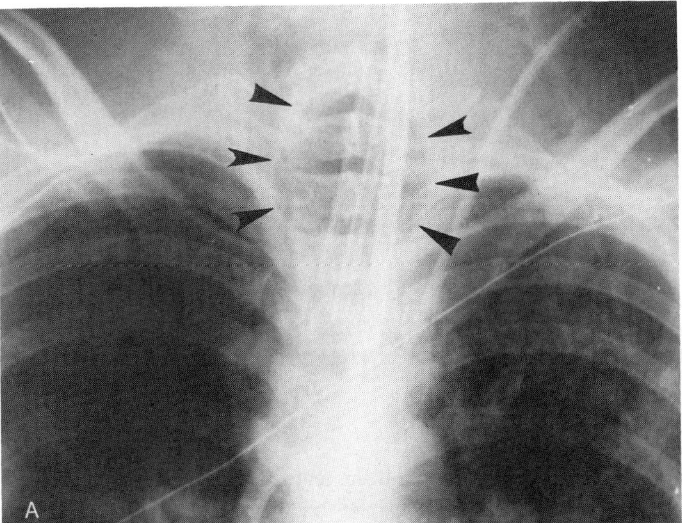

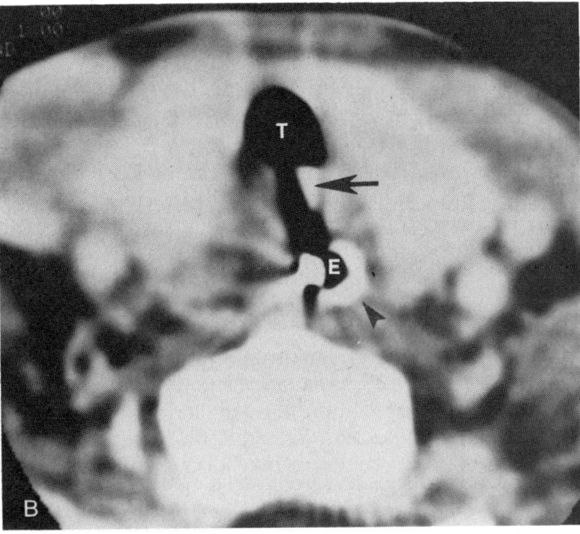

Figure 40–2. *A,* A coned-down anteroposterior view of the upper chest demonstrates overdistention of the radiolucent endotracheal tube cuff *(arrowheads)* that exceeds the diameter of the normal trachea. *B,* The patient subsequently developed signs and symptoms of recurrent aspiration, which prompted computed tomography evaluation. A transaxial image at the level of the thyroid gland reveals a fistulous communication *(arrow)* between the posterior wall of the trachea *(T)* and the esophagus *(E).* Note the nasogastric tube *(arrowhead).*

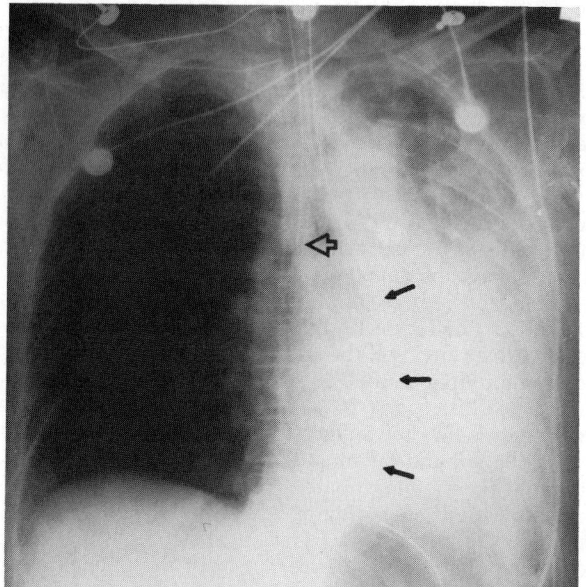

Figure 40–3. The tip of the ETT *(open arrow)* extends into the right mainstem bronchus, and hyperinflation of the right lung is present. Signs of volume loss of the left lung include increased opacity of the hemithorax with ipsilateral shift of the heart and mediastinal structures. Note the leftward displacement of the radiopaque nasogastric tube *(arrows)*.

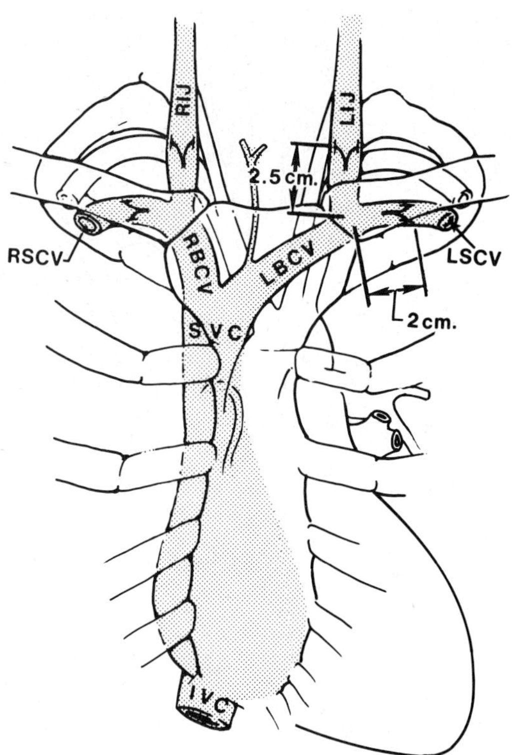

Figure 40–4. Diagram illustrating central venous anatomy. The most proximal venous valves (V) are located 2 to 2.5 cm from the origin of the left and right brachiocephalic veins (LBCV and RBCV, respectively), in the left and right internal jugular (LIJ and NIJ, respectively), and in the left and right subclavian veins (LSCV and RSCV, respectively) Central venous catheter tips should rest distal to these valves, optimally in the superior vena cava (SVC).

tracheal walls). Persistent acute angulation can damage the tracheal wall and erode into the mediastinum. Overdistention of the cuff may lead to mucosal ulceration or tracheostenosis.

Pneumomediastinum may be detected on the first postplacement radiograph, and close follow-up is indicated because a persistent pneumomediastinum may be the result of malposition or an ongoing air leak. A widened mediastinum should suggest the possibility of hemorrhage. Pneumothorax in the setting of recent TT placement is seen most commonly after inadvertent puncture of the apical pleura.

Central Venous Pressure Catheters

Single- and double-lumen central venous pressure (CVP) catheters are used routinely in the ICU setting. Insertion may be either by the subclavian or internal jugular veins; less commonly, the external jugular vein may be accessed. For accurate CVP readings, the catheter tip should rest beyond the most distal venous valves of the large central veins[13, 14] and optimally in one of the brachiocephalic veins or in the superior vena cava (Fig. 40–4). Suboptimal catheter positions are demonstrated in up to one third of PCXRs after catheter placement.[15] Insertion into the right atrium or ventricle is associated with an increased incidence of arrhythmias and cardiac perforation with hemopericardium and tamponade.[16, 17] An unusual-appearing catheter course may indicate an extravascular position, an arterial location (Fig. 40–5), or cannulation of a smaller venous vessel such as the internal thoracic or left superior intercostal vein. Variations in venous anatomy may also result in seemingly peculiar appearances.

Other complications related to CVP catheter placement (Fig. 40–6) are cited in Table 40–1, with pneumothorax foremost on the list, and present on as many as 6% of the immediate postinsertion PCXRs.[18]

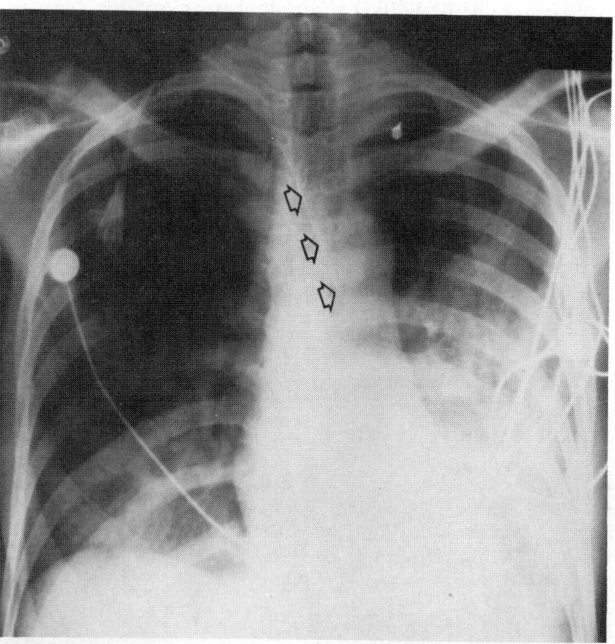

Figure 40–5. PCXR following central line placement presumably through the right internal jugular vein shows the catheter extending across the midline *(open arrows)* in a course more medial than expected. Although an extravascular location could not be excluded, arterial catheterization was confirmed by pressure readings.

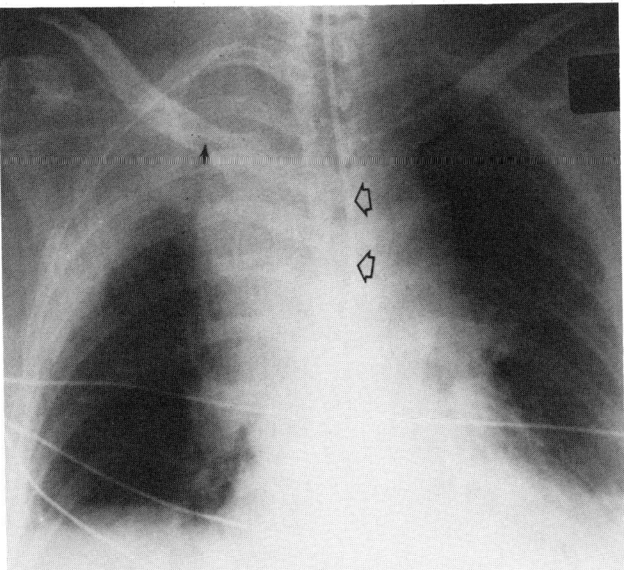

Figure 40–6. The tip of a right subclavian cordis sheath *(small arrow)* is faintly seen projecting over the medial right clavicle. Hemorrhage into the extrapleural space and mediastinum results in abnormal soft tissue density along the right lateral chest wall and lung apex as well as in marked mediastinal widening. Mass effect in the mediastinum is suggested by leftward deviation of the nasogastric tube *(open arrows).*

Swan-Ganz Catheters

The Swan-Ganz catheter (SGC) is used routinely to provide physiologic data regarding cardiac function by estimating left atrial pressure and left ventricular end-diastolic pressure when placed in the wedged position. Such measurements aid in distinguishing between cardiac and noncardiac causes of pulmonary edema.[19] It may also be used to determine cardiac output by the thermodilution technique. To achieve the most accurate pulmonary arterial wedge pressure reading, the catheter should be "floated" into the dependent, posterior lower lobe arterial branches, where it will lie at or below the level of the left atrium in the supine

TABLE 40–1. Radiographically Visible Complications of Central Catheter Placement

Malposition
Pneumothorax
Venous or arterial perforation with extrapleural, pleural, or mediastinal hemorrhage or ectopic infusion
Cardiac perforation
Retained introducer wire or catheter fragment
Knotted catheter
Air embolus

position (zone III).[20] Catheters directed into more anterior branches of the upper lobes or middle lobe (zones I and II) may reflect alveolar pressures and thereby give less precise readings (Fig. 40–7). Increasing PEEP will recruit a greater percentage of the pulmonary capillary bed to zones I and II, adding increased importance to this principle. When the balloon is deflated after a reading, the catheter tip should recoil back into its optimal position in a central pulmonary artery. An inflated balloon should never be observed on the PCXR.

The use of the SGC is not without risk. Complications include those mentioned in Table 40–1 and also problems that are unique to this particular device. If the catheter is left in a peripheral position, perforation and distal hemorrhage may result (Fig. 40–8).[21] Pulmonary artery rupture can also occur if the balloon is inflated in the wedged location. Excess catheter coiled in the sinus portion of the right ventricle predisposes to cardiac arrhythmias and sudden distal migration of the tip. Pulmonary artery pseudoaneurysm has been reported as a complication of SGC monitoring.[22]

Intra-Aortic Counterpulsation Balloon

The intra-aortic balloon pump is being used in patients with cardiogenic shock and in some cases as an assist device after cardiac surgery. The balloon, which is approximately 26 cm in length, is inflated with helium during diastole, thereby augmenting coronary artery perfusion.[23] Generally introduced through the common femoral artery, its radiopaque distal tip should be visible in the proximal descending thoracic aorta beyond the takeoff of the left subclavian artery

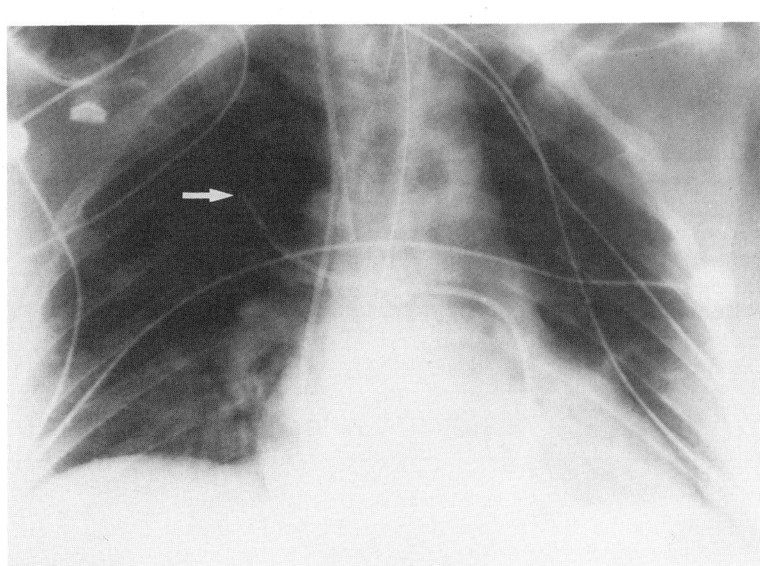

Figure 40–7. A Swan-Ganz catheter directed into an upper lobe branch of the right pulmonary artery *(arrow)* lies above the level of the left atrium and is, therefore, a less accurate predictor of LVEDP in this position.

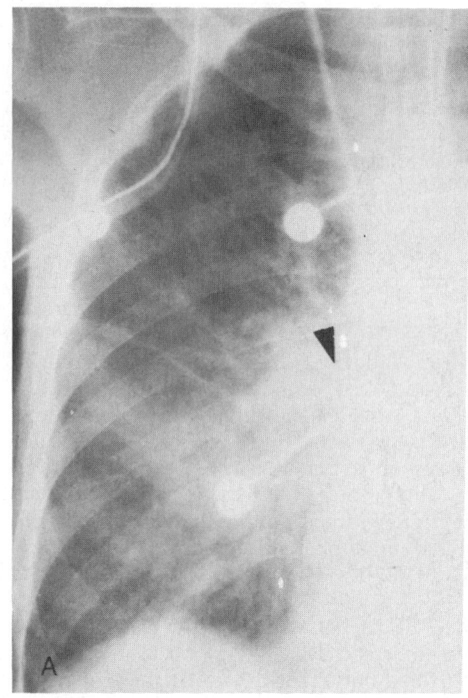

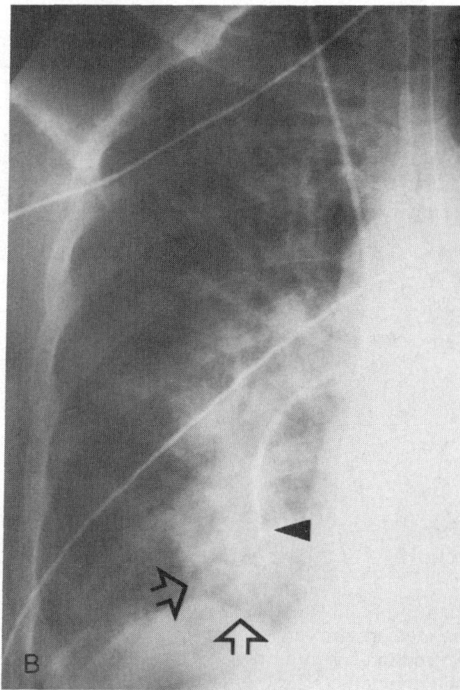

Figure 40–8. *A,* This coned-down view of the right hemithorax in a patient with cardiogenic pulmonary edema reveals vascular indistinctness and perihilar haze. The tip of the SGC *(arrowhead)* is faintly visible in the right pulmonary artery, above an overlying electrocardiograph electrode wire. *B,* One day later in this same patient, the SGC migrated peripherally *(arrowhead),* resulting in an area of hemorrhage distal to the catheter tip that is seen as a new opacity *(open arrows)* in the cardiophrenic angle.

and above the level of the left mainstem bronchus. If the PCXR is exposed during diastole, the elliptical radiolucency of the gas-inflated balloon may be visible (Fig. 40–9). When the tip extends more proximally into the aortic arch or into the left subclavian artery (Fig. 40–10), there is an increased risk of vascular complications. Dissection of the aortic wall has been described and reported as a subtle loss of definition of the descending thoracic aorta on the PCXR.[24] An intramural location can be confirmed with angiography.

PATTERNS OF PARENCHYMAL DISEASE

Abnormalities that result in increased opacity of the lung parenchyma have been divided into three radiographic patterns: (1) airspace, (2) interstitial, and (3) nodular.[25] The ability to classify an opacity into one of these categories may aid in the differential diagnosis in the ICU setting, where most processes are of an acute nature.

The airspace pattern is defined as increased parenchymal density involving the distal conducting airways and alveolar spaces.[25] Most often it is secondary to edema, infection, or hemorrhage. The constellation of radiographic signs that suggest this pattern includes (1) lobar or segmental distribution, (2) poor margination of the process, (3) tendency to coalesce, (4) air bronchogram, and (5) "butterfly" or "bat's wing" distribution.

For any given disease process, not all of these criteria will be met. For example, a butterfly pattern is seen more often in cases of edema and a lobar or segmental distribution with pneumonia or infarction. The presence of an air bronchogram is not disease specific; it is a common finding in adult respiratory distress syndrome (ARDS), pneumonia, and some forms of atelectasis (see later discussion).

The interstitial pattern is the radiographic correlate of disease in the connective tissue compartment of the lung. The radiographic signs of interstitial disease include (1) Kerley's lines, (2) perivascular and peribronchial cuffing, (3) hilar haze, (4) subpleural thickening, and (5) honeycombing. This is best exemplified in the ICU setting by Kerley's (septal) lines and peribronchial cuffing secondary to interstitial pulmonary edema. A reticular pattern consisting of a network of linear opacities may be noted throughout the lung fields. Some infectious processes such as atypical pneumonia may also present acutely with an interstitial pattern.

A nodular pattern may be seen with either an interstitial or an airspace process. Although metastatic pulmonary disease is commonly nodular, considerations in the ICU setting center on infectious causes such as viral or fungal pneumonia, miliary tuberculosis, or septic emboli. Pulmonary edema may occasionally appear nodular, particularly in patients with underlying obstructive pulmonary disease.

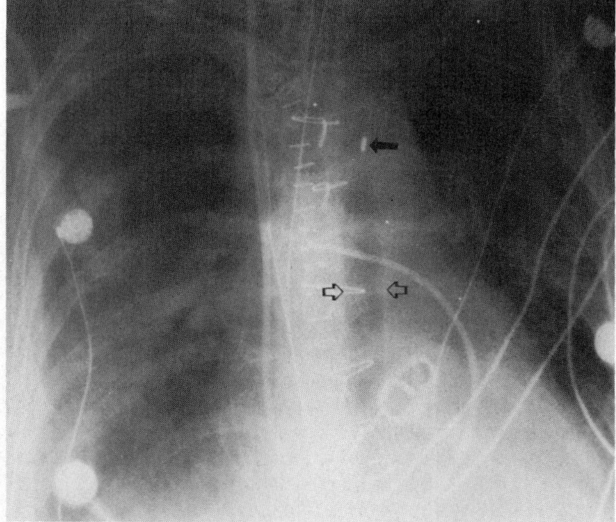

Figure 40–9. Note the radiopaque tip of the intra-aortic counterpulsation balloon *(arrow)* in the proximal descending thoracic aorta in appropriate position. Because the film was exposed during diastole, the inflated balloon can be seen as an elliptic lucency projecting to the left of the dorsal spine behind the cardiac silhouette *(open arrows).*

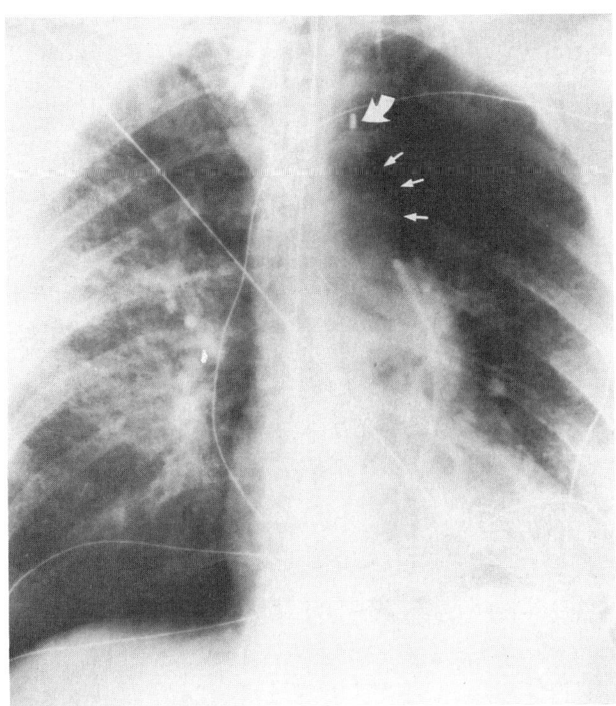

Figure 40–10. Suboptimal position of an intra-aortic counterpulsation balloon with the radiopaque tip *(curved arrow)* projecting above the aortic knob *(small arrows)* into the proximal left subclavian artery.

Patterns of Pulmonary Edema

Pulmonary edema has been broadly classified as being secondary to either increased hydrostatic pressure (cardiogenic pulmonary edema) or increased permeability (noncardiogenic pulmonary edema) at the capillary level. The most common cause of hydrostatic pulmonary edema is left ventricular dysfunction from ischemia or valvular disease[26] followed by obstructive lesions at the level of the left atrium. Increased capillary permeability edema is commonly seen with sepsis and after major trauma. Both mechanisms are likely contributory in cases of renal failure, neurogenic edema,[27] and edema associated with narcotic abuse.

Many radiographic signs have been used to classify pulmonary edema into one of these two categories because this differentiation influences patient management. There is a spectrum of radiographic changes demonstrated on the PCXR with increasing capillary hydrostatic pressures. The earliest sign, pulmonary vascular redistribution, is diagnosed only on films obtained with the patient in the erect position[26] and therefore rarely applicable in the ICU setting. In the erect position, the vessels perfusing the lower lobes are normally of larger diameter because of gravity-dependent flow. With increasing left ventricular failure, upper lobe vessels enlarge, and finally inversion of flow may be observed.

As capillary pressures continue to rise, interstitial edema develops. This is characterized by loss of definition of pulmonary vessels, perihilar haze, and peribronchial cuffing (Fig. 40–11*A*). In some cases, fluid in the interlobular septa is visible as fine linear opacities (Kerley's lines) best seen at the lung bases laterally (see Fig. 40–11*B*). Subpleural fluid is best seen along the fissural planes.

If edema progresses and fills the alveoli, airspace consolidation becomes evident. This tends to be bilateral and predominate in the central and lower lung zones. It is an interesting observation that air bronchograms are infrequently seen in patients with alveolar edema of cardiac cause.

The radiographic changes of cardiogenic pulmonary edema develop and clear rapidly after treatment. Heart size is generally increased except in some cases of pulmonary edema after acute myocardial infarction or cardiac arrhythmias. Although the overall heart size in patients with chronic obstructive lung disease may be within normal limits, comparison with a baseline film may show an interval increase. In this same patient population, the distribution of edema may be patchy or nodular. Pleural effusions are common in cardiogenic edema, may vary in size, and demonstrate a slight right-sided predominance.[28]

Unilateral pulmonary edema, secondary to either elevated hydrostatic pressures or increased capillary permeability, is an unusual occurrence and often not immediately included in the radiographic differential diagnosis of a unilateral interstitial or alveolar pattern. Conditions in the ICU setting that may present with ipsilateral edema are rapid thoracentesis of air or fluid (Fig. 40–12), pulmonary contusion, and prolonged lateral decubitus positioning.[29] Edema in the contralateral lung may be seen in patients with unilateral emphysema or massive unilateral pulmonary embolism and may appear asymmetric after lobectomy.

Noncardiogenic or capillary permeability edema is best exemplified by ARDS. ARDS can result from a variety of insults including septic or hemorrhagic shock, aspiration, severe trauma, acute pancreatitis, transfusion reaction, and virtually any clinical event that requires ICU admission. Regardless of the inciting condition, the clinical presentation and radiographic patterns are similar. The PCXR findings may lag behind the clinical onset by up to 12 hours[30] and may be minimal initially. However, serial films demonstrate patchy, diffuse, ill-defined, and often asymmetric airspace opacities. Over the next 24 to 48 hours, there is coalescence, which may progress to massive airspace consolidation with prominent air bronchograms (Fig. 40–13*A*). Heart size remains unchanged and pleural effusions and Kerley's lines are, as a rule, rare. As ventilatory support is increased, signs of barotrauma including pneumomediastinum, subcutaneous emphysema, and pneumothorax may develop. Even a seemingly small pneumothorax may have dramatic clini-

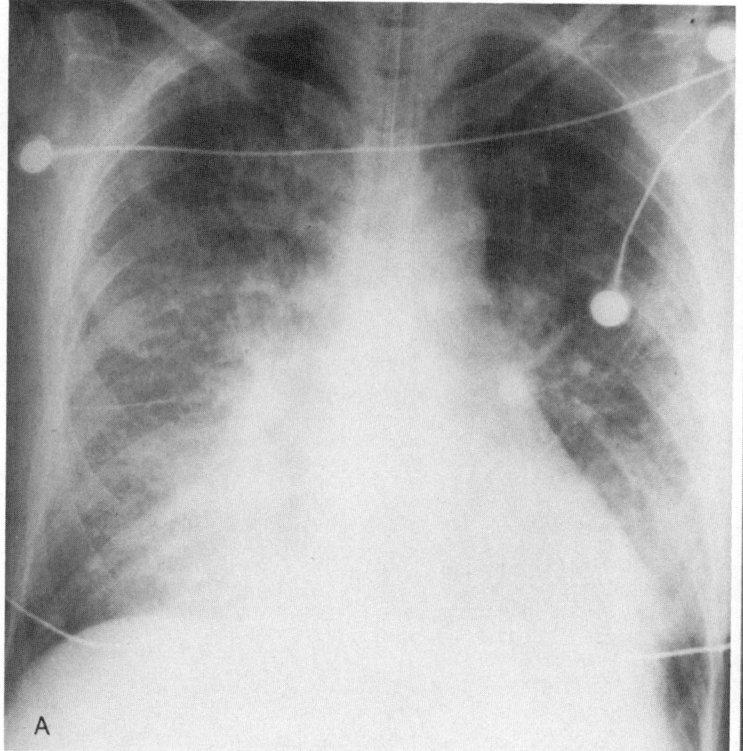

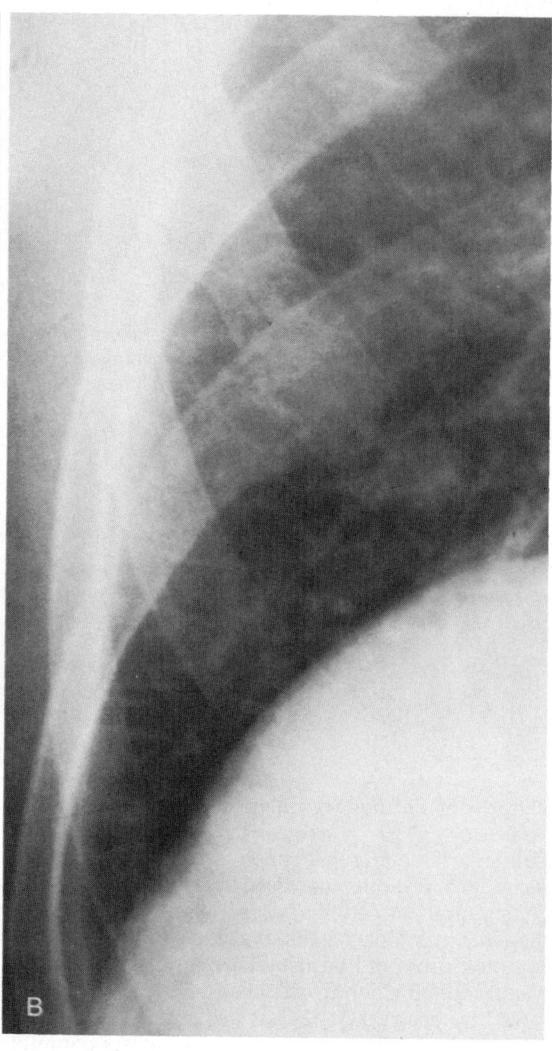

Figure 40–11. *A,* PCXR in a patient with cardiogenic pulmonary edema reveals mild cardiomegaly and signs of interstitial edema, including vascular indistinctness and perihilar haze. Subpleural edema fluid results in apparent thickening of the minor fissure. *B,* Fluid in the interlobular septae (Kerley's lines).

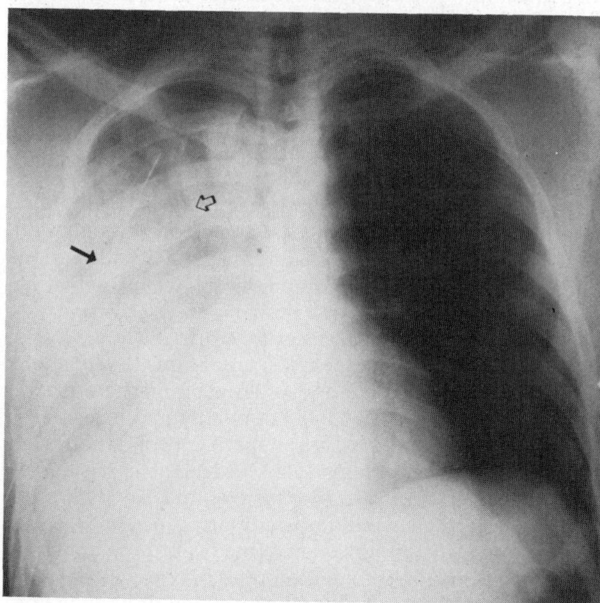

Figure 40–12. Following insertion of a chest tube *(arrow)* for a chronic right pleural effusion, the patient developed unilateral airspace pulmonary edema. Note the air bronchograms *(open arrow),* which are best visualized in the upper lung zone.

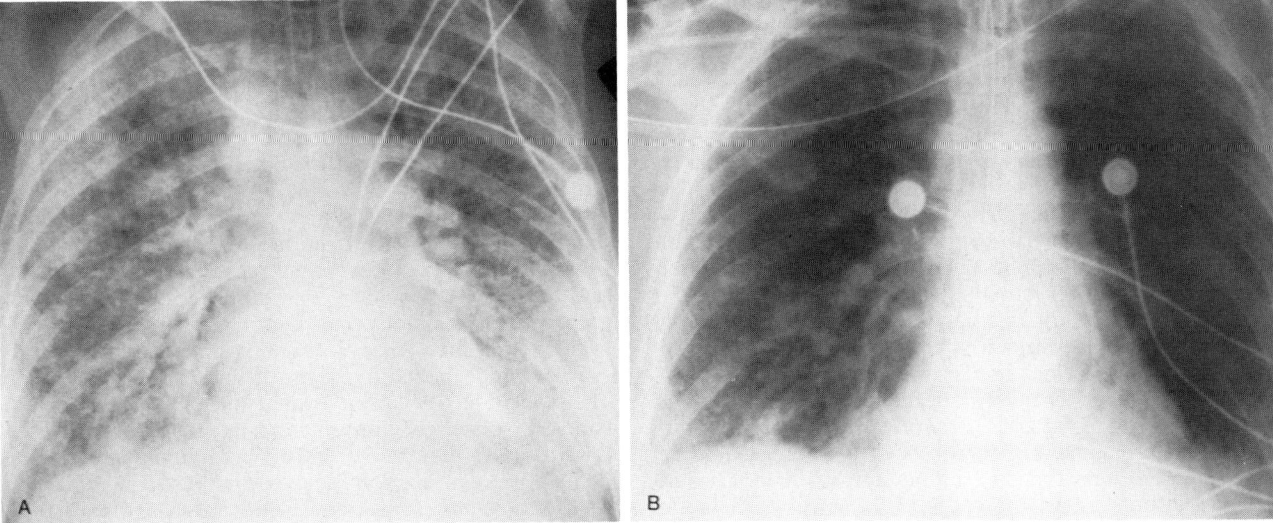

Figure 40–13. *A,* PCXR of a patient with clinical signs and symptoms of acute respiratory distress syndrome demonstrates bilateral airspace disease with extensive involvement of the lung periphery. Note the prominent central air bronchograms, normal heart size, and absence of pleural fluid. *B,* A film taken one week later with the patient still intubated shows residual interstitial opacities, particularly at the right lung base.

cal impact because the lungs are noncompliant and unable to fully collapse.

ARDS is slow to clear in contrast to cardiogenic pulmonary edema, and opacities may persist for days to weeks (see Fig. 40–13*B*). As resolution occurs, the parenchymal pattern often becomes more reticular in appearance.

The signs used to distinguish between cardiogenic and noncardiogenic causes of pulmonary edema on the PCXR have been controversial, with some overlap of the radiographic features, particularly if the edema is florid. A patchy, more peripheral distribution of edema and the presence of air bronchograms seem fairly specific for capillary permeability edema, whereas increased heart size, septal lines, and pleural fluid are more suggestive of cardiogenic edema.[31, 32] Interpretation of serial PCXRs in concert with knowledge of pulmonary capillary wedge pressures and ventilatory settings should lead to an accurate diagnosis in the majority of patients.

Pneumonia

Hospital-acquired pneumonia is a diagnostic challenge and is a significant cause of morbidity and mortality in the ICU population. Mortality rates have been estimated to be 20% to 35% in this setting and even higher in those patients with ARDS or multiple organ failure.[33]

Pneumonias have traditionally been divided into three types: lobar pneumonia, bronchopneumonia, and interstitial pneumonia. Radiographically, lobar pneumonia is suggested when there is a peripheral airspace opacity containing an air bronchogram. Consolidation tends to be relatively homogeneous and demarcated from adjacent aerated lung. Some pulmonary infections may be virulent, with rapid progression and involvement of an entire lung (Fig. 40–14). Bronchopneumonias typically have a more patchy appearance. Associated segmental atelectasis is common because of inflammatory exudate within the airways. Consequently, air bronchograms are less often seen. Complications such as abscess formation, empyema, and bronchopleural fistula may occur. Interstitial pneumonias frequently reflect atypical infection and initially present radiographically with a fine reticular or reticulonodular pattern. Progression to frank airspace consolidation may occur.

The radiographic diagnosis of a specific pneumonia is difficult, particularly in the ICU setting, where polymicrobial pneumonias and other superimposed processes such as edema are common. Therefore, the PCXR is only a moderately accurate predictor of nosocomial pneumonia.[34, 34a]

Aspiration

A common cause of airspace disease in the ICU is aspiration. Predisposing conditions include altered consciousness,

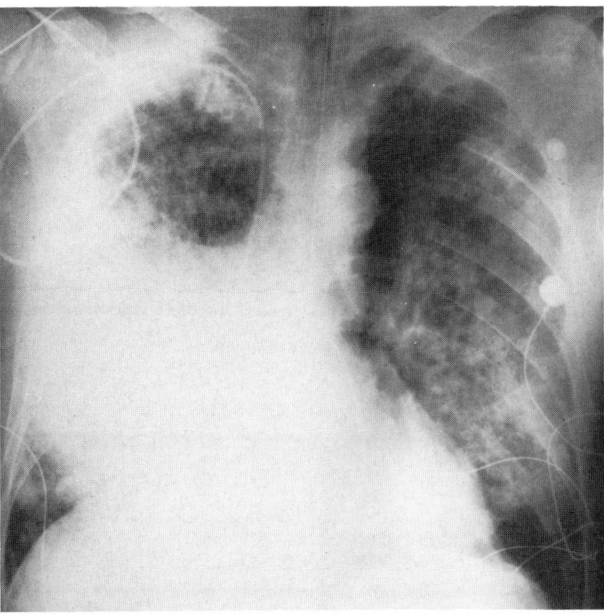

Figure 40–14. In this patient with fulminant pneumonia due to *Legionella,* an initial focus of airspace disease in the right lung progressed to dense consolidation with spread to the contralateral lung within a period of days.

esophageal immotility, and the presence of enteral or ventilatory tubes. A cuffed ETT or TT does not always protect the airway; in fact, both intratracheal tubes and nasogastric tubes may facilitate aspiration by causing disordered swallowing and altering esophageal sphincter function.

Bartlett and Gorbach[35] categorized aspiration into three syndromes: (1) aspiration of toxic fluids, (2) aspiration of bland fluids, and (3) aspiration of infected material. The aspiration may result in areas of consolidation in the gravity-dependent segments of the lung, including the posterior segments of the upper lobes and the superior and posterior segments of the lower lobes in the supine patient.

Aspiration of gastric contents has been termed *Mendelson's syndrome* and results in a chemical pneumonitis with the rapid onset of signs and symptoms. Radiographic abnormality is generally present on the first film and demonstrates an airspace pattern.[36] A perihilar or basilar distribution may be noted, or there may be more extensive consolidation depending on the amount of material aspirated. The process may progress in the ensuing 24 hours but should partially clear within the first 5 days unless complicated by bacterial pneumonia or ARDS (Fig. 40–15).

Bland fluid aspiration has a more limited course and may reveal no significant radiographic findings or only scattered areas of atelectasis. Aspiration of infected material may be unilateral or bilateral, and complications such as lung abscess or empyema are common.

Atelectasis

Atelectasis, or airlessness, occurs in the ICU patient from a variety of causes, including (1) malpositioned ETTs, (2) mucous plugging, (3) postoperative splinting and reduced ventilatory effort secondary to pain, (4) aspiration, (5) space-occupying pleural abnormality such as pneumo-, hydro-, or hemothorax, and (6) delayed presentation of a traumatic bronchial injury.

Four physiologic mechanisms have been proposed:[37] (1) passive atelectasis, which is seen when lung volume decreases secondary to an intrapleural collection of air or fluid, (2) resorption atelectasis, which occurs with airway obstruction and progresses 60 times faster when oxygen rather than air is inspired, (3) adhesive or nonobstructive type seen with inactivation of surfactant in respiratory distress syndrome and after bypass surgery, and (4) cicatrization atelectasis caused by fibrosis and best exemplified by chronic granulomatous processes.

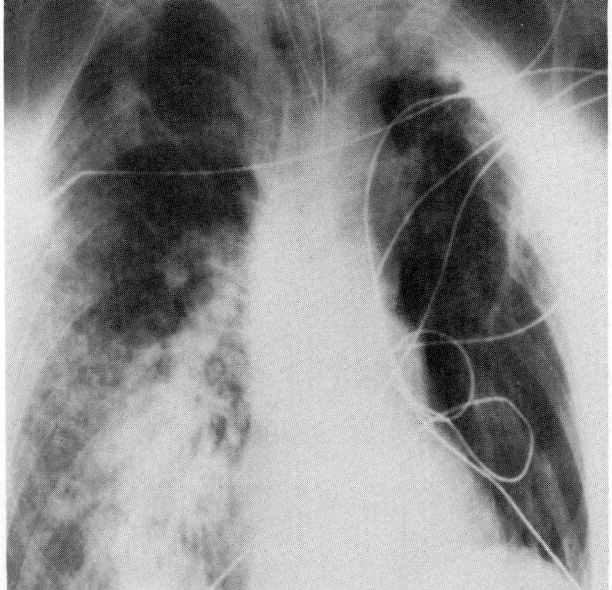

Figure 40–15. Following a witnessed episode of aspiration and respiratory distress, PCXR demonstrates airspace opacity in the right middle and lower lung zones. Aspiration pneumonia may be predominately unilateral (as in this case), or it may be bilateral.

The causal mechanism may vary, but the roentgenographic signs, both direct and indirect, that distinguish atelectasis from a space-occupying parenchymal process such as a lobar pneumonia are constant. The most direct radiographic sign is displacement of interlobar fissures. However, fissural identification is often difficult on PCXRs, and evaluation for the indirect signs of atelectasis should follow. These include a local increase in density, which may be band- or "platelike" or segmental, or involve an entire lobe (Fig. 40–16*A*). Elevation of the hemidiaphragm and mediastinal shift occur when volume loss is present in lobes adjacent to these structures (see Fig. 16*B* and *C*). Hilar displacement, compensatory overinflation, and rib approximation are additional indirect signs of atelectasis.

Pulmonary Embolism

Patients in the ICU are at high risk for the development of pulmonary embolism secondary to prolonged immobilization, obesity, poor cardiac function, and hypercoagulable states.

A normal PCXR does not exclude the possibility of pulmonary embolism, and, if clinical suspicion is high, the patient should undergo an additional diagnostic study such as a ventilation-perfusion radionuclide scan.

Signs of pulmonary embolism uncomplicated by infarction have been discussed extensively[38] and include (1) focal oligemia, otherwise known as Westermark's sign, (2) enlargement and abrupt termination of a central pulmonary artery, (3) loss of lung volume, and (4) cor pulmonale as manifested by right ventricular enlargement and enlargement of the azygos vein. In patients with left ventricular failure, asymmetric pulmonary edema with relative sparing of the hypoperfused segments may be observed.

If thromboembolism is accompanied by hemorrhagic edema, a peripheral parenchymal opacity ("infarct"), segmental in distribution and homogeneous in density, is observed. This bears the name *Hampton's hump* if it has a broad base at the visceral pleural surface and a rounded apex oriented toward the hilum (Fig. 40–17). An area of infarct will gradually diminish in size but will remain relatively homogeneous and appear to "melt away as would an ice cube." A true necrotic infarct will resolve similarly but over a longer period of time.[38]

Other PCXR features of thromboembolism are nonspecific and include pleural effusion (usually small and unilateral) and areas of platelike atelectasis.

PLEURAL DISEASE

Pneumothorax

Pneumothorax in the ICU is most often diagnosed in the setting of recent intervention such as central catheter placement or as a complication of barotrauma. The cardinal radiographic sign is visualization of a fine linear opacity paralleling the chest wall representing the visceral pleura outlined by intrapleural air on one side and aerated lung on the other. In the ambulatory patient for whom an upright, expiratory posteroanterior and lateral chest radiograph is

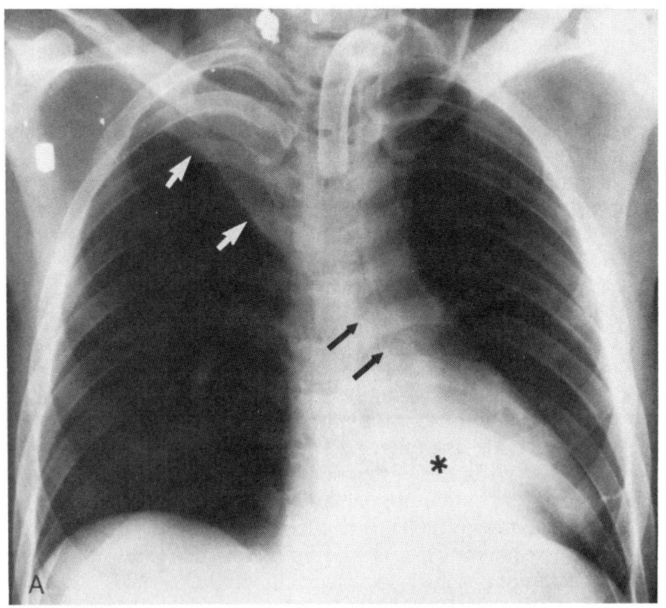

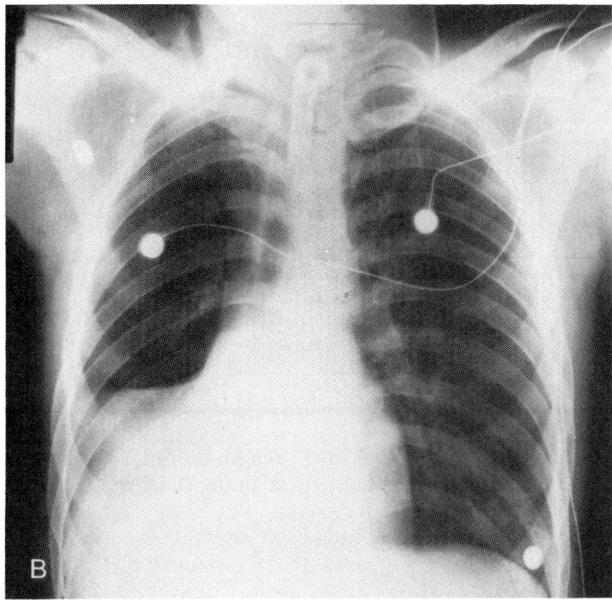

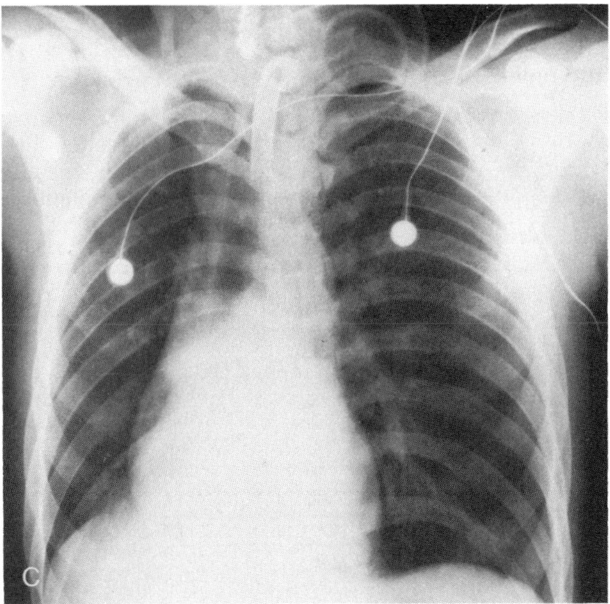

Figure 40–16. *A,* Features of right upper lobe collapse include upward displacement of the minor fissure *(white arrows)* and increased opacity of the airless lobe in the lung apex. Left lower lobe collapse is present as well, demonstrating indirect signs of atelectasis that include increased retrocardiac opacity *(asterisk)* and silhouetting of the medial portion of the left hemidiaphragm. The left mainstem bronchus is depressed *(black arrows),* and the shadow of the left proximal pulmonary artery is obscured. *B,* Combined collapse of the right middle and lower lobes presents as increased opacity at the lung base and as obscuration of the right border of the heart and hemidiaphragm. It can easily be mistaken for subpulmonic pleural effusion. However, note the additional evidence of volume loss with ipsilateral cardiac and mediastinal shift as well as hyperinflation of the aerated right upper lobe. *C,* Collapse of the right lower lobe results in ipsilateral shift of the heart and mediastinum and elevation of the hemidiaphragm. Increased opacity behind the right border of the heart and poor visualization of the descending interlobar pulmonary artery are additional secondary signs noted in this patient.

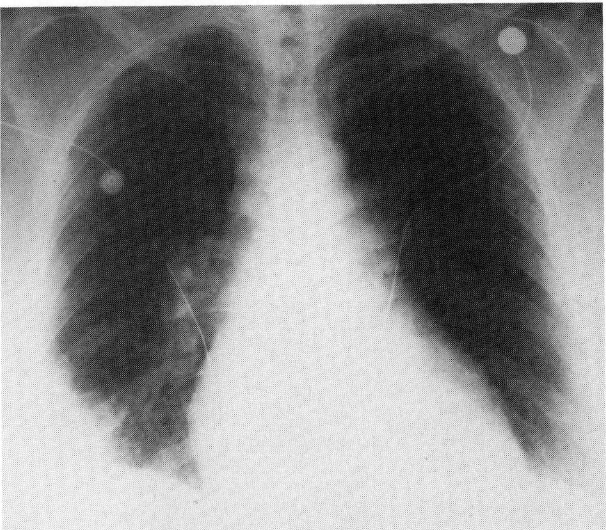

Figure 40–17. This PCXR in a patient with massive right pulmonary embolus demonstrates marked enlargement of the central right pulmonary artery. A peripheral, wedged-shaped opacity (Hampton's hump) obliterates the right costophrenic angle secondary to hemorrhagic edema.

the examination of choice, the pneumothorax is commonly demonstrated over the lung apex. In the ICU, where radiographs are obtained with patients in the supine or semierect position, air will collect along the lateral chest wall at the lung bases (Figs. 40–18 and 40–19), or medially, where it may simulate pneumomediastinum.[39] Skin folds and large bullae can be confused with pneumothorax. If the diagnosis cannot be made with certainty on the anteroposterior radiograph, an alternative examination is the lateral decubitus chest radiograph (Fig. 40–20).

Once the presence of a pneumothorax has been established, evaluation for radiographic signs of tension should follow. On a nonrotated frontal radiograph, these include (1) contralateral shift of the heart and mediastinal structures; (2) total or near-total collapse of the ipsilateral lung (although this may not be observed in the patient with a densely consolidated, noncompliant lung); and (3) flattening or inversion of the hemidiaphragm.

Pleural Effusion

The location and appearance of freely mobile pleural fluid depend on patient position. With patients in a supine position, fluid will layer posteriorly and appear as generalized haziness of the hemithorax without obscured vascular markings on the PCXR (see Fig. 40–19). If the effusion is large, the costophrenic angle may be blunted and an apical cap noted. However, sizable pleural effusions may go unrecognized on supine radiographs particularly if bilateral pleural fluid is present. The optimal plain radiographic examination in the ICU to evaluate for pleural effusion is the lateral decubitus, which, if adequately positioned and exposed, can demonstrate even a small quantity of a mobile effusion that will appear as a straightened fluid–lung interface along the dependent chest wall.[40]

When patients are in the erect position, pleural fluid may collect beneath the lung in a subpulmonic location and appear as an apparently elevated hemidiaphragm with a laterally shifted apex. Blunting of the lateral costophrenic angle may require an accumulation of 250 to 500 cc.[41]

Localized collections of fluid within an interlobar fissure, a pleural "pseudotumor," may simulate a parenchymal mass but can usually be differentiated by the abrupt appearance, fissural relationship, and shift in location on decubitus views.

Loculated fluid may present as focal or masslike pleural opacities when there are adhesions between the visceral and parietal pleurae. This appearance is seen more frequently in patients with previous pleural abnormality secondary to surgery, empyema, or hemothorax. The differentiation of a loculated fluid collection such as empyema from lung abscess[42, 43] directly affects patient management because infected fluid in the pleural cavity often requires drainage. An empyema appears lenticular in shape, making obtuse angles with the chest wall, whereas a peripheral lung abscess is spherical and forms acute angles with the chest wall. An air-fluid level, when present, will consequently be of discrepant length on orthogonal views with an empyema but will not vary in length with a spherical abscess.

Ultrasonography and computed tomography are additional imaging modalities of value in both detecting small effusions and guiding aspiration and chest tube drainage. Ultrasonography can be performed portably in critically ill patients and can suggest the presence of an exudative effusion when complex septated, complex nonseptated, or homogeneously echogenic patterns are present.[44]

Computed tomography has been advocated in patients who have an unexplained source of sepsis and a complex PCXR.[45, 46] It is the best modality for differentiating pleural from parenchymal abnormality and is frequently useful in resolving more complex problems (Fig. 40–21), provided the patient is stable enough to be transported to the radiology department.

AIDS-RELATED PULMONARY DISEASES

Infection

Pneumocystis carinii pneumonia (PCP) occurs in the clinical course of many patients with acquired immunodeficiency syndrome (AIDS) and is a frequent cause of death. The most typical radiographic appearance on initial presentation is that of bilateral, fairly symmetric, fine to medium reticular

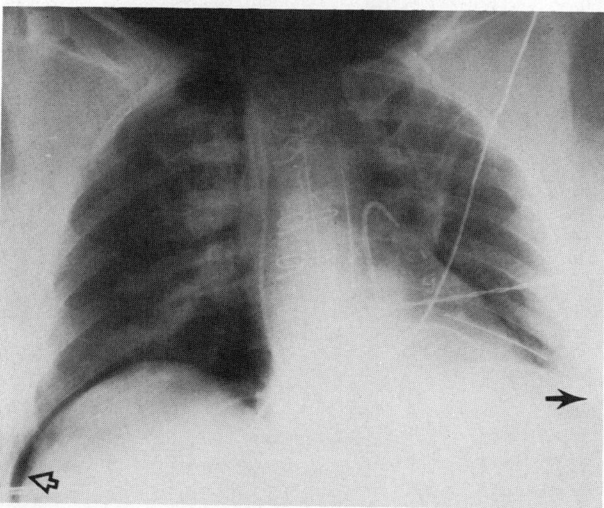

Figure 40–18. In this supine patient with multiple life support lines and tubes, a right basilar pneumothorax presents as a deep and lucent costophrenic angle *(open arrow)*. This is in contrast to the appearance of the normal left side *(black arrow)*.

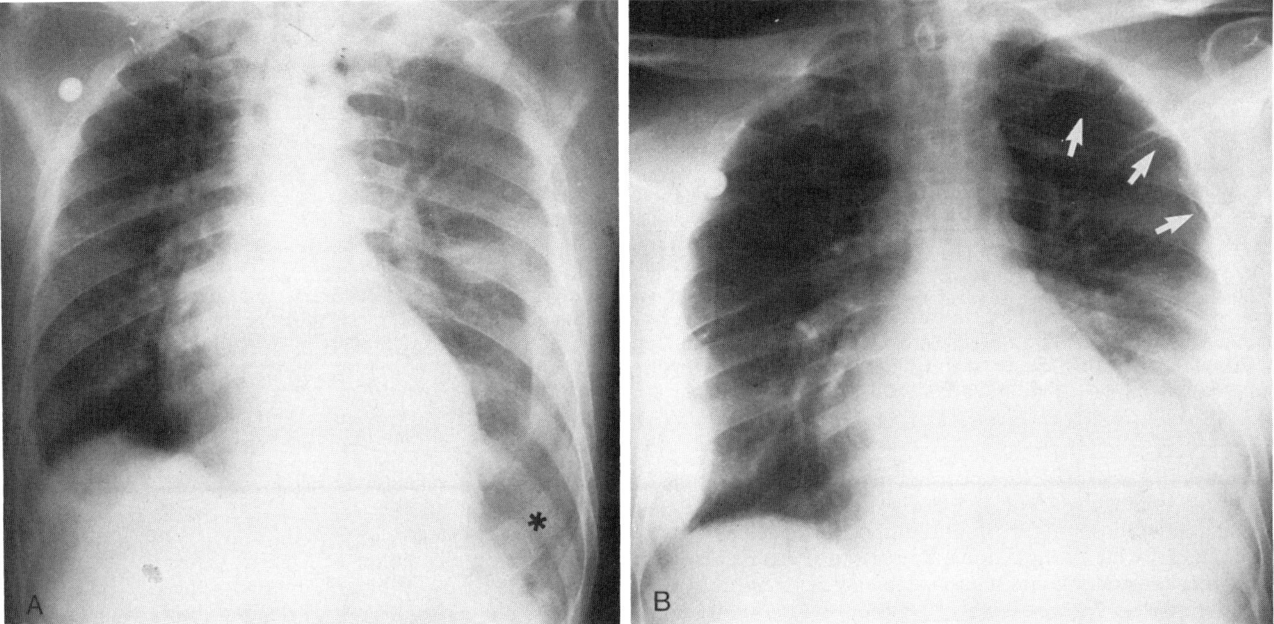

Figure 40–19. *A,* In this supine patient, detection of a left basilar pneumothorax is difficult owing to the presence of a moderately sized pleural effusion that creates an overall increase in the density of the left hemithorax. However, note the asymetric deepening and relative lucency of the costophrenic sulcus *(asterisk)* secondary to the presence of intrapleural air. *B,* When the same patient assumes the upright position, the visceral pleural edge *(arrows)* is now readily visible in the lung apex. Bilateral pleural effusions blunt the dependent costophrenic angles.

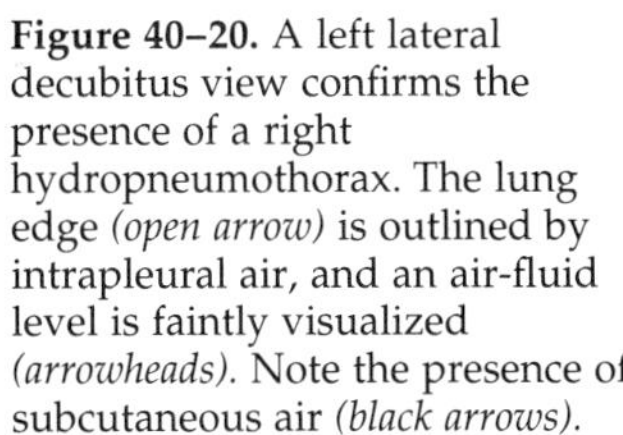

Figure 40–20. A left lateral decubitus view confirms the presence of a right hydropneumothorax. The lung edge *(open arrow)* is outlined by intrapleural air, and an air-fluid level is faintly visualized *(arrowheads).* Note the presence of subcutaneous air *(black arrows).*

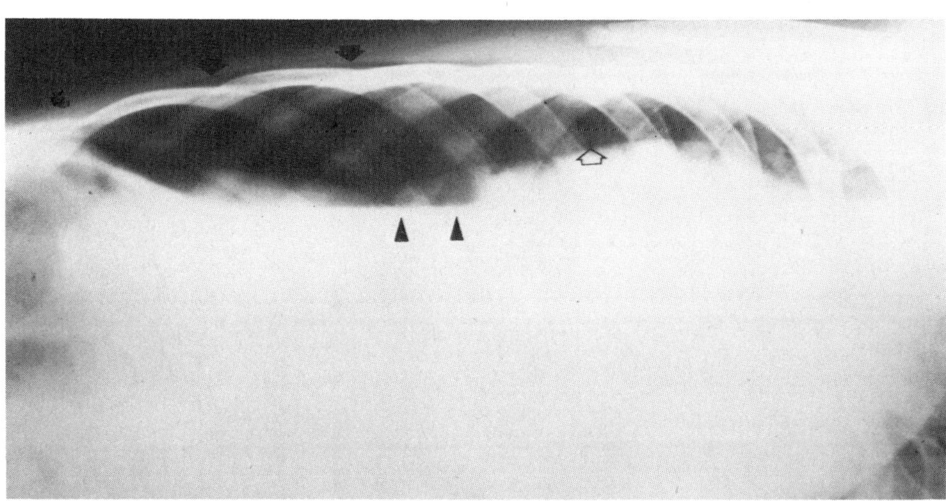

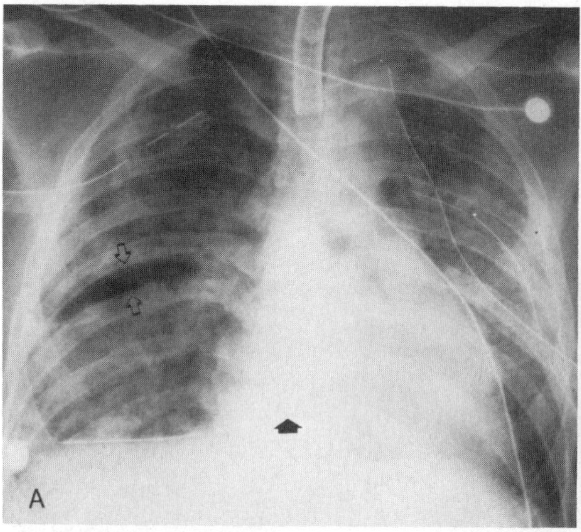

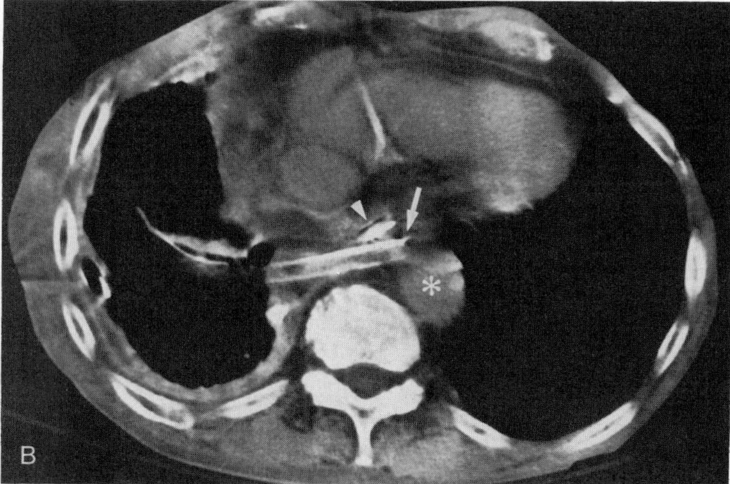

Figure 40–21. *A,* Bilateral chest tubes were required in this patient with acute respiratory distress syndrome and barotrauma. Note the presence of intrafissural air *(open arrows)* and of residual intrapleural air at the right lung apex. The right basilar chest tube was nonfunctional, and the tip projected across the midline *(arrow). B,* Computed tomography scan through the lower thorax confirmed malposition of the drainage catheter, which was located in the mediastinum with the tip *(arrow)* resting between the contrast-filled esophagus *(arrowhead)* and the descending thoracic aorta *(asterisk).*

opacities (Fig. 40–22). Not uncommonly, this may progress to frank homogeneous airspace disease. A less common presentation consisting of multiple nodular opacities may be confused with a fungal or malignant cause. An increased incidence of predominantly upper lobe involvement is now being reported with the use of aerosolized pentamidine, which is poorly distributed to the upper zones and therefore less effective in preventing reactivation in this area.[47]

Thin-walled pneumatoceles, often multiple and reaching diameters of up to 10 cm, may occur (Fig. 40–23). Spontaneous pneumothorax (Fig. 40–24), frequently but not always seen in association with visualized pneumatoceles or bullae, may result in persistent air leak and require multiple pleural drainage catheters.[48]

In uncomplicated cases of PCP, radiographic improvement is generally noted in 7 to 10 days. If initial clinical response is followed by an apparent relapse in 3 to 4 days, the possibility of volume overload secondary to the large quantity of fluid delivered with trimethoprim-sulfamethoxazole should be considered.

Recognition of pleural effusion and intrathoracic adenopathy is of practical importance in the radiographic differential diagnosis of AIDS-related thoracic diseases. Although rare in cases of isolated PCP, pleural fluid and/or adenopathy should suggest other superimposed neoplastic or inflammatory process such as lymphoma or mycobacterial

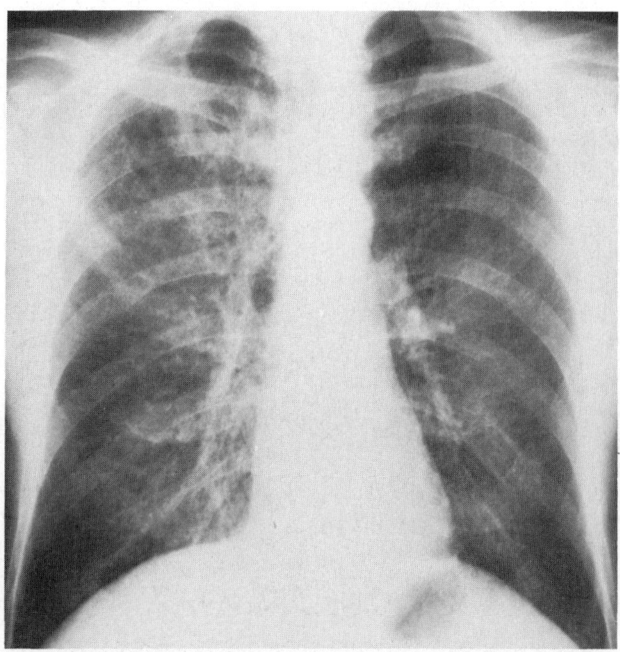

Figure 40–22. Typical radiographic appearance of *Pneumocystis carinii* pneumonia presenting as a diffuse interstitial pneumonia. Note the absence of adenopathy and pleural effusion.

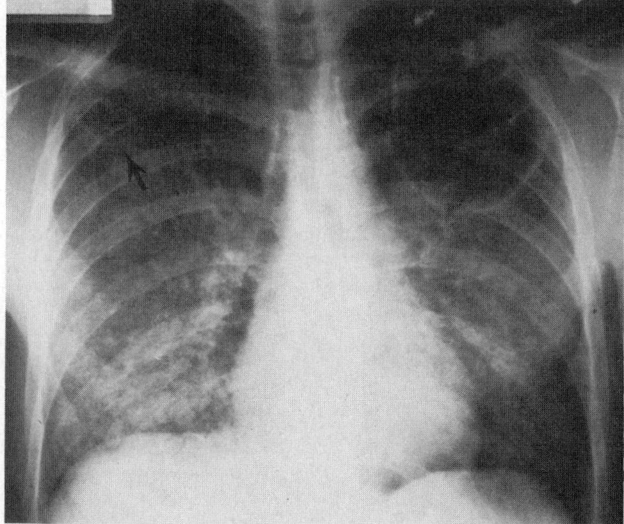

Figure 40–23. Chest radiograph of a young man with AIDS and *Pneumocystis carinii* pneumonia demonstrates bilateral interstitial and airspace disease. A large pneumatocele is present in the left upper lung zone, and a smaller cystic cavity is visible on the right *(arrow).*

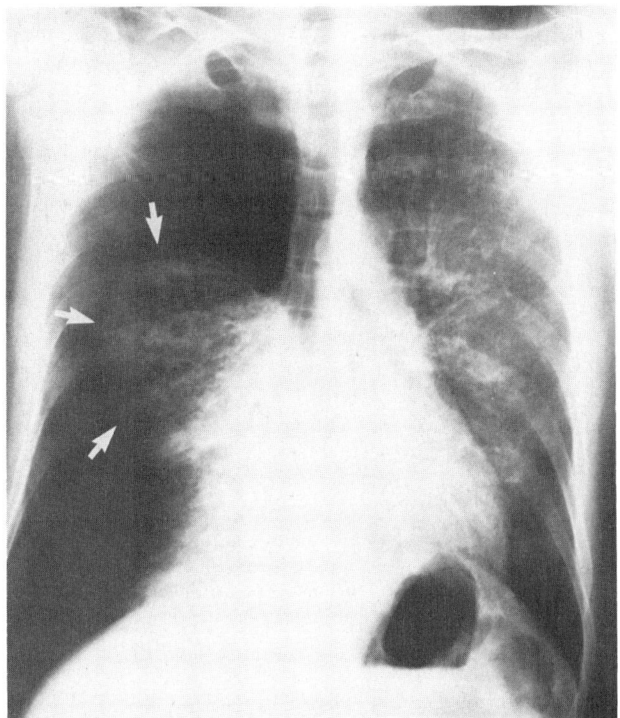

Figure 40–24. Same patient as in Figure 40–22 whose course was complicated by a right tension pneumothorax *(arrows).* Signs of tension seen here include contralateral shift of the heart and the mediastinum as well as depression of the right hemidiaphragm.

infection. Human immunodeficiency virus–positive patients are at greater risk for the development of community-acquired pyogenic pneumonias, especially those resulting from *Streptococcus pneumoniae* and *Haemophilus influenzae.* Several studies have shown a five- to sixfold increase in the annual incidence of community-acquired bacterial pneumonia when the seropositive population is compared with the general population.[49] In general, there are no distinctive radiographic features in this selected population.

Because of the increased incidence of AIDS among intravenous drug users, septic endocarditis may be suggested when there are multiple nodules with cavitation. These more focal opacities can coalesce and form a diffuse airspace pattern.

Disseminated fungal infection, particularly with *Cryptococcus, Histoplasma,* and *Coccidioides,* results in significant morbidity and mortality. When there is lung involvement in disseminated histoplasmosis, the majority of patients demonstrate diffuse reticulonodular opacities measuring up to 3 mm,[50] a pattern not dissimilar from that described with *Mycobacterium tuberculosis* or, occasionally, with *Cryptococcus.* Linear, irregular opacities represent the second most

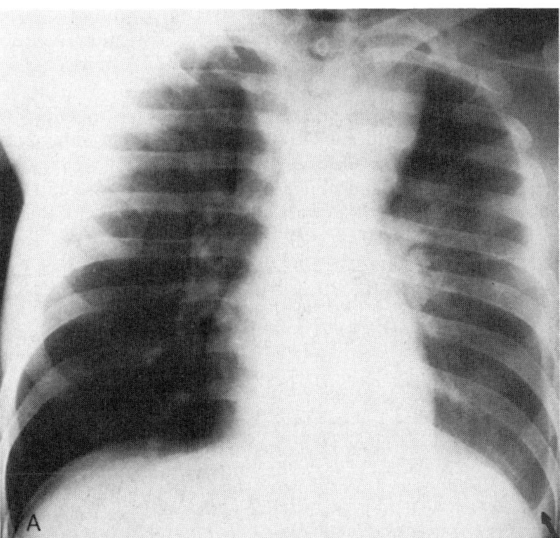

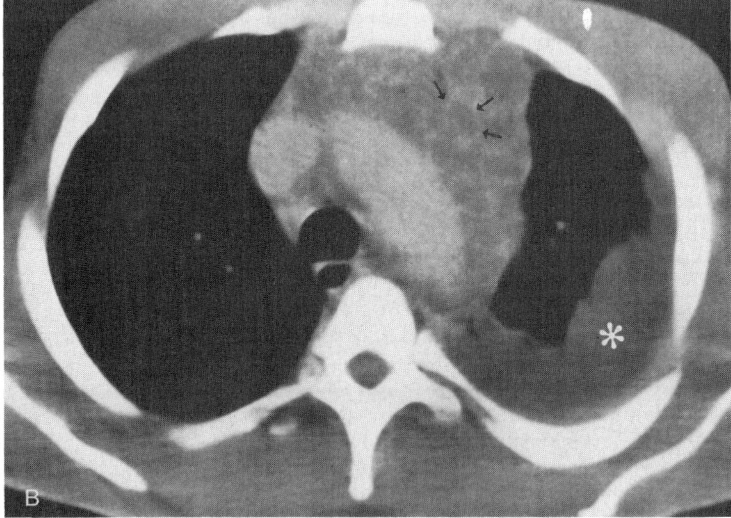

Figure 40–25. *A,* In this AIDS patient with disseminated mycobacterial infection, marked widening of the upper mediastinum and left perihilar airspace disease are demonstrated. A left pleural effusion layers posteriorly and blunts the costophrenic angle *(arrow). B,* This contrast-enhanced computed tomography scan at the level of the aortic arch demonstrates extensive prevascular adenopathy with areas of ringlike enhancement *(arrows).* Note the dependent left pleural effusion *(asterisk).*

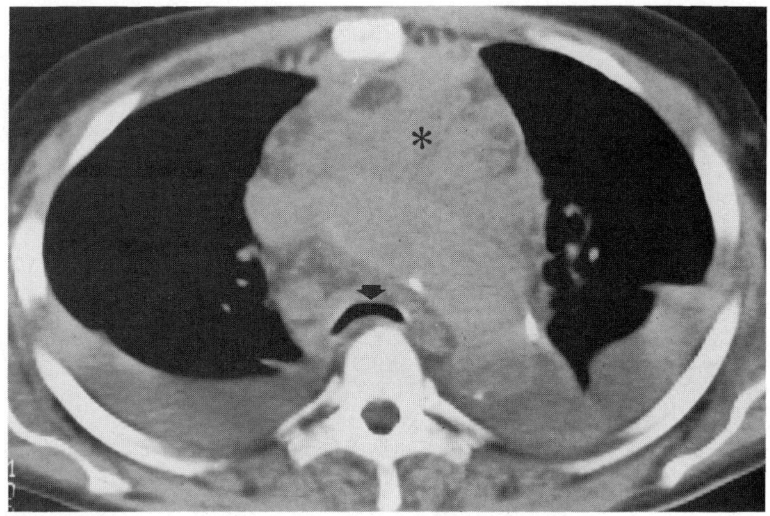

Figure 40–26. This computed tomography scan at the level of the aortic arch demonstrates extensive prevascular *(asterisk)* and precarinal adenopathy. Note the compression of the trachea *(arrow)*. Bilateral pleural effusions are present.

common presentation and may be indistinguishable from PCP, other fungal, or viral infections. Pulmonary cryptococcosis presents most commonly as interstitial opacities both on plain chest radiography and computed tomography scans. Segmental alveolar opacities and nodular densities may also be seen.[50a] Pulmonary cryptococcosis and coccidioidomycosis most often present with a diffuse reticulonodular pattern, although larger focal nodular opacities may be seen. Pleural effusion and adenopathy have been described with all three fungal organisms.[51]

M. tuberculosis and M. avium complex (MAC) are the two mycobacterial species that are frequently identified in the AIDS population. In the early stages, before profound immunosuppression, the radiographic pattern consists of parenchymal opacities in the posterior and apical segments of the upper lobes and the superior segment of the lower lobes, similar to the distribution that has classically been described in immunocompetent hosts. When the patient's immune status deteriorates, there is less lobar predominance and an increased incidence of adenopathy and pleural effusion (Fig. 40–25*A*).[52] The differential diagnosis includes lymphoma. Computed tomographic scan demonstrating enlarged lymph nodes with peripheral areas of enhancement and low-density centers suggests mycobacterial disease (Fig. 40–25*B*).[53, 53a] Infection with MAC exhibits no clear-cut radiographic distinction from *M. tuberculosis.*

Malignancy

Intrathoracic involvement with AIDS-related lymphomas (ARL) is seen in less than 10% of patients.[54] Patients may present with respiratory compromise secondary to large pleural effusions or airway compression from bulky mediastinal adenopathy (Fig. 40–26). Pulmonary parenchymal involvement may take the form of reticulonodular opacities or well-defined, rapidly enlarging nodules ranging in size from 0.5 to 5 cm.

Radiographic findings in patients with Kaposi's sarcoma include pulmonary nodules, adenopathy, and pleural effusion. The parenchymal nodules are characteristically poorly defined, a feature that helps to distinguish them from the opacities seen with ARL or fungal disease.[55] Autopsy studies have shown that metastatic Kaposi's sarcoma may involve the myocardium, epicardium, and pericardium and should therefore be considered in the differential diagnosis of cardiac dysfunction in this population.

References

1. Hall JB, White SR, Karrison T: Efficacy of daily routine chest radiographs in intubated, mechanically ventilated patients. Crit Care Med 1991; 19:689.
2. Bekemeyer WB, Crapo RO, Calhoon S, et al: Efficacy of chest radiography in a respiratory intensive care unit: A prospective study. Chest 1985; 88:691.
3. Greenbaum DM, Marshall KE: The value of routine daily chest x-rays in intubated patients in the medical intensive care unit. Crit Care Med 1982; 10:29.
4. Henschke CI, Pasternack GS, Schroeder S, et al: Bedside chest radiology: Diagnostic efficacy. Radiology 1983; 149:23.
5. Margolin SI, Rowberg AH, Godwin JD: Preliminary experience with portable digital imaging for intensive care radiography. J Thorac Imaging 1990; 5:49.
6. Niklason LT, Heang-Ping C, Cascade PN, et al: Portable chest imaging: Comparison of storage phosphor digital, asymmetric screen-film, and conventional screen-film systems. Radiology 1993; 186:387.
7. Sagel SS, Jost RG, Glazer HS, et al: Digital mobile radiography. J Thorac Imaging 1990; 5:36.
8. Brunel SW, Coleman DL, Schwartz DE, et al: Assessment of routine chest roentgenograms and the physical examination to confirm endotracheal tube position. Chest 1989; 96:1043.
9. Conrardy PA, Goodman LR, Lange R, et al: Alteration of endotracheal tube position: Flexion and extension of the neck. Crit Care Med 1976; 4:7.
10. Zwillich CW, Pierson DJ, Creagh CR, et al: Complications of assisted ventilation: A prospective study of 354 consecutive episodes. Am J Med 1974; 57:161.
11. Smith GM, Reed JC, Choplin RH: Radiographic detection of esophageal malpositioning of endotracheal tubes. Am J Roentgenol 1990; 154:23.
12. Zimmermann JE, Goodman LR, Shahvari MBG: Effect of mechanical ventilation and positive end expiratory pressure (PEEP) on chest radiograph. Am J Roentgenol 1979; 133:811.
13. Ravin CE, Putman CE, McLoud TC: Hazards of the ICU. Am J Roentgenol 1976; 126:423.
14. Williams PL, Warwick R, Dyson M, et al: Gray's Anatomy. 37th ed. New York, Churchill Livingstone, 1989.
15. Langston CS: The aberrant central venous catheter and its complications. Radiology 1971; 100:55.
16. Huygens L, Sennesael J, Verbeelen D, et al: Cardiothoracic complications of centrally inserted catheters. Acute Care 1985; 11:53.
17. Bone DK, Maddrey WC, Eagan J, et al: Cardiac tamponade: A fatal complication of central venous catheterization. Arch Surg 1973; 106:868.
18. Gibson RN, Hennessy OF, Collier N, et al: Major complications of central venous catheterization: A report of five cases and a brief review of the literature. Clin Radiol 1985; 36:205.

19. Brandstetter RD, Gitler B: Thoughts on the Swan-Ganz catheter. Chest 1986; 89:5.
20. West J, Dollery C, Naimack A: Distribution of blood flow in isolated lung: Relation to vascular and alveolar pressures. J Appl Physiol 1964; 19:713.
21. Sise MJ, Hollingsworth P, Brimm JE, et al: Complications of the flow-directed pulmonary artery catheter: A prospective analysis of 219 patients. Crit Care Med 1981; 9:315.
22. Dieden JD, Friloux LA III, Renner JW: Pulmonary artery false aneurysms secondary to Swan-Ganz pulmonary artery catheters. Am J Roentgenol 1987; 149:901.
23. Dunkman WB, Leinbach RC, Buckley MJ, et al: Clinical and hemodynamic results of intra-aortic balloon pumping and surgery for cardiogenic shock. Circulation 1972; 46:465.
24. Hyson EA, Ravin CE, Kelly MJ, et al: Intra-aortic counterpulsation balloon: Radiographic considerations. Am J Roentgenol 1977; 128:115.
25. Heitzman ER: The Lung. 2nd ed. St. Louis, CV Mosby, 1984, p 70.
26. Ravin CE: Pulmonary vascularity: Radiographic considerations. J Thorac Imaging 1988; 3:1.
27. Ell SR: Neurogenic pulmonary edema: A review of the literature and a perspective. Invest Radiol 1991; 26:499.
28. Armstrong P, Wilson AG, Dee P: Imaging of Diseases of the Chest. Chicago, Year Book Medical Publishers 1990, p 627.
29. Calenoff L, Kruglik GD, Woodruff A: Unilateral pulmonary edema. Radiology 1978; 126:19.
30. Morgan PW, Goodman LR: Pulmonary edema and adult respiratory distress syndrome. Radiol Clin North Am 1991; 29:943.
31. Aberle DR, Wiener-Kronish JP, Webb WR, et al: Hydrostatic versus increased permeability pulmonary edema: Diagnosis based on radiographic criteria in critically ill patients. Radiology 1988; 168:73.
32. Smith RC, Mann H, Greenspan RH, et al: Radiographic differentiation between different etiologies of pulmonary edema. Invest Radiol 1987; 22:859.
33. Smith RC, Mann H, Greenspan RH, et al: Radiographic differentiation between different etiologies of pulmonary edema. Invest Radiol 1987; 22:859.
34. Mock CN, Burchard KW, Hasan F, et al: Surgical intensive care unit pneumonia. Surgery 1988; 104:494.
34a. Winer-Muram HT, Rubin SA, Ellis JV, et al: Pneumonia and ARDS in patients receiving mechanical ventilation: Diagnostic accuracy of chest radiography. Radiology 1993; 188:479.
35. Bartlett JG, Gorbach SL: The triple threat of aspiration pneumonia. Chest 1975; 68:560.
36. Landay MJ, Christensen EE, Bynum LJ: Pulmonary manifestations of acute aspiration of gastric contents. Am J Roentgenol 1978; 131:587.
37. Fraser RG, Paré JAP, Paré PD, et al: Diagnosis of Diseases of the Chest. 3rd ed. Vol 1. Philadelphia, WB Saunders, 1991, p 472.
38. Fraser RG et al: Diagnosis of Diseases of the Chest. 3rd ed. Vol 3. Philadelphia, WB Saunders, 1991, p 1712.
39. Tocino IM, Miller MH, Fairfax WR: Distribution of pneumothorax in the supine and semirecumbent critically ill adult. Am J Roentgenol 1985; 144:901.
40. Moskowitz H, Platt RT, Schachar R, et al: Roentgen visualization of minute pleural effusion. Radiology 1973; 109:33.
41. Collins JD, Burwell D, Furmanski S, et al: Minimal detectable pleural effusions. Radiology 1972; 105:51.
42. Stark DD, Federle MP, Goodman PC, et al: Differentiating lung abscess and empyema: Radiography and computed tomography. Am J Roentgenol 1983; 141:163.
43. Hanna JW, Reed JC, Choplin RH: Pleural infections: A clinical-radiologic review. J Thorac Imaging 1991; 6:68.
44. Yang PC, Luh KT, Chang DB, et al: Value of sonography in determining the nature of pleural effusion. Am J Roentgenol 1992; 159:29.
45. Golding RP, Knape P, Strack van Schijndel RJ, et al: Computed tomography as an adjunct to chest x-rays of intensive care unit patients. Crit Care Med 1988; 16:211.
46. Mirvis SE, Tobin KD, Kostrubiak I, et al: Thoracic CT in detecting occult disease in critically ill patients. Am J Roentgenol 1987; 148:685.
47. Conces DJ Jr, Kraft JL, Vix VA, et al: Apical *Pneumocystis carinii* pneumonia after inhaled pentamidine prophylaxis. Am J Roentgenol 1989; 152:1192.
48. Feuerstein IM, Archer A, Pluda JM, et al: Thin walled cavities, cysts and pneumothorax in *Pneumocystis carinii* pneumonia: Further observations with histopathologic correlation. Radiology 1990; 174:697.
49. Selsyn PA, Feingold AR, Hartel D, et al: Increased risk of bacterial pneumonia in HIV-infected intravenous drug users without AIDS. AIDS 1988; 2:267.
50. Sarosi G, Johnson P: Progressive disseminated histoplasmosis in the acquired immunodeficiency syndrome: A model for disseminated disease. Semin Respir Infect 1990; 5:146.
50a. Sider L, Westcott MA: Pulmonary manifestations of cryptococcosis in patients with AIDS: CT features. J Thorac Imaging 1994; 9:78.
51. Murray J, Mills J: State of the art: Pulmonary infectious complications of human immunodeficiency virus infection. Am Rev Respir Dis 1990; 141:1356–1582.
52. Modelevsky T, Sattler F, Barnes PF: Mycobacterial disease in patients with human immunodeficiency virus infection. Arch Intern Med 1989; 149:2201.
53. Winer-Muram HT, Rubin SA: Thoracic complications of tuberculosis. J Thorac Imaging 1990; 5:46.
53a. Hartman TE, Primack SL, Muller NL, et al: Diagnosis of thoracic complications in AIDS: Accuracy of CT. AJR Am J Roentgenol 1994; 162:547.
54. Goodman PC: AIDS. *In:* A Radiologic Approach to Diseases of the Chest. Freudlich IM, Bragg DG (Eds). Baltimore, Williams & Wilkins, 1992, p 504.
55. Sivit CJ, Schwartz AM, Rockoff SD: Kaposi's sarcoma of the lung in AIDS: Radiologic-pathologic analysis. Am J Roentgenol 1987; 148:25.

CHAPTER 41

Chest Imaging in Pediatric Intensive Care

Stephanie E. Spottswood, MD, MSPH • Lakshmana Das Narla, MD • Elizabeth Hingsbergen, MD

Radiologic imaging of the pediatric chest contributes significantly to prompt diagnosis and appropriate management of infants and children with life-threatening cardiopulmonary disorders. Respiratory distress in the neonate can result from problems of prematurity, adverse perinatal events, and congenital malformations of the lung and heart. Respiratory distress in the older infant or child is most frequently due to acute airway disease or traumatic injury; chronic illness and surgical conditions are less frequently responsible.

New treatment modalities and advances in ventilator design and monitoring technology have led to the survival of progressively younger neonates. Sophisticated imaging techniques can provide important insight into thoracic pathologic processes. Ultrasonography, although limited by the poor transmission of sound waves through the air-filled chest, is useful for delineating fluid collections or evaluating the integrity of the diaphragm. Occasionally, computed tomography (CT) or magnetic resonance imaging may be used for further clarification of the cause or location of certain chest processes, whereas echocardiography is invaluable in the evaluation of congenital heart disease.

Critical to the successful management of these patients is the careful radiographic evaluation of the chest and the positioning of intrathoracic life-support devices. In most

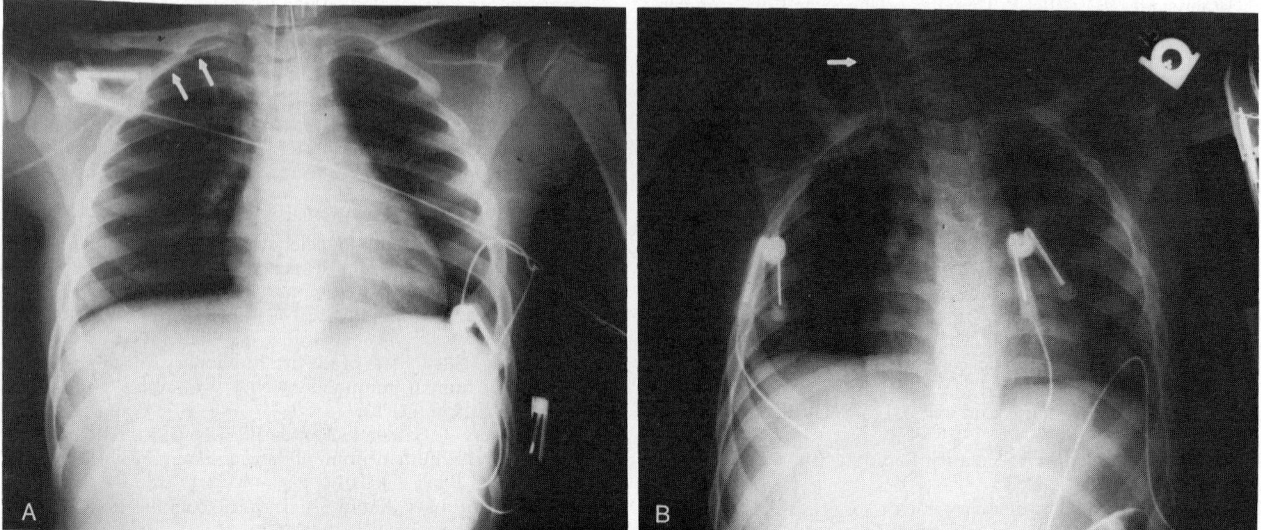

Figure 41–1. Migration of a subclavian catheter. *A,* A right subclavian catheter is in place *(arrows)* with its tip at the proximal margin of the superior vena cava. *B,* A follow-up radiograph shows the catheter in internal jugular vein *(arrow).* No interim manipulation of the catheter occurred.

cases, the frontal projection radiograph and an adequate clinical history are sufficient to establish the diagnosis, so that clinical treatment can be initiated and life-threatening complications monitored. In other cases, the radiologist can assess the need for additional radiologic evaluation and guide the intensivist in selecting the most appropriate study.

In this chapter, some of the more significant medical and surgical disorders of the pediatric chest are discussed.

PEDIATRIC MONITORING: CATHETERS AND TUBES

Central Venous Catheters: Malpositions and Complications

Intravenous catheter malposition or prolonged catheter placement may result in several complications, including intrathoracic infusion of fluids, intra-arterial placement, venous thrombosis, and thromboembolism. Consequently, regular monitoring of proper catheter positioning is important.

In infants, a small degree of arm movement or chest rotation can significantly distort catheter position or result in considerable dislocation of central venous catheters on sequential films. Figure 41–1*A* and *B* shows how a catheter may "travel" from the medial aspect of the subclavian vein to the internal jugular vein. The mechanism for this phenomenon is probably positional; it occurs frequently, and the clinician should be alert to the possibility.

Sometimes a catheter may appear to be intravenous when, in fact, it is not. When the catheter position is not clearly defined on the chest radiograph, a contrast study may be indicated (Fig. 41–2). Alternatively, a catheter may

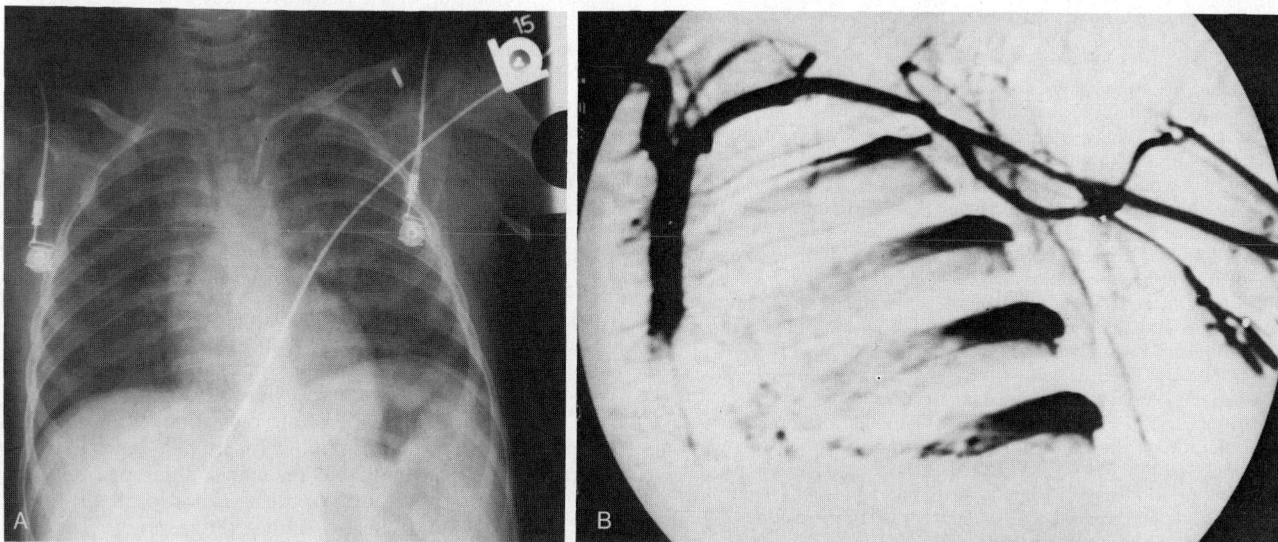

Figure 41–2. Malposition of a subclavian catheter. A subclavian catheter was placed intraoperatively for vascular access and was presumably positioned in the left subclavian vein. Postoperatively, the patient experienced a tingling sensation in the left arm, and a chest radiograph was obtained. The chest radiograph *(A)* suggested intra-aortic placement of the catheter. *B,* Contrast injection through the catheter shows opacification of the left subclavian artery, innominate artery, and descending aorta.

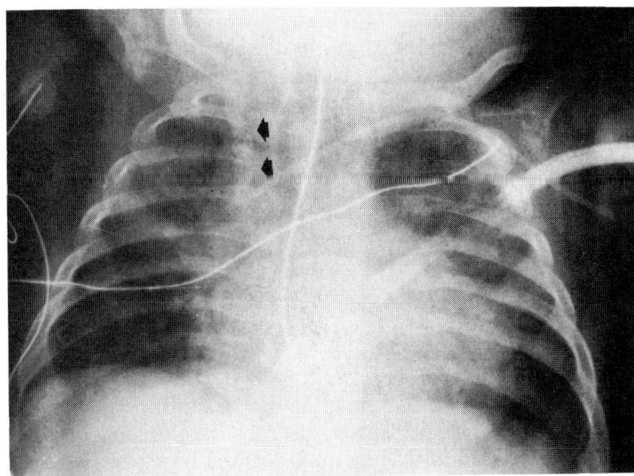

Figure 41–3. Calcified thrombus in the superior vena cava. A patient with prolonged catheter placement in the right internal jugular vein. Note the thickly calcified serpiginous structure outlining the superior vena cava. The thrombus propagated intravascularly, extending from the superior vena cava into the internal jugular vein, and intracranially, passing into the transverse sinus.

penetrate a vascular wall and enter the mediastinum, with extravasation of infused fluid into the mediastinal space.

Prolonged catheter placement can lead to venous thrombosis or thromboembolism. The thrombus may calcify and be visible radiographically (Fig. 41–3). Thrombus formed from central venous catheters may also travel intravascularly, from the superior vena cava into the internal jugular vein and as far cephalad as the transverse sinus.

Chest Tubes

Chest tubes require appropriate positioning to function properly. If the purpose is the evacuate a pneumothorax, the tube tip should be directed anteriorly and superiorly. If the function is to drain pleural fluid, the tube should be directed posteriorly and inferiorly. In all cases, the most distal tube side port must be positioned within the thoracic cavity. Inadvertent chest tube placement in the lung parenchyma occasionally occurs and may produce a bronchopleural fistula (Fig. 41–4).

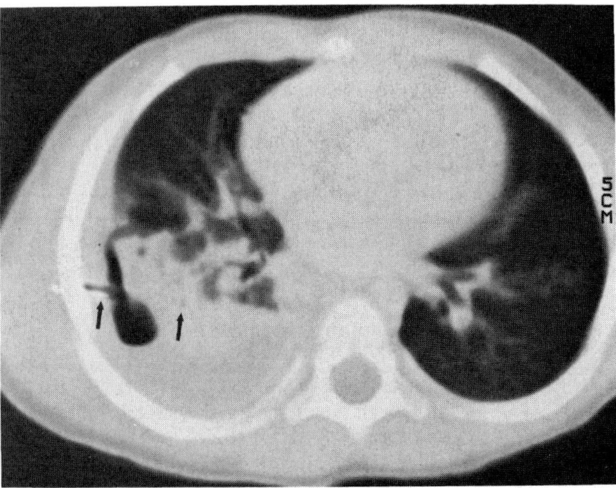

Figure 41–4. Malposition of a chest tube in a 16-month-old infant with right upper lobe pneumonia and right pleural effusion. The chest tube failed to drain the pleural fluid. Computed tomography (CT) of the chest reveals the intraparenchymal location of the tube *(arrows)* and the resultant bronchopleural fistula. Note the abnormal air collection in the right lateral hemithorax.

RESPIRATORY DISORDERS PRESENTING ACUTELY DURING THE FIRST FEW DAYS OF LIFE

Neonatal respiratory distress has numerous causes.[1] The more frequently encountered, requiring management in the neonatal intensive care unit (ICU), are listed in Table 41–1.

Common causes of neonatal respiratory distress include primary pulmonary processes such as respiratory distress syndrome, neonatal pneumonia, transient tachypnea of the newborn, and meconium aspiration syndrome. Congenital pulmonary anomalies make up another category of problems that compromise respiration as a result of mass effect or secondary pneumonitis. Cardiovascular anomalies usually cause respiratory distress from either cyanosis or congestive heart failure. Persistent pulmonary hypertension causes respiratory distress when, in the absence of cardiac anomalies, there is unrelenting hypoxemia despite aggressive oxygen therapy and ventilatory support.

Many extrathoracic problems can produce neonatal respiratory distress, such as congenital malformations of the oral cavity, upper airway, and neck. Central nervous system lesions and metabolic derangements can lead to respiratory

TABLE 41–1. Causes of Neonatal Respiratory Distress

Airway Obstruction
Choanal atresia
Macroglossia, micrognathia
Congenital subglottic stenosis
Laryngeal web or stenosis
Tracheomalacia
Primary Lung Disorders
Respiratory distress syndrome
Neonatal pneumonia
Transient tachypnea of the newborn
Meconium aspiration syndrome
Congenital Pulmonary Anomalies
Congenital diaphragmatic hernia
Congenital lobar emphysema
Pulmonary hypoplasia
Tracheoesophageal fistula
Congenital cystic adenomatoid malformation
Bronchogenic cyst
Neurenteric cyst
Pulmonary sequestration
Pulmonary agenesis
Jeune syndrome (asphyxiating thoracic dystrophy)
Congenital Cardiovascular Anomalies
Pulmonary atresia/severe pulmonic stenosis
Ebstein's anomaly
Tricuspid atresia
D-transposition of the great arteries
Hypoplastic left-heart syndrome
Critical aortic stenosis
Severe coarctation of the aorta
Interrupted aortic arch
Total anomalous pulmonary venous return, with obstruction
Other complex congenital heart lesions
Nonpulmonary Disorders
Metabolic derangement: acidosis, hypothermia, hypoglycemia
Central nervous system lesions: ischemia, hemorrhage
Other
Persistent pulmonary hypertension (persistent fetal circulation)

compromise. These processes have no specific chest radiographic findings and are not covered in this chapter.

The initial chest radiograph of the infant with respiratory distress is obtained to assist with the diagnosis, but it may not be specific. Serial films, however, are most helpful in recognizing improvement or deterioration of lung conditions and in identifying complications. In the following sections the clinical, pathophysiologic, and radiographic manifestations of some of the more important pulmonary processes presenting acutely in the neonatal period are reviewed.

PRIMARY LUNG DISORDERS

Respiratory Distress Syndrome

Respiratory distress syndrome (RDS) affects premature infants as a result of inadequate pulmonary surfactant. The major phospholipid component of surfactant, phosphatidylcholine, has begun to be synthesized and stored at 20 weeks' gestation.[1a] However, it is not clear when these lipids are secreted as surfactant or when surfactant is available in quantities sufficient for successful ventilation after birth. Absence of adequate amounts of surfactant causes neonatal respiratory distress, manifested pathologically by diffuse atelectasis, edema, and cellular injury, with protein and fluid leakage into the alveoli coalescing to form hyaline membranes.

The radiographic findings reflect the pathologic features, with hypoexpansion, and diffuse, fine reticulogranularity of the lungs, usually with air bronchograms. It is important to interpret as air bronchograms only those air-filled bronchi seen beyond the cardiac margins; those confined within the margins of the heart are seen normally because of the relative translucency of the neonatal mediastinum. If severe, the reticulogranular pattern may obscure the margins of the cardiac silhouette (Fig. 41–5). In these patients, the radiographic findings usually appear immediately after birth. In less severe cases, there may be as much as a 24-hour delay before the radiograph becomes diagnostic.

If the disease is mild to moderate in severity, it usually resolves within 4 to 7 days. Traditional treatment regimens include oxygen delivery with continuous positive airway pressure and mechanical ventilation with positive end-expiratory pressure. More recent treatment, used in conjunction with mechanical ventilation, includes surfactant replacement therapy. With the advent of surfactant, the frequency and severity of RDS have significantly decreased by both clinical and radiographic criteria.[2] Recent studies have shown that prophylactic surfactant therapy in newborns less than 30 weeks' gestation results in a higher survival rate (75%) than in neonates treated with rescue surfactant (52%).[3]

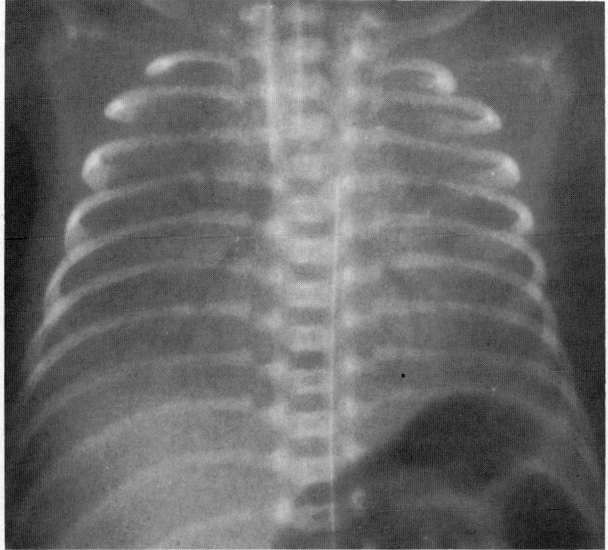

Figure 41–5. RDS in a premature newborn. The characteristic findings of diffuse granular infiltrate and air bronchograms are visualized.

Neonatal Pneumonia

Bacterial infections are a major cause of morbidity and mortality in the newborn. The agent most responsible for neonatal pneumonia is the group B β-hemolytic streptococcus (GBS). Infection with GBS is usually early in onset, most often resulting from exposure to infected amniotic fluid in utero or intrapartum exposure during vaginal transit. Maternal risk factors include premature labor and premature rupture of membranes. Histopathologic changes in the lungs bear some similarity to RDS with patchy hyaline membrane formation but with absence of the severe atelectasis seen with RDS. This is accompanied by inflammatory exudate mixed with cocci.[4]

Radiographically, patients with GBS exhibit features indistinguishable from RDS, with reticulogranularity and air bronchograms. Frequently, however, the lungs are normally expanded, and there may be a pleural effusion with GBS, which helps to distinguish this from RDS. In a retrospective study of infants who died from GBS, chest radiographs demonstrated pleural effusions in 67%. Pleural fluid was uncommon in both RDS and non-GBS neonatal sepsis.[5]

Treatment consists of broad-spectrum antibiotics and supportive care. Patients may have associated pulmonary hypertension. Survivors frequently have severe sequelae from septic shock and hypoxemia.

Transient Tachypnea of the Newborn

Transient tachypnea of the newborn (TTN), also known as wet lung disease or retained fetal fluid, is a common, self-limited condition characterized by tachypnea and mild cyanosis during the first several hours to days of life caused by delayed resorption of fetal lung fluid. There are several predisposing factors, including cesarean section, maternal diabetes, significant maternal sedation, precipitous delivery, and asphyxia. It is believed that the lack of the usual uterine squeeze is responsible for the delayed clearing of fluid from the lungs into the bronchial tree.

The radiographic findings are typically streaky, linear densities emanating from the hila and extending to the lung periphery, representing prominent vascular markings with hazy margins, caused by excessive perivascular interstitial fluid. These markings are often accompanied by a fluid-filled minor fissure or small pleural effusions, usually seen at the costophrenic sulcus (Fig. 41–6). The cardiac silhouette is normal in size. The chest film usually shows clearing within 48 to 72 hours. If findings are persistent beyond 72 hours, with normal heart size, the differential diagnosis should include neonatal pneumonia, obstructive total anomalous pulmonary venous return, or patent ductus arteriosus. Because the radiographic changes of TTN mimic those of other, more severe processes, it should be considered a diagnosis of exclusion.

Treatment is supportive with oxygen and parenteral fluids. The prognosis is excellent.

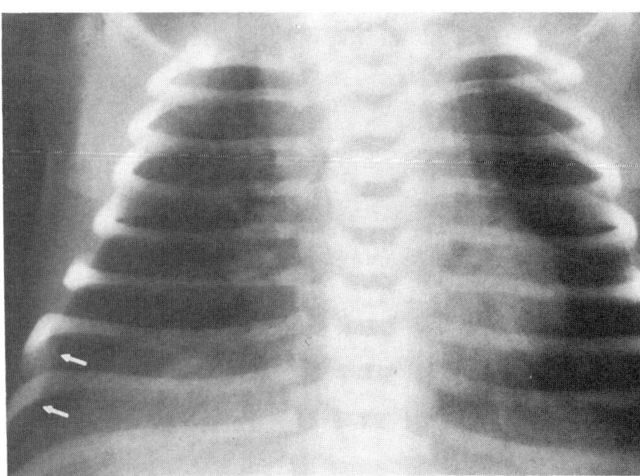

Figure 41–6. Transient tachypnea in a near-term neonate with increased respiratory rate. Note the prominent, hazy vascular markings and small right pleural effusion *(arrows)*.

Meconium Aspiration

Fetal distress can result in passage of meconium in utero; gasping respirations can then cause aspiration of meconium with bronchial obstruction, followed by postnatal interference with gas exchange, and severe respiratory distress. This occurs in as many as 62% of neonates born with meconium-stained amniotic fluid[6] and is seen in term and postmature infants who have experienced some degree of intrapartum hypoxia. Pulmonary hypertension may follow the meconium aspiration and contributes to the hypoxia.

The chest radiograph usually reveals hyperexpansion of the lungs with bilateral, coarse, patchy densities reflecting obstructive atelectasis and probable associated pneumonitis (Fig. 41–7). Complications of air-block phenomena (pneumothorax, pneumomediastinum, and so on) occur in approximately 25% and cause increased morbidity and possible mortality. The risk of these complications is increased with the barotrauma of mechanical ventilation.

Therapy with oxygen and mechanical ventilation is traditional. To this can be added drug therapy with pulmonary vasodilators and high-frequency ventilation. Failure here with noninvasive methods, as judged by the predetermined parameter of arterial–alveolar gradients and other such formulas, can logically lead to extracorporeal membrane oxygenation (ECMO), a form of cardiopulmonary bypass that may improve survival and reduce long-term morbidity. Patients with persistent progressive pulmonary hypertension and severe right-to-left shunting who are not responding to ventilator and pharmacologic manipulation may benefit from this therapy.

Persistent Pulmonary Hypertension

Persistent pulmonary hypertension, also known as persistent fetal circulation, is sustained, elevated pulmonary arterial pressure with right-to-left shunting, through a patent foramen ovale, a patent ductus arteriosus, or an extrathoracic shunt, occurring because the pulmonary vascular resistance exceeds systemic vascular resistance after transition to the neonatal circulation. It may be an isolated, idiopathic process, or it may be secondary to other pathophysiologic events, such as meconium aspiration, perinatal asphyxia, neonatal sepsis (including GBS pneumonia), or congenital diaphragmatic hernia.

The chest radiograph may show a variety of abnormalities, including the presence of interstitial fluid densities with or without cardiomegaly, or it may appear completely normal.

SELECTED CONGENITAL PULMONARY ANOMALIES

Pulmonary Hypoplasia

Pulmonary hypoplasia involves a spectrum of lung abnormalities characterized by pulmonary underdevelopment resulting from a variety of in utero insults. The process can be unilateral or bilateral. Unilateral pulmonary hypoplasia occurs when lung development is arrested; rudimentary pulmonary tissue is evident pathologically. Affected patients are usually asymptomatic. The chest radiograph reveals a small, radiodense affected hemithorax caused by reduced aeration.

Bilateral pulmonary hypoplasia most commonly occurs secondary to intrauterine compression of the fetal thorax, usually caused by oligohydramnios, resulting from severe bilateral renal disease or urinary outflow tract obstruction. Bony dysplasias of the thoracic cage (e.g., asphyxiating thoracic dystrophy), which restrict fetal respiratory movements, can also limit pulmonary growth, leading to bilateral hypoplasia. Intrathoracic masses that directly compress the lung, such as congenital diaphragmatic hernia or congenital cystic adenomatoid malformation, may be etiologic factors. Primary pulmonary hypoplasia, although less common, can also occur.

Clinically, patients with bilateral hypoplasia have severe respiratory distress and are prone to complications of pneumothorax and pneumomediastinum. The chest radiograph in bilateral hypoplasia demonstrates clear but small lungs. Spontaneous pneumothorax may be present at birth (Fig. 41–8).

Congenital Diaphragmatic Hernia

Congenital diaphragmatic hernia represents in utero herniation of abdominal contents into the chest, usually through the posteriorly located foramen of Bochdalek. The vast ma-

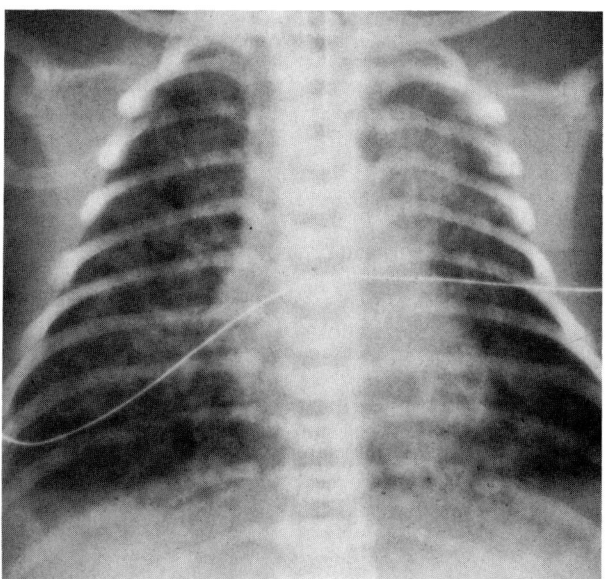

Figure 41–7. Meconium aspiration syndrome. This chest radiograph reveals coarse, asymmetric, and patchy bilateral opacities and hyperinflation.

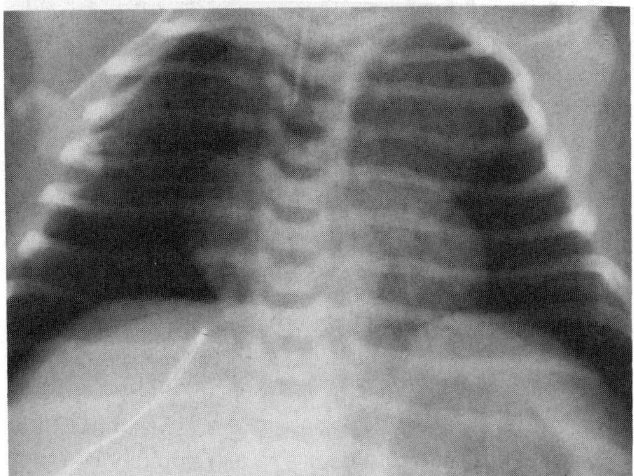

Figure 41–8. Pulmonary hypoplasia due to renal dysplasia. A chest radiograph obtained after intubation in this neonate with respiratory distress reveals bilateral pneumothoraces (lungs are collapsed medially). Note the small size of the thoracic cage.

jority occur on the left. Hernia contents can include bowel, stomach, spleen, liver, or omentum. The herniated abdominal structures exert considerable mass effect on the lungs, leading to long-standing compression and mediastinal shift in utero and resultant bilateral pulmonary hypoplasia. Both lungs are diminished in size, but the process is more marked on the ipsilateral side.

Clinically, the newborn may have a scaphoid abdomen, and bowel sounds may be auscultated in the chest. Large hernias cause severe and immediate respiratory distress because of respiratory compromise from pulmonary compression and hypoplasia.

The chest radiograph classically demonstrates multiple bubbly-appearing lucencies representing loops of intestine in the affected hemithorax, with pulmonary compression and shift of the mediastinum to the contralateral side (Fig. 41–9). Immediately after birth, before the infant has swallowed air into the gut, the herniated structures may be radiopaque, representing fluid-filled or collapsed bowel. There is usually a paucity or complete absence of abdominal bowel gas depending on the size of the hernia. This finding may be very important to the diagnosis if the bowel in the chest is gasless. Dilated, gas-filled, intra-abdominal bowel suggests bowel entrapment and obstruction.

In the newborn infant, the intrathoracic changes are radiographically similar to cystic adenomatoid malformation.[7] However, in the latter, the normal component of abdominal gas should be present.

The infant is resuscitated and stabilized before surgical correction, with measures including nasogastric intubation to relieve trapped air and positive-pressure ventilation. If there is relentless respiratory deterioration, the patient may benefit from the use of high-frequency (jet) ventilation or ECMO.

Congenital Lobar Emphysema

Congenital lobar emphysema is characterized by progressive hyperinflation and air trapping in one or more pulmonary lobes. The usually single hyperinflated lobe causes compression and atelectasis of the adjacent lobes or contralateral lung. Proposed causes include an obstructing lesion or congenitally insufficient bronchial cartilage leading to bronchial collapse. This results in a focal, ball-valve obstruction with air trapping, most commonly affecting the left upper lobe. The right middle and right upper lobes are next in order of frequency.

Clinically, there is acute or subacute respiratory distress in the newborn infant. Some neonates, however, are asymptomatic until older and then present with multiple respiratory infections and wheezing. Breath sounds are usually diminished over the involved lung.

The chest radiograph may initially demonstrate a large, radiopaque mass occupying one lobe and compressing adjacent aerated lobes. This mass is initially radiopaque because of delayed clearance of fetal lung fluid from the abnormal lobe.[7a] Later, after the fluid evacuates, the affected lobe becomes hyperlucent and hyperexpanded (Fig. 41–10*A*). There is compressive atelectasis of the adjacent lung parenchyma and mediastinal shift to the contralateral side. Similar findings are demonstrated on chest CT images (see Fig. 41–10*B*).

If the child is acutely symptomatic, surgical removal of the overinflated lobe with or without prior bronchoscopy is usually performed. However, there can be long-term improvement with conservative management. In one retrospective study of 12 children so treated, there was both symptomatic and radiologic improvement during an average follow-up of approximately 3 years.[7b] Nonoperative therapy can be anatomically assessed with both serial chest radiographs and CT, which can demonstrate a reduction in size of the emphysematous lobe. Gradual improvement in pulmonary function can be evaluated with nuclear medicine ventilation-perfusion imaging.

Esophageal Atresia/Tracheoesophageal Fistula

Esophageal atresia and tracheoesophageal fistula are congenital malformations in a spectrum of anomalies that may exist independently or in various combinations with each

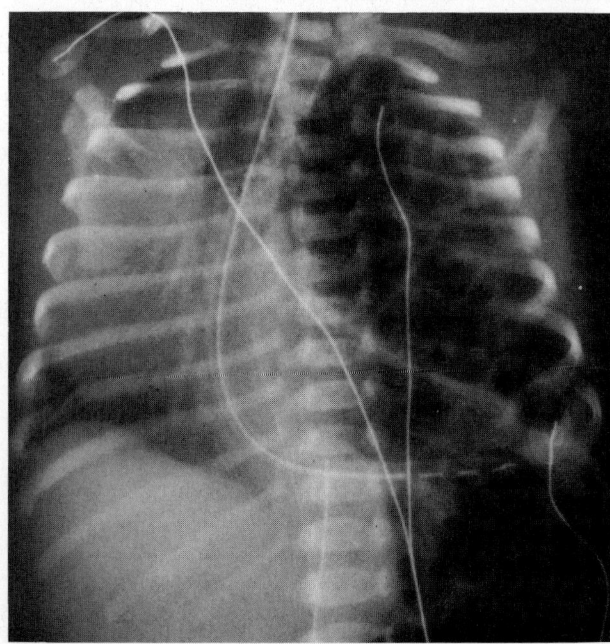

Figure 41–9. Congenital diaphragmatic hernia in a newborn infant with respiratory distress and a scaphoid abdomen. Multiple cystic lucencies are seen in the left side of the chest; the cysts exhibit mass effect and cause mediastinal shift to the right. Also note the abnormal position of the nasogastric tube, with the tip returning to the chest.

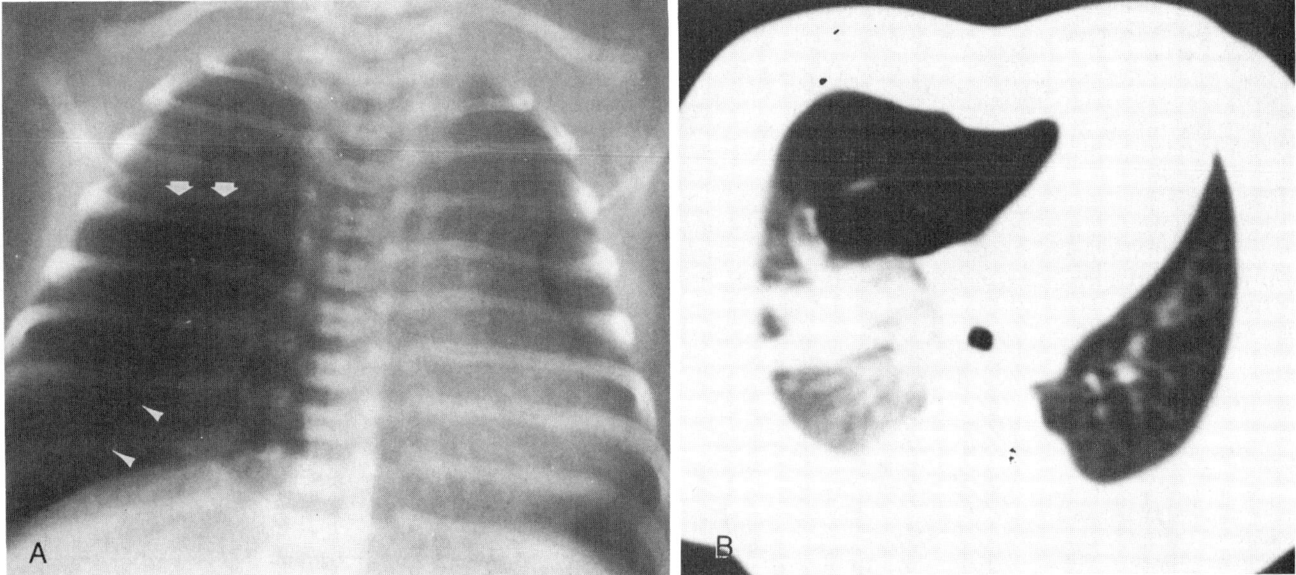

Figure 41–10. Congenital lobar emphysema. *A,* The right middle lobe is hyperlucent and hyperinflated, with resultant compression of the upper and lower lobes. Note the minor fissure *(arrows)* and the margin of right lower lobe *(arrowheads)*. *B,* A CT image demonstrates hyperexpansion of the middle lobe with vessel attenuation and compression of adjacent lung parenchyma. Note the shift of the heart to the left.

other. The malformations occur secondary to defective separation of the primitive trachea and esophagus. The result is an abnormal fistulous connection to the trachea from either an atretic segment of esophagus or from a nonatretic esophagus or complete atresia of the esophagus with no fistulous connection.

The most common variation is proximal atresia with distal tracheoesophageal fistula (85%). Saliva and feedings may pass into the trachea from above, and gastric contents may reflux into the trachea from below, pass through the fistula, and incite a severe aspiration pneumonitis.

In the case of esophageal atresia with or without a fistula, there is difficulty handling normal secretions, with drooling and choking. Resistance is encountered proximally during attempted passage of a nasogastric tube.

The chest radiographic appearance varies with the specific type of anomaly. With esophageal atresia, a dilated, gas-filled proximal esophageal pouch may be present. If this is an isolated finding with no fistula, there will be no gas present within the abdominal bowel loops (Fig. 41–11). When a fistula is present from the trachea to the distal esophagus, the abdominal bowel loops are gas filled and distended; there may be evidence of aspiration pneumonitis.

SELECTED CONGENITAL CARDIOVASCULAR ANOMALIES

Cardiovascular anomalies usually present with cyanosis or congestive heart failure and can be so classified. Table 41–2 lists congenital cardiac anomalies that occur during the neonatal period according to this classification, which is adapted from a functional approach to diagnosis by Gyepes and Vincent.[8] The selected lesions are seen in patients who are symptomatic at or shortly after birth.

Neonatal cardiovascular anomalies can also be characterized according to the features visualized on the chest radiograph.[8a] The cardiac configuration is usually abnormal in patients with congenital heart disease, but the heart can also appear completely normal with severe cardiac disease. Cer-

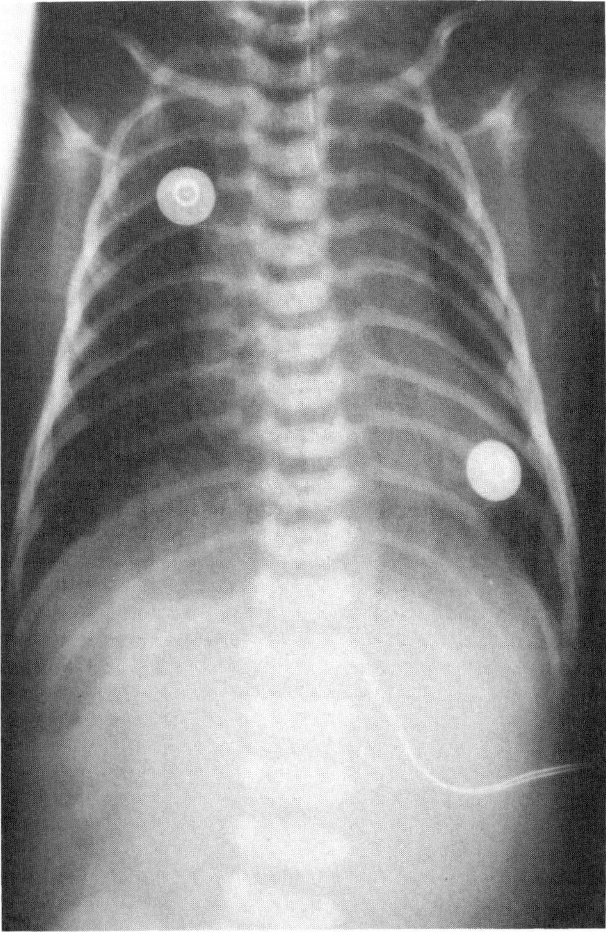

Figure 41–11. Esophageal atresia in a newborn with drooling and choking. The nasogastric tube could not be passed (note the tip at the T-3 vertebral level). No gas is present in the abdomen; this is consistent with esophageal atresia without fistula.

TABLE 41–2. Congenital Heart Disease in Neonates by Clinical Presentation

Diseases Presenting with Cyanosis
Pulmonary atresia/severe pulmonary stenosis with intact pulmonary septum
Pulmonary atresia/severe pulmonary stenosis with ventricular septal defect
Ebstein's anomaly
Tricuspid atresia
D-transposition of the great arteries
Diseases Presenting with Congestive Heart Failure
Hypoplastic left-heart syndrome
Critical aortic stenosis
Coarctation of the aorta: severe
Coarctation syndrome
Interrupted aortic arch
Total anomalous pulmonary venous return, with obstruction
Truncus arteriosus

(Data from Gyepes MT, Vincent WR: Severe congenital heart disease in the neonatal period: A functional approach to emergency diagnosis. Am J Roentgenol 1971; 116:490.)

TABLE 41–3. Congenital Heart Disease in Neonates by Radiographic Presentation

Decreased Pulmonary Vascularity
Pulmonary atresia/severe pulmonary stenosis with intact pulmonary septum
Pulmonary atresia/severe pulmonary stenosis with ventricular septal defect
Ebstein's anomaly
Tricuspid atresia
Pulmonary Venous Obstruction
Hypoplastic left-heart syndrome
Coarctation of the aorta: severe
Critical aortic stenosis
Coarctation syndrome
Interrupted aortic arch
Total anomalous pulmonary venous return, with obstruction
Initially Normal and Then Increased Pulmonary Vascularity
D-transposition of the great arteries
Atrioventricular canal
Truncus arteriosus
Single ventricle

tain cardiac configurations are characteristic for certain congenital anomalies. The oval or egg-on-a-string appearance is seen in D-transposition of the great arteries: The "string" represents the narrow superior mediastinum and results from the radiographically absent thymus and the anteroposterior relationship of the transposed aorta and main pulmonary artery (the pulmonary artery lies directly behind the aorta). A boot-shaped heart is seen with tetralogy of Fallot and is produced by the prominent, laterally displaced cardiac apex (caused by right ventricular hypertrophy) and the concave main pulmonary artery segment seen just superiorly. Marked cardiomegaly in the neonate is usually caused by right atrial enlargement (prominent rounded border of the right side of the heart) and should suggest either Ebstein's anomaly or pulmonary atresia/severe stenosis with intact ventricular septum.

Although these characteristic configurations may be helpful, a more useful radiologic clue to the cause of the cardiac anomaly can be derived from the appearance of the pulmonary vascular markings (Table 41–3).

Decreased pulmonary vascularity denotes diminished volume of blood flowing through the lungs with right-to-left shunting and clinical cyanosis. Decreased pulmonary blood flow is evident in obstructive lesions of the right side of the heart such as pulmonary atresia or severe stenosis, tricuspid atresia, or Ebstein's anomaly (Fig. 41–12). Tetralogy of Fallot, which usually presents later in infancy, can present in the newborn if the associated pulmonary stenosis is severe. Pulmonary venous obstruction indicates passive congestion of the pulmonary venous bed with transudation of fluid into surrounding perivascular interstitial tissues. This pattern is characterized radiographically by prominent vessels with indistinct margins. Pulmonary venous hypertension is associated with obstructive lesions of the left side of the heart such as hypoplastic left heart syndrome (Fig. 41–13), critical aortic stenosis, severe coarctation of the aorta, and total anomalous pulmonary venous return with obstruction (Fig. 41–14). The clinical presentation in these patients is usually congestive heart failure and diminished systemic perfusion.

Congestive heart failure can also present in the newborn secondary to perinatal events affecting the heart. These in-

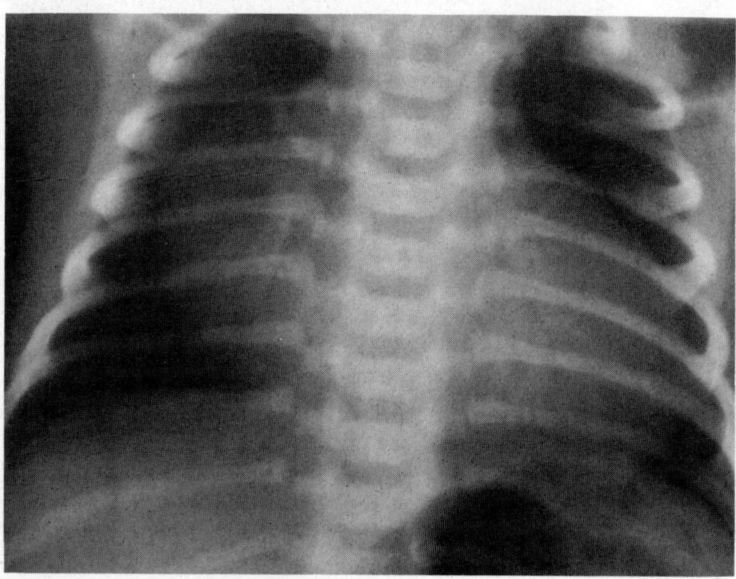

Figure 41–12. Ebstein's anomaly in a newborn with cyanosis and dyspnea. Severe cardiomegaly with marked right atrial enlargement is evident. The pulmonary blood flow is diminished.

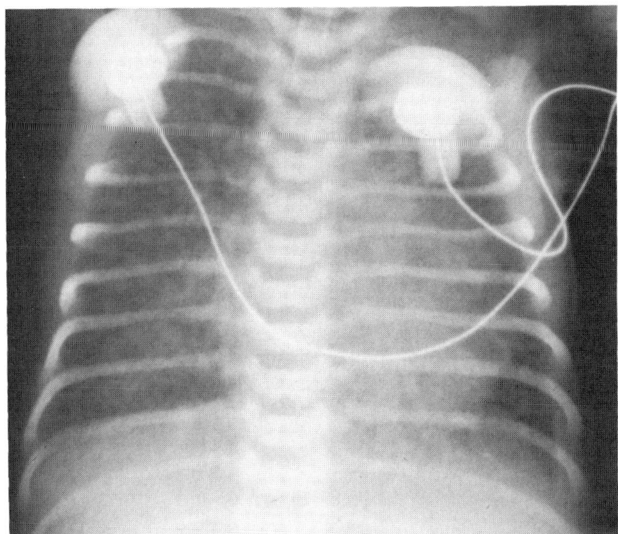

Figure 41–13. Hypoplastic left-heart syndrome in a newborn infant with grunting, poor systemic perfusion, and hepatomegaly. Cardiomegaly and marked pulmonary venous congestion are present. Note the small, bilateral pleural effusions.

clude transient myocardial ischemia as a result of perinatal asphyxia, myocarditis caused by perinatal infection, tachyarrhythmias, and conduction disturbances. Additional noncardiac causes of congestive heart failure in the neonate include high-flow states, as seen with arteriovenous malformations (vein of Galen malformation, hemangioendothelioma), and severe anemia; metabolic abnormalities, such as hypoglycemia and acidosis; severe infection; and hydrops.

Increased pulmonary vascularity is seen when there is more than the normal volume of blood flowing through the lungs and is present in conditions with left-to-right shunts. This radiographic finding is rarely present within the first few days of life because the degree of shunting is initially restricted by the high pulmonary vascular resistance in the transition period from fetal to neonatal life. Gradually, however, the neonate's pulmonary vascularity increases over time and appears excessive in patients with left-to-right shunts. At least a two to one shunt is required for radiographic recognition. Patients with admixture lesions such as tricuspid atresia, truncus arteriosus, and single ventricle usually present at birth because of severe cyanosis. Although not strictly considered an admixture lesion, D-transposition of the great arteries should be included in this group; it is the most common cause of cyanotic congenital heart disease in the newborn. During the first few days of life, the pulmonary vascularity on the normal neonate's chest radiograph is normal to slightly diminished because of high pulmonary vascular pressures. If there is also a cyanotic lesion, the pulmonary blood flow is markedly diminished, usually because of pulmonic stenosis. Later, as pulmonary vascular resistance decreases, shunting can occur across a patent foramen ovale, patent ductus arteriosus, or septal defect, and increased pulmonary blood flow is visualized (Fig. 41–15). Other left-to-right shunt lesions including atrioventricular canal defects and large ventricular septal defects present later in infancy with either a murmur or congestive failure from markedly increased pulmonary vascular flow. Patients with atrial septal defects rarely have severe cardiopulmonary problems during the first 30 days of life.

Another important consideration in the category of left-to-right shunts is the premature neonate with RDS who has persistent patency or reopening of a partially closed ductus arteriosus. The chest radiograph is often key to the diagnosis when the clinical picture is uncertain. Poorly defined pulmonary vessels caused by interstitial edema or diffuse airspace haziness from florid alveolar edema are the hallmarks (Fig. 41–16). The cardiac silhouette often enlarges, but this is not always evident. Visualization of flow through the ductus with color Doppler sonography is used to confirm the diagnosis.

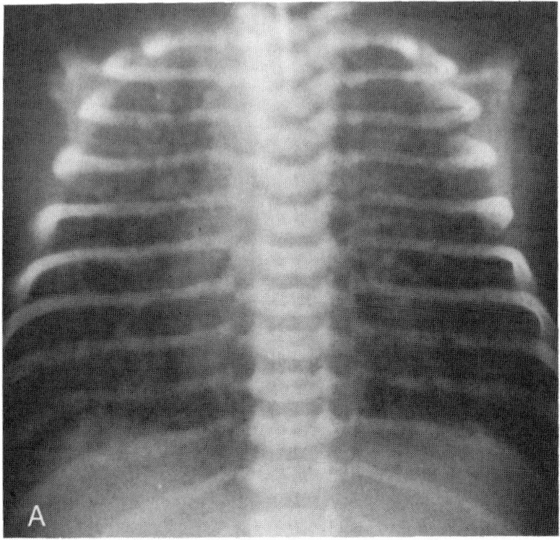

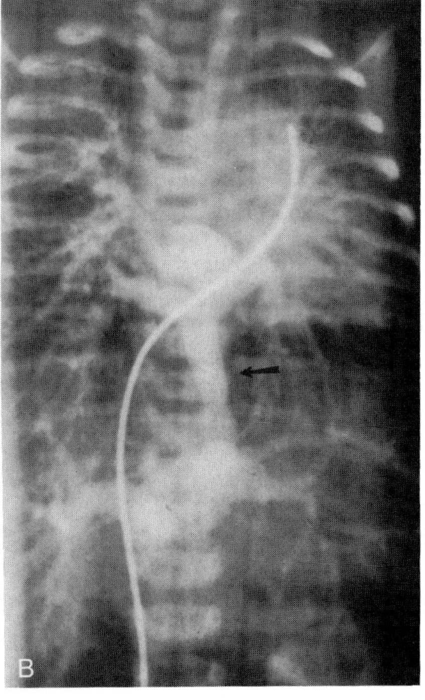

Figure 41–14. Total anomalous pulmonary venous return with subdiaphragmatic obstruction. *A,* This initial chest radiograph demonstrates prominent pulmonary vessels with indistinct margins, a finding consistent with venous congestion. Note that the heart is of normal size; this is typical for type III total anomalous pulmonary venous return. *B,* Venous phase of the pulmonary angiogram shows pulmonary veins converging to form an anomalous vessel *(arrow)* that travels subdiaphragmatically to enter the portal vein.

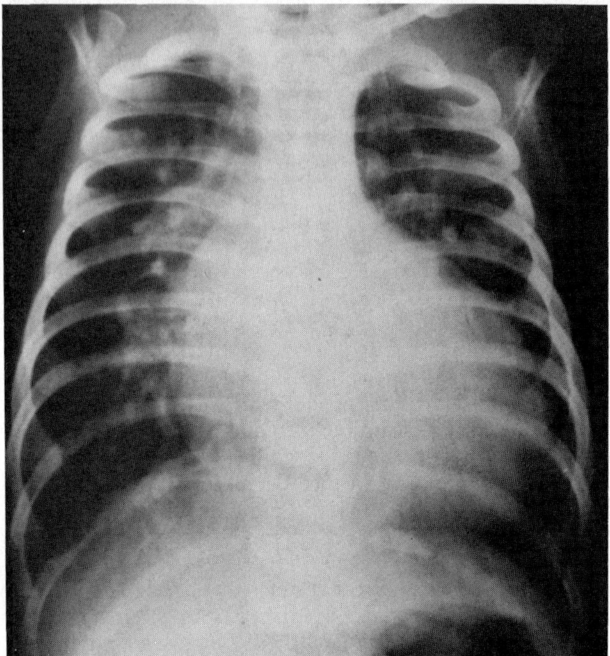

Figure 41–15. D-Transposition of the great vessels. This chest radiograph of an older infant illustrates markedly increased pulmonary blood flow. Note "egg-on-a-string" appearance of the cardiac silhouette, which occurs secondary to a narrow cardiac waist, enlarged heart, and inapparent aorta. The aorta and pulmonary artery are aligned more anteroposteriorly than usual, giving the appearance of a narrow mediastinum.

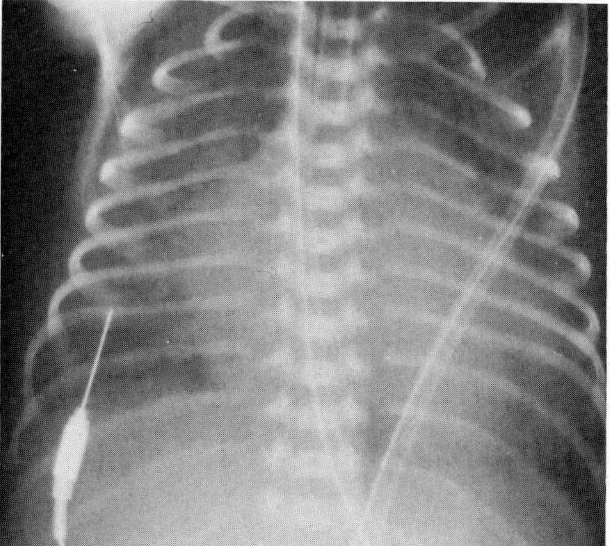

Figure 41–16. Patent ductus arteriosus in a premature neonate with RDS. The initial chest radiograph demonstrated a mild granular infiltrate, a finding consistent with RDS. Six days later, the patient became tachypneic. This follow-up chest radiograph reveals the development of cardiomegaly, indistinct pulmonary vascular margins, and diffuse lung opacity; these signs are consistent with pulmonary edema occurring secondary to patent ductus arteriosus.

Air-Block Phenomena in the Neonate

Air-block phenomena occur with high-pressure ventilation; escape of air from the terminal airspaces and dissection into the interstitial or pleural space creates fixed areas of abnormal inflation. Such processes occur frequently in the ventilated neonate when "excessive" or uneven ventilation exerts prolonged tension on alveolar walls. Other inciting conditions include the infant's own forceful, initial respiratory efforts, resuscitation procedures, and generalized or localized air trapping. The resulting pathologic air collections include pulmonary interstitial emphysema, pneumomediastinum, pneumothorax, pneumopericardium, and intravascular air embolism.

Pulmonary interstitial emphysema occurs when air dissects from a ruptured alveolus into the interstitium and becomes trapped. Lung compliance is significantly reduced, and there may be decreased chest excursion. Radiographically, the affected area is hyperinflated, and there are branching radiolucencies extending from the hila to the lung periphery that do not collapse on expiration and do not resemble air in branching bronchi. These lucencies can be linear or rounded and cystlike in appearance (Fig. 41–17). Conservative management for unilateral pulmonary interstitial emphysema is sometimes effective; the patient is positioned with the overinflated lung in the dependent position in an effort to decompress it through decreased ventilation. When more aggressive treatment is needed, selective intubation of the contralateral mainstem bronchus or selective balloon occlusion of the ipsilateral bronchus may be attempted. Other alternative therapies for severe, diffuse pulmonary interstitial emphysema include high-frequency (jet) ventilation and ECMO. Pulmonary interstitial emphysema may secondarily produce pneumomediastinum or pneumothorax.

Pneumomediastinum occurs when interstitial air from a ruptured alveolus escapes into the mediastinum. In the neonate, this follows barotrauma and traumatic intubation or occasionally can be seen spontaneously. Pneumomediastinum is seen most reliably on the lateral chest radiograph, which can be obtained in the cross-table lateral projection. The abnormal air collection is anterior to the heart in the

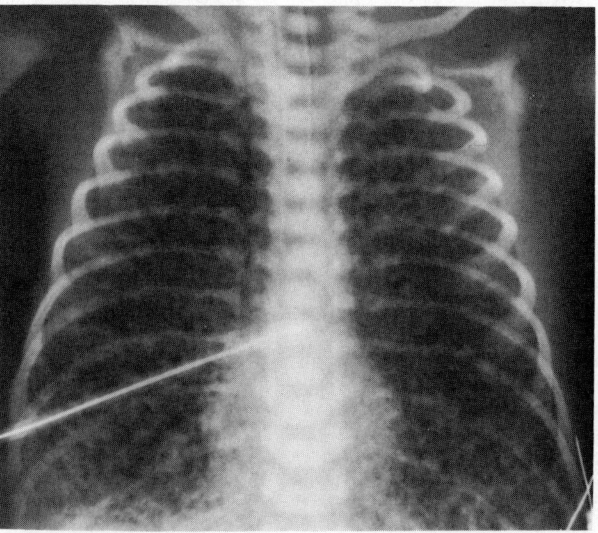

Figure 41–17. Pulmonary interstitial emphysema in a premature infant treated with mechanical ventilation for RDS. Both lungs are severely hyperexpanded, with linear and circular lucencies radiating from the hila to the periphery.

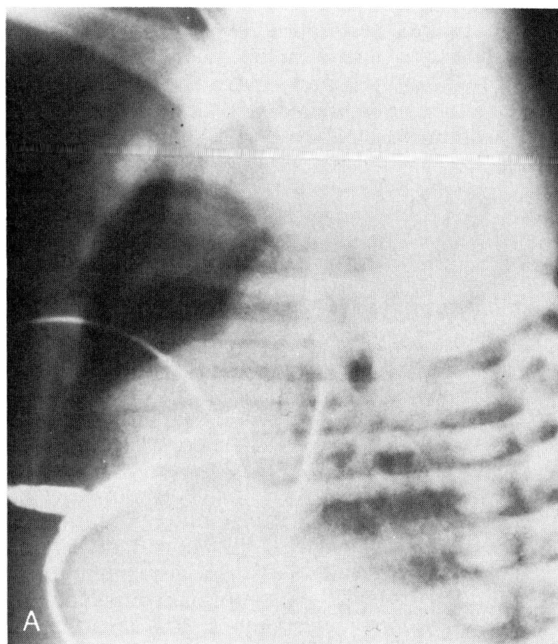

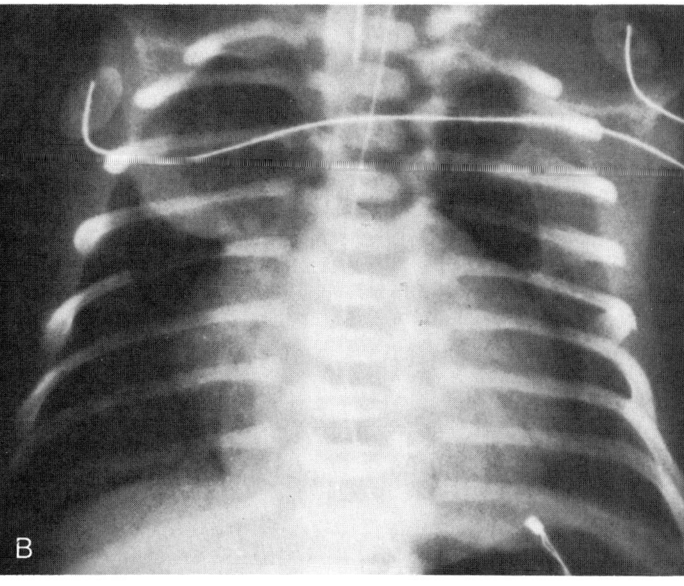

Figure 41–18. Pneumomediastinum. Lateral *(A)* and frontal *(B)* chest radiographs reveal lucency centered over the mediastinum superiorly and lifting of the thymus.

mediastinal space (Fig. 41–18*A*). The frontal view of the chest may also demonstrate the air collection elevating the thymus, creating the thymic "spinnaker sail" sign (see Fig. 41–18*B*). A linear area of radiolucency along the cardiac border or outlining the edge of the descending aorta is more subtle evidence of mediastinal air. Subcutaneous emphysema in the neck may be noted. Occasionally, a medially located pneumothorax may mimic pneumomediastinum. Differentiation can be made with a lateral decubitus film; a pneumothorax will move along the elevated portion of the thorax, whereas the pneumomediastinum will not.

Mediastinal air collections may decompress by dissecting into the fascial planes of the neck, with subcutaneous emphysema, or by tracking through the esophageal hiatus into the abdomen, leading to free retroperitoneal or intraperitoneal air. Collections can also be seen subpulmonically, loculated by or within the inferior pulmonary ligaments. Serious complications include rupture into the pericardial sac, with pneumopericardium, or disruption of the pulmonary venous system, and systemic air embolism.

There is no specific therapy for pneumomediastinum. It is important, nevertheless, to observe for the potentially serious complications mentioned previously.

Pneumothorax occurs when air dissects from a ruptured alveolus into the interstitium and escapes into the pleural space. Several risk factors for development of pneumothorax are well known: meconium aspiration, pulmonary hypoplasia caused by renal dysplasia, endotracheal intubation, resuscitation, and positive-pressure ventilation. The infant may exhibit signs of sudden deterioration, with severe respiratory distress. Breath sounds are diminished over the affected hemithorax. The chest radiograph will usually demonstrate lung collapse with an expanded pleural space on the ipsilateral side. If the pneumothorax is under tension (Fig. 41–19), there is associated mediastinal shift to the contralateral hemithorax. More subtle signs of pneumothorax include widened rib interspaces and depression of the ipsilateral hemidiaphragm, giving a "deep-sulcus" sign. Occasionally, the pneumothorax can accumulate medial to the lung. In this instance, if the diagnosis is not straightforward, a lateral decubitus view, with the suspected side up, will often reveal the abnormality. Chest tube placement is required in patients with tension pneumothorax, in patients with progressive accumulation of intrapleural air, and in patients receiving positive-pressure ventilation. Tube position is confirmed by frontal and lateral chest radiographs. When optimally placed, the tube is directed into the anterior pleural space, with the side port projecting within the confines of the chest wall.

Pneumopericardium occurs when air ruptures into the pericardial sac. This abnormal air collection is less common than those previously described, but because it has potentially severe consequences, accurate and rapid diagnosis is important. Symptomatic patients often have acute onset of

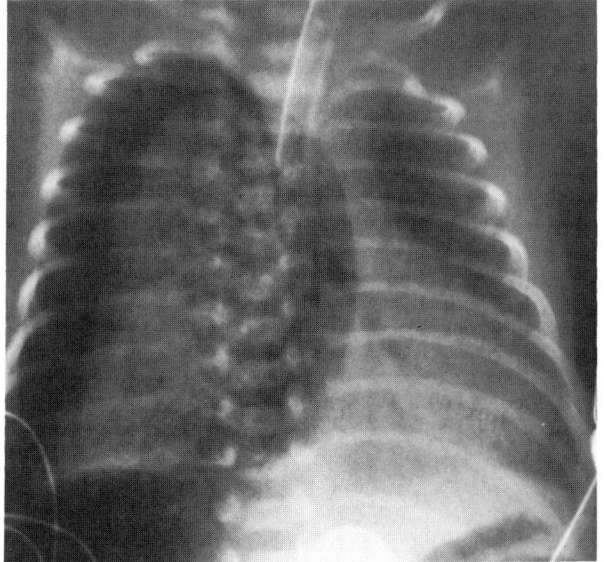

Figure 41–19. A right-sided tension pneumothorax in neonate treated for RDS.

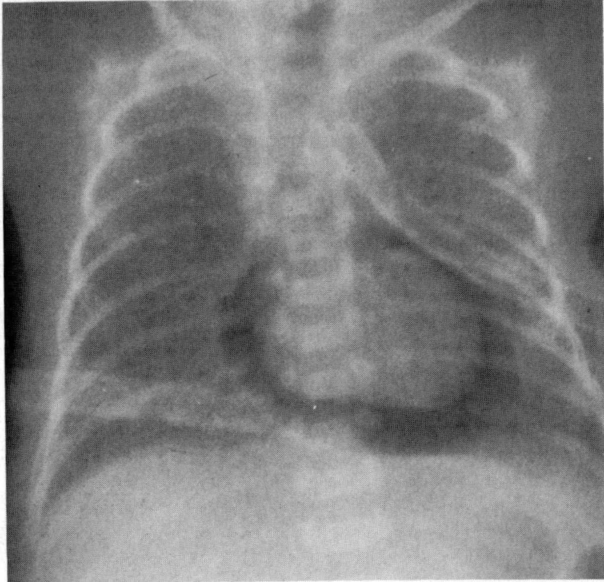

Figure 41–20. Pneumopericardium in an infant with RDS. Note the presence of radiolucent air encircling the heart that has occurred secondary to barotrauma. The endotracheal tube is high in position at the thoracic inlet.

hypotension, cyanosis, and decreased pulse pressure, and decreased breath sounds are auscultated on examination. The chest radiograph reveals a well-defined radiolucency encircling the heart (Fig. 41–20). The cardiac silhouette may be diminished in size if the process is under significant tension, with restricted venous return to the heart. Clinical signs of impaired cardiac output or cardiac tamponade require pericardiocentesis, sometimes with placement of a pericardial drainage catheter.

Pneumoperitoneum follows the decompression of intrathoracic air, such as pneumomediastinum, into the abdomen. The presumed mechanism is extension through a diaphragmatic hiatus into the retroperitoneum, into the bowel mesentery, and through the subserosal surface of the bowel with subsequent leak into the peritoneal cavity.[9] The importance of making this diagnosis is to differentiate the process from a ruptured viscus or from necrotizing enterocolitis with perforation. A ruptured viscus will demonstrate free intraperitoneal air without associated abnormal air collection in the chest. The hallmark of necrotizing enterocolitis is linear or circular lucencies within the bowel wall, sometimes accompanied by portal venous gas. If the pneumoperitoneum is sufficiently large, it may limit diaphragmatic movement and compromise respiration.

Intravascular air embolus is a rare but serious complication of positive-pressure–assisted ventilation. It often follows pulmonary interstitial emphysema and is usually massive, with air filling the heart and large vessels on the chest radiograph. The finding usually represents a terminal event in the treatment of RDS.

RESPIRATORY DISORDERS PRESENTING IN THE OLDER INFANT AND CHILD

Severe respiratory distress in children is a frequent indication for pediatric ICU admission. The causes are many; however, the mechanisms of lung injury are frequently similar. The most common pediatric respiratory problems requiring ICU management are acute airway disease and various types of trauma. Surgical conditions and complications of chronic illnesses make up the remainder. Current critical care management of these problems can be assisted by multiple imaging modalities, including plain films, ultrasonography, CT, and nuclear medicine scintigraphy.

Airway Disease

Bronchiolitis

Bronchiolitis is an acute inflammatory process of the respiratory epithelium in infants and small children whose airways are relatively small and highly susceptible to inflammatory narrowing. Pathophysiologically, edema and secretions obstruct the small bronchioles, creating airway narrowing, areas of irregular aeration, air trapping, and atelectasis. Affected children experience sudden onset of wheezing, caused by turbulent expiratory airflow traveling through narrowed air passages. There is frequently fever, cough, tachypnea, and tachycardia. Infants and children up to 2 years of age are usually affected. Children with bronchopulmonary dysplasia, congenital heart disease, or immunodeficiency syndromes especially are at increased risk for bronchiolitis and frequently need treatment in an acute care setting. Respiratory syncytial virus (RSV) is the most common etiologic agent, although a number of other viral pathogens have been incriminated. Hospitalization for RSV pneumonia is rarely required, but of those who are hospitalized, 11% may require intensive care and 8% may require intubation and ventilation.[10]

The chest radiograph (Fig. 41–21) typically demonstrates generalized hyperinflation of the lungs as a result of air trapping. Areas of focal hyperinflation alternate with patchy zones of atelectasis. As the disease develops, the areas of atelectasis may progress to complete segmental or lobar collapse. There may be perihilar linear opacities caused by bronchial wall thickening and peribronchial cuffing representing peribronchial inflammatory edema.

Sudden-onset wheezing can also occur with foreign body aspiration, an important differential diagnostic consideration. In this case, there is air trapping on the affected side, which is exaggerated on lateral decubitus views.

Asthma

Asthma is a chronic, intermittent, obstructive pulmonary process characterized by airway hyperactivity in response to a number of stimuli. Airway narrowing along with smooth-muscle spasm and inflammatory edema cause airflow obstruction and air trapping. The increased resistance to airflow leads to wheezing and hypoxemia. There is no specific cause, although allergens, emotional stress, and exercise seem to be common precipitating factors. Asthma behaves clinically like bronchiolitis, except that, unless complicated, there is no specific infectious agent. Usually, the two diseases are distinguished clinically by the age of presentation. Bronchiolitis occurs in children younger than 2 years; recurrent wheezing after this age is usually asthma.

The chest radiograph may be normal, or it may demonstrate increased aeration with increased perihilar markings and peribronchial cuffing. Patchy areas of atelectasis or infiltrate may be present, indicating complicated asthma. Atelectasis results from mucous plugging of the airway. Occasionally, the mucus-plugged bronchus can be visualized radiographically (Fig. 41–22). Patchy infiltrate may represent infection, usually viral in cause. The main pulmonary arteries may be enlarged, with normal-caliber peripheral vessels, reflecting transient pulmonary hypertension.[11]

The chest radiograph is obtained primarily to exclude

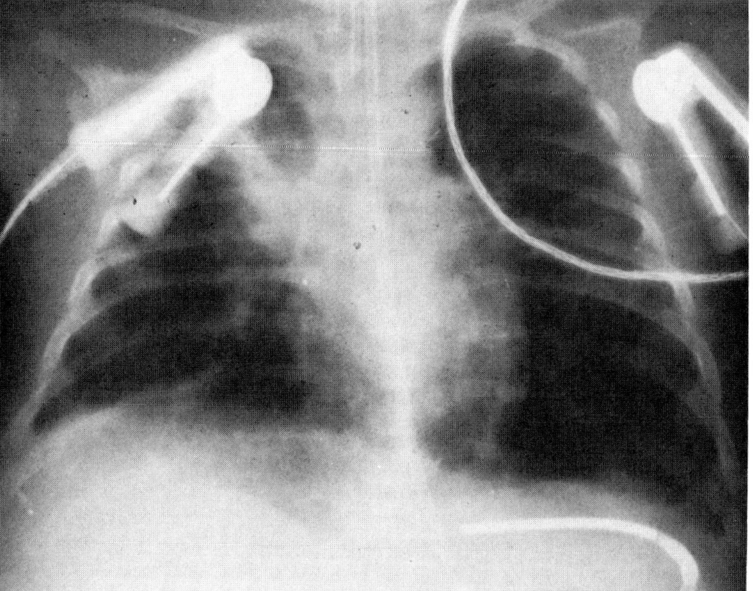

Figure 41–21. Bronchiolitis in an infant with fever and wheezing who was intubated for hypoxia. This chest radiograph shows the typical findings of airways pneumonia (bronchiolitis). Frequently, as in this patient, bronchiolitis is caused by respiratory syncytial virus. Visualized on this film are generalized hyperinflation, peribronchial thickening, and focal areas of hyperlucency (due to air trapping) that alternate with areas of increased density occurring secondary to atelectasis or pneumonitis.

other diagnoses and to look for complications, such as atelectasis secondary to mucus plugging, obstructive emphysema, air-block phenomena, and secondary pneumonia.

Pulmonary Insults Secondary to Accidental Injury

Near-Drowning

Near-drowning refers to submersion accidents that result in an outcome other than death (see Chapter 10). This occurs in a wide variety of locations, including bathtubs, hot tubs, pails of water, swimming pools, lakes, streams, rivers, and oceans. Lung injury is secondary to either aspiration of the submersion medium or stomach contents. Some researchers believe that seawater aspiration is more likely to produce pulmonary edema, whereas freshwater aspiration causes more damage to the pulmonary structures.[12–14] However, in a review of 20 cases of near-drowning, the composition of the aspirated fluid had no bearing on the biochemical changes occurring in the lung.[15] Of more practical importance in preventing secondary injury is the promptness with which treatment is initiated at the scene or during transport to a hospital.

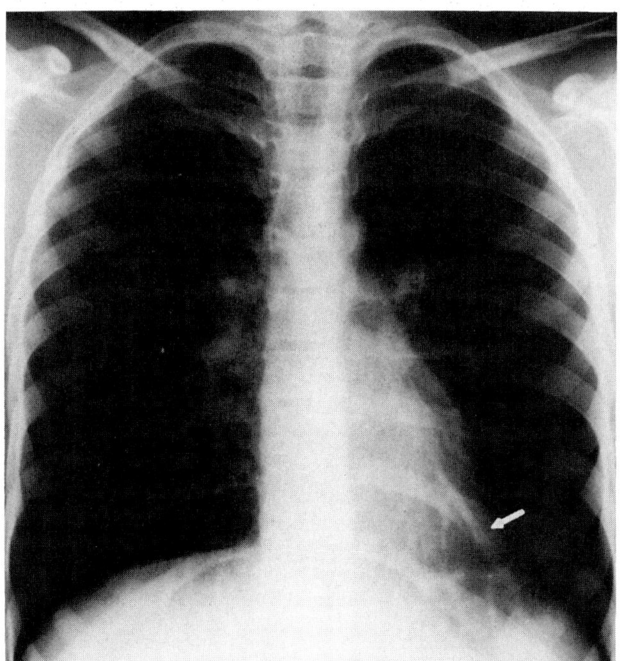

Figure 41–22. A 12-year-old boy with asthma. The chest radiograph demonstrates the typical findings of lung hyperinflation, peribronchial thickening, and increased perihilar markings. Note the thick, linear, obliquely oriented band of opacity in the left lower lobe that is consistent with a mucus-filled bronchus *(arrow)*.

Clinically, near-drowning victims are hypoxic with a metabolic acidosis, and pulmonary edema soon develops. The initial chest radiograph may be nonrevealing. However, within 24 to 48 hours, there are usually bilateral alveolar densities in a pattern reflecting noncardiogenic pulmonary edema (Fig. 41–23). Pulmonary edema results from increased permeability of the alveolocapillary membrane secondary to hypoxic injury. These changes may progress to diffuse airspace consolidation, pneumonia, abscess formation, or, rarely, adult respiratory distress syndrome (ARDS) (Fig. 41–24).[16] If the child survives, chronic pulmonary sequelae are uncommon.

Hydrocarbon Aspiration

Hydrocarbon pneumonia occurs when hydrocarbon-based materials such as kerosene and gasoline are accidentally ingested. Because of their low viscosity and surface tension, they are readily aspirated into the tracheobronchial tree. Table 41–4 lists hydrocarbon compounds that are frequently stored within the reach of young children and accidentally ingested. The aspiration of hydrocarbons incites an inflammatory reaction in the lung, with destruction of surfactant, bronchial wall edema, and necrosis.

The chest radiograph reveals patchy airspace disease in the medial, basilar portions of the lungs resembling pulmonary edema somewhat (Fig. 41–25). The radiographic changes are usually slow to resolve. Complications include pneumatocele formation, pleural effusion, air-block phenomena, and even frank necrosis.

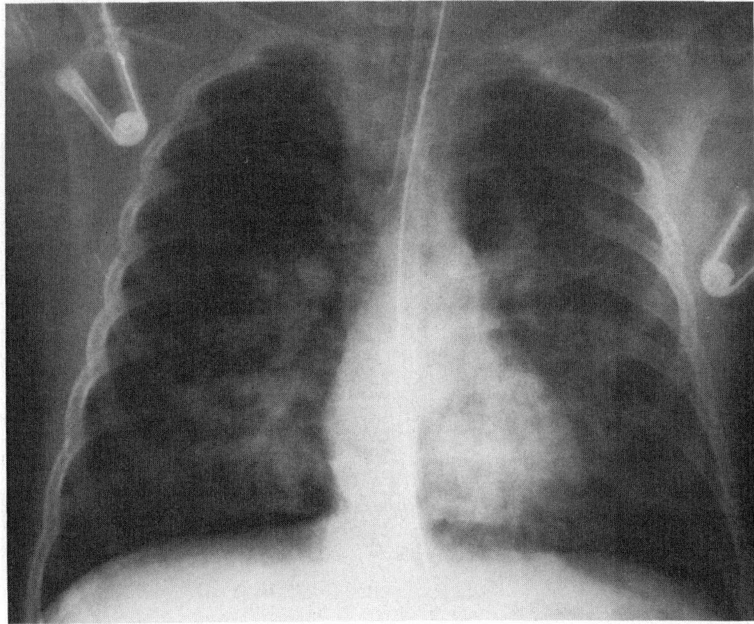

Figure 41–23. Near-drowning. A 5-year-old child was found facedown in a swimming pool containing chlorinated water. The child was intubated for hypoxia and acidosis. This chest film shows bilateral central "fluffy" alveolar infiltrates and a heart of normal size, findings typical for pulmonary edema and early adult respiratory distress syndrome (ARDS) due to near-drowning.

Smoke Inhalation

Smoke inhalation is a major cause of death in fires. The lung injury is believed to be produced primarily by the irritant effect of the combusted material inhaled and secondarily from upper airway burns. Airway irritation produces mucosal edema and sloughing, increased capillary permeability and extravascular lung water, decreased ciliary function, and altered surfactant production. These changes correlate well with the radiographic findings of airway obstruction, pulmonary interstitial edema, atelectasis, lung consolidation, and respiratory failure from ARDS (see Fig. 41–24).[17]

Chest Trauma

Chest trauma (see Chapter 159) in children is rare. When chest injuries occur, the cause is usually nonpenetrating or blunt trauma primarily from motor vehicle accidents. Blunt trauma to the chest can produce severe damage to intrathoracic organs without evidence of bony trauma to the thoracic cage. The ribs and other skeletal structures of the pediatric chest are often spared because of extreme pliability. However, even without recognizable fractures, a CT scan may reveal unsuspected intrathoracic injuries. In acute trauma, the head and abdomen are routinely evaluated with CT, whereas portable chest radiographs suffice for the chest and thus may underestimate or fail to demonstrate significant chest injuries. In a retrospective study of 512 children examined with CT after blunt abdominal trauma, in which several sections of the lower chest were included on the examinations, more than one third of the chest abnormalities seen on CT were underestimated or missed on the most recent chest radiograph.[18] Consequently, it is recommended that at least three or four images of the lower chest be included in the abdominal CT scan to assist in the early recognition of unsuspected intrathoracic injury.

When bony trauma is evident, the location can indicate other potential sites of injury. Fractures of the first three ribs are frequently associated with injury to the great vessels, trachea, and major bronchi. Posterior rib fractures in infants and toddlers, especially in several stages of healing, suggest

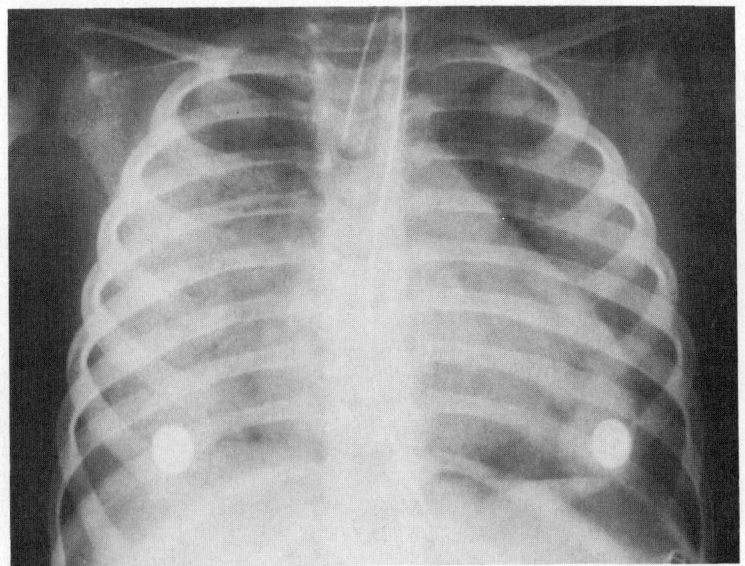

Figure 41–24. ARDS in a 15-month-old infant who was admitted to the emergency department with seizures, anemia, and shock of unknown etiology. He underwent massive volume resuscitation and then developed ARDS; the ARDS subsequently cleared. This chest radiograph shows a diffuse alveolar process and air bronchograms. Note the relative sparing of the medial aspects of the lungs, which is typical for ARDS.

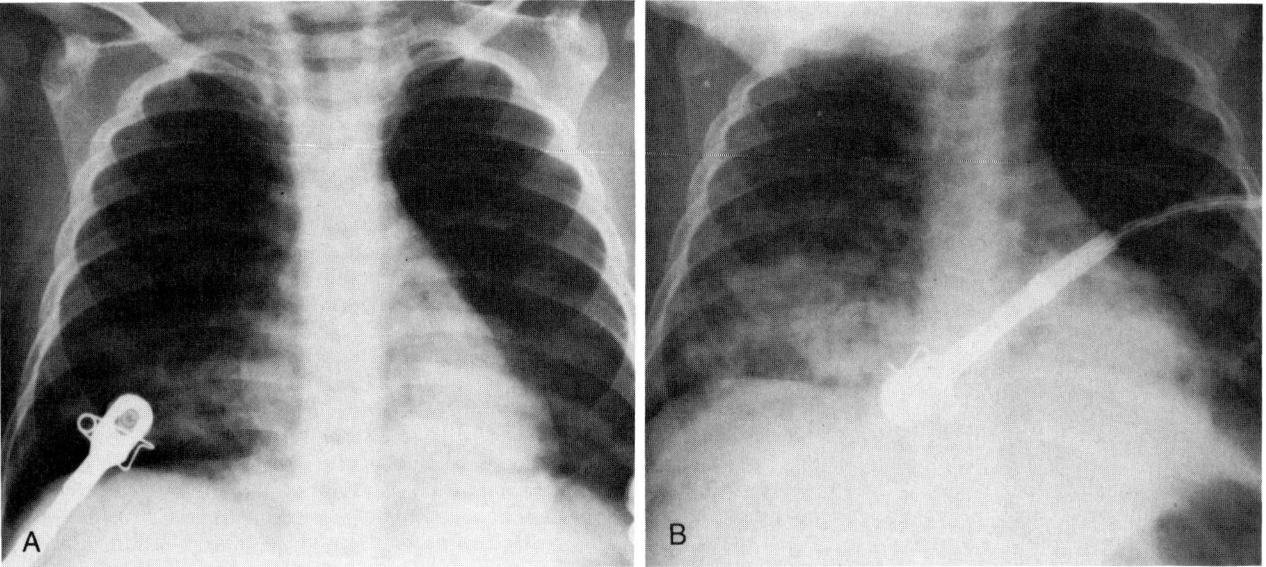

Figure 41–25. Hydrocarbon aspiration in an 8-month-old infant who ingested furniture polish. *A,* An early film demonstrates basilar patchy alveolar infiltrates. *B,* A film obtained 4 days later shows more extensive consolidation at the lung bases.

TABLE 41–4. Hydrocarbon Compounds Accidentally Ingested by Children

Gasoline
Kerosene
Floor wax
Furniture polish
Lighter fluid
Paint thinner
Acetone
Turpentine

the possibility of child abuse. Fractures of the lower ribs may indicate injury to the liver, spleen, or diaphragm. Sternal fractures may portend the presence of cardiac contusion or tamponade.

Nonpenetrating chest trauma can result in three types of pulmonary injury: pulmonary contusion, pulmonary hematoma, and traumatic pneumatocele. The basic mechanism for each is severe force applied to the chest wall, which is secondarily compressed, with transmission of the force to the underlying lung parenchyma. Additional, less common chest injuries produced by blunt trauma in children include traumatic tracheobronchial rupture, traumatic aortic rupture, traumatic diaphragmatic rupture, and traumatic lung torsion.

Pulmonary contusion is the most common injury from blunt chest trauma. It follows exudation of fluid and blood into the lung parenchyma. Chest radiographic findings are usually present soon after trauma, typically revealing either ill-defined, patchy areas of airspace consolidation or diffuse, homogeneous consolidation (Fig. 41–26). Contusions generally resolve within 24 to 48 hours, with complete clearing by 3 to 4 days.

Pulmonary hematoma is secondary to traumatic hemorrhage into the lung parenchyma from ruptured capillaries. It usually occurs after severe blunt trauma as in motor vehicle accidents. Children and young adults are susceptible to this injury because of greater flexibility of the chest wall. Pulmonary hematoma may be recognized soon after trauma; however, it can be first seen several hours to several

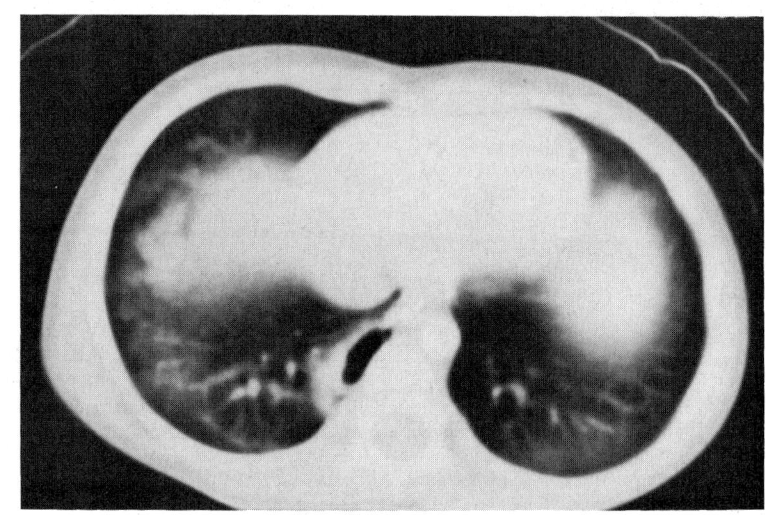

Figure 41–26. Chest trauma in a 2-year-old child run over by a car. This axial CT image demonstrates a right-sided radiopacity (representing lung contusion), a wedge-shaped radiolucency abutting the right margin of the heart (representing a right pneumothorax), and an oblong radiolucency in the right paraspinal area (consistent with a traumatic pneumatocele). Note the absence of rib fractures.

days later. It is frequently masked by surrounding pulmonary contusion; once the contusion resolves, the roentgenographic features of the hematoma become evident. On chest radiographs, hematomas are usually homogeneous, well-circumscribed radiodense masses, occasionally containing an air-fluid level. In contrast to pulmonary contusions, pulmonary hematomas heal slowly, usually resolving gradually over several months.

Traumatic pneumatoceles are acute, primary lesions resulting from laceration of the lung. The rupture of alveolar walls leads to dissection of air into a cavity, which assumes a spheric contour (see Fig. 41–26). Pneumatoceles may be round or oval, ranging in size from 2 to 14 cm. They can be single or multiple and may contain blood, often with an air-fluid level. When filled with blood, they may be characterized as pulmonary hematomas. They may not be recognized as cystic lesions until the blood is evacuated, which may take up to 12 hours.[19] The patient may experience hemoptysis for several days as the blood is expectorated. Although some pneumatoceles may persist for several weeks, most will clear completely in 2 to 3 weeks.

Traumatic fractures of the trachea and bronchi, although relatively uncommon, represent serious intrathoracic injuries from severe compression injury of the chest or a sharp blow to the anterior neck. Radiographic features include mediastinal and subcutaneous cervical emphysema and persistent segmental lung collapse; tension pneumothorax may be present. Often there is persistent air leak despite optimal positioning of a chest tube. Approximately 10% of children demonstrate no radiographic or physical evidence of intrathoracic injury.[20]

Traumatic diaphragmatic rupture is a difficult diagnosis. It must be differentiated from the more common hemothorax, diaphragmatic hemiparesis, or eventration. The latter two can be excluded with prior radiographs, if available. Rupture occurs more commonly on the left side primarily because of the protective effect of the liver on the right. Radiographic diagnosis can be made by recognizing an elevated hemidiaphragm and gas-filled bowel above the diaphragm with mediastinal shift to the contralateral hemithorax. Pleural fluid may be present if there is strangulated bowel. Confirmation of rupture can be made with identification of the distal portion of a nasogastric tube high in the left chest within herniated stomach or with an upper gastrointestinal study. If there is persistent diagnostic doubt, ultrasonography, CT, or nuclear medicine liver–spleen scan should confirm or refute the diagnosis.

Traumatic aortic rupture is exceedingly rare in children. Radiographic findings are the same as those identified in adults: mediastinal widening, poor visualization of the aortic knob, tracheal deviation, and hemorrhagic apical pleural fluid. Spouge and coworkers[21] recommended aortography when these findings are present in concert with additional signs of significant chest trauma. CT is useful in distinguishing a large thymus or vascular anomaly from traumatic vascular injury when no other signs of thoracic trauma are present.

Traumatic torsion of the lung is a rare complication of chest trauma that occurs predominantly in children. Children are believed to be susceptible to this injury because of the easily compressible thoracic cage. The lung is rotated 180°, which places the lung base superiorly in the upper hemithorax, with displacement of the lung apex inferiorly into the lower thorax. The chest radiograph reveals reversal of the pulmonary arterial markings. The injury results in compromise of the vascular supply, with airspace edema and hemorrhage. This diagnosis is considered a surgical emergency and is suggested clinically by the unilateral absence of breath sounds.

Pneumonia in the Pediatric Critical Care Patient

Pneumonia in the ICU setting can be classified as either community acquired or hospital acquired (nosocomial). Community-acquired infections can be transmitted by respiratory shedding from patients admitted to the ICU. The responsible organisms are either viral or bacterial in origin. Nosocomial infections occur at a high rate in the ICU partly because the patients have severe underlying disease and partly because of the many invasive and therapeutic proce-

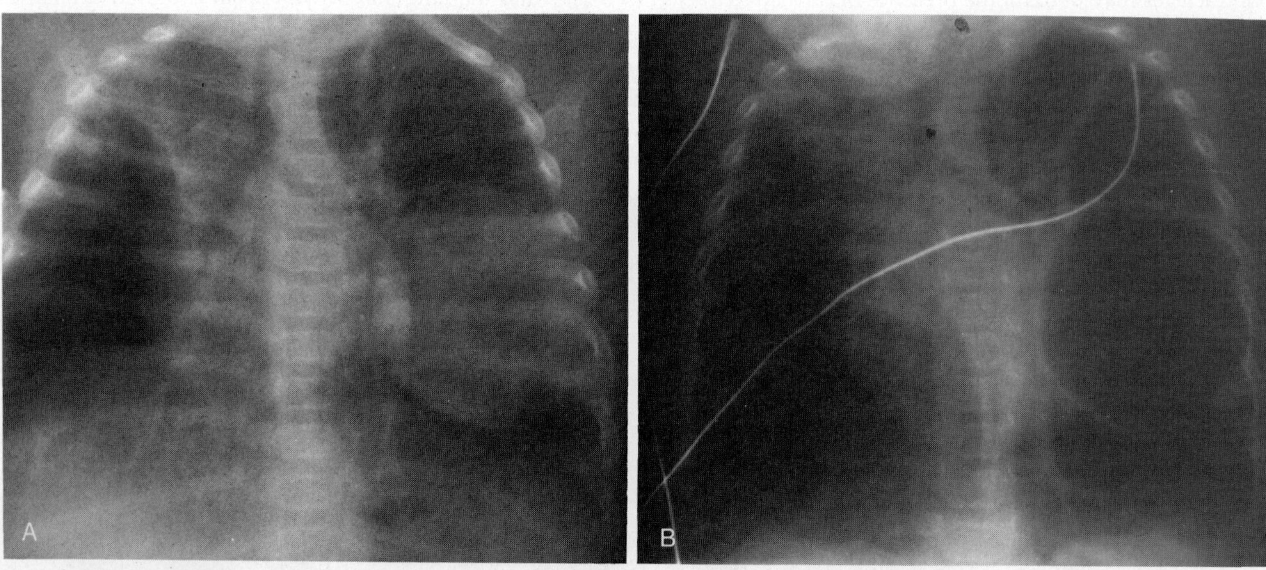

Figure 41–27. Staphylococcal pneumonia with pneumatocele formation. *A,* An initial supine radiograph shows a large, masslike area of consolidation in the left lower lobe and a central area of rounded radiolucency, findings consistent with abscess formation. Bilateral upper lobe atelectasis is present. *B,* A follow-up radiograph obtained 2 weeks later reveals a large, thin-walled, cystic area of radiolucency, representing pneumatocele formation in the prior region of consolidation. Note the generalized hyperinflation and the patchy areas of atelectasis bilaterally.

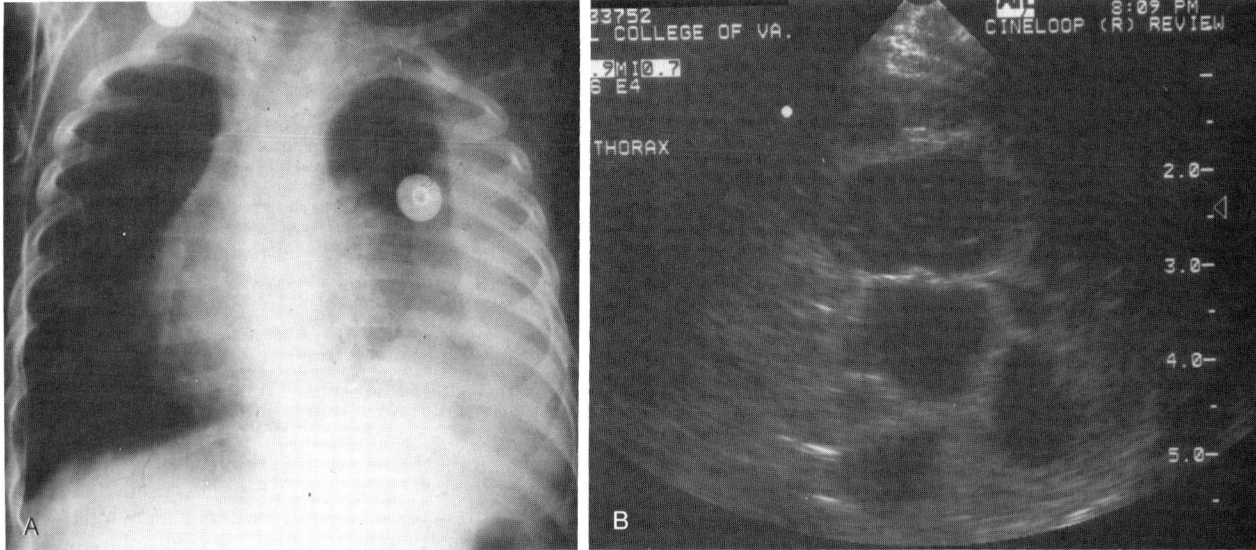

Figure 41–28. Streptococcal pneumonia with empyema. *A,* This chest radiograph demonstrates a large, homogeneous opacity along the left lateral chest wall that extends into the lower hemithorax; mediastinal shift to the right is also apparent. *B,* This sonogram of the left hemithorax reveals the loculated configuration of the empyema, with both cystic and solid components well visualized.

dures that are performed. Such infections are responsible for a high rate of morbidity among pediatric ICU patients. Lower respiratory tract infections are greatest in frequency and occur secondary to multiple pathogens, including *Klebsiella* species, *Pseudomonas aeruginosa, Staphylococcus aureus, Candida* species, and *Escherichia coli.*[22] Sources of respiratory infection in the ICU include transmission of organisms from contaminated personnel or equipment and aspiration pneumonia in obtunded patients who have difficulty handling oral secretions.

Chest radiographic features are variable depending on the organism. Staphylococcal pneumonia is a particularly virulent bronchopneumonia seen frequently in infants. It can secondarily invade the airways after influenza, and it is a relatively common nosocomial infectious agent. It initially affects the airways and then progresses to segmental consolidation (Fig. 41–27*A*) often complicated by pleural effusion, empyema, or lung abscess. Pneumatocele formation, relatively common with pediatric staphylococcal pneumonia, can occur during the healing phase (see Fig. 41–27*B*).

Streptococcus pneumoniae causes pneumonia in children with underlying illness, particularly those with sickle cell disease or immune deficiency. The usual radiographic pattern is homogeneous lobar consolidation, sometimes accompanied by pleural effusion or empyema (Fig. 41–28*A*). Ultrasonography may be of value in distinguishing between liquid effusion and loculated empyema[22a] (see Fig 41–28*B*). Additionally, it provides an assessment of the amount of fluid present and may be used to localize an anatomic point for thoracentesis.

Gram-negative organisms are also virulent agents that can cause dense lobar consolidation, bulging fissures, and abscess formation because of large amounts of inflammatory exudate. Abscess formation is characterized radiographically by air-fluid levels in cavitary lesions.

Pulmonary Problems Secondary to Systemic Diseases

Pneumonia in the Immunocompromised Host

Several underlying medical problems can place children at increased risk for opportunistic infection of the lungs. Some of these are listed in Table 41–5. Children with malignancies are at great risk for the development of pneumonia and may require hospitalization in the ICU. The cause of pneumonia in these children differs depending on whether the patient is neutropenic. In both neutropenic and non-neutropenic hosts, there is loss of cellular and humoral immunity, which leaves the child at risk for infection by both gram-positive and gram-negative pathogens (e.g., *S. pneumoniae, Haemophilus influenzae*). Neutropenic patients are additionally at risk for infection by opportunistic *(S. aureus, S. epidermidis)* or enteric gram-negative organisms as well as fungal agents. Notably, neutropenic patients cannot mount a normal inflammatory response, and the usual signs of infection may not be present. Leukemic and bone marrow transplant patients are also at risk for viral (e.g., cytomegalovirus) and protozoal *(Pneumocystis carinii)* infections.[23]

Children with human immunodeficiency virus (HIV) are at risk for a number of opportunistic pulmonary infections; the most common is *P. carinii* pneumonia, which occurs in some 40% to 50% of pediatric patients with acquired immunodeficiency syndrome.[24, 25] *P. carinii* has been classified as either a protozoan parasite or a fungus (Ascomycetes).

TABLE 41–5. Conditions Predisposing to Opportunistic Lung Infection

DiGeorge syndrome
Agammaglobulinemia
Immunoglobulin A deficiency
Severe combined immunodeficiency syndrome
Ataxia telangiectasia
Wiskott-Aldrich syndrome
Chronic granulomatous disease
Cystic fibrosis
Immotile cilia syndrome
Alpha$_1$-antitrypsin deficiency
Scimitar syndrome
Swyer-James syndrome
Organ transplantation with immunosuppressant therapy
Cancer chemotherapy
Steroid therapy

This organism invades the type I alveolar cells of the lung, inciting the development of foamy material within the alveoli and interstitial edema. Hypoxemia and decreased pulmonary compliance result, along with fever, dyspnea, and tachypnea. Symptoms can become severe enough to require ventilatory support. The majority of pediatric HIV infections are acquired either through transplacental exposure or by exposure to maternal blood during delivery.[26] Other less common means of transmission include contaminated blood products and sexual abuse.

The initial chest radiograph may be normal. Soon after presentation, however, patchy, localized or diffuse interstitial infiltrates appear. This appearance usually progresses to diffuse, patchy opacities that may rapidly coalesce, becoming more homogeneous. Secondary complications, including pneumomediastinum and pneumothorax, are not uncommon. It is not clear whether these air-block complications result from mechanical ventilation or the disease process itself.

Other commonly occurring pulmonary processes in children with HIV include lymphocytic interstitial pneumonitis, various recurrent bacterial infections, and a host of viral pneumonias, including, most commonly, cytomegalovirus and RSV.[27, 27a]

Sickle Cell Anemia: Acute Chest Syndrome

Acute chest syndrome is one of the vaso-occlusive crises seen in sickle cell disease. It is characterized by fever, pleuritic chest pain, cough, tachypnea, and hypoxemia. Radiographically, a focus of atelectasis or infiltrate is usually seen, sometimes accompanied by a pleural effusion (Fig. 41–29). Up to 25% of hospital admissions and deaths in sickle cell patients can be attributed to this syndrome.[28] The exact cause is not clear, but several theories have been proposed. Bacterial pneumonia is identified in 25% of patients[29] and was previously accepted by many as the cause. However, in those patients in whom bacterial infection is not found, alternative explanations have been considered for the pulmonary infiltrate.

Pulmonary infarction, although not always diagnosed by radiographic or scintigraphic criteria, has been accepted by many as the logical cause of the clinical syndrome of pain and pulmonary infiltrate.[30–32]

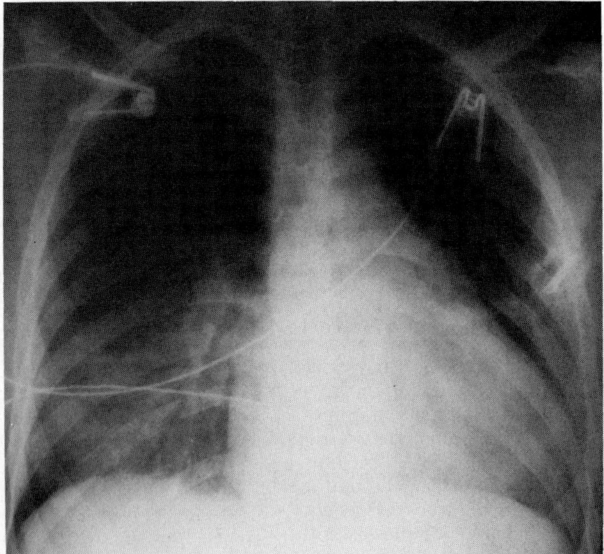

Figure 41–29. Acute chest syndrome in a 13-year-old girl with sickle cell anemia who presented with chest pain, fever, and tachypnea. This chest radiograph reveals cardiomegaly and infiltrate in the right lower lobe and the medial left lower lobe.

Rib infarction is another proposed mechanism. Rucknagel and coworkers[33] suggested that rib infarction with associated bone pain causes pleuritis and splinting, which leads to hypoventilation, atelectasis, and radiographic changes resembling pneumonia. They studied 10 sickle cell disease patients with chest pain and radiographic infiltrate and found, in each patient, evidence of rib infarction on radionuclide bone scans. They suggested that prevention of hypoventilation as well as pain control be considered as therapeutic goals. These findings, although convincing, await further confirmation.

An additional mechanism, proposed by Bhalla and colleagues[34] is microvascular pulmonary occlusion without overt infarction. Using thin-section CT, these researchers were able to detect with high sensitivity and specificity areas with a deficiency of visible arterioles and venules, indicating areas of hypoperperfusion. Parenchymal consolidation was the chest radiographic correlate of this finding. They suggested that timely diagnosis of acute chest syndrome using thin-section CT will permit early and appropriate treatment for improving perfusion. These findings as well await corroboration.

Pneumococcal pneumonia, although not specifically associated with acute chest syndrome, is often seen in sickle cell disease and has serious consequences when not treated.[35]

ADULT RESPIRATORY DISTRESS SYNDROME

ARDS is an acute, severe progressive inflammatory process that can occur secondary to a variety of underlying pulmonary and nonpulmonary conditions (Table 41–6). The syndrome, first described in adults, was derived from its similarity to the neontal RDS, with pathologic features of acute alveolar damage and formation of hyaline membranes. The syndrome does occur in children, but the incidence is not known.

Pathologically, the inciting condition causes injury to the alveolocapillary membrane, promoting fluid leakage and pulmonary edema. Three stages have been described.[36] Stage I reveals minimal fluid leakage, confined to the interstitial space. The lungs at this stage may be roentgenographically normal, or diminished lung volumes may be seen, as a result of microatelectasis and minimal interstitial edema. Stage II is a period of extensive fluid leakage, fibrin deposition, and hyaline membrane formation, causing a chest radiographic appearance of ill-defined, patchy opacities. These patchy areas of opacity coalesce rapidly to form large areas of alveolar consolidation (see Fig. 41–24). The appearance is frequently the reverse of the typical "bat's wing" pulmonary edema pattern in that the process begins more peripherally and progresses centrally, eventually becoming indistinguishable from cardiogenic pulmonary edema, with the exception that the heart size is usually normal. Pleural effusion is not characteristically present. Stage III is typified histologically by alveolar cell hyperplasia and collagen

TABLE 41–6. Adult Respiratory Distress Syndrome: Predisposing Conditions

Pneumonia
Sepsis
Pulmonary embolism: air, fat
Disseminated intravascular coagulation
Drug overdose
Trauma
Inhalation of noxious substances

deposition, with a less dense, more "ground-glass" radiographic appearance. Radiolucencies are believed to represent areas of ischemia that are ventilated but poorly perfused.

Radiographic evidence of healing can be seen 5 to 7 days after the onset of respiratory failure, with the homogeneous consolidation diminishing.[37] The lungs remain abnormal for a variable period of time thereafter, with a reticular appearance reflecting fibrosis.

The significance of distinguishing the diagnosis of ARDS from any underlying causative condition is that the patient may die from ARDS in spite of successful resolution of the underlying condition. The mortality rate in adults is greater than 50%.[38] An estimated mortality rate in pediatric patients is 59%.[39, 40] Despite the high mortality, studies in adults have shown that for those who survive the prognosis for recovery of pulmonary function is good.

EXTRACORPOREAL MEMBRANE OXYGENATION

ECMO is a type of arteriovenous cardiopulmonary bypass that provides support for patients with respiratory failure resulting from a potentially reversible cause. Candidates for ECMO are those who have persistent respiratory failure despite therapy with 100% oxygen, high-pressure ventilation, and appropriate pharmacologic agents; birth weight greater than 2 kg; gestational age greater than 34 weeks; and assisted ventilation for fewer than 10 days. Neonatal disease processes most commonly treated with ECMO are listed in Table 41–7. Also included are patients who have undergone surgical correction of congenital heart anomalies who fail removal from acute cardiopulmonary bypass.

The process usually involves cannulation of the right internal jugular vein and right common carotid artery. Venous blood is removed from the right atrium via the superior vena cava into the internal jugular cannula, and oxygenated blood is returned to the thoracic aorta via the common carotid cannula. The flow bypasses the heart and lungs, which allows an opportunity for the lungs to heal. Gas exchange is provided while the potential for oxygen toxicity and barotrauma are minimized. ECMO also alleviates right-to-left shunting in patients with persistent pulmonary hypertension.

The initial chest radiographs of ECMO patients usually demonstrate diffuse lung opacification with air bronchograms and a variable amount of basilar atelectasis (Fig. 41–30). The subcutaneous tissues may be expanded because of edema from an accumulation of fluid in the extravascular spaces. As the lungs improve clinically, there may be slower radiographic evidence of resolution. Daily radiographs are obtained to monitor the position of the ECMO cannulas and the other catheters and tubes and to monitor any complications, such as air-block phenomena.

ECMO is discontinued when the patient's lung function has recovered or when there is evidence of a serious complication, the most common of which is intracranial hemorrhage, monitored with cranial sonography. Cerebral infarction can also occur. ECMO results in improved survival and a lessened incidence of chronic lung disease.[41, 42]

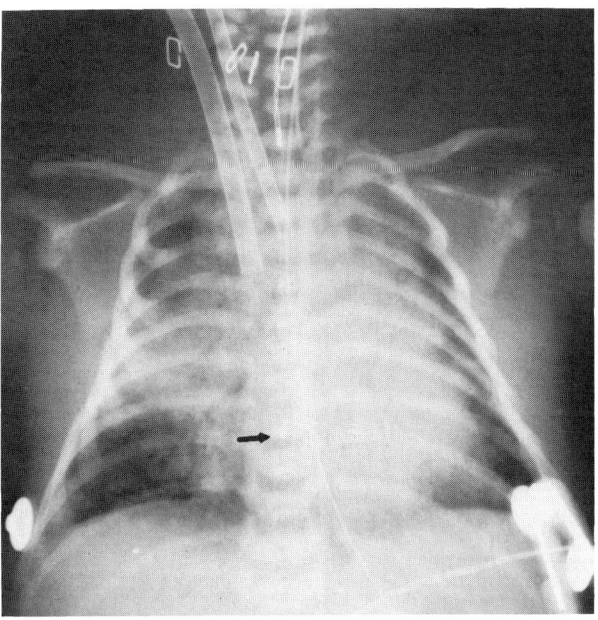

Figure 41–30. This patient was treated with ECMO for meconium aspiration. The arterial cannula tip is in the aortic arch. A radiopaque marker demonstrates the tip of the venous cannula in the right atrium *(arrow)*. Note the high position of the endotracheal tube.

TABLE 41–7. Neonatal Processess Treated with Extracorporeal Membrane Oxygenation

Meconium aspiration syndrome
Congenital diaphragmatic hernia
Perinatal asphyxia
Sepsis
Congenital pneumonia
Pulmonary hypoplasia
Persistent pulmonary hypertension from a variety of causes
Primary cardiac failure

References

1. Wood BP: The newborn chest. Radiol Clin North Am 1993; 31:667–676.

1a. Jobe AH: The respiratory system: Part one: The developmental biology of the lung. *In:* Neonatal-Perinatal Medicine—Diseases of the Fetus and Infant. 5th ed. Fanaroff AA, Martin RJ (Eds). St. Louis, Mosby-Year Book, 1992, pp 790–791.

2. Wood BP, Sinkin RA, Kendig JW, et al: Exogenous lung surfactant: Effect on radiographic appearance in premature infants. Radiology 1987; 165:11.

3. Kendig JW, Notter RH: A comparison of surfactant as immediate prophylaxis and as rescue therapy in newborns of less than 30 weeks' gestation. N Engl J Med 1991; 324:865.

4. Ablow RC, Driscoll SG, Effmann EL, et al: A comparison of early onset group B streptococcal neonatal infection and the respiratory distress syndrome of the newborn. N Engl J Med 1976; 294:65.

5. Weller MH, Katzenstein AA: Radiological findings in group B streptococcal sepsis. Radiology 1976; 118:385.

6. Wiswell TE, Tuggle JM, Turner BS: Meconium aspiration syndrome: Have we made a difference? Pediatrics 1990; 85:715.

7. Hernanz-Schulman M: Cysts and cystlike lesions of the lung. Radiol Clin North Am 1993; 31:631–633.

7a. Cleveland RH, Weber B: Retained fetal lung fluid in congenital lobar emphysema: A possible predictor of polyalveolar lobe. Pediatr Radiol 1993; 23:291–295.

7b. Kennedy CD, Habibi P, Mathew DJ, et al: Lobar emphysema: Long term imaging follow-up. Radiology 1991; 180:189.

8. Gyepes MT, Vincent WR: Severe congenital heart disease in the neonatal period: A functional approach to emergency diagnosis. Am J Roentgenol 1971; 116:490.

8a. Crowley JJ, Oh KS, Newman B, et al: Telltale signs of congenital heart disease. Radiol Clin North Am 1993; 31:573–582.

9. Leonidas JC, Berdon W: The neonate and young infant. *In:*

Caffey's Pediatric X-Ray Diagnosis. 9th ed. Silverman FN, Kuhn JP (Eds). St. Louis, CV Mosby, 1993, p 1987.
10. Green M, Brayer AF, Schenkman KA, et al: Duration of hospitalization in previously well infants with respiratory syncytial virus infection. Pediatr Infect Dis J 1989; 8:601.
11. Blair DN, Coppage L, Shaw C: Medical imaging in asthma. J Thorac Imaging 1986; 1:23.
12. Modell J, Moya F, Newby EJ, et al: The effects of fluid volume in seawater drowning. Arch Intern Med 1967; 67:68.
13. Yamamoto K, Yamamoto Y, Kikuchi H: The effects of drowning media on the lung water content: An experimental study on rats. Z Rechtsmed 1983; 90:1.
14. Orlowski JP, Abulleil MM, Philips JM: Effects of tonicities of saline solutions on pulmonary injury in drowning. Crit Care Med 1987; 15:126.
15. Putnam CE, Tummillo AM, Myerson DA, et al: Drowning: Another plunge. Am J Roentgenol 1975; 125:543.
16. Fine NL, Myerson DA, Myerson PJ: Near-drowning presenting as adult respiratory distress syndrome. Chest 1974; 65:347.
17. Spurrier EA, Spear RM, Munster AM: Burns, inhalational injury, and electrical injury. *In:* Textbook of Pediatric Intensive Care. 2nd ed. Rogers MC (Ed). Baltimore, Williams & Wilkins, 1992, p 1510.
18. Sivit CJ, Taylor GA, Eichelberger MR: Chest injury in children with blunt abdominal trauma: Evaluation with CT. Radiology 1989; 171:815.
19. Fagan CJ, Swischuk LE: Traumatic lung and paramediastinal pneumatoceles. Radiology 1976; 120:11.
20. Mahboubi S, O'Hara AE: Bronchial rupture in children following blunt abdominal trauma. Pediatr Radiol 1989; 10:133.
21. Spouge AR, Burrows PE, Armstrong D, et al: Traumatic aortic rupture in the pediatric population. Pediatr Radiol 1991; 21:324.
22. Merritt WT, Stephens M: Nosocomial infections in the pediatric intensive care unit. *In:* Textbook of Pediatric Intensive Care. 2nd ed. Rogers MC (Ed). Baltimore, Williams & Wilkins, 1992, p 30.
22a. Ben–Ami TE, O'Donovan JC, Yousefzadeh DK: Sonography of the chest in children. Radiol Clin of North Am 1993; 31:517–531.
23. Gordon JB, Yeager AM: Management of the child with malignant disease in the pediatric intensive care unit. *In:* Textbook of Pediatric Intensive Care. 2nd ed. Rogers MC (Ed). Baltimore, Williams & Wilkins, 1992, pp 1412–1416.
24. Caldwell MB, Rogers MF: Epidemiology of pediatric HIV infection. Pediatr Clin North Am 1991; 38:1.
25. Sanders-Laufer D, DeBruin W, Edelson PJ: *Pneumocystis carinii* infections in HIV-infected children. Pediatr Clin North Am 1991; 38:69.
26. Ambrosino MM, Genieser NB, Krasinski K: Opportunistic infections and tumors in immunocompromised children. Radiol Clin North Am 1992; 30:639.
27. Goodman PC: Pulmonary disease in children with AIDS. J Thorac Imaging 1991; 6:60.
27a. Berdon WE, Mellins RB, Abramson SJ, et al: Pediatric HIV infection in its second decade: The changing pattern of lung involvement—clinical, plain film, and computed tomographic findings. Radiol Clin North Am 1993; 31:453–563.
28. Bhalla M, Abboud MR, McLoud TC, et al: Acute chest syndrome in sickle cell disease: CT evidence of microvascular occlusion. Radiology 1993; 187:45.
29. Davies SC, Luce PJ, Win AA, et al: Acute chest syndrome in sickle cell disease. Lancet 1984; 1:36.
30. Barrett CE: Acute pulmonary disease in sickle cell anemia. Am Rev Respir Dis 1971; 104:159.
31. Sprinkle RH, Cole T, Smith S, et al: Acute chest syndrome in children with sickle cell disease. Am J Pediatr Hematol Oncol 1986; 8:105.
32. Poncz M, Kane E, Gill FM: Acute chest syndrome in sickle cell disease: Etiology and clinical correlates. J Pediatr 1985; 107:861.
33. Rucknagel DL, Kalinyak KA, Gelfand MJ: Rib infarcts and acute chest syndrome in sickle cell diseases. Lancet 1991; 337:831.
34. Bhalla M, Abboud MR, McLoud TC, et al: Acute chest syndrome in sickle cell disease: CT evidence of microvascular occlusion. Radiology 1993; 187:45.
35. Young RC, Castro O, Baxter RP, et al: The lung in sickle cell disease: A clinical overview of common vascular, infectious, and other problems. J Natl Med Assoc 1981; 73:19.
36. Greene R: Adult respiratory distress syndrome: Acute alveolar damage. Radiology 1987; 163:57.
37. Paré JAP, Fraser RG: Pulmonary hypertension and edema. *In:* Synopsis of Diseases of the Chest. Fraser RS, Paré JAP, Fraser RG, et al (Eds). Philadelphia, WB Saunders, 1983, pp 515–516.
38. Royal JA, Levin DL: Adult respiratory distress syndrome in pediatric patients: I. Clinical aspects, pathophysiology, pathology, and mechanisms of lung injury. J Pediatr 1988; 112:169.
39. Lyrene RK, Troug WE: Adult respiratory distress syndrome in a pediatric intensive care unit: Predisposing conditions, clinical course, and outcome. Pediatrics 1981; 67:790.
40. Effmann EL, Menten DF, Kirks DR, et al: Adult respiratory distress syndrome in children. Clin Pediatr 1983; 22:401.
41. Bartlett RH, Andrews AF, Toomasian CCP, et al: Extracorporeal membrane oxygenation for newborn respiratory failure: Forty-five cases. Surgery 1982; 92:2.
42. Krummel TM, Greenfield LJ, Kirkpatrick BV: Extracorporeal membrane oxygenation in neonatal pulmonary failure. Pediatr Ann 1982; 11:11.

CHAPTER 42

Critical Care Applications of Sonography

M. Leon Skolnick, MD

Ultrasonography is a noninvasive and noninjurious method of producing cross-sectional images of internal anatomy using high-frequency sound waves. Ultrasound images provide information about both anatomy and velocity of blood flow within tissues. The images are displayed in real time, negating the need for patients to suspend respiration. The equipment is portable; therefore, examinations may be conducted at the bedside.

Ultrasound images are produced by placing on the patient's skin a probe containing a piezoelectric crystal, a material that converts electric energy into sound energy and vice versa. Pulsing the crystal with high-frequency electric energy produces high-frequency bursts of sound energy (2.5–7.5 MHz) that are transmitted to the skin. When the ultrasound hits interfaces within the tissues, a small percentage of the transmitted ultrasound is reflected back from the interfaces to the crystal, where it is reconverted into electric signals. The instrument detects the depth at which the ultrasound reflections from different tissue interfaces have occurred and processes these data to produce images on a television monitor in real time as the ultrasound beam is swept across the face of the probe.

Sound is reflected from tissue interfaces when the acoustic impedance of the material on either side of the interface is different. Acoustic impedance is the product of the density of the material times the speed of sound through it. The greater the differences in acoustic impedance, the greater the reflection of sound from the interface. Although the mismatch between fluid and soft tissues or within soft tissues is only several per cent, the mismatch between fluid and air or fluid and bone is so large that the sound is reflected and none penetrates beyond the interface. Ultrasound is not useful for examining structures beneath air-filled bowel or lung or beneath bones. Therefore, it is primarily used for imaging fluid-filled or soft-tissue structures, such as the liver, spleen, kidneys, pancreas, gallbladder, urinary bladder, and vascular structures, providing no overlying gas-filled bowel or lung impedes the passage of sound to these organs. Ultrasound is also useful for detecting abnormal fluid collections within the pleural and peritoneal spaces or within soft-tissue organs. The total reflection of sound from air, bone, or bonelike structures such as stones can be used to an advantage in identifying abnormal collections of gas or stones within solid organs or fluid-filled structures. The presence of air or bone produces an absence of sound deep to the structure, called acoustic *shadowing*.[1, 2]

The higher the frequency of the ultrasound beam, the greater the resolution of the image but the less deep the beam can penetrate into tissue. Frequencies between 2.5 and 5.0 MHz are used for the abdomen and between 5 and 7.5 MHz for superficial structures.

In addition to producing cross-sectional images, some ultrasound scanners can also display blood flow within tissues using Doppler signal-processing techniques. Doppler detects motion when the frequency of the ultrasound beam reflected from moving red blood cells differs from the incident sound hitting them. The greater the velocity of the red blood cells, the greater the sound frequency shift between the incident and reflected beam. Although the frequency of both the incident and reflected beams lies within the megacycle range, the frequency shift is in the audible range. When red cells move toward the probe, the frequency shift increases, and when they move away, it decreases. Structures within the ultrasound Doppler beam that do not move produce no frequency shift and are not detected. Although the Doppler frequency shift can be presented as an audible sound, it is also displayed graphically, with velocity of moving cells on the y-axis and time on the x-axis (spectral Doppler).

Spectral Doppler displays blood velocity from a localized region within a blood vessel seen on a real-time ultrasound image that is defined by the placement of an electronic cursor. The spectral Doppler waveform is usually displayed together with the real-time image.

Color Doppler is a more sophisticated system that displays a colored map of moving blood superimposed on a real-time ultrasound gray scale image. By convention, a vessel colored red indicates flow toward the probe and a vessel colored blue indicates flow away from the probe. By knowing the color of the blood displayed in the vessel and the orientation of the vessel to the probe, one can determine the direction of blood flow in the vessel. Venous flow is usually unidirectional at a relatively low velocity (and therefore shows little change in intensity of the color), whereas arterial flow, because of the wider variation in velocity through the cardiac cycle, shows significant change in color intensity. Reversal of color (i.e., regions of blue in a predominantly red-appearing vessel) usually indicates regions of reversed flow, although it may occasionally be artifactual (see Fig. 42–18).

Real-time imaging alone is unreliable for detecting vascular thrombosis. Although echoes from within a vessel may denote a thrombus, they may also represent artifactual noise. The absence of echoes does not preclude a thrombus, because some thrombi may be anechoic, resembling liquid blood.

Color Doppler, by providing a two-dimensional display of blood flow, permits rapid identification of a specific region within a vessel for more detailed characterization of flow velocity by spectral Doppler.[3, 4]

Because the ultrasound probe easily fits within one's hand, the ultrasound examination should be viewed as an extension of physical diagnosis. The operator should tailor the examination to the patient's specific clinical problem and modify or expand the area of examination depending on what is initially found. More so than with other diagnostic imaging studies, the success of an ultrasound examination depends on the skill and knowledge of the operator. Because critically ill patients are often the most difficult ones to examine, one should choose the most sophisticated ultrasound scanner available and the most experienced operator in order to obtain the highest-quality images in the shortest time.

CLINICAL APPLICATIONS

In critically ill patients, the role of ultrasound should be primarily viewed as that of a clinical problem solver—an imaging modality designed to help resolve specific clinical uncertainties or assist in invasive procedures. Therefore, the clinical applications of ultrasound described in this chapter are presented from such a point of view.

Ultrasound examinations of critically ill patients are often performed under less than optimal conditions. The frozen images obtained during these studies, although of diagnostic value, may not be of appropriate technical quality for publication. Therefore, some of the illustrations used in this chapter were from noncritically ill patients with similar ultrasound findings.

Elevated Renal Function Values—Rule Out Obstructive Nephropathy

In renal failure, ultrasound can identify obstructive nephropathy, end-stage medical disease, and vascular occlusions as causes.[5] Hydronephrosis is usually appreciated because the dilated collecting system appears as an echo-free branching and connecting fluid-filled space within a central portion of the kidney (Fig. 42–1). The cortical mantle during hydronephrosis may be abnormally thin, yet it can return to more normal thickness after relief of the obstruction. Unless no cortical mantle is present at all, the thickness of the cortical mantle before relief of the obstruction may not accurately predict the amount of functional improvement after relief of the obstruction. The presence of blood (hemonephrosis) or pus (pyonephrosis) in the dilated collecting systems may make detection of hydronephrosis more difficult. Echoes from this material may be similar in intensity to adjacent renal tissue, making it difficult to appreciate the dilated collecting system, or may suggest an intrapelvic clot or tumor. However, a fluid-debris level confirms that material within the collecting system is liquid (Fig. 42–2).[6] Hydronephrosis should also be distinguished from multiple peripelvic cysts; the latter are spherical fluid spaces that do not connect.

Once hydronephrosis has been detected, causes should be sought. Dilatation of the collecting system or systems suggests processes obstructing both ureters (enlarged para-aortic nodes, a centrally placed bladder tumor blocking both ureterovesical junctions) or a bladder outlet obstruction (enlarged prostate). However, a distended bladder, even without the presence of output obstruction, may compress the distal ureters to produce proximal dilatation of the collecting systems. When a distended bladder is detected, therefore, the patient should be rescanned after the bladder is emptied to see if the hydronephrosis decreases or disappears.[7]

In the absence of hydronephrosis, ultrasound may suggest other causes of poor renal function. Bilaterally small kidneys (<8 cm in greatest length for adults), often with increased parenchymal reflectivity greater than adjacent

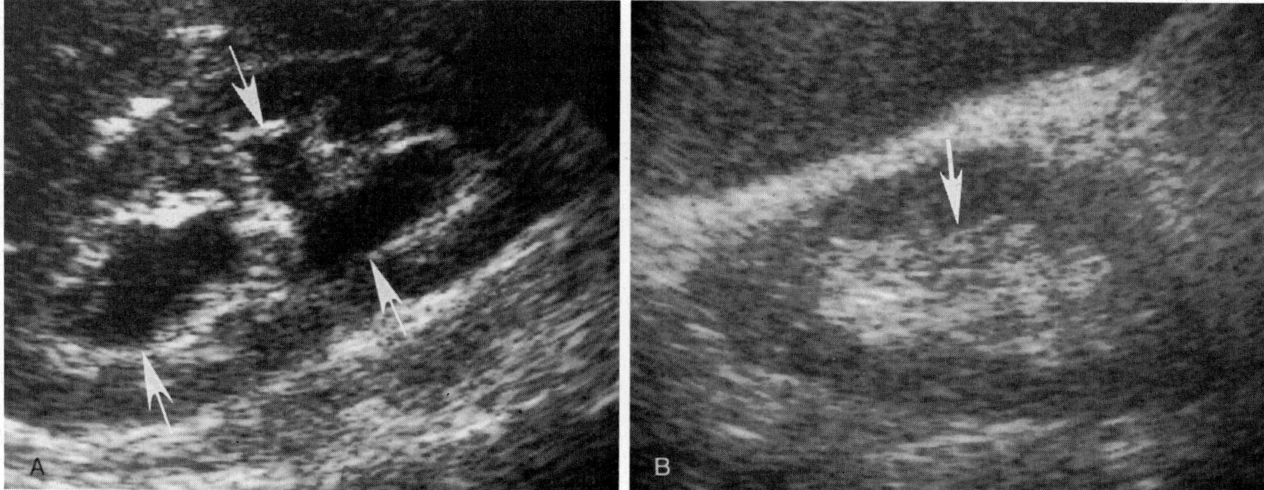

Figure 42–1. *A*, Hydronephrosis (sagittal view of the right kidney). The dilated collecting system *(arrows)* appears as an echo-free branching space in the central portion of the kidney. *B*, Normal left kidney (sagittal view). The central portion of kidney contains echogenic peripelvic fat *(arrow)*. The collecting system is collapsed and not visualized.

liver tissue (providing the liver is normal), imply generalized medical renal diseases (Fig. 42–3).[8] Acutely enlarged kidneys, which may be associated with reduced echogenicity (parenchymal edema), suggest renal vein thrombosis. Doppler ultrasound may demonstrate no flow in the main renal veins.[9] In renal artery occlusion, Doppler shows absence of main renal artery blood flow.

Right Upper Quadrant Pain—Rule Out Cholecystitis

Ultrasound examination of the gallbladder combines an imaging study with physical diagnosis—imaging to evaluate the appearance of the gallbladder and physical diagnosis to determine if pressure over the gallbladder produces localized tenderness. A thickened gallbladder wall, especially if the wall is irregular, in combination with localized tenderness over the gallbladder, fever, and increased white blood cell count, is suggestive of acute cholecystitis (Fig. 42–4*A*). In addition, stones may be noted within the gallbladder, as well as pericholecystic fluid, suggesting either a pericholecystic abscess or fluid accumulation in response to the inflammatory reaction in the gallbladder wall.[10]

A thickened gallbladder wall and possibly pericholecystic fluid may be seen in conditions other than cholecystitis. In acute hepatitis (Fig. 42–5), end-stage liver disease, or severe right heart failure, the gallbladder wall may be thickened and fluid may be seen around the gallbladder, either localized or as part of a more generalized intraperitoneal fluid accumulation. However, the gallbladder is usually not tender to localized pressure.[11] Radioisotope hydroxyiminodiacetic acid scanning may help distinguish acute cholecystitis from other causes of gallbladder wall thickening.[10] One may occasionally see what appears to be loculated collections of fluid surrounding the gallbladder in a patient with severe liver disease, often with portal hypertension. These spaces may actually be dilated pericholecystic varicosities, which can be demonstrated using color Doppler imaging.[12] In addition to the gallbladder, the common and intrahepatic ducts are examined to see if they are dilated or contain stones. These findings are described in the next section.

If a patient with the diagnosis of acute cholecystitis is too poor a risk to undergo surgery, a pigtail catheter can be

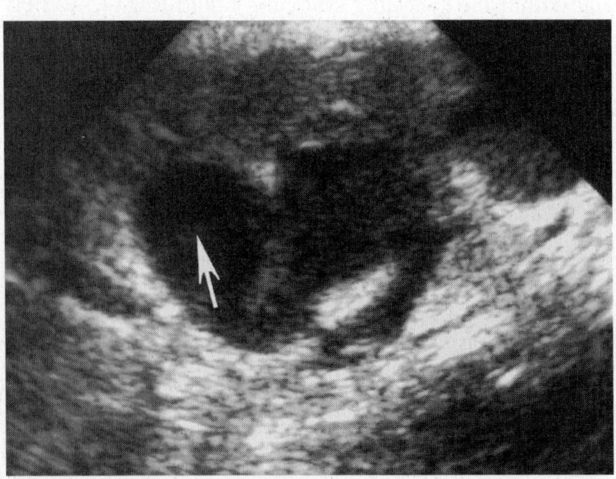

Figure 42–2. Pyonephrosis (sagittal view of the left kidney). Fluid-debris *(arrow)* level within dilated collecting system is visualized.

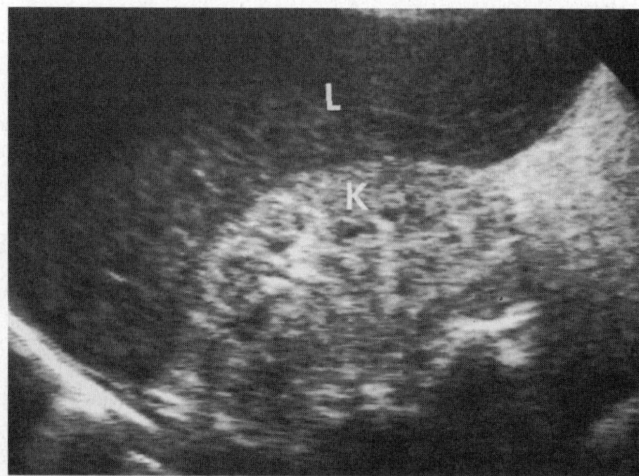

Figure 42–3. Medical renal disease (sagittal view of the liver [L] and right kidney [K]). The kidney is small and has general increased parenchymal reflectivity. The left kidney (not shown) appears similar.

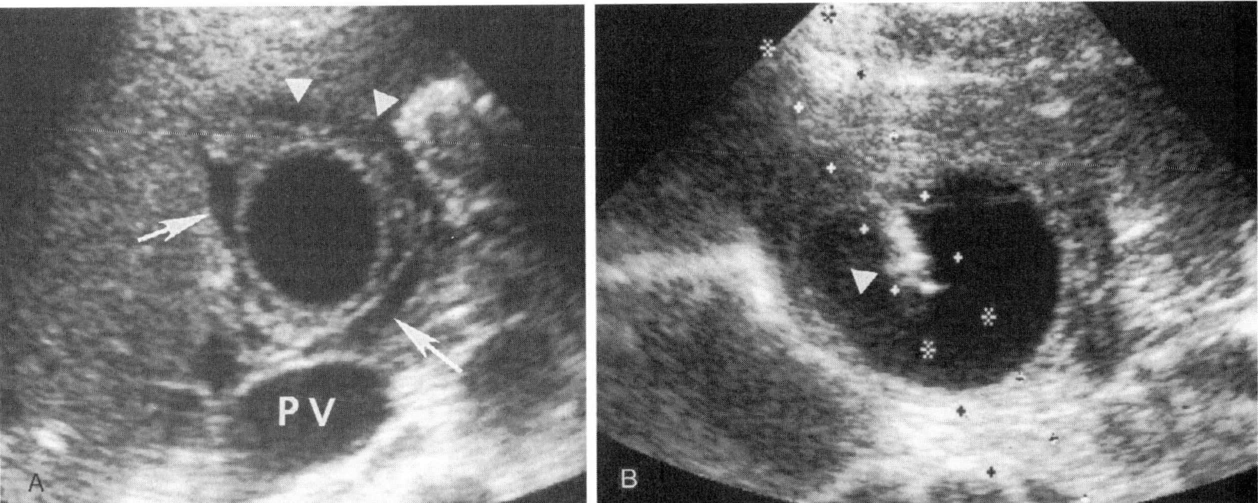

Figure 42–4. *A*, Acute acalculous cholecystitis (transverse view of gallbladder). The gallbladder wall is thickened *(arrowheads)*. Pericholecystic fluid is also visible *(arrows)*. *Abbreviation*: PV = portal vein. *B*, Ultrasonically guided percutaneous placement of a catheter in gallbladder of the patient in *A* for drainage (transverse view of gallbladder). A needle-pigtail catheter assembly (needle with pigtail catheter placed over it) is inserted through a needle guide attached to a probe. Parallel *dotted lines* on the screen define the path of the needle-pigtail catheter assembly. Bright echoes *(arrowhead)* indicate the tip of needle-catheter assembly within the gallbladder lumen. The needle is then removed, and the pigtail of the catheter re-forms within the gallbladder.

placed percutaneously in the gallbladder under ultrasound guidance to provide temporary bile drainage (see Fig. 42–4*B*).[13]

Examination of the right upper quadrant, especially when an ultrasonically normal-appearing and nontender gallbladder is identified, should not be limited to the gallbladder. Particular attention should also be paid to structures adjacent to the gallbladder, such as the common duct, the kidney, the pancreas, and the liver. Obstructive hydronephrosis, perinephric fluid abscesses or hematoma, pancreatitis, pancreatic pseudocysts, liver abscesses or tumors, or distention of the liver capsule from right heart failure, all of which can produce similar symptoms, may be appreciated by ultrasound.

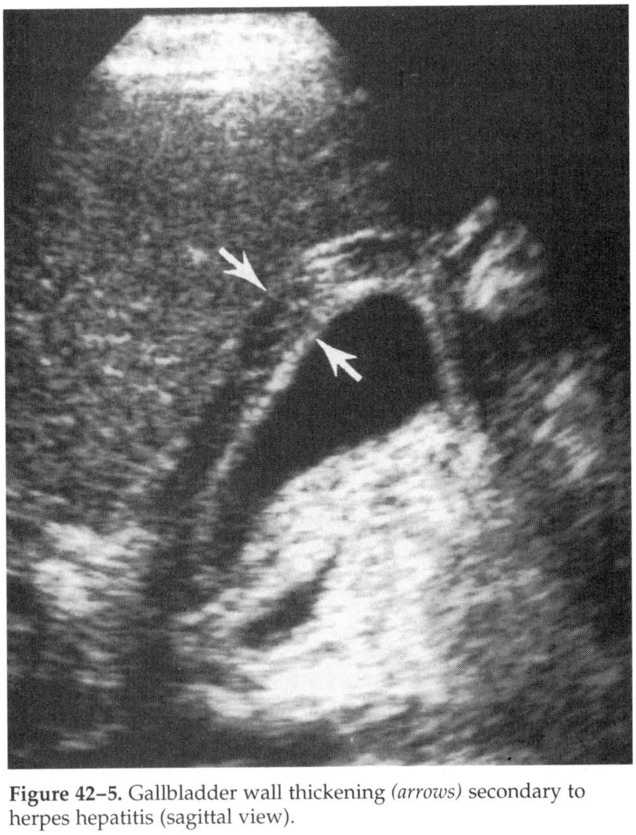

Figure 42–5. Gallbladder wall thickening *(arrows)* secondary to herpes hepatitis (sagittal view).

Elevated Liver Function Values—Rule Out Biliary Obstruction or Diffuse Liver Disease

Biliary Obstruction

The common duct, as it passes anterior to the portal vein, can usually be readily identified by ultrasound. The common duct should be distinguished from the hepatic artery, because in liver disease, the latter may have a greater diameter than the former and be mistaken for a dilated common duct. Doppler and particularly color Doppler examination provide such distinction.[14] A common duct greater than 8 mm in diameter is considered dilated (Fig. 42–6).[15] If a stone is seen within the common duct, it can be appreciated as an echogenic mass that usually produces distal shadowing similar to a stone in the gallbladder. Small-diameter stones may be symptomatic (pain and jaundice) because of intermittent obstruction, even though they do not dilate the common duct. A stone several millimeters in diameter may not cast an acoustic shadow if it does not completely block the ultrasound beam, because it is narrower than the width of the beam at the position of the stone (Fig. 42–7). The ability to visualize the common duct as it continues through the pancreas into the duodenum depends on this region being free of overlying gas-filled bowel. Although ultrasound is sensitive in detecting an abnormally dilated common duct, it may not demonstrate the cause of ductal dilatation if the region of obstruction cannot be appreciated. Unfortunately, in patients in an intensive care unit, many of whom have gas-distended bowel, the distal common duct often cannot be visualized.

Dilated intrahepatic bile ducts appear as tubular structures adjacent to the hepatic artery and portal vein branches. In the region of the porta hepatis, they may be appreciated

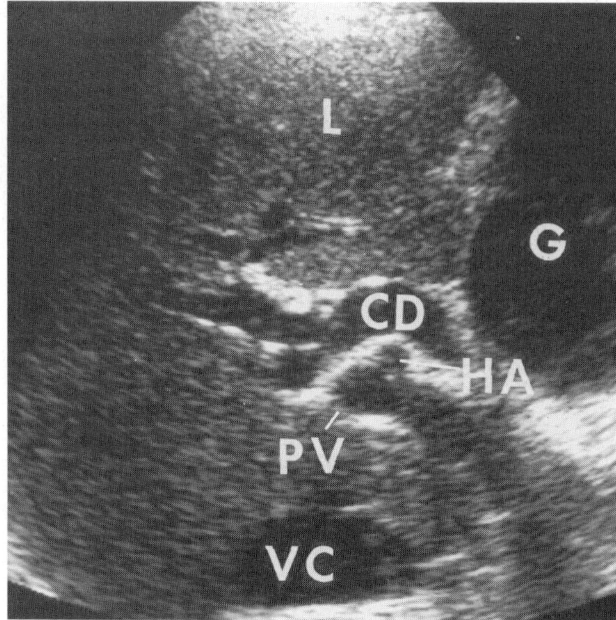

Figure 42–6. Dilated common duct (sagittal view). *Abbreviations*: CD = common duct; HA = hepatic artery; PV = portal vein; G = gallbladder; VC = vena cava; L = liver.

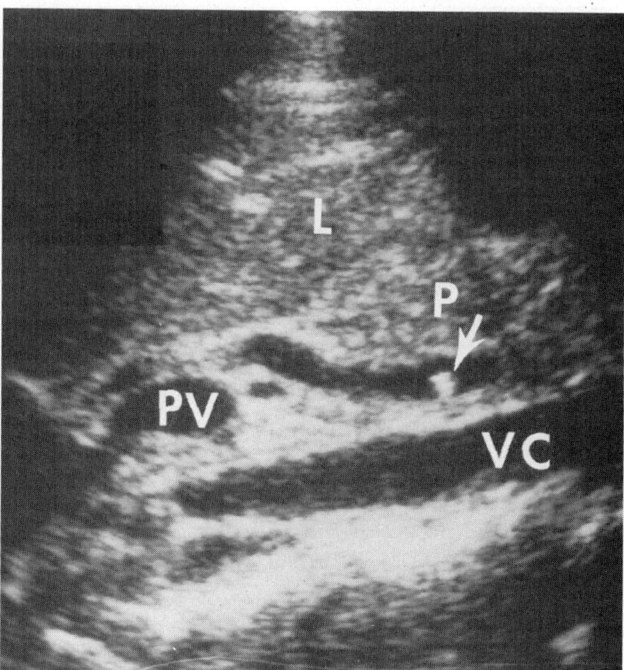

Figure 42–7. Nonobstructing stone *(arrow)* in distal common duct. Stone casts no acoustic shadow because its width is too narrow to completely block the ultrasound beam. *Abbreviations*: L = liver; P = head of the pancreas; PV = portal vein; VC = vena cava.

as an increased number of tubular structures adjacent to the main major branches of the portal veins (Fig. 42–8).[16] Visualization of peripheral intrahepatic bile ducts in portal triads does not necessarily imply dilatation, although the earlier ultrasound literature stated that this was the case. With modern higher-resolution ultrasound scanners, normal intrahepatic bile ducts 1 to 2 mm in diameter may be identified.[17] Furthermore, identification of two parallel tubular channels within the liver (parallel channel sign) does not imply that one represents a dilated bile duct adjacent to a portal vein branch. The channels may actually be the hepatic artery and portal vein. In patients with severe liver disease, the hepatic artery can be the main vascular supply to the liver. Arterial branches in the portal triads may become prominent and may be confused with dilated intrahepatic bile ducts unless Doppler or color Doppler examination is used to distinguish the arteries from the bile ducts.

Echogenic lines, often branching or associated with acous-

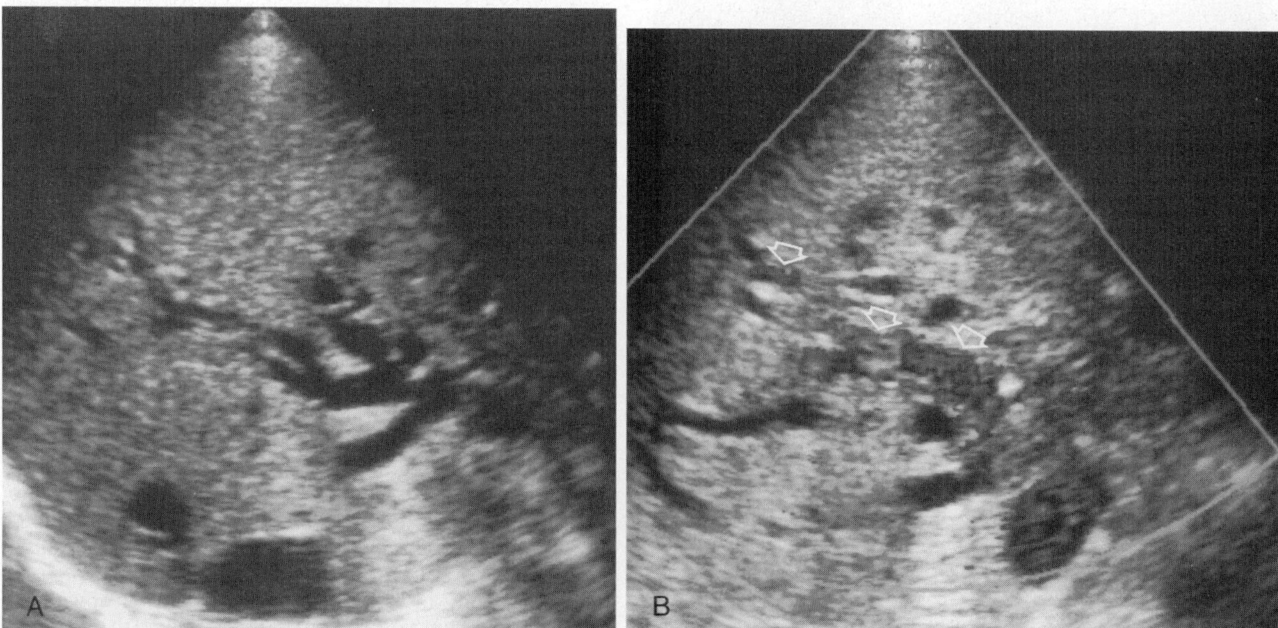

Figure 42–8. Dilated intrahepatic bile ducts in region of the porta hepatis. The transverse view *(A)* shows too many dilated and branching ducts in the region of the porta hepatis, whereas a color Doppler ultrasound image (displayed in black and white) *(B)* distinguishes a blood-containing portal vein *(arrows)* from dilated bile ducts.

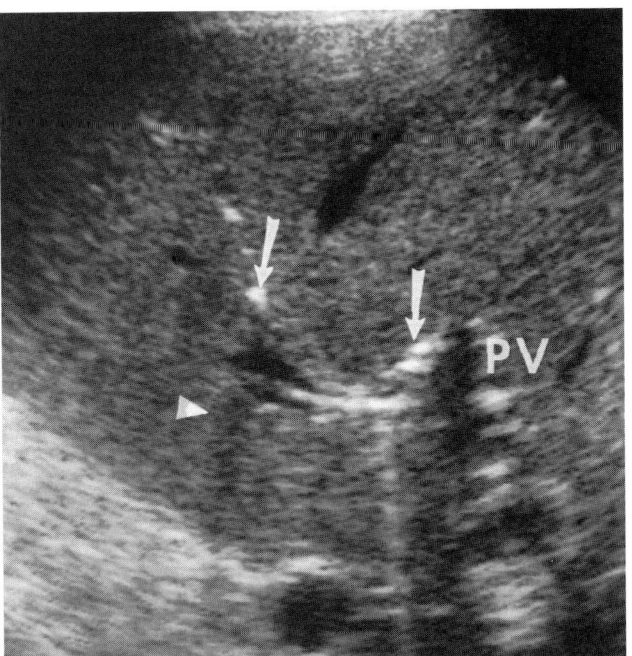

Figure 42–9. Gas in intrahepatic bile ducts following choledochojejunostomy in a patient with cadaveric liver transplant. Echogenic foci *(arrows)* with distal acoustic shadowing *(arrowhead)* represent the presence of gas in biliary ducts. During real-time ultrasound, one can see the gas bubbles move in the biliary system. *Abbreviation*: PV = portal vein branch.

tic shadowing, that lie parallel to portal vein branches represent air within the bile ducts. During real-time imaging, movement of the echogenic air bubbles may be seen. This pattern is usually an incidental finding in a patient who has undergone choledochojejunostomy (Fig. 42–9).

Liver Disease

Diffuse liver disease may be sonographically appreciated as generalized changes in parenchymal reflectivity. Increased reflectivity may occur in fatty liver and severe cirrhosis. In fatty liver, relatively uniform increased parenchymal reflectivity is usually noted. Loss of reflectivity from the diaphragm and from the walls of the portal veins is usually observed, because the increased parenchymal reflectivity of the liver parenchyma is similar to these structures, obscuring them (Fig. 42–10).[18] Although such infiltration is usually generalized, focal fatty infiltration may occasionally produce discrete areas of increased reflectivity.[19] The differential problem then becomes determining whether the areas of increased reflectivity are areas of fatty infiltration or focal masses. Noncontrast computed tomography is helpful; fatty infiltration has a reduced computed tomography number compared with tumor or normal liver.

Cirrhosis may also produce increased reflectivity of hepatic parenchyma, although often of a less uniform pattern than in fatty infiltration. The caudate lobe may be asymmetrically large, and the liver surface may be nodular. In severe disease, the liver may be small.[20] These parenchymal changes may hinder detection of hepatocellular carcinoma (which has an increased incidence in cirrhosis).[21] Signs of portal hypertension may also be present—reversed flow in the portal vein, portal vein thrombosis, cavernous transformation of the portal vein, patent umbilical vein, splenomegaly, and perisplenic varices. Doppler and particularly color Doppler are crucial to their evaluation.[22] Normally, portal vein flow is hepatopedal (Fig. 42–11); when reversed, flow is hepatofugal (Fig. 42–12). Portal vein thrombosis may be bland (nontumor) or secondary to hepatocellular carcinoma invading the portal vein (Fig. 42–13). In cases in which the tumor diffusely infiltrates the liver, the only ultrasonically visible sign of the tumor may be thrombus in the portal vein. Ultrasonically guided biopsy of the portal vein thrombus can differentiate bland thrombus from tumor thrombus.

Decreased parenchymal reflectivity occurs when the liver is swollen, such as in acute hepatitis.[23] The portal vessels become more prominent because of the greater difference in reflectivity between their walls and the adjacent edematous liver tissue. A similar pattern may also be seen in patients with congestive failure, when the liver becomes engorged because of poor venous return. In these patients, however, the hepatic veins and vena cava are abnormally distended and show a lack of caliber change with respiration because of the increased right atrial pressure.

Patients with the Budd-Chiari syndrome may have thrombosis of one or more hepatic veins, at times associated with reversed flow in other hepatic veins or thrombosis of the vena cava or portal vein. Doppler studies are required. Color Doppler is particularly useful. In severe liver disease due to various causes, hepatic veins may be narrowed or compressed. The veins may not be detectable on real-time imaging or spectral Doppler, but if flow is present, they can be seen with color Doppler.[24]

In patients who have portal hypertension and who are being considered for a transjugular intrahepatic portosystemic shunt (TIPS) procedure, establishing patency of the portal and hepatic veins is critical for success of the procedure. The direction of the portal vein is not important, however, as long as the main portal vein and its right branch are of adequate caliber to accept the shunt. Before TIPS, patients may have a reversed flow in the portal vein. After TIPS, the flow is normally from the portal to hepatic veins (Fig. 42–14). Deteriorating liver function test values and the

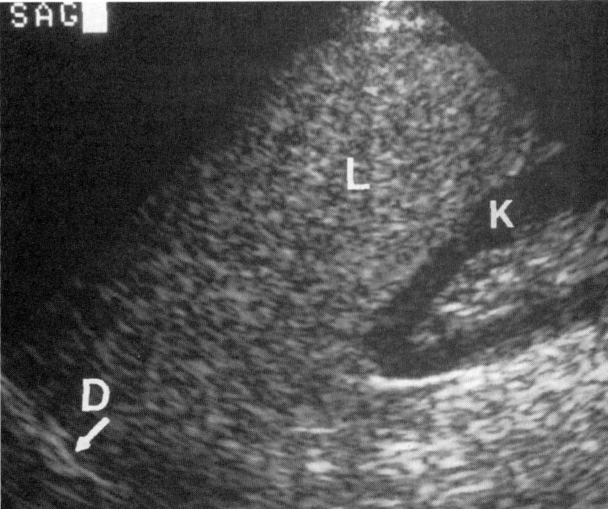

Figure 42–10. Diffuse fatty changes in the liver (sagittal view). The liver (L) shows a generalized increase in reflectivity. The renal cortex (K) appears unusually hypoechoic in comparison with liver tissue. Diaphragm (D) reflectivity is poorly distinguished from that of liver, whereas in the normal liver the diaphragm is much more reflective than liver parenchyma. (Compare with Figs. 42–3 and 42–8*A*.)

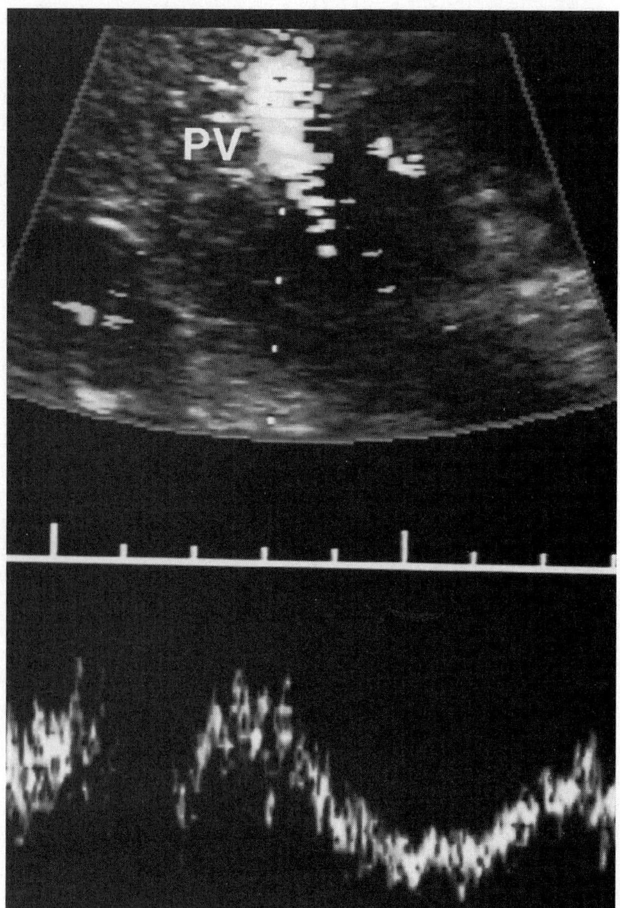

Figure 42–11. Normal direction of blood flow (hepatopedal) in the portal vein (PV). By convention, the flow appears as red with color Doppler ultrasound and above the baseline with spectral Doppler ultrasound when the direction of flow within the vessel is toward the probe. Hepatic artery flow also appears as red because it is too hepatopedal. (See Color Plate Section of this textbook.)

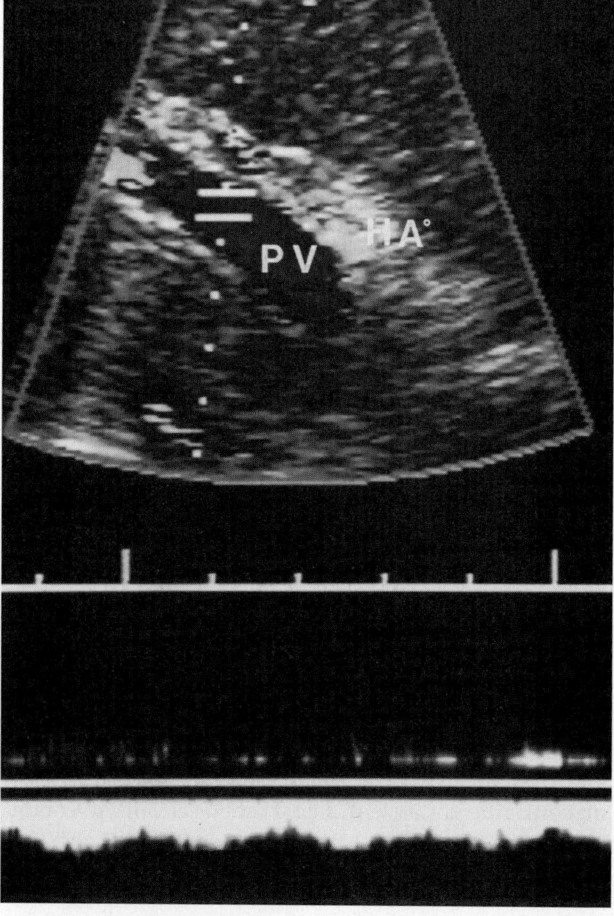

Figure 42–12. Reversed direction of blood flow (hepatofugal) in the portal vein. The blood visualized with color Doppler ultrasound and with spectral Doppler ultrasound below the baseline is blue because it flows away from the probe. However, hepatic artery (HA) flow remains red in appearance (hepatopedal). *Note*: Red/blue with color Doppler ultrasound or above/below the baseline with spectral Doppler ultrasound relate the direction of blood flow to the orientation of the Doppler ultrasound beam with respect to the blood vessel, not the absolute direction of blood flow. The operator has to be aware of the orientation of the Doppler ultrasound beam to the vessel to know the true direction of blood flow. (See Color Plate Section of this textbook.)

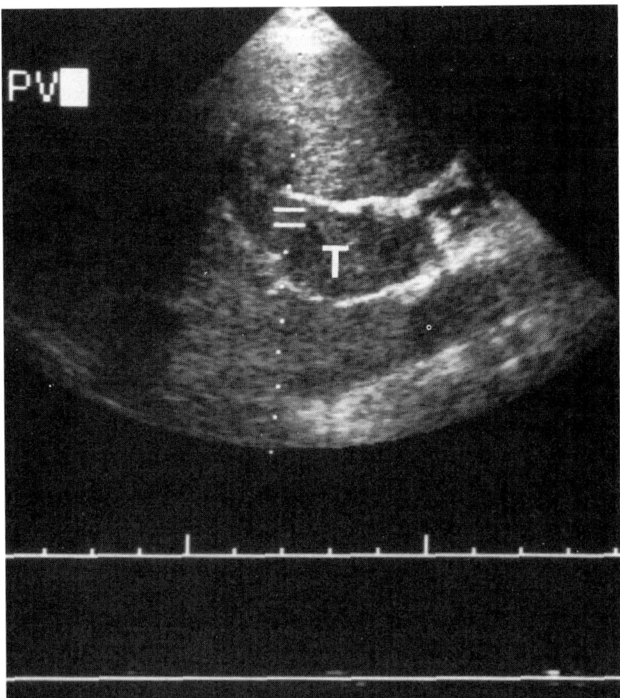

Figure 42–13. Hepatocellular tumor thrombus (T) occluding the portal vein (sagittal view). Spectral Doppler ultrasound shows no flow in the portal vein.

development of ascites after a TIPS procedure may represent a thrombosed (Fig. 42–15) or narrowed shunt channel.

In patients with portosystemic shunts (portocaval, splenorenal, and mesoatrial), color Doppler ultrasound may demonstrate the patency of the shunt.[25]

Among liver transplantation candidates, pretransplant assessment of the hepatic artery, vena cava, and especially the portal vein for patency is necessary. When no flow is observed in the portal vein, a venogram is usually indicated. It determines whether the portal vein is actually thrombosed or has flow that is so slow that it may not be appreciated by Doppler. If the vein is thrombosed, the venogram suggests alternate veins that are available for anastomosis to the donor liver.

Evaluation of Complications After Liver Transplantation

After liver transplantation, studies are most often performed to detect vascular thrombosis or stenosis. Of lesser importance is assessment of perihepatic fluid collections, because almost all patients in the acute postoperative period have perihepatic hematomas or seromas. However, detection of intrahepatic fluid collections (provided they are truly intrahepatic and not collections tracking along the falciform ligament or between lobes of the liver) is more significant. Bilomas may develop from bile duct ischemia as a result of hepatic artery stenosis or thrombosis.[26] If a patient is septic, fluid collections may be abscesses.

The hepatic artery is the vessel most prone to thrombosis or severe stenosis because of its small caliber. Although in most liver transplants a single donor common hepatic artery is anastomosed to the recipient hepatic artery or celiac axis, some transplanted livers may have separate right and left hepatic arteries with different anastomoses to recipient vessels. Therefore, it is important to demonstrate blood flow in the main hepatic artery and in both the right and left major

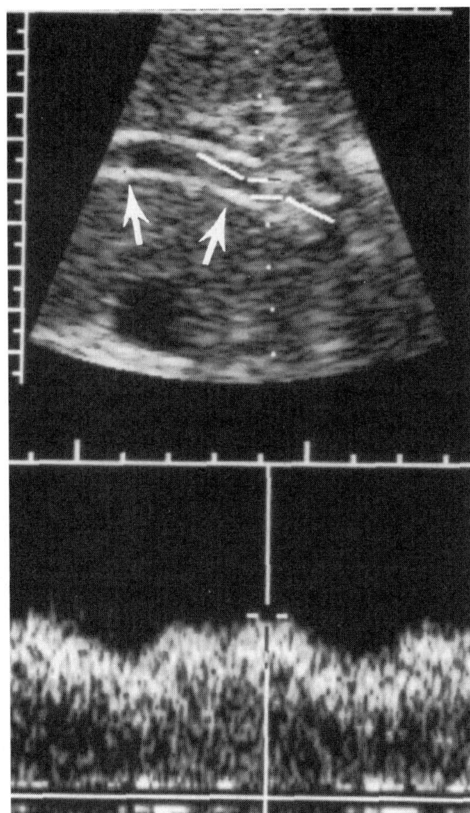

Figure 42–14. Patent TIPS *(arrows)*. Blood flow is from caudal to cephalad (from the portal to hepatic vein).

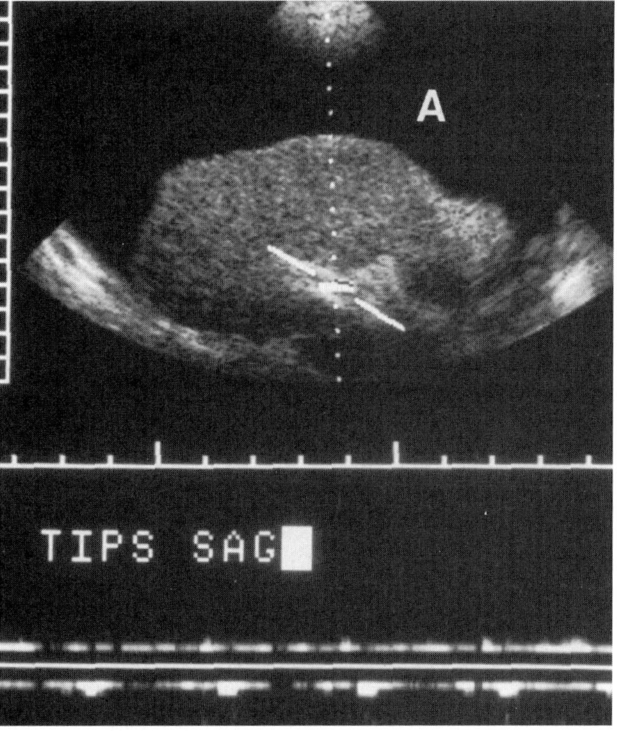

Figure 42–15. Occluded TIPS. Doppler ultrasound shows no flow. The patient developed ascites (A).

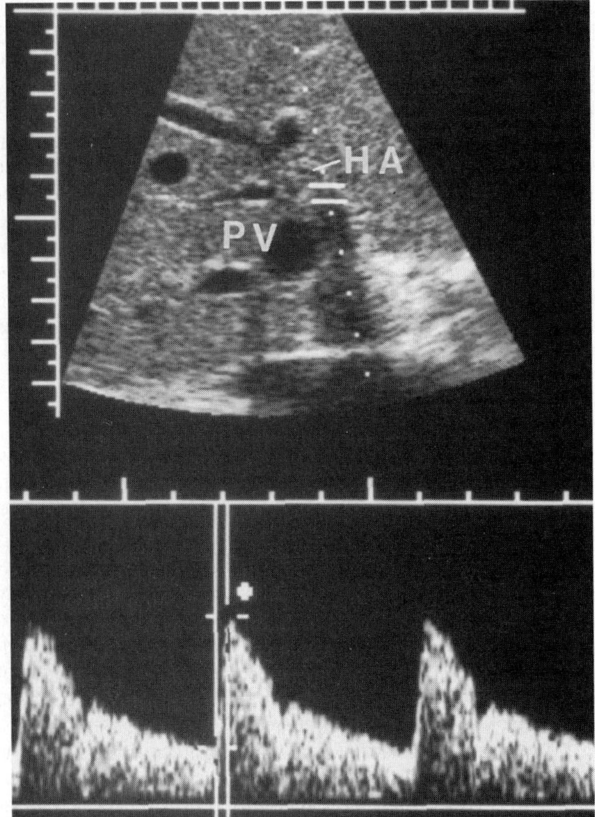

Figure 42–16. Normal hepatic artery with spectral Doppler ultrasound. Spectral Doppler ultrasound recording from the hepatic artery (HA) where it lies adjacent to the portal vein (PV). The spectral tracing shows rapid systolic upstroke (less than 0.1 s between end-diastole and peak systole and a resistive index of >0.5).

branch arteries. Color Doppler permits rapid identification of the hepatic artery, in both the intra- and extrahepatic locations, as well as detection of focal stenoses. Spectral Doppler is always used to characterize the flow velocity waveforms in order to identify abnormal flow patterns suggestive of a hepatic artery stenosis. The normal arterial waveform has a rapid systolic rise (<0.1 s between end-diastole and peak systole) (Fig. 42–16). The resistive index (peak systolic minus end-diastolic divided by peak systolic velocity) should be greater than 0.5. The blood flow is laminar, displayed as a Doppler wave in which the flow velocity follows the envelope of the wave. A resistive index (RI) less than 0.5, especially when coupled with a delayed systolic rise beyond 0.1 second in the main hepatic artery (where it crosses the portal vein) or in intrahepatic branch hepatic arteries, strongly suggests a more proximal hepatic artery stenosis (Fig. 42–17*A*), which is commonly at the anastomosis between the donor and recipient hepatic arteries. At the stenosis, the spectral Doppler waveform shows a high flow velocity (>2 m/s or greater than three times the peak systolic velocity of the artery proximal to the stenosis) and spectral broadening indicative of turbulent flow (Fig. 42–17*B*).[27] After recent transplantation, however, it may be difficult to visualize the more proximal hepatic artery because of the fresh skin suture line or intervening gas-filled bowel. Therefore, the findings of reduced RI and delay in systolic velocity rise time in the intrahepatic arteries are sufficient evidence to suspect a more proximal hepatic artery stenosis and warrant an arteriogram.

In the portal vein and vena cava, postoperative thrombosis rarely occurs; rather, the concern is stenosis at the anastomotic sites. Because venous blood is more uniform in its flow velocity than arterial blood, detection of venous stenosis with spectral and color Doppler depends on identifying high-velocity turbulent flow at the anastomosis. Visualizing the actual site of vascular narrowing on real-time images helps confirm the diagnosis. When the velocity of the blood at the anastomosis is at least three times greater than the velocity of the blood before reaching the anastomosis, a significant anastomotic stenosis is strongly suspected,[28] and venography may confirm the ultrasound findings (Fig. 42–18). Although the portal vein has only one anastomosis, the vena cava usually has two: the proximal anastomosis adjacent to the diaphragm and the distal near the inferior extent of the liver. If a "piggyback" caval anastomosis is performed, only one anastomosis is made—end-to-side donor to recipient close to the diaphragm.

Search for Abdominal Abscesses, Hematomata, Ascites

The three common clinical situations of (1) fever (rule out intra-abdominal abscess), (2) sudden decrease in hematocrit (rule out intra-abdominal hematoma), and (3) increasing abdominal distention (rule out ascites) are combined in one category because they all involve the search for intra-abdominal fluid collections.

Because detection of intra-abdominal fluid is limited by the physical properties of ultrasound—namely, its inability

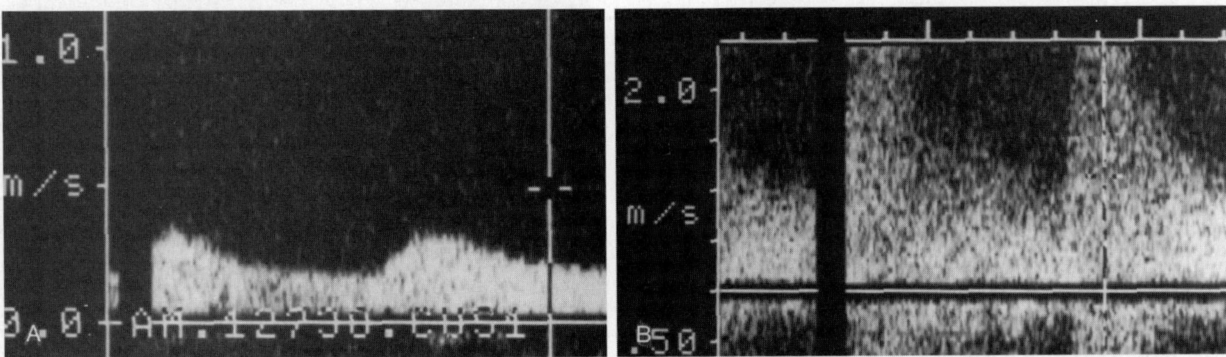

Figure 42–17. Stenosis of the hepatic artery at the anastomosis between the donor and recipient arteries. *A*, Spectral Doppler ultrasound of the main hepatic artery in the porta hepatis (distal to stenosis). The resistive index is reduced (0.3), and the rise to peak systole (0.15 s) is delayed; *B*, Spectral Doppler ultrasound at anastomotic stenosis. The flow velocity is turbulent and >2 m/s.

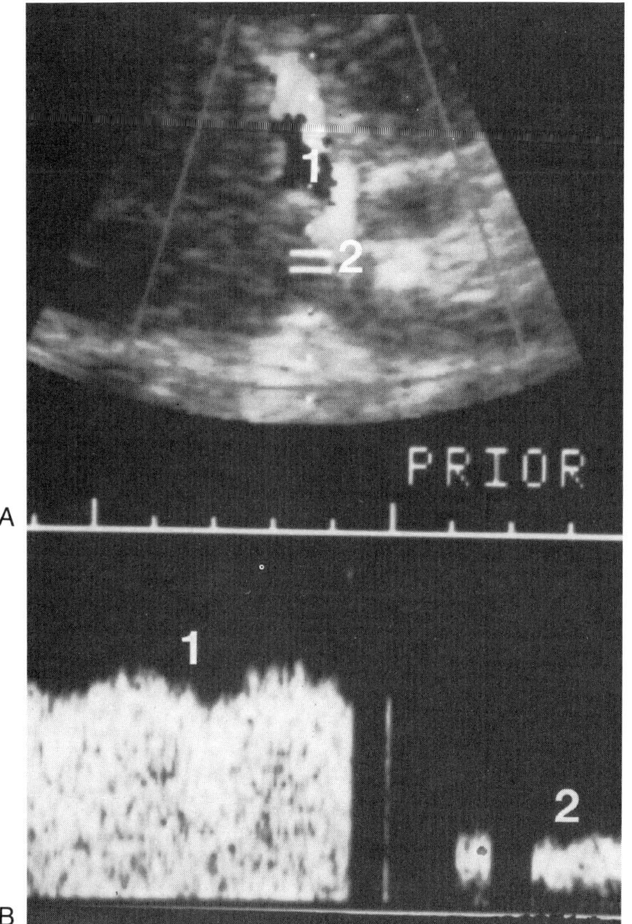

Figure 42–18. Portal vein stenosis following cadaveric liver transplant. The direction of flow is hepatopedal (red on color Doppler ultrasound). *A*, At the site of stenosis (1), where the velocity is greatest, the vein appears light red or yellow because the color of blood flowing toward the probe changes from dark red to bright yellow as velocity increases. However, if the velocities exceed the displayed range of the red scale, they are seen as shades of blue (the opposite end of the scale), progressing from dark to light with increasingly greater velocities. *B*, The spectral Doppler ultrasound tracing shows turbulent high-velocity flow from the site of stenosis (1) and low-velocity laminar flow prior to stenosis (2). (See Color Plate Section of this textbook.)

to penetrate through air- or gas-containing structures—the search for intra-abdominal fluid is restricted to regions of the abdomen where no gas-filled bowel intervenes between the skin and the region of interest. Accessible regions include the liver, gallbladder, and spleen in the upper abdomen; the kidneys and lateral retroperitoneal regions; the peritoneal cavity around the liver and spleen; along the lateral gutters; and in the pelvis, behind the urinary bladder. Fluid collections within the superficial tissues of the abdominal wall are also easily imaged. Pleural fluid accumulating in the inferior recesses of the chest can be seen above the diaphragms, adjacent to the liver or spleen. A collapsed segment of lower lung may appear within the fluid (Fig. 42–19). Periaortic and peripancreatic fluid is visible only when no gas-filled bowel covers these strictures or when probe pressure can displace or compress the bowel.

Within the peritoneal cavity, fluid that changes shape with localized pressure of the probe or a change of the patient's position from supine to lateral decubitus likely represents free fluid rather than loculated fluid. Fluid can be seen when it accumulates around the liver and spleen, in the deep lateral abdominal recesses, in the pelvis surrounding the uterus, and in Morison's pouch. As the quantity of ascitic fluid increases, the bowel is displaced toward the midline, making visualization of the central intra-abdominal and retroperitoneal structures more difficult. Fluid that is entirely echo free suggests a transudate (Fig. 42–20*A*). Diffuse echoes within a fluid collection suggest the presence of particulate material, which may be pus or blood (see Fig. 42–20*B*). Septa or echogenic strands within peritoneal fluid may be a sign of peritonitis.[29] A localized collection containing a spongelike or meshlike echogenic pattern suggests an organized hematoma. The spongelike pattern represents the fibrin strands, and the echo-free spaces between represent areas of more liquefied blood or serous fluid (see Fig. 42–20C).

In solid organs (liver, kidneys, spleen), both abscesses and hematomas can have a similar spectrum of ultrasound appearances.[30] Hypoechoic or anechoic collections can represent both abscesses (Fig. 42–21) and hematomas. They differ from cysts because they lack razor-sharp walls, are not usually completely echo free, and often do not have deep echo enhancement. Fresh hematomas, either intraparenchymal or subcapsular from percutaneous biopsy, may be echogenic (Fig. 42–22). Abscesses containing gas may display focal echogenic regions, some of which may produce acoustic shadowing (Fig. 42–23) (regions of absent image because the gas locally stopped the penetration of the sound beam). Clinical findings and, if necessary, percutaneous aspiration differentiate between them.

In patients with fluid-filled bowel, especially when the bowel is adynamic and the fluid does not demonstrate peristalsis, a bowel loop may be confused with a loculated intra-abdominal fluid collection unless plicae circulares or haustral markings are identified.

Evaluate Complications of Renal Transplantation

In the author's experience, a common reason for performing an ultrasound study is to evaluate reduced renal function; less frequently it is to assess unusual transplant tenderness,

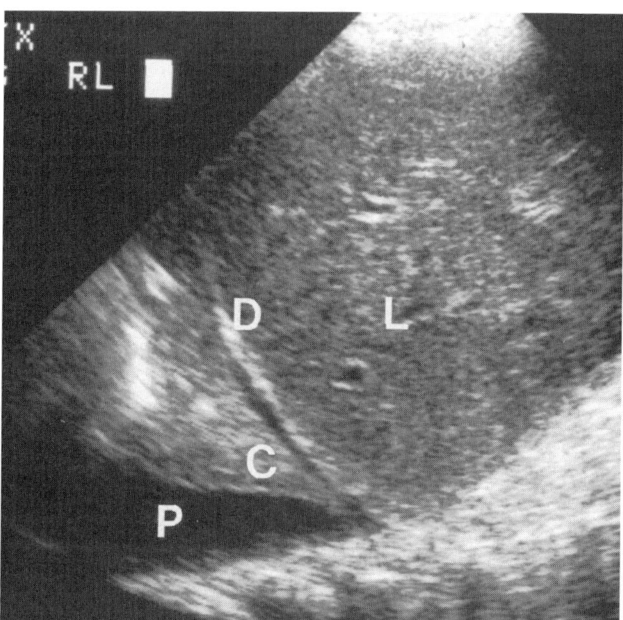

Figure 42–19. Pleural fluid and "tongue" of a collapsed right lower lung in posteroinferior right pleural recess (sagittal view, patient in supine position). *Abbreviations:* P = pleural fluid; C = collapsed lung; D = diaphragm; L = liver.

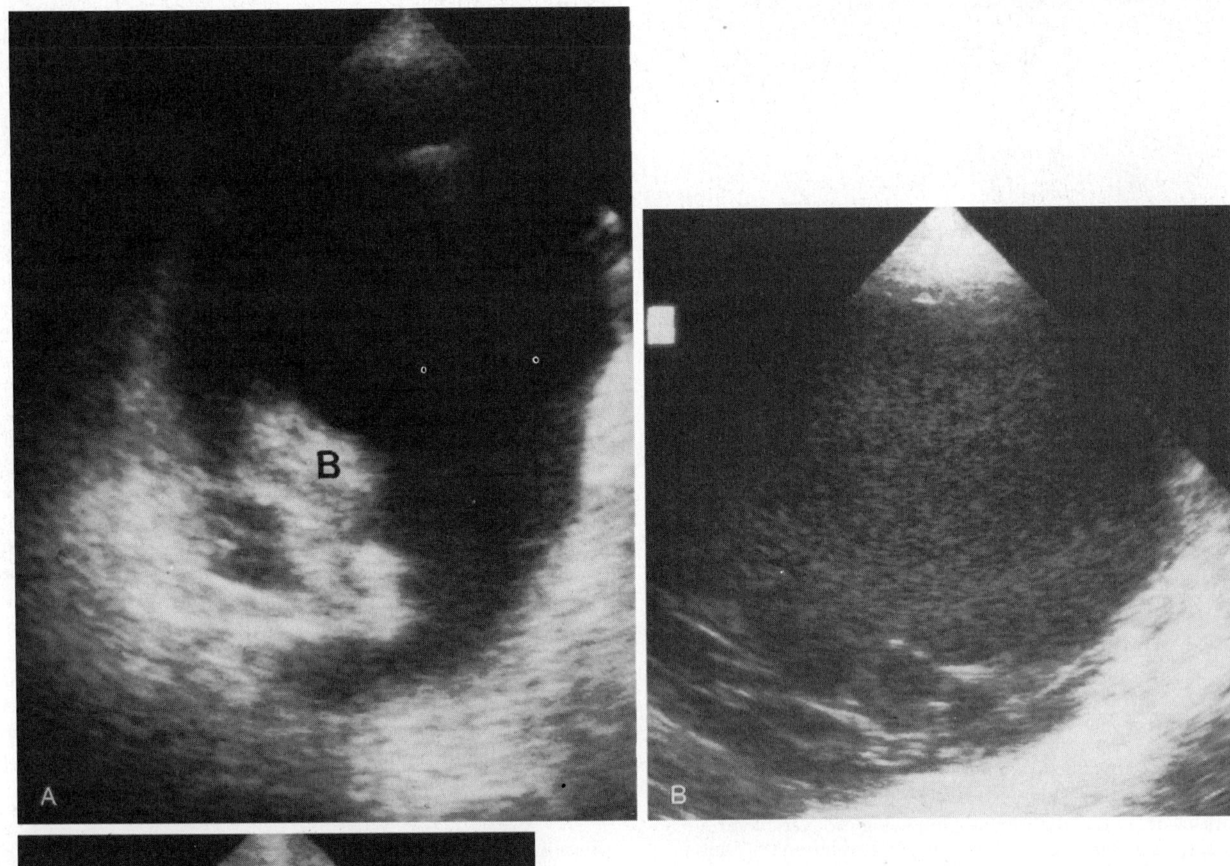

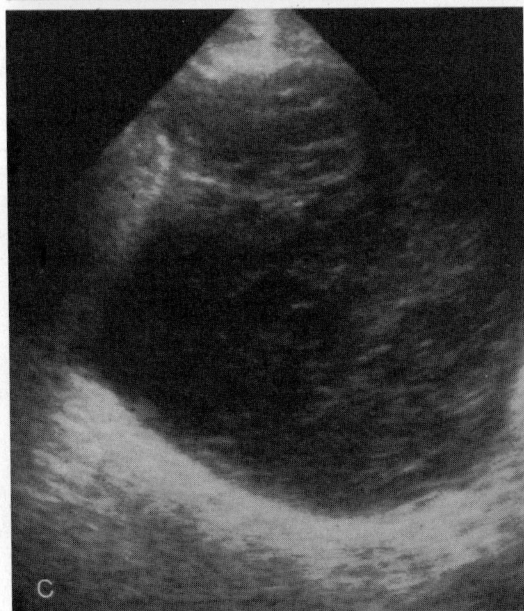

Figure 42–20. Three ultrasonic patterns of intraperitoneal fluid. *A*, Echo-free fluid: transudate is present in right lower quadrant, with gas-free bowel (B) lying in deeper region. *B*, Diffusely echogenic fluid: an abscess is present in the left upper quadrant. *C*, A spongelike pattern of echogenic septa and echo-free spaces: a hematoma is present in the left lower quadrant.

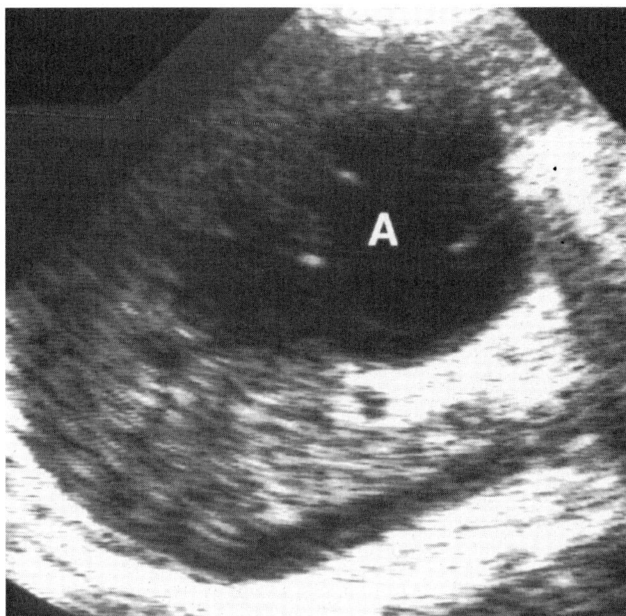

Figure 42–21. Liver abscess (A) (sagittal view, right lobe of the liver). An irregularly shaped mass without sharp margins and scattered low-intensity internal echoes is demonstrated. Percutaneous aspiration with ultrasound guidance obtained 10 mL of pus.

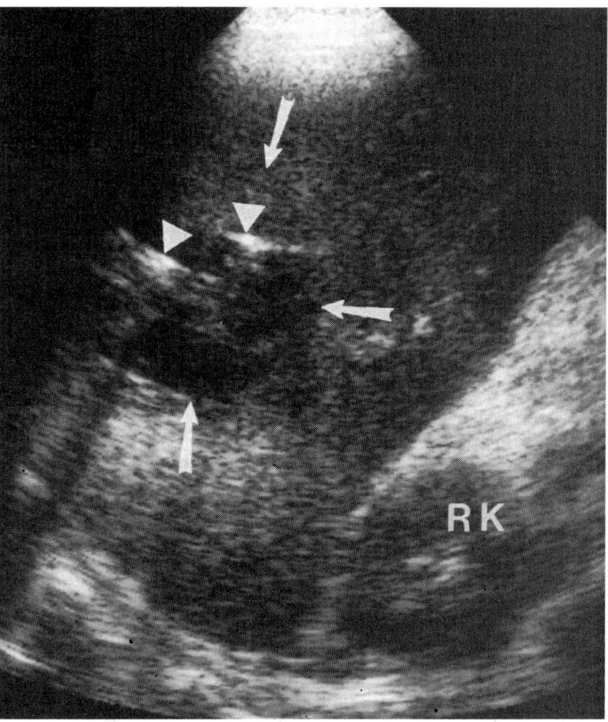

Figure 42–23. A gas-containing liver abscess (transverse view). The hypoechoic mass *(arrows)* is an abscess. Strongly echogenic foci within that mass shadow *(arrowheads)* represent the presence of gas within the abscess. *Abbreviation*: RK = right kidney.

sudden onset of hypertension, or a peritransplant mass. An attempt is made to distinguish causes for which there may be specific treatment versus nonspecific findings.

Ultrasound study of a renal transplant should combine both real-time imaging and Doppler flow velocity studies. Real-time imaging provides information about the size and architecture of the kidney, the presence or absence of hydronephrosis, and perinephric fluid collections. Doppler studies

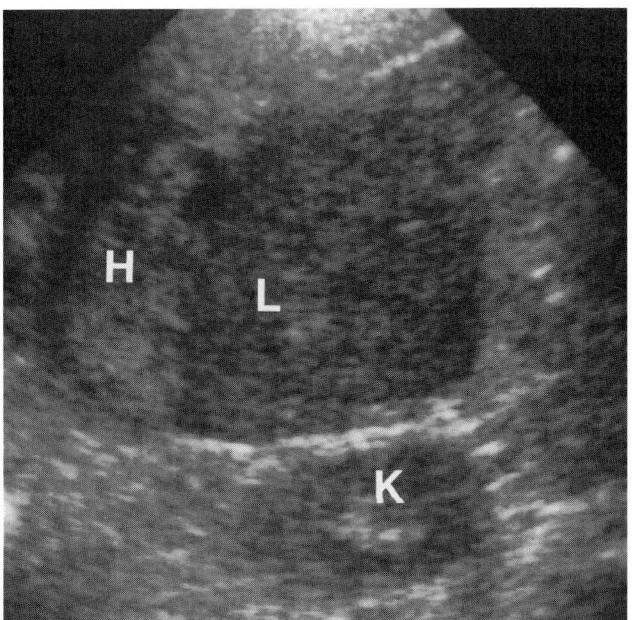

Figure 42–22. A subcapsular hematoma of right lobe of the liver (transverse view) seen several hours following needle biopsy of the liver (not performed with ultrasound guidance). *Abbreviations*: H = echogenic hematoma; L = liver; K = kidney.

can detect a stenosed or obstructed main renal artery or vein.

Generalized dilatation of the renal collecting system (hydronephrosis), especially if it is a new finding, suggests renal obstruction. When it is detected, specific causes should be sought. A urine-distended bladder may obstruct the ureter. Although most patients in intensive care units have bladder catheters, the catheter may have become temporarily obstructed. Perinephric fluid collections between the lower pole of the kidney and the urinary bladder may extrinsically compress and obstruct the ureter. An echo-free fluid collection in the recent postoperative period suggests a urinoma, whereas a similar fluid collection appearing several weeks later implies a lymphocele (Fig. 42–24).[31] An echogenic mass adjacent to the region of the ureter, especially if it has a spongelike internal architectural pattern, suggests a hematoma. A mass with more uniform low-level echogenicity could represent either hematoma or, in the appropriate clinical setting, an abscess.

Small echogenic masses, often crescent shaped, lying adjacent to the kidney are commonly seen in the immediate postoperative period, and if the patient is asymptomatic, these most often represent small hematomas. They usually produce no obstructive uropathy. A hematoma may occasionally be quite large, approximating the size of the transplant kidney. Although it produces no hydronephrosis, the hematoma may affect renal function by placing pressure on the kidney.[31] A large perinephric hematoma may at times have echogenicity so similar to that of the renal cortex that it is difficult to appreciate (Fig. 42–25).

Stenosis of the main renal artery, usually at its anastomosis with the iliac artery, can produce specific abnormal Doppler findings—a focal region of high-velocity turbulent blood flow. Color Doppler imaging greatly simplifies visualization of the anastomosis and detection of the high-veloc-

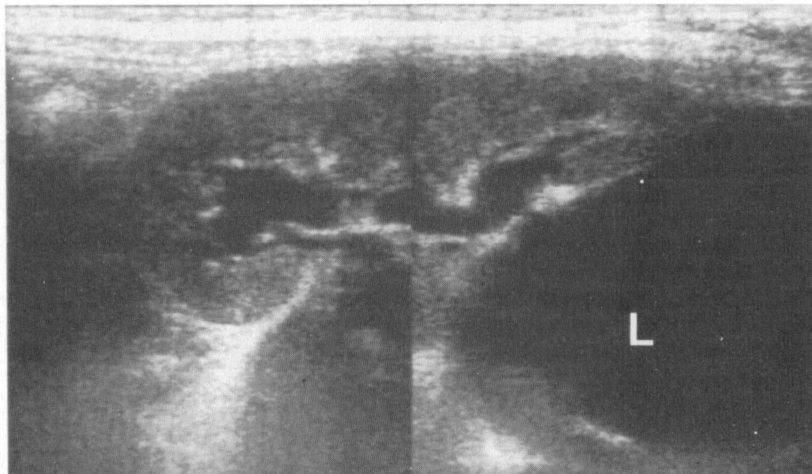

Figure 42–24. *A* and B, Hydronephrosis of a cadaveric renal transplant secondary to the occurrence of a large lymphocele (L), sagittal view.

ity flow at the stenosis. Spectral Doppler quantifies the increased velocity, which for a significant stenosis should be at least three times greater at the stenotic site than in the adjacent iliac artery. Main renal artery stenosis can also be suspected on the basis of the abnormal spectral Doppler waveform of intrarenal arteries. It shows a delayed onset of peak systolic velocity (>0.1 s), often with an RI less than 0.5 (similar to that seen with hepatic artery stenosis in liver transplant recipients) (Fig. 42–26).[32]

When a spectral Doppler arterial waveform demonstrating delayed peak systolic velocity rise and reduced RI is localized to one region of the kidney, a localized arteriovenous shunt is suggested. It is usually secondary to renal needle biopsy. Color Doppler may help identify the actual shunt site. Pseudoaneurysm is another complication of percutaneous renal biopsy that can be observed. On real-time imaging, it may appear as an echo-free mass simulating a renal cyst. The diagnosis of pseudoaneurysm is made either with spectral or color Doppler by demonstrating blood flow within the cavity.[32] Small, hemodynamically nonsignificant arteriovenous fistulas or small pseudoaneurysms often spontaneously resolve, although larger, symptomatic ones may require definitive treatment, either by angiographic occlusion or surgery. Extrarenal pseudoaneurysms and arteriovenous fistulas, although less frequent than their intrarenal counterparts, can be more serious because of the danger of rupture and exsanguination. They are commonly detected as incidental findings during renal scanning (nuclear or ultrasound scans) for other reasons, although they may occasionally cause symptoms of renal dysfunction as a result of renal compression or an arteriovenous fistula.[32]

The significance of an elevated interlobar or segmental artery RI is not clear. Although researchers initially believed that an elevated RI was specific for acute rejection, subsequent research showed that various other causes, including acute tubular necrosis and immunosuppressive medication toxicity, may elevate the RI.[33]

Ultrasound is very useful in guiding needle placement for percutaneous renal biopsy. At the author's institution, all such procedures are performed under ultrasound guidance. The biopsy specimens are taken from the renal cortex, preferably from a site in the lateral portion of the upper pole, to avoid major intrarenal vessels and portions of the collecting system (Fig. 42–27). Before biopsy, the site is imaged with color Doppler to see that no major vessels lie along the path of the needle. Immediately after biopsy, the site and needle tract are examined with color Doppler to search for bleeding (Fig. 42–28). If bleeding is seen, localized pressure is applied with the probe directly over the site to control it.

Invasive Ultrasonography

In addition to its diagnostic imaging capabilities, ultrasound may be used to percutaneously guide the insertion of a

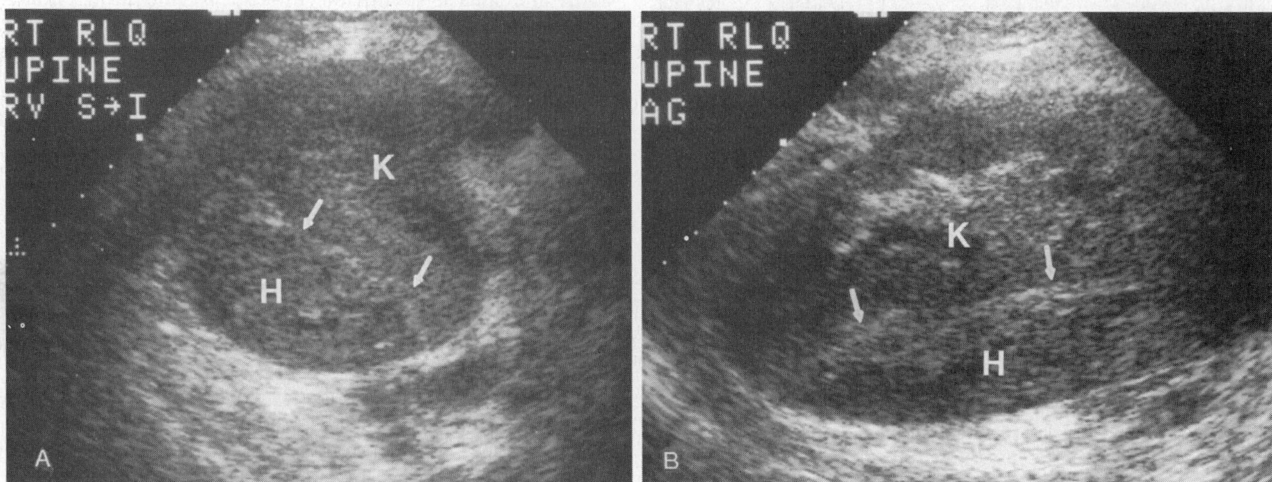

Figure 42–25. Large perinephric hematoma (H) is seen compressing a cadaveric renal transplant (K). Note the interface between the hematoma and the renal cortex *(arrows)*. (*A*, transverse view; *B*, sagittal view.)

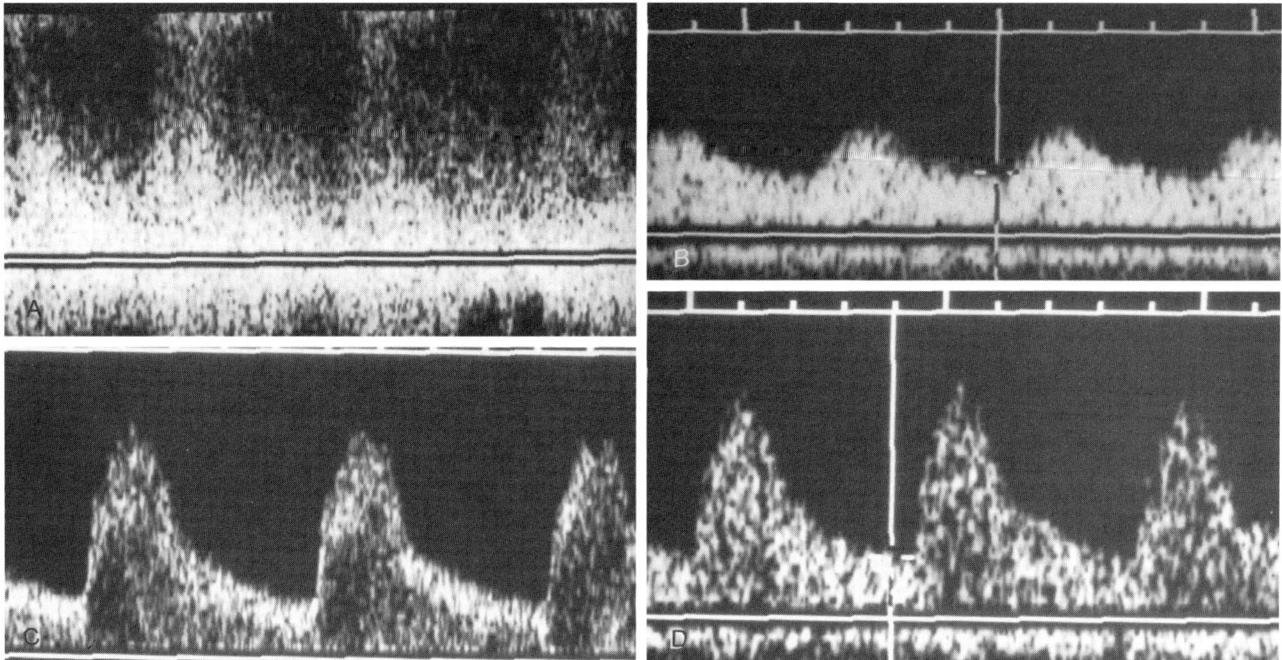

Figure 42–26. Cadaveric renal transplant with stenosis of the renal artery at anastomosis and with the iliac artery before and after arterial balloon dilatation. *A*, Spectral Doppler ultrasound at stenosis shows a velocity of >2 m/s with spectral broadening. *B*, A Doppler ultrasound tracing of the intrarenal artery demonstrates a reduced resistive index (0.43) and a prolonged time to peak systole (0.2 s). *C*, Following dilatation of the stenosis, the peak flow velocity at the anastomosis decreases to 0.8 m/s. *D*, The resistive index of segmental vessels increases to 0.71, with a time to peak systole of <0.1 s.

needle or catheter into a fluid collection (in the pleural, peritoneal, or retroperitoneal spaces) for sampling or drainage[34–36] or into a mass or organ for biopsy.[37, 38] Ultrasound guidance changes blind needle passage into a visually directed and monitored procedure. Both the target area and the needle, as it is directed to the target area, are under continuous ultrasound observation. The rapidity with which an ultrasonically guided invasive procedure can be performed is especially important in critically ill patients. The chances of bleeding from laceration from organ movement or vessel puncture are minimized, particularly in biopsy of a solid organ such as the liver, because the procedure is

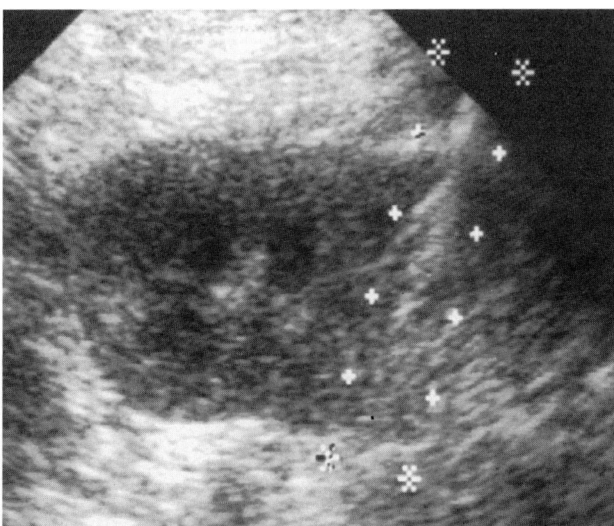

Figure 42–27. Ultrasonically guided biopsy of a left pelvic cadaveric renal transplant. *Dotted lines* (representing the path that the needle follows through kidney) are positioned through lateral cortex. Linear bright echoes from the path of an 18-gauge core needle immediately following biopsy confirm the correct site of the biopsy.

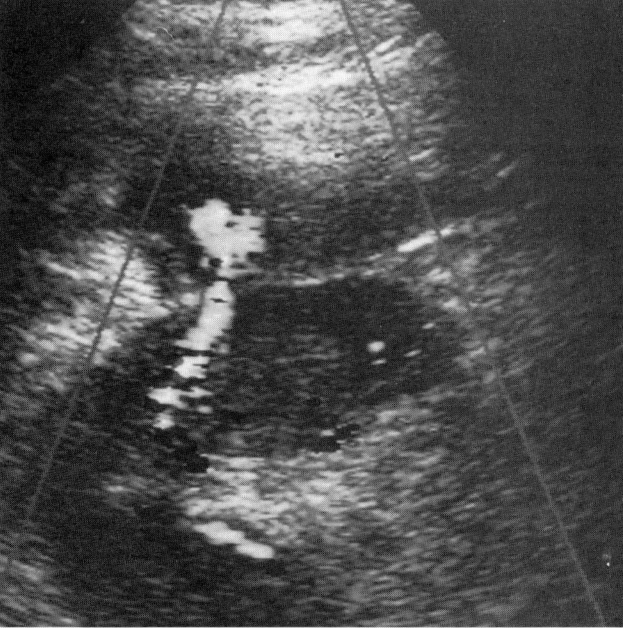

Figure 42–28. Color Doppler ultrasound imaging of a renal transplant biopsy site immediately following needle biopsy shows bleeding from the needle tract extending through the renal capsule. Several minutes of localized pressure with the ultrasound probe on the biopsy site stopped the bleeding. (See Color Plate Section of this textbook.)

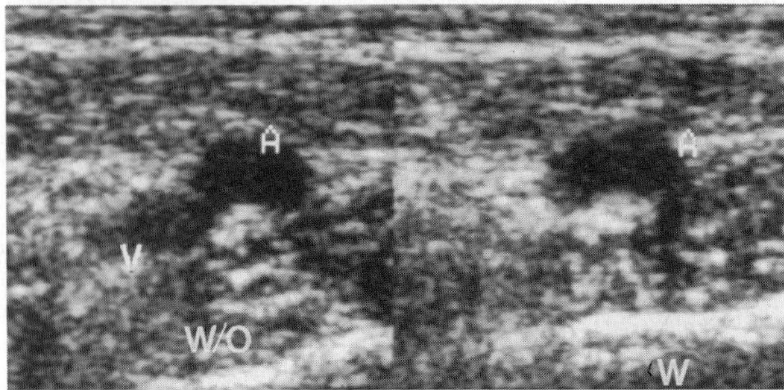

Figure 42–29. Normal superficial femoral vein (transverse views without [WO] and with [W] compression). During compression, the vein (V) collapses, whereas the artery (A) remains visible.

usually performed during a brief period of suspended respiration. Although the majority of ultrasound-guided invasive procedures can be performed with real-time imaging only, color Doppler may further reduce the risk of complications. Vessels overlying the target area are more easily identified, thus helping the operator avoid them. In addition, color Doppler can detect postbiopsy bleeding. When seen, bleeding can usually be stopped by pressure with the probe over the biopsy site, observing the region until the bleeding has ceased.

A 20- to 22-gauge needle is used to obtain a diagnostic sample from a fluid collection. To drain a fluid collection or gallbladder (see Fig. 42–4*B*), a catheter-sheathed trochar needle (a coaxial arrangement of a hollow needle containing a sharp inner trochar passed through a soft outer catheter) is inserted as a single assembly into the collection. The catheter forms a pigtail configuration after the needle is removed. For biopsy applications, if a core specimen is desired, a spring-loaded 18-gauge cutting needle is used, and for cytologic sampling, a 20- or 22-gauge needle is preferred.

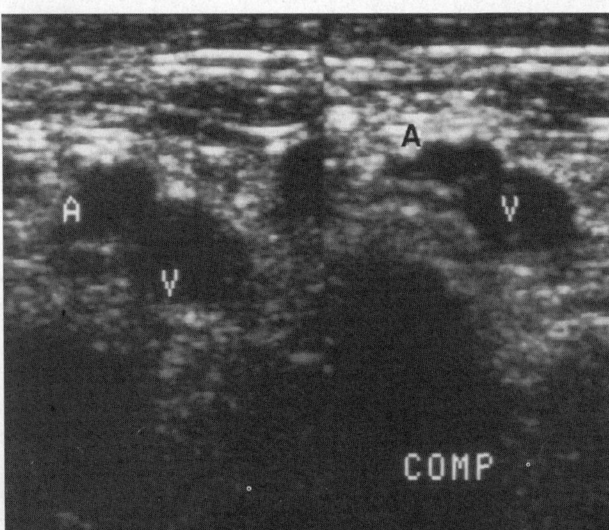

Figure 42–30. Thrombosed superficial femoral vein (transverse views). The vein (V) does not collapse with compression (COMP). However, the artery (A) shows flattening of its anterior wall from probe pressure, indicating that effective compressive force has been applied with the probe.

Vascular Ultrasound: Lower Extremities—Rule Out Femoral-Popliteal Deep Venous Thrombosis

The main critical care application of ultrasound examination of the lower extremities is for detecting thrombi within the femoral-popliteal venous system. A vein that is free of clot is one that completely collapses (the opposing walls touch each other) when pressure is applied on the skin over the vein (Fig. 42–29). When a vein contains clot, the two walls do not completely touch because of the intervening clot (Fig. 42–30).[39] Because the echogenicity of thrombi may vary considerably from being more reflective than blood to having a reflectivity similar to blood, imaging of the vessel without the use of compressive techniques is not satisfactory for determining the presence of intravascular thrombi. Doppler ultrasound supplements compression maneuvers. In a noncompressible vein, Doppler illustrates whether the clot is completely occluding (no blood flow) or partially occluding (flow detected). If the flow is too slow to be initially detected by Doppler, squeezing the limb distally (augmentation maneuver) may increase the cephalad flow enough to make it detectable by spectral or color Doppler. Color Doppler may be used in the same manner to differentiate occluding from nonoccluding clot and has the advantage of displaying the flow in the entire lumen of the vessel rather than in just one area where the spectral Doppler sensor is placed.[40]

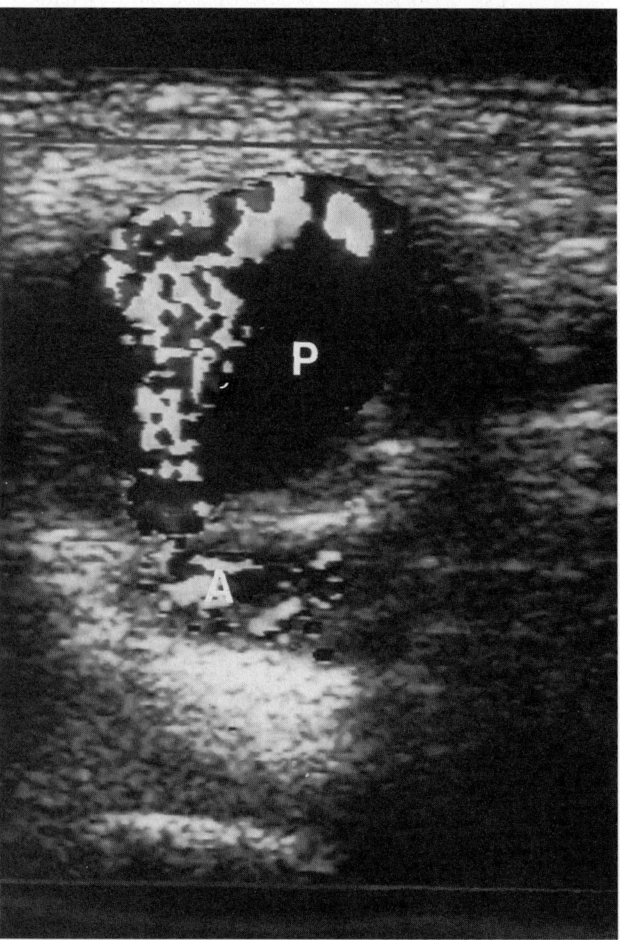

Figure 42–31. Pseudoaneurysm (P) of right femoral artery (A) following cardiac catheterization (transverse view, right groin). (See Color Plate Section of this textbook.)

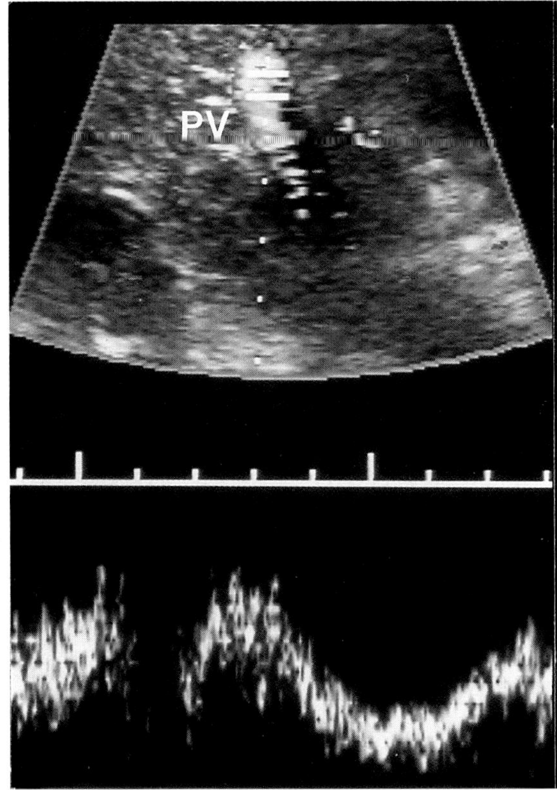

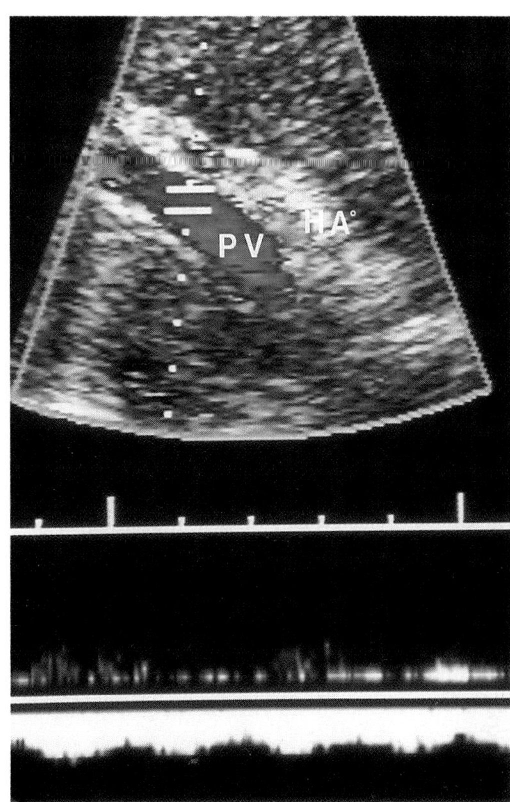

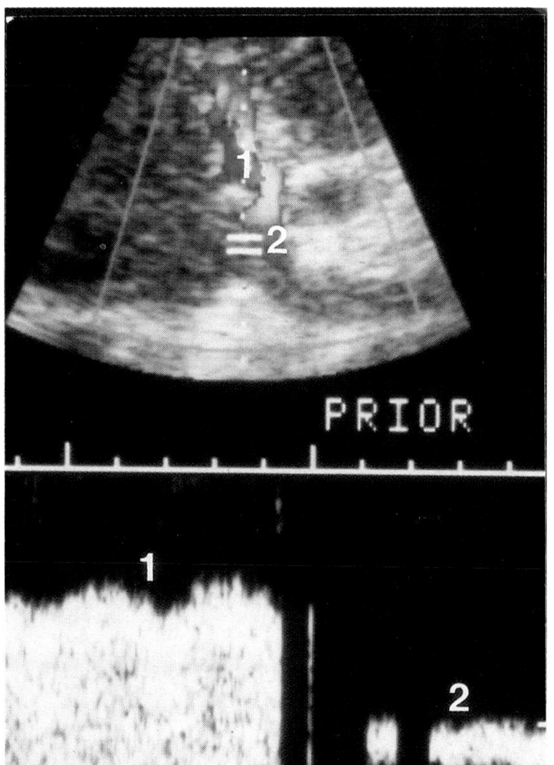

Figure 42–11. Normal direction of blood flow (hepatopetal) in the portal vein (PV). By convention, the flow appears as red with color Doppler ultrasound and above the baseline with spectral Doppler ultrasound when the direction of flow within the vessel is toward the probe. Hepatic artery flow also appears as red because it too is hepatopetal.

Figure 42–12. Reversed direction of blood flow (hepatofugal) in the portal vein. The blood visualized with color Doppler ultrasound and with spectral Doppler ultrasound below the baseline is blue because it flows away from the probe. However, hepatic artery (HA) flow remains red in appearance (hepatopetal). *Note*: Red/blue with color Doppler ultrasound or above/below the baseline with spectral Doppler ultrasound relate the direction of blood flow to the orientation of the Doppler ultrasound beam with respect to the blood vessel, not the absolute direction of blood flow. The operator has to be aware of the orientation of the Doppler ultrasound beam to the vessel to know the true direction of blood flow.

Figure 42–18. Portal vein stenosis following cadaveric liver transplant. The direction of flow is hepatopetal (red on color Doppler ultrasound). *A*, At the site of stenosis (1), where the velocity is greatest, the vein appears light red or yellow because the color of blood flowing toward the probe changes from dark red to bright yellow as velocity increases. However, if the velocities exceed the displayed range of the red scale, they are seen as shades of blue (the opposite end of the scale), progressing from dark to light with increasingly greater velocities. *B*, The spectral Doppler ultrasound tracing shows turbulent high-velocity flow from the site of stenosis (1) and low-velocity laminar flow prior to stenosis (2).

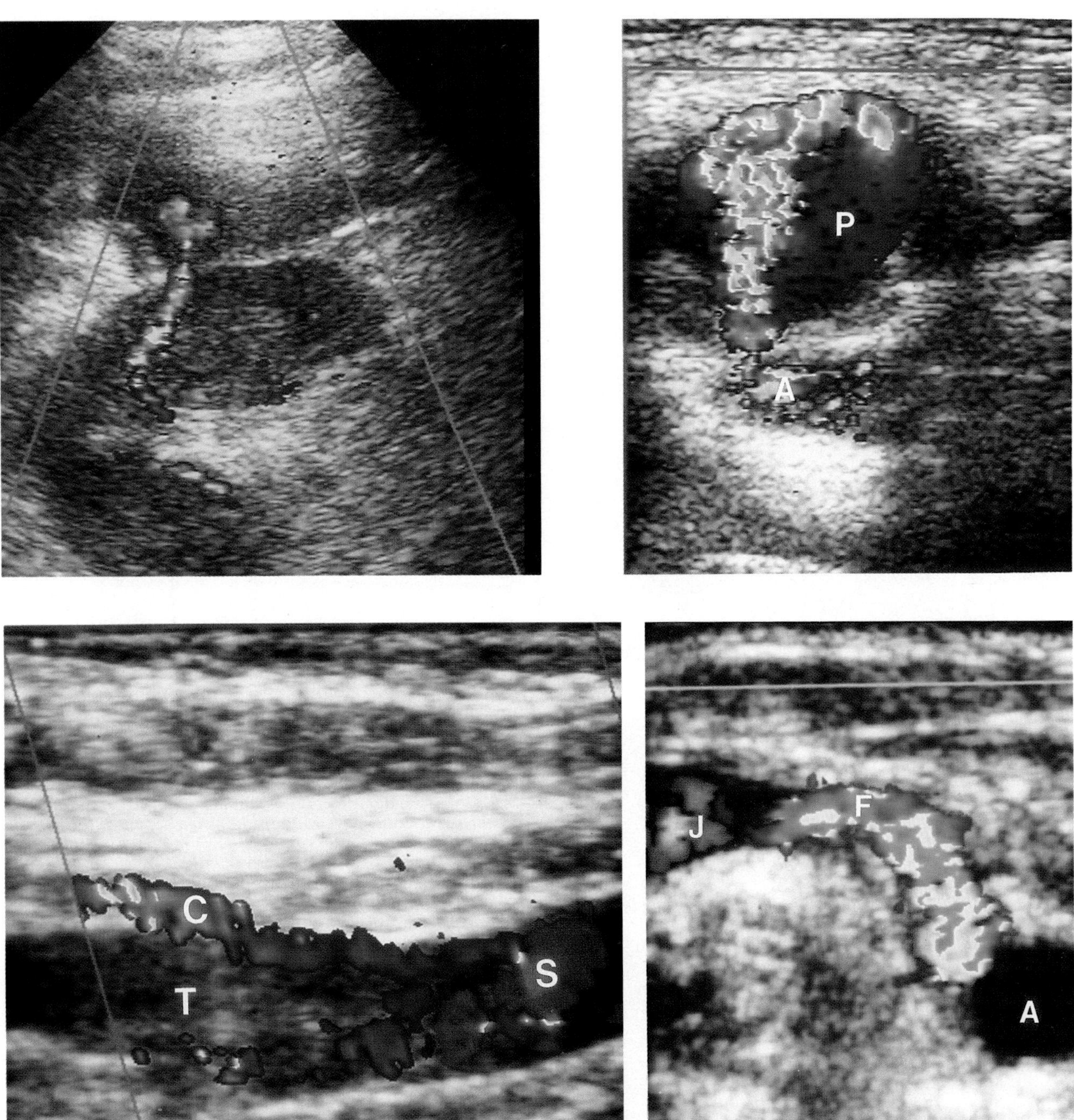

Figure 42–28. Color Doppler ultrasound imaging of a renal transplant biopsy site immediately following needle biopsy shows bleeding from the needle tract extending through the renal capsule. Several minutes of localized pressure with the ultrasound probe on the biopsy site stopped the bleeding.

Figure 42–31. Pseudoaneurysm (P) of right femoral artery (A) following cardiac catheterization (transverse view, right groin).

Figure 42–33. Swelling of right arm from a thrombus (T) within the right axillary vein. The cephalic vein (C) and the subclavian vein (S) are patent. The right axillary vein was cannulated for venous bypass during liver transplant surgery.

Figure 42–34. Carotid artery to jugular vein fistula. A 8.5-French sheath was inadvertently placed in the carotid artery during attempted cannulation of the jugular vein. A transverse view of right side of the neck is shown. *Abbreviations*: A = carotid artery; F = fistula; J = jugular vein.

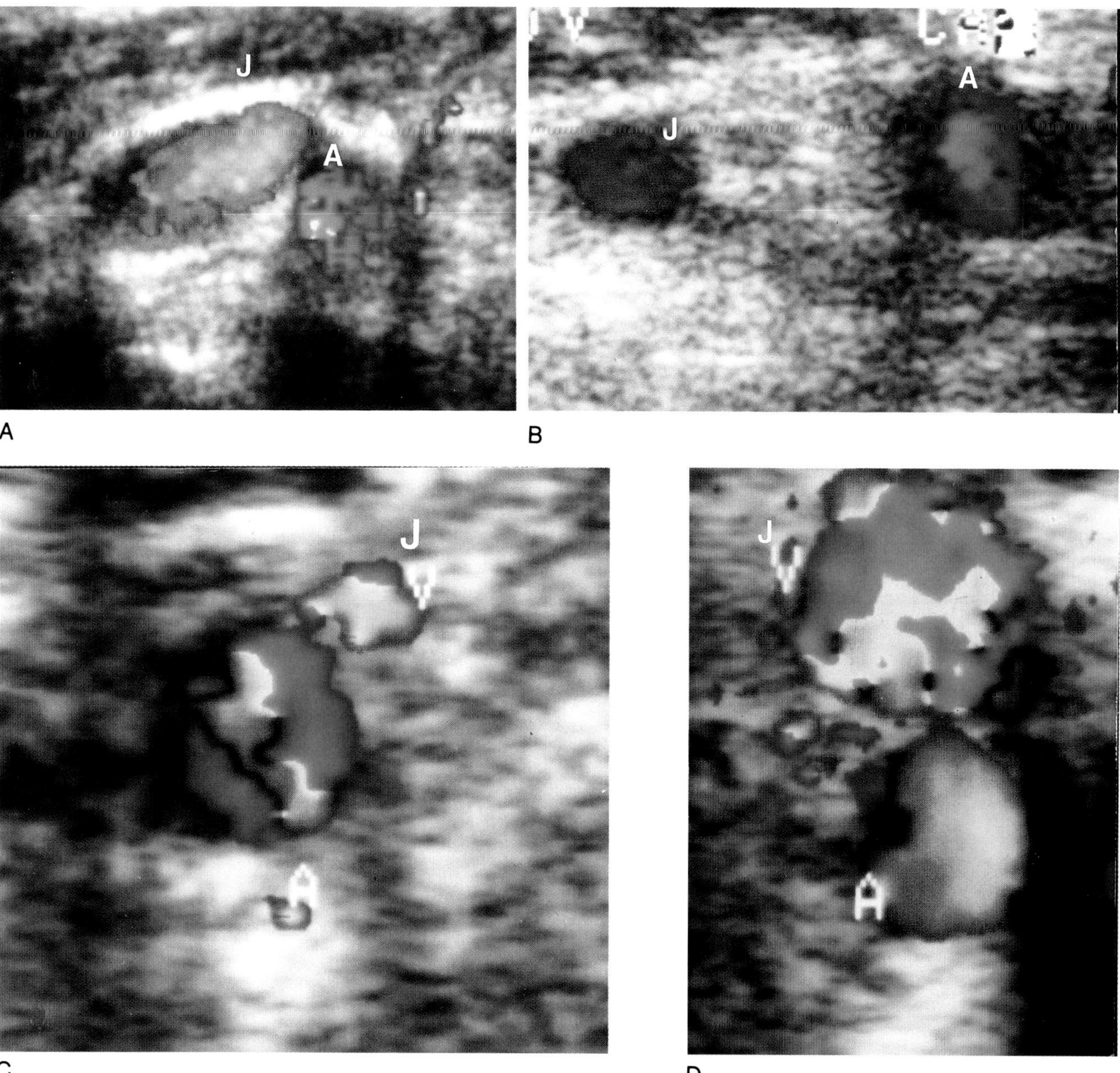

Figure 42–35. Varying anatomic positions of the jugular vein (transverse images). *A*, Right side of the neck—a normal jugular vein (J) lies just lateral to the carotid artery (A). *B*, Right side of the neck—the jugular vein is abnormally lateral to the carotid artery. *C*, Left side of the neck—an abnormally small jugular vein has a diameter that is less than the diameter of the carotid artery. *D*, Right side of the neck—the jugular vein lies directly anterior to the carotid artery; this increases the probability of carotid puncture.

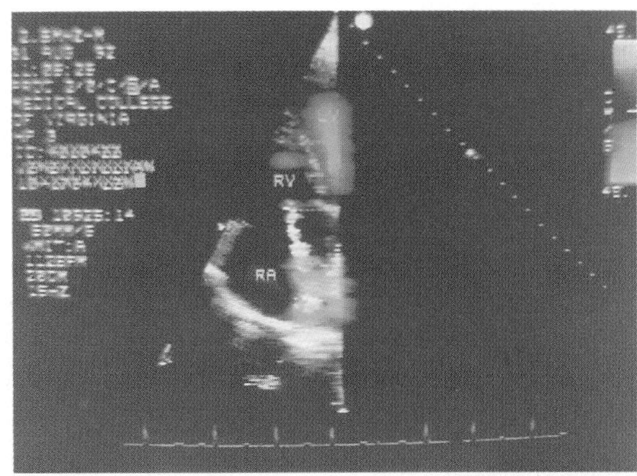

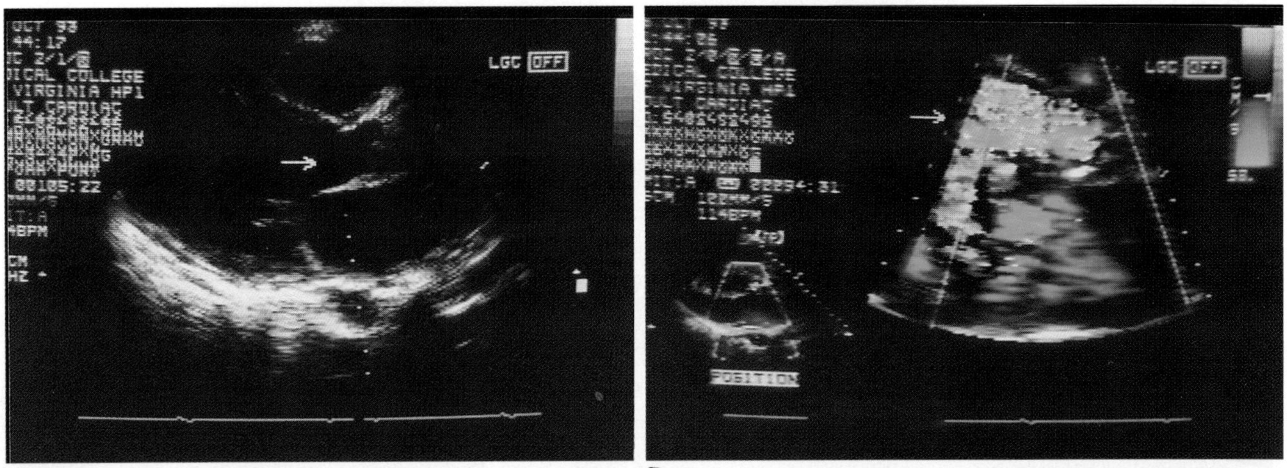

A

B

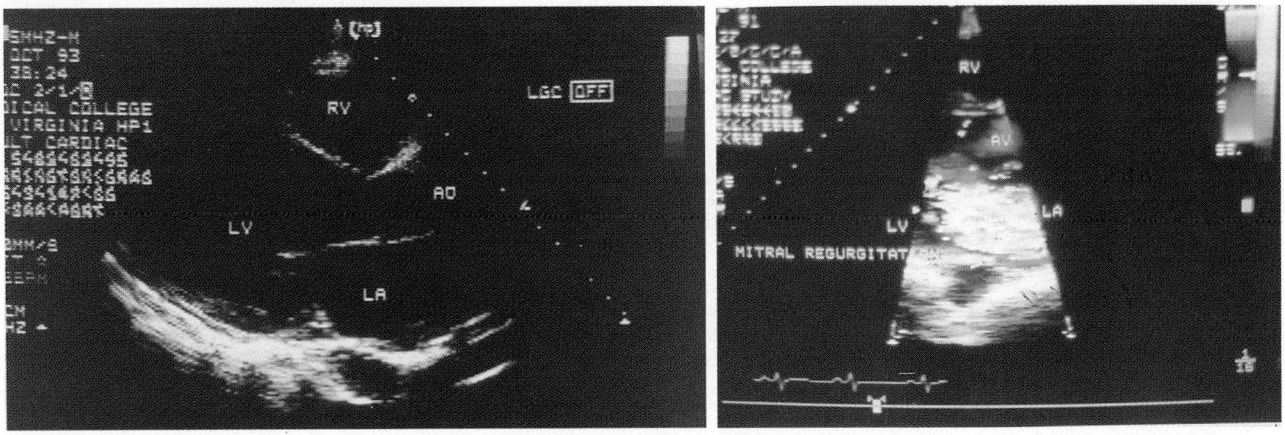

A

B

Figure 43–5. A color-flow Doppler echocardiogram in the apical four-chamber view showing tricuspid regurgitation.

Figure 43–11. *A,* A two-dimensional echocardiogram in the parasternal long-axis view in a patient with aortic regurgitation. *B,* A color-flow Doppler echocardiogram in the parasternal long-axis view showing severe aortic regurgitation in the same patient as in *A.*

Figure 43–12. *A,* A two-dimensional echocardiogram in the parasternal short-axis view showing left atrial enlargement in a patient with severe mitral regurgitation. *B,* A color-flow Doppler echocardiogram in the parasternal short-axis view showing severe mitral regurgitation in the same patient as in *A. Abbreviation*: AV = aortic valve.

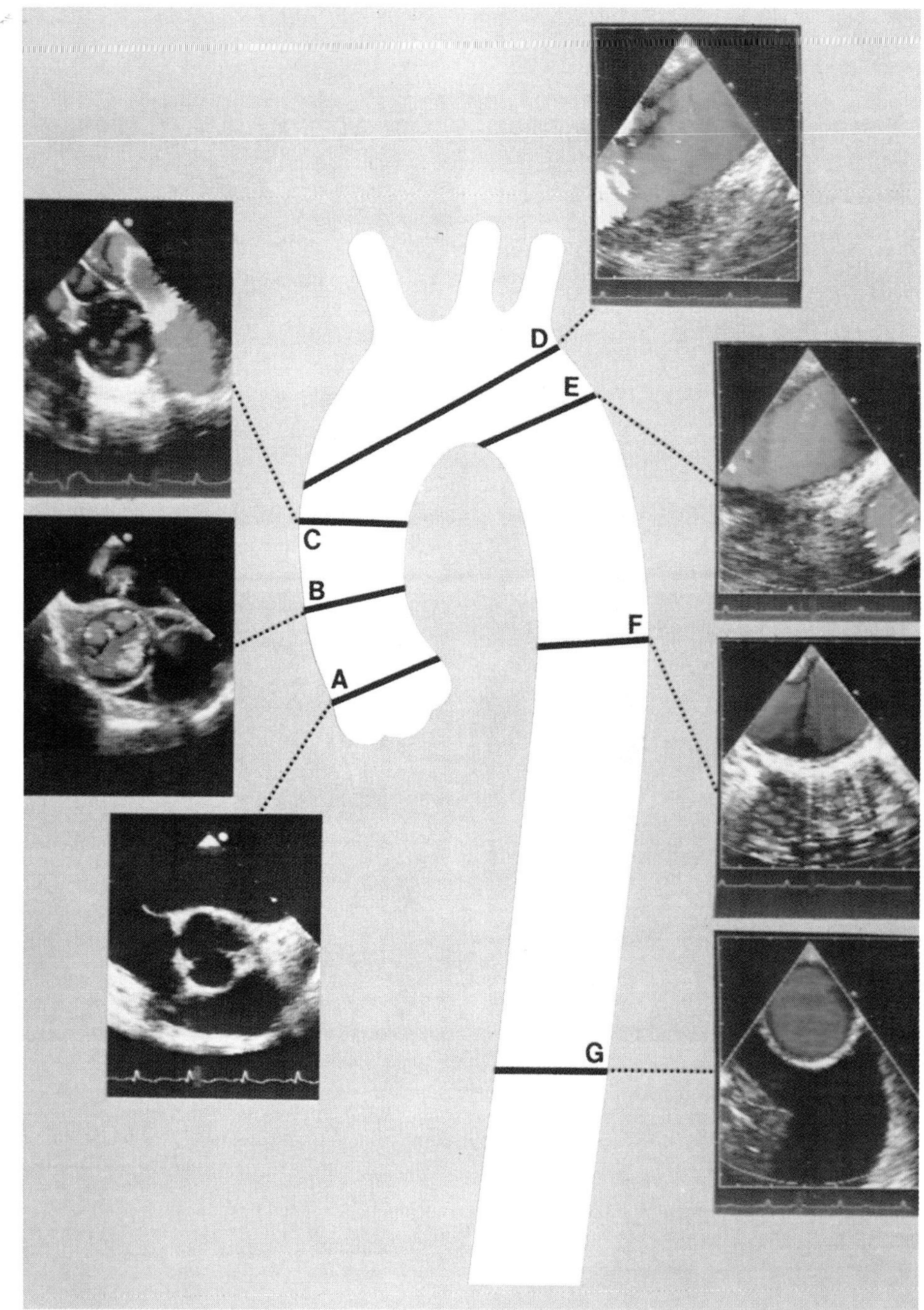

Figure 44–5. Thoracic aorta. Sequential transverse imaging of the ascending, arch, and descending thoracic aorta of normal anatomy with color flow Doppler echocardiography. (From Chandrasekaran K, Currie PJ: Transesophageal echocardiography in aortic dissection: Review. J Invasive Cardiol 1989; 1:333.)

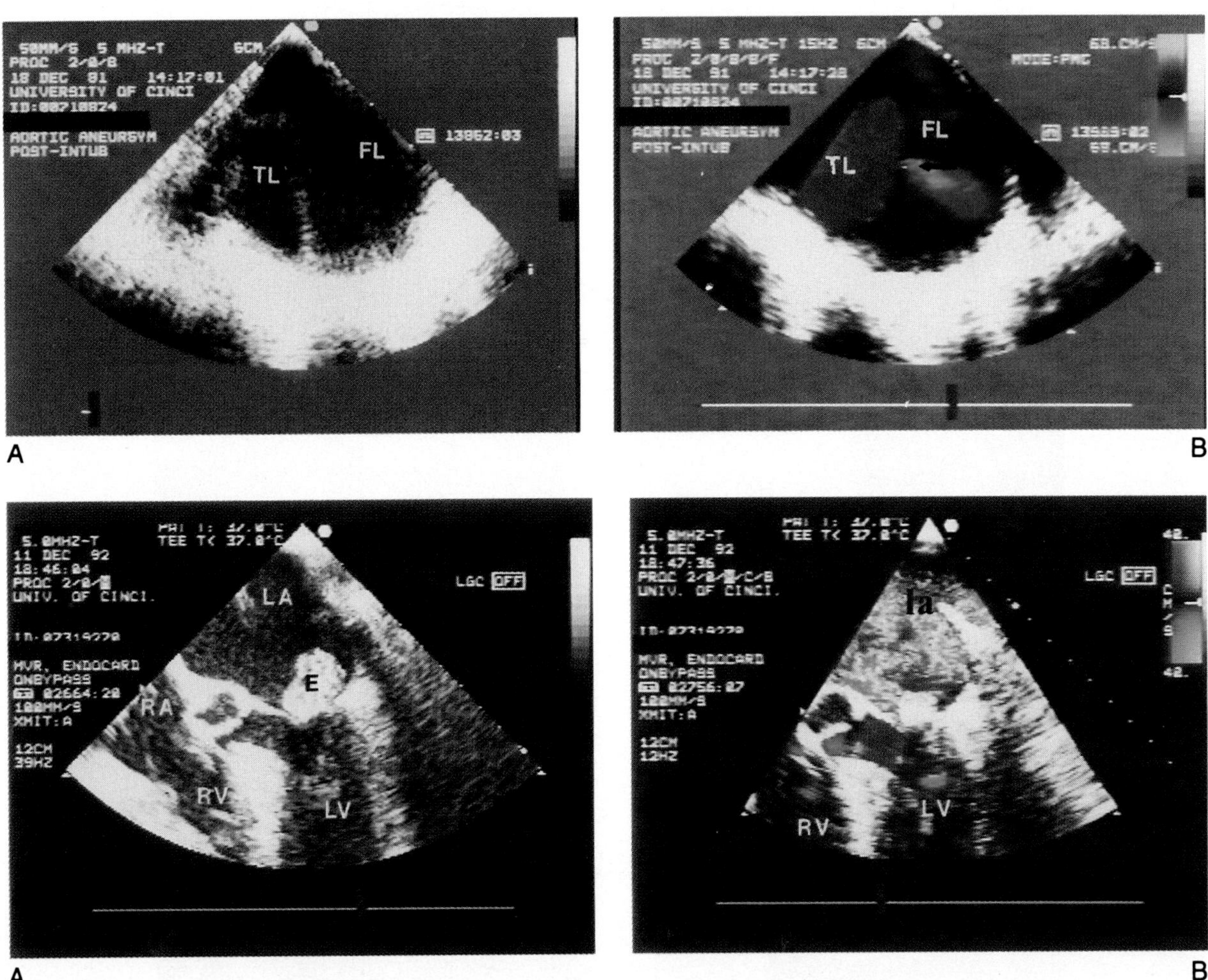

Figure 44–6. Aortic dissection. *A*, Transverse imaging reveals an intimal flap with a small true lumen and a larger false lumen. Spontaneous echo contrast is indicative of thrombus formation. *B*, Transverse imaging with color-flow Doppler echocardiography reveals a small true lumen and a larger false lumen with a jet crossing through the entry site into the false lumen. *Abbreviations*: FL = false lumen; TL = true lumen.

Figure 44–10. Endocarditis and mitral regurgitation. *A*, A 2.8 × 1.8-cm vegetation associated with an abscess attached to the posterior mitral valve leaflet (transverse view). *B*, The corresponding transverse view shows 4+ mitral regurgitation that enters the left superior pulmonary vein. *Abbreviation*: E = vegetation.

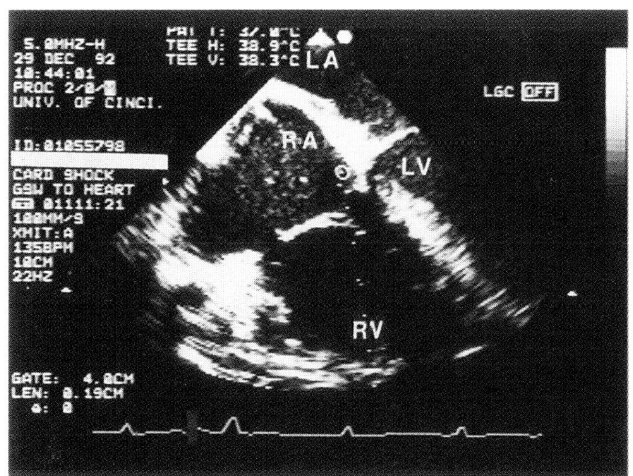

A

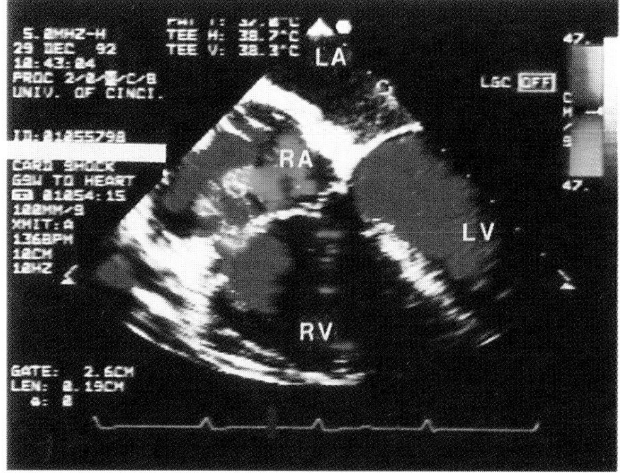

B

Figure 44–13. Acquired intracardiac shunt in an 18-year-old man in shock with a gunshot wound to the heart. *A*, After resuscitation and repair of the right ventricle and main pulmonary artery, a transverse image recorded the presence of a large defect of the anterior leaflet of the tricuspid valve. *B*, The corresponding transverse image with color-flow Doppler echocardiography revealed significant tricuspid regurgitation through the defect.

Figure 44–16. Continuous-wave Doppler echocardiography. TEE of a patient with congestive heart failure and rheumatic heart disease demonstrated mitral stenosis with a valve area of 1.13 cm^2, a mean gradient of 25.3 mm Hg, and a pressure half-time of 194 ms.

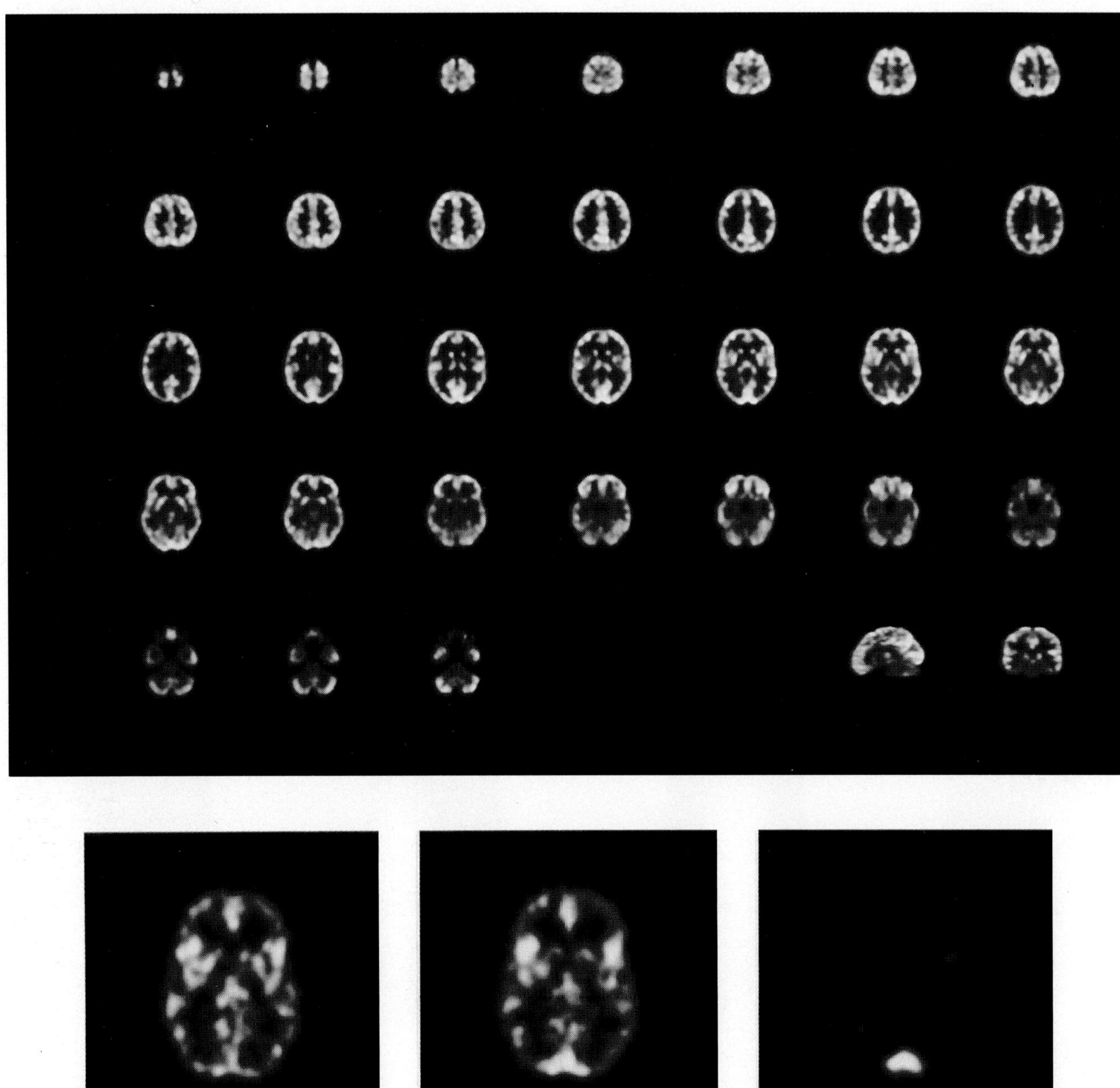

Figure 47–4. PET ^{18}F-labeled FDG brain images of a normal human subject using a Siemens 951/31 whole-body PET scanner. Starting with the most superior brain slice in the upper left corner, the 31 transaxial reconstructed slices are displayed (covering a 10.8-cm^2 field-of-view). The bottom right corner shows examples of the PET data resliced in a sagittal plane and in a coronal plane.

Figure 47–5. Example of PET activation method using ^{15}O-labeled water rCBF imaging in a normal human subject. *A*, Control state (cross-hair only). *B*, Visual stimulation state (with annular reversing checkerboard surrounding the cross-hair). *C*, Subtraction image (i.e., stimulus state minus control state) showing visual cortex activation.

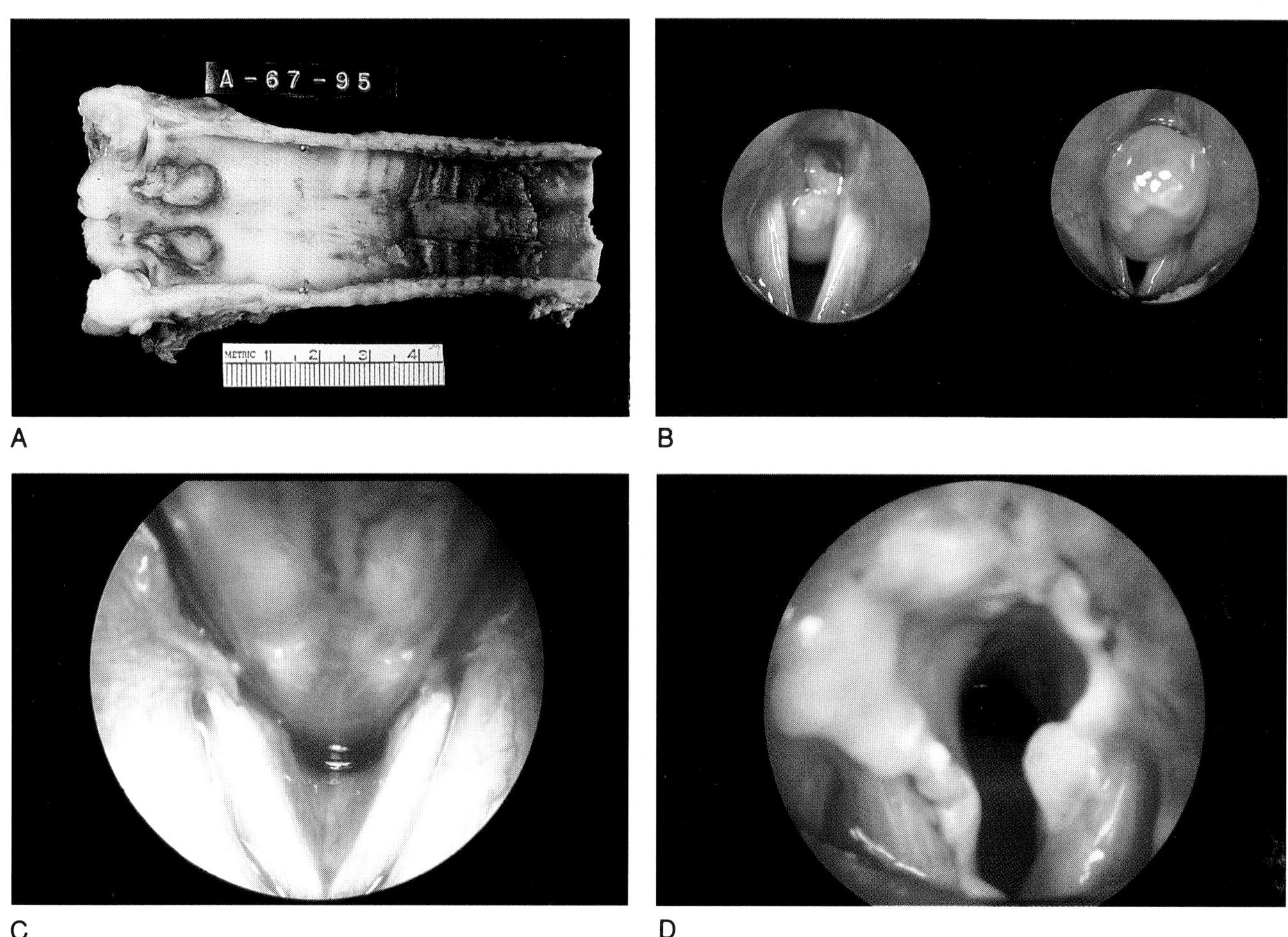

Figure 79–1. *A,* Laryngotracheal specimen, split along the anterior midline, showing necrotic lesions at the medial sides of the arytenoid cartilages and the cricoid plate. The lesions were caused by pressure from the tracheal tube and, further down the trachea, by the cuff. *B,* Endoscopic views of a pendular postintubation granuloma at the right medial region of the arytenoid cartilage. *C,* Endoscopic view of a tracheal tube that is too wide in relation to the size of the interarytenoid space. *D,* Close-up view of the larynx immediately after extubation. Pressure necrosis and inflammation posteriorly are present where the tracheal tube was located.

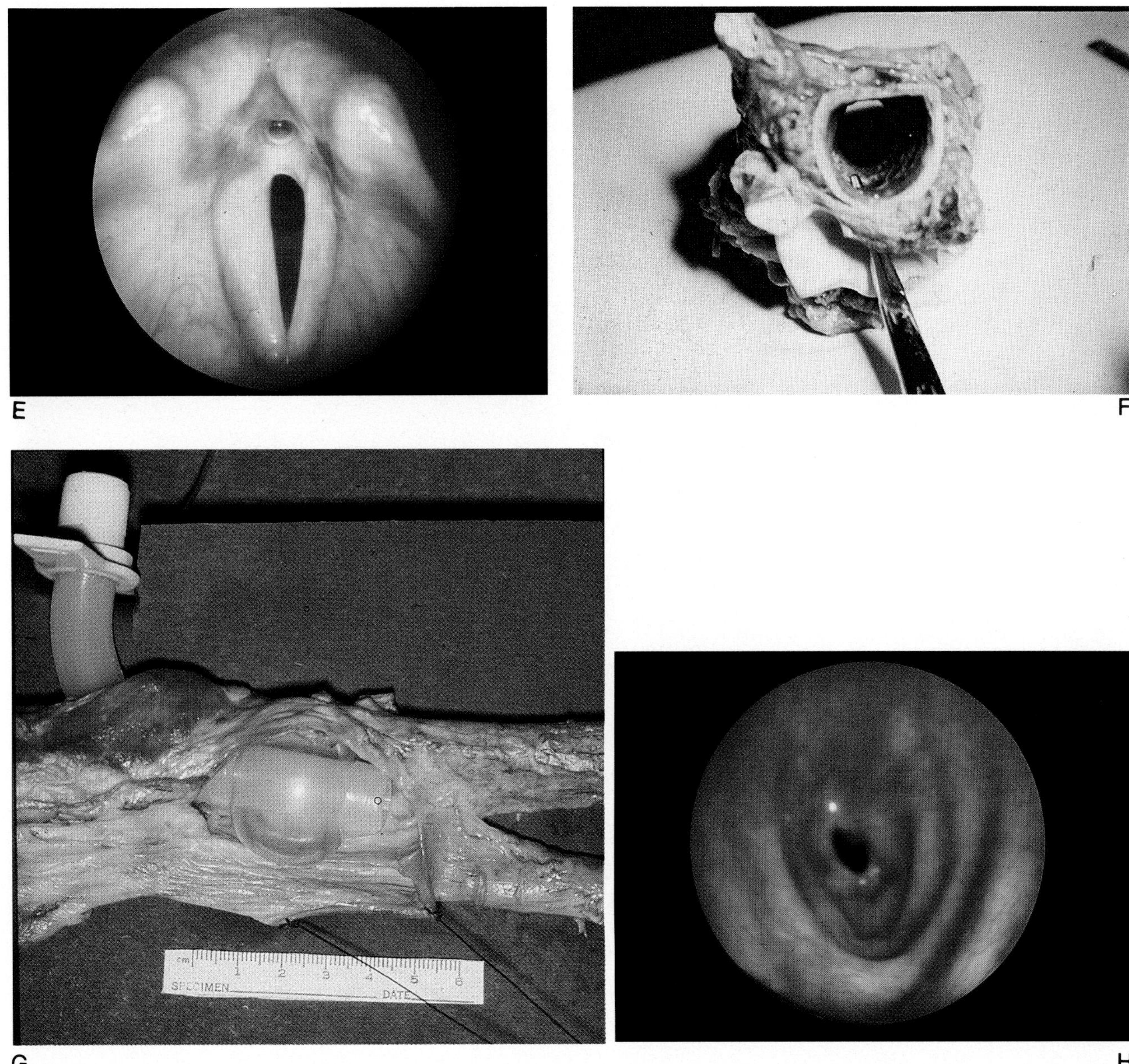

Figure 79–1 *Continued E,* Follow-up laryngeal view showing healing after prolonged intubation injury. Fibrous scarring is present between the arytenoid cartilages, and fixation of the vocal cords can be seen near the midline. The result was severe laryngeal stenosis. *F,* Autopsy specimen demonstrating a fistula (indicated by hemostat) between the trachea and the innominate artery. The fistula was caused by cuff erosion and resulted in lethal hemorrhage into the trachea. *G,* Specimen with a large tracheoesophageal fistula due to erosion by a low-volume, small-diameter, high-pressure cuff. *H,* Severe cuff-induced tracheal stenosis.

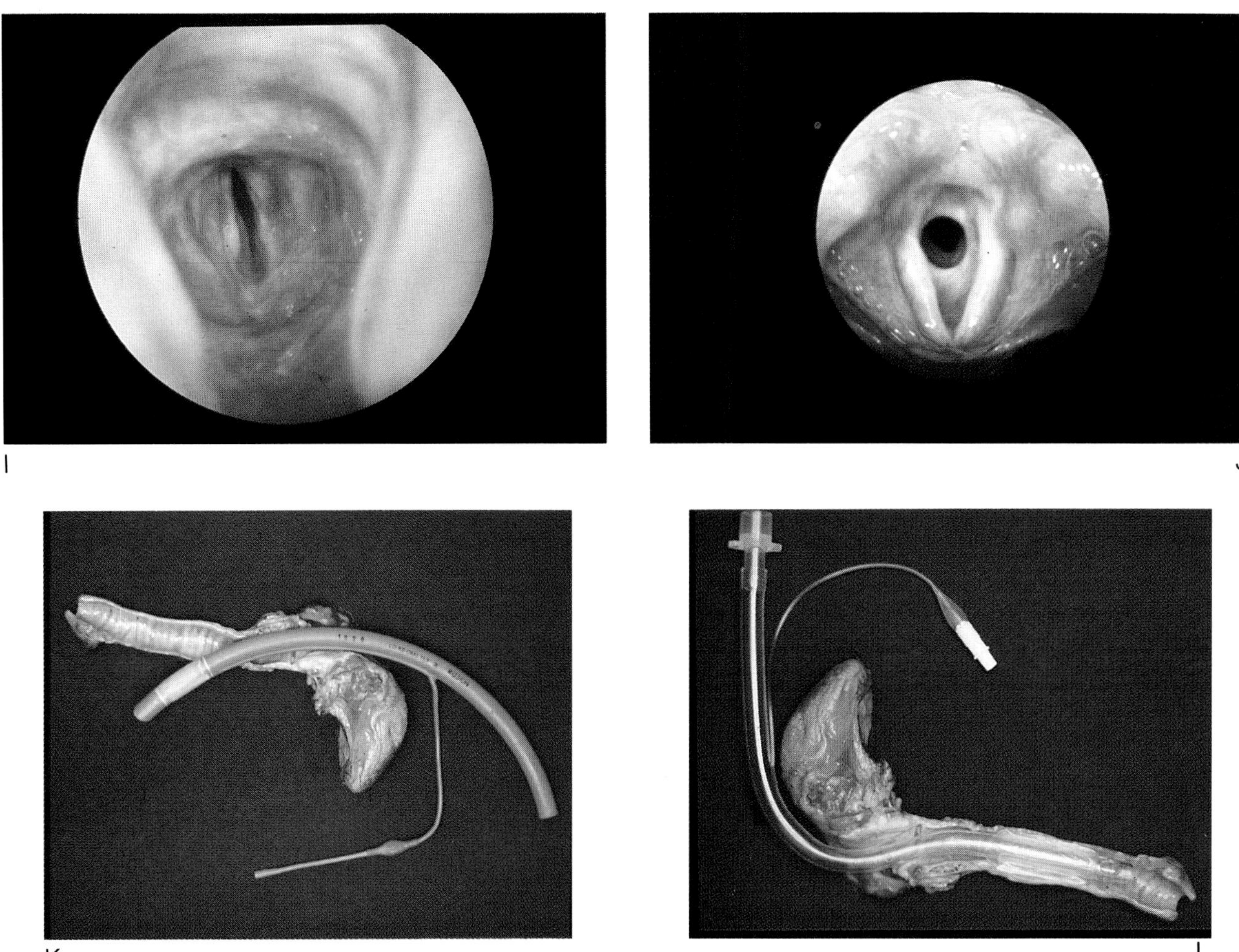

Figure 79–1 *Continued I,* Softening of the tracheal wall after healing of cuff pressure–induced necrosis and cartilage destruction (so-called "tracheomalacia") results in tracheal collapse during exhalation, air trapping in the lungs, and life-threatening respiratory failure. *J,* Endoscopic view of fibrous subglottic stenosis caused by circumferential pressure from a tracheal tube that was too large in relation to the size of the cricoid ring. *K,* An autopsy specimen of the tongue, larynx, and trachea, mainly in their in vivo positions, with a standard tracheal tube superimposed. The discrepancy between the size of the tube and that of the airway can be seen. *L,* The configuration of the anatomic Lindholm tube corresponds well to the shape of the natural human airway.

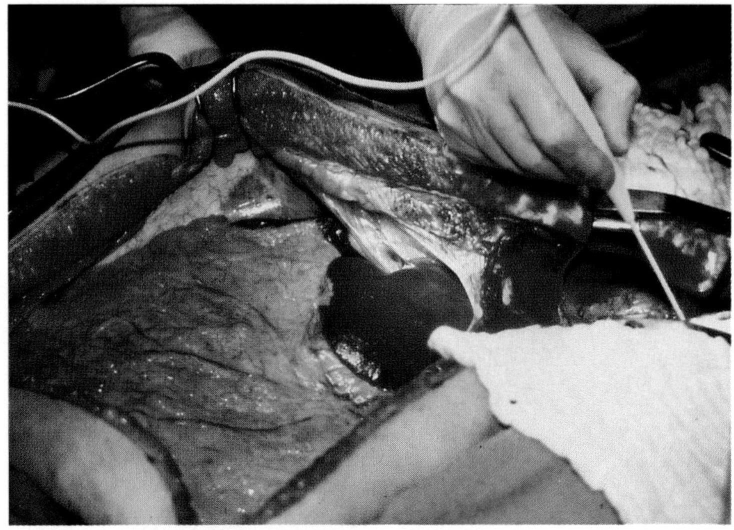

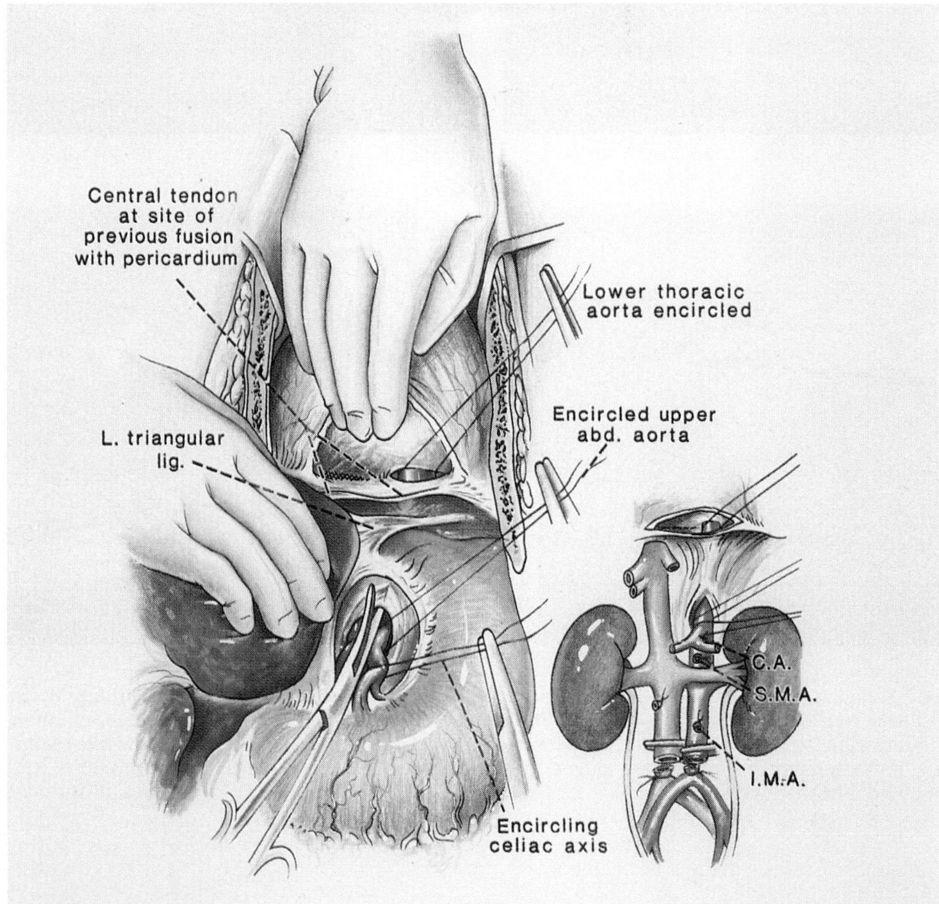

Figure 178–4. Intraoperative photograph showing the total midline incision used for multiple organ procurement. (Courtesy of Andrei Stieber, MD.)

Figure 178–5. The aorta is dissected and encircled just above (or, alternatively, just below) the diaphragm. *Abbreviations*: L. triangular lig. = left triangular ligament; Encircled upper abd. aorta = encircled upper abdominal aorta; C.A. = celiac axis; S.M.A. = superior mesenteric artery; I.M.A. = inferior mesenteric artery.

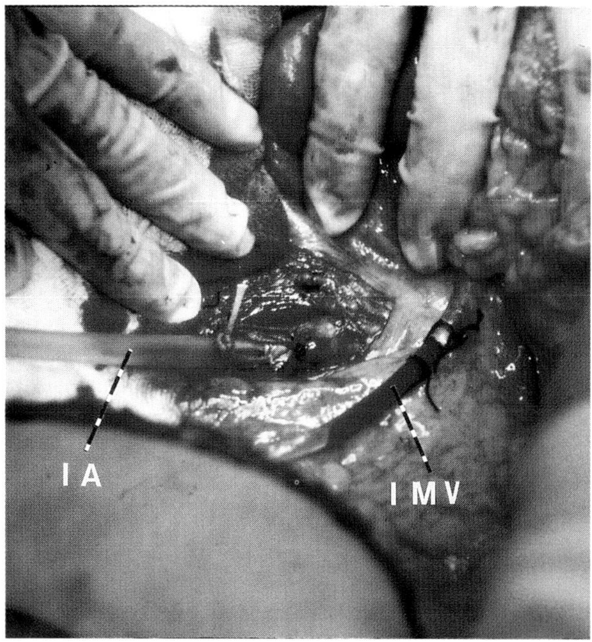

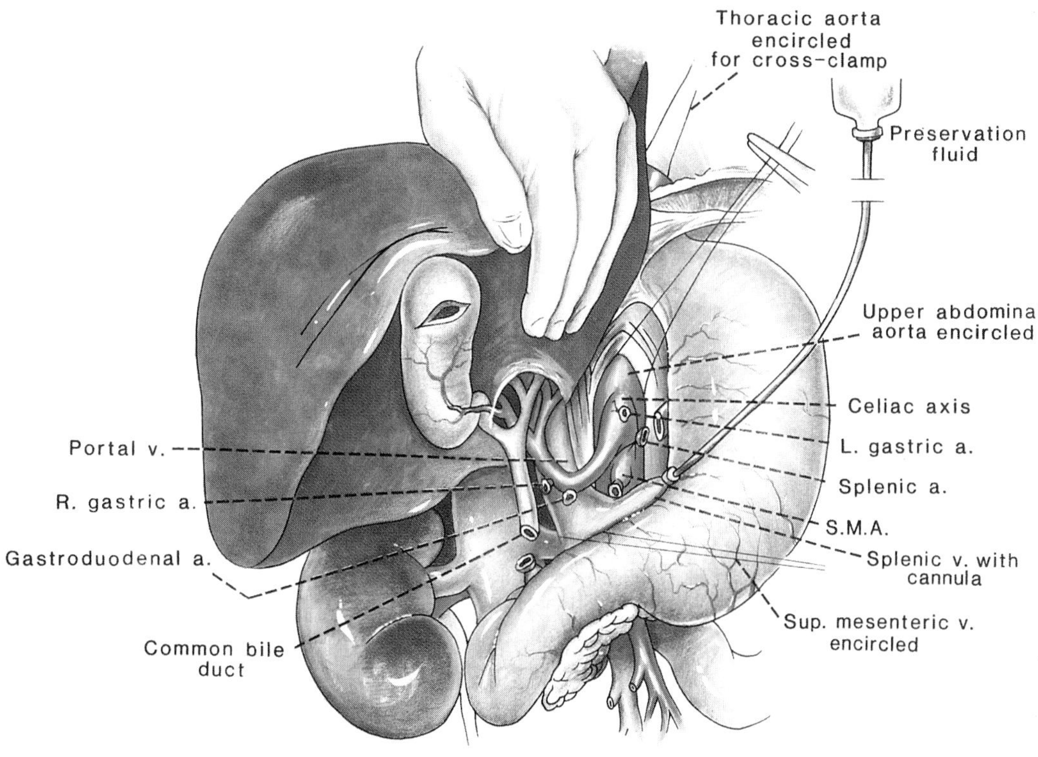

Figure 178–6. Intraoperative photograph showing the donor inferior mesenteric vein (IMV) and the infrarenal aorta (IA) dissected and cannulated for the cold perfusion. (Courtesy of Andrei Stieber, MD.)

Figure 178–7. Liver hilar dissection, transection of the common bile duct, and incision of the gallbladder fundus to prevent autolysis of the mucosa of the biliary tract. In this drawing, the splenic vein is cannulated; however, the inferior mesenteric vein can be cannulated alternatively, as shown in Figure 178–4. *Abbreviations*: Portal v. = portal vein; R. gastric a. = right gastric artery; Gastroduodenal a. = gastroduodenal artery; L. gastric a. = left gastric artery; Splenic a. = splenic artery; S.M.A. = superior mesenteric artery; Splenic v. with cannula = splenic vein with cannula; Sup. mesenteric v. encircled = superior mesenteric vein encircled.

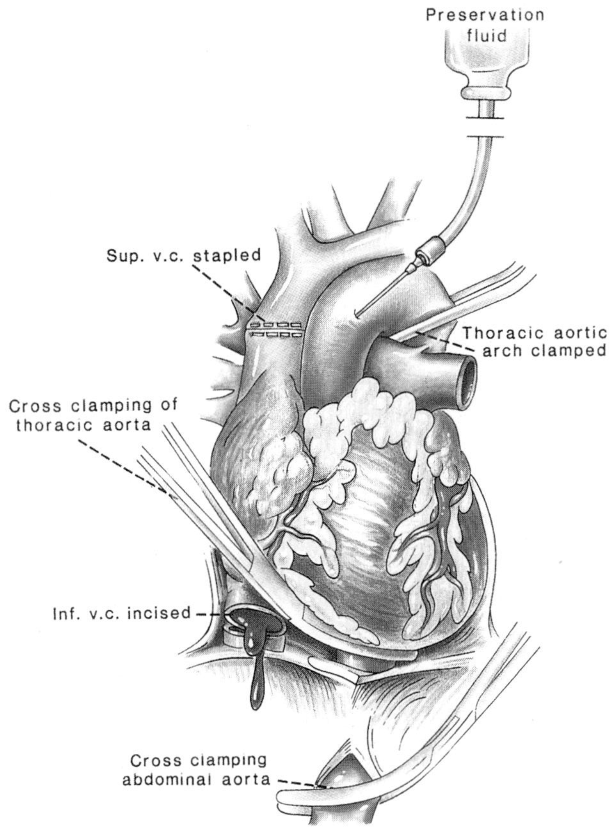

Figure 178–8. Occlusion of the superior vena cava inflow and simultaneous clamping of the aorta proximal to the innominate artery. The aorta is also simultaneously clamped just above or below the diaphragm. Cardioplegic solution infused through the ascending aorta is allowed to run only in the heart. *Abbreviations:* Sup. v.c. stapled = superior vena cava stapled; Inf. v.c. incised = inferior vena cava incised.

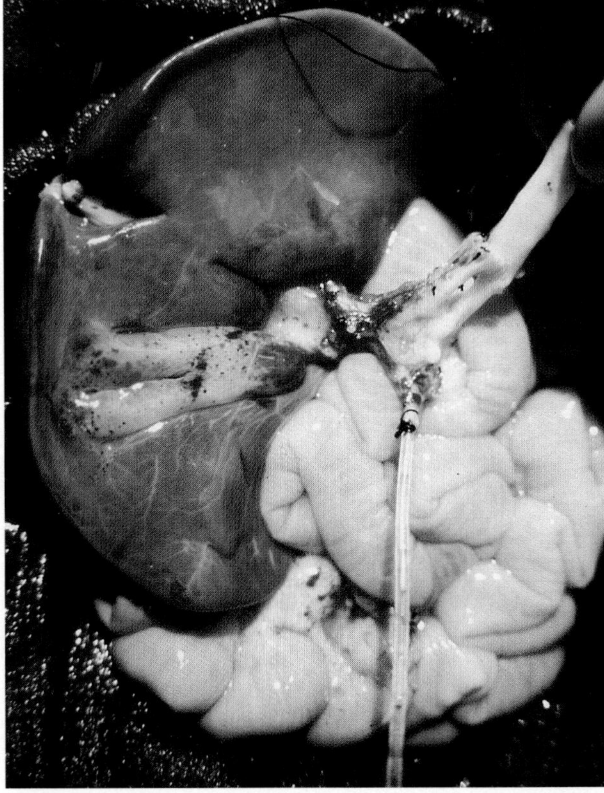

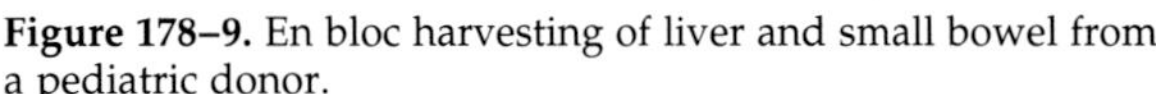

Figure 178–9. En bloc harvesting of liver and small bowel from a pediatric donor.

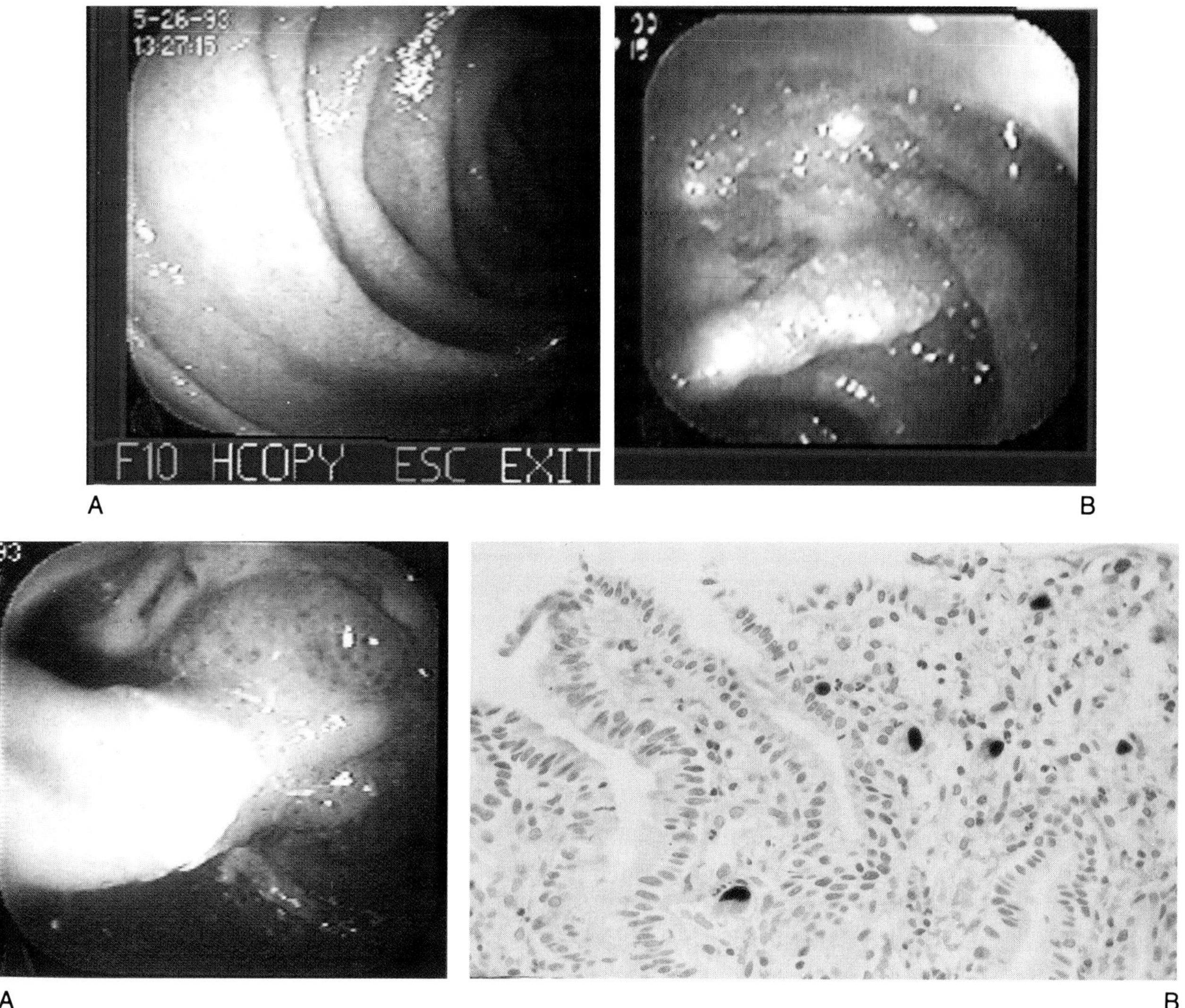

Figure 185–6. *A,* Normal endoscopic appearance of transplanted small intestine. *B,* Moderate acute cellular rejection of an intestinal allograft demonstrating diffuse edema and focal erythema.

Figure 185–8. *A,* Endoscopic appearance of cytomegaloviral enteritis is characterized by hyperemic erosions. *B,* The diagnosis was confirmed histologically by the presence of characteristic inclusions by staining for viral antigens, or both. Note the focal neutrophilic inflammation (immunoperoxidase for cytomegalovirus antigens, 350×).

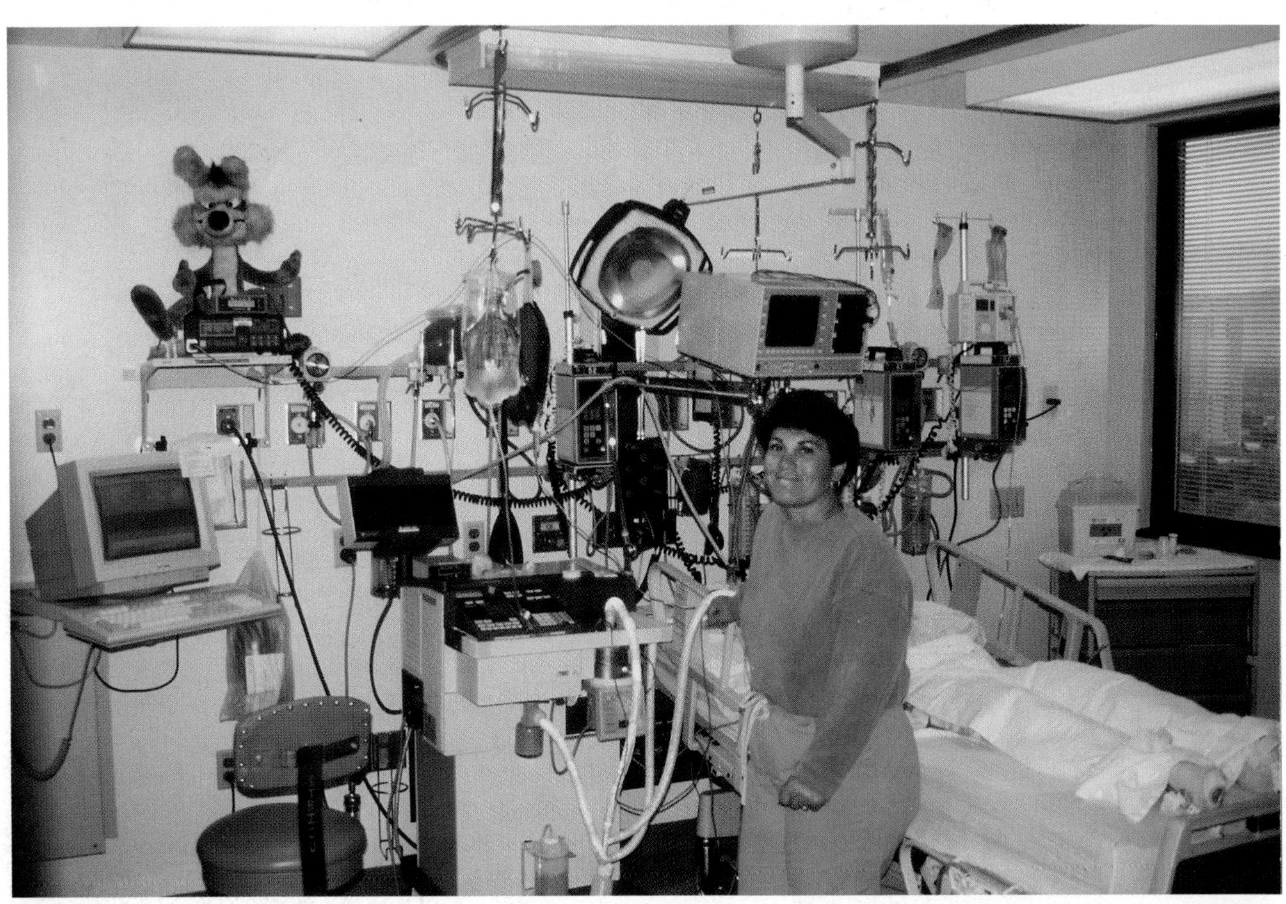

Figure 196–5. A photograph of a patient's room showing a computer terminal at each bedside. Also note the box in the center above the bed; this box is the Medical Information Bus bedside interface. Intravenous pumps, pulse oximeters, and ventilators are connected to the computer system through the Medical Information Bus.

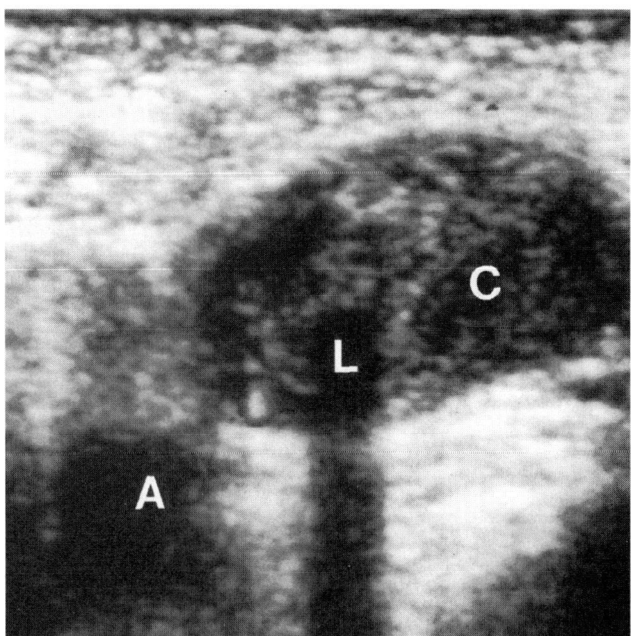

Figure 42–32. Thrombosed left jugular vein (transverse view). (See Plate X.) Echogenic clot (C) surrounds the central line (L) that lies along the posterior wall of vein and that casts acoustic shadow. *Abbreviation*: A = carotid artery.

Another application is for evaluating groin masses that may develop after cardiac catheterization or after surgery involving vascular bypass procedures used in heart, lung, and liver transplantation and in cardiac surgery. Doppler ultrasound, in particular color Doppler, can readily differentiate a hematoma from a pseudoaneurysm of the femoral artery (Fig. 42–31). The aneurysm may be occluded by applying direct local pressure over the neck of the aneurysm with the probe for 20 to 40 minutes. Continuous ultrasound monitoring is used to determine whether the aneurysm is occluded. Pressure should not be great enough to occlude the femoral artery. The chance for this maneuver to succeed is greater if the patient is not receiving anticoagulants or aspirin.[41]

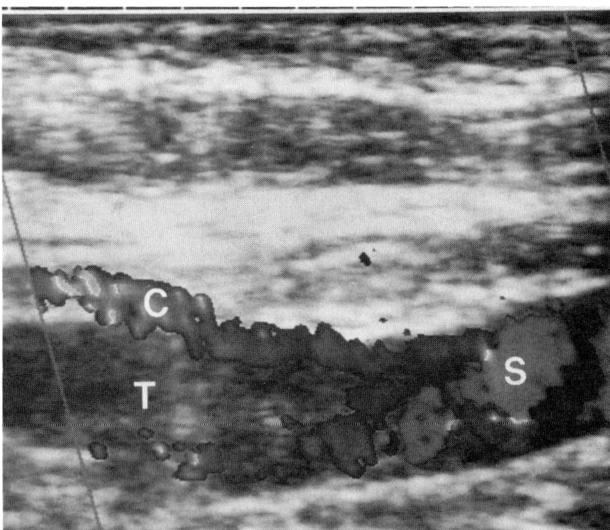

Figure 42–33. Swelling of right arm from a thrombus (T) within the right axillary vein. The cephalic vein (C) and the subclavian vein (S) are patent. The right axillary vein was cannulated for venous bypass during liver transplant surgery. (See Color Plate Section of this textbook.)

Jugular and Subclavian Veins—Problems Related to Central Venous Access

The jugular and subclavian veins are major routes of central venous access. Various complications have been reported (pneumothorax, hematoma from arterial puncture, stroke or death due to inadvertent puncture or cannulation of the carotid artery) when attempting to cannulate these veins using landmark techniques. Some of these problems may be secondary to prior catheterizations or attempts at such, and some may be secondary to aberrant anatomy.[42]

Frequent clinical requests for imaging ultrasound of the jugular and subclavian veins are to assess the jugular and subclavian veins for thrombi in a patient who has or has had prior central lines and requires a new one (Fig. 42–32); explain the cause of sudden upper extremity swelling (Fig. 42–33); explain why a subclavian or jugular vein could not be punctured after repeated attempts using landmark techniques (see Fig. 42–35*B* and *C*); and assess the extent of complications from inadvertent adjacent arterial (carotid artery) puncture (see Fig. 42–34).

The best way to preclude the presence of a thrombus in a vein is to demonstrate that the two walls can touch each other, thus completely obliterating the lumen (the same maneuver used in evaluating the femoral and popliteal veins).

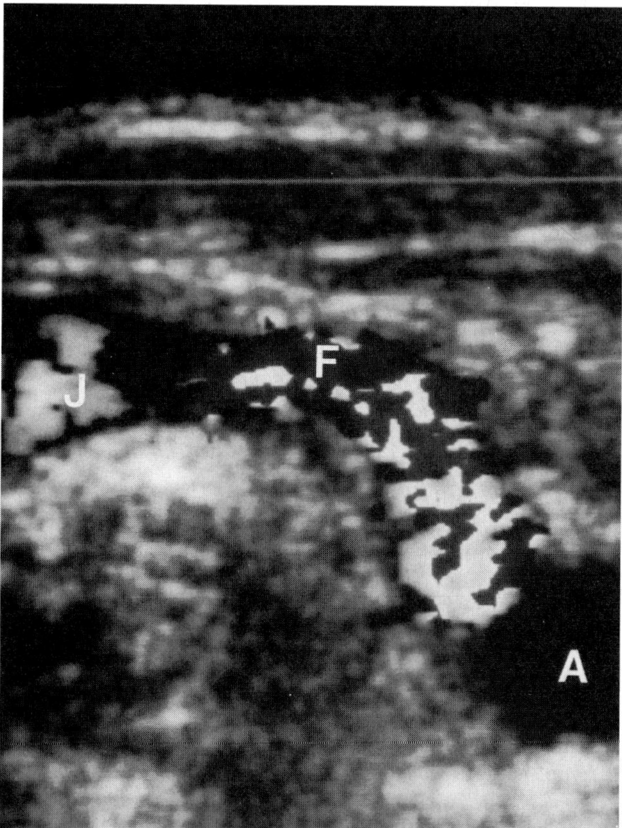

Figure 42–34. Carotid artery to jugular vein fistula. An 8.5-French sheath was inadvertently placed in the carotid artery during attempted cannulation of the jugular vein. A transverse view of right side of the neck is shown. *Abbreviations*: A = carotid artery; F = fistula; J = jugular vein. (See Color Plate Section of this textbook.)

In a normal jugular vein, usually only a slight increase in the pressure of the probe on the skin over the vein completely collapses it. The subclavian vein is also usually compressible, although it may require greater pressure than the jugular vein because of its greater depth. It may at times be difficult to apply enough probe pressure to compress a vein—either because the region is tender or swollen or because the vein, particularly the subclavian, is particularly deep. Doppler, especially color Doppler, is then effective in determining whether the vein is patent or contains a thrombus.

Failure to cannulate the jugular vein by landmark techniques may also occur because of aberrant anatomy. The normal position of the jugular vein is just lateral to the carotid artery (Fig. 42–35*A*).[43] The vein may be more laterally positioned in the neck (see Fig. 42–35*B*) or may be unusually small in diameter and therefore difficult to puncture (Fig. 42–35*C*), even if it lies in a normal location. When a jugular vein lies directly anterior to the carotid artery (Fig. 42–35*D*), the chance of arterial puncture and its associated complications is increased.

Use of ultrasound can not only determine whether the jugular vein is patent but can assist in its puncture. One may either direct the needle into the vein through a needle guide attached to the probe[44] or use a free-hand approach.[45, 46] In a study of jugular vein cannulation in 604 patients, half of which were by landmark technique and half by ultrasound guidance using a dedicated portable scanner with needle guide, ultrasound significantly improved success rate, reduced complications, and shortened the time to access the vein.[47] Ultrasound guidance has produced similar results with subclavian vein puncture.[48] With ultrasound guidance, the vein is often punctured more laterally—actually in the axillary vein. This site is usually lateral to the

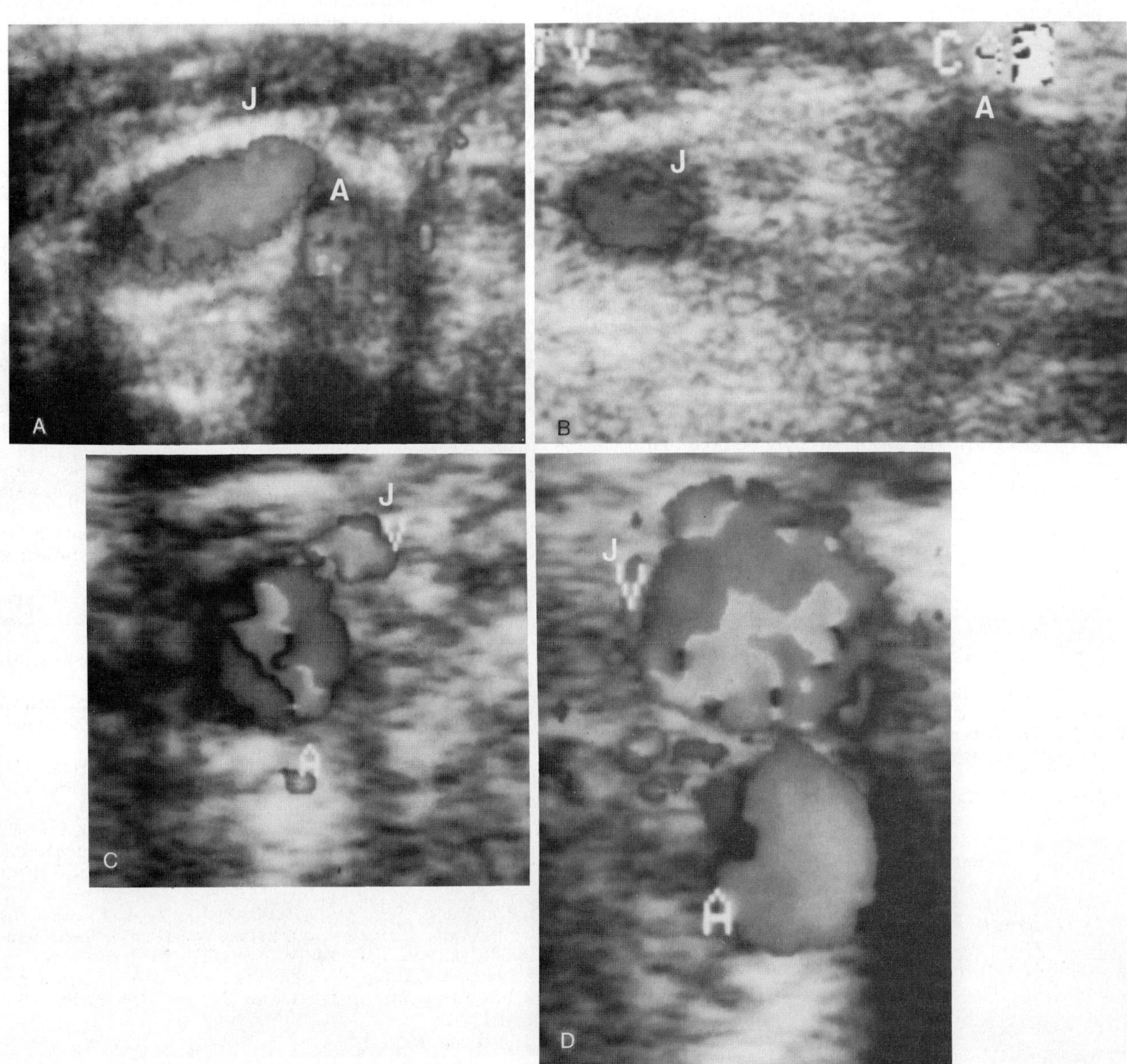

Figure 42–35. Varying anatomic positions of the jugular vein (transverse images). *A*, Right side of the neck—a normal jugular vein (J) lies just lateral to the carotid artery (A). *B*, Right side of the neck—the jugular vein is abnormally lateral to the carotid artery. *C*, Left side of the neck—an abnormally small jugular vein has a diameter that is less than the diameter of the carotid artery. *D*, Right side of the neck—the jugular vein lies directly anterior to the carotid artery; this increases the probability of carotid puncture. (See Color Plate Section of this textbook.)

lung, thus particularly minimizing the risk of causing a pneumothorax.[49]

References

1. Ziskin MC: Fundamental physics of ultrasound and its propagation in tissue. Radiographics 1993; 13:705–709.
2. Goldstein A: AAPM Tutorials. Overview of the physics of US. Radiographics 1993; 13:701–704.
3. Mitchell DG: Color Doppler imaging: Principles, limitations, and artifacts. Radiology 1990; 177:1–10.
4. Merritt CRB: AAPM Tutorial. Doppler US: The basics. Radiographics 1991; 11:109–119.
5. Lissoos I, Thomas RG: The value of ultrasound in the diagnosis of renal failure. Br J Urol 1986; 58:358–360.
6. Jeffrey RB, Laing FC, Wing VW, et al: Sensitivity of sonography in pyonephrosis: A reevaluation. AJR 1985; 144:71–73.
7. Mann MJ: Hydronephrosis secondary to bladder distension. J Diagn Med Sonogr 1990; 2:87–91.
8. Huntington DK, Hill SC, Hill MC: Sonographic manifestations of medical renal disease. Semin Ultrasound CT MR 1991; 12:290–307.
9. Rosenfield AT, Zeman RK, Cronan JJ, et al: Ultrasound in experimental and clinical renal vein thrombosis. Radiology 1980; 137:735–741.
10. Volgelzang RL, Nemcek AA: Percutaneous cholecystostomy: Diagnostic and therapeutic efficacy. Radiology 1988; 168:29–34.
11. Teefey SA, Baron RL, Bigler SA: Sonography of the gallbladder: Significance of striated (layered) thickening of the gallbladder wall. AJR 1991; 156:945–947.
12. West MS, Garra BS, Horii SC, et al: Gallbladder varices: Imaging findings in patients with portal hypertension. Radiology 1991; 179:179–182.
13. vanSonnenberg E, D'Agostino HB, Goodacre BW, et al: Percutaneous gallbladder puncture and cholecystostomy: Results, complications, and caveats for safety. Radiology 1992; 183:167–170.
14. Berland LL, Lawson TL, Foley WD: Porta hepatis: Sonographic discrimination of bile ducts from arteries with pulsed Doppler with new anatomic criteria. AJR 1992; 138:833–840.
15. Laing FC, Jeffrey RB, Wing VW, et al: Biliary dilatation: Defining the level and cause by real-time US. Radiology 1986; 160:39–42.
16. Laing FC, London LA, Filly RA: Ultrasonographic identification of dilated intrahepatic bile ducts and their differentiation from portal venous structures. JCU 1978; 6:90–94.
17. Bressler EL, Rubin JM, McCracken S: Sonographic parallel channel sign: A reappraisal. Radiology 1987; 164:343–346.
18. Scatarige JC, Scott WW, Donovan PJ, et al: Fatty infiltration of the liver: Ultrasonographic and computed tomographic correlation. J Ultrasound Med 1984; 3:9–14.
19. White EM, Simeone JF, Mueller PR, et al: Focal periportal sparing in hepatic fatty infiltration: A cause of hepatic pseudomass on US. Radiology 1987; 162:57–59.
20. Harbin WP, Robert NJ, Ferrucci JT: Diagnosis of cirrhosis based on regional changes in hepatic morphology. Radiology 1980; 135:273–283.
21. Dodd GD III, Miller WJ, Baron RL, et al: Detection of malignant tumors in end-stage cirrhotic livers: Efficacy of sonography as a screening technique. AJR 1992; 159:727–733.
22. Tessler FN, Gehring BJ, Gomes AS, et al: Diagnosis of portal vein thrombosis: Value of color Doppler. AJR 1991; 157:293–296.
23. Kurtz AB, Rubin CS, Cooper HS, et al: Ultrasound findings in hepatitis. Radiology 1980; 136:717–723.
24. Ralls PW, Johnson MB, Radin DR, et al: Budd-Chiari syndrome: Detection with color Doppler sonography. AJR 1992; 159:113–116.
25. Grant EG, Tessler JN, Gomes AS, et al: Color Doppler imaging of portosystemic shunts. AJR 1990; 154:393–397.
26. Campbell WL, Zajko AB: Better diagnosis improves transplant survival rates. Diagn Imaging 1989; 11:260–265.
27. Skolnick ML, Dodd GD: Doppler sonography in liver transplantation—pre- and post-transplant evaluation. *In*: Current Practice in Radiology. Thrall JH (Ed). Philadelphia, Mosby–Year Book, 1992, pp 161–178.
28. Dodd GD III: Sonographic diagnosis of vascular complications of hepatic and renal transplantation. Categorical Course Syllabus, ARRS 1993, San Francisco, 1993.
29. Edell SL, Gefter WB: Ultrasonic differentiation of types of ascitic fluid. AJR 1979; 133:111–114.
30. Kuligowska E, Connors SK, Shapiro JH: Liver abscess: Sonography in diagnosis and treatment. AJR 1982; 138:253–257.
31. Pozniak MA, Kelcz F, Dodd GD III. Renal transplant ultrasound: Imaging and Doppler. Semin Ultrasound CT MR 1991; 12:319–334.
32. Dodd GD III, Tublin ME, Shah A, et al: Imaging of vascular complications associated with renal transplants. AJR 1991; 157:449–459.
33. Genkins SM, Sanfilippo FP, Carroll BA: Duplex Doppler sonography of renal transplants: Lack of sensitivity and specificity in establishing pathologic diagnosis. AJR 1989; 152:535–539.
34. Reinhold C, Illescas FF, Atri M, et al: Treatment of pleural effusions and pneumothorax with catheters placed percutaneously under imaging guidance. AJR 1989; 152:1189–1191.
35. Yu C-Y, Yang P-C, Chang D-B, et al: Diagnostic and therapeutic use of chest sonography: Value in critically ill patients. AJR 1992; 159:695–701.
36. Ross GJ, Kessler HB, Clair MR, et al: Sonographically guided paracentesis for palliation of symptomatic malignant ascites. AJR 1989; 153:1309–1311.
37. Reading CC, Charboneau JW, James EM, et al: Sonographically guided percutaneous biopsy of small (3 cm or less) masses. AJR 1988; 151:189–192.
38. Matalon TAS, Silver B: US guidance of interventional procedures. Radiology 1990; 174:43–47.
39. Lensing WA, Prandoni P, Brandjes D, et al: Detection of deep-vein thrombosis by real-time B-mode ultrasonography. N Engl J Med 1989; 320:342–345.
40. Knighton RA, Priest DL, Zwiebel WJ, et al: Techniques for color flow sonography of the lower extremity. Radiographics 1990; 10:775–786.
41. DiPrete DA, Cronan JJ: Compression ultrasonography. Treatment for acute femoral artery pseudoaneurysms in selected cases. J Ultrasound Med 1992; 11:489–492.
42. Sznajder JI, Zveibil FR, Bitterman H, et al: Central vein catheterization: Failure and complication rates by three percutaneous approaches. Arch Intern Med 1986; 146:259–261.
43. Denys BG, Uretsky BF: Anatomical variations of internal jugular vein location: Impact on central venous access. Crit Care Med 1991; 19:1516–1519.
44. Denys BG, Uretsky BF: Portable ultrasound scanner for vascular access. Med Electron 1992; 23:82–86.
45. Denys BG, Uretsky BF, Reddy PS, et al: An ultrasound method for safe and rapid central venous access (Letter to the editor). N Engl J Med 1991; 324:566.
46. Troianos CA, Jobes DR, Ellison N: Ultrasound-guided cannulation of the internal jugular vein. A prospective, randomized study. Anesth Analg 1991; 72:823–826.
47. Denys BG, Uretsky BF, Reddy PS: Ultrasound-assisted cannulation of the internal jugular vein. A prospective comparison to the external landmark-guided technique. Circulation 1993; 87:1557–1562.
48. Lameris JS, Post PJM, Zonderland HM, et al: Percutaneous placement of Hickman catheters: Comparison of sonographically guided and blind techniques. AJR 1990; 155:1097–1099.
49. Mauro MA, Jaques PF: Radiologic placement of long-term central venous catheters: A review. J Vasc Interv Radiol 1993; 4:127–137.

CHAPTER 43

Echocardiography in Critical Care

Jiho Han, MD • J.V. Nixon, MD

Echocardiography has matured into a ubiquitously powerful and portable diagnostic and prognostic tool. Using high-frequency sound waves, it can image the structures of the heart and the great vessels and provide anatomic and physiologic information about myocardial performance. Because dilemmas in a critical care unit revolve around issues of hypotension and shock, echocardiography may differentiate cardiac and noncardiac causes of hypotension and provide a way to monitor therapeutic intervention (Table 43–1). In addition to anatomic information, through the use of Doppler and color-flow imaging, important physiologic data about valvular and myocardial function may be obtained. Because studies can be carried out at the bedside without significant risk to patients, echocardiography is convenient, may be performed serially, and avoids the dangers of transporting critically ill patients to other departments.

This chapter explores the uses and limitations of transthoracic Doppler echocardiography (TTE) in the critical care setting. Doppler echocardiography is approached within the framework of (1) the basic working principles of Doppler echocardiography, (2) the *diagnostic* utility of TTE in assessing critically ill patients, and (3) the use of TTE in *managing* critically ill patients with specific disorders. In addition to TTE, transesophageal echocardiography (TEE) is being increasingly used in the critical care setting.[1, 2] TTE and TEE are often complementary. TEE is addressed in Chapter 44.

GENERAL PRINCIPLES

Echocardiography is unique among medical imaging techniques because it uses reflected high-frequency sound waves to produce the picture. Unlike radiographic, magnetic resonance, or nuclear images, which depend on backprojection, ultrasound relies on the operator to direct the beam to the target of interest. Because sound waves are attenuated by tissue, image quality can vary greatly between patients and between operators. Therefore, echocardiography requires skilled personnel to perform the test and, more importantly, an experienced echocardiographer to interpret the study.

Two-dimensional (2-D) echo images are the result of computer processing of reflected signals from a multiple phased array of vibrating piezoelectric crystals. Various frequencies can be selected, with the general rule that higher-frequency transducers have better resolution at the expense of penetration. For adults, 2.5- to 3.5-MHz transducers are usually used.

Doppler echocardiography uses the principle that frequency of waves changes in relation to changing distance.

TABLE 43–1. Causes of Hypotension

Cardiac	Noncardiac
Tamponade	Hypovolemic
Acute LV dysfunction—MI	Septic
Acute RV dysfunction—MI	Neurologic
Pulmonary embolism	
Pulmonary embolism and RV failure	

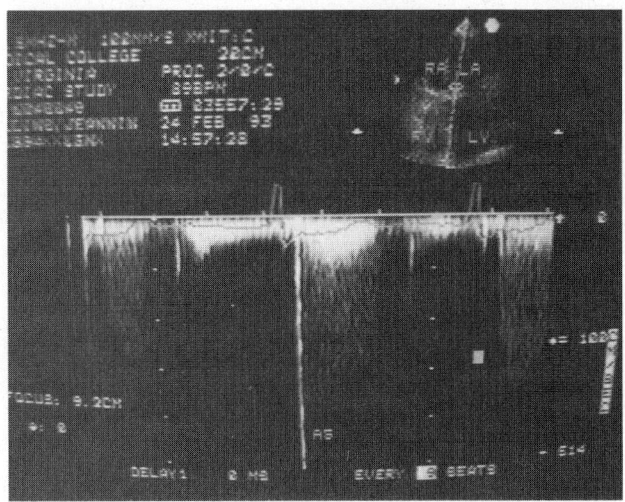

Figure 43–1. Continuous-wave Doppler echocardiography of a patient with severe aortic stenosis demonstrates the range ambiguity of the continuous-wave signal and its ability to detect high-velocity flows. *Abbreviations*: RA = right atrium; RV = right ventricle; LA = left atrium; LV = left ventricle.

The target of Doppler echocardiography is red blood cells. Because red cells are much smaller than the wavelength of ultrasound, backscattered waves (the impedance difference between red blood cells and plasma) are the subject of interrogation.[3]

Two different forms of Doppler echocardiography are available: continuous-wave and pulsed-wave Doppler. Continuous-wave Doppler is the older form and is immensely useful for detecting high-velocity jets typically seen with stenotic valves. Because two different transducers are used, one for projection and one for reception, continuous-wave Doppler is not subject to any limits in velocity but has range ambiguity (Fig. 43–1). Pulsed-wave Doppler uses the same transducer for sending and receiving the signal. Because the rate at which the transducer alternates between sending and receiving the signal is known, localization of the Doppler shift at a specific point is possible (range specificity). The operator can place the pulsed Doppler probe onto the 2-D image and "listen" for the presence of increased flow (Fig. 43–2). Pulsed-wave Doppler is used for detecting the extent of valvular regurgitation and the presence of abnormal blood flow, as in atrial septal defect. Pulse-wave Doppler is limited by its inability to record high-velocity jets where signal aliasing occurs.[4]

When the Doppler shift frequency exceeds one half of the pulse repetition frequency (the Nyquist limit), signal aliasing is present. Both continuous- and pulsed-wave Doppler data may be displayed as a plot of velocity plotted against time (x-axis) with the signal intensity reflected in the gray scale and the direction of flow on the ordinate (y-axis). In this spectral display, the signal can wrap around itself and artifactually appears to change direction (aliasing). Aliasing is an important clue that higher velocities are present.

Through computer quantification, blood flow patterns within the 2-D images can be displayed as a colored map. In Doppler color-flow imaging or mapping, the pulsed Doppler signal is color encoded with respect to velocity and direction.[5] The degree of color saturation quantifies velocity, and the direction of motion is reflected by different colors. These images are semi-quantitative estimates of blood flow. The presentation of flow data with respect to anatomy provides a graphic map of the heart and blood flow within it.

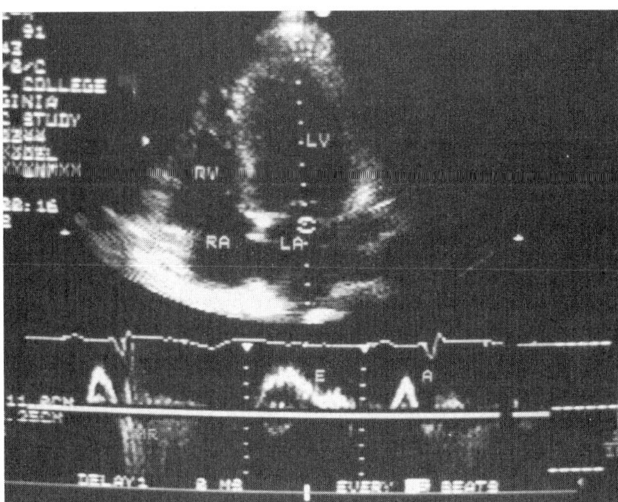

Figure 43–2. Pulsed-wave Doppler echocardiography of a patient with moderate mitral regurgitation demonstrates the range specificity of the pulsed-wave signal in detecting the presence of flow in a specific location. *Abbreviations*: E = early left ventricular filling velocity; A = atrial systolic filling velocity.

Confirmation with pulsed Doppler within these regions of color flow adds to sensitivity and specificity of detecting and quantifying the presence of valvular abnormalities. Doppler color-flow imaging is also bound by the Nyquist limit and cannot display the full Doppler spectrum.

TRANSTHORACIC ECHOCARDIOGRAPHY

TTE can be rapidly and serially performed at the bedside of critically ill patients. An average study takes about 10 to 15 minutes or less. Because infinite tomographic cuts can be made through selected windows, a standard approach is taken using five to six views (discussed next). The American Society of Echocardiography has devised a guide for quantifying left ventricle (LV) dimensions and wall motion based on a 16-segment model (Fig. 43–3).[6] Standardization has made reproducible measurements and comparable studies between centers and operators possible.

Parasternal long-axis views of the heart are usually obtained first (Fig. 43–4*A*). The right ventricle (RV) is seen anteriorly, and the whole of the septum is visualized with the LV below the septum. The aortic root and valve are on the right, with the left atrium (LA) below. The mitral valve is seen in cross section. The posterior wall of the LV is imaged along its length. This view is the basis of measuring LV, LA, and aortic root dimensions.

The *parasternal short-axis* view is obtained by rotating the transducer 90° (Fig. 43–4*B*). At the base of the heart, the aortic valve is seen in cross section along with the RV outflow tract and the pulmonic valve. By tilting the transducer toward the apex, successive short-axis views of the LV are obtained. The mitral valve orifice is observed below the aortic valve (Fig. 43–4C). Tilting the transducer more to the apex results in a cross section of the LV at the level of the papillary muscles. This level is important in assessing regional wall motion because all three coronary arteries supply this region.

The transducer is shifted to the apex, where *four-chamber* (RV, LV, right atrium [RA], RV) and *two-chamber* (LV, LA) views are obtained. The apical views are used to assess global function and to determine the integrity of valvular function. Although the intra-atrial and intraventricular septa are seen, dropout is often observed because these structures are parallel to the beam. Intracardiac masses may be detected in this view (Fig. 43–4*D*). The four-chamber view provides optimal Doppler studies of the mitral, tricuspid, and aortic valves. Color Doppler mapping can quantify the extent of mitral regurgitation. Aortic valve area may be estimated from Doppler studies of the aortic flow in the four-chamber view. Foreshortening and a more medial positioning of the transducer in the apical four-chamber view result in better images of the tricuspid valve and the RV. The presence of tricuspid regurgitation can be used to estimate pulmonary artery systolic pressures. Rotation of the transducer 90° provides the two-chamber apical long-axis view and is important in assessing true anterior and posterior wall motion (Fig. 43–4*E*).

The subcostal view is used consistently in critically ill patients and may be the only viable acoustic window (Fig. 43–4*F*). For patients who have emphysema or who are on high-volume positive-pressure ventilators, hyperinflation of the lungs results in poor parasternal and apical windows. The transducer is placed slightly right of the epigastrium, and the heart is imaged through the diaphragm. Four-chamber images can be obtained, and clockwise rotation 90° results in short-axis views of the LV. The intra-atrial septum is optimally seen in the subcostal view, and Doppler examination of the intra-atrial septum can be performed. The inferior vena cava, hepatic veins, and abdominal aorta can be imaged from this location.

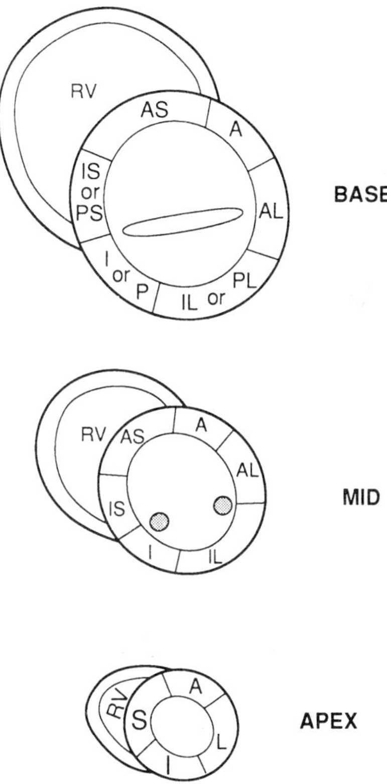

Figure 43–3. Sixteen-segment model for left ventricular wall motion analysis advocated by the American Society of Echocardiography. *Abbreviations*: A = anterior; AL = anterolateral; IL = inferolateral; I = inferior; IS = inferoseptum; AS = anterior septum; PL = posterior lateral; P = posterior; PS = posterior septum; L = lateral wall; S = septum. (From Schiller NB, Shah PM, Crawford M, et al: Recommendations for quantitation of the left ventricle by two-dimensional echocardiography. J Am Soc Echocardiogr 1989; 2:358.)

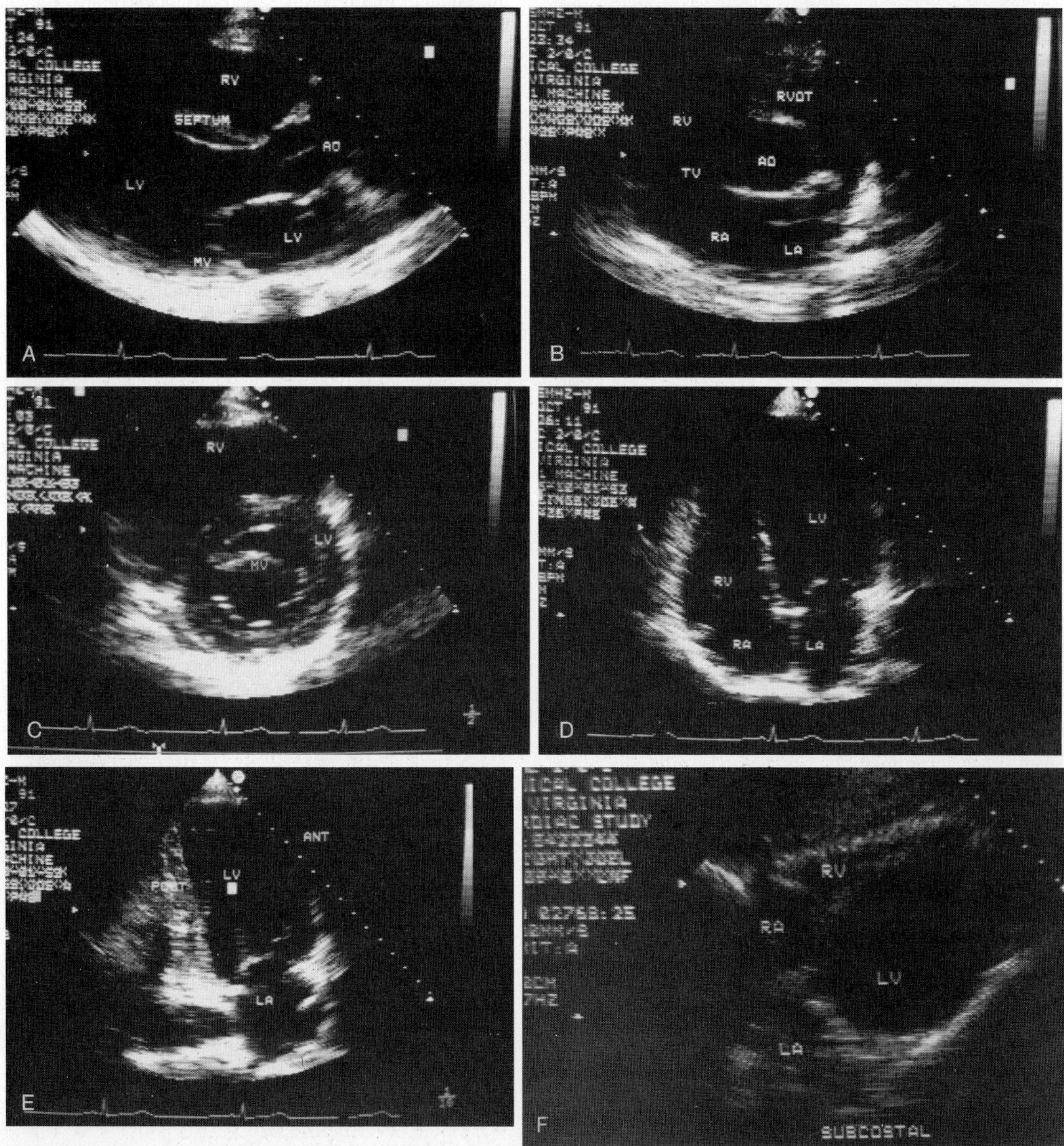

Figure 43–4. *A,* A normal two-dimensional echocardiogram in the parasternal long axis. *Abbreviations*: MV = mitral valve; AO = aortic root. *B,* A normal two-dimensional echocardiogram in the parasternal short-axis view at the level of the aortic root. *Abbreviations*: TV = tricuspid valve; RVOT = right ventricular outflow tract. *C,* A normal two-dimensional echocardiogram in the parasternal short-axis view at the level of the tips of the mitral valve leaflets. *D,* A normal two-dimensional echocardiogram in the apical four-chamber view. *E,* A normal two-dimensional echocardiogram in the apical two-chamber view. *Abbreviation*: ANT = anterior. *F,* A normal two-dimensional echocardiogram in the subcostal view.

The suprasternal position of the transducer allows visualization of the aorta, the aortic arch, and the origin of the brachiocephalic vessels and the descending aorta. The LA, the right pulmonary artery, and the aortic arch in cross section can be seen by rotating the transducer. The suprasternal view is useful in evaluating the aorta. Doppler assessment of the aortic valve may also be performed in this position.

HEMODYNAMIC USES OF ECHOCARDIOGRAPHY

Acutely ill patients often present with life-threatening hypotension. Clinical assessment gives clues to the cause of hypotension (see Table 43–1), as in the case of a patient with acute gastrointestinal hemorrhage and hypovolemic shock. However, a gastrointestinal bleed can cause myocardial infarction (MI) in an elderly patient, and fluid resuscitation can be hampered by pulmonary edema. Clinical presentations are often similar, but the medical therapy radically different. For instance, in patients presenting with hypotension, elevated jugular venous pressure, and a clear chest radiograph, the differential diagnosis includes pericardial tamponade, RV infarction, pulmonary embolism, and early acute LV infarction. If the patient has cardiac tamponade, volume resuscitation and pericardiocentesis are indicated. If RV infarction is the diagnosis, volume resuscitation with inotropic support would be needed to reverse hypotension. In acute LV infarction, fluid restriction and inotropic therapy are indicated. Two-dimensional echocardiography is immensely helpful in guiding radically different therapies in patients presenting with hypotension and similar clinical findings.[6a]

ESTIMATION OF PULMONARY ARTERY SYSTOLIC PRESSURE

In addition to providing anatomic data, Doppler echocardiography yields hemodynamic information previously gained only by invasive Swan-Ganz monitoring. Pulmonary artery systolic pressure can be derived from the simplified Bernoulli equation (Table 43–2, Equation 1). The RA pressure is estimated as 5 to 10 mm Hg and added to the RV systolic pressure to yield the pulmonary artery systolic pressure.[7] Because tricuspid regurgitation occurs in 17.4% of structurally normal hearts,[8] this method is widely applicable, is reproducible, and has been clinically validated (Fig. 43–5).[9, 9a]

ESTIMATION OF PULMONARY CAPILLARY WEDGE PRESSURE AND LEFT ATRIAL PRESSURE

Using the Bernoulli hydrodynamic principle, the velocity of mitral regurgitation has been used to assess LA pressure with excellent correlation in patients with congestive heart failure ($r^2 = 0.88$; Fig. 43–6).[10] Because brachial sphygmomanometry cuff pressure was used to estimate LV systolic pressure, mitral regurgitation cannot be used to estimate LA pressure by this method in patients with aortic stenosis, LV outflow tract obstruction, or subclavian artery diseases. However, especially when the LV compliance is acutely changing, as in postoperative cardiac surgery or in sepsis, pulmonary capillary wedge pressure may not accurately reflect LV end-diastolic volume.[11] In these instances, direct observation of myocardial function may be more useful to guide therapy.

LA pressure can qualitatively be assessed by the Doppler pulmonary venous flow patterns usually obtained during

TABLE 43–2. Equations

Equation 1. Bernoulli's equation
Change in pressure = 4 × (instantaneous velocity)^2
Equation 2. Estimation of cardiac output
Pulmonary artery cross-sectional area or aortic valve area × velocity flow integral = stroke volume
Cardiac output (L/min) = stroke volume (mL) × heart rate (bpm)

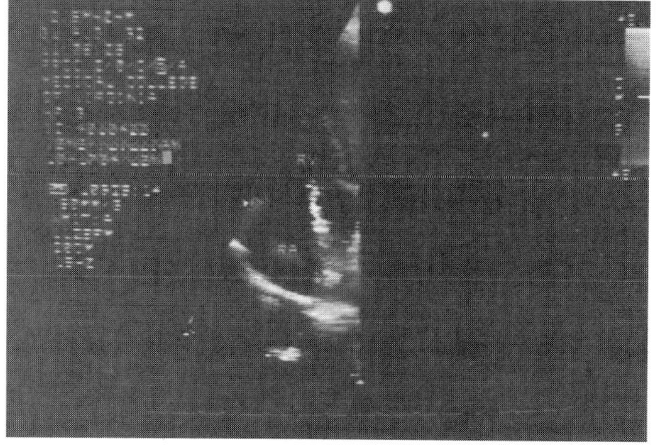

Figure 43–5. A color-flow Doppler echocardiogram in the apical four-chamber view showing tricuspid regurgitation. (See Color Plate Section of this textbook.)

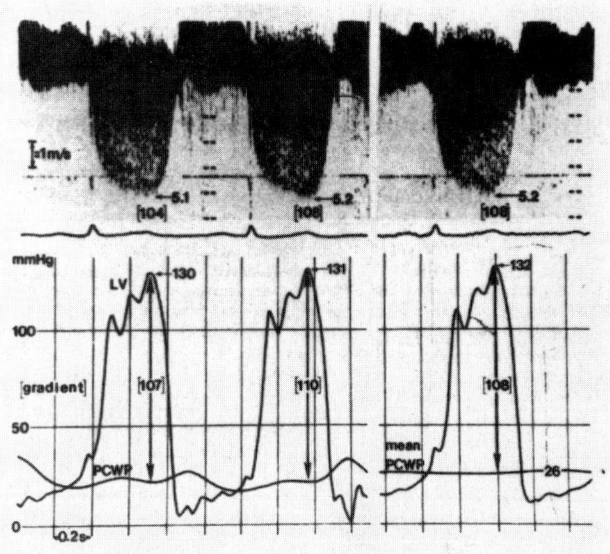

Figure 43–6. Simultaneous continuous-wave Doppler recordings of a mitral regurgitation jet and catheter recordings from the left ventricle and pulmonary capillary wedge positions in a patient with mitral regurgitation and mild mitral stenosis. The use of mild regurgitant flow velocity to estimate left atrial pressure is illustrated. Pressure gradients are shown in brackets. Simultaneous measurement of systolic blood pressure by cuff was 132 mm Hg; this value corresponds to an estimated left atrial pressure of 24 mm Hg, which correlates closely with the recorded mean pulmonary capillary wedge pressure (PCWP) at end-expiration of 26 mm Hg. (From Gorcsan J III, Snow FR, Paulsen W, et al: Noninvasive estimation of left atrial pressure in patients with congestive heart failure and mitral regurgitation by Doppler echocardiography. Am Heart J 1991; 121:858–863.)

TEE. The normal biphasic flow with a predominant systolic phase is reversed when the pulmonary capillary wedge pressure is greater than 15 mm Hg.[12] This measurement is usually not within the scope of TTE, although venous inflow can be determined in patients with good acoustic windows.

ESTIMATION OF CARDIAC OUTPUT

Velocity of blood flow across the aortic and pulmonic valves can be readily assessed by Doppler echocardiography. The flow-velocity integral (area under the spectral Doppler velocity plot) multiplied by the outflow tract diameter yields stroke volume. Cardiac output is the product of stroke volume and heart rate, and thus instantaneous right and left cardiac outputs can be measured[13] and have been validated (Table 43–2, Equation 2).[14]

PERICARDIAL DISEASE

Two-dimensional echocardiography is optimal for detecting and diagnosing pericardial effusion. The pericardium is a fibroserous membrane that is composed of anisotropic collagen fibrils that unite the heart into a working unit. Normally, as much as 50 mL of serous fluid can be present in the pericardial sac. Two-dimensional echocardiography may detect as little as 15 mL. Increasing pericardial effusion can develop as a response to injury, and its impact on myocardial performance is dependent on the amount of fluid and its rapidity of accumulation. Two-dimensional echocardiography can not only diagnose pericardial effusion but can assist in pericardiocentesis. Not all echo-free space represents pericardial effusion, because epicardial fat and fibrocalcific pericardial disease are indiscernible by 2-D echocardiography (Fig. 43–7*A*).[15]

Pericardial tamponade is a life-threatening clinical diagnosis defined hemodynamically as elevation of intrapericardial pressure with progressive limitation of diastolic filling that results in reduced stroke volume and ultimately systemic hypotension. The classic profile includes pulsus paradoxus, equalization of the LV and RV diastolic pressures, and depression of cardiac output. Tamponade may be difficult, especially in medical patients who do not present with Beck's classic triad of decline in blood pressure, elevated central venous pressure, and a small quiet heart.[16] Rather, nonspecific signs and symptoms such as dyspnea, tachycardia, and pulsus paradoxus are more common.[17]

Tamponade is now recognized as a continuum rather than a rigid "all-or-none" phenomenon. Tamponade is characterized by progressive increase in intrapericardial pressures, resulting in RA and RV impaired filling and collapse. Ultimately, impaired LV filling results in systemic hypotension.[18] Early RA and especially RV diastolic collapse can represent significant hemodynamic compromise (see Fig. 43–7*B*).[19] This sign is preload dependent and can be absent in patients with significant RV hypertrophy or in constrictive pericarditis or in patients who have a pericardiectomy and uncoupling of the RV and LV.[20] In patients with LV dysfunction, RA and RV collapse can occur with smaller pericardial pressures and absent pulsus paradoxus.[21] If RV collapse is present, longer duration of RV collapse in diastole may signify worsening hemodynamic compromise.[22]

Another sign of tamponade is movement of the interventricular septum toward the LV during inspiration, which is equivalent to the pulsus paradoxus noted on physical examination. Other nonspecific signs of cardiac tamponade include a reciprocal pattern of Doppler flow velocity across the tricuspid valve (E less than A),[23] pseudohypertrophy of the LV,[24] and a right-to-left shunt across a patent foramen ovale.[25]

Once a pericardial effusion has been detected and if pericardiocentesis needs to be performed, 2-D echocardiography can guide placement of the drainage catheter. The operator usually notes the depth to pericardial fluid and the necessary angle and approach. A needle guide can be mounted on the transducer, and the actual needle can be observed entering the pericardial space. In most cases, however, it is sufficient to locate the effusion and direct the operator with depth and orientation.

In patients with extensive chest trauma or in patients who have just undergone chest surgery, TTE may not be possible because of an inadequate acoustic window. TEE may be needed to detect a pericardial effusion.

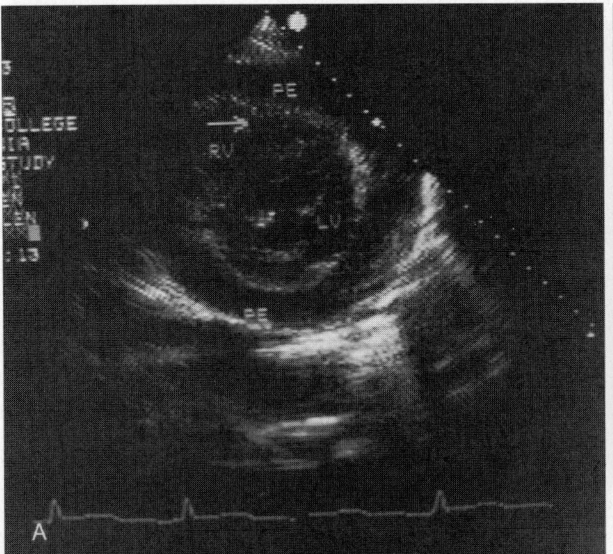

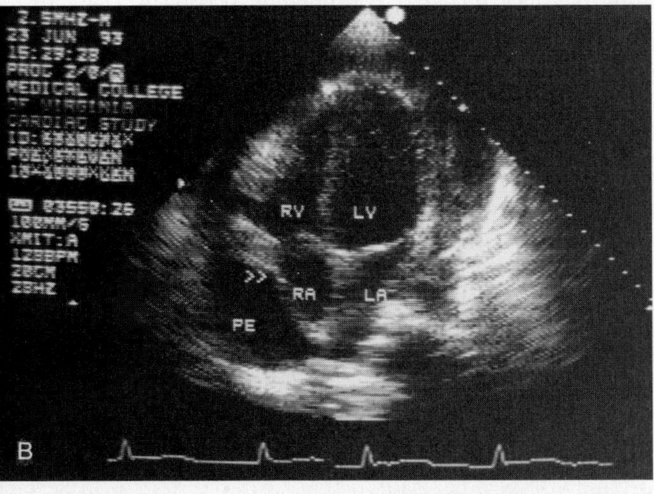

Figure 43–7. *A*, A two-dimensional echocardiogram in the parasternal short-axis view showing a circumferential pericardial effusion. *B*, A two-dimensional echocardiogram in the apical four-chamber view showing right atrial free-wall late diastolic collapse *(arrows)*, which is characteristically associated with cardiac tamponade. *Abbreviation*: PE = pericardial effusion.

No particular combination of echocardiographic signs is characteristic of constrictive pericarditis. Increased pericardial thickness behind the posterior wall may suggest thickening, but these measurements are not readily reproducible and are subject to gain error.[26] Some findings include mild LA enlargement with normal LV size,[27] dilatation of the vena cava, flattening of LV endocardial motion during mid and late diastole, and premature opening of the pulmonic valve.[28] Septal motion and Doppler flow of the mitral and tricuspid valves are abnormal during inspiration and expiration.[29, 29a]

MYOCARDIAL FUNCTION IN SEPSIS

LV systolic function is critical in evaluating the cause of hypotension. In addition to ischemic and valvular heart disease, the mediators released in the sepsis syndrome can cause transient myocardial dysfunction. Parrillo and coworkers have proposed a circulating "myocardial depressant factor" that causes decreased myocardial contractility in experimental rat myocyte preparations.[30] Furthermore, Parker and colleagues have noted transient LV dilatation and decreased LV function by radionuclide ventriculography (Fig. 43–8).[31] As a result of these observations, dobutamine is used as a pressor to increase oxygen delivery.[32] Because cardiac output is elevated in sepsis, 2-D echocardiography can help to guide and titrate dobutamine therapy.

In addition to LV dysfunction, RV dysfunction is noted in septic shock and in adult respiratory distress syndrome.[33] The RV is known to dilate rather than to develop wall-motion abnormalities when function is compromised, and this can readily be seen by 2-D echocardiography.[34] In the setting of RV infarction, dobutamine has been shown to improve RV function, and serial 2-D echocardiography may be helpful to guide therapy.

HYPOVOLEMIA

A small hypercontractile LV with a normal pulmonary venous inflow pattern and a prominent A wave mitral inflow pattern is seen in hypovolemia. When aggressive volume resuscitation fails to restore blood pressure, echocardiography can be useful to preclude other contributing factors such as cardiac tamponade, RV infarction, cardiogenic shock, or pulmonary embolism.

ACUTE PULMONARY EMBOLISM

Hypotension and atypical chest pain without pulmonary edema are a common presentation in patients with pulmonary embolism. Significant pulmonary emboli cause acute RV failure, and RV dilatation is seen on 2-D echocardiography.[35] An embolus can occasionally be seen in the pulmonary artery outflow tract or crossing the atrial septum owing to increased right heart pressures.[36] In a serial transesophageal study of patients with pulmonary emboli, 8 of 24 patients (33%) had thrombi in the pulmonary artery.[37] The mobility and expediency of 2-D echocardiography in precluding other causes of hypotension can be important in treating patients with pulmonary embolism.

RIGHT VENTRICULAR MYOCARDIAL INFARCTION

An important cause of hypotension that is often unrecognized is RV infarction, first described by Sanders in 1930.[38] Autopsy studies have shown an incidence from 1% to 43%, with variability attributed to diverse definitions of RV infarction, pathologic techniques, and different population samples.[39] When hemodynamic criteria are used, 15% to 20% of inferior wall MIs have RV involvement,[40] with severe hemodynamic derangement in 3% to 8% of the cases.[41] In patients with acute MI and hypotension, RV infarction is critical to recognize and differentiate from constrictive pericarditis and pericardial tamponade because patients commonly present with jugular venous distention, hypotension, and clear lungs on examination.[42] Diastolic equalization of pressures can be common to RV infarction, pericardial tamponade, and constriction.[43] Kussmaul's sign or inspiratory increase in venous pressure and prominent y descent are more specific and sensitive for RV infarction than is pericar-

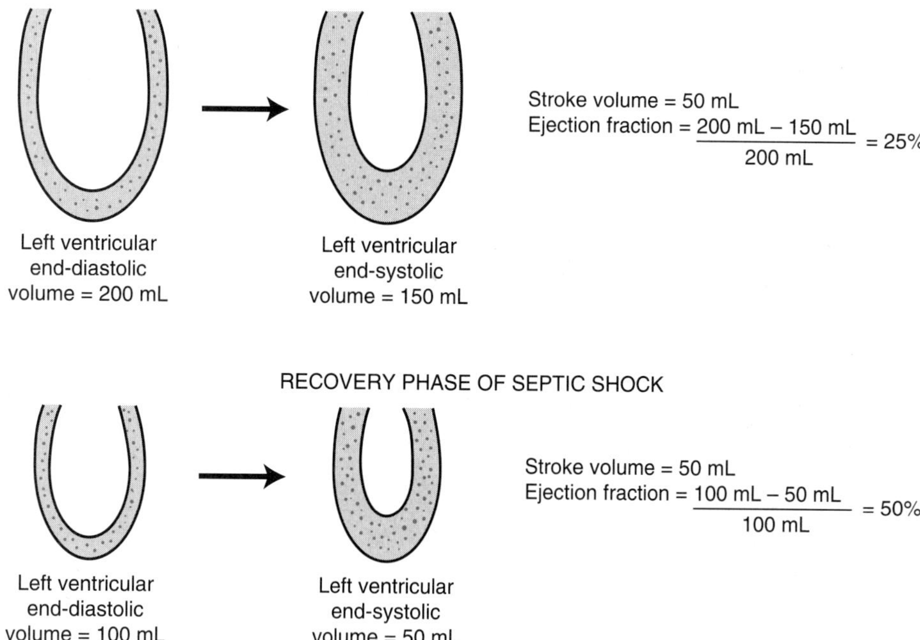

Figure 43–8. Reversible myocardial depression in survivors of septic shock—a schematic representation. (From Parker MM, Shelhamer JH, Bacharach SL, et al: Profound but reversible myocardial depression in patients with septic shock. Ann Intern Med 1984; 100:483–490.)

dial tamponade.[44] However, constrictive pericarditis and restrictive cardiomyopathy also exhibit Kussmaul's sign and exaggerated y descents with flattening diastolic filling pressures. Echocardiography is useful in rapidly differentiating between these three clinical entities.

Unlike in the LV, regional wall-motion abnormalities are seldom observed.[45] Rather, RV enlargement along with inferior LV wall-motion abnormalities connotes RV infarction. The RV dilates with ischemic injury, and the RV free wall may show diminished wall motion.[46] Caudal motion of less than 1.5 cm of the tricuspid annulus is also a marker of RV systolic dysfunction.[47] Another nonspecific sign of RV dysfunction is paradoxical septal motion.

The best view for assessment of RV wall motion is the subcostal view. When massive RV dilatation is present, the RV free wall may not be readily seen on the apical four-chamber view. Medial positioning of the transducer so that the apex is formed by the RV allows the free wall to be seen. Doppler echocardiography is rather nonspecific, but reversed peak velocities (normally early E greater than A atrial filling velocities) are a marker of RV dysfunction.[48]

If both RV infarction and pericardial tamponade coexist, the RV appears dilated and has less tendency to exhibit diastolic collapse. RA and RV collapse requires higher pericardial pressures and larger pericardial effusions and occurs later in diastole.[49] In addition to inferior LV infarction, anteroseptal MI can cause RV dysfunction owing to the commonly shared septum.[50, 51]

It is important to note that the echocardiographic signs of RV infarction are nonspecific and that increased RV afterload provokes these signs. LV dysfunction eventually causes RV dilatation and dysfunction. In patients with chronic heart failure, RV dilatation may be an independent predictor of mortality.[52]

ISCHEMIC HEART DISEASE

Regional wall motion develops in the LV within seconds of coronary occlusion (Fig. 43–9).[53–55] Diastolic dysfunction with thinning of the myocardium and bulging is seen on 2-D echocardiography with acute coronary occlusion. In a study of 180 patients presenting to the emergency department with chest pain, regional wall dysfunction on 2-D echocardiography identified patients with acute MI better than did conventional assessment (history and physical) and electrocardiographic criteria. Technically adequate studies in patients with acute MI range from 73% to 93.5%.[56] However, 2-D echocardiography is more conventionally used in this setting to determine prognosis and identify complications of acute MI (Table 43–3).

The presence of LV systolic dysfunction can predict a subset of patients at high risk during the hospital course and later.[57, 57a] However, regional wall motion is not specific for ischemic heart disease. Patients with idiopathic dilated cardiomyopathy, subarachnoid hemorrhage, and anorexia nervosa have been reported to have segmental LV wall-motion abnormalities.[58]

Immediate mechanical complications of acute MI include acquired ventricular septal defect, LV thrombi, ischemic mitral regurgitation, myocardial infarct expansion, and LV rupture. A patient who has a new systolic murmur and who develops hypotension or pulmonary edema may have rupture of the interventricular septum, ischemia, or rupture of the papillary muscle apparatus.[59] Acquired ventricular septal defects usually occur near the apex and are associated with a dilated cavity. The defect may be identified by 2-D echocardiography and confirmed by Doppler color-flow mapping or by contrast echocardiography.[60]

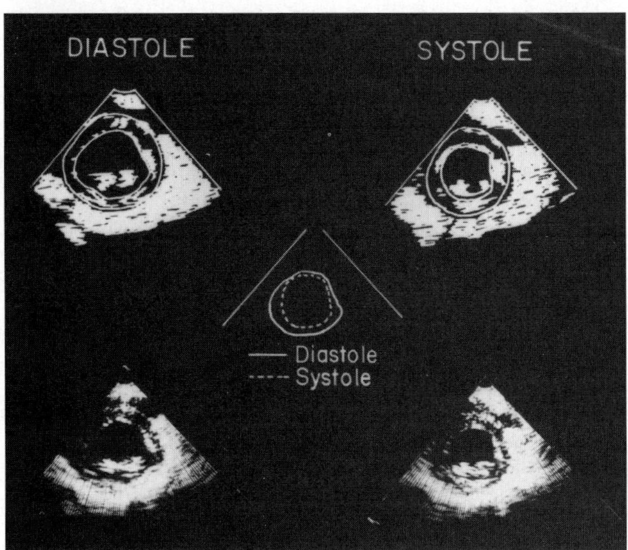

Figure 43–9. Two-dimensional echocardiograms in the parasternal short-axis views showing hypokinesia in the anterolateral segment in a patient with acute anterior myocardial infarction. (From Nixon JV, Narahara KA, Smitherman TC: Estimation of myocardial involvement in patients with acute myocardial infarction by two-dimensional echocardiography. Circulation 1980; 62:1248–1255.)

Two-dimensional echocardiography is ideally suited for detecting ventricular thrombi and is more sensitive than angiographic ventriculography.[61] The majority of patients with ventricular thrombi have anterior transmural MI.[62] Echocardiographic morphology of the thrombus can predict the possibility of systemic embolism. For example, thrombi that protrude into the LV cavity and that are mobile during the cardiac cycle have a higher risk of causing systemic embolization than thrombi that are sessile.[63] Patients with anterior MI and LV thrombi should receive anticoagulation, although other studies investigating the use of Persantine and aspirin or no therapy are ongoing.[64]

Papillary rupture is often catastrophic. It is secondary to disruption of the necrosed head of the papillary muscle and occurs in 1% of all MIs.[65] Massive mitral regurgitation is usually noted, with a flail leaflet. Because of size and blood supply, the posterior medial papillary muscle is often ruptured. The size of the infarction does not predict the propensity to have papillary rupture, because 50% of patients have small or non–Q wave MIs.[66] In acute mitral regurgitation, the murmur may be absent, and Doppler assessment can be falsely negative if there is no pressure gradient between the LA and the LV. This occurs in massive acute mitral regur-

TABLE 43–3. Mechanical Complications of Acute Myocardial Infarction

Mitral regurgitation
Papillary muscle dysfunction
Papillary muscle rupture
Chordal rupture
Cardiac rupture
Papillary muscle rupture 5%
Ventricular septal rupture 10%
Free-wall rupture 85%
LV aneurysm
LV pseudoaneurysm
LV thrombi
Infarct expansion

gitation because LV pressures are low and LA pressures are elevated as a result of rapid equilibration between the two chambers. A large regurgitant fraction producing a hyperdynamic LV wall may be the only echocardiographic sign. Prompt recognition with surgical intervention may be life saving. Mortality remains elevated, however, with 50% survival at 24 hours and 16% survival at 8 weeks.

Ischemic mitral regurgitation is a marker of adverse prognosis and is usually more a consequence of LV dysfunction than of isolated papillary ischemia.[67] On 2-D echocardiography, incomplete closure of the mitral valve is associated with ischemic regurgitation.[68] The murmur of mitral regurgitation is often absent on physical examination, even when ischemic mitral regurgitation is present.[69] Recognition is important, because future management with angiotensin-converting enzyme inhibitors and closer monitoring for heart failure may improve survival.

Infarct expansion occurs predominately in anterior wall transmural MI (35–42% of all anterior wall MIs).[70] Expansion is defined anatomically as fixed regional thinning and dilatation of the infarct zone caused by slipping of necrotic myofibrils. Two-dimensional echocardiography demonstrates regional cardiac dilatation. Infarct expansion is important to recognize because it predisposes to development of LV aneurysm and free-wall rupture. Prompt treatment with angiotensin-converting enzyme inhibitors can decrease infarct expansion.[71, 71a]

Free-wall rupture occurs in 1.5% to 8% of all heart attacks and accounts for 8% to 24% of infarct-related deaths.[72] Patients usually present catastrophically with chest pain, hypotension, distended neck veins, and electromechanical dissociation. Pericardial tamponade is invariably present, and this constellation of symptoms in a patient on the seventh or eight day of infarction should prompt heroic measures if the patient is to survive. Rarely, a patient may present subacutely, and corrective surgery is undertaken if the clinician is astute.

VALVULAR HEART DISEASE

Unknown murmurs in critically ill hypotensive patients can contribute to their hemodynamic demise. Doppler echocardiography allows possible physiologic assessment of valvular function in conjunction with structural function. In hemodynamically compromised patients, significant aortic stenosis/aortic regurgitation and mitral stenosis/mitral regurgitation can influence inotropic and hemodynamic management. For example, in elderly patients with heart failure and hypotension, the presence of aortic stenosis significantly affects their hemodynamic management and the choices of diuretic and vasodilator therapy. If the same patients develop sepsis, they may have a low cardiac output and artificially raised systemic vascular resistance even though they may be systemically vasodilated. In this case, they benefit from both dobutamine and dopamine inotropic therapy.

Two-dimensional echocardiography can assess the valves for congenital anomalies, calcification, vegetations, and masses. Doppler and color mapping graphically illustrate the results of any morphologic abnormality. Valvular stenosis (Tables 43–4 and 43–5) creates higher velocities of blood flow that can be detected by Doppler studies. Valvular regurgitation (Tables 43–6 and 43–7) produces reversed flow when compared with the cardiac cycle. For aortic and mitral stenosis (see Table 43–4), Doppler estimation of instantaneous gradients and calculated mean gradients correlate well with similar measurements obtained during cardiac catheterization.[73] The peak instantaneous gradient is higher than the mean gradient (two thirds of peak instantaneous gradient = mean gradient). The mean gradient can be derived by the integral of the spectral Doppler velocity envelope (Fig. 43–10). Because gradients are a function of the driving force (i.e., the cardiac output), the aortic valve area is calculated from the continuity equation, which compares the velocities of blood proximal and distal to the valve (see Table 43–2). The aortic valve area calculations are usually within 10% of cardiac catheterization–derived aortic valve areas.[74]

Aortic regurgitation can be accurately diagnosed by Doppler echocardiography (see Table 43–6). Color mapping demonstrates the regurgitant jet that is usually central, streaming into the LV during diastole (Fig. 43–11). The severity of aortic regurgitation may be quantitatively assessed. The width of the regurgitant jet, the length of the regurgitant jet, the area and slope of the spectral Doppler map,[75] and reversal of flow in the descending aorta have been used to quantify the regurgitation.[76] In the authors' experience, reversal of flow in the descending aorta and width of the regurgitant jet greater than 66% of the LV outflow tract correlate most closely with severe aortic regurgitation.

Mitral regurgitation is detected by color Doppler mapping of the LA (see Table 43–7; Fig. 43–12*A* and *B*). Pulsed Doppler is used to confirm the presence of retrograde flow

TABLE 43–4. Doppler Echocardiography and Stenotic Valvular Heart Disease

Mitral stenosis
- Abnormally high wedge values in patients with good LV ejection fraction and frequent pulmonary edema

Aortic stenosis
- Whether to institute vasodilator therapy in patient with congestive heart failure

TABLE 43–5. Obstruction in the Left Ventricular Outflow Tract

- Valvular—aortic stenosis
- Dynamic outflow obstruction
  - Interventricular—hypertrophic obstructive cardiomyopathy
  - Subaortic—discrete subaortic stenosis
  - Supravalvular
- Aortic arch interruptions
- Coarctation of the aortic isthmus

TABLE 53–6. Aortic Regurgitation

Chronic
- Rheumatic fever
- Healed infective endocarditis
- Degenerative calcified disease
- Bicuspid aortic valve
- Aortic root dilation
  - Hypertension
  - Marfan's syndrome
  - Cystic medial degeneration
  - Annuloaortic ectasia
  - Atherosclerosis
  - Syphilis
  - Systemic lupus erythematosus

Acute
- Acute infective endocarditis
- Traumatic rupture of aortic leaflet
- Rupture of myxomatous valve
- Aortic dissection (Stanford A)

TABLE 43–7. Mitral Regurgitation

- Congenital
  - Cleft mitral valve
  - Atrioventricular cushion defect
- Myxomatous degeneration
  - Mitral valve prolapse
- Rheumatic
- Infectious endocarditis
- Ischemic
- Calcific
  - Degenerative with mitral annular degeneration
  - Renal or hyperparathyroid diseases
- Traumatic
  - Chordal rupture due to nonpenetrating chest trauma
- Cardiomyopathy
  - Dilated
  - Hypertrophic
  - Restrictive
- Myocarditis
- Severe aortic regurgitation

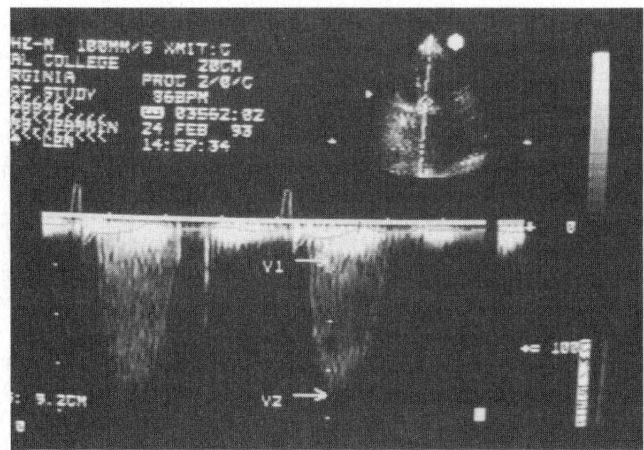

Figure 43–10. Continuous-wave Doppler echocardiographic recording of a patient with severe aortic stenosis. *Abbreviations:* V1 = flow velocity in left ventricular outflow tract; V2 = maximal flow velocity recorded along the cursor line, which reflects postvalvular velocity in the ascending aorta.

of blood during systole (see Fig. 43–2). Severe mitral regurgitation is present when flow retrograde to the pulmonary vein is seen by pulsed Doppler and when the regurgitant jet area is greater than 40% when compared with the LA area.[77] However, eccentric jets that impinge on the LA wall are underestimated by color Doppler imaging by as much as 40%.[78] These eccentric regurgitant jets can cause asymmetric pulmonary edema when selectively engaging the right pulmonary vein.[79]

Mitral stenosis can be reliably detected by 2-D echocardiography (see Table 43–4). The orifice of the mitral valve can be seen on parasternal short-axis view, and the area planimetered.[80] This measurement is less accurate when the valves are distorted, however, as in rheumatic heart disease. The pressure gradient during diastole is independent of cardiac output and is prolonged in the presence of mitral stenosis. Doppler interrogation of transmitral flow can measure the pressure half-time (time taken for the initial maximum diastolic gradient to drop to one half), and the mitral valve area (MVA) calculated from the relationship MVA equals 220/pressure half-time in milliseconds (Fig. 43–13).[81] This relationship holds true because the pressure half-time is 220 msec in patients who have an MVA of 1 cm^2. Compared with the Gorlin MVA derived by cardiac catheterization, the pressure half-time MVA derived by continuous-wave Doppler is in agreement within 0.2 cm^2.[82] Because flow across a stenotic valve is turbulent, color-flow mapping demonstrates a narrow candle-like jet. Color mapping can guide the optimal position of the Doppler probe to estimate the MVA.

AORTIC DISEASE

The proximal ascending aorta is well seen by TTE. Most of the aorta can be seen by combining the left and right parasternal, suprasternal, supraclavicular, and subcostal windows in 80% to 85% of patients.[83] Aortic root diseases such as sinus of Valsalva aneurysms and annuloaortic ectasia can be observed by 2-D echocardiography, and aortic root enlargement of greater than 6 cm has been used as a criterion for aortic root replacement.[84]

Dissection of the ascending aorta is a life-threatening condition in which early mortality can be as high as 1% per hour.[85] Prompt diagnosis and treatment are life saving. Surgical therapy benefits patients with ascending aortic involvement (Stanford A[86] or DeBakey I and II),[87] and recognition that aortic dissection is present leads to optimal

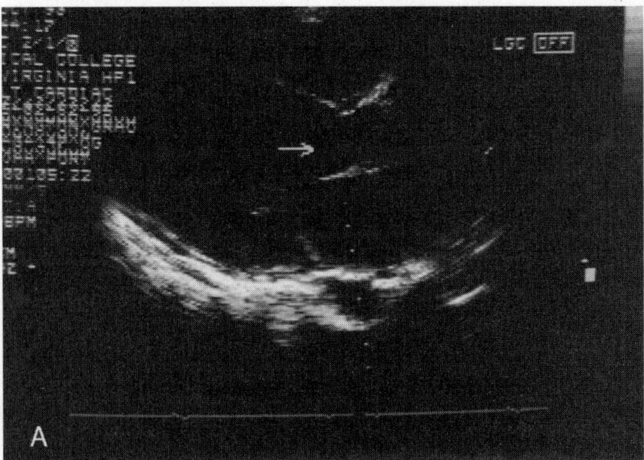

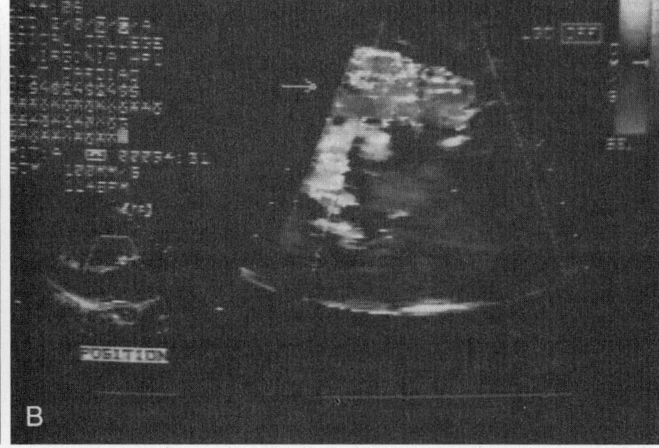

Figure 43–11. *A,* A two-dimensional echocardiogram in the parasternal long-axis view in a patient with aortic regurgitation. *B,* A color-flow Doppler echocardiogram in the parasternal long-axis view showing severe aortic regurgitation in the same patient as in *A.* (See Color Plate Section of this textbook.)

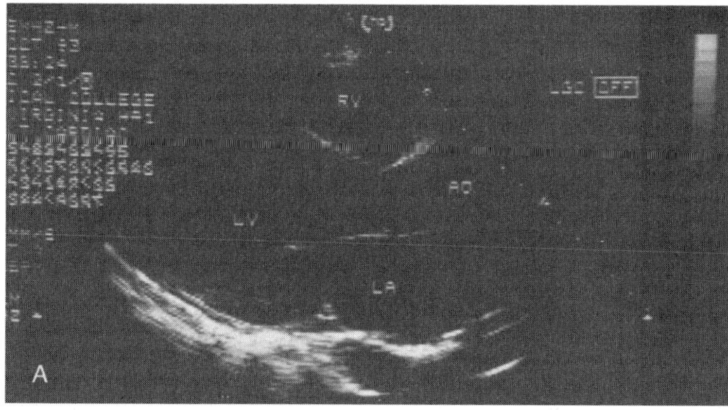

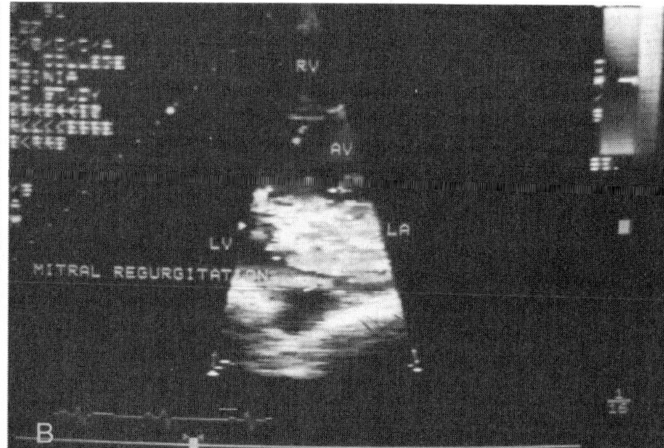

Figure 43–12. *A,* A two-dimensional echocardiogram in the parasternal short-axis view showing left atrial enlargement in a patient with severe mitral regurgitation. *B,* A color-flow Doppler echocardiogram in the parasternal short-axis view showing severe mitral regurgitation in the same patient as in *A*. *Abbreviation*: AV = aortic valve. (See Color Plate Section of this textbook.)

control of blood pressure, usually with Nipride and β-blockade to decrease shear forces.[88] TTE not only precludes other causes of acute chest pain but can identify aortic dissection, although TEE is warranted to fully rule out the diagnosis in hemodynamically unstable patients (Fig. 43–14*A* and *B*). The sensitivity of TTE in identifying the ascending aorta ranges from 78% to 100%,[89] though for the descending aorta it is only 55% to 31%.[90] TEE has 97.7% sensitivity and 76.9% specificity, but requires intubation of the esophagus and assistance from special personnel.[91]

INFECTIOUS ENDOCARDITIS

The diagnosis of infectious endocarditis is a clinical one based on history and examination, blood cultures, and serologic tests. Two-dimensional echocardiography is useful in improving the diagnostic acumen, with a 60% to 80% sensitivity in detecting vegetations (Fig. 43–15*A* and *B*).[92] More importantly, the absence of vegetations does not preclude endocarditis. Using TEE can improve the sensitivity to more than 90%, especially for detecting vegetations less than 0.5 cm (Fig. 43–15C).[93] The presence of valvular regurgitation and valvular stenosis, especially in prosthetic valves, can often give clues that endocarditis is present.

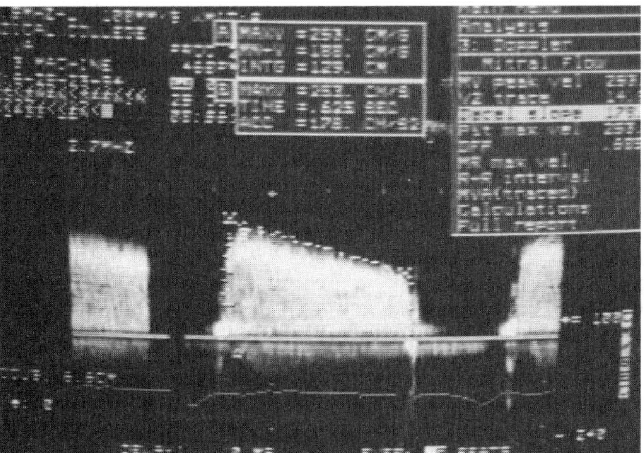

Figure 43–13. The spectral display of a continuous-wave Doppler echocardiogram in a patient with significant mitral stenosis. Quantification of the mitral stenosis may be performed with a number of spectral Doppler variables, including the deceleration slope.

Two-dimensional echocardiography is useful in monitoring the clinical course, especially in patients with left-sided endocarditis. Vegetation size exceeding 1 cm and aortic valve involvement correlate with the need for valve replacement and worse outcome.[94] For right-sided endocarditis, vegetation size exceeding 2 cm and increased RV size correlate with increased mortality and the need for valve replacement.

Vegetations can be difficult to visualize in prosthetic valve endocarditis owing to the metallic struts. For bioprosthetic valves, although the cusps can be seen, the quality of the images is poorer than for native valves. In addition to vegetations, valve ring abscesses indicate endocarditis. The presence of abnormal prosthetic valve rocking motion, thickening of the aortic root, and sinus of Valsalva aneurysm can signal a ring abscess.[95, 96] To evaluate the valve ring fully, TEE is probably indicated to assess prosthetic valve endocarditis more completely.

TRAUMATIC DISEASES

Penetrating trauma to the heart can involve the RV, LV, RA, and LA in order of greatest frequency.[97] Hemopericardium with tamponade leads to death unless the problem is recognized. Two-dimensional echocardiography can be immensely helpful in identifying this problem and in assisting with emergency drainage of tamponade. Furthermore, the extent of myocardial injury can be assessed in patients who are unstable, even after repair of free-wall perforations. Ventricular septal defects and valvular lacerations can be readily identified by Doppler color-flow studies.

Blunt trauma can cause myocardial contusion and aortic/mitral regurgitation. Myocardial contusion is a nebulous clinical entity. Although regional wall motion is possible,[98] most patients have unremarkable 2-D echocardiograms, and the presence of abnormalities on echocardiography is not predictive of morbidity or mortality.[99, 100] Although the presence of myocardial contusion may not be clinically evident by 2-D echocardiography, in hemodynamically unstable patients after trauma, timely 2-D echocardiography is mandated to preclude important pericardial and valvular abnormalities.

SUMMARY

Although echocardiography is a powerful diagnostic tool, a working understanding of the background principles is necessary to apply the findings to clinical practice. Because

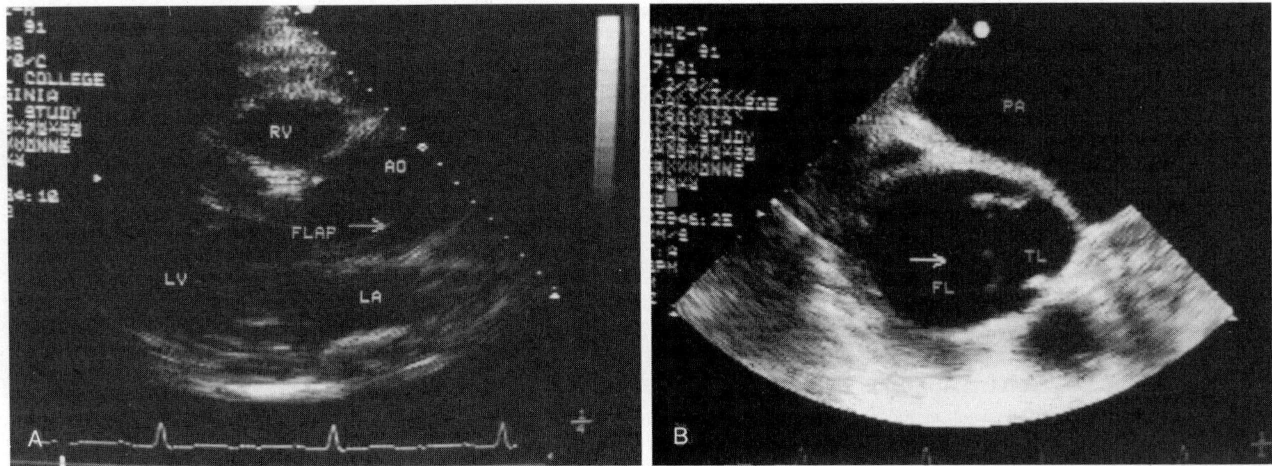

Figure 43–14. *A,* A transthoracic two-dimensional echocardiogram showing the flap in a type 1 dissection of the ascending aorta. *B,* A transesophageal two-dimensional echocardiogram of the same patient as in *A* showing the true lumen (TL) and the false lumen (FL) of this type 1 aortic dissection. *Abbreviations*: AO = aorta; PA = pulmonary artery.

technical expertise is needed to perform a thorough study and detailed understanding of cardiac anatomy and physiology is prerequisite to interpret the examination, familiarity with the echocardiography personnel and review of the examination are likely to enhance patient care. Echocardiography is useful in evaluating patients with shock because it graphically demonstrates myocardial performance and can help distinguish cardiac from noncardiac causes of hypotension. Because multisystem failure and sepsis syndrome influence myocardial function, echocardiography can help to make decisions about inotropic therapy. Echocardiography is diagnostic of effusive pericardial diseases and detects important valvular abnormalities. Echocardiography has the potential to provide hemodynamic data equivalent

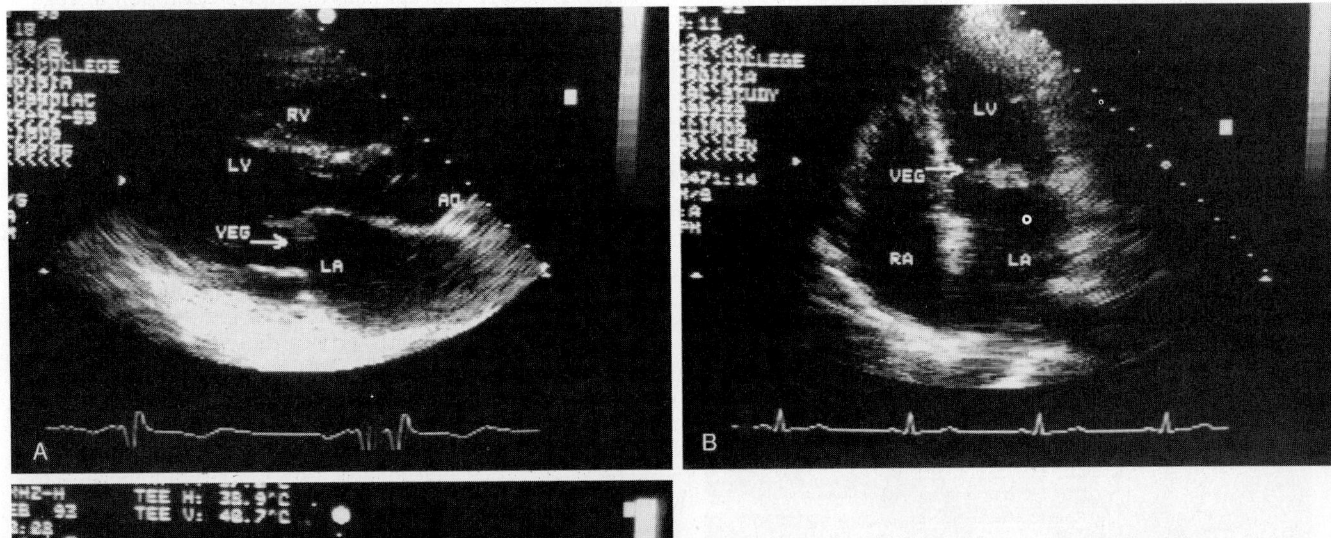

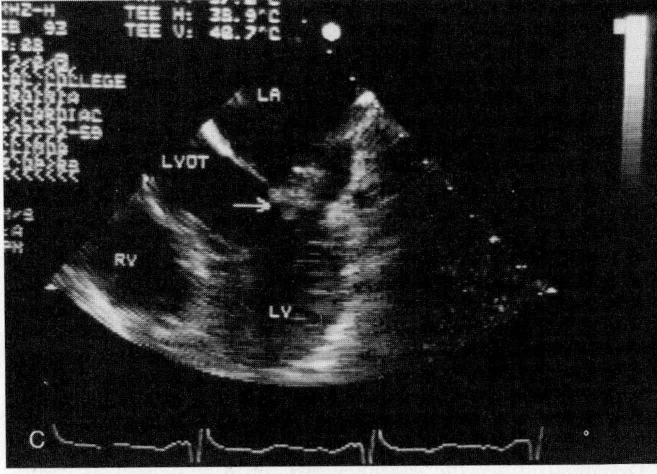

Figure 43–15. *A,* A transthoracic two-dimensional echocardiogram in the parasternal long-axis position of a vegetation attached to the anterior mitral leaflet of a patient with endocarditis. *B,* A transthoracic two-dimensional echocardiogram in the apical four-chamber view of the same patient as in *A* with endocarditis. *C,* A transesophageal two-dimensional echocardiogram showing the vegetation on the anterior leaflet of the mitral valve *(arrow)* in the same patient as in *A* and *B. Abbreviations*: VEG = vegetation on the anterior leaflet of the mitral valve; LVOT = left ventricular outflow tract.

to those of a Swan-Ganz catheter when determining cardiac output and pulmonary artery systolic pressures. Because echocardiography is easily performed at the bedside and in a timely manner, critically ill patients do not have to be transported out of the intensive care unit. Echocardiography will be increasingly used in all critical care units instead of just coronary care as the population ages and as more intensivists become familiar with the wealth of data that can be obtained.

ACKNOWLEDGMENT

The authors wish to thank Ms. Sylvia Converse for her assistance in the preparation of this chapter.

References

1. Fili EO, Labovitz AJ: Transesophageal echocardiography: Expanding indications for ICU use. J Crit Illness 1992; 7:85.
2. Pearson AC, Castello R, Labovitz AJ, et al: Safety and utility of transesophageal echocardiography in the critically ill patient. Am Heart J 1990; 119:1083.
3. Cannon SR, Richards KL: Principles and physics of doppler. *In*: Cardiac Imaging. Marcus ML, Schelbert HR, Skorton DJ, et al (Eds). Philadelphia, WB Saunders, 1991, pp 365–373.
4. Hatle L, Angelsen B (Eds): Doppler Ultrasound in Cardiology: Physical Principles and Clinical Applications. 2nd ed. Philadelphia, Lea & Febiger, 1985.
5. Sahn DJ: Real time two-dimensional Doppler echocardiographic flow mapping. Circulation 1985; 71:849.
6. Schiller NB, Shah PM, Crawford M, et al: Recommendations for quantitation of the left ventricle by two-dimensional echocardiography. J Am Soc Echocardiogr 1989; 2:358.
6a. Appleton CP, Gallowa JM, Gonzalez MS, et al: Estimation of left ventricular filling pressures using two dimensional and Doppler echocardiography in adult patients with cardiac disease: Additional value of analyzing left atrial size, left atrial ejection fraction and the difference in duration of pulmonary venous and mitral flow velocity at atrial contraction. J Am Coll Cardiol 1993; 22:1972.
7. Yock PG, Popp RL: Non-invasive estimation of right ventricular systolic pressure by Doppler ultrasound in patients with tricuspid regurgitation. Circulation 1984; 70:657.
8. Choong CY, Abascal VM, Weyman J, et al: Prevalence of valvular regurgitation by Doppler echocardiography in patients with structurally normal hearts by two-dimensional echocardiography. Am Heart J 1989; 117:636.
9. Laaban JP, Diebold B, Zelinski R, et al: Noninvasive estimation of systolic pulmonary artery pressure using Doppler echocardiography in patients with chronic obstructive pulmonary disease. Chest 1989; 6:1258.
9a. Seppanen MP, Kappa PO, Kero PO, et al: Doppler derived systolic pulmonary artery pressure in acute neonatal respiratory distress syndrome. Pediatrics 1994; 93:769.
10. Gorcsan J III, Snow FR, Paulsen W, et al: Noninvasive estimation of left atrial pressure in patients with congestive heart failure and mitral regurgitation by Doppler echocardiography. Am Heart J 1991; 121:858.
11. Rafferty T: Transesophageal two-dimensional echocardiography in the critically ill—is the Swan Ganz catheter redundant? Yale J Biol Med 1991; 64:375.
12. Kuecherer HF, Muhiudeen IA, Kusumot FM, et al: Estimation of mean left atrial pressure from transesophageal pulsed Doppler echocardiography of pulmonary venous flow. Circulation 1990; 82:1127.
13. Gardin JM, Burn CS, Childs WJ, et al: Evaluation of blood flow velocity in the ascending aorta and main pulmonary artery of normal subjects by Doppler echocardiography. Am Heart J 1984; 107:310.
14. Huntsmann LL, Stewart DK, Barnes SR, et al: Noninvasive Doppler determination of cardiac output in man—clinical validation. Circulation 1983; 67:593.
15. Clark JG, Berberich SN, Zager JR, et al: Echocardiographic findings of pericardial effusion mimicked by fibrocalcific pericardial disease. Echocardiography 1985; 2:467.
16. Beck CS: Two cardiac compression triads. JAMA 1935; 104:714.
17. Guberman BA, Fowler NO, Engel PJ, et al: Cardiac tamponade in medical patients. Circulation 1981; 64:633.
18. Reddy PS, Curtis E, Uretsky B: Spectrum of hemodynamic changes in cardiac tamponade. Am J Cardiol 1990; 66:1487.
19. Armstrong WF, Schilt BF, Helper DJ, et al: Diastolic collapse of the right ventricle with cardiac tamponade: An echocardiographic study. Circulation 1982; 65:1491.
20. Freeman GL: The effect of the pericardium on function of normal and enlarged hearts. Cardiol Clin 1990; 8:579.
21. Hoit BD, Gabel M, Fowler NO: Cardiac tamponade in left ventricular dysfunction. Circulation 1990; 82:1370.
22. Gaffney FA, Keller AM, Peshock RM, et al: Pathophysiologic mechanisms of cardiac tamponade and pulsus alternans shown by echocardiography. Am J Cardiol 1984; 53:1662.
23. Appleton CP, Hatle LK, Popp RL: Cardiac tamponade and pericardial effusion: Respiratory variation in transvalvular flow velocities studied by Doppler echocardiography. J Am Coll Cardiol 1988; 11:1020.
24. Segnni ED, Beker B, Arbel Y, et al: Left ventricular pseudohypertrophy in pericardial effusion as a sign of cardiac tamponade. Am J Cardiol 1990; 66:508.
25. Thompson RC, Finck SJ, Leventhal JP, et al: Right-to-left shunt across a patent foramen ovale cause by cardiac tamponade: Diagnosis by transesophageal echocardiography. Mayo Clin Proc 1991; 66:391.
26. Pandian NG, Skorton DJ, Kieso RA, et al: Diagnosis of constrictive pericarditis by two-dimensional echocardiography: Studies in a new experimental model and in patients. J Am Coll Cardiol 1984; 4:1164.
27. Tei C, Child JS, Tanaka H, et al: Atrial systolic notch on the interventricular septal echocardiogram: An echocardiographic sign of constrictive pericarditis. J Am Coll Cardiol 1983; 1:907.
28. Wann LS, Weyman AE, Dillon JC, et al: Premature pulmonary valve opening. Circulation 1977; 55:128.
29. Hatle LK, Appleton CP, Popp RL: Differentiation of constrictive pericarditis and restrictive cardiomyopathy by Doppler echocardiography. J Am Coll Cardiol 1988; 11:757.
29a. Oh JK, Hatle LK, Seward JB, et al: Diagnostic role of Doppler echocardiography in constrictive pericarditis. J Am Coll Cardiol 1994; 23:154.
30. Parrillo JE, Burch C, Shelhamer JH, et al: A circulating myocardial depressant substance in humans with septic shock: Septic shock patients with reduced ejection fraction have a circulating factor that depresses in vitro myocardial cell performance. J Clin Invest 1985; 76:1539.
31. Parker MM, Shelhamer JH, Bacharach SL, et al: Profound but reversible myocardial depression in patients with septic shock. Ann Intern Med 1984; 100:483.
32. Vincent JL, Roman A, Kahn RJ: Dobutamine administration in septic shock: Addition to a standard protocol. Crit Care Med 1990; 18:689.
33. Parker MM, McCarthy KE, Ognibene FP, et al: Right ventricular dysfunction and dilation, similar to left ventricular changes, characterize the cardiac depression of septic shock in humans. Chest 1990; 97:126.
34. Dell'Italia LJ, Starling MR, Crawford MH, et al: Right ventricular infarction: Identification by hemodynamic measurements before and after volume loading as assessed by two-dimensional echocardiography. J Am Coll Cardiol 1984; 4:931.
35. Kaul S: Doppler echocardiography in critically ill cardiac patients. Cardiol Clin 1991; 9:711.
36. Nelson CW, Snow FR, Barnett M, et al: Impending paradoxical embolism: Echocardiographic diagnosis of an intracardiac thrombus crossing a patent foramen ovale. Am Heart J 1991; 122:859.
37. Wittlich N, Erbel R, Todt M, et al: Detection of pulmonary artery thrombi in transesophageal echocardiography in patients with pulmonary embolism. Eur Heart J 1989; 10(Suppl):21.
38. Sanders AO: Coronary thrombosis with complete heart block and relative ventricular tachycardia: A case report. Am Heart J 1930; 6:820.

39. Nixon JV: Right ventricular myocardial infarction. Arch Intern Med 1982: 142:945.
40. Dell'Italia LJ, Starling MR, O'Rourke RA: Physical examination for exclusion of hemodynamically important right ventricular infarction. Ann Intern Med 1983; 99:608.
41. Cohn JN, Guiha NH, Broder MI, et al: Right ventricular infarction: Clinical and hemodynamic features. Am J Cardiol 1974; 33:209.
42. Lorell B, Leinbach RC, Pohost GM, et al: Right ventricular infarction: Clinical diagnosis and differentiation from cardiac tamponade and pericardial constriction. Am J Cardiol 1979; 43:465.
43. Lee WH, Fisher J: Right ventricular diastolic disorders. Arch Intern Med 1983; 143:332.
44. Williams JF: Right ventricular infarction. Clin Cardiol 1990; 13:309.
45. Jugdutt BI, Sussex BA, Sivaran CA, et al: Right ventricular infarction: Two dimensional echocardiographic evaluation. Am Heart J 1984; 107:505.
46. Jaffe CC, Weltin G: Echocardiography of the right side of the heart. Cardiol Clin 1992; 10:41.
47. Kaul S, Tei C, Hopkins JM, et al: Assessment of right ventricular function using two-dimensional echocardiography. Am Heart J 1984; 107:526.
48. Joseph G, Jose VJ: Right ventricular filling abnormalities in acute inferior wall myocardial infarction—a pulsed Doppler study. Indian Heart J 1990; 42:437.
49. Hoit BD, Fowler NO: Influence of acute right ventricular dysfunction on cardiac tamponade. J Am Coll Cardiol 1991; 18:1787.
50. Anderson HR, Falk E, Nielsen D: Right ventricular infarction: Frequency, size and topography in coronary heart disease: A prospective study comprising 107 consecutive autopsies from a coronary care unit. J Am Coll Cardiol 1987; 10:223.
51. Chuttani K, Sussman H, Pandian NG: Echocardiographic evidence that regional right ventricular dysfunction occurs frequently in anterior myocardial infarction. Am Heart J 1991; 122:850.
52. Lewis JL, Webber JD, Sutton LL, et al: Discordance in degree of right and left ventricular dilation in patients with dilated cardiomyopathy: Recognition and clinical implications. J Am Coll Cardiol 1993; 21:649.
53. Tennant R, Wiggers CJ: The effect of coronary occlusion on myocardial contraction. Am J Physiol 1935; 112:351.
54. Nixon JV, Narahara KA, Smitherman TC: Estimation of myocardial involvement in patients with acute myocardial infarction by two-dimensional echocardiography. Circulation 1980; 62:1248.
55. Nixon JV, Brown CN, Smitherman TC: Identification of transient and persistent segmental wall motion abnormalities in patients with unstable angina by two-dimensional echocardiography. Circulation 1982; 65:1497.
56. Visser A, Lie K, Kan G, et al: Detection and quantification of acute, isolated myocardial infarction by two-dimensional echocardiography. Am J Cardiol 1981; 47:1020.
57. Nishimura RA, Tajik AJ, Shub C, et al: Role of two-dimensional echocardiography in the prediction of in-hospital complications after myocardial infarction. J Am Coll Cardiol 1984; 4:1080.
57a. Fleischmann KE, Goldman L, Robiolio PA, et al: Echocardiographic correlates of survival in patients with chest pain. J Am Coll Cardiol 1994; 23:1390.
58. Pollick C, Cujec B, Parker S, et al: Left ventricular wall motion abnormalities in subarachnoid hemorrhage: An echocardiographic study. J Am Coll Cardiol 1988; 12:600.
59. Drobac M, Gilbert B, Howard R, et al: Ventricular septal defect after myocardial infarction: Diagnosis by two-dimensional echocardiography. Circulation 1983; 67:335.
60. Panidis IP, Mintz GS, Goel I, et al: Acquired ventricular septal defect after myocardial infarction: Detection by combined two-dimensional and Doppler echocardiography. Am Heart J 1987; 111:427.
61. Meltzer RS, Guthaner D, Rakowski J, et al: Diagnosis of left ventricular thrombi by two-dimensional echocardiography. Br Heart J 1979; 42:261.
62. Stratton JR, Lighty GW Jr, Pearlman AS, et al: Detection of left ventricular thrombus by two-dimensional echocardiography: Sensitivity, specificity, and causes of uncertainty. Circulation 1982; 66:156.
63. Visser CA, Kan G, Meltzer RS, et al: Embolic potential of left ventricular thrombus after myocardial infarction: A two dimensional echocardiographic study of 119 patients. J Am Coll Cardiol 1985; 5:1276.
64. Nihoyannopoulous P, Smith GC, Maseri A, et al: The natural history of left ventricular thrombus in myocardial infarction: A rationale in support of masterly inactivity. J Am Coll Cardiol 1989; 14:903.
65. Nishimura RA, Schaff HV, Shub C, et al: Papillary muscle rupture complicating acute myocardial infarction: Analysis of 17 patients. Am J Cardiol 1983; 51:373.
66. Wei JY, Hutchins GM, Bulkley BH: Papillary muscle rupture in fatal myocardial infarction. Ann Intern Med 1979; 90:149.
67. Kaul S, Spotnitz WD, Galsheen WP, et al: Mechanism of ischemic mitral regurgitation: An experimental evaluation. Circulation 1991; 84:2167.
68. Goodley RW, Wann S, Rogers EW, et al: Incomplete mitral leaf closure in patients with papillary muscle dysfunction. Circulation 1981; 63:565.
69. Lehmann KG, Francis CK, Dodge HT, et al: Mitral regurgitation in early myocardial infarction: Incidence, clinical detection, and prognostic implications. Ann Intern Med 1992; 117:10.
70. Weisman HF, Healy B: Myocardial infarct expansion, infarct extension, and reinfarction: Pathophysiologic concepts. Prog Cardiovasc Dis 1987; 30:73.
71. Pfeffer MA, Lamas GA, Vaughan DE, et al: Effect of captopril on progressive ventricular dilation after anterior myocardial infarction. N Engl J Med 1988; 319:80.
71a. Sutton MSJ, Pfeffer MA, Plappert T, et al: Quantitative two-dimensional echocardiographic measurements are major predictors of adverse cardiovascular events after acute myocardial infarction: The protective effects of captopril. Circulation 1994; 89:68.
72. Rasmussen S, Leth A, Kjoller E, et al: Cardiac rupture in acute myocardial infarction: A review of 72 consecutive cases. Acta Med Scand 1979; 205:11.
73. Currie PJ, Seward JN, Redder GS, et al: Continuous-wave Doppler echocardiographic assessment of severity of calcific aortic stenosis: A simultaneous Doppler-catheter correlative study in 100 adult patients. Circulation 1985; 71:1162.
74. Oh JK, Taliercio CP, Holmes DR, et al: Prediction of the severity of aortic stenosis by Doppler aortic valve area determination: Prospective Doppler catheterization correlation in 100 patients. J Am Coll Cardiol 1988; 11:1227.
75. Teague SM, Heinsimer JA, Anderson JL, et al: Quantification of aortic regurgitation utilizing continuous wave Doppler ultrasound. J Am Coll Cardiol 1986; 8:592.
76. Takenaka K, Dabestani A, Gardin JM, et al: A simple Doppler echocardiographic method for estimating severity of aortic regurgitation. Am J Cardiol 1986; 57:1340.
77. Abbasi AS, Allen MW, Decristofaro D, et al: Detection and estimation of the degree of mitral regurgitation by range-gated pulsed Doppler echocardiography. Circulation 1980; 61:143.
78. Chen C, Thomas JD, Anconian J, et al: Impact of impinging wall jet on color Doppler quantification of mitral regurgitation. Circulation 1991; 84:712.
79. Gurney JW, Goodman LR: Pulmonary edema localized in right upper lobe accompanying mitral regurgitation. Radiology 1989; 171:397.
80. Henry WL, Griffith JM, Michaelis LL, et al: Measurement of mitral valve orifice area in patients with mitral valve disease by real-time, two-dimensional echocardiography. Circulation 1975; 51:827.
81. Hatle L, Angelsen B, Tromsdal A: Noninvasive assessment of atrioventricular pressure half-time by Doppler ultrasound. 1979; 60:1096.
82. Motro M, Neufeld HN: Should patients with pure mitral stenosis undergo cardiac catheterization? Am J Cardiol 1980; 46:515.
83. Ewy GA, Appleton CP, De Maria AN, et al: ACC/AHA Guidelines for the clinical application of echocardiography: A report of the American College of Cardiology/American Heart

Association Task Force on assessment of diagnostic and therapeutic cardiovascular procedures (Subcommittee to develop guidelines for the clinical application of echocardiography). J Am Coll Cardiol 1990; 16:1505.
84. Gott VL, Pyeritz RE, Magovern GJ Jr, et al: Surgical treatment of aneurysms of the ascending aorta in the Marfan syndrome: Results of composite-graft repair in 50 patients. N Engl J Med 1986; 314:1070.
85. Hirst AE Jr, Johns VL Jr, Kime SW Jr: Dissecting aneurysm of the aorta: A review of 505 cases. Medicine 1958; 37:217.
86. Daily PO, Trueblood HW, Stinson EB, et al: Management of acute aortic dissection. Ann Thorc Surg 1970; 10:237.
87. DeBakey ME, Henly WS, Cooley DA, et al: Surgical management of dissecting aneurysms of the aorta. J Thorac Cardiovasc Surg 1965; 49:130.
88. Cigarroa JE, Isselbacher EM, DeSanctis RW, et al: Diagnostic imaging in the evaluation of suspected aortic dissection: Old standards and new directions. N Engl J Med 1993; 328:35.
89. Nienaber CA, Spielmann RP, von Kodolitsch Y, et al: Diagnosis of thoracic aortic dissection magnetic imaging versus transesophageal echocardiography. Circulation 1992; 85:434.
90. Nienaber CA, von Kodolitsch Y, Nicolas V, et al: The diagnosis of thoracic aortic dissection by noninvasive imaging procedures. N Engl J Med 1993; 328:1.
91. Nienaber CA, von Kodolitsch Y, Nicolas V, et al: The diagnosis of thoracic aortic dissection by noninvasive imaging procedures. N Engl J Med 1993; 328:1.
92. Mugge A, Daniel WG, Frank G, et al: Echocardiography in infective endocarditis: Reassessment of prognostic implications of vegetation size determined by the transthoracic and the transesophageal approach. J Am Coll Cardiol 1989; 14:631.
93. Erbel R, Rohman S, Drexler M, et al: Improved diagnostic value of echocardiography in patients with infective endocarditis by transesophageal approach: A prospective study. Eur Heart J 1988; 9:43.
94. Stewart JA, Silimperi D, et al: Echocardiographic documentation of vegetative lesions in infectious endocarditis: Clinical implications. Circulation 1980; 61:374.
95. Sanfilippo AJ, Picard MH, Davidoff R, et al: Prediction of risk for complications in patients with left sided infectious endocarditis. J Am Coll Cardiol 1989; 13(Suppl A):72A.
96. Arnett EN, Roberts WC: Prosthetic valve endocarditis: Clinicopathological analysis of 22 necropsy patients with comparison of observations in 74 necropsy patients with active infective endocarditis involving natural left-sided cardiac valves. Am J Cardiol 1976; 38:281.
97. Kissane RW: Traumatic heart disease. Circulation 1952; 6:421.
98. Hiatt JR, Yeatman LA Jr, Child JS: The value of echocardiography in blunt chest trauma. J Trauma 1988; 28:914.
99. Miller FB, Shumate CR, Richardson D: Myocardial contusion: When can the diagnosis be eliminated? Arch Surg 1989; 124:805.
100. Wisner DH, Reed WH, Riddick RS: Suspected myocardial contusion: Triage and indications for monitoring. Ann Surg 1990; 212:82.

CHAPTER 44

Transesophageal Echocardiography

David T. Porembka, DO, FCCP, FCCM • Keith L. Stein, MD, FCCM, FCCP • Morris I. Bierman, MD • Tom Masciangelo, MD

Advances in ultrasound technology have led to the development of transesophageal echocardiography (TEE) as a powerful diagnostic and monitoring tool for critical care physicians.[1–4a] TEE currently allows biplanar imaging of the heart and its contiguous structures and has capabilities for pulsed-wave and continuous-wave Doppler echocardiography.[5] Omniplanar and multiplanar imaging with TEE is also approaching the clinical arena.[10] Color-flow Doppler increased the utility and efficacy of TEE as a diagnostic tool. The standard TEE probe is either phase or annular array, with high-frequency transducers (5.0 or 7.5 MHz) that allow greater resolution but less tissue penetration than the standard two-dimensional transthoracic echocardiography (TTE) probe of 2.5 to 3.5 MHz. Pediatric probes, which can also be used for adults, are smaller and use a frequency of 7.5 MHz. Application of intraoperative and outpatient TEE has led to the next obvious venue, the intensive care unit (ICU).[2–4] This chapter addresses indications, contraindications, complications, and growing applications for TEE.

INDICATIONS

The indications for TEE vary between disciplines (medical, surgical, anesthesiology, or ICU). For example, TEE has been generally used for outpatient assessment. It is increasingly being used in the operating room (cardiac and noncardiac surgical patients), emergency room, and ICU. During operative management, the anesthesiologist uses TEE for evaluation of preload (structural assessment of chamber size) and function, especially for evaluation of new regional wall-motion abnormalities (RWMA) and valvular integrity during cardiac surgery (Table 44–1).

The indications for use in an ICU are for hemodynamic assessment: to evaluate ventricular chamber size and function, as well as valvular function (prosthetic and native); to search for intracardiac shunts, aortic pathology (aortic dissection or tear, aortic debris or thrombus), masses (thrombus and tumor), endocarditis and its complications (e.g., abscess); and to investigate complications of coronary artery disease, including RWMA.[1–4] Our indications for use in the ICU have expanded, especially in patients who have a confusing hemodynamic pattern seemingly discordant with their pathophysiologic disease state.

CONTRAINDICATIONS

TEE is contraindicated in patients with esophageal pathology, such as a history of esophageal surgery, strictures, varices, systemic sclerosis, esophagitis, or chest wall radiation. Upper gastrointestinal bleeding, dysphagia, and odynophagia are also contraindications.[1–5] A gastroenterologist should be consulted first for any patient suspected of having esophageal disease. In general, patients having elective operations should be fasting (nil per os) for 6 to 8 hours

TABLE 44–1. Uses for Transesophageal Echocardiography During Cardiac Surgery

Before Cardiopulmonary Bypass
Evaluation of valvular morphology to refine type of surgical repair, especially of the mitral valve
Emergent operations lacking complete preoperative assessment
After Cardiopulmonary Bypass
Evaluation for new or residual regurgitation after valve repair
Evaluation for new valvular stenosis after valve repair
Detection of dynamic left ventricular outflow tract obstruction after mitral valve repair
Detection of intraoperative myocardial ischemia/infarction (RWMA)
Detection of residual intracardiac shunting: atrial and ventricular septal defects, patent foramen ovale, penetrating trauma
Detection of periprosthetic regurgitation

before the procedure. Patients who are at risk for aspiration of gastric contents or who have a "full stomach" (e.g., pregnant women) are of concern but can be treated safely. Such "high-risk" patients should first receive prophylaxis such as histamine$_2$ antagonists or nonparticulate antacids. If marked sedation with midazolam or fentanyl is required, the airway must be adequately protected before insertion of a TEE probe.

COMPLICATIONS

Complications of the TEE examination are not uncommon (<1.0%).[6, 7] In a multicenter study of 10,419 TEE examinations including 88.7% conscious patients, the probe could not be successfully placed in only 201 of the cases because of poor patient cooperation or operator inexperience (98.5%) or anatomic reasons (1.5%).[7] After TEE placement, less than 1% of the examinations had to be interrupted because of patient's intolerance. One death occurred as a result of hematemesis due to unsuspected lung carcinoma that had eroded into the esophagus.[7] Other described complications include arrhythmias, angina, congestive heart failure, laryngospasm, bronchospasm, hypoxia, and temporary vocal cord dysfunction.[7]

In patients suspected of having esophageal disease, the incidence of esophageal perforation complicating flexible esophageal gastroscopy as low as 0.02% to 0.03%.[8] Only two esophageal tears or perforations have been reported with TEE.[7] Other mechanical complications include Mallory-Weiss tear,[9] transtracheal placement, bronchial obstruction, and aortic compression, particularly in children. Mechanical malfunction of the TEE probe was described in four patients, with buckling of its tip. Resistance in movement of the probe was the only initial sign.

The question arises, can prolonged use of the probe potentially cause injury? The authors have left the TEE probe in place for as long as 10 hours. This has been particularly helpful in critically ill patients with conflicting clinical hemodynamic data. In the author's opinion, esophageal damage is of minimal concern during this prolonged use. Studies of both animals and humans have shown that if the probe is not left in the locked position under tension for long periods, esophageal injury should not occur.[10]

Bacteremia has been associated with TEE in 3.2% to 12% of patients.[11] Routine antibiotic prophylaxis is not recommended for TEE by the American Heart Association. Several studies have confirmed the low incidence of bacteremia from which recommendations were founded.[12] Shyu and colleagues studied 135 patients with no incidence of bacteremia.[11a] Whether critically ill patients who have gram-negative or fungal colonization of the gut in an ICU are at higher risk has yet to be established.

ANATOMIC IMAGES

Major advantages of TEE are its ability to image the heart and contiguous structures, many of which are relatively inaccessible to TTE, and for high-resolution imaging from a retrocardiac position free from the intervening chest wall and lung parenchyma. Single-plane (transverse) TEE reveals the left atrial appendage, allows superior evaluation of mitral regurgitation in both prosthetic and native valves, and shows portions of the thoracic aorta, all invisible to TTE.[1] Biplanar (transverse and longitudinal) TEE provides a clearer view of the atrial septum (especially with a large aorta), right ventricular outflow tract (including conduits), mitral valve leaflets and its regurgitant jets, and the apical region of the left ventricle, as well as a short-axis view of the aortic valve and the number of aortic cusps. An ectatic aorta is better visualized with the longitudinal view.[5] We have noted limited views of the left ventricle with TEE in only two patients who had mediastinal emphysema and severe acute lung injury and required high levels of positive end-expiratory pressure (PEEP). Obvious considerations include the need for experienced TEE operators, the availability of echocardiography machines, and the inherent costs of this advanced technology.

Others have detailed the anatomic images possible with TEE.[1, 5] The three major transverse views are the basal short-axis view, four-chamber or frontal long-axis view, and short-axis view of the left ventricle (at the midpapillary region). Longitudinal views are at the midesophageal region (corresponding to the four chamber view) and the transgastric region. Additional longitudinal views include the base of the heart and the great vessels (corresponding to the position in the basal short-axis view with transverse imaging) (Figs. 44–1 to 44–4). Most of the thoracic aorta can be visualized with the transverse and longitudinal planes, but the ascending aorta and arch are not totally assessed (Fig. 44–5). Orientations of the longitudinal view depend on the operator's experience and institutional practice standards.

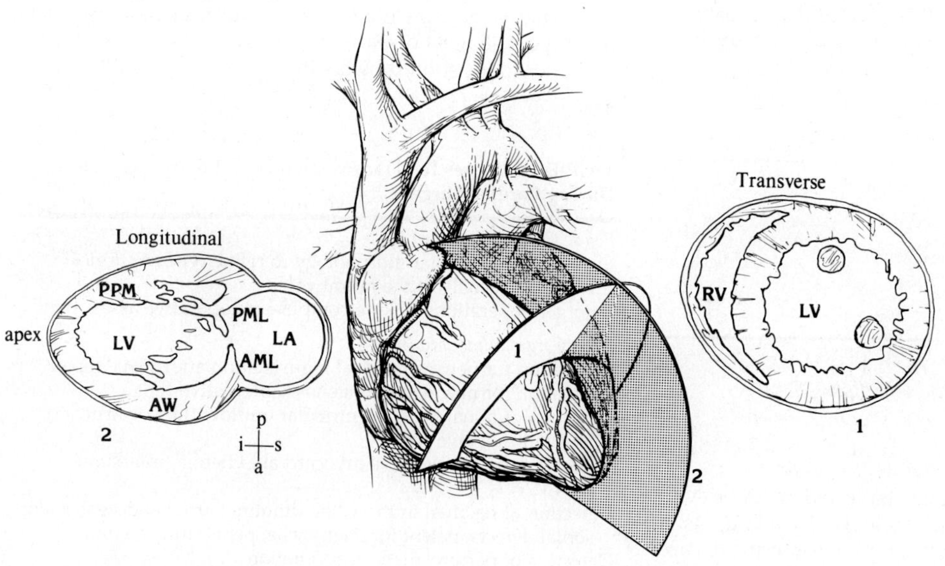

Figure 44–1. Transgastric view. Longitudinal and transverse imaging with transesophageal echocardiography. *Abbreviations*: a = anterior; AML = anterior mitral leaflet; AW = anterior wall; i = inferior; LA = left atrium; LV = left ventricle; p = posterior; PML = posterior mitral leaflet; PPM = posterior papillary muscle; RV = right ventricle; s = superior.

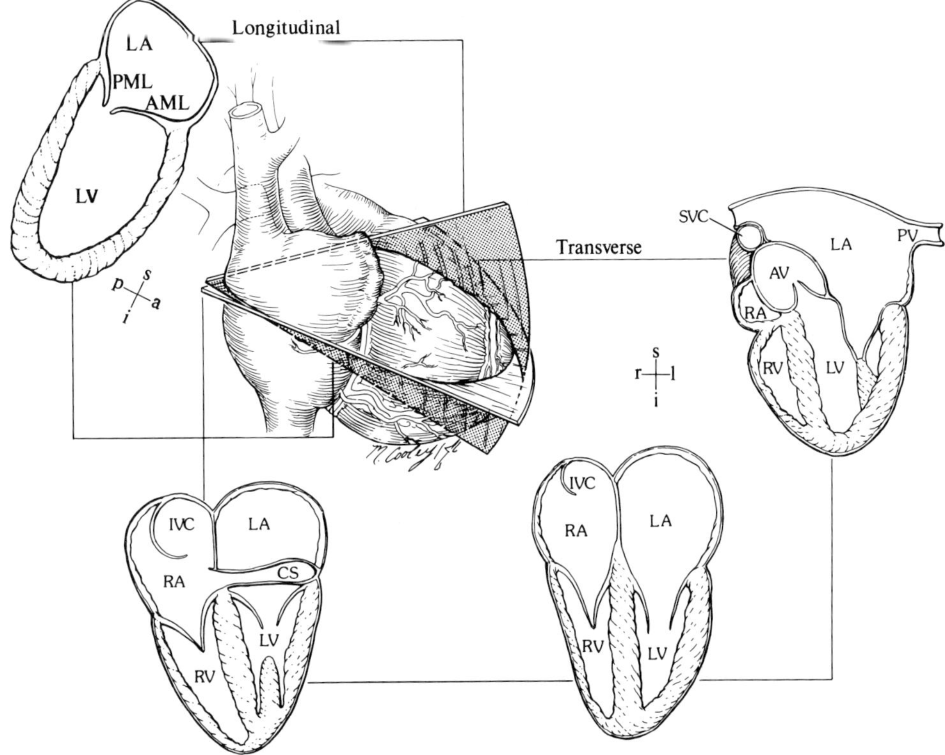

Figure 44–2. Midesophageal view. Longitudinal and transverse imaging with transesophageal echocardiography. *Abbreviations*: RA = right atrium; CS = coronary sinus; PV = pulmonary vein; IVC = inferior vena cava; SVC = superior vena cava; s = superior; l = left; r = right; i = inferior.

Figure 44–3. Base of the heart. Transverse imaging with transesophageal echocardiography. *Abbreviations*: AO = aorta; LAA = left atrial appendage; LLPV = left lower pulmonary vein; LUPV = left upper pulmonary vein; FO = fossa ovalis; LCA = left coronary artery; MPA = main pulmonary artery; PV = pulmonary vein; RAA = right atrial appendage; RCA = right coronary artery; RLPV = right lower pulmonary vein; RPA = right pulmonary artery; RUPV = right upper pulmonary vein.

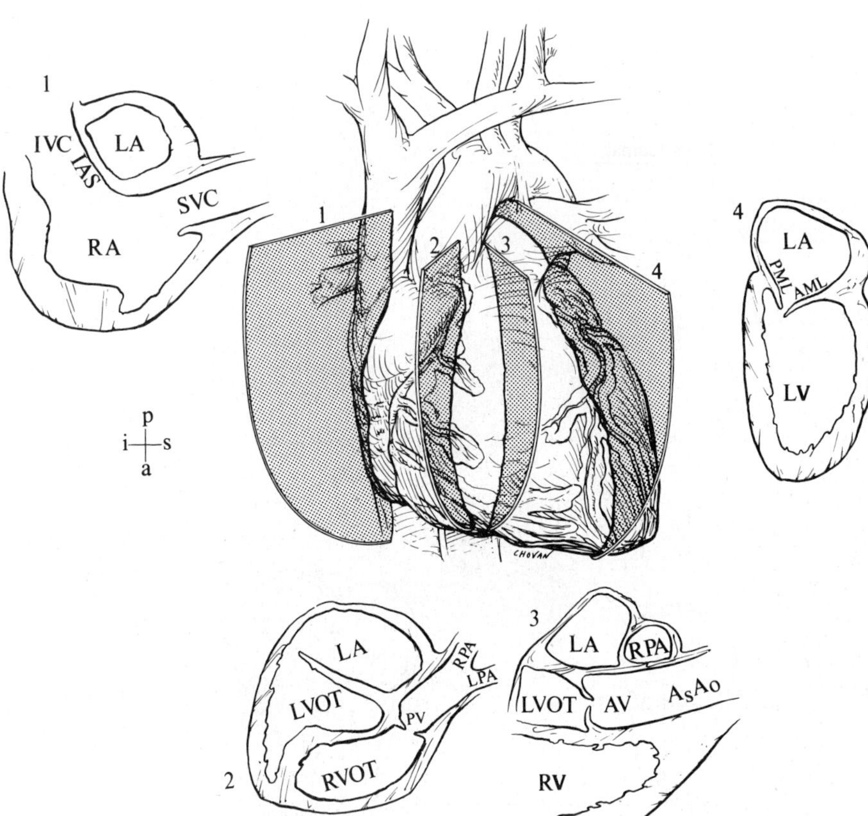

Figure 44–4. Base of the heart. Longitudinal views with transesophageal echocardiography. *Abbreviations*: ASAO = ascending aorta; AV = aortic valve; IAS = interatrial septum; LPA = left pulmonary artery; LVOT = left ventricle outflow tract; PV = pulmonary valve; RVOT = right ventricular outflow tract.

APPLICATIONS OF TRANSESOPHAGEAL ECHOCARDIOGRAPHY

Aortic Pathology

Aortic Dissection or Tear

TEE has demonstrated its benefit in diagnosing acute aortic dissection[12–21b] (Fig. 44–6, and Table 44–2). The technique has proved useful in evaluating the aorta for thrombus and atherosclerotic debris.[22–28] Correct identification of an acute aortic tear or dissection can be life saving.[15,21,22] Two-dimensional TEE has circumvented the limitations encountered earlier with the use of M-mode and TTE. Erbel and colleagues, in the European Cooperative Study, evaluated the efficacy of TEE for diagnosing acute aortic dissection compared with standard methods of computed tomography (CT) scanning and angiography.[13] The diagnosis of aortic dissection was confirmed by surgery or autopsy. The sensitivity for TEE was 99% and specificity 98%, compared with 88% and 94% for angiography and 83% and 100% for CT. In addition, aortic insufficiency and pericardial effusions can often be recognized. Hashimoto and coworkers, using TEE Doppler assessment for the diagnosis of dissecting aortic aneurysm, showed correct detection of the entry and intimal flap in all cases, compared with a 42% detection rate using conventional modalities.[14] Ballal and associates divided their cases into two groups: Group 1 consisted of 34 patients in whom the aortic dissection was proved by surgery, aortography, or autopsy; group 2 consisted of 27 patients with aortic dissection precluded by aortography.[16] CT was perfomed in 24 patients in group 1 and provided for a correct diagnosis in 67% of the patients but misclassified the type of dissection in 33% of the patients. TEE correctly identified the dissection in 29 of the 34 patients with a sensitivity of 97%, a specificity of 100%, and a positive and negative predictive value of 100% and 96%, respectively. In group 2, TEE correctly precluded aortic dissection in all 27 patients. Of particular interest was the echocardiographic identification of the coronary artery involvement with the aortic dissection in six of seven patients.[16]

TEE is useful for assessing repaired type A aortic dissection.[17] Upper ascending aortic diameter greater than 35 mm is considered to be highly pathologic. Patients have a higher survival rate (90%) when no flow is detected in the false lumen, easily assessed by color-flow Doppler. In addition, TEE assesses the integrity and function of the aortic and mitral valves, evaluates left ventricular function and volume, identifies pericardial effusion, and shows involvement of the coronary arteries. As with CT, TEE identifies prosthetic false aneurysms and sinus of Valsalva aneurysms.

TEE with color-coded Doppler flow imaging has been compared with magnetic resonance imaging (MRI) for diagnosing aortic dissection.[19,20] The sensitivities for both MRI and TEE were 100%. However, the specificities were lower with TEE (68.2%) than MRI (100%) because of false-positive results with TEE, particularly in evaluating the ascending aorta and arch. Thrombus formation in the false lumen of

TABLE 44–2. Transesophageal Echocardiographic Identification of Acute Aortic Dissection: Typical Findings

Small true lumen
Large false lumen
Entry site(s)
Communication between the lumina demonstrated by color-flow Doppler
Intimal flap with undulating motion
Accentuated color-flow Doppler in the true lumen
Thrombus in the false lumen and spontaneous echo

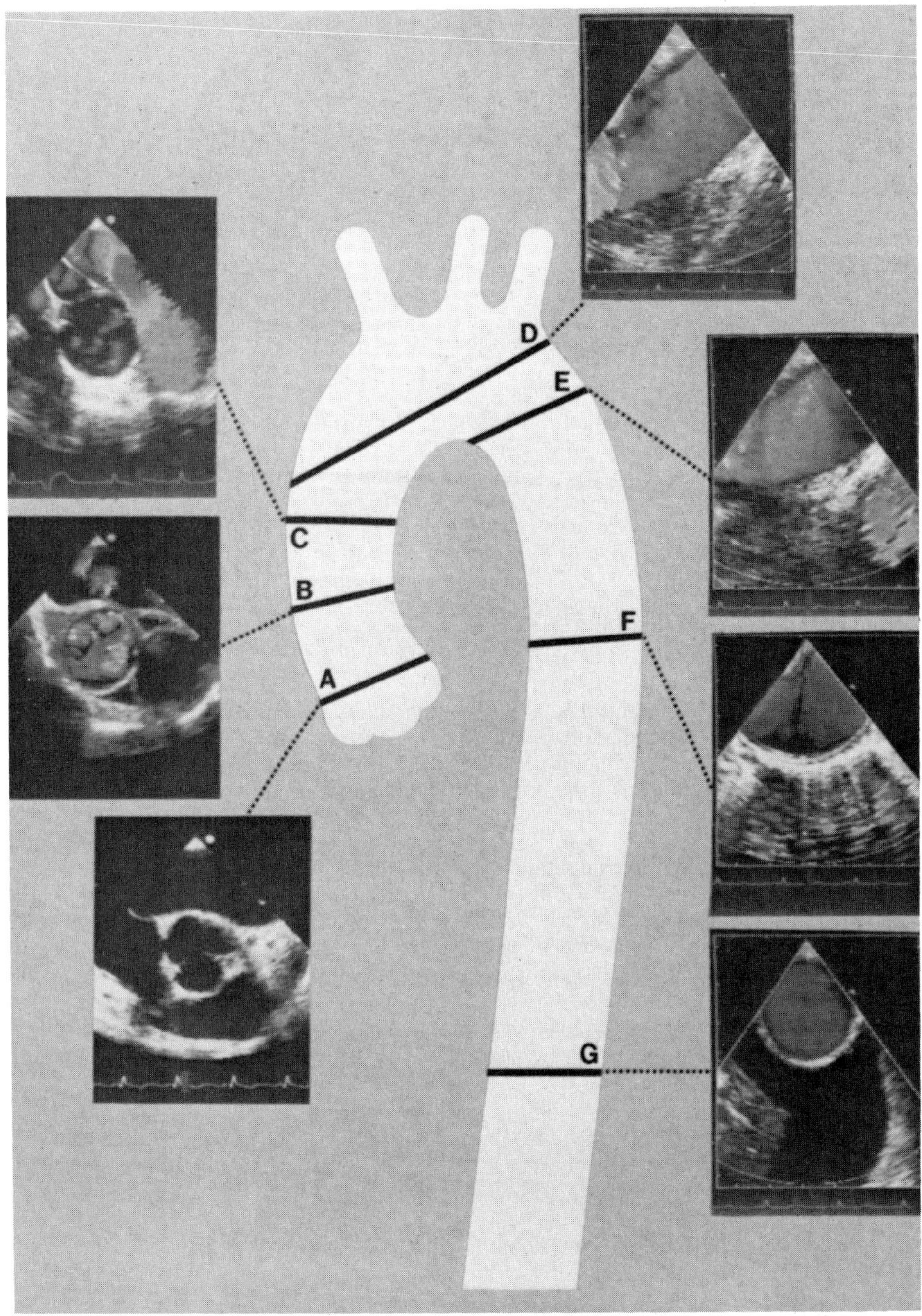

Figure 44–5. Thoracic aorta. Sequential transverse imaging of the ascending, arch, and descending thoracic aorta of normal anatomy with color flow Doppler echocardiography. (From Chandrasekaran K, Currie PJ: Transesophageal echocardiography in aortic dissection: Review. J Invasive Cardiol 1989; 1:333.) (See Color Plate Section of this textbook.)

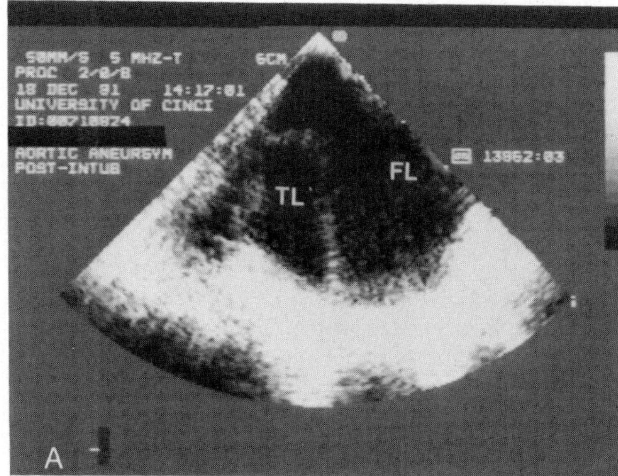

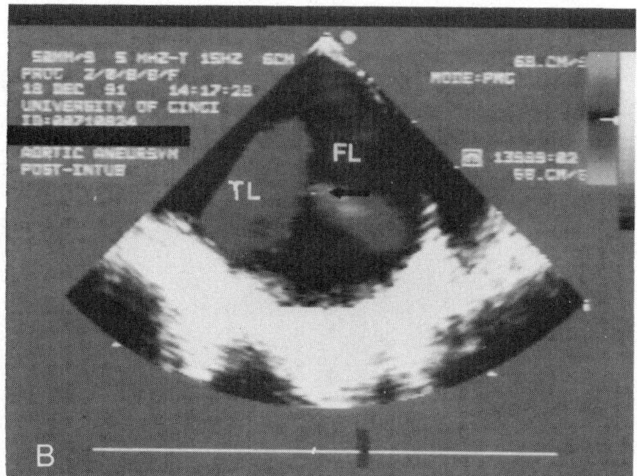

Figure 44–6. Aortic dissection. *A*, Transverse imaging reveals an intimal flap with a small true lumen and a larger false lumen. Spontaneous echo contrast is indicative of thrombus formation. *B*, Transverse imaging with color-flow Doppler echocardiography reveals a small true lumen and a larger false lumen with a jet crossing through the entry site into the false lumen. *Abbreviations*: FL = false lumen; TL = true lumen. (See Color Plate Section of this textbook.)

the aortic arch and the descending segments of the thoracic aorta was easily and consistently identified with MRI. The identification frequency of aortic regurgitation, pericardial effusion, and entry site of the dissection was the same with the two techniques. A follow-up study of aortic dissection by Nienaber and colleagues evaluated MRI, TEE, TTE, and CT.[20] The sensitivities of TTE, TEE, MRI, and CT were 59.3%, 97.7%, 98.3%, and 93.8%, respectively. The specificities were similar to their earlier study, with 83%, 76.9%, 97.8%, and 87.1%, respectively for TTE, TEE, MRI, and CT. False-positive results may occur with TEE, resulting from extensive plaque formation and echo reverberations in the ectatic vessel.[20] Biplanar images may further improve the evaluation of the ascending aorta and arch. Although MRI provides greater delineation of the pathology of the aorta, TEE should be used in the acute setting because it is much more convenient than MRI. Compared with the gold standard (angiography), TEE appears sufficient to evaluate and monitor patients with acute aortic dissection. TEE should be used for follow-up evaluation of postsurgical or medical management of aortic dissection and can be particularly helpful in delineating other causes of hemodynamic instability that mimic aortic dissection.[16] TEE is also useful for evaluating the aorta after a traumatic chest injury. One looks for an aortic wall hematoma associated with intimal tear or a pericardial effusion with intimal tear. In trauma cases, aortography may be too time consuming and provide only limited information. TEE, which is safe and prompt, provides an excellent imaging tool for diagnosis of traumatic aortic rupture or tear or a periaortic hematoma. If the diagnosis is questionable in any way, other modalities can then be used, depending on a patient's clinical status.

Aortic Thrombus and Debris

TEE has revealed the amount and extent of atheromatous debris in the aorta that can contribute to significant morbidity. Atherosclerotic debris in the aorta has now been associated with coronary artery disease. When the debris was mobile and penndunculated, the incidence of embolic event was increased.[21, 24] Some patients with transient ischemic attacks have been found to have plaques that were only visualized with TEE.[27] A significant increase in stroke postoperatively is noted in patients with mobile atheroma.[25] TEE can be used to identify debris in the ascending aorta and to alter the site of aortic cannulation and cross-clamping, in order to limit the extent of a cerebral event after cardiac surgery.[27a]

Also of concern to critical care physicians (in addition to

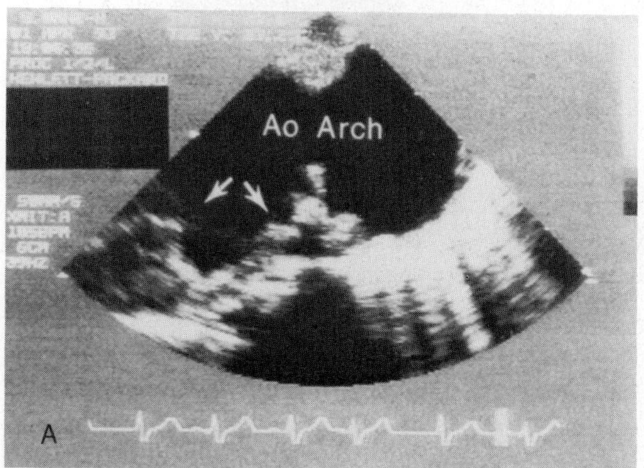

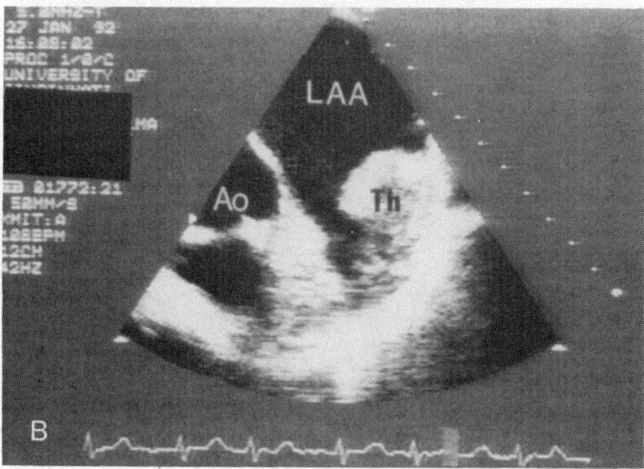

Figure 44–7. Extracardiac masses. *A*, Transverse image of the arch of the aorta with free-flowing pedunculated atherosclerotic debris. *B*, Transverse image of the left atrial appendage with thrombus. *Abbreviations*: Ao = aortic valve; LAA = left atrial appendage; Th = thrombus.

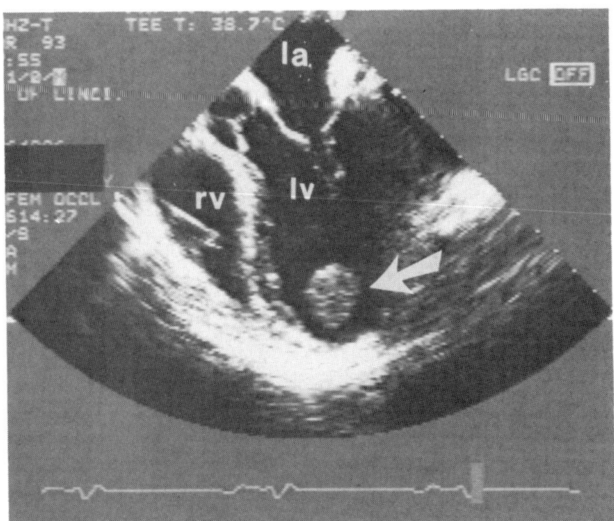

Figure 44–8. Intracardiac thrombus. Foreshortened long axis transverse view of the left ventricle identifying a 2.0 × 3.0-cm thrombus *(arrow)* in an 83-year-old woman who had undergone emergency surgery for an acute aortic femoral occlusion. *Abbreviations*: la = left atrium; lv = left ventricle; rv = right ventricle.

cerebral embolization of aortic debris) is peripheral embolization causing occult organ damage. For example, the authors identified a large thoracic thrombus in the descending thoracic aorta that caused multiple system organ failure in a previously healthy patient.[26] Other reports have also identified organ dysfunction from distal embolization of thoracic aortic debris.[27] In patients with occult single or multiple organ dysfunction or acute lower-extremity ischemia that cannot be explained, TEE can evaluate cardiac chambers and the aorta in search for the origin of emboli[28] (Figs. 44–7 and 44–8).

Endocarditis and Abscesses

Echocardiographic diagnosis of endocarditis in a patient who presented with typical signs and symptoms and a prosthetic mitral valve has often been difficult or inconclusive with TTE[29, 29a] (Fig. 44–9). The ability to see behind the mitral valve apparatus with TEE has helped considerably, because limitation with TTE was seen as acoustic shadowing from the prosthetic valve. The rate for identification of vegetations with TEE was 94%, compared with 40% with TTE. TEE has a sensitivity and specificity of 100% and 98%, respectively, and a positive and negative predictive value of 95% and 100%, respectively. The sensitivity and specificity with TTE were 63% and 98%, respectively.[30]

The size of vegetations affects the detection rate and the extent of morbidity. When the size of the vegetation is less than 5 mm, 6 to 10 mm, or greater than 11 mm, the detection rate with TEE is consistently 100%. In contrast, TTE detection rates are 25%, 70%, and 100%, respectively.[30] The prognostic implication of vegetation size by TEE is that when the size exceeds 10 mm, the incidence of an embolic event is 47%.[31]

Aortic valve endocarditis with abscess formation has a mortality rate of 23%[32] (Fig. 44–10). As in prior studies of endocarditis, TEE had a sensitivity and specificity of 87% and 94.6%, respectively, and positive and negative predictive values of 90.9% and 92.1%, respectively. With TTE, the sensitivity, specificity, and positive and negative predictive values were 28.3%, 98.6%, 92.9%, and 68.9%, respectively.[32] TEE may be limited in visualizing the tricuspid valve.[33] In patients with prosthetic or bioprosthetic aortic or mitral valves and endocarditis, TTE is of limited usefulness because of the acoustic shadowing from the prosthetic devices. TTE detects only 33% of endocarditis cases, whereas TEE detects vegetations in 82% of patients and thrombi in 100% of patients.[34]

TEE is particularly helpful in identifying pathology of subaortic structures such as the mitral-aortic intervalvular fibrosa area, difficult to see with TTE. In this area, an abscess or aneurysm can occur, then perforate and subsequently communicate with the left atrium, resulting in mitral regurgitation. Similarly, the ventricular surface of the anterior mitral leaflet can be easily visualized when looking for secondary infection. Patients who have eccentric jets of mitral regurgitation or unexplained congestive heart failure on TTE should undergo further evaluation with TEE to identify subaortic complications (which may be more common than previously recognized) and to evaluate these patients for future medical or surgical therapy.[35]

With longitudinal and omniplanar TEE imaging, the mi-

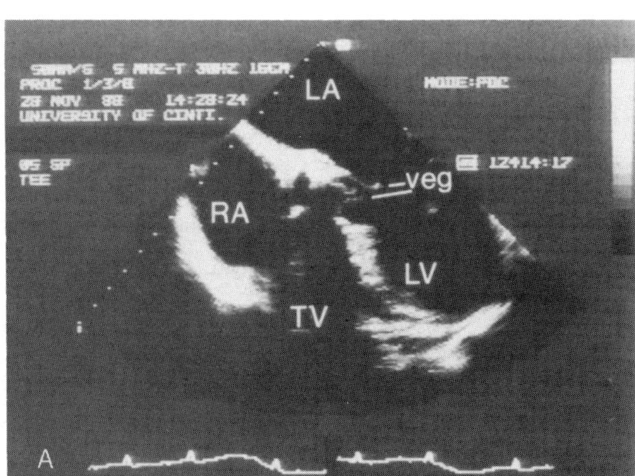

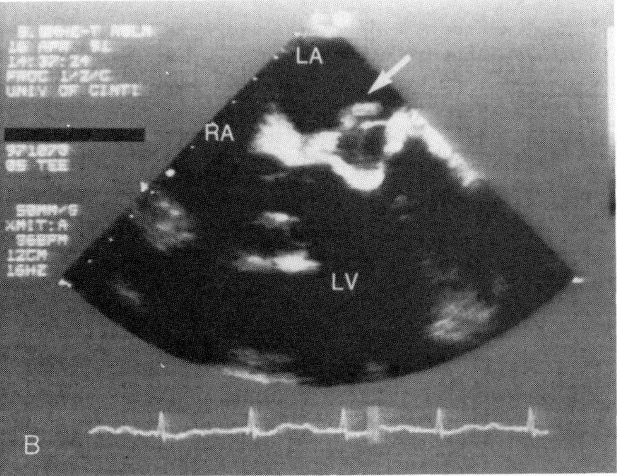

Figure 44–9. Endocarditis. *A*, Four-chamber transverse view identifying vegetations on the aortic valve that were not detected by transthoracic echocardiography. *B*, Foreshortened long axis view (transverse) of the mitral prosthetic valve apparatus *(arrow)*, a large mass that was not visualized with transthoracic echocardiography. *Abbreviation*: veg = vegetations.

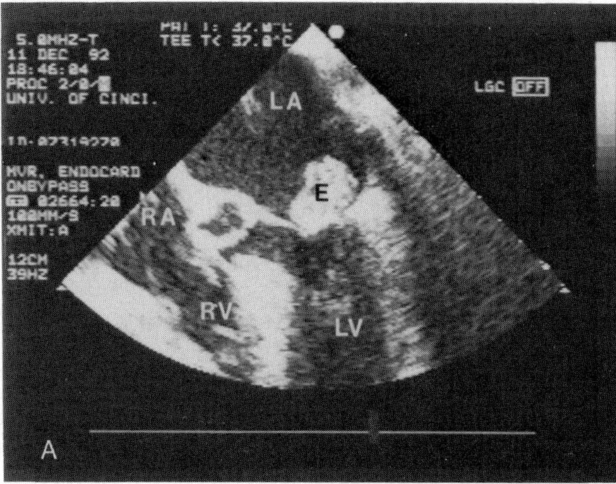

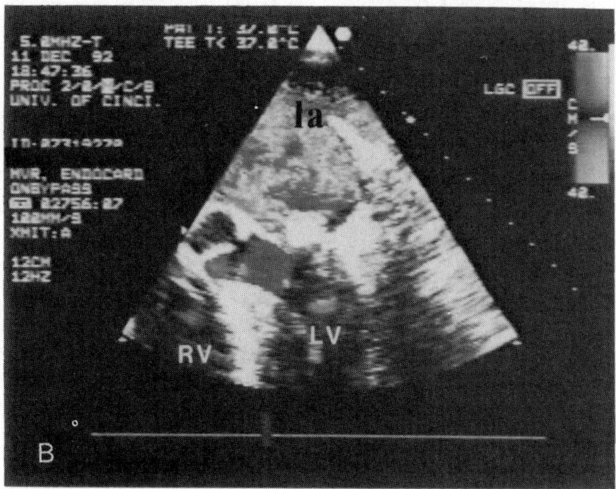

Figure 44–10. Endocarditis and mitral regurgitation. *A*, A 2.8 × 1.8-cm vegetation associated with an abscess attached to the posterior mitral valve leaflet (transverse view). *B*, The corresponding transverse view shows 4+ mitral regurgitation that enters the left superior pulmonary vein. *Abbreviation*: E = vegetation. (See Color Plate Section of this textbook.)

tral and pulmonic valves and adjacent structures are better visualized. In patients with right-sided cardiac lesions, TTE may not identify small vegetations. These patients should undergo TEE with biplanar imaging. Even in high-risk patients with previously negative TEE results looking for endocarditis, repeat TEE should be performed to identify any new endocarditis.[36] TEE can occasionally be used serially to evaluate disease progression of endocarditis treated conservatively with medical management.

Intracardiac and Extracardiac Masses

The cause of intracardiac masses can be either thrombus material or neoplastic tissue, associated with obstruction or systemic embolization.[37–40] The differential echocardiographic characteristics between thrombus and tumor have been described elsewhere.[38] TEE is particularly helpful when TTE evaluation is inconclusive, such as with small tumors and thrombi, laminated thrombi, thrombi limited to the left or right atrial appendage, or poor images.[39]

Faletra and colleagues compared TTE, TEE, MRI, and CT for evaluating mediastinal masses.[40] MRI and CT are excellent means for detecting them. In comparison with TTE, TEE is more accurate in identifying the mass, its structure, and its relationship to contiguous structures. Biplanar and omniplanar technology increases the capacity to delineate and define mediastinal masses.

An unsuspected extracardiac mass occasionally appears during examination of critically ill patients. This extracardiac mass can contribute to hypotension by compressing the pulmonary vein(s), thus decreasing left ventricular filling (Fig. 44–11*A*). Pericardiac neoplastic masses have been studied with TEE. Pulmonary venous obstruction is evaluated with Doppler flow characteristics and measurement of the diameter of the pulmonary vein. Peak velocities and time-velocity integrals in the obstructed pulmonary vein are increased, and the deceleration times of systolic flow are sometimes prolonged. After appropriate therapy, these characteristics normalize.

TTE can be inconclusive in diagnosing a mass, especially in the presence of prosthetic valves.[37] TEE overcomes this dilemma by having imaging ability posterior to the mechanical device and in the left atrial appendage (see Fig. 44–7*B*). Left atrial thrombus can be seen particularly in patients who

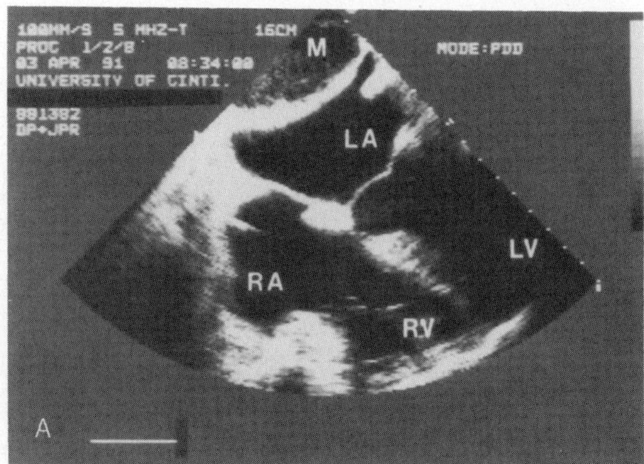

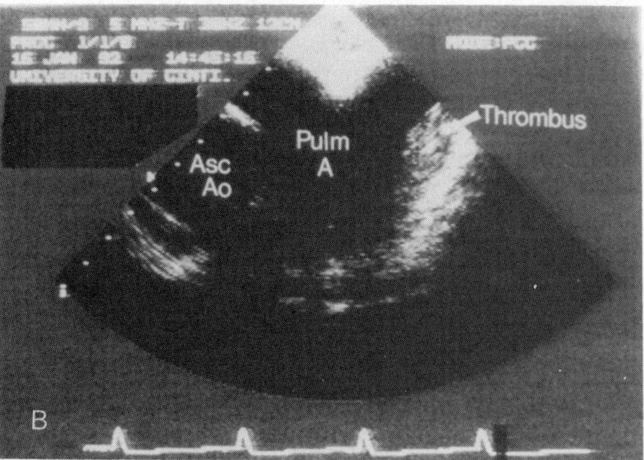

Figure 44–11. Extracardiac mass. *A*, TEE of a surgical patient with cardiac tamponade. Follow-up TEE (postexploration) revealed a large extracardiac mass posterior to the left atrium that was compressing the left atrium and the pulmonary veins (transverse view). *B*, Transverse image of the main pulmonary artery revealed a thrombus on the main and left pulmonary artery. *Abbreviations*: Asc Ao = ascending aorta; Pulm A = pulmonary artery.

have mitral stenosis or atrial fibrillation. A thrombus is occasionally visualized adjacent to central lines. Spontaneous contrast as a prelude to formation of a thrombus is usually seen with TEE but not with TTE, particularly when the left atrial end-systolic area exceeds 30 cm^2.[41] TEE should be used for assessing an atrial thrombus (especially in evaluating the atrial appendage), particularly if a patient has signs and symptoms of systemic embolization and is undergoing cardioversion, or mitral valve repair or replacement.[42] TEE visualized atrial thrombi in 13% of patients who had recent onset of atrial fibrillation and who were scheduled for elective cardioversion.[43] TEE evaluation may be considered to preclude a thrombus in patients who are in an ICU, have acute-onset atrial fibrillation, and are to be cardioverted. Before mitral valvuloplasty, TEE is similarly performed to rule out any thrombus in the atrium or appendage. During percutaneous mitral balloon valvulotomy, TEE has also helped in guiding insertion of the balloon catheter through the stenotic orifice of the mitral valve and evaluating the residual mitral regurgitation and intracardiac shunt.

TEE may be misleading in falsely identifying a mass.[44] For example, what appeared to be a right atrial mass in a patient undergoing replacement of the mitral valve was not. If a "mass" is found, other TEE views should always be used for complete definition. If a question persists, MRI or CT scan should be performed.

Pulmonary Embolism

TEE can be particularly beneficial during the acute resuscitative phase and the critical evaluation of a patient who is in shock or hypoxic condition. In addition to being able to assess left ventricular function and volume, the clinician can sometimes detect thrombi in the right atrium, ventricle, or pulmonary artery. If the diagnosis of pulmonary embolism can be made with TEE, an unstable patient may avoid the risks associated with pulmonary arteriography[45] (see Fig. 44–11*B*). A high index of suspicion for pulmonary embolism exists if TEE shows right ventricular dilatation or hypokinesis, reduced left ventricular dimensions and increased right ventricular–left ventricular diameter ratio, abnormal septal position and paradoxical systolic motion (compatible with increased right ventricular pressure and volume overload), unusual pulmonary or tricuspid regurgitation with increased flow velocity within regurgitant jets, or pulmonary artery dilatation.[46]

Intracardiac Shunts

Atrial Septal Defects

Intracardiac shunts, acquired and congenital, are occasionally noted in critically ill patients.[47] TEE correctly identifies all ostium secundum and ostium primum defects. The maximum color Doppler jet width of the flow across the atrial septal defect (ASD) only loosely correlates with the ASD size found at surgery but does reflect shunt flow volume. In comparison with cardiac catheterization, the calculated shunt flow volume and pulmonary-to-systemic blood flow ratio showed close correlation with TEE. In patients with sinus venosus ASD, TEE is superior to TTE and correctly identifies all defects; TTE demonstrates ASD in only 75% of these patients.

Patent Foramen Ovale

Paradoxical air embolism is a real phenomenon and is a concern for critical care physicians. The estimates of the prevalence of patent foramen ovale (PFO) defined by postmortem studies is 25% to 35%.[48] At basal in vivo conditions, the patency is 5% to 10% but increases to 18% to 22% after augmentation of the pressure differential in the atria by the Valsalva maneuver, coughing, or sudden release of positive intrathoracic pressure.[49–51] Detection of a PFO by contrast imaging using agitated saline with TEE is far superior to that of TTE.[49–51a] A Valsalva maneuver enhances the value of this "microbubble" test. This is particularly important in assessing cardiac patients and individuals with unexplained strokes. Hausmann and colleagues detected a PFO in 50% of patients who were younger than 40 years and who had an unexplained ischemic stroke.[50] Three groups were studied: group A, 74 patients with a history of unexplained ischemic stroke or peripheral embolic events; group B, 48 patients with embolic events explained by other cardiac abnormalities; and group C, patients who had no embolic events. The prevalence of a PFO by TEE in groups A, B, and C was 22%, 21%, and 22%, respectively. These results, when compared with TTE, revealed an overall detection rate of only 8%. Chen and associates found a PFO in 44% of patients during normal breathing and 63% during a Valsalva maneuver with contrast TEE during cardiac catheterization.[52] With contrast TTE, a shunt was found in only 25% of patients during normal breathing and 38% during Valsalva maneuver.[52]

Critical care physicians are concerned that PFO may allow a paradoxical embolic event leading to neurologic impairment or death. The possibility of creating a right-to-left shunt in patients with a PFO resulting in hypoxemia has been reported.[53] In patients with refractory hypoxemia, TEE is very useful in searching for an intracardiac cause. The authors diagnosed a large right-to-left interatrial shunt via a PFO as the cause of hypoxemia in a trauma victim who had isolated pulmonic valvular stenosis (Fig. 44–12). Such patients with acute lung injury may require high levels of PEEP to maintain adequate oxygenation.[54] The unidirectional flap-valve nature of the PFO permits shunt flow even with a transient interatrial pressure gradient or reversal of the normal left-to-right pressure differential. As described previously, the incidence of a PFO diagnosis is increased when maneuvers such as release of a Valsalva maneuver (cough) or PEEP are used in patients in an ICU. The shunt is accentuated by the release of PEEP. In a study of 30 critically ill patients, the authors detected a PFO incidence of 27% with TEE in a static or basal state.[55] If a clinician detects a significant atrial shunt in this type of critically ill patient who is hypoxemic, the question is whether this patient is a candidate for closure of the PFO.

Acquired Intracardiac Shunts

In addition to congenital shunts such as ASD or PFO, acquired intracardiac shunts can also easily be evaluated with TEE.[56, 57] Gunshot wounds to the chest may involve the right atrium and the left ventricle. Postoperatively, TTE did not detect any lesions because of subcutaneous emphysema, dressings, and chest tubes. In one case, however, TEE detected a defect of the septal leaflet of the tricuspid valve and an intraventricular septal defect.[56] Similarly, a patient arrived in the emergency department without any vital signs after a single gunshot to the right ventricle that exited the main pulmonary artery. TTE did not show any lesions, but TEE revealed a defect of the tricuspid valve, with significant tricuspid regurgitation visible on the transverse view (Fig. 44–13). The tract of the projectile was identified in the longitudinal view (Fig. 44–14). The authors evaluated a patient who had a penetrating knife injury to the left chest. A mural wound of the right ventricle was found intraoperatively. Three TTE examinations did not reveal any significant residual defects. However, postoperative TEE examinations discovered an aortic to right ventricular outflow tract lesion

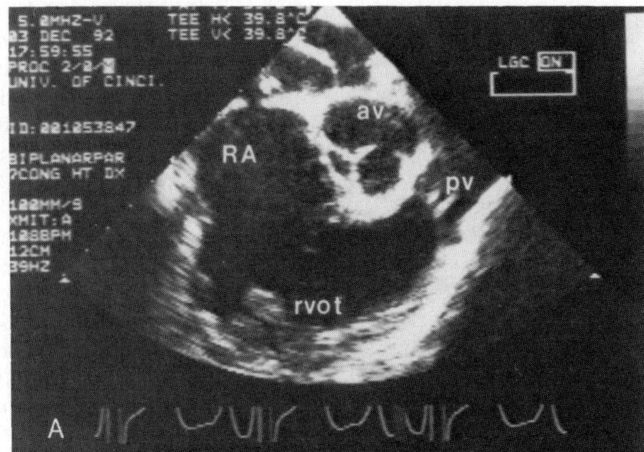

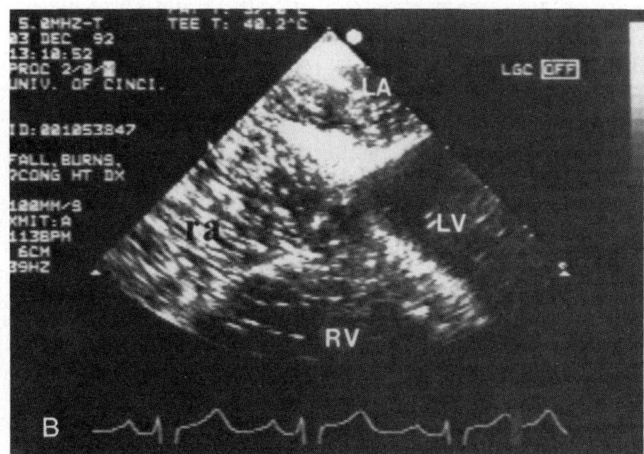

Figure 44–12. Congenital heart disease and patent foramen ovale in a 44-year-old man involved in a fall from a burning structure and with hypotension and severe hypoxia. *A*, A longitudinal image of the pulmonic valve revealed minimal movement and doming of the respective leaflets, which are indicative of isolated pulmonic valvular stenosis. The gradient across the pulmonary valve was 90 mm Hg. *B*, The corresponding transverse view of the right atrium, left atrium, and right ventricle (longitudinal view) revealed a large right-to-left shunt through a patent foramen ovale documented with the use of agitated saline as the contrast agent. *Abbreviation*: av = aortic valve; pv = pulmonic valve; rvot = right ventricular outflow tract.

that expanded over several days. The patient subsequently underwent repair of the defect, using cardiopulmonary bypass, and was discharged home without any untoward sequelae. Visualization of turbulence in the ascending aorta by color-flow Doppler offered the first clue to a defect.[57] In these patients, the initial lesions can be small, irregular, and occasionally multiple, and they are easily missed by TTE. These lesions are dynamic because patients are usually hypovolemic and underresuscitated initially, and the problem may not become apparent until later. After resuscitation, the use of TEE with color-flow Doppler echocardiography should thus be considered to evaluate any residual lesions from a penetrating injury to the heart and its contiguous structures.

Ischemic Heart Disease

A major role of TEE has been its use in identifying RWMA associated with myocardial ischemia. Myocardial ischemia, when unappreciated, can be life threatening. Identifying patients with signs of ischemia using TEE can be helpful, especially when the standard electrocardiogram (ECG) and hemodynamic measurements are not sufficiently sensitive diagnostic methods.[58] Standard ECG analysis is unreliable in the presence of left ventricular hypertrophy, left bundle branch block, drug effect (e.g., digitalis), lead placement, and patient movement or agitation. The earliest sign of myocardial ischemia is impaired ventricular relaxation. This is followed (in decreasing order of sensitivity) by the development of RWMA, impaired global systolic function, pressure-volume changes (compliance), ECG changes of the ST segment, and finally symptoms of angina.

TEE can evaluate RWMA or global function for early detection of myocardial ischemia in the distribution of each major coronary artery.[58] Extrapolation from canine studies shows that as flow is altered, the type of RWMA changes. The temporal relationship with ECG and echocardiography shows that with mild reduction of flow (<20%), echocardiography identifies ischemia as early as 15 seconds after reduction, compared with 10 minutes with ECG analysis.[59] A

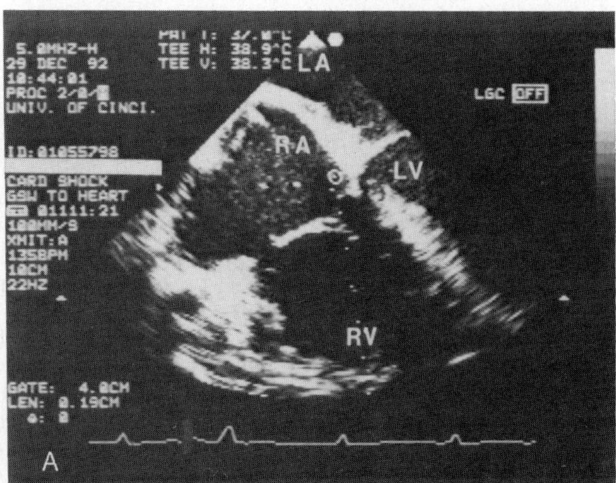

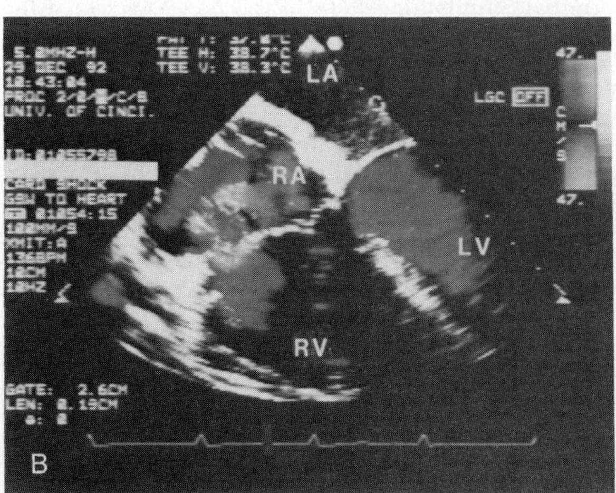

Figure 44–13. Acquired intracardiac shunt in an 18-year-old man in shock with a gunshot wound to the heart. *A*, After resuscitation and repair of the right ventricle and main pulmonary artery, a transverse image recorded the presence of a large defect of the anterior leaflet of the tricuspid valve. *B*, The corresponding transverse image with color-flow Doppler echocardiography revealed significant tricuspid regurgitation through the defect. (See Color Plate Section of this textbook.)

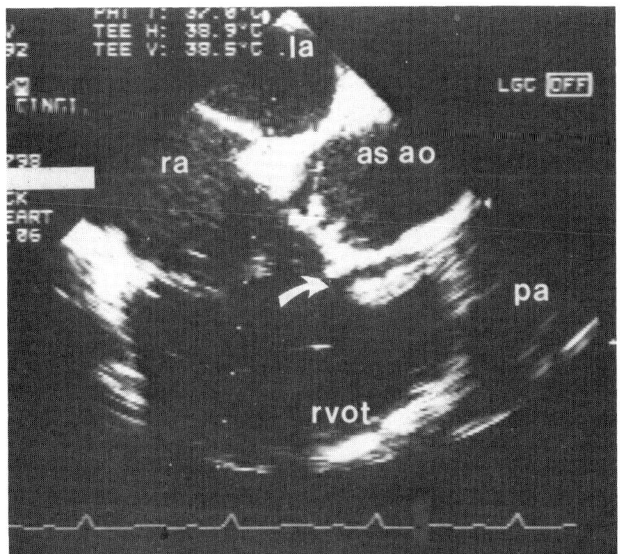

Figure 44–14. Acquired intracardiac shunt. This longitudinal image revealed the tract of the bullet from the right ventricle through the juncture of the ascending aorta and right ventricular outflow tract to the main pulmonary artery *(arrow)*. The tract was also identified with the use of agitated saline as a contrast agent. *Abbreviations*: asao = ascending aorta; la = left atrium; pa = main pulmonary artery; ra = right atrium.

representative scoring scheme for identification of RWMA is as follows: mild hypokinesis, evidenced by shortening of the left ventricular radius by less than 30% but with greater than 10% wall thickening (normal segmental contraction of the heart may be defined as shortening >30%, with associated wall thickening); severe hypokinesis, evidenced by less than 10% radial shortening and minimal wall thickening; akinetic segment, evidenced by no wall thickening during systole; and finally a dyskinetic segment, evidenced by thinning during systole and left ventricular wall bulging or displacement.

Not all RWMAs are caused by myocardial ischemia (which is one of the limiting factors of TEE). Intrinsic conditions that mimic ischemia include prior myocardial infarction with tissue fibrosis, premature ventricular contractions, ventricular paced rhythms, intraventricular conduction abnormalities due to bundle branch block, and shifting of the cardiac structures (i.e., translational rotation of the heart during cardiac and thoracic procedures). RWMA can also develop after bypass, when a decrease in septal thickening results from changes in the sequence of myocardial activation, in turn altering the velocity, timing, and systolic excursion of the endocardium. Extrinsic conditions, not related to myocardial ischemia, include abnormalities in the regional afterload, tethering of adjacent nonischemic segments, and the interaction of right and left heart chamber hemodynamics. Stunned myocardium has persistent RWMA. It would also be difficult to distinguish hibernating myocardium. Some patients who arrive in shock at the ICU with severe global left ventricular dysfunction experience total resolution in several days, as documented with TEE.

The use of peripheral hemodynamics and pulmonary artery occlusion pressure monitoring for identifying myocardial ischemia is insensitive and at times misleading.[60] Leung and colleagues evaluated the correlation between changes of hemodynamics and the development of new RWMA in 50 patients.[61] The increase in pulmonary artery diastolic pressure and heart rate and changes in systemic arterial blood pressure preceded any RWMA only 28% of the time, and 27% of the TEE episodes were associated with a decrease in mean arterial pressure/heart rate of less than 1 mm Hg per beat per minute. Seventy-two per cent of the TEE RWMA episodes occurred without *any* changes in the hemodynamics.[61]

One of the technical difficulties is that monitoring for new RWMA or myocardial ischemia, if carried out only at the midpapillary region or short axis of the left ventricle (with only transverse imaging), can miss apical involvement. This problem can be avoided if the TEE probe is manipulated throughout the procedure. Limited systolic wall thickness changes may be more reliable markers of ischemia than the identification of RWMA.[62] However, investigators continue to try to quantify wall thickening as a marker of ischemia because of interobserver variability. Also, it may be difficult to diagnose RWMA in patients with diffuse ischemic cardiomyopathy, thus explaining different reported sensitivities for detection of a myocardial infarction.[58] The clinical gold standard indicator for myocardial ischemia remains to be defined.

The prognostic importance of postbypass RWMA for patients undergoing coronary artery bypass has been investigated.[63] Forty-four per cent of patients had RWMA, 74% of which occurred in the areas grafted. ECG changes consistent with ischemia had concurrent echocardiography episodes in 18% of the patients. When no ischemia was identified with TEE after bypass or in the ICU period, the patients fared well. In contrast, patients with a poor outcome had a 38% incidence of an echocardiographic ischemia in the ICU and 33% incidence in the operating room after bypass.[63] In critically ill patients who are at high risk for ischemia, TEE may be a viable adjunctive diagnostic tool for early identification and follow-up of a new RWMA.

Experience with biplanar TEE imaging and cinememory loop comparison may increase the detection rate of myocardial ischemia (new RWMA).[64] The difficulties with studies to date lie in the evaluation of new RWMA presumably indicative of myocardial ischemia based on limited images taken in the ICU. Familiarity with the nuances of detection and diagnosis and an innovative operator are essential. Contrast agents are being investigated for assessment of coronary artery flow after completion of the bypass procedure.[65] With these advances, if it becomes technically feasible to evaluate patients for ischemia in the ICU "real time" (e.g., automated on-line subendocardial edge detection), morbidity and mortality might be decreased[66] (Fig. 44–15).

TEE Doppler color flow has also been used in guiding patient selection and surgical treatment of ischemic mitral regurgitation.[67] Identification and characterization of mitral regurgitation with TEE and color Doppler flow help clarify the surgical choices of isolated coronary bypass grafting without mitral valve surgery versus combined coronary bypass and mitral valve surgery.

Valvular Heart Disease

Evaluation of valvular heart disease with TEE includes Doppler echocardiography (pulsed and continuous wave) and two-dimensional ultrasound examination. Clinical expertise is essential for appreciation of normal findings in native and prosthetic valves. In evaluating valvular regurgitation, the actual spacial distribution of the regurgitant jet depends on its direction of flow and velocity, the regurgitant orifice size (shape, diameter, and number), and the chamber's size, compliance, and contractility. Various factors affect apparent spacial distribution, including color-flow gain and mapping algorithms, sector and depth, and transducer fre-

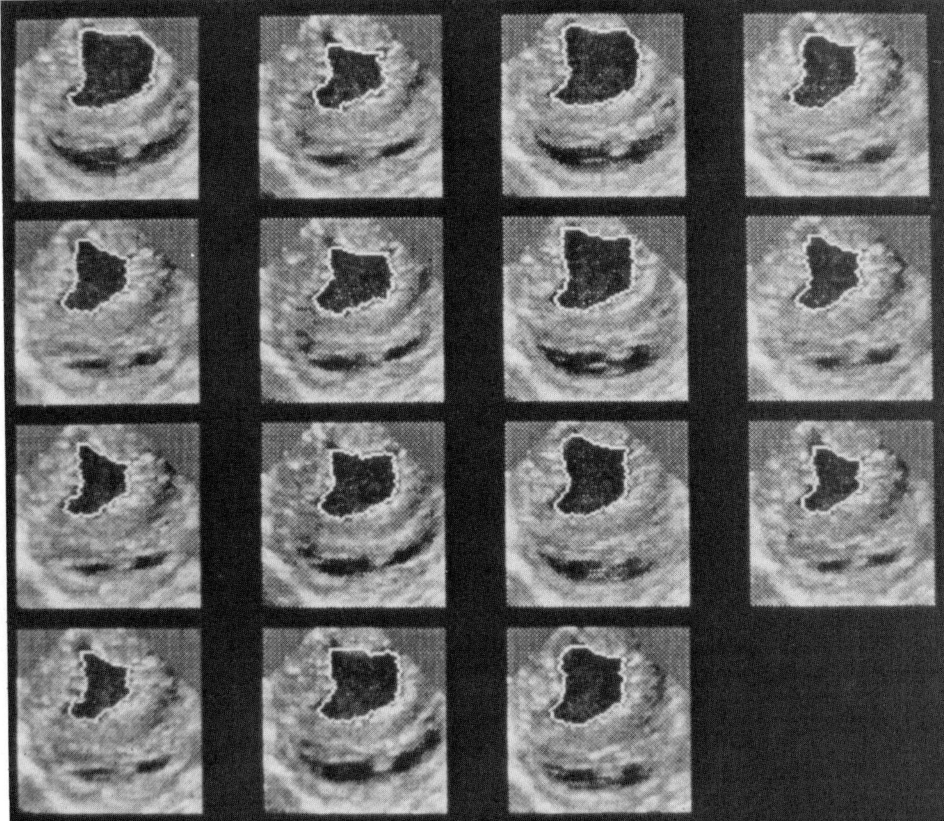

Figure 44–15. Computer edge detection application. Automated edge detection of the left ventricle through two cardiac cycles with computer methods of artificial intelligence tracking of the subendocardial edge of the ventricle. Technique application supported by the Society of Critical Care Medicine, Eli Lilly Research Grant 1991–1992.

quency, all of which can be manipulated by the operator.[68] In addition, different loading conditions influence the heart, such as anesthetics, positive-pressure ventilation, and vasoactive agents.

Characterization of the regurgitant jet (color-flow Doppler echocardiography) is important in planning for surgical repair of mitral valves.[68] Anteriorly directed jets occur with most posterior overriding, flailing, or prolapsing leaflets. Flailing leaflets have the most eccentric, anteriorly directed jets. Regurgitant jets that are directed posteriorly are from the anterior overriding, prolapsing, or flailing leaflets. When both leaflets are equally affected or annular dilatation is present, the regurgitant jets are centrally located. Different "normal jets" are noted with each type of prosthetic valve. All mechanical valve devices have early systolic closure backflow. With a St. Jude valve, three flamelike jets are usually noted. Tilting disk prostheses have small holosystolic jets. A single, early systolic regurgitant jet is seen with ball-cage valve (e.g., Starr-Edwards). Native valvular dysfunction due to rheumatic or ischemic causes results in central regurgitation of the mitral valve.[68]

Castello and colleagues attempted to quantify the severity of mitral regurgitation with Doppler color-flow mapping and angiography.[69] They found the closest correlation between angiography and the maximum regurgitant area (TEE single plane), r equals 0.90. The sensitivity and specificity were 96% and 100%, respectively, for mild mitral regurgitation when the maximum regurgitant area was less than 3.0 cm^2. For severe mitral regurgitation with a maximum regurgitant area exceeding 6.0 cm^2, the predicted sensitivity and specificity with angiography were 91% and 100%, respectively.[69]

Acute onset of cardiogenic pulmonary edema from ruptured chordae tendineae can occur. TTE is limited in providing accurate visualization, whereas TEE detects a ruptured chorda in 100% of these patients compared with 65% of patients when using TTE.[70] TTE also underestimates the severity of mitral regurgitation when compared with TEE.

The advent of biplanar TEE color-flow Doppler echocardiography has helped improve the assessment of mitral regurgitation. The closest correlation with angiography is obtained using transverse and longitudinal TEE imaging.[71] A maximum regurgitant jet area between 1.5 and 4.0 cm^2 is considered mild. A maximum jet area between 4.0 and 7.0 cm^2 predicts moderate mitral regurgitation with a sensitivity and specificity of 100% and 95%, respectively. In the prediction of severe mitral regurgitation, the maximum jet area is greater than 7.0 cm^2, with sensitivity and specificity of 83% and 100%, respectively.[71] To circumvent technical factors that can influence the character of regurgitant jets, Bargiggia and associates evaluated the flow convergence region proximal to the regurgitant orifice as a method for quantifying regurgitant flow rate according to the continuity principle.[72] Biplanar imaging has improved the analysis of the aortic valve in detecting aortic insufficiency, but this is still a qualitative study at this point. Steerable continuous-wave Doppler may help to evaluate stenosis, especially of the mitral valve[73] (Fig. 44–16).

The tricuspid valve occasionally is not visualized with TEE. Several studies using two-dimensional TTE have attempted to quantify tricuspid regurgitation with saline contrast enhancement or evaluation of the tricuspid valve annulus. The severity of tricuspid regurgitation correlates best in the apical four-chamber view during systole. An annular measurement of less than 3.2 cm in systole or less than 3.4 cm in diastole suggests the absence of significant tricuspid regurgitation. In addition to its use in evaluating mitral valve repair, TEE is also beneficial in assessing repair of aortic and tricuspid valves.[74]

Several studies have described and characterized the normal and pathophysiologic jets of prosthetic dysfunction.[69–79] Paravalvular mitral regurgitation may be noted in 24% of patients with a prosthetic mitral valve, as compared with 4% discovered by two-dimensional TTE.[76] With TEE, color-flow Doppler grading generally correlates well with angiography. Evaluation of the aortic prosthetic valve has been impaired by poor echo signal quality resulting from the marked attenuation of the signal from the mechanical valve itself. Evaluation is better for mitral valves.[69] A grading scale has been proposed as follows: Type 1 (physiologic) jet was described as holosystolic, narrow (<10 mm), short (<30 mm), and predominantly red; type 2 (pathologic) jet was described as holosystolic, broad (>10 mm), long (>30 mm), and multicolor. The type 1 jet is usually directed toward the center of the left atrium, whereas the type 2 jet is either directed eccentrically or centrally into the left atrium. TEE has increased sensitivity in description of the mitral regurgitant jet when compared with TTE, an overestimation of severity of approximately a mean area of 2.7 cm^2.[69] Smith and coworkers re-evaluated regurgitant jet size with TEE and TTE Doppler color-flow imaging.[75] Seventy-three lesions were visualized with TEE (34 mitral, 22 aortic, and 17 tricuspid valves). TTE revealed only 48 regurgitant jets (20 mitral, 16 aortic, and 12 tricuspid valves). Overall, agreement between TEE and TTE results was close.[75]

Analysis of pulmonary venous velocities from TEE color-guided pulsed Doppler imaging helps to quantify mitral regurgitation.[79] As the severity of mitral regurgitation increases, the peak systolic velocity and systolic velocity integral decrease while the diastolic velocity and diastolic velocity integral increase. The systolic flow becomes reversed in patients with severe mitral regurgitation. The sensitivity of reversed systolic flow is 90%, and specificity is 100%.[79] It must be remembered that in the operating room setting and ICU, alterations of loading conditions on the heart affect the size of the regurgitant jet and the characteristics of the pulmonary venous flow (PVF) patterns. Many factors are involved, including altered hemodynamics from different pathophysiologic disease states (e.g., sepsis), vasoactive medications, and positive-pressure ventilation. It is advantageous to have a baseline evaluation (two-dimensional and color Doppler flow echocardiography) in steady state to compare with results of subsequent studies during therapeutic manipulation

Left Ventricular Function

A frequent controversy is what constitutes adequate intravascular volume. TEE is useful for evaluating left ventricular size as an index of preload.[80–83] Misleading clinical findings and hemodynamic values are very common, especially in critically ill patients. In regard to left ventricular preload, many physiologic and technical factors influence the pulmonary artery occlusion pressure. Left ventricular pressure does not correlate with left ventricular end-diastolic dimensions or volume in states characterized by altered ventricular compliance and when the pressure surrounding the heart is increased (e.g., cardiac tamponade). Ventricular compliance is altered by the use of PEEP, by myocardial ischemia or infarction, by pathologic states with ventricular hypertrophy such as aortic stenosis, and in patients requiring inotropic or vasopressive agents. TEE short-axis imaging evaluates the end-diastolic and end-systolic area and area ejection fraction. TEE compares favorably with scintigraphic estimates of left ventricular end-diastolic volume index and ejection fraction.[80] The relationship between the end-diastolic area and left ventricular end-diastolic index is fair, and TEE may clarify the state of left ventricular preload.[80]

In patients with acute lung injury requiring increasing levels of PEEP, the estimation of adequate preload from the measurement of the pulmonary arterial occlusion pressure may be misleading. This estimation of preload is even more difficult in the presence of underlying cardiac dysfunction. TEE may be the ideal tool for estimating preload and myocardial function of both ventricles and for evaluating ventricular interaction or interdependency in these critically ill

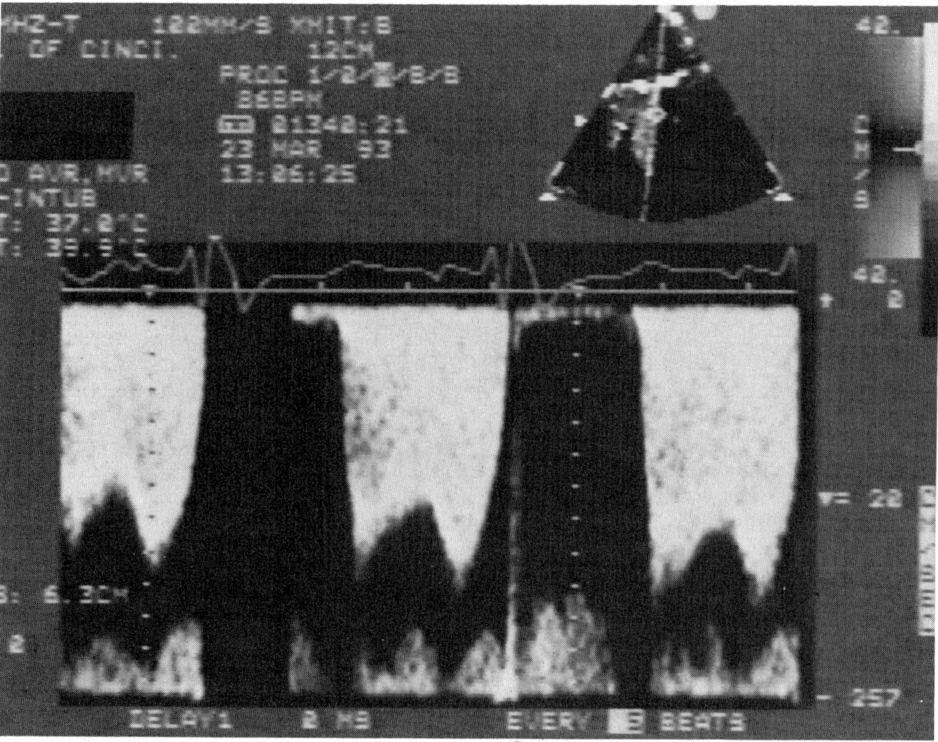

Figure 44–16. Continuous-wave Doppler echocardiography. TEE of a patient with congestive heart failure and rheumatic heart disease demonstrated mitral stenosis with a valve area of 1.13 cm^2, a mean gradient of 25.3 mm Hg, and a pressure half-time of 194 ms. (See Color Plate Section of this textbook.)

patients.[82] As PEEP is increased, the cardiac index, right ventricular filling, and end-systolic and end-diastolic area of the right atrium are decreased.[83] This decrease is associated with elevation of the right atrial pressure and static transmural pressure. Displacement of the septum to the left occurs with increasing levels of PEEP. Patients with severe ventricular failure may have an initial improvement of cardiac index with a corresponding decrease in the diastolic left ventricular area. Thus, in patients with normal left ventricular function, the addition of PEEP may result in relative hypovolemia (acute reduction of preload of the right ventricle). However, in patients with left ventricular dysfunction, the hemodynamics may improve until a critical level has been reached, after which ensues impairment of left ventricular filling. Echocardiography is more sensitive than the fast-response thermodilution technique for evaluation of right ventricular systolic function and area in patients with severe respiratory failure. During increasing levels of PEEP, the right ventricular end-diastolic volume and area do not change but right ventricular diastolic compliance decreases. At high levels of PEEP, the systolic function and preload markedly decrease. Thus, we recommend use of TEE to evaluate the interactions between the right and left sides of the heart when high levels of PEEP are required, particularly in patients who are hemodynamically unstable.

Computer Applications in Transesophageal Echocardiography

As much as 87% of the stroke volume is derived from fiber shortening, seen in the short-axis view of the left ventricle. However, ejection fraction is load dependent and cannot be assessed accurately in critically ill patients. Estimation of volume or preload based on dimensions of the cardiac chambers and myocardial function is offline and cumbersome. Computerized algorithms are being developed to improve qualitative analysis of the size and volume of the left ventricle.[84–87] When comparing angiography (the biplane area-length method) with echocardiography, close correlation was noted, with end-systole and end-diastole of r equals 0.96 and r equals 0.92, respectively.[64] Martin and associates, using in vivo studies, noted close correlation between ventricular volume and stroke volume with a multiplanar or three-dimensional TEE scanning method.[84] During a wide range of hemodynamic conditions in the in vivo study, the correlation coefficient was 0.92. Belohlavek and coworkers described acquisition of two-dimensional echocardiographic images in a sequential fashion.[85] Methods for a quick, accurate, on-line edge detection of the left ventricle for quantification of volume, RWMA, and myocardial performance are being developed.[66,86] Such new techniques will assist and improve our assessment of ventricular volumes and function (i.e., pressure-volume loops for assessment of contractility and diastolic compliance). It is just a matter of time until these will be applicable to clinical practice (see Fig. 44–15).

Pericardial Effusion and Cardiac Tamponade

Pericardial effusions can occur as a response to various injuries of the parietal pericardium (Figs. 44–17 and 44–18). Initially silent, effusions progress as the accumulation of the pericardial fluid increases cardiac compression. Tamponade can eventually result by elevation of pericardial pressure, progressive limitation of ventricular diastolic filling, and subsequent reduction in stroke volume. The increase of intrapericardial pressure depends on the absolute volume of the effusion, the rate of its development, and the physical characteristics of the pericardium itself. Pericardial effusion can be demonstrated after cardiac surgery in 56% to 85% of patients, whereas the incidence of cardiac tamponade is between only 1% and 2.5%.[87] Identifying a patient who has developed cardiac tamponade is lifesaving, because the outcome is directly related to prompt decompression. A diagnostic dilemma occurs with localized pericardial effusion, a relatively common finding in postoperative cardiac surgical patients. The typical findings of pulsus paradoxus and elevation and equalization of intracardiac pressures (right atrial, pulmonary artery diastolic, and pulmonary occlusion pressure) do not always occur. Although views with TTE are limited or suboptimal because of dressings, subcutaneous emphysema, pneumothoraces, body habitus, obesity, and chronic obstructive lung disease, TEE is an excellent diagnostic tool for identifying cardiac tamponade, particularly if it is loculated.[87] Hypotension (in cases with a loculated effusion) can be the result of compression not only of cardiac chambers but also of the venae cavae or the pulmonary veins. For example, an extracardiac mass compressing the right pulmonary veins contributed and exacerbated hypotension in one of the authors' patients (see Fig. 44–11*A*).

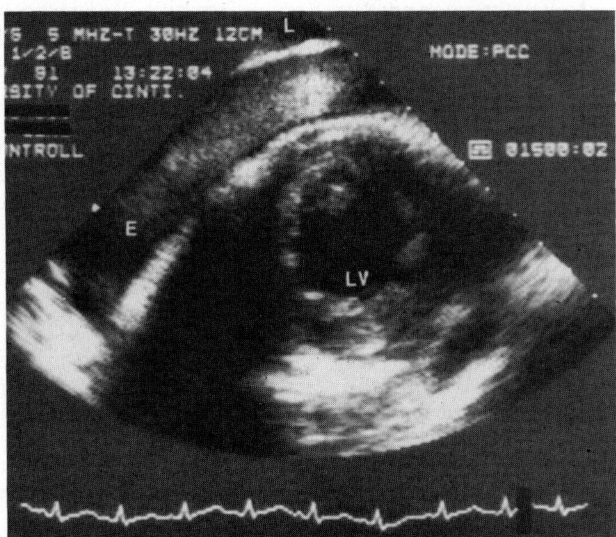

Figure 44–17. Cardiac tamponade. This previously healthy 26-year-old man was involved in a motor vehicle accident and sustained chest wall injuries that became hypotensive. A transgastric view of the left ventricle reveals a large pericardial effusion. *Abbreviation*: E = effusion.

Right atrial inversion is an early TEE finding suggesting cardiac tamponade. Early and late diastolic collapse of the right ventricle and atrium is also considered to be a reliable sign. However, it is highly dependent on the difference between the pericardial and intracardiac pressures. During the progression to cardiac tamponade, the right and left ventricular dimensions decrease. By Doppler echocardiography, an exaggerated respiratory variation is noted in mitral inflow velocities (MIV) across the mitral valve. A marked inspiratory increase (81%) in right-sided velocities with a corresponding decline in left-sided velocities has been described, as has marked inspiratory prolongation of the left ventricular isovolumetric relaxation.[88] With inspiration, the right ventricle expands and the septum shifts into the left ventricle. However, in patients with left ventricular dysfunction, the inspiratory decline of the systolic arterial pressure is less because filling occurs against common right and left ventricular diastolic pressures set by the pericardial pressure-volume relationship. An upward and leftward parallel shift occurs in the pericardial pressure-volume relationship such that right atrial and ventricular collapse occurs with smaller

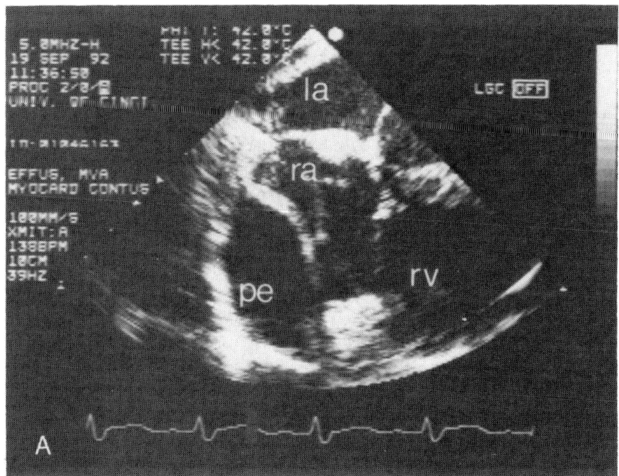

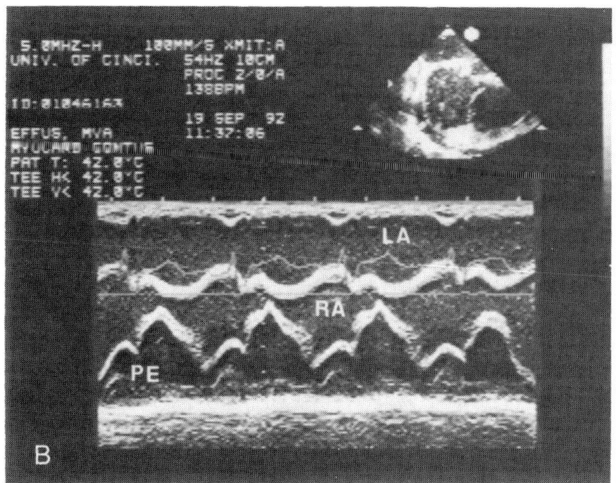

Figure 44–18. Cardiac tamponade. This previously healthy 26-year-old man was involved in a motor vehicle accident and sustained chest wall injuries that resulted in myocardial contusion, severe left ventricular dysfunction, and cardiac tamponade. *A*, Transview imaging of the left atrium and right atrium revealed a large pericardial effusion with right atrial diastolic collapse. *B*, Corresponding M-mode echocardiography through the left atrium, interatrial septum, and right atrium revealed inward displacement of the anterior wall of the right atrium in diastole. *Abbreviations*: pe = pericardial effusion; rv = right ventricle.

pericardial fluid volumes. With high left atrial pressure in this situation, left atrial collapse may not be visualized at all. The opposite can be seen with concomitant right ventricular dysfunction. Larger pericardial fluid volumes are required to evidence the echocardiographic findings of cardiac tamponade, and detection occurs later in the hemodynamic progression of tamponade. The filling of both ventricles is affected by the presence of the pericardium over a wide range of physiologic ventricular pressures and volumes.[89] TEE is an excellent technique for discriminating ventricular dysfunction from tamponade.

Pulmonary Venous Flow and Mitral Inflow Velocities

Because TEE imaging is retrocardiac, resolution of extracardiac structures such as the left superior pulmonary vein for analysis of pulmonary venous inflow is better than with TTE. TEE has afforded clinicians and investigators the opportunity for continuous evaluation of hemodynamic performance in critically ill patients. By evaluating PVF and MIV, a clinician can assess diastolic function.[89–90] Normal PVF signal has four phases: (1) systolic inflow due to atrial relaxation; (2) flow due to ventricular contractions with resultant "drop" of the mitral annulus toward the apex of the left ventricle; (3) diastolic inflow secondary to opening of the mitral valve; and (4) a negative signal secondary to atrial contraction. Analysis of PVF for systolic reversal has helped characterize the severity of mitral regurgitation.[79]

TEE has been used to evaluate MIV as an estimation of left ventricular diastolic function.[91] Left ventricular filling is determined by several factors: the interaction of the systolic and diastolic properties of the ventricles, the transmitral pressure gradient, atrial systole, right ventricular size, and preload. These interactions can be very complex, for example, in septic patients with acute lung injury requiring high levels of PEEP. Pulsed Doppler echocardiography (with TEE) provides a unique tool for direct evaluation of intracardiac blood flow patterns to assess left ventricular diastolic filling. Doppler-derived parameters that can be obtained are area or time velocity integral within the flow velocity profile curve during both atrial filling and early diastole, early diastolic deceleration time or pressure half-time, acceleration time, rate of decline of flow velocity in early diastole, isovolumetric relaxation time, peak filling rate, and peak early and late filling velocities. Evaluation of diastolic filling by Doppler echocardiography can be obtained from the mitral inflow portion of the left ventricle at the tips of the mitral valve leaflets using the four-chamber view, the long-axis view of the left ventricle, and the longitudinal view at the midesophageal position.

Maximum blood velocities should be obtained as parallel to the diastolic mitral inflow as possible. In general, the normal transmitral Doppler flow velocities are identified by two distinct filling peaks or waves (patients who are in sinus rhythm). The E wave (high initial velocity) represents the onset of rapid filling in early diastole and is followed by the decrease in velocity. The A wave, or second distinct peak, represents the onset of diastole and atrial contraction. In normal patients, the E wave is larger than the A wave. An E-A ratio (index of diastolic filling) less than 1.0 represents decreased ventricular relaxation.[91] However, in critically ill patients, the heart rate can be so high that the E and A waves appear as one wave. Other factors may also affect the absolute values derived from the transmitral patterns, such as preload, afterload, atrial systole, ventricular compliance, and aging. A normal E-A ratio does not necessarily imply normal ventricular diastolic function, because the Doppler filling patterns are a continuum.[91]

In diagnosing left ventricular diastolic dysfunction, two patterns are usually seen.[91] An abnormal relaxation pattern is associated with a prolonged isovolumic relaxation time and diastolic time of early filling. Observed are a decreased E-A ratio, normal or increased atrial systole (A) wave velocity, and a decrease in the early peak filling E velocity. These findings have been associated with myocardial ischemia, hypertension, left ventricular hypertrophy, myocardial injury, pulmonary hypertension, and some cardiomyopathies. The second characteristic pattern is described as a restrictive pattern (pronounced increases in early diastolic filling with shortened relaxation time). This pattern is associated with an increase in the E-A ratio, a normal or decreased late filling A velocity, a normal or increased E velocity, shortened diastolic time of peak filling, and decreased isovolumic relaxation time. Patients with increased left ventricular end-diastolic volume, increased left atrial pressure, and markedly impaired systolic function may have this pattern.[91]

PVF patterns may also be revealing in patients with dilated and hypertrophied hearts.[92] Peak velocity during systole is markedly decreased in patients with a dilated ventricle when compared with a hypertrophied or normal ventricle. In hypertrophied and dilated ventricles, the diastolic component of PVF is significantly decreased compared with normal controls. In hypertrophied ventricles, the ratio of the peak velocity of the diastolic component and the second phase of the systolic flow is lower than for normal controls. The second component of PVF in systole may be influenced by systolic ventricular function, and the diastolic component of PVF and atrial systole reversal may be influenced by diastolic dysfunction.

PVF and MIV respond to changes in loading conditions. When preload decreases, the initial E velocity is reduced and the deceleration time is prolonged. However, the effect on E velocity is variable when the preload is increased. Increasing the afterload increases E velocity and shortens the deceleration time. Hoit and colleagues studied the pericardial influence on the right and left ventricular interactions with volume loading.[89] In an animal model, after pericardiectomy, there was an increase in early mitral velocity, early peak diastolic pressure gradient, and E-A ratio, but the tricuspid inflow velocity showed no change in E, a decrease in E-A, and an increase in A. With volume loading, the pericardium has an equal restraining effect on right and left ventricular filling over a wide range of physiologic ventricular pressures and volumes.

TEE has been used for evaluating left ventricular diastolic function during increasingly inversed I-E ventilation ratio in patients (with no lung injury) subjected to increasing levels of PEEP.[92] Significant reductions of the total mitral valve velocity time integral and velocity-time integral of the E wave were noted. The ratio of E-A waves was decreased when 15 cm H_2O PEEP was added. With PVF, an increase of PEEP to 15 cm H_2O resulted in the increased ratio of the velocity time integral of systolic to diastolic waves from 2.0 to 2.4. The total velocity-time integral decreased from 16.9 to 12.5 cm. Both diastolic and systolic grade flow declined. This decrease in left ventricular function can be expected especially in patients who have compliant lungs. TEE should be performed to evaluate these changes in patients who have moderate to severe lung injury and who require increasing levels of PEEP and mean airway pressure.

TEE can be used as a tool for estimating left ventricular filling.[93] Pulmonary venous inflow allows estimation of left atrial pressure and pulmonary artery occlusion pressure. Klein and associates studied PVF in patients who had mitral regurgitation to determine the correlation between left atrial pressure A and V waves.[94] Pulmonary venous systolic to diastolic flow ratios corresponded to an increase in the V waves and a decrease in the left atrial pressure A-V ratios. However, with acute impairment of left ventricular function, PVF does not always reflect the left atrial pressure. Thus, more studies are needed to evaluate the clinical uses and efficacy of utilizing PVF and MIV as a reflection of left ventricular preload in critically ill patients.[95]

Transesophageal Echocardiography in the Pediatric Population

More experience is being gained with TEE in pediatric patients.[96] Congenital lesions that are often studied include tetralogy of Fallot, pulmonary atresia, atrioventricular canal, transposition of the great vessels, ventricular septal defect, tricuspid atresia, ASD, and hypoplastic left heart. In congenital heart disease, the hemodynamics are often complex and can be dependent on the relative resistances of the systemic and pulmonary vascular systems. Continuous- and pulse-wave Doppler techniques provide quantifiable and accurate hemodynamic data. Color Doppler flow imaging provides semi-qualitative or quantitative flow information about the physiology of congenital heart disease. In 40% of patients studied, additional anatomic or hemodynamic information can be obtained with TEE.[96] TEE is especially helpful in evaluating patients in the pediatric cardiac ICU if difficulty arises, searching for residual shunts across ventricular septal defects, ASDs, baffle leak after Mustard's procedure for transposition of the great vessels, residual outflow tract obstruction or insufficiency after critical aortic and pulmonic valve stenosis surgery, ductus arteriosus recanalization, aortic regurgitation after ASD or ventricular septal defect repair, and systemic-to-pulmonary artery shunt failure.[96] Stumper and coworkers prospectively studied 102 patients with TEE.[97] Treatment of these patients was assisted in 21% of the patients, and additional information was gained in 48% of the patients. The investigators found improved diagnostic insight in Fontan's circulation, systemic and pulmonary venous return, left ventricular outflow disease, atrial baffle function, and atrial ventricular junction abnormalities. The major limitations of the TEE technique are that it is semi-invasive and that sedation or general anesthesia is a requirement in the pediatric population.[97]

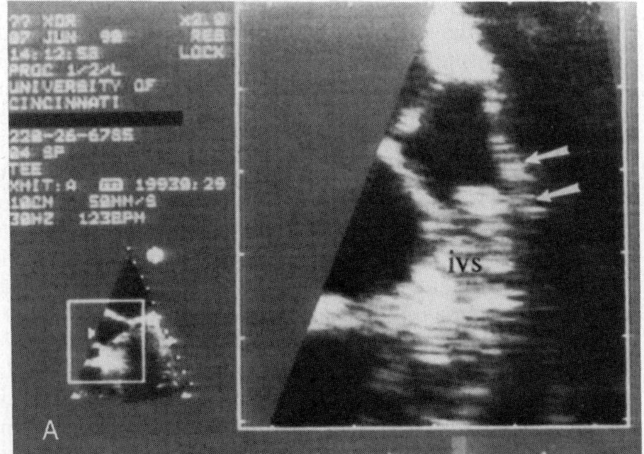

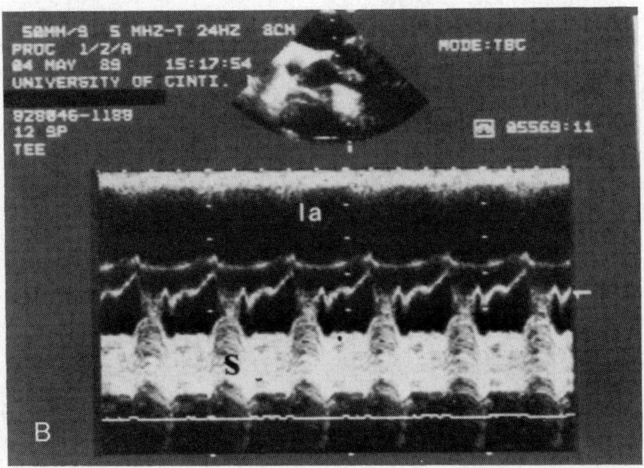

Figure 44–19. Systolic motion of the anterior mitral valve leaflet (SAM). *A*, Expanded transverse image of the left ventricular outflow tract and the short axis view of the aortic valve reveal SAM with obstruction in systole *(arrows)*. *B*, M-mode echocardiographic imaging through the septum, left ventricular outflow tract, anterior mitral valve leaflet, and left atrium reveal SAM with obstruction in a severely hypotensive patient after placement of a Carpenter's mitral valve ring. *Abbreviations*: ivs = intraventricular septum; S = septum.

Benefits of Transesophageal Echocardiography

TEE has had a significant impact during cardiac surgery in monitoring for new RWMAs and assessment of left ventricular volume and function. Especially during mitral valve surgery, TEE has been of major benefit in decision analysis for surgical repair versus replacement.[67, 69, 72, 79, 98] Sheikh and colleagues found that it influenced major decisions in 27% of 154 cardiac patients.[67] The surgical decision was altered in 40% of 64 mitral valve cases.[67] These results were later confirmed by others.[98] TEE has the opportunity to alter medical or surgical therapy, especially in critically ill patients. In Zabalgoitia and associates' study, TEE influenced the management decision in 82% of cases in which the TTE approach was inconsistent with the clinical findings or was not diagnostic.[99] The most frequent indication for TEE in Oh and coworkers' study is unexplained hemodynamic instability.[3] TEE often correctly identifies the cause of the clinical dilemma. What is most important is that TEE, because of its superior imaging capabilities, also precludes suspected abnormalities more definitely than TTE. TEE in critically ill patients is especially useful when the pulmonary artery occlusion pressure and peripheral hemodynamics are inconsistent with the clinical findings or when standard medical management has not resulted in expected improvement.

Finally, one of the major benefits of TEE has been to determine the cause of persistent or refractory hypotension in critically ill patients such as those with septic shock, traumatic injury, or severe acute lung injury requiring high levels of PEEP. One can evaluate the presence of intracardiac shunt, valvular dysfunction, papillary muscle rupture, pulmonary embolism, myocardial function and volume, and left ventricular outflow obstruction. For example, TEE has been an excellent tool for evaluating severe systolic anterior motion of the mitral valve apparatus (postrepair) (Fig. 44–19) and for facilitating resolution through hemodynamic manipulation. TEE has been beneficial for detection or preclusion of cardiac tamponade (particularly loculated effusion). As additional benefits, one can find pleural effusions and determine the position of an intra-aortic balloon and pulmonary artery catheter (Fig. 44–20).

As a new technology, TEE continues to evolve, with the development of smaller probes and multiplanar or omniplanar probes and incorporation of sophisticated computer algorithms. TEE is currently an adjunct to other existing technology. The team approach, combining the expertise of different disciplines in using TEE, is likely to improve patient care and outcome. Physicians should gain experience in TEE in the ICU and through collaboration with cardiology colleagues who are trained in Doppler echocardiography, cardiac anatomy, and TEE.[100, 101]

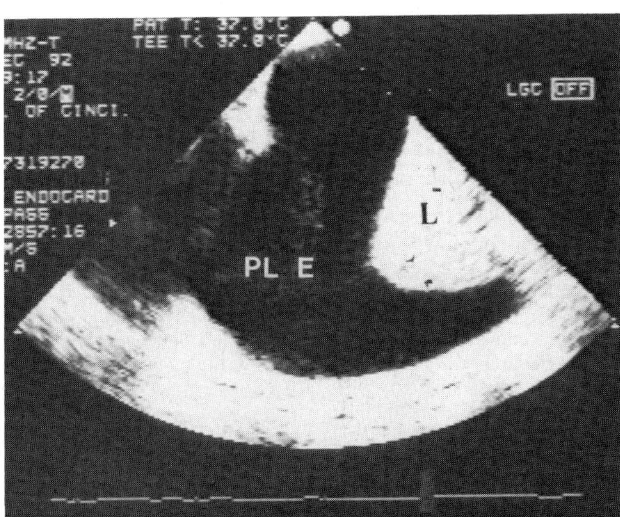

Figure 44–20. Pleural effusion. This transverse image from the transgastric position reveals a large right-sided pleural effusion. *Abbreviations*: L = liver, PLE = pleural effusion.

ACKNOWLEDGMENTS

The authors would like to thank Ms. Terri Emerson for her diligence, patience, and preparation of this manuscript. This manuscript is dedicated to Frank S. Porembka, Sr., for his continual loving support through the years.

References

1. Seward JB, Khandheria BK, Oh JK, et al: Transesophageal echocardiography: Technique, anatomic correlations implementation and cardiac applications. Mayo Clin Proc 1988; 63:6499.
2. Porembka DT, Hoit BD: Transesophageal echocardiography in the intensive care patient. Crit Care Med 1991; 19:826.
3. Oh JK, Seward JB, Khandheria BK, et al: Transesophageal echocardiography in critically ill patients. Am J Cardiol 1990; 66:1492.
4. Foster E, Schiller NB: The role of transesophageal echocardiography in critical care: USCF experience. J Am Soc Echocardiogr 1992; 5:368.

4a. Khoury AF, Afridi I, Quinones MA, et al: Transesophageal echocardiography in critically ill patients: Feasibility, safety, and impact on management. Am Heart J 1994; 127:1363.

5. Seward JB, Khandheria BK, Edwards WD, et al: Biplanar transesophageal echocardiography: Anatomic correlations, image orientation, and clinical applications. Mayo Clin Proc 1990; 65:1193.
6. Geibel A, Kasper W, Behroz A, et al: Risk of transesophageal echocardiography in awake patients with cardiac disease. Am J Cardiol 1988; 62:337.
7. Daniel WG, Kasper W, Erbel R: Safety of transesophageal echocardiography: A multicenter survey of 10,419 examinations. Circulation 1991; 83:817.
8. Dawson J, Cockel R: Oesophageal perforation at fiberoptic gastroscopy. Br Med J 1981; 283:583.
9. Dewhirst WE, Stragand JJ, Fleming BM: Mallory-Weiss tear complicating intraoperative transesophageal echocardiography in a patient undergoing aortic valve replacement. Anesthesiology 1990; 73:777.
10. O'Shea JP, Southern JF, D'Ambra MN, et al: Effects of prolonged transesophageal echocardiographic imaging and probe manipulation on the esophagus—an echocardiographic pathologic study. J Am Coll Cardiol 1991; 17:1426.
11. Pongratz G, Henneke K-H, von der Grun M, et al: Risk of endocarditis in transesophageal echocardiography. Am Heart J 1993; 125:190.

11a. Shyu KG, Hwang JJ, Lin SC, et al: Prospective study of blood culture during transesophageal echocardiography. Am Heart J 1992; 125:1541.

12. Erbel R, Engberding R, Daniel W, et al: Echocardiography in the diagnosis of aortic dissection. European Cooperative Study Group for Echocardiography. Lancet 1989; 1:457.
13. Erbel R, Engberding R, Daniel W, et al: Echocardiography in the diagnosis of aortic dissection. European Cooperative Study Group for Echocardiography. Lancet 1989; 1:457.
14. Hashimoto S, Kumada T, Osakada G, et al: Assessment of transesophageal Doppler echocardiography in dissecting aortic aneurysm. J Am Coll Cardiol 1989; 14:1253.
15. Adachi H, Kyo S, Takamoto S, et al: Early diagnosis and surgical intervention of acute aortic dissection by transesophageal color flow mapping. Circulation 1990; 82:IV–19.
16. Ballal RS, Nanda NC, Gatewood R, et al: Usefulness of transesophageal echocardiography in assessment of aortic dissection. Circulation 1991; 84:1903.
17. Roudaut RP, Marcaggi XL, Deville C, et al: Value of transesophageal echocardiography combined with computed tomography for assessing repaired type A aortic dissection. Am J Cardiol 1992; 70:1468.

18. Cigarroa JE, Isselbacher EM, DeSanctis R, et al: Diagnostic imaging in the evaluation of suspected aortic dissection. N Engl J Med 1993; 328:35.
19. Nienaber CA, Spielmann RP, von Kodolitsch Y, et al: Diagnosis of thoracic aortic dissection. Magnetic resonance imaging versus transesophageal echocardiography. Circulation 1992; 85:434.
20. Nienaber CA, von Kodolitsch Y, Nicholas V, et al: The diagnosis of thoracic aortic dissection by noninvasive imaging procedures. N Engl J Med 1993; 328:1.
21. Goarin JP, Le Bret F, Riou B, et al: Early diagnosis of traumatic thoracic aortic rupture by transesophageal echocardiography. Chest 1993; 103:618.
21a. Goldstein SA, Mintz GS, Lindsay J, et al: Aorta: Comprehensive evaluation by echocardiography and transesophageal echocardiography. J Am Soc Echocardiogr 1993; 6:634.
21b. Erbel R, Oelert H, Meyer J, et al: Effect of medical and surgical therapy on aortic dissection evaluated by transesophageal echocardiography. Circulation 1993; 87:1604.
22. Karalis DG, Chandrasekaran K, Victor MF, et al: Recognition and embolic potential of intraaortic atherosclerotic debris. J Am Coll Cardiol 1991; 17:73.
23. Sparks MB, Burchard KW, Marrin CAS, et al: Transesophageal echocardiography: Preliminary results in patients with traumatic aortic rupture. Arch Surg 1991; 126:711.
24. Katz ES, Tunick PA, Rusinek H, et al: Protruding aortic atheromas predict stroke in elderly patients undergoing cardiopulmonary bypass: Experience with intraoperative transesophageal echocardiography. J Am Coll Cardiol 1992; 20:70.
25. Horowitz DR, Tuhrim S, Budd J, et al: Aortic plaque in patients with brain ischemia: Diagnosis by transesophageal echocardiography. Neurology 1992; 42:1602.
26. Porembka DT, Johnson DJ, Fowl RJ, et al: Descending thoracic aortic thrombus as a cause of multiple system organ failure: Diagnosis by transesophageal echocardiography. Crit Care Med 1992; 20:1184.
27. Coy KM, Maurer G, Goodman D, et al: Transesophageal echocardiographic detection of aortic atheromatosis may provide clues to occult renal dysfunction in the elderly. Am Heart J 1992; 123:1684.
27a. Albeis GW, Comess KA, DeRook FA, et al: Transesophageal echocardiographic findings in stroke subtypes. Stroke 1994; 25:23.
28. Rubin BG, Barzilai B, Allen BT, et al: Detection of the source of arterial emboli by transesophageal echocardiography: A case report. J Vasc Surg 1992; 15:573.
29. Daniel WG, Schroder E, Nonnost-Daniel B, et al: Conventional and transesophageal echocardiography in the diagnosis of infective endocarditis. Eur Heart J 1987; 8:287.
29a. Yvorchuk KJ, Chan K: Application of transthoracic and transesophageal echocardiography in the diagnosis and management of infectious endocarditis. J Am Soc Echocardiogr 1994; 14:294.
30. Erbel R, Rohmann S, Drexler M, et al: Improved diagnostic value of echocardiography in patients with infective endocarditis by transesophageal approach. A prospective study. Eur Heart J 1988; 9:43.
31. Mugge A, Daniel WG, Frank G, et al: Echocardiography in infective endocarditis: Reassessment of prognostic implications of vegetation size determined by the transthoracic and transesophageal approach. J Am Coll Cardiol 1989; 14:631.
32. Daniel WG, Mugge A, Martin RP, et al: Improvement in the diagnosis of abscesses associated with endocarditis by transesophageal echocardiography. N Engl J Med 1991; 324:795.
33. Shively BK, Gurule FT, Roldan CA, et al: Diagnostic value of transesophageal compared with transthoracic echocardiography in infective endocarditis. J Am Coll Cardiol 1991; 18:391.
34. Daniel WG, Mugge A, Grote J, et al: Comparison of transthoracic and transesophageal echocardiography for detection of abnormalities of prosthetic and bioprosthetic valves in the mitral and aortic positions. Am J Cardiol 1993; 71:210.
35. Karalis DG, Bansal RC, Hauck AJ, et al: Transesophageal echocardiographic recognition of subaortic complications in aortic valve endocarditis. Clinical and surgical implications. Circulation 1992; 86:353.
36. Sochowski RA, Chan K-L: Implication of negative results on a monoplane transesophageal echocardiographic study in patients with suspected infective endocarditis. J Am Coll Cardiol 1993; 21:216.
37. Aschenberg W, Schluter M, Kremer P, et al: Transesophageal two-dimensional echocardiography for the detection of left atrial appendage thrombus. J Am Coll Cardiol 1986; 7:163.
38. Felner JM, Churchwell AL, Murphy DA: Right atrial thromboemboli: Clinical, echocardiographic and pathophysiologic manifestations. J Am Coll Cardiol 1984; 4:1041.
39. Reeder GS, Khandheria BK, Seward JB, et al: Transesophageal echocardiography and cardiac masses. Mayo Clin Proc 1991; 66:1101.
40. Faletra F, Ravini M, Moreo A, et al: Transesophageal echocardiography in the evaluation of mediastinal masses. J Am Soc Echocardiogr 1992; 5:187.
41. Vigna C, de Rito V, Criconia GM, et al: Left atrial thrombus and spontaneous echo-contrast in nonanticoagulated mitral stenosis. Chest 1993; 103:348.
42. Hwang J-J, Kuan P, Lin S-C, et al: Reappraisal by transesophageal echocardiography of the significance of left atrial thrombi in the prediction of systemic arterial embolization in rheumatic mitral valve disease. Am J Cardiol 1992; 70:769.
43. Manning WJ, Silverman DI, Gordon SPF, et al: Cardioversion from atrial fibrillation without prolonged anticoagulation with use of transesophageal echocardiography to exclude the presence of atrial thrombi. N Engl J Med 1993; 328:750.
44. Aronson S, Ruo W, Sand M: Inverted left atrial appendage appearing as a left atrial mass with transesophageal echocardiography during cardiac surgery. Anesthesiology 1992; 76:1054.
45. Yee LL, Williams GP, Gaitner NS, et al: Diagnosis of acute intraoperative pulmonary thromboembolism by transesophageal echocardiography. Am Heart J 1993; 125:262.
46. Come PC: Echocardiographic evaluation of pulmonary embolism and its response to therapeutic interventions. Chest 1992; 101:151S.
47. de Belder MA, Tourikis L, Griffith M, et al: Transesophageal contrast echocardiography and color flow mapping: Methods of choice for the detection of shunts at the atrial level? Am Heart J 1992; 124:1545.
48. Hagan PT, Scholz DG, Edwards WD: Incidence and size of patent foramen ovale during the first ten decades of life: An autopsy study of 965 normal hearts. Mayo Clin Proc 1984; 59:17.
49. Stoddard MF, Keedy DL, Dawkins PR: The cough test is superior to the Valsalva maneuver in the delineation of right-to-left shunting through a patent foramen ovale during contrast transesophageal echocardiography. Am Heart J 1993; 125:185.
50. Hausmann D, Mugge A, Becht I, et al: Diagnosis of patent foramen ovale by transesophageal echocardiography and association with cerebral and peripheral embolic events. Am J Cardiol 1992; 70:668.
51. Lechat PH, Mas JL, Lascault G, et al: Prevalence of patent foramen ovale in patients with stroke. N Engl J Med 1988; 318:1148.
51a. Stollberger C, Schneider B, Abzieher F, et al: Diagnosis of patent foramen ovale by transesophageal contrast echocardiography. Am J Cardiol 1993; 71:604.
52. Chen W-J, Kuan P, Lien W-P, et al: Detection of patent foramen ovale by contrast transesophageal echocardiography. Chest 1992; 101:1515.
53. Ravenscraft SA, Marinelli WA, Johnson T, et al: Profound hypoxemia precipitated by positive end-expiratory pressure: induction of an intracardiac shunt. Crit Care Med 1992; 20:434.
54. DeSio JM, Goodnough SR, Hajduczok ZD: The effect of positive end-expiratory pressure on right-to-left shunting at the atrial level as documented by transesophageal echocardiography. Anesthesiology 1992; 77:1033.
55. Porembka D, Valente J, Anderson G, et al: Postoperative detection of patent foramen ovale by transesophageal echocardiography. Crit Care Med 1993; 21:S269.
56. Brathwaite CEM, Weiss RL, Baldino WA, et al: Multichamber gunshot wounds of the heart. Chest 1992; 101:287.
57. Porembka DT, Johnson DJ, Hoit BD, et al: Penetrating cardiac trauma: A role for transesophageal echocardiography. Anesth Analg 1993; 77:1275.

58. Smith JS, Cahalan MK, Benefiel DJ, et al: Intraoperative detection of myocardial ischemia in high-risk patients: Electrocardiography versus two-dimensional transesophageal echocardiography. Circulation 1985; 72:1015.
59. Vatner SF: Correlation between acute reductions in myocardial blood flow and function in conscious dogs. Circ Res 1980; 47:201.
60. vanDaela M, Sutherland GR, Mitchell MM, et al: Do changes in pulmonary capillary wedge adequately reflect myocardial ischemia during anesthesia? A correlative preoperative hemodynamic, electrocardiographic, and transesophageal echocardiographic study. Circulation 1990; 81:865.
61. Leung JM, O'Kelly BF, Mangano DT: Relationship of regional wall motion abnormalities to hemodynamic indices of myocardial oxygen supply and demand in patients undergoing CABG surgery. Anesthesiology 1990; 73:802.
62. Voci P, Bilotta F, Aronson S, et al: Echocardiographic analysis of dysfunctional and normal myocardial segments before and immediately after coronary artery bypass graft surgery. Anesth Analg 1992; 75:213.
63. Leung JM, O'Kelly B, Browner WS, et al: Prognostic importance of post-bypass regional wall motion abnormalities in patients undergoing coronary artery bypass graft surgery. Anesthesiology 1989; 71:16.
64. Shah PM, Kyo S, Matsumura M, et al: Utility of biplane transesophageal echocardiography in left ventricular wall motion analysis. J Cardiothorac Vasc Anesth 1991; 5:316.
65. Aronson S, Lee BK, Wiencek JG, et al: Assessment of myocardial perfusion during CABG surgery with two-dimensional transesophageal contrast echocardiography. Anesthesiology 1991; 75:433.
66. Han CY, Lin KN, Porembka DT, et al: A knowledge-based image analysis for automated boundary extraction of transesophageal echocardiographic left-ventricular images. IEEE Trans Med Imaging 1991; 10:602.
67. Sheikh KH, Bengston JR, Rankin JS, et al: Intraoperative transesophageal Doppler color flow imaging used to guide patient selection and operative treatment of ischemic mitral regurgitation. Circulation 1991; 84:594.
68. Stewart WJ, Currie PJ, Salcedo EE, et al: Jet direction by color flow mapping accurately depicts the mechanism of mitral regurgitation. Circulation 1988; 78:434.
69. Castello R, Lenzen P, Aguirre F, et al: Quantitation of mitral regurgitation by transesophageal echocardiography with Doppler color flow mapping: Correlation with cardiac catheterization. J Am Coll Cardiol 1992; 19:1516.
70. Shyu K-G, Lei M-H, Hwang J-J, et al: Morphologic characterization and quantitative assessment of mitral regurgitation with ruptured chordae tendineae by transesophageal echocardiography. Am J Cardiol 1992; 70:1152.
71. Yoshida K, Yoshikawa J, Yamaura Y, et al: Assessment of mitral regurgitation by biplane transesophageal color Doppler flow mapping. Circulation 1990; 82:1121.
72. Bargiggia GS, Tronconi L, Sahn DJ, et al: A new method for quantitation of mitral regurgitation based on color flow Doppler imaging of flow convergence proximal to regurgitant orifice. Circulation 1991; 84:1481.
73. Gorcsan J III, Kenny WM, Diana P, et al: Transesophageal continuous-wave Doppler to evaluate mitral prosthetic stenosis. Am Heart J 1991; 121:911.
74. DeSimone R, Lange R, Saggau W, et al: Intraoperative transesophageal echocardiography for the evaluation of mitral, aortic, and tricuspid valve repair: A tool to optimize surgical outcome. Eur J Cardiothorac Surg 1992; 6:665.
75. Smith MD, Harrison MR, Pinton R, et al: Regurgitant jet size by transesophageal compared with transthoracic Doppler color flow imaging. Circulation 1991; 83:79.
76. Daniel LB, Grigg LE, Weisel RD, et al: Comparison of transthoracic and transesophageal assessment of prosthetic valve dysfunction. Echocardiography 1990; 7:83.
77. Herrera CJ, Chaudhry FA, DeFrino PF, et al: Value and limitations of transesophageal echocardiography in evaluating prosthetic or bioprosthetic valve dysfunction. Am J Cardiol 1992; 69:697.
78. Alton ME, Pasierski TJ, Orsinelli DA, et al: Comparison of transthoracic and transesophageal echocardiography in evaluation of 47 Starr-Edwards prosthetic valves. J Am Coll Cardiol 1992; 20:1503.
79. Castello R, Pearson AC, Lenzen P, et al: Effect of mitral regurgitation on pulmonary venous velocities derived from transesophageal echocardiography color-guided pulsed Doppler imaging. J Am Coll Cardiol 1991; 17:1499.
80. Urbanowicz JH, Shaaban J, Cohen NH, et al: Comparison of transesophageal echocardiographic and scintigraphic estimates of left ventricular end-diastolic volume index and ejection fraction in patients following coronary artery bypass grafting. Anesthesiology 1990; 72:607.
81. Reich DL, Konstadt SN, Nejat M, et al: Intraoperative transesophageal echocardiography for the detection of cardiac preload changes induced by transfusion and phlebotomy in pediatric patients. Anesthesiology 1993; 79:10.
82. Poelaert JI, Visser CA, Everaert JA, et al: Acute hemodynamic changes of pressure-controlled inverse ratio ventilation in the adult respiratory distress syndrome. Chest 1993; 104:214.
83. Schuster S, Erbel R, Weilemann LS, et al: Hemodynamics during PEEP ventilation in patients with severe left ventricular failure studied by transesophageal echocardiography. Chest 1990; 97:1181.
84. Martin RW, Bashein G, Detmer PR, et al: Ventricular volume measurement from a multiplanar transesophageal ultrasonic imaging system: An in vitro study. IEEE Trans Biomed Eng 1990; 37:442.
85. Belohlavek M, Foley DA, Gerber TC, et al: Three- and four-dimensional cardiovascular ultrasound imaging: A new era for echocardiography. Mayo Clin Proc 1993; 68:221.
86. Porembka D, Behbehani M, Wan L, et al: The implementation of artificial intelligence methods for automated edge detection of the left ventricle in a canine model. Crit Care Med 1993; 21:S269.
87. Berge KH, Lanier WL, Reeder GS: Occult cardiac tamponade detected by transesophageal echocardiography. Mayo Clin Proc 1992; 67:667.
88. Appleton CP, Hatle LK, Popp RL: Cardiac tamponade and pericardial effusion: Respiratory variation in transvalvular flow velocities studied by Doppler echocardiography. J Am Coll Cardiol 1988; 11:1020.
89. Hoit BD, Dalton N, Bhargava V, et al: Pericardial influences on right and left ventricular filling dynamics. Circ Res 1991; 68:197.
90. Castello R, Pearson AC, Lenzen P, et al: Evaluation of pulmonary venous flow by transesophageal echocardiography in subjects with a normal heart: Comparison with transthoracic echocardiography. J Am Coll Cardiol 1991; 18:65.
91. Nishimura RA, Abel MD, Hatle LK, et al: Assessment of diastolic function of the heart: Background and current applications of Doppler echocardiography. Part II: Clinical studies. Mayo Clin Proc 1989; 64:181.
92. Hoffmann R, Lambertz H, Jutten H, et al: Mitral and pulmonary venous flow under influence of positive end-expiratory pressure ventilation analyzed by transesophageal pulsed Doppler echocardiography. Am J Cardiol 1991; 68:697.
93. Kuecherer HF, Muhiudeen IA, Kusumoto FM, et al: Estimation of mean left atrial pressure from transesophageal pulsed Doppler echocardiography of pulmonary venous flow. Circulation 1990; 82:1127.
94. Klein AL, Stewart WJ, Bartlett J, et al: Effects of mitral regurgitation on pulmonary venous flow and left atrial pressure: An intraoperative transesophageal echocardiographic study. J Am Coll Cardiol 1992; 20:1345.
95. Porembka D, Hoit B, McMannis K, et al: Correlation of pulmonary artery occlusion pressure with pulmonary venous flow pattern by transesophageal echocardiography. Crit Care Med 1993; 21:S268.
96. Weintraub R, Shiota T, Elkadi T, et al: Transesophageal echocardiography in infants and children with congential heart disease. Circulation 1992; 86:711.
97. Stumper O, Kaulitz R, Elzenga NJ, et al: The value of transesophageal echocardiography in children with congenital heart disease. J Am Soc Echocargiogr 1991; 4:164.

98. Stewart WJ, Currie PJ, Salcedo EE, et al: Intraoperative Doppler color flow mapping for decision-making in valve repair for mitral regurgitation. Techniques and results in 100 patients. Circulation 1990; 81:556.
99. Zabalgoitia M, Gandhi DK, Evans J, et al: Transesophageal echocardiography in the awake patient: Its role in the clinical decision-making process. Am Heart J 1990; 120:1147.
100. Gardner CJ, Brown S, Hagen-Ansert S, et al: Guidelines for cardiac sonographer education: Report of the American Society of Echocardiography Sonographer Education and Training Committee. Am Soc Echocardiogr 1992; 5:635.
101. Fyfe DA, Ritter SB, Snider AR, et al: Guidelines for transesophageal echocardiography in children. J Am Soc Echocardiogr 1992; 5:640.

CHAPTER 45

Computed Tomography of the Abdomen in the Critical Care Patient

Raymond F. Austin, Jr., MD • Richard A. Szucs, MD • Steven M. Hall, MD

Patients in the intensive care unit (ICU) frequently develop signs or symptoms that require imaging evaluation. These include sepsis, unexplained abdominal pain, abdominal distention, diarrhea, and occult blood loss. Computed tomography (CT) of the abdomen has a central role in the evaluation of these patients because it can evaluate the gastrointestinal tract and solid organs of the abdomen as well as the mesentery and retroperitoneum.[1,2] CT can often establish the diagnosis or further direct the diagnostic work-up and is helpful in choosing between surgical and nonsurgical management. For example, when CT demonstrates a mass or adenopathy, CT-guided aspiration or biopsy can obtain cells or tissue for diagnosis. In cases of gastrointestinal perforation, when CT demonstrates pneumoperitoneum, it may suggest the likely source of perforation and help to direct the surgical approach.

Transporting critically ill patients to the CT suite is not without some potential risk. Indeck and colleagues[3] report that in 25% of their patients, transportation to radiology from the ICU resulted in a change in patient management. However, 68% of their patients experienced changes in their physiologic status that required therapeutic intervention. A number of studies demonstrate that significant changes in patient management were effected because of the information gained.[4–7]

It is imperative to perform an optimal CT examination on these patients. The entire abdomen and pelvis must be examined. Modern CT scanners with scan times of 5 seconds or less are essential because patients may not be able to control their respiration. Adequate bowel opacification with oral contrast material is particularly important for those in whom an abscess is being sought. Many patients have adynamic ileus with fluid-filled loops. Without proper oral contrast, it may be impossible to distinguish a fluid collection from fluid-filled loops of bowel. Intravenous contrast material is also important, particularly to demonstrate microabscesses in the liver and spleen and to define the enhancing rind of an intra-abdominal abscess. Patients must always be accompanied by critical care unit personnel for support during transport and examination.

Although magnetic resonance imaging (MRI) has a significant role in the assessment of brain and spinal cord abnormalities, the electronic monitoring devices and therapy pumps used to support the patients in critical care are incompatible with the magnetic fields of the MRI scanner. At present, nonferromagnetic devices are being developed for use in the MRI suite. The inordinate length of time required to examine the entire abdomen and pelvis using multiple sequences with MRI and the limited ability to aspirate and drain collections in the MRI suite are additional factors that continue to limit the use of MRI in the abdomen in the critical care setting.

This chapter reflects our experience with the use of CT in critical care patients. Immunocompromised patients and patients with pancreatitis present important and common problems. They are given special attention.

INTRA-ABDOMINAL INFECTION

The search for an intra-abdominal source of sepsis is the most frequent indication for CT evaluation of critically ill patients. The earlier an abscess is detected, the better the outcome. Mortality rates are reported to range from 30% in

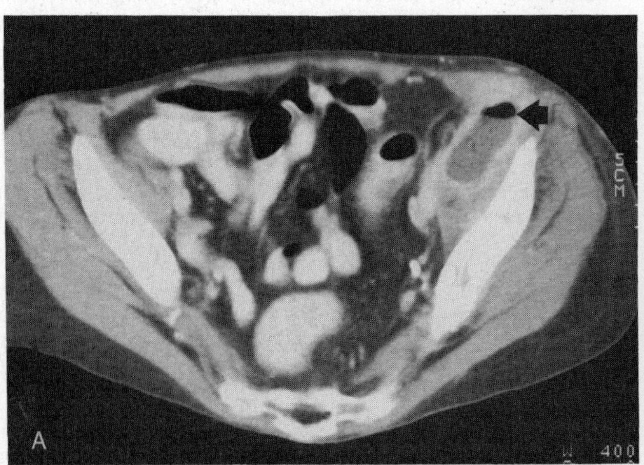

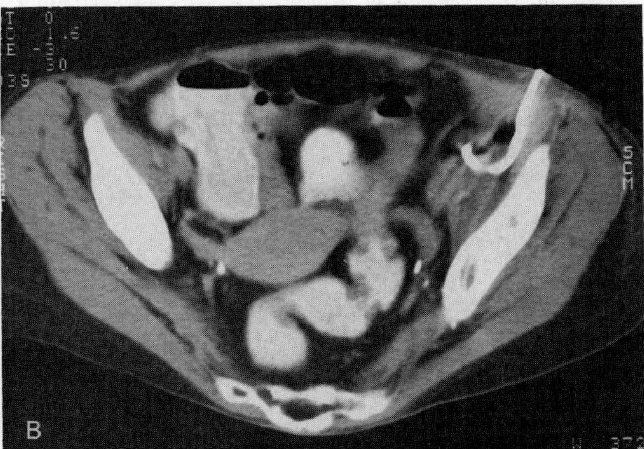

Figure 45–1. Diverticular abscess with drainage. A 57-year-old woman with Crohn's disease and breast cancer presented with left lower quadrant pain, fever, and leukocytosis. *A,* A collection with an air-fluid level *(arrow)* was located anterior to the left iliac muscle. Note the enhancing rind. *B,* The abscess was aspirated and subsequently drained with a catheter.

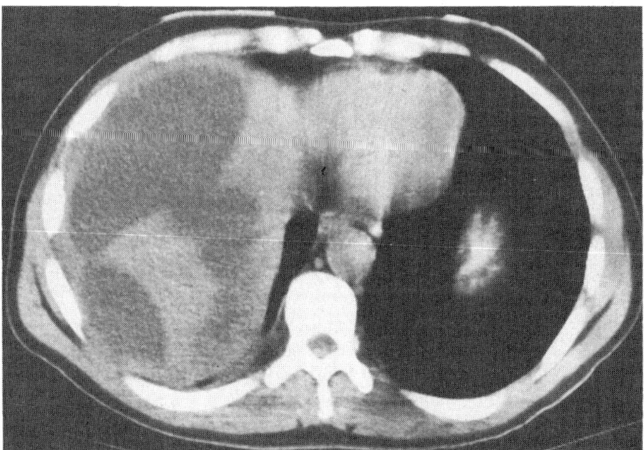

Figure 45–2. Infected biloma. A 49-year-old man with a liver laceration following a motor vehicle accident presented with persistent right upper quadrant pain, fever, and leukocytosis. A large subphrenic fluid collection extends from a major laceration of the liver. No evidence of gas within the fluid collection was present. The collection proved to be an infected biloma on subsequent aspiration and drainage.

operatively drained abscesses to as high as 100% for undrained abscesses.[7] CT has a 95% accuracy for detection of the presence of an abscess.[7] In the setting of sepsis, it is important to be very aggressive in aspirating and draining fluid collections at the time of diagnostic examination. The cure rate with percutaneous abscess drainage is reported to be between 64% and 90%.[8] When percutaneous drainage is not curative, patients may recover sufficiently to tolerate definitive surgery.

Abscesses are generally well-defined fluid collections with enhancing rinds (Fig. 45–1*A*). Aspiration for diagnosis and placement of drains into these collections (Fig. 45–1*B*) is recommended. The absence of gas does not preclude an infected collection (Fig. 45–2).

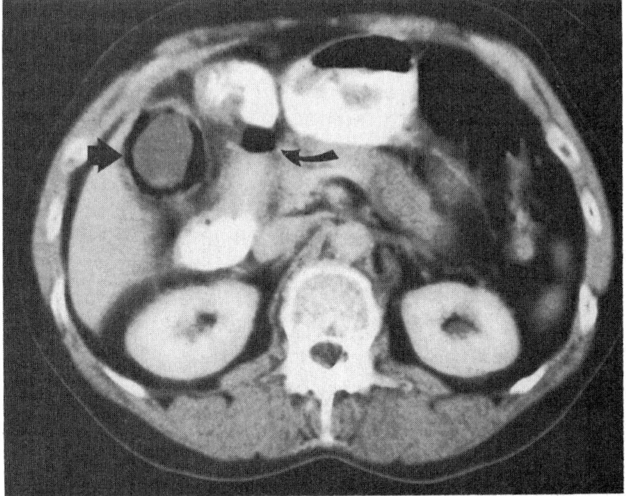

Figure 45–3. Emphysematous cholecystitis. A 42-year-old male with acute chest pain who had been admitted to rule out myocardial infarction developed atypical midepigastric pain after 2 days. The results of ultrasound examination were unclear. No right upper quadrant tenderness was present. The gallbladder wall was thickened and contained gas *(arrow)*. The gas posterior to the duodenal bulb *(curved arrow)* dissected the hepatoduodenal ligament. The findings were consistent with the presence of emphysematous cholecystitis.

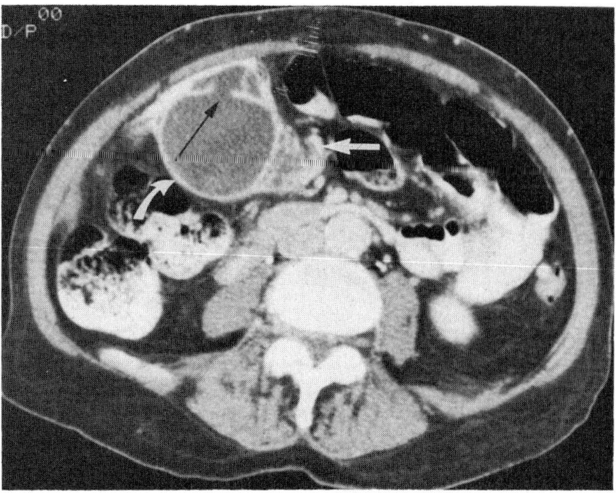

Figure 45–4. Acute acalculous cholecystitis. A 62-year-old man admitted following a motor vehicle accident with a liver laceration developed increasing right upper quadrant pain. His temperature and white blood cell count were normal. The gallbladder was distended and had an enhanced wall *(curved white arrow)*. A confined perforation was located anteriorly *(black arrow)*. Pericholecystic inflammatory change is visible *(white arrow)*. Surgery confirmed the diagnosis of acalculous cholecystitis.

Acute acalculous cholecystitis is not uncommon in this population. Risk factors include recent surgery, severe trauma or burns, total parenteral nutrition, and multiorgan failure.[9] Gangrene of the gallbladder is reported to afflict as many as 28% of these patients.[9] Patients with gangrene of the gallbladder may not have a Murphy sign. These patients may present with sepsis and no localizing signs, particularly if they are obtunded (Figs. 45–3 and 45–4). When acute acalculous cholecystitis is suspected, ultrasonography and hepatobiliary scanning are recommended as the first diagnostic imaging examinations.

Obtunded patients or patients insensitive to pain may present with an abdominal source of sepsis (Fig. 45–5).

More unusual causes of sepsis such as septic thrombi are

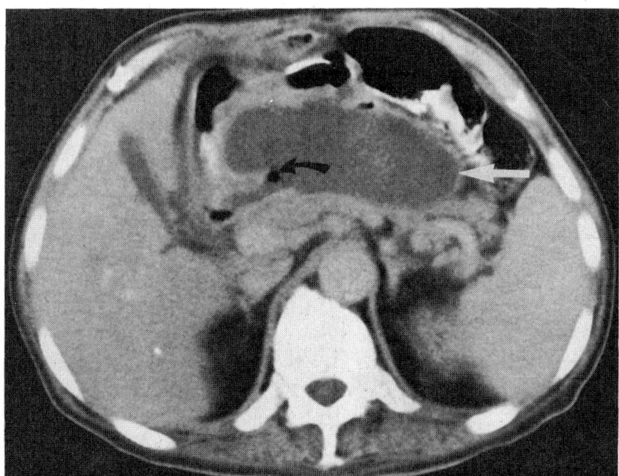

Figure 45–5. Lesser sac abscess. A 43-year-old quadriplegic man presented with abdominal distention, fever, and leukocytosis. The CT scan revealed a large fluid collection in the lesser sac *(straight arrow)*. A gas bubble was present within the collection *(curved arrow)*. The collection was successfully drained through the stomach. The patient was subsequently shown to have a perforated ulcer of the posterior gastric wall.

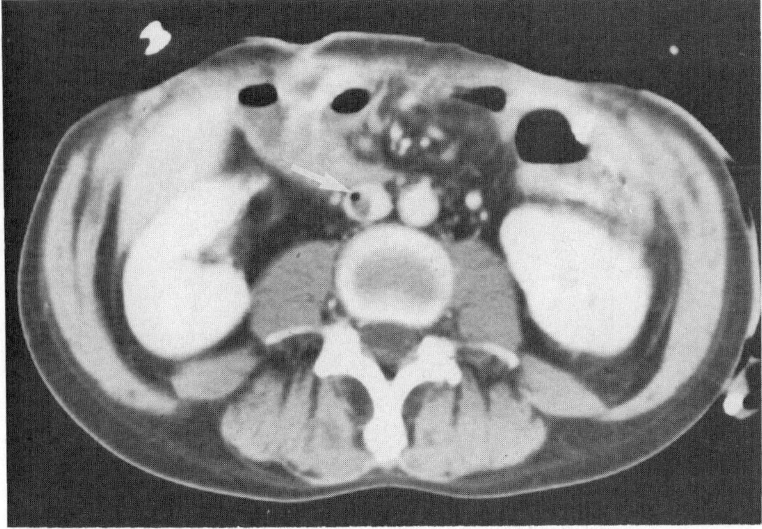

Figure 45–6. Infected thrombus in the inferior vena cava. A 47-year-old man with a long-standing history of Crohn's disease, multiple operations, recent surgery, and an indwelling right femoral catheter developed sepsis without focal abnormality. The CT examination revealed a clot containing a gas bubble *(arrow)* within the inferior vena cava. The femoral line had already been removed. A vena cava filter was placed through the jugular vein.

also demonstrated by CT (Fig. 45–6). Norwood and colleagues estimate that 50,000 catheter-related cases of septicemia occur annually.[10] In severely ill postpartum patients and patients with pelvic infection, ovarian vein thrombophlebitis must be considered (Fig. 45–7*A* and *B*).

Pseudomembranous colitis is most commonly encountered after use of clindamycin and ampicillin. It can occur as late as 3 weeks after antibiotics are discontinued. CT demonstrates a pancolitis (see Fig. 45–13), which may be indistinguishable from the severe infectious colitis afflicting immunosuppressed patients.

OCCULT BLOOD LOSS

Occult bleeding occurs most commonly after surgery (Fig. 45–8), after cardiac catheterization (Fig. 45–9), or in anticoagulated patients. A suspected ruptured abdominal aortic aneurysm (Fig. 45–10) can be confirmed by CT.

BOWEL ISCHEMIA

Bowel ischemia in critically ill patients may be nonocclusive and may be a delayed sequela of severe shock (Fig. 45–11). It is imperative to recognize the changes of bowel ischemia to undertake early intervention (Fig. 45–12). Unfortunately, the early signs of ischemia are nonspecific and the more specific signs are present only after the bowel has already infarcted (see Fig. 45–11).

COMPUTED TOMOGRAPHY OF THE ACUTE ABDOMEN IN AN IMMUNOCOMPROMISED HOST

Patients with the acquired immunodeficiency syndrome (AIDS) and patients receiving immunosuppressive therapy for cancer and autoimmune diseases as well as for organ transplantation are predisposed to various unique problems, including opportunistic infections[11] and unusual malignancies.[12] They may also have atypical presentations of common disorders and therefore present difficult problems in diagnosis and management.

Opportunistic Infection

The gastrointestinal tract is a frequent site of involvement by opportunistic infections.[13, 14] These include bacterial, fungal, viral, and protozoan infections. These patients usually

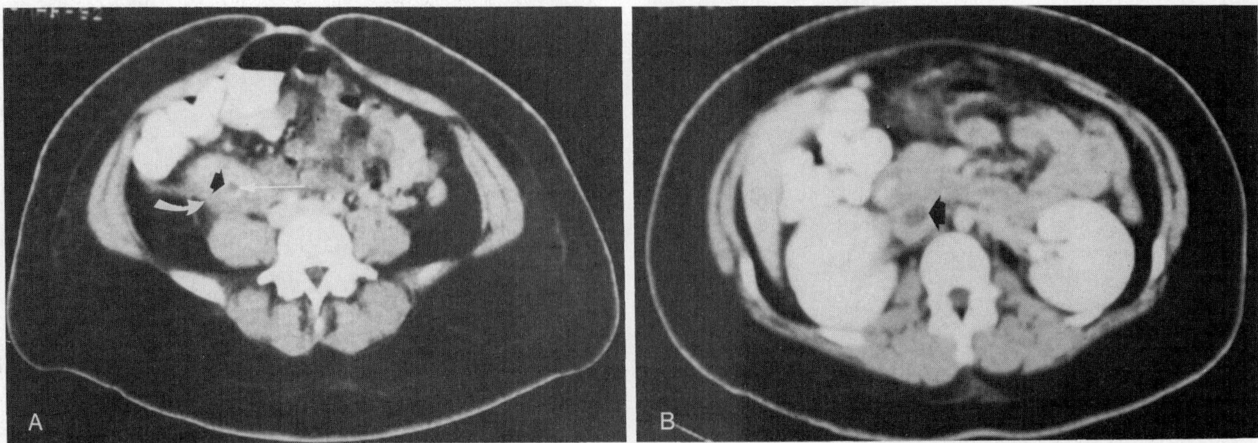

Figure 45–7. Thrombophlebitis of the right ovarian vein. A 28-year-old woman developed sepsis following cesarean section. *A,* An inflammatory mass *(curved white arrow)* surrounds the ovarian vein. The vein wall is enhanced *(black arrow)*, and a clot is present in the center of the vein *(straight white arrow)*. *B,* The clot extends into the inferior vena cava *(arrow)*. The patient underwent anticoagulation therapy and was treated with antibiotics.

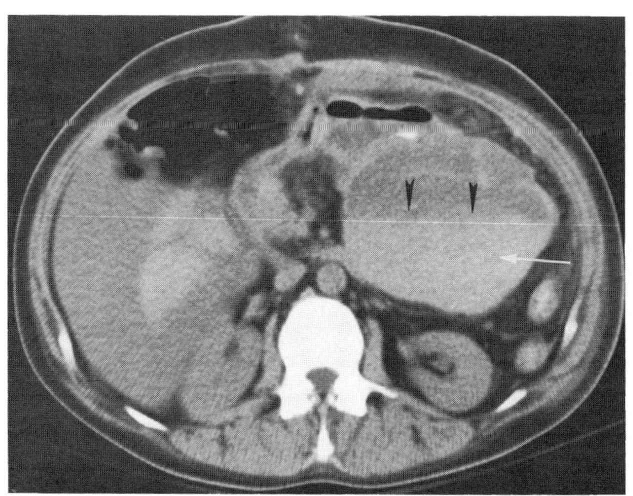

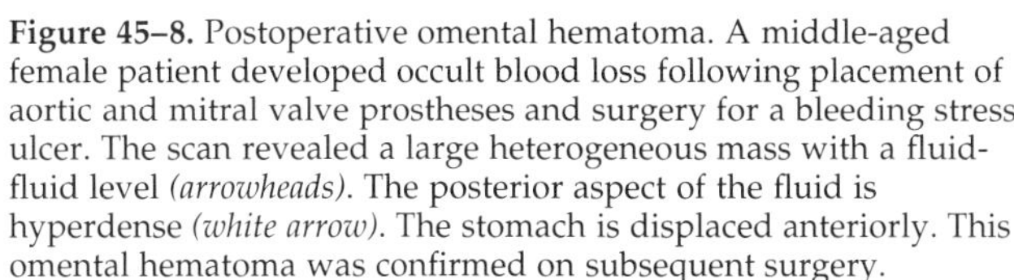

Figure 45–8. Postoperative omental hematoma. A middle-aged female patient developed occult blood loss following placement of aortic and mitral valve prostheses and surgery for a bleeding stress ulcer. The scan revealed a large heterogeneous mass with a fluid-fluid level *(arrowheads)*. The posterior aspect of the fluid is hyperdense *(white arrow)*. The stomach is displaced anteriorly. This omental hematoma was confirmed on subsequent surgery.

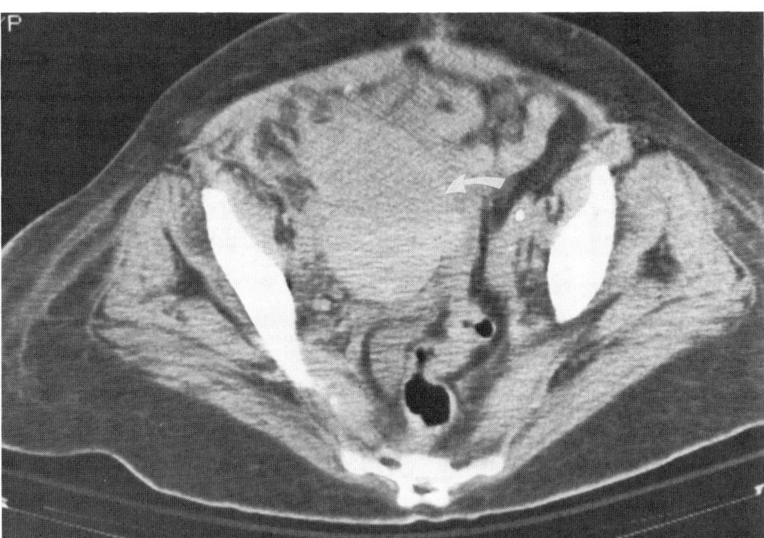

Figure 45–9. Retroperitoneal hematoma following coronary artery angioplasty. The scan revealed a large hyperdense hematoma along the right lateral pelvic wall *(curved arrow)*. The hematoma extended up to the level of the kidney. The patient required blood replacement and surgical closure of the lacerated femoral artery, which had been inadvertently punctured above the inguinal ligament.

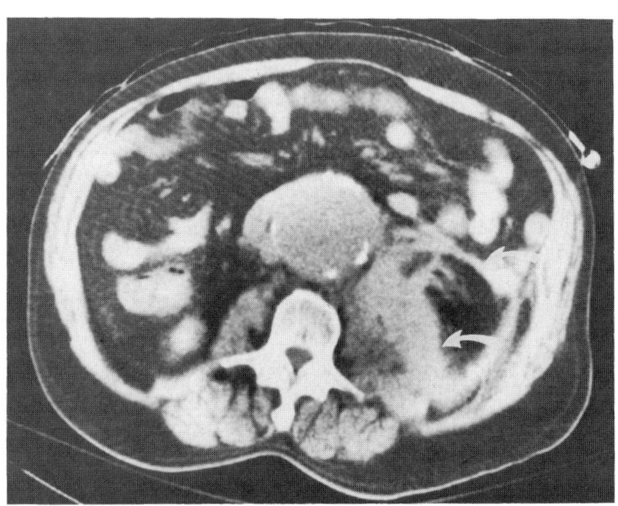

Figure 45–10. Ruptured abdominal aortic aneurysm. The patient presented with abdominal and back pain and with a pulsatile mass in the abdomen. The CT scan revealed the presence of an atherosclerotic abdominal aortic aneurysm with hyperdense fluid *(arrows)* extending into the anterior and posterior left pararenal spaces. The presence of a rupturing abdominal aortic aneurysm was confirmed at surgery.

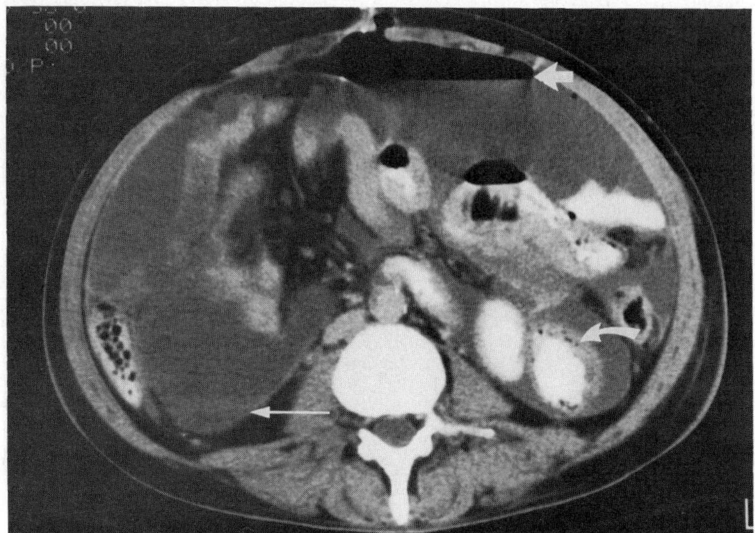

Figure 45–11. Small bowel infarction and perforation. A 69-year-old man suffered a motor vehicle accident with traumatic rupture of the thoracic aorta and left hemidiaphragm. The man experienced severe hypotension during surgery. Postoperative abdominal distention, pain, and leukocytosis developed. A large amount of fluid was present in the abdomen with an air-fluid level anteriorly *(short arrow)*. Note the fluid level in the right abdomen *(long straight arrow)*; this is orally administered contrast medium that has leaked from the bowel. Thickening of the small bowel wall and pneumatosis intestinalis are visible *(curved arrow)*. These changes represent extensive small bowel infarction with perforation due to severe shock and hypoperfusion of the bowel.

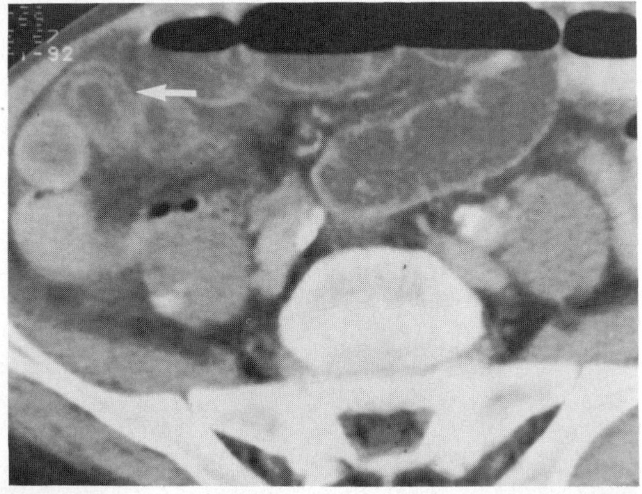

Figure 45–12. Closed-loop obstruction with small bowel ischemia. This patient was scanned 2 weeks following mitral valve annuloplasty. Lower abdominal pain developed acutely. The small bowel was markedly dilated with an air-fluid level and an enhancing wall *(arrow)*. Note the thickened wall of the bowel in the right lower quadrant with enhancement of the mucosa and marked edema of the wall. These are early changes of bowel ischemia but are nonspecific. At surgery, the patient was found to have a closed-loop obstruction. The bowel was edematous but viable.

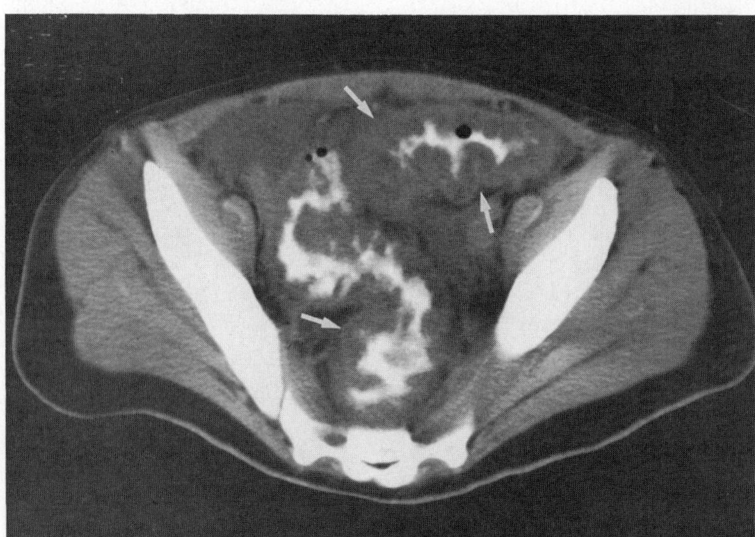

Figure 45–13. Cytomegalovirus colitis. A 36-year-old man with AIDS presented with a 1-week history of fever and watery diarrhea. CT demonstrated marked thickening and thumb printing of the colonic wall *(arrows)*. In this case, the wall thickening was much better seen after administration of rectal contrast medium. Culture of a rectal biopsy specimen produced cytomegalovirus. The patient was treated with ganciclovir.

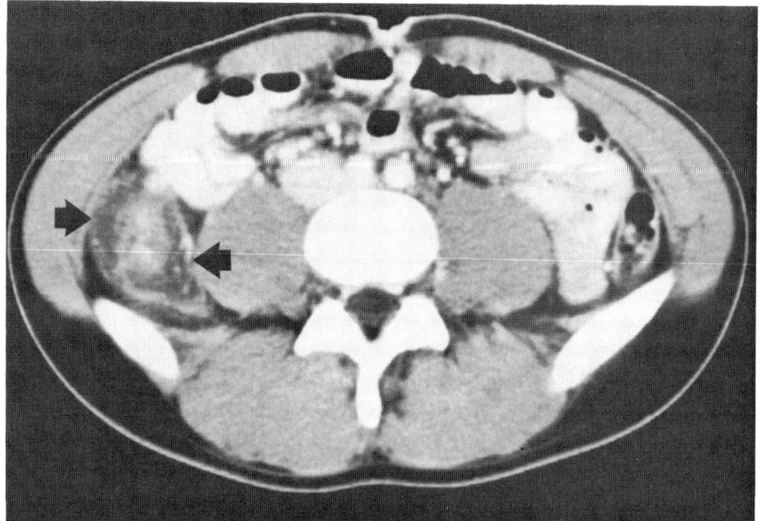

Figure 45–14. Neutropenic colitis. A 24-year-old HIV-positive white man with factor VIII deficiency presented with right lower quadrant tenderness and guarding and a total granulocyte count of 1100. CT demonstrated cecal wall thickening as well as low attenuation in the wall from edema *(arrows)*. The patient was treated with antibiotics, and his symptoms resolved.

present with gastrointestinal symptoms such as dysphagia, odynophagia, abdominal pain, or diarrhea. CT can demonstrate bowel wall thickening and lymphadenopathy in patients with opportunistic infections of the hollow viscera. Cytomegalovirus usually involves the esophagus, gastric antrum, and colon. CT in these patients may demonstrate striking bowel wall thickening (Fig. 45–13).[15, 16] *Cryptosporidium* and *Mycobacterium avium-intracellulare* usually involve the small bowel, resulting in dilated fluid-filled loops with thickened folds.[17] *Mycobacterium tuberculosis* characteristically involves the cecum and terminal ileum, with adjacent right lower quadrant adenopathy.[18, 19] Mycobacterial infections often produce caseation within lymph nodes, resulting in a characteristic CT appearance of adenopathy with central hypodensity. CT-guided aspiration of enlarged nodes may be helpful to establish the diagnosis and to distinguish these mycobacterial infections from AIDS-related malignancies such as Kaposi's sarcoma or lymphoma, which also produce lymphadenopathy.

Neutropenic colitis, also referred to as *typhlitis*, is an acute inflammation of the cecum that was initially described in children with leukemia, but it may also afflict patients with AIDS or immunosuppression after organ transplantation. Patients typically present with right lower quadrant tenderness. CT demonstrates thickening of the cecal wall, often with decreased attenuation due to edema (Fig. 45–14).[20] Early diagnosis and aggressive medical treatment are necessary to prevent transmural necrosis and perforation.

CT is the study of choice to evaluate for suspected abscess in immunocompromised patients with abdominal pain and fever. *Candida albicans*, the most common cause of opportunistic esophagitis, may also progress to hematogenous dissemination, with development of microabscesses in the liver, spleen, and kidneys.[21] CT demonstrates multiple low-attenuation foci in the involved organ (Fig. 45–15). CT-guided aspiration can establish the diagnosis. Immunocompromised patients may develop abscesses with all the usual pyogenic pathogens such as *Staphylococcus aureus* and *Streptococcus* species, as well as unusual opportunistic organisms such as *Aspergillus* (Fig. 45–16). CT can localize the abscess and guide percutaneous abscess drainage.

MALIGNANCIES

Patients with AIDS have an increased incidence of non-Hodgkin's lymphoma. AIDS-related lymphomas are highly

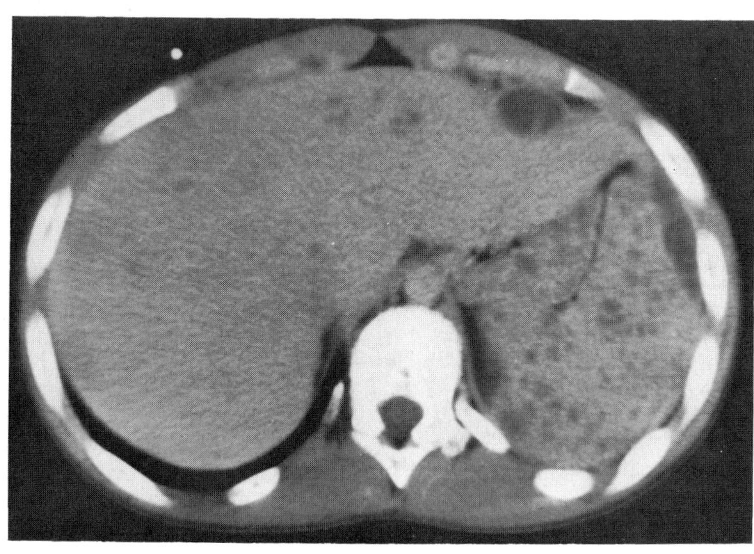

Figure 45–15. *Candida* microabscesses of the liver and spleen. A 14-year-old boy with acute myelocytic leukemia and neutropenia presented with fever and abdominal pain. CT revealed multiple hypodense lesions in the liver and spleen. CT-guided aspiration of the spleen produced a culture specimen that yielded *Candida albicans*. The patient was treated with amphotericin.

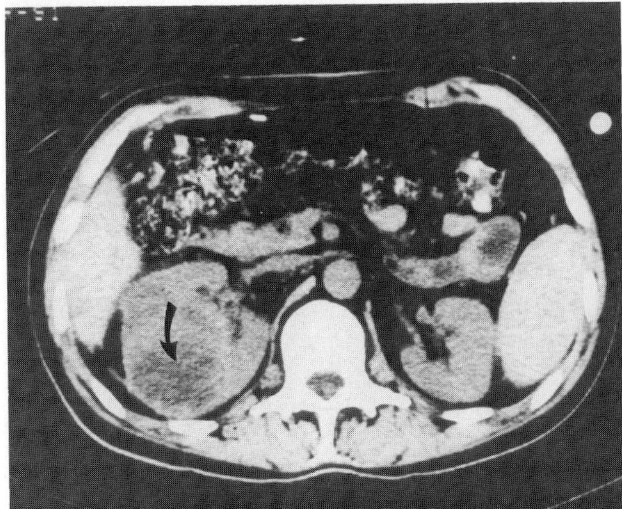

Figure 45–16. *Aspergillus* renal abscess. A 26-year-old man returned 8 months following orthotopic liver transplant with a 1-week history of fever, dysuria, and right flank tenderness. CT demonstrated the presence of a heterogeneous mass in the midportion of a markedly enlarged right kidney. The central portion of the mass was hypodense *(arrow)*; this suggested the presence of necrosis or fluid. The patient was being treated with cyclosporin; hence, intravenous contrast medium was not given because of the risk of nephrotoxicity. CT-guided catheter drainage was performed. The cultures yielded *Aspergillus fumigatus*. The patient was treated with amphotericin and subsequently underwent right-sided nephrectomy.

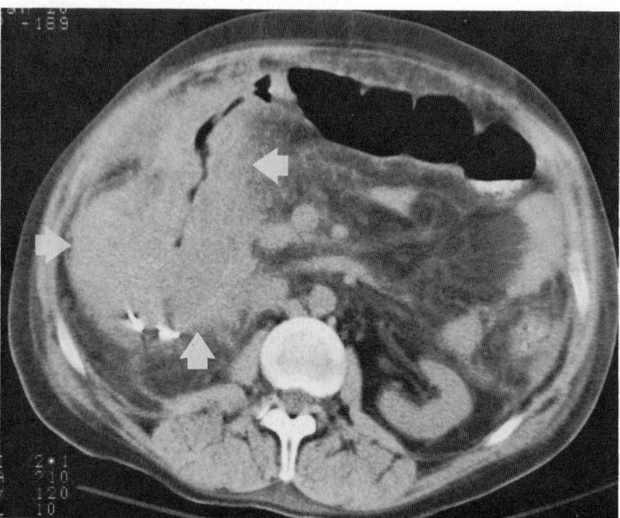

Figure 45–17. Post-transplantation lymphoma. A 47-year-old liver transplant patient presented 7 years after transplantation with a 2-week history of increasing abdominal distention in addition to nausea, vomiting, and dehydration. CT demonstrated the presence of ascites and marked thickening of the right colon as well as a mass that encased the colon *(arrows)*. Fluid obtained on paracentesis contained lymphoma cells, and open biopsy showed the presence of Burkitt's lymphoma.

aggressive tumors with poorly differentiated subtypes and have a poor prognosis. AIDS-related lymphoma may present as focal masses in the liver, spleen, gastrointestinal tract, or kidneys or as adenopathy or infiltration of the retroperitoneum or mesentery.[22, 23] Kaposi's sarcoma in patients with AIDS is an aggressive malignancy often involving the visceral organs, gastrointestinal tract, and lymph nodes.[24] Although CT demonstration of focal masses and adenopathy is nonspecific, CT-guided percutaneous aspiration can establish the diagnosis.

Transplant recipients have a 100-fold increased incidence of malignant neoplasms, including lymphomas and various types of carcinoma. Transplant recipients treated with cyclosporin, similarly to patients with AIDS, have an increased incidence of non-Hodgkin's B cell lymphomas because cyclosporin inhibits suppressor T cells.[25, 26] Malignant lymphomas in cyclosporin-treated transplant recipients occur relatively early and may be widespread at the time of diagnosis (Fig. 45–17).

IMAGING OF PANCREATITIS IN CRITICALLY ILL PATIENTS

Pancreatitis is an important entity in critical care patients, not only as a primary cause of ICU admission but also because of the susceptibility of these patients to develop pancreatitis secondarily. Drug therapy, hypotension with ischemia, infection, surgery, and ulcer formation all may lead to the development of pancreatitis in the critical care setting.

In most cases, the diagnosis is established on clinical grounds and no imaging is needed, particularly if a patient responds to conservative management. Imaging is reserved for patients with clinically severe pancreatitis to identify and evaluate the extent of local complications.[27, 28] CT is the method of choice because the entire abdomen and retroperitoneum can be evaluated. The major complications of acute pancreatitis include necrosis, hemorrhage, infection, and fluid collection. Other complications such as biliary obstruction, vascular thrombosis, and pseudoaneurysm formation can also be detected with CT.

Pancreatic necrosis is an important complication to recognize because of its frequently associated morbidity and mortality. Areas of pancreatic necrosis also have a high risk for subsequent infection. Dynamic CT with rapid infusion of intravenous contrast is the best method to identify pancreatic necrosis.[29] Necrotic areas are seen as regions of nonenhancement within the gland (Fig. 45–18). Infected necrosis requires surgical debridement, and the decision to

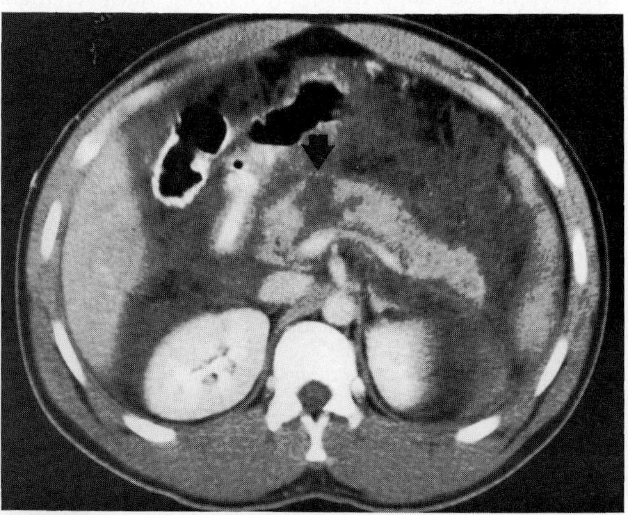

Figure 45–18. Focal pancreatic necrosis. A 24-year-old man with pancreatitis underwent CT examination for hypotension. This revealed a focal area of nonenhancement in the pancreatic neck consistent with an area of necrosis *(arrow)*.

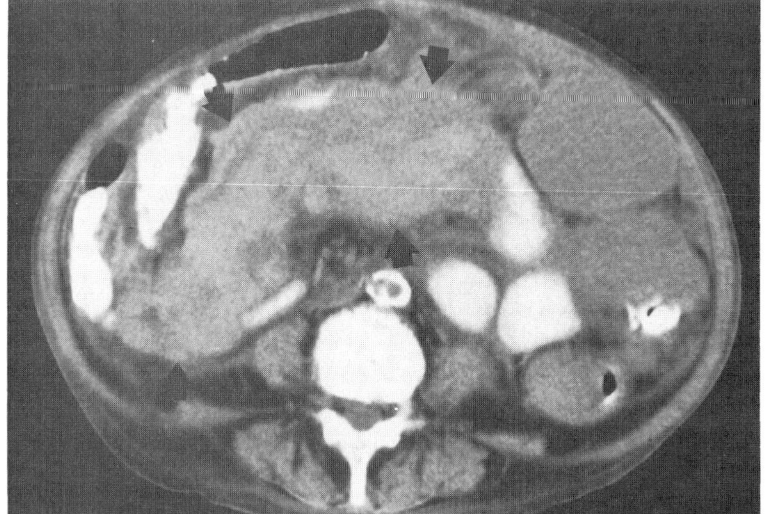

Figure 45–19. Hemorrhagic pancreatitis. A 61-year-old woman developed pancreatitis following ulcer surgery. CT revealed a large, mixed-attenuation hematoma in the small bowel mesentery *(arrows)*. Note the areas of increased density suggestive of acute hemorrhage.

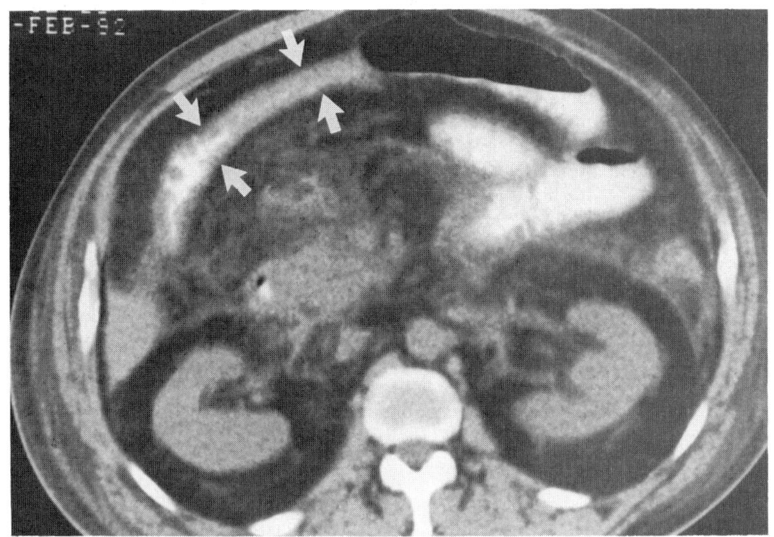

Figure 45–20. Ischemic colitis. A 55-year-old man with pancreatitis developed crampy abdominal pain and had bloody stools. CT examination revealed marked thickening of the transverse colon *(arrows)* that was consistent with the presence of ischemic colitis secondary to pancreatitis-induced arterial thrombosis.

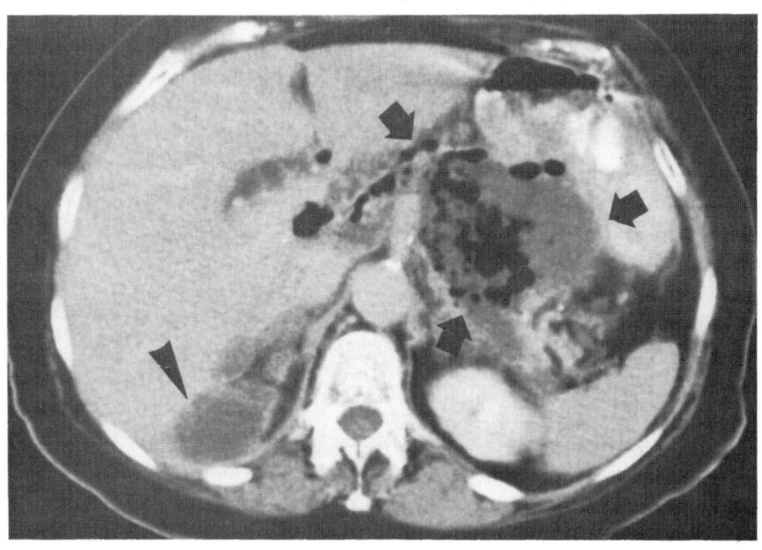

Figure 45–21. Pancreatic abscess. A 35-year-old black woman developed a fever and an elevated white blood cell count. CT demonstrated a gas-containing fluid collection in the lesser sac *(arrows)*. CT-guided aspiration confirmed the presence of a pancreatic abscess. Fluid collections are also present in the right anterior pararenal space *(arrowhead)*.

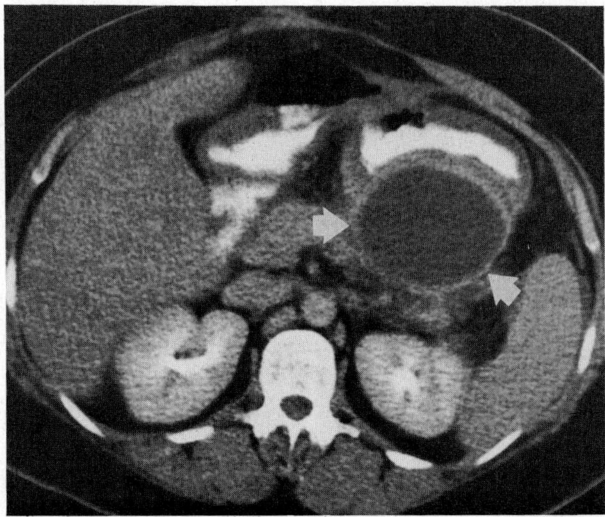

Figure 45–22. Pancreatic pseudocyst. A 30-year-old woman who developed pancreatitis following surgery complained of persistent left epigastric pain. CT revealed a well defined, encapsulated fluid collection *(arrows)* in the lesser sac with mass effect on the posterior gastric wall. The appearance is classic for the presence of a pseudocyst arising from the pancreatic tail.

operate on sterile necrosis is based on the clinical status of the patient.

Although diffuse hemorrhage into a pancreatic phlegmon is common, erosion into a large vessel may lead to formation of large focal hematomas (Fig. 45–19). These patients usually become hypotensive and have a poor clinical prognosis. Inflammatory changes can also cause arterial thrombosis with resultant bowel ischemia (Fig. 45–20), which may progress to frank bowel perforation. Other vascular complications include splenic vein thrombosis with subsequent formation of gastric varices and pseudoaneurysm formation of the splenic artery.

The development of fluid collections in pancreatitis is very common, occurring in up to 50% of patients in some series.[30] Most of these fluid collections, particularly if less than 6 cm in diameter, resolve spontaneously. It is estimated that fewer than 10% will become infected.[31] The accurate and early diagnosis of infection is critical because of the high morbidity and mortality associated with suppurative pancreatitis. The presence of infection cannot be reliably diagnosed on imaging criteria alone. Identification of gas within a collection is highly suggestive of infection (Fig. 45–21) but is not specific, because gas may be introduced secondary to a fistula from the gastrointestinal tract. Therefore, CT-guided fine-needle aspiration has a crucial role in detecting infection in patients with fluid collections. It is a safe and reliable method with a low false-negative rate.[28, 31]

The discovery of infection requires immediate intervention via either percutaneous drainage or surgery. It is important to distinguish infected fluid collections from infected necrosis, because the latter requires surgical debridement. Percutaneous drainage of pancreatic abscesses and chronic pseudocysts is playing an increasing part in the management of complicated pancreatitis with overall good success rates.[32, 33] The term *pseudocyst* should be used for chronic fluid collections that have an enhancing rim or remain unchanged for a prolonged period (Fig. 45–22). Pseudocysts usually require intervention if they become infected, are larger than 10 cm, or cause symptoms as a result of mass effect on adjacent structures.

References

1. Jeffrey RB: Abdominal imaging in the immunocompromised patient. Radiol Clin North Amer 1992; 30:579–596.
2. Kuhlman JE, Fishman EK: Acute abdomen in AIDS: CT diagnosis and triage. Radiographics 1990; 10:621–634.
3. Indeck M, Peterson S, Smith J, et al: Risk, cost and benefit of transporting ICU patients for special studies. J Trauma 1988; 20:1020.
4. Halber MD, Daffner FH, Morgan CL, et al: Intra-abdominal abscesses: Current concepts in radiologic evaluation. AJR 1979; 133:9.
5. Mueller PR, Simeone JF: Intra-abdominal abscesses: Diagnosis by sonography and CT. Radiol Clin North Am 1983; 21:425–443.
6. Roche J: Effectiveness of CT in the diagnosis of intra-abdominal abscess. Med J Aust 1981; 25:85–88.
7. Gerzof SG, Oates E: Imaging techniques for infections in the surgical patient. Surg Clin North Am 1988; 68:147–165.
8. Schurawitzki H, Karmel F, Stiglbauer R, et al: CT guided percutaneous drainage and fluid aspiration in intensive care patients. Acta Radiol 1992; 33:131–136.
9. Savoca PE, Longo WE, Zucker KA, et al: The increasing prevalence of acalculous cholecystitis in outpatients. Results of a seven year study. Ann Surg 1990; 211:433–437.
10. Norwood S, Ruby A, Scivetta J, et al: Catheter related infections and associated septicemia. Chest 1991; 99:968–975.
11. Smith PD, Quinn TC, Strober W, et al: Gastrointestinal infections in AIDS. Ann Intern Med 1992; 116:63–77.
12. Ioachim HL, Dorsett B, Cronin W, et al: Acquired immunodeficiency syndrome–associated lymphomas: Clinical, pathologic, immunologic, and viral characteristics of 11 cases. Hum Pathol 1991; 22:659–673.
13. Jones B, Fishman EK: CT of the gut in the immunocompromised host. Radiol Clin North Am 1989; 27:763–771.
14. Wall SD, Jones B: Gastrointestinal tract in the immunocompromised host: Opportunistic infections and other complications. Radiology 1992; 185:327–335.
15. Jacobson MA, Mills J: Serious cytomegalovirus disease in the acquired immunodeficiency syndrome (AIDS). Ann Intern Med 1988; 108:585–594.
16. Teixidor HS, Honig CL, Norsoph E, et al: Cytomegalovirus infection of the alimentary canal: Radiologic findings with pathologic correlation. Radiology 1987; 163:317–323.
17. Nyberg DA, Federle MP, Jeffrey RB, et al: Abdominal CT findings of disseminated *Mycobacterium avium-intracellulare* in AIDS. AJR 1985; 145:297–299.
18. Balthazar EJ, Gordon R, Hulnick D: Ileocecal tuberculosis: CT and radiologic evaluation. AJR 1990; 154:499–503.
19. Radin DR: Intraabdominal *Mycobacterium tuberculosis* vs *Mycobacterium avium-intracellulare* infections in patients with AIDS: Distinction based on CT findings. AJR 1991; 156:487–491.
20. Frick MP, Maile CW, Crass JR, et al: Computed tomography of neutropenic colitis. AJR 1984; 143:763–765.
21. Shirkhoda A: CT findings in hepatosplenic and renal candidiasis. J Comput Assist Tomogr 1987; 11:795–798.
22. Townsend RR: CT of AIDS-related lymphoma. AJR 1991; 156:969–974.
23. Nyberg DA, Jeffrey RB, Federle MP, et al: AIDS-related lymphomas: Evaluation by abdominal CT. Radiology 1986; 159:59–63.
24. Luburich P, Bru C, Ayuso MC, et al: Hepatic Kaposi sarcoma in AIDS: US and CT findings. Radiology 1990; 175:172–174.
25. Frick MP, Salomonowitz E, Hanto DW, et al: CT of abdominal lymphoma after renal transplantation. AJR 1984; 142:97–99.
26. Honda H, Barloon TJ, Franken EA, et al: Clinical and radiologic features of malignant neoplasms in organ transplant recipients: Cyclosporine-treated vs. untreated patients. AJR 1990; 154:271–274.
27. Moulton JS: The radiologic assessment of acute pancreatitis and its complications. Pancreas 1991; 6:513–522.
28. Fan ST, Choi TK, Chan FL, et al: Management of complicated acute pancreatitis: Impact of computed tomography. J Gastroenterol Hepatol 1990; 5:103–109.

29. London NJ, Leese T, Lavelle JM, et al: Dynamic computed tomography in acute pancreatitis: A prospective study. Br J Surg 1991; 78:1452–1456.
30. Kourtesis G, Wilson SE, Williams RA: The clinical significance of fluid collections in acute pancreatitis. Am Surg 1990; 56:796–799.
31. Stiles GM, Berne TV, Thommen VD, et al: Fine needle aspiration of pancreatic fluid collections. Am Surg 1990; 56:764–768.
32. Lee MJ, Rattner DW, Legemate DA, et al: Acute complicated pancreatitis: Redefining the role of interventional radiology. Radiology 1992; 183:171–174.
33. VanSonnenberg E, Wittich GR, Casola G, et al: Percutaneous drainage of infected and noninfected pancreatic pseudocysts: Experience in 101 cases. Radiology 1989; 170:757–761.

CHAPTER 46

Interventional Radiology in the Critically Ill

Jaime Tisnado, MD, FACR, FACC • Arthur M. Freedman, MD • Patricia E. Cole, PhD, MD

Time is an important factor in establishing a diagnosis and initiating temporary or definitive treatment of a life-threatening process in a critically ill patient. Diagnosis and treatment, which usually require several days, must take place within hours. Surgery can be catastrophic in these patients. The ability to diagnose critical diseases rapidly with cross-sectional imaging modalities has allowed safe and effective interventions by radiologists.

Improvements in radiographic equipment and guide wire and catheter technology have resulted in high rates of success and low rates of complications. Extensive diagnostic and interventional procedures can be performed using percutaneously introduced catheters without the risks of surgery and with minimum alteration of tissues. A protracted convalescence is thereby avoided. Lesions difficult to approach surgically can be accessed rapidly and easily. Frequently, an interventional procedure is temporary until a definitive procedure can be performed when a patient's condition improves.

This chapter presents a summary of the authors' experience in radiologic diagnosis and management of critically ill patients. A brief and practical discussion of the most frequently performed interventional procedures is provided.

A team approach by clinicians, surgeons, and radiologists is necessary for successful treatment of these patients. A serious commitment of time and resources is required. Nurses and radiologic technologists offer a supportive role to physicians. Specialized radiographic-angiographic laboratories with state-of-the-art equipment are needed to expedite interventional procedures. A single-plane (or a biplane) 14- or 16-in image intensifier with digital subtraction angiography is ideal. A 100-mm spot camera device enhances the capabilities of the room. Large-format (14 × 14 in) cut filming is now being replaced by totally digital fluoroscopy. A liberal supply of catheters, guide wires, needles, and other devices must be available to facilitate studies of seriously ill patients. Time, not cost, is usually the deciding factor in the success of these endeavors.

ACUTE GASTROINTESTINAL HEMORRHAGE

Acute gastrointestinal (GI) bleeding is divided into three basic categories: (1) upper GI bleeding from gastroesophageal varices, (2) upper GI bleeding of arterial or arteriolocapillary origin, and (3) lower GI bleeding (sites beyond the ligament of Treitz). Successful management of GI hemorrhage requires the joint effort of medical, surgical, and radiologic teams. Initially, the rate and quantity of blood loss are assessed and the patient stabilized. The source of bleeding is then localized to the upper or lower GI tract. As many as 75% of patients respond to conservative management.[1, 2] Angiographic diagnosis and transcatheter therapy become important management procedures when conservative medical and invasive endoscopic treatments fail.

Endoscopy, radionuclide scanning, and arteriography are used to demonstrate GI bleeding sites. Endoscopy is the initial procedure in upper GI bleeding. Radionuclide scans are important screening tests in lower GI bleeding. Either technetium 99m sulfur colloid (^{99m}Tc-SC) or ^{99m}Tc-labeled red blood cells (^{99m}Tc-RBC) are administered intravenously. Acute bleeding is diagnosed when radionuclide extravasates, with subsequent accumulation and movement through the GI tract (Fig. 46–1). Radionuclide scanning is more sensitive than angiography for detecting bleeding.[3]

Arteriographically, acute GI bleeding is demonstrated by extravasation of contrast material into the bowel lumen that persists and increases as the arterial phase progresses into the venous phase (see Fig. 46–1). A single site is typically identified, but multiple small sites of extravasation are sometimes seen. Arteriography is very sensitive and specific in localizing bleeding if the rate of hemorrhage is at least 0.5 mL/min.[4] Thus, patients with a persistently bloody nasogastric aspirate despite lavage and patients with continuing transfusion requirements are most likely to have positive arteriograms. Arteriography should not be performed emergently if active bleeding has stopped. However, emergent angiographic intervention may be indicated when the initial bleed was severe and the patient's ability to tolerate additional bleeding is low. In these cases, the purpose is either (1) transcatheter therapy of an endoscopically visualized lesion with bleeding not able to be treated endoscopically or (2) diagnosis and possible treatment of a previously unrecognized lesion.[2]

Transcatheter Therapy

Two types of transcatheter therapy are available: intra-arterial vasopressin infusion and embolization. Vasopressin controls hemorrhage by arteriocapillary vasoconstriction and by contraction of the muscular walls of the GI tract.[1] For upper GI bleeding, the catheter is positioned superselectively into the bleeding artery, usually the left gastric or gastroduodenal artery. For lower GI bleeding, placement of the catheter into the superior or inferior mesenteric artery is adequate. The initial dose of vasopressin is 0.2 unit/min. Arteriography is repeated after 20 minutes of infusion. The arteriographic endpoint is cessation of bleeding with mild vasoconstriction. The dose may be increased to a maximum of 0.4 unit/min if the initial dose does not control bleeding. If bleeding still persists, embolization or surgery is an alternative. The infusion is tapered gradually in decrements of 0.1 unit/min every 12 to 24 hours. Resumption of vasopressin therapy may be needed should bleeding recur.

For embolotherapy, the catheter is placed as closely as possible to the bleeding site and the artery is occluded with an embolic agent. Small pieces of Gelfoam are commonly used. Gelfoam resorbs in a few weeks, allowing recanalization after healing of the bleeding site. Small stainless-steel coils are used for permanent occlusion. Polyvinyl alcohol particles (Ivalon) are used for permanent control of tumor-related bleeding.

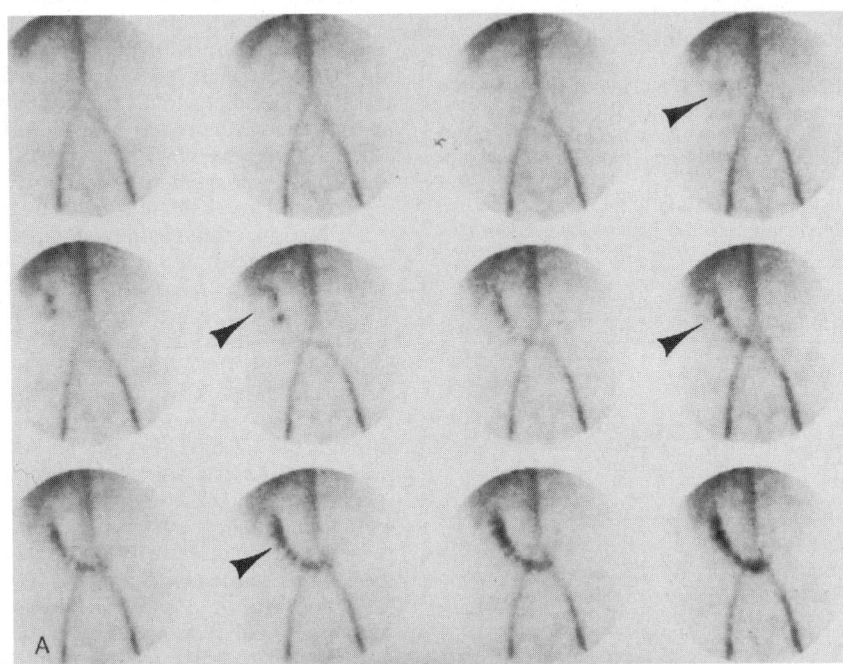

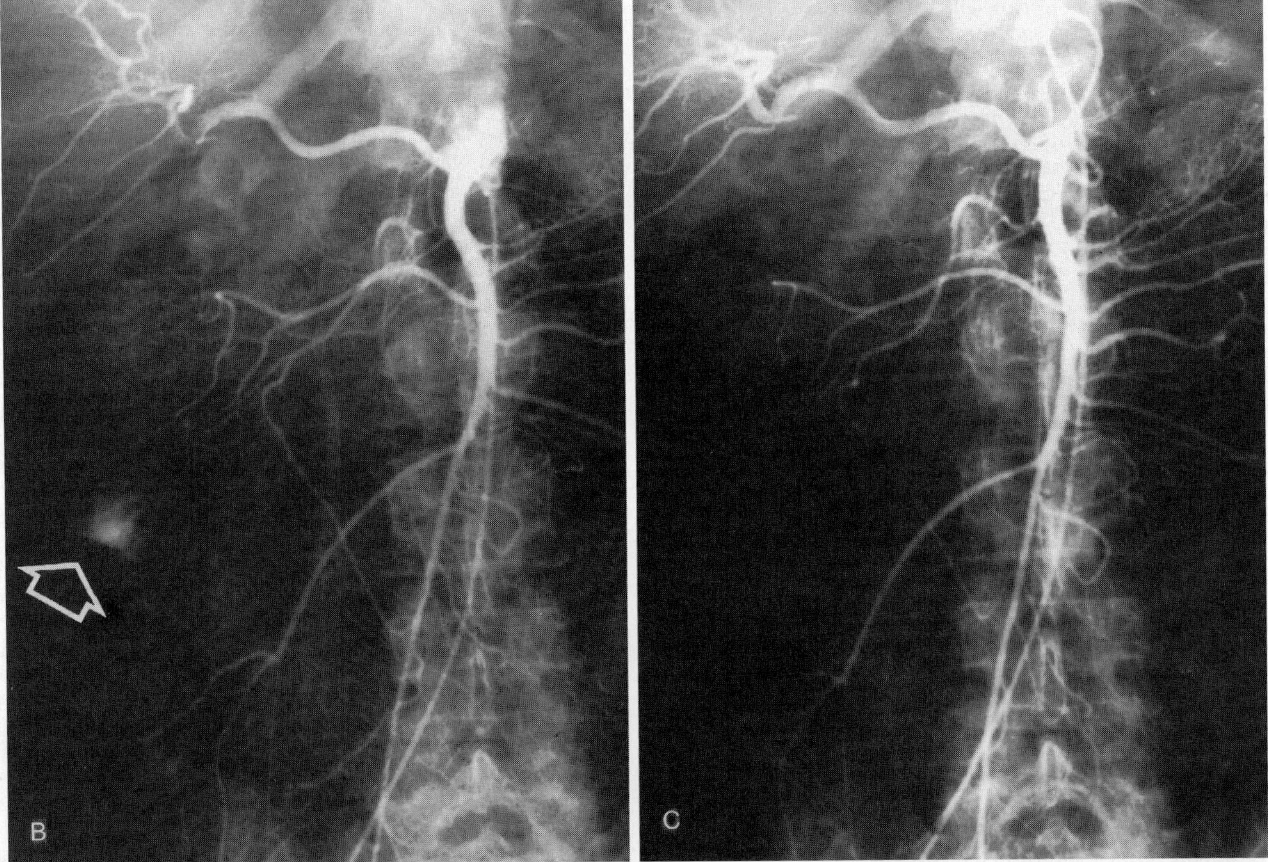

Figure 46–1. A 60-year-old woman with lower GI bleeding. *A,* This ^{99m}Tc-labeled–RBC radionuclide scan demonstrates colonic bleeding at the hepatic flexure *(arrowheads). B,* A superior mesenteric artery arteriogram demonstrates extravasation from a right colic branch *(arrow). C,* Arteriography after 20 minutes of vasopressin infusion at 0.2 U/min demonstrates cessation of bleeding and mild vasoconstriction. At surgery, multiple diverticula were found.

Variceal Hemorrhage

Endoscopy is the primary diagnostic modality for demonstration of GE variceal bleeding and for ruling out other sources of bleeding in patients with portal hypertension, because non-variceal causes account for more than 30% of bleeding episodes in this group. Intravenous vasopressin and endoscopic sclerotherapy are the therapeutic mainstays for variceal bleeding. Tamponade with a Sengstaken-Blakemore tube can be used as a 24 to 48 hour temporary measure. The definitive therapies are surgical portosystemic shunts, liver transplantation, or transjugular intrahepatic (nonsurgical) portosystemic shunt (TIPS). Because the surgical mortality in acutely bleeding patients is high (> 50%), these options are rarely used in acute bleeding management. In the past, if sclerotherapy or vasopressin failed, percutaneous transhepatic catheterization of the portal vein and embolization of coronary and short gastric varices was an alternate therapy. Because of its high rates of rebleeding and mortality, the procedure was only temporary to control bleeding for surgical shunt or liver transplantation to be performed.

A new interventional radiologic procedure, TIPS has become an option for nonsurgical radiologic control of variceal bleeding.[5] From the jugular vein approach, a long needle is placed into a hepatic vein and advanced through the liver parenchyma into the right or left portal vein. The intrahepatic tract is dilated with a balloon catheter, and a metallic mesh stent is placed to maintain new channel patency. The result is a portosystemic shunt that allows decompression of varices and a decrease in portal pressures (Fig. 46–2). TIPS is an effective and safe method for controlling acute variceal hemorrhage, even in patients who have failed sclerotherapy. Mortality of the procedure is less than 3%, and complications are uncommon. TIPS placement also improves control of ascites. Technical success is greater than 90%. Liver transplant is not precluded. The long-term efficacy of TIPS needs to be defined because the average follow-up is only in the 12- to 24-month range.[5a]

Upper Gastrointestinal Bleeding of Arterial or Arteriolocapillary Origin

Arteriography is indicated when endoscopy localizes a bleeding site that is unresponsive to conservative or invasive endoscopic management or when endoscopy is negative or inconclusive and significant bleeding persists. Initially, selective celiac arteriography is performed, followed by superselective left gastric and gastroduodenal arteriography. Superior mesenteric artery, splenic, or hepatic arteriography is occasionally needed.

Mallory-Weiss hemorrhage is treated successfully with vasopressin or embolization. Embolization controls more than 90% of cases. Hemorrhagic gastritis responds to vasopressin in more than 80% of cases. Pyloroduodenal ulcer bleeding is less effectively controlled by vasopressin, with success rates of 30% to 50%. Embolization is the initial transcatheter therapy for duodenal hemorrhage.[2] Aneurysms or pseudoaneurysms of visceral arteries are uncommon sources of serious upper GI hemorrhage.[1, 6] The most common sites are the splenic, gastroduodenal, hepatic, and pancreatic arteries. Although surgery has been the treatment of choice in the past for aneurysmal bleeding, embolotherapy with stainless-steel coils has become the initial therapy of choice[6] (Fig. 46–3).

Lower Gastrointestinal Bleeding

Only 10% of acute GI bleeding originates beyond the ligament of Treitz. Once rectal or anal causes have been ruled out by proctosigmoidoscopy, radionuclide scanning and arteriography are indicated for management. For massive continuous hemorrhage, arteriography is the initial study. For moderate or intermittent bleeding, a radionuclide scan is performed before arteriography. If the scan is nondiagnostic, arteriography is delayed until active bleeding recurs, or it is performed electively to diagnose other underlying lesions (tumors, angiodysplasias, arteriovenous malformations). If the scan is positive, selective superior and inferior mesenteric artery arteriography is performed based on information from the scan. Because scintigraphy is more sensitive than arteriography and GI bleeding is often intermittent, a positive scan may be followed by a negative arteriogram.[1, 2] In this case, further work-up depends on the clinical situation.

The major causes of colorectal bleeding are diverticulosis and angiodysplasia. Inflammatory/ischemic colitis, ulcers, tumors, and arteriovenous malformation are less common causes. Although diverticula are more frequent in the left colon, the majority of diverticular hemorrhages occur in the right colon (see Fig. 46–1).

The therapy for lower GI bleeding is vasopressin infusion into either the superior or inferior mesenteric artery (or both simultaneously if both vessels are involved). Bleeding is controlled in as many as 90% of cases; however, it recurs in 20% to 30% of cases. Embolization with Gelfoam is an alternate therapy if vasopressin fails. The rectum can be safely embolized because of its rich collateral supply. Embolization of jejunal, ileal, and colonic bleeding sites is successful but is controversial because of increased risk of infarction.

VENOUS VASCULAR ACCESS

Venous access is a routine requirement in critically ill patients. In the past, the role of the interventional radiologist has been in angiographic diagnosis of malfunctioning catheters, venographic definition of anatomy before catheter placement, retrieval of catheter fragments, unknotting of catheters, and repositioning of catheters.[7]

The role of the radiologist has expanded. Long-term central venous catheters and ports are now readily placed by radiologists in less than 24 hours to avoid surgery. With the aid of fluoroscopic and duplex Doppler ultrasonography, radiologists are highly successful in difficult central catheter placements.[8] Puncture complication rates are lower, and infection rates are comparable to surgically placed accesses. When a central access has been depleted, an inferior vena cava catheter can be placed by a percutaneous translumbar approach.[8]

Interventional radiologic techniques are also helpful in reestablishing vascular access. Thrombosed dialysis grafts can be lysed with urokinase and underlying stenoses relieved by angioplasty, extending the longevity of the access. In catheter-induced venous thromboses, local infusion of urokinase into the clot restores patency without catheter removal. Thus, indwelling catheters can be salvaged in patients with limited accesses. Metallic mesh stents are being investigated for the treatment of venous occlusions/stenoses. Because venous stenoses often respond poorly to balloon dilatation, stents are being successfully placed across stenoses or recanalized occlusions to maintain patency (Fig. 46–4).[9]

UROLOGIC INTERVENTIONS

Percutaneous nephrostomy placement is the primary nonvascular procedure performed on critically ill patients. Indications are supravesical urinary tract obstruction and uri-

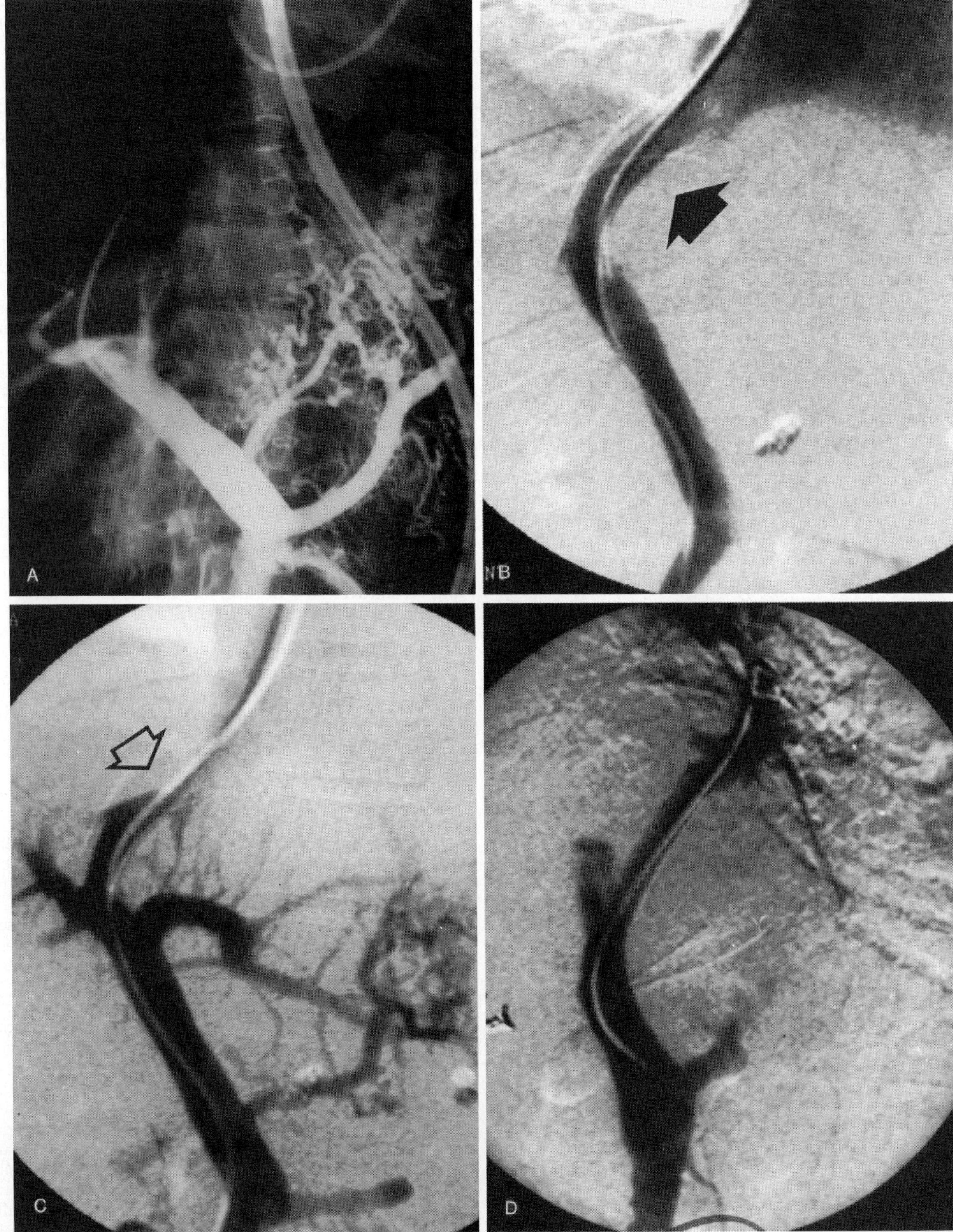

Figure 46–2. A 30-year-old man with alcoholic cirrhosis and recurrent variceal bleeding despite sclerotherapy. *A,* Splenoportography during TIPS shows left gastric varices. *B,* Post-TIPS splenoportogram. The 10-mm, metallic stented channel between the right hepatic and the right portal veins is evident *(arrow).* The left gastric varices are no longer filled. *C,* Follow-up portogram performed 12 months later. The shunt is nearly occluded owing to stenosis of the hepatic vein *(arrow).* The left gastric varices are again evident. *D,* Following balloon redilation and stent extension into the stenotic hepatic vein, good flow through the stent and nonopacification of varices are demonstrated.

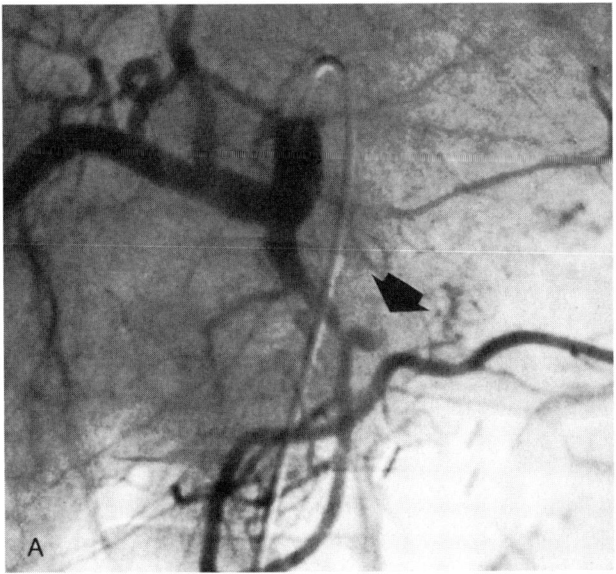

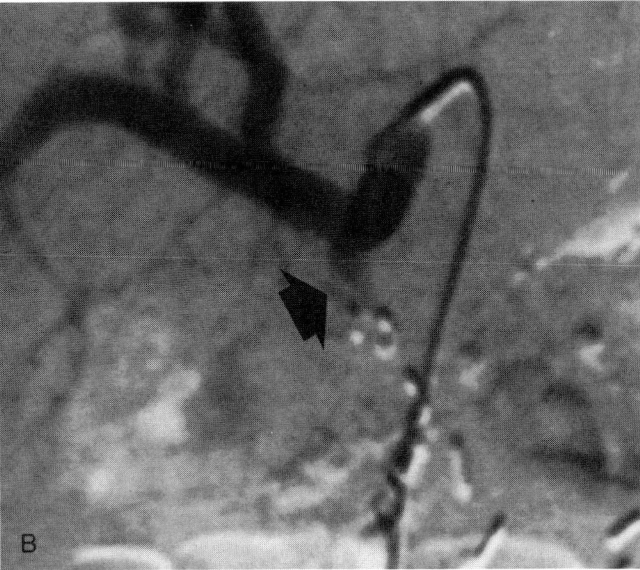

Figure 46–3. A 36-year-old man with severe pancreatitis and recurrent upper GI hemorrhage. *A*, Celiac arteriography demonstrates a small pseudoaneurysm *(arrow)* arising from the gastroduodenal artery. *B*, Stainless-steel coils were placed on either side of the pseudoaneurysm neck. Arteriography demonstrates occlusion of the gastroduodenal artery *(arrow)*. No further bleeding occurred.

nary leaks. Fluoroscopy or ultrasonography is used for guidance. If fluoroscopy is used, the anatomy is defined by direct injection of contrast material into the upper collecting system. With the patient prone, a 21- to 22-gauge Chiba needle is advanced from the posterolateral flank into a renal calyx or infundibulum. After guide wire placement and tract dilatation, a nephrostomy drainage catheter with a self-retaining locked loop is positioned in the renal pelvis to prevent catheter displacement. Before percutaneous nephrostomy placement, coagulopathy, if present, should be corrected and antibiotic therapy initiated if infection is present.[10, 10a]

When hydronephrosis is accompanied by signs of infection or a patient presents with sepsis and obstruction, prompt percutaneous nephrostomy placement is necessary. Retrograde cystoscopic placement of a ureteral stent may be attempted first in some nonseptic patients. Decompression of a noninfected kidney may be deferred for a few days if more critical problems exist. Immediate percutaneous nephrostomy placement is also indicated for uremia due to bilateral ureteral obstruction or obstruction of a solitary kidney.[10, 10a]

VASCULAR INTERVENTIONS

Mesenteric Ischemia

Mesenteric ischemia is considered only after other causes of acute abdominal disease have been excluded. Patients are elderly and often have multiple medical problems. They may present with acute onset of abdominal pain, nausea, vomiting, and diarrhea with or without blood. Rapid deterioration with sepsis, acidosis, hypotension, and death ensues. Even if mesenteric ischemia is properly diagnosed and treated, the mortality is 70%.[11] Occlusive ischemia is due to arterial embolism (60–80%) or thrombosis (20–30%). Nonocclusive ischemia, related to a low-flow state such as cardiogenic shock, occurs in 20% of cases.

The diagnosis of mesenteric ischemia is made by arteriography (Fig. 46–5). Biplane aortography is needed to evaluate the origins of the celiac, superior mesenteric, and inferior mesenteric arteries.

The treatment of occlusive ischemia varies. The presence of peritoneal signs mandates surgery and bowel resection for gangrene. Otherwise, interventional radiologic management consists of fragmentation of the thrombus with guide wires and catheters, transcatheter thrombolysis, suction embolectomy, or balloon thrombectomy followed by thrombolytic therapy.[11, 12] Lytic therapy is administered with 4000 units of urokinase per minute for 2 hours, then 2000 units per minute for 2 hours, followed by a lower dose for a longer infusion as necessary.

In nonocclusive mesenteric ischemia, infusion of vasodilators (papaverine or prostaglandin E_1) into the superior mesenteric artery is effective. The treatment should be discontinued only when significant clinical improvement is observed. If infarction of the bowel is present, bowel resection is necessary. Underlying medical problems such as heart failure and hypovolemia should also be corrected.

For severe chronic mesenteric ischemia, surgical revascularization is successful in 70% of cases and has a 3% to 8% mortality.[11] Focal stenotic lesions can be treated successfully with percutaneous transluminal angioplasty (PTA).[12] The long-term results of PTA are inferior to bypass grafting; however, the lower mortality and ease of repeating PTA offer an attractive alternative.

Peripheral Ischemia

Acute lower- or upper-extremity ischemia usually results from arterial thrombosis or embolism. Anteriography provides the diagnosis and allows transcatheter therapy with urokinase, followed by PTA. Atherectomy or stents sometimes are required. Thrombolysis or PTA can restore perfusion to the ischemic limb and permit surgical intervention nonacutely, thereby reducing morbidity and mortality (Fig. 46–6). Shorter and safer high-dose infusion is currently being used.[13] The choice of thrombolysis versus surgery depends on the degree of limb ischemia. Success rates of 100% and 84%, respectively, can be achieved in viable or threat-

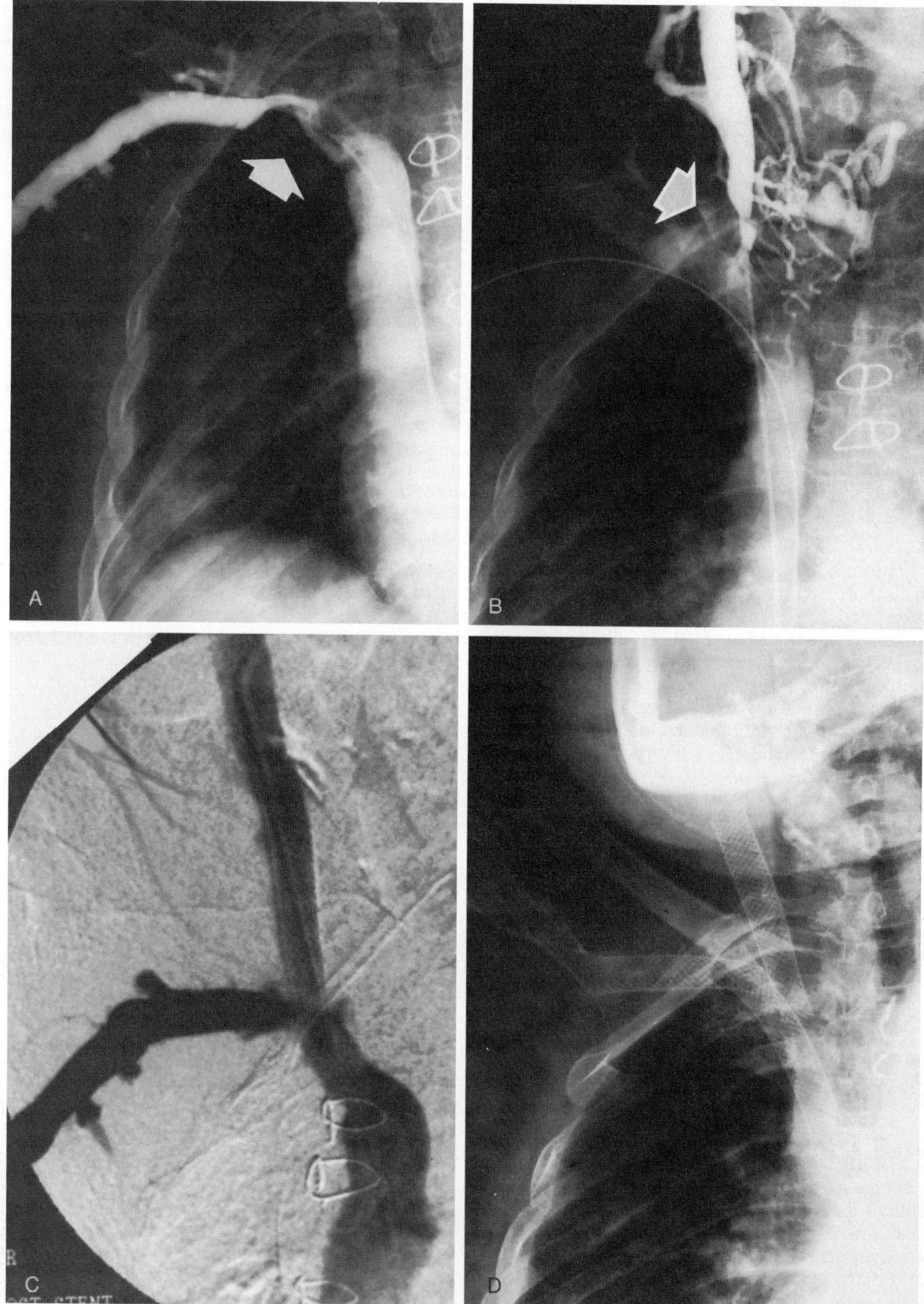

Figure 46–4. A 77-year-old woman with multiple failed dialysis catheter placements in the central veins. *A and B,* High-grade stenoses are present in the right internal jugular and subclavian veins at their confluence *(arrows)*. The stenoses were not adequately recanalized by percutaneous transluminal angioplasty, so metallic stents were placed. *C and D,* At 6 months' follow-up, the stented central vein remained patent, with excellent flow through the subclavian and internal jugular veins. Subsequently, a right-arm dialysis fistula was placed.

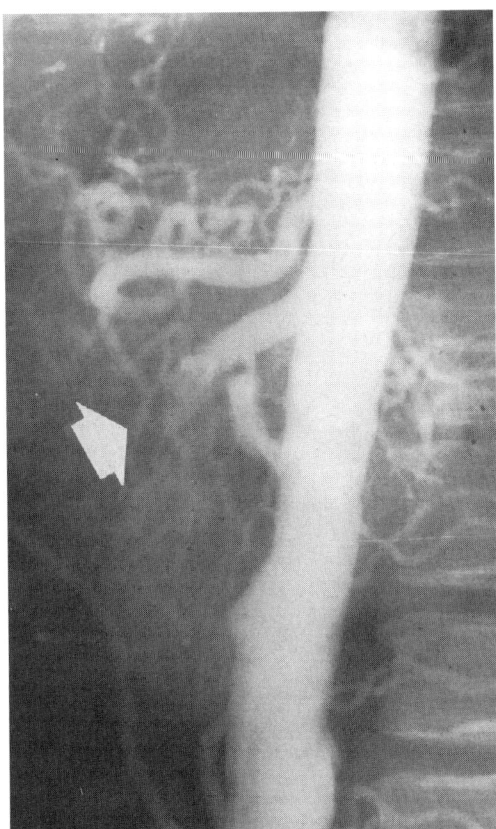

Figure 46–5. Lateral aortography reveals an embolus in the proximal superior mesenteric artery *(arrow)*.

ened limb states. However, in irreversible ischemia, a success rate of only 64% is expected. Thrombolysis also enables identification of an underlying flow-limiting stenosis that may have caused the thrombosis. Once antegrade flow is reestablished, PTA (or other interventions) may be performed (see Fig. 46–6).[13a]

Complications of thrombolysis are uncommon. Major bleeding complications occur in only 2% to 4% of patients, the majority at the puncture site.[13] The theoretic complications of central nervous system hemorrhage or distal embolization should not preclude therapy. Absolute contraindications include active GI or genitourinary bleeding, recent stroke or craniotomy (3–6 m), intracranial neoplasm, endocarditis, and irreversible ischemia with gangrene. Shorter, high-dose infusions have reduced the bleeding complications. Concomitant intravenous heparinization is responsible for some of the complications attending thrombolysis.

PTA provides recanalization of stenotic or occluded vessels by controlled injury to the arterial wall. A technical success of 85% to 96% and slightly lower clinical improvement may be expected.[14] Vascular stenting further enhances the success both angiographically and hemodynamically. At this time, only lesions in the iliac arteries are generally treated with stents. Long-term patency of as much as 93% at 5 years has been reported.[15]

Acute upper-extremity ischemia is a rare but serious problem. Causes include embolism, thrombosis, or an underlying collagen vascular disorder. Infusion of thrombolytic agents is very effective, even in the most severe occlusions.[16] Adjunctive vasodilators have an important role in the management of vasospastic disorders of the upper extremities.

Renal Ischemia

In dealing with renal ischemia, two emergencies may occur: acute hypertensive crisis secondary to renovascular hypertension and acute arterial occlusion with loss of function. The treatment options include surgical bypass or endarterectomy, PTA, thrombolysis, or medical therapy. PTA has a technical success rate of 81% to 97% and is clinically beneficial in 80% to 90% of cases, depending on the cause, location, and severity of stensosis, as well as a patient's under-

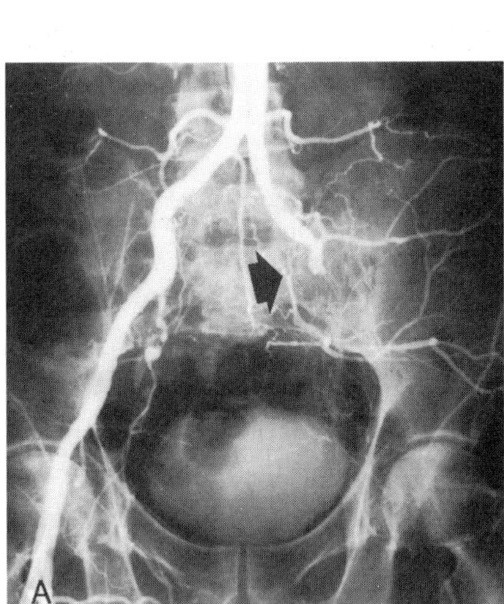

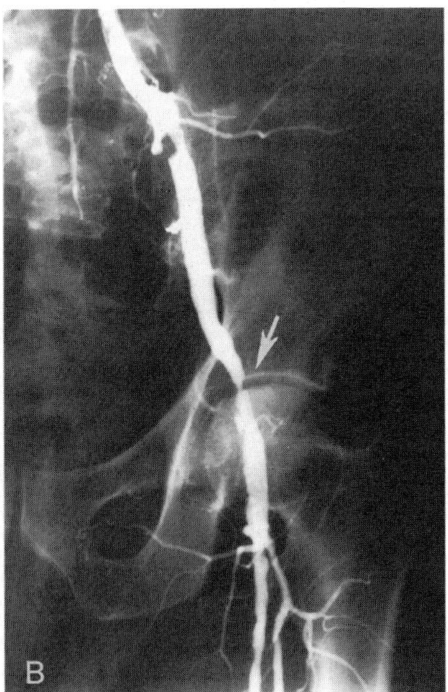

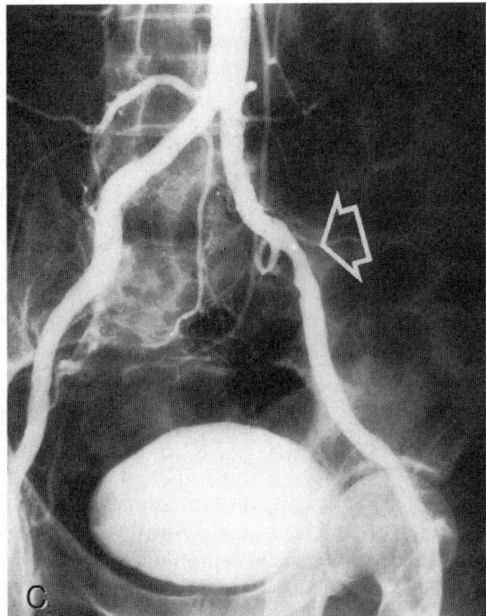

Figure 46–6. *A*, Acute thrombosis of the left external iliac and common femoral arteries *(arrow)*. *B*, Antegrade flow was restored after 40 hours of UK infusion. The underlying stenoses were identified and dilated *(arrow)*. *C*, At 1-month follow-up, continued patency was demonstrated *(arrow)*. The left external iliac artery remained patent 1 year later.

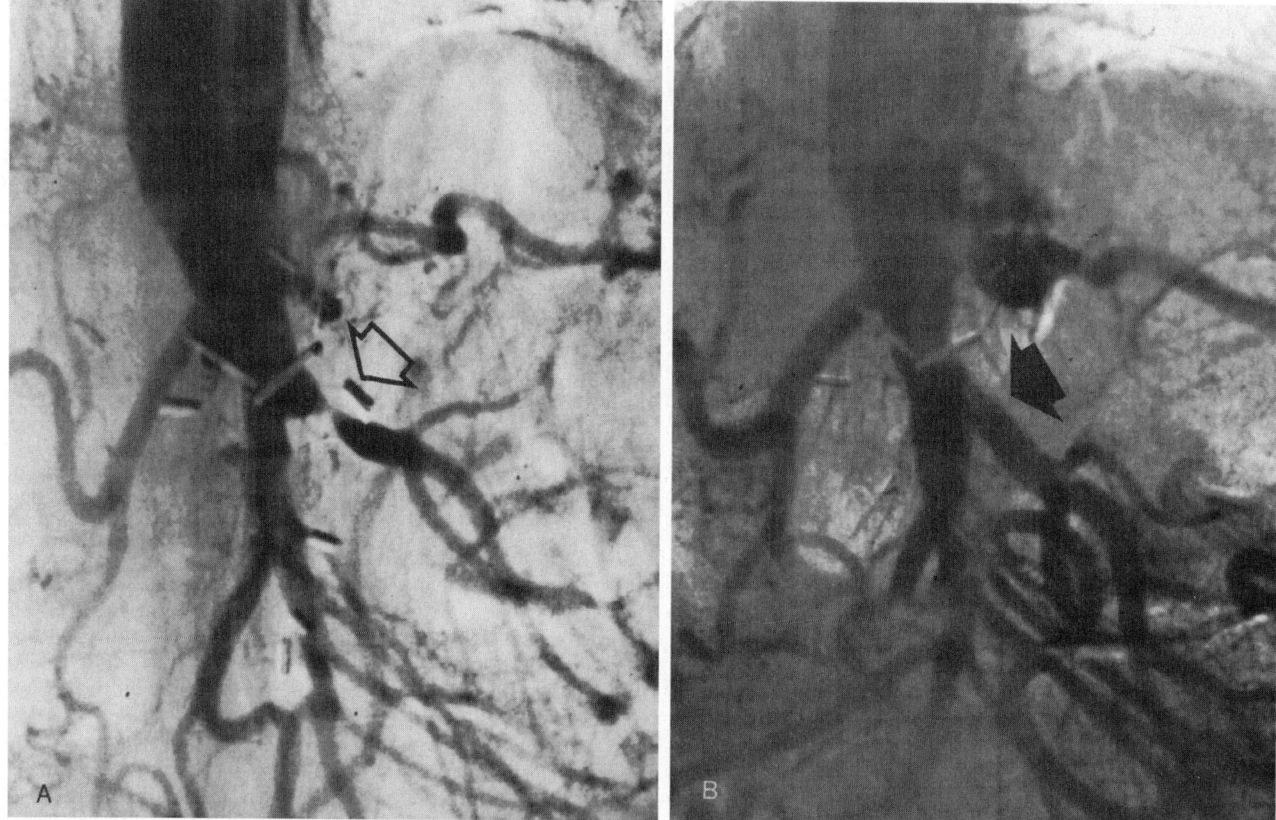

Figure 46–7. Pre-PTA *(A)* and post-PTA images *(B)* of a high-grade stenosis in a solitary kidney reveals an excellent result *(arrows)*. The patient's blood pressure was significantly improved.

lying clinical condition[17, 18] (Fig. 46–7). Ostial stenoses, previously believed to respond poorly to PTA, have been shown to have good long-term results but may require redilatation.[19] In acute renal failure, the clinical success of PTA is 30% to 50%, considered reasonable because of low invasiveness as compared with surgery. The overall complication rate of PTA is 5% to 10%, lower than with surgery (20%). The authors believe that PTA should be the first choice for revascularization of renal arteries.[18a]

Thrombolysis of acute renal artery thrombosis has not been widely implemented. An improvement in renal function is less likely, and the infusion must be initiated as early as possible.

PERCUTANEOUS NEEDLE BIOPSY

Percutaneous needle biopsy yields samples for either cytologic or histologic analysis. The risks are low if a safe computed tomography (CT) or ultrasonography guided pathway to the organ or lesion is available, a small-caliber needle is used, and coagulation abnormalities are corrected.[20] A 14-gauge cutting needle may be used to obtain core samples, and a 20- to 22-gauge Chiba needle is sufficient for cytologic sampling. The Chiba needle may be safely passed through stomach or bowel in order to sample deep, solid organs. The overall accuracy ranges from 79% for 1-cm or smaller masses to 98% for 2-cm or larger masses.[21]

Complications include hemorrhage, infection, inadvertent organ injury, pneumothorax, bile leakage, peritonitis, pancreatitis, and very rarely needle tract seeding of tumor cells.

Liver biopsy may be performed either percutaneously or by the transjugular venous route in patients with coagulopathy or ascites. Biopsy specimens of intravascular, urinary, or biliary tracts are routinely obtained using percutaneously guided forceps or brushes.

PERCUTANEOUS ASPIRATION AND DRAINAGE OF FLUID COLLECTIONS

The availability of CT and ultrasonography and the development of specialized catheters and guide wires have allowed percutaneous drainage of abscesses, cysts, hematomas, bilomas, urinomas, pseudocysts, lymphoceles, necrotic tumors, loculated ascites, and other fluid collections. The success rate of percutaneous drainage is 70% to 91%, with a mortality of 1% to 13%.[22, 23] The complication rate of 10% is lower than that for surgical drainage (22%). The risks of general anesthesia and extensive surgery are avoided. Aspiration of contents allows for immediate Gram staining as well. Placement of a drainage catheter, which may range in size from 5 to 24 French, also allows injection of specific agents into the cavity. Cysts may be ablated with alcohol, and infected hematomas lysed with thrombolytic agents. Aggressive antibiotic therapy, in addition to drainage, should be continued until the infection has disappeared. The catheter is best managed with serial CT scans, as well as gentle injections of contrast material under fluoroscopy (Figs. 46–8 and 46–9).

The only absolute contraindication to percutaneous drainage is the absence of a safe route to the collection. Traversal of contaminated structures, such as colon, should be avoided. Aspiration and drainage of a fluid collection is indicated only if a patient has fever, malaise, leukocytosis,

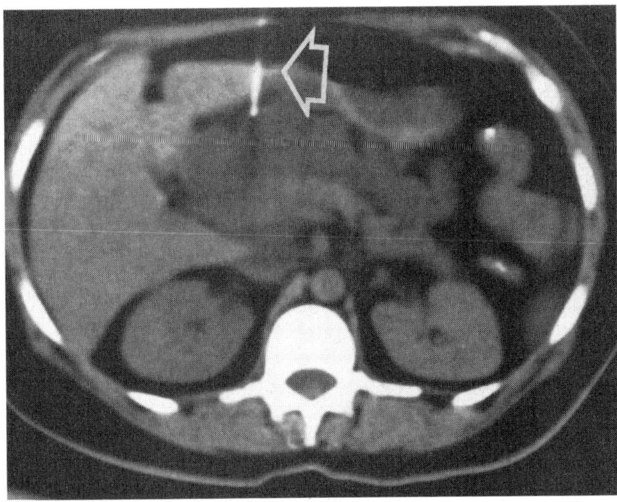

Figure 46–8. Transgastric aspiration and drainage of a lesser sac fluid collection. The Chiba needle traverses the fluid-filled gastric antrum *(arrow)*.

anorexia, or other evidence of infection. Complications include septicemia, contamination of an initially sterile collection, fistula to the bowel, hemorrhage, traversal of the pleural space, pneumothorax, and skin infection. Despite the high success rates of percutaneous drainage, it must be emphasized that when percutaneous drainage fails, surgery is the only alternative. Excessive delay in surgery and persistent sepsis may lead to multiple organ failure and death.

BILIARY TRACT INTERVENTIONS

Infection is the main reason for interventions in critically ill patients with obstructive biliary tract disease. Infection occurs in one third of malignant obstructions and two thirds of benign obstructions.[24] Obstruction is due to malignancy, sclerosing cholangitis, cholelithiasis, and postoperative or postendoscopic complications. Percutaneous transhepatic cholangiography (PTC), followed by percutaneous biliary drainage, is an effective, safe, and minimally invasive approach. Percutaneous biliary drainage may be performed either by the transhepatic route or by percutaneous cholecystostomy. Although either route may be used for drainage, the former is preferred for cholangitis and the latter for acute calculous or acalculous cholecystitis. The goal is stabilization of the patient for a definitive treatment, which can be percutaneous, endoscopic, or surgical. The success rate for establishing access to the biliary system by percutaneous techniques is greater than 95% in patients with ductal dilatation.[24, 25, 25a]

Immediate complications occur in 5% to 10% of cases and are related to pericatheter bile leak, hemorrhage, or infection. Delayed complications include cholangitis, peritonitis,

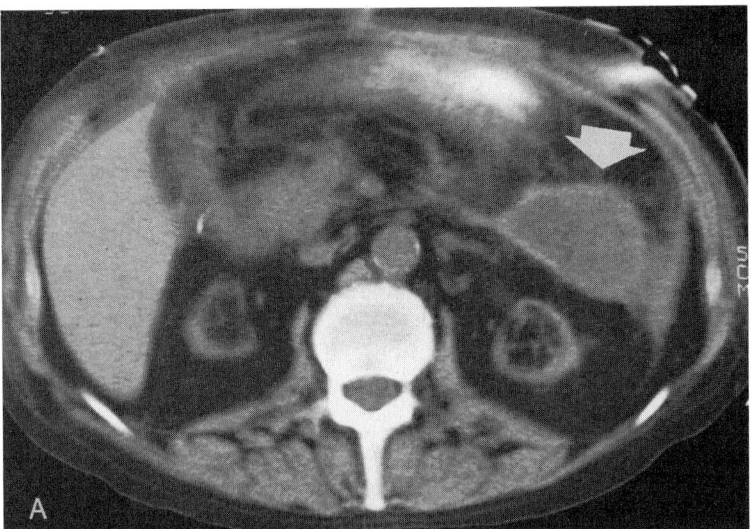

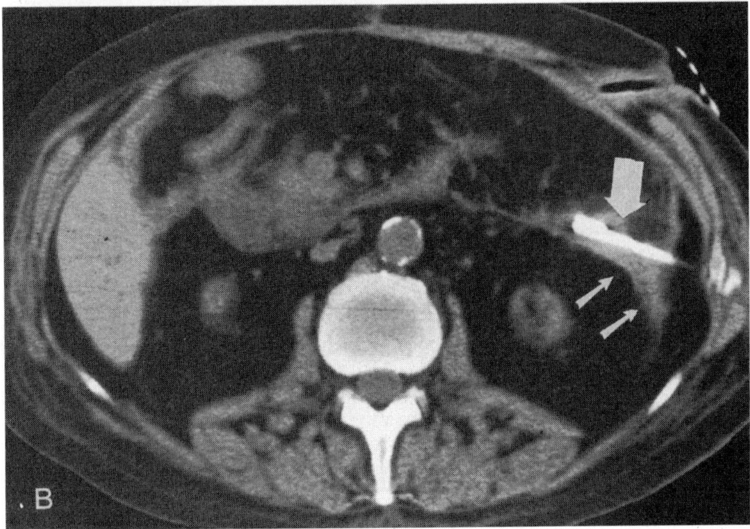

Figure 46–9. *A,* A fluid collection in the left anterior pararenal space is noted on the initial CT scan *(arrow)*. *B,* Two months following drainage, the cavity had disappeared. Some fatty inflammation *(thin arrows)* and the drainage catheter *(thick arrow)* are evident.

pancreatitis, pneumothorax, hemobilia, biliopleural fistula, and skin infection. Percutaneous biliary drainage is contraindicated in patients with multiple liver metastases, less than 2 weeks of life expectancy, and asymptomatic jaundice.

The treatment of acute cholecystitis or gallbladder empyema is cholecystectomy, which has a mortality rate of 0.5% to 1.8%. However, the mortality rate of emergency cholecystectomy in elderly patients is 13%, 10 times higher.[26] In critically ill patients, percutaneous cholecystostomy is an attractive alternative and is as effective as surgical cholecystostomy but has lower morbidity and mortality. Percutaneous cholecystostomy is very useful in acalculous cholecystitis because these patients do not require cholecystectomy once the inflammation subsides.[24]

Once the cholangitis or cholecystitis has subsided, the tract can be used for interventions such as retrieval or chemical dissolution of gallstones, dilation of benign strictures, stenting of malignant strictures, implantation of radioisotopes, and endoluminal biopsy.

Stones can be retrieved with a basket. Alternatively, the calculus may be dislodged and pushed into the duodenum with an occlusion balloon catheter. Retained common duct stones can be removed through a T-tube tract after 4 to 6 weeks to allow the tract to mature. Success of stone removal

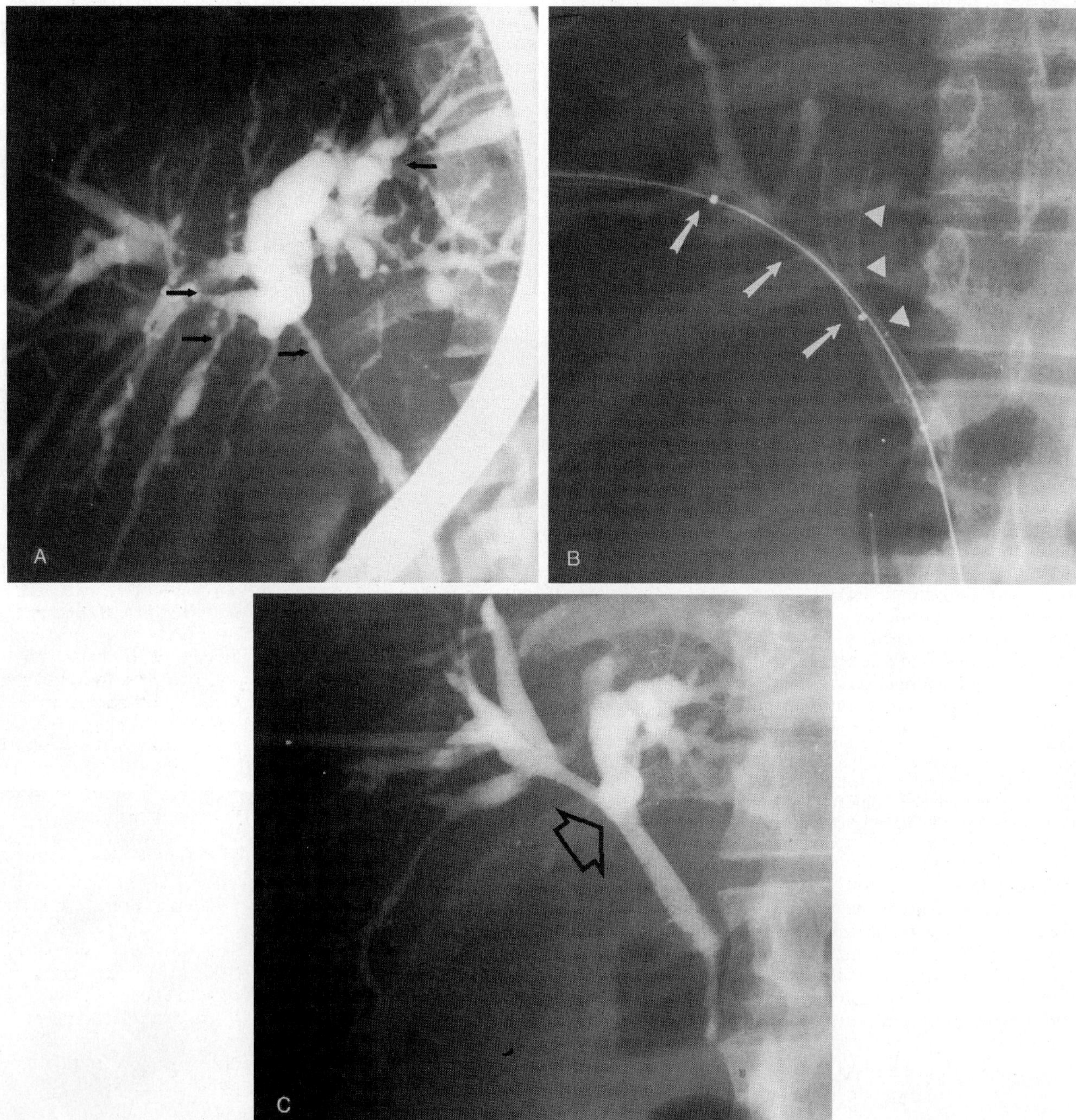

Figure 46–10. *A,* A cholangiogram reveals diffuse areas of narrowing and dilatation of the ducts *(arrows). B,* Following percutaneous transhepatic access, a partially opened Wallstent is seen during deployment into one of the right ducts *(arrows).* A completely opened Wallstent is already placed in one of the left ducts *(arrowheads). C,* A cholangiogram performed following stenting shows widely patent lumens *(arrow).*

is about 90% to 95%. Larger stones may be crushed with special baskets. Pure cholesterol gallstones can be dissolved with methyl tert-butyl ether or mono-octanoin. This topic is under investigation.

Benign strictures are best treated surgically. If this is not possible, balloon dilatation should be performed. The long term patency after dilatation is excellent, and the complications are low. Both surgery and balloon dilatation are successful in 70% to 80% of cases. If both procedures fail to maintain patency, an internal plastic endoprosthesis may be used.[27] Metallic stents cannot be removed, and therefore, their use must be carefully planned (Fig. 46–10).

In conclusion, percutaneous approaches to the biliary system provide the same temporizing effects as surgical approaches but with significantly lower morbidity and mortality.

PERCUTANEOUS GASTROSTOMY AND PLACEMENT OF ENTERAL FEEDING TUBES

Some patients with impaired swallowing function, neurologic disorders, extensive injuries, or terminal diseases require supplemental or complete intake other than by mouth. Short-term nutritional needs are met with nasoenteric tube feedings or total parenteral nutrition. However, aspiration may occur in many patients with nasogastric tubes.[28] In addition, total parenteral nutrition requires an indwelling catheter and may be complicated by infection, catheter thrombosis, or central venous thrombosis.

Gastrostomy or transgastric jejunal feeding tubes are alternatives for long-term feeding. These tubes are well tolerated and have a low complication rate. Peritonitis due to leakage of gastric contents around the tube is the most serious complication. The risk of aspiration may be greatly reduced by direct jejunal feeding. Furthermore, jejunal tubes permit feeding of patients with decreased gastric motility or with postoperative leakage from the upper GI tract.[29]

Surgical gastrostomy is associated with a high morbidity and a mortality of 1% to 6%.[30, 31] Endoscopic insertion of gastrostomy tubes is now possible. However, it is expensive, requires general sedation, may result in abdominal wall infection by oral flora, and is not possible in patients with esophageal obstruction.

Fluoroscopically guided percutaneous placement of gastrostomy and jejunostomy tubes is more attractive. The stomach is entered by percutaneous puncture of the abdominal wall. An 8- to 16-French tube is placed in less than 30 minutes, with a success rate of greater than 95%. The tubes are easily replaced once the tract has matured in about 2 weeks. Complications are rare. Peritonitis due to leakage around the catheter, before a mature tract forms between the stomach and the abdominal wall, is possible. Other complications are retrogastric hematoma, perforation of colon or small bowel, wound site infection, and hemorrhage from the gastrostomy site. However, only about 3% of these complications require treatment.[30, 31]

In conclusion, percutaneous placement of gastrostomy and gastrojejunostomy feeding tubes has an important role in the nutrition of critically ill patients. This approach is safe, simple, and highly successful.

PULMONARY THROMBOEMBOLISM AND DEEP VENOUS THROMBOSIS

Pulmonary embolism (PE) is the great simulator of other diseases. Previous reports have estimated a yearly incidence of 600,000. Pulmonary embolism is the third leading cause of death in the United States. About one fourth to one third of patients will die if the diagnosis is not made. The clinical diagnosis is difficult. Laboratory tests are not helpful. A high number of patients may have an abnormal chest radiograph, but the findings are nonspecific. Pulmonary arteriography is the definitive diagnosis for this entity. Ninety-five per cent of PE originate from deep venous thrombosis (DVT) of the lower extremities and pelvis. The rest (5%) originate from the superior vena cava and tributaries. Large emboli are frequently fatal. Small emboli may resolve spontaneously.[32–35]

DVT is a common clinical problem associated with significant morbidity and mortality and is an important cause of chronic disability. Venography is the gold standard for the diagnosis of DVT. Noninvasive methods are not as reliable or definitive as venography but can be used for screening. Duplex ultrasonography is being used with success and has replaced lower-extremity venography in many instances.[33]

The diagnosis of PE, a potentially fatal complication of DVT, is difficult. A high-probability ventilation-perfusion (V-Q) scan showing multiple segmental defects associated with normal ventilation is highly suggestive of PE. In this group, 87% of patients may have PE at pulmonary arteriography. A normal V-Q scan virtually rules out PE. However, 5% to 10% of patients in this category may have PE at pulmonary arteriography. The vast majority of patients undergoing lung scanning have indeterminate or intermediate findings on scans. The incidence of PE at pulmonary arteriography in this group is about 30%. Patients with low-probability V-Q scans may have a 10% to 15% incidence of PE at pulmonary arteriography.[32, 35]

Spiral CT and electron-beam CT are highly specific and sensitive methods for detecting large, central PE. These noninvasive modalities may eventually replace pulmonary arteriography for the diagnosis of PE. The aim of the diagnosis of PE should be to directly demonstrate the clot in the pulmonary arteries (pulmonary arteriography and CT), rather than the secondary effects of the clots in the pulmonary arteries and the airway (V-Q scanning).[32, 35]

The treatment of DVT (and its complication, PE) is intravenous heparin for 7 to 10 days and oral anticoagulation with warfarin (Coumadin) for 3 months. This treatment is safe and highly successful in preserving the function of the valves and reducing the risk of postphlebitic syndrome. Complications of heparin may occur in as many as 10% to 20% of patients. Oral anticoagulation with warfarin is also associated with a significant rate of complications, increasing in proportion to the duration of the therapy. Hemorrhagic complications may occur in 30% of patients after 2 years of therapy.

The objective of the treatment of PE is to prevent recurrent emboli. Anticoagulation prevents new thrombus formation or stops the progression of existing thrombi, but it does not lyse already formed thrombi. Thrombolytic therapy, on the other hand, either systemically or locally in the pulmonary arteries, in patients with massive thrombus and cardiopulmonary collapse lyses the existing clot (Fig. 46–11). Unfortunately, in many patients, anticoagulation is contraindicated. Other patients receiving anticoagulation develop complications requiring discontinuation of therapy. In addition, some patients develop recurrent PE despite adequate anticoagulation. Therefore, placement of a filter to mechanically interrupt the inferior vena cava is the procedure of choice to manage these patients (Fig. 46–12).

Low-dose fibrinolytic therapy has been administered to a selected group of patients with massive PE, with spectacular results. Systemic fibrinolytic therapy is also effective but is associated with a significant rate of hemorrhagic complications. In the past, these patients with unstable vital signs

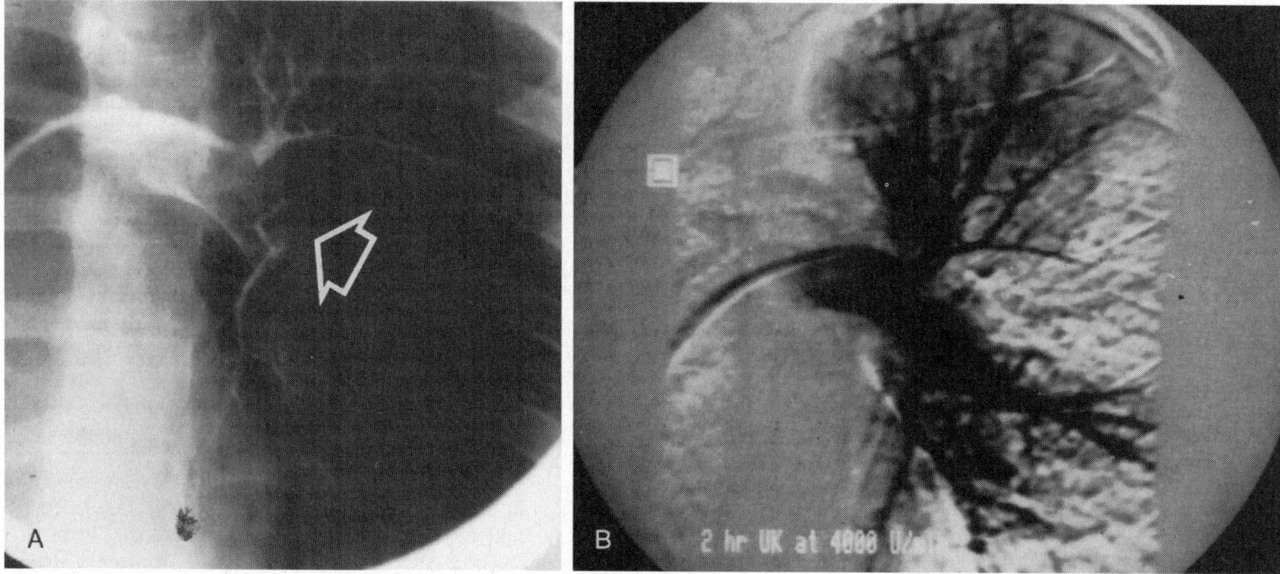

Figure 46–11. A young woman presented with shortness of breath and cardiovascular deficit. *A,* Complete occlusion of the left main pulmonary artery *(arrow)* occurred owing to massive embolism. *B,* Excellent recanalization was achieved after 2 hours of local, low-dose infusion of UK.

and hypotensive shock required open embolectomy. Transcatheter embolectomy with the Greenfield catheter is now an alternative.

Other vascular problems can be managed successfully with interventional radiologic techniques. Effort thrombosis of central veins and arteriovenous malformation and arteriovenous fistula causing serious disability are some examples (Fig. 46–13).[35a]

In summary, prevention of PE and its cause, DVT, is the goal. Early diagnosis and treatment of DVT prevent its serious consequences. The diagnostic and interventional radiologist has a major role in the treatment of patients with DVT and PE.

BRONCHIAL ARTERY EMBOLIZATION FOR MASSIVE HEMOPTYSIS

Massive hemoptysis, defined as bleeding of 300 to 600 mL in 24 hours, is a rare but life-threatening condition that requires emergent management. The mortality is 50% to

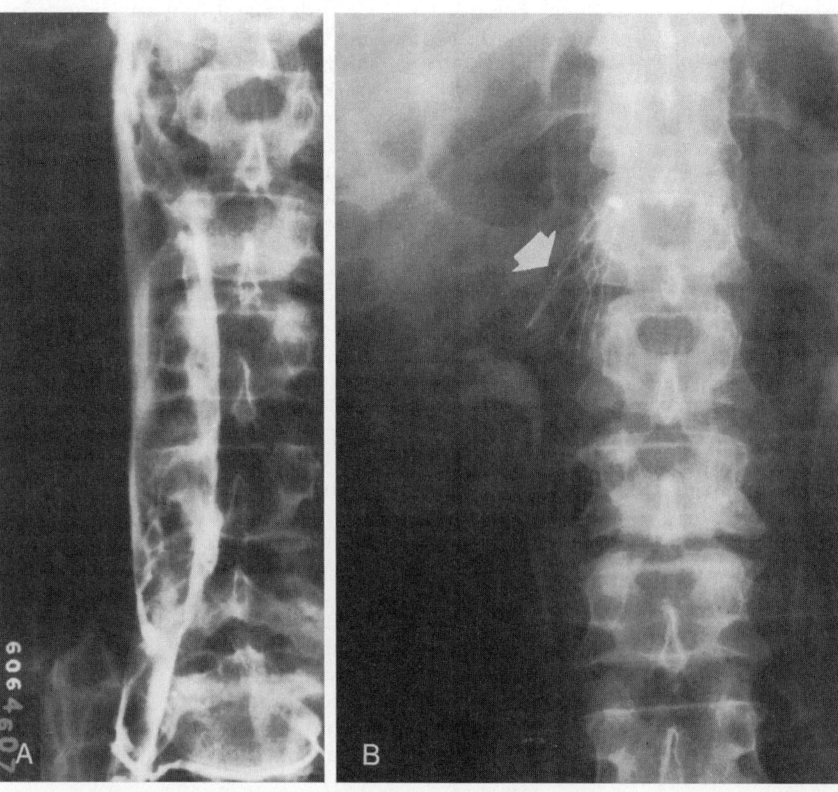

Figure 46–12. *A,* Massive thrombosis of the inferior vena cava to the level of the renal veins is demonstrated. *B,* A Greenfield filter *(arrow)* was placed in the suprarenal portion of the inferior vena cava.

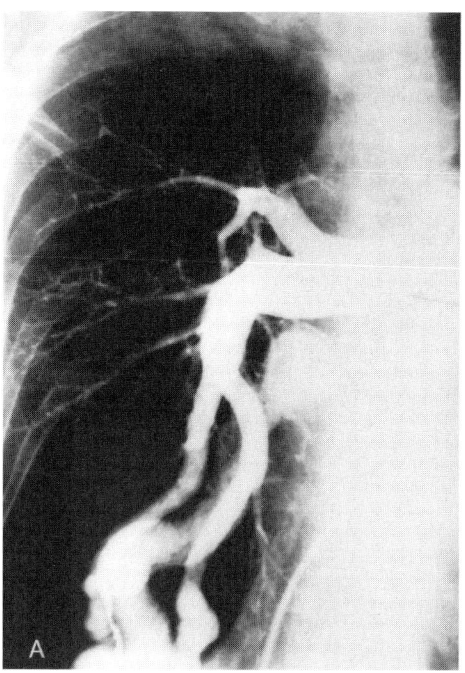

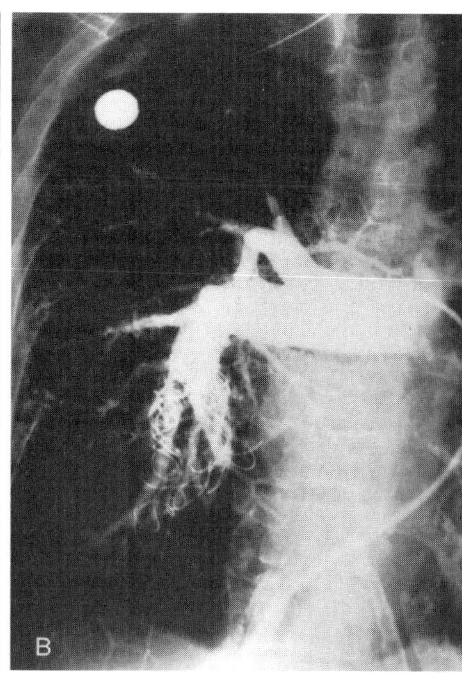

Figure 46–13. An elderly woman presented with severe cyanosis that she had had since childhood. *A*, This pulmonary arteriogram shows a huge arteriovenous malformation fed by two large arteries and drained by a massively dilated vein. *B*, Embolization with about 30 stainless-steel coils from 5 to 10 mm in size resulted in complete obliteration. The patient had an uneventful recovery.

80%, usually as a result of asphyxiation rather than exsanguination. A single expectoration can amount to 500 mL of blood. Hemoptysis almost always originates from hypertrophy of the bronchial arteries (90% of the cases). Rupture of the bronchial arteries into the lung parenchyma results in massive hemoptysis. Rupture of a mycotic aneurysm of the pulmonary arteries may occasionally be the cause. Pulmonary arteriovenous malformations and fistulas are very rare causes as well.[36–38] The most common causes of hemoptysis are tuberculosis and other granulomatous diseases, cystic fibrosis in young patients, and bronchiectasis, carcinoma of the lung, and fungal infections in older individuals.

Most patients with massive hemoptysis have poor respiratory reserve and therefore are poor surgical candidates. Furthermore, surgery requires resection of lung in these patients with borderline respiratory reserve. Bronchial artery embolization is the preferred method of therapy in these patients.

The initial radiologic study is a chest radiograph, followed by CT scanning to assess lung pathology. This frequently determines the side and lobe of hemorrhage. Bronchoscopy is performed next to determine the side and, ideally, the precise site of bleeding. Bronchoscopy is mandatory unless it is not available or not feasible because of the condition of the patient. Also, balloon occlusion of the nondiseased bronchus to prevent asphyxiation can be performed as a life-saving procedure.

Radiologic interventional management consists of selective bronchial arteriography followed by embolization of the bronchial arteries. The authors prefer Gelfoam and Ivalon particles to embolize peripheral arteries and sometimes use stainless-steel coils to occlude the proximal arteries[36–38] (Fig. 46–14).

Thorough knowledge of the bronchial arterial anatomy is important. Arteriography usually begins with a thoracic aortogram to identify the origins of the bronchial arteries and enlargement, if any, of other systemic arteries that may supply the affected areas. The bronchial arteries originate from the anterior or anterolateral aspect of the thoracic aorta at the level of T-3 to T-8. There are four common variations of anatomy: (1) two left and one right (41%); (2) one right and one left (21%); (3) two left and two right (21%); and (4) one left and two right (1%). The bronchial arteries can originate together with the intercostal arteries in some patients. The artery of Adamkiewicz originates from the left bronchial arteries or the intercostal arteries at the level of T-5 to L-3 and usually takes a hairpin turn. Identification of this artery on some occasions contraindicates embolization because of the high risk of permanent spinal cord injury.[36–38]

Gelfoam particles are used for benign processes. For malignant processes, permanent materials, such as Ivalon, are preferred. The authors avoid using powders or liquids (alcohol) because of the high risk of peripheral bronchial necrosis. Stainless-steel coils are used to embolize the main trunk of the bronchial arteries; however, this may preclude future re-embolizations. Embolization is highly effective in controlling hemoptysis in 80% to 90% of patients, with a recurrence rate of 10% to 15%. The complications are permanent spinal cord injury in about 1% of cases. Bronchial infarction is very rare. Peripheral embolization can be avoided with careful technique.

In conclusion, bronchial artery embolization is a safe and highly successful procedure to control life-threatening hemoptysis and is associated with few complications.

PERCUTANEOUS RETRIEVAL OF EMBOLIZED CATHETER FRAGMENTS AND OTHER IATROGENIC FOREIGN BODIES AND UNKNOTTING AND REPOSITIONING OF INTRAVASCULAR CATHETERS

Rupture and embolization of catheter fragments and other intravascular foreign bodies and formation of knots in catheters are serious complications of percutaneous catheterization techniques (central venous catheters and others such as ventriculoatrial, ventriculoperitoneal shunts, and others). Significant morbidity and a mortality rate as high as 75% have been reported if the catheters are not removed or unknotted. Death is related to thrombosis, sepsis, arrhythmias, myocardial necrosis, myocardial perforation, pericardial tamponade, endocarditis, and pulmonary thromboembo-

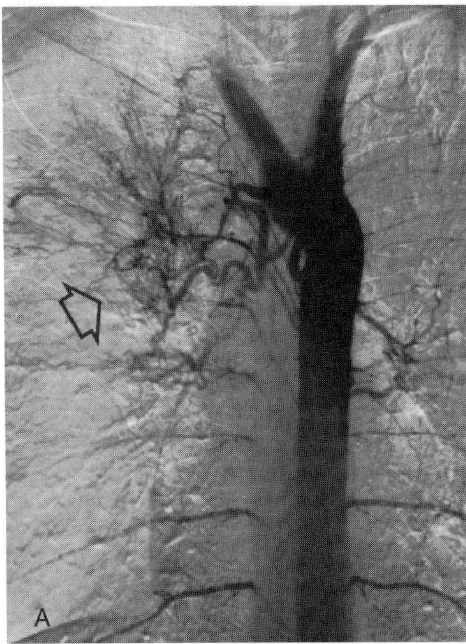

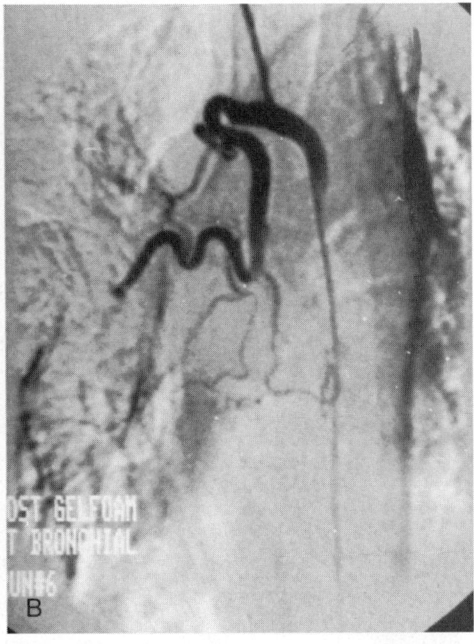

Figure 46–14. A young man with cystic fibrosis presented with massive hemoptysis. *A,* A thoracic aortogram shows marked enlargement of right bronchial arteries *(arrow).* A selective right bronchial arteriogram (not shown) demonstrated marked tortuosity and hypertrophy of the arterial branches. *B,* After embolization with Gelfoam particles, complete obliteration of bronchial arteries occurred. The hemorrhage stopped and did not recur.

lism, among others. However, if the catheter fragments are removed or the knots are untied, full recovery is expected.[7] (Fig. 46–15).

In the past, the only way to remove embolized catheters or intravascular foreign bodies or to unknot catheters was surgically. Because embolized catheters usually become lodged in the cardiac chambers or pulmonary arteries, removal by surgical means involves a thoracotomy and even open-heart surgery. With advances in angiographic techniques, removal of embolized catheter fragments and other intravascular foreign bodies and unknotting of intravascular catheter knots are relatively simple procedures accomplished with very low risk, on an outpatient basis, in a short time. In the authors' experience, this procedure can be accomplished in 10 to 15 minutes.[7]

Extreme care is needed during removal of catheters from the heart, particularly if the catheters have been lodged in cardiac chambers for a long time. Continuous electrocardiographic monitoring, vital sign assessment, and pulse oximetry are mandatory during attempts at retrieval. Arrhythmias, perforation of vessels or cardiac chambers, and myocardial or endothelial damage are possible during retrieval with stiff instruments such as stainless-steel forceps or baskets. Numerous instruments can be used for retrieval and unknotting of catheters. The authors prefer baskets, Curry loop snares, deflector wires, different types of angio-

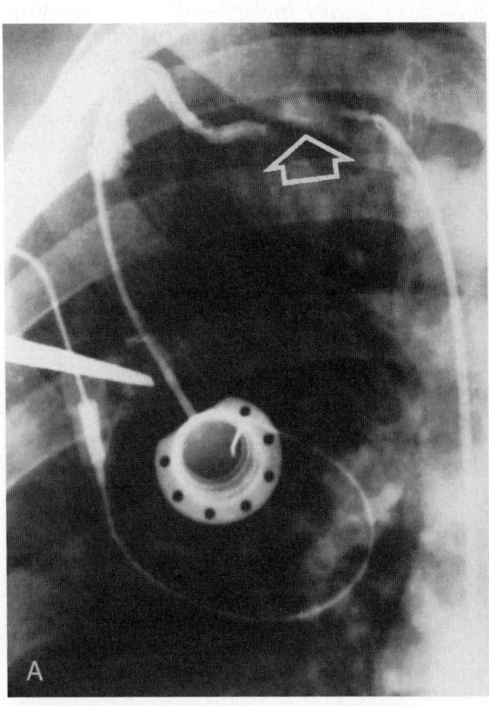

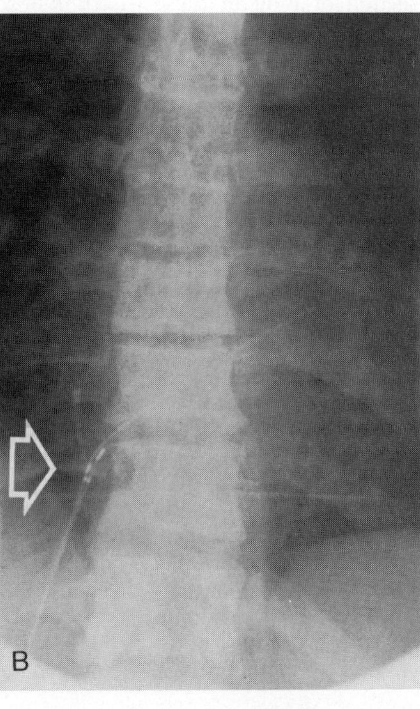

Figure 46–15. A young woman had a port-A-Cath placed for chemotherapy. *A,* A few weeks later, the catheter had broken at its entrance into the subclavian vein *(arrow).* The fragment embolized to the right atrium. *B,* During retrieval of the catheter fragment, the foreign body was snared with a basket and removed in 10 minutes *(arrow).*

graphic catheters, grasping and alligator forceps, and others.

Complications are migration of the fragments or foreign bodies peripherally into the pulmonary arteries, making removal almost impossible. Cardiac arrhythmias are common and can be prevented with lidocaine. Constant electrocardiographic monitoring is mandatory. Perforation of vessels or the heart is a serious but rare complication.[7]

In conclusion, vascular and interventional radiologists use different techniques for retrieval of intravascular catheter fragments and other iatrogenic foreign bodies and for unknotting of catheter knots. A major operation that could include open-heart surgery is avoided. These procedures are quick, simple, safe, and effective.

INTERVENTIONAL RADIOLOGY IN ACUTE TRAUMA

Trauma is the third leading cause of death in young people in the United States. It is the most common cause of death in people between 15 and 45 years of age. In the United States, more than 100,000 people died of trauma-related causes in 1988. More people die of trauma in 1 year than died in the Vietnam and Korean Wars together, yet little emphasis has been placed on the diagnostic and interventional aspects of trauma.

The authors' institution is a level I trauma center. This requires the presence of emergency medicine physicians, anesthesiologists, and trauma surgeons 24 hours a day. In addition, radiologists must be available for immediate consultation. Technologists experienced in diagnostic radiology, angiography, and CT must be available. Equipment required is CT, ultrasonography, radionuclide scanning, and a vascular and interventional radiology laboratory. This type of management of acutely traumatized patients has resulted in a significant decrease in morbidity and mortality and a faster recovery of patients.

Only three or four plain films, including lateral cervical spine, chest, abdomen, and pelvis, are necessary in the emergency room for the initial assessment and triage of acutely traumatized patients. Thereafter, patients either go to the operating room for an emergent surgical exploration or to the radiology department for an emergent radiologic or angiographic exploration. Appropriate triage is very important for reduction of mortality.[39–42]

Angiographic intervention can be the definitive treatment in certain instances. On other occasions, a necessary operation can be postponed and performed at a later date when a patient's condition improves. Angiographic intervention is frequently an adjunctive therapy to surgery enabling a major operation to be replaced by a minor or a smaller one. It is the authors' belief that an operation performed only for controlling hemorrhage in a severely traumatized patient is unnecessary if the bleeding can be controlled with angiographic intervention. Furthermore, in many instances, control of the hemorrhage must be angiographic rather than surgical. Moreover, surgical control of bleeding may preclude future angiographic interventions. The devastating consequences and long-term disability resulting from severe trauma can be improved.[39–42]

Head and Neck Trauma

The diagnostic and interventional management of traumatic vascular lesions of the head and neck is evolving. This topic is only mentioned here because it is the domain of neuroradiologists and is not pertinent to this chapter. A new subspecialty, surgical neuroradiology, is being developed. In the future, it will have a major role in treating victims of head and neck trauma.

Chest Trauma

About 25% of patients with acute trauma die of chest injuries. Acute traumatic rupture of the thoracic aorta is a catastrophic injury resulting from head-on automobile collisions. About 80% to 90% of patients die at the scene of the accident; however, 10% to 20% may survive the initial episode. Most of the survivors die if the diagnosis is not made. A chest radiograph has a very low predictive value for the diagnosis. The chest radiograph may appear normal in 5% of patients with aortic rupture. CT has been used by some to select patients for arteriography. However, we believe that arteriography should be performed in all patients with blunt chest trauma and suspected of having deceleration injury. The nature of the trauma dictates the need for arteriography. Liberal use of aortography results in increased survival of patients sustaining this potentially lethal injury[40–43] (Fig. 46–16).

The most common site of rupture is the aortic isthmus. Another site of injury is the distal aorta. Ruptures of the ascending aorta are usually fatal and therefore not seen at arteriography. Rupture of the brachiocephalic arteries occurs in about 15% of patients. Penetrating injuries to the chest are common in the authors' patient population. Transection of the brachiocephalic, internal mammary, and intercostal arteries is due to bullets or knives. Arteriography usually demonstrates occlusion but no extravasation, owing to spasm and retraction of the vessel. Interventional radiologic management prevents possible catastrophic bleeding. Embolization of the injured arteries is routinely performed with stainless-steel coils.[40–42]

Abdominal Trauma

Blunt and penetrating trauma to the abdomen is frequent. The spleen is most often injured. The liver is frequently injured as well. Injuries to hollow viscera are less common. Embolization is very effective in the treatment of vascular injuries of the spleen and liver. Embolization is also very effective in stopping the very rare instances of lumbar arterial bleeding. Major operations can be avoided (Fig. 46–17).[35a]

Pelvic Trauma

Blunt pelvic trauma is common in this era of high speeds and drunken driving. Pelvic fractures may lead to life-threatening bleeding because of the proximity of pelvic arteries to the bony pelvis. Pelvic arteriography and embolization is the management of choice in pelvic trauma. It is impossible to predict the presence or degree of pelvic hemorrhage based on plain films. Patients with severe pelvic fractures may have minor bleeding. Patients with minor fractures may have life-threatening hemorrhage.

Control of pelvic bleeding should be angiographic rather than surgical. Surgery, which involves ligation of the internal iliac arteries, does not control the bleeding owing to the extensive collateral circulation. Furthermore, ligation of the internal iliac arteries precludes future angiographic intervention.[39] Gelfoam is preferred for embolization. On occasion, the authors have used stainless-steel coils for central occlusion after peripheral embolization with Gelfoam. The authors prefer not to embolize the trunks of the internal iliac arteries so that repeat embolization can be performed if necessary (Fig. 46–18).

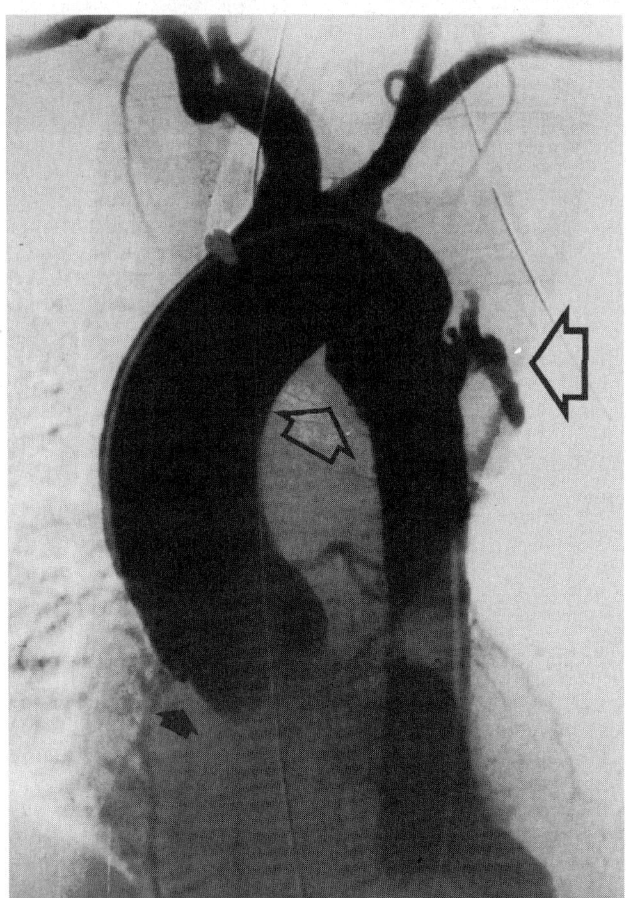

Figure 46–16. A thoracic aortogram in a young man involved in a head-on collision shows a pseudoaneurysm at the level of the aortic isthmus. Extravasation of contrast material is also noted *(arrows)*. An intimal injury in the ascending aorta is also present *(small arrow)*.

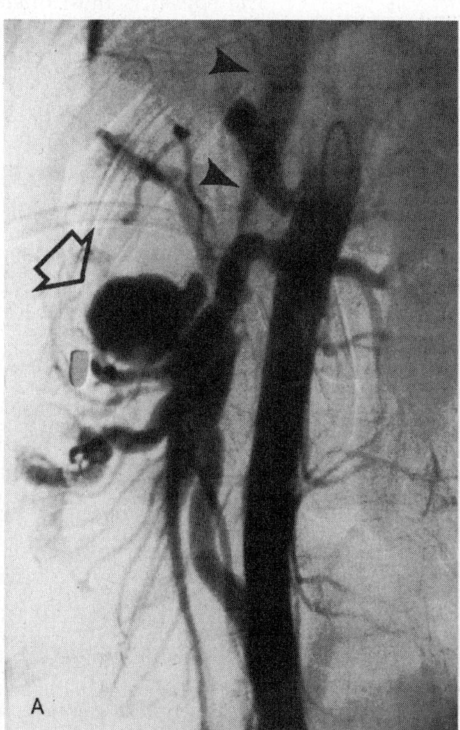

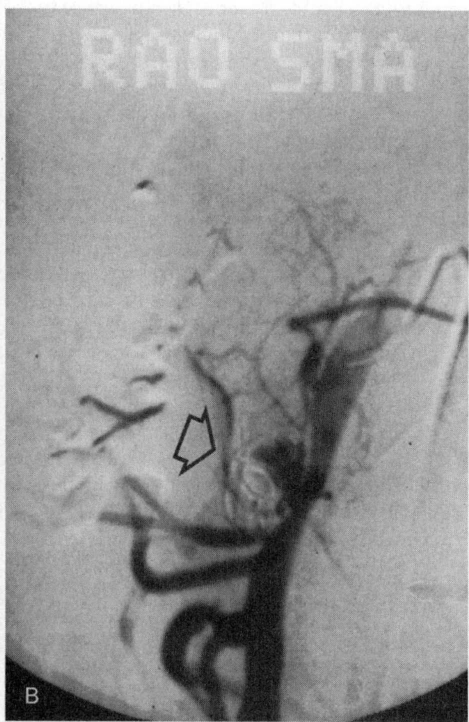

Figure 46–17. A young man sustained a bullet wound to the abdomen. *A*, An abdominal aortogram obtained after surgical exploration shows a large pseudoaneurysm from the superior mesenteric artery *(arrow)* associated with an arteriovenous fistula with the superior mesenteric vein and early opacification of the portal vein *(arrowheads)*. *B*, After embolization with several stainless-steel coils, a superior mesenteric arteriogram shows obliteration of the arteriovenous fistula and pseudoaneurysm *(arrow)*.

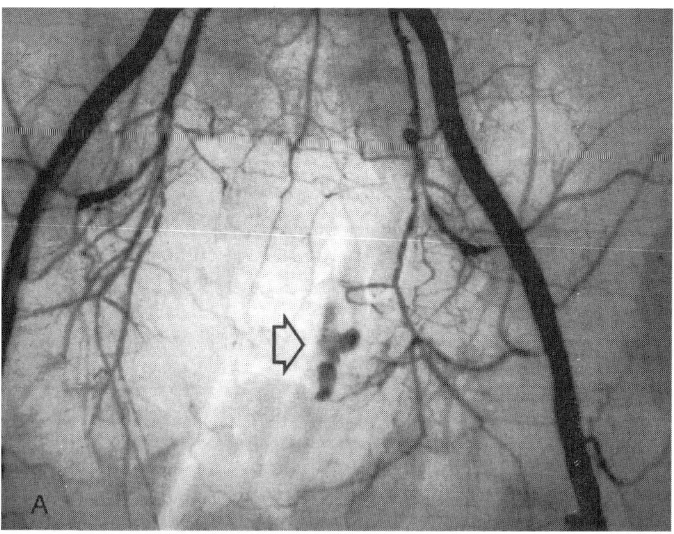

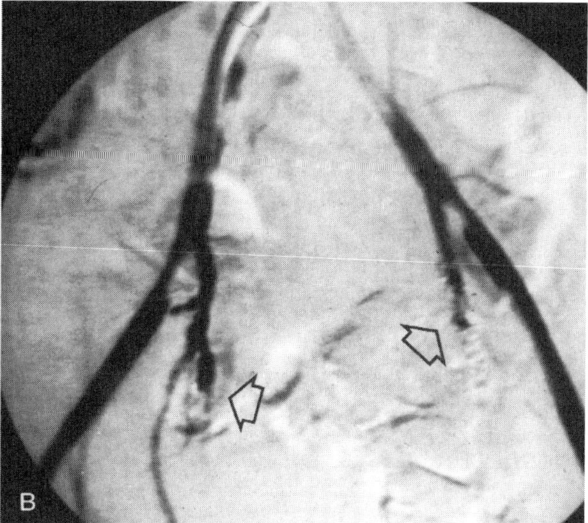

Figure 46–18. A pelvic arteriogram in a young patient who was involved in a severe automobile accident. *A*, Extravasation of contrast material from branches of the internal iliac arteries is evident *(arrow)*. *B*, Both internal iliac arteries *(arrows)* were embolized with Gelfoam particles. The patient recovered after a protracted hospitalization.

Extremity Trauma

Blunt and penetrating trauma to the limbs is common and may result in arterial injury. The brachial and popliteal arteries are more prone to injury. Arteriography is necessary in patients with expanding hematoma, bruit or thrill, acute bleeding from the wound, and diminished or absent pulses distally. Arteriography frequently illustrates positive findings in this setting. Arteriography performed only for "proximity" of injury results in very low yield of positive studies.

Arteriographic management of extremity vascular injuries is safe and effective. Operations performed specifically for controlling hemorrhage are unnecessary. Transcatheter embolotherapy is a better alternative. Arteriovenous fistulas and pseudoaneurysms can be controlled with embolization. Arteriography can be used to screen suspected vascular injuries. Surgical exploration is avoided if the arteriogram is nondiagnostic. If the arteriogram yields positive results, the exploration can be planned according to the angiographic findings.[40–42]

In conclusion, vascular and interventional radiologists are very important members of the team treating traumatized patients. In selected patients, angiographic management improves the outcomes. Severely traumatized patients must be cared for in level I trauma centers.

References

1. Reuter SR, Redman HC, Cho KJ: Gastrointestinal Angiography. 3rd ed. Philadelphia, WB Saunders, 1986, pp 282–338, 382–445.
2. Kadir S, Ernst CB: Current concepts in angiographic management of gastrointestinal bleeding. Curr Probl Surg 1983; 20:287–343.
3. Winzelberg GC, McKusick KA, Froelich JW, et al: Detection of gastrointestinal bleeding with ^{99m}Tc-labeled red blood cells. Semin Nucl Med 1982; 12:139–146.
4. Baum S: Angiography and the GI bleeder. Radiology 1982; 143:569–572.
5. Zemel G, Brown J, Becker GJ, et al: TIPS: Long-term follow-up. J Vasc Interv Radiol 1993; 4:44.

5a. Haskal ZJ, Scott M, Rubin RA, et al: Intestinal varices: Treatment with the transjugular intrahepatic portosystemic shunt. Radiology 1994; 191:183–187.

6. Mauro MA, Jacques P: Transcatheter management of pseudoaneurysms complicating pancreatitis. J Vasc Interv Radiol 1991; 2:527–532.
7. Cho SR, Tisnado J, Beachley MC, et al: Percutaneous unknotting and repositioning of intravascular catheters and percutaneous retrieval of embolized catheter fragments and other iatrogenic foreign bodies. *In*: Emergency Interventional Radiology. Neal MP, Tisnado J, Cho SR (Eds). Boston, Little, Brown and Company, 1989, pp 249–278.
8. Denny DF: Placement and management of long-term central venous access catheters and ports. AJR 1993; 161:385–393.
9. Dake MD, Semba CP, Enstrom RJ, et al: Percutaneous treatment of venous occlusive disease with stents. J Vasc Interv Radiol 1993; 4:42.
10. Leroy AJ: Percutaneous nephrostomy: Techniques and instrumentations. *In*: Clinical Urology, Pollack HM (Ed). Philadelphia, WB Saunders, 1990, pp 2725–2738.

10a. Lee WJ, Patel U, Patel S, et al: Emergency percutaneous nephrostomy: Results and complications. J Vasc Interv Radiol 1994; 5:135–139.

11. Wojtowycz M: Interventional Radiology and Angiography. Chicago, Year Book Medical Publishers, 1990, pp 110–112.
12. Mathias K: Angiographic management of intestinal ischemia. *In*: Interventional Radiology. Dondelinger RF, Rossi P, Kurdziel JC, et al (Eds). New York, Thieme Medical Publishers, 1990, pp 645–652.
13. McNamara TO, Bomberger RA, Merchant RF: Intra-arterial urokinase as the initial therapy for acutely ischemic lower limbs. Circulation 1991; 83(Suppl I):I-106–119.

13a. Clouse ME, Stokes KR, Perry LJ, et al: Percutaneous intraarterial thrombolysis: Analysis of factors affecting outcome. J Vasc Interv Radiol 1994; 5:93–100.

14. Wojtowycz M: Percutaneous angioplasty, recanalization, and vascular stents. Interventional Radiology and Angiography. Chicago, Year Book Medical Publishers, 1990, pp 162–188.
15. Palmaz JC, Laborde JC, Rivera FJ, et al: Stenting of the iliac arteries with the Palmaz stent: Experience from a multicenter trial. Cardiovasc Intervent Radiol 1992; 15:291–297.
16. Tisnado J, Bartol DT, Cho S-R, et al: Low-dose fibrinolytic therapy in hand ischemia. Radiology 1984; 150:375–382.
17. Tegtmeyer CJ, Kellum CD, Ayers C: Percutaneous transluminal angioplasty of the renal artery: Results and long-term follow-up. Radiology 1984; 153:77–84.
18. Martin LG, Price RB, Casarella WJ, et al: Percutaneous angioplasty in clinical management of renovascular hypertension; initial and long-term results. Radiology 1985; 155:629–633.

18a. Hennequin LM, Joffre FG, Rousseau HP, et al: Renal artery stent placement. Radiology 1994; 191:713–719.
19. Martin LG, Cork RD, Kaufman SL, et al: Long-term results of angioplasty in 110 patients with renal artery stenosis. J Vasc Interv Radiol 1992; 3:619–626.
20. Smith EH: Complications of percutaneous abdominal fine-needle biopsy. Radiology 1991; 178:253–258.
21. Charboneau JW: US-guided biopsy. *In*: Syllabus: A Categorical Course in Diagnostic Radiology. Interventional Radiology, Syllabus, Radiologic Society of North America categorical course Dec. 1–6, 1991. Meuller PR, van Sonnenberg E, Becker GJ (Eds). Oak Brook, IL, RSNA Publications, 1991, pp 9–16.
22. Kurdziel JD, Dondelinger RF: Intraperitoneal fluid collections. *In*: Interventional Radiology. Dondelinger RF, Rossi P, Kurdziel JC, et al (Eds). New York, Thieme Medical Publishers, 1990, pp 102–130.
23. Picus D, Marx MV: Peritoneal cavity, percutaneous drainage of intra-abdominal abscesses and fluid collections. *In*: Current Practice of Interventional Radiology. Kadir S (Ed). Philadelphia, BC Decker, 1991, pp 572–577.
24. Wojtowycz M: Interventional Radiology and Angiography. Chicago, Year Book Medical Publishers, 1990, pp 309–340.
25. Wittich GR, van Sonnenberg E, Simeone JF: Results and complications of percutaneous biliary drainage. Semin Interv Radiol 1985; 2:39–49.
25a. Harris VJ, Kopecky KK, Harman JT, et al: Percutaneous transhepatic drainage of the nondilated biliary system. J Vasc Interv Radiol 1994; 4:591–595.
26. Malone DE: Interventional radiologic alternatives to cholecystectomy. Radiol Clin North Am 1990; 28:1145–1156.
27. Lammer J, Klein GE, Kleinert R, et al: Obstructive jaundice: Use of expandable metal endoprosthesis for biliary drainage. Radiology 1990; 177:789–792.
28. Alzate GD, Coons HG, Elliott J, et al: Percutaneous gastrostomy for jejunal feeding: A new technique. AJR 1986; 147:822–825.
29. Ho C-S, Gray RR, Goldfinger M: Percutaneous gastrostomy for enteral feeding. Radiology 1985; 156:349–351.
30. Wojtowycz M: Interventional Radiology and Angiography. Chicago, Year Book Medical Publishers, 1990, pp 299–308.
31. Kandarpa K: Percutaneous gastrostomy and gastrojejunostomy tube placement. *In*: Handbook of Cardiovascular and Interventional Radiologic Procedures. Kandarpa K (Ed). Boston, Little, Brown and Company, 1989, pp 125–130.
32. Gurney JW: No fooling around: Direct visualization of pulmonary embolism. Radiology 1993; 188:619–620.
33. Gresham CL: Deep venous thrombosis. South Med J 1993; 86:438–440.
34. Dalen JE, Alpert JS: Natural history of pulmonary embolism. Prog Cardiovasc Dis 1975; 17:259–270.
35. Alderson PO, Martin EC: Pulmonary embolism: Diagnosis with multiple imaging modalities. Radiology 1987; 164:297–312.
35a. Coldwell M, Stokes KR, Yakes WF: Embolotherapy: Agents, clinical applications, and techniques. Radiographics 1994; 14:623–643.
36. Wholey MH, Smot S: Embolization of bronchial arteries in patients with hemoptysis. *In*: Emergency Interventional Radiology. Neal MP, Tisnado J, Cho SR (Eds). Boston, Little, Brown and Company, 1989, pp 123–138.
37. Mauro MA, Jaques PF, Morris S: Bronchial artery embolization for control of hemoptysis. Semin Interv Radiol 1992; 9:45–51.
38. Barth KH: Therapeutic Embolization in Thoracic Bleeding Emergencies (Abstract). Laguna Niguel, CA, Society of Thoracic Radiology, 1992.
39. Ben-Menachem Y, Coldwell DM, Young JWR: Hemorrhage associated with pelvic fractures: Causes, diagnosis and emergent management. AJR 1991; 157:1005–1014.
40. Ben-Menachem Y: Radiology. *In*: Early Care of the Injured Patient. Moore EE (Ed). Philadelphia, BC Decker, 1990, pp 84–90.
41. Ben-Menachem Y: Angiography in diagnosis of vascular trauma. *In*: Radiology: Diagnosis, Imaging, Intervention. Vol 2. Taveras JM, Ferrucci JJT (Eds). Philadelphia, JB Lippincott, 1988, pp 1–14.
42. Ben-Menachem Y: Logic and logistics of radiography, angiography and intervention in blunt trauma. Radiol Clin North Am 1981; 19:171–186.
43. Fisher RS, Chasen MH, Camki N: Diagnosis of injuries of the aorta and brachiocephalic arteries caused by blunt chest trauma: CT vs aortography. AJR Am J Roentgenol 1994; 162:1047–1052.

CHAPTER 47

Positron Emission Tomography: Basic Principles and Potential Applications in the Critically Ill

David J. Diehl, MD • Mark A. Mintun, MD

Positron emission tomography (PET) is a powerful imaging method that enables in vivo measurement of metabolism and other physiologic parameters in human beings. This type of imaging is termed *functional,* in contradistinction to the *structural* imaging methods described in the previous chapters. Since the first human PET study in 1979, PET has grown to have more than 60 imaging centers worldwide. PET studies have mostly focused on the brain and heart, although tumors and other organs (including the lungs, liver, and kidneys) have been investigated. PET imaging has been primarily a research tool, advancing the understanding of physiologic functioning in both normal and ill states. Researchers have also investigated clinical applications of PET, and although by no means routinely used, a few applications have emerged as helpful in clinical decision making (e.g., localization of seizure focus for epilepsy surgery).

This chapter begins with a summary of the basic principles of PET to give readers a sense of its capabilities and limitations. When appropriate, PET is compared with the other available method of tomographic functional imaging, single-photon emission computer tomography (SPECT). The second part of the chapter considers applications of PET imaging in critically ill patients. This section first reviews the relatively small literature on functional imaging of critically ill patients and then speculates on future directions. Throughout the chapter, the focus is on PET imaging of the *brain* because this is viewed as the area of greatest potential application in the critically ill.

BASIC PRINCIPLES

Physics and Instrumentation of Positron Emission Tomography

PET imaging involves intravenous injection of radiotracers labeled with positron-emitting nuclides. A positron is the antiparticle of an electron, having the same mass but the opposite charge (i.e., +1). When a positron is emitted in tissue, it travels up to a few millimeters before losing most of its energy and nearly coming to rest. At that point, the positron undergoes mutual annihilation with an electron in the tissue. The positron-electron annihilation results in the emission of two 511-keV γ-ray photons (thus obeying the law of conservation of energy). Furthermore, the photons are emitted in opposite directions (i.e., 180° apart) in accordance with the law of conservation of momentum. As described later, these 511-keV photons are what is detected by a PET scanner. (See Fig. 47–1 for a pictorial representation of positron decay.)

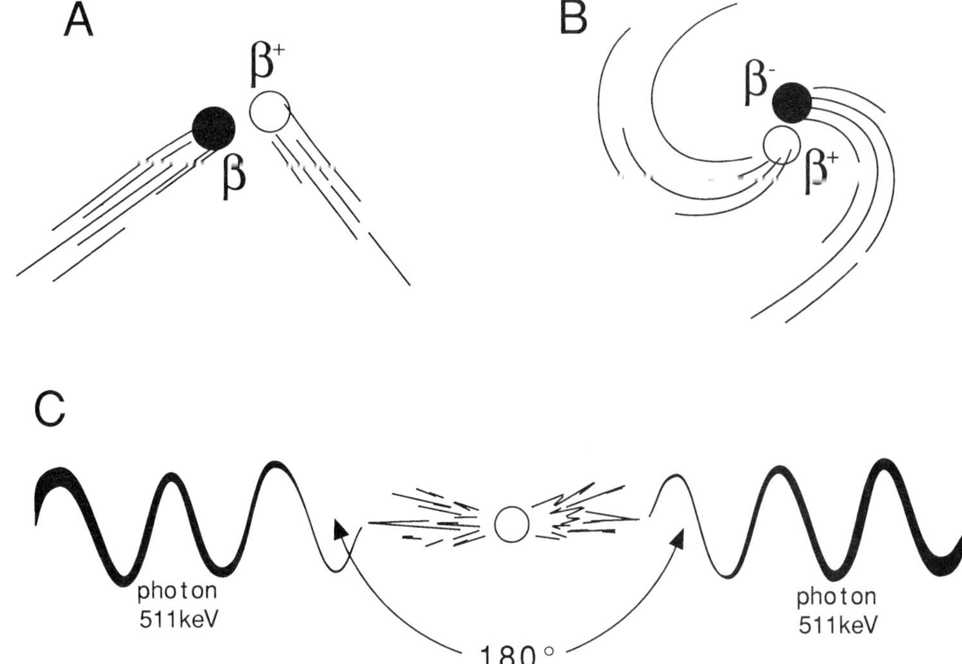

Figure 47–1. Pictorial representation of positron decay. *A*, A positron (β+) is emitted in tissue. *B*, The positron comes in contact with a nearby electron (β−). *C*, Mutual annihilation of the positron and electron results in the emission of two 511-keV gamma ray photons traveling in opposite directions.

PET scanners consist of parallel rings of detectors arranged transaxially around the field of view (Fig. 47–2). The detectors are electronically coupled as *coincidence circuits* so that the scanner only registers pairs of photons absorbed by two different detectors "simultaneously" (usually defined as < 6–15 nanoseconds). Thus, when two opposing detectors absorb 511-keV photons simultaneously, a positron annihilation event is assumed to have occurred along the line joining the two detectors (Fig. 47–3). The coincidence lines collected by the scanner are corrected for tissue attenuation of photons (using either calculated factors or a transmission scan) and then are reconstructed into transaxial images using filtered backprojection techniques (similar to those used in conventional x-ray computed tomography [CT]). These images reflect the quantitative in vivo distribution of the radionuclide. The spatial resolution of state-of-the-art PET scanners is 5 to 9 mm (full width at half maximum). The theoretically achievable resolution with PET is limited to approximately 2 to 3 mm because the positron travels a short distance before its annihilation (thus the site of annihilation differs from the location of the tracer) and the positron is not completely at rest at the time of annihilation (the net momentum results in a slight deviation of the usual 180° separation of the annihilation photons).

Coincidence detection confers important advantages over the radiation detection method used by SPECT. In the latter, single photons emitted by a radiotracer are absorbed by detectors placed as close to the body as possible. Lead collimators, interposed between the subject and the detectors, allow the detection of photons traveling in only a particular direction and thus enable the spatial distribution of the tracer to be determined. This detection method causes both the spatial resolution and sensitivity to decrease with increasing distance from the detector. On the other hand, with coincidence detection, the spatial resolution is independent of depth within the body, and the change in sensitivity with position in the body (due to tissue attenuation of photons) can be corrected by obtaining a transmission scan (i.e., a short period of imaging with a ring of radioactivity surrounding the body). Thus, PET generates a more accurate quantitative representation of radionuclide distribution and generally has a higher spatial resolution. Additionally, coincidence detection is intrinsically more efficient because lead collimation is not needed.

Positron Emission Tomography Radiochemistry

Conventional nuclear medicine studies, including SPECT, generally use radioisotopes of heavy elements (e.g., technetium 99m, indium 111, iodine 123) that have minimal biologic roles and thus are not naturally present in the organic compounds being labeled. The resulting radiotracers often have a different chemical behavior compared with their en-

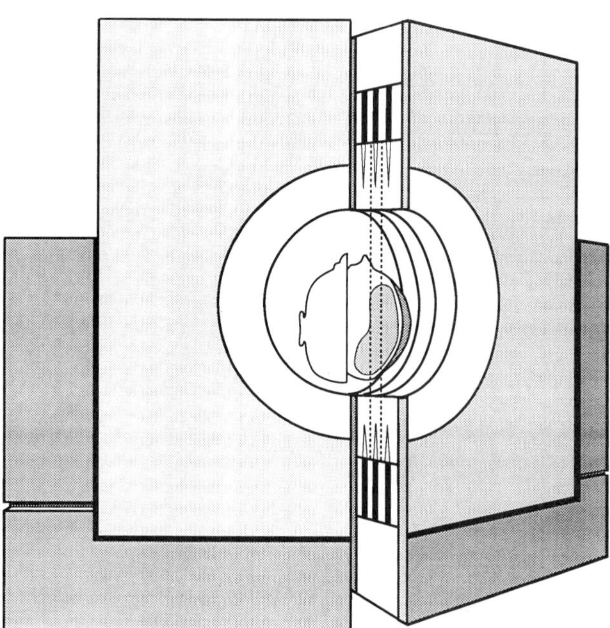

Figure 47–2. A cross-sectional view of a subject's brain in the typical axial field-of-view of a PET scanner. Note the parallel rings of detectors with lead septa positioned between adjacent rings.

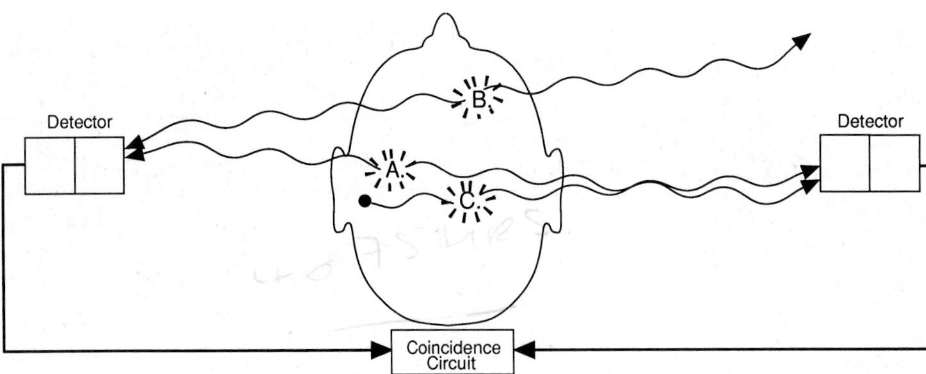

Figure 47–3. Coincidence detection method used in PET. *A*, Positron annihilation is detected because photons are absorbed by coincidence-paired detectors simultaneously. *B*, Positron annihilation is not detected because only one detector absorbs a photon. *C*, Positron annihilation is not detected because one photon is absorbed by the tissue (i.e., it is attenuated).

dogenous counterparts. On the other hand, positron-emitting radionuclides are isotopes of lighter elements (e.g., oxygen 15, carbon 11, nitrogen 13). Consequently, these radionuclides can be incorporated into organic compounds that are chemically similar to those present in the body. Additionally, the radionuclides used by PET afford a tremendous diversity of useful radiotracers that can potentially be synthesized.

The major limitation with the radioisotopes used in PET is their short physical half-life (Table 47–1) as compared with conventional nuclear medicine agents. This necessitates an on-site cyclotron for radiotracer production, which is a major factor contributing to PET studies' generally being more expensive than SPECT studies. It also challenges the ingenuity of radiochemists who have to devise rapid methods of incorporating the radionuclides into useful radiotracers. In some applications, a short half-life can be an advantage by allowing multiple studies in a single scanning session (see the later discussion of PET activation studies).

Measurable Physiologic Parameters with Positron Emission Tomography

As described previously, PET images reflect the quantitative in vivo distribution of the *radionuclide.* In order to convert these data into a useful physiologic measurement, one must know the physiologic disposition of the *radiotracer* (i.e., the compound labeled with the radionuclide) as well as its radionuclide-labeled metabolites. In practical application, a tracer kinetic model is developed to approximate the metabolic fate of the radiotracer and thereby facilitate calculation of the physiologic parameter of interest. Table 47–2 lists several of the physiologic parameters that have been successfully measured with PET, along with their respective radiotracers. These include the regional measurement of glucose metabolism, oxygen metabolism, blood flow, blood volume, and neuroreceptor concentration (Bmax) and binding affinity (K_d). In contrast, at the present time, SPECT can only measure blood flow and parameters of some neuroreceptor systems.

Glucose Metabolism

One of the most common PET measurements is the regional metabolic rate of glucose metabolism. This is most often accomplished using fluorine-18(^{18}F)–labeled fluorodeoxyglucose (FDG) as the radiotracer. FDG is a glucose analog that in most respects has a similar chemical behavior to glucose, including being a competitive substrate for the first step in the biochemical pathway of glucose metabolism (i.e., hexokinase-catalyzed phosphorylation to glucose-6-phosphate or FDG-6-phosphate). However, FDG differs from glucose in that FDG undergoes only this *first* metabolic step and then is essentially trapped in the cell (at least for the period of a typical FDG PET study). Thus, the amount of FDG-6-phosphate present in a given region is proportional to that region's rate of glucose metabolism. In FDG PET studies, scanning is usually started 30 to 45 minutes after injection of FDG, allowing most of the free FDG to wash out of the tissue (leaving the trapped FDG-6-phosphate). Therefore, the in vivo distribution of ^{18}F represented by the PET image is approximately proportional to the regional glucose metabolic rate. In order to calculate the absolute rate of regional glucose metabolism, one needs additional information, including the plasma concentration of glucose and the time-dependent radioactivity curves for plasma and tissue FDG.

The FDG PET method has been extensively used to study human brain function in both normal and pathologic conditions. Figure 47–4 shows the reconstructed PET brain images from an FDG study of a normal human subject. Examples of abnormal findings in pathologic conditions include interictal hypometabolism of the seizure focus in epilepsy, decreased temporal and parietal cortical metabolism in Alzheimer's disease, and reduced caudate metabolism in Huntington's disease.

TABLE 47–1. Decay Half-Lives of PET Radioisotopes

Radioisotope	*Half-Life (min)*
Oxygen 15 (^{15}O)	2.07
Nitrogen 13 (^{13}N)	9.96
Carbon 11 (^{11}C)	20.4
Fluorine 18 (^{18}F)	109.7

TABLE 47–2. Physiologic Parameters Measurable with PET

Measurement	*Radiotracers*
Blood flow	^{15}O-water
	^{15}O-carbon dioxide
	^{13}N-ammonia
Blood volume	^{15}O-carbon monoxide
	^{11}C-carbon monoxide
Glucose metabolism	^{18}F-fluorodeoxyglucose (FDG)
	^{11}C-deoxyglucose
Oxygen metabolism	^{15}O-oxygen
Protein synthesis	^{11}C-amino acids
	^{13}N-amino acids
Fatty acid metabolism	^{11}C-palmitate
Dopamine synthesis	^{18}F-fluorodopa
Dopamine receptors	^{11}C-raclopride
	^{11}C-*N*-methylspiperone (NMSP)
Opiate receptors	^{11}C-carfentanil
Cholinergic receptors	^{11}C-scopolamine

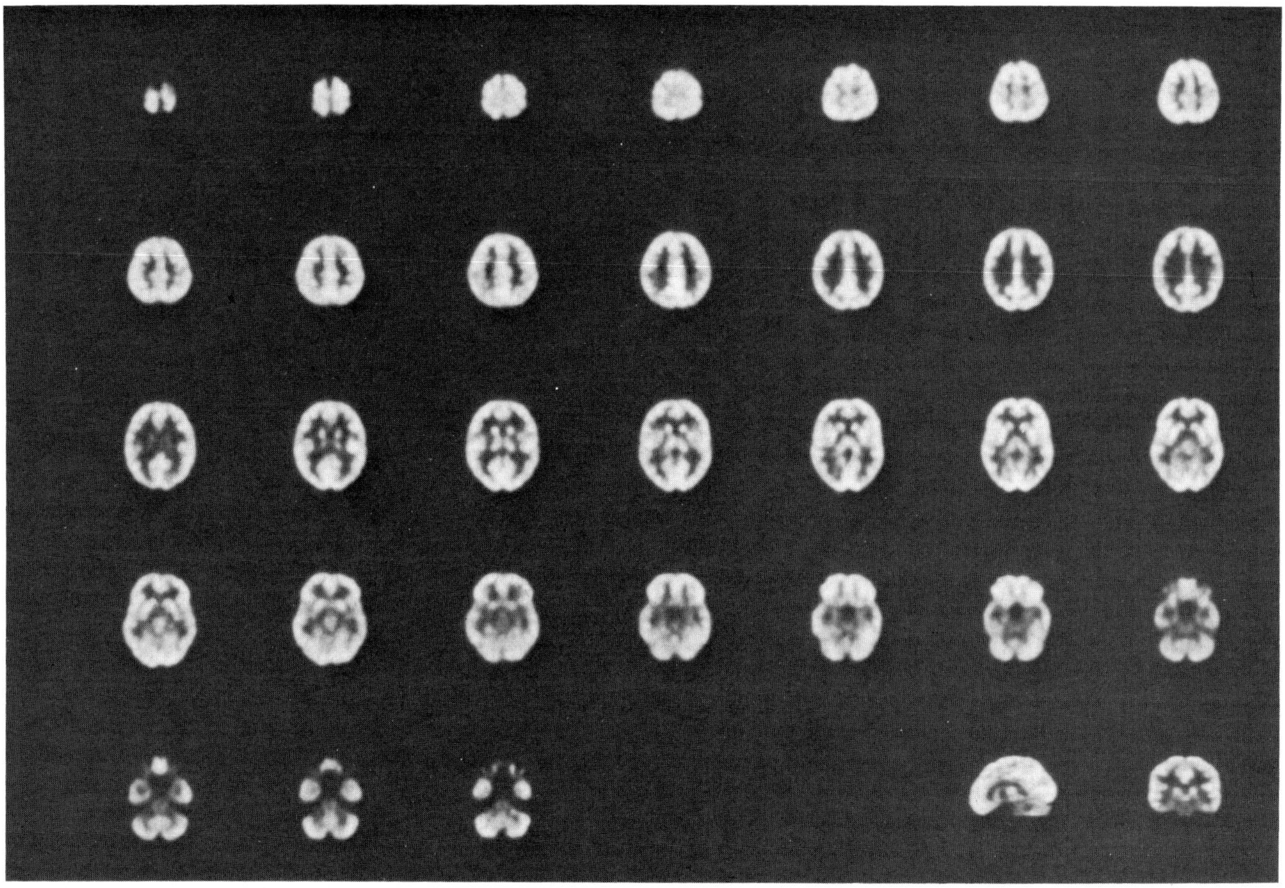

Figure 47–4. PET ^{18}F-labeled FDG brain images of a normal human subject using a Siemens 951/31 whole-body PET scanner. Starting with the most superior brain slice in the upper left corner, the 31 transaxial reconstructed slices are displayed (covering a 10.8-cm^2 field-of-view). The bottom right corner shows examples of the PET data resliced in a sagittal plane and in a coronal plane. (See Color Plate Section of this textbook.)

Blood Flow

Another common PET brain measurement is regional cerebral blood flow (rCBF). This can be accomplished using ^{15}O-labeled water. A typical scanning protocol consists of a bolus injection of ^{15}O-water followed by a 60-second scan started 15 to 20 seconds after the injection. The PET image reflects the in vivo distribution of ^{15}O-water, which is essentially proportional to rCBF. The concurrent determination of arterial ^{15}O-water radioactivity curves allows estimation of absolute rCBF. Because neuronal activity, glucose metabolism, and CBF are closely coupled under normal conditions, the ^{15}O-water rCBF technique is considered an indicator of local neuronal activity.

The ^{15}O-water rCBF method has particularly been used for PET activation studies. Such studies are used to map the functional organization of the brain by measuring changes in a physiologic parameter induced by a stimulus condition. This is achieved through the technique of paired-image subtraction (i.e., stimulus state minus control state), which removes brain areas not affected by the stimulus. ^{15}O-water is particularly well suited for activation studies because its short half-life (123 s) permits multiple scans under different conditions to be performed during a single scanning session. ^{15}O-water activation studies have successfully mapped functional systems ranging from vision to language. (Fig. 47–5 shows ^{15}O-water rCBF images including a subtraction image demonstrating visual cortex activation induced by a visual stimulus.) PET activation studies have also been carried out using measurements of oxygen and glucose metabolism.

Oxygen Metabolism

A third brain measurement is regional cerebral metabolic rate of oxygen (rCMRO_2) using ^{15}O-labeled oxygen gas. This is a more complex measurement than rCBF or glucose me-

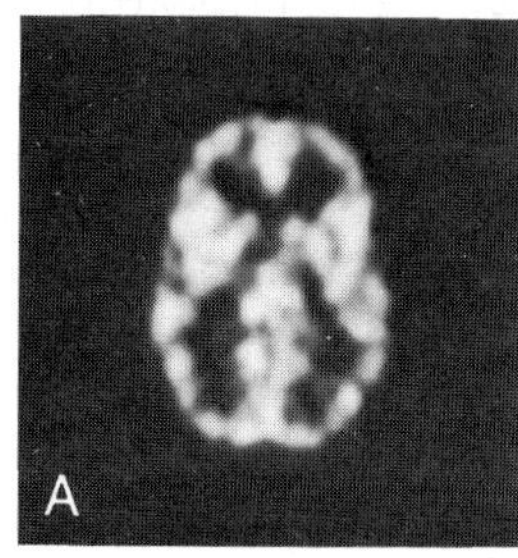

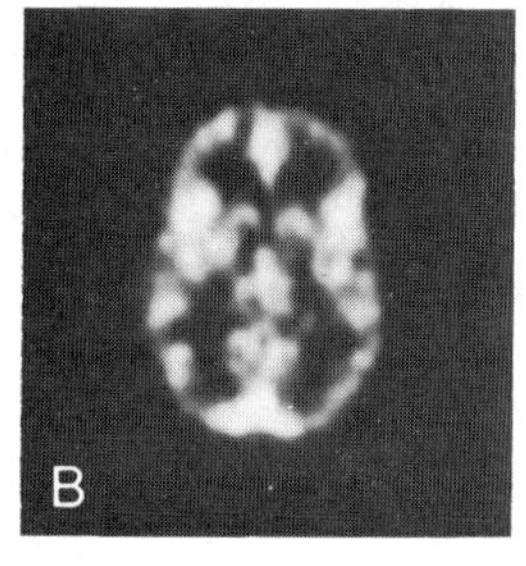

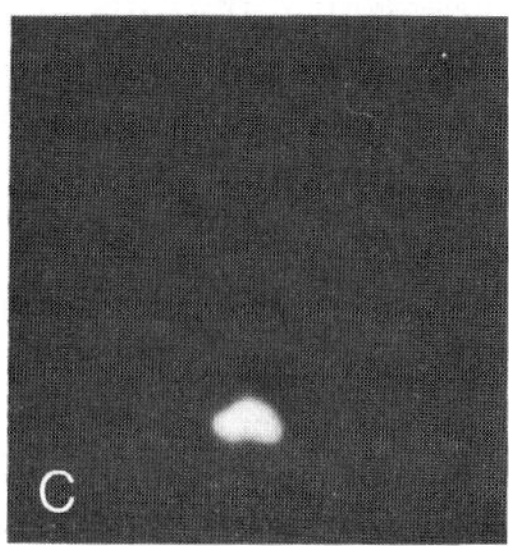

Figure 47–5. Example of PET activation method using ^{15}O-labeled water rCBF imaging in a normal human subject. *A*, Control state (cross-hair only). *B*, Visual stimulation state (with annular reversing checkerboard surrounding the cross-hair). *C*, Subtraction image (i.e., stimulus state minus control state) showing visual cortex activation. (See Color Plate Section of this textbook.)

tabolism and typically consists of three separate tracer administrations and scanning sequences. First, ^{15}O-labeled carbon monoxide inhalation and a 2- to 5-minute PET scan is used to measure the cerebral blood volume (because carbon monoxide tracer tightly binds to red blood cells). Second, ^{15}O-labeled water injection is used to measure CBF as described earlier. Third, ^{15}O-labeled oxygen gas inhalation is followed by a 1- to 3-minute PET scan. The regional cerebral blood volume and blood flow information is used to interpret the behavior of the ^{15}O-labeled oxygen gas by a tracer kinetic model that allows accurate calculation of the regional oxygen extraction fraction (rOEF). The $rCMRO_2$ is then calculated by the product of rOEF, rCBF, and the arterial oxygen content by blood gas analysis. Although the short half-lives of these ^{15}O tracers allow the three sequential PET studies to be accomplished in less than 45 minutes, the demanding technical nature of the $rCMRO_2$ measurement has greatly limited its use in brain research. A single-step approach to the $CMRO_2$ measurement has been described; this approach may increase its utility.

POTENTIAL APPLICATIONS OF POSITRON EMISSION TOMOGRAPHY IN THE CRITICALLY ILL

Summary of SPECT and PET Studies

During the past decade, several researchers have investigated the use of tomographic functional imaging in critically ill (and often comatose) patients. The majority of these studies have measured rCBF using SPECT with ^{99m}Tc-labeled hexamethylpropyleneamineoxime (^{99m}Tc-HMPAO) as the radiotracer. The PET studies have generally examined rCBF or regional cerebral metabolic rate of glucose (rCMRglu). The clinical population most often investigated has been patients who have sustained severe head trauma. Research goals have included elucidating the pathophysiology of severe brain injury, identifying predictors of clinical outcome, and aiding in the determination of brain death. Conclusions from almost all the studies described later are hindered by the heterogeneity of the patient samples and the variability in the time when the functional imaging was performed with respect to the time of the brain injury.

The most consistent finding in the head trauma studies has been that functional imaging is more sensitive to the extent and severity of pathology than the structural imaging methods of magnetic resonance imaging (MRI) and x-ray CT. Two SPECT rCBF studies involved primarily severely neurologically compromised patients who were mostly scanned within 2 to 3 days of their head injury.[1, 2] These studies found that SPECT revealed more lesions and demonstrated lesions at an earlier stage than CT. Goncalves and colleagues[3] investigated more stable patients (most with Glasgow Coma Scale [GCS] scores of at least 13) with focal neurologic deficits (primarily hemiparesis). They found that ^{99m}Tc-HMPAO SPECT was more likely than CT or MRI to demonstrate a lesion in the expected brain area (based on the type of neurologic deficit). Another SPECT rCBF study scanned patients 3 to 36 months after severe head injury and also found SPECT more sensitive than CT or MRI in detecting focal lesions.[4] Langfitt and associates[5] measured rCMRglu with PET in three head trauma victims and found that PET revealed regions of brain dysfunction not revealed by CT or MRI. Finally, a PET rCBF study investigated five patients 3 to 24 months after severe closed head injury and demonstrated that the PET but not the CT findings closely correlated with the site of cerebral dysfunction based on neurologic and behavioral examinations.[6]

Another area of investigation in victims of head injury has been identification of functional imaging correlates of the severity of brain injury. Using the xenon 133 CBF technique (a nontomographic method) and arteriovenous differences in oxygen concentration, the University of Pennsylvania research group found a positive correlation between global cerebral oxygen metabolism and GCS scores in 127 patients (i.e., more severe coma associated with lower oxygen metabolism) but did not find a correlation between CBF and coma severity. This group later used the FDG PET method and demonstrated a positive correlation between global CMRglu and GCS scores (see Alavi[7] for review of University of Pennsylvania studies). In a FDG PET study of seven patients in persistent vegetative states (PVS) and three "locked-in" patients (from various types of brain insults), Levy and coworkers[8] found that global CMRglu was less than half the normal value in PVS patients but only 25% reduced in locked-in patients. There have been no studies examining the relationship between severity of brain injury and *regional* cerebral metabolic decreases (e.g., in brain areas thought to have importance in arousal level).

Only two research reports have specifically addressed the question of whether functional imaging results can predict clinical outcome in patients with severe brain injury from head trauma. Oder and associates[9] performed SPECT rCBF in 12 PVS patients during their early rehabilitation (i.e., after the acute stage of injury). They found that globally decreased cortical CBF predicted poor longitudinal outcome, but the occurrence of only focal deficits did not reliably indicate a favorable outcome. Abdel-Dayem and associates[1] studied 14 comatose patients, measuring rCBF with SPECT (usually within 72 h of their head injury). Their results suggest that a poor prognosis is related to size, multiplicity, and location of lesions. The worst prognosis was associated with multiple large brain stem lesions.

The SPECT ^{99m}Tc-HMPAO method has been proposed as a possible aid in the diagnosis of brain death when other criteria are equivocal or when a prompt determination is important (e.g., organ donation). A finding of no brain uptake of HMPAO is taken as support of the diagnosis of brain death. It has been suggested that this method may be particularly helpful in patients under the effects of drugs (e.g., barbiturates) that may confound the usual diagnostic tests such as electroencephalogram and evoked potentials. De la Riva and colleagues[10] investigated this approach in 37 patients with severe brain injury. They demonstrated absence of HMPAO uptake in all patients meeting standard clinical criteria for brain death, whereas uptake (at least in the brain stem) was noted in all the remaining patients. Another SPECT HMPAO study confirmed clinical evidence of brain death in 15 of 17 patients.[11] However, it is not clear how much the SPECT data *add* to standard methods in the determination of brain death. Furthermore, establishment of criteria for brain death is a complicated area with medical, ethical, and legal aspects that need to be carefully considered before determining the role of SPECT in the diagnosis of brain death.

Future Directions

The foregoing summarized literature suggests promise for the use of functional brain imaging in the critically ill, particularly with respect to elucidating the pathophysiology of severe brain injury and assessing the prognosis of comatose patients (i.e., predicting the reversibility versus irreversibility of brain injury). PET has the most potential in this regard because of the diverse and specific nature of research and clinical questions that can be investigated. For example, one can measure regional CBF, $CMRO_2$, CMRglu, or a combination of these parameters (in a single scanning session) so that the relationship between two physiologic parameters can be determined in relevant brain areas.

The PET activation method described previously can also be used to address very specific research questions. Briefly, this technique involves measuring the regional changes in a physiologic parameter after an intervention. Thus, researchers could potentially design PET activation paradigms to test whether a particular brain region has the capacity to functionally respond to a relevant activation condition (e.g., pharmacologic or sensory). This will challenge critical care researchers to develop specific hypotheses and then to design practical activation paradigms. One research group has used PET to examine the changes in rCMRglu after an intervention. Momose and associates[12] imaged a single patient in a persistent vegetative state before and after 1 week of cervical spinal cord stimulation, which has been applied to comatose patients with promising results. This study found that the rCMRglu of the cerebral cortex increased after cervical spinal cord stimulation, particularly on the right side, where it had been most depressed at baseline.

An alternative line of investigation shows promise for prognostic assessment of brain viability in comatose patients. Nemoto and coworkers[13] have reported a method of measuring the basal and active components of $CMRO_2$ (i.e., $BCMRO_2$ and $ACMRO_2$, respectively). $ACMRO_2$ is the oxygen consumed to support spontaneous brain electric activity (i.e., synaptic transmission), and $BCMRO_2$ supports the energy-requiring processes of neurons in the resting state (e.g., from sodium ion leak). Nemoto and colleagues argue that spontaneous electric activity is the essence of brain viability, and thus the $ACMRO_2$ after cerebral insult is an estimate of brain viability. The components of $CMRO_2$ can be determined by first measuring the total $CMRO_2$ and then the $CMRO_2$ after administration of the barbiturate thiopental. Because thiopental specifically blocks spontaneous electric activity, the post-thiopental $CMRO_2$ is equivalent to $BCMRO_2$ and the $ACMRO_2$ can be calculated as total $CMRO_2$ minus $BCMRO_2$. Using whole-brain arteriovenous sampling methods in animals, these researchers have successfully measured $BCMRO_2$ and $ACMRO_2$ in both normal and pathologic (i.e., after global ischemia) conditions.[13, 14] In a clinical study with related methodology, Sari and colleagues[15] estimated the whole-brain CBF-$CMRO_2$ ratio (by measuring the arteriovenous oxygen content difference) in 11 comatose patients before and after barbiturate administration. The patients who eventually recovered showed a significant decrease in their CBF-$CMRO_2$ ratio with barbiturates, whereas this ratio did not change in the patients who failed to recover. PET offers the opportunity to extend this line of research by measuring $ACMRO_2$ and $BCMRO_2$ or the CBF-$CMRO_2$ ratio at a *regional* level in critically ill patients.

In conclusion, the use of PET in the investigation of critically ill patients is still in an early stage of development. The capability of PET to accurately measure diverse physiologic parameters makes it a potentially powerful method of studying this patient population. However, in order to realize this potential to the fullest, critical care researchers must carefully design studies that use the unique capabilities of PET to address specific hypotheses regarding the pathophysiology of severe brain injuries.

References

Recommended Reading on the Basic Principles of PET

Phelps ME, Mazziotta JC, Schelbert HR: Positron Emission Tomography and Autoradiography: Principles and Applications for the Brain and Heart. New York, Raven Press, 1986.

Cited References

1. Abdel-Dayem HM, Sadek SA, Kouris K, et al: Changes in cerebral perfusion after acute head injury: Comparison of CT with Tc-99m HM-PAO SPECT. Radiology 1987; 165:221–226.
2. Reid RH, Gulenchyn KY, Ballinger JR, et al: Cerebral perfusion imaging with technetium-99m HMPAO following cerebral trauma: Initial experience. Clin Nucl Med 1990; 15:383–388.
3. Goncalves JM, Vaz R, Cerejo A, et al: HM-PAO SPECT in head trauma. Acta Neurochir 1992; 55:11–33.
4. Newton MR, Greenwood RJ, Britton KE, et al: A study comparing SPECT with CT and MRI after closed head injury. J Neurol Neurosurg Psychiatry 1992; 55:92–94.
5. Langfitt TW, Obrist WD, Alavi A, et al: Computerized tomography, magnetic resonance imaging, and positron emission tomography in the study of brain trauma. J Neurosurg 1986; 64:760–767.
6. Rao N, Turski PA, Polcyn RE, et al: ^{18}F positron emission computed tomography in closed head injury. Arch Phys Med Rehabil 1984; 65:780–785.
7. Alavi A: Functional and anatomic studies of head injury. J Neuropsychiatry 1989; 1:S45–S50.
8. Levy DE, Sidtis JJ, Rottenberg DA, et al: Differences in cerebral blood flow and glucose utilization in vegetative versus locked-in patients. Ann Neurol 1987; 22:673–682.
9. Oder W, Goldenberg G, Podreka I, et al: HM-PAO-SPECT in persistent vegetative state after head injury: Prognostic indicator of the likelihood of recovery? Intensive Care Med 1991; 17:149–153.
10. de la Riva A, Gonzalez FM, Llamas-Elvira JM, et al: Diagnosis of brain death: Superiority of perfusion studies with ^{99m}Tc-HMPAO over conventional radionuclide cerebral angiography. Br J Radiol 1992; 65:289–294.
11. Schlake HP, Bottger IG, Grotemeyer KH, et al: Determination of cerebral perfusion by means of planar brain scintigraphy and ^{99m}Tc-HMPAO in brain death, persistent vegetative state and severe coma. Intensive Care Med 1992; 18:76–81.
12. Momose T, Matsui T, Kosaka N, et al: Effect of cervical spinal cord stimulation (cSCS) on glucose metabolism and blood flow in a vegetative patient assessed by positron emission tomography (PET) and single photon emission computed tomography (SPECT). Radiat Med 1989; 7:243–246.
13. Nemoto EM, Melick JA, Winter P: Active and basal cerebrometabolic rate for oxygen ($CMRO_2$) after complete global brain ischemia in rats. *In*: Oxygen Transport to Tissue X. Masaji M, Honig CR, Koyama T, et al (Eds). New York, Plenum Publishing, 1988, pp 391–396.
14. Nemoto EM, Lipin Y, Yonas Y, et al: Active and basal whole brain blood flow, oxygen and glucose metabolism in monkeys. *In*: Oxygen Transport to Tissue XIV. Erdmann W, Bruley DF (Eds). New York, Plenum Publishing, 1992, pp 695–699.
15. Sari A, Matayoshi Y, Yonei A, et al: Cerebral arteriovenous oxygen content difference during barbiturate therapy in patients with acute brain damage. Anesth Analg 1986; 65:1196–1200.

SECTION VI

CARDIOVASCULAR

Stephen M. Ayres

CHAPTER 48

Applied Cardiovascular Physiology in the Critically Ill

Peter W. Kakavas, MD • William J. Sibbald, MD, FRCP(C) • James E. Calvin, MD, FRCPS, FACC

A detailed appreciation of factors responsible for the alteration of cardiac function in critical illness requires knowledge of both the molecular basis of cardiac function and its influence on cardiac mechanics as it relates to both normal and pathologic conditions. Only then can therapeutics be rationally applied in the cardiovascular support of critically ill patients. This review characterizes both systolic and diastolic abnormalities at the cell and organ level and reviews how these are assessed at the bedside. Pressure-volume (P-V) loops and force velocity relationships are used in a theoretic sense to relate cellular mechanisms to abnormalities of cardiovascular function and the effects of various therapies in the critically ill.

CELLULAR PHYSIOLOGY OF MYOCARDIAL FUNCTION

Cellular Determinants of Contractility

The interaction of the proteins actin, myosin, and the troponin complex results in contractive activity of the myocardial muscle fibers. Engagement of actin and myosin occurs when calcium (Ca^{2+}) levels in the cytosol increase in the presence of adequate adenosine triphosphate (ATP). This process is regulated by a complex that consists of troponin C and other proteins. Troponin C contains a Ca^{2+}-specific binding site with variable affinity for Ca^{2+}.[1] When Ca^{2+} is bound to troponin C, tropomyosin (a protein bound to the troponin complex, which inhibits actin-myosin interaction in the absence of troponin C) undergoes a conformational change, allowing for actin-myosin interaction and contraction.

Removal of Ca^{2+} from the cytosol results in dissociation from troponin C, with subsequent cessation of actin-myosin cross-linkage. This event signals the end of contractile activity and the start of relaxation. This process is known as *inactivation*[2] and is later discussed further.

Calcium and Cyclic Adenosine Monophosphate

Alterations in the delivery, use, and myofibrillar sensitivity to and removal of Ca^{2+} from the myofibril and the myocyte cytosol constitute the biologic basis for the vast majority, if not all, of the abnormalities in both contractility and relaxation. Ca^{2+}, stored in the sarcoplasmic reticulum (SR), is released from storage sites via a number of mechanisms. In addition, Ca^{2+} entry from extracellular locations participates in the contractile process.

Entry of Ca^{2+} from extracellular locations occurs through voltage-dependent gated "slow channels," activated by membrane depolarization, or via sodium-calcium (Na-Ca^{2+}) exchange across the sarcolemma. This Ca^{2+}, rather than participating directly in activation of contraction, causes release of Ca^{2+} from the SR[3], so-called Ca^{2+}-dependent Ca^{2+} release. The Ca^{2+} released from the SR binds to troponin, with subsequent contractile activity.

In addition, elevated levels of cyclic adenosine monophosphate (cAMP), the major intracellular second messenger, cause increased Ca^{2+} influx by recruitment of additional voltage-dependent channels, previously dormant. This is accomplished by cAMP-mediated transfer of phosphates to phospholamban, a protein linked to the voltage-gated channels. Phospholamban, a protein within the SR, when phosphorylated by cAMP-dependent mechanisms, results in increased SR uptake of Ca^{2+}.[4, 5] This is noted to occur primarily after adrenergic stimuli (discussed later). All of these mechanisms result in increased contraction.

Altered Ca^{2+} kinetics are responsible for the increases in contractility observed in other circumstances. The increased contractility of postextrasystolic beats,[6, 7] increased heart rate (HR)[8, 9] and, during pharmacologic manipulation with cardiac glycosides, phosphodiesterase inhibitors,[10] sympathomimetic amines,[9] and caffeine[4] are dependent on changes in intracellular Ca^{2+} or cAMP levels.

Absolute blood Ca^{2+} levels (by raising cytosolic Ca^{2+} levels)[11] and hormonal changes such as hyperthyroidism increase contractility[12, 13] secondary to increased troponin C affinity for Ca^{2+}, increased ATPase activity with concomitant increased cAMP levels, and changes in intracellular Ca^{2+} handling.

Individual muscle units in the failing and hypertrophied ventricle have been found to have their function depressed.[14] The myocardial depression accompanying anoxia,[15] acidosis,[16] hypothyroidism,[12] barbiturate use, administration of local and general anesthetics, use of Ca^{2+} antagonists,[17] and ischemia[18] all result from abnormalities in the Ca^{2+}-dependent mechanisms described here.

Mediators of Contractility

Various mediators acting independently by linking stimulated α, β, or acetylcholine receptor to intracytoplasmic enzyme systems alter the contractile state of the myocardium. The most well-characterized of these systems, the *guanine nucleotide regulatory proteins*,[19, 20] are coupled to β, α, and acetylcholine receptors and possibly to receptors for nitric oxide and endothelins.

Beta Receptors and Guanine Nucleotide Regulatory Proteins

As alluded to earlier, adrenergic stimulation of cardiac myocytes is a very important regulator of both Ca^{2+} influx and cAMP levels within the cell (Fig. 48–1).[21] The predominant β receptor of myocytes, when stimulated, increases the manufacture of cAMP. This in turn, by the mechanisms described previously, results in increased Ca^{2+} influx. Ca^{2+}

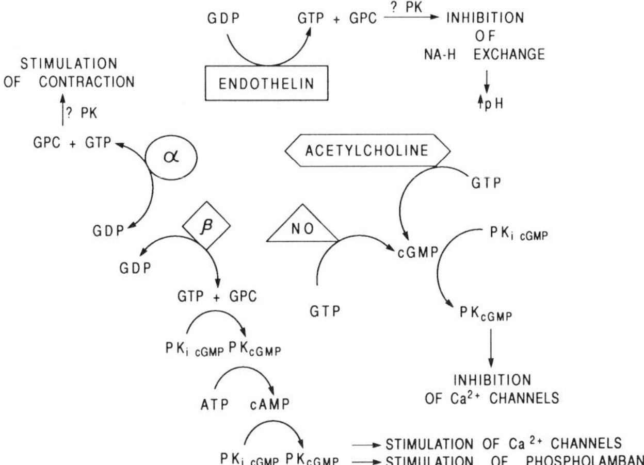

Figure 48–1. Receptors and intracellular signaling via G proteins (see text for discussion). *Abbreviations:* GDP = guanosine diphosphate; GTP = guanosine triphosphate; GPC = G protein complex; PK = active protein kinase; PK_i = inactive protein kinase; α = alpha receptor; β = beta receptor; NO = nitrous oxide receptor.

channels that are under the influence of β receptor–mediated increases in cAMP are known as *receptor-operated channels.*[22]

Stimulation of β receptors on the cell surface results in activation of adenylate cyclase (AC) and subsequent increases in cAMP levels. This results in increased Ca^{2+} influx with resultant increases in contractile force. The coupling between β receptors and AC occurs through guanine cyclic nucleotides, also known as *G proteins.*[23] G proteins have both stimulatory and inhibitory influences on AC. The G protein complex in its active form contains guanosine triphosphate (GTP). When present, this protein "couples" the β receptor to AC, and when β receptor adrenergic stimulation occurs, results in the formation of cAMP and subsequent increases in intracellular calcium. The G protein complex is capable of degrading its bound GTP to guanosine diphosphate (GDP) when β receptor stimulation ceases, thereby no longer stimulating AC.[24] G proteins also have a pivotal role in stimulation of cardiac contractility by α receptor stimulation through a cAMP-*independent* mechanism,[25] which results in increased contractility within a single heartbeat (see Fig. 48–1). Cyclic AMP–dependent mechanisms have demonstrated delays in response of 2 to 20 seconds, as opposed to G protein pathway delays in response of 150 msec. This allows alterations in Ca^{2+} flux within a single heartbeat, explaining the observed phenomenon of increased contractility immediately after increased sympathetic stimulation.

Inhibitory G proteins, when activated by stimulus acetylcholine receptors, have been shown to inhibit Ca^{2+} influx.[26] This has been demonstrated to occur via a cyclic guanosine monophosphate (cGMP)-mediated mechanism. A cGMP system, similar to the cAMP system outlined earlier, activates cGMP protein kinase (cGMP-PK), which inhibits calcium inward currents previously stimulated by cAMP.[27] Additionally, cGMP-mediated inhibition of Ca^{2+} channels has been demonstrated *not* to be a result of cAMP hydrolysis or a result of inhibition of cAMP-PK but a direct effect of cGMP-PK.

In addition to changes in receptor function, molecular alterations in β receptor production in various disease states have been shown to occur. In dilated cardiomyopathies, both β_1 receptor mRNA and absolute receptor levels were found to be depressed.[28] At the same time, β receptor kinase levels were elevated. β Receptor kinase, the molecule responsible for phosphorylation of β-adrenergic receptors, is elevated when β receptors are dysfunctional (uncoupled). This may provide an explanation for the catecholamine insensitivity observed in failing hearts as well as after cardiopulmonary bypass.[29]

Nitric Oxide

Nitric oxide has been shown to affect cardiac contractility. It has been found in many tissue types, including ventricular myocytes, where its physiologic effects are mediated via cGMP. Cholinergic myocardiac depressant effects, as evidenced by inhibition of the effect of the muscarinic agonist carbachol, were inhibited by antagonists of nitric oxide (methylene blue and oxyhemoglobin), as well as by L-arginine (the natural substrate of nitric oxide synthesis analogs), which inhibit nitric oxide. In addition, the positive inotropic action of the beta agonist isoproterenol is enhanced by nitric oxide inhibition. These data indicate that the effect of nitric oxide is to activate the inhibitory receptor cyclic nucleotide interaction through cGMP mechanisms (see Fig. 48–1).

Nitric oxide has been implicated in the myocardial response to sepsis. It has been well documented that myocardial depression in septic shock occurs secondary to a yet undefined substance. One potential substance, tumor necrosis factor-α, has been shown in vitro to depress the activity of spontaneously beating rat cardiomyocytes in tissue culture. Inhibition of nitric oxide synthesis by *N*-methyl-L-arginine blocked tumor necrosis factor–induced cardiomyocyte depression.[29a] Additionally, methylene blue, an inhibitor of guanylate cyclase,[30] prevented tumor necrosis factor–induced cardiomyocyte depression.

Although the cellular mechanism of the depression noted in septic myocardium has not yet been well characterized, it may be due to alterations in Ca^{2+} handling. Abnormalities of β receptor function as measured by decreased levels of cAMP in peripheral lymphocytes in septic patients have been elicited, as well as possible abnormalities in septic patients.[31] The exact cellular level of this defect, whether this abnormality of β receptor function is receptor down-regulation or reduced transcription of β receptor genes, has yet to be determined.

Endothelin

Endothelin-1, a 21-amino-acid vasoconstrictor peptide released from the vascular endothelium, was isolated by Yanagisawa and colleagues in 1988.[31a] Since that time, four additional isoforms and a closely related substance, vasoactive intestinal contractor, have been isolated. These substances have been found ubiquitously in mammalian tissues. Their intracardiac site of genesis is unknown but is believed to be the endothelium of the coronary arteries and microvasculature. Various vasodilator and vasoconstrictor substances released from the vascular endothelium alter blood flow and, in this way, indirectly affect cardiac contractility.[32] Of these locally elaborated paracrine substances, the endothelins have been most extensively studied.

High-affinity receptors for endothelins in mammalian atria and ventricles have been isolated. In vitro, these substances have been shown to be potent vasoconstrictors and positive inotropes, acting via a yet incompletely defined mechanism. Kelly and colleagues[32a] demonstrated that at constant cytosolic Ca^{2+} levels, using the Ca^{2+}-specific intracellular probe Fura-2, endothelins cause marked increases in the contractility of isolated rat ventricular myocytes. This observation suggests that endothelins may sensitize the myofibrils to calcium, although this finding has not been duplicated by others.

As previously discussed, an increase in intracellular pH results in increased myofibrillar sensitivity for Ca^{2+}, thereby increasing contractility. Endothelin causes an increase in intracellular pH with a subsequent increase in contraction when studied in rat ventricular myocytes. This effect is completely inhibited by pretreatment with amiloride, which inhibits sodium-hydrogen ion exchange across the sarcolemmal membrane and, hence, prevents increases in intracellular pH.[33] Furthermore, the effect of endothelin appears to be mediated via G proteins participating in signal transduction after binding of endothelin to its sarcolemmal receptor (see Fig. 48–1).

Cellular Determinants of Relaxation

Just as abnormalities of contraction have as their cellular basis derangements of Ca^{2+} handling, so too does relaxation. Cessation of the inward Ca^{2+} current (or inactivation) by closure of voltage-limited channels begins the period of relaxation at the myocyte level, with the rate and extent of Ca^{2+} removal affecting the rate and extent of relaxation. As alluded to earlier, inactivation signals the end of actin-myosin interaction. However, this single term does not adequately describe the interplay of processes that are occurring at the cellular level to facilitate relaxation. An SR Ca^{2+} pump, in the presence of adequate ATP, pumps Ca^{2+} into the SR from the cytosol. In addition, the Na-Ca^{2+} exchange pump (also ATP requiring), which allows influx of Ca^{2+} during contraction, also participates in the transport of Ca^{2+} out of the cell across the sarcolemma. The affinity of myofibril for Ca^{2+} also affects relaxation. As the myofibril shortens, its affinity for Ca^{2+} decreases, limiting Ca^{2+} effects.[34] All of these mechanisms are facilitated or inhibited by drugs or neurohumoral factors.

Little research has used critically ill patients to assess the cellular basis of relaxation in critical illness. However, these processes have been extensively studied in dilated cardiomyopathies, left ventricular (LV) hypertrophy, ischemia, and hypertrophic cardiomyopathy. Impairment of relaxation in these patients occurs secondary to increased levels of Ca^{2+} within the myocyte in diastole[35,36] owing to diminished function of the SR pump, decreased expression at the genetic level for this pump as evidenced by decreased messenger ribonucleic acid (mRNA) levels,[37] decreased phospholamban activity[38] or levels of phospholamban mRNA,[39] down-regulation or uncoupling of β receptors,[28,40] or inhibition of β receptor function by G protein inhibition.[41]

MECHANICS OF SYSTOLIC FUNCTION

Determinants of Stroke Volume

Systemic blood pressure (BP) is the product of cardiac output and total peripheral resistance; an increase in either results in an increase in BP, unless of course a compensatory depression occurs in the opposite variable. Disordered autoregulation of blood flow to microvascular beds disturbs the normal relationship of cardiac output, total peripheral resistance, and BP described earlier.[42] Therefore, determinants of central flow (cardiac output) assume greater importance. In addition, these same systemic illnesses can influence the cardiac output directly by altering the determinants of cardiac output—that is, HR and stroke volume (SV).

SV is defined as that portion of blood that is ejected from the ventricle by a single heartbeat. The magnitude of SV is determined by the following influences: (1) ventricular preload, (2) ventricular afterload, (3) and ventricular contractility.

Studies of isolated heart muscle preparations provided the basis for an understanding of both ventricular preload and afterload. From these studies, ventricular preload was initially related to the degree of myocardial fiber length at the onset of a contraction and could be varied by attaching different weights to one end of the muscle fiber. Because a change in muscle length was accompanied by changes in sarcomere length, the sarcomere was thereby recognized as the fundamental unit that defined contraction of cardiac muscle. The sarcomere, therefore, represents the ultrastructural basis for the *Starling law of the heart*, which states that the force of muscle contraction is dependent on initial muscle length.[43] In this context, Gordon and associates[44] first showed that the force of contraction developed in myocardial muscle was proportional to sarcomere length. The clinical expression of this relationship between muscle length and the force of a subsequent contraction is the observation that cardiac work increases as end-diastolic ventricular size or preload increases. Ventricular preload may therefore be assessed as end-diastolic stress, end-diastolic volume (EDV), or end-diastolic dimension (EDD). End-diastolic stress and EDD are clinically measured with cardiac ultrasonography. EDV can be measured by echocardiography or nuclear scintigraphic measurements. However, repeated measurements are time consuming. New catheters are being developed to allow these volumes to be measured repeatedly.

The most common and earliest measure of ventricular preload is the measurement of end-diastolic filling pressures. Early clinical studies reported ventricular preload as measured by end-diastolic filling pressures, such as the central venous pressure for the right ventricle (RV) and the pulmonary capillary wedge pressure (PCWP) for the left ventricle (LV)[45,46] Because end-diastolic pressure (EDP) does not relate to EDV by any linear function but rather exponentially,[47] an EDP cannot be adequately substituted as a measure of ventricular preload.[48]

Pertinent concepts that initially defined ventricular afterload also originated from studies of isolated heart muscle.[45] In these studies, afterload was defined as the weight the muscle fiber had to lift once contraction had been initiated. Clinically, however, the ventricle does not lift a weight. Rather, it ejects a viscous fluid load into a viscoelastic system. Therefore, the definition of afterload, described by experiments using isolated muscle preparations, does not adequately account for the load the ventricle must eject against in vivo.[49] In fact, any ideal definition of ventricular afterload should acknowledge several elements, including ventricular intracavitary pressure, wall thickness, chamber radius, and geometry. Although difficult to assess clinically, the afterload faced by either ventricle during ejection is probably best represented by systolic wall tension or stress.[50] Wall stress reflects an integration of the effects of two major loads, a vascular load and the load imposed by the ventricle itself. The vascular load is determined by the cross-sectional area of the vascular bed, the elasticity of the vascular wall, and the viscosity of the blood; all can be isolated in the laboratory by measuring vascular input impedance spectra.[51,52] The ventricular load represents the combined effects of the physiologic properties of cardiac muscle cells as well as ventricular shape and size.[45,53] However, ventricular afterload cannot be easily measured using this strict physiologic definition and is therefore clinically approximated by measuring the mean pressure that the ventricle is exposed to during ejection or by calculating the appropriate vascular resistance (i.e., systemic or pulmonary vascular resistance).[54] Independent ventricular afterload changes may profoundly influence ventricular muscle shortening and, hence, cardiac output and systemic oxygen transport.[55]

The third determinant of SV is ventricular contractility. The inotropic state of the heart refers to the vigor of ventricular contraction when both preload and afterload are known and held constant. Contractility is the most difficult determinant of SV to measure accurately, because almost every known index of contractility proposed has been found to be dependent to various degrees on ventricular preload or afterload,[56] as discussed later.

Pressure-Volume Loops

The interaction of these three determinants of SV (i.e., preload, afterload, and contractility) may be conceptualized in one of two ways. The first is by analysis of P-V loops for isolated cardiac beats,[57] and the second is by analysis of the force-velocity (F-V) relationship.[58] Understanding both these approaches to describing ventricular function further clarifies the interaction of the physiologic determinants of SV. Pressure-volume and force-velocity relations are particularly useful for describing the pathophysiology of clinical disorders encountered in the critically ill as well as mechanisms by which different therapeutic interventions might affect the ventricular stroke output in this patient population.

A ventricular P-V loop can be inscribed by continuously measuring ventricular volume and pressure (Fig. 48–2). At the end of ventricular contraction, the pressure within the ventricle falls. Ventricular filling is initiated when ventricular pressure has decreased below the atrial pressure (point A); with ventricular filling, diastole begins. Subsequently, activation of cardiac muscle by an action potential initiates isovolumic contraction at end-diastole (point B); isovolumic contraction continues until ventricular pressure exceeds aortic diastolic pressure when ejection begins (point C); at end-systole (point D), isovolumic relaxation is initiated. Joined together, points A, B, C, and D inscribe a single P-V loop, and the area within this loop reflects the stroke work performed by the ventricle during this one cardiac cycle. In this context, it is thereby intuitive that stroke work is made up of both volume and pressure work.

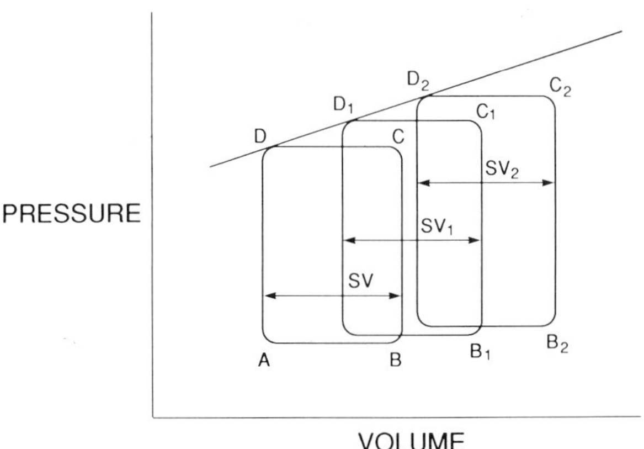

Figure 48–2. Ventricular pressure-volume loops. The loop bounded by points A, B, C, and D represents the resting pressure-volume relationship for an entire cardiac cycle. Diastole occurs between points A and B. Isovolumic contraction occurs between points B and C. At point C, the ventricular pressure exceeds the aortic pressure, and ejection commences. Ejection continues until the energy substrate is utilized by end-systole (point D). Isovolumic relaxation then occurs, and diastole starts when ventricular pressure drops below the atrial pressure. Increasing afterload (C_1, C_2) is compensated by increases in end-diastolic volume and pressure, as noted by points B_1 and B_2. The end-systolic points (D, D_1, D_2) for each of these loops all fall on a single line, which is called the *isovolumic pressure line* and which reflects the inotropic state.

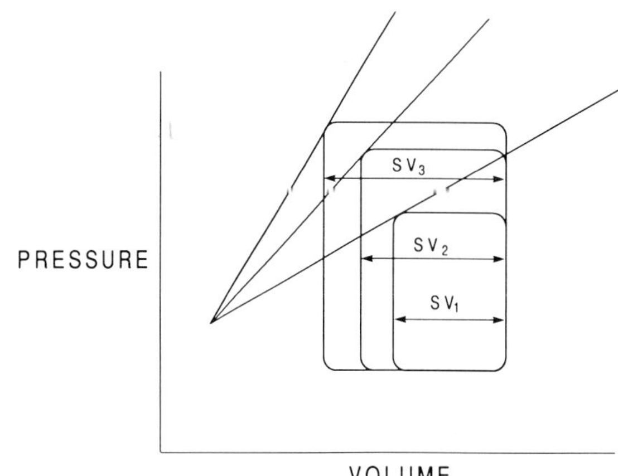

Figure 48–3. Ventricular pressure-volume loops at varying levels of contractility depicted by three different isovolumic lines. Note that end-diastolic pressure does not change but that stroke volume increases with increasing contractility (SV_1<SV_2<SV_3).

When ventricular afterload is increased at a constant inotropic state, as hypothetically represented by points C_1 and C_2 in Figure 48–2, new P-V loops are constructed because stroke work now increases proportional to the increase in afterload. Flow work or SV is maintained by a compensatory increase in EDV (B_1 and B_2). The end-systolic point of each loop (upper left corner of each loop, points D, D_1, D_2) falls along a single line, an *isovolumic pressure line,* the slope of which reflects the resting contractile or inotropic state.

This is further illustrated in Figure 48–3. The ventricle with depressed contractility is indicated by the P-V loop bounding stroke volume (SV_1). An inotrope given to this depressed ventricle would shift the isovolumic pressure line upward and to the left, resulting in larger SV for any given level of preload (SV_2 and SV_3).

The Frank-Starling mechanism or preload recruitable stroke work can now be described by the concepts that have been reviewed. At a constant inotropic and afterload state, increases in preload as represented by points B_1 and B_2 in Figure 48–4 result in increased SV (SV_1 to SV_2).

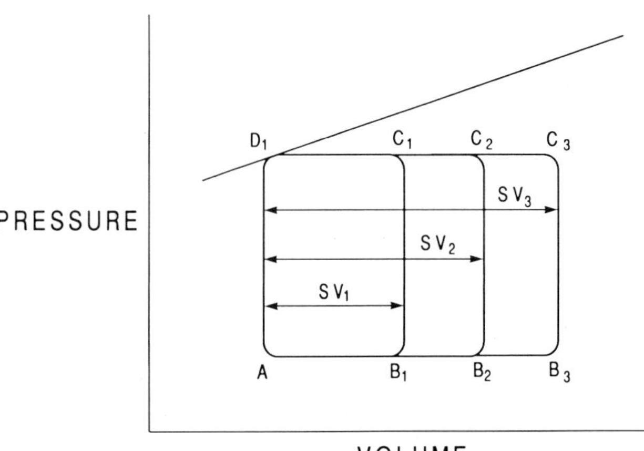

Figure 48–4. Ventricular pressure-volume loops at different preloads. Contractility and afterload are held constant. Increases in preload increase stroke volume and stroke work as a function of the Frank-Starling mechanism.

Force-Velocity Relationships

The F-V relationship (Fig. 48–5) is also a practical method to conceptualize the interaction of preload, afterload, and contractility in determining ventricular stroke output. The y-axis represents ventricular output, which could be either the SV, an ejection fraction, or the shortening fraction; the x-axis represents the vascular load (afterload), which is derived in the laboratory from impedance spectra and clinically has been described as a calculated vascular resistance or a measured mean pressure.[59] For a given inotropic state, the y-intercept is always similar and is referred to as Vmax. The relationship between afterload and ventricular output rotates up and to the right with an increase in ventricular preload and down and to the left with a decrease in ventricular preload. Point A represents a hypothetic normal resting state. An increase in ventricular afterload, not compensated for by any increase in preload, is described as point B and results in a decrease in ventricular output; the effect of an increase in afterload to depress stroke output can, however, be compensated for with an increase in ventricular preload. This compensatory action is shown in Figure 48–5 as point D; an augmented preload (rightward rotation) maintains ventricular output at the resting state, even though the vascular load or afterload has been increased.

A clinical example of the interaction between changes in afterload and ventricular stroke output may be observed in critically ill patients with acute pulmonary hypertension. A sudden increase in RV afterload noted with an acute pulmonary embolus[60, 61] would initially effect a fall in the RV stroke output (Fig. 48–5, point B). A sustained decrease in RV stroke output would result in RV failure, because this ventricle would no longer adequately subserve LV filling. With a consequent decrease in LV preload, cardiac output, oxygen transport, and BP would thereby fall. To reverse this sequence of events, augmentation of RV preload (i.e., to point D) should restore RV output and, hence, LV filling.[62] Conversely, Figure 48–5 also explains the potentially catastrophic systemic effects of a decrease in RV preload in a patient experiencing a sustained increase in ventricular afterload, illustrated as point C. Clinically, excessive diuresis in a patient with pulmonary hypertension secondary to chronic obstructive pulmonary disease would remove RV preload reserve (i.e., reduced to point C rather than point B), and a low output state ensues as the RV stroke output must thereby fall.[62]

Depressed contractility in the F-V relationship would be represented by a downward shift of the y-axis and a flatter slope (point C). Depressed contractility can be compensated for by either increasing preload (point F) or decreasing ventricular afterload (points G and E). Therefore, depressed ventricular contractility that characterizes ischemic heart disease is associated with a reduction of ventricular output; LV dilation (increased preload) or administration of vasodilators (afterload reduction) may preserve LV output and systemic oxygen transport, thereby delaying the emergence of a low cardiac output state.

Clinical Methods of Measuring Contractility

Traditionally, contractility was a measure of the overall vigor with which the ventricular geometry changed or by a rise in pressure over time (dp/dt) within the cavity of the LV. The most common measurement, the ejection fraction, measures a per cent change in the size of the LV in two dimensions by planimetry or by the difference in radionuclide counts between systole and diastole in the case of gated blood pool scanning. These methods, although convenient, do not control variables that affect contractility such as preload, HR, and afterload, making independent estimates of contractility impossible. So to does the dp/dt vary with HR, preload, and afterload.

Clinically, contractility might be most easily conceptualized as an increase in SV when preload, afterload, and HR are unchanged.[56] This situation is the ideal, however, and more precise measurement of contractility is often needed for clinical decision making and for research application.

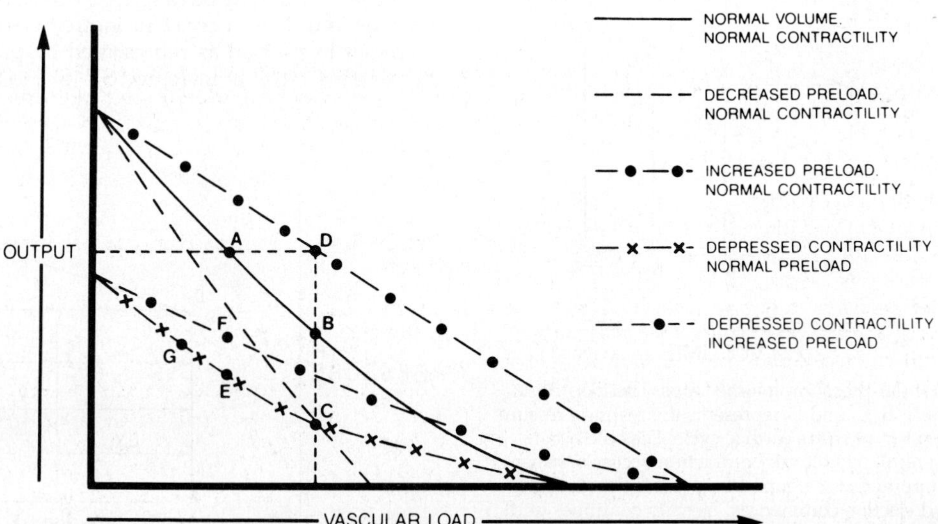

Figure 48–5. Conceptualized forced velocity relationship utilizing ventricular output and vascular load as the clinical variables that reflect both velocity and force, respectively. A normal patient operates at point A. With a reduced preload, the relationship is rotated toward the left; with an increased preload, the relationship is rotated toward the right. For a given inotropic state, the *y*-intercept is constant. A decrease in inotropic state results in a reduced *y*-intercept. An isolated increase in afterload results in the patient operating at point B with a resultant decrease in ventricular output. This can be compensated for by an increase in preload (point D). The output is normal at this point because preload and afterload are well matched. Depressed contractility results in decreased output for a given vascular load (point C). This can be compensated for by an increase in preload (point F) or by a decrease in afterload (points E and G).

An excellent load-independent measure of contractility, both in in vivo and ex vivo isolated heart preparations, is that of end-systolic P-V relations.[63] This is the point of the P-V curve at end-systole. As discussed earlier, alterations in afterload and preload without a change in contractility result in formation of a straight line with a constant volume intercept, the *isovolumic pressure line.* This slope of this line reflects the intrinsic contractility of the ventricle (see Figs. 48–2 and 48–3), and because the volume intercept does not change with alterations in preload and afterload, it is considered to be load independent. More recent studies, however, have shown that these relationships can be curvilinear with changes in load and inotropy. Furthermore, the isovolumic pressure line can be constructed only by pharmacologic intervention, nuclear or angiographic assessments of volume, and invasive pressure monitoring, limiting its use in clinical practice.

As stated earlier, almost all measures of contractility are to some extent dependent on loading conditions. The F-V curves described earlier require steady loading conditions.[64, 65] In addition, the measured points of the F-V curves are not measured at identical muscle lengths. Therefore, load is changing throughout the measurement, and the extrapolation to Vmax without consideration for the length of the muscle results in error.

A method for contractility evaluation that is independent of both preload, afterload, and HR has been described by Colan and colleagues.[66] The rate-corrected velocity of circumferential fiber shortening (Fig. 48–6) is a powerful measure of contractility with both research and clinical application. This measure describes the fractional shortening of the LV as measured by echocardiography from the parasternal short axis dimension (see Fig. 48–6, left upper panel and lower panel).

$$\frac{\left(\dfrac{EDD - ESD}{EDD}\right)}{ET_c}$$

where EDD is end-diastolic dimension, ESD is end-systolic dimension, and ET_c (the rate-corrected ejection time) is the ejection time (taken from external carotid pulse tracings) divided by the square root of the R-R interval.

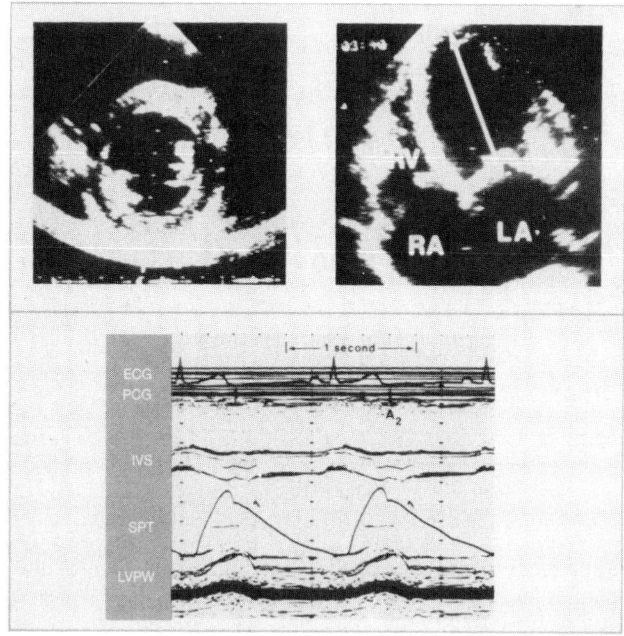

Figure 48–6. Noninvasively acquired data for determination of left ventricular (LV) force-velocity relations. The *upper left-hand panel* shows the two-dimensional short axis image through which the M-mode recording *(lower panel)* was obtained and the minor axis dimensions were measured. The *upper right-hand panel* shows an apical four-chamber, two-dimensional image from which long-axis measurements are made. The externally calibrated subclavian pulse tracing (SPT) is used to acquire simultaneous pressure data *(lower panel).* End-systole is identified by aortic valve closure (A_2) on the phonocardiogram (PCG). End-diastole is defined as the peak of the R wave on the electrocardiogram (ECG). *Abbreviations:* IVS = interventricular septum; LVPW = left ventricular posterior wall; RV = right ventricle; RA = right atrium; LA = left atrium. (From Borow KM, Marcus RH, Neuman A, et al: Modern noninvasive techniques for the assessment of left ventricular systolic performance. *In:* Heart Disease: A Textbook of Cardiovascular Medicine. 4th ed. Braunwald E [Ed]. Philadelphia, W. B. Saunders, 1982, p 31.)

MECHANICS OF DIASTOLE

Left Ventricular Compliance and the Diastolic Left Ventricular Pressure-Volume Relationship

The nonlinear relationship between pressure and volume during ventricular diastole is also depicted in Figure 48–2. The diastolic phase of the cardiac cycle extends from points A to B. A shift to the right in this diastolic pressure relationship is depicted by points B to B_1 and B_1 to B_2. These shifts reflect either a change in the operating chamber stiffness of the LV, as is normally noted with increased filling,[67] or these changes may occur as a result of various disease states (Fig. 48–7).[68]

Abnormal shifts in ventricular pressure at a given volume, reflecting a change in ventricular compliance outside of the norm (Fig. 48–8) where contractility is held constant,[67] is represented by a shift from the loop bounded by the broken line to that bounded by the solid line. The result of increased chamber stiffness (decreased compliance) is a decreased EDV for a given EDP. This nonlinear relationship of EDP and EDV is critically important in the clinical treatment of patients and is a source of significant error in hemodynamic manipulations.[48] Assessing EDV as EDP results in incorrect assumptions of the cause of decreased stroke work (area bounded by loops). The contractile state has not changed, as evidenced by the slope of the isovolumic pressure line, which, as previously stated, reflects the intrinsic contractile state of the myocardium. Rather, the cause of the decrease in stroke work has been the decrease in preload (EDV), which is not evident by measurement of EDP alone.

Factors That Affect the Diastolic Pressure-Volume Relationship

LV diastolic function is dependent on many factors, some *intrinsic* to the heart itself (e.g., the active energy-dependent process of relaxation and material properties of the myocardium) and some *extrinsic* to the LV (e.g., pericardial constraining forces and ventricular interaction). Furthermore, Gilbert and Glantz[68] have suggested that relaxation can be further divided into the *extent of relaxation* (i.e., the completeness of relaxation) and the *rate of relaxation.* Alterations in the extent, rate, or both characterize the abnormalities of relaxation and result in characteristic hemodynamic patterns (Fig. 48–9).[68]

Extent of Relaxation

The extent of relaxation is the major determinant of EDV and EDP, because these are measurements made at the end of the relaxation process. Abnormalities in extent of relaxa-

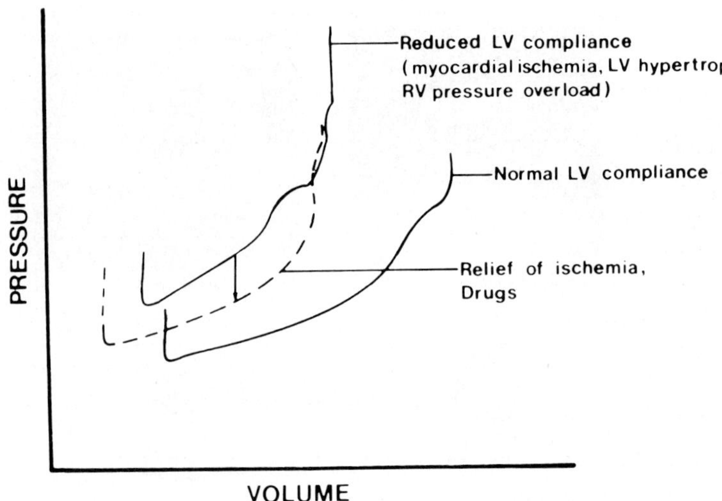

Figure 48–7. Causes of shifts in the LV diastolic pressure-volume relationship. Various factors can either increase or reduce compliance and shift the curve either upward and to the left or downward and to the right.

tion affect the end-diastolic P-V relationship in the greatest manner. Abnormalities in the rate of relaxation, however, tend to have minimum effect on the end-diastolic P-V relationship, because of the fact that they occur early in diastole and therefore do not alter EDP and EDV to any appreciable extent.

The extent of relaxation, as stated earlier, may be viewed as the compliance properties of the LV at the point where relaxation is complete (i.e., end-diastole). Alterations in the determinants of this relationship that are *intrinsic* to the myocardium result in shifts of the diastolic P-V curve. *LV geometry* (i.e., thickness, size, and chamber dimension) in large part determines the LV end-diastolic P-V relationship, as determined by mathematic approximations based on Laplace's law.[68] Alterations in the LV end-diastolic P-V relationship may occur secondary to the change in elastic properties as the ventricle stretches during filling. Changes in the diastolic P-V relationship that depend on the rate at which the LV deforms are known as *viscoelasticity*, a property that

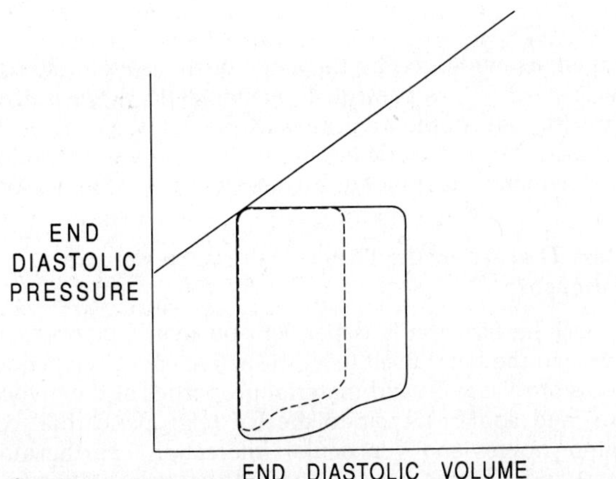

Figure 48–8. Effect of changes in compliance on stroke volume. Ventricular pressure-volume loops are constructed for two different conditions in the same heart. Contractility and ejection pressure do not change. The only change has been an upward shift to the left in the LV diastolic pressure-volume relationship of the loop bounded by the *broken line* caused by a decrease in the compliant properties of the myocardium. This results in a reduction both in end-diastolic volume at a given end-diastolic pressure and in the area enclosed by the loop (decreased stroke volume).

the myocardium shares with most biomaterials.[69] This property is manifested when filling rates are highest, occurring during the first half of diastole or after atrial contraction. Stress relaxation (a decrease in the distending pressure of the ventricle over time) and creep (a rightward shift in the diastolic P-V relationship) are two experimental manifestations of viscosity. The clinical importance of viscoelasticity has been disputed, however.

Other dynamic changes in relaxation that occur during ventricular filling are due to alterations in the elastic properties and the rate of relaxation of the myocardium mediated by changes in the load sensed by the LV during relaxation. These *load-dependent relaxation* phenomena cause instantaneous changes in LV compliance as well as in the rate of relaxation[2] that are independent of heart rate when LV muscle is abruptly stretched.

An additional determinant of the diastolic P-V relationship previously alluded to is *coronary vascular turgor.* The effect of this on the extent of relaxation is primarily through its erectile effect on LV stiffness.[70] This decreases LV diastolic compliance by increasing LV *wall* volume, resulting in a higher EDP for a given volume. This effect seems to be independent of pericardial influences and predominates in the late diastolic filling period, thereby influencing the extent of relaxation, albeit to a small degree. In addition, the constraining effect of the pericardium and the degree of ventricular interaction affect the extent of relaxation, as discussed later.

Clinical Examples of Alterations in Extent of Relaxation Secondary to Intrinsic Myocardial Disorders

LV hypertrophy results in abnormalities of relaxation that are characteristic of the manner in which the hypertrophy developed and of the type of hypertrophy formed.[71] Chronic volume overload, as in mitral or aortic insufficiency or due to physical conditioning, results in *eccentric* hypertrophy, characterized by increased ventricular volume but little or no change in elasticity. This results in little increase in pressure at increased volumes. In contrast, chronic pressure overload, as in aortic stenosis or chronic untreated hypertension,[72] results in hypertrophy of the *concentric* type, with increased elastic stiffness and an elevated EDP for a given volume. Geometrically, pressure overload or hypertrophy is characterized by additional myocytes in parallel with existing cells; volume overload (eccentric hypertrophy) results in increased length of existing myocytes. Alterations in Ca^{2+} metabolism, as discussed, result in elevated myocyte dia-

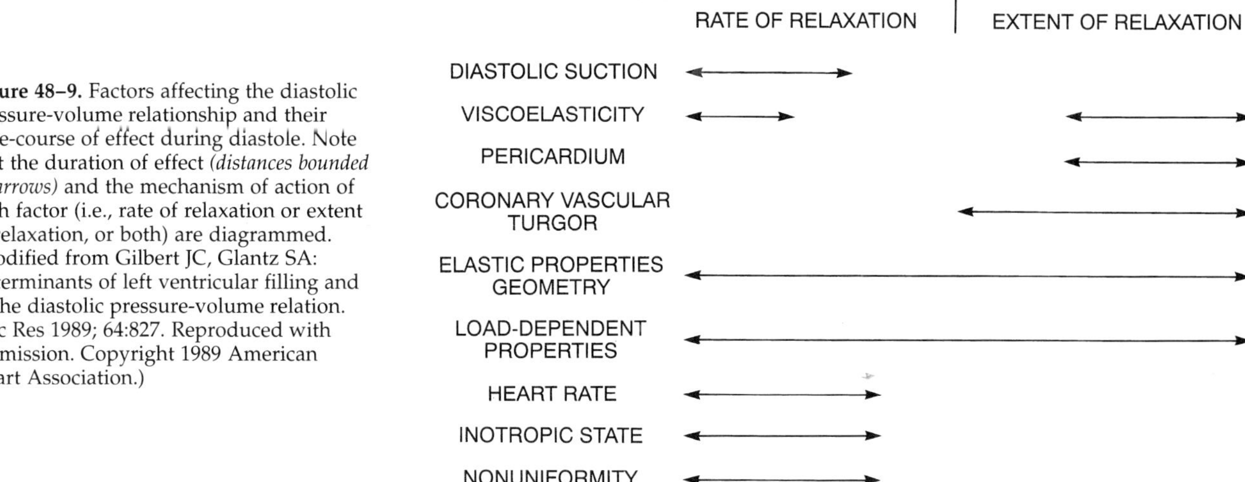

Figure 48–9. Factors affecting the diastolic pressure-volume relationship and their time-course of effect during diastole. Note that the duration of effect *(distances bounded by arrows)* and the mechanism of action of each factor (i.e., rate of relaxation or extent of relaxation, or both) are diagrammed. (Modified from Gilbert JC, Glantz SA: Determinants of left ventricular filling and of the diastolic pressure-volume relation. Circ Res 1989; 64:827. Reproduced with permission. Copyright 1989 American Heart Association.)

stolic Ca^{2+} levels. These factors account for the elevated EDP in chronic pressure overload hypertrophy.

Ischemia affects the extent of relaxation, as evidenced by upward shift in the end-diastolic P-V relationship when myocardial oxygen demand outstrips supply.[73, 74] Pacing-induced ischemia after the creation of a coronary stenosis in dogs results in such a shift in the P-V relationship at end-diastole (Fig. 48–10). These effects are independent of pericardial, RV, or lung interactions, implying a change in the intrinsic myocardial elastic properties. As previously discussed, changes in diastolic properties secondary to changes in myocardial Ca^{2+} handling,[44, 45] as well as in hydrogen ion accumulation[75] and repeated systolic stretch of the ischemia segment,[76] interact to produce the observed changes.

The changes in ventricular compliance seem to be restricted to the region of active ischemia.[76] Furthermore, uninvolved areas show evidence of a proportional increase in regional size and pressure (with a resultant constant diastolic P-V relation) to maintain SV by the Frank-Starling mechanism. Hence, during acute ischemia, the remaining normal areas of myocardium appear to use the Frank-Starling mechanism to maintain SV in compensation for the effects of abnormal contractility or an upward shift of the regional diastolic P-V relationship within the ischemic areas.

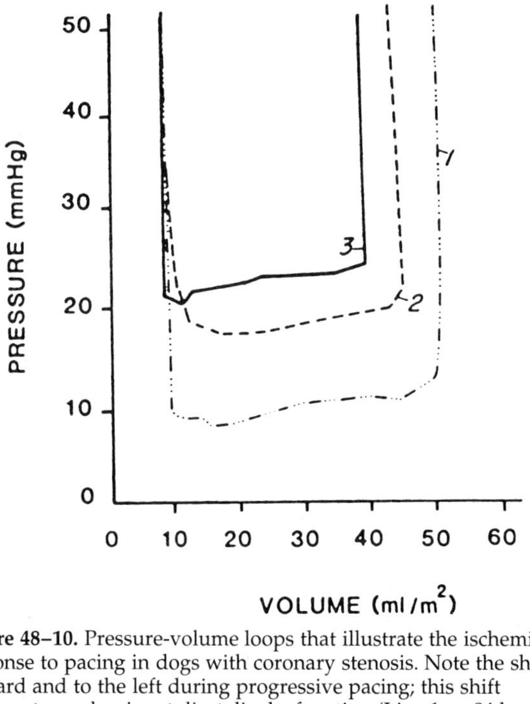

Figure 48–10. Pressure-volume loops that illustrate the ischemic response to pacing in dogs with coronary stenosis. Note the shift upward and to the left during progressive pacing; this shift represents predominant diastolic dysfunction (Line 1 = 84 beats per minute; line 2 = 110 beats per minute; line 3 = 135 beats per minute). (From Aroesty JM, McKay RG, Heller GV, et al: Simultaneous assessment of left ventricular systolic and diastolic function during pacing-induced ischemia. Circulation 1985; 71:889.)

Rate of Relaxation

The rate of relaxation, as stated earlier, results primarily in changes in the rate of diastolic early filling.[68] The determinants of relaxation rate are many, and their interactions complicated (see Fig. 48–9). Increases in *heart rate* and *inotropy*[99] result in increased rates of relaxation. Alterations in end-diastolic loading conditions result in changes in the rate of relaxation during experimental conditions.[2, 100] *Nonuniformity* of relaxation,[2] which describes a nonuniform distribution of load and electric inactivation during diastole in space and time, results in alterations in the rate of relaxation. *Ventricular suction,* or the ability of the ventricle to generate pressures below equilibrium diastolic pressures, may alter the rate and extent of LV filling.[99] Finally, ischemia can alter the rate as well as the extent of relaxation, as described earlier. Resolution of ischemia results in reversal of these changes.

Extrinsic Influences on the Diastolic Pressure-Volume Relationship

It is now apparent that external loads profoundly influence ventricular compliance properties. Specifically, the RV,[77] the pericardium,[78] and the lungs[79, 80] all may acutely induce shifts of the LV diastolic P-V relationship.

Pericardial Influences

The influence of the pericardium in the diastolic P-V relationship is a function of both its stiffness and its ability to constrain the entire heart.[81] An increase in size of one ventricle therefore causes an increase in the EDP for a given

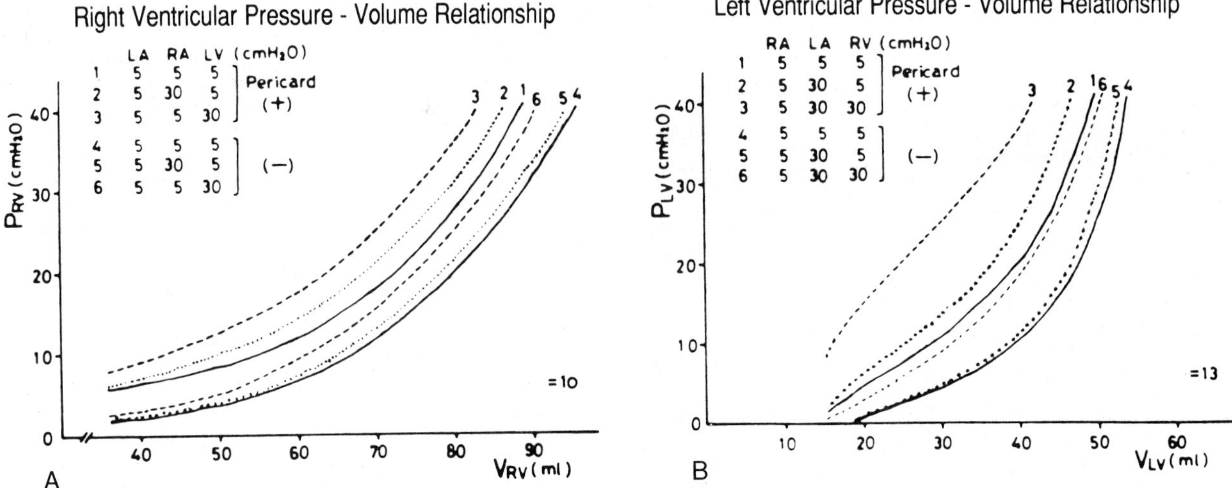

Figure 48–11. The effect of the pericardium on chamber pressure-volume relations. The ventricular pressure-volume relation of one ventricle is shifted upward when the pressure in one or more of the other chambers is increased. The pericardium causes this interaction to be more forceful. In addition, the direct interaction effect of the right ventricle on the left is greater than that of the left ventricle on the right, particularly with the pericardium on. The representative right *(A)* and left *(B)* ventricular pressure-volume curves from isolated, perfused dog hearts were obtained while holding the other three chambers at various pressures from 5 to 30 cm H_2O (4–22 mm Hg) with and without the pericardium. Curves 1, 2, and 3 in each situation were with the pericardium (pericard [+]). Curves 4, 5, and 6 were without the pericardium (pericard [−]). *Abbreviations:* PRV = right ventricular pressure; PLV = left ventricular pressure; VRV = right ventricular volume; VLV = left ventricular volume. (From Maruyama Y, Ashikawa K, Isoyama S, et al: Mechanical interactions between four heart chambers with and without the pericardium in canine hearts. Circ Res 1982; 50:86. Reproduced with permission. Copyright 1982 American Heart Association.)

volume (i.e., a shift upward in the P-V relationship) (Fig. 48–11). The constraining effect of normal pericardium is dependent on its intrinsic compliance and how it affects LV pressures. Just as dilatation of the RV affects the LV diastolic P-V relation (discussed later), dilatation of the LV (i.e., high LV filling pressure) amplifies the pericardium's influence. This has been demonstrated by measurement of the diastolic P-V relation before and after removal of the pericardium.[78, 82] Little normal pericardial effect is observed at normal filling pressures.

In addition, the intact pericardium allows interaction between the atria and the LV as well as between RV and LV. The effect of left atrial (LA) pressure was approximately one quarter that of the RV pressure in determining the LV diastolic pressure.[83]

Assessment of pericardial constraint in patients is very difficult. Experimental systems are too invasive, and measurement artifacts influence pressure measurements.[68] RV or right atrial (RA) pressure under normal conditions serves as a useful measurement of pericardial influence but may be of limited use in patients with RV hypertrophy, cor pulmonale, and pulmonary hypertension, as well as after drainage of chronic pericardial tamponade.

Right Ventricular Influences

Studies of RV influence on LV compliance[79, 84, 85] have demonstrated that an upward shift of the LV diastolic P-V curve (i.e., reduced compliance) accompanies RV volume increases at end-diastole (Fig. 48–12); although this effect is present with the pericardium open, the coupling is much stronger when it is closed.[78] Ventricular interaction is therefore an important mechanism underlying acute reductions in LV compliance, whether the RV is enlarged as a result of pressure or volume overload. Ventricular interaction may also be responsible for some of the improved LV compliance properties observed with the administration of vasoactive medications that reduce volume return to the RV (e.g., nitrates).[86]

The importance of appreciating the influence of RV pressure and volume overload, as well as the use of cardiotonic medications, on LV diastolic P-V relationship is apparent from clinical studies of patients with adult respiratory distress syndrome. This work, summarized in Table 48–1, described changes in the PCWP and LV preload in two clinical circumstances: (1) at three levels of pulmonary pressures, which thereby represented a progressive increase in RV afterload,[87] and (2) in patients in whom an inotrope was required to maintain adequate systemic oxygen transport.[88]

In patients with acute pulmonary hypertension, an in-

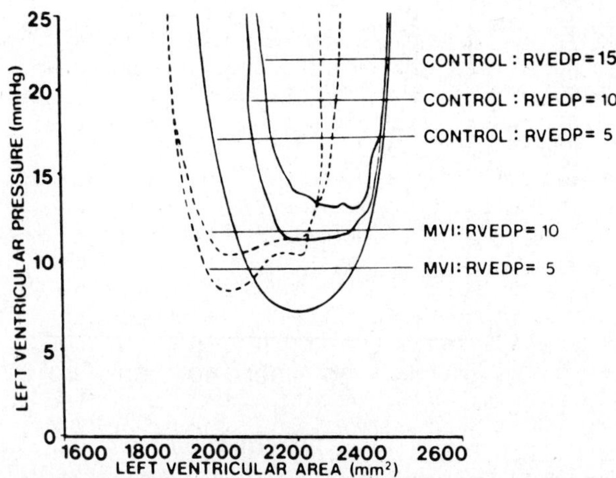

Figure 48–12. Effect of volume loading of the right ventricle on the LV diastolic pressure-volume (measured as area in square millimeters) relationship during control and with pulmonary hypertension induced by microvascular lung injury. Volume loading shifts the pressure-area relationship upward during both control *(solid lines)* and microvascular injury *(dashed lines)*. *Abbreviation:* RVEDP = right ventricular end-diastolic pressure. (From Calvin JE, Baer RW, Glantz SA: Pulmonary injury depresses cardiac systolic function through Starling mechanism. Am J Physiol 1986; 251:H722.)

TABLE 48–1. Effect of Pulmonary Hypertension and the Administration of Inotropes on Left Ventricular Compliance Properties (Mean ± SD Values)

	Mean BP (mm Hg)	*PCWP (mm Hg)*	*LV End-Diastolic Volume (mL/m²)*
Pulmonary hypertension			
Mean pulmonary artery pressure (mm Hg)			
Less than 20		5.0 ± 2*	87 ± 32
21–30		12.7 ± 4*	87 ± 31
Greater than 30		18.4 ± 4*	91 ± 27
Inotropes			
No inotropes	92 ± 15	12 ± 5	97 ± 31
Inotropes	78 ± 16†	15 ± 4†	96 ± 38

*$P < .5$, by analysis of variance between the three groups.
†$P < .5$, no inotropes vs. inotropes.

crease in the PCWP was found to be reflected by a constant LV EDV (preload), thereby demonstrating the effect of a pressure-overloaded RV to induce a depression in LV compliance properties. That is, LV chamber stiffness was altered with pulmonary hypertension so that the LV end-diastolic P-V curve was progressively shifted left with each successive increase in pulmonary artery pressure. Alterations in LV geometry were also noted with increasing pulmonary hypertension. The LV septal/free-wall axis appears disproportionately reduced when compared with either the base-to-apex or the anteroposterior axis.[77, 79] Acute pulmonary hypertension induced by glass bead embolization confirms that upward shifts in the LV diastolic P-V relationship occur with changes in RV afterload (i.e., a reduction in LV compliance) and that this effect is largely mediated by a reduction in the dimension of the LV septum to the free wall and an increase in intrapericardial pressure.[79] Similarly, during administration of inotropes, patients with adult respiratory distress syndrome demonstrated a higher mean PCWP than those without, although LV preload was again similar within the two groups (see Table 48–1). Hence, LV compliance was reduced in patients receiving inotropic support of systemic oxygen transport when compared with patients in whom inotropes were not used.

Reduced LV preload with RV dilation due to acute pulmonary hypertension may be the result of either the direct ventricular interaction described earlier resulting in reduced LV distensibility and a series interaction in which LV output falls because of reduced right ventricular output in both steady-state and transient conditions, especially with the pericardium in place. Slinker and Glantz[82] have determined that this series interaction is responsible for approximately one half of the RV-LV interaction with an intact pericardium. After removal of the pericardium, the dependence on series interaction of the RV and LV rises to four fifths. Other investigators have found conflicting results in this area[85, 89] but have failed to take into account the delay in RV input to LV input. Calvin and Ascah[90] have demonstrated a significant series interaction occurring in an open pericardial model of pulmonary hypertension consistent with the observation of Slinker and Glantz. Furthermore, LV hypertrophy results in far less dependence on direct but a greater series interaction either with or without the pericardium in place.[91]

The effects of RV pressure overload induced by glass bead embolization on the LV P-V relationship are diagrammatically illustrated in Figure 48–13.[84, 92] This figure demonstrates an upward shift in the LV diastolic P-V relationship after the induction of acute pulmonary hypertension, as well as a decrease in LV end-diastolic size. Stroke work is depressed because of the Frank-Starling relationship (Fig. 48–14).[79] Both direct and series interactions are likely present in this case. It has been shown, however, that volume loading[79] can restore LV preload to its baseline state. This observation suggests a dominance of the series interaction over the direct interaction in RV pressure overload.

The fall in preload-mediated LV stroke output that accompanies right heart failure[93] and acute RV pressure overload[94] reduces cardiac output and oxygen transport. Because BP also eventually falls, RV subendocardial ischemia[93, 95] develops further, contributing to the failure of the RV and exacerbating all of the events just described.

Patients with lung disease may, by a different mechanism than RV-LV interaction, produce a rise in the LV end-diastolic P-V relationship. Gomez and colleagues[96] have described global LV hypertrophic changes occurring as a result of chronic pulmonary hypertension secondary to experimentally induced chronic obstructive pulmonary disease in dogs. Previous investigators have also noted LV hypertrophy associated with RV pressure afterload secondary to pulmonary artery banding. It is postulated that sustained stress of the RV may lead to LV hypertrophy if the RV and LV myocardium act as a single structure. Alternatively, Gomez and coworkers postulated that a substance released by the RV as its hypertrophies may induce LV hypertrophy. Other investigators have postulated that in-

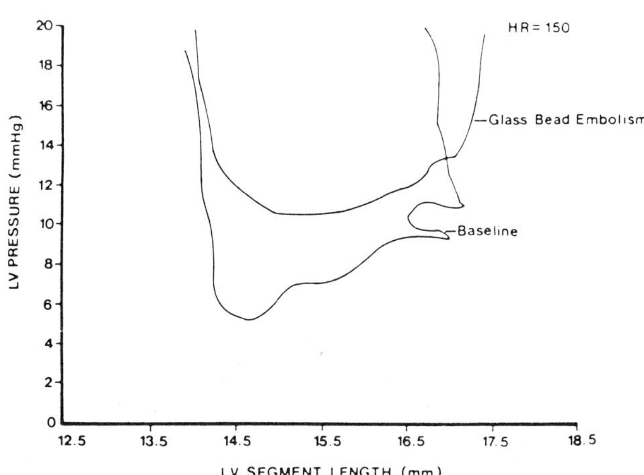

Figure 48–13. The LV diastolic pressure–segment length relationship during acute pulmonary hypertension at similar preloads and heart rate. Acute pulmonary hypertension shifts the relationship upwards. (From Calvin JE Jr, Langlois S, Garneys G: Ventricular interaction in a canine model of acute pulmonary hypertension and its modulation by vasoactive drugs. J Crit Care 1988; 3:43.)

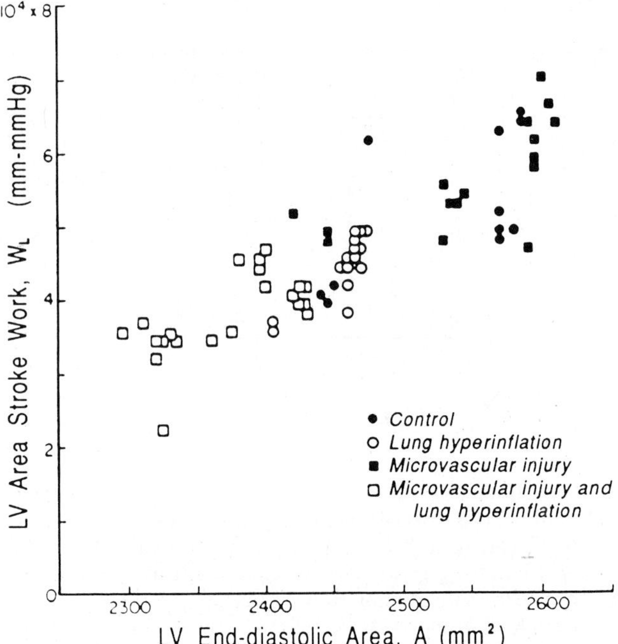

Figure 48–14. Relationship of LV area stroke work to LV end-diastolic area in an experimental model of dog. The acute pulmonary hypertension produced by a glass microvascular injury relationship is linear. Neither microvascular injury nor lung hyperinflation changed LV performance beyond the effect associated with the changes in end-diastolic LV size. (From Calvin JE, Baer RW, Glantz SA: Pulmonary injury depresses cardiac systole function through Starling mechanism. Am J Physiol 1986; 251:H722.)

creased RV wall tension, when sustained, results in LV hypertrophy.

The practical clinical significance of these two examples of ventricular interaction may then be summarized as follows: If the PCWP were used to define LV preload, volume resuscitation to support preload-dependent ventricular stroke output might be limited in patients with severe pulmonary hypertension or those on inotropes, before a normal LV preload is attained. That is, a normal LV preload in patients with severe pulmonary hypertension or in those concurrently receiving inotropic agents is likely reflected by a substantially higher PCWP than is found in those without these considerations. A depression in LV compliance that is observed with pulmonary hypertension or the use of the inotropic agents evokes a substantial increase in the hydrostatic pressure (i.e., PCWP) responsible for determining fluid flux across the pulmonary microvascular membrane at a constant LV preload. Therefore, the critical hydrostatic pressure within the pulmonary microvasculature, which if exceeded results in abnormal accumulation of extravascular lung water (i.e., pulmonary edema), is at a lower LV preload (hence, a lower preload-mediated stroke output) both in patients on inotropes and in those with pulmonary hypertension (Fig. 48–15, point b versus c).

Interactions between the LV and both the RV and RA are also extremely important in explaining the hemodynamics of low cardiac output states complicating RV wall infarction. Previous researchers have characterized the decrease in LV distensibility with RV ischemia and infarction.[97] Calvin[83] has demonstrated that upward shifts in the LV diastolic P-V relationships and decreased LV filling observed during RV infarction are related to both RV and RA interaction with the LV (Fig. 48–16).

Effect of Positive End-Expiratory Pressure on Left Ventricular End-Diastolic Pressure-Volume Relationship

A reduction in LV compliance has been observed with the institution of positive end-expiratory pressure (PEEP), further depressing ventricular preload beyond the decrease produced by the reduction in venous return. Jardin and associates[98] suggested that the cause of a depression in LV compliance with the use of PEEP was a leftward septal shift consequent to RV pressure overload (i.e., the concept of direct ventricular interaction due to a PEEP afterloading effect on the right ventricle, resulting in increased right-sided volume).

Others[79, 80] have, however, concluded that PEEP alters LV distensibility by increasing intrapericardial pressures through the external force it applies to the surface of the heart (Fig. 48–17). In one study, Calvin and colleagues[79] simulated PEEP by hyperinflation of the lung in an open-chest animal model. Although such a model would be expected to underestimate the PEEP effects, end-expiratory airway pressures of 15 mm Hg were maintained. A reduction in both RV and LV size resulted with this amount of positive airway pressure, primarily through a reduction in both RV and LV septal to free-wall dimensions. Despite the reduction in ventricular size, intracavitary pressures were unchanged from control. This observation defined that a primary effect of lung hyperinflation was to reduce ventricular compliance by the lungs' physically compressing both ventricles from the outside; there was no evidence that the RV dilated under the effects of the increased RV afterload. Hence, RV dilation could not be responsible for a leftward septal shift.

Using implanted radiopaque markers, Cassidy and Ramanathan[80] also noted that PEEP restricted outward expansion of the LV lateral wall during diastole; the position of the septum was not displaced by PEEP. It would therefore appear that PEEP is capable of causing a leftward shift in LV P-V relationships (i.e., reduction in compliance) by altering biventricular geometry because of direct compressive forces exerted on the heart surface with its use.

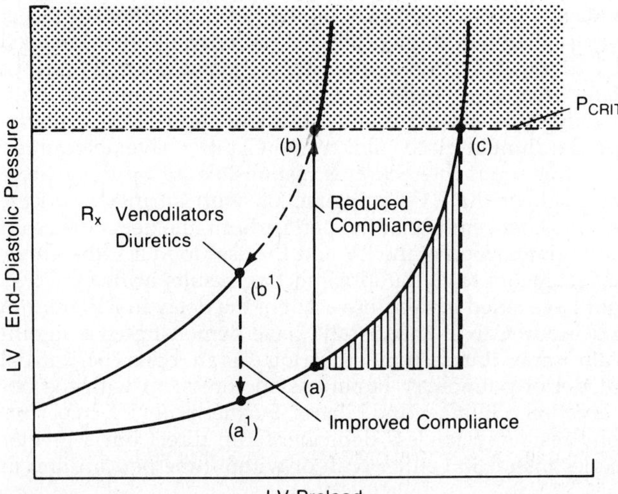

Figure 48–15. LV end-diastolic pressure-volume relationships. The critical hydrostatic pressure, P_{CRIT}, in the pulmonary microvascular membrane is exceeded at a lower preload when LV compliance is reduced by inotropes or by pulmonary hypertension. Treatment aimed at reducing pulmonary capillary hydrostatic pressure usually improves LV compliance.

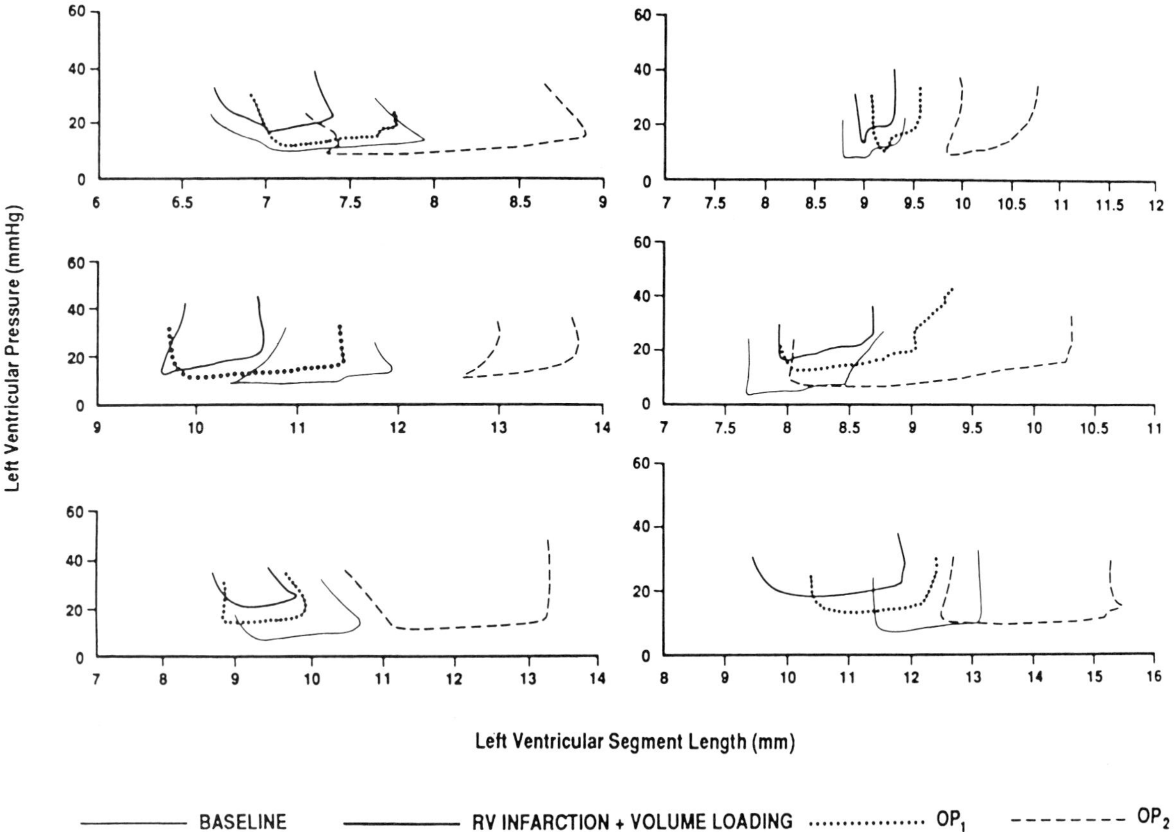

Figure 48–16. Plots of LV diastolic pressure–segment length relations in an experimental model of RV infarction. Volume loading after RV infarction shifted the relation further upward in all experiments. Partial opening of the pericardium (OP_1) shifted it downward, and complete opening of the pericardium (OP_2) returned it to baseline levels of pressure (although lengths increased). (From Calvin, JE: Optimal right ventricular filling pressures and the role of pericardial constraint in right ventricular infarction in dogs. Circulation 1991; 84:852.)

Clinical Measurement of Diastolic Abnormalities

The rate of relaxation is described by the time constant of relaxation (τ), which is exponentially related to the fall in LV pressure over time and can be measured by invasive experimental and clinical systems.[68] The time of isovolumic pressure decrease, beginning with the end of mechanical systole and lasting through mitral valve opening, is used to calculate the time constant of relaxation. The required cumbersome equations cannot be easily applied at the bedside but could be used to measure relaxation rates during coronary arteriography.[101]

Doppler filling velocity patterns provide an excellent noninvasive measurement of changes in the rate and extent of relaxation,[102] provided certain caveats are kept in mind. Alterations in chamber stiffness (e.g., a decrease in compliance

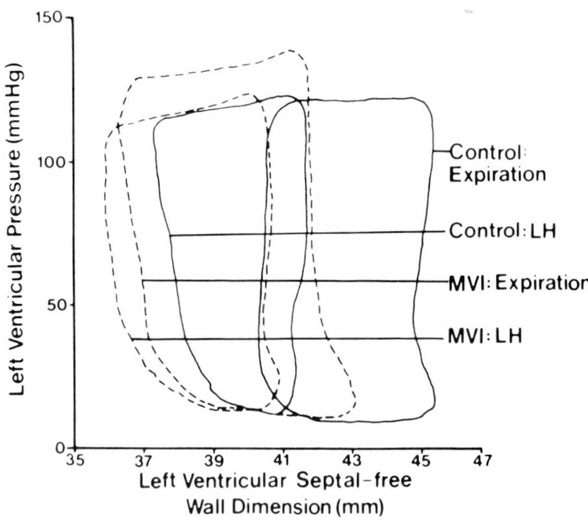

Figure 48–17. The ventricular septal free-wall pressure-dimension relationship during lung hyperinflation. End-expiratory loops during both a control period and a microvascular injury (MVI) are compared with loops taken during a lung hyperinflation, which is equivalent to an end-expiratory pressure of 15 mm Hg. Note the leftward shift of the end-diastolic points, which confirms a reduction in end-diastolic size or volume. Note also, however, that this shift occurs with very little decrease in end-diastolic pressure, which suggests that the lungs exerted an external force on the heart. (From Calvin JE, Baer RW, Glantz SA: Pulmonary injury depresses cardiac systolic function through Starling mechanism. Am J Physiol 1986; 251:H722.)

seen in various disease states) without alteration in relaxation rate result in changes in the pattern of Doppler filling time-velocity integrals, which have gained wide acceptance as indicators of diastolic compliance abnormalities. These changes are characterized by a decreased velocity of rapid filling (E wave) and augmented atrial contribution to filling (A wave) as the atrium contracts into a noncompliant ventricular chamber (Fig. 48–18, top panel).

This pattern has been noted in concentric LV hypertrophy,[103] in hypertrophic cardiomyopathy,[104] and with acute ischemia during angioplasty,[105] as well as in normal patients with increasing age and HR and with inspiration.[106] However, other studies of acute ischemic alterations of these filling patterns have failed to confirm these findings.

These disease states result in abnormalities in the Doppler filling pattern that characterize both the extent and rate of relaxation. The foregoing description represents the complex interaction of both early and late diastolic relaxation abnormalities, with early diastolic abnormalities predominating.[106] In those patients with unimpaired rates of relaxation and primary alterations in ventricular compliance, late diastolic filling, a reflection of the extent of relaxation, is primarily affected. The result is a decrease in atrial filling velocities, represented by a diminution in the A wave, which was seen in a subgroup of patients with coronary artery disease studied by Stoddard and coworkers (Fig. 48–18).[106] Conversely, alteration in the rate of relaxation (an early diastolic phenomenon) while chamber stiffness does not vary results in a diminution of the early filling of the ventricle and a larger atrial contribution (see Fig. 48–15). However, patients with elevated LA pressures secondary to significant mitral regurgitation exhibit maintained or exaggerated peak filling velocities, a manifestation of the increased driving force of the elevated LA pressure to ventricular early diastolic filling.[107] Even in patients with hypertrophic cardiomyopathy, this is not a reflection of impairment to late diastolic filling by atrial contraction, as might be surmised at first glance (Fig. 48–19). Therefore, assumptions based on Doppler-derived ventricular filling patterns need to be made in light of the overall hemodynamic picture, taking into account atrial pressure, valvular lesions, and age-adjusted normals.

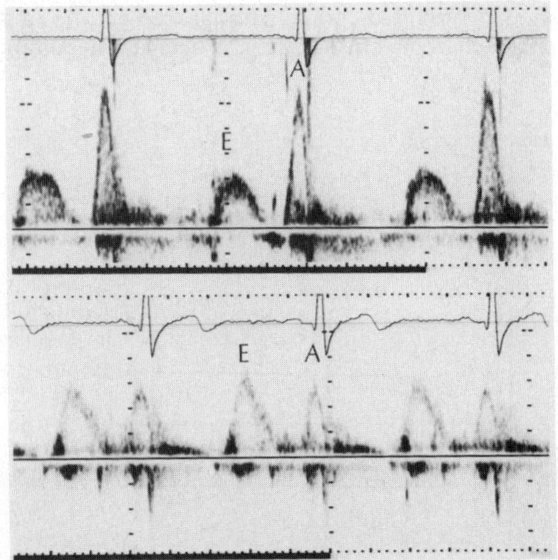

Figure 48–18. Pulsed Doppler mitral inflow velocities illustrating a diminished early filling velocity (E) and augmentation of atrial filling velocities (A) *(top panel)* compared with normal mitral inflow velocity patterns *(bottom panel).*

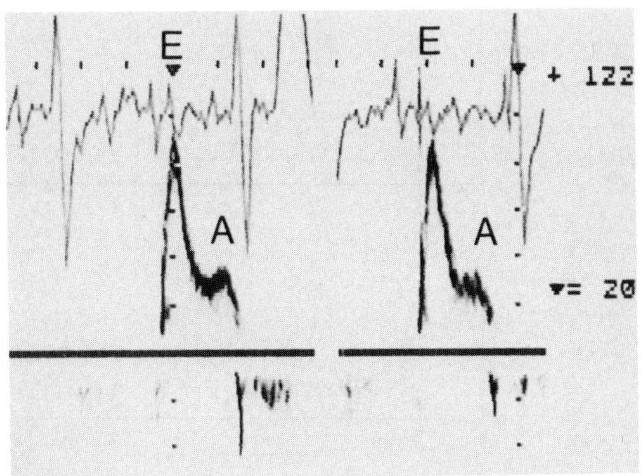

Figure 48–19. Pulsed Doppler mitral flow velocities demonstrating augmented early filling velocities (E) with blunted atrial filling patterns (A) that are characteristic of alterations in relaxation extent.

Nishimura and colleagues[107] reported their experience with noninvasive determination of τ by measuring continuous-wave Doppler velocities of mitral regurgitation and LVEDP. Correlation between τ measured invasively and LV pressure curves derived from Doppler velocity curves through application of a modification of the Bernoulli equation was obtained. This, however, required knowledge of the LVEDP, an invasively derived variable. A calculation approximation could be made with the addition of 20 mm Hg to the Doppler-derived atrioventricular pressure gradient, but according to the researchers, it is less accurate but acceptable.

SUMMARY

What has been presented here represents, we hope, a comprehensive review of current concepts put forth by many talented investigators in the field of ventricular performance. An understanding of the basic tenets of their detailed studies should, it is hoped, allow a more rational treatment plan to be devised for the critically ill patients attended to by our readers. Many of the subjects addressed cannot be directly measured or observed. However, their complex interaction in the production of such measured variables as HR, BP, SV, systemic vascular resistance peripheral vascular resistance, cardiac output, and PCWP can be better inferred, we believe, if a good grasp of what we have presented is achieved.

As a continued source of clinical "head scratching," the PCWP and its relationship to stroke output deserve special attention. As detailed earlier, the PCWP itself is not always indicative of optimal ventricular filling. Both the LV and RV are characterized by inherent stiffness properties, which in turn may be altered by various diseases affecting the ventricles themselves. The pulmonary circulation that joins them, as well as drugs and positive-pressure ventilation, used so frequently in the critically ill, establishes the well-appreciated difficulty in assessing ventricular preload by measuring end-diastolic filling pressure, such as the PCWP in the LV and the central venous pressure in the RV.

It is possible, however, to use information gained by following the trend in a measured PCWP or central venous pressure to make inferences with regard to ventricular compliance properties and to thereby appropriately define goal-

FLUID CHALLENGE

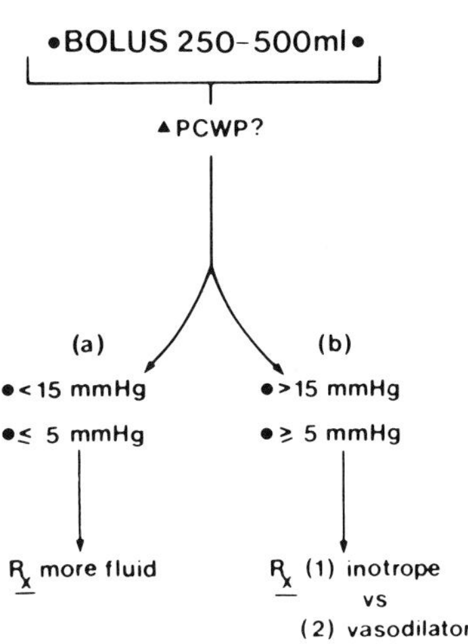

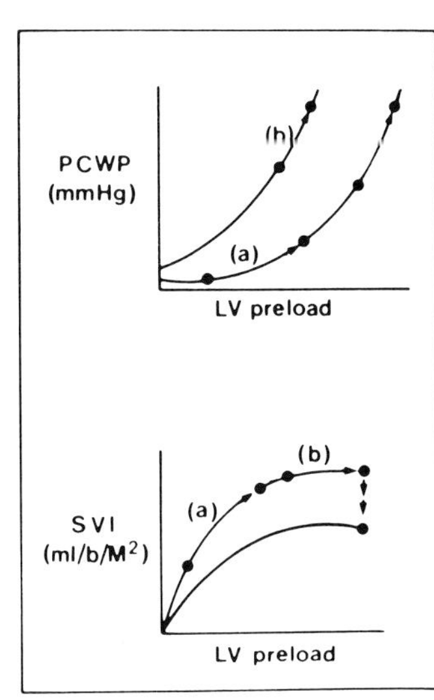

Figure 48–20. A clinical algorithm for volume loading in a critically ill patient. The absolute value of the WP and the magnitude of its change after a moderate volume load help dictate further therapy (see text).

directed therapy. When the goal of therapy is to match systemic oxygen with peripheral oxygen needs, the options to accomplish this are defined in the oxygen transport equation. To increase flow, fluid administration to enhance SV by augmenting preload is usually preferred if the PCWP is not so high that any further increase would risk a decrease in arterial oxygen content with the development or worsening of pulmonary edema. With a PCWP less than 10 to 12 mm Hg, a fluid challenge may be instituted; an increase in the PCWP of equal to or less than 5 mm Hg with a 250- to 500-mL fluid bolus implies that the LV is operating on the relatively flat portion of its diastolic P-V curve, and another fluid challenge may very well be attempted if further augmentation in SV is believed necessary to increase oxygen transport (Fig. 48–20). This process may be continued until the WP increases by an amount equal to or greater than 5 mm Hg, which would infer that the LV was now operating on the relatively steep ascending portion of the P-V curve. At this point, further fluid administration may simply increase the PCWP to approach the capillary hydrostatic pressure limit, without any significant effect on preload mediated SV (see Fig. 48–15). If an increase in oxygen transport is still required, the choices are now restricted to using inotropes or vasodilators to augment SV. If the BP is sufficiently stable to allow cautions titration of a vasodilator, the effect of this therapy may be to increase SV primarily as well as to improve LV compliance. The latter effect, a decrease in PCWP at a constant or slightly reduced preload, may then allow further fluid administration and, hence, an even greater increase in preload-mediated SV.

Without stability of systemic pressures sufficient to allow confidence in administration of a vasodilator, inotropes are the final alternative when the need is to increase SV and hence oxygen transport. By increasing contractility, inotropes indeed increase SV but potentially at the expense of reducing LV compliance (Table 48–2).

With the development of invasive techniques to measure ventricular diastolic filling as volume versus pressure, these interrelationships may become more clear in the day-to-day bedside practice of medicine. A volume-detecting catheter with the ability to measure both EDV and end-systolic volume as well as PCWP is currently being used clinically in our institution and may help evaluate difficult hemodynamic situations. We have found it to be of greatest use in those patients with RV disorders that traditionally have presented difficult hemodynamic assessments.

Echocardiographic measures of cardiac output have been shown to be highly accurate when properly applied but are often difficult to perform in critically ill patients and do not allow frequent sampling. Gated nuclear imaging, especially in patients with RV disorders and sepsis, when combined with thermodilution cardiac output monitoring or with continuous cardiac output monitoring, has allowed us to quantitate the cause of many hemodynamic derangements that are not obvious using conventional methods.

Finally, noninvasive measurement of contractility, as dis-

TABLE 48–2. Effect of Systemic Vasodilators in Cardiac Disease and Adult Respiratory Distress Syndrome

	Cardiac Disease		*Adult Respiratory Distress Syndrome*
	Phentolamine	*Nitroprusside*	*Nitroprusside*
Mean BP (mm Hg)	92 ± 14 → 82 ± 11†	92 ± 13 → 82 ± 14†	102 ± 16 → 84 ± 15†
Cardiac index	3.2 ± 0.8 → 3.7 ± 1.2†	3.7 ± 1.2 → 4.3 ± 1.3†	4.0 ± 1.1 → 4.1 ± 0.6
SV	38 ± 11 → 44 ± 10†	42 ± 15 → 47 ± 19†	38 ± 8 → 40 ± 5
PCWP	16 ± 6 → 11 ± 6†	17.5 ± 15 → 15 ± 4†	14 ± 5 → 14 ± 6
LVEDV	102 ± 39 → 124 ± 70	103 ± 40 → 110 ± 41	84 ± 29 → 78 ± 29

*See text for discussion.
†$P > .05$ by Student's T-test.

cussed earlier, by characterization of the fractional velocity of shortening corrected for heart rate, has proved useful in treating critically ill patients. However, these again are dependent on technical factors in image acquisition and the need for reproducibility requiring skilled personnel and interpretation of these images.

ACKNOWLEDGMENTS

The authors would like to thank Sharon Hines for her patience, expertise, and tireless effort in the preparation of this manuscript. Thanks to Gary Cummings for preparation of the figures included in the text. Thanks also to Alex Neumann and Peter Anagnos for contributing the echocardiographic tracings.

References

1. Housmans PR, Lee NKM, Blinks JR: Active shortening retards the decline of the intracellular calcium transient in mammalian heart muscle. Science 1983; 221:159.
2. Brutsaert DL, Rademakers FE, Sys SU: Triple control of relaxation: Implications in cardiac disease. Circulation 1984; 69:190.
3. Kohmoto O, Spitzer KW, Movsesian MA, et al: Effects of intracellular acidosis on [Ca^{2+}]i transients, transsarcolemmal C^{2+} fluxes, and contraction in ventricular myocytes. Circ Res 1990; 66:622.
4. Lee HC, Smith N, Mohabir R, et al: Cytosolic calcium transients from the beating mammalian heart. Physiol Sci 1987; 84:7793.
5. Hicks MJ, Shigekawa M, Katz AM: Mechanism by which cyclic adenosine 3':5'-monophosphate-dependent protein kinase stimulates calcium transport in cardiac sarcoplasmic reticulum. Circ Res 1979; 44:384.
6. Hoffman BF, Bindler E, Suckling EE: Postextrasystolic potentiation of contraction in cardiac muscle. Am J Physiol 1956; 185:95.
7. Ross J, Sonnenblick EH, Kaiser GA, et al: Electroaugmentation of ventricular performance and oxygen consumption by repetitive application of paired electrical stimuli. Circ Res 1965; 16:332.
8. Higgins CB, Vatner SF, Franklin D, et al: Extent of regulation of the heart's contractile state in the conscious dog by alteration in the frequency of contraction. J Clin Invest 1973; 52:1187.
9. Katz AM: Regulation of myocardial contractility 1958–1983: An odyssey. J Am Coll Cardiol 1983; 1:42.
10. Colluci WS, Wright RF, Braunwald E: New positive inotropic agents in the treatment of congestive heart failure (second of two parts). N Engl J Med 1986; 314:349.
11. Lang RM, Fellner SK, Neumann A, et al: Left ventricular contractility varies directly with blood ionized calcium. Ann Intern Med 1988; 108:524.
12. MacKinnon R, Gwathmey JK, Allen PD, et al: Modulation by the thyroid state of intracellular calcium and contractility in ferret ventricular muscle. Circ Res 1988; 63:1080.
13. Morkin E, Flink IL, Goldman S: Biochemical and physiologic effects of thyroid hormone on cardiac performance. Prog Cardiovasc Dis 1983; 25:435.
14. Braunwald E, Sommenblick EH, Ross J Jr: Mechanisms of cardiac contraction and relaxation in heart disease. *In:* A Textbook of Cardiovascular Medicine, 4th ed. Braunwald E (Ed). Philadelphia, WB Saunders, 1992, p 351.
15. Beierholm EA, Grantham RN, O'Keefe DD, et al: Effects of acid-base changes, hypoxia, and catecholamines on ventricular performance. Am J Physiol 1975; 228:1555.
16. Williamson JR, Schaffer SW, Ford C, et al: Contribution of tissue acidosis to ischemic injury in the perfused rat heart. Circulation 1976; 53:I-3.
17. Braunwald E: Mechanism of action of calcium-channel-blocking agents. N Engl J Med 1982; 307:1618.
18. Levine MJ, Harada K, Meuse AJ, et al: Excitation contraction uncoupling during ischemia in the blood perfused dog heart. Biochem Biophys Res Comm 1991; 179:502.
19. Gilman AG: G proteins: Transducers of receptor-generated signals. Annu Rev Biochem 1987; 56:615.
20. Spiegel AM, Gierschik P, Levine MA, et al: Clinical implications of guanine nucleotide-binding proteins as receptor-effector couplers. N Engl J Med 1985; 312:26.
21. Katz AM: Cyclic adenosine monophosphate effects on the myocardium: A man who blows hot and cold with one breath. J Am Coll Cardiol 1983; 2:143.
22. Homcy CJ, Graham RM: Molecular characterization of adrenergic receptors. Circ Res 1985; 56:635.
23. Neer EJ, Clapham DE: Roles of G protein subunits in transmembrane signalling. Nature 1988; 333:129.
24. Colucci WS, Wright RF, Braunwald E: New positive inotropic agents in the treatment of congestive heart failure (first of two parts). N Engl J Med 1986; 314:290.
25. Yatani A, Brown AM: Rapid β-adrenergic modulation of cardiac calcium channel currents by a fast G protein pathway. Science 1989; 245:71.
26. Mery PF, Lohmann SM, Walter U, et al: Ca^{2+} current is regulated by cyclic GMP-dependent protein kinase in mammalian cardiac myocytes. Proc Natl Acad Sci USA 1991; 88:1197.
27. Nawrath H: Cyclic AMP and cyclic GMP may play opposing roles in influencing force of contraction in mammalian myocardium. Nature 1976; 262:509.
28. Ungerer M, Bohm M, Elce JS, et al: Altered expression of β-adrenergic receptor kinase and β_1-adrenergic receptors in the failing human heart. Circulation 1993; 87:454.
29. Schranz D, Droege A, Broede A, et al: Uncoupling of human cardiac β-adrenoceptors during cardiopulmonary bypass with cardioplegic cardiac arrest. Circulation 1993; 87:422.
29a. Kumar A, Kosuri R, Kandula P, et al: Tumor necrosis factor–induced myocardial cell depression is mediated by nitric oxide and cyclic GMP generation. Crit Care Med 1994; 22:A191.
30. Schneider F, Lutun P, Hasselmann M, et al: Methylene blue increases systemic vascular resistance in human septic shock. Intensive Care Med 1992; 18:309.
31. Silverman HJ, Penaranda R, Orens JB, et al: Impaired β-adrenergic receptor stimulation of cyclic adenosine monophosphate in human septic shock: Association with myocardial hyporesponsiveness to catecholamines. Crit Care Med 1993; 21:31.
31a. Yanagisawa M, Kurihara H, Kimura S, et al: A novel potent vasoconstrictor peptide produced by vascular endothelial cells. Nature 1988; 332:411.
32. Kramer BK, Nishida M, Kelly RA, et al: Myocardial actions of a new class of cytokines. Circulation 1992; 85:350.
32a. Kelly RA, Eid H, Kramer BK, et al: Endothelin enhances the contractile responsiveness of adult rat ventricular myocytes to calcium by a pertussis toxin–sensitive pathway. J Clin Invest 1990; 86:1164.
33. Kramer BK, Smith TW, Kelly RA: Endothelin and increased contractility in adult rat ventricular myocytes: Role of intracellular alkalosis induced by activation of the protein kinase C-dependent Na^+-H^+. Circ Res 1991; 68:269.
34. Gwathmey JK, Slawsky MT, Hajjar RJ, et al: Role of intracellular calcium handling in force-interval relationships of human ventricular myocardium. J Clin Invest 1990; 85:1599.
35. Gwathmey JK, Copelas L, MacKinnon R, et al: Abnormal intracellular calcium handling in myocardium from patients with end-stage heart failure. Circ Res 1987; 61:70.
36. Limas CJ, Olivari M, Goldenberg IF, et al: Calcium uptake by cardiac sarcoplasmic reticulum in human dilated cardiomyopathy. Cardiovasc Res 1987; 21:601.
37. Mercadier J, Lompr' A, Duc P, et al: Altered sarcoplasmic reticulum CA^{2+}-ATPase gene expression in the human ventricle during end-stage heart failure. J Clin Invest 1990; 85:305.
38. Feldman MD, Copelas L, Gwathmey JK, et al: Deficient production of cyclic AMP: Pharmacologic evidence of an important cause of contractile dysfunction in patients with end-stage heart failure. Circulation 1987; 75:331.
39. Feldman AM, Ray PE, Silan CM, et al: Selective gene expression in failing human heart. Circulation 1991; 83:1866.
40. Bristow MR, Hershberger RE, Port JD, et al: β-adrenergic pathways in nonfailing and failing human ventricular myocardium. Circulation 1990; 82:I-12.

41. Feldman AM, Cates AE, Veazey WB, et al: Increase of the 40,000-mol wt pertussis toxin substrate (G protein) in the failing human heart. J Clin Invest 1988; 82:189.
42. Lang CH, Bagby GJ, Ferguson JL, et al: Cardiac output and redistribution of organ blood flow in hypermetabolic sepsis. Am J Physiol 1984; 246:R331.
43. Feldman T, Borow KM, Lang RM, et al: Differentiation of simultaneous changes in preload, afterload, peripheral resistance and left ventricular performance. Am J Noninvasive Cardiol 1987; 1:30.
44. Gordon AM, Huxley AF, Julian FJ: The variation in isometric tension with sarcomere length in vertebrate muscle fibres. J Physiol 1966; 184:170.
45. Milnor WR: Cardiac dynamics. *In:* Hemodynamics. Milnor WR (Ed). Baltimore, Williams & Wilkins, 1982, p 244.
46. Diamond G, Forrester JS: Effect of coronary artery disease and acute myocardial infarction on left ventricular compliance in man. Circulation 1992; 45:11.
47. Glantz SA, Parmley WW: Factors which affect the diastolic pressure-volume curve. Circ Res 1978; 42:171.
48. Calvin JE, Driedger AA, Sibbald WJ: Does the pulmonary capillary wedge pressure predict left ventricular preload in critically ill patients? Crit Care Med 1981; 9:437.
49. Kelly R, Fitchett D: Noninvasive determination of aortic input impedance and external left ventricular power output: A validation and repeatability study of a new technique. J Am Coll Cardiol 1992; 20:952.
50. Regen DM: Calculation of left ventricular wall stress. Circ Res 1990; 67:245.
51. Lloyd TR, Donnerstein RL: Afterload dependence of echocardiographic left ventricular ejection force determination. Am J Cardiol 1991; 67:901.
52. Nichols WW, Pepine CJ: Left ventricular afterload and aortic input impedance: Implications of pulsatile blood flow. Prog Cardiovasc Dis 1982; 24:293.
53. Grossman W, Jones D, McLaurin LP: Wall stress and patterns of hypertrophy in the human left ventricle. J Clin Invest 1975; 56:56.
54. Yin FCP, Liu Z: Estimating arterial resistance and compliance during transient conditions in humans. Am J Physiol 1989; 257:H190.
55. Takaoka H, Takeuchi M, Odake M, et al: Comparison of hemodynamic determinants for myocardial oxygen consumption under different contractile states in human ventricle. Circulation 1993; 87:59.
56. Starling EH. The Linacre Lecture on the Law of the Heart Given at Cambridge in 1915. London, Longmans, Green & Co, 1981.
57. Chatterjee K, Parmley WW: The role of vasodilator therapy in heart failure. Prog Cardiovasc Dis 1977; 19:301.
58. Ross J Jr: Cardiac function and myocardial contractility: A perspective. J Am Coll Cardiol 1983; 1:52.
59. Shoemaker WC, Czer LSC: Evaluation of the biologic importance of various hemodynamic and oxygen transport variables: Which variables should be monitored in postoperative shock? Crit Care Med 1979; 7:424.
60. Sibbald W, Myers ML, Calvin J, et al: Biventricular systolic and diastolic performance in ARDS. Crit Care Med 1982; 10:210.
61. Myers ML, Calvin JE, Driedger AA, et al: Myocardial dysfunction associated with massive pulmonary embolus as evaluated by radionuclide angiography. Crit Care Med 1982; 10:417.
62. Heinemann HO: Right-sided heart failure and the use of diuretics. Am J Med 1978; 64:367.
63. Sagawa K: The end-systolic pressure-volume relation of the ventricle: Definition, modifications and clinical use. Circulation 1981; 63:1223.
64. Mirsky I, Pasternac A, Ellison RC, et al: Clinical application of force-velocity parameters and the concept of a normalized velocity. *In:* Cardiac Mechanics. Mirsky I, Ghista DN, Sandler H (Eds). New York, John Wiley & Sons, 1974, p 293.
65. Grossman W, Haynes F, Paraskos JA, et al: Alterations in preload and myocardial mechanics in the dog and in man. Circ Res 1972; 31:83.
66. Colan SD, Borow KM, Neumann A: Left ventricular end-systolic wall stress-velocity of fiber shortening relation: A load-independent index of myocardial contractility. J Am Coll Cardiol 1984; 4:715.
67. Gaasch WH, Levine HJ, Quinones MA, et al: Left ventricular compliance: Mechanisms and clinical implications. Am J Cardiol 1976; 38:645.
68. Gilbert JC, Glantz SA: Determinants of left ventricular filling and of the diastolic pressure-volume relation. Circ Res 1989; 64:827.
69. Nikolic SD, Tamura K, Tamura T, et al: Diastolic viscous properties of the intact canine left ventricle. Circ Res 1990; 67:352.
70. Momomura S, Ingwall JS, Parker JA, et al: The relationships of high energy phosphates, tissue pH, and regional blood flow to diastolic distensibility in the ischemic dog myocardium. Circ Res 1985; 57:822.
71. Lorell BH, Grossman W: Cardiac hypertrophy: The consequences for diastole. J Am Coll Cardiol 1987; 9:1189.
72. Cuocolo A, Sax FL, Brush JE, et al: Left ventricular hypertrophy and impaired diastolic filling in essential hypertrophy and impaired diastolic filling in essential hypertension. Circulation 1990; 81:978.
73. Apstein CS, Grossman W: Opposite initial effects of supply and demand ischemia on left ventricular diastolic compliance: The ischemia-diastolic paradox. J Mol Cell Cardiol 1987; 19:119.
74. Paulus WJ, Grossman W, Serizawa T, et al: Different effects of two types of ischemia on myocardial systolic and diastolic function. Am J Physiol 1985; 248:H719.
75. Ikenouchi H, Kohmoto O, McMillan M, et al: Contributions of $[Ca^{2+}]i$, [Pi], and pHi to altered diastolic myocyte tone during partial metabolic inhibition. J Clin Invest 1991; 88:55.
76. Sasayama S, Nonogi H, Miyazaki S, et al: Changes in diastolic properties of the regional myocardium during pacing-induced ischemia in human subjects. J Am Coll Cardiol 1985; 5:599.
77. Stool EW, Mullins CB, Leshin SJ, et al: Dimensional changes of the left ventricle during acute pulmonary arterial hypertension in dogs. Am J Cardiol 1974; 33:868.
78. Glantz SA, Misbach GA, Moores WY, et al: The pericardium substantially affects the left ventricular diastolic pressure-volume relationship in the dog. Circ Res 1978; 42:433.
79. Calvin JE, Baer RW, Glantz SA: Pulmonary injury depresses cardiac systolic function through Starling mechanism. Am J Physiol 1986; 251:H722.
80. Cassidy SS, Ramanathan M: Dimensional analysis of the left ventricle during PEEP: Relative septal and lateral wall displacements. Am J Physiol 1984; 246:H792.
81. Tyson GS, Maier GW, Olsen CO, et al: Pericardial influences on ventricular filling in the conscious dog. Circ Res 1984; 54:173.
82. Slinker BK, Glantz SA: End-systolic and end-diastolic ventricular interaction. Am J Physiol 1986; 251:H1062.
83. Calvin JE: Optimal right ventricular filling pressures and the role of pericardial constraint in right ventricular infarction in dogs. Circulation 1991; 84:852.
84. Calvin JE Jr, Langlois S, Garneys G: Ventricular interaction in a canine model of acute pulmonary hypertension and its modulation by vasoactive drugs. J Crit Care 1988; 3:43.
85. Visner MS, Arentzen CE, O'Connor MJ, et al: Alterations in left ventricular three-dimensional dynamic geometry and systolic function during acute right ventricular hypertension in the conscious dog. Circulation 1983; 67:353.
86. Ludbrook PA, Byrne JD, McKnight RC: Influence of right ventricular hemodynamics on left ventricular diastolic pressure-volume relations in man. Circulation 1979; 59:21.
87. Sibbald WJ, Driedger AA: Right ventricular function in acute disease states: Pathophysiologic considerations. Crit Care Med 1983; 11:339.
88. Raper R, Cunningham D, Sibbald W: The influence of CAD on diastolic biventricular function in sepsis. Clin Invest Med 1985; 8:A69.
89. Olson CO, Tyson GS, Maiter GW, et al: Dynamic ventricular interaction in the conscious dog. Circ Res 1983; 52:85.
90. Calvin JE, Ascah KJ: Impact of leftward septal shift and potential role of ischemia in its production during experimental right ventricular pressure overload. J Crit Care 1992; 7:106.

91. Slinker BK, Chagas ACP, Glantz SA: Chronic pressure overload hypertrophy decreases direct ventricular interaction. Am J Physiol 1987; 253:H347.
92. Calvin JE, Baer RW, Glantz SA: Pulmonary artery constriction produces a greater right ventricular dynamic afterload than lung microvascular injury in the open chest dog. Circ Res 1985; 56:40.
93. Calvin JE, Quinn B: Right ventricular pressure overload during acute lung injury: Cardiac mechanics and the pathophysiology of right ventricular systolic dysfunction. J Crit Care 1989; 4:251.
94. Calvin JE: Right ventricular afterload mismatch during acute pulmonary hypertension and its treatment with dobutamine: A pressure segment length analysis in a canine model. J Crit Care 1989; 4:239.
95. Vlahakes GJ, Turley K, Hoffman JIE: The pathophysiology of failure in acute right ventricular hypertension: Hemodynamic and biochemical correlations. Circulation 1981; 63:87.
96. Gomez A, Unruh H, Mink SN: Altered left ventricular chamber stiffness and isovolumic relaxation in dogs with chronic pulmonary hypertension caused by emphysema. Circulation 1993; 87:247.
97. Goto Y, Yamamoto J, Saito M, et al: Effects of right ventricular ischemia on left ventricular geometry and the end-diastolic pressure-volume relationship in the dog. Circulation 1985; 72:1104.
98. Jardin F, Farcot J, Boisante L, et al: Influence of positive end-expiratory pressure on left ventricular performance. N Engl J Med 1981; 304:387.
99. Miyazaki S, Guth BD, Miura T, et al: Changes of left ventricular diastolic function in exercising dogs without and with ischemia. Circulation 1990; 81:1058.
100. Nikolic S, Yellin EL, Tamura K, et al: Effect of early diastolic loading on myocardial relaxation in the intact canine left ventricle. Circ Res 1990; 66:1217.
101. Kass DA, Midei M, Brinker J, et al: Influence of coronary occlusion during PTCA on end-systolic and end-diastolic pressure-volume relations in humans. Circulation 1990; 81:447.
102. Rokey R, Kuo LC, Zoghbi WA, et al: Determination of parameters of left ventricular diastolic filling with pulsed Doppler echocardiography: Comparison with cineangiography. Circulation 1985; 71:543.
103. Pearson AC, Labovitz AJ, Mrosek D, et al: Assessment of diastolic function in normal and hypertrophied hearts: Comparison of Doppler echocardiography and M-mode echocardiography. Am Heart J 1987; 113:1417.
104. Maron BJ, Spirito P, Green KJ, et al: Noninvasive assessment of left ventricular diastolic function by pulsed Doppler echocardiography in patients with hypertrophic cardiomyopathy. J Am Coll Cardiol 1987; 10:733.
105. Labovitz AJ, Lewen MK, Kern M, et al: Evaluation of left ventricular systolic and diastolic dysfunction during transient myocardial ischemia produced by angioplasty. J Am Coll Cardiol 1987; 10:748.
106. Stoddard MF, Pearson AC, Kern MJ, et al: Left ventricular diastolic function: Comparison of pulsed Doppler echocardiographic and hemodynamic indexes in subjects with and without coronary artery disease. J Am Coll Cardiol 1989; 13:327.
107. Nishimura RA, Schwartz RS, Tajik AJ, et al: Noninvasive measurement of rate of left ventricular relaxation by Doppler echocardiography: Validation with simultaneous cardiac catheterization. Circulation 1993; 88:146.

CHAPTER 49

The Coronary Arteries in Unstable Angina Pectoris, Acute Myocardial Infarction, and Sudden Coronary Death

William C. Roberts, MD

This chapter reviews and compares coronary arterial findings in patients with fatal unstable angina pectoris (UAP), acute myocardial infarction (AMI), and sudden coronary death (SCD).

AMOUNTS OF CORONARY ARTERIAL LUMINAL NARROWING IN THE THREE CORONARY SUBSETS

The amounts of coronary arterial narrowing observed at necropsy in patients with UAP, AMI, and SCD are generally enormous.[1] As shown in Table 49–1, from a necropsy study of 80 patients with these three coronary events (SCD in 31, AMI in 27, and UAP in 22), an average of 2.9 of the four major (right, left main, left anterior descending, and left circumflex) coronary arteries were severely (>75% decrease in cross-sectional area) narrowed at some points, and no significant differences were observed among the three coronary subsets.[1] The patients with UAP had a much higher frequency of severe narrowing of the left main coronary artery (10 of 22 patients [45%]) than did the AMI (3 of 27 patients [11%]) and SCD (3 of 31 patients [10%]) groups.

A more sophisticated approach to determining degrees of luminal narrowing is to examine the entire lengths of the four major epicardial coronary arteries. One technique involves incising each of the four major coronary arteries transversely at 5-mm intervals and then preparing a histologic section from each 5-mm segment. Normally, the total length of the four major arteries is about 27 cm (right, 10 cm; left main, 1 cm; left anterior descending, 10 cm; and left circumflex, 6 cm), and thus about 55 5-mm-long segments from each heart are available for examination. Studies using this approach in the patients with UAP, AMI, and SCD are summarized in Table 49–2.[1] Of the 4016 5-mm segments studied in the 80 patients, 38% were narrowed 76% to 100% in cross-sectional area by plaque alone (controls, 3%); 34% were narrowed 51% to 75% (controls, 3%); 34% were narrowed 51% to 75% (controls, 22%); 20% were narrowed 26% to 50% (controls, 44%); and only 7% were narrowed 25% or less (controls, 31%). Similar degrees of narrowing by plaque alone in all four categories of narrowing were observed in the groups with AMI and SCD; the patients with UAP had significantly more severe coronary narrowing than did the other two groups.

Thus, in general, patients with fatal UAP have more extensive severe narrowing by plaque alone of the four major epicardial coronary arteries than do patients with either AMI or SCD, and the patients with UAP compared with the other two groups have a significantly higher frequency of severe narrowing of the left main coronary artery.

COMPOSITION OF CORONARY ATHEROSCLEROTIC PLAQUES IN THE THREE CORONARY SUBSETS

Until recent years,[2, 3] no detailed information was available concerning the composition of atherosclerotic plaques in the

TABLE 49–1. Number of Major (Right, Left Main, Left Anterior Descending, and Left Circumflex) Coronary Arteries Narrowed >75% in Cross-Sectional Area by Atherosclerotic Plaque in Fatal Coronary Artery Disease

			Number of Four Arteries per Patient >75% Narrowed in Cross-Sectional Area by Plaque				
Coronary Event	*Patients (n)*	*Mean Age (years)*	*4*	*3*	*2*	*1*	*Mean*
Sudden coronary death	31	47	3	20	6	2	2.8
Acute myocardial infarction	27	59	3	14	10	0	2.7
Unstable angina pectoris	22	48	10	8	3	1	3.2
Totals	80	51	16 (20%)	42 (52%)	19 (24%)	3 (4%)	2.9
Controls	40	52	0 (0)	5 (5%)	12 (13%)	21 (23%)	0.7

epicardial coronary arteries of patients with fatal coronary events. Kragel and associates,[2, 3] using a computerized morphometry system, traced the various components of atherosclerotic plaques in histologic sections prepared from 1438 5-mm segments of the four major epicardial coronary arteries in 37 patients with fatal coronary artery disease (UAP in 10, AMI in 15, and SCD in 12 patients). The results are summarized in Table 49–3. The dominant component of the coronary atherosclerotic plaques in all three subsets of patients was fibrous tissue, accounting for about 80% of the plaques in each subset; extracellular lipid (pultaceous debris) and calcium each made up about 5% of the plaques, and several miscellaneous components formed the remainder of the plaques. The cellular component of the fibrous tissue occupied a larger portion of plaque in the patients with UAP and SCD, and the acellular (dense) component of fibrous tissue occupied a larger portion of the plaque in the AMI group. In all three subsets, the amount of dense fibrous tissue increased as plaque size increased (or as lumen size decreased) and the amount of cellular fibrous tissue decreased as plaque size increased.

FREQUENCY AND TYPES OF ACUTE LESIONS IN THE MAJOR CORONARY ARTERIES IN THE THREE CORONARY SUBSETS

Considerable effort has been directed toward understanding the acute coronary events that may be responsible for the development of UAP, AMI, and SCD. From angiographic, angioscopic, and necropsy studies, it has been speculated that plaque rupture and hemorrhage with overlying intraluminal thrombus, which are the acute lesions usually responsible for AMI, are also responsible for UAP and maybe SCD. Kragel and associates[4] examined 3101 5-mm segments of 268 epicardial coronary arteries of 67 patients with fatal coronary events (UAP in 14, AMI in 31, and SCD in 21 patients). The results of these detailed studies are summarized in Table 49–4. The frequency of *intraluminal thrombus* was similar in the UAP and SCD groups (29% in each) and significantly lower than that in the AMI group (69%). The thrombus was nonocclusive in the patients with UAP and in 5 of 6 patients with SCD but was nonocclusive in only 4 of the 22 patients with AMI. The composition of the nonocclusive and occlusive thrombi also was different: The nonocclusive thrombus consisted mainly of platelets, and the occlusive thrombus mainly of fibrin. Of the 32 patients with thrombus, plaque rupture was found in association with the thrombus in 17 patients (53%): in none of the 4 patients with UAP, in 2 of the 6 patients with SCD, and in 15 (83%) of the 22 patients with AMI. In the 15 patients with thrombus unassociated with plaque rupture, hemorrhage into the plaque at the site of thrombus was found in 7: in 3 of the 4 patients with UAP, in 2 of the 6 patients with SCD, and in 2 of the 32 patients with AMI.

Plaque rupture was found in 33 (49%) of the 67 patients. Its frequency was insignificantly different in the groups with UAP (36% [5 of 14] and SCD (19% [4 of 21]): In both groups the frequency was significantly less than in the group with AMI (75% [24 of 32]).

Plaque hemorrhage was observed in 27 (40%) of the 67 patients, and its frequency was significantly lower in the groups with UAP (21% [3 of 14]) and SCD (19% [4 of 21]) than in the group with AMI (63% [20 of 32]). Plaque hemorrhage was associated with plaque rupture or intraluminal thrombus in 20 (74%) of the 27 patients with plaque hemorrhage: in 4 of the 14 patients with unstable angina, in 4 of 21 with sudden death, and in 13 of the 32 with acute infarction.

Multiple small vascular channels were present in 60 (90%) of the 67 patients and with an insignificantly different frequency in each of the three patient groups (see Table 49–1). The frequency of multiluminal channels in each 5-mm-long segment of coronary artery was significantly higher in the group with UAP (12% [66 of 572]) than in either the SCD (7% [72 of 999]) or AMI groups (7% [107 of 1530]).

Thus, comparison of findings from examination of a histologic section from each of 3101 5-mm segments of 268 major epicardial coronary arteries from 67 patients with

TABLE 49–2. Amounts of Cross-Sectional Area Narrowing of Each 5-mm Segment of the Four Major (Right, Left Main, Left Anterior Descending, and Left Circumflex) Epicardial Coronary Arteries by Atherosclerotic Plaques in Subjects with Fatal Coronary Artery Disease

				Per Cent Segments Narrowed				
Subgroup	*Patients (n)*	*Mean Age (years)*	*Number of 5-mm Segments*	*0–25%*	*25–50%*	*51–75%*	*76–100%*	*Mean Score*
Sudden coronary death	31	47	1564	7%	23%	34%	36%	2.98
Acute myocardial infarction	27	59	1403	5%	23%	38%	34%	3.01
Unstable angina pectoris	22	48	1049	11%	12%	29%	48%	3.12
Totals	80	51	4016	7%	20%	34%	38%	3.02
Controls	40	52	1849	31%	44%	22%	3%	1.97

TABLE 49–3. Mean Composition of Coronary Arterial Atherosclerotic Plaques in the Four Major Epicardial Coronary Arteries

	Mean Per Cent of Plaque Containing Various Components in the Four Major Coronary Arteries (1438 Segments)		
Components of Plaque	*Unstable Angina Pectoris (n = 10)*	*Acute Myocardial Infarction (n = 15)*	*Sudden Coronary Death (n = 12)*
Dense fibrous tissue	35	46	29
Loose fibrous tissue	1	3	3
Cellular fibrous tissue	52	32	50
Calcium	4	4	8
Pultaceous debris	4	8	4
Foam cells	0	1	0
Foam cells and lymphocytes	3	4	6
Inflammatory infiltrates without significant numbers of foam cells	1	2	1

fatal coronary artery disease disclosed that the frequency of three acute coronary lesions (intraluminal thrombus, plaque rupture, and plaque hemorrhage) was similar in patients with UAP and SCD and that the frequency of each of these acute lesions was significantly higher in patients with a fatal first transmural AMI. Furthermore, although multiluminal channels (not acute lesions) within plaques were frequent in all three patient groups, these lesions were found significantly more often in 5-mm segments of coronary arteries in the group with UAP than in the groups with SCD and AMI, where their frequency was similar.

Several angiographic studies[5–9] have identified either intraluminal filling defects consistent with thrombus or specific morphologic lesions (eccentric narrowings with irregular borders) in patients with UAP, and these defects have been used to distinguish such patients from those with stable angina. Comparison of postmortem angiographic and histologic findings,[10] however, in patients with coronary artery disease (not necessarily UAP) has shown that these irregular eccentric lesions may represent not only sites of intraluminal thrombus but also plaque rupture, plaque hemorrhage, or organized thrombus. In addition, three angioscopic studies[11–13] have identified intraluminal thrombus and ulceration or rupture of plaque in patients with UAP. On the basis of these studies, it has been widely speculated that the lesion responsible for the development of UAP is an ulcerated plaque over which nonocclusive intraluminal thrombus develops.

Before accepting that this hypothesis is indeed true for all or most patients with UAP, the limitations of the previous studies[5–13] need to be considered. Interpretation of the significance of the eccentric irregular lesions seen angiographically in patients with UAP is based largely on the work of Levin and Fallon,[10] who compared postmortem coronary arteriograms and histologic sections of coronary artery narrowings in 39 patients who died either after coronary artery bypass surgery or of consequences of AMI. (Because the trauma of bypass surgery may be associated with plaque rupture or plaque hemorrhage or both, patients who had undergone this procedure were excluded from the study by Kragel and colleagues.[4]) Levin and Fallon identified 38 narrowings that had irregular borders or intraluminal lucencies on angiography. Of these, 8 (21%) were acute or organizing nonocclusive thrombi overlying atherosclerotic plaque, 6 (16%) were nonocclusive thrombi overlying sites of plaque rupture or hemorrhage, 10 (26%) were sites of plaque hemorrhage or rupture without thrombus, 6 (16%) contained recanalized thrombus (presumably multiluminal channels), and 21% showed narrowing of the segment by plaque without any complicating acute lesion. More than a third of the irregular eccentric lesions studied, therefore, showed no acute lesion that would account for the abrupt change in symptoms in the setting of UAP. In Kragel and coworkers' study, plaques containing multiluminal channels, although common to all three groups of patients, were found with greatest frequency in the group with UAP.

When interpreting reports of angiographic or angioscopic studies in patients with UAP, it is assumed that the patients did not have left ventricular necrosis (AMI) at the time of study, an assumption that may or may not be true. Guthrie and associates[14] studied 12 patients with UAP who died shortly after coronary artery bypass surgery. At autopsy, 4 of the 12 patients had AMI that histologically appeared to have occurred before the operation, and AMI was not suspected clinically in any of the 4 patients. Therefore, when studying living patients, it may be difficult to determine whether the patients have pure UAP or have combined UAP and AMI.

Information about coronary artery morphology in patients with UAP is scant, hard to obtain, and difficult to interpret for several reasons. UAP is rarely fatal, and those patients who do die during the period of UAP usually have

TABLE 49–4. Frequency of Acute Coronary Lesions and Multiluminal Channels at Necropsy in Patients with Unstable Angina Pectoris, Sudden Coronary Death, and Acute Myocardial Infarction

		Coronary Arteries			
Coronary Subset	*Number of Patients*	*Thrombus*	*Plaque Rupture*	*Plaque Hemorrhage*	*Multiluminal Channels*
Unstable angina pectoris	14	4 (29%)*	5 (36%)*	3 (21%)*	14 (100%)
Sudden coronary death	21	6 (29%)*	4 (19%)*	4 (19%)*	17 (81%)
Acute myocardial infarction	32	22 (69%)†	24 (75%)†	20 (63%)†	29 (90%)
Totals	67	32 (48%)	33 (49%)	27 (40%)	60 (90%)

*Versus † in same vertical column = $P < .02$.

had a coronary angioplasty or bypass procedure performed or have experienced an AMI shortly before death. In patients with AMI preceded by UAP, intracoronary lesions may not be representative of those occurring in patients with UAP not complicated by AMI.

Information about the acute coronary lesions in patients who died shortly after coronary artery bypass surgery has been provided in several studies. Guthrie and colleagues[14] described 12 patients and Roberts and Virmani[15] described 19 patients with unstable angina pectoris who died shortly after coronary bypass surgery. In both studies, the frequency of intraluminal thrombus was low (8% and 12%, respectively) when patients with AMI were excluded. In a separate report, Virmani and Roberts[16] described the frequency of extravasated erythrocytes and fibrin in the plaque of 17 of the 22 patients with UAP. Plaque hemorrhage (erythrocytes with or without fibrin) was identified in 94% of their patients. It is likely that surgical manipulation of the epicardial coronary arteries was responsible for the plaque hemorrhage in many of these cases.

In a study of UAP with fatal outcome, Falk[17] provided information about the frequency of acute lesions in the epicardial coronary arteries of patients with SCD, UAP, and AMI. He described necropsy findings in "25 patients, all of whom died of acute coronary thrombosis within 24 hours after the onset of acute symptoms." Of the 24 patients for whom clinical information was available, 15 clearly had UAP, 2 had an equivocal history of UAP, and 7 did not have UAP. Of these 25 patients, 15 had coagulative necrosis (AMI) that, as determined histologically, was compatible with an age of less than 24 hours. In these patients, he described lamellar thrombi (21 of 25 patients, including 14 of 15 with UAP), 81% of which were associated with plaque rupture and hemorrhage. Neither the frequency of plaque rupture nor the number of thrombotic episodes differed between the patients with and without UAP. Because all of these patients died suddenly (some with UAP and some with UAP complicated by AMI), the three ischemic syndromes cannot be analyzed individually.

Davies and associates[18] studied 90 patients who died suddenly outside the hospital within 6 hours of the onset of pain "or other symptoms." The data were presented in a report entitled "Intramyocardial platelet aggregation in patients with unstable angina suffering sudden ischemic cardiac death." Of their 90 patients, 36 (40%) had chest or arm pain at some time in the 2 weeks preceding death. The history of chest pain was obtained by a coroner's police officer from the next of kin who had been living with the patient. Thus, the history was not obtained from the patient or a physician. None of the 90 patients had been admitted to a hospital with increasing chest pain. No information about the presence or absence of chest pain at rest was available for any patient. Thus, in none of the 90 patients was the type, location, or severity of the pain known. Nevertheless, these patients were considered to have had UAP. Necropsy in the 90 patients disclosed the following: 31 (30%) had nonocclusive intracoronary thrombus, 22 (24%) had SCD associated with "regional coagulative necrosis" (AMI), and 23 (25%) had nontransmural necrosis. Of the 36 patients with chest or arm pain at some time in the 2 weeks before death, 35 had plaque rupture identified in one of the major epicardial coronary arteries. Of the 54 without chest pain in the 2 weeks before death, 51 had plaque rupture. Thus, whether the patients in that study had UAP is unknown. Some probably did have UAP, but some clearly had AMI, and most would fulfill most investigators' definition of SCD. Diagnosing UAP in persons not admitted to the hospital and with a history obtained by a nonphysician is difficult to say the least.

Multiluminal vascular channels were present in 90% of the 67 patients studied by Kragel and colleagues.[4] They most likely represented organized thrombus (the consequence of a previous nonfatal thrombotic event) and were usually at a site where the lumen was severely narrowed by plaque. Multiluminal channels were observed in a significantly higher percentage of the 5-mm coronary segments in the patients with UAP than in those with either SCD or AMI.

The lower frequency of plaque rupture and occlusive thrombus in the groups with UAP and SCD than in the group with AMI may be a reflection of differences in plaque composition between these groups. Likewise, the similarity in the frequency of these acute coronary lesions in patients with UAP and SCD may be a reflection of the similarity in plaque composition in these two groups. As described earlier, in all three types of patients, the mean percentage of dense fibrous tissue, calcific deposits, and pultaceous debris increases with increasing degrees of luminal narrowing and the mean percentage of cellular fibrous tissue decreases. Severely narrowed segments in the AMI group (those narrowed >75% in cross-sectional area) contained significantly more pultaceous debris and significantly less calcium and cellular fibrous tissue than did similarly narrowed segments in the UAP and SCD groups. Because occlusive thrombus is almost exclusively found in association with rupture of a lipid-rich plaque, the greater the amount of pultaceous debris, the greater is the frequency of plaque rupture and occlusive thrombus.

The characteristic lesion in patients with a fatal first AMI, then, is an occlusive thrombus overlying a ruptured plaque rich in pultaceous debris; in patients with UAP, it is a severely narrowed segment frequently containing multiluminal channels with or without a small nonocclusive thrombus; in patients with SCD without left ventricular necrosis, it is a segment of coronary artery with significant luminal narrowing by atherosclerotic plaque with or without platelet-rich nonocclusive thrombus. Thus, the frequency of acute coronary lesions (intraluminal thrombus, plaque rupture, and plaque hemorrhage) in patients with UAP (not complicated by AMI) and SCD (not complicated by AMI) is similar, and the frequency of these lesions is significantly lower than that observed in patients with AMI.

References

1. Roberts WC: Qualitative and quantitative comparison of amounts of narrowing by atherosclerotic plaques in the major epicardial coronary arteries at necropsy in sudden death, transmural acute myocardial infarction, transmural healed myocardial infarction and unstable angina pectoris. Am J Cardiol 1989; 64:324–328.
2. Kragel AH, Reddy SG, Wittes JT, et al: Morphometric analysis of the composition of atherosclerotic plaques in the four major epicardial coronary arteries in acute myocardial infarction and in sudden coronary death. Circulation 1989; 80:1747–1756.
3. Kragel AH, Reddy SG, Wittes JT, et al: Morphometric analysis of the composition of coronary arterial plaques in isolated unstable angina pectoris with pain at rest. Am J Cardiol 1990; 66:562–567.
4. Kragel AH, Gertz SD, Roberts WC, et al: Morphologic comparison of frequency and types of acute lesions in the major epicardial coronary arteries in unstable angina pectoris, sudden coronary death and acute myocardial infarction. J Am Coll Cardiol 1991; 18:801–808.
5. Cowley JM, DiSciasco G, Rehr RB, et al: Angiographic observations and clinical relevance of coronary thrombus in unstable angina pectoris. Am J Cardiol 1989; 63:108E–113E.
6. Gotoh K, Minamino T, Katoh O, et al: The role of intracoronary thrombus in unstable angina: Angiographic assessment and thrombolytic therapy during ongoing anginal attacks. Circulation 1988; 77:526–534.

7. Ambrose JA, Winters SL, Stern A, et al: Angiographic morphology and the pathogenesis of unstable angina pectoris. J Am Coll Cardiol 1985; 5:609–616.
8. Vetrovec GW, Leinbach RC, Gold HK, et al: Intracoronary thrombolysis in syndromes of unstable ischemia: Angiographic and clinical results. Am Heart J 1982; 104:946–952.
9. Holmes DR, Hartzler GO, Smith HC, et al: Coronary artery thrombosis in patients with unstable angina. Br Heart J 1981; 45:411–416.
10. Levin DC, Fallon JT: Significance of the angiographic morphology of localized coronary stenoses: Histopathologic correlations. Circulation 1982; 66:316–320.
11. Hombach V, Hoher M, Kochs M, et al: Pathophysiology of unstable angina pectoris: Correlations with angioscopic imaging. Eur Heart J 1988; 9 (Suppl N):40–45.
12. Forrester JS, Litvack F, Grundfest W: A perspective of coronary disease seen through the arteries of living man. Circulation 1987; 75:505–513.
13. Sherman CT, Litvack F, Grundfest W, et al: Coronary angioscopy in patients with unstable angina pectoris. N Engl J Med 1986; 315:913–919.
14. Guthrie RB, Vlodaver Z, Nicoloff DM, et al: Pathology of stable and unstable angina pectoris. Circulation 1975; 51:1059–1063.
15. Roberts WC, Virmani R: Quantification of coronary arterial narrowing in clinically-isolated unstable angina pectoris: An analysis of 22 necropsy patients. Am J Med 1979; 67:792–799.
16. Virmani R, Roberts WC: Extravasated erythrocytes, iron, and fibrin in atherosclerotic plaques in coronary arteries in fatal coronary heart disease and their relation to intraluminal thrombus: frequency and significance in 57 necropsy patients and in 2958 five-mm segments of 224 major epicardial coronary arteries. Am Heart J 1983; 105:788–797.
17. Falk E: Unstable angina with fatal outcome: Dynamic coronary thrombosis leading to infarction and/or sudden death. Circulation 1985; 71:699–708.
18. Davies MJ, Thomas AC, Knapman PA, et al: Intramyocardial platelet aggregation in patients with unstable angina suffering sudden ischemic cardiac death. Circulation 1986; 73:418–427.

CHAPTER 50

Management of Myocardial Infarction

Thomas Killip, MD

ETIOLOGY, PATHOLOGY, PATHOGENESIS

The etiology, pathology, and pathogenesis of myocardial infarction (MI) have been addressed in previous chapters. A brief review is in order, however, because current understanding of these matters has profoundly influenced current therapy. MI is generally a consequence of coronary atherosclerosis. Other causes may be invoked in fewer than 5% of cases, such as coronary spasm induced by drugs (especially cocaine) or of unknown cause, coronary embolization in the presence of aortic valve disease or bacterial endocarditis, or paradoxical embolism in the presence of a flow-patent foramen ovale.

Approximately 50% of patients presenting with first MI have only single-vessel disease. In acute Q wave infarction (transmural infarct characterized by ST segment elevation), the acute ischemia is often triggered by abrupt closure of a coronary artery that had previously been only moderately obstructed.[1] Instability of the atherosclerotic plaque initiates a sequence of events resulting in acute closure due to the thrombus formation.[2] Proliferation of smooth muscle in the media may have a role also.[3] Recognition of the significance of acute arterial occlusion in the development of transmural MI has provided a sound physiologic basis for the current emphasis on prompt treatment, be it thrombolysis or angioplasty, to relieve obstruction and achieve maximum flow in the culprit artery as promptly as possible.

The pathogenesis of acute non–Q wave (nontransmural ST segment depression) acute MI is less clear. Angiographic and pathologic studies suggest that complete occlusion of the culprit coronary artery by thrombus is uncommon.[4] Although thrombosis appears to have a role in the genesis of the infarct in many cases, clinical effectiveness after treatment with thrombolytic agents is less clear cut than with Q wave infarcts.[5] In both transmural and nontransmural MI, the majority of patients develop unstable angina before the acute event—clinical evidence that the process of occlusion, partial or complete, is a progressive event.[6] [In this chapter, the terms *Q wave* and *transmural* or *non–Q wave* and *subendocardial* or *nontransmural* are used interchangeably although it is understood that not all Q wave infarcts are truly transmural, nor are all non–Q wave infarcts only subendocardial.]

With the onset of infarction, time is of the essence if treatment is to be effective. Careful studies of animals as well as observations of humans indicate that within minutes of coronary occlusion, myocardial mitochondria begin to deteriorate. Contractility is sharply reduced in the infarct area, whereas noninvolved myocardium becomes hypercontractile. Myocyte death appears to be inevitable within 2 to 4 hours unless perfusion is restored.[7] In approximately 40% of transmural infarcts, ventricular remodeling develops during the following several weeks as hypercontractile normal myocardium stretches and thins the infarct area, increasing left ventricular wall tension (La Place) and reducing ventricular contractile efficiency.[8] Additionally, metabolic changes in ischemic or infarcted myocardium may trigger potentially lethal ventricular arrhythmia.

During both the acute phase and after recovery, the prognosis of MI is directly related to the volume of left ventricular myocardium infarcted. Studies in the prethrombolytic era documented that survival with 50% or more of infarcted left ventricular mass is unusual whether the damage occurs as one massive insult or a series of small events over time.[9]

DIAGNOSIS

Heart disease is the leading cause of death in the Western world, among both men *and* women.[10] A high index of suspicion must be maintained when any patient older than 35 years complains of persistent chest pain suggesting the possibility of myocardial ischemia lasting more than 20 minutes. After age 50 years, women have a rapidly increasing incidence of heart disease and MI yet may be more reticent in describing symptoms or seeking medical attention.[11] That chest pain in a woman may be due to myocardial ischemia should not be overlooked.

Rapid diagnosis and treatment of patients with acute MI are imperative; the sooner thrombolytic therapy is applied, if indicated, the more likely is myocardium to be salvaged. Physicians and emergency room personnel should have a target of triage, diagnosis, and initiation of the first dose of a thrombolytic agent within 20 to 30 minutes of initial contact. Time to first treatment in MI is an easily measurable index of quality that is the responsibility of all personnel involved.

After immediate and rapid clinical evaluation of a patient complaining of chest pain, an electrocardiogram (ECG) should be promptly obtained. Accuracy of the ECG in diagnosis of MI is influenced by the previous medical history. If the ECG was previously normal, sensitivity and specificity approach 80% to 85%; if the ECG was previously abnormal, and especially if the patient has had multiple past MIs, the diagnostic accuracy of the ECG is much reduced and may be indeterminant.[12]

Although various enzyme assays have been proposed, analysis of creatine kinase (CK) with measurement of the MB fraction has stood the test of time and remains the most widely available and reliable diagnostic tool. Both total CK and CKMB rise above normal values within 6 to 8 hours after infarction, reaching a peak at approximately 30 hours (or earlier after successful thrombolysis).[13] A useful routine is to obtain a CK measurement on first encounter and then every 8 hours for the first 24 hours. For greatest usefulness, it is important to have a responsive laboratory system that can provide a result within 1 to 2 hours of receipt of a specimen.

Chest Pain, Rule Out Myocardial Infarction

A diagnostic dilemma frequently encountered, especially in emergency departments of urban hospitals, is a middle-aged patient, often a woman, complaining of chest pain with atypical features. Although common syndromes often present, many individuals with MI are encountered with atypical features. Because of this, patients with atypical features must be taken seriously and carefully evaluated for the possibility of ischemic heart disease despite the fact that the majority of patients so presenting will prove not to have coronary artery disease. If the initial ECG is normal, the probability of acute MI averages about 3%, although unstable angina cannot be ruled out.[14] The presence or absence of MI can usually be established within 24 hours by triage to a monitoring unit, serial ECGs, CK determination every 8 hours, and judicious treatment of symptoms. If MI is ruled out, the patient can usually be discharged within 24 to 48 hours and further evaluation carried out on an ambulatory basis.

ADMISSION TO HOSPITAL VERSUS HOME TREATMENT

Earlier studies in Great Britain suggested that a proportion of patients with MI at low risk could be safely treated at home.[15] This approach has not found favor in the United States, where practice styles are different because of concern about accurately identifying low-risk patients and the belief that current hospital treatment is effective in limiting myocardial damage and reducing complications in many patients.

PROGNOSIS

Age is the single most important prognostic factor in MI. In patients age 70 or younger, hospital mortality of 3% to 6% has been reported, whereas in patients 85 years or older, the risk is 35% or higher. Although various other prognostic factors have been identified, outcome depends on the amount of left ventricle damage, a combination of acute infarction or scar, and the extent of coronary artery disease.[16] A large infarct with single-vessel coronary disease may be relatively well tolerated, yet a smaller infarction in the presence of old scar and extensive coronary atherosclerosis may be poorly tolerated.

A generation ago, Kimball and the author of this chapter described a simple system for bedside evaluation of left ventricular function based on the presence or absence of pulmonary rales, advanced left ventricular failure, or cardiogenic shock.[17] Despite the crudity of the physiologic evaluation, the classification has stood the test of time. Patients in class I, no evidence of heart failure, have an excellent prognosis. Those in class II, with pulmonary rales suggestive of early left ventricular failure, have a somewhat reduced prognosis. Patients in class III, pulmonary edema, or class IV, cardiogenic shock, have a sharply increased mortality. Indeed, cardiogenic shock remains a difficult therapeutic problem with minimal evidence of improved treatment during the past two decades. Evaluation of patients with MI on a daily basis according to our simple scheme provides useful prognostic information.

TREATMENT

Treatment is designed to (1) relieve symptoms, (2) limit the extent of myocardial damage, (3) reduce cardiac work and hence reverse ischemia, and (4) manage complications. About half of the mortality of acute MI occurs within the first 4 to 6 hours. Thus, management in an acute-care setting during the first few hours is critical. The most common factor limiting early treatment is denial. Although there is widespread public awareness of the significance of chest pain as a symptom of heart attack, delay in seeking medical aid is all too common, especially among women. Studies have shown that older women who live alone or are the functioning head of household often delay seeking medical help, with potentially severe consequences.[11] Because the major cause of early mortality is primary ventricular fibrillation—ventricular fibrillation occurring without significant premonitory ventricular ectopic beats—access to a monitoring unit as early as possible is essential.

Pain

The initial discomfort of MI may be agonizingly severe. Morphine, 2 to 4 mg IV, repeated as needed, is often highly effective in treating the pain of MI. Morphine has adverse effects, including respiratory depression, some decrease in myocardial contractility, bradycardia, and vasodilatation, so the response of the patient must be closely watched. The hypotensive effect of morphine often responds to simple elevation of the lower extremities. The ischemic pain of MI may also be relieved by nitroglycerin, which may be administered sublingually (0.4 mg repeated once or twice as necessary), followed by continuous intravenous drip if required (discussed later).

Oxygen

Increased left ventricular filling pressure consequent to myocardial dysfunction of acute MI raises pulmonary venous pressure, increases the work of breathing, and reduces pulmonary capillary oxygen tension and partial pressure of arterial oxygen. Hence, treatment with oxygen administered via nasal prongs at a rate of 4 to 6 L/min is reasonable for the first 36 to 48 hours in uncomplicated MI. More profound left ventricular dysfunction with pulmonary congestion may require more efficient means of oxygen delivery.

Aspirin and Platelet Dysfunction

Several studies have documented an association between increased platelet aggregability and coronary atherosclerosis.[18] Phasic alterations in platelet function correlate with the circadian rhythm for occurrence of MI in the waking hours and have been used to identify patients at high risk for recurrent ischemia or extension of infarction.

The Second International Study of Infarct Survival (ISIS-II) conclusively demonstrated that 162.5 mg of enteric coated aspirin administered immediately to patients with MI reduced hospital mortality by 23% compared with placebo.[19] The initial results have been confirmed and extended by other studies using aspirin in combination with various thrombolytic agents. Hence, all patients with suspected MI should receive aspirin in at least this dose immediately, chewed and swallowed for rapid effect, on first encounter and daily thereafter. Aspirin acetylates platelet cyclooxygenase for the life of the platelet, blocking synthesis of certain prostacyclines, especially thromboxane A_2, thus inhibiting aggregation in vivo. Doses less than 162.5 mg take several days to become effective and are probably less useful. Doses higher than 325 mg daily may produce adverse effects.

Restoration of Coronary Flow

DeWood and colleagues' angiographic demonstration that transmural MI is characterized by total coronary occlusion with subsequent spontaneous thrombolysis has been amply confirmed by subsequent studies.[20] Laboratory and clinical evidence supports the axiom that prompt restoration of coronary flow to the obstructed culprit artery preserves myocardium and reduces mortality in acute transmural MI. Flow may be restored mechanically or by treatment with thrombolytic agents. The currently available thrombolytic agents—streptokinase, urokinase, tissue plasminogen activator (t-PA), and anistreplase—effectively lyse coronary thrombi in patients with arterial occlusion. Issues currently debated are the choice of thrombolytic agent and the usefulness and route of administration of heparin.

Clinical trials have established that thrombolytic therapy reduces mortality, averaging about 25% overall, and salvages myocardium in patients with suspected acute MI characterized by ST segment elevation or bundle branch block, either right or left, on the initial ECG. The earlier the thrombolysin is administered, the greater the mortality reduction.[20a] Maximum effect—a 50% mortality reduction—was observed in GISSI-I (Gruppo Italiano per lo Studio della Supravivenza nel Infarcto Miocardico) when streptokinase was given within 1 hour of onset of symptoms.[21] Clear-cut effects are evident up to 6 hours and perhaps as long as 12 hours after onset of infarction. It was initially thought that mortality improvement was confined to anterior Q wave infarcts, but more recent analysis indicates improved mortality in inferior-posterior transmural infarcts also, although the gain is less striking.

Complications of thrombolysis are primarily related to bleeding, cerebral and locally at puncture sites. The incidence of cerebral hemorrhage averages about 3 to 6 per 1000 patients treated and has consistently been slightly higher in women and in trials involving t-PA. Thrombolysis converts an ischemic MI into a hemorrhagic infarct. Analysis of large trials has identified a slightly higher incidence of myocardial rupture and severe ventricular dysfunction, especially among the elderly, after administration of thrombolytic agents.[22] Fortunately, however, complications of thrombolysis are uncommon and the risk-benefit ratio remains favorable.

Three large clinical trials—GISSI-II,[23] ISIS-III,[24] and GUSTO-I (Global Utilization of Streptokinase and Tissue Plasminogen Activator to Treat Occluded Arteries)[25]—have compared the effectiveness of different thrombolytic agents. In GISSI-II and its international study extension, 20,891 patients with acute MI were randomized within 6 hours of onset of symptoms to either streptokinase (1.5 million units over 30–60 min) or t-PA (alteplase, 100 mg over 3 h). All patients received 325 mg of aspirin daily and were randomized to heparin (12,500 units SC twice daily) or to no heparin. No significant differences were noted in total mortality between t-PA and streptokinase and heparin or no heparin.

ISIS-III compared t-PA, streptokinase, and anisoylated plasminogen activator complex (APSAC). More than 41,000 patients were randomized. All patients received 162.5 mg of aspirin daily and were randomized to receive subcutaneous heparin (12,500 units SC twice daily) or no heparin. No advantage for heparin was observed. No mortality differences were noted among the three thrombolytic agents, and aside from a slight decrease in the reinfarction rate with patients receiving t-PA, no differences were found in the complication rates.

Many observers found these reports satisfying, because there is considerable cost differential among the agents. Streptokinase is relatively inexpensive, whereas t-PA costs six to seven times more. The studies suggested there was no need to use the more expensive agents.

The effective duration of action of t-PA is only about 5 to 10 minutes. Proponents have argued that in several trials, the dose was too low and that furthermore, intravenous heparin in proper dosage is required to maintain optimal patency of the infarct artery after t-PA–induced thrombolysis. The GUSTO trial was designed to determine whether the rapidity of return to coronary artery patency influenced mortality. Patients receiving "accelerated"* doses of t-PA and intravenous heparin with an anterior MI treated early had a 20% reduction in mortality compared with streptokinase. GUSTO also noted that intravenous heparin was not more effective than subcutaneous heparin in the streptokinase arm of the trial.

An angiographic substudy of GUSTO reported that culprit artery patency 90 minutes after therapy was highest in patients treated with t-PA and intravenous heparin.[26] Patients with open arteries had greater improvement in left ventricular function and lower mortality at 30 days. Interestingly, although the patency rate at 90 minutes was highest in the t-PA and heparin subset of patients, by 180 minutes, patency in all groups was similar, suggesting that the earlier the artery is opened, the better the prognosis. An open artery early after onset of symptoms appears to limit infarct size and improve mortality.

What does a practicing physician conclude from the multiple studies available? The following is a reasonable summary: (1) Effective thrombolysis reduces mortality and salvages myocardium in transmural MI by restoring coronary flow. (2) The sooner a patient is treated, the better the outcome. (3) Thrombolysis appears to be effective until at least 12 hours after onset of infarction. (4) An accelerated dose of t-PA combined with closely monitored intravenous heparin appears to be somewhat more effective than streptokinase with subcutaneous or intravenous heparin. (5) Complications of thrombolysis are mainly bleeding, both cranial and at puncture sites. (6) Tissue plasminogen activator has had a slightly higher risk of intracranial bleeds than the other agents, with an incidence averaging less than 1%. (7) Women appear to have a slightly higher risk of intracranial bleed. (8) Allergic reactions to streptokinase are rare, but second courses of treatment with this agent should probably be avoided.

Experience to date strongly supports the view that thrombolytic therapy should be offered to all patients strongly suspected of having acute transmural MI regardless of elec-

*Accelerated t-PA = IV bolus of 15 mg, then 0.75 mg/kg body weight over 30 minutes (maximum dose 50 mg) then 0.5 mg/kg over 60 minutes (maximum dose 35 mg).

trocardiographic location, in older patients perhaps up to age 80 years and older, and to those with a clinical syndrome suggesting infarction with a nondiagnostic ECG because of bundle branch block.

Heparin

Intravenous heparin is clearly effective in the management of unstable angina. In the United States, intravenous heparin is widely used in the management of MI, whereas in Europe, heparin is either not used or is administered subcutaneously, generally in a dose of 12,500 units twice daily. Early in the evaluation of thrombolytic agents, it was shown that intravenous heparin maintained a somewhat higher patency rate 24 hours or later after thrombolysis with t-PA. When streptokinase is the agent, no advantage for intravenous heparin can be demonstrated. The ISIS-III trial showed some modest advantage of heparin and aspirin over aspirin alone in the treatment of acute MI, but at the price of a small but medically important increase in the number and extent of bleeding episodes.[24] The GUSTO trial showed no advantage of streptokinase with intravenous heparin over standard doses of streptokinase with subcutaneous heparin.[25] As mentioned earlier, the accelerated t-PA protocol combined with prompt intravenous heparin in GUSTO revealed a mortality advantage, albeit small, over a standard dose regimen of streptokinase with subcutaneous heparin. Thus, despite a strong tradition for use of intravenous heparin in the management of acute MI, especially in the United States, there appears to be no advantage in combination with streptokinase but modest improvement in survival when combined with t-PA. Heparin therapy has many drawbacks, and other antithrombotic agents are under continued clinical and experimental evaluation.[25a]

Coronary Angiography and Angioplasty

In patients who are considered a good risk, after treatment with a thrombolytic agent, subsequent angiography and associated angioplasty do not contribute to further reduction in mortality when carried out in the first few hours after treatment.[27] If the principle of treatment is to open the occluded artery and restore coronary flow, why not do it immediately by mechanical means?[27–29a] Enthusiasts claim that restoration of flow during angiography is quicker, more effective, and potentially cheaper than thrombolysis and has a low rate of complication. It is unlikely that it can be quicker, because thrombolysis can and should be administered within a few minutes of a patient's arrival in the emergency department. Gearing up the catheterization laboratory and carrying out the procedure may take two or three times longer. In selected patients in certain institutions, immediate angioplasty appears to be a reasonable alternative to noninvasive treatment with thrombolytic agents. The problem is that it is simply not possible to maintain a nationwide network of skilled angiographers together with laboratory personnel on standby around the clock to provide this form of treatment to the population in need.

A number of anecdotal reports have convincingly documented the apparent effectiveness of angioplasty in patients who have massive infarction accompanied by cardiogenic shock and who appear to be moribund. Stabilization with the intra-aortic pulsating balloon or similar devices followed by angioplasty appears to have rescued jeopardized myocardium, restored reasonable myocardial function, and improved mortality in some moribund patients.[30]

Noninvasive therapy can quickly be made available at all hospitals. The challenge is to ensure that physicians and their associates diagnose MI quickly and initiate proper treatment as soon as possible. Increased public awareness of the importance of seeking medical attention when symptoms suggest the possibility of a heart attack is necessary. Limited trials are under way to evaluate the next step: Provide treatment outside the hospital. The ECG can be faxed from the ambulance to the dispatch center, symptoms and physical examination described via radio or telephone to a regional center, and a judgment made by an experienced physician about whether thrombolysis is indicated. Because time is of the essence, even a 30-minute advantage would likely translate into myocardium protected and mortality reduced.

Beta-Adrenergic Blockers

Beta-adrenergic blockade decreases heart rate, blood pressure, and cardiac work, with a consequent reduction in myocardial oxygen consumption. These agents also lower blood free fatty acids, possibly having a beneficial effect on cardiac arrhythmia. Results of randomized trials evaluating intravenous β-blockers early in MI have been variable. ISIS-I demonstrated a 15% reduction in mortality when intravenous atenolol was administered on average 5 hours after onset of MI.[31] Other studies have showed less certain results, but the trends have been favorable.[32]

Given these results, it is reasonable to recommend acute administration of a β-adrenergic blocker in treating acute MI, at least in patients with evidence of heightened sympathetic activity characterized by unexplained tachycardia or hypertension in the absence of contraindications such as heart failure or asthma. A useful regimen is metropolol, 5 mg IV every 2 to 4 minutes for three doses. If the drug is well tolerated, 50 mg PO is given every 12 hours, beginning 15 minutes after the last intravenous dose. The oral medication is continued for 48 hours and then changed to 100 mg daily as a single dose. Heart rate and blood pressure should be closely monitored, and the dosage adjusted if bradycardia or hypotension develops.

Nitrates

Nitrates decrease blood pressure, improve or reverse ischemia, and relieve cardiac pain. In addition, they may stabilize abnormal cardiac rhythm. The evidence suggests that nitrates may also reduce infarct size but do not reduce mortality.[23, 33] Intravenous nitroglycerin is often useful in the early treatment of evolving MI if the dose is carefully monitored and systolic blood pressure is not reduced more than 20 to 30 mm Hg. The possibility of right ventricular infarction, a frequent complication of inferior-posterior infarction, should be carefully evaluated before administration of nitroglycerin, because the drug's effect on the capacitance system may sharply reduce ventricular inflow, resulting in profound hypotension.

Nitroglycerin may be administered initially in the emergency room sublingually one to three times in a standard dose of 0.3 mg per tablet. Intravenous nitroglycerin is often initiated at a rate of 5 to 10 μg/min, and the dose increased by 5 to 10 μg every few minutes until the desired response is achieved.

Calcium Antagonists

Although useful in the management of hypertension, calcium antagonists have not been shown to reduce mortality in acute MI.[34] Diltiazem appears to have a modest long-term beneficial effect in some patients in the absence of heart failure but is associated with increased mortality in the presence of pulmonary congestion due to left ventricular failure.[35]

Glucose-Potassium-Insulin

Extensive literature describes the metabolic effects of various combinations of glucose, potassium, and insulin in MI in both experimental animals and humans.[36] Although improvements in ventricular function, reduction of cardiac arrhythmia, and favorable alterations of plasma fatty acids have been described, no randomized clinical trials have been carried out to demonstrate a mortality advantage.

Angiotensin-Converting Enzyme Inhibitors

In acute transmural MI, especially in anterior infarcts, ventricular remodeling with thinning and ballooning of the infarct segment inducing progressive ventricular enlargement and dysfunction occurs in as many as 40% of patients. The classic end result of this process, although uncommon, is ventricular aneurysm. Several clinical trials have clearly demonstrated that administration of angiotensin-converting enzyme inhibitors beginning 12 to 36 hours after onset of infarction can prevent or retard this process, with consequent preservation of ventricular function.[23, 37] Thus, serious consideration should be given to treating patients with a Q wave infarct, especially a large anterior infarct, with an angiotensin-converting enzyme inhibitor commencing within 1 to 2 days after admission.

Magnesium

Low serum magnesium levels potentiate ventricular arrhythmia. Several small clinical trials have suggested that administration of magnesium improved mortality after infarction.[38] However, a large randomized trial failed to document a mortality advantage for treatment with magnesium, and its routine use is not recommended.*

MYOCARDIAL STUNNING AND HIBERNATION

Two possible consequences of prolonged ventricular dysfunction—myocardial stunning and myocardial hibernation—have attracted considerable attention. In myocardial stunning, a contraction abnormality persists for a time after an episode of ischemia despite restoration of flow.[39] The hypocontractile state responds to positive inotropic drugs and is thought to be secondary to excess cytosolic calcium released from sarcoplasmic reticulum damaged by oxygen-derived free radicals. Stunning has been extensively investigated in experimental animals and probably occurs in humans in a number of situations, such as after thrombolysis following MI, after cardiopulmonary bypass, and possibly after exercise-induced ischemia.

Hibernating myocardium is defined as "persistent contractile dysfunction that is associated with reduced coronary flow but preserved myocardial viability."[39] The dysfunction is reversed when coronary flow is restored. Improved ventricular function has been observed after coronary bypass surgery and angioplasty in the apparent absence of recent ischemia, suggesting that hibernating myocardium had responded to revascularization. Clearly, unrecognized recurrent ischemia could induce changes in left ventricular function simulating hibernation.

Documenting the presence of stunned or hibernating myocardium or differentiating between the two conditions may be difficult clinically. These concepts imply, however, that not all ventricular dysfunction in patients with coronary artery disease is necessarily irreversible. Positron emission tomography scanning has been advanced as a diagnostic modality that can identify poorly functioning but viable myocardium to assist a clinician in evaluating whether revascularization in the presence of apparent chronic ventricular dysfunction might lead to significant contractile improvement.[40]

COMPLICATIONS OF MYOCARDIAL INFARCTION

Arrhythmia

During the first few days after MI, some arrhythmia is almost universal. Supraventricular arrhythmia including atrial tachycardia, atrial flutter, and atrial fibrillation occurs in about 5% of cases, similar to the incidence in the normal population. Patients with a previous history of heart failure and dilated left atrium are somewhat more likely to have a bout of atrial fibrillation or flutter. Treatment is generally focused on controlling heart rate. Intravenous β-blockers such as atenolol, esmolol, or metropolol may be given. Intravenous metropolol may be administered in doses of 5 mg every 3 to 5 minutes for three doses to slow the rate to an acceptable level, followed by oral doses as outlined earlier. If the rate is rapid and there is evidence of hemodynamic compromise, immediate direct-current cardioversion is indicated. Direct-current conversion is not applied routinely, however, because the atrial arrhythmia usually recurs in the first day or two. Spontaneous conversion to sinus rhythm after a few days is the rule.

First-degree heart block and Wenckebach's phenomenon commonly accompany posterior infarction in the first few hours after onset. These abnormalities are generally self-limited and subside within a few hours. If the ventricular rate slows because of excessive block, atropine in doses of 0.5 mg IV may be cautiously administered to a total dose of 1 to 2 mg. Complete heart block with a slow ventricular response usually denotes massive MI and is an ominous sign. Treatment with an intravenous pacemaker should be initiated, but technical problems not uncommonly occur, related in part to the difficulty of placing the pacemaker catheter in uninvolved ventricular muscle.

Ventricular arrhythmias are extremely common in the first 48 to 72 hours of MI. Within the first few hours of infarction, primary ventricular fibrillation may occur. Although the incidence of primary fibrillation appears to have declined during the past decade, this rhythm is the major immediate cause of the high early mortality in the first few hours after the onset of symptoms. The decreased occurrence may relate to changes in lifestyle, especially the decline in cigarette smoking among men, widespread use of β-blockers in patients with ischemic heart disease, the use of aspirin, and perhaps other measures.

Almost all patients with MI have some ventricular arrhythmia during the first 72 hours of monitoring. Many authorities have advocated the use of prophylactic lidocaine intravenously to prevent serious arrhythmia during the first 2 or 3 days of hospitalization. A review of clinical trials fails to show an advantage to prophylactic lidocaine.[41] Although it somewhat decreases the incidence of ventricular tachycardia or ventricular fibrillation, mortality due to all causes appears to be somewhat higher in patients receiving prophylactic lidocaine. Thus, treatment of ventricular arrhyth-

*Peer-reviewed published manuscript not available at this time.

mia on demand rather than prophylactic therapy is currently recommended.

Intravenous lidocaine is effective in the management of the majority of ventricular arrhythmias encountered as a complication of acute MI. An initial bolus of 1 mg/kg may be followed after 3 to 5 minutes by two subsequent doses of ½ mg/kg. When the arrhythmia responds to the acute dose, an intravenous drip of 3 mg/min is initiated. The infusion rate may be adjusted upward with additional intravenous boluses of drug or downward, depending on the response. Procainamide is also useful for both acute and long-term treatment of ventricular arrhythmia. In recurrent malignant arrhythmia, bretylium or amiodarone may be effective. It should be noted, however, that recurrent ventricular arrhythmia usually reflects ongoing ischemia in an unstable situation. Immediate revascularization may be an effective course of action.

Right Ventricular Infarction

Involvement of the right ventricle occurs in about 30% to 50% of posterior-inferior infarcts.[42] Loss of right ventricular propulsion is characterized by hypotension, low pulmonary capillary wedge pressure reflecting inadequate left ventricular filling, and intolerance of hypotensive agents such as nitroglycerin. Right ventricular infarct may be diagnosed with a high degree of certainty by examination of the QRS complex in V_{4R}. In patients who present with inferior infarction and hypotension, measurement of pulmonary artery and pulmonary capillary wedge pressure with the Swan-Ganz technique may be required to distinguish left ventricular forward failure or incipient cardiogenic shock, hypovolemia, or right ventricular infarction. In the presence of low capillary wedge pressure, administration of a volume load is helpful. In hypovolemia, volume administration should increase systemic pressure with maintenance of normal right ventricular hemodynamics. In right ventricular infarction, a high right ventricular filling pressure must be supported by administration of excess volume to maintain adequate left ventricular filling pressures.

Cardiogenic Shock

Although the incidence of cardiogenic shock appears to have declined during the past decade, mortality remains high, 75% or greater. Cardiogenic shock is almost always a reflection of infarction greater than 50% of left ventricular mass as a result of either a single acute event or a combination of old and new infarctions. Drug therapy with alpha or beta agonists may be temporarily effective. Dopamine is given intravenously with infusion rates of 0.5 to 1 $\mu g \cdot kg^{-1} \cdot min^{-1}$, and the dose gradually increased until a satisfactory response or a maximum infusion rate of 10 $\mu g \cdot kg^{-1} \cdot min^{-1}$ has been achieved. Higher doses induce vasoconstriction, which is deleterious. Dobutamine is most effective when the hypotension is secondary to low cardiac output. Dopamine and dobutamine are sometimes combined in parallel infusions. An intra-aortic counterpulsating balloon may provide temporary left ventricular assistance but does little to remedy the cause. Anecdotal evidence suggests that immediate revascularization by direct intracoronary thrombolysis, angioplasty, or emergency coronary artery bypass has been successful in some cases of refractory cardiogenic shock.[42] If facilities are available to attempt revascularization, it is helpful first to support the circulation and stabilize the patient by inserting an intra-aortic counterpulsating balloon or some other temporary ventricular assist device.

Mural Thrombus

Ventricular thrombus develops in about 30% of patients with apical-anterior transmural MI. In patients at risk, it is reasonable to obtain an echocardiogram between the third and fifth day. If thrombus is present, intravenous heparin is given for several days, followed by warfarin (Coumadin) therapy for 3 months. Serial echocardiography is used to monitor the status of the thrombus and guide the discontinuance of anticoagulants.

Pericarditis

A transient friction rub is not uncommon in the first few days after transmural MI. Surprisingly, thrombolytic therapy does not increase the incidence of hemorrhagic pericardial effusion, a rare complication of MI in the preanticoagulant era. The pericarditis is generally self-limited, although the symptoms may be confused with recurrent ischemia or peptic ulcer disease. If rub and pericardial pain are persistent, treatment with a nonsteroidal anti-inflammatory agent such as indomethacin may be useful.

PROGNOSIS AFTER MYOCARDIAL INFARCTION

Patients with uncomplicated MI may generally be discharged from the hospital in 7 to 10 days or even less. Long-term prognosis is influenced by the extent of coronary artery disease, preservation of left ventricular function, age, and coexisting morbid factors such as diabetes or the potential for malignant arrhythmia. After discharge, aspirin (165–325 mg daily) should be continued to reduce mortality and the risk of subsequent reinfarction.[43] Prophylactic administration of β-adrenergic blockers reduces postinfarct mortality by 20% to 30%, although the possible benefit in low-risk patients is controversial.[32] Maximum benefit occurs during the first year. Calcium channel blockers have not been shown to reduce postinfarct mortality in randomized clinical trials, although diltiazem may be of benefit in some low-risk groups with preserved left ventricular function.[35] Patients with ventricular extrasystoles do not benefit from treatment with class I antiarrhythmics; indeed, randomized trials suggest that mortality is actually increased.[44] Sustained ventricular tachycardia or recurrent cardiac arrest may require treatment with amiodarone or an implantable defibrillator.

Identification and modification of risk factors is a major component of postinfarct treatment.[43] Cessation of smoking, management of hypertension, and normalization of cholesterol abnormality improve outcome. Increasing evidence that successful cholesterol reduction retards progression and to some extent influences regression of atherosclerotic obstructive lesions should motivate both patients and doctors to maintain effective lipid-lowering therapy after infarction.[45] As mentioned earlier, angiotensin-converting enzyme inhibitors reduce ventricular modeling, especially in patients with large anterior transmural MI. When indicated, these drugs should be continued for at least a year after the initial attack.

Symptom-limited exercise testing can be performed safely within the first month after infarction and in some cases even before discharge from the hospital.[43, 45] Exercise testing provides important information about exercise capacity, blood pressure response, and the presence of reversible myocardial ischemia or arrhythmia. An abnormal result carries an adverse prognosis and may suggest the need for further studies to evaluate the presence of critical coronary artery obstruction. Revascularization may be indicated in the presence of continued ischemic symptoms or abnormal exercise response.

References

1. Davies MJ, Woolf N, Robertson WB: Pathology of acute myocardial infarction with particular reference to occlusive coronary thrombi. Br Heart J 1976; 38:659.
2. Fuster V, Badimon L, Badimon JJ, et al: The pathogenesis of coronary artery disease and the acute coronary synchromes. N Engl J Med 1992; 326:242–250, 310–318.
3. Flugelman MY, Virmani R, Correa R, et al: Smooth muscle cell abundance and fibroblast growth factors in coronary lesions of patients with nonfatal unstable angina. Circulation 1993; 88:2493–2500.
4. Buja LM, Willerson JT: Clinicopathologic correlates of acute ischemic heart syndromes. Am J Cardiol 1981; 47:343.
5. Simoons ML, Vos J, Tijssen JGP, et al: Long term benefit of early thrombolytic therapy in patients with acute myocardial infarction: 5 year follow-up of a trial conducted by The Interuniversity Cardiology Institute of the Netherlands. J Am Coll Cardiol 1989; 14:1609–1615.
6. Solomon H, Edwards A, Killip T: Prodromata in acute myocardial infarction. Circulation 1969; 40:463.
7. Jennings RB, Ganote CE: Structural changes in myocardium during acute ischemia. Circ Res 1974; 35(Suppl 3):156.
8. Pfeffer MA, Braunwald E: Ventricular remodeling after myocardial infarction. Circulation 1990; 81:1161.
9. Alonso DR, Scheidt S, Post M, et al: Pathophysiology of cardiogenic shock; quantification of myocardial necrosis, clinical, pathologic and electrocardiographic correlation. Circulation 1973; 48:588.
10. Wenger NK, Speroff L, Packard B: Cardiovascular health and disease in women. N Engl J Med 1993; 329:247–256.
11. Chesney MA: Behavioral barriers to cardiovascular health in women. *In*: Cardiovascular Health and Disease in Women. Proceedings of an NHLBI Conference. Wenger NK, Speroff L, Packard B (Eds). Greenwich, CT, Le Jacq Communications, 1993.
12. Cooperating investigators from the MILIS study group: Electrocardiographic, enzymatic and scintigraphic criteria of acute myocardial infarction as determined from a study of 726 patients (MILIS study). Am J Cardiol 1985; 55:1463.
13. Lee TH, Goldman L: Serum enzyme assays in the diagnosis of acute myocardial infarction. Recommendations based on a quantitative analysis. Ann Intern Med 1986; 105:221.
14. Rovan GW, Lee TH, Cook EF, et al: Clinical characteristics and outcome of acute myocardial infarction in patients with initially normal or nonspecific electrocardiograms. Am J Cardiol 1989; 64:1087–1092.
15. Hill JD, Hampton JR, Mitchell JRA: A randomized trial of home-versus-hospital management for patients with suspected myocardial infarction. Lancet 1978; 1:837.
16. Norris RM, Barnaby PF, Brandt PWT, et al: Prognosis after recovery from first acute myocardial infarction: Determinants of reinfarction and sudden death. Am J Cardiol 1984; 53:408.
17. Killip T, Kimball JT: Treatment of myocardial infarction in a coronary care unit. A two year experience with 250 patients. Am J Cardiol 1967; 20:457.
18. Coller BS: Platelets and thrombolytic therapy. N Engl J Med 1990; 322:33–42.
19. ISIS-2 Collaborative Group: Randomized trial of intravenous streptokinase, oral aspirin, both, or neither among 17, 187 cases of suspected acute myocardial infarction: ISIS-2. Lancet 1988; 8607:349–360.
20. DeWood MA, Spores J, Notske R, et al: Prevalence of total coronary occlusion during early hours of transmural myocardial infarction. N Engl J Med 1980; 303:897–902.

20a. Fibrinolytic Therapy Trialists' (FTT) Collaborative Group: Indications for fibrinolytic therapy in suspected acute myocardial infarction: Collaborative overview of early mortality and major morbidity results from all randomised trials of more than 1000 patients. Lancet 1994; 343:311–322.

21. GISSI: Effectiveness of intravenous thrombolytic treatment in acute myocardial infarction. Lancet 1986; 1:397–401.
22. Honan MB, Harrell FE, Reimer KA, et al: Cardiac rupture, mortality and the timing of thrombolytic therapy: A meta-analysis. J Am Coll Cardiol 1990; 16:359.
23. Gruppo Italiano per lo Studio della Sopravvivenza nell'Infarcto Miocardico, GISSI-2: A factorial randomized trial of alteplase versus streptokinase and heparin versus no heparin among 12,490 patients with acute myocardial infarction. Lancet 1990; 336:65–71.
24. ISIS-3 Collaborative Group. ISIS-3: A randomized comparison of streptokinase versus tissue plasminogen activator versus anistreplase and of aspirin plus heparin versus aspirin alone among 41,299 cases of suspected acute myocardial infarction. Lancet 1992; 339:753–770.
25. The GUSTO Investigators: An international randomized trial comparing four thrombolytic strategies for acute myocardial infarction. N Engl J Med 1993; 329:673–682.

25a. Cannon CP, McCabe CH, Henry TD, et al: A pilot trial of recombinant desulfatohirudin compared with heparin in conjunction with tissue-type plasminogen activator and aspirin for acute myocardial infarction: Results of the thrombolysis in myocardial infarction (TIMI) 5 trial. J Am Coll Cardiol 1994; 23:993–1003.

26. The GUSTO Angiographic Investigators: The effects of tissue plasminogen activator, streptokinase or both on coronary artery patency, ventricular functions, and survival after acute myocardial infarction. N Engl J Med 1993; 329:1615–1622.
27. The TIMI Study Group: Comparison of invasive and conservative strategies after treatment with intravenous tissue plasminogen activator in acute myocardial infarction. N Engl J Med 1989; 320:618–622.
28. Gibbons RJ, Holmes DR, Reeder GS, et al: Immediate angioplasty compared with the administration of a thrombolytic agent followed by conservative treatment for myocardial infarction. N Engl J Med 1993; 328:685–691.
29. Grines CL, Browne KF, Marco J, et al: A comparison of immediate angioplasty with thrombolytic therapy for acute myocardial infarction. N Engl J Med 1993; 328:673–679.

29a. De Boer MJ, Hoorntje JCA, Ottervanger JP, et al: Immediate coronary angioplasty versus intravenous streptokinase in acute myocardial infarction: Left ventricular ejection fraction, hospital mortality and reinfarction. J Am Coll Cardiol 1994; 23:1004–1008.

30. Lee L, Bates ER, Pitt B, et al: Percutaneous transluminal coronary angioplasty improves survival in acute myocardial infarction complicated by cardiogenic shock. Circulation 1988; 78:1345.
31. ISIS-1 Collaborative Group: Randomized trial of intravenous atenolol among 16,027 cases of unsuspected acute myocardial infarction: ISIS-1. Lancet 1986; 8498:57–66.
32. Yusuf S, Peto R, Lewis J, et al: Betablockade during and after myocardial infarction: An overview of the randomized trials. Prog Cardiovasc Dis 1985; 27:335–371.
33. Yusuf S, Collins R, MacMahon S, et al: Effect of IV nitrates on mortality in acute myocardial infarction: An overview of the randomized trials. Lancet 1988; 1:1088–1092.
34. Held PH, Yusuf S, Furberg CD: Calcium channel blockers in acute myocardial infarction and unstable angina: An overview. Br Med J 1989; 299:1187.
35. Multicenter Diltiazem Post-Infarction Research Group: The effect of diltiazem on mortality and reinfarction after acute myocardial infarction. N Engl J Med 1988; 319:385–392.
36. Oliver MF, Opie LH: Effects of glucose and fatty acids on myocardial ischemia and arrhythmias. Lancet 1994; 343:155–158.
37. Pfeffer MA, Braunwald E, Moye LA, et al: Effect of captopril on mortality and morbidity in patients with left ventricular dysfunction after myocardial infarction. Results of the survival and ventricular enlargement trial. N Engl J Med 1992; 327:669–677.
38. Yusuf S, Teo K, Woods K: Intravenous magnesium in acute myocardial infarction: An effective, safe, simple and inexpensive intervention. Circulation 1993; 87:2043–2046.
39. Bolli R: Myocardial stunning in man. Circulation 1992; 86:1671–1690.
40. Tillisch J, Brunken R, Marschall R, et al: Reversibility of cardiac wall motion abnormalities predicted by positron tomography. N Engl J Med 1986; 314:884–888.

41. Hine LK, Laird N, Hewitt P, et al: Meta-analysis evidence against prophylactic use of Lidocaine in acute myocardial infarction. Arch Intern Med 1989; 149:2694–2698.
42. Zehender M, Kasper W, Kander E, et al: Right ventricular infarction as an independent predictor of prognosis after acute inferior infarction. N Engl J Med 1993; 328:982–988.
43. Moss AJ, Benhorin J: Prognosis and management after a first myocardial infarction. N Engl J Med 1990; 322:743–753.
44. Teo KK, Yusuf S, Furberg CD: Effects of prophylactic antiarrhythmic drug therapy in acute myocardial infarction. JAMA 1993; 270:1589–1595.
45. Jain A, Myers H, Sapin P, et al: Comparison of symptom-limited and low level exercise tolerance tests early after myocardial infarction. J Am Coll Cardiol 1993; 22:1816–1820.

CHAPTER 51

Thrombolytic Therapy in Acute Myocardial Infarction

Nils U. Bang, MD

After 30 years of clinical trials with thrombolytic agents in acute myocardial infarction (MI),[1,2] much accelerated during the past decade,[3] the beneficial effect of this therapy is firmly established. In the majority of patients given tissue plasminogen activator (t-PA), the infarct-related artery is reperfused. Streptokinase (SK) also produces reperfusion, particularly when given very soon after the acute occlusion. SK and t-PA have been shown to reduce infarct size, improve myocardial performance, and reduce at least immediate and probably late mortality in MI. However, serious issues about thrombolytic therapy in acute MI remain. Successful thrombolysis is achieved with agents or combinations of agents that provide the highest rate of reperfusion with the lowest rate of reocclusion and the lowest rate of bleeding complications. During the past 5 to 10 years, we have seen a progression of increasingly successful outcomes, not via breakthroughs of new therapies but rather through optimizing existing regimens. On this basis, we can at this time establish some basic principles to which most cardiologists engaging in thrombolytic therapy will subscribe. We must also realize, however, that the introduction of new adjunctive agents may well change current recommendations within a very short time. Thus, this chapter has two aims: to provide readers with an up-to-date account of current recommendations for thrombolytic and adjunctive therapy in acute MI and to give a brief account of promising agents currently in clinical trial and likely to replace the agents recommended at this time.

CURRENT DATA BASE

Time to Reperfusion

The thrombolysis in myocardial infarction (TIMI-I) group[4] demonstrated that when t-PA was given at 100 mg over 3 hours (60, 20, and 20 mg/h after an initial bolus of 6 mg), reperfusion rates of 24% at 30 minutes, 57% at 60 minutes, and 71% at 90 minutes were obtained. When the dose was increased to 150 mg, earlier reperfusion was obtained in more patients (42% at 30 min, 68% at 60 min, and 76% at 90 min). Unfortunately, the incidence of intracranial hemorrhage at this high dose was subsequently observed in TIMI-II to be 1.6%,[5] more than twice that with the 100-mg dose. The higher dose was thus abandoned. TIMI-I[4] also demonstrated that SK given in the currently approved dose of 1.5 million units over 1 hour resulted in substantially lower reperfusion rates compared with t-PA at 30 minutes (8%), 60 minutes (23%), and 90 minutes (31%). It should be pointed out, however, that in TIMI-I, the interval between onset of symptoms and start of treatment averaged 4.7 hours. Although such delays in therapy do not affect reperfusion rates with t-PA, the efficacy of SK is profoundly reduced. Thus, in TIMI-I, the 90% reperfusion rate for patients treated with SK within 4 hours of the symptoms was twice that for patients treated after more than 4 hours.[4] It is clear that faster reperfusion of the infarct-related artery is beneficial. Both the empiric observation that thrombolytic therapy administered within the first hour of symptoms has marked survival advantages over later therapy[6] and the theoretic concern that 15% of myocardium at risk dies for every 30 minutes of persistent occlusion[7] strongly support the notion that faster reperfusion improves outcome.

The possibility that adjunctive anticoagulant or antiplatelet therapy may effect faster infarct-related artery thrombolysis is consistent with the hypothesis that coronary thrombolysis is accompanied by procoagulant events—that is, accretion of new platelets and fibrin onto the coronary thrombus takes place as thrombolysis proceeds (discussed later). Similarly, the observation that coronary thrombolysis is attended in some patients by intermittent patency[8] suggests a possible human equivalent to cyclic flow variations in animal models,[9] a platelet-dependent phenomenon. It was suggested from early trials that early reperfusion achieved by t-PA but not necessarily by SK might, in part, have been due to early administration of aspirin and heparin. Firm evidence for this hypothesis became available in large-scale clinical trials (discussed separately later).

Reperfusion/Patency Rate

Patency is typically defined as TIMI grade 2 or 3 patency of the infarct-related artery on a 90-minute angiogram. Unless one knows that the vessel was occluded before administration of the agent, the patency rate, not the reperfusion rate, is the variable examined. With t-PA, patency rates ranged from 61% to 79%,[10–14] and with intravenous SK a 90-minute patency rate of 55% has been documented.[14] In earlier studies, regardless of the intravenous thrombolytic regimen used, the infarct-related coronary artery remains occluded in at least 20% of patients on 90-minute angiograms (although reperfusion rates of 85% to 90% were reported early with the use of intracoronary thrombolytic regimens.[15–16]

Reocclusion

Reocclusion of the infarct-related artery after successful thrombolysis can be documented either angiographically or clinically. In angiographic studies, repeat cardiac catheterization is typically performed 24 hours to several days after thrombolytic administration. Because of the "time slice" nature of these observations and because spontaneous reperfusion is common (more than three fourths of placebo-treated patients in the European cooperative study group[14] trial had a patent index vessel at follow-up angiography 10–22 d after admission), it is impossible to know if a vessel may have at least transiently reoccluded and then recanalized. Thus, it is likely that angiographic reocclusion rates may underestimate the real incidence of this phenomenon. Clinically, reocclusion is taken as recurrent angina and particularly reinfarction in the same myocardial location as that observed on initial presentation. Clinical reocclusion rates are less than those angiographically documented, because many reocclusions are asymptomatic.

Angiographic reocclusion rates for native t-PA have been in the 5% to 24% range.[17] The infarction rates after thrombolytic therapy have been documented in numerous studies of patients receiving t-PA. This rate has ranged from 2.4% to 13% and for those receiving SK, from 2.8% to 12%.[17]

BLEEDING COMPLICATIONS

The rates of bleeding complications with the presumed fibrin-specific t-PA (discussed later) have been surprisingly high in all reported clinical studies. In fact, in all studies cited, t-PA caused bleeding complications at a rate that was not statistically different from the incidence of bleeding with SK. The incidence of major bleeding for t-PA ranges from 6.3% to 21% in the six studies listed in Table 51–1, and the incidence of all bleeds, major and minor, ranges from 30% to 45%. It should be emphasized that all the studies cited involved invasive procedures and that a large proportion of the bleeding complications encountered with either t-PA or SK occurred at arterial and venous puncture sites. Bleeding from puncture sites is extremely common with any thrombolytic agent, for reasons discussed later. It is not clear from the reports cited whether the concomitant administration of heparin or aspirin significantly contributed to bleeding complications.

THE LATER LARGE TRIALS: MORTALITY ESTIMATES

Many issues in thrombolytic therapy debated for many years have been resolved only recently, often in very large-scale clinical trials. The major issues under debate included optimal duration of therapy, choice of agent (SK, anisoylated plasminogen SK activator complex [APSAC], or t-PA), adjunctive therapy (aspirin, heparin) and "front loading" versus more protracted thrombolytic therapy.

The first "mega trial," GISSI-I from Italy, clearly established that SK treatment significantly reduced the mortality rate as compared with placebo infusion in some 12,000 patients.[6] A second very large trial, ISIS-II,[18] included more than 17,000 patients with acute MI randomized to placebo, SK, aspirin, and aspirin plus SK therapies. Five-week vascular mortality was reduced by 21% in those taking aspirin versus those taking placebo. SK alone also reduced the mortality by 23% relative to placebo, and when aspirin was given with SK, mortality was reduced by 42% compared with placebo, suggesting additive effects of SK plus aspirin.

The question of the early use of heparin was largely resolved in the heparin-aspirin reperfusion trial (HART).[19] This collaborative study compared early intravenous heparin with the use of oral aspirin as adjunctive treatment with recombinant t-PA (rt-PA) in coronary thrombolysis in acute MI. Two hundred fifty patients were randomly assigned to receive either immediate and then continuous intravenous heparin or immediate and then daily oral aspirin together with rt-PA (100 mg IV during a 6-h period). All patients were treated within 6 hours after the onset of symptoms. The patency of the infarct-related artery by angiography was evaluated 7 to 24 hours after beginning the rt-PA infusion, and the frequency of reocclusion of the artery by repeat angiography on day 7. At the time of the first angiogram, 82% of the infarct-related arteries in the patients assigned to heparin were patent, compared with only 52% in the aspirin group. Of the initially patent vessels, 88% remained patent after 7 days in the heparin group, compared with 95% in the aspirin group. The numbers of hemorrhagic events were similar in the two groups. Later and much larger trials (the t-PA–APSAC patency study [TAPS] and Global Utilization of Streptokinase and T-PA for Occluded Arteries [GUSTO-1]) confirmed the high incidence of reperfusion and low incidence of reocclusion with early intravenous heparin treatment.

The first study that compared SK and t-PA head to head was GISSI-II,[20] with the main endpoint of mortality rate. GISSI-II was a multicenter, randomized open trial with 2 × 2 factorial design comparing SK (1.5 million units IV infused over 30–60 min) and t-PA (100 mg IV infused over 3 hours) in patients with acute MI admitted to coronary care units within 6 hours of the onset of symptoms. The patients were also randomized to receive heparin (12,500 units SC twice daily until discharge from the hospital) starting 12 hours after the beginning of t-PA or the SK infusion. The patients (12,490) were randomized to four treatment groups: SK alone, SK plus heparin, t-PA alone, and t-PA plus heparin. No significant differences between the two thrombolytic agents were detected. Mortality rates were identical in the two groups (8.8% hospital mortality for the study population compared with approximately 13% in the control cohort of the GISSI-I trial. The rates of major in-hospital cardiac complications (reinfarction, postinfarction angina) were also similar. The incidence of major bleeds was significantly higher in SK- and heparin-treated patients. The overall incidence of stroke was similar in all four groups.

The second study to examine t-PA versus SK was the Third International Study of Infarct Survival (ISIS-III),[21] which entered 41,299 patients up to 24 hours (median 4 h) after the onset of suspected acute MI. Patients were randomized between SK, APSAC, and t-PA. All patients received aspirin from the time of admission, and half of all patients were randomly allocated subcutaneous heparin (12,500 IU starting at 4 h and given twice daily for 7 d or until discharge) in addition to aspirin, and the other half were to receive aspirin alone. There was no significant mortality difference during days 0 to 35 among all randomized patients, and no difference in 6-month survival was apparent. When reviewed with the very similar GISSI-II trials, the combined mortalities were exactly identical, 10% for t-PA and 10% for SK. The APSAC group was similar in all re-

TABLE 51–1. Incidence of Bleeding Complications in Reported Studies

			Incidence of Bleeding		
Study	*Treatment*	*No. of Patients*	*Major (%)*	*Minor (%)*	*Stroke (%)*
TIMI-1	SK + H	147	15.6	15.6	0
	rt-PA + H	143	15.4	17.5	0
ECSG-1	SK + H + A	65	7.7	2.3	1.5
	rt-PA + H	64	6.3	26.5	0
ECSG-2	Placebo + H + A	366	2.2	5.2	0
	rt-PA + H + A	355	10.2	29.3	1.7
TAMI-1	rt-PA* + H (± PCTA)	386	21	24	0.5
TAMI-2	rt-PA + H + A (±UK)	147	14	20	0.7
TAMI-3	rt-PA (±H)	175	14	22	1.2

(From Bang NU, Wilhelm OG, Clayman MD: After coronary thrombolysis and reperfusion, what next? J Am Coll Cardiol 1989; 14:837–849.)

*High dose = 150 mg.

Abbreviations: A = aspirin; ECSG = European Cooperative Study Group; H = heparin; PTCA = percutaneous transluminal coronary angioplasty; SK = streptokinase; TAMI = Thrombolysis and Angioplasty in Myocardial Infarction trial; TIMI = Thrombolysis in Myocardial Infarction trial; rt-PA = recombinant tissue type plasminogen activator; UK = urokinase.

spects to the SK group, with no statistically significant differences in treatment outcomes. The only significant differences were found in the rate of reinfarction, 3.26% for SK versus 2.80% for t-PA, and in the frequency of stroke, which was significantly higher among patients receiving t-PA (1.35%) than among patients receiving SK (1.00%). The addition of heparin to either SK, APSAC, or t-PA, as prescribed in the protocol (i.e., SC first dose 4 h after start of thrombolytic therapy) made no difference in any measured outcomes.

However, a theory that heparin contributed significantly to a favorable outcome, as was originally proposed in the HART study,[19] was confirmed in TAPS, conducted in Germany.[22] Two important new features were introduced: t-PA was front loaded, with the total dose of 100 mg given over 1.5 hour rather than the conventional 3 hours. Also, heparin was given intravenously at the same time t-PA or APSAC was given. Four hundred twenty-one patients with acute MI were randomized. Coronary angiography 90 minutes after the start of treatment revealed a patent infarct-related artery in 85% of 199 patients given t-PA versus 70.3% of patients given APSAC (P = .0007). The reocclusion rate was similar in the two groups. Five in-hospital deaths occurred (2.4% in the t-PA group and 8.1% in the APSAC group, P = .0095). More bleeding complications were noted after APSAC (45% versus 31%, P = .0019).

The latest and most exhaustive trial is GUSTO.[23] This trial was set up in 1990 as a direct consequence of the ISIS-III and GISSI-II trials having failed to show any improvement in mortality with t-PA compared with SK. Advocates of t-PA argued that these trials had not shown the advantage of the drug because it needed to be given with intravenous heparin to give early patency rates. In the GUSTO trial, 41,021 patients with MI were randomized within 6 hours of symptom onset to one of four treatments: (1) SK (1.5 million IU/60 min + SC heparin), (2) (1.5 million IU/60 min + IV heparin), (3) accelerated t-PA + IV heparin, or (4) a combination of SK (1 million IU/60 min and t-PA 1 mg/kg over 60 min, maximum dose 90 mg + IV heparin). All patients received aspirin, and 46% received intravenous β-blockade. The combination arm was included because this regimen was believed from limited data to be associated with a particularly low reocclusion rate. However, the combination arm did not do well, showing both higher mortality and stroke rates than were seen with t-PA alone. The mortality rates and stroke rates in the different groups are summarized in Table 51–2. The difference between the t-PA arm and the SK arms was statistically significant. The P value for 30-day mortality was .001 for t-PA versus the pooled SK arms. For 24-hour mortality, the P value for t-PA versus either SK arm was .01. As anticipated from the ISIS-III trial, the t-PA arm was associated with a higher incidence of stroke than was SK. Further analysis showed that t-PA remains significantly better than SK even when adverse effects like stroke are included in the assessment of net benefit.

The GUSTO results end the long debate about whether early patency is important, as suggested earlier by the TIMI trials, or whether the time to reperfusion or patency is irrelevant, as suggested by the GISSI-II and ISIS-III trials. The fact that GUSTO showed a correlation between early patency and lower mortality has substantial implications for future research. These include the need to improve early patency further. Even the best group had TIMI-III flow (open arteries) in only 53% of patients at 90 minutes. At this time, new regimens can be tested for their ability to produce higher patency rates (discussed later). Another issue raised by the GUSTO results is the possible increased role of primary angioplasty in place of thrombolysis. Primary angioplasty is one of the best methods of opening an artery quickly, giving 90-minute patency rates in the 80% range. It is not likely, however, that primary angioplasty will replace thrombolysis altogether because of the limited numbers of centers and physicians that can conduct the procedure.

TABLE 51–2. Gusto Trial Mortality Results

Mortality	*SK (SC)*	*SK (IV)*	*t-PA*	*Combination*
30-d	7.2%	7.4%	6.3%	7.0%
24-h	2.8%	2.9%	2.3%	2.8%

NEW APPROACHES TOWARD THROMBOLYTIC THERAPY

Some Theoretic Considerations

A basic understanding of the fibrinolytic enzyme system, the consequences of its activation, and certain features of the coagulation system are necessary to comprehend the relative advantages and risks of newer fibrinolytic agents, new anticoagulants, and new antiplatelet agents. Certain basic concepts pertaining to the mechanism of action of older agents as opposed to agents under development also need to be introduced.

The Fibrinolytic Enzyme System

An earlier published review[3] extensively discussed the biochemistry of the fibrinolytic enzyme system. For this review, the following points need to be re-emphasized as pertinent to the present discussion. The physiologic plasminogen activators are t-PA, single-chain urokinase-type plasminogen activator (scu-PA), and two-chain urokinase-type plasminogen activator (tcu-PA), usually referred to as urokinase (UK), a term used in this chapter. In addition to these physiologic plasminogen activators, the bacterial activator SK is widely used clinically. Tissue plasminogen activator and scu-PA preferentially activate the fibrinolytic proenzyme plasminogen adsorbed to fibrin; consequently, t-PA and scu-PA given at moderate doses do not significantly activate circulating plasma plasminogen. The older thrombolytic agents SK and UK, in contrast, activate plasminogen adsorbed onto fibrin and circulating plasma plasminogen with equal efficiency. Activation of plasma-plasminogen results in temporary hyperplasminemia and a profound multifactor coagulation defect. Although claimed to be fibrin specific, t-PA and scu-PA in some patients produce a serious coagulation defect, although less frequently than observed with SK and UK treatment. With respect to the fibrin specificity of t-PA, it should be emphasized that this activator is fibrin specific but not thrombus specific. Tissue plasminogen activator does not distinguish between the target thrombus and hemostatic plugs consisting of platelets and fibrin occurring any place in the circulation, including arterial and venous puncture sites. Therefore, the best fibrin-specific agents we may produce still possess a serious liability of causing bleeds from arterial and venous puncture sites and other potential bleeding sites, such as stress ulcers and small blood vessels in the cerebral circulation.

Another limitation to the efficacy of activators such as t-PA and UK is the presence of plasminogen activator inhibitors, particularly plasminogen activator inhibitor–I (PAI-I).[3] PAI-I is synthesized in and secreted by endothelial cells and megakaryocytes. It is found in plasma at varying concentrations, exists in platelets at high concentrations, and is released during platelet activation. Very large quantities of PAI-I have been demonstrated to be bound to subendothelial connective tissue. Plasminogen activator inhibitors are found at increased concentrations in patients with venous thromboembolism, in patients who have had an acute MI, and in patients with conditions predisposing to thromboembolic disease. PAI-I rapidly and efficiently inhibits t-PA as well as UK and PAI-I in plasma, in platelet-rich fibrin thrombi, and in subendothelial connective tissue, which may unfavorably change the therapeutic outcome of thrombolytic therapy in some patients.

Activation of Clotting and Platelets Through Activation of the Fibrinolytic Enzyme System

Administration of massive quantities of plasminogen activators results in activation of blood coagulation. The major enzyme systems in plasma—the clotting system, the fibrinolytic enzyme system, the kallikrein-kinin and the complement systems—are interdependent systems that are activators as well as inhibitors. The earlier steps of the intrinsic coagulation pathway involve Factor XII (Hageman factor) plus two proteins from the kallikrein-kinin system, prekallikrein and high-molecular-weight kininogen. Hageman factor on negatively charged surfaces is activated by plasmin or by kallikrein. Once Hageman factor is activated, the clotting cascade is set in motion via the intrinsic pathway, with activation of Factor XI to Factor XIa. It causes massive activation of prekallikrein to kallikrein, which works on kininogens to release kinins; activated Factor XIIa also activates clotting Factor VII and sets in motion the chain reaction resulting in clotting via the extrinsic pathway. Kallikrein also activates scu-PA to UK, which in turn results in additional activation of the fibrinolytic enzyme system. Thus, activation of the fibrinolytic enzyme system causes activation of clotting and activation of the kallikrein-kinin system, with a potential for hypotensive reactions, which do indeed occur when too much SK is given too fast. Activation of coagulation occurring during t-PA and SK therapy in acute MI has been shown unequivocally by Owen and colleagues,[24] who demonstrated a five- to seven-fold increase over baseline of fibrinopeptide A, a reliable marker for activation of the coagulation system. Eisenberg and colleagues[25] also measured fibrinopeptide A levels in a similar group of patients receiving SK. In their study, they found that increasing levels of fibrinopeptide A during SK therapy correlated with the occurrence of rethrombosis. It is of great interest in the study by Owen and associates[24] that elevations of fibrinopeptide A after either t-PA or SK administration occurred despite concurrent heparin therapy. The observation that thrombin generation occurs despite heparinization raises a possibility that thrombin generation occurs in pathways not generally recognized in the scheme of blood coagulation. Although never extensively commented on in the literature, it has been suspected by many authorities on the basis of animal experiments and clinical observations that heparin, although an extremely effective anticoagulant on the venous side of the circulation, is far less effective on the arterial side. According to a hypothesis that is being widely examined, α-thrombin, the final enzyme in the coagulation cascade, may exist as different molecular entities in relatively cell-poor venous thrombi and in arterial cell-rich thrombi. In venous thrombi, α-thrombin predominates. It is in free solution in plasma and is readily inhibited by heparin in consort with the heparin cofactor, antithrombin III. In arterial thrombi, the predominant form of thrombin appears to be meizothrombin.[26] Meizothrombin remains attached to cells and has thrombin activity that is not inhibited by heparin/antithrombin III. It has also been shown that the thrombus itself is the source of preformed thrombin.[27] Thrombin remains attached to fibrin, and clot-bound thrombin appears to be a significant factor in the extension of intravascular thrombi. Finally, thrombin can be liberated by plasmin digestion of the fibrin clot and can circulate in complex with fibrinogen/fibrin degradation products.

Activation of Platelets Associated with Fibrinolytic Therapy

It has been known for many years from in vitro experiments that activation of the fibrinolytic enzyme system results in activation of platelets. Activation of platelets was confirmed in vivo in patients receiving SK for the treatment of acute MI.[28] A 10- to 20-fold increase in urinary excretion of 2,3-dinor-thromboxane B_2 and plasma 11-dehydro-thromboxane B_2 was noted early during therapy. These prostaglandins are metabolites of thromboxane A_2, and the appearance of thromboxane A_2 in plasma reflects in vivo platelet activation. The implications of this finding are that new accretion of fibrin and platelets onto the thrombus can occur as thrombolysis is under way and that these events may contribute to reocclusion as well as delayed time to reperfusion.

NEW AGENTS AND STRATEGIES

Preliminary, Preclinical, and Clinical Results

APSAC has neither protease nor esterase activity, but when it interacts with human plasminogen, a one-to-one stoichiometric complex is formed and the proteolytically active serine of plasminogen exposed; this complex activates plasminogen. A special form of SK-plasminogen activator is prepared from such equimolar complexes of SK and human plasminogen in which the catalytic center of the plasminogen molecule is bound to an acyl group, resulting in an inactive complex. In aqueous solution, the acyl group is hydrolyzed and catalytic activity is regained. With the *p*-anisoyl derivative (APSAC), the in vivo deacylation half-life is about 90 to 110 minutes. Thus, APSAC can be considered a sustained-release SK activator preparation.[29] The drug has theoretic advantages. The temporary masking of the catalytic center of the activator complex does not interfere with the capacity of the molecule to bind to fibrin, because the location of the fibrin-binding sites of plasminogen, the kringle domains, are well separated from the catalytic site. Thus, relative fibrin specificity could be conferred, and this has been confirmed by in vitro experiments and by animal experiments in which APSAC proved more efficient in lysis of experimental thrombi and caused less fibrinogen depletion than did SK plasmin. However, at doses sufficient to cause coronary reperfusion in humans (30 mg as a bolus injection), APSAC causes considerable fibrinogen depletion and a rate of bleeding complications not apparently different from the rate with SK.[21] Furthermore, hypertensive reactions have occasionally been reported in patients. Although APSAC has been shown to bind less SK-neutralizing antibody than SK, the incidence of clinical anaphylactic reactions is similar to that observed with SK. The prolonged half-life for APSAC permits bolus administration. The sustained-release characteristics of APSAC also ensure relatively constant levels of SK throughout the treatment. Thus, excessive SK levels capable of completely depleting plasma plasminogen are not reached, perhaps explaining why reperfusion rates are generally somewhat higher with APSAC than with SK.

APSAC therapy, when instituted early after the onset of symptoms, has in several clinical studies led to a reperfusion rate of approximately 65% and a patency rate of approximately 75%. In the large placebo-controlled AIMS study,[30] APSAC administration in acute MI resulted in an impressive 47% reduction in mortality. Clot-specific thrombolysis by natural or recombinant scu-PA has been demonstrated in animal models of venous thrombosis or coronary artery thrombosis. In patients with acute MI, intravenous infusion of 40 to 70 mg/h resulted in coronary artery reperfusion in 75% of the patients, but pronounced fibrinogen depletion occurred in 25%. Synergistic combinations of t-PA with scu-PA or UK have worked well in animal experiments. Combinations of t-PA and scu-PA combinations have also been efficient in small uncontrolled studies of patients with acute MI. In a larger trial (evaluating the efficacy of t-PA–UK combined therapy),[10] only high doses of the two agents (1 mg/kg t-PA, 2 million units of UK) achieved patency rates at 90 minutes comparable to those achieved with t-PA alone (73% vs. 75%); additionally, the reocclusion rate was not statistically different in patients receiving the combination therapy from that in patients receiving t-PA alone. Thus, a combination of two plasminogen activators, as noted in these earlier studies and as also mentioned in the GUSTO trial, does not appear to offer clear advantages over t-PA alone.

Mutant Plasminogen Activators

Attempts to produce t-PA mutants aim at improving the following disadvantageous properties of the enzyme: (1) t-PA is a less catalytically efficient plasminogen activator than UK, even when it is bound to a fibrin clot; (2) the fibrin specificity, although considerable, is limited, as evidenced by the significant incidence of fibrinogen depletion in patients receiving high doses of t-PA; (3) the activity of t-PA is attenuated by several plasma inhibitors, mainly PAI-I; (4) t-PA, like all plasminogen activators, activates clotting as well as platelets; and (5) the biologic half-life of t-PA is very short, less than 5 minutes in humans. Considerable work and effort, much of it quite successful, have been invested in producing improved versions of the t-PA molecule through recombinant deoxyribonucleic acid technology. However, most of these efforts, particularly in industry, were abandoned after the GISSI-II and ISIS-III trials reported that t-PA itself had no advantage over the much cheaper SK. Thus, this line of research was largely abandoned for economic rather than scientific reasons. Several of the stated goals had already been achieved: t-PA variants with higher catalytic activity than the parent molecule had been produced, t-PA largely unreactive with PAI-I had been created, and t-PA variants with substantially prolonged half-lives were also a reality. Whether the results of GUSTO, which has established t-PA as a leading contender for the fibrinolytic market, will lead to re-examination of t-PA mutants remains to be seen.

Adjunctive Therapies

Antiplatelet Agents

THEORETIC CONSIDERATIONS. Platelets are activated in vivo and start adhering to subendothelial connective tissue and aggregate to each other through a series of complex and only partly interconnective events. Many agonists can cause platelet activation aggregation. These include thromboxane A_2 (a prostaglandin synthesized in the platelet), collagen, thrombin, adenosine diphosphate, serotonin, and epinephrine. Each has its own receptors on the platelet, and each causes receptor-linked signal transduction to activate several different pathways, resulting in platelet adhesion and aggregation. One can easily block one of the major pathways with a pharmacologic agent, but even if one pathway is blocked, other pathways may prevail so that it is extremely difficult through conventional pharmacologic monotherapy to block platelet activation completely.

A change in thinking occurred when it became apparent that a common final pathway exists.[30] It is now firmly established that platelets adhere to each other and adhere to the vessel wall, making use of "sticky proteins" contained in plasma irrespective of platelet activation. The structures in the platelet membranes that allow sticky proteins to attach themselves are receptor-like glycoprotein molecules of the so-called integrin family found in numerous cells. The integrins are of major general importance in bringing about cell-cell adhesion and promoting cell-cell interactions. On the platelet, a glycoprotein called Ib attaches the von Willebrand factor protein to the platelet. Von Willebrand's factor also sticks to subendothelial connective tissues, thereby allowing the platelet to adhere at the site of endothelial damage. Another integrin on the platelet is called glycoprotein IIb-IIIa, and it binds fibrinogen as well as von Willebrand's factor, thereby ensuring the sticking together of two or more platelets, resulting in platelet aggregation. A common motif in sticky proteins such as fibrinogen and von Willebrand's factor is the amino acid sequence Arg-Gly-Asp-X. The use of this knowledge has resulted in the construction of numerous peptide analogs containing the RGD sequence and peptidomimetic organic compounds capable of competing with fibrinogen or von Willebrand's factor for binding to the platelet IIb-IIIa complex or to the natural RGD sequence of the appropriate sticky proteins.

That platelets are important in the pathogenesis of coronary thrombi has long been suspected on the basis of two simple observations: (1) Coronary thrombi, like all arterial thrombi, are platelet rich and contain at least 10 to 20 times more platelets per unit mass than do venous thrombi; and (2) many coronary thrombi appear to originate at sites of ruptured atheromatous plaque exposing subendothelial connective tissue, allowing for platelet adhesion and aggregation.

ANTIPLATELET AGENTS CONSIDERED FOR ADJUNCT THERAPY. As mentioned, aspirin is now firmly established as adjunctive therapy in combination with any thrombolytic agent in acute MI. Aspirin is the cyclooxygenase inhibitor that works at the initial stages of the chain reaction resulting in thromboxane A_2 synthesis. Aspirin has the disadvantage that it also inhibits the cyclooxygenase enzyme contained in endothelial cells in addition to platelet cyclooxygenase. Blocking of cyclooxygenase in endothelial cells effectively blocks the synthesis of PGI_1, or prostacyclin. Whereas thromboxane A_2 is one of the most potent agonists of platelet aggregation and one of the most potent vasoconstrictors known, prostacyclin is an extremely potent inhibitor of platelet aggregation and a very potent vasodilator. Strategies aimed at developing specific thromboxane inhibitors include carefully titrating the dose of aspirin, which appears to have been successful in some series in which aspirin in doses as low as 50 mg daily has proved effective as adjunctive therapy. The synthesis of specific thromboxane synthetase inhibitors or thromboxane receptor antagonists has been partially successful but at present is untested or of unproven value in clinical medicine. Today, the most intensively studied agents are those that block platelet glycoprotein IIb-IIIa, thereby preventing aggregation independently of the pathway of activation of the platelets. Monoclonal antibodies with IIb-IIIa specificity (7E3 [CentoRx, Centocor,

Inc., Malvern, PA]) have proved highly effective in animal experiments. Proof of the concept of in vivo activity in humans has also been obtained in a trial that demonstrated the ability of 7E3 to reduce the incidence of abrupt closure in patients undergoing high-risk angioplasty.[31] The use of a IIb-IIIa monoclonal antibody in adjunctive therapy combined with a thrombolytic in acute MI is currently being seriously considered. One Arg-Gly-Asp–derived peptide (Integrelin, Cor Therapeutics) is currently undergoing clinical trials,[32] and other peptides and peptidol mimetics are soon to follow.

New Anticoagulants

Specific Antithrombins, Hirudin, and Hirudin Mimetic Peptides[33]

Hirudin derived from the salivary glands of the medicinal leech *Hirudo medicinalis* has been cloned and expressed. Recombinant hirudin has emerged today as an interesting candidate to replace heparin in adjunctive therapy to coronary artery thrombolysis. Hirudin is a relatively small peptide consisting of 65 amino acids and is a highly specific inhibitor of thrombin with little or no effect on other serine proteases. It is the most potent antithrombin known. The structure of hirudin and the interactions between hirudin and thrombin are well known. At the N-terminal end of the hirudin molecule is a tightly wound disulfide-linked bulky structure that covers and completely incapacitates the active site pocket of the enzyme; the C-terminal end of the hirudin molecule hooks up to a region in thrombin called the fibrinogen- or anion-binding exosite. This domain in thrombin possesses a high density of basic amino acids and positive charges, which effectively interact with complementary highly negatively charged domains in the natural substrate fibrinogen and in the highly negatively charged tail of the thrombin inhibitor hirudin.

Because of concerns (which turned out to be unwarranted) about the possible antigenicity of hirudin, Maraganore and colleagues[34] constructed a smaller hirudin derivative, hirulog, by linking an active site inhibitory sequence (D-Phe-Pro-Arg-Pro) to the 12 C-terminal amino acids of hirudin. That portion of the molecule is destined to bind into the anion-binding exosite of thrombin. The active site inhibitory sequence was hooked up to the hirudin tail via a glycine polymer spacer four amino acids long. Hirulog worked exactly as designed, and although it does not bind as tightly as hirudin, it appears to be a highly specific and potent thrombin inhibitor in vitro and in vivo.

In contrast to heparin, which requires cofactors (antithrombin III or heparin cofactor II) for activity, hirudin and hirulog are potent antithrombins without cofactor requirements. Another advantage of a growing number of direct antithrombins including hirudin and hirulog has become apparent as fibrin clots form, particularly on the arterial side of the circulation. Thrombin, as previously mentioned, is trapped in the fibrin network and remains active in that location. Fibrin-bound thrombin (like cell-bound meizothrombin) is poorly inhibited by heparin-antithrombin III but readily inhibited by "direct" antithrombins not requiring cofactors for inhibition.[27] These experimental observations may explain in part why hirudin and hirulog are far more effective than heparin in animal thrombosis models and so far in limited clinical trials. Among the hirudin group of direct thrombin inhibitors, hirulog has been shown to be significantly more potent than hirudin as an inhibitor of fibrin-bound thrombin. It is widely speculated, although not proved conclusively, that fibrin-bound thrombin, relatively inaccessible to natural inhibitors such as antithrombin III, has major pathophysiologic significance in acute MI in critical events such as thrombus extension and reocclusion after reperfusion achieved through physiologic or pharmacologic thrombolytic mechanisms.

The stage is set to define the clinical utility of hirudin as well as hirulog. Phase III trials are on the drawing board, and definitive results are anticipated to be available within the next year. The data available from phase II pilot trials are intriguing and promising for both compounds. In randomized, open-label, dose-ranging trials, recombinant hirudin versus heparin was given in conjunction with front-loaded t-PA and aspirin to 240 patients with acute MI. Patients receiving hirudin (all doses) had significantly fewer episodes of reocclusion (1% vs. 7%) in a strong trend toward early and more extensive reperfusion than did patients receiving heparin.[35] In a smaller study of 42 patients with acute MI, hirulog was given intravenously in combination with aspirin and 1.5 million units of SK.[36] Twenty-eight patients received hirulog, and 14 patients received heparin. In a randomized design, the study was double blind with single-blind administrations; angiographic data were analyzed blinding. Angiographic patencies at 90 and 120 minutes were strikingly improved in patients receiving hirulog compared with patients receiving heparin. Reperfusion at 120 minutes was achieved in 86% of patients receiving hirulog and in 43% of patients receiving heparin. The incidence of bleeding complications was not significantly different in the two groups. An incidence of 86% reperfusion with SK has not been achieved with any adjunctive therapy other than hirulog.

Smaller molecules that still retain high thrombin specificity (e.g., compounds of the general structure Phe-Pro-Argin*al*) look promising in animal models and in the early stages of phase II trials at this point, without any certain information available.

Although results with hirudin and hirulog give reason for guarded optimism, larger efficacy trials are clearly required to answer some crucial questions. Will these seemingly more potent arterial anticoagulants carry with them a greater bleeding liability than heparin? How readily can hirudin or hirulog in larger series be coadministered with other anticoagulants or antiplatelet agents in the setting of thrombolytic therapy? What is the therapeutic window? Will the concern of cerebrovascular hemorrhage so real with thrombolytic agents be further accentuated with antithrombin-type anticoagulants? The answers to these questions need to be clearly laid out before the determination can be made whether hirudin, hirudin mimetic peptides, and other pure antithrombins will assume a major role as antithrombotic agents, particularly in arterial thrombotic disorders.

Similar concerns can be expressed about the new and very potent antiplatelet agents, the IIb-IIIa–blocking agents. In all these areas, the pertinent clinical experiments are well under way, and answers to the questions and concerns should soon be available.

CONCLUSIONS

The results obtained with thrombolytic therapy in acute MI to date have been impressive. Nevertheless, results can clearly be improved in the area of time to reperfusion, reocclusion, and bleeding complications, with specific reference to intracerebral bleeds. The material included in this chapter strongly suggests that it is possible to design strategies, most likely through the introduction of improved adjunctive therapies, that would shorten the time to reperfusion, increase the incidence of reperfusion, and decrease the incidence of reocclusion. However, it is uncertain whether the incidence of bleeding complications can be reduced. Indeed, it is possible that some of these strategies will result in increased bleeding liability. It is certain, however, that through many of these strategies a new agent will be adequately tested clinically within a short period. At this time, we serve notice that the final chapter in the saga of thrombolytic therapy in acute MI is yet to be written.

References

1. Fletcher AP, Sherry S, Alkaersig N, et al: The maintenance of a sustained thrombolytic state in man. II. Clinical observation on patients with myocardial infarction and other thromboembolic disorders. J Clin Invest 1959; 38:111–119.
2. Duckert F: Thrombolytic therapy in myocardial infarction. Prog Cardiovasc Dis 1979; 21:342–350.
3. Bang NU, Wilhelm OG, Clayman MD: Thrombolytic therapy in myocardial infarction. Annu Rev Pharmacol Toxicol 1989; 29:605–610.
4. The TIMI Study Group: Comparison of invasive and conservative strategies after treatment with intravenous tissue plasminogen activator in acute myocardial infarction. N Engl J Med 1989; 320:618–626.
5. The TIMI Study Group: Immediate vs delayed catheterization and angioplasty following thrombolytic therapy for acute myocardial infarction. JAMA 1988; 260:2849–2858.
6. Gruppo Italiano per lo Studio della Streptochinasi Nell'Infarto Miocardico (GISSI): Effectiveness of intravenous thrombolytic treatment in acute myocardial infarction. Lancet 1986; 1:397–401.
7. Hugenholtz PG: Acute coronary artery obstruction in myocardial infarction: Overview of thrombolytic therapy. J Am Coll Cardiol 1987; 9:1375–1384.
8. Grines CL, Topol EJ, Bates ER, et al: Infarct vessel status after intravenous tissue plasminogen activator and acute coronary angioplasty: Prediction of clinical outcome. Am Heart J 1988; 115:1–7.
9. Golino P, Ashton JH, Glas-Greenwalt P, et al: Medication of reocclusion by thromboxane A_2 and serotonin after thrombolysis with tissue-type plasminogen activator in canine preparation of coronary thrombosis. Circulation 1988; 77:678–684.
10. Topol EJ, Califf RM, George BS, et al: Coronary arterial thrombolysis with combined infusion of recombinant tissue-type plasminogen activator and urokinase in patients with acute myocardial infarction. Circulation 1988; 77:1100–1107.
11. Verstraete M, Brower RW, Collen D, et al: Double-blind randomized trial of intravenous tissue-type plasminogen activator versus placebo in acute myocardial infarction. Lancet 1985; 2:965–969.
12. Topol EJ, George BS, Kereiakes DJ, et al: A randomized controlled trial of intravenous tissue plasminogen activator and early intravenous heparin in acute myocardial infarction. Circulation 1989; 79:281–286.
13. Verstraete M, Arnold AE, Brower RW, et al: Acute coronary thrombolysis with recombinant human tissue-type plasminogen activator: Initial patency and influence of maintained infusion on reocclusion rate. Am J Cardiol 1987; 60:231–237.
14. Verstraete M, Bory M, Collen D, et al: Randomized trial of intravenous recombinant tissue-type plasminogen activator versus intravenous streptokinase in acute myocardial infarction. Circulation 1989; 79:281–286.
15. Ganz W, Buchbinder N, Marcus H, et al: Intracoronary thrombolysis in evolving myocardial infarction. Am Heart J 1981; 101:4–13.
16. Markis JE, Malagold M, Parker JA, et al: Myocardial salvage after intracoronary thrombolysis with streptokinase in myocardial infarction. N Engl J Med 1981; 305:777–782.
17. Bang NU, Wilhelm OG, Clayman MD: After coronary thrombolysis and reperfusion, what next? J Am Coll Cardiol 1989; 14:837–849.
18. ISIS-2 (Second International Study of Infarct Survival) Collaborative Group: Randomised trial of intravenous streptokinase, oral aspirin, both, or neither among 17,187 cases of suspected acute myocardial infarction: ISIS-2. Lancet 1988; ii:349–360.
19. Hsia J, Hamilton WP, Kleiman N, et al: A comparison between heparin and low-dose aspirin as adjunctive therapy with tissue plasminogen activator for acute myocardial infarction. Heparin-Aspirin Reperfusion Trial (HART) Investigators. N Engl J Med 1990; 323:1433–1437.
20. GISSI-2: A factorial randomised trial of alteplase versus streptokinase and heparin versus no heparin among 12,490 patients with acute myocardial infarction. Gruppo Italiano per lo Studio della Sopravvivenza nell'Infarto Miocardico. Lancet 1990; 336:65–71.
21. ISIS-3: A randomised comparison of streptokinase vs tissue plasminogen activator vs anistreplase and of aspirin plus heparin vs aspirin alone among 41,299 cases of suspected acute myocardial infarction. Lancet 1992; 339:753–770.
22. Neuhaus KL, von Essen R, Tebbe U, et al: Improved thrombolysis in acute myocardial infarction with front-loaded administration of alteplase: Results of the rt-PA–APSAC patency study (TAPS). J Am Coll Cardiol 1992; 19:885–891.
23. The GUSTO Trial, American Federation for Clinical Research National Meeting, Washington, DC, April 30, 1993. Personal notes (NUB).
24. Owen J, Friedman KD, Grossman BA, et al: Thrombolytic therapy with tissue plasminogen activator or streptokinase induces transient thrombin activity. Blood 1988; 72:616–620.
25. Eisenberg PR, Sherman L, Rich N, et al: Importance of continued activation of thrombin reflected by fibrinopeptide A to the efficacy of thrombolysis. J Am Coll Cardiol 1986; 7:1255.
26. Krishnaswamy S, Mann KG, Nesheim, NE: The prothrombinase-catalyzed activation of prothrombin proceeds through the intermediate meizothrombin in an ordered, sequential reaction. J Biol Chem 1986; 261:8977.
27. Weitz JI, Hudoba M, Massel D, et al: Clot-bound thrombin is protected from inhibition by heparin-antithrombin III but is susceptible to inactivation by antithrombin III-independent inhibitors. J Clin Invest 1990; 86:385–391.
28. Fitzgerald DJ, Catella F, Roy L, et al: Marked platelet activation in vivo after intravenous streptokinase in patients with acute myocardial infarction. Circulation 1988; 77:142–150.
29. Smith RAG, Dupe RJ, English PD, et al: Fibrinolysis with acyl-enzymes: A new approach to thrombolytic therapy. Nature 1981; 290:505–508.
30. The AIMS Trial Study Group: Effects of intravenous APSAC on mortality after acute myocardial infarction: Preliminary report of a placebo-controlled clinical trial. Lancet 1988; 1:545–549.
31. The EPIC Investigators: Use of a monoclonal antibody directed against the platelet glycoprotein IIb/IIIa receptor in high-risk angioplasty. N Engl J Med 1994; 330:956–961.
32. Bang NU, Clayman MD: Antithrombotic agents from salivary glands of hematophagous animals. Trends Cardiovasc Med 1992; 2:183–188.
33. Bang NU: Hirudin and hirudin-mimetic peptides: A promising group of antithrombotic agents. ACC Current J Review 1993; Sept/Oct:43–45.
34. Maraganore JM, Bourdon P, Jablonski J, et al: Design and characterization of hirulogs: A novel class of bivalent peptide inhibitors of thrombin. Biochemistry 1990; 29:7095–7101.
35. Cannon CP, McCabe CH, Henry TD, et al: Hirudin reduces reocclusion compared to heparin following thrombolysis in acute myocardial infarction: results of the TIMI 5 trial. J Am Coll Cardiol 1993; 21:136A.
36. Lidón RM, Théroux P, Bonan R, et al: Hirulog as adjunctive therapy to streptokinase in acute myocardial infarction. J Am Coll Cardiol 1993; 21:419A.

CHAPTER 52

Interventional Therapies for Cardiogenic Shock

Geoffrey O. Hartzler, MD, FACC • Cres B. Miranda, MD, FACC

Acute myocardial infarction complicated by the clinical syndrome of cardiogenic shock (hypotension, oliguria, pulmonary edema, and/or mental obtundation) continues to be a most dreaded and deadly sequel of coronary artery disease. The reported incidence of cardiogenic shock ranged from 5% to 15% of those patients presenting with acute myocardial infarction in the 1950s through 1970s.[1–5] In fact, a community-wide analysis of 16 hospitals in Worcester, Massachusetts, identified a relatively constant frequency of shock at 7.5% between 1975 and 1988 and found no improvement over time of in-hospital and late survival.[6] The use of invasive monitoring,[7–9] pharmacologic inotropic support,[10–12] and vasodilator therapy[13] has not materially improved patient survival. Although contemporary thrombolytic therapy has reduced the relatively low mortality in low-risk subsets of patients with acute myocardial infarction, it has not improved survival in patients with congestive heart failure and cardiogenic shock.[14, 15]

Because conventional medical therapy has not benefited those patients with cardiogenic shock, more aggressive interventional techniques have been applied during the past decade. In this chapter, we review contemporary strategies for management of those patients with cardiogenic shock complicating acute myocardial infarction.

THROMBOLYTIC THERAPY

Mathey and colleagues[16, 17] first studied the use of thrombolytic therapy in acute infarction complicated by cardiogenic shock. They reported the survival of three patients in whom reperfusion was established by intracoronary streptokinase. In a later report by Kennedy and coworkers[18] for the Society for Cardiac Angiography's intracoronary streptokinase registry, 19 (43%) of 44 patients in shock had successful reperfusion and subsequent mortality of 42%, whereas 25 (57%) patients not achieving reperfusion had a doubling of mortality at 84%.

Because intravenous thrombolytic trials conducted in the 1980s uniformly excluded patients in cardiogenic shock, limited data exist characterizing this approach. However, the GISSI-1 investigators[14] reported the results of intravenous streptokinase administered to 280 patients presenting with Killip class IV congestive heart failure. In-hospital mortality was 69.9% (102/146) for those receiving streptokinase compared with 70.1% (94/134) for control patients. Similarly, the use of recombinant tissue plasminogen activator has failed to show benefit in shock patients.[19] Regardless of the lytic agent used by intravenous administration, the absence of patient benefit probably results, in part, from the low cardiac output state with reduced coronary perfusion impeding delivery of the lytic agent to the site of acute thrombosis,[20] further exposing the limitations of currently available lytic agents that under ideal hemodynamic circumstances, appear to effect reperfusion in only 50% to 80% of patients.

INTRA-AORTIC BALLOON COUNTERPULSATION

Mechanical hemodynamic support with intra-aortic balloon counterpulsation is based on relatively simple physiologic principles and has been widely used in critically ill patients for more than 20 years.[21] During left ventricular diastole (aortic valve closure), the intra-aortic balloon, which is situated in the upper descending thoracic aorta, expands and displaces blood to the systemic circulation while increasing coronary perfusion pressure and flow. When ventricular systole ensues (open aortic valve), the intra-aortic balloon collapses, leading to decreased left ventricular afterload, which augments ejection and cardiac output.

As a result, intra-aortic balloon counterpulsation reduces intrinsic systolic arterial pressure and left ventricular wall tension correlating with a decrease in myocardial oxygen requirements. Diastolic coronary perfusion pressure and blood flow are augmented not only to the infarct-related artery but importantly to non–infarct-related coronary arteries. Consequently, hemodynamic support may be of secondary benefit by contributing to the maintenance of perfusion pressure and flow in noninfarct arteries containing significant stenoses, thus contributing to global myocardial salvage and function.[22] Because severely ischemic myocardium may not recover immediately with reperfusion, intra-aortic balloon support can "buy time" for recovery within the infarct zone, assuming the occurrence of spontaneous or induced reperfusion within the infarct artery.

Unfortunately, the use of intra-aortic balloon pump counterpulsation has not correlated with improved in-hospital or late survival in patients with cardiogenic shock. In the 1970s, Scheidt and colleagues[23] described the results of a cooperative clinical trial in which 87 patients with cardiogenic shock underwent intra-aortic balloon pump counterpulsation for hemodynamic support. Short-term salutary clinical benefit was observed with a mean reduction in heart rate from 110 ± 24 beats per minute to 103 ± 21 beats per minute, augmentation of diastolic pressure from 53 ± 12 mm Hg to 83 ± 19 mm Hg, and an increase in cardiac output by approximately 500 mL per minute. In 18 of 19 patients undergoing metabolic studies, there was either decreased myocardial lactate production or increased lactate extraction, suggesting a reduction of ischemia. However, in-hospital mortality was 83% and after 1 year there were only eight survivors (91% mortality).

Intuitively, one might expect that intra-aortic balloon pump counterpulsation combined with intravenous thrombolytic therapy could lead to improved survival. However, this has not been the case; the combined treatments potentially result in increased bleeding complications. Although Goodwin and coworkers[24] observed no increase in hemorrhagic events relative to standard heparin therapy in 48 patients receiving intravenous streptokinase plus balloon pump counterpulsation, the Thrombolysis and Angioplasty in Myocardial Infarction (TAMI) investigators described a different experience.[25] Ohman and colleagues[25] observed increased hemorrhagic and vascular complications as well as death among 85 patients receiving combined lytic therapy and intra-aortic balloon pump counterpulsation. Although no deaths were directly attributed to the balloon pump itself, relentless progression of cardiogenic shock contributed to most deaths. Of interest, the TAMI investigators observed that no patient with initially successful thrombolysis experienced acute reocclusion while being supported by the intra-aortic balloon pump compared with a 13% reocclusion rate in nonsupported patients. Further, they observed that, in those shock patients who survived to have both early and late paired ventriculograms, there was a tendency toward improvement in resting left ventricular function, which was most pronounced in myocardial segments remote to the site of infarction. Regardless, in Ohman and colleagues' study, patients receiving lytic therapy plus intra-aortic balloon pumping experienced a 32% in-hospital mortality including more than 30% of study patients included in the analysis who were not in cardiogenic shock. Although a randomized controlled trial of intravenous lytic therapy with or without intra-aortic balloon pumping might show some survival benefit for the combined strategy, it is unlikely that this trial will be completed because of the critically ill and time-dependent nature of cardiogenic shock in addition to the increased potential for hemorrhagic and peripheral vascular complications.

Pathologic studies suggest that cardiogenic shock and fulminant cardiac failure result when approximately 40% of total left ventricular muscle mass is infarcted.[26–28] To maintain cardiac output, noninfarcted segments become hypercontractile in an attempt to compensate for the loss of infarcting myocardium. These segments eventually become dysfunctional, in part, resulting from high-energy adenosine triphosphate depletion combined with other metabolic abnormalities, especially in the setting of multivessel coronary disease. The time course of acute myocardial infarction and irreversible necrosis during cardiogenic shock is unknown and likely varies from patient to patient, depending on multiple factors including the presence or absence of additional coronary artery disease and collateral circulation. However, Gutovitz and coauthors[29] evaluated creatine kinase-MB (CK-MB) levels in patients with cardiogenic shock and found that, in the majority of patients, release of CK-MB evolved and persisted while paralleling clinical deterioration; peak CK-MB values were not only higher but were sustained relative to nonshock patients. Their finding suggests that, in shock patients, myocardial dysfunction and necrosis extend outside the territory of the infarct-related artery probably resulting from reduced coronary perfusion pressures in non–infarct-related arteries over time.

Because in cardiogenic shock the deleterious extension of left ventricular necrosis proceeds over a longer time course, the window of opportunity for revascularization may be greater compared with uncomplicated infarction. These nonacutely infarcting yet ischemic myocardial segments may be recoverable over a longer time course because of continued anterograde coronary flow induced by intra-aortic balloon pumping and/or the presence of collaterals.[30, 31] This observation is supported by the work of Dunkman[32] and Keon[33] and their colleagues, who performed coronary artery bypass grafting in patients with acute infarction complicated by cardiogenic shock. They found that patients responded favorably to reperfusion even if they were operated on late in the time course of their infarction. Lee and associates[34] performed coronary angioplasty in cardiogenic shock patients at a mean of 48 hours from symptom onset, still demonstrating a significant decrease in mortality compared with those treated with medical therapy alone. An indirect conclusion from these few and limited reports is that intra-aortic balloon counterpulsation in shock patients may decrease and prolong the attrition of myocardium in both the infarct and noninfarct zones and that reperfusion by bypass surgery or direct infarct angioplasty may confer a survival benefit.

The TAMI investigators' observation that acute infarct-artery reocclusion was decreased in patients with intra-aortic balloon pump counterpulsation is further supported by a report from Ishihara and coworkers.[35] In this study, 114 patients with acute anterior wall myocardial infarction were treated with emergency coronary angioplasty and then divided into two groups. One group of 48 patients had intra-aortic balloon support after angioplasty and the other group of 66 patients did not. Those patients with the balloon pump had a reocclusion rate of just 2.4% compared with 17.7% ($P < .05$) for those patients who were treated routinely. Further, the left ventricular ejection fraction improved 9.2% in the balloon pump group compared with 4.5% in the comparison group.

Regardless, in the absence of reperfusion, there has been no convincing evidence that intra-aortic balloon pump counterpulsation alone improves survival in patients with cardiogenic shock. Although data are limited, DeWood and associates[36] compared 21 patients with acute infarction and cardiogenic shock treated by balloon pumping alone with 19 patients treated with balloon pumping and emergency coronary artery bypass grafting. The long-term mortality was significantly better (47%) in the emergency bypass group compared with controls (71%), and the subset of patients treated with counterpulsation and bypass surgery at or before 16 hours from symptom onset had the lowest mortality (25%). These surgical data support the premise that counterpulsation with reperfusion is more effective than counterpulsation alone.

CARDIOPULMONARY BYPASS SUPPORT

Percutaneous femoral-femoral cardiopulmonary bypass in the cardiac catheterization laboratory has undergone initial evaluation in several medical centers.[37] The system consists of 18- to 20-French arterial and venous cannulas placed either by local cutdown or percutaneous insertion. Under fluoroscopic guidance, venous and arterial cannulas are placed at the junction of the right atrium and inferior vena cava and in the iliac artery, respectively. Other components of the system are a nonocclusive blood pump, heat exchanger, oxygenator, connecting catheters, and supporting hardware, including controllers and a transport cart. This active aspiration/reinfusion system can provide 4 to 6 L per minute of blood flow, improving system blood pressure and peripheral perfusion as assessed clinically, and by pulmonary capillary wedge pressure and mixed venous oxygen saturation.[37, 38] When used in the laboratory, enhanced systemic perfusion, particularly in patients in cardiogenic shock, can allow prolonged coronary instrumentation or balloon angioplasty.

Relative to intra-aortic balloon pump counterpulsation, benefits of cardiopulmonary bypass support include the fact that the system's output is independent of the patient's intrinsic cardiac function or rhythm. Consequently, it is entirely possible to maintain a patient's systemic perfusion, noncardiac organ function, and mentation despite ventricular tachycardia, fibrillation, or asystole. Systemic perfusion pressure and blood flow are more effectively maintained than with the intra-aortic balloon pump.[39] Regardless, several limitations of in-laboratory cardiopulmonary bypass exist, including the presence of iliofemoral disease preventing the placement of large cannulas, blood loss requiring transfusion, and the relatively high risk of vascular complications.[40] Most important, cardiopulmonary bypass does not provide antegrade coronary flow, and regional ventricular dysfunction is not relieved.[41] In general, the use of portable cardiopulmonary bypass is not recommended for longer than 8 hours. Finally, the distinct possibility exists that temporary cardiopulmonary bypass will maintain consciousness and noncardiac organ function in patients who do not have and cannot recover enough left ventricular function to survive without cardiac transplantation.[42]

Shawl and colleagues[38] described an experience with the use of cardiopulmonary bypass support in 8 patients experiencing acute myocardial infarction complicated by cardiogenic shock. Seven of these patients had coronary anatomies suitable for emergency coronary angioplasty, which was performed. All seven survived at a mean follow-up of 8.2 months. The late left ventricular ejection fraction in survivors ranged from 32% to 52%. Shawl and associates' limited report again suggests the importance of temporary hemodynamic support combined with reperfusion for the ultimate survival of patients in cardiogenic shock.[43]

An additional practical benefit of cardiopulmonary bypass compared with intra-aortic balloon pumping may relate to the reduction or avoidance of systemic lactic acidosis through better maintenance of systemic perfusion and oxygenation. As a consequence, the metabolic milieu for left ventricular recovery and patient survival may be optimized after reperfusion in patients supported with cardiopulmonary bypass. Laks and colleagues[44] described a surgical experience with 50 patients in cardiogenic shock. Of the 15 (30%) in-hospital deaths, 8 resulted from multiple organ failure, which was present preoperatively in 5 of the 8 patients. Only 4 (8%) of 50 patients died from progressive left ventricular failure. These observations suggest that support of the systemic circulation and the noncardiac organ systems through temporary cardiopulmonary bypass may further enhance patient survival.

Other systemic and coronary perfusion systems exist such as passive or active balloon catheter coronary perfusion,[45–47] passive and active coronary sinus retroperfusion,[48–50] transaortic valve turbine pumping,[51, 52] and percutaneous left ventricular assist devices.[53] However, experience with these systems in the care of patients with acute infarction complicated by cardiogenic shock is extremely limited.[54]

CORONARY ARTERY BYPASS SURGERY

Early surgical revascularization of patients presenting with cardiogenic shock has been performed since the 1970s. Laks and associates[44] summarized the results of nine such reports appearing before 1980 and identified an in-hospital survival rate of 35% to 59%; survival for fewer than 2 years' posthospitalization ranged from 27% to 55%. DeWood,[36] Berg,[55] and Phillips[56, 57] and their coworkers reported in-hospital survival rates of up to 83% and late survival of approximately 65% with cardiac catheterization, aggressive hemodynamic support, and early surgical revascularization from 5 to 16 hours after symptom onset. Guyton and colleagues,[58] described the results of emergency coronary bypass surgery in 17 patients with persistent hemodynamic instability whose initial therapy for cardiogenic shock included either thrombolytic therapy and/or coronary angioplasty. Although there were only two (12%) in-hospital deaths, 47% of patients experienced major complications including death, bleeding, infection, and congestive heart failure. No late deaths were reported at a mean follow-up of 21 months. As indicated by these retrospective reviews of unique experiences from separate medical centers, early surgical revascularization for cardiogenic shock can improve in-hospital and late survival in selected patients. However, the need for 24-hour on-call operating suites with skilled surgeons and support personnel, increasingly limited healthcare resources, and costs have precluded the widespread application of emergency surgery for patients in cardiogenic shock.

PERCUTANEOUS TRANSLUMINAL CORONARY ANGIOPLASTY

Preliminary reports by several clinician-investigators have implied a survival benefit for those patients in cardiogenic shock who receive emergency cardiac catheterization and coronary angioplasty (Table 52–1). Brown and associates[59] described a series of 28 patients treated with angioplasty and a resultant 43% mortality in those achieving successful reperfusion compared with 82% mortality in those who did not. Shani and colleagues[60] performed successful angioplasty in six of nine patients with acute infarction and cardiogenic shock and documented significant improvement in left ventricular filling pressures and cardiac output immediately after intervention. At a mean follow-up of 9.5 months, five of Shani's patients were symptom free. Heuser and associates[61] performed successful angioplasty in 6 of 10 patients in cardiogenic shock, 5 of whom were symptom free at a mean follow-up of 8.6 months. Verna and coworkers[62] performed successful angioplasty in six patients in cardiogenic shock who had not reperfused with thrombolytic therapy alone. Four of these six patients were alive at follow-up ranging from 6 months to 1 year. Shawl and coau-

TABLE 52–1. Summary of Survival Data Reported in PTCA Studies

Study	*No. Patients*	*PTCA Success*		*Survival*	
Brown et al[59]	28	17/28	(61%)	12/28	(43%)
Disler et al[80]	7	5/7	(71%)	3/7	(43%)
Eltchaninoff et al[81]	33	25/33	(76%)	21/33	(64%)
Gacioch and Topol[82]	25	18/25	(72%)	14/25	(56%)
Heuser et al[61]	10	6/10	(60%)	6/10	(60%)
Hibbard et al[83]	45	28/45	(62%)	25/45	(55%)
Lee et al[34]	24	13/24	(54%)	12/24	(50%)
Lee et al[65]	69	49/69	(71%)	38/69	(55%)
Meyer et al[84]	25	22/25	(88%)	13/25	(52%)
Moosvi et al[85]	38	29/38	(76%)	20/38	(52%)
O'Neill et al[86]	27	24/27	(88%)	19/27	(70%)
Shani et al[60]	9	6/9	(67%)	6/9	(66%)
Shawl et al[63]	8	7/8	(88%)	7/8	(87%)
Stack et al[64]	43	—	—	25/43	(58%)
Verna et al[62]	7	7/7	(100%)	6/7	(86%)
Present study	59	49/59	(83%)	33/49	(67%)
Total	457	305/414	(74%)	260/457	(57%)

Abbreviation: PTCA = percutaneous transluminal coronary angioplasty.

thors[63] performed successful angioplasty in seven of eight patients in cardiogenic shock while using percutaneous cardiopulmonary bypass support. All seven were alive at a mean follow-up of 8.2 months. Stack and colleagues[64] treated 43 patients in cardiogenic shock with combined intravenous thrombolytic therapy followed by emergency angioplasty. The in-hospital mortality was 42%.

In a retrospective comparison of 83 patients from the University of Michigan, Lee and colleagues[34] compared 24 patients treated with conventional medical therapy plus coronary angioplasty with 59 patients who were treated by conventional medical therapy alone. The group receiving angioplasty had a 30-day survival of 50%, whereas those treated with medical therapy alone had only a 17% survival. In a subsequent multicenter study, Lee and associates[65] retrospectively assessed 69 patients who were treated with emergency angioplasty for acute infarction complicated by shock. Outcomes were compared between a group of 49 patients (71%) who had successful angioplasty and a group of 20 patients (29%) in whom the procedure was unsuccessful. The median time from shock to reperfusion in the group with successful angioplasty was 5 hours. The in-hospital 7-day survival was 69% in those with successful reperfusion compared to 20% ($P < .0005$) in those with failed procedures. This survival advantage persisted over a mean follow-up of 32.5 months; 55% of patients with successful angioplasty were alive at follow-up, whereas only 20% with unsuccessful procedures were alive ($P < .002$).

On the basis of diagnostic catheterization data, the presence of multivessel disease is a predictor and strong correlate of long-term mortality[66, 67] and cardiac event–free survival.[68] Conversely, single-vessel disease is generally associated with a better prognosis.[68, 69] Of interest, Lee and colleagues[34, 65] showed that patients with successful angioplasty and improved survival had a higher prevalence of single-vessel coronary disease as opposed to a greater prevalence of multivessel coronary disease in nonsurvivors. It is likely that severe left ventricular dysfunction with reduced cardiac output is even more destructive in the setting of multivessel disease because reduced coronary perfusion and flow become inadequate to maintain coronary flow across significantly stenosed non–infarct-related arteries.

The authors have reviewed their experience at the Mid America Heart Institute with coronary angioplasty in 59 patients presenting with acute myocardial infarction complicated by cardiogenic shock. These 59 patients represented 7% of 888 consecutive patients with acute infarction treated with intra-aortic balloon counterpulsation and direct coronary angioplasty. Forty-nine (83%) of patients in shock had successful re-establishment of infarct artery patency at a mean time of 4.7 ± 3.4 hours from symptom onset. Of those patients with initially successful angioplasty, 60% (31/49) survived to hospital discharge. This is in contrast to a 20% (2/10) survival rate for those patients with unsuccessful procedures ($P < .001$). By multivariate analysis, independent negative correlates of in-hospital and late survival were the presence of multivessel coronary disease and prior coronary bypass surgery.

The risks of coronary angioplasty for acute myocardial infarction are increased when it is performed in the setting of antecedent intravenous thrombolytic therapy.[70–75] The systemic lytic state contributes to significantly increased bleeding complications and stroke but further compromises the ability to manage critically ill patients in shock who require intra-aortic balloon counterpulsation or cardiopulmonary bypass support, additional arterial and venous punctures, and potentially emergency bypass surgery. Further, there is pathologic evidence that the systemic lytic state may result in intimal, medial, and adventitial coronary artery hemorrhage in contrast to direct coronary angioplasty without antecedent thrombolytic therapy.[70] Conversion of an otherwise anemic or bland myocardial infarction to a more extensive hemorrhagic myocardial infarction after angioplasty has also been associated with antecedent thrombolytic therapy.[70] Because of the lack of measurable benefit to shock patients treated with thrombolytic therapy alone, the increased risks and compromised results of coronary angioplasty when performed in the setting of systemic lysis, and the clear patient-care advantages derived through catheterization in these critically ill patients, the authors and others[76–79] consider direct coronary angioplasty to be the optimal therapy for patients experiencing acute myocardial infarction but particularly those complicated by cardiogenic shock.[80–86]

Although no clinical or anatomic factors clearly predict the development of cardiogenic shock, perhaps a "typical" patient is an older man with a history of myocardial infarction, a new acute anterior wall infarction secondary to left anterior descending artery or graft occlusion, and underlying multivessel coronary disease. The prompt recognition of patients having this or other high-risk profiles should facilitate immediate triage to a center with the capability for cardiac catheterization and emergency coronary angioplasty. When used, this strategy allows for the possibility of emergency coronary bypass surgery if clinical circumstances and angiography support that decision. On the basis of limited, nonrandomized data (Fig. 52–1), angioplasty and bypass surgery appear to offer the highest likelihood of in-

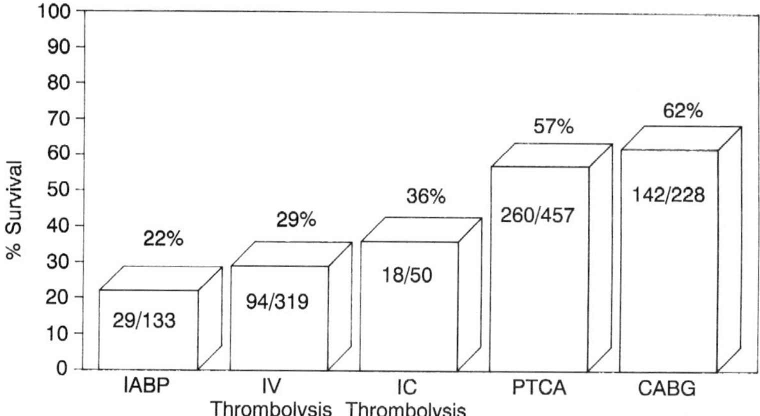

Figure 52–1. Comparison of pooled survival rates for various therapies utilized in cardiogenic shock. *Abbreviations:* IABP = intra-aortic balloon pump (references 23, 32, and 36); IV = intravenous thrombolysis (references 14 and 19); IC = intracoronary thrombolysis (references 16–18); PTCA = percutaneous transluminal coronary angioplasty (references 34, 59–65, and 81–86); CABG = coronary artery bypass grafting (references 32, 33, 36, 44, and 55–57).

hospital survival for those patients in cardiogenic shock. Regardless of primary therapy, strategies to decrease long-term mortality in hospital survivors of cardiogenic shock, particularly the subset of shock patients with multivessel disease, await further study.

CARDIOGENIC SHOCK CAUSED BY ACUTE RIGHT VENTRICULAR MYOCARDIAL INFARCTION

The clinical syndrome of right ventricular infarction has been well characterized in the literature.[87–91] Typically, right ventricular infarction occurs in association with inferior wall myocardial infarction, is recognized by clinical evidence of impedance to right ventricular filling, and is confirmed by cardiac catheterization. An even smaller subset of patients with right ventricular infarction present with or experience frank cardiogenic shock, usually resulting from concomitant left ventricular dysfunction. Reports of primary therapy with lytic agents alone are scant. However, a strategy of intravenous lytic therapy and delayed angioplasty has not been shown to enhance right ventricular function in this setting.[92]

We recently reviewed our experience at the Mid America Heart Institute with patients in cardiogenic shock in the setting of right ventricular infarction. This was an extremely uncommon mode of presentation, representing just 0.8% of all patients with acute myocardial infarction. Table 52–2 compares these seven patients with those experiencing cardiogenic shock, based solely on extensive left ventricular infarction, and with those not in cardiogenic shock at presentation. Despite the anticipated higher prevalence of right coronary artery occlusion in the patients in cardiogenic shock in the setting of right ventricular infarction compared with other groups, and despite a relatively low incidence of triple-vessel disease in the right ventricular infarction-shock group, the acute left ventricular ejection fraction in this subset was comparable to that in the left ventricular shock group. In-hospital mortality was also similar; three of the seven patients died (43%). Although patient numbers are small, these limited data suggest that cardiogenic shock in the presence of right ventricular infarction is associated with a prognosis comparable to that of predominantly left ventricular infarction and cardiogenic shock when treated with direct coronary angioplasty. Undoubtedly, this limited prognosis in part results from concomitant left ventricular dysfunction as reflected by the significantly reduced left ventricular ejection fraction at baseline in the right ventricular infarction group. Consequently, on clinical recognition of cardiogenic shock in the setting of right ventricular infarction and in the absence of a larger series of right ventricular infarction-shock patients shown to benefit from other therapies, the authors believe that this clinical syndrome should also be treated by intra-aortic balloon pump support, immediate catheterization, and direct coronary angioplasty in attempt to salvage both right and left ventricular function.

TABLE 52–2. Comparison of Left Ventricular (LV) and Right Ventricular (RV) Shock Versus Nonshock Patients

Variable	*LV Shock*	*RV Shock*	*Nonshock*
Number (%)	59 (7)	7 (0.8)	770 (92)
Anterior AMI (%)	63	0	41
AMI artery (%)	LAD (53)	RCA (71)	RCA (39)
3V CAD (%)	53	29	22
Mean LVEF (%)	30	34	48
Success (%)	83	100	95
In-hospital mortality (%)	44	43	5

Abbreviations: AMI = acute myocardial infarction; LAD = left anterior descending; RCA = right coronary artery; 3V CAD = three-vessel coronary artery disease; LVEF = left ventricular ejection fraction.

CONCLUSIONS

In the 1990s, cardiogenic shock is an unequivocal indication for immediate transfer to a facility with a catheterization laboratory and personnel and equipment available for emergency coronary angioplasty or bypass surgery. Percutaneous transluminal coronary angioplasty should be considered as the revascularization therapy of choice. Alternatively, emergency coronary artery bypass grafting when logistically possible, appears to result in at least comparable patient benefit and improvement in survival. Mechanical hemodynamic support by intra-aortic balloon pump counterpulsation or temporary cardiopulmonary bypass is an integral part of any acute care and revascularization strategy.

References

1. Binder MJ, Ryan JA, Marcus S, et al: Evaluation of therapy in shock following acute myocardial infarction. Am J Med 1955; 18:622–632.
2. Agress CM, Binder MJ: Cardiogenic shock. Am Heart J 1957; 54:458–477.
3. Kuhn LA. The treatment of cardiogenic shock: Part I. The nature of cardiogenic shock. Am Heart J 1967; 74:578–581.
4. Kimball T, Kimball JT: Treatment of myocardial infarction in a coronary care unit: A two year experience with 250 patients. Am J Cardiol 1967; 20:457–464.
5. Hands ME, Rutherford JD, Muller JE, et al: The in-hospital development of cardiogenic shock after myocardial infarction: Incidence, predictors of occurrence, outcome, and prognostic factors. J Am Coll Cardiol 1989; 14:40–46.
6. Goldberg RJ, Gore JM, Alpert JS, et al: Cardiogenic shock after acute myocardial infarction: Incidence and mortality from a community-wide perspective, 1975 to 1988. N Engl J Med 1991; 325:1117–1122.
7. Gunnar RM, Cruz A, Boswell J, et al: Myocardial infarction in shock: Hemodynamic studies and results of therapy. Circulation 1966; 33:753–762.
8. Scheidt S, Ascheim R, Kelley T: Shock after acute myocardial infarction: A clinical and hemodynamic profile. Am J Cardiol 1970; 26:556–564.
9. Ratshin RA, Rackley CE, Russell RO Jr: Hemodynamic evaluation of left ventricular function in shock complicating myocardial infarction. Circulation 1972; 45:127–139.
10. Shubin H, Weil MH: The hemodynamic effects of vasopressor agents in shock due to myocardial infarction (Abstract). Am J Cardiol 1965; 15:147.
11. Eichna LW: The treatment of cardiogenic shock: III. The use of isoproterenol in shock due to myocardial infarction. Am Heart J 1967; 74:848–852.
12. Talley RC, Goldberg LI, Johnson CE, et al: A hemodynamic comparison of dopamine and isoproterenol in patients in shock. Circulation 1969; 39:361–378.
13. Chatterjee K, Swan HJC, Kaushik VS, et al: Effects of vasodilator therapy for severe pump failure in acute myocardial infarction on short-term and late prognosis. Circulation 1976; 53:797–806.
14. GISSI (Gruppo Italiano per lo Studio della Streptochinasi nell'Infarto Miocardico): Effectiveness of intravenous thrombolytic treatment in acute myocardial infarction. Lancet 1986; 1:397–401.
15. Bates ER, Topol EJ: Limitations of thrombolytic therapy for acute myocardial infarction complicated by congestive heart failure and cardiogenic shock. J Am Coll Cardiol 1991; 18:1077–1084.

16. Mathey D, Kuck KH, Remmecke J, et al: Transluminal recanalization of coronary artery thrombosis: A preliminary report of its application in cardiogenic shock. Eur Heart J 1980; 1:207–212.
17. Mathey D, Kuck KH, Tilsner V, et al: Nonsurgical coronary artery recanalization in acute transmural myocardial infarction. Circulation 1981; 63:489–497.
18. Kennedy JW, Gensini GG, Timmis GC, et al: Acute myocardial infarction treated with intracoronary streptokinase: A report of the Society for Cardiac Angiography. Am J Cardiol 1985; 55:871–877.
19. The International Study Group: In-hospital mortality and clinical course of 20,891 patients with suspected acute myocardial infarction randomized between alteplase and streptokinase with or without heparin. Lancet 1990; 336:71–75.
20. Prewitt RM, Dounes AMT, Gu S, et al: Effects of hydralazine and increased cardiac output on recombinant tissue plasminogen activator induced thrombolysis in canine pulmonary embolism. Chest 1991; 99:708–714.
21. Kantrowitz A, Krakauer JS, Rosenbaum A, et al: Phase-shift balloon pumping in medically refractory cardiogenic shock. Arch Surg 1969; 99:739–743.
22. Mueller H, Ayres SM, Conklin F, et al: The effects of intra-aortic counterpulsation on cardiac performance and metabolism in shock associated with acute myocardial infarction. J Clin Invest 1971; 50:1885–1900.
23. Scheidt S, Wilner G, Mueller H, et al: Intraaortic balloon counterpulsation in cardiogenic shock: Report of a cooperative clinical trial. N Eng J Med 1973; 288:979–984.
24. Goodwin M, Hartmann J, McKeever L, et al: Safety of intraaortic balloon counterpulsation in patients with acute myocardial infarction receiving streptokinase intravenously. Am J Cardiol 1989; 64:937–938.
25. Ohman EM, Califf RM, George BS, et al: The use of intraaortic balloon pumping as an adjunct to reperfusion therapy in acute myocardial infarction. Am Heart J 1991; 121:895–901.
26. Scheidt S, Alonso DR, Post MR, et al: Quantification of myocardial damage in cardiogenic shock (Abstract). Circulation 1971; 44:11–46.
27. Page DL, Caulfield JB, Kastor JA, et al: Myocardial changes associated with cardiogenic shock. N Engl J Med 1971; 285:133–137.
28. Harnarayan C, Bennett MA, Pentecost BL, et al: Quantitative study of infarcted myocardium in cardiogenic shock. Br Heart J 1970; 32:728–732.
29. Gutovitz AL, Sobel BE, Roberts R: Progressive nature of myocardial injury in selected patients with cardiogenic shock. Am J Cardiol 1978; 41:469–475.
30. Vinten-Johansen J, Edwards H, Buckberg GD, et al: Effects of regional ischemia on the functional and metabolic state of the nonischemic segment. Physiologist 1982; 25:230.
31. Fujita M, Ohno A, Wada O, et al: Collateral circulation as a marker of the presence of viable myocardium in patients with recent myocardial infarction. Am Heart J 1991; 122:409–414.
32. Dunkman WB, Leinbach RC, Buckley MJ, et al: Clinical and hemodynamic results of intraaortic balloon pumping and surgery for cardiogenic shock. Circulation 1972; 46:465–477.
33. Keon WJ, Bedard P, Shankar KR, et al: Experience with emergency aortocoronary bypass grafts in the presence of acute myocardial infarction. Circulation 1973; 47:151–155.
34. Lee L, Bates ER, Pitt B, et al: Percutaneous transluminal coronary angioplasty improves survival in acute myocardial infarction complicated by cardiogenic shock. Circulation 1988; 78:1345–1351.
35. Ishihara M, Sato H, Tateishi H, et al: Intraaortic balloon pumping as the post angioplasty strategy in acute myocardial infarction. Am Heart J 1991; 122:385–389.
36. DeWood MA, Notske RN, Hensley MD, et al: Intraaortic balloon counterpulsation with and without reperfusion for myocardial infarction shock. Circulation 1980; 61:1105–1112.
37. Vogel RA, Shawl F, Tommaso C, et al: Initial report of the National Registry of Elective Cardiopulmonary Bypass Supported Coronary Angioplasty. J Am Coll Cardiol 1990; 15:23–29.
38. Shawl FA, Domanski MJ, Hernandez TJ, et al: Emergency percutaneous cardiopulmonary bypass support in cardiogenic shock from acute myocardial infarction. Am J Cardiol 1989; 64:967–970.
39. Smalling RW, Cassidy DB, Merhige M, et al: Improved hemodynamic and left ventricular unloading during acute ischemia using the hemopump left ventricular assist device compared to intraaortic balloon counterpulsation. J Am Coll Cardiol 1989; 13:160A.
40. Shawl FA, Domanski MJ, Punja S, et al: Percutaneous institution of cardiopulmonary (bypass) support: Technique and complications. J Am Coll Cardiol 1989; 13:159A.
41. Pavlides GS, Hauser AM, Stack RK, et al: Effect of peripheral cardiopulmonary bypass on left ventricular size, afterload and myocardial function during elective supported coronary angioplasty. J Am Coll Cardiol 1991; 18:499–505.
42. Kahn JK, Rutherford BD, McConahay DR, et al: Supported "high risk" coronary angioplasty using intraaortic balloon counterpulsation. J Am Coll Cardiol 1990; 15:1151–1155.
43. Phillips SJ, Ballantine B, Slonine P, et al: Percutaneous initiation of cardiopulmonary bypass. Ann Thorac Surg 1983; 36:223–225.
44. Laks H, Rosenkranz E, Buckbert GD: Surgical treatment of cardiogenic shock after myocardial infarction. Circulation 1986; 74:11–16.
45. Hinohara T, Simpson JB, Phillips HR, et al: Transluminal intracoronary reperfusion catheter: A device to maintain coronary reperfusion between failed coronary angioplasty and emergency coronary bypass surgery. J Am Coll Cardiol 1988; 11:977–982.
46. Lehmann KG, Atwood JE, Snyder EL, et al: Autologous blood perfusion for myocardial protection during coronary angioplasty: A feasibility study. Circulation 1987; 76:312–323.
47. Clemon M, Jaffee CC, Wohlgelernter D: Prevention of ischemia during percutaneous transluminal coronary angioplasty by catheter infusion of oxygenated Fluosol DA 20%. Circulation 1986; 74:555–562.
48. Drury JK, Yamazaki S, Fishbein MC, et al: Synchronized diastolic coronary venous retroperfusion: Results of a preclinical safety and efficacy study. J Am Coll Cardiol 1985; 6:328–335.
49. Corday E, Meerbaum S, Drury JK: The coronary sinus: An alternative channel for administration of arterial blood and pharmacologic agents for protection and treatment of acute cardiac ischemia. J Am Coll Cardiol 1986; 7:711–714.
50. Jacobs AK, Simon P, Hogfeldt V, et al: Increase in myocardial salvage by combining coronary sinus occlusion and retroperfusion. J Am Coll Cardiol 1989; 13:253A.
51. Smalling RW, Cassidy DB, Merhige M, et al: Improved hemodynamic and left ventricular unloading during acute ischemia using the left ventricular assist device compared to intra-aortic balloon counterpulsation. J Am Coll Cardiol 1989; 13:160A.
52. Lincoff AM, Popma JJ, Bates ER, et al: Successful coronary angioplasty in two patients with cardiogenic shock using the Nimbus Hemopump support device. Am Heart J 1990; 120:970–972.
53. Shani J, Hollander G, Nathan I, et al: Percutaneous left atrial-femoral artery bypass with a pulsatile pump: Initial experience in cardiogenic shock. J Am Coll Cardiol 1989; 13:53A.
54. Gacioch GM, Ellis SG, Lee L, et al: Cardiogenic shock complicating acute myocardial infarction: The use of coronary angioplasty and the integration of the new support devices into patient management. J Am Coll Cardiol 1992; 19:647–653.
55. Berg R Jr, Selinger SL, Leonard JL, et al: Immediate coronary artery bypass for acute evolving myocardial infarction. J Thorac Cardiovasc Surg 1981; 81:493–497.
56. Phillips SJ, Kongtahworn C, Skinner JR, et al: Emergency coronary artery reperfusion: A choice therapy for evolving myocardial infarction: Results in 339 patients. J Thorac Cardiovasc Surg 1983; 86:679–698.
57. Phillips SJ, Zeff RH, Skinner JR, et al: Reperfusion protocol and results in 738 patients with evolving myocardial infarction. Ann Thorac Surg 1986; 41:119–125.
58. Guyton RA, Arcidi JM Jr, Langford DA, et al: Emergency coronary bypass for cardiogenic shock. Circulation 1987; 76:22–27.
59. Brown TM, Iannone LA, Gordon DF, et al: Percutaneous myocardial reperfusion (PMR) reduces mortality in acute myocardial infarction complicated by cardiogenic shock. Circulation 1985; 72:309.

60. Shani J, Rivera M, Greengart A, et al: Percutaneous transluminal coronary angioplasty in cardiogenic shock. J Am Coll Cardiol 1986; 7:149A.
61. Heuser RR, Maddoux GL, Goss JE, et al: Coronary angioplasty in the treatment of cardiogenic shock: The therapy of choice. J Am Coll Cardiol 1986; 7:219A.
62. Verna E, Repetto S, Boscarini M, et al: Emergency coronary angioplasty in patients with severe left ventricular dysfunction or cardiogenic shock after acute myocardial infarction. Eur Heart J 1989; 10:958–966.
63. Shawl FA, Domanski MJ, Hernandez TJ, et al: Emergency percutaneous cardiopulmonary bypass support in cardiogenic shock from acute myocardial infarction. Am J Cardiol 1989; 64:967–970.
64. Stack RS, Califf RM, Hinohara T, et al: Survival and cardiac event rates in the first year after emergency coronary angioplasty for acute myocardial infarction. J Am Coll Cardiol 1988; 11:1141–1149.
65. Lee L, Erbel R, Brown TM, et al: Multicenter registry of angioplasty therapy of cardiogenic shock: Initial and long-term survival. J Am Coll Cardiol 1991; 17:599–603.
66. Muller DR, Topol EF, Ellis SG, et al: The Thrombolysis and Angioplasty in Myocardial Infarction (TAMI) Study Group: Multivessel coronary artery disease: A key predictor of short-term prognosis after reperfusion therapy for acute myocardial infarction. Am Heart J 1991; 121:1042–1049.
67. Miranda CP, Herbert WG, Dubach P, et al: Post-myocardial infarction exercise testing: Non Q-wave versus Q-wave correlation with coronary angiography and long-term prognosis. Circulation 1991; 84:2357–2365.
68. Schulman SP, Achuff SC, Griffith LSC, et al: Prognostic cardiac catheterization variables in survivors of acute myocardial infarction: A five-year prospective study. J Am Coll Cardiol 1988; 11:1164–1172.
69. Wilson WW, Gibson RS, Nygaard TW, et al: Acute myocardial infarction associated with single vessel coronary artery disease: An analysis of clinical outcome and the prognostic importance of vessel patency and residual ischemic myocardium. J Am Coll Cardiol 1988; 11:223–234.
70. Waller BF, Rothbaum DA, Pinkerton CA, et al: Status of the myocardium and infarct-related coronary artery in 19 necropsy patients with acute recanalization using pharmacologic (streptokinase, r-tissue plasminogen activator), mechanical (percutaneous transluminal coronary angioplasty) or combined types of reperfusion therapy. J Am Coll Cardiol 1987; 9:785–801.
71. Topol EJ, Califf RM, George BS, et al: A randomized trial of immediate versus delayed elective angioplasty after intravenous tissue plasminogen activator in acute myocardial infarction. N Engl J Med 1987; 317:581–588.
72. Simoons ML, Betriu A, Col J, et al: Thrombolysis with tissue plasminogen activator in acute myocardial infarction: No additional benefit from immediate percutaneous coronary angioplasty. Lancet 1988; 1:197–202.
73. The TIMI Research Group: Immediate vs. delayed catheterization and angioplasty following thrombolytic therapy for acute myocardial infarction: TIMI IIA results. JAMA 1988; 260:2849–2858.
74. Holmes DR Jr, Smith HC, Vlietstra RE, et al: Percutaneous transluminal coronary angioplasty alone or in combination with streptokinase therapy, during acute myocardial infarction. Mayo Clin Proc 1985; 60:449–456.
75. The TIMI Study Group: Comparison of invasive and conservative strategies after treatment with intravenous tissue plasminogen activator in acute myocardial infarction: TIMI II results. N Engl J Med 1989; 320:618–627.
76. O'Neill W, Timmis GC, Bourdillon PD, et al: A prospective randomized clinical trial of intracoronary streptokinase versus coronary angioplasty for acute myocardial infarction. N Engl J Med 1986; 314:812–818.
77. O'Neill WW, Topol EJ, Fung A, et al: Coronary angioplasty as therapy for acute myocardial infarction: University of Michigan experience. Circulation 1987; 76:79–86.
78. Stone GW, Rutherford BD, McConahay DR, et al: Direct coronary angioplasty in acute myocardial infarction: Outcome in patients with single vessel disease. J Am Coll Cardiol 1990; 15:534–543.
79. Kahn JK, Rutherford BD, McConahay DR, et al: Results of primary angioplasty for acute myocardial infarction in patients with multivessel coronary artery disease. J Am Coll Cardiol 1990; 16:1089–1096.
80. Disler L, Haitas B, Benjamin J, et al: Cardiogenic shock in evolving myocardial infarction: Treatment by angioplasty and streptokinase. Heart Lung 1987; 16:649–652.
81. Eltchaninoff H, Simpfendorfer C, Whitlow PL: Coronary angioplasty improves both early and 1 year survival in acute myocardial infarction complicated by cardiogenic shock. J Am Coll CArdiol 1991; 17:167A.
82. Gacioch GM, Topol EJ: Frontiers in cardiogenic shock management: Integration of angioplasty and new support devices. Circulation 1989; 80:624.
83. Hibbard MD, Holmes DR, Gersh BJ, et al: Coronary angioplasty for acute myocardial infarction complicated by cardiogenic shock. Circulation 1990; 82:511.
84. Meyer P, Blanc P, Baudouy M, et al: Treatment de choc cardiogenique primaire par angioplastie transluminale coronarienne a la phase aigue de l'infarctus. Arch Mal Coeur 1990; 83:329–334.
85. Moosvi AR, Villaneuva L, Gheorghiade M, et al: Early revascularization improves survival in cardiogenic shock. Circulation 1990; 82:308.
86. O'Neill WW, Erbel R, Laufer N, et al: Coronary angioplasty therapy of cardiogenic shock complicating acute myocardial infarction. Circulation 1985; 72:309.
87. Cohn JN, Guiha NH, Broder MI, et al: Right ventricular infarction: Clinical and hemodynamic features. Am J Cardiol 1974; 33:209–214.
88. Isner JM, Roberts WC: RV infarction complicating LV infarction secondary to coronary heart disease. Am J Cardiol 1978; 42:885–894.
89. Wackers FJT, Lie KI, Sokole EB, et al: Prevalence of right ventricular involvement in inferior wall infarction assessed with myocardial imaging with thallium-201 and technetium-99m pyrophosphate. Am J Cardiol 1978; 42:358–362.
90. Andersen HR, Falk E, Nielsen D: Right ventricular infarction: Frequency, size, and topography in coronary heart disease: A prospective study comparing 107 consecutive autopsies from a coronary care unit. J Am Coll Cardiol 1987; 10:1223–1232.
91. Sinha N, Ahuja RC, Saran RK, et al: Clinical correlates of acute right ventricular infarction in acute inferior myocardial infarction. Int J Cardiol 1989; 24:55–61.
92. Roth A, Miller HI, Kaluski E, et al: Early thrombolytic therapy does not enhance the recovery of the right ventricle in patients with acute inferior myocardial infarction and predominant right ventricular involvement. Cardiology 1990; 77:40–49.

CHAPTER 53

Congestive Heart Failure in Infants and Children

Bradley P. Fuhrman, MD • Lynn J. Hernan, MD • Michele C. Papo, MD • David M. Steinhorn, MD

Congestive heart failure (CHF) is a clinical syndrome. It is a circulatory state in which the heart (1) is unable to meet the demands of the body for blood flow, (2) cannot meet these demands without excessive use of compensatory mechanisms, or (3) meets these demands only at the expense of excessively high ventricular filling pressures. This crudely fashioned definition is purely operational and is not as concise as might be desired because cardiac decompensation is not an all-or-none phenomenon. It varies from absolute exhaustion of reserve (cardiogenic shock) to reliance on minor

TABLE 53–1. Processes Causing or Contributing to Congestive Heart Failure

Mechanism	*Example*
Ventricular volume overload	Ventricular septal defect
Vascular volume overload	Iatrogenic
Ventricular outflow obstruction	Aortic stenosis
Myocardial dysfunction	Myocarditis
Myocardial ischemia	Anomalous left coronary artery
Ventricular inflow restriction	Mitral stenosis
Arrhythmias	Paroxysmal atrial tachycardia
Anemia	Aplastic anemia
Hypoxia	Transposition of great vessels
Systemic hypermetabolism	Thyrotoxicosis

compensatory measures such as cardiac dilatation or hypertrophy at rest, with decompensation only on exertion.

CAUSES OF CONGESTIVE HEART FAILURE

Coronary vascular occlusion is generally not the cause of CHF in infants and children, although myocardial ischemia may be the confounding variable on which outcome depends.[1] Some general causes of CHF are listed in Table 53–1.

In congenital cardiac malformations, CHF is often the direct result of ventricular volume overload of the heart.[2] The infant with a ventricular septal defect, for example, may have so large a left-to-right shunt across the defect that only a small fraction of left ventricular inflow (left atrial return) is ejected to the aorta. A 75% left-to-right shunt, for instance, requires that the left ventricle pump 4 units of blood for every unit that enters the aorta. In such a patient, the left ventricular volume load is massive, perhaps four times normal. This requires an increase in left atrial pressure (preload) to achieve the requisite elevated left ventricular end-diastolic volume. Ultimately, the heart must hypertrophy to pump at this greater chamber circumference,[3] making it less compliant and further increasing requisite preload. Pulmonary edema and respiratory symptoms may occur. Any exertion that requires greater aortic flow will further elevate end-diastolic volume and left atrial pressure. In fact, for every additional liter of aortic flow demanded by the body, 4 L would have to be ejected by the left ventricle. The resultant limited ability of the heart to respond to an increased demand for oxygen delivery to tissues is manifest as "exercise intolerance."

Obstruction of a ventricle can cause CHF by exaggerating the ventricular work required to eject blood. When the metabolic cost of this work exceeds the potential of the coronary circulation to supply oxygen and substrate to the myocardium, coronary ischemia occurs.[4] Critical aortic stenosis, for instance, may present with CHF in infancy. Myocardial ischemia may lead to endocardial fibroelastosis, subendocardial infarction, and loss of myocardial function. Similarly, when the child with moderate aortic stenosis becomes an adult, calcification of the malformed valve causes progression of the obstruction and may cause ischemia, myocardial fibrosis, and CHF.[5]

Muscle dysfunction may be a primary cause of CHF in infants and children. In congenital cardiomyopathies and in myocarditis, muscle function is impaired and contractility is reduced. This limits the ability of the heart to use the Frank-Starling mechanism to augment stroke volume. Excessive preload may be required to generate even a subnormal stroke volume.

Primary myocardial ischemia may cause CHF. In anomalous origin of the left coronary artery from the pulmonary artery, coronary perfusion pressure may be inadequate to support left ventricular work.[6]

Inflow restriction may contribute to symptoms by elevating the preload required to fill even the normal ventricle, as in rheumatic mitral stenosis.[7] In this situation, even minor increases in left ventricular output or small decreases in cardiac filling time (associated with tachycardia) may inordinately elevate preload and precipitate pulmonary edema.

Other causes of CHF include arrhythmias (fast or slow), anemia, hypoxia, pathologic demand for oxygen delivery (e.g., thyrotoxicosis, pyrexia), and vascular volume overload.

These mechanisms may coexist and act synergistically to produce cardiac decompensation.

Table 53–2 lists conditions that may cause CHF in infants and children. This is not an exhaustive list but serves to illustrate the diversity of conditions that may be associated with CHF in this age group.

SIGNS AND SYMPTOMS

Because of the spectrum of decompensation encompassed by the term CHF and because of the age specificity of these manifestations, presenting findings are quite variable.[1] In all age groups, CHF implies cardiac enlargement, tachycardia, and tachypnea. In the neonate, because ventricular interdependence makes left- and right-sided heart failure virtually inseparable, hepatomegaly is virtually always present. Exercise intolerance may be manifest as dyspnea on exertion or as undue fatigue in the older child, or it may interfere with feeding in the infant. Hypoxia may be a sign of pulmonary edema, in which case it is generally responsive to oxygen administration, or it may represent an associated aspect of congenital cardiac disease such as right-to-left shunting of blood or admixture of systemic and pulmonary venous return.

Radiographic cardiomegaly may represent cardiac dilatation from ventricular volume overload in the patient with an atrial or ventricular septal defect and does not, in itself, establish the presence of CHF.[8] Poor contractility and reduced ejection fraction, documented by echocardiography or angiography, are often viewed as synonymous with CHF. When present, these findings clearly support a diagnosis of CHF. Their absence, however, cannot be interpreted as a guarantee that cardiac function is normal. The afterload reduction characteristic of mitral regurgitation, ventricular septal defect, or arteriovenous malformation may mask myocardial dysfunction and lend the appearance of normal contractility. Inotropic agents and sympathetic stimulation

TABLE 53–2. Causes of Congestive Heart Failure in Infants and Children

Congenital cardiac malformations
Congenital arteriovenous malformations
Anomalies of aortic arch
Endocardial fibroelastosis
Anomalous origin of left coronary artery
Cardiomyopathy
Myocarditis
Anemia
Congenital heart block
Tachyarrhythmias
Rheumatic fever
Kawasaki's syndrome
Endocarditis
Cardiac surgery

may also enhance ejection fraction and give the appearance of adequate myocardial function, although intrinsic compensatory mechanisms are no longer capable of supporting normal cardiac output.[9]

Frank cardiogenic shock is a common presentation of congenital cardiac disease. Metabolic acidosis, hypotension, poor perfusion, thready pulses, pallor, and diaphoresis are often presenting findings in ductus-dependent malformations such as coarctation, hypoplastic left-sided heart syndrome, interruption of the aortic arch, and critical aortic stenosis. This presentation is the hallmark of Galen's vein aneurysm. Cardiogenic shock is also an occasional presenting symptom in cardiomyopathy, anomalous origin of the left coronary artery, or myocarditis. In all age groups, sepsis may be accompanied by cardiogenic shock (low cardiac output, hypotension, and impaired cardiac contractility).

TREATMENT

Treatment of CHF in infants and children is not fundamentally different than it is in adults. (See also Chapter 48, Section VI.)

There are many components to the treatment of CHF. Some are quite specific, such as diuresis in iatrogenic volume overload, control of hypertension in hypertensive cardiomyopathy, transfusion in severe anemia, and balloon atrial septostomy in transposition of the great arteries. The generalities of treatment are, however, readily categorized (Table 53–3).

In general, myocardial dysfunction is treated by drug therapy directed at enhancement of contractility.[10] Myocardial dysfunction will occasionally respond to afterload reduction. Cautious vascular volume expansion (preload augmentation of ventricular work using the Frank-Starling mechanism) may improve cardiac output in the patient with cardiogenic shock and is a vital emergency measure. Reduction of myocardial workload is effective in all categories of CHF. This may be accomplished by bed rest, mechanical ventilation, or afterload reduction. Relief of the underlying cause of ventricular overwork should be immediately planned in the patient with surgically treatable CHF.

In certain situations, diuresis may be the mainstay of decongestive therapy. This is most commonly the case when pulmonary dysfunction contributes to symptoms and when edema, especially pulmonary edema, is itself troublesome.

Oxygen therapy is effective insofar as it enhances arterial oxygenation, relieves dyspnea, and reduces pulmonary vascular resistance.

Volume Expansion to Enhance Cardiac Output in Cardiogenic Shock

The infant or child with cardiogenic shock may exhaust the Frank-Starling mechanism reserve, but this is not always the case. Severe CHF may interfere with oral fluid intake or may occur quite suddenly (as in ductus-dependent cardiac defects). This may interfere with the natural tendency of the body to retain vascular volume in the face of low cardiac output. Excessive use of diuretics may pose a similar problem. Volume expansion is, therefore, a reasonable first line of treatment in cardiogenic shock unless preload is known to be adequate.

Overzealous volume expansion can cause pulmonary edema or anasarca. It may produce myocardial edema, which can interfere with diastolic function of the heart. Pulmonary edema generally responds to positive end-expiratory pressure (PEEP). Anasarca is of little acute significance. An initial trial of volume expansion is, therefore, safe in the patient with cardiogenic shock.

TABLE 53–3. Treatment of Congestive Heart Failure in Infants and Children

- Drugs that augment contractility
  - Digoxin
  - Catecholamines (dopamine, dobutamine, epinephrine, norepinephrine, isoproterenol)
  - Methylxanthines (theophylline)
  - Bipyridines (amrinone)
- Myocardial workload reduction
- Oxygen and positive end-expiratory pressure
- Diuretics
- Vascular volume expansion

Drugs That Enhance Myocardial Contractility

The general categories of inotropic agents are catecholamines, digitalis-like agents, and amrinone-like agents. Of these, the digitalis family has the longest tradition of use for cardiac inotropy.

Digoxin and related compounds inhibit activity of the membrane-bound sodium potassium adenosine triphosphatase. This raises intracellular sodium, which, in turn, slows the rate of exchange of intracellular calcium for extracellular sodium. The resultant rise in intracellular calcium augments contractility. This inotropic effect is not accompanied by a positive chronotropic effect. In fact, digoxin is vagomimetic and slows the heart. This may be beneficial because it lengthens diastole, allowing more time for cardiac filling. Digoxin is an effective short-term inotropic agent. Prolonged efficacy is more difficult to demonstrate. Digoxin has minimal vasomotor effects but is a modest systemic vasoconstrictor. In the critical care setting, digoxin has seen less use since the introduction of continuous catecholamine infusions because of its relatively long half-life, its predominant renal clearance, and its propensity to cause cardiac arrhythmias. This propensity of digoxin is exaggerated by hypokalemia. Diuretics, which may cause potassium depletion, add to this potential hazard of digoxin therapy.

Catecholamines act through the adrenergic receptor complex. These receptors are present in myocardium and in vascular and bronchial smooth muscle. Adrenergic receptors differ in their receptor specificity (α_1 or α_2 adrenergic, β_1 or β_2 adrenergic, and D_1 or D_2 dopaminergic). They also differ in the regulatory protein used to modify activity of membrane-bound adenyl cyclase (Gs, which stimulates cyclic adenosine monophosphate [cAMP] production, and Gi, which inhibits cAMP production). Intracellular levels of cAMP determine myocardial contractility, smooth-muscle tone, and rate of spontaneous action potential formation. For instance, a β_1 receptor linked to Gs regulatory protein allows a beta$_1$ agonist to raise intracellular cAMP. Such receptors are present in myocardium and in Purkinje's cells and, consequently, when stimulated, raise heart rate and enhance contractility.

The distribution of receptors is a primary determinant of the effect of an agonist. For instance D_1 receptors, which are stimulated by dopamine, are found primarily in kidney, viscera, and coronary arteries. When stimulated, they cause renal, splanchnic, and coronary blood flow to rise and yet have no detectable effect on skin perfusion because they are not present in skin.

Another determinant of agonist effect is relative potency at each kind of receptor (Table 53–4). For instance, norepinephrine is a potent alpha agonist and a weak beta agonist. Its effect is, therefore, predominantly to constrict systemic

TABLE 53–4. Adrenergic Receptors

Receptor	*Action*	*Order of Efficacy*
α_1	Vasoconstriction	Epi > NE > Dop
β_1	Inotropic, chronotropic	I, Epi, Dobut > Dop > NE
β_2	Vasodilatation & bronchodilation	I > Epi > Dobut > Dop > NE
D	Vasodilatation (renal)	Dop

Abbreviations: Epi = epinephrine; NE = norepinephrine; Dop = dopamine; Dobut = dobutamine; I = isoproterenol.

arterioles. It is a mild inotrope. Dopamine stimulates D_1 receptors at low, intermediate, and high doses, β_1 receptors at intermediate and high doses, and α_1 receptors only at high doses.

Some general comments concerning the use of catecholamines to manage CHF are warranted. First, when an inotropic agent causes the heart to pump more blood at constant aortic pressure (a desired effect), cardiac workload is increased. This requires augmentation of oxygen delivery to the myocardium. For this reason, catecholamine use may be associated with myocardial ischemia, even in nonischemic cardiac disease. Second, the commonly used catecholamines—epinephrine, norepinephrine, dopamine, dobutamine, and isoproterenol—all cause tachycardia. As the heart rate rises, diastole shortens proportionally more than does systole. This can interfere with cardiac filling, thereby worsening stroke volume. Third, catecholamines are intrinsically arrhythmogenic.

Methylxanthines (like theophylline) and bipyridines (like amrinone) augment contractility by elevating intracellular cAMP but using mechanisms independent of the adrenergic receptor. Theophylline inhibits activity of all phosphodiesterases: those that "degrade" cAMP (which augments contractility) and those that "clear" intracellular cyclic guanosine monophosphate (which is thought to decrease contractility). In the aggregate, theophylline is, nonetheless, a positive inotropic agent. Amrinone and its congeners inhibit activity of phosphodiesterase III, which degrades cAMP only. Amrinone raises intracellular calcium, is a positive inotrope, and is a systemic vasodilator. This combination, inotropic activity and afterload reduction, may have special value in low-output states and in situations in which myocardial workload should not be excessively increased.

Treatment of Congestive Heart Failure by Reducing Cardiac Work

The burden of the heart, to meet the needs of the body for systemic oxygen and substrate delivery while supporting its own metabolic requirements, can represent a conflict of interest.[11] In cardiogenic shock, when the heart is unable to bear this burden, forcing it to perform heroics will often cause myocardial necrosis. Other measures that are useful in infants and children focus on reducing cardiac work to allow the pump to recover. This is of special importance after cardiac operations, when the heart has been injured by myocardial incision, put at risk of air embolism by opening the heart, and subjected to coronary ischemia followed by reperfusion with blood. Several of these measures are listed in Table 53–5.

Foremost among them is mechanical ventilation with oxygen, coupled with sedation and, as appropriate, neuromuscular blockade.[12] Mechanical ventilation alleviates the work of breathing, which may be substantial if there is pulmonary edema or lung dysfunction. It protects the patient from risk of respiratory arrest when narcotics are used to relieve pain. Oxygen should be used to relieve arterial desaturation because desaturation wastes a fraction of the cardiac output; desaturated blood carries oxygen inefficiently. PEEP is often used to alleviate arterial desaturation in the patient with pulmonary edema. Sedation, pain relief, and neuromuscular blockade limit endogenous catecholamine secretion, reduce sympathetic vasoconstriction to pain, and prevent patient movement, which contributes to circulatory demand.

Prevention of fever reduces the metabolic demand that must be satisfied by activity of the heart. It also reduces heart rate, facilitates cardiac filling in diastole, and prevents or treats junctional ectopic tachycardia.

Pharmacologic treatment of excessive afterload may be used to reduce cardiac work to the extent that it does not impair organ perfusion, especially perfusion of the myocardium by the coronary circulation. Agents often used to reduce afterload include nitroprusside, calcium channel blockers, prostaglandin E_1, captopril, and enalapril. Myocardial work may also be limited using β-blockers, because cardiac output need not always be as great as the body appears to demand.

Devices to Support the Failing Heart

Aortic balloon counterpulsation is possible in very small children but becomes increasingly challenging as catheter size declines, heart rate rises, or myocardial function worsens. Arrhythmias interfere with this modality. However, fundamentally, the underlying limitation of aortic counterpulsion is that it pumps no blood. It reduces cardiac afterload and raises diastolic pressure but only by displacing blood that has been ejected by the left ventricle.

Infants and children, like adults, can be supported using extracorporeal devices if they suffer temporary or permanent myocardial devastation. Extracorporeal membrane oxygenation (ECMO) has been shown to be useful as a means of cardiac rescue after repair of congenital cardiac malformations.[13] Some postoperative patients are unable to support their circulation despite an adequate repair, and cardiogenic shock develops. Although ECMO raises afterload in this setting by restoring adequate blood pressure, it does relieve the heart of the burden of supporting the entire circulation. At the same time, it raises coronary artery diastolic pressure. ECMO, therefore, "rests" both right and left ventricles. When ECMO is used to "rest" the heart, it must be remembered that the left ventricle may find itself unable to eject at the higher afterload afforded by the extracorporeal pump. In this setting, left atrial return (flow through the ductus arteriosus, bronchial flow, residual anterograde flow across the pulmonary valve) may pool on the left side of the heart. Pressure could, in theory, rise in the left ventricle and atrium until it equaled aortic diastolic pressure.

TABLE 53–5. Modalities That May Be Used to Reduce Myocardial Work

Mechanical ventilation
Sedation
Pain relief
Neuromuscular blockade
Prevent fever
Pharmacologic afterload reduction
β-blockers
Aortic balloon counterpulsation
ECMO/ECLS, LVAD, RVAD

Abbreviations: ECMO = extracorporeal membrane oxygenation; ECLS = extracorporeal life support; LVAD = left ventricular assist device; RVAD = right ventricular assist device.

When this occurs to a clinically important degree, pulmonary edema develops. This scenario can be prevented by "venting" the left atrium to the venous return of the ECMO circuit, by administration of inotropic agents, or by atrial septectomy in selected patients. ECMO has been used with success in patients with myocarditis as well.

Other devices such as the left ventricular assist device and the right ventricular assist device can be used to move atrial return to the appropriate great cardiac vessel, completely or partially bypassing one ventricle. This does not require a membrane oxygenator and does not require systemic heparinization. In most infants and children, however, cardiogenic shock is a biventricular problem.

CONCLUSION

CHF is an unstable situation. Its presence implies very limited myocardial reserve. CHF demands prompt stabilization at all ages, although treatment may be quite age or cause specific.

References

1. Talner NS: Heart failure. *In*: Moss' Heart Disease in Infants, Children and Adolescents. 3rd ed. Adams FH, Emmanouilides GC (Eds). Baltimore, Williams & Wilkins, 1989, pp 890–911.
2. Sahn DJ, Vaucher Y, Williams DC, et al: Echocardiographic detection of large left to right shunts and cardiomyopathies in infants and children. Am J Cardiol 1976; 38:73–79.
3. Gaasch WH, Levine HJ, Quinones MA, et al: Left ventricular compliance: Mechanisms and clinical implications. Am J Cardiol 1976; 38:645–653.
4. Kubler W, Katz AM: Mechanisms of early pump failure in the ischemic heart: Possible role of ATP depletion and inorganic phosphate accumulation. Am J Cardiol 1977; 40:467–471.
5. Buckberg G, Eber L, Herman M, et al: Ischemia in aortic stenosis. Am J Cardiol 1975; 35:778.
6. Takahashi M, Lurie P: Abnormalities and diseases of the coronary vessels. *In*: Moss' Heart Disease in Infants, Children and Adolescents. 3rd ed. Adams FH, Emmanouilides GC (Eds). Baltimore, Williams & Wilkins, 1989, pp 630–635.
7. Rockley CE, Edwards JE, Karp RE: Mitral valve disease. *In*: The Heart. 7th ed. Hurst JW, Schlant RL, Rockley CE, et al. (Eds). New York, McGraw-Hill, 1989.
8. Freedom RM, Benson LN: Ventricular septal defect. *In*: Neonatal Heart Disease. Freedom RM, Benson LN, Smallhorn JF (Eds). London, Springer-Verlag, 1991, p 578.
9. Sanders SP: Echocardiography. *In*: Fetal and Neonatal Cardiology. Long WA (Ed). Philadelphia, WB Saunders, 1990, p 304.
10. Notterman DA: Pharmacology of the cardiovascular system. *In*: Pediatric Critical Care. Fuhrman BP, Zimmerman JJ (Eds). St. Louis, Mosby-Year Book, 1992, pp 323–338.
11. Fuhrman BP: Regional circulation. *In*: Critical Care: State of the Art. Vol 10. Fuhrman BP, Shoemaker WC (Eds). Anaheim, CA, Society of Critical Care Medicine, 1989, pp 338–339.
12. Fuhrman BP, Papo MC: Critical care after surgery for congenital cardiac disease. *In*: Pediatric Critical Care. Fuhrman BP, Zimmerman JJ (Eds). St. Louis, Mosby-Year Book, 1992, pp 345–358.
13. Dalton HJ, Siewers RD, Fuhrman BP, et al: Extracorporeal membrane oxygenation for cardiac rescue following surgery for congenital heart disease. Crit Care Med 1993; 21:1020–1028.

CHAPTER 54

Electrocardiography

Louis Rakita, MD, CM, FACP, FRCP(C), FACC
Thomas Vrobel, MD, FACP, FACC
Elizabeth S. Kaufman, MD, FACC

Electrocardiogram (ECG) interpretation and rhythm monitoring are essential in any unit devoted to the care of the critically ill. Standard and special lead ECGs are important in assessing the cardiac status of seriously ill patients. The purpose of ECG monitoring is to assess continuously cardiac rhythms and determine the presence or absence of myocardial ischemia. Abnormal cardiac rhythms (arrhythmias) can occur during any illness and are the most common mechanism of death. Similarly, myocardial ischemia (i.e., the inability to supply enough oxygen to the myocardial muscle) can occur in seriously ill patients even in the absence of primary coronary artery disease.

LEAD PLACEMENT

Before a skin electrode is attached, the skin must be lightly abraded and all hair removed. If skin preparation is inadequate, the large noise-signal ratio may cause a marked baseline instability and produce a noise artifact in the ECG tracing.

Correctly positioned electrodes produce large, easily recognized P waves and QRS complexes. Although a single lead may produce recognizable P, QRS, and T waves, two or more leads will allow determination of the wave orientation (Fig. 54–1). Potential electrode placements are shown in Figure 54–2.

Recording atrial activity is extremely helpful in some complicated arrhythmias. In some situations, this can be accomplished noninvasively by searching for atrial activity in standard leads (leads I, III, aVF, and V_1). Alternatively, modified leads such as those described by Lewis and Golub

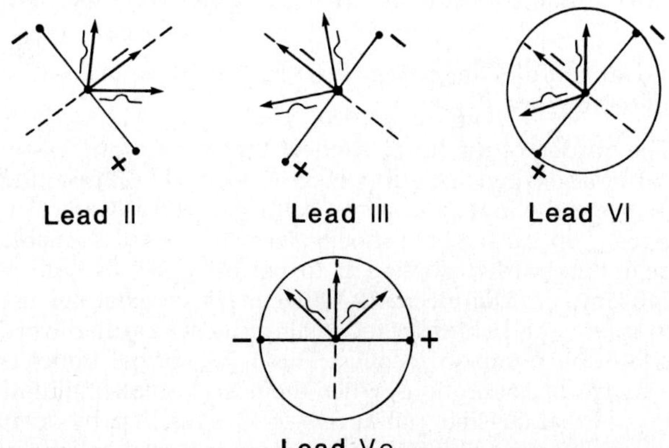

Figure 54–1. Leads II, III, V_1, and V_6 are each represented by the diagonal lines terminated by the positive and negative signs. The lines with the arrowheads represent vectors, and the discontinuous lines represent the perpendicular to the lead. The orientation of the vector with respect to the lead line determines whether the deflection is positive, negative, or isoelectric. Thus, several leads may be useful in the search for low-amplitude P waves.

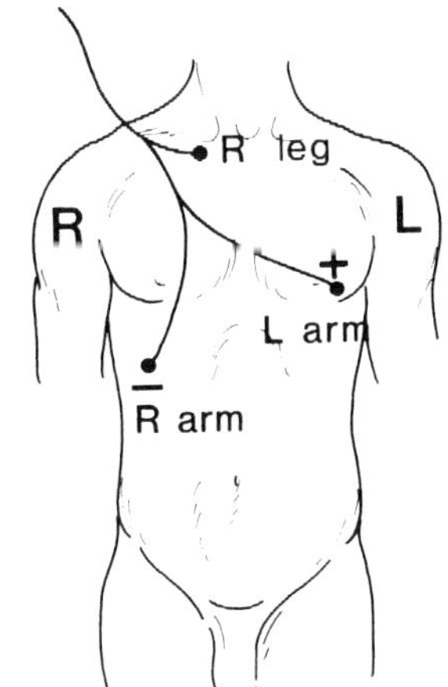

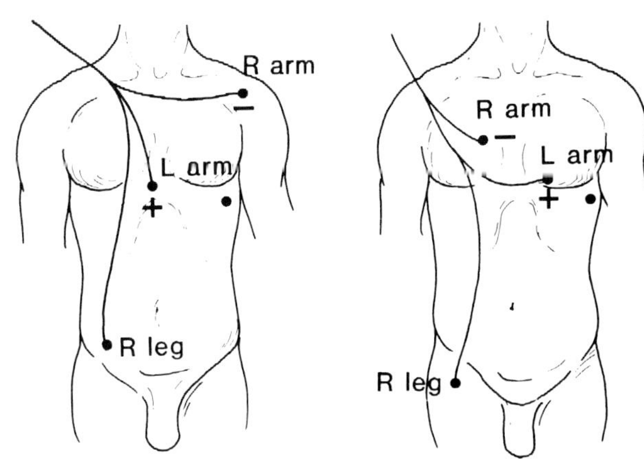

Figure 54–2. Various lead placements that are likely to give the most recognizable P and QRS deflections are illustrated. Modifications may have to be made for individual patients. The right (R) leg lead serves as a ground.

can reveal atrial activity. To record these, the right and left arm leads from a standard ECG machine are positioned in various locations over the right or left thorax, or both, and the ECG machine is run on lead I. If these are not helpful, an esophageal lead can be recorded. A cooperative patient can easily swallow a single-wire lead inserted in a capsule (Fig. 54–3). Alternatively, the same data can be provided by a right atrial lead inserted through a vein into the right atrium. Use of the esophageal or right atrial lead requires at least a two-channel recorder; one channel records the standard lead and the second channel records the esophageal/right atrial lead. QRS complexes and P waves are often confused in the latter two leads, which are closer to the heart, and the standard lead is, therefore, essential to distinguish the P wave from the QRS complex (Fig. 54–4).

Precordial leads recorded to the right of the sternum in positions usually recorded to the left may be helpful in delineating the presence of right ventricular infarction.

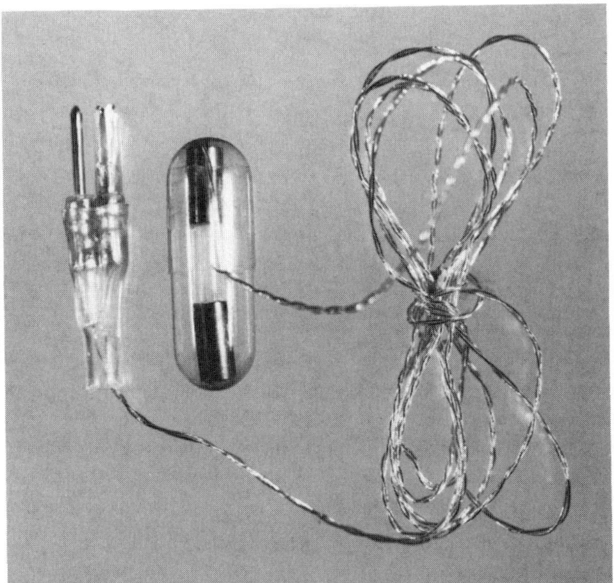

Figure 54–3. An esophageal lead (Arzco Medical Electronics, Iowa City, IA). The large capsule is difficult for some patients to swallow. Allowing the patient to consume liquids or soft food, such as bread or jellies, may facilitate swallowing.

INDICATIONS FOR CONTINUOUS ELECTROCARDIOGRAM MONITORING

Critically ill patients require continuous ECG monitoring. Arrhythmias are the most common cause of death in patients with acute myocardial infarction; therefore, acute myocardial infarction is an absolute indication for ECG monitoring, especially for the first 48 hours. With anterior infarction, recording two or more leads will facilitate detection of conduction defects.

Other indications for monitoring include known or suspected serious arrhythmias, syncope with suspected cardiac disease, electrolyte disorders, drug toxicity or potential proarrhythmia, temporary or new permanent pacemakers, cardiac trauma, unstable angina, and hypothermia. Patients whose conditions are unstable as a result of other acute cardiac or noncardiac problems may also be candidates for ECG monitoring. High-risk conditions include acute gastrointestinal bleeding, particularly with hypotension or shock; pulmonary embolism; acute pulmonary edema not immediately responsive to appropriate therapy; recovery from cardiac arrest; acute cardiac tamponade or hypertensive crisis; and recovery from cardiac surgery, noncardiac surgery, or burns.

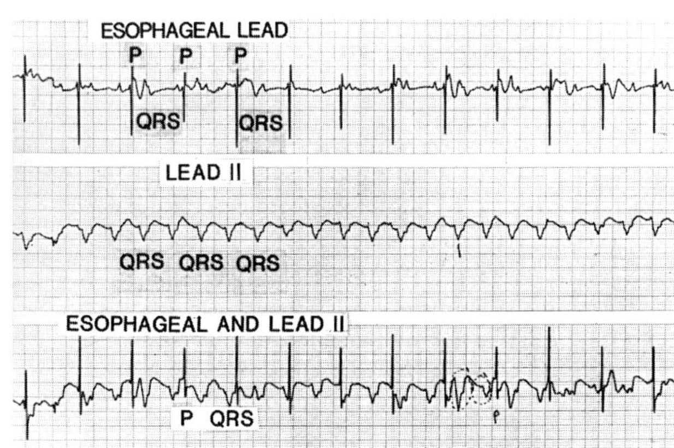

Figure 54–4. Esophageal lead and lead II. Note the large P waves and the small QRS complexes in the esophageal lead. Simultaneous recording of a limb lead is necessary to clearly separate P waves from QRS complexes.

MONITORING EQUIPMENT

ECG monitors at the bedside should be connected to a central station. The equipment should include alarm warnings for arrhythmias. The alarm sounding at the central station should preferably be shut off only at the bedside to ensure that the patient's condition is checked and that all connections are adjusted to limit false alarms. Most systems have at least some false alarms; however, these will be minimized if the system can be disconnected when electrodes are being changed or when the patient is being bathed or examined or is undergoing a procedure. The central station should have a strip recorder that is automatically activated by any alarm and identifies each tracing by the patient's name and time of day. Even better is a storage medium that can play back any or all (full disclosure) of the patient's ECG that is recorded during the previous 24 hours and that can record two different leads simultaneously for better identification of abnormal QRS and P waves. Many monitoring units use computers for arrhythmia diagnosis. Although these can assist in detecting abnormal rhythms, accurate arrhythmia detection requires continuous observation.

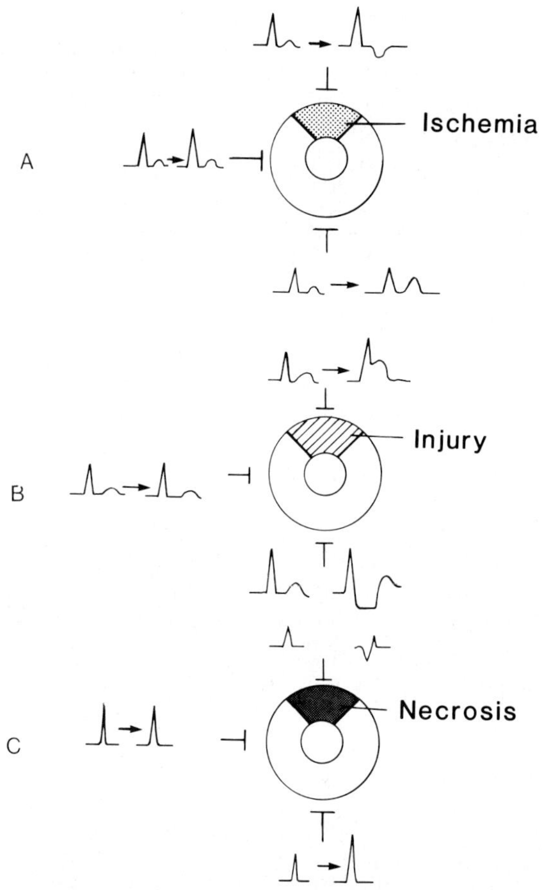

ELECTROCARDIOGRAPHIC DIAGNOSIS IN SPECIFIC CLINICAL CONDITIONS

Myocardial Ischemia and Infarction

The ECG is an important tool for diagnosing myocardial ischemia and infarction as well as associated cardiac arrhythmias. The ECG exhibits depolarization/repolarization patterns that vary with the severity of ischemia and infarction. Myocardial ischemia distorts the T wave (Fig. 54–5) by abruptly increasing its slope and amplitude (hyperacute peaking) and eventually changing its direction of repolarization so that the T-wave vector points away from the ischemic area (T-wave inversion). This pattern may or may not be reversible.

Prolonged ischemia causes myocardial injury that alters the ST segment (see Fig. 54–5). ST-segment elevation usually signifies the early phase of a myocardial infarction; however, it can also be a transient consequence of coronary artery spasm (Prinzmetal's angina). ST-segment depression and/or T-wave changes can often be reversible, without myocardial damage, but can also be associated with myocardial damage.

The final event in progressive ischemia is myocardial infarction or ischemic myocardial necrosis (see Fig. 54–5). This changes the direction of the initial depolarization and moves the mean 0.04-second vector away from the area of infarction. The result is Q-wave distortion, loss of R-wave voltage, an increased R wave, or no change in the QRS complex, depending on the relationship of the specific lead to the zone of necrosis produced by the infarction. Q-wave myocardial infarctions are preceded by the sequence of ECG patterns associated with the progression of ischemia to injury and then to necrosis. Typically, hyperacute T-wave alterations occur early after the onset of ischemia and last from minutes to hours. They are replaced by ST-segment alterations that depend on infarction site relative to lead placement. ST-segment elevations/depressions may return to baseline over a period of hours to days. During this transient period, the ECG may be fairly normal; this is referred to as the *paradoxic normalization phase.* T-wave inversions are usually seen in conjunction with the ST-segment changes and can last from a few days to many years. Depolarization abnormalities appear hours to days after the onset of infarction. Although they generally remain as a permanent marker of ischemic myocardial damage, they can disappear, especially in inferior wall myocardial infarctions, leaving the ECG with no evidence of the clinical event.

A Ischemia

B Injury

C Necrosis

Figure 54–5. Myocardial ischemia *A* causes abnormalities of the T wave. Leads directly over the involved area produce T wave inversion, whereas leads on the opposite wall may yield increases in T wave amplitude. Leads distant or perpendicular to the area of involvement result in no change in the T wave.

Myocardial injury *B* causes abnormalities of the ST segment. Transmural injury results in ST segment elevation in leads recorded directly over the involved area but causes ST segment depression in leads recorded over the opposite wall. Distant or perpendicular leads show no change.

Myocardial necrosis *C* causes abnormalities of the QRS complex (depolarization process). Q waves or loss of R wave amplitude develops in leads recorded over areas of myocardial necrosis. Increase in R wave amplitude develops in leads recorded over the opposite wall. Again, no change may occur in QRS configuration distant or perpendicular to the area of myocardial necrosis.

In *non–Q-wave* infarctions, the ECG shows persistent ST-segment depression and/or deep T-wave inversion in leads over the area of involvement. Although Q-wave infarctions tend to involve more myocardial necrosis, the presence or absence of Q waves does not infallibly distinguish between transmural and nontransmural infarctions identified anatomically.

The ECG depolarization/repolarization abnormalities that characterize ischemia and infarction are not unique to these disorders. Abnormal depolarization patterns consistent with myocardial infarction can also be produced by positional or orientational factors, left or right ventricular hypertrophy, other myocardial disease, pulmonary infarction, or conduction abnormalities. Early repolarization or juvenile T-wave inversion can produce repolarization ST-segment or T-wave patterns consistent with myocardial infarctions in otherwise normal patients. Other conditions that may have ECG patterns similar to that of myocardial infarction include acute pericarditis, numerous intra-abdominal processes, central nervous system processes (especially subarachnoid bleeding), ventricular strain, bundle branch block, mitral valve prolapse syndrome, hyperventilation, intrinsic and pacemaker-induced tachycardias, administration of pharmacologic agents such as digitalis, and certain metabolic abnormalities, especially those associated with abnormal potassium levels.

Although the ECG is a standard test for evaluating myocardial ischemia and infarction, there are marked limitations to its diagnostic usefulness. An absolute diagnosis should not be made solely on the basis of a single ECG; rather, the overall clinical picture should be carefully assessed together with serial ECGs. A 12-lead ECG obtained during an episode of pain can help to establish an otherwise uncertain diagnosis.

Patients with diagnosed or suspected acute myocardial infarction or with unstable angina should be electrocardiographically monitored for at least 48 hours to detect complicating arrhythmias. Ventricular arrhythmias are a frequent complication of myocardial infarction. Ventricular fibrillation and ventricular tachycardia may be preceded by premature ventricular complexes or may occur without warning. Sudden ventricular fibrillation occurs in up to 11% of acute myocardial infarctions. Supraventricular tachycardias are not as frequent, but their presence indicates a less favorable prognosis, and the associated rapid heart rate can precipitate or intensify the ischemic process.

Inferior wall myocardial infarction is often associated with sinus bradycardia, first-degree atrioventricular (AV) block, second-degree AV block, and/or third-degree AV block with a narrow-complex junctional escape rhythm at 40 to 60 per minute. The block is in the AV node, permitting normal antegrade bundle conduction. These conduction abnormalities almost invariably resolve within several days. If these conduction abnormalities are well tolerated, no specific therapy is needed. In contrast, in anterior wall myocardial infarctions complicated by heart block, the block may be sudden or rapid in progression, the escape rhythm is a slow, wide-complex, poorly tolerated idioventricular rhythm (because of infra-Hisian disease), and the prognosis is very poor.

Although there is some variation in terminology, the usual convention for infarction location is as follows. The infarct is in the inferior wall when leads II, III, and aVF are involved; the high lateral wall when leads I and aVL are involved; the anteroseptal wall when leads V_1 to V_4 are involved; the anterior wall when leads V_3 and V_4 are involved; and extensively throughout the anterior wall when leads V_1 to V_6 are involved. In true posterior infarction, the right precordial leads show ST-segment depression, T waves that are upright and tall, and an increase in R-wave voltage so that it exceeds the S-wave voltage.

Pericarditis

Although the ECG recording can be completely normal in patients with acute pericarditis, more frequently it progresses through four chronologic stages. The first, or acute, stage begins within days and lasts from a few days to about 2 weeks. Myocarditis of the epicardium partially depolarizes this layer so that the ST-segment vector points toward the epicardium. Thus, all leads not directed toward the cavity of the heart show ST-segment elevation, whereas leads that relate to the cavity potential, such as aVR and sometimes V_1, show ST-segment depression. Characteristically, the ST segment is concave upward. Occasionally, the PR segment is depressed probably because of epicardial atrial injury.

The second stage also may last up to 2 weeks. During the second stage, the ST segment returns to its baseline level, and the T wave remains concordant. In the third stage, injury to the subepicardial layer reverses the normal pattern of repolarization and inverts the T wave. Pericardial effusion may reduce the ECG voltage and/or cause current swings (electrical alternans), reflecting an effusion-induced swinging motion of the heart. This stage lasts from a week to several months. During the final stage, which may last months to years, T-wave changes gradually resolve.

The differentiation of pathologic acute pericarditis with ST-segment elevation from nonpathologic, early repolarization requires both clinical correlation and serial ECGs. The differential diagnosis also includes myocardial infarction or ischemia, myocarditis, hyperkalemia, acute cor pulmonale, cerebrovascular accidents, and pulmonary embolism.

Pericardial Tamponade

There are no specific ECG changes associated with pericardial tamponade; however, this condition should be considered in all hypotensive patients with low voltage and sinus tachycardia, or electrical alternans. Myocardial rupture may produce electromechanical dissociation with sinus bradycardia.

Congestive Heart Failure/Pulmonary Edema

The ECG should be carefully evaluated for evidence of ischemia, arrhythmias, and electrolyte disorders.

Pulmonary Embolism

Although the ECG is generally nonspecific in pulmonary embolism, it is useful in differential diagnosis. Right axis deviation, ST-segment depression in leads V_1 to V_4, new right bundle branch block and supraventricular tachycardias such as sinus tachycardia, atrial fibrillation, atrial flutter, and paroxysmal atrial tachycardia can suggest the presence of pulmonary embolism.

Respiratory Failure

The ECG can be helpful in determining whether chronic lung disease or complications such as myocardial ischemia are present during respiratory failure. Arrhythmias occur frequently during respiratory failure. Premature ventricular complexes, sinus tachycardia, and supraventricular tachycardia, including multifocal atrial tachycardia, are particularly common.

Hypothermia

Hypothermia produces diagnostically useful changes in the ECG. The decrease in body temperature progressively slows the sinus rate and prolongs the PR, QRS, and QT intervals. A distinctive ECG feature, the J wave or Osborn wave ("camel hump" sign), is a consistent sign of a body temperature below 25°C. The J wave produces an extra deflection in the early portion of the ST segment and is prominent and positive in leads facing the left ventricle. It increases with worsening hypothermia and can be associated with T-wave inversion. Atrial fibrillation and flutter can occur. Ventricular fibrillation can occur during rewarming.

Syncope

Loss of consciousness as a result of inadequate cerebral blood flow can be cardiogenic, usually the result of arrhythmias or obstructive cardiac lesions. Disturbances of cardiac rhythms that lead to syncope are complete heart block, the sick sinus syndrome, paroxysmal supraventricular tachycardia, and ventricular tachycardia. Aortic stenosis in patients with syncope is usually associated with left ventricular hypertrophy, evident on the ECG. Rare cardiac causes of syncope include acquired or congenital long QT syndrome, atrial myxomas, primary or secondary pulmonary hypertension, acute myocardial ischemia, and aortic dissection. These may be associated with distinct ECG abnormalities that can be helpful in the differential diagnosis.

Acute Abdominal Disease

Patients with acute abdominal disease may have complications such as myocardial ischemia and/or cardiac arrhythmias. However, primary repolarization changes such as ST depression or elevation and T-wave inversion can be a direct consequence of acute abdominal disease and do not necessarily indicate myocardial ischemia.

Shock

The ECG tracing can document the acute myocardial ischemia and/or arrhythmias causing cardiogenic shock. In patients with other forms of shock, ECG monitoring should be performed to detect complicating arrhythmias or myocardial ischemia produced by hypoperfusion of the myocardium.

Thoracic Trauma

Penetrating cardiac trauma, myocardial contusion, and cardiac laceration may or may not produce ECG changes. Myocardial contusion is the most likely lesion to cause ECG changes, which may be either nonspecific or similar to those produced by acute myocardial infarction. ECG monitoring is necessary to detect and assess complicating arrhythmias. Other cardiac complications, such as valve rupture or delayed pericarditis, also may produce ECG changes.

Cardiovascular and Thoracic Surgery

Serial ECGs and continuous ECG monitoring are essential in patients who have undergone thoracic surgery. Patients in whom the pericardium is opened can develop changes associated with acute pericarditis. Myocardial infarctions complicate the postoperative course of a small but distinct number of patients who undergo open-heart surgery, especially coronary revascularization. Ventricular and supraventricular arrhythmias are very common in patients recovering from thoracic surgery.

Drug Toxicity and Proarrhythmia

Digitalis toxicity is not uncommon, especially in the presence of renal insufficiency. It can produce a wide variety of arrhythmias, especially paroxysmal atrial tachycardia with block, junctional tachycardia with AV dissociation, sinus node dysfunction, second- and third-degree heart block, ventricular premature systoles (including bigeminy), ventricular tachycardia, and bidirectional tachycardia. Atrial fibrillation and flutter are rarely caused by digitalis intoxication.

Antiarrhythmic drugs such as quinidine, flecainide, propafenone, amiodarone, sotalol, and the tricyclic antidepressants can widen the QRS interval and cause varying degrees of AV block and asystole. These drugs, as well as other antiarrhythmic medications, can produce ventricular arrhythmias (proarrhythmias). Those with potassium channel-blocking properties (including quinidine, procainamide, disopyramide, tricyclic antidepressants, sotalol, and amiodarone) can cause prolongation of the QT interval and a

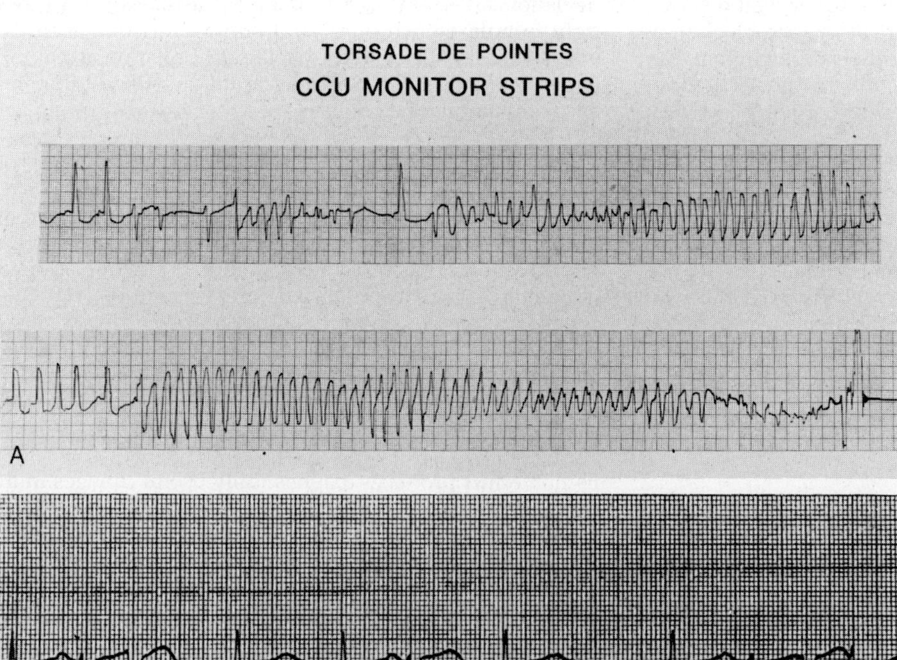

Figure 54–6. Polymorphous ventricular tachycardia (torsades de pointes). *A,* Paroxysms of multiform ventricular tachycardia are shown. *B,* Frequent premature ventricular complexes have been recorded. Supraventricular beats show a prolonged QT interval of 0.60 s. This is a frequent prelude to this type of arrhythmia.

TABLE 54–1. Major Causes of Torsades de Pointes (Delayed Repolarization with Prolonged QT and Polymorphous Ventricular Tachycardia)

1. Electrolyte disturbances
   - Hypokalemia
   - Hypomagnesemia
2. Drugs
   - Class Ia antiarrhythmics (quinidine, procainamide, disopyramide)
   - Class III antiarrhythmics (amiodarone)
   - Toxic dose of psychotropic drugs (phenothiazines, tricyclics)
3. Severe bradyarrhythmias
4. Congenital QT prolongation
5. Central nervous system disorders
   - Head trauma
   - Subarachnoid hemorrhage

distinctive polymorphous ventricular tachycardia called torsades de pointes (Table 54–1, and Fig. 54–6). This life-threatening arrhythmia typically occurs within the first few days of treatment and may occur even with therapeutic or subtherapeutic blood levels. Finally, cocaine and sympathomimetic drugs used to treat bronchospasm, nasal congestion, and hypotension can produce ECG evidence of myocardial ischemia and injury as well as arrhythmias, especially ventricular arrhythmias.

Electrolyte and Metabolic Disturbance

An increase in the serum potassium level causes the T wave to peak and narrow, widens the QRS interval, decreases and eventually eliminates the P wave, elevates the ST segment, and produces AV conduction defects, premature ventricular systoles, and, eventually, ventricular tachycardia, fibrillation, or standstill. A decrease in the serum potassium level depresses the ST segment, creates a pseudoprolongation of the QT interval (as a result of decreased T waves with prominent U waves), widens the QRS interval, and produces ventricular arrhythmias, especially those associated with digitalis toxicity or QT prolongation.

An increase in the serum calcium level shortens the QT interval, whereas a decrease in the serum concentration of this electrolyte prolongs the QT interval. Changes in serum calcium level rarely produce arrhythmias.

An abnormal level of magnesium in the blood cannot be detected by the ECG with certainty; however, hypomagnesemia can contribute to ventricular arrhythmias.

CHAPTER 55

Conduction Disturbances in the Critically Ill

Stephen Keim, MD • Patrick Tchou, MD

Bradycardia can arise from abnormal formation or propagation of electric impulses and is frequently poorly tolerated in the critically ill patient. Difficulty arises from the need to distinguish whether the problem relates to acute mechanical or pharmacologic injury or whether the conduction disturbance reflects the natural history of an acute or chronic pathologic process. We attempt to outline the structures involved in the genesis of effective myocardial contraction and the physiology of these structures as they relate to acute illness.

NORMAL PACEMAKER AND CONDUCTION SYSTEM OF THE HEART

The normal electrical impulses of the heart are initiated at the sinus node. The node is located at the anterosuperior junction of the superior vena cava with the right atrium. It is a spindle-shaped structure that lies on the epicardial side. It receives arterial supply via branches originating from the right coronary artery (55–60%) or the circumflex artery (40–45%).[1] Three types of cells are seen in the sinus node. The typical nodal cells, also called P cells, are probably responsible for the initiation of the sinus impulses. These impulses are then conducted to transitional cells, which, in turn, conduct to the normal-working atrial myocardium. The cells within the sinus node can generate spontaneous diastolic depolarizations, which result in slowly rising action potentials characteristic of calcium-dependent depolarization. The rate of spontaneous depolarization is modulated by sympathetic as well as a parasympathetic tone. The sinus node is richly innervated with neural fibers from the parasympathetic system. There are also sympathetic innervations to the sinus node. Intrinsic sinus node rates decline somewhat with age. In a teenager, the rate is 100 to 110 beats per minute, whereas in the 60- to 70-year age group, it declines to 70 to 80 beats per minute.[2,3] The reason for this decline is not clear but may be associated with age-related infiltration of fibrous tissue within the sinus node. In normal, healthy individuals, the resting heart rate is usually governed by the degree of parasympathetic tone and is thus slower than the intrinsic sinus rate. Because the parasympathetic system can respond quickly from hemodynamic feedback, this resting heart rate is frequently associated with a considerable amount of beat-to-beat variation. The sympathetic system, on the other hand, tends to modulate its tone more slowly. Therefore, a fast sinus rate that is driven by sympathetic tone tends to have little beat-to-beat variation in cycle length.

Once the impulse leaves the sinus node area, it is conducted to the rest of the atria via working atrial myocardium. The impulse travels more rapidly through the atrial myocardium primarily because of the fast upstroke of the atrial action potential, which is sodium dependent. Although there are preferential directions of conduction, there is no specific conduction system such as the His-Purkinje system in the ventricles. The preferential direction of conduction is related to orientation of muscle fibers. Impulse propagation occurs more rapidly along the longitudinal axis of the fibers than across the short axis.

Normally, electrical impulses in the atrium do not traverse the atrioventricular (AV) ring because of a discontinuity of myocardial cells along the ring. The sole site of AV conduction is via the AV nodal and His-Purkinje axis. The AV node consists of the compact node, which is located near the apex of the triangle of Koch in the atrial septum. The compact node is surrounded by a diffuse mesh of transitional nodal cells and atrial fibers that feed into the compact node from the anterior and posterior atrial septa. The transitional cells receive their inputs from atrial muscle and conduct the impulse to the compact node. Transitional cells, also called the AN cells, have slower rising action potentials that are calcium dependent and conduct the impulse at a much slower rate than atrial muscle. The impulse from the AN cells then enters the compact node and activates the N cells, which have an even slower upstroke to their action potential. As the compact node approaches the AV groove near the membranous septum, it becomes electrically isolated from the surrounding tissues by a fibrous layer. This fibrous layer surrounds the distal nodal cells, the NH cells, and the penetrating His bundle. The NH cells have much more rapid upstroke velocities to their action potential and thus conduct more rapidly. From the NH cells, the impulse conducts to the His bundle, the right and left bundles, and the Purkinje network. Ventricular activation occurs at the endocardial junction between Purkinje cells and ventricular myocardial cells. The His-Purkinje system has the most rapid conduction rates of all the myocardial tissues and, because of its treelike structure, allows rapid, relatively synchronized activation of the endocardium. This accounts for the observation that normal ventricular activation is associated with a "narrow" QRS complex. When ventricular activation does not proceed entirely through the His-Purkinje system, it becomes less synchronous because of slower impulse propagation via muscle conduction. Because the duration of the QRS complex represents the time of ventricular activation, myocardial conduction, which does not take advantage of the His-Purkinje system tree structure, causes the QRS to widen.

The normal conduction time from the atrium to the ventricle, represented on the surface ECG as the PR interval, consists of the intra-atrial conduction time, conduction time through AV nodal cells, and the conduction time along the His-Purkinje fibers. Conduction through the AV node can be modulated by cycle length as well as the autonomic nervous system. Short cycle length causes slowing of conduction through the AV node. The AV node is well innervated by both parasympathetic and sympathetic nervous systems. Parasympathetic tone slows AV nodal conduction, whereas sympathetic tone tends to accelerate this conduction. These conduction characteristics of the AV node explain why sinus tachycardia is usually not associated with a prolonged PR interval because the sympathetic tone that drives the sinus node also facilitates conduction via the AV node, whereas supraventricular tachycardias of other origins are frequently associated with prolonged PR intervals.

The AV conduction axis serves several functions. It creates an activation delay between the atria and the ventricles to allow atrial contraction to fill the ventricle. It serves as a "governor" that prevents rapid atrial arrhythmias, such as atrial fibrillation, from inciting ventricular fibrillation by blocking a proportion of atrial impulses from activating the ventricle. The tree structure of the His-Purkinje system allows relatively synchronous activation of the ventricles so as to obtain optimal mechanical function.

The ventricular myocardium is first activated at the endocardium. The impulse then traverses the myocardium to activate the epicardium. The basal portion of the subendocardium near the AV groove is not infiltrated by the Purkinje network and thus is also activated by muscle conduction. The first site of endocardial muscle activation is the left septum. The next site of activation is the right ventricular apex followed by the left and right ventricular free wall and then the base of the left ventricle and the right ventricular outflow tract. The time from the earliest activation in the septum until the depolarization of the base and outflow tract is normally in the range of 80 to 100 ms, accounting for the normal duration of the QRS complex. Widening of this duration usually occurs as a result of conduction block in certain areas of the His-Purkinje system or activation of the myocardium from an alternative pathway that does not take advantage of the His-Purkinje system structure. Generalized slowing of conduction in muscle caused by sodium channel blockade with drugs can also widen the QRS complex.

DISTURBANCES OF SINUS NODE FUNCTION

Activation of the sinus node is not readily appreciable on surface electrocardiogram (ECG). Although intra-atrial conduction disturbances are common, most frequently interpreted as atrial enlargement, it is distinctly unusual to have complete block within the atrial tissue. Therefore, the function of the sinus node is usually inferred from the P wave on ECG tracings. There can be considerable range in the sinus rate. However, it is unusual to have a pause of longer than 2 seconds.[4] The absence of P wave can result from primary failure of the sinus node to depolarize or failure of the sinus node to excite the atrium. Sinus arrest, the cessation of sinus node impulse formation, is identified as a sudden dropping or prolonged absence of P waves that occurs in an irregular pattern. Sinus node exit block, the failure of an impulse to excite the atrial tissue, usually occurs in an identifiable pattern such as a 2:1 or Wenckebach pattern. The cause of exit block or sinus arrest may be similar, and the treatment is the same.

The function of the sinus node is under considerable autonomic influences, and an increase in vagal tone or drug enhancement of parasympathetic effects probably accounts for the majority of transient sinus node conduction disturbances in the critically ill patient.[2] Ischemia, specifically with high-grade coronary occlusion in the right coronary artery, has been identified as another cause of sinus node dysfunction.[5] All of the pharmacologic agents listed in Table 55–1 can cause sinus slowing, arrest, or exit block and should be discontinued if hemodynamically detrimental bradycardia occurs. As with all tissues that spontaneously depolarize, the sinus node can be suppressed by being overdriven at a faster rate. A long pause may ensue when this faster rhythm terminates. This may be noted in its simplest form as a compensatory pause after an premature atrial beat. In its most dramatic form, it is noted as a prolonged pause at the termination of atrial fibrillation or flutter. These pauses can be exacerbated by all of the antiarrhythmic drugs and can represent either sinus arrest or sinoatrial exit block.

Sinus bradycardia may represent an acute change in the metabolic status of the patient. Careful attention to the arterial oxygen saturation and pH as well as potassium levels is necessary. Sinus node dysfunction may represent the natural history of a more generalized degenerative process within the atrium.[6] Sinus node dysfunction has been reported in most of the collagen vascular disorders, sarcoidosis, and infiltrative disorders such as amyloidosis. Unrecognized hypothyroidism may also be a cause. Cardiac

TABLE 55–1. Pharmacologic Agents That Inhibit Cardiac Conduction

Antiarrhythmics: quinidine, procainamide, disopyramide, lidocaine, mexiletine, diphenylhydantoin, flecainide, propafenone, sotalol, amiodarone
β-adrenergic blockers
Calcium channel blockers
Adenosine
Local anesthetics: bupivacaine, cocaine
$Histamine_2$ antagonists
Narcotics: morphine, fentanyl
Pancuronium
Nitroglycerin
General anesthetics: propofol, neostigmine/glycopyrrolate
Interleukin-2
Tricyclic antidepressants, lithium
Carbamazepine

transplantation is associated with sinus node dysfunction in 30% of patients. Its cause may be multifactorial, related to direct mechanical injury, to adenosine supersensitivity, to loss of autonomic control, or to modulators of immune injury.[6]

The significance of sinus node dysfunction is the hemodynamic consequences of pauses or loss of normal AV synchrony. If no subsidiary pacemaker assumes the role of spontaneous impulse generation, asystole will result and temporary pacing will be mandatory. If pauses are infrequent and the AV node provides an acceptable back-up rate, treatment of reversible causes is usually sufficient. Vagolytic therapy with atropine or sympathomimetic treatment with isoproterenol is usually the first approach to accelerate sinus rate. The AV junction is generally regarded as a reliable pacemaker, and temporary pacing for a junctional rhythm without hemodynamic compromise is not warranted, particularly if there is no other evidence for coexistent conduction disease. Cardiac output may be decreased by as much as 25% with the loss of AV synchrony. This may be seen in junctional rhythm or ventricular pacing with retrograde atrial activation. At times, atrial pacing can be used for patients without bradycardia when their cardiac outputs deteriorate with paroxysmal junctional rhythms. This can be seen in the setting of sepsis and postsurgical conditions requiring high cardiac outputs (e.g., liver transplantation).

Cardiac transplantation represents a special consideration. Because no vagal efferents exist in the graft, atropine will not increase the heart rate.[7] Catecholamines may support the rate acutely, and there are reports of both short- and long-term success with theophylline, an adenosine antagonist for the treatment of persistent sinus bradycardia.[8]

Bradycardia is very common after cardiopulmonary bypass.[9, 10] This may reflect sinus node injury when atrial surgery is involved (Fontan procedure) or injury from the placement of the superior vena cava cannula. Very high levels of potassium, adenine nucleotides, and free radicals accumulate during bypass and combine with atrial ischemia to make these bradycardias difficult to treat medically. Many centers place temporary atrial as well as ventricular epicardial pacing wires after cardiopulmonary bypass surgery as a prophylactic measure, especially if valve surgery has been performed.

Because the sinus node is somewhat vulnerable in the thin-walled atrium, it is frequently affected by processes that affect the atrial tissue. It is, therefore, common to have associated atrial tachyarrhythmias in conjunction with sinus node dysfunction (tachycardia-bradycardia syndrome). This combination usually mandates placement of a pacemaker because treatment of the tachyarrhythmias will exacerbate sinus dysfunction.

ATRIOVENTRICULAR BLOCK

Because every impulse initiating from the sinus node in the normal heart must pass through the AV node and His-Purkinje system to activate the ventricle, conduction block within these structures can cause bradycardia. Typically, conduction block through these structures is classified as first degree, second degree, or third degree. The normal conduction time of a sinus impulse from the atrium to the ventricle, measured as the PR interval on the surface ECG, is between 120 and 220 ms. Prolongation of the conduction time beyond this limit is described as *first-degree AV block,* even though every atrial impulse still conducts through to the ventricle. First-degree AV block is rarely a clinically significant problem and usually requires no therapy. On rare occasions, a long first-degree AV block (e.g., >300 ms) can result in suboptimal timing of AV contraction sequence. In a patient with very poor ventricular function, shortening the PR interval with artificial pacing may improve cardiac performance.

Second-degree AV block describes the condition in which atrial impulses do not always conduct to the ventricle. For example, every second beat may have AV block (2:1 AV block) or every third or fourth beat may have AV block (3:1 or 4:1 block, respectively). There are two types of second-degree AV block: Mobitz type I and Mobitz type II.

In Mobitz type I second-degree AV block, also called Wenckebach block, the block is in the AV node. The conduction pattern is most commonly characterized by progressive prolongation of the PR interval in sequential beats until AV block occurs in one beat. The next beat then resumes conduction with a comparatively short PR interval. This interval again prolongs on each subsequent beat until block occurs again. This pattern is usually repeated, but the number of conducted beats separating blocked beats may vary. The site of impulse block is in the AV node. The AV node has conduction characteristics that allow prolongation of the PR interval (sometimes quite marked), thus explaining the ability to generate progressively longer PR intervals before the blocked beat. This type of AV block is usually due to elevated vagal tone and is generally asymptomatic and benign. On occasion, Mobitz type I AV node block can occur in pathologic states such as an inferior myocardial infarction.[11] Symptomatic bradycardia resulting from second-degree Mobitz type I AV block during the acute phase of an inferior myocardial infarction can be treated with atropine or temporary pacing with a transvenous pacing electrode. Such blocks are usually short lived and resolve within 24 hours. In some cases, however, AV block may be more prolonged and may not respond to atropine. The lack of response to atropine may indicate ischemia of the AV node. Recovery of conduction may be delayed for several weeks. However, long-term pacing is almost never necessary.

Mobitz type II second-degree AV block is a more ominous type of rhythm. This is characterized by a marginally, if at all, prolonged PR interval with suddenly dropped ventricular beats indicating AV conduction block. There is usually very little prolongation of PR interval in sequential beats before the beat showing AV block. Other conduction abnormalities are common, such as a widened QRS from bundle branch block or conduction block within the Purkinje network. These findings indicate disease within the His-Purkinje network. Conduction block in this entity occurs in the diseased portion of the His bundle, bundle branches, or the Purkinje network. Because the His-Purkinje system has very little ability to produce conduction delay in the anterograde direction, PR-interval prolongation is not a prominent aspect of this type of conduction block. As a result of the disease within the His-Purkinje system, Mobitz type II second-degree AV block can quickly progress to complete AV block, a potentially life-threatening problem. Therefore, treatment of this type of AV block with permanent pacing is usually indicated. This type of AV block can be very sensitive to heart rate. AV conduction can change from first-degree to second-degree to high-grade AV block over a relatively narrow range of heart rate acceleration. For example, at a sinus rate of 60 beats per minute, a patient with a diseased His-Purkinje system may have 1:1 AV conduction. At a rate of 70 beats per minute, the conduction may be 2:1. At a rate of 80 or 90 beats per minute, there may be high-grade AV block.

The net effect is that ventricular rates may slow down

considerably in response to a relatively mild increase in atrial rate. When such a patient presents with 2:1 AV block, atropine should not be used because this drug has no effect on improving His-Purkinje system conduction but can accelerate sinus rhythm, possibly causing worsening of the AV block. Occurrence of Mobitz type II second-degree AV block during an acute anterior myocardial infarction, usually associated with new bundle branch block, is an ominous sign of impending complete AV block. Temporary pacing is indicated even in the asymptomatic patient when this occurs.[12]

The circumstance of 2:1 AV block deserves special mention. It is sometimes difficult to identify the type of block (type I or II) when every other sinus beat conducts to the ventricle. The typical Wenckebach pattern of progressively prolonging PR interval would not be apparent. However, other factors can be used to indicate the type of block. The presence of bundle branch block, especially left bundle branch block or bifascicular block, should raise the suspicion that the block is type II because it indicates the presence of disease within the His-Purkinje system. A narrow, normal-appearing QRS complex favors a type I block. Bedside maneuvers that manipulate the autonomic system can be of help. Vagal maneuvers may slow down sinus rhythm and improve conduction in a diseased His-Purkinje system; withdrawal of vagal tone should improve type I block.

Complete, or third-degree, AV block is the absence of conduction between the atrium and the ventricle. Third-degree AV block can be congenital or acquired. Congenital AV block is due to developmental abnormalities in the AV node. These patients usually have a reasonably good junctional escape rhythm coming from the proximal His bundle or the distal AV node. This type of junctional escape rhythm is quite stable, demonstrates rate response to sympathetic and parasympathetic tone, and usually has an adequate rate (50–70 beats per minute at rest) to generate appropriate cardiac output. Therefore, permanent pacemaker implant is not required in these patients unless they have symptomatic bradycardia. As patients age, however, the junctional escape rhythm has a tendency to slow down. These patients may become symptomatic when they are adults. A permanent pacemaker implant can readily correct this problem when it occurs.

Acquired forms of third-degree AV block are usually due to diseases affecting the heart, to iatrogenic causes secondary to surgery on the heart, or to deliberate ablation of the AV conduction system with catheter techniques to achieve control over atrial tachycardias. The site of conduction block is most commonly in the His bundle, bundle branches, or the Purkinje network. Permanent pacemaker implant is indicated with acquired third-degree AV block when it is not likely to be reversed. Although the lower AV node or the upper His bundle can sometimes have acceptably reliable pacemaker activity, acquired forms of AV block often interrupt conduction below this site of pacemaker activity. Pacemaker activity from sites lower in the His-Purkinje system are too slow and not reliable enough to act as the sole pacemaker for the human heart.

As mentioned earlier, atropine does not improve conduction when AV block is within the His-Purkinje system. It may actually be deleterious. Drugs such as isoproterenol can be tried with caution in an emergency because they can improve ventricular escape pacemakers, which can achieve adequate heart rate to maintain hemodynamic integrity. Temporary pacing should be instituted as soon as possible, followed by insertion of a permanent pacer when the patient's condition is stable.

Many diseases can affect AV conduction, resulting in third-degree AV block. Chronic ischemic disease from myocardial infarctions can damage the conduction system to such an extent as to cause third-degree AV block. Acute myocardial infarction can also cause AV block. Infiltrative diseases such as amyloidosis, sarcoidosis, sclerotic calcification of the valves, and malignancies can cause AV block by affecting the AV node or the His-Purkinje system. Inflammatory disorders such as rheumatic fever, myocarditis from various causes, and Lyme disease can also cause complete AV block. Certain skeletal muscular dystrophies can also affect the conduction system of the heart, resulting in AV block.

The case of third-degree AV block during myocardial infarction should be considered in view of the time of onset and site of myocardial infarction. With inferior wall myocardial infarction, prolonged (beyond 6 hours into the event) third-degree AV block is due to ischemia to the AV node. In many cases, there is an adequate junctional escape rhythm. Temporary pacing may be necessary if the patient is symptomatic from the junctional bradycardia or if proper AV sequence is important to preserve hemodynamic stability. More prolonged complete AV block in the setting of inferior myocardial infarction will usually resolve within a week but may take up to 3 weeks.[12] Therefore, permanent pacemaker implant should be delayed as long as possible. Earlier implantation of a permanent pacer may be necessary, however, to facilitate recovery and rehabilitation. This type of AV block is in contrast to the kind seen with anterior wall myocardial infarction, in which the block is more likely due to ischemic damage to the His-Purkinje system. The escape rates in the latter type of AV block are usually too slow to provide adequate cardiac output. Furthermore, damage to the His-Purkinje system is more likely to produce permanent heart block. The prognosis in such patients is poor because of the large associated infarction. Temporary pacing should always be instituted.[12] Although there are no definitive data for improved survival, we believe all patients in whom complete heart block develops during an anterior myocardial infarction, even if only transient, should undergo permanent pacemaker implantation.

Third-degree AV block (as well as lesser degrees) can be a toxic effect of certain medications such as digoxin, calcium channel blockers, and other antiarrhythmic medications. Underlying conduction system disease is frequently present, but the block can usually be reversed by allowing the offending drug to wash out of the body. Permanent pacing is not indicated under this circumstance if one-to-one AV conduction can be re-established. Temporary pacing may be necessary depending on the rate of the underlying escape rhythm and patient symptoms.

Drug therapy of bradycardia is indicated only for transient bradycardia or as a stopgap measure while a temporary or permanent pacemaker implant is being arranged. Sympathomimetics such as isoproterenol can be used to accelerate the intrinsic cardiac rhythm. Atropine can be used to block vagal effects if the cause of bradycardia is inappropriate parasympathetic tone. Temporary or permanent pacing is so readily available, safe, and effective that it should be the treatment of choice under most circumstances other than transient causes of bradycardia.

Other than withdrawal of potentially offending drugs and brief uses of intravenous atropine or isoproterenol, treatment of bradycardia caused by AV block usually means implantation of a temporary or permanent pacemaker. In emergent circumstances, external pacemakers can also be used. These devices essentially deliver transthoracic shocks to depolarize the heart and achieve myocardial contractions. This type of external pacing usually entails a significant discomfort to the patient and should be used only in life-threatening situations. Heavy sedation of the patient is usually required.

INTRAVENTRICULAR CONDUCTION DELAYS BUNDLE BRANCH BLOCK

The Purkinje network is one of the most durable electrical structures within the heart. Its diffusely arborizing structure lends itself to be partially damaged and yet maintain AV conduction. There is some decrement in cardiac function in patients with asynchronous ventricular contractions; however, this is only rarely clinically important. Therefore, the clinical importance of recognizing bundle branch blocks is in determining their likely relationship to the development of complete AV block, the extent of myocardial damage, and the concealment of such damage on the 12-lead ECG.

Using the traditional trifascicular concept, intraventricular conduction delay can be identified as right bundle branch block and left posterior and left anterior hemiblock. It is important to keep in mind that the QRS represents the sum of ventricular activation. Delay in the proximal His bundle, which produces equal delay in all the fascicles, will result in a normal QRS. When conduction is blocked or delayed in one of the bundle branches, the QRS is widened because the myocardium ipsilateral to the block is usually activated by the contralateral bundle.

Chronic complete left bundle branch block is usually associated with a structurally abnormal heart. A newly developed left bundle branch block can be associated with a 10-fold increase in mortality.[12] Isolated left anterior hemiblock is common and, like the less common isolated left posterior hemiblock, is not associated with increased mortality. Isolated right bundle branch block is probably the most frequent intraventricular conduction delay and is not necessarily associated with abnormal myocardial function. When right bundle branch block is combined with either of the hemiblocks, the incidence of coexistent cardiac abnormalities and mortality is increased.

As mentioned, the Purkinje network is sturdy both metabolically and structurally.[13] Therefore, the development of any new and persistent bundle branch block must be treated with considerable concern in the critically ill patient. Transient intraventricular conduction delays may represent "functional bundle branch block." This represents conduction delay as a result of normal physiologic variances. Phase 3 block, tachycardia-dependent conduction delay, results from a fast heart rate that impinges on the recovery of the bundle. By a 3:1 margin, tachycardia-dependent functional right bundle branch block is more common than left bundle branch block. It is characteristically associated with an abrupt acceleration in heart rate and resolves when the tachycardia subsides. Phase 4 block, bradycardia-dependent block, is associated with a slowing of the heart rate and results from partial diastolic depolarization of the bundle. It is almost exclusively associated with left bundle branch block and resolves when the heart rate accelerates.

Another type of functional block results from the interaction between the right and left bundles. If conduction block occurs in one fascicle for one beat, retrograde, concealed penetration may occur from the contralateral bundle and the block may persist. This block usually is transient and resolves with oscillation of the tachycardia rate, not necessarily with slowing of the tachycardia. Functional aberrancy by definition resolves, but it is important to distinguish from ventricular tachycardia as a cause of wide complex tachycardia. There is no additional morbidity associated with phase 3 block that occurs in normal hearts. Phase 4 block almost always implies myocardial disease, and the prognosis is related to the extent of myocardial injury.

Many of the pharmacologic agents listed in Table 55–1 can suppress conduction of the Purkinje network, causing a new persistent intraventricular conduction defect. This is different from the functional blocks because it is usually preceded by gradual QRS widening and persists over a wide range of heart rates. Recognition of diffuse conduction system disease (coexistent AV node disease or bifascicular block) should be a relative contraindication to starting these agents. Parasympathetic agonists or antagonists have little direct effects on the Purkinje system. However, acceleration and improvement of AV nodal conduction with atropine may, in fact, worsen infra-Hisian block. Adrenergic and calcium channel blockers usually do not worsen intraventricular conduction delays.

Myocardial injury should be assumed to be ongoing with the development of a new bundle branch block. It may be direct mechanical injury, such as with a pulmonary artery catheter, or electrolyte imbalance. The repolarization abnormalities with bundle branch blocks, especially left bundle branch block, obfuscate the changes associated with myocardial ischemia. Therefore, direct myocardial imaging techniques are usually required to rule out significant ongoing ischemia. Hypoxemia, acidosis, and hyperkalemia can all suppress conduction and be associated with a new bundle branch block.

Treatment of a newly acquired bundle branch block should be directed at reversible causes of myocardial injury. Placement of a right-sided catheter may injure the right bundle selectively without depressing myocardial function and, in the absence of conduction system disease in the left bundle, it is unusual to progress to higher grades of AV block. In patients with myocardial infarctions, complete AV block may occur without any preceding warning. It is generally not necessary to treat isolated bundle branch blocks directly, except when there is a likelihood to progress to high-grade AV block.

SPECIAL CONSIDERATIONS

Acute myocardial infarction can be associated with conduction disturbances in more than 30% of cases.[14] Frequently, pharmacologic agents used to limit infarction damage have direct depressant effects on cardiac conduction. Additionally, direct ischemic injury of the conduction system or the elicitation of vagotonic reflexes can cause bradycardia and heart block.[15] These bradyarrhythmias may reflect reperfusion, particularly in patients given thrombolytic agents. There is a special aspect of AV block and sinus bradycardia that is resistant to the effects of atropine. It is probably mediated by the depressant effects of local accumulation of adenosine in the AV and sinus nodes. These patients may well respond to aminophylline (100–200 mg). Because this conduction disturbance is frequently transient, in inferior infarctions this therapy may obviate the need for temporary pacing.[16]

The development of AV block or bundle branch blocks in the setting of acute myocardial infarction continues to be associated with marked increases in short- and long-term mortality.[17] General indications for prophylactic pacing in the setting of an acute myocardial infarction is the development of new bifascicular block.[18] The availability of transthoracic pacing, which is reliable and acceptable to patients, may obviate the need for prophylactic transvenous pacing, but there are no data to support this approach.

Myocardial infarction is almost always associated with some hemodynamic instability. Obviously, bradycardia from any mechanism that significantly reduces cardiac function should be paced. It is clear that AV sequential pacing, although technically more difficult, is associated with improved hemodynamics.[19]

Cardiac surgery by its very nature implies direct injury to the heart and, frequently, conduction system. Many cardioplegia solutions contain high concentrations of drugs that can suppress conduction, and these persist for several hours. As mentioned, atrial bradycardia is frequently associated with injury to the sinus node at the time of surgery, and many institutions practice the placement of prophylactic temporary pacing wires when this problem is anticipated.[9, 10] Surgery near the AV node and His bundle can cause high-grade AV block. This may persist for up to 2 weeks. Permanent pacing is usually recommended if AV conduction has not returned by this time. There is generally no specific treatment for newly acquired bundle branch blocks during surgery, and the majority of these will resolve. However, intraoperative myocardial infarction should be considered. Indications for permanent pacing are the same as for other conditions.

References

1. Kyriakidis MK, Kovrouklis CB, Papaioannu JT, et al: Sinus node coronary arteries studied with angiography. Am J Cardiol 1983; 51:749.
2. Jose AD, Collison D: The normal range and the determinants of the intrinsic heart rate in man. Cardiovasc Res 1970; 4:160.
3. Papanno A: Parasympathetic control of cardiac electrical activity. *In:* Cardiac Electrophysiology: From Cell to Bedside. Zipes DP, Jalife J (Eds). Philadelphia, WB Saunders, 1990, pp 271–276.
4. Brodsky M, Wu D, Denes P, et al: Arrhythmias documented by 24 hour continuous electrocardiographic monitoring in 50 male medical students without apparent heart disease. Am J Cardiol 1977; 39:390.
5. James TN, Nadeau RA: Sinus bradycardia during injections directly into the sinus node artery. Am J Physiol 1963; 204:9.
6. Rowland E, Morgado F: Sino-atrial node dysfunction, atrioventricular block and intraventricular conduction disturbances. Eur Heart J 1992; 13(Suppl H):130.
7. Ellenbogen KA, Thames MD, DiMarco JP, et al: Electrophysiological effects of adenosine in the transplanted human heart: Evidence of supersensitivity. Circulation 1990; 81:821.
8. Smith ML, Ellenbogen KA, Eckberg DL, et al: Subnormal parasympathetic activity after cardiac transplantation. Am J Cardiol 1990; 66:1243.
9. Goldman BS, Hill TJ, Wessel RD, et al: Permanent pacing after open heart surgery: Acquired heart disease. PACE 1984; 7:367.
10. Baerman JM, Kirsh MM, deBuitleir M: Natural history and determinants of conduction defects following coronary artery bypass surgery. Ann Thorac Surg 1987; 44:150.
11. Rotman M, Wagner GS, Wallace AGP: Bradyarrhythmias in acute myocardial infarction. Circulation 1972; 45:703.
12. Atkins JM, Leshin SJ, Blomqvist G, et al: Ventricular conduction block and sudden death in acute myocardial infarction. N Engl J Med 1973; 288:281.
13. Hecht HH, Kossman CE, Childers RW, et al: Atrioventricular and intraventricular conduction. Am J Cardiol 1973; 31:232.
14. O'Doherty M, Taylor DI, Quinn E, et al: Five hundred patients with myocardial infarction monitored within one hour of symptoms. Br Med J 1983; 286:1405.
15. Zipes DP: Clinical significance of bradycardia rhythms in acute myocardial infarction. Am J Cardiol 1969; 24:814.
16. Strasberg B, Bassevich R, Mager A, et al: Effects of aminophylline on atrioventricular conduction in patients with late atrioventricular block during inferior wall acute myocardial infarction. Am J Cardiol 1991; 67:5278.
17. Mullins CB, Atkins JM: Prognosis and management of ventricular conduction blocks in acute myocardial infarction. Mod Concepts Cardiovascular Dis 1976; 45:129.
18. Hindman MC, Wagner GS, Jaro M, et al: The clinical significance of bundle branch block complicating acute myocardial infarction. Circulation 1978; 58:689.
19. Rahimtoola SH, Ehsani A, Sinno MZ, et al: Left atrial transport function in myocardial infarction: Importance of its booster function. Am J Med 1975; 59:686.

CHAPTER 56

Diagnosis and Treatment of Cardiac Arrhythmias

Andrea Hastillo, MD • Michael L. Hess, MD

In every intensive care unit (ICU), monitoring of the heart rhythm is standard practice. Changes in heart rate may be harbingers of impending hemodynamic catastrophe. For instance, increasing heart rates may indicate worsening failure in the coronary unit, more blood loss in the trauma unit, or worsening hypoxia in the respiratory unit. Even small changes in the heart rate of a critically ill patient could produce dangerous hemodynamic changes. Thus, continuous observation of heart rate becomes an important part of the delivery of good critical care.

The major purpose of cardiac rhythm monitoring is to be able to detect abnormal rhythms as they develop to treat those that require intervention as soon as possible. This, it is hoped, will decrease the untoward outcomes that may result from perseverance of these rhythm abnormalities. Treatment response may be determined by constant monitoring. This may range from determining that an arrhythmia does not recur, that ectopic complexes decrease in number, or that ventricular rates in atrial fibrillation respond in a desired manner to deciding whether pacemakers are functioning properly.

ROUTINE SURVEILLANCE

Routine monitoring is accomplished by a single-lead display obtained at the bedside and displayed at the bedside and at a central monitor. If possible, the rhythm should also be displayed in other patients' rooms to increase the probability of early detection of arrhythmias.

A variety of leads may be used, but the one chosen should clearly display the P wave and the QRS complex. If the patient has an electronic pacemaker in place, one should select a lead that will maximize visualization of the pacemaker spike. The lead that is being used to monitor the rhythm should be documented. Any changes in the selected lead should be noted to avoid any confusion with other causes for axis shifts. "Patching into" other patients' rooms becomes critical because it is often difficult to have a constant monitor observer available, even in the ICU.

Electronic surveillance should include various warnings for high and low rates. These should always be set to supplement human surveillance in the detection of rhythm abnormalities. A good system should minimize artifact that initiates warning systems.

Rhythms should be permanently documented on admission and at the start of each shift. A rhythm strip should be obtained and placed in the patient's chart or on the bedside flow chart with interval measurements and diagnosis of the rhythm strip documented by the nurse or monitor observer. Any changes in rhythm should be further clarified with a 12-lead electrocardiogram (ECG) because a single-lead strip may not be adequate for a full rhythm interpretation. Because rhythm strips may be lost or questions about rhythms may arise later, the ability to obtain delayed printouts, as well as real-time strips, is very important.

Obtaining a good monitor strip will include adequate preparation of the skin to obtain good contact between the electrode and the skin. The diaphoretic patient can be problematic. Poor contact can lead not only to inadequate tracings but also to recurrent triggering of the alarm system, which could lead to frustration and perhaps eventual removal of the alarms or "tuning out" of the audible alarms.

It is important that the monitor be regularly checked to ensure that the paper speed is correct. This should be precise in ICUs, which deal with patients with electrophysiology problems and where, for example, rate changes of ventricular tachycardia (VT) may be important to determine whether an antiarrhythmic is affecting the rhythm.

SPECIAL TECHNIQUES

Frequently, the 12-lead ECG coupled with the monitor strip is inadequate to diagnose an arrhythmia. A Lewis lead or other variations of surface electrode placements can be tried to determine the rhythm. The Lewis lead is obtained by placing the right arm electrode in the second right intercostal space and the left arm electrode in the fourth right intercostal space. Lead I is selected. If this fails, one may then consider a more invasive approach: intra-atrial or esophageal electrocardiography. Both procedures will require ECG equipment that can record the surface ECG simultaneously with the intra-atrial or esophageal electrogram.

The intra-atrial lead is commonly placed through the jugular vein, sometimes the brachial vein, and, less commonly, the subclavian and femoral veins. One can determine the location of the intra-venous electrode by the configurations of the ECG, although fluoroscopy may be required.

Esophageal electrograms may be obtained by asking the patient to swallow a "pill" electrode. This may be facilitated by concomitantly swallowing water or gelatin. There are also catheters that may be passed much like a nasogastric tube.

LIMITATIONS OF SINGLE-CHANNEL MONITORING

There are various distinct limitations to single-channel monitoring:

It may not detect the full PR, QRS, or QT intervals.
The waveforms generated may be so small as to fail to consistently trigger the detection device.
Artifact may lead to overcounting of electrical events generated from the heart.
Positional changes may lead to severe axis shifts, which may be misleading if only one lead is being monitored.
Loose electrodes may create artifacts resembling ventricular fibrillation or asystole.
Other mechanical activity such as gastric suction or condensation in a delivery system may be responsible for creation of artifacts.

Whenever a question arises, and after quickly evaluating the patient for stability, a 12-lead ECG may be necessary for resolution. One must remember that a monitor system is designed to monitor rhythms, not to measure intervals, determine axis, detect ST-T changes, or diagnose hypertrophy or infarction. Although a monitor lead may suggest these abnormalities, a confirmatory 12-lead ECG is usually indicated.

MECHANISMS OF ARRHYTHMIAS

The depolarization sequence of the normal heart is initiated by spontaneous depolarization of the sinoatrial (SA) node, which leads to atrial depolarization, and then proceeds through the atrioventricular (AV) node, bundle of His, bundle branches, Purkinje system, and ventricular tissue. The direction and duration of various cardiac electrical events have been normalized for the adult ECG. Rhythm abnormalities evolve from disturbances involving three mechanisms: automaticity (impulse formation caused by spontaneous depolarization), re-entry (impulse formation caused by slowed or blocked conduction), and triggering activity (oscillations in membrane potential after an action potential results in impulse formation). It is important to develop an understanding of the mechanism of the arrhythmia because treatment may be determined by its cause.[1]

Automaticity

Certain cells in the normal heart have an inherent ability to depolarize spontaneously and discharge repetitively. These are the pacemaker cells of the heart and include the SA node, the AV node, and the His-Purkinje system. The SA node normally discharges faster than the other sites and is the dominant pacemaker of the heart. It normally discharges at a rate of 60 to 100 beats per minute (bpm). The AV nodal area's inherent rate is 40 to 60 bpm, and the His-Purkinje system's rate is 20 to 40 bpm. These subsidiary pacemakers are normally prematurely depolarized (relative to their inherent rate) by the faster SA node. Should the SA node fail to fire, be blocked, or slow to a level below the subsidiary pacemaker's inherent rate, the next faster subsidiary pacemaker, by default, assumes depolarization of the heart. Various disease states, drugs, and metabolic abnormalities may alter automaticity in cells normally possessing automaticity and may also bestow automaticity on nonpacemaker cells.

Changes in the cardiac action potential may alter automaticity and involve the following:

1. The membrane potential at the end of repolarization
2. The rate of phase 4 depolarization
3. The threshold potential for depolarization

By lowering the resting membrane potential, slowing phase 4 depolarization, or raising the threshold potential, automaticity will be decreased. Increased parasympathetic tone, hyperkalemia, hypothermia, and antiarrhythmic agents decrease automaticity. Automaticity is increased if the resting membrane potential is closer to the threshold membrane potential, if the threshold potential is lowered, or if the slope of phase 4 is increased. Clinically, increased sympathetic tone, hypokalemia, myocardial ischemia and necrosis, and cardiac stretching may increase automaticity.

Conduction

Many arrhythmias develop as a result of abnormalities of conduction. In these cases, depolarization may occur, but the impulse is not conducted normally. Conduction or propagation of the electrical impulse through the cardiac tissue depends on phase 0 and the amplitude of the action potential. If the rate of change of voltage slows or the height of the action potential lessens, the speed of conduction through the tissue decreases. This conduction delay may allow continued conduction but at a slower rate than normal. Conduction, however, may be so affected that it is totally blocked.

Many arrhythmias result from re-entry. Re-entrant arrhythmias arise as a result of abnormalities of conduction. For re-entry to occur, (1) an impulse must encounter two functionally or anatomically potential pathways exiting a common pathway, which then re-merge in a more distal common pathway; (2) the impulse must fail to conduct anterogradely down one pathway (unidirectional block); and (3) the impulse must conduct down the unblocked pathway but slowly enough that it finds the previously anterogradely blocked pathway now able to conduct retrogradely. When the impulse reaches the initial site where the common pathway first split, it then conducts anterogradely as previously and keeps re-establishing itself. Alternatively, the impulse may exit the proximal common path, quickly travel down the faster pathway, and not conduct retrogradely back up the slower pathway. However, because the impulse coming down the slower pathway is not blocked, it slowly conducts anterogradely and finds the faster, earlier depolarized pathway repolarized and able to conduct retrogradely. Thus, re-entrant loops are established.

The re-entrant pathway may be in the atrial tissue or may be limited to SA tissue. It may also occur at the level of the Purkinje fibers or be localized to nodal tissue. The Wolff-Parkinson-White syndrome epitomizes re-entrant arrhythmias by using two anatomically distinct pathways: the AV nodal tissue and an accessory pathway.[2]

Triggering

Afterdepolarizations are oscillations in voltage or the membrane potential that occur after or during an action potential. These afterpotentials may be early, occurring before the cell has completely repolarized during phase 3 (early afterdepolarization), or late, occurring after complete repolarization (delayed afterdepolarization). If the afterpotential reaches threshold for depolarization, spontaneous depolarization may result. Delayed afterdepolarizations associated with digitalis and catecholamines appear to be responsible for clinical arrhythmias. There is less information about the significance of early afterdepolarizations, although they have been incriminated as a mechanism for arrhythmias seen in ventricular hypertrophy, quinidine-associated torsades de pointes, and other ventricular arrhythmias.[3–8]

SPECIFIC CARDIAC RHYTHMS

Normal Sinus Rhythm

In the adult, normal sinus rhythm is due to the SA node depolarizing 60 to 100 times per minute. The P wave is depolarized in a leftward and inferior direction and should be normally directed to exclude other rhythms at this same rate, notably an accelerated junctional rhythm. Although considered normal, sinus rhythm at a rate of 60 to 100 bpm may be inappropriate in certain circumstances (e.g., in severe hypovolemia or with high fevers).

Sinus Tachycardia

Sinus tachycardia is a sinus rhythm with a rate increased to more than 100 bpm. The upper limit is about 200 bpm in most individuals. Sinus tachycardia usually is due to a problem other than increased automaticity of the SA node. Thyrotoxicosis, hyperthermia, volume depletion, heart failure, and certain drug toxicities should be suspected. Treatment to slow the tachycardia should take into consideration the cause and the role of the tachycardia in preserving cardiac hemodynamics.

Sinus Bradycardia

This is sinus rhythm with a rate lower than 60 bpm. It is often seen in healthy individuals, especially athletes. Many cardiac drugs including β-blockers and calcium channel blockers may cause sinus bradycardia. In the older individual, the sinus node's rate of discharge may slow, and in ischemia heightened vagal tone may precipitate sinus bradycardia. Sinus bradycardia is also seen in hypothyroidism and hypothermia. Sinus bradycardia may be normal, even desirable, and may be associated with no problems. If, however, sinus bradycardia is responsible for an inadequate resting cardiac output or ineffective increase in cardiac output manifested by dizziness, syncope, congestive failure, or weakness, treatment should be considered. In acute situations, intravenous atropine is usually successful. If this fails, or if the maximum dose is reached, the drug is not tolerated, or a longer treatment period is necessary, intravenous isoproterenol may be used. Electrical transvenous or external pacing may be needed. If there is no AV block, transvenous pacing may use the atrial rather than ventricular site to maximize stroke volume and cardiac output.

Sinus Arrhythmia

Sinus arrhythmia may be normal. The sinus rate is noted to vary about 10% over time with a pattern of rhythmically increasing and decreasing rates or PP intervals. If the variation in rate is due to respirations, the atrial rate should increase with inspiration and then decrease with exhalation. Respiratory sinus arrhythmia is often a normal phenomenon readily apparent in individuals with slower sinus rates or sinus bradycardia. Treatment is not indicated. If respirations are not causative, the sinus arrhythmia is nonrespiratory. The nonrespiratory sinus arrhythmia tends to occur in the older individual and is more likely to occur in the presence of cardiac disease. If related to digitalis toxicity, discontinuation of the drug is indicated.

Premature Atrial Contraction

Premature atrial contractions (PACs) are common and are characterized by a premature beat, which is preceded by a premature P wave. This premature P wave often displays a configuration different than the normal sinus P wave. Premature atrial contractions (PACs) usually conduct retrogradely to the SA node, causing the SA node to be depolarized prematurely. Hence, the PP interval surrounding the PAC is usually less than two times a normal sinus PP interval (noncompensatory pause). The QRS complex that follows the premature P wave is usually the same as the normal sinus-induced QRS complex. However, aberrancy may occur, and in this instance the QRS may resemble a right bundle branch block pattern. Premature P waves may not be followed by a QRS complex (blocked PAC). These may occur in healthy hearts because of a physiologic block when a very early P wave encounters refractoriness below the atrial tissue. Frequently, pauses in a rhythm are caused by blocked PACs, and these should be suspected. However, documentation may sometimes be difficult because the premature P wave may only minimally change the T wave on which it may superimpose. Importantly, a single monitor strip may not show the blocked PAC because of the P-wave vector, and this may confuse the interpretation. A blocked PAC may be differentiated from Mobitz type II second-degree AV block because in the latter instance the P wave that is blocked does not occur early.

The need for treatment of PACs is influenced by the presence of structural heart disease. If the ectopy relates to alcohol or stimulants, these should be avoided. If there is concern that the PACs are harbingers of atrial fibrillation or other potentially persistent atrial arrhythmias that might lead to hemodynamic compromise, prophylactic treatment may be considered. For example, the development of atrial fibrillation in significant hypertrophic cardiomyopathy or severe mitral stenosis could be followed by hemodynamic collapse. Digitalis and β-blockers could be considered to prevent a rapid ventricular response. Depending on the clinical situation, one might need to plan for the addition of class Ia antiarrhythmics if digitalis fails to achieve the desired response.

Premature Junctional Contraction

Similar to the PAC, the premature junctional contraction produces a premature QRS complex that resembles the normal sinus-induced QRS and is usually associated with a noncompensatory pause. A P wave may be visible or absent altogether. If a P wave occurs, it may be found before the QRS complex, in the QRS complex, or after the QRS complex. The P wave configuration differs from the normal sinus-induced P wave. It is important to recognize a P wave early before the QRS or even closely after the QRS complex to avoid misdiagnosing a wide QRS complex.

Junctional Escape Beats

Junctional escape beats may occur when AV block occurs, when the sinus node slows, or when the degree of AV block in atrial fibrillation is high. Failure to depolarize the junctional subsidiary pacemaker prematurely allows the focus to depolarize at its inherent rate. The junctional escape beat resembles the normal sinus-induced QRS complex and may be associated with an abnormal P wave within or contiguous with the QRS or with an absent P wave. The rate of the escape beat is less than 60 bpm. Treatment of the junctional escape beat itself is not indicated. Consideration of increasing the sinus rate or improving AV node conduction may be necessary if cardiac output is jeopardized.

Atrioventricular Nodal Re-entrant Tachycardia

The arrhythmias grouped together as paroxysmal supraventricular tachycardias (PSVTs) (a nonhomogeneous group mechanistically) include those resulting from a concealed AV bypass tract (15–50%), sinus node re-entry (3%), intra-atrial re-entry (6%), automatic atrial tachycardia, and AV nodal re-entry (50%).[9]

AV nodal re-entry requires dissociation of the AV node into two functionally different pathways that form the re-entrant loop. The onset of the arrhythmia is usually abrupt and initiated by a premature complex. Termination is also usually abrupt. The QRS is regular and the complex usually narrow in the absence of a preexisting bundle branch block or intraventricular conduction delay. The rate may range from 150 to 200 bpm, often in the higher range. P waves may be difficult to visualize and are often within the QRS complex (Fig. 56–1).

This arrhythmia often develops in persons with no underlying cardiac disease, and the patient may only describe chest or heart "fluttering" sometimes. However, at the onset of the tachycardia and before an adequate baroreceptor response occurs, dizziness or even syncope may occur. Prolonged episodes may result in compromised cardiac output and heart failure symptoms. With underlying cardiac disease, hemodynamic compromise may be severe and angina precipitated.

Treatment depends on the hemodynamic status, the cause, and the recurrence rate. Severe hemodynamic compromise may require emergency cardioversion using low energy settings (20–50 J). Vagal maneuvers to interrupt the re-entry pathway by slowing conduction, which leads to sudden termination of the arrhythmia, are usually the first line of treatment.

Valsalva's maneuver is used first. It may also be diagnostic should there be a question about the tachyarrhythmia. Sinus tachycardia may be transiently slow. Either AV nodal re-entry will stop or nothing will occur. Atrial flutter may demonstrate a transient increase in AV block, and the flutter waves may be readily visualized. Atrial tachycardia with block may demonstrate further AV block. Atrial fibrillation may demonstrate a transient increase in AV block. Occasionally, VT is included in the differential of AV nodal re-entry (with aberrancy); vagal maneuvers should not alter the ventricular rate. Carotid sinus massage, performed cautiously, carries more risk than Valsalva's maneuver (embolization of a plaque from the carotid artery, profound bradyarrhythmia, and asystole) but may be necessary to terminate the arrhythmia (see Fig. 56–1). The effect of carotid sinus massage on the other arrhythmias is the same as that of Valsalva's maneuver.

Adenosine is a short-lived drug that is very effective in terminating AV nodal re-entry tachyarrhythmias. Although the side effects of adenosine include sinus bradycardia, AV block, and sinus arrest, the effects are very transient (less than a minute). It is administered rapidly to maximize its negative dromotropic effect. Aminophylline is a competitive antagonist and prevents the action of adenosine. Verapamil may be used with caution and is quite effective in terminating most of the AV nodal re-entrant tachyarrhythmias. However, it is a negative inotropic as well as a negative dromotropic agent, and its side effects may include profound cardiovascular and hemodynamic collapse. Other treatment modalities may include β-blockers, digitalis, vasopressors, antiarrhythmics, edrophonium, and atrial or ventricular pacing to terminate the arrhythmia.[2, 10, 11]

Concealed Atrioventricular Bypass Tract Tachycardia

This is the second most common cause of PSVT and requires an accessory pathway that bypasses the AV node and conducts only retrograde. Retrograde conduction down the AV

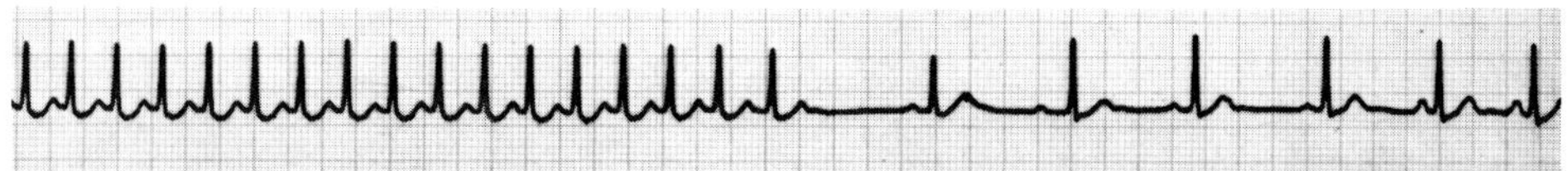

Figure 56–1. AV nodal re-entrant tachycardia usually fails to demonstrate a P wave because atrial depolarization and ventricular depolarization occur concomitantly. Sinus P waves become visible after carotid sinus massage is performed and abruptly stops the tachycardia.

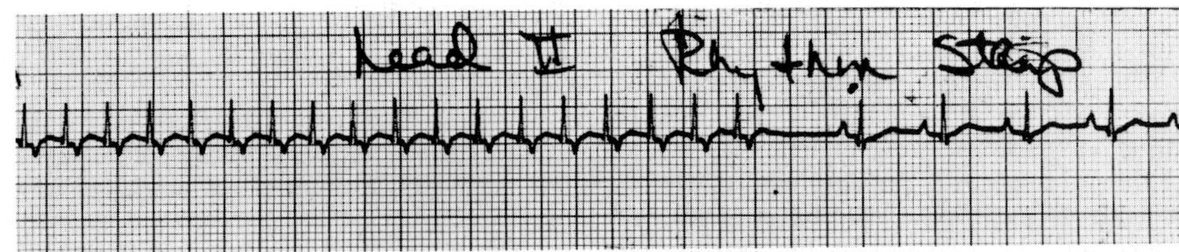

Figure 56–2. Orthodromic reciprocating tachycardia in which a concealed bypass tract is utilized for retrograde conduction often displays a retrograde P wave after the QRS complex. Carotid sinus massage interrupted the re-entrant loop by blocking conduction through the AV node. The retrograde P wave before restoration of sinus rhythm is not followed by a QRS complex owing to the AV block.

node through the bypass tract may result in a normal QRS complex with the upper rate limited by the AV node. The tachycardia requires anterograde conduction through the AV node, which leads to depolarization of the ventricle, and then retrograde conduction up the accessory pathway, leading to atrial depolarization. The atrial impulse then redepolarizes the AV node. This is also termed *orthodromic reciprocating tachycardia.* The onset of the tachycardia may be similar to that of AV nodal re-entry tachycardia. The rate may be faster than 200 bpm, and the P wave may be seen after the QRS wave, raising the suspicion of a bypass tract (Fig. 56–2). Termination of this arrhythmia may be due to interruption of the re-entrant loop at a variety of areas but most commonly at the AV node. The AV block results in a dangling retrograde P wave visible after the last QRS of the tachycardia (see Fig. 56–2).[2, 9, 12]

Depending on the clinical situation, treatment may require electrical cardioversion, or the situation may permit use of vagal maneuvers. Drugs used in this situation may include adenosine, verapamil, propranolol, and digoxin. Type Ia antiarrhythmics are sometimes used. Amiodarone has been successful when conventional therapy has failed.[2, 13]

Pre-Excitation Syndromes

Pre-excitation syndromes are characterized by early depolarization of ventricular myocardium. This is accomplished by use of pathways that avoid normal conduction through the AV node. This bypass tract or accessory pathway may connect various myocardial areas, but accessory bypass tracts, termed *Kent's bundles,* are the most common. These are involved in the Wolff-Parkinson-White syndrome, which is associated with tachyarrhythmias. Recognition of an accessory pathway is important because understanding of the pharmacologic effects of drugs on the pathways is critical to their selection for the arrhythmias associated with accessory pathways.[2, 14–16]

Wolff-Parkinson-White syndrome is diagnosed by the surface ECG when a short PR interval, wide QRS complex, and delta wave (a slur on the initial inscription of the QRS complex) is seen (Fig. 56–3). The delta wave represents early depolarization of ventricular myocardium resulting from the use of the accessory pathway. If conduction is through the AV node, one would expect a normal PR interval, normal QRS duration, and absence of a delta wave. Conduction through the accessory pathway may vary. At times, conduction through the AV node may be demonstrated; at other times, conduction may be through the accessory pathway; and yet at other times it may be through both. Conduction through the accessory pathway may be exceedingly rapid.

As described earlier, a re-entrant loop may be formed using the AV node and the bypass tract. Retrograde conduction down the AV node through the bypass tract may result in orthodromic reciprocating tachycardias with concealed conduction.

Atrial fibrillation associated with Wolff-Parkinson-White syndrome is usually characterized by conduction via the accessory pathway. The QRS is, therefore, widened and often quite bizarre as a result of the delta wave and the rapidity of conduction allowing for very rapid ventricular response (Fig. 56–4*A* and *B*). The mechanism for onset of the atrial fibrillation is not clearly understood. Some investigators implicate antidromic reciprocating tachycardia (re-entry with anterograde conduction via the accessory pathway and retrograde conduction via the AV nodal tissue) as a potential harbinger of atrial fibrillation, although there is ample evidence that orthodromic reciprocating tachycardia may also be followed by the development of atrial fibrillation with a rapid ventricular response. The stretch, hypoxia, and other factors following this tachycardia may help precipitate deterioration to atrial fibrillation. One of the major concerns about the development of atrial fibrillation with a rapid ventricular response is its obvious tendency to cause severe hemodynamic compromise. This is associated with a significant risk for deterioration into ventricular fibrillation. Atrial fibrillation in the hemodynamically unstable Wolff-Parkinson-White syndrome may require emergency cardioversion. Procainamide may be given intravenously in an attempt to slow anterograde conduction in the accessory pathway and terminate the atrial fibrillation as well.

Antidromic reciprocating tachycardia involves anterograde conduction through the accessory pathway with retrograde conduction through the AV node. The QRS complex is characteristic of pre-excitation. It is widened and may be confused with ventricular tachycardia. Multiple accessory pathways may occur in individuals with this arrhythmia. This pre-excited reciprocating tachycardia may

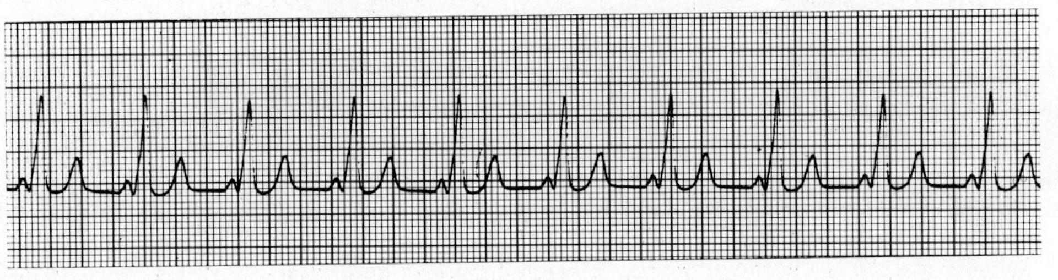

Figure 56–3. Lead II demonstrates the short PR interval, longer QRS complex, and the delta wave characteristic of WPW syndrome.

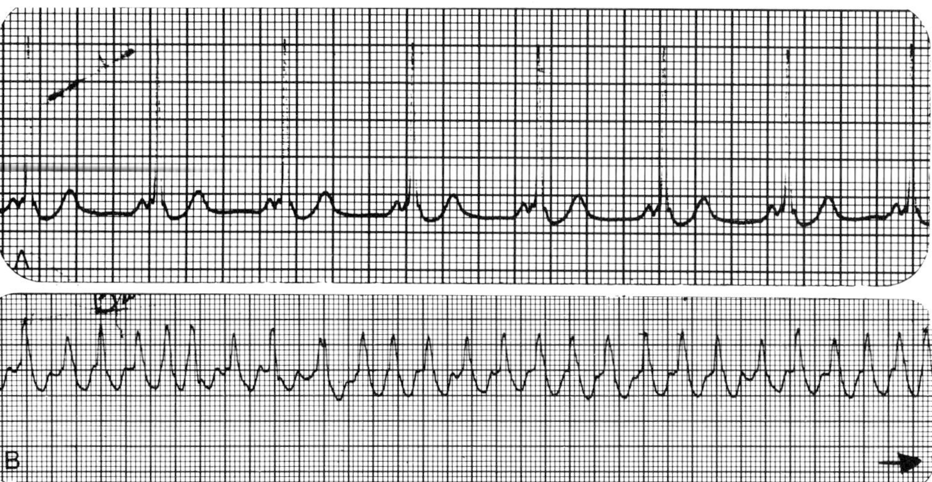

Figure 56–4. *A*, This is lead II of an individual with WPW syndrome. *B*, This is lead II of the same individual in Figure 56–4*A* after he developed spontaneous atrial fibrillation and conduction through the accessory pathway, achieving rapid ventricular responses (in this instance, about 200 beats per minute).

transform to atrial fibrillation followed by development of ventricular fibrillation.[15] Treatment includes cardioversion for emergency situations. Procainamide may be administered in certain situations.

Automatic Atrial Tachycardia

Automatic atrial tachycardia is due to increased automaticity and is often described in persons with cardiac or pulmonary disease, metabolic abnormalities, or digitalis toxicity. When the arrhythmia starts, it often demonstrates a warm-up as the rate of discharge gradually increases for a few beats. The P wave is usually visible and differs somewhat from the sinus-induced P wave because it is shorter in duration and more peaked. The rate of firing ranges from about 150 to 200 bpm. Treatment is difficult. If digitalis or another drug is incriminated as causative, it should be discontinued. Digitalis toxicity may require further treatment. Metabolic, cardiac, and pulmonary abnormalities should be treated. If the rhythm is still resistant and not due to digitalis, propranolol or digitalis may be considered if the ventricular rate needs to be slowed.[2]

Atrial Flutter

Atrial flutter is due to re-entry within the atrial tissue. It may, in fact, share a pathway with AV nodal re-entrant tachycardias in some individuals.[17] The usual clinical situation involves an individual with chronic obstructive pulmonary disease or decompensated heart failure. The flutter waves, appearing saw-toothed in the inferior leads (leads II, III, and aVF), occur at a regular frequency and with an unvarying height (Fig. 56–5). This characteristic helps to differentiate flutter wave from coarse atrial fibrillatory waves. In untreated instances, the flutter waves occur about 300 times per minute but vary between 220 and 350 bpm. In the absence of AV node disease or agents that slow AV node conduction, the ventricular response will be about 150 bpm. Every other flutter wave fails to conduct through the AV node because of the AV node's inherent conduction limits.

The more classic saw-toothed flutter with rates of 250 to 350 bpm is currently termed type I atrial flutter and is thought to represent a macroentrant mechanism. Type II atrial flutters are faster than 350 bpm and do not inscribe the classic saw-toothed pattern but have positive and regular deflections in the inferior leads. The QRS wave is usually normal in duration unless a previous bundle branch block or intraventricular conduction delay was present. Vagal maneuvers may be helpful if there is a question about the presence of atrial flutter. Valsalva's maneuver or carotid sinus massage may transiently increase block through the AV node, permitting flutter waves to be more readily visualized (Fig. 56–6).

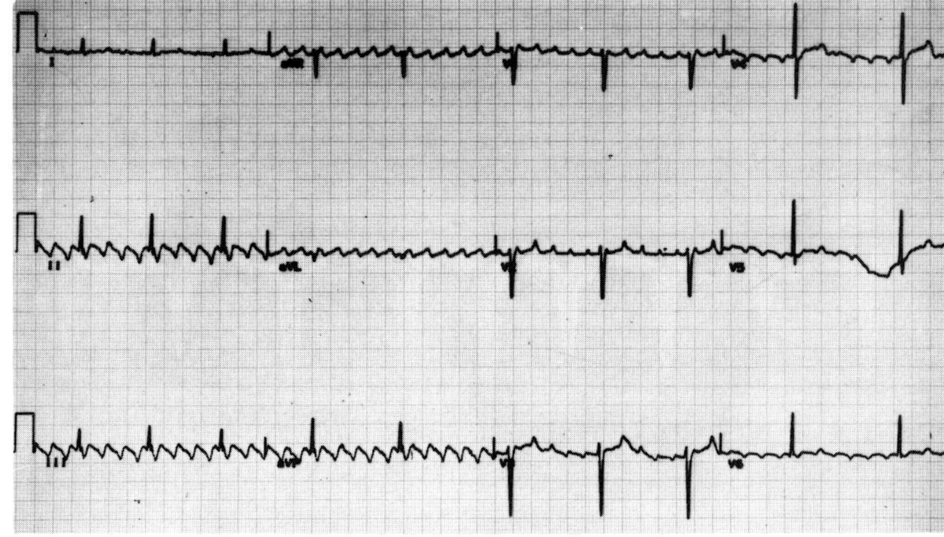

Figure 56–5. Typical atrial flutter demonstrates saw-toothed flutter waves in the inferior leads. Because the flutter rate is so rapid, physiologic block at the AV node usually prevents all flutter waves from conducting to the ventricles. In this instance, variable numbers of flutter waves fail to conduct to the ventricles; this phenomenon is termed "atrial flutter with variable AV block."

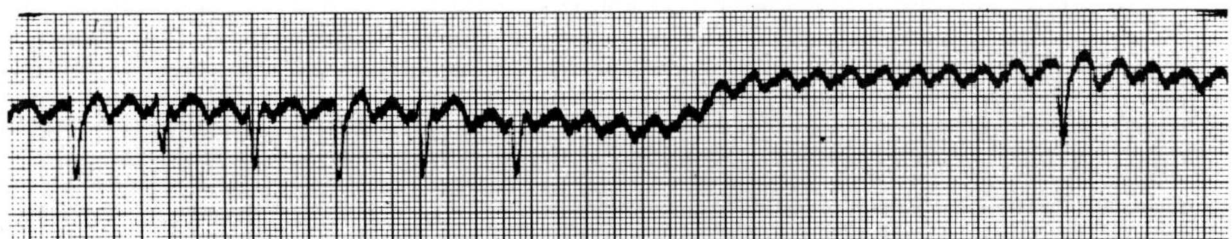

Figure 56–6. To help diagnose the underlying rhythm abnormality, carotid sinus massage was performed and led to profound AV block in this patient with atrial flutter. One should monitor the rhythm when vagal maneuvers are performed.

Severe hemodynamic compromise may require emergency electrical cardioversion at low energy levels of 20 to 50 J. Sometimes cardioversion of atrial flutter leads to atrial fibrillation, which may require a second shock at a higher level. Differentiation of type I from type II atrial flutter is important in the decision to attempt overdrive atrial pacing to terminate the atrial flutter. Type I may respond to atrial pacing, whereas type II does not. Atrial pacing requires placement of the electrode in the right atrium, preferably under fluoroscopic guidance. Care is needed to avoid dislodgement of the electrode into the right ventricle because pacing of the atrium requires 10 to 20 mA, which is quite high for endocardial ventricular pacing. Pacing starts at a rate just above the native flutter rate and is gradually increased until capture occurs, usually 20% to 30% faster than the native rate. The faster rate should be continued for 20 seconds and abruptly stopped to interrupt the atrial flutter. There are, however, different ways to perform atrial pacing to terminate atrial flutter. Rate of pacing, duration of pacing, and the method of terminating pacing will vary. Transesophageal pacing may be used as an alternative. One potential side effect of these modes of terminating atrial flutter is that atrial fibrillation may result. Drug therapy is also available for atrial flutter. Digitalis remains the mainstay. Beta-blockers, verapamil, quinidine, and amiodarone may also be used.[18–20]

Multifocal Atrial Tachycardia (Chaotic Atrial Rhythm)

Multifocal atrial tachycardia (MAT) is most commonly misinterpreted as atrial fibrillation because the RR intervals are so varied. MAT demonstrates an atrial rate greater than 100 bpm. At least three different P waves with three different PR intervals must be present, and no single focus predominates (Fig. 56–7). The presence of P waves may sometimes be misconstrued as fibrillatory waves, thus confusing the diagnosis. Increased automaticity is the underlying mechanism of MAT.

MAT is most commonly seen in individuals with severe decompensated lung disease. Chronic obstructive pulmonary disease and pneumonias may be complicated by this arrhythmia.

Treatment is difficult and usually excludes antiarrhythmic medications because these have been proven not to be helpful. Treatment is focused on improving the underlying pulmonary process. Digitalis may worsen the arrhythmia.[21, 22]

Atrial Fibrillation

Atrial fibrillation may occur as an intermittent, paroxysmal phenomenon or as the more typical chronic pattern. In atrial fibrillation, a variety of areas within the atrium are depolarizing in a random fashion, and re-entrant loops may develop, perpetuating the arrhythmia. Conduction through the atrial tissue, entry into the AV nodal region, and conduction through the AV node are, likewise, random. Thus, depolarization of the ventricle occurs in a sporadic fashion, with the QRS complexes characteristically occurring at irregular intervals. P waves are not visible because of the disorganized atrial depolarization, although the atrial activity noted on the surface ECG may reach such magnitude that the fibrillatory waves may resemble P waves. Unless aberrancy develops or a bundle branch block was preexisting, the QRS complex is narrow (Fig. 56–8). Aberrancy may occur, and usually the aberrated QRS complex is of a right bundle branch type. Characteristic of aberration in atrial fibrillation is Ashman's phenomenon; if a long RR interval is followed by a short RR interval, the QRS complex following the short RR interval may demonstrate aberrancy. This occurs because longer RR intervals (slower heart rates) are followed by longer recovery times. The subsequent shorter RR interval allows impulse conduction through the AV node but encounters a partially refractory right bundle, which allows conduction but at a slower than normal rate; hence, aberrancy results.

In some individuals, untreated atrial fibrillation may lead to hypotension, heart failure, and angina. Heart failure and hypotension may be partly due to the loss of the atrial contribution to ventricular filling, which leads to a decreased stroke volume, and to the decrease in diastolic fill-

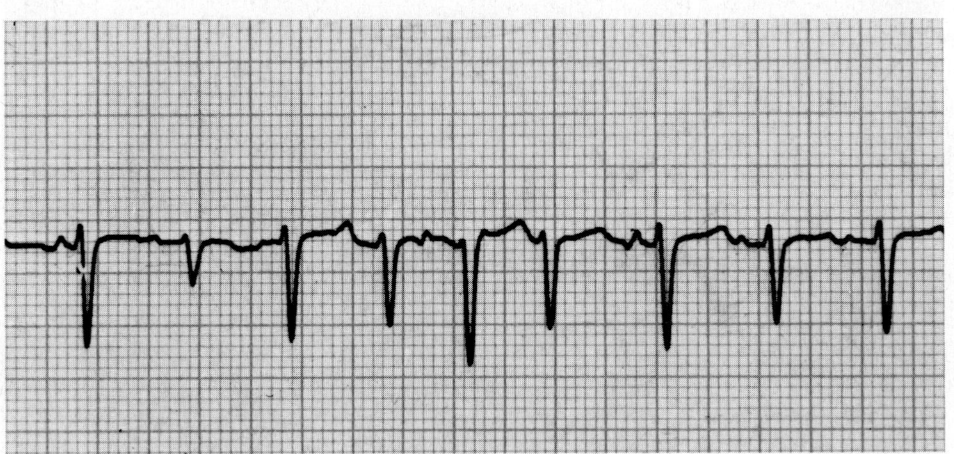

Figure 56–7. Multifocal atrial tachycardia demonstrates no predominant atrial focus. At least three different P waves with different PR intervals are present.

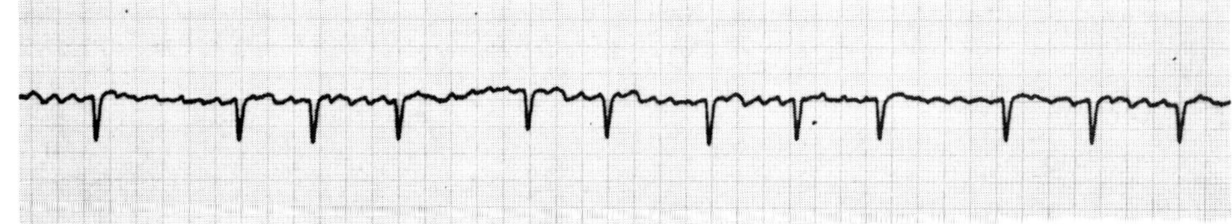

Figure 56–8. Atrial fibrillation.

ing time at high heart rates with a similar result. Angina may result from decreased diastolic filling time and the increased oxygen requirements caused by the increased ventricular rate.

The cause of atrial fibrillation is varied. Lone atrial fibrillation may occur without known heart disease. Systemic hypertension is the most common cause of atrial fibrillation. Other causes include atherosclerotic heart disease, valvular disease, cardiomyopathies, hyperthyroidism, and pulmonary disease. Hypoxia and a variety of drugs, including aminophylline, alcohol, and caffeine, may also precipitate atrial fibrillation.

Treatment may require emergency cardioversion in the acutely decompensated, life-threatening situation. In less critical situations, rapid slowing of the ventricular response with digitalis, β-blockers, and calcium channel blockers, for instance, may be indicated. After slowing of the ventricular response, pharmacologic attempts to convert the rhythm to sinus may be undertaken. The path that is taken will depend on the patient's hemodynamic status, cause of the atrial fibrillation, duration of atrial fibrillation, size of the left atrium, and associated diseases such as thyrotoxicosis, atrial clot, or recent stroke. Atrial fibrillation that occurs in Wolff-Parkinson-White syndrome and conducts down the Kent's bundle may be associated with intolerably rapid ventricular responses, which are associated with hypotension and even ventricular fibrillation. Treatment of the current arrhythmia and prevention of recurrence are mandatory.[23, 24]

Premature Ventricular Contraction

Premature ventricular contractions (PVCs) are characterized by the development of a premature QRS complex that is 0.12 seconds in duration or longer, different than the normal supraventricular-induced QRS complex, and associated with a compensatory pause. In most instances, the PVC does not conduct retrogradely through the atrium to reset the SA node. Thus, the PP interval is not interrupted, and the PP interval surrounding the premature QRS is two times the normal sinus-induced PP interval. This is a compensatory pause. Although the P wave (which occurs on time but is not conducted because of the refractory state induced by the PVC) may occasionally be seen on the surface ECG, it is normally "hidden" in the QRS complex of the PVC. PVCs may develop as a result of increased automaticity or reentry. They may occur in the absence of heart disease but are also commonly seen in individuals with atherosclerotic heart disease, cardiomyopathies, and nearly any form of cardiac disease. Common drugs such as caffeine, theophylline, and alcohol may induce PVCs. Infiltrative diseases must be considered and include tumors, infections, and sarcoidosis.

Treatment of isolated PVCs is complex and controversial. Over the last decade, treatment of PVCs has clearly decreased because the potential for severe side effects of antiarrhythmic drugs has been realized and because the efficaciousness of drug therapy is limited. Removal of precipitating factors is suggested. Treatment beyond this depends on the clinical situation and symptoms.[25–28]

Ventricular Tachycardia

The simplest definition of ventricular tachycardia (VT) is the occurrence of three PVCs in a row. The PVCs may be of the same configuration (monomorphic) or may vary (polymorphic), and the RR intervals may be similar or diverse. General terminology assigns the diagnosis of VT to instances in which the ventricular rate is 100 to 120 beats per minute or greater (Fig. 56–9). In instances of VT in which the rate is less than 100 to 120 bpm but greater than 50 to 60 bpm, the term *accelerated idioventricular rhythm* is used.

Long rhythm strips may demonstrate that the atrial and ventricular rates are firing independently of one another. The atrial rate is usually slower than the ventricular rate. Should a P wave occur at a time when the AV node and ventricular tissue is not totally refractory, conduction from the supraventricular focus may occur, leading to a normal QRS complex or to a fusion beat. This latter QRS complex often has a configuration that merges results of supraventricular conduction with ventricular conduction. When faced with the differential of a supraventricular tachycardia with aberration and VT, certain characteristics on the surface ECG as described by Wellens and colleagues will favor one diagnosis over the other.[29] Intra-atrial leads may be

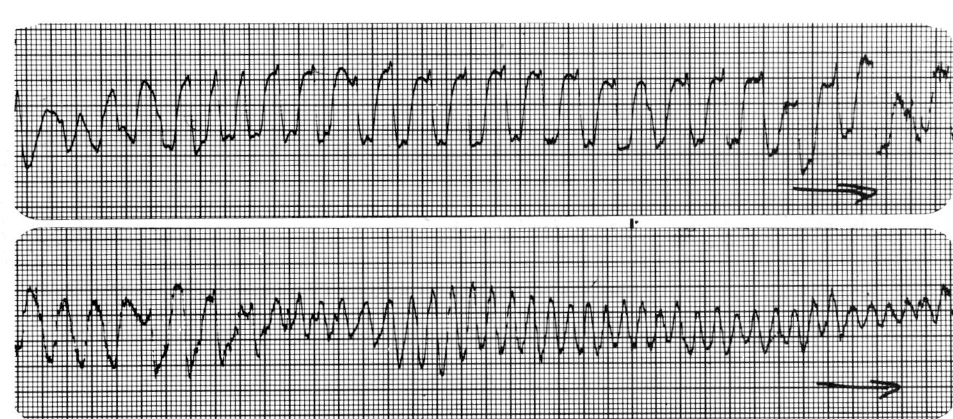

Figure 56–9. This continuous monitor strip demonstrates ventricular tachycardia that deteriorates to ventricular fibrillation.

extremely helpful in this situation. It is very important to differentiate supraventricular tachycardia from VT because misdiagnosis may lead to inappropriate treatment with a poor outcome.[30]

VT is associated with a number of diseases, commonly atherosclerotic heart disease and cardiomyopathy. Other abnormalities include hypoxia, hypokalemia, hypomagnesemia, and digitalis toxicity. Irritants such as right-sided heart catheters and ventricular pacemakers may also be culprits.

A variety of antiarrhythmic medications are available for treatment of VT. Selection and route of administration will depend on the patient's hemodynamic status and associated health problems. If the patient is hemodynamically unstable, electrical cardioversion may be first line of therapy. Symptomatic VT is an indication for immediate therapy. Acute situations may require, in addition to possible cardioversion, intravenous treatment with lidocaine, procainamide, or bretylium. Intravenous β-blockade and magnesium may be helpful.[26, 30–32]

Torsades de Pointes

Torsades de pointes is a specific form of ventricular arrhythmia manifest as a rapid VT with the QRS complex twisting on its axis (Fig. 56–10). The ventricular rate is variable. Initiation is often by a late premature ventricular beat in a person with a long QT interval. Although spontaneous termination occurs not infrequently, ventricular fibrillation may also develop. Torsades de pointes is often a side effect of antiarrhythmics, notably type I. It is seen in organophosphorus insecticide poisoning and has been associated with liquid protein diets.

Treatment requires removal of the offending agent. Isoproterenol infusion may be helpful by increasing the heart rate and shortening repolarization. Either atrial or ventricular pacing may be necessary to suppress the arrhythmia. Correction of magnesium and potassium deficits is warranted. Magnesium may be pivotal to understanding and treating torsades de pointes.[8, 33–40]

Accelerated Idioventricular Rhythm

Accelerated idioventricular rhythm (AIVR) abnormality is most often observed in acute myocardial infarction. The native rhythm is usually slow, allowing AIVR to develop. The VT is usually constrained to rates of 60 to 110 bpm. Fusion beats are common, and heart block is not present.

If necessary, treatment is aimed at carefully increasing the native rate rather than attempting to eradicate the AIVR via antiarrhythmic drugs. The latter could precipitate asystole.[26]

Ventricular Flutter

Ventricular flutter is fast VT with a rate of 300 or more. The QRS is usually regular but without the usual features of a QRS complex and approaching a sinusoid pattern (Fig. 56–11). This rhythm abnormality is of significant hemodynamic consequence and is associated with cardiac disease. Treatment is direct current countershock.

Ventricular Fibrillation

Ventricular fibrillation is a disorganized "rhythm." P waves are not visible. QRS complexes are not identifiable because there is no organized ventricular depolarization. Various areas of the ventricle are depolarizing, and subsequently small or even large deflections occurring at various heights and intervals are seen on the surface ECG (see Fig. 56–9). Untreated, the deflections become smaller, and eventually all electrical activity ceases or the electrical deflection becomes so small that the tracing demonstrates a flat line.

Ventricular fibrillation may occur de novo in acute myocardial infarction, or it may follow an ongoing episode of VT, ventricular flutter, or increased automaticity after treatment for asystole. It is also seen in patients who experience atrial fibrillation with Wolff-Parkinson-White syndrome and anterograde conduction through the accessory pathway.

Defibrillation is the first therapy. If this fails, Advanced Cardiac Life Support (ACLS) guidelines are implemented. Medications include epinephrine followed by lidocaine and then bretylium. If resuscitation is successful, an antiarrhythmic to prevent recurrence of ventricular arrhythmias should be started.

Ventricular Escape Beats

Ventricular escape beats resemble PVCs in that the QRS complex is wide and different than the QRS complex inscribed as a result of conduction from a supraventricular focus. The ventricular complex, however, is late and occurs when the ventricular focus is not depolarized before it can spontaneously depolarize. This is usually because the sinus node has slowed dramatically or there is AV block. Normally, the junctional escape focus, which has a faster rate of depolarization, will depolarize before the ventricular escape focus. Additionally, therefore, the junctional escape focus is suppressed or slowed. The ventricular escape rate is usually less than 60 bpm. Ventricular escape beats or rhythms are not suppressed. They have developed not because of increased automaticity but because they have not been suppressed by normal depolarization of a faster pacemaker. The treatment that is indicated must address the causes of the sinus slowing or AV block.

CONDUCTION ABNORMALITIES

First-Degree Atrioventricular Block

First-degree AV block is characterized by the presence of a prolonged PR interval (>0.20 seconds). Each P wave is fol-

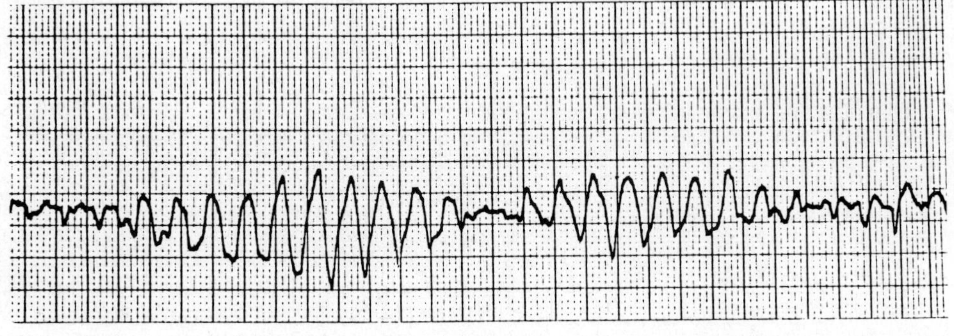

Figure 56–10. Twisting of the QRS axis around the isoelectric line with cyclic alternations in voltage characterizes torsades de pointes.

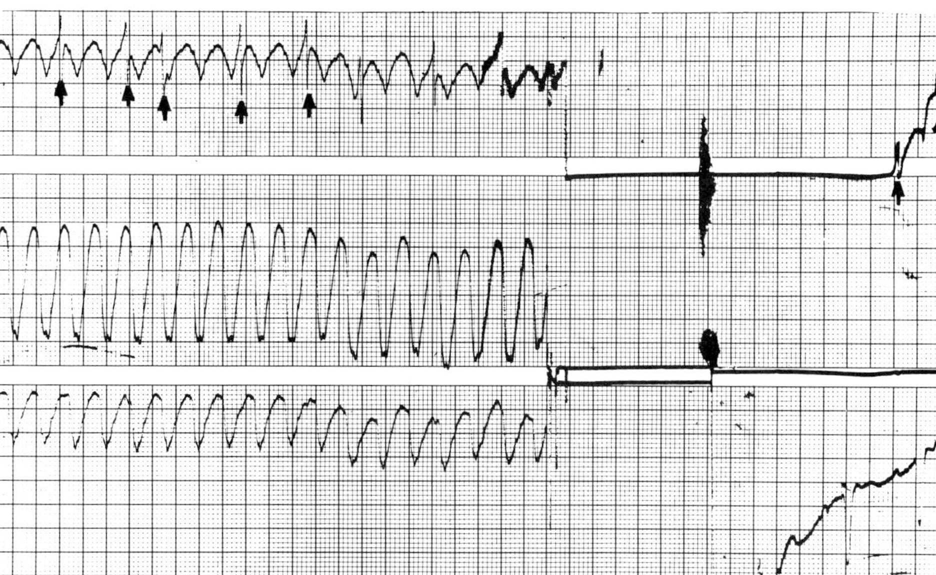

Figure 56–11. This three-channel tracing was obtained with the use of an intra-atrial electrode. The top tracing is intra-atrial, and the *arrows* point to the P waves generated by the underlying rhythm—multifocal atrial tachycardia. The middle and bottom tracings are from the surface electrode and represent the QRS complexes due to ventricular flutter. A precordial "thump" was delivered; this terminated the ventricular flutter and restored a supraventricular rhythm while P waves followed by a narrow QRS developed.

lowed by a conducted QRS complex. First-degree AV block may occur in healthy individuals but may also result from ischemia, high vagal tone, and a variety of drugs, most notably certain calcium channel blockers, β-blockers, and digitalis. Treatment is not needed. If first-degree AV block is due to drugs, dosages may need to be adjusted. In certain clinical situations such as endocarditis or acute myocardial infarction, the development of new first-degree AV block may alert one to potential worsening AV block. The selection of certain medications that cause AV block may be affected by preexisting first-degree AV block.[41, 42]

Second-Degree Atrioventricular Block

In second-degree AV block, some but not all P waves are conducted to the ventricles. It is imperative to demonstrate that the nonconducted P waves are not early to avoid confusion with blocked PACs. The failure to conduct may occur at various levels reflected in the PR interval (for instance, the atrial tissue, the AV node, and the His-Purkinje system) and is not always due to slowing of or failure to conduct solely at the AV node area.

Wenckebach Second-Degree Atrioventricular Block (Mobitz Type I)

This form of second-degree AV block is characterized by regular P wave activity, single P waves not followed by a QRS, and progressive PR prolongation, with subsequent failure to conduct while the RR intervals concomitantly shorten. The conduction block most frequently occurs within the AV node. The RR interval surrounding the nonconducted P wave is less than twice the RR interval of the last conducted P wave. (This is because the last PR interval before the nonconducted P wave is longer than the PR interval of the first conducted P wave.) The degree of AV block is expressed in a ratio of P waves to QRS complexes (i.e., 4:3 indicates that every fourth P wave is nonconducted). Mobitz type I AV heart block may be seen in healthy individuals. It is not uncommon in acute myocardial infarction, which involves the vessel supplying the blood to the AV node.

Treatment is usually not needed, but monitoring may be indicated in unstable situations that may progress, such as in acute myocardial infarction.

Mobitz Type II Second-Degree Atrioventricular Block

Mobitz type II second-degree AV block is seen less frequently than Mobitz type I and is viewed as potentially more dangerous. It may be associated with acute anterior wall myocardial infarctions and may be complicated by complete heart block with an unstable escape rhythm. Mobitz type II block demonstrates regular atrial activity with sudden failure to conduct one or more P waves. Often the QRS complex is wider than normal, consistent with the fact that the conduction delay occurs below the bundle of His. Because of this, the PR interval of conducted beats in Mobitz type II is usually normal.

Treatment is usually necessary because the conduction abnormality lies in the distal conduction system and is often progressive. A stable and reliable transvenous pacemaker is the usual form of treatment.

Sometimes second-degree AV block is simply that. If every other P wave is conducted, or blocked, one cannot label it as one of the usual two forms of second-degree AV block (Fig. 56–12). On the surface ECG, sustained 2:1 AV block fulfills the criteria for neither Mobitz type I nor Mobitz type II second-degree AV block. In reality, if the 2:1 AV block is characterized by a long PR interval and a narrow QRS complex, the block is probably intra-AV nodal and a Mobitz type I. If the PR interval is normal and the QRS wide, one should suspect block distal to the bundle of His (Mobitz type II block).

Third-Degree Atrioventricular Block

If the basic rhythm is sinus, third-degree AV block is diagnosed by the presence of an atrial rate that is faster than the ventricular rate, a regular ventricular rate that is less than or equal to 60 beats per minute, and the lack of any fixed PR interval. The atria fire independently of the ventricles, and the ventricular rate normally is controlled by an escape rhythm located below the atrium.

Common causes of complete or third-degree AV block include medications such as digitalis, selective calcium channel blockers and β-blockers, degenerative disease of the conduction system (Lev's disease and Lenegre's disease), and various cardiomyopathies. This may also develop in acute myocardial infarction. If third-degree AV block is due to inferior infarction, it is usually associated with a stable junctional escape rhythm, whereas the third-degree AV block resulting from acute anterior wall myocardial infarction is likely to be associated with an unstable and unreliable ventricular escape rhythm. Endocarditis, especially of the aortic valve, may be complicated by complete heart

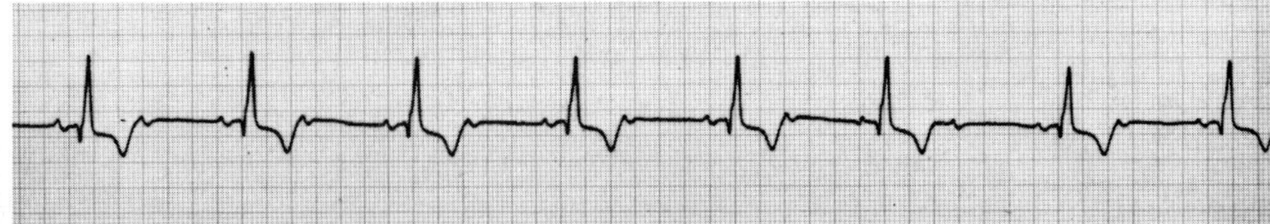

Figure 56–12. A 2:1 AV block in an elderly man with valvular and atherosclerotic heart disease. The PR interval is at the upper limits of normal, but the associated intraventricular conduction delay indicates a high probability of block distal to the Bundle of His. This man did develop higher-degree AV block, which warranted pacemaker insertion.

block as might valve replacement. Lyme disease may cause transient third-degree AV block.

Mechanisms of third-degree AV block may include increased vagal tone (inferior wall myocardial infarction), reversible slowing of conduction through the AV node (certain medications), and destruction of the conducting system (anterior wall infarction). In some instances, third-degree AV block is well tolerated at rest, although symptoms of inadequate cardiac output may occur with exercise because of the inability of the escape rhythm to accelerate properly. Other individuals may experience severe symptoms with third-degree AV block at rest.

Treatment, if indicated and depending on the urgency, may range from atropine to intravenous isoproterenol to electronic transvenous or external pacing.

Sinoatrial Exit Block

Similar to AV block, SA exit block may occur, causing pauses on the surface ECG. Because depolarization of the SA node does not cause any deflection on the surface ECG, determination of SA block is inferential. SA block is presumed to be the cause of a sudden pause if the PP interval surrounding the pause is an exact multiple of the normal sinus PP interval and, of course, no blocked PAC is present. SA exit block may be subdivided into two groups: type I (Wenckebach) SA exit block and type II SA exit block. Instead of measuring PR intervals, one measures PP intervals to determine that there is group beating, indicative of type I. The PP intervals should shorten, similar to the RR intervals in Mobitz I AV block, just before total block occurs. Pauses in the appearance of a P wave that do not fit into one of these types may be due to SA exit block, failure of the SA node to fire, or the inability of atrial tissue to depolarize. Causes of SA exit block include digitalis, atherosclerotic coronary disease, carotid sinus hypersensitivity, and high vagal tone.

NO RHYTHM

Asystole

In asystole, there is no cardiac electrical activity. If watching a monitor strip that suddenly becomes a straight line (especially if it is very flat), one must consider that an electrode has become dislodged. Very fine ventricular fibrillation may mimic asystole.

Treatment for asystole includes full cardiopulmonary resuscitation. Epinephrine is the first drug to be used for asystole, followed by atropine. Emergency pacing by various approaches should be considered early if the arrhythmia remains resistant to repeated medications. Attention to concomitant or precipitant drugs and metabolic abnormalities is also needed in an effort to restore a heart rhythm.

ACKNOWLEDGMENT

We thank Kathy Mulholland, RN, Samantha Lee Hastillo Hess, and Mark Wood, MD, for their invaluable help in preparing this chapter.

References

1. Wit AL, Rosen MR: Pathophysiologic mechanisms of cardiac arrhythmias. Am Heart J 1983; 106:798.
2. Josephson ME, Kastor JA: Supraventricular tachycardia: Mechanisms and management. Ann Intern Med 1977; 87:346.
3. Aronson RS: Mechanisms of arrhythmias in ventricular hypertrophy. J Cardiovasc Electrophysiol 1991; 2:249.
4. Baile DS, Inoue H, Kaseda S, et al: Magnesium suppression of early depolarizations and ventricular tachyarrhythmias induced by cesium in dogs. Circulation 1988; 77:1395.
5. Rosen MR: Cellular electrophysiology of digitalis toxicity. J Am Coll Cardiol 1985; 5:22A.
6. Zipes DP: Monophasic action potentials in the diagnosis of triggered arrhythmias. Prog Cardiovasc Dis 1991; 33:385.
7. Rosen MR, Anyukhovsky EP: Arrhythmias triggered by afterdepolarizations. *In:* Cardiac Electrophysiology and Arrhythmias. Fisch C, Surawica B (Eds). Amsterdam, Elsevier Science, 1991, pp 67–75.
8. Davidenko JM, Cohen L, Gooddrow R, et al: Quinidine-induced action potential prolongation, early afterdepolarization and triggered activity in canine Purkinje fibers. Circulation 1989; 79:674.
9. Josephson ME: Supraventricular tachycardias. *In:* Clinical Cardiac Electrophysiology. 2nd ed. Josephson ME (Ed). Philadelphia, Lea & Febiger, 1993, pp 181–274.
10. Waxman MB, Wald RW, Sharma A, et al: Vagal techniques for termination of paroxysmal supraventricular tachycardias. Am J Cardiol 1980; 46:655.
11. diMarco JP, Sellers TD, Lerman BB, et al: Diagnostic and therapeutic use of adenosine in patients with supraventricular tachyarrhythmias. J Am Coll Cardiol 1985; 6:417.
12. Kalbfleisch SJ, El-Atassi R, Calkins H, et al: Differentiation of paroxysmal narrow QRS complex tachycardias using the 12-lead electrocardiogram. J Am Coll Cardiol 1993; 21:85.
13. Feld GK, Nademanee K, Weiss J, et al: Electrophysiologic basis for suppression by amiodarone of orthodromic supraventricular tachycardia complicating preexcitation syndromes. J Am Coll Cardiol 1984; 3:1289.
14. Bauernfeind RA, Wyndham CR, Swiryn SP, et al: Paroxysmal atrial fibrillation in the Wolff-Parkinson-White syndrome. Am J Cardiol 1981; 47:562.
15. Bardy GH, Packer DL, German LD, et al: Preexcited reciprocating tachycardia in patients with Wolff-Parkinson-White syndrome: Incidence and mechanisms. Circulation 1984; 70:377.
16. Fujimura O, Klein GJ, Yee R, et al: Atrial fibrillation in the Wolff-Parkinson-White syndrome in atrial arrhythmias. *In:* Current Concepts and Management. Touboul P, Waldo AL (Eds). St. Louis, Mosby-Year Book, 1990, pp 262–269.
17. Interian A Jr, Cox MM, Jimenez RA, et al: A shared pathway in atrioventricular nodal reentrant tachycardia and atrial flutter: Implications for pathophysiology and therapy. Am J Cardiol 1993; 71:297.

18. Wells JL Jr, MacLean WA, James TN, et al: Characterization of atrial flutter: Studies in man after open heart surgery using fixed atrial electrodes. Circulation 1979; 60:665.
19. Waldo AL, MacLean WA, Karp RB, et al: Entrainment and interpretation of atrial flutter with atrial pacing. Circulation 1977; 56:737.
20. Boineau JP: Atrial flutter: A synthesis of concepts. Circulation 1985, 72.249.
21. Shine KI, Kastor JA, Yurchak PM: Multifocal atrial tachycardia: Clinical and electrocardiographic features. N Engl J Med 1968; 279:344.
22. Levine JH, Michael JR, Guarnieri T: Treatment of multifocal atrial tachycardia with verapamil. N Engl J Med 1985; 312:21.
23. Singer DH, Ten Eick RE: Aberrancy: Electrophysiologic aspects. Am J Cardiol 1971; 28:381.
24. Waldo AL: Mechanisms of atrial fibrillation, atrial flutter, and ectopic atrial tachycardia: A brief review. Circulation 1987; 75(Suppl III):37.
25. Vlay SC: How the university cardiologist treats ventricular premature beats: A nationwide survey of 65 university medical centers. Am Heart J 1985; 110:904.
26. Schamroth L: Ventricular extrasystoles, ventricular tachycardia, and ventricular fibrillation: Clinical-electrocardiographic considerations. Prog Cardiovasc Dis 1980; 23:13.
27. Kennedy HL, Whitlock JA, Sprague MK, et al: Long-term follow-up of asymptomatic healthy subjects with frequent and complex ventricular ectopy. N Engl J Med 1985; 312:193.
28. Hoffmann A, Schültz E, White R, et al: Suppression of high-grade ventricular ectopic activity by antiarrhythmic drug treatment as a marker for survival in patients with chronic coronary artery disease. Am Heart J 1984; 107:1103.
29. Wellens HJ, Bar FW, Lie KI: The value of the electrocardiogram in the differential diagnosis of a tachycardia with a widened QRS complex. Am J Med 1978; 64:27.
30. Stewart R, Bardy GH, Green HL: Wide complex tachycardia: Misdiagnosis and outcome after emergent therapy. Ann Intern Med 1986; 104:766.
31. Graboys TB, Lown B, Podrid PJ, et al: Long-term survival of patients with malignant ventricular arrhythmia treated with antiarrhythmic drugs. Am J Cardiol 1982; 50:437.
32. Follansbee WP, Michelson EL, Morganroth J: Nonsustained ventricular tachycardia in ambulatory patients: Characteristics and association with sudden cardiac death. Ann Intern Med 1980; 92:741.
33. Soffer J, Dreifus L, Michelson E: Polymorphous ventricular tachycardia associated with normal and long Q-T intervals. Am J Cardiol 1982; 49:2021.
34. Ludomirsky A: Q-T prolongation and polymorphous ("torsades de pointes") ventricular arrhythmias associated with organophosphorous insecticide poisoning. Am J Cardiol 1982; 49:1654.
35. Singh BN, Gaarder TD, Kanegae T, et al: Liquid protein diets and torsades de pointes. JAMA 1978; 240:115.
36. Arsenian MA: Magnesium and cardiovascular disease. Prog Cardiovasc Dis 1993; 35:271.
37. Tzivoni D, Keren A, Cohen AM, et al: Magnesium therapy for torsades de pointes. Am J Cardiol 1984; 53:528.
38. Kay GN, Plumb VJ, Arciniegas JG, et al: Torsade de pointes: The long-short initiating sequence and other clinical features: Observations in 32 patients. J Am Coll Cardiol 1983; 2:806.
39. Tzivoni D, Barrai S, Schuger C: Treatment of torsades de pointes with magnesium sulfate. Circulation 1988; 77:392.
40. Smith WM, Gallagher JJ: "Les torsades de pointes": An unusual ventricular arrhythmia. Ann Intern Med 1980; 93:578.
41. Dreifus LS, Wanatabe Y, Haiat R, et al: Atrioventricular block. Am J Cardiol 1971; 28:371.
42. Narula OS, Scherlag BJ, Samet P, et al: Atrioventricular block: Localization and classification by His bundle recordings. Am J Med 1971; 50:146.

Additional Readings

Josephson ME: Clinical Cardiac Electrophysiology. 2nd ed. Philadelphia, Lea & Febiger, 1993.

Vlay SC: Manual of Cardiac Arrhythmias. Boston, Little, Brown and Co, 1988.

CHAPTER 57

Pacemakers and Implantable Cardioverter Defibrillators in the Intensive Care Unit Setting

Michael K. Belz, MD • Mark A. Wood, MD
Kenneth A. Ellenbogen, MD

PACEMAKERS

General Description

The function of a pacemaker is to both sense intrinsic electrical cardiac events and provide electrical stimuli to excite the myocardium when they are absent. The pacemaker system consists of battery and logic circuits, lead(s) for electrical continuity between the generator and the heart, and an effective lead-myocardium interface (Fig. 57–1). For both sensing and pacing functions, there exist *threshold values* delineating the measured amplitude of the intracardiac electrical events (in millivolts) for sensing and the minimum energy required to stimulate the myocardium. These values depend primarily on characteristics of the lead system and its myocardial interface, lead position, and electrical properties of the myocardium.

The pacemaker coordinates sensed and paced cardiac events by means of an internal clock; thus, timing intervals between events are paramount to understanding pacemaker function. The lower rate interval is the time the pacemaker "waits" after sensed or paced events before emitting a pacing stimulus. The *upper rate interval* is the fastest the pace-

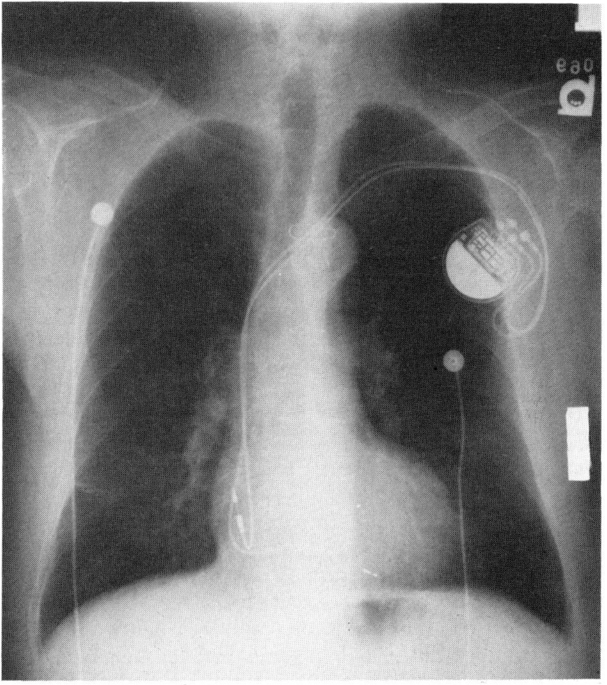

Figure 57–1. Posteroranterior chest radiograph showing a dual-chamber pacing system. The generator was implanted in the left pectoral fossa with a screw-in atrial lead in the right atrium and a tined ventricular lead in the right ventricular apex.

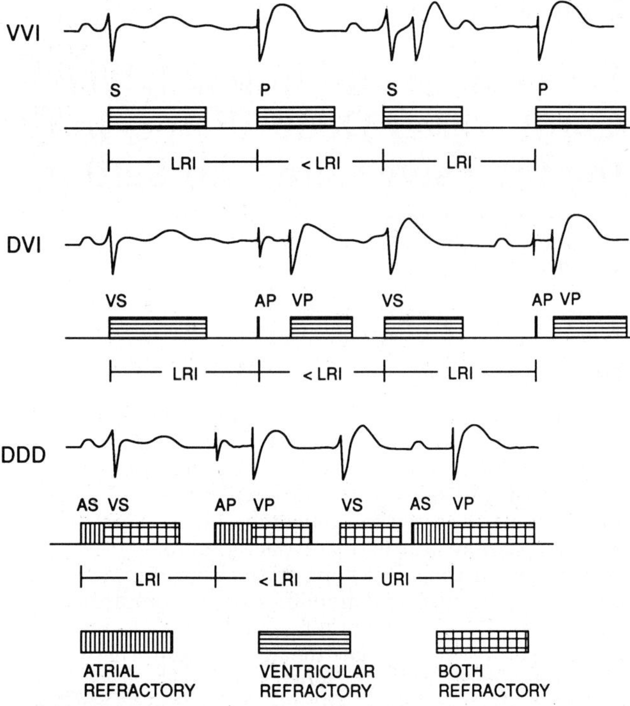

Figure 57–2. Common pacemaker modes with a surface lead, intracardiac events, and refractory periods noted. *Abbreviations:* LRI = lower rate interval; URI = upper rate interval; S = sense; P = pace; A = atrium; V = ventricle.

VVI: In this mode, only ventricular signals, native or paced, are sensed by the pacemaker. If the native rate is below the programmed lower rate interval, the pacemaker paces the ventricle at that rate. Ventricular signals that fall within the refractory period are not sensed (fourth complex).

DVI: Dual-chamber pacing with only ventricular sensing. The pacemaker is inhibited by ventricular signals but not by atrial signals.

DDD: DDD pacemakers pace both chambers and sense atrial and ventricular events. Additionally, a sensed atrial event triggers a ventricular pacing pulse if a ventricular signal is not detected within a programmed interval (the AV delay). Atrial or ventricular events that fall within their respective refractory periods are not sensed.

maker will pace in response to sensed events (e.g., atrioventricular [AV] sequential) or to sensor input in rate-responsive pacemakers. Following a sensed or paced event, atrial and/or ventricular sensing is turned off temporarily (e.g., *refractory period*) to prevent sensing far-field electrical events or repolarization artifacts. The AV delay establishes the electronic PR interval in dual-chamber pacing.

Each pacemaker has one or more programmable modes of operation summarized by a standardized five-letter code that describes the chamber(s) paced, chamber(s) sensed, response to sensed events, and special functions. Asynchronous pacing (SOO or DOO) paces constantly with no sensing occurring. This mode is activated in most pacemakers when exposed to an externally applied magnet. Single-chamber pacing modes are usually AAI or VVI and pace only when the intrinsic heart rate falls below the pacemaker's lower rate. Dual-chamber modes (e.g., DDD) can pace both the atrium and ventricle when the intrinsic heart rate is slower than the pacemaker's programmed lower rate interval but may follow sensed atrial events with ventricular pacing at heart rates between the programmed upper and lower rates (atrial tracking). Rate-responsive pacing uses sensors incorporated into the pacemaker circuitry to modulate heart rate in patients with chronotropic incompetence. These sensors may respond to body movement or vibration, respiratory rate, minute ventilation, blood temperature, or QT interval (catecholamines). A schematic illustration of common pacemaker operation modes is shown in Figure 57–2.

Evaluation of pacemaker function requires knowledge of the pacemaker manufacturer and model as well as its programmed settings. Pacemakers may be identified as to manufacturer and type by patient identification cards issued at implantation, by medical records from implantation, or by appearance and unique identification markings visible on an overpenetrated chest x-ray film (Fig. 57–3). Each manufacturer provides an electronic programmer to interrogate and reprogram the pacemaker. Programming units often display telemetry and marker channels, which are helpful in diagnosing various aspects of pacemaker function and malfunction (Fig. 57–4).

Troubleshooting

Failure to Pace with Pacing Stimuli Present

Failure to pace with pacing stimuli present (Table 57–1) is defined as the presence of pacemaker electrical output without capture of the myocardium. A rise in pacing threshold is seen during the first 4 to 6 weeks after a pacemaker is implanted secondary to tissue reaction at the lead-myocardium interface.[1] In some patients, the rise in threshold observed after implantation can exceed the maximum output of the generator. This is described by the term *exit block.* This may resolve with time (days to weeks), and one may elect to treat such patients with steroids in an attempt to hasten this resolution.[2] Pacemaker-dependent patients may require temporary transvenous pacing during this time. An abrupt rise in threshold or loss of capture within several days to weeks after implantation should arouse suspicion of lead dislodgement. This can also be suggested by a change in the paced QRS complex on 12-lead electrocardiogram

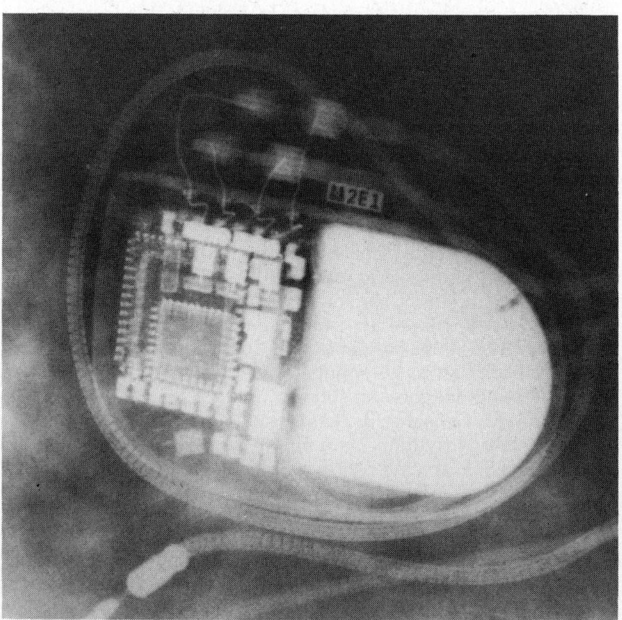

Figure 57–3. Detail of chest radiograph revealing a pacemaker's identification code. The symbol and numbers "2E1" identify this generator as an Elite model number #7084 (Reprinted by permission from Medtronic, Inc., Minneapolis, MN. © Medtronic, Inc.). Each manufacturer has its own unique symbol that can be seen with a well-penetrated magnified radiograph.

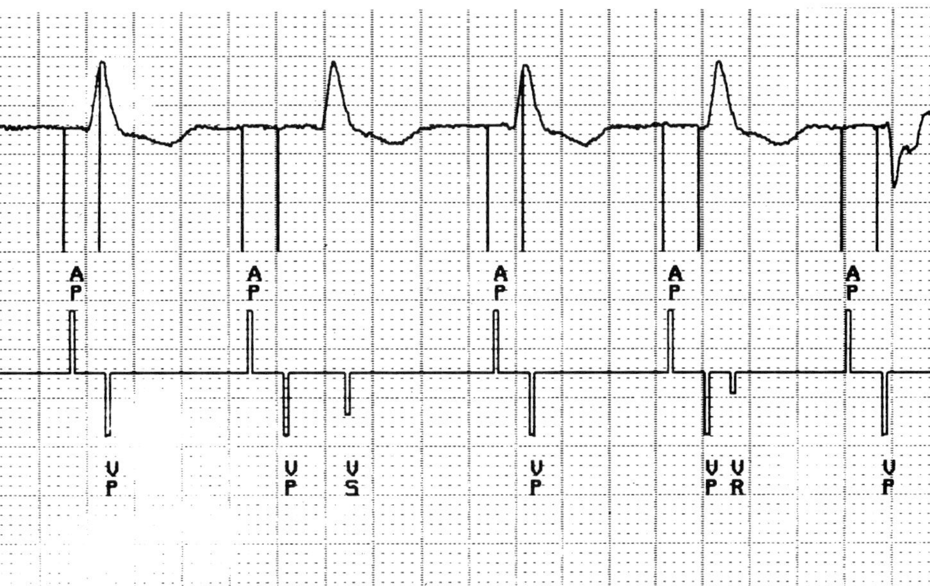

Figure 57–4. Telemetry strip that displays a surface lead and marker channels. This strip reveals intermittent loss of sensing and pacing. P waves are difficult to see in this lead. The first QRS complex is not sensed. The second and fourth ventricular output fail to capture. The second QRS complex is sensed appropriately, and the fourth is sensed in the ventricular refractory period. The fifth ventricular pacing spike captures. *Abbreviations:* AP = atrium paced; VP = ventricle paced; VS = ventricle sensed; VR = ventricle refractory.

(ECG), indicating the lead has moved, or by the pacing of a different chamber altogether (an atrial lead pacing the ventricle or vice versa). This can be confirmed with a posteroanterior and lateral chest x-ray film, noting displacement of the lead compared with the postimplant film. Another cause of loss of capture is lead perforation of the right ventricle or right atrium. This presents with high pacing threshold or complete loss of capture or abnormal sensing, or both. Chest x-ray film or echocardiography may reveal the lead outside the cardiac silhouette or a pericardial effusion, or both. Cardiac tamponade, signs of pericarditis, or diaphragmatic pacing may be present. Other causes of increased thresholds and failure to capture include myocardial infarction near the lead–myocardial interface; progressive myocardial fibrosis; electrolyte or metabolic derangements such as hyperkalemia, hyperglycemia, or acidemia; or certain pharmacologic agents, including antiarrhythmic drugs (especially class Ia, Ic, and III agents), mineralocorticoids, glucose with insulin, and hypertonic saline.[3–7] Thresholds can also increase after direct current (DC) cardioversion.[8] Correction of metabolic derangements or discontinuation of offending agents is remedial. Administration of ephedrine, epinephrine, glucocorticoids, or isoproterenol may acutely reduce pacing thresholds.[5] Elevated thresholds may also be overcome by increasing the energy output of the pacemaker generator or by using temporary pacing modalities.

Primary lead malfunction is another cause of loss of pacing. Leads can malfunction secondary to either an insulation defect or a conductor fracture.[9, 10] An insulation defect effectively shunts current away from the stimulating electrode. Thus, the output must be increased to deliver the same amount of current to the heart. Insulation defects may be associated with pectoral muscle stimulation and low measured impedance on pacemaker interrogation. This problem

TABLE 57–1. Loss of Capture During Transvenous Cardiac Pacing

Cause	*Evaluation*	*Solution*
Catheter dislodgment/perforation	Check position on chest x-ray, paced QRS morphology, or electrograms	Reposition catheter under fluoroscopy, increase output
Poor endocardial contact	Check position on chest x-ray, check electrograms	Reposition catheter, increase output
Local myocardial necrosis/fibrosis	Check electrograms, evaluate for previous infarction	Reposition catheter, possibly increase output
Local myocardial inflammation/edema	Document adequate catheter position (chest x-ray and electrograms)	Increase output, possibly reposition
Hypoxia/acidosis/electrolyte disturbance/drug effect (type Ia's and Ic's)	Check appropriate laboratory values/drug levels	Correct disturbance, reduce drug levels, increase output
Electrocautery/DC cardioversion damaging electrodes and/or tissue interface	Recent exposure to current source	Increase output, replace or reposition catheter, possibly replace generator
Lead fracture	Check unipolar pacing thresholds	Unipolarize functional electrode or replace catheter
Generator malfunction/battery depletion	Document adequate catheter position, check battery reserve	Replace batteries and/or generator
Unstable electrical connections	Document adequate catheter position, check connections	Secure connections

(From Wood M, Ellenbogen K, Haines D: *In:* Cardiac Pacing. Ellenbogen KA [Ed]. Boston, Blackwell Scientific Publications, 1992, p 187. Reprinted by permission of Blackwell Scientific Publications, Inc.)
Abbreviation: DC = direct current.

TABLE 57–2. Oversensing During Transvenous Cardiac Pacing

Cause	*Evaluation*	*Solution*
P-wave sensing	Catheter tip near tricuspid valve on chest x-ray, check electrograms	Reposition further into right ventricular apex, reduce sensitivity
T-wave sensing	Check electrograms	Reduce generator sensitivity, possibly reposition catheter
Myopotential sensing	Check electrograms during precipitating maneuvers	If unipolar, replace with bipolar system or reduce sensitivity
Electromagnet interference	Check proper electrical grounding and isolation of patient and pacer system, possibly check electrograms	Properly ground equipment, electrically isolate patient, turn off unnecessary equipment, reduce sensitivity
Intermittent electrical contacts, unstable connections, or lead fracture	Monitor sensing during manipulation connections/lead	Secure connections, replace lead

(From Wood M, Ellenbogen K, Haines D: *In:* Cardiac Pacing. Ellenbogen KA [Ed]. Boston, Blackwell Scientific Publications, 1992, p 189. Reprinted by permission of Blackwell Scientific Publications, Inc.)

may occur intermittently. Insulating material is radiolucent; therefore, a chest x-ray film will only rarely reveal a simple insulation defect, seen as a discontinuity in the lead. Lead conductor fractures may be incomplete and result in intermittent failure to pace. External manipulation of the lead or generator or motion of the ipsilateral arm and torso may reproduce the problem. Measured lead impedance may be elevated in this case, and chest x-ray film may demonstrate lead discontinuities.

Generator end of life will eventually result in noncapture as the battery is depleted. This usually follows several months of energy-conserving asynchronous pacing and/or slowing of pacing rate below programmed values. Battery depletion may be diagnosed by pacemaker interrogation or response to magnet application.

Failure to Pace with Stimuli Absent

To categorize a pacing system malfunction with stimuli absent, one must first ascertain that pacemaker output is truly absent. A 12-lead ECG is often necessary to confirm a lack of pacing stimuli because small pacemaker spikes may be overlooked on telemetry tracings or missed completely by some digital acquisition systems. With complete lead fractures or dislodgement of the lead from the generator, pacemaker spikes may be absent because of electrical discontinuity between the generator and the body. These conditions should be apparent on chest x-ray film.

Oversensing is the sensing of signals other than true intracardiac depolarizations (Table 57–2). This results in inappropriate inhibition of pacemaker output and thus failure to pace. Pectoral muscle potentials, diaphragmatic potentials, strong electrical fields (e.g., electrocautery), native T waves, pacemaker stimuli in opposing chambers in dual-chamber systems, and afterpotentials are examples of signals that may be inappropriately sensed.[11–16] Temporary pacemakers placed for dysfunctional permanent systems may be inhibited by subthreshold stimuli from the permanent system and vice versa. Decreasing the sensitivity of the system may eliminate these causes of oversensing, provided that intrinsic R waves continue to be sensed at the lower sensitivity setting. In triggered modes of pacing, including the DDD mode, oversensing may lead to inappropriate pacing, which is discussed later.

Lead problems can result in oversensing with inhibition of output. A break in the inner insulation of an in-line coaxial bipolar lead can lead to large electrical signals because of contact between the inner and outer conductors. These signals are typically extremely large, precluding a decrease in sensitivity as a management option. In the pacemaker-dependent patient, programming the system to the SOO of DOO mode may be the only option until the lead can be replaced.

Loss of Sensing

Loss of sensing (Table 57–3) is apparent as inappropriate pacing after intrinsic electrical cardiac events or failure to

TABLE 57–3. Loss of Sensing During Transvenous Cardiac Pacing

Cause	*Evaluation*	*Solution*
Lead dislodgment or perforation	Check position on chest x-ray, check unipolar or bipolar electrograms*	Reposition lead under fluoroscopy, increase sensitivity
Local tissue necrosis/fibrosis	Check unipolar or bipolar electrograms	Reposition lead, increase sensitivity
Electrodes perpendicular to depolarization wavefront, low amplitude electrograms and/or low dV/dt	Check unipolar or bipolar electrograms	Unipolarize lead or reposition
Lead fracture	Check unipolar electrograms from each electrode	Unipolarize functional electrode or replace lead
Electrocautery/DC current damaging electrode or tissue interface	Exposure to current source, check electrograms	Replace or reposition lead, increase sensitivity
Spontaneous QRS during refractory period of generator	Analyze appropriate ECG tracings	No intervention, or replace with generator having shorter refractory period
Generator malfunction	Confirm adequate electrograms and generator sensitivity settings	Replace generator or reset sensitivity
Unstable electrical connections	Confirm adequate electrograms	Secure connections

(From Wood M, Ellenbogen K, Haines D: *In:* Cardiac Pacing. Ellenbogen KA [Ed]. Boston, Blackwell Scientific Publications, 1992, p 188. Reprinted by permission of Blackwell Scientific Publications, Inc.)

*Connect bipolar intracardiac leads to right and left arm leads of ECG and monitor lead I.

Abbreviations: DC = direct current; dV/dt = slew rate; ECG = electrocardiogram.

track atrial activity in DDD systems. Factors that lead to high capture thresholds and loss of capture can also result in loss of sensing. These include lead dislodgement, lead maturation after implantation, perforation, metabolic derangements, antiarrhythmic drug therapy, primary myocardial processes, insulation defects, and conductor fractures.

When battery depletion reaches critical levels, most generators revert to asynchronous pacing modes to conserve energy. Similarly, pacing generators may revert to asynchronous modes in response to high levels of electromagnetic interference from Bovie cautery, magnet application, environmental noise, or DC cardioversion. These latter noise modes can be reprogrammed to other modes, whereas end-of-life behavior necessitates generator replacement.

True loss of sensing must be differentiated from the occurrence of intrinsic events during pacemaker refractory periods. Refractory period durations may be discovered by interrogation of the pacemaker.

Pacemaker-Mediated Tachycardias

Atrial tracking pacemakers will pace the ventricle up to the maximum tracking rate in response to supraventricular tachycardias such as atrial fibrillation, atrial flutter, sinus tachycardia, and ectopic atrial tachycardias.[17, 18] Lowering the maximum tracking rate or reprogramming to a nonatrial tracking mode may be needed until the arrhythmia can be controlled with cardioversion or antiarrhythmic drugs.

Originally the term *pacemaker-mediated tachycardia* (PMT) was used to describe the sensing of a retrograde P wave from a premature ventricular contraction or paced ventricular event by an atrial tracking (usually DDD) system.[19–23] The sensed retrograde P wave triggers a ventricular pacing pulse, leading to another sensed retrograde P wave and thus an endless-loop process. This form of PMT is diagnosed and terminated by reprogramming to an asynchronous mode briefly with magnet application or by termination of tachycardia with transient retrograde VA block. Recurrence is prevented by reprogramming the postventricular atrial refractory period and/or AV delay.

PMTs may also be caused by rate-adaptive pacemakers in response to sensor input. The two common sensors available are vibration sensors and minute ventilation sensors. Other less common sensors use temperature, QT interval, mixed venous oxygen saturation, stroke volume, evoked potential, or pH. These pacing systems respond to the particular parameter used as a sensor to increase paced rate in response to a perceived increase in metabolic demand. Inappropriate responses may result from body tremors stimulating increased rates with vibration sensors, hyperthermia in temperature sensors, and catecholamine administration with QT sensors. Respiratory-sensing pacemakers are invariably driven to higher rates by mechanical ventilation. Reprogramming the pacemaker to a non–rate-adaptive mode is frequently necessary to eliminate inappropriately paced tachycardias and is advisable for all patients with respiratory-sensing pacemakers during mechanical ventilation.

Miscellaneous

Damage to the generator as well as the leads of a pacing system can occur with external defibrillation shocks. Recently implanted leads can be dislodged by intense muscle contractions. Pacemakers may be reprogrammed to a different mode (usually VVI or VOO mode) by the defibrillation current. An acute rise in threshold may result from myocardial injury at the lead-myocardium interface from the defibrillation current. To minimize the risk of damage to the pulse generator, defibrillation paddles should be placed at least 10 cm from the generator, and the defibrillation current path should be perpendicular to the pacemaker current path (Fig. 57–5). Use of anteroposterior defibrillation patches may be useful. The pacemaker programmer should be immediately available if the need arises for reprogramming to an increased output. Pacemaker function should be monitored carefully after defibrillation or cardioversion. Thresholds should be checked immediately after cardioversion, 1 hour later, and 24 hours later.

Electrocautery can be sensed and thus inhibit or trigger pacemaker output and can damage the generator- or tissue-lead interface from high current flow if applied close to the generator or lead electrodes. Electrocautery can also trigger failure of output in devices that are near the end of battery life.

Temporary Cardiac Pacing

Temporary cardiac pacing is indicated for virtually any symptomatic or hemodynamically compromising bradyarrhythmia, except in the setting of hypothermia (wherein refractory ventricular tachyarrhythmias may be induced). Prophylactic temporary pacing is most frequently indicated in the setting of unstable escape rhythms or during acute myocardial infarction. In acute myocardial infarction, prophylactic pacing is generally indicated for new bifascicular or trifascicular block or alternating bundle branch block. Patients with new onset of two or more of first-degree AV block, Mobitz type I or II second-degree AV block, left anterior or posterior fascicular block, or right or left bundle branch block have a 25% to 36% risk of complete heart block in the setting of an acute myocardial infarction.[24]

The timing cycles, sensing, and pacing-threshold principles described for permanent pacing also apply to temporary pacing. There are several possible modes of temporary pacing including esophageal, transcutaneous, transvenous, and transthoracic (Table 57–4). Esophageal pacing is generally efficacious only for pacing the left atrium and is therefore of limited utility in emergency situations. Esophageal

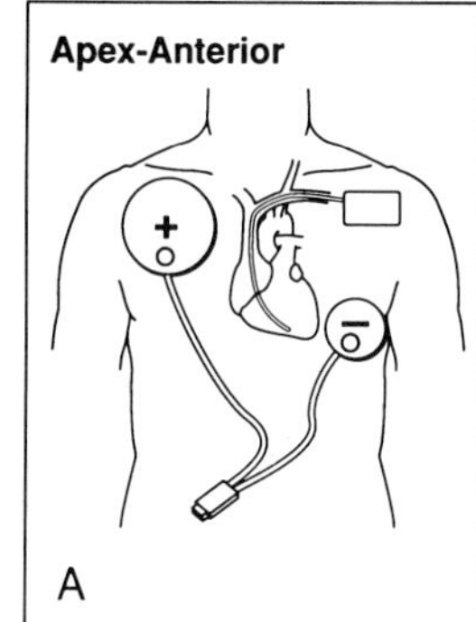

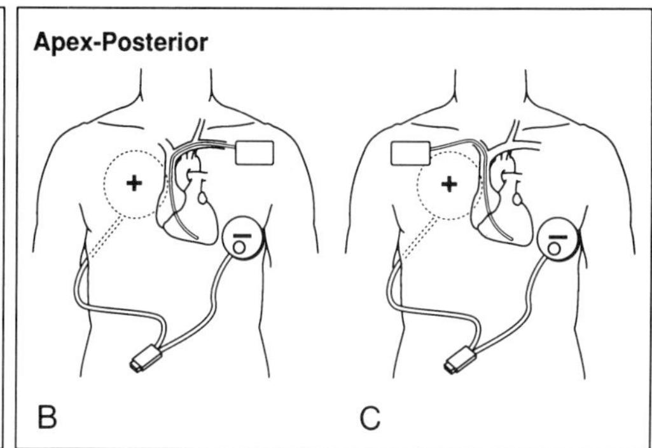

Figure 57–5. *A,* Schematic diagram of proper apical–right parasternal patch or paddle placement for external defibrillation in patients with pacemakers. Note that the axis of defibrillation current is perpendicular to the pacing lead. *B* and *C,* Apical-posterior patch placement. This is the preferred configuration for patients with right-sided pacemakers, as shown in *C.*

TABLE 57–4. Comparison of Temporary Pacing Techniques

Method	*Time to Initiate*	*Chambers Paced*	*Advantages*	*Disadvantages*	*Uses*
Transcutaneous	<1 minute	Ventricle	Simple, rapid, safe	Variable capture, patient intolerance	Arrest, prophylactic, maintenance
Transvenous	3–10 minutes	Atrium and/or ventricle	Most reliable, well tolerated long-term	Invasive, time-consuming, complications	Arrest, prophylactic, maintenance
Transthoracic	10–60 seconds	Ventricle	Extremely rapid, relatively simple	Complications, efficacy unproven	Arrest only
Transesophageal	Minutes	Atrium	Relatively simple, safe	Poor ventricular capture, patient tolerance	Prophylactic atrial pacing, diagnostics, termination SVT

(Adapted from Wood M, Ellenbogen K, Haines D: *In:* Cardiac Pacing. Ellenbogen KA [Ed]. Boston, Blackwell Scientific Publications, 1992, p 203. Reprinted by permission of Blackwell Scientific Publications, Inc.)

Abbreviation: SVT = supraventricular tachycardia.

pacing requires a high-output, long pulse-width generator that delivers current through special soft bipolar leads with electrode spacing of greater than 3 cm.

Transcutaneous pacing is a fast, simple, and generally effective initial method in bradyasystolic arrest situations. The large pacing electrodes are placed with the negative electrode on the anterior chest wall over the cardiac apex or chest lead V_3 position and the positive patch over the posterior chest wall between the right or left scapula and spine. The generator uses high current and long pulse widths and obscures unfiltered ECG monitors. Maximum current is recommended initially to ensure ventricular capture in urgent situations. Pacing thresholds are generally in the 40- to 80-mA range and are frequently uncomfortable for the patient. Transcutaneous pacemakers pace the ventricles with hemodynamics similar to endocardial VVI pacing. Transcutaneous pacing is very safe and especially useful for brief prophylactic pacing applications.

Transvenous pacing is the most reliable method of temporary pacing but requires more operator skill and time to institute than other methods. Temporary pacing leads are best positioned in the right ventricle from a right internal jugular or left subclavian approach. If the patient will eventually need a permanent pacemaker, the subclavian approaches should be reserved for the permanent pacemaker implantation. The leads are directed by fluoroscopic or ECG guidance. A defibrillator should always be immediately available during lead manipulation. Ideally, atrial and ventricular capture thresholds should be less than 1 mA and sensing thresholds greater than 1 mV and 6 mV, respectively. The pacing and sensing principles of temporary pacing generators are similar to those described for permanent pacemakers. Temporary generators are typically VVI or DVI. DDD units have recently become available. Patients suffering an acute myocardial infarction, valvular heart disease, left ventricular systolic dysfunction, or diastolic noncompliance and those recovering from cardiac surgery may benefit hemodynamically from temporary AV sequential pacing. Lead dislodgement is the most common cause of pacing or sensing malfunction or both. Troubleshooting is otherwise similar to that for permanent pacing systems. Complications include induction of ventricular tachyarrhythmias, vascular damage, myocardial perforation, thrombosis, and infection.

Transthoracic pacing is a rapid method of temporary ventricular pacing that is usable in emergent situations if other modes are not available. Electrode wires are introduced percutaneously into the ventricular myocardium via a subxiphoid or parasternal approach with a trocar introducer. The efficacy of this method has not been established. There are numerous potential complications including hemopericardium, pericardial tamponade, myocardial or coronary artery laceration, pneumothorax, and vascular or visceral laceration. Such wires should not be considered stable and should be replaced by transvenous pacing as soon as possible.

IMPLANTABLE CARDIOVERTER DEFIBRILLATORS

General Description

Implantable cardioverter defibrillators (ICDs) are designed to terminate malignant ventricular arrhythmias by delivering an electric shock or antitachycardia pacing to the heart. ICD systems are composed of defibrillation electrodes, sensing leads, and the generator hardware. The sensing and pacing aspects of ICDs are similar to those described for single-chamber pacemaker systems. Shock therapy is delivered through patch electrodes surgically positioned on the

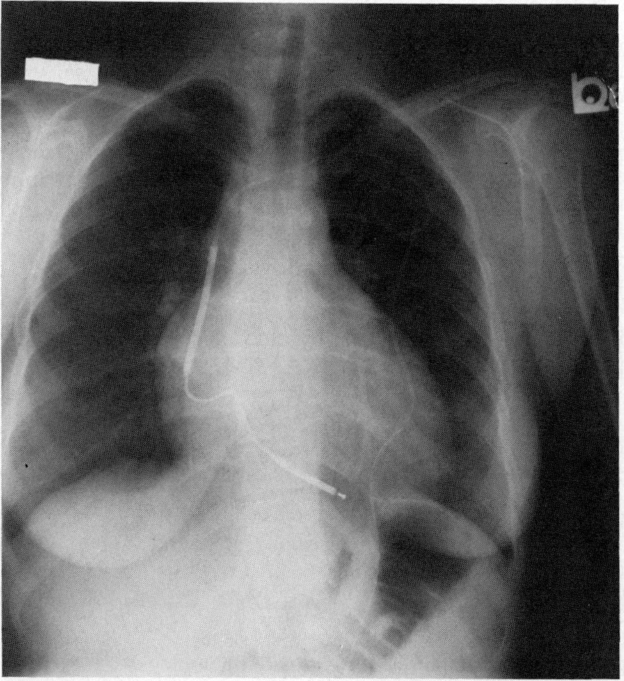

Figure 57–6. Posteroanterior chest radiograph from a patient with a transvenous endocardial cardioverter-defibrillator system without epicardial or subcutaneous patches. The generator is implanted in the abdomen and is not seen in this radiograph.

epicardium or through transvenous endocardial electrode systems with or without subcutaneous electrodes (Fig. 57–6). The generator contains the logic circuitry, charging capacitors, and the battery.

The detailed workings of each manufacturer's device vary; however, the general principles of tachycardia detection and therapy are similar. There is a sequence of events involving tachycardia detection, delay period, charging delay, therapy delivery, and monitoring for tachycardia termination. Heart rate is the primary and principally the sole discriminator of ventricular tachyarrhythmias used by ICDs. The device continuously monitors heart rate. Once the heart rate has exceeded a predetermined cutoff rate for a preprogrammed number of beats, the ICD will enter a therapy mode. There may be an initial delay of several seconds, during which time therapy may be aborted if the rhythm spontaneously terminates. After this delay, therapy will be initiated depending on the capabilities and programming of the device. Earlier "committed" devices will charge and then deliver a shock after detection criteria are fulfilled regardless of whether the tachycardia persists (Fig. 57–7*C*). "Noncommitted" devices will reconfirm the presence of tachycardia during charging and deliver therapy only if tachycardia persists. The time from tachycardia detection to therapy delivery may be 12 to 15 seconds.

There are two modes of therapy used by ICDs to terminate ventricular tachyarrhythmias. The first is delivery of an electric shock to the heart (see Fig. 57–7*A*). The energy required to defibrillate the heart is not an absolute value but rather follows a probability function.[25] The programmed energy delivered represents a threshold energy determined at the time of implant plus a safety factor (generally 10 J) to ensure a high likelihood of successful defibrillation. The defibrillation energy requirement at any particular time is influenced by characteristics of the device, impedance to current flow, and presence of ischemia, drugs, myocardial stretch, and other factors. In general, less energy is required to terminate ventricular tachycardia (VT) than ventricular fibrillation (VF). After a maximum of four to seven shocks are delivered without tachycardia termination, no further therapy is available until the device has sensed a heart rate below the tachycardia detection rate for a specified time period.

Newer devices have the capability to deliver antitachycardia pacing (ATP) as a means of terminating slower VT (see Fig. 57–7*B*). This may prevent delivery of electric shocks, improving patient comfort and prolonging ICD battery life. The heart rate that initiates ATP therapy, the number of pulses delivered, and the number of attempts are all programmable. If the rhythm persists or is accelerated by the pacing, shock therapy can be delivered.

For patients with ventricular arrhythmias of variable rate and hemodynamic stability, some devices deliver "tiered therapy" based on the rates of the various rhythms. For example, initial therapy for a well-tolerated, relatively slow VT could be ATP, followed by low-energy cardioversion if ATP failed and then high-energy cardioversion if low energy failed. Fast, less well tolerated VT or VF would initiate shock therapy immediately. Devices capable of ATP are also capable of VVI pacing for bradyarrhythmias, which may follow successful tachycardia termination, or for concomitant intrinsic bradyarrhythmias. Newer devices may have data-logging capabilities to store the time, date, rate, duration, and therapy delivered for each tachycardia detection. These data may greatly assist in evaluating the appropriateness of delivered therapy.

Evaluation of Recurrent Appropriate Therapy

Appropriate successful ICD shocks can be life saving but, if recurrent in a brief time period, are very uncomfortable for the patient and contribute to early battery depletion. Additionally, multiple episodes of ventricular tachyarrhythmias and multiple defibrillations can lead to myocardial ischemia, myocardial stunning, and worsening cardiac function.

Frequent appropriate shocks are best managed by suppression and treatment of the ventricular arrhythmia. Reversible causes of VT/VF should be investigated. Electrolyte abnormalities, especially hypokalemia or hypomagnesemia, should be aggressively treated. New or worsening heart failure can be a cause of more frequent arrhythmias and should be optimally managed. Myocardial ischemia or

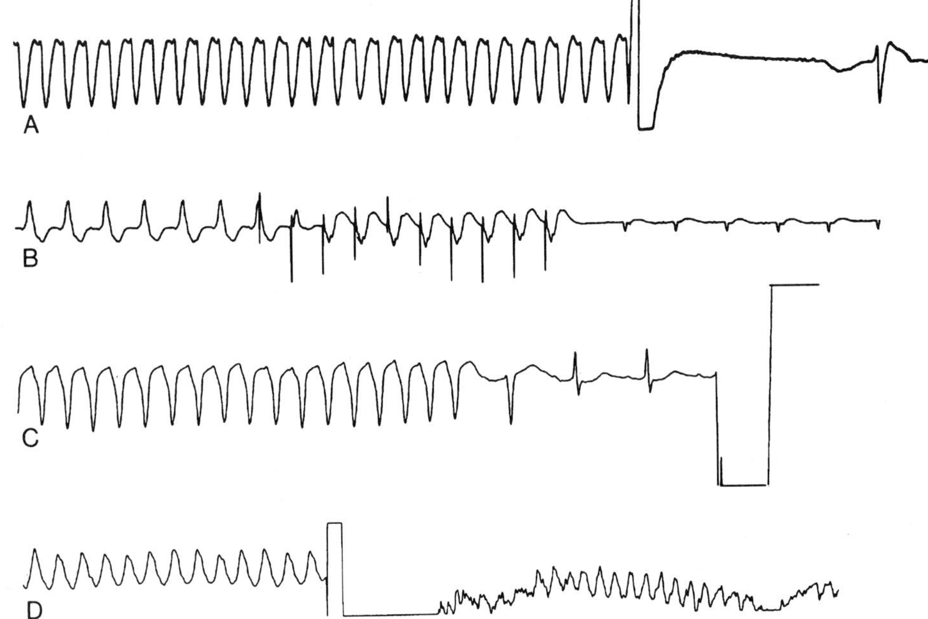

Figure 57–7. *A*, Ventricular tachycardia termination by ICD shock. Many telemetry units would not record the shock and termination because of their timed automatic cutoffs. *B*, Ventricular tachycardia successfully terminated by antitachycardia pacing. *C*, Shock delivered by ICD during sinus rhythm. This is appropriate function from a "committed" device (see text for explanation). *D*, Unsuccessful ICD shock delivered during ventricular tachycardia that precipitates ventricular fibrillation. The second ICD shock (not shown) was successful in terminating the ventricular fibrillation.

new infarction must be considered and treated. New antiarrhythmic drug therapy may be proarrhythmic, leading to multiple episodes of polymorphic VT. Treatment with tricyclics, phenothiazines, pentamidine, erythromycin, terfenadine, or astemizole[26–34] can lead to a prolonged QT interval in susceptible patients, precipitating torsades de pointes. Discontinuation of previously successful antiarrhythmic drug therapy may result in more frequent tachyarrhythmias.

Some patients will not have an identifiable cause for their multiple episodes of VT/VF. These patients require antiarrhythmic drug therapy to suppress frequent episodes. Specific antiarrhythmic drug therapy is usually empiric. Lidocaine, procainamide, and bretylium are easily administered, rapidly acting, and relatively effective in the short term in the intensive care unit setting. Patients should be monitored during the institution of antiarrhythmic drugs for proarrhythmia (both tachyarrhythmias and bradyarrhythmias). New antiarrhythmic drugs may cause an increase in defibrillation thresholds or slow the tachycardia rate below detection rates. Patients must therefore undergo repeat testing of their ICD after institution or change in antiarrhythmic drugs.

Inappropriate Therapy

Inappropriate therapy from ICDs may be in response to supraventricular tachyarrhythmias or electronic noise interpreted by the device as a ventricular tachyarrhythmia. Most ICDs use heart rate as the sole criterion to detect ventricular tachyarrhythmias. Any heart rate the device senses above its programmed cutoff rate is treated as VT. Thus, supraventricular tachyarrhythmias exceeding the rate cutoff will also initiate device therapy. Patients may receive inappropriate shocks for atrial fibrillation or flutter, paroxysmal supraventricular tachycardia, or even sinus tachycardia. This is not considered a device malfunction since the ICD is functioning as programmed within its limitations. Raising the cutoff rate for the detection of tachycardia may help prevent this problem. Some patients have overlap between their VT rate and their rates during atrial fibrillation, sinus tachycardia, or supraventricular tachycardia. Use of medications such as β-blockers, calcium channel blockers, or digoxin may be needed to slow the ventricular rates during these supraventricular rhythms. Some devices can incorporate heart rate stability and sudden-onset criteria into detection algorithms to discriminate atrial fibrillation and sinus tachycardia, respectively, from VT.

Committed therapy devices may also deliver shocks at inappropriate times after spontaneous termination of nonsustained VT (see Fig. 57–7*C*). Reprogramming to a noncommitted mode, if available, or extending the detection criteria or shock delay may prevent shocks for nonsustained VT.

If a discharge is observed in a patient in normal sinus rhythm with no preceding nonsustained tachycardia, system malfunction secondary to a lead or connector problem should be considered. Partial lead fractures or loose electrical connections among ICD generators, sensing leads, or adaptors may generate electrical noise that is interpreted by the device as tachycardia. In some devices, this can be diagnosed by placing a magnet over the generator, which elicits an audible beep with each sensed R wave. If manipulation of the device or leads brings out multiple beeps for each R wave, then the device may be sensing extraneous electrical signals (e.g., noise) and generally requires operative revision (see later discussion of double counting).

For frequent shocks from any cause, most ICDs can be deactivated by placing a strong doughnut or bar magnet over the device. Some devices (Cardiac Pacemakers, Inc.) are turned off by magnet application, confirmed by noting the disappearance of beeps with each sensed R wave and replacement by a continuous tone. Other devices are deactivated only as long as the magnet is over the generator. Bradycardia pacing is generally not affected by magnet application. Device deactivation is most often necessary in the patient with rapid supraventricular arrhythmias or lead/connector malfunction to prevent multiple inappropriate shocks. ICD inactivation should be done only in a carefully monitored situation with immediately available external defibrillation capability and after consultation with physicians trained in ICD management. ICDs may also respond to external electromagnetic interference from Bovie cautery, diathermy, and transcutaneous electrical nerve stimulation units. ICDs should generally be inactivated before surgical procedures with provisions for intraoperative external defibrillation.

Another important cause of inappropriate shocks is the sensing of pacing artifacts. In patients with temporary or permanent pacemakers and ICDs, the ICD may sense the atrial and/or ventricular pacing artifacts as QRS complexes leading to "double counting." The ICD will, therefore, sense a heart rate two or three times the actual heart rate. Double counting may also occur in patients with single-chamber ventricular pacemakers if the device senses both the pacing artifact and the paced QRS complex. Unipolar pacing (atrium or ventricle) is contraindicated in patients with ICDs because of the high likelihood of double counting. Bipolar pacing wires positioned in close proximity to the ICD endocardial sensing leads may also lead to double counting. T-wave sensing is another uncommon cause of this phenomenon. Double counting may be detected in some devices by placing a magnet over the device and hearing two beeps for each R wave. Repositioning temporary pacing wires, deactivation of the ICD, and reliance on external cardioversion or reprogramming the sensitivity of the ICD may eliminate many causes of double counting.

Failure to Respond

The time from detection of a ventricular tachyarrhythmia to the response by an ICD varies depending on the device and the programmed therapy. A long detection time or delay with charging for a maximum shock may take 20 seconds or longer to deliver therapy. Telemetry monitoring units may discontinue recording during this delay, leading to a misdiagnosis of failure to respond (see Fig. 57–7*A*). Noncommitted devices should not deliver therapy unless the VT persists for that time; failure to respond to nonsustained VT is appropriate.

A common reason for an ICD's failure to respond to sustained VT is that the VT rate is below the cutoff rate programmed for the device. This may be due to inappropriate programming or the emergence of a slower, previously unrecognized VT or previous VTs slowed by antiarrhythmic drug therapy. Reprogramming the rate cutoff may be necessary.

Electrical signals during VF may be extremely low in amplitude. A device that senses sinus rhythm or VT appropriately may fail to sense VF, leading to failure to deliver therapy. In a similar fashion, separate bradycardia pacemakers, temporary or permanent, may fail to sense VF. Therefore, they will not be inhibited by the VF signals and will continue to pace. The pacing artifacts, because of their relatively large size, may be sensed by the ICD as a normal slow rhythm, inhibiting tachycardia therapy.

ICDs must, of course, be turned on to respond. As described previously, magnets can turn off many devices in use. Patients who have come in contact with large industrial or military magnets or a magnetic resonance imaging magnet may have deactivated their device. Other uncommon sources of deactivation include high-fidelity stereo speakers, arc welding equipment, and power tools. Placing a magnet over the generator until beeps are heard with every sensed R wave will reactivate some devices.

In addition, after four to seven shocks without tachycardia termination, ICDs will not deliver further therapy until termination occurs. If unaware of previous failed therapy for a given episode, failure to respond may be misdiagnosed. Patients who fail to convert after the maximum number of shocks or whose devices fail to respond should undergo attempts at external defibrillation, coupled with cardiopulmonary resuscitative efforts, as in any patient. One should not wait for the ICD to complete its therapy before beginning resuscitative measures and external defibrillation. ICD patches may have an insulating effect to external shock, so different paddle positions, including anteroposterior and lateral-lateral, should be attempted if needed.

The increasing sophistication and complexity in pacemaker and ICD technology require greater knowledge and expertise to maintain competence in their management. There are, however, underlying common aspects to these devices that are relatively simple to comprehend. Understanding these basic principles allows the physician to manage the majority of patients with these devices in the acute setting.

References

1. Szabo Z, Solti F: The significance of the tissue reaction around the electrode on the late myocardial threshold. *In:* Advances in Pacemaker Technology. Schaldach M, Furman S (Eds). New York, Springer-Verlag, 1975, pp 273–285.
2. Beanlands DS, Akyurekli Y, Keon WJ: Prednisone in the management of exit block. *In:* Proceedings of the Fifth World Symposium on Cardiac Pacing. Meere C (ed). Montreal, Pacesymp, 1979, pp 18.
3. Lee D, Greenspan K, Edmands RE, et al: The effect of electrolyte alteration on stimulus requirement of cardiac pacemakers. Circulation 1968; 38:VI–124.
4. O'Reilly MV, Murnaghan DP, Williams MB: Transvenous pacemaker failure induced by hyperkalemia. JAMA 1974; 228:336.
5. Levick CE, Mizgala HF, Kerr CR: Failure to pace following high dose anti-arrhythmic therapy: Reversal with isoproterenol. PACE Pacing Clin Electrophysiol 1984; 7:252.
6. Dohrmann ML, Goldschlager N: Metabolic and pharmacologic effects on myocardial stimulation threshold in patients with cardiac pacemakers. *In:* Modern Cardiac Pacing. Barold SS (Ed). Mount Kisco, NY, Futura Publishers, 1985, pp 161–170.
7. Hughes JC Jr, Tyers GFO, Torman HA: Effects of acid-base imbalance on myocardial pacing thresholds. J Thorac Cardiovasc Surg 1975; 69:743.
8. Guarnieri T, Datorre SD, Bondke H, et al: Increased pacing thresholds after an automatic defibrillatory shock in dogs: Effects of class I and II antiarrhythmic drugs. PACE Pacing Clin Electrophysiol 1988; 11:1324.
9. Stokes K, Staffeson D, Lessar J, et al: A possible new complication of subclavian stick: Conductor fracture. PACE Pacing Clin Electrophysiol 1987; 10:748.
10. Levine PA: Clinical manifestations of lead insulation defects. J Electrophysiol 1987; 1:144.
11. Fetter J, Bobeldyk GL, Engman FJ: The clinical incidence and significance of myopotential sensing with unipolar pacemakers. PACE Pacing Clin Electrophysiol 1984; 7:871.
12. Gabry MD, Behrens M, Andrews C, et al: Comparison of myopotential interference in unipolar-bipolar programmable DDD pacemakers. PACE Pacing Clin Electrophysiol 1987; 10:1322.
13. Warnowicz-Papp MA: The pacemaker patient and the electromagnetic environment. Clin Prog Pacing Electrophysiol 1983; 1:166.
14. Sager DP: Current facts on pacemaker electromagnetic interference and their application to clinical care. Heart Lung 1987; 16:211.
15. Peter T, Harper R, Sloman G: Inhibition of demand pacemakers caused by potentials associated with inspiration. Br Heart J 1976; 38:211.
16. Barold SS, Ong LS, Falkoff MD, et al: Inhibition of bipolar demand pacemaker by diaphragmatic myopotentials. Circulation 1977; 56:679.
17. Levine PA, Seltzer JP: AV universal (DDD) pacing and atrial fibrillation. Clin Prog Pacing Electrophysiol 1983; 1:275.
18. Greenspan AJ, Greenberg RM, Frankk WS: Tracking of atrial flutter by DDD pacing, another form of pacemaker mediated tachycardia. PACE Pacing Clin Electrophysiol 1984; 7:955.
19. Levine PA, Selznick L: Prospective Management of the Patient with Retrograde Ventriculoatrial Conduction: Prevention and Management of Pacemaker Mediated Endless Loop Tachycardias. Sylmar, CA, Pacesetter Systems, Inc, 1990.
20. Luceri RM, Castellanos A, Zaman L, et al: The arrhythmias of dual chamber cardiac pacemakers and their management. Ann Intern Med 1983; 99:354.
21. Den Dulk K, Lindemans FW, Bar FW, et al: Pacemaker related tachycardias. PACE Pacing Clin Electrophysiol 1982; 5:476.
22. Rubin JW, Frank MJ, Boineau JP, et al: Current physiologic pacemakers: A serious problem with a new device. Am J Cardiol 1983; 52:88.
23. Furman S, Fisher JD: Endless loop tachycardia in an AV universal (DDD) pacemaker. PACE Pacing Clin Electrophysiol 1982; 5:486.
24. Lamas GA, Muller JE, Turi ZG, et al: A simplified method to predict occurrence of complete heart block during acute myocardial infarction. Am J Cardiol 1986; 57:1213.
25. Troup PJ: Implantable cardioverter defibrillators. Curr Probl Cardiol 1989; 14:785.
26. Crome P: Poisoning due to tricyclic antidepressant overdosage: Clinical presentation and treatment. Med Toxicol 1986; 1:261.
27. Raehl CL, Patel AK, LeRoy M: Drug-induced torsades de pointes. Clin Pharmacol 1985; 4:675.
28. Nattel S, Ranger S, Talajic M, et al: Erythromycin-induced long QT syndrome: Concordance with quinidine and underlying cellular electrophysiologic mechanism. Am J Med 1990; 89:235.
29. Mohahan BP, Ferguson CL, Killeavy ES, et al: Torsades de pointes occurring in association with terfenadine use. JAMA 1990; 264:2788.
30. Saviuc P, Danel V, Dixmerias F: Prolonged QT interval and torsades de pointes following astemizole overdose. J Toxicol Clin Toxicol 1993; 31:121.
31. Clark A, Love H: Astemizole-induced ventricular arrhythmias: An unexpected cause of convulsions. Int J Cardiol 1991; 33:165.
32. Honig PK, Woosley RL, Zamani K, et al: Changes in the pharmacokinetics and electrocardiographic pharmacodynamics of terfenadine with concomitant administration of erythromycin. Clin Pharmacol Ther 1992; 52:231.
33. Scott JL, Walls RM: QT interval prolongation. J Emerg Med 1985; 3:221.
34. Bigger JT Jr, Sahar DI: Clinical types of proarrhythmic response to antiarrhythmic drugs. Am J Cardiol 1987; 59:2E.

Additional Readings

Barold SS (Ed): Modern Cardiac Pacing. Mount Kisco, NY, Futura Publishers, 1985.

El-Sherif N, Samet P (Eds): Cardiac Pacing and Electrophysiology. 3rd ed. Philadelphia, WB Saunders, 1991.

Ellenbogen K (Ed): Cardiac Pacing. Boston, Blackwell Scientific Publications, 1992.

Troup PJ: Implantable cardioverter defibrillators. Curr Probl Cardiol 1989; 14:675.

CHAPTER 58

Hypertensive Crises: Emergencies and Urgencies

Janice L. Zimmerman, MD, FACP, FCCP, FCCM

Although chronic hypertension is common in the U.S. population, few patients present to critical care physicians with severe life-threatening elevations of blood pressure (BP). Emphasis on early detection and treatment of hypertension has resulted in a declining incidence of hypertensive crises, but it is imperative that physicians recognize situations requiring immediate intervention and choose therapy appropriately. Many patients with hypertensive crises require the expertise of critical care physicians and the supportive care of intensive care units (ICUs).

Various terminology has been used for adverse clinical conditions associated with severe hypertension. For the purpose of this chapter, hypertensive crises indicate the presence of severe hypertension that is potentially life threatening. The immediacy of lowering BP divides hypertensive crises into hypertensive emergencies or urgencies. In hypertensive emergencies, severe hypertension is associated with new or progressive end-organ damage of the neurologic, cardiovascular, and renal systems (Table 58–1). In these situations, BP should be lowered immediately to minimize organ dysfunction. In hypertensive urgencies, severe hypertension is present without evidence of immediate complications (Table 58–2). BP in urgent conditions can be lowered less rapidly, usually over 24 hours. When knowledge of prior end-organ dysfunction is not available, differentiating hypertensive emergencies from urgencies may be difficult. Accelerated hypertension is a hypertensive urgency characterized by the presence of retinal hemorrhages and exudates without papilledema. The term *malignant hypertension* has been used in discussions of hypertensive crises to refer to pathologic, fundoscopic, and/or clinical findings. Because of this confusion, malignant hypertension is not used in this chapter.

The physician should not rely on a specific BP level to differentiate a hypertensive emergency from a less urgent situation. The rate at which BP rises and the prior level of BP may be more important than the absolute level.[1, 2] Although most hypertensive emergencies are associated with a diastolic BP of greater than 120 mm Hg, a previously normotensive patient could experience end-organ dysfunction with a diastolic BP of 110 mm Hg. Conversely, patients with chronic hypertension may be asymptomatic with diastolic BP of greater than 120 mm Hg.

TABLE 58–1. Hypertensive Emergencies

Hypertensive encephalopathy
Acute myocardial ischemia syndromes
Unstable angina
Myocardial infarction
Acute left ventricular dysfunction
Acute aortic dissection
Acute renal insufficiency
Acute intracranial events
Hemorrhagic cerebrovascular accident
Thrombotic cerebrovascular accident
Subarachnoid hemorrhage
Excess catecholamine states
Pheochromocytoma crisis
MAOI–tyramine interaction
Antihypertensive withdrawal

Abbreviation: MAOI = monoamine oxidase inhibitor.

TABLE 58–2. Hypertensive Urgencies

Accelerated hypertension
Perioperative hypertension
Severe hypertension associated with the following:
Congestive heart failure
Stable angina
Transient ischemic attacks
Renal failure from other causes

PATHOPHYSIOLOGY

BP is a function of cardiac output and systemic vascular resistance (SVR). Several factors can thus influence the development of severe hypertension. Cardiac output is determined by heart rate, filling pressure (preload), and myocardial contractility. Tachycardia does not usually result in hypertension, but acute fluid overload can produce acute hypertensive crises. Fluid overload contributes to severe hypertension in patients with renal failure, overtransfusion, or excessive use of saline infusions. Many critically ill patients have limited ability to excrete salt and water loads, so fluid balance must be carefully evaluated. Increased myocardial contractility (i.e., cocaine abuse) may result in increased cardiac output and resultant hypertension. However, autoregulation usually limits the rise in pressure by a corresponding decrease in SVR.

An increase in SVR is the common denominator in the majority of hypertensive crises. This increase is mediated by increased levels of circulating catecholamines, increased α-adrenergic activity, and activation of the renin-angiotensin-aldosterone system.[2] The rise in arterial pressure increases renal perfusion and induces a pressure natriuresis. This is important to remember because most patients presenting with hypertensive crises tend to have relative hypovolemia. Baroreceptors are stimulated by the resultant decrease in effective arterial circulating volume and produce further increases in the α- and β-adrenergic tone.

Although many factors can precipitate hypertensive crises (Table 58–3), an acute rise in BP in patients with preexisting hypertension is most common. Other contributing factors that may impact on therapeutic management must also be considered.

CLINICAL MANIFESTATIONS

The clinical findings in patients with hypertensive crises are usually nonspecific and may be related to the underlying disease or to end-organ sequelae. The clinical assessment of the patient begins with confirmation of the BP measurement in both arms, using an appropriately sized cuff. This is followed by a rapid yet detailed evaluation of the organ systems most susceptible to damage from elevated BP: the central nervous system, the cardiovascular system, and the renal system.

Neurologic Assessment

Central nervous system involvement is suggested by complaints of headache, nausea, vomiting, visual disturbances, confusion, seizures, and focal neurologic deficits. Subtle abnormalities of mental status may be difficult to detect. A

TABLE 58–3. Precipitating Factors for Hypertensive Crises

Preexisting hypertension	Eclampsia
Progression of disease	Collagen vascular disease
Unrecognized hypertension	Systemic lupus erythematosus
Patient noncompliance	Progressive systemic sclerosus
Renovascular hypertension	Polyarteritis nodosa
Acute glomerulonephritis	Drugs
Parenchymal renal disease	Diet pills
Pheochromocytoma	Cocaine
Antihypertensive withdrawal	Amphetamines
Head injury	Oral contraceptives
Burns	Corticosteroids
MAOI–tyramine interactions	

Abbreviation: MAOI = monoamine oxidase inhibitor.

thorough examination requires inspection of the optic fundi for evidence of hypertensive retinopathy and papilledema. In the absence of other end-organ involvement, the presence of cotton-wool exudates or flame-shaped hemorrhages is compatible with a hypertensive urgency. A computed tomographic (CT) scan of the head is often necessary to rule out intracranial hemorrhage, stroke, or other lesions. Focal neurologic findings mandate early CT scan but can be associated with hypertensive encephalopathy.

Cardiovascular Assessment

The cardiovascular consequences of severe hypertension may precipitate symptoms of anginal chest pain, dyspnea, or severe, tearing chest pain associated with acute aortic dissection. Physical findings that suggest acute left ventricular dysfunction include rales, a third heart sound, jugular venous distension, and tachycardia. Findings that may be present with aortic dissection include pulse deficits, a new murmur of aortic insufficiency, and a pericardial friction rub. An electrocardiogram is necessary for evaluating possible ischemia or infarction. A chest radiograph may indicate pulmonary edema or the nonspecific finding of a widened mediastinum suggesting an aortic aneurysm.

Renal System Assessment

Renal involvement resulting from severe hypertension may be clinically silent with nonspecific symptoms of weakness, pedal edema, oliguria, polyuria, or hematuria. A complete assessment involves measurement of blood urea nitrogen and creatinine, as well as urinalysis with microscopic examination to detect proteinuria, hematuria, and the presence of cellular casts. The latter two findings are suggestive of glomerulonephritis as a secondary cause of hypertension. A complete blood count and electrolytes should also be obtained. A blood smear can be examined for evidence of microangiopathic hemolytic anemia, but this is a rare finding.

GENERAL PRINCIPLES OF TREATMENT

The goal of therapy in hypertensive crises is to effect a decrease in BP while maintaining organ perfusion and avoiding complications. Those patients likely to experience complications from severe hypertension are also at risk for complications of lowering BP. Three questions should be considered when making decisions for the treatment of severe hypertension: (1) Should the BP be lowered acutely?; (2) How much should the BP be lowered?; (3) Which medication(s) should be used to lower BP? The first question is the most important: Should the BP be lowered acutely? Although it is important to recognize clinical situations in which BP should be lowered immediately, it is also necessary to recognize when lowering the BP is not indicated. A rapid but thorough clinical evaluation of the central nervous system, cardiovascular system, and renal system should provide the necessary information. In the presence of new or progressive end-organ dysfunction, a hypertensive emergency exists and BP should be lowered promptly. This usually requires ICU admission and the use of parenteral agents to lower BP to safer levels in several hours. If end-organ dysfunction is not present or unchanged from baseline, severe hypertension may represent a hypertensive urgency (see Table 58–2). In these clinical situations, oral therapy can be used to lower the BP to safer levels over 24 hours. Asymptomatic patients with severe hypertension do not need immediate reductions of BP.[3] These patients are best served by instituting or reinstituting an appropriate antihypertensive regimen and ensuring adequate follow-up. Physicians should not be compelled to treat emergently an elevated BP in the absence of an appropriate indication.

Once the decision has been made to lower BP, the second question assumes great importance. Careful consideration in determining the extent of BP reduction may prevent complications. Excessive or precipitous lowering of BP can result in cerebral, cardiac, or renal ischemia. Cerebral blood flow is maintained constant at 50 mL/min per 100-g brain in normotensive patients over mean arterial pressures of 50 to 150 mm Hg by constriction and vasodilatation of cerebral arterioles. This autoregulatory mechanism adapts to higher pressures in patients with chronic hypertension because of structural changes in resistance vessels that allow toleration of elevated pressures without incurring cerebral damage (Fig. 58–1).[4] A shift to the right in the autoregulation of cerebral blood flow is also seen in elderly patients. Excessive reduction of BP could easily compromise cerebral perfusion and precipitate ischemic events in patients with altered cerebral autoregulation.[5] Similarly, coronary artery and renal blood flow can be compromised by overly aggressive BP reduction.

Although various recommendations for the extent of BP reduction have been proposed, each case must be individualized. A reasonable goal for most hypertensive emergencies is to lower the mean arterial pressure by approximately 25% or to reduce the diastolic BP to 100 to 110 mm Hg over

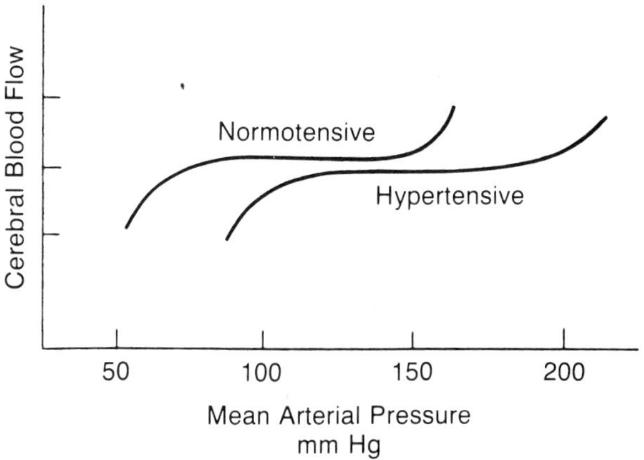

Figure 58–1. Cerebral blood flow remains constant over a wide range of pressures in normotensive individuals. This range is shifted to the right in the elderly and in individuals with chronic hypertension. (Courtesy of Leigh Thompson, MD, PhD.)

a period of several minutes to hours depending on the clinical situation. Although BP should be lowered to safer levels, it is not necessary to normalize BP in the first 24 to 48 hours of therapy in most situations. After the acute reduction of BP with parenteral agents in hypertensive emergencies, oral medications should be instituted within 12 to 24 hours and BP reduced to a normotensive level over the ensuing days to weeks.

The last question to consider is the choice of medications for lowering BP. The repertoire of drugs available to clinicians today has greatly expanded. The choice of optimal intervention in hypertensive emergencies and urgencies depends on several factors. Coexisting conditions such as coronary artery disease, congestive heart failure, pulmonary disease, and renal insufficiency influence drug selection. The desired extent and rate of BP reduction should be determined and appropriate drugs selected based on the pharmacology of the available agents. Important considerations in choosing antihypertensive agents include the onset of action, peak effect, and duration of action. In addition, the choice of specific therapy may depend on the availability of hospital facilities and personnel to implement therapeutic regimens and to safely monitor the patient. In the following sections, drugs that are available for hypertensive emergencies and hypertensive urgencies are described. Specific clinical situations are addressed later.

PHARMACOTHERAPY FOR HYPERTENSIVE EMERGENCIES

Parenteral drugs available for treatment of hypertensive emergencies are summarized in Table 58–4. The ideal agent for lowering BP in emergent situations should have the following characteristics: rapid onset of action, high potency, immediate reversibility, specific effect on resistance vessels without effects on other smooth-muscle or cardiac muscle, no central or autonomic nervous system effects, absence of tachyphylaxis, and minimal or no adverse effects. No drug currently meets all these desired characteristics. The challenge is to select the agent with the most favorable pharmacodynamic and adverse effect profile for the patient and the clinical circumstance.

SODIUM NITROPRUSSIDE

Nitroprusside has been the "gold standard" for treatment of most hypertensive emergencies.[6] Although the cellular mechanism of action remains unknown, sodium nitroprusside (NTP) causes relaxation of arterial and venous smooth muscle. A controlled reduction of BP is easily achieved because of the rapid onset of the hypotensive effect and the short duration of action. NTP has been used effectively for severe hypertension in encephalopathy, intracranial hemorrhage, myocardial ischemia, left ventricular failure, pheochromocytoma, dissecting aortic aneurysm, and postoperative hypertension.

The advantageous pharmacokinetic parameters of NTP can also result in excessive hypotension. An infusion pump must be used for administration and the BP should be closely monitored. Automated noninvasive BP devices can be used, but intra-arterial blood pressure monitoring is preferred. Infusion of NTP should be initiated at a very low rate (0.3 $\mu g \cdot kg^{-1} \cdot min^{-1}$) and titrated upward every few minutes.[7] If the BP falls below the desired level, discontinuation of NTP results in BP increases within 1 to 10 minutes.

Other potential adverse effects of NTP relate to its metabolism.[7] NTP is metabolized nonenzymatically by combining

TABLE 58–4. Parenteral Antihypertensive Agents

Drug	*Class*	*Route*	*Dose*	*Onset of Action*	*Peak Effect*	*Duration of Effect*
Sodium nitroprusside	Arteriolar and venous vasodilator	IV: infusion	0.3–10 $\mu g \cdot kg^{-1} \cdot min^{-1}$	Immediate	1–2 min	1–3 min
Labetalol	α- and β-adrenergic blocker	IV: bolus	20 mg, then 20–80 mg every 10 min	3–5 min	10–20 min	3–6 h
		IV: infusion	2 mg/min (max = 300 mg)			
Nitroglycerin	Venous >> arteriolar vasodilator	IV: infusion	5–300 μg/min	1–2 min	1–2 min	1–3 min
Nicardipine hydrochloride	Calcium channel blocker	IV: loading infusion	5–15 mg/h	1–3 min	5–20 min (dose dependent)	15–40 min
		IV: maintenance infusion	3–5 mg/h			
Enalaprilat	Angiotensin-converting enzyme inhibitor	IV: bolus	0.625–1.25 mg every 6 h	10–15 min	30 min–4 h	6–8 h
Diazoxide	Arteriolar vasodilator	IV: bolus	25–100 mg every 5–10 min	1–5 min	5 min	4–12 h
		IV: infusion	7.5–30 mg/min (total dose = 300 mg)		Variable	
Trimethaphan camsylate	Ganglionic blocker	IV: infusion	0.5–10 mg/min	1–2 min	1–2 min	5–10 min
Phentolamine mesylate	α-Adrenergic blocker	IV: bolus IV: infusion	5–10 mg 0.2–5 mg/min	1 min	3 min	10–30 min
Hydralazine	Arteriolar vasodilator	IV: bolus IV: infusion IM	5–20 mg 0.5–1 mg/min 10–40 mg	10–30 min	10–80 min	3–6 h

Abbreviations: IV = intravenous; IM = intramuscular; >> = greater than; q = every.

with hemoglobin to produce cyanmethemoglobin and cyanide ions. Rhodanase, a mitochondrial enzyme found predominantly in the liver, catalyzes the reaction of cyanide with thiosulfate to produce thiocyanate, which is excreted in the urine. Excess cyanide binds to cytochromes and inhibits oxidative metabolism. Renal failure can also result in thiocyanate toxicity with NTP use. Cyanide or thiocyanate toxicity usually does not pose a problem with use of NTP unless the infusion is maintained for more than 72 hours or at doses greater than 3 $\mu g \cdot kg^{-1} \cdot min^{-1}$. The maximum rate of 10 $\mu g \cdot kg^{-1} \cdot min^{-1}$ should not be maintained for more than 10 minutes. Patients with renal insufficiency or hepatic disease are prone to toxicity. Cyanide levels are not generally available, but thiocyanate levels are available through referral labs. In addition to close monitoring of the dose of NTP, the patient should be observed for clinical signs of cyanide toxicity such as metabolic (lactic) acidosis, confusion, or hemodynamic deterioration. Thiocyanate toxicity can manifest as abdominal pain, delirium, headache, nausea, muscle spasms, and restlessness. Some studies suggest that sodium thiosulfate infusion is effective for treating and preventing cyanide toxicity.[6] It decreases cyanide levels by acting as a sulfur donor and facilitating conversion of cyanide to thiocyanate. Hydroxycobalamine may also prevent toxicity when administered with NTP by combining with cyanide to form the nontoxic compound cyanocobalamin (vitamin B_{12}).[8] Hemodialysis is effective in eliminating thiocyanate.

Other adverse effects of NTP include rash, hypothyroidism, and, rarely, methemoglobinemia. Increased intracranial pressure has been noted in patients with mass lesions undergoing hypotensive surgery using NTP.

LABETALOL

Labetalol is an oral and parenteral α- and nonselective β-adrenergic blocker that reduces BP by decreasing SVR with little or no change in cardiac output or heart rate.[9] The β-blocking effect predominates 7:1 when labetalol is administered intravenously. A controlled reduction of BP is possible because of the rapid but not abrupt, peak effect with minimal further reduction of BP following an intravenous bolus or discontinuation of an infusion. Hypotension is infrequent provided the total dose remains below the recommended maximum of 300 mg. Selected cases may require prolonged infusions at reduced rates.[10] The β-blocking properties of labetalol contraindicate its use in patients with bronchospasm, severe sinus bradycardia (heart rate <50 beats/min), greater than first-degree heart block, or decompensated congestive heart failure. Minor side effects include nausea, vomiting, paresthesias such as scalp tingling, pain at the injection site, and headache.[9] Labetalol may be particularly advantageous when intensive care facilities and intra-arterial pressure monitoring are not readily available. Labetalol has been used effectively in lowering BP in hypertensive encephalopathy, myocardial ischemia, acute left ventricular dysfunction, acute neurologic syndromes, dissecting aortic aneurysm, pheochromocytoma, and eclampsia.[9, 11, 12] Labetalol is an excellent choice for control of severe hypertension associated with cocaine abuse.[13] An advantage of labetalol is the ability to convert to an oral form of the same drug.

NITROGLYCERIN

Nitroglycerin is a direct vasodilator, predominately venous, that also results in coronary artery vasodilatation. Higher doses are capable of producing arterial dilatation. The intravenous form is easily titrated because of the rapid onset of action and short duration of effect, but it is much less potent than other parenteral antihypertensive agents. The favorable effects of decreasing myocardial oxygen demand by reducing preload and afterload and increasing myocardial oxygen supply by dilating coronary arteries make it particularly useful in hypertensive patients with possible myocardial ischemia. Intravenous nitroglycerin has also been used for treatment of perioperative hypertension. Side effects include headache, nausea, vomiting, bradycardia, and hypotension.

NICARDIPINE HYDROCHLORIDE

Nicardipine is a dihydropyridine calcium channel blocker prepared as an oral or intravenous form. The intravenous form may be particularly suited for treatment of hypertensive emergencies because of its potency, rapid onset of action, titratability, and lack of toxic metabolites. It has a direct effect on vascular smooth muscle, resulting in systemic and coronary artery vasodilatation. Nicardipine has minimal or no negative inotropic effects and usually results in increased cardiac output and left ventricular ejection fraction. Heart rate is usually not significantly increased. Nicardipine is metabolized in the liver and excreted primarily in bile and feces. Caution should be exercised in the elderly or patients with liver disease who may have decreased hepatic metabolism. Most experience has been with loading infusions followed by maintenance infusions, but bolus administration has also been used.[14] Side effects are similar to those reported for other calcium channel blockers and include headache, flushing, lightheadedness, hypotension, tachycardia, nausea, and vomiting.[15, 16]

Most experience with intravenous nicardipine has been in the management of intraoperative and postoperative hypertension. Nicardipine is more effective than placebo [15, 17] and equally effective as nitroprusside.[18] Nicardipine effectively lowers BP in severe hypertension as a result of other causes, but reported experience in hypertensive emergencies is limited.[16, 19] Nicardipine may be an alternative to nitroprusside in many clinical situations.

ENALAPRILAT

Enalaprilat, an intravenously administered angiotensin-converting enzyme (ACE) inhibitor, is the active metabolite of the orally administered pro-drug enalapril. Inhibition of ACE results in vasodilation by decreasing angiotensin II vasopressor activity and decreasing aldosterone secretion. Patients with low renin hypertension may also respond to enalaprilat.[20] Side effects are similar to those observed with other ACE inhibitors: excessive hypotension (especially in sodium- or volume-depleted patients), angioedema, impaired renal function, hyperkalemia, and cough. Although enalaprilat has been used in patients with severe hypertension and hypertensive emergencies,[20, 21] limited experience precludes specific recommendations for use.

DIAZOXIDE

Diazoxide is a potent arterial vasodilator with little or no effect on venous capacitance. The duration of antihypertensive effect is measured in hours, but the short onset of action and short time to peak effect allow for a stepwise reduction of BP with repetitive bolus doses. Current recommendations of minibolus administration or continuous infusion offer greater control and safety.[22, 23] Previous recommendations for a rapid 300-mg bolus to overcome high protein binding were associated with precipitous drops of BP, leading to myocardial and cerebral ischemia. Diazoxide evokes a reflex tachycardia and should, therefore, not be used in patients with dissecting aortic aneurysm or coronary artery disease. Repetitive doses or prolonged administration may be associated with hyperglycemia, hyperuricemia, displacement of other protein-bound drugs, and salt and water retention, requiring the use of a loop diuretic. The solution is highly alkaline, so great care should be taken to avoid extravasation.

The current use of diazoxide for hypertensive emergencies is limited by serious potential adverse effects and the availability of other agents with better safety profiles. The use of a β-adrenergic blocker has been advocated to prevent the tachycardia that results from diazoxide,[24] but this combination offers no advantage over labetalol.

TRIMETHAPHAN CAMSYLATE

Trimethaphan is a titratable ganglionic blocking agent advocated for the treatment of hypertension associated with acute aortic dissection. Left ventricular ejection rate and heart rate are reduced. Adverse effects include urinary retention, paralytic ileus, mydriasis, and dry mouth. These effects, as well as tachyphylaxis, limit the use of trimethaphan.

PHENTOLAMINE MESYLATE

Phentolamine is an α-adrenergic blocker indicated for the management of hypertensive emergencies associated with excess catecholamine levels such as pheochromocytoma, monoamine oxidase inhibitor crises, and antihypertensive withdrawal syndrome. Side effects include hypotension, tachycardia, vomiting, and headache. Angina may also be provoked. Pheochromocytoma is rare, and the diagnosis may not be known at the time of a hypertensive emergency, but other parenteral agents such as NTP and labetalol can be used effectively.

HYDRALAZINE

Hydralazine is a direct arteriolar vasodilator that may be administered orally, intramuscularly, or intravenously. The parenteral form is used infrequently for hypertensive emergencies because the variable patient response and duration of action make reduction of BP unpredictable. Hydralazine is contraindicated in patients with myocardial ischemia or dissecting aortic aneurysm because of reflex tachycardia, increased cardiac output, and increased myocardial oxygen consumption. Hydralazine may still have a role in BP reduction in eclampsia because it improves uterine blood flow.

ESMOLOL

Esmolol is an ultra short-acting β_1-adrenergic blocker. It is currently indicated only for the treatment of supraventricular tachycardia but may have a role in the management of perioperative hypertension.[25, 26] The decline in BP results from a decrease in cardiac index, so it should not be used in patients with borderline or inadequate cardiac function. Other contraindications are the same as for labetalol. Esmolol may also be used in combination with nitroprusside to abrogate reflex tachycardia. It is unlikely that esmolol would be effective as a single agent for severe elevations of BP.

FENOLDOPAM MESYLATE

Fenoldopam is a parenteral postsynaptic dopamine-1 receptor agonist under development that has potential utility in hypertensive emergencies. Fenoldopam lowers BP by decreasing peripheral vascular resistance. A small increase in heart rate is observed and renal blood flow increases.[27] Fenoldopam has a rapid onset of action and short duration of effect (half-life = 10 minutes), which allow administration as a continuous infusion. No toxic metabolites accumulate, and renal dysfunction has minimal impact on the pharmacokinetic parameters. Adverse effects are minor and include flushing, headache, dizziness, hypotension, and tachycardia. The efficacy of fenoldopam has been favorably evaluated in patients with severe hypertension and hypertensive emergencies.[28] If fenoldopam becomes available, it may be another alternative to nitroprusside for management of hypertensive emergencies.

DIURETICS

Diuretics are not indicated in the acute treatment of hypertensive emergencies unless there is clinical evidence of volume overload. As mentioned previously, most patients have sodium and volume depletion, which can be further exacerbated by diuretic use.

PHARMACOTHERAPY FOR HYPERTENSIVE URGENCIES

Drugs frequently used for oral therapy of hypertensive urgencies are summarized in Table 58–5. Although patients with hypertensive urgencies do not usually require monitoring in an ICU, these drugs may be useful in patients hospitalized in critical care units for other reasons who require control of BP elevations. A brief review of these agents is presented. More detailed information is available in other reviews.[1, 29, 30]

NIFEDIPINE

Nifedipine is the oral calcium channel blocker used most often in the management of hypertensive urgencies. The reduction in SVR is associated with a mild increase in heart rate. Despite tachycardia, a simultaneous increase in coronary artery blood flow results in reduced myocardial oxygen consumption.[31] These hemodynamic effects make nifedipine potentially advantageous in selected patients with myocardial ischemia or known coronary artery disease. Administration in hypertensive urgencies is best accomplished by having the patient bite the capsule in half before swallowing because absorption is by gastric rather than buccal mucosa.[32] After treatment, the mean arterial pressure de-

TABLE 58–5. Oral Antihypertensive Agents

Drug	*Class*	*Route*	*Dose*	*Onset of Action*	*Peak Effect*	*Duration of Effect*
Nifedipine	Calcium channel blocker	Bite/swallow; oral	10 mg	5–15 min	15–30 min	3–5h
Clonidine	Central α-adrenergic agonist	Oral	0.1–0.2 mg, then 0.1 mg every 1 h (max = 0.8 mg)	30–60 min	2–4 h	3–8 h
Captopril	Angiotensin-converting enzyme inhibitor	Oral Sublingual	6.25–25 mg	15 min 5 min	60–90 min 10–15 min	4–6 h 2–3 h

creases approximately 25%.[31, 33] Side effects include headache, flushing, palpitations, dizziness, and hypotension.[33] Excessive hypotension may occur in the elderly, in patients receiving other vasodilators, and in hypovolemic patients.[31] Myocardial ischemia and cerebral ischemia have been reported after precipitous drops in BP during treatment of severe hypertension with nifedipine.[34, 35]

CLONIDINE

Clonidine is a central α-adrenergic agonist that decreases sympathetic outflow and leads to a reduction in SVR. It has been used extensively in the treatment of hypertensive urgencies.[31, 36] Precipitous drops in BP are less likely with clonidine compared with nifedipine. The sedative properties of clonidine may interfere with neurologic assessment of patients with encephalopathy or cerebrovascular events.[31] Other side effects include dry mouth, orthostasis, and bradycardia. A reduced dose or increase in dosing interval is necessary in the presence of renal insufficiency.

CAPTOPRIL

Captopril, an oral ACE inhibitor, has been used successfully in hypertensive urgencies.[30, 37] Hypotension after the initial dose may occur, especially in patients with sodium or volume depletion who concurrently use other antihypertensives and in those with renal vascular hypertension. Side effects with short-term use are minimal. Captopril should not be used in patients with suspected bilateral renal artery stenosis.

OTHER DRUGS

Minoxidil and prazosin have been used for the treatment of hypertensive urgencies, but their use is not recommended because of the side effect profiles and availability of better drugs. Oral labetalol has been used successfully in hypertensive urgencies, but experience is limited compared with that of other oral agents.[9, 38]

SPECIFIC CLINICAL CONSIDERATIONS

Hypertensive Encephalopathy

Cerebral dysfunction as a result of severe hypertension mandates rapid reduction of BP with a parenteral agent to prevent progression to coma and death.[39] Severe hypertension can exceed the upper limit of cerebral blood flow autoregulation and result in vasodilatation with cerebral edema. Nitroprusside is the drug of choice with labetalol, nitroglycerin, and diazoxide as potential alternatives. The lowering of BP is therapeutic as well as diagnostic, and mental status usually improves within hours. Cerebral dysfunction after the BP is decreased requires consideration of other conditions such as intracranial hemorrhage, cerebral infarction, a mass lesion, trauma, or infection. Appropriate diagnostic tests such as CT scan of the head and/or lumbar puncture should be performed.

Intracranial Hemorrhage, Ischemic Stroke, and Subarachnoid Hemorrhage

Treatment of severe hypertension in the setting of intracranial hemorrhage and ischemic stroke remains controversial.[39–41] The neurologic event may be the cause or consequence of elevated BP. No absolute guidelines exist concerning the decision to lower BP or the extent of BP reduction. Severe elevations of BP may cause further vascular damage, leading to increased hemorrhage, expansion of an infarct, or increased cerebral edema. However, reductions of BP can lead to inadequate cerebral perfusion and ischemia, particularly in areas of altered autoregulation or areas dependent on collateral flow.[42] Careful observation of patients with mild hypertension may be all that is necessary because BP often decreases spontaneously after the acute event.[43] Moderate hypertension can be controlled with oral agents over several days. In general, severe, sustained hypertension should be treated with a parenteral drug such as nitroprusside, nitroglycerin, or labetalol. Careful monitoring of the neurologic status is mandatory. If the neurologic examination worsens as BP is lowered, therapy must be discontinued or decreased and the BP allowed to rise.

Preexisting hypertension is an unfavorable prognostic factor in subarachnoid hemorrhage (SAH), but treatment of hypertension after hemorrhage has not been shown to be beneficial.[44] Current therapy of SAH includes use of the calcium channel blocker nimodipine, but the exact mechanism of the beneficial effect is unknown.[45] Guidelines recommended for the treatment of hypertension associated with SAH are similar to those for ischemic stroke and intracranial hemorrhage. The BP-lowering effects of nimodipine must be considered before instituting additional agents. Intravenous nicardipine may be an option.

Myocardial Ischemia

Sustained hypertension in patients with angina or myocardial infarction should be treated to reduce myocardial oxygen demand. Although hypertension may be initially present in one third of patients with myocardial ischemia, the BP usually falls within the first 6 hours of admission without specific antihypertensive therapy.[46] The initial therapeutic maneuver should be relief of pain with sublingual nitrates and/or morphine sulfate. If further intervention is necessary, nitroglycerin infusion addresses both hypertension and ischemia. Labetalol is another option with favorable hemodynamic effects in myocardial infarction.[12] If the hypertension is mild and a parenteral agent is not indicated, nifedipine is the oral agent of choice. Intravenous nicardipine is also a favorable antihypertensive agent for myocardial ischemia. Nitroprusside has been used safely to lower BP in myocardial ischemia, but concerns of coronary artery steal resulting in decreased collateral flow to ischemic areas make nitroglycerin and labetalol preferred agents.[47, 48] Diazoxide and hydralazine should be avoided because of reflex tachycardia.

Acute Left Ventricular Dysfunction

Acute elevations of BP result in decreased compliance of the left ventricle, with resultant inadequate diastolic filling and high filling pressures leading to pulmonary edema. Alternatively, primary myocardial failure caused by systolic dysfunction with low cardiac output can be associated with hypertension resulting from catecholamine-induced peripheral vasoconstriction. An echocardiogram, if readily available, may be helpful in distinguishing systolic and diastolic dysfunction. A significantly elevated diastolic BP and the presence of hypertensive retinopathy suggest a hypertensive emergency with cardiac end-organ dysfunction. Primary myocardial failure may be suggested by a mild to moderate increase in diastolic BP, absence of hypertensive retinopathy, and marked enlargement of the heart on chest radiograph. Although differentiation of the two clinical situations may be difficult, the choice of therapy, despite the different pathophysiology, is similar. Nitroglycerin or nitroprusside infusions may be used in most situations. If diastolic dysfunction is suspected, overzealous reduction of filling pressures may compromise left ventricular volume. Labetalol is contraindicated in primary myocardial failure, but it has been used successfully when left ventricular dysfunction is due to the acute rise in BP.

Acute Aortic Dissection

The initial treatment of a dissecting aortic aneurysm is BP reduction followed by definitive surgical or medical therapy. Proximal aortic dissections or distal dissections complicated by recurrent pain, expansion, vital organ compromise, or falling hematocrit indicate the need for surgical intervention. Distal aortic dissections without complications can be treated medically. The goal of antihypertensive therapy is to lower BP and reduce the shear force or rate of BP rise to prevent extension of injury. Blood pressure should be reduced to the lowest level that relieves pain and allows adequate organ perfusion, usually a systolic BP of 100 to 110 mm Hg. The most commonly used agents are nitroprusside in combination with intravenous propranolol.[49] Alternatives include labetalol and the combination of esmolol and nitroprusside. Trimethaphan is infrequently used because of potential adverse effects, but it may be necessary for patients who are unable to tolerate β-adrenergic blockers.

Eclampsia

Eclampsia can be considered a form of hypertensive encephalopathy in the pregnant patient. Therapy includes delivery, if possible, and intravenous magnesium sulfate to prevent seizures. Hydralazine has been the drug of choice for BP control because of the preservation of myometrial blood flow. Labetalol may be a safe and effective alternative agent.[12, 50] Because of the potential adverse effects on labor and the fetus, nitroprusside, trimethaphan, and diazoxide are contraindicated.

Perioperative Hypertension

Perioperative hypertension is classified as a hypertensive urgency, but in some circumstances emergent treatment may be required. Severe hypertension before surgery can usually be controlled with oral agents. If oral intake is precluded, parenteral agents such as labetalol and enalaprilat should be considered.

Intraoperative hypertension requires treatment to decrease the risk of myocardial ischemia, hemorrhage, or disruption of vascular anastomoses. The effects of analgesic and anesthetic agents will often decrease BP. If BP remains elevated, short-acting titratable agents such as nitroprusside and nitroglycerin are preferred, and hypotension must be judiciously avoided. Labetalol can be used, but lower initial doses (2–5 mg) should be selected. Nicardipine has also been effective in treating intraoperative hypertension.[17]

The incidence of postoperative hypertension depends on the preoperative history of hypertension and the type of surgery performed. It is usually self-limited (2–6 hours), but if untreated, it can lead to complications such as hemorrhage at the surgical site, disruption of vascular anastomoses, intracerebral hemorrhage, myocardial ischemia, and renal failure. Before antihypertensive therapy is instituted, each patient must be evaluated for the possible role of pain, anxiety, and hypothermia as a cause of elevated BP. Nitroprusside and nitroglycerin are routinely used for control of BP in the postoperative period. Both drugs are amenable for use in closed-loop, computer-controlled automatic administration.[51] Nitroprusside may have disadvantages after cardiac surgery because of increases in heart rate that may increase myocardial oxygen demand and a coronary artery steal phenomenon.[47, 48] Labetalol in low doses has been used effectively for control of BP after coronary artery bypass grafting.[52] Esmolol may also have a role in lowering BP in the postoperative period.[25, 26] Intravenous nicardipine has compared favorably with nitroprusside for control of postoperative hypertension after cardiac and noncardiac surgery.[18]

EXCESS CATECHOLAMINE STATES

Increased levels of catecholamines leading to severe hypertension are associated with pheochromocytoma, monoamine oxidase inhibitor interactions, clonidine withdrawal, and occasionally cocaine or amphetamine abuse. Phentolamine has been the traditional treatment of choice, especially in pheochromocytoma, but other drugs such as labetalol and nitroprusside are also effective. Hypertensive crises resulting from interactions of monoamine oxidase inhibitors with tyramine-containing foods or sympathomimetic amines have also been treated with nifedipine.

SUMMARY

Severe hypertension mandates a rapid clinical evaluation of the central nervous system, cardiovascular system, and renal system to determine whether a hypertensive emergency or urgency exists. If rapid reduction of BP is indicated, the choice of therapy and target BP should be individualized based on the clinical situation. Knowledge of the pharmacodynamics and adverse effects of available antihypertensive agents enables an appropriate selection for therapy. Careful monitoring is mandatory to avoid precipitous drops in BP and hypoperfusion of vital organs.

References

1. Houston MC: Hypertensive urgencies and emergencies: Pathophysiology, clinical aspects and treatment. *In:* Critical Care: State of the Art. Vol 7. Chernow B, Shoemaker WC (Eds). Fullerton, CA, Society of Critical Care Medicine, 1986, pp 151–246.
2. Houston MC: Pathophysiology, clinical aspects and treatment of hypertensive crises. Prog Cardiovasc Dis 1989; 32:99.
3. Zeller KR, Kuhnert LV, Matthews C: Rapid reduction of severe asymptomatic hypertension. Arch Intern Med 1989; 149:2186.
4. Strandgaard S: Autoregulation of cerebral circulation in hypertension. Acta Neurol Scand 1978; 57(Suppl 66):1.
5. Ledingham JGG, Rajagopalan B: Cerebral complications in the treatment of accelerated hypertension. Q J Med 1979; 48:25.
6. Cohn JN, Burke LP: Nitroprusside. N Engl J Med 1979; 91:752.
7. Physician's Desk Reference. 47th ed. Montvale, NJ: Medical Economics Data, 1993, pp 1999–2001.
8. Zerbe NF, Wagner BK: Use of vitamin B12 in the treatment and prevention of nitroprusside-induced cyanide toxicity. Crit Care Med 1991; 21:465.
9. MacCarthy EP, Bloomfield SS: Labetalol: A review of its pharmacology, pharmacokinetics, clinical uses and adverse effects. Pharmacotherapy 1983; 3:193.
10. Graves JW: Prolonged continuous infusion labetalol: A new alternative for parenteral antihypertensive therapy. Crit Care Med 1989; 17:759.
11. Wilson DJ, Wallin JD, Vlachakis ND, et al: Intravenous labetalol in the treatment of severe hypertension and hypertensive emergencies. Am J Med 1983; 75:95.
12. Renard M, Jacobs P, Melot C, et al: Effect of labetalol on preload in acute myocardial infarction with systemic hypertension. J Cardiovasc Pharmacol 1984; 6:90.
13. Gay GR, Loper KA: Control of cocaine-induced hypertension with labetalol. Anesth Analg 1988; 67:92.
14. Cheung DG, Gasster JL, Neutel JM, Weber MA: Acute pharmacokinetic and hemodynamic effects of intravenous bolus dosing of nicardipine. Am Heart J 1990; 119:438.

15. IV Nicardipine Study Group: Efficacy and safety of intravenous nicardipine in the control of postoperative hypertension. Chest 1991; 99:393.
16. Wallin JD, Fletcher E, Ram CVS, et al: Intravenous nicardipine for the treatment of severe hypertension. Arch Intern Med 1989; 149:2662.
17. Begon C, Dartayet B, Edouard A, et al: Intravenous nicardipine for treatment of intraoperative hypertension during abdominal surgery. J Cardiothorac Anesth 1989; 3:707.
18. Halpern NA, Goldberg M, Neely C, et al: Postoperative hypertension: A multicenter, prospective, randomized comparison between intravenous nicardipine and sodium nitroprusside. Crit Care Med 1992; 20:1637.
19. Wallin JD, Cook ME, Blanski L, et al: Intravenous nicardipine for the treatment of severe hypertension. Am J Med 1988; 85:331.
20. Evans RR, Henzler MA, Weber EM, DiPette DJ: The effect of intravenous enalaprilat (MK-422) administration in patients with mild to moderate essential hypertension. J Clin Pharmacol 1987; 27:415.
21. Rutledge J, Ayers C, Davidson R, et al: Effect of intravenous enalaprilat in moderate and severe systemic hypertension. Am J Cardiol 1988; 62:1062.
22. Ram CVS, Kaplan NM: Individual titration of diazoxide dosage in the treatment of severe hypertension. Am J Cardiol 1979; 43:627.
23. Garrett BN, Kaplan NM: Efficacy of slow infusion of diazoxide in the treatment of severe hypertension without organ hypoperfusion. Am Heart J 1982; 103:390.
24. Huysmans FTM, Thien TA, Koene RAP: Combined intravenous administration of diazoxide and beta-blocking agent in acute treatment of severe hypertension or hypertensive crisis. Am Heart J 1982; 103:395.
25. Smerling A, Gersony WM: Esmolol for severe hypertension following repair of aortic coarctation. Crit Care Med 1990; 18:1288.
26. Gray RJ: Managing critically ill patients with esmolol. Chest 1988; 93:398.
27. Weber RR, McCoy CE, Ziemniak JA, et al: Pharmacokinetic and pharmacodynamic properties of intravenous fenoldopam, a dopamine$_1$-receptor agonist, in hypertensive patients. Br J Clin Pharmacol 1988; 25:17.
28. Holcslaw TL, Beck TR: Clinical experience with intravenous fenoldopam. Am J Hypertens 1990; 3:120S.
29. DeVault GA: Hypertensive urgencies: Part 1. Sympatholytics, calcium antagonists. J Crit Illness 1991; 6:563.
30. DeVault GA: Hypertensive urgencies: Part 2. ACE inhibitors and vasodilators. J Crit Illness 1991; 6:935.
31. Houston MC: The comparative effects of clonidine hydrochloride and nifedipine in the treatment of hypertensive crises. Am Heart J 1988; 115:152.
32. McAllister RG: Kinetics and dynamics of nifedipine after oral and sublingual doses. Am J Med 1986; 81(Suppl 6A):2.
33. Houston MC: Treatment of hypertensive urgencies and emergencies with nifedipine. Am Heart J 1986; 111:963.
34. O'Mailia JJ, Sander GE, Giles TD: Nifedipine-associated myocardial ischemia or infarction in the treatment of hypertensive urgencies. Ann Intern Med 1987; 107:185.
35. Schwartz M, Naschitz JE, Yeshurun D, Sharf B: Oral nifedipine in the treatment of hypertensive urgency: Cerebrovascular accident following a single dose. Arch Intern Med 1990; 150:686.
36. Houston MC: Treatment of hypertensive emergencies and urgencies with oral clonidine loading and titration. Arch Intern Med 1986; 146:586.
37. Angeli P, Chiesa M, Caregaro L, et al: Comparison of sublingual captopril and nifedipine in immediate treatment of hypertensive emergencies. Arch Intern Med 1991; 151:678.
38. Zell-Kanter M, Leikin JB: Oral labetalol in hypertensive urgencies. Am J Emerg Med 1991; 9:136.
39. Phillips SJ, Whisnant JP: Hypertension and the brain. Arch Intern Med 1992; 152:938.
40. Spence JD, Del Maestro RF: Hypertension in acute ischemic strokes: Treat. Arch Neurol 1985; 42:1000.
41. Yatsu FM, Zivin J: Hypertension in acute ischemic strokes: Not to treat. Arch Neurol 1985; 42:999.
42. Meyer JS, Shimazu K, Fukuuchi Y, et al: Impaired neurogenic cerebrovascular control and dysautoregulation after stroke. Stroke 1973; 4:169.
43. Wallace JD, Levy LL: Blood pressure after stroke. JAMA 1981; 246:2177.
44. Wijdicks EFM, Vermeulen M, Murray GD, et al: The effects of treating hypertension following aneurysmal subarachnoid hemorrhage. Clin Neurol Neurosurg 1990; 92:111.
45. Pickard JD, Murray GD, Illingworth R, et al: Effect of oral nimodipine on cerebral infarction and outcome after subarachnoid haemorrhage: British aneurysm nimodipine trial. Br Med J 1989; 298:636.
46. Gibson TC: Blood pressure levels in acute myocardial infarction. Am Heart J 1978; 96:475.
47. Flaherty JT: Comparison of intravenous nitroglycerin and sodium nitroprusside in acute myocardial infarction. Am J Med 1983; 74(Suppl 6B):53.
48. Mann T, Cohn PF, Holman BL, et al: Effect of nitroprusside on regional myocardial blood flow in coronary artery disease. Circulation 1978; 57:732.
49. Shah PK: Acute aortic dissection: Part 2. Choosing among management options. J Crit Illness 1992; 7:1075.
50. Silver HM: Acute hypertensive crisis in pregnancy. Med Clin North Am 1989; 73:623.
51. McKinley S, Cade JF, Siganporia R, et al: Clinical evaluation of closed-loop control of blood pressure in seriously ill patients. Crit Care Med 1991; 19:166.
52. Sladen RN, Klamerus KJ, Swafford MWG, et al: Labetalol for the control of elevated blood pressure following coronary artery bypass grafting. J Cardiothorac Anesth 1990; 4:210.

CHAPTER 59

Hypertensive Emergencies in Infants and Children

Edward J. Ruley, MD

Acutely elevated blood pressure (BP) in the pediatric patient usually constitutes a medical emergency that can result in significant morbidity or mortality if unrecognized or improperly treated. Classically, several distinct patterns of acute hypertensive crisis have been described. *Malignant hypertension* is severe BP elevation associated with grade IV Keith-Wagener retinopathy (exudates, hemorrhages, arterial narrowing, and spasm with papilledema). The patient characteristically progresses rapidly to death or renal failure if untreated. *Accelerated hypertension* is marked BP elevation associated with grade III retinopathy (papilledema is absent). Malignant hypertension and accelerated hypertension usually occur as complications of chronic hypertension. *Hypertensive encephalopathy* refers to severe hypertension associated with central nervous system (CNS) dysfunction. Malignant hypertension and accelerated hypertension occur much less commonly in children than adults. Hypertensive encephalopathy is the most common severe manifestation of uncontrolled BP in children.

Prompt recognition of the clinical manifestations of uncontrolled BP and early implementation of individualized treatment regimens are of critical importance. Knowledge of the pathophysiology of hypertension and the pharmacology of various antihypertensive agents facilitates treatment decisions.

PATHOPHYSIOLOGY OF HYPERTENSIVE SYMPTOMS

The clinical manifestations of severe hypertension in pediatric patients are primarily neurologic and cardiovascular.

Development of symptoms is directly related to the premorbid BP and the suddenness and degree of BP elevation. Patients in whom hypertension has developed gradually may be asymptomatic in spite of very high sustained BP elevations. In contrast, symptoms may develop in the child who had previously been normotensive when the BP elevation is only modest. In this latter circumstance, the rapidity of BP elevation is more important than the absolute BP value.

Hypertensive encephalopathy is a serious but reversible condition that results from failed autoregulation of cerebral blood flow (CBF).[1-3] CBF is affected by a variety of factors including systemic BP, sympathetic adrenergic activity, and blood viscosity; however, arteriolar resistance, as determined by vessel radius, is the most important factor. Arteriolar diameter is autoregulated by local metabolic factors such as partial pressure of carbon dioxide (P_{CO_2}), and oxygen (P_{O_2}) and pH. An increase in P_{CO_2} or a decrease in pH or P_{O_2} cause vasodilatation, thereby increasing CBF. Opposite changes in P_{CO_2}, pH, and P_{O_2} produce vasoconstriction and a decrease in CBF. Animal experiments suggest that local concentrations of adenosine and potassium ion may also be important in autoregulation. Furthermore, changes in transmural pressure can cause change in smooth-muscle tension in the smaller cerebral arteries and arterioles. Thus, an increase in systemic BP will stimulate vasoconstriction, whereas a lower systemic BP produces vasodilatation. As seen by the solid line in Figure 59–1, the results of these autoregulatory changes are to keep the CBF constant over a wide range of mean arterial pressures (60–140 mm Hg in adults). However, if BP exceeds the upper limit of autoregulation, resultant hyperperfusion and plasma exudation will produce cerebral edema. These changes and the consequent decrease in CBF caused by compression of the capillaries by the cerebral edema are responsible for the symptoms of hypertensive encephalopathy.

Early symptoms of hypertensive encephalopathy include severe headache, nausea, and visual abnormalities such as blurring and diplopia. These may be followed by mental confusion, varying levels of consciousness, focal neurologic abnormalities, or seizures. Advanced Keith-Wagener retinal changes such as papilledema and hemorrhage occur less frequently in pediatric patients than in adults. Isolated cranial nerve palsies occur in up to 20% of children with severe

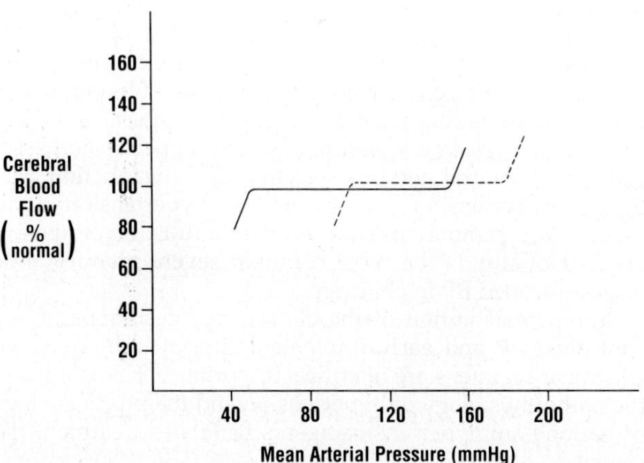

Figure 59–1. Autoregulation of cerebral blood flow at different systemic arterial mean blood pressures. *Solid line* = normal; *dashed line* = right shift with chronic hypertension. (From Ruley EJ: Hypertension. *In:* Textbook of Pediatric Critical Care. Holbrook PR (Ed). Philadelphia, W.B. Saunders, 1993, p 604.)

hypertension and are more common in chronic than acute hypertension.[4] Hypertensive encephalopathy must be distinguished from other syndromes of BP elevation and neurologic dysfunction, such as uremia, subarachnoid or intracerebral hemorrhage, subdural hematoma, thrombotic or embolic stroke, intracranial mass lesions, head trauma, encephalitis, cerebral vasculitis, and the postictal state.

In chronic hypertension, the limit of autoregulation and the pressure limit of brain hypoxia are shifted upward as part of the habituation process (dashed line in Fig. 59–1).[2] This explains why the child with slowly worsening chronic hypertension may be relatively asymptomatic even when the BP is markedly elevated. Lack of this shift in the pressure curve is why the previously normotensive child may become symptomatic after only moderate but sudden increases in BP.

Severely elevated arterial BP directly impairs the autoregulatory functions of other organs, particularly those of the kidney, heart, and eye. In the kidney, a moderate rise in arterial BP usually increases preglomerular and decreases postglomerular resistance, so that glomerular capillary flow rate and hydrostatic pressure are maintained within the normal range. However, severe hypertension can excessively elevate preglomerular resistance to cause glomerular hypoperfusion and the development of oliguria and azotemia. As with the brain, apparent habituation to these changes may cause a chronically hypertensive child to suffer a transient decrease in renal function when BP is lowered. More serious and permanent renal impairment is associated with necrotizing vasculitis, arteriolar thrombi, and fibrin deposits in glomerular vascular walls; these are typical pathogenic lesions of malignant hypertension, which progress unless the BP is controlled.[5]

Hypertension of any cause can increase cardiac work until congestive heart failure results. In these circumstances, control of BP is of paramount importance for the resolution of the heart failure. Children with underlying cardiac disease and newborns are particularly susceptible to congestive heart failure secondary to hypertension.

Besides subjective visual complaints of blurring and diplopia, permanent blindness as a result of optic nerve infarction has been reported in children with severe hypertension.[6] However, overly aggressive reduction of BP may contribute to the development of this lesion.

The early clinical manifestations of severe hypertension in the infant and neonate are more protean than those in the older child and include poor feeding, irritability, and vomiting. Cardiorespiratory symptoms, particularly tachypnea, cyanosis, and congestive heart failure, are the most common. The nonspecific clinical presentation and the difficulty of accurately measuring BP in infants make the diagnosis difficult and indicate the need for a high level of awareness and improved BP measurement technology.

Older children with an acute rise in BP may be asymptomatic or have nonspecific symptoms such as headache, anxiety, or dizziness. The most common severe manifestation of acute hypertensive emergency in this age group is hypertensive encephalopathy.

The pathogenesis of acute hypertension in children is related to the complex interaction of blood volume, cardiac output, and total peripheral resistance. In essence, BP is a function of circulating vascular volume and arteriolar vasoconstriction.[7] The former is largely determined by sodium balance, whereas the latter is a function of the renin-angiotensin system, catecholamines, and vascular autoregulation.[8,9] This highly simplistic model provides a framework for etiologic, prognostic, and therapeutic decisions.[9,10]

Severe hypertension in childhood is almost always secon-

TABLE 59–1. Causes of Severe Hypertension in Children

Renal
Acute glomerulonephritis (poststreptococcal, Henoch-Schönlein, etc.)
Hemolytic uremic syndrome
Chronic glomerulonephritis (all types)
Acute and chronic pyelonephritis
Congenital malformations (dysplasia, hypoplasia, cystic diseases)
Tumors (Wilms', leukemic infiltrate, etc.)
Post–renal transplantation with rejection
Oliguric renal failure
Trauma
Obstructive uropathy
After genitourinary surgery
Blood transfusions in children with azotemia
Cardiovascular
Coarctation of the aorta
Renal artery abnormalities (stenosis, thrombosis, etc.)
Takayasu's disease
Endocrine
Pheochromocytoma
Neuroblastoma
Adrenogenital disease
Cushing's syndrome
Hyperaldosteronism
Hyperthyroidism
Hyperparathyroidism
Iatrogenic
Intravascular volume overload
Sympathomimetic administration (epinephrine, ephedrine, isoproterenol, etc.)
Corticosteroid administration
Miscellaneous
Immobilization (fractures, burns, Guillain-Barré syndrome, etc.)
Hypercalcemia (hypervitaminosis D, metastatic disease, sarcoidosis, some immobilized patients, etc.)
Cocaine use
Hypernatremia
Stevens-Johnson syndrome
Increased intracranial pressure (any cause)
Dysautonomia
Postresuscitation

dary to identifiable renal, cardiovascular, endocrine, iatrogenic, or other disease (Table 59–1).[11, 12]

Renal Parenchymal Disease

Severe hypertension is commonly associated with acute nephritis and is particularly evident in acute poststreptococcal nephritis. Clinical and laboratory findings of acute poststreptococcal nephritis include periorbital edema, hematuria, cylindruria, hypocomplementemia, and positive streptococcal serology. Measurements of blood volume and plasma renin suggest that hypertension in acute nephritis is caused by an increase in total blood volume resulting from low glomerular filtration.[13, 14]

Hypertension occurs in up to one half of all patients with hemolytic uremic syndrome.[15] It may occur secondary to the renal disease or may be due to iatrogenic fluid overload in the child with oliguria.

Hypertension in chronic glomerulonephritis is related to the severity of glomerular involvement, and its pathogenesis is usually multifactorial. Many children with chronic glomerulonephritis have a gradually progressive BP elevation to which they accommodate; a sudden increase, however, may cause a hypertensive crisis. If renal failure and hypertension are undiagnosed before the sudden deterioration, the crisis may be perceived erroneously as an acutely acquired condition. The presence of cardiac hypertrophy and advanced Keith-Wagener funduscopic changes suggest chronic hypertension.

Chronic atrophic pyelonephritis secondary to renal parenchymal infection in children with vesicoureteral reflux may cause severe hypertension in children.[11, 16] It has been postulated that parenchymal ischemia of scarred renal tissue stimulates renin production, thereby producing hypertension.[17]

Hypertension may develop if blunt renal trauma produces a hematoma that compresses renal parenchyma or occludes a renal artery or vein. Transient renin-mediated hypertension is a frequent complication of trauma[18] and may be severe enough to require drug therapy. However, hypertension may not occur until months or years after the traumatic event, when renal artery stenosis develops in the injured arterial segment.[19]

Obstructive uropathy can cause hypertension, particularly in postoperative patients and those suffering from pyelonephritis. Usually, the BP elevation is mediated by the renin-angiotensin system and resolves with relief of the obstruction.[20]

Cardiovascular Disease

Hypertension is a cardinal feature of coarctation of the aorta. It has been suggested that the renin-angiotensin system mediates the BP elevation in a manner analogous to the one-kidney model of Goldblatt.[21] According to this theory, the kidneys produce renin in response to the decreased perfusion that results from obstruction of aortic pulsatile flow. The action of renin on plasma globulins generates angiotensin II, which stimulates the production of aldosterone. The ensuing increase in vascular volume causes hypertension, and the plasma renin stabilizes at near-normal values in the new hypertensive steady state. Patients with coarctation respond to sodium restriction and diuretic administration. After surgical coarctation repair, many children will have a sudden decrease in the degree of hypertension followed by a gradual return to normal values over months to years; this probably reflects re-equilibration of the cardiovascular system. Occasionally, so-called reactive or paradoxical hypertension occurs several days after successful coarctation repair. This may be related to the mesenteric arteritis syndrome, which results from sympathetic nerve stimulation and subsequent catecholamine and renin release.[22]

Renal artery stenosis in children is usually due to fibromuscular dysplasia. It may be an isolated finding associated with neurofibromatosis or the result of long-forgotten blunt trauma to the abdomen. The renin-angiotensin system elevates BP in response to the diminished perfusion distal to the stenotic lesion. Plasma renin values are increased in the child with two kidneys and unilateral arterial stenosis but may be normal in the child with a solitary kidney and renal artery stenosis.

Endocrine Disease

Although endocrine disease is not a frequent cause of pediatric hypertension, it is important because improper therapy may obscure its diagnosis or exacerbate the hypertension. In most cases, however, a diagnosis such as Cushing's syndrome, hyperthyroidism, or congenital adrenal hyperplasia is relatively obvious because of the multiple subjective and objective characteristics of the endocrine disease.

In contrast, pheochromocytoma may be associated with normal physical findings except for hypertension. BP elevation in this disease may be sustained or intermittent and is often associated with other symptoms of catecholamine excess including sweating, palpitations, weight loss, anxiety, fatigue, flushing, nausea, vomiting, and/or abdominal and chest pain.[23] Hypertensive crises can be precipitated by postural change, exercise, emotional stress, palpation of the area of the tumor, certain drugs (including general anesthesia), or the ingestion of food or alcohol. Currently, the diagnosis is confirmed by increased levels of catecholamines and their metabolites in the urine or blood.[24] Pharmacologic tests measuring BP reduction in response to α-adrenergic blocking agents are no longer indicated. Blood and urine specimens for catecholamine measurements should be collected before α-adrenergic blockade because the latter affects catecholamine excretion. Localization of the tumor before surgery is best done using newer radiographic techniques.[25, 26]

Miscellaneous Causes

Hypertension, sometimes severe enough to cause hypertensive encephalopathy, is seen in more than 50% of children immobilized for orthopedic reasons.[27, 28] The exact mechanism of BP elevation is unclear, and the elevation usually resolves with ambulation. The hypercalcemia of immobilization should always be considered in these patients. Children with burns also have a high incidence of hypertension; this may be due to increased peripheral resistance as a result of stimulation of the renin-angiotensin system, increased secretion of catecholamines, hypervolemia, or a combination of these factors.[29]

Cocaine exposure, either directly through illict use by the child or resulting from transplacental exposure from the substance-abusing mother, has been associated with hypertension.[30] Finally, increased intracranial pressure from causes such as intracranial hemorrhage or infection may be associated with hypertension. Differentiating elevated BP as a cause or effect of intracranial swelling and hemorrhage can be very difficult. The exact mechanism of hypertension from increased intracranial pressure is unknown, although elevated catecholamine values have been found in some patients.[31]

In general, a complete history, careful physical examination, and basic laboratory studies should allow the clinician to quickly decide the most likely cause of acute hypertension in the individual child.

GENERAL PRINCIPLES OF TREATMENT

In the child with acute hypertension, the determination of cause is less important than immediate BP control. More complicated diagnostic tests and transport of the patient to other departments for evaluation should not be done until the BP is adequately controlled.

The two most important general considerations in the treatment of hypertensive emergencies are probable cause and chronicity. Cause is primarily important in selecting the most effective antihypertensive treatment.

The chronicity of BP elevation indicates both the rapidity and degree by which BP should be reduced. BP reduction should be accomplished within minutes in children with acute hypertensive encephalopathy and within hours to days in children with chronic hypertension and no acute symptoms. Sudden BP reduction in a chronically hypertensive child may be associated with signs of cerebral hypoxia if cerebral autoregulation does not quickly adapt to the lower pressures. More gradual reduction obviates this problem.[32] The benefits of rapid BP reduction should be balanced against the risk, albeit small, of residual brain damage from relative hypotension. The question of how much to lower the BP remains controversial, although it appears that even chronically hypertensive patients will benefit from a BP reduction of 25% to 30% without untoward effects.

Severe acute hypertension usually mandates parenteral or sublingual therapy to reduce BP rapidly and predictably. Medications that can be titrated to control response (e.g., nitroprusside) are usually preferred over those with more unpredictable effects (e.g., parenteral hydralazine). Parenteral therapy should be supplemented and then replaced by oral therapy as soon as practicable.

The effectiveness of therapy in the severely hypertensive child should be monitored serially, ideally by direct intra-arterial measurement of BP. Serial neurologic evaluation is also important in the child with hypertensive encephalopathy. The signs and symptoms of hypertensive encephalopathy characteristically resolve with BP control, but there is minimal to no improvement in other syndromes of neurologic dysfunction and secondary hypertension. Likewise, serial assessment of cardiovascular variables in children with congestive heart failure resulting from hypertension also serves as a gauge of therapeutic effectiveness.

Pharmacologic Agents

Pharmacologic characteristics of the antihypertensive medications available for parenteral use are listed in Tables 59–2 and 59–3. Clinicians should consult the package insert for complete information on each agent.

Sodium nitroprusside is an extremely potent vasodilator whose rapid onset and short duration of action allow precise BP titration.[33] This agent should be administered by a constant infusion pump with continuous BP monitoring to ensure safety and efficacy. The reconstituted solution is stable for 24 hours and must be protected from exposure to light. Infusion should be started at a low dose (0.5 $\mu g \cdot kg^{-1} \cdot min^{-1}$) and increased cautiously to achieve the desired level of BP control. The use of nitroprusside is limited by the eventual development of thiocyanate toxicity. Although nitroprusside has been recommended as the drug of choice in severe hypertension or hypertensive encephalopathy, some investigators have suggested that it may further increase intracranial pressure by cerebral vasodilation.[34]

Labetalol is an adrenergic-receptor blocking agent that has selective α_1- and nonselective β-adrenergic blocking activity in a ratio of 1:7. When given intravenously in gradually increasing miniboluses, a prompt but gradual BP reduction can be achieved without the induction of reflex tachycardia or increased cardiac output, that which occurs with the use of direct arteriolar vasodilators.[35] Labetalol should be used with caution in patients with significant left ventricular dysfunction, pheochromocytoma, and bronchial asthma. Because a substantial fall in BP can occur with the assumption of an upright posture, patients should remain supine for at least 3 hours after receiving intravenous labetalol and should assume ambulation gradually. Although pediatric experience with labetalol is limited, it does seem to be effective, relatively safe, and easy to use.[36]

Diazoxide is a potent vasodilator that promptly reduces BP after rapid bolus intravenous injection.[37] Its effect is more prolonged but less controllable than that of nitroprusside;

Text continued on page 537

TABLE 59–2. Pharmacologic Characteristics of Antihypertensive Drugs Available for Parenteral and Sublingual Administration to Pediatric Patients

	Administration			Effect			Removal by Dialysis*				
Drug	*Route*	*Preparation*	*Dosage*	*Onset*	*Peak*	*Duration*	*H*	*P*	*Adverse Effects*	*Relative Contraindications*	*Comments*
Sodium nitroprusside**	IV infusion	50 mg of lyophilized powder in D5W	0.5 μg·kg^{-1}·min^{-1} titrated to a max of 10 μg·kg^{-1}·min^{-1}	Within 30 sec		Length of infusion	+	+	Nausea/vomiting Vasodilation sx† Neurologic sx‡ Apprehension restlessness	Hepatic insufficiency	Solution good for 24 h Photosensitive (wrap in foil) Monitor blood thiocyanate if used longer than 72 h (D/C for thiocyanate >10 mg/dL)
Labetalol HCl**	IV bolus injection	20 mL vial containing 100 mg (5 mg/mL)	Bolus: 0.5 mg/kg over 2 min. For nonresponse, double dose and repeat every 10 min to a max dose of 5 mg/kg	1–5 min	5 min	Variable	–	–	Postural hypotension Neurologic sx† Nausea/vomiting	Bronchial asthma CHF	Keep supine for 3 h after administering drug Ambulate gradually Use cautiously in pheochromocytoma and diabetes Synergistic with halothane (hypotension)
Diazoxide**	IV bolus injection	20-mL ampule containing 300 mg (15 mg/mL)	1–3 mg/kg repeated every 5–15 min until BP controlled (minibolus)	1–5 min	1–5 min	Variable Usually less than 12 h	+	+	Arrhythmias Hyperglycemia Sodium and water retention Vasodilation sx† Neurologic sx‡	Thiazide sensitivity Severe tachycardia Diabetes Coarctation	Ineffective in pheochromocytoma Give diuretics to decrease sodium retention Hypoproteinemia potentiates effects Prolonged use (weeks) often reinstates sensitivity to oral medications
Hydralazine	30-min IV infusion or IM	1-mL ampule containing 20 mg	0.15–0.2 mg/kg every 6 hr	10–20 min	10 min–1½ h	3–6 h	–	–	Headache Nausea/vomiting Tachycardia palpitation	Hypersensitivity to hydralazine ("hyperdynamic syndrome")	Undergoes color change in most infusion fluids, which does not indicate loss of potency
Nifedipine	Sublingual	10- and 20-mg capsules	0.25 mg/kg dose every 4–6 h	10–15 min	60–90 min	Variable, usually 2–4 h	–	–	Headache Vasodilation sx‡	Concomitant use of β-blocking drugs and cimetidine	Dose can be withdrawn from capsule with 1-mL syringe and squirted sublingually
Enalaprilat**	IV over 5 min	2-mL vials (1.25 mg/mL)	0.04–0.8 mg/kg dose Neonate 0.01 mg/kg dose	15 min	1–4 h	Variable	+	–	Hypotension when ECFV is contracted Hyperkalemia Oliguria	Renal failure Dehydration	Treat hypotension with volume expansion
Phentolamine	IV bolus injection	5 mg of lyophilized powder reconstituted with diluent	0.05–0.1 mg/kg	Within 30 sec	2 min	15–30 min			Tachycardia Arrhythmias Marked hypotension		Specific for pheochromocytoma

*Removal of drug for dialysis relates to the need to supplement a dose after dialysis. It does not apply to the use of dialysis to treat drug overdose.
**Manufacturer's warning: safety in children not established.
†Vasodilation symptoms include sweating, flushing, feelings of warmth, orthostatic hypotension, tachycardia, palpitations, nausea, and vomiting.
‡Neurologic symptoms include headache, blurred vision, dizziness, and lightheadedness.
Abbreviations: sx = symptoms; max = maximum; BP = blood pressure; D5W = 5% dextrose in water; H = hemodialysis; P = peritoneal dialysis; CHF = congestive heart failure; + = removed by dialysis; – = not removed by dialysis; IV = intravenous; D/C = discontinued; HCl = hydrochloride; IM = intramuscular; ECFV = extracellular fluid volume.

TABLE 59–3. Pharmacologic Effects of Antihypertensive Drugs Available for Parenteral and Sublingual Administration to Pediatric Patients

Drug	*HR*	*CO*	*SVR*	*RBF**	*GFR**
Nitroprusside	V (↑)	V (↓)	↓ ↓ ↓	NE	NE
Labetalol	V (↓)	V (↓)	↓	NE	NE
Diazoxide	↑ ↑	↑	↓ ↓	↓ then ↑	↓ then V
Hydralazine	↑ ↑	↑	↓	↑	V (→ ↑)
Nifedipine	V (↑)	↑	↓ ↓	NE	NE
Enalaprilat	NE	NE	↓ ↓	↑ ↑	↓

*May decrease if patient is dehydrated at time of treatment or if BP is excessively reduced.

Abbreviations: HR = heart rate; CO = cardiac output; SVR = systemic vascular resistance; RBF = renal blood flow; GFR = glomerular filtration rate; NE = no effect; V = variable (arrows in parentheses indicate the more commonly reported effects); ↓ / ↑ = slightly reduced/increased; ↓ ↓ / ↑ ↑ = moderately reduced/increased; ↓ ↓ ↓ = markedly reduced; → = no change.

TABLE 59–4. Pharmacologic Characteristics of Antihypertensive Drugs for Oral Administration to Pediatric Patients

	Administration		*Interval for Dose Increase*	*Removal by Dialysis*				
Drug	*Preparation*	*Dosage*		*H*	*P*	*Adverse Effects*	*Relative Contraindications*	*Comments*
β-Adrenergic Blocking Drugs								
Propranolol (Inderal/Wyeth-Ayerst)	Tablets: 10, 20, 40, 50 mg	0.5–1 $mg \cdot kg^{-1} \cdot d^{-1}$ ÷ every 6 h	3–6 d	–	–	Cardiovascular: bradycardia, congestive heart failure, intensification of AV block CNS: mental depression (insommia, lassitude, weakness, fatigue), visual disturbances, disorientation, emotional lability, hallucinations, nightmares) Respiratory: bronchospasm Gastrointestinal: nausea, vomiting, diarrhea	Asthma Congestive heart failure Sinus bradycardia Heart block greater than 1° Diabetes Active liver disease Pheochromocytoma (before α-blockade) Cardiogenic shock	Inhibits reflex tachycardia (exercise, posture, vasodilators) May mask signs of hyperthyroidism and hypoglycemia Action potentiated by diuretics
Atenolol† (Tenormin/Icl)	Tablets: 50, 100 mg	50 mg every day (adult dose)	7–14 d	+	–	Has the fewest side effects	Can be used cautiously in asthmatics	Relatively cardioselective
Metoprolol† (Lopressor/Geigy)	Tablets: 50, 100 mg	1 mg/kg every 12 h*	7 d			Same as β-blockers but less severe	Same as β-blockers but can be used in asthmatics	Same as β-blockers β_1 selectivity enhanced at low doses β-blocker of choice in asthmatics
Nadolol† (Corgard/Bristol)	Tablets: 40, 80, 120, 160 mg	1 mg/kg every 24 h*	3–7 d	+		Same as β-blockers but less severe, especially CNS	Same as β-blockers	Same as β-blockers Longer duration allows once-a-day dosage
Vasodilator Drugs								
Hydralazine (Apresoline/Ciba)	Tablets: 10, 25, 50, 100 mg (unstable in suspension)	0.75–3 $mg \cdot kg^{-1} \cdot d^{-1}$ ÷ 4–6 h to a maximum of 200 mg every 24 h	3–4 d	–	–	Vasodilation symptoms, sweating, flushing, feelings of warmth, orthostatic hypotension, tachycardia, palpitations, nausea, and vomiting	Tachycardia Hypersensitivity to hydralazine	Unstable in suspension Periodic LE prep and ANA should be done
Minoxidil (Loniten/Upjohn)	Tablets: 2.5, 10 mg	0.1–0.2 mg/kg every 8–24 h to a maximum of 50 mg less than 12 y; 100 mg more than 12 y	3 d (can be every 6 h with care)	+	+	Headache Vasodilation symptoms, sweating, flushing, feelings of warmth, orthostatic hypotension, tachycardia, palpitations, nausea, and vomiting Hypertrichosis Sodium retention Ascites Pericardial effusion	Pheochromocytoma	Always use with a diuretic May cause severe hypotension in patient on guanethidine Discontinue gradually

*Dose frequency may be decreased to twice daily after BP is controlled.

†Manufacturer's warning: Safety and effectiveness in children have not been established.

Abbreviations: H = hemodialysis; P = peritoneal dialysis; + = removed by dialysis; – = not removed by dialysis; AV = atrioventricular; CNS = central nervous system; LE = lupus erythematosus; ANA = antinuclear antibody.

TABLE 59–5. Pharmacologic Characteristics of Antihypertensive Drugs for Oral Administration to Pediatric Patients

Drug	Administration: Preparation	Administration: Dosage	Interval for Dose Increase	Removal by Dialysis: H	Removal by Dialysis: P	Adverse Effects	Relative Contraindications	Comments
Angiotensin Converting Enzyme Inhibitor Drugs								
Captopril (Capoten/Squibb)	Tablets: 25, 50, 100 mg (unstable in suspension)*	0.15 mg/kg dose (Infants: 0.05–0.1 mg/kg dose)	Dose to dose	+		Rash Hyperkalemia (patients with renal failure) Proteinuria Neutropenia	Renal artery stenosis Volume contraction	Presence of food decreases absorption by 30–40%: give a.c. Action potentiated by diuretics Causes false-positive urine acetone
Enalapril* (Vasotec/Merck, Sharp & Dohme)	Tablets: 2.5, 5, 10, 20 mg	2.5–5 mg every d (adult dose); may be given twice a day for more even control	2–3 d (takes weeks for full effect)	+		Same as captopril	Same as captopril	Absorption not affected by food
Calcium Channel–Blocking Drugs								
Nifedipine (Procardia/Pfizer)	Capsules: 10, 20 mg	0.25 mg/kg dose every 4–6 h	Dose to dose			Vasodilation Tachycardia Sweating Nausea Vomiting	Concomitant use of β-blocking drugs or cimetidine	Absorption unaffected by food
Nifedipine extended release (Nifedipine XL/Pfizer)	Tablets: 30, 60 mg	30 mg every day (adult dose)	7–14 d			Same as nifedipine	Same as nifedipine	Same as nifedipine
Verapamil (Calan/Searle)**	Tablets: 40, 80, 120 mg	4–10 $mg \cdot kg^{-1} \cdot d^{-1}$ ÷ three times a day	5–7 d			Same as nifedipine	Same as nifedipine	Absorption delayed by food
Central Adrenergic Stimulating Drugs								
Clonidine** (Catapres/Boehringer Ingleheim)	Tablets: 0.1, 0.2, 0.3 mg	0.05 mg/kg twice a day to a maximum of 2.4 mg every 24 h	1–4 d	–		Dry mouth Sedation/fatigue Retinal degeneration		Action potentiated by diuretics Rebound hypertension if D/C suddenly
α-Adrenergic Blocking Drugs								
Prazosin** (Minipress/Pfizer)	Capsules: 1, 2, 5 mg	1 mg to a maximum of 20 mg every 24 h†	2–3 d			Orthostatic hypotension Lethargy Sedation/fatigue	Patients already on minoxidil	Action potentiated by minoxidil and diuretic Acute orthostatic hypotension can occur with first dose
Phenoxybenzamine (Dibenzyline/SmithKline Beecham)	Capsules: 10 mg (unstable in suspension)*	0.2 mg/kg every 24 h	4 d			Nasal congestion Orthostatic hypotension		Specific for catecholamine excess

*Instability of this drug in suspension can be circumvented by dissolving tablets/capsules in a measured amount of water and administering immediately.
**Manufacturer's warning: No clinical experience for use in children.
†Dose frequency may be decreased to bid once BP is controlled.
Abbreviations: H = hemodialysis; P = peritoneal dialysis; + = removed by dialysis; – = not removed by dialysis; a.c. = before meals; D/C = discontinued.

TABLE 59–6. Pharmacologic Characteristics of Diuretic Drugs for Parenteral and Oral Administration to Pediatric Patients

	Administration							
Drug	*Preparation*	*Dosage*	*Onset*	*Peak*	*Duration*	*Adverse Effects*	*Relative Contraindications*	*Comments*
Furosemide (Lasix/Hoechst-Roussel)	Tablets: 20, 40, 80 mg Oral solution: 10 mg/mL; IV: 10 mg/mL	1–2 mg increased 1–2 mg/kg to a maximum of 6 mg/kg every 24 h	0–1 h IV* 5 min IV* 1 h (neonate)	1–2 h 30 min 1–2 h	4–6 h 2 h 5–6 h	Fluid and electrolyte depletion Hyperuricemia Hyperglycemia	Anuria Metabolic alkalosis Sulfonamide sensitivity	See ethacrynic acid Ototoxicity less than ethacrynic acid
Ethacrynic acid (Edacrin/Merck, Sharp & Dohme)	Tablets: 25, 50 mg IV: 50 mg (lyophilized powder reconstituted with D5W)	1 mg/kg increased to 25 mg every 24 hr	0–30 min IV: 15–30 min	2 h 45 min	6–8 h 3 h	Fluid and electrolyte depletion Hyperuricemia Hyperglycemia	Anuria Metabolic alkalosis	Periodic determination of serum electrolytes should be performed Ototoxicity with parenteral administration
Hydrochlorothiazide (HydroDIURIL/Merck, Sharp & Dohme)	Tablets: 25, 50, 100 mg	2 mg/kg twice daily	2 h	4 h	6–12 h	Electrolyte depletion Hyperuricemia Hyperglycemia	Anuria Sulfonamide sensitivity	Periodic determination of serum electrolytes should be performed
Spironolactone (Aldactone**/Searle)	Tablets: 25, 100 mg	1–3.3 mg/kg every 6, 8, or 12 h	Gradual	3 d	2–3 d	Hyperkalemia Gynecomastia	Anuria Rapidly decreasing renal function Hyperkalemia	Not effective alone, usually use with thiazide (Aldactazide)

*IV bolus injection should not exceed 4 mg/min to decrease ototoxicity risk.
**Manufacturer's warning: Safety and effectiveness in children have not been established.
Abbreviations: IV = intravenous; D5W = dextrose 5% in water.

however, minibolus administration reduces the incidence of hypotension and better controls BP reduction.[38] A diuretic may be used concomitantly with diazoxide to avoid sodium retention and, thus, to potentiate diazoxide's effects.

Phentolamine is used specifically for hypertensive crises caused by catecholamine excess. Its action is rapid in onset and brief in duration. It should be reserved for hypertensive crises (e.g., acute BP elevations during surgery) because prolonged BP control is better achieved by orally administered phenoxybenzamine.

Trimethaphan, a parenterally administered agent that lowers BP by decreasing peripheral resistance through ganglionic blockade, is not recommended because experience in children is limited, and it offers no advantages over other agents.

The pharmacologic characteristics of the more commonly used oral antihypertensive and diuretic agents are given in Tables 59–4 through 59–6. Selection of the appropriate antihypertensive medication is facilitated by understanding the pathophysiology of hypertension in an individual patient and the pharmacologic action of the various agents available for its treatment.

OUTCOME

The exact mortality of children with acute hypertension is unknown. However, the risk of death has been diminished by more widespread recognition of this problem in children and the availability of more efficacious drugs. Hypertension may spontaneously abate with resolution of the underlying condition, as in poststreptococcal glomerulonephritis; may be treated successfully by surgical intervention, as in renal artery stenosis; or may be incurable but controllable, as in chronic glomerulonephritis. Usually, the signs and symptoms of hypertensive encephalopathy or renal failure resolve or improve as BP is controlled; however, residual neurologic abnormalities such as seizure disorders, blindness, cranial nerve palsy, and hemiplegia may persist. In some children with preexisting renal disease, a slightly elevated BP may be necessary for adequate renal perfusion.[5, 39] More commonly, any further deterioration in renal function as BP is lowered will be transient and reversible.[40] The only predictor of transient deterioration is a clinical trial of BP normalization.

References

1. Dinsdale HB, Tobertson DM, Nag S: Cerebral consequences of acute and chronic hypertension: An overview. Clin Invest Med 1978; 1:181.
2. Strandgaard S, Olesen J, Skinhoj E, et al: Autoregulation of brain circulation in severe arterial hypertension. Br Med J 1973; 1:507.
3. Strandgaard S, MacKenzie ET, Jones JV, et al: Studies on the cerebral circulation of the baboon in acutely induced hypertension. Stroke 1976; 7:287.
4. Lloyd AVC, Jewitt DE, Still JD: Facial paralysis in children with hypertension. Arch Dis Child 1966; 41:292.
5. Weir MR: Hypertensive nephropathy: Is a more physiologic approach to blood pressure control an important concern for the preservation of renal function? Am J Med 1992; 93(S-2A):27S.
6. Hulse JA, Taylor DSI, Dillon MJ: Blindness and paraplegia in severe childhood hypertension. Lancet 1979; ii:553.
7. Laragh JH: Vasoconstriction–Volume analysis for understanding and treating hypertension. Am J Med 1973; 55:261.
8. Cowley AW: The concept of autoregulation of total blood flow and its role in hypertension. Am J Med 1980; 68:906.
9. Pickering TC, Laragh JH: Autoregulation as a factor in peripheral resistance and flow: Clinical implications for analysis of high blood pressure. Am J Med 1980; 68:801.
10. Bailie MD, Mattioli LF: Hypertension: Relationships between pathophysiology and therapy. J Pediatr 1980; 96:789.
11. Still JL, Cottom D: Severe hypertension in childhood. Arch Dis Child 1967; 42:34.
12. Londe S: Causes of hypertension in the young. Pediatr Clin North Am 1978; 25:55.
13. Eisenberg S: Blood volume in patients with acute glomerulonephritis as determined by radioactive chromium tagged red cells. Am J Med 1959; 27:241.
14. Powell HR, Rotenberg E, Williams AL, et al: Plasma renin activity in acute poststreptococcal glomerulonephritis and the haemolytic-uraemic syndrome. Arch Dis Child 1974; 49:802.
15. Mendoza SA, Mendoza G: Hemolytic uremic syndrome. West J Med 1975; 123:459.
16. Holland NH, Kotchen T, Bhathena D: Hypertension in children with chronic pyelonephritis. Kidney Int 1975; 8S:243.
17. Savage JM, Dillon MJ, Shah V, et al: Renin and blood pressure in children with renal scarring and vesicoureteric reflux. Lancet 1978; ii:441.
18. Elias AN, Anderson GH, Dalakos TG, et al: Renin angiotensin involvement in transient hypertension after renal injury. J Urol 1978; 119:561.
19. Grant RP, Gifford RW, Pudvan WR, et al: Renal trauma and hypertension. Am J Cardiol 1971; 27:173.
20. Munoz AI, Pascual JF: Arterial hypertension in infants with hydronephrosis. Am J Dis Child 1977; 131:38.
21. Alpert BS, Bain HH, Balfe JW: Role of the renin-angiotensin-aldosterone system in hypertensive children with coarctation of the aorta. Am J Cardiol 1979; 43:828.
22. Fox S, Pierce WS, Waldhausen JA: Pathogenesis of paradoxical hypertension after coarctation repair. Ann Thorac Surg 1980; 29:135.
23. Stackpole RH, Melicow MM, Uson AC: Pheochromocytoma in children. J Pediatr 1963; 63:315.
24. Bravo EL, Tarazi RC, Gifford RW, et al: Circulating and urinary catecholamines in pheochromocytoma. N Engl J Med 1979; 301:682.
25. Stewart BH, Bravo EL, Haaga J, et al: Localization of pheochromocytoma by computed tomography. N Engl J Med 1978; 299:460.
26. Sisson JC, Frager MS, Volk TW, et al: Scintigraphic localization of pheochromocytoma. 1981; 305:12.
27. Turner MC, Ruley EJ, Buckley KM, et al: Blood pressure elevation in children with orthopedic immobilization. J Pediatr 1979; 95:989.
28. Heij HA, Ekkelkamp S, Vos A: Hypertension associated with skeletal traction in children. Eur J Pediatr 1992; 151:543.
29. Popp MG, Silberstein EB, Srivastava LS, et al: A pathophysiologic study of the hypertension associated with burn injury in children. Ann Surg 1981; 193:817.
30. Horn PT: Persitent hypertension after prenatal cocaine exposure. J Pediatr 1992; 121:288.
31. Feibel JH, Baldwin CA, Joynt RT: Catecholamine-associated refractory hypertension following acute intracranial hemorrhage: Control with propranolol. Ann Neurol 1981; 9:340.
32. Bertel O, Marx B, Conen D: Effects of antihypertensive treatment on cerebral perfusion. Am J Med 1987; 82(S3B):29.
33. Gordillo-Paniagua G, Velasquez-Jones L, Martini R, et al: Sodium nitroprusside treatment of severe arterial hypertension in children. J Pediatr 1975; 87:799.
34. Davis RF, Douglas ME, Heenan TJ, et al: Brain tissue pressure measurement during nitroprusside infusion. Crit Care Med 1981; 9:17.
35. Cressman MD, Vidt DG, Gifford RW, et al: Intravenous labetalol in the management of severe hypertension and hypertensive emergencies. Am Heart J 1984; 107:980.
36. Bunchman TE, Lynch RE, Wood EG: Intravenously administered labetalol for treatment of hypertension in children. J Pediatr 1992; 120:140.
37. McCrory WW, Kohut EC, Lewy JE, et al: Safety of intravenous diazoxide in children with severe hypertension. Clin Pediatr 1979; 18:661.
38. Ram CVS, Kaplan NM: Individual titration of diazoxide dosage in the treatment of severe hypertension. Am J Cardiol 1979; 43:627.

39. Green TP, Nevins TE, Houser MT, et al: Renal failure as a complication of acute antihypertensive therapy. Pediatrics 1981; 67:850.
40. Adelman RD, Russo J: Malignant hypertension: Recovery of renal function after treatment with antihypertensive medications and hemodialysis. J Pediatr 1981; 98:776.

CHAPTER 60

Intra-Aortic Balloon Counterpulsation

Michael B. Kesselbrenner, MD, FACC, FACP • Howard M. Weinberg, DO • Keith Reemstma, MD • David Bregman, MD, FACC, FACS

The intra-aortic balloon (IAB) pump is currently the most widely used temporary circulatory assist device. The concept of counterpulsation, which is the basic physiologic principle underlying IAB pumping, was first described by Harken in 1958 and, as originally proposed, involved the removal of blood via the femoral route from the arterial tree during ventricular systole and the rapid reinfusion of the same blood during diastole to increase coronary perfusion pressure. By this method, in the normotensive preparation, one could decrease the work of the left ventricle and increase coronary blood flow.[1] Further pioneering work was done by Kantrowitz,[2,3] who surmised that poor left ventricle indexes could be improved by retarding the diastolic pressure.

Moulopoulos, Topaz, and Kolff[4,5] in 1962 suggested the use of a single-chambered IAB position in the descending thoracic aorta to accomplish the same purpose of counterpulsation but without the drawbacks of earlier methods used (Fig. 60–1). The balloon is inflated in diastole concurrently with closure of the aortic valve and is held in inflation until the onset of ventricular systole. The balloon is then rapidly deflated (Fig. 60–2). The inflation of the balloon displaces blood in the aorta (by an amount equal to the volume of the balloon) toward the coronary tree, thereby augmenting coronary perfusion pressure and blood flow. The collapse of the balloon creates a reduction in impedance to left ventricular ejection (i.e., decreased afterload) and consequently reduces left ventricular work.[6]

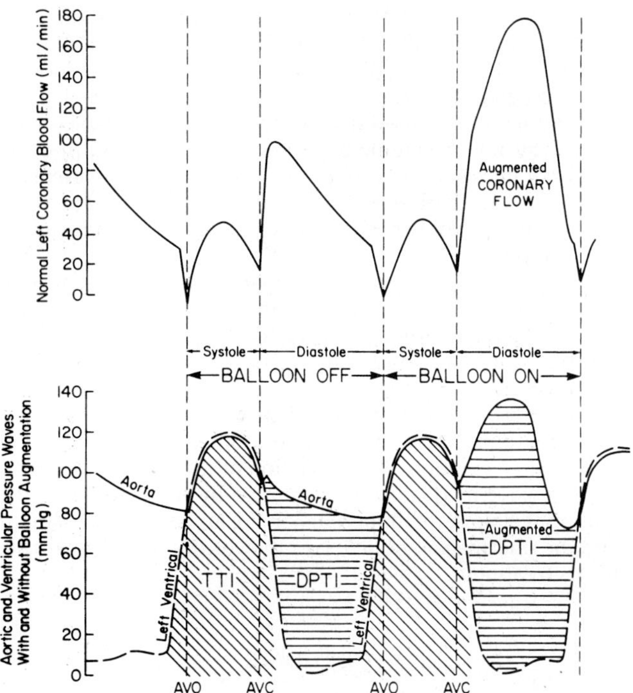

Figure 60–2. Schematic representation of coronary blood flow and aortic and left ventricular waves with and without intra-aortic balloon augmentation. *Top Panel,* Left coronary blood flow changes during the cardiac cycle. Peak flows occur during diastole when intraventricular pressures are decreased. Balloon augmentation of diastolic aortic root pressure produces further increases in coronary blood flow. *Bottom Panel,* The tension-time index (TTI) and the diastolic pressure-time index (DPTI) illustrated as the area under the left ventricular and aortic pressure curves during systole and diastole, respectively. Proper balloon inflation during diastole augments diastolic pressure and consequently increases coronary perfusion pressure as well as improves the relationship between myocardial oxygen supply and demand (DPTI:TTI ratio). (From Maccioli GA, Lucas WJ, Norfleet EA: The intra-aortic balloon pump: A review. J Cardiothorac Anesth 1988; 2:369.)

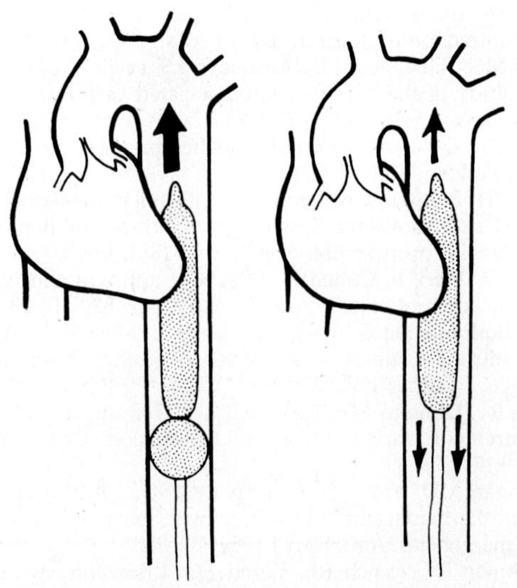

Figure 60–1. Intra-aortic balloon pumping action of omnidirectional (single-chambered) versus unidirectional (dual-chambered) balloons. (From Kesselbrenner M, Sack J, Saporito R, et al: Intra-aortic balloon counterpulsation. *In:* Techniques in Extracorporeal Circulation. Kay PH [Ed]. Oxford, Butterworth Heinemann, 1992, p 236.)

In 1968, Adrian Kantrowitz introduced the IAB pump to the clinical setting of cardiogenic shock. Careful follow-up of such patients showed that mortality remained largely unaltered.[7] However, the findings that counterpulsation decreased the extent and severity of ischemic injury[8–12] and opens dormant coronary vessels[11] suggest that perhaps counterpulsation ought to be applied in patients sustaining uncomplicated myocardial infarction. This then could minimize the quantity of myocardium that ultimately became necrotic,[13] theoretically preserving left ventricular function.

The applications and indications for intra-aortic balloon pumping have come a long way since the early days of counterpulsation. The current indications are listed in Table 60–1.

PRINCIPLES

The principle of counterpulsation is based on the assumption that the reduction of end-diastolic pressure improves

TABLE 60–1. Indications for Intra-Aortic Balloon Pumping

Medical	*Surgical*	*Expanding*
Cardiogenic shock	High-risk cardiac patients	Stunned myocardium
Acute anterior myocardial infarction	Patients undergoing noncardiac surgery	Septic shock
Mechanical complications of myocardial infarction	Adjunct to mechanical assistance	Drug-induced cardiac failure
Ventricular septal defect		Myocardial contusion
Acute mitral regurgitation		
High-risk angioplasty	Postoperative low cardiac output syndrome	Aortic stenosis
Angioplasty with acute myocardial infarction	Weaning from bypass open heart surgery	Pediatric applications
Unstable angina refractory to medical treatment		
In conjunction with thrombolysis		
Bridge to transport		
Ventricular arrhythmias secondary to ischemia		

left ventricular function. This is accomplished with improved stroke volume as created by the balloon. The balloon is positioned in the proximal descending thoracic aorta (Fig. 60–3). During diastole, it is rapidly inflated concurrently with closure of the aortic valve. Then, at the onset of systole, initiated via a sensing electrocardiogram, the balloon is rapidly deflated. This creates a vacuum effect, decreasing the afterload and augmenting ventricular outflow.

Thus, the mechanism of improved hemodynamics has two components. First, by raising diastolic pressures within the proximal aorta at balloon expansion, coronary perfusion pressure is increased, generating an increased myocardial oxygen supply, with concomitant bolstering of myocardial contractility. Second, with rapid balloon deflation, there is a sudden volume loss within the aorta (proportional to the volume of the balloon), effectively reducing the afterload against which the left ventricle must work. This decreases myocardial oxygen demand and, at the same time, increases cardiac output at any given level of filling pressure.[14]

The hemodynamic effects of IAB pumping are dependent on several factors: (1) the position of the balloon pump in the aorta, (2) the heart rate, (3) the volume of the balloon, (4) the heart rhythm, and (5) the compliance of the aorta and peripheral vascular bed. Additionally, the flow velocity generated in both the ascending and descending aortas is dependent on the rate of balloon inflation and deflation. This ultimately affects the pressure and perfusion to the myocardium. The mean arterial pressure generated and the change in the mean diastolic pressure are significantly influenced by the IAB volume (Fig. 60–4). Weber and Janicki defined several clinical variables affecting IAB counterpulsation (Table 60–2).[10]

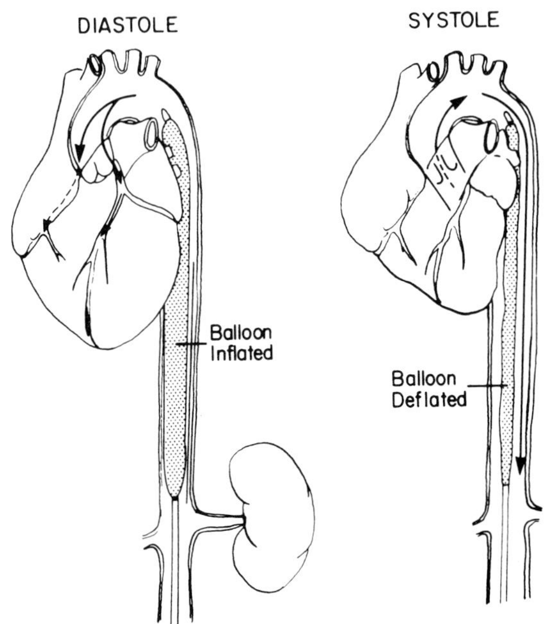

Figure 60–3. Proper positioning of the intra-aortic balloon below the left subclavian artery and above the renal arteries. With inflation of the balloon during diastole, blood is forced into the coronary ostia, resulting in increased coronary artery perfusion. During systole, deflation creates an intravascular void, allowing less impedance to ventricular ejection. (From Maccioli GA, Lucas WJ, Norfleet EA: The intra-aortic balloon pump: A review. J Cardiothorac Anesth 1988; 2:370.)

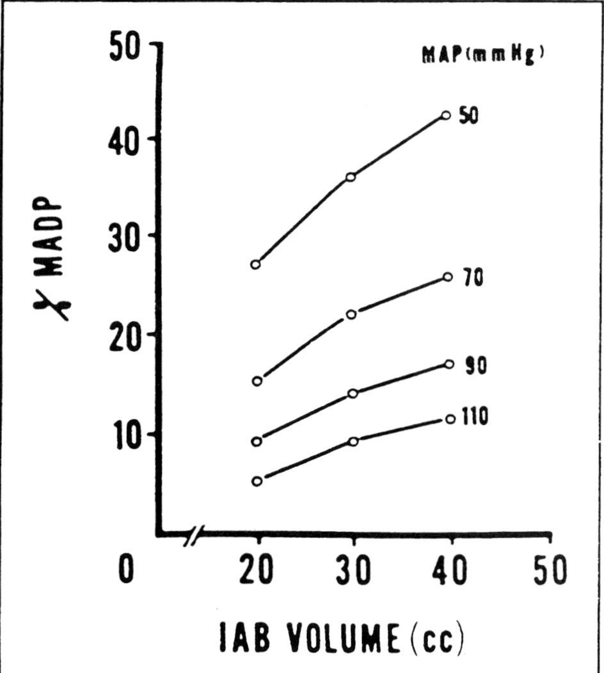

Figure 60–4. Augmentation of mean aortic diastolic pressure (MADP) as a function of IAB pump volume for four mean arterial pressure (MAP) levels. Increasing balloon volume increases MADP at every level of MAP, but the most at the lower levels. (From Weber KT, Janicki JS: Intra-aortic counterpulsation: A review of physiological principles, clinical results, and device safety. Ann Thorac Surg 1974; 17:602. Reprinted with permission from the Society of Thoracic Surgeons.)

TABLE 60–2. Clinical Variables Affecting Intra-Aortic Balloon Counterpulsation

Diastolic Pressure Augmentation	*Impedance and Work Reduction*
Physical variables	Physical variables
Position	Volume
Volume	Occlusivity
Diameter	Inflation duration
Occlusivity	Biologic variables
Configuration	Arterial pressure
Driving gas	Heart rate
Timing	Aortic pressure-volume relation
Biologic variables	Afterload reduction
Arterial pressure	Preload reduction
Heart rate	Augmented shortening
Aortic pressure-volume relation	

(From Weber KT, Janicki JS: Intra-aortic counterpulsation: A review of physiological principles, clinical results and device safety. Ann Thorac Surg 1974; 17:602.)

Weber and Janicki[10] also showed that with the IAB pump there is a decline in the end-diastolic left ventricular diameter, ejection time, and volume and a decrease in systolic pressure, resulting in a 18% and 19% reduction in developed and peak left ventricular wall stress, respectively. As left ventricular function is more depressed, the hemodynamic effects are more significant.

As seen in Figure 60–5, the collateral blood flow, as manifest by retrograde left anterior descending blood flow, is maximally augmented with the highest increase in the diastolic blood pressure.

Two additional advantages result from the use of either counterpulsation or IAB pumping. First, it has been demonstrated by Jacoby and colleagues[15] that, after a short period of counterpulsation, dormant intercoronary collateral beds are opened, and these channels remain open after termination of counterpulsation. Second, it has been demonstrated by several investigators[8, 13, 16] that early institution of IAB pumping decreases the size of the potential infarction after coronary occlusion.

BALLOON CONSTRUCTION AND SAFETY

Balloon Membrane

A single-chamber, dual-lumen balloon, the technology of the 1990s, is a single-cast tubular membrane of a specially formulated polyurethane polymer. Wall thickness is 3 to 4.25 mm. Figure 60–6 shows the behavior of a 4-mL cast of this polyurethane film subjected to increasing stress. In region 1, length changes very little with stress. Region 2 is an elastic zone; the molecular chains, normally folded and entangled, begin to straighten after the stress reaches the threshold value and the material stretches similar to a rubber band. When the chains are fully straightened, the curve then enters a saturation region, 3, and "locks" at its ultimate length. Sufficient force at region 4 will break the chain and then cause rupture. The single-chambered balloon is operated totally within region 1 for several reasons. The obvious reason is that we make use of a safety chamber and use only enough gas to "fill" but not "distend" the intra-aortic balloon. Because work equals force times distance, one can see that cyclic forces within region 1 cause very little distance change and consequently, very little work is expended on the balloon material, resulting in minimal fatigue.

Balloon Sizing

The standard adult balloon is 40 mL and 9.5 French. Currently, the IAB may be placed with or without a vascular sheath. In the last few years, the issue of balloon size has been amended to account for patient height (Table 60–3.)

However, the only catheter for sheathless insertion approved by the U.S. Food and Drug Administration is the 40-mL, 9.5-French dual lumen. All others need a sheath for placement.

CLINICAL SYSTEM FOR INTRA-AORTIC BALLOON PUMPING

In order for the IAB pump to perform its function of cardiac assistance, the timing of balloon inflation and deflation must be extremely accurate and responsive to changes in heart rate. The IAB console, therefore, had to undergo evolution along with the development of balloons with improved design.[17]

In its original concept, the console processed the patient ECG signal into an electrical output that commanded a solenoid valve to open, permitting the driving gas to inflate the balloon. At first, gas was supplied directly to the solenoid from the tank regulator. Balloon deflation was accomplished by closing the solenoid valve and permitting the balloon to vent to the atmosphere (Fig. 60–7). The console controlled only the point of balloon inflation, expressed as the delay after the R wave of the ECG (which served as an electronic triggering event), and the duration of inflation

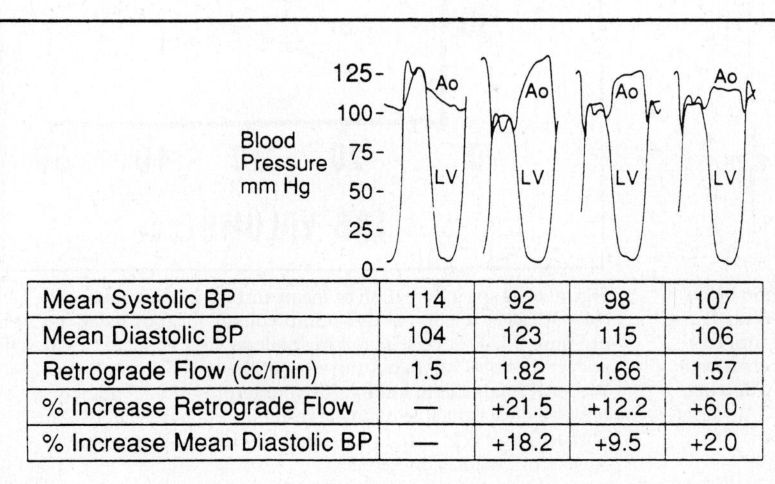

Mean Systolic BP	114	92	98	107
Mean Diastolic BP	104	123	115	106
Retrograde Flow (cc/min)	1.5	1.82	1.66	1.57
% Increase Retrograde Flow	—	+21.5	+12.2	+6.0
% Increase Mean Diastolic BP	—	+18.2	+9.5	+2.0

Figure 60–5. Hemodynamic tracings during IAB pumping coinciding with collateral perfusion represented by retrograde left anterior descending flow. Changes in aortic root pressure (Ao) and left ventricular pressure (LV) are for varying contributions to constant mean aortic blood pressure (BP) (107 mm Hg). The highest augmentation of retrograde flow (increased collateral flow) was associated with the maximal increase in diastolic blood pressure (123 mm Hg). (From Gundel WD, Brown BG, Gott VL: Coronary collateral flow studies during variable aortic root pressure waveforms. J Appl Physiol 1970; 29:579–586.)

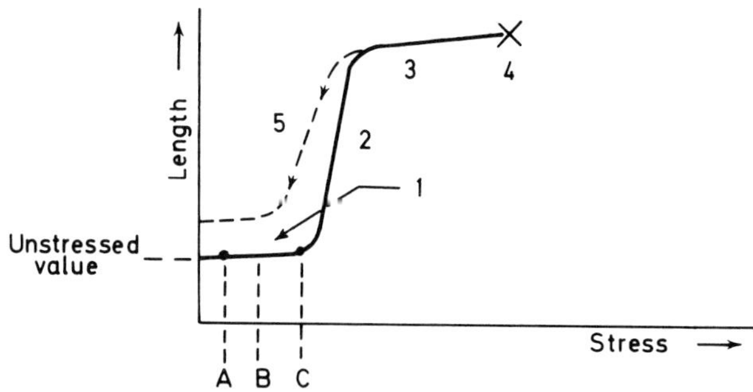

Figure 60–6. Stress/strain characteristics of polyurethane formula in a dual-chambered IAB. (From Kesselbrenner M, Sack J, Saporito R, et al: Intra-aortic balloon counterpulsation. *In:* Techniques in Extracorporeal Circulation. Kay PH [Ed]. Oxford, Butterworth Heinemann, 1992, p 240.)

over a given period of the cardiac cycle. Manual triggering was provided for use during cardiac resuscitation. Although the system worked well enough to introduce IAB pumping to the scientific community, it responded only to the basic needs of the balloon pump console.

Increasing experience led to continuing refinements and the introduction of Datascope System 80 and, ultimately, Datascope System 90. Fully automated prefilling of the safety chamber system and alarms to signal a loss of trigger, gas, or augmentation or to signal a kinked catheter were incorporated into the late model systems. In 1987, the Datascope System 90T was designed to allow continuous use of the balloon pump both at the community hospital and during transport to a tertiary care center.

In 1992, Datascope introduced System 95, which, in addition to all the features of the earlier systems, further improves balloon pump triggering with pacemakers and has improved pneumatic efficiency to track at high heart rates. This technology permits downloading of diagnostic information via a modem-telecom interface and offers an ultrasonic Doppler probe to monitor arterial pulsations.

EXPERIENCE WITH INTRA-AORTIC BALLOON PUMPING

The indications for IAB pumping are changing almost daily. However, the IAB pump remains especially useful for acute myocardial infarction and cardiogenic shock (Fig. 60–8).

All patients with an acute myocardial infarction diagnosed by the clinical picture, the ECG, and enzyme studies should be admitted to the coronary care unit.[18] Those patients who demonstrate systolic hypotension (systolic blood

TABLE 60–3. Guidelines for Balloon Sizing

	Patient Profile		
Variables	*<5′4″*	*5′4″–6′*	*>6′*
Balloon volume	34 mL	40 mL	50 mL
Balloon length	219 mm	263 mm	270 mm
Balloon diameter	14.2 mm	15 mm	16 mm
Catheter size	9.5 French	9.5 French	10.5 French

pressure <80 mm Hg or systolic blood pressure <100 mm Hg if formerly hypertensive) or, even without hypertension, a low output syndrome resulting in diminished tissue perfusion, peripheral cyanosis, cold and clammy skin, oliguria (urine output <20 mL/h, low sodium), and mental confusion or agitation are then evaluated for the possible effects of the following:

1. Drug depression
2. Arrhythmias
3. Metabolic disturbances
4. Volume depletion
5. Gram-negative sepsis

If the hypotensive or low-output state is not related to any of these disturbances or persists after one or more of the disturbances have been corrected, then the patient is described as suffering from cardiogenic shock as a result of myocardial infarction or ongoing myocardial ischemia.

Whether or not the patient is a candidate for thrombolytic therapy or emergency revascularization, initially, patients should receive standard supportive therapy, including medications for pain and cardiac failure as well as oxygen and the correction of acidosis. A central venous catheter should be inserted, a Swan-Ganz catheter positioned to monitor pulmonary artery wedge pressures, and a Foley catheter inserted. If the initial central venous pressure is less than 15 cm H_2O or the pulmonary capillary wedge pressure (PCWP) as measured with a Swan-Ganz catheter is less than 16 mm Hg, a volume infusion should be started and given in 100-mL increments of either normal saline or dextrose in water with or without salt-poor albumin added. If after a trial of volume expansion the systolic arterial pressure remains below 80 mm Hg or is less than 100 mm Hg in a formerly hypertensive patient or if the urine output remains below 20 mL/h, then initial cardiac output studies should be undertaken. While these are being arranged and performed, the patient should be given a therapeutic trial of inotropic agents, including dobutamine, amrinone, or dopamine. Isoproterenol should not be used in the setting of myocardial ischemia or infarction unless extreme bradycardia is present

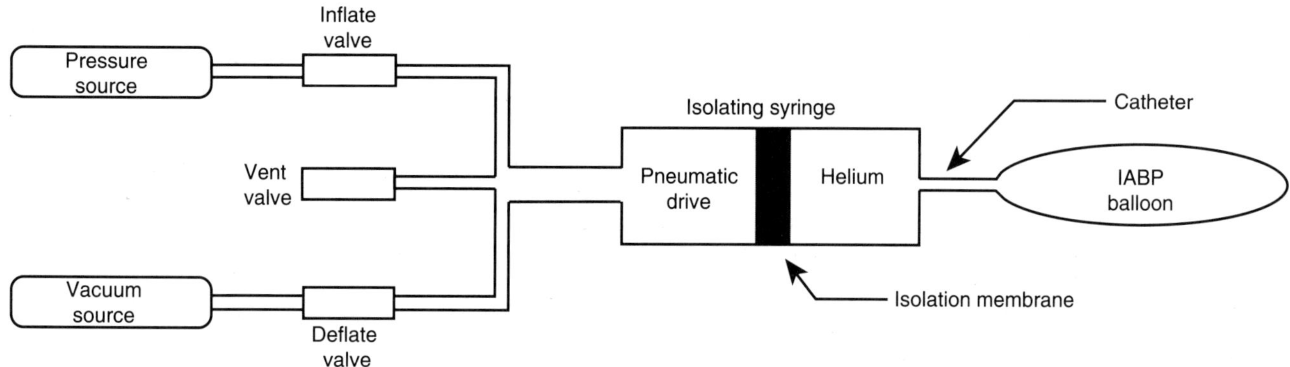

Figure 60–7. Schematic representation of IAB pneumatics. (Courtesy of Datascope Corporation, Paramus, NJ.)

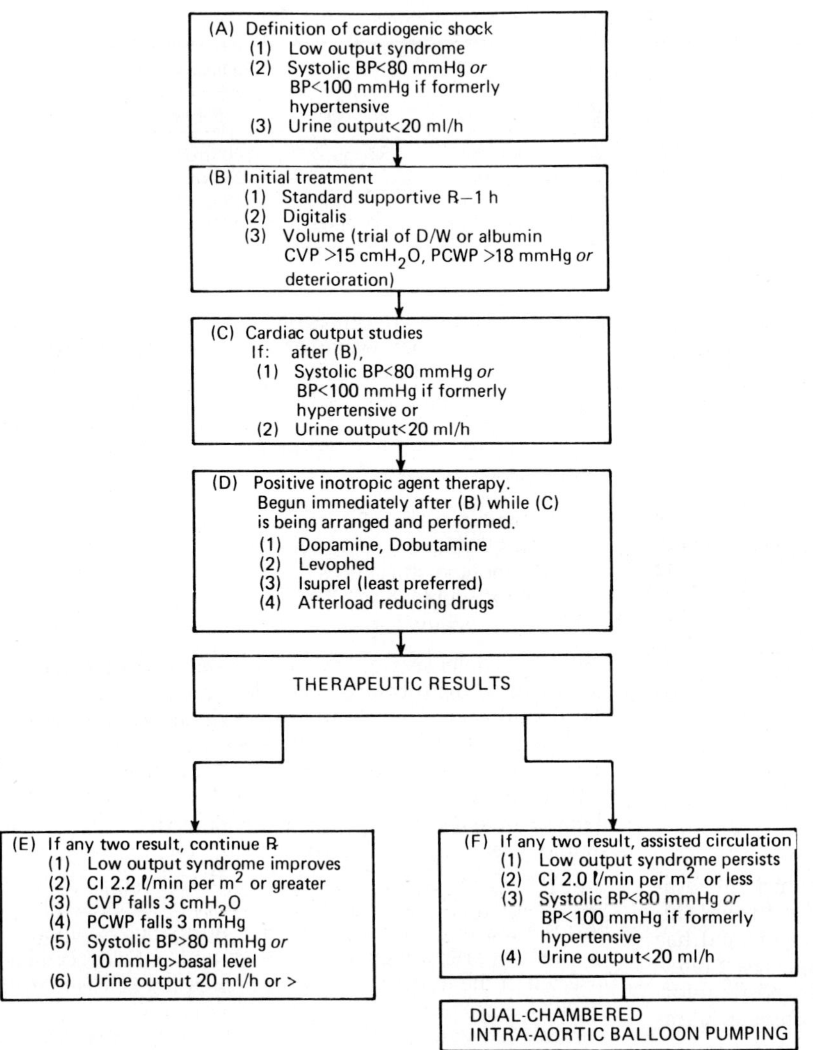

Figure 60–8. Management protocol for cardiogenic shock. (From Kesselbrenner M, Sack J, Saporito R, et al: Intra-aortic balloon counterpulsation. *In:* Techniques in Extracorporeal Circulation. Kay PH [Ed]. Oxford, Butterworth Heinemann, 1992, p 245.)

and the patient is unresponsive to atropine. In this case, a temporary pacemaker should be strongly considered. In addition, afterload reduction with sodium nitroprusside can be used alone or in combination with these inotropic agents.

Therapy should be considered temporarily successful and continued if any of two of the following measurements result from any agents:

1. There is improvement in the low output syndrome.
2. The cardiac index is 2.2 L/min · m^2 or greater.
3. The central venous pressure is lowered by 3 cm H_2O or more.
4. The PCWP falls by 3 mm Hg or more.
5. The systolic arterial blood pressure is greater than 80 mm Hg or shows an increase of 10 mm Hg from the prior basal level.
6. The urinary output is 20 mL/h or greater.

However, if any two of the following measurements apply, proceeding to IAB pumping should be strongly considered:

1. The low output syndrome clinically persists.
2. The cardiac index remains below 2.2 L/min · m^2.
3. The systolic blood pressure remains below 80 mm Hg (or 100 mm Hg in a previously hypertensive patient).
4. The urinary output persists at less than 20 mL/h (less than 0.5 mL·kg^{-1}·h^{-1}).

This entire diagnostic and therapeutic scheme can be performed in a short period of time.

Once the diagnosis of cardiogenic shock is established, these routine therapeutic procedures should be instituted as rapidly as possible because the earlier the patient is referred for circulatory assistance, the better the result will be. Surrounding the actual area of the infarct, or the area of frank myocardial necrosis, there is a significant area of marginal myocardial ischemia. It is this area of diminished myocardial perfusion that can be restored to viability by the early institution of IAB pumping. Hence, the earlier patients are referred for treatment, the higher the survival rate will be.

Metabolic Effects of Intra-Aortic Balloon Pumping

The metabolic effects of IAB pumping are now well described. Feola and colleagues[19] examined myocardial lactate metabolism with pacing-induced tachycardia in seven patients. They found that lactate production changed from 0.24 (±0.07 SD) extraction at rest to 0.94 (±0.01 SD) production after pacing ($P < .001$) without IAB pumping and from 0.10 (±0.003 SD) extraction at rest to 0.57 (±0.001 SD) production after pacing ($P < .001$) with IAB pumping. The difference between lactate production levels occurring with and without IAB counterpulsation was statistically significant ($P < .005$).

Previous studies have demonstrated that IAB pumping or arterial counterpulsation reduces myocardial oxygen consumption (MVO_2) in the normal circulation by diminishing heart rate, peak left ventricular systolic wall stress, and possibly, contractility.[20] Wall stress in the left ventricle, the major determinant of myocardial oxygen demand, can be decreased through a reduction of either peak systolic pressure or a reduction in left ventricular end-diastolic pressure and heart size.[22] Decreases in heart rate and a reduction in the frequency of ventricular ectopic beats suggest that IAB counterpulsation may reduce sympathetic tone and cardiac contractility through baroreceptor-mediated reflexes. This impression has been strengthened by observations of peripheral vasodilation[9] and increased frequency of discharge of the carotid sinus[23] during IAB pumping. The postulated reduction of sympathetic tone during IAB pumping is further supported in the present study by observation of a decrease in circulating arterial epinephrine and norepinephrine during IAB counterpulsation.

Contraindications to Intra-Aortic Balloon Pumping

There is an ever-expanding list of uses for the IAB pump. However, there remains only a few absolute contraindications. These include gross severe aortic insufficiency, acute aortic dissection, chronic end-stage heart disease (without the possibility of a transplant), and severe, irreversible brain damage. Minor aortic insufficiency should not be a deterrent.[24] The presence of an aortic aneurysm and a history of aortic surgery are only relative contraindications; their significance should be judged in view of the entire clinical picture.

The use of the IAB pump with cardiac standstill, especially in the setting of open heart surgery, remains controversial[25]; however, it never impairs survival when continued with closed-chest cardiopulmonary resuscitation.

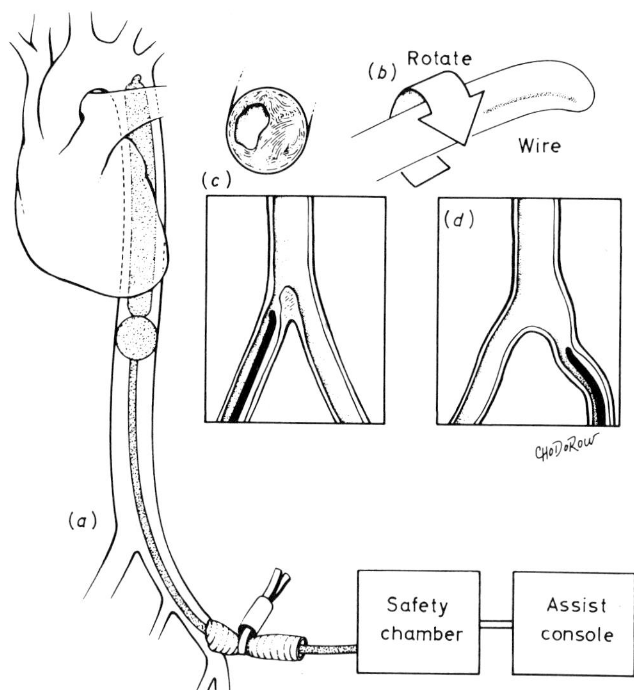

Figure 60–9. A proper position of a dual-chambered IAB just distal to left subclavian artery (a). Note that the balloon is inserted through a Dacron prosthesis that is snared; this permits perfusion of the distal extremity during the period of cardiac assist. Technique of blending and rotating a distal balloon catheter during insertion (b). Balloon negotiation of eccentric arteriosclerotic stenosis (c). Balloon passing through an arterial tortuosity (d). (From Kesselbrenner M, Sack J, Saporito R, et al: Intra-aortic balloon counterpulsation. *In:* Techniques in Extracorporeal Circulation. Kay PH [Ed]. Oxford, Butterworth Heinemann, 1992, p 248.)

Techniques of Intra-Aortic Balloon Pump Insertion

The initial description of IAB pump insertion was first outlined by Kantrowitz and coworkers (Fig. 60–9).[41] The common femoral artery is exposed through a vertical incision beginning high in the groin over the inguinal ligament. The vessel is then encircled by tapes for control. A 10-mm woven Dacron side arm graft is sutured on to the arterial site. Using bulldog clamps to control the blood flow above and below the arteriotomy site, the balloon catheter is inserted through the graft into the artery. An umbilical snare is used to secure the balloon catheter within the graft. The balloon catheter can now be advanced up into the descending and thoracic aorta.[26]

Transiliac Artery Insertion

Using the same technique, the balloon can be inserted into the common iliac artery. Exposure is obtained with a retroperitoneal approach using an oblique incision above the left inguinal ligament.[27]

Transaxillary Insertion

In the event of severe diffuse aortoiliac disease, tortuosity, or some other contraindication to femoroiliac insertion, the IAB pump catheter may be placed from the left subclavian artery. Surgical isolation of the vessel through the axilla allows advancement to the descending aorta. Although rarely required, this method may be ideal for the patient with an acute aortic dissection or aneurysm, when retrograde insertion of the IAB pump catheter may be possible.

Transthoracic Insertion

Yet another approach to circumvent peripheral vascular disease or anomalies is the transthoracic insertion. This is also advantageous if recent prior exposure to the aortic arch expedites access.[28–30] Pursestring sutures are embedded into the ascending aortic wall, lateral to the cannulation site, for catheter retention. The balloon may then be inserted and directed downward just below the left subclavian artery. Leaving the sternum unanchored, the catheter may exit at the inferior aspect of the midline incision. When balloon support is no longer necessary, the patient is returned to the operating room for balloon removal and aortic and sternal closure.

Although the method of arteriotomy is still widely used during cardiac surgery and is currently the procedure required during IAB pump insertion in infants and children, the most common insertion technique used today is the percutaneous method adapted by Bregman and Casarella.[31]

Percutaneous Intra-Aortic Balloon Pump

In 1979 a single-chambered 40-mL percutaneous IAB was constructed around a central wire.[32–34] The IAB was wrapped manually around the wire, which then allowed for percutaneous insertion into the femoral artery. A 12-French sheath-dilator assembly was previously inserted into the artery using the modified Seldinger technique.[35]

Difficulties with percutaneous insertion are sometimes encountered with the following circumstances:

1. Tortuous vessels
2. Weak femoral pulse
3. Dislodgement of atherosclerotic plaque on thrombus

A sheathless technique was introduced in November 1991. The advantage of this approach is that it allows a 30% reduction in the cross-sectional area of the artery punctured. By eliminating the 10-French sheath (11.5-French outer diameter), there have been fewer vascular complications. Nash and coworkers[36] reported a 10% incidence of limb ischemia, whereas prior studies cited rates as high as 31%.[37]

Technique of Percutaneous Insertion of the Intra-Aortic Balloon Pump

Using the modified Seldinger technique,[8] the 9.5-French Percor STAT DL percutaneous IAB is inserted in the following manner. First, the inguinal region is prepared and draped, and the common femoral artery is then punctured with an 18-gauge arterial needle (without puncturing the posterior wall of the artery). An 0.030-in (0.097-cm) Teflon-coated guide wire is introduced through the needle. The needle is then removed, and an 8-French dilator is passed over the guide wire to predilate the subcutaneous tissue and the arterial puncture site. The 8-French dilator is then removed, and a 10-French sheath-dilator combination is advanced over the guide wire. Allow approximately 1 in (2.5 cm) of the sheath to remain exposed because this acts to limit bleeding.

The percutaneous balloon should be prepared as follows. After removing the balloon from its sterile package under aseptic technique, connect the one-way valve to the IAB Luer-Lok connector and aspirate at least 30 mL with the 60-mL syringe. This allows any residual air to be removed from the balloon. At this point, remove the syringe from the one-way valve but leave the one-way valve connected to the IAB male Luer-Lok fitting. Vacuum is maintained on the balloon until the initiation of counterpulsation.

After balloon preparation, the IAB insertion should be carried out in the following sequence. First, measure the distance from Louis' angle to the umbilicus and then obliquely to the femoral insertion site. This allows a rough estimation of balloon positioning. Remove the inner stylet from the central lumen. Now the dilator is removed from the 10-French sheath, leaving the guide wire within the sheath. Some blood may leak after the dilator is removed. This is controllable by firmly pinching the exposed portion of the 10-French sheath. The 0.030-in guide wire is inserted into the central lumen of the IAB until it exits the female Luer-Lok fitting. The IAB is now advanced (ideally using fluoroscopy) over the guide wire into the descending aorta. The proper position of the IAB is approximately 2 cm distal to the left subclavian artery (Fig. 60–10). The 10-French sheath is pulled back somewhat to ensure that the entire membrane has exited the sheath; the amount of sheath exposed depends on the initial length used (6, 11, or 15 in).

At this point, the vacuum is released from the balloon by removing the one-way valve. The balloon catheter is attached to the balloon console, and counterpulsation commences once the system is operational (helium filled/balloon properly expanded). If the IAB pump was not able to be placed under fluoroscopy, a chest x-ray film is taken to visualize the radiopaque IAB tip to ensure proper placement. The patient should undergo immediate anticoagulation after insertion, and this should be maintained until the time of removal.

Although an IAB is placed more commonly with a 10-

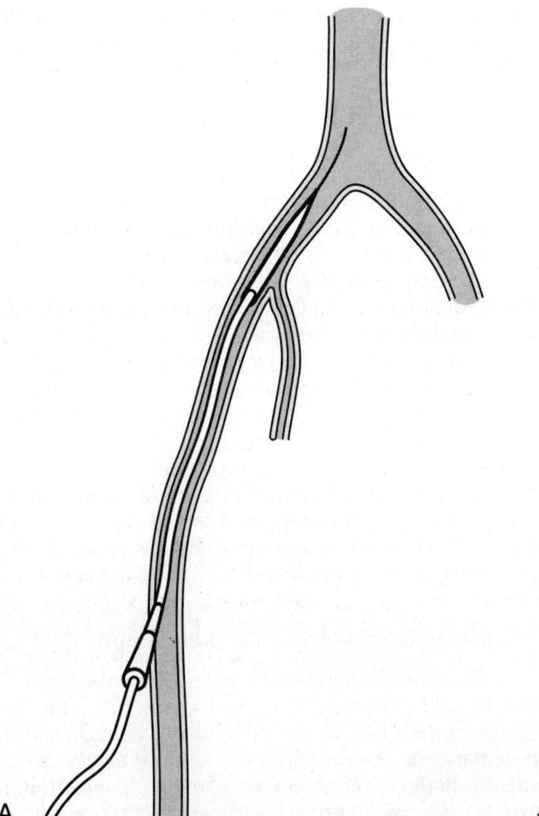

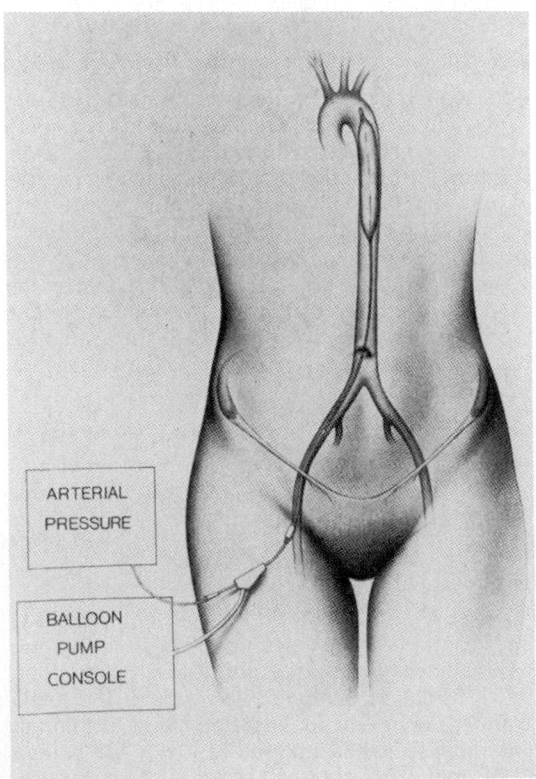

Figure 60–10. *A,* A single-chambered, dual-lumen IAB passing through the right iliac artery into the aorta. (From Kesselbrenner M, Bregman D: Mechanical support of the failing heart. *In:* Cardiopulmonary Bypass: Physiology, Related Complications and Pharmacology. Casthely PA, Bregman D [Eds]. Mount Kisco, NY, Futura, 1991, p 387.) *B,* Proper position of the IAB in the descending thoracic aorta. (From Kesselbrenner M, Sack J, Saporito R, et al: Intra-aortic balloon counterpulsation. *In:* Techniques in Extracorporeal Circulation. Kay PH [ed]. Oxford, Butterworth Heinemann, 1992, p 249.)

French sheath (outer diameter of 11.5 French), the technique gaining greater acceptance is the sheathless approach. This approach yields a 30% reduction in the cross-sectional area of the artery punctured. Nash[36] and Phillips[38] and their colleagues demonstrated significantly fewer vascular complications with this approach.

The technique for sheathless insertion is similar to the prior description. The artery is cannulated and a 0.030-in guide wire is passed into the descending aorta. A small incision is made at the exit site of the guide wire, and the skin and subcutaneous tissues are dilated with an 8-French or 9-French dilator. The dilator is removed, and firm pressure is applied to the area to control bleeding. Now the IAB (9.5-French) is advanced over the guide wire into the thoracic aorta, and counterpulsation is achieved in the usual fashion. Two modifications in the 9.5-French IAB has allowed for ease of insertion. First, a ballistic profile was incorporated into the catheter tip rather than the blunt design. Second, the ability to push was improved as the proximal end of the balloon was fused to the shaft more securely with a track weld.[36] Complications with this procedure have been kinking of the catheter and greater difficulty advancing the catheter through the soft tissues. However, the reduction in vascular complications appears to significantly outweigh the difficulties that may be encountered with insertion.

IDEAL BALLOON FUNCTION

The primary goals of IAB pumping are to implement the maximal increase in coronary blood flow during diastole and at the same time effect a decrease in left ventricular work.[6] Realization that these two beneficial effects are dependent on one another permits maximal benefit to be obtained from each factor in the following manner: The diastolic augmentation ordinarily begins at the dicrotic notch (Fig. 60–11) using an initial sequence of 1:3, whereby every third ventricular beat is augmented by the IAB. One can encroach on the dicrotic notch to begin balloon inflation slightly earlier in diastole. Provided the patient does not have premature ventricular contractions from this manipulation, it can be performed in patients who appear to be responding poorly to IAB pumping to give them additional benefit. The right-hand side or down slope of the augmentation is the part most intimately involved with the ventricular unloading aspect of IAB pumping. If the fall in left ventricular end-diastolic pressure is too great, the following sequence of events occurs. Excessive decrease in left ventricular end-diastolic pressure essentially means that the balloon has collapsed too soon before the aortic valve has opened. Because blood must flow to occupy the space of the formerly expanded balloon, it flows retrograde from all branches of the aorta, including the coronary arteries (if the decrease in left ventricular end-diastolic pressure is excessive).[6] Therefore, one must effect a compromise and have some, but not excessive, decrease in left ventricular end-diastolic pressure. Recent experimental and clinical work has indicated that this decrease in left ventricular end-diastolic pressure should not exceed 10 mm Hg.

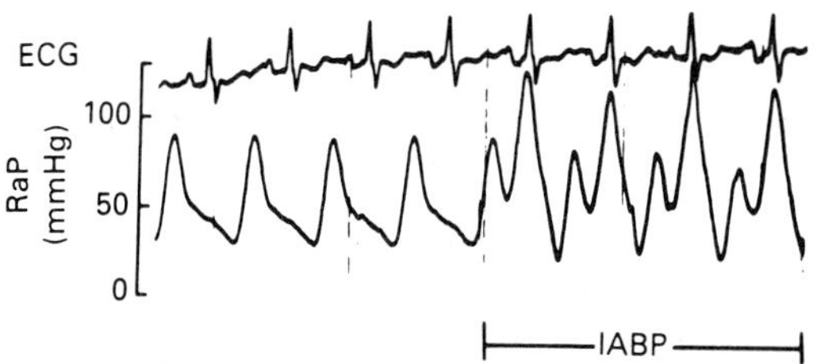

Figure 60–11. IAB pump function in a patient with cardiogenic shock. Note the fall in systolic pressure, large augmentation in diastolic pressure, and fall in end-diastolic pressure. (From Kesselbrenner M, Sack J, Saporito R, et al: Intra-aortic balloon counterpulsation. *In:* Techniques in Extracorporeal Circulation. Kay PH [Ed]. Oxford, Butterworth Heinemann, 1992, p 251.)

As far as the position of the balloon is concerned, we initially place the balloon as far proximally in the aorta as possible (i.e., with the tip of the balloon just distal to the left subclavian artery). Be sure to feel the pulse in the left arm so that the tip of the balloon is not the subclavian orifice and is not occluding the left subclavian inflow.

At rapid heart rates, there is more dead space in the safety chamber balloon. Therefore, one could increase the volume of carbon dioxide in the safety chamber balloon (e.g., to 45 mL with a 30-mL balloon) at heart rates of greater than 120 beats per minute. This will improve IAB function.[39]

In this clinical setting, heart rates of up to 140 beats per minute can usually be followed with the smaller balloon. If the rate is higher, it may be necessary to assist on 1:2 (every other beat) to achieve effective diastolic augmentation until the rate slows, when 1:1 assistance can be instituted.

If weaning a patient from IAB assistance is undertaken by changing from a 1:1 to a 1:2 or 1:3 assisting sequence, additional time will be present for the vacuum to build up, and augmentation may demonstrate a deep "sink"; the end-diastolic point may need elevation by a minor adjustment on the console.

Paramount for effective counterpulsation is the timing of balloon inflation and deflation. A pulse contour recorder within the central lumen or a radial arterial monitor will display a pressure waveform on the console screen. An electronic signal, which may be manually maneuvered within the cardiac cycle, then indicates balloon inflation and deflation.

For optimal augmentation of hemodynamics, the balloon should be deflated just before left ventricular ejection (i.e., at the QRS complex). Delay would present the ventricle with an obstruction to outflow. If deflated too early, the vacuum effect to enhance cardiac output not only is compromised but may actually hinder left ventricular ejection, thereby markedly decreasing cardiac output.

Inflation should take place during the dicrotic notch of the arterial pressure wave, corresponding to the peak of the T wave on the ECG. Early expansion creates increased afterload for the contracting ventricle. Delayed expansion will decrease coronary perfusion and create less diastolic augmentation. Most newer consoles will automatically collapse the balloon in case of timing errors.

Obviously, cardiac arrhythmias will also alter the efficiency of the IAB counterpulsation owing to the reliance of timing of balloon inflation and deflation on the surface ECG. Therefore, every effort should be made to suppress cardiac arrhythmias while the patient is on IAB support. Atrial arrhythmias, especially atrial fibrillation with a rapid ventricular response, may also lead to inadequate augmentation.

PERCUTANEOUS CLINICAL EXPERIENCE

Percutaneous IAB insertion was attempted in 202 patients from February 1979 to January 1985 at the Columbia-Presbyterian Medical Center (Table 60–4). Successful insertion was accomplished in 196 of 202 patients (97%). In 10 patients, the initial insertion attempt failed; however, 4 of the 10 patients eventually underwent successful IAB pump implantation when the 28-cm sheath-dilator combination was used.

TABLE 60–4. Experience with Percutaneous Intra-Aortic Balloon Pumping at Columbia-Presbyterian Medical Center 1979–1985*

Variable	*Successful Insertions*	*CCU*	*Cath Lab*
Preoperative	Unstable angina with general surgery	1	—
	Unstable angina with cardiac surgery	18 (3)	13 (2)
	Unstable angina—treated with medication	4 (1)	1
	Postinfarction angina—treated with medication	4 (2)	4 (1)
	Postinfarction angina with surgery	10 (1)	3
	Cardiogenic shock—treated with medication	2	4 (3)
	Cardiogenic shock with surgery	2	5 (2)
	Cardiac arrest	4 (3)	1
	Recurrent ventricular tachycardia—medication	1	—
	Failed Gruentzig procedure with emergency surgery	—	6 (2)
	Acute VSD with surgery	1	2 (1)
	Acute VSD without surgery	—	1 (1)
	Anesthesia support for open heart surgery	6 (1)	12 (1)
Perioperative	Low output—OR	71 (44)	
Postoperative	Low output	16 (9)	
	Cardiac arrest	4 (3)	
Total number assisted		196	
Total number discharged		116 (60%)	

*Parentheses indicate number of deaths.
Abbreviations: VSD = ventricular septal defect; OR = operating room; CCU = critical care unit; Cath = catheterization.

Indications in these patients were broadly divided among medical surgical groups. Of 196 patients, 91 received the IAB for a surgical indication. Surgical indications included intraoperative low cardiac output in 71, postoperative low output syndrome in 16, and cardiac arrest in 4. Medical indications for counterpulsation with the IAB included unstable angina refractory to medical management in 36, postinfarction angina in 21, cardiogenic shock in 13, acute ventricular septal defect complicating myocardial infarction in 4, and recurrent ventricular tachycardia in 1. Six patients received the IAB when hemodynamic decompensation occurred during transluminal coronary angioplasty. All six patients required surgical coronary revascularization. Only one patient received the IAB prophylactically for unstable angina before a general surgical procedure. This patient survived, and the balloon was removed in the immediate postoperative period.

The location of IAB pump insertion varied. Seventy-one patients had the balloon implanted in the operating room, 20 in the open heart surgery recovery room, 52 in the cardiac catheterization laboratory, and 53 in the cardiac intensive care unit.

Of the 105 patients in whom the IAB pump was successfully inserted for a medical indication (Fig. 60–12), 79 (75%) eventually underwent a cardiac surgical procedure, whereas 26 (25%) were treated medically. Only 13 of the 79 patients (16%) undergoing preoperative IAB support combined with a definitive surgical procedure died. In contrast, 56 of the 91 patients (61%) requiring intraoperative and postoperative IAB died.

COMPLICATIONS ASSOCIATED WITH INTRA-AORTIC BALLOONS

The nature of IAB insertion and function, as well as the critical status of those patients requiring its use, presents potential for major complications. Alcan and associates[40] collected data on 321 patients from 1974 to 1982 who required IAB counterpulsation for a variety of reasons under both emergent and controlled situations. They reported major complications in 9% of patients who had undergone IAB counterpulsation. Complications ranged from thrombosis and embolization, which accounted for greater than half of these, to aortic dissection in one patient. However, if a contingency exists, it is believed that risk factors include severity of peripheral vascular disease, extent of myocardial failure, significant long-standing hypertension, diabetes, female sex, and duration of use.

The principle complications associated with IAB pumping fall into six main categories:

1. Trauma to the arterial wall incurred while inserting and advancing the guide wire or balloon (laceration, dissection, subadventitial hematoma)
2. Limb ischemia associated with the position of the balloon catheter, which disappears with catheter removal
3. Dislodged thrombus created during balloon removal, resulting in distal embolization (peripheral, testicular, renal)
4. Hematologic (thrombocytopenia, red blood cell hemolysis, hemorrhage)
5. Balloon leak/rupture
6. Infection

The most extensive review of IAB pump complications was done by Kantrowitz and colleagues,[41] which includes more than 700 patients. Infectious and vascular complications were most common. There was an increased frequency of infectious complications when the IAB was not inserted in the operating room.

Additionally, the longer the balloon was left in place, the

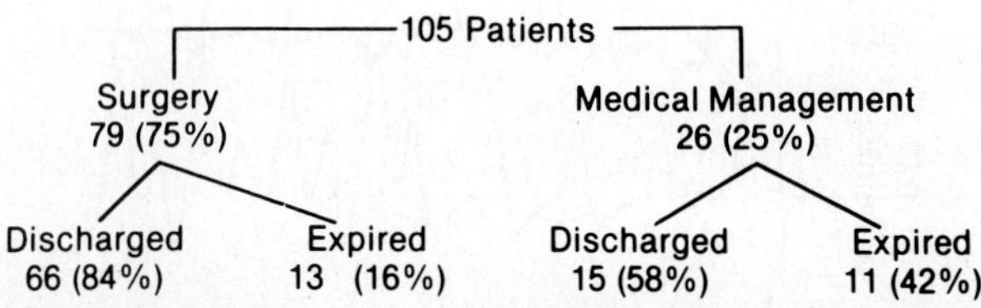

Figure 60–12. Results of the use of percutaneous IAB pumping for medical indications in 105 patients at the Columbia-Presbyterian Medical Center between 1979 and 1985. (From Kesselbrenner M, Sack J, Saporito R, et al: Intra-aortic balloon counterpulsation. *In:* Techniques in Extracorporeal Circulation. Kay PH [Ed]. Oxford, Butterworth Heinemann, 1992, p 253.)

greater was the incidence of infectious complications. Freed[42] reviewed the complications in patients requiring IAB pump support for 20 days or longer and found an increase in the infection rate of 67% versus 25%. Prolonged support in this same study showed more vascular (37 versus 15%) and more bleeding (26 versus 15%) complications. Freed concluded that prolonged support offered only a temporizing benefit (in patients with congestive heart failure) when a surgically correctable disease was lacking.

Despite the demonstrable technologic advances, vascular complications remain the major risk. Although the advent of the percutaneous insertion technique has allowed easier placement and expanded usage, there are clearly more vascular complications than with the surgical approach (31 versus 16%).[37] However, the sheathless percutaneous approach has significantly reduced this complication rate to as low as 10%.[36] The major risk factors for vascular complications are a history of peripheral vascular disease or diabetes mellitus, female gender, and a low ankle-brachial index.

The incidence of limb ischemia has been reported to range from 5% to 19%. The removal of the IAB pump from a compromised limb limits the development of permanent sequelae to 1% to 3%.[42, 43]

Isner and associates[44] found that 60% of the complications of the IAB appear to result from trauma associated with insertion of the catheter. These included aortoiliac dissection, arterial perforation, and dislodged atherosclerotic plaque. In addition, it was noted that the older the patient, the more likely it is that atherosclerotic disease will diminish the arterial lumen diameter, resulting in a greater potential for insertion damage. Along with these more common types of complications, several notable ones have appeared. For example, a patient presented with an improperly positioned IAB that intermittently occluded the origin of the superior mesenteric artery. The resulting abdominal pain was relieved on advancing the balloon to its "correct position."[45] Rodigas and Bridges[46] reported an occlusion of the left internal mammary artery by an improperly positioned balloon catheter. Busch and coauthors[47] reported a splenic infarction precipitated by IAB placement. In addition, there have been several instances of paraplegia related to balloon pumping.

BALLOON RUPTURE/LEAK

Balloon rupture is reported to occur in approximately 1% to 4% of patients. This incidence may approach 5% in patients at higher risk such as those who underwent reoperative coronary artery bypass grafting (CABG) and older patients secondary to atherosclerotic disease and plaque. Speculation as to the cause of balloon rupture centers around plaque abrasion. After prolonged usage, atherosclerotic plaque abrades the balloon membrane and may cause balloon leak and rupture. Stahl and associates[48] described a small series of patients in which IAB rupture occurred approximately 4.7 days after insertion. The patients found to be at risk for rupture were those with a history of hypertension, those with marked diastolic augmentation, and women. It is hypothesized that marked diastolic augmentation results from complete occlusion of the aorta in diastole and, therefore, greater coaptation of the balloon with the aortic wall. Inherently, this would allow more contact time for plaque to denude the balloon membrane and cause rupture/leak (Fig. 60–13).

Cox and colleagues[49] observed that female patients had an unusually high rate of IAB rupture. After microscopic examination of the balloon membrane, extensive plaque abrasion was found in the proximal portion. It was theorized that the IAB was more readily traumatized in the narrow portions of the aorta in these typically shorter patients (<65 in). Once the balloon size was changed from 40 mL to 34 mL in patients shorter than 65 in, no further ruptures were seen.

CLINICAL INDICATIONS

Myocardial Infarction with Shock

Initially, it was believed that the IAB balloon pump would be the physicians' salvation in the management of patients with acute myocardial infarction and shock. In fact, when a given patient who was in shock syndrome secondary to acute myocardial infarction was placed on IAB pump support, the patient invariably showed some clinical improvement. However, as the major experience has evolved throughout the world with support of cardiogenic shock patients on the IAB pump,[50–58] certain basic and consistent observations have been made. Offering balloon support to patients who have been in cardiogenic shock for extended periods of time is not practical.[59] Although frequently there is improvement in the patients' hemodynamic factors, organ function has often reached irreversible deterioration, and the ultimate outcome of these patients is uniformly fatal. Therefore, it appears more advisable to try to insert the IAB pump early in the course of cardiogenic shock.

A report by Hagemeijer and coauthors[60] involved 25 patients with New York Heart Association class III or IV acute myocardial infarction who were treated with IAB pumping during a 4-year period. Twenty of these patients were successfully weaned from the IAB pump; yet 6 died within 3 months, and 5 within the first 10 days of balloon weaning. Of the 14 patients who survived for more than 3 months, 13 were classified as functional class II. Six have resumed full

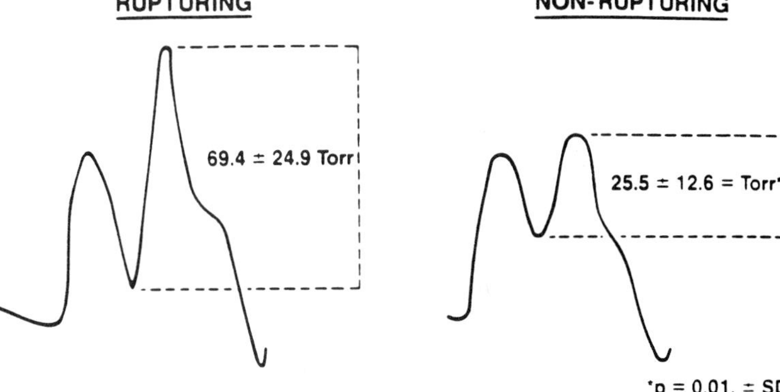

Figure 60–13. Diastolic augmentation in rupturing and nonrupturing IABs. Note that the augmentation in diastolic pressure was 2.5 times greater in patients with rupturing balloons than in patients with nonrupturing balloons. (From Stahl KD, Tortolani J, Nelson RL, et al: Intra-aortic balloon rupture. Trans Am Soc Artif Intern Organs 1988; 34:497.)

activity. This report indicates that the early application of IAB pumping during cardiac shock associated with acute myocardial infarction may improve patient survival. In addition, it is generally thought that enhanced coronary blood flow reduces the propensity for new clot formation and increases exposure of disrupted plaque to antiplatelet agents. By improving diastolic flow, IAB pumping may prove "protective" in the setting of preventing reocclusion of an infarct-related artery after a patient has received either percutaneous transluminal coronary angioplasty (PTCA) or thrombolytic therapy.

An overall survival rate of 30% to 85% has been reported for patients in cardiogenic shock secondary to either a mechanical defect complicating acute myocardial infarction or in patients with cardiogenic shock treated by the combination of IAB pumping and surgery.[61]

In a report of IAB use in 728 patients,[62] the rate of IAB pump-related mortality was only 0.8%, and the survival of a large number of patients with acute myocardial ischemia was attributed to the use of the IAB pump. The success of this treatment modality, coupled with its low mortality rate, has encouraged many authors[63–72] to advocate the earlier institution of IAB counterpulsation support for cardiogenic shock.

Still unresolved completely is the question of how to proceed after the institution of the counterpulsation. If the patient is completely stable on the IAB pump, it has been suggested that the maximal benefit from IAB counterpulsation will be achieved after 5 days of support. Accordingly, attempts should be made to wean the patient from balloon support at this time. Catheterization studies should be done if the clinical situation warrants. If the catheterization studies then indicate that the patient should undergo either CABG or PTCA, the definitive procedure should be performed during the same hospitalization period.

The patients who may best profit from this therapeutic route seem to be those who respond most promptly to the IAB and those who have major ischemic changes on their ECG that return to normal with the onset of IAB pumping.

The mortality rate for patients with cardiogenic shock who have an IAB placed early and ultimately undergo coronary revascularization surgery is being reported in excess of 50%.[14] It is clear that aggressive early revascularization with bypass surgery has led to a much higher survival rate.[73] However, if the patient becomes dependent on the IAB support and cannot be successfully weaned with the addition of pharmacologic maneuvers (i.e., inotropic support), this situation has uniformly led to a nearly 100% mortality, even when surgical intervention is attempted.

SAFETY WITH THROMBOLYTIC THERAPY

As alluded to previously, the safety record of the IAB pump when used in patients receiving thrombolytic therapy is encouraging. Goodwin and coworkers[74] retrospectively reviewed patients given streptokinase and IAB counterpulsation between 1985 and 1987. They found no statistically significant differences among three groups—those treated with streptokinase during acute myocardial infarction, those with acute myocardial infarction or unstable angina treated with IAB counterpulsation without thrombolysis, and those treated with streptokinase followed by IAB counterpulsation—with regard to requirement of surgical repair of the femoral artery, percentage of patients requiring transfusion, and number of units of packed red blood cells transfused (Fig. 60–14). They suggested that IAB pumping may be used safely and early in patients with acute myocardial infarction who receive thrombolytic therapy. Of note is that the complication rate of patients treated with thrombolysis and IAB pumping compared with that of patients treated with heparin alone was no greater.

Ohman and colleagues[75] prospectively evaluated 810 patients who were entered in the thrombolysis and angioplasty in myocardial infarction I, II, and III (TAMI) and urokinase trials. In these trials, 85 patients had an IAB pump inserted. This observational study supports the use of IAB counterpulsation with thrombolysis. Although there is a greater incidence of bleeding (59 versus 17%) and vascular trauma (12 versus 2%) with the IAB pump patients, these patients benefited from an absence of reocclusion of the infarct-related artery or reinfarction. Follow-up of these patients demonstrated a significant improvement in overall and noninfarct zone regional left ventricular function.

Although not definitely proven, the proposed physiologic mechanisms yielding these benefits may be as follows: (1) enhanced diastolic coronary artery perfusion pressure, (2) afterload reduction, allowing less myocardial oxygen demand, (3) improved and maintained collateral blood flow, and (4) improved flow to non–infarct-related myocardium (especially across a critical stenosis).

Even though the vascular complication rate was higher in the balloon pump group, it was within the accepted range of that for previously reported trials not using thrombolytic agents. Hence, the insertion of an IAB pump with thrombolysis (within the first 24 hours) is safe despite a small increase in bleeding and vascular complications. If an IAB pump is indicated after use of a thrombolytic agent, then the IAB pump should not be withheld.

Additionally, because these trials used an 11-French sheath, one would expect that as the sheathless approach is used more frequently (demonstrated to have less bleeding and vascular complication) after thrombolytic therapy, even fewer bleeding and vascular complications will result.

PREOPERATIVE INTRA-AORTIC BALLOON PUMPING IN HIGH-RISK CARDIAC PATIENTS

The risks of early infarction and death in patients with acute coronary insufficiency undergoing cardiac surgery are generally considered greater than those of patients with stable angina pectoris. The most appropriate therapy, however, and the timing of that therapy are points of controversy. Cooper and colleagues[76] reported on 63 high-risk myocardial revascularization patients who had preoperative IAB pumping. Only six patients required rapid institution of cardiopulmonary bypass after anesthesia induction despite a marked drop in blood pressure in 50% of the patients. There were two instances of postpump power failure, with two deaths in this series. The authors concluded from this experience that preoperative IAB pumping is a valid method of limiting morbidity associated with coronary surgery in high-risk patients.

Scully and associates[64] studied the effects of preoperative IAB pumping in 42 patients with acute coronary insufficiency complicated by abnormal left ventricular hemodynamics and refractory chest pain. Aggressive medical therapy had previously failed in all cases. The perioperative mortality rate, when compared with that of similar patients treated before and after the use of the IAB pump, was lowered from 25% to 8%.[63, 71, 77] In addition, inotropic support and duration of stay, both in the intensive care unit and in the hospital, were significantly decreased in the patients treated preoperatively with the IAB pump. Bolooki and colleagues[78] also reported a shorter time on cardiopulmonary bypass, and Feola and colleagues[79] noted an improvement in metabolic status as measured by decreased cardiac lactate production.

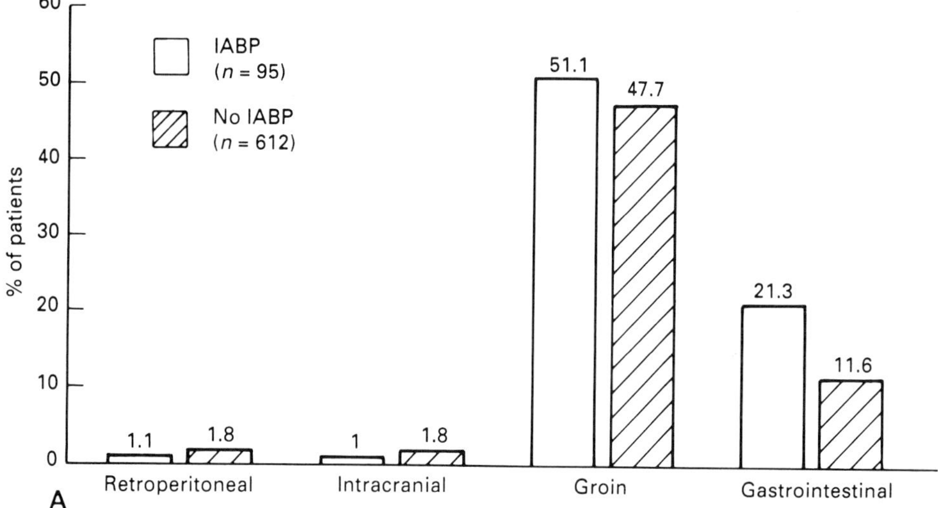

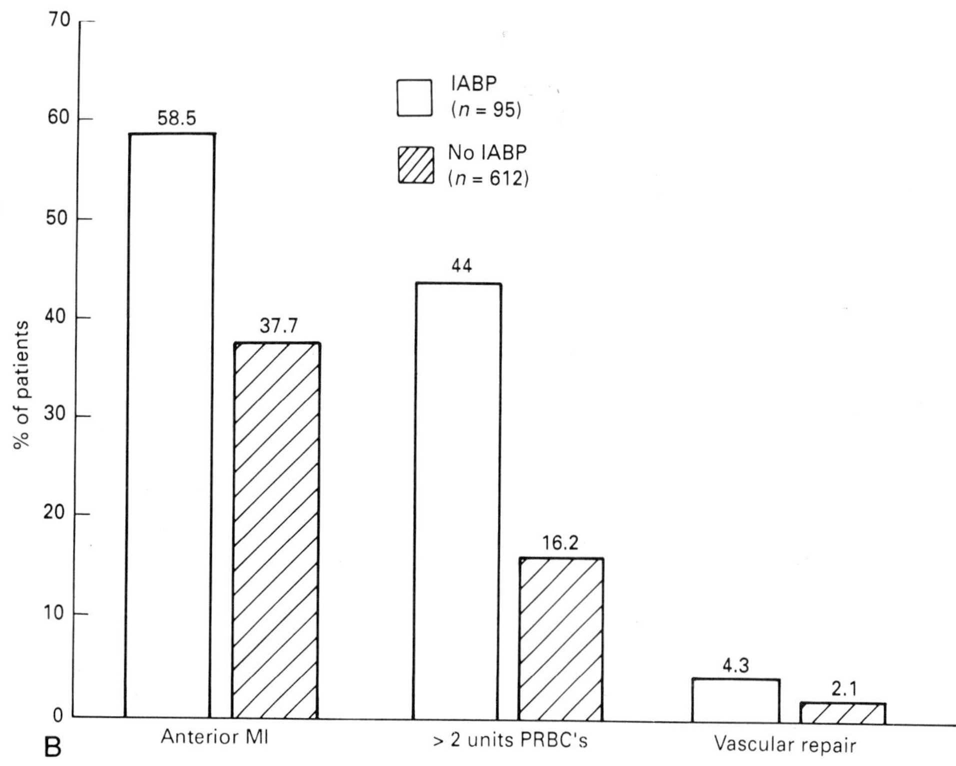

Figure 60–14. IAB pump use during the Thrombolysis and Angioplasty in Myocardial Infarction (TAMI) trials. *A,* No greater incidence of bleeding complications occurred in the group that received treatment with IAB pumps as compared with the group that did not. *B,* Although the IAB pump patients required more than 2 units of packed red blood cells (PRBCs) more often than the non-IAB pump patients, the difference between the two groups was not statistically significant. (From Kesselbrenner M, Sack J, Saporito R, et al: Intra-aortic balloon counterpulsation. *In:* Techniques in Extracorporeal Circulation. Kay PH [Ed]. Oxford, Butterworth Heinemann, 1992, p 258.)

INTRA-AORTIC BALLOON COUNTERPULSATION WITH "HIGH-RISK" ANGIOPLASTY

Several investigators reviewed the use of IAB pump counterpulsation with high-risk angioplasty. These include patients with poor left ventricular function, acute myocardial infarction, unstable angina, multiple vessel disease, advanced age, or advanced age (>70 years) patients with 40% to 50% of the myocardium jeopardized. Kahn and colleagues[80] reported on 28 high-risk patients over a 30-month period. They found a 96% initial PTCA success rate with no deaths or myocardial infarctions in the first 72 hours.

In examining the TAMI data, Califf and Ohman[81] discovered that only 7% of 85 patients who had undergone PTCA while on the IAB pump had reocclusion. More important, however, none of the reocclusions occurred while the IAB pump was in place. They further proposed the mechanism of prevention of reocclusion; as alluded to previously, improved diastolic blood pressures translates into improved coronary blood flow. This may reduce the propensity for clot formation while increasing the delivery time of antiplatelet agents and anticoagulants. In addition, improved coronary filling pressure may prevent closure of the initial flap made during PTCA against the opposing wall of the vessel.

Ishihara and colleagues[82] prospectively evaluated the role of the IAB pump in patients requiring emergent PTCA. This study included 116 patients with an acute anterior wall myocardial infarction. Of these patients, 66 were treated with conventional therapy after PTCA and 48 were treated with the IAB pump in addition to conventional therapy. The results of this study add support to prior reports[40, 74, 82] that the IAB pump is highly effective in patients undergoing revascularization. In this study, there was a 2.4% reocclusion rate with the IAB pump versus 17.7% without it (Fig. 60–15). The authors cited augmented diastolic pressures as the probable cause of sustained coronary perfusion and prevented reocclusion. This study also demonstrated a twofold increase in the left ventricular ejection fraction (Fig. 60–16). The suspected mechanisms for these improvements remain (1) prevention of reocclusion, (2) augmented diastolic pressure, (3) reduction in afterload-less myocardial oxygen consumption, and (4) potentially limiting infarct expansion and ventricular remodeling.

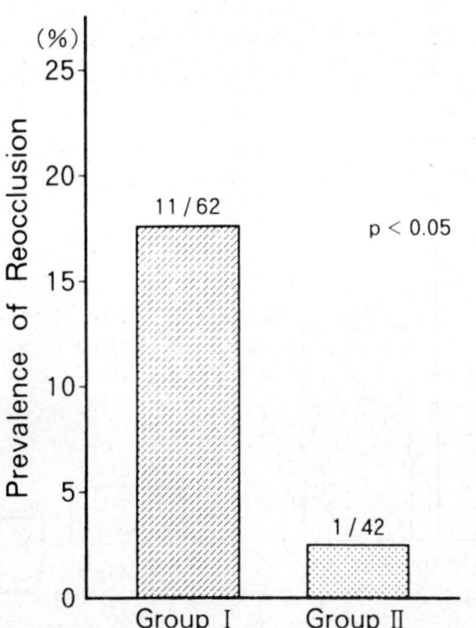

Figure 60–15. Incidence of reocclusion in two groups. Eleven of 62 patients in group I (no IAB pump) had reocclusion, whereas reocclusion occurred in only 1 of 42 patients in group II (IAB pump used) (17.7 versus 2.4%, $P < .05$). (From Ishihara M, Sato H, Tateishi H, et al: Intra-aortic balloon pumping as the postangioplasty strategy in acute myocardial infarction. Am Heart J 1991; 122:387.)

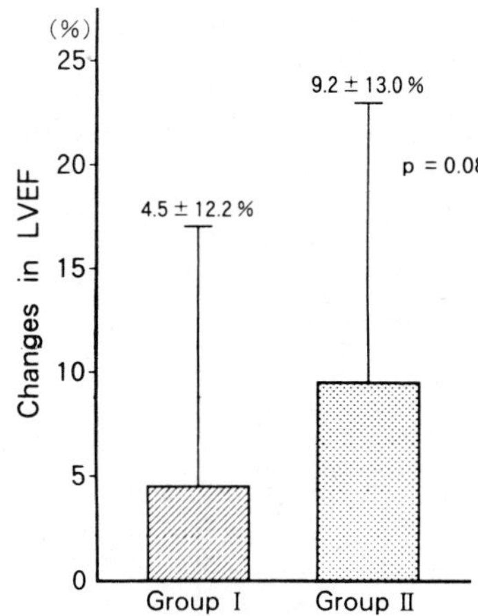

Figure 60–16. Changes in left ventricular ejection fraction (LVEF) as assessed by serial contrast ventriculography. Compared with group I, an increase in LVEF in group II attained marginal significance (4.5 ± 12.2% versus 9.2 ± 13.0%, $P = .08$). (From Ishihara M, Sato H, Tateishi H, et al: Intra-aortic balloon pumping as the postangioplasty strategy in acute myocardial infarction. Am Heart J 1991; 122:387.)

Anwar and coworkers[83] evaluated the role of IAB pump counterpulsation in elective high-risk PTCA patients. This was a two-center study involving a population with a left ventricular ejection fraction of less than 35% (26% with ejection fraction <25%), class III and class IV angina (92%), prior myocardial infarction (80%), and multivessel disease (81.5%). They reported an 85.6% (n = 83) success rate, with 82.5% (n = 80) being discharged from the hospital. Follow-up at 22 months (N = 72) showed that 72% (n = 52) sustained a myocardial infarction and were alive. Of the 20 deaths that occurred (28%), 4 were noncardiac and 16 were cardiac. The authors concluded that IAB pump counterpulsation is an attractive adjunct to the management of high-risk patients when considering PTCA. However, despite the early benefit, these patients still remain at high risk for late cardiac mortality.

TACHYARRHYTHMIA AND VENTRICULAR IRRITABILITY

The increase in coronary blood flow associated with the use of the IAB pump as well as the decrease in myocardial wall tension as a result of the acute reduction in left ventricular afterload is ideally suited for the treatment of refractory ventricular tachyarrhythmia both in the setting of the coronary care unit and in the postoperative surgical patient.[39] Unfortunately, although the treatment of tachyarrhythmia after open heart surgery with the IAB pump can frequently be definitive,[52] it is underused in this setting. Likewise, in the coronary care unit, many patients with ventricular irritability can be stabilized and the frequency of their arrhythmias decreased significantly. It is the policy of these authors to catheterize every medical patient on an IAB pump whose indication for insertion has been ventricular tachyarrhythmia so that the patient's anatomy can be defined and surgical intervention can proceed if indicated.

Mundth and colleagues[51] indicated that in the medical setting life-threatening, recurrent ventricular tachyarrhythmia in the acute postinfarction phase and in chronic coronary disease can be controlled initially with IAB pumping as a prelude to cardiac catheterization and cardiac surgery. Ten patients with recurrent ventricular tachyarrhythmia underwent cardiac surgery, and seven of those patients survived.

Williams and coauthors[84] reported success with IAB pumping therapy even when no surgically correctable lesion is present. They recommended the use of the IAB pump for all patients who experience ventricular arrhythmias and low nodal bradyarrhythmia that are refractory to standard medical therapy.

SEPTIC SHOCK

Initally, the physiologic response to sepsis is an increase in cardiac output, the limitation of which is posed by both Starling law and the functional cardiac reserve of the individual patient. Ultimately, the patient in septic shock will experience a low cardiac output state mediated by "myocardial depressant factors," and if the appropriate medical therapy fails, death will ensue. Berger and colleagues[14] reported on the fortuitous use of the IAB pump in a patient with septic shock who was initially thought to have a myocardial infarction with low-output state. The distinct improvement in this patient prompted the authors to use the IAB pump in another patient with septic shock. In both of these patients, cardiac output could be maintained while the appropriate treatment, including antibiotics and steroids, could be administered. Our experience has also justified the concept of IAB pumping in septic shock patients with low cardiac output syndrome. Indeed, Berger's two initial patients were ultimately discharged from the hospital. Since then, other investigators[71] considered septic shock an indication for use of the IAB pump.

MYOCARDIAL CONTUSION

Myocardial contusion complicates approximately 20% of cases of blunt anterior thoracic chest wall trauma.[85] Injuries caused by steering wheels are the most prevalent cause of myocardial contusion. Unfortunately, the diagnosis is frequently delayed or missed, complicating the treatment of myocardial contusion, which may, in turn, affect the treatment of associated injuries.

One of the most important physiologic consequences of myocardial contusion, which is always associated with severe blunt chest wall trauma, is decreased cardiac output. Proper treatment may be a major determinant of survival in some cases of myocardial contusion. Although clinical IAB pumping therapy for myocardial contusion has yet to be reported in the literature, Saunders and Doty[85] applied this technique in dogs with experimentally induced myocardial contusion. The results of their study show that IAB pumping does, in fact, improve left ventricular performance after myocardial contusion, especially when applied early after injury.

LONG-TERM SURVIVAL OF INTRA-AORTIC BALLOON PUMP PATIENTS

The ability of the IAB pump to hemodynamically support and stabilize the failing circulation is well established. However, does the short-term stabilization of patients by the IAB pump result in improved long-term survival for any group of patients? Because most of the patients requiring IAB counterpulsation would have otherwise succumbed in the short term, intuitively, the IAB pump has improved their long-term outlook. These patients most certainly would not have survived to hospital discharge had it not been for IAB pump support. One must consider this fact when reviewing the literature concerning long-term survival of IAB pump patients. Several investigators have studied this issue.

The first study of the long-term effect of balloon pumping was initiated by Bolooki and colleagues.[78] They examined 43 patients who required IAB pump support to be weaned off the cardiopulmonary bypass circuit. Twenty-three patients (53%) were discharged from the hospital and were living 4 months or longer. Golding and coworkers[86] at the Cleveland Clinic, studied 197 patients who underwent IAB pumping pre-, peri-, or postoperatively. Of the 197 patients, 143 (72.6%) were discharged from the hospital. The 2-year cardiac actuarial survival for the hospital survivors was 96% (n = 134). Eighty-five percent of the surviving patients remained asymptomatic during the follow-up period. Golding also reported that the survival statistics for patients who required IAB pumping in conjunction with myocardial revascularization were similar to those for patients who did not require IAB pump assistance. This becomes even more significant assuming that the patients requiring support, in general, are a sicker group of patients.

LONG-TERM SUPPORT BY INTRA-AORTIC BALLOON PUMP

There have been several instances in which patients have remained on the IAB pump for an extended period of time (greater than 3–5 days). Except for patient discomfort associated with a lengthy immobilization of the catheterized limb, no toxicity has been associated with long-term balloon pumping.[87] Brantigan, Grow, and Schoonmaker[88] reported on a woman with peripartum cardiomyopathy who was balloon dependent for 7 weeks and who improved during this period; she died 3 weeks after balloon removal.

The majority of patients on long-term balloon support can not be weaned off and are in fact balloon dependent. Most often, these are patients with end-stage coronary artery disease and cardiomyopathy, although several instances of septicemia with cardiogenic shock have been reported (Frazier et al., 1986).[89]

In 1978, Reemtsma and colleagues[90] reported successful heart transplantation in two patients maintained on the IAB pump. Both patients were discharged and survived for more than 1 year. Subsequent to this, Bregman[91] reported another four cardiac transplantations performed on balloon-maintained patients. These four patients survived the operation, with one living 12 months; the other three patients died within a month from acute transplant rejection.

References

1. Braunwald E, Covell JW, Maroko DR, et al: Effects of drugs and of counterpulsation on myocardial oxygen consumption. Circulation 1969; 38 and 40(Suppl IV):1–220.
2. Kantrowitz A, Mckinnon WM: The experimental use of the diaphragm as an auxiliary myocardium. Surg Forum 1958; 9:266.
3. Kantrowitz A: Experimental augmentation of coronary flow by retardation of the arterial pressure pulse. Surgery 1969; 34:678.
4. Moulopoulos SD, Topaz S, Kolff WJ: Diastolic balloon pumping (with carbon dioxide) in the aorta: A mechanical assistance to the failing circulation. Am Heart J 1962; 63:669.
5. Moulopoulos SD, Topaz S, Kolff WJ: Extracorporeal assistance to the circulation and intra-aortic balloon pumping. ASAIO Trans 1962; 8:85.
6. Corday E, Swan JC, Lang TW, et al: Physiologic principles in the application of circulatory assist for the failing heart. Am J Cardiol 1970; 26:595.
7. Bregman D, Bailin M, Bowman FO Jr, et al: A pulsatile assist

device (PAD) for improved myocardial protection during cardiopulmonary bypass. Ann Thorac Surg 1977; 24:574.
8. Nachlas HM, Sieband MP: The influence of diastolic augmentation on infarct size following coronary artery ligation. J Thorac Cardiovasc Surg 1967; 53:698.
9. Feola M, Limet RR, Glick G: Direct and reflex vascular effects of intra-aortic balloon counterpulsation in dogs at four levels of aortic pressure. Clin Res 1971; 19:313.
10. Weber KT, Janicki JS: Intra-aortic counterpulsation: A review of physiological principles, clinical results and device safety. Ann Thorac Surg 1974; 17:602.
11. Gold HK, Leinbach RC, Buckley MJ, et al: Refractory angina pectoris: Follow-up after intra-aortic balloon pumping and surgery. Circulation 1976; 54(Suppl III):41.
12. Johnson SA, Scanlon PL, Loeb HS, et al: Treatment of cardiogenic shock in myocardial infarction by intra-aortic balloon counterpulsation and surgery. Am J Med 1977; 62:687.
13. Maroko PN, Berstein EF, Lippy P, et al: Effects of intra-aortic balloon counterpulsation on the severity of myocardial ischemic injury following acute coronary occlusion. Circulation 1972; 45:1150.
14. Berger RL, Saini VK, Long W, et al: The use of diastolic augmentation with the intra-aortic balloon pump in human septic shock with associated coronary artery disease. Surgery 1973; 62:906.
15. Jacoby JA, Craddock LD, Wolf PS, et al: Clinical experience with counterpulsation in coronary artery disease. J Thorac Cardiovasc Surg 1968; 56:846.
16. Cox JL, McLaughlin VW, Flowers NC, et al: The ischemic zone surrounding acute myocardial infarction: Its morphology as detected by dehydrogenase staining. Am Heart J 1968; 76:650.
17. Wolvek S: The evolution of the intra-aortic balloon: The Datascope contribution. J Biomed Applications 1989; 3:527.
18. Bregman D: Management of patients undergoing intra-aortic balloon pumping. Heart Lung 1974; 3:916.
19. Feola M, Wiener L, Walinsky P, et al: Improved survival after coronary bypass surgery in patients with poor left ventricular function: Role of intra-aortic balloon counterpulsation. Am J Cardiol 1977; 39:1021.
20. Freed PS, Wasfie T, Zado B, et al: Intra-aortic balloon pumping for prolonged circulatory support. Am J Cardiol 1988; 61:554–557.
21. Summers DN, Kaplitt M, Morris J, et al: Intra-aortic balloon pumping: Hemodynamic and metabolic effects during cardiogenic shock in patients with triple coronary artery obstructive disease. Arch Surg 1969; 99:733.
22. American Heart Association: Heart Facts. New York, American Heart Association, 1981.
23. Norman NA, Kennedy JH: Arterial baroreceptor responses to intra-aortic balloon assistance. J Surg Res 1971; 11:396.
24. Yellin E, Levy L, Bregman D: Hemodynamic effects of intra-aortic balloon pumping in dogs with aortic incompetence. ASAIO Trans 1973; 19:389.
25. Bregman D: Intra-aortic balloon in open heart surgery. N Engl J Med 1971; 284:393.
26. Bregman D, Bolooki H, Malm JR: A simple method to facilitate difficult intra-aortic balloon insertions. Ann Thorac Cardiovasc Surg 1973; 15:636.
27. Lamberti JJ, Cohen LW, Collins JJ Jr: Iliac artery cannulation for intra-aortic balloon counterpulsation. J Thorac Cardiovasc Surg 1974; 67:976.
28. Pappas G: Intrathoracic intra-aortic balloon insertion for pulsatile cardiopulmonary bypass. Arch Surg 1974; 109:842.
29. Gueldner TL, Lawrence GC: Intra-aortic balloon assist through cannulation of the ascending aorta. Ann Thorac Surg 1975; 19:88.
30. Shirley AL, Loughridge BP, Lain KC: Insertion of the intra-aortic balloon through the aortic arch. Ann Thorac Surg 1976; 21:560.
31. Bregman D, Casarella WJ: Percutaneous intra-aortic balloon pumping: Initial clinical experience. Ann Thorac Surg 1979; 29:153.
32. Bregman D: A new percutaneous intra-aortic balloon. ASAIO Trans 1980; 26:8.
33. Bregman D: Intra-aortic balloon counterpulsation. *In:* Circulatory Assistance and the Artificial Heart. USA-USSR Joint Symposium. Tibilisi, USSR. Sept. 20–22, 1979. Pierce WS (Ed). Washington, DC, U.S. Department of Health and Human Services, Public Health Service, National Institutes of Health, 1980, pp 155–165.
34. Bregman D, Nicols AB, Weiss MB, et al: Percutaneous intra-aortic balloon insertion. Am J Cardiol 1980; 46:261.
35. Seldinger SL: Catheter replacement of the needle in percutaneous arteriography: A new technique. Acta Radiol 1953; 39:368.
36. Nash IS, Lorell BH, Fishman RF, et al: A new technique for sheathless percutaneous intra-aortic balloon catheter insertion. Cathet Cardiovasc Diagn 1991; 23:57–60.
37. Kern M: Intra-aortic balloon counterpulsation. Coronary Artery Dis 1991; 2:649–660.
38. Phillips SJ, Tannenbaum M, Zeff R, et al: Sheathless insertion of the intra-aortic balloon pump: An alternative method. Ann Thorac Surg 1992; 53:162.
39. Bregman D: Mechanical support of the failing heart. *In:* Current Problems in Surgery. Ravitch MM (Ed). Chicago, Year Book Medical Publishers, 1976.
40. Alcan KE, Stertzer SH, Wallsh E, et al: Current status of intra-aortic balloon counterpulsation in critical care cardiology. Crit Care Med 1984; 12:489.
41. Kantrowitz A, Tjonneland S, Freed PS, et al: Initial clinical experience with intra-aortic balloon pumping in cardiogenic shock. JAMA 1968; 203:113.
42. Freed R: The intra-aortic balloon pump system: Current roles and future directions. J Appl Cardiol 1991; 6:313–318.
43. Maccioli GA, Lucas WJ, Norfleet EA: The intra-aortic balloon pump: A review. J Cardiothorac Anesthesiol 1988; 3:365–373.
44. Isner JM, Cohen SR, Virmani R, et al: Complications of the intra-aortic balloon counterpulsation device: Clinical and morphologic observations in 45 necropsy patients. Am J Cardiol 1980; 45:260.
45. Karlson SB, Martin EC, Bregman D, et al: Superior mesenteric artery obstruction by intra-aortic balloon simulating embolism. Cardiovasc Intervent Radiol 1981; 4:236–238.
46. Rodigas PC, Bridges KG: Occlusion of the left internal mammary artery with intra-aortic balloon: Clinical implications. J Thorac Cardiovasc Surg 1986; 91:142–143.
47. Busch HN Jr, Cogbill TH, Gunderson AE: Splenic infarction: Complications of intra-aortic balloon counterpulsation. Am Heart J 1985; 109:383–385.
48. Stahl K, Tortolani A, Nelson R, et al: Intra-aortic balloon rupture. ASAIO Trans 1988; 34:496–499.
49. Cox P, Kellett M, Goran S, et al: Plaque abrasion and intra-aortic balloon leak. Poster presented by the American College of Chest Physicians, October, 1992.
50. Cohn LH: Intra-aortic balloon counterpulsation in the low cardiac output state. Surg Clin North Am 1975; 55:545.
51. Mundth ED, Buckley MJ, Daggett WM, et al: Intra-aortic balloon pump assistance and early surgery in cardiogenic shock: Integrated medical-surgical care in acute coronary artery disease. Adv Cardiol 1975; 15:159.
52. Willerson JT, Curry GC, Watson JT, et al: Intra-aortic balloon counterpulsation in patients with cardiogenic shock, medically refractory left ventricular failure and/or recurrent ventricular tachycardias. Am J Med 1975; 58:183.
53. Baron DW, O'Rourke MF: Long-term results of arterial counterpulsation in acute severe cardiac failure complicating myocardial infarction. Br Heart J 1976; 38:285.
54. Kveim M, Cappelen C Jr, Froysaker T, et al: Intra-aortic balloon pumping in the treatment of cardiogenic shock: Follow-up in open heart surgery. Scand J Thorac Cardiovasc Surg 1976; 10:231.
55. Bardet J, Rigaud M, Kahn JC, et al: Treatment of post-myocardial infarction angina by intra-aortic balloon pumping and emergency revascularization. J Thorac Cardiovasc Surg 1977; 74:299.
56. Ehrich DA, Biddle TL, Kronenburg MS, et al: The hemodynamic response to intra-aortic balloon counterpulsation in patients with cardiogenic shock complicating acute myocardial infarction. Am Heart J 1977; 93:274.
57. Jackson G, Cullum P, Pastellopoulos A, et al: Intra-aortic balloon assistance in cardiogenic shock after acute myocardial infarction or cardiac surgery. Br Heart J 1977; 39:598.

58. Johnson MD, Holub DA, Winston DS, et al: Retrospective analysis of 286 patients requiring circulatory support with the intra-aortic balloon pump: Cardiovascular disease. Bull Texas Heart Institute 1977; 4:428.
59. Scheidt S, Wilner G, Mueller H, et al: Intra-aortic balloon counterpulsation in cardiogenic shock: Report of a co-operative clinical trial. N Engl J Med 1973; 288:979.
60. Hagemeijer F, Laird JD, Haalebos MP, et al: Effectiveness of intra-aortic balloon pumping without cardiac surgery for patients with severe heart failure secondary to a myocardial infarction. Am J Cardiol 1977; 40:951.
61. Bourdarias JP, Gourgon R, Bardet J: Mechanical circulatory assistance by intra-aortic balloon pumping for the treatment of cardiogenic shock. Intens Care Med 1978; 4:29.
62. Mueller H, Ayres SM, Gianelli S Jr, et al: Effects of isoproterenol, 1-norepinephrine and intra-aortic counterpulsation on hemodynamics and myocardial metabolism in shock following acute myocardial infarction. Circulation 1972; 45:335.
63. Weintraub RM, Voukydis PC, Aroesty JM: Treatment of preinfarction angina with intra-aortic balloon counterpulsation and surgery. Am J Cardiol 1974; 34:809.
64. Scully HE, Gunstansen J, Williams WG, et al: Surgical management of complicated acute coronary insufficiency. Surgery 1976; 80:437.
65. Kuhn LA: Management of shock following acute myocardial infarction: Part I. Mechanical circulatory assistance. Am Heart J 1978; 95:789.
66. Bardet J, Masquet C, Kahn JC, et al: Clinical and hemodynamic results of intra-aortic balloon counterpulsation and surgery for cardiogenic shock. Am Heart J 1977; 63:280.
67. Bahn CH: Cardiac catheterization and intra-aortic balloon counterpulsation (Letter). Am J Cardiol 1978; 42:873.
68. Bregman D: Cardiac assist devices. *In:* Blades Surgical Diseases of the Chest. 4th ed. Effler DB (Ed). St. Louis, CV Mosby, 1978.
69. Cohn LH, Alpert J, Koster JH Jr, et al: Changing indications for the surgical treatment of unstable angina. Arch Surg 1978; 113:1312.
70. Leinbach RC, Gold HK, Harber RW, et al: Early intra-aortic balloon pumping for anterior myocardial infarction without shock. Circulation 1978; 58:204.
71. McEnany MT, Kay HR, Buckley MJ, et al: Clinical experience with intra-aortic balloon pump in 728 patients. Circulation 1978; 58(Suppl I):124.
72. Roberts AJ, Alonso DR, Combes JR, et al: Role of delayed intra-aortic balloon pumping in the treatment of experimental myocardial infarction. Am J Cardiol 1978; 41:1202.
73. Goldberg R, Gore J, Alpert J, et al: Cardiogenic shock after acute myocardial infarction: Incidence and mortality from a community-wide perspective, 1975–1988. N Engl J Med 1991; 325:1117–1122.
74. Goodwin M, Hartmann J, McKeever L, et al: Safety of intra-aortic balloon counterpulsation in patients with acute myocardial infarction receiving streptokinase intravenously. Am J Cardiol 1989; 64:973–974.
75. Ohman EM, Califf RM, George BS, et al: The use of intra-aortic balloon pumping as an adjunct to reperfusion therapy in acute myocardial infarction. Am Heart J 1991; 121:895–901.
76. Cooper GN Jr, Singh AK, Vargas LL, et al: Percutaneous intra-aortic balloon assist in high risk revascularization patients. Am J Surg 1977; 133:463.
77. Langon RA, Geha AS, Hammond GL: Surgical approach for patients with angina pectoris: Role of the response to initial medical therapy and intra-aortic balloon pumping in perioperative complications after aorta coronary bypass grafting. Am J Cardiol 1978; 42:629.
78. Bolooki H, Williams W, Thurer RJ, et al: Clinical and hemodynamic criteria for the use of the intra-aortic balloon pump in patients requiring cardiac surgery. J Thorac Cardiovasc Surg 1976; 72:756.
79. Feola M, Wiener L, Walinsky P, et al: Improved survival after coronary bypass surgery in patients with poor left ventricular function: Role of intraaortic balloon counterpulsation. Am J Cardiol 1977; 39:1021.
80. Kahn JK, Rutherford BD, McConahay DR, et al: Supported high-risk coronary angioplasty using intra-aortic balloon counterpulsation. J Am Coll Cardiol 1990; 15:1151–1155.
81. Califf R, Ohman EM: Reocclusion after thrombolytic therapy and percutaneous transluminal coronary angioplasty. Cardiac Assist 1990; 2:1–6.
82. Ishihara M, Sato H, Tateishi H, et al: Intra-aortic balloon pumping as the post angioplasty strategy in acute myocardial infarction. Am Heart J 1991; 122:385–389.
83. Anwar A, Mooney M, Stertzer S, et al: Intra-aortic balloon counterpulsation support for elective coronary angioplasty in the setting of poor ventricular function: A two center experience. J Invest Cardiol 1990; 2:175–180.
84. Williams EH, Tyers GF, Carter SL, et al: Ventricular arrhythmias following mitral valve replacement: Control with intra-aortic balloon counterpulsation. Chest 1975; 68:641.
85. Saunders CR, Doty DB: Myocardial contusion: Effect of intra-aortic balloon pumping on cardiac output. J Trauma 1978; 18:706.
86. Golding LA, Loop FD, Peter M, et al: Late survival following use of intra-aortic balloon pump in revascularization operations. Ann Thorac Surg 1980; 30:48.
87. Madras PN, Laird JD, Iatridis E, et al: Effects of prolonged intra-aortic balloon pump support. ASAIO Trans 1969; 15:400.
88. Brantigan CO, Grow JB Sr, Schoonmaker FW: Extended use of intra-aortic balloon pumping in peripartum cardiomyopathy. Ann Surg 1976; 183:1.
89. Frazier GH, Cooley DD, Okereke OJ, et al: Cardiac transplantation in a patient with septicemia after prolonged intra-aortic pump support: Implications for staged transplantation. Texas Heart J 1986; 13:13.
90. Reemtsma K, Drusin R, Edie R, et al: Cardiac transplantation for patients requiring mechanical circulatory support. N Engl J Med 1978; 29:670.
91. Bregman D: Percutaneous intra-aortic balloon pumping: A time for reflection. Chest 1982; 82:397.

CHAPTER 61

Ventricular Assist Devices and Artificial Hearts

Timothy J. Broderick, MD • Andrew S. Wechsler, MD

HISTORY

Mechanical assistance of the heart began with Gibbon's successful use of operative cardiopulmonary bypass in 1952.[1] Cardiopulmonary bypass was soon successfully used to treat ventricular dysfunction. For example, Stuckey and colleagues[2] used partial cardiopulmonary bypass to assist a patient with postinfarction cardiogenic shock in 1957, and Spencer and associates[3] used cardiopulmonary bypass to assist a postcardiotomy patient in 1963. In the midst of these successes, Dennis and coworkers[4] introduced percutaneous transseptal left-sided heart bypass. This system eliminated problems associated with the use of a bubble oxygenator, but hematologic dysfunction secondary to roller pump bypass and heparinization precluded successful long-term support. After further device refinement, DeBakey[5] successfully treated postcardiotomy shock with a rudimentary pneumatic left ventricular assist device (LVAD) in 1967. Concomitantly, Moulopoulos and colleagues[6] developed intra-aortic balloon (IAB) counterpulsation. Shortly thereafter, Kantrowitz and coauthors[7] successfully supported a postinfarction patient with the balloon pump. Nine years later, Reemtsma and others[8] bridged a patient to heart transplantation with short-term IAB counterpulsation.

Long-term mechanical support began when DeVries and colleagues implanted a total artificial heart (TAH) in 1982.[9]

Unfortunately, serious thromboembolic and infectious complications cluttered the 620 days that Dr. Barney Clark survived and dampened enthusiasm for permanent mechanical assistance. However, within 3 years, Portner and colleagues[10] successfully bridged a patient to transplantation with a Novacor pulsatile electric LVAD, and Copeland and others[11] successfully bridged a patient to transplantation with a TAH. Frazier and associates[12] introduced the percutaneous, intravascular Hemopump assist device for temporary treatment of cardiac dysfunction. Further refinement of device technology and application has continued to decrease the morbidity and mortality associated with ventricular assistance over the ensuing years (Table 61–1).

INDICATIONS

Currently, mechanical cardiac assistance is indicated in patients with cardiogenic shock refractory to maximal pharmacologic and intra-aortic counterpulsation therapy. The specific physiologic criteria routinely used to define refractory cardiogenic shock were initially determined by Norman and associates (Table 61–2).[13] Their retrospective analysis of cardiogenic shock patients determined that patients meeting these criteria have an extremely high mortality if mechanical support is not instituted. Subsequent clinical experience with ventricular assist devices (VADs) has confirmed these findings.

The metabolic cardiac insult of high doses of inotropic agents contrasts with the favorable decrease in myocardial work and oxygen consumption seen with mechanical assistance.[14–16] The decrease in myocardial oxygen consumption directly correlates with the degree of ventricular decompression and afterload reduction.[17] Moreover, increased mean intra-aortic pressure, decreased central venous pressure, and decreased ventricular wall tension augment myocardial perfusion and oxygen delivery. The increased myocardial oxygen supply and decreased oxygen demand seen with mechanical assistance promote recovery of stunned myocardium and limit infarct size.[16, 18, 19] Increased extracardiac organ perfusion also prevents systemic organ dysfunction.

Proper patient selection is the most important factor in minimizing the morbidity and mortality associated with mechanical assistance.[20, 21] Mechanical assistance is generally contraindicated for patients meeting any of the exclusion criteria listed in Table 61–3.

APPLICATIONS

Improving device technology and application have continued to decrease the morbidity and mortality associated with mechanical assistance. Currently, treatment of cardiogenic shock with mechanical assistance is indicated in the following populations: postcardiotomy, bridge to transplantation, acute myocardial infarction, orthotopic heart transplantation, and cardiac arrest. These patient populations are not mutually exclusive (Table 61–4).

TABLE 61–1. Successes in Mechanical Assistance

Year	*Description*
1952	Gibbon used operative CPB.
1957	Stuckey treated ischemic shock with partial CPB.
1961	Dennis introduced percutaneous left-sided heart bypass.
1963	Spencer treated postcardiotomy shock with CPB.
1967	DeBakey treated postcardiotomy shock with a LVAD.
1968	Kantrowitz treated ischemic shock with an IABP.
1977	Reemtsma bridged a patient to transplant with an IABP.
1982	DeVries implanted a TAH.
1984	Portner bridged a patient to transplant with a LVAD.
1985	Copeland bridged a patient to transplant with a TAH.
1988	Frazier supported patient with Hemopump.

Abbreviations: CPB = cardiopulmonary bypass; LVAD = left ventricular assist device; IABP = intra-aortic balloon pump; TAH = total artificial heart.

TABLE 61–2. Criteria for Institution of Mechanical Support

CI <1.8 L/m^2 per min
SBP <90 mm Hg
Atrial pressure(s) >20 mm Hg
Urine output <20 mL/h (adult)
SVR >2100 dyne·s·cm^{-5}
Metabolic acidosis
Adequate preload, maximum inotropic/IABP support, and inability to tolerate vasodilators without hypotension

(Modified with permission from Pennington DG, Swartz MT: Assisted circulation and mechanical hearts. *In:* Heart Disease: A Textbook of Cardiovascular Medicine. 4th ed. Braunwald E [Ed]. Philadelphia, WB Saunders, 1992, p 537.)

Abbreviations: CI = cardiac index; SBP = systolic blood pressure; SVR = systemic vascular resistance; IABP = intra-aortic balloon pump.

Postcardiotomy

Approximately 1% of the 300,000 patients undergoing cardiopulmonary bypass procedures annually in the United States are unable to be weaned from cardiopulmonary bypass despite maximal pharmacologic and counterpulsation therapy.[21, 22] Moreover, the mortality rate of the 1% to 7% of cardiotomy patients who require high-dose pharmacologic and IAB pump support is 65%.[21] Because the decision to institute mechanical assistance is routinely made when difficulty is encountered while weaning the patient from cardiopulmonary bypass, this group of patients represents a preselected population in whom lifesaving support could be easily instituted. Unfortunately, far less than 1% of all cardiotomy patients receive further mechanical support.[21, 23] Device unavailability and pessimism stemming from marginal improvement of patients in early clinical experience have deterred clinicians from instituting support. As a result of this prevailing attitude, morbidity and mortality in this group of patients are increased because of the coagulation problems associated with long periods of cardiopulmonary bypass before instituting mechanical support. However, improved devices and patient selection markedly decreased morbidity and mortality in later trials of postcardiotomy mechanical ventricular assistance.[23, 24] These clinically proven devices will soon become widely available.

Bridge to Transplantation

Transplant candidates are rigorously selected to maximize patient survival and donor organ utilization. Because pretransplant evaluation selects patients mostly with single organ cardiac disease, candidates in whom cardiogenic shock develops are ideally suited for mechanical assistance.[21, 25] In addition, 20% of patients on the cardiac transplant waiting

TABLE 61–3. Usual Contraindications to Mechanical Assistance

Age >70 years
Renal failure
Cerebrovascular insufficiency
Hepatic failure
Coagulopathy
Sepsis
Metastatic cancer

TABLE 61–4. Current Applications of Mechanical Assistance for Treatment of Cardiogenic Shock

Postcardiotomy
Bridge to transplantation
Acute myocardial infarction
Orthotopic heart transplantation
Cardiac arrest

list with medically controlled heart failure die from their cardiac disease before cardiac transplantation.[22, 25] Although current mechanical assist devices effectively bridge patients to transplantation, within the decade permanent assist devices could replace cardiac transplantation as the treatment of choice for some patients with end-stage cardiac disease.

Acute Myocardial Infarction

Current medical treatment of acute ischemic cardiogenic shock is associated with an 80% mortality.[26, 27] However, acute revascularization has been shown to improve survival. For example, infarct limitation with angioplasty within 12 hours of infarction reduces the in-hospital mortality of cardiogenic shock from 82% to 33%,[28] and coronary artery bypass grafting within 18 hours of the onset of the development of postinfarction shock decreases the mortality to 20% to 34%.[29]

Unfortunately, early studies of mechanical assistance failed to demonstrate an increase in survival of postinfarction shock patients treated with mechanical assistance. Scheidt and associates demonstrated that the balloon pump improved hemodynamics but did not significantly alter patient survival.[30] Later clinical trials with VADs demonstrated no increase in patient survival when these devices were not used in conjunction with orthotopic heart transplantation.[20, 26] However, these early trials did demonstrate a clear benefit when ventricular support was used as a bridge to cardiac transplantation.[20] (See Chapter 15.)

Recently, the percutaneous, intravascular Hemopump has been experimentally shown to improve regional myocardial blood flow and to limit infarct size.[16] Preliminary clinical studies of patients with acute ischemic shock have demonstrated that the Hemopump improves the hemodynamics and survival of cardiogenic shock patients.[31, 32] Table 61–5 depicts the authors' suggested algorithm for institution of mechanical support in the postinfarction patient with medically refractory cardiogenic shock.

Orthotopic Heart Transplantation

If without other perioperative complications, patients with cardiogenic shock after heart transplantation remain good candidates for ventricular assistance.[21] Early utilization is the most important factor in post-transplant mechanical assistance because it limits further myocardial insult by preventing distension injury of the acutely denervated heart.[21] Timely support also prevents severe secondary organ injury resulting from prolonged cardiogenic shock. Whereas short-term mechanical assistance decompresses the graft and promotes myocardial recovery, longer support can provide successful bridge to retransplantation.

Resuscitation from Arrest

Recent developments in percutaneous mechanical assist devices have rekindled interest in mechanical resuscitation of patients who have sustained cardiac arrest. Preliminary clinical trials have demonstrated improved survival of such patients treated with percutaneous cardiopulmonary bypass.[33–35] Moreover, these trials were conducted before the widespread availability of the Carmeda heparin-bonded cardiopulmonary bypass circuit. The biocompatibility of this circuit alleviates the need for full systemic heparinization and may reduce the side effects of extracorporeal membrane oxygenation (ECMO) support. Although the Hemopump has been experimentally shown to affect resuscitation from ventricular fibrillation favorably,[36] clinical evaluation of its benefit in the treatment of cardiopulmonary arrest is required.

Future Applications

In addition to the routinely accepted indications for mechanical support, initial clinical experience suggests that the Hemopump and percutaneous left-sided heart bypass may be of benefit in providing prophylactic hemodynamic support of complex angioplastic revascularizations.[37–40] As previously mentioned, totally implantable, minimally thrombogenic, permanent mechanical assist devices for the treatment of end-stage cardiac disease are projected to be ready for widespread clinical use within the decade.[33, 34, 41]

DEVICES

The number of different mechanical circulatory assist devices is continually increasing. Table 61–6 lists the devices currently available. The only systems approved for noninvestigational use are roller or centrifugal pump systems. The remainder of the assist devices have limited clinical availability. Because the IAB pump was thoroughly covered in Chapter 60, this device is not discussed here.

TABLE 61–5. Algorithm for Support of Patients with Refractory Cardiogenic Shock After Myocardial Infarction

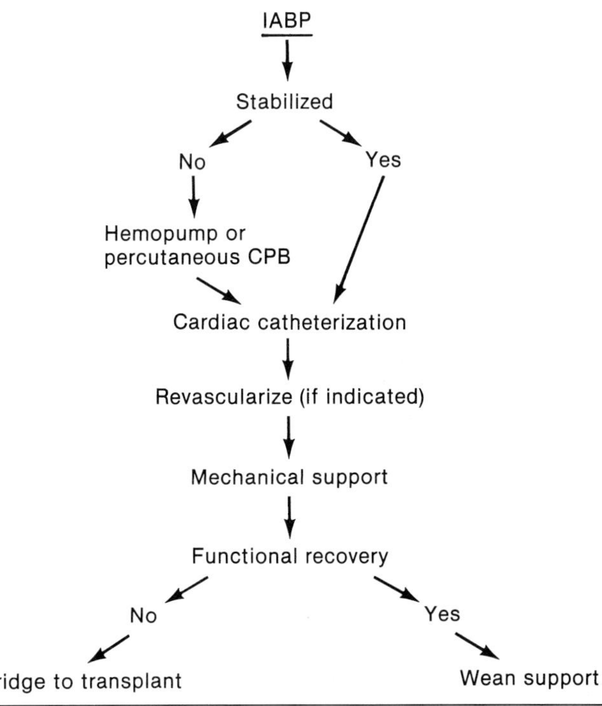

Abbreviations: IABP = intra-aortic balloon pump; CPB = cardiopulmonary bypass.

TABLE 61–6. Current Mechanical Assist Devices

Nonpulsatile
Extracorporeal
  Centrifugal (Biomedicus, Sarns, Aries)
  Roller pump
Intravascular
  Rotary (Hemopump)
Pulsatile
Paracorporeal
  Pneumatic (Thoratec VAD, Symbion AVAD, Abiomed 5000)
Heterotopic
  Pneumatic (Thermocardiosystems LVAS)
  Electric (Novacor LVAS)
Orthotopic
  Pneumatic (Symbion Jarvik 7)

Abbreviations: VAD = ventricular assist device; AVAD = acute ventricular assist device; LVAS = left ventricular assist system.

Nonpulsatile Assist Devices

The Biomedicus, Sarns, and Aries pumps are extracorporeal, vortex centrifugal pumps that can provide full circulatory support. Because these pumps are not considered VADs by the U.S. Food and Drug Administration (FDA), they are widely available for univentricular or biventricular support (BVS). The configuration for left ventricular support is left atrial or ventricular inflow and aortic outflow; the configuration for right ventricular support is right atrial inflow and pulmonary artery outflow. The nonthrombogenic, nonocclusive design of centrifugal pumps causes little hematologic activation and requires minimal anticoagulation. Although the Biomedicus pump has been previously used for up to 30 days, the recommended length of support for the centrifugal pumps is less than 1 week. Centrifugal pump applications include postcardiotomy assistance and short-term bridge to cardiac transplantation. Common complications include bleeding, renal failure, infection, and strokes. Many physicians familiar with these devices suggest concurrent IAB counterpulsation to alleviate end-organ dysfunction secondary to prolonged nonpulsatile flow. Smaller, totally implantable centrifugal pumps are currently under development.

Because roller pump bypass routinely provides intraoperative support during cardiac surgery, roller pump devices are also widely available. Current extraoperative adult applications of roller pump devices include postcardiotomy cardiogenic shock and resuscitation from arrest. Roller pumps and centrifugal pumps can be used interchangeably for these applications. Postcardiotomy roller pump support is routinely configured with ECMO and transthoracic right atrial inflow and aortic outflow. For resuscitation from arrest, percutaneous ECMO is configured with right atrial drainage (retrograde from the femoral vein) and femoral artery infusion. Recently, there has been renewed interest in percutaneous transseptal left atrium to femoral artery support of complex percutaneous coronary angioplasty. Common complications of roller pump support include bleeding, hemolysis, and renal failure. As previously mentioned, use of the Carmeda heparin-bonded bypass circuit can minimize the hematologic complications of ECMO support.

The Hemopump is an intravascular, Archimedean screw that rotates at 17,000 to 25,000 rpm within a cannula inserted through a femoral arteriotomy or aortotomy and passed retrogradely across the aortic valve into the left ventricle (Fig. 61–1). This relatively inexpensive device provides up to 3.5 L/min of flow regardless of the underlying cardiac rhythm. Of note, the Hemopump is very difficult to insert in patients with significant aortic valvular or aortoiliac occlusive disease. Similar to the IAB pump, use of the Hemopump severely limits patient mobility. Furthermore, device ejection from the left ventricle and drive-line fracture can cause temporary loss of Hemopump support. Primary applications of the Hemopump include postcardiotomy and postinfarction support of fewer than 14 days' duration. Limited clinical experience suggests that the Hemopump might also be of benefit in resuscitation of cardiac arrest patients and in support of complicated revascularizations. A larger extravascular ventriculoaortic device that could provide complete support is under development.

Pulsatile Assist Devices

The Pierce-Donachy Thoratec VAD is a paracorporeal, pneumatic pump that can provide up to 6 L/min of univentricular or biventricular support. It has a polyurethane pumping chamber with Bjork-Shiley inflow and outflow valves that ensure unidirectional flow. The configuration for left ventricular assistance is left atrial or ventricular inflow and aortic outflow; the configuration for right ventricular assistance is right atrial inflow and pulmonary artery outflow. The Thoratec can be operated in any of three modes: fixed rate, electrocardiogram synchronized, or volume activated. Common complications of its use include hemolysis and perioperative bleeding. Long-term warfarin sodium (Coumadin) therapy is required to minimize thromboembolism. Although the Thoratec has provided consistent postcardiotomy and pretransplant support for up to 81 days, the current device has a questionable future secondary to the cumbersome nature of its pneumatic drive system. However, a totally implantable, electric device with an inductively coupled transcutaneous energy-transfer system is currently under development. Figure 61–2 outlines the components of a totally implantable Thoratec. This schematic also adequately represents the basic design of most of the totally implantable systems currently under development.

The Symbion acute VAD (AVAD) is a paracorporeal, pneumatic biventricular assist device that is currently unavailable for use in the United States. Although this device has provided ventricular support for up to 163 days, serious

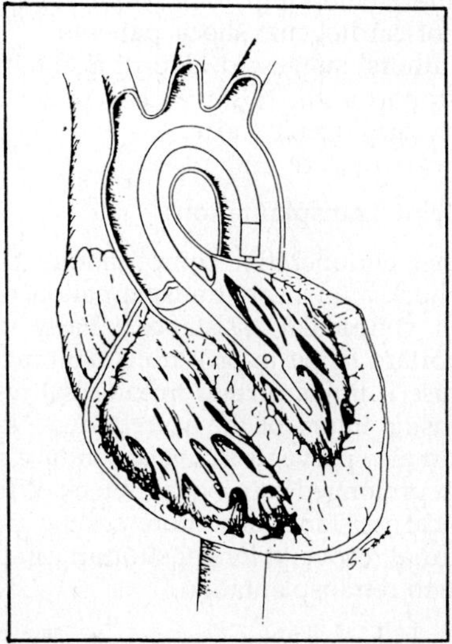

Figure 61–1. Hemopump configuration. (From Wampler RK, Frazier OH, Lansing AM, et al: Treatment of cardiogenic shock with the Hemopump left ventricular assist device. Ann Thorac Surg 1991; 52:506–513. Reprinted with permission from the Society of Thoracic Surgeons.)

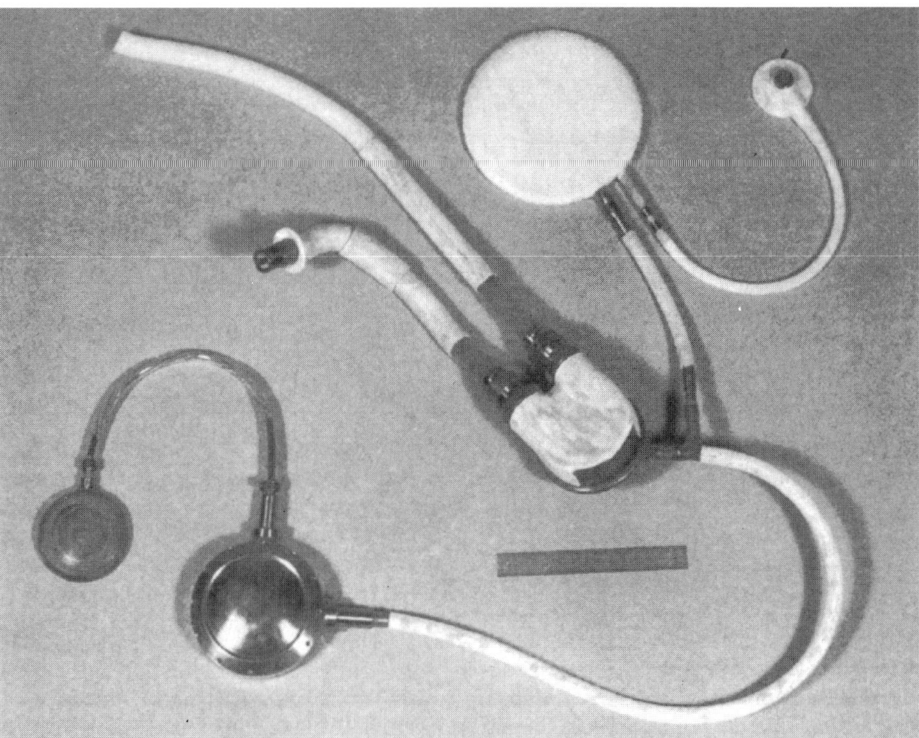

Figure 61–2. Representative totally implantable ventricular assist device (Thoratec, Berkeley, CA). (From Pierce WS, Snyder AJ, Rosenberg G, et al: A long term ventricular assist system. J Thorac Cardiovasc Surg 1993; 105:520–524.)

infection and thromboembolism plagued the patients who were supported with the Symbion AVAD. Further use of this device in the United States is unlikely.

The Abiomed BVS 5000 is an extracorporeal, gravity-filling, pneumatic pump that can provide full univentricular or biventricular support. The configuration for left ventricular assistance is left atrial inflow and aortic outflow; the configuration for right ventricular assistance is right atrial inflow and pulmonary artery outflow. Polyurethane valves are contained within the inflow and outflow cannulas to ensure unidirectional flow. Because direct left ventricular cannulation is not possible with the BVS 5000, support with this device does not completely unload the ventricle. Furthermore, decreased intraventricular flow during atrioaortic bypass can result in intraventricular thrombus formation. The cumbersome, gravity-filling Abiomed pumps require warfarin anticoagulation and severely limit patient mobility. Despite being the least expensive of all the pulsatile assist devices, the BVS 5000 has had limited clinical use. It has provided postcardiotomy and pretransplant support for up to 19 days. A promising totally implantable, electrohydraulic Abiomed device is currently under development.

Thermocardiosystems left ventricular assist system (LVAS) is heterotopically implanted and pneumatic. This device is implanted in the left upper quadrant and provides excellent long-term ventriculoaortic support. The unique textured polyurethane surface of this device promotes formation of a viable biologic membrane. Because this biologic membrane is nonthrombogenic, administration of aspirin and dipyridamole effectively prevents thromboembolism. Because insertion of the left ventricular cannula requires removal of a section of the ventricular apex, this device is primarily used for long-term support as a bridge to transplantation. Ventricular cannulation and high device outflow pressures can result in significant perioperative bleeding. The Thermocardiosystems LVAS has successfully supported patients for up to 280 days. Although the current model has a transcutaneous pneumatic drive system, a totally implantable electrical device is under development.

The Novacor LVAS is an implantable, heterotopic, electromagnetic solenoid pump with porcine unidirectional inflow and outflow valves. Implanted in the left upper quadrant, this device provides up to 7 L/min of long-term ventriculoaortic support. Because only an electric cord exits the patient, patient mobility is excellent. This device provides an effective bridge to transplantation and has successfully supported patients for up to 370 days. Novacor support requires long-term warfarin anticoagulation to prevent thromboembolism, and a common complication of its use is perioperative bleeding. A totally implantable long-term Novacor LVAS will soon be available for investigational use.

The Symbion Jarvik 7 is an orthotopic, pneumatic TAH. The Symbion TAH was initially considered to represent the future of biventricular assistance. Unfortunately, serious thromboembolic and infectious complications prompted the U.S. FDA to suspend clinical use of the Symbion TAH. Its future use within the United States seems unlikely. Table 61–7 summarizes the attributes of currently available VADs.

Biomechanical Assist Devices

Current biologic ventricular assist systems include dynamic cardiomyoplasty and skeletal muscle ventricles. These systems provide orthotopic or heterotopic assistance to the failing heart through use of conditioned skeletal muscle. Cardiomyoplasty provides ventricular assistance by stimulating a latissimus dorsi muscle that has been wrapped around the ventricle. Smooth-muscle ventricles provide support similar to that of other implantable VADs except the system is powered by a latissimus dorsi muscle wrapped around a prosthetic ventricle. Diastolic counterpulsation devices using skeletal muscle are also under investigation. Early experience with biologic ventricular assist systems has demonstrated that a few fundamental problems limit their ap-

TABLE 61–7. Description of Mechanical Circulatory Assist Devices

Device	Investigational*	Position	Support	Anticoagulation Required	Preferred Application	Duration
Biomedicus	No	Extracorporeal	Rt, L, B	Moderate	P, B-Tx	Short–intermediate-term
ECMO	No	Extracorporeal	B	Full	R	Short-term
Sarns/Centrimed	No	Extracorporeal	Rt, L, B	Moderate	P, B-Tx	Short–intermediate-term
Elecath	Yes	Extracorporeal	L	Full	R, P	Short-term
Abiomed BVS	Yes	Extracorporeal	Rt, L, B	Moderate	P, B-Tx	Short–intermediate-term
Pierce-Donachy VAD	Yes	Extracorporeal	Rt, L, B	Low	P, B-Tx	Intermediate–long-term
Symbion AVAD	Yes	Extracorporeal	Rt, L, B	Moderate	P, B-Tx	Intermediate–long-term
Sarns VAD	Yes	Extracorporeal	Rt, L, B	Low	P, B-Tx	Intermediate–long-term
Hemopump	Yes	Internal	L	Moderate	R, P	Short–intermediate-term
Novacor LVAS	Yes	Internal	L	Low	B-Tx	Intermediate–long-term
Symbion TAH	Yes	Internal	B	Moderate	B-Tx	Intermediate–long-term
Thermocardiosystems LVAS	Yes	Internal	L	Low	B-Tx	Intermediate–long-term

(From Pennington DG, Swartz MT: Assisted circulation and mechanical hearts. *In:* Heart Disease: A Textbook of Cardiovascular Medicine. 4th ed. Braunwald E [Ed]. Philadelphia, WB Saunders, 1992, p 538.)

*Investigational device exemption required from U.S. Food and Drug Administration.

Abbreviations: BVS = biventricular support system; ECMO = extracorporeal membrane oxygenation; LVAS = left ventricular assist system; VAD = ventricular assist device; AVAD = acute ventricular assist device; TAH = total artificial heart; Rt = right; L = left; B = biventricular; R = resuscitative; P = postcardiotomy; B-Tx = bridge to transplantation.

plicability. Of note, only dynamic cardiomyoplasty has been used clinically.

Although the concept of biologically driven mechanical assist systems is enticing, the construction of a functional biologic assist system requires a major operation and 6 weeks of postoperative skeletal muscle conditioning. Moreover, the orthotopic skeletal muscle wrap of the ventricle during cardiomyoplasty changes ventricular morphology and often decreases early postoperative ventricular function.[42, 43] Critically ill cardiac patients tolerate operations of this magnitude poorly, especially operations that further decrease ventricular function.[42] Heterotopic skeletal muscle ventricles do not limit postimplantation ventricular function, but the creation of a functional skeletal muscle ventricle still requires a major operation and 6 weeks of postimplantation muscle conditioning. The prosthetic cavity of the skeletal muscle ventricle also promotes thromboembolism.[44] Long-term skeletal muscle ischemia further limits both systems.[42–44] Continued evaluation of biologic systems is necessary to determine their future role.

GENERAL CONSIDERATIONS

Vigilant postimplantation care reduces complications. Common complications of mechanical assistance are listed in Table 61–8. The prevalence of these complications is device related.

Hematologic Dysfunction

Artificial surfaces provide continual stimulation of the humoral amplification system. Platelet activation, fibrin formation, fibrinolysis, and leukocyte activation continue throughout mechanical assistance. Not surprisingly, control of bleeding and thromboembolism remains problematic.[45]

Bleeding is a problem especially in patients requiring higher levels of anticoagulation, longer preimplant cardiopulmonary bypass, and treatment with amrinone before institution of mechanical assistance (amrinone-platelet dysfunction). High outflow device pressures and ventricular apex cannulation also predispose to bleeding.[45] Although perioperative mechanical bleeding demands reoperation, coagulopathy related to cardiopulmonary bypass and mechanical assistance can be controlled with judicious use of blood products. As soon as bleeding is under control, anticoagulation should begin. Of note, mediastinal tamponade is a relatively common occurrence that results in obstruction of inflow to the device and low outputs.

Thromboembolism is minimized by standardized anticoagulation regimens. Anticoagulation therapy is device specific and flow related. For example, thrombogenic devices such as the Novacor LVAS require intense anticoagulation with dipyridamole, postoperative heparin, and long-term warfarin. Aspirin is also added if the patient has a transient ischemic attack or other nonhemorrhagic neurologic event. In contrast, the biologic membrane that forms on the Thermocardiosystems LVAS requires minimal anticoagulation with dipyridamole, short-term dextran therapy, and long-term aspirin therapy.

Conditions that predispose to thrombus formation require increased anticoagulation. For example, ventricular fibrillation, distension, and hypokinesis promote intracardiac thrombosis during atrioaortic bypass. Kinked cannulas and increased ventricular function decrease device flow and increase intradevice thrombus formation.[45] Most importantly, low device flow during weaning from a device requires heparinization to prevent significant thromboembolism.

TABLE 61–8. Common Complications of Mechanical Assistance

Bleeding
Infection
Thromboembolism
Renal failure

TABLE 61–9. General Principles of Care for Mechanically Assisted Patients

Ensure adequate device support.
Extubate and remove indwelling catheters early.
Aggressively mobilize and rehabilitate patient.
Provide adequate nutrition (preferably enteral).
Use device-specific anticoagulation.
Treat infections with organism-specific antibiotics.
Minimize concurrent pharmacologic support.
Maximize oxygen delivery.

TABLE 61–10. Results of Ventricular Assistance in Postcardiotomy Cardiogenic Shock (from ASAIO/ISHT Registry)

Type of Support	*Number of Patients*	*Number Weaned*	*Number Discharged*
LVAD	494	254 (51.4%)	137 (27.7%)
RVAD	121	47 (38.8%)	31 (25.6%)
BVAD	350	132 (37.7%)	69 (19.7%)
Total	965	433 (44.9%)	237 (24.6%)

(With permission from Pae WE: Ventricular assist devices and total artificial hearts: A combined registry experience. Ann Thorac Surg 1993; 55:295–298.)
Abbreviations: ASAIO/ISHT = American Society of Artificial Internal Organs/International Society for Heart Transplantation; LVAD = left ventricular assist device; RVAD = right ventricular assist device; BVAD =biventricular assist device.

Infection

Implantation of a foreign body, multiple blood transfusions, invasive catheters, extensive surgery, nutritional compromise, and chronic illness predispose mechanically assisted patients to infection.[46] Although infection in these patients is usually at a site distant from the device, treatment of the infrequent device infection requires aggressive operative débridement and antibiotic therapy. Surprisingly, current support systems with transcutaneous cannulas do not have a large number of device infections presumably secondary to the ingrowth of tissue around the cannulas. The newer, totally implantable devices will not have these cannulas as a source of infection.

One regimen is to use perioperative antibiotic prophylaxis similar to that for routine cardiac operations. A cephalosporin begun immediately preoperatively and continued for 48 hours postoperatively usually suffices. Thereafter, organism-specific antibiotic therapy is used as necessary to treat clinically apparent infections. Importantly, candidal infections must be diagnosed and treated early and aggressively to prevent poor outcome.

Secondary Organ Dysfunction

Mechanical assistance commonly affects the renal, hepatic, pulmonary, and central nervous systems. Appropriate patient selection and early institution of mechanical assistance minimize preimplantation organ dysfunction. Intraoperative closure of a patent foramen ovale will prevent postoperative right-to-left shunting and severe peripheral desaturation in patients requiring isolated left ventricular support.[47] After implantation, volume restriction and α-adrenergic agonists remove venous hypertension as a cause of organ dysfunction. As necessary, continuous arteriovenous hemofiltration and albumin administration can control the profound edema that often develops in mechanically assisted patients with organ dysfunction. Most importantly, the intensivist should encourage metabolic recovery of the mechanically assisted patient by minimizing pharmacologic support while maximizing tissue oxygen delivery.[48]

Weaning

Weaning from mechanical assistance should not be attempted earlier than 24 hours after institution of support. Mechanical support is weaned by decreasing the output of the device while evaluating cardiac function with systemic and pulmonary arterial catheters and transesophageal echocardiography.[47] When ventricular function adequately supports the circulation without significant aid from the device, mechanical assistance can be safely discontinued. As previously mentioned, it is necessary to increase anticoagulation while weaning the device (Table 61–9).

RESULTS

The American Society of Artificial Internal Organs and the International Society for Heart Transplantation (ASAIO/ISHT) maintain a voluntary, international registry that represents the most complete data on mechanical assistance currently available. The ASAIO/ISHT results presented in this chapter reflect 6 years of mechanical assistance ending December 31, 1990.[20]

Postcardiotomy

Table 61–10 lists the results of postcardiotomy mechanical assistance. The mean duration of postcardiotomy support was 3.3 days with the range of support from 0 to 69 days. Not surprisingly, 90% of patients who were able to be weaned did so within 1 week of the institution of mechanical support. Overall, 45% of supported patients were weaned from mechanical assistance and 25% of supported patients were discharged from the hospital. Interestingly, weaning and discharge results were not related to the type of device used or the original operation performed. Retrospective analysis of mechanically assisted postcardiotomy patients showed that the following factors were associated with decreased survival: incomplete operation, perioperative myocardial infarction, biventricular failure, age greater than 65 years, uncontrolled hemorrhage, and cardiopulmonary bypass time greater than 4 to 6 hours.[20]

Although limited data are available, preliminary studies have demonstrated markedly improved survival in postcardiotomy shock patients supported with the Hemopump (Table 61–11).[24, 32] Mechanical assistance of postcardiotomy shock patients with the Hemopump salvaged 35% of postcardiotomy patients who would have otherwise died secondary to failure to wean from cardiopulmonary bypass.

Bridge to Transplantation

The results of mechanical support in bridging patients to transplantation are listed in Table 61–12. Of note, there are

TABLE 61–11. Results of Hemopump Support in the Treatment of Postcardiotomy Shock

Study	*Patients Supported*	*Patients Discharged*
Wampler et al[32]	17	4 (23.5%)
Burnett et al[24]	9	5 (55.5%)
Total	26	9 (34.6%)

TABLE 61–12. Results of Mechanical Assistance in Treating Cardiogenic Shock in the Bridge to Transplant Application (from ASAIO/ISHT Registry)

Device	*Number of Pts*	*Transplantation*	*Transplantation Pts Discharged*	*Bridge Pts Discharged*
RVAD	4	1 (25.0%)	1 (100%)	1 (25.0%)
LVAD	122	87 (71.3%)	76 (87.4%)	76 (62.3%)
BVAD	161	105 (65.2%)	73 (69.5%)	73 (45.3%)
TAH	189	135 (71.4%)	67 (49.6%)	67 (35.4%)
Total	476	328 (68.9%)	217 (66.2%)	217 (45.6%)

(With permission from Pae WE: Ventricular assist devices and total artificial hearts: A combined registry experience. Ann Thorac Surg 1993; 55:295–298.)
Abbreviations: ASAIO/ISHT = American Society of Artificial Internal Organs/International Society for Heart Transplantation; RVAD = right ventricular assist device; LVAD = left ventricular assist device; BVAD = biventricular assist device; TAH = total artificial heart.

no data available on the use of the Hemopump in this application.

The range of support was 0 to 438 days, and 69% of mechanically bridged patients received a transplant. Common reasons for removal from the transplant list were bleeding, biventricular failure, renal failure, respiratory failure, multiple system organ failure, and infection. Of note, patients supported before the transplant with biventricular devices and artificial hearts have significantly worse survival after the transplant than did patients supported with univentricular support. However, the 2-year survival of patients after univentricular mechanical assistance was equal to the 2-year survival of patients undergoing standard orthotopic heart transplant. Retrospective analysis of patients who were bridged toward transplantation reveals the following factors associated with decreased survival: increasing age, female gender, previous cardiac operation, and an elevated blood urea nitrogen level.[20] Interestingly, longer durations of mechanical support were not associated with decreased post-transplant patient survival.

Acute Myocardial Infarction

Table 61–13 lists the results of mechanical support of all registry patients temporarily supported with mechanical assist devices without the intention of subsequent cardiac transplantation. Unfortunately, there are no ASAIO/ISHT data available exclusively evaluating mechanical assistance of the postinfarction patient. Specifically, this table includes data collected during mechanical assistance of both postinfarction and post-transplant patients. Although these results are unimpressive, postinfarction Hemopump support provides much more effective postinfarction support than other implantable devices (Table 61–14).[31, 32]

Although these data represent preliminary investigation, the 45% survival of patients with postinfarction cardiogenic shock treated with Hemopump insertion compares favorably with the 20% survival of postinfarction shock patients treated with maximal pharmacologic and IAB pump therapy. Of note, none of the postinfarction Hemopump patients were acutely revascularized.

TABLE 61–14. Results of Percutaneous Mechanical Support in the Treatment of Cardiogenic Shock Secondary to Acute Myocardial Infarction

			Discharged		
Report	*N*	*No. with Successful Insertion*	*n*	*%*	*% with Successful Insertion*
Deeb et al[31]	8	5	3	60	38
Wampler et al[32]	21	17	7	41	33
Total	29	22	10	45	34

Abbreviation: N = total patients.

Orthotopic Heart Transplantation

There are limited data available for evaluation of mechanical assistance of cardiac allograft dysfunction. Table 61–15 lists results from the ASAIO/ISHT registry. In the ASAIO/ISHT registry, patients with rejection are considered candidates for retransplantation without the possibility of significant myocardial recovery, and patients without rejection are supported with hope of eventual myocardial recovery. Overall, 20% of patients requiring post-transplant mechanical assistance are discharged from the hospital. In this registry, ultimate discharge after post-transplant mechanical assistance is unrelated to the cause of allograft dysfunction and the need for subsequent retransplantation. Although anecdotal experience with the Hemopump suggests that it will be of benefit in the treatment of cardiac allograft dysfunction, further investigation is needed to support its use in this setting.

TABLE 61–13. Results of the Use of Mechanical Assist Devices Without the Intention for Later Heart Transplant (from the ASAIO/ISHT Registry)

Number of Patients	*Weaned*	*Discharged*
79	22 (28%)	8 (10%)

(With permission from Pae WE: Ventricular assist devices and total artificial hearts: A combined registry experience. Ann Thorac Surg 1993; 55:295–298.)
Abbreviation: ASAIO/ISHT = American Society of Artificial Internal Organs/International Society for Heart Transplantation.

TABLE 61–15. Results of Post-Transplant Mechanical Assistance (ASAIO/ISHT Registry)

Number of Patients	*Wean*	*2nd Tx*	*Discharge*
40 (rejection)	—	23 (58%)	8 (20%)
68 (nonrejection)	20 (29%)	—	13 (19%)

(With permission from Pae WE: Ventricular assist devices and total artificial hearts: A combined registry experience. Ann Thorac Surg 1993; 55:295–298.)
Abbreviations: ASAIO/ISHT = American Society of Artificial Internal Organs/International Society for Heart Transplantation; Tx = transplant.

TABLE 61–16. Results of Percutaneous Cardiopulmonary Bypass in Resuscitation from Arrest*

Report	*Number of Patients*	*Weaned*	*Discharged*
Dembitsky et al[35]	140	—	23 (26%)
Phillips et al[49]	14	9	4 (29%)
NCSR	187	—	40 (21%)

*Data compiled from Dembitsky et al,[35] Phillips et al,[49] and Hill et al.[34]
Abbreviation: NCSR = National Cardiopulmonary Support Registry.

Resuscitation from Arrest

The results of recent studies evaluating treatment of cardiopulmonary arrest with percutaneous cardiopulmonary bypass are summarized in Table 61–16. There have been no clinical studies evaluating the Hemopump in the resuscitation of cardiac arrest patients.

With percutaneous bypass, 20% to 30% of cardiac arrest patients are discharged from the hospital. This compares favorably with the 10% hospital discharge rate for cardiac arrest patients resuscitated without mechanical assistance.[33–35, 49] Improved selection criteria and use of the Carmeda bypass system may further increase patient survival after resuscitation from arrest. Additional evaluation of resuscitative cardiopulmonary bypass is underway.

References

1. Gibbon JH Jr: Application of a mechanical heart and lung apparatus to cardiac surgery. Minn Med 1954; 37:171.
2. Stuckey JH, Newman MM, Dennis C, et al: The use of the heart-lung machine in selected cases of acute myocardial infarction. Surg Forum 1957; 8:342.
3. Spencer FC, Eiseman B, Trinkle JK, et al: Assisted circulation for cardiac failure following intracardiac surgery with cardiopulmonary bypass. J Thorac Cardiovasc Surg 1965; 49:56–73.
4. Dennis C, Carlens E, Senning A, et al: Clinical use of a cannula for left heart bypass without thoracotomy. Ann Surg 1962; 156:623.
5. DeBakey ME: Left ventricular bypass pump for cardiac assistance: Clinical experience. Am J Cardiol 1971; 27:3.
6. Moulopoulos SD, Topaz S, Kolff WJ: Diastolic balloon pumping (with carbon dioxide) in the aorta: Mechanical assistance of the failing circulation. Am Heart J 1962; 63:669.
7. Kantrowitz A, Tjonneland S, Freed PS, et al: Initial clinical experience with intra-aortic balloon pumping in cardiogenic shock. JAMA 1968; 203:135.
8. Reemtsma K, Drusin R, Edie R, et al: Cardiac transplantation for patients requiring mechanical circulatory support. N Engl J Med 1978; 298:670–671.
9. DeVries WC, Anderson JL, Joyce LD, et al: Clinical use of the total artificial heart. N Engl J Med 1984; 310:273–278.
10. Portner PM, Oyer PE, Pennington DG, et al: Implantable electrical left ventricular assist system: Bridge to transplantation and the future. Ann Thorac Surg 1989; 47:142–150.
11. Copeland JG, Levinson MM, Smith R, et al: The total artificial heart as a bridge to transplantation: A report of two cases. JAMA 1986; 256:2991–2995.
12. Frazier OH, Wampler RK, Duncan JM, et al: First human use of the Hemopump, a catheter mounted ventricular assist device. Ann Thorac Surg 1990; 49:299–304.
13. Norman JC, Cooley DA, Igo SR, et al: Prognostic indices for survival during post-cardiotomy intra-aortic balloon pumping. J Thorac Cardiovasc Surg 1977; 74:709.
14. Emery RW, Joyce LD: Directions in cardiac assistance. J Cardiac Surgery 1991; 6:400–413.
15. Pennington DG, Swartz MT: Assisted circulation and mechanical hearts. *In:* Heart Disease: A Textbook of Cardiovascular Medicine. 4th ed. Braunwald E (Ed). Philadelphia, WB Saunders, 1992, pp 535–550.
16. Smalling RW, Cassidy DB, Barrett R, et al: Improved regional myocardial blood flow, left ventricular unloading, and infarct salvage using an axial-flow, transvalvular left ventricular assist device: A comparison with intra-aortic balloon counterpulsation and reperfusion alone in a canine infarction model. Circulation 1992; 85:1152–1159.
17. Watanabe K, Kabei N, MacRea J, et al: Continuous measurement of oxygen consumption (MVO_2) and hemodynamic response during transapical left ventricular bypass. ASAIO Trans 1975; 21:566.
18. Catinella FP, Cunningham JN, Glassman E, et al: Left atrium-to-femoral artery bypass: Effectiveness in reduction of acute experimental myocardial infarction. J Thorac Cardiovasc Surg 1983; 86:887–896.
19. Pennock JL, Pae WE, Pierce WS, et al: Reduction of myocardial infarct size: Comparison between left atrial and left ventricular bypass. Circulation 1979; 59:275–279.
20. Pae WE: Ventricular assist devices and total artificial hearts: A combined registry experience. Ann Thorac Surg 1993; 55:295–298.
21. Pennington DG, Farrar DJ, Loisance D, et al: Patient selection. Ann Thorac Surg 1993; 55:206–212.
22. Ott RA, Mills TC, Eugene J, et al: Clinical choices for circulatory assist devices. ASAIO Trans 1990; 36:792–798.
23. Pennington DG, Swartz MT: Temporary circulatory support in patients with postcardiotomy cardiogenic shock. *In:* Cardiac surgery: state of the art reviews. Vol 5. No 3. Spence PA, Chitwood WR (Eds). Philadelphia, Hanley and Belfus, 1991, pp 373–392.
24. Burnett CM, Vega JD, Radovancevic JL, et al: Improved survival after Hemopump insertion in patients experiencing postcardiotomy cardiogenic shock during cardiopulmonary bypass. ASAIO Trans 1990; 36:M626–M629.
25. Loisance DY, Deleuze PH, Houel R, et al: Pharmacologic bridge to cardiac transplantation: Current limitations. Ann Thorac Surg 1993; 55:310–313.
26. Moritz A, Wolner E: Circulatory support with shock due to acute myocardial infarction. Ann Thorac Surg 1993; 55:238–244.
27. Page DL, Caulfield JB, Kastor JA, et al: Myocardial changes associated with cardiogenic shock. N Engl J Med 1971; 285:133–137.
28. Lee L, Bates ER, Pitt B, et al: Percutaneous transluminal angioplasty improves survival in acute myocardial infarction complicated by cardiogenic shock. Circulation 1988; 78:1345–1351.
29. Allen BS, Rosenkranz E, Buckberg GD, et al: Studies on prolonged acute regional ischemia: IV. Myocardial infarction with left ventricular power failure: A medical surgical emergency requiring urgent revascularization with maximal protection of remote muscle. J Thorac Cardiovasc Surg 1989; 98:691–703.
30. Scheidt S, Wilner G, Mueller H, et al: Intra-aortic balloon counterpulsation in cardiogenic shock: Report of a cooperative clinical trial. N Engl J Med 1973; 288:979–984.
31. Deeb GM, Bolling SF, Nicklas J, et al: Clinical experience with the Nimbus pump. ASAIO Trans 1990; 36:M632–M636.
32. Wampler RK, Frazier OH, Lansing AM, et al: Treatment of cardiogenic shock with the Hemopump left ventricular assist device. Ann Thorac Surg 1991; 52:506–513.
33. Reichman RT, Joyo CO, Dembitsky WP, et al: Improved patient survival after cardiac arrest using a cardiopulmonary support system. Ann Thorac Surg 1990; 49:101–105.
34. Hill JG, Bruhn PS, Cohen SE, et al: Emergent applications of cardiopulmonary support: A multiinstitutional experience. Ann Thorac Surg 1992; 54:699–704.
35. Dembitsky WP, Moreno-Cabral RJ, Adamson RM, et al: Emergency resuscitation using portable extracorporeal membrane oxygenation. Ann Thorac Surg 1993; 55:304–309.
36. Schroder T, Hering JP, Uhlig P, et al: Efficiency of the left ventricle assist device Hemopump in cardiac fibrillation. Br J Anaesth 1992; 68:536–539.
37. Lincoff AM, Popma JJ, Ellis SG, et al: Percutaneous support devices for high risk or complicated coronary angioplasty. J Am Coll Cardiol 1991; 17:770–780.
38. Loisance D, Dubois-Rande JL, Deleuze D, et al: Prophylactic intraventricular pumping in high-risk coronary angioplasty. Lancet 1990; 335:438–440.
39. Babic UU, Grujicic S, Djurisic Z, et al: Percutaneous left atrial-aortic bypass with a roller pump (Abstract). Circulation 1989; 80(Suppl II):272.

40. Glassman E, Chinitz L, Levite H, et al: Partial left heart bypass support during high-risk angioplasty (Abstract). Circulation 1989; 80(Suppl II):272.
41. Hahn CJ, Pierce WS, Olsen DB, et al: Long-term biventricular assist. Ann Thorac Surg 1993; 55:227–232.
42. Moreira LF, Bocchi EA, Stolf NA, et al: Current expectations in dynamic cardiomyoplasty. Ann Thorac Surg 1993; 55:299–303.
43. Furnary AP, Magovern JA, Christlieb IY, et al: Clinical cardiomyoplasty: Preoperative factors associated with outcome. Ann Thorac Surg 1992; 54:1139–1143.
44. Lu H, Fietsam R, Hammond RL, et al: Skeletal muscle ventricles: Left ventricular apex to aorta configuration. Ann Thorac Surg 1993; 55:78–85.
45. Copeland JG, Frazier OH, McBride LR, et al: Anticoagulation. Ann Thorac Surg 1993; 55:213–216.
46. Hill JD, Griffith BP, Meli M, et al: Infections: Prophylaxis and treatment. Ann Thorac Surg 1993; 55:217–221.
47. Portner PM, Baumgartner WA, Cabrol C, et al: Internal pulsatile circulatory support. Ann Thorac Surg 1993; 55:261–265.
48. Pierce WS, Hershon JJ, Kormos RL, et al: Management of secondary organ dysfunction. Ann Thorac Surg 1993; 55:222–226.
49. Phillips SJ, Zeff RH, Kongtahworn C: Percutaneous cardiopulmonary bypass: Application and indication for use. Ann Thorac Surg 1989; 47:608–611.

CHAPTER 62

Pericardial Tamponade

William C. Shoemaker, MD

Pericardial tamponade is a condition caused by accumulation of pericardial fluid that constricts cardiac chambers by acutely increasing pericardial volume and pressure. It is an uncommon clinical condition produced by pericarditis with effusion or hemopericardium from penetrating trauma, central venous catheters, or cardiac instrumentation. The disorder may develop into life-threatening cardiogenic shock if it is not recognized and corrected rapidly.[1–7]

PERICARDIAL EFFUSION

The volume and significance of effusions vary widely. Effusions may be the cause of cardiogenic shock, a complication of constrictive pericarditis, or an incidental observation in acute pericarditis. Pericardial effusions may occur in a wide spectrum of disorders including (1) uremia; (2) neoplasms; (3) postmyocardial infarction (Dressler's syndrome); (4) post-cardiac surgery; (5) infection, including tuberculosis; and (6) systemic lupus erythematosus (SLE) and other rheumatologic disorders. Tamponade has been an infrequent observation in SLE, malignancies, benign teratoma, myeloid metaplasia, scleroderma, juvenile rheumatoid arthritis, and inflammatory bowel disease.[8–18] Pericarditis was reported in 75 of 395 (19%) SLE patients; tamponade occurred in 10 of these, 1 of whom died.[8]

The physiologic alterations produced by the effusion primarily depend on the volume of the effusion and the rate of its development. For example, small volumes that occur suddenly or large volumes in malignant disorders that take months to form may be well tolerated. In the latter instance, the relatively elastic pericardium will stretch over time to accommodate as much as 1000 mL of pericardial fluid.

Diagnosis

Symptoms and signs are not specific; they include distant heart sounds, "quiet precordium," increased area of cardiac dullness, or cardiac dullness percussed lateral to the apical impulse. These physical signs are more often seen rather late in the course of the disorder. The diagnosis is often suspected by serial chest radiography or electrocardiography (ECG) and confirmed by echocardiography, cardiac catheterization, or radionucleotide ventriculography. Early diagnosis is often suspected in patients with cancer of the lung or breast and leukemias, uremic patients on dialysis,[17] patients with unexplained increased central venous pressure (CVP), and patients with enlarged cardiac silhouette.

The ECG, which is sometimes suggestive of the diagnosis, may have low voltage and diffuse ST-segment elevation in most leads; the ST segments usually retain their normal concave appearance. There may also be PR depression. Chest radiograms that are nonspecific may reveal "water bottle" or globular shapes suggestive of an effusion. Echocardiography is the most sensitive test and can be used in the widest variety of situations. The M mode may show an echo-free space as the site of fluid collection. Two-dimensional echocardiography provides more accurate quantitation of the amount of effusion and its distribution, thickening of the pericardium, fibrinous adhesions, and the dimensions of the cardiac chambers. On occasion, ultrasonographic tests may suggest that an apparent cardiac enlargement may be accounted for by an effusion or that both may be present.[18, 19] The computed tomographic scan may demonstrate thickened pericardial sac walls.

Other laboratory tests of occasional usefulness include the sedimentation rate, which is usually elevated in acute viral or idiopathic pericarditis; leukocytosis (early) or lymphocytosis; cardiac enzymes, which are usually normal in pericarditis but elevated with acute myocardial infarction; and first-degree heart block or bundle branch block suggestive of widespread myocarditis.

Pericardiocentesis

Pericardiocentesis may be indicated for therapeutic reasons when there is rapid deterioration of hemodynamic function, when there is delay in operative decompression, and for diagnostic reasons in effusions of unknown cause. In the latter instance, the fluid is cultured for bacteria, fungi, mycobacteria; gram stained; and analyzed for hematocrit, cell count, cytology, glucose and protein levels, rheumatoid factor, antinuclear antibodies, and complement levels.

HEMOPERICARDIUM WITH TAMPONADE

Clinical Evaluation

The rate of development and severity of pericardial tamponade vary with its cause. Tamponade may abruptly occur after blunt trauma with rupture of the heart, penetrating cardiac injury, and cardiac catheterization or central venous catheterization. A rapidly forming tamponade is often fatal unless immediately corrected by pericardiotomy and decompression. This may be the case in tamponade after instrumentation during cardiac catheterization or placement of a central catheter because there is no route through the pericardium for spontaneous decompression of the pericardial fluid. With penetrating trauma, some of the pericardial blood initially may escape through the pericardial rent until clots obstruct this egress.

It is crucial to suspect tamponade from the clinical setting and to diagnose it promptly before shock or arrest occurs. Characteristically, the patient with acute tamponade is anxious, agitated, or even wildly disturbed, clawing the air like a caged animal and exhibiting air hunger. In later stages, there may be central nervous system depression, coma, and cardiac arrest. All patients with stab wounds of the chest and epigastrium, not excluding the back and right sides, must be suspected of having possible tamponade. Stab wounds of the right midaxillary line have been known to produce death from tamponade. Similarly, the diagnosis should be entertained in patients with gunshot wounds of the chest, back, or abdomen in whom the heart could have been in the direct line of the missile trajectory or could have been injured by the deflected missile. Tamponade should also be suspected in symptomatic patients who have recently undergone cardiac operations, catheterization, and placement of central venous catheters or pacing wires; radiographs should be taken after catheters are placed to document the position of the catheter tip. Finally, tamponade often occurs with significant hypovolemia as a result of blood loss into the pleural cavities from the rent in the pericardial sac; this often produces the typical picture of hypovolemic shock with hypotension, tachycardia, and low CVP. When volume is replaced, the CVP rises, but often hypotension and tachycardia persist.

Rarely, tamponade is also associated with blunt trauma or vigorous cardiopulmonary resuscitation that has fractured ribs. Pericardial tamponade produced by a penetrating chest injury may also occur within minutes, if rapid bleeding from the pierced heart produces clots that block the pericardial laceration and cause blood to accumulate in the pericardial sac. Alternatively, tamponade from a penetrating chest wound may develop over a period of days as blood from the lacerated heart slowly fills the pericardium and then leaks from the torn pericardial sac into the pleural space or mediastinum. This is in contrast to the temporal spectrum of pericardial effusions that produce tamponade slowly over weeks; the pericardial sac distends and may hold large volumes before clinical distress is manifest. In acutely developing tamponade, however, up to 250 mL usually is well tolerated, 250 to 450 mL produces moderately severe hemodynamic alterations, and hemopericardium greater than 450 mL produces severe hemodynamic changes, including shock and cardiac arrest.[10, 11]

Diagnosis

The clinical diagnosis of pericardial tamponade is based on Beck's triad of distant heart sounds, hypotension, and distended neck veins, the last of which reflects an elevated CVP (usually 18 cm H_2O and rising). In addition, there may be an increased area of cardiac dullness outside the apical point of maximum impulse and pulsus paradoxus. The latter is an exaggerated pulse variation with respiration, that is, decreased systolic pressure, pulse pressure, and heart rate during inspiration.[5, 6] It is evaluated as the patient breathes normally; the arm cuff is gradually deflated until the first sound is intermittently heard on auscultation at the brachial artery; this is pressure during expiration. The cuff is again deflated slowly until all beats are heard, especially during inspiration; differences in systolic pressures greater than 15 mm Hg indicate pulsus paradoxus.[20] Although measurable by sphygmomanometer, pulsus paradoxus is best illustrated by a continuous arterial pressure tracing. It is an inconsistent sign in acute tamponade from penetrating chest wounds but is seen more frequently when tamponade slowly develops with pericardial effusions.[3, 4] Conditions that increase intrathoracic pressure, such as chronic obstructive lung disease, obesity, and congestive failure, must be ruled out.

The incidence of tamponade after penetrating chest injury is only 2%.[1–4] Of those patients with proven cardiac tamponade, only about one third have the entire Beck's triad when first diagnosed. Characteristically, tamponade patients may appear to be stable for varying periods of time, but they may suddenly and rapidly deteriorate. It is most important to make an early diagnosis and give appropriate therapy rapidly during the early stage because, if treatment is delayed until all the classic signs of Beck's triad are present, cardiac arrest is likely to intervene. When hypotension occurs, it often leads rapidly to circulatory collapse and arrest. The mortality of patients with tamponade subjected to thoracotomy without delay is 15% to 25%; mortality increases to 60% after cardiac arrest occurs.[1]

Laboratory Diagnosis

Routine chest radiograph is rarely diagnostic. However, it may reveal hemothorax or hemomediastinum, which often occurs in tamponade from penetrating chest injuries when pericardial blood escapes into the chest cavity through the pericardial rent. Increased heart size is occasionally seen, and a water bottle–shaped heart may develop in patients with tamponade from pericardial effusion but is uncommon in acute tamponade from penetrating cardiac injuries.

Although rarely diagnostic of tamponade in penetrating wounds, echocardiography is necessary to rule out other cardiac disorders. Usually, there are nonspecific changes such as low voltage, depressed or altered ST segments suggestive of subepicardial ischemia, and, in some instances, alternating voltage of P and QRS complexes.

The diagnosis is confirmed if nonclotting blood is obtained by pericardiocentesis, but a negative tap does not rule out tamponade. About 20% of patients with tamponade have false-negative taps because the pericardial sac may be filled with blood clots, which obstruct needle aspiration of pericardial blood.[21, 22]

Echocardiography is a very informative, noninvasive test that can be rapidly performed. Normally, a single echo emanates from the posterior wall and moves synchronously with the heartbeat. Two distinct echoes from this area indicate the presence of pericardial fluid. The space between the two echoes reflects the amount of fluid in the pericardial sac.[18, 19]

In questionable cases when hemodynamic stability and time permit, cardiac catheterization and pulmonary angiography may confirm tamponade. Angiocardiography outlines the right atrial lumen by radiopaque dye. The volume of pericardial fluid is indicated by the thickness of the right atrial wall (i.e., the space between the inside and outside cardiac borders at the right atrium); thickness exceeding 6 mm is diagnostic of pericardial fluid.

Differential Diagnosis

Acute tamponade must be differentiated from other conditions with elevated CVP, including tension pneumothorax, acute right ventricular failure, chronic obstructive lung disease, constrictive pericarditis, acute exacerbation of chronic bronchitis, acute pulmonary embolism, and fat emboli. Also, the increased CVP associated with tamponade must be distinguished from the high CVP resulting from excessive or rapid administration of fluids, abdominal distension from ascites or ileus, acute renal failure, increased intrathoracic pressure from pneumothorax, hemothorax, airway obstruction or mechanical ventilation, administration of vasopressors, and clotted nonfunctioning CVP catheter or a CVP catheter that slipped into the right ventricle.

PATHOPHYSIOLOGY AND HEMODYNAMICS OF CARDIAC TAMPONADE

There are two important clinical questions: Does the patient have a hemodynamically significant tamponade? How urgently must thoracotomy be performed? The following section on hemodynamic physiology addresses these concerns and their corresponding therapeutic implications.

The Primary Physiologic Defect

As fluid accumulates in the pericardial space, pressure is exerted outward on the pericardial sac and inward on the cardiac wall. Because the cardiac wall is more compliant, it absorbs most of the increase in intrapericardial pressure and transmits it transmurally to increase atrial pressure and end-diastolic ventricular pressure. This decreases effective ventricular filling, which thereby directly limits stroke volume and reduces cardiac output without affecting ventricular contractility (Table 62–1).[6, 7, 20–23] Thus, reduced stroke volume is the primary hemodynamic effect of tamponade.

Tamponade decreases both cardiac output and coronary blood flow; the latter may lead to reduced myocardial performance from ischemia. Coronary blood flow occurs during diastole as it is driven by the aortic diastolic–ventricular end-diastolic pressure gradient. When intrapericardial pressure from tamponade approaches atrial and ventricular end-diastolic pressures, aortic pressure falls, but myocardial oxygen demands may increase from reflex tachycardia. The combination of reduced coronary perfusion pressure and increased myocardial oxygen demand leads to rapid myocardial failure, shock, and cardiac arrest.

When tamponade develops rapidly, there is a rapid restoration of blood pressure on opening the pericardium, but restoration of blood pressure may be delayed when the tamponade develops over several hours.

Compensatory Hemodynamic Responses

There are three compensatory mechanisms to the reduced stroke volume: increased peripheral resistance, increased CVP, and increased heart rate (Fig. 62–1).[22] The increase in peripheral resistance maintains arterial pressure when cardiac output begins to fall. CVP increases as intrapericardial pressure is transmitted across the cardiac wall into the atria.

TABLE 62–1. Hemodynamic Values of Patients with Hemopericardium and Tamponade at the Time of the Maximum Changes

Variable	*Normal Values*	*Hemopericardium*	P *Value*
Stroke index (mL/m²)	43 ± 3	27 ± 4	<.010
Cardiac index (L/min · m²)	3.2 ± 2	2.9 ± 0.4	NS
MAP (mm Hg)	90 ± 2	77 ± 4.5	<.025
CVP (cm H_2O)	4.4 ± 1	18.7 ± 2	<.001
Heart rate (beat/min)	90 ± 2	112 ± 4	<.001
Mean transit time (s)	14.4 ± .08	19.1 ± 1.7	<.025
Left ventricular stroke work (g · m/m²)	52 ± 5	30 ± 5	<.005

Abbreviations: MAP = mean arterial pressure; CVP = central venous pressure; NS = not significant.

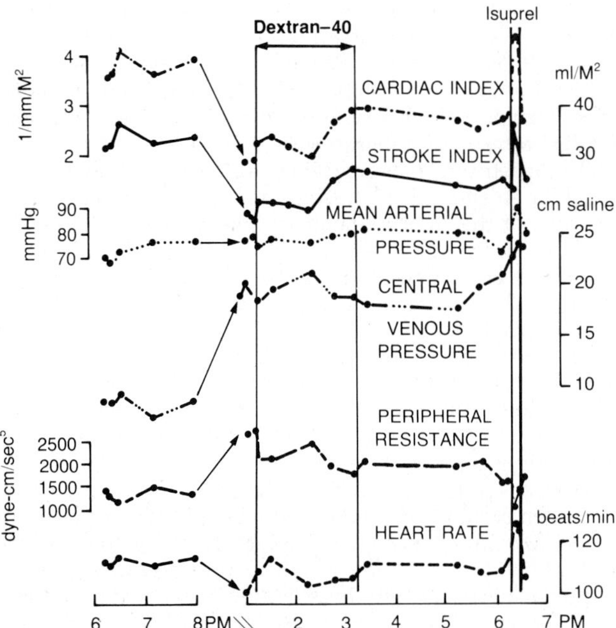

Figure 62–1. Early compensatory reactions to pericardial tamponade. A 22-year-old man was admitted to the intensive care unit 3 hours after being shot in the chest with a 22-caliber gun. The entrance wound was in the fifth intercostal space, just lateral to the midclavicular line; there was no exit wound. The findings on physical examination were otherwise normal. Radiography revealed the presence of a right hemothorax and a bullet in the posterior left side of the chest. A chest tube was placed, and 750 mL of blood was removed. After administration of 1 unit of whole blood and 750 mL of 5% plasma protein fraction, his blood pressure was 100/60 mm Hg, his heart rate was 110 beats per minute, and his CVP was 8 cm H_2O; other hemodynamic variables were essentially normal, except for the presence of tachycardia. Initially, it was believed that the bullet had missed the heart; however, over the next few hours, the complete hemodynamic picture of cardiac tamponade developed. The stroke index fell from about 36 to 18 mL/m², cardiac output decreased from about 4 to 2 L/min · m², and CVP rose from about 10 to 22 cm H_2O. The administration of 500 mL of colloid solutions improved the stroke index and cardiac index without appreciably increasing CVP. Mean arterial pressure was maintained by the compensatory increase in peripheral resistance; the high CVP increased the effective ventricular filling pressure, and the increased heart rates tended to partially maintain blood flow. Thus, volume therapy augmented the natural compensations and almost completely restored cardiac output during the short period when the patient was being prepared for surgery. Subsequently, surgery disclosed a small hole in the pericardium, which was filled with 250 mL of unclotted liquid blood and a large, 200-mL clot. The bullet had entered the anterior left ventricle and exited posterolaterally to lie free in the pericardial sac. The ventricular perforations were sutured, and the patient recovered without complications. (From Shoemaker WC, Carey JS, Yao ST, et al: Hemodynamic alterations in acute cardiac tamponade after penetrating injuries of the heart. Surgery 1970; 67:754.)

CVP is also elevated by venomotor constriction, an important compensation in which the increased venomotor tone returns more blood to the right side of the heart. The increase in heart rate is another early compensation that partially restores blood flow in the face of limited stroke volume.

The presence of these early compensatory responses to pericardial tamponade is indicated by CVP values between 12 and 18 mm Hg. Usually more than 250 mL of pericardial fluid does not produce hemodynamic effects, but as fluid accumulates the tamponade syndrome develops as a combination of the primary effects and their compensations. In time, the compensatory mechanisms preserving hemodynamic stability may become exhausted. Then decompensation occurs with decreased CVP and arterial pressures, circulatory deterioration, acidosis, exhaustion of the vasoconstrictive mechanisms, hypotension, shock, cardiac arrest, and, on occasion, death. By contrast, if the return of the elevated CVP value toward normal is associated with normotension, normal cardiac rate, and normal rhythm, the tamponade is no longer hemodynamically significant.

Therapeutic Management

The major problem is to correct the primary defect, hemopericardium, but a more immediate problem may be to maintain some degree of hemodynamic stability until the patient has definitive correction of the hemopericardium (Fig. 62–2).

Suspected cases of pericardial tamponade should undergo measurements of blood pressure, heart rate, and CVP every 5 to 15 minutes. Rising CVP and an increasing degree of hypotension indicate impending hemodynamic decompensation. Figure 62–3 illustrates a management protocol or clinical algorithm designed for the immediate treatment of patients suspected of having tamponade after penetrating (or blunt) trauma of the chest or upper abdomen; of those who exhibit neck vein distention or distress after thoracotomy, cardiac catheterization, or placement of a central venous catheter; and of patients with pericarditis, malignancies, or granulomatous diseases of the chest who become distressed or have increased neck vein distention.[24] The algorithm is primarily directed toward the sudden onset of life-threatening tamponade.

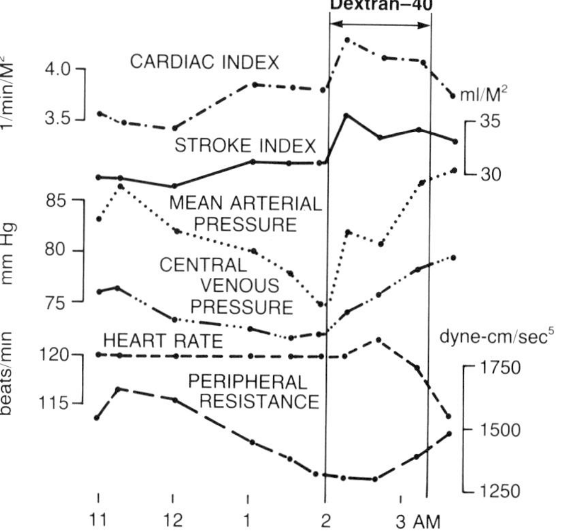

Figure 62–2. Decompensatory response to pericardial tamponade following initial improvement. A 49-year-old man was admitted to the intensive care unit 24 hours after sustaining a stab wound through the fourth intercostal space of the left anterior chest. On admission, his blood pressure was 125/70 mm Hg, his heart rate was 105 beats per minute, and his CVP was 17 cm H_2O. Chest radiographs revealed left hemothorax; a chest tube was placed, and 700 mL of blood was removed. Pericardiocentesis yielded only 9 mL of unclotted blood. Initially, hemodynamic measurements were stable: the cardiac index was slightly above normal, the stroke index was low, mean arterial pressure was 83 to 87 mm Hg, CVP was 18 cm H_2O, and the heart rate was 120 beats per min. However, as the pH fell from 7.4 to 7.2, decompensation gradually decreased peripheral resistance, arterial pressure, and CVP. Even though CVP values were still high, volume loading with 500 mL of colloid solutions restored the mean arterial pressure and increased both the stroke index and cardiac index while the patient was being prepared for definitive surgical correction of pericardial tamponade.

TABLE 62–2. Hemodynamic Changes Produced by Therapy

Variable	*Pericardiocentesis (n = 3)*	*Volume Load (n = 5)*	*Isoproterenol (n = 3)*
Stroke index (mL/m²)	+4	+8	+13
Cardiac index (mL/min · m²)	+0.9	+0.7	+2.3
Mean arterial pressure (mm Hg)	+7.0	+13	+11
Central venous pressure (cm H_2O)	−2.2	+5.7	+3
Heart rate (beat/min)	+14	−1	+18
Mean tension time (s)	−1	−1	−3
Left ventricular stroke work (g · m/m²)	+6	+16	+23

While the patient with suspected cardiac tamponade is being considered for operation, a trial of volume loading may improve hemodynamics and confirms that hypovolemia, myocardial insufficiency, or failure is not the major problem. Volume loading is not contraindicated by high venous pressures because tamponade is produced by inadequate ventricular filling as a result of high atrial pressure, not failure of myocardial performance (Table 62–2). Plasma volume expansion in patients with progressive reductions in stroke index improves stroke index, cardiac index, and arterial pressure.[21, 22] Fluid administration despite high venous pressures has a beneficial effect because contractility of the cardiac muscle is not initially impaired. Under these conditions, the heart is able to handle volume loads despite high venous pressures.

When sudden deterioration occurs, emergency thoracotomy may be indicated; if there is delay in operating for any reason, therapeutic pericardiocentesis may be lifesaving. It is not necessary to evacuate the entire pericardial contents; often, withdrawal of as little as 20 to 30 mL of nonclotting blood in acute hemopericardial tamponade may restore hemodynamic stability, because the difference between the amount of blood in compensated and decompensated hemopericardium may be small. Pericardiocentesis improves hemodynamics by reducing intrapericardial pressure; this increases venous return, cardiac output, and coronary perfusion. Additionally, preoperative pericardiocentesis reduces the risk of sudden deterioration and cardiac arrest during anesthesia induction. General anesthesia and positive-pressure ventilation lower cardiac output and blood pressure in tamponade patients, but pericardiocentesis reduces these effects. The goal of optimal therapy is urgently to remove hemodynamically significant pericardial fluid with appropriate expediency.

Complications

Recovery from tamponade after decompression and pericardial window is usually uneventful unless coronary vessels, septum, or cardiac valves have been injured by the penetrating injury. The pericardiotomy syndrome, which consists of fever, pain, and pericardial effusion, occurs in a small percentage of patients; this complication may respond to steroids or nonsteroidal anti-inflammatory drugs. Constrictive pericarditis is a rare complication.

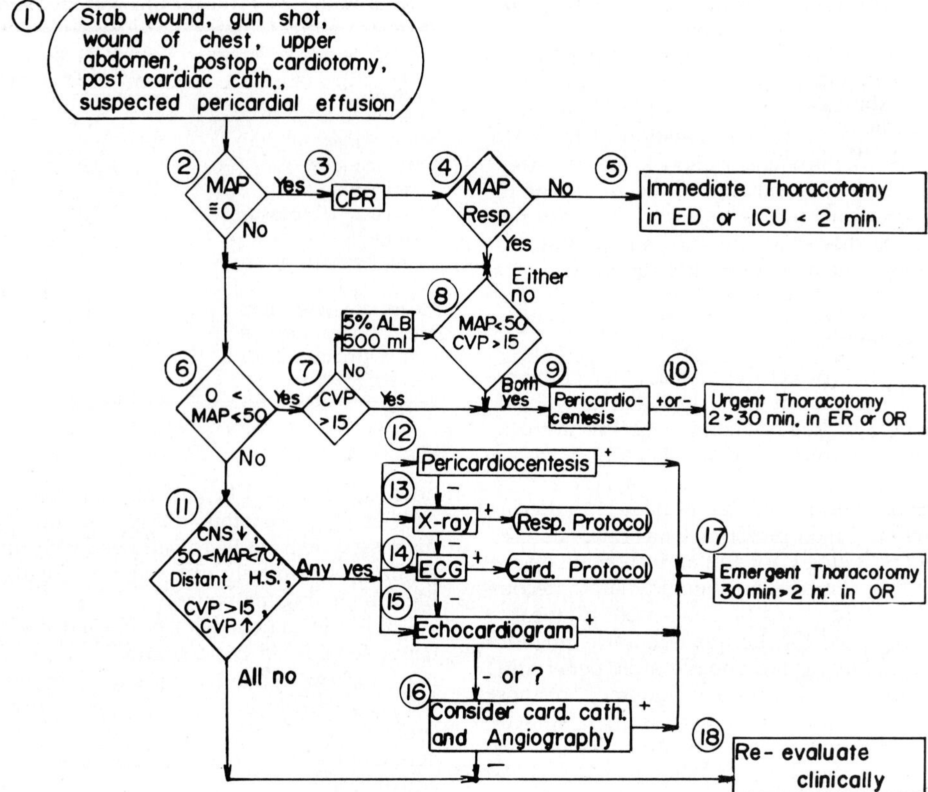

Figure 62–3. Algorithm for the management of cardiac tamponade.
Step 1: If mean arterial pressure (MAP) is zero or nearly zero, begin standard cardiopulmonary resuscitation (CPR) immediately with fluid and drug administration, airway management, and ECG.
Step 2: If blood pressure and pulse do not respond immediately to CPR, or if the response is not prompt and satisfactory (MAP >60 mm Hg), consider performing immediate thoracotomy, particularly in a trauma patient who is unresponsive to CPR. The decision to open the chest should be made within 2 to 5 minutes.
Step 3: If the patient has profound hypotension (MAP <50 mm Hg) on admission, or if severe hypotension persists after an initially successful CPR, measure CVP.
Step 4: If CVP >15 cm H_2O, perform therapeutic pericardiocentesis immediately; if CVP <15 cm H_2O, administer 500 mL of 5% albumin solution. This volume loading often restores hemodynamic stability and is safe even in the presence of high CVP.
Step 5: If MAP <50 mm Hg and CVP >15 cm H_2O in response to volume loading, consider a tentative diagnosis of tamponade if the patient has any of the following: 1) mild hypotension (50 mm Hg < MAP < 70 mm Hg); 2) disorientation, confusion, semicoma, or depressed CNS function; 3) distant or muffled heart sounds; 4) rising CVP, that is, from 12 to 15 cm H_2O; or 5) pulsus paradoxus.
Step 6: If any of the previous signs are observed, withdraw a small amount of pericardial fluid to check for the presence of nonclotting blood. Although the diagnostic removal of only a small portion of the pericardial fluid often restores hemodynamic stability to reverse an otherwise downhill course (Steps 4–7), usually a positive test result is an indication for emergent thoracotomy. Thoracotomy may be done in the emergency department, intensive care unit, or operating room, but should ideally be started in <30 minutes and, in all cases, within 2 hours. Timing is particularly critical in a hypotensive trauma victim with suspected tamponade.
Step 7: The normotensive patient should be re-evaluated clinically, his or her arterial and venous pressures should be monitored, and he or she should undergo any diagnostic procedures indicated by other associated findings. (Modified from Shoemaker WC, Carey JS, Yao ST, et al: Hemodynamic alterations in acute cardiac tamponade after penetrating injuries of the heart. Surgery 1970; 67:754.)

SUMMARY

The sequence of hemodynamic events in cardiac tamponade provides the basis for diagnosis as well as the rationale for preoperative management. The progressive rise in CVP in the presence of normotension is a compensatory response in the early stage of tamponade. A rise in CVP in the face of hypotension indicates compensations that are inadequate to maintain circulatory integrity (i.e., insufficient venomotor and metarteriolar constrictor responses to maintain normal pressure-flow relationships). The fall of CVP and arterial pressure indicates decompensation from failure of compensatory mechanisms and should warn of imminent cardiac arrest.

The immediate goal of therapy in suspected cases of tamponade is to support the compensatory responses during the time of diagnosis and allow time to institute definitive therapy. With penetrating cardiac wounds, it is essential to have the correct diagnosis and prompt operative intervention. In the rapidly deteriorating trauma patient with stab wounds of the chest, delayed diagnosis and therapy may lead to cardiac arrest.

References

1. Beall AC, Diethrich EB, Crawford HW: Surgical management of penetrating cardiac injuries. Am J Surg 1966; 112:686.
2. Naclerio EA: Penetrating wounds of the heart: Experience with 249 patients. Dis Chest 1964; 46:1.
3. Wilson RF, Bassett JS: Penetrating wounds of the pericardium and its contents. JAMA 1966; 195:513.
4. Yao ST, Vanecko RM, Printen KJ, et al: Penetrating wounds of the heart: A review of 80 cases. Ann Surg 1968; 168:67.
5. Sugg WL, Rea WJ, Ecker RR, et al: Penetrating wounds of the

heart: An analysis of 459 cases. J Thorac Cardiovasc Surg 1968; 56:531.
6. Sharp JT, Bunnel IL, Holland JF, et al: Hemodynamics during induced cardiac tamponade in man. Am J Med 1960; 29:640.
7. Carey JS, Yao ST, Kho LK, et al: Cardiovascular responses to acute hemopericardium, compression by balloon tamponade, and acute coronary artery occlusion. J Thorac Cardiovasc Surg 1967; 54:65.
8. Kohl LE: Spectrum of pericardial tamponade in systemic lupus erythematosus. Arthritis Rheum 1992; 11:1343.
9. Inase N, Enomoto N, Sakaino H, et al: Systemic lupus erythematosus presenting with pericardial tamponade and lupus pneumonitis. J Parenter Enteral Nutr 1989; 28:362.
10. Goldenberg DL, Leff G, Grayzel AI: Pericardial tamponade in systemic lupus erythematosus. NY State Med J 1975; 75:910.
11. Rinkevich D, Borovik R, Bendett M, et al: Malignant pericardial tamponade. Med Pediatr Oncol 1990; 18:287.
12. Probhakar G, Nigam BK, Williams WG: Benign mediastinal teratoma causing pericardial tamponade. Eur J Cardiothorac Surg 1987; 1:53.
13. Uhl GS, Koppes GM: Pericardial tamponade in systemic sclerosis (scleroderma). Br Heart J 1979; 42:345.
14. Greenberg JH, Lucher CL: Drug-induced systemic lupus erythematosus: A case with life-threatening pericardial tamponade. JAMA 1972; 222:191.
15. Vukman RB, Foy GJ: Juvenile rheumatoid arthritis with pericardial tamponade in an adult. Arch Intern Med 1981; 141:1078.
16. Breitenstein RA, Solel AF, Watson DW: Chronic inflammatory bowel disease: Acute pericarditis and pericardial tamponade. Ann Intern Med 1974; 81:406.
17. Merrill RH, Raab SO: Dialysis catheter-induced pericardial tamponade. Arch Intern Med 1982; 142:1751.
18. Feigenbaum H: Echocardiography. 2nd ed. Philadelphia, Lea & Febiger, 1976.
19. Asinger RW, Rourke T, Hodges M, et al: The role of echocardiography in emergencies. Minn Med 1980; 63:855.
20. Shabetai R, Fowler NO, Fenton JC: Pulsus paradoxus. J Clin Invest 1965; 44:1882.
21. Shoemaker WC, Carey JS, Yao ST, et al: Hemodynamic monitoring for physiologic evaluation, diagnosis, and therapy of acute hemopericardial tamponade from penetrating wounds. J Trauma 1973; 13:36.
22. Shoemaker WC, Carey JS, Yao ST, et al: Hemodynamic alterations in acute cardiac tamponade after penetrating injuries of the heart. Surgery 1970; 67:754.
23. Isaacs JP, Berglund E, Sarnoff SJ: Ventricular function: III. Pathologic physiology of acute cardiac tamponade studied by means of ventricular function curves. Am Heart J 1954; 38:66.
24. Shoemaker WC: Algorithm for early recognition and management of cardiac tamponade. Crit Care Med 1975; 3:59.

CHAPTER 63

Pulmonary Hypertension

Lewis J. Rubin, MD

The pulmonary circulation is a low-pressure circuit that accepts the entire right ventricular output at a resistance that is normally one tenth of that in the systemic circulation, even when cardiac output is increased severalfold with activity. Increases in pulmonary artery pressure lead to an increased impedance to right ventricular ejection. When afterload is increased either acutely or on a sustained basis, right-sided heart dysfunction ensues, producing symptoms that are a manifestation of the reduced cardiac output. *Cor pulmonale* is best defined as pulmonary hypertension in the setting of acute or chronic respiratory disease. Right-sided heart failure occurs relatively late in the course of cor pulmonale. Indeed, patients with acute cor pulmonale may manifest few of the signs of overt right-sided heart failure with which clinicians are familiar, such as edema, ascites, or hepatomegaly.

PATHOPHYSIOLOGY OF PULMONARY HYPERTENSION

Pulmonary hypertension can be classified on the basis of the primary anatomic site in which the vascular insult originates. Left ventricular failure and left-sided valvular disease produce pulmonary artery hypertension primarily by elevating the postcapillary (venous) pressure, resulting in an increased upstream pressure to maintain flow through the lung circuit. In this setting, the gradient between the pulmonary artery diastolic and pulmonary capillary wedge or left atrial pressures is relatively small (3–5 mm Hg) despite the presence of pulmonary hypertension. The total pulmonary resistance (TPR) is increased out of proportion to the pulmonary vascular resistance (PVR), and the histopathologic changes in the arterial tree are relatively mild and potentially reversible. In contrast, conditions in which the pulmonary arteries and arterioles are the primary site of disease are associated with an increased pulmonary arteriovenous pressure gradient and parallel increases in TPR and PVR. The vascular abnormalities in these conditions range from mild intimal proliferation to vascular obliteration and may be highly reversible or irreversible depending on the cause, severity, and duration.

The hemodynamic disparity in vascular resistances is helpful in differentiating the primary site and potential cause of disease in most cases, but there are two exceptions. The first is pulmonary veno-occlusive disease, which is characterized pathologically by obliteration of the small and medium-size pulmonary veins, yet the pulmonary capillary wedge pressure measured with a pulmonary artery flotation catheter may be normal. This occurs because the wedge pressure reflects downstream pressure in the large pulmonary veins, which drain blood largely from those capillary-venule networks that are unaffected and that do not readily communicate with diseased capillary-venule circuits. Thus, the PVR approximates TPR in the setting of postcapillary hypertension. An occasional clue to the presence of this disease may be the measurement of disparate wedge pressures in different regions of the lung. Second, many patients with mitral valve disease who undergo valve replacement surgery manifest a prompt fall in pulmonary artery pressure postoperatively because of the correction of the downstream obstruction to flow. However, long-standing pulmonary venous hypertension can result in persistent precapillary hypertension, characterized pathologically by extensive arterial remodeling, despite correction of the underlying cause.

Table 63–1 shows a classification of pulmonary hypertension based on cause. Pulmonary vascular diseases resulting from disorders that primarily alter the structure or function of the lung or diseases that affect the lung circulation as part of a systemic illness are considered to be secondary forms of pulmonary hypertension. Primary, or idiopathic, pulmonary hypertension (PPH) is a disorder in which pulmonary artery pressure is increased in the absence of a clinically demonstrable underlying cause.[1]

A variety of factors contribute to the development of pulmonary hypertension in the setting of respiratory disease and are depicted in Figure 63–1. Alveolar hypoxia is a common feature of many forms of acute or chronic respiratory disease and produces selective constriction of pulmonary

TABLE 63–1. Classification of Processes Causing Pulmonary Artery Hypertension

Diseases Affecting the Air Passages of the Lung and Alveoli
Chronic obstructive lung disease
Cystic fibrosis
Infiltrative or granulomatous diseases
Sarcoidosis
Idiopathic pulmonary fibrosis
Connective tissue diseases
Radiation
Pneumoconiosis
Upper airway obstruction
Congenital developmental defects
Adult respiratory distress syndrome
Diseases Affecting Thoracic Cage Movement
Kyphoscoliosis
Neuromuscular weakness
Sleep apnea syndrome
Idiopathic hypoventilation
Pleural fibrosis
Diseases Directly Affecting the Pulmonary Vasculature
Primary pulmonary hypertension
Granulomatous pulmonary hypertension
Toxin-induced pulmonary vascular disease
Anorectic agents
Intravenous drug use
L-tryptophan
Cocaine
Sickle cell disease
Thromboembolic disease
Pulmonary vasculitis
Pulmonary veno-occlusive disease
Congenital heart disease
Chronic portal hypertension
Human immunodeficiency virus infection
Diseases Affecting the Pulmonary Vasculature by Extrinsic Compression
Mediastinal tumors
Aneurysms
Granuloma
Mediastinal fibrosis
Left ventricular dysfunction and left atrial hypertension

arteries. Hypoxic pulmonary vasoconstriction appears to be an intrinsic property of pulmonary smooth-muscle cells and is dependent on both the availability of extracellular calcium and the state of the smooth-muscle cell membrane, voltage-gated calcium and potassium channels.[2] Hypercarbia and acidosis, which frequently accompany obstructive lung disease and may be particularly conspicuous in the setting of acute respiratory failure, potentiate the pulmonary vascular hypoxic pressor response. Although acute hypoxic pulmonary vasoconstriction is readily reversible on restoration of normal gas tensions, chronic hypoxia results in vascular remodeling, which is both slowly and incompletely responsive to correction of the derangements in ventilation and gas exchange. Mechanical compression of the vasculature by hyperinflated lungs may also play a role in the development of pulmonary hypertension in the setting of severe emphysema and may contribute to worsening pulmonary vascular dynamics during acute decompensations. The polycythemia that occurs in the setting of chronic hypoxemia to maximize oxygen delivery to the peripheral tissues can result in hyperviscosity, further impeding blood flow through the lung circulation. A loss of the cross-sectional surface area of the vasculature as a result of widespread destruction of normal lung parenchyma may also contribute to elevations in pulmonary arterial pressure in conditions such as advanced bullous emphysema or fibrotic diseases of the lung. Finally, thromboembolism can result in an acute decompensation in the setting of chronic cardiopulmonary disease by raising pulmonary artery pressure directly as a result of vascular obstruction by thrombus, by release of vasoactive substances at the site of thrombosis, or by worsening intrapulmonary gas exchange and potentiating hypoxic pulmonary vasoconstriction.

Elevations in pulmonary artery pressure occur frequently in patients with the adult respiratory distress syndrome (ARDS). In addition to the factors just listed, release of vasoactive mediators as a result of the underlying inflammatory process contributes to the pulmonary vascular process.[3]

A variety of connective tissue diseases can be complicated by the development of pulmonary hypertension either as part of a systemic vasculopathy or as the primary manifestation of the illness. Additionally, the vasculature may be secondarily involved as a result of parenchymal lung disease, such as pulmonary fibrosis in systemic sclerosis. Pulmonary vasospasm (pulmonary Raynaud's phenomenon) has been observed during right-sided heart catheterization in some patients with connective tissue diseases, particularly among those who experience typical peripheral Raynaud's phenomenon.

PPH is a condition of unknown cause in which the pulmonary vasculature appears to be the exclusive target of the disease process.[1, 4] A number of conditions have been associated with this disorder: Pulmonary hypertension may

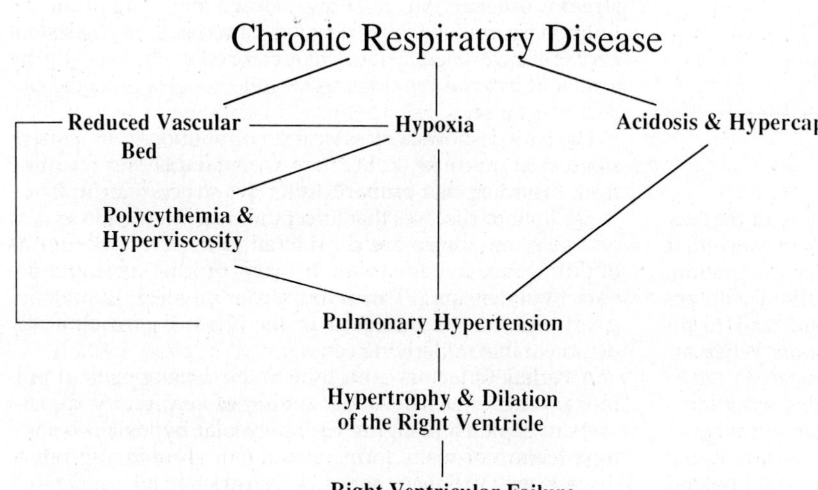

Figure 63–1. The pathogenesis of pulmonary hypertension in chronic respiratory disease (cor pulmonale).

complicate portal hypertension possibly because of an unidentified vasotoxin that bypasses hepatic metabolism and may injure the lung circulation. Pulmonary hypertension has resulted from the ingestion of diet suppressants, which are chemically similar to amphetamines, suggesting the possibility that these agents either induce vasoconstriction directly or may alter the metabolism of circulating vasoactive substances such as serotonin. This potential mechanism has also been suggested to cause the pulmonary vascular disease that has occurred in patients ingesting contaminated rapeseed oil (toxic oil syndrome) and contaminated L-tryptophan. Extracts from the plant species *Crotalaria,* which are used in parts of Africa and the Caribbean to make herbal tea, have also been implicated in the pathogenesis of PPH in several patients. Furthermore, the administration of the monocrotaline derivative of this plant to laboratory animals results in a severe necrotizing pulmonary arteritis and the subsequent development of chronic pulmonary vascular disease. Cocaine, which is known to possess potent vasoconstrictor properties, has been reported to produce pulmonary hypertension that is characterized pathologically by medial hypertrophy of the muscular pulmonary arteries. Pulmonary vascular disease that is pathologically identical to PPH has also been observed in patients who test positive for antibodies to the human immunodeficiency virus, even in the absence of evidence of substance abuse.

PPH occurs nearly twice as frequently in women as in men. Although individuals of any age may be affected, the disease is most common between the ages of 20 and 50 years. Less than 10% of patients have a family history of PPH, and it has been suggested that this disease may be transmitted genetically as an autosomal dominant trait with incomplete penetrance.

CLINICAL MANIFESTATIONS

Patients with pulmonary hypertension typically present with nonspecific and nondiagnostic symptoms. These include exertional dyspnea, fatigue, chest pain that is often described as a substernal pressure suggestive of angina pectoris, and syncope. The latter complaint is particularly noteworthy because it implies a markedly impaired cardiac output and is a poor prognostic sign. Similarly, edema or anasarca implies the presence of right-sided heart failure and portends a poor prognosis. Raynaud's phenomenon is reported to occur in up to 25% to 30% of patients with PPH, although it is far more common in pulmonary hypertension secondary to connective tissue diseases. Hoarseness may result from compression of the recurrent laryngeal nerve by massively dilated proximal pulmonary arteries. A chronic, nonproductive cough may also be evident and may be due to stimulation of interstitial irritant receptors as a result of vascular enlargement.

The physical examination may not only suggest the presence of pulmonary vascular disease but also provide important clues to its cause. Examination of the jugular venous pulse may demonstrate elevation of the venous pressure, suggesting right-sided heart volume overload as well as prominent a or cv waves, indicating altered right ventricular compliance and tricuspid regurgitation, respectively. Examination of the chest may disclose abnormalities that point to an underlying specific cause for pulmonary vascular disease, such as obstructive lung disease or restriction resulting from rib cage deformities. The findings on cardiac examination may vary depending on the cause and severity of the process. Patients with severe, chronic pulmonary hypertension usually manifest a prominent right ventricular impulse along the parasternal region; a right-sided fourth heart sound and pulmonic component to the second heart sound (P_2) may also be palpable. In contrast, the point of maximal cardiac impulse is frequently displaced to the subxiphoid region in patients with cor pulmonale resulting from severe obstructive lung disease. Auscultation of the heart may disclose an accentuated P_2, right-sided S_4 gallop, or a pulmonic ejection click. An S_3 gallop is indicative of right-sided heart failure and is a serious prognostic finding. The murmur of tricuspid insufficiency, audible along the lower right sternal border and increasing with inspiration, is a common finding in advanced pulmonary hypertension. On occasion, a murmur of pulmonic insufficiency may be heard at the left second intercostal space and the parasternal area. Fixed splitting of the second heart sound should raise suspicion of an unsuspected atrial septal defect. Short systolic bruits heard while auscultating the lungs may be a clue to the presence of partially occlusive thrombus in the larger pulmonary arteries.

Because a normal right ventricle can acutely increase systolic pressure only to a level of approximately 40 to 45 mm Hg in response to an acute vascular insult without resulting in overt right-sided heart failure and cardiogenic shock, the physical findings in acute pulmonary hypertension are usually less dramatic compared with the findings in established, long-standing hypertensive pulmonary vascular disease in which compensatory changes have occurred.

Peripheral cyanosis implies a markedly reduced cardiac output, whereas central cyanosis may indicate the presence of a right-to-left shunt, which may be due to congenital heart disease with Eisenmenger's physiology, pulmonary arteriovenous malformations, the opening of the foramen ovale caused by right atrial pressure and volume overload, or severe, acute lung injury. Digital clubbing does not occur in PPH, and its presence suggests that pulmonary hypertension is due to parenchymal lung disease, congenital heart disease, or hepatic cirrhosis.

DIAGNOSTIC APPROACH

A variety of laboratory tests are useful in establishing a diagnosis of pulmonary hypertension and determining its cause. Chest radiographs may disclose evidence of parenchymal lung disease or demonstrate right ventricular and pulmonary vascular prominence (Fig. 63–2). Kerley's B lines on the chest radiograph of a patient with unexplained pulmonary hypertension and a normal left side of the heart by cardiac catheterization or echocardiogram suggests the presence of pulmonary veno-occlusive disease. Electrocardiography (ECG) may show the characteristic signs of right ventricular hypertrophy, including a QRS axis greater than 110°, RSR′ complex in V_1 and V_2, and an incomplete right bundle branch block. The findings are generally much less prominent in patients with underlying lung disease because of the displacement of the heart in the thorax in patients with hyperinflation and the tendency for cor pulmonale to be a milder form of pulmonary hypertension than other causes. The presence of an $S_1Q_3T_3$ pattern on the ECG is strongly suggestive of an acute right ventricular pressure overload state, such as massive acute pulmonary thromboembolism. Prominent, peaked p waves in the inferior and right precordial leads (p pulmonale) are nonspecific findings on ECG and may appear and disappear in patients with acute, reversible airflow obstruction even in the absence of pulmonary hypertension. Echocardiography may demonstrate right-sided chamber enlargement, flattening of the interventricular septum during systole, or the presence of coexistent left ventricular or mitral valve disease (Fig. 63–3). A pericardial effusion may also be present and is sugges-

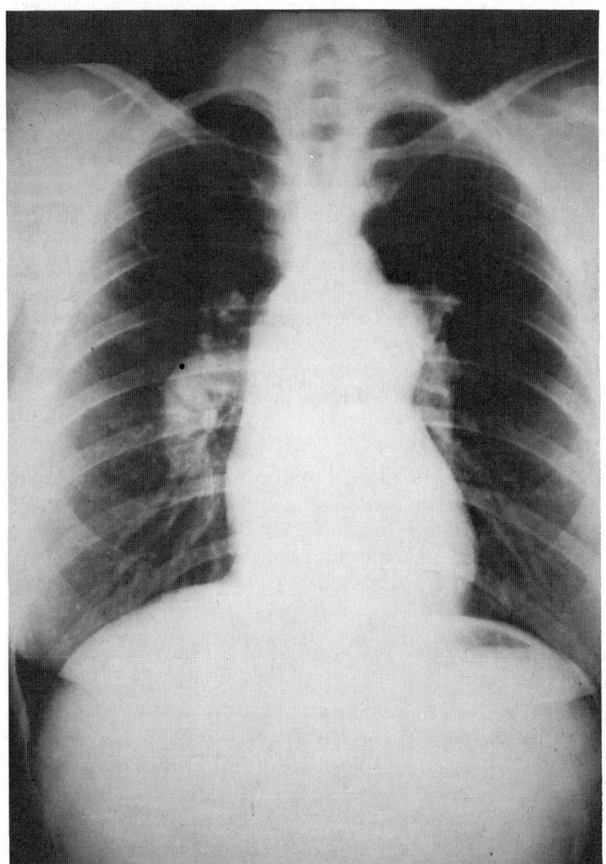

Figure 63–2. Posteroanterior chest radiograph from a patient with pulmonary hypertension. The proximal pulmonary arteries are enlarged, and the right ventricular configuration is prominent.

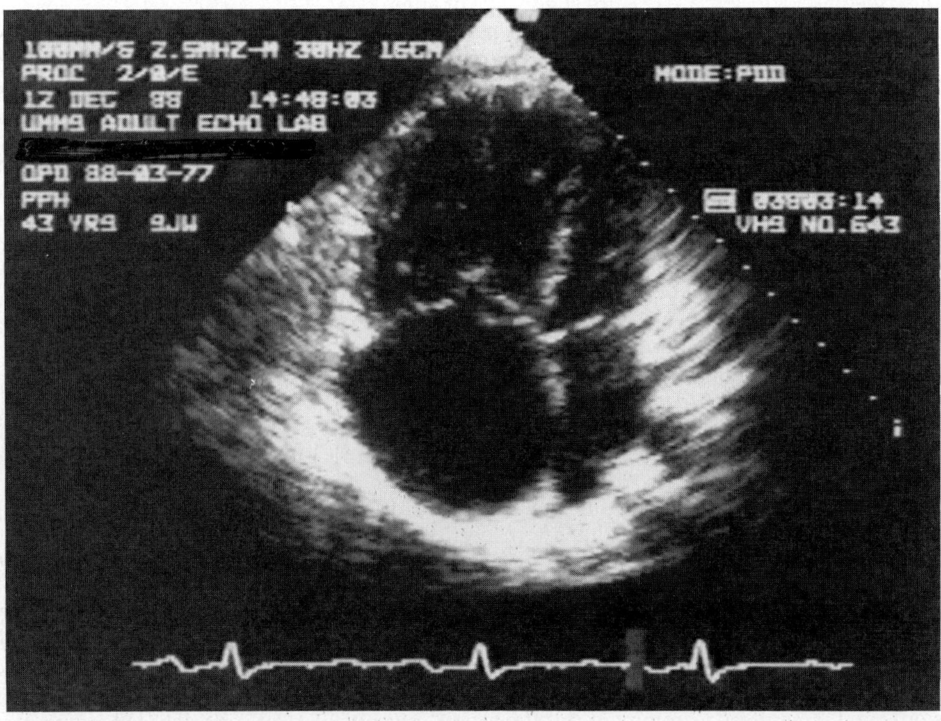

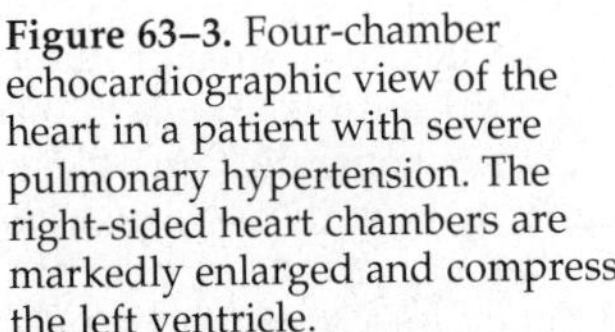

Figure 63–3. Four-chamber echocardiographic view of the heart in a patient with severe pulmonary hypertension. The right-sided heart chambers are markedly enlarged and compress the left ventricle.

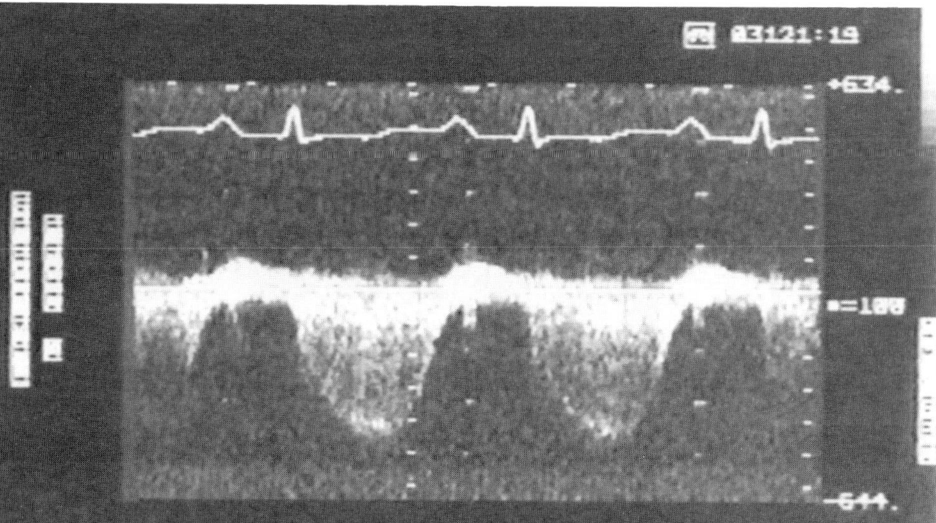

Figure 63–4. Doppler examination of the tricuspid valve showing a regurgitant jet, which can be used to estimate pulmonary artery systolic pressure.

tive of either a connective tissue disease or right atrial pressure overload. Doppler studies can be used to determine the presence and estimate the magnitude of tricuspid regurgitation, which may be useful in noninvasively estimating the pulmonary artery systolic pressure (Fig. 63–4). Intravenous injection of agitated saline or hydrogen peroxide during echocardiographic study may disclose the presence and site of an intracardiac shunt (Fig. 63–5).

The severity of pulmonary hypertension correlates closely with the degree of derangement in lung function in patients with chronic parenchymal lung disease. In general, patients with chronic airflow obstruction are likely to have concomitant pulmonary hypertension when the forced expiratory volume in 1 second falls below 1 L.[5] In chronic restrictive lung disease, pulmonary hypertension is usually present when the vital capacity or the diffusing capacity for carbon monoxide is below 50% of predicted. Patients whose partial pressure of arterial oxygen is below 55 mm Hg will generally have pulmonary hypertension, and the more severe the hypoxemia, the more severe the pulmonary hypertension is likely to be. Additionally, arterial blood gas measurements while the patient breathes ambient air may be important not only in establishing a cause but also in guiding the initial approach to therapy. Worsening pulmonary hypertension during acute exacerbations is likely in individuals with severe, chronic parenchymal disease.

Chronic thrombotic occlusion of the pulmonary vasculature should be considered in any patient with unexplained pulmonary hypertension because it is potentially treatable by thromboendarterectomy.[6] Radioisotope lung scanning is

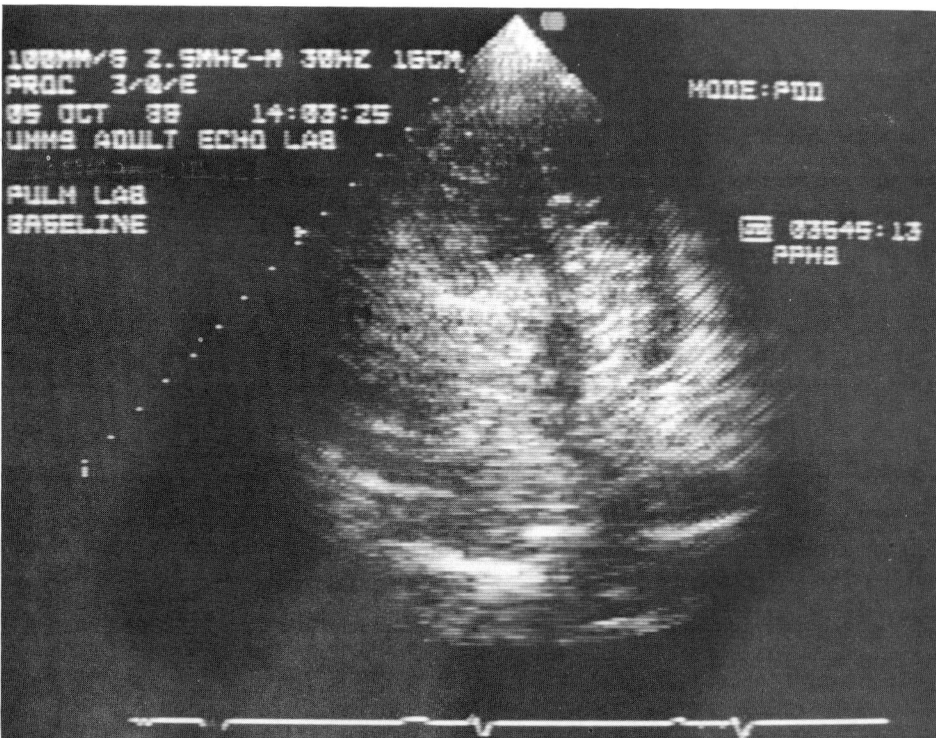

Figure 63–5. Saline contrast injection echocardiogram demonstrating the simultaneous appearance of echogenicity in both sides of the heart, indicating the presence of a right-to-left shunt.

a safe and reliable method to assess the distribution of ventilation and perfusion in the lungs, even in patients with severe pulmonary vascular disease. Patients with PPH usually manifest a homogeneous pattern of perfusion, whereas patients with chronic thromboembolism exhibit multiple perfusion defects of varying sizes. Scanning over the head or kidneys may demonstrate the presence of an unsuspected right-to-left shunt. Patients with veno-occlusive disease may have a mottled appearance on perfusion scan, although this is not always the case. Patients in whom a distinction between PPH and chronic thromboembolic disease cannot be made using noninvasive tests should undergo pulmonary arteriography. Similarly, consideration should be given to acute pulmonary thromboembolism in a patient with chronic cor pulmonale who experiences a sudden clinical deterioration in the absence of clear signs of exacerbation of the underlying parenchymal lung disease.

Patients with pulmonary vascular disease secondary to connective tissue diseases will usually have serologic studies that are abnormal and in high titers. Although some patients with PPH may have positive serologic studies as well, these are usually in nonspecific patterns and at low titers. Other studies that may be useful in the diagnostic work-up of unexplained pulmonary hypertension include high-resolution computed tomographic scanning of the chest to exclude occult interstitial disease, particularly when the chest radiograph is normal but pulmonary function is substantially impaired, magnetic resonance imaging to exclude fibrosing mediastinitis and proximal thrombosis of the pulmonary vasculature, and polysomnography to evaluate for the presence of sleep-disorder breathing.

Complete cardiac catheterization should be performed on patients with unexplained, severe pulmonary hypertension to exclude congenital heart disease, proximal or peripheral pulmonic stenosis, and valvular heart disease. The pulmonary artery pressure often approaches systemic levels in PPH, chronic thromboembolic disease, and connective tissue diseases and tends to be more modestly elevated in most forms of acute or chronic cor pulmonale. Hemodynamic monitoring in the critical care unit may also be useful in guiding the management of acute cor pulmonale.

In most cases, a cause for the pulmonary vascular disease can be ascertained on clinical grounds; however, in order for a definitive diagnosis to be made, it may be necessary to obtain a specimen of lung tissue from patients with severe pulmonary hypertension who have confusing evidence by physical examination or ancillary laboratory testing. Thoracoscopic-guided biopsy is the preferred approach. Although it carries an increased risk of complications in patients with severe pulmonary vascular disease, it can generally be performed safely in such patients and has a considerably lower risk and complication rate compared with traditional approaches. Transbronchial biopsy via the fiberoptic bronchoscope is not a suitable alternative to open lung biopsy in the setting of unexplained pulmonary vascular disease because the small size of the specimens precludes establishing a pathologic diagnosis.

APPROACH TO MANAGEMENT

The management of pulmonary hypertension should initially be directed at treating the underlying cause, if one exists. Improving gas exchange and airflow in patients with cor pulmonale resulting from chronic obstructive airways disease usually ameliorates the pulmonary hypertension to some degree. Patients with interstitial lung disease and pulmonary hypertension may show marked hemodynamic improvement when lung function is improved with corticosteroid or immunosuppressive therapy. Because hypoxia is a major contributor to both acute and chronic cor pulmonale, correcting hypoxemia is an important component of the therapeutic approach in affected patients. Although the hemodynamic effects of low-flow supplemental oxygen in patients with chronic obstructive lung disease are variable and slow in achieving their maximum,[7] survival is increased substantially when hypoxemia is corrected.[8] Patients with a stable PaO_2 of less than or equal to 55 mm Hg breathing ambient air or a PaO_2 less than or equal to 59 mm Hg *and* a hematocrit greater than 55%, p pulmonale on ECG or edema should be treated chronically with supplemental oxygen using flow rates sufficient to achieve a PaO_2 greater than 60 mm Hg. Flow rates may be increased for activity or at night in patients who experience arterial desaturation with exercise or sleep, respectively. In general, PPH patients with normal resting values for PaO_2 do not manifest hemodynamic improvement with oxygen therapy.[9] However, acute deteriorations caused by further compromise of cardiac function or lower respiratory tract infections can result in hypoxemia that is poorly tolerated and should be treated aggressively. Patients with a significant right-to-left shunt do not usually experience an improvement in oxygenation to an appreciable degree with supplemental oxygen therapy.

Polycythemia, resulting from the effects of chronic hypoxia in patients with severe parenchymal lung disease or congenital heart disease, may contribute to elevations in pulmonary vascular resistance by increasing blood viscosity. Although supplemental oxygen therapy usually results in a decrease in hematocrit in these patients, this response may be incomplete.[8] Isovolemic phlebotomy to a hematocrit of 50% to 55% may reduce the degree of hyperviscosity without compromising tissue oxygen delivery.[10]

OTHER THERAPEUTIC ALTERNATIVES

Vasodilator therapy for pulmonary hypertension is based on the premise that vasoconstriction is present in some forms of pulmonary vascular disease and that these drugs may exert their vasorelaxant properties in pulmonary as well as systemic vascular smooth muscle. Although vasodilator therapy may produce substantial hemodynamic and symptomatic improvement in some patients with chronic pulmonary hypertension, this effect is not universal, and serious adverse effects may also result. Thus, this approach to therapy should be individualized for each patient, and the patient's acute and long-term responses should be meticulously monitored.

A variety of systemic vasodilators have been shown to reduce pulmonary artery pressure in experimentally induced pulmonary hypertension, including hydralazine, calcium channel blockers (nifedipine, diltiazem, and verapamil), prostaglandins E_1 and I_2 (prostacyclin), adenosine, and nitrates (nitroglycerin and nitroprusside). These agents have also been used to treat selected patients with either primary or secondary pulmonary hypertension. A report from the National Institutes of Health–sponsored Registry on PPH suggests that approximately two thirds of patients manifest acute responses to vasodilator administration, which, if sustained, may be beneficial.[11]

The goal of vasodilator therapy is to reduce right ventricular afterload and increase cardiac output and systemic oxygen delivery. A substantial reduction in pulmonary arterial pressure concomitant with an increased stroke volume and an unchanged or minimally reduced systemic arterial pressure constitutes the optimal hemodynamic response to vasodilator administration and is frequently associated with evidence of regression of right-sided heart abnormalities by ECG, echocardiogram, or catheterization[12] and improved survival.[13] This "ideal" response is seen in only 25% to 30% of patients with PPH. In the remaining 30% to 40% of "responders," cardiac output is increased in the absence of any significant change in pulmonary artery or systemic blood pressures. The decision to institute long-term vasodilator therapy in these patients should be based on individual assessment.

The major adverse effects that may result from vasodilator administration include (1) systemic hypotension, which may result either from systemic vasodilation in the absence of any pulmonary vascular effect or from a reduced cardiac output caused by the negative inotropic properties of some drugs, (2) worsening pulmonary hypertension, which is due to an increased cardiac output flowing through a vascular bed with a fixed resistance, and (3) worsening hypoxemia caused by either an increased perfusion to poorly ventilated lung units (decreased ventilation-perfusion ratio) or increased right-to-left shunting if the systemic vascular effect predominates.[14] Patients with right-sided heart failure appear to be at the greatest risk for experiencing adverse effects with vasodilator administration;[11] however, there are no other demographic or clinical parameters that are reliable in predicting whether a patient will respond acutely or chronically to vasodilator therapy. Because the risk of sustained adverse effects is greatest with long-acting agents, the use of potent, short-acting, titratable vasodilators to test vasoreactivity has been advocated. Prostacyclin (prostaglandin I_2), prostaglandin E_1, adenosine, acetylcholine, nitroglycerin, and nitric oxide have all been used in this manner and appear to be well tolerated. The acute responses to prostacyclin have been useful in predicting responsiveness to orally active drugs.[15]

Patients with severe pulmonary hypertension are at risk for fatal pulmonary thromboembolic events because of their sedentary lifestyle, venous insufficiency, and dilated right-sided heart chambers with sluggish pulmonary blood flow. Even a small vascular thrombotic occlusion could be lethal to a patient with a compromised pulmonary vascular bed that possesses the capability to neither recruit unused vessels nor dilate functional vasculature in response to an acute insult. Accordingly, prophylactic anticoagulation has been advocated for patients with severe nonthrombotic pulmonary hypertension, and survival may be improved in patients receiving anticoagulants.[13, 16] However, anticoagulant therapy is not without risk in this setting, and life-threatening side effects, including hemoptysis from spontaneously ruptured pulmonary vessels, may occur. If therapy with warfarin is contemplated, the prothrombin time should be monitored frequently and maintained at a level 3 to 5 seconds above control. Adjusted-dose subcutaneous heparin may be a suitable alternative to warfarin, although it is more cumbersome to administer and its use should be reserved for patients who have a greater risk for complications with warfarin therapy. Acutely ill patients with nonthrombotic pulmonary hypertension should receive low-dose heparin subcutaneously during the acute illness.

Diuretics can be helpful in treating right-sided heart failure by reducing the degree of hepatic congestion and peripheral edema. In addition, patients with right-sided heart failure and hypoxemia resulting from a right-to-left shunt may experience improved oxygenation with diuresis owing to the reduction in the transatrial pressure gradient. However, diuretics should be used cautiously in this setting because decreasing right ventricular preload may result in a reduction in cardiac output. Additionally, diuretic-induced hypokalemia and alkalosis may be poorly tolerated.

There is little role for cardiac glycosides in the acute or chronic management of pulmonary vascular disease, with the exception of supraventricular tachyarrhythmias or biventricular failure.[17] Furthermore, patients with chronic respiratory disease are at an increased risk of experiencing toxicity with these agents.[18]

Combined heart-lung transplantation has been considered the surgical treatment of choice for severe pulmonary hypertension that is refractory to medical management.[19] However, the dearth of suitable organ donors and the limited number of centers with the expertise to perform this procedure have limited its availability. Early experience suggests that single lung transplantation may result in marked hemodynamic improvement in patients with isolated pulmonary vascular disease.[20] The greater availability of donor organs for lung transplantation may enable a larger number of seriously ill patients to undergo transplantation.

Because the course of pulmonary vascular disease is variable, it is difficult to determine the ideal time to consider transplantation in an individual patient. However, patients with symptoms that substantially limit their lifestyle and that are unresponsive to medical therapy may be suitable candidates for lung transplantation. Patients with evidence of severe and irreversible right-sided heart dysfunction, significant disease affecting the left side of the heart or coronary circulation, or complex congenital cardiac defects should be considered only for combined heart-lung transplantation. Organ rejection and opportunistic infections constitute the major causes of morbidity and mortality after transplantation. It is unknown whether idiopathic diseases such as PPH will recur in transplanted lungs.

At present, the average times on a waiting list for heart-lung transplantation and for single lung transplantation are approximately 18 to 24 months and 9 to 14 months, respectively. Prostacyclin delivered by a continuous intravenous infusion using a portable infusion pump has recently been used in patients with severe pulmonary hypertension and may be particularly helpful as a bridge to transplantation.[21]

The treatment of choice for chronic thrombotic pulmonary hypertension is pulmonary thromboendarterectomy.[6] However, only organized thrombus in the proximal vessels is approachable by this technique. Preoperative evaluation should include complete pulmonary angiography to determine the site and extent of thrombosis. Marked hemodynamic improvement frequently results from successful removal of organized thrombus. Patients with acute cor pulmonale caused by massive pulmonary embolism should be evaluated for emergent embolectomy if death is imminent and there is insufficient time for thrombolytic therapy to effect enough clot lysis to restore the integrity of the pulmonary vascular bed.

PROGNOSIS

In the settings of both chronic obstructive pulmonary disease and ARDS, the presence of cor pulmonale contributes significantly to a shortened survival.[3, 5] The 3-year survival in patients with severe airflow obstruction and a pulmonary vascular resistance three to four times normal is less than 10% to 15%.[5, 22] Survival is similarly influenced by the presence of pulmonary hypertension in chronic restrictive lung diseases and connective tissue diseases.

Mortality from PPH is, in large part, dependent on the state of the right ventricle. Patients with symptoms of severe right-sided heart dysfunction such as syncope and hemodynamic evidence of impaired right ventricular function such as a reduced cardiac output or mixed venous saturation and an elevated right atrial pressure usually succumb to the disease within 1 to 2 years.[23] Patients with milder symptoms and relatively well-preserved right-sided heart function survive longer, although the course is highly variable. The impact of therapy on survival has not been addressed in large-scale, prospective studies.

References

1. Rich S, Dantzker DR, Ayres SM, et al: Primary pulmonary hypertension: A national prospective study. Ann Intern Med 1987; 107:216–223.
2. Yuan XJ, Goldman WF, Tod M, et al: Hypoxia reduces potassium currents in cultured rat pulmonary but not mesenteric arterial myocytes. Am J Physiol 1993; 264:L116–L123.
3. Zapol WM, Rie MA, Frikker M, et al: Pulmonary circulation during adult respiratory distress syndrome. *In:* Acute Respiratory Failure. Zapol WM, Falke KJ (Eds). New York, Marcel Dekker, 1985, pp 241–273.
4. Rubin LJ, Barst RJ, Kaiser L, et al: Primary pulmonary hypertension: Report of the ACCP Consensus Panel. Chest 1993; 104:236–250.
5. Burrows B, Kettle LJ, Niden AH, et al: Patterns of cardiovascular dysfunction in chronic obstructive lung disease. N Engl J Med 1972; 286:912–918.
6. Moser KM, Dailey PO, Peterson K, et al: Thromboendarterectomy for chronic, major-vessel thromboembolic pulmonary hypertension. Ann Intern Med 1987; 107:560–565.
7. Timms RM, Khaja FU, Williams GW, et al: Hemodynamic response to oxygen therapy in chronic obstructive pulmonary disease. Ann Intern Med 1985; 102:29–36.
8. Nocturnal Oxygen Therapy Trial Group: Continuous or nocturnal oxygen therapy in hypoxemic chronic obstructive airways disease: A clinical trial. Ann Intern Med 1980; 93:391–398.
9. Morgan JM, Griffiths M, du Bois RM, et al: Hypoxic pulmonary vasoconstriction in systemic sclerosis and primary pulmonary hypertension. Chest 1991; 99:551–556.
10. Weisse AB, Moschos CB, Frank MJ, et al: Hemodynamic effects of staged hematocrit reduction in patients with stable cor pulmonale and severely elevated hematocrit levels. Am J Med 1975; 58:92–98.
11. Weir EK, Rubin LJ, Ayres SM, et al: The acute administration of vasodilators in primary pulmonary hypertension: Experience from the NIH registry on primary pulmonary hypertension. Am Rev Respir Dis 1989; 140:1623–1630.

11a. Rossaint R, Falke KJ, Lopez F, et al: Inhaled nitric oxide for the adult respiratory distress syndrome. N Engl J Med 1993; 328:399–405.

12. Rich S, Brundage BH: High-dose calcium channel blocking therapy for primary pulmonary hypertension: Evidence for long-term reduction in pulmonary arterial pressure and regression of right ventricular hypertrophy. Circulation 1987; 76:135–141.
13. Rich S, Kaufmann E, Levy P: The effect of high doses of calcium-channel blockers on survival in primary pulmonary hypertension. N Engl J Med 1992; 327:76–81.
14. Melot C, Naeije R, Mols P, et al: Effects of nifedipine on ventilation/perfusion matching in primary pulmonary hypertension. Chest 1983; 83:203–207.
15. Barst RJ: Pharmacologically induced pulmonary vasodilation in children and young adults with primary pulmonary hypertension. Chest 1986; 89:497–503.
16. Fuster V, Steele PM, Edwards WD, et al: Primary pulmonary hypertension: Natural history and the importance of thrombosis. Circulation 1984; 70:580–587.
17. Mathur PN, Powles P, Pugsley SO, et al: Effect of digoxin on right ventricular function in severe chronic airflow obstruction: A controlled clinical trial. Ann Intern Med 1981; 95:283–287.
18. Green LH, Smith TW: The use of digitalis in patients with pulmonary disease. Ann Intern Med 1977; 87:459–465.
19. Reitz BA, Wallwork JL, Hunt SA, et al: Heart-lung transplantation: Successful therapy for patients with pulmonary vascular disease. N Engl J Med 1982; 306:557–564.
20. Pasque MK, Trulock EP, Kaiser LD, et al: Single lung transplantation for pulmonary hypertension: Three month hemodynamic follow-up. Circulation 1991; 84:2275–2279.
21. Rubin LJ, Mendoza J, Hood M, et al: Treatment of primary pulmonary hypertension with continuous intravenous prostacyclin (epoprostenol). Ann Intern Med 1990; 112:485–491.
22. Traver GA, Cline MG, Burrows B: Predictors of mortality in chronic obstructive pulmonary disease. Am Rev Respir Dis 1979; 119:895–902.
23. D'Alonzo GG, Barst RJ, Ayres SM, et al: Survival in patients with primary pulmonary hypertension: Results from a national prospective registry. Ann Intern Med 1991; 115:343–349.

CHAPTER 64

Treatment of Massive Pulmonary Embolism

Graham F. Pineo, MD • Russell D. Hull, MBBS, MSc

Death from pulmonary embolism occurs in approximately 100,000 patients per year in the United States, and pulmonary embolism contributes to the death of another 100,000 patients.[1, 2] Pulmonary embolism represents the third most common cause of cardiovascular death after acute myocardial infarction and stroke[3] and is the most common preventable cause of death in hospitalized patients.[4] Although pulmonary embolism frequently develops in hospitalized patients with one or more comorbid disorders, this condition may develop in otherwise healthy individuals after orthopedic surgery or trauma or in pregnancy.[5–8] Effective prophylaxis is available for most of these situations,[9] but venous thromboembolism can occur unexpectedly in ambulant patients, particularly if they have been exposed to risk factors in the preceding months. When venous thromboembolism occurs, it is important that an accurate diagnosis be established by the use of the appropriate objective tests[10] so that treatment can be instituted immediately. The first indication that venous thromboembolism has occurred may be a massive pulmonary embolus that, unfortunately, can be fatal within a short time in up to one third of patients.[11, 12] This chapter is devoted to management of such patients with massive pulmonary embolism.

Patients with acute massive pulmonary embolism usually have a dramatic presentation: sudden onset of severe shortness of breath, hypoxemia, and right ventricular failure. Symptoms include central chest pain, often identical to angina, severe dyspnea, and frequently syncope, confusion, or coma. Examination reveals a patient in severe distress with tachypnea, cyanosis, and hypotension. The marked increase in pulmonary vascular resistance leads to acute right ventricular failure with the presence of large a waves in the jugular veins and a right ventricular diastolic gallop. With pulmonary hypertension, there is marked right ventricular dilatation with a shift of the intraventricular septum, decreasing cardiac output and further decreasing coronary perfusion, and this frequently results in cardiorespiratory arrest. If patients with a massive pulmonary embolus survive, they are acutely threatened by any further pulmonary thromboembolism.

The emergency management of massive pulmonary embolism includes the use of intravenous heparin (see Chapter 144); the use of oxygen with or without mechanical ventilation, which may include positive end-expiratory pressure; volume resuscitation; and the use of inotropic agents and vasodilators.[13] In addition to these supportive measures, specific treatment options for massive pulmonary embolism include (1) thrombolysis, (2) pulmonary thrombectomy with or without cardiopulmonary bypass support, (3) transvenous catheter embolectomy or clot dissolution, and (4) insertion of an inferior vena caval filter.

THROMBOLYTIC TREATMENT FOR MASSIVE PULMONARY EMBOLISM

Randomized clinical trials have demonstrated that the mortality rate from venous thromboembolism can be decreased by anticoagulant treatment.[11, 14, 15] A mortality rate of less than 5% should be achieved with intravenous heparin and oral anticoagulants, and this can be further reduced with the use of low-molecular-weight heparin.[16] However, patients who present with acute massive pulmonary embolism and hypotension have a mortality rate of approximately 20% despite the use of anticoagulants and other supportive measures. For such patients, the appropriate use of thrombolytic agents has a role. A high percentage of acute pulmonary emboli occur within 10 to 14 days of surgery[17–20]; therefore, they are excluded from treatment protocols using thrombolytic agents. These patients may be candidates for local infusion of low-dose thrombolytic agents.[20]

Several randomized clinical trials have compared thrombolytic drugs with heparin for the treatment of pulmonary embolism.[21–26] These trials compared urokinase (UK) with heparin,[21] streptokinase with heparin,[22, 23] or tissue plasminogen activator (t-PA) with heparin[24, 25] in different dosage regimens using either a bolus or chronic infusion up to 72 hours. Outcome measures for accelerated thrombolysis included quantitative measures on repeat pulmonary angiograms, quantitative scores on repeat pulmonary perfusion scans, and measures of pulmonary vascular resistance. Although all studies demonstrated superiority of thrombolysis (and in particular with t-PA) in terms of resolution of both radiographic and hemodynamic abnormalities when measured within the first 24 hours, this advantage was short lived. Repeat perfusion scans at 5 to 7 days revealed no significant difference between the patients treated with thrombolytic agents and those treated with heparin. Furthermore, the trials demonstrated a difference in neither mortality rate nor resolution of symptoms.

Measurement of diffusion capacity and capillary volumes at 2 weeks and 1 year after treatment showed that patients receiving thrombolytic therapy had higher diffusion capacity and lung capillary volumes compared with those receiving heparin.[27] Follow-up in the same group of 23 patients at an average of 7 years after thrombolytic treatment showed that patients treated with thrombolytic therapy had lower pulmonary artery pressure and pulmonary vascular resistance compared with patients who received heparin.[28] The clinical relevance of these findings, however, must await further prospective studies.

Several randomized clinical trials have compared different thrombolytic agents using different treatment protocols: streptokinase versus UK,[29] UK with UK,[30] t-PA with t-PA,[31] and t-PA with UK.[32] These studies again demonstrated resolution of angiographic and perfusion scan abnormalities as well as reduction of pulmonary pressure, but there was little or no difference between the regimens being compared. Again, the clinical relevance of the changes must await further study.

In weighing the risks and benefits of thrombolytic therapy, the main concern relates to bleeding. The incidence of major bleeding has decreased, particularly with the use of bolus or short-term infusions and newer thrombolytic agents, but intracerebral hemorrhage continues to occur more frequently than with heparin.[14, 17, 26, 33–35]

There does not appear to be a therapeutic advantage to any of the currently available thrombolytic agents, suggesting that a more modern approach to the use of streptokinase in a high-dose bolus fashion may be beneficial and less expensive. The addition of unfractionated or low-molecular-weight heparin does not enhance the effect of thrombolytic agents.[26, 36]

At this time, the role of thrombolytic agents in the management of acute massive pulmonary embolism still remains controversial. Although there is a more rapid dissolution of venous thromboemboli, the risk of serious bleeding remains a concern. Until there is a clearly demonstrated benefit in both morbidity and mortality from well-controlled, prospective, randomized clinical trials, the question of risk and benefit will remain.[37] In the meantime, the use of thrombolytic agents has become simpler with the use of high-probability ventilation-perfusion scans or echocardiography to confirm the diagnosis, the use of short-term or bolus infusion of thrombolytic agents into peripheral veins rather than into the pulmonary artery, the elimination of monitoring by laboratory tests, and treatment in the medical ward rather than in the intensive care unit. The fact that a high percentage of acute massive pulmonary emboli occur after surgery[8, 19, 20] despite the availability of effective prophylactic regimens against venous thromboembolism[9, 38] indicates that greater efforts must be taken to ensure that these prophylactic measures are being applied in a more uniform fashion.

Death from pulmonary embolism continues to remain high in North America and in Europe, and there are differences in mortality rate by sites and ethnic background, indicating that further epidemiologic studies are required.[39]

PULMONARY EMBOLECTOMY IN MASSIVE PULMONARY EMBOLISM

Pulmonary embolectomy is occasionally indicated in the management of massive pulmonary embolism. This is defined as the sudden occurrence of a massive embolus producing severe cardiovascular decompensation with severe hypotension, oliguria, and hypoxia refractory to aggressive treatment.[40] A somewhat more generous indication would be an obstruction of more than 50% of the pulmonary vasculature, arterial oxygen saturation less than 60 mm Hg, systolic blood pressure less than 90 mm Hg, and urine output of less than 20 mL per hour.[41] Patients who have contraindications to thrombolytic therapy or who have failed a trial of thrombolytic therapy in some centers are considered candidates for thrombectomy. On the other hand, others argue that a patient who survives the first 2 hours after an acute massive pulmonary embolus will probably survive with adequate medical management if no further pulmonary emboli occur. It is unlikely that it will be possible to perform a randomized trial comparing thrombolytic therapy with pulmonary embolectomy, and it is difficult to compare one case series of pulmonary thrombectomy with another because the case material is often not comparable.

Early experience with the Trendelenburg procedure revealed unacceptably high mortality rates (>50%).[12, 40] With the use of cardiopulmonary bypass (CPB) support, mortality rates between 16% and 57% have been reported.[42–50] In a review of 651 patients undergoing emergency pulmonary embolectomy, the survival rate was 59.3% with CPB support and 47.7% without CPB support.[40] Patients with chronic pulmonary hypertension, other medical disorders, or symptoms of more than 7 days' duration have higher mortality rates.[43, 48] Patients who have sustained a cardiac arrest before embolectomy have a higher mortality rate.[45] Greater care to avoid vasodilation at the initiation of anesthesia has decreased mortality rate.[13, 40] Pulmonary hemorrhagic infarction with reperfusion has been reported after pulmonary embolectomy.[50] Other causes of death after embolectomy include cardiogenic shock, infection, and hypoxic brain damage.[42] Pulmonary embolectomy is usually accompanied by insertion of a vena caval filter.

The role of pulmonary embolectomy remains unclear and will depend in part on the ready availability of a surgical team. Patients who are not candidates for thrombolysis (e.g., have had recent surgery) or who have not responded to maximal medical therapy may be candidates for pulmonary embolectomy. However, the report of successful thrombolysis with intrapulmonary UK in patients treated within 10 days of surgery casts further doubt on the need for this somewhat radical procedure.[20]

PERCUTANEOUS CLOT EXTRACTION OR DISRUPTION IN THE TREATMENT OF ACUTE MASSIVE PULMONARY EMBOLUS

Pulmonary embolectomy via a catheter suction device inserted into the jugular or femoral vein under local anesthetic has been used in the treatment of patients with acute massive pulmonary embolism who have contraindications to anticoagulants or thrombolysis.[51–55] Mortality rates of 27% and 28% were observed.[51, 54] The most common cause of death is cardiac arrest from ventricular arrhythmia, right-sided heart failure, and pulmonary hemorrhage.[51, 54] Some patients in whom clot extraction was not possible have gone on to successful pulmonary embolectomy on bypass. Inferior vena caval filters are used in conjunction with catheter embolectomy.[56]

Attempts have been made to fragment pulmonary emboli using conventional cardiac catheters[57] or a catheter guide wire in conjunction with pulmonary thrombolytic therapy.[58] Mechanical disruption of experimental pulmonary emboli in animals has been attempted using catheter-operated mechanical devices.[59, 60]

Catheter clot extraction is currently confined to use in a few centers with the required expertise, and this procedure cannot be used in patients who suffer cardiac arrest. The exact future role of catheter clot extraction is unclear.

INFERIOR VENA CAVAL INTERRUPTION IN THE TREATMENT OF PULMONARY THROMBOEMBOLISM

Early approaches to inferior vena caval interruption included ligation or plication using external clips.[61, 62] Both procedures were accompanied by an operative mortality rate of 12% to 14%, a recurrent pulmonary embolism rate of 4% to 6%, and an occlusion rate of 67% to 69%.[56] Also, many patients had chronic venous insufficiency after vena caval ligation. These complications gave rise to the development of catheter-inserted intraluminal filters.

Characteristics of an ideal filter include one that is easily and safely placed percutaneously, is biocompatible and mechanically stable, is able to trap emboli without causing occlusion of the vena cava, does not require anticoagulation, and is not ferromagnetic (does not cause artifacts on magnetic resonance images).[63–65] Although there is as yet no ideal filter, several of the available devices have proven useful. These include the Greenfield stainless-steel filter, titanium Greenfield filter, bird's nest filter, Vena Tech filter, and the Simon-Nitinol filter. In experienced hands, these devices can be quickly and safely inserted under fluoroscopic control. One novel filter can be inserted temporarily when needed, used in conjunction with thrombolytic therapy, and then removed.[66] With the available follow-up to date, the Greenfield filter has had the best performance record, and any future comparative studies should use this filter as the standard.[65]

The main indications for vena caval filters are when contraindications to anticoagulants exist, recurrent thromboembolism despite adequate anticoagulation, and prophylactic placement in high-risk patients. In the latter category are patients with cor pulmonale or a history of thromboembolism who are in high-risk situations (e.g., they have an acetabular fracture or have cancer). Patients who have had pulmonary embolectomy either surgically or via percutaneous catheters should have inferior vena caval filters inserted. As the filters have become safer and easier to implant, the indications have expanded somewhat. Their use in young individuals with a long life expectancy has been discouraged because it is unknown how well they will last in vivo. Complications of inferior vena caval filter placement include misplacement and tilting and occasional migration and perforation, but these complications are rare.[56]

FUTURE PROSPECTS

More efficient anticoagulation providing optimal therapeutic levels of heparin[67] or the use of low-molecular-weight heparin[16] has improved both the efficacy and safety of treatment of venous thromboembolism. Further experience with the newer thrombolytic agents using more efficient treatment protocols offers an expanded role for these agents with less serious bleeding than was seen in the past. With more efficient anticoagulation and thrombolysis, the need for pulmonary embolectomy should continue to diminish. There are a number of new antithrombotic agents on the horizon, some of which are coming to clinical trials.[68] The more widespread use of prophylaxis for venous thromboembolism[9] should diminish the incidence of thromboembolism after surgery and other high-risk situations. Nonetheless, the challenge confronting physicians managing patients with massive pulmonary embolism is the evidence that there has been little change in mortality rate over the past 30 years despite all of these efforts.[39]

References

1. Dalen JE, Alpert JS: Natural history of pulmonary embolism. Prog Cardiovasc Dis 1975; 17:259.
2. Anderson FA, Wheeler HB, Goldberg RJ, et al: A population-based perspective of the hospital incidence and case-fatality rates of deep vein thrombosis and pulmonary embolism: The Worcester DVT Study. Arch Intern Med 1991; 151:933.
3. Bell WR, Simon TL: Current status of pulmonary thromboembolic disease: Pathophysiology, diagnosis, prevention, and treatment. Am Heart J 1982; 103:239.
4. Morrell MP, Dunhill MS: The postmortem incidence of pulmonary embolism in a hospital population. Br J Surg 1968; 55:347.
5. Moser KM: Venous thromboembolism. Am Rev Respir Dis 1990; 141:235.
6. Coon WW, Willis PW, Keller JB: Thromboembolism and other venous disease in the Tecumseh community health study. Circulation 1978; 48:839.
7. Lindblad B, Sternby NH, Bergqvist D: Incidence of venous thromboembolism verified by necropsy over 30 years. Br Med J 1991; 302:709.
8. Hirsh J, Hull RD: Venous Thromboembolism: Natural History, Diagnosis and Management. Boca Raton, FL, CRC Press, 1987, p 17.
9. Hyers TN, Hull RD, Weg JG: Antithrombotic therapy for venous thromboembolic disease. Chest 1992; 102:391S.
10. Hull RD, Secker-Walker RH, Hirsh J: Diagnosis of deep vein

thrombosis. *In:* Hemostasis and Thrombosis, 2nd ed. Colman RW, Hirsh J, Marder VJ, Salzman EW (Eds). Philadelphia, JB Lippincott, 1987, p 1220.
11. Barritt DW, Jordon SC: Anticoagulant drugs in the treatment of pulmonary embolism: A controlled trial. Lancet 1960; 1:1309.
12. Donaldson GA, Williams C, Scannell JG, et al: A reappraisal of the application of the Trendelenburg operation to massive fatal embolism: Report of a successful pulmonary-artery thrombectomy using a cardiopulmonary bypass. N Engl J Med 1963; 268:171.
13. Dehring DJ, Arens JF: Pulmonary thromboembolism: Disease recognition and patient management. Anesthesiology 1990; 73:146.
14. Sevitt S, Gallagher NG: Venous thrombosis and pulmonary embolism: A clinicopathologic study in injured and burned patients. Br J Surg 1961; 48:475.
15. Hull RD, Delmore T, Genton E, et al: Warfarin sodium versus low-dose heparin in the long-term treatment of venous thrombosis. N Engl J Med 1979; 301:855.
16. Hull RD, Raskob GE, Pineo GF, et al: Subcutaneous low-molecular-weight heparin compared with continuous intravenous heparin in the treatment of proximal-vein thrombosis. N Engl J Med 1992; 326:975.
17. Goldhaber SZ, Morpurgo M: Diagnosis, treatment, and prevention of pulmonary embolism: Report of the WHO/International Society and Federation of Cardiology Task Force. JAMA 1992; 268:1727.
18. Goldhaber SZ: Recent advances in the diagnosis and lytic therapy of pulmonary embolism. Chest 1991; 99:173S.
19. Markel A, Manzo RA, Strandness Jr E: The potential role of thrombolytic therapy in venous thrombosis. Arch Intern Med 1992; 152:1265.
20. Molina JE, Hunter DW, Yedlicka JW, et al: Thrombolytic therapy for postoperative pulmonary embolism. Am J Surg 1992; 163:375.
21. The Urokinase Pulmonary Embolism Trial: A natural cooperative study. Circulation 1973; 47(Suppl II):II-1.
22. Tibbutt DA, Davies JA, Anderson JA, et al: Comparison by controlled clinical trial of streptokinase and heparin in treatment of life-threatening pulmonary embolism. Br Med J 1974; 1:343.
23. Ly B, Arnesen H, Eie H, et al: A controlled clinical trial of streptokinase and heparin in the treatment of major pulmonary embolism. Acta Med Scand 1978; 203:465.
24. The PIOPED Investigators: Tissue plasminogen activator for the treatment of acute pulmonary embolism. Chest 1990; 97:528.
25. Levine M, Hirsh J, Weitz J, et al: A randomized trial of a single bolus dosage regimen of recombinant tissue plasminogen activator in patients with acute pulmonary embolism. Chest 1990; 98:1473.
26. Dalla-Volta S, Palla A, Santolicandro A, et al: PAIMS 2: Alteplase combined with heparin versus heparin in the treatment of acute pulmonary embolism: Plasminogen activator Italian multicentre study 2. J Am Coll Cardiol 1992; 20:520.
27. Sharma GVRK, Burleson VA, Sasahara AA: Effect of thrombolytic therapy on pulmonary-capillary blood volume in patients with pulmonary embolism. N Engl J Med 1980; 303:842.
28. Sharma GVRK, Folland ED, McIntyre KM, et al: Longterm hemodynamic benefit of thrombolytic therapy in pulmonary embolic disease (Abstract). J Am Coll Cardiol 1990; 15:65A.
29. Urokinase-Streptokinase Embolism Trial: Phase 2 results. JAMA 1974; 229:1606.
30. The UKEP Study Research Group: The UKEP study: Multicentre clinical trial on two local regimens of urokinase in massive pulmonary embolism. Eur Heart J 1987; 8:2.
31. Verstraete M, Miller GAH, Bounameaux H, et al: Intravenous and intrapulmonary recombinant tissue-type plasminogen activator in the treatment of acute massive pulmonary embolism. Circulation 1988; 77:353.
32. Goldhaber SZ, Kessler CM, Heit JA, et al: Recombinant tissue-type plasminogen activator versus a novel dosing regimen of urokinase in acute pulmonary embolism: A randomized controlled multicentre trial. J Am Coll Cardiol 1992; 20:24.
33. Levine MN, Goldhaber SZ, Califf RM, et al: Hemorrhagic complications of thrombolytic therapy in the treatment of myocardial infarction and venous thromboembolism. Chest 1992; 102:364S.
34. Anderson DR, Levine MN: Thrombolytic therapy for the treatment of acute pulmonary embolism. Can Med Assoc J 1992; 146:1317.
35. Goldhaber SZ: Evolving concepts in thrombolytic therapy for pulmonary embolism. Chest 1992; 101:183S.
36. Werier J, Ducas J, Gu S, et al: Effect of low-molecular-weight heparin on recombinant tissue plasminogen activator-induced thrombolysis in canine pulmonary embolism. Chest 1991; 100:464.
37. Goldhaber SZ: Pulmonary embolism thrombolysis: A clarion call for international collaboration. J Am Coll Cardiol 1992; 19:246.
38. Collins R, Scrimgeour A, Yusuf S, et al: Reduction of fatal pulmonary embolism and venous thrombosis by perioperative administration of subcutaneous heparin. N Engl J Med 1988; 318:1162.
39. Lilienfeld DE, Chan E, Ehland J, et al: Mortality from pulmonary embolism in the United States: 1962–1984. Chest 1990; 98:1067.
40. del Campo C: Pulmonary embolectomy: A review. Can J Surg 1985; 28:111.
41. Sasahara AA, Sharma GVRK, Barsamian EM, et al: Pulmonary thromboembolism: Diagnosis and treatment. JAMA 1983; 249:2945.
42. Meyer G, Tamisier D, Sors H, et al: Pulmonary embolectomy: A 20-year experience at one center. Ann Thorac Surg 1991; 51:232.
43. Mattox KL, Feldtman RW, Geall AC, et al: Pulmonary embolectomy for acute pulmonary embolism. Ann Surg 1982; 195:726.
44. Bauer EP, Laske A, von Segesser LK, et al: Early and late results after surgery for massive pulmonary embolism. Thorac Cardiovasc Surg 1991; 39:353.
45. Clarke DB, Abrams LD: Pulmonary embolectomy: A 25 year experience. J Thorac Cardiovasc Surg 1986; 92:442.
46. Kieny R, Charpentier A, Kieny MT: What is the place of pulmonary embolectomy today? J Cardiovasc Surg 1991; 32:549.
47. Schmid C, Zietlow S, Wagner TOF, et al: Fulminant pulmonary embolism: Symptoms, diagnostics, operative technique, and results. Ann Thorac Surg 1991; 52:1102.
48. Satter P: Pulmonary embolectomy with the aid of extracorporeal circulation. Thorac Cardiovasc Surg 1982; 30:31.
49. Gray HH, Miller GAH, Paneth M: Pulmonary embolectomy: Its place in the management of pulmonary embolism. Lancet 1988; i:1441.
50. Brown S, Mulder D, Buckberg G: Massive pulmonary hemorrhagic infarction. Arch Surg 1974; 108:795.
51. Greenfield LJ, Langham MR: Surgical approaches to thromboembolism. Br J Surg 1984; 71:968.
52. Greenfield LJ: Vena caval interruption and pulmonary embolectomy. Clin Chest Med 1984; 5:495.
53. Greenfield LJ, Cho KJ, Proctor MC: Late results of suprarenal Greenfield vena cava filter placement. Arch Surg 1992; 127:969.
54. Timsit J-F, Reynaud P, Meyer G, et al: Pulmonary embolectomy by catheter device in massive pulmonary embolism. Chest 1991; 100:655.
55. Ponomar E, Carlson JE, Kindlund A, et al: Clot trapper device for transjugular thrombectomy from the inferior vena cava. Radiology 1991; 179:279.
56. Greenfield LJ: Evolution of venous interruption for pulmonary thromboembolism. Arch Surg 1992; 127:622.
57. Brady AJB, Crake T, Oakley CM: Percutaneous catheter fragmentation and distal dispersion of proximal pulmonary embolus. Lancet 1991; 338:1186.
58. Essop MR, Middlemost S, Skoularigis J, et al: Simultaneous mechanical clot fragmentation and pharmacologic thrombolysis in massive pulmonary embolism. Am J Cardiol 1992; 69:427.
59. Stein PD, Sabbah HN, Basha MA, et al: Mechanical disruption of pulmonary emboli in dogs with a flexible rotating-tip catheter (Kensey catheter). Chest 1990; 98:995.
60. Schmitz-Rode T, Günther RW: New device for percutaneous fragmentation of pulmonary emboli. Radiology 1991; 180:135.
61. Miles RM: Clinical evaluation of the serrated vena caval clip. Surg Gynecol Obstet 1971; 132:581.
62. Adams JT, DeWeese JA: Experimental and clinical evaluation

of partial vein interruption in the prevention of pulmonary emboli. Surgery 1965; 57:82.
63. King JN, Champlin AM, Ashby RN: Vena cava filters. West J Med 1992; 156:295.
64. Becker DM, Philbrick JT, Selby JB: Inferior vena cava filters; Indications, safety, effectiveness. Arch Intern Med 1992; 152:1985.
65. Grassi CJ: Inferior vena caval filters: Analysis of five currently available devices. Am J Roentgenol 1991; 156:813.
66. Thery C, Asseman P, Amrouni N, et al: Use of a new removable vena cava filter in order to prevent pulmonary embolism in patients submitted to thrombolysis. Eur Heart J 1990; 11:334.
67. Hull RD, Raskob GE, Rosenbloom D, et al: Optimal therapeutic level of heparin therapy in patients with venous thrombosis. Arch Intern Med 1992; 152:1589.
68. Salzman EW: Low molecular weight heparin and other antithrombotic drugs. N Engl J Med 1992; 326:1017.

CHAPTER 65

Diagnosis and Therapy of Emergent Vascular Diseases

Rodney A. White, MD

The vascular patient with peripheral, cerebrovascular, or myocardial ischemia frequently has diffuse atherosclerosis that increases the risk of death postoperatively and in the long term from vascular complications.[1] These patients often have a history of excessive smoking, diabetes mellitus, and/or a familial predisposition to vascular diseases (e.g., an inherited tendency to hyperlipidemia). Physical findings such as asymmetric extremities, fragile skin, hair loss, and xanthomas are suggestive of vascular disease. Careful palpation, auscultation, Doppler segmental pressure measurement of pulses, and pulse-volume recording can indicate the severity and distribution of vascular lesions. Contrast angiography is the most accurate method of diagnosing arterial and venous disease, although Doppler and ultrasound imaging techniques, computed tomography (CT), and magnetic resonance angiography are used increasingly for noninvasive diagnosis of vascular lesions.[2, 3] Treadmill exercise combined with electrocardiogram monitoring quantitates ischemic symptoms and is particularly useful to screen patients with peripheral vascular disease for concomitant coronary artery lesions that can be corrected by surgery.[4]

This chapter describes syndromes associated with acute and chronic vascular insufficiency, ischemic symptoms related to systemic inflammatory disease, complications of vascular reconstructions, and venous disorders.

ACUTE ARTERIAL INSUFFICIENCY

Acute arterial occlusion from trauma, embolus, or thrombosis frequently requires emergency surgery to prevent irreversible tissue loss. Symptoms are pain, analgesia or anesthesia, and discoloration of the ischemic tissue.

Embolic arterial occlusion produces symptoms that vary with the origin of the embolus. Emboli originating in the heart or ascending aorta cause central nervous system, visceral, or upper/lower-extremity symptoms, whereas emboli from the abdominal aorta and from iliofemoral or popliteal lesions affect only the lower extremities. The blue toe syndrome describes multiple bilateral ischemic areas in the lower leg caused by atheromatous debris showered distally from disease in aortoiliac vessels.[5] Ischemic paralysis and hypalgesia may develop in acutely ischemic limbs as a result of neurovascular compression from increased fascial compartment pressure. Compartmental compression syndromes require expedient decompression by fasciotomy to prevent irreversible neurovascular damage.[6] Embolic occlusion of visceral arteries may be insidious; pain, indigestion, or hematuria is often the only symptom.

Thrombotic arterial occlusion usually occurs as a result of decreased blood flow in progressively narrowed, atherosclerotic vessels. Acute thrombosis of diseased arteries may be due to hypovolemia or a sudden decrease in cardiac output. Frequently, elderly patients with cardiac failure or intraperitoneal disease have ischemic lower extremities, which simulates an aortic occlusion or a dissecting aneurysm. Appropriate attention to cardiac or intra-abdominal disease and restoration of blood volume often alleviate the ischemic symptoms. Axillary arterial thrombosis subsequent to intimal damage produced by repeated strain or trauma occurs in athletes, particularly baseball pitchers, and in individuals using crutches. Rarely, acute arterial thrombosis occurs in severely dehydrated children or in patients with hematologic disorders.

CHRONIC ARTERIAL INSUFFICIENCY

Although appropriate care is required to prevent complications, chronic arterial insufficiency caused by progression of atherosclerosis is infrequently a surgical emergency. Occlusion of major arteries may not cause tissue ischemia if hypertrophied collateral vessels provide adequate vascular supply. Chronic arterial occlusive disease is typically accompanied by insidious symptoms such as wasting of the extremity, hair loss, fragile skin, and pain with activity (claudication). Patients may complain of a burning or warm sensation in the affected extremity, which is actually cool or of normal temperature. Although nerve entrapment or inflammation also causes pain with activity,[7] claudication caused by chronic arterial insufficiency is distinguished by consistent and reproducible symptoms. Decreased exercise tolerance or prolonged recovery time suggests progression of the disease.

Because chronically ischemic limbs are easily ulcerated by local irritation, patients (especially diabetics) must be instructed in meticulous foot care, and any lesions should be aggressively treated. All patients with arterial insufficiency should be encouraged to quit smoking, control their diet, and immediately visit their physician if foot problems develop. Approximately 50% of patients with claudication will experience less pain on activity if they follow these recommendations and start a supervised exercise program. The onset of rest pain heralds complications and limb loss unless surgical intervention can restore adequate oxygenation.

Figure 65–1 summarizes the steps for diagnosing and treating arterial ischemia.

DISEASES OF THE AORTA

Improved techniques for reconstructing the thoracic aorta and its major arterial branches have increased the importance of early, accurate diagnosis of pathologic lesions. Too often, intrathoracic aortic lesions progress undiagnosed until they cause significant hemodynamic problems or symptoms from compression of adjacent structures.

Thoracic aortic aneurysms can frequently be visualized by chest x-ray films, ultrasonography, or CT; however, arteriography is the most reliable method of defining the ex-

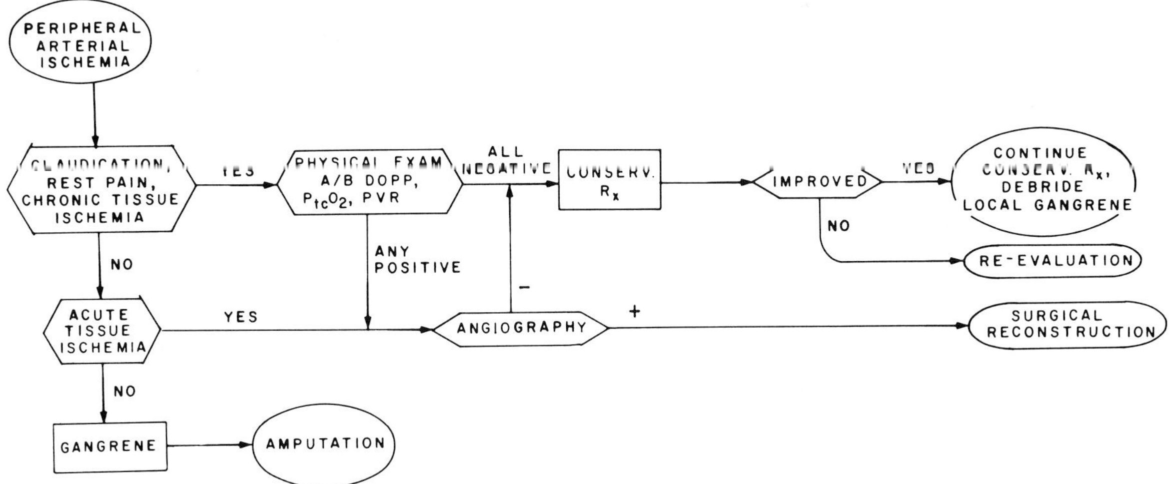

Figure 65–1. Claudication, rest pain, chronic or acute tissue ischemia, or gangrene suggests peripheral arterial ischemia. Patients with claudication, rest pain, or chronic tissue ischemia (Step 1) should have a physical examination, ankle/brachial artery Doppler pressure measurement (A/B Dopp), transcutaneous Po_2 ($Ptco_2$) determination, and pulse volume recording (PVR) performed (Step 2). Negative examination results rule out arterial disease; therefore, conservative therapy plus a search for other possible etiologies is required. If the patient's symptoms become worse (Step 3), re-evaluation is indicated. Any positive test result, (e.g., A/B Dopp $< .6$, $Ptco_2 < 70$ torr) or abnormal PVR, or patient presenting with acute tissue ischemia (Step 4) indicates arteriography (Step 5) to determine the cause and need for surgical reconstruction. Gangrene (Step 6) as the presenting symptom requires amputation of necrotic tissue.

tent of the lesions. Aneurysms may affect speech by irritating the recurrent laryngeal nerve, or they may cause dysphagia by compressing the esophagus.

Pain from a dissecting thoracic aneurysm may be substernal or referred to the intrascapular area. Migration of excruciating pain suggests extension of a dissection. Major arterial branches of the thoracic aorta may be occluded by extension of a subintimal dissection, causing a cerebrovascular accident or diminishing pulses in the upper extremity. Control of hypertension will frequently prevent further dissection. In unstable patients, immediate surgery may occasionally be the only chance for survival.

Atherosclerotic disease of the abdominal aorta and iliac arteries produces lesions that occur initially and are frequently most severe near the bifurcation of the aorta.[8] Symptomatic lesions can be reconstructed by aortoiliac or aortobifemoral bypasses using fabric prostheses that have 90% 10-year patency rates.[9] Approximately 5% of hypertensive patients can be cured by repairing renal artery obstructions. Transluminal balloon angioplasty of renal artery lesions, endarterectomy, and reconstruction are options for relief of hypertension and salvage of renal function.[10] Reduced blood flow to the hypogastric vessels has an important role in male impotence[11]; reconstructive procedures that increase flow to the pelvic vessels can restore sexual function in a significant number of patients.

Abdominal aortic aneurysms may rupture into the peritoneal cavity, a catastrophic event associated with rapid exsanguination, or they may rupture into an adjacent organ such as the vena cava, producing an aorta–vena caval fistula. Frequently, aneurysms perforate anteriorly between the renal vessels and aortic bifurcation or along the iliac artery into the retroperitoneum. Ruptured retroperitoneal aneurysms produce excruciating abdominal pain that may radiate to the groin and mimic renal colic.

Enlargement of an aneurysm to greater than 6 cm in diameter significantly increases the risk of its rupture in the near future;[12] thus, surgical correction is recommended if the patient's health is adequate. Ultrasonography accurately estimates the size of aortic aneurysms and is used to indicate the need for surgical correction. Surgery may also be indicated occasionally in postoperative patients because increased collagenase activity in the aneurysm wall of catabolic patients increases the risk of rupture.[13] Approximately 10% to 15% of abdominal aortic aneurysms extend above the renal vessels and require surgical reimplantation of the renal arteries into the prosthesis.

UPPER-EXTREMITY ISCHEMIA

Vascular ischemia of the upper extremity is caused by atherosclerosis, thoracic-outlet compression syndromes, trauma, and systemic or local inflammatory diseases. Upper-extremity ischemia from acute arterial occlusions causes limb loss in 10% of lesions in the subclavian artery, 15% in the axillary artery, and less than 5% in the proximal brachial artery.[14] Most acute arterial obstructions in the upper extremity are caused by trauma.

Thoracic-outlet compression syndrome is caused by impingement of adjacent structures on all or part of the neurovascular supply to the upper extremity. Common causes include a cervical rib, fibrocartilaginous bands, scalene or subclavius muscle hypertrophy, upper thoracic or cervical trauma, and repeated strenuous hyperabduction of the arm. Accurate diagnosis of the thoracic-outlet syndrome depends on reproducing symptoms with hand exercise when the arm is abducted and externally rotated. There may be tenderness to percussion over the clavicle or brachial plexus, an audible bruit over the subclavian artery, and reduction or obliteration of pulses when the arm is in an abducted position. However, these diagnostic maneuvers are only suggestive, and many normal individuals have the same findings. Objective tests include electromyography, nerve conduction velocity, and arteriography. Relief of symptoms often follows several months of a thoracic-outlet exercise program.[15] In severe cases, resection of a cervical rib or the first thoracic rib or scalenectomy may relieve symptoms. Occasionally, thoracic-outlet compression occurs with carpal tunnel syndrome.[16] This association should be suspected in patients with wasting of the intrinsic muscles of the hand, particularly if they have a systemic inflammatory disease.

Upper-extremity digital gangrene is infrequent but not

rare. Approximately 50% of patients with digital ischemia have a correctable aneurysm, traumatic lesion, or embolic source proximal to the hand. Digital ischemia may also appear as a symptom of vasospastic or obliterative arterial disease in patients with systemic inflammatory processes. Connective tissue disorders, particularly scleroderma, are associated with progressive occlusion of medium- and small-diameter arteries.

Many patients with inflammatory diseases experience Raynaud's syndrome before the onset of systemic symptoms.[17] Raynaud's syndrome is characterized by episodic cold or stress-induced digital cyanosis, coolness, and, in severe cases, ulceration. Sixty percent to 90% of patients with Raynaud's syndrome are young females with primarily vasospastic arterial disease. Older patients and males with Raynaud's syndrome typically have obstructive arterial disease. Certain occupations, particularly those using vibratory tools or involving prolonged exposure to cold temperatures, are associated with an increased incidence of Raynaud's syndrome. Therapy relies on identification and treatment of the underlying inflammatory process.

CEREBROVASCULAR INSUFFICIENCY

Atherosclerosis of the extracranial carotid artery (i.e., carotid stenosis or ulceration) can cause cerebrovascular insufficiency. Transient ischemic attacks (TIAs), visual disturbances, and contralateral weakness can often be relieved by carotid endarterectomy. Patients with less specific symptoms such as headaches, dizziness, or unusual distribution of sensory or motor abnormalities require extensive evaluation to document the relationship of neurologic symptoms to carotid stenosis. Patients with asymptomatic carotid lesions can be treated with antiplatelet medications instead of carotid endarterectomy; however, data suggest that endarterectomy reduces the incidence of subsequent stroke despite an initial elevation in morbidity and mortality related to surgery.[18]

Flow disturbance at the carotid bifurcation is postulated as the initial stimulus for the development of carotid atheroma.[19] Fibrous myointimal thickening is followed by hemorrhage beneath the lesion. The hematoma may significantly narrow the vessel lumen, causing an ischemic event. If the atheroma remains asymptomatic, it progressively thickens by a series of degenerative events; or the contents of the subintimal space may embolize, causing TIAs.[20] In the latter case, embolized atheromatous debris produces Hollenhorst's plaques on the retina, which are visible during funduscopic examination of the eye.[21] Release of the necrotic subintimal contents leaves an ulcerated plaque, which is the source of continued embolization. Arteriography may suggest an ulcerated plaque, although in some cases the ulcer endothelializes and is no longer a source of emboli. In many instances, repeated fibrosis, hemorrhage, and calcification of atheromatous lesions completely occlude the internal carotid artery lumen.

In all cases, intracerebral and vertebral artery lesions and any other possible cause of cerebrovascular insufficiency must be considered before implicating a carotid stenosis. For example, occlusion of the first portion of the subclavian artery can cause blood to flow retrograde from the vertebral artery to the axillary artery, precipitating cerebral ischemia during arm exercise (the subclavian steal syndrome).[22]

MESENTERIC ARTERIAL INSUFFICIENCY

Visceral ischemia is frequently not diagnosed until late in the clinical course. For this reason, reported mortality rates are between 55% and 100%.[23,24] Laboratory and noninvasive tests are not diagnostic, and the physician must always consider mesenteric insufficiency in the initial evaluation of severely ill patients with abdominal pain, particularly elderly cardiovascular patients. Expeditious establishment and maintenance of hemodynamic stability, as well as arteriographic documentation of mesenteric vascular occlusion, are required to reduce fatal complications.

Visceral ischemia may be acute or chronic. Acute insufficiency can cause nonspecific colicky pain and guaiac-positive stools, or it may produce sepsis, acidosis, and rapid hemodynamic deterioration. The symptoms of chronic intestinal ischemia are postprandial pain and weight loss. Approximately 40% of acute ischemic events are caused by emboli, 50% are associated with low-flow states and arterial thrombosis, and 10% or less are due to venous occlusion.[25]

If the vascular supply of the gut is otherwise normal, acute occlusion of the celiac or inferior mesenteric arteries is usually compensated for by extensive collateral circulation. In general, at least two of three mesenteric vessels must be significantly obstructed for occlusion of any one vessel to impair mesenteric blood flow markedly. Occasionally, acute occlusion of the inferior mesenteric artery by thrombosis or surgical ligation causes an ischemic colitis that is characterized by severe abdominal pain in the lower left quadrant, abdominal tenderness, and bloody stools.[26]

Although the superior mesenteric artery is subject to acute ischemia from either a thrombotic or embolic event, thrombosis usually results in more extensive ischemia because it occurs in severely diseased arteries and frequently involves the entire vessel. By contrast, emboli tend to lodge distal to the origin of the middle colic artery and may be found in otherwise normal intestinal vasculature. Mesenteric arterial emboli may only require embolectomy, whereas mesenteric thrombosis often requires resection of a large segment of devitalized intestine.

Thrombosis of the superior mesenteric veins is associated with low blood flow, hypercoagulation, portal vein thrombosis from portal hypertension, and/or splenic vein thrombosis from compression or invasion by malignancy, particularly pancreatic tumors. Splanchnic venous engorgement with edematous thickening of bowel loops produces a thumbprint pattern of gut folds, evident on upper gastrointestinal contrast radiography. Mesenteric venous thrombosis results in gut necrosis in 20% to 70% of patients. Mortality increases rapidly if therapy is delayed longer than 12 hours after the onset of symptoms and approaches 100% by 48 hours.[27] Frequently, acute mesenteric venous occlusion requires thrombectomy, resection of devitalized bowel, and anticoagulation.

COMPLICATIONS OF VASCULAR SURGERY

Immediate thrombotic or hemorrhagic complications of vascular reconstructions can frequently be corrected during the initial postoperative period. Long-term failures are related to progression of atherosclerosis, gradual thrombotic occlusion of prostheses, infection, deterioration of prosthetic grafts with false-aneurysm formation, perigraft hematoma accumulation, thrombosis from compression, or encroachment of a vascular reconstruction on adjacent organs. Many of the long-term failures are insidious because occlusion of a reconstruction may not produce ischemia if hypertrophied collateral circulation can provide adequate blood supply. Unfortunately, a significant number of long-term complications result in severe ischemia, sepsis, life-threatening hemorrhage, and/or compromised organ function.

Most long-term failures of vascular reconstructions are

related to progression of atherosclerosis or to a gradual thrombotic occlusion of a prosthetic segment. *Thrombosis of arterial repairs* is caused by narrowing of autogenous vein segments by arterialization of the vein wall, progressive thrombus accumulation in synthetic prostheses, infection, embolization of thrombotic deposits, and decreased flow in runoff vessels. Ankle Doppler pressure measurements every 3 months postoperatively can detect subclinical atherosclerotic or myointimal hyperplastic stenoses in lower-extremity vascular repairs. Many stenoses can be treated by surgery or transluminal balloon dilation before occlusion of the arterial reconstruction, thus restoring flow without compromising long-term patency.[28]

Graft infection frequently produces fever or sepsis and can be a life-threatening complication of vascular surgery, particularly if it occurs in synthetic or nonautogenous biologic vascular prostheses. In animals, tissue ingrowth decreases graft infection, but in humans, vascular prostheses do not completely heal,[29] and in most cases only superficial wound infections that do not involve the vascular prosthesis can be treated without removing the graft. Patients with cardiovascular implants undergoing invasive procedures or dental extractions should be prophylactically treated with antibiotics to avoid bacteremia.

Deterioration of vascular prosthetic materials may cause graft dilatation, false-aneurysm formation, suture-line disruption, or perigraft hematoma formation. In general, any change in the configuration of a vascular reconstruction should be investigated to prevent complications.

Extra-anatomic bypasses are vascular reconstructions remote from the anatomic course of the vessel. They are usually subcutaneous or subfascial.[30] Extra-anatomic reconstructions were originally developed to revascularize the lower extremities when repair of an aortoduodenal fistula required removal of an infected aortic bifurcation graft and ligation of the aorta below the renal vessels. Blood flow to one leg is restored by placing a prosthetic graft subcutaneously along the lateral chest wall, from the axillary artery to the ipsilateral femoral artery (i.e., axillofemoral bypass). Blood flow to the other leg is established through a second graft placed in a suprapubic subcutaneous position, from the axillofemoral reconstruction to the contralateral femoral artery (i.e., femoral-femoral bypass). Long-term function of axillobifemoral reconstructions is almost comparable to that of aortobifemoral interposition prostheses. An advantage of extra-anatomic bypasses is that these procedures can usually be performed with local or regional anesthesia in high-risk patients. A disadvantage is that subcutaneous prostheses are easily compressed while the patient is sleeping or unconscious, causing thrombosis of the graft and distal ischemia. Early recognition of thrombosis in an extra-anatomic bypass is essential because an acute thrombus can frequently be removed, restoring flow without affecting long-term patency.

Astute clinical judgment is required to detect symptoms caused by *encroachment of a vascular repair on adjacent structures*. Fibrous encapsulation and stiffening of a limb of an aortobifemoral prosthesis can obstruct the ureter, producing persistent flank pain from hydronephrosis or renal infection.[31] Compression of the iliac vein causes unilateral lower-extremity venous hypertension, swelling, and discomfort. Aortoduodenal fistula is a dramatic example of a vascular repair eroding into an adjacent organ.[32] Both infection and pulsation of the aortic anastomosis of an aortobifemoral reconstruction have been proposed as possible causes of the aortoduodenal communication. Aortoduodenal fistula should be suspected in patients with aortobifemoral bypasses who are experiencing massive upper gastrointestinal bleeding. These patients frequently have had a preliminary hematemesis within the previous 24 hours. Endoscopic confirmation of bleeding from the third portion of the duodenum requires immediate laparotomy to rule out this complication; aortography is usually contraindicated because it may not show the enteric communication and because immediate laparotomy is required to prevent exsanguination.

VENOUS DISEASES

Thrombophlebitis is venous thrombosis that follows inflammation of the vein wall and causes severe pain and swelling of the extremity. Venous thrombosis without inflammation of the vein wall may be asymptomatic except for mild discomfort and swelling. The incidence of venous thrombosis is increased by major injury or surgery, pregnancy, previous thrombosis, cancer, infection, varicose veins, obesity, and long periods of sitting or lying.[33] Thrombosis of the leg veins has been reported in 28% of elective surgical patients, 54% of hip fractures, and approximately 20% of patients treated for myocardial infarction.[34]

The three apparent causes of venous thrombosis are stasis, injury to the vessel wall, and increased coagulability of the blood (i.e., Virchow's triad). Fibrinogen radionuclide studies performed on hospitalized patients demonstrate that thrombi develop in areas of stasis and turbulent blood flow near venous valves.[35] Continued thrombosis occludes the vessel lumen and produces distal venous hypertension. Frequently, blood flow through the vein is restored by resorption and organization or embolization of the thrombus. However, organization of venous thrombosis destroys the valves, and recanalized veins are prone to subsequent thrombosis.

Chronic venous obstruction and valvular insufficiency are characterized by discoloration and induration of the overlying skin. If venous hypertension is greater than capillary diffusion pressure, edema develops. Tissue ischemia and venous gangrene develop if venous pressures exceed capillary perfusion pressure.

Superficial thromboses produce a bothersome lump or cord that can be treated with local care and, if necessary, excision. These thromboses are usually of no consequence unless caused by infection. By contrast, *deep venous thromboses* produce severe swelling of the extremity and without treatment can lead to long-term hemodynamic problems and significant (>1 cm in diameter) pulmonary emboli.[36] The soleal veins of the lower leg are the most frequent site of deep venous thromboses. Most soleal thromboses are asymptomatic, aside from mild calf pain; however, pain and swelling of the lower extremity increase if thrombi extend into the femoral and iliac veins. Femoral venous thrombosis produces massive swelling, pain, purpura, and a bluish discoloration of the leg called phlegmasia cerulea dolens. If iliofemoral thrombosis completely occludes venous outflow, venous pressure increases until venous gangrene and arterial spasm from local irritation result in a massively swollen and painful white leg, a condition known as phlegmasia cerulea albicans. This syndrome is usually associated with disseminated malignancies or sepsis. Isolated pelvic thrombi from pelvic inflammation or tumor invasion do not cause edema if the iliac vein remains patent.

Venous thrombosis of the upper extremity requires therapy if the deep veins are involved. Exertion, intravenous catheters, trauma, intravenous drug abuse, neoplastic disease, and congenital venous malformations have been described as causes of axillary-subclavian vein thromboses.[37] Intermittent subclavian vein obstruction and thrombosis can follow compression of the vein between the first rib and clavicle. Axillary-subclavian vein thromboses cause severe pain and swelling of the arm and hand, and frequently there is percussion tenderness over the clavicle and axillary vein. These thromboses can be a source of hemodynamically significant pulmonary emboli, particularly when associated with causes other than exertion.

A venous thrombosis may become infected, or it may be caused by infection. Infected thromboses are usually seen in intravenous drug abusers and in debilitated patients who have had multiple intravenous catheters. Infected thromboses may be the source of systemic sepsis, endocarditis, or septic emboli. Immediate excision of the entire vein is required to prevent complications.

Diagnosis and Therapy

Venography is the most accurate method for diagnosing significant venous thromboses, although a combination of Doppler ultrasound and impedance plethysmography has a 95% accuracy in detecting deep venous thrombosis of the leg.[38] A difference of 1.5 cm in diameter between a swollen leg and the contralateral leg offers corroborative physical evidence of venous thrombosis. Calf tenderness and Homans' sign are less reliable diagnostic signs.

Therapy for venous thrombosis ideally prevents propagation of the thrombosis, late sequelae related to destruction of venous anatomy, secondary infection, and pulmonary emboli. Destruction of the valves by the organizing thrombus increases venous pressures and ultimately leads to the postphlebitic syndrome, which is a debilitating and irreversible venous disease. There are few surgical alternatives, and therapy relies primarily on custom-fitted support stockings and meticulous skin care. Tortuous varicose veins can be removed if they are painful or unsightly, but varicosities frequently recur from persistent venous hypertension or primary venous degenerative disease. The superficial venous system should not be removed if there is deep vein occlusion, because in this instance the superficial veins are the only route for egress of blood from the extremity. Excision of varicose veins near stasis ulcers improves wound healing. In certain cases, valvuloplasty or crossover venous reconstructions can re-establish venous flow and reduce venous hypertension.[39]

FUTURE PERSPECTIVES

Vascular surgery has become a separate surgical subspecialty as direct surgical and pharmacologic approaches to therapy have developed. The pioneering vascular surgeons of the last 50 years discovered methods for disobliteration of occlusive atherosclerotic disease by incision of the vessel wall and surgical removal of obstructions or by use of tubular prosthetic bypasses to circumvent occluded segments. Concomitant advances in anesthetic technique, anticoagulation, and antibiotic therapy allowed reconstruction of smaller, lower flow arteries and veins with improved instrumentation, suture materials, and operative techniques. Subsequent advances included a redefinition of the indications for surgical interventions by establishing a natural history of occlusive lesions and the outcome of surgical interventions in the peripheral and coronary circulations. The careful follow-up of patients helped to establish the data base that serves as the "gold standard" for evaluation of new therapies.

Vascular therapy continues to evolve at a rapid rate, and the vascular surgeon is offered the opportunity to further advance the therapy of vascular diseases using new information about the biochemistry and genetics of pathologic lesions. This new information promises to enhance the understanding of the cause and development of vascular lesions and to improve the therapy for chronic ischemia and reperfusion syndromes.

Cardiovascular diagnosis and treatment are rapidly becoming less invasive. Ultrasound, CT scans, magnetic resonance imaging, and spectroscopy and positron emission tomographic scans all minimize the invasive nature of the procedure and maximize the accuracy of diagnosis.[40] Special applications of these technologies provide precise anatomic, hemodynamic, and biochemical information about vascular diseases and tissue metabolism, increasing the potential for early diagnosis and treatment of lesions. Therapeutic catheter-based interventions are being evaluated to expand the treatment while potentially replacing a significant percentage of conventional surgical procedures.[41]

This rapid evolution in vascular science and surgery exemplifies the effect that technologic development has on both medicine and science. Continued, controlled experimental and clinical investigations now have the potential to improve dramatically the successful treatment of many cardiovascular disorders. The influence of this rapid advance may be to redefine the prevention of some diseases and the therapy of others. It is the responsibility of the scientific-medical community to direct and apply our resources to maximize this evolution.

References

1. Loop FD: Combined cardiac and peripheral vascular disease. Contemp Surg 1981; 18:47.
2. Strandness DE Jr, Sumner DS, Mozersky DJ, et al: The use of ultrasonic arteriography for arterial visualization. Scand J Clin Lab Invest 1973; 31(Suppl 128):163.
3. Saloner D, Anderson C, Caputo G: Magnetic resonance imaging. *In:* Vascular Surgery: Basic Science and Clinical Correlations. White RA, Hollier L (Eds). Philadelphia, JB Lippincott, 1994, pp 477–486.
4. Stahler C, Strandness DE Jr: Ankle blood pressure response to graded treadmill exercise. Angiology 1967; 18:237.
5. Karmody AM, Powers SR, Monaco VJ, et al: "Blue toe" syndrome: An indication for limb salvage surgery. Arch Surg 1976; 111:1263.
6. Patman RD, Thompson JE: Fasciotomy in peripheral vascular surgery. Arch Surg 1970; 101:663.
7. Hines EA Jr: Some types of distress in the lower extremities simulating peripheral vascular disease. Med Clin North Am 1958; 42:991.
8. Perdue GD, Long WD, Smith RB III: Perspective concerning aortofemoral arterial reconstruction. Trans South Surg Assoc 1970; 82:330.
9. Ernst CB: Abdominal aortic aneurysm. N Engl J Med 1993; 328: 1167–1172.
10. Weibull H, Bergqvist D, Bergentz S, et al: Percutaneous transluminal renal angioplasty versus surgical reconstruction of atherosclerotic renal artery stenosis: A prospective randomized study. J Vasc Surg 1993; 18:841–852.
11. DePalma RG, Kedia K, Persky L: Surgical options in the correction of vasculogenic impotence. Vasc Surg 1980; 14:92.
12. Darling RC: Ruptured arteriosclerotic abdominal aortic aneurysms: Pathologic and clinical study. Am J Surg 1970; 119:397.
13. Busuttil RW, Abou-Zamzam Am, Machleder HI: Collagenase activity of the human aorta. Arch Surg 1980; 115:1373.
14. Brawley RK, Murray GR, Crisler C, et al: Management of wounds of the innominate, subclavian, and axillary blood vessels. Surg Gynecol Obstet 1970; 131:1130.
15. Peet RM, Henriksen JD, Anderson TP: Thoracic-outlet syndrome: Evaluation of a therapeutic exercise program. Proc Staff Mayo Clin 1956; 31:281.
16. Lord JW, Rosati LM: Thoracic outlet syndromes. Clin Symp 1971; 2(23):3.
17. Porter JM, Bardana EJ, Baur GM, et al: The clinical significance of Raynaud's syndrome. Surgery 1976; 80:756.

18. Thompson JE, Patman RD, Talkington CM: Asymptomatic carotid bruit: Long-term outcome of patients having endarterectomy compared with unoperated controls. Ann Surg 1978; 188:308.
19. Texon M, Imparato AM, Lord JW, et al: The experimental production of arterial lesions: Furthering the hemodynamic concept of atherosclerosis. Arch Intern Med 1962; 110:50.
20. Imparato AM, Riles TS, Gorstein F: The carotid bifurcation plaque: Pathologic findings associated with cerebral ischemia. Stroke 1979; 10:238.
21. Hollenhorst RW: Significance of bright plaques in the retinal arterioles. JAMA 1961; 178:23.
22. A new vascular syndrome—"The subclavian steal" (Editorial). N Engl J Med 1961; 265:912.
23. Bergan JJ, Dean RH, Conn J Jr: Revascularization in the treatment of mesenteric infarction. Ann Surg 1975; 182:430.
24. Pierce GE, Brockenbrough EC: The spectrum of mesenteric infarction. Am J Surg 1970; 119:233.
25. Ottinger LW: The surgical management of acute occlusion of the superior mesenteric artery. Ann Surg 1978; 188:721.
26. Marston A, Phiels MT, Thomas ML, et al: Ischemic colitis. Gut 1966; 7:1.
27. Warren S, Eberhard TP: Mesenteric venous thrombosis. Surg Gynecol Obstet 1935; 61:102.
28. Zarins CK, Lu C, McDonnell AE, et al: Limb salvage by percutaneous transluminal recanalization of occluded superficial femoral artery. Surgery 1980; 87:701.
29. Moore WS, Malone JS, Keown K: Prosthetic arterial graft material, influence of neointimal healing on bacteremic infectability. Arch Surg 1980; 115:1379.
30. Blaisdell FW: Symposium: Extra-anatomic vascular shunt. Contemp Surg 1979; 15:69.
31. Heard G, Hinde G: Hydronephrosis complicating aortic reconstruction. Br J Surg 1975; 62:344.
32. Kierman PD, Pairolero PC, Huber JP, et al: Aortic graft-enteric fistula. Mayo Clin Proc 1980; 55:731.
33. Coon WW, Coller FA: Some epidemiologic considerations in thromboembolism. Surg Gynecol Obstet 1959; 109:487.
34. Kakkar V: Prevention of fatal postoperative pulmonary embolism by low doses of heparin. Lancet 1975; ii:45.
35. Kakkar V: The diagnosis of deep vein thrombosis using the ^{125}I fibrinogen test. Arch Surg 1972; 104:152.
36. Barner HB, DeWeese JA: An evaluation of the sphygmomanometer cuff pain test in venous thrombosis. Surgery 1960; 48:915.
37. Harley D, White RA, Nelson RJ, et al: Pulmonary embolism secondary to upper extremity venous thrombosis. Am J Surg 1984; 147:221.
38. Sumner DS, Mattos MA: Diagnosis of deep vein thrombosis with real-time color and diplex scanning. *In:* Vascular Diagnosis. 4th ed. Bernstein EF (Ed). St. Louis, Mosby-Year Book 1993, 785–800.
39. Dale WA: Crossover graft for iliofemoral venous occlusion. *In:* Venous Problems. Bergen JJ, Yao JST (Eds). Chicago, Year Book Medical Publishers, 1978, pp 411–420.
40. Cavaye DM, White RA (Eds): A Text and Atlas of Arterial Imaging. London, Chapman & Hall, Ltd, 1994.
41. White RA, Cavaye DM: Endovascular surgery: History, arrest status and future perspectives. Int Angiology 1993; 12:245–255.

CHAPTER 66

Severe Heart Failure in Cardiomyopathy: Pathogenesis and Treatment

Clifford J. Kavinsky, MD, PhD • Joseph E. Parrillo, MD

The cardiomyopathies are a heterogeneous group of disorders, most often of unclear etiology, manifested as heart failure due to intrinsic disease of the cardiac muscle. The disease process is generally diffuse in character, involving all cardiac chambers. Chamber involvement is not necessarily uniform, however, and one chamber may display more extensive disease involvement than others. As a result, heart failure, the sine qua non of cardiomyopathy, may be predominantly right sided, left sided, systolic, diastolic, or a mixture thereof.[1]

Because cardiac dysfunction is considered to be a consequence of a primary myocardial disease process, heart muscle impairment occurring as a result of coronary artery disease (ischemic), hypertension, valvular heart disease, congenital disorders, or diseases of the pericardium would by definition not be grouped under the cardiomyopathy disease classification. Indeed, these disorders must effectively be ruled out when considering the diagnosis of cardiomyopathy. A comprehensive clinical assessment including a detailed history, physical examination, and judicious use of currently available diagnostic modalities including electrocardiography, chest radiography, radionuclide imaging, echocardiography, and cardiac catheterization with angiography usually allows one to identify patients with cardiomyopathies and exclude patients with other disorders. Two-dimensional and Doppler echocardiography are extremely useful in identifying patients with structural abnormalities such as congenital defects or valvular lesions. Examination of ventricular wall thickness often provides clues concerning long-standing hypertension, and findings of regional wall-motion abnormalities or aneurysm are suggestive of antecedent ischemic heart disease. Myocardial perfusion imaging may provide evidence for myocardial ischemia or previous infarction. Finally, cardiac catheterization with coronary angiography is believed by many to be an essential diagnostic component in precluding ischemic heart disease in patients with possible cardiomyopathy.

Cardiomyopathy has been classified using a number of different methods.[1, 2] The most commonly used, that adopted by the World Health Organization, refers to cardiomyopathies as diseases solely affecting heart muscle and lacking a clearly identifiable cause.[3] Other systemic illnesses of known cause (e.g., amyloidosis, muscular dystrophy) affecting the heart would not be referred to as cardiomyopathy but rather as *specific heart muscle diseases* despite a clinical presentation indistinguishable from cardiomyopathy.[4] Many refer to sole cardiac muscle dysfunction of unknown cause as *idiopathic* or *primary* cardiomyopathy and that due to specific disease affecting the heart in a manner consistent with a cardiomyopathic profile as *secondary* cardiomyopathy. Such a classification scheme is both useful and appropriate because it has important pathophysiologic, prognostic, and therapeutic implications.

The World Health Organization's classification scheme describes three general categories of cardiomyopathy based on clinical, structural, functional, and hemodynamic criteria

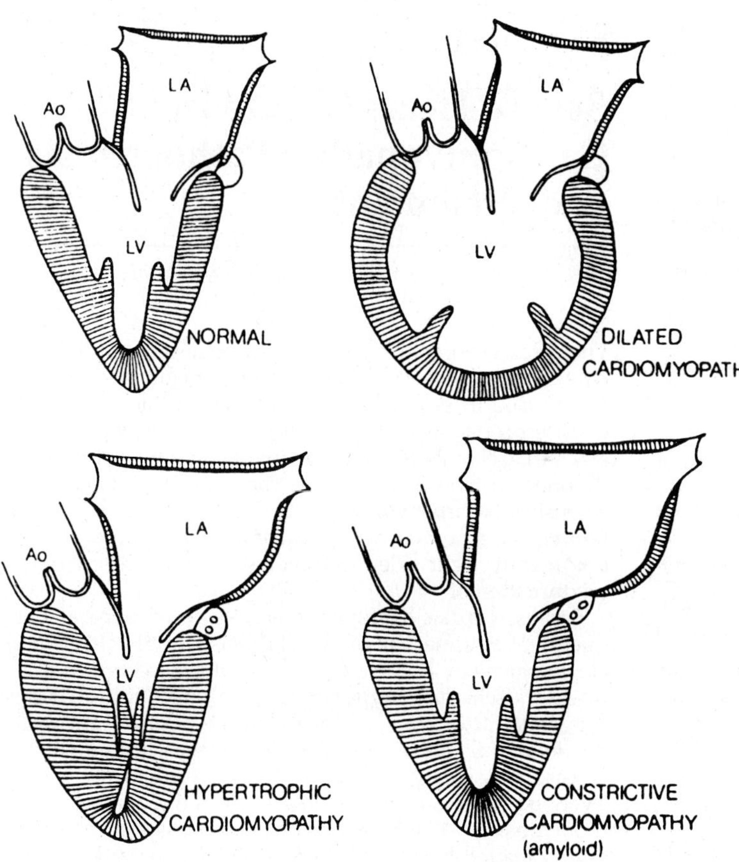

Figure 66–1. Schematic diagrams of the normal ventricle and the three types of cardiomyopathies. Table 66–1 also compares these different cardiomyopathies. (From Roberts WR, Ferrans VJ: Myocardial observations in cardiomyopathies. *In*: Myocardial Diseases. Fowler NO (Ed). New York, Grune & Stratton, 1973.)

(Fig. 66–1). Dilated cardiomyopathy, by far the most common form, is characterized by ventricular dilatation, impairment of systolic function as evidenced by a markedly reduced left ventricular ejection fraction, and often a clinical picture of congestive heart failure (Table 66–1). Distinguishing features of restrictive cardiomyopathy include normal left ventricular cavity dimensions, normal or only mildly reduced systolic function, and markedly reduced ventricular compliance often leading to signs and symptoms of biventricular heart failure. Restrictive cardiomyopathy exhibits many similarities to pericardial constriction, and differentiating the two disorders can often be difficult. The third category of cardiomyopathy is the hypertrophic form, which is due to inappropriate left ventricular hypertrophy. The hypertrophic form often involves the interventricular septum, leading to decreased compliance and impaired diastolic function. Septal hypertrophy in some cases may lead to a dynamic form of left ventricular outflow tract obstruction owing to contact between the anterior mitral valve leaflet and the hypertrophied septum, thus obstructing left ventricular outflow. This phenomenon may also be associated with systolic anterior motion of the mitral valve. Left ventricular cavity dimensions are usually normal or reduced with vigorous systolic function until late in the course of the disease. Most experts in the field believe that the cause of heart failure in hypertrophic cardiomyopathy relates more

TABLE 66–1. Classification of the Cardiomyopathies

			Hypertrophic	
	Dilated	*Restrictive*	*Nonobstructive*	*Obstructive*
Left ventricular end-diastolic pressure	↑ ↑	↑ ↑	↑ ↑	↑ ↑
Left ventricular end-diastolic volume	↑ ↑	nl or ↓	nl or ↓	nl or ↓
Diastolic compliance	↑	↓ ↓	↓ ↓	↓ ↓
Left ventricular ejection fraction	↓ ↓	nl or ↑ ↓ late	nl or ↑ ↓ late	nl, ↓, ↑
Echocardiography	↑ ↑ LV dimension ↓ ↓ Ventricular systolic function AV valve regurgitation	nl or ↓ LV dimension nl Ventricular systolic function ↑ LV wall thickness and mass	nl or ↓ LV dimension nl or ↑ Ventricular systolic function Localized ↑ LV wall thickness (septum)	LV outflow tract obstruction Systolic anterior motion of mitral valve Mitral regurgitation

Abbreviations: AV = atrioventricular; nl = normal; LV = left ventricle; ↑ = slightly increased; ↓ = slightly decreased; ↑ ↑ = greatly increased; ↓ ↓ = greatly decreased.

to impairment of ventricular diastolic relaxation (lusitropy) and decreased compliance rather than left ventricular dynamic outflow tract obstruction.[5,6]

As can be seen in Table 66–1, the classification scheme for the cardiomyopathies is far from arbitrary and highlights structural and hemodynamic differences that must be understood in order to evaluate and treat such patients properly, particularly when the clinical presentation is one of high acuity and hemodynamic instability. Patients with cardiomyopathy are generally treated as outpatients for chronic heart failure. Patients admitted to an intensive care unit (ICU) usually fall into two general categories. First, they may present with an acute exacerbation of heart failure, in which case it is incumbent on the critical care physician to identify both the cause of the patient's underlying chronic heart failure and the precipitating event leading to further deterioration of heart function. Such clinical information is essential for the intensivist in order to initiate effective treatment. The wrong therapeutic decision in a critically ill patient could yield disastrous results. Second, patients with cardiomyopathy may be admitted to the ICU in critical condition after developing a noncardiac illness. Such patients have unique management needs that must be anticipated by the critical care physician.

Whether because of increased physician awareness, improved diagnostic techniques, or a true increase in disease incidence, the number of hospitalizations and deaths attributed to cardiomyopathy is increasing.[7] The annual incidence of cardiomyopathy ranges from 0.7 to 7.5 cases per 100,000 population in developed countries.[1] In the present healthcare environment, in which cost-containment issues are assuming greater importance, proper recognition and treatment of cardiomyopathies and heart failure in the critical care setting are vital to optimizing outcome and efficiently using intensive care resources. This chapter reviews clinical, pathophysiologic, and diagnostic features of the cardiomyopathies. The management of patients with end-stage cardiomyopathies in an ICU is also addressed. In addition, newer therapeutic modalities including pharmacologic and surgical interventions are discussed, with an emphasis on improving symptoms and long-term survival.

USE OF ENDOMYOCARDIAL BIOPSY

Since Kono and Sakakibara introduced the percutaneous, transvenous technique for obtaining myocardial biopsy samples in 1962, physicians have realized that cardiac tissue samples can be obtained from patients with heart failure in a safe, nonsurgical manner.[8] The technique of transvenous endomyocardial biopsy (TEB) uses a specially designed catheter with small (1–2 mm diameter), sharp-edged, cup-like forceps situated on the end and controlled by manipulation of a scissors handle at the opposite end. The biopsy catheter is introduced via a sheath situated in the femoral or internal jugular vein and, using fluoroscopic or echocardiographic guidance, is advanced to the right ventricular side of the intraventricular septum, where multiple samples are taken (Fig. 66–2). Tissue thus obtained can then be prepared for routine histologic examination by light and electron microscopy as well as for application of immunochemical and molecular biology techniques.

In its original application, TEB was used largely to perform serial histologic evaluation of heart transplant recipients as a means of monitoring allograft rejection and the response to immunosuppressive therapy. This remains the most common and agreed-on indication for routine use of TEB. Endomyocardial biopsy is also extremely useful for monitoring the cardiotoxic effects of anthracycline chemotherapeutic agents. Endomyocardial biopsy has gained widespread use as an effective means for the diagnosis of myocarditis, particularly in patients with recent onset of symptoms of heart failure. Establishing myocarditis on biopsy specimens has been hindered in the past by interobserver variability, a lack of uniform guidelines in establishing the histologic diagnosis, and the frequently focal nature of the myocarditic process.[9] Adoption of histologic grading using the Dallas criteria may help standardize the diagnostic features of myocarditis; however, true knowledge of the value of biopsy requires prospective follow-up of a large number of patients with defined histologic myocardial inflammation.[10] The spectrum of specific diagnoses that can be established through use of TEB is summarized in Table 66–2.

The TEB can be an extremely useful diagnostic tool in evaluating and classifying patients with cardiomyopathy.[11]

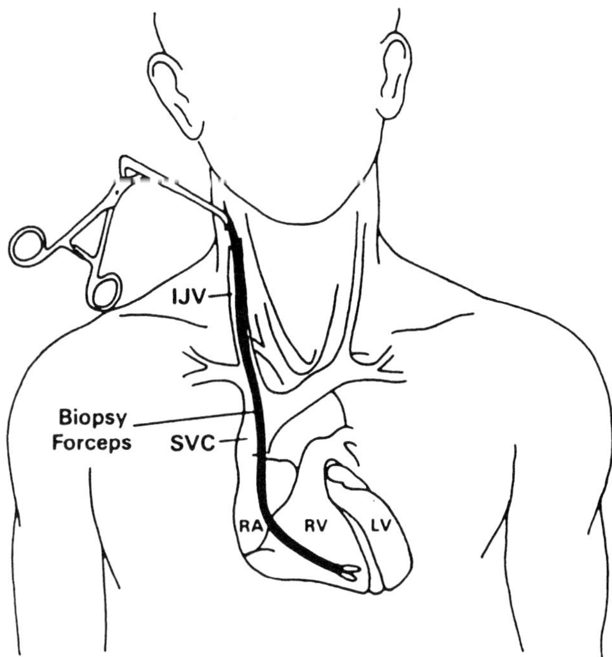

Figure 66–2. Schematic drawing of the right internal jugular vein approach to TEB of the right ventricle.

TABLE 66–2. Specific Diagnoses Made by Endomyocardial Biopsy

Cardiac allograft rejection	Cardiac tumors of cardiac origin
Myocarditis	Cardiac tumors of noncardiac origin
Giant-cell myocarditis	Kearns-Sayre syndrome
Doxorubicin cardiotoxicity	Cytomegalovirus infection
Cardiac amyloidosis	Toxoplasmosis
Cardiac sarcoidosis	Henoch-Schönlein purpura
Cardiac hemochromatosis	Rheumatic carditis
Endocardial fibrosis	Chagasic cardiomyopathy
Endocardial fibroelastosis	Chloroquine cardiomyopathy
Fabry's disease of the heart	Lyme carditis
	Carnitine deficiency cardiomyopathy
Carcinoid disease	Right ventricular lipomatosis
Irradiation injury	Hypereosinophilic syndrome
Glycogen storage disease	

(From Mason JW, O'Connell JB: Clinical merit of endomyocardial biopsy. Circulation 1989; 79:971.)

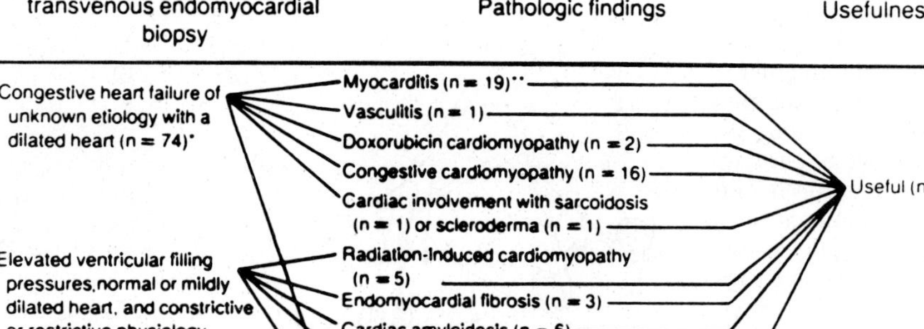

*Numbers in parentheses refer to the number of patients.
**Three patients had two diagnoses: one patient had amyloidosis and myocarditis, one patient had endomyocardial fibrosis with eosinophilic myocarditis, and one patient had vasculitis and myocarditis, so that the number of patients or indications totals 100 and the number of pathologic findings totals 103.

Figure 66–3. Flow diagram of the clinical indication, pathologic findings, and clinical usefulness of performing TEB in 100 patients. (From Parrillo JE, Aretz HT, Palacios I, et al: The results of transvenous endomyocardial biopsy can frequently be used to diagnose myocardial diseases in patients with idiopathic heart failure: Endomyocardial biopsies in 100 consecutive patients revealed a substantial incidence of myocarditis. Circulation 1984; 69:93.)

Two studies examining patients with restrictive cardiomyopathy using TEB resulted in specific diagnoses, most often amyloidosis, in a substantial proportion.[12, 13] Such information also assisted in differentiating restrictive cardiomyopathy from pericardial constriction. In this manner, TEB data aided in avoiding more invasive surgical procedures, guiding future diagnostic testing, and providing important prognostic information allowing for initiation of specific therapy.

The capacity for TEB to provide useful clinical diagnostic information has been further demonstrated in 100 consecutive patients referred for TEB for heart failure of undetermined cause.[14] The biopsies were performed to establish or preclude a potential specific cause of dilated (74%) or restrictive (26%) cardiomyopathy. Figure 66–3 summarizes the diagnostic results from these 100 consecutive heart biopsies. The pathologic diagnostic information obtained was judged to be useful in clinical decision making in 54 of these 100 patients.

More recently, the widespread application of TEB to patients with cardiomyopathy and unexplained heart failure has been disputed, particularly with respect to patients with dilated cardiomyopathy of long duration.[15] Critics of TEB argue that the yield of specific diagnostic information leading to effective therapy that improves outcome is low. It is the authors' opinion that patients with new onset of unexplained heart failure should be considered for TEB in addition to the conventional diagnostic tests discussed previously. Numerous studies report a significant incidence of active myocarditis in patients with idiopathic dilated cardiomyopathy.[16, 17] In the previously described study of 100 patients referred for TEB for unexplained heart failure, 26% presented evidence of myocarditis (see Fig. 66–3). Such patients may benefit from immunosuppressive therapy and would thus require TEB in order to identify this subset with inflammatory cardiomyopathy. In addition, cardiac biopsy also allows diagnosis of a number of other specific causes of cardiomyopathy (see Table 66–2).

DILATED CARDIOMYOPATHY

Clinical and Diagnostic Findings

Dilated cardiomyopathy is myocardial disease manifested as cardiac chamber dilatation with impairment of systolic function of one or both ventricles.[18] A multitude of widely divergent inflammatory, infectious, toxic, metabolic, hereditary, and vascular disorders are associated with development of dilated cardiomyopathy (Table 66–3). However, despite the diverse causes of this disorder, many and perhaps most cases do not have a clear discernible cause and are termed *idiopathic*. It is thought that dilated cardiomyopathy may represent the final common pathway resulting as a consequence of chronic recurrent myocardial damage from a wide variety of insults (Fig. 66–4).

Most patients present with heart failure. Ventricular arrhythmias may be the sole initial presentation in a small group of patients. Another presentation of cardiomyopathy is the unexpected finding of cardiomegaly on a patient's chest radiograph that was obtained for another indication. Subsequent cardiac evaluation documents a dilated, hypocontractile ventricle. Such patients eventually develop symptoms related to dilated cardiomyopathy, although it may take months or years. The overall prognosis for patients with dilated cardiomyopathy is considered later.

TABLE 66–3. Probable and Possible Causes of Dilated Cardiomyopathy

Idiopathic dilated cardiomyopathy	Metabolic/nutritional
Inflammatory/myocarditis	Uremia
Infectious	Hemochromatosis
Enterovirus	Carnitine deficiency
Human immunodeficiency virus	Selenium deficiency
Toxoplasma gondii	Thiamine deficiency
Trypanosoma cruzi	Electrolyte derangements
Trichinella spiralis	Endocrine
Noninfectious	Thyroid disease
Transplantation rejection	Cushing's disease
Autoimmune disease	Pheochromocytoma
Pregnancy	Hereditary
Sarcoid	Neuromyopathic disorders
Toxic	Familial cardiomyopathy
Alcohol	Miscellaneous
Catecholamines	Coronary microvascular spasm
Cocaine	Decreased coronary flow reserve
Anthracycline drugs	
5-Fluorouracil	
Azidothymidine	

Patients presenting with heart failure usually complain of symptoms related to low cardiac output, such as weakness, fatigue, and decreasing exercise tolerance. Shortness of breath, dyspnea on exertion, and orthopnea appear as pulmonary vascular congestion develops. Symptoms related to right heart failure such as increasing abdominal girth and peripheral edema generally appear late and connote a poor prognosis. Chest pain is observed in 25% to 50% of patients with idiopathic dilated cardiomyopathy. It is believed that decreased coronary flow reserve leading to subendocardial ischemia may be partly responsible for angina-type chest pain in these patients.[19] On physical examination, patients may demonstrate generalized wasting and pallor if the cardiomyopathy has been protracted. The systolic blood pressure may be low, with a narrow pulse pressure and pulsus alternans. Wheezing due to bronchospasm and engorgement of the bronchial vessels, as well as moist rales, is often noted on pulmonary examination of patients with decompensated heart failure. Pleural effusion, most often on the right side, may be detected as dullness to percussion. The apical impulse is displaced laterally. Heart sounds are often diminished, with an S_3 gallop noted at the apex. A murmur of mitral regurgitation due to left ventricular dilatation leading to nonapposition of mitral leaflets is frequently audible. With right heart dilation and failure, jugular venous distention with prominent a and v waves is present. The liver may be tender, enlarged, and pulsatile, with demonstrable hepatojugular reflux. Ascites and peripheral edema are usually found.

The heart failure of dilated cardiomyopathy is caused by a severe reduction in ventricular systolic function. Ejection fraction, a reliable measure of systolic function, is decreased (<40–45%) owing to impairment of contractility. Cardiac output is maintained by augmentation of heart rate and preload. Ventricular dilatation is thought to represent a compensatory response leading to increased preload and optimization of Starling forces.

A chest radiograph reveals generalized cardiomegaly and signs of pulmonary vascular hypertension. Kerley's lines, peribronchial cuffing, and interstitial and alveolar edema can also be seen. Pleural effusions are often present. The electrocardiogram may demonstrate sinus tachycardia as well as atrial or ventricular tachyarrhythmias. Conduction disturbances including atrioventricular block and bundle branch block are associated findings. Loss of anterior R wave forces and the presence of Q waves may resemble ischemic heart disease. ST segment and T wave abnormalities are the rule, and P wave changes consistent with left atrial enlargement may be noted. Twenty-four-hour Holter monitoring reveals ventricular arrhythmias, with approximately 50% of patients demonstrating nonsustained ventricular tachycardia.

Two-dimensional and Doppler echocardiography are extremely useful and gaining widespread application in the evaluation and follow-up of patients with dilated cardiomyopathy. Ventricular chamber dilatation is always present with a left ventricular end-diastolic diameter exceeding 2.7 cm/m². Ventricular wall thickness is normal or thin with global hypokinesis, with or without regional variation, and associated with percentage fractional shortening of less than 30%. Intracavitary thrombi may be present, usually at the apex. Doppler studies may reveal mitral or tricuspid regurgitation with pulmonary hypertension. Radionuclide ventriculography generally reveals increased end-diastolic and end-systolic volumes and diminished left ventricular ejection fraction. The right ventricle may also manifest chamber dilatation and reduced ejection fraction. Although involvement of the right ventricle is considered common in dilated cardiomyopathy, it is not always involved, and right ventricular involvement is not a reliable indicator of this disease. Indium 111 antimyosin scanning may aid in identifying subgroups of patients with active myocardial inflammation.[20]

Heart failure is commonly diagnosed hemodynamically by finding elevated filling pressures either by placement of a flow-directed pulmonary artery catheter in the ICU or during cardiac catheterization. Dilated cardiomyopathy produces a decreased stroke volume and increased left ventricular end-diastolic pressure. Mean left atrial pressure and pulmonary capillary wedge pressure (PCWP) are elevated to a degree corresponding to the extent of impairment of left ventricular systolic performance. Chronic elevation of left heart pressures may lead to moderate pulmonary vascular hypertension. Elevation of right ventricular end-diastolic and right atrial pressures signals the presence of right ventricular failure. Large V waves may be noted in the pulmonary capillary wedge tracing in patients with mitral regurgitation. In most patients with dilated cardiomyopathy, the resting cardiac output is normal or slightly decreased. Coronary angiography reveals no evidence of significant coronary artery disease. Contrast left ventriculography demonstrates global hypokinesia, sometimes with

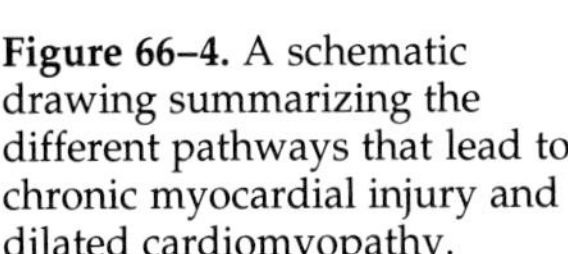

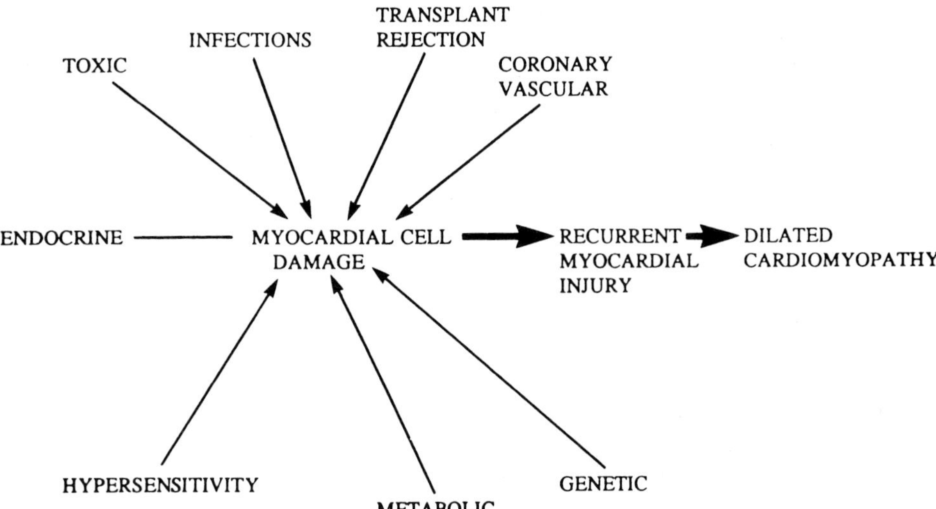

Figure 66–4. A schematic drawing summarizing the different pathways that lead to chronic myocardial injury and dilated cardiomyopathy.

segmental wall-motion abnormalities, chamber enlargement, decreased ejection fraction, and often mitral regurgitation.

Histologic examination of myocardial tissue specimens obtained either at autopsy or by TEB generally reveals areas of interstitial and perivascular fibrosis as well as myocyte degeneration.[21] Small focal areas of mononuclear cell infiltrate are often observed, along with various degrees of myocyte hypertrophy.[22]

Etiology and Natural History

When evaluating a patient with probable dilated cardiomyopathy, one should consider the specific diagnoses reviewed in Table 66–3. In most patients, however, a clear etiologic mechanism is not identifiable, and their cardiomyopathy is thus referred to as idiopathic. As previously mentioned, many investigators believe that dilated cardiomyopathy represents the end result of chronic recurrent myocardial insult due to a broad spectrum of causes (see Fig. 66–4). Dilated cardiomyopathy may result from myocardial inflammation due to viral infection (coxsackie B, echovirus, influenza, human immunodeficiency virus [HIV]), myocardial toxin (diphtheria), radiation, pharmacologic agents (Adriamycin, azidothymidine), metabolic disorders, or autoimmune collagen vascular disorders. Most bouts of myocardial inflammation due to any cause result in a self-limited illness that resolves. However, a small number of cases lead to immediate heart failure, or after a latent period, recurrent injury may lead to the late development of congestive heart failure and cardiomyopathy. Indeed, numerous studies of patients with dilated cardiomyopathy report biopsy evidence of myocarditis in a significant number of patients.[14, 16] Furthermore, enterovirus ribonucleic acid has been detected in myocardial biopsy specimens from patients with congestive cardiomyopathy using gene amplification by polymerase chain reaction.[23] Similarly, as many as 46% of patients with acquired immunodeficiency syndrome (AIDS) are found to have histologic evidence of myocarditis at necropsy.[24] Finally, biopsy specimens from patients with peripartum cardiomyopathy have revealed evidence of myocarditis in as many as 78%, further suggesting an acute inflammatory mechanism in this disorder.[25] Virus-induced myocardial inflammation injury may be mediated by various mechanisms, including virus-mediated cell lysis and humoral and cell-mediated autoimmunity directed against both normal myocytes (through shared epitopes) and virus-infected cardiac cells expressing structurally altered antigens or neoantigens, resulting in the development of a cardiomyopathic profile. Toxin-mediated myocardial cell injury may result in alteration of myocyte molecules, leading to formation of neoantigens to which the humoral and cell-mediated arms of the immune system respond. In addition, derangements in immune function have been reported in patients' with dilated cardiomyopathy. Certain human leukocyte antigens, specifically HLA-DR4, have been shown to be significantly more common in patients with dilated cardiomyopathy. Reduced suppressor and increased helper/inducer T cell subsets have been found in these patients.[26–28] Autoantibodies directed against cardiac tissue in general and the surface β-adrenoceptor in particular have been found in the sera of patients with dilated cardiomyopathy and may be partly responsible for immune-mediated injury in this illness.[29, 30]

Besides immunologic mechanisms, other molecular mediators of impairment of cardiac performance in patients with dilated cardiomyopathy have been reported. These include structural and functional alterations in the myosin heavy and light chains as well as other myofibrillar proteins,[31] abnormalities in intracellular calcium handling, decreased density and responsiveness of myocardial β-adrenoceptors,[32, 33] and alterations in the levels of the stimulatory and inhibitory subpopulations of regulatory guanine nucleotide-binding proteins.[34, 35]

Patients with idiopathic dilated cardiomyopathy generally present with symptoms secondary to heart failure, dysrhythmias, or thromboembolic phenomena. An asymptomatic patient is occasionally identified by finding impaired or dilated ventricles on routine diagnostic testing. Numerous retrospective studies have served to define the natural history of this disorder, as well as the prognostic factors associated with increased mortality.[36–39] Mortality rates for idiopathic dilated cardiomyopathy are approximately 20% per year, with a 5-year mortality of 50% to 75%. In a well-defined population of 169 patients with dilated cardiomyopathy, 1- and 5-year mortality rates were 28% and 57%, respectively (Fig. 66–5). The combination of progressive heart failure and sudden cardiac death accounts for the overwhelming majority of deaths. The 5-year point seems to define a subpopulation of patients with a more favorable long-term prognosis (see Fig. 66–5). These surviving patients, many of whom are alive after 10 years, generally have improvement in cardiac function to nearly normal. Thus, approximately 20% to 40% of patients with idiopathic dilated cardiomyopathy have a more favorable long-term survival, presumably because of improvement in cardiac function. Factors influencing survival in patients with idiopathic dilated cardiomyopathy (Table 66–4) generally reflect the severity of impairment in left ventricular performance and the presence of conduction abnormalities and ventricular dysrhythmias.

The presence of ventricular dysrhythmias is associated with a significantly increased risk of cardiac death in general and sudden cardiac death in particular. Pooled data indicate that approximately 28% of the deaths occurring in patients with idiopathic dilated cardiomyopathy were sudden and presumably arrhythmic in character.[40] Various degrees of ventricular ectopy are noted in virtually all patients with idiopathic dilated cardiomyopathy. Nonsustained ventricular tachycardia is encountered in 35% to 83% of patients and seems to correlate with degree of left ventricular dysfunction.[41–43] Although ambulatory monitoring, electrophysiologic testing, signal-averaged electrocardiography, and

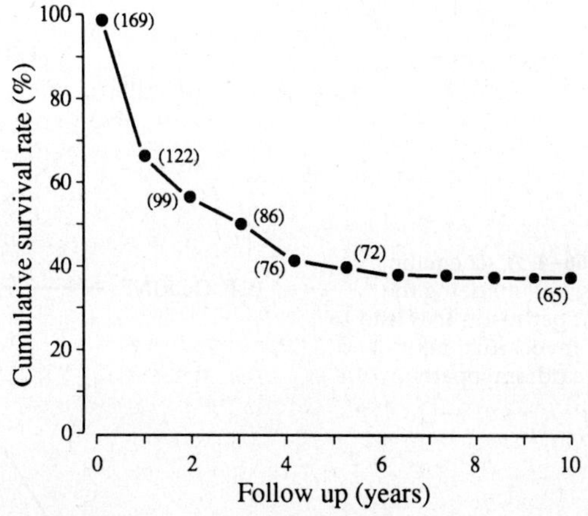

Figure 66–5. Ten-year survival curve of 169 patients with dilated cardiomyopathy. (From Diaz RA, Obasohan A, Oakley CM: Prediction of outcome in dilated cardiomyopathy. Br Heart J 1987; 58:393.)

TABLE 66–4. Factors Associated with Increased Mortality in Dilated Cardiomyopathy

Increased filling pressures	Ventricular arrhythmias
Decreased ejection fraction	Intraventricular conduction delay
Mitral regurgitation	Hyponatremia
Decreased peak oxygen consumption	Presence of S_3
Increased age	Thallium 201 perfusion defects
Functional class	
Requirement for intravenous inotropic support	Requirement for permanent pacemaker
Elevated serum norepinephrine levels	Severity of myocardial biopsy findings

Data from references 36–38, 44.

monitoring of heart rate variability have aided in identifying many patients at higher risk for arrhythmic death, none of these diagnostic techniques has proved itself superior in detecting all patients who have dilated cardiomyopathy and who are at risk for sudden death.

Treatment

In patients with dilated cardiomyopathy, irreversible myocardial injury leading to impairment of systolic performance with resultant decrease in ejection fraction and mean arterial blood pressure sets into motion a series of compensatory mechanisms directed at maintaining cardiac output and tissue perfusion. Initially, diminished systolic function associated with enhanced ventricular compliance allows for increased end-diastolic volume with nearly normal end-diastolic pressure, resulting in optimization of preload and maintenance of stroke volume. With continued deterioration of cardiac function, optimal compliance and Starling forces are exceeded, leading to elevation in left ventricular end-diastolic and PCWP and resultant pulmonary edema. Annular dilatation leads to mitrial regurgitation, further compromising forward stroke volume and exacerbating filling pressures. Reflex stimulation of the sympathetic nervous system tends to increase heart rate and systemic vascular resistance in an effort to maintain tissue perfusion. Systemic compensatory mechanisms such as activation of the renin-angiotensin system and increased vasopressin secretion lead to further fluid retention and vasoconstriction, which, though directed at maintaining mean arterial blood pressure, may worsen filling pressures, increase afterload, and result in increased wall stress, increased myocardial oxygen consumption, decreased stroke volume, and worsening mitral regurgitation. A cardiac index less than 2.5 L/min·m^2 and a left ventricular end-diastolic pressure greater than 27 mm Hg herald severe impairment of left ventricular function and a worse prognosis.[44]

The goals of therapy in idiopathic dilated cardiomyopathy are to improve symptoms related to heart failure and to prolong survival. In patients with decompensated heart failure in an ICU, therapy is directed at interrupting the vicious cycle of progressive deterioration of cardiac function outlined earlier. The various medical and surgical therapeutic modalities currently used for patients with dilated cardiomyopathy are summarized in Table 66–5.

Diuretics and digitalis preparations together represent the most common agents used in the treatment of heart failure. Diuretics inhibit renal tubular solute reabsorption and induce salt and water excretion. The result is decreased intravascular volume, which reduces ventricular filling pressures and promotes resolution of pulmonary edema as well as signs of right heart failure. Although potassium-sparing and thiazide diuretics can be effective, patients with significant decompensated heart failure usually require a loop diuretic. Metolazone, a thiazide diuretic, may exert a synergistic diuretic effect when combined with a loop diuretic. Potassium and magnesium losses with such therapy can be substantial, and care must be taken to avoid hypokalemia and hypomagnesemia, which may contribute to digitalis toxicity and ventricular dysrhythmias. Water restriction, particularly in the presence of hyponatremia, remains an important adjunct to diuretic therapy.

Digitalis glycosides have been used for more than 200 years for the management of congestive heart failure. Digitalis exerts both negative chronotropic and positive inotropic effects. Despite intensive debate that has spanned decades, digitalis preparations do appear to improve contractile function, augment left ventricular ejection fraction, and improve symptoms of heart failure.[45, 46] In those patients with heart failure and atrial fibrillation with a rapid ventricular response, digoxin is extremely effective in slowing the heart rate, improving diastolic filling, and augmenting ventricular systolic function. Although digitalis preparations have been shown to improve systolic performance and symptoms of heart failure, a survival benefit has not, to date, been demonstrated. Nevertheless, digitalis remains a mainstay of therapy for patients with chronic congestive heart failure.

Vasodilators, both venous and arterial, can produce significant improvement in hemodynamics as well as in signs and symptoms of congestive heart failure by favorably decreasing preload and afterload. Such therapy decreases filling pressures and wall stress and augments ejection fraction, stroke volume, and cardiac output.[47] Critically ill patients with severe congestive heart failure refractory to conventional oral medications may be treated with intravenous nitroprusside or nitroglycerin with improvement in clinical and hemodynamic parameters but without altering survival.[48] In patients with chronic congestive heart failure, the combination of isosorbide dinitrate and hydralazine when added to a conventional regimen of diuretics and digoxin has been shown to improve left ventricular function and long-term survival.[49] Angiotensin-converting enzyme inhibitors have gained widespread use and have now become an essential part of all medical regimens for the treatment of chronic congestive heart failure. These drugs inhibit formation of angiotensin II and aldosterone and result in decreased systemic vascular resistance. Prospective randomized trials of the addition of enalapril to conventional therapy for heart failure have demonstrated improvement in signs and symptoms of heart failure as well as prolonged survival.[50, 51] Newer vasodilators such as the dihydropyridine calcium channel blocker amlodipine and the direct-

TABLE 66–5. Therapeutic Modalities in Dilated Cardiomyopathy

- Diuretics
- Digitalis glycosides
- Vasodilators
  - Direct acting
  - Angiotensin-converting enzyme inhibitors
- Inotropic agents
- Beta-adrenergic blocking agents
- Immunosuppressive agents
- Anticoagulants
- Antiarrhythmic therapy including implantable defibrillators
- Cardiomyoplasty
- Mechanical circulatory support devices
- Heart transplantation

acting vasodilator flosequinan have been shown to exert beneficial effects in patients with refractory heart failure and are currently undergoing clinical evaluation.[52]

Short-term administration of inotropic agents can produce sustained improvement in hemodynamic and clinical parameters in patients with dilated cardiomyopathy in severe congestive heart failure. Dobutamine, a β_1-selective sympathomimetic agent, has positive inotropic and vasodilating properties and is widely used for severely decompensated heart failure. The phosphodiesterase inhibitors amrinone and milrinone have hemodynamic effects similar to those of dobutamine.[53] In addition, chronic long-term intermittent infusion of intravenous inotropic agents may be of value in treating patients with severe congestive heart failure despite maximum medical therapy. Because both dobutamine and milrinone have been associated with excess mortality, the authors favor using intermittent infusions of these agents in a monitored setting.[54] Newer oral inotropic vasodilator agents such as vesnarinone, coenzyme Q_{10}, and pimobendan are currently being evaluated for the treatment of chronic congestive heart failure and dilated cardiomyopathy.[55, 56] Vesnarinone has been shown to improve survival in a 60-mg dose; however, because the 120-mg dose increased mortality, further studies are needed to define its role.[57]

In 1975, Waagstein and colleagues reported beneficial effects of β-adrenergic blocking agents in patients with dilated cardiomyopathy, presumably by decreasing resting symptomatic tone and reversing the down-regulation of β-receptors produced by chronically elevated norepinephrine levels.[58] Widespread use of this therapy has been tempered by its potential to further suppress cardiac function owing to inherent negative inotropic effects. Nonetheless, randomized trials in patients with idiopathic dilated cardiomyopathy have demonstrated β-adrenergic blocker therapy to decrease filling pressures and improve cardiac function and exercise tolerance.[59] However, treatment with β-blockers has not yet been shown to improve survival, and their therapeutic role remains largely confined to symptomatic improvement in a subpopulation of patients with cardiomyopathy and resting tachycardia or only mild congestive heart failure.

The role of immunosuppressive agents in the treatment of idiopathic dilated cardiomyopathy is highly controversial. A prospective randomized trial of patients with idiopathic dilated cardiomyopathy and severe left ventricular dysfunction demonstrated a modest improvement in left ventricular ejection fraction in patients who had cellular infiltrates noted on myocardial biopsy and who were treated with prednisone.[60] This study provides controlled data that some patients with cardiomyopathy and a cellular infiltrate on myocardial biopsy have a corticosteroid-responsive inflammatory process in their myocardium.

Chronic anticoagulation in dilated cardiomyopathy is now widely advocated and is based on several retrospective studies suggesting an increased incidence of thromboembolic events in nonanticoagulated patients. The data are conflicting, however, and definitive resolution of this issue awaits a prospective randomized trial.[61] In the meantime, chronic warfarin administration in dilated cardiomyopathy should remain discretionary, and it is best prescribed for patients with severe atrial or ventricular dilatation, especially in the setting of atrial fibrillation.

Patients with symptomatic dilated cardiomyopathy have a 1-year mortality of 30% to 50%. Approximately half of these deaths are sudden and are believed to be secondary to malignant ventricular dysrhythmias. However, prospective identification of high-risk subsets of patients by diagnostic or clinical parameters has been disappointing. The risk of ventricular dysrhythmia and sudden death generally parallels the degree of left ventricular dysfunction. Electrolyte derangements, elevated catecholamine levels, and pharmacologic agents such as diuretics or digoxin can exacerbate ventricular arrhythmias in these patients. Several published studies suggest that electrophysiologic testing may be useful in detecting patients at increased risk for sudden death.[40] In patients with documented spontaneous sustained or symptomatic monomorphic ventricular tachycardia or aborted sudden death due to ventricular tachycardia or fibrillation, amiodarone or placement of an automatic implantable cardioverter-defibrillator may reduce arrhythmic death.[62] Conventional class Ia agents are generally contraindicated in these patients because of their significant negative inotropic and proarrhythmic effects. However, if antiarrhythmic drug therapy is used and renders a documented sustained monomorphic ventricular tachycardia noninducible on follow-up electrophysiologic testing, long-term survival is improved.[63]

For patients who have ejection fractions less than 25% and who are in severely decompensated heart failure despite maximal medical therapy, for patients with refractory ventricular dysrhythmias, and for patients dependent on intravenous inotropic agents or mechanical circulatory support devices, cardiac transplantation provides the only effective therapy for meaningful long-term survival. One- and 5-year post-transplant survival is approximately 80% and 60%, respectively. The major complications of this therapy are rejection, infection, and accelerated graft atherosclerosis. Mechanical circulatory support devices such as ventricular assist devices and the total artificial heart are currently being used in severely decompensated patients as a temporizing measure or as a bridge to transplantation. In patients who are not candidates for heart transplantation, the technique of cardiomyoplasty is currently being evaluated as a means of assisting cardiac function in severely impaired hearts. Several reports have demonstrated improvement in left ventricular function with a flap of synchronously contracting skeletal muscle wrapped around the failing heart.[64]

RESTRICTIVE CARDIOMYOPATHY

Of the different forms of cardiomyopathy, restrictive cardiomyopathy is the least common. As depicted in Figure 66–1 and Table 66–1, patients with restrictive cardiomyopathy frequently present with congestive heart failure, a small or only mildly enlarged heart, and relatively preserved left ventricular systolic function. The mechanism of heart failure in restrictive cardiomyopathy is related to reduced ventricular compliance and impaired diastolic relaxation, resulting in restricted ventricular filling, high ventricular filling pressures, and reduced stroke volume despite normal systolic contractile function. The pathophysiologic mechanism leading to impaired diastolic function is related to decreased ventricular distensibility limiting diastolic filling as a result of morphologic alterations in the myocardium.

Hemodynamic measurements in restrictive cardiomyopathy reveal elevation of pulmonary and systemic venous pressures. The ventricular pressure tracing exhibits a characteristic rapid diastolic filling phase followed by an early plateau as the limits of ventricular compliance are reached (Fig. 66–6). This diastolic dip-and-plateau or square root sign is also seen in pericardial constriction, making differentiation between the two disorders difficult at times. The restriction to diastolic filling may also be noted at the atrial level, where pressures are elevated and characterized by prominent x and y descents. In patients with mild forms of

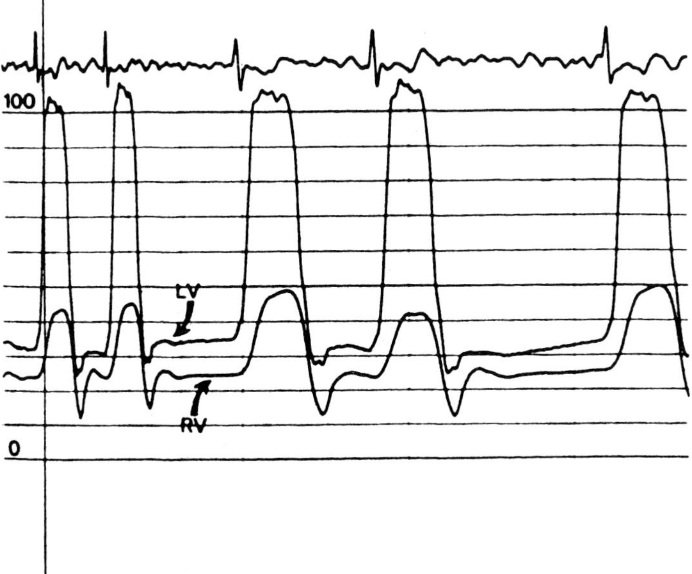

Figure 66–6. Simultaneous right and left ventricular pressure tracings from a patient with restrictive cardiomyopathy. Note the characteristic "dip-and-plateau" diastolic configuration. (From Hosenpud JD, Niles NR: Clinical, hemodynamic and endomyocardial biopsy findings in idiopathic restrictive cardiomyopathy. West J Med 1986; 144:303.)

the disease or in those whose intravascular volume is decreased secondary to diuretic therapy, the restrictive physiology described earlier may only be manifested after volume loading.

Most cases of restrictive cardiomyopathy are idiopathic. However, when evaluating a patient exhibiting restrictive physiology, one should keep in mind the secondary causes of restrictive cardiomyopathy listed in Table 66–6. Patients with restrictive cardiomyopathy generally relate symptoms of dyspnea, fatigue, or chest pain.[65] Physical findings including jugular venous distention, rales, S_3, S_4, ascites, and peripheral edema are common and due to biventricular failure. Echocardiography demonstrates small ventricular cavities with biatrial enlargement and normal or nearly normal ventricular systolic function. Atrioventricular valvular regurgitation is common. Late in the course of the disease, ventricular systolic function may deteriorate and the clinical picture may resemble that of a dilated cardiomyopathy.

In patients with suspected restrictive cardiomyopathy, pericardial constriction should be considered and effectively ruled out. Both conditions produce abnormal diastolic filling with high filling pressures and relatively spared systolic function, yet the treatment for these conditions is different. Constrictive pericarditis can be potentially cured by pericardiectomy, and restrictive cardiomyopathy can often be treated with tailored therapy directed at the underlying cause if known (e.g., amyloidosis, eosinophilic heart disease). A calcified pericardium seen on a lateral chest radiograph is suggestive of a constriction, whereas a speckled myocardium on two-dimensional echocardiography is consistent with cardiac amyloidosis. Cardiac catheterization can aid in differentiating these two disorders. Both conditions cause equalization of diastolic pressures to within 5 mm Hg of each other. The right ventricular and pulmonary artery systolic pressures are usually higher in restrictive cardiomyopathy, generally exceeding 45 mm Hg. Furthermore, the plateau of the right ventricular pressure is usually at least one third of the peak systolic pressure in pericardial constriction and less in myocardial restriction. In some cases, TEB may allow identification of a specific cause of restrictive cardiomyopathy, thereby aiding in differentiation from constrictive pericarditis. If TEB demonstrates only nonspecific changes or normal myocardium, then constrictive pericarditis becomes more likely. Diagnostic evaluation by computed tomography or magnetic resonance imaging can provide accurate estimates of pericardial thickness and aid in differentiating these diseases.[66, 67]

TABLE 66–6. Classification of the Restrictive Cardiomyopathies

Primary (idiopathic)	Endomyocardial
Secondary	Fibroelastosis
Myocardial	Eosinophilic heart disease
Amyloidosis	Carcinoid
Sarcoidosis	Radiation
Hemochromatosis	Cardiac transplant
Glycogen storage diseases	Anthracycline toxicity
Gaucher's disease	
Fabry's disease	
Tumor	

The prognosis for patients with restrictive cardiomyopathy is generally poor, with only approximately 10% of diagnosed patients alive at 10 years. Deaths are generally due to progressive heart failure, arrhythmias, or comorbid illness. Medical therapy is often supportive, targeted at the underlying hemodynamic diastolic abnormality. Judicious use of diuretics decreases filling pressures and improves symptoms but may do so at the expense of cardiac output. Nonetheless, diuretics represent an essential component of the therapeutic regimen for restrictive cardiomyopathy, particularly in those patients with congestive heart failure. Careful use of vasodilator agents or calcium channel antagonists may also provide some symptomatic benefit but may cause hypotension.

Some of the secondary forms of restrictive cardiomyopathy may be treated with more specific forms of therapy. For example, alkylating agents may be used in patients with amyloidosis, albeit with generally unsatisfactory results. Chelating agents such as desferoxamine can be effective in alleviating tissue iron deposition in hemochromatosis.

The hypereosinophilic syndrome is an uncommon cause of restrictive cardiomyopathy in which profound blood and bone marrow eosinophilia leads to multiorgan system disease presumably due to the toxic effects produced by release of eosinophil-granule products. Although many organs are involved, almost all patients who die do so because of severe heart failure. Cardiac involvement includes myocarditis associated with intense eosinophilic infiltration, myocardial thickening, endocardial thrombus formation, and progressive endocardial fibrosis. The dense endomyocardial fibrosis and scarring lead to a hemodynamic picture of restrictive cardiomyopathy. Signs of congestive heart failure often associated with a murmur of mitral regurgitation are noted.[68]

Patients with eosinophilic heart disease often have a beneficial response to administration of corticosteroids or cytotoxic agents, particular hydroxyurea. Such therapy may slow progression of the disease and improve symptoms as well as survival.[69] Chronic anticoagulation should be considered when ventricular thrombi are present. The course of the illness is variable. Patients with severe acute necrotizing myocarditis may rapidly drift into cardiogenic shock and death.[70] Most patients experience a more chronic, slowly progressive course of worsening heart failure.

HYPERTROPHIC CARDIOMYOPATHY

Myocardial hypertrophy occurring out of proportion to the hemodynamic load or in the absence of increased wall stress is characteristic of hypertrophic cardiomyopathy. The degree and extent of hypertrophy vary from patient to patient, with the septum and anterolateral wall involved more frequently than the posterior wall. A unique form of hypertrophic cardiomyopathy limited to the apical segments and associated with giant inverted precordial T waves is frequently encountered in patients of Japanese descent.[71] Genetic transmission of this disorder occurs in more than 50% of cases as an autosomal dominant trait with variable expression and penetrance. Myocardial hypertrophy leads to decreased ventricular cavity size and diminished lusitropic and compliance characteristics of the left ventricle, resulting in abnormal left ventricular diastolic filling. As a result, cardiac output is maintained at the expense of elevated filling pressures. Left ventricular systolic function is well preserved, and ejection fraction is often supernormal until late in the course of the disease, when approximately 10% of cases evolve to a profile more consistent with dilated cardiomyopathy.

In a minority of patients (25%), particularly those with predominant septal involvement (asymmetric septal hypertrophy), a dynamic obstruction to left ventricular outflow may exist in a way that allows a pressure gradient between the body of the left ventricle and the subaortic region during systole. The cause of the dynamic outflow obstruction is believed to be the close apposition of the hypertrophied septum and the anterior leaflet of the mitral valve. During vigorous ventricular contraction, systolic anterior motion of the mitral valve across the left ventricular outflow tract contracts the septum and impedes ventricular ejection. The obstruction to left ventricular outflow is labile and is increased by any alteration that augments ejection fraction or decreases left ventricular cavity dimension. Thus, increased contractility or decreased preload or afterload increases the outflow gradient and worsens the obstruction.

The cause of hypertrophic cardiomyopathy is unclear, but abnormal calcium regulation, genetic defects, and neurohormoral factors have been implicated.[72] Recombinant deoxyribonucleic acid techniques have identified mutations in the long arm of chromosome 14 coding for the myosin heavy chain in several families with hypertrophic cardiomyopathy.[73, 74] Whatever the cause, the morphologic end result is myocardial hypertrophy with gross disorganization of the muscle bundles and myofibrillar disarray along with fibrosis and scar formation. Myocardial ischemia is also believed to be an important pathophysiologic mechanism and is thought to be due to abnormal narrowing of small intramural coronary arteries, impairment of coronary vascular reserve, and reduced capillary density.

Most patients with hypertrophic cardiomyopathy are asymptomatic or only mildly symptomatic. Dyspnea, chest pain, fatigue, and syncope are the most common symptoms and generally correlate with the degree of hypertrophy but not the severity of the outflow tract obstruction. Physical findings vary but may include a hyperdynamic precordium, S_4, paradoxical splitting of S_2, and a bifid carotid pulse. The systolic murmurs of hypertrophic cardiomyopathy may reflect both turbulence at the outflow tract and associated mitral regurgitation.

Echocardiography is extremely useful in evaluating patients with suspected hypertrophic cardiomyopathy. The pattern and extent of left ventricular hypertrophy, narrowing of the left ventricular outflow tract, the magnitude of the outflow tract pressure gradient, and systolic anterior motion of the mitral valve can be readily assessed. The left ventricular cavity dimensions are often decreased and associated with vigorous systolic contraction. The atria are dilated as a result of chronically elevated filling pressures and atrioventricular valvular regurgitation. The septal left ventricular wall thickness is often 1.3 to 1.5 times the thickness of the posterior wall in patients with asymmetric septal hypertrophy. Mitral regurgitation and mitral valve prolapse are common associated features. Aortic insufficiency is noted in approximately one third of patients. Cardiac catheterization reveals elevated left-sided filling pressures due to decreased left ventricular compliance. A subaortic pressure gradient may exist between the left ventricle and the aorta during systole; it can be accentuated by maneuvers that increase contractility or decrease afterload or preload. The aortic pressure tracing exhibits the classic spike-and-dome configuration in patients with outflow tract obstruction.

Therapy in hypertrophic cardiomyopathy is aimed at improving symptoms and decreasing risk of death. Pharmacologic agents that decrease filling pressure, improve left ventricular diastolic relaxation, or reduce the magnitude of the left ventricular outflow tract pressure gradient improve symptoms in this disorder. Beta-adrenergic blocking agents are the mainstay of therapy in patients with hypertrophic cardiomyopathy. Such drugs slow heart rate and lengthen the diastolic filling period, thus improving the diastolic filling abnormality associated with this condition. Beta-adrenergic blocking agents also decrease myocardial oxygen consumption and improve ischemia. In patients with pulmonary congestion, careful use of diuretics may be beneficial. Calcium channel antagonists such as verapamil and to a lesser extent nifedipine and diltiazem have been postulated to improve left ventricular relaxation and ventricular diastolic filling in patients with hypertrophic cardiomyopathy with or without left ventricular outflow tract obstruction.[75] Disopyramide, presumably because of its negative inotropic effect, has also been shown to improve symptoms and exercise tolerance. These agents all must be used with caution because the potential for serious side effects such as bradycardia and hypotension is a genuine concern.

In one study, it was found that dual-chamber pacing carried out in patients who had hypertrophic cardiomyopathy and who failed conventional medical therapy resulted in improvement in symptoms, exercise tolerance, cardiac output, and the left ventricular outflow tract gradient.[76] Surgical therapy consisting of ventricular septal myotomy with or without myectomy has been shown to relieve the dynamic outflow tract obstruction, reduce systolic anterior motion of the mitral valve, reduce mitral regurgitation, and improve symptoms. However, because surgical therapy carries an operative risk of 5% to 8%, such therapy is generally reserved for patients with severe symptoms despite maximum medical therapy. Mitral valve replacement usually abolishes the subaortic gradient and may be helpful in certain patients.

Patients with hypertrophic cardiomyopathy exhibit an annual mortality rate of 2% to 3%, and about half the deaths are sudden and unexpected; sudden death may be the initial presenting event. Sudden death, the most ominous complication of hypertrophic cardiomyopathy, may be due to circulatory collapse in the presence of a severe outflow tract gradient but is most often thought to be secondary to malignant ventricular arrhythmias. Factors predisposing to sudden death include age less than 30 years, a family history of hypertrophic cardiomyopathy or sudden death, syncope, and evidence of ventricular tachycardia on ambulatory monitoring. The value of electrophysiologic testing in identifying high-risk individuals is unclear and currently being evaluated. Amiodarone may be of benefit in some patients with ventricular tachycardia. High-risk individuals with resuscitated cardiac arrest or documented sustained ventricular tachycardia should be considered for placement of an automatic implantable cardioverter-defibrillator.

Patients with hypertrophic cardiomyopathy are also susceptible to supraventricular tachycardia. The occurrence of atrial fibrillation may result in hemodynamic deterioration as a result of loss of the atrial contribution to left ventricular filling. Such patients benefit from aggressive treatment of their rhythm disturbance with rapid conversion to sinus rhythm.

Finally, for those patients with refractory heart failure or uncontrollable dysrhythmias, cardiac transplantation remains a final consideration.

CARDIOMYOPATHIES AND THE CRITICAL CARE ENVIRONMENT

As mentioned in the introduction, certain specific problems are frequently encountered when caring for critically ill patients with the various forms of cardiomyopathy discussed in this chapter. The pathogenetic mechanisms, diagnostic evaluations, and therapeutic modalities reviewed earlier represent a major body of information that must be well understood in order to effectively provide optimal care to these patients.

Management of Cardiomyopathy Using Invasive Hemodynamic Monitoring

Patients with severe decompensated heart failure due to cardiomyopathy are generally admitted to an ICU for diagnostic evaluation and treatment. Initially, a balloon-tipped, flow-directed pulmonary artery catheter should be placed to determine filling pressures, cardiac index, and systemic vascular resistance. Continued invasive hemodynamic monitoring aids in guiding therapy and optimizing cardiac performance.

Caring for patients with cardiomyopathy in the critical care unit requires a sophisticated understanding of fluid and pressor administration as well as the pathophysiology underlying the form of cardiomyopathy under evaluation. For example, a patient with hypertrophic cardiomyopathy with a severe dynamic outflow tract obstruction should not be treated with intravenous inotropic agents.

A first step to improving hemodynamics is to optimize preload in a way that obtains maximum cardiac index without exacerbating pulmonary edema. By using the PCWP, one can administer fluids until a PCWP of 15 to 20 mm Hg is achieved. When PCWP exceeds this level, pulmonary edema tends to occur. It should be emphasized that PCWP is a measurement of left ventricular diastolic pressure and does not necessarily reflect left ventricular volume. This is particularly true of patients with impaired diastolic relaxation or decreased compliance such as in restrictive or hypertrophic cardiomyopathy. In such patients, a small change in intravascular volume may produce a small change in ventricular volume but a large increase in ventricular filling pressure, leading to worsening pulmonary edema. These patients may best be served with treatment aimed at favorably altering lusitropic and compliance characteristics such as with β-adrenergic blockade, calcium channel antagonists, or vasodilators.

In dilated cardiomyopathy, ventricular compliance is usually increased, and one can give large amounts of fluid, increasing intraventricular diastolic volume, with a small or no change in PCWP. In these patients, one can continue to give fluid until the PCWP approaches 20 mm Hg, beyond which lung water begins to increase. Interestingly, some patients with dilated cardiomyopathy can be maintained at a higher PCWP without developing pulmonary edema, presumably because long-standing heart failure leads to increased lymphatic drainage of extravascular pulmonary fluid. In these patients, a higher end-diastolic volume and preload can be achieved by further intravascular volume expansion to a PCWP that is high by usual standards but is well tolerated.

Patients with restrictive or hypertrophic cardiomyopathy exhibit reduced compliance and abnormal ventricular diastolic relaxation. Such patients may generally achieve a PCWP of 20 mm Hg with very little fluid supplementation. However, a subgroup of these patients may not demonstrate an increased PCWP with continued fluid administration. The response of these patients to intravascular volume expansion cannot be predicted; therefore, each patient should be given a trial of fluid administration with careful hemodynamic monitoring. In addition, echocardiography is also helpful in assessing left ventricular systolic function and valvular regurgitation and ruling out pericardial effusion and tamponade.

Perhaps more important than the absolute value for filling pressure or cardiac index are trends or changes in PCWP, cardiac output, stroke volume, or systemic vascular resistance in response to therapeutic manipulations. For example, patients with dilated cardiomyopathy may exhibit an elevated PCWP that is well matched to achieve optimal cardiac index. A small decrease in this pressure may reflect a significant decrease in left ventricular end-diastolic volume and result in decreased cardiac performance. One should monitor these changes closely and target predetermined reasonable hemodynamic goals.

Patients who have cardiomyopathy with severe impairment of heart function may present with episodes of low cardiac output characterized by severe fatigue and hemodynamic embarrassment associated with low cardiac output and evidence of end-organ hypoperfusion. Such episodes are severe and potentially life threatening. They require admission to the ICU, invasive hemodynamic monitoring, and treatment with intravenous inotropic agents, vasopressors, diuretics, and vasodilators to prevent irreversible multiorgan system failure. Some patients improve, but others may exhibit further deterioration and become refractory to medical therapy. This latter group presents difficult ethical and practical issues regarding more aggressive means of cardiovascular support. Hemodynamic improvement can be obtained with mechanical circulatory support devices such as intra-aortic counterpulsation balloon pumping, ventricular assist devices, or the total artificial heart. However, it must be emphasized that such therapies are temporizing measures, and endpoints for therapy need to be decided on before mechanical circulatory assist devices are applied. Such patients should be urgently evaluated for heart transplantation, and if appropriate, mechanical circulatory assist devices may provide an effective bridge to transplantation therapy until such time that a donor becomes available. In the meantime, patients with cardiomyopathy and low-output states should be monitored with serial hemodynamic measurements, and their response to fluids, vasopressors, diuretics, and inotropic agents should be closely observed in an attempt to optimize blood flow to vital organs. Determinations of mixed venous oxygen saturation and serum lactate levels provide a reliable measure of tissue perfusion. Many patients, although considered to be refractory to conventional heart failure therapy, respond to an intensive tailored approach consisting of intravenous vasodilators and diuretics followed by oral therapy and meticulous attention to hemodynamics and fluid balance (Table 66–7).

IMPORTANT RHYTHM DISTURBANCES

Rhythm disturbances are another special problem encountered when treating patients with severe heart failure and cardiomyopathy. For example, patients with restrictive or hypertrophic cardiomyopathy may exhibit hemodynamic deterioration in the presence of atrial fibrillation owing to loss of the active atrial contribution to cardiac output. In such cases, aggressive measures to restore and maintain normal sinus rhythm should be implemented, including electric cardioversion and use of antiarrhythmic agents.

Recurrent ventricular arrhythmias also represent a serious problem for patients with cardiomyopathy. Type 1 antiarrhythmic agents are often poorly tolerated because of their negative inotropic and proarrhythmic effects. Care should be taken to avoid electrolyte derangements, myocardial ischemia, and drug toxicity, all of which can exacerbate ventricular arrhythmias in these patients. Amiodarone can be effective in treating both supraventricular and ventricular arrhythmias in patients with dilated cardiomyopathy.

TABLE 66–7. Tailored Therapy for Heart Failure Before Transplantation

1. Measurement of baseline hemodynamics
2. Intravenous nitroprusside and diuretics tailored to hemodynamic goals:
   - Pulmonary capillary wedge pressure $\leq$ 15 mm Hg
   - Systemic vascular resistance $\leq$ 1200 dyne·s/cm^5·m^2
   - Right atrial pressure $\leq$ 8 mm Hg
   - Systolic blood pressure $\geq$ 80 mm Hg
3. Definition of optimal hemodynamics by 24–48 h
4. Titration of high-dose vasodilators as nitroprusside weaned:
   - Captopril, hydralazine, isosorbide dinitrate
5. Monitored ambulation and diuretic adjustment for 24–48 h
6. Maintain digoxin levels 1.9–2.0 ng/dL if no contraindication
7. Detailed patient education
8. Flexible outpatient diuretic regimen including intermittent metolazone
9. Progressive walking program
10. Vigilant follow-up

(From Stevenson LW: Tailored therapy before transplantation for treatment of advanced heart failure: Effective use of vasodilators and diuretics. J Heart Lung Transplant 1991; 10:468.)

References

1. Abelmann WH, Lorell BH: The challenge of cardiomyopathy. J Am Coll Cardiol 1989; 3:1219.
2. Goodwin JF: Classification of nonhypertrophic cardiomyopathies. Prog Cardiol 1989; 2:3.
3. WHO:ISFC Task Force: Report of the WHO/ISFC Task Force on The Definition and Classification of Cardiomyopathies. Br Heart J 1980; 44:672.
4. World Health Organization: Cardiomyopathies: Report of a WHO Expert Committee. WHO Tech Rep Ser 1984; 697:7.
5. Stewart S, Mason DT, Braunwald E: Impaired rate of left ventricular filling in idiopathic hypertrophic subaortic stenosis and valvular aortic stenosis. Circulation 1968; 37:8.
6. Gaasch WH, Stauffer J-C: Diastolic dysfunction. Prog Cardiol 1989; 2:87.
7. Gillum RF: The epidemiology of cardiomyopathy in the United States. Prog Cardiol 1989; 2:11.
8. Kono S, Sakakibara S: Endomyocardial biopsy. Dis Chest 1963; 44:345.
9. Shanes JG, Ghali J, Billingham ME, et al: Interobserver variability in the pathologic interpretation of endomyocardial biopsy results. Circulation 1987; 75:401.
10. Aretz HT, Billingham ME, Edwards WD: Myocarditis. A histopathologic definition and classification. Am J Cardiovasc Pathol 1986; 1:3.
11. Starling RC, Unverferth DV: Value of endomyocardial biopsy: Indications and applications. Prog Cardiol 1989; 2:33.
12. French WJ, Siegel RJ, Cohen AH, et al: Yield of endomyocardial biopsy in patients with biventricular failure. Chest 1986; 90:181.
13. Schoenfeld MH, Supple EW, Dec WG, et al: Restrictive cardiomyopathy versus constrictive pericarditis: Role of endomyocardial biopsy in avoiding unnecessary thoracotomy. Circulation 1987; 75:1012.
14. Parrillo JE, Aretz HT, Palacios I, et al: The results of transvenous endomyocardial biopsy can frequently be used to diagnose myocardial diseases in patients with idiopathic heart failure. Circulation 1984; 69:93.
15. Mason JW, O'Connell JB: Clinical merit of endomyocardial biopsy. Circulation 1989; 79:971.
16. Dec WG, Palacios IF, Fallon JT, et al: Active myocarditis in the spectrum of acute dilated cardiomyopathies. N Engl J Med 1985; 312:885.
17. Vasiljevic JD, Kanjuh V, Seferovic P, et al: The incidence of myocarditis in endomyocardial biopsy samples from patients with congestive heart failure. Am Heart J 1990; 120:1370.
18. Manolio TA, Baughman KL, Rodcheffer R, et al: Prevalence and etiology of idiopathic dilated cardiomyopathy (summary of a national heart, lung, and blood institute workshop). Am J Cardiol 1992; 69:1458.
19. Cannon RO, Cunnion RE, Parrillo JE, et al: Dynamic limitation of coronary vasodilator reserve in patients with dilated cardiomyopathy and chest pain. J Am Coll Cardiol 1987; 10:1190.
20. Dec GW, Palacios I, Yasuda T, et al: Antimyosin antibody cardiac imaging: Its role in the diagnosis of myocarditis. J Am Coll Cardiol 1990; 16:97.
21. Roberts WC, Siegel RJ, McManus BM: Idiopathic dilated cardiomyopathy: Analysis of 152 necropsy patients. Am J Cardiol 1987; 60:1340.
22. Ferrans VJ: Pathologic anatomy of the dilated cardiomyopathies. Am J Cardiol 1989; 64:9C.
23. Jin O, Sole MJ, Butany JW, et al: Detection of enterovirus RNA in myocardial biopsies from patients with myocarditis and cardiomyopathy using gene amplification by polymerase chain reaction. Circulation 1990; 82:8.
24. Reilly JM, Cunnion RE, Anderson DW, et al: Frequency of myocarditis, left ventricular dysfunction and ventricular tachycardia in the acquired immune deficiency syndrome. Am J Cardiol 1988; 62:789.
25. Midei MG, DeMent SH, Feldman AM, et al: Peripartum myocarditis and cardiomyopathy. Circulation 1990; 81:922.
26. Sanderson JE, Koech D, Iha D, et al: T-lymphocyte subsets in idiopathic dilated cardiomyopathy. Am J Cardiol 1985; 55:755.
27. Limas CJ, Limas C: HLA antigens in idiopathic dilated cardiomyopathy. Br Heart J 1989; 62:379.

28. Eckstein R, Mempel W, Bolte H-D: Reduced suppressor cell activity in congestive cardiomyopathy and in myocarditis. Circulation 1982; 65:1224.
29. Caforio ALP, Bonifacio E, Stewart JT, et al: Novel organ-specific circulating cardiac autoantibodies in dilated cardiomyopathy. J Am Coll Cardiol 1990; 15:1527.
30. Limas CJ, Goldenberg IF, Limas C: Autoantibodies against beta-adrenoceptors in human idiopathic dilated cardiomyopathy. Circulation Res 1989; 64:97.
31. Margossian SS, White HD, Caulfield JB, et al: Light chain 2 profile and activity of human ventricular myosin during dilated cardiomyopathy. Identification of a causal agent for impaired myocardial function. Circulation 1992; 85:1720.
32. Ungerer M, Bohm M, Elce JS, et al: Altered expression of beta-adrenergic receptor kinase and $beta_1$-adrenergic receptors in the failing human heart. Circulation 1993; 87:454.
33. Sullebarger JT, Fan T-HM, Torres F, et al: Both cell surface and internalized beta-adrenoceptors are reduced in the failing myocardium. Eur J Pharmacol 1991; 205:165.
34. Morgan HE: Cellular aspects of cardial failure. Circulation 1993; 87(Supp IV): IV-4.
35. Feldman AM, Cates AE, Veazey WB: Increase of the 40,000-mol wt pertusis toxin substrate (G-protein) in the failing human heart. J Clin Invest 1988; 82:189.
36. Romeo F, Pelliccia F, Cianfroccia C, et al: Determinants of end-stage idiopathic dilated cardiomyopathy: A multivariate analysis of 104 patients. Clin Cardiol 1989; 12:387.
37. Saxon LA, Stevenson WG, Middlekauft HR, et al: Predicting death from progressive heart failure secondary to ischemic or idiopathic dilated cardiomygraphy. Am J Cardiol 1993; 72:62.
38. Diaz RA, Obasohan A, Oakley CM: Prediction of outcome in dilated cardiomyopathy. Br Heart J 1987; 58:343.
39. Fuster V, Gersh BJ, Giuliani ER, et al: The natural history of idiopathic dilated cardiomyopathy. Am J Cardiol 1981; 47:525.
40. Tamburro P, Wilber D: Sudden death in idiopathic dilated cardiomyopathy. Am Heart J 1992; 124:1035.
41. Holmes J, Kubo SH, Cody RJ, et al: Arrhythmias in ischemic and nonischemic dilated cardiomyopathy: Prediction of mortality by ambulatory electrocardiography. Am J Cardiol 1985; 55:146.
42. Huang SK, Messer JV, Denes P: Significance of ventricular tachycardia in idiopathic dilated cardiomyopathy: Observations in 35 patients. Am J Cardiol 1983; 51:507.
43. Olshausen KV, Shafer A, Mehmel HC, et al: Ventricular arrhythmias in idiopathic dilated cardiomyopathy. Br Heart J 1984; 51:195.
44. Stevenson LW: Dilated cardiomyopathy: Principles and prognosis. Prog Cardiol 1989; 2:51.
45. Captopril-Digoxin Multicenter Research Group: Comparative effects of therapy with captopril and digoxin in patients with mild to moderate heart failure. JAMA 1988; 259:539.
46. Gheorghiade M, Zarowitz BJ: Review of randomized trials of digoxin therapy in patients with chronic heart failure. Am J Cardiol 1992; 69:48G.
47. Parrillo JE: Pharmacologic Approach to the Critically Ill Patient. 2nd Ed. Baltimore, Williams & Wilkins, 1988, p 346.
48. Guiha MH, Cohn JN, Milkulic E, et al: Treatment of refractory heart failure with infusion of Nitroprusside. N Engl J Med 1974; 291:587.
49. Cohn JN, Archibald DG, Ziesche S, et al: Effect of vasodilator therapy on mortality in chronic congestive heart failure. Results of veterans administration cooperative study. N Engl J Med 1986; 314:1547.
50. The SOLVD Investigators: Effect of enalapril on survival in patients with reduced left ventricular ejection fraction and congestive heart failure. N Engl J Med 1991; 325:293.
51. The Consensus Trial Study Group: Effects of enalapril on mortality in severe congestive heart failure: Results of the cooperative North Scandinavian Enalapril Survival Study (Consensus). N Engl J Med 1987; 316:1429.
52. Barnett DB: Flosequinan. Lancet 1993; 341:733.
53. Marcus RH, Raw K, Patel J, et al: Comparison of intravenous amrinone and dobutamine in congestive heart failure due to idiopathic dilated cardiomyopathy. Am J Cardiol 1990; 66:1107.
54. Pickworth KK: Long-term dobutamine therapy for refractory congestive heart failure. Clinical Pharm 1992; 11:618.
55. Beck OM, Sorensen JD, Jensen MK, et al: Effects of long-term coenzyme Q_{10} and captopril treatment on survival and functional capacity in rats with experimentally induced heart infarction. J Pharm Exp Ther 1990; 255:346.
56. Katz SD, Kubo SH, Jessup M, et al: A multicenter, randomized, double-blind, placebo-controlled trial of pimobendan, a new cardiotonic and vasodilator agent, in patients with severe congestive heart failure. Am Heart J 1992; 123:95.
57. Feldman AM, Bristow MR, Parmley WW, et al: Effects of vesnarinone on morbidity and mortality in patients with heart failure. N Engl J Med 1993; 329:149.
58. Waagstein F, Hjalmarsou A, Varhauskus E, et al: Effect of chronic beta-adrenergic receptor blockage in congestive cardiomyopathy. Br Heart J 1975; 37:1022.
59. Waagstein F, Bristow MR, Swedberg K, et al: Beneficial effects of metoprolol in idiopathic dilated cardiomyopathy. Lancet 1993; 342:1441.
60. Parrillo JE, Connon RE, Epstein SE, et al: A prospective, randomized, controlled trial of prednisone for dilated cardiomyopathy. N Engl J Med 1989; 321:1061.
61. Dunkman WB, Johnson GR, Carson PE, et al: Incidence of thromboembolic events in congestive heart failure. Circulation 1993; 87(Suppl VI):VI-94.
62. Neri R, Mestroni TL, Salvi A, et al: Ventricular arrhythmias in dilated cardiomyopathy: Efficacy of amiodarone. Am Heart J 1987; 113:707.
63. Wilber PJ, Garan H, Finkelstein D, et al: Out-of-hospital cardiac arrest. Use of electrophysiologic testing in the prediction of long-term outcome. N Engl J Med 1982; 318:19.
64. Magovern JA, Magovern GJ, Maher TD, et al: Operation for congestive heart failure: Transplantation, coronary artery bypass, and cardiomyoplasty. Ann Thorac Surg 1993; 56:418.
65. Hosenpud JD, Niles NR: Clinical, hemodynamic and endomyocardial biopsy findings in idiopathic restrictive cardiomyopathy. West J Med 1986; 144:303.
66. Isner JM, Carter BL, Bankoff MS, et al: Differentiation of constrictive pericarditis from restrictive cardiomyopathy by computed tomographic imaging. Am Heart J 1983; 105:1019.
67. Sechtem U, Higgins CB, Sommerhoff BA, et al: Magnetic resonance imaging of restrictive cardiomyopathy. Am J Cardiol 1987; 59:480.
68. Parrillo JE, Borer JS, Henry WL, et al: The cardiovascular manifestations of the hypereosinophilic syndrome. J Med 1979; 67:572.
69. Parrillo JE, Fauci AS, Wolff SM: Therapy of the hypereosinophilic syndrome. Ann Intern Med 1978; 89:167.
70. Parrillo JE: Heart disease and the eosinophil. N Engl J Med 1990; 323:1560.
71. Webb JG, Sasson Z, Rakowski H, et al: Apical hypertrophic cardiomyopathy: Clinical follow-up and diagnostic correlates. J Am Coll Cardiol 1990; 15:83.
72. Maron BJ, Borow RO, Cannon RO, et al: Hypertrophic cardiomyopathy. Interrelations of clinical manifestations, pathophysiology, and therapy (first of two parts). N Engl J Med 1987; 316:780.
73. Jarcho JA, McKenna W, Pare P, et al: Mapping a gene for familial hypertrophic cardiomyopathy to chromosome 14q1. N Engl J Med 1989; 321:1372.
74. Geisterfer-Lowrance AA, Kass S, Tanigawa G, et al: A molecular basis for familial hypertrophic cardiomyopathy: A beta-cardiac myosin heavy chain gene missense mutation. Cell 1990; 62:999.
75. Maron BJ, Borow RO, Cannon RO, et al: Hypertrophic cardiomyopathy. Interrelations of clinical manifestations, pathophysiology, and therapy (second of two parts). N Engl J Med 1987; 316:844.
76. Fananapazir L, Cannon RO, Tripodi D, et al: Impact of dual-chamber permanent pacing in patients with obstructive hypertrophic cardiomyopathy with symptoms refractory to verapamil and beta-adrenergic blocker therapy. Circulation 1992; 85:2149.

CHAPTER 67

The Heart in Sepsis

Margaret M. Parker, MD

The changes in cardiovascular function that occur in septic shock have been the subject of intense investigation for more than 40 years. In the mid-1950s, Weil and colleagues reported that intravenous endotoxin given to dogs resulted in hypotension from a decrease in cardiac output, produced primarily by a reduction in venous return.[1] Early studies of humans with septic shock reported a decrease in cardiac output and increased systemic vascular resistance.[2, 3] In 1965, Wilson and coworkers reported that humans with septic shock usually have a hyperdynamic hemodynamic profile, characterized by an increased cardiac output and decreased systemic vascular resistance, in contrast to patients with cardiogenic or hypovolemic shock.[4] This hyperdynamic profile has subsequently been confirmed by many other investigators. During the ensuing decades, research efforts have been directed at further defining the pathophysiology of the cardiovascular changes that occur in septic shock and improving the hemodynamic management of patients with septic shock.

HEMODYNAMIC CHANGES

Clinicians and investigators have long been seeking to identify clinical or hemodynamic parameters that may be useful in determining the prognosis of patients with septic shock. From the earliest clinical studies, it was reported that the ability to maintain a normal or increased cardiac output was associated with a higher survival rate.[2, 5] Several studies, however, have documented that the initial hemodynamic profile does not differ between survivors and nonsurvivors.[6, 7] Baumgartner and associates reported that patients with an extreme hyperdynamic state after fluid resuscitation (cardiac index > 7.0 L/min·m²) had more severe metabolic abnormalities and a poorer prognosis than patients with a more moderate hyperdynamic state (cardiac index 3.5–7.0 L/min·m²).[8]

It is clear that septic shock is most commonly associated with a decrease in peripheral vascular resistance, which results in hypotension despite a normal or increased cardiac index. Most nonsurvivors of septic shock demonstrate persistent vasodilation and hence refractory hypotension.[7, 9] Failure of the peripheral vasculature may be one of the major determinants of mortality in septic shock.[10]

Serial hemodynamic parameters in 48 patients with septic shock were studied by Parker and colleagues to evaluate the relationship between the hemodynamic variables and outcome.[7] Patients were studied on presentation with septic shock and 24 hours later. The hemodynamic variables at both time points, as well as the change during the first 24 hours, were examined for predictive value. Table 67–1 shows the hemodynamic parameters found to be statistically significantly predictive of outcome. On initial presentation, a heart rate of less than 106 beats per minute was found to be predictive of survival. No other initial hemodynamic parameter was associated with outcome. At 24 hours, a heart rate less than 95 beats per minute or a systemic vascular resistance index of greater than 1529 dyne·s/cm⁵·m² was associated with recovery. Looking at the change in hemodynamic parameters during the first 24 hours, a decrease in heart rate of more than 18 beats per minute or a decrease in cardiac index of more than 0.5 L/min·m² predicted a positive outcome. These data indicate that normalization of the hemodynamic abnormalities during the first 24 hours after septic shock is associated with survival.

The significance of the type of organism producing the syndromes of sepsis and septic shock has been debated. Although Kwaan and Weil found that gram-negative organisms produced a different hemodynamic picture from gram-positive organisms,[11] several other investigators have not found any difference in the clinical syndrome or hemodynamic profile produced by various different organisms.[12–14] It is likely that the syndromes of sepsis and septic shock are produced by one or more common pathways of mediators that can be activated by various organisms, perhaps through different mechanisms. A discussion of the mediators producing sepsis is beyond the scope of this chapter.

MYOCARDIAL DEPRESSION

Despite the hemodynamic state found by measuring conventional hemodynamic parameters in patients with septic shock, significant reversible myocardial depression has been demonstrated using radionuclide heart scanning with simultaneous thermodilution hemodynamic studies.[15–20] Figure 67–1 shows the serial mean left ventricular ejection fraction and end-diastolic volume index in survivors and nonsurvivors of septic shock.[19] The survivors have an initially depressed ejection fraction with an increased end-diastolic volume index. These changes return toward normal as a patient recovers from septic shock (normal ejection fraction .50, normal end-diastolic volume index 90 mL/m²). The nonsurvivors have a minimally decreased ejection fraction that is not associated with ventricular dilation. Figure 67–2 shows in schematic form the changes in cardiac function that occur in septic shock.

Further data on ventricular function in septic shock are shown in Table 67–2.[18] The initial and final (within 24 hours of death in nonsurvivors, when hemodynamically stable in the survivors) left and right ventricular ejection fractions and end-diastolic indexes are shown for each group. In the

TABLE 67–1. Prognostic Hemodynamic Parameters in Human Septic Shock

Time	*Parameter*	*Cutoff Value*	*P Value*
Initial study	Heart rate (bpm)	106	<.05
24 h	Heart rate (bpm)	95	<.001
	Systemic vascular resistance Index (dyne·s/cm⁵·m²)	1529	<.01
Change during first 24 h	Heart rate	−18	<.001
	Cardiac index (L/min·m²)	−0.5	<.05

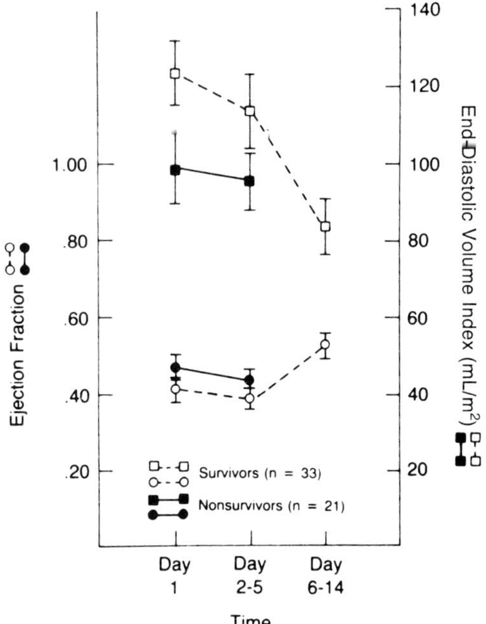

Figure 67–1. Serial mean left ventricular ejection fraction is plotted along the left axis, and end-diastolic volume index along the right axis for 33 survivors *(open symbols)* and 21 nonsurvivors *(closed symbols)* of septic shock. See text for explanation. (From Parker MM, Suffredini AF, Natanson C, et al: Responses of left ventricular function in survivors and nonsurvivors of septic shock. J Crit Care 1989; 4:19–25.)

survivors, both left and right ventricular ejection fractions are initially depressed and increase significantly toward normal with recovery. Both ventricles are initially dilated, decreasing in size toward normal with recovery. The nonsurvivors have a minimum decrease in biventricular ejection fraction and minimum increase in ventricular size, without significant change over time. The reason for the apparent paradoxically more severe myocardial dysfunction in the survivors than in the nonsurvivors is not clear at this time.

It is possible that the ability to develop ventricular dilation may represent a compensatory mechanism by which the survivors can maintain an adequate stroke volume (thereby maintaining cardiac output) despite significant depression of myocardial function and peripheral vascular dilation.[10, 15, 19] The reversible myocardial depression described using radionuclide studies has also been demonstrated echocardiographically in patients with septic shock.[21, 22] Ventricular dilation, however, has not been demonstrated using this technique, possibly because of differences in treatment of the patients or in the techniques used to calculate ventricular volumes. The role of ventricular dilation in the myocardial depression of septic shock requires further investigation.

PATHOGENESIS OF MYOCARDIAL DEPRESSION

Two possible mechanisms by which the myocardial depression of septic shock can be explained have been proposed in the literature, with support for each from animal models. Some investigators have postulated that a global decrease in myocardial blood flow produces diffuse ischemia and hence reversible myocardial depression. Other investigators have provided evidence supporting the theory that a circulating myocardial depressant substance is responsible for the changes in myocardial function observed in septic shock.

Two groups of investigators studied coronary blood flow in humans with septic shock. Cunnion and coworkers placed coronary sinus catheters in seven patients with septic shock and measured coronary sinus blood flow by the thermodilution technique.[23] Figure 67–3 shows the mean coronary sinus blood flow for the seven patients with septic shock compared with normal subjects. The coronary sinus blood flow was normal or increased in the patients with septic shock as compared with the normal subjects, when stratified for heart rate. Figure 67–4 shows the mean arterial and coronary sinus lactate values for each of the seven patients with septic shock. In each case, the arterial lactate level was greater than the coronary sinus lactate level, indicating net myocardial lactate extraction. In a similar study, Dhainaut and associates studied coronary sinus blood flow

ACUTE PHASE OF SEPTIC SHOCK

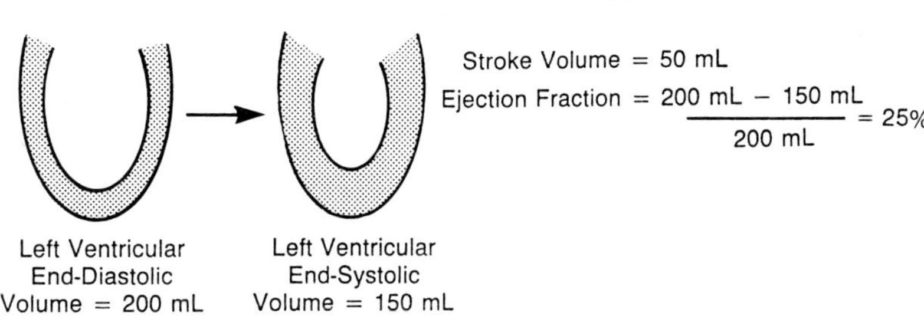

RECOVERY PHASE OF SEPTIC SHOCK

Stroke Volume = 50 mL

Ejection Fraction = $\frac{100 \text{ mL} - 50 \text{ mL}}{100 \text{ mL}}$ = 50%

Left Ventricular End-Diastolic Volume = 100 mL

Left Ventricular End-Systolic Volume = 50 mL

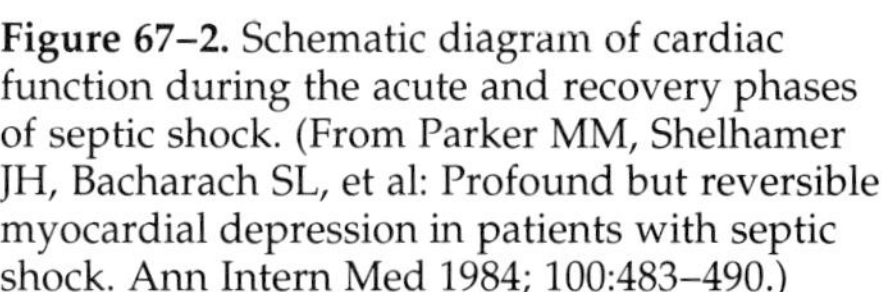

Figure 67–2. Schematic diagram of cardiac function during the acute and recovery phases of septic shock. (From Parker MM, Shelhamer JH, Bacharach SL, et al: Profound but reversible myocardial depression in patients with septic shock. Ann Intern Med 1984; 100:483–490.)

TABLE 67–2. Left and Right Ventricular Function in Septic Shock

	Survivors (n = 22)			*Nonsurvivors (n = 17)*		
Parameters	*Initial*	*Final*	*P**	*Initial*	*Final*	*P*
Left ventricular ejection fraction	.31	.47	.001	.40	.43	NS
Left ventricular end-diastolic volume index (mL/m^2)	145	106	.012	124	102	NS
Right ventricular ejection fraction	.35	.51	.001	.41	.39	NS
Right ventricular end-diastolic volume index (mL/m^2)	124	88	.03	120	114	NS

*Initial compared with final.
NS = not statistically significant

and myocardial metabolism in 40 patients with septic shock and confirmed the normal myocardial blood flow and increased myocardial lactate uptake.[24] These studies do not support the theory that myocardial depression in septic shock is produced by global myocardial ischemia.

Parrillo and colleagues developed an in vitro assay system to look for the presence of a myocardial depressant substance in serum from humans with septic shock.[25] Rat myocardial cells were grown in tissue culture, in which they would beat spontaneously (Fig. 67–5). The Petri dish was placed on a phase-contrast microscope and imaged by a television camera. The myocardial cell contraction was analyzed by a video area detector (Fig. 67–6). When the beating edge of a myocardial cell was placed in the video field, the area of the video field occupied by the cell varied according to the cell's contraction and was printed out as the per cent of the video area occupied by the cell. Figure 67–7 shows some representative examples of the effect that serum from patients with septic shock had on the extent of shortening and velocity of contraction of the myocardial cells in vitro. The assay was used to study serum from five different groups: (1) normal laboratory personnel, (2) patients with a decreased ejection fraction due to structural heart disease, (3) critically ill, nonseptic patients, (4) patients with septic shock in the acute phase, and (5) patients with septic shock after recovery or (in two cases) before the development of septic shock. Figure 67–8 shows the effect that the serum from each of these patient groups had on the extent of myocardial shortening. Serum from the control groups (groups 1–3) did not significantly depress myocardial cell contraction. In contrast, the serum from patients in the acute phase of septic shock produced significant depression of the extent and velocity of myocardial cell contraction in vitro. Serum from these same patients after recovery did not depress in vitro myocardial cell contraction. In a follow-up study, Reilly and associates demonstrated that the presence of the myocardial depressant substance (producing in vitro depression of rat myocardial cells) in serum from patients with septic shock was associated with myocardial dysfunction in vivo.[26] These studies are strongly supportive of the hypothesis that a circulating myocardial depressant substance is responsible for the reversible myocardial depression commonly noted in septic shock.

In addition to the foregoing studies, Silverman and associates studied myocardial responsiveness to catecholamines and found that patients with septic shock demonstrated im-

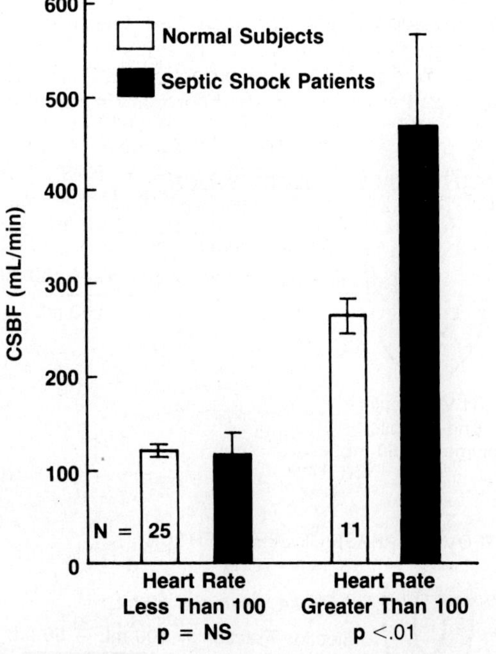

Figure 67–3. Coronary sinus blood flow in 7 patients with septic shock, stratified by heart rate (heart rate less than 100 beats per minute, n=3; heart rate greater than 100 beats per minute, n=4), compared with normal subjects. (From Cunnion RE, Schaer GL, Parker MM, et al: The coronary circulation in human septic shock. Circulation 1986; 73:637–644.)

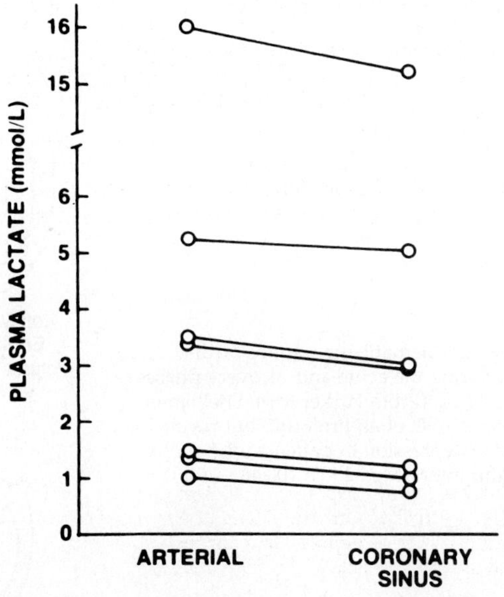

Figure 67–4. Mean arterial lactate and mean coronary sinus lactate concentrations for each of the 7 patients with septic shock discussed in Figure 67–3. (From Cunnion RE, Schaer GL, Parker MM, et al: The coronary circulation in human septic shock. Circulation 1986; 73:637–644.)

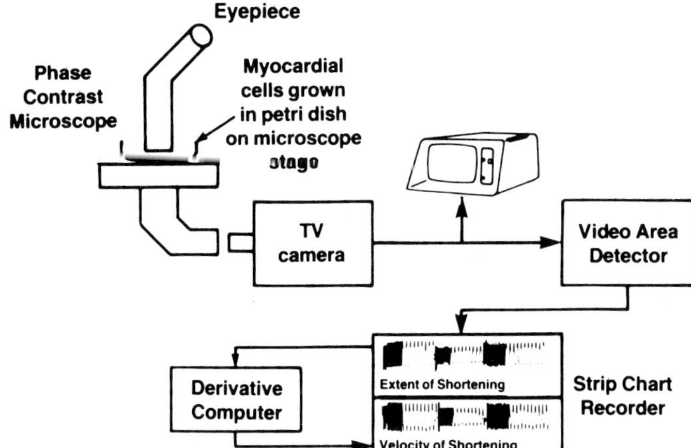

Figure 67–5. A schematic diagram of the myocardial cell contractility assay. See text for explanation. (From Parrillo JE, Burch C, Shelhamer JH, et al: A circulating myocardial depressant substance in humans with septic shock. J Clin Invest 1985; 76:1539–1553.)

paired β-adrenergic receptor stimulation of cyclic adenosine monophosphate, which was associated with decreased myocardial responsiveness to catecholamines.[27] Beta-adrenergic receptor dysfunction may contribute to the myocardial depression noted in septic shock.

MANAGEMENT

The initial treatment of patients with septic shock is fluid resuscitation. Although many studies have addressed the benefits of colloid versus crystalloid fluid resuscitation, clear advantage of one type of fluid over the other has not been demonstrated. The endpoint of fluid resuscitation has also been debated. Packman and Rackow reported hemodynamic data from 15 patients with septic or hypovolemic shock.[28] Figure 67–9 shows the response of left ventricular function as measured by stroke volume index, cardiac index, and left ventricular stroke work index to increases in pulmonary artery wedge pressure generated by fluid resuscitation. Cardiac function improved up to a pulmonary artery wedge pressure of approximately 12 mm Hg, with no further improvement at higher pressures. They suggest that the optimal left heart filling pressure for patients with hypovolemic or septic shock is not greater than 12 mm Hg.

Although volume infusion is widely accepted as the initial step in resuscitation of patients with septic shock, it must be remembered that ventricular performance is not normal and therefore the responses to volume infusion may not be as great as might be expected. Figure 67–10 shows the response in preload (end-diastolic volume index) and cardiac function (left ventricular stroke work index) that occurred in response to volume infusion given to increase the pulmonary artery wedge pressure in three groups of patients studied by Ognibene and colleagues.[29] They gave volume infusions to each of three patient groups: a control group of critically ill, nonseptic patients (n = 14), patients with sepsis without shock (n = 21), and patients with septic shock (n = 21). Before, during, and after volume infusion, conventional hemodynamic studies were performed with simultaneous radionuclide heart scans. From these measurements, the end-diastolic volume index and left ventricular stroke work index were calculated. The control group demonstrated the expected increases in end-diastolic volume index and left ventricular stroke work index. The patients with sepsis with or without shock had a lesser increase (although not statistically significant) in end-diastolic volume index than the control group in response to volume infusion. The patients with septic shock had a minimum increase in left ventricular stroke work index significantly less than that of the control group. This study demonstrated that patients with sepsis have an abnormal response of ventricular performance to volume infusion. The cardiac response to volume infusion was similarly studied by Schneider and coworkers, who demonstrated that some patients with septic shock do not develop an increase in end-diastolic volume or stroke volume index after volume loading.[30] Rackow and associates also used volume infusion to demonstrate depressed left ventricular performance in patients with septic shock.[31] From these studies, it is apparent that close hemodynamic monitoring during fluid resuscitation of patients with septic shock is important for optimal management.

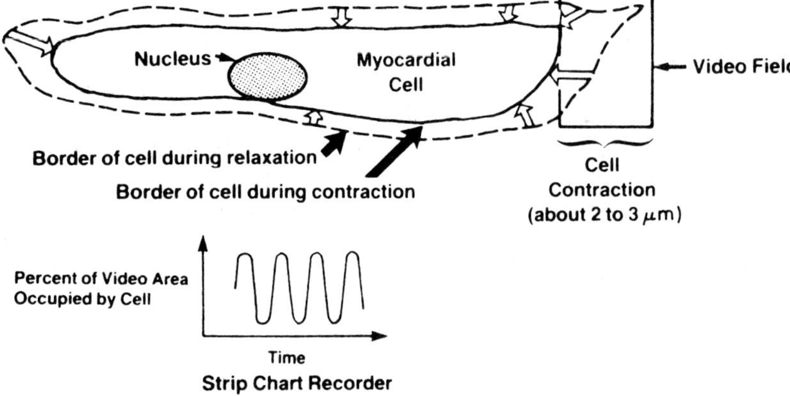

Figure 67–6. A schematic diagram of the variable area method of detecting cell movement. See text for explanation. (From Parrillo JE, Burch C, Shelhamer JH, et al: A circulating myocardial depressant substance in humans with septic shock. J Clin Invest 1985; 76:1539–1553.)

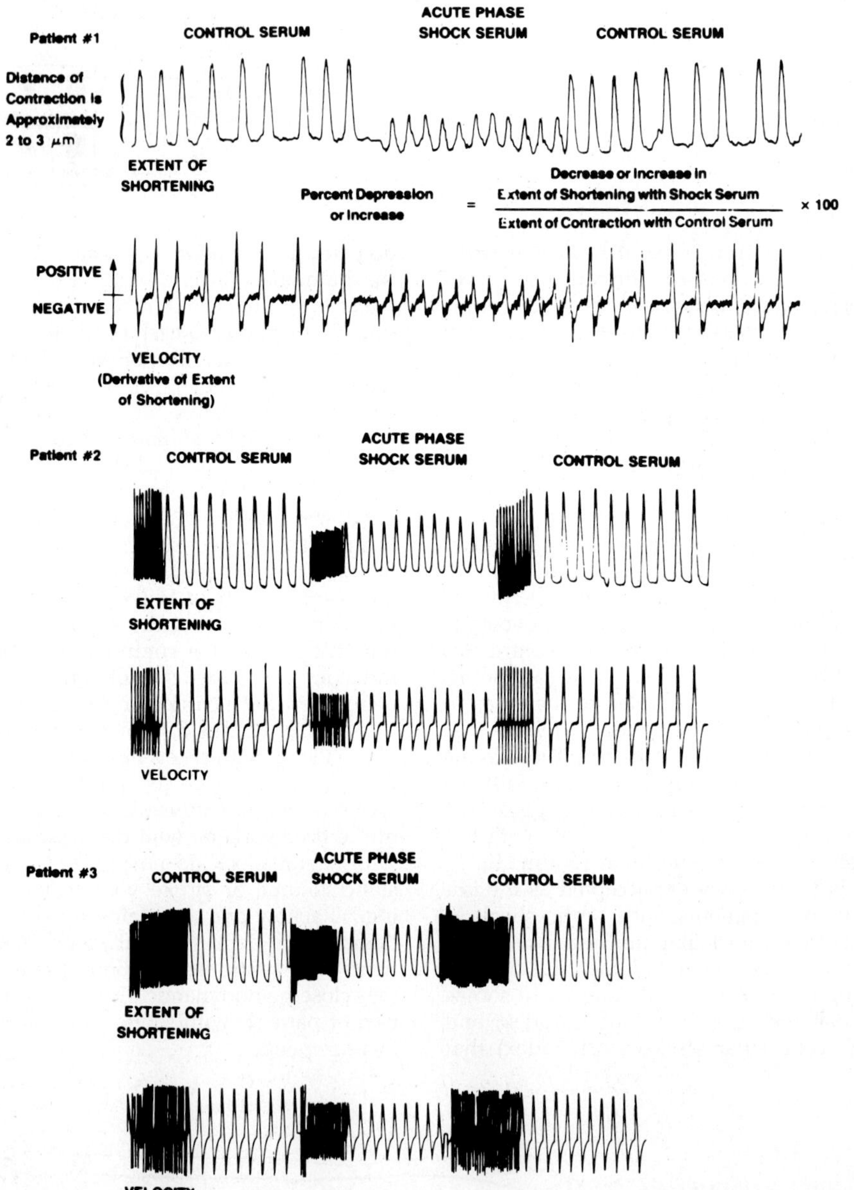

Figure 67–7. Representative samples of the effect of serum from patients with septic shock on the contraction of rat myocardial cells in vitro. (From Parrillo JE, Burch C, Shelhamer JH, et al: A circulating myocardial depressant substance in humans with septic shock. J Clin Invest 1985; 76:1539–1553.)

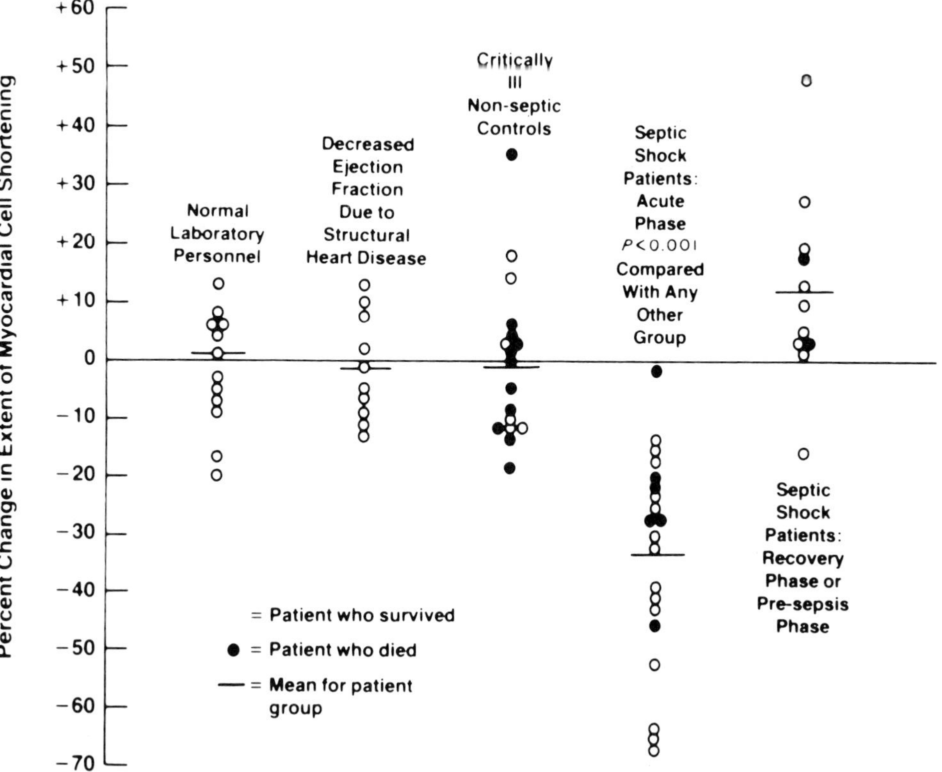

Figure 67–8. The effect of serum from control and septic shock patient groups on the extent of myocardial cell shortening in vitro. (From Parrillo JE, Burch C, Shelhamer JH, et al: A circulating myocardial depressant substance in humans with septic shock. J Clin Invest 1985; 76:1539–1553.)

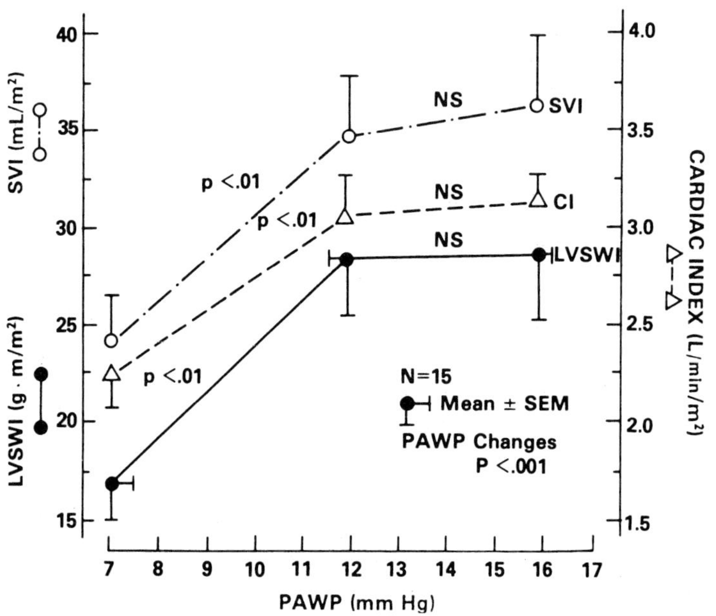

Figure 67–9. Changes in left ventricular stroke work index (LVSWI; *closed circles*), stroke volume index (SVI; *open circles*), and cardiac index *(triangles)* as pulmonary artery wedge pressure (PAWP) is increased during fluid resuscitation. *Abbreviation*: NS = not (statistically) significant. (From Packman MI, Rackow EC: Optimum left heart filling pressure during fluid resuscitation of patients with hypovolemic and septic shock. Crit Care Med 1983; 11:165–169.)

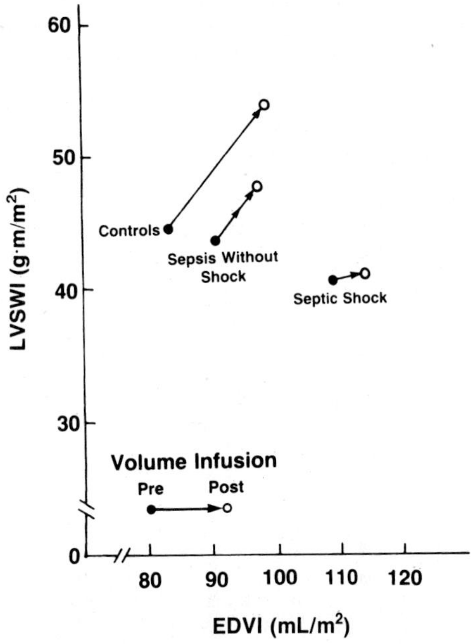

Figure 67–10. End-diastolic volume index (EDVI) versus left ventricular stroke work index (LVSWI) in control patients, patients with sepsis without shock, and patients with septic shock, in response to volume infusion. (From Ognibene FP, Parker MM, Natanson C, et al: Depressed left ventricular performance: Response to volume infusion in patients with sepsis and septic shock. Chest 1988; 93:903–910.)

Many studies have suggested that oxygen consumption is dependent on oxygen delivery in patients with septic shock.[32, 33] Accordingly, many clinicians and investigators have used increases in oxygen delivery or oxygen consumption as therapeutic goals in the management of patients with septic shock. It is not clear, however, that increasing oxygen delivery improves outcome from septic shock. Haupt and colleagues used fluid loading to increase oxygen delivery in 20 patients with septic shock.[34] Eight patients demonstrated an increase in oxygen delivery and in oxygen consumption. These patients had an initially elevated serum lactate level. Six patients had an increase in oxygen delivery without an increase in oxygen consumption. The remaining six patients had a decrease in oxygen delivery (with no change in oxygen consumption) that was attributed to hemodilution. In a similar study, with interventions designed to increase oxygen delivery, patients who received fluid or blood demonstrated an increase in oxygen consumption only if they had an elevated lactate level.[35] Patients who received catecholamines, however, demonstrated an increase in oxygen consumption regardless of the lactate level, suggesting that catecholamines may have a direct effect on oxidative metabolism. Edwards and coworkers treated 29 patients with septic shock using volume expansion followed by dopamine, dobutamine, or norepinephrine to meet predetermined hemodynamic goals.[36] Increases in delivery were associated with increases in oxygen consumption, but the overall survival rate was 52%, similar to that in most series in the literature. Tuchschmidt and associates randomized 25 patients with septic shock to standard management and 26 patients to management designed to meet specific hemodynamic goals.[37] No significant difference in mortality was noted between the two groups. Similar results were obtained in a study by Yu and colleagues.[37a] Thus, although one can clearly increase oxygen delivery and often oxygen consumption, it is not yet clear that therapy designed to meet specific hemodynamic endpoints will improve survival from septic shock. It does appear that patients who are able to reach a high oxygen delivery have a better prognosis.

If fluid resuscitation fails to reverse hypotension and inadequate organ perfusion, then treatment with inotropes or vasopressors must be considered. Dopamine is the most commonly used initial catecholamine.[6, 38] In low doses (1–5 $\mu g \cdot kg^{-1} \cdot min^{-1}$), it has positive inotropic effects as well as effects on the dopaminergic receptors in the kidneys. The latter effect is to improve renal blood flow, with the hope of decreasing the risk of renal failure, which is a common complication of septic shock. At higher doses (10 $\mu g \cdot kg^{-1} \cdot min^{-1}$ or more), dopamine becomes an α-adrenergic agonist and loses its dopaminergic renal effects. The α-adrenergic effects of dopamine may be useful in supporting blood pressure and perhaps organ blood flow in patients with septic shock who have a low systemic vascular resistance.

Dobutamine is a β-adrenergic agent with potent inotropic effects as well as vasodilating effects. The inotropic effects may be beneficial in patients with septic shock because of the myocardial depression that is present, and dobutamine is commonly used for that reason.[39, 40] In patients with high filling pressures or a relatively low cardiac index, dobutamine may be of particular value; however, it must be used with caution to ensure that the vasodilating effects do not worsen hypotension.[40] Dobutamine increases oxygen delivery; this may be of benefit in some patients with sepsis.[40a]

Norepinephrine is a potent vasoconstricting agent that is frequently used in treating patients with septic shock that has not responded to fluid resuscitation and low-dose dopamine. Many clinicians have been reluctant to use norepinephrine because of fear of reducing renal blood flow and precipitating acute renal failure. Renal function in patients who had septic shock and who were receiving norepinephrine was studied by Desjars and by Martin and their groups.[41, 42] Both studies demonstrated that the use of norepinephrine, either alone or in combination with dopamine or dobutamine, did not worsen renal function. The effects of dopamine and norepinephrine on hemodynamics, oxygen metabolism, and right ventricular performance were compared in 10 patients by Schreuder and colleagues.[43] Both drugs increased oxygen consumption, without decreasing right ventricular function. Dopamine increased oxygen delivery, and norepinephrine increased oxygen extraction. No difference in urine output was noted. Fukuoka and associates, however, reported that norepinephrine increased urine flow in patients with normal serum lactate levels but did not improve urine flow and decreased creatinine clearance in patients with elevated serum lactate levels.[44] Schaer and coworkers administered norepinephrine alone and norepinephrine plus low-dose dopamine to normal dogs.[45] The addition of low-dose dopamine to norepinephrine resulted in significantly higher renal blood flow and lower renal vascular resistance. This observation provides a rationale for the use of low-dose dopamine plus norepinephrine for the treatment of patients with septic shock and persistent hypotension related to decreased systemic vascular resistance.

Epinephrine has also been used in the management of septic shock. The hemodynamic effects of epinephrine are to increase heart rate, blood pressure, stroke volume index, cardiac index, and oxygen delivery and consumption, without changing systemic vascular resistance.[46] Some clinicians have reservations about using epinephrine because of the concern about precipitating myocardial ischemia by increasing myocardial oxygen demand. Nonetheless, epinephrine is a potentially useful drug in the treatment of patients with septic shock, especially younger patients.

Patients with septic shock may have highly variable courses and unpredictable responses to therapeutic maneuvers. Although one can set general therapeutic goals of supporting blood pressure, improving oxygen delivery, and improving tissue perfusion, no single management approach can be expected to work most of the time. Each patient must be closely monitored, and if the response to a therapeutic change is not the expected one or if a patient's condition changes, a change in therapeutic interventions should be made. By close monitoring and frequent reassessment, a physician has the greatest chance of a successful outcome in the management of septic shock.

References

1. Weil MH, MacLean LD, Visscher MB, et al: Studies on the circulatory changes in the dog produced by endotoxin from gram-negative micro-organisms. J Clin Invest 1956; 35:1191–1198.
2. Nishijima H, Weil MH, Shubin H, et al: Hemodynamic and metabolic studies on shock associated with gram negative bacteremia. Medicine 1973; 52:287–294.
3. Udhoji VN, Weil MH: Hemodynamic and metabolic studies on shock associated with bacteremia. Ann Intern Med 1965; 62:966–978.
4. Wilson RF, Thal AP, Kindling PH, et al: Hemodynamic measurements in septic shock. Arch Surg 1965; 91:121–129.
5. MacLean LD, Mulligan WG, McLean APH, et al: Patterns of septic shock in a man—a detailed study of 56 patients. Ann Surg 1967; 166:543–562.
6. Winslow EJ, Loeb HS, Rahimtoola SH, et al: Hemodynamic studies and results of therapy in 50 patients with bacteremic shock. Am J Med 1973; 54:421–432.
7. Parker MM, Shelhamer JH, Natanson C, et al: Serial cardiovascular variables in survivors and nonsurvivors of human septic shock: Heart rate as an early predictor of prognosis. Crit Care Med 1987; 15:923–929.
8. Baumgartner JD, Vaney C, Perret C: An extreme form of the hyperdynamic syndrome in septic shock. Intensive Care Med 1984; 10:245–249.
9. Groenveld ABJ, Bronsveld W, Thijs LG: Hemodynamic determinants of mortality in human septic shock. Surgery 1986; 99:140–152.
10. Groenveld ABJ, Nauta JJP, Thijs LJ: Peripheral vascular resistance in septic shock: Its relation to outcome. Intensive Care Med 1988; 14:141–147.
11. Kwaan HM, Weil MH: Differences in the mechanism of shock caused by bacterial infections. Surg Gynecol Obstet 1969; 128:37–45.
12. Wiles JB, Cerra FB, Siegel JH, et al: The systemic septic response: Does the organism matter? Crit Care Med 1980; 8:55–60.
13. Ahmen AJ, Kruse JA, Haupt MT, et al: Hemodynamic responses to gram positive versus gram-negative sepsis in critically ill patients with and without circulatory shock. Crit Care Med 1991; 19:1520–1525.
14. Parker MM, Ognibene FP, Rogers P, et al: Severe *Pneumocystis carinii* pneumonia produces a hyperdynamic profile similar to bacterial pneumonia with sepsis. Crit Care Med 1994; 22:50–54.
15. Parker MM, Shelhamer JH, Bacharach SL, et al: Profound but reversible myocardial depression in patients with septic shock. Ann Intern Med 1984; 100:483–490.
15a. Parker MM, Ognibene FP, Parrillo JE: Peak systolic pressure/end systolic volume index ratio, a load-independent measure of ventricular performance, is reversibly decreased in human septic shock. Crit Care Med 1994 (in press).
16. Ellrodt AG, Riedinger MS, Kimchi A, et al: Left ventricular performance in septic shock: Reversible segmental and global abnormalities. Am Heart J 1985; 110:402–408.
17. Kimchi A, Ellrodt AG, Berman DS, et al: Right ventricular performance in septic shock: A combined radionuclide and hemodynamic study. J Am Coll Cardiol 1984; 4:945–951.
18. Parker MM, McCarthy KE, Ognibene FP, et al: Right ventricular dysfunction and dilatation, similar to left ventricular changes, characterize the cardiac depression of septic shock in humans. Chest 1990; 97:126–131.
19. Parker MM, Suffredini AF, Natanson C, et al: Responses of left ventricular function in survivors and nonsurvivors of septic shock. J Crit Care 1989; 4:19–25.
20. Raper R, Sibbald WJ, Driedger AA, et al. Relative myocardial depression in normotensive sepsis. J Crit Care 1989; 4:9–18.
21. Ozier Y, Gueret P, Jardin F, et al: Two-dimensional echocardiographic demonstration of acute myocardial depression in septic shock. Crit Care Med 1984; 12:596–599.
22. Jardin F, Brun-Ney D, Auvert B, et al: Sepsis-related cardiogenic shock. Crit Care Med 1990; 18:1055–1060.
23. Cunnion RE, Schaer GL, Parker MM, et al: The coronary circulation in human septic shock. Circulation 1986; 73:637–644.
24. Dhainaut JF, Huyghebaert MF, Monsallier JF, et al: Coronary hemodynamics and myocardial metabolism of lactate, free fatty acids, glucose and ketones in patients with septic shock. Circulation 1987; 75:533–541.
25. Parrillo JE, Burch C, Shelhamer JH, et al: A circulating myocardial depressant substance in humans with septic shock. J Clin Invest 1985; 76:1539–1553.
26. Reilly JM, Cunnion RE, Burch-Whitman C, et al: A circulating myocardial depressant substance is associated with cardiac dysfunction and peripheral hypoperfusion (lactic acidemia) in patients with septic shock. Chest 1989; 95:1072–1080.
27. Silverman HJ, Penaranda R, Orens JB, et al: Impaired beta-adrenergic receptor stimulation of cyclic adenosine monophosphate in human septic shock: Association with myocardial hyporesponsiveness to catecholamines. Crit Care Med 1993; 21:31–39.
28. Packman MI, Rackow EC: Optimum left heart filling pressure during fluid resuscitation of patients with hypovolemic and septic shock. Crit Care Med 1983; 11:165–169.
29. Ognibene FP, Parker MM, Natanson C, et al: Depressed left ventricular performance: Response to volume infusion in patients with sepsis and septic shock. Chest 1988; 93:903–910.
30. Schneider AJ, Teule GJJ, Groenveld ABJ: Biventricular performance during volume loading in patients with early septic shock, with emphasis on the right ventricle: A combined hemodynamic and radionuclide study. Am Heart J 1988; 116:103–112.
31. Rackow EC, Kaufman BS, Falk JL, et al: Hemodynamic response to fluid repletion in patients with septic shock: Evidence for early depression of cardiac performance. Circ Shock 1987; 22:11–22.
32. Abraham E, Shoemaker WC, Bland RD, et al: Sequential cardiorespiratory patterns in septic shock. Crit Care Med 1983; 11:799–803.
33. Astiz ME, Rackow EC, Falk JL, et al: Oxygen delivery and consumption in patients with hyperdynamic septic shock. Crit Care Med 1987; 15:26–28.
34. Haupt MT, Gilbert EM, Carlson RW: Fluid loading increases oxygen consumption in septic patients with lactic acidosis. Am Rev Respir Dis 1985; 131:912–916.
35. Gilbert EM, Haupt MT, Madanas RY, et al: The effect of fluid loading, blood transfusion, and catecholamine infusion on oxygen delivery and consumption in patients with sepsis. Am Rev Respir Dis 1986; 134:873–878.
36. Edwards JD, Brown GCS, Nightingale P, et al: Use of survivors' cardiorespiratory values as therapeutic goals in septic shock. Crit Care Med 1989; 17:1089–1103.
37. Tuchschmidt J, Fried J, Astiz M, et al: Elevation of cardiac output and oxygen delivery improves outcome in septic shock. Chest 1992; 102:216–220.
37a. Yu M, Levy MM, Smith P, et al: Effect of maximizing oxygen delivery on morbidity and mortality rates in critically ill patients: A prospective, randomized, controlled study. Crit Care Med 1993; 21:830–838.
38. Wilson RF, Sibbald WJ, Jaanimagi JL: Hemodynamic effects of dopamine in critically ill septic patients. J Surg Res 1976; 20:163–172.
39. Jardin F, Sportiche M, Bazin M, et al: Dobutamine: A hemodynamic evaluation in human septic shock. Crit Care Med 1981; 9:329–332.
40. Vincent JL, Roman A, Kahn RJ: Dobutamine administration in

septic shock: Addition to a standard protocol. Crit Care Med 1990; 18:689–693.

40a. DeBacker D, Berre J, Zhang H, et al: Relationship between oxygen uptake and oxygen delivery in septic patients: Effects of prostacyclin versus dobutamine. Crit Care Med 1993; 21:1658–1664.

41. Desjars P, Pinaud M, Bugnon D, et al: Norepinephrine therapy has no deleterious renal effects in human septic shock. Crit Care Med 1989; 17:426–429.

42. Martin C, Eon B, Saux P, et al: Renal effects of norepinephrine used to treat septic shock patients. Crit Care Med 1990; 18:282–285.

43. Schreuder WO, Schneider AJ, Groenveld ABJ, et al: Effect of dopamine vs. norepinephrine on hemodynamics in septic shock. Chest 1989; 95:1282–1288.

44. Fukuoka T, Nishimura M, Imanaka H, et al: Effects of norepinephrine on renal function in septic patients with normal and elevated serum lactate levels. Crit Care Med 1989; 17:1104–1107.

45. Schaer GL, Fink MP, Parrillo JE: Norepinephrine alone versus norepinephrine plus low-dose dopamine: Enhanced renal blood flow with combination pressor therapy. Crit Care Med 1985; 13:492–496.

46. Moran JL, O'Fathartaigh MS, Peisach AR, et al: Epinephrine as an inotropic agent in septic shock: A dose-profile analysis. Crit Care Med 1993; 21:70–77.

CHAPTER 68

Postoperative Care of the Adult Cardiac Surgical Patient

Paul Corso, MD, FACS, FACC • Christopher Eager, MD

As a subset of surgical patients, few are potentially more critically ill than the more than 300,000 patients undergoing cardiac surgery using cardiopulmonary bypass (CPB) annually in the United States. Because of preoperative organ system dysfunction, intraoperative invasive monitoring, obligate transient myocardial ischemia with aortic cross-clamping, and the systemic effects of CPB, all such patients require critical care in the early postoperative period by physicians and nurses skilled in the management of every major organ system. It has therefore become customary to address care of cárdiac surgical patients system by system, remaining ever cognizant of issues involving the interface of these systems.

TRANSPORT AND INITIAL ASSESSMENT

When leaving the operating room for transport to the intensive care unit (ICU), cardiac surgical patients in their most fragile state must pass through a brief period when patient monitoring and control are at a minimum (see also Chapter 11). Transport is usually accomplished with a portable monitor displaying at least an electrocardiogram (ECG) tracing and arterial pressure waveform. Central pressures and arterial saturation may be included on more sophisticated modules. A kit including drugs commonly used for resuscitation, volume for intravenous infusion, a temporary pulse generator for pacing, and a defibrillator must accompany a patient. Despite these precautions, resuscitation of a moving patient in a hallway is inefficient at best.

Problems frequently encountered during transport include (1) hypotension due to cardiac dysfunction, volume shifts from patient movement, or vasomotor instability moderated by rewarming after systemic hypothermia; (2) hypertension secondary to sympathetic stimulation of movement or anesthetic emergence, which may result in anastamotic bleeding; (3) any of the atrial or ventricular arrhythmias encountered in the postoperative period; (4) accidental extubation; or (5) or accidental decannulation of arterial or venous catheters.

For these reasons, transfer of patients from the operating room table to stretcher to bed should be accomplished with extreme care and only after a period of hemodynamic stability, and transport should be as rapid as possible to an ICU that is optimally located adjacent to the operating room.

On arrival in the ICU, ECG leads from the bedside monitor should first be attached to the patient. If rhythm and blood pressure (BP) remain stable, the arterial pressure transducer should then be transferred from portable to bedside monitor and manual ventilation replaced by a bedside volume-cycled ventilator. After this, central venous, pulmonary artery, or atrial catheters should be transduced. Hypotension during this period should be treated first with volume expansion. If a response is not immediate or hypotension is severe (<70 mm Hg systolic), atrial pacing should be initiated at a rate of 90 to 100 if the intrinsic rate is substantially less than this. Simultaneous administration of 500 mg of calcium chloride or 50 mEq (1 ampule) of sodium bicarbonate or both if metabolic acidosis is suspected often transiently elevates arterial pressure, allowing time for more definitive hemodynamic assessment. Consideration should also be given to initiating or increasing an infusion of an inotropic agent. Breath sounds should be auscultated because hypoxia or hypoventilation during transport with resultant respiratory acidosis can result in hemodynamic instability. Mediastinal tube drainage should be checked, because mediastinal bleeding during the period of transport occasionally is massive enough to cause unexpected hypotension.

When heart rate and rhythm and BP are within desired norms, postoperative blood work, an ECG, and a portable chest radiograph can be obtained while the physician in charge of the patient's ICU management obtains a brief but pertinent verbal account from the anesthesiologist or surgeon. Included should be a report of the patient's preoperative history, intraoperative course, and current hemodynamic state, including use of any antiarrhythmic, inotropic, or vasoactive medications. This verbal transfer of patient information is essential for continuity of care in these complex cases. After this, a secondary survey of the patient should be undertaken, paying attention to the details of planned management of each organ system.

ANTICIPATED POSTOPERATIVE COURSE

The critical period in the postoperative recovery of most cardiac surgical patients is the first 24 hours. During this period, cardiovascular stability should re-establish itself, allowing for withdrawal or lowering of doses of inotropic support. Anesthetic emergence should permit extubation, and mediastinal bleeding should have ceased. On the first postoperative day, oral medications for preexisting conditions such as hypertension can be resumed, and most patients can be transferred to the surgical ward. However, it should be noted that the patient population undergoing cardiac procedures is changing. Age at operation, severity of coronary artery disease, and frequency of other organ system dysfunction all are increasing at a time when the incidence of more complex procedures such as reoperations and combined coronary artery bypass graft (CABG)–valve replacement is rising. Such patients often require prolonged cardiopulmonary support.

Recovery in the early postoperative period after cardiac surgery is dictated by those features of the operation unique to cardiac surgery: the use of prolonged high-dose narcotic anesthesia, CPB with systemic hypothermia, and aortic cross-clamping with attendant global myocardial ischemia. CPB produces a diffuse capillary leak leading to accumulation of water in the extravascular, extracellular space. The magnitude and duration of the capillary leak are directly proportional to the duration of CPB and may continue for 24 hours or more. Because patients are total-body water and salt overloaded after CPB, postoperative intravenous fluid administration is usually set at a rate substantially less than maintainance requirements. However undesirable, bolus administration of volume for plasma expansion is frequently necessary to maintain plasma volume and filling pressures, particularly in the first several hours after CPB, as capillary leak continues and rewarming from systemic hypothermia produces vasodilatation. When rewarming is complete and the capillary leak has ceased, further volume resuscitation is unnecessary, and diuresis occurs or may be stimulated. The physician caring for the patient should thus be aware of the total time of CPB as an indicator of potential need for postoperative volume expansion.

Various degrees of systemic hypothermia are used during CPB to reduce the metabolic demands of the heart and other organs and therefore protect them during the period of myocardial ischemia with aortic cross-clamping or during complete circulatory arrest. Systemic cooling is accomplished by a heat exchanger until rectal temperatures reach 28 to 32°C for routine CABG and valve replacement surgery. Cooling to a rectal temperature of 15°C may be used for complete circulatory arrest. Systemic rewarming to at least 35°C rectally is usually accomplished before separation from CPB. During chest closure and transport to the ICU, reperfusion of opening peripheral vascular beds redistributes core heat, and core temperature again declines. Patients arriving in the ICU frequently have rectal temperatures of 34 to 36°C. Residual hypothermia (1) mandates volume administration as a patient rewarms and vasodilates, sometimes precipitously; (2) increases myocardial oxygen (O_2) demand in the recovering postischemic heart by peripheral vasoconstriction, which increases systemic vascular resistance (SVR) (afterload); (3) induces shivering, which increases carbon dioxide (CO_2) production and places an unwanted metabolic demand on the recovering heart for O_2 delivery to skeletal muscle; (4) impairs coagulation; and (5) lowers the threshold for arrhythmia generation and propagation. For these reasons, attention should always be paid to patients' temperature and rate of rewarming. More profound hypothermia is treated with surface warming by overhead lamp or a heating blanket. Vasodilation with a fall in central filling pressures should be treated with volume expansion. Patients with impaired myocardial function, elevated SVR and an adequate BP should be administered an intravenous nitroprusside drip starting at 1 $\mu g \cdot kg^{-1} \cdot min^{-1}$ or less and titrated upward as needed as long as mean arterial pressure (MAP) remains greater than 70 mm Hg. Shivering may be treated with intravenous midazolam, diazepam, or meperidine. If these are ineffective, paralysis may be induced with a bolus of pancuronium followed by a constant intravenous infusion. Mediastinal bleeding exacerbated by hypothermia is treated with factor replacement as indicated by coagulation profiles and by aggressive rewarming. Arrhythmias are treated as outlined later in this chapter.

Aortic cross-clamping with global myocardial ischemia for various periods results in generalized myocardial depression in the early postoperative period. The length of cross-clamp time, of particular significance in patients with poor ventricular function, should always be noted. Myocardial depression typically worsens gradually during the first 6 to 12 hours after the ischemic period as the reperfusion injury progresses. The nadir of heart muscle function is then reached. Inotropic support may need to be added or increased during this period as dictated by the cardiac index. Thereafter, myocardial muscle function begins to recover, returning to preoperative baseline at 24 to 48 hours, assuming no permanent intraoperative injury. If increased or added inotropic support is necessary after the first 12 hours, ongoing ischemia, postoperative infarction, or other causes should be considered.

The use of high-dose narcotic anesthesia is principally limited to cardiac surgery. This technique ensures smooth induction and maintenance of anesthesia and minimizes myocardial depression and arrhythmias. However, variability of individual narcotic metabolic degradation rates and the need for a period of observation to ensure adequate hemodynamic performance in cardiac surgical patients usually preclude extubation on the day of operation. As anesthetic emergence progresses, patients are weaned from ventilator support in the intermittent mandatory ventilation mode if cardiac function is adequate, and extubation is accomplished on the first postoperative day. Exceptions may be made in younger, healthier patients with good myocardial function, leading to extubation in the first few hours after operation.

CARDIOVASCULAR SYSTEM

Low Cardiac Output Syndrome

The treatment of low cardiac output after cardiac surgery is central to the postoperative care of these patients. The object of treatment is to increase cardiac output to levels adequate for tissue perfusion while increasing myocardial O_2 consumption ($M\dot{V}O_2$) as little as possible. Interventions are always instituted with cost to heart muscle in mind.

Low cardiac output is defined as a cardiac index of less than 2.0 $L/min \cdot m^2$ with a normal left atrial pressure (<15 mm Hg) and heart rate (60–100 beats per minute). A cardiac index of 2.0 to 2.5 $L/min \cdot m^2$ is considered marginal and frequently indicates a need for intervention. The causes of low cardiac output are listed in Table 68–1 and include abnormalities of the four determinants of cardiac output, including preload, afterload, contractility, and heart rate and rhythm. Treatment of low cardiac output is always urgent and, if accompanied by hypotension, becomes emergent.

Surgically remediable causes of low cardiac output syndrome should always be considered when evaluating a patient's hemodynamic status. Hypovolemia from rapid mediastinal bleeding must be treated by reoperation. Tamponade should be suspected in the early postoperative period when significant mediastinal bleeding suddenly ceases. An increasing need for and declining response to inotropic support may represent development of tamponade. The measurable hallmark of tamponade, equalization of right and left heart pressures (central venous pressure equal to left atrial pressure) is often absent in postoperative tamponade secondary to mediastinal thrombus. If the diagnosis is uncertain and time permits, a bedside echocardiogram is 90% accurate, especially if a transesophageal method is used.[1] Tension pneumothorax is a rare cause of low cardiac output syndrome because lung injury during surgery producing an air leak is uncommon and air in a surgically

TABLE 68–1. Causes of Low Cardiac Output

Decreased Preload
- Hypovolemia
- PEEP
- Tamponade
- Tension pneumothorax

Increased Afterload
- Vasoconstriction
  - Hypothermia
  - Sympathetic stimulation (i.e., pain, anesthetic emergence)
  - Essential hypertension
  - Administration of alpha agonists
- Known uncorrected LV outflow tract obstruction

Reduced Contractility
- Impaired preoperative LV function
- Functional postoperative myocardial depression
- Myocardial edema, ischemia, or infarction
  - Poor intraoperative myocardial protection
  - Incomplete revascularization
  - Spasm
  - Stunning
  - Uncorrected valve lesions
- Metabolic abnormalities
  - Hypoxia
  - Acidosis
  - Hypocalcemia
- Pharmacologic
  - Anesthetic agents
  - Antiarrhythmics
  - Calcium channel blockade
  - β-Blockade
  - Protamine

Arrhythmias

entered pleural space is usually evacuated by mediastinal and pleural tubes. Maintenance of positive end-expiratory pressure (PEEP) at levels normally used in the postoperative period (5 cm H_2O) should not affect cardiac output, but with increasing levels of PEEP to correct hypoxia, cardiac output may decline, particularly with coexistent hypovolemia.

Low cardiac output due to increased afterload has surgical implications only in those rare patients with known uncorrected left ventricular (LV) outflow tract obstruction or malpositioned prosthetic aortic valves. Otherwise, increased afterload is a result of vasoconstriction, and treatment is thermal or pharmacologic. Hypothermia is treated with heating blankets and overhead lamps and judicious use of intravenous nitroprusside until rewarming is effected. Intravenous nitroprusside is also the treatment of choice in patients with essential hypertension until oral intake is resumed, at which time captopril or enalapril is started. Sympathetic stimulation due to anesthetic emergence may be poorly tolerated in the early postoperative period by patients with poor preoperative myocardial reserve or significant intraoperative muscle injury. Falling cardiac output in this setting should prompt administration of analgesics and sedation and sometimes mandates reparalysis.

Low cardiac output secondary to serious atrial or ventricular arrhythmias requires appropriate treatment as outlined later.

Most ominous is low cardiac output syndrome due to reduced myocardial contractility. Some causes of impaired contractility are amenable to simple interventions, such as metabolic abnormalities including hypoxemia, acidosis, and hypocalcemia. Native coronary artery or graft spasm is diagnosed by ECG and treated by intravenous nitroglycerin (10–200 μg/min) or sublingual nifedipine until ST segment changes revert to normal. Other causes imply a surgical solution such as an uncorrected valve lesion or ongoing ischemia secondary to incomplete revascularization. The latter occasionally prompts reoperation in the early postoperative period, but a valve lesion is most frequently left uncorrected intentionally when a longer period of operative ischemic arrest is believed to be dangerous. Reduced contractility producing low cardiac output syndrome most frequently is not amenable to direct intervention. Recovery is a function of time, and treatment in the form of inotropic agents is supportive. The etiology in such cases includes poor preoperative left ventricular function, functional postoperative myocardial depression, poor intraoperative myocardial protection and stunning, and persisting effects of various pharmacologic agents including anesthetics and preoperatively prescribed β-blockers or calcium channel blockers.

Treatment

The treatment of low cardiac output syndrome should be approached in a systematic fashion.

The first step is to preclude tamponade, tension pneumothorax, or PEEP as causes of low cardiac output. The second step is to optimize preload by correcting hypovolemia (pulmonary capillary wedge pressure [PCWP] <15) with crystalloid (lactated Ringer's solution or normal saline) or colloids such as 5% albumin or hetastarch, assuming an acceptable hematocrit (usually $>26\%$) and negligable bleeding. If the hematocrit is low or mediastinal hemorrhage is substantial, blood should be used for volume expansion. With active bleeding, whole blood with its coagulation factors is preferred but rarely available. Packed red blood cells are acceptable. In many institutions, shed mediastinal blood is now routinely collected postoperatively for filtered reinfusion and should be used first, keeping in mind that it is devoid of coagulation factors and may exacerbate bleeding by hemodilution or residual heparin activity. Volume expansion is most prolonged after blood administration, whereas only 20% of acutely infused crystalloid remains in the vascular compartment 90 minutes after administration. Five per cent albumin expands blood volume twice as long as salt solutions and may be the volume expander of choice.

The third step is to optimize heart rate and rhythm simultaneously. A sinus rate of approximately 90 is optimal in the early postoperative period and can be achieved by atrial pacing using the temporary atrial epicardial pacing wires placed at surgery and a portable temporary pulse generator. If atrioventricular (AV) nodal block is present, AV sequential pacing is initiated using the temporary ventricular pacing wires as well as the atrial wires. Ventricular pacing may be used if the atrial wires fail to capture, but it is less desirable because the loss of AV synchrony may reduce cardiac output as much as 25%. Atrial and ventricular arrhythmias that are affecting cardiac output should be treated as outlined later.

Afterload should then be reduced if calculated SVR is elevated. To the limits of systemic BP tolerance (MAP >70 mm Hg), SVR should be reduced to the low normal range (approximately 800 $dyne \cdot s/cm^5 \cdot m^2$). If the patient is hypertensive, this is accomplished with intravenous nitroprusside drip at 1 to 10 $\mu g \cdot kg^{-1} \cdot min^{-1}$. If hypothermia is present, rewarming with heating lamps and blankets may accompany nitroprusside administration. Sympathetic stimulation from anesthetic emergence is treated with analgesia and sedation or paralysis if the former is ineffective.

If cardiac output fails to respond to manipulations of preload, heart rate and rhythm, and afterload, myocardial contractility must then be enhanced with inotropic support, bearing in mind that improvement in contractile function is accompanied by increased $M\dot{V}O_2$.

The choice of inotrope used depends on the specific hemodynamic situation, local practice pattern, and personal preference. These agents are frequently used in combination, and variation in individual response is substantial.

Dopamine

Dopamine, a naturally occurring catecholamine, used in dosages of 1 to 20 $\mu g \cdot kg^{-1} \cdot min^{-1}$, is a frequent first choice as an inotrope postoperatively.[2] At doses less than 3 $\mu g \cdot kg^{-1} \cdot min^{-1}$, stimulation of dopaminergic receptors produces renal and splanchnic vasodilatation, increasing renal blood flow and glomerular filtration rate. Between 3 and 8 $\mu g \cdot kg^{-1} \cdot min^{-1}$, stimulation of β_1 receptors produces both an inotropic effect and a reduction in SVR. Above 7 $\mu g \cdot kg^{-1} \cdot min^{-1}$, α-adrenergic stimulation causes pulmonary and systemic vasoconstriction with increases in systemic and pulmonary artery pressures. Dopamine is most useful in low doses to increase renal perfusion and in moderate doses as an inotrope of first choice when a more potent agent is not indicated. It should not be used in patients with pulmonary hypertension because of its effect on pulmonary vascular resistance, and its use at any dose may be limited by its propensity to cause atrial tachyarrhythmias.

Dobutamine

Dobutamine is a synthetic catecholamine used in dosages of 1 to 20 $\mu g \cdot kg^{-1} \cdot min$. As a β_1-receptor stimulant, it has both inotropic and variable chronotropic effects. Also a β_2 agonist, it reduces SVR and as such is most useful in patients with mildly reduced cardiac output associated with an elevated SVR. Like dopamine, its use may be limited by atrial tachyarrhythmias.

Epinephrine

Epinephrine, the prototype catecholamine, is both an α and β receptor agonist. At dosages less than 2 $\mu g/min$, increased cardiac output and heart rate are accompanied by a reduction in SVR from its β_2 effects. At higher doses, β_1 effects predominate with a dose-dependent increase in cardiac output, systolic BP, and heart rate. At maximal doses, α-agonist properties produce marked vasoconstriction. Epinephrine is used in patients with marked impairment of ventricular contractility but at the expense of atrial and ventricular tachyarrhythmias, marked increase in $M\dot{V}O_2$, decreased renal blood flow and oliguria, and metabolic acidosis due to peripheral vasoconstriction. If any of these adverse effects becomes difficult to manage, every effort should be made to reduce the administered dose. Epinephrine is usually started in low doses as additive therapy after an inadequate response to dopamine, dobutamine, or amrinone.

Isoproterenol

Isoproterenol is a synthetic congener of epinephrine used in dosages of 0.5 to 10 $\mu g/min$. Although it is both a β_1 and β_2 agonist, augmentation of cardiac output is primarily mediated by a profound increase in heart rate (without change in stroke volume) because of pulmonary and peripheral vasodilation.[3] It is infrequently used in patients with coronary artery disease because of markedly increased $M\dot{V}O_2$ secondary to tachycardia. Isoproterenol is used clinically in right heart failure, in pulmonary hypertension, or as a temporizing measure to increase heart rate in hemodynamically significant bradycardias.

Norepinephrine

Norepinephrine is a catecholamine with both alpha and beta agonist effects used in dosages of 1 to 12 $\mu g/min$. Although at doses of 2 $\mu g/min$ it is a beta$_1$ agonist with little effect on SVR, it is used almost exclusively for its potent effect at higher doses when postoperative hypotension is mediated by a low SVR. It can be used as an inotrope in combination with nitroprusside, phentolamine, or nitroglycerin to ablate its alpha properties at higher doses.

Amrinone

The prototype of a new class of inotropic agents,[4] amrinone used in dosages of 5 to 10 $\mu g \cdot kg^{-1} \cdot min^{-1}$ after a bolus dose of 0.75 $\mu g/kg$ acts by inhibiting intracellular enzymatic degradation of cyclic adenosine monophosphate. If this agent has primary beta$_1$ agonist properties, they are modest at best.[5] Observed improvement in right and left heart function is likely due largely to afterload reduction (marked reduction in SVR and peripheral vascular resistance) unaccompanied by compensatory tachycardia. Because its use alone may cause severe hypotension, simultaneous use of agents with alpha agonist properties such as phenylephrine hydrochloride, norepinephrine, or epinephrine may be necessary. In contrast to other inotropes, it has a long half-life (3.6 h), and patients must be observed for hemodynamic deterioration occurring late after infusion is discontinued. Amrinone-induced thrombocytopenia is common and may prompt platelet transfusion or withdrawal of its use.

Calcium

Intravenous bolus administration of calcium can be used in urgent situations as a short-acting inotrope. Its effect is directly proportional to the degree of hypocalcemia. Hypocalcemia in the early postoperative period may be caused by CPB itself or by chelating agents in transfused blood. In addition, myocardial depression caused by calcium channel blockers may be overcome by intravenously administered calcium.

Inotrope Combinations

Although how an individual patient responds to any given agent or combination of agents cannot be predicted, a strategy for use of drugs is usually based on pharmacologic properties of individual agents and analysis of a patient's hemodynamic state.

Dopamine is thus frequently used initially after termination of CPB for its chronotropic as well as inotropic effects in patients with bradycardia and hypotension associated with reduced cardiac output. If tachycardia intervenes, SVR remains high despite rewarming, and cardiac index is still marginal, dobutamine is often added for afterload reduction as well as inotropic effect and dopamine is reduced to 2 to 3 $\mu g \cdot kg^{-1} \cdot min^{-1}$ to moderate the tachycardia while taking advantage of its salutary effect on renal blood flow.[6] If the addition of dobutamine does not produce the desired response, epinephrine is then added in low to moderate doses for its beta$_1$ inotropic effects while maintaining afterload reduction with dobutamine and renal blood flow with dopamine.

Another popular and rational combination for patients with more serious impairment of contractile function (particularly in the setting of right heart failure) is amrinone and epinephrine, the former used for its afterload reduction in both systemic and pulmonary vascular beds and the latter at low to moderate doses contributing its potent direct beta$_1$ inotropic effects.

Mechanical Support

When manipulation of preload, afterload, heart rate, and contractility fails to produce a stable hemodynamic state, intra- or postoperative addition of temporary mechanical support for the failing heart must be considered. Options currently available are the intra-aortic balloon pump (IABP) and various types of ventricular assist devices (VADs).[7] In clinical investigational use is the Hemopump.

Intra-Aortic Balloon Pump

In clinical use since 1969, the IABP (see Chapter 60) is a helium-filled balloon positioned in the descending thoracic aorta and attached to a bedside console that inflates and deflates the balloon with helium in synchrony with LV contraction. Formerly inserted by direct surgical exposure of the femoral artery, it is now almost always introduced into the common femoral artery through a sheath placed percutaneously using the Seldinger technique. Rarely, when severe iliofemoral atherosclerosis prohibits transfemoral insertion, it is positioned antegrade intraoperatively via the ascending aorta. Removal then requires reopening the sternotomy.

By inflation in diastole, the balloon augments MAP and thus also increases coronary blood flow. By rapid deflation just before systole, it increases cardiac output by reducing LV afterload.

It is indicated preoperatively for ischemic chest pain unresponsive to maximum medical therapy or cardiovascular collapse, most frequently after invasive coronary instrumentation. Intraoperatively, weaning from CPB is sometimes not possible without IABP assistance. Postoperatively, IABP insertion is indicated when low cardiac output syndrome fails to respond to maximum inotropic support, usually in the first 24 hours after surgery.

Complications of IABP use include aortic dissection or rupture; periaortic hematoma; distal atherosclerotic embolization to kidneys, viscera, or lower extremities; iliofemoral thrombosis with distal ischemia; focal ischemic neurologic compromise or paraplegia; thrombocytopenia secondary to mechanical trauma; false aneurysms of the femoral arteries; and so forth. For these reasons, intravenous heparin or dextran is used if the device remains in place for more than 2 days. Pedal pulses should be checked frequently and platelet counts obtained at least daily. The IABP should be weaned and removed as soon as hemodynamic stability permits.

Ventricular Assist Devices

If separation from CPB is still not possible despite maximum pharmacologic support and an IABP, the failing ventricle(s) may benefit from a period of total rest by use of a VAD (see Chapter 61).

A VAD is a generic term for an externally situated and driven pump that assumes the function of either ventricles or both. Cannulas positioned in the left atrium and ascending aorta or right atrium and pulmonary artery divert blood flow from and therefore "unload," respectively, the LV and right ventricle. Most commonly used as VADs are the same pump heads used for CPB, including the Biomedicus centrifugal pump or a simple roller pump. The Pierce-Donachy/Thoratec pulsatile device is available in some centers.[8]

After initial control of postoperative bleeding, patients must be heparinized to an activated clotting time of 150% of normal at full flow rates, reduced flow requiring higher levels of anticoagulation. Complete ventricular bypass is maintained for at least 48 hours, after which time pump flow is reduced to 500 mL/m^2 as hemodynamics permit over a period of at least 24 hours. Patients are then returned to the operating room for cannula removal. Although 50% of patients can be weaned from VADs, only half of these survive to hospital discharge.

Hemopump

The Hemopump is a new left VAD undergoing phase II clinical trials.[9] It consists of a small, cable-mounted, continuous axial flow pump driven at up to 46,000 rpm by an external electromechanical drive unit. It is inserted either via the ascending aorta at sternotomy or transfemorally; blood is drawn through an inflow port positioned in the LV apex and ejected from the pump itself positioned in the ascending aorta. Capable of flows of 5 L/min, it permits nearly complete unloading of the LV. As such, it can be used intraoperatively for coronary artery surgery without use of an oxygenator or perioperatively as a VAD.

Weaning of Pharmacologic and Mechanical Ventricular Assistance

As ischemic or stunned areas of myocardium recover function in the hours and days after operation, weaning of the various supportive modalities can begin, starting with devices or agents with the most potential adverse effects.

Thought should first be given to removing mechanical assist devices. A VAD should be surgically removed as soon as possible. An IABP should next be removed after weaning by reducing the frequency of augmented beat from 1:1 to 1:2 or 1:3. Concomitant weaning of inotropic support from maximum levels should optimally be in progress before device removal, so that subsequent unanticipated reduction in ventricular function can be managed by increased pharmacologic support.

Weaning of inotropes should begin with agents used at doses at which alpha agonist properties predominate. The vasoconstriction produced by high doses of epinephrine, norepinephrine, and dopamine maintains coronary and cerebral perfusion pressure at the expense of poor splanchnic and peripheral perfusion. The resulting ischemia in these vascular beds may lead to visceral infarction, renal failure, and lactic acidosis, which are difficult to control. When inotropes are reduced to doses at which primarily beta agonist activity remains, the most potent, usually epinephrine, is weaned first, followed by dobutamine and dopamine. Infusion of the latter is often maintained at 2 to 3 $\mu g \cdot kg^{-1} \cdot min^{-1}$ to facilitate continuous diuresis until management is possible with intermittent bolus diuretics.

Hypotension and Hypertension

The arterial BP necessary to maintain end-organ homeostasis in adults varies from individual to individual. In some adults, an MAP as low as 50 is sufficient, whereas an MAP of 60 or greater is generally necessary in patients with atherosclerotic cardiovascular disease. An MAP of 70 or greater is necessary to maintain adequate flow through an internal mammary artery graft through which flow is highly pressure dependent. For these reasons, hypotension in cardiac surgical patients is prudently defined as an MAP of less than 70 mm Hg.

Hypertension is not as well defined. Especially patients who have undergone cardiac surgery, incremental increases in BP above the minimum required for adequate organ perfusion are detrimental, incrementally increasing afterload and $M\dot{V}O_2$ and decreasing cardiac output. Secondarily, bleeding from exposed mediastinal surfaces and suture lines is exacerbated as arterial pressure rises.

Hypotension

Postoperative hypotension is frequently but erroneously equated with a low cardiac output. The latter may or may not be causally related to the former.

When hypotension is a result of low cardiac output, it may be due to decreased preload, reduced contractility, or arrhythmia (see Table 68–1). Treatment is dictated by the measures necessary to increase cardiac output (discussed earlier). Reduced preload secondary to hypovolemia is by far the most common cause of hypotension in the early postoperative period until patients are fully rewarmed with all vascular beds open. Thus, acute hypotension of uncertain cause in this period is first treated by volume administration without raising pulmonary artery diasotic pressure or PCWP above ~ 20 mm Hg. A rise in systemic pressure may or may not be diagnostic but usually affords the physician time for definitive etiologic assessment.

Hypotension may occur with a normal or elevated cardiac output when it is the result of reduced afterload (i.e., vasodilatation). Preload, contractility, and heart rate are adequate to maintain cardiac output, but the patient is hypovolemic relative to systemic capacitance. Postoperatively, this phenomenon may occur with rapid systemic rewarming; hyperthermia, which frequently occurs after CPB owing to transient impairment of hypothalamic thermoregulation; administration of $beta_2$ agonist agents such as nitroprusside and nitroglycerin; and spinal denervation following aortic surgery. Sepsis, unusual in the early postoperative period, must be considered as a possible cause. Hemodilution (hematocrit <22) may reduce afterload substantially secondary to decreased viscosity and responds rapidly to packed red blood cell transfusion. Otherwise, treatment of hypotension includes additional volume administration and intravenous infusion of alpha agonist agents such as phenylephrine hydrochloride or norepinephrine at 1 to 12 μg/min.

Hypertension

The incidence of hypertension after adult cardiac surgery varies with the definition used. Episodic hypertensive periods precipitated by anesthetic emergence, with pain shivering, hypoxia, or hypercarbia, are catecholamine mediated and occur in most patients in the first 24 hours after operation. Sustained hypertension with an MAP of greater than 120 or systolic BP greater than 160 occurs in previously hypertensive patients with good ventricular function but may be noted with significant hypothermia, a hyperdynamic LV, or combined procedures including carotid endarterectomy. Whether episodic or sustained, however, treatment is indicated to reduce the work of the recovering heart.

Thus in the 12- to 24-hour period usually required for cessation of mediastinal bleeding and substantial recovery of myocardial function, MAP is optimally maintained between 70 and 80 mm Hg. Thereafter, MAP is allowed to rise until pressures requiring treatment on a continuous basis are attained or until cardiac output falls. Treatment of episodic hypertension is directed at the cause. Anesthetic emergence with pain responds to narcotics and sedation, shivering is treated with muscle relaxants, and hypoxia and hypercarbia require appropriate ventilator adjustment. Sustained hypertension before extubation or before return of gastrointestinal (GI) motility in the first 24 to 48 hours is treated by afterload reduction with intravenous nitroglycerin at dosages of 10 to 200 μg/min or intravenous nitroprusside. Thereafter, angiotensin-converting enzyme (ACE) inhibitors are begun orally or by nasogastric tube at increasing doses until BP control permits withdrawal of intravenous infusions.

If ventricular function and cardiac output are adequate, hypertension may be treated with β-blockade using intravenous esmolol (500 μg/kg over 1 min, followed by a 50–200 $\mu g \cdot kg^{-1} \cdot min^{-1}$ drip) or labetalol (0.25 mg/kg over 2 min, 1–4 mg/min infusion). When oral medication can be taken, oral β-blockers or calcium channel blockers are started. Both classes of drugs have negative inotropic and chronotropic effects and must be used with caution when ventricular function is impaired.

Postoperative Arrhythmias

Although arrhythmias in postoperative cardiac surgical patients are morphologically no different from those in other circumstances, the cause, incidence, clinical implication, and treatment may not be the same. Apart from these patients' preexisting heart disease, frequently including a past history of specific arrhythmias, special consideration in postoperative patients must be given to promptly diagnosing and correcting causative mechanisms including postoperative ischemia or infarction, hypoxia, acidosis, and electrolyte abnormalities such as hypokalemia and hypomagnesemia.

Supraventricular Arrhythmias

Sinus Tachycardia

Sustained sinus tachycardia in cardiac surgical patients is undesirable because reduction of time in diastole reduces coronary flow to a heart already compromised by surgically induced ischemia and preexisting coronary artery disease.

Treatment is directed at correcting the underlying cause of this normal physiologic response, most commonly including pain, fever, and hypovolemia. After treatment or preclusion of such causes, β-blockade is the treatment of choice if ventricular function is adequate. Esmolol is currently popular because titration is simplified by its short duration of action.

Sinus Bradycardia

Most frequently caused by preexisting β-blockade, sinus bradycardia should be treated when it alters hemodynamic stability by reducing cardiac output or threatens a stable rhythm by ventricular escape beats.

Using the temporary epicardial wires placed at surgery, atrial pacing at a rate of 90 is attempted initially. If atrial capture is not achieved or capture interferes with native rhythm, ventricular pacing is frequently more successful. If AV nodal block is present, AV sequential pacing is attempted. If capture is not accomplished with any of the pacing wires, atropine (0.5–1.0 mg bolus) transiently increases heart rate in urgent circumstances, and a continuous infusion of isoproterenol produces a titratable chronotropic effect pending evaluation for invasive measures. Bradycardia unresponsive to the foregoing measures may mandate transvenous pacemaker placement and, if persistent, permanent pacemaker implantation.

Atrial Premature Beats

Atrial premature beats are extremely common postoperatively, and although they should not be ignored, isolated occurrences are usually of little significance. If frequent, atrial premature beats may herald the onset of atrial fibrillation, which may be poorly tolerated postoperatively, and consideration should be given to suppression.

In the early postoperative period, if the underlying sinus rate is less than about 80, atrial pacing at a faster rate is simple and frequently effective. Later postoperatively or if the sinus rate exceeds 80, digitalization is useful to reduce the frequency atrial premature beats, and suppress the ventricular response if fibrillation occurs. Quinidine, procainamide, or β-blockade may be added if digitalis is ineffective.

Atrial Fibrillation[10]

Most studies report a 30% to 40% incidence of atrial fibrillation postoperatively, although one study documented an 83% incidence. This arrhythmia is most likely secondary to a combination of atrial ischemia during aortic occlusion and postoperative inflammatory response to surgical trauma. Also implicated have been β-blocker withdrawal, atrial enlargement, and metabolic abnormalities.

When atrial fibrillation develops early postoperatively, the reduction in cardiac output as a result of loss of coordinated atrial systole (contributing as much as 30% to cardiac output) may result in marked hemodynamic instability. In addition, rapid ventricular response, as with any tachycardia, reduces coronary flow and may unmask ischemia. Atrial fibrillation developing later (after about 48 hours) is usually better tolerated.

Prevention of atrial fibrillation is the best approach. Prophylaxis with digoxin, β-blockers, or calcium channel blockers may reduce the incidence as much as 10% to 30%.

Historically, digitalization has been the treatment for atrial fibrillation in hemodynamically stable patients. Verapamil may be added to transiently reduce ventricular response,[11] but associated hypotension frequently limits its use. It is rarely used alone and converts only 10% of arrhythmias.

If ventricular response is rapid (>140) and moderate hypotension is developing, intravenous esmolol is effective and easily titratable. Intravenous diltiazem is becoming the drug of choice for ventricular rate control and conversion.

For marked (BP <90 systolic) or symptomatic hypotension, consideration should be given to electric cardioversion using an initial synchronized countershock of 50 J.

When control of ventricular response is established (rate <120), if cardioversion of a patient previously in normal sinus rhythm is not accomplished by digoxin, addition of procainamide or quinidine is indicated. Both of these agents may, however, be proarrhythmic.

Brief, hemodynamically insignificant bursts of atrial fibrillation may be left untreated.

Atrial Flutter

Atrial flutter is much less common than fibrillation; the causes and treatment are similar.

Paroxysmal Supraventricular Tachycardia

Paroxysmal supraventricular tachycardia (PSVT) is also uncommon after cardiac surgery. It may be converted to normal sinus rhythm, by rapid atrial overdrive pacing. Otherwise, PSVT is controlled initially with small, incrementally increasing intravenous bolus doses of verapamil (2.5–10 mg). Repetitive episodes of PSVT may be suppressed with continuous intravenous esmolol while a patient is digitalized.

Junctional Arrhythmias

A junctional rhythm in a postoperative patient usually represents a benign and self-limited conduction disturbance that resolves spontaneously, although digoxin toxicity should be an etiologic consideration. A slow junctional rate producing hemodynamic instability or ventricular escape beats may be treated with atrial or AV sequential pacing or intravenous isoproterenol if the epicardial wires are nonfunctional.

Ventricular Arrhythmias

Ventricular Premature Beats

Ventricular premature beats (VPBs) occur during the hospital course of almost all cardiac surgery patients and are usually of no significance. However, repetitive ventricular ectopy may have serious implications, particularly if the onset is sudden or early postoperatively.

Initial investigation includes determinations of pH, potassium, magnesium, and O_2 saturation. A surface ECG may reveal evidence of ischemia. After generic causes of ventricular ectopy alluded to earlier are precluded, VPBs may be observed if rare. If VPBs are common and the intrinsic sinus rate is less than 80, suppression by overdrive atrial pacing at a rate of 90 is often effective. Frequent or electrically arrhythmogenic VPBs occurring with higher sinus rates are treated with intravenous lidocaine. Intravenous procainamide or rarely bretylium may be necessary for refractory VPBs. All such antiarrhythmics, however, depress ventricular contractility.

Ventricular Tachycardia

A brief, single episode of nonsustained ventricular tachycardia (VT) in the later postoperative period should be investigated. A single episode of VT early after operation or repetitive runs of VT should be investigated and treated by the protocol established for VPBs. Sustained VT is treated immediately. In an asymptomatic patient, lidocaine or ventricular pacing may terminate the arrhythmia. Electric cardioversion is indicated if conversion to normal sinus rhythm is not rapid. If a patient is symptomatic with hemodynamic compromise, immediate cardioversion is indicated while lidocaine is being administered. Continued ectopy may require procainamide, bretylium, or amiodarone. Acute ischemia or infarction secondary to CABG occlusion must be considered.

Ventricular Fibrillation

Ventricular fibrillation is treated by immediate cardioversion while lidocaine and probably cardiopulmonary resuscitation are being administered.

Conduction Disturbances

Conduction disturbances occur in as many as 45% of patients after CABG[12] and 29% of those undergoing aortic valve replacements.[13] Most commonly encountered are complete and incomplete right bundle branch blocks, probably representing poor right ventricular preservation during the ischemia of aortic occlusion.[14] A postoperative right bundle brand block has no therapeutic implications and usually resolves in the first 24 hours.[15] Left bundle branch block is uncommon, occuring in about 4% of patients and perhaps representing intraoperative infarction. Complete heart block occurs in 4% of patients after CABG and 10% after valve replacement in which sutures are placed near the AV node. Temporary epicardial AV sequential pacing is indicated. If complete heart block fails to resolve after 5 to 7 days, a permanent transvenous pacemaker should be implanted.

Valve Surgery

Postoperative hemodynamic treatment of patients undergoing valve repair or replacement may be importantly altered by chronic changes in ventricular compliance. As shown in Figure 68–1, pressure in the normal LV initially rises slowly as diastolic filling proceeds. As LV volume increases, smaller increments of added volume produce larger increments of pressure rise. Changes in compliance accompanying chronic valvular heart disease shift this compliance curve to the right or left.

Aortic Stenosis

The hallmark of aortic stenosis is LV hypertrophy. The LV wall thickening increases $M\dot{V}O_2$, predisposing the subendocardium to ischemia, and shifts the compliance curve leftward.

Pressure in the noncompliant ventricle rises quickly with small increments of added preload. At a given filling pressure, ventricular volume is smaller than normal, or for a given rise in filling pressure, preload augmentation is reduced.

Higher filling pressures thus must be maintained in patients after valve replacement for aortic stenosis to maxi-

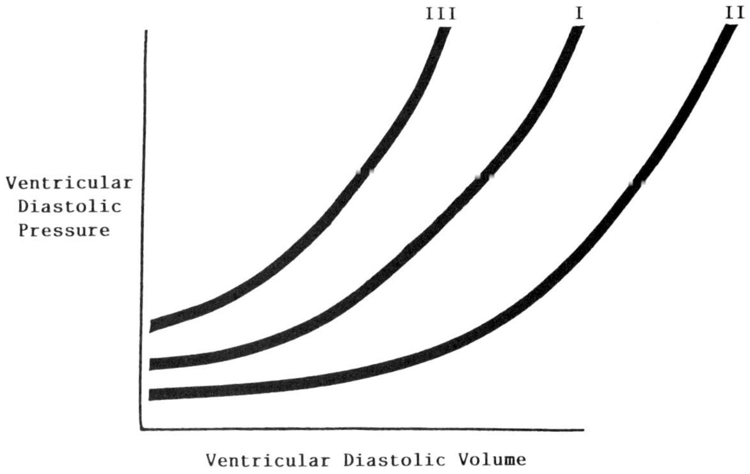

Ventricular Diastolic Pressure

III I II

Ventricular Diastolic Volume

Figure 68–1. Family of ventricular compliance curves. I = Normal ventricular compliance; II = increased ventricular compliance as in aortic and mitral insufficiency; III = reduced ventricular compliance as in aortic and mitral stenosis.

mize LV end-diastolic volume and therefore cardiac output. Special attention should be directed at maintaining AV synchrony, and systemic diastolic pressure is kept high to maintain coronary blood flow adequate to meet the increased demands of a thickened myocardium.

Aortic Insufficiency

The LV in aortic insufficiency is hypertrophied and dilated from chronic volume overload, and compliance is therefore increased. Maintenance of adequate intravascular volume and normal sinus rhythm is again important, but volume administration in these patients may produce little change in filling pressures. Overzealous fluid administration to treat a low PCWP in the presence of an adequate output may induce LV failure by volume overload.

Mitral Stenosis

In patients with mitral stenosis, the LV is protected by virtue of chronically low filling volumes. Compliance is thus reduced, and higher filling pressures must be maintained to produce an adequate cardiac output.

Mitral Insufficiency

LV hypertrophy and dilatation accompanying mitral regurgitation markedly increase compliance. Volume administration may little change filling pressures until the LV is on the verge of failure. Chronically elevated pulmonary vascular pressures result in right ventricular hypertrophy and dysfunction. Inotropic support in the form of amrinone achieves systolic unloading of both ventricles by pulmonary and systemic vasodilatation. Systemic afterload reduction with intravenous nitroprusside early and an ACE inhibitor such as captopril later is an important part of postoperative management.

Patients undergoing valve replacement or repair almost always receive some form of postoperative anticoagulation. Mechanical prostheses require lifelong anticoagulation with warfarin, which is usually started orally on the second postoperative day with or without a loading dose. Warfarin dosage is adjusted to maintain a prothrombin time of 1.6 to 2.2 times normal. Intravenous heparin may be also used with warfarin until the prothrombin time is therapeutic or alone beginning on the second day if a patient remains fasting. Patients with bioprostheses are similarly placed on warfarin for 3 months, at which time aspirin with or without dipyridamole may be substituted unless chronic atrial fibrillation is also present. Patients with bioprosthetic valves and containdications to warfarin may be maintained on aspirin and dipyridamole with acceptably low embolization rates. Patients with annuloplasty rings, which almost always accompany valve repairs, are treated similarly to those with bioprostheses.

RESPIRATORY SYSTEM

Mechanical ventilatory support of variable duration is almost always required after cardiac surgery owing to the use of neuromuscular blockade and high-dose narcotic anesthesia, which has an unpredictable duration of action.

Normal Postoperative Course

Initial Management

When an intubated and anesthetized patient arrives in the ICU, controlled mandatory ventilation is instituted at a rate of 10 to 12 breaths per minute with a tidal volume of 10 to 12 $mL \cdot kg^{-1} \cdot min^{-1}$ at an adequate fraction of expired O_2 (FIO_2) as judged by the patient's arterial blood gases in the operating room. PEEP of 5 cm H_2O is added to reduce atelectasis and therefore shunting, which impairs oxygenation. PEEP helps to preserve functional residual capacity, which is reduced by as much as 70% in these patients.

Arterial blood gas results are used to adjust the ventilator to maintain a pH of 7.35 to 7.45, a partial pressure of CO_2 (PCO_2) of 35 to 45, and a partial pressure of O_2 (PO_2) of 80 to 120. For most patients, FIO_2 can be immediately reduced substantially in increments down to 40% to 50%. Reliance on expensive arterial blood gas values during weaning can be safely reduced by monitoring arterial saturation with continuous pulse oximetry and ventilation with continuous end-tidal CO_2 ($PETCO_2$) monitors.

A chest radiograph is obtained and checked for (1) endotracheal tube position (2–3 cm above the carina), (2) complete lung expansion without pulmonary edema and the absence of pleural blood, (3) widening of the mediastinum or cardiac silhouette from accumulating hematoma, (4) position of all invasive lines and tubes and foreign bodies, and (5) extrathoracic pathology such as gastric dilatation.

A period of ventilatory stability may then follow, lasting from minutes to hours.

Rewarming and Awakening

As metabolic rate is reduced 10% for each degree centigrade that core temperature is below 37°C, rewarming from temperatures as low as 33°C on arrival in the ICU is accompanied by a substantial increase in CO_2 production. This rise is exacerbated by CO_2 production from shivering, which may be violent, and the voluntary muscle activity accompanying anesthetic emergence. The hypercapnea and resulting respiratory acidosis may cause tachycardia, hypertension, and arrhythmias.

In hemodynamically stable patients with adequate ventricular function, hypercapnea is treated by increasing the respiratory rate or tidal volume, and shivering is controlled, as noted earlier, with intravenous midazolam, diazepam, or meperidine. The metabolic stimulus to increase cardiac output accompanying shivering and mucular activity is poorly tolerated by patients with impaired LV function or hemodynamic instability. Such patients are best managed by reinduction of neuromuscular blockade with vecuronium. Intravenous narcotic analgesia must *always* be administered to paralyzed postoperative patients.[16]

Extreme rigidity with high peak inspiratory pressures, violent shivering, and rapid rise in P_{CO_2} or P_{ETCO_2} may represent the rare but sometimes lethal syndrome of fentanyl-induced chest wall rigidity. This syndrome is self-limited but must be treated by immediate paralysis.

Weaning and Extubation

When adequate anesthetic emergence is denoted by a consistently alert patient, weaning of ventilatory support is initiated by institution of intermittent mandatory ventilation. The number of machine-delivered breaths is then reduced by two or more per minute over a period of hours as tolerated down to an intermittent mandatory ventilation rate of four, from which most patients can be extubated. Some patients with marginal lung function, most often chronic obstructive pulmonary disease, may require weaning to an intermittent mandatory ventilation rate of two or continuous positive airway pressure and pressure support over a longer period before extubation.

Weaning to extubation is contraindicated in patients with hemodynamic instability, mediastinal bleeding, arrhythmias, or ventricular dysfunction requiring more than modest inotropic support. The presence of a transfemoral IABP does not per se contraindicate extubation.

Extubation may be accomplished the evening of operation in younger, stable, otherwise healthy patients but is more often achieved 12 to 24 hours after surgery. Arterial blood gases and respiratory mechanics should be determined on the final ventilator setting before extubation. Minimum criteria for extubation include an arterial P_{O_2} of greater than 70 or an F_{IO_2} less than or equal to 50%, a pH of 7.35 to 7.45, a P_{CO_2} of less than 50, a respiratory rate of less than 30 per minute, vital capacity greater than 10 mL/kg, and an inspiratory force of greater than -20 cm/H_2O.

Continuing Pulmonary Therapy

Impaired oxygenation due to increased lung water and atelectasis persists for days after surgery. Supplemental humidified O_2 is generally required after extubation, administered initially by 40% to 50% facemask, which is weaned to O_2 by nasal cannulas and then room air as dictated by pulse oximetry. Adjunctive therapy to maintain oxygenation and ventilation includes chest physiotherapy, inhaled bronchodilators, and intravenous or oral aminophylline. Nasotracheal suctioning may be required if secretions cannot be cleared by spontaneous effective coughing.

Potential Pulmonary Complications

PNEUMOTHORAX. Pneumothorax may occur postoperatively when the pleural space has been entered inadvertently or operatively placed mediastinal and pleural drainage tubes are ineffective. This is usually apparent on initial chest radiograph and is treated by tube thoracostomy in a mechanically ventilated patient. A delayed appearance of pneumothorax sometimes occurs but still may be due to intraoperative lung injury. Rising peak inspiratory pressure on a ventilator may be the first sign of accumulating pleural air. Pneumothorax may also occur after removal of mediastinal and pleural tubes. Observation is appropriate if the pneumothorax is small and the patient is asymptomatic.

ATELECTASIS. Microtelectasis and often radiographically apparent atelectasis in either or both lungs are unavoidable after cardiac surgery. However, dense atelectais of the left lower or right lobes accompanies left or right mammary artery harvest in a number of patients, possibly as a result of phrenic nerve palsy. Reaeration (on chest radiography) may take weeks to months.[17]

PLEURAL EFFUSION. Bilateral effusions may accumulate postoperatively secondary to cardiac failure, inflammation, or hypoproteinemia. A unilateral effusion almost always accompanies internal mammary artery harvest or an opened pleural space and should be aspirated or drained by tube thoracostomy only if symptomatic.

NONCARDIOGENIC PULMONARY EDEMA. Characterized by low left heart filling pressures and alveolar secretions with a protein content equal to that of plasma, this rare entity most often represents an anaphylactic allergic reaction to a drug (i.e., protamine) but may be encountered after prolonged CPB or valve surgery for endocarditis. Treatment is supportive, but antihistamines and steroids may be of value.

PROLONGED VENTILATORY SUPPORT. Mechanical ventilation beyond 48 hours after cardiac surgery is required in 9% of patients. Possible risk factors for ventilator dependency include age over 70 years, reoperation, coronary endarterectomy, severe chronic obstructive pulmonary disease, acute myocardial infarction, requirement for inotropic support or IABP, arrhythmias, LV dysfunction, postoperative bleeding, stroke, sternal infection, pneumonia, GI bleeding, and pulmonary embolus. Although complications of tracheostomy may exceed those of continued endotracheal intubation for up to 3 weeks, tracheostomy at 10 to 14 days postoperatively in the presence of anticipated continued need for ventilatory support has been recommended and is widely accepted.

RENAL SYSTEM

Cardiac surgery using CPB is a significant insult to the kidneys, reducing glomerular filtration rate by 50%.[18] Hypotension during CPB; nonpulsatile flow; the complex humoral response to anesthesia, surgery, and CPB; hypothermic vasoconstriction; and pump oxygenator microemboli and hemolysis all have a role in postoperative renal dysfunction. Nonetheless, it is uncommon for this dysfunction to become clinically apparent.

Normal Postoperative Function

A brisk diuresis of 100 to 400 mL of urine per hour typically is in progress as a cardiac surgical patient reaches the ICU. This is mediated by (1) the prophylactic addition of mannitol to the priming solution of the pump oxygenator to maintain urine output during CPB, (2) intraoperative administration of large volumes of crystalloid and furosemide, (3) hemodilution during CPB, and (4) a reduction in tubular salt and water reabsorption with rewarming from systemic hypothermia ("cold diuresis").

Urine volume then diminishes to 30 to 60 mL/h at normothermia as the effects of mannitol and diuretics wane.

The normal humoral response to surgical stress thereafter dictates urine volume (assuming normal renal perfusion). Elevated blood levels of epinephrine, norepinephrine, vasopressin, renin, angiotensin, aldosterone, and cortisol all lead to avid sodium and free-water retention. An ongoing capillary membrane leak for the first 24 hours and purposeful fluid restriction combined with judicious supplementation serve to maintain a plasma volume just adequate for organ perfusion but insufficient to generate higher urine volumes.

After 24 hours, the capillary leak seals, and after 48 hours, the humoral response to surgery abates. Plasma expansion then occurs by mobilization of the 2 to 10 L of free interstitial water gained during CPB (approximately 1 L/m^2 of body surface area per hour of CPB), and diuresis ensues.

Oliguria

In the vast majority of cases, postoperative oliguria (<0.5 mL$\cdot$kg$^{-1}\cdot$h^{-1}) reflects poor renal perfusion, not renal dysfunction or failure.

A systematic approach to oliguric patients first precludes a postrenal cause such as catheter obstruction or malposition.

Attention is then directed at cardiac function. Hypovolemia is the most common cause of postoperative oliguria. Left atrial hypotension reduces secretion of atrial natriuretic hormone and decreases renal blood flow by vasoconstriction. Judicious volume expansion rapidly increases urine volume. In the presence of normovolemia, an inadequate cardiac output due to impaired contractility must then be suspected and treated with appropriate inotropes and vasodilators to reduce afterload. If plasma volume and cardiac output are adequate, persisting oliguria is then treated with a continuous infusion of dopamine at "renal" doses (1–3 μg$\cdot$kg$^{-1}\cdot$min^{-1}). Older patients with peripheral vascular disease occasionally require higher systemic perfusion pressures to generate adequate urine flow and respond when systolic BP is raised.

The last therapeutic maneuver for oliguria after eliminating the foregoing causes is diuretic administration. Elderly patients may respond to a very small dose of furosemide (10 mg). Doubled successive doses up to 200 mg are administered, above which a response is unlikely. Bumetanide (0.5–5 mg IV), ethacrynic acid (50–100 mg IV), or a continuous furosemide drip (0.25–0.75 mg$\cdot$kg$^{-1}\cdot$h^{-1}) should then be tried, alone or in combination with metolazone (5–10 mg nasogastrically) or chlorothiazide (500 mg IV). Diuretic administration may be essential in those patients preoperatively dependent on these agents.

If renal dysfunction or failure is suspected, however, diuretics should be withheld if at all possible until diagnostic studies are obtained, because they alter test results.

Renal Failure

After cardiac surgery, 5% of patients develop clinically detectable renal dysfunction. Two per cent develop oliguric renal failure, with a mortality as high as 85%, but many more develop nonoliguric renal failure (which is transient and may be undiagnosed and unreported), which has only a 10% mortality.

Those at high risk for developing acute renal failure include patients with preexisting chronic renal disease, diabetes mellitus, significant peripheral vascular disease, congestive heart failure with diuretic treatment, advanced age (>75 y), and prior history of acute renal failure. Prolonged operation, prolonged CPB, LV dysfunction, exposure to contrast media, and certain drugs including aminoglycosides, nonsteroidal anti-inflammatory agents, and ACE inhibitors also have been implicated in the pathogenesis of acute renal failure.

Prophylaxis for those at high risk includes *preoperative* intravenous hydration, calcium channel blockade, intravenous dopamine infusion, and mannitol, furosemide, and allopurinol administration.

Evaluation of suspected renal dysfunction includes urine examination for cells or casts and serial determinations of blood urea nitrogen and creatinine. A 24-hour urine collection is obtained to calculate creatinine clearance and fractional excretion of sodium. Creatinine clearance of less than 15 mL/min and a rise in fractional excretion of sodium above 2% denote acute renal failure, or a free-water clearance of greater than -20 mL/h represents significant renal dysfunction.

Treatment of diagnosed, clinically apparent renal dysfunction is directed at maintaining renal perfusion and urine flow using the strategies outlined earlier for oliguria.

Patients with developing or established oliguric acute renal failure must be fluid restricted to output plus insensible losses. An oral diet or total parenteral nutrition should include only essential amino acids. Drug doses must be adjusted and potassium supplements avoided. Renal ultrasonography and possibly a renal scan are obtained to rule out obstructive and embolic causes, respectively.

Dialysis is necessary for hypervolemia, hyperkalemia, acidosis, or advancing uremia, but early dialysis may reduce mortality and should be considered. The several techniques available all have different indications, depending on hemodynamic stability of the patient, the duration of renal failure, and the volume of urine still produced. Hemodialysis is intermittent or continuous arteriovenous or venovenous. Hemofiltration may also be continuous arteriovenous or venovenous. Ultrafiltration is used primarily to treat volume overload in either its intermittent or continuous mode. Peritoneal dialysis is preferred for patients preoperatively using this modality or for those in whom hemodynamic instability prohibits vascular forms of dialysis.

GASTROINTESTINAL SYSTEM

Normal Postoperative Course

Nasogastric suction is initiated with intubation in the operating room to prevent gastric distention. The nasogastric tube is generally removed after extubation the day after operation, and oral intake is then resumed starting with clear liquids.

Complications

GI complications of cardiac surgery are most frequently related to low flow or low cardiac output states existing in the perioperative period.[19, 20] Although prolonged ileus is not uncommon, serious GI sequelae occur in only 0.5% to 2% of patients.

PROLONGED ILEUS. This may occur in otherwise nominally recovering patients but may be anticipated in those with low cardiac output syndromes postoperatively. Treatment is nasogastric suction until GI motility returns.

GASTROINTESTINAL ULCERATION, BLEEDING, AND PERFORATION. At one time, these sequelae were of great concern in all critically ill postoperative patients. Current incidences as low as 0.06% for bleeding duodenal ulceration following cardiac surgery have been reported. Patients with a history of duodenal ulcer are at greater risk. Attention to maintenance of gastric pH greater than 4.0 is responsible for the current rarity of this entity and has been facilitated by the introduction of parenteral $histamine_2$ blockers. Cytoprotective agents such as sucralfate may be preferable and help to decrease pathogenic GI colonization.

GASTROINTESTINAL ISCHEMIA, INFARCTION, AND PERFORATION. GI ischemia, associated with low cardiac output syndromes, vasopressor use, and digitalis use and sometimes manifested by prolonged ileus, may progress suddenly or insidiously to infarction and perforation. Atrial fibrillation with thromboembolism or atheroembolism (intraoperative or IABP related) are also etiologic considerations. An acute abdomen as always warrants immediate laparotomy.

HYPERBILIRUBINEMIA. Hyperbilirubinemia, afflicting 20% of patients after CPB, is associated with longer duration of CPB, multiple transfusions, and multiple valve replacement but also occurs after uncomplicated procedures. Resolution is spontaneous. A transfusion reaction must be considered.

CHOLECYSTITIS. Acalculous cholecystitis occurs in 2% of patients postoperatively. Ultrasonography of the gallbladder shows a dilated, edematous gallbladder. If conservative therapy fails, cholecystectomy is performed.[21]

PANCREATITIS. One third of cardiac surgical patients demonstrate a significant rise in serum amylase by the second postorerative day without clinical findings.[22] Ischemic pancreatic cellular injury is the presumed cause. Resolution is spontaneous.

Overt pancreatitis occurs in 2% of patients or less but may progress to lethal fulminant pancreatitis. Abdominal distress developing 3 days or more postoperatively should prompt serum amylase and lipase determinations and abdominal ultrasonography or computed tomography scan if indicated. Simple nasogastric suction with intravenous hydration usually is curative.

ENDOCRINE SYSTEM

Diabetes Mellitus

Diabetes mellitus is present in 30% to 60% of patients undergoing CABG and triples the total operative mortality in these patients. Specifically, diabetic patients may develop ketoacidosis and hyperosmolar states postoperatively; have impaired wound healing; are at higher risk for infections if hyperglycemic; have more diffuse coronary artery disease with poor runoff; and usually have more impaired LV function.

Preoperatively, one half to two thirds of the usual dose of intermediate-acting insulin is administered.[23] This dose usually results in modest hyperglycemia during and after operation.

The preferred method of intraoperative diabetic management is a continuous insulin infusion. Using a closed-loop system, one investigator has found mean insulin requirements (in U/h) perioperatively to be 1.0 preoperatively, 3.0 from incision to CPB, 5.0 during CPB, and 12.3 in the first 4 hours postoperatively.

Postoperatively, an initial blood glucose level of greater than 400 should be managed by insulin infusion starting at 0.1 $U \cdot kg^{-1} \cdot h^{-1}$. Hourly glucose determinations guide the infusion rate. Glucose is omitted from intravenous fluids until blood glucose level is less than 250 mg/dL.

If initial blood glucose is less than 400 mg/dL, intermittent bolus intravenous or subcutaneous insulin is administered on a sliding scale.

When adequate oral intake is resumed, intermediate-acting insulin is restarted at half the usual preoperative dose and subsequently adjusted upward.

Adrenal Dysfunction

Adrenal insufficiency is considered potentially present when exogenous steroids have been administered for 5 consecutive days within the year before surgery. The adrenal suppression thus induced may render the gland unable to respond to surgical stress (elevation of cortisol secretion from 37.5–300 mg/d). Cardiac surgery elevates urine cortisol excretion 15-fold.

Hydrocortisone succinate may be used for supplementation, administered as 100 mg IM on call to the operating room, 100 mg IV on induction, and 100 mg IV at the end of the procedure. Hydrocortisone, 100 mg IV, is then given every 6 hours initially and tapered over 3 to 4 days, at which time oral prednisone is substituted.

Preexisting undiagnosed adrenal insufficiency may lead to adrenal crisis postoperatively, recognized by unexplained hypotension unresponsive to catecholamines, hypothermia, hyponatremia, and hyperkalemia. Plasma cortisol levels are diagnostically low.

Rarely, intraoperative bilateral adrenal hemorrhage or infarction may occur.

Thyroid dysfunction

Hypothyroidism is common (8%) in the elderly patient population undergoing cardiac surgery but appears to confer little additional operative risk. Previously undiagnosed hypothyroidism should be considered in postoperative patients with low cardiac output, hypotension, and elevated SVR.

Interest has developed in the acute cardiovascular effects of T_3.[24, 25] Thyroid hormone increases O_2 consumption, cardiac output, myocardial contractility, and cardiac mass while reducing SVR. Circulating T_3 levels have been shown to be markedly depressed during CPB and for as long as 24 hours afterward. The potential role of acute T_3 administration during cardiac surgery for resuscitation from low cardiac output syndromes awaits further study.

NEUROPSYCHOLOGIC SYSTEM

Perhaps the most disturbing complication of cardiac surgery is postoperative central and peripheral nervous system dysfunction, ranging in presentation from subtle psychomotor abnormalities to depression, psychosis, hemiplegia, or fatal stroke.

Neurologic Complications

Frank stroke occurs in 1% to 5% of patients undergoing CABG, with a higher incidence reported for valve replacement. Fatal strokes occur in 0.3% to 2.0%.[26]

Etiologic mechanisms implicated include perioperative systemic hypotension or local cerebral hypotension secondary to cerebrovascular atherosclerosis and embolization of air, atherosclerotic debris, thrombus, or particulate matter. Thus, risk of neurologic injury is associated with age, known cerebrovascular disease, aortic atherosclerosis, hypotension, prolonged CPB, valve surgery, LV thrombus, and atrial fibrillation.

Presentation is determined by the location, extent, and duration of ischemic injury. Evaluation begins with a careful neurologic examination, carotid Doppler studies, and a noncontrast computed tomography scan of the head. Prognosis for recovery of those with limited focal deficits is favorable, but mortality is in excess of 50% for comatose patients.

Common peripheral neuropathies attributable to direct

local injury include (1) brachial plexus injuries secondary to sternal retraction, occurring in 5% to 25% of patients; (2) compressive ulnar nerve palsies due to inattentive arm positioning for surgery; (3) phrenic nerve palsies, related to the use of topical ice slush on the heart, inadvertent nerve division, or ischemia from internal mammary artery harvest; (4) femoral neuropathies secondary to groin cannulation; and (5) saphenous neuropathies associated with vein harvest.

Neuropsychologic Complications

Global encephalopathy or delerium has a reported incidence as high as 51%, but the pathogenesis is poorly understood.[27] It tends to occur in older, sicker patients who have preoperative organic impairments and who undergo prolonged, complex procedures. Postulated causes include metabolic derangements, cerebral microembolii, marginal intraoperative cerebral flow with ischemia but not infarction, red blood cell sludging, and sensory and sleep deprivation. Called *ICU psychosis* in one of its forms, this state is managed by transfer from the ICU if possible, adequate sleep, contact with friends and relatives, and haloperidol (1 mg IM or IV every 1–4 h until sedation is achieved).

Careful neuropsychologic testing of patients following CPB has documented a 16% to 100% incidence of deficits in concentration, memory, learning, and speed of psychomotor responses. The reported incidence appears to be related to the thoroughness of testing. Resolution of the deficits is spontaneous, although persistence of impairment at 2 months has been documented in 37%.

Psychiatric Complications

Postcardiotomy depression is most commonly encountered and most extensively studied, but normal and pathologic responses in postoperative patients include denial, anger, paranoia, confusion, and regression, among others. Psychotherapy may be indicated, depending on the severity and duration.

INFECTIOUS COMPLICATIONS

Infectious complications in cardiac surgery may be as mundane as local cellulitis in a leg wound or as catastrophic as exsanguination from an exposed suture line in an open, infected mediastinum. For fear of this latter complication, prophylactic antibiotics are administered to all patients undergoing cardiac surgery. A meta-analysis of 28 clinical trials involving use of prophylactic antibiotics in cardiac surgery during the past 25 years concluded that (1) antibiotic prophylaxis results in a fivefold reduction in wound infection rates, (2) the second-generation cephalosporins, cefamandole and cefuroxime, are superior to the commonly used cefazolin, and (3) prophylaxis beyond 48 hours (or after mediastinal tube removal) is not warranted.[28] The current use of vancomycin for prophylaxis in some institutions with a high prevalence of methicillin-resistant staphylococci has not been studied.

Normal Postoperative Course

CPB is normally terminated when core temperature reaches 35 to 37°C. Thereafter, core temperature drops again as heat is redistributed by dilating capillary beds to peripheral tissues. Rewarming in the ICU is often characterized by core temperature overshoot to 38 to 39°C, thought to be secondary to a temporary resetting of hypothalamic regulatory mechanisms or pyrogens in the CPB circuit. Low-grade fever in this range may persist for the first 48 hours postoperatively. Although as many as 75% of patients may have febrile episodes without evidence of infection even after the 6th postoperative day, a temperature greater than 38°C beyond 48 to 72 hours after surgery should be investigated.

Sternal Wound Infections and Mediastinitis

The reported incidence of sternal wound infections during the past 20 years ranges from 0.16% to 8.2%. This includes a wide spectrum of infectious complications, from minor wound abscesses responding to local wound care to mediastinitis requiring débridement by open sternotomy, the latter associated with a mortality rate of 14% recently to greater than 50% in the past. The organisms involved are usually staphylococci.

As many as 24 perioperative predisposing risk factors have been reported or hypothesized. Increased risk of sternal wound infection was correlated with operating room time, obesity, number of blood transfusions, and bilateral mammary grafting in diabetic patients in one study; another study implicated only operating times greater than 3 hours. The lowest reported rate of infection (0.16%) may be associated with very limited use of electrocautery.[29]

Superficial wound infections present as wound drainage or separation with or without cellulitis. Such infections are treated with wound incision and drainage, local care, and intravenous antibiotics.

Spiking fevers, leukocytosis, sternal wound drainage and cellulitis, and sternal instability are the hallmarks of mediastinitis, but a more indolent presentation consisting of low-grade fever, vague malaise, and substernal pain is not uncommon. Diagnosis is often clinical, but suprasternal or infrasternal aspiration and computed tomography scan may be helpful. Treatment consists of operative opening of the sternum, bone and mediastinal debridement, and irrigation. In early mediastinitis, the sternum is then closed over drainage tubes and an irrigation catheter through which 0.5% povidone-iodine or antibiotic solution is run at 1 to 2 $mL \cdot kg^{-1} \cdot h^{-1}$ for 7 to 14 days. Successful eradication of infection may be anticipated in three fourths of patients. If presentation is delayed and soft-tissue pliability poor, debridement is followed by immediate muscle flap reconstruction of the defect. Some surgeons prefer immediate muscle flap reconstruction in all cases.

Sterile sternal dehiscences occur occasionally and are closed primarily.

Leg Wound Infections

Leg wound infections occur in 1% to 2% of patients. Obesity, peripheral vascular disease, and diabetes mellitus are predisposing factors. Avoidance of large flaps of skin and subcutaneous tissue and undrained dead space is essential preventive surgical technique.

Such infections may consist of small areas of wound drainage or cellulitis, responding to local care and intravenous antibiotics. Large areas of skin flap necrosis may require plastic reconstruction.

Postoperative Prosthetic Valve Endocarditis

Although always of great concern in patients with fever after valve replacement, prosthetic valve endocarditis is rare (0.3%) with the use of prophylactic antibiotics.

Miscellaneous Infections

As with all critically ill patients, nosocomial pneumonia, intravenous catheter sepsis, and urosepsis are the most common infections unrelated to the surgical wounds.

POSTOPERATIVE HEMOSTATIC DYSFUNCTION

Mediastinal bleeding after cardiac surgery is a major concern in the first postoperative hours.[30]

Anticipated Perioperative Course

The use of CPB for cardiac surgery both requires and induces a coagulopathic state. Heparin is given to maintain an activated clotting time of usually greater than 400 to prevent intraoperative thrombogenesis. However, CPB itself results in a coagulopathy secondary to (1) hemodilution, (2) formed element and factor consumption, and (3) hypothermia, which produces a generalized suppression of the coagulation cascade. The consumptive element of this coagulopathy is multifactorial. Formed elements (i.e., platelets) are both quantitatively and qualitatively affected. The number of platelets is reduced by mechanical trauma, adherence to artificial surfaces, ongoing blood loss, and a subclinical disseminated intravascular coagulation induced by CPB. Remaining platelets are rendered dysfunctional by degranulation, which reduces aggregation. Similarly, proteins (i.e., factors) are denatured, traumatized, shed, and consumed. Factor activity is reduced 30% to 60% after CPB.

After termination of CPB, protamine is given to reverse the effects of heparin but the coagulopathic state induced by CPB persists. Therefore, mediastinal bleeding of 100 to 200 mL/h in the first 2 hours may be anticipated, thereafter tapering off to insignificant levels. Anticipated blood loss may be more substantial with prolonged CPB or reoperations with extensive adhesions.

Excessive Mediastinal Bleeding

In uncomplicated cases, persistent blood loss of greater than 2 $mL \cdot kg^{-1} \cdot h^{-1}$ is reason for concern. The following causes should be considered: (1) inadequate heparin reversal or the phenomenon of "heparin rebound," (2) quantitative or qualitative platelet defects, (3) factor deficiencies, (4) hypothermia, (5) hypertension, (6) inadequate surgical hemostasis, and (7) disseminated intravascular coagulation or primary fibrinolysis.

Clinical assessment of excessive bleeding involves observation and treatment of hypothermia and hypertension. A chest radiograph should be obtained to evaluate the mediastinum, cardiac silhouette, and pleural spaces for accumulation of thrombus or blood. A nonspecific clue to inadequate surgical hemostasis is consistent pulsatile movement of a column of saturated fresh blood up the mediastinal drainage tubes when elevated.

The cause of excessive bleeding other than that from the mediastinum is sought by coagulation laboratory study. At a minimum, a prothrombin time, partial thromboplastin time, and platelet count are included as a part of routine laboratory studies performed on arrival in the ICU. Many institutions also routinely include a postoperative thrombin time and fibrinogen assay. If available, activated clotting time and bleeding time determinations are useful and can be rapidly performed. Fibrin split product titration is obtained if disseminated intravascular coagulation is suspected. Factor assays are generally not readily available to be of use in such urgent situations. Interest in the perioperative use of thromboelastography has been stimulated by demonstration of its specificity and predictive potential.[31]

Treatment of excessive bleeding must often be initiated before the results of laboratory determinations are available. Initial maneuvers first and foremost consist of adequate replacement of ongoing blood loss with packed red blood cells to prevent hemodynamic instability. Reinfusion of shed blood by autotransfusion collection devices attached to mediastinal tubes reduces exogenous blood requirements. If the rate of bleeding is modest, this blood is defibrinated and may exaggerate bleeding by factor deficiency if infused in large quantity. Conversely, if the rate of bleeding is rapid, shed blood may not be defibrinated and clot formation makes reinfusion difficult. Cell Saver blood collected in the operating room is also frequently available but contains heparin and has no platelets or coagulation factors. Its use in large amounts also exacerbates bleeding. Attention must be paid to maintaining patency of the mediastinal tubes by gentle stripping to avoid tamponade. Hypertension must be controlled, usually with intravenous nitroprusside, to reduce the rate of bleeding. Aggressive rewarming should be instituted with heating blankets and overhead lamps if core temperature is less than 36°C. Increasing PEEP in 2.5-cm increments to hemodynamic tolerance may reduce bleeding by tamponade of open vessels. Consider empiric administration of protamine, platelets, and fresh frozen plasma if bleeding is rapid.

After laboratory results are available, therapy for bleeding can be accurately directed. Platelets are administered as 0.1 unit/kg if platelet count is less than 100,000. Each unit increases platelet count by 5000 to 10,000. However, bearing in mind that the platelets remaining after CPB are dysfunctional, active bleeding may warrant platelet transfusion, particularly if bleeding time (if measurable) is prolonged or aspirin has been used preoperatively.

Prolongation of both prothrombin time and partial thromboplastin time is noted with both heparin effect and factor deficiency. Maintenance of arterial catheter patency by heparinized infusions may produce spurious coagulopathy, precluded first by a sample drawn by direct puncture. Residual or rebound heparin effect from surgery is often reversed empirically with protamine given in 25-mg increments, up to 100 mg. Hypotensive protamine reactions of three different types may occur and are treated with volume administration, calcium, alpha agonists, and inotropes. Patients with diabetes, fish allergies, previous vasectomy, and previous protamine reaction are believed to be at higher risk and are pretreated with antihistamines and steroids. Coagulation factor deficiency is treated with fresh frozen plasma and cryoprecipitate. Doses of 10 to 15 mL/kg of fresh frozen plasma are necessary for factor replacement for hemostasis because one unit contains only about 8% of normal factor levels, and factor deficiencies exceeding 70% to 80% may be necessary to prolong the prothrombin time. However, cryoprecipitate must be given usually as 1 unit/10 kg to replace fibrinogen, Factors VIII and XIII, and von Willebrand's factor. One unit contains 50% of normal activity of the latter and 30% of normal adult Factors VIII and XIII and fibrinogen.

Desmopressin given as a single dose of 0.3 to 0.4 μg/kg releases von Willebrand's factor, necessary for platelet aggregation from endothelium, increasing levels by 50%.[32]

Fibrinolysis, either induced by CPB or a result of preoperative tissue plasminogen activator or streptokinase therapy, is inhibited by administration of ε-aminocaproic acid, 5 g followed by 1 g/h continuous infusion. Some institutions now routinely use ε-aminocaproic acid before bypass to reduce postoperative blood loss. Tranexamic acid has the same mechanism of action. A significant role may develop for aprotinin (recently approved by the Food and Drug Administration), which acts to reduce perioperative blood loss by preserving platelet function.

Mediastinal bleeding of a surgical nature is suggested if blood loss of 500 mL occurs in a single postoperative hour, 400 mL/h occurs for 2 hours, 300 mL/h for 3 hours, or 200 mL/h for 4 hours.

Cardiac surgical results have remained excellent in centers where an adequate volume is performed and the patients are taken care of in an ICU where the critical care team (physicians, nurses, and technicians) has a proactive protocol to handle the predictable occurrences, both normal and pathologic, occurring in the postoperative period. An algorithmic way of thinking ensures that small, predictable events do not become large disasters.

As the patient population has become older and sicker,[33] results have not changed appreciably, serving as testimony to the team of surgeons, anesthesiologists, intensivists, nurses, and technicians who apply a well-thought-out plan to each patient and communicate appropriately with each other.

References

1. Russo AM, O'Connor WH, Waxman HL: Atypical presentations and echocardiographic findings in patients with cardiac tamponade occurring early and late after cardiac surgery. Chest 1993; 104:71.
2. Goldberg LI, Rajfer SL: Dopamine receptors: Applications in clinical cardiology. Circulation 1985; 72:245.
3. Goldstein DS, Zimlichman R, Stull R, et al: Plasma catecholamine and hemodynamic responses during isoproterenol infusions in humans. Pharmacol Ther 1986; 40:233.
4. Alousi AA, Johnson DC: Pharmacology of the bipyridines: Amrinone and milrinone. Circulation 1986; 73:10.
5. Konstam MA, Cohen SR, Weiland DS, et al: Relative contribution of inotropic and vasodilator effects to amrinone-induced hemodynamic improvement in congestive heart failure. Am J Cardiol 1986; 57:242.
6. Richard C, Ricome JL, Rimailho A, et al: Combined hemodynamic effects of dopamine and dobutamine in cardiogenic shock. Circulation 1983; 67:620.
7. Golding LAP: Postcardiotomy mechanical support. Semin Thorac Cardiovasc Surg 1991; 1:29.
8. Pennington DG, McBride LR, Swartz MT, et al: Use of the Pierce-Donachy ventricular assist device in patients with cardiogenic shock after cardiac operations. Ann Thorac Surg 1989; 47:130.
9. Butler KC, Moise JC, Wampler RK: The Hemopump—a new cardiac prosthesis device. IEEE Trans Biomed Eng 1990; 37:193.
10. Lauer MS, Eagle KA, Buckley MJ, et al: Atrial fibrillation following coronary artery bypass surgery. Prog Cardiovasc Dis 1989; 31:367.
11. Ellenbogen KA: Role of calcium antagonists for heart rate control in atrial fibrillation. Am J Cardiol 1992; 69:36B.
12. Baerman JM, Kirsh MM, JeBuitleir M, et al: Natural history and determinants of conduction defects following coronary artery bypass surgery. Ann Thorac Surg 1987; 44:150.
13. Thompson R, Mitchell A, Ahmed M, et al: Conduction defects in aortic valve disease. Am Heart J 1980; 98:3.
14. Menaschle P, Subayi JB, Piwnica A: Retrograde coronary sinus cardioplegia for aortic valve operations: A clinical report on 500 patients (Discussion 563). Ann Thorac Surg 1990; 49:556.
15. Caspi Y, Safadi T, Ammar R, et al: The significance of bundle branch block in the immediate postoperative electrocardiograms of patients undergoing coronary artery bypass. J Thorac Cardiovasc Surg 1987; 93:442.
16. Coyle JP, Steele J, Cutrone F, et al: Patient controlled analgesia after cardiac surgery. Anesth Analg 1990; 70:51.
17. Large SR, Heywood LJ, Flower CD, et al: Incidence and aetiology of a raised hemidiaphragm after cardiopulmonary bypass. Thorax 1985; 40:444.
18. Paganini EP, Bosworth CR: Acute renal failure after open heart surgery: Newer concepts and current therapy. Semin Thorac Cardiovasc Surg 1991; 1:63.
19. Ohri SK, Desai JB, Gaer JA, et al: Intraabdominal complications after cardiopulmonary bypass. Ann Thorac Surg 1991; 52:826.
20. Johnston G, Vitikainen K, Knight R, et al: Changing perspective on gastrointestinal complications in patients undergoing cardiac surgery. Am J Surg 1992; 163:525.
21. Sessions SC, Scoma RS, Sheikh FA, et al: Acute acalculous cholecystitis following open heart surgery. Am Surg 1993; 59:74.
22. Svenson LG, Decker G, Kinsley RB: A prospective study of hyperamylasemia and pancreatitis after cardiopulmonary bypass. Ann Thorac Surg 1985; 39:409.
23. Elliott JH, Gill GV, Home PD, et al: A comparison of two regimens for the management of diabetes during open-heart surgery. Anesthesiology 1984; 60:364.
24. Hoogwerf BJ, Sheeler LR, Licata AA: Endocrine management of the open heart surgical patient. Semin Thorac Cardiovasc Surg 1991; 3:175.
25. Clark RE: Cardiopulmonary bypass and thyroid hormone metabolism. Ann Thorac Surg 1993; 56(Suppl 1):S35.
26. Reed GL, Singer DE, Picard EH: Stroke following coronary-artery bypass surgery. N Engl J Med 1988; 319:1246.
27. Mills SK, Prough DS: Neuropsychiatric complications following cardiac surgery. Semin Thorac Cardiovasc Surg 1991; 3:39.
28. Kreter B, Woods M: Antibiotic prophylaxis for cardiothoracic operations. J Thorac Cardiovasc Surg 1992; 104:590.
29. Nishida H, Grooters RK, Soltanzadeh H, et al: Discriminate use of electrocautery on the median sternotomy incision. J Thorac Cardiovasc Surg 1991; 101:488.
30. Ellison N, Campbell FW, Jobes DR: Postoperative hemostasis. Semin Thorac Cardiovasc Surg 1991; 3:33.
31. Spiess BD, Ivankovich AD: Thromboelastography: A coagulation monitoring technique applied to cardiopulmonary bypass. *In:* Effective Hemostasis in Cardiac Surgery. Ellison N, Jobes DR (Eds). Philadelphia, WB Saunders, 1988, p 163.
32. Rocha E, Llorens R, Paramo JA, et al: Does desmopressin acetate reduce blood loss after surgery in patients after cardiopulmonary bypass? Circulation 1988; 6:1319.
33. Naunheim KS, Fiore AC, Wadley JJ, et al: The changing profile of the patient undergoing coronary artery bypass surgery. J Am Coll Cardiol 1988; 11:494.

CHAPTER 69

Air Embolization

Steven L. Orebaugh, MD • Ake Grenvik, MD, PhD

Air embolism has become increasingly common and important as critical care medicine has come to focus on invasive procedures requiring vascular access, positive-pressure ventilation, and diagnostic sampling of fluid collections or parenchyma with large-bore needles. Entry of air or other gas into venous or arterial vessels with its attendant consequences requires a source of gas (usually the atmosphere), a breach in the vascular wall, and a pressure gradient that favors entry of gas into the vessel. Although the clinical consequences of venous air embolism (VAE) and arterial air embolism (AAE) are quite different, therapeutic interventions are in some ways similar.

Some aspects of tissue compromise caused by VAE and AAE share a common pathophysiology. When air is admitted into a blood vessel, bubbles form, as is the case when any gas enters a liquid in volumes exceeding its solubility. Once a bubble is blood borne, its fate is relatively predictable: It may be whipped into a froth or foam, it may coalesce into larger air bubbles, or it may fracture into smaller bubbles.[1] Typically, a lining forms around gas bubbles in blood, consisting of fibrin, plasma proteins, platelets, and phospholipids.[1, 1a] These aggregates represent foreign bodies, which may then lead to erythrocyte agglutination, microthrombi, platelet and leukocyte activation, altered blood viscosity, release of vasoactive substances, and altered capillary permeability.[1] The downstream consequence of such phenomena is obstruction to blood flow, altered hemodynamics (if occurring in the heart or pulmonary circulation), and ischemia of the end-organ affected (if arterial embolism occurs). The specific vascular beds affected determine the clinical manifestations of the VAE and AAE.

VENOUS AIR EMBOLISM

Etiology and Occurrence

As noted earlier, in order for VAE to occur there must be an open communication between the venous system and a source of gas, as well as a pressure gradient favoring ingress of the gas into the vessel. In the most direct example,[2] air is injected through a catheter into a peripheral vein or infused inadvertently via an improperly vented intravenous administration set, although this latter occurrence is infrequently reported. Likewise, air can enter the thoracic veins during insertion of a central catheter or during use of the catheter after placement, owing to the potential for subatmospheric intrathoracic venous pressure.[3–12] VAE has also been reported in penetrating head trauma[13] and during surgical procedures involving lung parenchyma.[14]

Neurosurgical and head/neck surgical procedures performed on patients in the sitting position and insufflation of air or other gases into the peritoneum are other situations in which VAE frequently has been described.[15–19a] Durant and colleagues[20] reported the occurrence of air embolism in the setting of maxillary sinus lavage, pneumothorax, and pneumoperitoneum. In total hip arthroplasty, VAE is more frequent than previously thought and is a possible cause of hemodynamic disturbances that formerly were attributed to the use of methylmethacrylate cement.[21–23] Hepatic surgery, including both liver resection and transplantation with venovenous bypass, has also resulted in VAE.[24–26] Use of the neodymium:yttrium-aluminum-garnet laser in uterine surgery has resulted in several deaths attributed to air embolism, because the instillation of air, carbon dioxide (CO_2), or nitrogen gas at high flow rates is required to cool the instrument's sapphire tip during the procedures.[27] VAE is known to occur in prostate surgery and in as many as 97% of cesarean sections.[28–30] It may occur in any surgical procedure in which a plexus of veins is opened. Both positive-pressure ventilation in infants with hyaline membrane disease and high peak airway pressure in mechanically ventilated adults have been reported to cause VAE.[31, 32, 32a] Vaginal insufflation of air during orogenital sex in pregnancy has also resulted in VAE.[33]

In the intensive care unit, VAE is most likely encountered during or after insertion of a central venous catheter (CVC). The occurrence rate of this problem is variable, reported as 1 in 47 CVC insertions[4] to none in 355.[34, 35] However, the mortality rate of VAE is significant. By 1987, only 79 cases related to CVC had been described in the world literature, but 25 (32%) of these cases had a fatal outcome.[4]

When a CVC is inserted, free communication may develop between the intrathoracic vasculature and the atmosphere. Admission of air then occurs whenever intravenous pressure decreases below ambient air pressure.[36] Negative intrathoracic venous pressure is most likely to occur with deep inspiration, dyspnea, or hypovolemia and in the upright position.[5] During strained breathing, thoracic vein pressure may decrease to 25 mm Hg below atmospheric pressure.[17]

Numerous case reports[3–12] of VAE related to CVCs exist in the medical and surgical literature. Air may enter the great veins directly after the needle is inserted, if the hub is not conscientiously occluded.[3, 5] However, the majority of cases occur not with the insertion of the catheter but during use of it.[3] CVC hub fracture or disconnection has been associated with 63% to 93% of VAEs.[5]

Pulmonary artery catheter introducers have been implicated as causes of VAE as well. Soon after these catheters came into widespread use, anesthesiologists noted a potential for air embolism through the introducers that were left in place for vascular access after removal of the catheter.[37, 38] However, changes made by manufacturers followed, and self-sealing valves in introducers became standard. Nonetheless, it is recommended that the introducer be removed along with the pulmonary artery catheter or that an obturator be used to occlude the introducer if left in situ.[38]

Pathophysiology and Pathology

Alterations in cardiovascular and pulmonary physiology resulting from admission of air into the venous system have been well studied in animals. In 1947, Durant and colleagues[20] reported that the most important factors in determining mortality after experimental VAE in dogs were (1) the amount of air entering the veins, (2) the speed with which it enters, and (3) the position of the body at the moment of embolization.

Adornato and coworkers[39] distinguished between the cardiovascular effects of bolus VAE and slow air infusion, as can occur with a separation of an intravenous line. With a massive bolus, the investigators noted an increase in central venous pressure, a decrease in pulmonary artery pressure, ST segment depression on the electrocardiogram, and shock. These changes were thought to be due to an "air lock" in the right ventricle, obstructing the outflow of blood. Slow, continuous infusion of air yielded an increase in central venous pressure and in pulmonary artery pressure, decreases in systemic vascular resistance and mean arterial pressure (MAP), and a surprising increase in cardiac output. Small bubbles lodge in pulmonary arterioles and create mechanical obstruction to flow, causing pulmonary arterial hypertension.[7, 40, 41] Pulmonary vasoconstriction results in further compromise of right heart function, as demonstrated by Berglund and colleagues[41] in a canine model subjected to slow air infusion.

Similar effects are evident in humans. Bedford and coworkers[42] evaluated 100 seated patients during neurosurgical procedures with both invasive hemodynamic and precordial Doppler ultrasound monitoring. They detected 80 episodes of air embolism. Of these patients, 36 demonstrated increased pulmonary arterial pressure, and a minority of these became hypotensive. Only those patients with an increase in pulmonary arterial pressure developed a fall in MAP.

Adornato and associates[39] found that air infusion rates of more than 1.8 $mL \cdot kg^{-1} \cdot min^{-1}$ were fatal in dogs. A bolus of more than 200 mL of air injected rapidly caused ventricular tachycardia and death in these animals. The researchers concluded that the amount of air and the speed of infusion are important factors affecting the mortality rate of VAE, affirming the earlier conclusions by Durant and colleagues.[20] The volume required to cause death decreases as the rate of air entry increases. In humans, the fatal dose of air is uncertain, but estimates vary between 300 and 500 mL at 100 mL/s.[7] Such flow rates are attainable through a 14-gauge needle if a pressure gradient of 5 cm H_2O exists.[8] However, as little as 20 mL of air may prove lethal to critically ill patients with compromised hemodynamics.

Microbubbles introduced into the pulmonary circulation result in significant ultrastructural changes and abnormalities of lung extravascular water content.[42–44] The bubbles themselves obstruct flow and increase pulmonary arterial pressure. On the bubbles' surfaces, a network of fibrin, platelets, red blood cells, and fat globules is constructed, serving to further restrict blood flow.[36] In sheep, Albertine and associates[44] demonstrated that neutrophils clumped around small air bubbles in pulmonary arterioles are attached to the endothelium of these vessels. This produces an increase in capillary leakage, lung lymphatic flow, and lymph protein concentration, also evident after infusion of 300-μm-diameter bubbles in sheep by Ohkuda and colleagues.[45] The important role of neutrophils in lung damage produced by VAE was further elucidated by Flick and coworkers.[46]

These histopathologic and ultrastructural changes lead to prominent abnormalities of pulmonary function. Lung compliance is reduced as a result of increased permeability and interstitial edema, and airway resistance is increased.[36] Abnormalities of pulmonary ventilation-perfusion matching result, with increases in physiologic dead space and pulmonary shunting after VAE. These aberrations underlie the hypoxemia universally found in victims of significant VAE, both human and animal.

Natural History

The natural history of VAE has been described in animal models[20, 41, 47] and humans.[48, 49] Adornato and associates[39] noted the changes in vital signs and venous pressures that occur with both graded venous air infusion and bolus introduction of air. The central venous, right atrial and pulmonary arterial pressure, and heart rate all increased in a dose-related fashion, with air infusion rates exceeding 0.4 $mL \cdot kg^{-1} \cdot min^{-1}$. At rates greater than 1.5 $mL \cdot kg^{-1} \cdot min^{-1}$, bradycardia supervened and cardiovascular decompensation occurred. No significant change occurred in the arterial pressure until a rate of 1.7 $mL \cdot kg^{-1} \cdot min^{-1}$ had been reached; thereafter, MAP decreased rapidly. When canines were subjected to intravenous boluses of air, the central venous pressure and heart rate again increased linearly with the dose of air, while MAP predictably decreased in a dose-related manner.

Presson and colleagues[43] described the effect of VAE in dogs by directly observing the pulmonary circulation with an *in vivo* microscopy technique while air was being infused into the animals. Microbubbles were observed to lodge in the pulmonary arterioles and underwent spontaneous resorption after 60 to 180 seconds. Larger doses of air take longer to resolve.

Clinical Manifestations

The clinical expression of VAE varies in both severity and in organs affected (Table 69–1). In canines[39] and humans,[36] a "gasp" has been reported to follow the initial infusion of air into the pulmonary circulation, possibly a reflex response. Intrathoracic pressure is thereby decreased, facilitating greater air entry into the venous system. Patients often complain of breathlessness, lightheadedness, chest pain, or a feeling of impending doom.[7, 36] In one series of 14 cases, all patients had sudden onset of dyspnea.[50]

Signs of air embolism are seldom specific for this entity. Significant embolism results in tachypnea, tachycardia, and frequently hypotension. The only sign specific for air embolism, the rare "mill-wheel" murmur, occurs late and is dependent on the presence of a large collection of air in the right ventricle.[29, 49] A harsh systolic murmur[17, 51] or normal heart sounds are more commonly found on examination. In a large proportion of patients, neurologic signs predominate. Kashuk and Penn[52] described a predominance of central nervous system (CNS) manifestations in 42% of 24 instances of VAE reviewed. These manifestations included altered mental status, frank coma, and focal deficits. Whether hypoxia, hypotension, paradoxical embolism, or some combination of these factors is responsible for this neurologic compromise is uncertain.

In some individuals, rales or wheezing can be detected on auscultation of the lung fields minutes to hours after air embolism occurs, indicating pulmonary edema.[52] In animal models and humans,[46, 53–55] the coexistence of increased pulmonary arterial pressure and pulmonary edema protein content with normal pulmonary artery occlusion pressures suggests that increased vascular permeability underlies the development of abnormal extravascular lung water.

TABLE 69–1. Clinical Manifestations of Venous Arterial Embolism and Arterial Air Embolism

System	*Venous Air Embolism*	*Arterial Air Embolism*
Cardiovascular	Chest pain Coarse systolic murmur Water mill-wheel murmur Tachycardia, arrhythmias Cardiovascular	Chest pain (if coronary embolism) Arrhythmias (if coronary embolism)
Neurologic	Altered level of consciousness Acute focal deficit (paradoxical embolism)	Sudden collapse or coma Acute focal deficit Subtle cognitive abnormalities
Pulmonary	Cough, dyspnea Hypoxemia Tachypnea Rales, wheezing Gasping	Lungs not usually affected unless pulmonary injury is source
Skin	No effects	Livedo reticularis Mottling
Mucous membranes	No effects	Partial or complete tongue ischemia

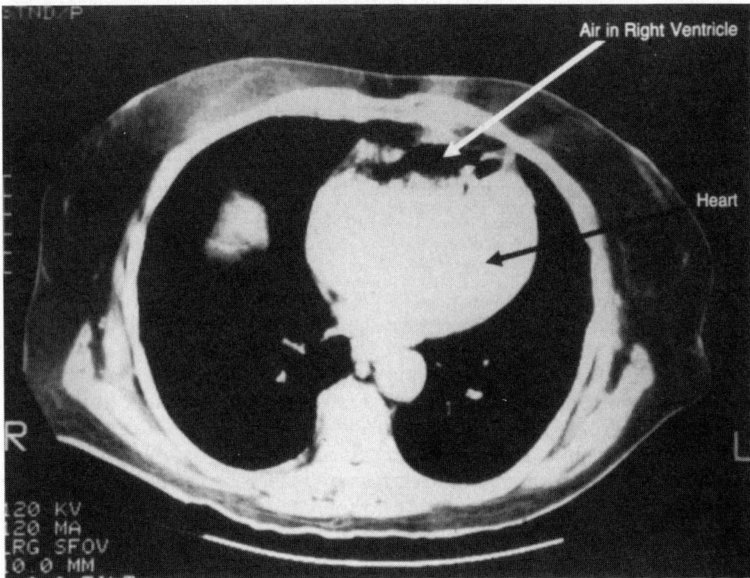

Figure 69–1. Computed tomography scan demonstrating air in the right ventricle. (From Oriscello RG, Robertello ME: Images in clinical medicine. N Engl J Med 1993; 328:855. Reprinted, by permission of the *New England Journal of Medicine.*)

Laboratory Data and Monitoring

Laboratory abnormalities vary with the severity of the embolism but lack specificity for this process. Electrocardiographic changes evident in canines include peaking of the P wave and ST segment depression.[20] Reports of VAE in humans describe sinus tachycardia, nonspecific ST segment and T wave changes,[12] and evidence of acute right heart strain.[56] In addition, atrial and ventricular dysrhythmias may be noted.[57] Findings on chest radiographs are usually normal initially but later may show evidence of noncardiogenic pulmonary edema.[53–55a] An air-fluid level in the central pulmonary artery or right ventricle is seen rarely (Fig. 69–1).[6] Arterial blood gases reflect abnormalities of matching of ventilation and perfusion, usually as hypoxia, which may be profound. Hypercarbia is occasionally present.

When used, invasive hemodynamic monitoring may provide further evidence of the clinically important air embolism. Increases in central venous and pulmonary arterial pressure are dose dependent in animals subjected to slow air infusion.[39] However, pulmonary arterial pressure may remain normal, with an increased central venous pressure, presumably due to a large air bubble trapped in the outflow tract of the right ventricle. This phenomenon occurs in animals with massive air embolism (>5 mL/kg). In one study of the occurrence of VAE in patients seated during neurosurgical procedures and monitored with CVCs, 10 of 40 patients had an increase in the central venous pressure.[51] In a similar population of 100 patients monitored with precordial Doppler technique, pulmonary artery catheters and end-tidal CO_2 monitors, Bedford and colleagues[42] described the occurrence in 80 patients of VAE detected by Doppler; nearly half of these patients developed an increased pulmonary arterial pressure.

The utility of end-tidal CO_2 monitoring to detect significant VAE is well described.[16, 17] In the previously noted study by Bedford and coworkers,[42] 30 of the 80 patients with VAE reportedly had a decrease in end-tidal CO_2 concentration, reflecting increased physiologic dead space. Airway pressure during mechanical ventilation may increase abruptly as end-tidal CO_2 falls in this situation.[58] Other useful indicators of VAE include aspiration of air or foam from an indwelling CVC or pulmonary artery catheter, as well as ultrasonography changes. Human and animal data have demonstrated the utility of Doppler ultrasound and precordial echocardiography. Transesophageal echocardiography, however, seems to be even more sensitive, detecting as little as 0.02 mL/kg of air in experimental scenarios,[59] and only this modality has proved useful in documenting paradoxical air embolism.[60]

Differential Diagnosis

VAE may present with a wide variety of signs and symptoms and spans a continuum of severity from clinically insignificant to life threatening, mandating consideration of various differential diagnoses (Table 69–2). When respiratory complaints and signs are evident, VAE must be differentiated from other causes of sudden pulmonary compromise, such as pulmonary clot embolism, pneumothorax, acute bronchospasm, and pulmonary edema. If signs of CNS compromise predominate, the clinician must consider focal or global brain ischemia, hemorrhage into the parenchyma or subarachnoid spaces, hypoxia, trauma, intoxication, and hypoglycemia.

In many cases, cardiovascular compromise dominates the clinical picture. This is usually in the form of hypotension, in which case VAE must be considered, along with other causes of obstructive shock, hypovolemia, primary cardiac dysfunction, and acute vasodilatory states such as septic shock. VAE has also been reported to manifest as electro-

TABLE 69–2. Differential Diagnoses of Venous Air Embolism

Predominant System Affected	*Differential Diagnoses*
Cardiovascular	Aortic dissection
	Pericardial tamponade
	Hypovolemia
	Myocardial infarction
Neurologic	Stroke
	Intracranial bleed
	Trauma
Pulmonary	Pulmonary thromboembolism
	Tension pneumothorax
	Acute bronchospasm
	Acute pulmonary edema

mechanical dissociation,[61] probably a result of right ventricular outflow obstruction, which reduces the cardiac output without initially disturbing cardiac electric activity. Therefore, one should consider this entity in the differential diagnosis of electromechanical dissociation when a patient is at risk for VAE.

Management of Venous Air Embolism

Identification of the source of air entry and immediate measures to counter this entry are the first priorities in the treatment of VAE. Subsequent management strategies are based on evidence derived from animal investigations and case reports in humans. Five areas of therapeutic intervention are discussed: patient positioning, cardiac massage, removal of air from the venous circulation, attenuation of bubble size, and miscellaneous measures (Table 69–3).

Durant and colleagues,[20] in their early work with air embolism in animals, demonstrated the importance of body positioning by showing that dogs had increased tolerance of air infusion when lying on their left side. Although not validated in clinical trials, placing patients with suspected VAE in this position remains a cornerstone of management today.[36, 51, 62] The head-down or Trendelenburg position is recommended as well, apparently with similar effects on right ventricular outflow obstruction.[7]

Closed-chest cardiac massage has been recommended as a means to force air out of the right ventricular outflow tract and into small pulmonary vessels, as it has been successfully used by Ericsson and colleagues[63] in resuscitating four of five patients sustaining VAE during neurosurgical procedures. External cardiac compression has been evaluated in dogs as therapy for VAE[62] and found to improve survival rate as effectively as use of the left lateral decubitus position or aspiration of air from the right atrium.

A more direct approach to the treatment of air embolism is withdrawal of air from the right side of the heart. A comparison of intracardiac aspiration from the right ventricle versus external cardiac massage and versus the left lateral decubitus position in therapy of VAE in dogs resulted in similar survival in all three groups but significantly more rapid resuscitation with air aspiration than with the other measures.[62] A greater proportion of injected air can be removed from the right atrium of dogs with VAE using a multiple-orifice CVC than by using either a pulmonary artery catheter or single-port CVC, resulting in a significantly improved survival rate.[64]

TABLE 69–3. Management of Venous Air Embolism

Positioning: Left lateral decubitus or Trendelenburg.
- Cardiac massage: Possibly useful in cardiac arrest due to venous air embolism.
- Air retrieval: If a central venous pressure or right atrial line is in place, a significant amount of air can sometimes be retrieved.
- Reduced bubble size: All patients should receive 100% oxygen. Case series support use of hyperbaric oxygen treatment for patients with severe CNS or cardiac manifestations.
- Miscellaneous: Fluorocarbon emulsions require further research to establish efficacy.

For patients in left-side-down lateral position.
- In cardiac arrest with secured VAE diagnosis, direct puncture of the right atrium via the parasternal fourth or fifth intercostal space with aspiration of air from the right atrium may be lifesaving. The possibility of subsequent cardiac tamponade is a significant risk.
- Consider emergency cardiopulmonary bypass in moribund patients.

Michenfelder and colleagues[51] evaluated the utility of air retrieval in humans via right atrial catheters in 23 episodes of VAE in seated patients undergoing neurosurgical procedures. Significant air retrieval with a favorable influence on resuscitation occurred in only eight cases. Other researchers have found that air retrieval from the right atrium has had minimal impact on improving hemodynamics.[42] Thus, withdrawal of air from the right atrium or ventricle is useful in VAE if a catheter is present but probably does not justify the time and effort necessary to insert a CVC in an acute situation, if not already in place.

To reduce the size of embolized bubbles, all patients with suspected VAE should receive 100% oxygen,[36] because this favors nitrogen diffusion out of the bubbles and into the alveoli (nitrogen "washout"). For patients under general anesthesia, it is imperative that nitrous oxide be discontinued, because it diffuses rapidly into all air-containing cavities in the body, including intravascular bubbles, significantly increasing their size and the obstruction they present to the circulation.[65]

For those patients not responding to these measures, hyperbaric oxygen (HBO) therapy should be considered. Although well-controlled, randomized trials comparing this therapy with other measures have not been conducted, many physicians advocate HBO use on the strength of numerous case reports[66–70] reflecting clinical improvement in cerebral air embolism (CAE) of venous or arterial origin after HBO therapy. This modality has long been used in the treatment of arterial gas emboli resulting from barotrauma in scuba divers.[71] HBO has more recently been applied to cerebral injury related to air embolism from therapeutic misadventures.[33, 48, 66, 67, 70] A review of the mechanisms and efficacy of HBO treatment is provided in Chapter 106.

HBO therapy must be carried out under the direction of a physician experienced and knowledgeable in this area. Despite the favorable anecdotal evidence cited, doubt has been expressed[72] about the efficacy of HBO in CAE. Indeed, scientifically valid data are needed in this area.

Several measures reported to be useful in the therapy of VAE have not yet been adopted in the treatment of humans. The protective effects of a perfluorocarbon emulsion as pretreatment in a canine model of VAE have been demonstrated.[73, 74] Cardiopulmonary bypass (CPB) has also been advocated in the therapy of VAE to reduce right heart strain and circumvent obstruction to cardiac output. This modality has not been systematically evaluated, however, and its utility remains dubious.

Prophylaxis

Most hospital episodes of VAE are related to CVCs, making preventive measures particularly important when these catheters are inserted, used, or removed. Patients to undergo catheterization of the central veins should be placed in the Trendelenburg position, which increases the central venous pressure and reduces the likelihood of air entry through the needle or catheter.[36] After entering the vein and before inserting the guide wire if using the Seldinger technique, one should occlude the needle hub, releasing to insert the wire only after asking the patient to perform a Valsalva maneuver, or timing the insertion of the wire to coincide with exhalation.[5] A through-the-plunger guide wire system may in the future reduce the risk of air embolism in this situation.[75]

Adequate hydration should be ensured before catheter insertion to mitigate against the low venous pressure of hypovolemia that encourages air entry. All connections to the central venous line should be tightly sealed using Luer-

Lok adapters. Placing an occlusive dressing over the catheter when in place and over the tract for 24 hours after removal also helps prevent air emboli.[5] As with insertion, removal of the catheter in a head-down position is recommended.

In the operating room, monitoring for air embolism during high-risk procedures using precordial Doppler and capnography has become the standard.[60] Avoiding procedures performed in the seated position should reduce the incidence of VAE. In particular, preoperative screening by echocardiography for the presence of a patent foramen ovale may alert the surgeon and anesthesiologists to those patients who are at risk for the severe consequences of paradoxical air embolism (PAE).[76] Gas insufflation for diagnostic purposes should be accomplished with CO_2, not air, because CO_2 has a low surface tension, is absorbed quickly, and causes less obstruction if embolism occurs.

Finally, if a patient experiencing air embolism can be ventilated with positive pressure, this procedure is preferable to spontaneous breathing because it reduces unfavorable pressure gradients permitting air entry (e.g., during insertion of CVCs). However, high peak inspiratory pressure causing barotrauma may, in itself, be a reason for VAE and must be avoided.[30, 31]

ARTERIAL AIR EMBOLIZATION

Arterial air embolization (AAE) was first reported in the medical literature by Morgagni in 1769.[77] This problem was not recognized as an iatrogenic complication until 1913, however, when it was observed with the irrigation of empyema cavities.[77] AAE in diving accidents was first described in the 1930s but was originally not distinguished from decompression sickness.[78] Scuba diving was not yet popular, and the accidents reported were related to military submarine escape training. In 30 years of Royal Navy submarine escape training, 91 cases of apparent AAE occurred in the United Kingdom.[79] In the United States, AAE among military divers has occurred with a frequency of approximately 7 in 100,000 dives.[80] When scuba diving accidents occurring in Hawaii during a 5-year period were analyzed, 42 cases of dysbaric AAE were evident.[81] In about half of these episodes, symptoms and signs could not reliably be distinguished from decompression sickness.[78, 80, 81] Approximately 750 cases of AAE requiring recompression therapy currently occur each year in the United States, with about 100 annual fatalities.[82]

Etiology and Occurrence

The two most common iatrogenic causes of AAE are the use of CPB and neurosurgical procedures performed with patients in the sitting position.[77] Arterial emboli related to use of CPB occur in 2% to 9% of patients, with 4% to 10% of these patients developing a major neurologic deficit.[83] In upright neurosurgical procedures, AAE occurs infrequently, contrary to the high incidence of VAE in this situation.[84]

CPB offers ample opportunity for entrainment of air into the arterial circulation. The most common source of air entry is the oxygenator itself. Because of the presence of a direct gas-blood interface, bubble oxygenators have contributed to this problem more often than the currently used membrane oxygenators.[85] Other sources of potential air entry during cardiac surgical procedures include cardiotomy suction blood return, cannulation of the ascending aorta, entrapment of air when closing the left ventricular or atrial chamber, the cavitation effect from the roller pump, and inadvertent direct injection of air through vascular catheters during the procedure.[86] During coronary artery bypass grafting (CABG), air may also be introduced directly into the coronary arteries themselves.[87] Interestingly, when the left ventricle is vented during CABG, negative intracavitary pressures encourage retrograde air entry into the aortic root from the open coronary arteriotomy sites, and from here it may embolize elsewhere after release of the aortic cross-clamp.[88]

Before the surge in popularity of sport diving, most AAE related to immersion occurred in submarine escape trainees.[77] Improvements in technique and apparatus have reduced the dangers of this training considerably. Therefore, scuba divers experience the majority of cases of noniatrogenic AAE treated in hyperbaric chambers.[77, 81] This can often be attributed to divers with exhausted air supply who panic and ascend too rapidly without the necessary exhalation en route,[78, 89] leading to expansion of pulmonary gas and eventual alveolar rupture with potential air admission into pulmonary veins. However, in many instances, no violation of safe diving principles is evident. Although inexperienced divers are more susceptible to AAE, this unpredictable occurrence strikes seasoned divers as well.[78] In one study of 117 episodes of AAE among divers, 43% had no predisposition and demonstrated no failure to comply with safe diving recommendations.[80]

Mechanical positive-pressure ventilation also places patients at risk for entry of air into the arterial system. Particularly in patients with inhomogeneous lung injury or chronic obstructive pulmonary disease, much of the positive-pressure inflation is directed away from the affected, poorly compliant alveoli into those that are more compliant.[90] These may rapidly overexpand, rupture, and release air into the interstitium, predisposing to pneumothorax[91] and entry of air into pulmonary capillaries or veins.[92, 93] This may occur with ventilator insufflations, spontaneous breaths from a positive-pressure circuit,[94] or manual bag ventilation.[93] Stiff lungs may predispose further to AAE by stenting open vascular channels disrupted by pressure, trauma, or inflammation.[92]

Other potential causes of iatrogenic AAE are operations on the head and neck,[95] lungs,[96] and aorta.[77] AAE has also been a result of fine-needle transthoracic lung biopsy,[97, 98] percutaneous transluminal coronary angioplasty,[99] catheter ablation of arrhythmia foci,[100] and penetrating lung injury,[101] especially stab wounds of the chest.[102, 103] The use of positive-pressure ventilation may worsen this situation by increasing the pressure gradient between the injured bronchus and the involved pulmonary vein.[104] In addition, AAE has been described as a consequence of hepatic surgery,[77] liver transplantation,[105] uterine surgery,[106] rupture of the gas-filled balloon of an intra-aortic balloon pump,[107] and laparoscopy.[108] In one case, compression and decompression during hyperbaric oxygen therapy for a nonhealing foot ulcer actually caused pulmonary barotrauma and AAE.[109] Finally, the dangers of intra-arterial catheters connected to high-pressure flush lines must be considered. On observing apparent cerebral embolism in critically ill patients after flushing radial arterial lines, Chang and colleagues described a primate model in which this hypothesis was evaluated.[110] The introduction of more than 2 mL of air into the radial artery while flushing the catheter resulted in retrograde passage of air to the cerebral circulation via the vertebral arteries.

Pathophysiology

Air may be introduced into the arterial system by three potential mechanisms: direct arterial air entry, venous air embolism with transgression of air to the arterial circulation via PAE, and entry of air into the pulmonary capillaries or veins by direct lung trauma.[76–81] After VAE, PAE may occur either by direct migration of air through the pulmonary vascular bed,[111] or by traversing intracardiac defects such as a patent foramen ovale or atrial septal defect.[112] The former occurrence is more likely in patients with a history of pulmonary hypertension.[111]

In addition to a communication between the left and right sides of the heart, a favorable pressure gradient must exist for air movement to the arterial side for the latter type of PAE to occur. During neurosurgery in the seated position, a gradient of 4 to 5 mm Hg favoring this transeptal migration of air can occur. Such gradients appear to be augmented by VAE and positive-pressure ventilation. Sudden changes in end-expiratory pressure may predispose to PAE, because the instantaneous gradient of right-to-left atrial pressure probably determines the occurrence and direction of air movement rather than mean pressures.[110] Attempts to identify patients at risk for PAE preoperatively using precordial echocardiography with provocative maneuvers to demonstrate a patent foramen ovale have not been uniformly successful; Valsalva maneuvers and positive end-expiratory pressure (PEEP) may not adequately re-create the hemodynamic effects that occur with actual VAE.[113]

As previously mentioned, air bubbles introduced into the bloodstream may coalesce into larger bubbles, fractionate into smaller ones and move more distally in the circulation, or form froth. Intravascular air bubbles are typically surrounded by a membrane of fibrin, platelets, lipids, red blood cells, cellular debris, and plasma proteins.[1] Such a coagulum developing about an intravascular air bubble becomes a foreign body, which provides a favorable setting for activation of the kinin, complement, coagulation, and fibrinolytic systems, all of which may contribute to end-organ injury in AAE.[114, 115] In animal models, arterial injection of gas may distribute to cerebral vessels, eventually occluding those of 30 to 60 μm diameter.[116, 117] This leads to patchy, intermittent ischemic neuronal damage.[118, 119] Increased capillary permeability and the loss of cerebral vascular autoregulation are prominent features of the response to air embolism.[120] However, not all models of CAE reveal evidence of vascular obstruction as a primary means of cellular compromise. In a rabbit model of CAE, no obstruction of pial vessels was observed in open brain studies, but a marked subsequent decline in local cortical blood flow and neuronal function was evident,[121] perhaps due to activation of damaging mediators and subsequent vascular response.

The immediate effects of AAE depend to some degree on the position of the individual.[77] In the supine position, coronary artery embolism is the likely result of air introduced into the pulmonary veins. Amounts smaller than 0.5 mL can be fatal. In such a situation, coronary embolism is a possible cause of death.[122] In the sitting position, air distribution to the brain is likely and results primarily in neurologic manifestations. In the head-down position, air migrates to the apex of the left ventricle, possibly delaying systemic air embolism.[77]

Pathology

The pathologic consequences of AAE are difficult to distinguish from other ischemic events. In the brain, astrocyte and neuron swelling, vacuolation, chromatolysis, hemorrhage, and necrosis identical to models of cerebral infarction are evident at necropsy.[77, 123–125] Pathologists may have difficulty distinguishing evidence of CAE from cerebral ischemic injury accompanying profound hypotension. Both cytotoxic and vasogenic edema may result.[126–128]

Natural History

The course of AAE is unpredictable. Patients typically develop maximum end-organ dysfunction within seconds to minutes. The deficit may remain profound, or spontaneous improvement may occur. In animal studies, bubbles of air may disappear within minutes from capillary beds or physically obstruct them for 48 hours or more.[79, 90] Fifty to 56% of divers with evidence of CAE recover partially or completely before definitive therapy is instituted.[80, 81] More profound deficits portend longer periods of recovery and less likelihood of resolution.[77]

Clinical Manifestations

In dysbaric diving accidents, the end-organ most commonly affected is the CNS. The most common sign reported in submarine escape training and among scuba divers is an abrupt loss of consciousness and collapse within seconds or minutes of surfacing. This occurs in 38% to 45% of those sustaining AAE.[80, 81, 89] The vast majority of episodes of loss of consciousness occur within 10 minutes of surfacing. Other evidence of CNS injury includes asymmetric multiple limb weakness,[81] sensory loss,[80] and frequent neuropsychiatric deficits.[89] Patients may present with cognitive abnormalities alone, and a thorough mental status examination is therefore imperative. Severe headache is common among divers sustaining AAE.[107] The manifestations of AAE are diverse and may overlap considerably with the neurologic signs and symptoms of decompression sickness, which may be expressed by spinal cord injury with symmetric limb weakness or sensory loss. These two entities frequently coexist in divers and have been referred to as the *dysbaric syndrome*.[97]

CPB may cause focal, obvious neurologic deficits as a result of air bubbles or cellular debris acting as emboli but is much more likely to result in subtle cognitive deficits. This occurs in up to 70% of patients.[83] In penetrating chest trauma, the creation of a bronchopulmonary venous fistula may be manifested by sudden cardiovascular collapse, hemoptysis, bloody foam emanating from a hole in the lung or great vessel, seizures, or direct visualization of air in the coronary arteries at thoracotomy.[101]

The frequency with which AAE occurs in mechanical positive-pressure ventilation is uncertain. The phenomenon is well documented in infants and children[129, 130] but less common in adults. Case reports describe the sudden, traumatic onset of arrhythmia, evidence of cerebral infarction, and livedo reticularis.[92]

Four signs of AAE have been described as pathognomonic of this entity: skin marbling, reduced perfusion of all or part of the tongue, bloody froth emanating from a wound or a needle-stick site, and air bubbles in the retinal vessels.[98, 131]

Laboratory Data and Monitoring

Unlike VAE, air emboli in the arterial circulation are detected largely by clinical acumen and produce few disturbances of laboratory or imaging modalities that would aid in establishing this diagnosis. However, transcranial ultrasonography has been used successfully in monitoring the occurrence of CAE during CABG procedures.[85, 132] Spencer and colleagues detected AAE in 38% of patients undergoing carotid endarterectomy, but most episodes remained clinically silent.[133] Electroencephalographic changes occur with CAE as well but are nonspecific and predict neurologic signs or symptoms in only half of the patients who develop them.[77] Both transthoracic and transesophageal echocardiography effectively identify VAE, as does precordial Doppler monitoring, but only the transesophageal probe can detect air that traverses the atrial septum or pulmonary circuit to end up in the left side of the heart en route to systemic embolism. If agitated saline is used as intravenous echocardiographic contrast, transthoracic echocardiography can also effectively image PAE.[134] Computed tomography scan of the brain performed within the first 24 hours after CAE may reveal foci of air density in the brain or decreased attenuation suggestive of cerebral infarction.[135]

Differential Diagnosis

Differential diagnosis of AAE depends on the end-organs affected and clinical manifestations thereby produced. The most common presentation is generalized neurologic compromise, which should lead to consideration of intracranial catastrophes such as subarachnoid hemorrhage, intracerebral bleeding, widespread infarction from thrombosis or atherogenic embolism, and the various causes of rapid deterioration of cardiac output. The difficulty in distinguishing AAE from decompression sickness in divers was mentioned earlier. Decompression sickness often results in spinal cord ischemia, but overlap in signs is common.[78] Metabolic, psychiatric, and infectious abnormalities as well as focal cerebrovascular events must also be considered along with AAE as potential causes of the subtle cognitive deficits that may occur after diving or CPB procedures.

Management of Arterial Air Embolism

The management of AAE varies somewhat with the setting in which it occurs. In CPB procedures, the sequence of interventions should begin immediately on detection of air embolism, including placing patients in head-down position, stopping air entry, compressing the carotid arteries, discontinuing administration of nitrous oxide, starting inhalation of 100% oxygen, and venting the aorta.[136] Limited data support the use of retrograde (venoarterial) circulation through the superior vena cava to help clear cerebral arterial air.[137–139] Otherwise, CPB may be carefully reinstituted along with cooling of the patient to profound hypothermia, which increases gas solubility.[140]

When penetrating chest trauma is complicated by AAE, head-down position and 100% oxygen administration should be accompanied by emergency thoracotomy and clamping of the entire hilum of the involved lung, vigorous open-chest cardiac massage, and aspirating the left ventricular apex for air or foam.[101] The coronary arteries can also be aspirated if bubbles are visible within them. Emergency CPB may be indicated, but no data exist to support use of this technique. Coronary artery air embolism occurring during percutaneous transluminal coronary angioplasty is generally managed with supportive care alone.[99]

Data supporting the use of HBO therapy in AAE and VAE are largely anecdotal.[140a–140c] No clinical trials have compared its efficacy with supportive measures or control groups. Clinical experience appears to have outstripped scientific knowledge in this area.[82] Still, available clinical and experimental evidence supports use of HBO, and it is considered the standard of care in circumstances in which a patient can be safely transported to a hyperbaric chamber. Ultimately, controlled trials will be necessary to confirm HBO efficacy. Details of HBO application are discussed in Chapter 106.

When AAE is suspected, the clinician should ensure that no secondary brain injury complicates the primary insult. Seizures, hyperthermia, hypoxia, and hypotension or hypertension must be carefully avoided.[77, 95] Other interventions supported by animal or experimental investigations but not yet accepted as standard management include infusion of dextran 40 to reduce blood viscosity,[141] perfluorocarbons to enhance oxygen-carrying capacity,[142] aspirin to reduce platelet aggregation,[77] and lidocaine infusion to reduce neuron damage.[143]

Prognosis

Complete resolution of neurologic deficits after AAE in divers occurs in 65% of patients treated with HBO. Two thirds of these patients reach baseline neurologic status within 25 minutes.[116] However, it is not uncommon for relapse to occur.[95] Initially, these patients are not distinguishable from those who achieve a lasting resolution of all deficits. Therefore, all patients with AAE must be considered for maximum therapy, including HBO.

Prophylaxis

Methods of preventing AAE vary with the clinical scenario. In surgical procedures using CPB, the perfusionist must be observant for evidence of air in the circuit facilitated by low blood level in the oxygenator. A low-level alarm and shutoff mechanism should be used[136] to signal this problem, which is a common cause of AAE.[137] The use of a 25- to 40-μm arterial filter has been demonstrated to reduce occurrence of gas emboli in the middle cerebral artery, as does the use of membrane instead of bubble oxygenators.[83]

After completion of cardiac valve or CABG surgery or heart or lung transplantation, retained intracardiac air is demonstrable by transesophageal echocardiography. It may occur in as many as 80% of valve replacements and 11% of CABG procedures.[144] In order to avoid AAE, air mobilization and removal is routinely performed (e.g., through aortic and left atrial venting), preferably before CPB is terminated.

It is possible to identify some patients to be subjected to upright neurosurgical procedures at high risk for PAE because of the presence of a foramen ovale. This is usually accomplished with transthoracic echocardiography with contrast material provided by rapid saline injection. A suitable maneuver is then used to increase right atrial pressure. Success has been variable, because no test is 100% sensitive in identifying patients at risk of paradoxical embolism.[113, 145] Nevertheless, a positive result allows the surgeon and anesthesiologist to carefully weigh the risks and benefits of the desired position during surgery.

In order to avert AAE related to the pulmonary dysbaric syndrome, scuba divers must be well acquainted with the physiology of compression and safe diving principles. Uncontrolled ascent must be avoided. Likewise, pulmonary overinflation with mechanical ventilation, usually manifested by high peak airway pressures, must not be allowed to occur, because the consequences of hypoventilation and respiratory acidosis are far less injurious than is pulmonary barotrauma, which may otherwise result.[92]

CONCLUSION

Air embolism in the venous or arterial circulation may have devastating consequences. Hemodynamic disturbances predominate with VAE, whereas CNS compromise is the most visible evidence of AAE. Presenting manifestations frequently are nonspecific. Identification of VAE or AAE depends on the knowledge and experience of the critical care physician, surgeon, or anesthesiologist and awareness of

TABLE 69–4. Risk Factors for Venous Air Embolism and Arterial Air Embolism in an Intensive Care Unit

Positive-pressure ventilation: mechanical ventilator or continuous positive airway pressure
Central venous catheter insertion, therapy, and maintenance
Postoperative state (especially after neurosurgery and procedures requiring cardiopulmonary bypass)
Hemodialysis and other forms of extracorporeal circulation
Intra-aortic balloon pumping
Trauma victims, especially penetrating chest trauma

those settings in which air embolism is likely (Table 69–4). Basic supportive measures and positioning are the cornerstones of therapy, along with stopping air entry and initiating HBO therapy when indicated and possible.

References

1. Butler BD: Biophysical aspects of gas bubbles in blood. Med Instrumentation 1985; 19:59–63.
1a. Thorsen T, Klausen H, Lie RT, et al: Bubble-induced aggregation of platelets. Undersea Hyperb Med 1993; 20:101–119.
2. Yeakel AE: Lethal air embolism from a plastic blood storage container. JAMA 1968; 204:175–177.
3. Borja A: Current status of infraclavicular subclavian vein catheterization. Ann Thorac Surg 1972; 13:615–622.
4. Seidelin PH, Thompson AM: Central venous catheterization and fatal air embolism. Br J Hosp Med 1987; 25:438–439.
5. Peters SG: Mediastinal air-fluid level and respiratory failure. Chest 1988; 94:1063–1064.
6. Gibson RN, Hennessy OF, Collier N, et al: Major complications of central venous catheterization. Clin Radiol 1985; 36:205–208.
7. Lambert MJ: Air embolism in central venous catheterization. South Med J 1982; 75:1189–1191.
8. Ordway CB: Air embolus via CVP catheter without positive pressure. Ann Surg 1974; 179:479–481.
9. Peter JL, Bradford R, Gelister JK: Air embolism. Intensive Care Med 1984; 10:261–262.
10. Puri VK, Carlson RW, Bonder JJ, et al: Complications of vascular catheterization in the critically ill. Crit Care Med 1980; 8:495–499.
11. Peters JL, Armstrong R: Air embolism occurring as a complication of central venous catheterization. Ann Surg 1978; 187:375–378.
12. Green HL, Nemir P: Air embolism as a complication during parenteral alimentation. Am J Surg 1971; 121:614–616.
13. Messmer JM: Massive head trauma as a cause of intravascular air. J Forensic Sci 1984; 29:418–424.
14. Cleveland JC: Fatal air embolism to the right side of the heart during pneumonectomy for carcinoma. Chest 1977; 71:556–557.
15. Tisovec L, Hamilton WK: Newer considerations in air embolism during operation. JAMA 1967; 201:376–377.
16. Campkin TV, Perks JS: Venous air embolism. Lancet 1973; ii:235–237.
17. Hybels RL: Venous air embolism in head and neck surgery. Laryngoscope 1980; 90:946–954.
18. Root B, Levy MN, Pollack S, et al: Gas embolism death after laparoscopy delayed by "trapping" in portal circulation. Anesth Analg 1978; 57:232–237.
19. Young ML, Smith DS, Murtagh F, et al: Comparison of surgical and anesthetic complications in neurosurgical patients experiencing venous air embolism in the sitting position. Neurosurgery 1986; 18:157–161.
19a. Williamson JA, Webb RK, Rursell WJ, et al: The Australian Incidence Monitoring Study: Air embolism—An analysis of 2000 incident reports. Anaesth Intensive Care 1993; 21:638–641.
20. Durant TM, Long J, Oppenheimer MJ: Pulmonary (venous) air embolism. Am Heart J 1947; 33:269–281.
21. Ngai SH, Stirchfeld FE, Triner L: Embolism during total hip arthroplasties. Anesthesiology 1974; 40:405–407.
22. Spiess BD, Sloan MS, Matz SD, et al: Incidence of venous air embolism in total hip arthroplasty. Anesthesiology 1974; 40:405–407.
23. Anderson KH, Halls A: Air aspirated from the venous system during hip replacement. JAMA 1984; 251:2720.
24. Hatano Y, Murakawa M, Segawa H, et al: Venous air embolism during hepatic resection. Anesthesiology 1990; 73:1282–1285.
25. Delva E, Sadoni N, Chandon M, et al: Air embolism during liver resection. Can Anesth Soc J 1986; 33:488–491.
26. Khoury G, Mann ME, Porot MJ, et al: Air embolism associated with veno-venous bypass during ortotopic liver transplantation. Anesthesiology 1987; 67:848–851.
27. Baggish MS, Daniell JF: Death caused by air embolism associated with neodymium:YAG laser surgery and artificial sapphire tips. Am J Obstet Gynecol 1989; 161:877–878.
28. Albin MS, Ritter RR, Reinhart R, et al: Venous air embolism during radical retropubic prostatectomy. Anesth Analg 1992; 74:151–153.
29. Robinson DA, Albin MS: Venous air embolism and cesarean sections. Anesthesiology 1987; 66:93–94.
30. Lew TWK, Tay DHB, Thomas E: Venous air embolism during cesarean section: More common than previously thought. Anesth Analg 1993; 77:448–452.
31. Bower FW, Chandra R, Avery GB, et al: Pulmonary interstitial emphysema with gas embolism in hyaline membrane disease. Am J Dis Child 1973; 126:117–118.
32. Chiu CJ, Golding MR, Linder JB, et al: Pulmonary venous air embolism: A hemodynamic reappraisal. Surgery 1967; 61:816–819.
32a. Morris WP, Butler BD, Tonnesen AS, et al: Continuous venous air embolism in patients receiving positive end-expiratory pressure. Am Rev Respir Dis 1993; 147:1034–1047.
33. Bernhardt TL, Goldmann RW, Thombs PA, et al: Hyperbaric oxygen treatment of cerebral air embolism from orogenital sex during pregnancy. Crit Care Med 1988; 16:729–730.
34. Ryan JA, Abel RM, Abbott WM, et al: Catheter complications in total parental nutrition. N Engl J Med 1974; 290:757–761.
35. Bernard RW, Stahl WM: Subclavian vein catheters: A prospective study. Ann Surg 1972; 173:184–190.
36. O'Quin RJ, Lakshminarayan S: Venous air embolism. Arch Intern Med 1982; 142:2173–2176.
37. Doblar DD, Hinkle JC, Fay ML, et al: Air embolism associated with pulmonary artery catheter introducer kit. Anesthesiology 1982; 56:307–309.
38. Kondo K, O'Reilly LP, Chiota J: Air embolism associated with an introducer for pulmonary artery catheters. Anesth Analg 1984; 63:871–872.
39. Adornato DC, Gildenberg PL, Gerrario CM: Pathophysiology of intravenous air embolism in dogs. Anesthesiology 1978; 49:120–217.
40. Anderson RM, Fritz JM, O'Hare JE: Pulmonary air embolism during cardiac surgery. J Thorac Cardiovasc Surg 1965; 49:440–449.
41. Berglund E, Josephson S, Ovenfors CO: Pulmonary air embolism. Physiologic aspects. Prog Respir Res 1970; 5:259–263.
42. Bedford RF, Marshall WK, Butler A, et al: Cardiac catheters for diagnosis and treatment of venous air embolism. J Neurosurg 1981; 55:610–614.
43. Presson RG, Kirk KR, Haselby KA, et al: Fate of air emboli in the pulmonary circulation. J Appl Physiol 1989; 67:1898–1902.
44. Albertine KH, Winer-Kronish JP, Koike K, et al: Quantification of damage by air emboli to lung microvessels in anesthetized sheep. J Appl Physiol 1984; 54:1360–1368.
45. Ohkuda K, Nakahara K, Binder A, et al: Venous air emboli in sheep. Reversible increase in lung vascular permeability. J Appl Physiol 1981; 51:887–893.
46. Flick ME, Perel A, Staub NC: Leukocytes are required for increased lung permeability after microembolization in sheep. Circ Res 1981; 48:344–351.
47. Gottdiener JS, Papademetriou V, Notargiacoma A, et al: Incidence and cardiac effects of systemic venous air embolism. Arch Intern Med 1988; 148:795–800.
48. Murphy BP, Harford FJ, Cramer FS: Cerebral air embolism resulting from invasive medical procedures. Ann Surg 1985; 101:242–245.

49. Maroon JC, Goodman JM, Horner TH, et al: Detection of minute venous air emboli with ultrasound. Surg Gynecol Obstet 1968; 157:1236–1238.
50. Coppa GF, Gouge TH, Hofstetter SR: Air embolism: A lethal but preventable complication of subclavian catheterization. JPEN 1981; 5:166–168.
51. Michenfelder JD, Martin JT, Allenburg BM, et al: Air embolism during neurosurgery. JAMA 1969; 208:1353–1358.
52. Kashuk JL, Penn I: Air embolism after central venous catheterization. Surg Gynecol Obstet 1984; 159:249–252.
53. Kuhn M, Fitting JW, Luenberger P: Acute pulmonary edema caused by venous air embolism after removal of subclavian catheter. Chest 1987; 92:362–365.
54. Clark MC, Flick MR: Permeability pulmonary edema caused by venous air embolism. Am Rev Respir Dis 1984; 129:633–635.
55. Perschau RA, Munson ES, Chapin JC: Pulmonary interstitial edema after multiple venous air emboli. Anesthesiology 1976; 45:364–367.
55a. Lam KK, Hutchinson RC, Gin T: Severe pulmonary edema after venous air embolism. Can J Anaesth 1993; 40:964–967.
56. Dasher WA, Weiss W, Bogen E: The electrocardiographic pattern in venous air embolism. Dis Chest 1955; 27:542–546.
57. Losasso TJ, Martino JD, Muzzi DA: Venous air embolism in the recovery room producing unexplained cardiac dysrythmia. Anesthesiology 1990; 72:203–205.
58. Sloan TB, Kimovec MA: Detection of venous air embolism by airway pressure monitoring. Anesthesiology 1986; 64:645–647.
59. Glenski JA, Cucchiara RF, Michenfelder JD: Transesophageal echocardiography and transcutaneous O_2 and CO_2 monitoring for detection of venous air embolism. Anesthesiology 1986; 64:541–545.
60. Cucchiara RF, Nugent M, Seward JB, et al: Air embolism in upright neurosurgical patients: Detection and localization by two-dimensional transesophageal echocardiography. Anesthesiology 1984; 60:353–355.
61. Gronert GA, Messick JM, Cucchiara RF, et al: Paradoxical air embolism from a patent foramen ovale. Anesthesiology 1979; 50:548–549.
62. Alvaran SB, Toung JK, Graff TE, et al: Venous air embolism: Comparative merits of external cardiac massage, intra-cardiac aspiration and left lateral decubitus position. Anesth Analg 1978; 57:166–170.
63. Ericsson JA, Gottlieb JD, Sweet RB: Closed-chest cardiac massage in the treatment of venous air embolism. N Engl J Med 1964; 270:1353–1354.
64. Colley PS, Artru AA: Bunegin-Albin catheter improves air retrieval and resuscitation from lethal venous air embolism in dogs. Anesth Analg 1987; 66:991–994.
65. Munson ES: Effect of nitrous oxide on the pulmonary circulation during venous air embolism. Anesth Analg 1971; 50:785–791.
66. Tomatis L, Nemiroff M, Riahi M, et al: Massive arterial air embolism due to rupture of pulsatile assist device. Ann Thorac Surg 1981; 32:604–608.
67. Baskin SE, Wozniak RF: Hyperbaric oxygen in the treatment of hemodialysis associated air embolism. N Engl J Med 1975; 293:184–185.
68. Bove AA, Clark JM, Simon AJ, et al: Successful therapy of cerebral air embolism with hyperbaric oxygen at 2.8 ATA. Undersea Biomed Res 1982; 9:75–80.
69. Catron PW, Dutka AJ, Biondi DM, et al: Cerebral air embolism treated by pressure and hyperbaric oxygen. Neurology 1991; 41:314–315.
70. Ireland A, Pounder D, Colin-Jones DG, et al: Treatment of air embolism with hyperbaric oxygen. Br Med J 1985; 291:106–107.
71. Arthur DC, Marguiles RA: A short course in diving medicine. Ann Emerg Med 1987; 16:689–701.
72. Layon AJ: Hyperbaric oxygen treatment for cerebral air embolism—where are the data? Mayo Clin Proc 1991; 66:641–646.
73. Tuman KJ, Spiess BD, McCarthy RJ, et al: Cardiorespiratory effect of venous air embolism in dogs receiving a perfluorocarbon emulsion. J Neurosurg 1986; 65:238–244.
74. Spiess BD, Braverman B, Woronowicz AW, et al: Protection from cerebral air emboli with perfluorocarbon in rabbits. Stroke 1986; 17:1146–1149.
75. Ellermeyer WP, Keifer P: Central venous cannulation: A new and efficient device. Anesthesiology 1986; 65:341–342.
76. Guggiari M, Lechat Ph, Garen-Colonne C, et al: Early detection of patent foramen ovale by two-dimensional contrast echocardiography for prevention of paradoxical air embolism during sitting position. Anesth Analg 1988; 67:192–194.
77. Peirce EC: Cerebral gas embolism (arterial) with special reference to iatrogenic accidents. HBO Rev 1980; 1:161–184.
78. Neuman TS, Bove AA: Combined arterial gas embolism and decompression sickness following no-stop dives. Undersea Biomed Res 1990; 17:429–435.
79. Broods GJ, Green RD: Pulmonary barotrauma in submarine escape trainees and the treatment of cerebral arterial air embolism. Aviat Space Environ Med 1986; 57:1202–1207.
80. Leitch DR, Green RD: Pulmonary barotrauma in divers and the treatment of cerebral arterial gas embolism. Aviat Space Environ Med 1986; 57:931–938.
81. Kizer KW: Dysbaric air embolism in Hawaii. Ann Emerg Med 1987; 16:535–541.
82. NHLBI Workshop Summary: Hyperbaric oxygenation therapy. Am Rev Respir Dis 1992; 144:1414–1421.
83. Padayachee TS, Parsons S, Theobold R, et al: The effect of arterial filtration on reduction of gaseous microemboli in the middle cerebral artery during cardiopulmonary bypass. Ann Thorac Surg 1988; 45:647–649.
84. Gilston A: Brain damage after cardiac arrest. Lancet 1986; 1:1323.
85. Deverall PB, Padayachee TS, Parsons S, et al: Ultrasound detection of microemboli in the middle cerebral artery during cardiopulmonary bypass surgery. Eur J Cardiothorac Surg 1988; 2:256–260.
86. Kurusz M: Gaseous microemboli: Sources, causes and clinical consideration. Med Instrum 1985; 19:73–77.
87. Murphy DA, Spencer KB: Intraventricular air during coronary operation. J Thorac Cardiovasc Surg 1984; 88:150–151.
88. Robicsek F, Duncan OD: Retrograde air embolization in coronary operations. J Thorac Cardiovasc Surg 1987; 94:110–114.
89. Dick AP, Massey EW: Neurologic presentation of decompression sickness and air embolism in sport divers. Neurology 1985; 35:667–671.
90. Snyder JV: Pulmonary physiology. *In:* Oxygen Transport in the Critically Ill. Snyder JV, Pinsky MR (Eds). Chicago, Year Book Medical Publishers, 1987, pp 304–305.
91. Haake R, Schlichtig R, Ulstad D, et al: Barotrauma. Chest 1987; 91:608–613.
92. Marini JJ, Culver BH: Systemic gas embolism complicating mechanical ventilation in the adult respiratory distress syndrome. Ann Intern Med 1989; 110:699–703.
93. Yamaki T, Ando S, Ohta K, et al: CT demonstration of massive cerebral air embolism from pulmonary barotrauma due to cardiopulmonary resuscitation. J Comput Assist Tomogr 1989; 13:313–315.
94. Ulyatt DB, Judson JA, Trubuhovich RV, et al: Cerebral arterial air embolism assocated with coughing on a continuous positive airway pressure circuit. Crit Care Med 1991; 19:985–987.
95. Dutka AJ: A review of the pathophysiology and potential application of experimental therapies for cerebral ischemia to the treatment of cerebral arterial gas embolism. Undersea Biomed Res 1985; 12:403–421.
96. Peachey T, Eason J, Mosham J, et al: Systemic air embolism during laser bronchoscopy. Anesthesia 1988; 43:872–875.
97. Worth ER, Burton RJ Jr, Landreneau RJ, et al: Left artrial air embolism during intraoperative needle biopsy of a deep pulmonary lesion. Anesthesiology 1990; 73:342–345.
98. Aberle DR, Gamsu G, Golden JA: Fatal systemic arterial air embolism following lung needle aspiration. Radiology 1987; 165:353.
99. Kahn JK, Hartzler GO: The spectrum of symptomatic coronary air embolism during balloon angioplasty: Causes, consequences and management. Am Heart J 1990; 119:1374–1377.
100. Lesh MD, Coggins DL, Ports TA: Coronary air embolism complicating transseptal radiofrequency ablation of left free-wall accessory pathway. PACE 1992; 15:1105–1108.

101. Estrera AS, Pass LJ, Platt MR: Systemic arterial air embolism in penetrating lung injury. Ann Thorac Surg 1990; 50:257–261.
102. Thomas AN, Stephens BG: Air embolism: A cause of morbidity and death after penetrating chest trauma. J Trauma 1974; 14:633–637.
103. Ponn RB, Zatarain G, Gerzberg L, et al: Systemic air embolism in experimental penetrating lung injuries. J Thorac Cardiovasc Surg 1977; 74:766–773.
104. Yee ES, Verrier ED, Thomas AN: Management of air embolism in blunt and penetrating thoracic trauma. J Thoracic Cardiovasc Surg 1983; 85:661–668.
105. Starzl TE, Schneck SA, Mazzone G, et al: Acute neurological complications after liver transplantation with particular reference to intraoperative cerebral air embolus. Ann Surg 1977; 187:236–240.
106. Rapin M, Goulon M, Nouailhat F: Four cases of postabortal neurologic accident treated with hyperbaric oxygenation. *In:* Proceedings of the Third International Conference on Hyperbaric Medicine. Brown IW Jr, Cox BG (Eds). Washington, DC, National Academy of Sciences, 1966, pp 455–462.
107. Frederiksen JW, Smith J, Brown P, et al: Arterial helium embolism from a ruptured intraaortic balloon. Ann Thorac Surg 1988; 46:690–692.
108. Wadhwa RK, McKenzie R, Wadhwa SJ, et al: Gas embolism during laparoscopy. Anesthesiology 1978; 48:74–76.
109. Wolf HK, Moon RE, Mitchell PR, et al: Barotrauma and air embolism in hyperbaric oxygen therapy. Am J Forensic Med Pathol 1990; 11:149–153.
110. Chang C, Dughi J, Shitabata P, et al: Air embolism and the radial arterial line. Crit Care Med 1988; 16:141–143.
111. Black M, Calvin J, Chan KL, et al: Paradoxical air embolism in the absence of an intracardiac defect. Chest 1991; 99:754–755.
112. Clayton DG, Evans P, Williams C, et al: Paradoxical air embolism during neurosurgery. Anaesthesia 1985; 40:981–989.
113. Cucchiara RF, Nishimura RA, Black S: Failure of preoperative echo testing to prevent paradoxical air embolism: Report of two cases. Anesthesiology 1989; 71:604–607.
114. Hallenbeck JM, Furlow TW Jr: Influence of several plasma fractions on post-ischemic microvascular reperfusion in the central nervous system. Stroke 1978; 9:375–382.
115. Hallenbeck JM, Bove AA, Elliott DE: The bubble as a nonmechanical trigger in decompression sickness. *In:* Proceedings of a Symposium on Blood-Bubble Interactions in Decompression Sickness. Ackles K (Ed). Downsview, Ontario, Canada, Defence and Civil Institute of Environmental Medicine, 1973, pp 129–139.
116. Babcock RH, Netsky MG: Respiratory and cardiovascular responses to experimental cerebral emboli. Arch Neurol 1960; 2:556–564.
117. Evans DE, Kobrine AI, Weathersby PK, et al: Cardiovascular effects of cerebral air embolism. Stroke 1981; 12:338–344.
118. Fischer E: Impaired perfusion following cerebrovascular stasis. Arch Neurol 1973; 29:361–364.
119. Ginsberg M, Myers RE: The topography of imparied microvascular perfusion in the primate brain following total circulatory arrest. Neurology 1972; 22:98–1011.
120. Chryssanthou C, Springer M, Lopschitz S: Blood-brain and blood-lung barrier alteration by dysbaric exposure. Undersea Biomed Res 1977; 4:117–128.
121. Helps SC, Parsons DW, Reilly PL, et al: The effect of air emboli on rabbit cerebral blood flow. Stroke 1990; 21:94–99.
122. Fries CC, Levowitz B, Adler S, et al: Experimental cerebral gas embolism. Ann Surg 1956; 145:461–469.
123. Hallenbeck JM, Bradley ME: Experimental model for systematic study of impaired microvascular reperfusion. Stroke 1977; 8:238–243.
124. Brierly JB: Neuropathological findings in patients dying after open heart surgery. Thorax 1963; 18:291–304.
125. Rapoport S, Thompson H: Osmotic opening of the blood-brain barrier in the monkey without associated neurologic deficits. Science 1973; 180:971–979.
126. Peirce EC II, Jacobson JH II: Cerebral edema. *In:* Hyperbaric Oxygen Therapy. Davis JC, Hunt TK (Eds). Bethesda, Undersea Medical Society, 1977, pp 287–301.
127. Warren BA, Philip RB, Inwood RJ: The ultrastructural morphology of air embolism. Br J Exp Pathol 1973; 54:163–169.
128. Waite CL, Massone WF: Cerebral Air Embolism. Basic Studies Naval Submarine Medical Center, 1967, p 493.
129. Kogutt MS: Systemic air embolism secondary to respiratory therapy in the neonate. AJR 1978; 131:425–429.
130. Brown ZA, Clark JM, Jung AL: Systemic gas embolism. Am J Dis Child 1977; 131:984–985.
131. Clarke DB: Arterial embolism. *In:* Hamilton Bailey's Emergency Surgery. McNair TJ (Ed). Bristol, John Wright, 1972, pp 87–88.
132. Albin MS, Hantler CB, Bunegin L, et al: Intracranial air embolism is detected by the transcranial Doppler during cardiopulmonary bypass procedures. J Neurosurg Anesth 1990; 2:223.
133. Spencer MP, Thomas HI, Nicholls SC, et al: Detection of middle cerebral artery emboli during carotid endarterectomy using transcranial Doppler ultrasonography. Stroke 1990; 21:415–423.
134. Stollberger C, Schneider B, Abzieher F, et al: Diagnosis of patent foramen ovale by transesophageal contrast echocardiography. Am J Cardiol 1993; 71:823–827.
135. Jensen ME, Lipper MH: CT in iatrogenic cerebral air embolism. Am J Neuroradiol 1986; 7:823–827.
136. Bayindir O, Parker T, Akpinar B, et al: A 58-year old man had a massive air embolism during cardiopulmonary bypass. J Cardiothorac Vasc Anesth 1991; 5:627–634.
137. Brown JW, Dierdorf SF, Moorthy SS, et al: Venoarterial cerebral perfusion for treatment of massive arterial air embolism. Anesth Analg 1987; 66:673–674.
138. Mills NL, Ochsner JL: Massive air embolism during cardiopulmonary bypass. J Thorac Cardiovasc Surg 1980; 80:708–717.
139. Hendriks F, Bogers AJ, De La Riviere AB, et al: The effectiveness of venoarterial perfusion in treatment of arterial air embolism during cardiopulmonary bypass. Ann Thorac Surg 1983; 36:433–436.
140. Diethrich EB, Koopot R, Maze A, et al: Successful reversal of brain damage from iatrogenic air embolism. Surg Gynecol Obstet 1982; 154:572–575.
140a. Kol S, Ammar R, Weisz G, et al: Hyperbaric oxygenation for arterial air embolism during cardiopulmonary bypass. Ann Thorac Surg 1993; 55:401–403.
140b. Bitterman H, Melamed Y: Delayed hyperbaric treatment of cerebral air embolism. Isr J Med Sci 1993; 29:22–26.
140c. Winter PM, Alvis HD, Gage AA: Hyperbaric treatment of cerebral air embolism during cardiopulmonary bypass. JAMA 1971; 215:1786.
141. Matthews WB, Oxbury JM, Grainger KM, et al: A blind controlled trial of Dextran 40 in the treatment of ischemic stroke. Brain 1976; 99:193–206.
142. Oda Y, Handa H, Nagasawa S, et al: Efficacy of a blood substitute (Fluosol-DA, 20%) on cerebral ischemia. Neurol Res 1982; 4:35–45.
143. Evans DE, Kobrine AI, Le Grys DC, et al: Protective effect of lidocaine in acute cerebral ischemia induced by air embolism. J Neurosurg 1984; 60:257–263.
144. Oka Y, Inoue T, Hong Y, et al: Retained intracardiac air. J Thorac Cardiovasc Surg 1986; 91:329–338.
145. Cucchiara FR, Seward JB, Nishimura RA, et al: Identification of patent foramen ovale during sitting position craniotomy by transesophageal echocardiography with positive airway pressure. Anesthesiology 1985; 63:107–109.

SECTION VII
PULMONARY

Ake Grenvik • Stephen M. Ayres

CHAPTER 70

The Structural Basis of Pulmonary Function

Curtis N. Sessler, MD • Alpha A. Fowler, III, MD

The human lung possesses many interacting cellular and tissue systems that act as an efficient unit, performing functions in near-automatic fashion. Low energy requirements for normal function leave the host largely unaware of the lung's ongoing metabolic activity. The transfer of oxygen from air into blood and its exchange with carbon dioxide is clearly of prime significance; however, the lung accomplishes many other tasks critical for host survival. Lung arteriolar and capillary beds autoregulate perfusion to maximize ventilation and perfusion. Lung capillaries act as "filtration devices" for systemic venous blood, preventing particulate debris from egressing to the systemic circulation. Varying cell populations in the vascular and interstitial spaces of lung are responsible for metabolism of vasoactive substances.

The lung's conducting airspaces (i.e., the trachea, bronchi, and bronchioles) and the vast network of alveoli are critical for the host's interaction with the environment. Respirable bacterial, viral, and parasitic organisms as well as dusts and other inorganic materials are effectively removed or neutralized in most instances by interaction with flowing mucus on ciliated epithelium or resident alveolar mononuclear phagocytes (i.e., alveolar macrophages).

Thus, the lung serves a complex array of functions to maintain homeostasis. Primary lung dysfunction or failure that results in the inability to perform these critical functions frequently leads to admission of a patient to the critical care unit. Patients initially admitted with single organ failure rapidly experience dysfunction or failure of multiple organs; this demands the rapid undertaking of therapeutic actions to support function of multiple organs and thereby prevent long-term organ impairment or death of the host. In many instances, deterioration or failure of non–pulmonary organ function seriously affects lung physiology, resulting in compromise of lung function that ultimately leads to respiratory failure. An understanding of basic concepts of lung function and physiology is therefore essential if a comprehensive approach to the care of the critically ill patient is to be implemented.

THE RESPIRATORY PUMP

Ventilation

Ventilation is the movement of air through the upper airways, trachea, and progressively smaller conducting airways to the gas exchange units followed by the flow of exhaled gases in the reverse direction. Inspiratory and expiratory bulk flow follows pressure gradients from high to low. Pressure gradients from the mouth to the alveoli that are necessary for inspiration are generated by the production of negative alveolar pressure relative to proximal airway pressure. At end-inspiration, elastic fibers in lung parenchyma produce a recoil pressure and generate positive pressure gradients from the alveoli to the mouth, resulting in passive exhalation of gas. Elastic fibers and collagen within lung tissue exert forces that favor collapse of the lung. Resting tension produced by diaphragm and chest wall musculature exerts outward forces on the lung-thorax unit. At the end of passive exhalation, opposing forces governing the movement of the lungs and thoracic cavity are balanced, resulting in intrathoracic pressure equal to ambient atmospheric pressure (assuming airway patency) and, thus, no net gas movement. This balanced state is called *functional residual capacity*, and it usually occurs at about 50% of total lung capacity.

The Thoracic Cage and Respiratory Muscles

The energy needed for lung ventilation is supplied by the contraction of the respiratory muscles. The "respiratory pump" consists of the rib cage and its related muscles, the diaphragm, and the abdominal muscles. The rib cage consists of thoracic vertebrae, ribs, costal cartilages, and the sternum. Figure 70–1 shows the anatomic relationships and actions of the principal inspiratory and expiratory muscles.

Tidal inspiration is achieved by coordinated contraction of the diaphragm and external intercostal muscles; this generates negative alveolar pressure of −2 to −3 cm H_2O.[1] The diaphragm is the primary muscle of inspiration. It is dome-shaped, with fibers radiating from a central tendon that inserts at the xiphoid process and the upper margins of the lower six ribs.[2] Abdominal contents help maintain the diaphragm's dome shape. Diaphragmatic contraction occurs craniocaudally rather than laterally. The diaphragm is innervated by phrenic nerves arising from cervical nerve roots C-3 to C-5. Upon contraction, diaphragmatic flattening forces abdominal contents downward, increasing intrathoracic volume. In diaphragms of adults, slow fatigue-resistant type I fibers predominate[3] and permit significant repetitive work against added loads without fatiguing. External intercostal muscles are innervated by the intercostal nerves arising between the 1st and 12th thoracic vertebrae. External intercostal muscles elevate the ribs during contraction; this increases the anteroposterior chest cavity diameter while accessory muscles of inspiration (i.e., the scalene and sternocleidomastoid muscles) splint open the upper thorax during periods of high minute ventilatory requirement.

Expiration usually occurs passively by recoil of the expanded lungs. During forced expiration, contraction of the internal intercostal and abdominal muscles produces increased intrathoracic pressure. Internal intercostal muscles are oriented at 90° to the external intercostal muscles, with contraction producing caudal rib movement. Contracting abdominal muscles produce inward movement of the abdominal wall and force the contents of the abdominal cavity

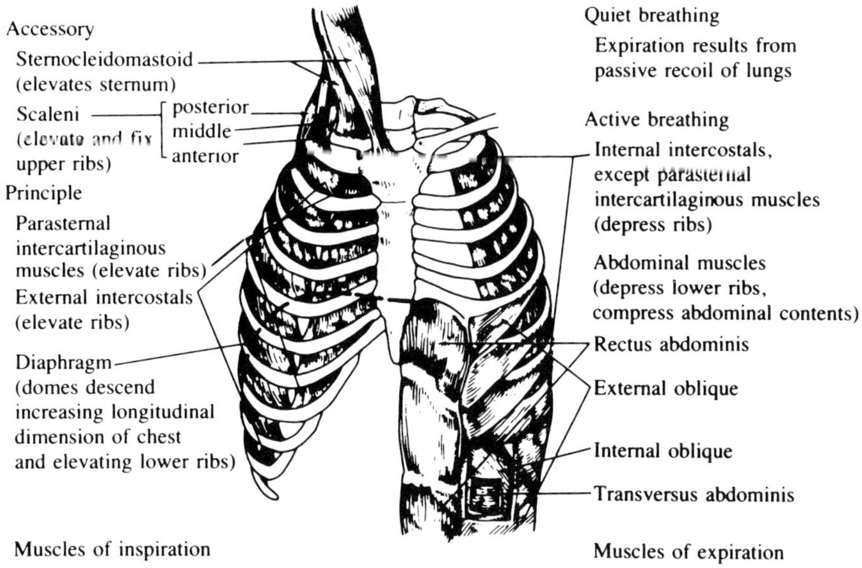

Figure 70–1. The anatomic relationship and actions of the principal inspiratory and expiratory muscles. (Adapted with permission from Garrity ER: Respiratory failure due to disorders of the chest wall and respiratory muscles. *In:* Respiratory Intensive Care. MacDonnell KF, Fahey PJ, Segal MS [Eds]. Boston, Little, Brown and Co, 1987, p 313.)

and the diaphragm cranially. This results in increased pleural pressure and decreased lung volume.[4]

Over most of the range of breathing capacity, the abdominal volume change is greater than rib cage volume change, and this is owing primarily to diaphragmatic contraction. The differences are more pronounced in supine rather than upright positions. At high lung volumes, however, alterations in rib cage volume predominate. With lung disease or neuromuscular dysfunction, paradoxical movement of the rib cage and abdomen occurs, and in extreme cases volume changes of other compartments must increase dramatically to compensate for the paradoxical motion and to achieve a normal tidal volume.[5]

Coupling of the Thorax and the Lung

The lungs and thoracic cage are coupled by a system that maintains close approximation of the structures, yet allows the smooth gliding of surfaces over one another; this minimizes frictional forces and, thus, the work of breathing. The pleura, a thin layer of mesothelium, lines the surface of the lung and the inner surface of the chest wall as well as the mediastinum and thoracic surface of the diaphragm. The "pleural space" between these structures contains a small amount of serous fluid and no air. The opposite resting forces of the lung (inward recoil from elastic fibers) and the chest wall (outward recoil due to tension in the muscles) create a negative pressure of -4 to -6 cm H_2O in the pleural space at functional residual capacity.[6] At end-inspiration, pressure in the pleural space may reach about -12 to -15 cm H_2O during quiet breathing and as much as -80 to -140 cm H_2O during maximum contraction of the inspiratory muscles.[7] During inspiration, negative pressure is transferred to the alveoli, creating the pressure drop required for airflow into the lungs.

AIRWAYS AND AIRFLOW

The Tracheobronchial Tree

Upon inspiration, air is filtered, warmed (37°C), and humidified by the nose, paranasal sinuses, mouth, pharynx, and larynx. Air passes through the trachea into a series of dichotomous branching bronchi and bronchioles, terminating in alveolar structures whose number is estimated at 300 million. Conducting airways, which contain no gas exchange units, include 13 generations of bronchi and bronchioles that conclude with terminal bronchioles. Conducting airways combined with the upper airway account for 25% to 30% of normal tidal breaths and is referred to as "anatomic dead space." Terminal bronchioles lead to 10 subsequent generations of gas-exchanging airways, which participate both as conduits for airflow and for gas exchange. These bronchioles include transitional and respiratory bronchioles, alveolar ducts, and alveolar sacs.[8]

Airway resistance is influenced by airway geometry, flow rate, and flow characteristics. The most important variable is the radius of the airway. Laminar airflow is found at low flow rates through straight tubes, and resistance under these conditions is proportional to tube length and gas viscosity and is inversely proportional to the fourth power of the radius. High flow rates or flow through irregular or branching airways produces turbulence, which causes resistance to vary with the fifth power of the airway radius. Airflow velocity is highest and most turbulent in larger airways and diminishes in smaller airways where laminar flow patterns predominate. However, marked increases in the number of airways with each successive generation yields large increases in total cross-sectional area and, thus, a progressive decrease in total airway resistance within distal airways. The highest airway resistances are found in large, proximal bronchi.

Airway Structure

Airway walls possess concentric layers, starting with epithelium on the luminal surface and followed by a basement membrane, lamina propria, submucosal and smooth muscle layers, and cartilage (in conducting airways only). The precise composition of airways (and thus their function) depends on the airway generation. Bronchial epithelium is primarily a pseudostratified, columnar epithelium that possesses apical cilia and goblet cells. Goblet cells, as well as mucous and serosal glands located in the submucosa, secrete a highly viscous material composed mostly of acid glycoproteins[9] that covers the luminal surface of the conducting airways. This mucus prevents desiccation of epithelium, clears inhaled particles, and performs antimicrobial functions.[10] Submucosal glands are confined to the bronchi, and even though goblet cells persist into the bronchioles, they are more sparse with successive airway generations. The mucous layer is continuously propelled by the synchronized, rhythmic beating of cilia up toward the pharynx where expectoration or swallowing occurs. Cilia diminish in number as airways diminish in caliber, becoming less dense and disappearing in the terminal or respiratory bronchioles. Clara cells account for about 15% of epithelial cells in the terminal and respiratory bronchioles of nonsmokers.[11] The many functions of Clara cells include (1) ion and liquid transport; (2) synthesis, storage, and secretion of lipids, proteins, and glycoproteins; (3) regeneration of new ciliated and new Clara cells; (4) metabolism of xenobiotic materials; and (5) secretion of bronchiolar surfactant.[12–14]

Structural support for airway patency includes cartilaginous plates in the bronchi, concentric smooth muscle, and the tethering action of radially arranged elastic fibers in the alveolar septa surrounding non–cartilage-containing bronchioles. The cartilages of the trachea and mainstem bronchi are horseshoe-shaped, whereas lobar and segmental bronchi are irregular and become smaller as the bronchial diameter diminishes. The amount and distribution of bronchial smooth muscle vary with airway caliber. In the trachea and large bronchi, muscles attach to the tips of the semicircular cartilaginous plates. In smaller bronchi, smooth muscle layers become separated from cartilage plates by loose connective tissue. In bronchioles, smooth muscle thickness diminishes as the airway caliber decreases.[15] In larger airways, muscle bundles are circular in configuration, whereas peripheral airways possess crisscrossing helical bands.

Airway smooth muscle and mucous glands are controlled by the parasympathetic nervous system and are supplied by vagus nerves.[16] Efferent nerve endings on submucosal glands include cholinergic, adrenergic, and peptidergic (e.g., vasoactive intestinal peptide) axonal profiles, with glandular secretions being stimulated more by muscarinic than by adrenergic agents.[11] Sensory receptors from the lung include large airway stretch receptors, irritant receptors, and juxtacapillary receptors, all of which are supplied by the vagus nerve. The lung also contains a component of the neuroendocrine system associated with the airways[17] that consists of neurons and amine precursor uptake and decarboxylation (APUD) cells and cell clusters termed *neuroepithelial bodies.* APUD cells contain vesicles rich in amine hormones (serotonin, dopamine, norepinephrine) and peptide hormones (vasoactive intestinal peptide, substance P, and others), however, the exact function of these hormones is unknown.

Conducting airways are supplied with blood from the bronchial circulation that originates at the thoracic aorta or upper intercostal arteries near the level of the lung hila. Venous blood from the trachea and proximal bronchi enter bronchial veins, which drain into the azygos or hemiazygos vein; venous blood from more distal airways enters pulmonary venules, which ultimately drain into the left atrium and contribute to venous admixture.

SURFACTANT SYSTEM

Surfactant Structure

To prevent widespread lung collapse at resting transpulmonary pressures and avoid alterations in ventilation and perfusion, alveolar structures throughout the lung parenchyma contain a thin film of surface active material known as *surfactant.* Surfactant is secreted by type II alveolar pneumocytes and is composed of phospholipids, neutral lipids, and surfactant-specific proteins designated SP-A, SP-B, and SP-C. Phospholipid components of surfactant are greater than 85% phosphatidylcholine.[18]

Surfactant's unique structure accounts for its surface active function. Saturated phosphatidylcholine is the phospholipid component in the surfactant milieu, whereas SP-A is the major surfactant protein constituent.[19] SP-A, a critically important component, is primarily secreted by type II alveolar pneumocytes as a large hydrophilic, multimeric protein.[20] SP-A binds to phosphatidylcholine, promoting formation of tubular myelinlike structures from newly secreted phospholipids. Furthermore, SP-A regulates secretion and uptake of surfactant between type II cells and alveolar structures. SP-B and SP-C promote accelerated adsorption and spreading of surfactant phospholipids along the air-liquid interface.

Surfactant Synthesis

Type II alveolar pneumocytes are critical to the synthesis and assembly of surfactant prior to its secretion into the alveolus. Figure 70–2 shows that surfactant phosphatidylcholine is synthesized in the endoplasmic reticulum of type II cells and transferred to lamellar bodies intracellularly. Lamellar bodies are then secreted into alveolar spaces in tightly bound, 1-μm structures.[21] Once they have reached the alveolus, the structures begin to "unravel" to form tubular myelin. These substances, now located in alveolar spaces, undergo a refinement process. Certain surfactant proteins initially present are likely removed with remaining surfactant composed of dipalmitoyl phosphatidylcholine, unsaturated phosphatidylcholine, and phosphatidylglycerol along with surfactant proteins. These components are necessary constituents for the promotion of adsorption of surfactant onto alveolar surfaces and for the spreading effect needed to produce a thin film across alveolar surfaces. The processes that control surfactant synthesis likely participate in its degradation and recycling phases as well. In the lungs of adults, approximately 50% of synthesized surfactant is recycled. The processes that control turnover or degradation of surfactant remain ill defined. Excursion (inflation and deflation) of the lung during the respiratory cycle likely promotes spreading of surfactant and modulates dynamic turnover processes as well. Type II alveolar pneumocytes in this schema of metabolism remain one of the major alveolar constituents responsible for the recycling of surfactant.[22]

Surfactant Failure

The consequences of surfactant failure as observed following the onset of acute lung injury (e.g., adult respiratory distress syndrome, widespread pneumonia) are (1) wide-

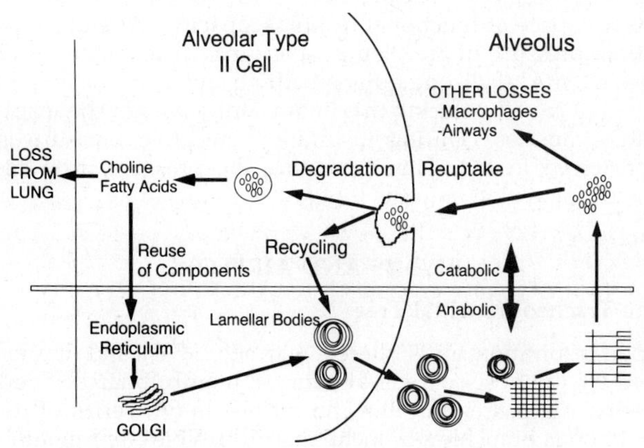

Figure 70–2. Surfactant synthesis, loss, and reuptake.

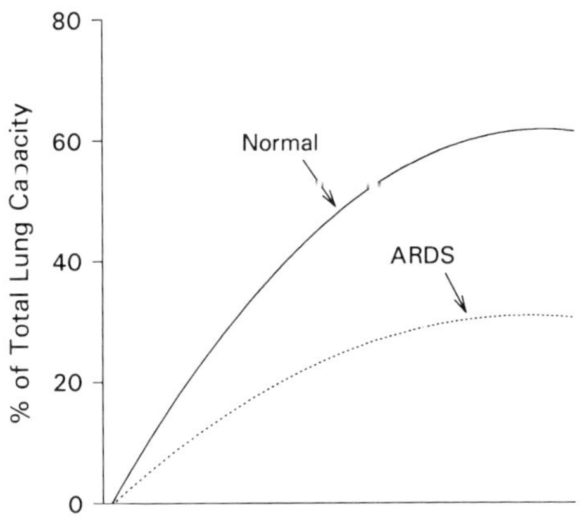

Figure 70–3. Pressure-volume curve for a person with normal lungs and for a person with lungs that contain damaged surfactant (in ARDS).

spread collapse of lung units, with resultant diffuse microatelectasis; (2) significant alterations of ventilation and perfusion with onset of arterial hypoxemia; and (3) increased work of breathing. Figure 70–3 shows a pressure-volume curve from normal lungs and one from lungs containing damaged surfactant. Line B shows the effects of altered compliance with a shifting of the pressure-volume curve downward and to the right. Thus, the physiologic effects of damaged lung surfactant is production of clinical circumstances in which significantly higher distending pressures are required to inflate the lungs to a percent that is nearly identical to predicted total lung capacity.

PULMONARY CIRCULATION

In contrast to the bronchial circulation, the pulmonary circulation is a low-pressure, high-volume system. Mean pulmonary arterial pressures average 15 mm Hg, with pulmonary vascular resistances that are one tenth of systemic vascular resistance. Whereas only 1% of systemic circulation reaches bronchial arteries, 100% of right ventricular output (5–6 L/min) flows through the pulmonary circulation. Pulmonary blood flow is distributed to the lungs via a dichotomous branching pulmonary arterial tree that is closely associated with the airways. In contrast, pulmonary veins are separated from airways and arteries until they reach the lung hilum. Pulmonary arterial walls are thin, reflecting the low-pressure circulation, and contain relatively little smooth muscle. Nevertheless, alteration in pulmonary vascular tone occurs with a wide variety of vasoactive substances capable of influencing pulmonary circulation. Potent pulmonary artery vasoconstrictors include histamine, serotonin, angiotensin II, and prostaglandins $F_2\alpha$ and E_2. Bradykinin, endothelial-derived relaxing factor, and prostacyclin produce vasodilatation. Alveolar hypoxia is a common, potent stimulus for pulmonary vasoconstriction. Reduction in alveolar oxygen tension to less than 60 to 70 mm Hg promotes vasoconstriction of precapillary pulmonary arterioles, permitting redistribution of blood flow away from hypoxic areas. At very low alveolar oxygen tensions, local pulmonary blood flow is virtually absent. In contrast to alveolar hypoxia, arterial blood hypoxemia does not provoke vasoconstriction. The role of circulating mediators in hypoxic vasoconstriction remains to be defined despite considerable work. Pulmonary arteries possess distensibility properties similar to those of systemic veins and are capable of acting as a blood reservoir for redistribution to the systemic circulation in response to hydrostatic, orthostatic, and vasoactive changes.[11]

Distribution of pulmonary vascular resistance differs from that of systemic vascular resistance. Arterial and venous resistances in lung are relatively low; this permits a proportionately larger fraction of total pulmonary vascular resistance (about 35–45%) to reside in alveolar capillaries at functional residual capacity.[11] An important mechanism for maintaining low pulmonary vascular resistance during periods of increased pulmonary arterial or venous pressure is the recruitment and distention of underperfused capillaries.[23] Blood volume in alveolar capillaries is capable of increasing three-fold above a baseline volume of 60 to 75 mL.[24] Contractile fibers and cells identified as *myofibroblasts* are present in pulmonary vasculature as far distally as the alveolar septa, where it is unclear whether they participate in the regulation of airway, vascular, or interstitial function. Alveolar pressure and lung volume may have a significant impact on pulmonary vascular resistance, with increases in resistances being observed in experimental models at low lung volumes as well as after inflation to high volumes. Compression of pulmonary capillaries with resultant increases in physiologic dead space is often present in patients subjected to high alveolar pressures. Positive-pressure ventilation with concomitant use of high levels of positive end-expiratory pressure produces this phenomenon.

PULMONARY INTERSTITIUM

The airspace compartment of the lung and the vascular spaces are separated anatomically by an interstitial space. The lung's "interstitium" is a region where fluid and protein continually pass in both directions—from microvasculature into the lung tissue and from the alveolar spaces into the vascular space. Hydrostatic and oncotic pressure gradients control the magnitudes of fluid and protein passage. Intravascular water and protein must pass across the vast interstitial space from areas with lower oncotic pressures to those with higher ones to bring oncotic pressure gradients to a state of equilibrium. The interstitial space is arranged in a series of loose, binding, connective tissue fibers that contain contractile fibroblasts, immune cellular constituents, and certain neural elements. With the structure of the interstitial space running continuously from the hilar regions of the lung to the alveolar septal structures, substantial surface area is available for fluid transport. A large majority of protein and fluid exchange occurring in the lung's interstitial space takes place in microvascular regions. The interstitial space completely surrounds lung microvasculature that is found in the alveolar septal spaces. Gas exchange across alveolar structures in terminal respiratory units can be greatly affected by the accumulation of interstitial fluid due to either increased left ventricular end-diastolic pressures or to primary injury to the lung's microvascular surfaces. Movement of fluid and protein across lung vascular endothelial surfaces is described by the Starling equation,

$$Qf = Kf(Pmv - Pis) - \sigma(\pi mv - \pi is)$$

where Qf is the rate of filtration over time, P is hydrostatic pressure, and π is the oncotic pressure of the pulmonary microvasculature (mv) and the interstitial space (is). Kf is a value for fluid conductance, whereas σ is the reflection coefficient, which is thought to be equivalent to zero for small molecules but equal to one for large proteins. This equation suggests that lung microvasculature is freely permeable to electrolyte-rich fluids but impermeable to large plasma proteins.

Pulmonary Edema

A negative hydrostatic pressure in the interstitial space combined with tight intercellular junctions and oncotic pressure gradients promotes fluid retention within the vascular spaces of the lung. Increased hydrostatic forces caused by left ventricular failure combined with associated increases in Pmv rapidly overcome these gradients and increase interstitial water content. Entry of low–protein-content, electrolyte-rich fluid is characteristic of this type of hydrostatic edema. When microvascular endothelial surfaces are injured and their integrity thus compromised, a protein-rich fluid moves into the interstitial and alveolar spaces. This type of increased-permeability pulmonary edema characteristic of adult respiratory distress syndrome also is frequently associated with the movement of cellular debris into the interstitial and alveolar spaces.

PULMONARY GAS EXCHANGE

The most important contribution of the lung is its exchange of oxygen (O_2) and carbon dioxide (CO_2) with the environment. Since human tissue possesses limited ability to store O_2 and CO_2, a continuous exchange of these gases with the environment is required to prevent tissue hypoxia and respiratory acidosis. Furthermore, gas exchange mechanisms must be able to compensate for wide variations in cellular requirements. For example, transfer of O_2 or CO_2 may increase from basal levels of from 150 to 250 mL/min to as great as 4000 mL/min during maximum exercise. To produce this range of gas exchange with minimum energy expenditure, gas and blood must be brought into apposition in volumes sufficiently great to permit rapid equilibration by means of diffusion.

The partial pressure of inspired O_2 (P_{IO_2}) is determined by the pressure of all gases (the barometric pressure), water vapor pressure (47 mm Hg at 100% saturation, as present within the airways), and the fraction of inspired gases that consists of O_2:

$$P_{IO_2} = 0.2093 \times (\text{Barometric pressure} - 47 \text{ mm Hg})$$

Barometric pressure is 760 mm Hg at sea level and diminishes with increases in altitude. Alveolar P_{O_2} (P_{AO_2}) is determined by the P_{IO_2} and an estimate of the amount of O_2 exchanged for arterial (a) CO_2:

$$P_{AO_2} = P_{IO_2} - \frac{P_{aCO_2}}{R}$$

R, the respiratory exchange ratio, equals the ratio of CO_2 production (V_{CO_2}) to O_2 consumption ($\dot{V}_{O_2}$) and typically ranges from 0.8 to 0.85. It is assumed that P_{aCO_2}, which can be measured, is equivalent to P_{ACO_2}.

The transfer of both O_2 and CO_2 across the alveolocapillary membrane is a passive process that is accomplished by diffusion. Diffusion is dependent on the physical characteristics of the membrane (it is directly proportional to the area and inversely proportional to membrane thickness), the characteristics of the gas (its diffusivity and solubility), and the difference in the partial pressure for that gas on either side of the membrane. Adult humans possess a total gas exchange surface of approximately 70 m^2 distributed among 300 million alveoli. Alveolocapillary membrane thickness averages 1.5 μm, and its thinnest measure is only 0.2 μm. Thus, gas exchange units are ideally suited for gas exchange with a massive, virtual sheet of capillary blood in close proximity to O_2-rich alveolar air. Diffusion of O_2 is estimated at 40 $mL \cdot min^{-1} \cdot mm\ Hg^{-1}$ and may increase more than threefold as increased pulmonary blood volume and pulmonary capillary recruitment improves conditions for gas diffusion.[25]

Diffusion may be impaired by (1) thickened alveolocapillary membranes, as present in pulmonary fibrosis; (2) diminished driving pressure (P_{AO_2}); and (3) reduced equilibration time (i.e., increased cardiac output during exercise or decreased number of pulmonary capillaries). Isolated diffusion abnormalities rarely impair gas exchange unless the problem is particularly severe. Exercise reduces the time for O_2 transfer by increasing blood flow through alveolar capillaries. When combined with a thickened alveolocapillary membrane, significant hypoxemia may result. Generally an increasing fraction of inspired oxygen (F_{IO_2}) easily overcomes diffusion-induced hypoxemia.

The ventilation-perfusion ratio ($\dot{V}/\dot{Q}$) is a major determinant of gas exchange. $\dot{V}/\dot{Q}$ may vary from zero in lung units that are unventilated but perfused (shunt) to infinity in lung units that are ventilated but not perfused (dead space). In young individuals, the mean $\dot{V}/\dot{Q}$ is 1.0.[26] Within the lungs of normal individuals, considerable regional variability in $\dot{V}/\dot{Q}$ exists as a consequence of the effects of gravity. Both ventilation and blood flow increase in more dependent lung regions. However, blood flow increases to a greater extent such that $\dot{V}/\dot{Q}$ is less than 1.0 in these dependent regions. At the apex of the lung in an upright individual, $\dot{V}/\dot{Q}$ exceeds 3.0 as blood flow falls more dramatically than ventilation.[27] Low $\dot{V}/\dot{Q}$ most commonly develops as a result of reduced ventilation from structural or functional abnormalities of the airways but may result from overperfusion of normally ventilated units, as is observed following pulmonary embolism.[28] High $\dot{V}/\dot{Q}$ results from underperfusion secondary to alveolar destruction or vascular obstruction. High $\dot{V}/\dot{Q}$ may be created artificially by mechanical ventilation that employs excessive positive end-expiratory pressure. During mechanical ventilation, increased $\dot{V}/\dot{Q}$ results in hypoxemia and hypercapnia if minute ventilation is maintained without change. However, in most clinical settings in which $\dot{V}/\dot{Q}$ mismatch occurs, hypercapnia is matched by increases in expired minute ventilation ($\dot{V}_E$), leading to normocapnia or even hypocapnia. The greater the degree of $\dot{V}/\dot{Q}$ inequality, the greater the $\dot{V}_E$ that must be produced to maintain normal or reduced P_{aCO_2}. Hypoxemia resulting from $\dot{V}/\dot{Q}$ inequality responds to a varying degree to increases in F_{IO_2}, depending on the severity of the $\dot{V}/\dot{Q}$ inequality present. When the $\dot{V}/\dot{Q}$ inequality is mild, P_{aO_2} increases almost linearly as F_{IO_2} is increased. As the degree of $\dot{V}/\dot{Q}$ inequality worsens, improving P_{aO_2} by O_2 administration becomes more difficult. Correction of hypercapnia requires an increase in alveolar ventilation.

The term *shunt* refers to blood entering systemic arteries without first flowing through ventilated lung units.[29] Small amounts of shunt are normally present. One per cent to 3% of venous return blood flows directly into the systemic circulation, through the bronchial and left thebesian vessels. A variety of conditions may produce considerably larger shunt fractions. Pathways for shunted blood may run through an anatomic channel, such as an atrial or ventricular septal defect, if pulmonary pressures are great enough to reverse the normal direction of blood flow. Rarely, blood may flow through pulmonary arteriovenous malformations. More commonly, however, shunts result from the passage of blood through pulmonary capillaries in contact with alveoli that are atelectatic or filled with fluid or inflammatory exudate. Increased shunt fractions result in hypoxemia, and hypercapnia rarely develops unless shunts are large and increased ventilation is prevented. Hypoxemia is relatively resistant to correction by means of the mere increase of F_{IO_2}, especially with larger shunts. With shunt fractions of 30% and greater, administration of O_2 in concentrations as high as 100% has a minimal impact on the Pa_{O_2}.

CONTROL OF VENTILATION

Despite large variations in O_2 consumption and CO_2 production and changing environmental conditions, the respiratory system normally maintains Pa_{O_2} and Pa_{CO_2} within narrow limits. These parameters are tightly regulated by the precise adjustment of ventilation that involves a complex network of feedback controls. The principal components of this network are (1) *sensors,* which gather information on blood chemistry (chemoreceptors) and mechanical actions of the lung and chest wall (mechanoreceptors); (2) a *central controller,* which processes this information and sends instructions for making short-term and long-term adjustments in accordance with metabolic needs; and (3) the *controlled system,* within which respiratory muscles contract and relax in a coordinated, efficient fashion to adjust alveolar ventilation.[30] The major elements of respiratory control are depicted in Figure 70–4. Pa_{CO_2} is the single most important factor in the control of ventilation under normal conditions. In the course of daily activity, Pa_{CO_2} is likely maintained within 3 mm Hg, although higher levels may occur during sleep. The effects of hypoxic ventilatory drive is minimal in the day-to-day control of ventilation, although it does become critically important in patients who suffer from severe lung disease and chronic hypercapnia.

Sensors

Chemoreceptors

Central chemoreceptors are the most important receptors involved in the minute-to-minute control of ventilation. These receptors are situated near the ventral surface of the medulla and respond to changes in the hydrogen ion (H^+) concentration of the surrounding brain and extracellular fluid. In conscious humans, central chemoreceptors account for 70% to 80% of the ventilatory response to hypercapnia.[31] Extracellular fluid acid-base homeostasis is governed by the cerebrospinal fluid, local blood flow, and local cellular metabolism. Cerebrospinal fluid is separated from blood by the blood-brain barrier; this barrier is relatively impermeable to H^+ and bicarbonate ions, but CO_2 diffuses across it readily. Carbon dioxide levels in blood regulate ventilation chiefly by affecting the H^+ concentration of cerebrospinal fluid. An increase in CO_2—and, thus, in extracellular fluid H^+ level—stimulates ventilation, whereas diminished levels inhibit ventilation. Increases in blood P_{CO_2} over a wide range cause a virtually linear increase in ventilation. Tidal volume increases first, and increases in respiratory frequency follow.

Peripheral chemoreceptors are located in carotid bodies at the bifurcation of the common carotid arteries and in aortic bodies near the aortic arch. Impulses from these chemoreceptors are carried by the 9th and 10th cranial nerves, respectively. Peripheral chemoreceptors respond primarily to hypoxemia, although carotid body receptors respond to a limited extent to hypercapnia and increased H^+ ion concentration. This response is particularly important with respect to the immediate increase in ventilation associated with metabolic acidosis.[30] Sensitivity to changes in Pa_{O_2} begins at around 50 mm Hg; however the maximum response occurs at a PaO_2 below of 50 mm Hg.[23] Patients undergoing bilateral carotid body resection have complete loss of hypoxic ventilatory drive.

Mechanoreceptors

Three types of respiratory mechanoreceptors exist: (1) stretch receptors present in airway smooth muscles, (2) irritant receptors in airway epithelium, and (3) J (juxtacapillary) receptors situated in the lung interstitium. Stretch receptors lie within airway smooth muscle and respond to lung distention. Impulses from stretch receptors travel along the vagus nerve via large myelinated fibers. The primary effects of activation are the inhibition of inspiration, promotion of expiration, and initiation of the Hering-Breuer reflex (a slowing of respiratory frequency due to increases in expiratory time).[31, 32] Stretch receptor activity is sustained during lung inflation. By promoting full expiration, stretch receptor activity helps to preserve inspiratory muscle function.

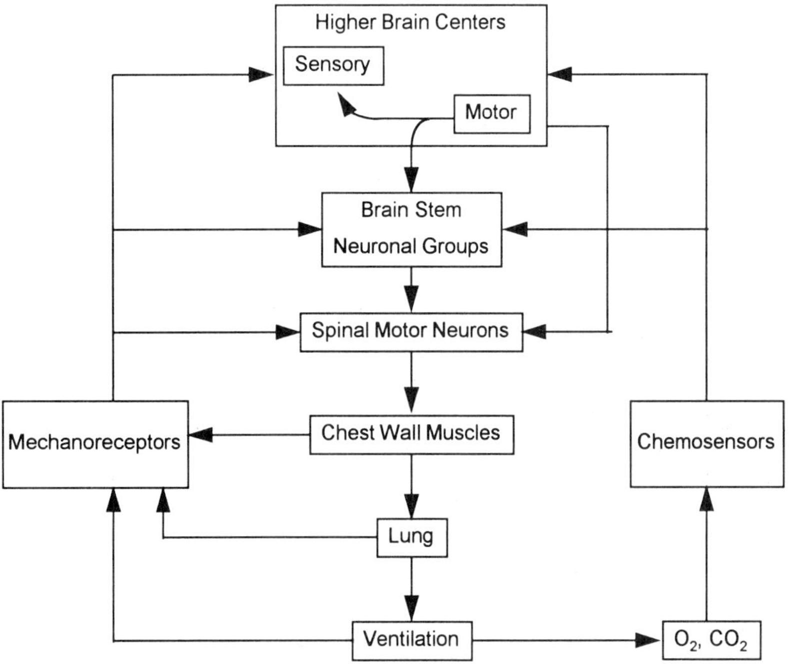

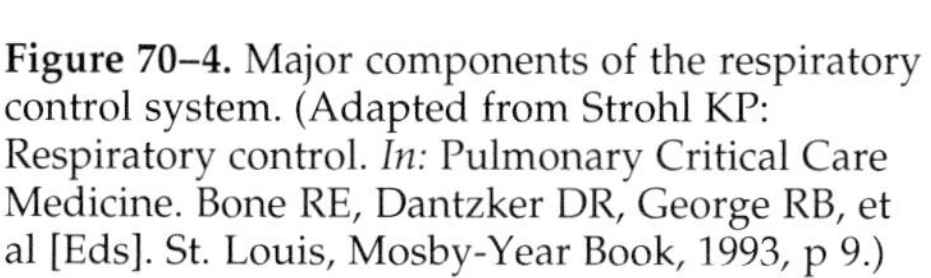
Figure 70–4. Major components of the respiratory control system. (Adapted from Strohl KP: Respiratory control. *In:* Pulmonary Critical Care Medicine. Bone RE, Dantzker DR, George RB, et al [Eds]. St. Louis, Mosby-Year Book, 1993, p 9.)

J receptors are believed to reside in alveolar walls near capillaries and to become activated in response to distention of pulmonary capillaries, increases in the interstitial fluid volume of alveolar walls, or to exposure to chemical agents such as histamine. J-receptor impulses travel up the vagus nerve in slowly conducting, nonmyelinated fibers and result in rapid, shallow breathing. Intense stimulation may produce apnea or laryngeal closure, or both. Investigators believe that J receptors play a significant role in the sensation of dyspnea associated with pulmonary edema and interstitial lung disease.

Irritant receptors lie between airway epithelial cells and are stimulated by noxious gases (e.g., nitrogen dioxide, sulfur dioxide, and ammonia), cigarette smoke, inhaled dusts, particulate matter, cold air, and mechanical traction such as atelectasis or reduced lung compliance. Impulses travel up the vagus nerve in myelinated fibers and rapidly (within seconds) induce bronchoconstriction, coughing, and rapid, shallow breathing. The resultant pattern of breathing, in combination with cough and airway constriction, may limit penetration of noxious agents into the lung.

Intercostal muscles and the diaphragm contain muscle spindles that sense elongation of the muscle tissue and reflexly control the strength of contraction. Joint receptors and tendon receptors in the chest wall also sense movement and thus help to control ventilation. These receptors may be involved in the sensation of dyspnea that accompanies large respiratory efforts. The mechanoreceptors associated with respiratory muscles are innervated by spinal nerves and monitor changes in joint movement and in the length and tension of the muscles themselves.

The Central Controller

The central controller is located in the pons and medulla and comprises three principal neuron groups: (1) the medullary respiratory center in the reticular formation of the medulla, which provides inherent rhythmicity; (2) the apneustic center in the lower pons; and (3) the pneumotaxic center in the upper pons, which regulates respiratory rate.[25] The interaction of cells primarily associated with inspiration and those associated with expiration produces the inherent rhythmicity of ventilation. In the event that all afferent stimuli are abolished, this rhythm continues, although somewhat irregularly.

Breathing is under voluntary control to a considerable extent, and the cortex can "override" the function of the brain stem respiratory centers within limits (i.e., with breath holding). The limbic system and hypothalamus may affect breathing patterns such as that present in highly emotional states (e.g., fear).

The Controlled System

The controlled system consists of the respiratory muscles and thoracic cage (discussed earlier). Controlled ventilation is the result of highly coordinated contraction and relaxation of these muscles. Ventilation is determined by tidal volume and frequency. Tidal volume can be varied by changing inspiratory time or the rate of lung inflation. Each of these factors are separately controlled. Both chemical and nonchemical input affect the rate of inspiratory activity (and, therefore, the rate of lung inflation). In contrast, pulmonary stretch receptors and higher central nervous system structures (but not chemoreceptors) influence the duration of inspiration.[27]

This complex system of checks and balances serves to maintain smooth, efficient ventilation and gas exchange during health yet also responds to sudden stresses and the crisis of disease. Multiple layers of feedback compensate for disruption in one or more afferent pathways. Conflicting demands or signals (or both) coming from different receptors may in part be responsible for the production of dyspnea.

LUNG DEFENSE

Continual assault by airborne particulate matter or infectious material demands that the lung possess well-developed defense mechanisms. Primarily, respirable particles deposited upon central or mainstem airways are subject to physical removal by sneeze or cough mechanisms. Secondarily, particles are subject to mucocilliary clearance that is accomplished by the continual beating of the ciliary ladder. Once impacted on ciliary structures that blanket the respiratory epithelium, particulate matter moves toward the mouth on a thin, electrolyte-rich film. Clearance of particulate material and microorganisms reaching beyond these areas to the terminal airways of the lung is performed by lung phagocytes, primarily resident macrophages, and neutrophils recruited to the airspaces.

Lung Mononuclear Phagocytes

Macrophages constitute the central phagocytic defenses of the lung and represent the key resident phagocytes of the alveoli and peripheral airways that interact with various cells and molecules. Macrophages arise from circulating blood monocytes and, when mature, possess the capability of secreting critical substances capable of controlling multiple aspects of lung host defense (Table 70–1). The interstitial space of the lung is occupied by populations of macrophages (i.e., interstitial macrophages) with slightly dissimilar functions. Macrophages are characterized by lobulated nuclei, vacuolated cytoplasm, numerous mitochondria, and lysosomes. Alveolar macrophages are heterogeneous cell populations that exhibit varied receptor expression and kinetically different enzyme and cytokine secretion.

Macrophages can be considered to be mobile scavengers that are attracted to an infected focus. Upon arrival at the focus, macrophages ingest non-self antigens, bacteria, viruses, and fungi. They are capable of inactivating viable, virulent encapsulated organisms. Alveolar macrophages phagocytose respirable particles from 0.5 to 3 μm in diameter. The presence of surface receptors to Fc fragments of several immunoglobulins (IgG1, IgA, IgE) and to the complement fragment C3b permits the recognition of microorganisms and are essential for phagocytosis. Through phagocytosis and the production of reactive oxygen intermediates (e.g., superoxide anion, O_2^-; hydrogen peroxide, OH•) and

TABLE 70–1. Secretory Products of Alveolar Macrophages

Enzymes	***Platelet Activating Factor***
Elastase	***Arachidonate Metabolites***
Plasminogen activator	Leukotrienes (LTB_4, LTC_4, LTD_4, and LTE_4)
Acid hydrolase	***Interferon-γ***
Oxygen Metabolites	***Cytokines***
Hydrogen peroxide	Interleukin-1
Superoxide anion	Tumor necrosis factor
Singlet oxygen	
Complement Components	
Enzyme Inhibitors	
$Alpha_2$-macroglobulin	

proteolytic enzymes, alveolar macrophages eliminate microorganisms and particles from distal airways.[33] Production of the oxygen-derived molecule hypochlorous acid (HClO) generated through the hydrogen peroxide–myeloperoxidase system greatly enhances the killing efficiency of alveolar macrophages once phagocytosis has been accomplished.

Susceptibility of Microorganisms to Alveolar Macrophage Killing

The ability of alveolar macrophages to eliminate microbes is a function of the inoculum size and of the strain of organisms reaching the distal airways. When activated by lymphokines, alveolar macrophages are extremely active against *Pneumocystis carinii,* cytomegalovirus, *Legionella pneumophila,* and *Cryptococcus neoformans* killing through the mechanisms cited earlier.[34] Organisms such as *Mycobacterium tuberculosis* and *M. avium–intracellulare,* once phagocytosed, can survive within macrophages, able to live for long periods in the alveolar space without the presence of bactericidal antibiotics and represent the nidus of eventual infection.[35] Certain pathogens do not appear to be affected by macrophage bactericidal activity. These organisms include *Escherichia coli, Listeria monocytogenes,* and protein A–positive staphylococci.

Recruitment of Neutrophils to the Alveolar Space by Macrophages

Following the onset of a high-inoculum infection, macrophages often recruit polymorphonuclear neutrophils (PMNs) from the circulation to boost host defenses. Macrophages promote PMN movement into the alveolar spaces by synthesizing and releasing lipid and peptide chemoattractant substances (Fig. 70–5). Cytokines secreted by alveolar macrophages, such as interleukin-1, interleukin-8, and tumor necrosis factor as well as the potent lipoxygenase metabolite leukotriene B_4, all serve to drive chemotaxis of PMN into a site of infection. During the process of migration, PMNs are activated to enhance bactericidal activity by many of these chemoattractant molecules; this provides a population of PMNs fully primed for bactericidal activity upon arrival.[36]

Role of Lymphocytes and Natural Killer Cells

Approximately 10% of nonmacrophage lung effector cells other than macrophages are lymphocytes. Five per cent of lymphocytes are plasma or B cells located in the lung parenchyma. B cells secrete IgG and IgA into the airways. These immunoglobulins play an important role in host defense. In its secretory form, IgA promotes clearance of microorganisms from the tracheobronchial tree, whereas IgG acts as an opsonic protein. Bacteria and fungi opsonized with specific IgG molecules and complement factor C3b are attacked and killed by alveolar macrophages. The factors that control the trafficking of lymphocytes to the lung are incompletely understood, and it is likely that lung macrophage populations recruit lymphocytes to the lung via the secretion of various lymphokines.

T cells are the largest population of lymphocytes in the lung. They comprise CD4 (helper) and CD8 (suppressor) cells in proportions similar to those present in the circulation. Following an infectious (bacterial, viral) or antigen challenge, T cells capable of nonspecific cytotoxicity represent a first line of defense killing in a specific fashion. If high antigen loads overwhelm these initial defenses, phagocytosis by alveolar macrophages is required. Antigen is then presented to T cells. Antigen presentation leads to the production of critical proinflammatory peptides (interleukin-1, interleukin-2, interferon-γ, tumor necrosis factor–α), which result in both expansion of the populations of specific cytotoxic lymphocytes and the recruitment of neutrophils from the circulation (Fig. 70–6). The complex orchestration of inflammatory events as described here promotes a specific response to both bacterial and viral targets.

Metabolic Functions of the Lung

It has become increasingly clear that the lung is an important site for the metabolism of circulating and locally produced substances as well as of exogenously administered agents. This metabolism results in these substances' alteration to substances with modified or enhanced activity or, in some cases, to inactive metabolites. As noted earlier, the lung is exposed to the entire blood volume and has continual exposure to inhaled gases and particulate matter. Pulmonary endothelial surfaces metabolize a number of biogenic, blood-borne substances, including prostaglandins of the E and F series, amines such as norepinephrine and serotonin, peptides such as angiotensin I and bradykinin, and adenine nucleotides and adenosine.[37] The lungs play an important role in the regulation of circulating levels of these substances. Experimental animal and human studies have applied changes in the pulmonary uptake of these substances to address questions regarding pulmonary vascular

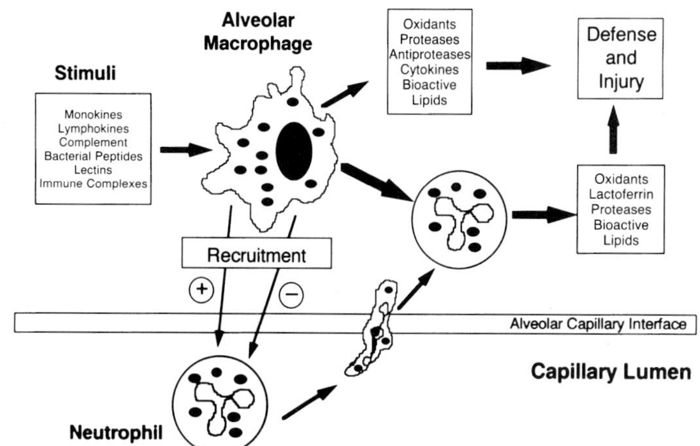

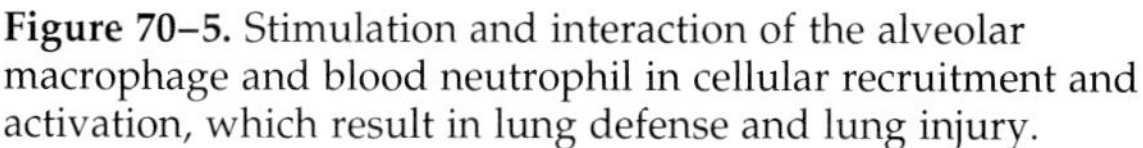
Figure 70–5. Stimulation and interaction of the alveolar macrophage and blood neutrophil in cellular recruitment and activation, which result in lung defense and lung injury.

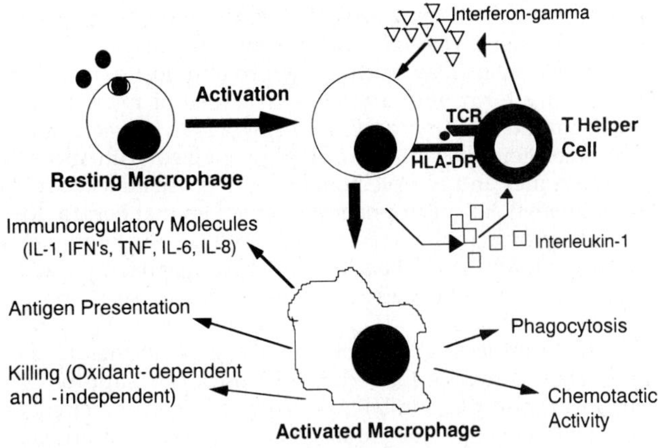

Figure 70–6. Central role of the alveolar macrophage in antigen presentation to T lymphocytes and in primary clearance of invading microorganisms. *Abbreviations:* IL = interleukin; IFN = interferon; TNF = tumor necrosis factor; TCR = T cell receptor; HLA-DR = human leukocyte antigen DR.

disease and endothelial injury; the observations made in these studies may become important in clinical settings.[38, 39] Uptake and metabolism of drugs such as anesthetics is of clinical importance. Surfactant metabolism is also highly important in health and disease.

A variety of xenobiotic—or foreign—agents can produce lung damage.[39] Among the most common are chemotherapeutic agents such as bleomycin and cyclophosphamide, antibiotics such as nitrofurantoin, and antiarrhythmics such as amiodarone. The mechanisms producing injury are varied and incompletely defined but include the generation of oxygen free radicals or the impairment of antioxidant systems. Lung metabolism and the production of oxygen free radicals are also important in other forms of lung injury, such as the ischemia-reperfusion involved in lung transplantation.[40]

References

1. Mecca RS: Pulmonary physiology. *In:* Respiratory Failure. Kirby RR, Taylor RW (Eds). Chicago, Year Book Medical Publishers, 1986, p 22.
2. Anderson WM, Zavecz JH: The chest wall, diaphragm, and mediastinum. *In:* Pulmonary and Critical Care Medicine. Bone RC, Dantzker DR, George RB, et al (Eds). St. Louis, Mosby-Year Book, 1993, pp 1–19.
3. Sieck GC: Diaphragm muscle: Structure and functional organization. Clin Chest Med 1988; 9:195.
4. DeTroyer A, Estenne M: Functional anatomy of the respiratory muscles. Clin Chest Med 1988; 9:175.
5. Rodarte JR: Mechanics of respiration. *In:* Pulmonary and Critical Care Medicine. Bone RC, Dantzker DR, George RB, et al (Eds). St. Louis, Mosby-Year Book, 1993, pp 1–16.
6. Agostoni E: Mechanics of the pleural space. Physiol Rev 1972; 52:57.
7. Comroe JH Jr: Physiology of Respiration. 2nd ed. Chicago, Year Book Medical Publishers, 1974.
8. Bastacky J, Hayes TL, Schmidt BV: Lung structure as revealed by microdissection. Am Rev Respir Dis 1983; 128:S7.
9. Basbaum CB, Finkbeiner WE: Mucus-producing cells of the airway. *In:* Lung Biology in Health and Disease. Massaro D (Ed). Cell Biology. New York, Marcel Dekker, 1989, p 37.
10. Albertine KH: Structure of the respiratory system, as related to its primary function. *In:* Pulmonary and Critical Care Medicine. Bone RC, Dantzker ER, George RB, et al (Eds). St. Louis, Mosby-Year Book, 1993, pp 1–22.
11. Widdicombe JG, Pack RJ: The Clara cell. Eur J Respir Dis 1982; 63:202.
12. Massaro D: Nonciliated bronchiolar epithelial (Clara) cells. *In:* Lung Biology in Health and Disease. Lung Cell Biology. Vol. 41. Massaro D (Ed). New York, Marcel Dekker, 1989, p 81.
13. Van Scott MR, Boucher RC: Current perspectives of Clara cell function. News Physiol Sci (NIPS) 1988; 3:13.
14. Walker SR, Williams MC, Benson B: Immunocytochemical localization of the major surfactant apoproteins in type II cells, Clara cells, and alveolar macrophages of rat lung. J Histochem Cytochem 1986; 34:1137.
15. Ebina M, Yaegashi H, Takahashi T, et al: Distribution of smooth muscles along the bronchial tree. Am Rev Respir Dis 1990; 141:1322.
16. Richardson JB: Recent progress in pulmonary innervation. Am Rev Respir Dis 1983; 128:S65.
17. Will JA, DiAugustine RP: Lung neuroendocrine cells and regulatory peptides: Distribution, functional studies, and implications. A symposium. Exp Lung Res 1982; 3:185.
18. Suzuki Y, Fujita Y, Kogishi K: Reconstitution of tubular myelin from synthetic lipids and proteins associated with pig pulmonary surfactant. Am Rev Respir Dis 1989; 140:75.
19. King RJ, Clements JA: Surface active materials from dog lung: Composition and physiological correlations. Am J Pathol 1972; 223:715.
20. Whitset JA, Hull W, Ross G, et al: Characteristics of human surfactant-associated proteins. Pediatr Res 1985; 19:501.
21. Ryan US, Ryan JW, Smith DS: Alveolar type II cells: Studies on the mode of release of lamellar bodies. Tissue Cell 1975; 7:587.
22. Wright JR: Clearance and recycling of pulmonary surfactant. Am J Pathol 1990; 259:1.
23. West JB, Wagner PD: Pulmonary gas exchange in bioengineering. *In:* Bioengineering Aspects of the Lung. West JB (Ed). New York, Marcel Dekker, 1977, p 361.
24. Weibel ER: Morphometry of the Human Lung. New York, Academic Press, 1963.
25. Dantzker DR: Pulmonary gas exchange. *In:* Pulmonary and Critical Care Medicine. Bone RC, Dantzker DR, George RB, et al (Eds). St. Louis, Mosby-Year Book, 1993, pp 1–13.
26. Wagner PD, Laravuso RB, Uhl RR, et al: Continuous distributions of ventilation-perfusion ratios in normal subjects breathing air and 100 per cent O_2. J Clin Invest 1974; 54:54.
27. West JB: Ventilation/Blood Flow and Gas Exchange. 3rd ed. Oxford, Blackwell Scientific Publications, 1977.
28. Dantzker DR, Brook CH, DeHart P, et al: Gas exchange in adult respiratory distress syndrome and the effects of positive end-expiratory pressure. Am Rev Respir Dis 1979; 120:1039.
29. West JB: Respiratory Physiology—The Essentials. 2nd ed. Baltimore, Williams & Wilkins, 1979.
30. Strohl KP: Respiratory Control. *In:* Pulmonary and Critical Care Medicine. Bone RC, Dantzker DR, George RB, et al (Eds). St. Louis, Mosby-Year Book, 1993, p 1–16.
31. Merrill EG, Lipski J, Kubin L, et al: Origin of the expiratory inhibition of nucleus tractus solitarius inspiratory neurons. Brain Res 1983: 263:43.
32. Gautier H, Boonora M, Gaudy M, et al: Breuer-Hering inflation reflex and breathing pattern in anesthetized humans and cats. J Appl Physiol 1981; 51:1162.
33. Johnson RB, Godzik CA, Cohn ZA: Increased superoxide anion production by immunologically activated and chemically elicited macrophages. J Exp Med 1978: 148:115.
34. Nathan CF, Murray HW, Wiebe ME, et al: Identification of interferon-gamma as the lymphokine that activates human macrophage oxidative metabolism and antimicrobial activity. J Exp Med 1983; 158:670.
35. Reynolds HY: Respiratory infections may reflect deficiencies in host defense mechanisms. Dis Mon 1985; 31:1.
36. Pennington JE, Rossing TH, Boerth LW, et al: Isolation and partial characterization of a human alveolar macrophage-derived neutrophil-activating factor. J Clin Invest 1985; 75:1230.
37. Dawson CA, Roerig DL, Linehan JH: Evaluation of endothelial injury in the human lung. Clin Chest Med 1989; 10:13.
38. Hart CM, Block ER: Lung serotonin metabolism. Clin Chest Med 1989; 10:59.
39. Duncan CA: Lung metabolism of xenobiotic compounds. Clin Chest Med 1989; 10:49.
40. Jenkinson SG: Free radical effects on lung metabolism. Clin Chest Med 1989; 10:37.

CHAPTER 71

Respiratory Muscle Failure in Critical Illness

Dudley F. Rochester, MD • Jonathan D. Truwit, MD

TYPES OF RESPIRATORY MUSCLE DYSFUNCTION

Weakness

The respiratory muscles are striated skeletal muscles that need to be stimulated in order to contract. Stimulation may be direct or via the nerve. The force of respiratory muscle contraction varies with the strength and the frequency of stimulation. For example, when the strength of external electrical stimulation is supramaximal, the force of diaphragmatic contraction is approximately 25%, 50%, and 90% of maximal, when the stimulation frequencies are 10, 20, and 35 Hz (impulses per second), respectively.

The weak muscle develops a subnormal contractile force in response to voluntary effort or external stimulation. Contractile force is lower than expected for any given stimulus strength and frequency. Muscle weakness can result from denervation, faulty transmission across the neuromuscular junction, and impairment of the contractile apparatus in the muscle. Weakness is not reversed by rest alone, in contradistinction to fatigue.

Respiratory Muscle Fatigue

Muscle fatigue is a particular form of weakness that is brought on by excessive work. It differs from other forms of weakness in that contractile force can be restored to normal by resting the muscle. Like weakness, fatigue also has multiple mechanisms, including reduction of central neural drive, impaired transmission of the neuromuscular junction, and dysfunction at several locations within the muscle cell.

Low-Frequency and High-Frequency Fatigue

Low-frequency fatigue is characterized by loss of force in response to stimulation at 10 to 20 Hz. Low-frequency fatigue of the diaphragm may be related to muscle injury caused by oxygen free radicals,[1] and recovery time is measured in hours. High-frequency fatigue is characterized by loss of force in response to stimulation rates of 50 to 100 Hz. It probably results from electrolyte shifts secondary to membrane depolarization, and recovery occurs within minutes. When the diaphragm is made to fatigue by effecting inspiration through a severe inspiratory resistance, both low-frequency and high-frequency fatigue are present.

Fatigue Threshold

When a muscle engages in static contraction such as weightlifting, it becomes fatigued when it sustains a contraction that requires more than 15% of its maximum force. In other words, the fatigue threshold for static contractions is 15% of maximum contractile force. In the case of rhythmically contracting muscles, the principle of the fatigue threshold is still valid, but both force and duration of contraction have to be taken into account.

The inspiratory pressure-time index (PTI) is used to assess the fatigue threshold for inspiratory muscles. The PTI is the product of Pbreath/PImax and TI/TTOT, where Pbreath is the pressure needed to inspire a breath, PImax is a measure of inspiratory muscle strength, TI is the duration of inspiration, and TTOT is the duration of the whole breath. Normally, Pbreath is −5 to −10 cm H_2O, and TI/TTOT is approximately 0.4. The normal value for PImax is −100 cm H_2O, and the normal value for PEmax is +150 cm H_2O. Roussos and coworkers showed that fatigue of the inspiratory muscles develops when Pbreath exceeded 40% of PImax,[2] and Bellemare and Grassino showed that diaphragmatic fatigue develops in normal subjects and in patients with chronic obstructive pulmonary disease (COPD) when the transdiaphragmatic PTI exceeds 0.15.[3,4]

It is important to recognize that overt fatigue does not develop immediately after the inspiratory muscles engage in a fatiguing pattern of contraction. The time to overt fatigue varies with the severity and duration of the contractile effort. For example, it would take 90 minutes to develop diaphragmatic fatigue when the transdiaphragmatic PTI is 0.15 compared with less than 10 minutes when the PTI is 0.30.

Respiratory Muscle Failure

We define respiratory muscle failure as a condition in which the contractility of the respiratory muscles is impaired to the point that the patient develops significant clinical respiratory dysfunction. The usual cause is severe respiratory muscle weakness, which is often associated with generalized muscle weakness; however, sometimes the respiratory muscles are fatigued. Respiratory muscle failure represents a state at which compensatory mechanisms can no longer offset the impact of global respiratory muscle dysfunction. As a result, ventilatory demands can be met only with excessive difficulty, and ventilatory failure (hypercapnic respiratory failure) ensues.

CLINICAL MANIFESTATIONS OF RESPIRATORY MUSCLE FAILURE

Prevalence in Critical Illness

Respiratory muscle weakness is widespread in critical illness. It exerts a pervasive influence on morbidity, the duration of mechanical ventilation, and a patient's length of stay in the intensive care unit. Many patients receiving mechanical ventilation for respiratory or ventilatory failure have extremely low values of PImax, often lower than 25% predicted,[5–7] and respiratory muscle weakness is an important determinant of weaning from mechanical ventilation.[8–10] Respiratory muscle weakness is a significant component of many neuromuscular diseases[11] as well as an important cofactor in the pathogenesis of ventilatory failure in COPD[12] and kyphoscoliosis.[13]

Kelly and associates found that PImax averaged −39 cm H_2O in a group of critically ill patients.[14] Jabour and colleagues found that mean PImax was −49 cm H_2O in 16 patients who were successfully weaned from mechanical ventilation compared with −35 cm H_2O in 22 patients who could not be weaned.[9] In both of these studies, approximately 40% of patients had values of PImax that were less than −30 cm H_2O. Truwit and Marini[15] and Burns and coworkers[16] assessed inspiratory muscle strength at the onset of weaning from mechanical ventilation in 61 intensive care unit patients at the University of Virginia and Vanderbilt University.[15,16] PImax was −10 to −40 cm H_2O in 39% of these patients (Fig. 71–1). Since respiratory muscle weakness severe enough to cause ventilatory failure occurs in one third or more of all critically ill patients, we recommend that respiratory muscle strength be evaluated routinely.

The prevalence of respiratory muscle fatigue is unknown. Efthimiou and associates reported that fewer than 10% of

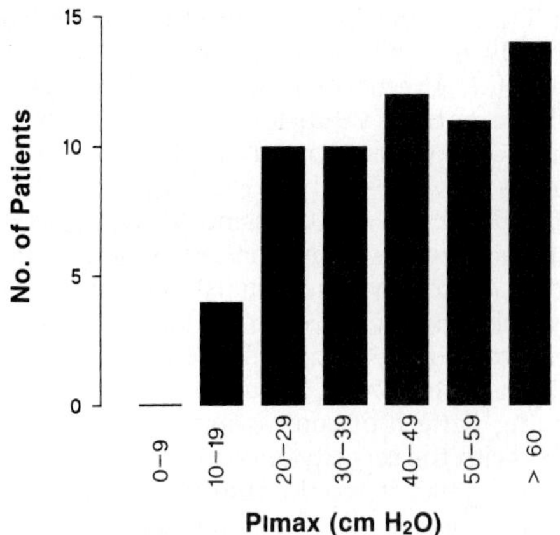

Figure 71–1. Histogram showing distribution of PImax in 61 critically ill patients.[15, 16] Note that PImax lies below 40 cm H_2O in 39% of patients.

patients with pulmonary disease admitted to a hospital for acute breathlessness had overt fatigue of the sternomastoid muscles on admission.[17] The respiratory muscles are frequently in a fatiguing pattern of contraction,[6, 9] but the pattern may not be sustained long enough for overt fatigue to develop.

Pattern of Breathing

Rapid, Shallow Breathing and Dyspnea

The principal manifestations of respiratory muscle failure are rapid, shallow breathing and dyspnea.[18, 19] These phenomena occur in many conditions and are certainly not specific to respiratory muscle failure. The mechanism may be as follows.[20] Weakness of the inspiratory muscles lowers PImax. Diseases of the airways, lungs, or chest wall increase Pbreath. When Pbreath/PImax reaches a threshold level of approximately 0.4, the patient tends to decrease the size of the breath (tidal volume [VT]), presumably in order to minimize dyspnea.

Recruitment of the Upper Airway, Neck, and Abdominal Muscles

Respiratory muscle failure is often accompanied by inspiratory flaring of the nostrils, which reflects the contraction of the alae nasi muscles, and by enhanced use of the neck (accessory) inspiratory muscles. In thin patients, contraction of the sternomastoid muscle may be visible as well as detectable by palpation. Contraction of the scalene muscles may be palpated in the supraclavicular space.

Another characteristic of respiratory muscle failure is asynchronous motion of the chest and abdomen, which results from recruitment of abdominal muscles. Abdominal muscle contraction assists expiration, and the subsequent relaxation at the onset of inspiration allows for substantial inspiratory air flow prior to the onset of inspiratory muscle contraction. Asynchronous movements of the chest and abdomen are often observed in patients being weaned from mechanical ventilation.[18, 21] Tobin and colleagues showed that this is more likely a response to an increase in ventilatory load than a manifestation of inspiratory muscle fatigue.[22] When the diaphragm is very weak or paralyzed, patients experience orthopnea and exhibit paradoxical inward displacement of the abdomen during inspiration.[23]

Contraction of the upper airway, neck, and abdominal muscles indicates that additional inspiratory muscles were recruited in response to an increase in Pbreath/PImax. Indeed, ventilatory drive as assessed by the mouth occlusion pressure ($P_{0.1}$) test is increased, not decreased, in most patients with ventilatory failure.[15, 20] Ventilatory drive is also increased with acute respiratory muscle weakness alone.[19]

Diagnosis of Respiratory Muscle Failure

It is important to identify respiratory muscle failure because it may be the component of a patient's clinical problem that is most amenable to therapy. The first step in diagnosis is to suspect that respiratory muscle failure is present. Clinical clues include unexplained dyspnea, rapid, shallow breathing, and the use of neck inspiratory and abdominal expiratory muscles in the absence of obstructive airways disease. Relief of these symptoms and signs by mechanical ventilation[24] is strong corroborating evidence for respiratory muscle failure. It is especially important to keep in mind that unexplained dyspnea, rapid, shallow breathing, and a low arterial partial pressure of oxygen (Pa_{CO_2}) are characteristic of impending ventilatory failure in patients with muscle weakness.[11]

Pulmonary function test manifestations of respiratory muscle weakness include reductions in vital capacity and maximum voluntary ventilation and an increase in the residual volume.[11] A tendency toward reduction in inspiratory capacity and total lung capacity exists, but these factors are not sensitive indicators of inspiratory muscle strength. Moreover, only vital capacity can be measured in the critical care setting.

The best test for respiratory muscle weakness is measurement of maximum static respiratory pressures (PImax and maximum pressure of expired gas [PEmax]) generated by maximum voluntary inspiratory and expiratory effort against a closed airway. In intensive care units, these parameters are often referred to as *negative inspiratory pressure* and *positive expiratory pressure*, respectively. Substantial errors are made when measuring PImax in critically ill patients[25]; however, it is possible to obtain reliable data,[9] especially when ventilatory drive is great.[15] In neuromuscular disease, PEmax is the most sensitive indicator of respiratory muscle weakness,[11, 26] and PEmax is a good predictor of a patient's ability to be weaned from mechanical ventilation.[27] To overcome the problem of uncertain patient effort, it would be desirable to measure transdiaphragmatic pressure responses to the stimulation of the phrenic nerves.[28] This technique requires considerable operator skill, and is not yet in general clinical use.

COMPLICATIONS OF RESPIRATORY MUSCLE FAILURE

Cough, Aspiration, and Pneumonia

Both inspiratory and expiratory muscle weakness affect the cough mechanism. The full inspiration needed for a good cough may be prevented by severe inspiratory muscle weakness.[29] The compressive and expiratory phases of cough depend mainly on the integrity of the expiratory muscles. Dynamic compression of large airways is essential for effective cough. It is recognizable from the transient spike increase in peak expiratory flow. When PEmax is less than 45 cm H_2O, which is less than one third of normal, bulk expiratory cough flow is relatively well preserved.[29, 30] However, the peak flow transients disappear, indicating that the cough mechanism is impaired. In addition to impaired cough capacity, patients with respiratory muscle weakness may have impaired mucociliary clearance,[31] and they are prone to the development of atelectasis.[32]

Ventilatory Failure

Severe respiratory muscle weakness leads to ventilatory failure (hypercapnic respiratory failure). Braun and coworkers showed that patients with proximal myopathies uncomplicated by lung disease do not retain carbon dioxide until respiratory muscle strength is less than 30% of the predicted normal value.[11] In such patients, respiratory muscle weakness of lesser degree is associated with modest hyperventilation and hypocapnia. When respiratory muscle weakness occurs concomitantly with lung disease, for example, as in COPD, then carbon dioxide retention occurs once respiratory muscle strength falls below 50% of the normal value.[12]

The mechanism of ventilatory failure lies in the altered pattern of breathing, which appears to be a response to an increase in the relative ventilatory load—that is, to an increase in Pbreath/PImax.[20] Although the reduction in VT ameliorates dyspnea, the small VT predisposes to carbon dioxide retention. The normal VT is 7 to 8 mL per kilogram of body weight at rest. When the lungs of patients with muscle weakness are relatively normal, they can tolerate VT as low as 3 to 4 mL per kilogram. However, when COPD and other lung diseases impair intrapulmonary gas exchange, then VT must be at least 5 to 6 mL per kilogram in order to maintain a normal level of Pa_{CO_2}.[9]

CAUSES OF RESPIRATORY MUSCLE WEAKNESS

Hypoxia and Hypercapnia, Acidosis, and Electrolyte Imbalance

The principal effect of hypoxia on the inspiratory muscles is to reduce their endurance for sustaining a contractile effort. When normal subjects developed fatigue of the diaphragm and intercostal muscles from breathing through a severe inspiratory flow-resistive load, the time to onset of overt fatigue was 60% shorter when subjects inspired 13% as compared with 21% oxygen.[33] However, hypoxia does not affect initial muscle strength.

By way of contrast, hypercapnia reduces both strength and endurance. Acute administration of carbon dioxide to normal human volunteers raised end-tidal P_{CO_2} (P_{ETCO_2}) to 53 mm Hg, and transdiaphragmatic pressure fell to 68% of control.[34] When P_{ETCO_2} was elevated to 64 mm Hg, transdiaphragmatic pressure decreased even further to 53% of control. Hypercapnia also shortens inspiratory muscle endurance time.[35] With carbon dioxide inhalation, electromyographic evidence of diaphragmatic fatigue during inspiratory resistive loading occurred much faster than when room air was breathed. In anesthetized dogs, respiratory acidosis has similar effects, whereas the effects of metabolic acidosis on diaphragmatic contractility are less pronounced.[36, 37]

Severe hypokalemia (serum potassium concentration <2 mEq/L) causes severe muscle weakness and acute myopathy[38] and may even precipitate ventilatory failure. Hypophosphatemia can cause severe respiratory muscle weakness[5] as well as ventilatory failure.[39]

Shock and Sepsis

Diaphragm muscle strips from rats with pneumococcal sepsis exhibited a 34% reduction in muscle strength and a 27% reduction in endurance compared with control muscle strips.[40] Transdiaphragmatic pressure is reduced to a similar degree in rats given endotoxin, and this is partially prevented by *N*-acetylcysteine.[41] Diaphragm failure in septic shock is accompanied by lactate production and glycogen depletion,[42] and it can be prevented by administration of superoxide dismutase.[43] Sepsis is associated with polyneuropathy in humans.[44] Chronic infection also causes severe weakness of the hamster diaphragm, mainly by inducing atrophy of type II muscle fibers.[45]

Spontaneously breathing animals in hemodynamic or septic shock die of respiratory arrest associated with diaphragmatic failure.[46, 47] Unlike the situation in congestive heart failure, respiratory muscle blood flow is well preserved in hemodynamic or septic shock alone[48–50] or together with pulmonary edema.[51] Total respiratory muscle blood flow in shock can be as much as 20% of the cardiac output.[48]

Malnutrition and Cachexia

Patients with COPD and acute ventilatory failure are poorly nourished as judged by serum albumin level, prealbumin concentration, or the creatinine height index, and the levels of these variables are lower in patients who require mechanical ventilation than in those who do not.[52] Kelly and associates showed that respiratory muscle weakness in other critically ill patients was correlated with body cell mass rather than with body weight.[14]

Body weight is an important indicator of undernutrition and impaired respiratory muscle function in some patients. Underweight patients whose body weight is approximately 75% of ideal have atrophy of the diaphragm, with a loss of over one third of its muscle mass.[53, 54] Underweight patients have respiratory muscle weakness that is out of proportion to the loss of muscle mass and correspondingly low values of maximum voluntary ventilation.[55] Some even develop ventilatory failure.[56] Values of maximum respiratory pressures in malnutrition and other medical conditions are summarized in Figure 71–2.

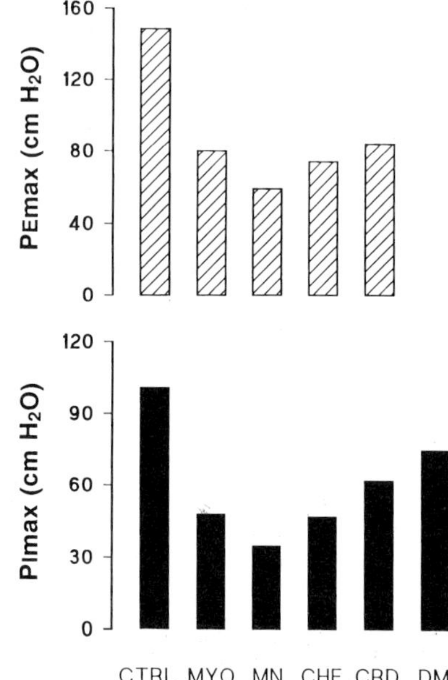

Figure 71–2. Bar graphs showing mean values for PEmax *(upper panel)* and PImax *(lower panel)* in various disorders. Moderate to severe respiratory muscle weakness is common in medical as well as in neurologic disease. *Abbreviations:* CTRL = control; MYO = proximal myopathy[11]; MN = malnutrition or cachexia[55]; CHF = congestive heart failure[57]; CRD = chronic renal disease[58]; DM = diabetes mellitus.[59]

Heart Failure, Renal Disease, and Diabetes

Respiratory as well as generalized muscle weakness is a prominent feature of congestive heart failure.[57] In patients with congestive failure, PImax was 42% and PEmax 50% of the values in age-matched normal subjects. In one third of the patients, PImax was less than 30 cm H_2O—that is, low enough to put them at risk for ventilatory failure. It is hypothesized that the respiratory and limb muscle dysfunction in heart failure results from cachexia or diminished muscle blood flow. Patients with chronic renal disease have a similar degree of inspiratory and expiratory muscle weakness.[58] Weakness in renal disease is correlated with hyperphosphatemia and may be severe enough to predispose to ventilatory failure. Patients with diabetes also have respiratory muscle weakness,[59] although on average this weakness is less severe than in patients with heart failure or renal disease.

Corticosteroids and Paralytic Agents

Patients with asthma or COPD are at risk of developing corticosteroid-induced proximal myopathy.[60] They excrete more creatinine in the urine and exhibit marked weakness of limb and respiratory muscles. A negative correlation exists between the level of PImax and the daily dose of steroid. Tapering of steroid dosage is associated with recovery of strength in several months. Corticosteroid myopathy is associated with high dosage and prolonged treatment. Normal volunteers who took 20 mg/d of prednisone for 2 weeks exhibited no loss of respiratory muscle strength.[61]

Patients with status asthmaticus treated with mechanical ventilation may develop severe muscle weakness consequent to treatment with corticosteroids and paralytic agents.[62, 63] This syndrome differs from conventional steroid myopathy in that its onset is faster and the muscle damage more severe. Suspected risk factors include administration of high doses of steroid given intravenously and the use of neuromuscular blockade.[62, 64] The mechanism is unknown but appears to be different from the neuropathy of critical illness, which also causes respiratory muscle weakness.[44] The impact of this syndrome is profound: patients have weakness of many muscle groups, receive mechanical ventilation for prolonged periods, are difficult to wean, and remain in intensive care units and hospitals for protracted periods of time.

Mechanical Disadvantage

Mechanical disadvantage lowers the effective pressures that can be generated by the respiratory muscles, even when the muscles are intrinsically healthy. Of all the respiratory muscles, the diaphragm is affected by mechanical disadvantage the most. The net effect is a reduction in PImax. Mechanical disadvantage to the diaphragm can come about in two distinct ways: (1) hyperinflation of the lung, which is characteristic of diffuse obstructive diseases of the airway, causes the diaphragm to be shorter than normal; and (2) abdominal distention, such as that which occurs with ileus and ascites, may overstretch the diaphragm.

Diaphragmatic Shortening

The optimal length for the diaphragm is at or near the length that the diaphragm has in a normal subject who is recumbent and breathing quietly. During an active inspiration to total lung capacity, the diaphragm shortens by approximately 30% from its normal resting length. Owing to the length-tension properties of the diaphragm, its ability to generate force at the end of a full inspiration is only one half of that at the normal breathing position.[12] When the lung is passively hyperinflated by air trapping, the diaphragm is shortened before it starts to contract. Acute hyperinflation, such as that which occurs in an asthma attack, causes the diaphragm to lose 25% to 50% of its force-generating capacity. However, in chronic hyperinflation, such as that in COPD, compensatory mechanisms allow the muscle to adjust to the new, shortened length.[65]

Diaphragmatic Lengthening

Sharp and associates found that obese patients with obstructive sleep apnea had impaired diaphragmatic contraction when they were supine and hypothesized that this was due to overstretching the diaphragm.[66] Ascites increases intra-abdominal hydrostatic pressure and decreases lung volume,[67] which indicates that the diaphragm is stretched. This was confirmed by finding that continuous ambulatory peritoneal dialysis decreases lung volume and increases diaphragm length beyond the normal operating length.[68] Diaphragmatic pressure-generating capacity is increased at these lengths with chronic abdominal distention but not with acute abdominal distention. This suggests that the diaphragm can also adapt its length to chronic overstretching. Finally, evidence exists to support that diaphragmatic fatigue occurs during obstetric labor.[69]

TREATMENT OF RESPIRATORY MUSCLE FAILURE

Respiratory Muscle Rest

The respiratory muscles can be rested by providing an appropriate level of mechanical ventilatory support. Most patients with ventilatory failure stop spontaneous ventilatory efforts when they receive mechanical ventilation, and their dyspnea also disappears.[24] During the first 2 days of treatment for acute ventilatory failure, mechanical ventilation offers several benefits. First, it provides rest to the respiratory muscles. Second, it allows for adequate oxygenation while correcting respiratory acidosis. Third, it permits the sleep-deprived patient to sleep. Finally, mechanical ventilation in shock can lower respiratory muscle blood flow and make more blood available for other vital organs.[48, 50]

Restoration of Normal Environment

The initial period of mechanical ventilation also serves to support a patient while other clinical abnormalities are addressed. These abnormalities include treatment of infection, correction of metabolic disarray, optimization of volume status, and treatment of arrhythmias. Oxygenation and correction of acid-base imbalance and of the other factors mentioned earlier restore a more normal internal environment in the body. Typically, this takes several days and benefits many organs, including the brain, heart, kidneys, and liver as well as the respiratory muscles. Because weaning from mechanical ventilation proceeds more smoothly when adverse influences have been eliminated, we prefer to defer aggressive weaning until such time as the abnormalities in the internal milieu have been corrected.

The second step in restoring the normal environment is reduction of the ventilatory load and restoration of as much mechanical advantage as possible. Measures to accomplish these goals are part of the overall management of the patient, but they have specific benefits to the respiratory muscles. Examples include bronchodilator therapy to reduce the work of breathing and lessen hyperinflation of the lungs, diuretic administration for pulmonary edema, thoracentesis for pleural effusion, and treatment of ileus to relieve abdominal distention. In addition, one must be sure that intubated patients have an adequate airway. Endotracheal or tracheostomy tubes that are too small or that become clogged with secretions clearly add to the burden of weak respiratory muscles.

Rebuilding the Contractile Apparatus

Nutritional Repletion

Nutritional repletion improves respiratory muscle function.[70] Total parenteral nutrition was found to increase body cell mass by 12% and PImax by 33% in 21 of 29 patients.[14] The reason for the eight treatment failures was the inability to control the underlying disease process. One would think that strengthening the inspiratory muscles would facilitate weaning from mechanical ventilation, and circumstantial evidence supports this concept.[70] However, we are unaware of a definitive prospective trial that tests the hypothesis.

As a rule, the resting energy expenditure (REE) of critically ill patients is 24 kcal per kilogram of bodyweight per 24 hours. This corresponds to an oxygen consumption level of 3.5 mL per kilogram of body weight per minute (1 metabolic equivalent). To preserve normal nutritional status, it is customary to prescribe caloric consumption to yield an energy expenditure that is 30% greater than the REE. However, for nutritional repletion, it is necessary to prescribe intake to attain an energy expenditure that is least 50% greater than the REE. Approximately 15% of calories are given as protein or amino acids, 50% as carbohydrate, and 35% as fat. Certain categories of patients, such as those with COPD, burn, trauma, or sepsis, have unusually high REEs and may require a caloric intake to yield more than twice the normal REE if nutritional repletion is to be achieved.

Excessive nutritional repletion has been associated with carbon dioxide retention,[70] but this problem has for the most part been solved by scaling caloric intake to energy expenditure. Nevertheless, one must take care not to overfeed critically ill patients with limited ventilatory reserve. This is especially important during the weaning process. High caloric intake either increases their spontaneous ventilation,[71] or it precipitates acute ventilatory failure.[72] It has been argued that patients with COPD should receive less carbohydrate and more fat, but the problem seems to be related more to the total caloric intake than to the distribution.[73]

Respiratory Muscle Training

Respiratory muscle training may be of benefit to the patient being weaned from mechanical ventilation. Examples of modalities include the use of voluntary hyperventilation to increase ventilatory endurance[74] and the application of inspiratory flow-resistive training to enhance respiratory muscle strength and endurance.[7] The results of such training must be confirmed by controlled clinical trials. In order for training or nutritional repletion to succeed, it is first necessary for the underlying disease to be controlled so that a change from muscle catabolism to anabolism is effected.

SUMMARY OF RESPIRATORY MUSCLE FAILURE

Prevalence and Clinical Relevance

Respiratory muscle weakness is widespread in critical illness, and it is severe enough to be considered respiratory muscle failure in at least one third of critically ill patients. The principal risk factor is severity of the underlying acute or chronic disease process. Respiratory muscle dysfunction is also common among neuromuscular diseases and in conditions that increase the work of breathing. Respiratory muscle failure predisposes to ventilatory failure, and it hinders weaning from mechanical ventilation. Respiratory muscle failure impairs the ability to cough effectively and thus increases the risk of aspiration and pneumonia. As a result, respiratory muscle failure prolongs a patient's length of stay in the intensive care unit and hospital.

Mechanisms and Recognition

Respiratory muscle weakness occurs with many complications of critical illness. The most serious are acid-base and electrolyte imbalance; hypoxemia and hypercapnia; shock; trauma and sepsis; and malnutrition and cachexia. Respiratory muscle weakness is also common in heart failure, renal disease, and diabetes. Weakness caused by mechanical disadvantage to the respiratory muscles is characteristic of hyperinflation of the lung and abdominal distention. Clues to the presence of respiratory muscle failure include rapid, shallow breathing, dyspnea, use of neck inspiratory muscles and abdominal expiratory muscles, flaring of the nostrils, and asynchronous movements of the chest and abdomen. Objective diagnosis is based on the measurement of maximum respiratory pressures (PImax and PEmax).

Treatment

To correct respiratory muscle failure in the critically ill patient, it is first necessary to control catabolic processes and to restore the muscles' normal working environment. This involves treatment of the underlying disease—with particular on the control of infection, blood pressure, and volume status—and correction of hypoxemia, acidosis, hypokalemia, or hypophosphatemia. One should reduce the ventilatory load and mechanical disadvantage as much as possible. Examples of modalities to achieve this include bronchodilator use to reduce the work of breathing and measures to relieve abdominal distention.

The contractile apparatus of the respiratory muscles can be rebuilt by nutritional repletion, provided that caloric intake provides approximately 1.5 of the REE. Excessive caloric intake should be avoided in patients with respiratory muscle failure because it may precipitate ventilatory failure, especially during weaning from mechanical ventilation. The application of respiratory muscle training appears promising in the weaning process, but its benefits have not yet been documented.

References

1. Anzueto A, Andrade FH, Maxwell LC, et al: Resistive breathing activates the glutathione redox cycle and impairs performance of rat diaphragm. J Appl Physiol 1992; 72:529–534.
2. Roussos C, Fixley M, Gross D, et al: Fatigue of inspiratory muscles and their synergic behavior. J Appl Physiol 1979; 46:897–904.
3. Bellemare F, Grassino A: Effect of pressure and timing of contraction on human diaphragm fatigue. J Appl Physiol 1982; 53:1190–1195.
4. Bellemare F, Grassino A: Force reserve of the diaphragm in patients with chronic obstructive pulmonary disease. J Appl Physiol 1983; 55:8–15.
5. Aubier M, Murciano D, Lecocguic Y, et al: Effect of hypophosphatemia on diaphragmatic contractility in patients with acute respiratory failure. N Engl J Med 1985; 313:420–424.
6. Pourriat JL, Lamberto CH, Hoang PH, et al: Diaphragmatic fatigue and breathing pattern during weaning from mechanical ventilation in COPD patients. Chest 1986; 90:703–707.

7. Aldrich TK, Karpel JP, Uhrlass RM, et al: Weaning from mechanical ventilation: Adjunctive use of inspiratory muscle resistive training. Crit Care Med 1989; 17:143–147.
8. Tobin MJ, Perez W, Guenther SM, et al: The pattern of breathing during successful and unsuccessful trials of weaning from mechanical ventilation. Am Rev Respir Dis 1986; 134:1111–1118.
9. Jabour ER, Rabil DM, Truwit JD, et al: Evaluation of a new weaning index, based on ventilatory endurance and the efficiency of gas exchange. Am Rev Respir Dis 1991; 144:531–537.
10. Conti G, De Blasi R, Pelaia P, et al: Early prediction of successful weaning during pressure support ventilation in chronic obstructive pulmonary disease patients. Crit Care Med 1992; 20:366–371.
11. Braun NMT, Arora NS, Rochester DF: Respiratory muscle and pulmonary function in polymyositis and other proximal myopathies. Thorax 1983; 38:616–623.
12. Rochester DF, Braun NMT: Determinants of maximal inspiratory pressure in chronic obstructive pulmonary disease. Am Rev Respir Dis 1985; 132:42–47.
13. Lisboa C, Moreno R, Fava M, et al: Inspiratory muscle function in patients with severe kyphoscoliosis. Am Rev Respir Dis 1985; 132:48–52.
14. Kelly SM, Rosa A, Field S, et al: Inspiratory muscle strength and body composition in patients receiving total parenteral nutrition therapy. Am Rev Respir Dis 1984; 130:33–37.
15. Truwit JD, Marini JJ: Validation of a technique to assess maximal inspiratory pressure in poorly cooperative patients. Chest 1992; 102:1216–1219.
16. Burns SM, Burns JE, Truwit JD: Comparison of five clinical wean indices: BWAP, WI, Fx/VT, CROP and NIP. Am J Crit Care 1994 (in press).
17. Efthimiou J, Fleming J, Spiro SG: Sternomastoid muscle function and fatigue in breathlessness patients with severe respiratory disease. Am Rev Respir Dis 1987; 136:1099–1105.
18. Cohen CA, Zagelbaum G, Gross D, et al: Clinical manifestations of inspiratory muscle fatigue. Am J Med 1982; 73:308–316.
19. Baydur A: Respiratory muscle strength and control of ventilation in patients with neuromuscular disease. Chest 1991; 99:330–338.
20. Rochester DF: Respiratory muscles and ventilatory failure: 1993 perspective. Am J Med Sci 1993; 305:394–402.
21. Krieger BP, Ershowsky P: Noninvasive detection of respiratory failure in the intensive care unit. Chest 1988; 94:254–261.
22. Tobin MJ, Perez W, Guenther SM, et al: Does rib-cage abdominal paradox signify respiratory muscle fatigue? J Appl Physiol 1987; 63:851–860.
23. Mier-Jedrzejowicz AK, Brophy C, Moxham J, et al: Assessment of diaphragm weakness. Am Rev Respir Dis 1988; 137:877–883.
24. Rochester DF, Braun NT, Laine S: Diaphragmatic energy expenditure in chronic respiratory failure. Am J Med 1977; 63:223–232.
25. Multz AS, Aldrich TK, Prezant DJ, et al: Maximal inspiratory pressure is not a reliable test of inspiratory muscle strength in mechanically ventilated patients. Am Rev Respir Dis 1990; 142:529–532.
26. Demedts M, Beckers J, Rochette F, et al: Pulmonary function in moderate neuromuscular disease without respiratory complaints. Eur J Respir Dis 1982; 63:62–72.
27. Younger DS, Braun NMT, Jaretzki A III, et al: Myasthenia gravis: Determinants for independent ventilation after transsternal thymectomy. Neurology 1984; 34:336–340.
28. Yan S, Gauthier AP, Similowski T, et al: Evaluation of human diaphragm contractility using mouth pressure twitches. Am Rev Respir Dis 1992; 145:1064–1069.
29. Arora NS, Gal TJ: Cough dynamics during progressive expiratory muscle weakness in healthy curarized subjects. J Appl Physiol 1981; 51:494–498.
30. Szeinberg A, Tabachnik E, Rashed N, et al: Cough capacity in patients with muscular dystrophy. Chest 1988; 94:1232–1235.
31. Mier A, Laroche C, Agnew JE, et al: Tracheobronchial clearance in patients with bilateral diaphragmatic weakness. Am Rev Respir Dis 1990; 142:545–548.
32. Schmidt-Nowara WW, Altman AR: Atelectasis and neuromuscular respiratory failure. Chest 1984; 85:792–795.
33. Jardim J, Farkas G, Prefaut C, et al: The failing inspiratory muscles under normoxic and hypoxic conditions. Am Rev Respir Dis 1981; 124:274–279.
34. Juan G, Calverley P, Talamo C, et al: Effect of carbon dioxide on diaphragmatic function in humans. N Engl J Med 1984; 310:874–879.
35. Ameredes BT, Clanton TL: Accelerated decay of inspiratory pressure during hypercapnic endurance trials in humans. J Appl Physiol 1988; 65:728–735.
36. Howell SJ: Acidosis and diaphragm dysfunction. Semin Respir Med 1991; 12:298–304.
37. Yanos J, Wood LDH, Davis K, et al: The effect of respiratory and lactic acidosis on diaphragm function. Am Rev Respir Dis 1993; 147:616–619.
38. Knochel JP: Neuromuscular manifestations of electrolyte disorders. Am J Med 1982; 72:521–535.
39. Newman JH, Neff TA, Ziporin P: Acute respiratory failure associated with hypophosphatemia. N Engl J Med 1977; 296:1101–1103.
40. Boczkowski J, Dureuil B, Branger C, et al: Effects of sepsis on diaphragmatic function in rats. Am Rev Respir Dis 1988; 138:260–265.
41. Van Surell C, Boczkowski J, Pasquier C, et al: Effects of *N*-acetylcysteine on diaphragmatic function and malonaldehyde content in *Escherichia coli* endotoxemic rats. Am Rev Respir Dis 1992; 146:730–734.
42. Hussain SNA, Graham R, Rutledge F, et al: Respiratory muscle energetics during endotoxic shock in dogs. J Appl Physiol 1986; 60:486–493.
43. Nashawati E, DiMarco A, Supinski G: Effects produced by infusion of a free radical–generating solution into the diaphragm. Am Rev Respir Dis 1993; 147:60–65.
44. Witt NJ, Zochodne DW, Bolton CF, et al: Peripheral nerve function in sepsis and multiple organ failure. Chest 1991; 99:176–184.
45. Drew JS, Farkas GA, Pearson RD, et al: Effects of a chronic wasting infection on skeletal muscle size and contractile properties. J Appl Physiol 1988; 64:460–465.
46. Aubier M, Trippenbach T, Roussos C: Respiratory muscle fatigue during cardiogenic shock. J Appl Physiol 1981; 51:499–508.
47. Hussain SNA, Simkus G, Roussos C: Respiratory muscle fatigue: A cause of ventilatory failure in septic shock. J Appl Physiol 1985; 58:2033–2040.
48. Viires N, Sillye S, Aubier M, et al: Regional blood flow distribution in dog during induced hypotension and low cardiac output: Spontaneous breathing versus artificial ventilation. J Clin Invest 1983; 72:935–947.
49. Scharf SM, Bark H, Einhorn S, et al: Blood flow to the canine diaphragm during hemorrhagic shock. Am Rev Respir Dis 1986; 133:205–211.
50. Hussain SNA, Roussos C: Distribution of respiratory muscle blood and organ blood flow during endotoxic shock in dogs. J Appl Physiol 1985; 59:1802–1808.
51. Rutledge FS, Hussain SN, Roussos Ch, et al: Diaphragmatic energetics and blood flow during pulmonary edema and hypotension. J Appl Physiol 1988; 64:1908–1915.
52. Laaban J-P, Kouchakji B, Dore M-F, et al: Nutritional status of patients with chronic obstructive pulmonary disease and acute respiratory failure. Chest 1993; 103:1362–1368.
53. Arora NS, Rochester DF: Effect of body weight and muscularity on human diaphragm muscle mass, thickness, and area. J Appl Physiol 1982; 52:64–70.
54. Arora NS, Rochester DF: COPD and human diaphragm muscle dimensions. Chest 1987; 91:719–724.
55. Arora NS, Rochester DF: Respiratory muscle strength and maximal voluntary ventilation in undernourished patients. Am Rev Respir Dis 1982; 126:5–8.
56. Ryan CF, Whittaker JS, Road JD: Ventilatory dysfunction in severe anorexia nervosa. Chest 1992; 102:1268–1288.
57. Hammond MJ, Bauer KA, Sharp JT, et al: Respiratory muscle strength in congestive heart failure. Chest 1990; 98:1091–1094.
58. Bark H, Heimer D, Chaimovitz C, et al: Effect of chronic renal failure on respiratory muscle strength. Respiration 1988; 54:153–161.
59. Wanke T, Formanek D, Auinger M, et al: Inspiratory muscle

performance and pulmonary function changes in insulin-dependent diabetes mellitus. Am Rev Respir Dis 1991; 143:97–100.
60. Decramer M, Stas KJ: Corticosteroid-induced myopathy involving respiratory muscles in patients with chronic obstructive pulmonary disease or asthma. Am Rev Respir Dis 1992; 146:800–802.
61. Wang Y, Zintel T, Vasquez A, et al: Corticosteroid therapy and respiratory muscle function in humans. Am Rev Respir Dis 1991; 144:108–112.
62. Douglass JA, Tuxen DV, Horne M, et al: Myopathy in severe asthma. Am Rev Respir Dis 1992; 146:517–519.
63. Griffin D, Fairman N, Coursin D, et al: Acute myopathy during treatment of status asthmaticus with corticosteroids and steroidal muscle relaxants. Chest 1992; 102:510–514.
64. Kupfer Y, Namba T, Kaldawi E, et al: Prolonged weakness after long-term infusion of vecuronium bromide. Ann Intern Med 1992; 117:484–486.
65. Similowski T, Yan S, Gauthier AP, et al: Contractile properties of the human diaphragm during chronic hyperinflation. N Engl J Med 1991; 325:917–923.
66. Sharp JT, Druz WS, Kondragunta VR: Diaphragmatic responses to body position changes in obese patients with obstructive sleep apnea. Am Rev Respir Dis 1986; 133:32–37.
67. Hanson CA, Ritter AB, Duran W, et al: Ascites: Its effect upon static inflation of the respiratory system. Am Rev Respir Dis 1990; 142:39–42.
68. Prezant DJ, Aldrich TK, Karpel JP, et al: Adaptations in diaphragm's in vivo force-length relationship in patients on continuous ambulatory peritoneal dialysis. Am Rev Respir Dis 1990; 141:1342–1349.
69. Nava S, Zanotti E, Ambrosino N, et al: Evidence of acute diaphragmatic fatigue in a "natural" condition. Am Rev Respir Dis 1992; 146:1226–1230.
70. Rochester DF: Nutritional repletion. Semin Respir Med 1992; 13:44–52.
71. Laaban J-P, Lemaire F, Baron JF, et al: Influence of caloric intake on the respiratory mode during mandatory minute volume ventilation. Chest 1985; 87:67–72.
72. Dark DS, Pingleton SK, Kerby GR: Hypercapnia during weaning: A complication of nutritional support. Chest 1985; 88:141–143.
73. Talpers SS, Romberger DJ, Bunce SB, et al: Nutritionally associated increased carbon dioxide production: Excess total calories vs high proportion of carbohydrate calories. Chest 1992; 102:551–555.
74. Belman MJ: Respiratory failure treated by ventilatory muscle training (VMT): A report of two cases. Eur J Respir Dis 1981; 62:391–395.

CHAPTER 72

The Work of Breathing

John W. Kreit, MD • Robert M. Rogers, MD

The primary function of the respiratory system, which consists of the lungs and chest wall, is to supply oxygen to and remove carbon dioxide from the mixed venous blood entering the lungs. For this to occur, two interrelated processes are essential: (1) *gas exchange,* which is the transfer of oxygen and carbon dioxide between the alveolar gas and the pulmonary capillary blood; and (2) *ventilation,* which is the repetitive movement of gas into and out of the lungs. Ventilation delivers the oxygen and removes the carbon dioxide that is exchanged across the alveolocapillary interface.

For ventilation to occur, the respiratory system must alternately expand above and then return to its equilibrium position. This is possible only when sufficient force is provided to overcome two opposing forces, elastic recoil and flow resistance. The elastic recoil of the respiratory system is measured under static conditions as the pressure required to maintain the passive thorax at a given volume. During inspiration and expiration, additional pressure must be provided to overcome frictional or flow-resistive forces that are produced primarily by the flow of gas in the airways but also by the movement of the lung parenchyma and chest wall.

The respiratory muscles normally provide the force required for inspiration. Expiration is usually passive, with expiratory flow driven by the elastic recoil of the respiratory system. However, in the setting of high ventilation requirements or increased airway resistance, expiratory muscles may also become active. The respiratory muscles, therefore, normally perform the work of breathing. Here, the term "work" is used in a generic sense because, as discussed in the next section, this term has a very specific definition. When the respiratory muscles are unable to generate sufficient force to provide adequate ventilation, respiratory failure occurs, and the work of breathing must be partially or completely assumed by a mechanical ventilator. This chapter discusses the measurements used to quantify the work of breathing or, more accurately, the activity of the respiratory muscles. It also reviews our current knowledge about respiratory muscle activity in critically ill patients during both spontaneous and mechanical ventilation.

MEASURES OF RESPIRATORY MUSCLE ACTIVITY

Work

By definition, work has been performed when a force results in the movement of an object. The work (W) is calculated as the product of force (F) and the length (L) or distance that the object was moved: $W = F \cdot L$. This definition can be extended to refer to fluid-filled or air-filled systems (e.g., the respiratory system) by noting that force equals the product of pressure (P) and area, and area multiplied by length equals volume (V). Work then becomes equal to $P \cdot V$ or $\int PdV$ (the d indicates that pressure is being integrated with respect to volume).[1]

In practice, the work performed on the respiratory system is calculated either by computerized integration of pressure and volume measurements obtained at a high-frequency or by actual measurement of the area enclosed by pressure-volume curves. Work is expressed in a variety of units, with joules (J) being the most popular in clinical studies ($1\ J = 10\ cm\ H_2O \cdot L$). Values may be listed as work per liter of ventilation (J/L) or work per minute (J/min). Work expressed per unit time is referred to as *power.*

The work performed on the respiratory system is calculated by measuring the transstructural pressure gradient and the volume change produced by it. If pleural pressure is estimated by means of an esophageal balloon, the work required to inflate the lungs (W_L) and expand the chest wall (Wcw) can be calculated separately from the following equations:

$$W_L = \int (Paw - Pes)\, dV \quad \text{[Equation 1]}$$

$$Wcw = \int (Pes - Patm)\, dV \quad \text{[Equation 2]}$$

where Paw, Pes, and Patm are central airway, esophageal, and atmospheric pressure, respectively. The total work performed on the respiratory system is then the sum of these two values. It is important to emphasize that work can be calculated only when Equations 1 and 2 contain the pressure gradients that actually produce the observed change in volume. Because of this requirement, the actual techniques used to measure the work performed by the respiratory muscles vary, depending on whether a patient is breathing spontaneously or receiving assisted mechanical ventilation. Since expiratory work is usually of relatively low magnitude and is not commonly measured in clinical studies, only the work performed during inspiration is discussed in this chapter.

Spontaneous Ventilation

During spontaneous breathing, the force required for ventilation is provided entirely by the respiratory muscles. Since the pressure acting to distend the lungs is Paw − Pes, W_L can be calculated by using Equation 1. The work required to inflate the lungs alone is shown in Figure 72–1 as the area enclosed by the esophageal pressure–volume curve. Total work may be divided into the components used to overcome elastic recoil and flow-resistance either mathematically, by measuring Pes during stepwise inflation (when Pes equals the elastic recoil pressure of the lungs), or graphically by connecting the points of zero flow.[1]

During spontaneous ventilation, the work performed on the chest wall cannot be directly measured. This is because the pressure gradient across the chest wall (Pes − Patm) is not acting to distend it. In fact, this value progressively decreases as the chest wall expands during a spontaneous inspiration. The work performed on the chest wall can, however, be estimated by measuring Pes during stepwise increases in the volume of the relaxed respiratory system. Alternatively, in intubated patients, Pes may be measured continuously during a passive (controlled) mechanical inflation under these conditions. Pes progressively increases, Pes − Patm becomes the relevant transstructural pressure, and the work required to expand the chest wall may be calculated using Equation 2. The work of chest wall expansion is illustrated in Figure 72–2. Note that work is performed on the chest wall only when Pes becomes positive. When Pes is negative, the outward elastic recoil of the chest wall actually assists inspiration.[1]

The total work performed by the respiratory muscles during spontaneous ventilation is, therefore, calculated by measuring Pes during both active and passive inflation. Graphically, total work is equal to the area between these two esophageal pressure-volume curves (Fig. 72–3). Note in this illustration that, because of the elastic recoil of the chest wall, the work required to expand the entire respiratory system is less than the work needed to inflate the lungs alone.

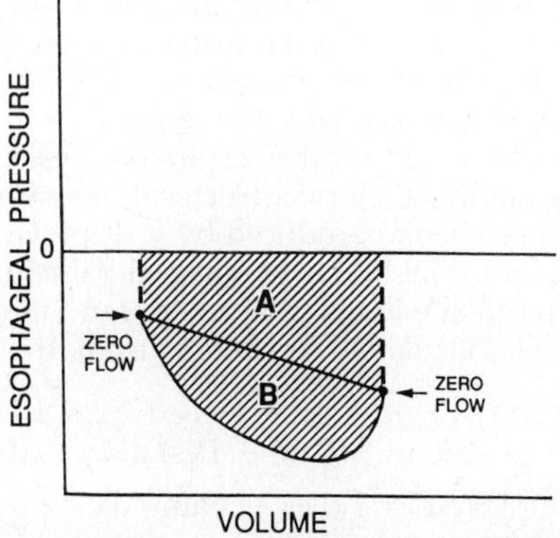

Figure 72–1. Schematic diagram of esophageal pressure versus volume during a spontaneous inspiration. The total work performed to inflate the lungs alone is defined by the *cross-hatched area.* A line connecting the points of zero flow divides total work into the portions required to overcome the elastic recoil *(area A)* and flow-resistance *(area B)* of the lungs and airways.

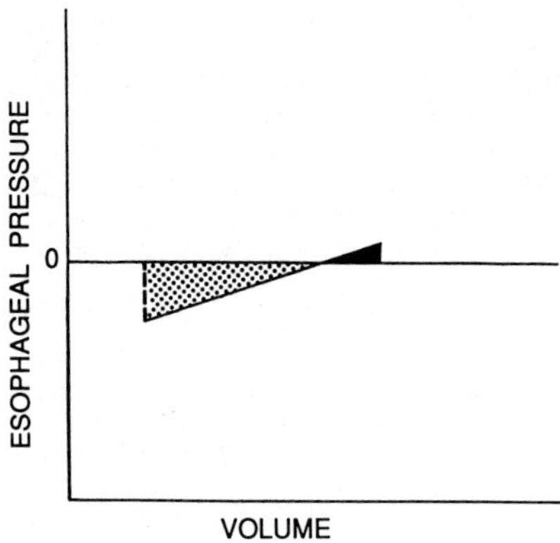

Figure 72–2. Plot of esophageal pressure (Pes) and volume during a controlled mechanical inflation. Work is performed on the chest wall *(solid area)* only when it is expanded beyond its equilibrium position (Pes > 0). When esophageal pressure is negative, the outward elastic recoil of the chest wall assists with the work of inflating the respiratory system *(stippled area).*

Assisted Mechanical Ventilation

In this chapter, the term "assisted mechanical ventilation" is used to denote those modes of mechanical support in which inspiration is triggered by patient effort. The more commonly used assisted mechanical ventilation modes are assist-control ventilation, synchronized intermittent mandatory ventilation, and pressure support ventilation. During assisted mechanical ventilation, the pressure required for ventilation is generated jointly by the ventilator and the respiratory muscles. Two methods are available for calculating the work performed by the patient. The first is identical to the technique described earlier—that is, the work performed by the respiratory muscles on the lungs and chest wall is equal to the area enclosed by plots of esophageal pressure and volume during assisted and controlled mechanical breaths. The second method is applicable only to the assist-control ventilation and synchronized intermittent mandatory ventilation modes. During a mechanical inflation, Paw − Pes and Pes − Patm are the relevant pressures acting to distend the lungs and chest wall respectively.

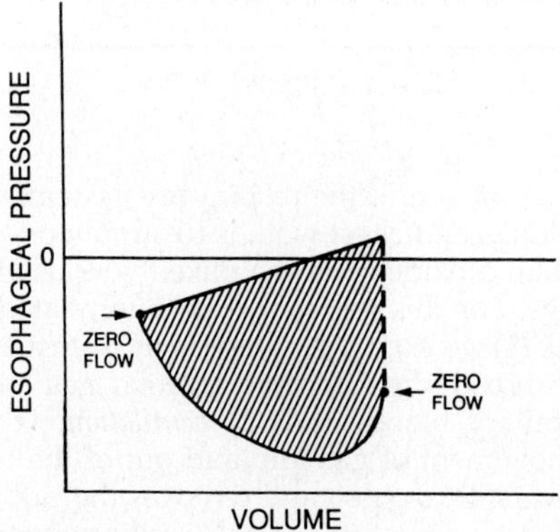

Figure 72–3. The work performed on the entire respiratory system during a spontaneous inspiration. This figure combines the esophageal pressure curves shown in Figures 72–1 and 72–2.

Equations 1 and 2 can, therefore, be added together to yield an expression for the total work performed by the ventilator (Wv):

$$Wv = \int (Paw - Pes)\, dV + \int (Pes - Patm)\, dV \quad \text{[Equation 3]}$$

or

$$Wv = \int (Paw - Patm)\, dV \quad \text{[Equation 4]}$$

If Patm is considered to be zero, Equation 4 can be reduced to

$$Wv = \int Paw\, dV \quad \text{[Equation 5]}$$

The work performed by the ventilator is, therefore, equal to the area enclosed by the airway pressure-volume curve. During a controlled mechanical inflation, the respiratory muscles are assumed to be at rest, and Wv equals the total work required to inflate the respiratory system. During an assisted, volume-set (volume-cycled) mechanical breath, airway pressure and the work required of the ventilator will be lowered by an amount that is dependent on the patient's inspiratory effort. The work performed by the patient should then be the difference between the ventilator work performed during controlled and assisted mechanical breaths of identical tidal volume and flow rate.[2, 3]

These two methods are illustrated in Figure 72–4. During assist-control ventilation and synchronized intermittent mandatory ventilation, patient work is equal to the area enclosed by either airway or esophageal pressure-volume curves obtained during assisted and controlled mechanical breaths.

During pressure support ventilation, all breaths are patient initiated (i.e., there are no controlled breaths), and airway pressure does not vary significantly with patient effort. With this mode of ventilation, therefore, patient work of breathing can be calculated only by measuring esophageal pressure.

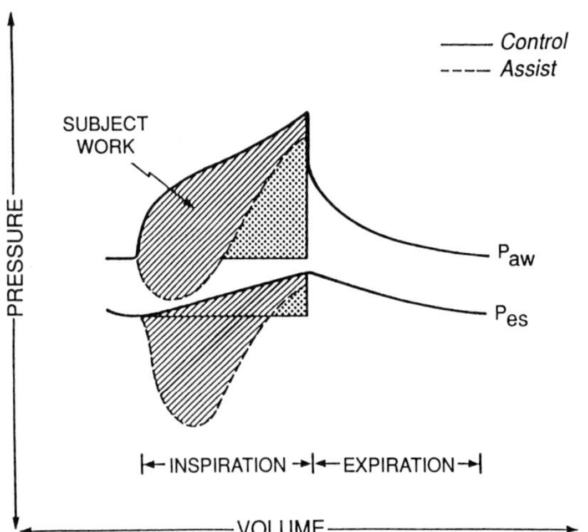

Figure 72–4. Schematic diagram of airway (Paw) and esophageal (Pes) pressure-volume curves obtained during performance of assisted and controlled mechanical breaths having equal tidal volumes and flow rates. The total work performed by the patient during inspiration *(cross-hatched area)* may be calculated using either Paw or Pes. (Modified from Marini JJ: Monitoring during mechanical ventilation. Clin Chest Med 1988; 9:73.)

Respiratory Muscle Efficiency

Although work is the most commonly used measure of patient respiratory effort, the activity of the respiratory muscles is, in fact, best equated with the energy expended during contraction. The ratio of work performed to energy consumed (e) is defined as the muscle efficiency (E): E = W/e. Thus, work is a fixed proportion of energy expenditure and normally provides a good indication of respiratory muscle activity and patient effort. When the efficiency of the respiratory muscles is abnormally low, however, work measurements correlate poorly with respiratory muscle activity. The most common example of this is the effect of hyperinflation on diaphragm function. As end-expiratory lung volume increases, the diaphragm flattens and its muscle fibers shorten. Both of these effects decrease efficiency—the former by reducing the inspiratory action of the diaphragm on the chest wall, and the latter by decreasing the tension developed by muscle contraction. To perform a required amount of work, the diaphragm must, therefore, increase its energy expenditure.

Isometric muscle contraction represents the most extreme example of the dissociation between work and muscle activity. Since, by definition, work is performed on the respiratory system only when there is a change in volume, muscle contraction without shortening results in patient effort and energy expenditure but no work, and muscle efficiency is zero. Isometric contraction of the respiratory muscles occurs in a variety of settings; these are discussed in later sections of this chapter.

Because work measurements do not always correlate with patient effort and energy expenditure, other measures have been used to assess the activity of the respiratory muscles. The most commonly used are measures of oxygen consumption and the pressure-time product.

Oxygen Consumption

Like all muscles, the energy required for contraction of the diaphragm and of the other respiratory muscles is liberated during the hydrolysis of adenosine triphosphate (ATP):

$$ATP + H_2O \rightarrow ADP + P + Energy$$

Unlike other skeletal muscles, however, respiratory muscle function is almost entirely aerobic. This means that ATP must be continuously replenished through the complete oxidation of substrates, primarily glucose and amino acids, through a process known as *oxidative phosphorylation:*

$$O_2 + ADP + Substrate \rightarrow CO_2 + H_2O + ATP$$

Since, under steady-state conditions, the rates of ATP hydrolysis and production must be equal, oxygen consumption should very accurately reflect the rate at which ATP (and energy) is consumed and should provide an excellent measure of respiratory muscle activity and of a patient's respiratory effort.

The oxygen consumed by a particular muscle (in milliliters of oxygen per minute) may be directly measured with the use of the Fick principle. That is, the rate of oxygen consumption ($\dot{V}O_2$) is equal to muscle blood flow ($\dot{Q}$) multiplied by the difference between the oxygen content of blood entering (CaO_2) and leaving (CvO_2) the muscle:

$$\dot{V}O_2 = \dot{Q}\,(CaO_2 - CvO_2) \quad \text{[Equation 6]}$$

This technique obviously requires invasive monitoring and has been used exclusively in animal studies. In addition, it allows oxygen consumption to be measured only in individual muscles (usually the diaphragm). The total oxygen cost of breathing cannot be determined.

An indirect approach that avoids these problems has been used to measure respiratory muscle oxygen consumption in humans. Total body $\dot{V}O_2$ is measured at baseline and after a stress has been applied to the respiratory system, and the difference between the two is assumed to be the amount of oxygen consumed by the respiratory muscles. In critically ill patients, respiratory muscle $\dot{V}O_2$ is typically calculated by measuring total $\dot{V}O_2$ during controlled mechanical ventilation (no respiratory muscle activity) and during assisted mechanical ventilation or spontaneous ventilation.

Although theoretically attractive as an indicator of respiratory muscle activity, measurement of respiratory muscle oxygen consumption is technically difficult and may be inaccurate for several reasons. First, total $\dot{V}O_2$ may be extremely variable, especially in critically ill patients, and the oxygen consumed by the respiratory muscles is often small in proportion. This produces a very unfavorable "signal-to-noise" ratio.[1] Second, during active breathing, $\dot{V}O_2$ may reflect not only increased respiratory muscle activity but also catecholamine-induced increases in energy consumption by nonrespiratory skeletal muscles and by the heart.[1] Finally, since random measurement errors are amplified as the fraction of inspired oxygen increases, measurement of $\dot{V}O_2$ is inaccurate in patients who receive high concentrations of oxygen.[4]

Pressure-Time Product

In theory, the product of pressure and time should provide a better measure of respiratory muscle activity and patient effort than the product of pressure and volume (work) because it takes into account isometric muscle contraction. Since it was first described in 1961,[5] the pressure-time product has been calculated in a variety of ways. This has led to confusion about its exact definition and is responsible, at least in part, for the uncertainty about its clinical usefulness. The pressure-time product is now most commonly calculated as the area enclosed by plots of esophageal pressure and time ($\int$Pes dT) during both assisted (or spontaneous) and controlled mechanical breaths.[6,7] This technique is analogous to the one used to measure work. However, the pressure-time product is also often calculated without taking chest wall expansion into account[8] and with the substitution of transdiaphragmatic pressure[9,10] and even airway pressure[11,12] for Pes.

The role of the pressure-time product in assessing respiratory muscle activity remains unclear. Several studies have shown respiratory muscle $\dot{V}O_2$ to correlate better with the pressure-time product than with work measurements.[5,8] Others, however, have reached the opposite conclusion.[11] These conflicting results are probably due to differences in experimental design and, as noted earlier, to different methods of calculating the pressure-time product.

RESPIRATORY MUSCLE ACTIVITY IN PATIENTS WITH ACUTE RESPIRATORY FAILURE

During the past decade, many studies have evaluated respiratory muscle activity in patients with acute respiratory failure through the measurement of respiratory work, $\dot{V}O_2$, and the pressure-time product. These studies have been performed both in spontaneously breathing intubated patients and in patients receiving assisted mechanical ventilation. In this section, the results of these studies are reviewed and their implications for patient management are discussed.

Spontaneous Ventilation

In normal subjects during quiet breathing, the oxygen consumption of the respiratory muscles is approximately 0.25 to 0.50 mL of oxygen per liter of ventilation or about 1% to 2% of total body oxygen consumption.[13] In intubated, spontaneously breathing, postoperative patients with normal pulmonary function, the mean oxygen cost of breathing has been found to range between 11% and 13% of total $\dot{V}O_2$.[14,15] The oxygen consumed by the respiratory muscles has been found to be even higher in intubated, spontaneously breathing patients with respiratory failure. In stable patients being weaned from mechanical ventilation, mean respiratory muscle oxygen consumption has varied between 16% and 27% of total $\dot{V}O_2$[10,16,17] and has been found to exceed 50% in individual patients.[17]

In normal subjects, the mean inspiratory work of spontaneous breathing is probably somewhere between 0.38 and 0.72 J/L.[1,18] As expected, inspiratory work is much greater in patients with acute respiratory failure who are breathing spontaneously through the ventilator circuit and has been found to average 1.39 J/L and 1.62 J/L in two studies by Marini and colleagues.[3,7]

There are several reasons why spontaneously breathing, intubated patients have a high level of respiratory muscle activity. First, patients with lung disease typically have abnormal respiratory mechanics. Increased flow-resistance or elastic recoil, or both, force the respiratory muscles to generate high pressures to inflate the respiratory system, and reduced respiratory muscle efficiency requires that more energy be expended to generate a given level of pressure. Second, an additional burden is placed on the respiratory muscles by the endotracheal tube and by the ventilator and its connecting tubing. Airway resistance is dramatically increased by the presence of the endotracheal tube. Tube resistance is inversely related to the fourth power of its radius and increases with flow.[19] Airway resistance is increased even further by the ventilator tubing and the exhalation valve.[20] The ventilator itself contributes to the respiratory muscle load because of the presence of the inspiratory demand valve. During both spontaneous and assisted mechanical ventilation, most ventilators provide inspiratory airflow only after the patient lowers airway pressure by an amount equal to the set trigger sensitivity. Thus, a lag exists between the onset of inspiratory muscle contraction and inspiratory airflow. The presence of a demand valve has been shown to lead not only to isometric muscle contraction but also to increased respiratory drive, which results in forceful and sustained contraction even after inspiration begins.[2] The detrimental effect of the demand valve has been clearly demonstrated in several studies. In comparison with circuits that provide continuous flow past the endotracheal tube (continuous-flow systems), the presence of a demand valve (demand-flow systems) significantly increases respiratory muscle oxygen consumption,[21] respiratory muscle work,[22,23] and the pressure-time product.[9]

In an attempt to decrease the extra burden imposed on spontaneously breathing patients by the demand valve, a modified continuous-flow system called "flow-by" has recently become available. In this system, gas continuously flows through the ventilator circuit but at a much slower rate (5–20 L/min) than in conventional continuous-flow systems. The rate of gas flow (base flow) is set by the operator and is continuously monitored at the exhalation port of the ventilator. When a patient inhales, gas flowing past the endotracheal tube immediately enters the lungs, and this decreases the measured base flow. When a clinician-selected decrease in base flow is detected (sensitivity), additional inspiratory airflow is immediately provided by the ventilator. Therefore, this system should both eliminate isometric muscle contraction and reduce the work of breathing. In fact, studies have demonstrated that flow-by, when compared with demand flow systems, significantly reduces respiratory muscle work and the pressure-time product to levels comparable with those produced by conventional continuous-flow systems.[6, 23]

Assisted Mechanical Ventilation

Pressure Support Ventilation

Pressure support ventilation is a mode of assisted mechanical ventilation in which a clinician-selected level of airway pressure is maintained throughout a patient-initiated inspiration. Unlike volume-cycled modes of ventilation, pressure support ventilation allows the patient to exert considerable control over the inspiratory flow rate, inspiratory time, and tidal volume.

Pressure support ventilation is used primarily to augment spontaneous ventilation in stable patients, often during the process of weaning from mechanical support. At relatively low levels (e.g., 5–10 cm H_2O), pressure support has been shown to compensate for the additional work imposed by the endotracheal tube, ventilator circuit, and demand valve.[24, 25] When compared with spontaneous ventilation through either a continuous-flow or a demand-flow system, low-level pressure support ventilation has been shown to decrease the oxygen consumption of the respiratory muscles,[10, 14] patient work,[17, 26] and the pressure-time product.[6, 9, 10] As the level of pressure support is increased, respiratory muscle activity continues to fall. In one study,[17] mean patient work decreased from 1.58 to 0.39 J/L, and respiratory muscle oxygen consumption fell from 27% to 1.5% of total $\dot{V}O_2$ as pressure support was increased from 0 to 20 cm H_2O. Thus, at high pressure levels, pressure support ventilation can provide almost complete ventilatory support.

Assist-Control and Synchronized Intermittent Mandatory Ventilation

It is commonly believed that respiratory muscle activity is minimal during assisted, volume-cycled mechanical ventilation. It is assumed that after the demand valve has been opened and inspiration has been triggered, the respiratory muscles relax and allow the lungs to be passively inflated by the ventilator. However, several studies by Marini and colleagues have demonstrated that significant muscular effort can persist throughout a mechanically assisted breath. With the assist-control mode, patient inspiratory work was found to average 0.78 J/L. This was 63% of the work performed by these patients during spontaneous ventilation on a demand-flow system.[3] During synchronized intermittent mandatory ventilation, patient work during mechanically assisted breaths was also found to be a large fraction of the work performed during totally spontaneous ventilation. In addition, as the set respiratory rate was changed to provide 100% to 20% of the patient's ventilatory requirements, patient work and the pressure-time product progressively increased during both assisted and spontaneous breaths. As the set rate was decreased, patient work during mechanical breaths increased from 0.69 J/L to 1.19 J/L.[7]

It is important to note that these results were obtained with the use of early-generation ventilators in acutely ill patients and that they may not be applicable to all patients and to all ventilators. One study has in fact demonstrated much lower levels of work in chronically ill patients supported by later-generation ventilators.[27] However, it is evident that the respiratory muscles do not relax immediately after the triggering of an assisted mechanical breath. Instead, muscle contraction continues for a variable period of time after inspiratory flow begins. Respiratory muscle activity and patient effort during assisted mechanical ventilation have been shown to be dependent on two major factors—respiratory drive and respiratory muscle strength.[2, 3, 7] Respiratory drive is augmented when minute ventilation requirements are increased, when trigger sensitivity is reduced, and when the delivered inspiratory flow is less than the patient's spontaneous flow requirement. Because of these multiple determinants, respiratory muscle activity varies from patient to patient. However, in some patients the respiratory muscles can be taxed, even when these patients are receiving assisted, volume-cycled mechanical ventilation.

The Effect of Intrinsic Positive End-Expiratory Pressure

During either spontaneous or mechanical ventilation, when insufficient time is allowed for complete exhalation, the respiratory system does not return to its equilibrium position. Thus, at the onset of inspiratory effort, lung volume is increased and the elastic recoil pressure of the respiratory system remains positive. This positive end-expiratory pressure (PEEP) is referred to as "intrinsic PEEP" (PEEPI)[28] or "auto-PEEP"[29] to distinguish it from "extrinsic PEEP" (PEEPE) applied through the ventilator.

When exhalation is incomplete, inspiration can occur only after the inspiratory muscles have generated sufficient force to balance the elastic recoil of the respiratory system. That is, expiratory airflow must be completely stopped before inspiration can begin. In mechanically ventilated patients, the inspiratory muscles must also generate sufficient additional pressure to trigger inspiratory flow. Hence, PEEPI like the inspiratory demand valve, acts as a threshold load on the respiratory muscles. The inspiratory muscles contract but do not shorten (or perform work) until a critical pressure is generated. Once this pressure has been reached and inspiratory airflow begins, respiratory muscle work and energy expenditure are increased by the volume-related rise in elastic recoil of the lungs and chest wall.

PEEPI and its associated respiratory muscle load are diminished by interventions that promote more complete exhalation. These include the reduction of expiratory resistance (e.g., with bronchodilators, secretion clearance, use of a large-diameter endotracheal tube) and, in mechanically ventilated patients, an increase in the inspiratory flow rate (which allows a longer expiratory time). Several studies have investigated the use of extrinsic PEEP or continuous positive airway pressure in patients with PEEPI.[30–32] The rationale for this seemingly counterproductive and dangerous maneuver is based on the fact that many patients with PEEPI have expiratory flow limitation during passive exhalation. That is, they have critical narrowing of the airways such that increasing expiratory effort does not increase flow. In such patients, expiratory flow is driven by the pressure difference between the alveolus and the site of critical airway narrowing (Pcrit), not the pressure at the airway opening (Paw). Therefore, increases in Paw (such as that produced by PEEPE) should have no effect until Pcrit is exceeded. This was confirmed by Ranieri and coworkers in a study of nine pharmacologically paralyzed, mechanically ventilated patients with chronic obstructive pulmonary disease and PEEPI.[30] They found that the addition of PEEPE had no effect on expiratory flow, end-expiratory lung volume, total end-expiratory pressure, peak inspiratory pressure, or cardiac index until it reached approximately 85% of PEEPI. Higher levels were associated with further hyperinflation, increased inspiratory and expiratory pressures, and hemodynamic compromise.

The advantage of substituting PEEPE for PEEPI is that this maneuver decreases the load on the inspiratory muscles. The addition of positive expiratory pressure establishes a new equilibrium position for the respiratory system. Thus, at the same end-expiratory lung volume, elastic recoil is largely balanced by PEEPE, and the respiratory muscles must generate much less force to initiate inspiratory flow. That is, the effective trigger sensitivity of the ventilator is improved. In fact, studies have shown that PEEPE is effective in decreasing respiratory drive, respiratory work, and the pressure-time product in patients with expiratory flow limitation during both spontaneous[31] and mechanical ventilation.[32] Two important points must be made. First, PEEPE is merely being substituted for PEEPI. Total end-expiratory pressure is not changed. Second, the addition of positive pressure is detrimental rather than beneficial in patients without expiratory flow limitation. Mechanically ventilated patients may have incomplete exhalation and PEEPI owing to high expiratory resistance or high ventilation requirements, even though they do not have critical airway narrowing. In these patients, the rate of expiratory flow is determined by the pressure gradient between the alveoli and the airway opening. Added expiratory pressure, therefore, increases end-expiratory lung volume, total end-expiratory pressure, and peak and mean airway pressure and thereby increases the risk of hemodynamic compromise and barotrauma. Even in patients with evidence of expiratory flow limitation, areas of the lungs that are not flow limited are likely to be present. The addition of PEEPE would increase the volume and pressure of alveoli in these areas and increase the risk of barotrauma. Because of its potentially detrimental effects and uncertain clinical benefits, the role of PEEPE in patients with PEEPI remains poorly defined and cannot currently be recommended.

Clinical Considerations

From the information presented, it is evident that patient effort and respiratory muscle energy expenditure persist to a variable but often significant degree in mechanically ventilated patients. It is unknown, however, what the ideal level of respiratory muscle activity is. For example, too much activity may lead to chronic respiratory muscle fatigue, whereas too little might result in muscle atrophy. Both conditions could lead to inability to wean from mechanical ventilation. Although data are lacking, it is likely that the optimal level of respiratory muscle activity varies with the clinical circumstances. For example, early in the course of acute respiratory failure, it would seem reasonable that most or all of the work of breathing be assumed by the ventilator and that the respiratory muscles be allowed to rest. As recovery proceeds, however, the activity of the respiratory muscles should probably be allowed to gradually increase until it is sufficient to maintain spontaneous ventilation. If these assumptions are true, the data presented in this chapter have several therapeutic implications.

During the initial management of acute respiratory failure, respiratory muscle activity can be minimized by placing the patient on the assist-control mode and by taking steps to reduce respiratory drive. The trigger sensitivity of the ventilator should be set at a low level ($\leq$2 cm H_2O), and an inspiratory flow rate that exceeds the patient's spontaneous requirements should be selected. PEEPI, if present, should be minimized by interventions that allow more complete exhalation. Pain relief and mild sedation can be effective in efforts to reduce respiratory drive further. During recovery, synchronized intermittent mandatory ventilation or pressure support ventilation with decreasing levels of support or spontaneous trials of increasing duration should allow a gradual resumption of respiratory muscle activity and facilitate weaning from mechanical ventilation. During spontaneous breathing trials, the adverse effects of the ventilator demand valve should be eliminated through the use of a continuous-flow system (T tube, flow-by). Alternatively, the additional work imposed by the endotracheal tube and ventilator can be counterbalanced by the addition of low levels of pressure support.

CONCLUSION

The work of breathing or, to use a more appropriate term, the activity of the respiratory muscles, can be assessed on the basis of measurements of work, oxygen consumption, and the pressure-time product. Although all three have drawbacks, work is the one most commonly determined because of its clear definition and its relative ease of measurement. Numerous studies have demonstrated that the endotracheal tube, the ventilator tubing, and the ventilator itself impose a significant burden and that respiratory muscle activity can persist at high levels even in patients receiving assisted, volume-cycled mechanical ventilation. Since both too much and too little respiratory muscle activity can lead to failure to wean from mechanical ventilation, it is essential that critical care physicians attempt to optimize patient respiratory effort throughout the course of acute respiratory failure.

References

1. Roussos C, Campbell EJM: Respiratory muscle energetics. *In:* Handbook of Physiology. Fishman AP (Ed). Bethesda, MD, American Physiological Society, 1986, pp 481–509.
2. Marini JJ, Capps JS, Culver BH: The inspiratory work of breathing during assisted mechanical ventilation. Chest 1985; 87:612.
3. Marini JJ, Rodriguez RM, Lamb V: The inspiratory workload of patient-initiated mechanical ventilation. Am Rev Respir Dis 1986; 134:902.
4. Ultman JS, Bursztein S: Analysis of error in the determination of respiratory gas exchange at varying FIO_2. J Appl Physiol 1981; 50:210.
5. McGregor M, Becklake MR: The relationship of oxygen cost of breathing to respiratory mechanical work and respiratory force. J Clin Invest 1961; 40:971.
6. Sassoon CSH, Light RW, Lodia R, et al: Pressure-time product during continuous positive airway pressure, pressure support ventilation, and T-piece during weaning from mechanical ventilation. Am Rev Respir Dis 1991; 143:469.
7. Marini JJ, Smith TC, Lamb VJ: External work output and force generation during synchronized intermittent mechanical ventilation. Am Rev Respir Dis 1988; 138:1169.
8. Field S, Sanci S, Grassino A: Respiratory muscle oxygen consumption estimated by the diaphragm pressure-time index. J Appl Physiol 1984; 57:44.
9. Brochard L, Pluskwa F, Lemaire F: Improved efficacy of spontaneous breathing with inspiratory pressure support. Am Rev Respir Dis 1987; 136:411.
10. Annat GJ, Viale JP, Dereymez CP, et al: Oxygen cost of breathing and diaphragmatic pressure-time index. Chest 1990; 98:411.
11. Collett PW, Perry C, Engel LA: Pressure-time product, flow, and oxygen cost of resistive breathing in humans. J Appl Physiol 1985; 58:1263.
12. Dodd DS, Collett PW, Engle LA: Influence of inspiratory flow rate and frequency on O_2 cost of resistive breathing in humans. J Appl Physiol 1988; 65:760.
13. Roussos C: Energetics. *In:* The Thorax. Roussos C, Macklem PT (Eds). New York, Marcel Dekker, 1985, pp 437–492.
14. Viale JP, Annat GJ, Bouffard YM, et al: Oxygen cost of breathing in post-operative patients. Chest 1988; 93:506.
15. Thung N, Herzog P, Christlieb II, et al: The cost of respiratory effort in post-operative cardiac patients. Circulation 1963; 28:552.

16. Field S, Kelly SM, Macklem PT: The oxygen cost of breathing in patients with cardiorespiratory disease. Am Rev Respir Dis 1982; 126:9.
17. Brochard L, Harf A, Lorino H, et al: Inspiratory pressure support prevents diaphragmatic fatigue during weaning from mechanical ventilation. Am Rev Respir Dis 1989; 139:513.
18. Sharp JT, Henry JP, Sweany SK, et al: The total work of breathing in normal and obese men. J Clin Invest 1964; 43:728.
19. Rossi A, Gottfried SB, Higgs BD, et al: Respiratory mechanics in mechanically ventilated patients with respiratory failure. J Appl Physiol 1985; 58:1849.
20. Marini JJ, Culver BH, Kirk W: Flow resistance of exhalation values and positive end-expiratory pressure devices used in mechanical ventilation. Am Rev Respir Dis 1985; 131:850.
21. Henry WC, West GA, Wilson RS: A comparison of the oxygen cost of breathing between a continuous-flow CPAP system and a demand-flow CPAP system. Respir Care 1983; 28:1273.
22. Beydon L, Chasse M, Harf A, et al: Inspiratory work of breathing during spontaneous ventilation using demand values and continuous flow systems. Am Rev Respir Dis 1988; 138:300.
23. Sassoon CSH, Lodia R, Rheeman CH, et al: Inspiratory muscle work of breathing during flow-by, demand-flow, and continuous-flow systems in patients with chronic obstructive pulmonary disease. Am Rev Respir Dis 1992; 145:1219.
24. Fiastro JF, Habib MP, Quan SF: Pressure support compensation for inspiratory work due to endotracheal tubes and demand continuous positive airway pressure. Chest 1988; 93:499.
25. Brochard L, Rua F, Lorino H, et al: Inspiratory pressure support compensates for the additional work of breathing caused by the endotracheal tube. Anesthesiology 1991; 75:739.
26. Van de Graaff WB, Gordey K, Dornseif SE, et al: Pressure support-changes in ventilatory pattern and components of the work of breathing. Chest 1991; 100:1082.
27. Kreit JW, Capper MW, Eschenbacher WL: Patient work of breathing during pressure support and volume-cycled mechanical ventilation. Am J Respir Crit Care Med 1994; 149:1085.
28. Rossi A, Gottfried SB, Zocchi L, et al: Measurement of static compliance of the total respiratory system. Am Rev Respir Dis 1985; 131:672.
29. Pepe PE, Marini JJ: Occult positive end-expiratory pressure in mechanically ventilated patients with airflow destruction. Am Rev Respir Dis 1982; 126:166.
30. Ranieri VM, Giuliani R, Cinnella G, et al: Physiologic effects of positive end-expiratory pressure in patients with chronic obstructive pulmonary disease. Am Rev Respir Dis 1993; 147:5.
31. Petrof BJ, Legare M, Goldberg P, et al: Continuous positive airway pressure reduces work of breathing and dyspnea during weaning from mechanical ventilation. Am Rev Respir Dis 1990; 141:281.
32. Smith TC, Marini JJ: Impact of PEEP on lung mechanics and work of breathing in severe airflow obstruction. J Appl Physiol 1988; 65:1488.

CHAPTER 73

Assessment of Pulmonary Function in Critically Ill Patients

Charles G. Alex, MD • Martin J. Tobin, MD

The detailed assessment of pulmonary function has become essential in the evaluation of ambulatory patients with respiratory disease.[1] In contrast, the functional assessment of critically ill patients has remained relatively rudimentary and frequently is omitted or limited to the measurement of arterial blood gases. It is becoming increasingly clear that tests of lung mechanics and respiratory muscle function are important in the optimal management of patients on mechanical ventilation and play a major role in determining the ease with which a patient can resume spontaneous respiration after a period of mechanical ventilation.[2]

The assessment of pulmonary function in the critically ill patient is of particular importance in (1) deciding whether mechanical ventilation is indicated, (2) assessing response to therapy, (3) optimizing ventilator management, and (4) deciding whether a weaning trial is indicated. In addition, management of a surgical patient frequently is enhanced by a knowledge of the patient's preoperative pulmonary function.

CLINICAL ASSESSMENT

Helpful clues regarding pulmonary performance can be derived from a detailed history and physical examination. Examination of the respiratory system is often focused on auscultatory findings; however, considerable information can be obtained from careful inspection and examination of the pattern of breathing. An elevated respiratory rate has been shown to be a sensitive indicator of respiratory dysfunction and is important in the diagnosis of impending respiratory failure.[3] Some idea of the work of breathing in relation to the patient's arterial carbon dioxide tension ($Pa{CO_2}$) is very helpful when it is necessary to make decisions regarding the institution or discontinuation of mechanical ventilation. Work of breathing is calculated as the product of the changes in lung volume and transpulmonary pressure (alveolar pressure minus pleural pressure). Unfortunately, clinical estimation of tidal volume is extremely inaccurate,[4] but the extent of suprasternal and intercostal space recession provides helpful indirect evidence of increased pleural pressure swings.[5] In addition, recruitment of the accessory muscles of respiration, especially the sternomastoid muscles, indicates increased patient effort. Finally, observing the pattern of rib cage abdominal motion provides useful information.[6] Normally, both the rib cage and abdomen expand and deflate in phase with each other during inspiration and expiration, respectively. If one compartment moves in an opposite direction to the other, *paradoxic breathing* is said to occur. It has been shown that the degree of rib cage–abdominal paradox is a direct reflection of the level of respiratory load against which a patient is breathing.[7] In addition, the induction of marked hyperinflation in healthy volunteers did not result in clinically significant abnormal rib cage–abdominal motion.[8] Thus, noting the respiratory rate, the extent of suprasternal and intercostal recession, the presence of accessory muscle recruitment, and the degree of rib cage–abdominal paradox provides good insight into the work of breathing being performed by a patient.

VITAL CAPACITY

In the intensive care unit (ICU), vital capacity (VC) is the only lung volume that is commonly measured. VC is the greatest volume of gas that a subject is able to exhale after maximum inspiration (Fig. 73–1). When performed as a forced maneuver, it is termed *forced vital capacity* (FVC) and is the difference between total lung capacity (the point of maximum inspiration) and residual volume (the point of maximum expiration). The size of the VC indicates a patient's ability to inspire deeply and to cough. Reduction in VC is observed in obstructive lung disease owing to an increase in residual volume; a decrease in total lung capacity is responsible for the decrease in VC in restrictive lung disease (see Fig. 73–1). A decrease in VC is also observed with poor patient effort or with neuromuscular disease that involves the respiratory muscles. In a recent study of pa-

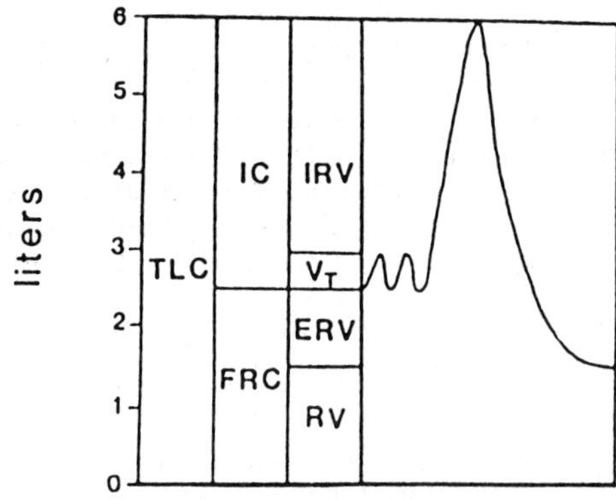

Figure 73–1. Lung volumes and capacities. *Abbreviations:* TLC = total lung capacity; IC = inspiratory capacity; FRC = functional residual capacity; IRV = inspiratory reserve volume; VT = tidal volume; ERV = expiratory reserve volume; RV = residual volume. A vital capacity maneuver is displayed on the right.

tients with the Guillain-Barré syndrome, the VC measurement was found to be a reliable predictor of respiratory failure hours before actual intubation.[9] Timed measurements of VC, such as the forced expiratory volume in 1 second (FEV_1), are very helpful in the diagnosis of obstructive airway disease, in which the ratio of FEV_1 to FVC (FEV_1/FVC) is less than 0.7 (Fig. 73–2). However, FEV_1/FVC is rarely measured in critically ill patients because suboptimal patient effort and the frequent presence of an endotracheal tube may contribute to erroneous results.

Normal VC is usually between 65 and 75 mL/kg, and it has been suggested that a VC of 10 mL/kg[10] or greater is essential for spontaneous ventilation to be sustained. These values are commonly employed as outcome predictors when patients receiving mechanical ventilation are being considered for a weaning trial.[11] However, in a prospective study of 47 patients who were weaned and extubated, Tahvanainen and coworkers[12] found that a VC of 10 mL/kg was falsely positive in 18% of patients (predicted success but actual failure) and falsely negative in 50% of patients (predicted failure but actual success).

FUNCTIONAL RESIDUAL CAPACITY

Functional residual capacity (FRC) is the volume of gas remaining in the lungs when the respiratory muscles relax at the end of a normal expiration. From a physiologic standpoint, it is an important index for several reasons: (1) it is the equilibrium point between the elastic recoil of the lung and that of the chest wall; (2) it is a major reservoir of oxygen (O_2), containing about one third of the body's O_2 stores, and thus minimizes fluctuation in arterial oxygen tension (PaO_2) during breathing; and (3) it determines the resting length of the muscles of respiration and thus determines their force-generating ability. Although measurement of FRC is easily obtained in the pulmonary function laboratory, it is very difficult to obtain in mechanically ventilated patients; presently, measurements of FRC are restricted to research studies.[13] However, a change in FRC over brief time periods can be assessed by noting the change in the end-expiratory level of an inductive plethysmography signal (Fig. 73–3).

BEDSIDE MEASUREMENT OF THORACIC COMPLIANCE

To achieve adequate ventilation, it is necessary to overcome the elasticity of both the lungs and the chest wall. Physiologically, this elasticity is defined in terms of *compliance,* which is calculated as the change in volume for a given change in distending transthoracic pressure. Since this is measured at a time of zero gas flow, it is termed the *static compliance.* During normal spontaneous breathing, the change in thoracic volume is caused by the decrease in intrathoracic pressure consequent to respiratory muscle contraction; in contrast, in patients receiving mechanical ventilation, an increase in intrathoracic pressure is responsible for the volume change. Lung compliance in a healthy adult is approximately 200 mL/cm H_2O, indicating that a change of 1 cm H_2O in transpulmonary pressure causes the lungs to expand by 200 mL. The compliance of the relaxed chest wall is also approximately 200 mL/cm H_2O; thus, in order to expand both the lungs and the chest wall, it is necessary to generate 1 cm H_2O of intrathoracic pressure for each component (i.e., a total of 2 cm H_2O). Therefore, the total thoracic compliance is 100 mL/cm H_2O.

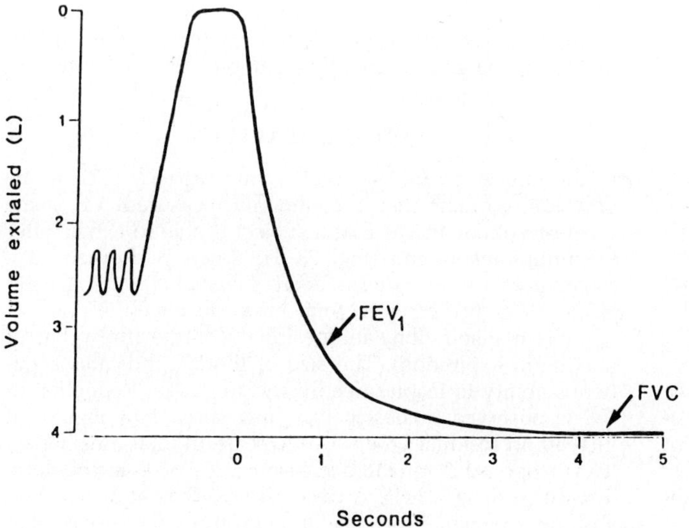

Figure 73–2. The normal spirogram. The forced expiratory volume in 1 second (FEV_1) and forced vital capacity (FVC) are indicated. (From Tobin MJ: Essentials of Critical Care Medicine. New York, Churchill Livingstone, 1989, p 141.)

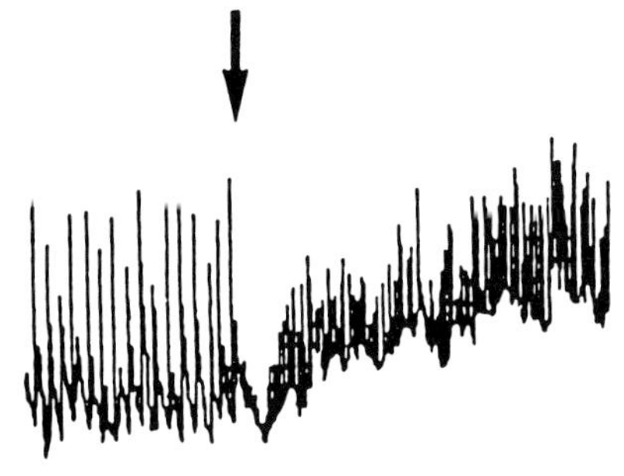

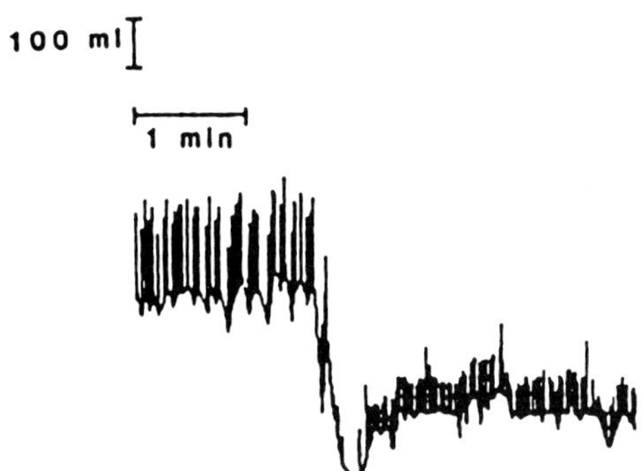

Figure 73–3. A compressed microprocessor plot of breathing pattern, measured with a calibrated respiratory inductive plethysmograph, in two patients who failed a weaning trial. Each *vertical line* represents the volume of a single breath; alterations in the baseline or end-expiratory level represent the changes in FRC. The *arrow* represents the point at which spontaneous breathing resumed following the discontinuation of mechanical ventilator use. The patient whose plot is in the upper panel developed an increase in respiratory frequency of 20 breaths per minute over the ventilator rate associated with an increase in FRC. This dynamic hyperinflation presumably occurred because the shortening of expiratory time allowed insufficient time for the complete emptying of lung units with long time constants. Conversely, another patient, whose plot is shown in the lower panel, also developed an increase in respiratory frequency of 20 breaths per minute that was associated with a decrease in the FRC. (From Tobin MJ, Perez W, Guenther SM, et al: The pattern of breathing during successful and unsuccessful trials of weaning from mechanical ventilation. Am Rev Respir Dis 1986; 134:1111.)

Manual Measurement

In patients receiving mechanical ventilation and making no respiratory effort, total thoracic compliance can be estimated by dividing the volume delivered (tidal volume [VT]) by the distending thoracic pressure (measured as the pressure difference between the airway opening and atmospheric pressure). Conditions of zero gas flow to permit measurement of total thoracic compliance can be achieved by employing "inspiratory hold" or by occluding the expiratory port long enough to allow airway pressure to reach a constant value (usually 1 to 2 seconds) (Fig. 73–4). This pressure, commonly termed "plateau" pressure, represents the static elastic recoil pressure of the total respiratory system at end-inflation volume. Any applied positive end-expiratory pressure (PEEP) or the presence of auto-PEEP (vide infra) must be subtracted from the plateau pressure to yield the correct distending pressure. If volume measurements are not made at the connection port of the endotracheal tube, then a correction for compression volume must be made. The compression volume is a function of the internal volume of the ventilator, the in-line humidifier volume, and the volume and compliance of the circuit tubing.[14] The compression volume of commercially available circuit tubing ranges from 0.3 mL/cm H_2O (in the presence of high compliance) to 4.5 mL/cm H_2O (in the presence of low compliance) at peak airway pressure. Thus, total thoracic compliance is calculated as follows:

$$\text{Compliance} = \frac{\text{Volume delivered} - (P_{plateau} - \text{PEEP}) \cdot \text{CV}}{P_{plateau} - (\text{PEEP} + \text{auto-PEEP})}$$

where $P_{plateau}$ equals plateau pressure, and CV equals the correction factor for volume compressed in the circuit tubing. Calculations of compliance should be based on at least three breaths. In many ICU patients, reproducibility of the measurement is usually no better than 10%, and a 20% to 30% difference between breaths may be observed.[15] The normal range of total thoracic compliance in adult patients receiving mechanical ventilation is generally reported to be from 60 to 100 mL/cm H_2O. It is important to note that the pressure-volume curve is not linear, and thoracic compliance may vary enormously at the extremes of VC within an individual patient. However, over the range of normal VT, the pressure-volume curve of the lungs and chest wall is approximately linear.[16]

A decrease of thoracic compliance is observed in patients with disorders of the thoracic cage or with a reduction in the number of functioning lung units (e.g., due to resection, bronchial intubation, pneumothorax, pneumonia, atelec-

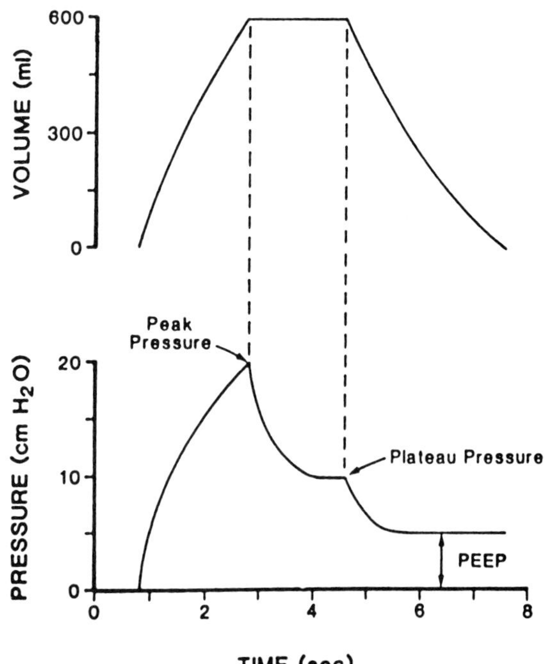

Figure 73–4. Relationship between VT and airway pressure in a patient receiving mechanical ventilation. The inspiratory plateau in the volume tracing is achieved by temporary occlusion of the expiratory tubing. During this period, airway pressure falls from a peak of 20 cm H_2O to a static pressure of 10 cm H_2O. These readings allow the calculation of static and dynamic thoracic compliance. *Abbreviation:* PEEP = positive end-expiratory pressure. (From Tobin MJ: State of the art: Respiratory monitoring in the intensive care unit. Am Rev Respir Dis 1988; 138:1625.)

tasis, or pulmonary edema). Total thoracic compliance also has been proposed as a predictor of weaning outcome, with the attraction that it is less dependent on patient cooperation than are other indices. It is thought that a successful weaning outcome is unlikely in patients with a compliance that is less than 25 mL/cm H_2O because the associated increase in the work of breathing makes it difficult to sustain a level of ventilation adequate for satisfactory gas exchange.

As with any measurement, care is required to avoid erroneous results. First, the volume-measuring device of the ventilator may be inaccurate at extremes of flow—that is, it underestimates volume at low flow rates and overestimates it at high flow rates. Second, adequate tracheal cuff pressure should be ensured to avoid gas leaks. Third, part of the volume generated by the ventilator expands the connecting tubing and is not delivered to the patient. The compliance of this tubing varies with its structure, diameter, length, and brand.[14] This factor may result in significant measurement errors in patients with very stiff lungs, who typically have high airway pressures and low VT. Fourth, the respiratory muscles should be relaxed at the time that measurements are being made. If the patient is actively inspiring, the pressure developed by the ventilator is less than the total pressure required for thoracic inflation, and a falsely high compliance will be obtained. Conversely, if the patient is "fighting" the ventilator, the total pressure developed by the ventilator is greater than that necessary to inflate the relaxed respiratory system, and a falsely low compliance will be measured. Finally, it is important to check for auto-PEEP.[17, 18] Use of the plateau pressure in calculating static compliance is valid only if the elastic recoil pressure reaches zero at end-expiration, indicating that the elastic equilibrium point of the respiratory system has been attained. Failure to account for the level of auto-PEEP may lead to an understimation of thoracic compliance of up to 48%.[18] Accordingly, it is necessary to divide the delivered VT by the difference between the plateau pressure and the total level of PEEP (i.e., the combination of extrinsically applied PEEP and auto-PEEP). An example of the development of dynamic hyperinflation following discontinuation of mechanical ventilation is seen in Figure 73–3.

Effective dynamic compliance is derived by dividing the ventilator-delivered volume by the peak (rather than the plateau) airway pressure (minus total PEEP). This index is not a measure of true thoracic compliance because the peak airway pressure also includes a resistive component, so that disorders of either the airways or the lung parenchyma (or chest wall) may cause a reduction in effective dynamic compliance. If effective dynamic compliance falls to a greater extent than static compliance, an increase in airway resistance has occurred (e.g., due to bronchospasm, mucous plugging, saturated in-line filter, or kinking of the endotracheal tube). The ventilator flow rate at the time of measurement should be noted, since this also alters dynamic compliance. It is difficult to state a normal range of dynamic compliance, since the values are dependent not only on respiratory mechanics and flow rate but also on the diameter of the endotracheal tube and the presence of tubing adapters. In general, effective dynamic compliance is approximately 10% to 20% lower than the compliance measured at plateau pressure[15, 19] (i.e., approximately 50–80 mL/cm H_2O). In practice, alterations in the difference between the peak and plateau airway pressures probably provide the best indication of change in airway resistance.[19]

A lack of change in compliance may also be helpful diagnostically. If a patient develops hypoxemia with no change in compliance, pulmonary embolism should be suspected.[20]

Automated Measurement

The manual measurement of thoracic compliance depends on the visualization of a single point on the ventilator pressure gauge, which means that the chance of error is considerable. Furthermore, sudden changes in the respiratory status of severely ill patients may be missed by intermittently performed manual measurements. Accordingly, on-line continuous monitoring of pulmonary mechanics has been advocated in the hope that such measurement might provide clues of impending respiratory failure, improve the management of ventilator performance, and aid in the critical transition between the discontinuation of ventilator support and the resumption of spontaneous breathing.[21, 22]

Continuous monitoring of pulmonary compliance (or resistance) requires continuous measurement of pressure and volume. Airway pressure recordings are sufficient to calculate total thoracic compliance, but calculations of pure lung compliance or resistance require a measure of pleural pressure. Esophageal pressure is usually employed as a measure of pleural pressure, and nasogastric tubes containing an attached balloon to facilitate such measurement have become available.[23]

The use of an esophageal catheter to measure pleural pressure is problematic in the supine patient and requires careful attention to detail.[24, 25] Lung volume is usually measured with a spirometer, but the spirometer is a cumbersome instrument, and the additional problem of rebreathing makes it unsuitable for use in the ICU. By contrast, a pneumotachograph, which measures flow, can be inserted easily into the ventilator circuit, and integration of the signal provides a continuous measure of volume. Most automated systems whose intended use is for measuring pulmonary mechanics in the ICU have included a pneumotachograph. The Fleisch pneumotachograph, the prototype of other models, consists of a bundle of parallel metal tubes that provide a fixed resistance and ensure laminar flow. By recording the pressure gradient across this resistance, it is possible to derive a measure of flow. This instrument is unsatisfactory in the ICU, however, because condensation of moist gases and the presence of mucus easily clog the narrow columns and thus alter the resistance. To circumvent this problem, Osborn[26] developed a variable-orifice flowmeter in which the resistance consists of a plastic flap that contains a V-shaped orifice. As flow is increased, the flap opens progressively, thus maintaining a direct relationship between pressure and flow. However, additional problems arise with the use of a pneumotachograph in patients who are receiving mechanical ventilation. The pressure drop across the resistance not only is influenced by flow but also depends on gas viscosity and thus gas composition and temperature. Substituting 100% O_2 for room air causes an approximately 16% change in calibration.[15] Alteration in body temperature (fever or hypothermia) or the use of a heated humidifier leads to measurement errors. The humidity and moisture of the normal airway cause problems because water vapor has a markedly lower viscosity than does dry air.[27] Thus, it is important to ensure that the pneumotachograph is calibrated under the same clinical conditions in which measurements are going to be obtained. Finally, problems with the differential transducers used to measure pressure gradients across the resistive element of a pneumotachograph may arise. The sudden application of high pressure during mechanical ventilation causes the two transducer chambers to have different frequency responses, thus resulting in erroneous measurement.[27–29] Recent work has shown that this problem may be minimized in spontaneously breathing patients through the application of digital compensation.[30]

Despite the shortcomings of using the pneumotachograph in the mechanically ventilated patient, such instrumentation has been employed by a number of investigators to monitor pulmonary compliance and resistance.[21, 22, 22a] However, it has not been shown that on-line measurements of compliance and resistance lead to improvements in patient care.

RESPIRATORY CENTER FUNCTION

An abnormality of the respiratory control system should be suspected when hypercapnia exists in the following settings: (1) when FEV_1 is persistently greater than 1.3 L, (2) when the alveolar-arterial O_2 gradient is normal, (3) when correction to normocapnia is possible after voluntary hyperventilation, and (4) when respiratory muscle weakness is absent (i.e., a patient has the ability to generate a sufficient negative inspiratory pressure).[31] One parameter that can be measured at the bedside is airway occlusion pressure, which is the negative pressure generated by an isometric contraction of the inspiratory muscles against an occluded airway. It is directly related to the intensity of the respiratory neural drive.[32] The occlusion pressure is performed by transiently and occluding the airway (without warning to patient) during early inspiration and by measuring the change in airway pressure after 0.1 second ($P_{0.1}$) before the patient reacts to the occlusion.[33] A pneumotachograph is usually included in the circuit to provide a simultaneous measure of airflow (Fig. 73–5).

Although $P_{0.1}$ values represent negative pressures, it is customary to report them in positive units; in the normal resting subject during relaxed breathing, the range is 0.93 ± 0.48 (SD) cm H_2O.[34] Most recently, $P_{0.1}$ has been used as a predictor of outcome for weaning from mechanical ventilation. A high $P_{0.1}$ during acute respiratory failure indicates increased respiratory drive and neuromuscular activity and, if sustained, may result in inspiratory muscle fatigue. In studies examining the use of $P_{0.1}$ measurements during weaning, an elevated $P_{0.1}$ was found to predict a poor weaning outcome.[35] However, Montgomery and coworkers[36] found that $P_{0.1}$ values were similar in patients who were successfully weaned and those who failed a weaning trial. In addition, they found that $P_{0.1}$ measurements during hypercapnic challenge were similar in the weaning success and weaning failure groups but that hypercapnic augmentation of $P_{0.1}$ (expressed as the ratio of the CO_2-stimulated $P_{0.1}$ to the baseline $P_{0.1}$) was greater in the patients who were successfully weaned. This technique is complex and primarily relegated to research work but may soon have a clinical role in the ICU.

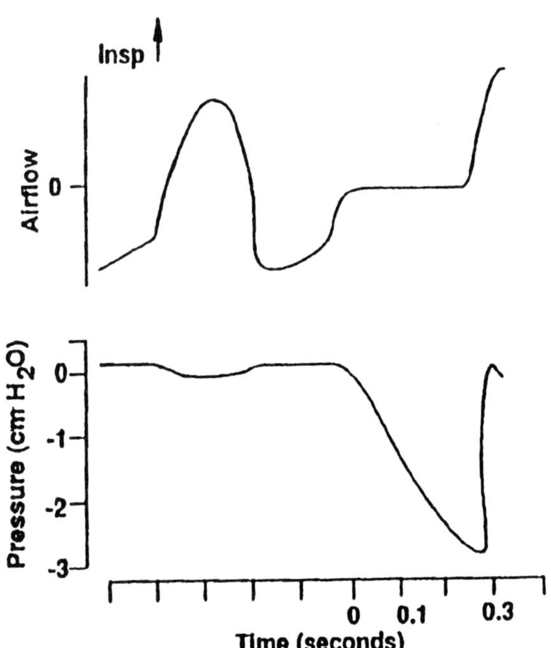

Figure 73–5. Measurement of airway occlusion pressure. The airway occlusion pressure is the pressure generated at 0.1 second ($P_{0.1}$) after inspiration begins against an occluded airway. Inspiration (Insp) is denoted by the airflow tracing. (From Tobin MJ, Walsh JM: Respiratory neuromuscular function. *In:* Respiratory Monitoring. Tobin MJ [Ed]. New York, Churchill Livingstone, 1991, p 139.)

MAXIMUM RESPIRATORY PRESSURES

An increased awareness of the importance of respiratory muscle function has developed over the last decade. Respiratory muscle fatigue is now considered to be an important contributor to ventilatory failure, particularly in critically ill patients. Unfortunately, a satisfactory diagnostic test to detect respiratory muscle fatigue does not exist, and assessment of respiratory muscle function in the ICU is currently limited to measurement of maximum respiratory pressures.[37, 38] These pressures provide a global assessment of the strength of the entire respiratory musculature in patients with neuromuscular disease at a time when spirometric values remain normal.[38, 39]

Respiratory muscle strength is assessed by measuring the maximum inspiratory and maximum expiratory pressure (PImax and PEmax, respectively) generated against an occluded airway. In the ICU setting, these measurements can be obtained readily with an inexpensive aneroid manometer.[6] The best of three efforts is usually selected. As with other skeletal muscles, the maximum force that can be generated by the respiratory muscles is related to their degree of stretching. Inspiratory muscles generate less force as their length is decreased, such as occurs at high lung volumes in obstructive lung disease.[40] Therefore, it is important to control the lung volume at which the measurements are made. PImax is usually measured after expiration to residual volume.[28] Because of the absence of respiratory system recoil at FRC, measurements at this volume may be preferable.[40] PEmax should be measured after inspiration to total lung capacity, when the expiratory muscles are maximally stretched. In the ICU, however, the PEmax is usually not measured because it is difficult to be confident that a patient has inhaled to total lung capacity.

Published normal values for PImax and PEmax show considerable variation among reports. This variation may depend on the cohorts employed to establish the normal range and on the method used to make the measurement. Black and Hyatt[37] described a technique using a tube connected to pressure gauges that allows a small air leak to minimize the contribution of the facial muscles to expiratory pressure. Lower values for PImax and PEmax have been found when a flanged mouthpiece is used instead of a simple rubber tube mouthpiece.[41] When the flanged mouthpiece is used, PImax and PEmax in healthy adult males are approximately 111 ± 34 (SD) and 151 ± 68 cm H_2O, respectively.[41–43] Values are lower in females (PImax is 72 ± 26, and PEmax is 93 ± 30 cm H_2O). In addition, strength tends to decrease with age:

PImax values are 6%, 25%, and 32% lower in men who are from 31 to 35, from 40 to 60, and from 61 to 75 years old, respectively, compared with healthy subjects who are from 16 to 30 years old.[44]

In ambulatory patients with neuromuscular disease but who are free of lung disease, hypercapnia is likely to develop when PImax is reduced to one third of the normal predicted value.[45] In patients with chronic obstructive pulmonary disease, hypercapnia is observed with less severe reductions in PImax (less than one half normal) because of the additional problems of abnormal gas exchange and increased work of breathing.[40]

PImax has been a standard measurement for the prediction of weaning outcome in mechanically ventilated patients. Traditionally, PImax values more negative than −30 cm H_2O are predictive of weaning success, whereas values no lower than −20 cm H_2O are predictive of weaning failure.[11] However, more recent work has undermined the reliability of this measurement in ventilated patients by showing that true muscle strength is grossly underestimated.[12, 46]

Attention has been redirected to standardizing the method of measuring PImax in critically ill patients. Using a valve attached to the airway to ensure that inspiration begins at a low volume and standardizing the period of occlusion to 20 seconds, Marini and associates[47] obtained PImax values that were approximately 33% more negative than nonstandardized measurements. Multz and colleagues[46] examined the reproducibility of this method of measuring PImax. Triplicate measurements were obtained in 14 ventilator-dependent patients by 5 experienced investigators. Measurements of PImax obtained at a single sitting by a single investigator showed good reproducibility (coefficient of variation: 12±1%). However, significant variation existed among PImax measurements obtained by different investigators studying the same patient on the same day (coefficient of variation: 32±4%). Since true inspiratory muscle strength must be equal to or greater than the highest recorded PImax, the variation in values obtained by different investigators indicates that PImax values, even when obtained in a standardized manner, commonly underestimate true strength.

It should be noted that PImax is an indicator of muscle strength rather than of endurance and, thus, provides limited information about fatigue, which is more related to endurance. *Endurance* is the capacity of a muscle to sustain a contractile force and depends on muscle capillary and mitochondrial density and overall oxidative enzyme capacity.[48] The converse of endurance is *fatigue,* which can be defined in operational terms as the inability of a muscle to generate and sustain a required contractile force.[49] Respiratory muscle fatigue can be divided into central, transmission, and contractile fatigue.[49, 50] Central fatigue is considered present when a voluntary contraction generates less force than does electrical stimulation. In a cooperative subject, the force generated by voluntary contraction should be the same as that resulting from electrical stimulation.[49, 50] Although central fatigue has been demonstrated in some healthy subjects breathing against high respiratory loads,[51] whether central fatigue has any relevance to ventilatory failure remains unclear.[50] Transmission fatigue is thought to be due to impaired neuromuscular transmission, which is manifested by a decrease in the electromyographic response to phrenic nerve stimulation. The clinical significance of transmission fatigue has yet to be established. Contractile fatigue is characterized by a decrease in the contractile response to neural stimulation. This decrease in contractile response or force can occur over different frequencies of neural stimulation. Usually, contractile fatigue is subdivided into high-frequency fatigue and low-frequency fatigue.[50] It appears that only low-frequency fatigue has any clinical significance, since it occurs at the nerve firing frequency of normal daily activities (10–20 Hz). During very brief voluntary efforts (2–3 seconds in duration), nerve firing frequencies are high, with the result that force-generating ability is little affected by low-frequency fatigue.[52] Consequently, measurements of maximum effort, such as PImax or VC, may not be decreased despite the presence of low-frequency fatigue. A number of techniques, such as phrenic nerve stimulation, power spectral analysis of the electromyogram, and calculation of the pressure-time product and of the relaxation rate of respiratory pressures, have been used to detect the presence or development of muscle fatigue.[34] However, their utility in the ICU setting remains to be determined.

MINUTE VENTILATION AND ITS SUBSETS

The relationship between minute ventilation ($\dot{V}_E$) and Pa_{CO_2} provides a good indication of the demands that are placed on the respiratory system. In the resting healthy adult subject, $\dot{V}_E$ is usually about 6 L/min,[53] and a value of less than 10 L/min (in the presence of normocapnia) is desirable in patients being considered for participation in a weaning trial. Since Pa_{CO_2} is determined by the relationship between alveolar ventilation and CO_2 production, a high $\dot{V}_E$ in the presence of hypercapnia indicates the presence of either increased CO_2 production or increased dead space ventilation. Conversely, hypercapnia associated with a low $\dot{V}_E$ (a less common occurrence) should arouse suspicion of decreased respiratory center drive, structural abnormality of the thoracic cage, or respiratory muscle dysfunction.

To obtain meaningful measurements of ventilation, every attempt should be made to collect data in an unobtrusive manner. Measurements of $\dot{V}_E$ are easily obtained in intubated patients with a Wright or similar type of spirometer attached to the endotracheal tube. Calibration of spirometric devices is flow dependent; thus, caution is required when measurements are obtained in patients with very high or very low flow rates. The measurement of $\dot{V}_E$ should be partitioned into its V_T and respiratory frequency (f) components. In healthy subjects, V_T is approximately 400 mL,[53] and higher values are observed usually under conditions of physiologic stress. The presence of a V_T that is less than 200 to 300 mL suggests that a weaning trial undertaken at that time is unlikely to have a successful outcome.[54] Such a low V_T is commonly combined with a high f (i.e., rapid shallow breathing) and usually is associated with hypercapnia due to increased dead space ventilation (Fig. 73–6). As a way to quantitate rapid shallow breathing, an index has been devised by calculating the ratio of f to V_T. In a prospective study of 100 patients,[55] it was found that a ratio lower than 100 breaths per minute per liter was the best predictor of successful weaning. Even in the absence of V_T or $\dot{V}_E$ measurements, detecting a high f (>22 breaths per minute) is an extremely helpful sign of respiratory distress, as tachypnea may be evident for 24 to 48 hours before the clinical diagnosis underlying this sign is established.[3] Although highly sensitive, an increased f is nonspecific, and further investigation is required to determine the nature of the underlying disturbance. Despite the simplicity of the measurement, nursing records of f are frequently inaccurate; this has led to underestimation of this measurement's clinical value.[56]

Problems arise when measurement of $\dot{V}_E$ and V_T is attempted in spontaneously breathing patients who do not have an endotracheal tube in place. Critically ill patients have a low tolerance for devices that require the use of a mouthpiece or mask. Furthermore, these devices themselves

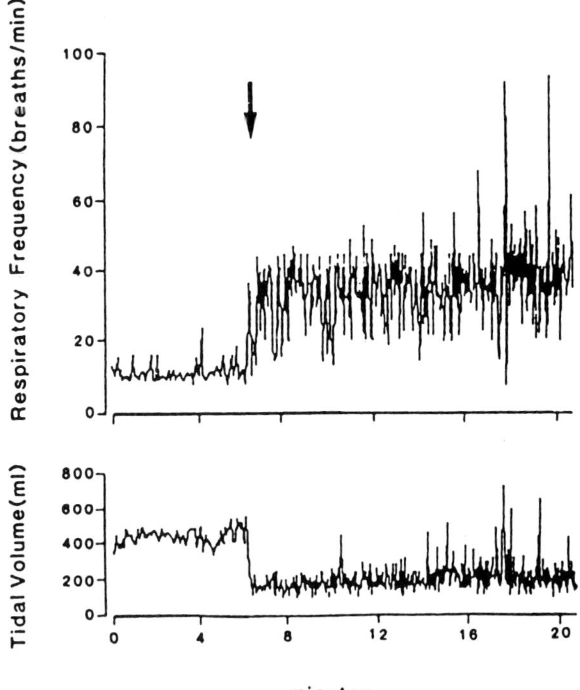

Figure 73–6. A time-series, breath-by-breath plot of respiratory frequency and VT in a patient who failed a weaning trial. The *arrow* indicates the point of resumption of spontaneous breathing following discontinuation of ventilator support. Rapid shallow breathing developed almost immediately, suggesting the prompt establishment of a new steady state. Although it has been considered that rapid shallow breathing may reflect the presence of respiratory muscle fatigue, its almost instantaneous development without subsequent progression is difficult to reconcile with the development of respiratory muscle fatigue. (From Tobin MJ, Perez W, Guenther SM, et al: The pattern of breathing during successful and unsuccessful trials of weaning from mechanical ventilation. Am Rev Respir Dis 1986; 134:1111.)

produce spurious alterations in the breathing pattern, causing VT to increase and f to fall.[57] Consequently, several devices have been developed to measure ventilation indirectly.[58] The most experience has been gained with magnetometry and inductive plethysmography, both of which provide measurements of ventilation by recording motion of the rib cage and abdomen (Fig. 73–7). It has been demonstrated that accurate ventilatory measurements can be obtained with inductive plethysmography in patients who require mechanical ventilation.[59] By recording ventilation on a breath-by-breath basis in this manner, additional information of physiologic interest can be derived from a more detailed analysis of the respiratory cycle. For example, VT divided by the inspiratory time (TI), termed the *mean inspiratory flow rate* (VT/TI), provides a measure of respiratory center drive.[60, 61] A crude measure of airway obstruction can be obtained by calculating the ratio of TI to the time of a single or total respiratory cycle (TTOT), termed the *fractional inspiratory time* (TI/TTOT).[62] Since the respiratory muscles are usually active only during inspiration, TI/TTOT has also been termed the *duty cycle* of the respiratory system, and it is an important determinant of the amount of stress being placed on the respiratory muscles. Bellemare and Grassino[63, 64] have shown that TI/TTOT and the amplitude of transdiaphragmatic pressure swings are of equal importance as determinants of respiratory muscle fatigue. Finally, since magnetometers and inductive plethysmographs record motion of the rib cage and abdomen, it is possible to detect the paradoxical motion of these two compartments (Fig. 73–8). Paradoxical motion of the abdomen was once believed to represent diaphragm fatigue; however, the abnormal motion has been shown to reflect increased respiratory load rather than fatigue.[7] In a study of 17 ventilated patients undergoing weaning trials, abdominal paradox was found to be a poor predictor of weaning outcome.[65] It was noted that abnormal motion of the rib cage and abdomen was observed in these patients regardless of their outcome. Patients who failed their weaning trials, however, displayed more severe asynchrony and paradox than those who underwent successful weaning. This study demonstrated that weaning outcome could be better predicted by analyzing the ratio of the maximum compartment amplitude (MCA) to VT.[65] This index represents the arithmetic sum of the absolute values of rib cage and abdomen excursions, regardless of their phase relationship, to the algebraic sum signal (represented by VT) (see Fig. 72–7). When the rib cage and abdomen signals are in phase with the sum (VT), MCA/VT equals one. When the rib cage and abdomen signals are out of phase with each other, MCA/VT is greater than one. Therefore, values closer to one indicate less respiratory system load and predict better weaning outcome.

MAXIMUM VOLUNTARY VENTILATION

Maximum voluntary ventilation (MVV) is the volume of air that can be inhaled and exhaled with maximum effort over 1 minute. It is usually measured over 15 seconds and then multiplied by four. Normal values range from 50 to 250 L/min. Since the value achieved depends not only on lung mechanics but also on muscle strength, coordination, and patient cooperation, calculation of MVV may be a more sensitive test of overall pulmonary function than simple spirometry. The relationship between resting $\dot{V}_E$ and MVV indicates the degree of reserve available for further respiratory demands. A resting $\dot{V}_E$ of 10 L/min or less and the capability of doubling this value during an MVV maneuver have been commonly employed as a predictor of weaning success. Sahn and Lakshminarayan[11] found that the combination of these two indexes had a high discriminating value in predicting the outcome of a weaning trial, although Tahvanainen and coworkers[12] found them to be relatively poor predictors. It should be clear that a patient requiring a high $\dot{V}_E$ (50–60% of MVV or greater) and who is on a ventilator to maintain a satisfactory Pa_{CO_2} will be unable to prevent the development of hypercapnia upon removal of the ventilator because of his or her poor ventilatory reserve and the predictable onset of respiratory muscle fatigue.

WORK OF BREATHING

To achieve normal ventilation, work needs to be performed to overcome the elastic and frictional resistances of the lungs and chest wall. In the physical sense, work is calculated as force multiplied by distance; in the pulmonary context, this is translated into the product of the pressure and the volume of the air moved into and out of the lungs. In the presence of increased airway resistance or decreased lung compliance, increased transpulmonary pressure is required to achieve a given VT and a consequent increase in the work of breathing. A problem arises in obtaining measurements of the work of breathing in patients with marked discoordination of rib cage–abdominal motion in that the measured external work of breathing does not take into account this extra internal work being performed by the respiratory system.

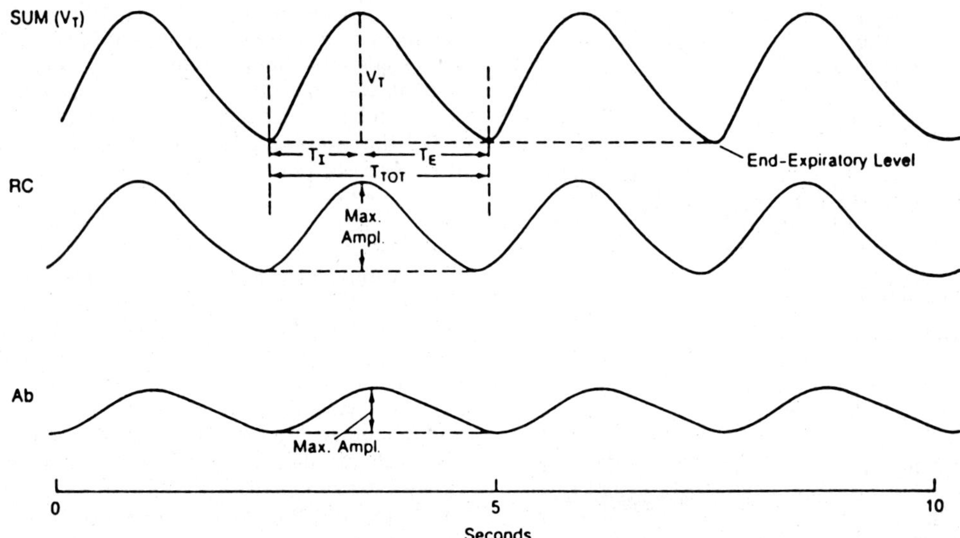

Figure 73–7. Schematic recording of the respiratory cycle depicting the points of reference for computation of the various breathing pattern parameters. The signals have been obtained with a respiratory-inductive plethysmograph, thus SUM indicates VT that has been calibrated to spirometry and represents the algebraic sum of the rib cage (RC) and abdominal (Ab) excursions. TI represents inspiratory time, TE is expiratory time, TTOT is time of a total breath, VT/TI is a mean inspiratory flow rate, and VT/TE is the mean expiratory flow rate. Alterations in the end-expiratory level represent changes in FRC, provided that movement artifact is absent. Maximum amplitude is the trough-to-peak amplitude of the rib cage and abdominal excursions, irrespective of their phase relationship to the SUM (VT) signal; their arithmetic sum, designated the maximum compartmental amplitude, is equivalent to the algebraic sum signal (VT) when the rib cage and abdomen move in phase. (From Tobin MJ: State of the Art: Respiratory monitoring in the intensive care unit. Am Rev Respir Dis 1988; 138:1625.)

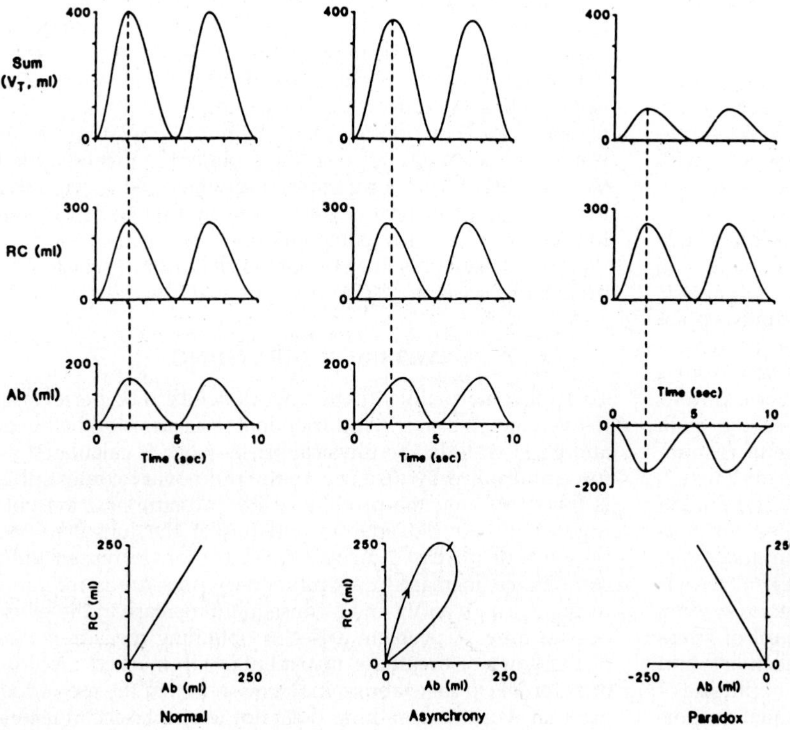

Figure 73–8. Schematic representation of rib cage and abdomen motion and their sum signal (VT) during normal breathing *(left panel),* asynchronous breathing *(middle panel),* and abdominal paradox *(right panel).* The pattern of rib cage motion is identical in each panel; the *vertical dashed line* represents maximum inspiration on the sum signal. The respective XY (Konno-Mead) plot for each type of motion is shown below the time tracings. Normal or synchronous breathing results in a straight line (actually a closed loop) with a positive slope. Asynchronous breathing produces an open loop, with the *arrow* indicating the direction of inspiration, and the *tick mark* indicating the point of end-inspiration. Paradoxical motion of the abdomen (i.e., movement in a direction opposite to the sum signal) results in a straight line (closed loop) with a negative slope. (From Tobin MJ: State of the Art: Respiratory monitoring in the intensive care unit. Am Rev Respir Dis 1988; 138:1625.)

The metabolic cost of work of breathing at rest constitutes only 1% to 3% of total O_2 consumption in healthy subjects. This may be increased considerably in patients with pulmonary disease. In a study of patients being weaned from mechanical ventilation, the average O_2 cost of breathing was 24% of the total O_2 consumption, and in some patients was greater than 50%.[66] This high metabolic cost of breathing curtails the delivery of O_2 to other tissues and is one of the reasons that mechanical ventilation is beneficial in pulmonary disease patients. As in the case of FRC, measurement of work of breathing is still largely restricted to research studies and is rarely performed for clinical use.

ASSESSMENT OF THE SURGICAL PATIENT

Pulmonary complications are observed commonly after surgery.[67] Of the risk factors associated with pulmonary complications, the site of the surgical incision has long been recognized to be of major importance. In a landmark study published in 1927, Churchill and McNeil[68] detected a 75% decrease in VC in the first 24 hours after cholecystectomy and a 40% to 50% decrease in VC after lower abdominal surgery; in contrast, lung function remained unchanged after peripheral (nonthoracic, nonabdominal) surgery. Lung volume returned gradually to the preoperative value over the next 14 days. The second and possibly more important risk factor is the presence of preexisting lung disease, which is associated with a 3-fold to 20-fold increase in the incidence of pulmonary complications.[69] Accordingly, preoperative assessment of pulmonary function is considered advisable in cigarette smokers and in patients with pulmonary symptoms, especially if they are undergoing thoracic or upper abdominal surgery. Such assessment identifies the high-risk patient and allows careful planning of perioperative respiratory care.[70] Table 73–1 lists the important pulmonary function criteria used to identify high-risk patients undergoing either abdominal or lung resection surgery.[71]

It is natural to expect a decrease in lung volume after resectional lung surgery. Although surgery is usually undertaken for a localized lesion, many lung resection patients also have evidence of diffuse pulmonary disease; thus, accurate prediction of postoperative pulmonary function is desirable. Because the lung being resected varies considerably in its contribution to total pulmonary function, special attempts have been made to assess separately the function of each lung so that postoperative pulmonary function can be more accurately predicted. Several methods of assessing split pulmonary function have been employed, including bronchospirometry (i.e., the lateral position lung function test) and the vascular pressure response to temporary occlusion of the pulmonary artery, but quantitative split perfusion lung scanning is now the method most commonly employed.[72, 73] Multiplying the preoperative pulmonary function values by the percentage of perfusion to the lung that is not to be resected has been shown to provide a reasonably accurate prediction of postoperative pulmonary function. Based on data obtained with this and other techniques, it is considered that patients with an FEV_1 of at least 2 L usually tolerate pneumonectomy. If the preoperative FEV_1 is less than 2 L, split lung function studies are required. If predicted postoperative FEV_1 is expected to be 0.8 L or greater, he or she is considered to be a suitable candidate for pneumonectomy.[72, 73]

TABLE 73–1. Pulmonary Function Criteria Predicting High Risk in Abdominal and Thoracic Surgery

	Abdominal	*Thoracic*
FVC	<50% predicted	<50% predicted
FEV_1	<70% predicted	<2 L
FEV_1/FVC	<65%	<50%
MVV	<50% predicted	<50% predicted
P_aCO_2	>45 mm Hg	>45 mm Hg
$\dot{V}O_2$	—	$<15 \text{ mL} \cdot \text{kg}^{-1} \cdot \text{min}^{-1}$

Abbreviations: MVV = maximum voluntary ventilation; $\dot{V}O_2$ = oxygen consumption.

SUMMARY

The assessment of pulmonary function in the ICU differs from that undertaken in the hospital laboratory with respect to the nature and range of tests performed, with less concentration on lung volume subdivisions and flow rates and greater emphasis on respiratory pressures, compliance, and breathing patterns. In addition, it is becoming more evident that the continuous trending of pulmonary function in the critically ill patient is more useful then intermittent measurement. The predictive power of many pulmonary function test results is somewhat low; however, when combined with the results of careful physical examination, they provide a better understanding of the pathophysiologic nature of a patient's pulmonary disease. As with other diagnostic techniques in the ICU, such as pulmonary artery catheterization for pressure measurement, it is difficult to demonstrate whether pulmonary function tests are cost effective or save lives. Hopefully, as we gain greater insight into the physiologic determinants of patient morbidity and outcome, present tests will be modified and additional tests with greater sensitivity and specificity will be introduced.

References

1. Wanner A: Interpretation of pulmonary function tests. *In:* Diagnostic Techniques in Pulmonary Disease. Part 1. Sackner MA (Ed). New York, Marcel Dekker, 1980, pp 353–426.
2. Tobin MJ, Skorodin M, Alex CG: Weaning from mechanical ventilation. *In:* Critical Care: State of the Art. Taylor RW, Shoemaker WC (Eds). The Society of Critical Care Medicine, 1991, pp 373–415.
3. Browning IB, D'Alonzo GE, Tobin MJ: Importance of respiratory rate as an indicator of respiratory dysfunction in patients with cystic fibrosis. Chest 1990; 97:1317.
4. Semmes BJ, Tobin MJ, Snyder JV, et al: Subjective and objective measurement of tidal volume in critically ill patients. Chest 1985; 87:577.
5. Tobin MJ, Jenouri GA, Watson H, et al: Noninvasive measurement of pleural pressure by surface inductive plethysmography. J Appl Physiol 1983; 55:267.
6. Tobin MJ: State of the art: Respiratory monitoring. Am Rev Respir Dis 1988; 138:1625.
7. Tobin MJ, Perez W. Guenther SM, et al: Does rib cage–abdominal paradox signify respiratory muscle fatigue? J Appl Physiol 1987; 63:851.
8. Jubran A, Tobin MJ: The effect of hyperinflation on rib cage–abdominal motion. Am Rev Respir Dis 1992; 146:1378.
9. Chevrolet J-C, Deléamont P: Repeated vital capacity measurements as predictive parameters for mechanical ventilation need and weaning success in the Guillain-Barré syndrome. Am Rev Respir Dis 1991; 144:814.
10. Bendixen HH, Egbert LD, Hedley-Whyte J, et al: Respiratory Care. St. Louis, CV Mosby, 1965, p 149.
11. Sahn SA, Lakshminarayan S: Bedside criteria for discontinuation of mechanical ventilation. Chest 1973; 63:1002.
12. Tahvanainen J, Salenpera M, Nikki P: Extubation criteria after weaning from intermittent mandatory ventilation and continuous positive airway pressure. Crit Care Med 1983; 11:702.
13. Weaver LJ, Pierson DJ, Kellie R, et al: A practical procedure for

measuring functional residual capacity during mechanical ventilation with or without PEEP. Crit Care Med 1981; 9:873.

14. Hess D, McCurdy S, Simmons M: Compression volume in adult ventilator circuits: A comparison of five disposable circuits and a nondisposable circuit. Respir Care 1991; 31:1113.
15. Fallat RJ, McQuitty JC: Bedside testing and intensive care monitoring of pulmonary function. *In:* Pulmonary Function Testing: Guidelines and Controversies. Clausen JL (Ed). Orlando, Grune & Stratton, 1984, pp 293–310.
16. Comroe JH, Forster RE, Dubois AB, et al: The Lung: Clinical Physiology and Pulmonary Function Tests. Chicago, Year Book Medical Publishers, 1962, pp 162–203.
17. Pepe PE, Marini JJ: Occult positive end-expiratory pressure in mechanically ventilated patients with airflow obstruction. Am Rev Respir Dis 1982; 126:166.
18. Rossi A, Gottfried SB, Zocchi L, et al: Measurement of static lung compliance of the total respiratory system in patients with acute respiratory failure during mechanical ventilation: The effect of intrinsic positive end-expiratory pressure. Am Rev Respir Dis 1985; 131:672.
19. Fallat RJ: Bedside pulmonary function and ICU monitoring: Indications and interpretation. *In:* Pulmonary Function Testing: Indications and Interpretations. Wilson AF (Ed). Orlando, Grune & Stratton, 1985, pp 293–309.
20. Bone RC: Monitoring ventilatory mechanics in acute respiratory failure. Respir Care 1983; 28:597.
21. Osborn JJ, Beaumont JO, Raison JCA, et al: Measurement and monitoring of acutely ill patients by digital computer. Surgery 1986; 64:1057.
22. Wilson RS: Monitoring the lung: Mechanics and volume. Anesthesiology 1976; 45:135.

22a. Fernandez R, Blanch L, Artigas A: Inflation static pressure-volume curves of the total respiratory system determined without any instrumentation other than the mechanical ventilator. Intensive Care Med 1993; 19:33.

23. Marini JJ: Monitoring the mechanics of the respiratory system. *In:* Respiratory Monitoring: Management in Critical Care. Tobin MJ (Ed). New York, Churchill Livingstone, 1992, pp 163–196.
24. Baydur A, Berakis PK, Zin WA, et al: A simple method for assessing the validity of the esophageal balloon technique. Am Rev Respir Dis 1982; 126:788.
25. Higgs BD, Berakis PK, Bevan DR, et al: Measurement of pleural pressure with esophageal balloon in anesthetized humans. Anesthesiology 1983; 59:340.
26. Osborn JJ: A flowmeter for respiratory monitoring. Crit Care Med 1978; 6:349.
27. Sykes MK, Vickers MD, Hill CJ: Principles of Clinical Measurement. Oxford, Blackwell Scientific Publications, 1981, p 197.
28. Mortimer AJ, Sykes MK: Monitoring of ventilation. *In:* Recent Advances in Critical Care Medicine. Vol 2. Ledingham I, Hanning CD (Eds). Edinburgh, Churchill Livingstone, 1983, pp 5–28.
29. Churches AE, Loughman J, Fisk GC, et al: Measurement errors in pneumotachography due to pressure transducer design. Anaesth Intensive Care 1977; 5:19.
30. Renzi PE, Giurdanella CA, Jackson AC: Improved frequency response of pneumotachometers by digital compensation. J Appl Physiol 1990; 68:382.
31. Alex CG, Tobin MJ: Noninvasive respiratory monitoring. *In:* Pulmonary Disease in the Elderly Patient. Mahler DA (Ed). New York, Marcel Dekker, 1993, pp 27–60.
32. Lopata M, Lourenço R: Evaluation of respiratory control. Clin Chest Med 1980; 1:33.
33. Whitelaw WA, Derenne JP: Airway occlusion pressure. J Appl Physiol 1993; 74:1475.
34. Tobin MJ, Laghi F, Walsh JM: Monitoring of respiratory neuromuscular function. *In:* Principles and Practice of Mechanical Ventilation. Tobin MJ (Ed). New York, McGraw-Hill, 1994, pp 945–966.
35. Sassoon C, Te TT, Mahutte CK, et al: Airway occlusion pressure: An important indicator for successful weaning in patients with chronic obstructive pulmonary disease. Am Rev Respir Dis 1987; 135:107.
36. Montgomery AB, Holle RHO, Neagley SR, et al: Prediction of successful ventilatory weaning using airway occlusion pressure and hypercapnic challenge. Chest 1987; 91:496.
37. Black LF, Hyatt RE: Maximal respiratory pressures: Normal values and relationship to age and sex. Am Rev Respir Dis 1968; 99:696.
38. Black LF, Hyatt RE: Maximal static respiratory pressure in generalized neuromuscular disease. Am Rev Respir Dis 1971; 103:641.
39. Baydur A: Respiratory muscle strength and control of ventilation in patients with neuromuscular disease. Chest 1991; 99:330.
40. Rochester DF, Braun NMT: Determinants of maximal inspiratory pressure in chronic obstructive pulmonary disease. Am Rev Respir Dis 1985; 132:42.
41. Koulouris N, Mulvey DA, Laroche CM, et al: Comparison of two different mouthpieces for the measurement of Pimax and Pemax normal and weak subjects. Eur Respir J 1988; 1:863.
42. Vincken W, Ghezzo H, Cosio NG: Maximal static respiratory pressures in adults: Normal values and their relationship to determinants of respiratory function. Bull Eur Pathophysiol Respir 1987; 23:435.
43. Wilson SH, Cooke NT, Edwards RHT, et al: Predicted normal values for maximal respiratory pressures in Caucasian adults and children. Thorax 1984; 39:535.
44. Chen H-I, Kuo C-S: Relationship between respiratory muscle function and age, sex, and other factors. J Appl Physiol 1989; 66:943.
45. Braun NMT, Arora NS, Rochester DF: Respiratory muscle and pulmonary function in polymyositis and other proximal myopathies. Thorax 1983; 38:616.
46. Multz AS, Aldrich TK, Prezant DJ, et al: Maximal inspiratory pressure is not a reliable test of inspiratory muscle strength in mechanically ventilated patients. Am Rev Respir Dis 1990; 142:529.
47. Marini JJ, Smith TC, Lamb V: Estimation of inspiratory muscle strength in mechanically ventilated patients: The measurement of maximal inspiratory pressure. J Crit Care 1986; 1:32.
48. Faulkner JA, Maxwell LC, Ruff GL, et al: The diaphragm as muscle: Contractile properties. Am Rev Respir Dis 1979. 119(Suppl):89.
49. Aldrich TK: Respiratory muscle fatigue. *In:* The Respiratory Muscles. Tobin MJ (Ed). Philadelphia, JB Lippincott, 1990, pp 329–342.
50. Moxham J: Respriatory muscle fatigue: Mechanisms, evaluation and therapy. Br J Anaesth 1990; 65:43.
51. Bellemare F, Bigland-Ritchie B: Central components of diaphragm fatigue assessed by phrenic nerve stimulation. J Appl Physiol 1987; 62:1307.
52. Green M, Moxham J: The respiratory muscles. Clin Sci 1985; 68:1.
53. Tobin MJ, Chadha TS, Jenouri G, et al: Breathing patterns: 1. Normal subjects. Chest 1983; 84:202.
54. Tobin MJ, Perez W, Guenther SM, et al: The pattern of breathing during successful and unsuccessful trials of weaning from mechanical ventilation. Am Rev Respir Dis 1986; 134:1111.
55. Yang KL, Tobin MJ: A prospective study of indexes predicting the outcome of trials of weaning from mechanical ventilation. N Engl J Med 1991; 324:1445.
56. Krieger B, Feinerman D, Zaron A, et al: Continuous noninvasive monitoring of respiratory rate in critically ill patients. Chest 1986; 90:632.
57. Perez W, Tobin MJ: Separation of factors responsible for change in breathing pattern induced by instrumentation. J Appl Physiol 1985; 59:1515.
58. Tobin MJ: Noninvasive evaluation of respiratory movement. *In:* Noninvasive Respiratory Monitoring. Nochomovitz ML, Cherniack NS (Eds). New York, Churchill Livingstone, 1986, pp 29–57.
59. Tobin MJ, Jenouri G, Lind B, et al: Validation of respiratory inductive plethysmography in patients with pulmonary disease. Chest 1983; 83:615.
60. Clark FJ, von Euler C: On the regulation of depth and rate of breathing. J Physiol 1972; 222:267.
61. Lind FG, Truve AB, Lindborg BPO: Microcomputer-assisted online measurement of breathing pattern and occlusion pressure. J Appl Physiol 1984; 56:235.
62. Tobin MJ, Chadha TS, Jenouri G, et al: Breathing patterns: 2. Diseased subjects. Chest 1983; 84:286.
63. Bellemare F, Grassino A: Effect of pressure and timing of con-

traction on human diaphragm fatigue. J Appl Physiol 1982; 53:1190.
64. Bellemare F, Grassino A: Evaluation of human diaphragm fatigue. J Appl Physiol 1982; 53:1199.
65. Tobin MJ, Guenther SM, Perez W, et al: Konno-Mead analysis of ribcage-abdominal motion during successful and unsuccessful trials of weaning from mechanical ventilation. Am Rev Respir Dis 1987; 135:1320.
66. Field S, Kelly SM, Macklem PT: The oxygen cost of breathing in patients with cardiorespiratory distress. Am Rev Respir Dis 1982; 126:9.
67. Proceedings, Perioperative Respiratory Care Conference: Parts 1 and 2, Vail, Colorado. Respir Care 1984; 29:459,603.
68. Churchill ED, Mcneil D: Vital capacity following operations: The reduction in vital capacity following operation. Surg Gynecol Obstet 1927; 44:483.
69. Wightman JAK: A prospective survey of the incidence of postoperative pulmonary complications. Br J Surg 1968; 55:85.
70. Stein M, Cassara EL: Preoperative pulmonary evaluation and therapy for surgery patients. JAMA 1970; 211:787.
71. Gass GD, Olsen GN: Postoperative pulmonary function testing to predict postoperative morbidity and mortality. Chest 1986; 89:127.
72. Olsen GN, Block AJ, Tobias JA: Prediction of post-pneumonectomy pulmonary function using quantitative macroaggregate lung scanning. Chest 1974; 66:13.
73. Boysen PG, Block AJ, Olsen GN, et al: Prospective evaluation for pneumonectomy using the 99m technetium quantitative perfusion lung scan. Chest 1977; 72:422.

CHAPTER 74

Regulation of Capillary Exchange of Fluid and Protein

Aubrey E. Taylor, PhD • W. Keith Adkins, MD, PhD
Peter Wilson, MD • Pavel L. Khimenko, MD, PhD

Critical care physicians must understand the physiology and biophysics of transcapillary water and solute exchange if they are to apply effectively and on a daily basis various forms of fluid therapy in clinical situations in patients with burns, shock, sepsis, and emboli. Over the past 80 years, physiologists and clinicians have evaluated the exchange of fluid and molecules between the tissues and plasma using a wide variety of experimental models, and a great deal of new information has emerged. This chapter has been designed to review the important factors responsible for the physiology and biophysics of the transcapillary exchange of fluid and solute across normal and abnormal capillary barriers, and it specifically focuses on ischemia-reperfusion injury in lungs as it relates to pulmonary edema formation and on how certain interventions can reverse the endothelial damage and resolve pulmonary edema.

STRUCTURE OF THE CAPILLARY WALL

The capillary walls are usually defined as having continuous, fenestrated, or discontinuous endothelial barriers, as shown schematically in Figure 74–1. The anatomy of the microcirculation varies in different organs, but as a general rule, small arteries with radii less than 40 μm divide into smaller arteries that finally divide into blood vessels with radii of 7 to 10 μm. The last of these form capillary beds that have huge surface areas that promote the rapid exchange of small molecules and water between the plasma and intestinal fluid. Actually, solute and solvent can also leave or enter the microcirculation in small arteries and veins, but because the capillaries are so great in number as compared with other small blood vessels, physiologists refer to the portion of the microcirculation where water and solute leak as "capillaries." *Continuous capillaries,* with their dense and continuous basement membrane, are found in muscle, the lungs, subcutaneous tissue, the kidneys, the heart, and the brain, and a few are found in most organs of the body.[1,2] The intercellular clefts, designated as 2 in Figure 74–1, are highly permeable to small solutes such as sodium chloride, glucose, and water. However, only the transendothelial channels (designated as 3 in Figure 74–1) are sufficiently large to allow the larger proteins in plasma to pass across the capillary wall. These transendothelial channels likely represent the capillary "pores" as determined in many physiologic studies. In addition, physiologists have postulated that large molecules may cross the capillary membrane in vesicles (designated as 1 in Figure 74–1). However, these vesicles must be sensitive to increased capillary filtration and must also be selective to the various proteins in plasma, since it is well known that the transcapillary movement of macromolecules increases when large quantities of fluid are filtered across capillary walls. In addition, the blood-tissue barrier is also selective to all plasma proteins with molecular radii that range from 3.7 nm (albumin) to 12.0 nm (beta-lipoprotein)—that is, small proteins cross capillary walls with less restriction than do large proteins. In addition, when electron micrographs are made in series through endothelial cells, they indicate that endothelial vesicles do not communicate with the plasma and interstitium. However, a few transendothelial channels, which are formed by fused vesicles, are present in the endothelial cells. In fact, these fused plasmalemmal vesicles are both the small and large pores of 4 to 5 nm and with 12.0- to 15.0-nm radii that have been identified in many organs by physiologic measurement. When the transendothelial channels are covered by diaphragms, they have the biophysical characteristics of the small pore system (4–5-nm radius), whereas the endothelial channels without diaphragms have dimensions similar to the large-pore system (20.0-nm radius).

Fenestrated capillaries are found in the gastrointestinal tract, glomerular capillaries, and many glands. The major difference between this type of capillary wall barrier and the continuous endothelial barriers is the presence of diaphragms that cover the fenestrae (designated as 4 in Figure 74–1). Fenestrated capillaries are always found in organs in which large amounts of small solutes and fluid move into or out of the microcirculation, for example, in glomeruli and gastrointestinal tract capillaries. In some organs, the fenestrae are not always covered by diaphragms; this gives the endothelial barrier the appearance of a very leaky barrier. However, these capillaries are not overtly leaky to plasma proteins as assessed by physiologic measures, indicating that basement membranes may be a substantial barrier to macromolecule exchange between plasma and the interstitium.[1]

The third type of capillary shown in Figure 74–1 is the *discontinuous capillary.* This type of capillary wall has huge gaps between endothelial cells that measure from 100 to 1000 nm and has no basement membranes. Discontinuous capillaries are highly permeable to plasma proteins and exchange freely all constituents of plasma, including plasma proteins, with an organ's interstitial space. These types of capillaries are found in the liver, spleen, and some glands, and the protein concentration in the tissues is equal to that found in the plasma.

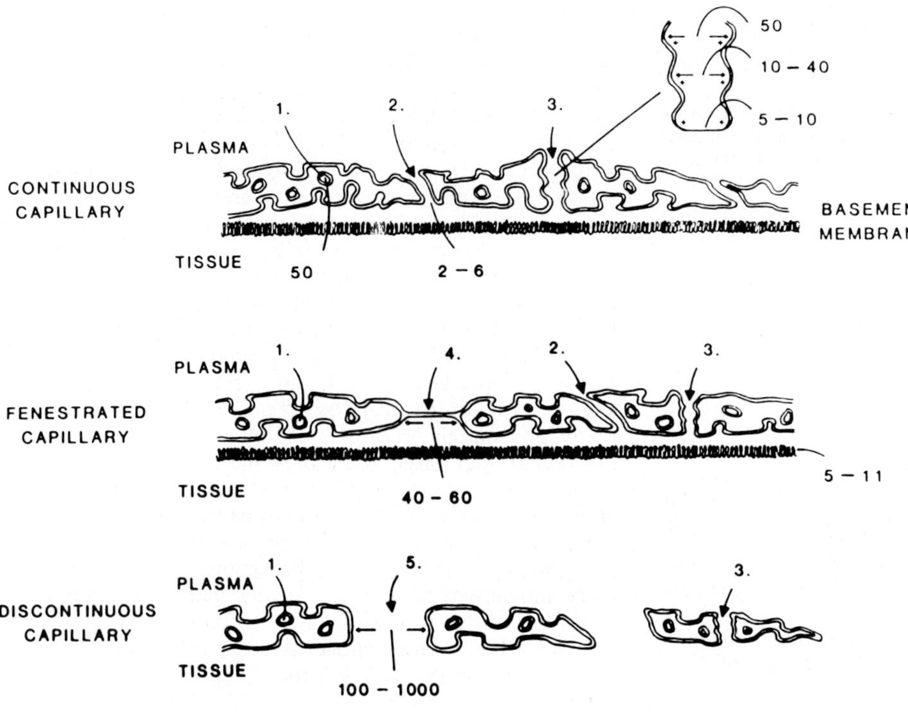

Figure 74–1. Diagrammatic representation of continuous, fenestrated, and discontinuous capillaries. *Key:* 1. = plasmalemmal vesicles; 2. = interendothelial channels; 3. = transendothelial channels (expanded in right upper insert); 4. = diaphragms; 5. = large gaps in discontinuous capillaries. The numbers at each site show predicted radii in nanometers. (From Taylor AE: Microvascular fluid and solute exchange. *In:* Encyclopedia of Human Biology. Vol 5. Dulbecco R [Ed]. Orlando, Academic Press, 1991, p 34.)

In summary, continuous and fenestrated capillaries are very selective barriers to plasma proteins, and little protein escapes these capillaries to enter the tissues; however, fenestrated capillaries have extremely high permeabilities to water and small solutes as compared with the continuous capillaries. Discontinuous capillaries are extremely permeable to plasma proteins and offer little or no restriction to their movement into tissues.[2]

BIOPHYSICS OF CAPILLARY PROTEIN AND SOLVENT EXCHANGE

Starling[3] was the first to postulate that fluid moved between the plasma and tissues as a function of the difference between the hydrostatic and protein osmotic forces that operate across the capillary wall. He defined the pressure gradient responsible for moving fluid across the capillary wall as the difference between the capillary pressure (P_c) and tissue hydrostatic pressure (P_t) gradient; and the protein osmotic (or oncotic) pressure gradient acting across the capillary wall, which is the plasma protein osmotic pressure (π_p) minus the tissue protein osmotic pressure (π_t). He used this relationship to define the Starling law of capillary exchange—that is, $P_c - P_t$ equals $\pi_p - \pi_t$ in physiologic ranges of P_c, since $P_c - P_t$ causes fluid to leave the capillaries, whereas $\pi_p - \pi_t$ tends to hold fluid in the capillary.

This equation describing Starling's hypothesis of capillary fluid exchange was actually first written by Iverson and Johansen[4] in its familiar form:

$$P_c - P_t = \pi_p - \pi_t$$

This equation assumes, as had Starling, that the plasma protein and fluid loss into the interstitium was small—that is, that the hydrostatic and protein osmotic forces were balanced. However, Starling knew that these assumptions were not correct, since under normal physiologic conditions fluid and proteins leak into the tissue and leave the tissues as lymph. Under normal conditions, the transcapillary loss of fluid and protein is small, and this small amount of fluid and protein is totally returned into the circulation by the lymphatic system. The net result is the maintenance of an almost constant interstitial fluid volume.

In the late 1950s, the classic papers by Kedem and Katchalsky[5] described the irreversible thermodynamics of solute and water movement across biologic barriers. Their work resulted in the development of the following equations that describe solvent[6] and solute[7] transport across capillary walls:

$$J_v = K_{fc}(\Delta P_c - \sigma\Delta\pi_c) \quad \text{[Solvent Flux Equation]}$$

$$J_s = (1 - \sigma)J_vC_p + (x/e^x - 1)(PS\Delta C) \quad \text{[Solute Flux Equation]}$$

In these equations, J_v is the net volume flow (or capillary filtration) occurring across the capillary walls. In most organs, J_v contains all of the small molecules in plasma at concentrations that are almost identical to those in plasma; however, J_v contains only small amounts of plasma proteins. K_{fc} is the filtration coefficient of the capillary wall[8] and describes how easily fluid is filtered across the capillary wall. K_{fc} is a function both of the permeability of the capillary wall to fluid and of the surface area of the capillaries. ΔP_c is the difference between P_c and P_t, and it is sometimes defined as the *capillary filtration pressure.* $\Delta\pi_c$ is the difference between π_p and π_t. The osmotic reflection coefficient (σ) equals 1.0 when the capillary wall is impermeable to a protein molecule and equals zero when the protein can move freely out of the capillaries without being restricted by the capillary wall. The effective protein osmotic pressure acting across the capillary wall is $\sigma(\pi_p - \pi_T)$ and is defined as the *capillary absorptive force.* The hydrostatic pressure operating across the capillary wall has been defined as merely $P_c - P_t$, but this is an oversimplification of a very complicated exchange system. P_c and P_t are known to differ in the various parts of the microcirculation and in the tissues, respectively. In addition, all of the proteins in plasma have been represented as having a single π and a single σ—that is, total plasma protein osmotic pressure has been used to describe the biophysics of solute and solvent movement in this presentation. However, several different proteins are present in plasma, and they should be considered separately if an exact analysis of transcapillary exchange is needed.

In the solute flux equation, J_s is net protein flux and C_p is the total protein concentration in the plasma. PS is the permeability–surface area product of the plasma proteins and is a function of the permeability of the capillary wall to plasma proteins and of the surface area available for exchange. Note that the solute flux equation is used to describe the flux of proteins. This equation can also be used to describe small solute flux, but small molecules are not important in transcapillary fluid exchange because their σ values are small and their permeabilities large. ΔC is the protein concentration difference acting across the capillary wall (i.e., the difference between plasma $[C_p]$ and tissue protein $[C_t]$ concentrations). x is equal to $(1 - \sigma)J_v/PS$ and has been defined as a Peclet number. Proteins can move across capillary walls by convection (first term) and diffusion (second term). Diffusion predominates at low J_v because the first term is small, but convection predominates when transcapillary filtration is large.[1]

These two equations define the capillary wall–protein–solvent system in terms of only three variables: σ, PS, and K_{fc}. Unfortunately, they can only describe interstitial protein and fluid movement in very general terms, since several different proteins are present in plasma and because P_c, P_t, and π_t vary within an organ system because of pressure drops that occur in the circulation, different types of capillaries within an organ, different capillary permeabilities at different portions of the microcirculation, different hydrostatic pressures operating down the length of the capillaries, hydrostatic gradients existing within tissues (e.g., gravity-induced differences in lung vascular and interstitial pressures), and different π_t and P_t in the interstitium caused by nonuniform capillary permeability and lymphatic drainage. Any analysis of fluid and protein exchange occurring across capillary walls must always consider the implications and limitations of assigning a single value to microcirculatory permeability or to capillary pressures, especially in the critically ill patient. However, a simplified analysis, such as that presented in this chapter, is sufficient to predict how a particular clinical intervention will affect transcapillary fluid movement in a patient.

TRANSVASCULAR PROTEIN AND FLUID MOVEMENT

In many tissues, the fluid and protein movement occurring across capillary walls can be described by a capillary-tissue-lymphatic system as shown in Figure 74–2. The capillaries in this system continuously filter fluid and leak plasma proteins into the interstitium. Normally, this volume is returned to the circulation by the lymphatics, and the tissues neither shrink nor swell. In the lung, gastrointestinal tract, and bronchial tissues, the lymphatics drain the tissues, but fluid can spill into the alveoli, the peritoneal cavity, or the airways, respectively, when the volume of fluid leaving the capillary exceeds the ability of the interstitial tissue spaces to swell and the ability of the lymphatics to remove interstitial fluid.

It is now known that the interstitium is composed of large proteoglycans (e.g., hyaluronate) and collagen in addition to interstitial fluid and that tissue protein concentrations are lower than plasma levels. Studies have indicated that hyaluronate is in a dynamic state in the tissue, and an increased capillary filtration results in the removal of large amounts of this important tissue component. The effect of the presence of large amounts of edema fluid on the constituents of the interstitium is not well known, and the interested reader

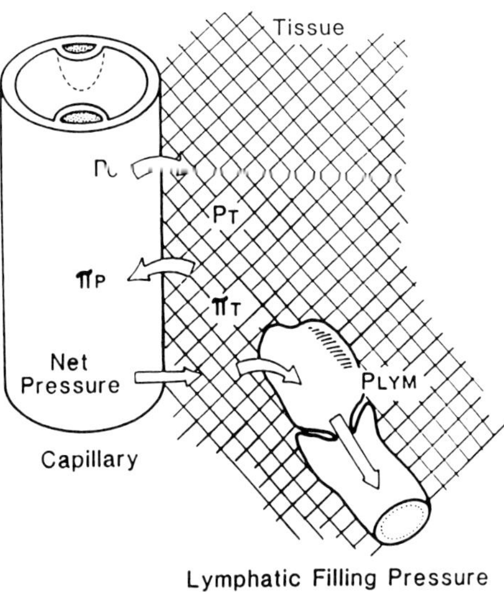

Figure 74–2. Diagrammatic representation of a capillary-tissue-lymphatic system. (From Taylor AE: Microvascular fluid and solute exchange. *In:* Encyclopedia of Human Biology. Vol 5. Dulbecco R [Ed]. Orlando, Academic Press, 1991, p 36.)

should consult a review by Aukland and Reed[9] that addresses this important topic. Needless to say, it can no longer be assumed that the interstitium is a static system that does not respond to physiologic events, and future studies should concentrate on evaluating the effects of the removal of tissue proteoglycans on wound healing and edema resolution.

Most tissues, with the exception of those of the brain and ocular system, have extensive lymphatic systems. The tissues have small initial lymphatics (or lymphatic capillaries) into which the interstitial fluid enters without any restrictions with respect to molecular size. The next segment of the lymphatics contains valves, which cause lymph to always flow away from the tissues. These larger lymphatics have smooth muscle and act as small "lymphatic hearts." Their contraction propels lymph away from the tissues. In addition to this intrinsic pumping ability of the lymphatics, tissue motion accelerates lymph flow.[10] The lymph finally drains into the large veins in the thorax. The lymphatic system is very extensive: all albumin contained in plasma crosses the capillary walls, enter the tissues, and is carried back into the circulation by the lymphatic system within a 24-hour period.

TISSUE FLUID PRESSURE, THE EFFECTIVE OSMOTIC PRESSURE, AND LYMPH FLOW

When the capillaries filter fluid into the interstitium, tissue fluid pressure increases (Fig. 74–3). Small changes in P_c produce only small changes in interstitial fluid volume, yet this small amount of filtration causes marked increases in the interstitial fluid pressure. However, when the tissues swell to some critical volume, only small changes in tissue pressure occur, and large amounts of fluid began to accumulate in the tissues. Normally, hydrated tissues are very compact and rigid; that is, they demonstrate a very low compliance $(\Delta V_t/\Delta P_t)$; however, when the tissues become edematous or if an overflow system opens, P_t cannot change to any significant level, even with continuous edema formation, because the tissue compliance is high.[11, 12] This

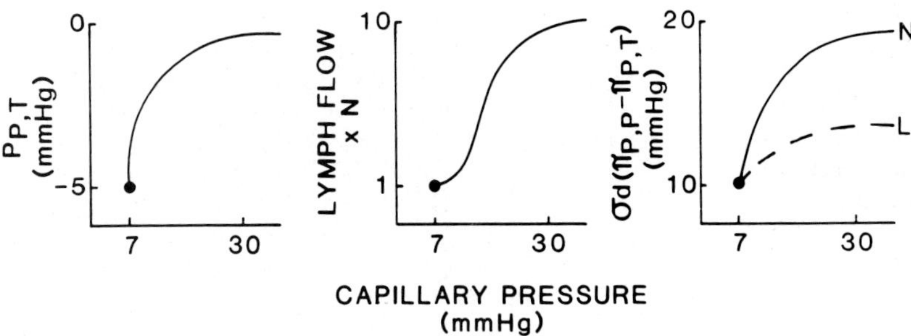

Figure 74–3. Effect of increasing capillary pressure on pulmonary tissue fluid pressure (P_{PT}), lymph flow times normal, and the absorptive force ($\sigma_d[\pi_p - \pi_T]$) for normal (N) and leaky (L) capillaries. (From Taylor AE, Barnard JW, Barman SA, et al: Fluid balance. *In:* The Lung: Scientific Foundation. Crystal RG, West JB [Eds]. New York, Raven Press, 1991, p 157.)

change in tissue compliance occurs because the tissues become less rigid, expand more easily, and produce less retarding pressures when interstitial fluid volume increases or when fluid spills into a potential space such as the alveoli in the lung and the peritoneal cavity in the intestine. A few tissues such as ocular, brain, and muscle tissues have restricted swelling, so continued edema formation causes interstitial pressures to become so large that blood flow to these tissues is greatly compromised.

When capillaries with normal permeability characteristics (i.e., low protein permeability) filter large volumes of fluid (designated as N in Fig. 74–3), π_t decreases to a limiting value that is a function of the permeability of the capillary walls. For most capillary walls, π_t approaches 5% to 10% of the π_p at high capillary filtration rates, and the osmotic gradient ($\sigma[\pi_p - \pi_t]$) becomes almost equal to the plasma colloid osmotic pressure. However, when the capillary walls become more permeable to plasma proteins, π_t does not decrease to low levels because more protein leaks into the tissues as the capillary filters (as shown by the dashed line [L] in Fig. 74–3). The osmotic reflection coefficient also decreases. The reflection coefficient can decrease to values as low as 0.5 to 0.4 in severely damaged capillaries; this results in a decrease in the absorptive force to 40% to 50% of the measured difference between π_p and π_t,[10, 11] since the effective protein osmotic pressure gradient is $\sigma(\pi_p - \pi_t)$.

In most capillary beds, lymph flow steadily increases with net capillary filtration and plateaus as the lymphatic system saturates (Fig. 74–3, middle panel). In the lung, intestine, and bronchial tissues, lymph flow actually declines as fluid enters the alveoli, the intestinal lumen, and airways, respectively. The importance of lymph flow in removing excess capillary filtration is not well understood, and certainly varies from tissue to tissue. For many years, physiologists thought that the lymphatic system was not important because lymph flow was low. However, the lymphatics' ability to remove capillary filtrate is not just a function of flow (LF) but is also related to the filtration characteristics of both the capillary wall and the interstitium (K_{LF}) is a function of the K_{fc} of the capillary wall and the conductance of the tissues ($K_{F,TISS}$):

$$\text{Lymphatics' abilty to remove fluid} = \frac{\text{Total lymph flow}}{K_{LF}}$$

Thus, if K_{LF} is small, even small lymph flows remove sufficient fluid to oppose excessive fluid accumulation. However, when K_{LF} is large, then even large lymph flows do not represent an important tissue volume removal system. It seems that the resistance of fluid movement within the interstitium, and not capillary wall permeability, may be the most important factor in determining the lymphatic system's ability to remove capillary filtrate in nonedematous tissues.[10, 12–16] However, the lymphatics represent the only means by which plasma proteins can reenter the plasma once they have leaked into the interstitium. Obviously, if proteins can leave the circulation, then a lymphatic system or some type of drainage system must be present to remove the tissue proteins; otherwise, their concentrations in the interstitium would eventually equal those within the plasma.

For many years, physiologists assumed that tissues with high protein concentrations in lymph contained highly permeable capillaries. This is not necessarily true, since the concentration of proteins in the tissues is a function of the protein concentration of plasma, the capillary filtration, the permeability of the capillary wall, and lymph flow. At very high transcapillary volume flows, the ratio of the protein concentration in tissues to plasma approaches 1.0 minus the reflection coefficient, and this relationship has been used extensively to define σ for various plasma proteins in many different organs.[1] The process by which proteins cross capillary walls and finally gain access to the lymph is a very complex mechanism, but the concept of a single osmotic reflection coefficient (σ) and a single protein osmotic pressure difference ($\Delta\pi$) has proved to be an extremely useful tool for predicting the movement of plasma proteins and water between plasma and interstitium under many experimental conditions.[1]

PERMEABILITY PROPERTIES OF CAPILLARIES IN DIFFERENT ORGANS

Tables 74–1 and 74–2 present predicted pore sizes, the permeability surface area products (PS), the reflection coefficients (σ) for sodium chloride, glucose, and albumin, and the filtration coefficient of the capillary in several different organs. These pore analyses were determined through the measurement of the reflection coefficient of various plasma proteins in lymph (C_L) by increasing venous pressure until σ could be calculated by $1 - C_L/C_p$ for each protein contained in plasma (C_p).[1, 17] Note that most capillary beds appear to contain a large number of small pores (~5 nm) that are sufficiently large for albumin to escape into the interstitium but are too small to permit the passage of the larger plasma proteins into the tissues. However, a small number of large pores (~20 nm) are present in most capillaries, and all plasma proteins can pass through these pores into the interstitium. The major exceptions to this are in the liver, whose capillaries have only two sets of very large pores, and the lung, whose capillaries appear to have small pores with radii of 70 to 80 nm. The large-pore system is very similar in all organs and may be present to allow large gamma globulins to gain access to the tissues to deliver various metabolic substrates and hormones to parenchymal cells.

The PS products sodium chloride and glucose presented in Table 74–2 are large in all tissues except those of the brain, where they cannot cross the capillary wall and where PS equals zero. These molecules have very low σ values in other tissues because they are not greatly restricted. Albu-

TABLE 74–1. Predicted Pore Sizes for Capillary Walls in Selected Tissues

Tissue	*Small Pore (nm)*	*Large Pore (nm)*	*Ratio of Large to Small Pores*
Subcutaneous	5.0	20.0	1:3000
Skeletal muscle	6.0	22.0	1:3600
Brain	0.4	—	—
Intestine	4.6	20.0	1:6400
Liver	9.5	33.0	1:50
Lung	8.0	20.0	1:200

(Reproduced from Taylor AE: Molecular fluid and solute exchange. *In:* Encyclopedia of Human Biology. Vol 5. Dulbecco R [Ed]. Orlando, Academic Press, 1991, p 35.)

min is much less permeable in all tissues, and, of course, it cannot enter the interstitial spaces of the brain. The σ for albumin in skeletal muscle, intestine, glomerular membrane, and subcutaneous tissue capillaries is close to one and is equal to one in brain. Interestingly, the lung and cardiac muscles have relatively lower σ values (0.75 and 0.45, respectively, for albumin). The smaller σ values in these tissues may reflect an underestimation of the reflection coefficient or a higher protein permeability. The higher protein permeability in lung and heart tissues provides lipid "shuttles" for metabolism and surfactant production in the parenchymal cells of these organs' tissues, respectively. K_{fs} values are high in tissues in which large amounts of fluid are filtered. This occurs because of either large solvent permeability (kidney) or high surface areas (lung), or both. It appears that assuming a reflection coefficient of one does not greatly affect most predictions of transcapillary solvent movement over a short period of time in organs with normal capillary permeability, since PS determines the length of time required for proteins to leave the circulation. When PS is increased because of capillary damage, the magnitude of transcapillary fluid flux is grossly underestimated when assuming that σ for plasma proteins is equal to one owing to the rapid vascular loss of the protein.

PHYSIOLOGY OF SOLVENT EXCHANGE, AND THE DEFINITION OF STARLING FORCES

Figure 74–4 shows schematically how fluid is thought to move across capillary walls.[18] For many years, it was believed that fluid was filtered at the arterial end of the capillary and was reabsorbed on the venous end (Landis'[18a] capillary fluid exchange hypothesis). This was thought to occur because the hydrostatic pressure on the arterial ends of the capillaries is about 30 mm Hg, but that at the venous ends of the capillaries was 10 mm Hg. Since only small amounts of fluid filter across the capillary wall, π_p remains almost constant as the fluid traverses the capillary. The difference in hydrostatic and osmotic forces inside the capillary at the arterial and venous ends of the capillary would be $P_c - \pi_p = +1$ and $P_c - \pi_p = -19$ respectively, if π_p were 29 mm Hg. This assessment of capillary filtration forces assumes that π_t and P_t are near zero in the tissues surrounding the capillary wall. However, this simple capillary model fails to consider that P_t and π_t will be different in the tissues surrounding the capillary walls at the arterial and venous ends of the capillary. If P_c is greater than π_p on the arterial end of the capillary, then fluid filters, causing π_t to decrease and P_t to increase. This causes an imbalance of Starling forces of only 1 mm Hg, which act at the arterial portion of the capillary—that is, $(30 - 0) - (29 - 0) = 30 - 29 = +1$. At the venous end of the capillary, the absorption of fluid causes P_t to become more subatmospheric (-10) and π_t to increase because of interstitial volume removal. This results in an imbalance of Starling forces of +1 mm Hg at the venous end of the capillary—that is, $10 - (-10) - (29 - 10) = 20 - 19 = +1$. This is a simplistic model of transcapillary fluid exchange, but it does illustrate the importance of knowing all capillary and tissue forces when estimation of transcapillary fluid flux is attempted. The force balance in the lung is even more complicated because of the hydrostatic gradients existing in capillary and tissue pressures from the apex to the base of the lung. The interested reader is directed to reviews by Staub[15] and by Taylor and colleagues[13] for a more in-depth analysis of the heterogeneous capillary and tissue forces that operate in lung tissue.

All recent data and theoretic analyses indicate that capillary filtration within physiologic limits is self-regulating; that is, if P_c increases, then P_t increases and π_t decreases to oppose filtration; if P_c decreases, then P_t decreases and π_t increases to halt absorption. This is just a restatement of the Starling law of capillary exchange: capillary filtration within normal physiologic limits is self-regulating ($P_c - P_t = \pi_p - \pi_t$).

Table 74–3 lists P_c, P_t, π_p and π_t colloid osmotic pressures, LF, and the imbalance in Starling forces (ΔP) for several organs, where

$$\Delta P = (P_c - P_t) - (\pi_p - \pi_t)$$

For instance, in the intestine, the imbalance of these forces in a *nonabsorbing intestine* is

$$\begin{aligned}\Delta P &= (16 - 2) - (23 - 10)\\ &= 14 - 13\\ &= +1 \text{ mm Hg}\end{aligned}$$

TABLE 74–2. Permeability Surface Area Product Reflection Coefficients, and Filtration Coefficients for Selected Tissues*

	PS (mL • min⁻¹ per 100g)		σ_d		K_{fc}
Tissue	*NaCl*	*Glucose*	*NaCl*	*Albumin*	*(mL • min⁻¹ • mm Hg per 100 g)*
Subcutaneous	15	15	0.002	0.90	0.020
Skeletal muscle	15	16	0.002	0.94	0.015
Brain	0.01	0	1.0	1.0	0.000001
Intestine	1400	80	0.0004	0.92	0.085
Liver	1500	1500	0.0	0.0	1.00
Lung	200	150	0.002	0.75	0.200
Cardiac muscle	100	50	0.020	0.45	0.70
Kidney	150	150	0.0	0.999	2.00

(Modified from Taylor AE: Molecular fluid and solute exchange. *In:* Encyclopedia of Human Biology. Vol 5. Dulbecco R [Ed]. Orlando, Academic Press, 1991, p 39.)

*The molecular radius of both sodium chloride (NaCl) and glucose is about 0.5 nm, and albumin's molecular radius is 3.7 nm.

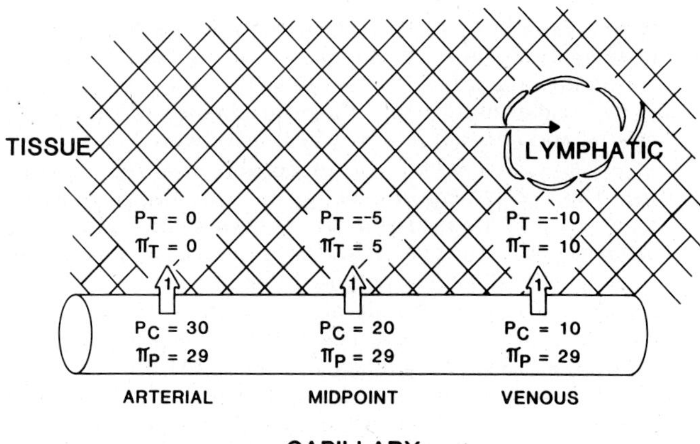

Figure 74–4. Capillary forces (P_c and π_p) in the arterial, midpoint, and venous ends of the capillary and their corresponding tissue forces (P_t and π_t). (From Taylor AE, Townsley MI: Evaluation of the Starling fluid flux equation. News Physiol Sci 1987; 2:37.)

A positive value means that the capillaries are filtering and forming lymph. In an *absorbing small intestine,* the imbalance of forces is

$$\Delta P = (16 - 3) - (23 - 5) = 13 - 18 = -5 \text{ mm Hg}$$

The negative value for the imbalance of forces indicates that the capillary is absorbing fluid from the interstitium. These examples indicate that the physical forces acting at the capillary wall are very dynamic and that capillaries filter fluid when P_c and protein permeability are increased and reabsorb when P_c is small and $\sigma(\pi_p - \pi_t)$ is large. The reader should evaluate the balance of forces for all tissues listed in Table 74–3 to gain a better understanding of the basic phenomenon of transcapillary fluid exchange in different organs.

STARLING FORCE ANALYSIS DURING EDEMA FORMATION

Tissue edema safety factor is an abstract term that reflects the ability of P_t, $\sigma(\pi_p - \pi_t)$, and lymph flow to increase when P_c is increased.[19–20] The tissue edema safety factors act to limit tissue edema formation until P_c becomes excessively high, as shown in Figure 74–3.[11, 16] Table 74–4 lists the per cent change in these three safety factors following an increase in P_c of about 20 mm Hg in several organs. This pressure change does not cause observable edema, yet only a small increase in P_c above this level causes excessive edema formation. Changes in the protein osmotic gradient provide the major opposition to capillary filtration in most organs unless π_t is initially small (subcutaneous and muscle) or capillary permeability is very high (e.g., in the capillaries of the liver and heart). The lymphatics' ability to remove capillary filtrate has recently been shown to be an important tissue volume reducer when the capillaries are damaged or following large plasma volume expansions with saline,[21] but substantial interstitial edema must occur before the lymphatic safety factors can attain their maximum capacity to remove capillary filtrate. P_t is an important safety factor in lung, small intestine, hind limb tissues; it is especially important in liver and heart tissues, since $\sigma(\pi_p - \pi_t)$ is very small or equal to zero in these two tissues.[20] It appears that all tissues can buffer changes in capillary pressures of 10 to 20 mm Hg without significant edema formation, but the mechanisms responsible for this effect are not the same in all tissues.

EDEMA FORMATION IN THE LUNGS

Hydrostatic Edema

The tissue safety factors buffer changes in P_c to prevent edema formation until P_c exceeds 25 to 30 mm Hg in normal lungs, as shown diagrammatically by the solid line in Figure 74–5. The solid line represents either interstitial edema (IE) or alveolar edema (AE) associated with increasing P_c. Note that P_c increases to 25 to 30 mm Hg before alveolar edema develops. P_t, $\sigma(\pi_p - \pi_t)$, and lymph flow increase to oppose

TABLE 74–3. Starling Forces for Selected Tissues

Tissue	P_c	P_t *(mm Hg)*	π_p	π_t	*LF (mL • min⁻¹ per 100 g)*	*ΔP* (mm Hg)*
Subcutaneous	13	−5	21	4	0.015	+1
Skeletal muscle	9	−3	20	8	0.005	0
Brain	11	7	14	0	—	−10
Intestine (normal)	16	2	23	10	0.08	+1
Intestine (absorbing)	16	3	23	5	0.10	−5
Liver	7	6	22	20	0.10	−1
Lung	7	−5	23	12	0.10	+1
Cardiac muscle	23	15	21	13	0.12	0
Glomerular	50	15†	28	0†	2.0	+7
Renal peritubular	25	7	32	7	2.0	−7

(Modified from Taylor AE: Molecular fluid and solute exchange. *In:* Encyclopedia of Human Biology . Vol 5. Dulbecco R [Ed]. Academic Press, 1991, p 35.)
*ΔP is the sum of the forces $[(P_c - P_t) - (\pi_p - \pi_t)]$ and represents filtration when negative. A sum of zero indicates no filtration or absorption.
†This represents tubular pressures rather than renal interstitial pressure.

TABLE 74–4. Safety Factors in Various Dog Tissues*

Tissue	*Increased* $\sigma_d(\pi_p - \pi_t)$	*Increased LF*	*Increased* P_t
Lung	50	17	33
Hind paw	14	24	62
Small intestine	45	20	35
Colon	52	4	44
Liver	0	42	58
Heart	7	12	81

(Modified from Taylor AE: Molecular fluid and solute exchange. *In:* Encyclopedia of Human Biology. Vol 5. Dulbecco R [Ed]. Orlando, Academic Press, 1991, p 35.)

*The values are shown as a per cent of the total safety factor measured when P_c was increased 20 mm Hg above control values.

P_c, as demonstrated in Figure 74–3. However, once these forces attain their maximum changes, interstitial lung edema develops; this is followed by alveolar flooding. Obviously, much research in this area with modern assessments of P_c, P_t, and π_t is needed. It is important to know how effectively the safety factors can buffer alterations in the pulmonary capillary pressures of critically ill patients, since different plasma volume expanders and drugs must always be used to maintain proper oxygen delivery to tissues and because overhydration can result in pulmonary edema, which decreases oxygen exchange in the lungs.

Permeability Edema

The tissue's maximum ability to buffer acute increases in P_c or decreases in plasma colloid osmotic pressure can become greatly impaired by any pathologic condition that causes capillaries to become abnormally leaky to plasma proteins (see Fig. 74–5, dashed line labeled "permeability"). This inability of the safety factors to adequately respond is mainly due to the failure of $\sigma(\pi_p - \pi_t)$ to increase when capillaries are damaged, since π_t approaches the value of π_p and σ is also decreased; thus, an increase in P_c does not produce any significant increase in $\sigma(\pi_p - \pi_t)$. Damaged capillaries have a high filtration coefficient, and the tissue resistance also decreases; this results in a decreased lymphatic safety factor, since the lymphatic edema safety factor is inversely related to the capillary wall and tissue conductances (K_{LF}).[11, 15, 19, 20] However, as discussed later in this chapter, the high lymph flows that occur after interstitial edema forms provide an additional safety factor that opposes alveolar edema formation.

An analysis of the lymphatic safety factor by Taylor[21] indicates that large plasma volume expansions with saline and damaged capillary endothelium cause lymph flow to increase to astronomic levels in edematous tissues. The reason for this high lymph flow response is not known, but it is likely that some compound or compounds released by endothelial cells cause the lymphatic flow to increase to levels never observed in the absence of edema. Further research is greatly needed in this area because lymph flow has the ability to increase to levels that can accommodate large transvascular fluid fluxes; however, the mechanisms by which this occurs are unknown. If this factor is considered in Figure 74–5 (as shown by the larger dashed line labeled "actual"), then intra-alveolar edema does not develop in the lungs at moderate P_c elevations, although interstitial edema is present.

Relevance to Critical Care Medicine

Since capillary fluid and protein exchange is a much more complex phenomenon than has been presented in the previous section, how can the physician use this information to treat edema, especially pulmonary edema? From the present analysis, it is clear that $\sigma(\pi_p - \pi_t)$ is a most important regulator of lung interstitial fluid volume. However, if the capillaries are abnormally leaky to proteins, then albumin administration will not be an effective treatment for the reduction of edema. How to increase cardiac output while maintaining proper lung function is a problem that always faces the clinician. Colloids and plasma proteins expand blood volume and usually increase pulmonary P_c. If the lung capillaries are abnormally leaky to proteins, then the effective osmotic pressure gradient acting across the capillary wall is small, and the use of colloids if P_c increases will actually accelerate interstitial fluid accumulation. This occurs because P_c is increased by the removal of interstitial fluid from the large muscle and subcutaneous tissue spaces secondary to an increase in protein osmotic pressure in plasma.[24] In a lung injury study,[25] the amount of pulmonary edema decreased when left atrial pressures were controlled with dextran therapy; however, when left atrial pressure was allowed to increase, the amount of pulmonary edema greatly increased. Unfortunately, it is not always possible to determine exactly to what degree pulmonary capillaries are damaged in different disease states. Brigham and associates[26] have shown promising results in this area by estimat-

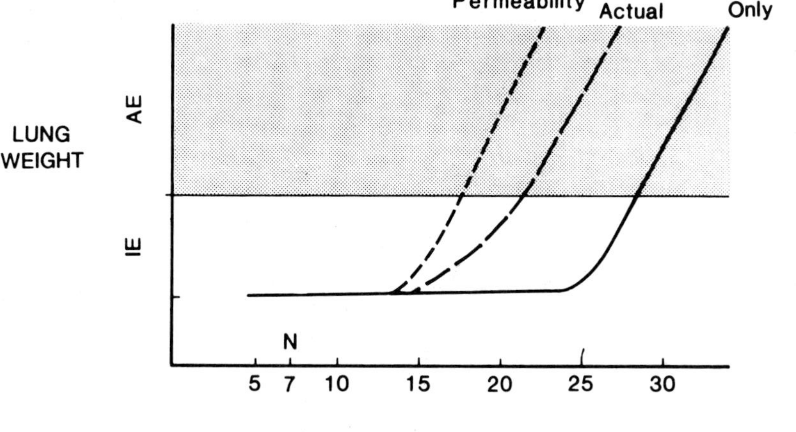

Figure 74–5. Lung weight as a function of capillary pressure. IE and AE refer to interstitial and alveolar edema, respectively. The *solid line* represents normal lungs subjected to only hydrostatic pressure increase (e.g., left-sided heart failure), the *dashed line* refers to damaged capillaries (permeability), and the *large dashed line* refers to the actual gain in lung weight in the presence of damaged capillaries. (Reprinted from Taylor AE: Pulmonary edema: Ischemia reperfusion endothelial injury and its reversal by c-AMP. Proc Natl Sci Counc Repub China [B] 1991; 15:192, with kind permission from Elsevier Science Ltd, The Boulevard, Langford Lane, Kidlington 0×5 1GB, UK.)

ing endothelial damage using urea and sodium ion clearance as indices of vascular permeability in the pulmonary circulation. In addition, radioactive markers can be used to measure leakage across the pulmonary circulation in intact human lungs.[27] Modern imaging techniques, such as positron emission tomography, are also quite useful in determining the leakiness of the pulmonary capillary beds with respect to proteins.[28] When the lungs are more permeable to plasma proteins, then an accurate estimate of P_c becomes an important measure in the critically ill patient, since even slight elevations of P_c can cause severe pulmonary edema.

The Role of Oxygen Radicals in Lung Damage

It is now well known that pulmonary vascular walls can be damaged by the release of oxygen radicals that are toxic to tissues. The classic work of Granger and associates clearly showed that a period of ischemia followed by reperfusion causes excessive damage to endothelial cells in the small intestine.[29] Granger postulated that tissue oxygen level, which increased as the tissues were reperfused, caused the formation of superoxide anion (O_2^-). This phenomena has been confirmed in many studies.[30] The O_2^- formed at reperfusion is reduced by superoxide dismutase to produce hydrogen peroxide (H_2O_2). The tissues contain several different peroxidases and catalases that reduce H_2O_2 to water and molecular oxygen. These chemical reactions are shown schematically in Figure 74–6. Superoxide anion and H_2O_2 do not always cause tissue damage because of their low reactivity and their inactivation by enzymes, but when O_2^- and H_2O_2 combine in the presence of iron (Fe^{3+}), a very reactive compound, the hydroxyl radical is formed (OH·). In fact, many forms of tissue injury are now known to be caused by periods of ischemia followed by reperfusion and the formation of the OH· radicals.[31] Leukocytes (most likely neutrophils) are now known to be responsible for oxygen radical production in ischemia-reperfusion. As leukocytes adhere to the vascular endothelium, they release these oxygen radicals; the endothelial membranes are damaged, and the leukocytes disrupt the capillary barrier as they migrate from the capillaries into the tissues. In effect, the endothelial damage associated with ischemia-reperfusion is an exaggerated inflammatory response that is superimposed on ischemic tissue damage.[30] In order to describe the most recent developments in endothelial injury associated with ischemia-reperfusion, we will present our lung studies in the next section of this chapter; similar studies of other organs have been conducted and have shown similar results.

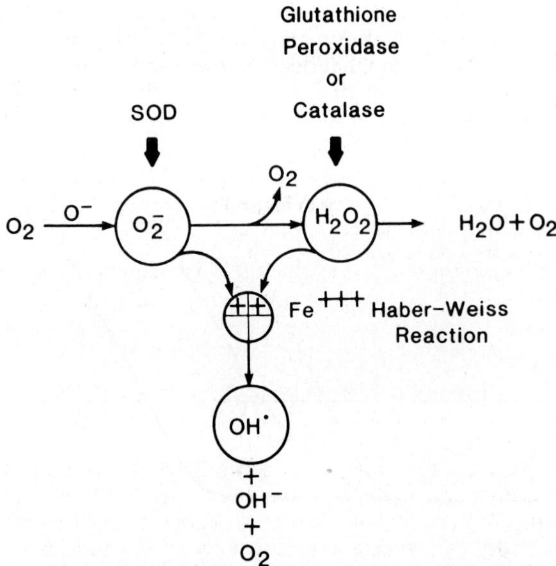

Figure 74–6. Oxygen radical formation. (From Taylor AE, Rehder K, Hyatt RE, et al: *In:* Clinical Respiratory Physiology. Taylor AE, Rehder K, Hyatt RE, et al [Eds]. Philadelphia, W.B. Saunders, 1989, p 22.)

ROLE OF OXYGEN RADICALS IN LUNG INJURY

Effects of Antioxidants and Neutrophils

Figure 74–7*A* shows the effect of ischemia-reperfusion on endothelial permeability as measured by K_{fc} in isolated rabbit lungs. This damage can be prevented by pretreating the lung with superoxide dismutase and catalase. Catalase totally prevented the ischemia-reperfusion endothelial injury, whereas superoxide dismutase only lessened the damage.[32] Figure 74–7*B* shows the effects of blocking xanthine oxidase by means of the institution of a diet that causes this enzyme to be inactivated as well as the effects of allopurinol, which blocks this enzyme activity, on the prevention of the endothelial damage associated with ischemia-reperfusion. Note that blocking xanthine oxidase totally inhibits this endothelial damage. Menadione, which is an inhibitor of aldehyde oxidase, was ineffective at preventing the endothelial damage. Importantly, IB_4, which inhibits leukocyte adherence to endothelial cells by blocking the CD11/CD18 integrins, also prevents ischemia-reperfusion injury in lung tissue.[33] These studies clearly indicate that ischemia followed by reperfusion causes endothelial damage associated with oxygen radical formation (likely hydroxyl radicals) in the lung. Xanthine oxidase is required for the production of these radicals, and leukocyte (likely neutrophil) adherence and transcapillary migration is required for ischemia-reperfusion to damage the endothelial barrier. The lung appears to behave similarly to the small intestine and to muscle with respect to these phenomena.[31]

EFFECT OF INTRACELLULAR MESSENGERS

In order to gain a better understanding of the cellular mechanisms involved in the production of ischemia-reperfusion damage, we evaluated the effects of increasing intercellular cyclic AMP (cAMP) on ischemia-reperfusion lung injury.[33] We chose to study cAMP because it had been established that isoproterenol prevents endothelial cell damage associated with histamine release in the systemic circulation.[34] However, the protective effect of cAMP on the pulmonary capillary barrier had not yet been studied in the lung. Figure 74–7*C* shows the effects of increasing cAMP with isoproterenol, forskolin, and dibutyryl cAMP on the endothelial damage associated with ischemia-reperfusion in rabbit lungs.[33] Note that ischemia-reperfusion severely damaged the endothelial cells in untreated lungs compared with those of controls; however, when cAMP level was elevated, the damage failed to occur. These studies indicate that cAMP prevents the endothelial damage associated with ischemia-reperfusion by either an endothelial cell or leukocyte effect. To understand the effect of activated leukocytes in producing endothelial damage, a phorbol ester (phorbol myristate) was used to activate leukocytes in isolated dog lung.[35] Activation of circulating leukocytes causes extensive lung damage and pulmonary edema, but when adenosine, was given prior to the cell activation, the damage was totally prevented. Since adenosine has been implicated in leukocyte activation and adhesion, we further evaluated adenosine's effect on phorbol myristate neutrophil activation as shown in Figure 74–7*D*.[36] When adenosine was present and the

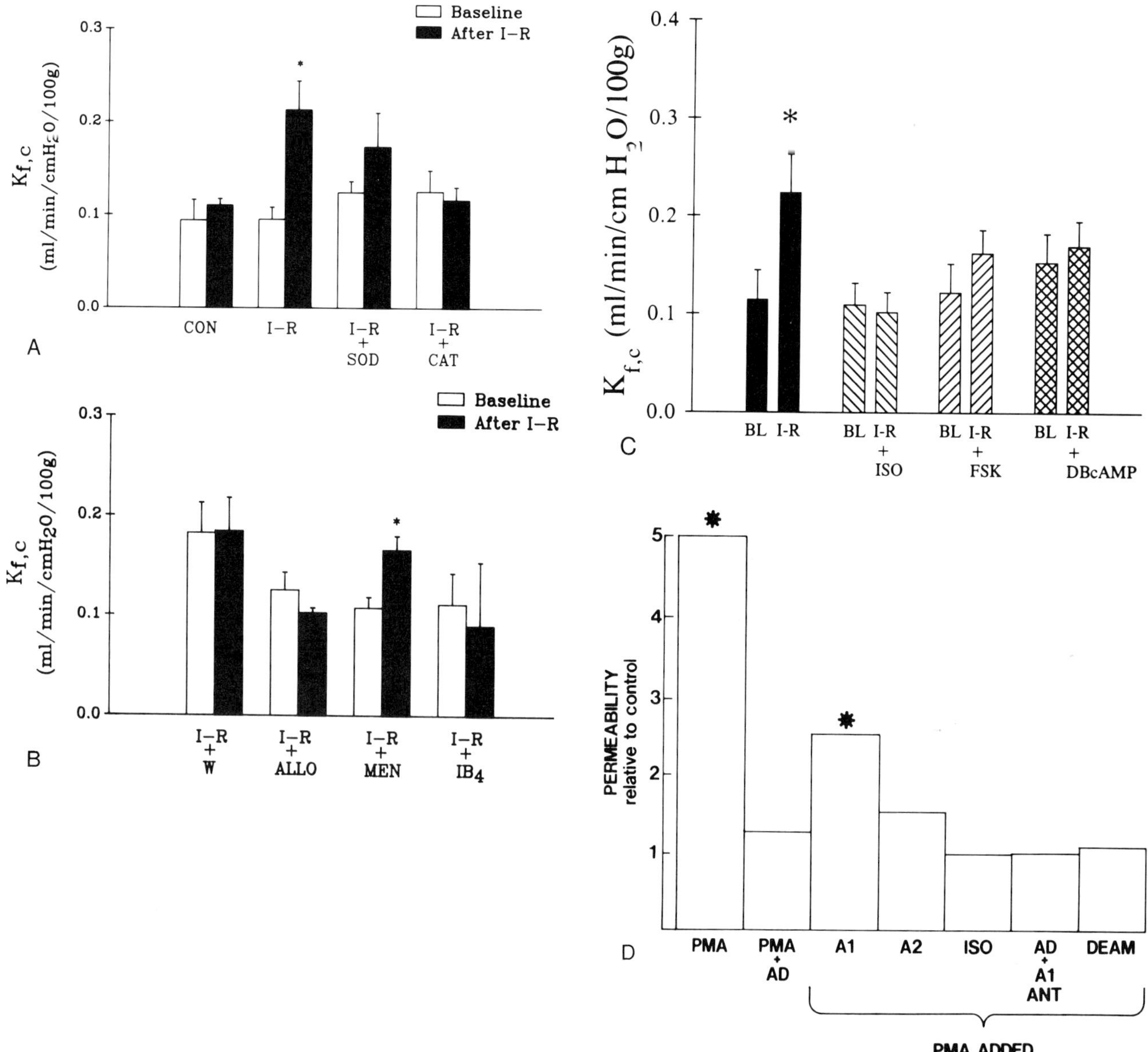

Figure 74–7. *A,* Permeability changes ($K_{f,c}$) associated with ischemia-reperfusion injury (I-R) and the effects of superoxide dismutase (SOD) and catalase (CAT) on I-R. (From Adkins WK, Taylor AE: Role of xanthine oxidase and neutrophils in ischemia-reperfusion injury in rabbit lung. J Appl Physiol 1990; 69:2044.) *B,* Effect of altering xanthine oxidase on the permeability change associated with ischemia-reperfusion using a diet (W) that inactivates xanthine oxidase; allopurinol (ALLO), which blocks xanthine oxidase; an aldebide oxidase inhibitor (MEN); and inhibition of leukocyte adherence (IB_4). (From Adkins WK, Taylor AE: Role of xanthine oxidase and neutrophils in ischemia-reperfusion injury in rabbit lung. J Appl Physiol 1990; 69:2016.) *C,* Permeability ($K_{f,c}$) following I-R in the presence of isoproterenol (ISO), forskolin (FSK), and dibutyryl cAMP (DBcAMP). (From Adkins WK, Barnard JW, May S, et al: Compounds that increase c-AMP prevent ischemia-reperfusion pulmonary capillary injury. J Appl Physiol 1992; 72:494.) *D,* Effect of adenosine (AD), A_1 and A_2 agonists, isoproterenol (ISO), an A_1 antagonist, and adenosine deaminase (DEAM) on preventing damage associated with phorbol myristate activation (PMA) of leukocytes. (Modified with permission from Adkins WK, Barnard JW, Moore TM, et al: Adenosine prevents PMA-induced lung injury via an A_2 receptor mechanism. J Appl Physiol 1993; 74:984.)

leukocytes were activated, no endothelial damage occurred. When an adenosine A_1 agonist was given, the damage occurred; however, an adenosine A_2 agonist and an A_1 antagonist totally prevented the damage. In addition, adenosine deaminase and a protein kinase C, inhibitor (not shown in Figure 74–7*D*) blocked the damage associated with phorbol myristate. These studies in animal lungs indicate that (1) the activation of neutrophils causes endothelial damage in ischemia-reperfusion because oxygen radicals are produced by leukocytes (likely neutrophils), (2) cAMP protects the endothelial cells, and (3) adenosine and adenosine A_2 receptors as well as the inhibition of adenosine A_1 receptors prevent the endothelial cell damage associated with the phorbol myristate activation of leukocytes.

The model as proposed in Figure 74–8 shows how the activation of stimulatory proteins (G_s) and inhibitory proteins (G_i) can activate or inhibit the action of adenylcyclase, respectively. Activating adenylcyclase causes the level of cAMP to increase; this can either inactivate some protein kinase C or activate protein kinase A in the neutrophils or endothelial cells. This would both prevent neutrophils from adhering and migrating and promote polymerization of mi-

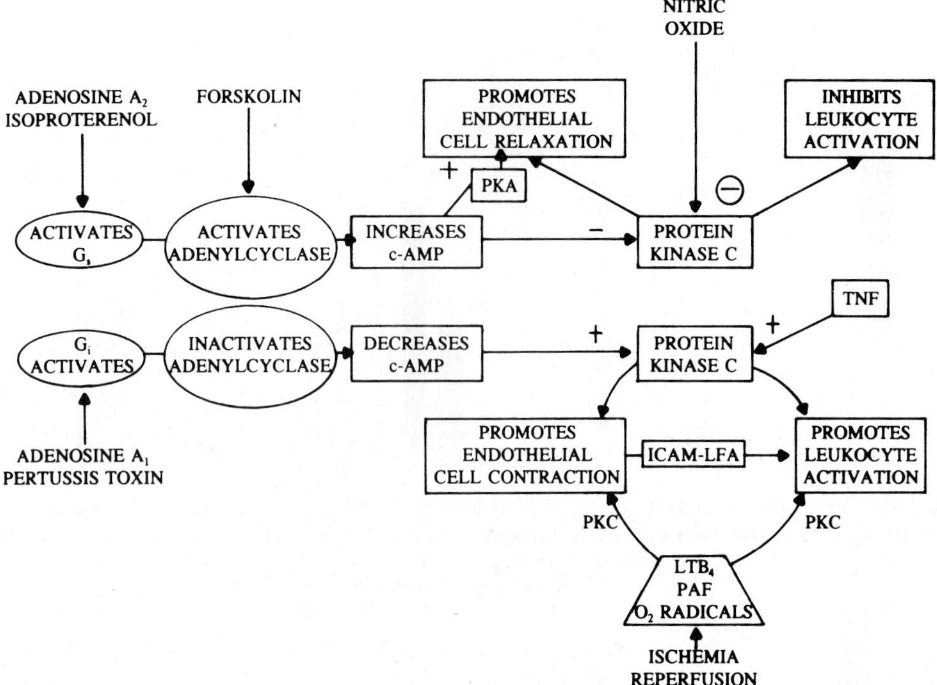

Figure 74–8. Flow diagram showing the possible mechanisms involved with the cAMP and adenosine affects on neutrophil activation and endothelial cell contraction.

crofilaments, which relaxes the endothelial cells. Activating the G_i protein inhibits adenylcyclase activity, which decreases cAMP level, and activates a protein kinase C which disrupts endothelial microfilaments, resulting in endothelial contraction and promotion of neutrophil activation and migration into tissue. Adenosine could exert its effect in this system in two ways: (1) the A_1 receptor activation caused by the release of tissue adenosine during ischemia could directly activate protein kinase C in leukocytes, causing them to adhere[37]; or (2) the A_2 adenosine receptors inactivate protein kinase C or activate protein kinase A to block the neutrophil migration and promote endothelial cell relaxation. Basically, the schematic representation in Figure 74–8 explains the protective effects of cAMP and adenosine on ischemia-reperfusion via the alteration of neutrophil activation and oxygen radical production and the promoting endothelial cell relaxation. The following data indicate that endothelial cell cAMP effects are probably independent of their neutrophil effects, and one study has shown a dramatic experimental finding: that the pulmonary edema associated with ischemia-reperfusion is actually resolved by an elevation of cAMP level.

RESOLUTION OF PULMONARY EDEMA

Figure 74–9*A* shows recent data from the work of Siebert and associates.[38, 39] The permeability of an isolated rat lung preparation (K_{fc}) was used to assess endothelial damage following ischemia of 45 minutes' duration followed by reperfusion. After 30 minutes of reperfusion, the endothelial permeability was again measured. Note that considerable endothelial damage had occurred since the permeability factor had increased threefold to fourfold above normal values. At this time, after the endothelial damage had occurred, forskolin (which activates adenycyclase), isoproterenol (which activates adenylcyclase through a β receptor effect), and a cAMP analog (dibutryl cAMP) were added to the perfusate of the damaged lung. In the lungs not receiving cAMP-elevating compounds, the permeability continued to increase to levels fivefold to sixfold greater than that in the controls (line labeled "I/R"). However, postinjury treatment actually *reversed* the endothelial damage—that is, the permeability decreased *below* the values measured 30 minutes after reperfusion. If only the neutrophils had been inhibited, then the cAMP-elevating compounds would have prevented additional damage but not returned the permeability of the endothelial cells back to normal levels. Another important finding from these studies is presented in Figure 74–9*B*. Figure 74–9*B* shows wet/dry weight ratios compared with normal lung values (left scale and hatched histogram) and the number of alveoli filled with alveolar fluid (right scale and clear histogram). One hour following the introduction of isoproterenol and forskolin into the damaged lung, most of the *alveolar edema fluid had been removed*. This is the first study to show such rapid removal of edema fluid in isolated lungs and indicates that cAMP elevation should be studied as a possible clinical means of resolving pulmonary edema. Similar studies have been conducted using a phosphodiesterase inhibitor. The effects were similar to the activity of adenylcyclase, and tissue levels of cAMP correlate with the levels of the drug.[39a]

Our basic hypothesis is that the damaged endothelial cell barrier must be "repaired" and that the epithelial transport system must be stimulated before such a rapid resolution of alveolar edema can occur. This is an exciting finding that will certainly stimulate new studies, but it also emphasizes the importance of maintaining a low capillary pressure and normal endothelial permeability in critically ill patients so as to remove the fluid that is transported out of the airways by the alveolar epithelium. Although the exact mechanisms that cause cAMP to reverse the endothelial damage and promote the almost complete removal of alveolar fluid are not understood, there is absolutely no doubt that elevating cAMP causes these effects in animal models and that the effect may be due to the cytoskeleton changes.[40] Hopefully, studies on human lungs to evaluate the effect of cAMP elevation on pulmonary edema resolution can be conducted in the future. We believe that these findings explain why

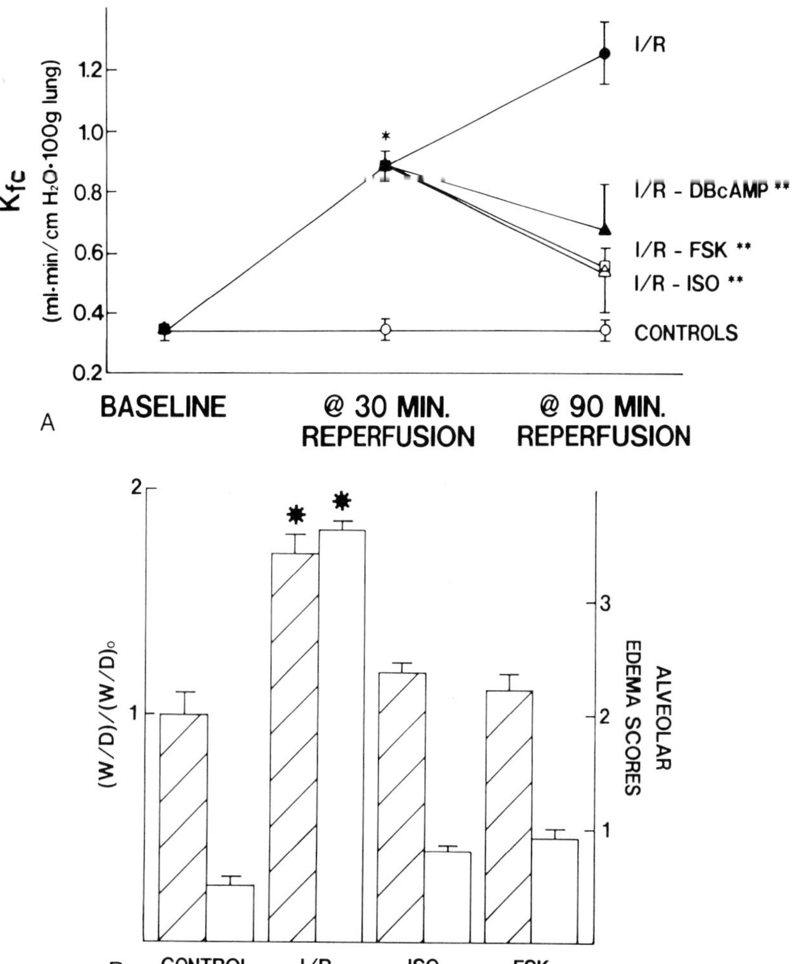

Figure 74–9. *A,* Permeability (K_{fc}) following ischemia-reperfusion (I/R) in isolated rat lungs. After reperfusion, DB-cAMP, FSK, and ISO were placed into the perfusate. Note that these interventions actually "reversed" the damage. (From Seibert AF, Thompson WJ, Taylor A, et al: Reversal of increased microvascular permeability associated with ischemia-reperfusion: Role of cAMP. J Appl Physiol 1992; 72:390.) *B,* Wet-to-dry (W/D) after I-R and treatment relative to control W/D weight ratios *(left ordinate)* and an anatomic estimate of fluid-filled alveoli *(right ordinate).* Note that the edema fluid present after the ischemia-reperfusion period was almost totally reabsorbed 1 hour after treatment. (From Taylor AE, Adkins WK, Moore TM: Ischemia reperfusion lung injury: Repair of endothelial damage by adenosine and cAMP. *In:* Yearbook of Intensive Care Medicine. Vincent JL [Ed]. Berlin, Springer-Verlag, 1993, p 17.)

some patients show rapid removal of edema fluid, whereas others have persistant edema. The rapid resolution of edema may occur both because the vascular damage is "repaired" by the release of epinephrine and because the epithelial cell transport system must be "up-regulated" if alveolar edema is to be cleared in an efficient manner.

MEASURE OF PULMONARY CAPILLARY PRESSURE

Because P_c is the most important determinant of edema formation (see Fig. 74–5), P_c should be monitored in patients in intensive care situations when pulmonary arterial Swan-Ganz catheters are in place. Most physicians use pulmonary arterial wedge pressure, which has been misdefined as the *capillary* wedge pressure, whereas others average systolic and diastolic pressures to estimate pulmonary capillary pressures (P_{pc}). We have developed a simple and reproducible way to assess P_{pc} in animals. Figure 74–10 shows the physical principles on which a clinical estimate of P_{pc} is based.[41] The pulmonary vascular circuit is defined as two resistances, the arterial (r_a) and venous (r_v) resistances, in series with a large capacitor located in the capillary compartment. When a catheter is wedged into the arterial side of the pulmonary circulation, the catheter tip pressure rapidly decreases to the pressure present on the large capacitor (i.e., to the existing P_c). Then, the pressure slowly approaches the wedge pressure, which in most cases is the left atrial pressure. The largest capacitance of the pulmonary circulation is located at the filtration midpoint as well as the anatomic midpoint of the alveolar capillaries.[42] This arrangement allows capillary pressure to be estimated with a great deal of accuracy with occlusion of a Swan-Ganz catheter, even if the actual system is more complex than that shown in the electrical analog of Figure 74–10.[43, 44] The major requirement to estimate P_{pc} from the pressure transient is that any precapillary compliance is small relative to the

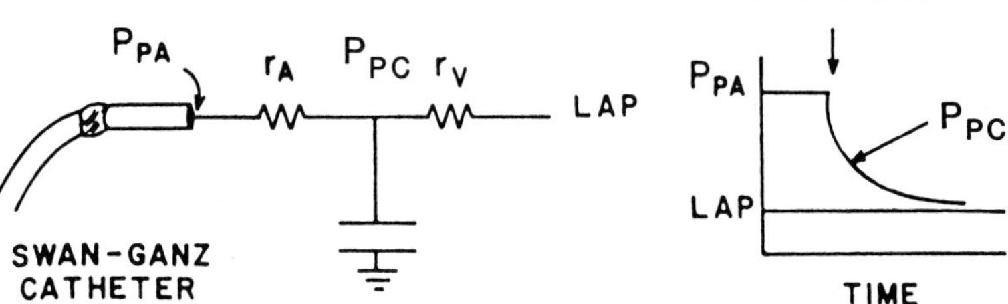

Figure 74–10. Schematic representation of the pulmonary arterial occlusion method for determining capillary pressure. A simple two-resistance, single-capacitance electrical model is shown on the right, and a pressure tracing observed after balloon occlusion of the pulmonary artery is shown on the left.

central or capillary compliances. This assumption has been validated in many experimental conditions.[45] The P_c can be estimated by simply identifying the inflection point at which the pressure changes from a rapid to the slow component of the P_{pa} tracing, which approaches the left atrial pressure as shown in the right panel of Figure 74–10.

In an extensive review of capillary pressure measurements in animal and human lungs, Cope and colleagues[45] described a useful method to determine the P_c using Swan-Ganz catheters in animal and human lungs. Figure 74–11*A* shows a computer prediction of an electrical model[43, 44] of a complex electrical model of pulmonary circulation that contains three vascular capacitances (arterial, capillary, and venous) and four segmental vascular resistances (large artery, small artery, large vein, and small vein). This more extensive model of the pulmonary circulation was used to evaluate the effects of altering large and small vessel compliances and resistances on the measures of P_{pc}, using known values for the four resistances and the three capacitances determined in experimental animals. Figure 74–11*A* shows the pulmonary arterial pressure transient that was present after the arterial input was clamped (upper solid line, labeled

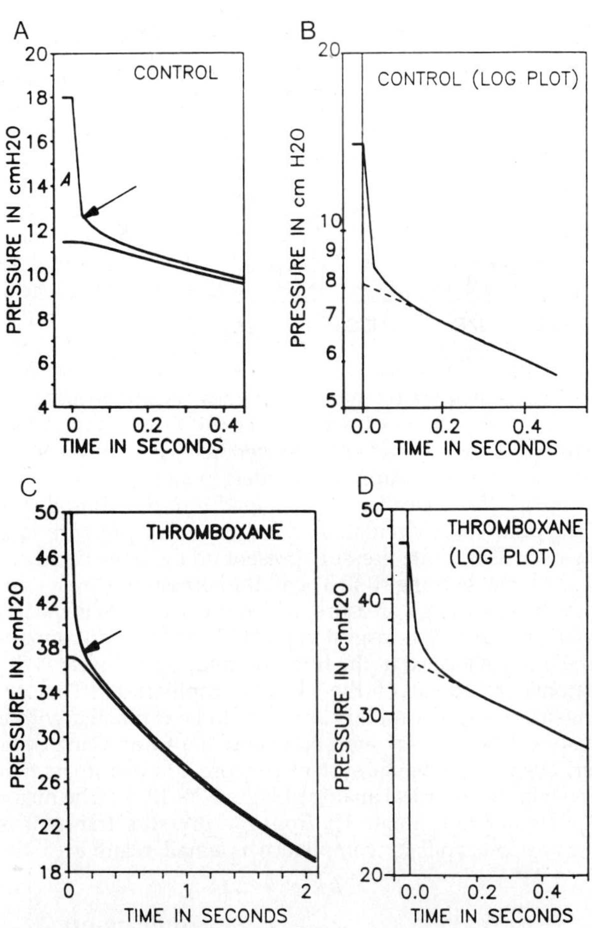

Figure 74–11. Model predictions of a four-resistance, three-compliance model following occlusion of a Swan-Ganz catheter in the pulmonary artery. *A,* The *upper curve* is the P_{pa}, and the *lower curve* is the existing capillary pressure. *B,* In this panel, $P_{pa} - P_{p,wedge}$ is shown as a function of time, and the extrapolation of the slow component to zero time is presented *(dashed line)*. Panels *C* and *D* show the same curves as in *A* and *B* with the exception that P_{pc} was elevated by thromboxane infusion. (From Cope DK, Grimbert F, Downey JM, et al: Pulmonary capillary pressure: A review. Crit Care Med 1992; 20:1048.)

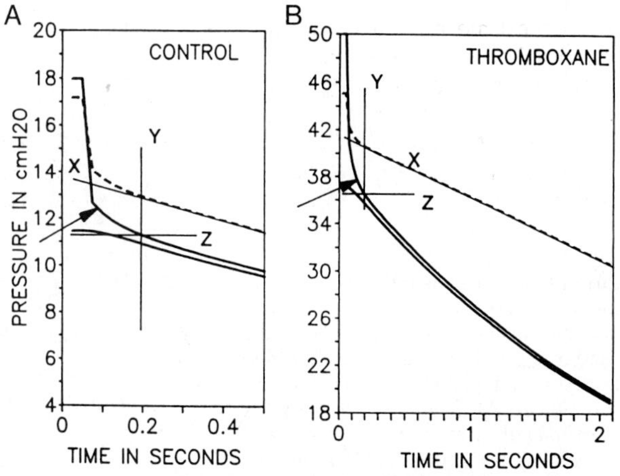

Figure 74–12. A more exact method for determining capillary pressure. *A,* The arterial pressure tracing after occlusion of the pulmonary artery *(solid curve)*. The *dashed curve* is $P_{pa} - P_{p,wedge}$, whereas the *solid line* (X) is used to identify the time when P_{pa} becomes linear. The line Y is then dropped to the P_{pa} curve, and the line Z is drawn perpendicular to Y in order to obtain a P_{pc}. Note that this method predicts the P_{pc} that is the existing capillary pressure. *B,* The same analysis is used with the exception that thromboxane was used to elevate capillary pressure. (From Cope DK, Grimbert F, Downey JM, et al: Pulmonary capillary pressure: A review. Crit Care Med 1992; 20:1049.)

"A"). Note that the inflection point in this curve (at the arrow) occurs at about 13 cm H_2O, whereas the P_c used in the model was 12.5 mm Hg. This indicates that a reasonable estimate of the existing P_{pc} (lower solid line) can be made by inspection. Figure 74–11*B* shows the $\log(P_{pa} - P_{wedge})$ plotted as a function of time (a method introduced by Holloway and coworkers[41] to estimate capillary pressure in dog lungs). The zero extrapolation of the slow pressure transient component intercepts the $P_{pa} - P_{wedge}$ at 8 cm H_2O, which, when added to the P_{wedge} of 4 cm H_2O, yields a P_c of 12 cm H_2O. Again, this more rigorous mathematical treatment produces a good estimate of the existing P_c. When thromboxane was used to elevate pulmonary vascular resistance (see Fig. 74–11*C* and *D*), the inflection point (arrow) yielded a P_c of about 38 cm H_2O, whereas the actual P_c in the model was 37 cm H_2O. When the $\log(P_{pa} - P_{wedge})$ is plotted as a function of time, the extrapolated value of the slow component to zero time (dashed line) intercepts the ordinate at 35 cm H_2O. When this intercept is added to the P_{wedge} of 4 cm H_2O, a P_{pc} of 39 cm H_2O is estimated. Both methods yield excellent approximations of the existing P_{pc} of 37 cm H_2O.

However, evaluation is problematic when the P_{pa} curve can be represented as a single exponential function approaching the wedge pressure, and simple identification of the inflection point as the pressure curve changes to the slower component may be too subjective. To eliminate these problems, Cope and colleagues developed a more accurate method to determine the existing P_c. Figure 74–12*A* and *B* shows how this analysis can be used to measure a P_{pc} that is unbiased by the observer.[45] Figure 74–12*A* shows the pulmonary arterial pressure curve obtained in a normal lung after the balloon on a Swan-Ganz catheter (solid line) is inflated. Remembering that this curve contains two distinct components, the $\log(P_{pa} - P_{wedge})$ was plotted as a function of time (dashed curve), but its magnitude was expanded to determine more precisely the time at which the P_{pa} curve becomes linear (solid line designated as "X" drawn on the dashed $\log[P_{pa} - P_{wedge}]$ curve). The lower solid line in Figure 74–12*A* represents the existing P_c in the modeled data.

When the time at which the $\log(P_{pa} - P_{wedge})$ plot attained linearity is extrapolated to the P_{pa} tracing (Y), an almost exact capillary pressure can be estimated, as seen by the Z line in comparison with the existing P_c. Figure 74–11*B* shows that the same analysis as applied to a lung in which thromboxane was used to increase vascular resistance and P_c. The solid line X indicates the linear portion of $\log(P_{pa} - P_{wedge})$, which is shown as a dashed line. When the time at which this linearity occurs is determined (line Y) and is extrapolated to the original P_{pa} curve (Z), a P_c of 36 to 37 cm H_2O is estimated; this estimate is almost equal to the existing P_{pc}.

Although this approach for evaluating P_{pc} is more exact than other methods, its major importance is that it can easily be computerized to estimate P_{pc} to a high degree of accuracy. However, the P_c can easily be estimated by simply observing the inflection point at which the P_{pa} curve changes to the slower component (arrow on curves). A computerized approach for estimating the P_c using the method of Cope and colleagues can easily be applied to any measure of a Swan-Ganz catheter–determined pulmonary arterial wedge pressure. However, the reader is urged to simply observe the P_{pa} pressure tracing after inflating the balloon to estimate P_{wedge} in his or her own clinical setting. If P_{pa} drops rapidly toward the P_{wedge}, then the resistance is precapillary; if it decreases slowly to the P_{wedge}, then the resistance is mostly postcapillary. Perhaps this is all the information that the reader requires when assessing a certain clinical intervention that affects the pulmonary circulation.

IMPORTANCE OF CAPILLARY PRESSURE MEASUREMENTS

The most important reason for determining P_c is to evaluate whether precapillary or postcapillary pressures are increased by a clinical intervention. Consider the following equation:

$$P_{pc} = P_{p,wedge} + \frac{r_v}{r_T}(P_{pa} - P_{p,wedge})$$

where r_T is the total vascular resistance ($r_a + r_v$) and $P_{p,wedge}$ is the pulmonary wedge pressure. This equation was developed by Gaar and associates to estimate P_c in their classic 1967 study.[46] From that study, r_v/r_T was determined to be 0.4; this reduces the above equation to:

$$P_{pc} = P_{p,wedge} + 0.4(P_{pa} - P_{p,wedge})$$

This equation has been used to estimate P_c in human lungs when P_{pa} and $P_{p,wedge}$ are measured. However, when the equation is used, it is assumed that r_v/r_T equals 0.4. This may be true in some conditions, but this assumption is not always correct. For the data used in the models presented in Figures 74–11 and 74–12, we can compare the P_{pc} predicted using an $r_v/r_a + r_v = 0.4$ with that measured using Cope and colleagues[45] more exact analysis:

In control:	P_{pc}	$= 4.1 + 0.4\ (18 - 4.1)$
		$= 4.1 + 5.6$
		$= 9.7$ mm Hg
	Error	= Actual − Calculated
		$= 11.5 - 9.5$
		= 2 (a 17% error)
For thromboxane:	P_{pc}	$= 4.1 + 0.4\ (50 - 4.1)$

These calculations clearly show that P_c should always be estimated from the P_{pa} pressure tracing rather than through the use of the distribution of r_a and r_v determined by Gaar and associates[45] to represent an undefined resistance distribution in lungs. Figure 74–13 shows P_c values as estimated in human lungs by Cope and colleagues.[44] In this figure, the ratio of P_{pc} to $P_{p,wedge}$ was evaluated in patients undergoing coronary artery bypass, aortic valve replacement, and mitral valve replacement. Note that the measured $P_{pc}/P_{p,wedge}$ was about 1.10 for all three measurements before the surgery but that r_v/r_T was only 0.25. This indicates that $P_{p,wedge}$ was a good indicator of P_{pc}, being in error by only 10% in these patients. Even after surgery, the $P_{pc}/P_{p,wedge}$ values for the coronary bypass and aortic valve replacement patients were similar to those recorded preoperatively. However, the P_c after the replacement of the mitral valve was 30% higher than the $P_{p,wedge}$, and r_v/r_T acutely fit the data of Gaar and associates better than did the control data (equaling 0.35). The best way to estimate P_{pc} to any degree of certainty is to use the methods developed by Cope and colleagues.[45] The P_{pc} is such an important determinant of transcapillary fluid flux that it should be routinely measured when $P_{p,wedge}$ is monitored in critically ill patients.

PLASMA VOLUME EXPANSION WITH ALBUMIN

Table 74–5 shows the half-time ($t_{1/2}$) for albumin equilibration between plasma and tissues in normal (control) lungs, lungs with elevated capillary pressure, and lungs with a damaged endothelial barrier. The initial $\Delta\pi$ was calculated for each condition using the concentrations of protein found in plasma and lung lymph. The measured $\Delta\pi$ was multiplied by σ to obtain the effective osmotic pressure. A σ of 0.7 was used for controls, and one of 0.4 was used for damaged capillaries. The maximum effect reflects the addition of protein to the plasma in an amount that increased the plasma protein osmotic pressure by 10 mm Hg. Δ (expressed in millimeters of mercury) is the actual change of $\sigma\Delta\pi$ associated with each experimental condition. On addition of the albumin to the normal condition, the protein osmotic pressure is $0.7 \times 20 = 14$; however, $\Delta\pi$ was 7

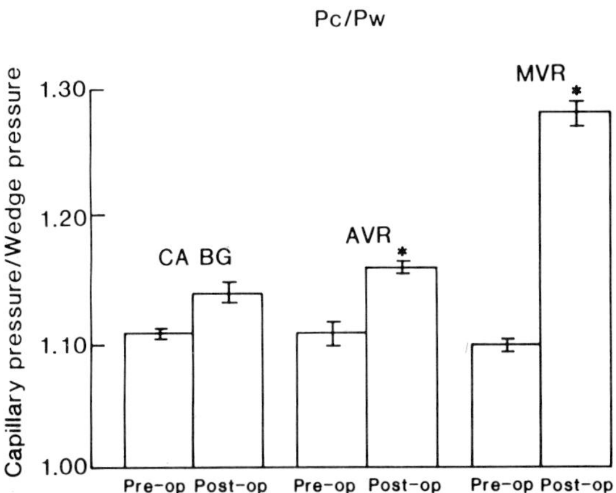

Figure 74–13. Plot of pulmonary capillary pressure divided by the wedge pressure for patients undergoing coronary bypass (CABG), aortic valve replacement (AVR), and mitral valve replacement (MVR). Pre-op and Post-op refer to before and after the operative procedure, respectively. (From Taylor AE, Cope DK, Allison RC, et al: Capillary pressure measurement. *In:* Human Lungs. Zapol WA, Lemaire F [Eds]. New York, Marcel Dekker, 1991, p 364.)

TABLE 74–5. Effects of Albumin Infusions on Lung Fluid Balance

		Control			*After Adding 10 mm Hg Colloid*			
Condition	$t^{1/2}$ *(h)*	*Equilibration Time (h)*	*Measured* $\Delta\pi$ *(mm Hg)*	$\sigma\Delta\pi$ *Actual (mm Hg)*	*Measured* $\Delta\pi$ *(mm Hg)*	*Actual* $\sigma\Delta\pi$ *(mm Hg)*	Δ *Difference (mm Hg)*	Δ *(3 h) (mm Hg)*
Normal (σ = 0.7)	2.9	18.0	10	7	20	14	7	3.5
Increased P_c (σ = 0.7)	2.0	12.0	20	14	30	21	7	2.6
Damaged endothelium (σ = 0.4)	0.8	4.8	10	4	20	8	4	1.0

Note: Δ = final actual colloid osmotic pressure minus initial actual colloid osmotic pressure (e.g., for Normal, Δ = 14−7).

before the addition, so that a change of only 7 mm Hg actually resulted. This addition would provide a greater absorptive force in the circulation of 7 mm Hg; however, in 18 hours, this gradient would be dissipated. In fact, after 3 hours, the effect is reduced to only 3.5 mm Hg as the albumin leaks into the interstitium! When vascular pressure was elevated, $\sigma\Delta\pi$ increased to 14 mm Hg; after the addition of protein, $\sigma\Delta\pi$ is $0.7 \times 30 = 21$ mm Hg, which also increased $\Delta\pi$ by only 7 mm Hg. After 3 hours, though, the remaining effect is only 2.6 mm Hg because the $t_{1/2}$ of protein loss from the capillary was decreased substantially when capillary filtration was increased. Therefore, for both normal and increased vascular pressures, the addition of protein could be beneficial in removing extravascular water, but the effect lasts for only a very short period of time.

Increasing plasma proteins when the capillary endothelium is damaged provides almost no absorptive effect, since the $t_{1/2}$ of protein leakage into the interstitium is extremely short—that is, in 3 hours, almost no effect remains. When $\sigma\Delta\pi$ is calculated ($0.4 \times 20 = 8$), the maximum net change is small (4 mm Hg), and since protein leaks from the circulation rapidly, only a small osmotic pressure gradient is present after 2 to 3 hours.

Table 74–5 does not reflect that both pulmonary capillary and pulmonary arterial wedge pressures usually increase with albumin (or colloid) infusions. The changes in P_{pc} must also be considered when the tendency for fluid to enter the lungs is predicted. Obviously, when capillary walls are damaged, wedge pressures may increase by more than the effective $\Delta\pi$, and edema can actually become more severe following colloid usage.

When crystalloid solutions are infused into the circulation, cardiac output changes transiently, and fluid rapidly leaves the circulation. Even if $\Delta\pi$ is reduced to near zero, lung interstitial volume would not increase greatly unless P_{pc} also increased (see Fig.74–5). However, since $\Delta\pi$'s ability to change with increased P_{wedge} is eliminated, the only safety factors left to oppose edema formation are the lymph flow and the tissue pressure. Therefore, if pulmonary arterial wedge pressure is elevated much above normal values during saline infusions, pulmonary edema can develop. Obviously, P_c is the critical factor that determines the state of lung water, especially during plasma volume infusions. This effect is clearly demonstrated in the study of Rutili and coworkers, which shows that dextran 70 actually removed water transiently from the lungs when capillaries were damaged only when P_{wedge} was not allowed to change.[25] When the $P_{p,wedge}$ was allowed to increase, the lungs gained more edema fluid. Of course, the measurement of choice with fluid therapy in critically ill patients is of P_{pc}, since the $P_{p,wedge}$ may not always predict the prevailing P_{pc}, as is shown in the previous section.[45]

The choice of colloid or crystalloid solutions as plasma volume expanders is a matter of critical importance in the maintenance of adequate blood flow in the critically ill patient. When colloid or crystalloid solutions are used in patients with either normal or leaky capillaries, P_c must be maintained at the minimum possible level adequate oxygenation is to be provided. For instance, if colloid solutions are infused into a patient with normal lungs and if the rise in P_c exceeds the change in $\Delta\pi$, a greater tendency for edema to develop in the lungs exists. If the lung capillaries are also leaky, then severe edema will occur if only small increases in P_c occur. Also, if $\Delta\pi$ is reduced to low levels and P_c increases by more than 10 to 15 mm Hg above control values after either crystalloid or colloid solution infusions, then severe edema can result, since the $\Delta\pi$ safety factor is no longer operative. Crystalloid volume replacement causes fewer lung problems simply because P_{pc} values do not remain elevated for long periods of time and because lymph flows can increase to extremely high levels. Colloid therapy can elevate P_{pc} for several hours because of the retention of fluid absorbed from the large tissue spaces in skin and muscles, and it can actually promote rather than resolve pulmonary edema.

SUMMARY

Our understanding of fluid and protein leakage across the microcirculation is expanding at a rapid rate, but more basic research is required to assess the problems associated with fluid therapy. P_{pc} is certainly the most important determinant of lung water accumulation in critically ill patients, even in those patients so-called with "leaky capillary" syndromes. Estimation of P_{pc} by the principles described in this chapter reflects capillary filtration pressure more accurately than does simple P_{wedge} measurement; however, valid Starling force analysis in any tissue requires measurement of several forces. Although new techniques are becoming available, no complete Starling force studies have been conducted in isolated tissues, much less in the critically ill patient. However, using a simple model of fluid dynamics coupled with a measure of P_c provides the sufficient insight needed to assess proper fluid therapy in the critically ill patient. Finally, it is now clear that ischemia-reperfusion damages the capillary membranes of lungs and that this process is caused by neutrophil and endothelial cell activation. The damage can be "reversed" by using compounds that activate protein kinase A and prevent protein kinase C activation in neutrophils and endothelial cells; future therapy for ischemia-reperfusion injury will certainly be directed toward alteration of intracellular messengers in the critically ill patient.

References

1. Taylor AE, Granger DN: Exchange of macromolecules across the microcirculation. *In*: Microcirculation: Physiological Handbook Series. Renkin EM, Michel CC (Eds). Bethesda, American Physiological Society, 1985, pp 462–520.

2. Taylor AE: Microvascular fluid and solute exchange. *In*: Encyclopedia of Human Biology. Vol 5. Orlando, Academic Press, 1991, pp 31–42.
3. Starling EH: On the absorption of fluid from the connective tissue spaces. J Physiol (Lond) 1896; 19:312.
4. Iversen P, Johansen EH: Pathogenese und Resorption von Trans- und Exsudaten in der Pleura. Klin Wochenschr 1929, 8:1311.
5. Kedem O, Katchalsky A: Thermodynamic analysis of the permeability of biological membranes to non-electrolytes. Biochim Biophys Acta 1958; 27:229.
6. Landis EM, Pappenheimer JR: Exchange of substances through the capillary walls. *In*: Handbook of Physiology. Vol 2. Hamilton WF, Dow P (Eds). Baltimore, Williams & Wilkins, 1963, pp 961–1034.
7. Wendt RP, Klein E, Bresler EH, et al: Sieving properties of hemodialysis membranes. J Membr Sci 1979; 5:23.
8. Krogh A, Landis EM, Turner AH: The movement of fluid through the human capillary wall in relation to venous pressure and to the colloid osmotic pressure in the blood. J Clin Invest 1932; 11:63.
9. Aukland K, Reed R: Interstitial-lymphatic mechanisms in the control of extracellular fluid volume. Physiol Rev 1993; 73:1–78.
10. Benoit JN: Relationship between lymphatic pump flow and total flow in the small intestine. Am J Physiol 1991; 261:H1970–H1978.
11. Guyton AC, Taylor AE, Granger HJ: Circulatory Physiology: Dynamics and Control of the Body Fluids. Vol 2. Philadelphia, WB Saunders, 1975, pp 18–52.
12. Granger HJ: Role of the interstitial matrix and lymphatic pump in regulation of transcapillary fluid balance. Microvasc Res 1979; 18:209.
13. Taylor AE, Parker JC, Granger DN, et al: Assessment of capillary permeability using lymphatic protein flux: Estimation of the osmotic reflection coefficient. *In*: Microcirculation. Effros RM, Schmid-Schonbein H, Ditzel J (Eds). New York, Academic Press, 1981, pp 19–31.
14. Nicoll PA, Taylor AE: Lymph formation and flow. Ann Rev Physiol 1977; 39:73.
15. Staub NC: Pulmonary edema. Physiol Rev 1974; 54:678.
16. Taylor AE, Gibson WH, Granger HJ, et al: The interaction between intracapillary and tissue forces in the overall regulation of interstitial fluid volume. Lymphology 1973; 6:192.
17. Granger DN, Taylor AE: Permeability of intestinal capillaries to endogenous macromolecules. Am J Physiol 1980; 238:H457.
18. Taylor AE, Townsley MI: Evaluation of the Starling fluid flux equation. Int News Physiol Sci 1987; 2:48–57.
18a. Landis EM: Microinjection studies of capillary permeability: II Relationship between capillary pressure and the ratio at which fluid passes through the walls of single capillaries. Am J Physiol 1927; 82:217.
19. Taylor AE: Capillary fluid filtration: Starling forces and lymph flow. Circ Res 1981; 49:557–575.
20. Granger HJ, Laine GA, Barnes GE, et al: Dynamics and control of transvascular fluid exchange. *In*: Edema. Staub NC, Taylor AE (Eds). New York, Raven Press, 1984, pp 189–227.
21. Taylor AE: The lymphatic edema safety factor: Role of edema-dependent safety factors (EDLF). Lymphology 1990; 23:111–123.
22. Granger DN, Kvietys PR, Wilborn WH, et al: Mehcanism of glucagon-induced intestinal secretion. Am J Physiol 1980; 239:G30.
23. Rutili G, Kvietys P, Parker JC, et al: Increased pulmonary microvascular permeability induced by ANTU. J Appl Physiol 1982; 52:1316.
24. Taylor AE, Parker JC: The pulmonary interstitial spaces and lymphatics. *In*: Handbook of Physiology: Non-respiratory Functions and Pulmonary Circulation. Fishman AP, Fisher AB (Eds). Bethesda, American Physiological Society, 1985, pp 162–230.
25. Rutili G, Parker JC, Taylor AE: Fluid balance in ANTU-injured lungs during crystalloid and colloid infusions. J Appl Physiol 1984; 56:993.
26. Brigham KL, Harris TR, Owen PJ: C14 urea and C14 sucrose as permeability indicators in histamine pulmonary edema. J Appl Physiol 1977; 43:99.
27. Gorin AB, Kohler J, DeNardo G: Noninvasive measurement of pulmonary transvascular protein flux in normal man. J Clin Invest 1980; 66:869.
28. Schuster DP: Positron emission tomography: Theory, and its application to the study of lung disease. Acta Physiol Scand Suppl 1986; 548:87–99.
29. Granger DN, Rutili G, McCord JM: Superoxide radical in feline intestinal ischemia. Gastroenterology 1981; 81:22.
30. Granger DN: Role of xanthine oxidase and granulocytes in ischemia-reperfusion injury. Am J Physiol 1988; 255:H1260–H1275.
31. Taylor AE, Matalon S, Ward P: The Physiology of Oxygen Radicals. Baltimore, Williams & Wilkins, 1986.
32. Adkins WK, Taylor AE: Role of xanthine oxidase and neutrophils in ischemia-reperfusion injury in rabbit lung. J Appl Physiol 1990; 69:2012–2018.
33. Adkins WK, Barnard JW, May S, et al: Compounds that increase cyclic-AMP prevent ischemia-reperfusion pulmonary capillary injury. J Appl Physiol 1992; 72:492–497.
34. Marciniak DL, Dobbins DE, Grega GJ, et al: Antagonism of histamine edema formation by catecholamines. Am J Physiol 1978; 234:H180–H185.
35. Allison RC, Hernandez EW, Prasad VR, et al: Protective Effects of O_2 Radical Scavengers and Adenosine in PMA-Induced Lung Injury. J Appl Physiol 1988; 64:2175–2182.
36. Adkins WK, Barnard JW, Moore TM, et al: Adenosine prevents PMA-induced lung injury via an A_2 receptor mechanism. J Appl Physiol 1993; 74:982–988.
37. Cronstein BN, Levin RI, Belanoff J, et al: Adenosine: An endogenous inhibitor of neutrophil-mediated injury to endothelial cells. J Clin Invest 1986; 78:760–770.
38. Seibert AF, Thompson WJ, Taylor A, et al: Reversal of increased microvascular permeability associated with ischemia-reperfusion: Role of cAMP. J Appl Physiol 1992; 72:389–395.
39. Seibert AF, Haynes J, Taylor A: Ischemia-reperfusion injury in the isolated rat lung: Role of flow and endogenous leukocytes. Am Rev Respir Dis 1993; 147:270–275.
39a. Barnard JW, Siebert AF, Prasal VR, et al: Reversal of pulmonary capacity ischemia-reperfusion injury by rolipram, a cyclic AMP phosphodiesterase inhibitor (in press).
40. Shasby DM, Shasby SS, Sullivan JM, et al: Role of endothelial cell cytoskeleton in control of endothelial permeability. Circ Res 1982; 51:657–661.
41. Holloway H, Perry M, Parker JC, et al: Estimation of pulmonary capillary pressures in intact dog lungs. J Appl Physiol 1983; 54:846.
42. Bhattacharya J, Staub NC: Direct measurement of microvascular pressures in the isolated perfused dog lung. Science 1980; 210:327.
43. Dawson CA, Bronikowwski TA, Linehan JH, et al: On the estimation of pulmonary capillary pressure from arterial occlusion. Am Rev Respir Dis 1989; 140:1228–1232.
44. Cope DK, Allison RC, Parmentier JC, et al: Using pulmonary arterial pressure profile after occlusion. Crit Care Med 1986; 14:16.
45. Cope DK, Grimbert F, Downey JM, et al: Pulmonary capillary pressure: A review. Crit Care Med 1992; 20:1043–1056.
46. Gaar KA, Taylor AE, Owens LJ, et al: Pulmonary capillary pressure and filtration coefficient in the isolated perfused lung. Am J Physiol 1967; 213:910–914.

CHAPTER 75

Increased Lung Vascular Permeability: Mediators and Therapies

Gordon R. Bernard, MD • Kenneth L. Brigham, MD

BASIC PATHOPHYSIOLOGY OF LUNG FLUID BALANCE

Although the lung is anatomically unique, the forces affecting movement of fluid and solutes across the walls of microvessels into the lung interstitium are similar to those in other organs. Because of the seminal work by Ernest Starling in the late 19th century describing the relationships in capillaries that determine the transmural filtration of fluid, the physical forces affecting filtration are generally called *Starling forces.* The concept presented by Starling is often written as the equation:

$$\text{Net filtration} = Kf(Pmv - Ppmv) - \sigma(mv - pmv) \quad \text{[Equation 1]}$$

where Kf is the capillary filtration coefficient and is the protein osmotic reflection coefficient, Pmv is microvascular pressure, Ppmv is perimicrovascular pressure, mv is plasma oncotic pressure; pmv is perimicrovascular oncotic pressure; and σ is the protein osmotic reflection coefficient.

For many years, it was believed that no filtration occurred from lung microvessels under normal conditions. This concept was based on the fact that microvascular pressure in the lung is lower than plasma oncotic pressure. Thus, ignoring any extravascular forces, under normal conditions, the net Starling forces should be in the direction of absorption. Because pulmonary edema (i.e., accumulation of excess water in the lungs) does not occur in experimental animals until left atrial pressure exceeds plasma oncotic pressure,[1] this concept seemed correct. In fact, the difference between pulmonary arterial wedge pressure and plasma oncotic pressure is still often used as an index of tendency toward development of pulmonary edema.[2]

Work done in a variety of laboratories in the last 20 years has clearly shown that, contrary to the concept just described, extravascular forces play an important role in influencing lung fluid balance under normal conditions and also provide important protection against the tendency for fluid accumulation in the lung.[3, 4] This work has centered around measurements of lung lymph flow and lung lymph protein concentrations. Because lymph flows from the normal lung and the principal origin of lymph is as a filtrate of exchange vessels in any organ, transvascular filtration must be occurring in the lung microcirculation under normal conditions.[3,4] Hydrostatic pressure around exchange vessels (Ppmv) is unknown, but many investigators believe that the pressure may be negative.[5] Extravascular forces appear to play an important role in protecting the lung against edema when hydrostatic pressures in the microcirculation are increased. For instance, when pressure is increased in the lung microcirculation, lung lymph flow increases, thus draining away the excess filtered fluid.[3, 4]

A major protective mechanism for dealing with increased hydrostatic pressure is that as lung lymph flow increases with increased capillary pressure, lung lymph protein concentration falls relative to that in plasma. This plus the reported rise in perivascular hydrostatic pressure[6] opposes the effects of increased capillary hydrostatic pressure on filtration. These factors (i.e., increasing lung lymph flow, decreasing perimicrovascular oncotic pressure, and increasing interstitial hydrostatic pressure) have been called *safety factors* against pulmonary edema.[7]

There are two general ways in which pulmonary edema may develop. First, there may be an imbalance of the physical forces affecting filtration. In theory, this could be any one or all of the four factors in the Starling equation, but, in fact, it is usually caused by an increase in capillary pressure in the lung resulting from heart failure. This kind of edema has been called *high-pressure edema* or *secondary pulmonary edema* because it originates from abnormalities extrinsic to the lung.[8] It is now clear that pulmonary edema may also develop in the face of normal Starling forces. This results from increased permeability of exchange vessels so that they leak excessive fluid and protein.[8, 9] This is thought to be a basic pathogenetic abnormality in the group of diseases commonly referred to clinically as the adult respiratory distress syndrome (ARDS). Edema of this sort has been called *increased permeability edema* or *primary pulmonary edema* because it results from abnormalities intrinsic to the lung.[8] The result is that these normally important safety factors are severely stressed and the tendency for the accumulation of fluid is great.[10, 11] Although this sequence of events has not been clearly demonstrated in human ARDS, maintenance of a low circulating volume through the use of fluid restriction and diuretics is often advocated. In contrast, the deleterious effects of decreased left ventricular loading volume with subsequent reduction in cardiac output and oxygen delivery have been clearly demonstrated, as is discussed more fully later.

ROLE OF METABOLITES OF ARACHIDONIC ACID IN LUNG EDEMA CAUSED BY INCREASED MICROVASCULAR PERMEABILITY

There are several reasons to suspect that metabolites of arachidonic acid produced or released within the lung, or both, may mediate abnormalities in function of the lung, which occur in primary pulmonary edema.[12] Cells within the lung produce prostaglandins and other arachidonate metabolites; these substances may affect vascular and airway function, and production or release of these substances is increased in some experimental conditions in which lung vascular permeability is increased.[13] Figure 75–1 is an abbreviated scheme of arachidonic acid metabolism, listing some known actions of arachidonate metabolites that might contribute to respiratory failure. As Figure 75–1 shows, in response to injury, phospholipids containing arachidonic acid are released from cell membranes. Through the action of phospholipases, arachidonic acid is liberated from phospholipids, and free arachidonate may then be metabolized through a cyclooxygenase enzyme to prostaglandins and thromboxanes or through lipoxygenase enzymes into leukotrienes and other compounds.[12] The classic prostaglandins, E_2 and F_2, are pulmonary vasoconstrictors as is free arachidonic acid.[14] There is substantial indirect evidence that thromboxane, a potent smooth-muscle constrictor, constricts pulmonary blood vessels and perhaps airways as well. In contrast, prostacyclin (PGI_2) is a potent smooth-muscle relaxer and therefore is a pulmonary vasodilator.[15] In fact, PGI_2 is the most potent known pulmonary vasodilating substance on a weight basis. Other actions of thromboxane and PGI_2 that may be important in the pathogenesis of primary pulmonary edema include their effects on platelets and perhaps on circulating white blood cells. Lipoxygenase metab-

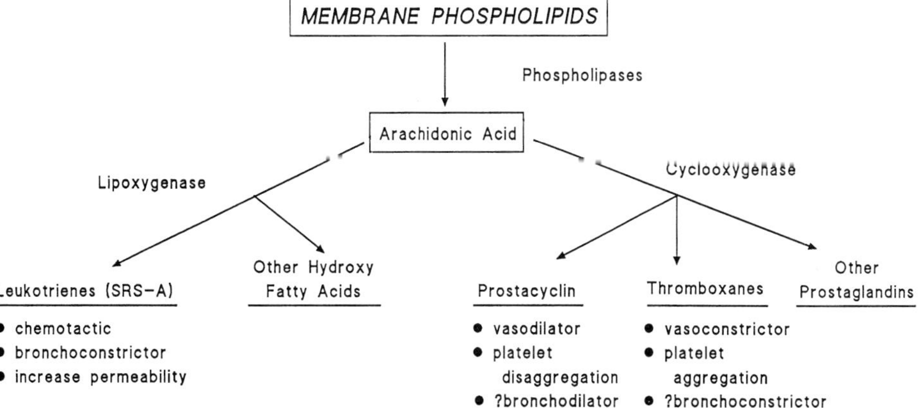

Figure 75–1. Abbreviated metabolic scheme of arachidonic acid metabolism showing some of the biologic activities of arachidonic acid metabolites.

olites of arachidonate also may have profound effects on lung function,[16] which include chemotactic activity for granulocytes.[17]

It has been supposed that the therapeutic effects of aspirin, indomethacin, ibuprofen, and meclofenamate result from the inhibition of arachidonate cyclooxygenase. The effects of cyclooxygenase inhibitors on the lungs' response to insults that produce primary pulmonary edema have been studied in experimental animals. The pulmonary response of the pig and the sheep to gram-negative endotoxemia has been extensively studied.[9, 18] Because the changes that occur in these animal models are similar to those seen in humans with ARDS and the syndrome commonly occurs in humans in the setting of gram-negative sepsis, the animal model approximates the clinical situation.[18, 19] There is other evidence in experimental animals indicating that the loss of the normal pulmonary vasoconstriction in response to alveolar hypoxia occurring after endotoxemia[20] or pulmonary oxygen toxicity[21] can be restored by arachidonate cyclooxygenase inhibitors. The loss of hypoxic vasoconstriction in those circumstances appears to result from endogenous production of the potent vasodilator PGI_2.[20, 21] Studies in the canine lobar atelectasis model show that, even in the "normal" lung, hypoxic vasoconstriction can be enhanced and that the weaker the initial hypoxic response, the more effective meclofenamate is in improving the response to subsequent hypoxic challenge.[22]

There appears to be increased production of lipoxygenase metabolites of arachidonate after endotoxemia in animals, and this increased production or release, or both, seems to be specifically attributable to the lung.[23] Several of the lipoxygenase products are potent chemotaxins for granulocytes.[17] The possible interaction between these substances and circulating granulocytes in mediating injury to the lung is discussed later. There is some evidence that slow-reacting substance of anaphylaxis may itself cause increased capillary permeability in a peripheral vascular bed.[24] One additional piece of evidence that may implicate lipoxygenase products of arachidonate in mediating capillary injury in the lung is the demonstration in experimental animals that high doses of corticosteroids will inhibit both the pulmonary vasoconstriction and the increase in lung microvascular permeability following gram-negative endotoxemia.[25] One of the effects of corticosteroids is inhibition of the release of arachidonate-containing phospholipids from cell membranes. This effect might prevent increased generation of both cyclooxygenase and lipoxygenase products of arachidonic acid. Unfortunately, steroids may have a host of other effects, so that their inhibition of endotoxin-induced lung injury in animals does not necessarily implicate arachidonate metabolites as mediators.

ROLE OF GRANULOCYTES IN MEDIATING INCREASED LUNG MICROVASCULAR PERMEABILITY

In vitro, granulocytes may mediate membrane injury to cultured endothelial cells.[26] The bulk of evidence suggests that this in vitro injury results from close approximation of granulocytes to the endothelial cells and the generation of superoxide, other free radicals, and proteolytic enzymes by the activated granulocytes.[27, 28] Further evidence that free radicals produced by granulocyte activation is revealed through experiments with free radical scavengers such as N-acetylcysteine. When N-acetylcysteine is given in pharmacologic doses to sheep before endotoxin infusion, the magnitude of most aspects of the response, especially that of the lymph, is attenuated.[29] There is some evidence that a sizable marginated pool of granulocytes exists in the normal lung.[30] Additional evidence in both animals and humans suggests that granulocytes accumulate in microvessels in the lung in response to a variety of injuries. Some of the same interventions (e.g., high doses of corticosteroids) prevent the in vitro and in vivo responses. Recent studies in experimental animals have implicated granulocytes as obligate participants in injury to the lung produced by gram-negative endotoxemia,[31] extensive air microembolization,[32] and pulmonary oxygen toxicity.[33] The infusion of substances that activate granulocytes into experimental animals results in lung vascular injury that is pathophysiologically similar to ARDS in humans.[34] It is not yet clear whether the interaction of circulating granulocytes with the lung microcirculation is a common denominator for all injuries to the lung that result in increased vascular permeability. However, such a hypothesis seems tenable, at least at the moment, if not in mediating the initial reaction then in amplifying the injury.[28] Although there is little direct evidence for it, granulocytes may also play a role in lung repair, especially with regard to their phagocytic properties. A number of clinical settings in which ARDS occurs are accompanied by intravascular activation of complement. Complement activation can cause activation of granulocytes, resulting in margination into the lung circulation and increased lung microvascular permeability.[35] Whether all circumstances of pulmonary leukostasis and injury require complement activation as a prerequisite is not yet known. It remains possible that granulocytes are a pathogenetic common denominator but that complement activation may simply represent one mechanism by which granulocytes may be activated.

INTERACTIONS BETWEEN ARACHIDONIC ACID AND GRANULOCYTES

Several of the lipoxygenase products are potent granulocyte chemotaxins. For example, it has been demonstrated that granulocytes, activated in vitro, produce leukotriene B_4, a potent chemotaxin, activating other granulocytes.[17] This provides a kind of positive feedback in which granulocyte activation may perpetuate itself. Although it has been demonstrated that lipoxygenase products of arachidonic acid are produced in abnormally high quantities in the lung in animal models when lung vascular permeability is increased,[23] it is not yet clear whether these substances originate from granulocytes trapped within the lung microcirculation or from other cells in the lung. If cells other than granulocytes residing in the lung produce these substances, this could account for pulmonary leukostasis, the activation of marginated granulocytes, and the subsequent chain of events resulting in injury to lung microvessels. In animal models of acute lung injury, leukopenia and pulmonary leukostasis precede the increase in vascular permeability. Inhibitors of arachidonate cyclooxygenase (e.g., indomethacin, ibuprofen, and meclofenamate) do not prevent the leukopenia caused by these substances but do prevent the initial pulmonary vasoconstriction.[36, 37] Further, cyclooxygenase inhibitors do not prevent the increase in lung vascular permeability caused by the infusion of the agents that activate granulocytes. Thus, analogous to the endotoxin reaction, in vivo activation of granulocytes appears to cause pulmonary hypertension mediated by cyclooxygenase products of arachidonic acid (most likely thromboxane A_2) and a later increase in vascular permeability, which is mediated some other way.

What do activated granulocytes do in the lung microcirculation to increase vascular permeability? There are at least two possibilities. First, activated granulocytes generate superoxide and other free radicals. These highly labile species are very toxic to cell membranes and, in in vitro systems, appear to be responsible for endothelial cell injury.[27] It is not yet known which of these possible mechanisms of injury is most important in the damage to lung microvessels resulting from pulmonary leukostasis and granulocyte activation. On the basis of what is known about the role of metabolites of arachidonic acid and the role of granulocytes in the lungs' response to insults that may cause primary pulmonary edema, it is possible to construct a hypothetical sequence of events involving the interaction of these two systems (Table 75–1).

TABLE 75–1. Proposed Sequence of Events in Endotoxin-Induced Lung Injury

Pathophysiologic Response	*Implicated Mediator*
Granulocyte sequestration	Leukocyte adhesion molecules Cytokines Leukotrienes
Bronchoconstriction	Products of arachidonic acid (thromboxane)
Pulmonary hypertension	Products of arachidonic acid (thromboxane)
Loss of hypoxic vasoconstriction	Products of arachidonic acid (prostacycline, thromboxane)
Increased endothelial permeability	Activated granulocytes (free radicals of oxygen, proteolytic enzymes) Direct toxic effects of endotoxin on endothelium Complement activation

THERAPEUTIC IMPLICATIONS IN HUMANS

Therapy Aimed at Pulmonary Edema Reduction

It should be emphasized that failure of the lung, that is, failure of oxygenation in ARDS, is not due solely to pulmonary edema. There are marked abnormalities in airways function,[38] and there may be loss of hypoxic vasoconstriction, both of which could result in mismatching of ventilation and perfusion and hypoxemia out of proportion to the amount of fluid in the lung. It has been demonstrated in both animal models of the syndrome and in humans with ARDS that the magnitude of gas exchange abnormality does not correlate with the amount of measurable extravascular lung water.[39] Furthermore, although some studies have attempted to relate fluid therapy to intensive care outcome for patients with ARDS, none are conclusive. That is, it has not been conclusively shown that a reduction in circulating volume is of benefit in ARDS patients who do not have excessively high pulmonary artery wedge pressure.[40, 41] Indeed, concern has been expressed that a decrease in circulating volume to effect a decrease in microvascular pressure may worsen multiple system organ failure by reducing cardiac output and oxygen delivery. Thus, although pulmonary edema is an important part of the pathophysiology in ARDS, therapies aimed only at the edema may not be very effective in correcting the gas exchange abnormality.

From a pharmacologic standpoint, there are several agents that, on the basis of in vitro or animal studies, appear promising in the therapy of ARDS. The most common drug used clinically is methylprednisolone, but its use has be-

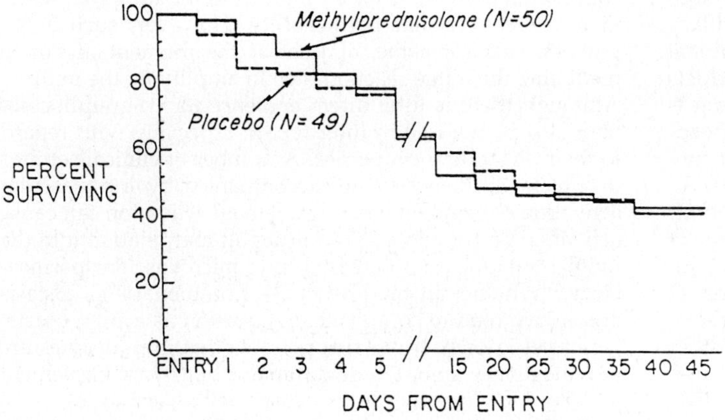

Figure 75–2. Comparison of the survival of patients with ARDS over the first 45 days after entry into the study, according to treatment with methylprednisolone or placebo. No significant differences in survival were observed at any time during the 45-day follow-up period (P = .77). (From Bernard GR, Luce JM, Sprung CL, et al: High-dose corticosteroids in patients with Adult Respiratory Distress Syndrome. N Engl J Med 1987; 317:1565–1570. Reprinted, by permission of the *New England Journal of Medicine.*)

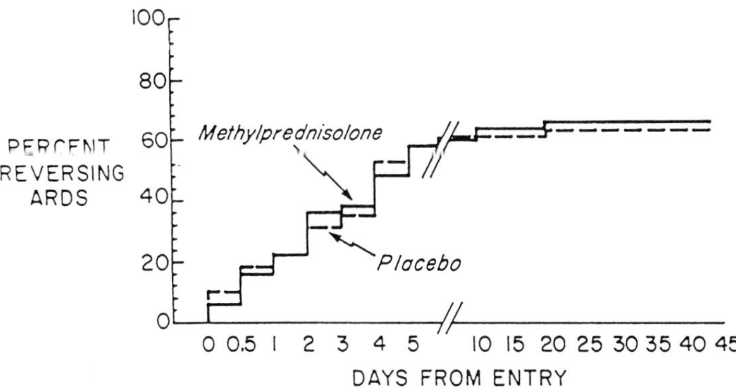

Figure 75–3. Comparison of the percentage of patients in whom ARDS was reversed through reversal of the arterial blood gas criteria alone after treatment with either methylprednisolone (N = 50) or placebo (N = 49). No significant differences in the reversal rates between the two groups were observed at any point during the 45-day follow-up period (P = .74). (From Bernard GR, Luce JM, Sprung CL, et al: High-dose corticosteroids in patients with Adult Respiratory Distress Syndrome. N Engl J Med 1987; 317:1565–1570. Reprinted, by permission of the *New England Journal of Medicine.*)

come very controversial on the basis of a large clinical trial of high-dose methylprednisolone. Although the use of methylprednisolone in ARDS has been extensively reported, there is only one well-designed study using pharmacologic doses in the literature.[42] In this prospective, placebo-controlled trial, patients meeting a stringent definition of ARDS were randomized to receive 30 mg/kg of methylprenisolone intravenously every 6 hours for 48 hours or placebo. Figure 75–2 shows that the mortality of patients in each treatment group was similar. A closer examination of the patients also shows that ARDS did not reverse any more rapidly with methylprednisolone than with placebo (see Fig. 75–3). Finally, the patients in each group were observed closely for changes in chest radiograph edema score, gas exchange, and static lung compliance, and again no differences were found (Fig. 75–4).[42] Although the debate will likely continue, there appears to be no reliable evidence that corticosteroids are effective in the treatment of established ARDS in humans.[43]

On the basis of animal data described earlier, there is a rationale for the use of inhibitors of arachidonate cyclooxygenase (e.g., indomethacin, meclofenamate, or ibuprofen) in ARDS, particularly if induced by sepsis.[38] If loss of hypoxic vasoconstriction is an important cause of ventilation-perfusion mismatching and hypoxemia, animal studies suggest that arachidonate cyclooxygenase inhibition might restore hypoxic vasoconstriction and therefore improve oxygenation. Such therapy would not be aimed specifically at the increased intravascular permeability because these drugs do not prevent or reverse such abnormalities, but the drugs could be effective in cases of refractory hypoxemia. At least one prospective, double-blind trial of a cyclooxygenase inhibitor has been performed in patients with sepsis, a high-risk group for the development of ARDS. This study established that cyclooxygenase products of arachidonic acid, specifically thromboxane and PGI_2, are present in dramatically increased concentrations in septic patients; these concentrations were readily reduced to near normal by treatment with ibuprofen; and there were physiologic responses as a consequence of this intervention, including decreased tachycardia, normalization of body temperature, decrease in peak airway pressure, and a trend toward stabilized blood pressure and improvement in oxygenation.

Other drugs that in the future might prove useful include those that oppose the effects of free radicals.[44] It should be emphasized that all specific pharmacologic therapies aimed at treating lung abnormalities remain speculative, and demonstration of their efficacy will depend on further research in experimental animals as well as carefully designed clinical studies. At this time, there is no specific or nonspecific pharmacologic intervention in patients with ARDS that has been demonstrated in humans to reverse the abnormalities in lung function or structure.

At present, therapy in humans with this syndrome remains largely supportive. The administration of oxygen and the use of positive end-expiratory airway pressure (PEEP) are clearly beneficial in maintaining oxygenation. Because

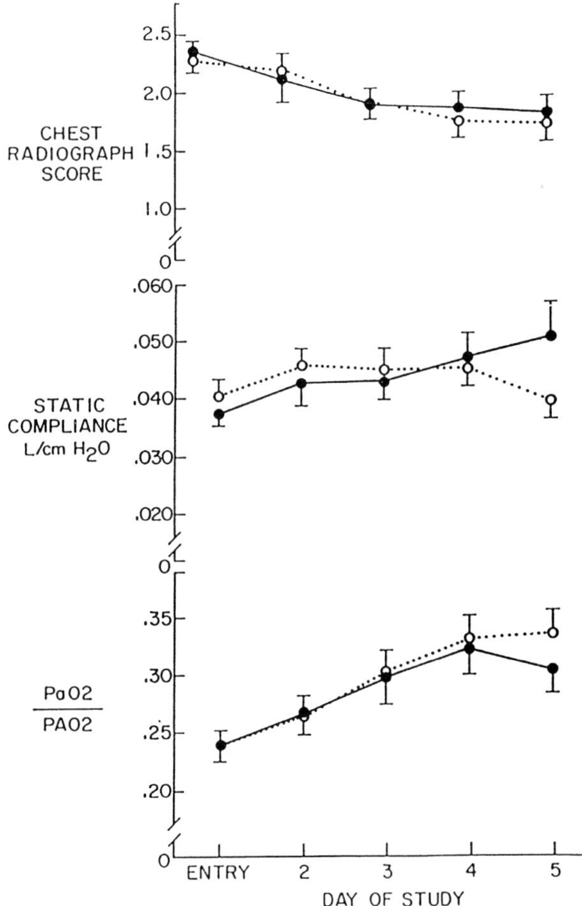

Figure 75–4. Comparison of patients treated with methylprednisolone (*solid line,* N = 50) or placebo (*dotted lines,* N = 49), according to chest radiograph score (0 denotes normality, 1 mild, 2 moderate, and 3 severe pulmonary edema), effective total thoracic static lung compliance (static compliance), and the ratio of arterial to alveolar partial oxygen pressures (PaO_2/PAO_2). No significant differences between the methylprednisolone and placebo groups were observed at the time of entry or during the 5 days immediately following entry ($P > .05$). (From Bernard GR, Luce JM, Sprung CL, et al: High-dose corticosteroids in patients with Adult Respiratory Distress Syndrome. N Engl J Med 1987; 317:1565–1570. Reprinted, by permission of the *New England Journal of Medicine.*)

estimation of left ventricular filling pressure by physical examination or chest radiograph is difficult, imprecise, and often inaccurate, the flow-directed pulmonary artery catheter has become a very important tool in the fluid management of the ARDS patient. Pulmonary pressures derived in this way give reasonable estimates of microvascular filtration pressure and left ventricular filling pressure.[45] Knowledge of filtration pressure is especially useful because of the potential problems brought on by the combination of wide swings in volume status and increased permeability often seen in these patients. Microvascular pressure data must be interpreted in the context of plasma oncotic pressure (i.e., acceptably low microvascular pressure might be offset by a very low serum albumin). Although the pulmonary artery wedge pressure reasonably estimates left ventricular diastolic filling pressure, in many cases filling pressure does not correlate with left ventricular end-diastolic volume, the latter being the important determinant of cardiac output according to Starling's law of the heart. This is especially true in patients with ARDS receiving PEEP because high levels of PEEP effectively decrease left ventricular filling for any given pulmonary wedge pressure.[46]

As discussed earlier, oxygenation and lung water content do not correlate, so maintenance of a relatively low circulating volume, although generally desirable, should not be pursued at the expense of cardiac output and oxygen delivery. There continue to exist two schools of thought in the issue of volume resucitation in patients with ARDS. One theory is that reduction in circulating volume will improve outcome in ARDS[40, 41] by reducing pulmonary edema, improving oxygenation, and reducing time on mechanical ventilation. The other theory does not necessarily refute this idea; it simply suggests that high oxygen delivery should be the goal in these patients and that fluid resuscitation should be used as needed to maintain higher cardiovascular filling pressures to achieve that goal.[47] There is no consensus, so a firm recommendation cannot be made at this time. In the meantime, it seems that moderation is in order, that is, fluid resuscitation should be used as needed to maintain a normal to slightly high oxygen delivery. If intravascular volume must be reduced, administration of diuretics and central vasodilators may be useful. Most vasodilators, especially nitroprusside, can increase pulmonary shunt and therefore should be used with caution. The best agent to use when volume replacement is required to maintain adequate cardiac output has not been clearly established. The controversy between colloid and crystalloid has been persistent, with a massive literature supporting both sides of the issue. Use of colloid (e.g., albumin) seems logical because an increase in intravascular colloid pressure would be expected to favor fluid resorption from the interstitium of the lung. The problem with this line of reasoning is that, under conditions of increased permeability, albumin readily crosses from the intravascular space to the interstitial space, thus canceling the expected beneficial effect. Crystalloid solutions seem to offer no advantage over colloid solutions except that these agents are substantially less expensive,[48] and some animal studies suggested that colloid actually increases interstitial edema.[49, 50]

PROGNOSIS

The mortality of ARDS is generally reported to be in the range of 50% to 70%, but this figure should be interpreted in the context of the mortality of the underlying disease process. In one report,[51] overall mortality was 56% but remained high (28%) even if ARDS reversed. ARDS in patients with high pulmonary permeability (measured by single-pass, multiple-indicator dilution methods) and low static compliance tended not to reverse and was associated with very high mortality. Interestingly, when measured at the time of ARDS onset, neither the degree of oxygenation defect, whether measured by total shunt calculation or alveolar-arteriolar difference in partial pressure of oxygen, nor the amount of extravascular lung water predicted whether ARDS would reverse (Table 75–2). Several studies have shown that pulmonary abnormalities persist for several months after clinical resolution of ARDS and in some cases after resolution of the oxygenation defect. Generally, these reports indicate mild to moderate restriction with persistent oxygenation defects. It is well established that many patients experience normalization of pulmonary function, gas exchange, and chest radiographs over a period of months.[52]

TABLE 75–2. Predictors of Reversal of Adult Respiratory Distress Syndrome (ARDS) in Patients with Established ARDS

Indicators of Poor Prognosis	*Neutral Indicators*
Elevated pulmonary artery pressure	Cardiac output
Elevated pulmonary vascular resistance	Shunt
Decreased compliance	Chest radiograph
Multiple system organ failure	Extravascular lung water
Sepsis	
Indicators of Good Prognosis	
Low permeability—surface area product	
Normal systemic blood pressure	
Single organ failure	
Treatable infection	

SUMMARY

The lung accumulates fluid in response to either elevated pressures in exchange vessels or increased permeability in those vessels because transvascular filtration of fluid within the lung microcirculation exceeds the ability of lung lymphatics to drain the fluid away. The normal safety factors protecting against edema, including increasing lymph flow, decreasing perimicrovascular oncotic pressure, and possibly increasing interstitial fluid pressure, are operative in secondary pulmonary edema (i.e., edema resulting from heart failure) but are severely compromised in primary pulmonary edema (increased permeability edema). Increases in lung vascular permeability in a variety of experimental models of infection or ischemia reperfusion require the presence of circulating granulocytes and presumably result from the interaction of activated granulocytes with the walls of microvessels in the lung. Because several cyclooxygenase and lipoxygenase products of arachidonic acid are potent chemotaxins or have other effects that make them likely mediators of abnormal lung function, it is quite possible that these substances are important in the pathogenesis of respiratory failure. There are adequate experimental data to construct a hypothetical sequence of events in primary pulmonary edema in which there is an initial production of cyclooxygenase products of arachidonic acid. These mediators cause pulmonary vasoconstriction, airway constriction, and intravascular activation of granulocytes resulting in pulmonary leukostasis. The further generation of lipoxygenase products of arachidonate by activated granulocytes results in the perpetuation of granulocyte activation. Lung microvessels are injured by the generation of superoxide, by release of lysosomal enzymes, and perhaps directly by lipoxygenase products of arachidonate. Failure of the oxygenation function of the lung in ARDS is due to not only pulmonary edema but also abnormalities in airway function and possibly loss of hypoxic pulmonary vasoconstriction.

Although no specific or nonspecific pharmacologic therapy has been proven efficacious in this syndrome, there is an experimental basis for inferring that a number of pharmacologic interventions may favorably affect its outcome, but clinical tests have failed to prove corticosteroids useful in human ARDS. A variety of other possible interventions that might prove useful in the future include the use of inhibitors of arachidonate cyclooxygenase (which could restore hypoxic pulmonary vasoconstriction and improve oxygenation) and the use of agents that would oppose the effects of free radicals. Until specific therapy becomes available, the mainstay of ARDS management remains supportive. Treatment of the underlying disease process and maintenance of respiratory support through use of oxygen, PEEP, and mechanical ventilation to overcome the excessive work of breathing is basic. Additional support by way of hemodynamic monitoring and maintenance of appropriate volume status is essential. The high mortality of ARDS is related not so much to the inability to oxygenate the patient but to the invasive nature and length of aggressive support required to allow the patient to recover lung function adequately to eliminate the need for life-support equipment. The mainstay of therapy at this time remains supportive. The use of supplemental oxygen and PEEP and the maintenance of intravascular pressures below levels known to produce pulmonary edema in normal lungs are the only measures that seem unequivocally beneficial.

ACKNOWLEDGMENTS

This work is supported by grants Nos. HL 19153 and HL 07123 from the National Institutes of Health, National Heart, Lung and Blood Institute.

References

1. Guyton A, Lindsey A: Effect of elevated left atrial pressure and decreased plasma protein concentration on the development of pulmonary edema. Circ Res 1959; 7:649–657.
2. Puri V, Freund U, Carlson RW, et al: Colloid osmotic and pulmonary wedge pressures in acute respiratory failure following hemorrhage. Surg Gynecol Obstet 1978; 147:537–540.
3. Erdmann AJ, Vaughn T, Brigham K, et al: Effect of increased vascular pressure on lung fluid balance in unanesthetized sheep. Circ Res 1975; 37:271–284.
4. Parker R, Roselli R, Harris T, et al: Effects of graded increases in pulmonary vascular pressures on lung fluid balance in unanesthetized sheep. Circ Res 1981; 49:1164–1172.
5. Harris T, Roselli R: A theoretical model of protein, fluid and small molecule transport in the lung. J Appl Physiol 1981; 50:1–14.
6. Taylor A, Gibson W, Granger H, et al: The interaction between intracapillary and tissue forces in the overall regulation of interstitial fluid volume. Lymphology 1973; 6:192–208.
7. Parker J, Falgout H, Parker R, et al: The effect of fluid volume loading on exclusion of interstitial albumin and lymph flow in the dog lung. Circ Res 1979; 45:440–450.
8. Bernard GR, Artigas A, Brigham KL, et al: The American-European consensus conference on ARDS: Definitions, mechanisms, relevant outcomes, and clinical trial coordination. Am J Respir Crit Care Med 1994; 149:818–824.
9. Brigham K, Bowers R, Haynes J: Increased sheep lung vascular permeability caused by *E. coli* endotoxin. Circ Res 1979; 45:292–297.
10. Brigham K, Harris T, Bowers R, et al: Lung vascular permeability: Inferences from measurements of plasma to lung lymph protein transport. Lymphology 1979; 12:177–190.
11. Bernard GR, Pou NA, Coggeshall JW, et al: Comparison of the pulmonary dysfunction caused by cardiogenic and non-cardiogenic pulmonary edema. Chest 1994; (in press).
12. Brigham K: Mechanisms of lung injury. Clin Chest Med 1982; 3:9–24.
13. Frolich J, Ogletree M, Brigham K: Pulmonary vascular response to endotoxemia in sheep. Pulmonary hypertension correlated to pulmonary thromboxane synthesis. Adv Prostaglandin Thromboxane Res 1980; 7:745–750.
14. Oletree M, Brigham K: Arachidonate increases pulmonary vascular resistance without changing lung vascular permeability in unanesthetized sheep. J Appl Physiol 1980; 48:581–586.
15. Ogletree M, Brigham K: Prostaglandin PGI2 and PGE1 produce opposite effects on sheep lung vascular permeability. Fed Proc 1979; 38:1266.
16. Samuelsson B, Hammarstrom S: Nomenclature for leukotrienes. Prostaglandins 1980; 19:645–648.
17. Bernard GR, Korley V, Chee P, et al: Persistent generation of peptide leukotrienes in patients with the adult respiratory distress syndrome (ARDS). Am Rev Respir Dis 1991; 144:263–267.
18. Kopolovic R, Thrailkill KM, Martin DT, et al: Effects of ibuprofen on a porcine model of acute respiratory failure. J Surg Res 1984; 36:300–305.
19. Bernard GR, Reines HD, Halushka PV, et al: Prostacyclin and thromboxane A_2 formation in human sepsis syndrome: Effects of cyclooxygenase inhibition. Am Rev Respir Dis 1991; 114:1095–1101.
20. Weir K, Miczoch J, Reeves J, et al: Endotoxin and the prevention of hypoxic pulmonary vasoconstriction. J Lab Clin Med 1976; 88:975–983.
21. Newman J, McMurtry I, Reeves J: Oxygen toxicity blunts hypoxic vasoconstriction in rat lungs: Possible role of prostaglandins. Prostaglandins 1981; 22:20.
22. Garrett RC, Thomas HM: Meclofenamate uniformly decreases shunt fraction in dogs with lobar atelectasis. J Appl Physiol 1983; 54:284–289.
23. Ogletree M, Brigham K, Oates J, et al: Increased flux of 5-HETE in sheep lung lymph during pulmonary leukostasis after endotoxin. Fed Proc 1981; 40:757.
24. Williams T, Piper P: The action of chemically pure SRS-A on the micro-circulation in vivo. Prostaglandins 1980; 19:779–789.
25. Brigham K, Bowers R, McKeen C: Methylprednisolone prevention of increased lung vascular permeability following endotoxemia in sheep. J Clin Invest 1981; 67:1103–1110.
26. Jacob H, Craddock P, Hammerschmidt D, et al: Complement induced granuloctye aggregation: An unsuspected mechanism of disease. N Engl J Med 1980; 302:789–803.
27. Sacks T, Moldow C, Craddock P, et al: Oxygen radicals mediate endothelial cell damage by complement-stimulated granulocytes: An in vitro model of immune vascular damage. J Clin Invest 1978; 61:1161–1167.
28. Bernard GR, Lucht WD, Niedermeyer ML, et al: Effect of N-acetylcysteine on the pulmonary response to endotoxin in the awake sheep and upon in vitro granulocyte function. J Clin Invest 1984; 73:1772–1784.
29. Fantone JC, Ward PA: Role of oxygen-derived free radicals and metabolites in leukocyte-dependent inflammatory reactions. Am J Pathol 1982; 107:397–418.
30. Bone RC: The pathogenesis of sepsis. Ann Intern Med 1991; 115:457–469.
31. Heflin C, Brigham K: Prevention by granulocyte depletion of increased vascular permeability of sheep lung following endotoxemia. J Clin Invest 1981; 68:1253–1260.
32. Flick M, Peril A, Staub N: Leukocytes are required for increased lung microvascular permeability after microembolization in sheep. Circ Res 1981; 48:344–351.
33. Fox R, Hoidal J, Brown J, et al: Mechanism of pulmonary oxygen toxicity: Hyperoxia damaged alveolar macrophages release factors which attract polymorphonuclear leukocytes and stimulate their release of superoxide. Clin Res 1980; 28:528A.
34. Johnson K, Chapman W, Ward P: Immunopathology of the lung. Am J Pathol 1979; 95:795–844.
35. Watts FL, Bernard GR, Harris TR, et al: Effects of hemodialysis on pulmonary permeability surface area product. Am Rev Respir Dis 1986; 133:A131.
36. Brigham K, Loyd J, Newman J, et al: Granulocytes in acute lung

vascular injury in unanesthetized sheep. Chest 1982; 81:56S–57S.
37. Fountain S, Martin B, Busclow CE, et al: Pulmonary leukostasis and its relationship to pulmonary dysfunction in sheep and rabbits. Circ Res 1980; 46:175–180.
38. Snapper JR, Hutchison AA, Ogletree ML, et al: Effects of cyclo-oxygenase inhibitors on the alterations in lung mechanics caused by endotoxemia in the unanesthetized sheep. J Clin Invest 1983; 72:63–76.
39. Brigham KL, Kariman K, Harris TR, et al: Correlation of oxygenation with vascular permeability-surface area but not with lung water in humans with acute respiratory failure and pulmonary edema. J Clin Invest 1983; 72:339–349.
40. Humphrey H, Hall J, Sznajder I, et al: Improved survival in ARDS patients associated with a reduction in pulmonary capillary wedge pressure. Chest 1990; 97:1176–1180.
41. Eisenberg PR, Hansbrough JR, Anderson D, et al: A prospective study of lung water measurements during patient management in an intensive care unit. Am Rev Respir Dis 1987; 136:662–668.
42. Bernard GR, Harris T, Luce JE, et al: High dose corticosteroids in patients with the adult respiratory distress syndrome: A randomized double-blind trial. N Engl J Med 1987; 317:1565–1570.
43. Flick MR, Murray JF: High-dose corticosteroid therapy in the adult respiratory distress syndrome. JAMA 1984; 251:1054–1056.
44. Bernard GR: N-acetylcysteine in experimental and clinical acute lung injury. Am J Med 1991; 91(Suppl 3C):54s–59s.
45. Swan HJC, Ganz W, Forrester J, et al: Catheterization of the heart in man with use of a flow-directed balloon-tipped catheter. N Engl J Med 1970; 283:447–451.
46. O'Quin R, Marini JJ: Pulmonary artery occlusion pressure: Clinical physiology, measurement, and interpretation. Am Rev Respir Dis 1983; 128:319–326.
47. Yu M, Levy MM, Smith P, et al: Effect of maximizing oxygen delivery on morbidity and mortality rates in critically ill patients: A prospective randomized, controlled study. Crit Care Med 1993; 21:830–838.
48. Erstad BL, Gales BJ, Rappaport WD: The use of albumin in clinical practice. Arch Intern Med 1991; 151:901–911.
49. Wood LDH, Prewitt RN: Cardiovascular management in acute hypoxemic respiratory failure. Am J Cardiol 1981; 47:963–972.
50. Holcroft JW, Trunkey DD: Extravascular lung water following hemorrhagic shock in the baboon: Comparison between resuscitation with Ringer's lactate and plasmanate. Ann Surg 1974; 180:408–417.
51. Bernard GR, Rinaldo J, Harris T, et al: Early predictors of ARDS reversal in patients with established ARDS. Am Rev Respir Dis 1985; 131:A143.
52. Snyder LS, Hertz MI, Peterson MS, et al: Acute lung injury: Pathogenesis of intraalveolar fibrosis. J Clin Invest 1991; 88:663–673.

CHAPTER 76

Approach to the Patient with Acute Respiratory Failure

John W. Kreit, MD • Robert M. Rogers, MD

The respiratory system, which consists of the lungs, chest wall, and respiratory muscles, performs the vital function of gas exchange. Oxygen is transported through the upper airways to the alveoli, diffuses across the alveolocapillary membrane, and enters the capillary blood. It then combines with hemoglobin and is transported by the arterial blood to the tissues. In the mitochondria, oxygen is essential for the production of adenosine triphosphate, which provides the energy required for all metabolic processes. The major byproduct of cellular metabolism is carbon dioxide. Carbon dioxide diffuses from the tissues into the capillary blood, where much of it is reversibly hydrated to form carbonic acid. It is then transported to the lungs by the venous blood, diffuses from the pulmonary capillary blood into the alveoli, and is exhaled into the atmosphere. It is evident, then, that the exchange of oxygen and carbon dioxide at the alveolocapillary interface is essential to meet the metabolic demands of the body and to prevent the development of life-threatening acidosis.

Respiratory failure may be defined as a significant impairment in the capacity of the respiratory system to perform gas exchange and is recognized by the presence of arterial hypoxemia and/or hypercapnia. On the basis of the duration of impaired gas exchange, respiratory failure may be classified as either acute or chronic. Chronic respiratory failure, which most commonly results from chronic obstructive pulmonary disease (COPD), is accompanied by physiologic adaptations that return systemic oxygen delivery and blood pH toward normal. For this reason, the terms *acute* and *chronic* also imply differences in clinical manifestations and in the urgency of therapy. Patients with chronic respiratory failure may, of course, experience an intercurrent illness that leads to acute decompensation (acute on chronic respiratory failure).

This chapter focuses on the evaluation and management of the patient with acute respiratory failure. This abrupt impairment of gas exchange represents a threat to the life of the patient and must be rapidly diagnosed and aggressively and effectively treated. We begin with a brief overview of the mechanisms of abnormal gas exchange. This topic is discussed in detail in Chapter 87.

MECHANISMS OF ABNORMAL GAS EXCHANGE

The effectiveness of the lungs in transferring both oxygen and carbon dioxide is determined by three factors: (1) the rate at which fresh air is supplied to the alveoli (alveolar ventilation); (2) the degree to which ventilation and perfusion are matched in each of the gas-exchanging units of the lungs; and (3) the extent to which oxygen and carbon dioxide equilibrate between the alveolar gas and the pulmonary capillary blood. A disturbance in any of these processes could, therefore, be expected to result in arterial hypoxemia and hypercapnia. Except in the setting of extensive parenchymal and pulmonary capillary destruction (e.g., severe interstitial fibrosis), equilibration of oxygen and carbon dioxide across the alveolocapillary interface is virtually always complete. Diffusion impairment is, therefore, rarely a cause of hypoxemia in patients with respiratory failure and probably never results in hypercapnia. This leaves two major mechanisms of abnormal pulmonary gas exchange: ventilation-perfusion imbalance and alveolar hypoventilation. The partial pressure of oxygen and carbon dioxide in the arterial blood (Pa_{O_2}, Pa_{CO_2}) are also influenced by the fractional concentration of oxygen (FI_{O_2}) in the inspired gas and by the partial pressure of oxygen (P_{O_2}) and carbon dioxide (P_{CO_2}) of the venous blood entering the lungs. These factors are not discussed further in this chapter.

Ventilation-Perfusion Imbalance

The P_{O_2} and P_{CO_2} of the gas contained in each alveolus, and therefore of the capillary blood leaving it, are determined primarily by the ventilation-perfusion ratio ($\dot{V}/\dot{Q}$) of that alveolus.[1] This concept is illustrated by the oxygen–carbon dioxide diagram shown in Figure 76–1. As the ratio between ventilation and perfusion decreases, the P_{O_2} of the end-

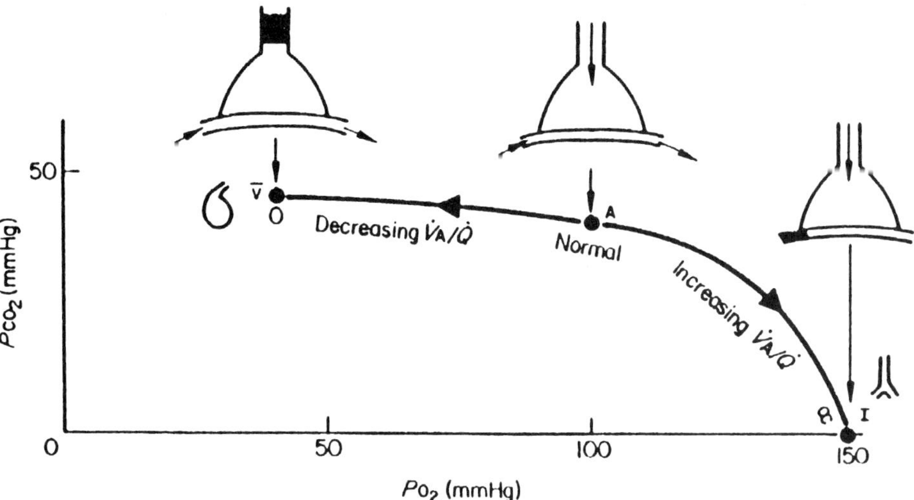

Figure 76–1. The oxygen–carbon dioxide diagram. The P_{O_2} and P_{CO_2} of the gas contained in an alveolus and of the blood leaving it is determined by the alveolar ventilation–perfusion ratio ($\dot{V}_A/\dot{Q}$). As the ratio increases from zero (no ventilation) to infinity (no perfusion), the alveolar gas composition progressively changes from that of mixed venous blood (v̄) to that of inspired air (I). (From West JP: Ventilation/Blood Flow and Gas Exchange. 5th ed. Oxford, Blackwell Scientific Publications, Ltd, 1990, p 35.)

capillary blood falls and the P_{CO_2} rises. The opposite occurs as $\dot{V}/\dot{Q}$ increases. In the normal lung, ventilation and perfusion are closely matched so that a narrow and symmetric distribution of ratios exists around a value of approximately 1.0. Figure 76–2 shows the distribution of $\dot{V}/\dot{Q}$ in a young, healthy man. Any disorder that affects the airways, parenchyma, or vasculature of the lungs, however, will cause an imbalance between ventilation and perfusion, and this will produce abnormally high and low $\dot{V}/\dot{Q}$. The extent to which gas exchange is impaired depends on both the values of the $\dot{V}/\dot{Q}$ and the shape of their distribution.[1] It is important to recognize, however, that arterial hypoxemia and hypercapnia will result only from regions of the lungs with low $\dot{V}/\dot{Q}$. High $\dot{V}/\dot{Q}$ regions increase the amount of "wasted ventilation" (see later discussion) but do not adversely affect the arterial blood gas tensions.

Ventilation-perfusion imbalance interferes with oxygen transfer in the following way: Areas of the lung with low $\dot{V}/\dot{Q}$ contribute blood with an abnormally low P_{O_2} to the pulmonary venous and systemic arterial blood. Coexisting lung regions with high $\dot{V}/\dot{Q}$ contribute blood with a high P_{O_2}. However, these high and low $\dot{V}/\dot{Q}$ regions, even if equal in number, do not counterbalance each other for two reasons. First, low $\dot{V}/\dot{Q}$ areas typically receive more blood flow than high $\dot{V}/\dot{Q}$ areas and therefore make a proportionately larger contribution to the arterial blood. Second, because of the nonlinear shape of the oxygen-hemoglobin dissociation curve, the higher P_{O_2} of blood leaving high $\dot{V}/\dot{Q}$ regions does not translate into a proportionate increase in hemoglobin saturation and oxygen content and therefore provides little extra oxygen to the arterial blood. This concept is illustrated in Figure 76–3.

As shown by the oxygen–carbon dioxide diagram in Figure 76–1, when no ventilation reaches perfused alveoli ($\dot{V}/\dot{Q}$ = 0), mixed venous blood passes unchanged through the lung. This is a right-to-left intrapulmonary shunt. This extreme form of ventilation-perfusion imbalance causes hypoxemia simply by the addition of venous blood to the arterial circulation.

Although it is well recognized that ventilation-perfusion inequality and shunt impair oxygen transfer and produce arterial hypoxemia, it is less well appreciated that they also interfere with the removal of carbon dioxide.[1, 2] This occurs because regions of the lungs with low $\dot{V}/\dot{Q}$ contribute blood with an elevated P_{CO_2} to the arterial circulation (see Fig. 76–1). The shift of ventilation from low to high $\dot{V}/\dot{Q}$ regions simultaneously produces an increase in alveolar dead space (see later discussion). Ventilation-perfusion imbalance usually does not lead to hypercapnia because chemoreceptors increase minute ventilation to maintain the Pa_{CO_2} in the normal range. Hypercapnia will occur, however, if an increase in ventilation is limited by respiratory depression, neuromuscular disease, or excessive work of breathing (e.g., end-stage lung disease).

The severity of ventilation-perfusion imbalance may be assessed by several different measurements. All are based

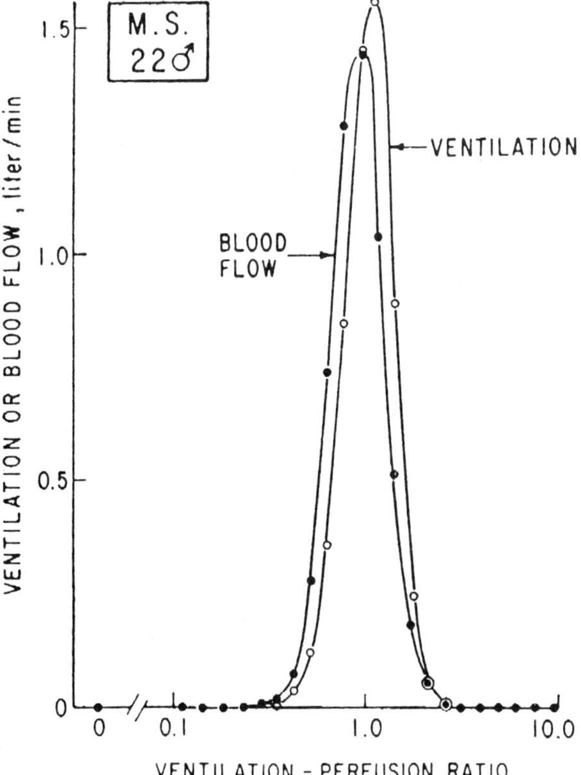

Figure 76–2. The distributions of ventilation and blood flow in a young, healthy man. Both distributions are narrow, symmetric on a log scale, and positioned about a $\dot{V}/\dot{Q}$ ratio of approximately 1.0. (From Wagner PD: Continuous distributions of ventilation-perfusion ratios in normal subjects breathing air and 100% O_2. J Clin Invest 1974; 54:54.)

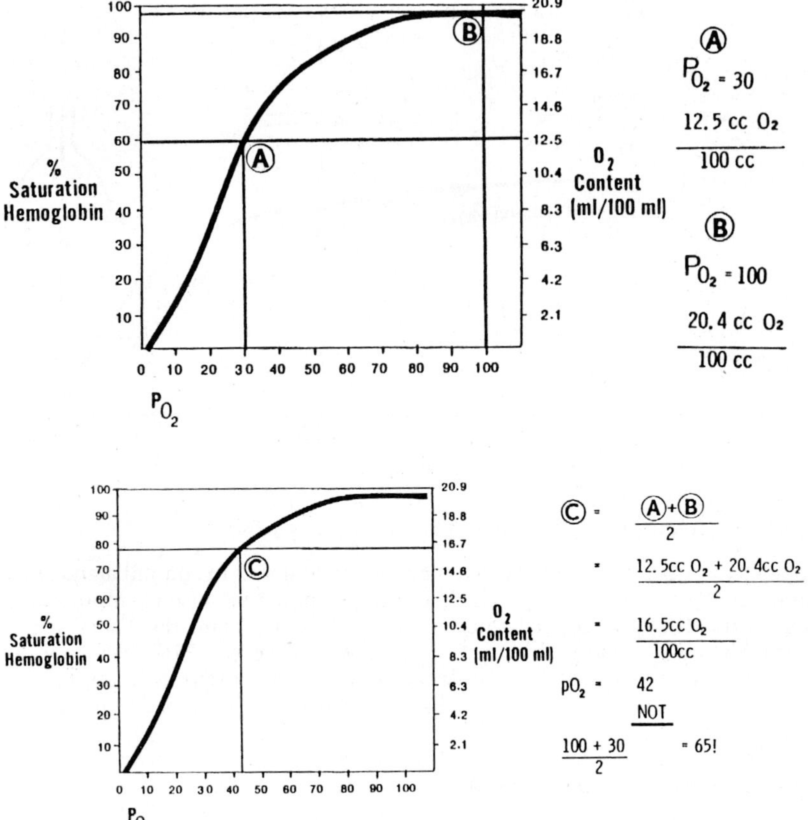

Figure 76–3. The mechanism by which $\dot{V}/\dot{Q}$ imbalance produces arterial hypoxemia. If a low $\dot{V}/\dot{Q}$ lung unit contributes blood with a PO_2 of 30 mm Hg *(Point A)* and if a high $\dot{V}/\dot{Q}$ lung unit provides an equal quantity of blood with PO_2 of 100 mm Hg *(Point B)*, the final PO_2 will *not* be the average of the two values (i.e., 65 mm Hg). Rather, the resultant PO_2 *(Point C)* is determined by the average of the oxygen contents (16.5 cc O_2/100 cc) or of the hemoglobin saturations (78%). Therefore, the final PO_2 is 42 mm Hg.

on the composition of "ideal" alveolar gas, which represents mixed alveolar gas in the absence of any ventilation-perfusion imbalance. The ideal alveolar PO_2 (PAO_2) is calculated from a modification of the alveolar gas equation:

$$PAO_2 = (PB - PH_2O)\ FIO_2 - PaCO_2/R$$

[Equation 1]

where PB is the barometric pressure, PH_2O is the partial pressure of water in the alveoli (47 mm Hg at body temperature), and R is the respiratory quotient (assumed to be 0.8). The PCO_2 of ideal alveolar gas is assumed to be equal to the $PaCO_2$.

One commonly used measure of ventilation-perfusion imbalance is the difference between the PAO_2 and the PO_2 of arterial blood ($PA-aO_2$). This value varies directly with the number and severity of low $\dot{V}/\dot{Q}$ lung units and with the fraction of the cardiac output (CO) that passes through unventilated regions (shunt fraction).

Another measure of the contribution of low $\dot{V}/\dot{Q}$ lung units and shunt to the arterial blood is the venous admixture. For this calculation, we assume that the difference between the oxygen content of "ideal" pulmonary capillary blood (no ventilation-perfusion imbalance) and arterial blood is due solely to the addition of mixed venous blood to the arterial circulation. The venous admixture ($\dot{Q}va$) is expressed as a fraction of total CO:

$$\frac{\dot{Q}va}{\dot{Q}t} = \frac{(CIO_2 - CaO_2)}{(CIO_2 - C\bar{v}O_2)}$$

[Equation 2]

where CIO_2, CaO_2, and $C\bar{v}O_2$ are the oxygen content of ideal capillary blood (calculated using the alveolar gas equation), arterial blood, and mixed venous blood, respectively. When the FIO_2 is increased to 1.0, the contribution of low $\dot{V}/\dot{Q}$ lung units is removed, and $\dot{Q}va/\dot{Q}t$ measures the shunt fraction ($\dot{Q}s/\dot{Q}t$).

The volume of inspired air that reaches areas of the lungs with either high $\dot{V}/\dot{Q}$ or no perfusion at all does not contribute optimally to gas exchange. This is referred to as *wasted ventilation* or *physiologic dead space* and provides a measure of the number and severity of high $\dot{V}/\dot{Q}$ lung units. The physiologic dead space (V_{DS}) is calculated by assuming that the difference between the PCO_2 of ideal alveolar gas (estimated by the $PaCO_2$) and the PCO_2 of mixed exhaled gas ($PECO_2$) is due to the addition of inspired air that does not participate in gas exchange. Expressed as a fraction of the tidal volume (V_T), V_{DS} is calculated from the Bohr equation:

$$\frac{V_{DS}}{V_T} = \frac{PaCO_2 - PECO_2}{PaCO_2}$$

[Equation 3]

The V_{DS} reflects both the volume of the conducting airways (anatomic dead space) and the amount of wasted ventilation to high $\dot{V}/\dot{Q}$ lung units (alveolar dead space). Anatomic dead space can be estimated as 1 mL per pound of (ideal) body weight. The dead space ventilation ($\dot{V}_{DS}$) is the total volume of air entering the lungs each minute that does not contribute to gas exchange.

Unfortunately, the clinical usefulness of these three measurements is limited by the fact that all are influenced by factors other than the amount of ventilation-perfusion imbalance and shunt.[1, 2] Venous admixture and V_{DS}/V_T are affected by changes in both minute ventilation and cardiac output. In addition, venous admixture varies inversely with the FIO_2 unless a large shunt fraction is present. The $PA - aO_2$ is by far the easiest of the measurements to perform and is unaffected by changes in minute ventilation. These advantages have made the $PA - aO_2$ the most commonly

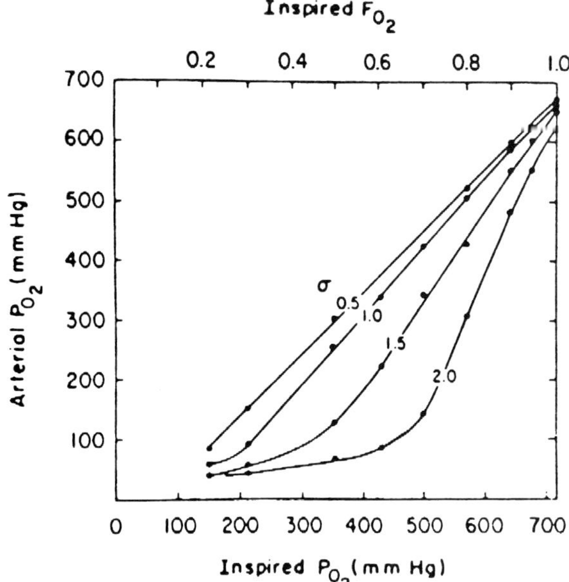

Figure 76–4. The relationship between PaO_2 and FIO_2 with varying distributions of $\dot{V}/\dot{Q}$. The value of σ equals the standard deviation of the distribution. Increasing σ indicates worsening $\dot{V}/\dot{Q}$ imbalance. (From West JB, Wagner PD: Pulmonary gas exchange. *In*: Bioengineering Aspects of the Lung. West JB [Ed]. New York, Marcel Dekker, 1977, p 389. Reprinted by courtesy of Marcel Dekker, Inc.)

used method for assessing the severity of ventilation-perfusion imbalance. The major limitation of this measurement is that it varies unpredictably as the FIO_2 is changed. This occurs because, in the presence of ventilation-perfusion imbalance, the PaO_2 rises relatively slowly with initial increases in FIO_2 but increases rapidly when high concentrations of oxygen are reached. As shown in Figure 76–4, the greater the imbalance between ventilation and perfusion, the higher the FIO_2 that is required to produce a significant increase in the PaO_2. Because the PAO_2 varies directly with oxygen concentration, the $PA - aO_2$ initially increases by an amount

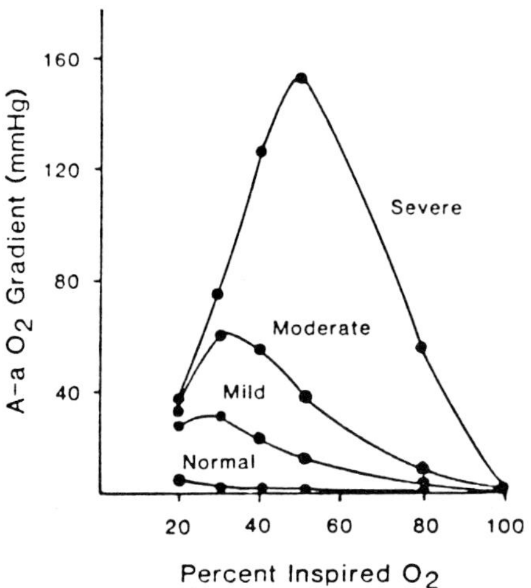

Figure 76–5. The relationship between $PA - aO_2$ and FIO_2 in a normal lung and in lungs with mild, moderate, and severe ventilation-perfusion imbalance. (From Dantzker DR: Mechanisms of hypoxemia and hypercapnia. *In*: Critical Care: A Comprehensive Approach. Bone RC [Ed]. Chicago, American College of Chest Physicians, 1984, pp 1–14.)

dependent on the extent of ventilation-perfusion imbalance and then falls as the FIO_2 is progressively increased. This is illustrated in Figure 76–5. The $PA - aO_2$ also increases with age (as the PaO_2 falls). In a young patient breathing room air, the $PA - aO_2$ should be less than 10 but may increase to as much as 20 in an elderly patient.[3, 4]

Alveolar Hypoventilation

The alveolar ventilation ($\dot{V}A$) is the volume of air entering the lungs each minute that actually participates in gas exchange. It is, therefore, the difference between the minute ventilation ($\dot{V}E$) and $\dot{V}DS$:

$$\dot{V}A = \dot{V}E - \dot{V}DS \qquad \text{[Equation 4]}$$

The $PaCO_2$ is determined by the $\dot{V}A$ and by the rate of carbon dioxide production ($\dot{V}CO_2$):

$$PaCO_2 = K\frac{\dot{V}CO_2}{\dot{V}A} \qquad \text{[Equation 5]}$$

or

$$PaCO_2 = K\frac{\dot{V}CO_2}{\dot{V}E - \dot{V}DS} \qquad \text{[Equation 6]}$$

where K is a constant.

By definition, alveolar hypoventilation is present whenever the $PaCO_2$ rises above normal. As illustrated by equation 6, if carbon dioxide production is constant, an increase in the $PaCO_2$ must be associated with either a decrease in $\dot{V}E$ or an increase in $\dot{V}DS$ (without a compensatory rise in $\dot{V}E$). As predicted by the alveolar gas equation, an increase in the $PaCO_2$ will, in turn, result in a fall in the PaO_2. If the rise in $PaCO_2$ is due to a fall in $\dot{V}E$, the $PA - aO_2$ will remain constant. When alveolar hypoventilation is associated with an increase in alveolar dead space, however, low ventilation-perfusion lung units must have also increased. The PaO_2 falls by more than the amount predicted by the alveolar gas equation, and the $PA - aO_2$ increases.

CLASSIFICATION OF RESPIRATORY FAILURE

On the basis of the underlying mechanism of abnormal gas exchange, respiratory failure may be divided into three types (Table 76–1). Type 1, or oxygenation failure, is characterized by an abnormally low PaO_2 and a normal or low $PaCO_2$. It may be caused by any disorder that produces ventilation-perfusion imbalance or a right-to-left intrapulmonary shunt. The abnormally high and low $\dot{V}/\dot{Q}$ result in a fall in the PaO_2 and an increase in the $PA - aO_2$, venous admixture, and VDS/VT. Minute ventilation increases to compensate for the elevated alveolar dead space, and therefore the $PaCO_2$ remains normal or falls. Type 1 respiratory

TABLE 76–1. Classification of Respiratory Failure

Type	PaO_2	$PaCO_2$	$PA - aO_2$
1: Oxygenation failure	↓	NL-↓	↑
2: Ventilation failure	↓	↑	NL
3: Combined failure	↓	↑	↑

Abbreviations: PaO_2 = arterial partial pressure of oxygen; $PaCO_2$ = arterial partial pressure of carbon dioxide; $PA - aO_2$ = alveolar-arterial difference in partial pressure of oxygen.

TABLE 76–2. Causes of Type 1 (Oxygenation) Failure

Adult respiratory distress syndrome
Asthma
Atelectasis
Cardiogenic pulmonary edema
Chronic obstructive pulmonary disease (including bronchiectasis and cystic fibrosis)
Interstitial fibrosis
Pneumonia (infectious or chemical)
Pneumothorax
Pulmonary embolism
Pulmonary hypertension

failure can be caused by any disorder that affects the airways, parenchyma, or vasculature of the lung. The most common causes are listed in Table 76–2.

Type 2, or ventilation failure, occurs when a primary fall in $\dot{V}_E$ results in alveolar hypoventilation. The resulting rise in the Pa_{CO_2} is accompanied by a decrease in the Pa_{O_2} as predicted by the alveolar gas equation, and therefore the $PA - aO_2$ does not increase. Type 2 respiratory failure can be caused by any disorder that decreases central respiratory drive, interferes with the transmission of signals from the central nervous system, or impedes the ability of the respiratory muscles to expand the lungs and chest wall. A partial list is provided in Table 76–3.

Type 3, or combined oxygenation-ventilation failure, occurs when $\dot{V}_E$ cannot be increased sufficiently to maintain a normal Pa_{CO_2} in the presence of marked ventilation-perfusion imbalance. Type 3 respiratory failure is, therefore, characterized by a low Pa_{O_2}, an elevated Pa_{CO_2}, and an increased $PA - aO_2$, venous admixture, and V_{DS}/V_T. In theory, any disorder causing type 1 can also cause type 3 respiratory failure. In fact, however, only a few of these disorders commonly result in carbon dioxide retention. These are listed in Table 76–4.

DIAGNOSIS

The diagnosis of respiratory failure is based on the presence of hypoxemia and/or hypercapnia and, therefore, relies primarily on arterial blood gas analysis. Although the exact values are somewhat arbitrary, respiratory failure is typically defined as a Pa_{O_2} less than 60 mm Hg (breathing room air) and/or a Pa_{CO_2} greater than 46 mm Hg. Hypercapnia in the setting of acute respiratory failure will be accompanied by an uncompensated respiratory acidosis.

In recent years, oximetry has become increasingly available and popular as a means of noninvasively measuring

TABLE 76–3. Causes of Type 2 (Ventilation) Failure

Disorders Affecting Central Respiratory Drive
Brain stem infarction or hemorrhage
Brain stem compression from supratentorial mass
Drug overdose (e.g., narcotics, benzodiazepines, tricyclics)

Disorders Affecting Signal Transmission to the Respiratory Muscles
Amyotrophic lateral sclerosis
Guillain-Barré syndrome
Multiple sclerosis
Myasthenia gravis
Spinal cord injury

Disorders of the Respiratory Muscles or Chest Wall
Muscular dystrophy
Polymyositis/dermatomyositis
Flail chest

TABLE 76–4. Causes of Type 3 (Combined Oxygenation-Ventilation) Failure

Adult respiratory distress syndrome
Asthma
Chronic obstructive pulmonary disease (including bronchiectasis and cystic fibrosis)

arterial hemoglobin saturation (Sa_{O_2}). Inaccurate readings may be obtained, however, when the Sa_{O_2} is low[5] and in the presence of jaundice,[6] dark skin pigmentation,[7] and elevated levels of carboxyhemoglobin.[8] In addition, oximetry provides no information about the Pa_{CO_2}. Significant hypercapnia and acidosis may be present without an abnormally low hemoglobin saturation, especially if supplemental oxygen is being administered. Oximetry should, therefore, never be used as a substitute for arterial blood gas measurement in the initial assessment of the patient suspected of having respiratory failure. Oximetry may be used to follow the Sa_{O_2} provided that periodic validation is obtained via blood gas analysis.

Arterial blood gas measurements will be obtained, of course, only if the diagnosis of respiratory failure is suspected on clinical grounds. Patients with acute respiratory failure will have manifestations of the underlying disease and may also have symptoms and signs of hypoxemia and/or hypercapnia. Hypoxemia may be accompanied by tachypnea, tachycardia, and hypertension. Cerebral hypoxia produces changes in mentation that can range from mild confusion (with a characteristic loss of recent memory) to delirium. Cyanosis of the nail beds may be evident. Hypercapnia exerts its major effect on the central nervous system. Patients typically progress through the stages of lethargy, stupor, and finally coma as the Pa_{CO_2} rises. At high Pa_{CO_2} levels, brain stem depression leads to slowing of the respiratory rate and finally to apnea. Although hypoxemia and hypercapnia may be associated with many clinical manifestations, these symptoms and signs may not occur until long after gas exchange is markedly and dangerously impaired. For example, significant increases in heart rate, respiratory rate, and blood pressure may not occur until the arterial hemoglobin saturation falls below 70% to 80%.[9] Cyanosis will occur only when the concentration of deoxygenated hemoglobin in the capillary blood exceeds 5 g/dL.[10] Even under optimal conditions, therefore, cyanosis will be present only when the Pa_{O_2} falls to approximately 45 mm Hg. In fact, cyanosis is often detected only at much lower levels.[9] This is especially true in the presence of anemia.[10] In addition, the clinical manifestations associated with hypoxemia and hypercapnia are nonspecific and may occur in the absence of respiratory failure. Physicians must then remain vigilant for even subtle symptoms and signs of respiratory insufficiency and have a very low threshold for obtaining arterial blood gas measurements.

EVALUATION

Once the diagnosis of respiratory failure is made, a search must be made for its cause. This evaluation is based on arterial blood gas measurements and the history, physical examination, and chest x-ray films.

Arterial Blood Gas Analysis

As shown in Table 76–1, measurement of the Pa_{O_2} and Pa_{CO_2} and calculation of the $PA - aO_2$ can be used to place patients with respiratory failure into one of three categories.

Once this classification has been made, the diagnostic possibilities become more limited (see Tables 76–2 to 76–4).

History

The medical history must include information about both pulmonary and extrapulmonary symptoms and signs. The presence or absence of cough, sputum production, hemoptysis, pleuritic or nonpleuritic chest pain, fever, paroxysmal nocturnal dyspnea, orthopnea, weakness, and sensory disturbances must be noted. The duration of symptoms, any events or circumstances associated with the onset of symptoms (e.g., surgery, trauma, drug or alcohol ingestion), and the presence of prior pulmonary or extrapulmonary disease must also be determined.

Physical Examination

The physical examination must be thorough, but particular attention should be directed toward the respiratory, cardiovascular, and neuromuscular systems. The pulmonary examination must detect the presence of stridor, wheezing, rales, rhonchi, bronchial breath sounds, a pleural rub, a prolonged expiratory time, diminished or absent breath sounds, and dullness or hyperresonance to percussion. The cardiovascular examination must include an assessment of jugular venous pressure and a careful search for cardiac murmurs and an S_3 gallop. The neurologic examination must detect altered mentation, sensory loss, and weakness of both the skeletal muscles and the diaphragm. The presence of paradoxical inward movement of the anterior abdominal wall during inspiration is very suggestive of paralysis or weakness of the diaphragm and is a key, but often overlooked, physical finding.

Chest X-Ray Examination

The chest x-ray examination is useful for further narrowing the differential diagnosis or for solidifying or confirming a presumptive diagnosis based on the history and physical examination. The presence of interstitial or airspace disease, bullae, atelectasis, pleural effusion, pneumothorax, chest wall deformity, and high or low lung volumes provides important information about the underlying disease process. It should be noted that some causes of respiratory failure may be associated with a normal-appearing chest x-ray film. These include pulmonary embolism, asthma, upper airway obstruction, and most disorders producing respiratory center depression or weakness of the respiratory muscles.

On the basis of the information provided by arterial blood gas analysis and the history, physical, and chest x-ray examination, a specific diagnosis can often be made. For example, the previously healthy patient with several days of fever, chills, productive cough, and dyspnea who has bronchial breath sounds on physical examination and a focal area of airspace disease on chest x-ray films has pneumonia. The patient who experiences the acute onset of dyspnea, hemoptysis, and a pleural rub several days after surgery must be strongly suspected of having a pulmonary embolus. In the patient with a history of coronary artery disease who experiences substernal chest pain and dyspnea, has rales and an S_3 gallop on examination, and has interstitial densities on chest x-ray examination, myocardial infarction with congestive heart failure is the most likely diagnosis. The patient with a history of suicide attempts who presents with a markedly depressed mental status, shallow and slow respirations, an otherwise normal examination, and a normal chest x-ray film should be suspected of having drug-induced respiratory depression.

MANAGEMENT

The management of every patient with respiratory failure, regardless of the cause, has four essential components: (1) establish a patent airway; (2) maintain sufficient ventilation; (3) ensure adequate oxygen delivery to the tissues; and (4) treat the underlying cause of respiratory failure.

Airway Management

All patients with respiratory failure must be assessed for the presence of upper airway obstruction. Signs of partial obstruction are inspiratory snoring or stridor accompanied by a diminished tidal volume. Complete obstruction is indicated by lack of airflow in the presence of sustained and often vigorous inspiratory efforts. Patients may have upper airway obstruction as the primary cause of respiratory failure (e.g., food or foreign body aspiration, laryngeal edema) or as a secondary event. For example, hypoventilation from central nervous system depression or neuromuscular disease may be exacerbated by airway obstruction at the level of the oropharynx as a result of loss of muscle tone. Secondary airway obstruction can often be relieved by lifting the mandible or by inserting an oropharyngeal airway. In all cases of upper airway obstruction, however, translaryngeal intubation or tracheostomy must be performed if airway patency cannot be rapidly established. Additional indications for endotracheal intubation are listed in Table 76–5 and include loss of laryngeal reflexes that prevent aspiration, inability to clear pulmonary secretions adequately, and inadequate oxygenation or ventilation (see following discussion).

Ventilation

As previously discussed, hypercapnia signifies the presence of alveolar hypoventilation. This may result from either a fall in $\dot{V}_E$ or an inadequate ventilatory response to an increase in low $\dot{V}/\dot{Q}$ lung units and alveolar dead space. An abrupt rise in the Pa_{CO_2} will, in turn, lead to an acute respiratory acidosis. Mechanical ventilation is used to treat acute, severe hypoventilation. Traditionally, this has required endotracheal intubation. Recently, however, several studies have suggested that noninvasive mechanical ventilation using a nasal or full facemask is an effective alternative in a small number of patients.[11, 12, 12a] Mechanical ventilation, including noninvasive ventilatory assistance, is discussed in detail in Chapters 97 to 104. In this chapter, we discuss only a few general but very important aspects of mechanical ventilatory support.

Guidelines for the institution of mechanical ventilation are shown in Table 76–6. As a general rule, mechanical ventilation should be initiated when hypercapnia results in an arterial pH less than or equal to 7.25. Note that hypercapnia by itself is not an indication for mechanical ventilation.

TABLE 76–5. Indications for Endotracheal Intubation

Upper airway obstruction
Loss of protective reflexes
Impaired secretion clearance
Refractory hypoxemia
Requirement for mechanical ventilation

TABLE 76–6. Guidelines for the Initiation of Mechanical Ventilation

Guideline	
Ventilation Failure	
Respiratory acidosis with pH $\leq$7.25	
Evidence of progressive or impending ventilation failure	
Rising partial pressure of carbon dioxide	
Tachypnea with air hunger	
Diaphragmatic weakness or fatigue	
Paradoxical movement of the abdominal wall	
Vital capacity <15 mL/kg	in patients with neuromuscular disease
Maximum inspiratory pressure ≥ -30 cm H_2O	in patients with neuromuscular disease
Maximum expiratory pressure $\leq$30 cm H_2O	in patients with neuromuscular disease
Oxygenation Failure	
Refractory hypoxemia	

Many patients with chronic ventilation failure have a relatively normal pH as a result of metabolic compensation. It is the acidosis, not the hypercapnia, that must be corrected. This guideline is, however, not meant to be strictly applied. For example, intubation and mechanical ventilation might be appropriately delayed if a patient with an arterial pH of less than 7.25 has ventilation failure from a process that is potentially rapidly reversible (e.g., narcotic overdose, some cases of asthma). On the other hand, patients with evidence of worsening ventilation failure or impending failure of the respiratory muscles should be electively intubated rather than waiting until intubation becomes an emergency procedure. Patients with progressive hypercapnia, marked tachypnea, or signs of diaphragmatic fatigue should, therefore, be intubated and mechanically ventilated long before the arterial pH reaches 7.25. Elective intubation and ventilation have been advocated for patients with neuromuscular disease when the vital capacity falls below 15 mL/kg or when the maximum inspiratory and expiratory pressure decreases to ± 30 cm H_2O.[13, 14]

Several modes of mechanical support are available on modern ventilators. When selecting a mode of ventilation for a patient with acute respiratory failure, several principles should be kept in mind. First, the ventilator should relieve most of the patient's work of breathing and allow the respiratory muscles to rest. This can be best accomplished by selecting the assist-control mode or the synchronized intermittent mandatory ventilation (SIMV) mode with the set respiratory rate close to the patient's spontaneous rate. SIMV with a low set rate should not be used in the initial management of acute respiratory failure because it may not significantly reduce the work of breathing and may perpetuate or even worsen respiratory muscle fatigue.[15] Second, the mode of ventilation selected should guarantee the patient a minimum safe or back-up minute ventilation. Once again, the assist-control and SIMV modes meet this requirement. Pressure-set modes of ventilation do not and should be used only with great caution in patients with acute respiratory failure. During pressure support ventilation, for example, the tidal volume delivered with each mechanical breath depends not only on the set pressure but also on the patient's inspiratory effort and on the compliance and resistance of the respiratory system. In addition, all pressure-supported mechanical breaths must be triggered by the inspiratory efforts of the patient. Therefore, the tidal volume, $\dot{V}E$ and, most importantly, the $PaCO_2$ and pH may vary significantly over time even on the same ventilator settings. Pressure control ventilation may be beneficial in some patients with ARDS that is refractory to conventional ventilatory management.[16, 16a] Again, because the tidal volume is variable and not set, the $\dot{V}E$ and $PaCO_2$ must be closely monitored when this mode of ventilation is used.

In addition to the mode of ventilation, the clinician must also select the tidal volume, respiratory rate, and FIO_2 to be provided by the ventilator. Tidal volume should be based on body size and should be in the range of 8 to 12 mL/kg (ideal body weight). As previously mentioned, the set respiratory rate should produce a $\dot{V}E$ that will meet most of the patient's ventilatory requirements. An initial rate of 10 to 16 breaths per minute is typically required. Intubated patients with oxygenation failure should initially receive an FIO_2 of 1.0. This will either rapidly correct the hypoxemia or allow for the early institution of therapy with positive end-expiratory pressure (see later discussion). Changes in these initial ventilator settings should be based on serial blood gas analysis.

Oxygenation

One of the cornerstones in the management of acute respiratory failure must be to provide sufficient oxygen to the tissues of the body. Although arterial hypoxemia must be corrected, it is important to realize that the PaO_2, inasmuch as it determines the SaO_2, is only one determinant of the amount of oxygen delivered to the tissues. Oxygen delivery ($\dot{D}O_2$) is also dependent on the concentration of hemoglobin (Hb) and the CO.

$$\dot{D}O_2 = 1.34 \times Hb \times \frac{SaO_2}{100} \times CO \times 10$$

[Equation 7]

Tissue oxygen delivery can, therefore, be improved not only by increasing the SaO_2 but also by correcting anemia and increasing the CO.

In the patient with arterial hypoxemia, sufficient supplemental oxygen should be provided to increase the PaO_2 to approximately 60 to 70 mm Hg. Because of the shape of the oxygen-hemoglobin dissociation curve (see Fig. 76–3), at a PaO_2 below 60 mm Hg, relatively small increases will result in a significant improvement in SaO_2 and $\dot{D}O_2$. As the PaO_2 is increased further, however, there is little additional increase in SaO_2.

The initial concentration of oxygen chosen should be based on the underlying mechanism of impaired gas exchange. Diseases associated with the mismatching of ventilation and perfusion (e.g., asthma, COPD) produce hypoxemia that is usually responsive to relatively low levels of supplemental oxygen. Depending on the initial PaO_2, patients with these conditions can usually be treated with oxygen concentrations ranging from 0.24 to 0.40 using a Venturi or aerosol mask or with oxygen flow rates of 1 to 4 L/min via a nasal cannula. It is well known that some patients with COPD experience hypercapnia and respiratory acidosis when given supplemental oxygen. For many years, this was believed to be due to loss of the hypoxic respiratory drive with consequent fall in $\dot{V}E$. It has recently been shown, however, that hypercapnia in this setting is due primarily to worsening ventilation-perfusion imbalance.[17, 18] Regardless of its mechanism, fear of this complication often results in inadequate oxygen administration to patients with acute respiratory failure. Several important points must be emphasized. First, oxygen-induced hypercapnia occurs almost exclusively in patients with severe airflow obstruction and chronic carbon dioxide retention.[17, 18] Second, the rise in $PaCO_2$ is minimized by administering just enough oxygen to eliminate arterial hypoxemia.[17, 19] In this group of patients, then, it is best to start with lower levels of supplemental oxygen (FIO_2 of 0.28 or 1 to 2 L/min). Third, although controlled oxygen administration may cause worsening hypercapnia, the development of significant respiratory acidosis is uncommon[19] and in our experience is often due to sedative- or narcotic-induced central respiratory depression. Finally, it is essential to remember that hypoxemia must be corrected even if the $PaCO_2$ rises. If necessary, hypercapnia and acute respiratory acidosis can be managed with mechanical ventilation.

Hypoxemia caused primarily by intrapulmonary shunting will improve but only partially correct, even with the administration of high concentrations of oxygen. Therefore, patients with pneumonia, cardiogenic pulmonary edema, ARDS, and other diseases producing extensive alveolar filling should initially receive the highest possible concentration of oxygen. In nonintubated patients, this can be achieved by using a non-rebreather mask or a high-flow aerosol mask. The all-too-common practice of beginning with low fractional concentrations of oxygen and "working upward" as repeated blood gas measurements show a persistently low PaO_2 can delay the correction of life-threatening tissue hypoxia for several hours.

Not uncommonly, patients with a large intrapulmonary shunt have hypoxemia that is not corrected even by the highest FIO_2 achievable with a facemask. In a few patients, hypoxemia may be corrected by the administration of continuous positive airway pressure via a facemask.[20] In most cases, however, refractory hypoxemia is managed by endotracheal intubation and mechanical ventilation. Intubation allows the delivery of higher concentrations of oxygen to the alveoli, and mechanical ventilation reduces oxygen consumption by decreasing patient work of breathing. Patients with ARDS will usually also require the addition of PEEP. In this group of patients, PEEP has been shown to increase the PaO_2 by opening atelectatic alveoli and by redistributing lung water from the alveoli to the interstitium.[21, 22] Unfortunately, PEEP often produces a decrease in CO primarily through its effect on venous return. It may, therefore, increase the PaO_2 and SaO_2 and yet cause a fall in $\dot{D}O_2$ to the tissues. For this reason, serial measurements of $\dot{D}O_2$, not just PaO_2, are essential when PEEP is used in patients with acute respiratory failure.

Therapy of the Underlying Disease

Once a stable airway and adequate ventilation and oxygenation have been established, therapy can be focused on the cause of acute respiratory failure. The management of specific disorders is beyond the scope of this chapter but is discussed in detail in subsequent chapters in this section.

CONCLUSION

Acute respiratory failure represents a sudden, severe disturbance in the exchange of oxygen and carbon dioxide between the environment and the cells of the body. It is, therefore, a medical emergency and a very real threat to the life of the patient. A large number of diseases may lead to acute respiratory failure, and many have specific therapies. However, the diagnosis, evaluation, and initial management of this disorder are the same regardless of the underlying cause. The approach to the patient with acute respiratory failure must be thorough and systematic and based on an understanding of the mechanisms of normal and abnormal gas exchange.

References

1. West JB: Ventilation-perfusion relationships. Am Rev Respir Dis 1977; 116:919.
2. West JB: Ventilation-perfusion inequality and overall gas exchange in computer models of the lung. Respir Physiol 1969; 7:88.
3. Harris EA, Kenyon AM, Nisbet HD, et al: The normal alveolar-arterial oxygen tension gradient in man. Clin Sci 1974; 46:89.
4. Sorbini CA, Grassi V, Solinas E, et al: Arterial oxygen tension in relation to age in healthy subjects. Respiration 1968; 25:3.
5. Severinghaus JW, Naifeh KH: Accuracy of response of six pulse oximeters to profound hypoxemia. Anesthesiology 1987; 67:551.
6. Chaudhary BA, Burki NK: Ear oximetry in clinical practice. Am Rev Respir Dis 1978; 117:173.
7. Zeballos RJ, Weisman IM: Reliability of noninvasive oximetry in black subjects during exercise and hypoxia. Am Rev Respir Dis 1991; 144:1240.
8. Barker SJ, Tremper KK: The effect of carbon monoxide inhalation on pulse oximetry and transcutaneous PO_2. Anesthesiology 1987; 66:677.
9. Comroe JH, Botelho S: The unreliability of cyanosis in the recognition of arterial anoxemia. Am J Med Sci 1947; 214:1.
10. Blount SG. Cyanosis: Pathophysiology and differential diagnosis. Prog Cardiovasc Dis 1971; 13:595.
11. Meduri GU, Abou-Shala N, Fox RC, et al: Noninvasive face mask mechanical ventilation in patients with acute hypercapnic respiratory failure. Chest 1991; 100:445.
12. Pennock BE, Kaplan PD, Carlin BW, et al: Pressure support ventilation with a simplified ventilatory support system administered with a nasal mask in patients with respiratory failure. Chest 1991; 110:1371.

12a. Hill NS: Noninvasive ventilation. Am Rev Respir Dis 1993; 147:1050.

13. Ropper AH, Kehne SM: Guillain-Barré syndrome: Management of respiratory failure. Neurology 1985; 35:1662.
14. Gracey DR, Divertie MB, Howard FM: Mechanical ventilation for respiratory failure in myasthenia gravis. Mayo Clin Proc 1983; 58:597.
15. Marini JJ, Smith TC, Lamb VJ: External work output and force generation during synchronized intermittent mandatory ventilation. Am Rev Respir Dis 1988; 138:1169.
16. Marcy TW, Marini JJ: Inverse ratio ventilation in ARDS. Chest 1991; 100:494.

16a. Blanch PB, Jones M, Layon AJ, Cammer N: Pressure-preset ventilation. Chest 1993; 104:590, 904.

17. Aubier M, Murciano D, Milic-Emili J, et al: Effects of the administration of O_2 on ventilation and blood gases in patients with chronic obstructive pulmonary disease during acute respiratory failure. Am Rev Respir Dis 1980; 122:747.
18. Sassoon CSH, Hassell KT, Mahutte CK: Hyperoxic-induced hypercapnia in stable chronic obstructive pulmonary disease. Am Rev Respir Dis 1981; 124:26.
19. Degaute JP, Domenighetti G, Naeije R, et al: Oxygen delivery in acute exacerbation of chronic obstructive pulmonary disease. Am Rev Respir Dis 1981; 124:26.
20. Bersten AD, Holt AW, Vedig AE, et al: Treatment of severe cardiogenic pulmonary edema with continuous positive airway pressure delivered by face mask. N Engl J Med 1991; 325:1825.
21. Sassoon CSH, Mahutte CK, Light RW: Ventilator modes: Old and new. Crit Care Clin 1990; 6:605.
22. Malo J, Ali J, Wood LDH: How does positive end-expiratory pressure reduce intrapulmonary shunt in canine pulmonary edema? J Appl Physiol 1984; 57:1002.

CHAPTER 77

Principles of Respiratory Care

Robert M. Kacmarek, PhD, RRT • James K. Stoller, MD

Many technologies are used in the intensive care unit (ICU) to maintain the integrity of the respiratory system and to support gas exchange. Normally, most attention is directed toward positive-pressure therapy or mechanical ventilation. In this chapter, we address those other facets of respiratory care that play an important role in the management of patients breathing spontaneously, with or without artificial airways, as well as of those requiring mechanical ventilatory support. Specifically, oxygen therapy, humidification, aerosolized pharmacologic agents, and suctioning are discussed.

OXYGEN THERAPY

Historically, approaches to oxygen therapy have been divided into two broad categories: high-flow and low-flow systems.[1] The basis for this division is the ability of the gas delivery system to provide a conditioned gas volume sufficient to meet the patient's total ventilatory demand. High-flow systems are capable of meeting these high ventilatory demands, whereas low-flow systems are not.

High-Flow Systems

These systems provide a precise and consistent fraction of inspired oxygen (FIO_2) independent of alterations in patient ventilatory pattern. In order to ensure this, high-flow systems must provide a flow of gas exceeding patient demand. This requires a system flow greater than the patient's peak inspiratory flow rate, or at least four times the patient's minute volume.[2] However, because peak inspiratory flows during marked cardiopulmonary stress may exceed 80 to 100 L/min, it is doubtful that any gas delivery system applied to a nonintubated patient is capable of meeting ventilatory demands under all circumstances; on the other hand, in relatively stable patients, peak inspiratory flows average about 40 L/min.[3] Thus, systems classified as high-flow systems for adults must be capable of delivering at least 40 L/min of conditioned gas to the patient's face.

Many high-flow systems use air entrainment not only to enhance volume of gas delivered to the airway but also to regulate FIO_2 precisely. Entrainment occurs by the jet drag effect, whereby a rapid flow of one gas creates a shearing effect, which entrains a second gas (Fig. 77–1). All gas delivery devices that include entrainment function by the jet drag effect. Table 77–1 lists oxygen/air entrainment ratios, minimal oxygen flow, total output, and resulting FIO_2, with various entrainment settings.

Low-Flow Systems

All of the common oxygen delivery systems are classified as low-flow systems: nasal cannula, simple mask, and mask with a reservoir. With these devices, the FIO_2 is dependent on (1) the flow of oxygen into the device; (2) the size of the equipment reservoir (e.g., volume of the facemask); (3) the size of the anatomic reservoir (volume of the oral and nasal pharynx); (4) the capability of filling the reservoir during the transition between expiration and inspiration; and (5) the ventilatory pattern of the patient.[1] Because all these factors determine FIO_2, it is virtually impossible to predict the precise FIO_2 that a patient is receiving with a low-flow system. Nor is it possible to state that the FIO_2 stays constant over time in spite of the use of a consistent low-flow system at a single set flow rate. In general, FIO_2 and minute ventilation are inversely related with any low-flow system. Table 77–2 lists estimated FIO_2 ranges with low-flow systems.

Selection of an Oxygen Delivery Device

When deciding which oxygen delivery system to use, the following questions should be addressed:[4] (1) What FIO_2 is needed? (2) Are consistency and accuracy of FIO_2 required? (3) Is there a need for high humidity? (4) Is an artificial airway present? (5) Is tolerance and compliance a problem? In the ICU setting, patient compliance should not be as much of a problem as on the general medical/surgical floors because of the constant monitoring by nurses and therapists of the patient's critical status.

When low FIO_2 (<40%) is needed, we generally recommend either a nasal cannula or an air entrainment mask (frequently referred to as a Venti mask) depending on the need for a precise FIO_2 and the stability of the ventilatory pattern. If an FIO_2 of greater than 40% is required, we prefer either a high-flow aerosol or a large-volume humidifier system. With either approach, system flows of up to 100 L/min can be achieved at any FIO_2 and with gas either cool or heated. These systems are normally applied with an aerosol mask, a tracheostomy mask, or a Briggs adapter with reservoir via large-bore tubing. Because of inconsistency in delivered FIO_2, we rarely recommend using simple oxygen masks or masks with reservoirs in the ICU setting.

HUMIDIFICATION OF INHALED GAS

Inspired gas is normally conditioned by the upper respiratory tract and the trachea, ensuring that gas entering the

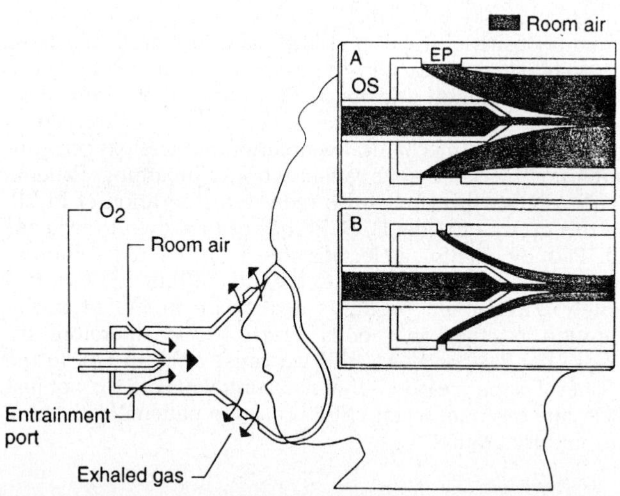

Figure 77–1. Operational principle of an air entrainment device. Pressurized O_2 is forced through a nozzle (constricted orifice); the increased gas velocity distal to the orifice creates a jet drag or shearing effect that causes room air to be drawn through the entrainment ports. The high flow of gas fills the mask, allowing both exhaled and delivered gas to escape. In this illustration, the size of the entrainment port (EP) determines the amount of room air to be entrained; a large port results in a relatively low FIO_2 because of high volume entrainment (A), whereas a small port results in a higher FIO_2 (B). Other systems vary entrainment by varying the size of the nozzle. *Abbreviation*: OS = O_2 source. (From Shapiro BA, Kacmarek RM, Cane RA, et al: Clinical Application of Respiratory Care. 4th ed. St. Louis, Mosby-Year Book, 1991, pp 123–150.)

TABLE 77–1. Entrainment Ratios and Outputs of Specific Air Entrainment Systems*

O_2/Air Entrainment Ratio	Minimal O_2 Flow	Total Flow†	F_{IO_2}
1:25	4	104	0.21
1:10	4	44	0.28
1:7	6	48	0.31
1:5	8	48	0.35
1:3	8	32	0.40
1:1.7	12	32	0.50
1:1	12	24	0.60
1:0.6	12	19	0.70

(From Kacmarek RM: In-hospital O_2 therapy. *In:* Current Respiratory Care. Kacmarek RM, Stoller JK [Eds]. Toronto, BC Decker, 1988, pp 1–8).

*Variations in delivered F_{IO_2} may occur because systems are disposable.

†For the system to be classified high flow, ≥40 L/min must be provided.

Abbreviation: F_{IO_2} = fraction of inspired oxygen; O_2 = oxygen.

lower respiratory tract is 100% saturated with water vapor at body temperature (37°C, 100% relative humidity, 43.8 mg/L absolute humidity, 47 mm Hg water vapor pressure).[5,6] The exact location at which these conditions are reached may be as much as 5 cm beyond the carina during normal breathing and is called the *isothermic saturation boundary.* The precise location of this boundary depends primarily on the condition of the inspired gas.[7] That part of the airway above the isothermic saturation boundary acts as a heat and moisture exchanger, adding heat and moisture to inspired gas and extracting it from exhaled gas.

Normally, inspired gas is heated by convection, and water vapor is added by evaporation in the upper respiratory tract. Under normal conditions, 570 mL of water and 54,456 J of heat are required daily to change room air (15°C and 50% relative humidity) to alveolar conditions (37°C and 100% relative humidity). Of these amounts, 320 mL of water and 52,986 J of heat are returned to the upper airway during exhalation. Therefore, about 250 mL of water and 1470 J of heat are lost from the lungs each day,[8] causing a humidity deficit. During health, systemic hydration provides the water necessary to meet this humidity deficit. However, during disease, when therapeutic gases are administered and the upper airway is bypassed by artificial airways, the humidity deficit created may tax the body's ability to meet this deficit. As a result, secretions may be dried, leading to (1) impairment of ciliary activity; (2) impairment of mucus movement; (3) inflammatory changes and necrosis of ciliated pulmonary epithelium; (4) retention of viscid, tenacious secretions with secondary encrustation; (5) bacterial infiltration; (6) atelectasis; and (7) pneumonia.[1,9] Whether or not inspired gas should be conditioned before inhalation depends on the delivery method, the liter flow, and the presence of an artificial airway.

Spontaneous Breathing

Conditioning gas during spontaneous breathing without an artificial airway is normally performed by a simple bubble-through humidifier, a large-volume unheated humidifier, or an aerosol generator. With low-flow oxygen therapy via a mask, a simple bubble-through humidifier is always used. During nasal cannula therapy, a humidifier is needed only when gas flow exceeds 4 L/min.[10,11] At flows less than or equal to 4 L/min, the volume of inspired dry gas is insufficient to affect the humidity deficit.

Artificial Airways

Generally, all patients with acutely placed artificial airways require the addition of water to the gases they inspire because the gas conditioning portion of the respiratory tract is largely bypassed. Although there is consensus that gas administered to patients with artificial airways should be humidified, there is ongoing debate whether the gas should be heated. Heat loss from the respiratory tract results from raising the temperature of inspired gases to body temperature and from loss of heat of vaporizations when the inspired gases are humidified. Air has a low specific heat (1008 J/kg),[8] whereas the latent heat of vaporization for water is relatively high (2450 J/kg); each gram of vaporized water results in a loss of 580 calories.[12] Thus, most of the potential heat loss from the respiratory tract results from humidifying inspired gases. Adequate humidification of the inspired gas may be important in maintaining body temperature.[13–15] However, heat loss from mechanisms other than respiration are usually more important for temperature homeostasis.[16] As a result, if large-volume nebulizers are used to humidify inspired gas via an artificial airway, heating of the system is normally unnecessary unless the patient requests heating for comfort or temperature homeostasis is crucial. On the other hand, heating is necessary if large-volume humidifiers are used. Without heating, these devices can only saturate gas at system temperature. When gas flow through the humidifier is rapid, gas temperature may only be 15°C and absolute humidity may be 15 to 20 mg/L.

Mechanical Ventilation

During mechanical ventilation, gas is inspired exclusively from the ventilator circuit and must be fully conditioned before entering the patient's airway. Gas conditioning is normally performed using heated humidifiers (with or without heated circuits) or by the use of artificial noses. Aerosol generators (large-volume jet nebulizers) are normally avoided in this setting because of problems with nosocomial infection,[17] the cost of daily circuit changes, and the potential for overhydrating the airway.[18,19]

Ideally, a device used to provide humidification during mechanical ventilation should be able to reproduce normal gas conditioning at the point of gas entry into the respiratory system. According to standards set by the American National Standards Institute,[20] a humidifying device should provide a minimum of 30 mg of water per liter of delivered

TABLE 77–2. Estimated F_{IO_2} with Low-Flow Systems*

System	Flow (L/Min)	F_{IO_2}
Nasal cannula	1	0.24
	2	0.28
	3	0.32
	4	0.36
	5	0.40
	6	0.44
Mask		
Simple	≥5	0.40–0.60
Partial rebreathing	≥8	≥0.60
Non-rebreathing	≥10	≥0.80

*Values are estimated based on a tidal volume of 500 mL, respiratory rate of 20 breaths per minute, inspiratory time of 1 s, and an anatomic reservoir of 50 mL.

Abbreviation: F_{IO_2} = fraction of inspired oxygen.

gas at a temperature of at least 30°C during mechanical ventilation. Characteristics of an ideal humidifier include ability to deliver adequate heat and moisture, safety (electrical), protection against transmitting infection, and convenience and economy.[21]

Heated Humidifiers

High-flow heated humidifiers can provide relative humidity of 100% at body temperature. However, continuously monitoring the temperature at the patient's airway is necessary whenever these devices are used. Specific devices include passover, cascade, wick, and vapor phase humidifiers. The humidifying efficiency of all these devices is generally comparable. Many are manufactured with closed water-feed systems, thereby reducing the risk of reservoir contamination from repeated opening. These continuous-feed systems avoid fluctuations in the temperature of delivered gas, as can occur when a bolus of cold water is added. In addition, because the level of fluid in the humidifier is kept constant, the compressible volume of the ventilator circuit is kept constant.

Many heated systems are servo humidifier–controlled. With these units, a thermistor is placed at the patient's proximal airway. The desired gas temperature at the thermistor is set, and the system maintains that delivered temperature. These thermistors have a relatively slow response and only reflect the average temperature of the inspired gas. Actual temperatures may fluctuate above and below the average temperature with cyclic gas flow, as occurs in a ventilator circuit.

To maintain a desired temperature at the patient end of the ventilator circuit, the temperature in the humidifier reservoir is typically greater than that of gas delivered to the patient. Cooling of the gas between the humidifier and the patient causes condensation ("rain out"). Water that collects in the tubing can serve as a source of nosocomial infection.[22] This water can also produce in accidental lavage of the patient's airway. Water that condenses in the tubing should be collected in a water trap. This water should be considered contaminated and should not be drained into the humidifier reservoir.

The tubing that carries gas from the humidifier to the patient can also be heated. This prevents a temperature drop in the tubing, permitting a more precise control of gas temperature delivered to the patient. By heating the inspiratory and expiratory limbs, a heated circuit also decreases or eliminates the amount of condensation in the tubing. Whenever the temperature of the tubing is less than the temperature of the gas leaving the humidifier, condensation occurs in the tubing. On the other hand, if the temperature of the tubing is greater than the temperature of the gas leaving the humidifier, the relative humidity of the gas will drop. This decrease in relative humidity with heated circuits has been shown to produce drying of secretions.[23, 24]

Another issue regarding types of humidifiers is the point in the ventilator circuit at which patient effort is sensed. If patient effort is sensed on the inspiratory side of the circuit internal to the ventilator, using a cascade-type (bubble-through) humidifier can markedly increase patient effort required to trigger the ventilator.[25] Thus, with all ventilators that sense patient effort on the inspiratory side, a passover humidifier should be used (Fig. 77–2).[26]

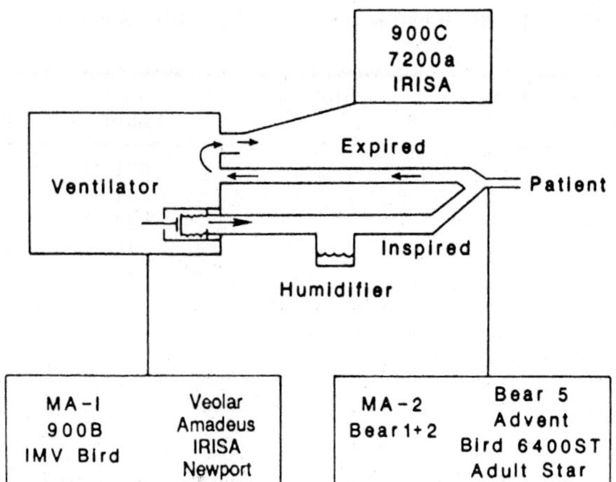

Figure 77–2. Pressure sensing sites of select commercially available mechanical ventilators. (From Branson RD: Enhanced capabilities of current ICU ventilators: Do they really benefit patients? Respir Care 1991; 36:362–376.)

Artificial Noses

All of the aforementioned devices actively add water to inspired gas, whereas the artificial nose passively humidifies inspired gas. A number of different types of artificial noses are currently available: heat and moisture exchangers (HME), heat and moisture exchanging filters (HMEF), hygroscopic condenser humidifiers (HCH), and hygroscopic condenser humidifying filters (HCHF).

The simplest but least efficient of these devices is the HME. It consists of an aluminum insert and may have an additional fibrous element. Because aluminum rapidly exchanges temperature, condensation forms between layers of aluminum during exhalation. The retained heat and moisture are then returned during the next inhalation. The HMEF was originally marketed as a bacterial filter. It contains a fibrous insert that is hydrophobic and thus repels water and traps heat and moisture on the patient side of the insert. The HCH uses a hygroscopically treated insert that allows efficient exchange of heat and moisture. The hygroscopic insert in these devices is usually polypropylene or paper that is treated with lithium chloride or calcium chloride. The HCHF uses a hygroscopically treated paper roll with a bacterial filter between the insert and the source of inspired gas.

Most heat and moisture exchangers can provide 22 to 28 mg/L of water to the airway,[27, 28] with the most efficient devices delivering up to 30 mg/L. They are ideally suited for transport and during anesthesia.[29–32] There is increasing interest in the long-term use of these devices, although controversy surrounds this issue.[29–32] If artificial noses are used for prolonged periods of time, the patient should be assessed for signs of inadequate humidification. In general, as long as there are no contraindications to using an artificial nose (Table 77–3), these devices provide safe and effective humidification for most patients who are ventilated for a short term (48–72 h).

Finally, the resistance to flow across artificial noses requires a 1- to 4-cm H_2O pressure gradient (Table 77–4).[33] The magnitude of this pressure gradient increases after 24 hours.[33] Although this resistance may not represent a concern in most patients, in patients with poor ventilatory drive, when it is considered in series with auto–positive end-expiratory pressure (auto-PEEP), the artificial airway, and triggering of the ventilator, the artificial nose may contribute to an overwhelming resistance to gas flow.

Artificial noses should not be used in conjunction with heated humidifiers or nebulizers because they cause excessive resistance to flow through the device. However, the use

TABLE 77–3. Clinical Situations in Which Artificial Noses Are Contraindicated

Copious amounts of secretions; partial occlusion of device common
Small tidal volumes (<0.15 L); the device dead space (10–90 mL) may lead to carbon dioxide retention
Large tidal volume (>1.0 L); beyond the capacity of the device to humidify
Low SIMV rate; imposed work when spontaneously breathing through the device
Expired VT less than 70% of inspired VT; device cannot function properly unless inhaled and exhaled VT constant
Hypothermia (<32°C)
During aerosolized delivery of pharmacologic agents

Abbreviations: SIMV = synchronized intermittent mandatory ventilation; VT = tidal volume.

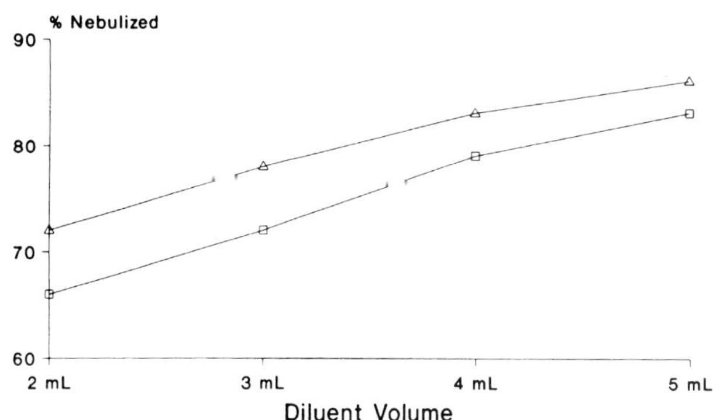

Figure 77–3. Effects of flow and diluent volume on nebulizer dead volume. *Open square* = 6 L/min; *open triangle* = 8 L/min. (From Hess D, Horney D, Snyder T: Medication-delivery performance of eight small-volume, hand-held nebulizers: Effects of diluent volume, gas flow rate, and nebulizer model. Respir Care 1989; 34:717–723.)

of an artificial nose with an unheated humidifier has been reported to improve the efficiency of the artificial nose.[34]

AEROSOLIZED PHARMACOLOGIC AGENTS

Patients in ICUs commonly require aerosolized bronchodilators and steroids as part of their respiratory care management regardless of whether they are breathing spontaneously or are mechanically ventilated. Two general approaches are used to deliver aerosolized pharmacologic agents: small-volume nebulizers (SVNs) and metered dose inhalers (MDIs). A third method, dry powder inhalers, although being used increasingly in non-ICU settings and with outpatients, is not designed for administration to mechanically ventilated patients.

Small-Volume Nebulizers

The efficacy of drug delivery with SVNs is influenced by the solution volume, nebulizer flow rate, intermittent versus continuous nebulization, and nebulizer design.[35] Regardless of nebulizer design, some of the solution (dead volume) remains in the nebulizer after completion of a treatment. The dead volume varies from about 0.5 to 1.0 mL[36] and represents the solution adhering to the walls, cap, and connections between the nebulizer and the patient (i.e., corrugated tubing and mouthpiece or mask). The quantity of the medication remaining in solution in the dead volume depends primarily on the total volume of solution and the nebulizer flow rate (Fig. 77–3). Many studies[37–39] demonstrated that the use of a large solution volume (4 mL) and a nebulizer flow rate of 6 to 8 L/min maximizes the delivery of actual drug to the patient.

Aerosols from SVNs should be inhaled via the mouth rather than the nose to minimize deposition of the drug in the nose and nasopharynx (Table 77–5). Upper airway deposition is increased with nasal breathing because of the tortuous route the aerosol must follow and the high resistance to gas flow. Many patients prefer delivery via facemask, and the use of a facemask may improve compliance, although patients should concentrate on mouth breathing.

Intermittent activation of the SVN (vs. continuous nebulization) increases the quantity of the drug actually delivered to the respiratory tract, although intermittent activation requires cooperation and coordination by the patient. On the other hand, intermittent nebulization greatly prolongs the treatment time and may adversely affect compliance. Thus, continuous nebulization may be the only practical alternative for many patients. Ventilatory pattern does influence deposition of nebulized aerosols in the lower respiratory tract. Although some controversy exists over the ideal ventilatory pattern, a slow inspiratory flow (0.5 L/min) at normal tidal volume, with an occasional inspiration to total

TABLE 77–4. Effect of Peak Inspiratory Flow Rate and Duration of Use on Pressure Gradient Necessary Across Various Artificial Noses Currently in Common Use*

	0.50 L/s		*0.75 L/s*		*1.00 L/s*	
Device	*Init*	*24 H*	*Init*	*24 H*	*Init*	*24 H*
Portex HCH	1.13 ± 0.11	1.59 ± 0.16	2.20 ± 0.22	2.89 ± 0.28	3.54 ± 0.35	4.36 ± 0.43
Siemens 150 HCH	0.54 ± 0.05	1.47 ± 0.14	1.05 ± 0.10	2.86 ± 0.28	1.16 ± 0.16	4.58 ± 0.45
Siemens 151 HCH	1.11 ± 0.11	2.29 ± 0.23	2.45 ± 0.24	4.76 ± 0.47	4.29 ± 0.42	7.98 ± 0.78
NCC HCH	0.85 ± 0.08	0.98 ± 0.10	1.66 ± 0.16	1.79 ± 0.18	2.52 ± 0.25	2.76 ± 0.27
Engstrom HCH	0.93 ± 0.09	1.25 ± 0.12	1.71 ± 0.17	2.30 ± 0.23	2.64 ± 0.26	3.54 ± 0.35
Pall HCH	1.14 ± 0.11	1.73 ± 0.17	2.22 ± 0.22	3.16 ± 0.31	3.54 ± 0.35	4.83 ± 0.47

(Modified with permission from Ploysongsang Y, Branson R, Rashkin MC, et al: Pressure flow characteristics of commonly used heat-moisture exchangers. Am Rev Respir Dis 1988; 138:675–678.)

*Values represent mean ± SD in cm H_2O pressure.

Abbreviations: Init = Initial setup of artificial nose; 24 H = after 24 hours of continuous use; HCH = hygroscopic condenser humidifier.

TABLE 77–5. Technique for Use of SVN During Spontaneous Breathing

- Place drug in nebulizer.
- Dilute with physiologic saline (0.9%) to 4 mL total volume.
- Incorporate a finger port into the driving gas system to provide intermittent nebulization during inspiration only.
- Set driving gas flow at 6–8 L/min.
- Connect patient to SVN via a mouthpiece or mask (in some patients a nose clip may be necessary).
- Instruct patient to inspire through open mouth if using a mask or to close lips around mouthpiece.
- Have patient inhale slowly (0.5 L/s) at normal tidal volume.
- Have patient occasionally inspire to total lung capacity and incorporate a 4- to 10-s breath hold.
- Tap sides of nebulizer to minimize dead volume.
- Continue treatment until no aerosol is produced.
- Monitor patient for presence of side effects (e.g., tachycardia or tremor) and beneficial effects (e.g., improved breath sounds, peak flow, and FEV_1).

(Modified with permission from Kacmarek RM, Hess D: The interface between patient and aerosol generator. Respir Care 1991; 36:952–976.)
Abbreviations: SVN = small-volume nebulizer; FEV_1 = forced expiratory volume in 1 s.

lung capacity (TLC) and an inspiratory hold, is recommended.[40]

Metered Dose Inhalers

MDIs are available for administering bronchodilators, anticholinergics, and steroids and have compared favorably with SVNs in a number of recent studies.[41, 42] As with SVNs, approximately 9% to 11% of the drug deposits in the lower respiratory tract.[43] However, in marked contrast to SVNs, in which 2% of the inhaled drug is deposited in the stomach and mouth, about 80% of the drug from an MDI is deposited in the mouth and stomach. With SVNs, many of the large aerosol particles impact in the nebulizer and mouthpiece or mask because of the low velocity at which the aerosol moves. Thus, most of the drug is deposited in the apparatus (66%), whereas with MDIs little is deposited in the apparatus (5–10%) because of the very high velocity of the MDI flow. As a result, side effects may be higher, especially with steroids, when MDIs without spacers are used.

Much controversy exists over the technique that should be followed when an MDI is used. Differences of opinion exist over the lung volume at which the MDI should be actuated, the position of the MDI in relationship to the mouth during actuation, the length of a postinhalation breath hold, and the inspiratory flow rate. Table 77–6 summarizes these data and includes the technique we recommend for using MDIs.[35] As noted, in the ICU we recommend the use of a spacer whenever an MDI is used for nonintubated patients unless the patient has prior experience with an MDI. This recommendation stems from data indicating that differences in response between SVNs and MDIs are normally related to technique.[44–46] In the ICU, it is particularly difficult to teach proper MDI technique and to ensure that this technique is always used. In addition to eliminating the need for hand-breath coordination, spacers greatly reduce the deposition of large aerosol particles in the upper airway.[47] Avoiding upper airway deposition is of particular concern during inhalation of steroids but may also reduce the side effects associated with bronchodilators.

The technique for using an MDI with a spacer (see Table 77–6) is essentially the same as that for an MDI alone, except that (1) after warming, shaking, and assembling the apparatus and positioning it for use, the MDI is actuated, after which inspiration begins; and (2) because inspiration should continue to TLC and because spacer volume is relatively small (normally less than 500 mL), a tight lip seal about the spacer is relaxed as inspiration continues, allowing for the inspiration of room air.[35] As a result, a second inspiration from the spacer is recommended with some units (Inspir-Ease) after an appropriate breath hold. This ensures that all of the aerosol from a single actuation is inspired. With other units (AeroChamber), this is not recommended. As with the MDI alone, inspiration should be slow (<0.5 L/s) and complete, beginning at functional residual capacity and continuing to TLC.

Delivering Aerosolized Drugs to Spontaneously Breathing Patients

In the nonintubated ICU patient, both SVNs and MDIs appear to be equally efficacious, provided the MDI can be used properly. As a result, if MDIs are used in this setting, it is our opinion that they should always be used with a spacer. Table 77–7 presents a comparison of the advantages and disadvantages between SVNs and MDIs in spontaneously breathing patients.

Delivering Aerosolized Drugs During Mechanical Ventilation

As during spontaneous breathing, aerosolized drugs may be delivered by either an SVN or an MDI during mechanical ventilation. Unfortunately, factors affecting delivery during mechanical ventilation differ greatly from those affecting delivery during spontaneous breathing. In addition, data comparing the use of SVNs and MDIs during mechanical ventilation are much more limited.

Small-Volume Nebulizers

During spontaneous breathing, approximately 12% of the drug that is nebulized reaches the lower respiratory tract. Administration during mechanical ventilation results in only about 2.9% to 4.8% of the drug deposited in the lower airway.[48, 49] Factors affecting this decreased delivery include endotracheal tube size, the use of continuous versus intermittent nebulization, and the precise location of nebulizer placement in the ventilator circuit. The size of the endotracheal tube appears to be directly related to the volume of drug depositing in the lower airway. With neonatal-size

TABLE 77–6. Technique for Use of MDI with Spacer During Spontaneous Breathing

- Warm MDI to body temperature.
- Shake canister vigorously.
- Hold canister upright.
- Actuate MDI.
- Place mouthpiece in mouth.
- Close lips about mouthpiece.
- Inspire slowly (≤0.5 L/s) from spacer.
- Continue to inspire to total lung capacity.
- Hold breath 4–10 s.
- Repeat inspiration with breath hold if indicated by spacer manufacturer.
- Wait 3–10 min between subsequent actuations.
- Monitor patient for presence of side effects (e.g., tachycardia or tremor) and beneficial effects (e.g., improved breath sounds, peak flow, and FEV_1).

(Modified with permission from Kacmarek RM, Hess D: The interface between patient and aerosol generator. Respir Care 1991; 36:952–976.)
Abbreviations: MDI = metered dose inhaler; FEV_1 = forced expiratory volume in 1 s.

TABLE 77–7. Advantages and Disadvantages of the Use of Small-Volume Nebulizers (SVN) and Metered Dose Inhalers (MDI)

Advantages	*Disadvantages*
SVN	
Less patient coordination required	Expensive
High doses possible (even continuous)	Wasteful
No chlorofluorocarbon release	Not all medications available
	Pressurized gas source required
	More time required
MDI	
Convenient	Patient coordination required
Inexpensive	Patient activation required
	Results in pharyngeal deposition
	Has potential for abuse
	Difficult to deliver high doses
	Not all medications available
	Dependent on ozone-depleting chlorofluorocarbons
MDI with Auxiliary Device	
Less patient coordination required	More complex process for patient than MDI alone
	More expensive than MDI alone
	Less portable than MDI alone

(Modified with permission from Kacmarek RM, Hess D: The interface between patient and aerosol generator. Respir Care 1991; 36:952–976.)

endotracheal tubes in animal models, only about 1.5% of the drug reaches the lower respiratory tract.[50]

As with spontaneously breathing patients, intermittent nebulization is ideal, because up to two thirds of the drug is lost via the exhalation valve during continuous nebulization. However, the single most significant factor affecting volume of drug deposited beyond the endotracheal tube is the position of the nebulizer in the ventilator circuit. Ideally, the SVN should be placed at least 18 inches (45 cm) from the endotracheal tube.[51] Hughes and Saez[51] evaluated the amount of aerosol presented to the endotracheal tube of a lung model under four conditions: (1) continuous nebulization at the Y-piece; (2) intermittent nebulization at the Y; (3) continuous nebulization at the ventilator circuit manifold; and (4) intermittent nebulization at the ventilator circuit manifold. The highest percentage of aerosol presented to the endotracheal tube (68.3 ± 1.2%) occurred during intermittent nebulization at the manifold, whereas the lowest percentage (30 ± 2.0%) occurred during continuous nebulization at the Y. Others have found that bypassing the humidifier during aerosol therapy and extending the inspiratory time increase the volume of drug deposited in the lower respiratory tract.[52]

In spite of the fact that little specific information is available regarding the optimal technique for the use of SVN via ventilator circuits, observations by Hughes and Saez[51] and O'Riordan and colleagues[52] and the information presented earlier on SVN technique during spontaneous breathing (see Table 77–5) allow us to establish guidelines for using SVNs in ventilator circuits (Table 77–8). All SVNs should be placed at least 18 inches from the Y and powered intermittently through the ventilator (if possible). The volume of solution nebulized should be 4 mL and, if powered by a gas source external to the mechanical ventilator, a flow of 6 to 8 L/min should be used.

While administering SVNs to spontaneously breathing patients, a periodic deep breath and a breath hold are recommended. Although we realize that this may be impossible for many mechanically assisted patients, it is encouraged. To maximize distribution and establish a more ideal ventilatory pattern during SVN treatments, we recommend delivering volume-limited mechanical breaths at a rate of 4 to 8 per minute or more, with tidal volumes set at 12 mL/kg or greater unless contraindicated in a given patient. Patients on continuous positive airway pressure should be changed to synchronized intermittent mandatory ventilation (SIMV) or assist-control ventilation during therapy, and patients receiving pressure support ventilation (PSV) with an SIMV back-up rate less than 8 per minute should have the PSV trigger rate carefully monitored. If the PSV rate decreases, a back-up SIMV rate of 8 per minute should be set. As noted by Beaty and associates,[53] using continuous nebulizer flow increases the pressure gradient that patients must overcome to trigger PSV. In patients with marginal respiratory efforts, significant hypoventilation has been noted.

Metered Dose Inhalers

As with SVNs, the addition of an artificial airway decreases the quantity of MDI-delivered drug that deposits in the lower respiratory tract. Although limited, data available on deposition beyond the distal tip of the endotracheal tube indicate up to about 50% less deposition than during spontaneous breathing, or 4% to 6% of the actuated aerosol exits the endotracheal tube.[54,55] Crogan and Bishop,[55] using a lung model, reported a greater percentage of the aerosol exiting the endotracheal tube as size increased (3.0 ± 1.9% for a 6.0-mm tube and 6.5 ± 4.4% for a 9.0-mm tube). They also reported more aerosol exiting the endotracheal tube if actuation occurred just after the start of a mechanical tidal volume delivery than if actuation began before onset of the mechanical breath.

Adapters designed to interface MDIs with the ventilator circuit can be classified as (1) modified tracheal swivel adapters (Fig. 77–4), (2) circuit inspiratory limb adapters (Fig. 77–5), and (3) circuit inspiratory limb spacers (Fig. 77–6). However, few data are available to determine which of

TABLE 77–8. Technique for Use of Small-Volume Nebulizer During Mechanical Ventilation

- Place drug in nebulizer.
- Dilute with physiologic saline (0.9%) to 4 mL total volume.
- Insert nebulizer into inspiratory limb of ventilator circuit at least 18 inches from "Y".
- Use intermittent nebulizer flow from ventilator if available.
- If continuous flow is used, set at 6–8 L/min.
- Set ventilator rate at 4–8 breaths per minute or higher if not contraindicated.
- Lengthen inspiratory time if tolerated and not contraindicated.
- Set tidal volume at 12 mL/kg or more unless contraindicated. If PSV rate drops, add back-up SIMV rate.
- With children, adjust ventilator flow to ensure that total flow is unchanged during pressure-limited ventilation.
- With children (and some adults), readjust tidal volume during continuous-flow nebulization to maintain constant tidal volume and peak airway pressure.
- Tap sides of nebulizer to minimize dead volume.
- Continue treatment until no aerosol is produced.
- Remove equipment from ventilator circuit.
- Return ventilator to pretreatment settings.
- Monitor patient for presence of side effects (e.g., tachycardia or tremor) and beneficial effects (e.g., improved breath sounds, peak flow, and FEV_1).

(Modified with permission from Kacmarek RM, Hess D: The interface between patient and aerosol generator. Respir Care 1991; 36:952–976.)

Abbreviations: PSV = pressure support ventilation; SIMV = synchronized intermittent mandatory ventilation; FEV_1 = forced expiratory volume in 1 s.

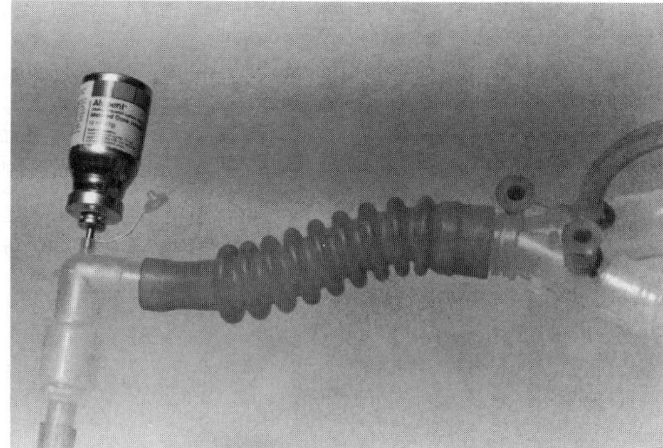

Figure 77–4. MDI and modified tracheal swivel adapter.

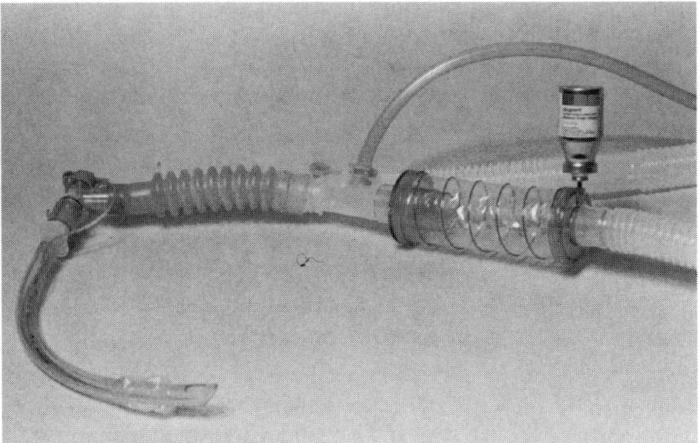

Figure 77–6. MDI and circuit inspiratory limb spacer (AeroChamber).

the adapters is most effective in depositing aerosol beyond the distal tip of the endotracheal tube and producing maximum patient response. More recently, catheters extending to the tip of the endotracheal (ET) tube have been used by Taylor and Lerman[56] and Niven and coworkers[57] to increase the delivery of metered dose drugs beyond the endotracheal tube. In a lung model, Taylor and Lerman demonstrated 97% delivery of actuated salbutamol beyond the ET tube when a 19-gauge catheter attached to the MDI was positioned at the tip of the ET tube. Also using a lung model, Niven and colleagues[57] demonstrated that use of a 16-gauge, 30-cm intravenous catheter attached to the MDI and positioned in a tracheal swivel adapter resulted in delivery of 80% of the MDI-generated aerosol beyond the ET tube. These preliminary data suggest an exciting alternative for MDI delivery in intubated patients, but additional research is required before recommending application. The data available on the placement of MDIs in ventilator circuits are too limited at this time to allow a recommendation for the best approach.

Little information derived specifically from the evaluation of MDI use during mechanical ventilation is available to assist in defining the ideal technique for MDI administration of drugs. However, it seems reasonable to extrapolate from the abundant information available on the use of MDIs during spontaneous breathing. Table 77–9 presents preliminary guidelines for MDI drug administration during mechanical ventilation. Ideally, a large tidal volume delivered at moderate flow rates of 30 to 60 L/min and held in the lungs for at least 2 to 3 seconds is recommended. Whether this ventilatory pattern should be performed by manual or mechanical ventilation has not been determined. As with nonintubated, spontaneously breathing patients, a pause between actuations is probably ideal, although this has not been studied extensively. Unless a true in-line spacer is used (AeroVent), actuation of the MDI should occur immediately after the beginning of a mechanical breath. If the AeroVent is used, actuation should occur 1 to 2 seconds before the beginning of the mechanical breath or at the end of exhalation depending on the patient–mechanical ventilator rate.

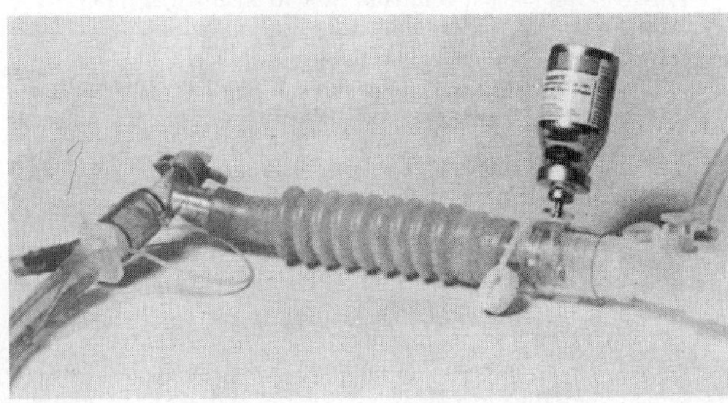

Figure 77–5. MDI and circuit inspiratory limb adapter.

Metered Dose Inhaler Versus Small-Volume Nebulizer

Little information comparing the efficacy of SVN and MDI during mechanical ventilation is available.[58–61] Recently, Gay and coauthors[58] demonstrated no difference administering 170 μg (three puffs via MDI) and 2.5 mg of albuterol in a 3.5-mL solution volume via SVN. Changes in passive expiratory flow at respiratory system recoil pressures of 6 to 10 cm H_2O were the same in both arms of this single-blinded, randomized, crossover comparison. Similar results have been reported in abstracts by Hess and colleagues[59] and Gutierrez and Nelson[60] in series of mechanically ventilated patients, whereas Fernandez and associates[61] noted no differences between the effects of MDI-administered ipratropium bromide or salbutamol and intravenous aminophylline in a series of 20 mechanically ventilated chronic obstructive pulmonary disease patients. From these limited data and our clinical experience, it is our opinion that equal

TABLE 77–9. Technique for Use of MDI During Mechanical Ventilation

- Place MDI adapter into circuit.
- Adjust ventilator to deliver volume-limited breaths or use a manual ventilator.
- Warm MDI to body temperature.
- Shake MDI vigorously.
- Place MDI in circuit.
- Actuate MDI immediately after the beginning of a mechanical breath; if spacer is used, actuate 1–2 s before mechanical breath or near end-exhalation, depending on the rate.
- Apply a 2- to 3-s inflation hold, if not contraindicated.
- Wait 1 min between actuations.
- Return ventilator to pretreatment settings.
- Monitor patient for presence of side effects (e.g., tachycardia or tremor) and beneficial effects (e.g., improved breath sounds, peak flow, and FEV_1).

(Modified with permission from Kacmarek RM, Hess D: The interface between patient and aerosol generator. Respir Care 1991; 36:952–976.)

Abbreviations: MDI = metered dose inhaler; FEV_1 = forced expiratory volume in 1 s.

efficacy can be obtained with either an MDI or an SVN during mechanical ventilation. However, because of the infection control issues with SVNs and issues regarding intermittent administration of SVNs, we generally prefer the use of MDIs.

Dosing

Appropriate dosing is of major concern when delivering aerosolized pharmacologic agents during mechanical ventilation. On the basis of the data regarding lung deposition that have already been presented, standard drug doses should be doubled to deliver a dose equivalent to that during spontaneous breathing. More importantly, dosing should be tailored to patient response[62] such that many patients may require doses that are three or four times greater than standard doses or even more. Responses to bronchodilators during mechanical ventilation can be evaluated using flow-volume loops or by calculating changes in expiratory resistance.[63]

AIRWAY SUCTIONING

Because of their inability to mobilize secretions effectively, all ICU patients with artificial airways require airway suctioning. In addition, as a result of difficulty swallowing, especially when endotracheal tubes are in place, the mouth and the oral pharynx must also be periodically suctioned. Because this procedure has potentially serious side effects, suctioning should not be performed on a scheduled basis but only when physical examination reveals the presence of secretions in the airway.

Complications of Suctioning

Table 77–10 lists complications that may accompany airway suctioning and that can be minimized by attention to correct technique.

Hypoxemia

The most likely complication of airway suctioning is hypoxemia.[64] The best method of avoiding suctioning-associated hypoxemia is to establish a suctioning technique that minimizes those factors that affect the development of hypoxemia (interruption of oxygenation, PEEP, and mechanical ventilation; aspiration of gas from the respiratory tract; entrainment of room air into the lungs; and prolonged duration of the procedure and atelectasis formation). The most effective way to avoid hypoxemia during suctioning is to hyperoxygenate before and after the procedure.[65, 66] This can be accomplished by administering 100% oxygen through the ventilator or by ventilating with a manual ventilator delivering 100% oxygen and appropriate PEEP. The easiest and best method is use of the 100% oxygen suction control button, which is available on some but not all ventilators. The concern about elevating the ventilator F_{IO_2} setting is that the F_{IO_2} is not reset after the procedure. In addition, many ventilators have large washout volumes. That is, because of internal reservoirs, it may take minutes before the delivered F_{IO_2} actually reaches 100%.[67]

There are advantages and disadvantages to using a manual ventilator. On the one hand, the clinician has a feel for the presence and movement of secretions with a manual ventilator. Also, because controlled sigh breaths can be delivered to hyperinflate the lungs, the clinician can coordinate ventilatory assistance with the patient's effort. On the other hand, four disadvantages are noteworthy. First, if appropriate flow of oxygen is not delivered to the bag or the proper PEEP applied, hyperoxygenation may not be accomplished. Second, several studies[68–70] indicate that most practitioners deliver a smaller than expected volume when compressing a manual ventilator. Thus, instead of achieving hyperinflation, hypoinflation may be occurring. Third, because volume and pressure are normally not measured during manual ventilation, the risk of barotrauma may be increased. Fourth, manual ventilators may be a source of airway contamination because the attachment to the airway is frequently open to atmosphere and is moist while sitting at the bedside for days. Ideally, the port for attaching the manual ventilator to the patient should be capped when not in use. We use a cap that moves from the Y-piece of the ventilator circuit to the manual ventilator depending on which is in actual use.

Atelectasis

Problems with atelectasis can be avoided by using a properly sized catheter, by appropriately setting suctioning pressure, and by performing the suction procedure as quickly as possible. During suctioning, gas is simultaneously drawn from the lower and upper airway. If too large a catheter is used, gas cannot be drawn into the lung from the atmosphere. Generally, a suction catheter should be no larger than one half the internal diameter (ID) of the artificial airway. Appropriate suction catheter size (using the French sizing system) can be estimated by dividing the ID of the airway by 2 and then multiplying it by 3.[71]

$$\text{Catheter size (French)} = \text{ID}/2 \times 3$$

Generally, for adults, a 14-French catheter is appropriate. Suction pressure should also be limited to minimize atelectasis risk. With adults, a suction regulator setting at a maximum of 120 to 150 mm Hg is recommended (80–100 mm Hg for infants and 100–120 mm Hg for children).[72]

The total amount of time that the catheter is within the airway should also be limited to avoid atelectasis; a maximum of 15 seconds has been recommended.[71] Finally, suction should not be applied while the catheter is lodged in a bronchus. Ideally, the catheter should be advanced to its maximum length and then pulled back slightly while suction is only applied during removal of the catheter.

Cardiac Arrhythmias

Bradyarrhythmias are the most common arrhythmias during suctioning,[73, 74] usually resulting from hypoxemia or vagal stimulation. However, more serious arrhythmias have been observed, including ventricular fibrillation with cardiac arrest.[75]

Airway Trauma

It is well recognized that suctioning is traumatic to the airway.[76, 77] Decreased mucociliary transport, mucosal ulceration, hemorrhage, hyperemia, and airway edema have all been reported. Generally, adherence to appropriate technique (Table 77–11) will minimize the risk of trauma. Also, properly sized catheters, appropriate vacuum setting, intermittent (rather than continuous) suctioning, and an overall "gentle" approach are helpful in avoiding trauma.

TABLE 77–10. Complications of Endotracheal Suctioning

Hypoxemia
Airway trauma
Cardiac arrhythmias
Atelectasis
Infection
Increased intracranial pressure
Coughing and bronchospasm

TABLE 77–11. Artificial Airway Suctioning Technique

Preoxygenate (100% oxygen).
Assemble suction catheter (use sterile technique).
Insert catheter until resistance is met.
Pull back slightly.
Apply suction while removing catheter from airway.
Reoxygenate (100% oxygen).
Limit total procedure time (≤15 s).

Increased Intracranial Pressure

Increased intracranial pressure (ICP) usually occurs in patients who cough excessively or who become markedly agitated during the procedure. In patients for whom even transient increases in ICP are problematic, hyperventilation and pharmacologic support before the procedure may be helpful.

Off- Versus On-Ventilator Techniques

Suctioning can be accomplished while the patient is connected to the mechanical ventilator or while disconnected briefly. With the off-ventilator technique, the patient is disconnected from the ventilator during the procedure and reconnected after each pass of the suction catheter or after reoxygenation with a manual ventilator. This approach is generally tolerated well, although there is a subset of patients who become markedly unstable if the rhythmic pattern of ventilation or PEEP is disrupted.

There are two variations of on-ventilator suction techniques. One is to simply use the tracheal swivel adapter that has a port allowing suctioning while mechanical ventilation continues.[78] The other is to use a closed-system suction catheter, which is actually part of the ventilator circuit, and changed every 24 hours. Several studies evaluated whether such closed-system catheters maintain adequate oxygenation during suctioning[79–81] and suggest that oxygenation during suctioning was similar using closed-system and off-ventilator techniques. Thus, although head-to-head comparisons suggest equivalence of the techniques (and therefore approach), the most critically ill patients have not been included in these studies. On the basis of this critical review of available literature and our experience, we continue to recommend a closed suctioning technique when the patient's oxygenation is tenuous and when momentary discontinuation of PEEP or mechanical ventilation is poorly tolerated.

References

1. Shapiro BA, Kacmarek RM, Cane RA, et al: Clinical Application of Respiratory Care. 4th ed. St. Louis, Mosby-Year Book, 1991, pp 123–150.
2. Kacmarek RM: In-hospital O_2 therapy. *In*: Current Respiratory Care. Kacmarek RM, Stoller JK (Eds). Toronto, BC Decker, 1988, pp 1–8.
3. Nunn JF: Applied Respiratory Physiology. 2nd ed. London, Butterworths, 1977.
4. Kacmarek RM: Supplemental oxygen and other medical gas therapy. *In*: Foundations in Respiratory Care. Pierson DJ, Kacmarek RM (Eds). New York, Churchill Livingstone, 1992, pp 859–889.
5. McFadden ER Jr: Respiratory heat and water exchange: Physiological and clinical implications. J Appl Physiol 1983; 54:331–336.
6. McFadden ER Jr, Pichurko BM, Bowman HF, et al: Thermal mapping of the airways in humans. J Appl Physiol 1985; 37:887–890.
7. Dery R: The evaluation of heat and moisture in the respiratory tract during anesthesia with a non-rebreathing system. Can J Anesth 1973; 20:296–309.
8. Kapadia FN, Shelly MP: Normal mechanisms of humidification. Prob Respir Care 1991; 4:395–402.
9. Benson DM: Systemic and pulmonary changes with inhaled humid atmospheres. Anesthesiology 1969; 30:199–206.
10. Campbell EJ, Baker D, Cites-Silver P: Subjective effects of humidification of oxygen delivery by nasal cannula: A prospective study. Chest 1988; 93:289–293.
11. American College of Chest Physicians, National Heart, Lung, and Blood Institute: National Conference on Oxygen Therapy. Respir Care 1984; 29:922–935.
12. Nolan DM: Problems of inadequate humidification. Prob Respir Care 1991; 4:413–417.
13. Tausk HC, Miller R, Roberts RB: Maintenance of body temperature by heated humidification. Anaesthesia 1976; 55:719–723.
14. Stone DR, Downs JB, Paul WL, et al: Adult body temperature and heated humidification of anesthetic gases during general anesthesia. Anesth Analg 1981; 60:736–741.
15. Fonkalsrud EW, Calmes S, Barcliff LT, et al: Reduction of operative heat loss and pulmonary secretions in neonates by use of heated and humidified anesthetic gases. J Thorac Cardiovasc Surg 1980; 80:718–723.
16. Chalon J, Patel C, Ali M, et al: Humidity and the anesthesized patient. Anesthesiology 1979; 50:195–198.
17. Pierce AK, Sanford JP: Bacterial contamination of aerosols. Arch Intern Med 1973; 131:156–162.
18. Modell JH, Giammona ST, Davis JH: Effect of chronic exposure to ultrasonic aerosols on the lung. Anesthesiology 1967; 28:680–688.
19. Graff TD: Humidification: Indications and hazards in respiratory therapy. Anesth Analg 1975; 54:444–448.
20. American National Standards Institute (ANSI): Standard for humidifiers and nebulizers for medical use. ANSI Z79;9-1979. New York, ANSI, 1979.
21. Shelly MP: Inspired gas conditioning. Respir Care 1992; 37:1070–1080.
22. Craven DE, Goularte TA, Make BJ: Contaminated condensate in mechanical ventilator circuits. Am Rev Respir Dis 1984; 129:625–628.
23. Miyao H, Hirokawa T, Miyasaka K, et al: Relative humidity, not absolute humidity, is of great importance when using a humidifier with a heating wire. Crit Care Med 1992; 20:674–679.
24. O'Hagan M, Reid E, Tarnow-Mordi WO: Is neonatal inspired gas humidity accurately controlled by humidifier temperature? Crit Care Med 1991; 19:1370–1373.
25. Nishimura M, Nishijima M, Okada T, et al: Comparison of low-resistive work load due to humidifying devices. Chest 1990; 97:600–604.
26. Branson RD: Enhanced capabilities of current ICU ventilators: Do they really benefit patients? Respir Care 1991; 36:362–376.
27. Ploysongsang Y, Branson RD, Rashkin MC, et al: Effect of flowrate and duration of use on the pressure drop across six artificial noses. Respir Care 1989; 34:902–907.
28. Eckerbom B, Lindholm CE: Laboratory evaluation of heat and moisture exchangers: Assessment of the draft international standard in practice. Acta Anesthesiol Scand 1990; 34:291–295.
29. MacIntyre NR, Anderson HR, Silver RM, et al: Pulmonary function in mechanically-ventilated patients during 24-hour use of hygroscopic condenser humidifier. Chest 1983; 34:560–564.
30. Conti G, DeBlasi RA, Rocco M, et al: Effects of heated moisture exchangers on dynamic hyperinflation of mechanically-ventilated COPD patients. Intensive Care Med 1990; 16:441–443.
31. Roustan JP, Kienlen J, Aubas P, et al: Comparison of hydrophobic heat and moisture exchangers with heated humidification during prolonged mechanical ventilation. Intensive Care Medicine 1992; 18:97–100.
32. Perch SA, Realey AM: Effectiveness of the Servo SH 150 "artificial nose" humidifier: A case report. Respir Care 1984; 29:1009–1012.
33. Ploysongsang Y, Branson R, Rashkin MC, et al: Pressure flow characteristics of commonly used heat-moisture exchangers. Am Rev Respir Dis 1988; 138:675–678.

34. Suzukawa M, Usuda Y, Numata K: The effects on sputum characteristics of combining an unheated humidifier with a heat-moisture exchanging filter. Respir Care 1989; 34:976–984.
35. Kacmarek RM, Hess D: The interface between patient and aerosol generator. Respir Care 1991; 36:952–976.
36. Hess D, Horney D, Snyder T: Medication-delivery performance of eight small-volume, hand-held nebulizers. Effects of diluent volume, gas flow rate, and nebulizer model. Respir Care 1989; 34:717–723.
37. Wood JA, Wilson RSE, Bray C: Changes in salbutamol concentration in the reservoir solution of a jet nebulizer. Br J Dis Chest 1986; 8:164–169.
38. Clay MM, Pavia D, Newman SP, et al: Factors influencing the size distribution of aerosols from jet nebulizers. Thorax 1983; 38:755–759.
39. Douglas JG, Leslie MJ, Brompton GK, et al: Is the flow rate used to drive a jet nebuliser clinically important? (Letter). Br Med J (Clin Res) 1985; 290:29.
40. Newman SP, Woodman G, Clarke SW: Deposition of carbenicillin aerosols in cystic fibrosis: Effects of nebulizer system and breathing pattern. Thorax 1988; 43:318–322.
41. Gomm SA, Keaney NP, Hunt LP, et al: Dose response comparison of ipratropium bromide from a metered dose inhaler and by jet nebulization. Thorax 1983; 38:197–301.
42. Christensson P, Arborelius M, Lilja B: Salbutamol inhalation in chronic asthma bronchiale: Dose aerosol vs jet nebulizer. Chest 1981; 79:416–419.
43. Newman SP, Pavia D. Moren F, et al: Deposition of pressurized aerosols in the human respiratory tract. Thorax 1981; 36:52–55.
44. Epstein SW, Manning CPR, Ashley MJ, et al: Survey of the clinical use of pressurized aerosol inhalers. Can Med Assoc J 1979; 120:813–816.
45. Orehek J, Gayrard P, Grimand CH, et al: Patient error in the use of bronchodilator metered aerosols. Br Med J 1976; 1:76–77.
46. Shim C, Williams MH: The adequacy of inhalation of aerosol from canister nebulizers. Am J Med 1980; 69:891–896.
47. Dolovich M, Ruffin R, Corr D, et al: Clinical evaluation of a simple demand inhalation MDI aerosol delivery device. Chest 1983; 84:36–41.
48. MacIntyre NR, Silver RM, Miller CW, et al: Aerosol delivery in intubated, mechanically ventilated patients. Crit Care Med 1985; 13:81–85.
49. Fraser I, DuVall A, Dolovich M, et al: Therapeutic aerosol delivery in ventilator systems (Abstract). Am Rev Respir Dis 1981; 123:107.
50. Cameron D, Clay M, Silverman M: Evaluation of nebulizers for use in neonatal ventilator circuits. Crit Care Med 1990; 18:866–870.
51. Hughes JM, Saez J: Effects of nebulizer mode and position in a mechanical ventilator circuit on dose efficiency. Respir Care 1987; 32:1131–1135.
52. O'Riordan TG, Greco MJ, Perry RJ, et al: Nebulizer function during mechanical ventilation. Am Rev Respir Dis 1992; 145:1117–1122.
53. Beaty CD, Ritz RH, Benson MS: Continous in-line nebulizers complicate pressure support ventilation. Chest 1989; 96:1360–1363.
54. Hess D, Beener C, Kacer Watson K: An evaluation of the effectiveness of metered dose inhaler (MDI) use with mechanical ventilation (Abstract). Respir Care 1988; 33:910–914.
55. Crogan SJ, Bishop MJ: Delivery efficiency of metered dose aerosols given via endotracheal tubes. Anesthesiology 1989; 70:1008–1010.
56. Taylor RH, Lerman J: High efficiency delivery of salbutamol with a metered-dose inhaler in narrow tracheal tubes and catheters. Anesthesiology 1991; 74:360–363.
57. Niven RW, Kacmarek R, Brain D, et al: Small bore nozzle extensions to improve the delivery efficiency of drugs from metered dose inhalers: Laboratory evaluation. Am Rev Respir Dis 1993; 147:1590–1594.
58. Gay PC, Patel HG, Nelson SB, et al: Metered dose inhalers for bronchodilator delivery in intubated, mechanically ventilated patients. Chest 1991; 99:66–71.
59. Hess D, Fillman D, Daugherty A, et al: Use of metered dose inhalers in intubated patients (Abstract). Respir Care 1989; 34:1027.
60. Gutierrez CJ, Nelson R: Short-term bronchodilation in mechanically ventilated patients receiving metaproterenol via SVN and MDI (Abstract). Respir Care 1988; 33:910.
61. Fernandez A, Lazaro A, Garcia A, et al: Bronchodilators in patients with chronic obstructive pulmonary disease on mechanical ventilation. Am Rev Respir Dis 1990; 141:164–168.
62. American Association for Respiratory Care: Aerosol consensus statement. Respir Care 1991; 36:916–921.
63. Hess D, Murray R, Rexrode WO: Bronchodilator response during mechanical ventilation. Chest 1992; 102:82S.
64. Karem E, Yatsiv I, Goitein KJ: Effect of endotracheal suctioning on arterial blood gases in children. Intensive Care Med 1990; 16:95–99.
65. Barnes CA, Kirchoff KT: Minimizing hypoxemia due to endotracheal suctioning: A review of the literature. Heart Lung 1986; 15:164–176.
66. Buchanan LM, Baun MM: The effect of hyperinflation, inspiratory hold, and oxygenation on cardiopulmonary status during suctioning in a lung-injured model. Heart Lung 1986; 15:127–134.
67. Benson MS, Pierson DJ: Ventilator wash-out volume: A consideration in endotracheal suction preoxygenation. Respir Care 1979; 24:832–835.
68. Crabtree Goodnough SK: The effects of oxygen and hyperinflation on arterial oxygen tension after endotracheal suctioning. Heart Lung 1985; 14:11–17.
69. Preusser BA, Stone KS, Gonyon DS, et al: Effects of two methods of preoxygenation on mean arterial pressure, cardiac output, peak airway pressure, and postsuctioning hypoxemia. Heart Lung 1988; 17:290–299.
70. Baker PO, Baker JP, Koen PA: Endotracheal suctioning techniques in hypoxemic patients. Respir Care 1983; 28:1563–1568.
71. Shapiro BA, Kacmarek RM, Cane RA, et al: Clinical Applications in Respiratory Care. 4th ed. St. Louis, Mosby-Year Book, 1991, pp 177–195.
72. Curran JF, Stanek KS, Kacmarek RM: Portable airway-suction systems: A comparison of performance. Respir Care 1991; 36:259–265.
73. Walsh JM, Vanderwarf C, Hoscheit D, et al: Unsuspected hemodynamic alterations during endotracheal suctioning. Chest 1989; 95:162–165.
74. Cabal LA, Siassi B, Blanco C, et al: Cardiac rate and rhythm changes during airway suctioning in premature infants with RDS. J Calif Perinatal Assoc 1984; 4:45–48.
75. Fineberg C, Cohn HE, Gibbon JH: Cardiac arrest during nasotracheal aspiration. JAMA 1960; 174:410–412.
76. Amikam B, Landa J, West J, et al: Bronchofiberscopic observations of the tracheobronchial tree during intubation. Am Rev Respir Dis 1972; 105:747–755.
77. Landa JF, Chapman GA, Sackner MA: Effects of suctioning on mucociliary transport. Chest 1980; 77:202–207.
78. Brown SE, Stansbury DW, Merrill EJ, et al: Prevention of suctioning-related arterial oxygen desaturation. Chest 1983; 4:621–627.
79. Craig KC, Benson MS, Pierson DJ: Prevention of arterial oxygen desaturation during closed-airway endotracheal suction: Effect of ventilator mode. Respir Care 1984; 29:1013–1018.
80. Carlon GC, Fox SJ, Ackerman NJ: Evaluation of a closed-tracheal suction system. Crit Care Med 1987; 15:522–525.
81. Clark AP, Tyler DO, White KM: Effects of endotracheal suctioning on mixed venous oxygen saturation and heart rate in critically ill patients. Heart Lung 1990; 19:552–557.

CHAPTER 78

Conventional Airway Access

Donna A. Castello, DO • Howard S. Smith, MD • Philip D. Lumb, MBBS, FCCM

HISTORY

Airway patency and breathing have long been recognized to be vital for life. Vesalius is credited with the earliest reports of tracheal intubation (through a tracheotomy opening) for resuscitation.[1] The translation of his 1543 experiment is "Life may in a matter of speaking be restored . . . an opening must be attempted in the trunk of the trachea into which a reed or cane should be put; you will then blow into this so that the lung may rise again."[2] A similar experiment was performed by Robert Hooke in 1667,[3] in which he kept a dog alive by the "reciprocal blowing up of his lungs with bellows." He found that "upon ceasing the blast and suffering the lungs to fall and lie still, the dog would immediately fall into dying convulsing fits; but was soon revived again by renewing the fullness of his lungs with the constant blast of fresh air."[3] John Mayow, a physiologist, wrote in 1674 "on the suppression of respiration . . . the beating of the heart and, consequently, the flow of blood to the brain will necessarily be interrupted and death will ensue . . . so it appears that the air is that without which the movements of the heart cannot go on at all."[2, 4]

The first recognized account of tracheal intubation through the glottis was Macewen's work in 1880,[2, 5] although both nasal and oral tactile blind intubation of the trachea is probably the oldest method used and was practiced by Kite in 1785.[6, 7] Desault in the early 1800s proposed blind nasal intubation for protection of the airway in patients with laryngeal disease.[2] It was later that Kuhn described and favored nasotracheal intubation as a means of airway maintenance.[8]

Indirect laryngoscopy, developed by Manuel Garcia[6, 7] (a singing teacher), did not alleviate the difficulty of endotracheal tube (ETT) placement but did familiarize physicians with the anatomy of the pharynx and laryngeal inlet. These principles are used today with fiberoptic bundles to provide illumination of the field (fiberoptic bronchoscope and Bullard laryngoscope).

Unlike Macewen, whose work was intended for the administration of anesthesia, Joseph O'Dwyer[9] publicized his extensive use of tracheal intubation during the diphtheria epidemics of the late 1800s. He developed ETTs that were positioned over a curved introducer, which was then removed (a forerunner of the stylet). His success prompted others such as Maydl, Eisenmenger, Dorrance, and Van Stockum[10] to devise ETTs with cuffs. Originally, cuffs were "milked" onto the tubes.[10] A tube with an inflatable cuff was constructed by Rowbotham in 1944.[11] Later, cuffed ETTs were used for prolonged intubation during the poliomyelitis epidemics of the 1950s and 1960s. These early cuffs led to tracheal injury such as tracheomalacia, stenosis, and tracheoesophageal fistula. Modern ETTs may vary in their construction but most commonly are constructed of polyurethane with a low-pressure, high-volume inflatable cuff.

Direct laryngoscopy developed as the need to overcome the technical difficulty of ETT insertion was recognized in the early 1900s. Several individuals developed the laryngoscope, most notably Chevalier Jackson in 1913, who streamlined the apparatus and expounded the merits of examining the larynx before intubation.[12] As Elsberg, Janeway, Miller, MacIntosh, and a host of others practiced this technique and introduced adaptations and variations of laryngoscopes, endotracheal, and nasotracheal tubes, tracheal intubation became commonplace.[6]

ANATOMY

Successful management of the airway and the potential complications related to procedures undertaken to ensure its patency requires an understanding of basic anatomic features.[13, 14]

Two external openings lead to the human airway. The nose leads to the nasopharynx and the mouth to the oropharynx. These are separated anteriorly by the palate but join posteriorly (Fig. 78–1*A*). The nasal septum divides the nasal cavity into two pyramids that contain bone, cartilage, and sinus openings and receive innervation from both the olfactory (cranial nerve [CN] I) and the trigeminal (CN V) nerves. The roof of the nose is formed by the nasal and frontal bones, the cribriform plate of the ethmoid, and the body of the sphenoid bone. The floor is formed by the maxilla and palatine bones. The medial wall is formed by septal cartilage, the vomer, and the perpendicular plate of the ethmoid (see Fig. 78–1*A*). The septum, if deviated, creates asymmetry of the nasal passages. This should be noted when planning a nasal intubation, because success will probably be greatest when attempts are made via the larger nasal passage. The lateral wall contains a portion of the ethmoid bone with three turbinate bones: superior, middle, and inferior with the openings of the paranasal sinuses and nasolacrimal duct (see Fig. 78–1*B*). Any foreign body (nasotracheal or nasogastric tube) in close proximity to these sinus openings can provoke serious infection in the intensive care unit (ICU) patient and should be removed if this occurs.

The nasal cavity receives its blood supply from the anterior and posterior branches of the ophthalmic artery and branches of the maxillary and facial arteries. Its venous plexus drains into sphenopalatine, facial, and ophthalmic veins. The mucous membranes that line the turbinates are extensively vascularized, and careless manipulation can lead to severe hemorrhage.

The mouth is bounded by the lips and cheeks externally, the gums and teeth internally, the hard and soft palate superiorly, and the mucosa inferiorly, which is connected to the tongue. The tongue, especially if large, may impede attempts at laryngeal visualization and intubation and must be swept to the left with the laryngoscope blade to afford an optimal view.

The pharynx is subdivided into the nasopharynx, oropharynx, and laryngopharynx. The nasopharynx follows directly from the nasal cavity above the soft palate. The oropharynx begins at the soft palate and extends to the tip of the epiglottis. It contains the pillars of the fauces (the lateral walls of the oropharynx) between which the palatine tonsils lie, an important landmark in the airway classification of Mallampati, which is described later.[15]

The laryngopharynx extends from the epiglottis to the cricoid cartilage. It is separated laterally from the larynx by the aryepiglottic folds. These lateral portions are the piriform recesses in which the inferior laryngeal nerve lies.

The laryngeal skeleton consists of several cartilages: the thyroid, cricoid, epiglottic, arytenoids, corniculate, and cuneiform cartilages (the latter three are paired) (Fig. 78–2). The thyroid cartilage is a shield-shaped structure that does not project posteriorly and consists of right and left laminae

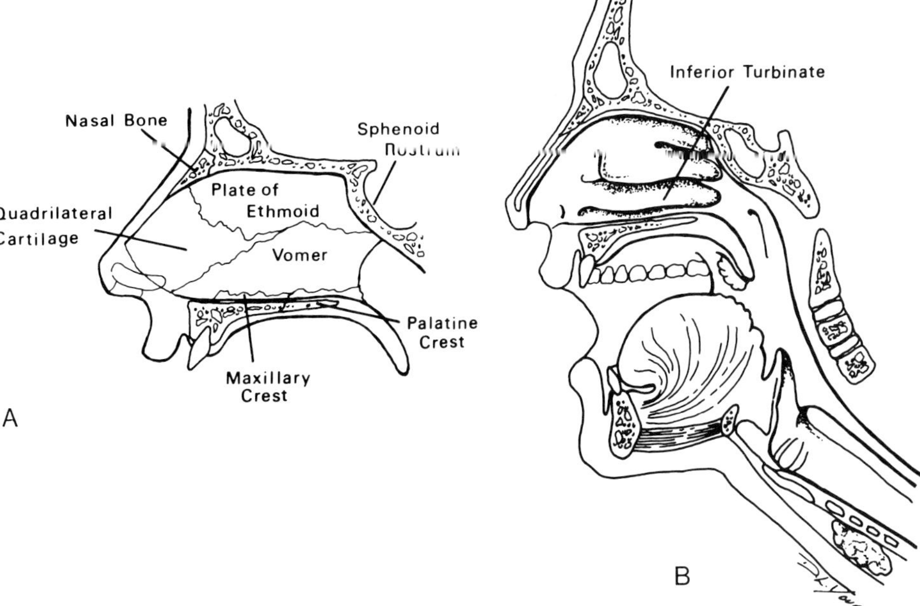

Figure 78–1. *A,* Sagittal view of the bone structure of the nose. *B,* Sagittal view of the oral and nasal airway anatomy. Note the communication of the nasopharynx and the oropharynx. (Courtesy of the Stratton Veterans Administration Medical Center, Albany, NY.)

that meet in the midline forming the thyroid notch and thyroid prominence. The superior projections (horns) are connected to the hyoid bone, an important landmark for the performance of a superior laryngeal nerve block. Inferiorly, its attachment is the cricoid cartilage via the cricothyroid membrane.

The cricoid cartilage is signet ring shaped and is connected to the first tracheal ring. Curry in 1915, and later Sellick, described posterior cricoid pressure as a useful maneuver. Curry found it useful to limit the entry of air into the esophagus during resuscitation attempts,[16] whereas Sellick noted its ability to prevent passive regurgitation of gastric contents.[17]

The epiglottis is leaf shaped and covered with a membranous surface innervated by the superior laryngeal nerve (internal branch). The reflection of its membranous surface forms the depression known as the vallecula. It is here that the curved laryngoscope blade is placed to elevate the epiglottis and allow visualization of the laryngeal entrance. The aryepiglottic folds join the epiglottis with the paired pyramidal-shaped arytenoids. They have a synovial articular surface with the superolateral aspect of the cricoid, and each has an anterior vocal process to which attaches the vocal ligament of the cords. Disarticulation of this joint during traumatic intubation can lead to adduction of the vocal cord involved, resulting in changes in phonation as well as a decrease in the size of the airway opening.

The corniculate cartilages rest on the apex of each arytenoid cartilage along with the cuneiform cartilage and tubercle. The arytenoids are returned to their resting position after abduction, which is facilitated by the elastic recoil of the corniculate and cuneiform cartilages. The cuneiform and corniculate tubercles can often be seen during direct laryngoscopy and may provide a landmark to the opening of the trachea when it is impossible to bring the vocal cords into view.

The glottis consists of the vocal cords and space between them (rima glottidis) (Fig. 78–3). In the adult, this is the narrowest portion of the airway. The true vocal cords are covered by stratified squamous epithelium, which gives them a pearly white color when illuminated. The subglottic area begins below the vocal cords and is the narrowest area in infants and children.

The muscles of the larynx protect its entrance and produce changes in the quality of phonation. The extrinsic muscles elevate, depress, and constrict the pharynx. The intrinsic muscles are important for abduction, adduction, and changes in tension of the vocal cords. The only muscle that abducts the cords is the posterior cricoarytenoid muscle. Branches of the vagus (CN X) innervate the muscles of the larynx. The superior laryngeal nerve supplies only the cricothyroid muscle and provides sensory innervation to the

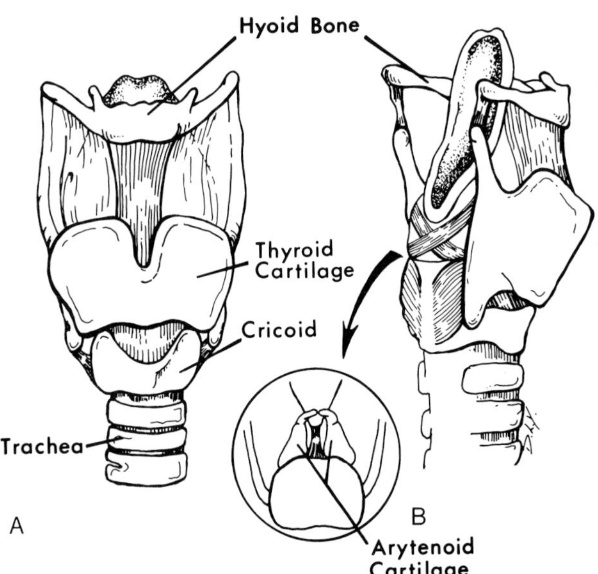

Figure 78–2. Laryngeal cartilages. *A,* Anterior view. *B,* Posterolateral view. Magnified view from the anterior aspect of the laryngeal inlet. The cuneiform and corniculate cartilages sit atop the arytenoid cartilages and are a useful landmark for identification of the glottic opening. (Courtesy of the Stratton Veterans Administration Medical Center, Albany, NY.)

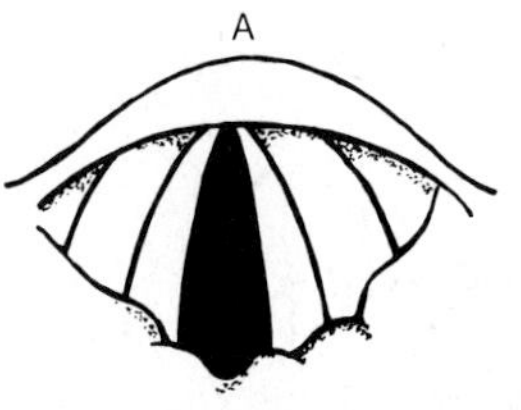

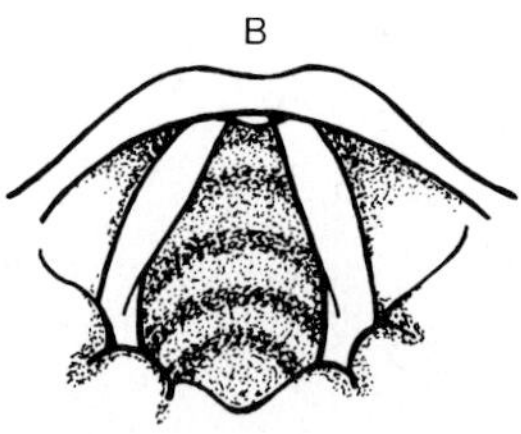

Figure 78–3. Laryngoscopic view of the glottis. *A,* Position on expiration (cadaveric position; also seen in living patients with the use of muscle relaxants or in those with bilateral cord paralysis). *B,* Position of the vocal cords during inspiration. Note the humplike projections of the corniculate cartilages, which may provide the only landmark in identifying the laryngeal inlet in a patient with a difficult airway. (Courtesy of the Stratton Veterans Administration Medical Center, Albany, NY.)

entire mucosal surface of the larynx, the piriform recess, vallecula, and base of the dorsal tongue posteriorly. Stimulation without adequate anesthesia may reflexly provoke laryngospasm. Afferent impulses transmitted to the central vagal nuclei are then carried by efferents to the intrinsic muscles of the larynx, which protect its entrance.[16, 18] Application of positive pressure with a mask and bag-valve device may relieve spasm in some cases. A tight mask seal is imperative for its proper application. If unsuccessful, a short-acting muscle relaxant may be administered by those skilled in it uses and complications. Because a patient may be unable to be ventilated as a result of laryngospasm followed by the use of muscle relaxants, properly trained individuals should be present to proceed quickly with alternative means of airway control whenever needed.

The recurrent laryngeal nerve provides motor supply to the rest of the intrinsic muscles of the larynx and sensory supply to the larynx below the vocal cords. Injury to this nerve results in paralysis of the ipsilateral vocal cord, which then lies in the cadaveric position near the midline. Bilateral paralysis of this nerve leads to vocal cord paralysis, with the cords remaining in the cadaveric position. They are seen in midline with bowing (see Fig. 78–3*A*) and not in complete opposition. This results in almost complete loss of phonation. Often, the cords become less bowed over time and voice improves, but the airway opening narrows and obstruction may ensue.

The trachea extends from its attachment to the cricoid cartilage to the carina where the mainstem bronchi begin. It is composed of 16 to 20 C-shaped cartilages with connective tissue between them and the tracheal muscle posteriorly, which is then in apposition to the esophagus. Obstruction of the airway may arise here from compression (mediastinal and esophageal tumors, postoperative hematoma) and foreign body ingestion.

Tracheomalacia and esophageal scarring may result from ischemic injury secondary to either trauma during intubation or overinflated cuffs. Tracheostenosis may also result from airway manipulation and postoperative changes. In the pediatric patient, lack of air leak around the ETT indicates an excessively tight fit that may lead to ischemic subglottic and tracheostenosis.

AIRWAY ASSESSMENT

A rapid assessment of the airway should be performed when management decisions involve the maintenance of airway patency and gas exchange. This should include knowledge of patient disease that may alter airway anatomy and its related structures (e.g., acromegaly, connective tissue disease, and other systemic diseases). Consideration of surgical and traumatic deformities of the maxillofacial bones and tissues, surgical scarring and fibrosis, laryngeal trauma and edema, congenital anomalies, airway tumors and abscesses, cervical spine instability, immobility, and acute injury (hematoma, paravertebral swelling), teeth and jaw structure or abnormalities (temporomandibular joint syndrome, mandibular fracture, large or loose teeth, dentures), and those diseases that may affect the airway in their pathologic destruction is a vital component of the initial assessment.[19]

In those patients with obvious disease that may make ventilation and/or intubation difficult, it is prudent to assemble the equipment for alternative means of airway control and intubation as well as to summon those personnel with expertise in airway management.

Potential difficulties in intubation may be subtle, and unless careful initial assessment has been performed before attempts at intubation, serious complications may result, including loss of the airway, cardiac arrest, and death. In any case, the individual responsible for maintaining the airway should have an understanding of failed intubation drills (Fig. 78–4) because morbidity from the interruption of gas exchange as well as from directly mediated deleterious laryngeal reflexes (cardiovascular instability, vomiting, laryngospasm) may ensue if corrective action is not taken expediently.

Several indicators of anatomically difficult airways have been described.[15, 20–23] Of these, three are easy to perform (with certain exceptions in the ICU patient) and may together provide a reliable index for predicting difficulty in intubation.[19]

Visual grading of tongue to pharyngeal size is simple in the awake, cooperative patient. The patient should be sitting upright, with the head in the neutral position, the mouth opened as widely as possible, and the tongue protruded maximally. The airway is then classified according to the structures visible to the observer[15] (Fig. 78–5):

class I: soft palate, fauces, uvula, anterior and posterior tonsillar pillars
class II: soft palate, fauces, uvula
class III: soft palate, base of uvula
class IV: soft palate only

The ease or difficulty of laryngoscopy and subsequent intubation has been correlated with these views (Fig. 78–6). A class I airway most often provides a laryngoscopic view that includes the entire laryngeal aperture.[15, 22, 24] Patients with intermediate Mallampati airway classifications were found to have all grades of laryngoscopic view by one group of investigators.[25] The majority of those patients with class IV airways on laryngoscopy provided very limited or no exposure of the laryngeal opening, with difficult intubation conditions. However, taken alone, especially in the ICU patient with the usual array of coexisting disease that may alter airway anatomy, this classification may not be clearly predictive of the degree of difficulty in intubation. The supine position, arched tongue, and phonation (patient says "Ah") may alter the view.[19]

A second bedside examination, evaluation of atlanto-occipital extension, requires a cooperative patient without cervical spine injury. Patients with unstable cervical spine injuries at C-1 and C-2 may experience neurologic damage after neck flexion or extension.[26] The patient should sit with head erect and facing forward and then extend the atlanto-occipital joint with little extension of the remainder of the

Difficult Airway Algorithm

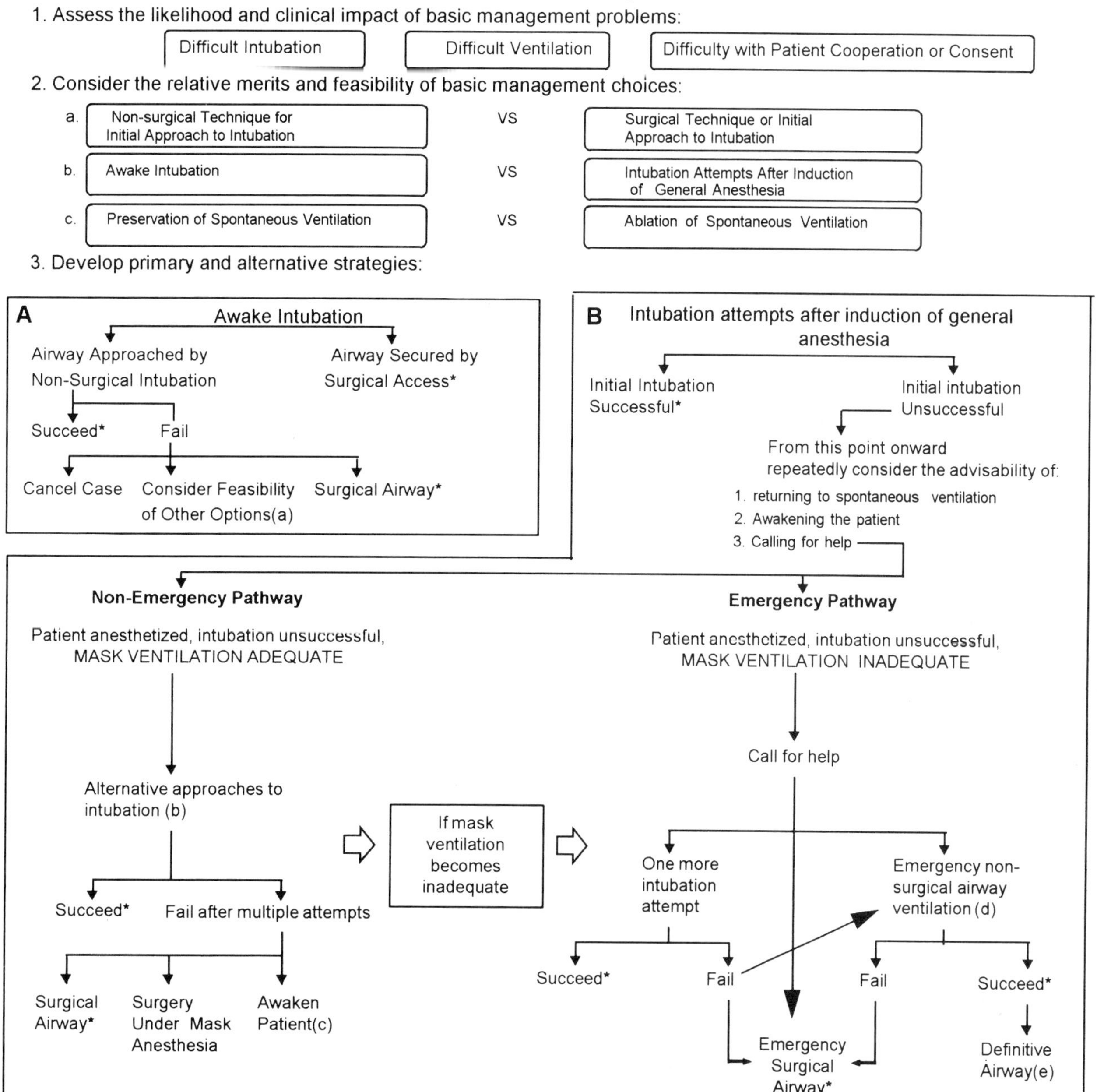

*** Confirm intubation with exhaled CO_2**

(a) Other options include (but are not limited to): surgery under mask anesthesia, surgery under local anesthesia infiltration or regional nerve blockade, or intubation attempts after induction of general anesthesia.

(b) Alternative approaches to difficult intubation include (but are not limited to): use of different laryngoscope blades, awake intubation, blind oral or nasal intubation, fiberoptic intubation, intubating stylet or tube changer, light wand, retrograde intubation, and surgical airway access.

(c) See awake intubation

(d) Options for emergency non-surgical airway ventilation include (but are not limited to): transtracheal jet ventilation, laryngeal mask ventilation, or esophageal-tracheal combitube ventilation.

(e) Options for establishing a definitive airway include (but are not limited to): returning to awake state with spontaneous ventilation, tracheotomy, or endotracheal intubation.

Figure 78–4. Algorithm developed by the American Society of Anesthesiologists Task Force. (From the American Society of Anesthesiologists Task Force on Management of the Difficult Airway: Practice Guidelines for Management of the Difficult Airway. Anesthesiology 1993; 78:597–602.)

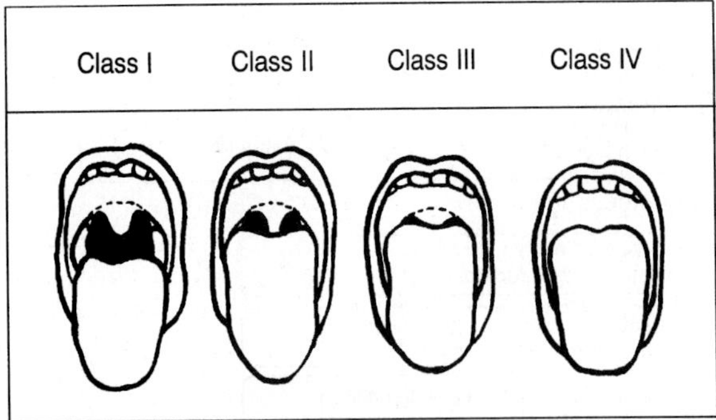

Figure 78–5. Mallampati classification of the airway. A class I airway affords view of the soft palate, fauces, uvula, and anterior and posterior tonsillar pillars, a class II airway—a view of the soft palate, fauces, and uvula, a class III airway—a view of the soft palate and base of the uvula, and a class IV airway—a view of the soft palate only. (From Mallampati SR, Gatt SP, Gugino LD, et al: A clinical sign to predict difficult tracheal intubation: A prospective study. Can J Anaesth 1985; 32:429–435.)

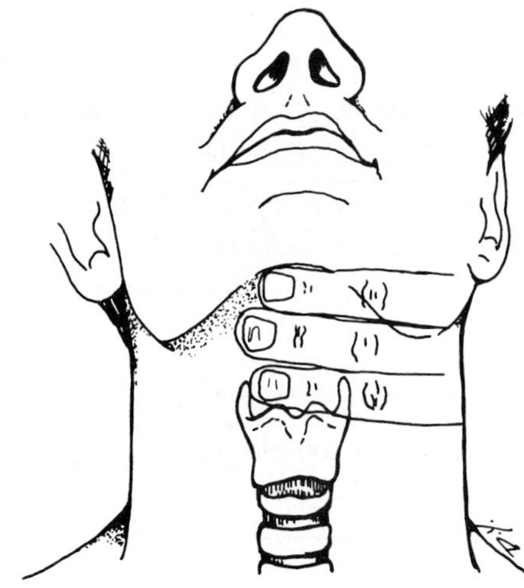

Figure 78–7. Assessment of thyromental distance. The fingers are placed such that one is touching the point of the chin and another the thyroid cartilage. The number of fingers or centimeters that span the mandibular space is the thyromental distance. (Courtesy of the Stratton Veterans Administration Medical Center, Albany, NY.)

cervical spine. An estimate of the angle is made by the occlusal surface of the upper teeth with the occlusal surface of the lower teeth, which should be horizontal and parallel to the ground. Thirty-five degrees of atlanto-occipital extension are possible if no disease exists. Bellhouse and Doré graded the reduction in joint extension and then correlated this with tongue size using a two-variable analysis to predict the difficulty in intubation.[20]

Additionally, the mandibular space can be measured as the thyromental distance (Fig. 78–7), which grades the space anterior to the larynx, is described as the number of fingerbreadths (or centimeters) between the thyroid cartilage and point of the chin, and determines the acuity of the laryngopharyngeal axis. The more acute the angle, the greater the difficulty in alignment of these axes despite adequate atlanto-occipital extension.

There is a strong inverse correlation between the adequacy of the mandibular space and the pharyngeal class (Mallampati class). A low pharyngeal class coupled with a thyromental distance greater than 6 cm and/or horizontal mandibular length greater than 9 cm has been shown to provide a low-grade direct laryngoscopic view.[21, 23, 27]

The obstetric patient deserves special mention because physiologic changes of pregnancy may make mask ventilation and intubation difficult. Of particular concern is the higher rate of failed intubation in the obstetric population undergoing cesarean section[28] when compared with the general surgical patient.[29] In fact, the inability to intubate the trachea of these patients is a leading cause of maternal death.[30]

Increased extracellular fluid and plasma volume during pregnancy resulting from greater mineralocorticoid activity[31] leads to airway mucosal edema, friability, and bleeding with minimal trauma.[32] These changes are exacerbated in patients with preeclampsia and those given tocolytic agents.[33] Intubation criteria examined by one group of investigators included the pharyngeal class and tongue size, mandibular space, short neck, protruding incisors, obesity, facial edema, and swollen tongue.[34] Using multivariable analysis, these investigators found a direct correlation between the difficulty in intubation and increasing pharyngeal class, short neck, receding mandible, and protruding incisors. No correlation between facial edema and swollen tongue was found.

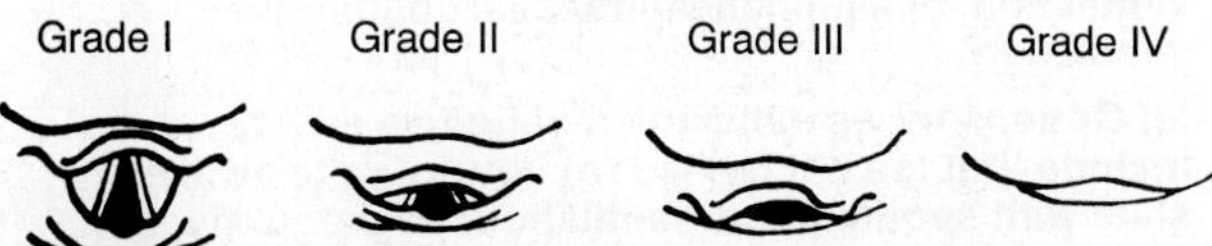

Figure 78–6. Laryngoscopic views of the laryngeal inlet. Grades I through IV show a progressive decrease in the number of structures visible. A grade I view allows inspection of the epiglottis, vocal cords, and surrounding structures. A grade IV view permits inspection of the epiglottis only. (From Cormack RS, Lehane J: Difficult tracheal intubation in obstetrics. Anaesthesia 1984; 39:1105.)

Parturients are at a greater risk for gastric aspiration as gastric acid secretion increases,[35] and in late pregnancy, gastric emptying is delayed, lower esophageal sphincter tone decreases, and intragastric pressure increases. If mask ventilation is performed, cricoid pressure should be maintained until the trachea is intubated and the tracheal tube cuff inflated.[33]

It is important to recognize that obesity and pregnancy both contribute to a decreased functional residual capacity. In the parturient, oxygen consumption increases as well. These factors combine to lead to the rapid development of hypoxia with apnea of even short duration.

As stated previously, these criteria may be difficult to assess in some ICU patients. Nevertheless, a rapid evaluation should be performed as equipment and personnel are assembled and plans made for alternative means of airway control and patency.

AIRWAY CONTROL

Airway maintenance remains the highest priority for those involved in acute patient care. In those patients who are obtunded or unconscious with sudden airway obstruction, attempts to open the airway should be initiated immediately using the triple-airway maneuver.[36]

Head tilt with anterior displacement of the mandible (chin lift) and jaw thrust should be attempted except in the management of patients with known or suspected cervical spine instability. Although there are no outcome studies examin-

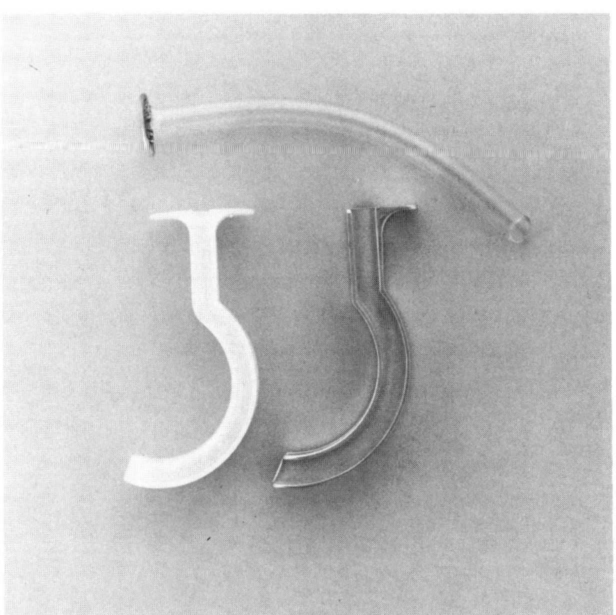

Figure 78–8. Nasopharyngeal and oral airways. *Top,* A nasopharyngeal airway. Note the angulation of the distal end. The opening should face the medial wall of the nares as the airway is inserted and advanced. *Left,* A conventional plastic oral airway. *Right,* A metal airway for use during fiberoptic bronchoscopic intubation. Note that the opening allows passage of a bronchoscope.

ing these maneuvers, chin lift with jaw thrust and head tilt may lead to untoward neurologic sequelae in those patients.[27] These maneuvers should be practiced until expertise is gained and repracticed at intervals to maintain the skill.

Oropharyngeal and nasopharyngeal airways (Fig. 78–8) are important adjuncts to airway control. They are designed to hold the tongue away from the posterior wall of the pharynx and should be inserted by properly trained individuals. Oral airway placement is performed either by inserting it directly convex side up with anterior tongue displacement or with the convex side down and then rotating it 180°, with care taken to avoid rough handling of the teeth and gums. If improperly placed, the airway will increase airway obstruction by downward displacement of the tongue into the pharynx. In patients with intact upper airway reflexes, the placement of a rigid oral airway may provoke laryngospasm, vomiting, coughing, and bronchospasm.

Nasal airways are softer and better tolerated by conscious patients. Contraindications for their use are the same as those for nasotracheal intubation (Table 78–1). Insertion should be preceded by topical vasoconstrictors (i.e., phenylephrine or oxymetazoline nasal spray) and topical lidocaine. The tip should be aimed perpendicularly to the plane of the face, with the opening facing the septum and advanced with gentle downward pressure until it reaches the oropharynx. Advancement should proceed until airflow is optimal. This can be tested by listening over the airway, auscultating the neck near the larynx, or feeling the flow with a hand held above the airway. Head tilt is necessary (jaw thrust may also be required) to hold the tongue away from the posterior pharyngeal wall between the airway and the laryngeal aperture;[37] therefore, these devices may not be helpful in patients with cervical spine instability.

The laryngeal mask airway (LMA) is a cuffed pharyngeal airway developed by Brain in 1981[38] to obtain a direct connection with the patient's airway. Its use, as well as that of the esophageal obturator airway (EOA) and pharyngotracheal lumen airway (PTLA) in the intensive care setting, is described in another chapter.

TABLE 78–1. Contraindications to Nasal Intubation

Coagulopathy
Systemic anticoagulation
Severe intranasal disease
Basilar skull fracture
Head trauma with cerebrospinal fluid leak

Masks

Masks are an essential component of the airway apparatus (Fig. 78–9). Clear masks allow early visualization of regurgitation. The correct size varies from individual to individual, and a tight seal may be extremely difficult in edentulous and bearded patients. Placement of the mask over the nose and mouth while holding it in place with one hand and providing downward pressure with the thumb and first finger, at the same time raising the mandible with gentle pressure along its bony prominences (taking care not to exert pressure on the soft tissues), allows the other hand freedom for other tasks (e.g., inflation of a self-refilling bag-valve device).

Bag-Mask-Valve Units

The self-refilling bag-mask-valve unit was developed by Ruben[39] after devices by Kreiselman,[40] Macintosh,[41] and the anesthesia bag-mask units.[42] It may be used with a mask, ETT, EOA, esophageal gastric tube airway (EGTA), PTLA, combination esophagotracheal tube, tracheostomy tube, and LMA.

These units can deliver 100% oxygen if the reservoir is at least as large as the bag volume and the oxygen inflow rate at least equals the delivered minute volume. The bag should be squeezed and then quickly released to allow for complete passive exhalation. With excessive flow rates and slow re-

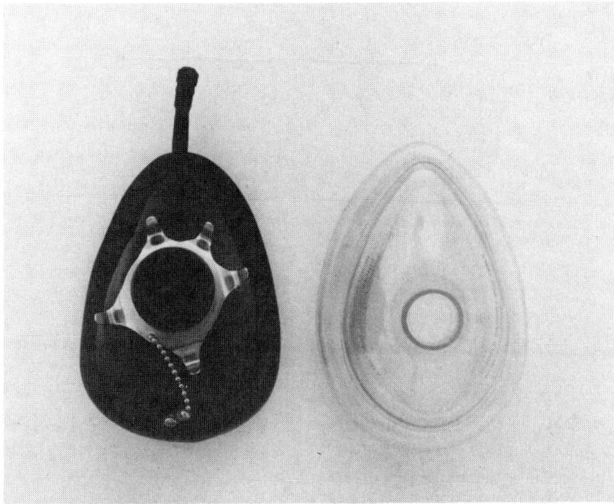

Figure 78–9. Anatomic masks. *Left,* A rubber (Saratoga) mask. Note that in this adaptation of the standard rubber mask, a chain is connected to a cover to provide for the passage of a fiberoptic scope. *Right,* A clear plastic mask that makes possible early visualization of regurgitation.

lease, the valve may lock in the inspiratory position and lead to both barotrauma and decreased venous return to the heart.[37] A similar situation develops with hyperventilation and associated air trapping (auto–positive end-expiratory pressure generation), which are often seen in transport.

EQUIPMENT

Once an indication (Table 78–2) has been met for endotracheal intubation, the equipment must be available immediately and checked before use to ensure proper functioning (Table 78–3). Patient monitoring is essential and should include a continuous visible electrocardiogram, a manual or automated blood pressure device, and continuous pulse oximetry. Peripheral intravenous access should be obtained rapidly.

As the patient is prepared for intubation (i.e., if conscious or semiconscious, a brief explanation of the plans should be conveyed to him or her), the bed is locked and positioned optimally for the laryngoscopist, topical local anesthetics and vasoconstrictors as needed are applied, and drugs for resuscitation are prepared. Ancillary personnel should assist in providing adequate oxygenation and necessary equipment as previously outlined.

The equipment should be checked by the person who will assume responsibility for the initial attempt at intubation and arranged at the bedside for easy visualization and accessibility. Suction (with a Yankauer tip) should be on at 120 mm Hg negative pressure to facilitate pharyngeal suctioning as needed.

Laryngoscopes

A laryngoscope consists of a handle and blade. The blade contains the light source, a bulb, which should fit securely and tightly in its socket. Proper placement of the blade onto the handle results in an audible snap. The bulb should illuminate when the laryngoscope is in its position of function. Replacements should be available in case of malfunction.

TABLE 78–2. Indications for Endotracheal Intubation*

Respiratory or Ventilatory Failure
Cardiac arrest
ARDS
Pulmonary edema or embolism
Atelectasis
Neuromuscular disease or weakness (muscle relaxants, insecticides)
Pleural effusion
Near-drowning

Acute Airway Obstruction
Trauma
Tumor
Abscess
Infection (i.e., epiglottitis)
Coma
Tracheostenosis
Laryngeal edema

Airway Protection
Trauma to upper airway
CNS depressant overdose
Cerebrovascular accident
Status epilepticus
Upper airway burn or inhalation injury

Pulmonary Toilet

*This list is not all inclusive.
Abbreviations: ARDS = adult respiratory distress syndrome; CNS = central nervous system.

TABLE 78–3. Equipment for Intubation

Mandatory Equipment
1. Suction
    Yankauer tip (large-bore tonsil tip)
    Suction catheters (sized to permit passage through ETT tube)
2. Oxygen source
3. Bag-valve device
4. Masks (at least two sizes)
5. Oral and nasal airways
6. ETTs (include sizes smaller than anticipated)
7. Laryngoscope handle and blade (various sizes)
8. Syringe for cuff inflation
9. Stylet
10. Method of securing ETT (i.e., tape)
11. Monitors on: ECG, pulse oximetry, blood pressure cuff/device
12. Resuscitation drugs
13. Stethoscope

Highly Suggested Equipment
1. Tongue depressors
2. Local anesthetics (for topical application)
3. Topical vasoconstrictors
4. Lubricants
5. Intravenous access
6. End-tidal CO_2 monitoring

Abbreviations: ETT = endotracheal tubes; ECG = electrocardiogram; CO_2 = carbon dioxide.

The two major classes of laryngoscope blades are curved and straight: MacIntosh[43] and Miller,[44] respectively (Fig. 78–10). The tip of the curved blade should be placed in the vallecula and the epiglottis raised to expose the glottis. The straight blade lifts the epiglottis by lying under it. The choice of blade should depend on the experience of the laryngoscopist. Conscious patients may tolerate the MacIntosh blade better because, when correctly positioned in the vallecula, minimal CN X and CN XII stimulation occurs. The short-handled laryngoscope[45] and the adjustable-angle laryngoscope[46] may be helpful in obese patients and in patients with large breasts and short necks. The blade lock allows adjustable positioning of the blade at various angles to the handle. This is extremely useful for patients in whom the standard laryngoscope handle abuts the chest on attempts to insert it.

The Bullard intubating laryngoscope (Circon ACMI, Stamford, CT) is a fiberoptic endoscope that uses the principles of indirect laryngoscopy to facilitate oral or nasal intubation. It has a broad, anatomically designed curved blade and introducing stylet (preshaped and easily attached to the laryngoscope), which allows easier visualization and intubation of the larynx.

The tip of the blade is placed at the base of the tongue in the vallecula or under the epiglottis, and force (minimal) is directed along the axis of the handle to obtain the desired view. The ETT can then be advanced off the intubating stylet through the glottis or, during nasotracheal intubation, advanced forward with forceps into the trachea. It is useful in patients with unstable cervical spines because it requires no neck extension or flexion[47] and in one author's experience was extremely useful for intubation of patients with airway abnormalities.[48] It must be recognized that skills necessary for its use have to be acquired but are easily attained by those already experienced in direct laryngoscopy.[49]

Stylets

Stylets have been an aid to endotracheal intubation since the curved introducers of O'Dwyer.[9] The standard stylet is composed of a malleable substance (Fig. 78–11) and is in-

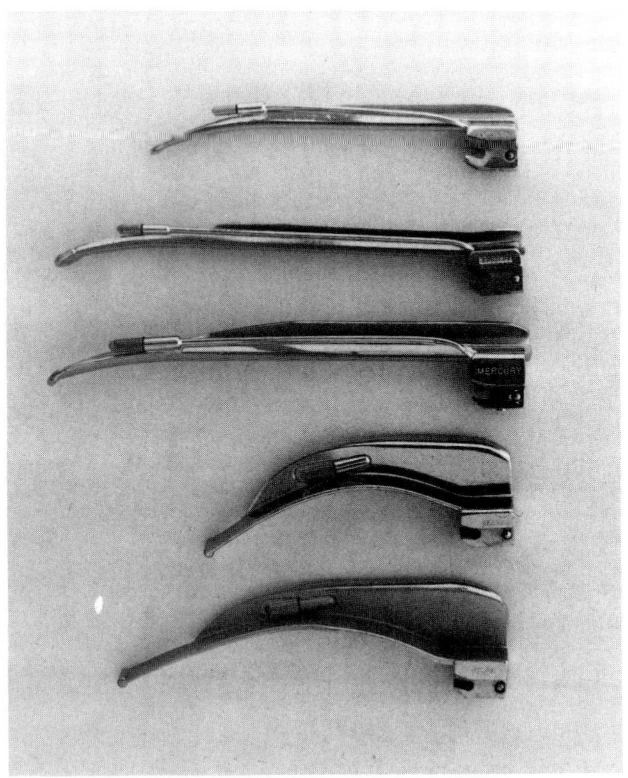

Figure 78–10. An assortment of laryngoscope blades. *From top to bottom,* Miller blades sizes 2, 3, and 4, and MacIntosh blades sizes 3 and 4.

serted into the ETT and designed to maintain its curve. Its distal end should be proximal to the Murphy's eye of the ETT and its proximal end curved over the tube to prevent inadvertent forward slippage.

Several modifications of the stylet exist and include the Flex-guide (Scientific Sales International, Kalamazoo, MI), which has a proximal thumb ring to flex its distal end, guiding it through the glottic opening,[50] and the Eschmann Introducer, a gum elastic bougie introducer (Sims Surgical Inc., Keene, NH) whose distal end enters the laryngeal inlet followed by ETT advancement over it.[50, 51]

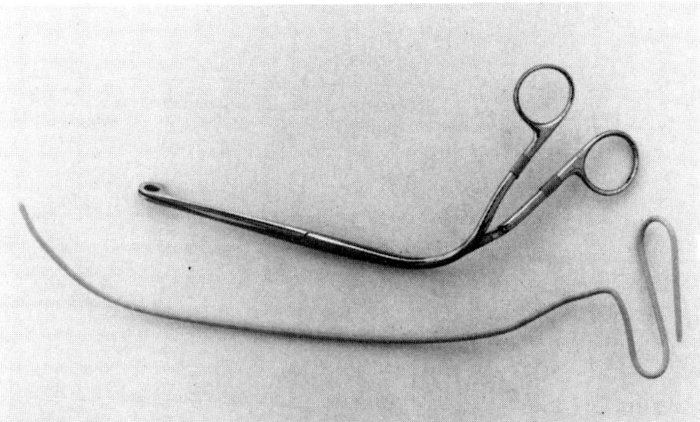

Figure 78–11. *Top,* Magill forceps. This instrument is used to advance the endotracheal tube into the trachea during orotracheal or nasotracheal intubation under direct laryngoscopy. *Bottom,* A malleable stylet. The stylet should be placed inside the endotracheal tube proximal to the Murphy eye. The tube can then be manipulated into the desired position.

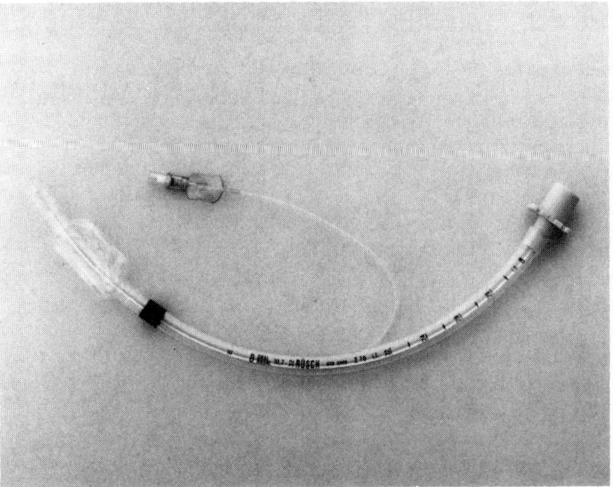

Figure 78–12. An endotracheal tube. Note the standard 14-mm adapter on the proximal end, the pilot balloon, and the cuff.

The illuminating intubating stylet was introduced in 1985[52] and is a unique adjunct to intubation techniques. The Steward Tracheal Light Wand may possess advantages over its predecessors.[53] With proper position, just before entering the trachea, a glow seen in the anterior neck is diminished if the esophagus is intubated.[50] Ellis and colleagues found that tracheal intubation using a lighted stylet was as fast as direct laryngoscopy and easily learned.[54]

Endotracheal Tubes

Most ETTs (Figs. 78–12 and 78–13) are composed of sterile, nontoxic polyvinylchoride and are marked with IT (implant tested) or Z-79 (Z-79 Committee of the American National Standards Institute) to indicate that there has been no evidence of toxicity found on testing. The internal diameter in millimeters and lengthwise centimeter markings are imprinted along the side of each tube. The selection of internal diameter should be based on the age and/or gender of the patients (Table 78–4) to avoid excessive pressure on the tracheal mucosa.

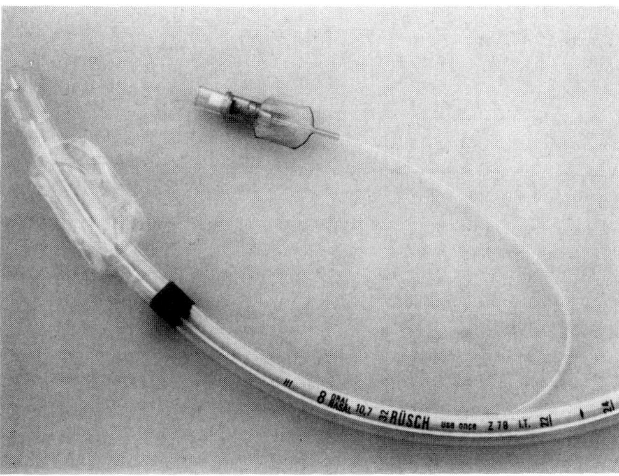

Figure 78–13. Magnification of markings on an endotracheal tube. Note that the size (internal diameter) is marked in millimeters and expressed as a size French. The lengthwise markings indicate distance between the distal end in the midtrachea and the final secured position at the lips or teeth.

TABLE 78–4. Commonly Used Endotracheal Tube Sizes

Age	*Distance from Midtrachea* to Lips/Teeth (cm)*	*Internal Diameter (mm)*	*French Gauge*
Adult male	23–25	10.0	42
Adult male	23–25	9.5	40
Adult male	23–25	9.0	38
Adult male	21–25	8.5	36
Adult female	21–23	8.0, 7.5, 7.0, (6.5†, 6.0†)	34, 32, 30 (28, 26)

*Add 3 cm for nasal tubes.
†Should be available in all obstetric patients and patients with known tracheostenosis or suspected laryngeal edema.

High-volume, low-pressure cuffs adapt to the tracheal contour as intracuff and tracheal wall pressure equilibrate, forming a leak-free seal when inflated.[55] Excessive cuff pressure causing tracheal mucosal ischemia, although less likely than with earlier cuffs (low volume), can still occur if the cuff is inflated beyond the point of no leak. Typically, 4 to 6 mL of air is sufficient to just reach the no-leak point, but tracheal cuff pressure should be obtained and the cuff volume adjusted to maintain intracuff pressure less than 25 cm H_2O.

Once the ETT is placed, the cuff inflated, and initial verification of placement performed (discussion follows), the tube should be secured. The lengthwise markings determine the distance from the end of the ETT to a landmark such as the lips or teeth (see Table 78–4).[56]

Esophagotracheal Double-Lumen Tube (Combitube)

The EOA and PTLA may be obsolete with the development of the esophagotracheal double-lumen tube (Combitube). Improvement of the Combitube design has minimized previous problems with the EOA.[57] The Combitube is a disposable double-lumen cuffed tube with two balloons.[58, 59] Tube no. 2 (shorter clear tube) has an open distal end, and tube no. 1 (longer blue tube) has a blind distal end with pharyngeal side holes.

The Combitube is introduced blindly through the mouth, entering either the trachea or the esophagus (Fig. 78–14). It is advanced until the two proximal black rings are located between the upper and lower teeth. The pharyngeal balloon is inflated with 100 mL of air, occluding the pharynx, and the distal cuff is inflated with about 15 mL of air occluding either the tracheal or esophageal lumen.[60] Wissler recommended placing the Combitube into the esophagus under direct vision using a laryngoscope.[57]

Ventilation is initiated through tube no. 1. If the lungs inflate (bilateral chest expansion) and carbon dioxide is present by capnography and bilateral breath sounds by auscultation, all without auscultation of gastric insufflation, then ventilation is continued because the tube is properly placed in the esophagus (see Fig. 78–14*A*). When the Combitube is in the esophagus, tube no. 2 may be used for passage of a suction catheter into the stomach.[60]

If the lungs do not inflate (no chest expansion) and there is no evidence of carbon dioxide exhalation or breath sounds but auscultation of gastric insufflation, then the tube is in the trachea and ventilation should immediately be switched to tube no. 2 (see Fig. 78–14*B*). Wissler[57] recommended titrating additional air to the proximal balloon (to a total of 160 mL)[61] to seal the upper pharynx and then attempt to achieve adequate ventilation before switching to ventilation through tube no. 2.

Contraindications to use of the Combitube include the following:

1. Patients younger than 16 years and shorter than 5 feet
2. Responsive patients with an intact gag reflex
3. Patients with known esophageal disease
4. Patients who have ingested caustic substances

The Combitube has been used in patients with cardiac arrest[58, 59] and in cases of difficult intubation[62–65] and may be a reasonable option in certain cases in which an ETT is unable to be placed.

AWAKE INTUBATION

Awake intubation should be considered in unfasted ("full-stomach") patients and in anticipated difficult airways. This approach is generally the safest option. In the awake state, spontaneous respiration and normal resting muscle tone protect the airway from aspiration. Under direct visualization the awake-state airway structures clearly stand out

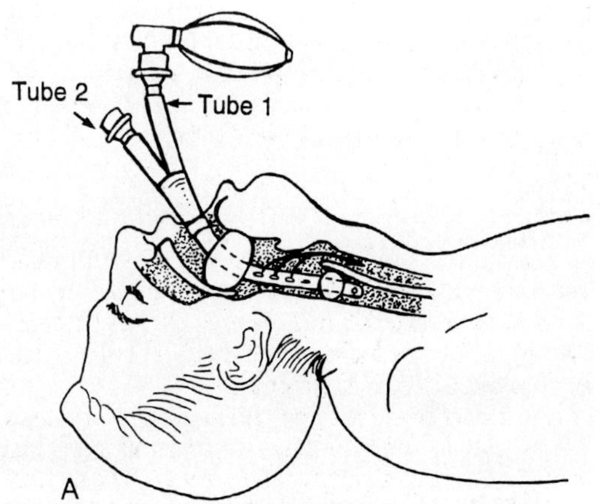

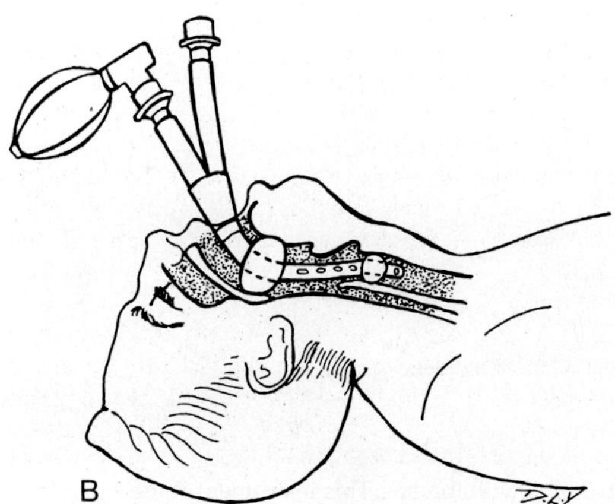

Figure 78–14. Placement of an esophageal-tracheal double-lumen tube (see text for details). *A*, Placement of the tube in the esophagus with the pharyngeal and distal cuffs inflated. Ventilation proceeds via the lumen of tube 1. *B*, Placement of the tube in the esophagus with the cuffs inflated. Ventilation proceeds through the lumen of tube 2. (Courtesy of the Stratton Veterans Administration Medical Center, Albany, NY.)

from one another. Although safe, it may take more time and be more uncomfortable for the patient. Discomfort can be minimized with psychologic and airway preparation.[19] This includes a well-delineated explanation to the patient, topical and nerve block anesthesia, and the use of an agent that minimizes orotracheal secretions.

The need for sedation should be carefully assessed individually. In preventing possible aspiration, intubation with local anesthesia preparation (limited to the supraglottic region) of the airway without sedation is safer than intubation using sedation without local anesthesia.[66] If sedation is used, it should be titrated to effect. Additionally, one agent should be used and its antagonist should be immediately available (e.g., midazolam and flumazenil). One should recognize that if the use of an antagonist becomes necessary, the protective reflexes may be lost during the time required for reversal.

Various approaches of awake intubation may be used. The techniques of oral, nasal (blindly under direct laryngoscopy or with fiberoptic endoscopy), and retrograde intubation are described in the following sections.

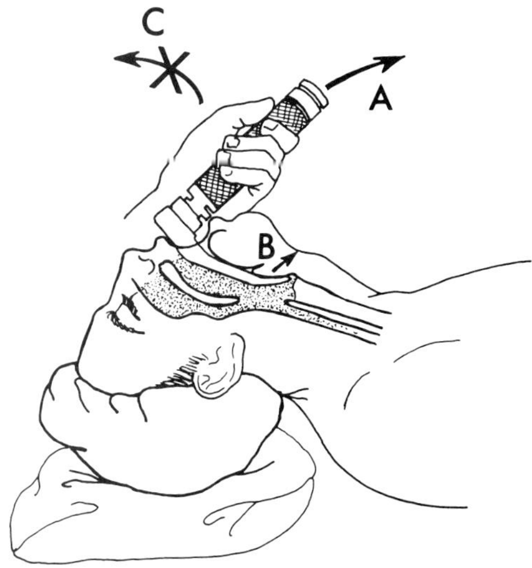

Figure 78–15. Correct alignment of the oral, pharyngeal, and laryngeal axes, with elevation of the head on a pad and head extension. The direction of force should follow the *arrows A* and *B*. If the laryngoscope force is positioned in the direction of *arrow C*, tooth damage and inadequate laryngoscopic view may result. (Adapted with permission from Roberts JT: Fundamentals of Tracheal Intubation. New York, Grune & Stratton, 1983, p 78.)

Orotracheal Intubation

Different techniques of orotracheal intubation include the following:

1. Blind orotracheal intubation
2. Orotracheal intubation under direct laryngoscopy
3. Orotracheal intubation with fiberoptic bronchoscopy

Orotracheal intubation should be used in patients who have absolute or relative contraindications to nasal intubation (see Table 70–1). Additionally, because of the potential for nasal bleeding, the oral route is generally used in pediatric and obstetric populations. The importance of head and neck positioning cannot be overemphasized. The "sniffing position" in the supine patient is an attempt to align the axes of the mouth, pharynx, and larynx. The head is elevated about 10 cm on a pad, the base of the neck is flexed slightly, and the head is extended. Oral tubes tend to be larger than those used nasally and are advantageous in patients with excessive secretions or with a need for endotracheal toilet.

Blind Orotracheal Intubation

Blind orotracheal intubation by digital technique (without a laryngoscope) and blind orotracheal intubation with a laryngoscope (but without direct visualization of anatomic landmarks) are alternatives best reserved for experienced personnel familiar with these techniques. These techniques may be helpful in difficult intubations, especially in trauma victims (i.e., gunshot wound to face) and in cases in which all visual anatomic landmarks are obscured (e.g., by blood). If the patient is breathing spontaneously, then listening to exhaled air passing from the proximal end of the ETT may aid the clinician as it can with blind nasal intubations.

Orotracheal Intubation Under Direct Laryngoscopy

The laryngoscope is generally held in the left hand, and the blade is introduced into the right side of the patient's mouth. The blade is advanced posteriorly and toward the midline, sweeping the tongue to the left and holding it away from the visual path to the larynx. When the tonsillar fossa is reached with a curved blade, the blade is slipped into the vallecula. Traction along the axis of the laryngoscope handle will lift the base of the tongue, thereby exposing the larynx (Fig. 78–15). The upper incisors must not be used as a fulcrum. If the epiglottis is seen overhanging the larynx, advance the tip of the blade further into the vallecula. If the esophagus is seen, withdraw the blade until the larynx comes into view.

A straight blade should be slipped under the epiglottis. If the laryngeal aperture is obscured by a large floppy epiglottis, it may be helpful to pass the blade intentionally into the esophagus and then slowly withdraw it until the vocal cords are seen.

If the larynx is anterior and not well seen, the application of gentle pressure dorsally on the thyroid cartilage by an assistant may help bring the vocal cords fully into view.

The glottic opening is triangular and is bounded by the true vocal cords. Often only epiglottic cartilage or the cuneiform/arytenoid projections are observed. Downward and cephalad pressure on the thyroid cartilage may bring the vocal cords into view. This position can be held by an assistant as the ETT is advanced and secured in place. In bearded patients, cloth ties ("umbilical tape") or Velcro straps may be used instead of adhesive tape.[50]

Although variation exists, the adult trachea is approximately 15 cm long.[13] The proper position of the ETT tip is roughly the middle third of the trachea with the head in a neutral position.[67] Conrady and associates demonstrated that the tip of the ETT advances distally about 1.9 cm with neck flexion and is withdrawn proximally about 1.9 cm with neck extension.[67]

Orotracheal Intubation with Fiberoptic Bronchoscopy

Orotracheal intubation and nasotracheal intubation with fiberoptic bronchoscopy are similar; however, the oral route is usually more difficult. Therefore, oral fiberoptic intubation is chosen as a preferred method only when it is necessary to avoid the nasal route.

Use of the oral route permits passage of a larger ETT and is associated with less tissue trauma and bleeding,[19] although it is technically more difficult. If assisted ventilation is required, fiberoptic bronchoscopy can be continued with the use of an endoscopic mask that includes a port through which the fiberoptic bronchoscope (FOB) is passed[19] (see Fig. 78–9).

Careful airway preparation/anesthesia is achieved as with a nasal fiberoptic intubation (excluding the nasal passages). An airway intubator is then gently placed into the midline of the mouth (see Fig. 78–8). The ETT must be smaller than the airway intubator (e.g., an 8-mm endotracheal tube or smaller should be used with a no. 9 airway intubator). The FOB is threaded through the ETT, which sits at the external end of the FOB.[19]

The FOB and light source should be checked thoroughly and lubricated with clear lubricating fluid. An antifog agent should be applied to the lens, and the instrument should then be focused before use.[50] To enable movement of the tip, the FOB is held in an anteroposterior axis.[19] The FOB is then inserted through the airway intubator. A constant flow of oxygen maintained through the operating channel provides a higher inspired oxygen concentration and at the same time pushes mucus, blood, and secretions away from the lens.[50] Local anesthetic can be sprayed onto the vocal cords through the same channel of the FOB. The airway intubator facilitates the path to the larynx.[19] After the FOB is passed through the airway intubator, the epiglottis or vocal cords may be in view. The FOB must be maneuvered just posterior to the epiglottis and then back anteriorly until the vocal cords are in the center of the field.[50] Maintaining this view, the FOB is advanced between the vocal cords into the trachea. The ETT is passed over the FOB until it is in proper position in the trachea. The FOB is then used to confirm proper ETT position before it is removed.

Complications associated with fiberoptic bronchoscopy include hypoxemia (usually lasting between 1 and 4 hours), arrhythmias, and increased resistance to airflow.

Nasotracheal Intubation

The decision to place a nasotracheal tube in an ICU patient may be related to the presence of traumatic and surgical deformities (fractured mandible, maxillofacial surgery). Personal bias (i.e., level of comfort) of the clinician is influential, although no clear advantage in level of patient comfort or nursing care exists with nasotracheal intubation.[68, 69] Before this decision is made, contraindications to nasotracheal intubation should be reviewed (see Table 78–1).

Nasotracheal intubation can be performed in the awake or anesthetized patient using blind, direct laryngoscopic or fiberoptic (bronchoscope or Bullard laryngoscope) guidance. Awake techniques with use of nerve blocks and supplemental topical anesthesia are discussed.

After proper psychologic and sedative preparation of the conscious patient, the nasal mucosa should be anesthetized. This can be accomplished with the use of soaked cotton-tip applicators or pledgets. If cocaine is used, a vasoconstrictor need not be applied. If not, a topical vasoconstrictor in spray form should be used after adequate absorption of the local anesthetic is ensured.

The glossopharyngeal nerve (lingual branch) and the superior laryngeal nerve (internal branch) can be blocked effectively, permitting intubation with minimal patient discomfort and hemodynamic alteration. These procedures are time consuming and may have to be forgone in the emergency setting.

The superior laryngeal nerve can be blocked by either one of two techniques: internal or external. The internal block is performed by coating each piriform fossa with local anesthetic–soaked pledgets.[19] The external approach[70] involves sterile preparation of the extended neck. The hyoid bone is then palpated, displaced laterally toward the side to be blocked as a 25-gauge needle is placed on the greater cornu of this bone, walked off inferiorly, and advanced through the thyrohyoid membrane. A slight loss of resistance is felt, and 3 mL of local anesthetic is injected on either side of the membrane after negative blood aspiration. This block should be performed bilaterally. The laryngeal epiglottis, vallecula, vestibule, aryepiglottic folds, and rima glottidis are anesthetized if this block is properly performed.

Additionally, the lingual branch of the glossopharyngeal nerve can be blocked by injection of local anesthetic into the palatoglossal arch, where it meets the base of the tongue using a 25-gauge spinal needle.[19] Two milliliters of 2% lidocaine should be injected in incremental doses after negative aspiration of blood. This should be repeated on the contralateral side. If effective, the posterior third of the tongue and the pharyngeal surface of the epiglottis (vallecula) will be anesthetized with all protective airway reflexes intact. If performed alone, care should be taken to anesthetize the larynx adequately either by spray or nebulized inhalation of local anesthetic solution, which anesthetizes the trachea as well. Care should be taken to quantify the amount of local anesthetic used to avoid systemic toxicity.

Blind nasotracheal intubation is performed through the larger naris. A tube 1 mm (internal diameter) smaller than that used for orotracheal intubation is selected and placed with the bevel facing the nasal septum. A lubricant placed on the tube will ease its passage as it is guided posteriorly and caudad into the pharynx. Slight resistance may be met as the tube passes the inferior turbinate bone of the naris. Breath sounds can be heard as the tube is advanced. As the patient reaches late inspiration, the tube should be placed through the laryngeal aperture. If the patient is breathing spontaneously and breath sounds cease during this maneuver, the tube should be withdrawn until breath sounds are again heard and then readvanced. Flexion of the neck and lateral bending toward the side of nasotracheal intubation may guide the tube into the trachea.[16]

If not contraindicated, direct laryngoscopy or indirect laryngoscopy with the laryngeal retraction blade (Bullard laryngoscope) may facilitate nasotracheal intubation. The tube should first be guided into the pharynx as stated previously. Then, the laryngoscope is placed in the mouth, with the techniques already described, a view of the laryngeal aperature is obtained, and the tube is advanced into the trachea. Magill forceps (see Fig. 78–11) may be used to grasp the distal end of the tube and guide it through the glottis. As in all endotracheal intubations, correct placement should be confirmed (see later discussion)

Intubation of the trachea with flexible fiberoptic bronchoscopy is useful for patients with known or anticipated difficult airways or patients in whom airway and associated structured abnormalities may obscure a view of the larynx. The same preparation should precede initiation of this technique. Once completed, the lubricated FOB is inserted through the ETT, which has been placed in the oropharynx. It is then advanced into the trachea, the ETT is passed over the FOB into the trachea, the FOB is removed, and the ETT adapter is returned to its proper position. Again, confirmation of the placement should follow. This technique takes well-practiced skill and should not be performed in the emergency setting. Further descriptions of the technique are beyond the scope of this chapter.

Retrograde Intubation

The technique of retrograde intubation is suitable for the management of the difficult airway in a spontaneously breathing patient in the nonfasted state. It requires preparation and time to perform and is not ideal for emergency airway access. As always, the patient should be prepared for awake intubation (see previous discussion).

The cricothyroid membrane is punctured with an 18-gauge needle after sterile preparation of the field and skin infiltration with a local anesthetic. The bevel should be directed cephalad at an angle of approximately 45°. On entering the trachea confirmed by aspiration of air, a flexible guide wire is threaded retrogradely between the vocal cords, into the pharynx, and out through the mouth. The needle is removed, and the guide wire is clamped at the skin.

The guide wire is held taut, and the ETT is advanced over the guide wire, with rotation if necessary, until it has passed between the cords into the larynx. The wire is withdrawn, and the ETT is advanced further into the trachea.

To make the guiding system effectively stiffer and larger in diameter, a nasogastric tube can be passed anterogradely over the wire.[71]

An FOB can be used in a similar manner. The guide wire is threaded through the suction channel of the FOB, which has been passed through an ETT. The tube is positioned under direct vision and the guide wire removed via the proximal port of the FOB suction channel.[72]

Confirmation of Endotracheal Tube Placement

Confirmation of ETT placement is crucial. An incorrectly placed ETT is usually not a problem if it is immediately recognized.

Every tracheal intubation needs to be assessed by clinical methods. Several maneuvers and techniques make up the clinical assessment of correct ETT placement. Direct visualization of the ETT passing between the vocal cords followed by inspection, palpation, and auscultation of the chest is necessary. The chest wall should rise and fall with equal excursion bilaterally. Auscultation of bilateral breath sounds in the lung apices laterally is mandatory after intubation. Placement of the stethoscope bell behind the pectoralis major muscle in the axilla where chest wall mass is minimal may be preferable, especially in obese patients. Sounds may be transmitted elsewhere, yielding false-positive results. Auscultation over the epigastrium to confirm no air movement is also indicated. Visualization of water vapor with exhalation and "the feel of the bag" cannot be relied on but are part of the picture of proper tube placement, as is maintenance or improvement of preintubation oxygenation.

Clinical assessment must also be accompanied by verification of exhaled carbon dioxide. Continuous exhaled carbon dioxide detection is the "gold standard" of proper ETT placement and must accompany every tracheal intubation! End-tidal carbon dioxide may be assessed with capnography (the best method), capnometry, or disposable colorimetric indicators, which change color when exposed to carbon dioxide. These disposable devices can be attached to the proximal end of the endotracheal tube and are used during active ventilation.

Extremely low cardiac output states may yield false-negative results because inadequate carbon dioxide is transported to the lungs to be detected in the exhaled air. Recent ingestion of carbonated fluids may yield false-positive results because carbonation may be detected as carbon dioxide. However, the signal and waveform will not be maintained.

Additional techniques to confirm intubation include the use of fiberoptic bronchoscopy and the lighted stylet. An FOB passed through the ETT yields confirmation of correct placement if the tracheal rings and carina are observed. A lighted stylet advanced through the ETT to the level of the suprasternal notch will transilluminate the anterior neck if the tube is in its proper position.

In 1988 Wee described an esophageal detector device to help assess correct ETT placement.[73] It is a 60-mL syringe with a catheter tip and an airtight attachment to a standard catheter mount with a 15-mm fitting. The 15-mm fitting is attached to the ETT, and aspiration with the syringe is initiated. Easy flow with minimal resistance is supportive of proper position in the trachea. Resistance to aspiration may indicate incorrect placement.[53]

Radiologic confirmation must always be performed but should not be relied on because the deleterious effects of an incorrectly placed tube will have already begun and may be irreversible before its completion. All methods to confirm ETT placement are fallible; therefore, the total picture of maintained adequate oxygenation, continuous carbon dioxide detection, and clinician assessment needs to be considered. If the clinician is uncertain of correct ETT placement, then it should be removed and the patient ventilated by mask before any reattempts at intubation.

SPECIAL CONSIDERATIONS

Nonfasting (Full-Stomach) Patient

Parturients, the morbidly obese, diabetics with gastroparesis, patients who have just eaten, patients with known gastroesophageal reflux and hiatal hernia, patients with bowel obstruction, upper gastrointestinal hemorrhage, peritonitis, active nausea/vomiting, or incompetent lower esophageal sphincter, trauma and head-injury patients, and those who have diminished bowel transit time (possibly secondary to pain, narcotics, disease processes, and so on) are all considered in this category. These patients are at increased risk for pulmonary aspiration of gastric contents and therefore require either a sedative-assisted/topical anesthetic "awake" intubation or a rapid-sequence induction. The extent of lung injury from aspiration is more extensive with fecal or bacterial material, particulate matter, volumes greater than 25 mL (or 0.4 mL/kg), and more acidic pH (<2.5). Pharmacologic premedication before attempting airway management has included nonparticulate antacids (e.g., 30 mL of 0.3 mol/L sodium citrate),[74] histamine (H_2) receptor antagonists,[75] and metoclopramide (a dopamine antagonist)[76] alone or in combination.[75,77] Metoclopramide acts as an antiemetic, accelerates gastric emptying, and increases lower esophageal sphincter pressure.

The best airway protection is afforded by a properly placed cuffed ETT. The LMA, EOA, EGTA, and PTLA do not provide adequate airway protection from regurgitation of gastric contents in the full-stomach patient.

Rapid Sequence Induction

After checking all equipment (as discussed earlier and listed in Table 78–3) and availability of a trained assistant, the clinician may proceed with preoxygenation for at least 3 minutes at high oxygen flow. If time does not permit 3 minutes of preoxygenation, four vital capacity breaths of 100% oxygen can be substituted, but this is not as effective.[78] A rapidly acting induction agent and rapidly acting muscle relaxant are administered, in sequence, and cricoid pressure is applied (Sellick's maneuver).[17] This maneuver is the application of pressure by a trained assistant with the thumb and index finger pushing on the cricoid cartilage with a dorsal and cephalad force against the sixth cervical vertebra to occlude the esophagus and prevent passive regurgitation of stomach contents. If intubation cannot be accomplished, the patient should immediately be ventilated while still holding cricoid pressure until proper ETT placement is confirmed or the patient is awake. Cricoid pressure is believed to be effective in preventing passive regurgitation of gastric contents with gastric pressures as high as 50 to 94 (mean of 74) cm H_2O.[79]

Cricoid pressure should not be released until the cuff is inflated and there is confirmation of proper ETT placement unless there is active regurgitation at which point cricoid pressure is released and the patient is placed in Trendelenburg's position with the head turned to the side and suctioned. If intubation and ventilation cannot be accomplished (cannot intubate–cannot ventilate situation), the clinician should proceed immediately with alternative methods of securing an airway (see Fig. 78–4).[80]

Endotracheal Tube Exchange

If an ETT needs to be changed, it is prudent to use a jet stylet (especially with a difficult airway), which does not need to be removed to confirm proper ETT placement.[81] Any semirigid hollow catheter can be used as a jet stylet (e.g., tube exchanger). It is inserted through the ETT, and after the ETT is removed, the hollow catheter can be used for jet ventilation.[19] This technique can be invaluable when changing an ETT or extubating a patient with a difficult airway.[19, 82] An FOB may be used effectively as a jet stylet.[83] The FOB serves as a reintubation stylet, allowing for jet ventilation, airway suctioning, and continuous oxygen administration. The FOB may also be used in a similar manner for extubation of patients in whom there is suspicion of airway injury or edema or of patients in whom access to the upper airway is limited (e.g., by halo traction).[83]

Pharmacologic Approaches to Blunt the Cardiovascular Response to Laryngoscopy/Intubation

Numerous pharmacologic agents are used to attempt attenuation of the hemodynamic responses to laryngoscopy and intubation. These include fentanyl,[84] intravenous lidocaine,[85] esmolol bolus[86] or infusion,[87] sodium nitroprusside,[88] intravenous nitroglycerin,[89] captopril,[90] labetalol,[91] alfentanil,[92] or combinations of these agents.

The Difficult Airway

Lack of gas exchange leads to morbidity and mortality, and in cases of acute airway obstruction with inability to ventilate or intubate, a plan of corrective action must progress rapidly. A difficult airway is defined as "the clinical situation in which a conventionally trained anesthesiologist experiences difficulty with mask ventilation, difficulty with tracheal intubation or both."[84]

Preparation, well-maintained airway management skills and knowledge of the algorithm that the clinician should follow for airway maintenance are essential to the intensivist. Figure 78–4 is the ASA Task Force's algorithm developed to guide all clinicians who perform tracheal intubation in their medical practice. Additionally, well-developed skill in other methods of airway access must be maintained.

CONCLUSION

The maintenance of a patent airway and the ability to ventilate with adequate gas exchange is crucial. Airway control must be achieved rapidly to sustain a neurologically intact patient. Currently, there are no adequate methods available for effective rapid intravenous oxygenation. All clinicians should be familiar with the many aspects of airway management and should have a preplanned strategy when faced with emergency airway problems.

ACKNOWLEDGMENT

We thank Ms. Jae Brady, secretary, Department of Anesthesiology, Albany Medical Center, for her excellent work with an earlier version of this chapter. We also thank Donna L. Youmans, medical illustrator, Department of Medical Media, Stratton V.A. Medical Center, Albany, NY, for her illustrations.

References

1. Vesalius A: De Humani Corporis Fabrica Libri Septem. Basel, Oporinus, 1543, p 658.
2. Faulconer A Jr, Keys TE: Foundations in Anesthesiology. Springfield, IL, Charles C Thomas, 1965, pp 10–11.
3. Hooke R: Philosophical Transactions of the Royal Society of London 1667; 2:539–540.
4. Mayow J: Tractatus Quinque Medico-Physici. Edinburgh, The Alembic Club, 1907, pp 183–210.
5. Macewen W: Clinical observations on the introduction of tracheal tubes by the mouth instead of performing tracheotomy or laryngotomy. Br Med J 1880; 2:122–124, 163–165.
6. Sykes WS: Essays on the First Hundred Years of Anaesthesia. 2nd ed. Edinburgh, Livingstone, 1982, pp 96–98.
7. Davison MH, Meredith HA: The Evolution of Anaesthesia. London, Williams & Wilkins, 1905.
8. Kuhn F: Die Pernasale Tubage. Munchener Medizinische Wochenschrift 1902; 49:1456–1457.
9. O'Dwyer J: Med Record 1887; 32:557.
10. Gillespie NA: Endotracheal Anesthesia. 2nd ed. Madison, WI, University of Wisconsin Press, 1948, pp 8–11, 75.
11. Rowbotham ES: An inflatable pharyngeal tube. Lancet 1944; II:15.
12. Jackson C: The technique of insertion of intratracheal insufflation tubes. Surg Gynecol Obstet 1913; 17:507–509.
13. Ellis H, Feldman S: Anatomy for the Anaesthetist. London, Blackwell Scientific Publications, 1988.
14. Hollinshead WH: Textbook of Anatomy. 3rd ed. Hagerstown, MD, Harper & Row, 1974.
15. Mallampati SR, Gatt SP, Gugino LD, et al: A clinical sign to predict difficult tracheal intubation: A prospective study. Can J Anaesth 1985; 32:429–435.
16. Roberts JT: Fundamentals of Tracheal Intubation. New York, Grune & Stratton. 1983.
17. Sellick B: Cricoid pressure to control regurgitation of stomach contents during induction of anesthesia. Lancet 1961; ii:404–406.
18. Rex M: A review of the structural and functional basis of laryngospasm and a discussion of the nerve pathways involved in the reflex and its clinical significance in man and animals. Br J Anaesth 1970; 42:891–899.
19. Benumof JL: Management of the difficult adult airway: With special emphasis on awake tracheal intubation. Anesthesiology 1991; 75:1087–1110.
20. Bellhouse CP, Doré C: Criteria for estimating likelihood of difficulty of endotracheal intubation with Macintosh laryngoscope. Anaesth Intensive Care 1988; 16:329–337.
21. Mathew M, Hanna LS, Aldrete JA: Preoperative indices to anticipate a difficult tracheal intubation. Anesth Analg 1989; 68:51–87.
22. Samsoon GLT, Young JRB: Difficult tracheal intubation: A retrospective study. Anaesthesia 1987; 42:487–490.
23. Finucane BT, Santora AH: Evaluation of the Airway Prior to Intubation, Principles of Airway Management. Philadelphia, FA Norris, 1988, pp 69–83.
24. Cohen SM, Zaurito CE, Segil LJ: Oral exam to predict difficult intubations: A large prospective study (Abstract). Anesthesiology 1989; 71:A937.
25. Cormack RS, Lehane J: Difficult tracheal intubation in obstetrics. Anaesthesia 1984; 39:1105–1111.
26. Hastings RH, Marks JD: Airway management for trauma patients with potential cervical spine injuries. Anesth Analg 1991; 73:471–482.
27. Patil VU, Stehling LC, Zauder HL: Techniques of Endotracheal Intubation, Fiberoptic Endoscopy in Anaesthesia. Chicago, Year Book Medical Publishers, 1983, p 79.

28. Lyons G: Failed intubation: Six years experience in a teaching maternity unit. Anaesthesia 1985; 40:759–762.
29. King TA, Adams AP: Failed tracheal intubation. Br J Anaesth 1990; 65:400–414.
30. Morgan M: Anaesthetic contribution to maternal mortality. Br J Anaesth 1987; 59:842.
31. Ueland K: Maternal cardiovascular dynamics VII: Intrapartum blood volume changes. Am J Obstet Gynecol 1976; 126:671.
32. Bonica JJ: Principles and Practice of Obstetric Analgesia and Anesthesia. Philadelphia, FA Davis, 1967.
33. Santos AC, Pedersen H, Finster M: Obstetric anesthesia. *In*: Clinical Anesthesia, 2nd ed. Barash PG, Cullen BF, Stoelting RK (Eds). Philadelphia, JB Lippincott, 1992, p 1278.
34. Rocke DA, Murray WB, Rout CL, et al: Relative risk analysis of factors associated with difficult intubation in obstetric anesthesia. Anesthesiology 1992; 77:67–73.
35. Murray FS, Eiskine JP, Fielding J: Gastric secretion in pregnancy. J Obstet Gynecol Br Common 1957; 64:373.
36. Morikawa S, Safar P, DeCarlo J: Influence of head position upon upper airway patency. Anesthesiology 1961; 22:265.
37. Safar P, Bircher-Nicholas G: Cardiopulmonary Cerebral Resuscitation. Philadelphia, WB Saunders, 1984.
38. Brain AIJ: The laryngeal mask airway: A possible new solution to airway problems in the emergency situation. Arch Emerg Med 1984; 1:229–232.
39. Ruben H: Combination resuscitator aspirator. Anesthesiology 1958; 19:408.
40. Kreiselman J: A new resuscitation apparatus. Anesthesiology 1943; 4:608.
41. MacIntosh RR: Oxford inflating bellows. Br Med J 1953; ii:202.
42. Hingson RA: Western Reserve anesthesia machine, oxygen inhalator and resuscitator. JAMA 1958; 167:1077.
43. MacIntosh R: A new laryngoscope. Lancet 1943; i:914.
44. Miller R: A new laryngoscope. Anesthesiology 1941; 2:318.
45. Datta S, Briwa J: Modified laryngoscope for endotracheal intubation of obese patients. Anesth Analg 1981; 60:120–121.
46. Patil VU, Stehling LC, Zauder HL: An adjustable laryngoscope handle for difficult intubations. Anesthesiology 1984; 60:609.
47. Saunders PA, Geisecke AH: Clinical assessment of the adult Bullard™ laryngoscope. Can J Anesth 1989; 36:S118–S119.
48. Gorback MS: Management of the challenging airway with the Bullard laryngoscope. J Clin Anesth 1991; 3:473–477.
49. Borland LM, Caselbrant M: The Bullard laryngoscope: A new indirect oral laryngoscope (pediatric version). Anesth Analg 1990; 70:105–108.
50. Stehling LC: Management of the airway. *In*: Clinical Anesthesiology. 2nd ed. Barash PG, Cullen BF, Stoelting RK (Eds). Philadelphia, JB Lippincott, 1992.
51. Kidd JF, Dyson A, Latto IP: Successful difficult intubation: Use of the gum elastic bougie. Anaesthesia 1988; 43:437–438.
52. Vollmer TP, Stewart RD, Paris PH, et al: Use of a lighted stylet for guided orotracheal intubation in the prehospital setting. Ann Emerg Med 1985; 14:324–328.
53. Baskett PJF: Difficult and impossible intubation in the anaesthetic crisis. Fisher MMcD (Ed). Baillieres Clinical Anesthesiology 1993; 7:261–280.
54. Ellis DG, Jakvmec A, Kaplan RM, et al: Guided orotracheal intubation in the operating room using a lighted stylet: A comparison with direct laryngoscopic technique. Anesthesiology 1986; 64:823–826.
55. Dorsch JA, Dorsch SE: Understanding Anesthesia Equipment. Baltimore, MD, Williams & Wilkins, 1984, pp 353–400.
56. Owen RL, Cheney FW: Endobronchial intubation: A preventable complication. Anesthesiology 1987; 67:255–257.
57. Wissler RN: The esophageal-tracheal Combitube. Anesth Rev 1993; 20:147–152.
58. Frass M, Frenzer R, Zdrahal F, et al: The esophageal tracheal Combitube: Preliminary results with a new airway for CPR. Ann Emerg Med 1987; 16:768–772.
59. Frass M, Frenzer R, Rauscha F, et al: Ventilation with the esophageal tracheal Combitube in cardiopulmonary resuscitation. Promptness and effectiveness. Chest 1988; 93:781–784.
60. Sheridan Catheter Corp: Argyl, NY. Sheridan Catheter Corp. Package insert for the esophageal tracheal double lumen tube.
61. Frass M, Johnson JC, Atherton GL, et al: Esophageal tracheal Combitube (ETC) for emergency intubation: Anatomical evaluation of ETC placement by radiography. Resuscitation 1989; 18:95–102.
62. Frass M, Frenzer R, Zahler J, et al: Ventilation via the oesophageal tracheal Combitube in cases of difficult intubation. J Cardiothorac Anaesth 1987; 1:565–568.
63. Bigenzahn W, Pesau B, Frass M: Emergency ventilation using the Combitube in cases of difficult intubation. Eur Arch Otorhinolaryngol 1991; 248:129–131.
64. Eichinger S, Schreiber W, Heinz T, et al: Airway management in a case of neck impalement: Use of the oesophageal tracheal Combitube airway. Br J Anaesth 1992; 68:534–535.
65. Klauser R, Roggla G, Pidlich J, et al: Massive upper airway bleeding after thrombolytic therapy: Successful airway management with the Combitube. Ann Emerg Med 1992; 21:431–433.
66. Kopriva CJ, Eltringham RJ, Siebert PE: A comparison of the effects of intravenous Innovar and topical spray on the laryngeal closure reflex. Anesthesiology 1974; 40:596–598.
67. Conrady PA, Goodman LR, Lainge F, et al: Alteration of endotracheal tube position. Crit Care Med 1976; 4:7–12.
68. Stone DJ, Bogdonoff DL: Airway considerations in the management of patients requiring long-term endotracheal intubation. Anesth Analg 1992; 74:276–287.
69. Stauffer JL, Olson DE, Petty TL: Complications and consequence of endotracheal intubation and tracheostomy. Am J Med 1981; 70:65–76.
70. Wedel DJ, Brown DL: Nerve blocks. *In*: Anesthesia. 3rd ed. Miller RD (Ed). New York, Churchill Livingston, 1990, p 1429.
71. King HK, Wang LF, Khan AK, et al: Translaryngeal guided intubation for difficult intubation. Crit Care Med 1987; 15:869–871.
72. Lechman MJ, Donahoo JS, MacVaugh H: Endotracheal intubation using percutaneous retrograde guide wire insertion followed by antegrade fiberoptic bronchoscopy. Crit Care Med 1986; 14:589–590.
73. Wee MYK: The oesophageal detector device. Anaesthesia 1988; 43:27–29.
74. Gibbs CP, Spohr L, Schmidt D: The effectiveness of sodium citrate as an antacid. Anesthesiology 1982; 57:44–46.
75. Hodgkinson R, Glassenberg R, Joyce TH III, et al: Comparison of cimetidine (Tagament) with acidity before elective cesarean section. Anesthesiology 1983; 59:86–90.
76. Murphy DF, Nally B, Gardiner J, et al: Effect of metoclopramide on gastric emptying before elective and emergency cesarean section. Br J Anaesth 1984; 56:1113–1116.
77. Manchikanti L, Marrero TC, Roush JR: Preanesthetic cimetidine and metoclopramide for acid aspiration prophylaxis in elective surgery. Anesthesiology 1984; 61:48–54.
78. Gambee AM, Hertzka RE, Fisher DM: Preoxygenation techniques: Comparison of three minutes and four breaths. Anesth Analg 1987; 66:468–470.
79. Fanning GL: The efficacy of cricoid pressure in regurgitation of gastric contents. Anesthesiology 1970; 32:553–555.
80. American Society of Anesthesiologists Task Force on Management of the Difficult Airway: Practice guidelines for management of the difficult airway. Anesthesiology 1993; 78:597–602.
81. Goskowicz R, Gaughan S, Benumof JL, et al: It is not necessary to remove a jet stylet to determine tracheal tube location. J Clin Anesth 1992; 4:42–44.
82. Bedger RC, Chang JL: A jet stylet catheter for difficult airway management. Anesthesiology 1987; 66:221–223.
83. Wheeler S, Fontenot R, Gaughan S, et al: Use of a fiberoptic bronchoscope as a jet stylet. Anesthesiol Rev 1993; 20:16–17.
84. Martin DE, Rosenberg H, Aukburg SJ, et al: Low dose fentanyl blunts circulatory responses to tracheal intubation. Anesth Analg 1982; 61:680.
85. Splinter WM, Cervenko F: Haemodynamic responses to laryngoscopy and tracheal intubation in geriatric patients: Effects of fentanyl, lidocaine and thiopentone. Can J Anaesth 1989; 36:370.
86. Ebert TJ, Bernstein JS, Stowe DF, et al: Attenuation of hemodynamic responses to rapid sequence induction and intubation in healthy patients with a single bolus of esmolol. J Clin Anesth 1990; 2:243–252.
87. Ebert JP, Peason JD, Gelman S, et al: Circulating responses to laryngoscopy: The comparative effects of placebo, fentanyl and esmolol. Can J Anaesth 1989; 36:301.

88. Stoelting RK: Attenuation of blood pressure response to laryngoscopy and tracheal intubation with sodium nitroprusside. Anesth Analg 1979; 58:116.
89. Grover VK, Sharma S, Mahajan RP: Low-dose intranasal nitroglycerine attenuates pressor response (Letter). Anesthesiology 1987; 66:722.
90. McCarthy GJ, Hainsworth M, Lindray K, et al: Pressor responses to tracheal intubation after sublingual captopril: A pilot study. Anaesthesia 1990; 45:243.
91. Bernstein JS, Ebert TJ, Stowe DF, et al: Partial attenuation of hemodynamic responses to rapid sequence induction and intubation with labetalol. J Clin Anesth 1989; 1:444–451.
92. Martineau RJ, Tousignant CP, Miller DR, et al: Alfentanil controls the haemodynamic response during rapid-sequence induction of anaesthesia. Can J Anaesth 1990; 37:755–761.

CHAPTER 79

Laryngotracheal Injury from Prolonged Tracheal Intubation

Rade B. Vukmir, MD • Ake Grenvik, MD, PhD • Carl-Eric Lindholm, MD, PhD

FREQUENCY AND TYPES OF COMPLICATIONS

The complications of airway intubation are inevitable, as suggested by a study of 1000 patients extubated after standard operative intervention demonstrating a 6% rate of severe lesions including hematoma, mucous membrane laceration, and subluxation of the arytenoid cartilages.[1] Diabetic females and patients with burns are especially predisposed to injuries from prolonged intubation.[2, 3] This higher prevalence in females is demonstrated by another study in which both laryngeal dysfunction (48% vs. 18%) and structural lesions (23% vs. 13%) occurred more commonly in women than in men perhaps because of the tracheal tube size[4] and the narrower larynx in women.[5]

Mucosal ulcerations are common and are usually found on the posteromedial areas of the vocal cords, over the arytenoid cartilages, and posteriorly in the larynx in the interarytenoid area and over the cricoid plate (Fig. 79–1*A*). These lesions occur even after short duration of intubation and are caused by pressure from the tracheal tube. Most resolve spontaneously,[6] but laryngeal granulomas and scarring stenoses are not infrequently formed (see Fig. 79–1*B*). The late lesions associated with endotracheal intubation are primarily laryngostenosis of the glottic and subglottic regions, whereas tracheostomy may result in tracheostenosis. Observed lesions are related to duration of intubation and the presence of chronic conditions such as diabetes mellitus, atherosclerotic heart disease, and immunosuppression.[7] The complication rate in healthy, young, head-injury patients was as high as 61% for prolonged intubation in one study but only 20% for early tracheostomy.[7] Pediatric head-trauma patients, on the other hand, demonstrated a higher complication rate with tracheostomy (26%) than orotracheal (10%) or nasotracheal (11%) intubation.[8] Using long-term artificial airway, adult patients with closed head injury have a greater complication rate, mainly sinusitis, vocal cord paralysis, laryngotracheostenosis, and tracheomalacia.[9] The overall complication rate is perhaps highest in those with severe medical illness, equivalent for prolonged intubation and tracheostomy in incidence of laryngotracheal injury (95% vs. 91%) but more common than tracheostenosis in those with tracheostomy (19% vs. 65%).[10]

The complication rate of prolonged intubation is related to duration. For those intubated for periods of 1 week or less the rate was 37%, whereas for those intubated longer than 1 week the complication rate was 52%.[11] These complications may be as subtle as hoarseness and are found in even larger proportion (77%) in those receiving tracheostomy after a period of prolonged intubation.[11] Problems reported by patients are diverse and include dysphonia (57%), aspiration (25%), dysphagia (23%), odynophagia (21%), dyspnea (21%), stridor (17%), and hoarseness (14%).[12]

Adverse sequelae of endotracheal intubation and tracheostomy may be delineated in incidence (i.e., common vs. rare) (Table 79–1). Infection is often encountered during prolonged intubation. Most of these problems occur in the first 2 weeks and more often with nasal (40%) than oral (20%) intubation.[13] Predisposition is established by the presence of a tracheal tube; the cuffed variety decreases mucus flow in the trachea more so than the uncuffed variety.[14] The low-volume, small resting diameter cuff is causing deeper damage to the tracheal mucosa; hence, healing takes longer and a defective mucociliary transport may exist for weeks. This decrease in mucociliary clearance is enhanced by the administration of anesthetic agents[14] and inadequate humidification.[15] Nosocomial infection of the tracheobronchial tree often implicates gram-negative bacilli and is somewhat lessened by adequate humidification.[16] Culture identification of *Klebsiella pneumoniae, Staphylococcus aureus, Escherichia coli, Proteus mirabilis,* and *Pseudomonas aeruginosa* helps to differentiate infection from colonization.[4] The incidence of pneumonia, mostly resulting from aspiration, is highest after emergency intubation (45%), often occurring within 72 hours but without changing outcome.[17]

PATHOPHYSIOLOGY

Aphonia is the result of decreased vocal cord adduction ability often caused by subluxation of the arytenoid cartilages (see Fig. 79–1*C*), ulceration of this area (see Fig. 79–1*D*), and cricoarytenoid ankylosis after long-term endotracheal intubation.[18] Vocal cord immobility may be caused by interarytenoid fibrosis specifically involving the vocal processes and posterior commissure[17, 19] (Fig. 79–1*E*). Vocal cord paralysis suggests dysfunction of the recurrent laryngeal nerve, which may be injured if the cuff is inflated in the

TABLE 79–1. Complications Associated with Prolonged Intubation*

Common	*Rare*
Infection	Cricoarytenoid subluxation
Hemorrhage	Cricoarytenoid fixation and scarring
Aspiration	Vocal cord paralysis
Air leak	Tracheal necrosis
Subcutaneous emphysema	Tracheal rupture
Pneumomediastinum	Paratracheal abscess
Pneumothorax	Tracheoinnominate artery fistula
Atelectasis	Tracheoesophageal fistula
Laryngeal edema	
Laryngeal ulceration	
Laryngeal granuloma	
Laryngotracheostenosis	
Tracheomalacia	

*For details, see Hsu et al,[12] Chilla and Gabriel,[18] Cavo,[20] Gibbin and Eggington,[21] Levin,[22] Bein et al,[23] Heath and Peirce,[24] Abbey et al,[25] Rinecker and Schvet,[26] Payne et al,[27] Bishop et al.[28]

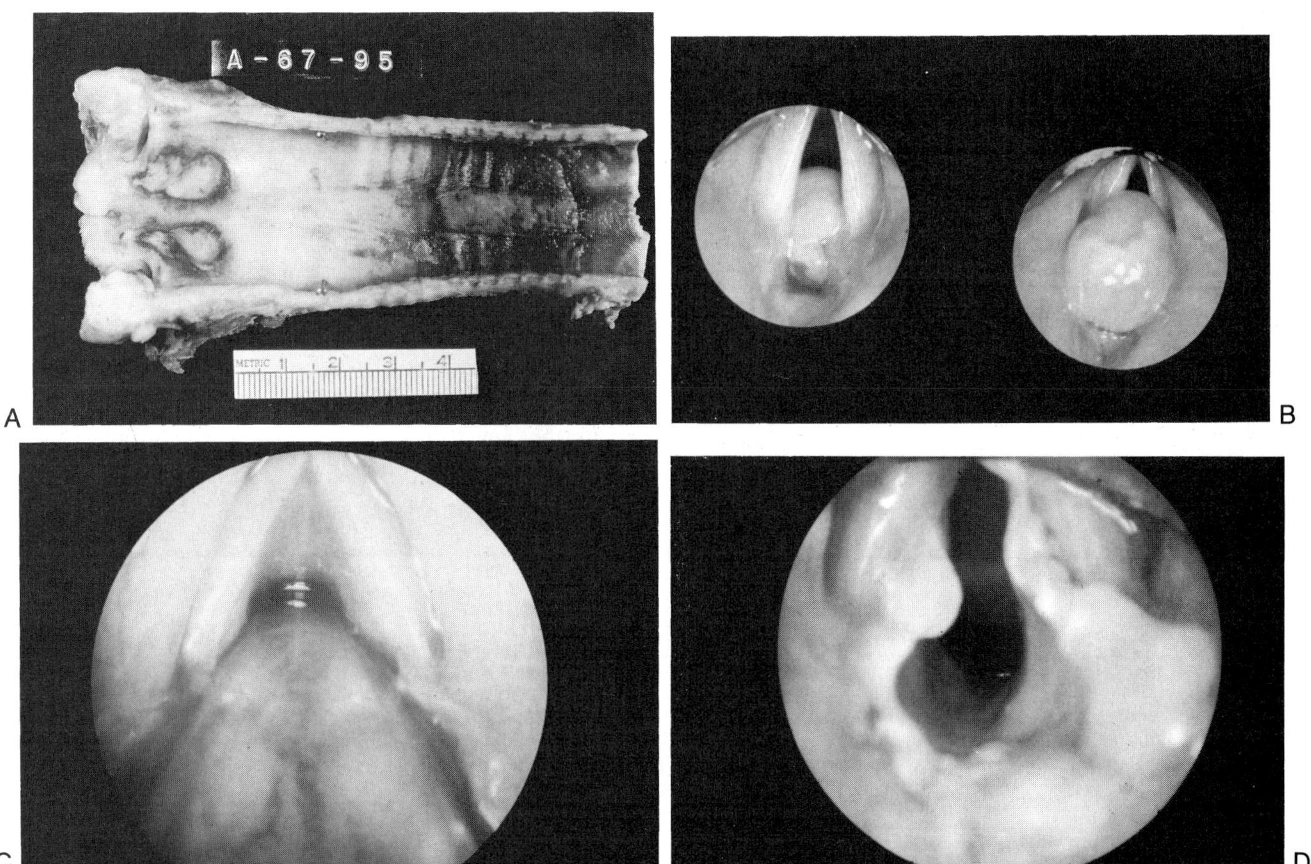

Figure 79–1. *A,* Laryngotracheal specimen, split along the anterior midline, showing necrotic lesions at the medial sides of the arytenoid cartilages and the cricoid plate. The lesions were caused by pressure from the tracheal tube and, further down the trachea, by the cuff. *B,* Endoscopic views of a pendulating postintubation granuloma at the right medial region of the arytenoid cartilage. *C,* Endoscopic view of a tracheal tube that is too wide in relation to the size of the interarytenoid space. *D,* Close-up view of the larynx immediately after extubation. Pressure necrosis and inflammation posteriorly are present where the tracheal tube was located. (See Color Plate Section of this textbook.)

Illustration continued on following page

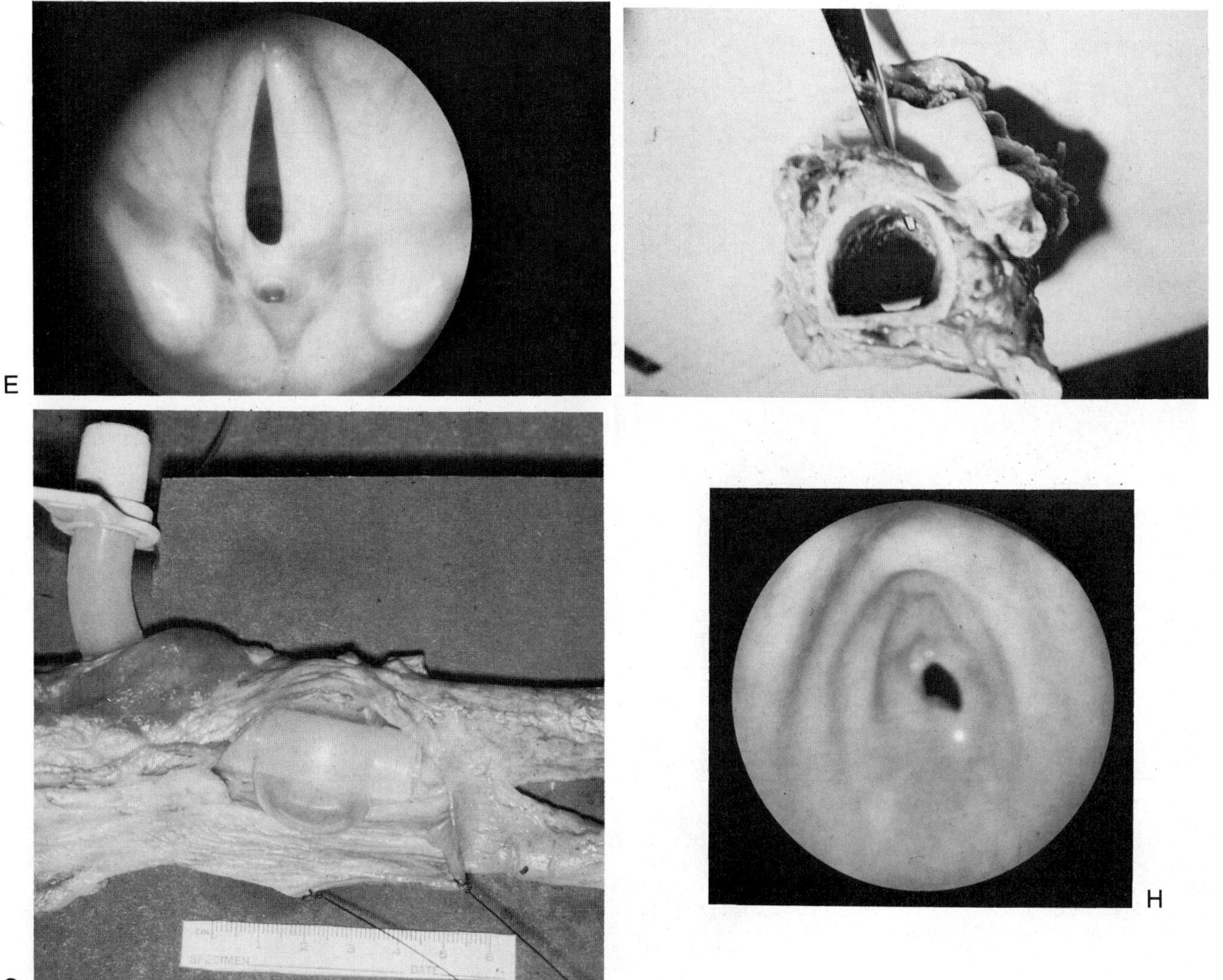

Figure 79–1 *Continued E,* Follow-up laryngeal view showing healing after prolonged intubation injury. Fibrous scarring is present between the arytenoid cartilages, and fixation of the vocal cords can be seen near the midline. The result was severe laryngeal stenosis. *F,* Autopsy specimen demonstrating a fistula (indicated by hemostat) between the trachea and the innominate artery. The fistula was caused by cuff erosion and resulted in lethal hemorrhage into the trachea. *G,* Specimen with a large tracheoesophageal fistula due to erosion by a low-volume, small-diameter, high-pressure cuff. *H,* Severe cuff-induced tracheal stenosis. (See Color Plate Section of this textbook.)

larynx with the nerve interposed between the tracheal tube cuff and thyroid cartilage below the vocal cords.[20] This vocal cord paralysis may be unilateral or bilateral.[21] Function may return because this neuropraxia is sometimes only temporary.

Catastrophic complications include perforations in the hypopharynx, posterior to the cricopharyngeal muscle, or in the piriform sinus, which require early surgical repair.[22] Tracheal rupture may be found in those predisposed by musculoskeletal conditions such as the rigid spine syndrome.[23] Retropharyngeal abscesses are found after lacerations caused by emergency nasotracheal intubation and are indicated by rapid onset of fever and odynophagia.[24] Massive tracheal necrosis has been found in patients with hypoperfusion, infection, and excessive cuff pressure.[25]

The tracheoarterial erosion syndrome involving the brachiocephalic trunk often results in rapid patient demise as a result of massive bleeding into the trachea (see Fig. 79–1*F*).[26] Tracheoesophageal fistulas (see Fig. 79–1*G*) can be found acutely in those with traumatic injury, including iatrogenic lesions during tracheostomy, whereas chronically ventilated patients may demonstrate a more indolent course.[27] These conditions require a high index of suspicion to avoid further patient compromise. However, the most germane issue for routine intensive care practice is an immediate diagnosis of tracheostomy-induced pneumothorax, either unilateral or bilateral. Complications of prolonged airway support are better understood by analysis of pathologic findings. Most long-term complications are attributed to the tube or cuff components (see Fig. 79–1*A*). The presence of an endotracheal tube segment affixed in a canine larynx caused erythema at 24 hours, progressing to severe mucosal ulceration and loss of normal architecture by 1 week.[28] Cuff-induced complications, usually stenosis (see Fig. 79–1*H*) or tracheomalacia (Fig. 79–1*I*), occur most commonly below the first tracheal cartilage.[29] Initial changes are functional, with slowing or complete interruption of tracheal mucus transportation. The superficial respiratory epithelium may undergo squamous metaplasia.[30] The epithelium may begin this alteration after as few as 4 hours of intubation. These early

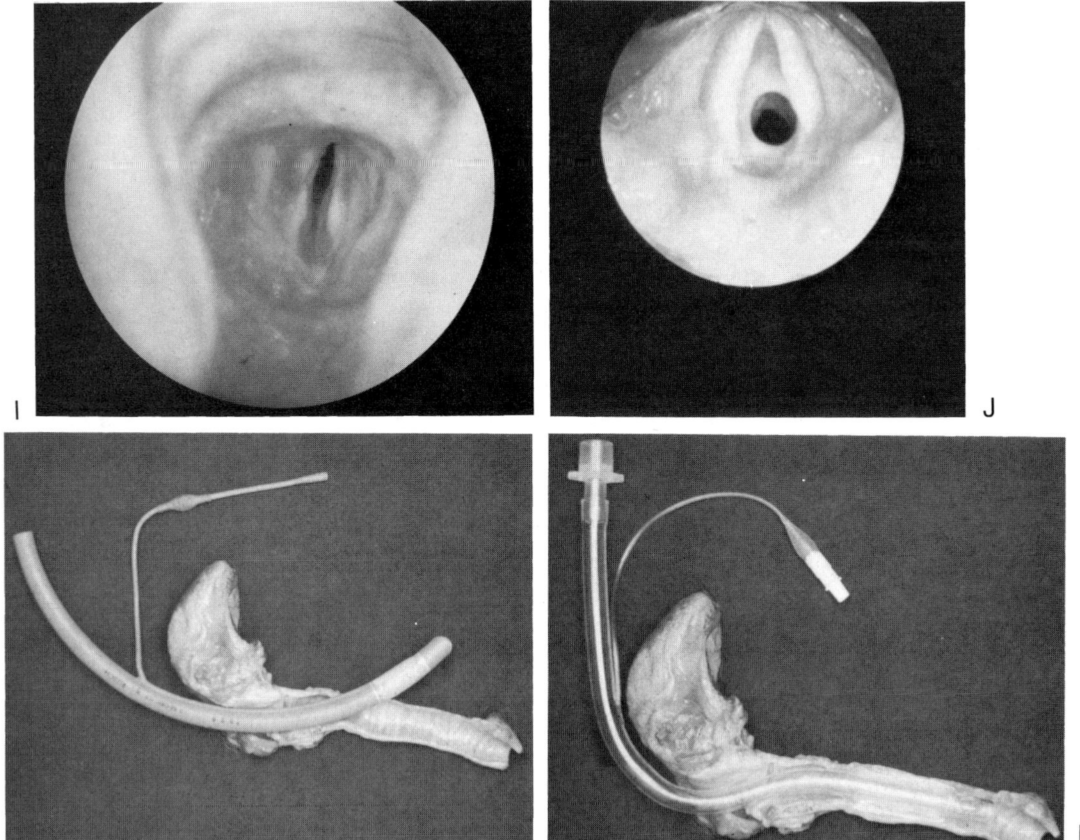

Figure 79–1 *Continued I,* Softening of the tracheal wall after healing of cuff pressure–induced necrosis and cartilage destruction (so-called "tracheomalacia") results in tracheal collapse during exhalation, air trapping in the lungs, and life-threatening respiratory failure. *J,* Endoscopic view of fibrous subglottic stenosis caused by circumferential pressure from a tracheal tube that was too large in relation to the size of the cricoid ring. *K,* An autopsy specimen of the tongue, larynx, and trachea, mainly in their in vivo positions, with a standard tracheal tube superimposed. The discrepancy between the shape of the tube and that of the airway can be seen. *L,* The configuration of the anatomic Lindholm tube corresponds well to the shape of the natural human airway. (See Color Plate Section of this textbook.)

changes consist of flattening, fusion, and erosion of respiratory epithelial cells with ciliary disappearance or compromised function resulting from mechanical abrasion and ischemia (Fig. 79–2).[31] The presence of cuff irritation also results in constriction of smooth muscle of the trachea.[32]

The tracheal arterioles are located in the submucosa and are circumferentially oriented anteriorly between the cartilages and longitudinally in the posterior membranous portion.[33] Capillary perfusion pressure, estimated at 22 mm Hg (30 cm H_2O), is inversely proportional to cuff tracheal wall pressure. Studies using an endoscopic photographic technique suggest continued tracheal blood flow at a cuff pressure of 25 cm H_2O, but the mucosa becomes pale at 40 cm H_2O and blanched at 50 cm H_2O, and flow is absent at 60 cm H_2O.[33] Thus, consideration of cuff to tracheal wall pressure suggests that flow is initially affected at cuff pressure levels of 30 cm H_2O, with complete occlusion at 50 cm H_2O of intracuff pressure.[33] These results have been reproduced by radioactive hydrogen clearance testing, suggesting decreased flow at cuff to tracheal wall pressure of 30 mm Hg (41 cm H_2O) with a practical limit for intracuff pressure of 20 mm Hg (27 cm H_2O).[34] However, at least in rabbit experiments, there is a biphasic response in which normal tracheal blood flow (0.3 mL/min per gram of tissue) is increased 10-fold by the tube irritation because of histamine relaxation of arterioles.[35] Nonetheless, cuff pressure of 30 mm Hg or even levels between 20 and 30 mm Hg may cause significant ischemia of mucosa localized over the tracheal cartilages if a low-volume, small-diameter cuff is used.[35] With a high-volume, large-diameter, thin-walled cuff, the safety margin is greater before total mucosal ischemia over the cartilages occurs.[35] The endpoint of mucosal ischemia is necrosis and infection followed by scarring and stenosis.[19] Subglottic stenosis was found in a canine model after 2 weeks of intubation in which ulceration was followed by granulomatous tissue and scar formation.[36]

In one study, 33% of patients intubated more than 24 hours healed with granuloma formation and concomitant hoarseness, but at 3 months' follow-up only 10% of these granulomas persisted and necessitated removal.[37] Human studies in neonates reveal a 1% to 8% incidence of such lesions in the subglottic region at the cricoid cartilage ring beginning with mucosal necrosis and progressing to full-thickness erosion, perichondritis, and scar formation proportional to the duration of intubation.[19]

Another outcome study demonstrated that 78% of laryngeal intubation lesions re-epithelialized and healed by 8 weeks. Only 7% were left with residual granuloma.[38] Retrospective autopsy observations include inflammation of the perichondrium of the vocal cord processes and arytenoid and cricoid cartilages as well as bacterial invasion beginning at 48 hours and progressing to ulceration by 96 hours.[39] In a prospective study of patients intubated for a mean of 48 hours, most patients had mucosal ulcerations over the ary-

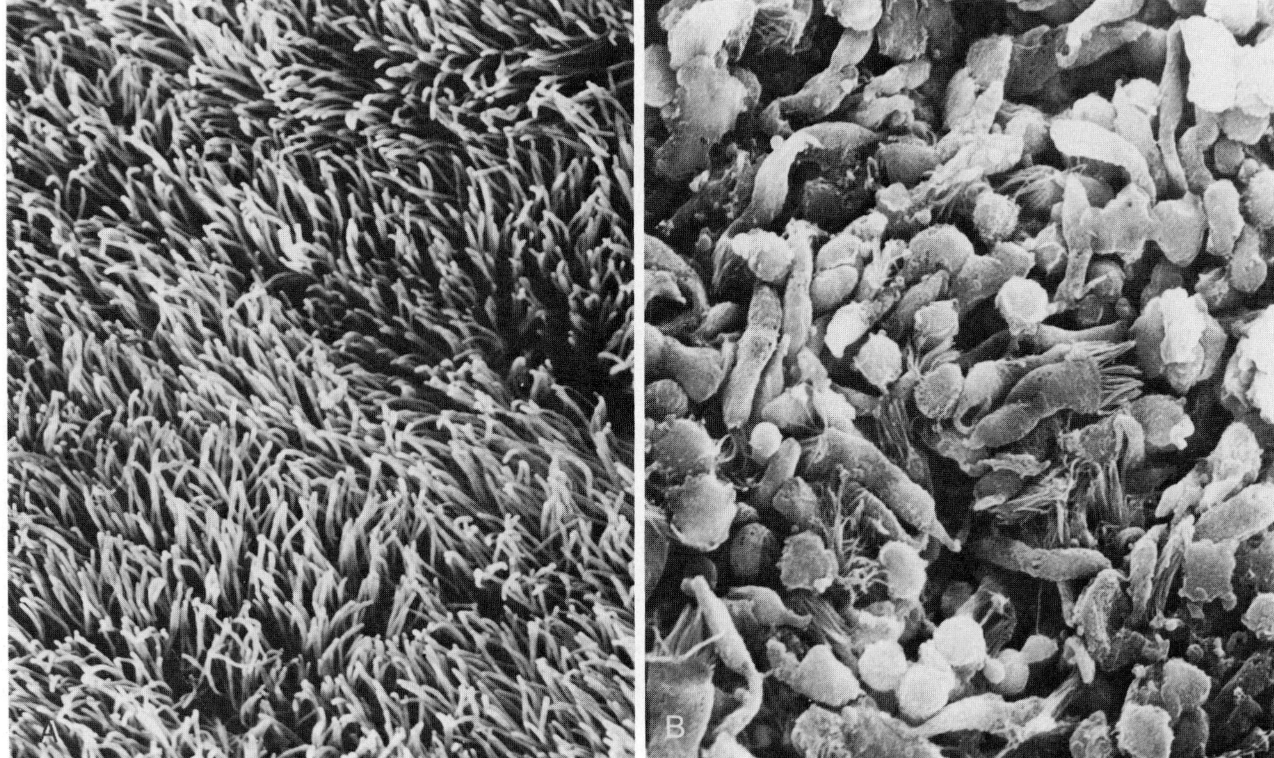

Figure 79–2. Scanning electronic micrograph of the respiratory epithelium. *A*, Normal endothelium (the cells are covered by cilia). *B*, Respiratory cells that have lost their cilia due to erosion by the tracheal tube cuff.

tenoid and cricoid cartilages.[37] Comprehensive endoscopic evaluation suggests inflammation of the true vocal cords in 68%, posterior commissure in 29%, false vocal cords in 29%, glottis in 21%, closed folds in 18%, and arytenoid cartilage area in 11% of the patients examined.[20] Using a grading scale, such lesions have been described as mild in 36%, moderate in 24%, severe in 22%, and complete subglottic obstruction in 15%.[11]

Tracheal Tube Problems

Complications of tracheal intubation can be attributed to the separate tube and cuff components. The presence even of a cuffless tube has resulted in severe laryngeal injury, discovered at autopsy.[40] These effects may be due to tracheal tube characteristics such as size, tip design, rigidity, position, shape, or other distinguishing qualities.[19] There is a clear association between endotracheal tube diameter and complications (Table 79–2).[41] The tracheal tube injury is primarily localized to the posterior glottis, where pressures of 200 to 400 mm Hg are exerted by the elastic recoil force of regular polyvinylchloride (PVC) tubes, somewhat lessened by a narrower tube. The nondeformable round tube exerts lateral pressure on the arytenoid cartilages, where it is wedged between the vocal cords (see Fig. 79–1*C* and *D*).[42] This relationship depends on the external diameter of the tube compared with the available distance between the arytenoid cartilages. The narrowest rigid portion of the larynx is found at the cricoid cartilage, the only solid complete ring of the airway. Particularly in children, a tracheal tube that is too wide will result in circumferential necrosis, healing with serious stenosis, which is difficult to treat surgically (see Fig. 79–1*J*). Thus, even a 7-mm internal diameter (ID) tube is sometimes too large for women, whereas an 8-mm ID tube is often acceptable for the larger interarytenoid space in men. Clinical examination of tubes of various sizes suggests that, although laryngeal wall pressure is decreased by smaller tubes, the sealing cuff pressure required for effective ventilation may increase as tube diameter decreases. Because the smaller tubes have a smaller cuff resting diameter in relation to the trachea, they fail to act as large-diameter, high-volume cuffs.[43] Thus, the most effective regimen

TABLE 79–2. Tracheal Tube Sizes

Inner Diameter (mm)	*Approximate Outer Diameter (mm)*	*Length (mm)*
2.0	3.0	140
2.5	3.6	140
3.0	4.3	160
3.5	4.9	180
4.0	5.6	200
4.5	6.2	220
5.0	6.9	240
5.5	7.5	270
6.0	8.2	280
6.5	8.9	290
7.0	9.5	300
7.5	10.2	310
8.0	10.8	320
8.5	11.4	320
9.0	12.1	320
9.5	12.8	320
10.0	13.5	320

(Modified with permission from International Standards Organization: International standard 5361-2: Tracheal tubes: Part 2. Orotracheal tubes of Magill type [plain and cuffed]. Geneva, Switzerland, International Standards Organization, 1993.)

is to use an appropriately sized tube based on laryngeal diameter with a cuff diameter of more than 30 mm in adults, which is required for an effective seal at approximately 25 cm H_2O of intracuff pressure.

Conventionally shaped, semicircular tubes do not conform with the patient's airway anatomy and exert undue high pressure posteriorly in the larynx (see Fig. 79–1*K*). A most promising new development in minimizing the complication rate inherent to the tube itself is the anatomically shaped tube (see Fig. 79–1*L*). This tube design uses an anteroposterior configuration that conforms with the human airway anatomy and minimizes those posterior deformation forces that result in laryngeal damage.[44] This relationship was first explored by Lindholm, who suggested that deformation forces were minimal with an anatomically shaped tube (30–41 g) compared with PVC (230–296 g) and red rubber (1000 g) tubes. These differences were accentuated as tracheal tube size increased.[45, 46]

Recently, laboratory viscoelastic tests to predict the mechanical consequences of intubation were described by a French group that mainly confirmed previous findings (see Table 79–2).[47] Furthermore, when used clinically, the anatomic tube resulted in a decreased incidence of moderate and severe laryngeal injury and less postintubation complaints of hoarseness and sore throat.[48, 49] Use of soft tracheal tubes composed of silicone rubber also results in decreased posterior laryngeal pressure.[46] However, one clinical trial suggested equivalent isolated arytenoid and tracheal damage (mainly because of tube diameter and cuff pressure), but posterior laryngeal damage to the interarytenoid area and over the cricoid plate is still minimized by the Lindholm tube.[15] This is crucial because these lesions posteriorly at the arytenoid cartilages and the upper part of the cricoid cartilage are the cause of laryngeal scarring, fixation, and stenosis.[19] Such sequelae are almost impossible to correct and lead to lifelong impairment of breathing and phonation. It is the authors' opinion that the result of a peg board test giving the approximate value of the recoil pressure at the cricoid cartilage should be provided by tracheal tube manufacturers so that the clinicians may choose the least traumatizing tube for each situation.[46]

The limiting factor in minimizing tube size is the increasing respiratory gas flow resistance, imposing increased work for the patient with each spontaneous breath. There is a linear relationship between the pressure gradient and flow. The pressure gradient required is decreased with a larger diameter, shorter, and straighter tube. The position of the tube in the airway is also significant; a concentric intratracheal location sufficiently above the carina to prevent obstruction is clearly advantageous.[50] The resistance of gas flow may be quantified as work of breathing, which is inversely proportional to the tube diameter. Thus, the work of breathing is greater with tubes of 6- to 7-mm ID, sometimes used for nasal or emergency intubation, compared with tubes of 8- to 9-mm ID.[51] In other words, one must balance the more traumatizing effect of larger tubes against increased work of breathing through narrower tubes.

The next significant correlate is the tube composition. These intubation devices are tested for safety and designated IT (implantation tested) according to the U.S. Pharmacopeia XVII or Z79-certified by the American National Standards Institute.[52]

The issues regarding the nasotracheal intubation route are complex, with a clear dichotomy between those that support or reject its use. The most common complication is bleeding, occurring in roughly 45% of nasotracheally intubated patients, usually without adequate nasal mucosa preparation.[53] However, in the intensive care unit (ICU), the most important issue is iatrogenic sinusitis. Among the causes is decreased nasal mucociliary clearance, which can be detected after extubation by a radiopaque disk method with correlation to difficult or prolonged intubation, resulting in mechanical trauma to the surface of the epithelium.[54] The incidence of sinusitis is considerably higher with nasal (43%) than with oral (2%) tubes.[55] Infection occurs on the ipsilateral side in 42% and on the contralateral side in 27% of patients. Sinusitis may require drainage but does not seem to affect mortality.[55] Nasotracheal intubation is most often associated with maxillary or sphenoid sinusitis, followed by ethmoid and frontal sinus problems.[56] The incidence is related to the duration of intubation, with about 33% affected after 3 days and 100% of patients involved after 1 week. However, the majority of cases (88%) resolve within 1 week of extubation.[56]

The clinical significance of sinusitis needs to be examined in the context of bacteremia and sepsis. The incidence of bacteremia is common with nasotracheal intubation but rarely occurs with orotracheal intubation.[57] True sepsis occurs in 7% of those with paranasal sinusitis and more commonly after emergency intubation than elective cases.[58] Patients are predisposed by a history of diabetes mellitus or steroid use. Diagnosis is achieved by computed tomography or plain radiography. A decision must be made whether to extubate, change to orotracheal intubation, or tracheotomize. Topical decongestants, antihistamines, and antibiotics are indicated in these cases.

The debate concerning the advisability of nasal intubation remains active. Some investigators believe that the nasal route may be safe for long-term (3–63 days) intubation and may be associated with half the laryngeal damage of oral intubation.[59] However, others suggest that nasal intubation takes two and one-half times longer to perform than oral intubation and has a significant rate of bleeding (45%) and septicemia (9%). Were it not for greater comfort and less laryngeal injury, it would offer no significant advantage.[53] The development of laryngeal injuries caused by tracheal tubes has been summarized by Benjamin (Fig. 79–3).[19]

Cuff Problems

Traditionally, the cuff of the tracheal tube has caused more severe complications than the tube itself. However, these cuff problems have decreased, both in frequency and severity, with the common, almost exclusive use of large-diameter, large-volume cuffs with soft, moderately compliant, thin walls. These are inflated to 25 cm H_2O at the end of exhalation. The intracuff pressure should be monitored frequently or continuously to avoid tracheal mucosal injury and, as mentioned previously, should not be allowed to exceed 30 cm H_2O. During the inspiratory phase of positive-pressure ventilation, the cuff pressure will passively increase to or just above peak airway pressure. The cuff volume simply decreases with a concomitant elevation of pressure, but the cuff still expands its diameter to seal the trachea because of excess cuff resting diameter.

Standard monitoring uses a three-way stopcock and a mercury sphygmomanometer to sense cuff pressure (Portex, Keene, NH), a simple system that is 99% accurate to within $\pm$ 2 mm Hg.[60] Direct cuff to tracheal wall pressure sensing has been described in research protocols using a Teflon envelop positioned between the cuff and tracheal wall, which is able to document pressures as low as 1 to 2 mm Hg.[61]

The effect of peak airway pressure is usually not appreciated as an important factor in cuff-induced mucosal injury if only exhalation cuff pressure is considered.[50] In addition, the monitored proximal airway pressure does not reflect

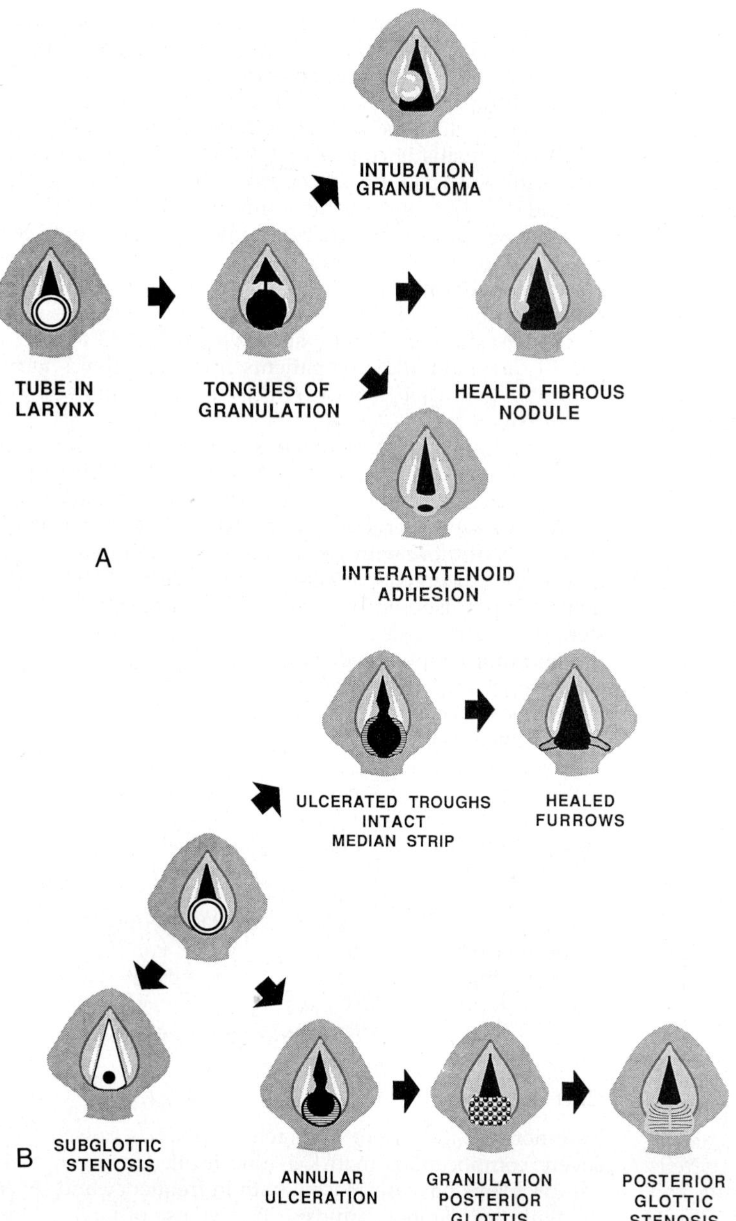

Figure 79–3. *A,* Development of three types of sequelae following endotracheal tube–induced laryngeal injury. Tongues of granulation may cause vocal cord granulomas or fibrous nodules, which are easy to remove without causing functional impairment. As long as interarytenoid adhesions leave the posterior commissure intact, it is usually possible to resect the fibrous band and restore adequate laryngeal function. *B,* Prolonged tracheal intubation may also lead to the formation of ulcerated troughs. Trough healing results in the creation of "furrows," which may cause a problem referred to as "leaking voice," which occurs when air loss causes phonation difficulties. A circumferential subglottic stenosis as well as posterior glottic stenosis are conditions that are extremely difficult to correct surgically. (From Benjamin B: Prolonged intubation injuries of the larynx: Endoscopic diagnosis, classification, and treatment. Ann Otol Rhinol Laryngol Suppl 1993; 160:1.)

actual distal airway pressure (below the tube), which is different (i.e., lower during inspiration and higher during exhalation).[62] Furthermore, an awake patient often fights the ventilator with a significant increase in airway pressure at oral suctioning (twofold), endotracheal suctioning (threefold), coughing, and movement.[63]

Cuff damage initially manifests itself clinically as tracheal dilatation with onset after 4 to 8 days, especially with small-diameter, high-pressure, low-compliance cuffs.[64] Scanning electron microscopy of canine trachea from autopsy sections documents complete absence of cilia after short use of an inflated small-diameter cuff. Mucous membrane damage occurs, especially over the tracheal cartilages with minimal cuff inflation already after 2 hours.[65] In dogs, these changes are partially reversed after 2 days and completely resolved by 1 week. Similar observations have been made in human anatomic specimens using standard tracheal tubes and cuffs.[65]

The first tracheal tube cuffs used were of the low-volume, high-pressure variety. Currently, the standard is a large-diameter, high-volume, low-pressure cuff, which causes a lower and more evenly distributed cuff to tracheal wall pressure with less mucosal damage (Fig. 79–4). A canine model suggests that a low-pressure cuff demonstrates minimal gross or microscopic lesions compared with the high-pressure variety, which, with prolonged use, causes circumferential erosion, mucosal ulceration, and cartilage destruction.[66] Tracheal wall pressure is due to a complex interaction of tracheal diameter and compliance versus cuff diameter, compliance, inflation pressure, and symmetry.

Intubated ICU patients are at risk for further complications after general anesthesia, including use of nitrous oxide (N_2O), which results in spontaneous elevation of cuff pressure. This effect occurs when oxygen and N_2O diffuse into the air-filled cuff. Partial gas pressures inside the cuff will equilibrate with the outside, causing a progressive increase in cuff volume and pressure. Clinical trials have suggested that this effect is minimized in low-pressure, high-volume

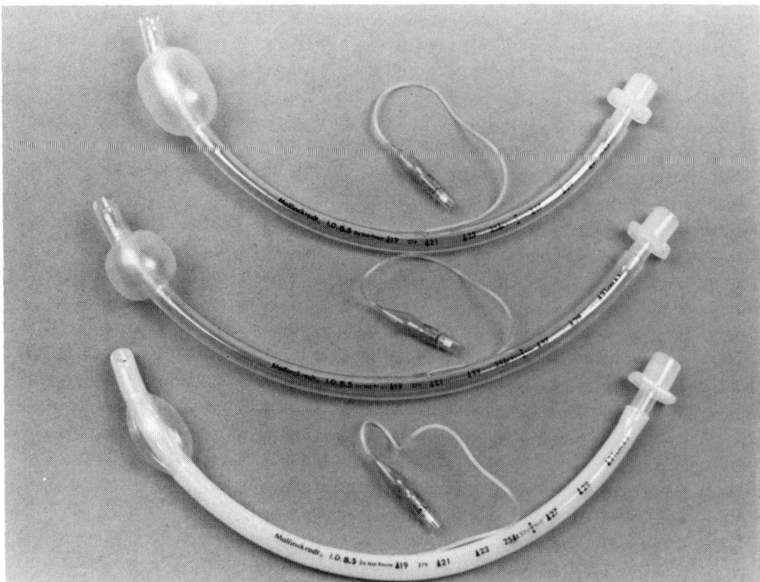

Figure 79–4. Different cuff designs. *Top,* A large-diameter, high-volume, low-pressure cuff. *Middle,* An intermediate-diameter, -volume, and -pressure cuff. *Bottom,* A small-diameter, low-volume, high-pressure cuff.

cuffs and may be prevented by filling the cuff with the used anesthetic gas mixture. Cuff pressure has been monitored and has demonstrated a fivefold increase during general anesthesia with N_2O inhalation. Modern tracheal tubes may reach cuff pressures of 30 to 100 mm Hg within 2 to 3 hours.[67] Gas diffusion is governed by N_2O concentration, wall thickness, and compliance of the cuff. The "rediffusion system" allows cuff-resorbed N_2O to diffuse into a high-compliance pilot balloon in which reversed diffusion takes place, resulting in reduction of cuff pressure toward the original setting.[68]

Lomholt tested different resting-diameter cuffs in a tracheal model with a compliance similar to that of the human trachea. The lung model was ventilated with different peak airway pressures up to 6 kPa (60 cm H_2O).[69] The lateral wall pressure (LWP) at end-expiration was registered when the cuff achieved a leak of 10 mL ± 1 mL per inspiration. For cuffs with a resting diameter of 31 mm or greater, a seal was present below 3 kPa LWP at end-expiration even when peak airway pressures reached 6 kPa. These cuffs could be regarded as true low-pressure, high-volume, large-diameter cuffs. Cuffs with diameters of 25 to 29 mm had to be inflated to an LWP of more than 3 kPa to provide a seal at peak airway pressures exceeding 3 kPa. These cuffs acted similarly to high-pressure, low-volume, small-diameter cuffs. Lomholt concluded that the minimum diameter for a low-pressure, large-volume cuff should be approximately one and one-half times the tracheal diameter when high inflation pressures are used.[69]

More moderate approaches suggest that the best cuff may be the intermediate-volume variety. However, it is not possible to rely on monitored intracuff pressure as an indication of cuff to tracheal wall pressure if the cuff diameter is too small for such pressure equilibrium in patients with a wide trachea. Both large- and small-volume cuffs may cause experimental damage.[50, 70] The risk of cuff herniation between the vocal cords with a malpositioned large-volume cuffed tube has also been described.[71] Although the enlarged surface area of a large-volume, thin-walled cuff results in less severe damage than the low-volume, high-pressure cuff, large-volume, thick-walled cuffs may still cause specific lesions as a result of redundant excessive cuff folds.[72] The current consensus is that large-diameter, large-volume cuffs should be used in most patients, although occasional individuals may benefit from use of an intermediate-volume cuff or, in rare circumstances, even a low-volume cuff.

In canine trials, the foam cuff has demonstrated a decreased incidence of mucosal ischemia, ulceration, and cartilage damage.[73] This foam cuff (Bivona, Gary, IN) establishes a tracheal seal from recoil pressure of the foamy material, generating a tracheal wall pressure of approximately 15 cm H_2O, but only if a cuff diameter is chosen that is optimal in relation to the size of the trachea (Fig. 79–5). The seal persists at atmospheric airway pressure, thus preventing aspiration without tracheal damage.[72] Trials of foam cuffs compared with high-volume, low-pressure cuffs suggest less mucosal damage with the former.[74]

Mucosal damage caused by the cuff is also minimized by regulation of pressure compared with monitoring alone. The Lanz pressure-limiting device, for instance, allows maximal cuff pressures of 25 cm H_2O (see Fig. 79–5). If overinflated, cuff volume decreases as excess air moves into the more compliant pilot balloon.[33, 75]

Another significant cuff-related complication is aspiration. Secretions pooled above the cuff may slowly and gradually leak into the trachea, causing subsequent infection.[76] Interestingly, mechanical ventilation compared with spontaneous breathing is protective, with aspiration decreasing from 100% to 55%.[77] The addition of positive end-expiratory pressure further decreases aspiration.[77] Similarly, a cuff system that permits removal of subglottic secretions pooling above the cuff (HiLo evacuation tube, Mallinkrodt) decreases tracheal colonization and the incidence of pneumonia.[78]

Clinical evaluation of cuff design demonstrates that the highest rate of aspiration occurs with the high-volume, low-pressure cuff (56%) followed by the intermediate cuff (39%) and the low-volume, high-pressure (20%) design.[79] The most likely explanation for these results is incorrect intermittent monitoring of intracuff pressure. If the manometer is attached to the cuff inflation tube while reading zero, the cuff pressure will drop momentarily because of the dead space in the measuring device, and aspiration may occur. Although the high-volume, low-pressure cuff minimizes mucosal damage, the aspiration rate may be substantial if the cuff pressure is not maintained at all times.

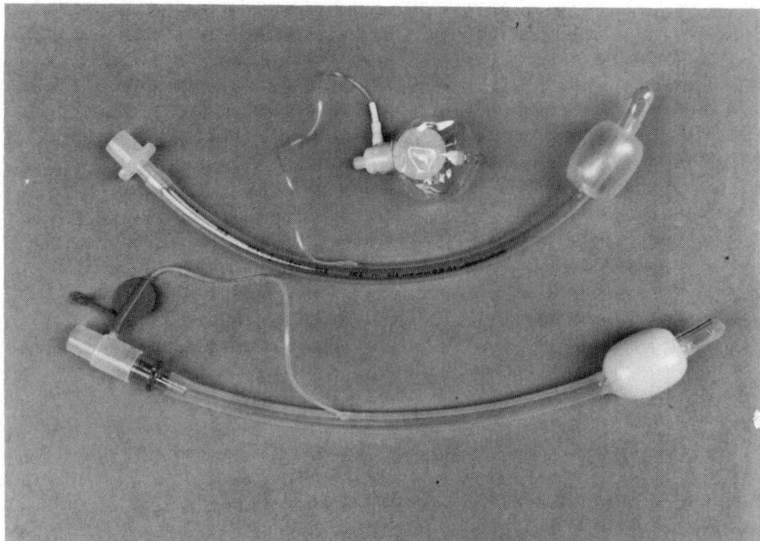

Figure 79–5. Cuff pressure regulating system. *Top,* A Lanz device. *Bottom,* Foam cuff connected to main airway.

SPECIAL TUBES

The double-lumen tube was first described by Carlens.[80] Robertshaw modified the original design because of difficulty with placement and increased resistance with Carlens' tube.[81] Advantages of the double-lumen tube include avoidance of contamination of the unaffected lung from contralateral abscess or hemorrhage during surgery.[82] Double-lumen tubes are increasingly used in patients who undergo single (or bilateral sequential) lung transplantation. Gross difference in compliance between the remaining native and transplanted lung is an indication for continued use of the double-lumen tube postoperatively in the ICU. Disadvantages are due to tube rigidity and include the presence of two cuffs with increased risk of laryngeal and tracheobronchial injury. Air leak and even mainstem bronchial rupture have been reported.[82]

Correct positioning of the double-lumen tube is crucial to its intended function. There are two types of tubes—left sided and right sided—depending on into which mainstem bronchus the distal of the two lumina will enter. With the left-sided tube, positioning is easier because of the longer mainstem bronchus on that side. The distance between the distal opening of the tube and lower cuff margin is 30 mm.[83] The right-sided tube is more complex in its design because the distance between the carina and the right upper lobe bronchus is only about 15 mm. Therefore, this cuff configuration is not symmetric because of the necessary side opening in the distal tube component to permit ventilation of the right upper lobe. This intermediate opening is located 10 to 20 mm from the tube tip. Thus, the right-sided tube has a total of three distal openings, whereas the left-sided tube has only two.

Cadaver studies have revealed an estimated length of the right mainstem bronchus of only 15 versus 19 mm and of the left mainstem bronchus of 44 versus 49 mm in females and males, respectively.[83] Consequently, fiberoptic bronchoscopy confirmation of tube position is essential to minimize complications. It has been recommended to place the left-sided tube with its distal tip 29 cm ± 1 cm from the teeth with 1 cm added or subtracted for each 10-cm height difference from a 170-cm normal height.[84] The right-sided tube has a decreased margin of safety for anatomic reasons discussed previously. Therefore, the left-sided double-lumen tube is favored in most situations. The double-lumen tube has been used in 48,000 anesthetic procedures with a 0.4% rate of tracheal rupture in patients predisposed for this complication as a result of tuberculosis or bronchitis.[85] The left-sided tube has been associated with acute right mainstem bronchus obstruction by the distal cuff if the tube tip is too close to the carina.[86] Tracheal rupture has also been reported with PVC tubes.[82] Clinical evaluation further reveals that other complications such as unsuccessful intubation, dislodgement, and malposition manifested as hypoxemia are more common with the Carlens (50%) and Robertshaw (23%) tubes than the newer PVC tubes (4%).[87]

The right-sided endobronchial blocker tube (Portex, Ltd., Hythe Kent, UK) has been found to have an efficacy equivalent to that of the standard double-lumen tube.[88] This tube is also used postoperatively for independent lung ventilation with separate regulation of ventilatory parameters in cases of different lung compliance.[89]

TUBE POSITION AND FIXATION

Complications may be minimized by attention to detail concerning tracheal tube position and fixation. Laryngeal damage is worsened in those who undergo head extension positioning, excessive suctioning, and states of agitation.[90] The extent of damage is partly due to the amount of movement of the tube shaft relative to the arytenoid cartilages and posterior cricoid plate. Furthermore, the tube tip may be directed into the anterior tracheal wall.[91]

Initial tube position may be estimated from various anatomic landmarks. The following distances are of importance: from teeth to vocal cords (12–15 cm), from vocal cords to carina (10–15 cm), and from tube tip to carina (2–6 cm).[49, 92] Clinically, Goodman's criteria suggest a 5 cm ± 2 cm tracheal tube tip distance to carina, which has demonstrated no accidental extubation and only 1% endobronchial intubation.[91] Essential to intensive care is the dynamic description of tube variability in which head flexion moves the tube tip approximately 2 cm closer to the carina, extension moves it approximately 2 cm away from the carina, and lateral rotation moves it 1 cm away from carina, suggesting that the appropriate tube tip position is in the middle third of the trachea.[93] However, this means that part of the cuff sometimes is located in the lower half of the larynx because the distance from the tube tip to the upper end of the cuff

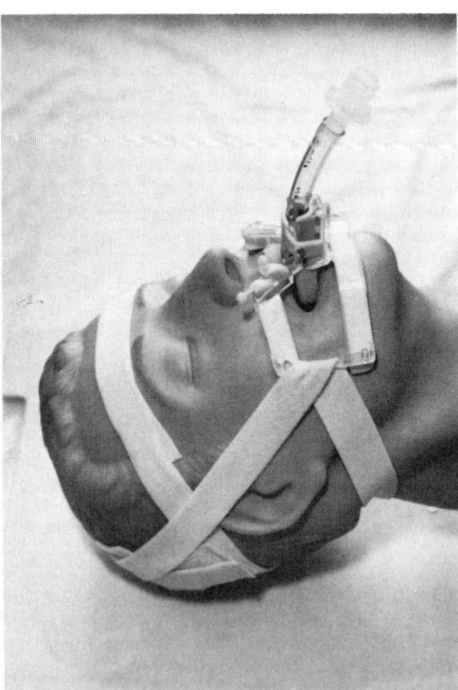

Figure 79–6. The ReviveEasy PtL Airway used with the Secure Easy endotracheal tube holder. (Courtesy of Respironics, Murrysville, PA, and of IPI Medical Products, Chicago, IL, respectively.)

in most tubes is 5 to 6 cm. Therefore, it might be safer to place the tube tip at the border between the lower and middle thirds of the trachea (i.e., 3–4 cm above the carina).

Tracheal tube fixation should be stable and comfortable and allow emergency access to the patient. The most stable fixation is provided by buccal or oral devices used in oral and maxillofacial surgery, but these systems are uncomfortable to the patient.[94] The emergency situation is addressed by tube fixation using various adhesive tape strategies. The Secure Easy fixation device (IPI Medical Products, Chicago, IL) is composed of a Velcro wrap and plastic tube holder (Fig. 79–6). This device has proven superior to adhesive tape in preventing tube displacement, as measured clinically and radiographically.[95] However, cutaneous breakdown may still occur as with adhesive tape.

ASSESSMENT OF INJURIES AND THERAPEUTIC INTERVENTION

The most simplistic analysis of complications may be addressed by monitoring of cuff size on routine chest radiography.[64] The appearance of an overdistended cuff often precedes tracheal dilatation, subcutaneous emphysema, or pneumomediastinum.[96] The most sensitive diagnostic tool is bedside video laryngoscopic assessment, which has been used in the ICU setting, demonstrating vocal cord ulceration or subtle motion abnormalities or paresis.[97] Historically, xerotomography and tracheography have been supplanted by computed tomography, with the capability of diagnosing a wide variety of conditions including fracture or dislocation of laryngeal cartilages and subcutaneous emphysema.[98]

The management of immediate postextubation tracheostenosis includes both medical and surgical approaches. Medical therapy includes inhaled beclomethasone, intralesional triamcinolone, and systemic methylprednisolone, resulting in edema resolution and improved inspiratory and expiratory flow.[99, 100] However, large granulomas must be removed endoscopically. In patients with significant postintubation fibrotic tracheostenosis, surgical therapy has been most successful with resection and end-to-end anastomosis of the trachea.[101] If the stenosis also involves the lower larynx, partial cricoid resection may be combined with tracheal resection. However, endoscopic laser surgery is becoming increasingly common in less pronounced tracheostenosis and in different types of laryngostenosis.[100]

TIMING OF TRACHEOSTOMY

One of the most controversial issues in intensive care medicine is the timing of tracheostomy to avoid complications from prolonged intubation. The incidence of complications is strongly correlated with duration of translaryngeal intubation, but prolonged intubation has been tolerated by the nasal route for up to 63 days and oral route for as much as 155 days and even longer in occasional patients.[59, 102] The optimal timing for tracheostomy has been suggested to range from 24 hours to 3 weeks of translaryngeal intubation based on incidence of complications, with no clear consensus.[103, 104] It has to be emphasized that the less traumatizing the tube, the longer that tracheal intubation may be tolerated. Thus, it is not possible to provide specific time limits for all kinds of tubes. Tube size and configuration play important roles regarding the advisable period of intubation in each individual case. Analysis of tracheostomy timing suggests that 3% of patients are intubated for fewer than 3 days, 29% for 3 to 7 days, 50% for 7 to 14 days, 10% for 14 to 21 days, and 6% for longer than 21 days.[105] Prospective clinical trials demonstrate fewer infection complications in patients with early tracheostomy (within 5 days).[106] Mechanical complications are increased in those patients who remain intubated for more than 7 days.[107] This mechanical complication rate is minimized for those tracheotomized immediately, with most laryngeal damage occurring after 1 week.[108] However, an early tracheostomy trial (3 days) revealed an eightfold increase in the frequency of infectious complications.[109]

We must realize that the complication rate of prolonged intubation may decrease because of improved airway care and tube design. Laryngeal damage of tracheal intubation must also be balanced against the early bacterial colonization and subsequent airway infection associated with tracheostomy. Recommendations suggesting a specific duration of tracheal intubation with the least traumatizing tube followed by tracheostomy should be individualized according to the patient's diagnosis, condition, predicted clinical outcome, and laryngeal appearance at repeated examination.

Clinical trials of available tracheal tubes allow us to draw some conclusions. An evaluation of 500 intubated patients revealed that use of low-cuff pressure, PVC tube composition, and an N_2O diffusion system results in fewer complications, such as voice change or odynophagia with an incidence of 51% and 24%, respectively.[110] Furthermore, the addition of a cuff pressure regulation system results in less tracheal damage and aspiration compared with a high-volume, low-pressure cuff without such pressure regulation system. Thus, the ideal tracheal tube cuff should be thin walled and of moderate compliance with a resting diameter that is 50% wider than the trachea. According to the International Standards Organization, the cuff resting diameter should be indicated on the unit package to allow proper choice.[111]

References

1. Kambic V, Radsel Z: Intubation lesions of the larynx. Br J Anaesth 1978; 50:587.
2. Gaynor EB, Greenberg SB: Untoward sequelae of prolonged intubation. Laryngoscope 1985; 95:1461.
3. Atalic MR, Burke JF: Severe low-pressure cuff tracheal injury in burn patients. Intensive Care Med 1981; 7:89.
4. Realini E: Vocal and laryngo-tracheal sequelae of prolonged intubation at the university medical clinic of the cantonal hospital at Lausanne. ORL J Otorhinolaryngol Relat Spec 1976; 38(Suppl 1):94.
5. Tonkin JP, Harrison GA: The effect on the larynx of prolonged endotracheal intubation. Med J Aust 1966; 2:581.
6. Colice GL, Stukel TA, Dain B: Laryngeal complications of prolonged intubation. Chest 1989; 96:877.
7. Lanza DC, Parnes SM, Koltai PJ: Early complications of airway management in head-injury patients. Laryngoscope 1990; 100:958.
8. Orlowski JP, Ellis NG, Amin NP, et al: Complications of airway intrusion in 100 consecutive cases in a pediatric ICU. Crit Care Med 1980; 8:324.
9. Nowak P, Cohn AM, Guidice MA: Airway complications in patients with closed-head injuries. Am J Otolaryngol 1987; 8:91.
10. Stauffer JL, Olsen DE, Petty TL: Complications and consequences of endotracheal intubation and tracheotomy: A prospective study of 150 critically ill adult patients. Am J Med 1981; 70:65.
11. Sellery GR, Worth A, Greenway RE: Late complications of prolonged tracheal intubation. Can Anaesth Soc J 1978; 25:140.
12. Hsu S, Dreisbach JN, Charlifue SW: Glottic and tracheal stenosis in spinal cord injured patients. Paraplegia 1987; 25:136.
13. Boles JM: Upper respiratory tract infections in patients with tracheal intubation. Rev Praticien 1990; 40:2341.
14. Forbes AR, Gamsu G: Lung mucociliary clearance anesthesia with spontaneous and controlled ventilation. Am Rev Respir Dis 1979; 120:857.
15. Eckerbom B, Lindholm CE, Alexopoulos C: Airway lesions caused by prolonged intubation with standard and with anatomically shaped tracheal tubes: A post-mortem study. Acta Anaesthesiol Scand 1986; 30:366.
16. Comer PB, Gibson RL, Weeks DB, et al: Airway maintenance in patients with long-term endotracheal intubation. Crit Care Med 1976; 4:211.
17. Lowy FD, Carlisle PS, Adams A: The incidence of nosocomial pneumonia following urgent endotracheal intubation. Infect Control 1987; 8:245.
18. Chilla R, Gabriel P: The arthritis of the cricoarytenoid joint: A rare postintubation complication and its novel treatment. Laryngol Rhinol Otol (Stuttg) 1976; 55:389.
19. Benjamin B: Prolonged intubation injuries of the larynx: Endoscopic diagnosis, classification, and treatment. Ann Otol Rhinol Laryngol (Suppl) 1993; 160:1.
20. Cavo JW Jr: True vocal cord paralysis following intubation. Laryngoscope 1985; 95:1352.
21. Gibbin KP, Eggington MJ: Bilateral vocal cord paralysis following endotracheal intubation. Br J Anaesth 1981; 53:1091.
22. Levin PA: Hypopharyngeal perforation: An untoward complication of endotracheal intubation. Arch Otolaryngol 1980; 106:578.
23. Bein T, Lenhart FP, Berger H, et al: Rupture of the trachea during difficult intubation. Anaesthesist 1991; 40:456.
24. Heath LK, Peirce TH: Retropharyngeal abscess following endotracheal intubation. Chest 1977; 72:776.
25. Abbey NC, Green DE, Cicale MJ: Massive tracheal necrosis complicating endotracheal intubation. Chest 1989; 95:459.
26. Rinecker H, Schvet T: Arterio-tracheal fistula during long-term intubation of an awake patient. Anaesthesist 1979; 28:180.
27. Payne DK, Anderson W, Romero MD, et al: Tracheoesophageal fistula formation in intubated patients: Risk factors and treatment with high-frequency jet ventilation. Chest 1990; 98:161.
28. Bishop MJ, Hibbard AJ, Fink BR: Laryngeal injury in a dog model of prolonged endotracheal intubation. Anesthesiology 1985; 62:770.
29. Windsor HM, Shanahan MX, Cherian K: Tracheal injury following prolonged intubation. Aust N Z J Surg 1976; 46:18.
30. Belson TP: Cuff induced tracheal injury in dogs following prolonged intubation. Laryngoscope 1983; 93:549.
31. Schmidt WA, Schaap RN, Mortensen JD: Immediate mucosal effects of short-term, soft-cuff, endotracheal intubation: A light and scanning electron microscopic study. Arch Pathol Lab Med 1979; 103:516.
32. Nishino T, Sugimori, Hiraga, et al: Effects of tracheal irritation and hypercapnia on tracheal smooth muscle in humans. J Appl Physiol 1990; 69:419.
33. Seegobin RD, van Hasselt GL: Endotracheal cuff pressure and tracheal mucosal blood flow: Endoscopic study of effects of four large volume cuffs. Br Med J 1984; 288:965.
34. Joh S, Matsuura H, Kotani Y, et al: Change in tracheal blood flow during endotracheal intubation. Acta Anaesthesiol Scand 1987; 31:300.
35. Nordin U, Lindholm CE, Wolgast M: Blood flow in the rabbit tracheal mucosa under normal conditions and under the influence of tracheal intubation. Acta Anaesthesiol Scand 1977; 21:81.
36. Gould SJ, Howard S: The histopathology of the larynx in the neonate following endotracheal intubation. J Pathol 1985; 146:301.
37. Lindholm CE: Prolonged endotracheal intubation. Acta Anaesthesiol Scand (Suppl) 1970; 33:1.
38. Colice GL: Resolution of laryngeal injury following translaryngeal intubation. Am Rev Respir Dis 1992; 145:361.
39. Donnelly WH: Histopathology of endotracheal intubation: An autopsy study of 99 cases. Arch Pathol 1969; 88:511.
40. Trim CM: Complications associated with the use of the cuffless endotracheal tube in the horse. J Am Vet Med Assoc 1984; 185:541.
41. Santos PM, Afrassiabi A, Weymuller EA Jr: Prospective studies evaluating the standard endotracheal tube and a prototype endotracheal tube. Ann Otol Rhinol Laryngol 1989; 98:935.
42. Weymuller EA, Bishop MJ, Hibbard AW, et al: Quantification of intralaryngeal pressure exerted by endotracheal tubes. Ann Otol Rhinol Laryngol 1983; 92:444.
43. Lee TS: Routine monitoring of intracuff pressure. Chest 1992; 102:1309.
44. Alexopoulos C, Larsson SG, Lindholm CE: Anatomical shape of the airway. Acta Anaesthesiol Scand 1983; 27:185.
45. Lindholm CE, Carroll RG: Evaluation of tube deformation pressure in vitro. Crit Care Med 1975; 3:196.
46. Steen JA, Lindholm CE, Brdlik CG: Tracheal tube forces on the posterior larynx: Index of laryngeal loading. Crit Care Med 1982; 10:186.
47. Gustin B, G'Sell C, Cochelin B, et al: Influence of the instrinsic viscoelastic properties of the tube on the forces undergone by the anatomic structures during an endotracheal intubation. *In*: Tracheal Intubation. Anne-Marie Cros, Gerard Janvier (Eds). Baltimore, MD, Williams & Wilkins, 1992.
48. Alexopoulos C, Lindholm CE: Airway complaints and laryngeal pathology after intubation with an anatomically shaped endotracheal tube. Acta Anaesthesiol Scand 1983; 27:339.
49. Lindholm CE: Experience with a new orotracheal tube. Acta Otolaryngol 1973; 75:389.
50. Homi J, Notcutt W, Jones JJ, et al: A method for comparing endotracheal cuffs: A controlled study of tracheal trauma in dogs. Br J Anaesth 1978; 50:435.
51. Shapiro M, Wilson RK, Casar G, et al: Work of breathing through different sized endotracheal tubes. Crit Care Med 1986; 14:1028.
52. Stetson JB, Guess WL: Causes of damage to tissues by polymers and elastomers used in the fabrication of tracheal devices. Anesthesiology 1970; 33:635.
53. Depoix JP, Malbezin S, Videcoq M, et al: Oral intubation v. nasal intubation in adult cardiac surgery. Br J Anaesth 1987; 59:167.
54. Elwany S, Mekhamer A: Effect of nasotracheal intubation on nasal mucociliary clearance. Br J Anaesth 1987; 59:755.
55. Saylord F, Gaussorgues P, Marti-Flich J, et al: Nosocomial maxillary sinusitis during mechanical ventilation: A prospective comparison of orotracheal versus the nasotracheal route for intubation. Intensive Care Med 1990; 16:390.

56. Fassoulaki A, Pamouktsoglou P: Prolonged nasotracheal intubation and its association with inflammation of paranasal sinuses. Anesth Analg 1989; 69:50.
57. Cannon LA, Gardner W, Treen L, et al: The incidence of bacteremia associated with emergent intubation: Relevance to prophylaxis against bacterial endocarditis. Ohio Med 1990; 86:596.
58. Deutschman CS, Wilton P, Sinow J, et al: Paranasal sinusitis associated with nasotracheal intubation: A frequently unrecognized and treatable source of sepsis. Crit Care Med 1986; 14:111.
59. Glumcher FS, Treshchinskii AI, Kravchenko EP, et al: Clinical use of long-term nasotracheal intubation. Anesteziol Reanimatol 1989; 1:42.
60. Bouvier JR: Measuring tracheal tube cuff pressures: Tool and technique. Heart Lung 1981; 10:686.
61. Lomholt N: A device for measuring the lateral wall cuff pressure of endotracheal tubes. Acta Anaesthesiol Scand 1992; 36:775.
62. Badenhorst CH: Changes in tracheal cuff pressure during respiratory support. Crit Care Med 1987; 15:300.
63. Ao EL: Continuous dynamic record of intracuff pressure in endotracheal intubated patients. Kao-Hsiung I Hsueh o Hsueh Tsa Chih 1991; 7:1.
64. Honig EG, Francis PB: Persistent tracheal dilatation: Onset after brief mechanical ventilation with a "soft-cuff" endotracheal tube. South Med J 1979; 72:487.
65. Klainer AS, Turndorf H, Wu W, et al: Surface alterations due to endotracheal intubation. Am J Med 1975; 58:674.
66. Cooper JD, Grillo HC: Experimental production and prevention of injury due to cuffed tracheal tubes. Surg Gynecol Obstet 1969; 129:1235.
67. Revenas B, Lindholm CE: Pressure and volume changes in tracheal tube cuffs during anaesthesia. Acta Anaesthesiol Scand 1976; 20:321.
68. Brandt L, Pokar H, Ren D, et al: Cuff pressure changes due to diffusion of nitrous oxide: A contribution to the question of the in vivo-diffusion: Area of the cuff. Anaesthesist 1982; 31:345.
69. Lomholt N: Personal communication, 1993.
70. Homi J, Notcutt W, Jones J, et al: A method for comparing endotracheal cuffs. Br J Anaesth 1978; 50:435.
71. Treffers R, de Lange JJ: An unusual case of cuff herniation. Acta Anaesthesiol Belg 1989; 40:87.
72. Loeser EA, Hodges M, Gliedman J, et al: Tracheal pathology following short-term intubation with low- and high-pressure endotracheal tube cuffs. Anesth Analg 1978; 57:577.
73. Weymuller EA Jr: Laryngeal injury from prolonged endotracheal intubation. Laryngoscope 1988; 98:1.
74. Kamen JM, Wilkinson CJ: A new low-pressure cuff for endotracheal tubes. Anesthesiology 1971; 34:482.
75. McGinnis GE, Shively JG, Patterson RL, et al: An engineering analysis of intratracheal tube cuffs. Anesth Analg 1971; 50:557.
76. Whiffler K, Andrew WK, Thomas RG: The hazardous cuffed endotracheal tube: Aspiration and extubation. S Afr Med J 1982; 61:240.
77. Janson BA, Poulton TJ: Does PEEP reduce the incidence of aspiration around endotracheal tubes? Can Anaesth Soc J 1986; 33:157.
78. Mahul P, Auboyer C, Jospe R, et al: Prevention of nosocomial pneumonia in intubated patients: Respective role of mechanical subglottic secretions drainage and stress ulcer prophylaxis. Intensive Care Med 1992; 18:20.
79. Spray SB, Zuidema GD, Cameron JL: Aspiration pneumonia: Incidence of aspiration with endotracheal tubes. Am J Surg 1976; 131:701.
80. Carlens E: A new flexible double-lumen catheter for bronchospirometry. J Thorac Surg 1949; 18:742.
81. Robertshaw FL: Low resistance double lumen endobronchial tubes. Br J Anaesth 1962; 34:576.
82. Joos D, Zeiler D, Muhrer K, et al: Bronchial rupture: Diagnosis and therapy of a rare complication of the use of double-lumen tubes. Anaesthesist 1991; 40:291.
83. Benumof JL, Partridge BL, Salvatierra C, et al: Margin of safety in positioning modern double-lumen endotracheal tubes. Anesthesiology 1987; 67:729.
84. Brodsky JB, Benumof JL, Ehrenwerth J, et al: Depth of placement of left double-lumen endobronchial tubes. Anesth Analg 1991; 73:570.
85. Lobo Sanchez M, Reinaldo Lapuerta JA, Tamame Tamame C, et al: Tracheobronchial lesions due to anesthetic procedures: Report of 2 cases. Rev Esp Anestesiol Reanim 1991; 38:51.
86. Homann B: Acute right bronchial blockade following intubation with a left-swing Robertshaw tube. Anaesthesist 1985; 34:91.
87. Burton NA, Watson DC, Brodsky JB, et al: Advantages of a new polyvinyl chloride double-lumen tube in thoracic surgery. Ann Thorac Surg 1983; 36:78.
88. Trazzi R, Nazari S: Clinical experience with a new right-sided endobronchial tube in left main bronchus surgery. J Cardiothorac Anesth 1989; 3:461.
89. Gallagher TJ, Banner MJ, Smith RA: A simplified method of independent lung ventilation. Crit Care Med 1980; 8:396.
90. Schultz-Coulon HJ: Prolonged endotracheal intubation or tracheostomy in children. HNO 1976; 24:283.
91. Neumann OG: Parameters of trauma at posterior subglottic region by long term translaryngeal intubation. Praktische Anaesthesie, Wiederbelebung Und Intensivtherapie 1975; 10:135.
92. Stone DJ, Bogdonoff DL: Airway considerations in the management of patients requiring long-term endotracheal intubation. Anesth Analg 1992; 74:276.
93. Conrardy PA, Goodman LR, Lainge F, et al: Alteration of endotracheal tube position. Crit Care Med 1976; 4:8.
94. Richard P, Perier JF, Marsol P, et al: Intrabuccal fixation technic for oral intubation catheters. Rev Stomatol Chir Maxillofac 1986; 87:402.
95. Tasota FJ, Hoffman LA, Zullo TG: Evaluation of two methods used to stabilize oral endotracheal tubes. Heart Lung 1987; 16:140.
96. Rollins RJ, Tocino I: Early radiographic signs of tracheal rupture. Am J Roentgenol 1987; 148:695.
97. Alessi DM, Hanson DG, Berci G: Bedside videolaryngoscopic assessment of intubation trauma. Ann Otol Rhinol Laryngol 1989; 98:586.
98. Vukanovic S, Sidani AH, Ducommun JC, et al: Tracheal and subglottic lesions following long-standing intubation: A radiological and clinical study. Diagn Imag 1982; 51:224.
99. Braidy J, Breton G, Clement L: Effect of corticosteroids on post-intubation tracheal stenosis. Thorax 1989; 44:753.
100. Maniglia AJ: Conservative surgical management of tracheal stenosis. Otolaryngology 1978; 86:380.
101. Grillo HC: Congenital lesions, neoplasms, and injuries to the trachea. *In*: Surgery of the Chest. 5th ed. Sabiston DC, Spencer FC (Eds). Philadelphia, WB Saunders, 1990.
102. Rashkin MC, Davis T: Acute complications of endotracheal intbuation: Relationship to reintubation, route, urgency, and duration. Chest 1986; 89:165.
103. Berlauk JF: Prolonged endotracheal intubation vs. tracheostomy. Crit Care Med 1986; 14:742.
104. Marsh HM, Gillespie DJ, Baumgartner AE: Timing of tracheostomy in the critically ill patient. Chest 1989; 96:190.
105. Pippin LK, Short DH, Bowes JB: Long-term trachea intubation practice in the United Kingdom. Anaesthesia 1983; 38:791.
106. Aass AS: Complications to tracheostomy and long-term intubation: A follow-up study. Acta Anaesthesiol Scand 1975; 19:127.
107. Whited RE: A prospective study of laryngotracheal sequelae in long-term intubation. Laryngoscope 1984; 94:367.
108. Fuchs HH, Flugel KA, Druschky KF: Tracheotomy or intubation? Problems with long-term intensive care patients. Dtsch Med Wochenschr 1981; 106:1022.
109. El-Naggar M, Sadagopan S, Levine H, et al: Factors influencing choice between tracheostomy and prolonged translaryngeal intubation in acute respiratory failure: A prospective study. Anesth Analg 1976; 55:195.
110. Lipp M, Brandt L, Daublander M: Frequency and severity of throat complaints following general anesthesia with the insertion of various endotracheal tubes. Anaesthesist 1988; 37:758.
111. International Standards Organization: International standard 5361-2. Tracheal tubes: Part 2: Oro-tracheal tubes of Magill type (plain and cuffed). Geneva, Switzerland, International Standards Organization, 1993.

CHAPTER 80

Surgical Airway, Cricothyroidotomy, and Tracheotomy: Procedures, Complications, and Outcome

Rade B. Vukmir, MD • Ake Grenvik, MD, PhD • Carl-Eric Lindholm, MD, PhD

Emergency laryngotracheal intubation is efficacious in approximately 97% of cases.[1] Thus, a surgical airway is needed in only 3% of such emergencies.[2] A summary of indications and contraindications for choice of airway access is presented in Table 80–1.

The need for an immediate surgical airway is evaluated in light of difficulties associated with emergency intubation (e.g., presence of laryngotracheal trauma or a foreign body lodged in the pharyngolaryngeal area). The surgical airway is also considered emergently in cases of suspected cervical spine fracture or severe anatomic deformity associated with oromaxillofacial or laryngeal trauma. Preoperative intubation of patients with known cervical fracture under optimum conditions in one investigation demonstrated new neurologic deficits in 1% to 2% of the patients with no differences based on technique (awake vs. with induction) or route (oral vs. nasal).[3] According to one report,[4] most cervical fractures encountered today occur in motor vehicle accidents (61%), with the following distribution: C-1, 7.1%; C-2, 12%; C-3, 5.7%; C-4, 15.0%; C-5, 29.2%; C-6, 27.0%; C-7, 3.5%. These patients were intubated in the operating room by nasal (71%) or oral (22%) routes, in the emergency department (6%), or in the prehospital realm (1%), all successfully without new neurologic deficit.[4] In another study of blunt trauma, the incidence of cervical fracture was approximately 6% of all patients; 49% of these patients were intubated orally and 47% were intubated nasally, leaving 4% who were treated with cricothyroidotomy.[5]

The presence of severe laryngotracheal trauma may require immediate establishment of a surgical airway. Such trauma occurs more commonly with penetrating injury (65%) and is associated with airway compromise (43%) and significant mortality (12%).[6] The neck injury may be localized to the larynx itself, presenting with stridor and/or dysphonia as a result of edema, hematoma, laceration, and vocal cord dysfunction. Injury to the cervical trachea often presents with subcutaneous emphysema. Rupture of the intrathoracic trachea is suspected in the presence of pneumomediastinum or hemoptysis. Laryngeal injury is a relative contraindication to cricothyroidotomy and both oral and nasal intubation for extended periods. This situation remains the only indication for "emergency" tracheostomy, a procedure that is often time consuming even in expert hands.[6] Therefore, preceding tracheal intubation to provide a guaranteed patent airway, if possible, is preferred even for this type of emergency tracheostomy.

When surgical airway is required emergently, cricothyroidotomy is the procedure of choice, except in patients with laryngeal trauma. Cricothyroidotomy has a higher success rate compared with tracheostomy and better patient neurologic outcome based primarily on less time required for the procedure.[7] However, as a group, patients requiring an emergency surgical airway have a relatively high mortality.[8]

LARYNGEAL ANATOMY

The thyroid cartilage is the most readily identified laryngeal structure; it is located superior to the cricoid cartilage, to which it is connected by the cricothyroid joints and membrane (Fig. 80–1). This cricothyroid membrane occupies a trapezoidal area of approximately 3 cm^2 and has a 5- to 12-mm vertical height.[9, 10] Adjacent vascular structures may include the overlying pyramidal lobe from the thyroid isthmus and small branches of the superior thyroidal arteries. Through another short, fibrous connection, the cricoid cartilage is united with the first tracheal cartilage. Sensory innervation to the larynx is provided mainly by the superior

TABLE 80–1. Artificial Airway Categories

Intubation	*Surgical Cricothyroidotomy*	*Percutaneous Catheter Cricothyroidotomy or Tracheotomy*	*Surgical Tracheotomy*
Indications			
General anesthesia	Failed intubation	Failed intubation	Failed cricothyroidotomy
Respiratory arrest	Upper airway obstruction	Cervical fracture	Upper airway obstruction
Airway obstruction	Secretion retention	Partial airway obstruction	Long-term mechanical ventilation
Respiratory distress	Medium-term mechanical ventilation	Pharyngeal foreign body	Difficult weaning
Hemorrhage	Respiratory failure after recent sternotomy		ETT laryngeal injury
Secretion retention	Cervical fracture		Speech capability
Pulmonary contusion	Facial trauma (severe)		Need for oral intake
Facial trauma (moderate)	Emergency airway		Psychosocial benefit
Penetrating neck trauma			Oromaxillofacial trauma
Cardiac instability			Pharyngeal/glottic edema
Cardiac arrest			Nasal/oral/laryngeal hemorrhage
Coma			Neurologic deficit
Contraindications			
Anatomic difficulty	Laryngeal infection	Complete airway obstruction	Recent sternotomy
Coagulopathy (nasal)	Laryngeal trauma	Pediatric patients (relative)	Emergency airway
Facial fracture (nasal)	Intubation (>3 days)	Laryngeal trauma (relative)	
Cervical spine fracture (relative)	Pediatric patients (relative)		
	Coagulopathy		

Abbreviation: ETT = endotracheal tube.

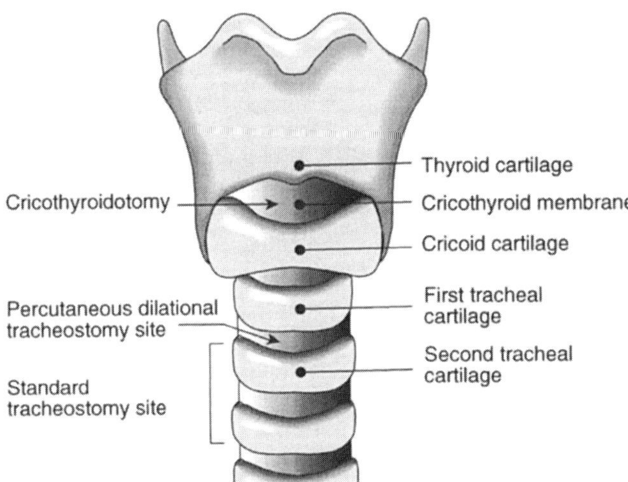

Figure 80–1. The laryngeal anatomy.

laryngeal nerves, whereas the recurrent laryngeal nerves provide motor innervation to the small laryngeal muscles except the cricothyroid muscles, which are supplied by the motor branches of the superior laryngeal nerves.

CRICOTHYROIDOTOMY

Historic Background

The modern history of cricothyroidotomy begins with the classic works of Chevalier Jackson, whose 30-year experience in treatment of laryngostenosis indicated that 93% of all complications occurred with what he referred to as "high tracheostomy" but with only 20% involving the cricothyroid membrane.[11] Thus, this valuable surgical airway technique was viewed with disfavor until the important review of cricothyroidotomy published by Brantigan and Grow in 1976. They reported a complication rate of only 6% in a large series, none of which was severe.[12]

Indications

The indications for cricothyroidotomy vary, but the technique is useful in any condition in which conventional intubation is not immediately successful. The technique is suitable for both emergent and elective situations (see Table 80–1). Contraindications are relative because most of these patients are in dire need of airway control. The procedure itself is simple to perform but optimized by meticulous technique (e.g., as follows):

PROCEDURE

1. *Position:* Neck hyperextension is desirable using a towel roll beneath the shoulders. The head must remain supported by the operating room table.
2. *Stabilization:* The nondominant hand stabilizes laryngeal cartilage with the index finger in the superior notch and the thumb and forefinger laterally.
3. *Cutaneous incision:* Although a horizontal incision is preferred when anatomic structures are easily identified, a vertical incision performed in the midline allows better landmark identification, greater chance of locating the cricothyroid membrane, and less bleeding, but healing is cosmetically inferior to the horizontal incision.
4. *Cricothyroid incision:* A horizontal stab incision through the cricothyroid membrane is performed with the knife directed slightly upward to avoid unintentional injury of the posterior tracheal wall.
5. *Stabilization:* An assistant with superior and inferior skin hooks will optimize visualization.
6. *Dilatation:* "Once in, stay in." Replace the scalpel blade with a Trousseaux dilator or curved hemostat.
7. *Insertion:* Insert a 6-mm tracheostomy (or tracheal) tube or a special cricothyroidostomy tube (Rusch, Germany).
8. *Confirmation:* Assess air and suction catheter passage through the tube. Obtain a chest radiograph, noting the tube position and the presence of any pneumothorax.
9. *Fixation:* Stabilize the tube with cloth, tracheal ties, and sutures or tape around the tube.

Emergency Aspects

The experience with emergency cricothyroidotomy suggests that adequate ventilation is achieved in most cases. Careful attention to depth and angle of penetration minimizes complications. With proper training, the procedure is easily and rapidly performed and is the emergency airway procedure of choice, especially in life-threatening airway obstruction.[13] The clinical efficiency of cricothyroidotomy has been demonstrated particularly in trauma centers whenever a difficult intubation is encountered.

Prehospital indications for cricothyroidotomy in one large series included severe facial trauma (40%), failed oral intubation (35%), and potential cervical fracture (5%), with an 88% rate of success reported.[14] When the procedure fails, the outcome usually is not good; patients in cardiac arrest demonstrated particularly poor survival or neurologic devastation.[14] In another study, the most common indications for a surgical airway were oromaxillofacial trauma (67%) and failed intubation (20%). A surgical airway was required in 2% to 3% of prehospital airway emergencies; a surprisingly high success rate of 98% was reported.[15]

Patients have undergone cricothyroidotomy secondarily to failed intubation (e.g., resulting from emesis or hemorrhage).[16] The survival rate was 32% in a reported material with significant difficulties encountered, such as misplacement of the tube (33%), insertion time longer than 3 minutes (26%), unsuccessful procedure (20%), hemorrhage (13%), and thyroid cartilage fracture (7%).[16]

Rapid cricothyroidotomy performed in the trauma setting allowed survival of 59% of such patients in one study.[17] Minor complications occurred in 27% at subsequent conversion to conventional tracheostomy, whereas major complications were more common with immediate tracheostomy.[17] Emergency cricothyroidotomy was predisposed to particularly poor outcome if instituted late in the course of respiratory failure.

Elective Utilization

The elective indications for cricothyroidotomy include the need for secretion clearance and prolonged mechanical ventilation. Because of the high risk of mediastinitis, cricothyroidostomy has been recommended instead of tracheostomy in patients after recent cardiac surgery via midline sternotomy. Cricothyroidotomy has a complication rate of 1% to 9% in patients predisposed by preceding endotracheal intubation of 7 days or more, which, therefore, is a relative contraindication.[18] However, more recent clinical experience has documented that patients converted from endotracheal intubation to cricothyroidostomy after 7 days demonstrated only 5% of minimal side effects (e.g., laryngeal granulation tissue and stenosis).[19]

Cricothyroidostomy has also been explored for the management of secretions postoperatively with very high effi-

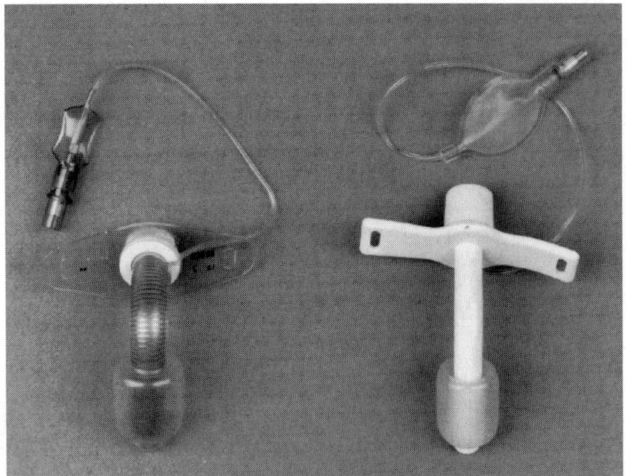

Figure 80–2. *Left,* A No. 7 cricothyroidotomy cannula. The cannula lumen is rounded at the end but ovally shaped (6 × 8 mm ID) in the part that penetrates the cricothyroid membrane (Courtesy of Willy Rüsch, Kernen-Rommelshausen, Germany). *Right,* Standard No. 6 tracheostomy tube without an inner cannula (Courtesy of Shiley Tracheostomy Products, Mallinckrodt Medical, Irvine, CA.)

cacy and a low complication rate of 3% to 8% manifested mostly as minor bleeding. Such "minitracheostomy" established through a cricothyroidotomy has an 87% success rate when maintained for approximately 10 days, enabling effective secretion removal via a narrow suction catheter.[20] Cricothyroidotomy and cannulation with a small adult or pediatric tracheostomy tube (Fig. 80–2) will prevent cricothyroid cartilage separation. This technique may also be used for prolonged management of mechanically ventilated patients, who preferably have been intubated for a duration shorter than 1 week and are without bleeding diathesis.

Complications

Difficulties encountered in emergency cricothyroidotomy are often related to massive neck swelling obscuring the thyroid cartilage. This emergent setting results in complications in 18% to 32% of the patients.[16, 17] These complications include hemorrhage, tube occlusion from debris, tube misplacement, and late subglottic stenosis.[21] Tube misplacement may occur outside of the cricothyroid space in one third of such cases (e.g., into the pretracheal tissue). Unintentional passage of the tube upward into the pharynx instead of downward into the trachea may be avoided if the cricothyroidostomy tube is inserted over a guide wire, catheter, or dilating probe, which is directed to enter the trachea. Insertions through the thyroid cartilage, into the pharynx, or even intraesophageally have also been described.[22, 23]

Elective cricothyroidotomy is technically easier than tracheotomy and has only minor adverse sequelae; voice change is the most common and minimal evidence of subglottic stenosis is less common.[24] Patients predisposed to complications are those with cricothyroidostomy for more than 30 days, preceding intubation greater than 7 days, diagnosis of diabetes mellitus, and advanced age.[25, 26] Another strong correlate is the presence of stomal infection, causing formation of subglottic granulation tissue and subsequent cartilaginous injury and stenosis.[27] Thus, the procedure is associated with some morbidity manifested as moderate to severe perichondrial inflammation but only minimal stenosis. Mortality has been identified as a covariable of patients in poor condition.[28] Major complications have been reported in 7% and include subglottic stenosis resulting from granulation tissue formation, whereas minor complications occurred in 30% and usually were located at the cuff site.[29]

The most sensitive indication of dysfunction after airway intubation is temporary voice change, demonstrated in 50% to 75% of the patients.[30] Also, cricothyroid muscle dysfunction occurs by an unknown mechanism with normal electromyogram and muscle biopsy but manifested as diminished voice range with lower pitch.[31] The most specific measure of iatrogenic trauma induced by cricothyroidostomy is subglottic stenosis. This problem may occur in as many as 12% of patients.[29, 30] However, most modern comparisons suggest that cricothyroidotomy performed under optimal conditions without active infection or prolonged preceding intubation has a lower rate of subglottic stenosis compared with endotracheal intubation.

PERCUTANEOUS CRICOTHYROIDOTOMY

The "cut and poke" cricothyroidotomy (using a knife blade with rubber limit followed by cannula insertion) was described by Safar and Penninckx in 1967.[9] A "last-ditch airway" was reported in 1979, performed with a scalpel blade and insertion of an intravenous tubing spike connected to pressurized oxygen for ventilation.[32] However, none of these techniques has gained significant utilization.

The first large clinical trial used the Minitrach (Portex) system consisting of a 4-mm internal diameter (ID) pediatric tube placed over an introducer through a cricothyroid membrane incision. The technique has been used in post-thoracotomy patients for up to 45 days, providing satisfactory removal by suction of retained secretions in these patients (Fig. 80–3, *left*).[33] The Minitrach II System (Portex) was reevaluated for pulmonary toilet, demonstrating significant efficacy manifested as earlier discharge from the intensive care unit (ICU) in 88% after limited therapy (4 days). Minor bleeding in 7% was the only significant side effect.[34] Compared with control, this technique also demonstrated a decrease in the frequency of postoperative atelectasis, and fewer patients required bronchoalveolar lavage for secretion management.[35] One study, however, cited therapeutic failure in one third of its patients.[36]

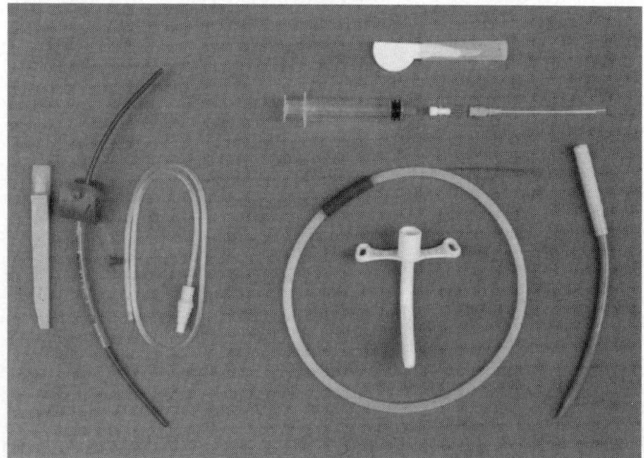

Figure 80–3. Percutaneous cricothyroidotomy kits. *Left,* The Minitrach II minitracheotomy kit, which includes a scalpel, an introducer with a 4-mm-ID cannula, and a suction catheter (Courtesy of Concord Portex, Keene, NH). *Right,* A scalpel; an 18-gauge catheter-over-needle attached to a syringe; a guide wire; a dilator; and a 6-mm-ID cannula (Courtesy of Cook Critical Care, Bloomington, IN).

The Nutrake System (International Medical Devices, Northridge, CA) has demonstrated rapid placement and high success rate after video instruction of trainees,[37] but the equipment is sharp, rigid, and potentially harmful. The use of minitracheostomy postoperatively in thoracic surgery patients, in whom a 20-French pediatric tracheostomy tube was placed as a cricothyroidostomy cannula for removal of retained secretions, resulted in a 99% success rate and significant decrease in the need for bronchoscopy.[38] Complications were minimal, with minor bleeding in a few patients. Subglottic stenosis was not demonstrated.[38] This procedure has minimal documented mortality but may occasionally be difficult or impossible to perform in elderly patients because of cricothyroid membrane calcification.[39]

The Seldinger technique using a guide wire may be more amenable to use by nonsurgeons. A percutaneous method has been described in which needle placement and guide wire insertion are followed by dilatation with a nasal speculum-like dilator and placement of a 6-mm tracheostomy tube. Although cumbersome, this method suggests the use of instruments readily available to the critical care physician.[39] However, use of the so-called Quicktrach device resulted in longer insertion time compared with open technique and a complication rate of up to 27% related to the operator's level of experience.[40]

The Melker percutaneous dilatational cricothyroidotomy kit (Cook, Bloomington, IN) allows cricothyroid membrane needle puncture, guide wire placement, and insertion of a unitized, anatomically conformed tube and dilator in a single step, minimizing the risk of malposition and cartilage damage (Fig. 80–3, *right*). This appears to be a safe and effective technique. Prior devices have been difficult to insert, often resulting in paratracheal cannula placement and subcutaneous emphysema.[41] Correct position is verified by fiberoptic bronchoscopy, but suction catheter passage, unobstructed airflow, or normal end-tidal carbon dioxide concentration may suffice.[41]

Percutaneous cricothyroidotomy, as described previously, allows placement of a definitive airway in the routine or emergency setting by practitioners of all specialties. However, some available kits provide dangerously traumatic equipment. The procedure may also lead to significant complications in patients with anatomic distortion and bleeding diathesis or when placed by an inexperienced operator. Therefore, the technique should be included in the educational airway repertoire of all critical care medicine physician trainees.

SURGICAL TRACHEOTOMY

Historic Background

Although tracheotomy was a procedure practiced already in ancient Egypt, little is known about the technique used. However, Vesalius in 1555 published a compendium illustrating a tracheotomy performed by cherubs on a cow, hinting at potential complications of the procedure itself. His description of performing a tracheotomy reads "but that life may in a manner of speaking be restored to the animal, an opening must be attempted in the trunk of the trachea into which a reed or cane should be put; you will then blow into this so that the lung may rise again and the animal takes in air."[42]

Use of the tracheotomy procedure resurfaced during the diphtheria epidemic of the 19th century. Trousseau described its use to prevent asphyxia and airway obstruction. Jackson, in his classic publication of 1921, discussed how poor tracheotomy technique caused laryngeal stenosis, specifically with a hasty operation; general anesthesia; "high tracheotomy"; cricoid cartilage division; tight wound suture closure; poor postoperative care; cannula of improper size, shape, or material; and neglect of ordering decent cleanliness in weaning from the cannula.[11] The best described complication in diphtheria survivors is subglottic stenosis. "The difficulties and dangers, experienced in so many cases on attempting after the pulmonary disease had subsided, removal of the cannula [sic] from the trachea in which it has remained for some time, is well known in many. Chief among these are the sudden attacks of asphyxia, which occur at this period."[43]

Indications

The indications for tracheostomy are diverse. The only contraindication is the necessity for an emergency airway because this procedure is time consuming and requires significant expertise. Comparison of emergent versus elective tracheotomy reveals a twofold complication rate with the former because of longer time spent isolating the trachea as a result of commonly occurring bleeding.[44] The procedure requires attention to detail and is truly an operative intervention that preferably should be performed in the operating suite and be followed by intensive care, if conditions so warrant.

PROCEDURE

1. *Setting:* An operative suite is preferred.
2. *Position:* The head and neck are extended, using a towel roll beneath the shoulders but with the head still resting against the operating table.
3. *Anesthesia:* General anesthesia is preferred with preceding orotracheal or nasotracheal intubation.
4. *Skin incision:* A transverse incision is made 1 to 2 cm below the cricoid cartilage in the triangle formed by the medial sternocleidomastoid heads and cricoid cartilage.
5. *Dissection:* Dissection must be adequate to identify fascial planes. Strap muscles in the midline are separated.
6. *Laryngeal nerves:* Avoid lateral tracheal dissection, which may cause injury to the recurrent laryngeal nerves.
7. *Thyroid isthmus:* Transect with suture ligature. If this area is not divided, occlusion can occur at accidental decannulation.
8. *Tracheal incision:* A tracheal incision is done at the second to third or third to fourth tracheal cartilage. Midline division (not the horizontal stab method) is used.
9. *Tracheal resection:* A tracheal fenestration wider than 5 mm should be avoided. A wide vertical flap or excessively large tracheal window causes risk of stenosis formation after decannulation.
10. *Stabilization:* Skin hooks (or Allis Clamp) superiorly and inferiorly are used.
11. *Tracheal stoma:* If a tracheal stoma is used, suture the inverted tracheal flap to the subcutaneous tissue. Use lateral tracheal stay sutures, exteriorized, and taped to skin.
12. *Cannulation:* The tube is 50% to 75% of the diameter of the trachea. Insert the tube at a right lateral angle and rotate caudad. The sizing is as follows: males, 7- to 8-mm ID; females, 6- to 7-mm ID.
13. *Confirmation:* Correct position of tracheostomy tube is confirmed by free airflow, suction catheter passage, or radiography.
14. *Fixation:* Tracheal sutures are placed for identification of stoma in case of early tube dislocation, and around-the-neck straps are placed for fixation.
15. *Incision closure:* The skin is loosely approximated to prevent subcutaneous emphysema.

Technique

Tracheostomy success and complications are dependent on surgical technique and the equipment used. If an inverted horseshoe flap technique is used, the flap is sutured to the subcutaneous tissue. This technique was designed by Bjork

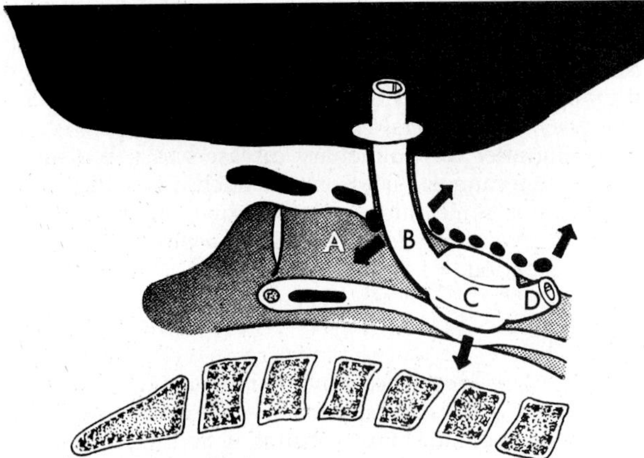

Figure 80–4. Schematic illustration of tracheostomy-induced lesions. A = Too high area for tube position; B = stoma damage area; C = cuff pressure–induced lesion; D = anterior lesion caused by the tube tip.

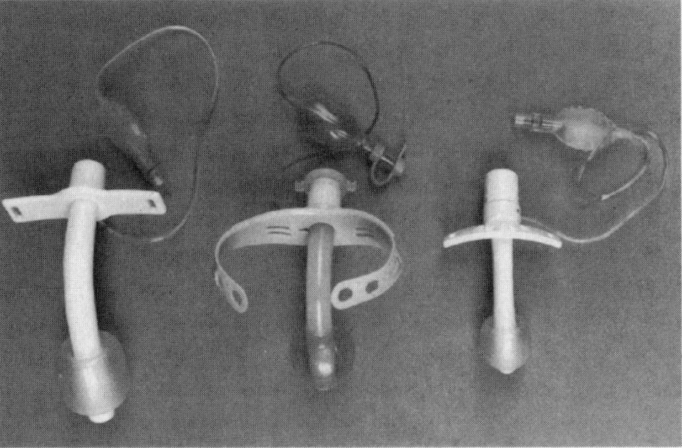

Figure 80–5. Tracheostomy tubes. *Left,* Soft tube without inner cannula (Courtesy of Shiley Tracheostomy Products, Mallinckrodt Medical, Irvine, CA). *Middle,* Soft tube without inner cannula (Courtesy of Concord Portex, Keene, NH). *Right,* Rigid tube with inner cannula (Courtesy of Shiley Tracheostomy Products, Mallinckrodt Medical, Irvine, CA).

and Engstrom to avoid pretracheal insertion after early dislocation of the tracheostomy tube.[45] The oval tracheal window with a diameter of one half of the tracheal width has been suggested for optimal tube placement.[46] However, resection of less than 5-mm width is sufficient for reinsertion of an accidentally dislodged tracheostomy tube. The different methods compared clinically in a pediatric model suggest that the lowest rate of stenosis occurs with the vertical tracheal incision followed by the horizontal H technique, and the most significant rate of stenosis occurs with the inverted-U flap.[47]

The design characteristics of the tracheostomy tube are also important. Pressure necrosis occurring between the posterior tracheal wall and vertical body of the tube at the thoracic inlet may be minimized by tube shape (i.e., modification of length and curvature) as well as stable tube fixation (Fig. 80–4).[48] Longer tracheostomy tubes may impact against the carina or result in a right mainstem bronchus intubation.[49] Thus, the tracheostomy tube should be soft but resilient and straight in the intratracheal position, resist torque, and be of appropriate length (Table 80–2, Fig. 80–5).

For the spontaneously breathing patient, the fenestrated tube allows use of the larynx for speech and better respiratory toilet. However, position of the fenestration is crucial to avoid obstruction. Individualizing its placement and using tubes with multiple small openings compared with one large fenestration are advantageous techniques (Fig. 80–6).[50]

The ideal tracheostomy cuff should have a sufficiently large sealing surface area and be of the large-diameter, high-volume, low-pressure variety.[51] Prevention of cuff complications is best addressed by cuff inflation to a maximum of 25 cm H_2O pressure and frequent monitoring unless preset automatic cuff pressure technique is used (Fig. 80–7).

TABLE 80–2. Tracheostomy Tube Size

Tracheostomy Tube Size (French)	*Inner Diameter (mm)*	*Outer Diameter (mm)*
5	5.0	7.0–8.5
6	6.0	8.1–9.9
7	7.0	9.6–11.3
8	8.0	10.9–12.6
9	9.0	12.1–14.0
10	10.0	13.3–13.5

Emergency Versus Elective Tracheotomy

The emergency indications for tracheostomy are few but occur when endotracheal intubation is impossible and cricothyroidotomy is precluded by high-grade upper airway obstruction, massive neck swelling, or laryngeal injury. When those conditions are encountered, a finder needle on a saline-filled syringe is helpful in locating the trachea.

Tracheostomy has a high associated morbidity and significant mortality from different complications occurring after prolonged intubation.[52] However, the mortality of ICU patients caused by underlying disease must be separated from that caused by the procedure itself.[6]

Tracheostomy complications such as bleeding or pneumothorax usually present early (i.e., during tracheotomy or within 2 days). Tracheobronchopulmonary infections occur late and with high frequency in critically ill patients.[53] The tracheotomy procedure has been performed safely at the

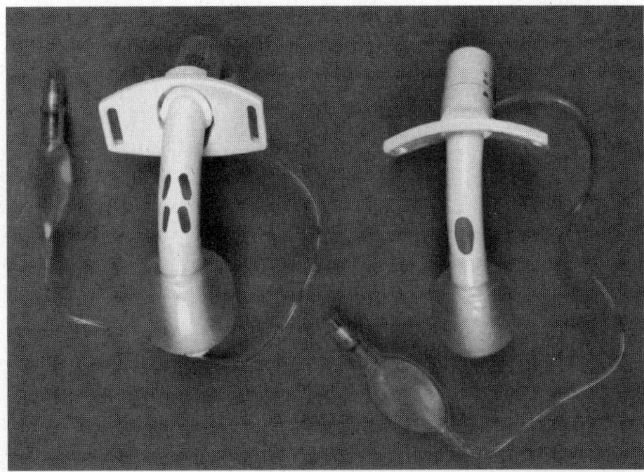

Figure 80–6. Fenestrated tracheostomy tubes. *Left,* Multiple fenestrations (Courtesy of Shiley Tracheostomy Products, Mallinckrodt Medical, Irvine, CA). *Right,* Single fenestration (Courtesy of Shiley Tracheostomy Products, Mallinckrodt Medical, Irvine, CA).

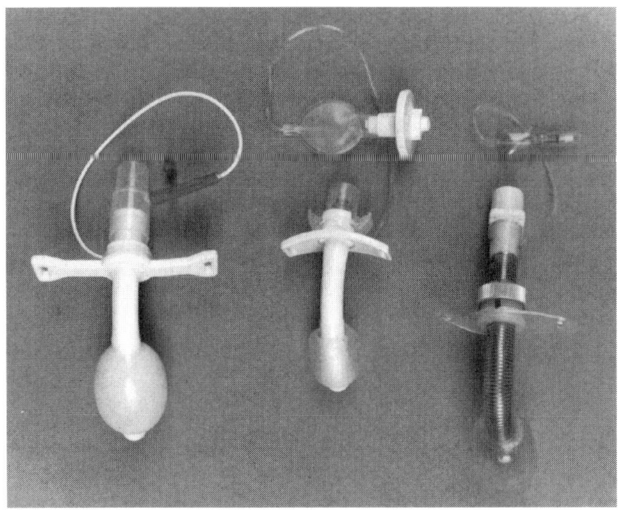

Figure 80–7. Modified tracheostomy cannulas. *Left,* Foam cuff tube (Courtesy of Bivona, Gary, IN). *Middle,* Tube with a cuff regulating device (Courtesy of Shiley Tracheostomy Products, Mallinckrodt Medical, Irvine, CA). *Right,* Tube allowing variable length of insertion (Courtesy of Willy Rüsch, Kernen-Rommelshausen, Germany).

bedside in selected patients under local anesthesia and intravenous sedation without significant complications, avoiding the risk of operating room transfer.[54] Timing strategies for tracheotomy are numerous and should be individualized. One clinical trial examined tracheotomy performed in burn patients on day 1 (7%), day 8 (17%), and day 14 (58%), with the tracheostomy maintained for 1 to 208 days without clear correlation to complications.[55] Tracheostomy within 4 days has been recommended in trauma patients, resulting in a decreased mechanical ventilation requirement and improved pulmonary toilet with less airway and pulmonary infections.[56] Similarly, early tracheostomy (within 7 days) has proven superior based on a shorter period of mechanical ventilation and length of ICU and hospital stay.[57] However, another study of trauma patients showed no difference in laryngotracheal complications between early (fewer than 2 weeks) and late (more than 2 weeks) tracheostomy.[58]

Current recommendations are based on clinical evaluation. There are isolated data to suggest that nasal intubation is equivalent to tracheostomy in the incidence and onset of laryngeal complications.[59] Tracheostomy may be superior to translaryngeal tracheal intubation in specific patient populations, such as those with burns, who have an increased incidence of laryngotracheal granuloma formation and stenosis.[60] The preponderance of evidence suggests that tracheostomy (14%) is associated with less laryngeal trauma than nasotracheal or orotracheal intubation (57%).[61] Patients also find tracheostomy more comfortable, and it allows them to communicate. It simplifies airway nursing care, and in one study 92% of the patients preferred this technique for artificial airway requirements of more than 10 days.[61]

Complications

Most initial perioperative tracheostomy complications are minor, including hemorrhage and subcutaneous emphysema. Major early complications such as loss of airway control, obstruction, or excessive blood loss are uncommon. Mediastinal emphysema and/or unilateral or bilateral pneumothoraces may suddenly develop if the patient has an occluded airway during the procedure and is struggling to breathe. When the pretracheal fascia is transected, the excessive negative intrapleural pressure may create a pressure gradient large enough to rupture the pleura with air entering the pleural cavity from the outside. Whenever possible, tracheotomy should be performed with preceding tracheal intubation. The reported overall complication rate of tracheostomy varies between 6% and 48%, which is still less than that encountered with prolonged endotracheal intubation.[58, 62, 63]

The most often discussed complication is tracheostenosis. The most significant lesions are found at the cuff site, where high tracheal wall pressure may cause circumferential ulceration, ischemic necrosis, and subsequent scarring.[64] The incidence of this complication has decreased from 6% in the 19th century to between 1% and 2% today.[6, 43, 62] These lesions are mainly caused by a cuff pressure that is too high with a distinct pathogenesis and outcome. However, removal of too much of the tracheal wall and excessive movement of the tracheostomy tube may also cause stenosis at the stoma level.

The most common complication is infection with far-reaching sequelae (Table 80–3). Those with tracheostomy have a higher rate of lower respiratory tract colonization (76%) with gram-negative rods, such as *Pseudomonas aeruginosa,* often causing tracheobronchitis.[65] The bacteria that colonize the respiratory tree at the time of tracheostomy subsequently may grow in number and pathogenic properties.[66] More severe infections include necrotizing tracheitis associated with purulent stomal drainage and difficult mechanical ventilation caused by air leak and peristomal cavitation.[67] Critically ill patients are predisposed to these complications, if colonized with *Pseudomonas, Enterobacter,* or *Klebsiella.*[67] Paratracheal mediastinal abscess formation has been described as being associated with upper lobe consolidation and septicemia.[68] Tracheal soft-tissue injury is usually localized to the posterior wall (e.g., in cases of mucosal rigidity associated with radiation therapy or infection).[67] Massive dissecting emphysema can occur when the tracheostomy tube is malpositioned into the pretracheal space with positive-pressure ventilation applied.[69]

Life-threatening hemorrhage involving the brachiocephalic trunk (innominate artery) and resulting from tube tip or cuff erosion,[70] has been found in 1% of patients. It occurs especially with cuff overdistention, low-lying tracheostomy, or pretracheal soft-tissue infection.[70, 71] Acute hemostasis is achieved by cuff hyperinflation and pretracheal digital compression of the innominate artery, followed by emergency exploration for brachiocephalic trunk division and suture ligation, which, when successful, is associated with good neurologic outcome.[71]

Vascular erosion may also present as a fistula. An innominate artery fistula may be caused by the extratracheal portion of the tracheostomy tube, whereas the intratracheal fis-

TABLE 80–3. Complications Associated with Tracheostomy* (In Approximate Order of Frequency)

Pneumonia	Mediastinal emphysema
Tracheobronchitis	Tracheal-innominate artery fistula
Hemorrhage	Necrotizing tracheitis
Stomal infection	Paratracheal abscess
Tracheostenosis	Posterior wall laceration
Tracheomalacia	Tracheoesophageal fistula
Subcutaneous emphysema	

*For details see Holley and Jordan,[4] Minard et al,[6] Boyd and Benzel,[62] Miller and Kapp,[63] Snow et al,[67] Cole and Kerr,[68] Arola et al,[76] Adolfsson et al,[71] Takano et al,[72] Schachner et al.[108]

tula is caused by the tube tip or cuff.[72] Patients are predisposed by low-lying tracheostomy (below the fourth tracheal cartilage), high innominate artery position, infection, and steroid use.[72] Thus, an extratracheal innominate artery fistula may present with exsanguination and hemodynamic instability, whereas a tracheoinnominate fistula may present with less bleeding (100–150 mL) but instead life-threatening airway obstruction and asphyxia.[73]

Tracheoesophageal fistula occasionally occurs secondary to compression between an overdistended cuff or the posterior convex contour of a curved rigid tracheostomy tube and nasogastric tube.[74] This complication occurs late in patients with poor prognosis, is difficult to treat, and is usually lethal.[75]

The institution of a tracheostomy requires constant vigilance and frequent assessment of complications. Prospective laryngotracheal examination has demonstrated asymptomatic stomal narrowing in 16%, bleeding in 10%, and miscellaneous problems in an additional 17%. Sellery and colleagues reported tracheostenosis severe enough to require tracheal resection in 8% of patients.[76] Follow-up of such patients should include routine bronchoscopic surveillance.[76] Video technique is especially helpful in the diagnosis of phonation difficulty and aspiration problems, which are often caused by laryngeal nerve or vocal cord dysfunction.[77] Conventional tomography of the larynx has been replaced by computed tomography in the diagnosis of glottic abnormalities.[27] The need for therapeutic intervention of subglottic stenosis may be related to the higher likelihood of survival with current resuscitation techniques.[78] Patients are predisposed for tracheostomy complications by abnormal neck anatomy or low-lying tracheostomy.[79]

Medical therapy includes the use of topical and systemic antibiotics because stenosis is related to an acute inflammatory and infectious phase.[80] The use of systemic corticosteroids has been explored to address the reactive scarring phase.[81] Progressive balloon dilatation has been described initially in this condition.[82] Surgical repair is required for patients with tracheal diameter narrowing of greater than 50%.[83] Laryngostenosis occurs most commonly at the cricoid cartilage level, the narrowest part of the upper airway.[84] Tracheostenosis results from endotracheal trauma most often because of a cuff pressure that is too high. As previously indicated, the surgical approach includes primary resection with end-to-end anastomosis[75] or multistage endoscopic laser resection.[78]

PERCUTANEOUS TRANSTRACHEAL CATHETERIZATION

Historic Background

Transtracheal artificial ventilation was described by Reed and colleagues in 1954 in a canine model using a tapered 13-gauge steel needle and a flow system of 15 L per minute for 30 minutes.[85] This technique allowed adequate oxygenation but inadequate ventilation, with increasing hypercarbia and resultant respiratory acidosis causing hemodynamic depression with decreasing mean arterial pressure and heart rate and increasing central venous pressure.[85] Therefore, the pressure-flow characteristics of resuscitation needles were analyzed. The 13-gauge needle with 88 cm H_2O pressure was found to permit 200 mL/s of gas flow.[86] However, the normal adult at rest has a peak inspiratory flow of about 400 mL/s. Therefore, the described system was capable of maintaining adequate ventilation in an apneic model only for a few minutes.[86] This method was further explored, and the authors concluded that 18-gauge and 16-gauge catheters are too narrow as emergency airways, with survival limited to 5 to 15 minutes.[5] The 13-gauge system allowed survival up to 60 minutes in dogs, but in calves survival was limited to 16 minutes.[5] A cannula size of 13 to 14 gauge necessitates a high-pressure (40–50 psi) jet insufflation system for adequate ventilation (Fig. 80–8).

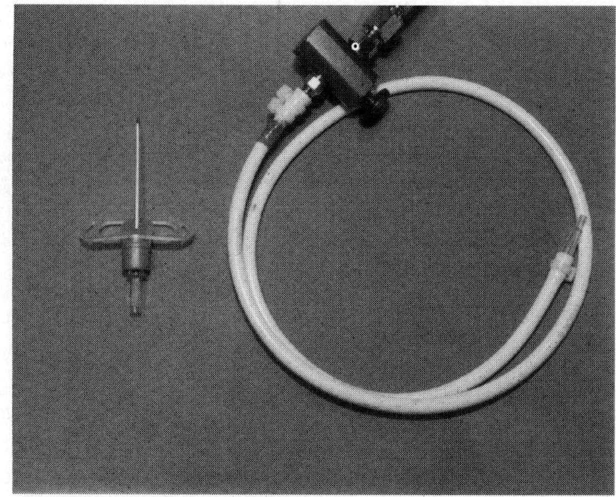

Figure 80–8. *Left,* Cricothyroidotomy catheter device with wings (for fixation) mounted onto a needle for insertion (Courtesy of CVM Medizintechnic, Sulz/Neckar, Germany). *Right,* Manual activation jet ventilation system designed to provide a pressure of 50 psi. The system is suitable for ventilation with the catheter to the left.

PROCEDURE

Percutaneous transtracheal catheterization is indicated for failed intubation as the procedure of choice in partial airway obstruction, but success depends on operator experience. There are some contraindications to the procedure, including operator inexperience, severe coagulopathy, and complete airway obstruction (e.g., caused by laryngeal trauma), with possibilities for inadequate exhalation (see Table 80–1).

1. *Position:* Extend the neck (if there is no cervical spine trauma) with the face directed straight anteriorly (not turned to the side).
2. *Stabilization:* The nondominant hand holds thyroid cartilage.
3. *Palpation:* The index finger guides to cricoid cartilage.
4. *Apparatus:* Use a saline-filled syringe, catheter-over-needle assembly, connector, and oxygen source (50 psi).
5. *Entry:* The catheter/syringe is directed 45° caudad and inserted cautiously into the upper trachea while avoiding lesions of the posterior tracheal wall. A free airflow indicates correct position.
6. *Connection:* Withdraw the needle, and connect the tubing from the oxygen source (50 psi).
7. *Ventilation:* An inspiration-expiration ratio of 1:4 to prevent air trapping is used.
8. *Stabilization:* Always retain control of the catheter until it is permanently secured in the neck.
9. *Monitoring:* Look for indications of barotrauma, such as hypotension or subcutaneous emphysema.
10. *Confirmation:* Chest radiograph should be taken to check for catheter position and absence of pneumothorax and/or subcutaneous air.

Mechanics

The most critical issue regarding efficacy of ventilation is the diameter of the catheter, where turbulent flow varies inversely with the radius to the fourth power according to the law of Poiseuille. The minimum catheter size should be 14 gauge, which permits a flow 10 times greater than a 22-

gauge catheter.[87] A 14-gauge catheter is readily available in most hospitals. However, it is too narrow for passive exhalation, which must take place through the patient's natural airway.

The flow delivery system is next in importance when determining ventilatory efficacy. The minimum pressure gradient required to generate flow through a small-diameter cannula is 0.1 to 0.5 psi (7–35 cm H_2O).[88] However, the pressure gradient required to achieve adequate ventilation is far greater, easily provided by a 50-psi (3500 cm H_2O) source, but not by a manual bag-valve or demand-valve system generating a pressure of less than 60 cm H_2O.[87] The previously described model with a 14-gauge cannula using a 50-psi jet system instead of manual bagging provided a flow five times greater (235–1034 mL/s) (i.e., enough to achieve adequate ventilation).[87] The lower flow systems of 15 L/min may provide adequate oxygenation, but ventilation is inadequate and survival is limited to 1 to 2 hours before lethal hypercarbia and respiratory acidosis occur.[89, 90]

The percutaneous transtracheal ventilation (PTV) system has been described as a life-support adjunct in 80 patients treated at the accident site.[91] Using PTV, a canine hemorrhagic shock model demonstrated adequate oxygenation and ventilation (partial pressure of carbon dioxide of 21 mm Hg) but still serious metabolic acidosis (pH 7.14).[92]

The indications for emergency use include the presence of partial airway obstruction. If this obstruction is due to a laryngotracheal foreign body, PTV may assist in expelling the object.[93] However, complete airway obstruction does not provide for adequate exhalation, resulting in air trapping and hyperinflation. In such cases, barotrauma becomes a concern, with the possibility of bilateral tension pneumothorax, cardiac arrest, and death.

Emergency percutaneous transtracheal catheterization has been used for treatment of airway obstruction with reasonable success, but complications including catheter displacement, total expiratory obstruction, and barotrauma were encountered.[94] Used cautiously, this technique has been explored for difficult intubation with no adverse effects on morbidity or mortality.[95] The technique has proven effective in providing more adequate oxygenation than ventilation.[96] Clinical evaluation using a commercially available emergency infusion device (Arrow International, Reading, PA), with an 8.5-gauge catheter resulted in adequate ventilation in partial-obstruction models.[97] A 13-gauge angulated catheter with side holes placed between the tracheal cartilages has also been used successfully in patients.[98] Further, the Minitrach II System (Portex) has been adapted for jet ventilation, proving efficacious in patients.[99]

Complications

High-frequency jet ventilation (HFJV) at a rate of 250 to 400 per minute has been provided via transtracheal catheters, but airway inflammation occurs in all such cases and is manifested as mucosal erosion and leukocyte infiltration at the catheter tip. This HFJV injury is greater than with conventional intubation and high-frequency ventilation at a lower rate (150/min) as well as traditional ventilation frequency (20/min).[100] Tracheal mucosal hemorrhage may occur secondary to catheter trauma. Posterior tracheal wall perforation has also been reported.[100]

Cardiac sequelae are related to the presence of air trapping often caused by auto–positive end-expiratory pressure (PEEP) resulting from obstructed exhalation. Increasing PEEP is productive to a point with increased peak airway and mean arterial pressures, improved oxygenation, and reduced shunt fraction.[101] However, at levels greater than 20 cm H_2O, this auto-PEEP also becomes a limiting factor, decreasing cardiac output and increasing intracranial pressure.[101] The hypovolemic patient, in particular, will improve when switched to low-frequency ventilation.[102]

The pulmonary complications of PTV include barotrauma manifested as unilateral or bilateral pneumothorax, pneumomediastinum, and subcutaneous emphysema.[103, 104] This interstitial emphysema may also dissect along the great vessels and secondarily rupture into the abdominal cavity, forming pneumoperitoneum,[105] which has led to unnecessary laparotomy because of suspected gastrointestinal perforation.

PERCUTANEOUS DILATATIONAL TRACHEOSTOMY

Historic Background

Percutaneous tracheostomy using a large-bore needle and guide wire was described in 1976 for emergency use.[106] Current discussion centers on the use of this technique in the ICU at the bedside. This percutaneous tracheostomy technique has been used for treatment of excess secretions, in patients with prolonged intubation for mechanical ventilation, and in patients with neurologic dysfunction. It has been performed electively (77%), urgently (28%), or as an occasional emergency procedure (5%).[107] This technique proved successful in 90% of patients when performed in the emergency department and in 70% of those done in the ICU or operating room, all with minimal morbidity.[107]

PROCEDURE

1. *Position:* The neck is hyperextended.
2. *Anesthesia:* Local anesthesia is preferable.
3. *Landmarks:* A minimal horizontal incision is made midway between the cricothyroid membrane and the sternal notch.
4. *Puncture:* Intercartilage membrane is punctured at a 45° caudad angle, avoiding the posterior tracheal wall.
5. *Aspiration:* Intratracheal position is confirmed by aspiration of air into a saline-filled syringe.
6. *Catheter:* Advance the catheter over the needle with air aspiration reconfirmation.
7. *Guide wire:* The wire is inserted and the catheter removed.
8. *Dilatation:* Progressively larger dilators are passed.
9. *Tracheostomy tube:* The tube is passed over the largest dilator, which is subsequently removed.
10. *Confirmation:* Position is confirmed by air entry and suction catheter passage.
11. *Stabilization:* Around-the-neck straps are placed for fixation.

Equipment

The described procedure is simplified by use of a commercially available kit (Fig. 80–9; Cook, Bloomington, IN). The technique is safe but relatively slow. Modifications for rapid placement include the Rapitrach System (Premier Medical, Norristown, PA), which uses a hinged device as a dilator for effective placement[108, 109] of the tracheostomy tube. The Nutrach System (International Medical Device, Northridge CA) includes a steel cannula that has been used for both cricothyroidostomy and tracheostomy. The original progressive dilator technique was described by Ciaglia and colleagues in 1985 and stressed entry between the cricoid cartilage and first tracheal cartilage to reduce the incidence and severity of complications.[110] A clinical trial comparing the Rapitrach and Cook devices with conventional tracheostomy demonstrated procedure times of 5, 15, and 60 minutes, respectively (see Fig. 80–9).[111] However, the highest complication rate was found with the Rapitrach System.[109]

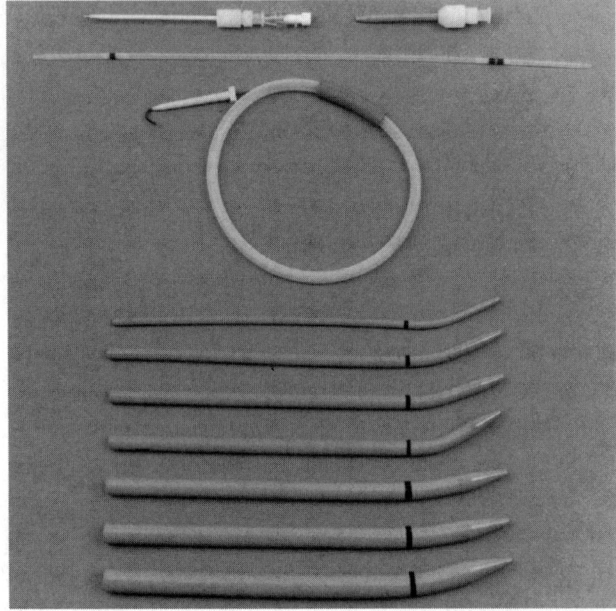

Figure 80–9. Percutaneous dilational tracheostomy kit (Courtesy of Cook Critical Care, Bloomington, IN). From *top* to *bottom:*
Step 1: A catheter-over-needle is used to puncture the trachea.
Step 2: After needle removal, a plastic guide is inserted through the catheter.
Step 3: The catheter is removed, and a guide introducer is inserted over the plastic guide, which is replaced by a guide wire.
Step 4: The introducer is removed, and progressively larger dilators are inserted; finally, a tracheostomy cannula is inserted over the dilator.

The Cook device offered an appropriate compromise in the rapidity of the technique and complication rate.

Complications

The complication rate of this dilatational tracheostomy technique is minimal, and the mortality has been reported at only 1%.[107, 112, 113] This low complication rate of the dilatational technique (mainly hemorrhage) compares favorably with the standard procedure, in which obstruction, hemorrhage, pneumothorax, and wound infection occur frequently.[81] However, occasional cases of life-threatening hemorrhage as well as pneumothorax have also been reported with the percutaneous technique.[114] Tomography confirms the advantage of percutaneous versus open tracheostomy with a lower frequency of overall complications using the former technique.[115] The incidence of complications may be minimized by endoscopic guidance of the percutaneous technique confirming intratracheal placement and, if necessary, guiding insertion of the tracheostomy tube.[116] However, such endoscopy is not a practical choice in emergency situations.

CONCLUDING REMARKS

The success of the percutaneous cricothyroidostomy and tracheostomy techniques includes appropriate patient selection. There is a reported failure rate of 22% in percutaneous tracheostomy of patients with "non-ideal anatomy."[117] The best of circumstances allows the percutaneous cricothyroidotomy procedure to be performed in 30 seconds instead of several minutes for a tracheostomy.[112] The percutaneous dilatational tracheostomy procedure is slow but has a 94% success rate, although the failure rate has been cited to be higher when performed by nonexperienced operators.[118] However, the postoperative result has been optimal (95%) with decannulation possible in most patients.[113]

References

1. Redan JA, Livingston DH, Tortella BJ, et al: The value of intubating and paralyzing patients with suspected head injury in the emergency department. J Trauma 1991; 31:371.
2. Murphy-Macabobby M, Marshall WJ, Schneider C, et al: Neuromuscular blockade in aeromedical airway management. Ann Emerg Med 1992; 21:664.
3. Suderman VS, Crosby ET, Lui A: Elective oral tracheal intubation in cervical spine-injured adults. Can J Anaesth 1991; 38:785.
4. Holley J, Jorden R: Airway management in patients with unstable cervical spine fractures. Ann Emerg Med 1989; 18:1237.
5. Hughes RK: Needle tracheostomy. Arch Surg 1966; 93:834.
6. Minard G, Kudsk KA, Croce MA: Laryngotracheal trauma. Am Surg 1992; 58:181.
7. Steinert R, Lullwit E: Failed intubation with case reports. HNO 1987; 35:439.
8. Goldberg J, Levy PS, Morkovin V, et al: Mortality from traumatic injuries: A case-control study using data from the National Hospital Discharge survey. Med Care 1983; 21:692.
9. Safar P, Penninckx J: Cricothyroid membrane puncture with special cannula. Anesthesiology 1967; 28:943.
10. Caparosa RJ, Zabatsky AR: Practical aspects of the cricothyroid space. Laryngoscope 1959; 67:577.
11. Jackson C: High tracheotomy and other errors: The chief causes of chronic laryngeal stenosis. Surg Gynecol Obstet 1921; 32:392.
12. Brantigan CO, Grow JB Sr: Cricothyroidotomy: Elective use in respirator problems requiring tracheotomy. J Thorac Cardiovasc Surg 1976; 71:72.
13. Plummer WB: The cricothyroidotomy: A lifesaving adjunct in acute obstructive asphyxia. J Georgia Dent Assoc 1969; 43:8.
14. Spaite DW, Joseph M: Prehospital cricothyrotomy: An investigation of indications, technique, complications, and patient outcome. Ann Emerg Med 1990; 19:279.
15. Boyle MF, Hatton D, Sheets C: Surgical cricothyrotomy performed by air ambulance flight nurses: A 5-year experience. J Emerg Med 1993; 11:41.
16. McGill J, Clinton JE, Ruiz E: Cricothyrotomy in the emergency department. Ann Emerg Med 1982; 11:361.
17. DeLaurier GA, Hawkins ML, Treat RC, et al: Acute airway management: Role of cricothyroidotomy. Am Surg 1990; 56:12.
18. Boyd AD, Romita MC, Conlan AA, et al: A clinical evaluation of cricothyroidotomy. Surg Gynecol Obstet 1979; 149:365.
19. O'Connor JV, Reddy K, Ergin MA, et al: Cricothyroidotomy for prolonged ventilatory support after cardiac operations. Ann Thorac Surg 1985; 39:353.
20. Pedersen J, Schurizek BA, Melsen NC, et al: Minitracheotomy in the treatment of postoperative sputum retention and atelectasis. Acta Anaesthesiol Scand 1988; 32:426.
21. Nugent WL, Rhee KJ, Wisner DH: Can nurses perform surgical cricothyrotomy with acceptable success and complication rates? Ann Emerg Med 1991; 20:367.
22. Slobodkin D, Topliff S, Raife JH: Retrograde intubation of the pharynx: An unusual complication of emergency cricothyrotomy. Ann Emerg Med 1992; 21:220.
23. Ryan DW, Dark JH, Misra U, et al: Intraesophageal placement of minitracheotomy tube. Intensive Care Med 1989; 15:538.
24. Holst M, Hedenstierna G, Kumlien JA, et al: Five years experience of coniotomy. Intensive Care Med 1985; 11:202.
25. Kuriloff DB, Setzen M, Portnoy W: Laryngotracheal injury following cricothyroidotomy. Larngoscope 1989; 92:125.
26. Weymuller EA Jr, Cummings CW: Cricothyroidotomy: The impact of antecedent endotracheal intubation. Ann Otol Rhin Laryngol 1982; 91:437.
27. Holst M, Veress B: The healing of cricothyroidostomy in pigs: A morphological study. Acta Otolaryngol 1989; 107:300.
28. Greisz H, Qvarnstorm O, Willien R: Elective cricothyroidotomy: A clinical and histopathological study. Crit Care Med 1982; 10:387.

29. Sise MJ, Shackford SR, Cruickshank JC: Cricothyroidotomy for long-term tracheal access: A prospective analysis of morbidity and mortality in 76 patients. Ann Surg 1984; 200:13.
30. Gleeson MJ, Pearson RC, Armistead S, et al: Voice changes following cricothyroidotomy. J Larynogol Otol 1984; 98:1015.
31. Holst M, Halbig I, Persson A, et al: The cricothyroid muscle after cricothyroidotomy: A porcine experimental study. Acta Otolaryngol 1989; 107:136.
32. Fisher JA: A "last ditch" airway. Can Anaesth Soc J 1979; 25:225.
33. Matthews HR, Hopkinson RB: Treatment of sputum retention by minitracheotomy. Br J Surg 1984; 71:147.
34. Mastboom WJB, Wobbes TH, van den Dries A: Bronchial suction by minitracheotomy as an effective measure against sputum retention. Surg Gynecol Obstet 1991; 173:187.
35. Randell TT, Tierala EK, Lepantalo MJ, et al: Prophylactic minitracheostomy after thoracotomy: A prospective, random control, clinical trial. Eur J Surg 1991; 157:501.
36. Clancy MJ: A study of the performance of cricothyroidotomy on cadavers using the Minitrach II. Arch Emerg Med 1989; 6:143.
37. Ravlo O, Bach V, Lybecker H, et al: A comparison between two emergency cricothyroidotomy instruments. Acta Anaesthesiol Scand 1987; 31:317.
38. Au J, Walker WS, Inglis D: Percutaneous cricothyroidostomy (minitracheostomy) for bronchial toilet: Results of therapeutic and prophylactic use. Ann Thorac Surg 1989; 48:850.
39. Ciaglia P, Brady C, Graniero D: Emergency percutaneous dilatational cricothyroidostomy: Use of modified nasal speculum. Am J Emerg Med 1992; 10:152.
40. Frei FJ, Meier PY, Lang FJ, et al: Cricothyrotomy using the Quicktrach coniotomy instrument set. Anasth Intensivther Notfallmed 1990; 25(Suppl 1):44.
41. Randell T, Kalli I, Lindgren L, et al: Minitracheotomy: Complications and follow-up with fibreoptic tracheoscopy. Anaesthesia 1990; 45:875.
42. Vesalius A: DeHumani Corporis Fabrica Libri Septem. Basel, 1555.
43. Colles CJ: On stenosis of the trachea after tracheotomy for croup and diphtheria. Ann Surg 1886; 3:499.
44. Kato I, Uesugi K, Kikuchihara M, et al: Tracheostomy: The horizontal tracheal incision. J Laryngol Otol 1990; 104:322.
45. Bjork VO, Engstrom CG: The treatment of ventilatory insufficiency after pulmonary resection with tracheostomy and prolonged artificial ventilation. J Thorac Surg 1955; 20:151.
46. Bercic J, Pocajt M, Drzecnik J: The influence of tracheal vascularization on the optimum location, shape and size of the tracheostomy in prolonged intubation. Resuscitation 1978; 6:131.
47. Fry TL, Jones RO, Fischer ND, et al: Comparisons of tracheostomy incisions in a pediatric model. Ann Otol Rhinol Laryngol 1985; 94:450.
48. Leverment JN, Milne DM: Tracheo-graft fistulae following pharyngo-laryngo-oesophagectomy: A cause and its prevention. J Laryngol Otol 1979; 93:293.
49. Fairshter RD, Liff MO, Wilson AF: Complications of long tracheostomy tubes. Crit Care Med 1976; 4:271.
50. Snyder GM: Individualized placement of tracheostomy tube fenestration and in-situ examinations with the fiberoptic laryngoscope. Respir Care 1983; 28:1294.
51. Klausen NO, Lomholt N, Qvist J: Dilatation of the trachea treated with the NL-tracheostomy tube. Crit Care Med 1982; 10:52.
52. Gunawardana RH: Experience with tracheostomy in medical intensive care patients. Postgrad Med J 1992; 68:338.
53. Goldstein SI, Breda SD, Schneider KL: Surgical complications of bedside tracheotomy in an otolaryngology residency program. Laryngsocope 1987; 97:1407.
54. Hawkins ML, Burrus EP, Treat RC, et al: Tracheostomy in the intensive care unit: A safe alternative to the operating room. South Med J 1989; 82:1096.
55. Hunt JL, Purdue GF, Gunning T: Is tracheostomy warranted in the burn patient? Indications and complications. J Burn Care Rehabil 1986; 7:492.
56. Lesnik I, Rappaport W, Fulginiti J, et al: The role of early tracheostomy in blunt, multiple organ trauma. Am Surg 1992; 58:346.
57. Rodriguez JL, Steinberg SM, Luchetti FA, et al: Early tracheostomy for primary airway management in the surgical critical care setting. Surgery 1990; 108:655.
58. Dunham CM, LaMonica CA: Prolonged tracheal intubation in the trauma patient. J Trauma 1984; 24:120.
59. Desjardins R, Desjardins G, Blanc VF, et al: Nasotracheal intubation and tracheostomy in acute epiglottitis and laryngotracheal bronchitis. J Otolaryngol 1978; 7:230.
60. Lund T, Goodwin CW, McManus WF: Upper airway sequelae in burn patients requiring endotracheal intubation or tracheostomy. Ann Surg 1985; 201:374.
61. Astrachan DI, Kirchner JC, Goodwin WJ Jr: Prolonged intubation vs. tracheostomy: Complications, practical and psychological considerations. Laryngoscope 1988; 98:1165.
62. Boyd SW, Benzel EC: The role of early tracheotomy in the management of the neurosurgical patient. Laryngoscope 1992; 102:559.
63. Miller JD, Kapp JP: Complications of tracheostomies in neurosurgical patients. Surg Neurol 1984; 22:186.
64. Cooper JD, Grillo HC: The evolution of tracheal injury due to ventilatory assistance through cuffed tubes: A pathologic study. Ann Surg 1969; 169:334.
65. Neiderman MS, Ferranti RD, Zeigler A, et al: Respiratory infection complicating long-term tracheostomy. Chest 1984; 85:39.
66. Neiderman MS, Merrill WW, Ferranti RD, et al: Nutritional status and bacterial binding in the lower respiratory tract in patients with chronic tracheostomy. Ann Internal Med 1984; 100:795.
67. Snow N, Richardson JD, Flint LM: Management of necrotizing tracheostomy infections. J Thorac Cardiovasc Surg 1981; 82:341.
68. Cole AGH, Kerr JH: Paratracheal abscess after tracheostomy. Intensive Care Med 1983; 9:345.
69. Rubio PA, Sharman TL, Farrell EM: Tracheostomy tube insertion in the pretracheal fascia. Int Surg 1982; 67(Suppl):418.
70. Arola M, Inberg MV, Sotarauta M, et al: Tracheo-arterial erosion complicating tracheostomy. Ann Chir Gynaecol 1979; 68:9.
71. Adolfsson R, Winblad B, Ostberg: Survival after haemorrhage from the brachiocephalic truncus following tracheostomy. Acta Otolaryngol 1975; 80:312.
72. Takano H, Ihara K, Sato S: Tracheo-innominate artery fistula following tracheostomy: Successful surgical management of a case. J Cardiovasc Surg 1989; 30:860.
73. Nunn DB, Sanchez-Salazar AA, McCullagh JM, et al: Tracheainnominate artery fistula following tracheostomy: Successful repair using an innominate vein graft. Ann Thorac Surg 1975; 20:698.
74. Wood DE, Mathisen DJ: Late complications of tracheotomy. Clin Chest Med 1991; 12:597.
75. Grillo HC: Congenital lesions, neoplasms, and injuries to the trachea. *In*: Surgery of the Chest. 5th ed. Sabiston DC, Spencer FC (Eds). Philadelphia, WB Saunders, 1990, pp 335–371.
76. Sellery GR, Worth A, Greenway RE: Late complications of prolonged tracheal intubation. Can Anaesth Soc J 1978; 25:140.
77. Woo P, Kelly G, Kirshner P: Airway complications in the head injured. Laryngoscope 1989; 99:725.
78. Oeken FW: Tracheostomy: Late complications and their treatment. Zentralblatt Chir 1978; 103:1169.
79. Jones JW, Reynolds M, Hewitt RL, et al: Tracheo-innominate artery erosion: Successful surgical management of a devasting complication. Ann Surg 1976; 184:194.
80. Sasaki CT, Horiuchi M, Koss N: Tracheostomy: Related subglottic stenosis: Bacteriologic pathogenesis. Laryngoscope 1979; 89:857.
81. Hsu S, Dreisbach JN, Charlifue SW: Glottic and tracheal stenosis in spinal cord injured patients. Paraplegia 1987; 25:136.
82. Lebowitz PW, Geller E, Andeweg SK: Endotracheal balloon cuff dilatation of tracheostomal stenosis. Anesthesiology 1982; 57:323.
83. Grillo HC, Mathisen DJ: Surgical management of tracheal strictures. Surg Clin North Am 1988; 68:511.
84. Rose KG: Cicatricial stenosis in the crico-tracheal region: A new surgical approach. HNO 1982; 30:285.
85. Reed JP, Kemph JP, Hamelberg W, et al: Studies with transtracheal artificial respiration. Anesthesiology 1954; 15:28.
86. Bougas TP, Cook CD: Pressure-flow characteristics of needles

suggested for transtracheal resuscitation. N Engl J Med 1960; 262:511.
87. Yealy DM, Plewa MC, Stewart RD: An evaluation of cannulae and oxygen sources for pediatric jet ventilation. Am J Emerg Med 1991; 9:20.
88. Dallen LT, Wine R, Benumof JL: Spontaneous ventilation via transtracheal large-bore intravenous catheters is possible. Anesthesiology 1991; 75:531.
89. Mackenzie CF, Barnas GM, Smalley J, et al: Low-flow endobronchial insufflation with air for 2 hours of apnea provides ventilation adequate for survival. Anesth Analg 1990; 71:279.
90. Slutsky AS, Watson J, Leith DE: Tracheal insufflation of O_2 (TRIO) at low rates sustains life for several hours. Anesthesiology 1985; 63:278.
91. Smith RB, Babinski M, Klain M, et al: Percutaneous transtracheal ventilation. JACEP 1976; 5:765.
92. Jorden RC, Moore EE, Marx JA: A comparison of PTV and endotracheal ventilation in an acute trauma model. J Trauma 1985; 25:978.
93. Tan SS, Dhara SS, Sim CK: Removal of a laryngeal foreign body using high frequency jet ventilation. Anaesthesia 1991; 46:741.
94. Weymuller EA Jr, Pavlin EG, Paugh D: Management of difficult airway problems with percutaneous transtracheal ventilation. Ann Otol Rhinol Laryngol 1987; 96:34.
95. Lassa RE, Habal MB, Ross N, et al: Rapid access airway: Surgical device and technique. Int Surg 1978; 63:152.
96. Schein B, Orko R, Orsback C: Ventilation through a minitracheostomy: An experimental study in pigs. Ann Chir Gynaecol 1987; 76:327.
97. Campbell CT, Harris RC, Cook MH, et al: A new device for emergency percutaneous transtracheal ventilation in partial and complete airway obstruction. Ann Emerg Med 1988; 17:927.
98. Ravussin P, Freeman P: A new transtracheal catheter for ventilation and resuscitation. Can Anaesth Soc J 1985; 32:60.
99. Matthews HR, Fischer BJ, Smith BE: Minitracheostomy: A new delivery system for jet ventilation. J Thorac Cardiovasc Surg 1986; 92:673.
100. Mammel MC, Ophoven JP, Lewallen PK, et al: High-frequency ventilation and tracheal injuries. Pediatrics 1986; 77:608.
101. Shuptrine JR, Auffant RA, Gal TJ: Cerebral and cardiopulmonary responses to high-frequency jet ventilation and conventional mechanical ventilation in a model of brain and lung injury. Anesth Analg 1984; 63:1065.
102. Wei HF, Jin SA, Bi HS: Hemodynamic effects of high frequency jet ventilation during acute hypovolemia. J Tongji Med Univ 1991; 11:174.
103. Lindholm P, Outzen KE: Pneumothorax during jet ventilation in laryngobronchoscopy. Ugesk Laeger 1991; 153:199.
104. Bourreli B, Bigot A, Wesoluch M, et al: Pneumomediastinum and subcutaneous emphysema after translaryngeal jet ventilation. Ann Fr Anesth Reanim 1984; 3:377.
105. Yealy DM, Plewa MC, Reed JJ, et al: Manual translaryngeal jet ventilation and the risk of aspiration in a canine model. Ann Emerg Med 1990; 19:238.
106. Golden GT, Fox JW, Edlich RF: Emergency tracheostomy. Am J Surg 1976; 131:766.
107. Ivatury R, Siegel JH, Stahl WM, et al: Percutaneous tracheostomy after trauma and critical illness. J Trauma 1992; 32:133.
108. Schachner A, Ovil Y, Sidi J, et al: Percutaneous tracheostomy: A new method. Crit Care Med 1989; 17:1052.
109. Bodenham A, Cohen A, Webster N: A clinical evaluation of the "Rapitrach:" A bedside percutaneous tracheostomy technique. Anaesthesia 1992; 47:332.
110. Ciaglia P, Firsching R, Syniec C: Elective percutaneous dilatational tracheostomy: A new simple bedside procedure: Preliminary report. Chest 1985; 87:715.
111. Leinhardt DJ, Mughal M, Bowles B, et al: Appraisal of percutaneous tracheostomy. Br J Surg 1992; 79:255.
112. Toye FJ, Weinstein JD: Clinical experience with percutaneous tracheostomy and cricothyroidotomy in 100 patients. J Trauma 1986; 26:1034.
113. Ciaglia P, Graniero KD: Percutaneous dilatational tracheostomy: Results and long-term follow-up. Chest 1992; 101:464.
114. Hutchinson RC, Mitchell RD: Life-threatening complications from percutaneous dilational tracheostomy. Crit Care Med 1991; 19:118.
115. Hazard P, Jones C, Benitone J: Comparative clinical trial of standard operative tracheostomy with percutaneous tracheostomy. Crit Care Med 1991; 19:1018.
116. Paul A, Marelli D, Chiu RC, et al: Percutaneous endoscopic tracheostomy. Ann Thorac Surg 1989; 47:314.
117. Fisher EW, Howard DJ: Percutaneous tracheostomy in a head and neck unit. J Laryngol Otol 1992; 106:625.
118. Bodenham A, Diament R, Cohen A, et al: Percutaneous dilational tracheostomy: A bedside procedure on the intensive care unit. Anaesthesia 1991; 46:570.

CHAPTER 81

Proximal Airway Disorders in the Pediatric Patient

Richard E. Weibley, MD, MPH

Airway pathology is a common problem for physicians caring for pediatric patients. The proximal airway from the nares to the carina is often involved. Although the number of different disorders that can occur in the proximal airway of pediatric patients is large, careful attention to history and physical findings coupled with an understanding of anatomy and pathophysiology should allow a clinician to localize the lesion generally and begin treatment while investigating and defining the specific diagnosis.

ANATOMY

The processes of development as well as absolute size differences are important for understanding the causes of proximal airway failure and their appropriate treatment in infants, children, and adolescents. Because newborn infants have a relatively small mandible and a large tongue that crowds and fills the oropharynx, infants are primarily obligate nose breathers during quiet respiration.[1] As the midface and mandible grow, the relative difficulties of oropharyngeal breathing in infancy disappear.

The epiglottis in infancy is relatively long and stiff, U or V shaped, and angulated approximately 45° from the anterior pharyngeal wall owing to the close proximity of the hyoid bone and thyroid cartilage.[2] As growth occurs, separation of the hyoid and the thyroid cartilage results in a more erect position of the epiglottis. By adolescence, the epiglottis assumes the flattened and flexible adult anatomy, positioned parallel to the base of the tongue.

The laryngeal structures also change with growth, moving lower in the neck with age.[1] In term infants, the laryngeal inlet is at the level of the cervical vertebral interspace C3-4, whereas in adults it rests at interspace C4-5. As an infant grows, the vocal cords change direction and shape with increasing length, primarily as a result of growth of the anterior ligamentous portion. In adults, the narrowest portion of the respiratory tract is generally the laryngeal inlet, whereas in infants and young children it is usually the laryngeal outlet, the inferior ring portion (arch) of the cricoid cartilage. With growth the ring enlarges, the cricoid plate assumes a more vertical position, and this anatomic point of narrowing disappears.

The histologic characteristics of the larynx remain constant from infancy to adulthood. Squamous epithelium covers the upper epiglottis, the lateral walls of the vestibule, and the vocal cords. Ciliated columnar epithelium lines the ventricle, the inferior portion of the vestibules, and the entire laryngeal cavity below the laryngeal inlet. Attached by loose connective tissue, the columnar epithelium becomes easily infiltrated with edema when irritated, an important process in the pathophysiology of several obstructive disorders.

Although airway diameter decreases progressively with branching of the conducting airways, total airway area steadily increases at each successive level of the tracheobronchial tree.[3] Little decrease in individual airway diameter occurs with branching distal to the bronchiole. As the airstream moves peripherally, increases in cross-sectional area sharply reduce airflow velocity, with important physiologic implications for the distribution of airway resistance in normal and disease states.

NORMAL AND ABNORMAL PHYSIOLOGY

The proximal airway performs many functions, including filtering, warming, and humidifying air in its passage from the atmosphere to the alveoli. Perhaps the most critical physiologic characteristic of the proximal airway is its substantial contribution to total functional resistance secondary to tissue and gas movements.[4] This has implications for both acute and chronic disease states, especially in infants and young children.

Airway resistance is affected by changes in airway dimension, number, pressure, and flow. A simple formula for resistance is

$$\text{Resistance} = \frac{\text{change in pressure}}{\text{flow}}$$

Thus, resistance is directly proportional to pressure changes and inversely proportional to flow changes. Poiseuille's law describes the pressure produced by laminar gas flow through a tube.[3, 4] The radius, raised to the fourth power in the denominator of the equation, is the most important determinant of pressure and thus resistance.

Airway resistances normally change at differing lung volumes.[3, 4] At large volumes, the airways are distended and resistance is low. After forced expiration and near residual volume, resistance becomes infinitely high as pleural pressures close airways and flow ceases. Estimates of total lung resistance (airway and tissue) have been obtained using dynamic pressure-volume curves and plethysmography.[4, 5] Measurements in children younger than 2 years are 6 to 20 times those in adults at resting lung volumes. An infant's average nasal resistance by indirect measurements is nearly half of total respiratory resistance. Because of the rapid increase in total cross-sectional area with successive branching of conducting airways, nearly all airway resistance occurs proximal to small bronchioles. Hence, even modest reductions in the size of the most proximal airways significantly increase airway resistance, producing signs and symptoms of obstruction. This is particularly important in the smallest and youngest patients.

Abnormalities associated with proximal airway obstruction may be either acute or chronic in character. They include changes in respiratory rate, depth, inspiratory-expiratory ratio, nasal flaring, retractions, wheezing or stridor, right or left heart failure, and pulmonary edema. In severe obstruction, patients may exhibit agitation, irritability, confusion, or somnolence. Cyanosis, hypercarbia, and uncompensated respiratory or metabolic acidosis signal imminent collapse.

Normal breathing is not audible because even during maximum inspiration and exhalation, linear airflow velocity is too low to produce sound. Breathing becomes audible when narrowed air passages change the linear velocity and airflow characteristics, creating turbulence and noise. Stridor and wheezing are the hallmarks of respiratory obstruction.[6] Understanding their pathophysiology helps a clinician to localize an obstructive lesion and direct therapy most effectively.

Supracarinal lesions commonly reveal symmetric changes throughout the respiratory cycle, whereas obstructive pathology beyond the carina creates evidence of unilateral signs and symptoms. Similarly, lesions of the extrathoracic airway are evident during the inspiratory phase of respiration, and those of an intrathoracic conducting airway during exhalation. A useful general rule is that lesions causing stridor are found above the clavicle (thoracic inlet) whereas those associated with wheezing are located below the clavicle (intrathoracic). In rare circumstances, an inspiratory wheeze or expiratory stridor may be described. Generally, a careful physical examination coupled with a thorough history allow localization of the obstructive site.

Stridor may be loud or soft, high pitched or low, musical or harsh. It occurs overwhelmingly in the proximal airway between the laryngeal inlet and the thoracic inlet of the trachea. In this portion of the airway, the individual forces of a relatively positive atmospheric pressure and negative intraluminal airway pressure combine to collapse the airway and obstruct airflow at the site of pathology during inspiration. The resulting airflow turbulence creates the characteristic noise termed *stridor.*

Wheezing, most often associated with asthma and reactive airway disease, is predominately an expiratory sound related to obstruction of the intrathoracic conducting airways. In contrast to the dynamics of the extrathoracic airway during inspiration, the intrathoracic airways are collapsed and obstructed by positive thoracic pressures and tissue elastic forces during exhalation. Wheezing is not synonymous with bronchospasm because it also arises from other obstructive airway pathologies.

Chronic obstruction of proximal airways was linked to cardiac disease in 1965. Several investigators[7, 8] reported the finding of cor pulmonale in patients with various types of chronic airway obstruction such as hypertrophied lymphoid tissue or laryngotracheomalacia (LTM). Other researchers even reported on finding left heart failure due to airway obstruction.[9, 10] In all cases, the patient had experienced airway obstruction for many months before evaluation. Relief of the obstruction improved the heart failure in all cases.

Pulmonary edema has also been described in association with acute airway obstruction.[11] In the 1970s and 1980s, pulmonary edema was reported in association with croup or epiglottitis,[12] strangulation,[13] laryngospasm or laryngeal edema,[14] and foreign bodies.[14, 15] The presence of the pulmonary edema was noted both before and after relief of the obstructive lesion. Whether it is often present (but not recognized) before the airway obstruction is relieved is of some controversy.[16] It is clear that acute pulmonary edema may be a complicating factor of both acute and chronic airway obstruction.

Chronic airway obstruction can also lead to pulmonary hypertension. As the right ventricle hypertrophies, encroachment of the left ventricle occurs via ballooning of the interventricular septum. Left ventricular end-diastolic pressures may be followed by elevated left atrial pressures, resulting in biventricular failure and pulmonary edema.[13]

DIFFERENTIAL DIAGNOSIS AND TREATMENT

Congenital Problems

Airway obstruction in pediatric patients can be easily categorized into acquired and congenital causes (Table 81–1).[17]

TABLE 81–1. Common Causes of Obstruction in Pediatric Patients

Congenital
Choanal atresia
Craniofacial dysmorphologic features (with micrognathia and glossoptosis)
Pierre Robin syndrome
Treacher Collins syndrome
Macroglossia
Beckwith's syndrome
Congenital hypothyroidism
Down's syndrome
Laryngotracheomalacia
Subglottic stenosis
Vocal cord paralysis
Laryngotracheoesophageal webs
Vascular rings and slings
Tracheal anomalies
Tumors and cysts
Metabolic: hypocalcemia
Neurogenic: reflex laryngospasm
Acquired Obstruction
Infectious
Supraglottitis
Laryngotracheobronchitis
Retropharyngeal abscess
Bacterial tracheitis
Trauma
Foreign bodies
Iatrogenic
Postextubation
Postinstrumentation
Postoperative
External trauma
Thermal and chemical burns
Neoplasia
Laryngeal papillomatosis
Miscellaneous tumors and nodes

Among the congenital lesions, three craniofacial anomalies occur most frequently: choanal atresia, Pierre Robin anomaly, and Treacher Collins syndrome.

Bilateral choanal atresia, evident in neonates who develop respiratory distress when their mouth is closed, is easily diagnosed by failure of a suction catheter to pass from the naris through the nasopharynx and into the posterior pharynx. Treatment involves the placement of an oral airway followed by surgical removal of the obstructing tissue or bony plate. Both Pierre Robin and Treacher Collins syndrome cause airway obstruction owing to mandibular hypoplasia and relative macroglossia with posterior positioning of the tongue into the nasopharynx and oropharynx. Management goals are to maintain an adequate airway until mandibular growth occurs.[18] In the most severely affected infants, tracheostomy may be necessary to prevent the development of cor pulmonale.

LTM, also called *congenital laryngeal stridor,* is a common, transient, and generally self-limited cause of stridor due to cartilaginous immaturity and laxness in the laryngeal framework and epiglottis. The stridor gradually resolves with growth. Endotracheal intubation or tracheostomy is rarely necessary, although symptoms may worsen dramatically with the occurrence of otherwise trivial viral upper respiratory tract infections. LTM reportedly accounts for as much as 75% of congenital laryngeal pathology; however, it is probably overdiagnosed as a result of a lack of precise diagnostic criteria.[17] Patients with LTM with persistent symptoms not resolving with growth and maturation or with severe symptoms should be carefully evaluated for alternative pathology.

Congenital subglottic stenosis usually has its most significant point of narrowing in the area of the cricoid cartilage, 2 to 3 mm below an infants glottis. Inflammation and swelling from secondary causes superimposed on the fixed lesion further decrease airway diameter. In airways of this size, as little as 1 mm of uniform edema can reduce the airway cross-sectional area 70%, seriously limiting a child's ability to breathe.[2]

Congenital vocal cord paralysis may account for as many as 10% of congenital laryngeal disorders.[17] Bilateral or unilateral paralysis generally corresponds to central or peripheral nerve pathology. The left recurrent laryngeal nerve is more susceptible to damage associated with surgery or other congenital lesions, often cardiovascular. Bilateral vocal cord paralysis is associated with increased intracranial pressure as a result of caudal brain stem displacement and nerve root traction.[1, 17] Birth trauma may also be responsible, although in most cases the cause remains unknown. Of importance, congenital vocal cord paralysis has a favorable prognosis for spontaneous recovery.

Aberrant aortic arch remnant vessels create vascular rings and slings with secondary compression of the esophagus or trachea.[17, 19–20] These may be present as either intermittent or persistent wheezing or stridor, often in association with eating. Surgical correction is necessary for lesions causing moderate to severe obstruction associated with recurrent pneumonia, atelectasis, or failure to thrive.[4] Preoperatively, an endotracheal tube provides a secure airway.

Acquired Pathology

Infection

After the newborn period, infectious causes of upper-airway obstruction are most common. Adenoidal and tonsillar hypertrophy may cause acute or chronic obstruction.[21–24] Potential spaces defined by fascial places serve as sites for abscess formation and airway obstruction. These occur most commonly in children older than 1 to 2 years and are generally bacterial, although a notable exception is the lymphoid hypertrophy associated with Epstein-Barr virus infection.[22–23] Acute epiglottitis (AE), laryngotracheobronchitis (LTB), and bacterial tracheitis (BT) are the most common presenting infectious causes of upper-airway obstruction (Table 81–2).

AE, also called *supraglottitis,* is most often due to *Haemophilus influenzae* type B but also includes viral agents and group A beta-hemolytic streptococci. Widespread vaccination of infants against *H. influenzae* appears to be dramatically lowering the incidence of life-threatening disease, including epiglottitis.[25] The clinical picture of AE is classically one of extreme respiratory distress, high fever, drooling, and dysphagia, all of abrupt onset. Unfortunately, supraglottic infections may not present with the classic picture; symptoms often mimic LTB or BT.[26–28]

The unacceptably high mortality and morbidity associated with failure to diagnose AE have led to a systemized approach to diagnosis and treatment in suspected cases.[29] Patients should not be left unattended by someone skilled in airway management. The use of radiologic procedures such as lateral neck films should only be used for exceptional cases. At present, the accepted plan is to take the child to the operating room for visual inspection of the airway and nasotracheal intubation. Cultures of the epiglottis and blood should be obtained after the airway is secured, and antibiotics instituted, ensuring coverage against β-lactamase–positive *H. influenzae.* Other sites of infection due to *H. influenzae* should also be screened, such as the lungs, joints, and rarely the central nervous system.[30]

After intubation, patients should remain in an intensive

TABLE 81–2. Comparison of Laryngotracheobronchitis, Acute Epiglottis, and Bacterial Tracheitis

	LTB	*AE*	*BT*
History			
Age	2 mo–3 y	3–7 y (usually)	All ages
Onset	Gradual	Rapid	Gradual
Respiratory disease	None to moderate	Marked	Moderate–marked
Symptoms			
Dysphagia	0	2+	+1−
Dyspnea	+1−	2–3+	2+−
Sore Throat	+1−	4+	+1−
Signs			
Sound	Bark, stridor	Muffed, guttural	Bark, stridor
Secretions	Normal for age	Drooling	Normal for age
Position	Lying, sitting, standing	Sitting, leaning	Sitting
Temperature	37–38° C	38° C+	38° C+
Facies	Normal	Anxious, distressed, toxic	Anxious

care unit where proper maintenance of the airway can be accomplished. An issue of some controversy is when to extubate patients and whether to visualize the epiglottis to aid in the decision. Although numerous studies have addressed this issue, none has really provided evidence of the need for or predictive value of visualization.[31] Resolution of airway obstruction does not appear to correlate with resolution of fever[31] or the size of the epiglottis.[31, 32]

LTB is usually a mild illness not requiring critical care services. The clinical features are well recognized (see Table 81–2). For those with symptoms severe enough to warrant hospital admission, the use of a scoring system provides an objective measure of the degree of respiratory difficulty. Several different scoring systems have been developed.[33, 34] A relatively simple one is found in Table 81–3.

A host of viral agents cause LTB. Parainfluenza viruses account for most cases; adenoviruses, respiratory syncytial virus, influenza virus, and measles virus are other identifiable agents. Viral LTB usually has a less rapid onset, lower fever, and less toxic appearance than AE. It also tends to occur in younger infants and children, primarily 3 months to 5 years of age.

Treatment of viral LTB is symptomatic. Mist therapy, although historically used, has never been shown to be beneficial.[35, 36] Oxygen is indicated if hypoxemia is present. The use of α-adrenergic agents, primarily racemic epinephrine, is common and beneficial although associated with rebound of symptoms.[37] Corticosteroid therapy has been debated for the past 25 years and still remains controversial.[33, 38, 39] Helium and oxygen mixtures have been used for LTB and other obstructive lesions.[40, 41] Of lower viscosity than nitrogen and oxygen mixtures, heliox reduces airway resistance and work of breathing. At least one study has suggested a risk of hypoxemia in small infants.[41] Antibiotics are of no benefit in uncomplicated viral LTB.

Bacterial tracheitis, with features that overlap both LTB and AE (see Table 81–2), probably represents a bacterial superinfection complicating viral LTB.[42–44] Clinical symptoms begin with gradual onset of upper respiratory tract complaints progressing to fever, toxicity, and marked distress. Laryngoscopy reveals a normal epiglottis with mucopurulent edema and copious thick secretions requiring tracheal intubation for airway toilet and relief of obstructive symptoms. The usual pathogens are *Staphylococcus aureus*, *H. influenzae*, or alpha-hemolytic streptococci. A few patients have been reported to develop toxic shock syndrome,[43, 45] and BT may occur more frequently in children with trisomy 21, a population with underlying airway anatomic and immunologic differences.[46] *Aspergillus* tracheobronchitis with symptomatic upper airway obstruction is an emerging problem in HIV-infected or other immunocompromised patients.[46a, 46b] Despite the concern about BT, antibiotics should not be used routinely as prophylaxis in patient with LTB.

Trauma

Trauma follows infection as the second most common cause of upper respiratory tract obstruction in the pediatric population.[47] Included are such injuries as foreign bodies, iatrogenic instrumentation injury to the laryngeal airway or recurrent laryngeal nerve, facial and laryngeal impact injuries, and chemical or thermal burns. Foreign bodies and iatrogenic, postextubation obstructive symptoms are most common.

Foreign bodies in children lodge most commonly in the major bronchi.[48, 49] Nuts, especially peanuts, and miscellaneous food particles are frequent offenders. Toddlers are most often affected, although foreign bodies may be found from 6 months of age on into adulthood. Obstruction distal to the larynx usually does not cause stridor but wheezing. Esophageal foreign bodies produce stridor or wheezing by secondary airway compression.[49, 50] When no aspiration history is obtained, tracheal foreign bodies often are initially misdiagnosed as viral LTB.

Foreign body removal requires close teamwork between the intensivist, pulmonologist or surgeon, and anesthesiologist. The use of inhaled bronchodilators, postural drainage, and percussion is not recommended for removal of foreign bodies, because dislodgement of a distal object into the subglottic space may cause severe or total airway occlusion, a life-threatening complication.[48, 51]

The mechanical trauma associated with intubation, instrumentation, and surgery usually causes stridor due to localized mucosal edema. Less commonly, ulceration, granuloma formation, webs, membranes, stenosis, necrosis, infection, or vocal cord paralysis occurs.[52] Facial blows and neck injuries can precipitate acute respiratory difficulty through dislocation of the cricoarytenoid cartilage, hematoma or soft-tissue swelling and airway compression, and laryngeal or trachea edema or disruption.[53]

Acute upper-airway obstruction due to laryngeal and tracheal edema follows ingestion of acids, alkalis, and corrosive chemical substances, as well as inhalation of hot air, steam, smoke, or chemicals.[54] Patients should be admitted to the hospital for observation in a setting where they can

TABLE 81–3. Croup Severity Scoring System

Sign	*0*	*1*	*2*	*Individual Score*
Inspiratory breath sounds	Normal	Harsh rhonchi	Delayed	________
Stridor	None	Inspiratory	Inspiratory and expiratory	________
Cough	None	Hoarse cry	Seal-like bark	________
Retractions/ nasal flaring	None	Nasal flaring Suprasternal retractions	Flaring suprasternal intercostal retractions	________
Cyanosis	None	In room air	In 40% oxygen	________
			Total score	________

be closely monitored for signs or symptoms of airway compromise. Endoscopic examination of the airway and esophagus may be indicated in selected patients. Intravenous fluids, oxygen, and racemic epinephrine may relieve obstructive symptoms and alleviate the need for mechanical airway support. Corticosteroids, although used by some clinicians, are probably of no benefit.

Tumors

Children with tumors may present with symptoms of airway obstruction due to extrinsic compression from a mass lesion.[20, 21, 55] Airway support is often necessary until radiation or chemotherapy can be instituted to shrink the tumor size.

Early intubation is recommended before edema or obstruction becomes life threatening as a result of any proximal airway lesion in childhood. It is important to realize that laryngoscopy in infants demonstrates a larynx located superiorly, a large tongue, and a hyoid bone positioned to depress the epiglottis.[3] The epiglottis is relatively large, stiff, and U shaped, and the airway's narrowest portion is not the glottic inlet but the subglottic space in the region of the cricoid cartilage. An endotracheal tube that passes easily between the vocal cords but not through the cricoid ring should be replaced with a smaller tube to avoid irritating the mucous membranes, a precipitating factor in the development of postextubation stridor and obstruction. In selected circumstances, flexible fiberoptic bronchoscopy may be the method of choice for intubation and evaluation of the airway.[56]

References

1. Hengerer AS, Newburg JA: Congenital malformations of the nose and paranasal sinuses. *In*: Pediatric Otolaryngology. 2nd ed. Bluestone CD, Stool SE (Eds). Philadelphia, WB Saunders, p 727, 1990.
2. Eckenhoff JE: Some anatomic considerations of the infant larynx influencing endotracheal anesthesia. Anesthesiology 1951; 12:401.
3. Brody JS, Thurlbeck WM: Development, growth and aging of lung. *In:* Handbook of Physiology. Section 3: The Respiratory System. Fishman AP (Ed). Bethesda, MD, American Physiological Society, 1986.
4. Wohl MEB, Mead J: Age as a factor in respiratory disease. *In*: Kendig's Disorders of the Respiratory Tract. 5th ed. Chernick V (Ed). Philadelphia, WB Saunders, 1990, pp 175–181.
5. Bryan AC, Wohl MD: Respiratory mechanics in children. *In*: The Respiratory System: Handbook of Physiology. Section 3. Vol 3. American Physiologic Society. Fishman AP (Ed). Baltimore, Williams & Williams, 1986.
6. Respiratory noises. *In*: Respiratory Illness in Children. 2nd ed. Phelan PD, Landau LI, Olinsky A (Eds). Boston, Blackwell Scientific Publications, 1982, pp 104–131.
7. Cox MA, Schiebler GL, Taylor WJ, et al: Reversible pulmonary hypertension in a child with respiratory obstruction and cor pulmonale. J Pediatr 1965; 67:192.
8. Menashe VD, Farrchi C, Miller M: Hypoventilation and and cor pulmonale due to chronic upper airway obstruction. J Pediatr 1965; 67:198.
9. Luke MJ, Mehrizi A, Golger EH, et al: Chronic nasopharyngeal obstruction as a cause of cardiomegaly, cor pulmonale and pulmonary edema. Pediatrics 1966; 37:762.
10. Levin DL, Muster AJ, Pachman LM, et al: Cor pulmonale secondary to upper airway obstruction—cardiac catheterization, immunologic and psychometric evaluation in nine patients. Chest 1975; 68:166.
11. Timby J, Reed C, Zeilander S, et al: "Mechanical" causes of pulmonary edema. Chest 1990; 98:973.
12. Travis KW, Todres ID, Shannon DC: Pulmonary edema associated with croup and epiglottitis. Pediatrics 1977; 59:695.
13. Ladbrook PA, Byrne JD, McKnight RC: Influence of right ventricular hemodynamics on left ventricular diastolic pressure-volume relations in man. Circulation 1979; 59:21.
14. Oudjhane K, Bowen A, Oh KS, et al: Pulmonary edema complicating upper airway obstruction in infants and children. Can Assoc Radiol J 1992; 43:278.
15. Izsak E: Pulmonary edema due to acute upper airway obstruction from aspirated foreign body. Pediatr Emerg Care 1986; 2:235.
16. Kanter RK, Wacehko JF: Pulmonary edema associated with upper airway obstruction. Am J Dis Child 1984; 138:356.
17. Maze A, Bloch E: Stridor in pediatric patients. Anesthesiology 1979; 50:132.
18. Bull MJ, Given DC, Sandove AM, et al: Improved outcome in Pierre Robin sequence: Effect of multidisciplinary evaluation and management. Pediatrics 1990; 86:294.
19. Fletcher BD, Cohn RC: Tracheal compression and the innominate artery. MR evaluation in infants. Radiology 1989; 170:103.
20. Colquhoun IW, Pollock JC: Distal tracheal stenosis in two children with double aortic arch and associated tracheomalacia. Eur J Cardiothorac Surg 1990; 4:287.
21. Kraus DH, Rehm SJ, Orlowski JP, et al: Upper airway obstruction due to tonsillar lymphadenopathy in human immunodeficiency virus infection. Arch Otolaryngol Head Neck Surg 1990; 116:738.
22. Woolf DC, Diedericks RJ: Airway obstruction in infectious mononucleosis. A case report. S Afr Med J 1989; 75:584.
23. Kielmovitch IH, Keleti G, Bluestone CD, et al: Microbiology of obstructive tonsillar hypertrophy and recurrent tonsillitis. Arch Otolaryngol Head Neck Surg 1989; 115:721.
24. Sofer S, Weinhouse E, Tal A, et al: Cor pulmonale due to adenoidal or tonsillar hypertrophy or both. Chest 1988; 93:119.
25. Black SB, Shinefield HR, and the Kaiser Permanente Pediatric Study Group: Immunization with oligosaccharide conjugate *Hemophilus influenzae* type b (HbOC) vaccine on a large health maintenance organization population: Extended follow-up and impact on *Hemophilus influenzae* disease epidemiology. Pediatr Infect Dis J 1992; 11:610.

25a. Gorelick MH, Baker MD: Epiglottitis in children, 1979 through 1992: Effects of *Hemophilus influenzae* type b immunization. Arch Pediatr Adolesc Med 1994; 148:47.

25b. Beck RA, Kambiss S, Bass JW: The retreat of *Hemophilus influenzae* type b invasive disease: Analysis of an immunization program and implications for OTO-HNS. Otolaryngol Head Neck Surg 1993; 109:712.

26. Shackleford GD, Siegel MJ, McAllister WH, et al: Subglottic edema in acute epiglottitis in children. Am J Roentgenol 1978; 131:603.
27. Brilli RJ, Benzing G, Cotcamp DH: Epiglottitis in infants less than two years of age. Pediatr Emerg Care 1989; 5:16.
28. Gershan WM, Gillman K, Baxter M, et al: Acute airway obstruction in a seven month old infant with epiglottitis. Pediatr Emerg Care 1988; 4:197.

28a. Cressman WE, Myer CM 3rd: Diagnosis and management of croup and epiglotittis. Pediatr Clin North Am 1994; 41:265.

29. Bass JW, Fajardo JE, Brien JH, et al: Sudden death due to acute epiglottitis. Pediatr Infect Dis 1987; 4:447.
30. Friedman EM, Healy GB, Damioh J, et al: Sypraglottitis and concurrent hemophilus meningitis. Ann Otol Rhinol Laryngol 1985; 94:470.
31. Rothstein P, Lister G: Epiglottitis—duration of intubation and fever. Anesth Analg 1983; 62:785.
32. Rowe LD: Advances and controversies in the management of supraglottitis and laryngotracheobronchitis. Am J Otholaryngol 1980; 1:235.
33. Leipzig B, Oski FA, Cummings CW, et al: A prospective randomized study to determine the efficacy of steroids in croup. J Pediatr 1979; 94:194.
34. Taussig LM, Castro O, Beaudry AC: The respiratory status of children with croup. J Pediatr 1975; 81:1068.
35. Bourchier D, Dawson KP, Fergusson DM: Humidification in viral croup: A controlled trial. Aust Pediatr J 1984; 20:289.
36. Henry R: Moist air in the treatment of laryngotracheitis. Otolaryngol Head Neck Surg 1980; 88:207.
37. Fogel, JM, Berg IJ, Gerber MA, et al: Racemic epinephrine in treatment of croup: Nebulization alone versus nebulization with intermittent positive pressure breathing. J Pediatr 1982; 101:1028.

38. Martinez-Fernandez A, Sanchez-Gonzalez E, Rica-Etxebarria I, et al: Randomized double-blind study of treatment of croup with adrenaline and/or dexamethasone in children. An Esp Pediatr 1993; 38:29.
39. Tibballs J, Shann FA, Landau LI: Placebo-controlled trial of prednisolone in children intubated for croup. Lancet 1992; 340:745.
40. Skrinkas GJ, Hyland RH, Hutcheon MA: Using helium-oxygen mixtures in the management of acute airway obstruction. Can Med Assoc J 1983; 128:555.
41. Butt WW, Koren G, England S, et al: Hypoxia associated with helium-oxygen therapy in neonates. J Pediatr 1985; 106:474.
42. Edwards KM, Dundon MC, Altemeier WA: Bacterial tracheitis as a complication of viral croup. Pediatr Infect Dis 1983; 2:390.
43. Donnelly BW, McMillan JA, Weiner LB: Bacterial tracheitis: Report of eight new cases and review. Rev Infect Dis 1990; 12:729.
44. Dubin AA, Tholji A, Rambaud-Cousson A: Bacterial tracheitis among children hospitalized for severe obstructuve dyspnea. Pediatr Infect Dis J 1990; 9:293.
44a. Eckel HE, Widemann B, Damm M, et al: Airway endoscopy in the diagnosis and treatment of bacterial tracheitis in children. Int J Pediatr Otorhinolaryngol 1993; 27:147.
45. Chenaud M, Leclere F, Martinot A: Bacterial croup and toxic shock syndrome. Pediatrics 1986; 145:306.
46. Caut AJ, Gibson PJ, West RJ: Bacterial tracheitis in Down's syndrome. Arch Dis Child 1987; 62:962.
46a. Kemper CA, Hostetler JS, Follansbee SE, et al: Ulcerative and plaque-like tracheobronchitis due to infection with *Aspergillus* in patients with AIDS. Clin Infect Dis 1993; 17:344.
46b. Tait RC, O'Driscoll BR, Denning DW: Unilateral wheeze caused by pseudomembranous *Aspergillus* tracheobronchitis in the immunocompromised patient. Thorax 1993; 48:1285.
47. Kissoon N, Dreyer J, Walia M: Pediatric trauma: Differences in pathophysiology, injury patterns and treatment compared with adult trauma. Can Med Assoc J 1990; 142:27.
48. Lima JA: Laryngeal foreign bodies in children: A persistent, life-threatening problem. Laryngoscope 1989; 99:415.
49. Freidman EM: Foreign bodies in the pediatric aerodigestive tract. Pediatr Annu 1988; 17:640.
50. Adachi K, Hayashida M, Toyoshima K: Airway obstruction in a child with esophageal achalasia. Acta Pediatr Jpn 1989; 31:600.
51. Humphries CT, Wagener JS, Morgan WJ: Fatal prolonged foreign body aspiration following an asymptomatic interval. Am J Emerg Med 1988; 7:669.
52. Koka BV, Jeon IS, Andre JM, et al: Postintubation croup in children. Anaest Analg 1977; 56:501.
53. Fitz-Hugh GS, Powell JB: Acute traumatic injuries of the oropharynx, laryngopharynx, and cervical trachea in children. Otolaryngol Clin North Am 1970; 3:375.
54. Charnock EL, Meehan J: Postburn respiratory injuries in children. Ped Clin North Am 1980; 27:661.
55. Pelton JJ, Ratner IA: A technique of airway management in children with obstructed airway due to tumor. Ann Thorac Surg 1989; 48:301.
56. Baines DB, Goodrick MA, Beckenham EJ, et al: Fiberoptically guided endotracheal intubation in a child. Anaesth Intensive Care 1989; 17:354.

CHAPTER 82

Distal Airway Disorders in Infants and Children: Bronchiolitis and Asthma

John B. Downes, MD • Sharon L. Pilmer, MD

Disorders of the lower airways, those airways distal to the carina, account for much of the morbidity and mortality associated with pulmonary disease in postneonatal infants and children. Bronchiolitis and asthma rank among the leading causes of acute, reversible respiratory failure in infancy and childhood. Infants with bronchopulmonary dysplasia (BPD), a chronic lung disease of infancy involving significant small airway obstruction, when experiencing a viral respiratory tract infection such as tracheobronchitis or bronchiolitis, often develop acute respiratory failure. Together, these disorders account for significant resource utilization in a busy pediatric intensive care unit.

PULMONARY DEVELOPMENT

Important maturational changes in respiratory system structure and function occur in the first 6 years of life.[1–3] In utero development of the lungs normally results in formation of the permanent bronchovascular framework of the airways from the carina to the terminal bronchioles at approximately the 16th branching generation, by 16 weeks' gestation. Between 16 and 25 weeks of gestation, distal to the terminal bronchioles, the respiratory zone develops, with branching respiratory bronchioles, alveolar ducts, and alveolar sacs. Blood vessels accompany these structures, including a capillary mesh that becomes adjacent to the future respiratory epithelium. By approximately 25 weeks' gestation, this process has advanced sufficiently that when accompanied by some surfactant secretion, gas exchange compatible with extrauterine survival is possible. Rapid growth of the respiratory airways, alveolar sacs, and apposed capillaries occurs distal to the terminal bronchiole, until approximately 2 years of postnatal age. Thereafter, additional branching of airways appears to be limited, although the airways increase in size as the thorax and lungs grow. Enlargement of alveolar surfaces and further alveolar septal invagination with an enclosed capillary network progressively increase the gas exchange membrane surface until age 8 to 12 years. From then until full thoracic and cardiopulmonary development in adolescence, lung growth consists primarily of enlargement of existing structures.

A fetus at term has approximately 30 million saccules with few true alveoli and, therefore, a less efficient gas exchange surface than an adult. The total lung volume and functional residual capacity are only slightly smaller in relation to body mass than in a normal 8- to 10-year-old child.[3, 4] A child of 8 years should have nearly a full adult complement of approximately 300 million alveoli.[4] Neonates and young infants, however, have an oxygen consumption, carbon dioxide production, and caloric expenditure, in relation to body mass, approximately double that of an 8-year-old child and young adult. These features underlie the propensity of young infants to develop respiratory failure more often and more precipitously when afflicted with pulmonary disorders than older children or young adults. Available data suggest that throughout infancy and childhood, the gas exchange surface enlarges proportionately to meet the increasing demand for gas exchange associated with growth and activity.

The centrally integrated control of breathing has not fully developed in a normal newborn, even at term.[3] This immaturity of ventilatory control in term infants consists of ventilatory depression or a failure to hyperventilate in the presence of hypoxia. In preterm infants, a depressed ventilatory response occurs with both hypoxia and hypercarbia. Abnormal patterns of ventilatory control, including prolonged apnea, also occur in young infants with severe acute pulmonary disorders such as bronchiolitis.

In infancy and childhood, growth occurs in length and diameter of both the proximal and distal airways. Between 6 months and 5 years of age, small-airway growth surpasses proximal airway growth by as much as 30%.[3] Although airways resistance in infants, when indexed to lung volume (functional residual capacity), is comparable to adult values, pathologic processes that lead to minimum mucosal edema or excessive secretions impede gas flow because of the airway's diminutive size, especially beyond the fourth order of branching. Airway smooth-muscle fibers extend from the terminal bronchiole at birth to the terminal ducts in an adult, permitting regional redistribution of gas at the intra-acinar level. Pores of Kohn and Lambert's channels develop later in childhood; their scarcity may explain in part an infant's propensity to develop atelectasis.[3]

A number of factors render an infant's thoracic cage, diaphragm, and other muscles of respiration less able to meet the demands of cardiopulmonary illness than those of an adult. First, the horizontal projection of an infant's ribs from the vertebral bodies imparts a circular configuration to an infant's thorax. Unlike an adult, an infant is unable to increase thoracic volume by raising the ribs in a "bucket-handle" movement. Compared with an older child and adult, an infant's diaphragm is composed of less mature muscle fibers and is flatter, thereby limiting excursions. Finally, the highly compliant cartilaginous chest wall of an infant is easily deformed during diaphragmatic contraction, especially in pathologic states. Together these structural features diminish an infant's inspiratory reserve volume in relation to metabolic rate and body mass.

Not only an infant's diaphragm but also the accessory muscles of breathing perform less effectively than in an older child under pathologic conditions that impair lung compliance or airways resistance. Respiratory muscle fiber composition changes in the first year of life, however, with intercostal and diaphragmatic muscles containing 30% slow-twitch high-oxidative (type I) fibers at term, increasing to 60% by the end of the first year. Respiratory muscle endurance has been related directly to the density of type I muscle fibers. Respiratory muscle power increases with age, as manifested by increasing maximum inspiratory and expiratory pressures.[3]

In summary, an infant faces the following physiologic compromises in comparison with an older child and adult:

1. A higher metabolic rate and oxygen consumption but a comparable functional residual capacity, which, when combined with the normally lower blood hemoglobin concentration, results in a relatively diminished body oxygen reserve
2. Diminished total alveolocapillary surface for gas exchange
3. Less mature and less powerful muscles of ventilation
4. Very small absolute diameters of the distal airways
5. Higher compliance of the chest wall and thus diminished chest wall stability, especially in infants younger than 6 months

These physiologic liabilities account in great measure for the predisposition of infants with lower airways disorders to develop acute respiratory failure.

BRONCHIOLITIS

Bronchiolitis is a form of bronchopneumonia, usually of viral etiology, occurring in infants and toddlers up to age 2 years but most profoundly affecting infants younger than 6 months. Although healthy full-term infants older than 3 months can suffer life-threatening acute respiratory failure from bronchiolitis, those most at risk of death or severe respiratory failure are former preterm infants of less than 3 months postnatal age and those with BPD.

Clinical Presentation

Initial findings include signs of an upper respiratory tract infection such as coryza, cough, otitis media, and fever. As the disease progresses over 1 to 2 days, the infant develops tachypnea (rates exceeding 40 breaths per minute), retractions, and wheezing unresponsive to bronchodilators. Hypoxemia is common in sicker infants who are hospitalized. Nonobstructive apnea occurs, often as a presenting problem, in approximately 20% of the hospitalized infants, most commonly in young former preterm babies.[5] The mechanism of apnea remains unclear.

A typical chest roentgenogram usually shows considerable hyperinflation, often with peribronchial thickening, but also may appear normal. Infiltrates, indistinguishable from atelectasis, signify more severe pulmonary infection and greater morbidity. Fever (38.5–39.0°C), malaise, and hyperventilation may combine to dehydrate these infants. Although the disease usually runs its course in 3 to 10 days, acute respiratory failure and occasionally prolonged respiratory insufficiency lasting for months can occur.[6] Follow-up studies suggest that 20% to 50% of infants continue to have reactive airway disease from 1 to 8 years after bronchiolitis.[7,8] Infants with congenital heart disease or neuromuscular disease, as well as those with BPD, may have an unusually severe or protracted illness and are prone to acute respiratory failure.

Etiology

Estimates of the overall incidence of bronchiolitis and of the percentage of children requiring hospitalization vary greatly because uniform diagnostic criteria are lacking. Respiratory syncytial virus (RSV) is the etiologic agent in 50% to 75% of infants hospitalized with bronchiolitis, cases of which number approximately 100,000 each year in the United States.[9] A rapid enzyme-linked immunosorbent assay or immunofluorescent RSV antigen test of nasopharyngeal secretions confirms this etiology. Other organisms associated with bronchiolitis include parainfluenza virus, adenovirus, rhinovirus, mumps virus, influenza virus, and *Mycoplasma pneumoniae,* as well as coinfection with bacteria, especially *Streptococcus pneumoniae* and *Haemophilus influenzae.*[10]

Rapid and extensive nosocomial spread of RSV infections, which can affect more than half of exposed hospitalized infants as well as hospital staff, can continue for 8 to 10 days after onset.[9] Isolation with universal precautions is necessary throughout the illness but especially in the first week.

Pathophysiology

The bronchospasm and mucosal edema associated with RSV bronchiolitis may be induced by a reaction to immunoglobulin E,[11] as well as to mediators released from neutrophils such as thromboxane B_2.[12] The small airways of infants dying of RSV bronchiolitis show necrosis of respiratory epithelium. Indeed, the term *syncytia* refers to a multinucleated mass of protoplasm produced by the merging of cells, the consequence of the epithelial cell necrosis induced by RSV. Extensive terminal bronchiolar and alveolar occlusion occurs because of intraluminal eosinophilic debris and peribronchiolar lymphocytic infiltration and edema. Syncytial giant cells may adhere to alveolar walls, and inclusion bodies can be found in the epithelial lining of the alveoli, bronchioles, and bronchi.[9]

Because collateral ventilation of lung units is less efficient in infants than in older children and adults, the ensuing obstruction of small airways causes atelectasis and hyperinflation, thereby profoundly decreasing dynamic compliance and mean tidal volume while mean minute volume increases owing to tachypnea. The decrease in dynamic compliance that follows is augmented by uneven distribution of resistance in small peripheral airways. Although elevations in both inspiratory and expiratory resistance contribute to the increased stiffness of the lungs and chest wall, the increase in expiratory resistance is greater, suggesting dynamic narrowing of airways on expiration. This leads to a considerable increase in the work of breathing.

The observed inverse relation between arterial carbon dioxide tension ($Paco_2$) and arterial oxygen tension (Pao_2) during air breathing suggests that alveolar hypoventilation contributes to the characteristic arterial hypoxemia, which results primarily from the mismatching of ventilation and perfusion (V-Q abnormalities) in bronchiolitis. Alveolar hypoventilation results from an increase in the ratio of wasted ventilation (physiologic dead space) to tidal volume. An infant initially compensates by increasing both tidal volume and respiratory rate. This occurs in the presence of the increased work of breathing, and the airways eventually open or the infant fatigues and respiratory failure ensues.

Differential Diagnosis

Although the diagnosis of bronchiolitis on the basis of a careful history, physical examination, and roentgenographic evaluation usually proves straightforward, clinicians also should consider other disorders that produce similar findings. The most common of these is asthma. A history of repeated attacks of wheezing provides the key fact indicating the likelihood of asthma and differentiating the two entities. If this is the first such episode, a brisk dilator response of the airways to a $beta_2$-agonist bronchodilator by aerosol or to a single subutaneous injection of epinephrine (0.01 mL/kg of 1:1000 dilution) combined with a familial history of atopy or asthma strongly suggests the diagnosis of asthma. The intense wheezing episode may have been induced by a viral or bacterial respiratory infection. Other entities to be considered as causes of acute intense wheezing in infants include pertussis, foreign body aspiration, tracheal compression by a vascular ring or sling with superimposed tracheitis, cardiac failure, and inhalation of toxic fumes.

Routine Management

All infants hospitalized with bronchiolitis should be administered humidified oxygen in concentrations sufficient to overcome hypoxemia as determined by pulse oximetry and direct Pao_2 determinations. Increasing the Pao_2 to normal or above does not depress ventilation in these children. We consider radial artery cannulation for sequential determination of pH and gas tensions in infants with intense wheezing, respiratory rates exceeding 60 per minute, and no response to bronchodilators. Oral feedings initially should be withheld. Intravenous fluid therapy initially should correct any deficits to establish a urine output of 1 to 2 $mL \cdot kg^{-1} \cdot h^{-1}$.

Ribavirin, a nucleoside analog administered by aerosolization, in some infants may modestly reduce the duration and severity of bronchiolitis if administered early in the course of the disease.[13, 14] Administered for 3 to 5 days, the drug acts by limiting the replication of virus within the cell and is associated with minimum toxicity. Its administration requires diligence because the solutions can interfere with equipment during the 3 to 5 days of therapy.[15] Broad-spectrum antibiotics are usually administered even when clinical evidence suggests a viral cause because of the extraordinary hazards of pulmonary bacterial infection in these patients and the uncertainity about secondary bacterial infection.[16] Intravenous corticosteroids, used in large studies during the past 20 years, appear to be of no benefit in the treatment of bronchiolitis[17] but may reduce airway reactivity due to mediators of anaphylaxis in infants with a prior history of wheezing espisodes (e.g., probable asthmatics) or with underlying BPD.

Although the data regarding the efficacy of sympathomimetic drugs administered by nebulization are somewhat conflicting, we advocate a clinical trial of aerosolized albuterol (salbutamol), which has proved beneficial in clinical trials and a double-blind randomized study.[18, 19] Chest physiotherapy does not appear to be of benefit for unintubated children with bronchiolitis.[20]

Management of Respiratory Failure

Acute respiratory failure occurs in infants with bronchiolitis as a result of central apnea[5] or, more commonly, by progressive airways obstruction with increasing hypercapnia. The clinical signs of acute respiratory failure consist of (1) apnea, (2) increasing respiratory rate to 60 to 90 breaths per minute (until exhaustion, when apnea may ensue), (3) increasing subcostal retractions, (4) persistent hyperinflation, (5) diminished breath sounds, and (6) diminished alertness and reactivity. Apneic episodes or the other signs combined with a rising $Paco_2$ to levels exceeding 50 mm Hg despite the supportive therapy outlined earlier call for tracheal intubation and increased ventilatory support.[21–23] Large pediatric centers report an incidence of severe respiratory failure requiring treatment with tracheal intubation and mechanical ventilation varying from 7%[21] to 38%.[23]

Although some reports cite the benefits of continuous positive-pressure breathing applied nasally or after tracheal intubation,[21, 24] we recommend proceeding directly with intermittent positive-pressure mechanical ventilation to take over most of the work of breathing and augment alveolar ventilation. Volume preset pediatric ventilators ensure the delivery of the selected tidal volume against a high and varying airway impedance. Sedation of infants with a combination of morphine or fentanyl and midazolam may provide satisfactory coordination of the smaller infants with the ventilator. In most patients, however, the addition of a continuous intravenous infusion of muscle relaxant such as vecuronium proves necessary to improve chest wall compliance, minimize the peak inflating pressures, and provide the coordination required for optimal ventilation. Slow inspiratory flow rates with an inspiratory-expiratory time ratio of 1:2 gradually reduce $Paco_2$. Mechanical ventilation may be complicated by barotrauma, bacterial pneumonia, and sepsis, although these are uncommon.[21–23] Mechanical ventilation is ordinarily needed for 3 to 5 days (range 1–18 days[21–23]), after which a trial of spontaneous ventilation for several hours with continuous positive airway pressure at 2 to 3 cm H_2O usually indicates whether or not an infant will ventilate adequately after tracheal extubation.

Sequelae of Bronchiolitis

Mortality is approximately 2% for hospitalized children with proven RSV infection but is much higher in immunosuppressed infants or those with congential heart disease.[25] Although most children recover from episodes of acute bronchiolitis within 2 to 4 weeks after hospital discharge, former preterm infants with mild to moderate BPD often develop more severe disease that waxes and wanes for many months. The major long-term sequelae of bronchiolitis include an increased incidence of lower respiratory tract symptoms, hyperactive airways disease, and asthma.[7, 26] Increases in thoracic gas volumes and airways resistance, abnormalities in gas exchange, and lowered mean peak expiratory flow rate have been observed 8 to 10 years after bronchiolitis.[26] Whether these abnormalities are permanent and what role they have in the development of asthma and chronic pulmonary disease in older children or adults remain unknown.

SEVERE ASTHMA AND RESPIRATORY FAILURE

Asthma, the most common chronic disease of childhood, has been defined in various ways through the centuries because of its protean and episodic manifestations. The U.S. Public Health Service–National Institutes of Health Expert Panel Report on Guidelines for the Diagnosis and Management of Asthma states that "Asthma is a lung disease with the following characteristics: (1) airway obstruction that is reversible (but not completely so in some patients) either spontaneously or with treatment; (2) airway inflammation; and (3) increased airway responsiveness to a variety of stimuli."[27] The term *reactive airways disease* has been applied to infants with recurrent episodes of wheezing or other evidence of peripheral airways obstruction when suffering an acute upper respiratory tract infection, as well as to older children and adolescents who experience cough and dyspnea with inhalation of cold air or the onset of vigorous exercise. Such persons generally are included in the overall spectrum of "asthma" for diagnostic and therapeutic purposes.[28]

The term *status asthmaticus* formerly denoted a severe asthmatic attack in which the intense wheezing failed to respond to routine medication as well as to two doses of subcutaneous epinephrine (0.01 mg/kg) given within a 30-minute period. During the past decade, the term has been applied less specifically or abandoned in favor of the more flexible term *acute severe asthmatic episode* (or *attack*). This term implies that intense wheezing persists despite frequent application of aerosolized beta agonists in conjunction with intravenous corticosteroids and sometimes systemic bronchodilators such as subcutaneous terbutaline or intravenous aminophylline. For the purposes of this chapter, the term *status asthmaticus* is replaced in most contexts by *severe acute asthmatic episode*, which implies a lack of response to conventional emergency therapy. The term *acute respiratory failure* refers to a severe acute asthmatic episode that leads to significant hypercapnia with a progressively rising $PaCO_2$ above 45 mm Hg (the upper limit of normal for children 7 years and older). Most children suffering an acute asthmatic episode also have hypoxemia while breathing air but have hypocapnia rather than carbon dioxide retention. Hypercapnia subsequently develops as a result of further impairment of gas flow and eventual muscular fatigue[29] (discussed later).

Epidemiology

The prevalence of asthma in the total population increased 29% from 1980 to 1987. The most striking increment, however, occurred in the age group younger than 20 years, in whom the incidence rose 43%, from 35 to 50 per 1000 population.[27] This represents approximately 12.5 million children and adolescents in the United States with asthma or reactive airways disease of some degree. Hospitalization rates for children younger than 15 years during this same period also increased 43%, from 20 to 28 per 10,000 population, and remained significantly higher than that of older asthmatic patients (16 to 18 per 10,000 population).[27]

After a decline in overall mortality from asthma in the 1970s, the mortality rate for all ages increased during the 1980s but was highest for the age group 5 to 14 years, with an average increase of 10% per annum.[30] Causes of these increases remain speculative. Race and socioeconomic status have a role; the prevalence, hospitalization rates, and mortality of asthma for all ages consistently prove to be many times higher among non-whites and the urban poor.[27, 30, 31]

Nonetheless, mortality from childhood asthma is relatively low, although among severely asthmatic children it may reach 1% to 2%. In all likelihood, most of these deaths are preventable by (1) appropriate education of the child and family, (2) diligent outpatient medical care, (3) attention by all involved to the warning signs of a severe acute episode, and (4) aggressive emergency and intensive care of severe acute attacks when they develop.

Sudden Death

Sudden death due to asthma in children and young adults appears to be increasing, although it remains a rare event. Case studies of these tragic events reveal characteristics that tend to distinguish children at higher risk of sudden death from other comparably severe asthmatic patients[32, 33]: (1) a history of abrupt onset of intense bronchospasm with hypoxic seizures, (2) a history of at least one progressively severe attack culminating in acute respiratory failure, (3) self-management problems including failure to acknowledge worsening symptoms, (4) patient and family failure to adhere to the medical plan including symptom monitoring and physician notification, (5) recent tapering or withdrawal of corticosteroids, (6) unrecognized pneumonia, and (7) major psychologic stress or depression. These deaths occur most often but not exclusively in children who have had at least one intensive care unit admission for an acute severe asthmatic episode. The time interval from onset of the attack to death may vary from minutes (sudden death) up to 2 hours (termed slow onset–late arrival).[34, 35] The fatal hypoxic event usually occurs at home or apart from a medical facility, and emergency resuscitation proves futile. Therefore, physicians caring for survivors of asthma with respiratory failure or children with the other risk factors need to ensure that the family is properly informed of this risk of sudden death and has access to comprehensive outpatient care including medication, education, and psychologic support.

Pathophysiology

The fundamental mechanisms producing a severe asthmatic episode with unresponsiveness of bronchomotor smooth muscle to catecholamines remain unclear. Any proposed theory must account for the contribution of various interacting factors, including (1) a strong familial tendency for atopy, (2) an associated immunoglobulin E response to various allergens, (3) the action of potent bronchoconstrictors released by mast cells such as histamine and the leukotrienes, and (4) the levels of cyclic adenosine monophosphate (cAMP) in airway smooth-muscle cells.[27]

These factors appear to exert their effect through cyclic nucleotides, which have a central role in regulating cell functions that modulate the asthmatic response. Decreased metabolic responses to stress and to adrenergic agents as well as bronchomotor spasm have been attributed to β-adrenergic blockade and impaired cAMP formation induced by the mediators of the allergenic response. Direct β_2-adrenergic stimulation, through administration of agonist agents, which overcome the β-blockade, relaxes bronchomotor smooth muscle and improves airway conductance. This constitutes the central treatment goal in dealing with severe asthmatic episodes.

Viral respiratory infections appear to be an important inciting factor in many acute asthmatic episodes. Studies show an overall 24% to 54% incidence of acute exacerbations of asthma asociated with concurrent viral respiratory tract infections.[36] Viral infections of the airways induce local and systemic inflammatory cell responses, including enhanced pulmonary (most cells) and plasma mast cells, as well as basophil release of histamine and other bronchoconstrictor mediators. In addition, infections cause an intensified late-phase response, 4 to 8 hours after onset of wheezing, with an influx into the airways of inflammatory cells in response to the chemotactic factors released by mast cells. Viral infections also seem to enhance β-adrenergic blockade, increase cholinergic activity, and directly damage airway epithelium. Cold inspired gas, air pollutants, exercise, and emotional factors act alone or in combination to exaggerate bronchoconstrictor responses.

Atopic phenomena, with or without infection, cause contraction of bronchial and bronchiolar smooth muscle, hypertrophy of the mucous glands and smooth muscle, and inflammatory cell infiltration and edema within the mucosa and submucosal structures. Bronchoconstriction may be direct and local or may be widespread and mediated by the vagus nerve. It involves the lung in a nonuniform fashion, causing maldistribution of gas with respect to pulmonary capillary blood flow. The small peripheral airways respond differently from the large central airways to various stimuli. In adult humans, peripheral airways dilate in response to aerosolized isoproterenol but not atropine, whereas the central airways are dilated by atropine but respond minimally to isoproterenol. In nonsmoking adults, histamine inhalation constricts the peripheral airways, with little effect on the central airways. The airway lumen in an asthmatic patient often becomes further narrowed or occluded by viscid secretions.

In children with severe asthma, the peripheral airways are markedly obstructed by goblet-cell hyperplasia, mucous plugging, eosinophilic and neutrophilic cell infiltration, and increased collagen under the airway mucosa basement membrane. These cause significant changes from pre-episode pulmonary function, including increased total airways resistance (mean 370%) and residual volume (mean 301%) and decreased forced expiratory volume in 1 second (mean 29%) and compliance (mean 52%)[37] (Fig. 82–1). Comparable information in children with severe asthma and respiratory failure is not available, but we can safely assume the deviations in pulmonary function are significantly worse than in a less severe acute episode.

Pressure from gas trapped below the obstructed airways combines with persistent inspiratory muscle activity during expiration and a supranormal nonchemical respiratory drive to increase residual volume and hyperinflate the chest. These changes increase both the elastic and flow-resistant components of the work of breathing. This increase, in combination with the rising minute ventilation observed early in the asthmatic episode,[38] leads to excessive inspiratory as well as expiratory efforts. The increased respiratory effort and sensation of extreme dyspnea produce fear and even terror in a child.

An infant or child with status asthmaticus has abnormalities in gas exchange and acid-base balance (Fig. 82–2).[38] Segmental regional hyperinflation with impaired pulmonary capillary flow significantly increases physiologic dead space (wasted ventilation), as reflected in physiologic dead space-tidal volume ratios of 0.4 to 0.6 or higher.[38] An early increase in minute ventilation, averaging two and one-half times normal resting levels, initially overcompensates for the increase in wasted ventilation and slightly reduces Pa_{CO_2}. Pa_{O_2} concomitantly falls from normal levels of 90 to 100 mm Hg to about 60 mm Hg. Hypoxemia results from maldistribution of gas with respect to blood flow within the lungs and by venoarterial shunting of blood through atelectatic lung segments.

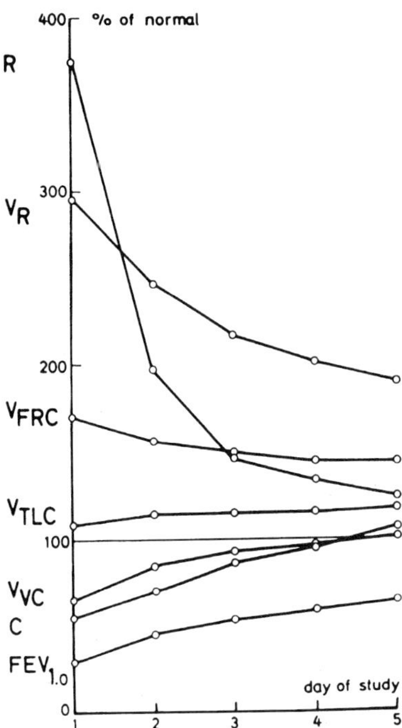

Figure 82–1. Mean values for pulmonary function tests expressed as a per cent of predicted normal values during and for 4 days following an acute asthmatic episode. *Abbreviations*: R = total airways resistance; V_R = residual volume; V_{FRC} = functional residual capacity; V_{TLC} = total lung capacity; V_{VC} = vital capacity; C = total pulmonary compliance; FEV_1 = forced expiratory volume in 1 second. (From Engstrom I: Respiratory studies in children. XI: Mechanics of breathing lung volumes, and ventilator capacity in children from attack to symptom-free status. Acta Paediatr Suppl 1964; 155:1–60.)

Most severe asthmatic episodes begin with moderate wheezing and various degrees of malaise. Dehydration, lack of adequate food intake, and exogenous catecholamines can result in ketonemia as well as small elevations in arterial lactate and pyruvate levels. These anions, perhaps with other organic acid anions, produce a moderate to severe nonrespiratory acidosis in 75% of children with an acute severe asthmatic attack. Acidosis and ketonemia tend to be greater in patients younger than 4 years.

Unless airway resistance and wasted ventilation are decreased, the excessive work of breathing and the demand for a high minute volume as well as hypercapnia[29] cause respiratory muscle fatigue. The minute volume then falls toward normal resting levels, resulting in progressively severe hypercapnia (Pa_{CO_2} rising over 50–65 mm Hg), central nervous system irritability followed by depression, and respiratory failure[38] (see Fig. 82–2). Progressive hypercapnia, in conjunction with a nonrespiratory acidemia and progressive arterial hypoxemia, can lead to severe asphyxia, Pa_{CO_2} levels in excess of 100 mm Hg, and an arterial pH of less than 7.00.[38] If alveolar ventilation is not restored, the severe acidosis and hypoxia result in cardiovascular depression, arrhythmias, and cardiopulmonary arrest. In our experience, this sequence of events more commonly occurs and is more likely to be lethal in children with chronic severe asthma requiring maximum maintenance therapy.

Diagnosis of Severe Acute Asthma and Respiratory Failure

A child with an acute, intense asthmatic episode that may lead to respiratory failure demonstrates marked dyspnea,

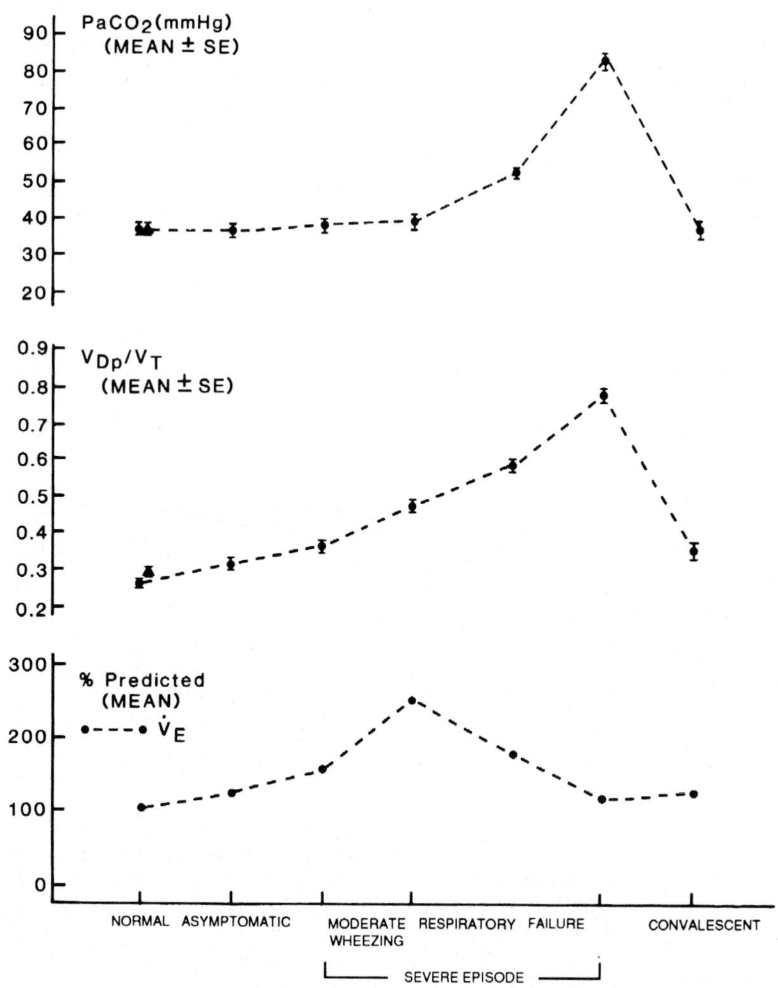

Figure 82–2. Changes in mean $Pa{CO_2}$, the ratio of physiologic dead space to tidal volume (V_{Dp}/V_T), and minute ventilation ($\dot{V}_E$) (as a per cent of predicted) in children in various stages of an asthmatic episode compared with normal children of the same age group (7–14 years). The child with a severe asthmatic attack initially maintains $Pa{CO_2}$ at normal (compensated) levels, despite significant increases in V_{Dp}/V_T, by increasing $\dot{V}_E$ (range: 135–350% above predicted normal level). Acute respiratory failure ($Pa{CO_2} > 45$ mm Hg) occurs when V_{Dp}/V_T approaches 0.6; respiratory muscle fatigue causes $\dot{V}_E$ to fall toward normal resting levels despite continued increases in $\dot{V}_{Dp}/V_T$. (*Normal values [means]* from Levison H, Featherby EA, Weng TR: Arterial blood gases, alveolar-arterial oxygen difference, and physiologic dead space in children and young adults. Am Rev Respir Dis 1970; 101:972; *Asthmatic values [means]* from Downes JJ, Heiser MS: Status asthmaticus in children. *In*: Respiratory Failure in the Child. Gregory G [Ed]. New York, Churchill Livingstone, 1981, p 114.)

intractable bilateral wheezing, thoracic hyperinflation, the use of accessory muscles of ventilation, and pulsus paradoxus. These clinical signs are ordinarily associated with a significantly elevated clinical asthma score in any of the scoring systems used, with a score of 4 or more in our institution (Table 82–1). Children with a severe asthmatic attack should undergo a complete history evaluation and physical examination to detect preexisting infection, record the type and dosage of both immediate and long-term medications, and describe the course of events in any previous severe asthmatic episode. A chest roentgenogram obtained at the time of hospital admission usually demonstrates considerable pulmonary hyperinflation with depression or flattening of the diaphragm as well as occasional infiltrates (atelectasis or pneumonitis) or barotrauma. A complete blood count, urinalysis, and determination of blood glucose and serum electrolyte levels aid in defining associated infection and metabolic disorders. If a patient has been receiving aminophylline, a serum theophylline level should be obtained, regardless of whether this drug will continue to be used, in order to assess the patient's resistance to bronchodilator therapy, preclude potentially toxic theophylline blood levels, and properly begin additional theophylline therapy if indicated.

Acute respiratory failure usually results in the following signs: cyanosis despite administration of 40% inspired oxygen; decreased or absent breath sounds; maximum use of the accessory respiratory muscles; intense, high-pitched wheezing; and depressed consciousness or coma. These clinical signs are ordinarily associated with a $Pa{CO_2}$ well in excess of 45 mm Hg and frequently between 65 and 100 mm Hg.

Patients with severe asthma often experience widely diverse degrees of wheezing and differ in their reactions to bronchodilators. Assessment of a child's response to therapy requires frequent observation of clinical signs and repeated determinations of arterial pH and blood gas tensions. Estimates of clinical severity and the response to therapy also can be facilitated by sequential determination of the clinical asthma score (see Table 82–1). If the $Pa{CO_2}$ consistently exceeds 45 mm Hg, the child should be admitted to an intensive care unit. Sternocleidomastoid and scalene muscle contraction and supraclavicular retraction correlate well with the severity of airway obstruction.

Continuous electrocardiogram (ECG) monitoring provides for early detection of the cardiac arrhythmias that can accompany severe hypercapnia or hypoxemia. Progressively severe airway obstruction may produce pulsus paradoxus with limited right ventricular filling. Arterial hypotension usually is the presenting sign of tension pneumothorax, although some of these children are moderately hypovolemic and become severely hypotensive with the initiation of positive-pressure mechanical ventilation.

Management of the Severe Asthmatic Episode

The treatment goals are to (1) increase airway conductance by relaxing airway smooth muscle, decreasing the viscosity

TABLE 82–1. Clinical Asthma Score

	Score		
Clinical Signs	*0*	*1*	*2*
Oxygenation	In air	In air	In 40% oxygen
Pa_{O_2}	65–100 mm Hg	<70 mm Hg	<70 mm Hg
Sp_{O_2}	90–97%	<90%	<90%
Inspiratory breath sounds	Normal	Unequal	Decreased to absent
Use of accessory muscles	None	Moderate	Maximum
Expiratory wheezing	None	Moderate	Marked
Cerebral function	Normal	Depressed or agitated	Coma

Acute respiratory failure = Score >5, Pa_{CO_2} >45 mm Hg after intermittent aerosol bronchodilator and intravenous corticosteroid therapy.

(Adapted from Wood DW, Downes JJ, Lecks HI: A clinical scoring system for the diagnosis of respiratory failure. Am J Dis Child 1972; 123:227. Copyright 1972, American Medical Association.)

and volume of secretions, and reducing mucosal edema and (2) support vital functons until an effective and sustained bronchomotor response to bronchodilators returns. This requires (1) elevated concentrations of humidified oxygen to alleviate hypoxemia, (2) correction of systemic dehydration with intravenous fluids, (3) restoration of the arterial pH to the range of 7.25 to 7.30 with intravenous sodium bicarbonate to prevent profound acidemia in the event of sudden hypercarbia and to elevate the threshold for cardiac arrhythmias, (4) an attempt to overcome the β_2-adrenergic blockade with continuous aerosolized beta agonists such as albuterol, and (5) intravenous infusion of corticosteroids to reduce inflammation and enhance responsiveness to the beta agonists (Table 82–2).

Correction of hypoxemia with oxygen constitutes the most important factor in preventing cardiac arrest and major central nervous system damage in a child suffering a severe asthmatic attack. Elevated inspired oxygen concentrations must be maintained throughout the asthmatic episode, including periods in the radiology department and during transport. Hypoxic encephalopathy continues to be a major complication and cause of death in children with a severe asthmatic episode and unrecognized respiratory failure.[39]

TABLE 82–2. Management of Severe Acute Asthmatic Episodes: Fundamental Therapy

Oxygen (with humidity)
Maintain Pa_{O_2} between 90 and 120 mm Hg (Sp_{O_2} 95–99%), fraction of inspired oxygen usually 0.30–0.50
Intravenous Fluids
Up to twice maintenance rates until urine flow ≥ 2 mL · kg^{-1} · h^{-1}; then maintenance rates
Bronchodilators
Primary
Albuterol aerosolized 0.15–0.25 mg/kg per dose every 1–2 h (0.03–0.05 mL/kg per dose in 2 mL saline)
Secondary
Aminophylline (IV), 3–6 mg/kg initially, 0.5–1.5 mg · kg^{-1} · h^{-1} continuous infusion; target serum level 15 μg/L
Corticosteroids
Methylprednisolone (sodium succinate) IV, 1–2 mg · kg^{-1} · 6h^{-1} for 24h; then 1–2 mg · kg^{-1} · d^{-1} in 3 divided doses
Buffers
Intravenous sodium bicarbonate ($NaHCO_3$), 1–2 mEq/kg initially, followed by doses adjusted according to base deficit and administered as necessary to maintain arterial pH >7.30*
Antibiotics
If bacterial infection suspected (fever, pulmonary infiltrates)

*Dose $NaHCO_3$ (mEq) = base deficit × 0.3 (body weight in kilograms).

Bronchodilators used widely in the initial treatment of severe asthmatic episodes in children include various aerosolized beta$_2$ agonists such as albuterol[40] and terbutaline,[41] as well as intravenous aminophylline.[41–43] These drugs act in part by enhancing cAMP synthesis and thereby relaxing the airway smooth muscle; these agents also inhibit mast-cell degranulation and release of pathogenic mediators. Prior treatment with beta agonists, however, may decrease the responsiveness of an asthmatic patient to that class of drugs.[27] Nonetheless, there are no effective therapeutic options to directly relieve airways obstruction other than these agents plus corticosteroids.

The age at which children develop bronchomotor responsiveness to beta agonists has not been clearly defined. Many infants younger than 6 months show little if any clinical response. Some infants between 6 and 20 months may respond to these agents, whereas children older than 20 months consistently respond to inhaled beta agonists with a decrease in wheezing and an improvement in airway conductance. Intermittent positive-pressure breathing does not enhance this response, but aerosol droplet size ranging from 0.5 to 2 μm diameter is essential for proper drug deposition.

With the availability of more effective pediatric aerosol delivery systems and beta$_2$ agonists such as albuterol, intravenous aminophylline has been used less frequently as a mainstay of therapy, although some groups still use it routinely.[39] The details of intermittent and continuous albuterol aerosol therapy are summarized in Tables 82–2 and 82–3. Table 82–2 also outlines the occasionally used supplemental therapy with intravenous aminophylline. The sequence of management for progressive respiratory failure appears in Table 82–3.

Children suffering a severe asthmatic episode have limited inspiratory capacity and flow rates and thus may not

TABLE 82–3. Management of Severe Acute Asthmatic Episodes: Respiratory Failure Management

Continuous albuterol aerosol inhalation (0.5 mg · kg^{-1} · h^{-1}) *or*
Intravenous isoproterenol infusion (0.1 μg · kg^{-1} · min^{-1} to maximum of 6.0 μg · kg^{-1} · min^{-1}) *or*
Mechanical ventilation

- Tracheal intubation
- Volume-preset ventilator
- Neuromuscular blockade (pancuronium infusion)
- Sedation:
  Morphine, 0.1–0.3 mg · kg^{-1} · h^{-1}, *or*
  Fentanyl, 2–5 μg · kg^{-1} · h^{-1}, *and*
  Diazepam, 0.2–0.3 mg · kg^{-1} · h^{-1}
- Continuous beta$_2$ agonist by aerosol or intravenous infusion

effectively inhale drugs delivered by a metered, gas-propelled aerosol. Furthermore, the dose per inhalation from such devices remains fixed and therefore may be inadequate for a 50-kg child but excessive for one weighing 10 kg. A beneficial response depends on an appropriate concentration of the drug and a sufficient peak inspiratory flow rate to permit dispersion and deposition of an effective dose in the lower airways. The duration of bronchodilation in a child with a severe asthmatic episode responding to a 5- to 10-minute aerosol treatment varies widely. Despite these drawbacks, intermittent or continuously nebulized beta agonists diluted in saline and delivered at an appropriate gas flow rate and inspired oxygen concentration via facemask have proved effective in most children during a severe, acute asthmatic episode[40, 41] (see Table 82–2).

Intravenous aminophylline, now only a secondary drug for acute asthma, has a half-life in children of approximately 3.5 hours, significantly shorter than the 4.6 hours observed in adults. An initial loading dose followed by a continuous infusion appears to produce a stable, effective serum level (15–20 μg/ml). When used in conjunction with aerosolized beta$_2$ agonists and corticosteroids, it appears to further improve pulmonary function in some patients.[28] The side effects of aminophylline include gastrointestinal symptoms (nausea, vomiting, or hematemesis), tachycardia, cardiac arrhythmias, and heightened central nervous system irritability that may culminate in seizures.[28, 44] These effects are infrequent and mild in most patients, provided the serum theophylline level is maintained below 20 μg/ml.

Ipratropium bromide, a derivative of atropine that has twice the potency, 50% longer duration of bronchodilator effects, and does not cross the blood-brain barrier, may be beneficial in some children as an adjunctive aerosol with beta$_2$ agonists for treatment of a severe acute asthmatic episode.[45] Experience with this drug has been limited in asthmatic children with an acute attack, although it may prove useful also as an adjunct to maintenance therapy.

Correction of acidemia with intravenous sodium bicarbonate should raise the threshold for cardiac arrhythmias and possibly enhance bronchomotor responsiveness to aminophylline and beta$_2$ agonists. In addition, maintenance of arterial pH levels at 7.30 or greater provides some protection against extreme acidemia in the event of sudden respiratory failure and severe hypercapnia. In our experience, the transient mild elevation of Pa_{CO_2} associated with a 30-minute infusion of sodium bicarbonate reverts to the preinfusion level in less than 30 minutes, but the plasma bicarbonate level remains elevated; the expected elevation of plasma bicarbonate level secondary to hypercapnia-induced renal compensation takes 12 to 24 hours to occur.

Intravenous corticosteroids have been used routinely in the treatment of status asthmaticus in children for 30 years, and controlled studies support their use.[46] Corticosteroids enhance cAMP formation, and their anti-inflammatory action justifies their short-term use in every child with status asthmaticus. Intravenous methylprednisolone in a dose of 2 $mg \cdot kg^{-1} \cdot 6h^{-1}$ appears to be more effective than other corticosteroids in ameliorating airway obstruction in asthmatic children. This may be because of the drug's greater penetration into the airway epithelium and longer mean residence time in this tissue, as shown in carefully controlled animal studies.[47]

Increased potassium excretion by the kidneys is the only consistent undesirable side effect of short-term corticosteroids that we have observed. However, the hypokalemia is intensified by concurrent administration of aerosolized or intravenous beta$_2$ agonists, which themselves have a potent kaluretic effect. Therefore, serum potassium levels should be determined at least every 12 hours, and appropriate intravenous supplementation provided.

Antibiotics should be reserved for children with clinical evidence of bacterial infection such as a fever, a pulmonary infiltrate, or a history strongly suggestive of infection. When bacterial infection seems a reasonable possibility, nasopharyngeal and blood cultures should be obtained and a broad-spectrum intravenous antibiotic initiated.

Intravenous Isoproterenol and Other Beta$_2$ Agonists

In approximately 5% of children hospitalized for severe acute asthma, fundamental therapy including continuous aerosolized beta$_2$ agonist inhalation fails to relieve the intense airways obstruction and extraordinary work of breathing, and respiratory failure develops with Pa_{CO_2} rising progressively to levels of 45 to 55 mm Hg.[38, 39] In many such patients, overcoming the apparent β_2 airways receptor blockade with high systemic blood levels of beta$_2$ agonists has proved effective in relieving airways obstruction and reducing hypercarbia. Three such agents used intravenously in children are isoproterenol, albuterol, and terbutaline. Intravenous albuterol has been used in Canada[38, 48] but is unavailable in injectable form in the United States. Intravenous terbutaline[49] rarely has been used. Thus, most experience in the United States has been and continues to be with intravenous isoproterenol in children, despite its undesirable side effects in some patients.[50] Evidence of permanent myocardial ischemic damage is lacking, and even continuous nebulized albuterol can cause transient elevations in the isoenzyme creatine phosphokinase MB fraction (CPK-MB).[51]

In our practice, intravenous isoproterenol is indicated for patients with intractable airways obstruction, characterized by an asthma score of 5 or greater (see Table 82–1) and a progressively rising Pa_{CO_2} exceeding 45 to 55 mm Hg.[38] Isoproterenol has a half-life of only 2.5 to 5.0 minutes in children. It reduces airway resistance, Pa_{CO_2}, and the excessive work of breathing, usually within 2 hours. The systemic arterial hypertension that frequently accompanies the hypercapnia also declines with Pa_{CO_2} and gives a child a feeling of considerable relief.

However, because of the hazard of hypoxemia, arrhythmias, and progressive hypercapnia, intravenous isoproterenol should be used only in an intensive care unit, where continuous ECG monitoring, equipment and drugs for cardioversion, and personnel skilled in resuscitation are immediately available. The authors believe that aminophylline infusion, if in use, should be discontinued because of its potential additive cardiac arrhythmogenic effect in the presence of isoproterenol. Because of the need for frequent arterial blood sampling and the advantage of continuous arterial pressure monitoring, peripheral artery cannulation is advocated for these patients.

Infusion dosage and duration the authors have used vary from 0.1 to 7.0 $\mu g \cdot kg^{-1} \cdot min^{-1}$ and from 8 hours to 5 days, respectively. The effective dose may approach toxic levels, particularly after extended prior use of aerosolized bronchodilators. Because the infusion rate of a gravity drip is neither consistent nor precise, isoproterenol should be administered with a constant-infusion pump. Although the average alveolar-arterial oxygen tension difference is not affected by the infusion of isoproterenol, transient serious decreases in Pa_{O_2} at 30% to 40% inspired oxygen develop in about 4% of patients, requiring oxygen concentrations of 60% to 85%.[38]

The authors recommend an initial dose of 0.1 $\mu g \cdot kg^{-1} \cdot min^{-1}$, with determination of arterial pH and blood gas tensions at approximately 20-minute intervals. The dose is increased in increments of 0.2 to 0.4 $\mu g \cdot kg^{-1} \cdot min^{-1}$ until

(1) Pa_{CO_2} falls below 50 mm Hg or decreases at least 10% from its preinfusion levels; (2) heart rate exceeds 200 beats per minute; or (3) an arrhythmia develops. An average dosage of 0.3 $\mu g \cdot kg^{-1} \cdot min^{-1}$ produces initial, concomitant decreases in clinical score and Pa_{CO_2}; normocapnia (Pa_{CO_2} < 45 mm Hg) is achieved at an average dosage of 0.7 $\mu g \cdot kg^{-1} \cdot min^{-1}$. Heart rate tends to stabilize or decrease after an initial rise, suggesting tachyphylaxis. Tachycardia exceeding 200 beats per minute rarely occurs and decreases when the isoproterenol dosage is lowered. When the Pa_{CO_2} has stabilized below 45 mm Hg and the clinical score is less than 4, the dosage may be decreased by 0.2 $\mu g \cdot kg^{-1} \cdot min^{-1}$ at hourly intervals; the Pa_{CO_2} should be determined after each change. A dosage of 0.2 to 0.5 $\mu g \cdot kg^{-1} \cdot min^{-1}$ usually needs to be maintained for 24 to 40 hours and then decreased gradually until the infusion can be discontinued. Attempts to decrease the dosage before the infusion has continued at least 12 hours are usually futile. After a dosage decrement, if the Pa_{CO_2} exceeds 45 mm Hg or the wheezing recurs (score increases by 1 or more), the dosage should be increased by 0.1 to 0.2 $\mu g \cdot kg^{-1} \cdot min^{-1}$.

Intravenous isoproterenol, if administered at sufficient dosage levels, reverses hypercapnia and respiratory failure in more than 90% of infants and children with severe asthma and respiratory failure. Patients who fail to achieve a sustained reduction in Pa_{CO_2} with isoproterenol infusion usually have a preinfusion Pa_{CO_2} exceeding 65 mm Hg, fever, or radiographic evidence of pulmonary infiltrates. These patients require tracheal intubation, neuromuscular blockade, and mechanical ventilation.[38]

ECG evidence suggestive of myocardial ischemia has been reported during isoproterenol infusion in children with status asthmaticus.[50] We also have found abnormal (> 2 mm) elevation or depression of the ST segment during isoproterenol infusion in 3 of 24 episodes (15 patients), a 12% incidence, when monitoring with a multiple-lead ECG. The CPK-MB, determined in six of these patients, was elevated in only one of the children with an abnormal ECG. The ECG and enzyme abnormalities quickly reverted to normal in all patients once the isoproterenol was discontinued. None of these patients complained of anginal pain, and none experienced systemic arterial hypotension or cardiac arrhythmias. Because of the concern about myocardial ischemia, the authors and others[50] advocate preinfusion and daily or more frequent 12-lead ECGs and determination of serial serum CPK-MB isoenzyme levels in children receiving an isoproterenol infusion. Unless clear evidence of progressive ischemia emerges, the authors advocate continuing with an isoproterenol infusion in patients whose Pa_{CO_2} is persistently rising above 50 mm Hg despite ST segment changes. Follow-up ECG and CPK-MB levels quickly revert to normal once isoproterenol is stopped. The authors believe that the well-established risks of tracheal intubation and mechanical ventilation in asthmatic children[39] probably exceed those of possible transient myocardial ischemia in children.

Mechanical Ventilation

Infants and children with severe asthma and respiratory failure who are experiencing life-threatening acute asphyxia or are unresponsive to conventional thereapy and intravenous isoproterenol require tracheal intubation and mechanical ventilation for a minimum of 12 hours and an average of 24 hours.[38] In an acutely asphyxiated asthmatic child, cyanosis, cardiac arrhythmias, or coma that fails to improve with manually assisted ventilation and oxygen calls for immediate trancheal intubation; otherwise, tracheal intubation can usually be deferred until experienced personnel and optimal equipment are present. The authors advocate a rapid intravenous sequence with ketamine and succinylcholine plus cricoid pressure for laryngoscopy and orotracheal intubation. During mechanical ventilation, continued infusion of isoproterenol in an appropriate dosage partially relieves airway obstruction, thereby reducing the mean and peak inspiratory airway pressures required for adequate ventilation. *However, initial treatment of these patients should emphasize correction of hypoxemia, if present, and ensurance of sustained, adequate delivery of oxygen to the brain and heart. Reduction of Pa_{CO_2} remains a secondary and subsequent goal.*

When arterial blood gas tensions and pH demonstrate that pulmonary gas exchange and acid-base balance have improved, a nasotracheal tube may be inserted. The nasal route provides greater security, does not hinder mouth care, and may cause less gagging and coughing on reversal of neuromuscular block. An adequate tracheal seal permits the development of the high intratracheal pressures (usually > 50 cm H_2O) needed to restore adequate alveolar ventilation. In patients younger than 8 years, an adequate seal can be achieved with uncuffed tubes, but older patients require a tube with a large-volume low-pressure cuff, inflated sufficiently to prevent an audible tracheal air leak until the airway pressure exceeds 50 to 60 cm H_2O.

A volume-preset ventilator compensates more reliably than pressure-preset or time-flow cycled ventilators for changes in airway resistance and total pulmonary compliance, thus ensuring more consistent alveolar ventilation. A long inspiratory time with a large tidal volume minimizes the turbulence of inspiratory gas flow and tends to distribute gas more uniformly throughout the lungs. An inspiratory-to-expiratory time ratio of 1:2 maximizes the emptying of lung segments distal to severely obstructed airways. If the expiratory time is inadequate, progressive gas trapping in the lungs or occult positive end-expiratory pressure increases the hazard of pneumothorax. An initial delivered tidal volume of 15 to 18 mL/kg (corrected for internal compliance) and a ventilator frequency that is approximately 50% of the predicted respiratory rate for age (approximately 8–12/min) should produce a substantial and sustained reduction in Pa_{CO_2} within 6 to 12 hours.[38] Limiting peak inspiratory pressure to 60 cm H_2O reduces the incidence of barotrauma but does not eliminate it. An inspired oxygen concentration at the minimum level required to maintain Pa_{O_2} between 90 and 120 mm Hg usually permits some nitrogen to remain in the alveoli, thus reducing the likelihood of alveolar collaspse and atelectasis distal to obstructed airways.

Controlled hypoventilation, which provides appropriate oxygen delivery yet allows Pa_{CO_2} to remain elevated, may reduce the incidence of barotrauma.[52, 53] In some patients, however, a Pa_{CO_2} exceeding 70 mm Hg from low tidal volumes (10–12 mL/kg) can cause intracellular acidosis, elevates both pulmonary and systemic arterial pressures, and raises intracranial pressure. The authors advocate attempting to reduce the Pa_{CO_2} over several hours to levels below 70 mm Hg in extremely hypercapnic asthmatic children by adjusting ventilation and bronchodilator therapy.

Neuromuscular blockade serves to coordinate patients with the ventilator so that adequate alveolar ventilation can be achieved with minimum airway pressures. This also prevents coughing, thereby reducing the risk of barotrauma. An initial intravenous dose of pancuronium, 0.1 mg/kg, followed by continuous intravenous infusion of 0.1 $mg \cdot kg^{-1} \cdot h^{-1}$ has proved effective for this purpose. Amnesia, sedation, and analgesia should be provided with intravenous narcotics (morphine, 0.1–0.3 mg/kg) and sedatives (diazepam, 0.2–0.3 mg/kg) at 3 to 4-hour intervals. Morphine does not appear to cause symptoms associated with histamine release in these children who probably have undergone maximum histamine release. Because of its negative inotropic effect on the myocardium, barbiturate sedation is less desirable.

Chest physiotherapy, tracheobronchial toilet with repeated saline instillations, and changes in body position facilitate the removal of tracheobronchial secretions and may help expand previously collapsed, atelectatic lung segments, especially during the resolution phase. Gentle, slow manual ventilation with 100% oxygen before and after chest physiotherapy and tracheobronchial toilet prevents arterial hypoxemia during these procedures, which initially should be performed approximately every 4 to 6 hours. As airway obstruction subsides and the bronchomotor response to catecholamines returns, mobilization of thick and voluminous secretions often requires hourly tracheobronchial toilet and chest physiotherapy. In the authors' experience, bronchoscopy in these patients ordinarily offers no advantage over tracheal intubation with frequent tracheobronchial toilet and chest physiotherapy.

Reliable physiologic criteria for determining when to decrease and stop mechanical ventilation have yet to be established. Because attempts at assisted ventilation in asthmatic children result in poor coordination of patients with a ventilator, a trial of spontaneous breathing with assisted or intermittent mandatory ventilation is not recommended. Instead, the following criteria have been found to indicate that a patient can achieve pulmonary gas exchange without mechanical ventilation: (1) a sustained bronchomotor response to a low dose (< 0.1 $\mu g \cdot kg^{-1} \cdot min^{-1}$) of intravenous isoproterenol, as indicated by decreased wheezing and a reduction in peak airway pressure for more than 12 hours; (2) a chest radiograph showing reduced hyperaeration with minimal or no atelectasis; (3) a Pa_{CO_2} less than 45 mm Hg at a delivered minute volume less than 150% of the predicted normal; and (4) a Pa_{O_2} greater than 200 mm Hg at 50% inspired oxygen. Tracheal extubation can be performed within 2 to 6 hours after spontaneous unassisted ventilation is resumed. If intravenous isoproterenol is being used concurrently with mechanical ventilation, it should be continued for at least 6 to 8 hours after extubation in order to ensure bronchodilatation.

Complications

Various complications may occur in children suffering a severe acute asthmatic episode, yet most of these are transient and, if appropriately managed, without permanent sequelae. However, severe hypoxemia and acidosis can lead to cardiac arrest, hypoxic encephalopathy, and death.[54]

Overdose with oral or intravenous aminophylline has been implicated in some deaths associated with status asthmaticus. In a review of 65 children suffering theophylline toxicity,[44] serum theophylline levels in excess of 20 mg/L were associated with vomiting, hematemesis, tachycardia, tremors and agitation or lethargy, and abdominal pain. At serum levels exceeding 30 mg/L, these symptoms intensified, and headache, hallucinations, seizures, and premature ventricular contractions (at serum concentrations of 50–102 mg/L) occurred. None of the children died despite the fact that seven had attempted suicide with aminophylline ingestion and developed serum theophylline levels as high as 102 mg/L. Thus, despite all the warnings, aminophylline appears to be a relatively safe, albeit unpleasant, drug for children with severe asthma.

In patients who have previously received long-term corticosteroid therapy, acute adrenocortical insufficiency can develop during the stress of an asthmatic episode if supplemental corticosteroids are not given. Experience demonstrates that acute respiratory failure and cardiac arrest often have been preceded by a 50% or greater decrease in maintenance corticosteroid medication in the month immediately before hospital admission for status asthmaticus.[55] As many as 70% of asthmatic children receiving intravenous corticosteroids and aerosolized or intravenous beta$_2$ agonists experience hypokalemia (< 3.5 mEq/L) despite some supplementary potassium infusion.[39] Thus, in children with respiratory failure, it is necessary to monitor serum potassium closely and infuse additional potassium as indicated.

Radiographic evidence of spontaneous extrapleural air accumulation is observed in 1% of children with status asthmaticus. Mechanical ventilation in children with preexisting pneumothorax or pneumomediastinum may result in tension pneumothorax or cardiac tamponade, with subsequent cardiac arrest. If mechanical ventilation proves necessary in these patients, the pneumothorax must first be treated with a thoracostomy tube, underwater seal, and high-volume suction; extensive tension pneumomediastinum requires tracheostomy and mediastinostomy.

Tracheal intubation with mechanical ventilation in asthmatic children without previously detected barotrauma is associated with a 10% to 20% incidence of pneumothorax or pneumomediastinum, even with intentional alveolar hypoventilation with gradual reduction in Pa_{CO_2}.[39] In the authors' experience, the inspiratory pressure may need to reach a level of 70 to 80 cm H_2O to accommodate a tidal volume sufficient to ensure *adequate arterial oxygen content* and to gradually reduce and maintain Pa_{CO_2} at or below 70 mm Hg; this has been associated with an incidence of ventilator-related barotrauma of 10% to 15% during the past 30 years.[38]

Acute respiratory failure recurred in 30% of asthmatic children who experienced one episode of status asthmaticus requiring intravenous isoproterenol, and 16% of these patients had more than two recurrences of respiratory failure.[38] Others have observed similar rates of recurrent respiratory failure requiring mechanical ventilation in children who had severe chronic asthma with a history of corticosteroid dependence and frequent hospital admissions.

Anesthetic Agents

The profound systemic arterial hypotension and cardiac arrhythmias observed to develop with halothane in acidotic asthmatic patients lead the authors to conclude that inhalation anesthesia is unsuitable for management of severe asthma with respiratory failure. Despite numerous anecdotal case reports advocating anesthesia with halothane, isoflurane, or ketamine in status asthmaticus, the bronchodilator effects of anesthetics at safe blood levels appear to be considerably less than that of intravenous isoproterenol, which does not cause hypotension and rarely results in arrhythmias.

References

1. Murray JF (Ed): The Normal Lung. Philadelphia, WB Saunders 1986, pp 1–24.
2. Weibel ER (Ed): The Pathway for Oxygen. Cambridge, MA, Harvard University Press, 1984, pp 175–210.
3. Scarpelli EM (Ed): Pulmonary Physiology: Fetus, Newborn, Child and Adolescent. 2nd ed. Philadelphia, Lea and Febiger, 1990, pp 215–232, 257–280.
4. Burri PH: Development and growth of the human lung. *In*: Fishman AP (Ed): Section 3—The Respiratory System. Hand-

book of Physiology. Bethesda, American Physiological Society, 1985, pp 1–46.

5. Anas N, Boettrich C, Hall CB, et al: The association of apnea and respiratory syncytial virus infection in infants. J Pediatr 1982; 101:65.
6. Hodges IGC, Milner AD, Groggins RC, et al: Causes and management of bronchiolitis with chronic obstructive features. Arch Dis Child 1982; 57:495.
7. Hall CB, Hall WJ, Gala CL, et al: Long-term prospective study in children after respiratory syncytial virus infection. J Pediatr 1984; 105:358.
8. Stokes GM, Milner AD, Hodges GC, et al: Lung function abnormalities after acute bronchiolitis. J Pediatr 1981; 98:871.
9. Ruuskanen O, Ogra PL: Respiratory syncytial virus. Curr Probl Pediatr 1993; 23:50.
10. Korppi M, Leinonen M, Koskela M, et al: Bacterial coinfection in children hospitalized with respiratory syncytial virus infections. Pediatr Infect Dis J 1989; 8:687.
11. Welliver RC, Sun M, Rinaldo D, et al: Predictive value of respiratory syncytial virus—specific IgE responses for recurrent wheezing following bronchiolitis. J Pediatr 1986; 109:776.
12. Faden H, Kaul TN, Ogra PL: Activation of oxidative and arachidonic acid metabolism in neutrophils by respiratory syncytial virus antibody complexes: possible role in disease. J Infect Dis 1983; 148:110.
13. Taber LH, Knight V, Gilbert BE, et al: Ribavirin aerosol treatment of bronchiolitis associated with respiratory syncytial virus infection in infants. Pediatrics 1983; 72:613.
14. Smith DW, Frankel LR, Mathers LH, et al: A controlled trial of aerosolized ribavirin in infants receiving mechanical ventilation for severe respiratory syncytial virus infection. N Engl J Med 1991; 325:24.
15. Frankel LR, Wilson CW, Demers RR, et al: A technique for the administration of ribavirin to mechanically ventilated infants with severe respiratory syncytial virus infection. Crit Care Med 1987; 15:1051.
16. Tristram DA, Miller RW, McMillan JA, et al: Simultaneous infection with respiratory syncytial virus and other respiratory pathogens. Am J Dis Child 1988; 142:834.
17. Springer C, Bar-Yishavy E, Uwayyed K, et al: Corticosteroids do not affect the clinical or physiological status of children with bronchiolitis. Pediatr Pulmonol 1990; 9:181.
18. Schuh S, Canny G, Reisman JJ, et al: Nebulized albuterol in acute bronchiolitis. J Pediatr 1990; 117:633.
19. Klassen TP, Rowe PC, Sutcliffe T, et al: Randomized trial of salbutamol in acute bronchiolitis. J Pediatr 1991; 118:807.
20. Webb MS, Martin JA, Cartlidge PHT, et al: Chest physiotherapy in acute brochiolitis. Arch Dis Child 1985; 60:1078.
21. Outwater KM, Crone RK: Management of respiratory failure in infants with acute viral bronchiolitis. Am J Dis Child 1984; 138:1071.
22. Frankel LR, Lewiston NJ, Smith DW, et al: Clinical observations on mechanical ventilation for respiratory failure in bronchiolitis. Pediatr Pulmonol 1986; 2:307.
23. Lebel MH, Gauthier M, Lacroix J, et al: Respiratory failure and mechanical ventilation in severe bronchiolitis. Arch Dis Child 1989; 64:1431.
24. Beasley JM, Jones SF: Continuous positive airway pressure in bronchiolitis. Br Med J 1981; 283:1506.
25. MacDonald NE, Hall CB, Suffin SC, et al: Respiratory syncytial viral infection in infants with congenital heart disease. N Engl J Med 1982; 307:397.
26. McConnochie KM, Roghmann KJ: Bronchiolitis as a possible cause of wheezing in childhood: New evidence. Pediatrics 1984; 74:1.
27. Sheffer AL (Chair): Expert panel report—guidelines for the diagnosis and management of asthma. US Department of Health and Human Services, Public Health Service. National Institutes of Health Publication 91-3042, 1991, pp 1–15, 26, 30–31.
28. Larsen GL: Asthma in children. N Engl J Med 1992; 326:1540.
29. Yanos J, Wood LDH, Davis K, et al: The effect of respiratory and lactic acidosis on diaphragm function. Am Rev Respir Dis 1993; 147:616.
30. Weiss KB, Wagener DK: Changing patterns of asthma mortality—identifying target populations at high risk. JAMA 1990; 264:1683.
31. McFadden ER, Gilbert IA: Asthma. N Engl J Med 1992; 327:1928.
32. Kravis L, Kolski GB: Unexpected death in childhood asthma—a review of 18 deaths in ambulatory patients. Am J Dis Child 1985; 139:558.
33. Strunk RC, Mrazek DA, Fuhrmann GSW, et al: Physiologic and psychological characteristics associated with deaths due to asthma in childhood. JAMA 1985; 254:1193.
34. Strunk RC: Death due to asthma (Editorial). Am Rev Respir Dis 1993; 148:550.
35. Sur S, Crotty TB, Kephart GM, et al: Sudden-onset fatal asthma. Am Rev Respir Dis 1993; 148:713.
36. Cypcar D, Stark J, Lemanske RF: The impact of respiratory infections on asthma. Pediatr Clin North Am 1992; 39:1259.
37. Engstrom I: Respiratory studies in children XI. Mechanics of breathing, lung volumes, and ventilator capacity in children from attack to symptom-free status. Acta Paediatr Suppl 1964; 155:1–60.
38. Downes JJ, Heiser MS: Status asthmaticus in children. *In*: Respiratory Failure in the Child. Gregory G (Ed). New York, Churchill Livingstone, 1981, p 107–133.
39. Stein R, Canny GJ, Bohn DJ, et al: Severe acute asthma in a pediatric intensive care unit: Six years' experience. Pediatrics 1989; 83:1023.
40. Schuh S, Parkin P, Rajan A: High versus low-dose, fequently administered, nebulized albuterol in children with severe acute asthma. Pediatrics 1989; 83:513.
41. Moler FW, Hurwitz ME, Custer JR: Improvement in clinical asthma score and $Pa{CO_2}$ in children with severe asthma treated with continuously nebulized terbutaline. J Allerg Clin Immunol 1988; 81:1101.
42. Hendeles L, Weinberger M, Szefler S: Safety and efficacy of theophylline in children with asthma. J Pediatr 1992; 120:177.
43. Ward AJM, McKenniff M, Evans JM: Theophylline—an immunomodulatory role in asthma? Am Rev Respir Dis 1993; 147:518.
44. Baker MD: Theophylline toxicity in children. J Pediatr 1986; 3:538.
45. Reisman J, Goldes-Sebaldt M, Fazim F, et al: Frequent administration by inhalation of salbutamol and ipratropium bromide in the initial management of severe acute asthma in children. J Allerg Clin Immumol 1988; 81:16.
46. Younger RE, Gerber PS, Herrod HG, et al: Intravenous methylprednisolone efficacy in status asthmaticus of childhood. Pediatrics 1987; 80:225.
47. Greos LS, Vichyanond P, Bloedow DC: Methylprednisolone achieves greater concentrations in the lung than prednisolone. Am Rev Respir Dis 1991; 144:586.
48. Bohn D, Kalloghlian A, Jenkins J: Intravenous salbutamol in the treatment of status asthmaticus in children. Crit Care Med 1984; 12:892.
49. Fuglsang G, Pedersen S, Borgstrom L: Dose-response relationships of intravenously administered terbutaline in children with asthma. J Pediatr 1989; 114:315.
50. Maguire JF, O'Rourke PP, Cohen SD, et al: Cardiotoxicity during treatment of severe childhood asthma. Pediatrics 1991; 88:1180.
51. Katz RW, Kelley HW, Crowley MR, et al: Safety of continuous nebulized albuterol for bronchospasm in infants and children. Pediatrics 1993; 92:666.
52. Darioli R, Perret C: Mechanical controlled hypoventilation in status asthmaticus. Am Rev Respir Dis 1984; 129:385.
53. Cox RG, Barker GA, Bohn DJ: Efficacy, results and complications of mechanical ventilation in children with status asthmaticus. Pediatr Pulmonol 1991; 11:120.
54. Newcomb RW, Akhter J: Respiratory failure from asthma—a marker for children with high morbidity and mortality. Am J Dis Child 1988; 142:1041.
55. Ruberstein S, Hindi R, Moss RB, et al: Sudden death in adolescent asthma. Ann Allergy 1984; 53:311.

CHAPTER 83

Life-Threatening Asthma

Walter J. O'Donnell, MD • Jeffrey M. Drazen, MD

The incidence of asthma and deaths due to asthma is increasing worldwide.[1, 2] Although most patients with asthma never experience life-threatening asthma, the care of individuals with severe asthma—usually young and otherwise healthy individuals with impending or actual respiratory failure—presents a challenge to intensivists. Appropriate treatment often but not always results in a salutary therapeutic outcome, whereas inappropriate treatment can lead to a complicated course or death.

DEFINITIONS

Asthma: is a clinical syndrome characterized by increased responsiveness of the tracheobronchial tree to various stimuli, manifested as variable airways obstruction. Obstruction may resolve spontaneously or as a result of administration of a bronchodilator.[3]

Status asthmaticus: is variously defined but can be summarized as evidence of persistent severe airways obstruction and asthmatic symptoms despite a standard course of acute asthma therapy.

Life-threatening asthma: (also called *near-fatal asthma* or *potentially fatal asthma*) may be defined as asthmatic airway obstruction with ventilatory failure manifested as relative hypercapnia.

PATHOPHYSIOLOGY OF ASTHMA

Asthma as an Inflammatory Syndrome

Immunohistochemical evaluation of endobronchial biopsy samples obtained from volunteers with mild asthma, as well as careful morphometric examination of the lungs of patients dying of status asthmaticus, has established that the airways of even mildly asthmatic patients are inflamed; some data suggest that asthma severity parallels the degree of inflammation.[4, 5] In severe asthma, the airway inflammation is associated with the presence of thick, inspissated secretions in the airway lumen. As shown in Table 83–1, airway inflammation in asthma has three distinct components.

Alterations in Airway Constitutive Cells

It is now well established that in asthma, both hyperplasia and hypertrophy of the cells in the airway wall result in wall thickening.[6, 7] Within the epithelial layer are increased numbers of surface secretory cells as well as mucous glandular hypertrophy and hyperplasia.[8, 9] The airway smooth-muscle layer thickens.[10, 11] Mast cells increase in number, with a proinflammatory phenotype in the airway epithelium and in the subepithelial connective tissue.[12, 13] The combined effect is not only to thicken the airway wall, promoting airway hyper-responsiveness on a simple mechanical basis,[14, 15] but also to allow for enhanced production of prophlogistic mediators through activation of mast cells.

TABLE 83–1. Airway Inflammation in Asthma

Alterations in Airway Constitutive Cells
Cells such as airway epithelial cells and mast cells, ordinarily present in the airway wall, become more abundant and are thought to adopt a proinflammatory phenotype.

Increased Numbers of Infiltrating Cells
Cells such as eosinophils and TH_2 lymphocytes are found in the airway wall in increased numbers.

Changes in the Noncellular Component of the Airway Wall
The airway wall is thickened beyond what can be accounted for on the basis of the infiltrating cells alone. Noncellular structural alterations occur in the airway wall, such as changes in the basement membrane.

Infiltration by Inflammatory Cells

The airway wall is known to be infiltrated by T lymphocytes bearing the TH_2 phenotype.[16] These cells have the capacity to produce interleukin-3, interleukin-4, interleukin-5, and granulocyte–macrophage colony-stimulating factor. Although the primary signals resulting in infiltration of the asthmatic airways by this lymphocyte subset have not been identified, their net effect is to promote synthesis of immunoglobulin E, to enhance the differentiation of mast cells, and to stimulate the differentiation and migration of eosinophils.[17, 18] Indeed, infiltration by eosinophils is now recognized to be a critical component of the airway inflammation associated with asthma.[4, 19]

Thickening of the Noncellular Component of the Airway Wall

The airway wall is thickened in asthma. Some of the thickening can be ascribed to the cellular components noted earlier, but other aspects of thickening are not cellular in character. The basement membrane is increased in thickness, with alterations in the structure of its collagen components.[7, 20, 21] The specific cellular events responsible for this thickening and the mechanism of their accumulation are not known.

Potential Schema Linking Airway Inflammation and Asthma Pathobiology

Although the anatomic alterations in the airway wall are well established, the links between the cells now known to be resident in the airway and asthma pathobiology remain speculative. A potential schema linking the known anatomic alterations with the clinical observations is illustrated in Figure 83–1.

As described earlier, an unknown stimulus results in accumulation in the airways of lymphocytes bearing the TH_2 phenotype. The cytokines elaborated by these cells favor the synthesis of immunoglobulin E and promote the recruitment of primary effector cells, most notably mast cells and eosinophils. When activated, these cells elaborate mediators of inflammation, including histamine, leukotrienes, platelet-activating factor, and various proteases, into the local microenvironment.[22–26] These *primary effector molecules* have the capacity to stimulate airway smooth muscle, to alter microvascular permeability, and to promote the release of mucins from airway glands and surface secretory cells. In addition, primary effector molecules can contribute to the inflammatory nature of the lesion; for example, platelet-activating factor[25, 26] and leukotriene B_4[27, 28] are potent chemoattractants for eosinophils. As eosinophils undergo apoptosis, they release toxic proteins, further damaging airway epithelium. Primary effector molecules can also stimulate sensory nerve fibers within the airway, leading to the release of *secondary effector molecules,* most notably substance P and neurokinin A. Nerve stimulation also initiates the release of both vaso-

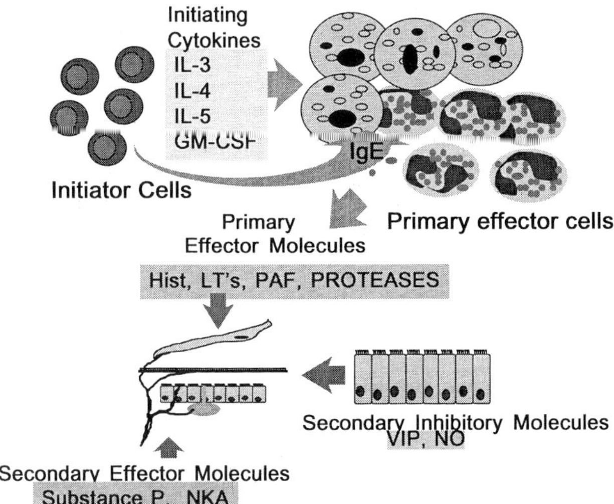

Figure 83–1. Schema linking potential airway inflammation and airway obstruction. Abbreviations: IL = interleukin; GM-CSF = granulocyte macrophage colony–stimulating factor; Hist = histamine; LT's = leukotrienes; PAF = platelet activating factor; NKA = neurokinin A; VIP = vasoactive intestinal peptide; NO = nitric oxide.

active intestinal peptide and nitric oxide.[29, 30] These molecules, termed *secondary inhibitory molecules,* ameliorate the effects of the effector species noted earlier.

Airway inflammation, as exists in status asthmaticus, is marked by not only more primary effector cells and hence more primary and secondary effector molecules but also epithelial disruption, which prevents the function of endogenous inhibitory mechanisms such as the formation of nitric oxide[31] or the cleavage of contractile neuropeptides.[32] Indeed, the primary immunologic trigger and the series of events that follow could account for both the rapid onset of effects and the slow response to treatment that characterize this disorder.

CLINICAL PRESENTATION

History

PRECIPITANTS. The most common precipitant of an acute asthmatic exacerbation is an upper respiratory tract infection, presumably viral in origin.[33] Other potential infectious causes include *Chlamydia pneumoniae* infection, which has been linked by serologic surveys to episodes of wheezing in asthmatic and nonasthmatic individuals,[34] and tracheobronchitis due to Herpes simplex, which has been reported as a cause of refractory bronchospasm in previously nonasthmatic individuals.[35]

DURATION. Before an episode of status asthmaticus, most patients describe several days to weeks of worsening asthma control and an increasing need for treatment with a beta-agonist inhaler; abuse of beta-agonist therapy often occurs, with many patients using inhaled treatment almost continuously. A subgroup of patients with a syndrome of *sudden asphyxic asthma* has been described; these patients, mainly young males, develop the abrupt onset of asthma symptoms, present with a "silent chest" on auscultation, and progress to severe hypercapnic respiratory failure requiring mechanical ventilation within minutes to hours.[36]

ASSOCIATED SYMPTOMS. Other symptoms of deteriorating asthma control include increasing nocturnal awakenings with breathlessness, as well as more profound wheezing with less exertion. More atypical presentations include those with a primary feature of hoarseness, cough, or nocturnal dyspnea alone.

Physical Examination

During an episode of status asthmaticus, patients prefer to sit bolt upright and refuse to lie supine; they may be too breathless to furnish a history. The respiratory rate is usually 25 to 30 breaths per minute, with a markedly prolonged expiratory phase. Characteristically, the accessory respiratory muscles including the sternocleidomastoid muscles, intercostal muscles, and abdominal muscles may be recruited during both inspiration and expiration; nasal flaring may be evident. With more severe attacks, retractions of these muscle groups and abdominal paradox (inward rather than outward movement at the onset of inspiration) may herald respiratory muscle fatigue and incipient respiratory failure.[37]

The cardiovascular examination is notable for tachycardia and pulsus paradoxus. The degree of pulsus paradoxus correlates with the severity of airways obstruction.[33, 38] Auscultation of the chest reveals diffuse expiratory and inspiratory wheezes. In patients with severe bronchospasm, airflow may be so minimal that an absence of wheezes results. More atypical auscultatory findings include rhonchi (most likely representing mucus hypersecretion and plugging) and focal crackles or egophony in the rare case of bacterial pneumonia.

Examination of the extremities may demonstrate eczema. In a severe hypoxemic episode, the fingernails may be cyanotic, but in simple asthma, digital clubbing should not be present. In patients who have received chronic systemic corticosteroid therapy, cushingoid stigmata may be evident, including round facies, centripetal fat deposition, thin extremities, and thin, easily bruised skin.

Laboratory Findings

BLOOD TESTS. Blood eosinophilia is common.[39] Hypokalemia may occur as a result of beta-agonist abuse or therapy.[40] Hypophosphatemia may also be noted, also typically in the setting of treatment; potential causes include beta-agonist therapy and resolution of respiratory acidosis.[41] Hyponatremia due to inappropriate antidiuretic hormone release has been reported.[42] Serum creatine phosphokinase levels, generally of the MM isozyme, may be elevated in severe asthma and appear to reflect the extreme muscular exertion required of the ventilatory muscles.[43]

PULMONARY FUNCTION TESTS. In inadequately controlled asthma, the peak flow rate is significantly depressed and demonstrates marked diurnal variation,[44] which resolves as asthma control improves. Patients who regularly measure and record their daily peak flow usually document several days to weeks of depressed values before presentation. Spirometry on presentation typically evinces low flow rates, including a depressed forced expiratory volume in the first second (FEV_1), a low ratio of the FEV_1 to the forced vital capacity, and a low maximum midexpiratory flow rate. Plethysmographic or gas dilution measurements of lung volumes, although imperfect methods in this patient subgroup, show evidence of hyperinflation, with an increased total lung capacity, functional residual capacity, and residual volume.[45] Bronchodilator responsiveness, measured as an increase in FEV_1 after inhalation of a beta-agonist aerosol, may also be decreased or absent. It should be noted that in status asthmaticus, patients may be so critically ill that they cannot adequately perform the maneuvers needed to measure these indexes of lung function. Also, bronchoprovocation challenge testing has no role in acute asthma management, except perhaps as part of a research protocol.

ARTERIAL BLOOD GASES. Mild hypoxemia (i.e., an arterial partial pressure of oxygen between 65 and 85 mm Hg and an increased alveolar-arterial gradient for oxygen) is common, even in mild to moderate asthma.[46] These findings have been attributed to ventilation-perfusion mismatching caused by mucous plugging and bronchospasm. The degree of hypoxemia roughly correlates with the severity of airway obstruction and shows a slower rate of resolution than does the obstructive element.[33, 47] Beta-agonist therapy can aggravate rather than ameliorate this hypoxemia, probably by reversing hypoxic vasoconstriction and worsening ventilation-perfusion mismatching.[48]

Most patients presenting with asthma are mildly hypocapnic, with a mild acute respiratory alkalosis. Hypercapnia usually occurs only in the setting of severe obstruction (an FEV_1 <20% of predicted).[46] In status asthmaticus, hypercapnia (or even eucapnia) and acute respiratory acidosis on presentation or early in the course of treatment may portend an increased risk of respiratory failure. Nonetheless, a recent report suggests that with aggressive therapy and close monitoring, patients in status asthmaticus presenting with normocapnia rarely develop respiratory failure; fewer than 10% of patients presenting with hypercapnia may require mechanical ventilation, and the resolution of hypercapnia generally occurs within 8 hours in the absence of mechanical ventilation.[49] Metabolic acidosis can occur in severe status asthmaticus; this disorder is mainly attributable to lactic acidosis from a combination of tissue hypoxemia, increased work of breathing, and intracellular alkalosis, but hyperventilation-related hyperchloremic acidosis may also contribute.[50]

SPUTUM EXAMINATION. The sputum of an asthmatic patient in the throes of an acute attack is often laden with thick, tenacious brownish plugs. A Gram's stain of this material should be performed to exclude the possibility of a concomitant bacterial infection, particularly in febrile patients with a productive cough. Other potential findings in the sputum include *Aspergillus* in a patient with allergic bronchopulmonary aspergillosis, Charcot-Leyden crystals (crystallized eosinophil lysophospholipase), bronchiolar casts (Curschmann's spirals) comprising cells and mucus, and Creola's bodies (clusters of epithelial cells often with intact beating cilia).[51]

THORACIC IMAGING. In hospitalized patients with asthma, the most common finding on the chest radiograph is hyperinflation, but clinically significant abnormalities can include pneumonia, congestive heart failure, atelectasis, pneumothorax, or pneumomediastinum.[52]

ELECTROCARDIOGRAM. Sinus tachycardia is the most common electrocardiographic finding in status asthmaticus. Other possible findings include right-axis deviation, clockwise rotation, right bundle branch block, ST segment and T wave abnormalities, P-pulmonale, and ventricular ectopic activity.[33] This test is particularly important in evaluating the middle-aged or older asthmatic patients to exclude the possibility of concomitant myocardial ischemia.

MANAGEMENT

General Principles

The treatment of status asthmaticus focuses on administration of bronchodilators to treat the airway smooth-muscle spasm and anti-inflammatory agents to reduce the acute local inflammatory response. The condition is labile, requiring frequent clinical and laboratory reassessment for evidence of improvement or deterioration.

Primary Therapies

β-ADRENERGIC AGONISTS. Current data show that aerosol delivery of β-adrenergic agonists, either by nebulizer or metered-dose inhaler (MDI), is more effective and less toxic than other routes of administration.[53] Hand-held jet nebulizers are the most common method of aerosol delivery, in conventionally used doses (for adults) of any one of several beta-agonist nebulizer solutions: albuterol (0.5 mL diluted in 2–2.5 mL normal saline), isoetharine (0.5 mL in 2 mL normal saline), isoproterenol (0.5 mL of a 1:200 solution in 2 mL normal saline), or metaproterenol (0.3 mL diluted in 2.5 mL normal saline) delivered at intervals of 20 to 30 minutes for moderately severe cases and by continuous nebulization for patients in extremis. Several studies, each involving small numbers of patients, have shown that patients presenting to the emergency room with mild to moderate asthma exacerbations can be treated effectively with a combination of an MDI and spacer device.[54] However, in the authors' experience, patients with asthma severe enough to warrant hospital admission often have difficulty with the instructions and maneuvers required to use an MDI-spacer combination. For patients who are intubated and receiving mechanical ventilation, adapters are available to deliver either inhaled beta agonists by nebulizer or by MDI.

For intubated patients who have status asthmaticus and who require dangerously high ventilatory pressures, the authors have found that direct endotracheal administration of 1 mL of a 1-mg/mL isoproterenol solution can be used to treat refractory bronchoconstriction when all other measures have failed; this treatment should *not* be repeated. Subcutaneous injection of epinephrine or terbutaline or a continuous intravenous infusion of isoproterenol for the control of bronchospasm can precipitate adverse cardiac events in adults, such as ventricular arrhythmias and myocardial infarction, and is not recommended in routine management. Frequent or even continuous nebulization is preferred over these systemic routes; it is at least equally effective and carries less risk.

CORTICOSTEROIDS. Systemic corticosteroid therapy is a well-established component of the treatment regimen for status asthmaticus. Because of the high doses required and the uncertainty of oral absorption in the acute setting, these agents should be administered intravenously. Both intravenous hydrocortisone and intravenous methylprednisolone have been demonstrated to be very effective agents in status asthmaticus. Although no comparative trials have been undertaken, there appears to be no clinical difference in the efficacy of these two agents. Methylprednisolone does have the theoretic advantage of less severe mineralocorticoid side effects and can be administered by intermittent intravenous bolus rather than as a continuous intravenous drip.

The optimal dose of intravenous corticosteroids to be used in status asthmaticus is undefined.[55] The authors prefer a regimen consisting of methylprednisolone, 80 to 125 mg IV every 8 hours. Only when a patient is stable and otherwise ready to be discharged is a switch to oral prednisone, 0.5 to 1 mg/kg a day, indicated.

The acute adverse effects of high-dose corticosteroid therapy include gastrointestinal upset, worsening gastroesophageal reflux, hyperglycemia, and mental status changes including anxiety and psychosis. The chronic side effects are those of hypercortisolism.

OXYGEN THERAPY. The hypoxemia noted in status asthmaticus is usually mild and transient. Because supplemental oxygen promotes absorption atelectasis and has the potential to adversely affect ventilation-perfusion matching,[56] the amount of oxygen administered should be titrated to yield an arterial blood oxygen saturation *just over 90%*. Patients who develop severe hypercapnia and respiratory acidosis in the setting of hyperoxic therapy should be treated with intubation and mechanical ventilation rather than discontinuation of oxygen therapy.

Adjunctive Therapies

METHYLXANTHINES. The conventional rationale for the use of these methylxanthines in the treatment of acute asthma is for their bronchodilator effects; however, theophylline is at best a modest bronchodilator, with minimum additive effects to adequate inhaled beta-agonist therapy. Methylxanthines have been found to have other potentially salutary properties, including inhibition of spasmogenic mediator release, improved diaphragmatic contractility, increased mucociliary transport and clearance of mucus plugs, and decreased pulmonary arterial pressures.[57] Because this class of drugs has a very narrow therapeutic-toxic ratio, serum concentration monitoring is required. Furthermore, to avoid the uncertainties of absorption in critically ill patients, delivery must be by continuous intravenous infusion. The toxicity of theophylline increases significantly when the serum level exceeds 20 μg/mL but can occur at much lower serum concentrations. Gastrointestinal side effects—nausea, vomiting, gastroesophageal reflux, and diarrhea—have been documented to occur even below a serum level of 10 μg/mL. Central nervous system side effects include tremulousness and anxiety; seizures may occur, especially in the setting of overdose. Cardiac side effects include supraventricular and ventricular tachyarrhythmias, as well as increased atrioventricular conduction rates in patients with atrial fibrillation. An individual patient may not have a predictable progression of symptoms from gastrointestinal to central nervous system to cardiac adverse effects.

In patients not already taking theophylline, a loading dose of 5.6 mg/kg should be administered as a bolus, followed by immediate institution of a continuous intravenous drip at a rate of 0.5 to 0.9 mg/kg (Table 83–2). In patients already receiving theophylline, the loading dose may be omitted; a determination of serum theophylline concentration should be taken before beginning an intravenous drip.

Because theophylline's primary locus of metabolism is the liver, other commonly used drugs can influence its rate of disappearance from the circulation. Factors known to increase theophylline clearance include use of tobacco or marijuana cigarettes or treatment with rifampin, barbiturates, phenytoin, cimetidine, fluoroquinolone antibiotics, erythromycin, propranolol (although this drug should not be administered to any patient with asthma), or antiepileptic agents. Disease states that impair theophylline clearance and increase the risk of toxicity include infection, congestive heart failure, and hepatic disease.[58] Advanced age is also a factor.

ANTICHOLINERGIC AGENTS. Inhaled atropine, 0.5 to 1 mg given via a nebulizer in 2 to 3 mL of a saline solution, has been reputed to be beneficial, particularly in patients with mucus hypersecretion or an overtly neurogenic component to their bronchoconstriction. However, studies of inhaled atropine[59] and inhaled ipratropium bromide[60] suggest that anticholinergic agents contribute little to the benefits of aggressive beta-agonist therapy in the treatment of status asthmaticus.

MAGNESIUM SULFATE. Several uncontrolled trials suggest that intravenously administered magnesium sulfate, even to patients with no evidence of serum magnesium deficiency, may have an additive benefit to inhaled beta agonists in the treatment of status asthmaticus. However, a randomized controlled clinical trial suggested minimal if any additive benefit of this treatment, and it is not recommended.[61]

TABLE 83–2. Intravenous Maintenance Dose of Aminophylline

Patient Population	*Age (y)*	*Aminophylline Infusion Rate to Achieve Target Concentration of 10 μg/mL (mg/kg Body Weight Per h)*
Young children	1–9	1.0
Older children	9–12	0.9
Adolescents (cigarette/marijuana smokers)	12–16	0.9
Adolescents (nonsmokers)	12–16	0.6
Adults (otherwise healthy cigarette/marijuana smokers)	16–50	0.9
Adults (otherwise healthy nonsmokers)	>16	0.5
Cardiac decompensation, cor pulmonale, or liver dysfunction (or a combination of these factors)	>16	0.3

**Note:* Loading doses of aminophylline average 5.6 mg/kg of lean body weight for adult patients not currently taking methylxanthine preparations (up to 9 mg/kg of lean body weight may be needed for children not currently taking methylxanthine preparations) and are administered intravenously over 20 to 30 minutes.

(Adapted from Hendeles L, Weinberger M: Theophylline: A "state-of-the-art" review. Pharmacotherapy 1983; 3:2.)

OTHER TREATMENT. Routine antibiotic administration in the setting of status asthmaticus, unlike exacerbations of chronic obstructive pulmonary disease, is not indicated. As mentioned, most patients usually have bronchoconstriction precipitated by a nonbacterial infection. It is conceivable that future studies may demonstrate a contributory role for *C. pneumoniae;* if so, routine administration of doxycycline or erythromycin may then be indicated. Obviously, in the rare asthmatic patient found to have pneumonia, antibiotic therapy directed by Gram's stain and sputum culture is indicated.

Mucolytic agents like *N*-acetylcysteine can cause severe endobronchial irritation and in the setting of maximum bronchial hyperreactivity could aggravate bronchoconstriction. The authors favor the use of more standard therapies such as humidification of inspired air and ensurance of adequate patient hydration rather than the use of so-called mucolytic agents. Although the use of acute bronchoscopic lavage for removal of mucous plugs and "cleansing of the airways" has been advocated, the procedure carries a significant risk of worsened bronchospasm, barotrauma, and pneumonia and is not recommended.

Antihistamines, α-adrenergic antagonists, nitroglycerin, calcium channel antagonists, cromones, and inhaled loop diuretics (e.g., furosemide) all have been found to have antibronchoconstrictor effects in the clinical laboratory setting. As of this writing, they have no proven clinical role in the management of status asthmaticus.

RESPIRATORY FAILURE: INTUBATION AND MECHANICAL VENTILATION

Epidemiology

Fewer than 5% of patients admitted with an acute asthmatic attack require intubation and mechanical ventilation.[62]

However, the proper treatment of these patients is critical, because this group has the greatest risk of morbidity and mortality.

General Principles of Management

Intubation and mechanical ventilation should be undertaken for a combination of clinical and laboratory data that suggest either deterioration in a patient's status or prolonged failure of a patient to improve with standard therapy.

Intubation is best performed in an awake patient in a nonemergent setting rather than in the setting of acute cardiopulmonary collapse. Transoral rather than transnasal tracheal intubation is the preferred approach in patients with status asthmaticus; the larger endotracheal tubes permitted by this route impose less expiratory resistance to flow and should thereby have the least adverse effects on airway mechanics predisposing to automatic positive end-expiratory pressure (auto-PEEP[63]) (discussed later). Because the duration of mechanical ventilatory support is usually short, the potential for airway complications due to the larger-diameter endotracheal tube should be minor.

Ventilatory support should be undertaken to provide an adequate (but not necessarily "normal") level of ventilation, enabling the therapies described earlier to relieve the bronchoconstriction. The severe limitation of expiratory flow in these patients, when matched with an inadequate exhalation time (either patient or physician generated), can result in dynamic hyperinflation, also known as intrinsic PEEP or auto-PEEP. The adverse cardiopulmonary effects of this hyperinflation include depression of cardiac output, hypotension, hypercapnia, weaning failure, and in extreme cases cardiac arrest with electromechanical dissociation.[64, 65] To minimize the level of auto-PEEP, the authors favor tidal volumes of 8 to 10 mL/kg, frequencies of 11 to 14 breaths per minute, and peak inspiratory flow rates of 80 to 100 L/min as initial ventilator settings, based on the work of Williams, Tuxen, and others[66, 67] and their own experience. These relatively low levels of minute ventilation permit a strategy of permissive hypercapnia or controlled hypoventilation and likely result in continued respiratory acidosis. This acidosis can be compensated for by administration of sodium bicarbonate to bring the arterial pH above 7.3,[68] although this entails the risk of overshoot alkalosis; in one large series, controlled hypoventilation and hypercapnia without bicarbonate loading were associated with no mortality.[69]

Sedation and temporary *paralysis* are often required after institution of mechanical ventilation for status asthmaticus, to minimize the problems of patients' discomfort during controlled hypercapnia, patient-ventilator dyssynchrony, and respiratory muscle overactivity. In many cases, maximum sedation alone is often sufficient to allow safe and effective mechanical ventilation and obviates the need to resort to neuromuscular blockade. Continuous infusion of an intravenous benzodiazepine such as midazolam might theoretically be preferable to intravenous narcotics, given the potential of morphine sulfate to cause mast-cell degranulation and exacerbate bronchoconstriction. However, judicious addition of narcotics decreases the sensation of air hunger in these patients.

Neuromuscular blockade with a nondepolarizing muscle relaxant such as vecuronium may be necessary within the first 24 to 48 hours of intubation to abolish any chest wall or respiratory muscle resistance to ventilation and attain an adequate level of ventilation at the lowest possible peak airway pressure. Pharmacologic paralysis, if necessary, should be instituted only after profound sedation is established. Vecuronium and pancuronium are preferred over metocurine, tubocurarine, and possibly even atracurium, because these first two do not cause significant histamine release. Once a patient is paralyzed, the degree of paralysis should be titrated either by allowing the patient to recover movement partially before the next dose is administered or preferably by using a peripheral nerve stimulator. At least one or two twitches rather than total paralysis with no response should be obtained from a train-of-four stimulus protocol at all times.[70, 71] Prolonged neuromuscular blockade may occur in patients with renal impairment, owing to delayed clearance of these agents and their active metabolites. More importantly, severe myopathy may occur even with careful monitoring. Special caution is needed in patients with status asthmaticus; nearly all the patients affected in these reports of myopathy were also receiving high-dose corticosteroids, in addition to more than 2 days of aminosteroid neuromuscular-blocking agents (e.g., vecuronium and pancuronium).[72] Because barotrauma and hypotension due to hyperinflation generally occur in the first 24 hours after mechanical ventilation is begun,[66] more than 2 days of neuromuscular blockade to reduce the risk of these complications should rarely be required and should be avoided.

The addition of extrinsic PEEP has no demonstrated beneficial role in status asthmaticus; indeed, the known deleterious effects of intrinsic PEEP and the demonstrated adverse effects of applied PEEP in the setting of acute airways obstruction[73] lead the authors to advise against the use of this modality in status asthmaticus.

HYPOTENSION. A transient drop in systolic blood pressure is common after endotracheal intubation. This hypotension can be attributed in part to the sedating and paralytic medications used in intubations. However, dynamic hyperinflation also renders these patients extremely sensitive to reductions in preload as occurs at the initiation of positive-pressure ventilation. A useful maneuver to rapidly diagnose and stabilize such a hypotensive, hyperinflated patient is described by Corbridge and Hall; they recommend removing a patient from the ventilator, administering three or four breaths per minute with a fraction of inspired oxygen of 1.0 using a self-inflating anesthesia bag and watching for the hemodynamic improvement to occur within 1 minute or so, followed by intravenous fluid resuscitation with normal saline as needed.[74] If hemodynamic improvement is noted, strategies to reduce dynamic hyperinflation should be instituted.

OTHER MEASURES. Anesthetics such as halothane[75] and intravenous thiopental[76] have been reported to have efficacy in refractory status asthmaticus, based on several case reports. The potential mechanism of action is unclear but most likely involves profound sedation and perhaps direct bronchial smooth-muscle relaxation. Their role in the acute management of life-threatening asthma remains undefined.

Monitoring

MEASUREMENT OF RESPIRATORY SYSTEM MECHANICS. The peak-to-plateau pressure difference (peak inspiratory pressure minus end-inspiratory pressure, measured after a 0.5- to 1.0-second end-inspiratory pause) provides only a crude index of ongoing bronchoconstriction. The degree of dynamic hyperinflation should be closely monitored; auto-PEEP can be measured by occluding the expiratory port of the ventilator at end-expiration in a nonspontaneously breathing patient and reading the value on the ventilator manometer,[64] or it can be estimated by examination of real-time expiratory flow waveforms. Measurement of the end-expiratory volume is an alternative method of assessing dynamic hyperinflation; this is done by measuring the total volume of gas exhaled (the end-inspiratory volume) by a nonspontaneously breathing patient during a 20- to 40-second apneic period; end-expiratory volume can then be obtained by subtracting tidal volume from the end-inspiratory volume.[77]

INDWELLING RADIAL ARTERIAL LINE. Fluctuations and trends in blood pressure and in the degree of pulsus paradoxus, as well as repeated blood gas measurements to determine the degree of hypercapnia, often necessitate the placement of an intra-arterial cannula, preferably in the radial artery.

OXIMETRY. Pulse oximetry allows careful titration of supplemental oxygen to treat the common mild to moderate hypoxemia. This noninvasive method can reduce the need for frequent phlebotomy to obtain direct arterial blood gas measurements.

CAPNOMETRY. End-tidal carbon dioxide monitoring is unreliable in patients with obstructive lung disease, because of increased physiologic dead space and nonuniform regional ventilation. This modality may markedly underestimate the degree and, more importantly, the trend of hypercapnia[78] and cannot be recommended for routine monitoring.

SERUM CHEMISTRIES. Serum electrolytes and phosphorus levels should be monitored during aggressive beta-agonist administration. If intravenous theophylline is used, serum theophylline levels should be monitored to adjust the dosing.

CHEST RADIOGRAPHY. Chest radiographs should be obtained on a frequent basis to ensure proper endotracheal tube position and to detect barotrauma, atelectasis/mucous plugging, and pneumonia. Emergency chest films are likewise important in patients with hypotension to determine whether pneumothorax is present.

PULMONARY ARTERIAL CATHETERIZATION. In the management of a typical patient with status asthmaticus and no evidence of cardiac disease, routine use of this invasive monitoring device cannot be recommended.

Course/Prognosis

WEANING. Most asthmatic patients intubated for status asthmaticus improve rapidly within 24 to 48 hours; several reports suggest a mean duration of intubation of 3 to 5 days.[62, 79] A trial of weaning and possible extubation should be considered when airway pressures and auto-PEEP have fallen, secretions are minimum, bronchospasm is managed with intermittent nebulized beta-agonist treatments, and there is no evidence of neuromuscular deficits.

MORTALITY. The mean mortality rate for intubation in the setting of status asthmaticus is 13.0%,[66] and although several centers have reported large series with no mortality, at least one series reported a mortality rate of 22%.[79] Of note, the centers reporting no mortality for intubated patients with status asthmaticus had a large number of patients with profound hypercapnia managed with aggressive care short of intubation; the greatest number of complications occurred in the intubated patients.

FOLLOW-UP. Status asthmaticus severe enough to warrant admission to an intensive care unit marks a patient as being in a high-risk group for recurrent admission and possibly even death due to asthma. Therefore, counseling and outpatient management need to be carefully arranged.

References

1. Gergen PJ, Weiss KB: The increasing problem of asthma in the United States. Am Rev Respir Dis 1992; 146:823–824.
2. Whitelaw WA: Asthma deaths. Chest 1991; 99:1507–1510.
3. American Thoracic Society: Standards for the diagnosis and care of patients with chronic obstructive pulmonary disease (COPD) and asthma. Am Rev Respir Dis 1987; 136:225–244.
4. Bousquet J, Chanez P, Lacoste JY, et al: Eosinophilic inflammation in asthma. N Engl J Med 1990; 323:1033–1039.
5. Holgate ST, Roche WR, Church MK: The role of the eosinophil in asthma. Am Rev Respir Dis 1991; 143:S66–S70.
6. Pare PD, Wiggs BR, James A, et al: The comparative mechanics and morphology of airways in asthma and in chronic obstructive pulmonary disease. Am Rev Respir Dis 1991; 143:1189–1193.
7. Brewster CE, Howarth PH, Djukanovic R, et al: Myofibroblasts and subepithelial fibrosis in bronchial asthma. Am J Respir Cell Mol Biol 1990; 3:507–511.
8. Jeffery PK: Morphology of the airway wall in asthma and in chronic obstructive pulmonary disease. Am Rev Respir Dis 1991; 143:1152–1158.
9. Aikawa T, Shimura S, Sasaki H, et al: Marked goblet cell hyperplasia with mucus accumulation in the airways of patients who died of severe acute asthma attack. Chest 1992; 101:916–921.
10. Ebina M, Yaegashi H, Chiba R, et al: Hyperreactive site in the airway tree of asthmatic patients revealed by thickening of bronchial muscles. A morphometric study. Am Rev Respir Dis 1990; 141:1327–1332.
11. Rodger IW: Asthma. Airway smooth muscle. Br Med Bull 1992; 48:97–107.
12. Heard BE, Jeffery PH, Kay AB: Quantitation of mast cells and eosinophils in the bronchial mucosa of symptomatic atopic asthmatics and healthy control subjects using immunohistochemistry. Am Rev Respir Dis 1991; 143:1200–1201.
13. Galli SJ: New concepts about the mast cell. N Engl J Med 1993; 328:257–265.
14. Moreno RH, Hogg JC, Pare PD: Mechanics of airway narrowing. Am Rev Respir Dis 1986; 133:1171–1180.
15. Wiggs BR, Bosken C, Pare PD, et al: A model of airway narrowing in asthma and in chronic obstructive pulmonary disease. Am Rev Respir Dis 1992; 145:1251–1258.
16. Robinson DS, Hamid Q, Ying S, et al: Predominant TH2-like bronchoalveolar T-lymphocyte population in atopic asthma. N Engl J Med 1992; 326:298–304.
17. Sanderson CJ: Interleukin-5, eosinophils, and disease. Blood 1992; 79:3101–3109.
18. Renz H, Gelfand EW: T-cell receptor V elements regulate murine IgE production and airways responsiveness. Allergy 1992; 47:270–276.
19. Bradley BL, Azzawi M, Jacobson M, et al: Eosinophils, T-lymphocytes, mast cells, neutrophils, and macrophages in bronchial biopsy specimens from atopic subjects with asthma: Comparison with biopsy specimens from atopic subjects without asthma and normal control subjects and relationship to bronchial hyperresponsiveness. J Allergy Clin Immunol 1991; 88:661–674.
20. Djukanovic R, Lai CK, Wilson JW, et al: Bronchial mucosal manifestations of atopy: A comparison of markers of inflammation between atopic asthmatics, atopic nonasthmatics and healthy controls. Eur Respir J 1992; 5:538–544.
21. Roche WR, Beasley R, Williams JH, et al: Subepithelial fibrosis in the bronchi of asthmatics. Lancet 1989; 1:520–524.
22. Schwartz LB: Cellular inflammation in asthma: Neutral proteases of mast cells. Am Rev Respir Dis 1992; 145:S18–S21.
23. Holgate ST: Mast cell activation in asthma. Agents Actions 1989; 28(Suppl):57–66.
24. Nadel JA: Biologic effects of mast cell enzymes. Am Rev Respir Dis 1992; 145:S37–S41.
25. Page CP: Mechanisms of hyperresponsiveness: Platelet-activating factor. Am Rev Respir Dis 1992; 145:S31–S33.
26. Smith LJ: The role of platelet-activating factor in asthma. Am Rev Respir Dis 1991; 143:S100–S102.
27. Shindo K, Matsumoto Y, Hirai Y, et al: Measurement of leukotriene B4 in arterial blood of asthmatic patients during wheezing attacks. J Intern Med 1990; 228:91–96.
28. Wardlaw AJ, Hay H, Cromwell O, et al: Leukotrienes, LTC4 and LTB4, in bronchoalveolar lavage in bronchial asthma and other respiratory diseases. J Allergy Clin Immunol 1989; 84:19–26.
29. Lei DF, Barnes PJ, Rogers DF: Regulation of NANC neural bronchoconstriction in vivo in the guinea-pig—involvement of

nitric oxide, vasoactive intestinal peptide and soluable guanylyl cyclase. Br J Pharmacol 1993; 108:228–235.
30. Belvisi MG, Stretton CD, Yacoub M, et al: Nitric oxide is the endogenous neurotransmitter of bronchodilator nerves in humans. Eur J Pharmacol 1992; 210:221–222.
31. Dupuy PM, Shore SA, Drazen JM, et al: Bronchodilator action of inhaled nitric oxide in guinea pigs. J Clin Invest 1992; 90:421–428.
32. Nadel JA, Borson DB: Modulation of neurogenic inflammation by neutral endopeptidase. Am Rev Respir Dis 1991; 143:S33–S36.
33. Rebuck AS, Read J: Assessment and management of severe asthma. Am J Med 1971; 51:788–799.
34. Hahn DL, Dodge RW, Golubjanitkov R: Association of *Chlamydia pneumoniae* (strain TWAR) with wheezing, asthmatic bronchitis, and adult-onset asthma. JAMA 1991; 266:225–230.
35. Sherry MK, Klainer AS, Wolff M, et al: Herpetic tracheobronchitis. Ann Intern Med 1988; 109:229–233.
36. Wasserfallen J-B, Schaller M-D, Feihl F, et al: Sudden asphyxic asthma: A distinct entity? Am Rev Respir Dis 1990; 142:108–111.
37. Cohen CA, Zagelbaum G, Gross D, et al: Clinical manifestations of inspiratory muscle fatigue. Am J Med 1982; 73:308–316.
38. Rebuck AS, Pengelly LD: Development of pulsus paradoxus in the presence of airways obstruction. N Engl J Med 1973; 288:66–69.
39. Horn BR, Robin ED, Theodore J, et al: Total eosinophil counts in the management of bronchial asthma. N Engl J Med 1975; 292:1152–1155.
40. Gelmont DM, Balmes JR, Yee A: Hypokalemia induced by inhaled bronchodilators. Chest 1988; 94:763–766.
41. Laaban J-P, Waked M, Laromiguiere M, et al: Hypophosphatemia complicating management of acute severe asthma. Ann Intern Med 1990; 112:68–69.
42. Baker JW, Yerger S, Segar WE: Elevated plasma antidiuretic hormone levels in status asthmaticus. Mayo Clin Proc 1976; 51:31–34.
43. Burki NK, Diamond L: Serum creatine phosphokinase activity in asthma. Am Rev Respir Dis 1977; 116:327–331.
44. Hetzel MR, Clark TJH, Branthwaite MA: Asthma: Analysis of sudden deaths and ventilatory arrests in hospital. Br Med J 1977; 1:808–811.
45. McFadden ER Jr, Kiser R, DeGroot WJ: Acute bronchial asthma. Relations between clinical and physiologic manifestations. N Engl J Med 1973; 288:221–225.
46. McFadden ER Jr, Lyons HA: Arterial-blood gas tension in asthma. N Engl J Med 1968; 278:1027–1032.
47. Ferrer A, Roca J, Wagner PD, et al: Airway obstruction and ventilation-perfusion relationships in acute severe asthma. Am Rev Respir Dis 1993; 147:579–584.
48. Gazioglu K, Condemi JJ, Hyde RW, et al: Effect of isoproterenol on gas exchange during air and oxygen breathing in patients with asthma. Am J Med 1971; 50:185–190.
49. Mountain RD, Sahn SA: Clinical features and outcome in patients with acute asthma presenting with hypercapnia. Am Rev Respir Dis 1988; 138:535–539.
50. Mountain RD, Heffner JE, Brackett NC, et al: Acid-base disturbances in acute asthma. Chest 1990; 98:651–655.
51. Hogg JC: Pathology of asthma. J Allergy Clin Immunol 1993; 92:1–5.
52. White CS, Cole RP, Lubetsky H, et al: Acute asthma. Admission chest radiography in hospitalized adult patients. Chest 1991; 100:14–16.
53. Pierce RJ, Payne CR, Williams SJ, et al: Comparison of intravenous and inhaled terbutaline in the treatment of asthma. Chest 1981; 79:506–511.
54. Idris AH, McDermott MF, Rauci JC, et al: Emergency department treatment of severe asthma. Chest 1993; 103:665–672.
55. McFadden ER Jr: Dosages of corticosteroids in asthma. Am Rev Respir Dis 1993; 147:1306–1310.
56. Rodriguez-Roisin R, Ballester E, Roca J, et al: Mechanisms of hypoxemia in patients with status asthmaticus requiring mechanical ventilation. Am Rev Respir Dis 1989; 139:732–739.
57. Milgrom H, Bender B: Current issues in the use of theophylline. Am Rev Respir Dis 1993; 147:S33–S39.
58. Bukowskyj M, Nakatsu K, Munt PW: Theophylline reassessed. Ann Intern Med 1984; 101:63–73.
59. Karpel JP, Appel D, Breidbart D, et al: A comparison of atropine sulfate and metaproterenol in the emergency treatment of asthma. Am Rev Respir Dis 1986; 133:727–729.
60. Summers QA, Tarala RA: Nebulized ipratropium bromide in the treatment of acute asthma. Chest 1990; 97:430–434.
61. Green SM, Rothrock SG: Intravenous magnesium for acute asthma: Failure to decrease emergency treatment duration or need for hospitalization. Ann Emerg Med 1992; 21:260–265.
62. Braman SS, Kaemmerlen JT: Intensive care of status asthmaticus. A 10-year experience. JAMA 1990; 264:366–368.
63. Scott LR, Benson MS, Bishop MJ: Relationship of endotracheal tube size to auto-PEEP at high minute ventilation. Respir Care 1986; 31:1080–1082.
64. Pepe PE, Marini JJ: Occult positive end-expiratory pressure in mechanically ventilated patients with airflow obstruction. The auto-PEEP effect. Am Rev Respir Dis 1982; 126:166–170.
65. Rosengarten PL, Tuxen DV, Dziukas L, et al: Circulatory arrest induced by intermittent positive pressure ventilation in a patient with severe asthma. Anaesth Intensive Care 1991; 19:118–120.
66. Williams TJ, Tuxen DV, Scheinkestel CD, et al: Risk factors for morbidity in mechanically ventilated patients with acute severe asthma. Am Rev Respir Dis 1992; 146:607–615.
67. Tuxen DV, Williams TJ, Scheinkestel CD, et al: Use of a measurement of pulmonary hyperinflation to control the level of mechanical ventilation in patients with acute severe asthma. Am Rev Respir Dis 1992; 146:1136–1142.
68. Menitove SM, Goldring RM: Combined ventilator and bicarbonate strategy in the management of status asthmaticus. Am J Med 1983; 74:898–901.
69. Darioli R, Perret C: Mechanical controlled hypoventilation in status asthmaticus. Am Rev Respir Dis 1984; 129:385–387.
70. Isenstein DA, Venner DS, Duggan J: Neuromuscular blockade in the intensive care unit. Chest 1992; 102:P1258–1266.
71. Wheeler AP: Sedation, analgesia, and paralysis in the intensive care unit. Chest 1993; 104:566–577.
72. Hansen-Flaschen J, Cowen J, Raps EC: Neuromuscular blockade in the intensive care unit. Am Rev Respir Dis 1993; 147:234–236.
73. Tuxen DV: Detrimental effects of positive end-expiratory pressure during controlled mechanical ventilation of patients with severe airflow obstruction. Am Rev Respir Dis 1989; 140:5–9.
74. Corbridge T, Hall JB: Status asthmaticus in the adult: Assessment, drug therapy, and mechanical ventilation. Respir Management: 21:119–126.
75. Rosseel P, Lauwers F, Baute L: Halothane treatment in life-threatening asthma. Intensive Care Med 1985; 11:241–246.
76. Grunberg G, Cohen JD, Keslin J, et al: Facilitation of mechanical ventilation in status asthmaticus with continuous intravenous thiopental. Chest 1991; 99:1216–1219.
77. Tuxen DV, Lane S: The effects of ventilatory pattern of hyperinflation, airway pressures, and circulation in mechanical ventilation of patients with severe air-flow obstruction. Am Rev Respir Dis 1987; 136:872–879.
78. Morley TF, Giamo J, Maroszan E, et al: Use of capnography for the assessment of alveolar ventilation during weaning from mechanical ventilation. Am Rev Respir Dis 1993; 148:339–344.
79. Mansel JK, Stogner SW, Petrini MF, et al: Mechanical ventilation in patients with acute severe asthma. Am J Med 1990; 89:42–48.
80. Hendeles L, Weinberger M: Theophylline: A "state of the art" review. Pharmacotherapy 1983; 3:2.

CHAPTER 84

Pulmonary Aspiration of Stomach Contents

Philip G. Boysen, MD, FACP, FCCM • Jerome H. Modell, MD

Acid is the main cause of severe pulmonary injury after aspiration of stomach contents.[1–6] However, although clear liquid aspirates with a pH greater than 2.5 can be essentially innocuous in small quantities, even nonacidic aspirates, particularly those containing foodstuff, can produce severe pulmonary insufficiency.[2,7]

PATHOLOGY

Most experimental work in this area has been performed with aspirates having a pH of 1.0 to 2.5. After aspiration, acid rapidly spreads throughout the lungs and produces diffuse damage that is characterized by epithelial degeneration of the bronchi, pulmonary edema, hemorrhage, isolated areas of atelectasis, necrosis of type I alveolar cells, and the presence of free laminated inclusion bodies in the pulmonary transudate.[8] Within 4 hours, acute infiltration by polymorphonuclear cells and fibrin can be seen in the alveolar space. Degeneration of type II alveolar cells and further necrosis of type I cells with detachment from the basement membrane have also been noted. Within the next 24 to 36 hours, alveolar consolidation is seen, and some of the airways show mucosal sloughing. After 48 hours, hyaline membranes appear.[8] The lung appears boggy, edematous, and hemorrhagic on gross examination. By 72 hours, resolution has begun, with regeneration of bronchial epithelium, proliferation of fibroblasts, and a decrease in acute inflammation.[9]

When clear liquids with a pH greater than 2.5 are aspirated, pulmonary edema, diapedesis of erythrocytes, separation of endothelial cells from basement membranes, and peribronchial neutrophilic infiltration may occur. Compared with the aspiration of highly acidic liquid, however, aspiration of nonacidic liquids causes little necrosis of alveolar cells and minimal neutrophilic infiltration. Also, the duration of injury is significantly shorter if a patient survives the acute hypoxia caused by the initial aspiration.[10]

Correlation of laboratory data with clinical aspects of pH and volume of gastric contents has been the subject of investigation.[11] Although increasing volume and decreasing pH may be problematic and associated with the degree of pulmonary damage, critical values for each variable are not easily determined. Particularly for children, methods to reduce the risk of aspiration have come into question. Having a child fast for a long time to achieve gastric emptying is not always efficacious and may, in itself, lead to intravascular volume depletion and other problems. Similar untoward effects may occur in adult patients. For the trauma patient, there is usually little time to manage such problems. Therefore, as an index of increased severity of parenchymal lung damage after acid aspiration, it is generally agreed that the more acidic the aspirated fluid and the greater its volume, the greater will be the lung damage. This implies that morbidity and mortality after aspiration can also be similarly related. Administration of a variety of agents has been suggested as a way to alter both gastric pH and gastric volume.[12]

Experimental acid aspiration of variable volumes with a pH of 1.0 has been studied in primates.[13] Aspiration of 0.4 to 0.6 mL/kg produced mild to moderate clinical and chest radiographic changes, but not death. Aspiration of volumes greater than 0.8 mL/kg produced increasingly severe pneumonitis, and 50% of the monkeys succumbed. Extrapolation of these values to adult humans approximates the critical aspirated volume of 50 mL at a pH 1.0. Although this analysis of severity in relation to the volume and acidity of gastric aspirate might considerably reduce the number of patients thought to be "at risk," the values of pH less than 2.5 and volumes greater than 25 mL have been promulgated by some as indicators of severe lung damage and of a protracted clinical course.

Large particulate aspirates obstruct major airways. Aspiration of neutral stomach contents containing small, nonobstructing food particles can produce a prolonged inflammatory response similar to that caused by acid.[2, 14] Within 6 hours of aspiration, extensive hemorrhagic pneumonia may occur, with erythrocytes, granulocytes, and macrophages invading the alveoli and bronchi. A widespread granulomatous reaction with numerous macrophages and giant cells is present within 48 hours, and the alveolar walls are thickened by edema and infiltrating mononuclear cells. Obstruction of airways by food particles does not appear to cause the reaction described above, although obstructive bronchiolitis is caused by inflammatory exudate. Within 5 days, focal areas resembling hard granulomas are present in large numbers; food particles can be identified at the center of many of these granulomas. In some cases, the smaller pulmonary vessels are occluded and have adjacent areas of hemorrhagic infarction.[7]

PHYSIOLOGY

Although any aspirated fluid may obstruct the airway and interfere with normal ventilation-perfusion patterns, the chemical burn induced by acid aspiration appears to be the most severe problem. It causes a loss of alveolocapillary integrity and an exudation of fluid and protein into the interstitial spaces, the alveoli, and the bronchi.[8] The exudation causes pulmonary edema, a decrease in pulmonary compliance, an increase in lung weight, and significant intrapulmonary shunting or venous admixture.[8, 15, 16] Sufficient fluid may be lost from the circulation to deplete intravascular volume and cause hypotension.[8, 15, 17]

Perhaps the most immediate and severe physiologic problem is the hypoxemia that occurs within minutes of acid aspiration.[4, 8, 9, 15, 17, 18] This hypoxemia most likely is secondary to several events: reflex airway closure in response to the aspiration of fluid[16, 19, 20]; destruction or alteration of normal surfactant activity[4, 20]; and migration of fluid and protein into the damaged tissues, which causes interstitial edema and, thus, further pulmonary embarrassment. Even after the acute lesion has subsided, the exudate may remain in the form of hyaline membranes.

The aspiration of acid also affects the pulmonary vasculature and can cause pulmonary hypertension. Pulmonary vascular resistance (PVR) increases,[8, 21, 22] and marked constriction of pulmonary arterioles has been demonstrated arteriographically[23] and histologically after aspiration.[18] If pulmonary artery pressure is not elevated, the cause may be low intravascular volume or low cardiac output, or both.[24]

The change in PVR can be attributed to multiple factors. Hypoxemia, an intense stimulus to the pulmonary vascular tree, results in vasoconstriction. Immediately after aspiration, when gastric contents flow into the pharynx, trachea, and lung, prolonged apnea may occur. Not only does this aggravate the hypoxemia, but the resultant hypercarbia and acidosis increase the stimulus to the pulmonary vasculature and, thus, also cause vasospasm. Accumulation of extravascular lung water results in a loss of lung volume, whether or not alveolar fluid accumulates. Such a lung not only is stiff and noncompliant but also evidences a lower alveolar gas volume and functional residual capacity. The end result is impingement of the pulmonary microvasculature due to mechanical forces and the increase in PVR. If atelectatic, edematous areas can be re-expanded with reclamation of lung volume, the PVR may return toward normal. Overexpansion of the lungs similarly causes pressure (transmitted alveolar pressure) on the pulmonary microvasculature, which elevates PVR (see *Treatment* later in this chapter). This indicates the strong relationship between lung volume and PVR.[12]

If PVR is elevated, for whatever reason, hemodynamic consequences are usually immediate and severe. The right ventricle, which operates against a low impedance or pressure under normal conditions, can maintain ejection of a significant volume in order to match left ventricular output. Acute elevations in PVR overload the right ventricle, a heart chamber ill-equipped to handle such changes, and may precipitate right ventricular dilatation, a decrease in right ventricular ejection fraction, and right ventricular failure.

If clear liquid with a pH greater than 2.5 is aspirated, the extent of the resultant lesion may not be as severe as if a highly acidic liquid had been aspirated. However, reflex airway closure,[20] pulmonary edema, and changes in the surface tension characteristics of the lung still may occur.[25]

In summary, the aspiration of significant amounts of stomach contents into the lung causes acute respiratory insufficiency regardless of the nature of the aspirate. If the aspirate is small in volume, has a pH greater than 2.5, is free of particulate matter, and has normal tonicity, recovery may be rapid.[26] If the fluid has a pH less than 2.5, is hypertonic, or contains food particles or irritating liquid food, the inflammatory response may be prolonged. The reaction is primarily hemorrhagic, granulocytic, and necrotizing when the aspirate is acid; it is mononuclear and granulomatous when the aspirate contains food. The nature, volume, and distribution of the aspirate are all important in determining the degree of respiratory embarrassment. Although volume for volume acidic aspirates cause the most damage, aspiration of any material from the stomach, even those of a neutral pH, can be life-threatening.

THERAPY

Prophylaxis

In many cases, aspiration of stomach contents can be avoided. The risk of aspiration in the unconscious patient may be reduced by careful observation and by positioning the patient in a semi-prone position with his or her head down. Emergency surgery perhaps entails the greatest risk. The incidence of aspiration in this setting can be reduced by the use of regional anesthetics when appropriate or by awake endotracheal intubation before induction of general anesthesia. If awake intubation is not possible, rapid induction of anesthesia with simultaneous application of cricoid pressure and intubation of the trachea with a cuffed endotracheal tube is appropriate to protect the patient's airway. Before the endotracheal tube is removed, the patient should be awake and have normal laryngeal reflexes to protect the airway.

When sufficient time is available to prepare a patient for anesthesia and surgery, other therapeutic interventions may be of benefit, and concepts are changing. Although implementation of a nil per os (NPO) regimen has been a longstanding practice before the administration of an anesthetic, this requirement may not reduce gastric contents. Administration of clear fluids may be beneficial rather than harmful. Liberal intake of clear fluids in the 6 hours before surgery results in residual gastric volume that is similar to that after 6 hours of fasting (22 mL and 19 mL, respectively).[27] Additionally, the pH of gastric fluid was reported to be higher in those allowed to consume fluids than in a control group of fasting subjects (2.64 compared with 1.57).[27] As might be expected, patients receiving clear fluids had lesser preoperative thirst and a lesser tendency toward dehydration. Apple juice has been commonly used in clinical studies as the preferred clear liquid to administer to patients before surgery.[28, 29]

A variety of drugs have been studied and recommended as efficacious in altering residual gastric volume and pH.[30–32] This includes the histamine$_2$ receptor antagonists (e.g., cimetidine and ranitidine), particulate and nonparticulate antacids, cholinergic receptor agonists (e.g., metoclopramide), and proton pump inhibitors (e.g., omeprazole). Ranitidine is also available as an oral liquid that can be given to children. The goal of histamine$_2$ receptor therapy is to reduce gastric volume and pH. Metoclopramide facilitates gastric emptying and has a central antiemetic effect. To achieve synergism, it has been recommended that these drugs be given together. The peak effect of these drugs is between 2 and 4 hours after administration.[28] A newer histamine$_2$ receptor–blocking agent, roxatidine, has a longer duration of action; a single, oral bedtime dose has an effect for 8 to 12 hours.[33] Famotidine has similarly been recommended for children.[34] When ranitidine and metoclopramide are given to adults who are given clear fluids up until 2 hours before surgery, these adults remain at low risk for aspiration.[35]

Proton pump inhibitors prevent secretion of hydrogen ion into the stomach and, thus, lessen gastric acidity and raise pH. For a group of pregnant women about to undergo cesarean section, a single oral dose of 80 mg of omeprazole resulted in a pH greater than 2.5 and a residual gastric volume less than 50 mL in 80% of patients.[36]

The preoperative use of oral particulate antacids to reduce gastric acidity has often been recommended,[1, 37–40] although this practice has not been proved to reduce morbidity or mortality. Further, if the antacid itself is aspirated, a severe persistent pulmonary lesion occurs; microscopic evidence of the antacid compound can be seen in the lungs for several weeks after aspiration.[41] Orally administering either two antacid tablets (e.g., Alka-Seltzer) in 30 mL of water or a 0.3-mol/L sodium citrate solution, 30 mL, both of which are nonparticulate, also effectively buffers stomach acid without risking severe pulmonary insufficiency if the solution is aspirated.[42, 43] Since cimetidine or ranitidine, or both, decrease the volume of gastric fluid and increase gastric pH, preoperative use of these compounds might be worthwhile for patients at risk.[43, 44]

Endotracheal Suctioning

If aspiration has occurred, the trachea should be suctioned, if possible. This stimulates coughing, may remove some of the aspirated material, and may aid in confirming the diagnosis. Since liquid and small particulate aspirates disperse rapidly and damage the lung almost instantaneously, suctioning can only remove a portion of the aspirate and, therefore, is only the first step in therapy.

Mechanical Ventilatory Support

Severe intrapulmonary shunting causes significant venous admixture and arterial hypoxemia that must be treated immediately. Positive-pressure ventilation with positive end-expiratory pressure (PEEP) or the administration of continuous positive airway pressure (CPAP) reduces blood gas abnormalities and increases the rate of survival after acid aspiration. If the patient is alert and further aspiration is not a risk,[15, 30, 45–48] CPAP applied by mask may reinflate alveoli, increase functional residual capacity, and decrease the intrapulmonary shunt. If the patient is obtunded, cannot maintain a patent airway, or is at risk of further aspiration, intubation of the trachea with a high-volume, low-pressure cuffed endotracheal tube is indicated. Optimal CPAP minimizes the intrapulmonary venous admixture without compromising the circulation.[49]

The concept of optimal PEEP or CPAP has been elusive because of the combined and variable effects of PEEP on pulmonary and cardiac physiology. PEEP is meant to increase lung volumes, diminish shunt, and improve oxygenation. Cardiac output must be preserved to maintain oxygen delivery. As PEEP or CPAP is increased, the resultant increase in lung volume decreases PVR as functional residual capacity returns toward normal and as oxygenation and gas exchange improve. This has the effect of decreasing impedance on the right ventricle, which improves right ventricular performance. If PEEP or CPAP results in lung hyperinflation, PVR will again increase but by another mechanism. In this case, lung overdistention has resulted in the mechanical transmission of alveolar pressures to the pulmonary vasculature. The end result is right ventricular dilatation, decreased right ventricular ejection fraction, and eventual impingement of left ventricular geometry due to shift of the intraventricular septum.

Further complicating therapeutic assessment is the observation that excessively high peak airway pressure may cause parenchymal lung damage that may persist and, thus, prolong supportive therapy.[50, 51] For this reason, mean airway pressure has been monitored as an indication of the simultaneous effect on lung inflation and alteration of hemodynamic function. Increasing inflation times to the point of reversing the normal inspiratory-to-expiratory ratio has been recommended as a means of increasing mean airway pressure and of avoiding high peak airway pressure while minimizing the end-expiratory pressure necessary to improve oxygenation. The patient with severe adult respiratory distress syndrome due to gastric aspiration may be included in the group recommended for low-frequency positive-pressure ventilation (with a small tidal volume) and simultaneous extracorporeal removal of carbon dioxide by venovenous bypass.[52] Under such conditions, oxygenation is maintained by using a low level of PEEP and by performing simultaneous tracheal insufflation of oxygen. Low-frequency ventilation (2–4 breaths per minute) with small tidal volume avoids high peak airway pressure, which is thought to be deleterious to lung healing. To avoid hypercapnia, extracorporeal carbon dioxide removal is accomplished by venovenous bypass. Although good conceptual and theoretic data support these concepts, improved outcome has yet to be demonstrated with their use. In an experimental study of severe acid aspiration in the rabbit, conventional mechanical ventilation with PEEP was compared with inverse-ratio ventilation.[53] No difference in morbidity or mortality could be demonstrated.

Bronchoscopy and Lavage

If a patient is suspected of having aspirated large particulate matter, and especially if clinical and radiographic signs of lung volume loss are present, bronchoscopy should be performed. However, bronchoscopy for a patient in severe respiratory distress after aspiration of stomach contents is a formidable and hazardous procedure. Some physicians have advocated pulmonary lavage with neutral or alkaline solutions to neutralize acid, but damage to the lung by acid is almost instantaneous, and lavage is not useful unless particulate aspiration has been observed or is strongly suspected.[26] If bronchoscopy is performed, only small amounts of saline should be used to clear the airway of secretions or aspirated material. Large-volume lavage may actually further compromise pulmonary function.

Corticosteroids

Theoretically, steroid administration should decrease inflammation, stabilize lysosomal membranes,[54, 55] prevent platelet and leukocyte agglutination,[56] and improve the peripheral release of oxygen from erythrocytes by shifting the oxyhemoglobin dissociation curve.[57] However, no conclusive clinical or experimental data document that steroids are beneficial for patients with aspiration pneumonitis.[26] In fact, steroids administered after aspiration of food particles may interfere with normal healing.[7] For this reason, we do not recommend their use.

Antibiotics

Infection in the patient who has aspirated frequently is difficult to document. Fever, leukocytosis, the presence of pulmonary infiltrates, and production of thick tenacious sputum are nonspecific responses to uncomplicated chemical pneumonitis. Cultures of sputum may be misleading because samples can be contaminated by oropharyngeal flora. In general, patients with lung abscess, empyema, and pneumonia after aspiration are more likely to have organisms that reflect the oropharyngeal flora, especially anaerobic bacteria.[58, 59] Patients with severe respiratory failure who require ventilatory support frequently harbor aerobic bacteria such as *Staphylococcus* and *Pseudomonas* species.[60, 61] The effectiveness of prophylactic antibiotics is dubious; they may lead to superinfections with resistant organisms. Antibiotics should be withheld until clinical evidence of infection can be produced. Treatment can then be based on analysis of well-controlled smear and culture specimens.

Particular attention has been paid to those patients who aspirate gastric contents while in the hospital, especially to critically ill patients who are in the intensive care unit.[62] In hospitalized patients, pharyngeal colonization by gram-negative rods, which are often resistant to antibacterial therapy, develops. The bacterial flora also change during a patient's hospitalization, particularly in critically ill patients and especially in those with immune dysfunction. A gastropulmonary route of infection is thus postulated. Elevation of gastric pH during ulcer prophylaxis creates a tendency toward gastric bacterial colonization. Thus, in some patients, the stomach is a bacterial reservoir independent of changes in the oropharynx. The potential for reflux and aspiration amplifies the risk of parenchymal damage with a potential for superinfection.[33] In the intubated intensive care patient, the risk of aspiration is increased owing to gastroduodenal reflux and regurgitation of gastric contents. Instead of gastric alkalization for prolonged periods, administration of cytoprotective antiulcer medication—for example, sucralfate—may prevent infection. Aquisition of adequate culture information remains the best means of choosing appropriate antibiotic therapy when aspiration pneumonitis occurs.[58]

Fluids

Proper use of fluids is clinically important in patients with severe aspiration. Intravascular volume lost through pulmonary edema must be restored. Furthermore, if high levels of PEEP or CPAP are necessary, particularly combined with mechanical ventilatory breaths, venous return may decrease; this accentuates the physiologic effects of hypovolemia, and cardiac output may decrease markedly, in turn decreasing oxygen delivery. Therefore, these patients must be monitored carefully, and the use of a properly placed pulmonary artery catheter or the performance of transesophageal echocardiography, or both, frequently are indicated.

SUMMARY

The simplest and most efficient therapy for aspiration of stomach contents is prevention. If aspiration does occur, the following steps are recommended:

Suction the trachea.
Analyze arterial blood for gas tensions and pH.
Apply aggressive mechanical ventilatory support, particularly with CPAP or PEEP, and document its effectiveness by measuring blood gas parameters and shunt.
Ensure adequate fluid replacement.
Perform bronchoscopy if large particulate aspirates obstruct airways.

We do not recommend the use of corticosteroids, prophylactic antibiotics, or pulmonary lavage with large volumes of neutral or alkaline solutions.[43]

References

1. Mendelson CL: The aspiration of stomach contents into the lungs during obstetric anesthesia. Am J Obstet Gynecol 1946; 52:191.
2. Teabeaut JR II: Aspiration of gastric contents: An experimental study. Am J Pathol 1952; 28:51.
3. Taylor G, Pryse-Davies J: Evaluation of endotracheal steroid therapy in acid pulmonary aspiration syndrome (Mendelson's syndrome). Anesthesiology 1968; 29:17.
4. Awe WC, Fletcher WS, Jacob SW: The pathophysiology of aspiration pneumonitis. Surgery 1966; 60:232.
5. Bannister WK, Sattilaro AJ: Vomiting and aspiration during anesthesia. Anesthesiology 1962; 23:251.
6. Vandam LD: Aspiration of gastric contents in the operative period. N Engl J Med 1965; 273:1206.
7. Wynne JW, Reynolds JC, Hood CI, et al: Steroid therapy for pneumonitis induced in rabbits by aspiration of foodstuff. Anesthesiology 1979; 51:11.
8. Greenfield LJ, Singleton RP, McCaffree DR, et al: Pulmonary effects of experimental graded aspiration of hydrochloric acid. Ann Surg 1969; 170:74.
9. Downs JB, Chapman RL Jr, Modell JH, et al: An evaluation of steroid therapy in aspiration pneumonitis. Anesthesiology 1974; 40:129.
10. Alexander IG: The ultrastructure of the pulmonary alveolar vessels in Mendelson's (acid pulmonary aspiration) syndrome. Br J Anaesth 1968; 40:408.
11. Rocke DA, Brock-Utne JG, Rout CC: At risk for aspiration: New critical values of volume and pH (Letter)? Anesth Analg 1993; 76:666.
12. Goresky GV, Finley GA, Bissonnette B, et al: Efficacy, duration, and absorption of a paediatric oral liquid preparation of ranitidine hydrochloride. Can J Anaesth 1992; 39:791.
13. Raidoo DM, Rocke DA, Brock-Utne JG, et al: Critical volume for pulmonary acid aspiration: Reappraisal in a primate model. Br J Anaesth 1990; 65:248.
14. Moran TJ: Experimental food-aspiration pneumonia. Arch Pathol 1951; 52:350.
15. Cameron JL, Caldini P, Toung JK, et al: Aspiration pneumonia: Physiologic data following experimental aspiration. Surgery 1972; 72:238.
16. Davidson JT, Rubin S, Eyal Z, et al: A comparison of the pulmonary response to the endotracheal instillation of 0.1 N hydrochloric acid and Hartmann's solution in the rabbit. Br J Anaesth 1974; 46:127.
17. Lewis RT, Burgess JH, Hampson LG: Cardiorespiratory studies in critical illness: Changes in aspiration pneumonitis. Arch Surg 1971; 103:335.
18. Hamelberg W, Bosomworth PP: Aspiration pneumonitis: Experimental studies and clinical observations. Anesth Analg (Cleveland) 1964: 43:669.
19. Halmagyi DF, Colebatch HJ, Starzecki B: Inhalation of blood, saliva, and alcohol: Consequences, mechanism, and treatment. Thorax 1962; 17:244.
20. Colebatch HJ, Halmagyi DF: Reflex airway reaction to fluid aspiration. J Appl Physiol 1962; 17:787.
21. Toussaint GP, Chiu CJ, Hampson LG: Experimental aspiration pneumonia: Hemodynamics, ventilator and membrane oxygenator support. J Surg Res 1974; 16:324.
22. Fisk RL, Symes JF, Aldridge LL, et al: The pathophysiology and experimental therapy of acid pneumonitis in ex vivo lungs. Chest 1970; 57:364
23. Booth DJ, Zuidema GD, Cameron JL: Aspiration pneumonia: Pulmonary arteriography after experimental aspiration. J Surg Res 1972; 12:48.
24. Morgan BC, Abel FL, Mullins GL, et al: Flow patterns in cavae, pulmonary artery, pulmonary vein, and aorta in intact dogs. Am J Physiol 1966; 210:903.
25. Giammona ST, Modell JH: Drowning by total immersion: Effects on pulmonary surfactant of distilled water, isotonic saline and sea water. Am J Dis Child 1967; 114:612.
26. Wynne JW, Modell JH: Respiratory aspiration of stomach contents. Ann Intern Med 1977; 87:466.
27. Phillips S, Hutchinson S, Davidson T: Preoperative drinking does not affect gastric contents. Br J Anaesth 1993; 70:6.
28. Ghignone M, Calvillo O, Quintin L: Anesthesia and hypertension: The effect of clonidine on perioperative hemodynamics and isoflurane requirements. Anesthesiology 1987; 67:3.
29. Vincent RD Jr, McNeil TJ, Spaid CL, et al: Does 360 mL of apple juice ingested before elective surgery worsen volume and acidity in patients given acid aspiration prophylaxis? J Clin Anesth 1991; 3:285.
30. Maltby JR, Sutherland AD, Sale JP, et al: Preoperative oral fluids: Is a 5-hour fast justified prior to elective surgery? Anesth Analg 1986; 65:1112.
31. Pandit SK, Kothary SP, Pandit UA, et al: Dose-response study of droperidol and metoclopramide as antiemetics for outpatient anesthesia. Anesth Analg 1989; 68:798.
32. White PF: Pharmacologic and clinical aspects of preoperative medication. Anesth Analg 1986; 65:963.
33. Tryba M, Wruck G, Thole H, et al: The use of roxatidine acetate in fasting patients prior to induction of anaesthesia as prophylaxis against the acid aspiration syndrome. Drugs 1988; 35(Suppl 3):20.
34. Jahr JS, Burckart G, Smith SS, et al: Effects of famotidine on gastric pH and residual volume in pediatric surgery. Acta Anaesthesiol Scand 1991; 35:457.
35. Strunin L: How long should patients fast before surgery? Time for new guidelines (Editorial). Br J Anaesth 1993; 70:1.
36. Moore J, Flynn RJ, Sampaio M, et al: Effect of single-dose omeprazole on intragastric acidity and volume during obstetric anaesthesia. Anaesthesia 1989; 44:559.
37. Roberts RB, Shirley MA: Reducing the risk of acid aspiration during cesarean section. Anesth Analg (Cleveland) 1974; 53:859.
38. Taylor G, Pryse-Davies J: The prophylactic use of antacids in the prevention of the acid-pulmonary-aspiration syndrome (Mendelson's syndrome). Lancet 1966; i:288.
39. Lahiri SK, Thomas TA, Hodgson RM: Single-dose antacid therapy for the prevention of Mendelson's syndrome. Br J Anaesth 1973; 45:1143.
40. Peskett WGH: Antacids before obstetric anaesthesia: A clinical evaluation of the effectiveness of mist, magnesium trisilicate BPC. Anaesthesia 1973; 28:509.
41. Gibbs CP, Schwartz DJ, Wynne JW, et al: Antacid pulmonary aspiration in the dog. Anesthesiology 1979; 51:380.
42. Gibbs CP, Spohr L, Schmidt D: The effectiveness of sodium citrate as an antacid. Anesthesiology 1982; 57:44.
43. Gibbs CP, Modell JH: Aspiration pneumonitis. *In:* Anesthesia.

2nd ed. Vol 3. Miller RD (Ed). New York, Churchill Livingstone, 1986, pp 2023–2050.
44. Maliniak K, Vakil AH: Pre-anesthetic cimetidine and gastric pH. Anesth Analg (Cleveland) 1979; 58:309.
45. Chapman RL Jr, Downs JB, Modell JH, et al: The ineffectiveness of steroid therapy in treating aspiration of hydrochloric acid. Arch Surg 1974; 108:858.
46. Cameron JL, Sebor J, Anderson RP, et al: Aspiration pneumonia: Results of treatment by positive-pressure ventilation in dogs. J Surg Res 1968; 8:447.
47. Chapman RL Jr, Modell JH, Ruiz BC, et al: Effect of continuous positive-pressure ventilation and steroids on aspiration of hydrochloric acid (pH 1.8) in dogs. Anesth Analg (Cleveland) 1974; 53:556.
48. Pontoppidan H, Geffin B, Lowenstein E: Acute respiratory failure in the adult. N Engl J Med 1972; 287:690.
49. Downs JB, Modell JH: Patterns of respiratory support aimed at pathophysiologic conditions. *In:* ASA Refresher Courses in Anesthesiology. Vol 5. Hershey SG (Ed). Philadelphia, JB Lippincott, 1977, pp 71–85.
50. Kolobow T, Moretti MP, Fumagalli R, et al: Severe impairment in lung function induced by high peak airway pressure mechanical ventilation: An experimental study. Am Rev Respir Dis 1987; 135:312.
51. Dreyfuss D, Bassett G, Soler P, et al: Intermittent positive-pressure hyperventilation with high inflation pressures produces pulmonary microvascular injury in rats. Am Rev Respir Dis 1985; 132:880.
52. Gattinoni L, Pesenti A, Maicolin R, et al: Extracorporeal support in acute respiratory failure. Intensive Care 1988; 5:42.
53. Sohma A, Brampton WJ, Dunnill MS, et al: Effect of ventilation with positive end-expiratory pressure on the development of lung damage in experimental acid aspiration in the rabbit. Intensive Care Med 1992; 18:112.
54. Janoff A, Weissmann NG, Zweifach BW, et al: Pathogenesis of experimental shock: IV. Studies on lysosomes in normal and tolerant animals subjected to lethal trauma and endotoxemia. J Exp Med 1962; 116:451.
55. Starling JR, Rudolf LE, Ferguson W, et al: Benefits of methylprednisolone in the isolated perfused organ. Ann Surg 1973; 177:566.
56. Wilson JW: Treatment or prevention of pulmonary cellular damage with pharmacologic doses of corticosteroid. Surg Gynecol Obstet 1972; 134:675.
57. Bryan-Brown CW, Baek S, Makabali G, et al: Consumable oxygen: Availability of oxygen in relation to oxyhemoglobin dissociation. Crit Care Med 1973; 1:17.
58. Bartlett JG, Gorbach SL, Finegold SM: The bacteriology of aspiration pneumonia. Am J Med 1974; 56:202.
59. Lorber B, Swenson RM: Bacteriology of aspiration pneumonia: A prospective study of community- and hospital-acquired cases. Ann Intern Med 1974; 81:329.
60. Arms RA, Dines DE, Tinstman TC: Aspiration pneumonia. Chest 1974; 65:136.
61. Bynum LJ, Pierce AK: Pulmonary aspiration of gastric contents. Am Rev Respir Dis 1976; 114:1129.
62. Atherton ST, White DJ: Stomach as a source of bacteria colonising respiratory tract during artificial ventilation. Lancet 1978; ii:968.

CHAPTER 85

Fiberoptic Bronchoscopy in Critical Care Medicine

R. Phillip Dellinger, MD, MSc

The value of fiberoptic bronchoscopy (FOB) in the intensive care unit (ICU) has been recognized and described.[1–5] This chapter addresses the comprehensive use of the flexible fiberoptic bronchoscope (FFB) in multidisciplinary critical care medicine.

TECHNIQUE

Intubation is recommended in most critically ill patients undergoing FOB, as the procedure may worsen oxygenation and ventilation, especially in the nonintubated patient.[6] Intubation facilitates delivery of high oxygen concentrations and allows volume ventilation during FOB in the intubated patient. The presence of an endotracheal (ET) tube during FOB is essential if removal of the FFB is anticipated during the procedure to collect specimens (biopsy, brush) and remove viscid inspissated mucous plugs with traction through the suction port of the FFB, or if large amounts of blood or thick secretions are expected. The latter invariably leads to loss of visual field and necessitates FFB removal for cleaning. The timing of intubation depends on the urgency of the situation and on the immediate availability of FOB equipment. If intubation is done before FOB (5-mm FFB), an 8-mm or larger ET tube should be used to ensure that ventilation is not compromised during FOB. Alternatively, intubation can be accomplished over the FFB at the time of the procedure. An 8-mm ET tube can be utilized with either a nasal or oral route of insertion. Ovassapian and coworkers[7] demonstrated that greater than 95% of elective intubations could be accomplished by the nasotracheal (NT) route with an 8-mm or larger ET tube. It must be remembered that the NT route should not be used for intubation in patients with clotting disorders because of the risk of severe nasal hemorrhage. Swivel adaptors allow insertion of the FFB into the ET tube or tracheostomy (TO) tube while adequate seal and mechanical ventilation are maintained.[8] Current models are simplified and disposable. An assistant is necessary to support the ET tube upright during the procedure to facilitate easy passage of the FFB in and out of the ET tube. To facilitate FFB passage, a clear gel is applied generously to the FFB and to the entrance of the swivel adaptor's one-way valve. Silicone spray may also be used and is less likely to obstruct the visual field. A common cause of fiberoptic bundle damage is forcing of the FFB through a curved ET tube against resistance.

In elective situations, the patient should be nil per os (NPO) for 6 to 8 hours. This is not a consideration in emergencies or in most mechanically ventilated patients. Routine FOBs are done with a wide variety of premedication and anesthesia. Usually, the elective patient receives a parenteral analgesic (narcotic or non-narcotic), intramuscular atropine (to decrease secretions and as prophylaxis for vasovagal phenomenon), and an antianxiety agent such as intramuscular hydroxyzine or an intravenous benzodiazepine. In the critically ill nonintubated patient, narcotics or other potential respiratory depressant medications should generally be avoided, particularly if intubation is not to be performed as part of the procedure. Most ICU patients require little or no premedication before FOB, particularly if an ET tube is already in place. Similarly, intramuscular atropine should be avoided or used with caution in patients with dysrhythmia or angina. Since anticholinergics in vitro have a secretion-drying effect, atropine premedication might predispose a patient to secretion inspissation. This does not seem to be a clinically significant problem. Urgency of intubation may dictate omission of all or part of premedication and anesthetic technique.

If time allows, topical lidocaine can be delivered with a hand-held nebulizer in the nonintubated patient and applied directly through the suction channel of the FFB in both the intubated and nonintubated patient. Lidocaine dosage in the adult should be limited to 200 to 300 mg.[9] In a patient receiving continual lidocaine infusion, a significant reduction in the recommended maximum dosage of topical lidocaine is warranted.

Assuming that the tube size is adequate, compromised ventilation is not a problem with FOB. With a volume ventilator, the set tidal volume is delivered at the expense of increased airway pressure. Inspiratory pressures distal to the ET tube should remain essentially unchanged. More problematic is the increase in resistance to expiration, which may induce intrinsic positive end-expiratory pressure (PEEP) in susceptible patients. Chest excursion, tidal volume, and PEEP should be monitored.

The potential for FOB to lower the arterial partial pressure of oxygen (PaO_2), particularly in the nonintubated patient, should be realized. A pulse oximeter should therefore be utilized. An arterial line is ideal for monitoring mean arterial pressure. Periodic measurement with an automated cuff is an alternative. When oxygen saturation drops below a predetermined value (usually 90%), the procedure is terminated temporarily until acceptable saturation returns. During the FOB, the fraction of inspired oxygen (FIO_2) is adjusted to higher levels (if possible) to compensate for the potential decreased oxygenation. Increasing the FIO_2 to a value of 1.0 is reasonable. In the nonintubated patient, oxygen can be delivered by nasal catheter or nasal prongs directed intranasally or held in the patient's mouth. Alternatively, oxygen can be delivered with a disposable facemask with a hole cut for the FFB.[10] An additional option is to deliver oxygen through the suction channel of the FFB. This has the advantage of making secretion-induced obstruction of the fiberoptic visual field less likely. This may be a particularly valuable technique when the smaller-diameter FFB is utilized, since oxygen insufflation into the suction port will maintain a clearer visual field than suctioning through the small-diameter port. Oxygen delivery through the suction channel is best accomplished with a three-way stopcock, which allows alternatively suction, delivery of fluids, or oxygen delivery through the channel.[11]

A capable assistant should monitor cardiac rhythm, blood pressure, and oxygen saturation. Observation for dysrhythmias is imperative because their persistence indicates the need to abandon the procedure and begin specific antidysrhythmic treatment.

USE WITH ENDOTRACHEAL AND TRACHEOSTOMY TUBES

Intubation

The FFB or flexible fiberoptic laryngoscope (FFL) can be used to overcome intubation difficulties in many patient groups (Table 85–1). The reduced length of the FFL facilitates manipulation; however, the length is inadequate to establish position of the ET tube relative to the carina after the intubation. Some FFLs also lack suction capability.

TABLE 85–1. Considerations for Fiberoptic Bronchoscopy Intubation

Upper airway obstruction suspected	Fiberoptic bronchoscopy planned immediately after intubation
Morbidly obese patients	History of previous difficult intubations
Patients with short thick neck	
Oropharyngeal tumors	Known or suspected cervical fractures
Tongue cellulitis	
Congenital or acquired maxillofacial deformities	Head and face trauma
	Arthritic ankylosis of cervical vertebrae
Ankylosis of temporomandibular joints	
	Spondylitis
	Trismus

Intubation with the FFB is contraindicated in the apneic patient in whom the pharynx tends to collapse; direct laryngoscopic intubation is more expeditious. Likewise in the patient with extreme ventilatory difficulty, laryngoscopic intubation is more appropriate.

FOB intubation may be accomplished by the following steps: (1) placing the ET tube over the FFB, pushing it to the FFB's most proximal end; (2) employing oral or nasal FOB with localization of the vocal cords; (3) inserting FFB through the vocal cords and into a midtracheal position; and (4) using the FFB as an obturator, advancing the ET tube into the trachea. For nasal FOB intubation, it is desirable to insert the ET tube into the posterior pharynx before insertion of the FFB through the tube.

The nasal route offers a less angled approach to the vocal cords; in the conscious or semiconscious patient, this approach is less dependent on cooperation. When intubating with a pediatric FFB (3.5-mm) and an adult ET tube, it is possible to push a loop of FFB and the ET tube down the esophagus.[12] This can be minimized by holding constant the position of the bronchoscope while the ET tube is advanced. During oral FOB intubation, the conscious patient may bite down, thus causing difficulty in passage of and damage to the bronchoscope. This problem may be minimized with a bite block. Owing to the acute angle the ET tube must take as it passes over the posterior area of the tongue and through the vocal cords during oral over-the-FFB intubation, an increased incidence of ET tube tip hang-up on the vocal cords is experienced.[13]

For nonemergency nasal insertion, topical vasoconstrictors and anesthetics help to facilitate passage of the ET tube. These same medications also facilitate passage of the FFB through the nasopharynx when intubation is not to be accomplished. The use of increasingly larger nasopharyngeal airways lubricated with anesthetic jelly progressively dilates the nasopharyngeal passage. Application of lidocaine solution directly through the in-place nasopharyngeal airway also directs anesthesic to the glottic area. For oral insertion, larger ET tube sizes can be used, and a bite block is recommended. An 8.0- to 9-mm ET tube is ideal for oral intubation, and an 8.0-mm tube is ideal for nasal intubation in most adults. During the insertion procedure, supplemental oxygen should be given either transnasally, transorally, or through the FFB channel.

If the outer diameter (OD) of the FFB approaches the internal diameter (ID) of the ET tube, ventilation is likely to be compromised; however, ET tube tip hang-up on the vocal cords becomes less likely. If resistance to insertion is felt during attempts to pass the ET tube through the vocal cord area, the tube should be slightly withdrawn and minimally rotated, and the attempt repeated (Fig. 85–1). This rotation procedure is repeated in small increments until passage is achieved. Once the ET tube is within the trachea, the FFB is used to position the ET tube in its desired location above the carina. The ET tube cuff is then inflated, and the FFB is withdrawn. If bronchoscopy is to follow, then the FFB is withdrawn, and a T adaptor is inserted for use with either supplemental oxygen or ventilation before FFB reinsertion. If active bleeding into the posterior pharynx occurs, intubation may be difficult, even with the use of a large suction channel FFB.

Shinnick and Freedman[14] and Ovassapian[15] described techniques for insertion of the double-lumen endobronchial tube. The technique entails first insertion of the double-lumen tube into the trachea with the rigid laryngoscope until the cuff is beyond the larynx. The tracheal cuff is then inflated, and ventilation is resumed. A pediatric FFB (3.5-

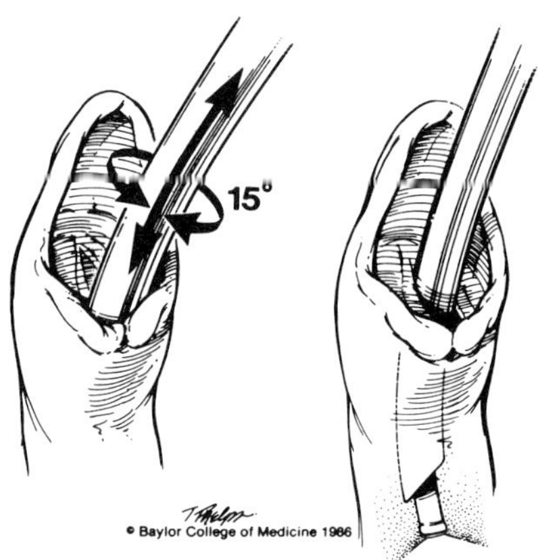

Figure 85–1. Procedure for correcting hang-up of the endotracheal tube on the vocal cords during FOB intubation. If resistance is met during passage of the endotracheal tube over the bronchoscope and into trachea, the tube should be withdrawn slightly and rotated in 15° increments *(left)*, either clockwise or counterclockwise, followed by readvancement until resistance is no longer met *(right)*.

mm OD) is introduced through the endobronchial lumen of the tube and guided into the appropriate mainstem bronchus. The FFB is withdrawn and inserted into the tracheal lumen to position the bronchial cuff 1 cm distal to the carina. This should place the tracheal cuff in the desired position and orient the tracheal lumen exit toward the left mainstem bronchus. During non-FOB placement of double-lumen tubes, inadequate positioning and complications such as tracheal rupture have been reported.[16]

The FFB can also be used to change ET tubes in critically ill patients.[17] Two techniques are available. One technique involves the insertion of the FFB with the new ET tube placed proximally (as described earlier in this section) through the right nares, left nares, or mouth, depending on which is not presently occupied by the ET tube to be changed. Nasogastric (NG) and enteral feeding tubes often limit nasal alternatives in the ICU as do previous nasal mucosa trauma from intubation, NG or enteral feeding tubes, and NT suctioning. One method of FOB ET tube change is performed as previously outlined for FOB intubation, with the exception that after the FFB is fixed just above the vocal cords, the present ET tube is removed, the FFB is advanced through the vocal cords, and the intubation is accomplished over the FFB. Problems with this technique are that at the time of removal of the pre-existing ET tube, patient movement, cough, or gag or the presence of secretions may lead to loss of visual field, making FFB insertion into the trachea difficult or delayed. The second method, which is safer and preferred, utilizes the standard FOB intubation technique through an alternative orifice but with the FFB (3.5-mm or 5.0-mm) passed through the vocal cords and outside of the present ET tube. Available space between the present ET tube and vocal cords is usually adequate. Any bronchoscopist who uses either of the above two techniques for ET tube changes must be competent in back-up alternatives for airway control, including direct laryngoscopy and, ideally, emergency tracheostomy and cricothyroidotomy (adults only).

Diagnostic Applications

The FFB is an excellent tool for airway inspection before extubation or to document complications of prolonged or difficult intubation. After prolonged or difficult intubation, an increased risk exists for complications such as mucosal erosions, mucosal edema, hematoma, and tracheomalacia.[18, 19] Tracheoesophageal fistula or tracheovascular fistula may be suspected. Tube position may also be questioned. By inserting the FFB through the ET tube, deflating the cuff after proper suctioning, and withdrawing the ET tube, all areas of the trachea can be inspected. After abnormalities are diagnosed and located, the physician may then elect to change tube position, change the tube itself, or proceed to a tracheostomy (TO) tube. Movement of the ET tube slightly up and down may decrease further cuff damage at that site.

Another valuable use of the FFB is to rule out upper airway obstruction (UAO) during extubation in patients with (1) prolonged ET intubation, (2) suspected tracheal damage secondary to a difficult intubation, (3) a previous or current history suggestive of a UAO as the etiology of the patient's acute respiratory failure, or (4) at the time of removal of the TO tube, or (5) conversion to a fenestrated TO tube. With the TO tube, routine oral or transnasal FOB is accomplished to inspect superglottic, glottic, and subglottic areas. To inspect for UAO at the time of ET tube removal, the FFB is inserted through the ET tube at the time of extubation. Adequate pharyngeal suction is maintained, and the cuff is deflated. The ET tube is then withdrawn carefully, and the patient observed for any evidence of UAO. If the patient is noted to have symptoms or findings of tracheal edema, tracheal stenosis, or vocal cord edema that might compromise the airway, the tube is readvanced over the FOB and returned to its previous position.

Patil and associates[20] used the FFB inserted through the ET tube at the time of tracheostomy to ensure proper placement of the TO tube under direct ET vision. Adequate visualization involves retracting the ET tube and FFB to above the tracheostomy site with the FFB just outside the ET tube. FOB can also be used to diagnose or rule out aspiration around the ET tube cuff. This can be further facilitated by adding colored dye to secretions or to the enteral feeding solution.

It is important to understand the relationship of ET tube ID to FFB relative to ventilatory constraints. In 1974, Grossman and Jacobi[21] computed the smallest ET tube through which the 5-mm FFB could be inserted without reducing critically the effective ventilation area of the ET tube. Assuming 7 mm is the minimal acceptable ID without an FFB in place, they computed that insertion of a 5-mm FFB through an 8.5-mm ID ET tube correlated with the use of a 6.9-mm ET tube without a bronchoscope. They therefore concluded that all 5-mm FFBs be done with at least an 8.5-mm tube. Lindholm and Grenvik[22] stated that an FFB with a 5.7-mm diameter occupies approximately 10% of the tracheal cross-sectional area when an ET tube is not inserted. However, with insertion through an 8-mm ID ET tube, the lumen is more than 50% occluded. They therefore recommended that a 5.7-mm FFB not be used with any tubes with an ID less than 8 mm. Note that this is more liberal than standards published by Grossman and Jacobi. The current 5.0-mm adult FFB should be used (with the possible exception of brief use as an intubation guide) with an ET tube with an ID of no less than 8 mm and, ideally, with one with an ID of 8.5 mm.

ATELECTASIS

There is much anecdotal literature on the value of FOB for acute lobar collapse. When FOB is compared with vigorous pulmonary toilet, its value is controversial.

Therapeutic FOB for atelectasis employs standard FOB technique. The tracheobronchial tree is inspected for mucous plugs or retained secretions. Suction is performed in attempts to extract the mucus. Saline is usually required to extract tenacious mucus. If the plug or mucus cannot be cleared with saline alone, 10% *N*-acetylcysteine may be utilized. Sometimes gentle probing of the mucous plug with the unopened biopsy forceps may also be of value. However, care must be taken with the technique to ensure that the biopsy forceps are advanced only under direct visualization and when no significant resistance is felt. To attempt FOB removal of mucous secretions in the absence of an ET tube is not recommended. The need to remove the FFB frequently to clear the visual field and the capability to remove a large mucous plug through the ET tube while fixing it to the distal end of the FFB with suction are essential.

In patients with atelectasis, there have been multiple reports of improvement in oxygenation, radiography, and peak inspiratory pressures after fiberoptic removal of retained secretions.[23, 24] The major concern in studies demonstrating the efficacy of FOB for atelectasis is the lack of a control group and failure to compare with other therapeutic methods. In 1979, Marini and colleagues[25] performed a prospective randomized study comparing (1) FOB followed by respiratory therapy (RT) with (2) RT alone. No difference between the two groups with regard to reversal of volume loss was noted after the first treatment or at 24 and 48 hours. Both groups, however, had an 80% resolution of volume loss. If an air bronchogram was present, neither treatment was successful; however, the atelectasis seemed to clear slowly over time. In this study, RT consisted of therapy at 4-hour intervals that included (1) repeated deep breaths to total lung capacity for 3 minutes with incentive spirometry or, if a patient was intubated, multiple 1- to 2-liter inflations using an anesthesia bag; (2) coughing (tracheal suctioning if cough was judged ineffective or if the patient was intubated); (3) beta agonist nebulizer treatment; and (4) chest percussion and postural drainage. FOB was performed transnasally (in nonintubated patients) or through the ET tube. Although the clinical study was small (14 patients in the RT group and 17 in the FOB group followed by the RT group), the authors concluded that there was no significant difference in the benefits between these two regimens. Significant points from this study are as follows: (1) air bronchograms should make one reluctant to approach volume loss with FOB, and (2) the initial treatment for lobar atelectasis in most cases should be intensive RT. If RT fails to clear atelectasis, FOB would seem to be a reasonable next step. FOB for atelectasis will only be effective if central mucous plugging or retained secretions are noted on direct endoscopic examination and are cleared. One exception to RT as the initial therapy is in symptomatic whole-lung collapse, in which FOB is reasonable as the initial therapy. Vigorous pulmonary toilet may be difficult to accomplish in the left tracheobronchial tree, where passage of the suction catheter is complicated by the acute angle of the left mainstem bronchus. When FOB is done for therapy of atelectasis, the FFB with the largest suction channel is preferred. One must remember that FOB does not treat the cause of the atelectasis and is therefore a temporizing measure only. As long as the patient continues to have risk factors for atelectasis, it is essential that FOB be followed by intensive RT to prevent recurrence. If follow-up RT is not done, one can expect multiple repeat FOBs to be necessary until predisposing factors are corrected. The inability to perform adequate RT may be encountered in patients with multiple rib fractures, cervical spine injury, multiple plaster casts, or traction devices. These patients may require repeated FOBs for recurrent atelectasis.

Use of the FFB with a balloon cuff for direct re-expansion of areas of refractory atelectasis has been reported.[26] This technique involves inserting the FFB into the involved segmental bronchus and occluding that bronchus with a balloon cuff attached around the distal end of the bronchoscope. Air is then directed down the suction channel and insufflation of the atelectatic area is attempted. Harada and coworkers[26] showed radiographic clearing in 13 of 15 patients in whom this technique was utilized. All had failed to respond to conventional RT. In six patients, atelectasis recurred and retreatment was again successful.

During FOB performed for atelectasis, the instillation of saline and *N*-acetylcysteine in combination with frequent suctioning may lower PaO_2. In the patient with compromised oxygenation and ventilation, supplemental oxygen and comprehensive monitoring during the procedure are essential. Pulse oximetry is recommended.

UPPER AIRWAY OBSTRUCTION

Causes of UAO in the adult include epiglottitis, bilateral vocal cord paralysis, laryngeal edema, and a foreign body. FOB should be diagnostic in all of these conditions, and FOB intubation should be therapeutic in all except foreign body UAO, in which rigid bronchoscopy or tracheostomy may be more appropriate. In the pediatric patient, laryngeal edema with acute epiglottitis as well as subglottic stenosis secondary to croup must be considered. FOB may also be useful for diagnosis and therapeutic intubation in UAO secondary to burn and smoke injuries as well as to trauma.

In patients who present with stridor or unexplained dyspnea with known predisposing factors for UAO, FOB affords not only immediate direct visualization of the upper airways for diagnosis but also, with the ET tube placed proximally on the FFB, expeditious intubation if UAO is noted. Guidice and associates[27] reported their experience with 22 adult patients referred to them for suspected acute UAO. They utilized a 5.2-mm FFB and the transnasal approach. An 8.0-mm nasotracheal tube was placed proximally on the FOB and was readily available if intubation was necessary. Eight patients were found to have life-threatening UAO and all were successfully intubated with FOB. There was no mortality and no significant morbidity. Three patients did have slight bleeding in the nares secondary to mucosal trauma. The average time of the procedure was 15 minutes. The nasotracheal approach is preferred in this situation owing to (1) patient tolerance, (2) the less angled approach to the glottic area, and (3) decreased likelihood of irritation or trauma exacerbation of UAO.

FOB incorporates immediate and direct visualization of the upper airway and offers potential definitive treatment if necessary in acute UAO. It is better accepted by the patient and less traumatic to the tissues than laryngoscopic examination. When done in the sitting position, it theoretically avoids posterior displacement of the epiglottis over the compromised upper airway, which may occur with laryngoscopic examination in the supine position. General anesthesia is not required, and it represents the diagnostic approach of choice for UAO in children and adults unless foreign body obstruction is definitely known or highly suspected to be the etiology before FOB.

ACUTE INHALATION INJURY

Pulmonary complications of burns can be classified as heat-induced or chemical-induced, and as upper airway injuries or lower airway injuries. Except when caused by steam, thermal injury is confined to the upper airways. Both upper and lower airway injuries can be diagnosed with FOB.

The location and extent of injury depend on the amount and caustic nature of the gases and particles, duration of

TABLE 85–2. Considerations for Fiberoptic Bronchoscopy in Acute Inhalation Injury

1. Singed nasal hairs
2. Facial burns about nose or mouth
3. Oral or nasopharyngeal burns
4. Carbonaceous sputum
5. Physical examination or review of systems results suggestive of UAO (wheezing, sore throat, hoarseness)
6. Steam inhalation

exposure, and solubility of gases. There are multiple possibilities of upper and lower airway injury with burn and smoke inhalation injuries. It has been recommended that regardless of symptoms at the time of evaluation, there are signs and risk factors that necessitate the use of FOB to rule out upper airway damage.[28] Prophylactic intubation would follow if mucosal damage was considerable. Table 85–2 lists considerations for FOB in acute inhalation injury.

If FOB reveals evidence of significant glottic or tracheal edema or mucosal damage, then intubation is accomplished prophylactically using the FFB. Airway edema may not be evident for 24 hours after burn injury, but FOB should demonstrate some abnormal findings (hyperemia, erythema, carbon particles). This may warrant a repeat FOB in 24 hours or as symptoms indicate to re-evaluate for edema.[29]

FOB is a good predictor of lower airway damage as well. If mucosal changes are noted at the segmental level or lower, patients are at increased risk for acute respiratory failure. In cases of documented or suspected lower airway damage, prophylactic intubation and PEEP therapy have been recommended.[30] This option is controversial.

DIAGNOSIS OF BACTERIAL PNEUMONIA WITH FIBEROPTIC BRONCHOSCOPY

It is known that sputum culture is unreliable for the diagnosis of a specific cause of bacterial pneumonia (and, therefore, for diagnosis of bacterial pneumonia itself) in the critically ill patient. This is true for the culture of coughed sputum, induced sputum, and endotracheal suction sputum. This is also the case for traditional FOB techniques in which bacterial contamination of lower airways by introduction of upper airway secretions, both on and around the FFB, make routine bronchial washing or suction channel culture results (for bacteria that might colonize the posterior oropharynx in the absence of infection) unreliable.[31] The specificity of bronchial washings is further compromised by bacterial tracheobronchial tree colonization in the absence of pneumonia in critically ill patients. Although the sensitivity of bronchial washings may be greater than the sensitivity of sputum culture, specificity is a problem in both circumstances. Data does support that preparing FOB washings with Gram's stain is a more reliable indicator of a specific bacterial cause.[32] This is also true for sputum analysis. In both circumstances such staining, showing predominantly lower respiratory tract cells with intracellular organisms and few squamous epithelial cells, may be used to provide Gram's classification and morphologic character of the organism.

Two more validated techniques that use quantitative cultures of lower tract secretions obtained with FFB—protected brush catheter (PBC) and bronchoalveolar lavage (BAL)—offer more reliable culture information for identifying a specific causative organism or organisms of bacterial pneumonia and for differentiating between infectious and noninfectious infiltrates. This is particularly important to the critical care physician, since the diagnosis of ICU pneumonia based on clinical acumen and radiographic appearance is frequently in error.[33, 34] Many ICU patients with diffuse infiltrative disease have fever that may or may not be related to pulmonary infection. These FOB quantitative culture techniques may be helpful in clinical decision making in these circumstances.[75]

Fiberoptic Bronchoscopy with Protected Brush Catheter

The PBC was developed by Wimberly and associates for use with the FFB to increase pneumonia diagnostic capability.[36] Since its introduction, numerous clinical investigators have demonstrated the value of specimens obtained with this tool when these specimens are subjected to quantitative culture.[37–46] The PBC is a telescoping double-catheter brush system with a distal occluding wax plug. The outer catheter has within it a recessed sterile inner catheter. The inner catheter is protected with a wax plug that occludes the orifice of the outer catheter. Within the inner catheter is a recessed sterile brush capable of advancement. The plug is dispelled when the inner catheter is advanced (accomplished immediately prior to advancing the sterile brush into a subsegmental orifice for sampling). Once sampling has occurred, the process is repeated in reverse, and the device is removed from the bronchoscope. Administration of lidocaine through the suction port of the FFB is minimized or avoided because this may instill oropharyngeal bacteria into the lower airways. It may also decrease recovery of lower tract organisms through its bacteriostatic effect. When the area sampled is a focal process, the sampling occurs in the segment identified on chest radiography or other radiographic study. Use of fluoroscopy may facilitate the sampling of focal infiltrates. Although most bronchoscopists attempt to sample the area with the greatest quantity of radiographically identifiable infiltrates, this may not be necessary.[38] When the infiltrative process is diffuse, multiple segments are usually sampled. Even with meticulous PBC technique, contamination still can occur; therefore, quantitative culture technique of the specimen is required. Following removal of the sampling apparatus, the brush is exposed, severed from the apparatus using sterile technique, and placed in 1 mL of nonbacteriostatic sterile saline. The container is mixed using a Vortex mixer, and 0.1 mL of the solution is plated for quantitative culture counts. Any organism growing in a concentration of 10^3 colonies per cubic millimeter or greater is more likely to be the causative agent, whereas those growing in colonies with counts less than this number are more likely to be contaminants. Although better than sputum analysis, this technique offers neither 100% sensitivity or specificity. Sensitivity is decreased by the prior administration of antibiotics and by the presence of diffuse infiltrates (because of sampling error). Decreased sensitivity is also judged to be potentially problematic because the decision to withhold therapy based on false-negative results from quantitative cultures could produce considerable morbidity. Another problem with PBC clinical studies relates to the gold standard to which comparison is made. Pleural fluid culturing, although infrequently yielding positive results, serves as a legitimate gold standard as would fine-needle aspirate,[47] a technique not traditionally used for comparison in clinical studies. Decreased sensitivity is also a problem with fine-needle aspiration.[48] Data from immediately performed autopsy would also be a legitimate standard. Blood cultures from a pneumonia source are usually assumed to be positive when that clinical diagnosis exists; however, other sources are possible, especially in the critically ill ICU patient. Chastre and coworkers[40] validated PBC culture results with simultaneous open-lung biopsy at the time of patient demise in the

ICU. Moser and coworkers,[42] Higuchi and associates,[43] and Johanson and colleagues[44] have also demonstrated the effectiveness of PBC using reliable standards for the diagnosis of pneumonia. Villers and coworkers showed good correlation with this technique, utilizing reasonable reference methods for bacterial pneumonia diagnosis in the intubated, mechanically ventilated patient and, in addition, used a control group without clinical evidence of pneumonia to show the absence of false-positive results.[45] Torzillo and associates[46] have utilized PBC for management decisions with good results.

Although PBC may offer clinical utility, its current impact would be greatest in clinical research in which data analysis is dependent on a more valid diagnosis of bacterial pneumonia than on traditional clinical and radiographic criteria. PBC may also have significant utility in the clinical practice of medicine when in the hands of an experienced bronchoscopist with appropriate technique for gathering and handling of specimens and with adequate laboratory support and appropriate quantitative culturing.[49] In this circumstance, PBC is ideally accomplished prior to initiation of antibiotic therapy, which dictates that it be done shortly after the diagnosis of pneumonia is suspected. Potential limits and drawbacks of the PBC technique include decreased sensitivity in diffuse lung injury and the potential for yielding false-positive and false-negative results.[50] As mentioned earlier, false-negative results are particularly problematic. Traditional PBC technique also fails to provide immediate information with which to guide therapy because culture results are not available for 24 to 48 hours. New developments in PBC technique include protected brushing using a nonbronchoscopic method in which a catheter is directed through an endotracheal tube usually under fluoroscopy.[51–53]

Bronchoalveolar Lavage with Quantitative Cultures

BAL has become the preferred method for diagnosing opportunistic infections in the immunocompromised patient (see later) and, when the quantitative culture technique is used, offers utility similar to that of the PBC technique for the diagnosis of bacterial pneumonia.[39, 54–61] When BAL is performed the bronchoscope is wedged into a subsegmental bronchus, and multiple aliquots (30–50 mL) of saline are instilled into the lung segment and removed (ideally by manual suction). Quantitative culture is performed in a manner similar to that for the PBC specimen. A cutoff of 10^4 to 10^5 colonies per cubic millimeter is used to suggest differentiation between contaminants–tracheobronchial tree colonizers and the causative organism. The limitations listed previously for PBC are also true for BAL. The sensitivity of this BAL technique is perhaps better than that of PBC because the area sampled is greater than that with PBC technique.[39, 58] Contamination potential is also greater.[59, 60] Meduri and colleagues have utilized a protected transbronchoscopic balloon technique (protected BAL) to avoid contamination by organisms in the suction channel during BAL.[37, 54] Other investigators have shown that specificity is enhanced when more than 1% of squamous epithelial cells are used to predict heavy contamination by oropharyngeal flora.[61]

Clinical validation with BAL is not as strong or as extensive as with PBC. In addition, BAL is more likely to be associated with significant hypoxemia than PBC, although FOB used for both procedures may produce hypoxemia.[55, 62, 63] A refinement in BAL diagnostic capability is the usefulness of the microscopic examination of fluid for organisms.[64] Cytocentrifuged specimen is stained and examined for the percentage of cells that contain intracellular organisms as a further correlate to specificity of positive quantitative culture results. Some impairment of oxygenation should be anticipated with BAL as well as with PBC procedures.[64a]

PULMONARY INFECTION IN THE IMMUNOCOMPROMISED HOST

The value of FOB in the diagnosis of opportunistic pulmonary infection is of major import in critically ill patients,[65–67] including transplant patients receiving immunosuppressive drugs, patients receiving long-term, high-dose steroid therapy, patients on chemotherapy for leukemia or lymphoma, and patients with acquired immune deficiency syndrome (AIDS). Although bronchial washings, transbronchial brushing, BAL, and, in selected cases, transbronchial biopsy are all valuable resources for identifying potential or definite pathogenic organisms, BAL has become the standard because of its sensitivity and risk-benefit ratio. The BAL technique is particularly valuable for the identification of organisms that do not colonize the tracheobronchial tree in the absence of infection, which include *Pneumocystis, Histoplasma, Blastomyces, Mycobacterium tuberculosis, Coccidioides, Nocardia,* and *Mucor* species. Initial clinical diagnosis is ideally made based on staining of centrifuged BAL fluid but may be made only by culture. Transbronchial brushings and biopsies (ideally obtained under fluoroscopy) increase the diagnostic yield for opportunistic infections but also increase the complication rate; this is especially the case for transbronchial biopsy, which is contraindicated in patients with bleeding diathesis and is usually avoided in patients who are at high risk for barotrauma (high-peak airway pressure and significant PEEP). Although transbronchial biopsy has been shown to increase diagnostic yield with some organisms, such as mycobacteria[35] and *Pneumocystis* species,[36] with recent advances in staining techniques for *Pneumocystis* organisms, there is minimal additional clinically significant yield in this disorder. Transbronchial biopsy is of value if it shows organisms in tissue that may colonize the upper airway without tissue invasion; such organisms include *Aspergillus,* atypical *Mycobacterium, Candida,* and *Cryptococcus* species. Although *Aspergillus* and *Cryptococcus* may colonize the upper airway in the absence of disease, the presence of these organisms in the appropriate clinical situation warrants therapy without a biopsy specimen showing tissue invasion.

The use of FOB in the diagnosis of suspected *Pneumocystis* infection in the ICU AIDS patient is an area worthy of particular emphasis. As mentioned earlier, FOB with BAL has become the standard diagnostic technique for diagnosing pneumocystis pneumonia in AIDS patients. Although transbronchial biopsy was added to BAL in the past (when no contraindication existed), this practice is uncommon currently. BAL and new staining techniques such as fluorescent antibody against *Pneumocystis carinii* have increased yield when compared with previous staining techniques such as those that use silver methenamine and Gomori methenamine silver.[68–70] Diagnostic yield of close to 95% is now expected. Considering the high yield without utilizing transbronchial biopsy, biopsy is typically reserved for those patients in whom chest radiography, although potentially indicating a diagnosis of pneumocystis pneumonia, could mean the presence of other opportunistic infections in which transbronchial biopsy would normally increase yield. Although some investigators have reported increased yield by performing BAL bilaterally in suspected AIDS-related pneumocystis pneumonia,[67] yield with unilateral sampling is clinically satisfactory in most circumstances. Upper lobe BAL may increase yield in suspected pneumocystis pneumonia in patients undergoing inhaled pentamidine prophylaxis because organism burden may be greater in the upper lobes.[72, 73]

ASTHMA

Credle[74] showed that laryngospasm in the asthmatic patient could occur either during ET insertion before FFB insertion or with direct FFB passage. FOB in the nonintubated asthmatic patient, especially with active bronchospasm, should have solid indications and no alternatives that carry less risk. If FOB is indicated in the patient with active asthma who is not yet intubated, an ET tube should be inserted on the proximal bronchoscope for introduction into the airway if laryngospasm develops.

In the nonintubated asthmatic, premedication with nebulized atropine[75] and nebulized beta agonist is indicated. This regimen would also seem reasonable for intubated asthmatic patients as well. Intravenous steroids are given, depending on activity of disease and medication history. With proper premedication, the chance of laryngospasm is unlikely, and exacerbation of bronchospasm is unusual. Intravenous lidocaine[76, 77] (but not nebulized[78] lidocaine) has been shown efficacious in preventing mechanical stimulation–induced laryngospasm.

The poor prognosis and increased ventilator complication rate in ventilated status asthmaticus patients have been well described.[79] If the ventilated asthmatic patient fails to respond to vigorous and intensive drug therapy, one is faced with less traditional choices for additional therapy. General anesthesia and intensification of subcutaneous or aerosolized beta agonists are considerations. Bronchopulmonary lavage is another alternative. This technique was popularized for the treatment of pulmonary alveolar proteinosis.[80] Bronchopulmonary lavage with both the rigid and fiberoptic instrumentation has been used in the severe asthmatic patient refractory to standard therapy.[81, 82] Lavage has been utilized in acute and chronic asthmatic patients both on and off the ventilator. Solutions for irrigation have included various combinations of saline, acetylcysteine, beta agonists, and steroids. There have been no prospective controlled studies done in this area. Lavage solutions have consisted of (1) 30 mL of 20% *N*-acetylcysteine solution; (2) 250 mg of methylprednisolone; and (3) 2 mL of isoetharine, all combined in 600 mL of normal saline.[81] It would appear that the substitution of a more beta-2 selective agent such as albuterol instead of isoetharine would be advantageous if this technique is employed.

If bronchopulmonary lavage is planned in the mechanically ventilated asthmatic patient suspected of having peripheral mucous plugging associated with asthma, the FFB seems the most rational approach to lavage. During the procedure, it is recommended that the FIO_2 be increased to 0.9 to 1.0 and that either transcutaneous or ear oximetry oxygen saturation be monitored continuously. Use of bronchopulmonary lavage in the severely ill mechanically ventilated asthmatic patient remains controversial and unproven, and the rise in airway pressures and likelihood of worsened oxygenation make this technique poorly tolerated.

HEMOPTYSIS

It is important to remember that since hemoptysis causes morbidity and mortality by its effect on oxygenation and not from blood loss, it is blood remaining in the tracheobronchial tree that is of greatest concern, and not the blood that is expectorated and quantitated. However, these two values usually correlate.

Although the FFB is the instrument of choice in the diagnosis of nonmassive hemoptysis (less than 200–600 mL in 24 hours)[83] because of comfort to the patient and ability to examine the distal bronchial tree, its use in massive hemoptysis is controversial.[84] Traditionally, the rigid bronchoscope has been preferred in this circumstance. The rigid bronchoscope is an open-ended metal tube with a light source and suction capabilities. Although success in flexible fiberoptic localization of bleeding sites in patients with massive hemoptysis has been reported,[85] rigid bronchoscopy allows greater suction capability, facilitates ventilation through its large rigid chamber, and remains the procedure of choice. If an ET tube is in place, however, the rigid bronchoscope cannot be passed and the FFB becomes the only instrument for diagnosis and therapeutic use (if the ET tube is to remain in place). Even with newer, larger suction channels, FOB diagnosis of the segmental area of hemoptysis is difficult when bleeding is brisk. Segmental lavage has been used in an attempt to increase diagnostic yield[85] and offers greatest usefulness between episodes of massive hemoptysis when old blood obscures endobronchial pathology. Maintenance of the visual field for FOB intubation in the setting of brisk hemoptysis is difficult.

FFB-directed endobronchial tamponade through an ET tube has been successful in controlling massive hemoptysis.[86] A 4-French, 100-cm Fogarty balloon is guided to the segmental orifice under direct vision with the aid of forceps passed through the biopsy channel of the FFB. This technique requires that an ET tube be in place.

In life-threatening hemoptysis, FFB-directed double-lumen endobronchial tube insertion may be accomplished to isolate the bleeding left or right lung from the nonbleeding contralateral lung. Inadequate visual field may, however, complicate its use. Similarly, a single-lumen ET tube can be inserted orally (for adequate length), and with FFB guidance, into the bronchus of the nonbleeding lung to isolate it from massive contralateral lung hemorrhage.

PEDIATRIC FIBEROPTIC BRONCHOSCOPY

In older children, the 5-mm FFB is used with essentially the same indications as in the adult. In younger children, the airways are small and delicate, patients are less cooperative and less able to communicate, and the margin for error may be small. Still, FOB can be very useful in pediatric critical care.

The two most important considerations are the small caliber of neonatal and pediatric airways (including the nares) and the lack of cooperation in most younger pediatric patients, thus making oral FOB more difficult. Sedation should generally be avoided in nonmechanically ventilated infants younger than 4 months of age.

Wood and Sherman[87] published their pediatric experience with the FFB (3.5-mm) in 211 patients with ages varying from less than 1 month to 14 years. Minimal ET tube ID was 4.5 mm. Diagnoses included mucous plugging in 46 patients, bronchial stenosis or compression in 25, tracheomalacia in 15, and inflammation in 13. No diagnosis was made in 33. Of 29 infants weighing less than 2800 g undergoing FOB for atelectasis, 25 had radiographic resolution within 1 hour. There were three complications: laryngospasm in one patient, pneumothorax in one patient, and seizure in one patient occurring 1 hour after FOB. There were no deaths or long-lasting sequelae related to the procedure.

Vauthy and Reddy[88] used FOB for evaluation and treatment of UAO in infants and children. The fiberoptic instrument was preferred because direct laryngoscopic examination may distort and irritate upper airway anatomy. Using the 3.2-mm FFB without suction capability, they were able to differentiate between epiglottitis, subglottic croup, foreign body aspiration, and other less common causes of airway obstruction. The procedure was easily performed, well tolerated, and usually performed in the upright position in older children. Small infants were restrained by a blanket wrapped around the body, and children under 5 years of age by a papoose board (head elevated 40–45%). The most common cause of acute UAO in infants was laryngomalacia. Vocal cord trauma, congenital abnormalities, vocal cord web, and polyps were additional causes. In older children, the most common cause was epiglottitis and croup. When a foreign body was found to be the etiology, it was diagnosed and removed subsequently by rigid bronchoscopy. They preferred the transnasal FOB route and demonstrated the value of FOB intubation in this group.

The new ultrathin FFB (Olympus 1.8-mm) has its greatest application in defining tube position but can also be used for intubations in small infants.[89] With this instrument, an ET tube as small as 3 mm can be inserted over the FFB or FOB safely performed through a 3-mm ET tube already in place. Tracheal insertion of the ultrathin FFB may be difficult if the ultrathin FFB lacks flexion-extension (no tip control). Without flexion-extension or a suction channel, it is also less useful for other therapeutic purposes. This is in contrast to the pediatric FFB, which has both flexion-extension and suction capabilities (Olympus 3.7-mm). Some ultrathins (Olympus 2.5-mm) have a 0.5-mm suction channel but no tip control, and others have tip control but no suction (Olympus 2.7-mm).

MISCELLANEOUS INDICATIONS

Foreign bodies may be a significant problem in ventilated patients. As the patient is already intubated and rigid bronchoscopy is not possible, FOB may be useful in retrieving smaller foreign bodies from the tracheobronchial tree. Basket forceps, backloading grasping forceps, or four-pronged forceps may be utilized.

High-frequency jet ventilation can be delivered through the suction channel of the FFB. Smith and coworkers[90] demonstrated successful delivery of high-frequency jet ventilation through the FFB in six dogs and eight adult human subjects. This technique has subsequently been successfully used for airway examination of both critically ill children[91] and adults.[92] High-frequency jet ventilation in combination with FOB has potential advantages if ventilation and direct airway inspection are both paramount needs in the critically ill patient.

FOB is the procedure of choice to diagnose traumatic tears of the tracheobronchial tree. In the patient with significant face or neck trauma, FOB can be utilized to diagnose and treat UAO.

Lee and Wright[93] successfully used a pulmonary artery catheter inserted through a 2.6-mm FFB suction channel to reinflate persistently collapsed lobes after the surgical repair of a tear in the tracheobronchial tree. In this older child, the balloon was inflated to occlude the bronchus and air delivered through the distal port of the pulmonary artery catheter. Various FOB techniques have been used to facilitate diagnosis and management of bronchopleural fistula.[94]

FOB can be used to expedite insertion of nasal or oral gastric and enteral tubes. Through the use of a direct-vision pediatric FFB as obturator or of grasping forceps, passage is facilitated.

COMPLICATIONS

ICU patients often have limited pulmonary and cardiac reserve. Therefore, effects on cardiopulmonary function, even when minimal, may be clinically significant. Systemic disease, drug therapy, and treatment regimens may predispose to or increase the severity of complications. Examples are increased airway pressure in mechanically ventilated patients that predisposes to barotrauma and coagulopathies, making bleeding complications more likely.

HYPOXEMIA

When performing FOB, especially in the presence of acute or chronic lung disease, desaturation may occur. In the mechanically ventilated patient, removal of oxygenated tracheal gas by prolonged suction (1) decreases tidal volume and therefore minute ventilation, (2) decreases functional residual capacity, and (3) lowers PEEP effect. These effects may lead to an increase in intrapulmonary shunt as well as in procedure zones with a low ventilation-perfusion ratio. Extensive use of irrigating or anesthetic solutions has an adverse effect on ventilation both as airspace-occupying substances and as surfactant diluents. Hypoxemia during and immediately after FOB has been substantiated both in the mechanically ventilated and in the nonintubated patient.[95, 96]

Increased PaO_2 during FOB in critically ill, mechanically ventilated patients has been reportedly attributed to the beneficial effect of FOB-induced PEEP. Although suction may decrease the PEEP effect, the additional intra-airway expiratory resistance of the FOB may increase the PEEP effect. In patients undergoing FOB during mechanical ventilation, the following are recommended: (1) use of a tube no smaller than 8.0 ID; (2) monitoring for increased PEEP; (3) increasing FIO_2; (4) monitoring tidal volume or observing for adequate chest excursions; (5) suctioning for short periods only; (6) monitoring oxygenation; and (7) obtaining a post-procedure chest x-ray to rule out pneumothorax. If expiratory airway resistance is a greater factor than suctioning, PEEP setting should be titrated down to maintain the same level of PEEP. Saturation should be monitored with an oximeter. One study has documented the safety of FOB with BAL in most patients with the acute respiratory distress syndrome.[97]

Arrhythmias

Ventricular and supraventricular arrhythmias may occur in critically ill patients undergoing FOB. Hypoxemia less than 60 mm Hg correlates with arrhythmia occurrence.[98] Katz and associates[99] reported a significant decrease in PaO_2 in 68% of FOB patients that persisted for more than 1 hour after FOB and correlated with the frequency of arrhythmias. Hemodynamic changes during FOB included an increase in mean arterial pressure, heart rate, and cardiac index.[100] The increase in rate-pressure product was attributed to a reflex sympathetic discharge caused by mechanical irritation of the airways.

Complications Secondary to Fiberoptic Bronchoscopy Transbronchial Brushing and Biopsy

Although there is abundant literature on FOB transbronchial lung biopsy in nonventilated patients, there are minimal published data concerning transbronchial biopsy in the ventilator-dependent patient and perhaps none in patients receiving PEEP. Moser and associates[101] in 1982 used a canine model with unilateral *Streptococcus pneumoniae* to evaluate the sensitivity, specificity, and risk of diagnostic procedures. Data from 15 dogs indicated that catheter brushing and transbronchial biopsy were not associated with pneumothorax or significant hemorrhage. They also studied 20 additional dogs that were mechanically ventilated and again showed that transbronchial biopsy and catheter brush sampling were not associated with pneumothorax formation. Transthoracic needle aspiration was associated with pneumothorax formation in both groups. They postulated that although pneumothorax did not occur with a catheter brush or transbronchial biopsy in these ventilated dogs, this could reflect biopsy or brushing of densely consolidated lung parenchyma and careful avoidance, with fluoroscopy, of inadvertent visceral pleural biopsy. Other considerations such as coagulopathy or pulmonary hypertension, which did not exist in their model, might also predispose the ICU patient to increased incidence of pulmonary hemorrhage. Moser[102] in 1984 summarized diagnostic procedures done in patients with acute pulmonary infiltrates. He believed that patients with undiagnosed roentgenographic infiltrates deserve an aggressive, early invasive approach that includes, if warranted, FOB with washings, PTC brushing, and transbronchial biopsy, regardless of the patients' ventilator status. His opinion concerning fine-needle lung aspiration was similar if this was the procedure of choice; however, he recommended that it not be done in the patient on PEEP. Transbronchial biopsy, if the procedure of choice for diagnosis, should not be contraindicated in patients on a ventilator. Although PEEP may be a relative contraindication for transbronchial biopsy, any pneumothorax that may develop can be treated with chest-tube drainage, which would be required after open-lung biopsy in any event.

Although there are no studies addressing hemorrhagic complications specifically in critically ill patients, work by Zavala[103] in critically ill patients shows an extremely low rate of life-threatening hemorrhage. Fluoroscopy is ideal to ensure that the biopsy forceps are peripheral to decrease biopsy of larger vessels but not so peripheral as to increase the chance of visceral pleural biopsy and pneumothorax. Several techniques can decrease hemorrhage complications. Coagulopathy should be corrected before the procedure. Platelets should be administered to those patients who have a platelet count less than 50,000 or bleeding with thrombocytopenia. If this platelet-related bleeding diathesis cannot be corrected by supplemental platelet therapy, then transbronchial biopsy is contraindicated. Dialysis, desmopressin, or estrogen therapy may decrease bleeding risk in patients with uremia. Fresh frozen plasma should be given to correct abnormal clotting times. Epinephrine solution 1:1000 (up to 1 mL diluted in 9 mL normal saline) can be instilled into subsegmental orifices before or after biopsy if the patient is at increased risk of hemorrhage or develops hemorrhage. If epinephrine is used prophylactically in patients with coronary artery disease, risks should be considered. In those patients who develop significant brisk hemorrhage, it is advisable to quickly wedge the tip of the FFB into the bleeding segment's orifice, hopefully tamponading the bleeding area until hemostasis is achieved. Once the FFB is backed away from the segmental orifice and significant hemorrhage occurs, it is difficult to regain an adequate visual field for reinsertion of the FFB tip into that segment.

Fever and Pneumonia

Fever greater than 101°F and parenchymal infiltration have been noted within 72 hours after performance of transnasal FOB. Data do not support pneumonia as the etiology of these infiltrates (no increase in white blood cell count, no bacteremia, and resolution without therapy).[104]

Topical Anesthesia

The most commonly used topical anesthetic in FOB is lidocaine, which is less toxic than either tetracaine or cocaine. Cocaine also shrinks mucosa, facilitating passage of the FFB, but creates problems relative to inappropriate access for abuse as an illicit substance. In the tracheobronchial tree, it is not recommended. Local anesthetics applied topically to the posterior pharynx, larynx, and tracheobronchial mucosa are rapidly absorbed. Peak venous blood levels occur 10 to 15 minutes after application. Signs of toxicity include tremulousness, shivering, dizziness, or sedation. This may be followed by unconsciousness, convulsions, respiratory arrest, or cardiovascular collapse. Various ceilings have been published as recommendations for maximum lidocaine topical application. The adult should be limited to 200 to 300 mg.[9]

SUMMARY

The value of FOB in critical care medicine seems greatest in intubation and in ET tube management. Diagnosis of airway damage, insertion of specialized ET tubes, and ET tube changing are all facilitated by FOB. It offers capability for simultaneous diagnosis and treatment of UAO. FOB also has potential for therapy of atelectasis not responding to vigorous chest physiotherapy or if chest physiotherapy is contraindicated. Although controversial, in the ICU patient with bacterial pneumonia, FOB with PTC brush culture may allow narrowing of the spectrum of antibiotic coverage. In intubated patients, it offers an alternative to rigid bronchoscopy for identifying the cause of hemoptysis. Ultrathin and pediatric FFBs have increased the pediatric capability of FOB. The critical care specialist should have the knowledge to recognize appropriate indications for FOB and in most circumstances both the skill and training to perform emergent FOB, particularly in intubated patients. It is essential that the bronchoscopist understand indications, limitations, potential complications, and necessary precautions for this procedure.

References

1. Lindholm CE, Ollman B, Snyder J, et al: Flexible fiberoptic bronchoscopy in critical care medicine. Crit Care Med 1974; 2:250.
2. Feldman NT, Huber GL: Fiberoptic bronchoscopy in the intensive care unit. Heart Lung 1981; 10:1037.
3. Lindholm CE, Grenvik A: Flexible fiberoptic bronchoscopy and intubation in intensive care. *In:* Recent Advances in Intensive Therapy. Ledingham IM (Ed). London, Churchill Livingstone, 1977, pp 47–66.
4. Stevens RP, Lillington GA, Parson GH: Fiberoptic bronchoscopy in the intensive care unit. Heart Lung 1981; 10:1037.
5. Fulkerson WJ: Fiberoptic bronchoscopy. N Engl J Med 1984; 311:511.
6. Lindholm CE, Ollman B, Snyder JV, et al: Cardiorespiratory effects of flexible fiberoptic bronchoscopy in critically ill patients. Chest 1978; 74:362.
7. Ovassapian A, Yelick SJ, Dykes MHM, et al: Fiberoptic nasotracheal intubation: Incidence and causes of failure. Anesth Analg 1983; 62:692.
8. Burgin WW Jr, Blumer RB, McCabe J: Simplified ventilator bronchoscopy. Chest 1975; 67:501.
9. Perry LB: Topical anesthesia for bronchoscopy. Chest 1978; 73:691.
10. Britton RM, Nelson KG: Improper oxygenation during bronchofiberscopy. Anesthesiology 1974; 40:87.
11. Patil UU, Stehling LC, Zuder HL: Fiberoptic Endoscopy in Anaesthesia. Chicago, Year Book Medical Publishers, 1983.
12. Moorthy SS, Dierdorf SF: An unusual difficulty in fiberoptic intubation. Anesthesiology 1985; 63:229.
13. Sia RL, Edens ET: How to avoid problems when using the fiberoptic bronchoscope for difficult intubations. Anaesthesia 1981; 36:74.
14. Shinnick JP, Freedman AP: Bronchofiberscopic placement of a double-lumen endotracheal tube. Crit Care Med 1982; 10:544.
15. Ovassapian A: Fiberoptic bronchoscope and double-lumen tracheal tubes. Anaesthesia 1983; 38:1104.
16. Wagner DL, Gammage GW, Wong ML: Tracheal rupture following the insertion of a disposable double-lumen endotracheal tube. Anesthesiology 1985; 63:698.
17. Rosenbaum SH, Rosenbaum LM, Cole RP, et al: Use of the flexible fiberoptic bronchoscope to change endotracheal tubes in critically ill patients. Anesthesiology 1981; 54:169.
18. Stauffer JL, Olson DE, Petty TL: Complications and consequences of endotracheal intubation and tracheotomy. Am J Med 1981, 70:65.

19. Amikam B, Landa J, West J, et al: Bronchofiberscopic observations of the tracheobronchial tree during intubation. Am Rev Respir Dis 1972; 105:747.
20. Patil VU, Stehling LC, Zuder HL: Another use for the fiberoptic bronchoscope. Anesthesiology 1981; 55:484.
21. Grossman E, Jacobi AM: Minimal optimal endotracheal tube size for fiberoptic bronchoscopy. Anesth Analg 1974; 53:475.
22. Lindholm EC, Grenvik A: Tracheal tube and cuff problems. Int Anesthesiol Clin 1982; 20:103.
23. Wanner A, Landa JF, Nieman RE Jr, et al: Bedside bronchofiberscopy for atelectasis and lung abscess. JAMA 1983; 224: 1281.
24. Groitl H: The flexible bronchofiberscope in the intensive care unit (ICU): The optimal postoperative care for the bronchial system. Endoscopy 1981; 13:100.
25. Marini JJ, Pierson DJ, Hudson LD: Acute lobar atelectasis: A prospective comparison of fiberoptic bronchoscopy and respiratory therapy. Am Rev Respir Dis 1979; 119:971.
26. Harada K, Mutsuda T, Saoyama N, et al: Re-expansion of refractory atelectasis using a bronchofiberscope with a balloon cuff. Chest 1983; 84:725.
27. Guidice JC, Komansky H, Gordon R, et al: Acute upper airway obstruction—Fiberoptic bronchoscopy in diagnosis and therapy. Crit Care Med 1981; 9:878.
28. Cahalane M, Demling RH: Early respiratory abnormalities for smoke inhalation. JAMA 1984; 251:771.
29. Hunt JL, Agee RN, Pruitt BA Jr: Fiberoptic bronchoscopy in acute inhalation injury. J Trauma 1975; 15:641.
30. Venus B, Matsuda T, Copiozo J, et al: Prophylactic intubation and continuous airway pressure in the management of inhalation injury in burn victims. Crit Care Med 1981; 9:519.
31. Bartlett JG, Alexander J, Mayhew J, et al: Should fiberoptic bronchoscopy aspirates be cultured? Am Rev Respir Dis 1976; 114:73.
32. Flatauer FE, Chabalko JJ, Wolinsky E: Fiberoptic bronchoscopy in bacteriologic assessment of lower respiratory tract secretions. JAMA 1980; 244:2427.
33. Wunderink RG, Woldenberg LS, Zeiss J, et al: The radiologic diagnosis of autopsy-proven ventilator-associated pneumonia. Chest 1992; 101:458–463.
34. Pingleton SK, Fagon JY, Leeper KV: Patient selection for clinical investigation of ventilator-associated pneumonia. Chest 1992; 102:553S–556S.
35. Leeper KL: Diagnosis and treatment of pulmonary infections in adult respiratory distress syndrome. New Horizons 1993; 1:550.
36. Wimberly N, Faling LJ, Bartlet JG: A fiberoptic bronchoscopy technique to obtain uncontaminated lower airway secretions for bacterial culture. Am Rev Respir Dis 1979; 119:337–343.
37. Meduri GU: Ventilator-associated pneumonia in patients with respiratory failure. Chest 1990; 97:1208–1219.
38. Marquette CH, Herengt F, Saulnier F, et al: Protected specimen brush in the assessment of ventilator-associated pneumonia. Chest 1993; 103:243–247.
39. Violan JS, Castro FR, Luna JC, et al: Comparative efficacy of bronchoalveolar lavage and telescoping plugged catheter in the diagnosis of pneumonia in mechanically ventilated patients. Chest 1993; 103:386–390.
40. Chastre J, Viau F, Brun P, et al: Concise clinical studies: Prospective bacteriologic diagnosis of nosocomial pneumonia in primates. Am Rev Respir Dis 1984; 130:924.
41. Fagon JY, Chastre J, Hance AJ, et al: Detection of nosocomial lung infection in ventilated patients. Am Rev Respir Dis 1988; 137:253–255.
42. Moser KM, Maurer J, Jassy L, et al: Sensitivity, specificity, and risk of diagnostic procedures in a canine model of *Streptococcus* pneumonia. Am Rev Respir Dis 1982; 25:436–442.
43. Higuchi JH, Coalson JJ, Johanson WG: Bacteriologic diagnosis of nosocomial pneumonia in primates: Usefulness of the protected specimen brush. Am Rev Respir Dis 1982; 125:53–57.
44. Johanson WG, Seidenfeld JJ, Gomez P, et al: Bacteriologic diagnosis of nosocomial pneumonia following prolonged mechanical ventilation. Am Rev Respir Dis 1988; 137:259–264.
45. Villers D, Derriennic M, Raffi R, et al: Reliability of the bronchoscopic protected catheter brush in intubated and ventilated patients. Chest 1985; 88:527.
46. Torzillo PH, McWilliam DB, Young IH, et al: Use of protected telescoping brush system in the management of bacterial pulmonary infection in intubated patients. Br J Dis Chest 1985; 79:125.
47. Torres A, Jiménez P, Puig de la Bellacasa J, et al: Diagnosis value of nonfluoroscopic percutaneous lung needle aspiration in patients with pneumonia. Chest 1990; 98:840–844.
48. Zavala DC, Schoell JE: Ultrathin needle aspiration of the lung in infectious and malignant diseases. Am Rev Respir Dis 1981; 123:125–131.
49. Baselski VS, El-Torky M, Coalson JJ, et al: The standardization of criteria for processing and interpreting laboratory specimens in patients with suspected ventilator-associated pneumonia. Chest 1992; 102:571S–579S.
50. Torres A, Bellacasa J, Albert A, et al: Diagnostic value of quantitative cultures of bronchoalveolar lavage and telescoping plugged catheters in mechanically ventilated patients with bacterial pneumonia. Am Rev Respir Dis 1989; 140:306–310.
51. Torres A, Bellacasa J, Rodriguez-Roisin R, et al: Diagnostic value of telescoping plugged catheters in mechanically ventilated patients with bacterial pneumonia using the Metras catheter. Am Rev Respir Dis 1988; 138:117–120.
52. Zucker A, Pollack M, Kate R: Blind use of the double-lumen plugged catheter for diagnosis of respiratory tract infections in critically ill children. Crit Care Med 1984; 12:867–870.
53. Papazian L, Martin C, Meric B, et al: A reappraisal of blind bronchial sampling in the microbiologic diagnosis of nosocomial bronchopneumonia. Chest 1993; 103:236–242.
54. Meduri GU, Wunderink RG, Leeper KV: Management of bacterial pneumonia in ventilated patients. Chest 1992; 101:500–508.
55. Guerra LF, Baughman RP: Use of bronchoalveolar lavage to diagnose bacterial pneumonia in mechanically ventilated patients. Crit Care Med 1990; 18:169–173.
56. Meduri GU, Baselski V: The role of bronchoalveolar lavage in diagnosing non-opportunistic bacterial pneumonia. Chest 1991; 100:179–190.
57. Chastre J, Fagon JY, Lamer CH: Procedures for the diagnosis of pneumonia in ICU patients. Intensive Care Med 1992; 18:S10–S17.
58. Reynolds HY: Bronchoalveolar lavage. Am Rev Respir Dis 1987; 135:250–263.
59. Kahn FW, Jones JM: Diagnosing bacterial respiratory infection by bronchoalveolar lavage. J Infect Dis 1987; 155:862–869.
60. Chastre J, Fagon JY, Soler P, et al: Diagnosis of nosocomial bacterial pneumonia in intubated patients undergoing ventilation: Comparison of the usefulness of bronchoalveolar lavage and the protected specimen brush. Am J Med 1988; 85:499–506.
61. Kahn FW, Jones JM: Diagnosing bacterial respiratory infection by bronchoalveolar lavage. J Infect Dis 1987; 155:862–869.
62. Trouillet JL, Guiguet M, Gibert C, et al: Fiberoptic bronchoscopy in ventilated patients: Evaluation of cardiopulmonary risk under midazolam sedation. Chest 1990; 97:927–933.
63. Guerra LF, Baughman RP: Use of bronchoalveolar lavage to diagnose bacterial pneumonia in mechanically ventilated patients. Crit Care Med 1990; 18:169–173.
64. Chastre J, Fagon JY, Soler P, et al: Quantification of BAL cells containing intracellular bacteria rapidly identifies ventilated patients with nosocomial pneumonia. Chest 1989; 95:190–192.
64a. Papazian L, Colt HG, Scemama F, et al: Effects of consecutive protected specimen brushing and bronchoalveolar lavage on gas exchange and hemodynamics in ventilated patients. Chest 1993; 104:1548.
65. Tobin MH, Grenvik A: Nosocomial lung infection and its diagnosis. Crit Care Med 1984; 12:191.
66. Olopade CO, Prakash UR: Bronchoscopy in the critical care unit. Mayo Clin Proc 1989; 64:1255.
67. Repsher LH, Levin DC, Matthay RA, et al: Transbronchial lung biopsy via the fiberoptic bronchoscope in the diagnosis of diffuse pulmonary infiltrates in the immunocompromised host. Natl Cancer Inst Monogr 1976; 43:127.
68. Weldon-Linne CM, Rhone DP, Bourassa R: Bronchoscopy specimens in adults with AIDS. Chest 1990; 98:24–28.
69. Griffiths MH, Kochan G, Miller RF: Diagnosis of pulmonary disease in human immunodeficiency virus infection: Role of

transbronchial biopsy and bronchoalveolar lavage. Thorax 1989; 44:554–558.
70. Homer KS, Wiley EL, Smith AL: Monoclonal antibody to *Pneumocystis carinii.* Am J Clin Pathol 1992; 97:619–624.
71. Meduri GU, Stover DE, Nash T: Bilateral bronchoalveolar lavage in the diagnosis of opportunistic pulmonary infections. Chest 1991; 100:1272–1276.
72. Read CA, Cerrone F, Busseniers AE, et al: Differential lobe lavage for diagnosis of acute pneumocystic carinii pneumonia in patients receiving prophylactic aerosolized pentamidine therapy. Chest 1993; 103:1520–1523.
73. Baughman RP, Dohn MN, Shipley R: Increased *Pneumocystis carinii* recovery from the upper lobes in pneumocystis pneumonia. Chest 1993; 103:426–432.
74. Credle WF Jr: Complications of fiberoptic bronchoscopy. Am Rev Respir Dis 1974; 109:67.
75. Sahn SA, Scoggins C: Fiberoptic bronchoscopy in bronchial asthma. Chest 1976; 69:39.
76. Kingston HCG, Hirshman CA: Perioperative management of the patient with asthma. Anesth Analg 1984; 63:844.
77. Downes H, Gerber N, Hirshman CA: I.V. lignocaine in reflex and allergic bronchoconstriction. Br J Anaesth 1980; 52:873.
78. Downes H, Hirshman CA: Lidocaine aerosols do not prevent allergic bronchoconstriction. Anesth Analg 1981; 60:28.
79. Williams MH Jr: Life-threatening asthma. Arch Intern Med 1980; 140:1604.
80. Brach BB, Harrell JH, Moser KM: Alveolar proteinosis. Chest 1976; 69:224.
81. Millman M, Goodman AH, Goldstein IM, et al: Status asthmaticus: Use of acetylcysteine during bronchoscopy and lavage to remove mucous plugs. Ann Allergy 1983; 50:85.
82. Shridharani M, Maxson TR: Pulmonary lavage in a patient in status asthmaticus receiving mechanical ventilation: A case report. Ann Allergy 1982; 49:157.
83. Garzon AA, Gourin A: Surgical management of massive hemoptysis. Ann Surg 1978; 178:267.
84. Khan MA, Whitcomb ME, Snider GL: Flexible fiberoptic bronchoscopy. Am J Med 1976; 61:151.
85. Imgrund SP, Goldberg SK, Walkenstein MD, et al: Clinical diagnosis of massive hemoptysis using the fiberoptic bronchoscope. Crit Care Med 1985; 13:438.
86. Saw EC, Gottlieb LS, Yokoyama T, et al: Flexible fiberoptic bronchoscopy and endobronchial tamponade in the management of massive hemoptysis. Chest 1976; 70:589.
87. Wood RE, Sherman JM: Pediatric flexible bronchoscopy. Ann Otol 1980; 89:414.
88. Vauthy PA, Reddy R: Acute upper airway obstruction in infants and children: Evaluation by the fiberoptic bronchoscope. Ann Otol 1980; 89:417.
89. Vigneswaran R, Whitfield JM: The use of a new ultra-thin fiberoptic bronchoscope to determine endotracheal tube position in the sick newborn infant. Chest 1981; 80:174.
90. Smith RB, Lindholm CE, Klain M: Jet ventilation for fiberoptic bronchoscopy under general anesthesia. Acta Anaesth Scand 1976; 20:111.
91. Dalens B, Labbe A, Haberer JP: Respiratory assistance secured by jet-ventilation during broncho-fiberscopy in forty-nine infants. Anesthesiology 1982; 57:551.
92. Satyanarayana T, Capan L, Ramanathan S, et al: Bronchofiberscopic jet ventilation. Anesth Analg 1980; 59:350.
93. Lee TS, Wright BD: Selective insufflation of collapsed lung with fiberoptic bronchoscope and Swan-Ganz catheter. Intensive Care Med 1981; 7:241.
94. Pierson DJ: Management of bronchopleural fistula in the adult respiratory distress syndrome. New Horizons 1993; 1:521.
95. Arai T, Hatano Y, Komatsu K, et al: Real-time analysis of the change in arterial oxygen tension during endotracheal suction with a fiberoptic bronchoscope. Crit Care Med 1985; 13:855.
96. Dubrawsky C, Awe RJ, Jenkins DE: The effect of bronchofiberscopic examination on oxygenation status. Chest 1975; 67:137.
97. Steinberg KP, Mitchell DR, Maunder RJ, et al: Safety of bronchoalveolar lavage in patients with adult respiratory distress syndrome. Am Rev Respir Dis 1993; 148:556
98. Shrader DL, Lakshminarayan S: The effect of fiberoptic bronchoscopy on cardiac rhythm. Chest 1978; 73:721.
99. Katz AS, Michelson EL, Stawicki J, et al: Cardiac arrhythmia frequency during fiberoptic bronchoscopy and correlation with hypoxemia. Arch Intern Med 1981; 141:603.
100. Montravers P, Ganzitt R, Dombret MC, et al: Cardiopulmonary effects of bronchoalveolar lavage in critically ill patients. Chest 1993; 104:1541.
101. Moser KM, Maurer J, Jassy L, et al: Sensitivity, specificity, and risk of diagnostic procedures in a canine model of *Streptococcus pneumoniae* pneumonia. Am Rev Respir Dis 1982; 125:436.
102. Moser KM: Diagnosis of acute, diffuse pulmonary infiltrates. JAMA 1984; 252:2044.
103. Zavala DC: Pulmonary hemorrhage in fiberoptic transbronchial biopsy. Chest 1976; 70:584.
104. Pereira W, Kovnat DM, Khan MA, et al: Fever and pneumonia after flexible fiberoptic bronchoscopy. Am Rev Respir Dis 1975; 112:59.

CHAPTER 86

Life-Threatening Hemoptysis

John C. Wain, MD

Hemoptysis is a frequent finding in patients with a variety of cardiopulmonary disorders. In most instances, it is a nonspecific, self-limited symptom whose origin is in the bronchial arterial system. The term *life-threatening hemoptysis* is applied to bleeding in a subpopulation of patients in whom hemoptysis is a potentially fatal occurrence. Blood in the airway rapidly coagulates and, in these patients, obstructs the main branches of the tracheobronchial tree, leading to asphyxiation and death. Death from exsanguination via the airway is a very rare occurrence in any patient.[1, 2]

An expectorated volume of blood ranging from 200 to 500 mL over a 24-hour period has been arbitrarily defined as *massive hemoptysis* in various reports. This amount of blood loss is generally considered to be life-threatening in any patient. The *rate* of bleeding is perhaps even more important, as it has been shown to correlate directly to mortality. The term *exsanguinating hemoptysis* has been used to identify patients losing more than 600 mL in 16 hours, or more than 1000 mL at a rate greater than 150 mL per hour. This group of patients has a 75% mortality rate if aggressive surgical intervention is not undertaken.[3, 4]

Although the rate and amount of bleeding are significant factors in the classification of life-threatening hemoptysis, the outcome of the event may relate as much to patient-specific factors as it does to the actual volume of expectorated blood. Additional risk factors include the presence of preexisting pulmonary insufficiency, ineffective cough, obtundation or muscular weakness, preexisting anticoagulation, and fistulization to a nonbronchial systemic artery (Table 86–1). Expeditious diagnostic and therapeutic management of all patients with life-threatening hemoptysis,

TABLE 86–1. Factors Contributing to Life-Threatening Massive Hemoptysis

Rate of blood loss
Volume of blood loss
Baseline pulmonary function
Efficacy of cough
Antecedent disease states
Anticoagulation
Mechanism of bleeding

particularly when such additional risk factors are present, is critical if a satisfactory clinical outcome is to be obtained.

ETIOLOGY

Life-threatening hemoptysis has its source in a bronchial artery in 95% of patients. The most common precipitating factor for bronchial artery bleeding is inflammatory lung disease, particularly tuberculosis.[1, 2, 4] In patients in whom a nonbronchial source is identified, either in the pulmonary circulation or a nonbronchial systemic artery, a wide variety of both intrapulmonary and extrapulmonary causes have been reported (Table 86–2).

Bronchial Artery

The bronchial arteries are visceral branches of the descending thoracic aorta and are distributed throughout the lung along the major bronchi as well as within the vasa vasorum of the larger pulmonary arteries. Typically, two or three arteries arise at the fifth or sixth thoracic vertebral level. Several patterns of origin have been described, with the most common being one artery leading to each lung (type 1) and the second most common consisting of one trunk to the right lung and two vessels to the left lung (type 2). The right bronchial artery most commonly arises, in either type, as a common trunk with an intercostal artery. In the type 1 pattern, this common trunk also supplies a second branch to the left bronchial tree in the subcarinal region.[5]

Bronchial arteries leading to regions of inflamed, bronchiectatic, or abscessed lung tissue undergo progressive enlargement, tortuosity, and proliferation.[6] Similar changes are noted in patients with congenital cardiovascular anomalies that result in a diminished pulmonary blood flow (e.g., tetralogy of Fallot, pulmonary atresia). Because of the presence of anastomoses between the bronchial arterial and pulmonary circulations, the bronchial arteries may become the main source of blood to the lung tissue. It is postulated that mural disruption of a dilated, thin-walled bronchial vessel by cough, direct inflammatory involvement, or aneurysmal rupture is the precipitating event in most cases of life-threatening hemoptysis. Owing to the aortic origin of the bronchial arteries, the bleeding is supported by systemic arterial pressure and may respond to interventions that either lower systemic blood pressure (e.g., antihypertensive agents) or induce contraction of the muscular arterial wall (e.g., cold saline lavage).

TABLE 86–2. Etiology of Life-Threatening Hemoptysis

Bronchial Artery (95%)
- Inflammatory lung disease
  - Tuberculosis, cavitary (70%) or acute (30%)
  - Histoplasmosis
  - Aspergillosis
  - Bronchiectasis
  - Lung abscess
  - Necrotizing pneumonia
  - Broncholithiasis
  - Pneumoconiosis
- Neoplasm
  - Bronchogenic carcinoma
  - Endobronchial carcinoid tumor
  - Endobronchial metastases
- Cryptogenic hemoptysis

Pulmonary Circulation (<5%)
- Flow-directed pulmonary artery catheterization
- Pulmonary infarction
- Pulmonary embolism
- Postresectional bronchovascular fistula
- Pulmonary arteriovenous fistula
- Rasmussen's aneurysm

Nonbronchial Systemic Artery (<1%)
- Penetrating trauma
- Tracheoinnominate artery fistula
- Thoracic aortic aneurysm
- Post-traumatic aortic pseudoaneurysm
- Subclavian artery aneurysm

Pulmonary Circulation

The low-pressure, thin-walled vessels of the pulmonary circulation are the origin of massive hemoptysis in fewer than 5% of patients. The most common cause of bleeding from this site is flow-directed pulmonary artery (Swan-Ganz) catheterization. Hemoptysis occurs in 1 of every 500 Swan-Ganz catheter insertions. Injury to the pulmonary artery by these catheters is due to perforation by the tip of the catheter, which can be avoided by limiting advancement of the catheter from the insertion site. Abnormalities of balloon inflation (e.g., abnormal contour or configuration or overinflation), which also can lead to perforation, can be avoided by judicious observation of waveforms during balloon inflation and by verifying balloon deflation between wedge pressure measurements.[7, 8]

Other causes of pulmonary circulation hemoptysis include arteriovenous fistulas,[9, 10] fistulization at the site of prior parenchyma-sparing pulmonary and airway resection (e.g., sleeve lobectomy), Rasmussen's aneurysm[11] and postembolic pulmonary infarction,[12] particularly in patients receiving systemic anticoagulants (see Table 86–2). Despite the infrequent occurrence of these, a reasonable index of suspicion for a pulmonary circulation source of bleeding should be maintained, particularly when the standard therapeutic measures, directed primarily at management of bronchial bleeding sites, are ineffective.

Systemic Artery (Nonbronchial)

The most infrequent etiology of life-threatening hemoptysis is fistulization of the bronchial tree with a nonbronchial systemic artery. Such an occurrence may be related to concurrent or preexisting vascular trauma, aneurysmal erosion of the airway, or inflammatory fistulization induced by surgical maneuvers (e.g., post-tracheostomy tracheoinnominate artery fistula; see Table 86–2). In all cases, hemorrhage into the airway is likely to be massive and acute, with the patient at risk for *both* asphyxiation and exsanguination. Successful therapeutic intervention at the time of such hemoptysis is rare because of the nature of the underlying causes in these cases. However, most patients have premonitory, self-limited "herald" hemorrhages that are characterized by an abrupt and projectile nature, which may alert the clinician to the need for intervention prior to the potential manifestation of massive hemoptysis. As compared with therapy at the time of massive bleeding, intervention at this juncture has a reasonable opportunity for success.[13–15]

DIAGNOSIS

Diagnostic and therapeutic efforts are closely interrelated in the management of massive hemoptysis. The most significant factor in the treatment of life-threatening hemoptysis is the ability to localize the site of bleeding, either to a single lung or, preferably, to a specific location within that lung. Localization of the bleeding site is, of course, an intrinsic component of the diagnostic process. Diagnostic modalities are therefore the initial steps in the management of massive hemoptysis.

History and Physical Examination

The most common history related by a patient with massive hemoptysis is a previous episode of hemoptysis, usually within 3 months of presentation. Such an event can be identified in over 40% of patients. Underlying infection, typically tuberculosis, is ultimately identified in three fourths of patients. A prior history of tuberculosis or of exposure to infected individuals is important. Neoplasms, most commonly bronchogenic carcinoma, are identified in 5% of patients, and a history of significant risk factors should be identified.[4] Finally, a history of familial disorders (e.g., cystic fibrosis) or of pharmaceutical ingestion (e.g., anticoagulants) should be elicited.

Few pertinent findings are identified on physical examination. On occasion, a patient may identify a gurgling sensation on the side of bleeding prior to the episode of hemoptysis; this may be useful in lateralizing the bleeding site. More importantly, the character and amount of bleeding should be recorded. The appearance of the expectorated blood (bright versus dark red) relates more to the rapidity with which bleeding is occurring than to the specific site of origin (bronchial versus pulmonary). The volume of blood should be estimated as accurately as possible for outpatients and should be an integral part of monitoring for inpatients. All expectorated blood should be collected in a single container. Deceptively small intermittent volumes may indicate significant hemoptysis; a hospital sputum cup has a volume of over 400 mL and may be filled by a typical patient within several hours.

Radiographic Studies

A chest radiograph should be obtained for all patients with massive hemoptysis; ideally, both posteroanterior and lateral films should be obtained if the clinical context allows. The aim of radiography is to attempt to identify the bleeding site in the lung. A diffuse abnormality presenting as prominent interstitial alveolar infiltrates in both lungs is typical when aspiration of blood throughout the tracheobronchial tree has occurred.

Computed tomography of the chest has a limited role in patients with life-threatening hemoptysis. Regions of bronchiectasis or cavitation (which are not evident on plain radiographs) or parenchymal abnormalities characteristic of neoplastic or inflammatory processes (e.g., calcification that signifies broncholithiasis) can be identified.[16] However, in most patients, the supine positioning and cessation of respiration required for computed tomographic examination are not well tolerated and may place the patient at significant risk for clinical deterioration.

Bronchoscopy

Evaluation of the tracheobronchial tree by bronchoscopy is the pivotal examination in patients with life-threatening hemoptysis. Bronchoscopy allows evaluation of both the cause and site of the bleeding and provides information useful in determining the most appropriate form of definitive management. Rigid bronchoscopy and flexible fiberoptic bronchoscopy are both useful in such patients.

The rigid bronchoscope is the instrument of choice for the patient with active bleeding or a tenuous airway. It is a wide conduit that allows adequate ventilation, rapid aspiration of blood, and clots and a stable field of vision. The rigid bronchoscope allows passage of various interventional devices via its lumen (e.g., balloon catheters) and also may provide snug cannulation of the bronchus for ventilation of the nonbleeding lung. Although it may be passed after application of a topical anesthetic, its insertion and use are better performed with general anesthetic techniques in an operating room environment.

Flexible bronchoscopy is the most sensitive diagnostic method available to localize the site of bleeding. The ability to visualize segmental bronchial orifices, especially in the upper lobes of the lung, where most bleeding originates, makes it an extremely useful tool. In addition, its ease of insertion (with the use of topical anesthetics or passage via an endotracheal tube) facilitates its adaptation to a variety of clinical settings. A flexible bronchoscope may be easily inserted through a rigid bronchoscope to optimize diagnostic visualization in patients with massive bleeding. The major disadvantages of flexible bronchoscopy include its inability to provide ventilatory assistance, the limitations of the suction channel in aspirating large volumes of blood or clot, and the frequent loss of the visual field due to obscuration of the optics by blood. Design modifications to flexible bronchoscopes that incorporate a 4- to 5-mm suction channel have helped to resolve the last two of these problems. However, the use of flexible bronchoscopy in patients with life-threatening hemoptysis should be generally limited to patients with minimum ongoing hemoptysis or cessation of active bleeding or to application as an adjunct to rigid bronchoscopy.

MANAGEMENT

Management of life-threatening hemoptysis follows several basic principles. First, the airway and ventilation of nonbleeding lung tissue must be maintained. Second, the bleeding site must be localized as specifically as possible. Third, the bleeding site must be isolated from the other portions of the tracheobronchial tree and lung. Finally, the source of the bleeding should be controlled (Table 86–3). The specifics of the clinical circumstance dictate the time-course for achieving these objectives, but each portion of the algorithm must be addressed to successfully manage these patients.

Initial Intervention

The initial approach to the patient with massive hemoptysis should include a rapid assessment of the rate and amount of bleeding as well as of the other factors that contribute to a life-threatening circumstance. Potential causes should be rapidly evaluated simultaneously with an assessment of a patient's respiratory status. In most patients, spontaneous ventilation and coughing is the most effective method of maintaining airway patency. Endotracheal intubation eliminates glottic closure and its positive effects on the generation of a cough and the maintenance of functional residual capacity, and it creates a fixed, high-resistance lumen for expectoration that is smaller than the native airway. Therefore, intubation should be reserved for patients with overwhelming hemoptysis of rapid onset or for patients with evidence of impending respiratory failure (e.g., respiratory rate >30 breaths per minute, partial pressure of carbon dioxide >60 mm Hg). An uncut endotracheal tube with a

TABLE 86–3. Principles of Management of Life-Threatening Hemoptysis

Maintenance of airway
Preservation of ventilation in nonbleeding lung
Identification of bleeding site
Isolation of bleeding site
Control of source of bleeding

diameter of 8.0 mm or greater should be used for intubation of normal adult patients.

Sputum specimens should be collected for microbiologic study. In addition to cultures for routine, acid-fast, and fungal organisms, immediate Gram's staining, acid-fast bacillus analysis, and fungal smears should be completed. Additional sputum should undergo cytologic evaluation. Blood samples for typing and crossmatching, coagulation studies, and arterial blood gas analysis should be obtained. A large-bore, intravenous line should be inserted in the upper extremity. If the possibility of a nonbronchial systemic arterial source is likely (e.g., a tracheoinnominate artery fistula), a similar line should be placed in the lower extremity as well.

Patients with massive hemoptysis should be placed in a semi-Fowler position and confined to bed while initial evaluations are being carried out. If a site of origin for the hemoptysis can be identified, the patient should be positioned so that the bleeding lung is dependent, so as to prevent soilage of the nonbleeding lung by blood in the airway. Humidified oxygen should be applied to optimize arterial saturation and maintain hydration of tracheobronchial secretions. Administration of mild antitussive medications may be of benefit in that they prevent intractable coughing episodes, which may further aggravate bleeding. A low level of sedation achieved with the administration of anxiolytic agents such as midazolam (0.5–1.5 mg IV every 1–2 hours) may be similarly useful. If significant systemic arterial hypertension persists after these measures have been taken, additional antihypertensive measures may be instituted based on a presumption of a bronchial artery bleeding source. More commonly, however, systemic hypertension and tachycardia are indicative of relative hypercarbia and impending respiratory failure. Finally, grossly purulent sputum or a clinical context suggestive of tuberculosis are indications for the initiation of pre-emptive antimicrobial therapy while other measures are being undertaken.

Patients with massive hemoptysis require careful monitoring of vital signs. Placement of electrocardiographic leads and use of an oxygen saturation monitor and blood pressure monitor (noninvasive or arterial line) are mandatory. Frequent assessment and recording of electrocardiographic changes, oxygen saturation, and blood pressure as well as of respiratory rate and of the amount of blood expectorated are required. Typically, this level of observation and skilled assessment requires placement of these patients in an intensive care unit or a postanesthesia care unit. In all cases, urgent thoracic surgical evaluation and an assessment of available operating room facilities should be performed.

Bronchoscopy should be undertaken early in all patients, following initial evaluation and stabilization. Rigid bronchoscopy should be performed initially in all actively bleeding patients to optimally control the airway and evacuate endobronchial blood. A singular exception can be made for the hemodynamically unstable, intubated patient in whom flexible bronchoscopy may be the only measure rapidly available to perform emergent management of the bleeding. Bronchoscopy provides diagnostic information and allows for institution of initial measures to preserve ventilation in the nonbleeding lung and to isolate and control the hemorrhage.

Endobronchial Control Measures

Endobronchial control measures are intended to isolate the bleeding site from the remainder of the airway and lung. These are instituted at the time of bronchoscopy after the initial evacuation of blood from the airway and determination of the site—or, at a minimum, the side—of bleeding.

Selective Bronchial Intubation

Selective bronchial intubation is achieved by advancing an *uncut* endotracheal tube into the appropriate mainstem bronchus. The tube is directed into the nonbleeding lung; this serves to isolate the lung from the bleeding site and to direct all ventilation to it. Frequently, a flexible bronchoscope passed through the endotracheal tube and directed into the appropriate orifice is helpful in accomplishing this maneuver. Both the right and left main bronchi in an adult easily accommodate an 8.0-mm tube. However, because of the early takeoff of the right upper lobe bronchus from the right mainstem bronchus, it is frequently difficult to stabilize an endotracheal tube at this site and to maintain ventilation of the right upper lobe in patients with left-sided bleeding. This technique is most valuable for the control of bleeding from the right lung, with placement of the tube in the left mainstem bronchus, or in intubated patients who present with acute hemoptysis (e.g., following Swan-Ganz catheterization). Placement of double-lumen endotracheal tubes should only be performed in rare circumstances. Although these tubes offer the advantages of isolation and independent ventilation of the bleeding and nonbleeding lungs, their placement demands skill and time not ordinarily available in urgent circumstances. In addition, the lumens available for aspiration and ventilation are relatively small. Finally, pulmonary separation is not always maintained; one study reported loss of lung isolation and subsequent death in 60% of patients managed with double-lumen tubes.[17]

Endobronchial Balloon Tamponade

Endobronchial balloon tamponade is perhaps the most useful method for controlling massive hemoptysis. Fogarty-type embolectomy catheters can be positioned in the mainstem, lobar, and segmental bronchi, with subsequent inflation to occlude the bleeding bronchus. This approach works equally well for both right-sided and left-sided bleeding sites. An 8-French catheter is used for mainstem bronchi, and a 4- or 5-French catheter is used for lobar or segmental bronchi. These catheters may be placed through a rigid bronchoscope or may be positioned with a flexible bronchoscope in intubated patients. When used in intubated patients, the catheter is placed intratracheally outside of the endotracheal tube. The inflated cuff of the endotracheal tube helps to maintain the position of the catheter. The balloon should only be inflated under direct bronchoscopic vision, and inflation should only proceed to the point at which the selected airway is occluded. Once positioned, the catheter should be fixed in place and the balloon not be deflated for at least 12 hours.

Deflation or dislocation of the balloon and recurrent bleeding are the main drawbacks to the use of this approach. Should hemoptysis recur after catheter placement, repeat bronchoscopy should be performed for assessment of the cause and the source of bleeding. Empiric repositioning of the catheter should not be carried out. Some authors have suggested that radiopaque material be instilled into the balloon to aid confirmation of catheter position on a plain radiograph. Even with this approach, however, catheter repositioning should only be performed under bronchoscopic visualization.

Balloon tamponade serves to isolate the bleeding site for a period of time so that hemostasis can be achieved by the coagulation cascade. It is a temporizing measure that allows further diagnostic and functional evaluation and provides time to optimize function in the nonbleeding lung, which is frequently compromised by aspiration of blood. Cessation of active bleeding is followed by catheter removal. However, without subsequent definitive intervention directed toward the bleeding site, recurrent bleeding will occur in over 35% of patients.

Endobronchial Iced Saline Lavage

Endobronchial iced saline lavage is a technique used to temporarily control bleeding by the induction of hypothermic vasospasm of the likely bronchial artery source. Systematic instillation of iced saline in 50-mL aliquots into the bleeding lung via a rigid bronchoscope, alternating with ventilation of the nonbleeding lung via the rigid bronchoscope, is carried out.[18] Although in most instances bleeding is controlled with instillation of up to 1000 mL of saline, this technique is a temporizing measure only. It is not appropriate for patients with very rapid bleeding (e.g., because of a nonbronchial systemic source) in whom bronchial isolation or balloon tamponade is more appropriate.

Endobronchial Packing

Endobronchial packing with tamponade material soaked in vasoconstrictive substances (most commonly epinephrine at 1:20,000 dilution) has an extremely limited role in the management of life-threatening hemoptysis. Typically, the bleeding source is not accessible to topical application of medication, and the drugs most frequently used are likely to cause systemic arterial hypertension, which may actually exacerbate the hemorrhage. The tamponade material also has the potential for subsequent dislodgement, migration, and airway obstruction. Although useful for the control of excessive bleeding from parenchymal or endobronchial biopsies, this technique should be used for patients with life-threatening hemoptysis only when other effective therapy is not available.

Surgery

Surgical resection of site of bleeding is the primary form of definitive therapy in patients with life-threatening hemoptysis. Surgical resection is performed in patients in whom the bleeding source can be identified as specifically as possible by bronchoscopic or radiographic evaluation. Exsanguinating hemoptysis or bleeding from a nonbronchial systemic arterial source requires emergent surgical intervention. In most other cases, resection is carried out after a patient has been stabilized and is free of active bleeding for several days to allow return of optimal pulmonary function in the nonbleeding lung. Surgery is usually undertaken in those patients with nonterminal disease states and in those patients with sufficient pulmonary reserve to enable return to a functional lifestyle postoperatively. However, persistent episodic bleeding or a recurrent episode of massive hemoptysis may require a more urgent surgical approach, despite potential compromise of nonbleeding parenchyma.

Typically, resection involves lobectomy or, occasionally, segmentectomy. Pneumonectomy is rarely necessary unless a major bronchovascular connection is present or unless extensive parenchymal destruction is present throughout the lung. Endobronchial isolation of the nonbleeding lung is an absolute requirement for successful resection in these patients. If necessary, intraoperative bronchoscopy should be performed to confirm lung isolation and to aspirate any residual blood or secretions from the nonoperative lung. The surgical approach is via a posterolateral thoracotomy. Technical modifications to a standard pulmonary resection include the use of extrapleural dissection of the lung when severe inflammatory adhesions have obliterated the pleural space and early identification and division of the appropriate bronchus to prevent further contamination of the tracheobronchial tree.

Transcatheter Vessel Embolization

Occlusion of the bleeding vessel by transcatheter embolization may be applied for the management of massive hemoptysis from either bronchial artery or pulmonary circulation sources.[19, 20] Typically, this method is used either as an alternative to surgery in patients who are poor candidates for resection or as a means of preoperative stabilization after initial endobronchial control of the bleeding.[21] A transfemoral approach is used, and a variety of 5- to 7-French catheters are advanced through an introducer sheath. The catheters are advanced into the descending thoracic aorta, and the bronchial arteries are identified. The angiographer is directed to the bleeding lung by the results of the bronchoscopic examination. Dilation and tortuosity of the bronchial vessels are commonly noted; extravasation of contrast medium is rarely seen angiographically. Embolization is usually performed with surgical gelatin pledgets and polyvinyl alcohol in small aliquots, with frequent visualization and use of contrast material to confirm positioning of the catheter in the appropriate artery.

A major risk of bronchial artery embolization relates to the proximity of the spinal cord vasculature. The anterior and posterior spinal arteries receive contributions from the descending thoracic aorta. The posterior spinal artery receives segmental branches from the dorsal rami of the intercostal arteries. The anterior spinal artery commonly anastomoses with a thoracic aortic branch arising between the third and seventh thoracic levels on the right. In addition, the bronchial arteries may distribute branches to the spinal artery in 60% of patients.[5] Both contrast media and embolic material may therefore have effects on the spinal cord circulation during bronchial arteriography. Nonionic contrast media, iohexol, and iopamidol are used because of their lower risk of neurotoxicity, compared with standard ionic contrast media.[21] In addition, the angiography is directed by bronchoscopic findings to the bleeding lung, and embolization is frequently limited to those arteries on the side of the bleeding site. Finally, the angiographic catheter is securely seated in the bronchial artery so that delivery of the embolic material does not result in catheter displacement and aberrant embolization. Use of these maneuvers has led to an overall incidence of spinal cord injury of less than 0.5% following this procedure. However, inability to obtain secure catheter positioning remains an absolute contraindication to bronchial artery embolization.

Aberrant embolization to systemic vessels other than the spinal arteries may also occur, usually in fewer than 1% of patients. Reports of embolization to the gastrointestinal tract and extremities have been made. Careful technique and attention to warning signs, such as the development of abdominal tenderness or acute changes in peripheral pulses, serve to minimize the incidence and morbidity of these complications. Other complications such as bronchial infarction or bronchopleural fistula are very rare, although all patients do develop a self-limited febrile response to the embolization procedure.[19, 20]

Although the majority of patients have a bronchial artery source for bleeding, a similar technique may be used for control of massive hemoptysis from a pulmonary circulation source. The risk for spinal cord injury or systemic embolization, however, is much lower in these patients. Conversely, larger embolic elements (e.g., coils, detachable balloons) may be required for satisfactory control.[11, 20]

OUTCOME

The mortality from life-threatening hemoptysis among hospitalized patients is 10%.[2, 4] No significant difference in hospital mortality exists between patients undergoing surgical resection and those having nonsurgical management (i.e., vessel embolization) as definitive therapy.

The success rate of therapy for life-threatening hemoptysis varies, according to the underlying cause. For the majority of patients, the bleeding has a bronchial artery source in the context of inflammatory or neoplastic lung disease. In these patients, the success of surgical resection, as determined by control of hemoptysis and the prevention of rebleeding, is between 98% and 100%.[1, 3, 6] By comparison, vessel embolization is successful in controlling bleeding in from 85% to 90% of patients, but rebleeding occurs in 25% of patients.[19–21] In patients who are managed expectantly after initial control of their hemoptysis without surgery or embolization, the rate of recurrent bleeding is 40% within 6 months.[4]

For patients with a pulmonary circulation source of bleeding, which is most commonly due to Swan-Ganz catheterization, catheter removal after endobronchial control measures have been instituted provides definitive therapy in nearly all cases. In rare instances of persistent bleeding or if other causes of pulmonary circulation bleeding are present, surgical resection of the involved pulmonary region provides complete control.

Finally, for patients with life-threatening hemoptysis from a nonbronchial systemic artery, emergent surgical intervention offers the only possibility of control. Unfortunately, the rapidity of bleeding in most instances results in mortality before surgical control can be achieved.[14, 15] Assessment and intervention are generally successful only when performed pre-emptively at the time of "herald" hemorrhages in this group of patients.[13]

References

1. Conlan AA, Hurwitz SS, Krige L, et al: Massive hemoptysis: Review of 123 cases. J Thorac Surg 1983; 85:120.
2. Garzon AA, Cerruit MM, Golding ME: Exsanguinating hemoptysis. J Thorac Cardiovasc Surg 1982; 84:829.
3. Crocco JA, Rooney JJ, Frankushen DS, et al: Massive hemoptysis. Arch Intern Med 1968; 12:495.
4. Knott-Craig CJ, Oostuizen JG, Rossouw G, et al: Management and prognosis of massive hemoptysis. J Thorac Cardiovasc Surg 1993; 105:394–397.
5. Ulflaker R, Kaemmerer A, Neves C, et al: Management of massive hemoptysis by bronchial artery embolization. Radiology 1983; 146:627.
6. Marchand P, Gilroy JC, Wilson VH: An anatomical study of the bronchial vascular system and its variations in disease. Thorax 1950; 5:207.
7. Boyd KD, Thomas SJ, Gold J, et al: A prospective study of complications of pulmonary artery catheterizations in 500 consecutive patients. Chest 1983; 84:245.
8. Barash PG, Nardi D, Hammond G, et al: Catheter-induced pulmonary artery perforation: Mechanisms, management, and modifications. J Thorac Cardiovasc Surg 1981; 82:1.
9. Hoffman WS, Weinberg PM, Ring E, et al: Massive hemoptysis secondary to pulmonary arteriovenous fistula: Treatment by a catheterization procedure. Chest 1980; 77:697.
10. Hayakawa K, Soga T, Hamamoto K, et al: Massive hemoptysis form a pulmonary sequestration controlled by embolization of aberrant pulmonary arteries: Case report. Cardiovasc Intervent Radiol 1991; 14:345–348.
11. Remy J, Smith M, Lemaitre L, et al: Treatment of massive hemoptysis by occlusion of a Rasmussen aneurysm. AJR 1980; 135:605.
12. Dalen JE, Haffajee CI, Alper JS, et al: Pulmonary embolism, pulmonary hemorrhage and pulmonary infarction. N Engl J Med 1977; 296:1431.
13. Cooper JD: Trachea-innominate artery fistula: Successful management of 3 consecutive patients. Ann Thorac Surg 1977; 24:439.
14. Dickens P, Pittaluga S, Chau CH: Sudden death presenting as massive hemoptysis due to ruptured intrapulmonary aortic aneurysm. Forensic Sci Int 1993; 60:121–125.
15. Wu MH, Lai WW, Lin MY, Chou NS: Massive hemoptysis caused by ruptured subclavian artery aneurysm. Chest 1993; 104:612–613.
16. McLean TR, Beal AC, Jones JW: Massive hemoptysis due to broncholithiasis. Ann Thorac Surg 1991; 52:1173–1175.
17. Gourin A, Garzon AA: Control of hemorrhage in emergency pulmonary resection for massive hemoptysis. Chest 1975; 68:120.
18. Conlan AA, Hurwitz SS: Management of massive hemoptysis with the rigid bronchoscope and cold saline lavage. Thorax 1980; 35:901.
19. Remy J, Arnaud A, Fardou H, et al: Treatment of hemoptysis by embolization of bronchial arteries. Radiology 1977; 122:33–37.
20. Rabkin J, Astafjev V, Gothman L, et al: Transcatheter embolization in the management of pulmonary hemorrhage. Radiology 1987; 163:361–365.
21. Denham JS, Athanasoulis CA: Massive hemoptysis control with transcatheter vessel embolization. *In*: Current Therapy in Cardiothoracic Surgery. Grillo HC, Auston WG, Wilkins EW, et al (Eds). Philadelphia, BC Decker, 1989, pp 176–178.

CHAPTER 87

Pulmonary Gas Exchange, Transport, and Delivery

Christopher W. Bryan-Brown, MD, FCCM • *Guillermo Gutiérrez, MD, PhD, FCCM*

The process of ventilation provides a mechanism for replacing the alveolar gas with fresh gas from the ambient atmosphere. This is done by a process involving conduction, convection, and, in the smallest airways and alveoli, diffusion. The control of ventilation is normally set to exchange the alveolar gas at a rate sufficient to provide for the gas requirements of metabolism (Table 87–1) that is, maintaining a sufficiently high oxygen (O_2) tension and a sufficiently low carbon dioxide (CO_2) tension for these gases to be exchanged adequately to meet the needs of aerobic metabolism. This chapter reviews the factors that influence the gas exchange between the alveolus and the blood in the pulmonary circulation, the transport of the gases between the lungs and the tissues, and the delivery of arterial blood to the tissues.

GAS EXCHANGE IN THE LUNG

The major physical determinants of any gas exchange are the *solubility coefficient* of the gas in any particular phase

TABLE 87–1. Basal Gas Exchange*

	$\dot{V}O_2$		$\dot{V}CO_2$	
	mL	*mmol*	*mL*	*mmol*
Per minute	250	11	200	9
Per hour	15,000	670	12,000	539
Per day	360,000	16,079	288,000	12,938

*For a 70-kg resting man.

(e.g., fat, water, and blood) and the *partial pressure* gradient of the gas between phases. The solubility coefficient is the volume of gas that dissolves in a given volume of fluid at a given temperature and for a given unit of pressure—for example, $mL \cdot dL^{-1} \cdot mm\ Hg^{-1}$ at 37°C. (Système Internationale [SI] units are $mmol \cdot L^{-1} \cdot kPa^{-1}$ at 37°C.) The *partial pressure* gradient is expressed in millimeters of mercury (the SI unit of measure is the kilopascal [kPa]).

Henry's law, which is based on experimental observation, holds that the amount of gas dissolved in a given liquid is directly proportional to the pressure of the gas.[1] Furthermore, the higher the temperature of the liquid, the smaller the amount of gas that dissolves. The normal gradients for O_2 and CO_2 between the alveolus and the arterial blood in the pulmonary microcirculation are approximately 60 mm Hg and 4 to 6 mm Hg (8 and 0.5–0.8 kPa), respectively. The constitution of alveolar gas is therefore a driving force in gas exchange. At 37°C, the partial pressure of water vapor is 47 mm Hg. At one atmosphere, this leaves 713 mm Hg for the other alveolar gases. The tension of the CO_2 in the alveolus (P_ACO_2) is the product of the flow of carbon dioxide diffusing into the alveolus ($\dot{V}CO_2$) divided by the alveolar ventilation ($\dot{V}_A$):

$$P_ACO_2 = (\dot{V}CO_2/\dot{V}_A) \times 713 \text{ mm Hg} \quad \text{[Equation 1]}$$

Thus, if the $\dot{V}CO_2$ is 200 mL/min and the $\dot{V}_A$ 3565 mL/min, then the P_ACO_2 is 40 mm Hg. Also, the P_ACO_2 is inversely proportional to the $\dot{V}_A$.

The alveolar O_2 tension (P_AO_2) is dependent on the replenishment of O_2 uptake in the alveolus ($\dot{V}O_2$) by the $\dot{V}_A$ and the inspired O_2 tension (P_IO_2). In the normal fasting and resting man, the *respiratory quotient* (RQ) ($\dot{V}CO_2$:$\dot{V}O_2$) is about 0.8. When more O_2 is taken up by the lung than CO_2 is excreted into it, if another gas is present (e.g., nitrogen), its tension rises; this diminishes the P_AO_2. When RQ is 1.0 at sea level,

$$P_AO_2 = (F_IO_2 \times 713) - P_ACO_2 \text{ mm Hg} \quad \text{[Equation 2]}$$

When the respiratory quotient is other than 1.0,

$$P_AO_2 = (F_IO_2 \times 713) - P_ACO_2 \times \left[\frac{F_IO_2 + (1 - F_IO_2)}{RQ}\right] \quad \text{[Equation 3]}$$

The F_IO_2 is the inspired O_2 fraction (e.g., for air it is 0.21). Also, note that the arterial CO_2 tension ($PaCO_2$) is usually used instead of the P_ACO_2 because these two values are not significantly different until pulmonary arteriovenous admixture is approximately 25%.[2]

From the previous equations, it can be deduced that an increase in $\dot{V}_A$ will be very effective at making a major reduction in P_ACO_2 and that a modest increase in ventilation could double the diffusion gradient between the pulmonary arterial and alveolar tensions of CO_2. Alveolar hyperventilation makes an incremental change in the P_AO_2 that is proportional to the reduction in P_ACO_2. Although this is of great importance for producing a margin for the survival of high altitude mountaineers,[3] it is of little useful clinical importance in the critically ill. The effective way to increase the O_2 diffusion gradient is to increase F_IO_2. The different methods of augmenting the exchange of O_2 and CO_2 have led to the clinical introduction of *permissive hypercapnia.* High inspiratory pressures appear to cause further pulmonary damage in patients with the adult respiratory distress syndrome.[4] These high pressures are necessary to provide sufficient ventilation in lungs that are compromised by the low compliance induced by the disease state. If a $PaCO_2$ much higher than normal can be well tolerated by a patient (which is often possible), then the $\dot{V}_A$ required to remove the metabolic production of CO_2 can be reduced; this lessens the destructive effects of high intrapulmonary pressures.[5] The effects of the higher P_ACO_2 and diminished $\dot{V}_A$ on oxygenation can be overcome by increasing the F_IO_2, at least to the limits of O_2 toxicity (usually considered to be >60% at sea level).

The artificial lung, or membrane oxygenator, can also decrease the need for ventilation to remove CO_2. With a blood flow of just over 1 L/min and a 12-L/min fresh gas flow, this device could eliminate normal carbon dioxide production without the complications of full extracorporeal membrane oxygenation support and avoid much pulmonary barotrauma as ventilatory requirements are reduced. Results from initial studies with this technique are encouraging.[6,7] Because of the labor-intensive management of long-term bypass circulation, permissive hypercapnia seems to be rapidly gaining popularity.

Within the alveolus, the low molecular weight of O_2 allows it to diffuse about 1.2 times faster than CO_2 ($\sqrt{44}/\sqrt{32} \approx 1.2$). Moreover, because mixed venous CO_2 tension ($P\bar{v}CO_2$) is around 40 mm Hg (5.3 kPa) and P_ACO_2 is about 44 to 46 mm Hg (6 kPa), the diffusion gradient of O_2 (about 60 mm Hg [12 kPa]) is 12-fold that of CO_2 (about 5 mm Hg [0.7 kPa]). The combination of these factors should cause O_2 to diffuse about 14-fold more quickly than CO_2. However, the blood/gas solubility coefficient of CO_2 is about 24-fold that of O_2; thus, CO_2 diffuses in and out of blood about 1.7-fold more quickly than does O_2.

Pulmonary perfusion maintains blood for gas exchange, which is increased when cardiac output increases. The uptake of a gas can also be increased by raising its inspired concentration, such as in the administration of a high F_IO_2, an anesthetic vapor, or a gas.[8] All gas exchange between the alveolus and the blood depends on the continuous restoration of the plasma-alveolar diffusion gradient. The alveolar gases are maintained at appropriate tensions by ventilation and therapeutically by alteration of the inspired mixture. The diffusion of O_2 is enhanced only to the extent that deoxyhemoglobin is present to be saturated. The "hemoglobin sink" maintains a low plasma O_2 tension in the pulmonary microcirculation until the hemoglobin is saturated. When this happens, only a marginal increase in O_2 uptake occurs. When the hemoglobin is saturated, the only way to increase the oxygen level in the blood is to elevate the P_AO_2. A subject breathing air normally has a P_AO_2 of about 100 mm Hg (13.3 kPa). The solubility of O_2 in blood at 37°C is $0.00314\ mL \cdot dL^{-1} \cdot mm\ Hg^{-1}$. Therefore, the amount carried in solution is a little more than 0.3 mL/dL. During breathing of 100% O_2, it is possible to increase the PaO_2 to over 600 mm Hg (80 kPa) and the dissolved arterial O_2 content to about 2.0 mL/dL. The clinical importance of this marginal increase is debatable, but above-normal PaO_2 levels may be helpful in the process of wound healing and promote the "killing" power of macrophages.[9–11]

Hyperbaric oxygenation was revived in the 1940s by Boerema when he demonstrated that piglets could survive without red blood cells in 3 atmospheres absolute ATA of O_2. However, the hyperoxygenation of tissues with hyperbaric O_2 has not had the expected impact on O_2 transport and delivery. The theoretic basis of hyperbaric oxygenation is that the PaO_2 is increased to as much as 1800 mm Hg (240 kPa) by increasing the ambient pressure around a patient with an F_IO_2 of 1.0. This may make the diffusion of O_2 from the microcirculation to the tissues sufficiently greater to oxygenate hypoxic regions. It also may increase the concentration of O_2 in solution to such an extent that hemoglobin becomes unnecessary for O_2 transport. Augmented oxygenation may fail because of the compensatory development of an increasing systemic vascular resistance and of a concomitant reduction of blood flow.[12] Tissue acidosis is also a possibility because less deoxyhemoglobin is present; this interferes with CO_2 transport because the carbamino compound is reduced and because oxyhemoglobin is a less effective recipient of hydrogen ions (protons) than deoxyhemoglobin. This may be compensated for by hyperventilation. The application of hyperbaric oxygenation is discussed in Chapter 106.

Alterations in ventilation acutely affect CO_2 elimination. If the $\dot{V}A$ is increased, the elimination of carbon dioxide is also increased; this lowers the $PACO_2$. Because the alveolus has a very rapid turnover, a new $PaCO_2$ is clinically established in 9 to 12 minutes (three time constants). On the other hand, if $\dot{V}A$ is decreased, CO_2 is retained as the venous-alveolar tension difference is decreased. The $PACO_2$ rises slowly as the whole-body content (about 120 L as CO_2 and bicarbonate ion in a normal man) is replenished at the metabolic production rate of 200 mL/min^{-1}; some of what is produced is removed by ventilation. Establishment of a new steady state may take well over an hour.[13] As body stores of O_2 are approximately two orders of magnitude less than those of CO_2, O_2 values change very rapidly when either ventilation or the inspired O_2 concentration is changed. The implication for respiratory care is that when blood for an arterial blood gas measurement is drawn, most changes resulting from increases in the ventilation or from alteration of the FIO_2 can be assessed in a few minutes, whereas the $PaCO_2$ may continue to increase for over an hour following a reduction in minute volume.

The exchange of O_2 and CO_2 in the lungs and tissues is augmented by a complex buffering system in which both gases interact (Fig. 87–1*A* and *B*). Hemoglobin transports O_2 in loose chemical combination and CO_2 as carbamino compound. Until the hemoglobin is nearly saturated with O_2 in the lungs, the alveolocapillary plasma diffusion gradient is maintained, and hemoglobin is responsible for over 98% of the arterial O_2 transport ($\dot{D}O_2$). As carbamino compound level decreases, a process accelerated by the oxygenation of hemoglobin, the oxyhemoglobin dissociation curve is shifted to the left, that is, the avidity of hemoglobin for O_2 is increased. As oxyhemoglobin is more acid than is deoxyhemoglobin, the additional hydrogen ion release also increases the breakdown of bicarbonate into CO_2 and water, augmenting the capillary CO_2 tension.

The effect of the position of the oxyhemoglobin dissociation curve on the rate of O_2 uptake in the lungs and of delivery to the tissues can be summarized as follows: a leftward shift decreases and a rightward shift increases O_2 transfer rates in the tissues, but the opposite occurs in the lungs. The hemoglobin molecule is a tetramer with four heme subunits, each of which is capable of combining with an oxygen molecule. The factor 1.39 is used as a stoichiometric number to calculate in milliliters the quantity of O_2 that binds to 1 g of hemoglobin; however, the maximum binding capacity may be considerably less than this. Nunn[14] suggested that as the measurement of hemoglobin is validated by comparison with the International Cyanmethaemoglobin Standard, which includes the iron content of methemoglobin and other erythrocyte non–oxygen-combining pigments, the actual hemoglobin concentration seems decreased. Therefore, the observed combining capacity is less than 1.39 mL/dL. Newer methods of hemoglobinometry give a value of about 1.31, which may be more accurate than previously proposed values.[15] As each heme subunit

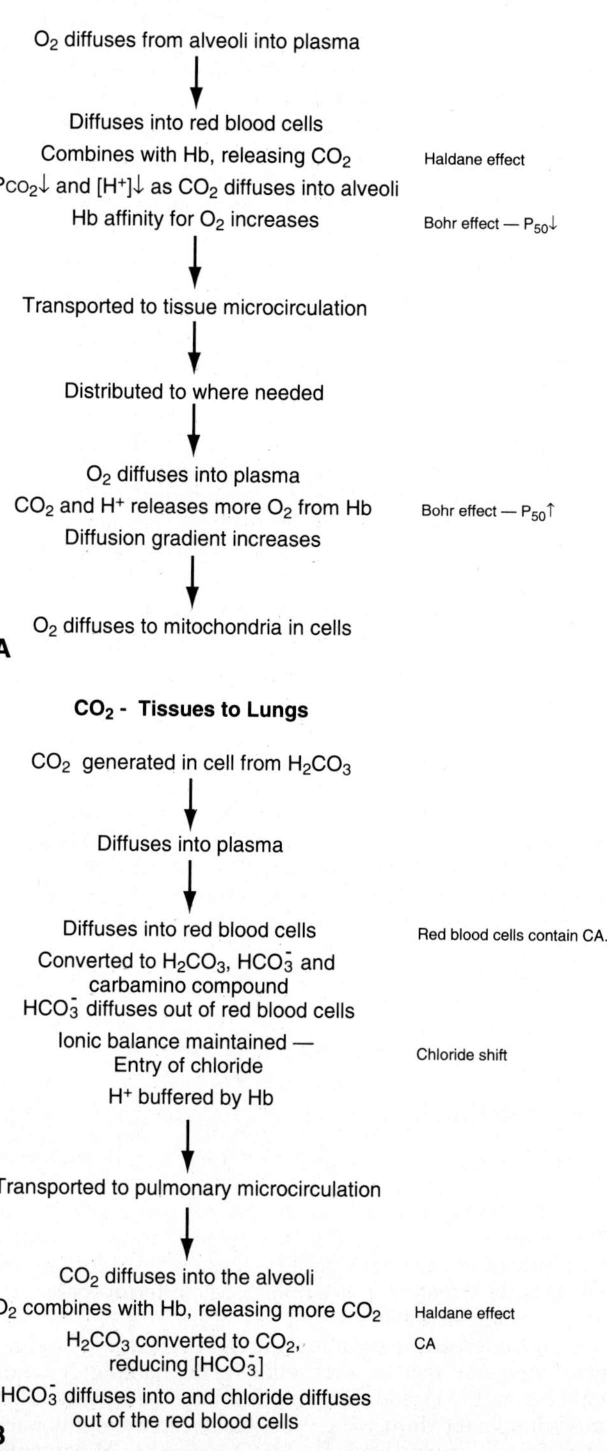

Figure 87–1. *A and B,* Flowcharts showing the processes involved in O_2 and CO_2 exchange between tissues and alveoli. Note the interactions that assist the uptake and elimination of gases in the tissues and lungs. *Abbreviations*: P_{50} = oxygen tension when hemoglobin is half-saturated; CA = carbonic anhydrase.

sequentially binds O_2, the spatial arrangement of the molecule is altered. This increases the O_2 affinity of the other heme groups and results in the sigmoid shape of the oxyhemoglobin dissociation curve.[16] Therefore, reduced hemoglobin (deoxyhemoglobin) has a lower affinity for O_2 than does oxygenated hemoglobin (oxyhemoglobin). Hemoglobin's ability to alter its O_2 affinity makes it an excellent O_2 carrier. The binding of O_2 to hemoglobin is facilitated in the pulmonary capillaries, whereas dissociation is favored at the lower O_2 tensions found in the systemic capillaries. Hydrogen ions, CO_2, and 2,3-diphosphoglycerate can combine with oxyhemoglobin, altering its affinity and making the combining sites for O_2 less available. Changes in temperature alter the conformation of hemoglobin; this also affects the O_2 affinity. The influence of these factors on O_2 affinity varies inversely with the degree of hemoglobin saturation and is greater when fewer heme groups are occupied by O_2. When hemoglobin binds with O_2, the tetramer relaxes to expose other heme sites; thus, hemoglobin's oxygen affinity is increased while hydrogen ions, CO_2, and 2,3-diphosphoglycerate are released. This interaction is shown in Figure 87–1.

Although experimental evidence might indicate that shifting the oxyhemoglobin dissociation curve can aid the O_2 loading and unloading of hemoglobin in the lungs and tissues,[17, 18] this has never been convincingly demonstrated to have any clinical effect on the outcome of critically ill patients.[19]

CARBON MONOXIDE

The affinity of hemoglobin for carbon monoxide (CO) is over 200-fold greater than its affinity for O_2; therefore, 0.1% CO in air eventually gives rise to 50% carboxyhemoglobin (COHb). At COHb saturations of greater than 40%, heme-heme interactions are far more pronounced in COHb than in oxyhemoglobin.[20] Thus, the patient with a COHb saturation of greater than 40% has both affinity (leftward shift of the oxyhemoglobin dissociation curve) and anemic hypoxias. The other possible damaging effects, such as the combination of CO with the heme of the cytochrome oxidase and cytochrome P_{450} systems, are probably of less immediate consequence than the hypoxia.

Chronic exposure to CO, as may occur in heavy smokers, road traffic tunnel workers, and even taxi drivers,[21] can cause compensatory polycythemia, decrease exercise tolerance, induce angina, and possibly increase the incidence of myocardial infarction. Acute CO poisoning follows accidental inhalation of high CO concentrations (e.g., inhalation of internal combustion engine exhaust in an enclosed space). Acute severe CO poisoning results in severe nonrespiratory acidosis due to anaerobic metabolism. Usually, if a poisoned patient is unconscious, COHb saturation is greater than 50%. Moderate or high COHb saturation (COHb $> 40\%$) increases the hydrogen ion Bohr effect to greater than that found with oxyhemoglobin.[20] The ensuing acidemia increases O_2 release, and the compensatory hypocarbia changes the hemoglobin-O_2 affinity only as much as it alters the hydrogen ion concentration. Therefore, it is not prudent to blindly correct pH with sodium bicarbonate until COHb levels are lowered.

The primary treatment for CO poisoning is to ventilate the patient with as high an F_{IO_2} as possible so that a competitive release of CO from hemoglobin is initiated. With air breathing, the COHb reduction takes about 4 hours; this can be decreased to 40 minutes by allowing the patient to breathe pure O_2. Administration of hyperbaric O_2 (at 3 ATA) reduces this to 20 minutes and increases arterial O_2 content to an amount that is nearly 5 mL/dL more in solution than when O_2 is breathed at normal pressures.[22]

DECOMPRESSION SICKNESS AND AIR EMBOLISM

The physiologic relationship between gas pressure and solubility is seen in decompression sickness (the "bends"). Inert gases are absorbed and distributed in the body according to tissue solubility and perfusion. If a sudden reduction of ambient pressure occurs, as does with nonpressurized flying or an ascent from diving, the partial pressure of gas in blood or tissue may exceed the solubility coefficient, and bubbles are formed. The blood/fat partition coefficient is approximately .55 for helium and .19 for nitrogen, the two common diving gases. If the body fat is partially loaded or saturated with these gases, as tissues decompress, they unload helium or nitrogen into the blood. If decompression is very sudden, gas may come out of solution in blood and form bubbles, especially in the fatty tissue. The most severe form of decompression sickness is central nervous system bends. Nervous system tissue has a high lipid content and, because the blood supply to the spinal cord than to other regions is relatively reduced, central nervous system bends are frequently seen in divers.

Bubbles in the blood probably originate in the distal venous system, where intravascular pressure is low, and then travel to the pulmonary capillary system. The bubbles cause an immediate microvascular embolus, tissue distortion, or clotting in the venules and small veins.[23, 24] An apparent consumption coagulopathy and elaboration of edema fluid occur, often with a marked reduction of plasma volume. The goal of therapy is to "recompress" the patient so that the bubbles are again dissolved. Because small bubbles have high internal pressures, the increase in pressure to drive a bubble back into solution can be more than the reduction in pressure that was required to make it. The shortcoming of recompression is that a further increased loading with inert gas takes place. Oxygen breathing may speed the absorption of bubbles, since the lungs clear the inert gas (i.e., nitrogen) more quickly if the inspired concentration is reduced. This, in turn, lowers tissue tensions more rapidly. However, pure O_2 is too toxic for prolonged breathing at recompression pressures.

Following proper decompression procedures minimizes the danger of serious bends and diminishes the hazard of minor decompression sickness. Slowly reducing ambient pressure allows tissues with a low blood flow and high solubility coefficient to unload excess gas without appreciable bubble formation. Decompression can be rapid when exposure to increased pressure is short and must be prolonged if exposure has allowed tissues to become saturated.

Arterial air embolism can occur with very rapid decompression or when an air cyst in the lung ruptures into the pulmonary venous system. This can give rise to a very rapid and fatal cerebrovascular blockage. In clinical practice, the two most common sources of venous air embolism are posterior fossa neurosurgery and central venous catheter placement and use.[25] When air embolism occurs over an extended period, a moderate consumption of coagulation factors occurs. Massive amounts of air may compromise right ventricular or pulmonary function. Elevated pulmonary artery pressure may increase right atrial pressure and reopen a functionally closed foramen ovale, admitting air to the systemic circulation.[26] The treatment involves positioning the supine patient on his or her left side with the head lowered so as to minimize central nervous system embolization, giving 100% O_2 to breathe, and the retrieval of air from the heart if a central venous catheter is in place. Systemic air embolism should be treated in a recompression chamber.

The transport of gas bubbles in the venous blood usually ends in the lungs, where they embolize and are eliminated in the alveoli. The microemboli in the lung can be recognized by an increase in dead space, which results in an evanescent fall in end-tidal CO_2 tension and in an elevation of pulmonary vascular resistance combined with a rise in pulmonary arterial pressure. In the case of air embolism in the anesthetized patient, nitrogen can be detected in the expired gas.[27] Experimental work shows that in acute air embolism this may be the first detectable sign.[28] Clinical observation has shown that venous air embolism can result in "paradoxical" cerebral air embolism in the absence of a patient or probe-patent foramen ovale.[29] It has become increasingly evident that a sufficient amount of air injected into the venous system may reach the arterial system via the pulmonary capillaries[30] and that this may account for some of the embolic phenomena seen in decompression sickness. Lung surfactant appears to migrate from the alveoli to line microbubbles in the pulmonary capillaries. Reduced surface tension allows these emboli to be pushed through the pulmonary circulation by the increase in the pulmonary arterial pressure.[31] In the dog, a threshold intravenous infusion of 0.35 $mL \cdot min^{-1} \cdot kg^{-1}$ has to be reached before arterial bubbles can be detected.[32] The pulmonary arterial pressure is about doubled at this point.[33] The filtration by the lung can be shown to break down at a lower threshold with aminophylline[29] or halothane[34] administration and oxygen toxicity, and it can be increased by nitrous oxide anesthesia.[35] Nitrous oxide acts as a bubble amplifier because it moves into air-filled spaces much more quickly than nitrogen moves out. Clinically, air embolism is reported to be a worse condition when nitrous oxide is present,[36] but this observation has to be confirmed experimentally.

CARBON DIOXIDE TRANSPORT

Carbon dioxide is transported in the blood in solution as bicarbonate and is combined with amino groups (particularly on hemoglobin) as carbamino compound. The steps in the bulk flow of CO_2 from the tissues to the lungs is shown in Figure 87–1*B*.

The normal resting venoarterial CO_2 tension difference ($P[\bar{v}-a]CO_2$) is 4 to 6 mm Hg (0.7 kPa), and the content difference is ($C[\bar{v}-a]CO_2$) is about 4 mL/dL. In arterial blood at a $PaCO_2$ of 40 mm Hg (13.3 kPa) and with a hematocrit of 44%, 2.5 mL/dL of CO_2 is carried in solution, 1.3 mL/dL as carbamino compound, and 43 mL/dL as bicarbonate. During changes in CO_2 content, the greatest amount of change occurs in the bicarbonate.

For CO_2 to be cleared from the lungs, its mobilization from bicarbonate occurs with the inactivation of hydrogen ion:

$$H^+ + HCO_3^- \rightleftarrows H_2O + CO_2 \qquad \text{[Equation 4]}$$

When the clearance of CO_2 is diminished in the tissues, such as during low-flow states or resuscitation from cardiac arrest, the CO_2 tension builds up in the tissues; this creates respiratory acidosis, which is reflected in a high $P\bar{v}CO_2$ and frequently in a low or normal $PaCO_2$.[37] The administration of sodium bicarbonate increases the $P\bar{v}CO_2$. The reasoning that this may portend a higher tissue intracellular CO_2 tension and, therefore, an increased hydrogen ion concentration has to be regarded with circumspection unless the $PaCO_2$ is elevated. The sodium bicarbonate is usually administered intravenously between the tissues and the mixed venous blood sampling site. The best therapeutic measure for the treatment of this type of tissue acidosis would seem to be to produce arterial hypocarbia with hyperventilation.

TISSUE OXYGENATION

The transport of O_2 from the atmosphere to a cell's mitochondria is an exceedingly complex process that involves the convection of O_2 into the alveoli, its diffusion across the alveolocapillary membrane into the red blood cells, its binding to hemoglobin, its transport in blood by the pumping action of the heart, its dissociation from hemoglobin in the peripheral capillaries, and, finally, its diffusion across the endothelium into the cell mitochondria. Under normal physiologic conditions, this transport system provides each cell in the body with an adequate supply of O_2.

An important aspect of tissue oxygenation is the distribution of cardiac output to the various organs according to their metabolic needs. This is determined by the coordinated action of neurogenic control mechanisms—which are responsible for arteriolar tone—acting in concert with microvascular mechanisms inherent to every capillary bed.[38] Large-scale alterations in blood flow distribution, such as those that occur during a patient's transition from the supine to the standing position, are coordinated by neurogenic mechanisms that act through α and β vascular receptors. The finer control of cellular perfusion, also known as *autoregulation,* is effected through the release of endothelial derived factors (e.g., nitric oxide or adenosine) that act on the microvasculature to produce the phasic movement of the red blood cells through the capillaries.

It is nearly impossible to describe and even more so to quantify the process of cellular O_2 delivery. However, we can establish a first-order model of tissue oxygenation by measuring systemic $\dot{D}O_2$ and total-body O_2 consumption in critically ill patients. Systemic $\dot{D}O_2$ is defined as the product of the cardiac output ($\dot{Q}$) and the arterial O_2 content (CaO_2):

$$\dot{D}O_2 = \dot{Q} \times CaO_2 \qquad \text{[Equation 5]}$$

where

$$CaO_2 = 1.34 \times [Hb] \times SaO_2 + 0.003\ PaO_2 \qquad \text{[Equation 6]}$$

where [Hb] is the concentration of hemoglobin in arterial blood (grams per 100 mL), SaO_2 is the fraction of hemoglobin saturated with O_2, and PaO_2 is the partial pressure of O_2 in arterial blood.

Since cellular energy demand is an unmeasurable quantity, systemic $\dot{V}O_2$ has been used as an estimate of tissue energy utilization. This parameter gives an approximate indication of energy utilization in critically ill patients but sometimes may be difficult to interpret. Under normoxic conditions, cellular energy requirements are met exclusively by aerobic metabolism, and $\dot{V}O_2$ approximates the rate of cellular energy generation. However, when cellular O_2 supply is compromised, as occurs during hypoxia, anaerobic energy sources are needed to supplement aerobic metabolism, and $\dot{V}O_2$ no longer reflects total energy utilization but only that portion of adenosine triphosphate that is produced aerobically.

The preferred technique to measure systemic $\dot{V}O_2$ is direct analysis of the inspired and expired gases. This can be accomplished routinely in the intensive care unit with commercially available devices. The error of this measurement increases in direct proportion to the FIO_2, and it becomes unreliable at an FIO_2 greater than 0.60. In patients with a pulmonary artery catheter in place, it is often more practical to calculate $\dot{V}O_2$ using Fick's equation:

$$\dot{V}O_2 = \dot{Q} \times (CaO_2 - C\bar{v}O_2) \qquad \text{[Equation 7]}$$

where $C\bar{v}O_2$ is the mixed venous O_2 content.

Another useful parameter in defining the state of tissue oxygenation is the O_2 extraction ratio (ERO_2), which is defined as follows:

$$ERO_2 = \dot{V}O_2/\dot{D}O_2 = CaO_2/(CaO_2 - C\bar{v}O_2) \qquad \text{[Equation 8]}$$

THE RELATIONSHIP OF OXYGEN DELIVERY TO OXYGEN CONSUMPTION

The relationship of $\dot{D}O_2$ to $\dot{V}O_2$ was initially described by Stainsby and Otis[39] in isolated skeletal muscle. This relationship is also found in animals at rest that are exposed to progressive decreases in whole-body DO_2 (Fig. 87–2). Decreases in $\dot{D}O_2$ from the normal resting state are not accompanied by changes in $\dot{V}O_2$, which remains relatively constant for a wide range of $\dot{D}O_2$ values. The portion of the $\dot{D}O_2$-$\dot{V}O_2$ graph corresponding to a constant $\dot{V}O_2$ is the *O_2 supply–independent* region. $\dot{V}O_2$ does not decrease in concert with $\dot{D}O_2$ because the vasculature adapts to hypoxia by redistributing cardiac output from overperfused organs to those with higher energy requirements. Also, the number of open capillaries in a given tissue bed increases, and this shortens the diffusion distance from capillary to cell. As more capillaries open up and are perfused, lower values of capillary O_2 tension are needed to maintain the O_2 flux into the tissues. The concept of capillary-tissue O_2 diffusion can be expressed in terms of the following equation[40]:

$$\dot{V}O_2 = \text{Cellular } O_2 \text{ flux} = K\,(Pc O_2 - \text{Pmito } O_2) \qquad \text{[Equation 9]}$$

where K is a diffusion term accounting for tissue composition and geometry, PcO_2 is the capillary O_2 tension, and $PmitoO_2$ is the O_2 tension in the mitochondria. By recruiting capillaries, the tissues increase K; this allows smaller O_2 tension gradients to provide a constant O_2 flux to the same number of cells. Eventually, microvascular adaptations to hypoxia are not sufficient to maintain the flux of O_2 into the cells at a constant rate, and $\dot{V}O_2$ begins a steady decline until death occurs. The portion of the $\dot{D}O_2$-$\dot{V}O_2$ diagram where $\dot{V}O_2$ decreases as a function of $\dot{D}O_2$ is the *O_2 supply–dependent* region. The level at which $\dot{V}O_2$ becomes a function of $\dot{D}O_2$ is the *critical $\dot{D}O_2$*.[41] In the supply-independent region, cellular energy requirements are satisfied aerobically. In the supply-dependent region, the tissues must resort to anaerobic sources of adenosine triphosphate production. This, in turn, results in lactate production and in cellular acidosis.

PATHOLOGIC OXYGEN SUPPLY DEPENDENCY

Critically ill patients, especially those with sepsis syndrome or adult respiratory distress syndrome, do not display a biphasic curve having a clearly defined critical $\dot{D}O_2$. Instead, a linear $\dot{D}O_2$-$\dot{V}O_2$ relationship appears to be the rule for these patients, a pattern that has been as labeled as *pathologic supply dependency*. The reason why critically ill patients exhibit a linear $\dot{D}O_2$-$\dot{V}O_2$ function, as opposed to the biphasic function observed in experimental animals, is the subject of intense debate.

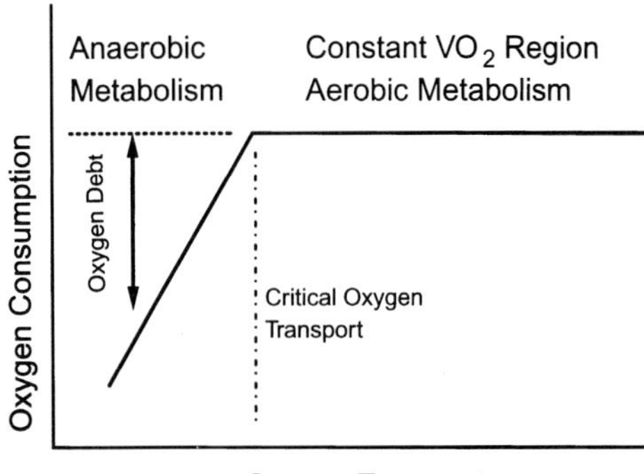

Figure 87–2. The relationship of O_2 delivery to O_2 consumption in experimental animals subjected to progressive decreases in $\dot{D}O_2$.

A possible explanation for the phenomenon of pathologic O_2 supply dependency is that mathematic coupling of measured data results in a linear function. The cardiac output term forms part of the calculation of both $\dot{D}O_2$ and $\dot{V}O_2$ (when Fick's equation is used to calculate $\dot{V}O_2$). Therefore, random errors in the measurement of cardiac output by thermodilution raise or lower $\dot{V}O_2$ and $\dot{D}O_2$ in a proportional manner, giving rise to a spurious linear function. This problem was analyzed by Moreno and coworkers,[42] who concluded that mathematic coupling probably plays a minor role in the genesis of the linear $\dot{D}O_2$-$\dot{V}O_2$ function. Other studies comparing measurements of $\dot{V}O_2$ obtained with the expired gases method with simultaneous calculations of $\dot{V}O_2$ obtained with Fick's equation show that O_2 supply dependency disappears when directly measured $\dot{V}O_2$ is plotted as a function of $\dot{D}O_2$.[43]

Another possibility is that measurements of $\dot{V}O_2$ obtained at different times change with the clinical condition of the patient. For example, a point describing a certain $\dot{V}O_2$ and $\dot{D}O_2$ when the patient is asleep moves upward and to the right of the graph if the next measurement is taken when the patient is awake and agitated. Therefore, the linear relationship found under these circumstances is not the result of an O_2 deficit. Instead, it represents the physiologic response to increases in activity, which are similar to those that occur during exercise. Dantzker and associates[44] examined this issue by compiling data from critically ill patients and from normal subjects during exercise. They noted that the ERO_2 in patients experiencing declines in $\dot{D}O_2$ does not increase to the same levels as those seen during exercise. They concluded that the critical ERO_2 in normal humans may lie close to the normal resting ERO_2 and that a $\dot{V}O_2$ plateau may be difficult to establish.

Perhaps the most popular interpretation of the linearity of the $\dot{D}O_2$-$\dot{V}O_2$ relationship is the one proposed by Cain.[45] He reasoned that critically ill patients have higher cellular energy needs and a greater basal $\dot{V}O_2$ (e.g., as the result of fever or inflammation). Also, the ability of the tissues to extract O_2 from blood may be impaired by the maldistribution of cardiac output to organs with low O_2 requirements and the development of so-called "functional peripheral shunts." The latter are not true anatomic shunts but rather develop as microcirculatory heterogeneity increases that result in a mismatch between capillary perfusion and cellular O_2 requirements. The combination of greater O_2 requirements and decreased critical ERO_2 results in a higher $\dot{V}O_2$ plateau and a greater critical $\dot{D}O_2$. This is shown in Figure 87–3, in which the "pathologic" curve has been superimposed onto the curve representing the normal response of the O_2 delivery system. A popular corollary to this theory is that patients may reach the supply-independent region when increases in $\dot{D}O_2$ are induced pharmacologically. This theory has been the basis of numerous studies aimed at eliminating "supply dependency" in critically ill patients. The hypothesis of pathologic supply dependency is supported by the findings of Gutiérrez and Pohil[46] in a series of critically ill patients. The subjects were separated into those capable of maintaining $\dot{V}O_2$ constant (supply independent; 30% mortality) and those whose $\dot{V}O_2$ declined with decreases in $\dot{D}O_2$ (supply dependent; 70% mortality). Another study supporting the theory of pathologic supply dependence is that of Bihari and colleagues[47] who infused prostacyclin—a potent peripheral vasodilator—in patients with sepsis. They noted that $\dot{V}O_2$ increased in a subset of patients, all of whom subsequently died. This was regarded as evi-

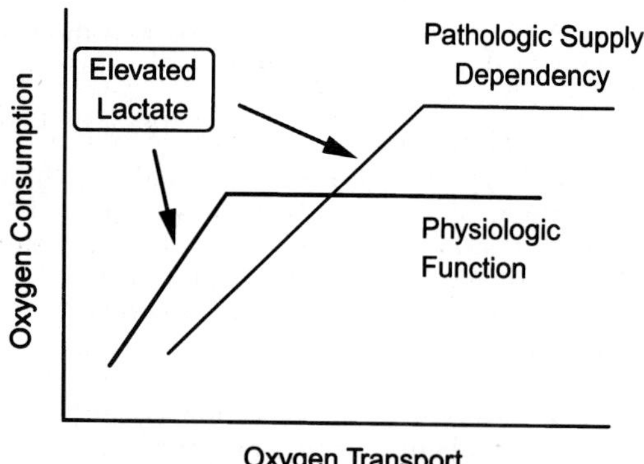

Figure 87–3. The physiologic behavior of the $\dot{D}O_2$–$\dot{V}O_2$ relationship found in experimental animals compared with the condition of pathologic supply dependency. The pathologic curve is characterized by a flatter O_2 extraction slope and by a higher $\dot{V}O_2$ plateau.

dence that inadequate oxygenation of the peripheral tissues is often unrecognized. These authors proposed the use of an "O_2 flux" test, whereby acute increases in $\dot{D}O_2$ are used to unmask covert tissue hypoxia. Increases in $\dot{V}O_2$ in response to the O_2 flux test suggest that a patient is in a "supply-dependent" state and may benefit from sustained increases in $\dot{D}O_2$.

Increases in $\dot{D}O_2$ beyond the normal physiologic levels have been advocated as therapy to prevent the development of an O_2 deficit in the tissues. Much of the work in this field stems from the observation of Shoemaker and coworkers,[48] who found improved postoperative survival rates in patients in whom pulmonary artery catheters were used to help maximize cardiac output, $\dot{V}O_2$, and $\dot{D}O_2$. In a prospective randomized study, they compared three groups: one treated according to information derived from central venous lines (CVP-control), another in which pulmonary artery catheters were used to achieve normal values of oxygenation parameters as therapeutic goals (PA-control), and a protocol group in which patients with PA catheters were treated with fluids and catecholamines (mainly dobutamine) in efforts to reach supranormal levels of $\dot{V}O_2$ and $\dot{D}O_2$ as therapeutic endpoints (PA-protocol). Hospital mortalities were 38%, 23%, and 4% for the CVP-control, PA-control, and PA-protocol groups, respectively. These data offer proof that prevention of the development of an O_2 debt improves survival in postoperative patients.[49]

In addition to dobutamine, other pharmacologic agents have been used in an attempt to induce increases in $\dot{D}O_2$. Epinephrine infusions have been reported to increase $\dot{D}O_2$ and $\dot{V}O_2$ in patients with sepsis who were still hypotensive despite the fact that they received fluids and dopamine.[50] Similarly, in a case report by Bouffard and associates,[51] cardiac index and $\dot{V}O_2$ increased following infusion of norepinephrine in a patient with sepsis who is unresponsive to other catecholamines. Dopexamine hydrochloride is a new synthetic catecholamine with α_2-adrenergic and dopaminergic properties. Doses up to 5 $\mu g \cdot kg^{-1} \cdot min^{-1}$ result in significant increases in cardiac index and decreases in systemic vascular resistance. The hemodynamic effects of intravenous dopexamine hydrochloride administration in sepsis are still not well defined. Colardyn and associates[52] studied a group of 10 patients with sepsis and found a dose-dependent increase in cardiac index and heart rate and a dose-dependent decrease in systemic vascular resistance with dopexamine hydrochloride use. In the long term, however, these effects seemed to wane, implying that the patients developed a tolerance to this drug.

REGIONAL OXYGENATION

Systemic measurements of $\dot{D}O_2$ and $\dot{V}O_2$ offer little information regarding the adequacy of O_2 supply to individual organs. This is an important consideration, since disturbances in tissue perfusion occur commonly in patients with adult respiratory distress syndrome. Hypoperfusion and the accompanying decreases in tissue oxygenation set in motion a cascade of local regulatory responses that results in the redistribution of the cardiac output to different organs according to their metabolic need, with those organs having the highest metabolic rate receiving the greatest fraction of the cardiac output. Also, some organs are better prepared to regulate tissue perfusion than are others. An example is skeletal muscle, whose capillary density can increase 20- to 30-fold during exercise; skeletal muscle tissue is also capable of withstanding protracted periods of systemic hypoxia. This type of blood flow regulation is not available to other organs (e.g., the gut and kidneys) that depend heavily on autonomic reflex regulation.

Few techniques are available with which to monitor the adequacy of regional oxygenation. The tonometric measurement of intestinal or gastric mucosal pH (pH_i) has been used to obtain metabolic information about the gut mucosa—a tissue that is very sensitive to decreases in oxygenation. Tonometry involves insertion of a Silastic balloon filled with saline inside the intestines or the stomach. The CO_2 in the outer layers of the gastric or intestinal mucosa comes into equilibrium with the CO_2 in the saline inside the Silastic balloon. An approximation to the mucosal pH is obtained by applying the Henderson-Hasselbalch equation to concurrently measured mucosal CO_2 tension and arterial HCO_3 levels. The sensitivity of the intestinal and gastric mucosa to decreases in O_2 transport and sepsis has been demonstrated in several experimental studies.[53, 54] A low gastric pH_i is predictive of morbidity[55, 56] and of mortality. Doglio and colleagues[57] prospectively followed 80 consecutive patients, measuring gastric pH_i upon their admission to the intensive care unit and then again 12 hours later. They found the lowest mortality in those patients with normal pH_i at both measuring periods (29%). Conversely, the highest mortality was noted in patients with low pH_i at admission and during the first 12 hours in the intensive care unit (87%).

In a multicenter prospective randomized study, Gutierrez and coworkers[58] measured gastric pH_i in 260 critically ill patients. Decreases in pH_i below 7.35 were treated with therapy aimed at increasing $\dot{D}O_2$, including fluid administration, blood transfusion, and the infusion of dobutamine. They found that patients admitted with a pH_i less than 7.35 did not benefit from this resuscitation protocol. On the other hand, patients admitted with a pH_i greater than or equal to 7.35 in whom pH_i-guided resuscitation was actively pursued whenever pH_i decreased below 7.35 had a 58% survival rate (compared with 42% for patients in the control group).

CONCLUSIONS

The exchange of O_2 and CO_2 between the tissues and the atmosphere is often disrupted in critically ill patients. Global oxygenation indicators, such as $\dot{D}O_2$ and $\dot{V}O_2$ provide a first-order approximation of the adequacy of tissue oxygenation, but optimal manipulation of these variables requires further insight into the mechanisms that regulate regional tissue perfusion and cellular oxygenation.

References

1. Henry W: Experiments on the quantity of gases absorbed by water at different pressures, and at different temperatures. Philos Trans R Soc 1803; 93:29.
2. Kowabara S, Duncalf D: The effect of anatomic shunt on physiologic dead space–to–tidal volume ratio: A new equation. Anesthesiology 1969; 31:575.
3. West JB, Hackett PH, Maret KH, et al: Pulmonary gas exchange on the summit of Mt Everest. J Appl Physiol: Respir Environ Exerc Physiol 1983; 54:678.
4. Parker JC, Hernandez LA, Peevy KJ: Mechanisms of ventilator-induced lung injury. Crit Care Med 1993; 21:131.
5. Marini JJ, Kelson SG: Retargeting ventilatory objectives in adult respiratory distress syndrome. Am Rev Respir Dis 1992; 146:2.
6. Gattinoni L, Presenti A, Kolobow T, et al: A new look at therapy of adult respiratory distress syndrome: Motionless lungs. *In*: European Advances in Intensive Care. Geiger K (Ed). Boston, Little, Brown and Co, 1983, pp 97–117.
7. Hickling KG: Extracorporeal CO_2 removal in severe adult respiratory distress syndrome. Anaesth Intensive Care 1986; 14:46.
8. Eger EI II: Anesthetic Uptake and Action. Baltimore, Williams & Wilkins, 1974, pp 77–98, 113–121.
9. Chang N, Goodson WH III, Gotrup F, et al: Direct measurement of wound and tissue oxygen tension in postoperative patients. Ann Surg 1983; 179:470.
10. Knighton DR, Halliday B, Hunt TJ: Oxygen as an antibiotic: The effect of inspired oxygen on infection. Arch Surg 1984; 119:199.
11. Jonsson K, Hunt TJ, Mathes SJ: Oxygen as an isolated variable influences resistance to infection. Ann Surg 1988, 208:783.
12. Plewes JL, Fahri LE: Peripheral circulatory response to hyperoxia. Undersea Biomed Res 1983; 10:123.
13. Nunn JF: Applied Respiratory Physiology. London, Butterworth's, 1987, pp 226–228.
14. Nunn JF: Applied Respiratory Physiology. 4th ed. Boston, Butterworth's, 1993, p 271.
15. Gregory IC: The oxygen and carbon monoxide capacities of foetal and adult blood. J Physiol 1974; 236:625.
16. Perutz MF: Regulation of the oxygen affinity hemoglobin: Influence of structure of the globin on the heme. Ann Rev Biochem 1979; 48:327.
17. Bryan-Brown CW, Baek SM, Makabali G, et al: Consumable oxygen: Oxygen availability in relation to oxyhemoglobin dissociation. Crit Care Med 1973; 1:17.
18. Gutiérrez G: The rate of oxygen release and its effect in capillary O_2 tension: A mathematical analysis. Respir Physiol 1986; 63:79.
19. Klocke RA: Oxygen transfer from the red cell to the mitochondrion. *In*: New Horizons II: Oxygen Transport and Utilization. Bryan-Brown CW, Ayres SN (Eds). Fullerton, CA, Society of Critical Care Medicine, 1987, p 239.
20. Hlastala MP, McKenna HP, Franada RL: Influence of carbon monoxide on hemoglobin-oxygen binding. J Appl Physiol 1976; 41:893.
21. Jones RD, Commins BT, Cernik AA: Blood level and carboxyhaemoglobin level in London taxi drivers. Lancet 1971; ii:302.
22. Pace N, Strajman E, Walker EL: Acceleration of carbon monoxide elimination in man by high pressure oxygen. Science 1950; 111;652.
23. Hemmpelman HV: Decompression theory: British practice. *In*: The Physiology of Diving and Compressed Air Work. Bennett PD, Elliott DH (Eds). Baltimore, Williams & Wilkins, 1975, p 331.
24. Hallenbeck JM, Bove AA, Moquin RB, et al: Accelerated coagulation of whole blood and cell free plasma by bubbling *in vitro*. Aerospace Med 1973; 44:712.
25. Burri C, Ahnefeld FW: The Caval Catheter. New York, Springer-Verlag, 1978.
26. Gronert GA, Messick JM, Cucchiara RF, et al: Paradoxical air embolism from a patent foramen ovale. Anesthesiology 1979; 50:458.
27. Brechner VL, Bethune RWM: Recent advances in monitoring pulmonary air embolism. Anesth Analg 1971; 50:255.
28. Matjasko J, Petrozza P, MacKenzie CF: Sensitivity of end-tidal nitrogen in venous air embolism in dogs. Anesthesiology 1985; 63:418.
29. Marques J, Sladen A, Gendell H, et al: Paradoxical air embolism without an intracardiac septal defect. J Neurosurg 1981; 55:997.
30. Butler BD, Bryan-Brown CW, Hills BA: Paradoxical air embolism: The transcapillary route. Crit Care Med 1983; 11:837.
31. Butler BD, Hills BA: Role of lung surfactant in cerebral decompression sickness. Aviat Space Environ Med 1983; 54:11.
32. Butler BD, Hills BA: The lung as a filter for microtubules. J Appl Physiol 1979; 47:537.
33. Butler BD, Hills BA: Transpulmonary passage of venous air emboli. J Appl Physiol 1985; 59:453.
34. Katz J, Luehr S, Hills BA, et al: Halothane decreases pulmonary filtration of venous air emboli. Anesthesiology 1985; 63:A523.
35. Butler BD, Luehr S, Hills BA, et al: Nitrous oxide and pulmonary air embolism. Anesthesiology 1985; 63:A422.
36. Munson ES: Transfer of nitrous oxide into body cavities. Br J Anaesth 1974; 46:202.
37. Weil MH, Rackow EC, Trevino R, et al: Difference in acid-base state between venous and arterial blood during cardiopulmonary resuscitation. N Engl J Med 1986; 315:153.
38. Kreuzer F, Cain SM: Regulation of the peripheral vasculature and tissue oxygenation in health and disease. Crit Care Clin 1985; 1:453.
39. Stainsby WN, Otis AB: Blood flow, oxygen tension, oxygen uptake, and oxygen transport in skeletal muscle. Am J Physiol 1964; 206:858–866.
40. Wagner PD: An integrated view of the determinants of maximum oxygen uptake. Adv Exp Med Biol 1988; 227:245.
41. Cain SM: Supply dependency of oxygen uptake in ARDS: Myth or reality? Am J Med Sci 1984; 288:119.
42. Moreno LF, Stratton HH, Newell JC, et al: Mathematical coupling of data: Correction of a common error for linear calculations. J Appl Physiol 1986; 60:335.
43. Ronco JJ, Phang T, Walley KR, et al: Oxygen consumption is independent of changes in oxygen delivery in severe adult respiratory distress syndrome. Am Rev Respir Dis 1991; 143:1267–1273.
44. Dantzker DR, Foresman B, Gutiérrez G: Oxygen supply and utilization relationships. Am Rev Respir Dis 1991; 143:675.
45. Cain SM: Assessment of tissue oxygenation. Crit Care Clin 1986; 2:536.
46. Gutiérrez G, Pohil RJ: Oxygen consumption is linearly related to O_2 supply in critically ill patients. J Crit Care 1986; 1:45.
47. Bihari D, Smithies M, Gimson A, et al: The effects of vasodilation with prostacyclin on oxygen delivery and uptake in critically ill patients. N Engl J Med 1987; 317:397.
48. Shoemaker W, Appel P, Kram H, et al: Prospective trial of supranormal values of survivors as therapeutic goals in high-risk surgical patients. Chest 1988; 94:1176.
49. Shoemaker W, Appel P, Kram H: Tissue oxygen debt as a determinant of lethal and nonlethal postoperative organ failure. Crit Care Med 1988; 16:1117.
50. Bollaert P, Bauer P, Audibert G, et al: Effects of epinephrine on hemodynamics and oxygen metabolism in dopamine resistant septic shock. Chest 1990; 98:949.
51. Bouffard Y, Tissot S, Viale J, et al: The effects of norepinephrine infusion on oxygen consumption in a patient with septic shock. Intensive Care Med 1990; 16:133.
52. Colardyn NF, Vandenbogaerde J, Vogelaers D, et al: Use of dopexamine hydrochloride in patients with septic shock. Crit Care Med 1989; 19:999.
53. Grum CM, Fiddian-Green RG, Pittenger GL, et al: Adequacy of tissue oxygenation in intact dog intestine. J Appl Physiol 1984; 56:1065.
54. Fink MP, Cohn SM, Lee PC, et al: Effect of lipopolysaccharide on intestinal mucosal hydrogen concentration in pigs: Evidence of gut ischemia in a normodynamic model of septic shock. Crit Care Med 1989; 17:641.
55. Fiddian-Green R, Baker S: Predictive value of the stomach wall pH for complications after cardiac operations: Comparison with other monitoring. Crit Care Med 1987; 15:153.

56. Gys T, Hubens A, Neus H, et al: Prognostic value of gastric intramural pH in surgical intensive care patients. Crit Care Med 1988; 16:1222.
57. Doglio G, Pusajo J, Egurrola M, et al: Gastric mucosa pH as a prognostic index of mortality in critically ill patients. Crit Care Med 1991; 19:1037.
58. Gutiérrez G, Palizas F, Doglio G, et al: A controlled study of gastric intra-mucosal pH as a therapeutic index of tissue oxygenation in critically ill patients. Lancet 1992; 339:195.

CHAPTER 88

Oxygen Therapy and Toxicity

Robert M. Jackson, MD

The availability of compressed oxygen (O_2) and equipment with which to administer it greatly influenced medical practice during the past century. The rationale for administering therapeutic O_2 was not obvious before it became possible to estimate tissue oxygenation by measuring arterial O_2 saturation or the partial pressure of O_2 in plasma. Such analytic techniques confirmed the ability to increase arterial O_2 content from 19.5 (breathing room air) to 22.2 (breathing 100% O_2) volumes per cent in individuals with normal gas exchange. Increases in the O_2 content of mixed venous blood, although apparently small, could also cause significant increases in capillary partial pressures of O_2 (PO_2), the force that drives O_2 into tissues and determines cellular oxygenation.

In 1939, Boothby and colleagues summarized indications and methods for O_2 administration, which had previously been a therapy of last resort.[1] Surgical indications included the application of 100% O_2 to speed resorption of nitrogen and decompress obstructed bowel. It was recognized that gas gangrene and tetanus were caused by anaerobic organisms, the growth of which could be inhibited by 100% O_2. Medical indications included the administration of 100% O_2 for headache due to encephalography, migraine, or alcoholic hangover. Therapeutic effects of O_2 in pneumonia, pulmonary edema, and heart disease were also noted at that time.

The therapeutic uses of O_2 have a sound theoretic basis. Oxygen breathing increases both the O_2 content and partial pressure of arterial blood (PaO_2), thus increasing tissue delivery of O_2, and a high partial pressure of O_2 in capillary blood increases the distance through which O_2 diffuses into tissues.[2] Oxygen may also improve the function of a number of O_2-dependent cellular systems, including the granulocyte reduced form of nicotinamide-adenine dinucleotide phosphate (NADPH) oxidase, which is critical to maintenance of host defense and NO• synthase, which regulates vasodilation. A number of microsomal enzymes depend on O_2 as a coreactant, including some of the cytochrome P_{450} system responsible for metabolism of toxic xenobiotic compounds.[3]

EFFECTS OF OXYGEN IN DISORDERED GAS EXCHANGE

Although it is possible to predict that increased inspired PO_2 will increase alveolar PO_2 (PAO_2), O_2 delivery to the tissues depends on O_2 content of blood, O_2-hemoglobin binding characteristics, cardiac output, and undefined factors controlling distribution and diffusion of O_2 from capillary blood. Until it becomes possible to monitor intracellular PO_2 in cells perfused by the vascular bed of clinical interest, dose (fraction of inspired O_2 [FIO_2])–response (intracellular PO_2) relationships will remain assumptions. However, general relationships exist between inspired PO_2 (PIO_2) and changes in PaO_2 based on knowledge of the intrapulmonary mechanisms of hypoxemia.

If ventilation-perfusion ($\dot{V}/\dot{Q}$) relationships remain normal during alveolar hypoventilation owing to sedation or neuromuscular disease, PAO_2 will increase directly with PIO_2. The alveolar gas equation then can be used to predict PaO_2. Patients with decompensated chronic bronchitis and emphysema are often admitted to an intensive care unit with respiratory failure characterized by both hypoxemia and hypercapnia. In that situation, relatively small increases in FIO_2, often to less than 0.4, substantially correct PAO_2 and permit maintenance of 90% O_2 saturation of hemoglobin. However, the PaO_2 response varies greatly from patient to patient, depending on the pattern of breathing and the underlying disorder causing $\dot{V}/\dot{Q}$ mismatching.[4] In one group of such patients with respiratory failure, the 24% Venturi mask increased PaO_2 from 9 to 15 mm Hg (mean 11 mm Hg) and the 35% Venturi mask an average of 30 mm Hg.[5] In this situation, $PaCO_2$ may increase after starting O_2 therapy because of increased dead space, although neither minute ventilation nor respiratory drive decreases. Similarly, diffusion impairment can be overcome by increased FIO_2 with improvement in PaO_2 because the rate of O_2 transfer from the lungs to the blood in that situation is a function of PAO_2.

PaO_2 is less responsive to increased FIO_2 when anatomic dead space is present or when portions of the lung have extreme $\dot{V}/\dot{Q}$ mismatching, the functional equivalent of shunt. In this context, however, application of supplemental O_2 therapy may also improve systemic O_2 delivery by increasing the O_2 content of arterial blood. Thus small increases in PaO_2 may be amplified as large increases in O_2 content, which can favorably affect mixed venous PO_2 and tissue oxygenation. Oxygen therapy may also be of some benefit in disease states characterized by systemic hypoperfusion (e.g., hemorrhagic or cardiogenic shock) even in the absence of hypoxemia, but the increase in O_2 delivery due to increased dissolved O_2 in plasma is incremental.[6]

OXYGEN DELIVERY EQUIPMENT

Equipment currently in use in a critical care unit allows delivery of increased levels of inspired O_2 concentration ranging from a few per cent above that in room air to pure O_2 at atmospheric pressure. Oxygen therapy equipment available for nonintubated patients and indications for the use of each are listed in Table 88–1. Although less commonly used for hypoxemia in the absence of ventilatory failure, mechanical ventilators with which the FIO_2 can be varied from 0.21 to 1.00 may be required to treat hypoxemic states refractory to O_2 therapy by facemask.[7,7a]

MECHANISMS OF OXYGEN TOXICITY

An overview of the pathogenesis of pulmonary O_2 toxicity is presented in Figure 88–1. Normal cellular respiration produces partially reduced, reactive O_2 metabolites. Most molecular O_2 used by mitochondria is reduced completely to water, with addition of four electrons by the mitochondrial respiratory chain.[8] A fraction of the O_2 used metabolically undergoes the addition of a single electron, a process that occurs mainly in the ubiquinone–cytochrome B region of the electron transport chain to form superoxide anion (O_2^-).

TABLE 88–1. Oxygen Delivery Equipment for Spontaneous Breathing

Target FIO_2*	*Device*	O_2 *Flow (L/min)*
0.21–0.40	Nasal cannula	1–6
0.35–0.50	Facemask	5–10
0.50–0.90	Reservoir mask (rebreathing)	5–15
0.50–0.90	Reservoir mask (nonrebreathing)	5–15
0.24–0.40	Venturi	4–10
0.50–1.00	Continuous positive airway pressure†	10–15

(Data summarized from references 4–7.)
*FIO_2 is approximate and depends on mask fit and ventilatory pattern.
†Tight mask seal, high gas flow rate, and expiratory resistance required to maintain positive airway pressure.

Production of incompletely reduced O_2 increases as intracellular PO_2 rises. At physiologic pH, superoxide is protonated to form the perhydroxyl radical ($O_2H^•$), a stronger oxidant that diffuses through cell membranes. Superoxide formed within mitochondria may interact with cellular constituents directly, but most reacts further, forming hydrogen peroxide (H_2O_2) and reactive hydroxyl radicals ($OH^•$), a process that occurs by redox cycling in the presence of catalytic iron or copper.[8a]

In hyperoxia, an elevated intracellular PO_2 and the law of mass action dictate that excess superoxide is formed in mitochondria and other intracellular organelles.[9] Iron is normally present in low-molecular-weight complexes, and the production of excess superoxide results in the iron-catalyzed formation of hydroxyl radicals. These highly reactive radicals are believed to engage in destructive oxidation and reduction reactions with cell components.[9a]

ANTIOXIDANT SYSTEMS

Production of free radicals and H_2O_2 is a normal aspect of cellular metabolism, and intracellular enzymes usually eliminate the most toxic products.[10] The prototypes of these antioxidant enzymes are metalloproteins termed *superoxide dismutases* (SOD), which catabolize superoxide by extremely rapid conversion to H_2O_2.[11] Catalase (found in peroxisomes and mitochondria) and glutathione peroxidase (found in cytosol and mitochondria) sequentially degrade H_2O_2 to water. Glutathione peroxidase removes products of lipid peroxidation as well as H_2O_2. Two related cytoplasmic enzymes, glutathione reductase (NADPH dependent) and glucose-6-phosphate dehydrogenase (NADPH producing) participate in antioxidant defense by generating intracellular reduced glutathione. Glutathione is the primary, nonprotein sulfhydryl intracellular antioxidant.[12] Other nonenzymatic antioxidants, including vitamin A, alpha-tocopherol, ascorbate, cysteine, ceruloplasmin, urate, and hemoglobin, are present within cells and extracellular fluid.[13–16a] It is noteworthy that several of these depend directly on the nutritional state of the patient.

PHYSIOLOGIC RESPONSES TO OXYGEN

Physiologic responses to O_2 are defined as being completely reversible on resumption of air breathing. They differ in their functional character from those resulting in the pathologic changes of O_2 toxicity. The most evident physiologic responses to O_2 occur in the cardiovascular system.

Cardiovascular responses to hyperoxia are typical but inconsistent from subject to subject. Oxygen breathing for approximately 30 minutes results in decreased pulse rate and pressure, whereas diastolic blood pressure increases significantly but only slightly.[17] Significant decreases in cardiac index have been observed and are usually accompanied by increases in peripheral vascular resistance as well as systolic and diastolic blood pressures. The heart rate response to O_2 is abolished by atropine, indicating vagal control of the bradycardia.[18] Regional circulations appear to respond differently to hyperoxia, but in general blood flow decreases with the rise in venous O_2 saturation. Patients with acute myocardial infarction breathing 40% O_2 had increases in systemic blood pressure and detectable decreases in cardiac output, so the increase in blood pressure appeared to be a result of increased peripheral vascular resistance.[15] During administration of O_2 to individuals with normal coronary arteries or coronary artery disease, coronary sinus blood flow decreases owing to an increase in coronary vascular resistance, and net lactate extraction increases in some cases. The overall beneficial effects of O_2 appear to be due to increasing coronary PaO_2 and reducing myocardial O_2 consumption.

SYMPTOMS AND PHYSIOLOGIC MANIFESTATIONS

Pulmonary O_2 toxicity was only slowly recognized as a clinical problem after the introduction of O_2 into clinical and operational medicine. Before the Second World War, Becker-Freyseng and Clamann found that vital capacity was

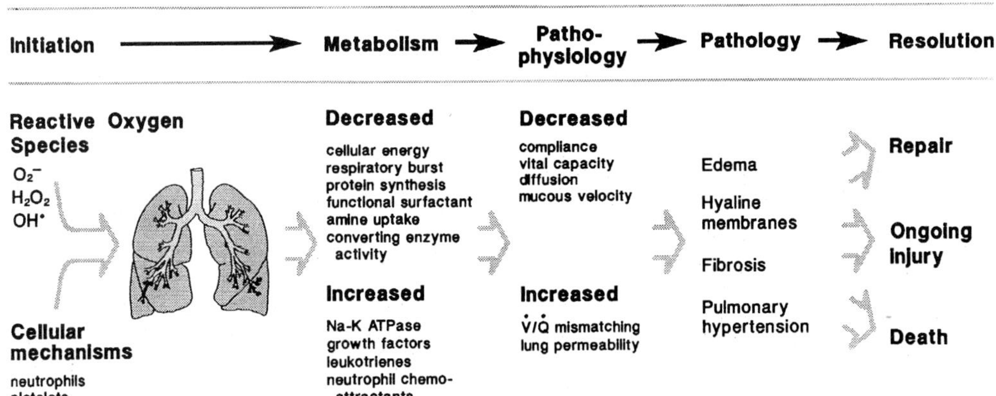

Figure 88–1. Pathogenesis of pulmonary oxygen toxicity. Oxygen toxicity is initiated by reactive oxygen metabolites and inflammatory mediators derived from granulocytes and platelets. Initially detectable as impaired cellular metabolism, oxygen toxicity evolves through stages in which physiologic or pathologic manifestations predominate. The lung injury may resolve or be perpetuated as fibrosis.

reduced in normal men who breathed 90% O_2 for 65 hours.[20] A clear demonstration of clinical O_2 toxicity was provided by Comroe and colleagues.[21] The most prominent symptom in the subjects was substernal discomfort, which varied from mild to severe pleuritic pain. Cough and nasal congestion appeared in nearly half of those breathing O_2; subjects also had significantly decreased vital capacities, but the decreases did not correlate with the severity of substernal distress. Subsequently, Caldwell and associates performed one of the most comprehensive studies of O_2 toxicity in humans.[22] Four normal men remained in 98% O_2 for periods ranging from 30 to 74 hours. During this time, O_2 toxicity became clinically evident as symptoms affecting both the respiratory and nervous systems. Cough and chest pain occurred in all four, and paresthesias and anorexia occurred in three. A progressive, statistically significant fall in vital capacity occurred in all subjects. In all but one, vital capacity quickly returned to normal; the remaining subject, however, had a delayed recovery lasting weeks. Diffusing capacity decreased during the O_2 exposure but returned to normal in the follow-up period.

Although some investigators have found hyperoxia to cause no changes in pulmonary compliance, those trials involved short periods of O_2 breathing interrupted by hyperinflation. Burger and Mead tried to differentiate the direct toxic effects of O_2 from atelectasis in a study of six normal patients exposed to O_2 for short times.[23] They measured static volume-pressure relationships in the lungs after various O_2 exposures. Most of the subjects had chest pain or coughing after the exposure. The volume-pressure curves were altered in the direction of decreased volume for a given pressure compared with the control subjects breathing air. When this change was found, it was most marked at higher inflation volumes. Some of the subjects could not inhale to total lung capacity and seemed unable to generate maximum transpulmonary pressure. One proposed explanation was that nonuniform behavior of the lung after atelectasis led to disproportionate receptor firing and an early inhibition of inflation. Similar changes in lung mechanics were evaluated by Fisher and coworkers in studies of normal men breathing O_2 at 2 atm.[24] All of their subjects had decreased vital capacity, along with a slight decrease in lung compliance that occurred without major changes in airway resistance.

CLINICAL MANIFESTATIONS

A major study of O_2 toxicity in hospitalized patients was performed by Barber and colleagues, who studied 10 patients with irreversible brain damage.[25] Five who were ventilated with pure O_2 developed significantly worse lung function than did controls. Gas exchange worsened, and a progressive decrease in PaO_2 was noted. Both intrapulmonary shunt and the ratio of dead space to tidal volume (reflecting $\dot{V}/\dot{Q}$ ratio abnormalities) increased significantly in the group exposed to pure O_2. Their lungs showed radiographic evidence of edema and were heavier at autopsy.

In a less extreme experiment, patients who had undergone cardiac surgery were randomized to receive either pure O_2 or an FIO_2 sufficient only to maintain a PaO_2 between 80 and 120 mm Hg[26] for 24 to 48 hours. During this time, no difference in intrapulmonary shunt, respiratory system compliance, or the ratio of dead space to tidal volume could be detected. Within these time limits, high FIO_2 appeared safe in critically ill postoperative patients.

Detection of pulmonary O_2 toxicity by traditional physiologic testing is, however, insensitive.[27] Nine normal individuals who breathed 100% O_2 for 6 to 12 hours had no significant changes in alveolar-to-arterial oxygen gradient, pulmonary shunt, pulmonary artery pressure, total pulmonary resistance, cardiac output, or extravascular lung water.[28] One very early manifestation of O_2 toxicity appears to be decreased tracheal mucus velocity, which can be assessed by direct observation through a fiberoptic bronchoscope. Sackner and colleagues found that tracheal mucus velocity decreased after 6 hours of oxygen breathing but could be restored by beta-agonist therapy.[29] This occurred in the absence of any significant changes in vital capacity or any other pulmonary function index, but the clinical significance of this early change remains unclear. Davis and associates studied changes in bronchoalveolar lavage constituents in normal subjects who were exposed to O_2 for approximately 17 hours.[30] An increase in albumin and transferrin was detected in lavage fluid from these subjects. No changes were detected in the lung cells recovered by lavage, but cultured alveolar macrophages from subjects exposed to O_2 released increased amounts of fibronectin and alveolar macrophage–derived growth factor for fibroblasts. The changes had reversed when the subjects were studied 2 weeks later, but they did indicate that very early in O_2 exposure, functional abnormalities may occur and would later initiate fibrosis of the alveolar wall. The course of oxygen toxicity in humans is summarized in Table 88–2.

TABLE 88–2. Time Course of Pulmonary Oxygen Toxicity in Humans

Manifestation	*Time (hours)*
Decreased tracheal mucus velocity	6
Tracheobronchitis	12
Physiologic changes (forced vital capacity, lung compliance [C_{Lung}])	24–48
Gas exchange abnormalities	30
Edema	72–96
Fibrosis	>96

(Data summarized from references 21–32.)

HUMAN STUDIES

Acceptance of O_2 toxicity as a pathologically and clinically distinct syndrome in humans was delayed. When mechanical ventilation became available, it was noted that the pulmonary function of many patients so supported underwent gradual deterioration. Nash and coworkers studied a group of 70 patients who required prolonged artificial ventilation.[31] Most patients in that study were ventilated with pressure-limited, O_2-driven ventilators, which resulted in a mean O_2 concentration exceeding 90%. Patients exposed to the highest concentrations of O_2 for long periods had heavier and more consolidated lungs. Microscopic study also showed many more fibrin membranes and evidence of early fibrosis. One patient who was ventilated with 100% O_2 for 4 days was found to have acute exudative changes involving congestion, edema, and hyaline membranes lining the alveolar septal spaces. Another patient who was ventilated with 90% to 100% O_2 for 45 days before death had proliferative changes described in animal studies: Lung sections showed both fibroblast proliferation and collagen deposition along with prominent alveolar lining cells. This clearly demonstrated an early exudative phase characterized by congestion, alveolar edema, intra-alveolar hemorrhage, and a fibrin exudate along with prominent alveolar membranes. Later, a proliferative phase characterized by alveolar and septal edema and fibroblast proliferation occurred along with fibrosis and hyperplasia of alveolar lining cells. These morphologic changes were directly correlated with the prolonged use of a ventilator delivering a high F_{IO_2}.

Fifteen patients who clinically were said to have the "respirator lung" syndrome were studied.[32] They had been exposed to 40% to 100% O_2 for periods of up to 30 days. The earliest changes again involved alveolar type I cells and endothelial cells. Septal edema was noted, and endothelial sloughing followed by fibrin thrombus formation occurred. Hyaline membranes were found after about 7 days of exposure, and re-epithelialization of the alveoli occurred by proliferation of granular pneumocytes. After 10 days, septal proliferation and deposition of interstitial collagen, elastin, and fibrosis occurred.

Detailed studies on the morphology and time course of O_2 toxicity in baboons have clarified the time course of injury in primates. The earliest detectable injury includes endothelial injury, followed by neutrophil aggregation and thickening of the alveolar interstitium. Later phases of the injury are characterized by loss of alveolar type I cells, denudation of basement membranes, and proliferation of alveolar type II cells.[33]

Similar acute changes that progressed to fibrosis have been noted after cutaneous burns and following smoke inhalation, influenza pneumonia, thoracic irradiation, and ingestion of toxins such as paraquat.[34] The histologic resemblance of pulmonary O_2 toxicity with hyaline membranes to diffuse alveolar injury due to other causes has led some investigators to propose that O_2 toxicity is a major cause of the adult respiratory distress syndrome.[35, 36] However, the near uniformity of O_2 administration to patients with respiratory failure due to diverse causes makes isolation of O_2 as the primary cause of adult respiratory distress syndrome problematic.[37] The pathologic progression of O_2 toxicity is summarized in Table 88–3.

DRUG INTERACTIONS

Many drugs used clinically affect O_2 tolerance, frequently enhancing O_2 toxicity. These fall into several broad categories: drugs that increase tissue O_2 consumption, drugs that undergo redox cycling or produce free radicals during metabolism, and drugs that affect endogenous antioxidant systems. Potentially deleterious interactions between drugs and O_2 are summarized in Table 88–4.

Epinephrine, norepinephrine, thyroid hormone, and hyperthermia all increase sensitivity to pulmonary O_2 poisoning.[38] A common mechanism appears to be increased cellular metabolism. No studies have investigated effects of more commonly used adrenergic agents such as dopamine or dobutamine in adult patients receiving hyperoxic mechanical ventilation. In addition to increasing cellular O_2 use, thyroxine lowers lung glutathione content. In distinction, dimethylthiourea, a sulfhydryl compound, protects rats from O_2 toxicity.[39] Corticosteroids are administered frequently to patients with acute respiratory failure. Mice pretreated with methylprednisolone (10 $mg \cdot kg^{-1} \cdot d^{-1}$ for 7 d) suffer significantly greater mortality in hyperoxia than do control mice.[40] Steroid pretreatment inhibited phospholipid synthesis in lung slices, suggesting that methylprednisolone has an unfavorable effect on the mature lungs' surfactant system. However, the timing of corticosteroid administration in acute lung injury appears critical. Methylprednisolone decreases survival time of adult rats in hyperoxia and minimizes adaptive increases in lung SOD. In contrast, when dexamethasone is administered to rats near the end of a 72-hour hyperoxia exposure (when lung inflammation is most pronounced), survival may be improved and lung damage is minimized.[41, 42]

Bleomycin, a chemotherapeutic agent, causes acute and chronic lung damage that is attributed in part to formation of hydroxyl radicals in the vicinity of cell nuclei. Lung damage due to bleomycin is synergistic with a number of other chemotherapeutic agents. Simultaneous administration of bleomycin and high F_{IO_2} predictably produces accelerated lung injury and progressive pulmonary fibrosis.[43] Despite isolated clinical reports to the contrary, in animal models, administration of bleomycin well before O_2 exposure results in less rather than more lung injury.[44–48] This discrepancy is due partially to differences in the acute and chronic effects of bleomycin on lung antioxidant defenses.[49, 50] Lung antioxidant enzymes initially decrease after intratracheal bleomycin administration but increase later to account for increased tolerance to O_2. Cyclophosphamide and 1,3-bis-(2-chloroethyl)-1-nitrosourea similarly increase hyperoxic lung injury while decreasing antioxidant defenses.[44–45] Many other agents used clinically have been investigated in experimental animal models of O_2 toxicity, but they may not apply directly to human patients. However, it is quite unlikely that similar studies will ever be conducted in humans, so they form the only available data base. Indomethacin has no protective effect in rabbits exposed to 95% O_2 for 65 hours, but it did decrease lung lavage 6-keto-$PGF_{1\alpha}$, a metabolite of prostacyclin.[51] Similarly meclophenamate had no protective effect on rats exposed to hyperoxia.[52, 53] Aminophylline is administered almost universally to patients in respiratory failure; fortunately, it has no detectable effect on the severity of O_2 toxicity in rats. Nitrofurantoin increases hyperoxic lung injury because reduction of the nitro- group

TABLE 88–3. Pathology and Time Course of Pulmonary Oxygen Toxicity

Feature	*Time* (hours)*
Edema	48–72
Interstitial	
Alveolar	
Endothelial cytolysis	40
Alveolar type II cell proliferation	72
Fibrin thrombi and septal fibrosis	72–96
Hyaline membranes	72–96
Pulmonary hypertension	96

(Data summarized from references 31–37.)
*Approximate time of onset in rodent and nonhuman primate models.

TABLE 88–4. Potential Oxygen-Drug Interactions

Drug	*Effect*	*Reference*
Catecholamines		
Epinephrine	Decrease survival	38
Norepinephrine		
Corticosteroids		
Methylprednisolone	Increase lung injury	40, 42
Dexamethasone	Decrease survival	41
Chemotherapeutics		
Bleomycin	Increase lung injury	45–48
Cyclophosphamide		49
1,3-bis(2-chloroethyl)-1-nitrosourea		50
Antibiotics		
Nitrofurantoin	Increase lung injury	54

of the antibiotic in the presence of O_2 leads to intracellular formation of both superoxide and H_2O_2.[54, 55] A metabolite of disulfiram inhibits SOD and accelerates O_2 toxicity in rats.[56]

PHARMACOLOGIC MODULATION OF OXYGEN TOXICITY

No effective therapeutic modality has to date been introduced to minimize O_2 toxicity in adult humans ventilated with high FIO_2. Laboratory studies suggest several potentially useful approaches, however. Pretreatment of rats with low-dose endotoxin very effectively improved survival in greater than 95% O_2 while minimizing both acute and chronic lung injury.[57–59] Interstitial edema and neutrophil infiltration occurred in rats pretreated with endotoxin in 100% O_2 but was much less than in nonpretreated controls.[60] Progressive stepwise increases in FIO_2, which are common clinically, result in accelerated mortality of rats in 95% O_2, an effect that can also be ameliorated by endotoxin.[61] Endotoxin, however, does not prevent lung injury due to hyperbaric O_2. The therapeutic index of endotoxin can be improved significantly by induction of endotoxin tolerance with progressively increasing doses, which do not decrease its protective effects.

Endotoxin is hypothesized to be protective primarily because it induces lung antioxidant enzyme activities.[61a] Many studies have shown that after endotoxin pretreatment during hyperoxic exposure, lung SOD, glutathione peroxidase, and catalase activities increase rapidly. This response is rather specific for rats, because similar protection does not occur in mice or other rodents. Possible molecular mechanisms of endotoxin's protective effects have been investigated. Endotoxin increases synthesis of CuZnSOD in rat lung slices that have been exposed to hyperoxia.[62] It also stimulates monocyte production of interleukin-1 and tumor necrosis factor–α, each of which individually protects rats from O_2 toxicity with similar efficiency. Interleukin-1 induces synthesis of mitochondrial manganese containing SOD in human melanoma cells and fibroblasts.[63] Increases in lung antioxidant enzymes, analogous to those observed in endotoxin-pretreated rats, occur after interleukin-1 and tumor necrosis factor–α pretreatment in hyperoxia.

Antioxidant enzyme proteins can be encapsulated in lipid vesicles produced in the laboratory.[11] Liposome-encapsulated antioxidant enzymes can be used to increase intracellular SOD or catalase activities, and they protect endothelial cells from O_2 toxicity. Intravenous injection of liposome-encapsulated SOD and catalase improves survival of adult rats maintained in 100% O_2 but does not completely eliminate lung injury. The protective effect is also apparent when liposome-encapsulated SOD and catalase are administered intratracheally.[64]

Conjugation of antioxidant enzyme proteins to a high-molecular-weight alcohol, polyethylene glycol, significantly increases circulating lifetime and cell permeability. Exposure of cultured endothelial cells to polyethylene glycol–SOD and polyethylene glycol–catalase increases intracellular SOD and catalase activities and makes the cells more resistant to damage from reactive O_2 species.[65] Rats pretreated with polyethylene glycol–SOD and polyethylene glycol–catalase are protected to an extent from pulmonary O_2 toxicity. Such rats maintained more normal lung glutathione levels and had less pulmonary edema in 100% O_2 than did rats pretreated with polyethylene glycol–conjugated inactivated antioxidant enzymes.[66] Decreased immunogenicity, increased circulating half-lives, and cell permeation could make polyethylene glycol–conjugated antioxidant enzymes potentially useful clinical anti-inflammatory agents.

Because O_2 toxicity impairs the surfactant system, attempts have been made to minimize O_2 toxicity by administration of exogenous surfactant.[66a] Intratracheal administration of exogenous surfactant significantly protects rabbits from O_2 toxicity.[67] This therapy may prove most useful in neonatal respiratory distress syndrome, which is characterized by endogenous surfactant deficiency and which requires prolonged high FIO_2. Trials of its efficacy are also under way in patients with adult respiratory distress syndrome, who commonly require hyperoxic therapy.

References

1. Boothby W, Margo C, Lovelace W: One hundred percent oxygen. Indications for its use and methods of administration. JAMA 1939; 113:477.
2. Connett R, Honig C, Gayefski T, et al: Defining hypoxia: A systems view of VO_2, glycolysis, energetics, and intracellular PO_2. J Appl Physiol 1990; 68:833.
3. Gillette J, Brodie B, La Du B: The oxidation of drugs by liver microsomes: On the role of TPNH and oxygen. J Pharmacol Exp Ther 1957; 119:532.
4. Mithoefer J, Karetzky M, Mead G: Oxygen therapy in respiratory failure. N Engl J Med 1967; 277:947.
5. Schiff M, Massaro D: Effect of oxygen administration by a Venturi apparatus on arterial blood gas values in patients with respiratory failure. N Engl J Med 1967; 277:950.
6. Snider G, Rinaldo J: Oxygen therapy in medical patients hospitalized outside of the intensive care unit. N Engl J Med 1980; 122(5, Part 2):29.
7. Lewis D, Barnes T, Beattie K, et al: Oxygen therapy in the acute care hospital. Respir Care 1991; 36:1410.

7a. Lin Y, Jamieson D: Effect of humidity on hyperoxic toxicity. J Appl Physiol 1993; 75:1980.

8. Fridovich I: The biology of oxygen radicals. Science 1978; 201:875.

8a. Suzuki Y, Ford G: Mathematical model supporting the superoxide theory of oxygen toxicity. Free Radic Biol Med 1994; 16:63.

9. Freeman B, Rosen G, Barber M: Superoxide perturbation of the organization of vascular endothelial cell membranes. J Biol Chem 1986; 261:5690.

9a. Gladstone I, Levine R: Oxidation of proteins in neonatal lungs. Pediatrics 1994; 93:764.

10. Mustafa M, Tierney D: Biochemical and metabolic changes in the lung with oxygen, ozone, and nitrogen dioxide toxicity. Am Rev Respir Dis 1978; 118:1001.
11. Freeman B, Young S, Crapo J: Liposome-mediated augmentation of superoxide dismutase in endothelial cells prevents oxygen injury. J Biol Chem 1983; 258:12534.
12. Asbeck A, Hoidal J, Schwartz B, et al: Insufflated red cells protect lungs from hyperoxic damage: Role of red cell glutathione in scavenging toxic O_2 radicals. Trans Assoc Am Physicians 1984; 97:365.
13. Cohen-Addad N, Bollinger R, Chou J, et al: Vitamin A deficiency and pulmonary oxygen toxicity: Morphometric studies in the murine lung. Pediatr Res 1988; 23:76.
14. Deneke S, Gershoff S, Fanburg B: Potentiation of oxygen toxicity in rats by dietary protein or amino acid deficiency. J Appl Physiol 1983; 54:147.
15. Jenkinson S, Lawrence R, Grafton W, et al: Enhanced pulmonary toxicity in copper deficient rats exposed to hyperoxia. Fund Appl Toxicol 1984; 4:170.
16. Jenkinson S, Long R, Lawrence R: Endotoxin protects selenium-deficient rats from hyperoxia. J Lab Clin Med 1984; 103:143.

16a. Kennedy K, Lane N: Effect of in vivo hyperoxia on the glutathione system in neonatal rat lung. Exp Lung Res 1994; 20:73.

17. Eggers G, Paley H, Leonard J, et al: Hemodynamic responses to oxygen breathing in man. J Appl Physiol 1962; 17:75.
18. Daly W, Bondurant S: Effects of oxygen breathing on the heart rate, blood pressure, and cardiac index of normal men—resting, with reactive hyperemia, and after atropine. J Clin Invest 1962; 41:126.
19. Ganz W, Donoso R, Marcus H, et al: Coronary hemodynamics and myocardial oxygen metabolism during oxygen breathing

in patients with and without coronary artery disease. Circulation 1972; 45:763.

20. Becker-Freyseng H, Clamann H: Zur frage der sauerstoffvergifturg. Klin Wochenschr 1939; 18:1382–1385.
21. Comroe J, Dripps R, Dimke P, et al: Oxygen toxicity. The effect of inhalation of high concentrations of oxygen for twenty-four hours on normal men. JAMA 1945; 128:710.
22. Caldwell P, Lee W, Schildkraut H, et al: Changes in lung volume, diffusing capacity, and blood gases in men breathing oxygen. J Appl Physiol 1996; 21:1477.
23. Burger E, Mead J: Static properties of lungs after oxygen exposure. J Appl Physiol 1969; 27:191.
24. Fisher A, Hyde R, Puy R, et al: Effect of oxygen at 2 atmospheres on the pulmonary mechanics of normal man. J Appl Physiol 1968; 24:529.
25. Barber RE, Lee J, Hamilton W: Oxygen toxicity in man. A prospective study in patients with irreversible brain damage. N Engl J Med 1970; 283:1478.
26. Singer MM, Wright F, Stanley L, et al: Oxygen toxicity in man. A prospective study in patients after open heart surgery. N Engl J Med 1970; 283:1483.
27. Erdmann A, Huttemeier P, Landolt C, et al: Pure oxygen breathing increases sheep lung microvascular permeability. Anesthesiology 1983; 58:153.
28. Vandewater J, Kagey K, Miller T, et al: Pulmonary effects of oxygen breathing. A six-hour study in normal men. Ann Intern Med 1975; 82:40.
29. Sackner M, Landa J, Hirsch J, et al: Pulmonary effects of oxygen breathing. A six-hour study in normal men. Ann Intern Med 1975; 82:40.
30. Davis W, Rennard S, Bitterman P, et al: Pulmonary oxygen toxicity. Early reversible changes in human alveolar structures induced by hyperoxia. N Engl J Med 1983; 309:878.
31. Nash G, Blennerhassett JB, Pontoppidan H: Pulmonary lesions associated with oxygen therapy and artificial ventilation. N Engl J Med 1967; 276:368.
32. Gould V, Tosco R, Wheelis R, et al: Oxygen pneumonitis in man. Ultrastructural observations on the development of alveolar lesions. Lab Invest 1972; 26:499.
33. Fracica P, Knapp M, Crapo J: Pattern of progression and markers of lung injury in rodents and subhuman primates exposed to hyperoxia. Exp Lung Res 1989; 14:869.
34. Katzenstein A, Bloor C, Leibow A: Diffuse alveolar damage. The role of oxygen, shock, and related factors. Am J Pathol 1976; 85:210.
35. Pratt P: Pathology of adult respiratory distress syndrome: Implications regarding therapy. Semin Respir Med 1982; 4:79.
36. Pratt P, Vollmer R, Shelburne J, et al: Pulmonary morphology in a multihospital collaborative extracorporeal membrane oxygenation project. Am J Pathol 1979; 95:191.
37. Sevitt S: Diffuse and focal oxygen pneumonitis. A preliminary report on the threshold of pulmonary oxygen toxicity in man. J Clin Pathol 1974; 27:21.
38. Gerschman R, Gilbert D, Nye S, et al: Effects of autonomic drugs and adrenal glands on oxygen poisoning. Proc Soc Exp Biol Med 1955; 88:617.
39. Yam J, Roberts R: Pharmacological alteration of oxygen-induced lung toxicity. Toxicol Appl Pharmacol 1979; 47:367.
40. Gross N, Smith D: Methylprednisolone increases the toxicity of oxygen in adult mice. Mechanical and biochemical effects on the surfactant system. Am Rev Respir Dis 1984; 129:805.
41. Koizumi M, Frank L, Massaro D: Oxygen toxicity in rats. Varied effect of dexamethasone treatment depending on duration of hyperoxia. Am Rev Respir Dis 1985; 131:907.
42. Halpern P, Teitelman U, Lanir A: Effect of methylprednisolone on normobaric pulmonary oxygen toxicity in rats. Respiration 1985; 48:153.
43. Hay J, Haslam P, Turner-Warwick M, et al: The effects of iron and desferrioxamine on the lung injury induced by intravenous bleomycin and hyperoxia. Free Radic Res Commun 1987; 4:109.
44. Berend N: The effect of bleomycin and oxygen on rat lung. Pathology 1984; 16:136.
45. Matalon S, Harper W, Goldinger J, et al: Modification of pulmonary oxygen toxicity by bleomycin treatment. J Appl Physiol 1985; 58:1802.
46. Fantone J, Phan S: Oxygen metabolite detoxifying enzyme levels in bleomycin-induced fibrotic lungs. Free Radic Biol Med 1988; 4:399.
47. Rinaldo J, Goldstein R, Snider G: Modification of oxygen toxicity after lung injury by bleomycin in hamsters. Am Rev Respir Dis 1982; 126:1030.
48. Tryka A, Godleski J, Brain J: Differences in effects of immediate and delayed hyperoxia exposure on bleomycin-induced pulmonary injury. Cancer Treat Rep 1984; 68:759.
49. Hakkinen P, Morse C, Martin F, et al: Potentiating effects of oxygen in lungs damaged by methylcyclopentadienyl manganese tricarbonyl, cadmium chloride, oleic acid, and antitumor drugs. Toxicol Appl Pharmacol 1983; 67:55.
50. Kehrer J, Paraidathathu T: Enhanced oxygen toxicity following treatment with 1,3-bis(2-chloroethyl)-1-nitrosourea. Fundam Appl Toxicol 1984; 4:760.
51. Hageman J, Babler S, Lee S, et al: The early involvement of pulmonary prostaglandins in hyperoxic lung injury. Prostaglandins Leukot Med 1986; 25:105.
52. Hageman J, Zemaitis J, Holtzman R, et al: Failure of non-selective inhibition of arachidonic acid metabolism to alleviate hyperoxic lung injury. Prostaglandins Leukot Essent Fatty Acids 1988; 32:145.
53. Smith L, Summers E, Hunt C, et al: Hyperoxic lung injury in mice: A possible protective role for prostacyclin. J Lab Clin Med 1986; 108:479.
54. Boyd M, Catignani G, Sasame H, et al: Acute pulmonary injury in rats by nitrofurantoin and modification by vitamin E, dietary fat, and oxygen. Am Rev Respir Dis 1979; 12:93.
55. Michaels C, Remack J: Quantitative study of antioxidant systems for cellular nitrofurantoin toxicity. Biochim Biophys Acta 1988; 967:341.
56. Forman H, York J, Fisher A: Mechanism for the potentiation of oxygen toxicity by disulfiram. J Pharmacol Exp Ther 1980; 212:452.
57. Frank L, Nerishi K: Endotoxin treatment protects vitamin E-deficient rats from pulmonary O_2 toxicity. Am J Physiol 1984; 247:R520.
58. Frank L, Roberts R: Oxygen toxicity: Protection of the lung by bacterial lipopolysaccharide (endotoxin). Toxicol Appl Pharmacol 1979; 50:371.
59. Frank L, Roberts R: Endotoxin protection against oxygen-induced acute and chronic lung injury. J Appl Physiol 1979; 47:577.
60. Thet L, Wrobel D, Crapo J, et al: Morphologic aspects of the protection by endotoxin against acute and chronic oxygen-induced lung injury in adult rats. Lab Invest 1983; 48:448.
61. Frank L: Endotoxin reverses the decreased tolerance of rats to $>95\%$ O_2. J Appl Physiol 1981; 51:577.
61a. Hamburg D, Tonoki H, Welty S, Geske R, et al: Endotoxin induces glutathione reductase activity in lungs of mice. Pediatr Res 1994; 35:311.
62. Hass M, Frank L, Massaro D: The effect of bacterial endotoxin on synthesis of (Cu,Zn) superoxide dismutase in lungs of oxygen-exposed rats. J Biol Chem 1982; 257:9379.
63. Masuda A, Longo D, Koboyashi K, et al: Induction of mitochondrial manganese superoxide dismutase by interleukin-1. FASEB J 1988; 2:3087.
64. Padmanabhan R, Gudapaty R, Liener I, et al: Protection against pulmonary oxygen toxicity in rats by the intratracheal administration of liposome encapsulated superoxide dismutase or catalase. Am Rev Respir Dis 1985; 132:164.
65. Beckman J, Minor, Freeman B: Augmentation of antioxidant enzymes in vascular endothelium. J Free Radic Biol Med 1986; 2:359.
66. White C, Jackson J, Abuchowski A, et al: Polyethylene glycol attached antioxidant enzymes decrease pulmonary oxygen toxicity in rats. J Appl Physiol 1989; 66:584.
66a. Gilliard N, Heldt GP, Loredo J, Gasser H, et al: Exposure of the hydrophobic components of porcine lung surfactant to oxidant stress alters surface tension properties. J Clin Invest 1994; 93:2608.
67. Matalon S, Holme B, Notter R: Modification of pulmonary hyperoxic injury by administration of exogenous surfactant. J Appl Physiol 1987; 62:756.

CHAPTER 89

Pulmonary Edema

Anton I. Kidess, MBBS, MD • D. Robert McCaffree, MD

Pulmonary edema is a manifestation of a potentially serious and life-threatening disorder. Prompt recognition and management of this common clinical problem can improve outcome in the majority of patients. This chapter presents a review of the current literature as it affects the treatment of patients with pulmonary edema. A more thorough review of certain aspects of pulmonary edema can be found in Chapters 74 and 75.

DEFINITIONS

Pulmonary edema is a clinical syndrome characterized by excessive accumulation of extravascular fluid in the lungs, leading to alveolar flooding, hypoxemia, and increased work of breathing.[1] Pulmonary edema is classically categorized into hydrostatic and permeability pulmonary edema based on the underlying pathophysiologic mechanism. Hydrostatic *(high-pressure, transudative,* or *cardiogenic)* pulmonary edema is characterized by increased pulmonary microvascular pressure that leads to transudation of fluid across the endothelium into the pulmonary interstitium and subsequently into the alveolar space. In permeability *(low-pressure, exudative,* or *noncardiogenic)* pulmonary edema, injured microvascular endothelium enables protein-rich fluid to enter the extravascular space.[2]

PATHOPHYSIOLOGY

The alveolar space is lined by type I epithelial cells, which cover 98% of the alveolar surface, interspersed with larger polygonal type II epithelial cells. Together, these cells form a complete epithelial layer that impedes the movement of fluid and proteins across its surface. The pulmonary capillaries are lined by nonfenestrated endothelial cells, which, in contrast to epithelial cells, are more permeable to water and electrolytes.[3] The movement of fluid across the capillary endothelium is governed by Starling's law of transcapillary exchange and is expressed in the Starling equation:[4]

$$F = K_f[(P_{CAP} - P_{ISF}) - \sigma(\pi_{CAP} - \pi_{ISF})]$$

where F is the rate of fluid filtration, K_f is the hydraulic filtration coefficient, P_{CAP} is capillary hydrostatic pressure, P_{ISF} is interstitial fluid hydrostatic pressure, σ is the osmotic reflection coefficient, π_{CAP} is plasma oncotic pressure, and π_{ISF} is interstitial fluid oncotic pressure.

According to this equation, fluid movement out of the capillary occurs whenever the difference between capillary and interstitial hydrostatic pressure is greater than the difference between capillary and interstitial oncotic pressure. The oncotic pressure gradient is modified by the reflection coefficient (σ), which is a function of endothelial cell permeability to proteins. A barrier that is completely impermeable to protein molecules would have a σ of one, whereas a freely permeable one would have a σ that is equal to zero. In the lung, σ is estimated to be approximately 0.9 for the endothelium of the pulmonary capillaries and close to 1 for the alveolar epithelium.[5, 6]

In *hydrostatic pulmonary edema,* the principal factor leading to interstitial and alveolar fluid accumulation is an increase in capillary hydrostatic pressure, usually as a result of left ventricular failure or fluid overload (Table 89–1). The specific pathways for movement of fluid and proteins into the interstitial space and eventually into the alveolar space are not totally understood. Studies suggest that hydrostatic pulmonary edema does not follow a simple uniform membrane model of passive fluid movement along pressure gradients. In an excised rabbit lung model of hydrostatic pulmonary edema, Bachofen and coworkers[7, 8] found evidence of epithelial cell disruption and marked inhomogeneity between alveolar interstitial edema and adjacent alveolar flooding. The regional distribution of hydrostatic pulmonary edema was not solely gravity dependent, and striking inequalities in the density of proteinaceous fluid pools were present, suggesting local differences in the sieving properties of the alveolar epithelial barrier.

Permeability pulmonary edema is a consequence of diffuse injury to the alveolocapillary units, allowing greater permeability of capillary endothelium and alveolar epithelium to large molecules, such as proteins. This injury accompanies a multitude of disease states such as sepsis and gastric fluid aspiration (see Table 89–1). The lungs respond to injury in a nonspecific but predictable manner regardless of the precipitating factor.[9–12] Clinically, acute lung injury manifests as a constellation of symptoms and signs that are often referred to as the *adult respiratory distress syndrome* (ARDS). Histologically, the damage appears to change with time and is conveniently divided into three interrelated and overlapping phases that correlate with the clinical evolution of the disease.[13] The onset *(stage I* or *exudative phase)* is characterized by extravasation of protein-rich fluid into the interstitial and alveolar spaces. As the disease process evolves, edema is overshadowed by an intense cellular response associated with hemorrhage, cellular necrosis, hyperplasia of type II pneumocytes, fibrin deposition, and thrombotic vas-

TABLE 89–1. Causes of Pulmonary Edema

Hydrostatic Pulmonary Edema
Left ventricular failure
Volume overload
Mechanical obstruction of left outflow tract (e.g., mitral stenosis)
Overperfusion
Lymphatic insufficiency
Subsequent to lung transplantation
Lymphangiectatic carcinomatosis
Fibrosing lymphangitis
Permeability Pulmonary Edema
Infectious: Pneumonia (bacterial, viral, fungal, or parasitic)
Sepsis (most commonly gram-negative sepsis)
Toxins (e.g., smoke, ozone, phosgene, chlorine, nitrogen dioxide, cadmium)
Trauma and burns
Aspiration of acidic gastric contents
Acute radiation pneumonitis
Disseminated intravascular coagulation
Hypersensitivity pneumonitis
Pancreatitis
Drug related (e.g., thiazides, salicylates, interleukin-2, colchicine, chlordiazepoxide)
Near-drowning
Air, thrombotic, or amniotic fluid emboli
Multiple transfusion
Mixed or Incompletely Understood Pathogenesis
High-altitude pulmonary edema
Neurogenic pulmonary edema
Re-expansion pulmonary edema
Narcotic overdose
Tocolytic therapy
Uremia

cular occlusion *(stage II* or *proliferative phase)*. In patients who survive the acute insult, the reparative process is characterized by fibrosis and thickening of the alveolar septa, resulting in irregular enlargement of the air spaces and vascular obliteration *(stage III* or *fibrotic phase)*.

The mechanism of lung injury in most forms of permeability pulmonary edema is not known.[14] A complex cascade of inflammatory mediators triggered by the acute insult leads to activation and recruitment of macrophages, neutrophils, and lymphocytes. In addition, cytotoxic mediators, free oxygen radicals, proteases, and arachidonic acid metabolites are released, leading to endothelial and epithelial cell damage. The result is increased conductance of the alveolocapillary barrier to fluids and proteins.

Pulmonary Edema of Mixed or Incompletely Understood Pathogenesis

Although it is convenient to categorize pulmonary edema into hydrostatic and permeability pulmonary edema, it should be understood that these are not two mutually exclusive or distinct entities. There is significant overlap in the clinical presentation, pathophysiology, and treatment of both forms of pulmonary edema.

High-Altitude Pulmonary Edema

High-altitude pulmonary edema (HAPE) develops within the first few days after rapid ascent to altitudes above 2500 m (7644 ft). The frequency of HAPE depends on the elevation, gain in altitude, speed of ascent, and individual susceptibility. HAPE develops in 0.5% to 15% of young individuals who ascend rapidly to high altitude and engage in strenuous exercise before they have become acclimatized.[15–17] A recurrence rate of more than 60% has been reported.[18] Restoring the partial pressure of oxygen to sea level values early in the course of the illness results in rapid and complete recovery. A mortality rate of up to 50% has been reported in the Himalayan expeditions in which descent was impossible and supplemental oxygen was not available.

The pathogenesis of HAPE is not known. Hypoxia increases pulmonary vascular resistance, which might lead to overperfusion of the alveolocapillary bed, leading to the development of pulmonary edema.[15] The pulmonary capillary wedge pressure (PCWP) is usually normal,[19] but pulmonary artery pressure is consistently elevated. Prophylactic administration of nifedipine leads to a reduction in pulmonary arterial pressure and prevents HAPE in some patients.[20] Schoene and colleagues[21] reported that climbers with HAPE had bronchoalveolar fluid that was protein rich and contained an increased number of alveolar macrophages.

Rapid descent and supplemental oxygen, which promptly reverses HAPE, remains the treatment of choice. In addition to nifedipine, acetazolamide and dexamethasone have been found of value in preventing HAPE in some patients.[15]

Neurogenic Pulmonary Edema

Pulmonary edema may occur in conjunction with various central nervous system insults, such as head trauma, central nervous system bleeding, seizures, and neurosurgical procedures. It may present acutely, within minutes to hours of the precipitating event, or insidiously, over several days.[22] The pathogenesis of neurogenic pulmonary edema is not completely understood.[23] Increased centrally mediated sympathetic discharge can lead to generalized vasoconstriction that may result in increased PCWP. This increase in PCWP is transient, and most patients have persistent edema even after normalization of the PCWP. In addition, edema fluid protein concentration is usually increased,[24] suggesting an increase in the permeability of the alveolar epithelium. It appears that both hydrostatic and permeability pathophysiologic mechanisms have a role to various degrees in the development of neurogenic pulmonary edema.[22, 25]

Re-Expansion Pulmonary Edema

Pulmonary edema occasionally develops after rapid re-expansion of a collapsed lung.[26–28] Most cases are unilateral, but a few cases of contralateral pulmonary edema have been reported.[29] The pathogenesis of re-expansion pulmonary edema is not completely understood. An imbalance in the Starling forces due to the generation of high negative intrathoracic pressure during external suctioning may lead to pulmonary edema.[27] Ratios of edema fluid to serum protein are usually increased, and PCWP is normal.[30–32] Animal studies suggest that re-expansion pulmonary edema is a result of alveolar damage mediated by activated inflammatory cells triggered by reperfusion of the ischemic collapsed lung.[31–34]

Pulmonary Edema Associated with Narcotic Overdose

Pulmonary edema is a well-described complication of narcotic overdose.[35–40] Opiates are respiratory depressants and can lead to hypoxemia, hypercarbia, and respiratory acidosis. Cerebral edema and opiate-mediated hypothalamic dysfunction may lead to neurogenic pulmonary edema. Severe hypoxemia can cause reversible left ventricular dysfunction; however, PCWP is usually normal[41] and pulmonary edema protein concentration is increased, suggesting increased pulmonary capillary permeability.[39] Impurities in illicit drugs can have a direct toxic effect on the lungs,[42, 43] but pharmacologic narcotic preparations can also cause pulmonary edema.[44] In addition, heroin and morphine have been shown to increase plasma histamine levels.[45]

Pulmonary Edema Associated with Tocolytic Therapy

Pulmonary edema is a serious complication of tocolytic therapy. It occurs in as many as 4% of pregnant women who receive β-sympathomimetic agents to inhibit preterm labor.[46] The pathophysiology of this syndrome remains poorly understood. It is thought that the combination of volume overload, decreased colloid oncotic pressure, and the physiologic alterations caused by pregnancy and tocolysis produce pulmonary edema. Discontinuation of tocolytic therapy, diuresis, and administration of supplemental oxygen usually result in prompt clinical improvement.

Resolution of Pulmonary Edema

The processes involved in resolution of pulmonary edema are not completely understood.[11, 47] Excess fluid in the interstitial space is removed by the bronchial and pulmonary circulation as well as the pulmonary lymphatics. The pleural space is also an important route for clearance of interstitial edema.[48, 49] Protein-rich fluid that leaks into the alveolar space during acute lung injury must be actively absorbed by alveolar epithelial cells into the interstitium before being returned to the intravascular compartment.[3] Studies have confirmed that cultured alveolar epithelium can actively transport sodium into the interstitial space.[3, 11, 50–52] Matthay and Wiener-Kronish studied the protein concentration of pulmonary edema fluid in patients with both hydrostatic and permeability pulmonary edema.[47] They found that resolution of pulmonary edema was associated with an increase in edema fluid protein concentration that sometimes even exceeded plasma protein concentration, thus confirming that active transport of fluid across the epithelial barrier occurs during the resolution of pulmonary edema.

DIAGNOSIS

History and Physical Examination

The clinical manifestations of pulmonary edema can vary, depending on the severity, acuteness, and underlying pathophysiology of the precipitating condition. Dyspnea is the most prevalent symptom of pulmonary edema, but patients with chronic pulmonary edema may present with nonspecific symptoms such as fatigue and nonproductive cough. Patients with acute onset of pulmonary edema typically appear ill and complain of severe dyspnea, orthopnea, and cough that may be productive of frothy and blood-tinged sputum. Apprehension, cyanosis, tachypnea, and tachycardia may be present. Rales, rhonchi, and wheezes are frequently heard throughout the chest.

Pulmonary edema is usually a manifestation of a serious underlying disorder (see Table 89–1), which frequently results in a constellation of symptoms and signs that lead an astute physician to the proper diagnosis. Symptoms of myocardial ischemia in association with signs of left ventricular failure suggest the diagnosis of hydrostatic pulmonary edema, whereas a history of gastric fluid aspiration and a hyperdynamic cardiovascular response suggest permeability pulmonary edema.

Stevenson and Perloff[53] prospectively compared physical signs with hemodynamic measurements in 50 patients with known chronic heart failure being evaluated for cardiac transplantation. Rales, edema, and elevated mean jugular venous pressure were absent in 18 of 43 patients with PCWP greater than or equal to 22 mm Hg. The combinations of these signs had a 58% sensitivity and a 100% specificity in their highly selected population. In a similar study, Chakko and associates[54] found that the absence of orthopnea, edema, rales, third heart sound, or elevated jugular venous pressure had a poor predictive value in precluding significantly elevated PCWP. They found a group of patients with marked elevation of PCWP without clinical evidence of pulmonary edema. In addition to the inaccuracy of physical signs in the diagnosis of pulmonary edema, physicians' ability to detect these signs might be variable. Ishmail and colleagues[55] studied the interobserver variability among four trained clinicians asked to recognize a third heart sound. They found that the agreement between clinicians varied between 48% and 73% and concluded that physicians cannot agree reliably about the presence or absence of a third heart sound.

Chest Roentgenograms

The earliest radiographic sign of *hydrostatic pulmonary edema* is redistribution of pulmonary blood flow.[56] Initially, equalization of apical and basilar pulmonary vessel size is noted, followed by pulmonary vascular redistribution. This occurs especially in chronic left ventricular failure and may not be present in cases of acute left ventricular failure.

With increasing interstitial fluid, the interlobular septa are thickened and may become radiographically visible as fine linear opacities known as *septal lines* or *Kerley's lines*. Kerley's B lines (Fig. 89–1) are perpendicular lines seen laterally and anteriorly at the lung bases and extending to the pleural surface. Kerley's A lines are longer linear lines seen in other parts of the lung. Kerley's C lines are fine, randomly distributed reticular opacities. Septal lines are neither specific nor sensitive for hydrostatic pulmonary edema.

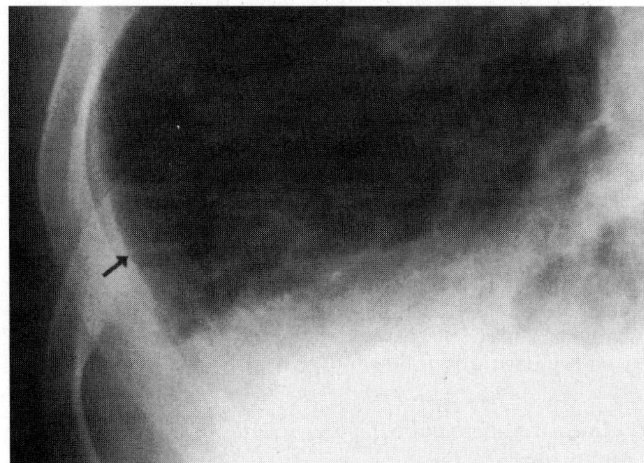

Figure 89–1. Kerley's B lines. (Courtesy of Thomas Johnson, MD, Department of Veterans Affairs Medical Center, Oklahoma City, OK.)

Persistent pulmonary venous hypertension causes fluid to escape into the alveolar air spaces, resulting in acinar shadows that become confluent, creating irregular, poorly defined areas of consolidation. These opacities are generally bilateral, symmetric, and more prominent in the dependent areas of the lung.

Cardiomegaly, pleural effusions, and increased pulmonary vascular pedicle width are common associated features. In an autopsy study of patients with congestive heart failure, Race and associates[57] found that 72% of patients had pleural effusions with volumes greater than 250 mL. A total of 88% of those patients had bilateral effusions, 8% had a right-sided unilateral effusion, and 4% had a left-sided effusion. More recent reports[58] confirm these findings. The width of the pulmonary vascular pedicle (Fig. 89–2), which is defined as the distance along the horizontal axis between the point at which the superior vena cava crosses the right mainstem bronchus and the point of takeoff of the left subclavian artery from the aorta,[59] correlates with total blood volume and is increased in patients with congestive heart failure.[60]

The radiographic appearance of *permeability pulmonary edema*, as seen in ARDS, is commonly divided into three stages.[56] During the first 12 to 24 hours (stage 1), no radiographic abnormalities are detected. This is followed by alveolar flooding (stage 2), which appears as patchy, acinar infiltrates that progress to become confluent and result in a radiographic appearance that is quite similar to hydrostatic pulmonary edema. In many patients, ARDS evolves into a chronic phase (stage 3), during which consolidations become less confluent and diffuse reticular infiltrates predominate.

The ability to differentiate the various types of pulmonary edema by using a plain chest radiograph is controversial.[56, 60–62] Milne and colleagues[60] studied 216 chest radiographs obtained on 119 patients with pulmonary edema; 61 of these patients had cardiac disease, 30 had overhydration or renal failure, and 28 had permeability pulmonary edema. Three principal and seven ancillary radiographic features were identified, allowing two independent observers to differentiate the three major categories of pulmonary edema with high accuracy (Table 89–2). The highest accuracy (91%) was obtained in distinguishing permeability pulmonary edema from all other varieties. The radiographic features that were most reliable were the width of the pulmonary vascular pedicle, the distribution of the blood flow, and

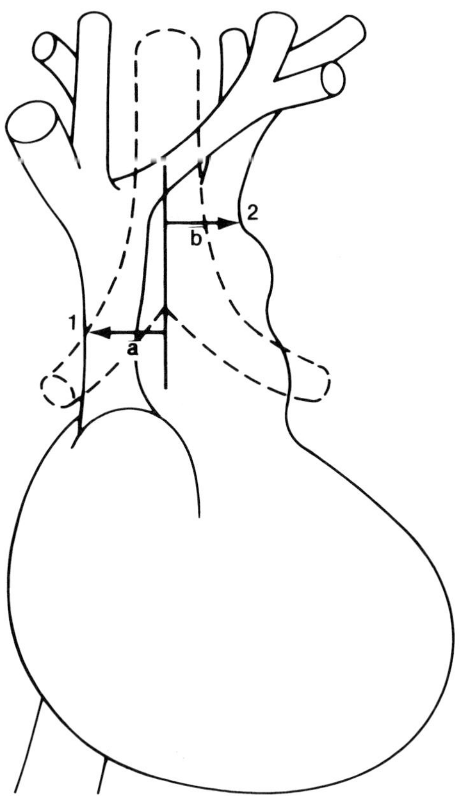

Figure 89–2. The vascular pedicle width is the distance along the horizontal axis (a + b) between the point at which the superior vena cava crosses the right mainstem bronchus (1) and the point of takeoff of the left subclavian artery from the aorta (2). The mean value for the vascular pedicle width is 48 ± 5 mm (this value ranges from 38 mm for thin and short patients to 58 mm for tall and obese patients).

pulmonary edema. Less specific radiographic features included an assessment of pulmonary blood volume, peribronchial cuffing, septal lines, pleural effusions, air bronchograms, lung volume, and cardiac size. *Permeability edema* was characterized by a patchy, peripheral, nongravitational distribution of edema; normal distribution of pulmonary blood flow; normal vascular pedicle width; and normal cardiac size. Septal lines were not seen. Peribronchial cuffing

TABLE 89–2. Radiographic Features of Pulmonary Edema

Radiographic Features	*Hydrostatic Edema*	*Permeability Edema*
Vascular pedicle width*	Normal or increased	Normal
Pulmonary blood flow distribution*	Inverted or balanced	Normal or balanced
Regional distribution of pulmonary edema*	Peripheral and symmetric	Patchy and asymmetric
Blood volume and heart size	Normal or increased	Normal
Septal lines, peribronchial cuffs, and pleural effusions	Common	Uncommon

(Adapted from Milne EN, Pistolesi M, Miniati M, et al: The radiologic distinction of cardiogenic and noncardiogenic edema. Am J Roentgenol 1985; 144:879–894.)
*Principal features.

and pleural effusions were rare. *Hydrostatic edema* was characterized by an inverted pattern of pulmonary blood flow, a symmetric distribution of pulmonary edema, cardiomegaly, pleural effusions, peribronchial cuffing, and an enlarged pulmonary vascular pedicle.

The patients studied by Milne and colleagues had early or mild pulmonary edema and were imaged in the upright position. When patients with more severe pulmonary edema were studied, Milne's criteria became less sensitive and less specific. Aberle and associates[63] studied 45 patients with severe pulmonary edema. Overall, 87% of patients with hydrostatic pulmonary edema but only 60% of patients with permeability pulmonary edema were correctly identified. A patchy peripheral distribution of edema was the single most specific criterion, occurring in 13% of patients with hydrostatic and 50% with permeability pulmonary edema. Using Milne's criteria, Rocker and colleagues[62] were unable to differentiate pulmonary edema of renal or cardiac origin but were more successful in identifying patients with permeability pulmonary edema.

Other radiographic procedures such as computed tomography and ultrasonography may be useful in selected cases. Computed tomography is not superior to conventional radiography, yet it may provide additional information in complicated cases.[64, 65]

Hemodynamic Measurements

Since its introduction in 1970 by Swan and Ganz,[66] bedside right heart catheterization with a flow-directed, balloon-tipped catheter has assumed a major role in the evaluation of patients with pulmonary edema.[67] Despite its widespread use, no controlled studies have proved its efficacy in improving survival, and its use continues to stimulate passionate debate among intensivists.[68–70]

Invasive hemodynamic monitoring may be associated with potentially serious complications.[68, 69, 71] In addition, collection and interpretation of the data can be distorted by technical difficulties.[72] When invasive hemodynamic monitoring is used in the appropriate setting by trained physicians aware of the potential risks and limitations, the hemodynamic data obtained may be invaluable in the clinical evaluation and treatment of patients with pulmonary edema.[68, 73–75]

Arterial Pressure Response to Valsalva's Maneuver

In 1944, Hamilton and colleagues[76] reported that the strain phase of the arterial waveform response to the Valsalva maneuver is related to the PCWP. McIntyre and coworkers[77] developed a noninvasive sensing and recording system that provides a reproducible estimate of arterial response to the Valsalva maneuver at the bedside. Preliminary data indicated that this noninvasive method may accurately predict PCWP. If further studies confirm these initial observations, the cardiovascular response to the Valsalva maneuver could be valuable in evaluating patients with pulmonary edema.

Pulmonary Edema Fluid Protein Concentration

Fein and colleagues[78] measured pulmonary edema protein concentration and compared it with plasma protein concentration in patients with hydrostatic and permeability pulmonary edema (the diagnosis was based on the clinical picture and PCWP values). They found that patients with a PCWP less than 20 mm Hg had a ratio of edema fluid to plasma protein that exceeded 0.6, whereas the mean ratio in patients with increased PCWP (>20 mm Hg) was 0.46.

Similar findings were reported by several other investigators.[79–82]

Sprung and associates[82] simultaneously collected pulmonary edema fluid and serum samples from patients with clinically diagnosed hydrostatic and permeability pulmonary edema. Proteins were separated into nine fractions by electrophoresis based on their size. They found that patients with hydrostatic pulmonary edema had a higher fractional content of small proteins and a lower fractional content of large proteins in edema fluids than did patients with permeability pulmonary edema.

Matthay and Wiener-Kronish[47] measured total protein and albumin concentrations in sequential samples of pulmonary edema fluid from patients with both hydrostatic and permeability pulmonary edema. They noted no change in pulmonary edema fluid protein concentration from the initial edema fluid protein concentration, obtained within 15 minutes of endotracheal intubation, in patients who did not clinically improve. However, patients who clinically improved showed an increase in the final edema protein concentration compared with their initial edema protein concentration, suggesting that active transport is important for resolution of pulmonary edema.

Despite initial enthusiastic reports, assessment of alveolocapillary barrier function by analysis of the protein concentration in edema fluid has not achieved widespread clinical use.[83–86] Results are not always diagnostic; edema liquid cannot always be sampled, and sequential edema protein changes were not appreciated until recently, making analysis of pulmonary edema fluid concentration of little value in evaluating individual patients with pulmonary edema.

Double Indicator Techniques for Measurement of Extravascular Lung Water

These techniques use two indicators, one that diffuses across the capillary endothelium and into the surrounding tissue, providing a measure of intravascular and extravascular lung volume, and a second indicator that remains in the intravascular space. Both indicators are injected into or near the right atrium, and the indicators are sampled in the distal aorta. Indicator dilution curves are generated, and from these, extravascular lung water can be calculated.[87, 88] A cold indocyanine green dye solution usually is injected into the right atrial port of a pulmonary artery catheter. A special catheter, introduced through the femoral artery and advanced into the descending aorta, is used to detect the change in temperature and concentration of indocyanine. Because heat is dissipated across the endothelium into the surrounding lung tissue, its dilution curve reflects both the intravascular and extravascular compartments. Indocyanine green stays in the intravascular compartment and provides an estimate of the intravascular compartment. This method has several limitations, including the invasive nature of the test and variable accuracy.[87] Although several investigators have advocated its use in the management of pulmonary edema,[89] its routine use requires further investigation.

Other techniques for evaluation of the alveolar-microvascular injury include tracer protein equilibration, nuclear magnetic resonance, positron emission tomography, multiple indicator dilution studies (e.g., carbon 14–urea permeability), and clearance of aerosolized technetium 99m–labeled diethylenetriamine pentaacetate. These techniques have given us a better understanding of the pathophysiology of the various forms of pulmonary edema, but none has proved practical and reliable enough to be of use in the evaluation of individual patients with pulmonary edema.[86, 90]

THERAPY

Acute pulmonary edema is a medical emergency that requires prompt evaluation and appropriate therapy. While supportive measures are being provided, clues to the underlying pathophysiologic mechanism of a patient's illness should be sought in order to institute specific therapeutic interventions.

Hypoxemia is common in patients with pulmonary edema, and administration of supplemental oxygen is an essential therapeutic intervention. In mild cases, oxygen may be administered by nasal cannula or facemask. Continuous positive airway pressure (CPAP), administered by a traditional or nasal mask,[91, 91a] is helpful in selected patients, but intubation, mechanical ventilation, and the use of positive end-expiratory pressure (PEEP) may be necessary in severe cases.

Pulmonary edema is characterized by an increase in extravascular lung water (EVLW). Therapeutic interventions directed at reducing EVLW have long been accepted modalities in the treatment of patients with hydrostatic pulmonary edema. Reports suggest that this strategy might also be appropriate in patients with permeability pulmonary edema.

Simmons and colleagues[92] studied the effect of fluid balance on survival in patients with ARDS. They found that survivors lost weight and had lower cumulative fluid balance than nonsurvivors. Eisenberg and coworkers[93] studied EVLW in patients with pulmonary edema and found that patients with initially high EVLW (twice normal) had a higher mortality than patients with lower EVLW. In a retrospective analysis of the survival of patients with ARDS, Humphrey and associates[75] found that patients who had at least a 25% reduction in their PCWP had an improved survival compared with patients who had a lower decrease or an increase in PCWP. In a prospective randomized trial to evaluate the effect of a fluid management protocol that emphasized diuresis and fluid restriction in patients with pulmonary edema, Mitchell and colleagues[89] found that this approach was safe. They found that lower positive fluid balance was associated with reduced EVLW, fewer days on a ventilator, and a shorter stay in the intensive care unit. Schuller and coworkers retrospectively analyzed the data from the same study[94] and concluded that a positive fluid balance was an independent predictor of mortality in their patients.

Based on the foregoing studies, it is prudent to conclude that achieving the lowest EVLW in patients with both hydrostatic and permeability pulmonary edema that preserves tissue perfusion may improve patients' outcome. This strategy should be carefully monitored, because restricting fluid intake and diuresis without maintaining cardiac output and tissue oxygenation is potentially dangerous.

In some situations, improving myocardial performance using inotropic agents or vasodilators may be beneficial. These approaches are discussed more completely in Chapters 49 and 50.

PROGNOSIS

Goldberger and colleagues[95] monitored 94 patients with *hydrostatic pulmonary edema* and reported an in-hospital mortality of 17% and an overall 1-year mortality of 51.2%. Fedullo and coworkers[96] retrospectively evaluated the outcome of patients with cardiogenic pulmonary edema that required mechanical ventilation. They reported a mortality rate of 56% and found that the degree of compromise in left ventricular function correlated with mortality.

Patients with *permeability pulmonary edema* have an overall poor prognosis. Montgomery and associates analyzed the

TABLE 89–3. Mortality Rates (%) of Adult Respiratory Distress Syndrome by Year

Year	83	84	85	86	87	88	89	90	91	92
Total number	67	98	87	71	69	90	73	109	87	76
Overall mortality	54	67	69	56	62	60	56	48	48	40
Sepsis	71	67	77	66	64	66	68	57	59	30
Trauma	43	55	71	48	48	32	50	31	25	44
Other	48	74	63	46	81	70	50	50	51	42

(Adapted from Mitchell DR, Milberg JA, Steinberg LD, et al: Trends in adult respiratory distress syndrome [ARDS] fatality rates from 1983–1992 [Abstract]. Am Rev Respir Dis 1993; 147:A348.)

causes of death in 47 consecutive patients with ARDS.[97] The overall mortality was 68%, compared with 34% in a control group of 160 patients who were at risk for developing ARDS but did not. Only 16% of deaths were caused by irreversible respiratory failure. Most deaths in the first 3 days were due to the underlying illness or injury. Late deaths were related to sepsis. When compared with nontraumatic causes of ARDS, patients with trauma had a lower mortality than patients with other underlying illness. In an update from the same institution, Steinberg, Mitchell, and colleagues[98, 99] reported an improved overall outcome of patients with ARDS (Table 89–3). This trend has been reported by other institutions.[100] Survivors of ARDS have a good prognosis,[100a] as their pulmonary function tests improve considerably in the first 3 months after extubation.[100b]

References

1. Allison RC: Initial treatment of pulmonary edema: A physiological approach. Am J Med Sci 1991; 302:385–391.
2. Crapo JD: New concepts in the formation of pulmonary edema (editorial; comment). Am Rev Respir Dis 1993; 147:790–792.
3. Staub NC: Alveolar flooding and clearance. Am Rev Respir Dis 1983; 127:S44–S51.
4. Bayliss WM, Starling EH: Observation on venous pressures and their relationship to capillary pressures. J Physiol (Lond) 1894; 16:159–202.
5. Taylor AE, Granger DN: Exchange of macromolecules across the microcirculation. *In*: Microcirculation, Physiological Handbook Series. Renkin EM, Michel CC (Eds). Bethesda, American Physiological Society, 1985, pp 462–520.
6. Matthay MA: Pathophysiology of pulmonary edema. Clin Chest Med 1985; 6:301–314.
7. Bachofen H, Schurch S, Weibel ER: Experimental hydrostatic pulmonary edema in rabbit lungs. Barrier lesions. Am Rev Respir Dis 1993; 147:997–1004.
8. Bachofen H, Schurch S, Michel RP, et al: Experimental hydrostatic pulmonary edema in rabbit lungs. Morphology [see comments]. Am Rev Respir Dis 1993; 147:989–996.
9. Beer DJ: ARDS: Evolving concepts of a systemic disease. Hosp Pract 1992; 27:57–60, 64, 69–80.
10. Matthay MA: The adult respiratory distress syndrome. New insights into diagnosis, pathophysiology, and treatment (Clinical conference). West J Med 1989; 150:187–194.
11. Matthay MA: Resolution of pulmonary edema. New insights (Clinical conference). West J Med 1991; 154:315–321.
12. Bernard GR, Brigham KL: Pulmonary edema. Pathophysiologic mechanisms and new approaches to therapy. Chest 1986; 89:594–600.
13. Bachofen M, Weibel ER: Structural alterations of lung parenchyma in the adult respiratory distress syndrome. Clin Chest Med 1982; 3:35–56.
14. Rinaldo JE, Christman JW: Mechanisms and mediators of the adult respiratory distress syndrome. Clin Chest Med 1990; 11:621–632.
15. Tso E: High-altitude illness. Emerg Med Clin North Am 1992; 10:231–247.
16. Sophocles AM Jr: High-altitude pulmonary edema in Vail, Colorado, 1975–1982. West J Med 1986; 144:569–573.
17. Sophocles AM Jr, Bachman J: High-altitude pulmonary edema among visitors to Summit County, Colorado. J Fam Prac 1983; 17:1015–1017.
18. Siefkin AD, Nichols BG: Noninvasive lung water quantitation by 1H nuclear magnetic resonance spectroscopy. Am Rev Respir Dis 1986; 134:509–512.
19. West JB, Mathieu-Costello O: High altitude pulmonary edema is caused by stress failure of pulmonary capillaries. Int J Sports Med 1992; 13(Suppl 1):S54–S58.
20. Bartsch P, Maggiorini M, Ritter M, et al: Prevention of high-altitude pulmonary edema by nifedipine. N Engl J Med 1991; 325:1284–1289.
21. Schoene RB, Hackett PH, Henderson WR, et al: High-altitude pulmonary edema. Characteristics of lung lavage fluid. JAMA 1986; 256:63–69.
22. Colice GL: Neurogenic pulmonary edema. Clin Chest Med 1985; 6:473–489.
23. Simon RP: Neurogenic pulmonary edema. Neurol Clin 1993; 11:309–323.
24. Maron MB: Analysis of airway fluid protein concentration in neurogenic pulmonary edema. J Appl Physiol 1987; 62:470–476.
25. Malik AB, Horgan MJ: Mechanisms of thrombin-induced lung vascular injury and edema. Am Rev Respir Dis 1987; 136:467–470.
26. Matsuura Y, Nomimura T, Murakami H, et al: Clinical analysis of reexpansion pulmonary edema. Chest 1991; 100:1562–1566.
27. Timby J, Reed C, Zeilender S, et al: "Mechanical" causes of pulmonary edema. Chest 1990; 98:973–979.
28. Zwaveling JH, Gans SJ: A one-sided affair? Myocardial infarction with pulmonary edema and forward failure. Chest 1989; 95:673–675.
29. Ragozzino MW, Greene R: Bilateral reexpansion pulmonary edema following unilateral pleurocentesis. Chest 1991; 99:506–508.
30. Sprung CL, Loewenherz JW, Baier H, et al: Evidence for increased permeability in reexpansion pulmonary edema. Am J Med 1981; 71:497–500.
31. Jackson RM, Veal CF: Re-expansion, re-oxygenation, and rethinking. Am J Med Sci 1989; 298:44–50.
32. Jackson RM, Veal CF, Beckman JS, et al: Polyethylene glycol-conjugated superoxide dismutase in unilateral lung injury due to re-expansion (re-oxygenation). Am J Med Sci 1990; 300:22–28.
33. Jackson RM, Veal CF, Alexander CB, et al: Re-expansion pulmonary edema. A potential role for free radicals in its pathogenesis. Am Rev Respir Dis 1988; 137:1165–1171.
34. Doerschuk CM, Allard MF, Oyarzun MJ: Evaluation of reexpansion pulmonary edema following unilateral pneumothorax in rabbits and the effect of superoxide dismutase. Exp Lung Res 1990; 16:355–367.
35. Steinberg AD, Karliner JS: The clinical spectrum of heroin pulmonary edema. Arch Intern Med 1968; 122:122–127.
36. Bogartz LJ, Miller WC: Pulmonary edema associated with propoxyphene intoxication. JAMA 1971; 215:259–262.
37. Bruera E: Narcotic-induced pulmonary edema. J Pain Symptom Management 1990; 5:55–58.
38. Bruera E, Miller MJ: Non-cardiogenic pulmonary edema after narcotic treatment for cancer pain. Pain 1989; 39:297–300.
39. Katz S, Aberman A, Frand UI, et al: Heroin pulmonary edema. Evidence for increased pulmonary capillary permeability. Am Rev Respir Dis 1972; 106:472–474.
40. Turturro MA, O'Toole KS: Oxycodone-induced pulmonary edema (Letter). Am J Emerg Med 1991; 9:201–203.
41. Gpinathan K, Saroja D, Spears RJ, et al: Hemodynamic studies in heroin-induced acute pulmonary edema. Circulation 1970; XLI:S-III-44.
42. Frand UI, Shim CS, Williams MH Jr: Heroin-induced pulmonary edema. Sequential studies of pulmonary function. Ann Intern Med 1972; 77:29–35.
43. Karliner JS, Steinberg AD, Williams MH Jr: Lung function after pulmonary edema associated with heroin overdose. Arch Intern Med 1969; 124:350–353.
44. Fraser DW: Methadone overdose. Illicit use of pharmaceutically prepared parenteral narcotics. JAMA 1971; 217:1387–1389.

45. Brashear RE, Kelly MT, White AC: Elevated plasma histamine after heroin and morphine. J Lab Clin Med 1974; 83:451–457.
46. Pisani RJ, Rosenow EC: Pulmonary edema associated with tocolytic therapy. Ann Intern Med 1989; 110:714–718.
47. Matthay MA, Wiener-Kronish JP: Intact epithelial barrier function is critical for the resolution of alveolar edema in humans. Am Rev Respir Dis 1990; 142:1250–1257.
48. Wiener-Kronish JP, Broaddus VC, Albertine KH, et al: Relationship of pleural effusions to increased permeability pulmonary edema in anesthetized sheep. J Clin Invest 1988; 82:1422–1429.
49. Broaddus VC, Wiener-Kronish JP, Staub NC: Clearance of lung edema into the pleural space of volume-loaded anesthetized sheep. J Appl Physiol 1990; 68:2623–2630.
50. Mason RJ, Williams MC, Widdicombe JH, et al: Transepithelial transport by pulmonary alveolar type II cells in primary culture. Proc Natl Acad Sci USA 1982; 79:6033–6037.
51. Castranova V, Jones GS, Wright JR, et al: Transport properties of isolated type II alveolar epithelial cells. Am Rev Respir Dis 1983; 127:S28–S33.
52. Mason RJ, Williams MC, Widdicombe JH: Fluid and electrolyte transport across monolayers of alveolar type II cells in vitro. Am Rev Respir Dis 1983; 127:S24–S28.
53. Stevenson LW, Perloff JK: The limited reliability of physical signs for estimating hemodynamics in chronic heart failure. JAMA 1989; 261:884–888.
54. Chakko S, Woska D, Martinez H, et al: Clinical, radiographic, and hemodynamic correlations in chronic congestive heart failure: Conflicting results may lead to inappropriate care. Am J Med 1991; 90:353–359.
55. Ishmail AA, Wing S, Ferguson J, et al: Interobserver agreement by auscultation in the presence of a third heart sound in patients with congestive heart failure. Chest 1987; 91:870–873.
56. Morgan PW, Goodman LR: Pulmonary edema and adult respiratory distress syndrome [published erratum appears in Radiol Clin North Am 1991;29:ix]. Radiol Clin North Am 1991; 29:943–963.
57. Race GA, Schiefley CH, Edwards JE: Hydrothorax in congestive heart failure. Am J Med 1957; 22:83–89.
58. Peterman TA, Brothers SK: Pleural effusions in congestive heart failure and in pericardial disease (Letter). N Engl J Med 1983; 309:313.
59. Milne EN, Pistolesi M, Miniati M, et al: The vascular pedicle of the heart and the vena azygos. Part I: The normal subject. Radiology 1984; 152:1–8.
60. Milne EN, Pistolesi M, Miniati M, et al: The radiologic distinction of cardiogenic and noncardiogenic edema. AJR Am J Roentgenol 1985; 144:879–894.
61. Milne EN: Hydrostatic versus increased permeability pulmonary edema (Letter). Radiology 1989; 170:891–894.
62. Rocker GM, Rose DH, Manhire AR, et al: The radiographic differentiation of pulmonary oedema. Br J Radiol 1989; 62:582–586.
63. Aberle DR, Wiener-Kronish JP, Webb WR, et al: Hydrostatic versus increased permeability pulmonary edema: Diagnosis based on radiographic criteria in critically ill patients. Radiology 1988; 168:73–79.
64. Stark P, Jasmine J: CT of pulmonary edema. Crit Rev Diagn Imag 1989; 29:245–255.
65. Forster BB, Muller NL, Mayo JR, et al: High-resolution computed tomography of experimental hydrostatic pulmonary edema. Chest 1992; 101:1434–1437.
66. Swan HJ, Ganz W: Guidelines for use of balloon-tipped catheter (Letter). Am J Cardiol 1974; 34:119–120.
67. King EG, Sibbald WJ: The territorial imperative (Editorial). Chest 1988; 93:1121–1122.
68. Fein AM, Goldberg SK, Walkenstein MD, et al: Is pulmonary artery catheterization necessary for the diagnosis of pulmonary edema? Am Rev Respir Dis 1984; 129:1006–1009.
69. Gore JM, Dalen JE: Pulmonary artery catheters (Letter). Chest 1988; 93:1115.
70. Staub NC: Pulmonary edema: "Whodunit?" Clin Invest Med 1985; 8:176–184.
71. Robin ED: Warning about pulmonary artery (Swan-Ganz) flow catheters (Letter). Ir Med J 1987; 80:330–331.
72. Staub NC: New concepts about the pathophysiology of pulmonary edema. J Thorac Imaging 1988; 3:8–14.
73. Connors AF Jr, McCaffree DR, Gray BA: Evaluation of right-heart catheterization in the critically ill patient without acute myocardial infarction. N Engl J Med 1983; 308:263–267.
74. Connors AF Jr, Dawson NV, McCaffree DR, et al: Assessing hemodynamic status in critically ill patients: Do physicians use clinical information optimally? J Crit Care 1987; 2:174–180.
75. Humphrey H, Hall J, Sznajder I, et al: Improved survival in ARDS patients associated with a reduction in pulmonary capillary wedge pressure. Chest 1990; 97:1176–1180.
76. Hamilton WF, Woobury RA, Harper HT Jr: Arterial, cerebrospinal, and venous pressures in man during cough and strain. Am J Physiol 1944; 141:42–50.
77. McIntyre KM, Vita JA, Lambrew CT, et al: A noninvasive method of predicting pulmonary-capillary wedge pressure. N Engl J Med 1992; 327:1715–1720.
78. Fein A, Grossman RF, Jones JG, et al: The value of edema fluid protein measurement in patients with pulmonary edema. Am J Med 1979; 67:32–38.
79. Carlson RW, Schaeffer RC Jr, Michaels SG, et al: Pulmonary edema fluid. Spectrum of features in 37 patients. Circulation 1979; 60:1161–1169.
80. Sprung CL, Rackow EC, Fein IA, et al: The spectrum of pulmonary edema: Differentiation of cardiogenic, intermediate, and noncardiogenic forms of pulmonary edema. Am Rev Respir Dis 1981; 124:718–722.
81. Carlson RW, Schaeffer RC Jr, Carpio M, et al: Edema fluid and coagulation changes during fulminant pulmonary edema. Chest 1981; 79:43–49.
82. Sprung CL, Long WM, Marcial EH, et al: Distribution of proteins in pulmonary edema. The value of fractional concentrations. Am Rev Respir Dis 1987; 136:957–963.
83. Staub NC, Hogg JC: Conference report of a workshop on the measurement of lung water. Crit Care Med 1980; 8:752–759.
84. Staub NC, Hogg JC: Clinical measurement of lung water content (Editorial). Chest 1981; 79:3–4.
85. Staub NC: Clinical use of lung water measurements. Report of a workshop. Chest 1986; 90:588–594.
86. Staub NC, Hyde RW, Crandell E: Workshop on techniques to evaluate lung alveolar-microvascular injury. Am Rev Respir Dis 1990; 141:1071–1077.
87. Allison RC, Carlile PV Jr, Gray BA: Thermodilution measurement of lung water. Clin Chest Med 1985; 6:439–457.
88. Oppenheimer L, Elings VB, Lewis FR: Thermal-dye lung water measurements: Effects of edema and embolization. J Surg Res 1979; 26:504–512.
89. Mitchell JP, Schuller D, Calandrino FS, et al: Improved outcome based on fluid management in critically ill patients requiring pulmonary artery catheterization. Am Rev Respir Dis 1992; 145:990–998.
90. Bshouty Z, Ali J, Younes M: Arterial occlusion versus isofiltration pulmonary capillary pressures during very high flow. J Appl Physiol 1987; 62:1174–1178.
91. Bersten AD, Holt AW, Vedig AE, et al: Treatment of severe cardiogenic pulmonary edema with continuous positive airway pressure delivered by face mask. N Engl J Med 1991; 325:1825–1830.
91a. Lapinsky SE, Mount DB, Mackey D, et al: Management of acute respiratory failure due to pulmonary edema with nasal positive pressure support. Chest 1994; 105:229–231.
92. Simmons RS, Berdine GG, Seidenfeld JJ, et al: Fluid balance and the adult respiratory distress syndrome. Am Rev Respir Dis 1987; 135:924–929.
93. Eisenberg PR, Hansbrough JR, Anderson D, et al: A prospective study of lung water measurements during patient management in an intensive care unit. Am Rev Respir Dis 1987; 136:662–668.
94. Schuller D, Mitchell JP, Calandrino FS, et al: Fluid balance during pulmonary edema. Is fluid gain a marker or a cause of poor outcome? Chest 1991; 100:1068–1075.
95. Goldberger JJ, Peled HB, Stroh JA, et al: Prognostic factors in acute pulmonary edema. Arch Intern Med 1986; 146:489–493.
96. Fedullo AJ, Swinburne AJ, Wahl GW, et al: Acute cardiogenic pulmonary edema treated with mechanical ventilation. Factors determining in-hospital mortality. Chest 1991; 99:1220–1226.
97. Montgomery AB, Stager MA, Carrico CJ, et al: Causes of mortality in patients with the adult respiratory distress syndrome. Am Rev Respir Dis 1985; 132:485–489.

98. Steinberg KP, McHugh LG, Hudson LD: Causes of mortality with the adult respiratory distress syndrome (ARDS): An update (Abstract). Am Rev Respir Dis 1993; 147:A347.

99. Mitchell DR, Milberg JA, Steinberg LD, et al: Trends in adult respiratory distress syndrome (ARDS) fatality rates from 1983–1992 (Abstract). Am Rev Respir Dis 1993; 147:A348.

100. Suchyta MR, Clemmer TP, Orme JF Jr, et al: Increased survival of ARDS patients with severe hypoxemia (ECMO criteria). Chest 1991; 99:951–955.

100a. Elliott CG, Rasmusson BY, Crapo RO, et al: Prediction of pulmonary function abnormalities after adult respiratory distress syndrome (ARDS). Am Rev Respir Dis 1987: 135:634–638.

100b. McHugh LG, Milberg JA, Whitcomb ME, et al: Recovery of function in survivors of the acute respiratory distress syndrome. Am J Respir Crit Care Med 1994; 150:90–94.

CHAPTER 90

Pathophysiologic Features of Infant and Adult Respiratory Distress Syndromes

Jacqueline J. Coalson, PhD

Hyaline membrane disease (HMD) and *adult respiratory distress syndrome* (ARDS) are nonspecific terms for illnesses associated with edema and hyaline membrane formation in the lungs of infants and adults.[1,2] HMD is also labeled *idiopathic respiratory distress of the newborn* or *pulmonary syndrome of the newborn,* whereas ARDS has been called *shock lung, respiratory lung,* or *congestive atelectasis.* The term used in pathology to express the tissue findings of ARDS is *diffuse alveolar damage* (DAD). For comparison purposes in this chapter, the syndrome in infants is referred to as HMD and the syndrome in adults referred to as DAD or ARDS. Likewise, *alveoli* is used to describe the lung saccules (primitive alveoli) in infants when comparisons are made with adults.

HYALINE MEMBRANE DISEASE

On gross inspection, the lungs in HMD are airless, plum colored, and liverlike in consistency. These features are reflected microscopically by widespread atelectasis; hyaline membranes at the respiratory bronchiolar, alveolar duct, and air saccular levels (Fig. 90–1); pulmonary edema; and usually striking lymphatic dilation. The edema fluid occasionally stains poorly with eosin, reportedly because of its inadequate fixation with formalin. Edema occurs within the first few hours, but hyaline membranes have not been found earlier than 2 hours after birth. Electron microscopic studies of infants dying of HMD reveal endothelial cell changes and interstitial edema. Epithelial cells of the respiratory bronchioles and alveolar ducts may be necrotic and covered with hyaline membranes containing cellular debris, fibrillar and amorphous proteinaceous material, and occasionally fibrin.[3] These descriptive histologic criteria of HMD appear unchanged even in the lower-birth-weight infants who have failed surfactant treatment and eventually developed HMD.

Before the improvements in obstetric and neonatal care that occurred during the past 20 years, premature infants who did not experience resolution of their HMD within 72 hours and thus required prolonged therapy developed a lesion called *bronchopulmonary dysplasia* (BPD).[4] The pathologic features of BPD in these infants include alveolar and bronchiolar necrosis followed by bronchial epithelial metaplasia and interstitial fibrosis (Fig. 90–2). Changes are noted in the bronchial and bronchiolar mucosae, the pulmonary interstitium, the lymphatics, and the inflation pattern.[5] In the "healed" stage of BPD, alveolar septal fibrosis is the main residual feature.[6] Many of these chronic tissue responses correlate with those in the reparative phase of DAD. Better clinical care, the development of new technologies, and the use of surfactant therapy have led to increased survival of extremely low-birth-weight infants of

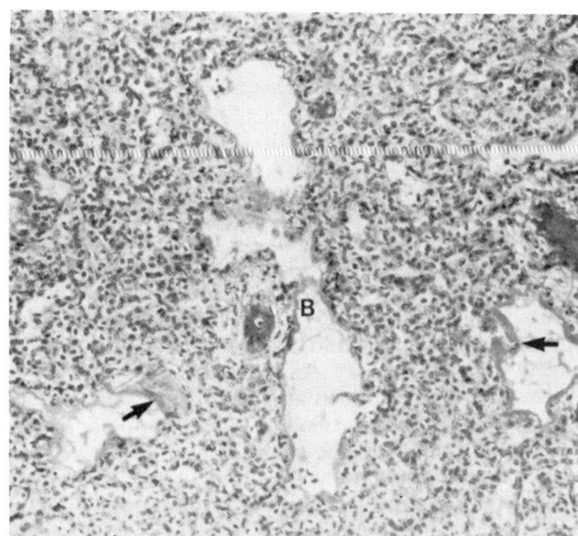

Figure 90–1. Premature baboon model of HMD. This low-power micrograph depicts severe alveolar atelectasis with hyaline membranes *(arrows)* in the expanded respiratory bronchioles (B), surrounding alveolar ducts and air saccules (hematoxylin and eosin, ×150).

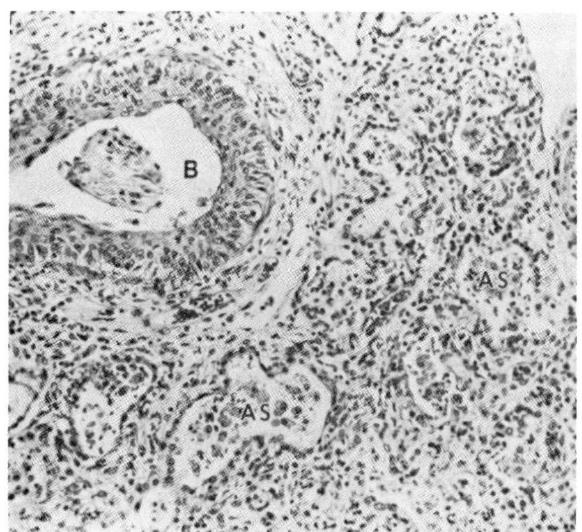

Figure 90–2. Human infant BPD. The terminal bronchiole (B) is seen on the left of this micrograph. Marked epithelial hyperplasia with early squamoid differentiation is present. The peribronchiolar fibrosis merges into interstitial fibrosis between distal air saccules. Alveolar macrophages and inflammatory cells are scattered within the thickened saccular walls and spaces (AS) (hematoxylin and eosin, ×150).

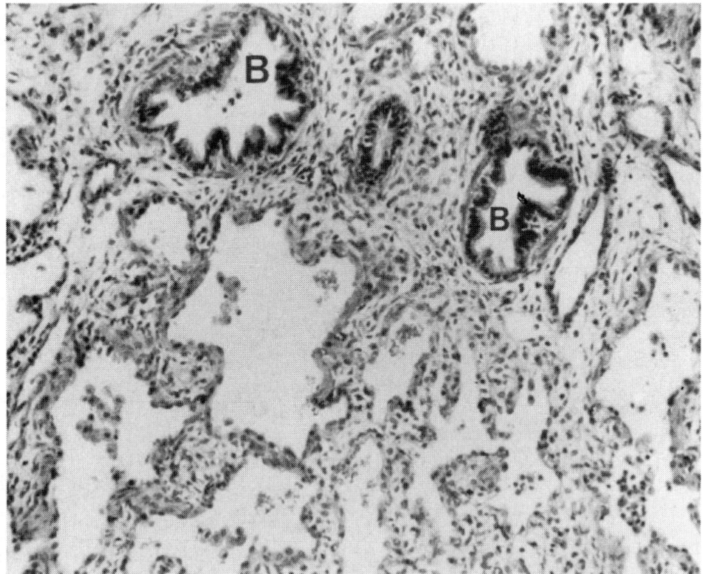

Figure 90–3. Human lung biopsy. This specimen is from a 25-day-old infant born at between 24 and 25 weeks' gestation. Note the lack of severe hyperplastic/metaplastic lesions in the bronchioles (B). The saccular walls are irregularly thickened and hypercellular, and the capillary network is not well visualized. The lung still has a saccular appearance; few alveoli are present (hematoxylin and eosin, ×140).

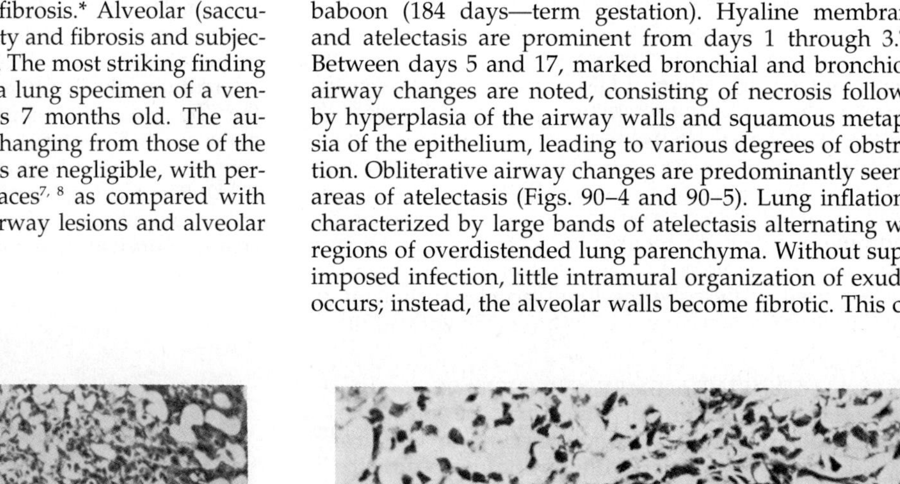

less than 28 weeks' gestation and 1000 g birth weight. In these infants, a new pattern of chronic lung disease has emerged. In ongoing clinical studies, open lung biopsies from low-birth-weight, ventilator-dependent infants with BPD reveal less airway epithelial damage, peribronchial fibrosis, and widespread alveolar fibrosis.* Alveolar (saccular) walls show increased cellularity and fibrosis and subjectively fewer capillaries (Fig. 90–3). The most striking finding is a lack of alveolization even in a lung specimen of a ventilator-dependent infant who was 7 months old. The autopsy findings also appear to be changing from those of the 1970s.[7, 8] Changes in small airways are negligible, with persistence of simple terminal airspaces[7, 8] as compared with the earlier pathology of severe airway lesions and alveolar emphysema or fibrosis.[5, 8]

*Personal observation.

The use of baboon models has allowed induction of both mild and moderately severe lesions of HMD-BPD.[9–10] The moderately severe model of BPD is elicited with treatment including positive-pressure ventilation and 100% oxygen for periods of 10 to 17 days in the 140-day cesarean-delivered baboon (184 days—term gestation). Hyaline membranes and atelectasis are prominent from days 1 through 3.[9, 10] Between days 5 and 17, marked bronchial and bronchiolar airway changes are noted, consisting of necrosis followed by hyperplasia of the airway walls and squamous metaplasia of the epithelium, leading to various degrees of obstruction. Obliterative airway changes are predominantly seen in areas of atelectasis (Figs. 90–4 and 90–5). Lung inflation is characterized by large bands of atelectasis alternating with regions of overdistended lung parenchyma. Without superimposed infection, little intramural organization of exudate occurs; instead, the alveolar walls become fibrotic. This cor-

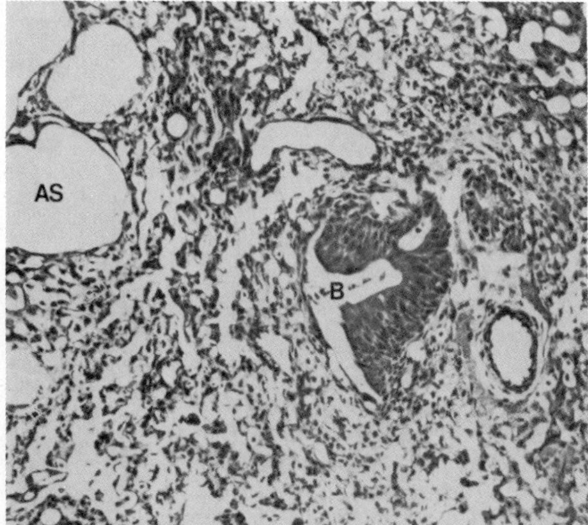

Figure 90–4. Baboon model of BPD. This specimen with vascular perfusion shows a bronchiole (B) with striking epithelial hyperplasia. To the left, some air saccular/alveolar expansion (AS) is visible; to the right, atelectasis is seen (Masson-Verhoeff's connective tissue stain, ×150).

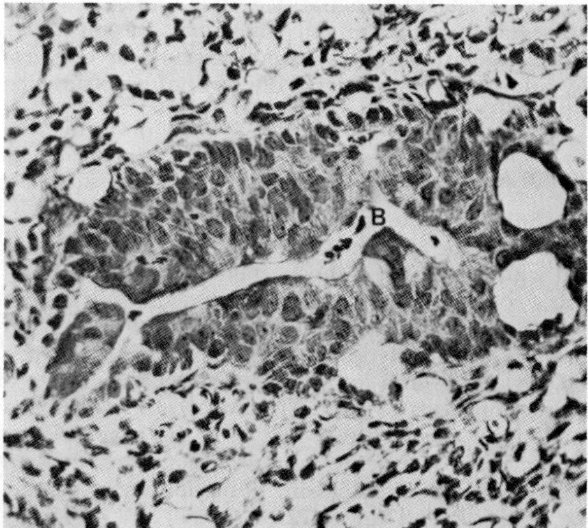

Figure 90–5. Baboon model of BPD. Bronchiolar (B) epithelial changes are highly magnified. The epithelium is markedly thickened from its usual single layer, and intercellular spaces are seen. Surrounding alveoli/air saccules show atelectasis. (Masson-Verhoeff's connective tissue stain, ×400.)

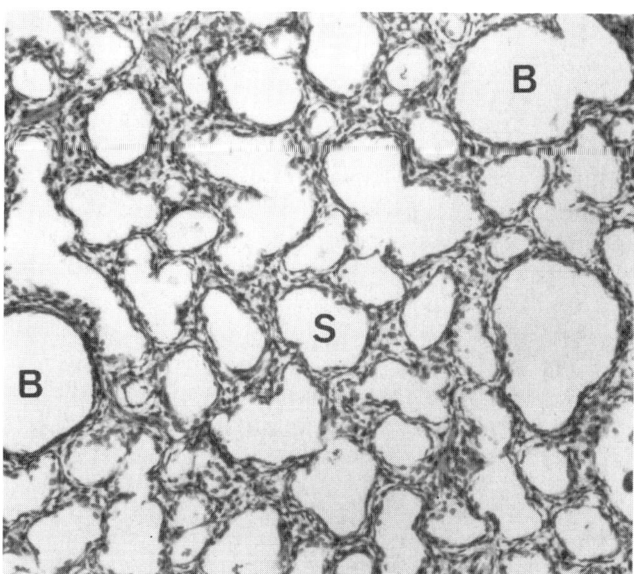

Figure 90–6. Control lung of a baboon delivered following 125 days' gestation. The lung shows primitive saccules (S) separated by thick saccular walls that contain undifferentiated cells and abundant mesenchyme. Several bronchioles are evident (B) (hematoxylin and eosin, ×90).

relates with the finding that sustained fibrinolytic activity is present in these animals, blocking intra-alveolar fibrin deposition.[11]

A milder lesion of BPD, developed to assess long-term changes in survivors, is produced by ventilating premature baboons delivered at 140 days of gestation for 21 days with 100% oxygen for the first 7 days and then 80% oxygen for 14 days.[11] This protocol elicits a lesion with less severe airway damage and alveolar fibrocellular deposition when compared with the 10- to 17-day model. When these animals are weaned at 21 days and allowed to survive to 33 weeks of age, light microscopic morphometry demonstrates a decrease of alveoli when these animals are compared with premature controls that were ventilated with appropriate oxygen for 21 days and that survived.[11a] This observation is important because the expected lung development of a 33-week-old baboon is comparable to that of a 2-year-old human infant, the age at which alveolarization in the lungs is complete.[12]

A new model of BPD has been developed in a 125-day premature baboon delivered by cesarean section.[13] This animal was treated with surfactant, maintained on appropriate oxygen, and ventilated for a period of 2 weeks, comparable to a very low-birth-weight infant (<1000 g) who requires surfactant therapy and ventilatory support. The pathology is identical to the new BPD pathology in humans and consists of arrested alveolar development, thickened saccular walls, and little airway disease (Figs. 90–6 and 90–7).

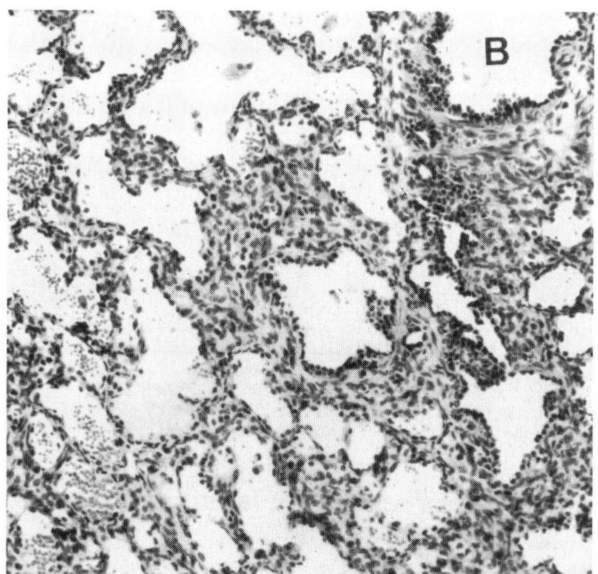

Figure 90–7. Specimen from a baboon of 125 days' gestation at 2 weeks post-treatment. Following treatment with surfactant, appropriate oxygen, and mechanical ventilation for 14 days, the lungs show irregularly thickened and hypercellular saccular walls. Foci of extravasated red blood cells are present in saccular spaces. Bronchiolar (B) epithelium does not show severe hyperplastic or metaplastic changes. Note that these findings are similar to those of the human BPD lung shown in Figure 90–3 (hematoxylin and eosin, ×90).

Unique Features of Hyaline Membrane Disease

In addition to the lack of adequate surfactant, the developmental state of the lungs probably contributes to the atelectasis of the syndrome in infants. Undeveloped human lungs lack pores of Kohn and well-developed bronchiolar-to-bronchiolar connections, so that collateral channels cannot support ventilation distal to obstructed airways. The lack of collateral ventilatory mechanisms may also decrease elastic recoil, increase airway resistance, or promote pulmonary interdependence to produce the overdistended, emphysematous lung regions found in BPD.

A second feature is the extraordinary compliance of a neonate's chest wall. This is not a feature of DAD, except in adults with massive flail chest injury. The seesaw pattern of respiration in infants with HMD is induced by the increased negativity of the inspiratory pleural pressure. This distorts the markedly complaint chest wall so that the lung adjacent to the rib cage may in fact diminish in volume. During expiration, the compliance of the chest wall does not provide a recoil pressure to counter the elastic recoil of the lung, allowing the surfactant-deficient lung to collapse.[14]

Retention of the fetal circulatory components also influences the evolution of HMD.[14] Pulmonary vascular resistance (PVR) normally drops precipitously at birth, thus allowing a major increase in pulmonary blood flow. Simultaneously, extrapulmonary fetal shunts close and sys-

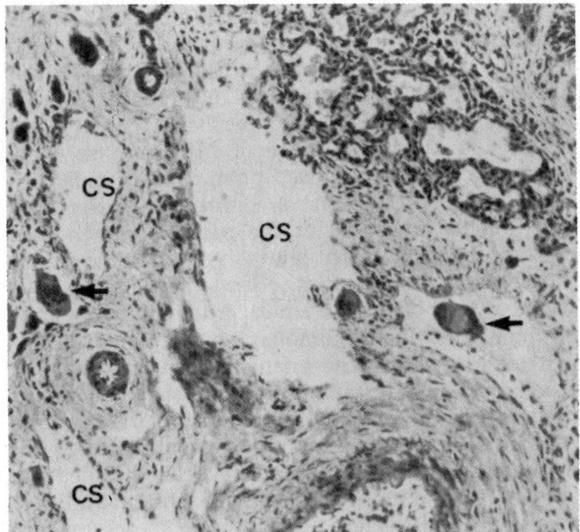

Figure 90–8. Human infant PIPE: The dilated cystic spaces (CS) represent the foci of interstitial emphysema. Note the multinucleated giant cells *(arrows)* within the connective tissue surrounding the cysts and within the cyst wall or along the border of the wall (hematoxylin and eosin, ×150).

temic vascular resistance increases with the removal of the placental circulation. In a premature infant, pulmonary circulation may remain vasoconstricted owing to hypoxia and acidosis, and the pulmonary vascular resistance may remain high. High pulmonary vascular resistance causes retention of the fetal components of circulation, and right-to-left shunts through the ductus arteriosus and foramen ovale further aggravate arterial hypoxemia. Such shunts may be 20% to 80% of cardiac output. It is unclear whether persistent patent ductus arteriosus is a primary cause of BPD or a secondary reflection of the compromised pulmonary vascular characteristics. ARDS has no counterparts to the patent ductus arteriosus or the patent foramen ovale; however, intrapulmonary shunts secondary to ventilation-perfusion abnormalities, edema, and atelectasis desaturate arterial blood to a similar extent.[15]

Chronic interstitial emphysema, a manifestation of barotrauma, is much more severe in infants than in adults. The lesion of interstitial emphysema in infants can result in persistent interstitial pulmonary emphysema or pneumatosis pulmonalis.[16] It follows the rupture of alveoli, during which air penetrates alveolar walls and traverses through the sheaths of blood vessels and bronchi to the mediastinum or the pericardium. If dissection occurs toward the periphery of the lung, rupture into the pleural space produces a pneumothorax. Affected infants usually have BPD and concomitantly develop numerous air-filled interstitial cysts, lined fully or in part by multinucleated giant cells (Fig. 90–8). The origin of the giant cells in these interstitial cystic lesions is uncertain. They may be histiocytes, alveolar cells displaced following rupture, or cells from the pulmonary lymphatics. Persistent interstitial pulmonary edema has not been described in the ARDS literature.

DIFFUSE ALVEOLAR DAMAGE

The clinical syndrome of acute respiratory failure due to noncardiogenic pulmonary edema (i.e., ARDS) can result from a host of insults, such as sepsis syndrome, pulmonary aspiration, disseminated vascular coagulation, severe pneumonia, bacteremia, long bone or pelvic fractures, hypertransfusions, and others.[17] Experimental models of ARDS have been produced by hydrochloric acid instillation, microemboli, oleic acid, and intravenous endotoxin and live bacterial infusions. The suspected mediators of the pulmonary microvascular injury include cellular (polymorphonuclear leukocytes, platelets, lymphocytes, macrophages) and humoral (complement activation, lipid mediators, coagulation/fibrinolytic system, kallikrein-kinin system, cytokine release, and histamine release) systems.[17, 18]

The pathologic hallmark of ARDS is the presence of DAD. Gross pathologic findings of DAD include heavy, beefy lungs that ooze fluid on cutting. Pathologic alterations include hyaline membrane formation, pulmonary edema, interstitial mononuclear cell infiltration, and resultant secondary changes.[2] These alterations represent the lung's nonspecific response to various agents, including noxious gas/fume exposures, shock due to various causes, toxic oxygen concentrations, and drugs.

DAD can be separated histopathologically into exudative and reparative (proliferative) phases.[2] The early stage of exudative DAD involves degeneration or necrosis of alveolar lining cells and endothelium; this increases the permeability of blood vessels and produces proteinaceous exudates. These proteinaceous exudates, plus the fragmented lining cells, are the origin of the nonhomogeneous structures of hyaline membranes. Microscopic findings during the 1- to 6-day exudative phase include pulmonary edema, hyaline membranes, alveolar wall edema, and microatelectasis (Figs. 90–9 and 90–10). Hyaline membranes are present at the respiratory bronchiolar and alveolar levels and particularly at the alveolar duct level (Fig. 90–11). Polymorphonuclear leukocytes appear in the edematous alveolar walls and alveolar spaces within 24 to 36 hours after injury. After 6 days, the reparative phase of DAD has usually begun and is characterized by hyperplasia of epithelial type II cells, an interstitial mononuclear inflammatory infiltrate, and the aggregation of hyaline membranes by mural application or encirclement with alveolar macrophages. Increased numbers of fibroblasts are noted in thickened alveolar walls and

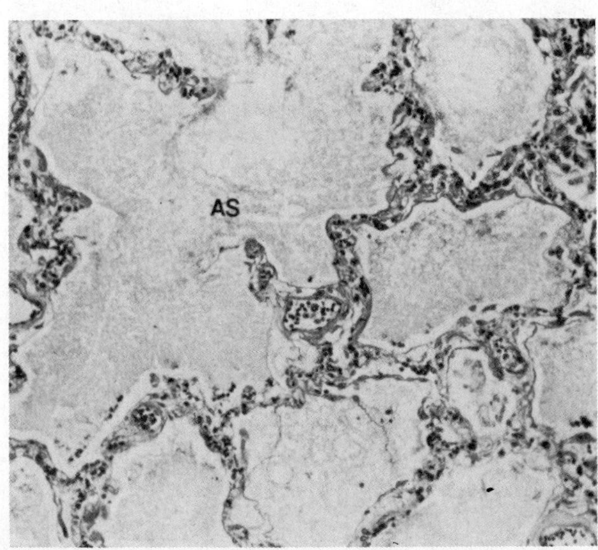

Figure 90–9. Adult patient material: Pulmonary edema is reflected by air spaces (AS) filled with proteinaceous material. The underlying alveolar walls are edematous, and the capillaries are congested (hematoxylin and eosin, ×150).

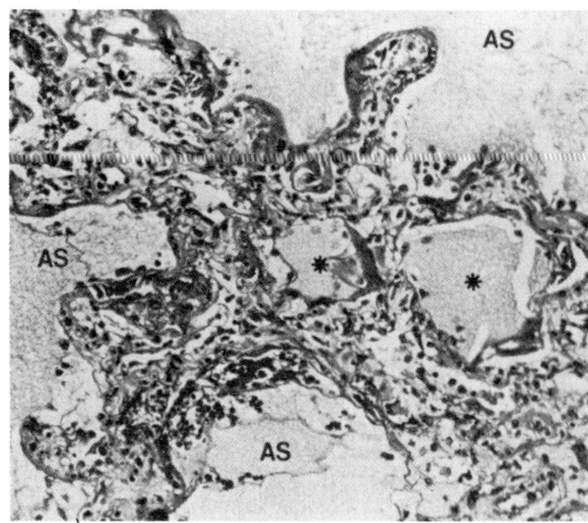

Figure 90–10. Adult patient material. Microatelectasis is characterized by nonuniformly sized air spaces, two of which have hyaline membranes *(asterisks)*. Surrounding alveolar ducts and dilated alveoli (AS) are lined by hyaline membranes. The walls of the collapsed alveoli show edema and an infiltrate of inflammatory cells (hematoxylin and eosin, ×150).

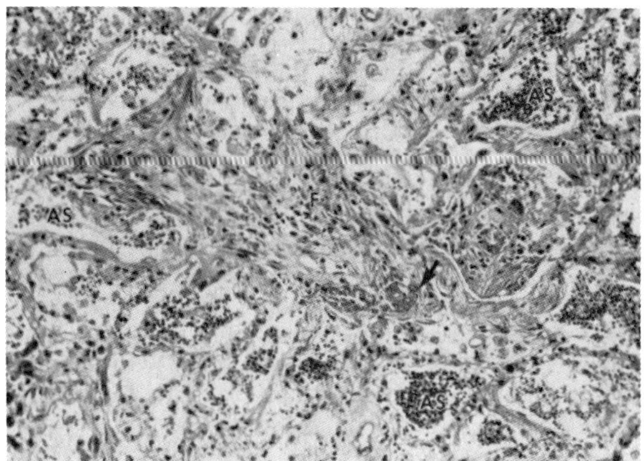

Figure 90–12. Adult patient material. In the reparative phase of DAD, the fibrin *(arrow)* is enmeshed in the fibroblastic proliferation (F). Several of the alveolar spaces (AS) contain extravasated red blood cells. The normal pulmonary architecture is distorted (hematoxylin and eosin, ×150).

in organizing alveolar exudates (Figs. 90–12 and 90–13). Fibrin is invariably found in those lesions with prominent fibroplasia. Fibrin strands are found within the damaged alveolar wall and free within the alveolar space, frequently forming a major component of the hyaline membrane. If the reparative phase is arrested, the lesion resolves. The reparative phase persists in a subset of patients in whom widespread fibrosis can ensue.

Because of the diverse and multiple factors that can elicit DAD in an adult, underlying damage may occur to either endothelial or alveolar epithelial cells. The edema of DAD has been characterized as protein-rich fluid resulting from increased permeability rather than increased hydrostatic pressure.[15] Idell and colleagues have demonstrated that the bronchoalveolar lavage fluids of patients with ARDS have an increase in total protein and procoagulant activity.[19] The procoagulant activity is attributed to the expression of tissue factor associated with Factor VII (the extrinsic activation complex). Conversely, fibrinolytic activity is depressed, favoring tissue fibrin deposition and retention.

Baboon models have been used to study the development of experimental respiratory failure in adult nonhuman primates.[20] An intravenous injection of oleic acid followed by ventilation with 100% oxygen or 100% oxygen only for 5 to 7 days produces acute, diffuse lung injury. Intrapulmonary shunting reduces lung compliance and causes hypoxemia. Histologic studies reveal endothelial injury, pulmonary edema, hyaline membranes (Fig. 90–14), an influx of polymorphonuclear leukocytes after 24 hours, and a reparative response of epithelial type 2 hyperplasia and intra-alveolar organization of fibrinous exudate in animals surviving 5

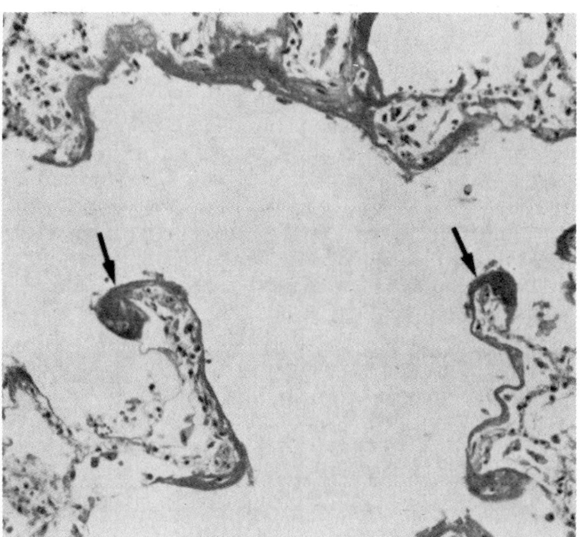

Figure 90–11. Adult patient material. At the alveolar duct site, hyaline membranes are plastered against underlying wall structures *(arrows)*. The pulmonary parenchyma is edematous (hematoxylin and eosin, ×150).

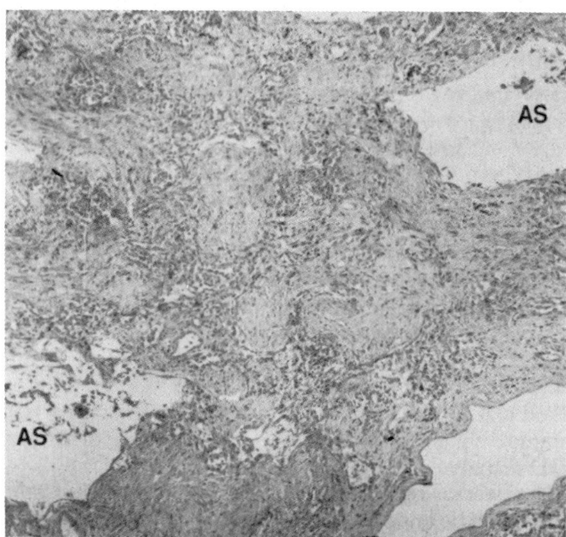

Figure 90–13. Adult patient material. Normal pulmonary architecture is absent in this markedly fibrotic specimen. Only a few cystic air spaces (AS) are present; the remainder is fibrotic tissue and scattered inflammatory cells (hematoxylin and eosin, × 100).

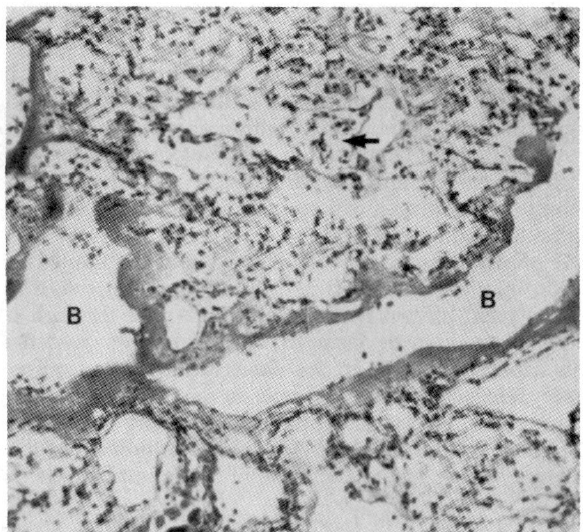

Figure 90–14. Adult baboon model of DAD. This oleic acid–induced lesion shows underlying alveolar wall edema *(arrow)*. The respiratory bronchioles (B) are covered with hyaline membranes (hematoxylin and eosin, ×150).

days or more. This histopathologic finding of intramural organization of exudate correlates well with the coagulation and fibrinolytic findings in bronchoalveolar lavage fluids, which are comparable to those of humans with ARDS.[21] Unlike infants with BPD, the fibrinolytic system in adults remains impaired; thus, the intra-alveolar coagulum is not lysed and undergoes fibrocellular organization and fibrosis.[19]

The atelectasis of DAD is predominantly microscopic; a diffuse but focal reduction in the size of alveolar spaces is observed, rather than the large, confluent loss of air-containing spaces characteristic of HMD.

FACTORS AFFECTING BOTH HYALINE MEMBRANE DISEASE–BRONCHOPULMONARY DYSPLASIA AND DIFFUSE ALVEOLAR DAMAGE

Oxygen

For years, investigators have incriminated oxygen treatment as the primary injurant responsible for the development of BPD. The important role of oxygen in the lesions in infants and adults is no doubt the recruitment of white blood cells from the vascular stream into the alveolar space through release of chemotactic factors,[17] especially from alveolar macrophages.[18] The resulting accumulation of neutrophils shows evidence of activation, and the cells generate elevated levels of oxygen metabolites that are widely thought to induce cellular damage. Susceptibility to oxygen injury is documented to vary with development and among species.[22] These findings have been explained by the lack of an antioxidant enzymatic response. Data now exist to refute that a human fetal lung is more sensitive to oxygen than is an adult's lung. Normal human infants and infants with respiratory distress syndrome have comparable superoxide dismutase activities in lungs and blood,[23] despite the use of oxygen therapy in the infants with HMD, which would have been expected to increase superoxide dismutase activity. Strange and associates described similar expression of antioxidant enzyme levels in human premature infants and in adults,[24] negating the argument that infants with HMD have an increased susceptibility to oxygen toxicity. In the baboon models of HMD-BPD, the neonates show induction of antioxidant enzymes and have an increased resistance to oxygen injury when compared with comparably treated adults.[9, 20]

The decreasing order of susceptibility to oxygen injury appears to be endothelial cells, type I cells, and then type II cells.[25] Because a premature infant's lungs are lined more extensively with alveolar type II cells than are an adult's lungs, a premature lung may show fewer epithelial changes. Oxygen can produce DAD lesions and is frequently used to produce animal models of ARDS. The time of onset of edema, atelectasis, and evident cellular injury varies from species to species, but the histology of the lesions is usually similar.[22, 26] In addition to directly causing DAD, oxygen toxicity increases mortality or cellular damage in animals with DAD of multiple causes (viral pneumonia, paraquat toxicity, hemorrhagic shock, ozone, butylated hydroxytoluene, and bleomycin). In mice, oxygen toxicity leads to necrotizing bronchiolitis,[27] similar to that described in baboons with BPD.[9] Although barotrauma could have been an additive component to the severity of the airway lesions described by Northway and colleagues (positive end-expiratory pressure was not widely used until the 1970s),[4] the lack of marked airway changes in the BPD now noted may primarily reflect the more judicious use of oxygen. The author's newborn baboon models have always been ventilated with positive end-expiratory pressure, so the striking airway lesions are thought to represent primarily an oxygen-induced lesion. Several species when exposed to elevated oxygen concentrations for weeks to months have emphysema with underlying extensive fibrosis.[9] The findings are similar to the pattern of alternating overdistention and fibrosis described in BPD.

Several studies have attempted to define safe concentrations of oxygen that do not interfere with the reparative regeneration of alveolar epithelial cells or that retard the development of lung fibrosis.[28, 29] This is especially problematic for prematurely delivered infants because of the hypoxic in utero environment (arterial partial pressure of oxygen of 25–35 mm Hg), so room air probably represents a hyperoxic exposure.

Infection

Bronchopulmonary infection may affect the underlying pathology of both HMD and DAD. Gram-negative nosocomial pneumonias in human adults are usually preceded by upper respiratory tract colonization,[30] which alters respiratory tract epithelial cell adherence properties. Upper respiratory epithelial cells of seriously ill patients avidly bind gram-negative bacilli to their surfaces, whereas cells from normal individuals do not.[31] The occurrence of pneumonia, usually due to gram-negative bacteria in the setting of acute respiratory failure, is frequent[30] and greatly complicates patient care and outcome. A lung injured by DAD has a diminished capacity for antimicrobial defense.[32]

In the 1980s, bacterial colonization of neonates was dominated by coagulase-negative staphylococci, which can be associated with infection but usually do not cause life-threatening infections. When neonatal patients become colonized and then infected with gram-negative organisms, comparable clinical management problems and serious pneumonias occur, comparable to those in adult patients.[33]

Baboon models of BPD and ARDS have documented a sequential pathogenetic pattern of colonization and infection. Colonization of the upper respiratory tract simultaneously occurs with colonization of the trachea, or the nose or pharynx is colonized initially followed by colonization of the trachea. Of those organisms isolated in the trachea, one or more are found in the lungs of animals at autopsy, indicating that microaspiration of tracheal secretions occurred.[34, 35] In adults, gram-negatives dominate as the colonizing and infective microbes.[34] In infants, coagulase-negative staphylococci dominate the colonization pattern, and gram-negatives are acquired later in the hospital course.[35]

The exact incidence of pneumonia in either HMD or DAD is difficult to establish. In our series of 77 necropsies in DAD nonsurvivors, 72% had histologic evidence of pneumonia.[36] In a group of 27 patients reviewed in detail, the clinical diagnosis of pneumonia or the diagnosis of only DAD was in error 30% of the time because virtually all the patients had fever, leukocytosis, radiographic infiltrates, and pathogenic bacteria in respiratory secretions.[37] In patients with HMD or DAD, the effects of nosocomial pneumonia on the repair of the injured lung are not known, although an association between lung infection and the occurrence of lung fibrosis after DAD has been suggested.[38, 39] Pneumonia alone can cause pulmonary fibrosis; however, this is an unusual outcome of pyogenic pneumonia. The exact incidence of pneumonia in infants with HMD-BPD has not been documented.

The influence of infection on a damaged lung has been assessed in the baboon model. Ventilation of adult baboons with 80% oxygen for 11 days induces a mild lung lesion, whereas ventilation with 80% oxygen for 6 days followed by an inoculation of *Pseudomonas aeruginosa* and further ventilation for 5 days with 50% oxygen results in physiologic, morphologic, and morphometric changes comparable to a severe 100% oxygen insult.[20] This synergistic effect of hyperoxia and infection very likely reflects the frequent evolution of ARDS in patients in intensive care units.

The potential additive or synergistic effect of infection on a BPD-injured lung has not been quantitatively studied in a clinical setting. Vapaavuori and Krohn[40] correlated clinical symptoms with pathology in 27 premature infants treated with intermittent positive-pressure ventilation. A histologic diagnosis of pneumonia was confirmed in 10 patients, 6 of whom had bacterial cultures revealing gram-negative bacilli. The diagnosis of pneumonia had been clinically suspected in nine of the cases. The role of *Ureaplasma* organisms in the pathogenesis of BPD has received attention, but only association with BPD and not causation has yet been determined.[41]

It is now recognized that most patients with ARDS die as a result of infection combined with multiple organ failure, not respiratory failure.[36, 42, 43] The lung and abdomen have been identified as troublesome sources of infection in patients with ARDS.[42, 43] Additional prospective studies are needed to properly assess the suspected, though unproven, role of infection in the evolution of BPD.

Mechanical Ventilation

At this time, there is enormous interest in unraveling the potentially deleterious effects of mechanical ventilation on lungs of both infants and adults.[44, 45] Much of this renewed interest in barotrauma-induced lung disease results from the development of new ventilatory modalities such as high-frequency ventilation. In this era, barotrauma-induced lung disease not only includes the gross air-leak problems of interstitial pulmonary edema, pneumothorax, pneumomediastinum, and so forth but also implies a microscopic lesion of epithelial disruption and a resulting permeability edema lesion.[44, 45] An emerging consensus is that any ventilatory modality or maneuver that induces any form of overinflation is the underlying genesis of the lung injury, so-called volutrauma.[44] Finding ways to monitor lung volumes rather than just the airway pressure may be the key to preventing damage to healthy lungs and avoiding further injury to diseased lungs.

Regardless of these conceptual aspects, the use of positive-pressure ventilation is associated with the development of interstitial emphysema or air leak problems in infants and adults. It is strongly implicated in the development of BPD in infants with HMD.[46] Persistent abnormalities in lung function after recovery from HMD correlate more closely with the use of intermittent positive-pressure ventilation than with oxygen exposure.[47]

An ARDS study reported a positive correlation between the magnitude of applied airway pressure and the amount of collagen deposited in the lungs.[48] The role of volutrauma in the initiation and propagation of lung injury and repair needs extensive study.

Other Factors

Infants and adults in respiratory failure share the risk of fluid overload.[49, 50] Both HMD-BPD and DAD are associated with injury of the pulmonary vasculature and fluid loading, which increases hydrostatic pressure in the vascular bed and increases fluid loss into the interstitial and alveolar spaces. This concept is supported by the shock and trauma literature discussing possible hazards of massive crystalloid replacement during resuscitation[51] and by the experimentally increased accumulation of water in the lungs of oleic acid–injured dogs.[52]

Other factors that may influence HMD and DAD are the coagulation, fibrinolytic, kallikrein-kinin, arachidonic acid cascade, and angiotensin systems, as well as prostaglandins. The kallikrein-kinin system apparently is activated at birth to assist in closure of the ductus arteriosus. It decreases pulmonary vascular resistance, increases umbilical vascular resistance, and accelerates coagulation and fibrinolysis. Fibrinolytic activity is increased in the intrapartum and early postpartum periods. Premature infants have low blood plasminogen levels and high titers of plasmin inhibitors.[14] In infants with HMD, an inhibitor of plasminogen activation may prevent normal fibrinolytic processes, allowing fibrin to accumulate in the hyaline membranes. Also, alpha$_1$-antitrypsin, a potent plasmin inhibitor, is low in the cord blood of infants who develop HMD; its plasma level is inversely correlated with the severity of the illness. Whether the deficiency of this protein in blood is a cause or a result of HMD is unclear, because alpha$_1$-antitrypsin has been demonstrated in the hyaline membranes of the affected infants.[14]

Coagulation abnormalities are commonly found in patients with ARDS[53] and have been recognized for many years as a common problem in sepsis. There are no definitive data to indicate whether the coagulopathy alone can cause DAD or whether the factor that elicited the injury activates the clotting system. It is probable that the kallikrein-kinin system and its role in the multiple cascades will be important in clarifying the consequences of lung injury. Many of the potent enzymes found in these various cascades are processed in the lungs, and it is still unclear how effectively a damaged endothelium can properly perform this function.

OUTCOMES OF HYALINE MEMBRANE DISEASE–BRONCHOPULMONARY DYSPLASIA AND DIFFUSE ALVEOLAR DAMAGE

The advent of better ventilatory techniques, the antenatal administration of glucocorticoid, and the intratracheal instillation of surfactants have changed the morbidity of infants born at 32 weeks or more of gestation. Previously, infants who survived the first 72 hours of HMD improved dramatically and had no evident pulmonary impairment;[1] however, a small percentage have abnormal results of pulmonary function tests during the first year after recovery, as well as more frequent respiratory tract infections.[54] Children who have had HMD and who have lived for 5 to 10 years after their disease appear to have nearly complete recovery.[55] The low-birth-weight infants who survive respiratory distress syndrome have a low maximum expiratory flow at age 8 to 10 years.[56]

In those infants with HMD who develop BPD, bronchial hyperreactivity, increased small-airway resistance, and abnormal blood gas levels have been identified during the first year after recovery in survivors who are 7 to 9 years old and in young adults.[57] Northway and colleagues have reported the late pulmonary sequelae of BPD in 26 young adults born between 1964 and 1973.[58] Mean values for all tests of airway function were reduced by 25% to 50%, and more than half the group had physiologic evidence of obstruction of the airways. Low-birth-weight infants will in all likelihood have substantial sequelae, because the lungs are so immature. Twenty-eight weeks' gestation marks the beginning of the saccular period of lung development, during which secondary crests arise from airspace walls to form the primitive alveoli (saccules). Alveolarization usually begins at 32 weeks, and at normal completion of gestation, approximately one fourth to one half are formed, with the remainder added during infancy and probably completed by age 2.[12, 59] This timetable readily points out that the chronic lung injury of very immature infants who are now being treated in neonatal intensive care units will undoubtedly interfere with the lungs' program for future growth and development. Functionally, the impairment will probably be manifested at the alveolar level rather than at that of the airway.

In adults who survive an episode of ARDS, lung function usually shows little or no long-term impairment.[60] Approximately one third of adult survivors may demonstrate some abnormality in diffusing capacity, vital capacity, or total lung capacity. Peters and colleagues[60] demonstrated that long-term abnormalities of pulmonary function in ARDS survivors are not related to initial lung impairment but are directly related to persistence of impaired lung function during the acute episode.

There are few data correlating the pathologic findings of DAD with the clinical outcome of ARDS. Lung biopsy specimens are similar in both survivors and nonsurvivors of shock-lung syndrome. ARDS survivors show little or no functional impairment after recovery, but the possibility of residual lung damage cannot be precluded. In baboons, lung function is severely impaired after induction of DAD with oleic acid, but functional abnormalities disappear as the reparative processes resolve over 6 months.

SUMMARY

HMD and DAD have many common histologic characteristics; however, there are significant differences. The fetal parenchyma is characterized by thick-walled saccules with capillaries directly beneath the epithelium on both sides. Pulmonary arteries are thick walled, and the prominent intra-alveolar septa contain relatively large lymphatic vessels. The inflation pattern in HMD is characterized by rather uniform atelectatic involvement.[3] Before the use of surfactant treatment in HMD, infants who developed BPD consistently had an altered inflation pattern of atelectasis and overinflation. In adults, the inflation pattern has more uneven atelectatic involvement of alveolar units;[38] areas of microatelectasis may be separated by histologically normal alveoli.

HMD is initiated by a deficiency in surfactant, resulting in high surface tension forces at the terminal sac or alveolar level and failure of airspace expansion.[1] In DAD, either epithelial or endothelial cell injury increases permeability, with resultant edema formation and hyaline membrane deposition; some surfactant abnormalities may result, but DAD is not a primary surfactant-deficiency disease. However, various insults associated with HMD, such as asphyxia, meconium aspiration, or shock, may elicit a DAD response—albeit with modifications due to differences in the structure and function of the immature lung.

Thus, HMD-BPD and DAD are characterized by an increased permeability lesion that gives rise to pulmonary edema and hyaline membrane formation; however, fibrinolytic activity is evident in infants, and it yields a different reparative pattern of fibroplasia. Both HMD-BPD and DAD are affected by high oxygen concentrations, which no doubt influence the evolution of HMD-BPD and DAD. Mechanical ventilation is now thought to have an even more important role in potentiating and aggravating lung injury. Pulmonary infection severely complicates both syndromes, and infection or its complications are the leading cause of death in patients with ARDS. The role of various mediators and other plasma proteins in the evolution of these processes is worthy of intense investigation. Continued research efforts to identify the cause of the permeability damage associated with these syndromes should be accompanied by clinical prevention of amplifying factors, especially infection.

References

1. Avery ME, Fletcher BP, Williams RG: The Lung and Its Disorders in the Newborn Infant. 4th ed. Philadelphia, WB Saunders, 1981, pp 222–274, 284–302.
2. Katzenstein AA, Askin FB: Surgical pathology of non-neoplastic lung disease. *In*: Major Problems in Pathology. 2nd ed. Vol 13. Bennington JL (Ed). Philadelphia, WB Saunders, 1990, pp 9–57.
3. Singer DB: Morphology of hyaline membrane disease and its pulmonary sequelae. *In*: Hyaline Membrane Disease Pathogenesis and Pathophysiology. Stern L (Ed). New York, Grune & Stratton, 1984, pp 63–96.
4. Northway WH Jr, Rosan RC, Porter DY: Pulmonary disease following respirator therapy of hyaline-membrane disease: Bronchopulmonary dysplasia. N Engl J Med 1967; 276:357.
5. Bonikos DS, Bensch KG, Northway WH Jr, et al: Bronchopulmonary dysplasia: The pulmonary pathologic sequel of necrotizing bronchiolitis and pulmonary fibrosis. Hum Pathol 1976; 7:643.
6. Stocker JT: Pathologic features of long-standing "healed" bronchopulmonary dysplasia. Hum Pathol 1986; 17:943.
7. Chambers HM, Van Velzen D: Ventilator-related pathology in the extremely immature lung. Pathology 1989; 21:79.
8. Van Lierde S, Cornelis A, Devlieger H, et al: Different patterns of pulmonary sequelae after hyaline membrane disease: Heterogeneity of bronchopulmonary dysplasia? Biol Neonate 1991; 60:152.
9. Coalson JJ, Kuehl TJ, Prihoda TJ, et al: Diffuse alveolar damage in the evolution of bronchopulmonary dysplasia in the baboon. Pediatr Res 1988; 24:357.
10. Coalson JJ, Winter VT, Idell S, et al: Pathophysiologic, morphometric and biochemical studies in the premature baboon with bronchopulmonary dysplasia. Am Rev Respir Dis 1992; 145:872.
11. Idell S, Koenig KB, et al: Pathways of fibrin turnover in lavage of premature baboons with hyperoxic lung injury. Am J Respir Crit Care Med 1994; 149:767–775.

11a. Coalson JJ, Winter VT, deLemos RA: Decreased alveolarization in long-term baboon survivors with bronchopulmonary dysplasia. Pediatr Res 1994; 35:329A.

12. Thurlbeck WM: Postnatal human lung growth. Thorax 1982; 37:564.

13. Seidner S, McCurnin D, Coalson J, et al: A new model of chronic lung injury in surfactant-treated preterm baboons delivered at very early gestations. Clin Res 1992; 40:825A.
14. Stalcup SA, Mellins RB: Acute respiratory distress in the newborn infant. *In*: Pulmonary Diseases and Disorders. Fishman AP (Ed). New York, McGraw-Hill, 1980, pp 1653–1666.
15. Connors AF, McCaffree DR, Rogers RM: The adult respiratory distress syndrome. Disease-a-Month 1981; 27:1.
16. Stocker JT, Madewell JE: Persistent interstitial pulmonary emphysema: Another complication of the respiratory distress syndrome. Pediatrics 1977; 59:847.
17. Simon RH, Ward PA: Adult respiratory distress syndrome. *In*: Inflammation: Basic Principles and Clinical Correlates. 2nd ed. Gallin JI, Goldstein IM, Snyderman R (Eds). New York, Raven Press, 1992, pp 999–1016.
18. Sibille Y, Reynolds HY: Macrophages and polymorphonuclear neutrophils in lung defense and injury. Am Rev Respir Dis 1990; 141:471.
19. Idell S, Gonzalez K, Bradford H, et al: Procoagulant activity in bronchoalveolar lavage in the adult respiratory distress syndrome: Contribution of tissue factor associated with factor VII. Am Rev Respir Dis 1987; 136:1466.
20. Coalson JJ, King RJ, Winter VT, et al: O_2 and pneumonia-induced lung injury. I. Pathological and morphometric studies. J Appl Physiol 1989; 67:346.
21. Idell S, Peters J, Gonzalez K, Fair D, et al: Local abnormalities of coagulation and fibrinolytic pathways which promote alveolar fibrin deposition in the lungs of baboons with diffuse alveolar damage. J Clin Invest 1989; 84:181.
22. Frank L: Effect of oxygen on the newborn. Fed Proc 1985; 44:2328.
23. Autor AP, Frank L, Roberts RJ: Developmental characteristics of pulmonary superoxide dismutase: Relationship to idiopathic respiratory distress syndrome. Pediatr Res 1976; 10:154.
24. Strange RC, Cotton W, Fryer AA, et al: Lipid peroxidation and expression of copper-zinc and manganese superoxide dismutase in lungs of premature infants with hyaline membrane disease and bronchopulmonary dysplasia. J Clin Lab Med 1990; 116:666.
25. Frank L, Massaro D: The lung and oxygen toxicity. Arch Intern Med 1979; 139:347.
26. Pratt PC: Pathology of pulmonary oxygen toxicity. Am Rev Respir Dis 1974; 110(Suppl):51.
27. Ludwin SK, Northway WH, Bensch KG: Oxygen toxicity in the newborn. Necrotizing bronchiolitis in mice exposed to 100 per cent oxygen. Lab Invest 1974; 31:425.
28. Hackney JD, Evans MJ, Spier CE, et al: Effect of high concentrations of oxygen on reparative regeneration of damaged alveolar epithelium in mice. Exp Mol Pathol 1981; 34:338.
29. Cheney FW, Huang TW, Gronka R: The effects of 50% oxygen on the resolution of pulmonary injury. Am Rev Respir Dis 1980; 122:373.
30. Johanson WG Jr, Pierce AK, Sanford JP, et al: Nosocomial respiratory infections with gram-negative bacilli: The significance of colonization of the respiratory tract. Ann Intern Med 1972; 77:701.
31. Johanson WG Jr, Higuchi JH, Chaudhuri TR, et al: Bacterial adherence to epithelial cells in bacillary colonization of the respiratory tract. Am Rev Respir Dis 1980; 121:55.
32. Harris GD, Johanson WG Jr, Pierce AK: Determinants of lung bacterial clearance in mice after acute hypoxia. Am Rev Respir Dis 1977; 116:671.
33. Hensey OJ, Hart CA, Cooke RWI: Serious infection in a neonatal intensive care unit: A two-year survey. J Hyg (Lond) 1985; 95:289–297.
34. Crouch TW, Higuchi JH, Johanson WG Jr: Pathogenesis and prevention of nosocomial pneumonia in a nonhuman primate model of acute respiratory failure. Am Rev Respir Dis 1984; 130:502.
35. Coalson JJ, Gerstmann DR, Winter VT, et al: Bacterial colonization and infection studies in the premature baboon with bronchopulmonary dysplasia. Am Rev Respir Dis 1991; 144:1140.
36. Coalson JJ: Pathology of sepsis, septic shock and multiple organ failure. *In*: New Horizons: Perspectives on Sepsis and Septic Shock. Sibbald WJ, Spring CL (Eds). Fullerton, CA, Society of Critical Care Medicine, 1986, pp 27–59.
37. Andrews CP, Coalson JJ, Smith JD, et al: Diagnosis of nosocomial bacterial pneumonia in acute, diffuse lung injury. Chest 1981; 80:254.
38. Lamy M, Fallat RJ, Koeniger E, et al: Pathologic features and mechanisms of hypoxemia in adult respiratory distress syndrome. Am Rev Respir Dis 1976; 114:267.
39. Ashbaugh DC, Petty TL: Sepsis complicating the acute respiratory distress syndrome. Surg Gynecol Obstet 1972; 135:865.
40. Vapaavuori EK, Krohn K: Intensive care of small premature infants. II. Postmortem findings. Acta Paediatr Scand 1971; 60:49.
41. Holtzman RB, Hageman JR, Yogev R: Role of *Ureaplasma urealyticum* in bronchopulmonary dysplasia. J Pediatr 1989; 114:1061.
42. Bell RC, Coalson JJ, Smith JD, et al: Multiple organ system failure and infection in adult respiratory distress syndrome. Ann Intern Med 1983; 99:293.
43. Montgomery AB, Stager MA, Carrico CJ, et al: Causes of mortality in patients with the adult respiratory distress syndrome. Am Rev Respir Dis 1985; 132:485.
44. Dreyfuss D, Saumon G: Barotrauma is volutrauma, but which volume is the one responsible? Intensive Care Med 1992; 18:139–141.
45. Parker JC, Hernandez LA, Peevy KJ: Mechanisms of ventilator-induced lung injury. Crit Care Med 1993; 21:131–143.
46. Taghizadeh A, Reynolds EOR: Pathogenesis of bronchopulmonary dysplasia following hyaline membrane disease. Am J Pathol 1976; 82:241.
47. Stocks J, Godfrey S, Reynolds EOR: Airway resistance in infants after various treatments for hyaline membrane disease: Special emphasis on prolonged high levels of inspired oxygen. Pediatrics 1978; 61:178.
48. Collins JF, Smith JD, Coalson JJ, et al: Variability in lung collagen amounts after prolonged support of acute respiratory failure. Chest 1984; 85:641.
49. Sladen A, Laver MB, Pontoppidan H: Pulmonary complications and water retention in prolonged mechanical ventilation. N Engl J Med 1968; 279:448.
50. Brown ER, Stark A, Sosenko I, et al: Bronchopulmonary dysplasia: Possible relationship to pulmonary edema. J Pediatr 1978; 92:982.
51. Shoemaker WC, Hauser CJ: Critique of crystalloid versus colloid therapy in shock and shock lung. Crit Care Med 1979; 7:117.
52. Prewitt RM, McCarthy J, Wood LDH: Treatment of acute low pressure pulmonary edema in dogs: Relative effects of hydrostatic and oncotic pressure, nitroprusside, and positive end-expiratory pressure. J Clin Invest 1981; 67:409.
53. Rodvien R: Hematologic observations made in patients with acute respiratory distress syndrome in the Cooperative ECMO Project. Artif Organs 1978; 2:12.
54. Outerbridge EW, Nogrady MB, Beaudry PH, et al: Idiopathic respiratory distress syndrome. Recurrent respiratory illness in survivors. Am J Dis Child 1972; 123:99.
55. Stahlman M, Hedvall G, Lindstrom K, et al: Role of hyaline membrane disease in production of later childhood lung abnormalities. Pediatrics 1982; 69:572.
56. Tammela OKT, Linna OVE, Koivisto ME: Long-term pulmonary sequelae in low birthweight infants with and without respiratory distress syndrome. Acta Paediatr Scand 1991; 80:542.
57. Wohl MEB: Bronchopulmonary dysplasia in adulthood. N Engl J Med 1990; 323:1834.
58. Northway WH Jr, Moss RB, Carlisle KB, et al: Late pulmonary sequelae of bronchopulmonary dysplasia. N Engl J Med 1990; 323:1793.
59. Langston C, Kida K, Reed M, et al: Human lung growth in late gestation and in the neonate. Am Rev Respir Dis 1984; 129:607.
60. Peters JI, Bell RC, Prihoda TJ, et al: Clinical determinants of abnormalities in pulmonary functions in survivors of the adult respiratory distress syndrome. Am Rev Respir Dis 1989; 139:1163.

CHAPTER 91

Surfactant Physiology, Metabolism, Function, and Replacement Therapy

Kristine M. McCulloch, MD • Dharmapuri Vidyasagar, MD

Understanding the role of surfactant in pulmonary physiology and disease is important for the appropriate use of surfactant replacement therapy in critical care medicine.

SURFACTANT PHYSIOLOGY

The unique contributions of surfactant to the respiratory system are functions of its composition, physical behavior, and chemical properties.

Surfactant is a complex mixture of components. The chemical composition of surfactant from various mammalian species is quite similar (Table 91–1). Surfactant can be prepared from lung homogenates and from the fluid obtained by bronchoalveolar lavage (BAL). The latter represents surfactant that has been secreted into the alveoli. Surfactant usually is isolated by differential centrifugation. It comprises approximately 90% lipid, approximately 10% protein, and very small quantities of carbohydrate. Approximately 50% by weight of surfactant lipid is fully saturated phosphatidylcholine, mostly dipalmitoyl phosphatidylcholine (DPPC). Unsaturated phosphatidylcholines and acidic phospholipids, such as phosphatidylglycerol (PG) and phosphatidylinositol (PI), are present in smaller amounts. Approximately 10% by weight of total lipid is neutral lipid, mostly cholesterol.[1–4] Approximately two thirds of the protein in surfactant is derived from serum.[5] Four lung-specific nonserum proteins, SP-A, SP-B, SP-C, and SP-D, have been found in close association with surfactant phospholipids (Table 91–2).[4, 6, 7]

Pulmonary gas exchange occurs at the interface between alveolar air and the extracellular fluid subphase of the alveolar lining. Surface tension is the contractile force on the alveolar surface produced by attractive forces between the molecules of the fluid subphase. The problem of alveolar stability may be understood by the Laplace relationship for a sphere. Surface pressure (P) is directly related to twice the surface tension (T) and inversely related to the radius (R):

$$P = 2T/R$$

The alveolar surface pressure that is generated by its surface tension is mechanically opposed by transpulmonary pressure. During expiration, transpulmonary pressure decreases and the radius and surface area of the alveolus become smaller. Unless surface tension is lowered during expiration, the pressure on the alveolar surface exceeds transpulmonary pressure and the alveolus collapses.[8, 9] Surfactant coats the alveolar surface area as a monomolecular film that is capable of decreasing its molecular surface area as the alveolus contracts during expiration. The reduction of molecular surface area decreases the alveolar surface tension, thereby preventing the alveolar collapse that would be predicted from the Laplace relationship. Surface balance measurements confirm that when a film of surfactant is compressed, surface tension decreases as surface area decreases.[2, 3, 8]

The upper limit of alveolar surface tension consistent with alveolar stability at end-expiration was calculated by King and Clements using transpulmonary pressure and the rate of change of surface area with change in volume and was determined to be 10 dyne/cm. These investigators demonstrated in vitro at 37°C that surfactant lowers surface tension to less than 10 dyne/cm, shows small surface compressibility, and exhibits rapid rates of movement from a liquid subphase and of adsorption onto the air-liquid interface.[1] These properties account for the ability of the lungs to expand from a collapsed state after just a few inflations and to maintain a residual volume at low pressures.

DPPC is the only component of surfactant with enough molecular compressibility to lower alveolar surface tension adequately and with a sufficiently slow rate of monolayer collapse to keep surface tension low and alveoli open for the duration of the respiratory cycle. The choline moiety is in the polar head group of the DPPC molecule, which is hydrophilic and thus aligns on the aqueous side of the air-liquid interface. The two fully saturated palmitic acid residues are on the opposite, nonpolar end of the DPPC molecule, which is hydrophobic and points toward the gaseous phase. The very straight, fully saturated palmitic acid chains allow close packing of the DPPC molecules. As surface area decreases, less compressible molecules may be forced out of the surface film, leaving concentrated amounts of DPPC.[2, 3, 10] Thus, DPPC is the surfactant component responsible for lowering alveolar surface tension and preventing alveolar collapse.

The ability of surfactant to form a surface film also depends on its rates of diffusion through the liquid subphase and of spread onto the air-liquid interface. By itself, DPPC diffuses and spreads slowly.[2] Thus, other surfactant components must be responsible for its rapid adsorption in vivo and in vitro. Unsaturated phosphatidylcholines, neutral lipids, and surfactant-associated proteins SP-A, SP-B, and SP-C all appear to promote adsorption of DPPC to the air-

TABLE 91–1. Biochemical Composition of Pulmonary Surfactant

Component	
Lipid	85–90%
Phospholipids	75–85%
PC	60–70%
DSPC	40–45% (DPPC >90%)
PG, PI, PE	10–15%
Lyso-PC, SM	5–10%
Neutral lipids	5–10% (predominantly cholesterol)
Protein	5–10%
Carbohydrate	5%

Abbreviations: PC = phosphatidylcholine; DSPC = disaturated phosphatidylcholine; PG = phosphatidylglycerol; PI = phosphatidylinositol; PE = phosphatidylethanolamine; Lyso-PC = lysophosphatidylcholine; SM = sphingomyelin; DPPC = dipalmitoylphosphatidylcholine.

TABLE 91–2. Surfactant Proteins

Type	*Monomer Size (Da)*	*Predominant Oligomer*
SP-A	30,000–36,000	Trimer
SP-B	8000	Dimer
SP-C	3800	Dimer
SP-D	43,000	Trimer

liquid interface.[2, 4, 7] The poor adsorption velocity of pure DPPC may be due to the fact that it exists in the gel state at 37°C, whereas its phase transition to the liquid state occurs at 41°C. Unsaturated phosphatidylcholines and neutral lipids have phase transition temperatures of less than 37°C, and they may cause the surfactant mixture to be in the liquid phase at 37°C, thereby increasing its adsorption rate in vivo.[2, 9] SP-A also may enhance surfactant adsorption by favoring the transition of its lipids to the liquid phase at lower temperatures.[7, 9]

Surfactant is found in the type II alveolar cells in storage and secretory organelles called *lamellar bodies*. Surfactant phospholipids and surfactant-associated proteins are packed in folded layers that surround a proteinaceous core. The lamellar bodies are enclosed by a limiting membrane that participates in the exocytotic process of surfactant secretion. The limiting membrane of the lamellar body fuses with the plasma membrane of the type II cell, and surfactant is released into the extracellular fluid subphase of the alveolar lining.[2, 3, 8] After secretion, some of the lamellae are converted to tubular myelin by a calcium-dependent process of aggregation of phospholipids that is markedly enhanced by SP-A and SP-B. It is from tubular myelin that surfactant is believed to move to the air-liquid interface to form a surface film.[4, 5, 7]

The surfactant-associated proteins are found in type II alveolar cells and in the nonciliated bronchiolar cells, or Clara cells. These proteins are involved in various ways in surfactant physiology. SP-A is a water-soluble protein whose structure includes a collagen-like region and a carbohydrate-binding C-terminal. SP-A does not lower surface tension. It promotes surface adsorption when added to DPPC with SP-B or SP-C or both but has no significant effect on phospholipid adsorption by itself. In the presence of calcium, SP-A enhances lipid aggregation, and thus it can promote the transformation of lamellar body contents into tubular myelin. SP-A has been shown to increase the phagocytosis of bacteria by alveolar macrophages, a function that may involve the carbohydrate-binding portion of its structure. SP-B and SP-C are hydrophobic proteins. SP-B and, to a lesser extent, SP-C enhance the ability of phospholipids to reduce surface tension. SP-B or SP-C promotes surfactant adsorption. SP-B acts with SP-A to convert lamellae to tubular myelin. SP-D is water soluble and is structurally similar to SP-A. Thus, it may also have a role in the clearance of bacteria from the lower airway.[4, 6, 7]

SURFACTANT METABOLISM

Surfactant Phospholipid Synthesis

Synthesis of surfactant phospholipids occurs only in type II alveolar cells. The initial compound is glycerol-3-phosphate, which is formed from dihydroxyacetone phosphate in an adult or from glycogen in a fetus. New fatty acids may be synthesized from lactate, or circulating fatty acids can be used. Acylation of glycerol-3-phosphate by glycerol-3-phosphate acyltransferase produces palmitoyl-sn-glycerol-3-phosphate, which is further acylated by 1-acylglycerol-3-phosphate acyltransferase to phosphatidic acid, from which diacylglycerols are formed. When palmitoyl-CoA is the principal acyl donor, disaturated phosphatidic acid predominates.

Choline is taken up efficiently by type II cells and is acted on sequentially by choline kinase and phosphocholine cytidyltransferase to form cytidine-diphosphocholine (CDP-choline). Phosphatidylcholines are formed from diacylglycerols and CDP-choline by cholinephosphotransferase. DPPC may be formed de novo by the type II cell from disaturated phosphatidic acid and CDP-choline. DPPC also can be produced by the remodeling of unsaturated phosphatidylcholines through deacylation by phospholipase A, followed either by transacylation by lysophosphatidylcholine acyltransferase or by reacylation with palmitoyl-CoA.

The precursor for both PG and PI is CDP-diacylglycerol. It is formed from cytidine triphosphate and phosphatidic acid by phosphatidate cytidyltransferase. Phosphatidylglycerolphosphate, formed by CDP-diacylglycerol glycerolphosphate phosphatidyltransferase, is dephosphorylated to form PG. Conversion of CDP-diacylglycerol by CDP-diacylglycerol inositol phosphatidyltransferase produces PI.[9–11] During gestation, the relative amounts of these acidic phospholipids in pulmonary surfactant show predictable changes that have been useful in assessing fetal lung maturity. The relative quantity of PG is much lower than that of PI until about 36 weeks' gestation in a human fetus, when a sudden increase in PG synthesis causes a marked change in the ratio. This change is delayed in infants of diabetic mothers. Normally, the PG:PI ratio increases from 0.04 at 35 weeks' gestation to 1.75 at term. One reason for this change may be a decline in the amount of inositol available for synthesis of PI. Another possible explanation is that the cytidine monophosphate, formed from increased phosphatidylcholine synthesis at term, may enhance the conversion of PI to inositol and CDP-diacylglycerol, which then is available for PG synthesis. In vitro studies of human fetal lung cells have shown that glucocorticoids with prolactin or insulin increase the ratio of the rates of lamellar body synthesis of PG:PI from 0.4 to 1.6. Increased amounts of PG in pulmonary surfactant result in detectable PG in amniotic fluid, in amounts that correlate with fetal lung maturity.[10, 12]

Newly synthesized surfactant phospholipids are transferred from the endoplasmic reticulum to the Golgi apparatus. From the Golgi complex, they must be moved to the lamellar bodies. This may be accomplished by vesicular transport, in which small, dense lamellar bodies carry phospholipid from the Golgi apparatus to the large, less dense lamellar bodies.[3, 11]

Hyaline membrane disease (HMD) is primarily a result of surfactant deficiency in prematurely born infants. The developmental regulation of surfactant phospholipid synthesis is relevant to the occurrence of HMD. As in other mammals, the human fetus does not synthesize and secrete surfactant until gestation is approximately 80% complete. Although lamellar bodies are seen by 20 to 22 weeks and become numerous after 25 weeks, surfactant can be detected in amniotic fluid only after 30 to 32 weeks' gestation. Glucocorticoids increase the activities of phosphatidylcholine cytidyltransferase, cholinephosphotransferase, and possibly lysophosphatidylcholine acyltransferase and thus increase the synthesis of DPPC. Thyroid hormones, cyclic adenosine monophosphate (cAMP), prolactin, estrogen, and growth factors all have been shown to increase phospholipid synthesis by fetal lung cells. In rat, rabbit, and human fetuses, glucocorticoids and triiodothyronine (T_3) have additive or synergistic effects on phosphatidylcholine synthesis. Glucocorticoids plus cAMP analog or glucocorticoids plus theophylline (which increases cellular cAMP) are supra-additive in enhancing the rate of DPPC synthesis by fetal lung cells. In clinical practice, the incidence of HMD in premature infants can be decreased by giving glucocorticoids to pregnant women in preterm labor. Because infants of diabetic mothers are at increased risk for HMD, studies of the effects of insulin are of interest. One study demonstrated that glucocorticoids with prolactin or insulin stimulated DPPC synthesis and surfactant secretion by human fetal lung cells better than did each hormone by itself. However, other investigators have shown that insulin antagonizes the enhancement of DPPC synthesis by glucocorticoids.[10, 12]

Surfactant Protein Synthesis

Surfactant-associated proteins are synthesized in type II cells and possibly in Clara cells. Genes encoding for human SP-A, SP-B, and SP-C are located on chromosomes 10, 2, and 8, respectively. Precursor proteins are produced in the endoplasmic reticulum. Post-translational products then undergo extensive modification. The proteins are completely processed by the time they reach the lamellar bodies.[4, 11] The lipid and protein components of surfactant probably are integrated in the lamellar bodies and secreted simultaneously into the extracellular fluid subphase.[3, 9, 10]

In vitro studies of fetal lung cells demonstrate that the developmental regulation of surfactant protein synthesis is multifactorial. Low concentrations of glucocorticoids have been shown to stimulate SP-A synthesis, whereas higher concentrations are inhibitory. By contrast, glucocorticoids consistently increase SP-B and SP-C messenger ribonucleic acid (mRNA) production in a dose-dependent manner. Induction of SP-A synthesis by prostaglandin E_2 is believed to be mediated by cAMP. Analogs of cAMP and substances that increase cellular cAMP (e.g., methylxanthines, forskolin, terbutaline) increase SP-A mRNA and SP-A gene transcription. These agents have smaller, if any, effects on SP-B and SP-C synthesis. Epidermal growth factor increases SP-A mRNA and SP-A synthesis. The effect of insulin on SP-A synthesis is inhibitory and dose dependent. A combination of insulin and inhibitory concentrations of glucocorticoids decreases SP-A synthesis more than does either hormone individually. In diabetic pregnancies, amniotic fluid contains significantly less SP-A than does fluid from nondiabetics. Inhibition of SP-A synthesis by insulin may contribute to the increased risk of HMD among infants of diabetic mothers. Transforming growth factor-β also has been shown to be an inhibitor of SP-A synthesis.[13]

Surfactant Secretion

The process of surfactant secretion that has been studied most extensively is the regulated release of assembled, stored surfactant from type II cells. Studies of excised lungs have shown that the phospholipid content of BAL fluid increases when lung volume is increased. Associated decreases in lamellar body density indicate that inflation-induced increases in phospholipids result from stimulation of surfactant secretion. Studies demonstrating that a single stretch applied to cultured type II cells results in phosphatidylcholine secretion provide further evidence that mechanical factors can stimulate surfactant secretion. Increases in cellular cAMP are known to enhance surfactant secretion, and stimulatory factors that probably act through this mechanism include β-adrenergic agents (endogenous catecholamines, isoproterenol, metaproterenol, terbutaline), methylxanthines, and adenosine compounds. Calcium ionophores, protein kinase C activators, arachidonic acid metabolites, leukotrienes, histamine, vasopressin, and intracellular alkalosis all have been shown to stimulate surfactant secretion.[13] Both baseline and stimulated surfactant secretion by type II cells are inhibited in a calcium-dependent manner by SP-A in vitro.[4, 13]

Surfactant Clearance

Clearance of secreted surfactant may occur by recycling, degradation, or removal. SP-A, SP-B, SP-C, and PG stimulate the endocytotic uptake of intact, previously secreted phospholipids by type II cells. SP-A appears to be involved in the intracellular movement of these lipids to the lamellar bodies, from which they then are resecreted. Such phospholipid recycling seems to be more efficient in newborn than in adult animals. Secreted SP-A can be taken up from the fluid subphase by type II cells, but it is not clear whether it is resecreted.[4, 11, 13] It appears that very little surfactant is degraded in the extracellular fluid subphase. Surfactant components can be phagocytosed by alveolar macrophages, and degradation may then occur. Type II cells can degrade surfactant phospholipids, and radiolabeling studies have shown that these degradation products subsequently are incorporated into other lipids. Surfactant components and their degradation products have been found in very small quantities in the blood, lymph, and respiratory mucus. Radiolabeling studies have shown that some degradation products later appear in nonsurfactant lipids in the lungs or in other organs. Clearance of surfactant may be enhanced by some of the same factors that stimulate secretion, including hyperventilation and β-adrenergic agents.[13] However, SP-A enhances surfactant clearance but inhibits surfactant secretion. Thus, it has been suggested that SP-A may be an important regulator of feedback inhibition in surfactant metabolism and, as such, a prime controller of size of the surfactant pool of the extracellular fluid subphase.[4, 6, 13]

Ranges of values for surfactant flux have been calculated by Wright and Clements. They estimate that type II cells secrete 11% to 47% of the lamellar body surfactant pool per hour. At steady state, an equal amount of surfactant must be cleared from the alveoli. Thus, in 1 hour, 9% to 40% of the DPPC content of BAL fluid is removed from the alveoli and replaced by newly synthesized phospholipid.[3, 13]

Using radiolabeled glucose and palmitate, the half-life of DPPC initially was estimated to be 14 hours. Subsequent estimates of surfactant half-life have ranged from 17 to 90 hours and appear to vary with the phospholipid, the radiolabel, and the age and species of animal studied. Estimates of phosphatidylcholine turnover time have ranged from 3.8 to 11.1 hours and thus are more consistent with the rapid, active metabolism suggested by the surfactant flux estimates of Wright and Clements.[3, 8, 13] Pulmonary surfactant is a dynamic, continuously self-renewing system.

SURFACTANT FUNCTION

The primary function of pulmonary surfactant is to lower alveolar surface tension. As previously discussed, lowered surface tension decreases the pressure on the alveolar surface at end-expiration when alveoli are smallest and transpulmonary pressures are lowest and thus prevents alveolar collapse. The compliance of a lung determines the volume to which it may be expanded at a given pressure. Lowering alveolar surface tension reduces the pressure needed to inflate alveoli in accordance with the Laplace relationship ($P = 2T/R$). Pulmonary surfactant raises compliance by lowering the pressure needed to inflate the lung to a desired volume. The reduction of alveolar surface tension by surfactant also prevents transudation of fluid from pulmonary capillaries into the alveolar airspaces. Normally, capillary colloid oncotic pressure and intra-alveolar air pressure oppose capillary hydrostatic pressure, preventing movement of fluid into the alveoli. In the absence of surfactant, high alveolar surface tension can raise capillary hydrostatic pressure above its opposing pressures, resulting in pulmonary edema and hemorrhage. An additional function of surfactant may be a role in the immune defense of the lungs attributable to the ability of SP-A and possibly SP-D to enhance the phagocytosis of opsonized bacteria by pulmonary macrophages, as already mentioned.[6, 8, 10]

SURFACTANT REPLACEMENT

Hyaline Membrane Disease

In HMD, surfactant is not present in sufficient quantity to perform the functions just discussed. Surfactant deficiency results in the widespread atelectasis, poor compliance, edema, and hemorrhage that characterize the lungs of infants with HMD. The feasibility of replacing the deficient surfactant in HMD has been of great interest to physiologists and clinicians. Initial clinical trials of exogenous artificial surfactant in human infants with HMD used aerosolized DPPC and were not successful, probably because of the poor adsorption velocity of pure DPPC that was discussed earlier. Two other exogenous artificial surfactants, a dry mixture of DPPC and PG in a 7:3 ratio and a mixture of DPPC and high-density human serum lipoprotein in a 10:1 ratio, produced inconsistent results in four and one clinical trials, respectively, again probably as a result of adsorption rates inferior to natural surfactant. In premature animal models of HMD, excellent therapeutic effects were demonstrated with direct tracheal instillation of natural surfactant isolated by centrifugation of BAL fluid from mature lungs. Successful clinical trials in human infants with HMD have used exogenous natural surfactant from the following sources: human amniotic fluid; bovine lung homogenates supplemented with PG or with DPPC, palmitic acid, and tripalmitoylglycerol (surfactant TA); neonatal bovine BAL fluid (calf lung surfactant extract, or CLSE, and Infasurf) and porcine lung homogenates (Curosurf). Survanta is a Food and Drug Administration–approved bovine lung–derived, reconstituted surfactant. Efforts to develop an effective synthetic surfactant continued because of concern about possible immune sensitization of infants to foreign animal proteins present in heterologous natural surfactants. Clinical trials using a synthetic surfactant consisting of DPPC supplemented with hexadecanol and tyloxapol (Exosurf) have shown good results.[14–16] So far, only Survanta and Exosurf are approved by the Food and Drug Administration for clinical use in the United States (Table 91–3).

Immediate beneficial effects of surfactant therapy include improved oxygenation, lowered mean airway pressure, and improved aeration on chest radiographs. Meta-analyses of the outcome differences between surfactant-treated and control infants from the reports of 35 randomized controlled trials revealed that surfactant was associated with a 30% to 40% reduction in neonatal mortality, a marked decrease in the occurrence of pneumothorax, and a decrease in the combined outcomes of bronchopulmonary dysplasia or death at 28 days. However, there were no overall decreases in the incidence of bronchopulmonary dysplasia, patent ductus arteriosus, or intracranial hemorrhage.[16, 17, 17a–c] Although a concern has been that improved survival in premature infants with HMD might be associated with increased long-term morbidity, several follow-up studies have shown that surfactant treatment is associated with similar or improved late pulmonary and neurodevelopmental function in comparison with untreated controls (Table 91–4).[14–18, 18a, b]

TABLE 91–3. Exogenous Surfactants Currently Approved for Use in Human Infants in the United States

Surfactant	*Components*	*Dose*
Exosurf	DPPC Cetyl alcohol Tyloxapol	5 mL/kg
Survanta	Bovine lung extract DPPC Palmitic acid Tripalmitin	4 mL/kg

Abbreviation: DPPC = dipalmitoylphosphatidylcholine.

TABLE 91–4. Clinical Outcomes of Surfactant Trials for Hyaline Membrane Disease* (Prophylaxis and Rescue; Synthetic and Natural)

Mortality	↓
BPD or death at 28 days	↓ †
BPD	+ / − †
Pneumothorax	↓
PDA	No effect
IVH	No effect
Long-term morbidity	No effect

*Cumulative data from 35 clinical trials[16, 17] expressed in a simplified way.

†Although the combination of BPD or death at 28 days was definitely influenced by surfactant replacement, a reduction in BPD alone was not found consistently in all trials analyzed.

Abbreviations: BPD = bronchopulmonary dysplasia; PDA = patent ductus arteriosus; IVH = intraventricular hemorrhage.

The earliest clinical trials of exogenous surfactant involved administering it to infants in whom the diagnosis of severe HMD had already been established. Studies using this therapeutic approach have been termed *treatment* or *rescue* trials. However, animal studies showed that instillation of surfactant before the onset of ventilation resulted in better outcomes. Thus, in clinical trials, surfactant was administered in birthing areas to infants at high risk of developing HMD. Studies using this treatment strategy are called *prophylaxis* or *prevention* trials. In prophylaxis studies, the incidence of HMD among treated infants becomes an outcome variable. Because not all at-risk infants actually develop HMD, the prophylaxis approach leads to unnecessary treatment of some infants, the proportion increasing with gestational age. However, using the treatment strategy, HMD may be quite advanced and infants may receive significant exposure to high oxygen concentrations and ventilator trauma before surfactant is given. Because results of studies comparing prophylaxis and treatment have differed, the issue of which strategy is better remains unresolved.[18c] Initial trials involved single-dose treatment, but because only transient improvement often occurred, later trials usually allowed multiple doses. Response to treatment is not 100%. Although about 80% of treated infants respond immediately with a rise in arterial partial pressure of oxygen, others may not. Causes for treatment failure include extreme prematurity, preexisting severe hypoxia, hypotension, and acidosis. In clinical practice, it is widely acknowledged that repeat doses may be required, but whether re-treatment should be scheduled or based on severity of symptoms is controversial. In the United States, a number of surfactant preparations were approved for open trials and thus became widely used in 1989. Exosurf was licensed for treatment of HMD in 1990, and Survanta (a modified bovine surfactant) in 1991.[14, 16] During 1990, the United States infant mortality rate decreased 6%. This was twice the annual average rate of decrease that occurred between 1980 and 1989. The large decrease in 1990 resulted from a 36% decrease in the mortality from HMD, which in turn was attributed to the widespread clinical use of surfactant replacement therapy.[19]

Other Neonatal Respiratory Conditions

Infants with gestational ages of 34 weeks or more may be treated with extracorporeal membrane oxygenation (ECMO) for respiratory failure that is not responsive to usual medical management. Among the various conditions that can lead to respiratory failure requiring ECMO, meconium aspiration syndrome (MAS) is common but HMD is not. ECMO survivors were shown to have tracheal aspirate ratios of SP-A to total protein that increased at the same time that measurements of pulmonary compliance and aeration on chest radiographs were improving and weaning from ECMO was being accomplished. Ratios of SP-A to total protein remained low in infants who could not be weaned. The investigators speculated that ratios of tracheal aspirate SP-A to total protein reflected surfactant production in the study infants.[20] A subsequent study demonstrated that during weaning from ECMO, tracheal aspirate protein concentrations decreased whereas the concentrations of SP-A, total phospholipids, and disaturated phosphatidylcholine increased. Again it was concluded that increased surfactant production contributed to recovery from the respiratory failure that had necessitated ECMO.[21] In a blind, randomized, controlled trial of Survanta in full-term infants with respiratory failure and receiving ECMO, surfactant-treated infants had significantly shorter ECMO durations, better pulmonary compliance measurements, higher ratios of SP-A to total protein in tracheal aspirates, and a lower incidence of complications after ECMO.[22] In an uncontrolled trial, multiple doses of CLSE were given to full-term newborn infants who had respiratory failure and who were not receiving ECMO. Half of the infants had underlying MAS, and half had pneumonia. Surfactant treatment was associated with improved oxygenation and lower mean airway pressures. None of the study infants died, subsequently required ECMO, developed pneumothorax, or required oxygen for longer than 2 weeks.[23]

MAS follows the aspiration of amniotic fluid that contains particulate meconium. One of the pathologic features of MAS is atelectasis, traditionally explained as secondary to small-airway obstruction by particles of meconium. However, several experimental observations indicate that atelectasis in MAS might also be due to surfactant deficiency or inactivation and thus lend support to the use of exogenous surfactant therapy in MAS. Classic animal experiments performed by Johnson and coworkers demonstrated that when fluid was instilled and ventilated into degassed portions of the lung in vivo, later pressure-volume and surface activity studies of the excised lung showed evidence of high surface tension and low surface activity in the fluid-instilled portions. These investigators concluded that fluid in the alveoli could displace or inactivate endogenous surfactant.[24] Later studies showed that endobronchial instillation of a filtered meconium solution caused changes in the pressure-volume relationships of excised lungs, consistent with decreased surface activity.[25] Other investigators demonstrated increased surface tension measurements of animal lung extracts after the addition of meconium, an ether extract of meconium, or meconium free fatty acids in vitro. In vivo instillation of each of these meconium derivatives was associated with reduced oxygenation, increased mean airway pressures, and decreased pulmonary compliance measurements. Extracts from the atelectatic portions of the lungs of the experimental animals had high minimum values when assayed for surface tension.[26] Another in vitro study showed that inhibition of the surface activity of CLSE by meconium solutions could be overcome by increasing CLSE concentrations.[27] All of this investigative work suggests that exogenous surfactant may have a place in the management of MAS.

Adult Respiratory Distress Syndrome

First described in 1967, adult respiratory distress syndrome (ARDS) comprises a clinical pattern of dyspnea, tachypnea, hypoxemia despite supplemental oxygen, and poor pulmonary compliance; diffuse alveolar infiltrates on chest radiographs; and histologic findings of atelectasis, edema, hemorrhage, and hyaline membranes. ARDS was noted always to occur in association with another illness (e.g., severe trauma, viral infection). Several findings in the original series of patients with ARDS were recognized as being similar to features of infants with HMD—namely, hypoxemia and acidosis before the onset of respiratory distress, low measured values for total dynamic compliance, improved oxygenation with positive end-expiratory pressure, alveolar atelectasis and hyaline membranes on autopsy, and high values for minimum surface tension of lung homogenates from patients. The authors of this early report speculated that ARDS was associated with loss of pulmonary surfactant.[28]

Many now believe that respiratory failure in ARDS is primarily due to pulmonary edema that is the result of increased alveolocapillary permeability. It has been proposed that complement activation leads to neutrophil aggregation. Aggregated neutrophils then generate oxygen radicals, proteases, and cytokines that cause endothelial injury.[29, 30] Studies have shown that several of the components of edema fluid are capable of inhibiting the function of pulmonary surfactant.[31] Comparisons of BAL fluid from patients with ARDS and controls have shown decreased quantities of SP-A and qualitative differences in surfactant phospholipids, consisting of relative decreases in phosphatidylcholine and PG, in ARDS.[32–34] BAL samples from patients with ARDS demonstrate abnormally low surface activity, and measurements made on serial samples show that surface activity decreases as ARDS worsens.[30, 33]

Although the relative importance of surfactant abnormalities in the pathogenesis of ARDS still must be established, functional inactivity of surfactant probably at least contributes to the poor pulmonary compliance and atelectasis that characterize ARDS. The effect of exogenous surfactant therapy has been studied extensively in various animal models of acute lung injury. In controlled trials, exogenous surfactant has resulted in improvements in animals that have been subjected to lung lavage, bilateral cervical vagotomy, infusion of antilung serum, hyperoxia, injection of *N*-nitroso-*N*-methylurethane, acid aspiration, viral pneumonia, or infusion of oleic acid.[30, 31] Among human patients with acute lung injury, tracheal instillation of exogenous surfactant has produced inconsistent results. In a controlled clinical trial in patients with sepsis-induced ARDS, aerosolized Exosurf was associated with improved oxygenation and survival.[30] Future clinical trials may determine when and how exogenous surfactant should be used to reduce the severity and mortality of ARDS.

References

1. King RJ, Clements JA: Surface active materials from dog lung. II. Composition and physiological correlations. Am J Physiol 1972; 223:715.
2. King RJ: The surfactant system of the lung. Fed Proc 1974; 33:2238.
3. Wright JR, Clements JA: Metabolism and turnover of lung surfactant. Am Rev Respir Dis 1987; 135:426.
4. Weaver TE, Whitsett JA: Function and regulation of expression of pulmonary surfactant-associated proteins. Biochem J 1991; 273:249.
5. Hawgood S, Benson BJ, Hamilton RL Jr: Effects of a surfactant-associated protein and calcium ions on the structure and surface activity of lung surfactant lipids. Biochemistry 1985; 24:184.
6. Weaver TE: Surfactant proteins and SP-D. Am J Respir Cell Mol Biol 1991; 5:4.
7. Hawgood S, Shiffer K: Structures and properties of the surfactant-associated proteins. Annu Rev Physiol 1991; 53:375.

8. Morgan TE: Pulmonary surfactant. N Engl J Med 1971; 284:1185.
9. King RJ: Pulmonary surfactant. J Appl Physiol 1982; 53:1.
10. Harwood JL: Lung surfactant. Prog Lipid Res 1987; 26:211.
11. Haagsman HP, van Golde LMG: Synthesis and assembly of lung surfactant. Annu Rev Physiol 1991; 53:111.
12. Mendelson CR, Boggaram V: Hormonal control of the surfactant system in fetal lung. Annu Rev Physiol 1991; 53:415.
13. Wright JR, Dobbs LG: Regulation of pulmonary surfactant secretion and clearance. Annu Rev Physiol 1991; 53:395.
14. Vidyasagar D, Adeni S, Uhing MR: Surfactant replacement therapy. Perspect Crit Care 1990; 3:69.
15. Yee WFH, Scarpelli EM: Surfactant replacement therapy. Pediatr Pulmonol 1991; 11:65.
16. Jobe AH: Pulmonary surfactant therapy. N Engl J Med 1993; 328:861.
17. Soll RF, McQueen MC: Respiratory distress syndrome. *In*: Effective Care of the Newborn Infant. Sinclair JE, Bracken MB (Eds). Oxford, England, Oxford University Press, 1992, pp 327–358.
17a. Horbar JD, Wright EC, Onstad L, et al: Decreasing mortality associated with the introduction of surfactant therapy: An observational study of neonates weighing 601 to 1300 grams at birth. Pediatrics 1993; 92:191.
17b. Schwartz RM, Luby AM, Scanlon JW, et al: Effects of surfactant on morbidity, mortality, and resource use in newborn infants weighing 500 to 1500 g. N Engl J Med 1994; 330:1476.
17c. Kari MA, Hallman M, Eronen M, et al: Prenatal dexamethasone treatment in conjunction with rescue therapy of human surfactant: A randomized placebo-controlled multicenter study. Pediatrics 1994; 93:730.
18. Abbasi S, Bhutani VK, Gerdes JS: Long-term pulmonary consequences of respiratory distress syndrome in preterm infants treated with exogenous surfactant. J Pediatr 1993; 122:446.
18a. Ferrara TB, Hoekstra RE, Couser RJ, et al: Survival and follow-up of infants born at 23 to 26 weeks of gestational age: Effects of surfactant therapy. J Pediatr 1994; 124:119.
18b. Survanta Multidose Study Group: Two-year follow-up of infants treated for neonatal respiratory distress syndrome with bovine surfactant. J Pediatr 1994; 124:962.
18c. Egberts J, de Winter JP, Seden G, et al: Comparison of prophylaxis and rescue treatment with Curosurf in neonates less than 30 weeks' gestation: A randomized trial. Pediatrics 1993; 92:768.
19. Centers for Disease Control: Infant mortality—United States, 1990. MMWR 1993; 42:161.
20. Lotze A, Whitsett JA, Kammerman LA, et al: Surfactant protein A concentrations in tracheal aspirate fluid from infants requiring extracorporeal membrane oxygenation. J Pediatr 1990; 116:435.
21. Bui KC, Walther FJ, David-Cu R, et al: Phospholipid and surfactant protein A concentrations in tracheal aspirates from infants requiring extracorporeal membrane oxygenation. J Pediatr 1992; 121:271.
22. Lotze A, Knight GR, Martin GR, et al: Improved pulmonary outcome after exogenous surfactant therapy for respiratory failure in term infants requiring extracorporeal membrane oxygenation. J Pediatr 1993; 122:261.
23. Auten RL, Notter RH, Kendig JW, et al: Surfactant treatment of full-term newborns with respiratory failure. Pediatrics 1991; 87:101.
24. Johnson JWC, Permutt S, Sipple JH, et al: Effect of intra-alveolar fluid on pulmonary surface tension properties. J Appl Physiol 1964; 19:769.
25. Chen CT, Toung TJK, Rogers MC: Effect of intra-alveolar meconium on pulmonary surface tension properties. Crit Care Med 1985; 13:233.
26. Clark DA, Nieman GF, Thompson JE, et al: Surfactant displacement by meconium free fatty acids: An alternative explanation for atelectasis in meconium aspiration syndrome. J Pediatr 1987; 110:765.
27. Moses D, Holm BA, Spitale P, et al: Inhibition of pulmonary surfactant function by meconium. Am J Obstet Gynecol 1991; 164:477.
28. Ashbaugh DG, Bigelow DB, Petty TL, et al: Acute respiratory distress in adults. Lancet 1967; 2:319.
29. Rinaldo JE, Rogers RM: Adult respiratory-distress syndrome. N Engl J Med 1982; 306:900.
30. Lewis JF, Jobe AH: Surfactant and the adult respiratory distress syndrome. Am Rev Respir Dis 1993; 147:218.
31. Holm BA, Notter RH: Surfactant therapy in adult respiratory distress syndrome and lung injury. *In*: Surfactant Replacement Therapy. Shapiro DL, Notter RH (Eds). New York, Alan R Liss, 1989, pp 273–304.
32. Hallman M, Spragg R, Harrell JH, et al: Evidence of lung surfactant abnormality in respiratory failure. J Clin Invest 1982; 70:673.
33. Gregory TJ, Longmore WJ, Moxley MA, et al: Surfactant chemical composition and biophysical activity in acute respiratory distress syndrome. J Clin Invest 1991; 88:1976.
34. Pison U, Obertacke U, Seeger W, et al: Surfactant protein A (SP-A) is decreased in acute parenchymal lung injury associated with polytrauma. Eur J Clin Invest 1992; 22:712.

CHAPTER 92

Adult Respiratory Distress Syndrome

Steven J. Trottier, MD • Robert W. Taylor, MD

DEFINITION

Adult respiratory distress syndrome (ARDS) is a broad term for catastrophic acute respiratory failure of diverse etiology and high mortality. It is commonly associated with sepsis and the multiple organ dysfunction syndrome. ARDS is generally characterized by a violent and apparently chaotic immunologic reaction leading to diffuse alveolar damage, pulmonary microvascular thrombosis, aggregation of inflammatory cells, and stagnation of blood flow through the lungs. This chain reaction gives rise to increased pulmonary capillary permeability and excessive extravascular lung water. Once started, the pathophysiologic cascade leads to intense arterial hypoxemia, pulmonary arterial hypertension, radiographic evidence of pulmonary edema, and stiff, noncompliant lungs. Implicit in the foregoing description is that ARDS is *not* a single disease but rather a pathophysiologic syndrome. Patients with increased pulmonary capillary filtration pressures causing "cardiogenic" pulmonary edema and those with chronic lung disease are characteristically excluded from this grouping for epidemiologic reasons. Experience has taught us, however, that patients with heart failure or chronic lung disease are not "protected" from ARDS, and indeed the conditions can coexist.

Ashbaugh and Petty and their colleagues drew attention to this syndrome and are credited with the acronym ARDS.[1, 2] However, many highly accurate and interesting clinical descriptions of this syndrome may be found from the early 1900s.[3–6] During the years, this form of acute respiratory failure has been referred to by many colorful and descriptive names[7] (Table 92–1). Grouping acute lung injury due to diverse causes under a single name has been questioned.[8–10] Some suggest that use of the term ARDS oversimplifies, creates ambiguity, and hampers research.[11] Patients fulfilling clinical criteria for ARDS might on the surface appear similar but may in fact have distinctly different pathophysiologic underpinnings. There is little question that use of the term is commonplace in critical care settings. The authors believe that the term ARDS has clinical utility because it creates a conceptual framework on which supportive care may be based. Clinicians are advised to be mindful

TABLE 92–1. Synonyms for Adult Respiratory Distress Syndrome

Adult hyaline membrane disease	Post-traumatic pulmonary insufficiency
Adult respiratory insufficiency syndrome	Progressive pulmonary consolidation
Congestive atelectasis	Progressive respiratory distress
Da Nang lung	Pump lung
Hemorrhagic atelectasis	Shock lung
Hemorrhagic lung syndrome	Transplant lung
Hypoxic hyperventilation	Traumatic wet lung
Postperfusion lung	Wet lung
Post-traumatic atelectasis	White lung

(From Taylor RW, Duncan CA: The adult respiratory distress syndrome. Res Medica 1983; 1:17.)

that the pathophysiology of this syndrome is incompletely understood and may vary according to the cause.

Accepted clinical definitions generally contain the following elements:

1. Severe arterial hypoxemia
2. Bilateral radiographic infiltrates consistent with pulmonary edema
3. Reduced lung compliance
4. Presence of a definable catastrophic event or risk factors

Criteria for the diagnosis of ARDS used in clinical trials vary.[11a] Much of the controversy surrounding this syndrome stems from the lack of a more precise clinical definition. The severity of ARDS is variable, and a useful lung injury scoring system incorporating radiographic appearance, degree of hypoxemia, level of positive end-expiratory pressure used, and respiratory system compliance has been described[12] (Table 92–2).

Elevation of the MB isoenzyme of creatine kinase is a rather sensitive and specific biochemical marker for the diagnosis of acute myocardial infarction. Likewise, marked elevations of aminotransferases establish the diagnosis of hepatocellular damage. Unfortunately, no such test exists to diagnose or predict the outcome of ARDS. Measurement of pulmonary endothelial protein permeability has been studied but is rather cumbersome and poorly predictive of progression to ARDS.[13] Several markers of endothelial damage have been studied, including C5a,[14] terminal complement complex,[15] and von Willebrand's factor antigen.[16] Various confounding problems have hindered interpretation of elevations of these markers. Although no simple biochemical test exists to diagnose ARDS convincingly or to predict outcome, perhaps as the molecular biology of this syndrome is further unraveled, a useful diagnostic marker will surface.

INCIDENCE

The incidence of ARDS is unknown. In 1972, the National Heart and Lung Institute estimated 150,000 cases per year in the United States (75 cases per 100,000 population).[17] A more recent study found a much lower incidence of 1.5 to 3.5 cases per 100,000 population.[18] Part of the problem is lack of a precise definition. If strict criteria are established for diagnosis, then of course the incidence appears lower than if criteria for diagnosis are relaxed.

On the practical side, the syndrome occurs frequently enough to consume much of a critical care practitioner's time, energy, and resources.

ETIOLOGY

Numerous, varied conditions have been causally related to ARDS (Table 92–3). Most of our therapy for ARDS remains supportive; however, in many cases, specific, targeted therapy is essential, making a thorough search for the cause critical. Risk factors for ARDS have been identified.[19] Those that seem to place patients at greatest risk include sepsis (especially gram-negative septic shock), aspiration of gastric contents, pulmonary contusion, and multiple transfusions. Pepe and coworkers reported an additive effect of risk factors.[20] ARDS developed in 25% of patients with a single risk factor, in 42% of patients with two risk factors, and in 85% of patients with three.

Important questions remain. Do these varied causes result in the same disease? Are the conditions listed in Table 92–3 directly causal, or do some of them represent epiphenomena? Is the pulmonary edema caused by aspiration of gastric contents the same disease as neoplastic pulmonary emboli? Is ARDS in the setting of gram-negative septic shock the same ARDS associated with heroin injection? Subsets of this syndrome with distinct molecular biologic, immunologic, and pathophysiologic features certainly exist.

IMPORTANT CAUSES OF ADULT RESPIRATORY DISTRESS SYNDROME

Sepsis and Multiple Organ Dysfunction

The pathophysiology of sepsis, septic shock, multiple organ dysfunction syndrome, and ARDS is closely linked. Many believe that what we call ARDS is simply the pulmonary manifestation of a systemic inflammatory response gone askew.[21] The biology of the initiators and mediators is cur-

TABLE 92–2. Components and Individual Values of the Lung Injury Score

Component		*Value*
Chest roentgenogram score		
No alveolar consolidation		0
Alveolar consolidation confined to 1 quadrant		1
Alveolar consolidation confined to 2 quadrants		2
Alveolar consolidation confined to 3 quadrants		3
Alveolar consolidation in all 4 quadrants		4
Hypoxemia score		
PaO_2/FIO_2	>300	0
PaO_2/FIO_2	225–299	1
PaO_2/FIO_2	175–224	2
PaO_2/FIO_2	100–174	3
PaO_2/FIO_2	<100	4
PEEP score (when ventilated)		
PEEP	≤5 cm H_2O	0
PEEP	6–8 cm H_2O	1
PEEP	9–11 cm H_2O	2
PEEP	12–14 cm H_2O	3
PEEP	≥15 cm H_2O	4

The final value is obtained by dividing the aggregate sum by the number of components that were used

	Score
No lung injury	0
Mild to moderate lung injury	0.1–2.5
Severe lung injury (ARDS)	>2.5

(From Murray JF, Matthay MA, Luce JM, et al: An expanded definition of the adult respiratory distress syndrome. Am Rev Respir Dis 1988; 138:720.)

Abbreviations: PaO_2/FIO_2 = ratio of arterial oxygen tension to inspired oxygen concentration; PEEP = positive end-expiratory pressure.

TABLE 92–3. Conditions Associated with the Adult Respiratory Distress Syndrome

Shock	Metabolic
Septic	Renal failure
Hemorrhagic	Hepatic failure
Cardiogenic	Diabetic ketoacidosis
Anaphylactic	Miscellaneous
Aspiration of gastric contents (especially with a pH <2.5)	Pancreatitis
Trauma	Extracorporeal circulation
Systemic inflammatory response syndrome	Cardioversion
Pulmonary contusion	Multiple transfusions
Nonthoracic trauma (especially head trauma)	Disseminated intravascular coagulation
Near-drowning	Leukoagglutinin reaction
Burns	Eclampsia
Fat embolism	Chorioamnionitis
Crush injury	Amniotic fluid emboli
Infection	Air emboli
Bacterial (especially gram-negative sepsis)	Bowel infarction
Viral	Neoplastic pulmonary emboli
Fungal	High-dose irradiation
Mycobacterial (miliary tuberculosis)	Hanging
Parasitic	Airway obstruction
Inhalation of toxic gases and fumes	High altitude
Oxygen (high concentration)	Autologous bone marrow transfusion
Smoke	Suction lipectomy
Nitrogen dioxide	Acute myocardial infarction
Ammonia	Volume overload
Chlorine	Baby powder inhalation
Sulfur dioxide	Still's disease
Cadmium	Systemic lupus erythematosus
Phosgene	Mixed essential cryoglobulinemia
Drug and poisons	
Cocaine	
Heroin	
Methadone	
Barbiturates	
Ethchlorvynol	
Thiazides	
Fluorescein	
Propoxyphene	
Salicylates	
Chlordiazepoxide	
Colchicine	
Dextran 40, 70	
Ergotamine	
Organophosphates	
Paraquat	
Ritodrine	
Cystosine arabinoside	
Bleomycin	
Contrast medium	

(Modified from Taylor RW, Duncan CA: The adult respiratory distress syndrome. Res Medica 1983; 1:17.)

rently under intense investigation. ARDS develops in about 25% of patients with gram-negative sepsis and has been reported in 90% of patients with gram-negative septic shock.[22, 23]

Trauma

Severely injured patients are at high risk for development of ARDS.[24] Both thoracic and extrathoracic trauma are associated. Multiple factors are operative: direct lung contusion, hemorrhagic shock, multiple transfusion, aspiration of gastric contents, head injury, infection, and long bone fractures with associated fat embolization.[25, 26, 27]

Aspiration of Gastric Contents

Thirty-four per cent of patients with witnessed aspiration of gastric contents develop ARDS.[19] This is a particularly important cause of ARDS if the pH of the aspirated material is less than 2.5;[28, 29] however, ARDS also occurs in the absence of severe acidity.[30]

Blood Transfusions

Transfusion-related acute lung injury may be caused by pulmonary microembolism with platelet-fibrin microaggregates, leukoagglutination reactions, or incorrectly cross-matched blood.[31–33] Many patients who have massive transfusion requirements may have one or more additional risk factors for ARDS, such as hemorrhagic shock, making it difficult to confidently implicate blood transfusion as the sole cause.

PATHOPHYSIOLOGY

The Inflammatory Response

Despite the multiple causes of ARDS, the pathophysiologic consequences are remarkably uniform. An intense inflammatory response causing acute alveolar and endothelial damage; increased vascular permeability, lung water, and protein; and deterioration in gas exchange set the stage for development of ARDS (see Chapter 74).

The initiators and mediators of the systemic inflammatory response syndrome are currently being carefully scrutinized (see Chapter 75).[34] Macrophages have an important role in recognizing initiators such as endotoxin, releasing cytokines, and modulating the inflammatory response (Table 92–4). Abundant evidence suggests that the inflammatory mediators act to recruit neutrophils to the pulmonary microcirculation during the early stages of ARDS.[35–37a] Indeed, the chemotactic response of neutrophils in patients with ARDS is more than twice normal.[38] Neutrophils are believed to release many histotoxic agents in patients with ARDS[39] (Table 92–5).

Histologic Changes

Alveolar gas is separated from capillary hemoglobin by a very thin alveolocapillary membrane. The alveolar cells are supported by a basement membrane, as are the capillary endothelial cells. Between the basement membranes lies the interstitial space, containing interstitial fluid, connective tissue, and scattered fibroblasts. When acute lung injury occurs, the endothelium becomes increasingly permeable to fluid and protein (see Chapter 90). Interstitial fluid accumulates and soon overwhelms the lymphatic drainage system. Interstitial edema is followed by alveolar flooding. Alveolar surface cells (type I) are sensitive to insult, and many are destroyed in the first hours to days after injury. Within several days, the denuded alveolar basement membrane is covered with proliferating alveolar type II cells. Plasma proteins, cellular debris, fibrin, and surfactant remnants aggregate to form hyaline membranes that cover the bare basement membrane of alveoli and alveolar ducts. The normally thin alveolocapillary membrane widens with the accumulation of more fluid, proliferating fibroblasts, plasma cells, leukocytes, and histiocytes during the course of the next week. After a week to 10 days, hyaline membrane, alveolar septum, and alveolar duct fibrosis may occur.[40]

These histologic changes do not occur in their entirety in all patients. In some, the process is arrested midstream and resolves. Why one case resolves and another progresses is not known but probably relates to the nature and severity of the original insult. Even patients with extensive fibrosis may have partial resolution of the damage.[41]

Surfactant

Surfactant is critical in maintaining normal lung function. It is secreted by alveolar type II cells and decreases surface tension as it coats the alveolar lining. This serves to keep alveoli open and participating in gas exchange. Various surfactant abnormalities occur in ARDS, including an alteration in the amount of surfactant made as well as its chemical composition (see Chapter 91). Furthermore, serum proteins found in the alveolar space in ARDS inactivate surfactant. Although these surfactant abnormalities are not primary in ARDS, they promote alveolar collapse and contribute to altered gas exchange.[42, 43]

TABLE 92–4. Inflammatory Mediators in Adult Respiratory Distress Syndrome

Cytokines	Prostaglandins
Interleukins	Leukotrienes
Tumor necrosis factor	Vasoactive peptides
Interferons	Serotonin
Complement proteins	Histamine
Contact activation proteins	Platelet-activating factors
Bradykinin	
Coagulation proteins	
Thrombin	
Fibrin degradation products	

(From Taylor RW, Norwood S: The adult respiratory distress syndrome. *In:* Critical Care. 2nd ed. Civetta JM, Taylor RW, Kirby RR [Eds]. Philadelphia, JB Lippincott, 1992, pp 1237–1247.)

TABLE 92–5. Histotoxic Neutrophil Products

Oxidants and radicals
Superoxide anion
Hydrogen peroxide
Hydroxyl radical
Hypochlorous acid
Chloramines
Nitric acid
Proteolytic enzymes
Elastase
Gelatinase
Collagenase
Cathepsin
Lysozyme
Neuraminidase
Heparanase
Others
Cationic proteins

(From Zimmerman G, Renzetti A, Hill R: Functional and metabolic activity of granulocytes from patients with adult respiratory distress syndrome. Am Rev Respir Dis 1983; 127:290.)

Lung Mechanics and Gas Exchange in Adult Respiratory Distress Syndrome

Alveolar flooding coupled with qualitative and quantitative surfactant abnormalities leads to widespread atelectasis. Reduced functional residual capacity is a hallmark of ARDS. Fluid-filled and collapsed alveoli are difficult to expand, thus explaining the reduction in lung compliance noted in this syndrome.[44] Furthermore, increased airway resistance to gas flow has been described in some patients.[45] The severe hypoxemia that occurs in ARDS most certainly results from advanced alveolar flooding and alveolar collapse, leading to intrapulmonary shunting and areas of low ventilation-perfusion ($\dot{V}/\dot{Q}$).[46]

Extrapulmonary Organ Failure in Adult Respiratory Distress Syndrome

As previously stated, ARDS likely represents the pulmonary expression of a systemic inflammatory process that causes dysfunction of many other organ systems[47] (Table 92–6). The mechanisms of multiple organ dysfunction are incompletely understood. Many of the mediators that lead to acute lung injury (see Table 92–4) probably are also operative in other organ dysfunction. Leading hypotheses suggest that mediators lead to altered tissue blood flow by various mechanisms. Overperfusion of tissues with low oxygen extraction ratios may coexist with areas of relative underperfusion. Arteriovenous shunting may increase in some tissue beds, leaving affected organs underperfused. The ability to recruit capillaries at the tissue level may also be lost or diminished, further impairing the ability to adjust to local tissue needs. Direct endothelial or parenchymal injury may result in organ edema and may increase diffusion distances for oxygen and substrate delivery. Under these circumstances, the gut mucosal barrier to bacteria may be compromised, resulting

TABLE 92–6. Complications Associated with Adult Respiratory Distress Syndrome

Pulmonary	Complications attributable to intubation and extubation
Pulmonary emboli	Prolonged attempt at intubation
Pulmonary barotrauma	Intubation of a mainstem bronchus
Pulmonary fibrosis	Premature extubation
Oxygen toxicity	Self-extubation
Gastrointestinal	Complications associated with endotracheal/tracheostomy tubes
Gastrointestinal hemorrhage	Tube malfunction
Ileus	Nasal necrosis
Gastric distention	Paranasal sinus infection
Pneumoperitoneum	Tracheal stenosis
Renal	Tracheomalacia
Renal failure	Polyps
Fluid retention	Erosion
Cardiovascular	Fistulas
Invasive catheters	Airway obstruction
Arrhythmia	Hoarseness
Hypotension	Complications attributable to operation of the ventilator
Low cardiac output	Machine failure
Infection	Alarm failure
Sepsis	Alarms silenced
Nosocomial pneumonia	Inadequate nebulization or humidification
Hematologic	Complications occurring during positive airway pressure therapy
Anemia	Alveolar hypoventilation
Thrombocytopenia	Alveolar hyperventilation
Disseminated intravascular coagulation	Massive gastric distention
Other	Barotrauma
Hepatic	Atelectasis
Endocrine	Pneumonia
Neurologic	Hypotension
Psychiatric	
Malnutrition	

(From Taylor RW: The adult respiratory distress syndrome. *In*: Respiratory Failure. Kirby RR, Taylor RW [Eds]. Chicago, Year Book Medical Publishers, 1986, pp 208–244.)

in translocation of bacteria or bacterial products from the gut lumen to the systemic circulation. Thus, once initiated, the systemic inflammatory response may be perpetuated and amplified by various mechanisms.

CLINICAL FEATURES

Many of the specific clinical features of ARDS depend on the cause. Tachypnea and tachycardia usually develop in the first 12 to 24 hours after the initial insult. A clinically apparent increase in work of breathing becomes obvious. High-pitched end-expiratory crackles are heard throughout the lung fields during auscultation.

Radiographic changes become evident early in the course. An increase in interstitial markings gives way to more dense "alveolar" infiltrates as alveolar flooding occurs (Fig. 92–1). The infiltrates are typically seen diffusely; however, they may start as a focal process and then generalize.[48, 49] Several scoring systems have been developed to help quantify the increased lung water.[50, 51] Computed tomographic scanning of patients with ARDS has given us a different view of distribution patterns. Although a plain chest radiograph might suggest diffuse and uniform distribution of pulmonary edema, a computed tomographic scan suggests a more patchy distribution of infiltrates favoring the dependent portions of the lung.[52–54]

As the syndrome progresses and diffuse fibrosis ensues, the chest radiograph may take on a patchy or nodular appearance. The application of positive-pressure ventilation and positive end-expiratory pressure (PEEP) alters the radiographic appearance. PEEP does not decrease lung water but rather increases functional residual capacity making the lungs on a chest radiograph appear better aerated. Careful search of the chest radiograph should be made for mediastinal emphysema, subcutaneous emphysema, and pneumothorax (Fig. 92–2). A normal-sized cardiac silhouette sometimes helps to distinguish ARDS from "cardiogenic" pulmonary edema. Chest radiographic findings return to normal in as many as 80% of patients who survive.

MANAGEMENT OF ADULT RESPIRATORY DISTRESS SYNDROME

ARDS is an entity manifested in various clinical settings. Effective treatment of this syndrome requires resolution of the original underlying process. To date, no therapeutic interventions convincingly prevent or alter the progression of ARDS once initiated. Therefore, treatment of patients with ARDS remains supportive. Therapeutic goals include alleviation of hypoxemia, provision of cardiovascular and nutritional support, treatment of secondary infections, and avoiding iatrogenic complications.

Mechanical Ventilation

The first and most immediate therapy is supplemental oxygen. Most patients with ARDS become refractory to supplemental oxygen and require positive-pressure ventilation.[2] These patients classically have decreased lung volumes and compliance, $\dot{V}/\dot{Q}$ mismatching, and right-to-left intrapulmonary shunting. The goals of positive-pressure ventilation are to restore arterial oxygenation, maintain systemic oxygen delivery, and avoid complications associated with mechanical ventilation (see Chapter 97). Conventional recommendations for the initial settings for volume-controlled ventilation (i.e., synchronized intermittent mandatory ventilation or assist control ventilation) are a tidal volume in the range of 10 to 15 mL/kg, a fractional inspired concentra-

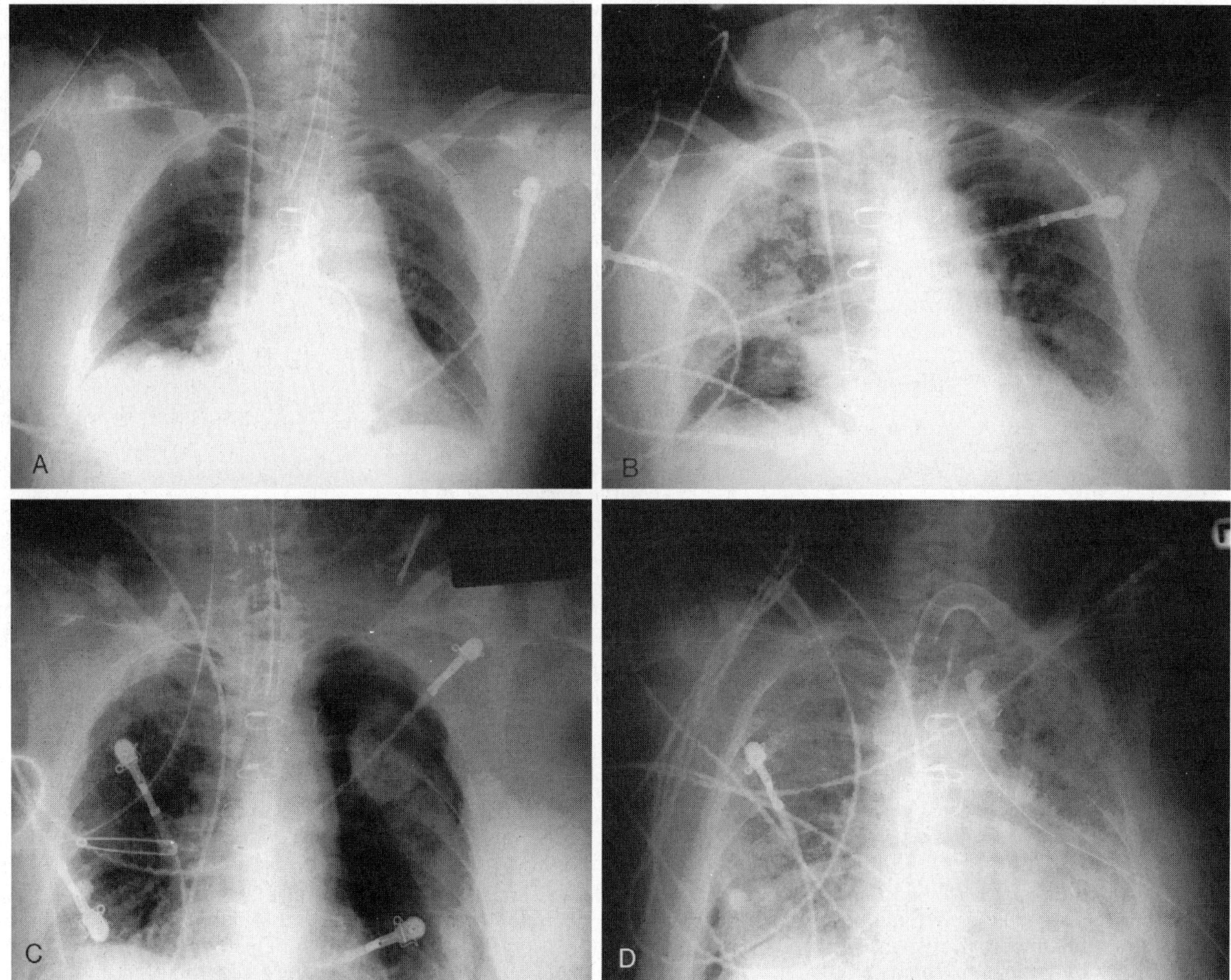

Figure 92–1. Many of the common radiographic feature of ARDS are shown in chest radiographs. All radiographs are portable (anteroposterior projection). *A*, A 62-year-old woman with a prior history of coronary artery bypass surgery underwent abdominal aortic aneurysm resection. This relatively unremarkable chest radiograph was obtained on the day of the operation immediately upon her arrival in the ICU. She was extubated during the morning of the first postoperative day. *B*, Because of her increasing respiratory difficulty, this radiograph was obtained during the afternoon of the first postoperative day. Interstitial and alveolar infiltrates can be seen throughout the right lung field and in the left base. *C*, This radiograph was obtained on the 13th postoperative day. The patient remains intubated and mechanically ventilated. Diffuse infiltrates are seen throughout, and a large left pneumothorax is present. *D*, This radiograph was obtained on the 23rd postoperative day. Dense infiltrates are seen throughout all lung fields. The left lung is expanded. A left thoracostomy tube is in place. A tracheostomy tube is also in place. A small pneumothorax is present in the right costophrenic sulcus.

tion of oxygen (FIO_2) of 1.0 atm, and a PEEP of 3 to 5 cm H_2O. Data have demonstrated that the lung injury occurring in ARDS is a heterogeneous process.[55] The use of large tidal volume may be deleterious to areas of spared alveoli. Large tidal volume causes acute lung injury in animals.[56] In the setting of ARDS, the use of tidal volume in the range of 7 to 10 mL/kg may be more appropriate.

The FIO_2 should be titrated downward as soon as possible to avoid oxygen toxicity (see Chapter 88). Continuous pulse oximetry may facilitate this process. The exact threshold of oxygen toxicity in an injured lung remains unknown. Pulmonary endothelial cells replicate less effectively at an FIO_2 greater than 0.50 atm; therefore, this level may be an appropriate therapeutic goal.[57] If the arterial saturation remains less than 90% at an FIO_2 greater than 0.50 atm, then PEEP should be increased.

Ashbaugh described the use of PEEP in the management of ARDS more than 25 years ago.[1] Since then, the clinical difficulties associated with the use of PEEP have been multiple. This becomes apparent when looking at the array of adjectives (i.e., best, optimal, preferred, and least) used to describe the most effective level of PEEP. The most appropriate level of PEEP for patients with ARDS is controversial and should be individualized. PEEP improves oxygenation by restoring lung volumes, decreasing intrapulmonary shunting, and improving $\dot{V}/\dot{Q}$ mismatch (see Chapter 98). PEEP does not decrease lung water but may cause a redistribution of lung water from the intra-alveolar space to the interstitial space.[58] From a practical standpoint, the application of PEEP should be applied every 10 to 15 minutes while monitoring arterial saturation and systemic perfusion. PEEP frequently increases intrathoracic pressure, which in turn decreases venous return and may compromise cardiac output and oxygen delivery. Hypovolemic states exaggerate this effect, as is often noted early in ARDS, owing to prior diuretic therapy or a systemic vascular leak phenomenon.

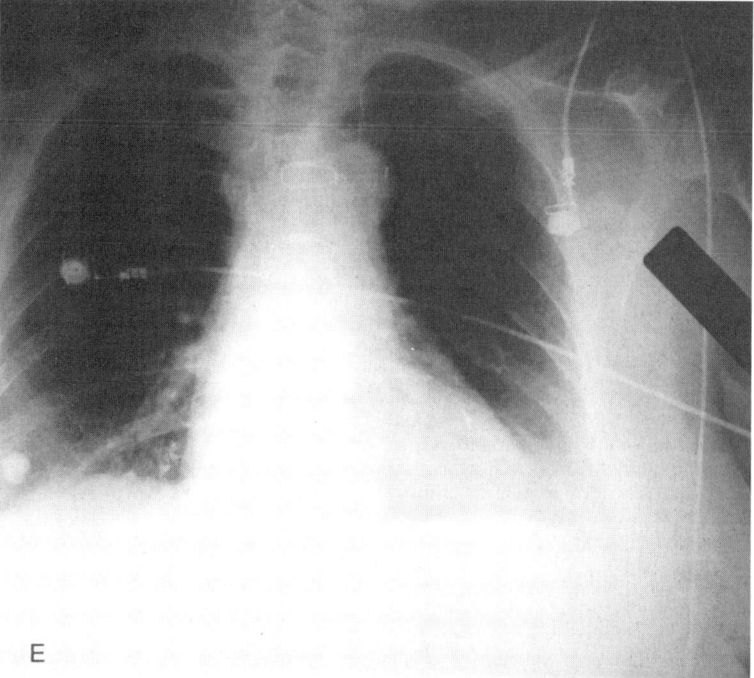

Figure 92–1 *Continued E,* This radiograph was obtained on the 110th postoperative day. Mechanical ventilation had been discontinued, and the tracheostomy tube had been removed. The appearance of the chest radiograph returned to baseline. One year later this patient enjoyed an active and independent lifestyle.

Judicious fluid administration usually restores venous return. At levels of 10 to 15 cm H_2O of PEEP, the hemodynamic effects are less predictable and more complex. PEEP may overdistend alveoli, causing increased pulmonary vascular resistance, increased right ventricular afterload, and altered ventricular geometry, compromising left ventricular function.[59] In this setting, hemodynamic monitoring with a pulmonary artery catheter is warranted.

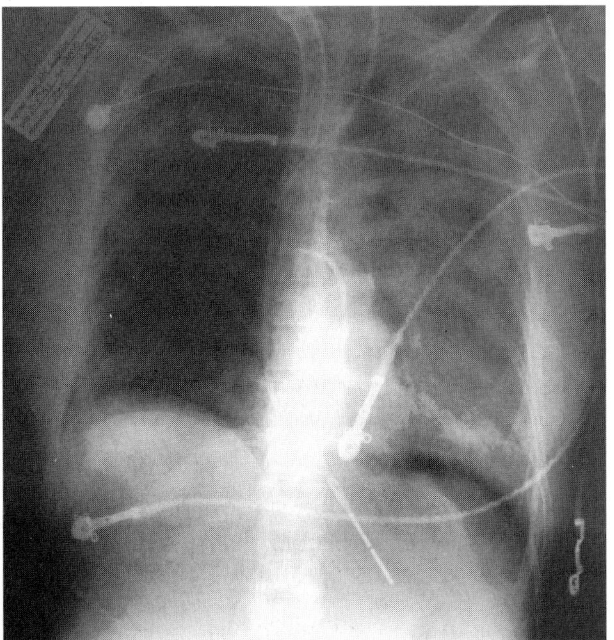

Figure 92–2. A 47-year-old woman developed ARDS in association with intra-abdominal sepsis. This portable chest radiograph was taken with the patient in the supine position. Diffuse infiltrates appear more prominent on the left. Hyperlucency overlying the left upper abdominal quadrant represents gas (pneumothorax) in the anterior costophrenic sulcus. Gas often rises to this most superior portion of the pleural space when a patient is in the supine position (deep sulcus sign).

In patients who remain difficult to oxygenate, efforts to minimize oxygen demand should ensue. Optimizing hemoglobin and cardiac output, maintaining normothermia, addressing infections, and using sedation and, if necessary, neuromuscular-blocking agents have been recommended.

Patients failing to respond despite the foregoing measures should be considered candidates for less conventional modes of mechanical ventilation. Inverse-ratio ventilation, high-frequency jet ventilation, and airway pressure-release ventilation have been studied in the setting of ARDS.[60–62] These modes of mechanical ventilation have been successfully used to oxygenate and ventilate patients with lung injury but have not altered complications or outcomes. To date, there have been no randomized controlled trials demonstrating the optimal approach to oxygenate or ventilate patients with ARDS.

Hemodynamic Monitoring and Fluid Balance

Myocardial function may be altered as a result of the underlying pathophysiology or secondarily as a result of treatment (i.e., mechanical ventilation). From a diagnostic and therapeutic standpoint, hemodynamic monitoring has become an important aspect of care for patients with ARDS.[63] Difficult decisions about oxygen transport and fluid balance may be facilitated by the use of pulmonary artery catheters. The focus on the pathologic dependence of oxygen uptake on oxygen delivery in ARDS is intriguing, yet the clinical implications of this phenomenon are at present unknown[64] (Fig. 92–3). At a minimum, oxygen delivery should be maintained within the normal range, optimizing arterial saturation ($\geq$0.90), hemoglobin (10–11 g/dL), and cardiac output with the use of fluids or inotropes such as dobutamine. Whether increasing the oxygen delivery beyond the "normal" range affects the incidence of organ failure or alters outcome is an area of ongoing study.[64a]

Fluid balance remains a controversial issue in ARDS (see also Chapter 94). At the onset of ARDS, patients frequently

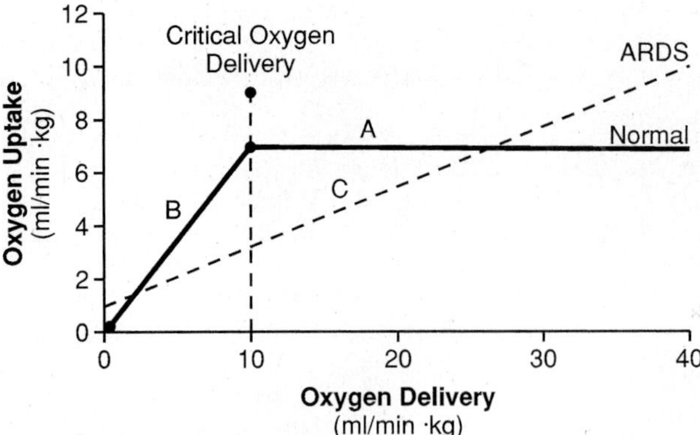

Figure 92–3. Under normal circumstances (A), oxygen uptake is constant over a wide range of oxygen delivery rates. This is referred to as flow-independent oxygen uptake. The body consumes only the oxygen it needs. This activity is controlled to a large extent by local regulation of the microvasculature. If oxygen delivery falls below a critical level, compensatory mechanisms are exhausted, and oxygen uptake decreases as oxygen delivery decreases (B). In patients with ARDS and in patients with sepsis (C), oxygen uptake is dependent on oxygen delivery. This pathologic condition is referred to as "flow-dependent oxygen consumption" and suggests the presence of deregulation of the microvasculature. (From Dorinsky PM, Gadek JE: Mechanisms of nonpulmonary organ failure in ARDS. Chest 1989; 96:885.)

require fluid resuscitation to maintain hemodynamic stability, especially those patients requiring increasing levels of PEEP. After achieving stability, minimizing fluid intake to maintain the lung as "dry" as possible has physiologic appeal, provided systemic oxygen delivery is not compromised. Patients remaining in persistent positive fluid balance may have a worse outcome.[65] Judicious administration of diuretics must be balanced with the adequacy of systemic perfusion.

Furthermore, the type of fluid administered—crystalloid versus colloid—is an area of unresolved debate.[66] Colloid advocates argue that less volume is required with colloids and that lung water may be minimized by maintaining colloid osmotic pressure. Crystalloid proponents argue that colloids may actually exacerbate pulmonary edema by traversing leaky pulmonary membranes. Adequate administration of either agent can effectively resuscitate patients. Numerous studies have failed to favor either agent in terms of outcome, but cost analysis favors the use of cystalloids.

Nutrition

Early institution of enteral feedings is an essential aspect of care in patients with ARDS. These patients characteristically are hypermetabolic and quickly become malnourished. Parenteral supplementation may be required until full needs are met through the enteral route.[66a] Translocation of bacteria or bacterial products through the gastrointestinal tract may be one of the pivotal causes of persistent hypermetabolic states and multiple organ dysfunction.[67] Enteral feedings may help to maintain gastrointestinal mucosal integrity.[68] Postoperative patients have fewer septic complications when provided nutritional support enterally, compared with parenteral administration.[69] Whether this observation translates to a decreased incidence of multiple organ dysfunction or improved outcome in ARDS is unknown.

Extracorporeal Membrane Oxygenation

The first prospective randomized controlled trial involving extracorporeal membrane oxygenation (ECMO) in the management of ARDS was reported in 1979.[70] Ninety patients entered the study, 48 randomized to conventional mechanical ventilation and 42 randomized to conventional mechanical ventilation supplemented with partial venoarterial bypass. Survival for these groups was 8.3% and 9.5%, respectively. Enthusiasm for ECMO waned until 1986, when Gattinoni reported an impressive 49% survival in an uncontrolled trial using low-frequency positive-pressure ventilation and extracorporeal carbon dioxide removal (venovenous LFPPV-ECCO$_2$R) with apneic oxygenation.[71] The National Institutes of Health recently reported the results of a prospective randomized controlled trial of conventional mechanical ventilation, pressure-controlled inverse-ratio ventilation, and LFPPV-ECCO$_2$R with apneic oxygenation. The investigators found equivalent survival rates between groups and recommended that extracorporeal support for ARDS should be restricted to clinical trials.[72, 73]

Controversies in Management of Adult Respiratory Distress Syndrome

The optimal approach to positive-pressure ventilation in ARDS remains unknown. Literature has drawn attention to the possibility of iatrogenic lung injury secondary to mechanical ventilation administered at high pressures and volumes[56, 74] (Fig. 92–4). The suggested solution is to decrease tidal volumes (6–8 mL/kg), maintain transalveolar pressures at 35 cm H_2O or less, and limit PEEP to 7 to 15 cm H_2O.[75] Improvements in oxygenation can be achieved by increasing mean airway pressure. This can be accomplished by changing the inspiratory pressure waveform, increasing PEEP or minute ventilation, or extending the inspiratory time fraction. In one study, the limitation of airway pressures took precedence over ventilation, allowing for carbon dioxide retention (permissive hypercapnia).[76] It is hoped

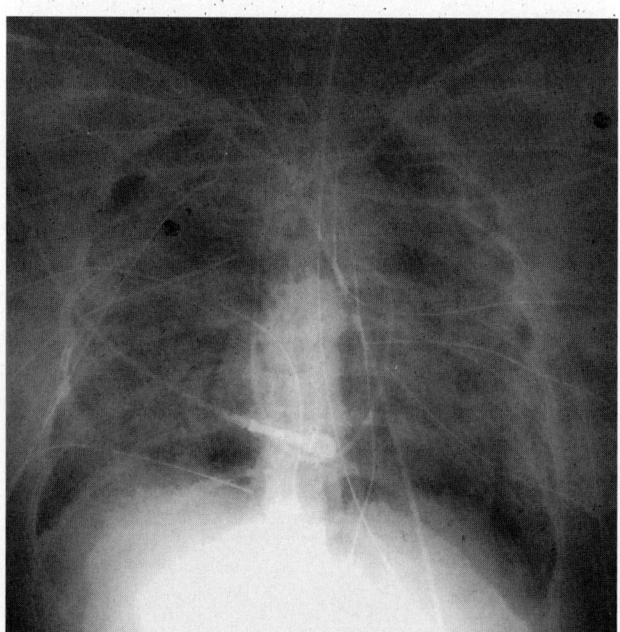

Figure 92–4. A 30-year-old woman with Crohn's disease developed ARDS following a small bowel perforation and peritonitis. High peak and mean airway pressures were required. She sustained devastating barotrauma with multiple pneumothoraces. Large bronchopleural fistulas developed. A total of eight chest tubes were inserted over time in an attempt to expand her lungs. This patient died subsequent to single-organ system failure. She is one of the few patients in whom all attempts to achieve adequate oxygenation and ventilation have failed.

that future research will clarify whether or not these manipulations are beneficial in the management of ARDS.

Secondary infections are a major cause of mortality in ARDS, with pneumonia occurring in more than 60% of patients.[77] Gastrointestinal tract decontamination decreases the incidence of pneumonia in mechanically ventilated patients but does not improve survival.[78] Gastrointestinal tract decontamination has not been specifically addressed in the setting of ARDS.

At present, no therapy prevents or alters the course of ARDS after its onset. However, multiple agents have been investigated. Administration of corticosteroids to prevent or halt the progression of ARDS has been ineffective.[79, 80] The use of corticosteroids for the fibroproliferative phase of ARDS may have promise, but more data are required.[81, 82] Administration of prostaglandins to patients with ARDS decreases pulmonary vascular resistance without enhancing survival.[83] A study of inhaled nitric oxide demonstrated improved oxygenation and decreased pulmonary artery pressure. No systemic side effects were noted. Further studies are warranted.[84, 84a] Whether administration of monoclonal antibodies or modulation of cytokines can positively affect patients with sepsis and ARDS is under investigation. Exogenous surfactant administered to neonates with respiratory distress syndrome has resulted in improved lung function and increased survival.[85] Ongoing prospective randomized trials of aerosolized exogenous surfactant in ARDS will potentially define surfactant's role in these patients.

Complications

Numerous potential complications are associated with the treatment of patients with ARDS[86] (see Table 92–6). The staff caring for these patients must be cognizant of these complications and respond promptly to them. Preventive measures such as deep vein thrombosis prophylaxis and stress ulcer prophylaxis are strongly encouraged.

OUTCOME

Despite an accumulation of research and experience during the past 25 years, the mortality of ARDS remains greater than 50%. Death occurring within 3 days after the onset of ARDS is usually related to the underlying illness.[87] Later mortality in ARDS frequently results from sepsis or multiple organ failure. Irreversible respiratory failure accounts for 16% of deaths in ARDS, although a recent report describes an increasing incidence of mortality secondary to respiratory failure.[88] The majority of patients who survive an episode of ARDS have normal or mildly impaired pulmonary function 1 year later. Symptoms are not associated with impairment of pulmonary function test results[89] (Fig. 92–5). Improvement in pulmonary function has been documented for up to 1 year after ARDS.

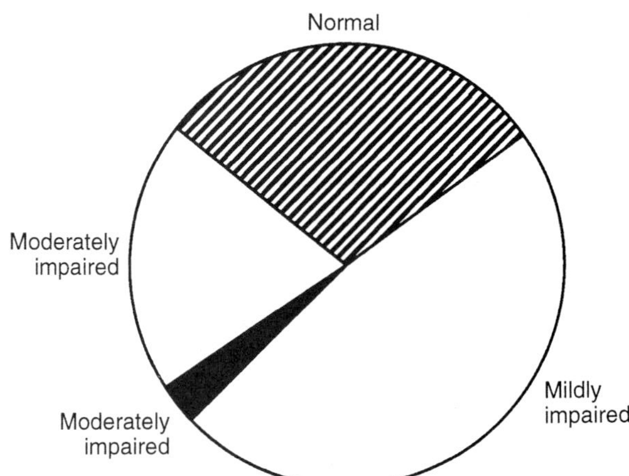

Figure 92–5. Most patients who survive ARDS have normal or mildly impaired pulmonary function when studied 1 year after development of the disorder. In this group of patients, symptoms did not correlate with pulmonary function. (Modified from Ghio AJ, Elliott CG, Crapo RO, et al: Impairment after adult respiratory distress syndrome: An evaluation based on American Thoracic Society recommendations. Am Rev Respir Dis 1989; 139:1158.)

References

1. Ashbaugh DE, Bigelow DB, Petty TL, et al: Acute respiratory distress in adults. Lancet 1967; 2:319.
2. Petty TL, Ashbaugh DG: The adult respiratory distress syndrome: Clinical features, factors influencing prognosis and principles of management. Chest 1971; 60:233.
3. Montgomery BA: Early description of ARDS. Chest 1991; 99:261.
4. Sloggett AT (Ed): Memorandum of the Treatment of Injuries in War. London, Harrison and Sons, 1915, pp 115–122.
5. Pasteur W: Massive collapse of the lung. Br J Surg 1914; 1:587.
6. Bradford JR: Massive collapse of the lung as a result of gunshot wounds with special reference to wounds of the chest. Q J Med 1919; 12:217.
7. Taylor RW, Duncan CA: The adult respiratory distress syndrome. Res Medica 1983; 1:17.
8. Fishman AP: Shock lung (a distinctive non-entity). Circulation 1973; 47:921.
9. Murray JF: The adult respiratory distress syndrome (may it rest in peace). Am Rev Respir Dis 1975; 111:716.
10. Petty TL: The adult respiratory distress syndrome: Confessions of a "lumper." Am Rev Respir Dis 1975; 111:713.
11. Rocker GM, Wiseman MS, Pearson D, et al: Diagnostic criteria for adult respiratory distress syndrome: Time for reappraisal. Lancet 1989; 1:120.
11a. Bernard GR, Artigas A, Brigham KL, et al: The American-European consensus conference on ARDS definitions, mechanisms, relevant outcomes, and clinical trial coordination. Am J Respir Crit Care Med 1994; 149:818.
12. Murray JF, Matthay MA, Luce JM, et al: An expanded definition of the adult respiratory distress syndrome. Am Rev Respir Dis 1988; 138:720.
13. Jones DK: Markers for impending adult respiratory distress syndrome. Respir Med 1990; 84:89.
14. Hammerschmidt D, Weaver L, Hudson C, et al: Association of complement activation and elevated plasma-C5a with the adult respiratory distress syndrome: Pathophysiologic relevance and possible prognostic value. Lancet 1980; 1:947.
15. Langlois PF, Gawryl MS: Accentuated formation of the terminal C5b-9 complement complex in patient plasma precedes development of the adult respiratory distress syndrome. Am Rev Respir Dis 1988; 138:368.
16. Carvalho ACA, Bellman SM, Saullo VJ, et al: Altered factor VIII in acute respiratory failure. N Engl J Med 1982; 307:1113.
17. Lung Program, National Heart and Lung Institute: Respiratory Diseases: Task Force on Problems, Research, Approaches, Needs. US Department of Health, Education and Welfare, publication No. (NIH) 73–432, 1972, p 171.
18. Villar J, Slutsky AS: The incidence of the adult respiratory distress syndrome. Am Rev Respir Dis 1989; 140:814.
19. Fowler AA, Hamman RF, Good JT, et al: Adult respiratory distress syndrome: Risk with common predispositions. Ann Intern Med 1983; 98:593.
20. Pepe PE, Potkin RT, Reus DH, et al: Clinical predictors of the adult respiratory distress syndrome. Am J Surg 1982; 144:124.
21. Welbourn CR, Young Y: Endotoxin, septic shock and acute lung injury: Neutrophils, macrophages and inflammatory mediators. Br J Surg 1992; 79:998.
22. Kaplan RL, Sahn SA, Petty TL: Incidence and outcome of the respiratory distress syndrome in gram-negative sepsis. Arch Intern Med 1979; 139:867.

23. Martin MA, Silverman HJ: Gram-negative sepsis and the adult respiratory distress syndrome. Clin Infect Dis 1992; 14:1213.
24. Fulton RL, Jones CE: The cause of post-traumatic pulmonary insufficiency in man. Surg Gynecol Obstet 1975; 140:179.
25. Shoemaker WC, Appel P, Czer LSC, et al: Pathogenesis of respiratory failure (ARDS) after hemorrhage and trauma. Crit Care Med 1980; 8:504.
26. Lewis FR, Blaisdell W, Schlobohm RM: Incidence and outcome of post-traumatic respiratory failure. Arch Surg 1977; 112:436.
27. Horovitz JH, Carrico CJ, Shires GT: Pulmonary response to major injury. Arch Surg 1974; 108:349.
28. Mendelson CL: The aspiration of stomach contents into the lungs during obstetric anesthesia. Am J Obstet Gynecol 1946; 52:191.
29. Wynne JW, Modell JH: Respiratory aspiration of stomach contents. Ann Intern Med 1977; 87:466.
30. Schwartz DJ, Wynne JW, Gibbs CP, et al: Pulmonary consequences of aspiration of gastric contents at pH values greater than 2.5. Am Rev Respir Dis 1980; 121:119.
31. Popovsky MA, Chaplin HC Jr, Moore SB: Transfusion-related acute lung injury: A neglected, serious complication of hemotherapy. Transfusion 1992; 32:589.
32. Barrett J, Davidson I, Dhurandhar HN, et al: Pulmonary microembolism associated with massive transfusion: II. The basic pathophysiology of its pulmonary effects. Ann Surg 1975; 182:52.
33. Grindlinger GA, Vegas AM, Churchill WH, et al: Is respiratory failure a consequence of blood transfusion? J Trauma 1980; 20:627.
34. Horn JK, Lewis FR: Acute lung injury: Pathophysiology and diagnosis. *In*: Critical Care: State of the Art. Vol 12. Taylor RW, Shoemaker WC (Eds). Fullerton, CA, Society of Critical Care Medicine, 1991, pp 1–31.
35. Taylor RW, Norwood S: The adult respiratory distress syndrome *In*: Critical Care. 2nd ed. Civetta JM, Taylor RW, Kirby RR (Eds). Philadelphia, JB Lippincott, 1992, pp 1237–1247.
36. Rinaldo JE, Rogers RM: Adult respiratory distress syndrome: Changing concepts of lung injury and repair. N Engl J Med 1982; 306:900.
37. Tate RM, Repive JE: Neutrophils and the adult respiratory distress syndrome. Am Rev Respir Dis 1983; 128:552.
37a. Hasegawa N, Husari AW, Hart WT, et al: Role of the coagulation system in ARDS. Chest 1994; 105:268.
38. Zimmerman G, Renzetti A, Hill R: Functional and metabolic activity of granulocytes from patients with adult respiratory distress syndrome. Am Rev Respir Dis 1983; 127:290.
39. Donnelly SC, Haslett C: Cellular mechanisms of acute lung injury: Implications for future treatment in the adult respiratory distress syndrome. Thorax 1992; 47:260.
40. Hasleton PS: Adult respiratory distress syndrome—review. Histopathology 1983; 7:307.
41. Lakshminarayan S, Stanford RL, Petty TL: Prognosis after recovery from adult respiratory distress syndrome. Am Rev Respir Dis 1976; 113:7.
42. Pison U, Seeger W, Buckhorn R, et al: Surfactant abnormalities in patients with respiratory failure in multiple trauma. Am Rev Respir Dis 1989; 140:1033.
43. Gregory T, Longmore W, Moxley M, et al: Surfactant chemical composition and biophysical activity in acute respiratory distress syndrome. J Clin Invest 1991; 65:1976.
44. Lamy M, Fallat RJ, Koeniger E, et al: Pathologic features and mechanisms of hypoxemia in adult respiratory distress syndrome. Am Rev Respir Dis 1976; 114:267.
45. Wright PE, Bernard GR: The role of airflow resistance in patients with the adult respiratory distress syndrome. Am Rev Respir Dis 1989; 139:1169.
46. Dantzker DR, Brook CH, DeHart P, et al: Gas exchange in adult respiratory distress syndrome and the effects of positive end-expiratory pressure. Am Rev Respir Dis 1979; 120:1039.
47. Dorinsky PM, Gadek JE: Mechanisms of nonpulmonary organ failure in ARDS. Chest 1989; 96:885.
48. Johnson TH, Altman AR, McCaffree RD: Radiologic considerations in the adult respiratory distress syndrome treated with positive end-expiratory pressure (PEEP). Clin Chest Med 1982; 3:89.
49. Altman AR, Johnson TH: Roentgenographic findings: PEEP therapy, indicators of pulmonary complications. JAMA 1979; 242:727.
50. Pistolesi M, Miniati M, Milne ENC, et al: The chest roentgenogram in pulmonary edema. Clin Chest Med 1985; 6:315.
51. Halperin BD, Feeley TW, Mihm FG, et al: Evaluation of portable chest roentgenogram for quantitating extravascular lung water in critically ill adults. Chest 1985; 88:649.
52. Peruzzi W, Garner W, Bools J, et al: Portable chest roentgenography and computed tomography in critically ill patients. Chest 1988; 93:727.
53. Golding RP, Knape P, Strack Van Schijndel RJM, et al: Computed tomography as an adjunct to chest x-rays of intensive care unit patients. Crit Care Med 1988; 16:211.
54. Bombino M, Gattinoni L, Pesenti A, et al: The value of portable chest roentgenography in adult respiratory distress syndrome: Comparison with computed tomography. Chest 1991; 100:762.
55. Maunder RJ, Shuman WP, McHugh JW, et al: Preservation of normal lung regions in the adult respiratory distress syndrome. JAMA 1986; 255:2463.
56. Dreyfuss D, Soler P, Basset G, et al: High inflation pressure pulmonary edema: Respective effects of high airway pressure, high tidal volume, and positive end-expiratory pressure. Am Rev Respir Dis 1988; 137:1159.
57. Martin WJ, Kachel DL: Oxygen-mediated impairment of human pulmonary endothelial cell growth: Evidence for a specific threshold of toxicity. J Lab Clin Med 1989; 113:413.
58. Pave PD, Warriner B, Baile EM, et al: Redistribution of pulmonary extravascular water with positive end-expiratory pressure in canine pulmonary edema. Am Rev Respir Dis 1983; 127:590.
59. Pinsky MR: The effects of mechanical ventilation on the cardiovascular system. Crit Care Clin 1990; 6:663.
60. Rasanen J, Cane RD, Downs JB, et al: Airway pressure release ventilation during acute lung injury: A prospective multicenter trial. Crit Care Med 1991; 19:1234.
61. Carlon GC, Howland WS, Ray C, et al: High-frequency jet ventilation: A prospective randomized evaluation. Chest 1983; 84:551.
62. Shanholtz C, Brower R: Should inverse ratio ventilation be used in adult respiratory distress syndrome? Am J Respir Crit Care Med 1994; 149:1354.
63. Broaddus CV, Berthiaume Y, Biondi JW, et al: Hemodynamic management of the adult respiratory distress syndrome. J Intensive Care Med 1987; 2:190.
64. Schumaker PT, Samsel RW: Oxygen supply and consumption in the adult respiratory distress syndrome. Clin Chest Med 1990; 11:715.
64a. Russell JA, Phang TP: The oxygen delivery/consumption controversy approaches to management of the critically ill. Am J Respir Crit Care Med 1994; 149:533.
65. Simmons RS, Bordine GG, Seidenfeld JJ: Fluid balance and the adult respiratory distress syndrome. Am Rev Respir Dis 1987; 135:924.
66. McConachie I: The ARDS and fluid therapy controversy. What we need and don't need. Intensive Crit Care Dig 1991; 10:59.
66a. DeBiasse MA, Wilmore DW: What is optimal nutritional support? New Horizons 1994; 2:122.
67. Mainous MR, Deitch EA: Bacterial translocation and its potential role in the pathogenesis of multiple organ failure. J Intensive Care Med 1992; 7:101.
68. Wilmore DW, Smith RJ, O'Dwyer ST: The gut: A central organ after surgical stress. Surgery 1988; 104:917.
69. Moore FA, Feliciano DV, Andrassy RJ, et al: Early enteral feeding, compared with parenteral, reduces postoperative septic complications. Ann Surg 1992; 216:172.
70. Zapol WM, Snider MT, Hill OJ, et al: Extracorporeal membrane oxygenation in severe acute respiratory failure. JAMA 1979; 242:2193.
71. Gattinoni L, Pesenti A, Mascheroni D, et al: Low-frequency positive-pressure ventilation with extracorporeal CO_2 removal in severe acute respiratory failure. JAMA 1986; 256:881.
72. Morris AH, Wallace CJ, Menlove RL, et al: Randomized clinical trial of pressure-controlled inverse ratio ventilation and extracorporeal CO_2 removal for adult respiratory distress syndrome. Am J Respir Crit Care Med 1994; 149:295.
73. Petty TL, Bone RC, Gee MH, et al: Contemporary clinical trials in acute respiratory distress syndrome. Chest 1992; 101:550.

74. Tsuno K, Prato P, Kolobow T: Acute lung injury from mechanical ventilation at moderately high airway pressures. J Appl Physiol 1990; 69:956.
75. Marini JJ: New approaches to the ventilatory management of the adult respiratory distress syndrome. J Crit Care 1992; 7:256.
76. Hickling KG, Henderson SJ, Jackson R: Low mortality associated with low pressure limited ventilation with permissive hypercapnia in severe adult respiratory distress syndrome. Intensive Care Med 1990; 16:372.
77. Seidenfeld JJ, Pohl DF, Bell RC, et al: Incidence, site, and outcome of infections in patients with the adult respiratory distress syndrome. Am Rev Respir Dis 1986; 134:12.
78. Vandenbrouke-Grauls CM, Vandenbrouke JP: Effect of selective decontamination of the digestive tract on respiratory tract infections and mortality in the intensive care unit. Lancet 1991; 338:859.
79. Luce JM, Montgomery AB, Marks JD, et al: Ineffectiveness of high-dose methylprednisolone in preventing parenchymal lung injury and improving mortality in patients with septic shock. Am Rev Respir Dis 1988; 138:62.
80. Bernard GR, Luce JM, Sprung CL, et al: High-dose corticosteroids in patients with the adult respiratory distress syndrome. N Engl J Med 1987; 317:1565.
81. Hooper RG, Kearl RA: Established ARDS treated with a sustained course of adrenocortical steroids. Chest 1990; 97:138.
82. Meduri VG, Belenchia JM, Estes RJ, et al: Fibroproliferative phase of ARDS: Clinical findings and effects of corticosteroids. Chest 1991; 100:943.
83. Bone RC, Slotman G, Maunder R, et al: Randomized double-blind, multicenter study of prostaglandin E, in patients with adult respiratory distress syndrome. Chest 1989; 96:114.
84. Rossaint R, Falke KJ, Lopez F, et al: Inhaled nitric oxide for the adult respiratory distress syndrome. N Engl J Med 1993; 328:399.
84a. Gaston B, Drazen JM, Loscalzo J, et al: The biology of nitrogen oxides in the airways. Am J Respir Crit Care Med 1994; 149:538.
85. Lewis JF, Jube AH: Surfactant and the adult respiratory distress syndrome. Am Rev Respir Dis 1993; 147:218.
86. Taylor RW: The adult respiratory distress syndrome. *In*: Respiratory Failure. Kirby RR, Taylor RW (Eds). Chicago, Year Book Medical Publishers, 1986, pp 208–244.
87. Montgomery AB, Stager MA, Carrico CJ, et al: Causes of mortality in patients with the adult respiratory distress syndrome. Am Rev Respir Dis 1985; 132:485.
88. Suchyta MR, Clemmer TP, Elliot CG, et al: The adult respiratory distress syndrome: A report of survival and modifying factors. Chest 1992; 101:1074.
89. Ghio AJ, Elliott CG, Crapo RO, et al: Impairment after adult respiratory distress syndrome: An evaluation based on American Thoracic Society recommendations. Am Rev Respir Dis 1989; 139:1158.

CHAPTER 93

Acute Parenchymal Disease in Childhood

Robert Katz, MD

Disorders of respiratory system structure and function with subsequent respiratory failure are a frequent cause for the admission of children to the pediatric intensive care unit. In a recent survey of 160 pediatric intensive care units, respiratory failure accounted for 31% of all admissions.[1] Although the management of acute parenchymal processes in infants and children is based on the same principles as that for adults, differences in physiology, etiologic agents, and technical needs exist between pediatric and adult patients; these differences are emphasized in this chapter.

ASSESSMENT OF RESPIRATORY STATUS

The manifestations of respiratory failure are not always evident, and precise assessment of a patient's ventilatory status must be based on both clinical and laboratory values. Attention should first be devoted to respiratory rate and to the pattern of breathing. The respiratory rate decreases with age and shows its greatest variability in newborn and young infants (Table 93–1). Tachypnea may be the first manifestation of respiratory distress in infants. With respect to the pattern of breathing, objective signs that indicate respiratory distress include chest wall retractions, visible use of accessory muscles, flaring of the alae nasi, and paradoxical respiratory movements. Visible contraction of the sternocleidomastoid muscles and the drawing in of the supraclavicular fossa are among the most reliable clinical signs of airway obstruction. Grunting is produced when premature glottic closure accompanies active chest wall contraction during early expiration. Infants and children grunt to increase airway pressure and, thus, functional residual capacity.

Clinical criteria also include the effects that alterations of arterial blood gas tensions and pH have on other organ systems. These may include restlessness, irritability, mood changes that progress to seizures, and coma. Cardiovascular effects range from tachycardia to bradycardia, blood pressure changes, and cardiac arrest. General fatigue and excessive sweating may also be useful clinical indicators of acute respiratory failure.

Arterial blood gas measurements are almost always necessary if an accurate assessment of a child's ventilatory status is to be made. Numerous studies (mainly in adults) have shown that clinical estimation of arterial oxygen and carbon dioxide partial pressures are often unreliable. Any patient who has unexplained signs such as confusion or cyanosis, is in an obtunded or comatose state, or has symptoms such as dyspnea, anxiety, or restlessness may have respiratory failure, and his or her arterial blood gases should be measured.

INDICATIONS FOR INTUBATION AND MECHANICAL VENTILATION

The decision to intubate and commence mechanical ventilation should be based on assessment of clinical parameters, serial measurement of arterial blood gases, and knowledge of the natural histories of the disease process affecting a particular child.

Clinical criteria should include the status of a patient's central nervous system, hemodynamic stability, and adequacy of the work of breathing and of the overall capacity of a patient to maintain sufficient respiratory effort. Clinical signs of significant deterioration include uncontrolled rest-

TABLE 93–1. Normal Respiratory Rates

Age	*Breaths per Minute*
Newborn (after 7 d)	30
6 mo	28
1 y	24
3 y	22
5 y	20
8 y	18
12 y	16
15 y	14

lessness, anxious expression, lack of response to physical stimuli, and limpness. Severe changes in heart rate or blood pressure, which are indicative of hemodynamic instability, are also signs that cardiopulmonary collapse may be imminent. Significant changes in the respiratory system such as marked decrease in breath sounds, loss of the ability to cry, and apnea are indications for securing of the airway and for providing ventilatory assessment.

Serial evaluation of arterial blood gases provides invaluable information when it must be decided whether mechanical ventilation is indicated. In general, blood gas criteria for initiating mechanical ventilation in infants and children are similar to those in adults. Arterial carbon dioxide partial pressures that are greater than 50 to 60 mm Hg (in the absence of chronic lung disease) or that rise at a rate greater than 5 mm Hg/h as well as a partial pressure of oxygen less than 60 mm Hg or a fraction of inspired oxygen greater than 60% are generally accepted criteria for assisting ventilation.

Initiating mechanical ventilation in a critically ill child may be difficult for the physician who does not treat children on a regular basis. Since uncuffed tubes are used in most infants and children, an air leak that can result in significant volume loss in the compressible spaces in the ventilator is usually present.

An approach to the initiation of mechanical ventilation in the infant and child is outlined in Figure 93–1*A* and *B*. A fraction of inspired oxygen from 0.90 to 1.0 minimizes the risk of hypoxia. Providing positive end-expiratory pressure (PEEP) of from 3 to 5 cm H_2O tends to maintain functional residual capacity and improve oxygenation. Maintenance of an inspiratory time of at least 0.75 seconds provides even distribution of ventilation while limiting peak airway pressure. The frequency of assisted breaths depends on the age of the child: 20 to 25 breaths is appropriate for infants younger than 2 years of age; 15 to 20 for children 2 to 10 years; and 10 to 15 for patients older than 10 years. Initial tidal volume is best selected on the basis of clinical judgment, which includes observation of adequate chest wall excursion and audible air entry. Maintenance of adequate minute ventilation should reduce a patient's work of breathing and dyspnea. Peak pressures usually range from 20 to 35 cm H_2O, depending on the severity of the pulmonary process. Immediately after stabilization with the ventilator has been achieved, adequacy should be assessed based on data from arterial blood gas measurement or from noninvasive modalities such as pulse oximetry and end-tidal carbon dioxide monitoring.

PARENCHYMAL DISEASES

Viral Pneumonia

Respiratory viruses are responsible for most pediatric lower respiratory tract infections, including pneumonia. It is estimated that about 80% to 85% of cases of pediatric pneumonia are caused by viruses following direct invasion of the lower respiratory tract. Epidemiologic factors, such as the time of year and the age of a child, may aid the clinician in differentiating viral from bacterial pneumonia. However, these factors do not provide much assistance in differentiating the sporadic bacterial infections that occur throughout the respiratory disease season. This becomes important when the clinician is deciding whether to initiate antibiotic therapy in a child with pneumonia.

In general, bacterial infections produce infiltrates that are well defined, involve only one lobe, and are more likely to be located in the medial or peripheral lung field. Fluid in the pleural space and abscess or pneumatocele formation are considered characteristic of bacterial infection. In contrast, infiltrates that result from viral infections are likely to be poorly defined, involve more than one lobe, and be located in the perihilar areas. Scattered areas of atelectasis or right upper lobe atelectasis is usually associated with viral infections.

Respiratory syncytial virus (RSV) is the most important nonbacterial pathogen to infect the respiratory tract during early life. It may cause bronchiolitis, pneumonia, or upper airway obstruction. Most cases of RSV infection occur in the first 3 years of life and occasionally in patients aged 5 to 7 years. At particular high risk for RSV are premature infants and infants with congenital heart disease or bronchopulmonary dysplasia. The usual illness begins with a low-grade fever and signs of upper respiratory tract infection. Coughing increases over the first 3 days of illness, and wheezing may also be present. More severe involvement develops for about 1% of infants during the first year of life and is evidenced by intercostal retractions and tachypnea.

Diagnosis of RSV infection may be made on the basis of clinical grounds in addition to knowledge of the presence of the virus in the community. Fluorescent antibody slide tests for rapid diagnosis are performed in most laboratories. This factor has become more important now that antiviral therapy is available for RSV. The drug ribavirin (Virazole) is available for use in infants with moderate to severe infections. Most reports in infants infected with RSV with and without underlying disease have reported a moderate beneficial effect from the drug. Ribavirin is administered in a nebulized form for 18 hours per day for 3 to 5 days and should be considered for all infants with underlying cardiopulmonary disease and for normal infants who are moderately to severely ill.[2] Bronchospasm is frequently noted in infants infected with RSV. Recent studies have indicated that the status of many of these infants improves after administration of inhaled $beta_2$ agonists such as albuterol.[3] The usual initial dose of albuterol is 0.15 mg/kg by nebulization; administration of this dose may be repeated every 20 minutes if necessary.

Parainfluenza viruses account for about the same total morbidity as does RSV. Parainfluenza virus type 3, like RSV, may produce serious lower respiratory tract infection in infants. The clinical course and radiographic findings for patients with parainfluenza pneumonia are similar to those for RSV.

Influenza viruses are the most important causes of pneumonia that leads to hospitalization of school-age children. The morbidity rates for infants and preschool-age children with influenza viruses are also considerable and rank just behind those for RSV and parainfluenza viruses. The clinical course of influenza virus infection is usually more abrupt and intense than the course of other respiratory viral infections. A high fever is common; older children complain of myalgia and headache. A dry, hacking cough usually precedes the development of pneumonitis. Chest radiography findings include the presence of multiple areas of atelectasis and of infiltrates that involve multiple lobes.

Influenza A virus infections can be treated with amantadine hydrochloride. Several studies have demonstrated that therapy with this drug shortens the course of uncomplicated influenza infection in otherwise healthy young adults and children if it is instituted within the first 48 hours of illness. Amantadine is not effective for the treatment of influenza B virus infections.

Adenoviruses are an uncommon cause of pneumonia in infants and children. However, adenoviruses types 7, 14, and 21 are associated with severe necrotizing pneumonia and respiratory failure. Mortality rates from infections with these adenoviruses range from 10% to 17%. Most infants

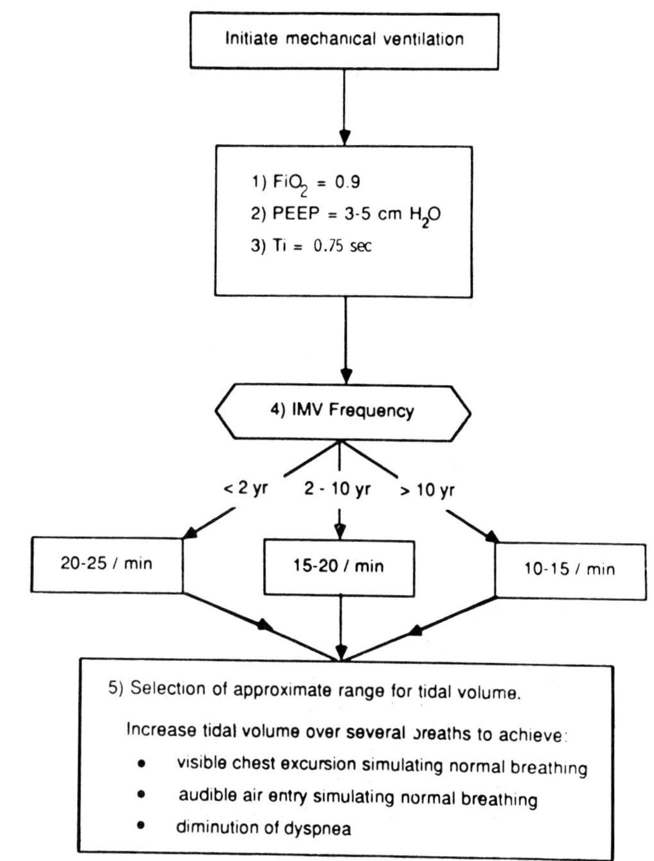

Figure 93–1. Algorithm for the initiation of mechanical ventilation in the pediatric patient. (From Kanter RK: Evaluation and stabilization of the critically ill child. Clin Chest Med 1987; 8:576–577.)

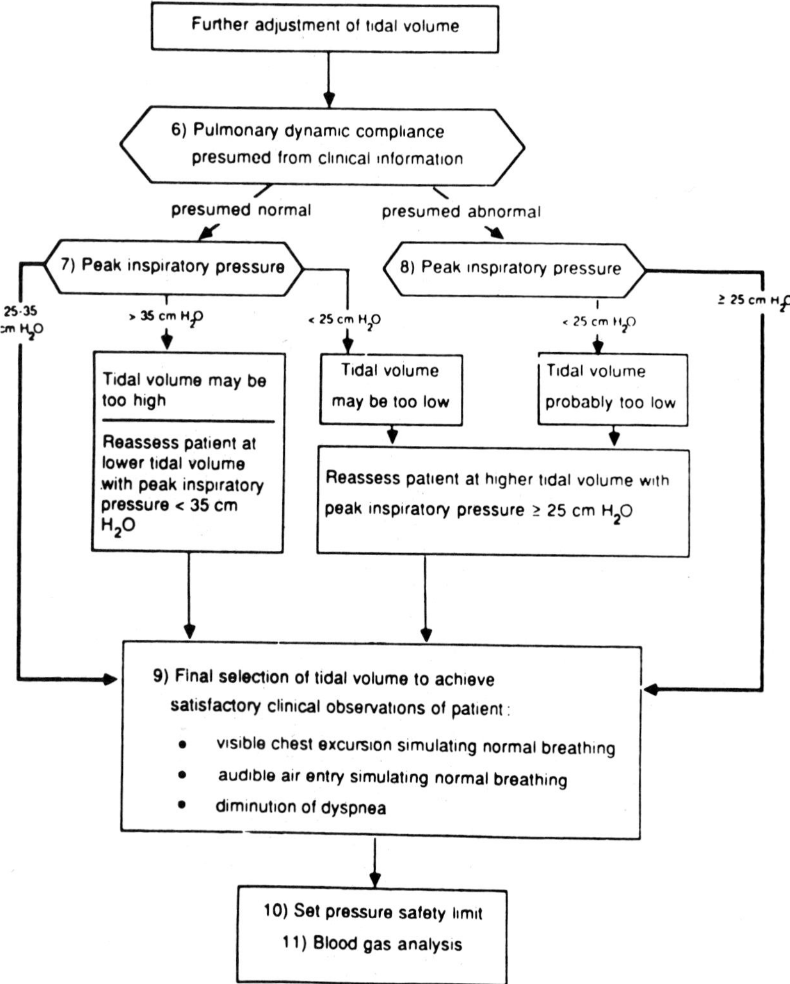

with severe disease are younger than 18 months of age. Clinically, the course can be very protracted, with tachypnea, cough, and wheezing persisting for weeks. Treatment is supported with mechanical ventilation, if necessary. Patients with adenovirus infections have a high incidence of residual pulmonary function abnormalities and bronchiectasis.[4]

Viral infections of the lung follow certain clinical and epidemiologic patterns; knowledge of these patterns is useful in determining proper management for the patient with pneumonia. The course of viral pneumonia is not altered by the administration of antibiotics, and bacterial superinfections are so uncommon (especially in patients with RSV infections) that the routine use of antimicrobial agents is not warranted. Most children with viral pneumonia who require intensive care are younger than 3 years of age. It is unusual for older children with viral pneumonia (except those with chronic cardiopulmonary disease) to require ventilatory assistance.

Bacterial Pneumonia

The bacterial pathogens causing pneumonia vary with the age of a patient as well as with the patient's immune status and environmental conditions. The most common of these pathogens in newborns are group B streptococci followed by gram-negative enteric bacilli and chlamydiae. In children between the ages of 1 month and 6 years, *Streptococcus pneumoniae* and *Haemophilus influenzae* B are the most common pathogens. The latter is especially likely in children between the ages of 4 months and 2 years and often is associated with bacteremia. In adolescents, *Mycoplasma pneumoniae* and *S. pneumoniae* are the most common causative agents. However, much overlap exists, and the age of the child is only one factor in elucidating the cause of the pneumonia.

It is difficult to determine the per cent of pneumonia cases that are caused by bacteria. Unless a patient is bacteremic, has pleural empyema, or has antigenuria, opportunities to establish a cause are limited. It is estimated that a causative agent is defined in less than one fourth of hospitalized children with pneumonia.[5]

Although the blood culture is a specific method for establishing a cause, its results are positive only in 10% to 15% of cases and mainly in younger children with pneumonia caused by *H. influenzae, Staphylococcus aureus,* or *S. pneumoniae.* Because of the associated risks of bacteremia, cultures should be performed for any child with suspected bacterial pneumonia before antibiotic therapy is initiated. A diligent search should be made for other sites of infection (e.g., joints, pleural space, meninges), and the appropriate fluids should be collected for culture. Counterimmunoelectrophoresis for pneumococcal or *H. influenzae* type B antigen in the urine may increase the percentage of positively identified causative agents.

Diagnostic lung aspiration should be considered in any severely ill child in whom a prompt diagnosis is essential, such as one with progressive disease who has responded poorly to therapy or one with underlying immunodeficiency in whom empiric, broad-spectrum treatment is hazardous because of the risk of superinfection and other adverse effects.

Staphylococcal pneumonia in infants usually develops as a primary infection of the respiratory tract or as part of a septicemic infection. Infection of the respiratory tract may rapidly produce severe distress characterized by tachypnea, grunting respirations, retractions, and cyanosis. Many infants with staphylococcal pneumonia are often gravely ill.

Diagnosis is based on a patient's history, radiography findings, and positive culture results. The radiography ray findings of staphylococcal pneumonia distinguish it from other types of pneumonia, especially in infants. Within a few hours, radiography findings can change from small infiltrative lesions to patchy consolidation, to pneumatocele and empyema formation. Pneumothorax, pyopneumothorax, and bronchopleural fistula are not uncommon. Blood culture results are positive in 9% to 25% of cases.[6] Empyema is almost universal, and cultures of pleural fluid invariably yield positive results.

Staphylococcal pneumonia is an acute medical emergency that requires early, maximum, and prolonged antibiotic therapy if tissue necrosis and the tendency for bacterial persistence, which provide a potential focus for relapse, are to be avoided. Initial treatment should be with a parenteral β-lactamase–resistant antibiotic such as nafcillin or methicillin. Chest radiography performed daily is necessary to watch for possible pneumothorax, pneumatocele, empyema, or pyopneumothorax. Pneumatoceles usually resolve spontaneously and do not require needle aspiration or surgical intervention. However, if the bullae mechanically compress the trachea or mainstem bronchi, aspiration or excision may be necessary. Early closed-chest tube drainage is the preferred treatment for empyema or pyopneumothorax. This procedure is much more effective than repeated aspirations.

Despite the use of effective antimicrobial agents and the availability of intensive care, the mortality associated with staphylococcal pneumonia remains high, with most deaths occurring in infants younger than 1 year of age. For the surviving children, abnormalities revealed on radiography may persist for weeks or months; however, the prognosis for pulmonary function is excellent.

Pneumococcal pneumonia is caused by *S. pneumoniae,* the organism most frequently responsible for bacterial pneumonia. The incubation period is 1 to 3 days, and the onset of pneumonia is heralded by coughing, severe shaking, chills, and high fever. Patchy bronchopneumonia is more common than lobar consolidation, particularly during the first year of life. About 25% to 33% of patients develop pneumococcal bacteremia; this worsens the prognosis because it introduces extrapulmonary complications, including empyema, pericarditis, and meningitis. However, most infants with pneumococcal pneumonia do not require intensive care unless these complications develop. The treatment of choice is therapy with penicillin.

H. influenzae is an important etiologic agent of pneumonia in children between the ages of 3 months and 2 years.[6] Radiography demonstrates consolidative pneumonia in most patients. The incidence of pleural effusions, particularly empyema, appears to be high, as does the incidence of positive blood culture results. Extrapulmonary infection sites are common, and *H. influenzae* may be recovered from cerebrospinal fluid, joint fluid, or pericardial fluid in affected children. Clinically, it may be difficult to differentiate pneumonia caused by *H. influenzae* from pneumococcal or, occasionally, staphylococcal infections. About 25% of *H. influenzae* type B strains in the United States are β-lactamase producers.[7] Therefore, standard initial therapy consists of administration of one of the third-generation cephalosporins such as cefuroxime, cefotaxime, or ceftriaxone.

Adult Respiratory Distress Syndrome

Adult respiratory distress syndrome (ARDS) is a major cause of death in children receiving intensive care for sepsis and has been associated with mortality rates of from 50% to 90%.[8–10] Septic shock, pneumonia, and near-drowning are the most common precipitating events. ARDS has been described in neonates as well.[11]

Children who are at risk for ARDS should be carefully monitored in a pediatric intensive care unit. Respiratory rates should be compared with age-related normal values (see Table 93–1). Respiratory rates consistently above normal may indicate increasing atelectasis and worsening compliance. Serial evaluation of arterial blood gases is essential if incipient pulmonary dysfunction is to be detected. The use of pulse oximeters for the continuous monitoring of saturation is extremely helpful in this setting. Indications for intubation are similar to those described previously in this chapter.

Respiratory assistance remains the keystone of supportive care for the patient with ARDS; however, despite many technologic improvements in this form of therapy, mortality rates remain high. The optimal mode of ventilation in ARDS patients is still a matter of debate. Although intermittent mandatory ventilation has become popular over the last 10 years, none of the advantages of this ventilatory mode has proved to alter the outcome in patients with ARDS.[12] However, assisted mechanical ventilation in rarely used in pediatric patients, since sensitivity is difficult to adjust and hyperventilation is frequent. Thus, most pediatric patients are at least initially treated with intermittent mandatory ventilation. However, even this approach is not without difficulties. Many new ventilators with built-in intermittent mandatory ventilation circuits are not continuous-flow systems; often, a demand valve must be activated if gas is to flow to the patient. For small children and even some adults, this mechanism may significantly increase the work of breathing.[13] In addition, significant differences exist in the sensitivity of these demand valves among ventilators; these differences may be important when a child with severe respiratory failure is ventilated.[14] The addition of 10 to 15 cm H_2O of pressure support decreases the work of breathing associated with the inspiratory phase of ventilation.

The application of PEEP improves oxygenation in most patients with ARDS. The improvement in arterial oxygen partial pressure is usually due to a decrease in shunt perfusion, with occasional decreases in blood flow to areas with a low area ventilation-perfusion ratio.[15] Despite this effect of PEEP, considerable controversy exists regarding the level of PEEP to be used for ARDS patients. Although a variety of endpoints have been suggested, no data prove that one is better than another.[16] However, it is clear that the response to any PEEP increment cannot be predicted from the characteristics of the patient or of gas exchange before the application of PEEP. It is important to apply PEEP in a controlled manner (e.g., in 3- to 5-cm H_2O increments), with arterial blood gas measurements performed 15 to 20 minutes after each increase. Ideally, 90% saturation should be achieved with a fraction of inspired oxygen of less than 0.6. It has been demonstrated that with the judicious use of fluids or inotropes, cardiac function can be maintained in children subjected to high PEEP levels.[17] In fact, their highly compliant chest walls should lessen the transmission of positive airway pressure to the heart and great vessels.[18]

If low PEEP levels are sufficient to achieve satisfactory gas exchange and if a patient is hemodynamically stable, the frequent monitoring of routine vital signs and arterial blood gas parameters will probably ensure adequate oxygen delivery. A pulmonary artery catheter should be placed and more sophisticated variables monitored if a child with respiratory failure has clinical evidence of hemodynamic instability, an uncertain blood volume status, or a PEEP greater than 10 to 15 cm H_2O. The bedside placement of pulmonary artery catheters in children can be done easily and with a minimum of complications. Catheterization allows direct measurement of cardiac output ($\dot{Q}t$) by thermodilution and the calculation of oxygen delivery ($\dot{Q}t$ multiplied by arterial oxygen concentration). In addition, access to mixed venous blood permits calculation of the intrapulmonary shunt fraction ($\dot{Q}sp/\dot{Q}t$), which is a more accurate assessment of the degree of lung injury than are alveolar-arterial pressure gradient ratios of arterial oxygen tension to inspired fraction of oxygen. In addition, the use of catecholamines or afterload-reducing agents can have complex effects on arterial oxygen tension, intrapulmonary shunt fraction, and oxygen delivery ($\dot{D}O_2$).

Chest radiographs should be obtained daily to assess the evolution of the disease, ensure the proper placement of all centrally placed lines, and monitor for pulmonary barotrauma. Barotrauma and pneumothorax are possible complications associated with high PEEP (>15 cm H_2O).[19] However, patients with ARDS appear to have an increased risk of pneumothorax if they are not treated with PEEP (no study has clearly found a high incidence of pneumothorax in patients receiving PEEP). The incidence of pneumothorax and pneumomediastinum in ventilated infants without hyaline membrane disease is comparable to that found in the adult series.[19]

A decrease in venous admixture in ARDS patients often precedes substantial clearing of the infiltrates on chest radiographs. A patient's compliance will probably be improved and peak pressures on the ventilator will be reduced with such a decrease. PEEP can then be reduced in 3- to 5-cm H_2O increments, with arterial blood gas parameters checked 15 to 20 minutes after each change to ensure continued satisfactory oxygenation. If the arterial oxygen tension decreases substantially, PEEP should be returned to its original level.

Weaning small infants and children from mechanical ventilation is complicated by the scant information available on the reliability of mechanical variables of patients in this age group. Most reports in this area have addressed weaning from mechanical ventilation after cardiovascular surgery in infants without severe parenchymal disease. Because vital capacity, peak negative pressure, and tidal volume do not usually reflect the ability to wean, intermittent mandatory ventilation is very useful in weaning these patients. Ventilator breaths should be reduced three to five at a time, and serial evaluations of respiratory rate, breathing patterns, and blood gases should be performed. A marked increase in respiratory rate, development of carbon dioxide retention, or metabolic acidosis secondary to an increase in the work of breathing is an indication that weaning should be stopped and the ventilatory rate increased. At all times, 3- to 5-cm H_2O PEEP should be used, as the absence of this physiologic level may lead to decreases in functional residual capacity and hypoxemia.

PULMONARY CONTUSION

The types of thoracic injury that children suffer depend on the age of the children and on the pediatric population studied. Blunt chest injury tends to be an injury of infancy and early childhood, whereas penetrating trauma is more common in adolescents. In a series of 199 patients, the incidence of blunt trauma far exceeded that of other types of trauma until the age of 13 years was reached.[20] In children older than 13 years of age, penetrating injury was more frequent and followed the adult pattern. In a series of 94 children with chest trauma reviewed by Smyth,[21] 86 had closed-chest injury and only 8 sustained penetrating injuries. The most frequent cause of closed-chest injury was road traffic accident. In 70 cases of such an accident, 68 children were pedestrians and only 2 were passengers in vehicles.

A pulmonary contusion is a blunt parenchymal injury

that produces edema, hemorrhage, or desquamative alveolitis. Microscopically, the changes found in pulmonary contusion vary in degree and distribution, depending on the severity of the injury. Minimal damage produces only focal areas of interstitial edema, whereas severe injury causes a rapid intra-alveolar extravasation of blood with consolidation of the lungs.

Clinically, pulmonary contusion may lead to hypoxemia, tachypnea, reduced pulmonary compliance, and, ultimately, acute respiratory failure. Because a child's thorax is more elastic than the adult's, fractured ribs are generally less common in children than in adults, even if a severe, crushing force has been exerted. Some series have documented higher mortality in patients without rib fractures; it has been postulated that fractures of the sternum or ribs expend a portion of the force applied to the chest wall and, thus, reduce injury to the underlying lung. Flail chest is also less common in children than in adults owing to the lower prevalence of rib fractures.

Significant thoracic injury is frequently a component of multisystemic injuries; therefore, management must consider the possibility of multiple organ failure. Mortality is related to the number of organs injured. In Smyth's study,[21] 10 of the 13 deaths reported were due to nonthoracic trauma; chest trauma was the cause of death in only 3 children. Other studies of children have reported mortality rates from pulmonary contusion of 4% to 15%.

Initially, the clinical and radiographic appearance of the child with pulmonary contusion may be misleading. Some patients are asymptomatic and have normal chest radiographs or minimal patchy consolidation. Pulmonary contusion may be easily overlooked in the absence of rib fractures or when multiple injuries—especially those of the head or the abdomen—demand urgent attention. Concomitant pneumothorax or hemothorax may mask the underlying parenchymal damage. Auscultation of the chest may only reveal a few rales. In more severe cases, the sputum may be blood tinged.

All children who have suffered thoracic or multiple injuries should be carefully monitored in an intensive care unit. The value of initial and serial arterial blood gas determinations cannot be overemphasized; often, the severity of insult is not appreciated until blood gas analyses are performed. Although initial chest radiographs may be unremarkable, parenchymal injury, if present, is readily apparent within 24 hours. Criteria for intubation and aspects of ventilatory management are the same as those described earlier in this chapter.

Secondary bacterial pneumonias are common in patients with pulmonary contusions. Infection should be suspected in patients who initially respond to treatment with an improvement in gas exchange but then deteriorate. Tracheal secretions should be obtained for Gram's staining and culturing, and appropriate antibiotics should be administered. Prophylactic antibiotic administration appears to be of little value in preventing infection following blunt or penetrating trauma.[22]

References

1. Groeger J, Guntupalli K, Strosberg M: Descriptive analysis of critical care units in the United States: Patient characteristics and intensive care unit utilization. Crit Care Med 1993; 21:279–291.
2. Hall CB, McBride JT, Gala CL, et al: Ribavirin treatment of respiratory syncytial viral infection in infants with underlying cardiopulmonary disease. JAMA 1985; 254:3047.
3. Schuh S, Ganny C, Reisman J: Nebulized albuterol in acute bronchiolitis. J Pediatr 1990; 117:633–637.
4. Becroft DM: Histopathology of fatal adenovirus infection of the respiratory tract in young children. J Clin Pathol 1967; 20:561.
5. Grossman M, Klein J, McCarthy P: Consensus: Management of presumed bacterial pneumonia in ambulatory children. Pediatr Infect Dis 1984; 3:497.
6. Yeto SD, Heller R: Acute respiratory infections. Pediatr Clin North Am 1974; 21:683.
7. Freij B: Pneumonia of known etiology. *In*: Current Therapy in Pediatric Infectious Disease. Nelson JD (Ed). New York, BC Decker, 1986, pp 25–34.
8. Lyrene R, Truog W: Adult respiratory distress syndrome in a pediatric intensive care unit: Predisposing conditions, clinical course and outcome. Pediatrics 1981; 67:790.
9. Holbrook PR, Taylor GT, Pollack MM, et al: Adult respiratory distress syndrome in children. Pediatr Clin North Am 1980; 27:677.
10. Timmons OD, Dean JM, Vernon DD: Mortality rates and prognostic variables in children with adult respiratory distress syndrome. J Pediatr 1991; 199:896–899.
11. Pfenninger J, Tschaeppeler H, Wagner BP: The paradox of adult respiratory distress syndrome in neonates. Pediatr Pulmonol 1991; 10:18–24.
12. Weisman JM, Rinaldo JE, Rogers RN, et al: Intermittent mandatory ventilation. Am Rev Respir Dis 1985; 127:641.
13. Christopher KL, Niff TA, Bowan JS: Demand and continuous flow intermittent mandatory ventilation systems. Chest 1985; 87:625.
14. Cox D, Niblett DJ: Studies on continuous positive airway pressure breathing systems. Br J Anaesth 1984; 56:905.
15. Ralph DD, Robertson HT, Weaver JL, et al: Distribution of ventilation and perfusion during positive and expiratory pressure in the adult respiratory distress syndrome. Am Rev Respir Dis 1985; 131:54.
16. Albert RK: Least PEEP: Primum non nocere. Chest 1985; 7:2.
17. Katz R, Pollack M, Spady D: Cardiopulmonary abnormalities in severe acute respiratory failure. J Pediatr 1984; 194:357.
18. Bryan AC, Mansell AL, Levison H: Development of the mechanical properties of the respiratory system. *In*: Development of the Lung. Hodson WA (Ed). New York, Marcel Dekker, 1977, pp 445–468.
19. Pollack MM, Fields AL, Holbrook PR: Pneumothorax and pneumomediastinum during pediatric mechanical ventilation. Crit Care Med 1979; 7:536.
20. Sinclair MC, Moore TC: Major surgery for abdominal and thoracic trauma in childhood and adolescence. J Pediatr Surg 1974; 9:155.
21. Smyth BT: Chest trauma in childhood. J Pediatr Surg 1979; 14:41.
22. Mandal AK, Montano J, Ihadepalli H: Prophylactic antibiotics and no antibiotics compared in penetrating chest trauma. J Trauma 1985; 25:639.

CHAPTER 94

Pathophysiology and Management of Adult Respiratory Distress Syndrome

William C. Shoemaker, MD

The purpose of this chapter is to summarize the temporal relationship among blood volume, hemodynamics, oxygen transport, and cytokine patterns occurring in postoperative patients before and after the onset of adult respiratory distress syndrome (ARDS) in order to develop a more complete mechanistic evaluation of its pathophysiology and to propose more rational therapeutic strategies. Time relationships of circulatory patterns that have pathogenic importance have not been well studied. The data reviewed indicate that hypovolemia, reduced or uneven blood flow, inadequate delivery of oxygen ($\dot{D}O_2$), and insufficient consumption of oxygen ($\dot{V}O_2$) precede the appearance of ARDS and are primary precipitating physiologic events of this disease.

This observation is contrary to conventional thinking, which emphasizes capillary leak and fluid overload as the primary causes of ARDS. The conventional approach ignores events antecedent to ARDS that produce hypoxia of the lung tissue and that result in pulmonary vasoconstriction and increased pulmonary shunt. Therapy to prevent or rapidly treat these antecedent events has been shown to prevent or attenuate postoperative and post-traumatic ARDS.

THE COMMON CLINICAL SETTING OF ARDS

ARDS is a frequent complication of trauma and surgery. The syndrome is defined clinically as hypoxemia (arterial oxygen tension [PaO_2] < 55 when room air is breathed) that is unresponsive to conservative management and that necessitates use of mechanical ventilation with increased fraction of inspired oxygen (FIO_2) for life support for more than 24 hours.[1,2] Chest radiography may reveal the existence of basal infiltrates. The diagnosis is confirmed by a PaO_2/FIO_2 less than 200, a pulmonary venous admixture (shunt) greater than 20%, and reduced chest compliance.[3–8] It most frequently occurs in the postoperative or post-traumatic patient who may have had hypotension, unstable hemodynamics, or shock during or shortly after surgery or sepsis. The patient is usually treated with sufficient amounts of crystalloid solutions to restore blood pressure and urine output to normal ranges. Radiographic evidence of pulmonary congestion or edema, which indicates the presence of excess fluid in the lung, is often interpreted as overadministration of fluids. Fluid restriction and diuretics are often used for the postoperative patient who has developed ARDS even after physicians had made an attempt to "keep the patient on the dry side."

This chapter describes the temporal patterns of blood volume, hemodynamics, and oxygen transport measurements that precede the development of ARDS with the goal of reevaluating pathogenic mechanisms that contribute to this syndrome. Hypovolemia and inadequate or maldistributed blood flow were uniformly observed before the onset of ARDS in patients treated inadequately or with delays in treatment. Frequently hypotension, oliguria, and other superficial signs of shock were corrected, but the underlying tissue perfusion deficiencies usually were not adequately corrected in a timely manner.

THE CONVENTIONAL APPROACH TO ADULT RESPIRATORY DISTRESS SYNDROME

Conventional Pathophysiology

Pulmonary edema resulting from the increased permeability of the alveolocapillary membrane is traditionally regarded as the physiologic basis of ARDS. Increases in intravascular and extracellular water volumes with reductions in protein flux produce pulmonary interstitial and alveolar edema, which in turn produce hypoxemia owing to their interference with gas exchange.[4–12] Evidence in support of the concept of increased endothelial permeability or capillary leak as the primary event in ARDS are usually based on three arguments. First, experimental pulmonary edema has been produced in sheep and other animals by intravenous administration of live bacteria or endotoxin.[9,10]

Second, pulmonary edema is widely invoked as the principle mechanism produced in septic shock patients without cardiac problems or excessive fluid administration.[11] However, direct measurements of the presence and amount of capillary leak are not available under clinical conditions. Nevertheless, capillary leak is often presumed from the clinical and radiologic appearance of pulmonary edema. Patients whose initial resuscitation and subsequent fluid therapy had solely been the administration of large volumes of crystalloid solutions may have immediate improvement with fluid restriction and use of diuretics.[13] It is not surprising that an overly distended interstitium occurring after resuscitation with massive crystalloid therapy may be improved after diuretic therapy, particularly if the plasma volume is not concomitantly reduced; this only means, however, that diuretics may partially correct an untoward effect of therapy, and not the underlying disease. Some authors have actually defined increased capillary permeability as pulmonary edema without cardiac failure or fluid overload.[9] Stated in its simplest form, this concept tends to resemble "circular" reasoning: capillary leak causes pulmonary edema and, therefore, pulmonary edema is due to capillary leak.

Third, evidence for capillary leak as the primary event in ARDS has been demonstrated in studies of biopsy and necropsy specimens. However, maldistribution of body fluids from increased permeability or capillary leak usually occurs in the middle or late stages of ARDS. Capillary leak at this time may be inferred from, but not proven by, the failure to sustain blood volume and adequate hemodynamics with fluid therapy. The crucial problems facing efforts to objectively define capillary leaks clinically are the development of measurable criteria of leaks and the time relationships between the appearance of the leaks and the onset of ARDS. Lung biopsies describe early anatomic changes immediately after the onset of respiratory failure. After hemorrhagic shock in conscious animals on the day that the diagnosis of ARDS is established, small patchy areas of round cell infiltration, perivascular hemorrhage, atelectasis or hyperaerated alveoli, and thickening of the alveolocapillary membrane are observed; the lesions are confined to areas constituting as little as 5% to 10% of the lung fields.[14] Subsequently, on the second and third days, these areas become larger and more confluent.[15,16] Not until the late stage of ARDS or at the time of autopsy does red or gray "hepatization" occur. At this time, capillary leak is obvious because alveoli are filled with pink proteinaceous fluid. In essence, capillary leak in biopsy and autopsy specimens is evidenced by pink proteinaceous fluid in the alveoli.[5,17–19] The problem with this argument is that late, terminal, or postmortem histologic findings may reflect the results of ARDS, and not necessarily its cause.

The Conventional Therapeutic Approach to Fluid Therapy

The conventional aims of resuscitation in acute illness and ARDS are the attainment of normal vital signs, hematocrit, urine output, and blood gas measurements while pulmonary artery occlusion pressure is maintained as low as possible. After normal vital signs are achieved, the goal of therapy in ARDS consists of fluid restriction and diuretic administration, which prevent or minimize pulmonary edema by maintaining low pulmonary artery occlusion pressures. Justification for "drying the patient out" is based on (1) input/output records of large amounts of fluids given before the diagnosis of ARDS was made; (2) clinical evidence of excessive fluid retention, such as peripheral edema;

(3) clinical and radiologic evidence of pulmonary congestion and edema; and (4) improvement in arterial blood gas values after administration of diuretics.

The conventional approach maintains the patient "on the dry side."[4, 8, 9, 12] However, this is more a philosophic statement of intent rather than a useful operational therapeutic rule.[12] Explicit physiologic criteria for this approach that can be used to make clinical management decisions are either lacking or have not been developed as guidelines or protocols.

Critique of the Conventional Approach

Several major problems are associated with conventional concepts of fluid restriction in ARDS. The diagnosis of capillary leak is based solely on clinical or radiologic evidence of pulmonary congestion, not on direct measurement of increased capillary permeability. This is usually interpreted as the result of excessive fluid administration and that the excessive fluids have leaked into the lungs and caused pulmonary edema, which interferes with gas exchange. However, Bishop and coworkers[13] and Johnson and associates[14] have demonstrated that trauma patients resuscitated to optimal supranormal $\dot{D}O_2$ and $\dot{V}O_2$ values are given more fluids and accumulate greater fluid balances but have improved survival with fewer lung and other organ failures compared with the control group treated with conventional therapy. However, pulmonary edema may result from (1) cardiac failure, (2) capillary leak, (3) excessive infused volumes of crystalloid solutions, (4) hemorrhage with massive crystalloid solution replacement, (5) low oncotic pressure from nutritional failure, and (6) hypoxia of the lung tissue itself. Pulmonary edema, therefore, may be produced by many conditions; in postoperative and septic patients, it is more often the effect than the cause of ARDS.

Pulmonary edema has been observed when no fluids were given in patients with high-altitude sickness, sepsis, decompression injury after diving, head injury, nutritional failure (e.g., kwashiorkor), and postcardiac arrest states. Combat casualties with head injuries who died on the battlefield without having received any fluid therapy were found at autopsy to have pulmonary edema. Most commonly, it is seen in the high-risk postoperative patient resuscitated with massive crystalloid infusions. Under these conditions, pulmonary edema is due to overexpansion of the interstitium, and not to plasma volume overload. In essence, peripheral and pulmonary edema reflects an increase in interstitial fluid volumes due to, for example, maldistribution of body water, massive crystalloid infusions, low plasma oncotic pressure, nutritional failure, increased endothelial permeability (capillary leak), lung hypoxia, or anaphylactoid reactions. In any case, fluid overload in the sense of overexpanded blood volume is usually not a causative factor. However, the most disturbing evidence against the application of fluid restriction and diuretics is the admission of Bartlett and coworkers[6] that 15 years of this approach has not reduced mortality rate of patients with ARDS. Depending on associated diseases and organ failures, 50% to 70% of ARDS patients still die. With each additional organ failure, mortality increases: among those patients with one other organ failure, 54% died; of those with two, 72% died; of those with three, 84% died; and of those with four other organ failures, 100% died.[6]

TEMPORAL DESCRIPTION OF PHYSIOLOGIC PATTERNS

The pathogenesis of ARDS should be based on objective physiologic evidence, and not on plausible theories. The concept that ARDS is caused by antecedent tissue hypoxia is evidenced by the demonstration of oxygen debt from circulatory deficiencies as the earliest physiologic event associated with high-risk surgical operations, major trauma, and hypovolemia. ARDS does not just materialize as a new entity; rather, it is the end-organ failure of an antecedent postoperative or post-traumatic shock in which blood pressure and other superficial signs of shock were corrected but in which the underlying tissue perfusion defect persisted. If this is indeed the precipitating event of ARDS, then the present conventional approach to ARDS therapy is inappropriate or even counterproductive.

A crucial factor in the determination of causality is time. Unfortunately, this is the parameter most often ignored in the pathophysiologic evaluation of ARDS. When event A occurs before event B, A may or may not be the cause of B, but B can be excluded as the cause of the antecedent A. By separating events in time, an appropriate hypothesis regarding pathogenesis may be developed using temporal descriptions that allow primary events to be separated from secondary and terminal events.

The following section briefly summarizes physiologic data and other evidence obtained before the onset of ARDS.

Blood Volume Measurements

Studies have reported the results of blood volume measurement with iodine 125–labeled albumin in critically ill surgical intensive care unit patients.[20, 21] Table 94–1 summarizes blood volume measurements in 48 survivors and 47 nonsurvivors of ARDS at times before and after the onset of this syndrome. At the time that diagnostic criteria of ARDS were met, the mean blood volume deficit was greater in the nonsurvivors than in the survivors of ARDS. Similarly, nonsurviving ARDS patients had greater blood volume deficits at the initial observation and at the time when maximum blood volume was observed. The data document major blood volume deficits in postoperative ARDS patients 1 to 4 days before the time that criteria for diagnosis of ARDS were met. The hypovolemia was of greater intensity and lasted longer in patients who died of ARDS. Postoperative patients who did not develop ARDS had minimal or no blood volume deficits.

Temporal Hemodynamic and Oxygen Transport Patterns Before, During, and After High-Risk Surgical Operations

The hemodynamic and oxygen transport patterns of 708 high-risk patients were analyzed before, during, and after surgical operations in an effort to describe the temporal responses to life-threatening trauma under conditions in which hemodynamic and oxygen variables could be measured with reasonably satisfactory reproducibility.[22] The major findings were intraoperatively reduced circulatory function after the early postoperative period followed by increased circulatory functions as manifested, primarily, by

TABLE 94–1. Blood Volume Deficits in Adult Respiratory Distress Syndrome Patients Before and at the Time of Their Diagnosis*

Blood Volume Deficit	*Survivors (mL/m²)*	*Nonsurvivors (mL/m²)*
Initial	518 ± 51	722 ± 56
Maximum	713 ± 56	981 ± 52
At onset of ARDS	401 ± 67	620 ± 58

*Values are mean ± SEM.

increases in cardiac index (CI), $\dot{D}O_2$, and $\dot{V}O_2$. The postoperative increases in CI and $\dot{D}O_2$ values were greater in patients who survived their hospitalization than in those who did not, particularly when these patterns were related to their own preoperative baseline values. The temporal patterns of survivors and nonsurvivors in each of the following stratifications were described in patients with and without associated cardiovascular disease: baseline CI values were normal in patients without cardiovascular disease; patients with sepsis, trauma, stress, and late cirrhosis had high preoperative baseline CI values; and patients with hemorrhage, dehydration, hypovolemia, and cardiac conditions had low preoperative values for CI, $\dot{D}O_2$, and $\dot{V}O_2$. The data indicate that the increases in CI and $\dot{D}O_2$ are compensatory mechanisms against prior circulatory deficits that produce tissue hypoxia and organ dysfunction during and immediately after surgical trauma.

Therapeutic goals for patients with high-risk criteria were empirically determined as the median values of CI, $\dot{D}O_2$, and $\dot{V}O_2$ at their maxima for survivors of high-risk surgery in their early postoperative course.[23, 24] These values were observed to be as follows: CI greater than 4.5 L/min · m^2; $\dot{D}O_2$ greater than 600 mL/min · m^2; $\dot{V}O_2$ greater than 170 mL/min · m^2; and blood volume 500 mL greater than normal (i.e., 3.2 L/m^2 for men, and 2.7 L/m^2 for women). Optimal goals are higher for patients with severe trauma and for those with sepsis. These values should be reached within the first 8 to 12 hours postoperatively.

Prospective Clinical Trials

The basic hypothesis that therapeutic goals should be the supranormal values empirically observed in survivors was supported in an initial trial of 252 high-risk patients. They were grouped by services, with normal values as the goals for the control service patients and with supranormal values as the therapeutic goals of a protocol service. Then, a randomized trial preoperatively allocated patients to (1) a central venous pressure (CVP) catheter group (CVP group) with normal values as goals; (2) a pulmonary artery (PA) catheter group (PA-control group) with normal values as goals of therapy; and (3) a PA catheter group (PA-protocol group) with supranormal values as goals.[23] No significant differences in outcome were observed between the CVP group and the PA-control group, both of which had normal values as their goals. This suggests that when the therapeutic intent is to maintain normal values, no real advantages are gained from the use of the PA catheter. Compared with the PA-control group, the PA-protocol group had reduced mortality (4% versus 33%, $P < .02$), fewer ventilator days (2.4 ± 0.5 versus 9.4 ± 3.4 [SEM] days, $P < .05$), fewer hospital days (19.3 ± 2.4 versus 25.2 ± 3.4 days), and fewer days in the intensive care unit (10.2 ± 1.6 versus 15.8 ± 3.1, $P < .05$) as well as an about 25% reduction in hospital costs (Table 94–2).[23] In the PA-protocol group, the goals were achieved with fluid therapy alone in two thirds of the patients, using an average of about 6 to 7 L of crystalloid solutions and about 3 L of colloid solutions, principally albumin. The remaining one third also were given dobutamine for inotropic support, and two patients (7%) required a vasodilator because of sudden hypertensive episodes on recovery from anesthesia. The control group received about the same amount of crystalloid solutions and packed red blood cells but about one third as much colloid solutions in order to maintain normal values.[23, 24] This concept has been corroborated by the results of a number of subsequent studies.[22, 25–37]

A higher incidence of organ failure, sepsis, and disseminated intravascular coagulopathy was observed in patients with normal values as therapeutic goals than in those with supranormal values as goals; however, no significant differences were seen in the incidence of other common complications.[24]

Tissue Hypoxia as the Primary Event in Postoperative Shock and Organ Failure

Data from the previously discussed prospective randomized trials indicate poor tissue perfusion and tissue hypoxia are occasioned by inadequate or maldistributed peripheral blood flow in the face of increased metabolic demands from inflammatory responses, postoperative wound healing, and fever as well as prior tissue hypoxia associated with hypovolemia, anesthesia, and surgical trauma. Progressively increasing tissue hypoxia may result in multiple vital organ failure, which is the major proximate cause of death in intensive care unit patients. This corollary hypothesis was tested by measuring the preoperative $\dot{V}O_2$ and by extrapolating this value, corrected for the effects of anesthesia and temperature changes, as the estimated amount of oxygen need for the first 48 hours postoperatively.[35] Yu and coworkers and Boyd and associates originally developed this approach to estimating oxygen need in experimental hemorrhagic shock. The oxygen debt was calculated from the observed $\dot{V}O_2$ subtracted from the estimated oxygen need. The net cumulative oxygen debt was calculated from the rate of oxygen deficit integrated over time. Guyton and colleagues[36, 37] demonstrated that dogs who developed an oxygen debt greater than 140 mL/kg all died, whereas those with an oxygen debt less than 100 mL/kg all survived; the halfway mark between survivors and nonsurvivors was 120 mL/kg.

TABLE 94–2. Clinical Data of Prospective Randomized Clinical Trial

	Nonrandomized (n = 45)	*CVP Group (n = 30)*	*PA-Control Group (n = 30)*	*PA-Protocol Group (n = 28)*
Age (y)	56.9 ± 25	55.2 ± 30	53.4 ± 2.5	56.4 ± 3.1
Sex, men/women (%)	45/55	64/36	39/61	75/25
Hospital days	21.9 ± 1.7	22.2 ± 2.8	25.2 ± 3.4	19.3 ± 2.4
Intensive care unit days	14.0 ± 1.7	11.5 ± 1.7	15.8 ± 3.1	10.2 ± 1.6*
Ventilator days	6.5 ± 1.3	4.6 ± 1.4	9.4 ± 3.4	2.3 ± 0.5*
Intraoperative deaths	0	0	1	0
Postoperative deaths, n (%)	17 (38%)	7 (23%)	10 (33%)	1 (4%)*
Organ failures	41	22	31	1
Other complications	7	9	8	10
Average costs	$31,438	$30,748	$37,335	$27,665
Average cost per survivor	$50,525	$40,106	$58,950	$28,690

*$P < .05$.

Hemodynamic and Oxygen Transport Patterns Before and After Adult Respiratory Distress Syndrome

Hemodynamic patterns for 96 hours before the diagnostic criteria for ARDS were met are listed in Table 94–3 and illustrated in Figure 94–1.[38] Prior to the onset of ARDS, the CI was at the upper range of normal in nonsurvivors; the CI values were slightly greater than normal but less than the values of critically ill postoperative survivors who did not develop ARDS; CI was significantly elevated (4 L/min · m²) in survivors of ARDS but did not reach the mean optimal values of postoperative patients (4.5 L/min · m²). In postoperative patients with sepsis, the CI was higher; in postoperative ARDS patients without sepsis, it was 3.92 ± 0.18 L/min · m², whereas the postoperative ARDS patients with sepsis had CIs of 4.21 ± 0.15 L/min · m² in the 96-hour period before ARDS onset.[38–40]

Before the onset of ARDS, the mean PA wedge pressures were within acceptable limits; none of the patients had PA wedge pressures greater than 20 mm Hg, and the mean PA pressures were well within acceptable limits for critically ill postoperative patients. In essence, based on blood volume, hematocrit, mean arterial pressure, central venous pressure, and pulmonary artery occlusion pressure, none of the patients were plasma-volume overloaded before the onset of ARDS.[38–40] Oxygen delivery patterns were decreased prior to the time of ARDS diagnosis. Oxygen consumption was at the upper range of normal in the nonsurvivors and slightly above normal but not optimal in most of the survivors. Pulmonary shunt increased to more than 20% at the time of ARDS diagnosis.

After the onset of ARDS, hemodynamic variables tended to improve, especially CI and mean arterial pressure. Pulmonary arterial pressures tended to remain elevated, but the pulmonary vascular resistance index decreased as the CI increased. The pulmonary artery wedge pressure remained at acceptable levels. CI, $\dot{D}O_2$, and $\dot{V}O_2$ tended to increase after mechanical ventilation, maintenance of high FIO_2 levels, and the administration of additional fluids and inotropic agents. Pulmonary shunt was over 30% to 40% most of the time after the onset of ARDS. In general, the pattern of pulmonary shunt values was slightly higher in nonsurvivors than in the survivors.

In essence, the physiologic changes that preceded the clinical diagnosis of ARDS include (1) hypovolemia made manifest by reduced blood volume, red blood cell mass, and hematocrit; (2) inadequate myocardial performance as indicated by a suboptimal increase in CI response to administration of fluids and inotropic agents; (3) inadequate tissue perfusion as indicated by suboptimal $\dot{D}O_2$ and $\dot{V}O_2$; and (4) increased pulmonary vasoconstriction as indicated by increased mean pulmonary arterial pressure and pulmonary vascular resistance index.[38–40]

TABLE 94–3. Hemodynamic and Oxygen Transport Values in Survivors and Nonsurvivors of Postoperative Adult Respiratory Distress Syndrome

		Time Period (h)			
		−48 to −24	*−24 to 0*	*0*	*0 to 24*
MAP (mm Hg)	Survivors	95 ± 17*	89 ± 17	92 ± 19	90 ± 17
	Nonsurvivors	89 ± 19	87 ± 22	83 ± 22	83 ± 20
MPAP (mm Hg)	Survivors	20 ± 5	23 ± 7	24 ± 8	26 ± 7
	Nonsurvivors	23 ± 8	24 ± 10	25 ± 9	28 ± 8
PAOP (mm Hg)	Survivors	10 ± 5	13 ± 7	14 ± 7	14 ± 5
	Nonsurvivors	13 ± 6	14 ± 6	14 ±7	16 ± 5
CI (L/min · m²)	Survivors	3.8 ± 1.0	3.9 ± 1.2	4.3 ± 1.4	4.5 ± 1.3
	Nonsurvivors	3.5 ± 1.5	3.6 ± 1.7	4.0 ± 1.6	4.1 ± 1.3
SI (mL/min · m²)	Survivors	35 ± 11	37 ± 15	39 ± 12	39 ± 12
	Nonsurvivors	34 ± 14	33 ± 14	37 ± 14	37 ± 14
LVSW (g · m/m²)	Survivors	45 ± 15	44 ± 19	48 ± 20	49 ± 19
	Nonsurvivors	46 ± 21	42 ± 21	42 ± 20	42 ± 20
SVRI	Survivors	1989 ± 711	1712 ± 633	1629 ± 667	1491 ± 460
(dyne · s/cm⁵ · m²)	Nonsurvivors	1785 ± 913	1907 ± 1024	1588 ± 903	1489 ± 685
PVRI	Survivors	224 ± 142	211 ± 151	198 ± 144	221 ± 124
(dyne · s/cm⁵ · m²)	Nonsurvivors	241 ± 217	264 ± 186	244 ± 196	260 ± 179
SaO_2 (%)	Survivors	97.6 ± 1.6	97.2 ± 2.9	94.8 ± 4.8	95.9 ± 2.9
	Nonsurvivors	97.0 ± 3.0	97.1 ± 3.0	93.4 ± 5.9	94.3 ± 4.9
SvO_2 (%)	Survivors	70.0 ± 9.1	69.9 ± 10.3	70.3 ± 9.2	71.9 ± 8.3
	Nonsurvivors	70.4 ± 10.9	67.4 ± 13.2	67.8 ± 11.4	69.0 ± 10.2
$\dot{Q}sp/\dot{Q}t$ (%)	Survivors	14 ± 5	17 ± 5	32 ± 10	29 ± 9
	Nonsurvivors	14 ± 8	18 ± 8	34 ± 12	32 ± 12
PaO_2/FIO_2	Survivors	332 ± 67	277 ± 88	154 ± 48	176 ± 71
	Nonsurvivors	341 ± 107	285 ± 89	153 ± 55	162 ± 73
$\dot{D}O_2$ (mL/min · m²)	Survivors	524 ± 165	556 ± 197	610 ± 210	643 ± 199
	Nonsurvivors	476 ± 217	507 ± 254	528 ± 222	564 ± 191
$\dot{V}O_2$ (mL/min · m²)	Survivors	151 ± 38	152 ± 49	153 ± 47	157 ± 40
	Nonsurvivors	140 ± 43	133 ± 74	133 ± 53	146 ± 45
O_2 extr. (%)	Survivors	29.7 ± 9.2	29.6 ± 10.5	26.7 ± 8.3	25.8 ± 7.8
	Nonsurvivors	29.1 ± 9.9	31.8 ± 12.1	28.2 ± 10.3	27.8 ± 9.1

*Values are mean ± SD.

Abbreviations: MAP = mean arterial pressure; MPAP = mean pulmonary arterial pressure; PAOP = pulmonary artery occlusion pressure; CI = cardiac index; SI = stroke volume index; LVSW = left ventricular stroke work; SVRI = systemic vascular resistance index; PVRI = pulmonary vascular resistance index; SaO_2 = arterial oxygen saturation; SvO_2 = venous oxygen saturation; $\dot{Q}sp/\dot{Q}t$ = shunt fraction; $\dot{D}O_2$ = oxygen delivery; $\dot{V}O_2$ = oxygen consumption; O_2 extr. = oxygen extraction.

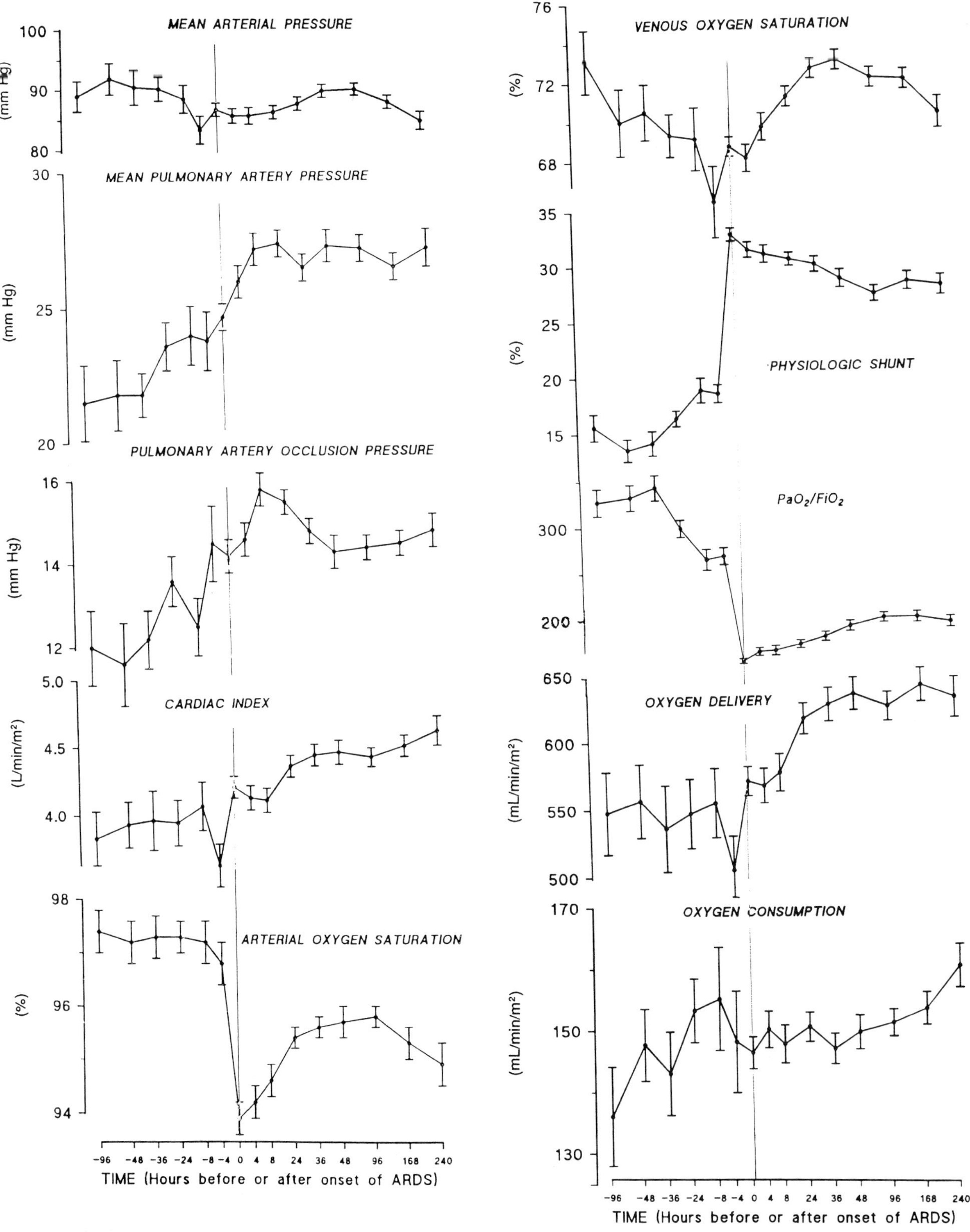

Figure 94–1. Data describing temporal patterns of mean arterial pressure, mean PA pressure, PA occlusion pressure, CI, and arterial oxygen saturation *(left panel)*; mixed venous oxygen saturation, physiologic shunt, PaO_2/FIO_2, $\dot{D}O_2$, and $\dot{V}O_2$ *(right panel)* for 402 consecutive, monitored postoperative ARDS patients from 96 hours before until 10 days after diagnosis of ARDS. (From Shoemaker WC, Appel PL, Bishop MH: Temporal patterns of blood volumes, hemodynamics, and oxygen transport in pathogenesis and therapy of postoperative adult respiratory distress syndrome. New Horizons 1993; 1:530. Copyright Williams & Wilkins, 1993.)

Oxygen Delivery–Oxygen Consumption Relationships in Postoperative Patients

The patterns of $\dot{D}O_2$ plotted against their corresponding $\dot{V}O_2$ values have been studied during relatively short periods of $\dot{D}O_2$ increase. A region of increasing $\dot{D}O_2$ associated with increasing $\dot{V}O_2$ values suggests supply-dependent $\dot{V}O_2$, whereas increasing $\dot{D}O_2$ values associated with relatively constant $\dot{V}O_2$ values suggest supply-independent $\dot{V}O_2$.[38, 41–53] The tissues' capacity to maintain $\dot{V}O_2$ while $\dot{D}O_2$ is decreasing represents a compensatory peripheral circulatory response that preserves $\dot{V}O_2$ via maintenance of greater oxygen extraction rates. Several small series have found good correlations in ARDS patients but poor correlations in critically ill patients without ARDS.[40–42] $\dot{V}O_2$ was found to be supply-dependent at $\dot{D}O_2$ values below 21 mL/min·kg in 10 patients with ARDS but supply-independent at $\dot{D}O_2$ values above this level.[27] This concept has been confirmed in several other small series[41–49]—for example, Appel and coworkers[51] studied supply-dependent $\dot{V}O_2$ in a series of 127 consecutive, acute, postoperative ARDS patients. In 50 of the ARDS patients, sufficient measurements were obtained over a short period of time to make possible an evaluation of the presence or absence of a plateau: 29 of the 50 patients (58%) had plateaus at or near the upper end of their $\dot{D}O_2$ range, indicating supply-independent $\dot{V}O_2$ and suggesting that substantial oxygen debts had been present.

Recently, the relationships of $\dot{D}O_2$ to $\dot{V}O_2$ values were evaluated in a consecutive series of 238 ARDS patients before and after disease onset.[52–55] Supply-dependent $\dot{V}O_2$ was observed in 166 of the 238 patients (69%) who had sufficient numbers of increasing $\dot{D}O_2$ values. When $\dot{D}O_2$ was further increased with therapy, a plateau of sorts that suggested supply-independent $\dot{V}O_2$ was identified in 72% of these patients (Fig. 94–2). The plateau suggested that tissue oxygen needs, which were previously rate-limited by inadequate oxygen supply, had been met and that no further increases in $\dot{V}O_2$ were needed; in essence, the patients had become $\dot{V}O_2$ supply–independent.[55]

Mathematic Coupling of Oxygen Delivery and Oxygen Consumption Values

The mathematic coupling of $\dot{D}O_2$ values with $\dot{V}O_2$ values is potentially problematic because CI is a common term for the calculations of both $\dot{D}O_2$ and $\dot{V}O_2$. Obviously, if there is a spuriously increased CI, then the calculated $\dot{D}O_2$ and $\dot{V}O_2$ values also will be incorrectly high. Although this is theoretically possible, it is unlikely to be a frequent or a consistent error if careful trouble-shooting and quality controls are routinely performed.

In a number of clinical conditions, changes in $\dot{D}O_2$ are not associated with similar changes in $\dot{V}O_2$, as would be the case if $\dot{D}O_2$ and $\dot{V}O_2$ were linked: (1) in the preterminal stages of nonsurvivors, fluid volume infusions and inotropes may produce appreciable $\dot{D}O_2$ changes and minimal $\dot{V}O_2$ changes, which are consistent with an oxygen debt that has become irreversible; (2) severe cardiac conditions with limited CI responses to fluids and inotropes but reasonable good $\dot{V}O_2$ responses are indicative of significant oxygen debt that was at least partly reversible despite limited cardiac responsiveness; (3) in some late-stage sepsis, postoperative, and cardiac patients, small $\dot{D}O_2$ changes were associated with large $\dot{V}O_2$ responses, which are suggestive of large oxygen debts; (4) early postoperative patients may have major $\dot{D}O_2$ increases with minimal $\dot{V}O_2$ changes, which are suggestive of good cardiac responsiveness but only small oxygen debts; (5) infusion of packed red blood cells often stimulates major $\dot{V}O_2$ changes with minimal or insignificant CI changes; and (6) normal unstressed or preoperative patients also may have large $\dot{D}O_2$ increases with little or no $\dot{V}O_2$ responses because they had little or no oxygen debt. In essence, when $\dot{D}O_2$ and $\dot{V}O_2$ increase together, supply-dependent $\dot{V}O_2$ or an error due to coupling may be present. However, coupling cannot explain the supply-independent oxygen values; a nearly horizontal line of $\dot{D}O_2$ values plotted against their corresponding $\dot{V}O_2$ values would not be possible if $\dot{D}O_2$ and $\dot{V}O_2$ were linked (see Fig. 94–2).

When carefully obtained direct Fick measurements (using measured inspired and expired oxygen concentrations together with tidal volumes) were compared with concomitant thermodilution values recorded using pulmonary artery catheters with arterial and mixed venous blood gas analysis to calculate $\dot{D}O_2$ and $\dot{V}O_2$, the indirect thermodilution–calculated $\dot{V}O_2$ values closely approximated the direct Fick $\dot{V}O_2$ measurements. Confirmation of the validity of these two approaches was reported by Hankeln and associ-

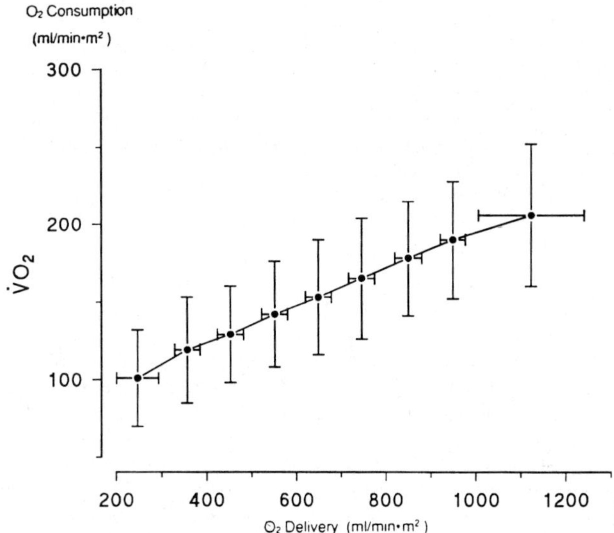

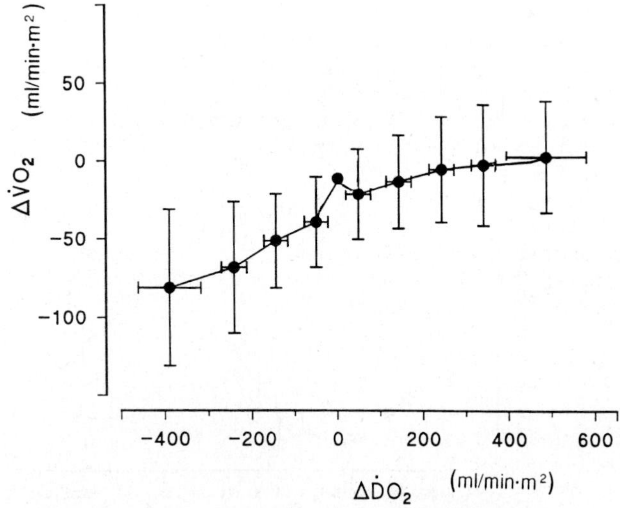

Figure 94–2. *Upper panel,* $\dot{D}O_2$ values of postoperative ARDS patients plotted against their corresponding $\dot{V}O_2$ values during periods when both were increasing (suggesting supply dependency). *Lower panel,* Changes in $\dot{D}O_2$ values plotted against their corresponding changes in $\dot{V}O_2$ values during periods when increasing $\dot{D}O_2$ values did not increase $\dot{V}O_2$ values, resulting in supply-independent $\dot{V}O_2$. *Vertical lines* are SDs to indicate degrees of variation in the values. (From Shoemaker WC, Appel PL, Bishop MH: Temporal patterns of blood volumes, hemodynamics, and oxygen transport in pathogenesis and therapy of postoperative adult respiratory distress syndrome. New Horizons 1993; 1:532. Copyright Williams & Wilkins, 1993.)

ates[25] and others who found good agreement between $\dot{V}O_2$ values as measured with both methods.

It should be noted that the direct Fick method, which calculates $\dot{V}O_2$ from inspired and expired oxygen concentrations, measures a different $\dot{V}O_2$ than that calculated with the thermodilution method. The former includes the metabolism of the lung itself and is particularly susceptible to error from high FIO_2 values; FIO_2 values greater than 0.6 have calculations based on small differences between large inspiratory and expiratory oxygen values. Furthermore, the direct Fick measurement is not reliable in rapidly changing (nonsteady) metabolic states. In such conditions, changes in the size of the oxygen pool are misinterpreted as $\dot{V}O_2$ changes. Finally, calibration of metabolic charts is time consuming and fraught with major technical problems.

Oxygen Debt and Its Relationship to Mortality and Organ Failure

When increases in $\dot{D}O_2$ produce increases in $\dot{V}O_2$, supply-dependent $\dot{V}O_2$ suggests that an oxygen debt was present. Since oxygen cannot be stored, the increased $\dot{V}O_2$ indicates greater utilization of oxygen as the body restores normal metabolism after an accumulated reversible oxygen debt. The extent of the oxygen debt is estimated from the $\dot{V}O_2$ need based on preoperative $\dot{V}O_2$ measurements extrapolated to the intraoperative and to the first 48-hour postoperative period after corrections for anesthesia and temperature have been made.[22] Estimation of the oxygen debt in high-risk surgical operations is calculated from the difference between the actual measured $\dot{V}O_2$ and the estimated $\dot{V}O_2$ need calculated from the preoperative $\dot{V}O_2$ corrected for the effects of anesthesia and temperature. The net cumulative oxygen debt at any given time is calculated from the integrated area between the actual $\dot{V}O_2$ and the estimated $\dot{V}O_2$ need. Greater oxygen debts were observed in patients with organ failure than in those without organ failure, and greater oxygen debts were seen in those who died (all of whom had organ failure) than in those who survived with or without organ failure (Fig. 94–3).

Prospective,[25–27, 29, 31–35] randomized[24, 28, 30, 36, 37] trials demonstrated that attainment of supranormal values empirically observed in survivors significantly reduced oxygen debt, organ failure, and death in high-risk surgical patients. The data indicate that the oxygen debts of postoperative patients with organ failure (especially ARDS) were larger than were those of patients without organ failures; even larger debts were found in patients who died with organ failure. Furthermore, optimal values of CI, $\dot{D}O_2$, and $\dot{V}O_2$ in prospective trials reduce oxygen debt and thus decrease organ failure and death.[24] The evidence indicates that oxygen debt from inadequate tissue perfusion is the primary event and that ARDS as well as other organ failures are the end-organ consequence of postoperative and septic shock.

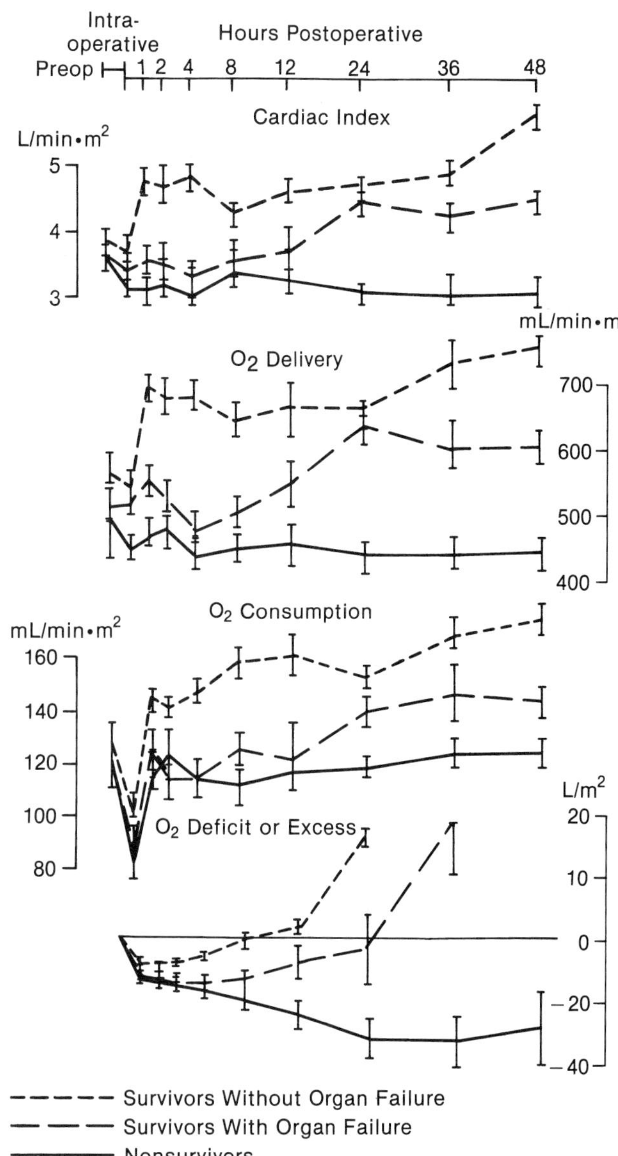

Figure 94–3. Serial measurements of CI, $\dot{D}O_2$, $\dot{V}O_2$, and net cumulative oxygen debt of surviving patients with and without organ failure and nonsurviving patients with organ failure. Values were taken during preoperative *(extreme left)*, intraoperative *(second measurement to left)*, and postoperative periods. *Dots* are mean values, and the *vertical lines* are SEM.

Various mediators, such as interleukin-6 and interleukin-8, as measured by plasma levels do not *precede* the occurrence of the diagnostic features of ARDS but may accelerate and augment the disorder as it is occurring. That is, the levels of these mediators increase along with the developing patterns of post-traumatic ARDS, but their maximum plasma concentrations do not occur before the time that the patients attained diagnostic criteria.[54]

In the complex multifactorial array of physiologic problems of shock states, it is difficult to distinguish primary from secondary and tertiary events or precipitating causes from subsequent responses. Temporal patterns may be used to elucidate pathophysiology by describing events that contribute to death; for example, the therapy that prevents or rapidly corrects a given pathogenic event should be favorably reflected by improved outcome. However, since shock is a multifactorial problem, it is rarely reversed with the use of a single therapeutic agent; it usually requires that all relevant pathogenic mechanisms be addressed if satisfactory results are to be obtained. On the other hand, the effects of specific therapy may be used to evaluate the responsiveness of compensations in terms of the degree and duration of the action required to restore body metabolism.[55]

THERAPY

Effectiveness of Fluid Restriction and Diuretic Therapy

Conventional therapy focuses on the restriction of fluids and diuretics as well as on the avoidance of colloid solution infusions. The latter measure is based on the assumption that with increased endothelial permeability, the colloid solutions would leak into the lung and drag water into the lung tissue, thus worsening the ARDS. We have been unable to find documentation of this occurring before or in the early period of ARDS.

Restriction of fluids and diuretic therapy have not proved to be effective in the overall management of ARDS. The mortality rate of 66% reported by Bartlett and coworkers[6] for a multi-institutional study was not appreciably different from the rates reported during the previous 15 years or earlier. Although patients now may be more ill than those reported in previous studies, the conventional fluid restriction approach has nevertheless not led to major improvement in outcome; two thirds of ARDS patients still die. Therefore, it is appropriate to reconsider the effectiveness of diuretic and fluid restriction with respect to the underlying pathophysiology of ARDS based on analysis of the responses to therapy.

Comparison of Hemodynamic and Oxygen Transport Responses to Colloid and Crystalloid Solutions in Early Adult Respiratory Distress Syndrome

Therapeutic goals for postoperative patients are designed to prevent tissue hypoxia and oxygen debts that lead to shock and shock lung. However, once ARDS occurs, the question of whether albumin produces capillary leak arises. Evidence of increased capillary permeability may be observed in the physiologic responses to fluid administration at successive time periods. In prospective, controlled, random-ordered crossover studies, the physiologic effects of the infusion of 1000 mL of crystalloid solutions were compared with those of the infusion of 100 mL of 25% albumin solution in 23 studies on 11 postoperative surgical patients who had developed ARDS in the previous 24 to 48 hours.[56] All patients had unmistakable evidence of respiratory distress, with shunt flow greater than 20%, alveolar-arterial difference in oxygen tension greater than 200 mm Hg, radiologic evidence of pulmonary infiltration, and mechanical ventilation as a required life-support measure for more than 48 hours. Each patient was given each fluid in random order. The 100 mL of 25% albumin solution increased plasma volume 450 mL by dragging 350 mL of interstitial water into the intravascular space. In essence, the albumin solution did not leak.

By contrast, 1000 mL of lactated Ringer's solution given to the same patients expanded blood volume by less than 200 mL at the end of the infusion; that is, 80% of the crystalloid solution left the vascular space during the 1-hour infusion, and 40 minutes later, most of the remaining 200 mL had left the intravascular space.[56] Thus, crystalloid solutions rapidly distribute predominantly in the interstitium and, when given in large quantities, lead to both peripheral and pulmonary edema. This author concluded that in the first day or two after the diagnosis of ARDS has been made, capillary leak, if present, does not limit hemodynamic and oxygen transport responses to colloid solutions; in the middle period—48 hours to 6 days after onset of ARDS—a less pronounced but significant hemodynamic and oxygen transport response occurred to colloid solutions. However, in the terminal stage of nonsurvivors (defined as the last 48 hours of life), no significant response occurred to the infusion of colloid solutions, packed red blood cells, whole blood, or crystalloid solutions. In any case, crystalloid solutions rapidly equilibrate into the interstitial space and provide only small transient plasma volume expansion and hemodynamic support. Moreover, they may deter tissue oxygenation by increasing the diffusion pathway through the expanded interstitium as well as by increasing the diffusion time of oxygen as it passes from the erythrocytes to cell mitochondria.

Effects of Colloid and Crystalloid Solutions on the Distribution of Body Water

If colloid solutions are deleterious and may actually cause ARDS, as has been purported by some clinicians, then plasmapheresis to remove plasma proteins and their replacement with the crystalloid solutions should be undertaken. However, this has already been done under rigorous experimental conditions by Guyton and Lindsey,[57] who demonstrated the importance of maintaining plasma protein levels. They depleted dogs of plasma proteins by instituting protein-deficient diets and plasmapheresis. They observed that pulmonary edema occurred at mean left atrial pressures of 13 mm Hg in depleted dogs with increasing afterload, but pulmonary edema did not occur in control dogs until atrial pressures had reached 20 mm Hg.

Exogenously administered albumin does not act on pulmonary capillaries differently from the patient's own endogenous albumin. Rather, the infused albumin mixes in and expands the miscible albumin pool; this increases oncotic pressure and produces physiologic effects on hemodynamics, blood volume, and body water distribution. By contrast, saline infusions mix with the plasma and interstitial fluid pools; however, because capillary membranes are freely permeable to salt under normal conditions, the added saline solution rapidly equilibrates, predominately in the interstitial space. Measured with the use of radiolabeled bromide, sodium, or chloride, in the average man weighing 70 kg, the interstitial fluid volume averages about 14 L, or 200 mL/kg, and the plasma volume about 3 L, or 4 mL/kg.[58]

In major trauma, massive crystalloid infusions have been advocated in amounts up to 1 L or more per hour for the first 2 days. This inevitably leads to as much as a threefold expansion of the interstitium that may be tolerated in young, previously healthy combat casualties or street fighters. However, it is difficult to understand how this approach would benefit an elderly cardiac patient on a diet having 1 g of salt per day. If massive amounts of crystalloid solutions are given to such a patient, demise is likely to be attributed to the patient's trauma rather than to the inappropriateness of the therapy.

When patients given massive crystalloid infusion develop ARDS, it is likely that some improvements in arterial blood gas values occur with diuretics administration and fluid restriction, not because the ARDS improved, but because the overexpansion of the interstitium was corrected.

SUMMARY

An Alternative Hypothesis of Adult Respiratory Distress Syndrome Pathogenesis and Therapy

An alternative hypothesis has been presented for the pathogenesis and therapy of ARDS based on the temporal physiologic patterns observed before the appearance of ARDS in patients who are destined to develop ARDS after severe high-risk surgery or massive trauma. In essence, hypovolemia, low blood flow, and maldistribution of blood flow produce inadequate tissue perfusion made manifest by inadequate $\dot{D}O_2$ and $\dot{V}O_2$. Insufficient $\dot{D}O_2$ needed to maintain body metabolism is reflected by suboptimal $\dot{V}O_2$. There also are common precipitating physiologic events that produce tissue hypoxia and oxygen debts, which in turn cause postoperative shock, shock lung, and other organ failures. Hypoxia to the lung per se increases pulmonary artery pressures, pulmonary vascular resistance, and pulmonary shunting by neural mechanisms; this response is similar to the well-known response of the hypoxic neonate. These events take place before the clinical appearances of ARDS and are not the result of ARDS.

In essence, ARDS is not a new disease that begins with clinical manifestations of arterial hypoxemia and the need for mechanical ventilation with high FIO_2. Rather, it is the same old set of postoperative circulatory deficiencies: hypovolemia, maldistribution of blood flow in the microcirculation, and inadequate $\dot{D}O_2$ and $\dot{V}O_2$, which, when protracted, lead to postoperative shock and shock lung.

The underlying concept is that the increased CI, $\dot{D}O_2$, and $\dot{V}O_2$ empirically observed in survivors represent compensations for the basic physiologic problem of postoperative shock. Without compensatory increases in tissue perfusion and tissue oxygenation, local hypoxic areas progress to organ dysfunction and ultimately to organ failure. The interacting mechanisms of circulatory problems that contribute to lethal patterns include hypovolemia, a reduction in CI, anemia, hypoxemia, neural and neurohumoral components of the pituitary-adrenal stress response, various cascades of biochemical initiators and mediators, length of time in shock or low-flow state, and the amount of tissue hypoxia and oxygen debt accumulated.

References

1. Ashbaugh DG, Bigelow DB, Petty TL, et al: Acute respiratory distress in adults. Lancet 1967; ii:319–323.
2. Hudson LD: Causes of ARDS: Clinical recognition. Clin Chest Med 1988; 138:720–723.
3. Murray JF, Mathay MA, Luce J, et al: An expanded definition of the adult respiratory distress syndrome. Am Rev Respir Dis 1988; 138:720–723.
4. Pepe PE: The clinical entity of adult respiratory distress syndrome: Definitions, prediction and prognosis. Crit Care Clin 1986; 2:377–403.
5. Katzenstein A-LA, Askin FB: Acute lung injury patterns. *In*: Surgical Pathology of Non-neoplastic Lung Disease. Bennington JL (Ed). Philadelphia, WB Saunders, 1990, pp 9–57.
6. Bartlett RH, Morris AH, Fairley B, et al: A prospective study of acute hypoxic respiratory failure. Chest 1986; 89:684–689.
7. Murray JF: Mechanisms of acute respiratory failure. Am Rev Respir Dis 1977; 115:1071–1078.
8. Fein AM, Lippman M, Holzman H, et al: Risk factors, incidence and prognosis of adult respiratory distress syndrome following septicemia. Chest 1978; 83:40–42.
9. Staub NC: Pulmonary edema: Physiologic approaches to management. Chest 1978; 74:559–564.
10. Brigham KL: Mechanisms of lung injury. Clin Chest Med 1982; 3:9.
11. Montgomery AB, Stager MA, Carrico CJ, et al: Causes of mortality in patients with the adult respiratory distress syndrome. Am Rev Respir Dis 1984; 132:485–489.
12. Staub NC: Pulmonary edema: Physiologic approaches to management. Chest 1978; 74:559–564.
13. Bishop M, Shoemaker WC, Appel PL, et al: Relationship between supranormal circulatory values, time delays and outcome in severely traumatized patients. Crit Care Med 1993; 21:57.
14. Johnson KS, Bishop MH, Stephen CM, et al: Temporal patterns of radiographic infiltration in severely traumatized patients with and without adult respiratory distress syndrome. J Trauma (in press).
15. Pontoppidan H, Geffin B, Lowenstein B: Acute respiratory failure in the adult. N Engl J Med 1972; 287:690.
16. Schuster DP: The case for and against fluid restriction and occlusion pressure reduction in adult respiratory distress syndrome. New Horizons 1993; 1:478.
17. Tiefenbrun J, Dikeman S, Shoemaker WC: The correlation of sequential changes in the distribution of pulmonary blood flow in hemorrhagic shock with the histopathologic anatomy. Surgery 1975; 76:618.
18. Katzenstein A-LA, Askin FB: Acute lung injury patterns. *In*: Surgical Pathology of Non-neoplastic Lung Disease. Bennington JL (Ed). Philadelphia, WB Saunders, 1990, pp 9–57.
19. Hogg JC, Katzenstein A-LA: Pulmonary edema and diffuse alveolar injury. *In*: Pathology of the Lung. Turlbeck WM (Ed). New York, Thieme, 1990.
20. Shippy, Appel PL, Shoemaker WC: Reliability of clinical monitoring to assess blood volume in critically ill patients. Crit Care Med 1984; 12:107–112.
21. Suzuki F, Baker RJ, Shoemaker WC: Red cell and plasma volume alterations after hemorrhage and trauma. Ann Surg 1964; 160:263.
22. Shoemaker WC, Appel PL, Kram HB: Role of oxygen debt in the development of organ failure, sepsis, and death. Chest 1992; 102:208–215.
23. Shoemaker WC, Appel P, Kram HB, et al: Prospective trial of supranormal values of survivors as therapeutic goals in high-risk surgical patients. Chest 1988; 94:1176–1186.
24. Shoemaker WC, Kram HB, Appel PL, et al: Efficacy of central venous pulmonary artery catheters and therapy based upon them in reducing mortality and morbidity. Arch Surg 1990; 125:1332–1338.
25. Hankeln KB, Gronemeyer R, Held AM, et al: Use of continuous noninvasive measurement of oxygen consumption in patients with ARDS following shock of various etiologies. Crit Care Med 1991; 119:642–649.
26. Edwards JD, Brown GCS, Nightingale P, et al: Use of survivors' cardiorespiratory values as therapeutic goals in septic shock. Crit Care Med 1969; 17:1098–1103.
27. Tuchschmidt J, Obitors D, Fried JC: Oxygen consumption in sepsis and septic shock. Crit Care Med 1991; 19:664–671.
28. Tuchschmidt J, Fried JC, Astiz M, et al: Elevation of cardiac output and oxygen delivery improves outcome in septic shock. Chest 1992; 102:216–220.
29. Creamer JE, Edwards JD, Nightingale P: Hemodynamic and oxygen transport variables in cardiogenic shock secondary to acute myocardial infarction. Am J Cardiol 1990; 65:1287–1291.
30. Berlauk JF, Abrams JH, Gilmour IJ, et al: Preoperative optimization of cardiovascular hemodynamics improves outcome in peripheral vascular surgery. Ann Surg 1991; 214:289–297.
31. Cryer HM, Richardson JD, Longmire-Cook S, et al: Oxygen delivery in patients with adult respiratory distress syndrome who undergo surgery. Arch Surg 1989; 124:1378–1385.
32. Edwards JD: Oxygen transport in cardiogenic and septic shock. Crit Care Med 1991; 19:658–663.
33. Scalea TM, Simon HM, Duncan AO: Geriatric blunt multiple trauma: Improved survival with early invasive monitoring. J Trauma 1990; 39:129–136.
34. Fleming AW, Bishop MW, Shoemaker WC, et al: Prospective trial of supranormal values as goals of resuscitation in severe trauma. Arch Surg (in press).
35. Hayes MA, Yan EHA, Timmons AC, et al: Response of critically ill patients to treatment aimed at achieving supranormal oxygen delivery and consumption in relation to outcome. Chest 1993; 103:886.
36. Yu M, Levy MM, Smith P, et al: Effect of maximizing oxygen delivery on morbidity and mortality rates in critically ill patients. Crit Care Med 1993; 21:530.
37. Boyd O, Grounds M, Bennett D: Perioperative increase of oxygen delivery reduces mortality in high risk surgical patients. JAMA (in press).
38. Shoemaker WC, Appel PL, Bishop MH: Temporal patterns of blood volume, hemodynamics, and oxygen transport in pathogenesis and therapy of postoperative adult respiratory distress syndrome. New Horizons 1993; 1:522.
39. Shoemaker WC, Appel PL, Czer LS, et al: Pathogenesis of respiratory failure after hemorrhage and trauma. Ann Surg 1964; 160:172.
40. Shoemaker WC, Appel PL: Pathophysiology of adult respiratory distress syndrome following sepsis and surgical operations. Crit Care Med 1985; 13:166–172.
41. Shubitani K, Komatsa T, Kubal K, et al: Critical level of oxygen delivery in anesthetized man. Crit Care Med 1983; 11:640.

42. Danek SJ, Lynch JP, Weg JD, et al: The dependence of oxygen uptake on oxygen delivery in adult respiratory distress syndrome. Am Rev Respir Dis 1985; 132:109.
43. Mohsenifar Z, Goldbach P, Tashkim DP, et al: Relationship between oxygen delivery and oxygen consumption in adult respiratory distress syndrome. Chest 1983; 84:267.
44. Gutierrez G, Pohil RJ: Oxygen consumption is linearly related to O_2 supply in critically ill patients. J Crit Care 1986; 1:336.
45. Bihari D, Smithies M, Gimson A, et al: The effects of vasodilation with prostacyclin on oxygen delivery and uptake in critically ill patients. N Engl J Med 1987; 317:397.
46. Mohsenifar Z, Amin D, Jasper AC, et al: Dependence of oxygen consumption on oxygen delivery in patients with chronic congestive heart failure. Chest 1987; 92:447.
47. Kariman K, Burns SR: Regulation of tissue oxygen extraction is disturbed in adult respiratory distress syndrome. Am Rev Respir Dis 1985; 132:109.
48. Brent BN, Matthay RA, Mohler DA, et al: Relationship between oxygen uptake and oxygen transport in stable patients with chronic obstructive pulmonary disease. Am Rev Respir Dis 1984; 129:682.
49. Dorinsky PM, Costello JL, Godek JE: Relationships of oxygen uptake and oxygen delivery in respiratory failure not due to adult respiratory distress syndrome. Chest 1988; 93:1013.
50. Arnal G, Viole JP, Percival C, et al: Oxygen delivery and uptake in adult respiratory distress syndrome. Am Rev Respir Dis 1986; 133:999.
51. Appel PL, Shoemaker WC: Relationship of oxygen consumption and oxygen delivery in surgical patients. Chest 1992; 102:906.
52. Shoemaker WC, Appel PL, Kram HB: Oxygen transport measurements to evaluate tissue perfusion and titrate therapy. Crit Care Med 1991; 19:672.
53. Shoemaker WC, Appel PL, Kram HB: Hemodynamic and oxygen transport responses in survivors and nonsurvivors of high risk surgery. Crit Care Med 1993; 21:977.
54. Meade P, Shoemaker WC, Donnelly TJ, et al: Temporal patterns of hemodynamic oxygen transport, cytokine, and complement activity in the development of adult respiratory distress syndrome after severe injury. J Trauma (in press).
55. Shoemaker WC, Appel PL, Bishop MH: Temporal patterns of blood volume, hemodynamics, and oxygen transport in pathogenesis and therapy of postoperative adult respiratory distress syndrome. New Horizons 1993; 1:522.
56. Hauser CJ, Shoemaker WC, Turpin I, et al: Oxygen transport responses to colloids and crystalloids in critically ill surgical patients. Surg Gynecol Obstet 1990; 150:811–818.
57. Guyton AC, Lindsey AW: Effect of elevated left atrial pressure and decreased plasma protein concentration on the development of pulmonary edema. Circ Res 1959; 7:649.
58. Moore FD, Olesen KH, McMurrey JD, et al: The Body Cell Mass and Its Supporting Environment: Body Composition in Health and Disease. Philadelphia, WB Saunders, 1963.

CHAPTER 95

Acute Respiratory Failure in Chronic Obstructive Pulmonary Disease

Michael Donahoe, MD • Robert M. Rogers, MD

The management of patients with chronic obstructive pulmonary disease (COPD) is a frequent challenge for the critical care practitioner. COPD exacerbations are a common short-term and long-term (chronic mechanical ventilation) management problem in medical intensive care units (ICUs). Likewise in surgical units, the course of many postoperative patients is complicated by exacerbations of underlying obstructive airways disease. Epidemiologic investigations suggest this clinical problem is likely only to increase in magnitude.[1]

The term *COPD* has been defined as a process characterized by the presence of chronic bronchitis or emphysema, which may lead to the development of airways obstruction; airways obstruction need not be present at all stages of the process, and the airways obstruction may be partially reversible.[2] This definition conforms to the more common use of this term by clinicians. It excludes patients with completely reversible airways obstruction (i.e., asthma) and yet includes patients with combined, partially reversible, and fixed obstructive airways disease (Fig. 95–1).

The diagnosis of acute respiratory failure especially in this population requires careful consideration of terminology. Respiratory failure is defined on the basis of arterial blood gas criteria. The absolute values are somewhat arbitrary, but generally a partial pressure of arterial oxygen (Pa_{O_2}) of less than 60 mm Hg and a partial pressure of arterial carbon dioxide (Pa_{CO_2}) greater than 50 are chosen by conventional criteria to define respiratory failure. Stable, ambulatory outpatients with COPD will frequently meet these diagnostic criteria, however. A more appropriate definition of acute respiratory failure for the COPD patient is a condition in which the Pa_{O_2} is less than or the Pa_{CO_2} is greater than the usual range of values expected for that individual.[3]

The majority of acute COPD exacerbations are mild in

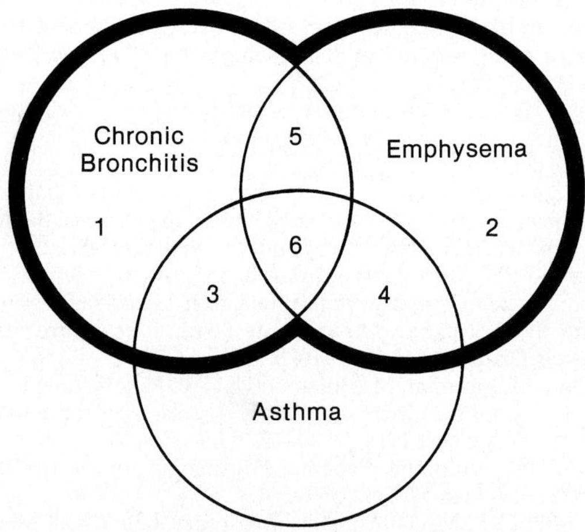

Figure 95–1. Schematic drawing illustrating the relationship between disorders characterized by airflow obstruction. A nonproportional Venn diagram illustrates the clinical overlap of patients with chronic bronchitis, emphysema, and asthma who can present with respiratory failure. Patients in subset 1 have chronic bronchitis without emphysema, whereas patients in subset 2 have emphysema without chronic bronchitis. Patients in subsets 3 and 4 have a reversible component of obstructive lung disease in the setting of chronic cough or emphysema. Patients in subsets 5 and 6 represent the most common patients who present for medical care. These patients have a combination of chronic bronchitis and emphysema with variable elements of reversible airflow obstruction. Patients who fall within the *hatched border* are typically considered as having COPD as the etiology of acute respiratory failure. (Modified from Snider G: Chronic obstructive pulmonary disease: a definition and implications of structural determinants of airflow obstruction for epidemiology. Am Rev Respir Dis 1989; 140:53–58.)

nature and can be managed in the outpatient setting. Despite this fact, COPD has been reported as the discharge diagnosis in more than 13% of all hospitalizations.[1] Pontoppidan and colleagues, in their published series, suggest COPD accounts for up to 15% of all cases of respiratory failure.[4] This range is likely to underestimate the true incidence because COPD patients are often included in other diagnostic categories.

PRECIPITATING FACTORS IN CHRONIC OBSTRUCTIVE PULMONARY DISEASE EXACERBATIONS

The inciting agent leading the clinically stable COPD patient to experience the signs and symptoms of progressive respiratory failure is not always identified. Although a significant number of precipitating factors have been described, the relative frequency of each cause is unknown. Most of these factors are unlikely to produce respiratory failure in the absence of significant underlying obstructive airways disease. Those precipitating factors with particular relevance to the management of the hospitalized patient with acute respiratory failure are reviewed (Table 95–1).

Infection

Infection is believed to represent the most common cause of COPD exacerbations. Pathogenic bacteria have been cultured from the lower airways in more than 80% of patients with chronic bronchitis in one series.[5] The most common isolates are *Streptococcus pneumoniae* and *Haemophilus influenzae. Streptococcus viridans* and *Branhamella catarrhalis* have been noted in some series.[6] *Chlamydia pneumoniae* strain TWAR, recognized as an important etiologic agent in community-acquired pneumonia, appears to be uncommon.[7] *Mycoplasma pneumoniae* and numerous viral agents have also been reported.[8]

The causal relationship between infection and COPD exacerbations has been difficult to prove. Macroscopic examination of the sputum can be misleading because both neutrophils and eosinophils can produce purulent sputum in the absence of infection. The presence of bacteria or viral agents in airway secretions does not necessarily imply a causative role, because organisms are frequently isolated during stable intervals, suggesting airway colonization rather than infection.[8, 9] Inferential evidence could be gained from studies of the response to antibiotic therapy, yet conflicting information has been reported in this area also.[10, 11] Despite these limitations, most clinicians still approach the treatment of COPD with attention to airway secretions and include antibiotic treatment based on culture results or on empiric data.

TABLE 95–1. Precipitating Factors for Chronic Obstructive Pulmonary Disease Exacerbations

Infection
Bacterial
Viral
Cardiac disease
Cardiac arrhythmia
Coronary artery disease
Cor pulmonale
Environmental
Allergens
Occupational irritants
Humidity
Air pollution
Primary or secondary smoke exposure
Medications
Beta-blocking agents
Narcotics/sedatives
Oxygen therapy
Pneumothorax
Pulmonary thromboembolic disease
Respiratory muscle fatigue

Cardiac Disease

Decompensation in the patient with stable COPD can occur secondary to a number of cardiac causes including superimposed coronary artery disease, cardiac arrhythmia, and cor pulmonale.

A reduction in pulmonary function is an independent risk factor for coronary artery disease. This relationship is at least partially attributable to the common risk factor of cigarette smoking. The significance of this problem is highlighted by the estimate that 27% of patients with COPD die from coronary artery disease rather than the pulmonary disorder.[12] Underlying coronary artery disease is aggravated by the hypoxemia and/or hypercarbia produced by the pulmonary disorder.

Cardiac arrhythmias have been reported in a high percentage of COPD patients undergoing long-term cardiac monitoring. Both supraventricular and ventricular arrhythmias are reported; however, in acute respiratory failure, up to 80% of arrhythmias are supraventricular in origin.[13] The propensity to arrhythmias may be aggravated by accompanying hypoxemia and/or hypercarbia as well as medications. Theophylline preparations, in particular, have been associated with an arrhythmogenic potential.[14]

Multifocal atrial tachycardia is recognized in a high proportion of COPD patients with respiratory failure and is often confused with other supraventricular arrhythmias such as atrial fibrillation (Fig. 95–2).[15] Why COPD patients with respiratory failure are predisposed to this arrhythmia is unclear. The combination of hypoxemia, hypercarbia, acidosis, electrolyte disturbances, and adrenergic medications is believed to promote ectopic atrial foci and sustain the arrhythmia.

Cor pulmonale is an alteration in right ventricular structure or function secondary to pulmonary hypertension resulting from pulmonary parenchymal or vascular disease. COPD is the most frequent cause of this disorder. Pulmonary hypoxic vasoconstriction is believed to play a major causative role in its development. Pulmonary vascular resistance in COPD patients is not typically elevated to the degree seen in primary pulmonary hypertension, however. Cardiac output, therefore, is often maintained at near-normal values until late in the disease course. However, the ability to elevate cardiac output in the face of factors that limit tissue oxygen delivery, such as hypoxemia, may be compromised. The increased metabolic workloads associated with the work of breathing or infection also may not be met through simple augmentation of oxygen delivery.[16] Evidence suggests that the ability of COPD patients with right ventricular dysfunction to vary tissue oxygen delivery in response to oxygen demand may be limited and has important prognostic implications.[17]

Medications

Commonly used medications can exacerbate underlying obstructive airways disease. Beta-blocking agents, in particular, have been associated with disease exacerbation. Beta$_1$-selective agents, such as metoprolol, are less likely to produce bronchospasm at lower dosages, but this advantage is

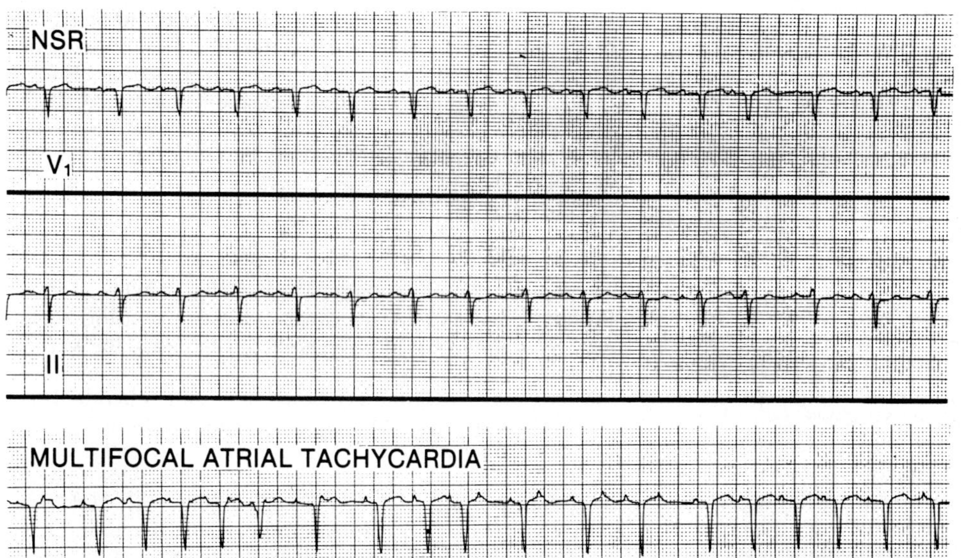

Figure 95–2. Continuous electrocardiographic rhythm strips illustrating the contrast between normal sinus rhythm (NSR) and MAT. Note the characteristic morphologically distinct P waves and variable RR, PP, and PR intervals in MAT. (Courtesy of Edward Curtiss, MD.)

not present in the higher dosage range. Likewise, topical β_1 agents used for the treatment of glaucoma, such as timolol, have been associated with disease flares.[18]

Sedative-hypnotic medications invariably produce some element of respiratory depression as a secondary manifestation of the drug action. These medications are contraindicated in patients with COPD, and inappropriate prescription can lead to acute respiratory decompensation.

Oxygen Therapy

Oxygen administration is the single therapeutic item that has been clearly demonstrated to benefit COPD patients with hypoxemia. However, excessive oxygen administration in susceptible patients, primarily those with chronic hypercapnia, can lead to progressive hypercapnia and respiratory acidosis. Although unlikely to precipitate respiratory failure, inappropriate oxygen administration can aggravate the disease course.

On the basis of revised physiologic measurements, the proposed mechanism for oxygen-induced hypercapnia has undergone significant change. The hypercapnic drive in COPD patients was previously believed to be reduced and the hypoxic drive was believed to play a prominent role in regulating minute ventilation. Supplemental oxygen was believed to suppress the hypoxic drive and promote hypercapnia in the setting of a reduced carbon dioxide response. Recent investigations, however, have documented that, despite the occurrence of arterial hypercapnia, resting minute ventilation is maintained in hypercapnic COPD patients after the administration of supplemental oxygen.[19]

If partial pressure of carbon dioxide (P_{CO_2}) increases after the administration of supplemental oxygen without a change in the measured expired volume per unit of time ($\dot{V}_E$), then a change in dead space–tidal volume (V_{DS}/V_T) ratio must be hypothesized. This could be explained by changing ventilation-perfusion ($\dot{V}/\dot{Q}$) relationships in response to oxygen administration. The mechanism for this change remains to be elucidated.

Pneumothorax

Pneumothorax is a recognized complication of COPD that can precipitate acute respiratory failure. The clinical diagnosis may be complicated by clinical signs (decreased breath sounds, hyperresonance) and radiographic findings (absent lung markings) that are present in emphysema patients without pneumothorax. Patients with alpha$_1$-antitrypsin deficiency and large lower lobe bullae are at particular risk for misdiagnosis of pneumothorax. Loculated pneumothoraces can be especially difficult to diagnose, and additional radiographic studies (i.e., computed tomographic scan) may be necessary. Despite the theoretical risk of hyperinflation and high transpulmonary pressures in COPD patients, the risk of spontaneous pneumothorax in one reported series was very low.[20]

Pulmonary Embolism

At autopsy examination, up to 50% of COPD patients had evidence of pulmonary thromboembolic disease.[21] COPD patients may have an abnormal predisposition to thromboembolic disease on the basis of abnormal platelet function promoting a hypercoagulable state.[22] Clinicians are faced with very similar clinical presentations of pulmonary embolism and uncomplicated COPD exacerbations. Documented pulmonary embolus was seen in only 19% of patients suspected of having this complication in one series.[23] The majority of patients have $\dot{V}/\dot{Q}$ scans with an intermediate probability for pulmonary embolism, confirming the difficulty with interpretation of these tests in the setting of COPD. Clinical features do not appear to reliably distinguish the disorders. The clinician is forced to rely on interpretation of clinical signs and risk factors to diagnose pulmonary embolism in the COPD patient until more reliable diagnostic tools are identified.

Respiratory Muscle Fatigue

Respiratory muscle fatigue exists when the muscles lose the capacity to develop force and/or velocity in response to a load and the loss of force is reversible by rest.[24] The ability to recover a previously sustained muscle force distinguishes fatigue from muscle weakness in which a target force can never be achieved. Fatigue results when the energy demand of the muscle exceeds the energy supply. COPD subjects are predisposed to heightened respiratory muscle energy requirements based on an increased ventilatory demand, high inspiratory workload, and reduced mechanical efficiency. The reversal of muscle fatigue generally requires a period of rest for recovery of muscle function. Therefore, the ability to track the onset and progression of muscle fatigue in COPD patients would have major therapeutic implications.

Respiratory muscle fatigue has been clearly documented under controlled laboratory conditions of inspiratory muscle loading.[25] Fatigue during weaning from mechanical ventilation has also been suggested.[26] However, the relationship between the onset of respiratory failure and fatigue in COPD patients is less clear.[27, 28] Much of the confusion in this area relates to the lack of precise definitions regarding the type of fatigue as well as the lack of a simple methodology to identify specific fatigue states.

At present, respiratory muscle fatigue is best viewed as a continuous process rather than a single event.[29] The process begins when the respiratory muscles are subjected to an excessive mechanical load, leading to a series of changes within the neuromuscular command chain. Part of this change includes a reduction in the central stimulation frequency of the fatigued respiratory muscle. The rate of progression to complete respiratory muscle task failure will depend on the relationship between the supply and demand variables in any single patient. The clinician should focus therapeutic efforts on this relationship. Therapy that reduces the mechanical workload will obviously reduce energy demand. On the supply side, a number of metabolic factors influence respiratory muscle capacity and deserve attention (Table 95–2). These metabolic factors are not expected to precipitate respiratory failure in normal individuals, and yet they can lead to early fatigue in the setting of a high ventilatory demand.

Electrolyte abnormalities including hypokalemia, hypophosphatemia, hypocalcemia, and hypomagnesemia are recognized to affect respiratory muscle function adversely. Hypophosphatemia is a particularly common complication of COPD management, being seen in up to 28% of COPD patients presenting with respiratory infections.[30]

Recent attention has focused on the potential adverse effects of corticosteroids on respiratory muscle function. Changes noted in animal models include muscle fiber atrophy and loss of muscle strength and endurance.[31] Frequent use of these agents in the COPD patient population would place these patients at high risk for this potential complication.

Hypoxia and hypercapnia are frequent gas exchange disorders characteristically seen in the patient with acute respiratory failure. Both disorders are recognized to affect respiratory muscle function adversely. Likewise, the reduced tissue oxygen delivery characteristic of shock states can be associated with respiratory failure secondary to primary respiratory muscle dysfunction.[32]

TABLE 95–2. Nonmechanical Factors That Contribute to Respiratory Muscle Failure in the Subject with Chronic Obstructive Pulmonary Disease

Drug therapy
Sedatives
Paralytics
Electrolyte abnormalities
Hypocalcemia
Hypokalemia
Hypophosphatemia
Hypomagnesemia
Endocrine disorders
Hypo- and hyperthyroidism
Glucocorticoid excess (including exogenous administration)
Gas exchange abnormalities
Hypoxemia
Hypercapnia
Nutritional status
Oxygen delivery

Protein-calorie malnutrition (PCM) results in a progressive reduction in body weight and skeletal muscle mass. Human autopsy studies confirm that the changes witnessed in animal models also occur in the human diaphragm in relation to body composition changes.[33] PCM also results in biochemical changes within skeletal muscle that are independent of changes in muscle fiber dimensions. Intracellular electrolytes, including magnesium and phosphate, and intracellular energy stores are abnormal in malnourished COPD patients.[34] Abnormal respiratory muscle cellular energy metabolism is characteristic of COPD patients with respiratory failure and may relate to nutritional deprivation.[35] Biopsies of both intercostal and quadriceps muscles reveal reduced energy stores in the form of adenosine triphosphate and phosphocreatine. The importance of these biochemical changes relative to the muscle atrophy is not firmly established but is expected to add to the loss of muscle power.

These physiologic effects of nutritional deprivation on muscle are manifested by reductions in force generation primarily at high stimulation frequencies. In the setting of nutritional deprivation, additional changes in muscle function include decreased muscle endurance and prolonged relaxation time.[36] Studies of nutrition support suggest that positive energy balance improves respiratory muscle strength. It is unclear whether the therapeutic benefit results from improved muscle bulk or reversal of the previously described biochemical changes associated with malnutrition.

While our understanding of the mechanisms and nature of respiratory muscle fatigue continues to evolve, it is clear that a number of clinical factors contribute to optimal function in the setting of respiratory failure. Successful treatment of the COPD patient requires recognition of these factors and efforts to reverse their potential adverse effects.

PATHOPHYSIOLOGY OF RESPIRATORY FAILURE IN CHRONIC OBSTRUCTIVE PULMONARY DISEASE PATIENTS

Respiratory failure in COPD patients is defined by the presence of systemic hypoxemia and possibly hypercapnia. The primary mechanism of hypoxemia in these patients results from a $\dot{V}/\dot{Q}$ mismatch.[37] Both high and low $\dot{V}/\dot{Q}$ units are recognized in COPD subjects. The correlation among $\dot{V}/\dot{Q}$ abnormalities, physiologic indexes (i.e., forced expiratory volume in 1 second [FEV_1]), and arterial blood gas parameters is poor, however. This lack of correlation suggests that the severity of gas exchange derangement in any patient is determined by multiple variables including the level of total alveolar ventilation, total pulmonary vascular perfusion, and the match of these variables within individual alveolar units. Shunt physiology appears to play an insignificant role.

The dispersion of $\dot{V}/\dot{Q}$ units results in inefficient gas exchange, leading to a higher ventilatory requirement in COPD subjects than in normal subjects to maintain arterial oxygenation and P_{CO_2}. The ability of COPD patients to augment ventilation is significantly limited, however, by the presence of expiratory airflow obstruction.

Expiratory airflow obstruction is the cardinal feature of COPD exacerbations. The morphologic basis of reduced expiratory airflow includes obstructive changes in the peripheral conducting airways (i.e., bronchitis) as well as destructive changes in the terminal respiratory bronchioles (i.e., emphysema). These morphologic changes lead to the physiologic equivalents of increased expiratory airflow resistance and reduced lung elastic recoil.

During resting tidal breathing, normal subjects use only a small fraction of their volume and flow maximums. During extreme exercise, they augment ventilation by increasing inspiratory and expiratory flow rates and reducing end-expiratory lung volume. COPD patients, in contrast, have been shown to exceed their maximum forced expiratory flow capacity during resting minute ventilation (Fig. 95–3).[79] In the face of this marked reduction in ventilatory reserve, COPD patients have limited options to increase their ventilatory capacity.

The ability to increase expiratory airflow is markedly limited. Reduced driving pressure (reduced elastic recoil) and increased airways resistance enhance the loss of airway distending pressure during expiration and favor dynamic airway collapse. Increased expiratory effort produces more positive pleural pressure during expiration and serves only to promote further airway collapse. Dynamic airway collapse in the COPD patient with respiratory failure leads to values of average expiratory airways resistance that significantly exceed inspiratory resistance and promotes hyperinflation.

Faced with a fixed rate of expiratory airflow, the COPD patient is limited to increasing inspiratory flow rate or lung volume in response to heightened ventilatory demands. An increase in V_T at a constant resting lung volume can be achieved only with an increase in inspiratory flow rate to allow adequate time for expiration. In a similar manner, an increase in respiratory frequency shortens the total breath duration while expiratory time remains unchanged. If V_T is to remain constant, a marked increase in inspiratory flow rate must occur.

Alternatively, COPD patients can attempt to raise expiratory flow rates by increasing end-expiratory lung volumes. Expiratory airflow increases with hyperinflation as elastic recoil pressure increases and airways resistance decreases secondary to lung distention. Either an increase in inspiratory flow rates or an increase in resting lung volume places a significant demand on the inspiratory muscles. As a result, the expiratory "mechanical load" of COPD results in adaptations that place a significant burden on the inspiratory muscles.

The elastic work of ventilation increases at higher lung volumes. Further, hyperinflation in the setting of dynamic airway collapse increases the end-expiratory elastic recoil pressure of the respiratory system (Prs). This positive end-expiratory pressure (PEEP) has been variously termed auto-PEEP or intrinsic PEEP. Under normal conditions, the Prs at

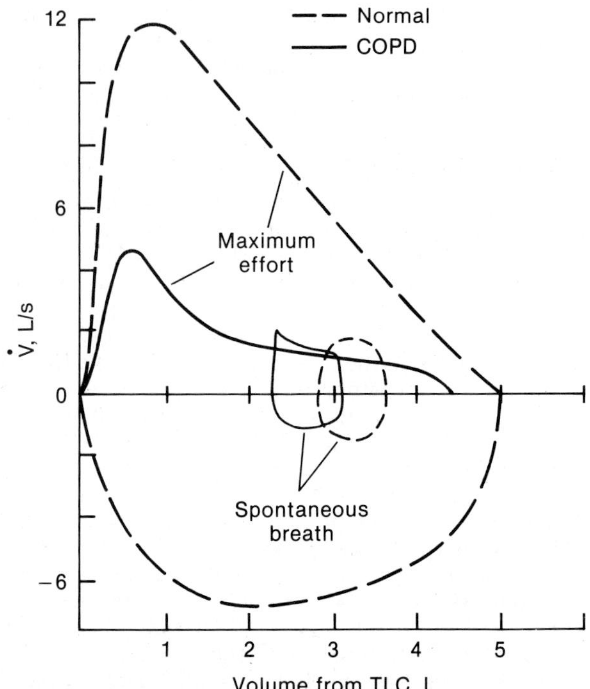

Figure 95–3. Maximum expiratory flow-volume curves in normal subjects *(dashed line)* and in subjects with COPD *(solid line)*. Note that COPD patients can exceed their maximum expiratory flow capacity during resting spontaneous breathing. (From Hubmayr R, Rodarte J: Cellular effects and physiologic responses: Lung mechanics. *In*: Chronic Obstructive Pulmonary Disease. Cherniak N [Ed]. Philadelphia, WB Saunders, p 85.)

end-expiration reaches its equilibrium point (zero), and the patient must initiate only a small negative inspiratory effort to produce inspiratory airflow. In the presence of dynamic airway collapse and hyperinflation, however, the Prs remains positive at end-expiration, favoring continued expiratory airflow. The patient must generate a negative inspiratory force equal and opposite to the the level of Prs at end-expiration before inspiratory airflow begins. This dynamic hyperinflation in effect places an additional "threshold" load on the process of inspiration, which can contribute to respiratory distress, respiratory muscle fatigue, and failure to cycle mechanical ventilation. The positive Prs at end-expiration must be overcome either by the respiratory muscles (spontaneous ventilation) or by the ventilator for inspiratory airflow to begin.

Potential complications of dynamic hyperinflation are threefold: (1) an increased work of breathing during spontaneous breathing and patient-cycled mechanical ventilation, (2) cardiovascular compromise secondary to elevated intrathoracic pressures, and (3) an increased risk for barotrauma. In addition, the interpretation of compliance measurements and hemodynamic information may be in error if this condition is not recognized.

Hyperinflation has additional adverse effects on the inspiratory muscles. The pressure-generating ability of the diaphragm at higher lung volumes is reduced. Structural changes, including reduced dimensions of type I and II fibers as well as reduced enzymatic activity of these fibers, have been described.[38] Alterations in geometry (flattening) and orientation of the diaphragm muscle fibers further reduce the force-generating capacity of this muscle. To compensate, increased activity of the intercostal muscles, scalene, and sternomastoid muscles occurs in the setting of acute respiratory failure.

In summary, ventilatory demands are increased in COPD subjects secondary to alterations in gas exchange. For any given level of ventilation, the work of breathing is increased secondary to elevated airways resistance. Mandated increases in inspiratory flow rate in the face of high inspiratory resistance further increase the mechanical load. Dynamic hyperinflation secondary to fixed airflow obstruction results in an increased elastic load. This combination of factors explains the abnormal relationship between minute ventilation and respiratory muscle energy requirements in COPD patients (Fig. 95–4).

To maintain adequate alveolar ventilation in the face of these mechanical changes, efferent neural drive to the respiratory muscles must be increased. The majority of COPD patients in acute respiratory failure, even in the presence of hypercapnia, demonstrate sustained levels of minute ventilation and higher respiratory control center output compared to more stable intervals.[39] The pattern of ventilation is altered, however. Patients in respiratory failure with normal or elevated levels of minute ventilation tend to breathe using higher respiratory rates and smaller V_T. An increase in V_T and reduction in breathing frequency is associated with the recovery phase. The reduction in V_T increases the dead space fraction of each breath (V_{DS}/V_T), effectively reducing alveolar ventilation. The mechanism of this abnormal breathing pattern is likely multifactorial. During disease exacerbations, the patient may adopt this breathing pattern to reduce the ventilatory workload of the inspiratory muscles. Alternatively, airway receptors have been hypothesized to respond to bronchoconstriction, airway secretions, and edema to alter the respiratory pattern.

Cardiovascular changes in COPD and acute respiratory failure are dominated by the presence of pulmonary hypertension. While chronic pulmonary hypertension is frequently present, it is worsened during acute exacerbations. The change in mean pulmonary artery pressure is related to

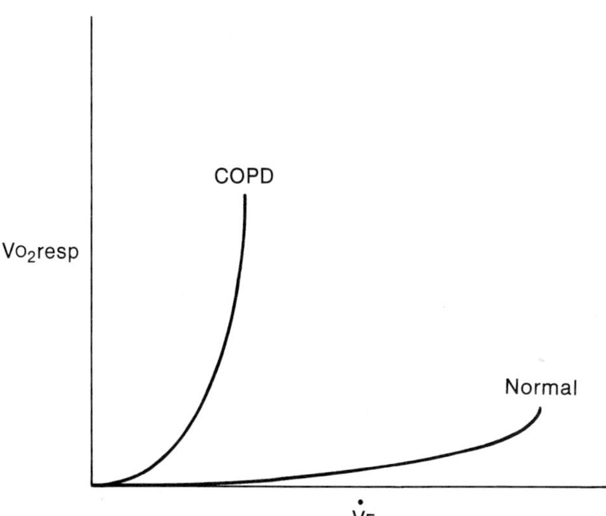

Figure 95–4. Relationship between resting minute ventilation and respiratory muscle energy requirements in COPD patients and normal subjects. Whereas only small changes in energy requirements are noted with increased ventilation in normal subjects, marked increases in respiratory muscle energy requirements occur secondary to small changes in ventilation in the COPD patients. *Abbreviations:* $\dot{V}_E$ = minute ventilation; $\dot{V}O_2resp$ = oxygen consumption of the respiratory muscles.

the degree of hypoxemia and often returns to baseline values once the exacerbation subsides.[40] Secondary changes in right ventricular function include a reduced ejection fraction. Positive pleural pressure, seen with dynamic hyperinflation, can limit systemic venous return, further limiting right ventricular function. Measurements of pulmonary capillary wedge pressure (PCWP) in this setting can falsely overestimate left ventricular filling pressure if the effects of dynamic hyperinflation are not recognized.

CLINICAL PRESENTATION

The primary clinical symptom in patients with COPD and acute respiratory failure is dyspnea. The majority of patients will complain of a progressive rather than acute onset. Additional complaints typically include cough and sputum production to varying degrees. The cough may have changed in character from baseline with increased sputum volume and/or purulence.

Early clinicians recognized a distinctive pattern to the clinical presentation of the COPD patient based on body habitus and gas exchange parameters. The patient with predominant emphysema, labeled the "pink puffer," is recognized to suffer from predominant dyspnea, marked hyperinflation, and body wasting. Mild hypoxemia is the primary gas exchange disorder, with hypercapnia appearing only late in the disease course. Alternatively, the "blue bloater" presents with recurrent bouts of bronchitis. Hypercapnia and hypoxemia are present early in the disease course with clinical signs of right-sided heart failure. Many patients present with an "overlap" of these two patterns.

Additional signs and symptoms may be present in relation to precipitating factors. Most commonly, a change in sputum characteristics to a yellow or green color with increased volume suggests an infectious exacerbation. A history suggesting an environmental trigger should be sought. Orthopnea and/or chest pain suggest the possibility of complicating left ventricular dysfunction. Clinical symptoms such as diaphoresis, alterations in mental status, headache, asterixis, and tremors are usually manifestations of the associated gas exchange defect rather than the underlying disorder.

Physical findings can provide important clues to the presence of impending ventilation failure and the need for mechanical ventilation. Early findings of progressive respiratory failure include tachycardia, tachypnea, and a reduction in the resting V_T. More progressive signs of abnormal respiratory muscle activation include an asynchronous respiratory pattern (chest and abdomen moving together with a time lag), use of accessory muscles, or paradoxical motion (chest and abdomen moving in opposite directions).[41] However, some caution is indicated. Atypical breathing patterns can be seen in COPD patients at rest during stable intervals. Monitoring of arterial blood gases becomes an integral component in the evaluation of the patient with COPD and acute respiratory failure.

TREATMENT

The majority of patients with an acute COPD exacerbation do not require mechanical ventilation. The associated risks related to artificial airway management, potential barotrauma, nosocomial infection, and chronic ventilator dependence dictate that mechanical ventilation should be avoided, if possible. However, the principles of treatment remain similar independent of whether mechanical ventilation is required (Table 95–3).

TABLE 95–3. Principles in the Treatment of Chronic Obstructive Pulmonary Disease Exacerbations

Correct gas exchange defects
- Supplemental oxygen
- Respiratory stimulants
- Mechanical ventilation

Minimize airflow resistance
- Bronchodilators
  - $Beta_2$ agonists
  - Anticholinergic agents
  - Theophylline
- Corticosteroids
- Vigorous cough/chest physiotherapy

Treat the precipitating cause

Correction of Gas Exchange Defects

The initial step in the management of acute COPD exacerbations is correction of gas exchange abnormalities, especially hypoxemia. Hypoxemia carries significant risks of cardiac arrhythmia, ischemia, and acidosis and should not go untreated for fear of precipitating progressive hypercapnia and respiratory acidosis. Oxygen administration in these patients must achieve two simultaneous goals: correcting hypoxemia while minimizing oxygen-induced hypercapnia. This can generally be accomplished through rapid, yet cautious, titration upward of the inspired oxygen concentration. The administration method is less critical (i.e., Venturi mask versus nasal cannula) than careful monitoring of oxygen therapy to achieve an oxygen saturation of approximately 90%. The immediate use of high oxygen concentrations (i.e., 10–15-L facemask), often advocated for the patient with other types of respiratory failure, should be avoided. The titration is best accomplished with the use of serial arterial blood gas measurements.

Although pulse oximetry has become a favored noninvasive method of gas exchange monitoring, it must be used with caution in the COPD patient. The shape of the oxyhemoglobin dissociation curve dictates that minor changes in measured saturation will occur with marked increases in the PaO_2 above 55 to 60 mm Hg. In the setting of excessive supplemental oxygen (PaO_2 > 55–60 mm Hg), secondary hypercapnia will go undetected using pulse oximetry as the sole monitoring tool. Pulse oximetry does not assess the adequacy of ventilation, which becomes the primary indication for mechanical ventilatory support in these patients. Further, the accuracy of the pulse oximeter is compromised in the presence of significant carboxyhemoglobin, which may be seen in COPD patients who continue to smoke.

The hypercapnia seen in COPD exacerbations may reflect a chronic disease process or may result from superimposed acute ventilatory failure. These two states can best be distinguished by careful examination of the relationship between the $PaCO_2$ and the arterial pH. Respiratory acidosis (carbon dioxide retention) sustained for more than 6 to 12 hours will stimulate urinary excretion of acid and a net retention of bicarbonate ion (HCO_3^-) buffer. In the face of this buffering effect, the hydrogen ion (H^+) concentration changes less for a given PCO_2 change. In acute conditions, the H^+ concentration will "account for" approximately 80% of the measured change in PCO_2.[42] Therefore, a 10-mm Hg rise in the measured PCO_2 will lead to a reduction in the measured pH of approximately 0.08 units.

Under chronic conditions of PCO_2 retention, the change in H^+ concentration is approximately 30% of the change in PCO_2. For example, a chronic 10-mm Hg rise in the measured PCO_2 will lead to a reduction in the measured pH of only 0.03 units. Renal HCO_3^- retention in association with ammonium ion (acid) excretion results in a net chloruresis and an associated hypochloremia of chronic respiratory acidosis.[43] The renal compensation to a chronic sustained respiratory acidosis is incomplete, and normalization of the pH is not expected.

The degree of hypercapnia has been implicated in the mental status changes associated with progressive respiratory failure. This state, described as *carbon dioxide narcosis,* has been demonstrated in normal subjects during the rebreathing of carbon dioxide. However, all clinicians recognize the late-stage COPD patient with marked hypercapnia who is mentally intact. For the COPD patient, buffered hypercapnia without hypoxemia appears to have minimal effects. It is likely that the degree of systemic acidemia is the primary determinant of the patient's mental status.

Respiratory stimulants have been used in the setting of acute COPD exacerbations to correct the gas exchange defects. This category of medications includes methylxanthines, narcotic antagonists (naloxone), progesterone, acetazolamide, doxapram, and almitrine. The use of these agents remains controversial. Two of these agents, doxapram and almitrine, have been used to prevent the worsening of hypercapnia with the use of supplemental oxygen.

Doxapram acts to stimulate ventilation through both peripheral (low-dose) and central (high-dose) mechanisms. Investigators suggested that the use of this agent in hypercapnic patients increases minute ventilation, lowers $PaCO_2$, and increases PaO_2.[44, 45] The concern associated with the use of respiratory stimulants is that the majority of patients with COPD in respiratory failure already show evidence for high control center output. Hypercapnia is viewed as an "adaptive" event by some researchers to decrease the workload of a stressed neuromuscular system. Further stimulation of ventilation with pharmacologic agents may be detrimental in this setting.

Almitrine bimesylate acts on peripheral chemoreceptors to stimulate respiration in normal subjects. In patients with COPD, improvements in gas exchange exceed those attributable to ventilation changes alone, suggesting additional beneficial effects on $\dot{V}/\dot{Q}$ matching within the lung. In the setting of acute respiratory failure, the effect of this agent on gas exchange is not uniformly beneficial.[46, 47] Concerns regarding a reported increase in pulmonary vascular resistance have also limited its general acceptance.

The decision to initiate mechanical ventilation is based on a complete evaluation of the patient rather than any specific level of pH or PCO_2. The patient's hemodynamic stability, mental status, and response to initial therapy are often used as factors that will determine the need for mechanical support.

Minimize Expiratory Airflow Obstruction

Bronchodilator therapy becomes the focus of efforts to reduce airways resistance. The mainstays of early bronchodilator therapy are the $beta_2$ agonists. Medications available in the United States include metaproterenol, salbutamol, terbutaline, pirbuterol, and bitolterol. These agents are generally preferred over epinephrine or isoproterenol because of a more selective $beta_2$ action and limited toxicity. This class of medication acts through β_2 receptors in the airway mucosa to stimulate adenylate cyclase and promote increased intracellular cyclic adenosine monophosphate, leading to bronchodilatation. Although these agents can be administered orally, subcutaneously, or via inhalation, the inhalational route is favored because of the more rapid onset of activity and reduced toxicity.[48] As a general rule, this class of drugs has an onset of action typically within 3 to 6 minutes and a duration of action of 4 to 6 hours.[48] Metaproterenol is reportedly associated with a shorter onset and duration in comparison to salbutamol and terbutaline; however, this is of questionable clinical significance. Pirbuterol and bitolterol are newer agents with a reported prolonged duration of action.

The administration of these agents by the inhalation route may occur via either an updraft nebulizer or a metered dose inhaler (MDI). Comparative studies suggest the therapeutic effectiveness is equivalent regardless of whether or not the patient is on mechanical ventilation.[49–51] Caution is indicated, however, in the interpretation of these investigations. For spontaneously breathing patients, the importance of using the correct technique for MDI administration is essential. A spacer device may be required to assist the patient with proper drug administration. In addition, the majority of studies have used a single mechanical measure of therapeutic efficacy such as the FEV_1 for spontaneously breathing patients or inflation pressures for mechanically ventilated patients. Whether these isolated measures reflect all the potential benefits of $beta_2$ agonist therapy is unclear. Patients not clearly responsive to one method of drug administration may benefit from the alternative method.

Parasympathetic activity in the trachea and bronchi influences bronchomotor tone and irritant response. Anticholinergic agents act to inhibit parasympathetic activity and therefore promote bronchodilatation. Atropine sulfate and glycopyrrolate, delivered by the aerosol route, and ipratropium bromide, delivered by MDI or aerosol, are the currently available agents in the United States. Both agents are effective bronchodilators; however, ipratropium bromide is preferred because of reduced mucosal absorption, which minimizes the potential systemic anticholinergic side effects. It has been stated that the $beta_2$ agonists have a more rapid time to maximum effect than do the anticholinergic agents. However, published response curves show that greater than 75% of the effect is present in 30 to 60 minutes.[52] In COPD patients with exacerbations, there is a delay to peak effect for both metaproterenol and ipratropium bromide, the former being 60 minutes and the latter being 90 minutes in this situation.[53]

Comparison studies between $beta_2$ agonists and anticholinergic agents have suggested similar bronchodilator efficacy when given in appropriate doses in both acute and stable COPD patients.[54] A study of long-term use in COPD subjects (90 days) favored the use of ipratropium bromide in these patients, suggesting that tachyphylaxis to this agent, unlike $beta_2$ agonists, does not occur.[55] The likelihood of additive benefits when the two classes of bronchodilators are used simultaneously is less clear. Conflicting results have been reported when a second agent is added after the first bronchodilator is used to maximum therapeutic efficacy.[56, 57] Whereas $beta_2$ agonists have been associated with a reduction in the measured PaO_2 during acute administration, this effect has not been seen with anticholinergic agents.[53]

The correct dosing frequency for these agents is also controversial. Clinicians frequently recommend a dose of two puffs every 4 to 6 hours for both categories of inhaled bronchodilators. However, this level of drug administration is believed by most investigators to be significantly less than what is needed, especially in the setting of acute respiratory failure.

On the basis of the available scientific investigation, $beta_2$ agonists should be used in the acute management of COPD patients because of their rapid onset. Acute nebulizer or MDI therapy may be provided every 15 to 20 minutes, depending on patient tolerance for three to four doses to provide early symptomatic relief as long as the patient is monitored for signs of adrenergic stimulation. After acute stabilization, a more appropriate dosing frequency is selected (every 2–4 hours). Ipratropium bromide is added to provide a second bronchodilating agent in the acute setting for patients responding poorly to $beta_2$ agonists.

Few areas in medicine have generated the same degree of controversy as seen regarding the use of theophylline compounds in the acute and chronic management of COPD patients. As a bronchodilator, theophylline has been shown to provide only slight additive benefit to the use of inhaled agents.[58] Other proposed benefits to the administration of this agent include improvements in respiratory muscle strength, ventricular contractility, and mucociliary clearance.[58a] The clinical significance of these effects is unclear. Clinical trials have examined the role of this agent during acute disease exacerbations and have suggested minimal benefit from its use in the face of adequate inhaled bronchodilator therapy.[59]

For clinicians who elect to use theophylline compounds in the acute management of COPD patients, recognition of the complexity of dosing and potential drug toxicities is essential. The optimal therapeutic range remains undefined; however, the risk of toxicity is certainly associated with higher serum levels. The need for continuous intravenous administration has not been justified.

Corticosteroids are frequently used in the acute management of COPD exacerbations. This category of agents reduces airway inflammation and enhances the responsiveness to catecholamine bronchodilators. The use of corticosteroid therapy in stable outpatients with COPD remains controversial because a large number of conflicting studies exist. In contrast, few studies are available regarding the use of these agents in hospitalized patients with COPD exacerbations.[59a] A randomized clinical trial of methylprednisolone (0.5 mg/kg every 6 hours) suggested a benefit as assessed by measurements of the FEV_1.[60] This benefit is not seen in the initial 12 to 18 hours because the effects of corticosteroid administration are delayed. If corticosteroids are needed for the management of the COPD population, they should be started early in recognition of this delayed onset. Further, they should be converted to the oral form (i.e., prednisone, 40–60 mg per day) and tapered as quickly as possible (less than 2 weeks). No studies currently exist to select patients for corticosteroid therapy in the acute setting, although it seems plausible that patients with recognized disease reversibility (i.e., an asthma component) would be most likely to benefit.

Attention to secretion management is also warranted. Coughing is the most effective method of secretion clearance. Patients should be encouraged to perform forced expiratory coughing in the upright or sitting position, as necessary. Dehydration should be avoided, although overhydration to "loosen" secretions is not advised. Mucolytic agents have no clear benefit, and *N*-acetylcysteine carries the risk of significant bronchospasm when administered by aerosol. Chest percussion can assist secretion clearance in the difficult patient, although there are few data to suggest that this technique is advantageous over vigorous coughing. Aggravation of hypoxemia during chest physiotherapy has been described in relation to body position.[61]

Treatment of the Precipitating Cause

The evaluation and treatment of the patient with COPD and respiratory failure are often dominated by considerations of the underlying disease process. A careful history and physical examination are indicated in every patient to identify factors that might precipitate disease activity and require therapeutic intervention.

Drug toxicities must be identified and corrected. For patients with difficult arrhythmias in the setting of theophylline use, this medication is best withheld given its less than favorable benefit-risk ratio. Beta-blockers and sedative medications should also be withdrawn, if possible.

Because infection is thought to be a frequent precipitating cause, the role of routine antibiotic use for this disorder has received much attention. Certainly, the patient with complicating pneumonitis secondary to bacterial infection deserves therapy. Less clear are the indications for antibiotic therapy in patients with only mild to moderate sputum production (i.e., bronchitis). Although sputum Gram's stains and cultures are often positive, this is also true during periods of disease stability. A double-blind, placebo-controlled investigation studied 362 COPD exacerbations and found that routine use of antibiotic therapy resulted in more prompt resolution of symptoms, earlier improvements in peak flow measurements, and a reduced rate of hospitalization.[10] The benefit was most significant in patients presenting with strong clinical features suggestive of bronchitis, including increased dyspnea, increased sputum volume, and sputum purulence. Of note, the investigators chose three routine oral antibiotics for use: amoxicillin, doxycycline, and trimethoprim-sulfamethoxazole. The selection appeared to be based primarily on physician preference rather than culture and sensitivity data.

The results of this investigation are in contrast to those of other studies that have described no benefit. A possible explanation of these contradictory findings is that the benefit to routine use of antibiotic therapy is small and is seen only in investigations with large sample sizes. However, especially for patients with evidence of inflammatory bronchitis in the setting of acute respiratory failure, the benefit-risk ratio seems favorable.

Respiratory muscle function should be optimized. A search for and correction of electrolyte deficiencies is indicated. Correction of hypoxemia and/or hypercarbia will improve muscle function. For the patient with complicating cardiac dysfunction, correction of volume expansion, control of arrhythmias, and reversal of myocardial ischemia are essential. Weaning studies in COPD patients suggest that complicating cardiac dysfunction can be a major limiting factor to success.[62]

For the patient who is unable to maintain caloric intake (i.e., because of mechanical ventilation), consideration of supplemented intake is indicated usually via a small-bore nasogastric or nasojejunal feeding tube. Parenteral nutrition should be avoided at all costs because the potential risk of pneumothorax associated with central venous access can be disastrous in this patient group. Caloric requirements can be estimated at approximately 25 to 30 kcal/kg or determined using available prediction formulas.[63] Typical protein requirements for this mildly to moderately stressed population are in the range of 1.2 to 1.5 g of protein per kilogram of body weight per day.

The target of nutritional therapy in the acute setting is the maintenance of caloric balance and correction of obvious deficiencies. Despite the frequent presence of marked malnutrition in COPD patients who progress to respiratory failure, aggressive attempts to feed these patients can be hazardous. Caloric intake that far exceeds energy demand results in heightened carbon dioxide production and increased ventilatory requirements.[64] Excess energy provision is generally converted to fat stores without significant expansion of lean tissue mass during short-term nutritional repletion.

Mechanical Ventilation

When deciding to initiate mechanical ventilation, one must now consider the mode of support as well as the method of delivery. The development of soft, leak-proof nasal and oral facemasks has allowed the use of noninvasive ventilation applied at the nose and/or mouth as a means of support. Noninvasive ventilatory support delivered via this method has been successfully used for the treatment of COPD exacerbations.[65] This method of support is limited to awake, oriented patients without secretion clearance problems or markedly elevated respiratory impedance. Patients must be able to tolerate the tight-fitting facemask associated with this form of support. A secure patient-mask interface is essential to ensure no loss of pressure during assisted ventilation and to maximize the benefits of therapy. Problems with secretion management and provision of caloric support occur in relation to the nasal/oral facemask. In general, nasogastric tubes are not routinely required in the absence of caloric intake during the period of noninvasive ventilation. Although studies have suggested that this form of therapy can be used to "avoid" endotracheal intubation, the criteria for patient selection require further definition. Noninvasive ventilation has not yet been shown to be beneficial for hospitalized COPD patients compared with the use of conventional therapy in a single clinical trial.[65a]

For the patient who requires mechanical ventilation with endotracheal intubation, a wide range of ventilator assistance modes exists. A full discussion of this topic is beyond the scope of this review. A few items specific to the COPD population are reviewed, dividing the ventilator management into the acute and chronic phase of ventilatory support.

Acute Phase

Early in the resuscitation period, a mode should be selected that adequately "unloads" the work of the respiratory muscles. For most patients, this mode will be a form of volume-cycled ventilation (assist-control or synchronized intermittent mandatory ventilation [SIMV]). Pressure-cycled modes provide variable levels of minute ventilation depending on the patient's effort and respiratory impedance and, therefore, are less desirable. This is especially true for the acute management of the COPD patient in whom variable degrees of bronchospasm, airway secretions, and response to therapeutic intervention may provide a changing airways resistance.

A V_T of approximately 10 mL/kg of body weight is typically used in the early management period. Further adjustments are based on patient response and additional arterial blood gas monitoring. A rough rule of thumb is that the machine-supported minute ventilation should be adjusted to approximately two thirds of the spontaneous minute ventilation in the acute phase. Normalization of the P_{CO_2} is not the target of ventilatory assistance; rather, a level of minute ventilation that "rests" the neuromuscular system and corrects acidosis is desired. Normalization of the P_{CO_2} in a patient with chronic hypercapnia should be avoided because this can lead to a significant posthypercapnic respiratory alkalosis. Early complications of this acid-base disorder include cardiac arrhythmias and seizures, whereas late complications include a complicated weaning course resulting from the increased ventilatory demand in the setting of lost buffering capacity. The inspired oxygen concentration is usually set at 0.80 to 0.90 until the patient is stabilized. Further adjustments in this parameter may be guided by arterial blood gas data or pulse oximetry.

Attention to timing parameters, specifically cycle length, inspiratory-expiratory time ratios, and peak inspiratory flow rate, is essential. A peak inspiratory flow rate that is five to six times the resting minute ventilation will generally meet inspiratory flow demands without causing excessively high peak cycling pressures. The increased airways resistance and reduced elastic recoil characteristic of COPD patients provide a requirement for prolonged expiratory duration. An elevated VDS increases ventilatory requirements, which is most frequently met through tachypnea, leading to a short cycle length. The combination of short cycle length and prolonged expiratory phase places the patient at high risk for dynamic hyperinflation if inspiratory flow characteristics are not adjusted properly.

To compensate for dynamic hyperinflation, clinicians have studied the use of external expiratory airway pressure as a means of unloading the inspiratory muscles. Externally applied PEEP or continuous positive airway pressure (CPAP) is used in this setting to offset the positive Prs at end-expiration, which favors continued expiratory airflow. A series of studies have now documented that external PEEP or CPAP can reduce the work of breathing on patient-cycled breaths in the setting of hyperinflation.[66–69] Critical to this observation is the selection of an external PEEP level that does not exceed the end-expiratory Prs.[68] External PEEP in excess of end-expiratory Prs (auto-PEEP) will lead to further hyperinflation, elevation of peak cycling pressures, and increased work of breathing. The nonuniformity of expiratory airflow obstruction across all alveoli suggests that Prs at end-expiration will vary within individual lung units. Application of external PEEP may adversely affect those individual lung units with low end-expiratory Prs, although the mean end-expiratory Prs will not be changed. This factor should limit the use of external PEEP in COPD subjects to only those patients with specific problems (i.e., inability to cycle mechanical ventilation) that cannot be addressed with careful attention to reducing minute ventilation and airflow obstruction.

The elevated end-expiratory intrathoracic pressure of dynamic hyperinflation, similar to externally applied PEEP, can lead to impedance of venous return and reduction in cardiac output. Transmission of this intrathoracic pressure to the intrathoracic vasculature can lead to elevation in measured hemodynamic variables, including the PCWP. This can adversely result in fluid restriction or vasopressor use in the severely obstructed patient if this complication is not recognized.

Because of its significant risks, dynamic hyperinflation or auto-PEEP should be carefully sought in all patients with obstructive airways disease. A number of techniques for the measurement of these parameters have been described (Table 95–4). Each of these methods offers particular advantages and limitations. When correctly applied, the variable techniques appear to give similar information. Because of inherent measurement variability, complementary techniques are often used to confirm measured values.

When present, the most important treatment goals for dynamic hyperinflation are directed toward relieving expiratory airflow obstruction and reducing total minute ventilation. Adjustments in inspiratory timing through manipulation of peak flow measurements can be helpful and should be used early in the treatment course, as necessary.

Reducing the minute ventilation requirements, in addition to positive benefits with respect to hyperinflation, can significantly reduce the work of breathing. As previously mentioned, the relationship between augmented ventilation and energy consumption is hyperbolic in these patients. Small increments in ventilation require disproportionate increases in resting oxygen consumption. Hypermetabolism secondary to fever or agitation must be reduced. Treatable causes of high VDS (i.e., volume depletion or lung overdistention) should be identified and reversed if possible.

A number of strategies have been described to deal with progressive hypercapnia and high inflation pressures in the setting of COPD. These include controlled hypoventilation and tracheal gas insufflation. Alternative strategies for mechanical ventilation in this setting are discussed more completely in Chapters 98 and 104.

For the patient with COPD, the decision to initiate mechanical ventilation should be based on physiologic criteria, with appropriate recognition of the patient's therapeutic goals. The outcome for COPD patients who require mechanical ventilation is not uniformly poor. Yet a significant number of patients will progress to chronic ventilator dependence and/or require prolonged ICU care. The patient's premorbid clinical status appears to be the major determinant of outcome. Discussions between the clinician and patient regarding therapeutic goals and the use of life-support measures should be initiated before the acute episode. Providing the patient with knowledge regarding the potential outcomes from the use of ventilatory support allows an informed decision regarding life-support measures. Understanding who the patient wishes to participate in decision making should that be necessary is also important. A trusting physician-patient relationship is essential for the management of chronic obstructive lung disease to clarify treatment goals and preserve patient autonomy.

TABLE 95–4. Techniques for the Assessment of Dynamic Hyperinflation or Auto-PEEP in the Patient with Chronic Obstructive Pulmonary Disease

Technique	*Description*
Occlusion	The expiratory valve at end-expiration is occluded before the next inflation. In the closed system, alveolar pressure transmitted to the airway opening and the ventilator manometer reflects Prs at end-expiration.
Counterbalance	In the presence of auto-PEEP, inspiratory airway pressure must exceed the Prs at end-expiration before inspiratory airflow can begin. The level of airway pressure at which inspiratory airflow begins is equivalent to Prs. The use of an esophageal balloon to measure pleural pressure provides a high degree of accuracy.
Spirometer/flowmeter	Expiratory lung volume/flow is monitored during each exhalation. Failure of the spirometer volume to reach a stable end-expiratory volume or zero flow before the next inspiration suggests the possibility of dynamic hyperinflation.
Exhaled gas	The volume of gas expired after a ventilator disconnect or apnea interval is measured as an index of the end-expiratory lung volume above the true resting lung volume.
Thoracic gas volume	The change in thoracic gas volume, determined by inductance plethysmography, is assessed in response to progressive increments of external PEEP. The point of increasing thoracic gas volume in response to external PEEP is equivalent to the Prs at end-expiration.

Abbreviations: PEEP = positive end-expiratory pressure; Prs = pressure of the respiratory system.

Chronic Phase

Mechanical support is usually continued for a minimum of 24 to 48 hours while therapy directed at the underlying pathophysiologic processes is instituted. The focus for COPD patients on more long-term ventilation must be to minimize the risk of complications associated with this support.

Barotrauma is a recognized complication of mechanical ventilatory support in COPD patients. The incidence of this complication relates at least in part to the level of ventilator cycling pressures. Efforts to maintain peak airway pressure less than 40 cm H_2O are appropriate but will be compromised by the need for higher resting minute ventilations and inspiratory flow rates in COPD patients. Reducing the inspiratory flow rate can be counterproductive because it will shorten the time for expiration and increase the risk of dynamic hyperinflation. A slightly reduced VT (7–10 mL/kg) and therapy directed at reducing minute ventilation and airways resistance are most helpful.

The COPD patient who requires mechanical ventilation is predisposed to a long list of potential complications.[70] Complications of acute respiratory failure have been described for almost every organ system either secondary to the disease process or as a result of therapy. Particularly common problems in the COPD patient include gastrointestinal bleeding and nosocomial infection, including chronic airway infection (bronchitis). The approach to these clinical problems is discussed in other chapters.

For the more alert COPD patient on mechanical ventilation, the management of anxiety becomes a major issue. Anxiety can provoke periods of panic during the weaning phase, leading to hyperventilation, dynamic hyperinflation, and worsening dyspnea. Although sedation is often necessary early in the treatment phase to minimize ventilatory requirements, regular sedation can interfere with the normal weaning process. Patients on more chronic ventilatory support appear to benefit from a regular daily schedule. Nighttime intervals are best conducted with full ventilatory support to allow adequate rest periods. The addition of regular physical therapy, including ambulation on mechanical ventilation if possible, appears to also be helpful. If patients understand the goals for the weaning process and actively participate in the daily program, often anxiety can be minimized and the need for pharmacologic intervention eliminated. The use of specific biofeedback techniques in the weaning process has been reported and may be beneficial.[71]

The mode of mechanical ventilation selected for weaning remains a matter of physician preference. Randomized studies comparing ventilator weaning methods are few and inconclusive. However, special attention to the "external" workload associated with the ventilator system is warranted, especially in the COPD patient, because small changes in minute ventilation or mechanical work produce large changes in respiratory muscle energy requirements. The resistance of the endotracheal tube increases exponentially in relation to reductions in tube size. The use of smaller endotracheal tubes (<8 mm) in the COPD patient can limit secretion clearance and significantly increase the work of breathing. The use of low levels of pressure support (3–5 cm H_2O) during spontaneous breaths on mechanical ventilation can limit the effects of endotracheal tube resistance.

Demand valves associated with an SIMV circuit can require a significant reduction in airway pressure by the patient to initiate airflow. This factor, combined with the lack of instantaneous delivery of gas flow, can cause a significant increase in the mechanical workload of ventilation.[72] Ventilator circuits that incorporate a continuous flow design may serve to minimize this workload. Finally, the importance of matching ventilator sensitivity and flow rates to patient inspiratory flow demands should be emphasized. Significant amounts of respiratory work can be performed by the patient, even in the assist mode of ventilation, if these variables are adjusted incorrectly.[73]

A number of physiologic parameters have been examined in an effort to predict the likelihood of success in weaning the COPD patient from mechanical ventilation. Traditional indexes developed for postoperative patients, including an adequate negative inspiratory force ($\leq$30 cm H_2O), an appropriate level of minute ventilation ($\leq$10 L/min), and significant reserve capacity (ability to double $\dot{V}$E), have shown poor sensitivity and specificity when applied to the COPD population.

A measurement of the inspiratory pressure generated during the first 100 ms of partial airway occlusion during inspiration (P_{100}) reflects the motor output of the respiratory neurons in response to the mechanical demands of the ventilatory apparatus. The measurement is independent of lung and chest wall mechanics, although the value is influenced by muscle strength and lung volume. The measurement can be obtained during spontaneous breathing trials or after a period of carbon dioxide rebreathing. COPD patients with a high level of respiratory motor output at rest (P_{100} > 6.0 cm H_2O) and/or a value that fails to increase during periods of carbon dioxide–stimulated ventilation are unlikely to be weaned.[74] Despite these findings, it is not clear that the regular measurement of this parameter in COPD subjects would alter clinical decision making. Further, the measurement is limited by the need for technical expertise and specialized equipment.

A clinical trial of ventilation at reduced mechanical support (or spontaneous breathing) remains a reasonable approach to identify patients who can progress in weaning from mechanical ventilation. Careful attention to the breathing pattern including the identification of small VT and/or high respiratory rates appears to be as reliable in identifying weaning "failures" as more sophisticated measurements.[75]

Prognosis

The prognosis for patients with COPD and acute respiratory failure is unclear from published series. Reported hospital mortality rates have ranged from 5% to 38%.[45, 76] The requirement for mechanical ventilation has ranged from less than 5% to more than 50% of patients admitted with this diagnosis in published series. It is unlikely that this wide variability reflects the true biologic behavior of this disorder. Rather, many of the investigations in this area suffer from retrospective analyses, small sample sizes, variable definitions for COPD and respiratory failure, and limited long-term follow-up. Despite these limitations, a few general conclusions are suggested.

The short-term mortality rate for respiratory failure secondary to COPD is significantly less compared with that of other causes of acute respiratory failure.[45, 76, 77] The majority of patients do not require assisted ventilation for management.[45, 76] Further, the development of respiratory failure does not always predict an adverse prognosis for individual patients.[76] Adverse prognostic variables suggested for COPD patients with respiratory failure include reduced premorbid clinical status, reduced serum albumin, and the severity of acidemia on presentation.[45, 78] The degree of hypoxemia and hypercarbia was not an important prognostic variable in one series.[44] The clinical usefulness of these indexes is limited by the lack of prospective validation in a larger series of patients.

SUMMARY

Management of the COPD patient with acute respiratory failure requires an understanding of the pathophysiologic changes associated with expiratory airflow obstruction. Our knowledge of risk factors and mechanisms that trigger typical COPD disease exacerbations remains incomplete and limits further progress in this area. Therapeutic efforts directed at reversal of the airflow obstruction are the foundation of the treatment plan. For the majority of patients, careful management, even in the setting of respiratory failure that requires mechanical ventilation, can allow a satisfactory patient outcome.

References

1. Feinleib M, Rosenberg H, Collins J, et al: Trends in COPD morbidity and mortality in the United States. Am Rev Respir Dis 1989; 140:S9.
2. Snider G: Chronic obstructive pulmonary disease: A definition and implications of structural determinants of airflow obstruction for epidemiology. Am Rev Respir Dis 1989; 140:S3–S8.
3. Murray J: Pathophysiology of acute respiratory failure. Respir Care 1983; 28:531.
4. Pontoppidan H, Geffin B, Lowenstein E: Acute respiratory failure in the adult (part 1). N Engl J Med 1972; 287:690.
5. Bjerkestrand G, Digranes A, Schreiner A: Bacteriological findings in transtracheal aspirates from patients with chronic bronchitis and bronchiectasis: A preliminary report. Scand J Respir Dis 1975; 56:201.
6. Christensen J, Gadeberg O, Bruvn B: *Branhamella catarrhalis*: Significance in pulmonary infections and bacteriologic features. Acta Pathol Microbiol Immunol Scand 1986; 94(Section B):89.
7. Blasi F, Legnani D, Lombardo V, et al: *Chlamydia pneumoniae* infection in acute exacerbations of COPD. Eur Respir J 1993; 6:19.
8. Buscho R, Saxtan D, Shultz P, et al: Infections with viruses and *Mycoplasma pneumoniae* during exacerbations of chronic bronchitis. J Infect Dis 1978; 137:377.
9. Haas H, Morris J, Samson S, et al: Bacterial flora of the respiratory tract in chronic bronchitis: Comparison of transtracheal, fiber-bronchoscopic, and oropharyngeal sampling methods. Am Rev Respir Dis 1977; 16:41.
10. Anthonisen N, Manfreda J, Warren C, et al: Antibiotic therapy in exacerbations of chronic obstructive pulmonary disease. Ann Intern Med 1987; 106:196.
11. Nicotra N, Rivera M, Awe R: Antibiotic therapy of acute exacerbations of chronic bronchitis: A controlled study using tetracycline. Ann Intern Med 1982; 97:18.
12. Kuller L, Ockene J, Townsend M, et al: The epidemiology of pulmonary function and COPD mortality in the multiple risk factor intervention trial. Am Rev Respir Dis 1989; 140:S76.
13. Sideris D, Katsadoros D, Valianos G, et al: Type of cardiac dysrhythmias in respiratory failure. Am Heart J 1975; 89:32.
14. Bittar G, Friedman H: The arrhythmogenicity of theophylline. Chest 1991; 99:1415.
15. Varriale P, David W, Chryssos B, et al: Multifocal atrial arrhythmia: A frequent misdiagnosis? A correlative study using the computerized ECG. Clin Cardiol 1991; 15:343.
16. Donahoe M, Rogers RM: Is loss of body weight in COPD secondary to low tissue oxygenation? Respiration 1992; 24:33.
17. Kawakami Y, Kishi F, Yamamoto H, et al: Relation of oxygen delivery, mixed venous oxygenation, and pulmonary hemodynamics to prognosis in chronic obstructive pulmonary disease. N Engl J Med 1983; 308:1045.
18. Charan N, Lakshminarayan S: Pulmonary effects of timolol. Arch Intern Med 1980; 140:843.
19. Sassoon C, Hassell K, Mahutte C: Hyperoxic-induced hypercapnia in stable chronic obstructive pulmonary disease. Am Rev Respir Dis 1987; 135:907.
20. Dines D, Clagett O, Payne W: Spontaneous pneumothorax in emphysema. Mayo Clin Proc 1970; 45:481.
21. Moser K, Lemoine J, Nachtwey F, et al: Deep venous thrombosis and pulmonary embolism. JAMA 1981; 246:1422.
22. Cordova C, Musca A, Violi F, et al: Platelet hyperfunction in patients with chronic airways obstruction. Eur J Respir Dis 1985; 66:9.
23. Lesser B, Leeper K, Stein P, et al: The diagnosis of acute pulmonary embolism in patients with chronic obstructive pulmonary disease. Chest 1992; 102:17.
24. Macklem P: The importance of defining respiratory muscle fatigue. Am Rev Respir Dis 1990; 142:274.
25. Bellemare F, Grassino A: Force reserve of the diaphragm in patients with chronic obstructive pulmonary disease. J Appl Physiol 1983; 55:8.
26. Brochard L, Harf A, Lorino H, et al: Inspiratory pressure support prevents diaphragmatic fatigue during weaning from mechanical ventilation. Am Rev Respir Dis 1989; 139:513.
27. Efthimiou J, Fleming J, Spiro S: Sternomastoid muscle function and fatigue in breathless patients with severe respiratory disease. Am Rev Respir Dis 1987; 136:1099.
28. Kongragunta V, Druz W, Sharp J: Dyspnea and diaphragmatic fatigue in patients with chronic obstructive pulmonary disease. Am Rev Respir Dis 1988; 137:662.
29. Moxham J: Respiratory muscle fatigue: Mechanisms, evaluation and therapy. Br J Anaesth 1990; 65:43.
30. Fisher J, Magid N, Kallman C, et al: Respiratory illness and hypophosphatemia. Chest 1983; 83:504.
31. Lewis M, Monn S, Sieck G: Effect of corticosteroids on diaphragm fatigue, SDH activity, and muscle fiber size. J Appl Physiol 1992; 72:293.
32. Hussain S, Simkus G, Roussos C: Respiratory muscle fatigue: A cause of ventilatory failure in septic shock. J Appl Physiol 1985; 58:2033.
33. Arora N, Rochester D: Effect of body weight and muscularity on human diaphragm muscle mass, thickness, and area. J Appl Physiol 1982; 52:64.
34. Fiaccadori E, Canale SD, Coffrini S, et al: Muscle and serum magnesium in pulmonary intensive care unit patients. Crit Care Med 1988; 16:751.
35. Gertz I, Hedenstierna G, Hellers G, et al: Muscle metabolism in patients with chronic obstructive pulmonary disease and acute respiratory failure. Clin Sci Mol Med 1977; 52:396.
36. Jeejeebhoy K: Bulk or bounce: The object of nutritional support. JPEN J Parenter Enteral Nutr 1988; 12:539.
37. Wagner P, Dantzker D, Deuck R, et al: Ventilation-perfusion inequality in chronic obstructive pulmonary disease. J Clin Invest 1977; 59:203.
38. Sanchez J, Derenne J, Debesse B, et al: Muscle fiber types in costal and crural diaphragm in normal men and in patients with moderate chronic respiratory diseases. Bull Eur Physiopathol Respir 1985; 21:351.
39. Aubier M, Murciano D, Fournier M, et al: Central respiratory drive in acute respiratory failure of patients with chronic obstructive pulmonary disease. Am Rev Respir Dis 1980; 122:191.
40. Abraham A, Cole R, Green I, et al: Factors contributing to the reversible pulmonary hypertension in patients with respiratory failure studied by serial observations during recovery. Circ Res 1969; 23:51.
41. Tobin M, Perez W, Guenther S, et al: Does rib cage-abdominal paradox signify respiratory muscle fatigue? J Appl Physiol 1987; 63:851.
42. Brackett N, Wingo C, Muren O, et al: Acid-base response to chronic hypercapnia in man. N Engl J Med 1969; 280:124.
43. Narins R, Emmett M: Simple and mixed acid-base disorders: A practical approach. Medicine 1980; 59:161.
44. Moser K, Luchsinger P, Adamson J, et al: Respiratory stimulation with intravenous doxapram in respiratory failure: A double-blind cooperative study. N Engl J Med 1973; 288:427.
45. Jeffrey A, Warren P, Flenley D: Acute hypercapnic respiratory failure in patients with chronic obstructive lung disease: Risk factors and use of guidelines. Thorax 1992; 47:34.
46. Bardsley P, Tweney J, Morgan N, et al: Oral almitrine in treatment of acute respiratory failure and cor pulmonale in patients with exacerbation of chronic obstructive pulmonary disease. Thorax 1991; 46:493.
47. Castaing Y, Manier G, Guenard H: Improvement in ventilation-perfusion relationships by almitrine in patients with chronic obstructive pulmonary disease during mechanical ventilation. Am Rev Respir Dis 1986; 134:910.

48. Popa V: Beta-adrenergic drugs. Clin Chest Med 1986; 7:313.
49. Fernandez A, Lazaro A, Garcia A, et al: Bronchodilators in patients with chronic obstructive pulmonary disease on mechanical ventilation. Am Rev Respir Dis 1990; 141:164.
50. Berry R, Shinto R, Wong F, et al: Nebulizer vs spacer for bronchodilator delivery in patients hospitalized for acute exacerbations of COPD. Chest 1989; 96:1241.
51. Gay P, Patel H, Nelson S, et al: Metered dose inhalers for bronchodilator delivery in intubated mechanically ventilated patients. Chest 1991; 99:66.
52. Le Doux E, Morris JF, Temple WP, et al: Standard and double dose ipratropium bromide and combined ipratropium bromide and inhaled metaproterenol in COPD. Chest 1989; 95:1013.
53. Karpel J, Pesin J, Greenberg D: A comparison of the effects of ipratropium bromide and metaproterenol sulfate in acute exacerbations of COPD. Chest 1990; 98:835.
54. Karpel J: Bronchodilator responses to anticholinergic and beta-adrenergic agents in acute and stable COPD. Chest 1991; 99:871.
55. Taskin D, Asotosh K, Bleeker E, et al: Comparison of anticholinergic bronchodilator ipratropium bromide with metaproterenol in chronic obstructive pulmonary disease: A 90 day multicenter study. Am J Med 1986; 81(Suppl 5A):81.
56. Easton P, Jadue C, Dhingra S, et al: A comparison of the bronchodilating effects of a beta-2 adrenergic agent (albuterol) and an anticholinergic agent (ipratropium bromide) given by aerosol or in sequence. N Engl J Med 1986; 315:735.
57. Lefcoe N, Gross N, Skorodin M: Role of the parasympathetic nervous system in airway obstruction due to emphysema. N Engl J Med 1984; 311:421.
58. Lloberes P, Ramis L, Alarcon J, et al: Effect of three different bronchodilators during an exacerbation of chronic obstructive pulmonary disease. Eur Respir J 1988; 1:536.
58a. Kirsten DK, Wegner RE, Jorres RA, et al: Effects of theophylline withdrawal in severe chronic obstructive pulmonary disease. Chest 1993; 104:1101–1107.
59. Rice K, Leatherman J, Duane P, et al: Aminophylline for acute exacerbations of chronic obstructive pulmonary disease. Ann Intern Med 1987; 107:305.
59a. Rubini F, Rampulla C, Nava S: Acute effect of corticosteroids on respiratory mechanics in mechanically ventilated patients with chronic airflow obstruction and acute respiratory failure. Am J Respir Crit Care Med 1994; 149:306–310.
60. Albert R, Martin T, Lewis S: Controlled clinical trial of methylprednisolone in patients with chronic bronchitis and acute respiratory insufficiency. Ann Intern Med 1980; 92:753.
61. Connors A, Hammon W, Martin R, et al: Chest physical therapy: The immediate effect on oxygenation in acutely ill patients. Chest 1980; 78:559.
62. Lemaire F, Teboul J, Cinotti L, et al: Acute left ventricular dysfunction during unsuccessful weaning from mechanical ventilation. Anesthesiology 1988; 69:171.
63. Moore J, Angelillo V: Equations for the prediction of resting energy expenditure in chronic obstructive lung disease. Chest 1988; 94:1260.
64. Talpers S, Romberger D, Bunce S, et al: Nutritionally associated increased carbon dioxide production. Chest 1992; 102:551.
65. Brochard L, Isabey D, Piquet J, et al: Reversal of acute exacerbations of chronic obstructive lung disease by inspiratory assistance with a face mask. N Engl J Med 1990; 323:1523.
65a. Bott J, Carroll MP, Conway JH, et al: Randomized controlled trial of nasal ventilation in acute ventilatory failure due to chronic obstructive airway disease. Lancet 1993; 341:1555–1557.
66. Gay P, Rodarte J, Hubmayr R: The effects of positive expiratory pressure on isovolume flow and dynamic hyperinflation in patients receiving mechanical ventilation. Am Rev Respir Dis 1989; 139:621.
67. Smith T, Marini J: Impact of PEEP on lung mechanics and work of breathing in severe airflow obstruction. J Appl Physiol 1988; 65:1488.
68. Ranieri V, Giuliani R, Cinnella G, et al: Physiologic effects of positive end-expiratory pressure in patients with chronic obstructive pulmonary disease during acute ventilatory failure and controlled mechanical ventilation. Am Rev Respir Dis 1993; 147:5.
69. Petrof B, Legare M, Goldberg P, et al: Continuous positive airway pressure reduces work of breathing and dyspnea during weaning from mechanical ventilation in severe chronic obstructive pulmonary disease. Am Rev Respir Dis 1990; 141:281.
70. Pingleton S: Complications of acute respiratory failure. Am Rev Respir Dis 1988; 137:1463.
71. Holliday J, Hyers T: The reduction of weaning time from mechanical ventilation using tidal volume and relaxation biofeedback. Am Rev Respir Dis 1990; 141:1214.
72. Gibney R, Wilson R, Pontoppidan H: Comparison of work of breathing on high gas flow and demand valve continuous positive airway pressure systems. Chest 1982; 82:692.
73. Marini J, Capps J, Culver B: The inspiratory work of breathing during assisted mechanical ventilation. Chest 1985; 87:612.
74. Montgomery A, Holle R, Neagley S, et al: Prediction of successful ventilator weaning using airway occlusion pressure and hypercapnic challenge. Chest 1987; 4:496.
75. Yang K, Tobin M: A prospective study of indexes predicting the outcome of trials of weaning from mechanical ventilation. N Engl J Med 1991; 324:1445.
76. Martin T, Lewis S, Albert R: The prognosis of patients with chronic obstructive pulmonary disease after hospitalization for acute respiratory failure. Chest 1982; 82:310.
77. Gillespie D, Marsh H, Divertie M, et al: Clinical outcome of respiratory failure in patients requiring prolonged (> 24 hours) mechanical ventilation. Chest 1986; 90:364.
78. Menzies R, Gibbons W, Goldberg P: Determinants of weaning and survival among patients with COPD who require mechanical ventilation for acute respiratory failure. Chest 1989; 95:398.

CHAPTER 96

Pulmonary Host Defense and Inflammatory Lung Disease

John William Christman, MD

Gas exchange is the primary physiologic function of the respiratory system that is essential for survival. The conducting airways and alveoli are constantly exposed to potentially contaminated atmospheric gases. Normal pulmonary function depends on the lung's ability to defend itself against pathogens and maintain a sterile subglottic environment. Pulmonary host defense is an extremely effective system composed of many overlapping layers rife with redundancy. A first level of host defense consists of related physical mechanisms that prevent penetration of bacteria into the lung and subsequent subglottic colonization. Beyond the bronchiolus, the lung is arduously defended by alveolar macrophages (AM). These AMs are capable of essential antibacterial operations that prevent most bacterial infections and are especially effective against gram-positive bacteria. AM antibacterial actions, in some cases, are augmented by the recruitment of granulocytic phagocytes into the lung through the elaboration of chemotactic agents. Neutrophil recruitment appears to be most essential for the containment of gram-negative bacteria. A new class of cytokines, which are now referred to as chemokines, has recently been defined and has potent chemotactic activity for acute inflammatory cells. Interleukin (IL)-8 is a potent chemoattractant for neutrophils and is thought to have a pivotal role in regulating neutrophilic inflammation in both infectious and noninfectious inflammatory lung disease.

In this chapter, I review pulmonary host defense strategies, with emphasis on the role of resident and recruited phagocytes. I focus primarily on the mechanisms of pulmonary host defense that pertain to the development and resolution of gram-negative nosocomial pneumonia in mechanically ventilated critically ill patients. I emphasize a comparison between the cellular containment of gram-negative organisms and pathogenesis of noninfectious inflammatory lung disease. In this regard, focus is maintained on the syndrome of idiopathic pulmonary fibrosis (IPF), which is an infrequent but important cause for admission to a critical care unit.

SCOPE OF THE PROBLEM

Pneumonia remains a common complication in patients treated with endotracheal intubation and mechanical ventilation and continues to have a significant impact on the mortality of these patents. Pneumonia is both a frequent admitting diagnosis to the intensive care unit (ICU)[1] and a common complication of airway instrumentation and intensive care.[2–13] Nosocomial pneumonia is defined as a lower respiratory tract infection that develops in hospitalized individuals in which the infection was either not present or not incubating at the time of admission and occurs beyond 72 hours of hospitalization. Although the incidence of nosocomial pneumonia is only 0.5% to 5% in patients treated outside a critical care setting, the incidence of nosocomial pneumonia in mechanically ventilated patients is 11% to 21%.[13] In long-term ventilated patients, the incidence of nosocomial pneumonia is at least 50% to 70%. This high incidence, coupled with a reported mortality between 25% to 55%, catapults pneumonia as the leading cause of death from nosocomial infections.[9, 10] Nosocomial pneumonia has a tremendous impact on healthcare resources because its occurrence is associated with a significantly longer hospital stay and an increase in total hospital costs.[14] A possible pathophysiologic sequence involved in the development of nosocomial pneumonia is shown in Table 96–1 and is subsequently discussed in detail.

The bacteria that cause nosocomial pneumonia differ from those that cause community-acquired pneumonia (Table 96–2). Although many nosocomial pneumonia infections are determined to be polymicrobial,[3] certain species may predominate or be difficult to treat with antibiotics. Gram-negative bacilli are a rare cause of community-acquired pneumonia but represent two thirds of nosocomial pneumonia cases; *Pseudomonas aeruginosa, Serratia marcescens,* and *Acinetobacter* spp are prominent bacterial species. In some published series, *Staphylococcus aureus* makes up approximately 25% of nosocomial pneumonia, in which the incidence of methicillin-resistance species appears to correlate with prior antibiotic treatments.[2, 6, 7] Staphylococcal pneumonia may account for as much as 55% of nosocomial pneumonia in younger individuals after multiple trauma or neurosurgery.[6, 7] Some pathogens, like *Branhamella catarrhalis, Streptococcus pneumoniae,* and *Haemophilus influenzae,* are generally thought to be community-acquired pneumonia[1] but may also account for 10% to 20% of nosocomial pneumonia. *Legionnella pneumophila* is an important cause of nosocomial infections in which the incidence is contingent on respiratory therapy practices and hospital water purity.[15–18] Before rigorous control practices, *Legionella* pneumonia accounted for up to 30% of nosocomial pneumonia in some hospitals.

TABLE 96–1. Possible Pathophysiologic Sequence Involved in the Development of Nosocomial Pneumonia

1. Gastric colonization
2. Oropharyngeal colonization
3. Aspiration
4. Depressed cough and sneeze reflexes
5. Inactive mucociliary escalation
6. Tracheobronchial colonization
7. Sufficient bacterial burden and virulence
8. Overwhelmed resident and recruited phagocytic defense
9. Pneumonia

TABLE 96–2. Bacterial Species That Are Commonly Associated with Nosocomial Pneumonia

Pseudomonas aeruginosa
Staphylococcus aureus
Klebsiella pneumoniae
Legionella pneumophila
Acinetobacter calcoaceticus
Streptococcus pneumoniae
Haemophilus influenzae
Enterobacter cloacae
Serratia marcescens
Escherichia coli

DIAGNOSIS OF NOSOCOMIAL PNEUMONIA

Typically, pneumonia is associated with fever, leukocytosis, a radiographic infiltrate, purulent sputum, and the presence of a pathogen. None of these findings are diagnostic because fever and leukocytosis may result from extrapulmonary infections, and a wide variety of radiologic shadows can occur in the absence of infection. Winer-Muram[19] carefully evaluated the diagnostic utility of portable chest radiographs for diagnosing pneumonia. The author reported that conventional radiologic criteria for pneumonia could not identify pneumonia on bedside portable films compared with rigid clinical and bronchoscopic diagnostic criteria.

Evaluation of tracheal secretions remains the initial step in identifying the cause of the pneumonia but is frequently misleading. The diagnostic utility of stained sputum is probably best for diagnosing community-acquired pneumonia. In a febrile patient with a lobar infiltrate associated with respiratory failure, a Gram's-stained sputum showing gram-positive diplococci may be diagnostic. However, the diagnostic specificity of stained sputum decreases after prolonged intubation. Although purulent sputum develops at some point during the transition from airway colonization to tracheobronchitis and lower respiratory tract infections, there is no generally agreed-on point at which antimicrobial intervention is indicated. Purulent secretions are also characteristic of reactive airway disease and can be particularly copious during recovery from an asthmatic attack. Salata and colleagues[18] performed quantitative cultures on tracheal secretions of mechanically ventilated patients suspected of having pneumonia and found that patients with nosocomial pneumonia had a higher concentration of colony-forming units (CFUs) (1.37×10^6 versus 1.29×10^4) and were more likely to have elastin degradation fragments (52 versus 9%). This and other studies seem to indicate that a threshold exists in the number of airway organisms that separates colonization from infection. One major problem has been the difficulty in obtaining airway secretions that reflect disease in the distal lung. Many laboratories exclude sputum with upper airway squamous cells because routine surveillance of these secretions has not been proved useful in predicting or diagnosing pneumonia. Because of these technical limitations, there is intense interest in the identification of more efficient modalities for the accurate diagnosis of nosocomial pneumonia in mechanically ventilated patients. A standardized and generally agreed-on approach is essential for future epidemiologic and intervention studies. There is no "gold standard" because studies that use open lung biopsy are not feasible in critically ill patients, and autopsy studies are few. Two fiberoptic bronchoscopic techniques, protected specimen brushing (PSB) and bronchoalveolar lavage (BAL), have been studied extensively and have shown promising results.

A landmark animal study of the accuracy of various techniques in diagnosing pneumonia was reported by Johanson and associates.[3] These authors evaluated the sensitivity and specificity of BAL, PSB, lung aspirates, and cultures of lung homogenate in 35 baboons that were mechanically ventilated for at least 1 week. In this study, quantitative cultures of BAL fluid provided the best reflection of the lung's bacterial burden. Large, prospective, multicenter trials using standardized techniques have not been reported, but a growing number of small series have evaluated the practical application of PSB and BAL with quantitative cultures in diagnosing pneumonia in mechanically ventilated patients. Fagon and coworkers studied the utility of PSB with quantitative cultures in 147 mechanically ventilated patients and found a true positive diagnostic accuracy of 75%, an uncertain diagnosis in 15%, and a false-positive diagnostic rate of only 11%.[20] Remarkably, a quantitative culture of less than 10^3 CFUs accurately excluded the diagnosis of pneumonia in 102 patients. The type of PSB catheter used does not appear to be an essential factor because there is no difference in diagnostic accuracy between double- and single-lumen plugged catheters.[21]

Chastre and colleagues directly compared PSB to BAL in 21 mechanically ventilated patients who had new pulmonary infiltrates and purulent tracheal secretions.[22] Quantitative cultures from PSB were greater than 10^3 CFUs in 5 of 5 patients with subsequently confirmed pneumonia but negative in 13 of 13 patients without bacterial pneumonia. There was no diagnostic value to BAL total and differential cell counts, but the presence of intracellular bacteria in more than 25% of the BAL cells identified all 5 patients with pneumonia and excluded those 13 patients without pneumonia. Guerra and Baughman obtained BAL for quantitative bacterial culture in 30 ventilated patients with suspected pneumonia and 24 in whom BAL was performed for other reasons.[23] With a criterion of 10^4 CFUs, 89% of pneumonia patients were identified, but none of the nonpneumonia patients had a positive BAL quantitative culture. Future studies are necessary to make specific recommendations regarding diagnostic techniques for nosocomial pneumonia.

THE AIRWAY DEFENSE BARRIER

Passive Upper Airway Mechanisms

Bacteria reach the lung by one of four routes: inhalation of infectious droplets, hematogenous seeding from distant sites of infection, direct contiguous spread, and aspiration of contaminated secretions from a colonized upper airway. The conducting airways are ideally designed to repel and remove bacteria. In mechanically ventilated patients, bacteria typically penetrate the lung by either aspiration of infected material or inhalation of contaminated aerosolized droplets. Pneumonia results when a sufficient number of virulent organisms take hold in a permissive microenvironment.

In hospitalized patients, the normal pharyngeal bacterial flora seen in healthy individuals is gradually replaced by potentially pathologic gram-negative bacteria. Infected liquids in the upper airway may be aerosolized as the result of positive-pressure ventilation. Aerosolized particles are deposited in the lung by either inertial impaction at airway branching points or sedimentation. The point of deposition in the lung depends on the aerodynamic size and velocity of the droplet particles. The initial high linear velocity of inspired air slows as air movement progresses toward the alveoli, where the gas is dispersed over a much greater total cross-sectional area. In the very small bronchi and alveoli, air movement approaches that which would result from random brownian movement alone. Particles with an average aerodynamic size of greater than 10 μm are deposited on the sticky surfaces of the nasal turbinate and nasopharynx, where there is a bend in the air stream. Mid-range particle sizes, 5 to 10 μm, are deposited in the medium to large airways, where they can be actively removed by mucociliary transport. Smaller particles, 0.5 to 2 μm, reach the bronchiolar and alveolar surfaces, where they are deposited by inertial impaction at sites of small-airway bifurcation. Very small particles, less than 0.2 μm, may be inhaled and exhaled without being deposited in the distal lung. Endotracheal intubation and mechanical ventilation alter particle deposition by allowing all sizes of droplets to have unimpeded access to the distal lung.

Reflexes

Passive upper airway defense is augmented by the sneeze and cough reflexes. Sneezing is a forceful, explosive exhalation triggered by receptors in the nose and nasopharynx. Coughing is a sudden and forceful expulsion of air from the lungs triggered by stimulation of the epipharynx, larynx, and tracheobronchial tree. These reflexes actively clear foreign particles from the nose, pharynx, and large airways. These reflexes also require an intact glottic function so that intrathoracic positive pressure can be generated and suddenly released. Endotracheal intubation blocks an effectual cough reflex by decreasing the peak attainable intrathoracic pressure. Further, depressed central nervous system function as a result of disease and/or sedation may decrease the cough and sneezing reflex.

Mechanical Lower Airway Mechanisms

Another active airway defense mechanism for the clearance of inhaled particles is the mucociliary escalator. This system consists of an overlying mucous layer that is propelled toward the glottis by an underlying pseudo-stratified ciliated epithelial network. The mucus is secreted by submucosal glands and goblet cells of the upper and lower airways. Mucus is a complex substance composed of electrolytes, amino acids, lipids, carbohydrates, nucleic acids, mucin, immunoglobulin, enzymes, and albumin. These molecules interact to determine the rheologic (flow viscosity) properties of mucus. The rheologic properties of the overlying mucus are important in that they influence the underlying ciliary movement of the epithelial cells that line the airways down to the distal bronchioles. Ciliary movement directs overlying mucus-containing particles toward the pharynx, where they can be swallowed or expectorated. Cilia beat at a frequency of 1000 to 1500 cycles per minute, propelling the overlying mucus at progressively increasing rates up the airways. The linear velocity of mucus transport increases from the distal to the proximal airways. As a result, particles that are deposited in the tracheal and major bronchi can be removed by mucociliary transportation in 30 to 60 minutes, whereas those particles deposited more deeply can be potentially cleared in 1 to 24 hours.

Immunologic Lower Airway Mechanisms

BAL fluid from normal individuals contains proteins that are derived from active or passive transport from the vascular space and from local secretion by airway or alveolar tissue. This protein fraction is composed of approximately 45% albumin and 17% immunoglobulins (Ig).[24] The Ig fraction is composed of approximately 55% IgG, 44% IgA, and 1% IgM. The role of airspace Ig in lung defense is not fully defined. IgG appears to be the principal opsonic antibody in BAL fluid. IgA is less abundant and has much less opsonic activity than IgG. IgM occurs in minimal amounts and probably does not play an important role in homeostasis. Other molecules contained in epithelial lining fluid, including complement components, may have additional opsonic activity. Opsonin-coated bacteria are more easily phagocytized by macrophages.

THE IMPACT OF MECHANICAL VENTILATION ON AIRWAY COLONIZATION AND THE DEVELOPMENT OF NOSOCOMIAL PNEUMONIA

Colonization of the Oropharynx

Bacteria that enter the respiratory tract encounter an elaborate and effective host defense system. The location of possible bacterial infections of the respiratory tract traces the passage of air from the environment to alveoli; the most serious infections occur in the distal lung. Recent studies indicate that bacterial colonization of the oropharynx routinely precedes the occurrence of lower respiratory tract infections. The incidence of oropharyngeal colonization appears to be related to the severity and duration of illness. Oropharyngeal colonization is defined as the persistence of a potential pathogen above the vocal cords. Lower respiratory tract colonization is the presence of any bacteria in the normally sterile environment between the vocal cords and terminal bronchi. Bacterial colonization represents an equilibrium state in which pulmonary host defense is adequate to prevent bacterial invasion but insufficient to eradicate the bacteria completely. Colonization exists without obvious adverse effects to the host. In contrast, bacterial infection is associated with both tissue invasion and a prominent host reaction.

Endotracheal intubation bypasses all host defense mechanisms proximal to the vocal cords by disarming the epiglottis, disrupting the cough reflex, and interrupting mucociliary escalation and thus predisposes to bacterial colonization and subsequent infection. In intubated patients, bacteria can potentially colonize the lower airways directly without first colonizing the upper airway. Positive-pressure ventilation rhythmically insufflates the lungs with warm, moist air, which can become contaminated and lead to the deposition of bacteria directly into the alveoli. In spite of meticulous sterile technique and frequent circuit changes, the condensate that collects in dependent portions of ventilator tubing can become contaminated. If condensate is inadvertently dumped into the airway, pneumonia can follow. The inflated cuff of an endotracheal tube is an effective physical barrier to mucociliary transport. The chronic irritating effects of an endotracheal tube cuff may result in pressure necrosis of the tracheal mucosa, which can serve as a nidus for a bacterial foothold that can be disseminated distally.

Chronic inflammation and infection may also result in various amounts of mucopurulent secretions with altered rheologic properties, which may contribute to ciliostasis stasis and depressed mucociliary function. Patients are dependent on caregivers for removal of secretions from their airways, yet frequent high negative-pressure endotracheal suctioning can result in ulceration of the epithelial surfaces and may play a role in the development of bacterial colonization. Deppe and colleagues reported a twofold increase in the incidence of tracheal colonization (but not pneumonia or mortality) when a closed in-line suction devise was used compared with conventional single-use suction catheter (67 versus 39%).[8] Although endotracheal intubation prevents massive aspiration, it may facilitate microaspiration of infected upper airway secretions. A stagnant column of potentially infected secretions collects between the low-pressure endotracheal cuff and the larynx. This pool of material may gradually leak into the trachea and bronchi, where positive-pressure ventilation may propel these secretions distally. This idea is supported by the observation that specially designed endotracheal tube cuffs that allow removal of the stagnant subglottic pool of secretions have been shown to reduce the incidence of lower respiratory tract colonization and nosocomial pneumonia.[25]

Bacterial Factors That Predispose to Colonization

Both bacterial and host factors predispose to colonization and pulmonary infections. Bacterial factors are related to the size of the inoculum and virulence of the organism, whereas host factors generally relate to the degree of immunity impairments. Various bacteria have a spectrum of invasive capacity and subsequent infectivity. *P. aeruginosa* accounts for 10% to 15% of all nosocomial pneumonia[11] and is notoriously virulent, with a reported overall mortality of established infections ranging from 70% to 90%.[4, 5] The reported incidence of *Pseudomonas* pneumonia is at least 30% for mechanically ventilated patients,[4] which is attributed to increased severity of illness and airway instrumentation. Approximately 40% of patients who are colonized with *Pseudomonas* will ultimately acquire a nosocomial infection.[5] *Pseudomonas* has a great propensity to bind to damaged respiratory epithelial surfaces. Silver and associates reported that *Pseudomonas* pneumonia was seen more often in chronically ventilated patients in whom the increased morbidity and mortality were not influenced by the adequacy or duration of antibiotic treatment.[5] Fick showed altered lower airway humoral immunity to *Pseudomonas,* which results in inadequate formation of opsonins and phagocytic clearance.[26] Altered phagocytic clearance may predispose to bacterial infection. Martin and coauthors reported that a deficiency in membrane receptors existed on neutrophils and monocytes recovered from 32 ICU patients with nosocomial pneumonia.[27] Other factors that influence the adherence of gram-negative bacteria to the bronchial epithelium include cellular variables, bacterial surface characteristics and exoproducts, and the microenvironmental conditions of the airway surface. Airway secretions contain adhesion blocking factors, such as secretory IgA and fibronectin, which prevent gram-negative organisms from attaching to bronchial mucosa. Endotracheal intubation can result in an enhanced capacity of tracheobronchial cells to bind gram-negative species, an effect that favors airway colonization and subsequent pneumonia. Minor injury to the airway can create potential sites for adherence of bacteria by causing sloughing of the pseudo-stratified ciliated epithelial cells with disruption of the mucociliary conduction system and by exposing the basement membrane of the bronchi and creating bacterial binding sites.

Host Factors That Predispose to Colonization

The rate of colonizations with gram-negative species appears to parallel the extent and duration of systemic illness. Although only 6% of healthy hospitalized individuals are colonized by gram-negative organisms, this increases to 70% to 80% in ICU patients. In one study, more than 80% of bacterial pneumonia cases were preceded by gram-negative upper airway colonization. The incidence of colonization of the oropharynx is related to underlying disease, nutritional status, prior exposure to antibiotic therapy, endotracheal and gastric intubation, and gastric colonization. Other factors that influence the incidence of bacterial colonization include advanced age, altered consciousness, hemodynamic instability, presence of lung disease, and incidence of renal failure.

Role of Gastric Colonization in the Development of Nosocomial Pneumonia

The gastrointestinal tract may serve as a reservoir for bacteria, and retrograde pharyngeal colonization by organisms from the stomach has recently been recognized as an important contributor to the pathogenesis of nosocomial pneumonia. The normally low pH of the stomach contents provides an effective barrier to bacterial colonization. When gastric acid is absent, the risk of infection and gastric colonization is increased. Treatments with histamine$_2$ (H_2) blockers, which decrease hydrochloric acid secretion by parietal cells, appear to promote gram-negative bacterial colonization of the upper gastrointestinal tract and increase the incidence of nosocomial pulmonary infections. Gastric organisms can be transmitted to the airway and result in tracheal colonization and nosocomial pneumonia. Migration of bacteria from the stomach to the trachea probably involves prior colonization of the oropharynx and subsequent pulmonary aspiration. Several factors may facilitate this process, including the presence of nasogastric tube, method of nutrient delivery, patient position, and gastric motility.

The gastropulmonary hypothesis has been indirectly supported by a large number of small clinical studies that show that the incidence of gram-negative pneumonia is decreased in patients treated with sucralfate compared with H_2 blocking drugs. Sucralfate is thought to have a cytoprotective effect on the gastric mucosa, which prevents stress ulceration while maintaining the normal low pH gastric environment. Driks and associates first reported that agents that elevate gastric pH were associated with an increased incidence of oropharyngeal and tracheal colonization.[28] In this study, the incidence of nosocomial pneumonia was not significantly increased in patients given antacids and H_2 blockers but sparked a controversy that has spawned a great number of small studies. Tryba and Heyland studied the available literature and concluded that sucralfate, an agent that is effective in preventing stress gastric bleeding without raising the pH, minimized the risk of nosocomial pneumonia in long-term ventilated patients.[29–31] Some investigators suggested that continuous nasogastric tube feeding may provide gram-negative bacterial prophylaxis as a beneficial side effect of nutritional management. Although the incidence of stress ulceration appears to be decreased in patients given tube feedings, the rate of nosocomial infections is not reduced.[32] Patients fed by jejunal tube have been shown to have a lower rate of pneumonia than those fed by continuous gastric tube infusion.[33]

Fiddian-Green and Baker suggested that ischemic gastrointestinal mucosal injury with translocation of enteric bacteria might also be important in the pathogenesis of nosocomial pneumonia.[34] This is not a widely accepted mechanism of infection but may result in the release of endotoxin directly into the bloodstream and generate a sepsislike picture. Nevertheless, selective decontamination of the gastrointestinal tract by administering nonabsorbable antibiotics has been advocated as an intervention that decreases the incidence of nosocomial pneumonia,[35] but conclusive evidence of efficacy is lacking.

OTHER RISK FACTORS FOR THE DEVELOPMENT OF NOSOCOMIAL PNEUMONIA

The triad of endotracheal intubation, altered mental status, and presence of a nasogastric tube is associated with the highest incidence of nosocomial pneumonia.[11] Patients undergoing upper abdominal or thoracic surgery are at increased risk for the development of nosocomial pneumonia,[10, 12, 13] although this may be a study selection bias. The elderly are particularly at risk for pneumonia,[10–12] especially if they are unable to defend their airway from oropharyngeal secretions, have deteriorating health, and are treated with a nasogastric tube.[12] Hanson and coauthors reported a twofold increase in the incidence of pneumonia in patients older than 65 years compared with a similar group of patients aged 25 to 50 years.[36] In this study, the older patients had more than twice the number of identifiable risk factors, with a significant predictive relationship found for a low serum albumin, diagnosis of neuromuscular disease, and endotracheal intubation. Celis and colleagues reported that the typical patient who dies with a nosocomial pneumonia is older than 60 years, is being mechanically supported for respiratory failure, has bilateral radiographic infiltrates, and has been on an "inappropriate antibiotic regimen."[10] Fagon and colleagues found that prior antibiotic therapy appears to increase the risk of pneumonia caused by *P. aeruginosa*, *Acinetobacter*, and methicillin-resistant *Staphylococcus*.[4] Interestingly, some antibiotics have been shown to paradoxically impair host immunity. For example, Nelson and associates demonstrated a dose-related suppression of antibacterial defenses by erythromycin administration in mice.[37] These observations underscore the necessity for selective and judicious antibiotic usage in critically ill patients. Other drugs may have adverse side effects on pulmonary host defense. For example, Eberhardt and colleagues reported a dose-related increase in the rate of pneumonia in patients receiving barbiturates for brain edema.[38]

A wide variety of systemic illnesses predispose to pulmonary infections by their association with depressed pulmonary host defense. These diseases include conditions in which host defense is abnormal, such as malnutrition, cancer, renal failure, and cirrhosis of the liver. Several studies indicated that the mortality from nosocomial pneumonia is related to nutritional status.[9] Gorse and coworkers retrospectively compared 45 patients with nosocomial infections with 45 matched control patients.[39] These authors found a significant relationship between various nutritional parameters and the development of pneumonia, urinary tract infections, and bacteremia. Skerrett and others detected an abnormality in the release of arachidonic acid metabolites by AM recovered from protein-starved rats.[40] These two studies, taken together, indicate that malnutrition is associated with a predilection to infection that is possibly caused by alteration in macrophage function. A prospective study is expected to show that the frequency of nosocomial infections can be minimized by attention to nutritional status of critically ill patients.

Patients with chronic bronchitis, bronchiectasis, and cystic fibrosis may be predisposed to certain types of pulmonary infections. Other diseases, such as congestive heart failure and adult respiratory distress syndrome (ARDS), may promote infections by their association with abnormal lung areas as a result of alveolar edema, hemorrhage, and atelectasis. Alcoholics are prone to aspiration because of the attendant alterations of mental status that are associated with their addiction. A similar propensity for aspiration exists in patients who have attempted suicide by ingesting sedatives/hypnotics. Alcoholics appear to be more prone to experiencing community-acquired gram-negative infections such as *Klebsiella* pneumonia. Dorio and Foreman reported that ethanol inhibits AM production of superoxide, which could alter bactericidal capacity and could explain the increased sensitivity of alcoholics to pneumonia.[41] A summary of risk factors for the development of nosocomial pneumonia is provided in Table 96–3.

RESIDENT PHAGOCYTIC DEFENSE MECHANISMS

The cellular defense mechanism becomes the first effective line of defense when the adequacy of the physical defense mechanism is breached by the supportive appliances used in the management of critically ill patients. Small to medium-sized droplets, which may contain bacteria, routinely reach the bronchioles and alveoli, where they may result in infection. The AM is the resident phagocyte that has the capacity to eradicate invading bacteria by three fundamental processes: directional locomotion, phagocytosis, and generation of reactive oxygen species (ROS) with associated bactericidal activity.[42, 43]

AMs, like other tissue macrophages, are primarily derived from progenitors in the bone marrow. The direct precursor to the AM appears to be an interstitial cell derived from circulating monocytes. In the lung, the monocyte develops the functional and metabolic features characteristic of AMs. The AM varies from 15 to 45 μm in diameter and commonly has a nuclear-cytoplasmic ratio of about 1:4. Nucleoli are frequently visible, and many cells are multinucleated. Occasionally, the cells appear to have "foamy" cytoplasm, although the significance of this finding is not clear. AMs contain cytoplasmic lysosomes that are rich in enzymes, including acid phosphatase, cathepsin, lysozyme, β-glucuronidase, and β-galactosidase. These hydrolytic enzymes can be transferred to phagocytic vesicles during phagocytosis.

AMs contain contractile proteins that can be activated and result in directed chemotactic movement into areas of infection or inflammation. The chemotactic gradients that drive AM movement are incompletely characterized, but a macrophage chemotactic protein-1 (MCP-1) has been described.[44] MCP-1, also known as monocyte chemotactic and activating factor, is produced by a wide variety of cell types such as monocytes/macrophages, fibroblasts, B lymphocytes, endothelial cells, and smooth-muscle cells. The human MCP-1 complementary deoxyribonucleic acid encodes for a 99–amino acid residue precursor protein that is cleaved during cellular secretion to generate the 76–amino acid residue mature protein. Peripheral blood monocytes have a specific cell-surface receptor for MCP-1 that initiates the chemotactic process, contributing to the movement of monocytes into the lung interstitium, where they differentiate into tissue macrophages. Apart from its chemotactic activity on monocytes, MCP-1 can stimulate monocytes to release superoxide anions, lysosomal enzymes, and inflammatory cytokines. The biologic role played by MCP-1 in host defense is not yet completely understood but is likely to be important.

AMs phagocytize any particles, including bacteria, that reach the alveoli and terminal bronchi. Phagocytosis is an energy-dependent process that involves particle recognition, adhesion of the particle to the cytoplasmic membrane, assembly of pseudopodia, particle engulfment, and fusion of the pseudopodia to form an intracellular phagocytic vacuole.[45] Opsonization of bacteria appears to be required for maximal phagocytosis. Subsequent to phagocytosis, the phagocytic vacuole fuses with a lysosome to form a phagolysosome, which is a sequestered compartment in which bacterial killing can occur. When activated by phagocytosis and other stimuli, AMs generate hydrogen peroxide, hydroxyl radicals, and oxygen radicals. These molecules are derived from atmospheric oxygen and are collectively referred to as ROS. In conjunction with lysosomal hydrolytic and proteolytic enzymes, ROS results in bactericidal activity within the phagocytic vacuole that is sufficient to kill most bacteria.[46]

TABLE 96–3. Risk Factors for the Development of Nosocomial Pneumonia

Endotracheal intubation
Altered consciousness or coma
Nasogastric tube
Gram-negative pharyngeal colonization
Advanced age
Poor nutrition
Witnessed aspiration
Treatment with antacids/histamine$_2$ blockers
Upper abdominal or thoracic surgery
Multiple trauma
Barbiturate treatment

RECRUITED PHAGOCYTIC DEFENSE MECHANISM

Although AMs are formidable antibacterial effector cells, in certain infectious diseases they manifest insufficient bactericidal activity to control the exponential growth of bacteria.[46, 46a] In these situations, AMs have been implicated as a source of chemotactic cytokines (chemokines), which play a central role in the regulation of neutrophilic lung inflammation (NLI).[47, 48] Neutrophils appear to be required for effective clearance of gram-negative organisms, and effective pulmonary host defense is at least partially dependent on mechanisms involved in mounting an acute neutrophilic inflammatory reaction.[49, 50] This hypothesis has been supported by many in vitro studies including the observation that the phagocytic activity of neutrophils for *P. aeruginosa* is higher than that of AMs.[49]

Chemokines direct the movement of blood neutrophils into the lungs, where they assist in eradication of the bacterial infection. IL-8 is the best described chemotactic protein for neutrophils.[44] Rodriguez and colleagues detected immunoreactive IL-8 in the bronchial secretions of 105 of 151 mechanically ventilated patients within 36 hours of admission.[51] The presence of IL-8 was associated with a 66% incidence of nosocomial pneumonia and greater pulmonary dysfunction,[51] indicating a possible involvement of IL-8 in the pathogenesis of pneumonia. IL-8 was purified and cloned in 1988, and since this time a great deal of information has accumulated regarding its synthesis, regulation, and role in neutrophilic inflammation.[52] IL-8 is synthesized as a 99–amino acid precursor and secreted as a 79–amino acid mature molecule with a molecular weight of 8383 ds. This protein probably undergoes extracellular processing to yield a 72–amino acid variant. IL-8 is a heparin binding protein, resistant to heat, pH extremes, and some proteases, which may account for its persistence in inflamed tissues. X-ray crystallography indicates that IL-8 is prone to dimerization. IL-8 has three unique interactions with peripheral blood neutrophils that result in chemotactic movement, exocytosis of granular enzymes, and induction of respiratory burst activity with generation of ROS.

Many cell types can be stimulated in vitro to express IL-8 messenger ribonucleic acid (mRNA) and release biologically active IL-8.[47] Peripheral blood monocytes and AMs can be stimulated with endotoxin or by phagocytosis to release IL-8. Because the AMs can move into areas of infection, their role may be to imitate and localize inflammation. Mesenchymal cells such as fibroblasts and smooth-muscle cells are also a source of IL-8. These matrix cells may increase inflammation when stimulated by tumor necrosis factor (TNF) or IL-1. Recently, neutrophils have been shown to be a potential source of IL-8. It is possible that IL-8 secreted by neutrophils in an area of inflammation may serve to amplify, intensify, or localize the inflammatory process.[53] Paradoxically, endothelial cells may secrete IL-8 into the circulation, where it may prevent movement of neutrophils into the airspace and serve a regulatory anti-inflammatory role.[54] The potentially important role of IL-8 in regulating NLI is depicted in Figure 96–1.

CHEMOKINE SUPERGENE FAMILY

IL-8 and MCP-1 belong to the same cytokine supergene family that is referred to as the *intercrine supergene family*.[55] All intercrines have four conserved cysteine residues forming two disulfide bridges, which are important for tertiary structure and function. IL-8 is the prototypic member of the intercrine α subfamily, where the first two cysteines are separated by a single amino acid (CXC). MCP-1 is the prototypic member of the intercrine β subfamily, where the first two cysteines are adjacent (C-C). Members of both intercrine subfamilies have pleotrophic biologic activities, but the subfamily distinction is associated with different types of target cells. The α subfamily members are characteristically potent chemoattractants for neutrophils, whereas β subfamily members exhibit relatively selective chemotactic activity for monocytes. The description of the intercrine supergene family is rapidly expanding. For example, other related molecules have been described with potent chemotactic properties for neutrophils including neutrophil-activating peptide-2 (NAP-2), melanoma growth stimulatory activity protein/gro (MGSA/gro), and epithelial cell–derived peptide (ENA-78).

Chemotaxis is the directional movement of cells toward a chemical concentration gradient. This biologic response is mediated by specific cell-surface receptors. Two IL-8 receptors (IL-8R) have been identified that are referred to as types I and II. Type I IL-8R has a high affinity for IL-8 and other intercrine family members, including NAP-2 and MGSA, whereas the type II IL-8R binds only IL-8. This difference may have a regulatory function that has not yet been defined. In general, cytokine receptors have an extracellular portion that contains a specific binding domain for a particular cytokine, a transmembrane domain that orients and anchors the receptor to the cell surface, and an intracellular domain that is responsible for initiating signal transduction or the generation of second messengers. Many cytokine receptors are susceptible to proteolytic cleavage of the extracellular binding domain, which can function as a circulating inhibitor by preventing interactions between cytokine- and membrane-anchored receptors. Types I and II IL-8R differ from typical cytokine receptors by having a serpiginous structure containing seven transmembrane domains. Circu-

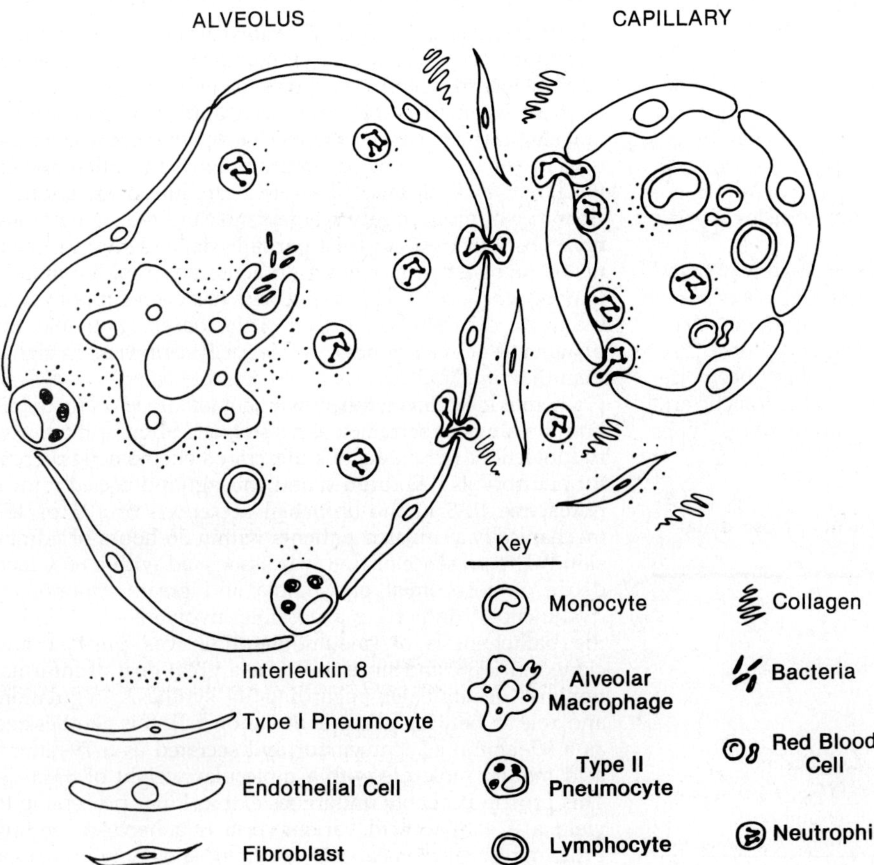

Figure 96–1. The potentially important role of IL-8 in regulating neutrophilic lung inflammation. Multiple cell types, including the alveolar macrophage, can produce IL-8 when stimulated with endotoxin, tumor necrosis factor, or IL-1. When a concentration gradient is established, neutrophils attach to the endothelial surface of pulmonary capillaries and migrate through the interstitium and into alveoli.

lating receptors for IL-8 that have binding capacity have not been described and are unlikely because of this complex structure. Chemotactic movement results when IL-8 binds to the IL-8R and initiates the activation of cytoplasmic contractile proteins, which are associated with a locomoid-shape change and oscillatory assembly/disassembly of actin fibers. This results in protrusion and retraction of lamellipodia, which cause cell movement toward a concentration gradient of IL-8. This process is shown schematically in Figure 96–2.

Cytokine Network Theory

There is increasing evidence that cytokines play a major role in the response to infection.[56] The development of lung inflammation is thought to involve a series of events that are controlled by a variety of mediators. The process of inflammation appears to be regulated by the release of counterbalanced cytokines, which are involved in the initiation and resolution of inflammation. The cytokine network theory is based on the idea that cytokines are released in a coordinated manner in which the production of one cytokine is dependent on the synthesis of another. This dynamic process may be initiated by endotoxemia or other bacterial products. Endotoxemia is associated with the appearance of TNF, IL-1, and IL-6 in the peripheral circulation.[57] TNF and IL-1 are potent stimuli for the release of IL-8 by a variety of cell types. The production of IL-8 by different cell types may be a mechanism that regulates inflammation because the stimulus specificity and regulatory sequences may differ between cell types. The cell of origin may also contribute to the sequestration or compartmentalization of inflammatory process. This cascade mechanism may allow for precise regulation of inflammation by incorporating a series of checks and balances that are susceptible to regulation at a number of levels. Paradoxically, the synthesis and release of cytokines can lead to an explosive inflammatory response that may be difficult to control.

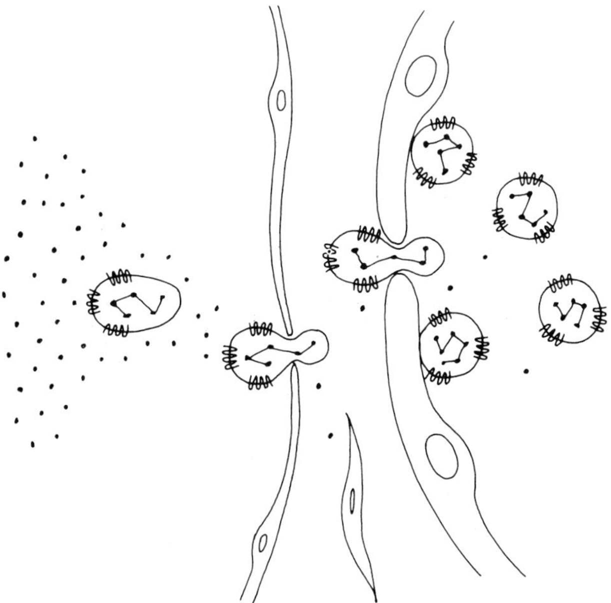

Figure 96–2. The process of chemotaxis. Intravascular neutrophils *(left)* have an even distribution of surface receptors for IL-8. When IL-8 binds to these receptors, the neutrophil develops a locomoid morphology and migrates toward a positive concentration gradient of IL-8 in the alveolus *(right)*. See Figure 96–1 for a key to the cell types.

Noninfectious Inflammatory Lung Disease

Although the process of inflammation is a fundamental component of pulmonary host defense, it also plays a role in the pathogenesis of a wide variety of pulmonary disorders. A partial list of noninfectious pulmonary disorders that might present with acute respiratory failure and mimic infection are included in Table 96–4. It is difficult to describe each of these disorders in sufficient detail within the confines of this chapter. One of these disorders, IPF, has been best studied and is the focus of the final portion of this chapter.

Clinical Aspects of Idiopathic Pulmonary Fibrosis

IPF, also known as usual interstitial fibrosis and cryptogenic fibrosing alveolitis, is an interstitial lung disease of uncertain cause with an estimated prevalence of 5 per 100,000 population.[58] Some studies have suggested a relationship between the development of IPF and cigarette smoking,[59] although no formal case-control studies have been reported. Typically, IPF occurs in the fifth decade of life with a slight male predominance. Patients usually present with increasing dyspnea on exertion, which typically evolves over years but the course is variable. The original reports of IPF by Hamman and Rich described a group of patients with a rapidly progressive disease that was fatal within a few months.[60] More recently, Ashbaugh and Maier reported a group of patients with IPF who presented with acute respiratory failure and were initially thought to have an ARDS-like syndrome.[61] Olson and colleagues suggested that this type of IPF be renamed acute interstitial pneumonia to emphasize the fulminant clinical course.[62]

The reported mean length of survival is 3 to 5 years, but the course is quite variable. Because of the insidious nature of this disease, it is not uncommon for patients to present with advanced conditions. Some patients have a rapidly deteriorating course and may present with severe hypoxemia. Most patients experience episodes of increased dyspnea, decreased exercise capacity, worsened hypoxemia, or other decline in functional level during the course of their illness. Panos and associates examined the reported causes of death in 326 patients with IPF.[63] The leading causes of death were progressive respiratory failure (39%), heart failure (14%), bronchogenic carcinoma (10%), and ischemic heart disease (10%).

The most prevalent physical finding of IPF is symmetric, coarse, Velcro-sounding crackles heard best over the bases of the lungs. Clubbing is frequently present, and advanced disease may be associated with findings of right ventricular failure. Pulmonary functions are consistent with restrictive lung disease with reduced static lung volume and diffusion capacity. A common finding is the presence of a widened alveolar-arterial gradient with stress or exercise. Severe hy-

TABLE 96–4. Noninfectious Inflammatory Lung Disorders That Might Present with Acute Respiratory Failure

Idiopathic pulmonary fibrosis
Sarcoid alveolitis
Goodpasture's syndrome
Hypersensitivity pneumonitis
Acute eosinophilic pneumonia
Systemic lupus erythematosus
Adult respiratory distress syndrome

poxemia can result from the physiologic stress of an extrapulmonary infection and may precipitate clinical deterioration. Resting hypoxemia, when present, is usually refractory to oxygen therapy. Hypercapnia develops late in the course and usually is associated with a rapid clinical decline and poor prognosis. The radiologic features of IPF are not diagnostic but show progressive interstitial infiltrates with volume loss, which can be confused with features of congestive heart failure. The most characteristic radiologic feature of IPF is that of small, irregular shadows predominantly in the bases of the lung. End-stage disease is associated with a honeycomb radiographic pattern. High-resolution computed tomography enhances the ability to detect early disease but has not been evaluated prospectively.[64, 65]

Pathophysiology of Idiopathic Pulmonary Fibrosis

Because of sampling errors and the absence of unique diagnostic features, an open lung biopsy is the preferred diagnostic approach.[66, 67] The histopathologic features of IPF are classified by the relative degrees of inflammation and fibrosis. Early-stage disease is thought to be characterized by intra-alveolar and interstitial inflammation and minimal fibrosis, whereas late-stage disease characteristically has severe fibrosis and little inflammation. The sequence of inflammation progressing to fibrosis is supported by the reports of Carrington and colleagues, who noted that a cellular inflammatory pattern on open lung biopsy was associated with a mean survival of 12.2 years, whereas a fibrotic pattern was associated with a mean survival of only 5.6 years.[68] Typically, IPF has a heterogenous histologic distribution with varying degrees of inflammation and fibrosis existing at different locations in the same individual. The inflammatory component of IPF involves accumulations of a variety of inflammatory cell types including neutrophils, eosinophils, lymphocytes, and plasma cells. Increased numbers of fibroblasts are seen with a parallel increase in collagen matrix. An interesting feature is the presence of cells referred to as myofibroblasts because of phenotypic similarities to smooth-muscle cells and fibroblasts. The myofibroblast has well-formed actin-filament bundles that might have an active contractile role in altering lung compliance and/or remodeling of the lung.[69]

BAL has been used to evaluate IPF patients. The cellular constituents usually reveal increased numbers of neutrophils, eosinophils, and lymphocytes.[59, 70, 71] Increased BAL eosinophil counts correlate with worse disease[71] and are predictive of future deterioration.[70] Abnormalities have also been identified in the BAL fluid including alteration in surfactant protein A,[72] changes in lipid profile, and increased amounts of N-terminal type III procollagen peptides.[73] BAL neutrophil counts are uniformly increased in BAL from IPF patients, yet the intensity of neutrophilic inflammation does not clearly correlate with histopathologic changes or future response to treatment.[70] The link between inflammation and fibrosis has not been fully identified, but activated AMs and PMNs appear to play a cardinal role in the pathogenesis of IPF.

A currently prevailing hypothesis is that neutrophils are attracted to the lung by chemotactic gradients, where they potentiate the production of ROS and release tissue-damaging proteases. A number of investigators have studied AM function in IPF patients, including the evaluation of bactericidal capacity[74] and the release of ROS.[75] AMs appear to have a role in the generation of a neutrophil chemotactic gradient. Three studies indicated that BAL fluid contains increased concentrations of IL-8 and AMs from IPF patients have increased expression of IL-8 mRNA.[76–78] Other cytokines may also play a role in the pathogenesis of IPF. For example, MCP-1 may have a role in attracting or activating peripheral blood monocytes. Epithelial cells from IPF patients have been shown to have an increased expression of MCP-1 mRNA by in situ hybridization and immunohistochemical staining of MCP-1.[79] Activated AMs are also a potential source of growth factors that may play a role in stimulating fibroblast proliferation and collagen production.

Treatment of Idiopathic Pulmonary Fibrosis

A number of drugs have been used in an attempt to reverse the inflammatory component of IPF, including corticosteroid, cyclophosphamide, and azathioprine. Johnson and colleagues reported a randomized controlled study of high-dose prednisolone versus combined cyclophosphamide/low-dose prednisolone.[80] Overall, there was little difference in these treatments, and only 12 of 43 patients initially improved. Baughman and Lower evaluated the efficacy of intermittent, intravenous cyclophosphamide in an uncontrolled study.[81] In this study, 9 of 33 patients had higher BAL neutrophil counts and died within 6 months of diagnosis. Those who survived more than 6 months had a small improvement in measured vital capacity. O'Donnell and coworkers reported, in a small series, that cyclophosphamide, but not prednisone, was effective in reducing BAL neutrophil counts but not in improving survival.[82] Raghu and colleagues evaluated the effects of prednisone and placebo versus azathioprine and low-dose prednisone in a blinded, randomized, controlled trial of 27 patients with newly diagnosed IPF.[83] Their data suggested an advantage to combination treatment but were inconclusive. Lung transplantation is the best current hope for prolonged survival after the diagnosis of IPF is established. Egan and associates reported that 20% of referrals for lung transplantation have a primary diagnosis of IPF.[84]

References

1. Potgieter PD, Hammond JM: Etiology and diagnosis of pneumonia requiring ICU admission. Chest 1992; 10:199.
2. Rello J, Quintana E, Ausina V, et al: Incidence, etiology and outcome of nosocomial pneumonia in mechanically ventilated patients. Chest 1991; 100:439.
3. Johanson WG, Seidenfield JJ, Gomez P, et al: Bacteriologic diagnosis of nosocomial pneumonia following prolonged mechanical ventilation. Am Rev Respir Dis 1988; 137:259.
4. Fagon JY, Chastre J, Domart Y, et al: Nosocomial pneumonia in patients receiving continuous mechanical ventilation: Prospective analysis of 52 episodes with use of a protected specimen brush and quantitative culture techniques. Am Rev Respir Dis 1989; 139:877.
5. Silver DR, Cohen IL, Weinberg PF: Recurrent *Pseudomonas aeruginosa* pneumonia in an intensive care unit. Chest 1992; 101:194.
6. Rello J, Ausina V, Castella J, et al: Nosocomial respiratory tract infections in multiple trauma patients: Influence of level of consciousness with implication for therapy. Chest 1992; 102:525.
7. Rello J, Quintana E, Ausina V, et al: Risk factors for *Staphylococcus aureus* nosocomial pneumonia in critically ill patients. Am Rev Respir Dis 1990; 142:1320.
8. Deppe SA, Kelly JW, Thoi LL, et al: Incidence of colonization, nosocomial pneumonia, and mortality in critically ill patients using a Trach Care closed suction system versus an open-suction system: Prospective, randomized study. Crit Care Med 1990; 18:1389.
9. Louie M, Dyck B, Parker S, et al: Nosocomial pneumonia in a Canadian tertiary care center: A prospective surveillance study. Infect Control Hosp Epidemiol 1991; 12:356.
10. Celis R, Torres A, Gatell JM, et al: Nosocomial pneumonia: A multivariate analysis of risk and prognosis. Chest 1988; 93:318.
11. Joshi N, Localio AR, Hamory BH: A predictive risk index for nosocomial pneumonia in the intensive care unit. Am J Med 1992; 93:135.

12. Harkness GA, Bentley DW, Roghmann KJ: Risk factors for nosocomial pneumonia in the elderly. Am J Med 1990; 89:457.
13. Nielsen SL, Roder B, Magnussen P, et al: Nosocomial pneumonia in an intensive care unit in a Danish university hospital: Incidence, mortality, and etiology. Scand J Infect Dis 1992; 24:65.
14. Boyce JM, Potter-Bynoe G, Dziobek L, et al: Nosocomial pneumonia in Medicare patients: Hospital costs and reimbursement patterns under the prospective payment system. Arch Intern Med 1991; 151:1109.
15. Marrie TJ, MacDonald S, Clarke K, et al: Nosocomial legionnaires' disease: Lessons from a four year prospective study. Am J Infect Control 1991; 19:79.
16. Mastro TD, Fields BS, Breiman RF, et al: Nosocomial legionnaires' disease and use of medication nebulizers. J Infect Dis 1991; 163(3):667.
17. Roig J, Aguilar X, Ruiz J, et al: Comparative study of legionella pneumophilia and other nosocomial-acquired pneumonia. Chest 1991; 99:344.
18. Salata RA, Lederman MM, Shlaes DM, et al: Diagnosis of nosocomial pneumonia in intubated, intensive care unit patients. Am Rev Respir Dis 1987; 135:426.
19. Winer-Muram HT, Rulsin SA, Ellis JV, et al: Pneumonia and ARDS in patients receiving mechanical ventilation: Diagnostic accuracy of chest radiography. Radiology 1993; 188:479–485.
20. Fagon JY, Chastre J, Hance AJ, et al: Detection of nosocomial lung infection in ventilated patients: Use of a protected specimen brush and quantitative culture techniques in 147 patients. Am Rev Respir Dis 1988; 74:110.
21. Pham LH, Brun-Buisson C, Legrand P, et al: Diagnosis of nosocomial pneumonia in mechanically ventilated patients: Comparison of a plugged telescoping catheter with the protected specimen brush. Am Rev Respir Dis 1991; 143:1055.
22. Chastre J, Fagon JY, Soler P, et al: Diagnosis of nosocomial pneumonia in intubated patients undergoing ventilation: Comparison of the usefulness of bronchoalveolar lavage and the protected specimen brush. Am J Med 1988; 85:499.
23. Guerra LF, Baughman RP: Use of bronchoalveolar lavage to diagnose bacterial pneumonia in mechanically ventilated patients. Crit Care Med 1990; 18:169.
24. Bronchoalveolar Lavage Cooperative Group: Bronchoalveolar lavage constituents in healthy individuals, idiopathic pulmonary fibrosis, and selected comparison groups: 7. Proteins in bronchoalveolar lavage fluid. Am Rev Respir Dis 1990; 141:S183.
25. Mahul P, Auboyer C, Jospe R, et al: Prevention of nosocomial pneumonia in intubated patients: Respective role of mechanical subglottic secretions drainage and stress ulcer prophylaxis. Intensive Care Med 1992; 18:20.
26. Fick RB: Lung humoral response to *Pseudomonas* species. Eur J Clin Microbiol Infect Dis 1989; 8:29.
27. Martin C, Bongrand P, Sauz P, et al: Abnormalities of some phagocyte membrane receptors during nosocomial infections. Crit Care Med 1987; 15:467.
28. Driks MR, Craven DE, Celli BR, et al: Nosocomial pneumonia in intubated patients given sucralfate as compared with antacids or histamine type 2 blockers: The role of gastric colonization. N Engl J Med 1987; 317:1376.
29. Tryba M: Sucralfate versus antacids or H_2-antagonists for stress ulcer prophylaxis: A meta-analysis on efficacy and pneumonia rate. Crit Care Med 1991; 19:942.
30. Tryba M: Risk of acute stress bleeding and nosocomial pneumonia in ventilated intensive care unit patients: Sucralfate versus antacids. Am J Med 1987; 83:117.
31. Heyland D, Mandell LA: Gastric colonization by gram-negative bacilli and nosocomial pneumonia in the intensive care unit patient: Evidence for causation. Chest 1992; 101:187.
32. Pingleton SK, Hinthorn DR, Liu C: Enteral nutrition in patients receiving mechanical ventilation: Multiple sources of tracheal colonization include the stomach. Am J Med 1986; 80:827.
33. Montecalvo MA, Steger KA, Farber HW, et al: Nutritional outcome and pneumonia in critical care patients randomized to gastric versus jejunal tube feedings. Crit Care Med 1992; 20:1377.
34. Fiddian-Green RG, Baker S: Nosocomial pneumonia in the critically ill: Product of aspiration or translocation? Crit Care Med 1991; 19:763.
35. Stoutenbeek CP, van Saene JKF: Prevention of pneumonia by selective decontamination of the digestive tract (SDD). Intensive Care Med 1992; 18:S18.
36. Hanson LC, Weber DJ, Rutala WA: Risk factors for nosocomial pneumonia in the elderly. Am J Med 1992; 92:161.
37. Nelson S, Summer WR, Terry PB, et al: Erythromycin-induced suppression of pulmonary antibacterial defenses: A potential mechanism of superinfection in the lung. Am Rev Respir Dis 1987; 136:1207.
38. Eberhardt KE, Thimm BM, Spring A, et al: Dose-dependent rate of nosocomial pulmonary infection in mechanically ventilated patients with brain edema receiving barbiturates: A prospective case study. Infection 1992; 20:12.
39. Gorse GJ, Messner RL, Stephens ND: Association of malnutrition with nosocomial infection. Infect Control Hosp Epidemiol 1989; 10:194.
40. Skerrett SJ, Henderson WR, Martin TR: Alveolar macrophage function in rats with severe protein calorie malnutrition: Arachidonic acid metabolism, cytokine release, and antimicrobial activity. J Immunol 1990; 144:1052.
41. Dorio RJ, Foreman HJ: Ethanol inhibition of signal transduction in superoxide production by rat alveolar macrophage: A proposed mechanism for ethanol related pneumonia. Ann Clin Lab Sci 1988; 18:190.
42. Hocking WG, Golde DW: The pulmonary alveolar macrophage. N Engl J Med 1979; 301:580, 639.
43. Reynolds HY: Host defense impairments that may lead to respiratory infections. Clin Chest Med 1987; 8:339.
44. Leonard EJ, Yoshimura T: Human monocyte chemoattractant protein-1. Adv Exp Med Biol 1991; 305:47–56.
45. Stossel TP: Phagocytosis. N Engl J Med 1974; 290:717–723, 774, 833.
46. Babior BM: Oxygen-dependent microbial killing by phagocytes. N Engl J Med 1978; 298:659, 721.
46a. Levi MH, Pasculle AW, Dowling JN: Role of the alveolar macrophage in host defense and immunity to *Legionella micdadei* pneumonia in the guinea pig. Microb Pathog 1987; 2:269.
47. Kunkel SL, Standiford T, Kasahara K, et al: Interleukin-8 (IL-8): The major neutrophil chemotactic factor in the lung. Exp Lung Res 1991; 17:17.
48. Strieter RM, Chensue SW, Basha MA, et al: Human alveolar macrophage gene expression of interleukin-8 by tumor necrosis factor-alpha, lipopolysaccharide, and interleukin-1 beta. Am J Respir Cell Mol Biol 1990; 2:321.
49. Ozaki T, Maeda M, Hayashi H, et al: Role of alveolar macrophages in the neutrophil-dependent defense system against *Pseudomonas aeruginosa* infection in the lower respiratory tract: Amplifying effect of muramyl dipeptide analog. Am Rev Respir Dis 1989; 140:1595.
50. Sordelli DO, Djafari M, Garcia VE, et al: Age-dependent pulmonary clearance of *Pseudomonas aeruginosa* in a mouse model: Diminished migration of polymorphonuclear leukocytes to N-formyl-methionyl-leucylphenylalanine. Infect Immun 1992; 60:1724.
51. Rodriguez JL, Miller CG, DeForge LE, et al: Local production of interleukin-8 is associated with nosocomial pneumonia. J Trauma 1992; 33:74.
52. Baggiolini M, Clark-Lewis I: Interleukin-8: A chemotactic and inflammatory cytokine. FEBS Lett 1992; 307:97.
53. McCain R, Dessypris M, Christman JW: Granulocyte/macrophage colony-stimulating factor stimulates human polymorphonuclear leukocytes to produce interleukin-8 in vitro. Am J Respir Cell Mol Biol 1993; 8:28–34.
54. Luscinskas FW, Kiely JM, Ding H, et al: In vitro inhibitor effect of IL-8 and other chemoattractants on neutrophil-endothelial adhesive interactions. J Immunol 1992; 149:2163–2171.
55. Oppenheim JJ, Zachariae COC, Mukaida N, et al: Properties of the novel proinflammatory supergene "intercrine" cytokine family. Annu Rev Immunol 1991; 9:617.
56. Bellomo R: The cytokine network in the critically ill. Anaesth Intensive Care 1992; 20:288.
57. Christman JW, Wheeler A, Bernard G. Cytokines and sepsis: What are the therapeutic implications? J Crit Care 1991; 6:172.

58. Crystal RG, Bitterman PB, Rennard SI, et al: Interstitial lung disease of unknown cause: Disorders characterized by chronic inflammation of the lower respiratory tract. N Engl J Med 1984; 310:154.
59. Schwartz DA, Helmers RA, Dayton CS, et al: Determinants of bronchoalveolar lavage cellularity in idiopathic pulmonary fibrosis. J Appl Physiol 1991; 71:1688.
60. Hamman L, Rich AR: Acute diffuse interstitial fiborosis of the lung. Bull Johns Hopkins Hosp 1944; 74:177.
61. Ashbaugh DG, Maier RV: Idiopathic pulmonary fibrosis in adult respiratory distress syndrome. Arch Surg 1985; 120:530.
62. Olson J, Colby TV, Elliott CG: Hamman-Rich syndrome revisited. Mayo Clin Proc 1990; 65:1538.
63. Panos RJ, Mortenson RL, Niccoli SA, et al: Clinical deterioration in patients with idiopathic pulmonary fibrosis: Causes and assessment. Am J Med 1990; 88:396.
64. Bessis L, Callard P, Gotheil C, et al: High-resolution CT of parenchymal lung disease: Precise correlation with histologic findings. Radiographics 1992; 12:45.
65. Nishimura K, Kitaichi M, Izumi T, et al: Usual interstitial pneumonia: Histologic correlation with high-resolution CT. Radiology 1992; 182:337.
66. Hyde DM, King TE Jr, McDermott T, et al: Idiopathic pulmonary fibrosis: Quantitative assessment of lung pathology: Comparison of a semiquantitative and a morphometric histopathologic scoring system. Am Rev Respir Dis 1992; 146:1042.
67. Cherniack RM, Colby TV, Flint A, et al: Quantitative assessment of lung pathology in idiopathic pulmonary fibrosis: The BAL Cooperative Group Steering Committee. Am Rev Respir Dis 1991; 144:892.
68. Carrington CB, Gaensler EA, Coutu RE, et al: Idiopathic pulmonary fibrosis: Clinical, histologic, radiologic, physiologic, scintigraphic, cytologic, and biochemical aspects. Ann Intern Med 1976; 86:801.
69. Kuhn C, McDonald JA: The roles of the myofibroblast in idiopathic pulmonary fibrosis: Ultrastructural and immunohistochemical features of sites of active extracellular matrix synthesis. Am J Pathol 1991; 138:1257.
70. Watters LC, Schwarz MI, Cherniack RM, et al: Idiopathic pulmonary fibrosis: Pretreatment bronchoalveolar lavage cellular constituents and their relationships with lung histopathology and clinical response to therapy. Am Rev Respir Dis 1987; 135:696.
71. Hallgren R, Bjermer L, Lundgren R, et al: The eosinophil component of the alveolitis in idiopathic pulmonary fibrosis: Signs of eosinophil activation in the lung are related to impaired lung function. Am Rev Respir Dis 1989; 139:373.
72. McCormack FX, King TE Jr, Voelker DR, et al: Idiopathic pulmonary fibrosis: Abnormalities in the bronchoalveolar lavage content of surfactant protein A. Am Rev Respir Dis 1991; 144:160.
73. Low RB, Giancola MS, King TE Jr, et al: Serum and bronchoalveolar lavage of N-terminal type III procollagen peptides in idiopathic pulmonary fibrosis. Am Rev Respir Dis 1992; 146:701.
74. Savici D, Campbell PA, King TE Jr: Bronchoalveolar macrophages from patients with idiopathic pulmonary fibrosis are unable to kill facultative intracellular bacteria. Am Rev Respir Dis 1989; 139:22.
75. Strausz J, Muller-Quernheim J, Steppling H, et al: Oxygen radical production by alveolar inflammatory cells in idiopathic pulmonary fibrosis. Am Rev Respir Dis 1990; 141:124.
76. Lynch JP, Standiford TJ, Rolfe MW, et al: Neutrophilic alveolitis in idiopathic pulmonary fibrosis: The role of interleukin-8. Am Rev Respir Dis 1992; 145:1433.
77. Ozaki T, Hayashi H, Tani K, et al: Neutrophil chemotactic factors in the respiratory tract of patients with chronic airway diseases or idiopathic pulmonary fibrosis. Am Rev Respir Dis 1992; 145:85.
78. Carre PC, Mortenson RL, King TE, et al: Increased expression of the interleukin-8 gene by alveolar macrophages in idiopathic pulmonary fibrosis: A potential mechanism for the recruitment and activation of neutrophils in lung fibrosis. J Clin Invest 1991; 88:1802.
79. Antoniades HN, Neville-Golden J, Galanopoulos T, et al: Expression of monocyte chemoattractant protein 1 mRNA in human idiopathic pulmonary fibrosis. Proc Natl Acad Sci USA. 1992; 89:5371.
80. Johnson MA, Wan SK, Snell NJC, et al: Randomized controlled trial comparing prednisolone with cyclophosphamide and low dose prednisolone in combination in cryptogenic fibrosing alveolitis. Thorax 1989; 44:280.
81. Baughman RP, Lower EE: Use of intermittent, intravenous cyclophosphamide for idiopathic pulmonary fibrosis. Chest 1992; 102:1090.
82. O'Donnell K, Keogh B, Cantin A, et al: Pharmacologic suppression of the neutrophil component of the alveolitis in idiopathic pulmonary fibrosis. Am Rev Respir Dis 1987; 136:288.
83. Raghu G, Depaso WJ, Cain K, et al: Azathioprine combined with prednisone in the treatment of idiopathic pulmonary fibrosis: A prospective double-blind, randomized, placebo-controlled clinical trial. Am Rev Respir Dis 1991; 144:291.
84. Egan TM, Trulock EP, Boychuk J, et al: Analysis of referrals for lung transplantation: The Washington University Lung Transplantation Group. Chest 1991; 99:867.

CHAPTER 97

Principles of Mechanical Ventilation

Robert A. Smith, MS, RRT, FCCM

Mechanical ventilation has not been observed to significantly blunt or reverse pathophysiology associated with human acute respiratory insufficiency, but mechanical ventilatory support may promote further damage of injured lung[1] and injure remaining healthy lung.[2–4] Modern mechanical ventilators provide myriad modes and operator-controlled variables to clinicians for administering full or partial ventilatory support. Modes of mechanical ventilation are presented in Chapter 98. Cognizance of functional characteristics of operator-controlled variables will enable clinicians to balance potentially detrimental ventilatory support with desired physiologic goals appropriately. Operator-controlled variables of positive-pressure ventilators introduced in the past decade are emphasized in this chapter.

OPERATOR CONTROL OF MECHANICAL INSUFFLATION

Basic elements of a mechanical ventilator and breathing circuit are illustrated in Figure 97–1. Compressed air and oxygen are regulated to a uniform pressure and piped to the insufflation mechanism. Insufflation mechanisms using one electromechanical valve are supplied with respiratory gas of a selected fraction of inspired oxygen (F_{IO_2}) piped either directly from an air and oxygen blending system or from a reservoir of blended air and oxygen. Insufflation mechanisms using two electromechanical valves proportion air and oxygen independently to achieve selected F_{IO_2}. F_{IO_2} is adjustable from 0.21 to 1.0, with a precision of approximately 0.02 to 0.04 depending on the mechanical ventilator model. F_{IO_2} should be measured with an oxygen analyzer after each change and when arterial blood is sampled for oxygen tension analysis.

Inspiratory valves are used to modulate gas flow rate ($\dot{V}$) function as variable resistors (RVs) with a pressure gradient determined by a normally constant working pressure (PW) and variable breathing circuit pressure (PC).[5] Inspira-

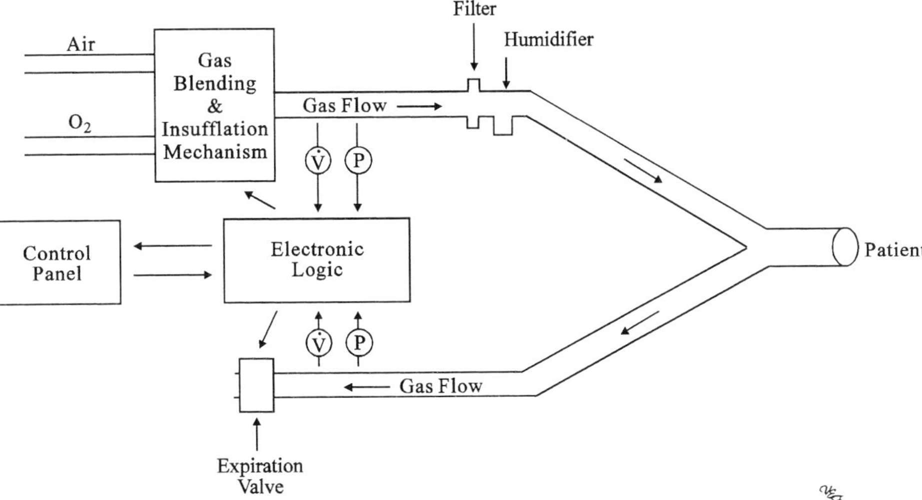

Figure 97–1. Schematic illustration of the basic elements of a mechanical ventilator and breathing circuit.

tory valve resistance is modulated by the electronic logic, and $\dot{V}$ into the breathing circuit is determined by the following relationship:

$$\dot{V} = (PW - PC) / RVs \quad \text{[Equation 1]}$$

Gas flow from the inspiratory valve is regulated by the electronic logic according to selected control panel variables and data received from inspiratory and expiratory gas flow and pressure sensors (i.e., servocontrolled valve events). Electronic logic circuitry includes electronic comparators and/or programmed devices. Details of valve events regulated by programmed control incorporating exchangeable programmable read-only memory devices, erasable programmable read-only devices, and nonvolatile (e.g., "bubble") memory devices programmed by the operator using a keyboard on the control panel are described in Chapter 101. Control of the expiratory valve is also directed by the electronic logic according to selected control panel variables and data based on the PC sensor.

Gas from the inspiratory valve passes through a bacterial filter and humidifier into the breathing circuit. These bacterial filter and humidification devices should not pose significant resistance to gas flow. See Chapter 77 for a discussion of humidification of inspiratory gas and humidification devices.

During mechanical insufflation, gas flows along a pressure gradient from the inspiratory valve into the inspiratory limb of a breathing circuit, through the artificial airway, and into the patient's lungs. Gas flow from the inspiratory valve during mechanical insufflation is controlled for volume or pressure by the electronic logic according to operator-selected variables.

Volume-Controlled Mechanical Insufflation

Volume-controlled mechanical insufflation may include a dynamic and static component (Fig. 97–2). Operator-selected variables during the dynamic insufflation may include initiation and termination mechanism, tidal volume (V_T) or minute ventilation ($\dot{V}_E$), and $\dot{V}$ characteristics. A static component of mechanical insufflation is included by activating a postinsufflation pause.

Each volume-controlled mechanical insufflation may be initiated automatically or synchronized with spontaneous inspiration (Fig. 97–3). A timing mechanism provides automatic mechanical insufflation at intervals independent of spontaneous breathing (e.g., controlled mechanical ventilation, intermittent mandatory ventilation). Timed sequencing of mechanical insufflation is selected with a rate control (breaths per minute). The selected rate of breaths per minute establishes the total time (T_T) of mechanical ventilation cycle (see Fig. 97–2). For example, if the selected rate is six breaths per minute, then T_T is 10 seconds. Mechanical insufflation may be initiated when data from a gas flow sensor and/or gas pressure sensor to the electronic logic indicate spontaneous inspiration (e.g., assisted mechanical ventilation, synchronized intermittent mandatory ventilation). The gas flow rate threshold for initiating mechanical insufflation may be factory or operator selected. When the gas flow initiation mechanism is activated, a precisely controlled continuous flow of gas is generated by the inspiratory valve. The threshold of gas flow change required to start mechanical insufflation is a set difference between gas flowing through sensors located near the inspiratory and expiratory valves (i.e., the expiratory valve $\dot{V}$ is less than inspiratory valve $\dot{V}$ by a set amount). A threshold of pressure change to begin mechanical insufflation is usually selected at the least possible value while avoiding autoinitiation.

Volume-controlled mechanical insufflation may be terminated after a selected time (time cycled) has elapsed or volume (volume cycled) is delivered. The time of mechanical insufflation (T_I) may be selected directly, usually in seconds, or indirectly as a fraction of T_T (T_I/T_T). Mechanical insufflation is volume cycled when the selected V_T is delivered through a sensor (e.g., a gas flow sensor). The V_T is calculated using the electronic logic by integrating the gas flow measured with a sensor located either within the ventilator near the inspiratory valve or at the proximal airway between the breathing circuit and artificial airway. During volume-cycled, volume-controlled mechanical insufflation, T_I is indirectly determined when V_T and a constant $\dot{V}$ are selected and may be estimated with the following expression:

$$T_I \text{ (second)} \approx V_T \text{ (L)} / \dot{V} \text{ (L/s}^{-1}\text{)} \quad \text{[Equation 2]}$$

where s is time in seconds and L is volume in liters.

As a safety precaution, an upper limit of acceptable pressure associated with mechanical insufflation is selected, and if achieved, gas from the inspiratory valve is automatically terminated, the expiratory valve opens, and an alarm activates. The expiratory valve remains open until the gas pressure decreases in the breathing circuit to the selected base-

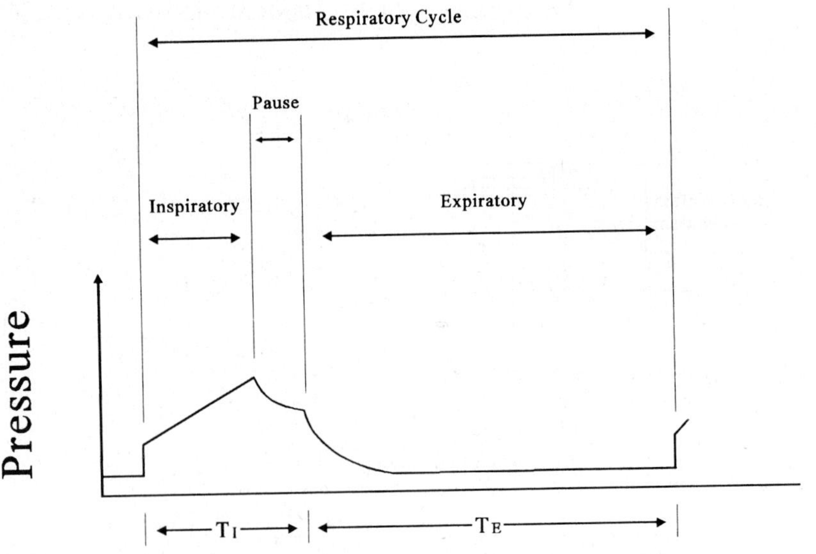

Figure 97–2. Idealized pressure and flow patterns illustrating the inspiratory (TI) and expiratory (TE) time phases of one complete respiratory cycle. The inspiratory phase includes a dynamic inspiratory and static pause component.

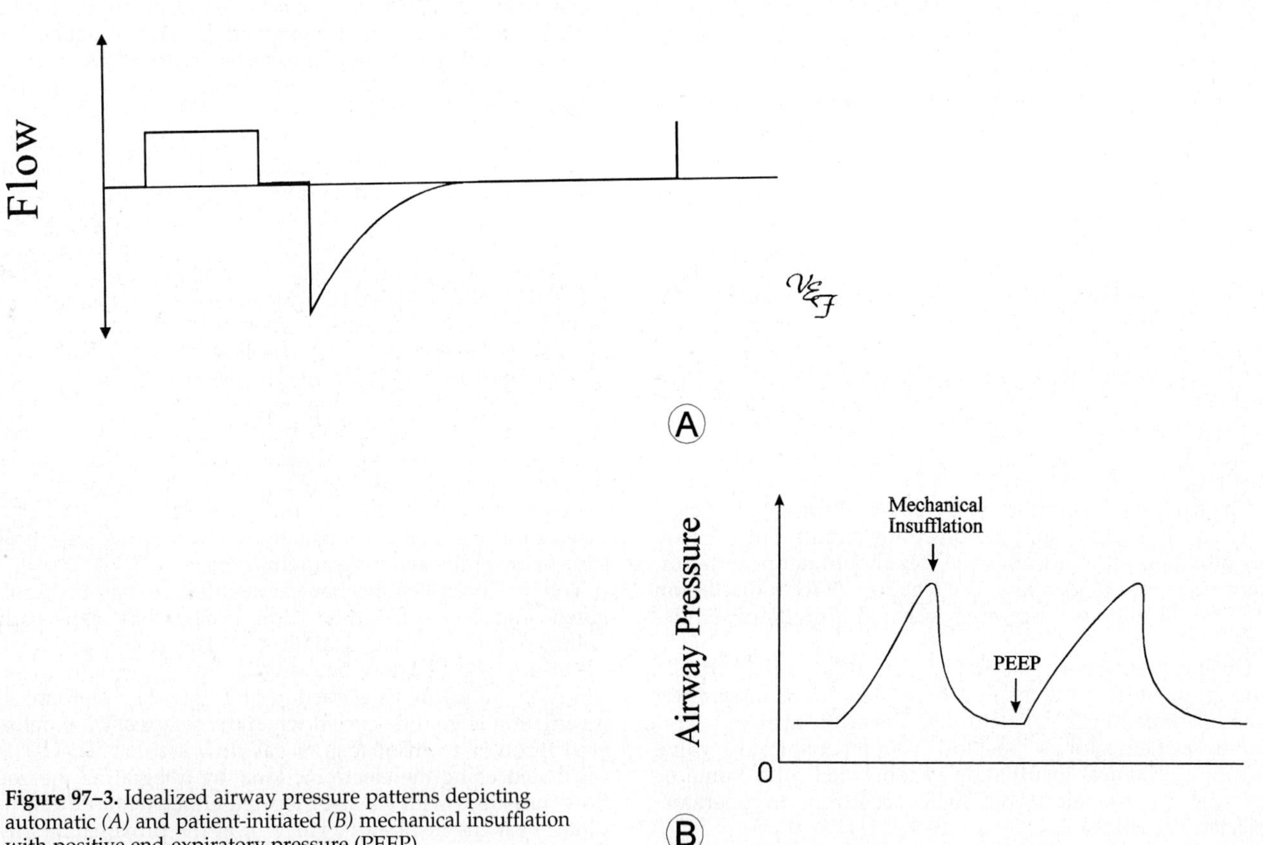

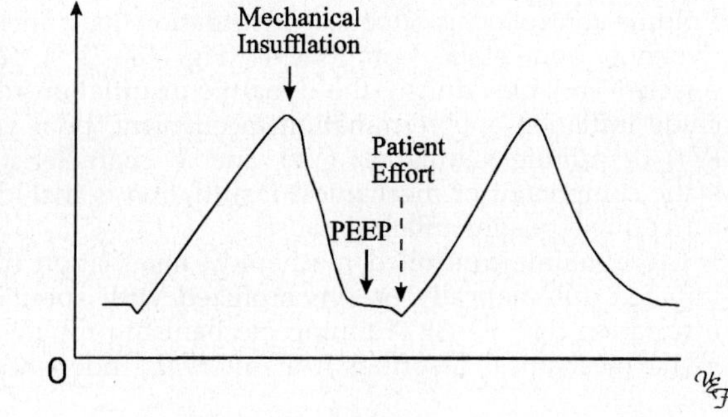

Figure 97–3. Idealized airway pressure patterns depicting automatic *(A)* and patient-initiated *(B)* mechanical insufflation with positive end-expiratory pressure (PEEP).

line pressure (atmospheric pressure or positive end-expiratory pressure [PEEP]) or a mechanical insufflation is initiated.

Tidal volume may be selected directly or indirectly by selecting ventilator rate and ($\dot{V}$E). Tidal volume during normal spontaneous breathing is approximately 5 mL/kg of body weight (BW). During positive-pressure ventilation, alveolar dead space is increased, and selected VT is usually greater than 5 mL/kg BW (e.g., 8–12 mL/kg BW). Optimizing VT under conditions of varied lung disease is discussed in Chapters 92, 93, 97, 98, 99, 100, and 101. The distribution of the selected VT between the breathing circuit and patient's lungs depends not only on the patient's pulmonary compliance but also on the compliance of the breathing circuit and change of breathing circuit pressure. For example, if the change of breathing circuit pressure is 20 cm H_2O during mechanical insufflation of a VT of 500 mL via a breathing circuit with a compliance of 5 mL/cm H_2O, then the distribution of VT to the lungs would be 400 mL. Breathing circuit compliance varies with equipment used (e.g., 2.0–7.0 mL/cm H_2O) and can be estimated with the patient disconnected. Selecting a VT of 100 mL and cycling mechanical insufflation while occluding the patient connector and observing the change in circuit pressure will provide the breathing circuit compliance as the quotient of 100 mL and the change in pressure. Some mechanical ventilators permit automatic circuit compliance compensation. A compliance factor, calculated as described previously, is programmed from the control panel, and as pressure rises the electronic logic modulates flow to add inspired volume to compensate for volume remaining in the circuit because of equipment compliance. Where automatic compensation for circuit compression volume is provided, selected VT delivery to the lungs remains constant during mechanical insufflation despite alterations of impedance in the patient's respiratory system. Airway pressure fluctuates independently of operator control if the patient's respiratory system impedance changes during normal volume-controlled mechanical ventilation.

The gas flow during volume-controlled mechanical insufflation may be constant (Fig. 97–4), sinusoidal (Fig. 97–5), or decelerating (Fig. 97–6). Depending on the type of ventilator, the peak $\dot{V}$ or TI will change when the $\dot{V}$ pattern is altered with a given VT. During time-cycled ventilation when VT and TI are selected, $\dot{V}$ required to produce a constant pattern is computed by the electronic logic in the following manner:

$$\dot{V}\ (L/s) = V_T\ (L)/T_I\ (s) \qquad \text{[Equation 3]}$$

and peak gas flow will be higher when nonconstant flow patterns are used. During volume-cycled ventilation, TI required for complete insufflation is a function of the mean gas flow rate and VT:

$$T_I\ (s) = V_T\ (L)/\dot{V}\ (L/s) \qquad \text{[Equation 4]}$$

Mean $\dot{V}$ is less during nonconstant versus constant flow; thus, TI is longer when VT is delivered with nonconstant versus constant flow.

Because mechanical insufflation may cause regional and intraregional pulmonary maldistribution of VT, manipulation of $\dot{V}$ or gas pressure pattern has been advocated to improve the efficiency of mechanical ventilation.[6,7] The Engström 300 and Emerson 3PV piston ventilators were designed specifically to generate a sinusoidal flow pattern because it was thought to approximate physiologic airflow and would minimize maldistribution of VT. Numerous investigations incorporating lung models, animals, or humans and showing advantages of one or another inspiratory $\dot{V}$

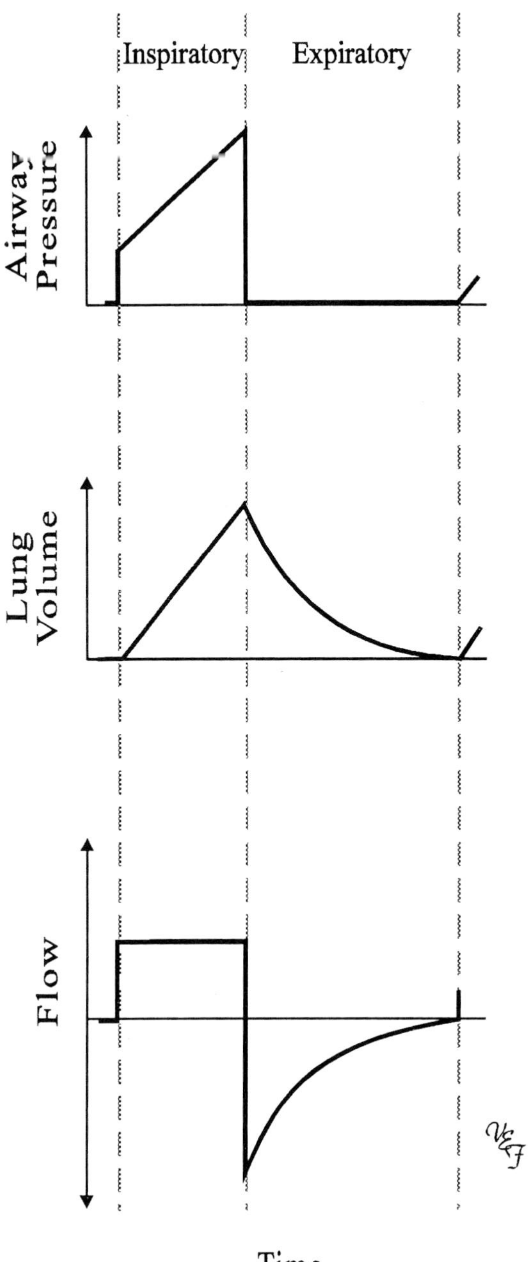

Figure 97–4. Schematic illustration of pressure, volume, and flow during mechanical insufflation with a constant flow. Nearly constant respiratory system compliance is assumed.

trajectory have been published.[8–15] Deceleration versus acceleration of gas flow during mechanical insufflation of animals with experimental lung injury produced significantly lower dead space and peak airway pressure and significantly greater partial pressure of arterial oxygen.[12] However, there is no convincing physiologic evidence that inspiratory gas flow pattern at a given VT and TI affects alveolar ventilation. Because $\dot{V}$ rapidly approaches zero as VT is partitioned within the extensive, dichotomous branching of the airways of the respiratory system ending in a cul-de-sac, it seems unlikely that a particular $\dot{V}$ pattern would significantly influence alveolar ventilation. Ventilating efficiency of a given VT is more likely improved with maneuvers increasing the duration of potential mixing of VT and resi-

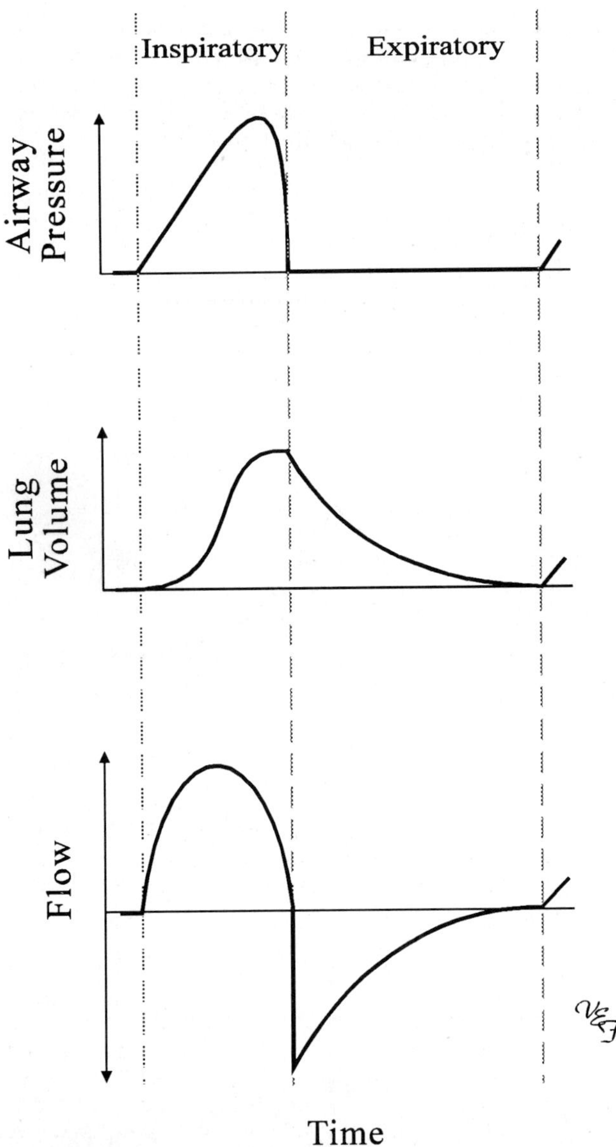

Figure 97–5. Schematic illustration of pressure, volume, and flow during mechanical insufflation with a sinusoidal flow. Nearly constant respiratory system compliance is assumed.

dent lung volume rather than choice of a particular $\dot{V}$ profile.

A selected gas flow rate during patient-initiated, volume-controlled mechanical insufflation should equal or slightly exceed the patient's intrinsic $\dot{V}$ requirement. The appropriate $\dot{V}$ may be approximated by the quotient of the selected V_T and estimation of the patient's intrinsic inspiratory time. The appropriate $\dot{V}$ may also be estimated by quadrupling measured $\dot{V}_E$. Inadequately selected $\dot{V}$ is tantamount to partial obstruction of airway. When the patient's intrinsic $\dot{V}$ requirement exceeds that of mechanical insufflation, work of breathing may significantly increase and the patient may experience "iatrogenic dyspnea" (Fig. 97–7). Grossly inappropriate $\dot{V}$ may be assessed by observing acute decreases in pressure via the airway pressure manometer or pressure bar graph during mechanical insufflation, and/or the patient may exhibit clinical signs of dyspnea. Some mechanical ventilators are designed to "sense" (usually via a pressure sensor) inadequacy of a selected $\dot{V}$ and automatically increase the $\dot{V}$.

Some ventilators permit gradual increase of an initial $\dot{V}$ to a selected or computed final $\dot{V}$ during volume-controlled mechanical insufflation. The time for increase of the $\dot{V}$ from onset of mechanical insufflation to the final $\dot{V}$ may be selected from 0% to 10% of the total respiratory cycle (inspiratory rise time) (Siemens 300). When inspiratory rise time is 0%, $\dot{V}$ (i.e., electronic logic computed $\dot{V} = V_T/T_I$) is immediately generated and sustained throughout mechanical insufflation, thus producing a constant $\dot{V}$. As the inspiratory rise time is increased from 0%, the slope of the $\dot{V}$ trajectory is decreased as the initial $\dot{V}$ accelerates to the final $\dot{V}$. Care should be taken to match initial $\dot{V}$ with intrinsic $\dot{V}$ of the patient when using an inspiratory rise time greater than 0%. Otherwise, similar problems as those discussed with inadequate $\dot{V}$ during patient-initiated, volume-controlled insufflation may manifest.

Activating a postinsufflation pause mechanism (i.e., static

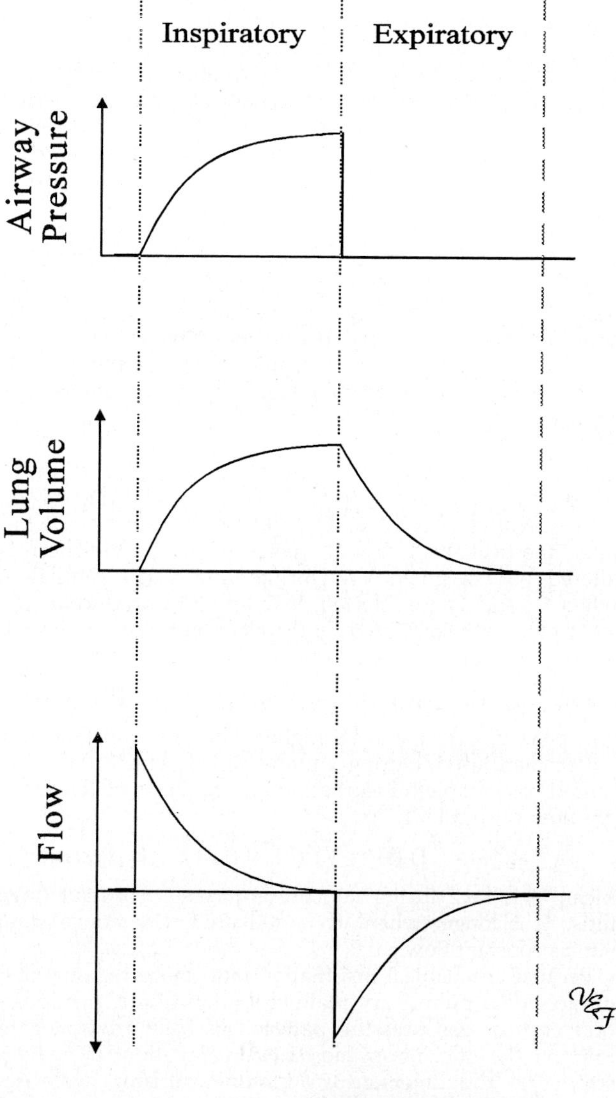

Figure 97–6. Schematic illustration of pressure, volume, and flow during mechanical insufflation with a decelerating flow. Nearly constant respiratory system compliance is assumed.

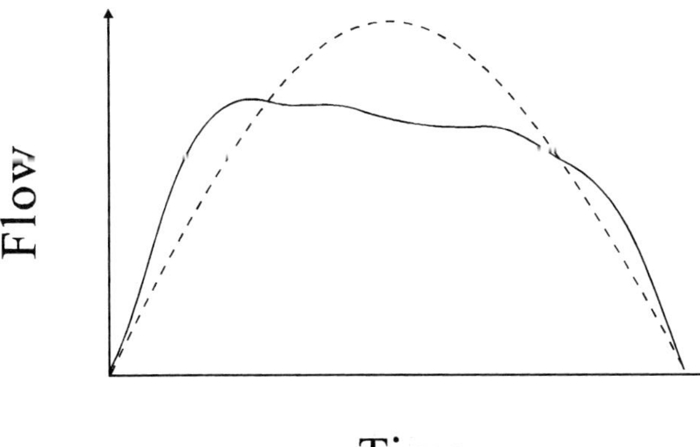

Figure 97–7. Schematic representation of inspiratory gas flow patterns typical for a spontaneously breathing patient with acute lung injury *(solid line)* and with mechanical insufflation delivered with a sinusoidal flow pattern *(broken line).*

phase of mechanical insufflation) delays opening of the expiratory valve after a normally volume- or time-cycled mechanical insufflation when the gas flow has ceased and V_T has been delivered (see Fig. 97–2). The postinsufflation pause is time cycled and selected either directly by a time control or indirectly as a percentage of the total mechanical ventilation cycle time. A postinspiratory pause provides a period of quasi-static mechanical inspiration, which increases the opportunity for mixing of V_T and resident lung volume.[11, 16, 17] A postinsufflation pause may reduce the dead space to tidal volume ratio (V_{DS}/V_T) and improve carbon dioxide removal, thus permitting a reduction of $\dot{V}_E$ with consequent reduction of pressure intervention. Clinical utility of postinsufflation pause should be evaluated individually. A postinsufflation pause should be titrated in increments (e.g., 0.2 second) and, when effective, should increase carbon dioxide excretion per exhaled breath and decrease partial pressure of arterial carbon dioxide tension without causing abnormal hemodynamics or patient-ventilator asynchrony. However, patient-ventilator asynchrony may limit the use of postinsufflation pause. Airway pressure during a postinsufflation pause may be used to quantify quasi-static recoil pressure of the respiratory system.

Pressure-Controlled Mechanical Ventilation

Operator-selected variables for pressure-controlled ventilation may include the initiation and termination mechanism, mechanical insufflation pressure (P_I), and P_I characteristics. Pressure-controlled mechanical insufflation may be initiated automatically or synchronized with spontaneous inspiration. A timing mechanism provides automatic mechanical insufflation at intervals independent of spontaneous breathing (e.g., pressure-controlled ventilation). Timed sequencing of mechanical insufflation is selected with a rate control (breaths per minute). Mechanical insufflation may be initiated (e.g., pressure support ventilation) when data from a gas flow sensor and/or gas pressure sensor to the electronic logic indicate spontaneous inspiration. The gas flow rate threshold for initiating mechanical insufflation may be factory or operator adjusted. A precisely controlled continuous flow of gas is generated via the inspiratory valve. The threshold of gas flow change required to initiate mechanical insufflation is a set difference between gas flowing through sensors located near the inspiratory and expiratory valves (i.e., expiratory valve $\dot{V}$ less than inspiratory valve $\dot{V}$ by a set amount). The threshold of pressure change to initiate mechanical insufflation is usually selected at the least possible value while avoiding inadvertent initiation.

Pressure-controlled mechanical insufflation may be terminated after a selected interval (time cycled) or when $\dot{V}$ declines to a factory-selected level (flow cycled). Mechanical insufflation during time-cycled, pressure-controlled ventilation (e.g., pressure-controlled ventilation and pressure-controlled–inverse ratio ventilation) is terminated after a selected time has elapsed. Insufflation time is selected either directly, usually in seconds, or indirectly as a percentage of the total mechanical ventilation cycle time (vide supra). Mechanical insufflation during flow-cycled, pressure-controlled mechanical insufflation (e.g., pressure support ventilation) is terminated when the gas flow rate decreases to a given level (e.g., 5 L/min or 25% of initial $\dot{V}$). As a safety measure, mechanical insufflation terminates when the factory-set or operator-selected upper limit of circuit pressure is reached. Pressure support ventilation may be used independently or in association with modes incorporating volume-controlled mechanical insufflation (e.g., synchronized intermittent mandatory ventilation).

During time-cycled, pressure-controlled ventilation, the gas flow rate into the lungs is determined with the following relationship:

$$\dot{V} = (P_I - P_A)/Raw \qquad \text{[Equation 5]}$$

where P_A is alveolar pressure at onset of mechanical insufflation and Raw is airway resistance (i.e., resistance to $\dot{V}$ posed by the artificial airway and the patient's airways).[5, 18] At equilibrium at the end of insufflation ($P_A = P_I$), V_T may be estimated as:

$$V_T \approx P_I \cdot Crs, \qquad \text{[Equation 6]}$$

where Crs is compliance of the patient's respiratory system. For example, if P_I is 10 cm H_2O and Crs is 50 mL/cm H_2O, then V_T is 500 mL. Equilibration of P_A and P_I is confirmed when $\dot{V}$ is 0 L/min (Fig. 97–8). When inspiration time does not permit equilibration of P_A and P_I, $\dot{V}$ continues at the end of insufflation and V_T will be less than the product of P_I and Crs. Contrary to volume-controlled mechanical insufflation, V_T fluctuates with alterations of respiratory system impedance during pressure-controlled mechanical ventilation.

When P_I is constant during pressure-controlled ventilation, $\dot{V}$ is initially maximal and declines as P_A approaches P_I (Equation 5 and Fig. 97–8). However, some ventilators permit a gradual increase of pressure toward the selected P_I. Time for increase from P_{zero} to P_I may be selected with inspiratory rise time control (Siemens 300). Inspiratory rise time during pressure-controlled ventilation functions similarly as during volume-controlled mechanical insufflation except that selected P_I rather than computed gas flow rate is the endpoint. Phasic application of airway pressure provides a predictable airway pressure envelope determined by selected baseline pressure (atmospheric or supra-atmospheric), P_I, and T_I. Depending on the type of mechanical ventilator, fresh gas may be available for spontaneous breathing during phased levels of airway pressure.[19] For example, airway pressure release ventilation (APRV) is a technique to augment $\dot{V}_E$ of spontaneously breathing patients with intermittent reduction and restoration of airway pressure.[20] See Chapter 98 for details about regarding APRV and other modes of mechanical ventilation using time cycling of varied levels of airway pressure.

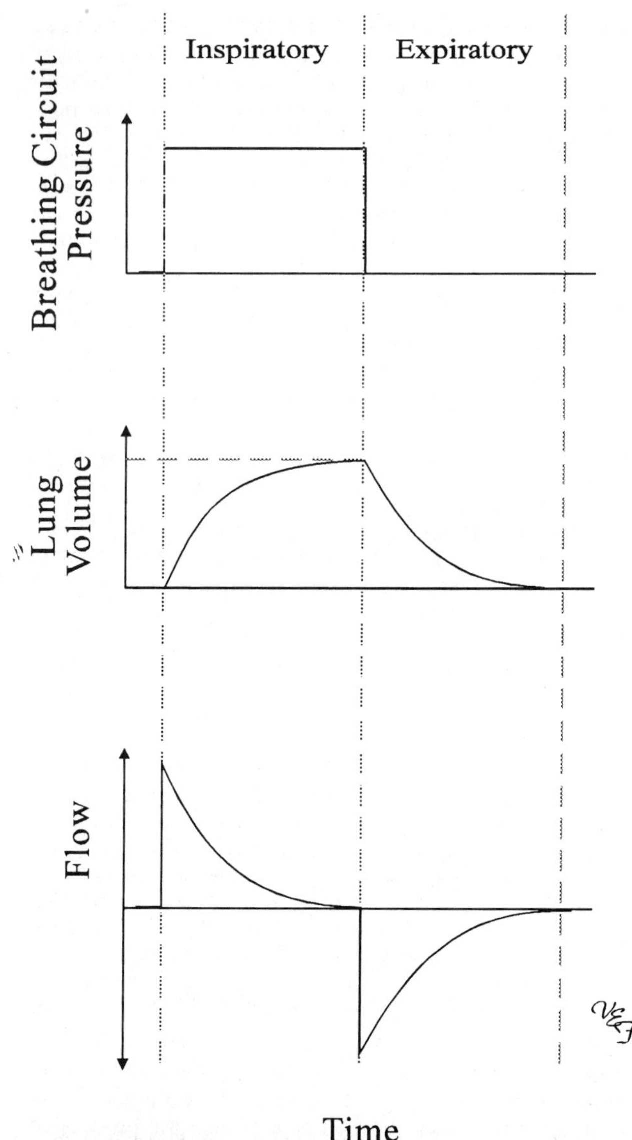

Figure 97–8. Idealized breathing circuit pressure, lung volume, and flow patterns during the inspiratory and expiratory phase of time-cycled, pressure-controlled ventilation.

Automatic Pressure-Regulated Ventilation

Selected VT or minute volume may be achieved with automatic regulation of PI. An example of automated PI-regulated ventilation is pressure-regulated, volume-controlled ventilation (Siemens 300). A test breath is delivered at PI of 5 cm H_2O, and Crs (mL/cm H_2O) is estimated by electronic logic as the dividend of actual VT and PI. An estimation of required PI to achieve selected VT is computed by electronic logic in the following manner:

$$P_I = Crs/V_T \qquad \text{[Equation 7]}$$

The subsequent three mechanical insufflations are delivered at a PI of 75% of estimated PI needed to produce selected VT. Inspiratory pressure of subsequent mechanical insufflations is regulated to a level determined by estimated Crs for previous mechanical insufflations versus selected VT. Automatic regulation of PI is never altered more than 3 cm H_2O among mechanical insufflations, and PI is adjusted between baseline pressure (i.e., atmospheric pressure or PEEP) and 5 cm H_2O less than the selected upper pressure limit. If actual VT exceeds selected VT, PI is automatically decreased in a similar fashion. As a safety feature, if VT reaches 150% of selected value, mechanical insufflation is terminated (i.e., volume cycled). Another technique of automatic regulation of PI permits the operator to select an anticipated spontaneous breathing rate and minimum VT and $\dot{V}_E$ (volume support ventilation) (Siemens 300). Inspiratory pressure is automatically titrated as during pressure-regulated, volume-controlled ventilation (vide supra). However, mechanical insufflation is terminated when $\dot{V}$ has decreased to 5% of initial $\dot{V}$ or after 80% of selected total mechanical cycle time. Total mechanical cycle time is determined by the selected estimated breathing frequency. Selected VT will be sustained even when an increased breathing rate increases actual $\dot{V}_E$ above selected $\dot{V}_E$. If the spontaneous breathing rate is less than anticipated, the electronic logic automatically calculates a "new" target VT to sustain selected minimum $\dot{V}_E$. If the calculated new VT is 150% of selected VT, PI is not increased. Some ventilators will automatically decrease PI. Thus, VT is decreased when actual $\dot{V}_E$ exceeds selected $\dot{V}_E$. A reduction of VT coincident with increased breathing frequency is undesirable and may be detected by adjusting the high $\dot{V}_E$ alarm threshold to a value slightly greater than selected $\dot{V}_E$.

OPERATOR CONTROL AFTER MECHANICAL INSUFFLATION IS CYCLED OFF

During passive expiration, the gas flow is approximately laminar and proportional to the pressure gradient between the alveoli and expiration valve. The pressure gradient is related to the volume of the lungs in excess of passive relaxation volume, assuming near-constant respiratory system compliance.[5, 18] As a result, there is a relationship between the rate of emptying of the lungs and the volume of the lungs in excess of passive relaxation volume, and it is commonly expressed with an exponential model using a washout function of the form:

$$V_T = V_L \cdot e^{(-t/Crs \cdot Raw)} \qquad \text{[Equation 8]}$$

where VT is expired tidal volume, VL is volume in the lungs in excess of relaxation volume, and e is base of natural logarithm (Fig. 97–9).[5, 18] According to the exponential model, when VT reaches steady-state, t/Crs · Raw is 0, the time must be infinite. Although the model provides a reasonable approximation of reality, from a practical standpoint, expiration does "cease" in a finite time. A convenient unit of time measurement may be obtained by letting the exponent of e = −1 and solve for t:

$$t = Crs \cdot Raw \qquad \text{[Equation 9]}$$

The product of Crs and Raw is defined as the time constant (τ) of the exponential function. For example, if Crs is 0.05 L/cm H_2O and Raw is 6 cm H_2O/L · second, then τ is 0.3 second. Thus, expiration would be completed in 0.3 second if the initial rate of lung emptying was sustained. However, during passive expiration, the initial rate of emptying is not sustained and progressively decreases according to the washout function (Equation 7 and Fig. 97–9). Approximately 63%, 86%, 95%, 98%, or 99% of VT is washed out in one, two, three, four, or five time constants, respectively.[5] Thus, knowing τ facilitates estimation of adequate expiratory time. For example, when τ is 0.3 second, an expiratory time of 1.2 seconds would permit 98% emptying of VT.

When mechanical insufflation is terminated, expired gas is vented to the environment through an electromechanical

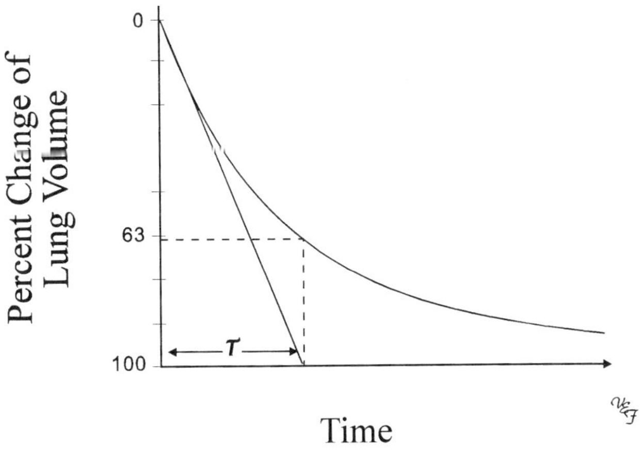

Figure 97–9. Schematic representation of the per cent change of lung volume during passive expiration. Approximately 63% of the tidal volume is expired in one time constant (τ). See text for details.

or pneumatic balloon valve. Ideally, an expiration valve should permit rapid reduction of breathing circuit pressure to atmospheric pressure or a selected level of supra-atmospheric pressure (PEEP). The portion of the mechanical ventilation cycle electronically partitioned for expiratory time (TE) is determined by the inspiratory time and total cycle time in the following manner:

$$T_E = T_T - T_I \qquad \text{[Equation 10]}$$

Some ventilators permit selection of expiratory pause hold (e.g., Siemens 300) to determine end-expiratory lung pressure. End-expiratory lung pressure should equal baseline pressure (i.e., atmospheric pressure or selected level of PEEP) to avoid increasing air trapping. See Chapters 95, 98, 99, 100, and 102 for discussion of the physiologic consequences of air trapping. When the end-expiratory lung pressure is greater than the selected baseline pressure, corrective measures to increase expiratory time should be instituted. Increasing TE while preserving optimized VT may be accomplished by decreasing cycling frequency and/or decreasing TI (i.e., directly or by increasing gas flow rate).

Selected PEEP is developed when the electronic logic closes the expiration valve and interrupts relief of pressure in the breathing circuit after mechanical insufflation is cycled off according to data from the pressure sensor and control panel. PEEP is generally applied to recruit or sustain recruitment of alveoli otherwise collapsed by hydrostatic forces.[21] PEEP may be administered in conjunction with mechanical insufflation initiated automatically or synchronized with patient effort (see Fig. 97–3). Detailed discussions of PEEP are presented in Chapters 92, 95, 98, 99, 100, and 102.

PEEP may be used during spontaneous breathing and is usually administered as continuous positive airway pressure (CPAP). During normal spontaneous breathing, airway opening pressure is constant (atmospheric pressure), availability of gas is virtually infinite (atmospheric air), and gas flow impedance of the patient's respiratory system is minimal. When an artificial airway is inserted, the resistance to gas flow and load on inspiratory muscles are increased.[5, 18] During spontaneous inspiration, a reduction of pressure at the distal end of the tracheal tube exceeding 5 cm H_2O indicates either insufficient gas flow or significant added resistance of the breathing circuitry. A significant reduction of airway pressure during spontaneous inspiration may in and of itself precipitate further deterioration of pulmonary function and gas exchange.[22, 23] Application of pressure support ventilation of 5 cm H_2O will significantly reduce respiratory muscle work associated with the resistive load imposed by the breathing apparatus.[24]

During spontaneous breathing, minimal fluctuation of airway pressure is desirable. See Chapter 72 for a detailed discussion of the work of breathing. Gas for spontaneous breathing is provided in the same manner as during patient-initiated, volume- or pressure-controlled mechanical insufflation (vide supra). The gas flow from the inspiratory valve is modulated by the electronic logic according to a selected level of airway pressure (i.e., CPAP equal to or greater than atmospheric pressure) and data from gas pressure and/or flow sensors. As the patient breathes, CPAP is regulated by modulation of gas flow and tension of the expiration valve.

TECHNICAL CONSIDERATIONS OF MECHANICAL VENTILATOR MONITORING

Monitoring functional performance of the mechanical ventilator is essential to substantiate its performance and to improve patient safety.

Electronic Source

Some ventilators incorporate a rechargeable battery or capacitor to activate an audible alarm if internal electronics or the alternating current (AC) power source malfunctions. Because human activity around ventilated patients is quite often heavy, power cord disconnection can occur easily. For these reasons, battery competence must be established before ventilator use and checked periodically. This is accomplished by activating the main power switch and disconnecting the cord from the wall outlet. Capacitor-powered alarm function is tested by removing the external AC source while the ventilator power switch is turned on after a 15- to 20-minute warm-up period. A fully charged battery/capacitor should provide sufficient audible tone for at least 5 minutes.

Pneumatic Source

Pressurized air and oxygen are supplied to respective inlets. Each gas source is monitored independently by an electronic switch and the pressure displayed via the inlet pressure gauge. If oxygen or air pressure decreases below a critical level (e.g., 20–30 psi depending on the specific system), the appropriate pressure switch activates an audible alarm and visual pressure indicator. Because pressure rather than gas concentration is sensed, absence of a pneumatic source alarm does not guarantee correct gas composition.

Oxygen Concentration

The oxygen concentration of respiratory gas from the flow valve is usually monitored by a polarographic or galvanic fuel cell. Periodic calibration of this monitor is necessary to compensate for drift in the electrical circuitry and sensor. The oxygen monitor should be recalibrated at least every 12 hours. Pressure and humidity can alter displayed oxygen concentration. Increased pressure (above atmospheric) causes a greater number of oxygen molecules, and proportional current generated produces a higher displayed oxygen concentration when system pressure increases during positive-pressure inspiration. Theoretically, this amounts to approximately 1% per 10 cm H_2O above atmospheric pressure. This phenomenon also holds true during application of PEEP. The alteration in partial pressure of inspired oxygen (P_{IO_2}) is, of course, real, but at routine clinical pressure this produces little if any significant effect (e.g., in gas exchange calculations using P_{IO_2}). Most oxygen-monitoring systems incorporated in ventilators include an audible alarm and visual indicator. Both activate when the delivered oxygen concentration deviates from the selected threshold. A range of acceptable fluctuations is usually established by adjusting low and high alarm limits (e.g., ±2%).

Gas Flow and Volume Monitoring

Hypoventilation may result from mechanical ventilator failure or leaks in the patient-ventilator interface. Continuous monitoring of inspired and expired gas flow may be performed with a hot-wire anonemeter or more often with a pneumotachometer. A hot-wire (e.g., platinum) anonemeter quantifies a decrease of temperature that is proportional to the gas flow over the wire. One type of pneumotachometer consists of a tube with a pressure port on either side of a hydraulic resistance or variable orifice. The variable orifice is achieved by a hinged membrane. During ventilation, the variable orifice increases or decreases corresponding to the gas flow. The pressure gradient across the membrane is proportional to the gas flow rate. An algorithm in the electronic logic converts differential pressure to flow and integrates flow against time to calculate inspired gas volume. Another pneumotachometer design incorporates ultrasonic detection. Vortices are waves generated by gas tumbling over a strut placed in the air stream. The tube-strut combination is designed to generate one beat, or vortex, each time a milliliter of gas passes the strut. An electronically powered crystal transducer continuously transmits ultrasonic sound waves across the gas stream. The vortices intermittently alter the ultrasonic beam. These variations are detected and converted to electrical signals directly proportional to flow, and the electronic logic integrates the signal against time to derive gas volume. The respiratory rate may be calculated by the electronic logic with data from a gas flow sensor. A detected breath matched with the volume permits electronic logic to partition mechanical insufflation and spontaneous breath frequency.

Sensor position determines whether indicated volume includes gas volume compressed in the breathing circuit. Respirometers located at the outlet valve measure compression volume of the breathing circuit and respired gas volume. However, respirometers located between the ventilator tubing and artificial airway will only measure volume to and/or from lungs.

Alarms

Alarms may be adjusted to indicate low $\dot{V}_E$ and/or V_T and high $\dot{V}_E$ and/or V_T. Low-V_T threshold is usually adjusted to monitor the breathing pattern providing predominant contribution to effective ventilation (i.e., mechanical versus spontaneous breathing) (Fig. 97–10). When a selected threshold is not maintained, an audible alarm and visual indicator activate, which is presumptive evidence that a condition of hypoventilation exists and warrants immediate attention. In general, when an adult patient is receiving mechanical ventilation at a frequency greater than 6 breaths per minute, preselected machine-delivered V_T should be monitored. However, when $\dot{V}_E$ provided via volume- or pressure-controlled mechanical insufflation is less than 50% of combined $\dot{V}_E$, spontaneous V_T should be monitored. Because V_T is a critical parameter, it must be meticulously monitored with sensitive and specific alarm thresholds.

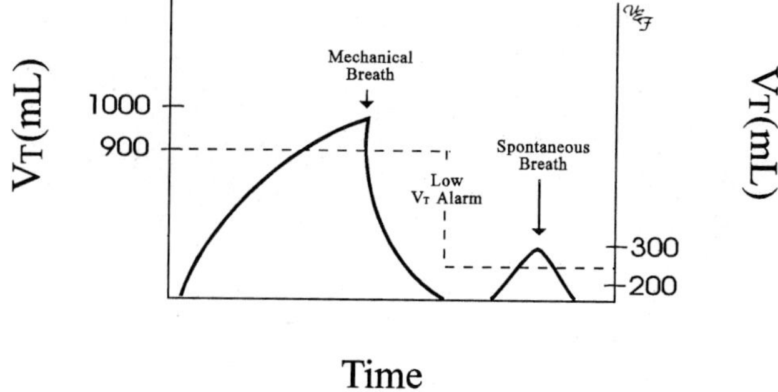

Figure 97–10. Schematic illustration indicating low V_T alarm threshold selection for a mechanically or spontaneously produced breath.

Airway Pressure Monitoring

Gas pressure is a type of stress characterized by its uniformity in all directions, and it is measured as force per unit area. Numerous units are used to measure gas pressure including pounds per square inch, millimeters of mercury, centimeters of water, kilopascals, and atmospheres. Atmospheric (ambient) pressure at sea level or 1 atm is equivalent to 14.7 psi, 760 mm Hg, 1033 cm H_2O, or 101 kPa. Physiologic pressure is quantified as gauge pressure (i.e., with reference to atmospheric pressure). In the United States, source gas pressure is commonly measured in psi, whereas patient circuit pressure is expressed in either centimeters of water or millimeters of mercury.

Transduced airway pressure can be displayed on the control monitor or externally recorded from analog outputs (e.g., a cathode ray tube screen may be an integral component of the control panel, thus permitting breath-by-breath evaluation of airway pressure patterns). Pressure transducers are usually calibrated at sea level. Correction factors for use at altitudes above sea level are published in the operator's manual.

Once selected V_T delivery is verified, peak airway pressure (Paw) should be noted. Some ventilators permit adjustment of the peak Paw limit and provide a low inspiratory pressure alarm and a loss of PEEP/CPAP alarm. The peak Paw and low inspiratory pressure alarm ranges should be set to 5 to 10 cm H_2O above and below initial peak Paw, respectively. An abrupt decrease in peak Paw of greater than 5 to 10 cm H_2O may be indicative of a circuit leak or exhalation valve malfunction, which may predispose to subsequent hypoventilation. An acute peak Paw elevation of greater than 5 to 10 cm H_2O pressure may signify a number of problems including accumulation of airway secretions, significant water condensate in hoses of the delivery circuit, bronchospasm, kinked tracheal tube, tension pneumothorax, patient-ventilator phasing problems, or improper valve function. Loss of PEEP/CPAP alarm threshold should be set 3 to 5 cm H_2O below end-expiratory pressure to provide leak detection when spontaneous breathing is the dominant contribution of $\dot{V}_E$. A low-pressure alarm may also activate during patient-initiated mechanical inspiration modes. This may be due to improper adjustment of the sensor used to cycle-on mechanical inspiration or too long response time of gas pressure generator or gas flow generator or inadequate gas source pressure.

Monitoring functional and operational characteristics of equipment used for ventilatory support is of paramount importance to ensure patient safety. However, surveillance systems are only as good as their sensitivity. Alarm thresholds must be selected to monitor critical parameters adequately and should be individualized to patients, equipment, and changing clinical circumstances. Expanding the threshold range because of frequent alarm activation ("nuisance alarms") may severely compromise patient safety. Often, these irritating alarm conditions are symptomatic of an impending problem. Inappropriately adjusted alarm thresholds may result in failure to detect changes in ventilatory status, proving lethal or damaging to vital organ function. Automatic alarm ranging may be available. By initiating the auto-set program, the electronic logic evaluates current ventilator-patient interface conditions and then invokes suitable alarm ranges for each monitored parameter.

Equally important to sophistication and sensitivity is the ability to ascertain monitor/alarm status rapidly. Critical ventilation variables (VT, respiratory rate, Paw) and alarm thresholds must be conveniently indicated. Modern ventilators provide real-time (i.e., breath by breath) and trend monitoring. Analog signals from gas pressure and flow sensors provide information to a printer, central monitoring, or a computerized equipment/patient data management systems. Computer-generated, time-sequenced "hard copies" of ventilator performance, ventilatory function, selected alarm thresholds, and alarm conditions may become the standard of practice for documenting patient care. A centralized monitoring system may optimize alarm detection and response time by clinical personnel (see Chapter 101).

ACKNOWLEDGMENT

Valerie Fumea prepared the medical illustrations, and Mauricio León, M.D., provided invaluable editorial assistance.

References

1. Pratt PC, Vollmer RT, Shelburne JD: Pulmonary morphology in a multihospital collaborative extracorporeal membrane oxygenation project: Light microscopy. Am J Pathol 1977; 95:191.
2. Barsch J, Bibara C, Eggers GWN, et al: Positive pressure as a cause of respirator induced lung disease. Ann Intern Med 1970; 72:810.
3. Greenfield LJ, Ebert PA, Benson DW: Effects of positive pressure ventilation on surface tension properties of lung extracts. Anesthesiology 1984; 25:312.
4. Dreyfuss D, Basset G, Soler P, et al: Intermittent positive pressure hyperventilation with high inflation pressures produces pulmonary microvascular injury in rats. Am Rev Respir Dis 1985; 132:880.
5. Mushin WW, Rendell-Baker L, Thompson PW, et al: On Automatic Ventilation of the Lungs. 3rd ed. Oxford, England, Blackwell Scientific Publications, 1980, p 68.
6. Froese AB, Bryan AC: Effects of anesthesia and paralysis on diaphragmatic mechanics in man. Anesthesiology 1974; 41:242.
7. Rehder K, Sessler AD, Rodarte JR: Regional intrapulmonary gas distribution in awake and anesthetized-paralyzed man. J Appl Physiol 1977; 42:391.
8. Herzog P, Norlander OP: Distribution of alveolar volume with different types of positive pressure gas-flow patterns. Opuscula Med 1968; 13:26.
9. Lyager S: Influence of flow pattern on the distribution of respiratory air during intermittent positive pressure ventilation. Acta Anaesthesiol Scand 1968; 12:191.
10. Johansson H: Effects of different inspiratory gas flow patterns on thoracic compliance during respirator treatment. Acta Anaesthesiol Scand 1975; 19:89.
11. Dammann JF, McAslan TC, Maffeo CJ: Optimal flow pattern for mechanical ventilation of the lungs: II. The effect of a sine versus square wave flow pattern with and without an end-inspiratory pause on patients. Crit Care Med 1978; 6:293.
12. Modell HI, Cheney FW: Effects of inspiratory flow pattern on gas exchange in normal and abnormal lungs. J Appl Physiol 1979; 46:1103.
13. Epstein RA, Epstein MAF: Flow to lung compartments with different time constants: Effect of choice of model. Acta Anaesthesiol Scand 1981; 25:39.
14. Al Saady N, Bennett ED: Decelerating inspiratory flow waveform improves lung mechanics and gas exchange in patients on intermittent positive-pressure ventilation. Intensive Care Med 1985; 11:68.
15. Smith RA, Venus BV: Cardiopulmonary effect of various inspiratory flow profiles during controlled mechanical ventilation in a porcine lung model. Crit Care Med 1988; 16:769.
16. Fulheihan S, Wilson R, Pontoppidan H: Effect of mechanical ventilation with end-inspiratory pause on blood gas exchange. Anesth Analg 1976; 55:122.
17. Lindahl S: Influence of end inspiratory pause on pulmonary ventilation, gas distribution, and lung perfusion during artificial ventilation. Crit Care Med 1979; 7:540.
18. Comroe JH: Physiology of respiration. 2nd ed. Chicago, Year Book Medical Publishers, 1974, p 94.
19. Smith RA: Respiratory care: mechanical. *In:* Anesthesia, 2nd ed. Vol 3. Miller R (Ed). New York, Churchill Livingstone, 1986, p 2188.
20. Downs JB, Stock MC: Airway pressure release ventilation: A new concept in ventilatory support. Crit Care Med 1987; 15:459.
21. Gattinoni L, D'Andrea L, Pelosi P, et al: Regional effects and mechanism of positive end-expiratory pressure in early adult respiratory distress syndrome. JAMA 1993; 269:2122.
22. Schlobohm RM, Falltrick RT, Quan SF, et al: Lung volumes, oxygenation during spontaneous positive-pressure ventilation: The advantage of CPAP over EPAP. Anesthesiology 1981; 55:416.
23. Quan SF, Falltrick RT, Schlobohm RM: Extubation from ambient or expiratory positive airway pressure in adults. Anesthesiology 1981; 55:53.
24. Christie JM, Smith RA: Pressure support ventilation decreases inspiratory work of breathing during general anesthesia and spontaneous ventilation. Anesth Analg 1992; 75:167.

CHAPTER 98

Airway Pressure Therapy

Jukka Räsänen, MD • John B. Downs, MD

The evolution of airway pressure therapy has resulted in a confusing array of modalities and techniques designed to augment alveolar ventilation, decrease the work of spontaneous breathing, and improve the oxygenation of arterial blood. Many of these techniques are closely related both physically and physiologically and, therefore, are not expected to produce different outcomes. In the absence of results from large-scale comparative studies, it is left to the clinician to decide whether to adopt or reject a given modality. This decision is not insignificant, given the financial and intellectual investment required to initiate a new form of therapy and the commercial and professional pressures to stay abreast of modern developments. This discussion attempts to clarify the principles of different forms of airway pressure therapy and their expected and observed physiologic effects. The clinical use of these therapeutic modalities in different disease states is covered in chapters addressing the specific disease. For a discussion of the physical principles of airway pressure therapy, the reader is referred to Chapter 97. Details of high-frequency ventilation, independent lung ventilation, and the hemodynamic effects of positive airway pressure therapy are presented in separate chapters.

CLASSIFICATION OF AIRWAY PRESSURE THERAPY

Airway pressure therapy is used to accomplish two goals: (1) static alteration in transpulmonary pressure to change resting lung volume for the duration of the therapy and (2) dynamic, cyclic alteration in transpulmonary pressure to augment alveolar ventilation artificially. An increase in transpulmonary pressure can be accomplished either by increasing airway pressure or by decreasing intrathoracic pressure; transpulmonary pressure can be decreased either by decreasing airway pressure or by increasing intrathoracic pressure. A static decrease in transpulmonary pressure and lung volume below normal is detrimental. In contrast, a static increase in transpulmonary pressure is used commonly to bring reduced resting lung volume closer to normal functional residual capacity (FRC). A sustained increase in transpulmonary pressure is usually effected by applying continuous positive pressure to the airway.

Mechanical ventilatory support techniques operate by producing a dynamic increase or decrease in transpulmonary pressure. Depending on how transpulmonary pressure is altered, four classes of mechanical ventilatory support are formed: (1) ventilation by decrease in intrathoracic pressure, (2) ventilation by increase in airway pressure, (3) ventilation by increase in intrathoracic pressure, and (4) ventilation by decrease in airway pressure. All of these four principles have been used at least experimentally in an attempt to augment alveolar ventilation (Table 98–1).

The interfacing of spontaneous breathing and mechanical ventilation can be arranged by modulating either minute ventilation or tidal volume. Minute ventilation is modulated by adding mechanical breaths to spontaneous breathing without an effort to provide mechanical support of each spontaneous respiratory cycle. Intermittent mandatory ventilation (IMV) is a typical example of a ventilatory technique that primarily supports minute volume. This type of interfacing does not require complex triggering mechanisms, and it provides a minimum minute ventilation regardless of spontaneous respiratory drive. However, it leaves some or all spontaneous respiratory efforts unsupported and does not respond to an increase in ventilatory demand unless the ventilator settings are changed. Tidal volume modulation (e.g., pressure support ventilation [PSV]) provides breath-to-breath support of each spontaneous respiratory cycle. If the patient's ventilatory rate increases in response to increased ventilatory demand, the mechanical ventilatory support increases proportionately.[1] However, tidal volume modulation requires sensitive synchronizing mechanisms and reliable spontaneous respiratory efforts if it is to be used as the patient's only support modality.

In Table 98–1, the three characteristics—method of altering transpulmonary pressure, magnitude of tidal volume, and patient-ventilator interface—have been used to separate physiologically dissimilar ventilatory techniques from each other. In discussing the various modalities, it is recognized that a "ventilatory support technique" is a technically unique method that is capable of providing full or partial support of alveolar ventilation. Therefore, among the most widely used methods that utilize an increase in airway pressure to deliver conventional tidal volume, only three separate entities can be distinguished: IMV, extended mandatory minute ventilation (EMMV), and PSV. For example, conventional controlled mechanical ventilation and IMV represent different levels of ventilatory support using the same technique. IMV and PSV are different techniques in the same physiologic group, the difference being the method of interfacing between spontaneous breathing and mechanical ventilation.

STATIC AIRWAY PRESSURE THERAPY: POSITIVE END-EXPIRATORY PRESSURE AND CONTINUOUS POSITIVE AIRWAY PRESSURE

Sustained elevation in lung volume can be accomplished by applying positive end-expiratory pressure (PEEP) or continuous positive airway pressure (CPAP) to the airway. If resting lung volume is reduced by an acute parenchymal disease process or by loss of negative intrathoracic pressure, restoring lung volume usually improves the ventilation-perfusion ($\dot{V}/\dot{Q}$) relationships and the mechanical characteristics of the respiratory system. The improvement in the $\dot{V}/\dot{Q}$ matching will alleviate hypoxemia and allow a decrease in inspired oxygen concentration. Optimizing the mechanical function of the lung will decrease the work of breathing often to the extent that mechanical ventilatory support may be reduced or discontinued. According to current nomenclature, positive expiratory airway pressure is called PEEP when the patient is receiving mechanical ventilation and CPAP is used when the patient is breathing spontaneously.

TABLE 98–1. Classification of Ventilatory Modalities

	Conventional VT (VT > VDS)		
Method of Lung Inflation	*Tidal Volume Modulation*	*Minute Volume Modulation*	***Low VT (VT < VDS): Minute Volume Modulation***
Decrease in intrathoracic pressure	Pneumatic chamber (1926)	Iron Lung (1920s)	NPO (1986)
Increase in intrathoracic pressure	Assisted exhalation	Resuscitation (1700s)	HFTTV (1986)
Increase in airway pressure	AMV (1970s), PSV (1982), PAV (1992)	CMV (1555) IMV (1973)	HFPPV (1967), HFJV, HFFI, HFO, CFAV
Decrease in airway pressure	IMPRV (1990)	IRV (1960s) APRV (1987)	

Abbreviations: NPO = negative-pressure oscillation; HFTTV = high-frequency transthoracic oscillation; AMV = assist-mode ventilation; PSV = pressure support ventilation; PAV = proportional assist ventilation; IMPRV = intermittent mandatory pressure release ventilation; CMV = control mode ventilation; IMV = intermittent mandatory ventilation; HFPPV = high-frequency positive-pressure ventilation; HFJV = high-frequency jet ventilation; HFFI = high-frequency flow interruption; HFO = high-frequency oscillation; CFAV = continuous flow apneic ventilation; IRV = inverse ratio ventilation; APRV = airway pressure release ventilation; VT = tidal volume; VDS = volume of dead space.

Therefore, any perceived differences between the physiologic effects of PEEP and CPAP can be traced to the level of mechanical ventilation.

Ventilation, Perfusion, and Positive End-Expiratory Pressure

The majority of gas exchange between the lungs and blood occurs during the expiratory phase of the respiratory cycle. Consequently, when arterial hypoxemia is secondary to a decrease in $\dot{V}/\dot{Q}$, effective improvement of arterial blood oxygenation requires correction of $\dot{V}/\dot{Q}$, primarily during exhalation. Mechanical ventilation usually is not effective in improving hypoxemia in acute lung injury because it increases the $\dot{V}/\dot{Q}$ only during the inspiratory phase of the respiratory cycle. In fact, Zarins and associates[2] observed a lower partial pressure of arterial oxygen (Pa_{O_2}) in baboons receiving controlled mechanical ventilation than in those receiving partial ventilatory support with IMV, with the same level of PEEP, suggesting that mechanical ventilation promoted a decrease in $\dot{V}/\dot{Q}$ and an increase in venous admixture.[2] The application of PEEP effects an improvement in $\dot{V}/\dot{Q}$ relationships during exhalation by augmenting ventilation in poorly aerated alveoli and by recruiting previously collapsed alveoli into effective gas exchange.[3] Thus, it alleviates the effects of the two major causes of hypoxemia associated with acute lung injury: $\dot{V}/\dot{Q}$ mismatching and intrapulmonary shunting of blood. Additionally, an increase in alveolar volume and oxygen tension may have a beneficial effect on diffusion-related hypoxemia. Improvement in arterial blood oxygenation in response to PEEP in patients with acute lung injury is well established in experimental and clinical literature. Radiographic imaging studies indicate that the best correlate to the improvement in oxygenation is the amount of recruitable lung tissue.[3, 4]

Despite its beneficial effects, the addition of PEEP to mechanical ventilation may increase physiologic dead space and actually decrease effective alveolar ventilation because of overinflation of the lungs during a positive-pressure inspiration. Therefore, to minimize $\dot{V}/\dot{Q}$ mismatching in all lung regions, it is important to allow spontaneous ventilation to persist at a level comfortable to the patient, while mechanical ventilation is used to prevent acidemia and excessive work of breathing.

The effect of PEEP and CPAP on oxygenation is closely tied to oxygen therapy both in a therapeutic and diagnostic sense. The presence of an increased oxygen concentration in areas of lung with low, but finite, $\dot{V}/\dot{Q}$ may lead to absorption atelectasis, which may not be prevented even by the application of PEEP.[5] On the other hand, evaluating pulmonary gas exchange and the appropriate airway pressure therapy in patients breathing increased concentrations of oxygen might lead to incorrect conclusions because administration of as little as 30% oxygen may mask the hypoxemia, producing effect of areas with low $\dot{V}/\dot{Q}$. For example, a patient breathing 40% oxygen with a Pa_{O_2} of 70 mm Hg might be thought to have adequate pulmonary gas exchange. The clinician might then decide to wean the patient from mechanical ventilation and PEEP. However, ventilation and perfusion could be mismatched to such a degree that breathing only 30% oxygen might decrease Pa_{O_2} to 50 mm Hg. Were the clinician aware of this abnormality, it is likely that PEEP would be increased rather than decreased. Such evaluations of pulmonary gas exchange and the rational application of PEEP are possible only when the inspired oxygen concentration is low. The lowest possible inspired oxygen concentration to maintain an acceptable arterial blood–oxyhemoglobin saturation maximizes alveolar nitrogen concentration, minimizes absorption atelectasis and right-to-left intrapulmonary shunting, and may decrease the need for PEEP. To minimize the potentially toxic oxygen therapy, proper PEEP must be used to make the maximum number of alveoli accessible to oxygen. Therefore, PEEP and oxygen therapy should be considered together in the treatment of patients with arterial hypoxemia.

Work of Breathing

If patients with respiratory failure are to breathe spontaneously, the work of breathing must be maximally efficient. Few clinical studies have attempted to quantify the work of breathing in patients with respiratory failure perhaps because quantification of work requires techniques that are not readily available.[6] For this discussion, only a graphic representation of the elastic work of inspiration is considered. A normal volume-pressure curve for the lung-thorax system is shown in Figure 98–1. When the distending pressure of the lung-thorax system is zero, as occurs when airway pressure is ambient, the lung volume is the FRC. As a result of a small pressure change, normal tidal breathing from FRC occurs along the volume-pressure curve. The elastic work of inspiration can be estimated by the shaded areas under the curve. Any alteration in the volume-pressure relationship of the lung can alter the work of breathing. This point is critical for a full understanding of the pathophysiology of respiratory failure and its therapy.

In patients with acute lung injury, a shift in the volume-pressure curve not only decreases FRC, but can increase the work of breathing. When FRC is decreased, the required pressure change may be increased for the same tidal volume (see Fig. 98–1). When the required pressure change is increased, the area under the curve representing work also is increased. If this occurs, the patient will decrease tidal volume and increase respiratory rate in an effort to minimize total work. Because of these changes, clinicians often have assumed the work of breathing for the patient by instituting mechanical ventilation. However, an increase in FRC and compliance also may decrease the patient's work of breathing to an acceptable level.

Restoration of FRC can be accomplished by applying PEEP to increase distending pressure (Fig. 98–2). Each volume-pressure curve will require a different level of PEEP to restore FRC and minimize the work of breathing. Therefore, PEEP must be individualized, titrated for each patient, and reassessed frequently.[7] If PEEP is applied to meet these goals, FRC will be increased and often will lie on a favorable portion of the volume-pressure curve, where the required change in pressure to produce a tidal volume will be smaller. Thus, lung compliance will be improved and work of breathing reduced.

Application of PEEP also may be useful in the reduction of respiratory work related to increased upper airway resistance. An increased intraluminal pressure in the airways will enlarge their caliber both directly by elevating the transmural pressure and indirectly by increasing lung volume.[8] CPAP with a nasal mask is now used widely in patients with nocturnal upper airway obstruction, and the application of facemask or nasal CPAP has been successful in children with tracheobronchomalacia.[9, 10] In these cases, the effect of CPAP is simply that of splinting a collapsible airway with an increase in transmural pressure.

Studies of the use of PEEP in patients with peripheral airways disease have produced variable results.[11] Anecdotal reports of a beneficial effect of a high level of PEEP in patients with severe asthma were followed by a consistent detrimental effect in a later controlled study.[12, 13] However,

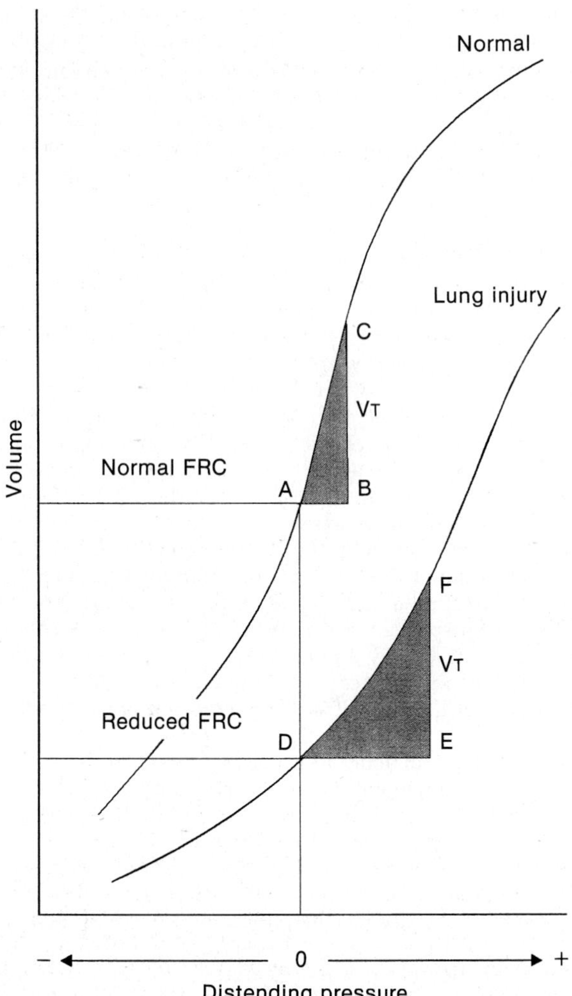

Figure 98–1. Schematic respiratory system pressure volume curves under normal conditions and during acute lung injury. When distending pressure is zero, the expanding tendency of the chest wall and the collapsing tendency of the lungs are in equilibrium, and lung volume is at functional residual capacity (FRC). When the lungs are healthy, inspiration of a tidal volume (VT; BC) requires an increase in distending pressure (AB) and elastic work that can be estimated from the area under the pressure volume curve (ABC). The injured lung operates at reduced FRC and requires a considerably larger change in distending pressure (DE > AB) for a normal VT (EF) and more work during inspiration ($Area_{DEF} > Area_{ABC}$) than does a healthy lung. See text for further details.

some patients who have chronic airflow obstruction with dynamic hyperinflation and expiratory flow limitation have been shown to respond to low levels of PEEP with improved efficiency of ventilation and decrease in dyspnea without side effects.[14, 15] In these patients, the application of PEEP may decrease expiratory resistance by opposing external compressive forces at the site of obstruction and decrease the inspiratory muscle work required to overcome the resting pressure gradient between the alveoli and the airway opening.[11] The application of PEEP in excess of the positive pressure distal to the airway obstruction (intrinsic PEEP) is expected to lead to further hyperinflation and both ventilatory and circulatory compromise. Evidence of reduced gas trapping with carefully titrated PEEP also has been noted in patients with acute lung injury,[16] even though directly measured airway flow resistance has been observed to increase.[17]

Continuous Positive Airway Pressure Therapy

Spontaneous respiration with elevated airway pressure was recognized six decades ago to decrease pulmonary edema in patients with congestive heart failure.[18] A motor-driven blower provided an inspiratory gas source, and airway pressure was elevated with a facemask and an expiratory valve for constant positive-pressure breathing (CPPB). Shortly thereafter, CPPB was used to treat pulmonary edema secondary to traumatic lung injury[19] and pulmonary contusion in patients with flail chest injuries.[20] Thus, there is ample historic precedent for applying elevated airway pressures to spontaneously breathing patients. Much later, mechanical ventilation was emphasized for the treatment of lung injuries and spontaneous breathing when CPPB was abandoned.[21] Because of the early emphasis on mechanical ventilation, discontinuation of mechanical ventilatory support often is attempted only after the need for PEEP has been alleviated. This may not be the most rational approach.

Lung compliance and arterial oxygenation are decreased

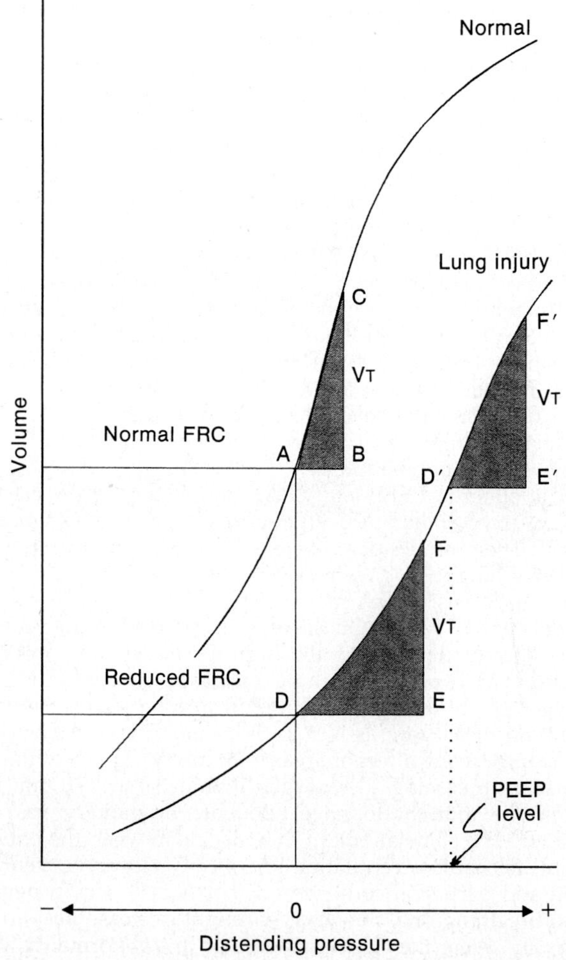

Figure 98–2. Schematic respiratory system pressure volume curves under normal conditions and during acute lung injury. When the resting volume of the injured lung is increased with PEEP, the change in distending pressure required for a normal VT decreases (D′E′ < DE), and the elastic work is reduced ($Area_{D'E'F'} > Area_{DEF}$). See text for further details.

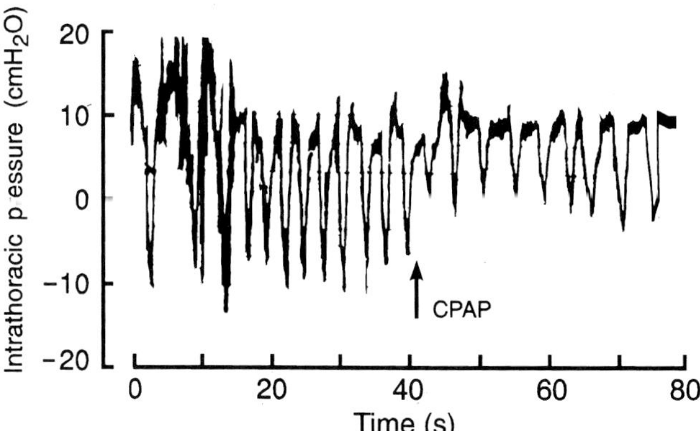

Figure 98–3. Directly recorded intrathoracic pressure tracing in a patient with cardiogenic pulmonary edema before and after institution of 7.5 cm H_2O CPAP *(arrow)*. Within one respiratory cycle from the application of the CPAP mask, the ventilatory rate and the inspiratory fall in intrathoracic pressure decrease dramatically.

and work of breathing is increased in patients with acute lung injury. In fact, it is often the increased work of breathing that leads many clinicians to institute mechanical ventilation. By application of CPAP, resting lung volume and compliance can be increased. The increase in lung volume will improve $\dot{V}/\dot{Q}$ and arterial oxygenation. Increased compliance will decrease the work of breathing (Fig. 98–3). Thus, CPAP may reduce the requirement for mechanical ventilation and inspired oxygen supplementation. Because application of CPAP also may alleviate many problems associated with the mechanical ventilator and oxygen, we prefer to wean patients from mechanical ventilation and oxygen before removing CPAP.

After application of positive airway pressure to restore resting lung volume, a reduction in the work of breathing will occur only if the inspiratory drop in airway pressure is small.[22, 23] To maintain unchanged airway pressure during spontaneous breathing, gas must flow at a rate equal to or greater than the patient's inspiratory flow rate. This is particularly important in patients with impaired left ventricular function.[24] As lung compliance decreases, intrapleural pressure change is greater because the stiff lung requires a greater intrapleural pressure change to accomplish tidal breathing. The associated increase in left ventricular afterload may lead to acute cardiopulmonary decompensation (see Chapter 102). Because our goal must be to minimize the patient's work of breathing, proper functioning of breathing circuits used in spontaneously breathing patients should be carefully monitored.

CPAP therapy in patients with intact protective airway reflexes does not necessitate tracheal intubation. Equipment for the delivery of CPAP with a mask covering the nose and mouth or the nose only have been commercially available for two decades. The adverse effects of facemask CPAP are minimal in a conscious, cooperating patient, even when the duration of the treatment is several days.

Practical Aspects of Positive End-Expiratory Pressure/Continuous Positive Airway Pressure Therapy

Several methods have been recommended in the literature for finding the optimum level of positive airway pressure for a given patient. Oxygenation of arterial blood, venous admixture, oxygen delivery, lung compliance, and dead space ventilation have all been suggested as endpoint variables for the adjustment of PEEP and CPAP therapy.[25–27] However, considering the multiple and interconnected desirable and undesirable effects of PEEP, it seems obvious that no one variable adequately reflects the physiologic effects of PEEP. Therefore, the assessment of PEEP therapy must evaluate pulmonary gas exchange, lung mechanics, and circulatory function simultaneously. Pulse and pulmonary artery oximetry can be used to monitor both pulmonary gas exchange and total body oxygen extraction continuously.[28] This technique has been shown to be comparable in accuracy to titrating PEEP using full cardiopulmonary profiles with repeated off-line blood gas analysis.[7]

After initiation of respiratory therapy with sufficient supplemental oxygen and mechanical ventilatory support, the appropriate level of PEEP or CPAP should be determined and instituted immediately. Subsequently, oxygen supplementation and ventilatory support are reduced to the levels that afford adequate oxygenation and arterial blood with a comfortable level of ventilatory work. Thereafter, PEEP therapy needs to be frequently re-evaluated and readjusted in response to the course of the patient's pulmonary disease. Infrequent re-evaluation of PEEP therapy may result in considerable overtreatment, "bureaucratic" PEEP, which may unnecessarily prolong the patient's stay in the intensive care unit.[7]

Adverse Effects of Sustained Positive Airway Pressure

Improper application of PEEP and CPAP may have adverse effects on pulmonary and circulatory function. Excessive PEEP will effect overinflation of the lungs, with a resultant increase in dead space ventilation and impairment of pulmonary and systemic blood flow. The spontaneous respiratory work will increase because of the low compliance of the distended respiratory system, and the respiratory muscles will be forced to operate at an unfavorable length-tension range. However, when evaluating the pros and cons of properly applied PEEP therapy, one must carefully consider whether the side effects are likely to occur because of the PEEP or the associated mechanical ventilation. In fact, the reduction in mechanical ventilatory support and inspired oxygen concentration afforded by proper use of PEEP or CPAP frequently decreases the overall impairment in cardiopulmonary function attributable to respiratory therapy.

To the extent that mean intrathoracic pressure is elevated by the application of sustained positive airway pressure, venous return and cardiac preload will decrease. Patients who have high lung compliance and low chest wall compliance (i.e., enhanced transmission of airway pressure into the intrathoracic space) are particularly susceptible to circulatory impairment from elevated airway pressure. On the other hand, such adverse effects are unlikely to occur in patients with poorly compliant lungs, especially if the chest wall is distensible, because transmission of airway pressure in these patients is attenuated.

The decrease in venous return is caused by a reduction in the transmural pressure of the intrathoracic veins as the pressure around them increases. Therefore, restoration of venous return will occur at the expense of an elevated systemic venous pressure. An impairment in venous and lymphatic drainage, coupled with possible decrease in arterial pressure, flow, and oxygen transport, has been reported to affect the function of several extrapulmonary tissues and organs, including the central nervous system, the kidney, the gut, the pancreas, and the liver.[29–33] Experimental studies indicate that neural and humoral mechanisms also may mediate impairment in systemic and regional blood flow during PEEP therapy. Finally, deleterious effects of PEEP on end-organ function also depend on disease-related factors such as metabolic state, circulatory performance, and capillary permeability.

The effect of intrathoracic pressure on the forward flow from the right ventricle depends largely on lung volume, which is a major determinant of pulmonary vascular resistance. The effect of elevated intrathoracic pressure on left ventricular output depends on venous return and right ventricular function for its preload and is additionally influenced by the effect of pleural pressure on left ventricular afterload. An elevation in intrathoracic pressure effects a decrease in left ventricular afterload. For a detailed discussion of cardiopulmonary interaction, the reader is referred to Chapter 102.

Application of positive airway pressure to an injured lung could easily be construed to result in further structural damage to the respiratory system. However, complications such as pneumothorax, pneumomediastinum, and interstitial pulmonary emphysema, which are seen in patients receiving mechanical ventilatory support, are rare in patients who breathe spontaneously with positive airway pressure. Therefore, in looking for a connection between positive airway pressure therapy and pulmonary trauma, the more logical culprit is the mechanical ventilation, not the expiratory airway pressure per se.[34, 35] Application of PEEP will definitely lead to an increase in end-inspiratory airway pressure and lung volume achieved during the mechanical breaths if mechanical ventilatory support is maintained unchanged. However, if PEEP is applied appropriately, the associated improvement in lung mechanics should allow a reduction in mechanical ventilatory support with fewer positive-pressure cycles, which should reduce the risk of respiratory therapy-related lung damage.

An analogous reasoning applies to the derangement in $\dot{V}/\dot{Q}$ matching that can be induced by overinflating the lung with positive airway pressure. Mechanical positive-pressure breaths have been shown to be inherently inefficient in augmenting gas exchange because of the propensity of the mechanical tidal volume to be distributed to the nondependent, least perfused regions of the lung.[36, 37] Although this tendency can be aggravated by simultaneous application of PEEP, $\dot{V}/\dot{Q}$ matching will improve if the improvement in lung mechanics effected by PEEP allows a reduction in mechanical ventilatory support and an increase in spontaneous breathing activity without excessive work of breathing.

In cases of severe, distinctly localized pulmonary parenchymal disease, application of positive airway pressure may not cause improvement in the $\dot{V}/\dot{Q}$ relationships of the affected area. Instead, overinflation of the unaffected regions of the lung may shift perfusion toward the nonventilated lung units. Consequently, arterial blood oxygenation may not respond to the application of PEEP but may actually be impaired by it.[38]

MECHANICAL VENTILATORY SUPPORT

Partial and Total Ventilatory Support

Considerable variability exists in the application of ventilatory support among institutions, disciplines, and individual practitioners. Most often, however, the techniques used allow administration of variable levels of ventilatory support. Partial ventilatory support has been traditionally seen as an independent ventilatory technique; hence, for instance, controversy results between controlled mechanical ventilation and IMV. In reality, conventional controlled mechanical ventilation and IMV are merely different levels of ventilatory support administered by using the same basic technique. Fortunately, modern respiratory care considers partial ventilatory support as a necessary feature of any useful ventilatory modality.

Mechanical ventilatory support in patients with acute respiratory failure provides symptomatic treatment of alveolar hypoventilation or increased respiratory work. Ventilator therapy reverses respiratory acidemia and relieves the patient of ventilatory work, but it does not correct the primary cause of ventilatory failure. In fact, the application of a high level of mechanical ventilatory support usually induces some impairment in cardiopulmonary function. Controlling ventilation beyond a comfortable level of spontaneous work of breathing and adequate alveolar ventilation has not been shown to be advantageous to the patient. Differences in hemodynamic performance between total and partial ventilatory support have not been shown, even in patients with ischemic heart disease and left ventricular dysfunction, a patient group that would likely benefit from high airway and intrathoracic pressure.[39] Therefore, controlled ventilation should be seen as an extreme on the spectrum of ventilatory support, and its use should be justified for each individual patient.

Control of ventilation is possible only in a patient whose intrinsic drive to breathe has been extinguished or whose neuromuscular impulse transmission has been blocked. Respiratory drive can be removed by lowering the arterial blood carbon dioxide tension below the effective apneic threshold. To avoid respiratory alkalemia, sedatives are often used to raise the apneic threshold so that ventilation can be controlled while the patient still is normocapnic. However, deep sedation and prolonged neuromuscular blockade are not without side effects. Sedatives may adversely affect cardiovascular performance, and prolonged use of muscle relaxants has been reported to cause longstanding abnormalities of neuromuscular function.[40] Furthermore, loss of muscle tone and motion requires intense nursing care to prevent complications related to immobilization, and loss of spontaneous breathing activity makes accidental disconnection from the ventilator life threatening within minutes. To avoid deep sedation and muscle paralysis, hyperventilation and respiratory alkalosis are frequently necessary if ventilation is to be controlled. Unfortunately, respiratory alkalosis is associated with a decrease in systemic oxygen delivery while simultaneously increasing oxygen consumption. A decrease in cerebral blood flow and bronchospasm may constitute additional hazards to critically ill patients.[41] A patient who, to some extent, is allowed to breathe spontaneously will usually regulate the arterial pH to normal.[42, 43] When a sufficient level of partial ventilatory support is given, side effects of deep sedation and muscle relaxation are avoided without the need to induce respiratory alkalemia.

The lower efficiency of gas exchange and the increased ventilatory requirement during mechanical positive-pressure ventilation compared with spontaneous breathing has been referred to earlier and is discussed in detail in Chapter 102. Controlled mechanical ventilation of long duration has been reported to reduce respiratory muscle strength and cause uncoordinated breathing when spontaneous ventilation is resumed.[44] Impaired strength and coordination of the respiratory system may lead to prolongation of ventilatory insufficiency and protracted weaning to spontaneous breathing long after the initial cause of respiratory failure has disappeared. Maintenance of some spontaneous breathing activity during the course of ventilator therapy is likely to maintain better respiratory muscle strength and coordination than complete artificial control of ventilation. However, because excessive workload also may decrease muscle strength, ventilatory support sufficient to maintain spontaneous work of breathing within tolerable range must always be provided.[45]

From a theoretical standpoint, the decrease in intrathoracic pressure during spontaneous breathing with partial ventilatory support should be detrimental to patients with left ventricular dysfunction, because the fall in intrathoracic pressure increases left ventricular afterload. Moreover, the dilated, failing ventricle may not respond favorably to increased filling secondary to augmented venous return. Several studies emphasize the urgent need for adequate ventilatory support and CPAP in patients with cardiogenic respiratory failure.[39, 46] However, studies in patients with acute myocardial infarction and heart failure have shown that even patients with heart failure can tolerate normal work of breathing and that control of ventilation is not indicated to support circulatory function.[39]

Although the exact association between structural pulmonary damage and mechanical ventilator support remains obscure, it stands to reason that trauma secondary to hyperinflation or overpressurization of the respiratory system would be minimized during spontaneous breathing and maximized when ventilation is controlled using positive-pressure ventilation with high tidal volume. Some substantiation of this claim is offered by clinical studies that show an association between high peak airway pressure and pulmonary barotrauma.[34] The possible significance of a reduced number of positive-pressure lung inflations is suggested by a study in which partial ventilatory support with IMV appeared to lower the incidence of barotrauma in adult patients.[35] The most convincing evidence of ventilator-related lung injury comes from studies showing reduced risk of bronchopulmonary dysplasia in neonates with respiratory failure undergoing cardiopulmonary support with extracorporeal membrane oxygenation.[47] Avoidance of ventilator-induced pulmonary injury would, therefore, favor the use of the least necessary amount of partial ventilatory support. Whether ventilatory modalities other than conventional positive-pressure ventilation are associated with reduced risk of respiratory system trauma at the same level of support remains to be seen.

Use of partial ventilatory support is the basis of weaning the patient from the ventilator. The flexibility of partial support allows gradual reduction rather than sudden discontinuation of ventilatory support and is an essential feature of a clinically useful modern ventilatory support technique. Opposition to weaning with partial support instead of a "T-piece trial" has over the years turned into a tendency to apply slow tapering of mechanical ventilation with frequent blood gas analysis even to postoperative patients with normal pulmonary function recovering from general anesthesia.[48–50] Although inappropriate and cost ineffective, this practice probably is not dangerous. However, to discontinue full ventilatory support abruptly in a patient recovering from cardiogenic respiratory failure would be both highly inappropriate and extremely dangerous.[39] The proper use of partial ventilatory support in weaning is discussed in detail in Chapter 103.

VENTILATION WITH AN INCREASE IN AIRWAY PRESSURE

Three major ventilatory techniques rely on increase in airway pressure to generate tidal volume: IMV, mandatory minute ventilation (MMV), and PSV. They differ from one another primarily in the method of interfacing spontaneous breathing and mechanical ventilation. From a physiologic standpoint, when used to provide near-total ventilatory support, these techniques are very similar. It is noteworthy that PSV cannot be used to provide full ventilatory support because the mechanical breaths are triggered by spontaneous effort.

Assisted mechanical ventilation (AMV) and inverse inspiratory-expiratory ratio ventilation (IRV) are frequently viewed as independent modes of ventilatory support. However, neither technique is capable of providing adjustable ventilatory support; therefore, these techniques cannot be used independently. Actually, they represent special cases of PSV and airway pressure release ventilation (APRV), respectively. They are discussed separately here for historic reasons.

Intermittent Mandatory Ventilation

During IMV, positive-pressure breaths are delivered with an operator-adjusted mechanical rate, while unassisted spontaneous breathing is allowed to occur simultaneously. The mechanical breaths can be synchronized to be triggered by spontaneous breathing efforts. The mechanical breaths can be cycled or limited in any way. Mechanical ventilatory support during IMV may vary from 0% to 100% of total minute ventilation or ventilatory work. If full control of ventilation is desired, the frequency of mandatory breaths is increased until the arterial blood carbon dioxide tension decreases below the apneic threshold and the patient stops breathing spontaneously. Weaning is accomplished by decreasing the frequency of mechanical breaths gradually to zero.

IMV remains the ventilatory technique most widely used in critically ill patients at present. Considering the range of ventilatory support that can be provided with IMV, there are few patients whose ventilatory support cannot be managed with IMV alone. There are no scientific data available to indicate that a more favorable outcome would result in any patient group from the use of an alternative ventilatory modality. Therefore, IMV will likely remain as the basic ventilatory technique well into the future.

Mandatory Minute Ventilation

MMV provides conventional positive-pressure mechanical ventilatory support in a fashion similar to the function of an on-demand cardiac pacemaker. The original MMV circuit of Hewlett consisted of separate gas reservoirs for spontaneous breathing and for the ventilator, which received fresh gas from a common source.[51] The total flow of gas to these reservoirs was adjusted to the desired minute ventilation. If spontaneous minute ventilation was lower than the fresh gas flow, the excess gas flow was diverted to the ventilator reservoir and delivered to the patient with a mandatory positive-pressure breath. Therefore, a patient whose spontaneous ventilation matches the desired level receives no mechanical ventilation, whereas an apneic patient receives the predetermined minute volume in a fashion indistinguishable from conventional controlled mechanical ventilation. If the patient breathes spontaneously less than the preset minute volume, the ventilator provides for the difference. The term *EMMV* is used by some ventilator manufacturers to denote a modification that allows spontaneous breathing beyond the set minute ventilation.

Inverse Ratio Ventilation

IRV is mechanical ventilation with an inspiratory-expiratory time ratio greater than 1. The extended inspiration is designed to maintain mean alveolar pressure to maximally recruit alveolar units with long time constants without generating a high peak airway pressure. IRV can be applied either with a volume-controlled (VC) or pressure-controlled (PC) technique. During VC-IRV, inspiratory time is extended with slow inspiratory flow, an end-inspiratory pause, or decelerating inspiratory flow. During PC-IRV, constant pressure applied to the airway for the duration of the inspiration results in a decelerating gas flow into the lungs. Several practical differences exist between VC-IRV and PC-IRV.[52] VC-IRV allows control of minute ventilation and inspiratory flow but requires careful monitoring of the airway and alveolar pressures. PC-IRV permits exact adjustment of airway pressure but may result in considerable variation in tidal volume and minute ventilation. Almost any ventilator can be adjusted to deliver VC-IRV, whereas PC-IRV requires a ventilator specifically designed to deliver this modality. Nevertheless, most of the data regarding the use of IRV in adults have been generated with PC-IRV. PC-IRV is identical to APRV when APRV is used to control ventilation. The relationship between PC-IRV and APRV is similar to that between conventional controlled positive-pressure ventilation and IMV, and, from a physiologic standpoint, the two may be viewed as different levels of one ventilatory technique.

Assisted Mechanical Ventilation

AMV is a ventilatory modality in which the ventilator responds to each spontaneous breathing effort with a positive-pressure mechanical breath. The triggering event usually is a small decrease in airway pressure at the beginning of a spontaneous inspiration. The ventilator breath may be delivered using any type of cycling with or without positive expiratory airway pressure. Ventilation with AMV relies on a spontaneous drive to breathe, and full ventilatory support cannot be delivered using this technique. Consequently, a back-up modality must be provided for patients who may become apneic (assist-control ventilation). The tidal volume delivered from the ventilator depends on the ventilator settings and is not sensitive to the patient. Therefore, AMV does not provide a method for transition from mechanical ventilation to spontaneous breathing. Weaning is accomplished by simply discontinuing mechanical ventilation or by switching to another technique.

AMV was developed in an attempt to allow better synchronization between the ventilator and the patient. Because the patient controls the ventilatory rate during AMV, this technique was believed to allow nearly full ventilatory support without the need for massive sedation or hyperventilation. However, studies by Marini and colleagues have since demonstrated that a patient receiving AMV usually continues the spontaneous breathing effort throughout the mechanical cycle and contributes significantly to total ventilatory work.[53, 54] Under favorable conditions, the patient's respiratory work amounts to 33% to 50% of the energy required for passive lung-thorax inflation and may, under less favorable conditions, even exceed that of passive lung inflation. Therefore, AMV provides an uncontrolled and variable amount of breath-to-breath partial ventilatory support.

Pressure Support Ventilation

PSV, also termed *inspiratory assist* or *assisted spontaneous breathing,* originally was developed as an adjunct to MMV to augment spontaneous tidal volume and, in particular, to overcome high circuit resistance during spontaneous breathing.[55] Inefficient, rapid, shallow, spontaneous respiration that contributed little to alveolar ventilation was sensed by the MMV ventilators as part of the MMV, which resulted in inadequate ventilatory support. To avoid this, some ventilators were modified to provide additional gas flow up to an adjustable pressure limit during spontaneous inspiration. Hansen and associates used PSV without conventional positive-pressure breaths as a weaning technique, thus initiating its use as a new ventilatory support modality.[56]

During PSV, the patient's spontaneous inspiration triggers the ventilator to provide a variable gas flow that increases until airway pressure reaches a preselected level above baseline. A servocontrolled mechanism adjusts the flow to keep inspiratory airway pressure constant. When the patient's inspiratory effort wanes, flow decreases. When patient demand for inspiratory flow is sufficiently reduced, flow terminates and airway pressure returns to baseline. Thus, during each spontaneous respiratory effort, the patient receives assisted ventilation with a mechanism that is pressure limited and flow cycled. The amount of inspiratory work of breathing performed by the ventilator during PSV depends on the pressure level and the patient's respiratory mechanics and cannot be determined directly. If the pressure support level is elevated sufficiently, most of the respiratory work is performed by the ventilator, and the ventilatory mode is similar to conventional assisted positive-pressure ventilation.[56, 57] The major theoretical advantage of PSV is adjustable breath-to-breath ventilatory assistance, in which each respiratory cycle is similar in configuration and equally assisted by the ventilator. This may facilitate adaptation of the patient to the ventilator and weaning from ventilatory support. Because the patient controls respiratory rate and the duration of inspiration, the development of respiratory alkalosis, frequently seen during AMV, should be less likely.

The level of pressure support is normally adjusted to achieve a desired tidal volume, ventilatory rate, and patient comfort. During successful weaning from PSV, the patient maintains an adequate tidal volume and acceptable ventilatory rate by increasing relative spontaneous ventilatory effort as the pressure support level is gradually decreased to zero or to a level that represents work done against the resistance of the breathing circuit.

Appropriate use of PSV requires that it be recognized as a method of administering variable positive-pressure mechanical ventilatory support and not a form of spontaneous breathing. Although the patient triggers all PSV breaths and the progression of the assisted breath is dependent on the patient continuing to perform ventilatory work, high levels of pressure support provide nearly full ventilatory assistance. Even low levels of pressure support may contribute significantly to the patient's tidal volume and minute ventilation. A patient with a respiratory system compliance of 100 mL/cm H_2O receives a 500-mL mechanical contribution to tidal volume when receiving 5 cm H_2O of pressure support. Adequate alveolar ventilation with these settings does not guarantee that the patient will be able to maintain full unsupported spontaneous ventilation.

Proportional Assist Ventilation

Proportional assist ventilation (PAV) was described by Younes in 1992.[58] Like PSV, this technique provides breath-to-breath ventilatory assistance with positive airway pressure. However, the amount of airway pressure support during PAV is effort dependent. The PAV ventilator applies positive airway pressure support of inspiration that is proportional to the instantaneous inspiratory flow and volume generated by the patient (Fig. 98–4). The response of the

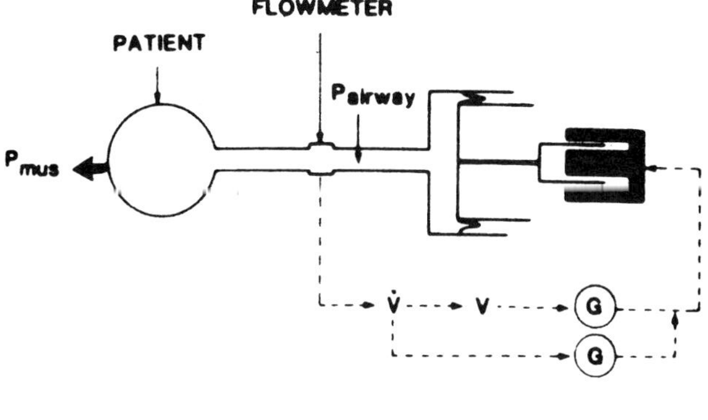

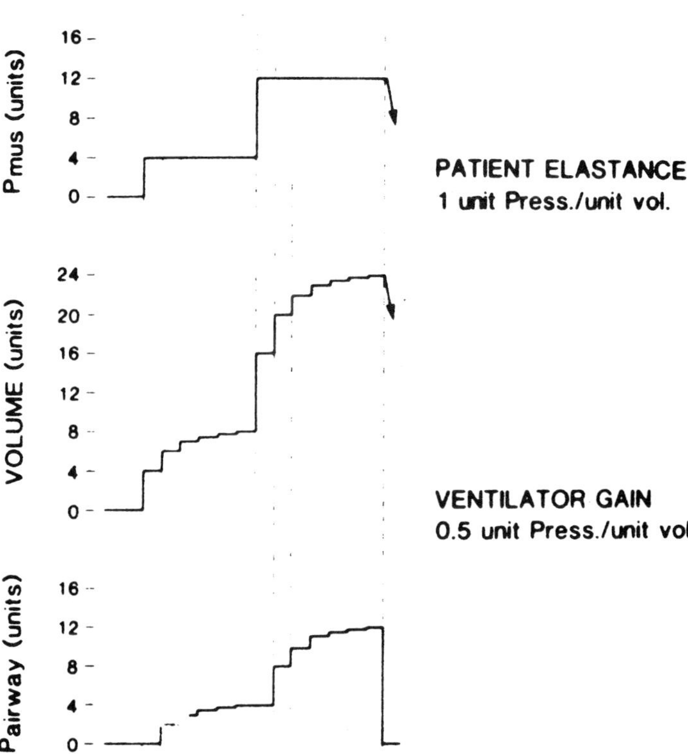

Figure 98–4. *Top,* Schematic diagram of a PAV delivery system. *Abbreviations:* Pmus = a patient's inspiratory effort; V̇ = instantaneous flow; V = instantaneous volume; G = gain controls. *Bottom,* A schematic representation of events during a PAV-supported inspiration. For the purposes of illustration, events are shown to occur in discrete steps, and all units are arbitrary. Resistance is assumed to be zero. With the ventilator gain set to 50% of the patient's respiratory system elastance, an increment of volume results in an increase in airway pressure support equivalent to one half of the muscle pressure required by the patient to generate that volume. At the left side of the graphs, the volume increment is generated by the patient with 4 units of muscle pressure. The ventilator responds with 2 units of pressure, which produce an additional 2 units of volume. The ventilator continues to respond to the volume change it generated with diminishing increments in airway pressure (because the ventilator gain is lower than the patient's elastance) until an increase in the patient's effort calls for further support. (From Younes M: Proportional assist ventilation, a new approach to ventilatory support: Theory. Am Rev Respir Dis 1992; 145:114.)

ventilator can be altered by adjusting two separate gain controls: one that responds to an increase in flow and another that responds to an increase in volume. Therefore, the type of ventilator assistance can be weighted to reduce workloads secondary to altered resistance or elastance.

Initial results from investigation applying PAV with an experimental ventilator to four normal individuals during rest and exercise and to five stable ventilator-dependent patients have been reported by Younes and colleagues.[59] On average, the normal subjects responded to PAV by decreasing ventilatory effort, while maintaining ventilation and breathing pattern relatively unchanged. However, some subjects appeared to use the assistance preferentially to reduce muscle pressure, whereas others maintained a relatively strong spontaneous effort and let PAV augment flow and volume. In ventilator-dependent patients, PAV resulted in a 54% average decrease in peak airway pressure compared with synchronized IMV. Peak airway pressure was frequently lower during PAV even for ventilatory cycles with a tidal volume equivalent to or larger than that delivered by the IMV. An acceptable tidal volume and ventilatory rate was achieved with PAV in each patient; ventilation and oxygenation were comparable to those recorded during IMV and remained unchanged during the 1- to 3-hour PAV trial. The feasibility of providing effort-related support with PAV could be confirmed by the investigators both in normal subjects and in ventilator-dependent patients (Fig. 98–5). The technique was well accepted by all subjects, and no complications occurred.

The potential advantages of PAV result from patient control of the ventilator throughout the ventilatory cycle. Because the ventilator adjusts its output according to instantaneous patient effort, fighting the ventilator and the need for sedation should be minimized. Synchronization of patient and ventilator effort allows delivery of flow and volume with minimum increases in airway pressure, and maintenance of patient control throughout the cycle should preserve natural ventilatory control mechanisms and decrease the likelihood of hypocapnia.

PAV augments tidal ventilation with positive airway pressure and is, therefore, associated with the circulatory and respiratory side effects common to ventilatory modalities of its general class. Like other breath-to-breath support techniques, PAV depends on the patient's ventilatory drive and does not provide ventilation to an apneic patient. From the effort-related assistance, it also follows that PAV does

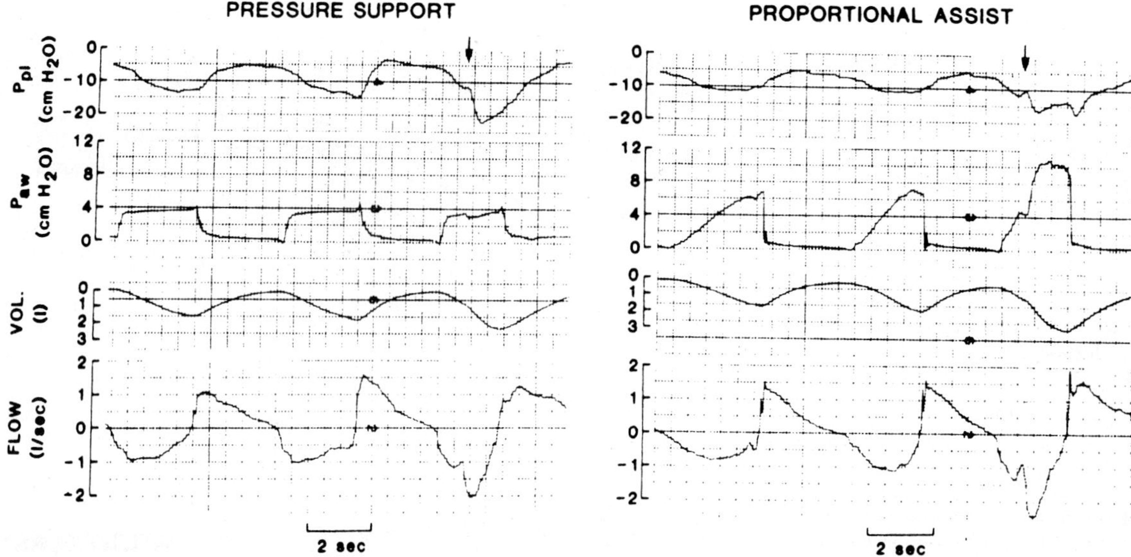

Figure 98–5. Intrathoracic pressure (Ppl), airway pressure (Paw), volume (V), and flow tracings of a patient during ventilation with PSV and PAV. Increase in the patient's respiratory effort *(arrow)* is not met with a response from PSV. However, PAV participates in the effort by augmenting airway pressure and ventilatory assistance, which results in increased inspiratory flow and VT with only a small change in intrathoracic pressure. (From Younes M, Puddy A, Roberts D, et al: Proportional assist ventilation: Results of an initial clinical trial. Am Rev Respir Dis 1992; 145:121.)

not rapidly correct hypoventilation resulting from an inadequate ventilatory drive. On the other hand, augmentation of the effects of any ventilatory stimuli by PAV may lead to manifestation of periodic breathing in susceptible patients.[59] Because the breathing pattern during PAV is controlled by the patient, and not the ventilator, the application of PAV or increasing the level of support may not normalize the pattern. For example, as pointed out by Younes,[58] rapid, shallow breathing may be normalized with PAV if it is secondary to a derangement in pulmonary mechanics, but it may be unaffected if it is a consequence of abnormal reflex activity.

To determine the significance of the potential advantages and limitations of PAV requires investigations on a larger scale. The interaction between the patient and the ventilator is poorly developed in currently used ventilatory techniques. Therefore, some aspects of PAV are likely to be quickly adopted to ventilatory care.

VENTILATION BY DECREASE IN AIRWAY PRESSURE

Airway Pressure Release Ventilation

Stock, Downs, and Frolicher introduced APRV in 1987.[60] It was the first ventilatory technique that produced augmentation of alveolar ventilation by decrease in airway pressure and lung volume. The APRV ventilator consists of a CPAP circuit that maintains baseline airway pressure above ambient. Alteration in lung volume is accomplished using intermittent release of CPAP (Fig. 98–6). To accomplish a rapid release of positive airway pressure, a release valve is situated in the expiratory limb of the CPAP circuit. The release valve must have sufficiently low flow resistance to allow adequate emptying of the lungs during pressure release. The release valve is controlled with a timer that allows adjustment of the duration and frequency of pressure release. APRV is designed to augment alveolar ventilation as an adjunct to spontaneous breathing with CPAP.[61] Therefore, it is assumed that the patient who is to receive APRV has parenchymal lung injury that requires CPAP therapy and that the CPAP therapy has been optimized to produce the lung volume associated with the best available lung mechanics and gas exchange. Augmentation of alveolar ventilation during APRV is determined by the APRV rate and tidal volume. The tidal volume depends on lung compliance, airway resistance, release time, and the difference between CPAP and the airway pressure during the release phase. The patient can breathe freely at any time during the APRV cycle. If the release frequency and tidal volume are sufficient to lower the patient's arterial blood carbon dioxide below apneic threshold, controlled ventilation will result. Weaning from APRV entails lowering the release frequency

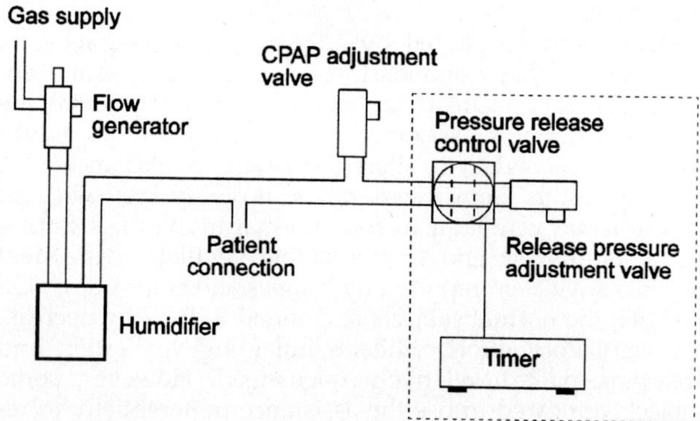

Figure 98–6. Diagram of the original APRV circuit modified from a high-flow CPAP assembly by the addition of a timer-controlled airway pressure release valve and of a second threshold resistor valve to the circuit *(dotted box)*. A high flow of humidified gas is provided to the breathing circuit to maintain a nearly constant level of CPAP during spontaneous inspiration and during exhalation. To assist breathing, CPAP is interrupted briefly by opening a pressure release valve; this allows a transient decrease in lung volume to a level determined by the release pressure valve. After closure of the pressure release valve, FRC is reestablished.

until the patient is breathing with CPAP without any APRV breaths.

Initial experimental and clinical investigations showed that alveolar ventilation and arterial oxygenation can be maintained effectively using APRV.[60, 62] Experimental studies comparing APRV and conventional positive-pressure ventilation found no significant differences in oxygenation or ventilation in animals with normal lung function when the two ventilatory modalities were delivered using similar airway pressure, tidal volume, and ventilator rate. However, in dogs with oleic acid–induced lung injury, the use of APRV resulted in significantly lower arterial blood carbon dioxide tension and higher arterial blood oxygen tension compared with PPV. These results suggested that the airway pressure pattern of APRV may favor a more uniform distribution of ventilation than PPV in injured lungs. A study comparing spontaneous breathing, APRV, and PPV using a similar level of CPAP in dogs with oleic acid–induced lung injury revealed that ventilatory failure and arterial desaturation that existed during spontaneous breathing could be effectively corrected by either APRV or PPV.[63] In this study, arterial blood oxygenation was significantly better and venous admixture lower during PPV. The differences in oxygenation may have reflected mean transpulmonary pressure that, by design, was lower during APRV, or it may have resulted from reduction and redistribution of pulmonary blood flow during PPV. Nevertheless, systemic oxygen delivery was far superior during APRV because it preserved circulatory function even when ventilation was controlled by hyperventilating the animal.

By design, peak airway pressure during APRV equals the CPAP level (Fig. 98–7). Augmentation of alveolar ventilation with low peak airway pressure and without overdistention of the lung parenchyma appears to be a consistent major advantage of APRV. Changeover from positive-pressure ventilation to APRV has been shown to allow a 30% to 75% reduction in peak airway pressure both in experimental and clinical studies.[63–65] The peak airway pressure reduction depends on lung mechanics and on whether APRV and positive-pressure ventilation have been adjusted to a similar mean airway pressure or to a similar level of CPAP.

Not surprisingly, no differences in circulatory function have been observed between APRV and PPV in studies that have used similar levels of mean airway pressure.[60, 62, 64, 65] This has been the case regardless of the presence or absence of acute lung injury or the volume status of the experimental animal or the patient. However, APRV originally was designed to be used as an adjunct to CPAP therapy. When APRV and PPV are added to existing CPAP therapy, the hemodynamic advantages of APRV become obvious. An experimental investigation in dogs with induced lung injury revealed that ventilation could be controlled using APRV, with no depression of stroke volume, cardiac output, and tissue oxygen delivery compared with spontaneous breathing with CPAP. When positive-pressure ventilation was used in a similar fashion, stroke volume decreased by 42%, oxygen delivery diminished by 32%, and the oxygen utilization coefficient increased by 33%.[63]

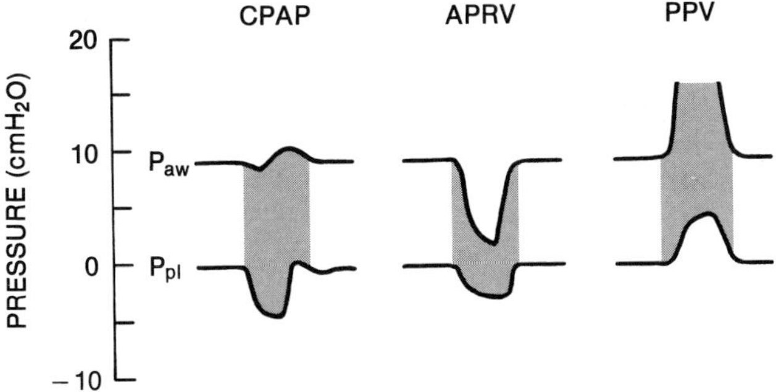

Figure 98–7. Changes in Paw and Ppl during spontaneous breathing with CPAP, during APRV, and during conventional positive pressure ventilation (PPV). Note the similarity in the intrathoracic pressure pattern between spontaneous breathing and APRV, the decrease in transpulmonary pressure *(dotted area)* during APRV, and the high peak airway pressure during PPV. (From Räsänen J, Downs JB, Stock MC: Cardiovascular effects of positive pressure ventilation and airway pressure release ventilation. Chest 1988; 93:911–915.)

The usefulness of APRV in providing ventilatory support to patients has been addressed in four clinical studies. Garner and colleagues compared APRV and positive-pressure ventilation with similar mean airway pressures in patients with mild acute lung injury after cardiopulmonary bypass and found the two modalities to be equally effective in providing ventilation and oxygenation.[62] Peak airway pressure, however, was significantly reduced during APRV; no differences in circulatory function were detected. All patients were weaned successfully from ventilatory support using APRV without complications. In a prospective short-term study, 47 of 50 adult patients with moderate to severe acute respiratory failure were adequately ventilated with APRV.[64] Institution of APRV effected a reduction in peak airway pressure by $55 \pm 17\%$ compared with conventional ventilation. No significant effects on oxygenation or circulatory function were documented. Apart from inadequate alveolar ventilation in three patients, likely resulting from inadequate adjustment of APRV, no complications were reported. Cane and associates reported data from 18 adult patients with severe acute respiratory failure, sequentially ventilated with conventional positive-pressure ventilation and APRV.[65] APRV provided effective ventilatory support to 17 of the 18 patients, with peak airway pressure significantly lower than that during positive-pressure ventilation. One patient experienced unexplained cardiopulmonary decompensation after initiation of APRV; six patients who initially responded well to APRV were later returned to positive-pressure ventilation because of lobar atelectasis (two), hypoxemia (two), and inadequate ventilation (two). The authors attributed the development of atelectasis to the volume-variable nature of APRV. Valentine and coworkers, in comparing APRV, IMV, and PSV in eight patients recovering from open heart operations, found that APRV provided adequate ventilation with the lowest peak airway pressure and dead space ventilation (Table 98–2).[66] No differences in oxygenation of arterial blood and no complications were seen during APRV.

Airway pressure levels of at least 20 cm H_2O can be maintained safely using a tight-fitting mask in most patients who have intact protective airway reflexes. Because airway pressure during APRV never exceeds the CPAP level, it may be clinically feasible to commence APRV in a patient receiving mask CPAP therapy without tracheal intubation. Jousela and associates described a patient with myasthenia gravis in whom postoperative weaning from mechanical ventilation and removal of the tracheal tube was accomplished successfully by using APRV with a mask CPAP circuit.[67]

Available experimental and clinical data indicate that a marked lowering of peak airway pressure is a major advantage of APRV. Depending on the method of application, mean airway and mean intrathoracic pressure may be reduced as well. Consequently, the use of APRV may lower the incidence of airway pressure or lung volume–related pulmonary trauma and the severity of circulatory impairment associated with mechanical ventilatory support. The

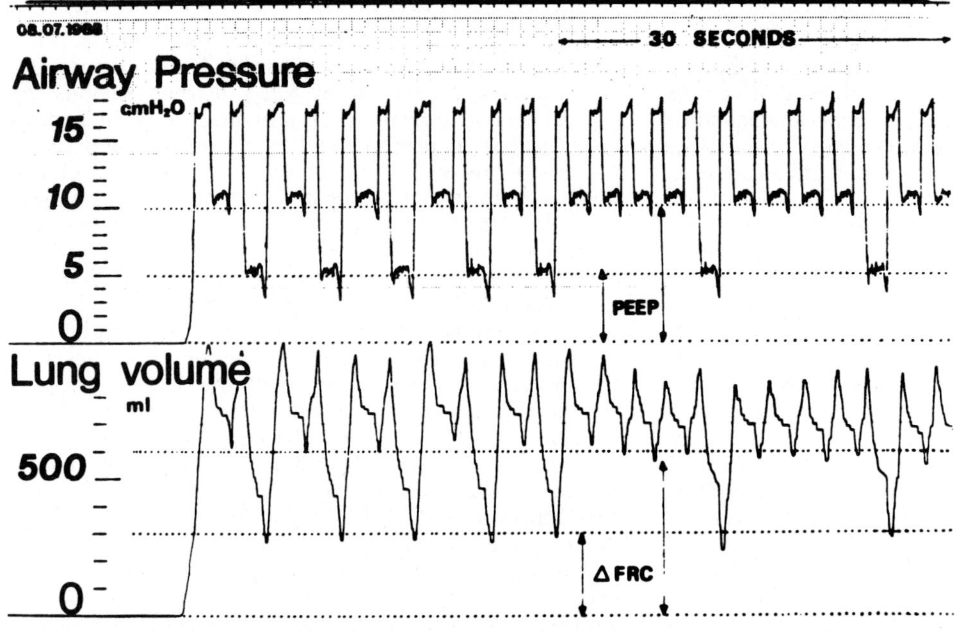

Figure 98–8. Simultaneous changes in airway pressure and lung volume in a patient under IMPRV (CESAR ventilator). PEEP is released from 11 to 5 cm H_2O, and an inspiratory pressure support of 6 cm H_2O is used. First, PEEP is released every two spontaneous respiratory cycles and, later, every five spontaneous respiratory cycles. The increase in lung volume above apneic functional residual capacity (ΔFRC) oscillates with PEEP release from 300 mL to 600 mL. ΔFRC changes are not modified by decreasing the rate of PEEP release. (From Rouby JJ: Pressure release ventilation. *In:* Update in Intensive Care Medicine. Vincent JL [Ed]. Vol. 10. Berlin, Springer-Verlag, 1990, pp 185–195.)

low airway pressure during APRV may allow this form of ventilation to be delivered effectively without tracheal intubation in some cases. Sufficient data are not available to assess the effect of APRV on cardiopulmonary function over several days of ventilatory support or to define clearly the optimum pressure levels and the duration of pressure release during ventilation with APRV. However, APRV may offer clinically important advantages and improve the care of patients requiring ventilatory support. Therefore, further development of this technique deserves attention.

Intermittent Mandatory Pressure Release Ventilation

Intermittent mandatory pressure release ventilation (IMPRV)[68] combines PSV with CPAP and APRV. The IMPRV cycle begins with a pressure support breath, which is followed by airway pressure release below the initial level of CPAP (Fig. 98–8). The desired amount of mechanical ventilatory support is given by adjusting the ratio of spontaneous and IMPRV breaths. Breath-to-breath ventilatory support, synchronization of mechanical breaths to spontaneous breathing, and the ability to alter airway pressure independently above and below CPAP are potential advantages of IMPRV over APRV.[69] IMPRV requires a microprocessor-controlled ventilator that is programmed to deliver this mode of ventilation and thus contrasts with the simplicity and low cost of APRV. The feasibility of IMPRV has been demonstrated in patients with acute respiratory failure.[70] Results of comparisons between IMPRV and other modalities of mechanical ventilatory support are not yet available.

TABLE 98–2. Pulmonary Mechanics, Blood Gas Values, and Inert Gas Data from Nine Patients Ventilated with Synchronized IMV, PSV, and APRV after Cardiac Operations*

Variable	*SIMV*	*PSV*	*APRV*
Peak Paw	32.8 ± 1.3	19.4 ± 2.1†	14.3 ± 1.0†
(cm H_2O)	9.6 ± 1.1	8.4 ± 1.0	11.0 ± 0.7‡
Mean Paw	9.4 ± 0.6	9.0 ± 0.5	7.5 ± 0.7
(cm H_2O)	102.0 ± 7.0	98.0 ± 8.0	94.0 ± 8.0
$\dot{V}$E (L/min)	33.0 ± 2.0	39.0 ± 2.0†	40.0 ± 2.0†
Pa_{O_2} (mm Hg)	15.4 ± 1.7	18.2 ± 2.7	19.9 ± 2.3†
Pa_{CO_2} (mm Hg)	36.2 ± 1.5	37.1 ± 2.7	30.1 ± 1.7†
Shunt (%)			
Dead space (%)			

(Modified with permission from Valentine DD, Hammond MD, Downs JB, et al: Distribution of ventilation and perfusion with different modes of mechanical ventilation. Am Rev Respir Dis 1991, 143:1262.)

*Values represent mean ± standard error of the mean.

†$P < .05$ v. SIMV.

‡$P < .05$ v. PSV.

Abbreviations: Paw = airway pressure; $\dot{V}$E = expired minute volume; SIMV = synchronized intermittent mandatory ventilation; PSV = pressure support ventilation; APRV = airway pressure release ventilation; Pa_{O_2} = partial pressure of arterial oxygen; Pa_{CO_2} = partial pressure of arterial carbon dioxide.

CONCLUDING REMARKS

Despite the large number of ventilatory modalities already available, new techniques are still being introduced. With the development of sophisticated controlling techniques to adapt ventilator function to the patient's needs better, some improvements in ventilatory therapy may indeed occur. However, it would be reasonable to expect that the clinical value of a new ventilatory technique is demonstrated scientifically by showing its superiority in therapeutic efficacy, safety, ease of operation, or cost in the patient group for which it is intended. The development of mechanical ventilation clearly has not proceeded according to these criteria, and considerable research is needed to establish the basis for the clinical use of most already existing ventilatory modalities and for any new techniques yet to come.

References

1. Räsänen J, Leon MA, Cane RD: Adaptation of pressure support ventilation to increasing ventilatory demand during experimental airway obstruction and acute lung injury. Crit Care Med 1993; 21:562.
2. Zarins CK, Bayne CG, Rice CL, et al: Does spontaneous ventilation with IMV protect from PEEP induced cardiac output depression? J Surg Res 1977; 22:299.

3. Gattinoni L, Pesenti A, Bombino M, et al: Relationships between lung computed tomographic density, gas exchange, and PEEP in acute respiratory failure. Anesthesiology 1988; 69:824.
4. Gattinoni L, D'Andrea L, Pelosi P, et al: Regional effects and mechanism of positive end-expiratory pressure in early adult respiratory distress syndrome. JAMA 1993; 269:2122.
5. Douglas ME, Downs JB, Dannemiller FJ, et al: Change in pulmonary venous admixture with varying inspired oxygen. Anesth Analg 1976; 55:688.
6. Gherini S, Peters RM, Virgilio RW: Mechanical work on the lungs and work of breathing with positive end-expiratory pressure and continuous positive airway pressure. Chest 1979; 76:251.
7. Räsänen J, Downs JB: Optimum versus clinically established continuous positive airway pressure in respiratory therapy. J Clin Monit 1988; 4:235.
8. Cormier Y, Couture J, Desmeules M: Changes in upper airway resistance with lung inflation and positive airway pressure. J Appl Physiol 1990; 68:1075.
9. Sotomayor JL Godinez RL, Borden S et al: Large-airway collapse due to acquired tracheobronchomalacia in infancy. Am J Dis Child 1986; 140:367.
10. Ferguson GT, Benoist J: Nasal continuous positive airway pressure in the treatment of tracheobronchomalacia. Am Rev Respir Dis 1993; 147:457.
11. Marini JJ: Should PEEP be used in airflow obstruction? Am Rev Respir Dis 1989; 140:1.
12. Qvist J, Anderson JB, Pemberton M, et al: High-level PEEP in severe asthma. N Engl J Med 1982; 307:1347.
13. Tuxen DV: Detrimental effects of positive end-expiratory pressure during controlled mechanical ventilation of patients with severe airflow obstruction. Am Rev Respir Dis 1989; 140:5.
14. Smith TC, Marini JJ: Impact of PEEP on lung mechanics and work of breathing in severe airflow obstruction. J Appl Physiol 1988; 65:1488.
15. Petrof BJ, Legare M, Goldberg P, et al: Continuous positive airway pressure reduces the work of breathing and dyspnea during weaning from mechanical ventilation in severe chronic obstructive pulmonary disease. Am Rev Respir Dis 1990; 141:281.
16. Dall'ava-Santucci J, Armaganidis A, Brunet F, et al: Mechanical effects of PEEP in patients with adult respiratory distress syndrome. J Appl Physiol 1990; 68:843.
17. Pesenti A, Pelosi P, Rossi N, et al: The effects of positive end-expiratory pressure on respiratory resistance in patients with the adult respiratory distress syndrome and in normal anesthetized subjects. Am Rev Respir Dis 1991; 144:101.
18. Barach AI, Martin J, Eckman M: Positive pressure respiration and its applications to the treatment of acute pulmonary edema. Ann Intern Med 1938; 12:754.
19. Burford TH, Burbank B: Traumatic wet lung: Observations on certain physiologic fundamentals of thoracic trauma. J Thorac Surg 1945; 14:415.
20. Jensen NK: Recovery of pulmonary function after crushing injuries of the chest. Dis Chest 1952; 22:319.
21. Ashbaugh DG, Petty TL, Bigelow DG, et al: Continuous positive-pressure breathing (CPPB) in adult respiratory distress syndrome. J Thorac Cardiovasc Surg 1969; 57:31.
22. Douglas ME, Downs JB: Cardiopulmonary effects of PEEP and CPAP (Special correspondence). Anesth Analg 1978; 57:347.
23. Sturgeon CL Jr, Douglas ME, Downs JB, et al: Cardiopulmonary effects during spontaneous ventilation. Anesth Analg 1977; 56:633.
24. Scharf SM, Bianco JA, Tow DE, et al: The effects of large negative intrathoracic pressure on left ventricular function in patients with coronary artery disease. Circulation 1981; 63:871.
25. Downs JB, Klein EF Jr, Modell JH: The effect of incremental PEEP on PaO_2 in patients with respiratory failure. Anesth Analg 1973; 52:210.
26. Suter PM, Fairley HB, Isenberg MD: Optimum end-expiratory airway pressure in patients with acute pulmonary failure. N Engl J Med 1975; 292:284.
27. Kirby RR, Downs JB, Civetta JM, et al: High level positive end expiratory pressure (PEEP) in acute respiratory insufficiency. Chest 1975; 67:156.
28. Räsänen J, Downs JB, Hodges MR: Continuous monitoring of gas exchange and oxygen use with dual oximetry. J Clin Anesth 1988; 1:3.
29. Cooper KR, Boswell PA, Choi SC: Safe use of PEEP in patients with severe head injury. J Neurosurg 1985; 63:552.
30. Marquez JM, Douglas ME, Downs JB, et al: Renal function and cardiovascular responses during positive airway pressure. Anesthesiology 1979; 50:393.
31. Arvidsson D, Almquist P, Haglund U: Effects of positive end-expiratory pressure on splanchnic circulation and function in experimental peritonitis. Arch Surg 1991; 126:631.
32. Kahle M, Lippert J, Willemer S, et al: Effects of positive end-expiratory pressure (PEEP) ventilation on the exocrine pancreas in minipigs. Res Exp Med 1991; 191:309.
33. Matuschak GM, Pinsky MR, Rogers RM: Effects of positive end-expiratory pressure on hepatic blood flow and performance. J Appl Physiol 1987; 62:1377.
34. Petersen GW, Baier H: Incidence of pulmonary barotrauma in medical ICU. Crit Care Med 1983; 11:359.
35. Mathru M, Rao TL, Venus B: Ventilator-induced barotrauma in controlled mechanical ventilation versus intermittent mandatory ventilation. Crit Care Med 1983; 11:359.
36. Froese AB, Bryan AC: Effects of anesthesia and paralysis on diaphragmatic mechanics in man. Anesthesiology 1974; 41:242.
37. Wolff G, Brunner JX, Grädel E: Gas exchange during mechanical ventilation and spontaneous breathing. Chest 1986; 89:11.
38. Hawker FH, Torzillo PJ, Southee AE: PEEP and "reverse mismatch": A case where less PEEP is best. Chest 1991; 99:1034.
39. Räsänen J, Nikki P, Heikkilä J: Acute myocardial infarction complicated by respiratory failure: The effects of mechanical ventilation. Chest 1984; 85:21.
40. Hansen-Flaschen J, Cowen J: Neuromuscular blockade in the intensive care unit: More than we bargained for. Am Rev Respir Dis 1993; 147:234.
41. Kilburn KH: Shock, seizures, and coma with alkalosis during mechanical ventilation. Ann Intern Med 1966; 65:977.
42. Culpepper JA, Rinaldo JE, Rogers RM: Effect of mechanical ventilator mode on tendency towards respiratory alkalosis. Am Rev Respir Dis 1985; 132:1075.
43. Hudson LD, Hurlow RS, Craig KC, et al: Does intermittent mandatory ventilation correct respiratory alkalosis in patients receiving assisted mechanical ventilation? Am Rev Respir Dis 1985; 132:1071.
44. Pontoppidan H, Geffin B, Lowenstein E: Acute respiratory failure in the adult. N Engl J Med 1972; 287:743.
45. Roussos C: Respiratory muscle fatigue and ventilatory failure. Chest 1990; 97:89S.
46. Räsänen J, Heikkilä J, Downs JB et al: Continuous positive airway pressure by face mask in the treatment of cardiogenic pulmonary edema. Am J Cardiol 1985; 55:296.
47. Bartlett RH, Toomasian JM, Roloff DW, et al: Extracorporeal membrane oxygenation (ECMO) in neonatal respiratory failure: 100 cases. Ann Surg 1986; 204:236.
48. Downs JB, Douglas ME: Intermittent mandatory ventilation: Why the controversy? Crit Care Med 1981; 9:622.
49. Petty TL: IMV vs. IMC. Chest 1975; 67:630.
50. Weisman IM, Rinaldo JE, Rogers MH: Intermittent mandatory ventilation. Am Rev Respir Dis 1983; 127:641.
51. Hewlett AM, Platt AS, Terry G: Mandatory minute volume: A new concept in weaning from mechanical ventilation. Anaesthesia 1977; 32:163.
52. Marcy TW, Marini JJ: Inverse ratio ventilation in ARDS: Rationale and implementation. Chest 1991; 100:494.
53. Marini JJ, Capps JS, Culver BH: The inspiratory work of breathing during assisted mechanical ventilation. Chest 1985; 87:612.
54. Marini JJ, Rodriguez RM, Lamb V: Bedside estimation of the inspiratory work of breathing during mechanical ventilation. Chest 1986; 89:56.
55. Norlander O: New concepts of ventilation. Acta Anaesth Belg 1982; 33:221.
56. Hansen J, Wendt M, Lawin P: Ein neues weaning-Verfahren (inspiratory flow assistance—IFA). Anaesthesist 1984; 33:428.
57. Banner MJ, Kirby RR: Similarities between pressure support ventilation and intermittent positive-pressure ventilation. Crit Care Med 1985; 13:997.
58. Younes M: Proportional assist ventilation: A new approach to ventilatory support: Theory. Am Rev Respir Dis 1992; 145:114.

59. Younes M, Puddy A, Roberts D, et al: Proportional assist ventilation: Results of an initial clinical trial. Am Rev Respir Dis 1992; 145:121.
60. Stock MC, Downs JB, Frolicher DA: Airway pressure release ventilation. Crit Care Med 1987; 15:462.
61. Downs JB, Stock MC: Airway pressure release ventilation: A new concept in ventilatory support. Crit Care Med 1987; 15:459.
62. Garner W, Downs JB, Stock MC, et al: Airway pressure release ventilation (APRV): A human trial. Chest 1988; 94:779.
63. Räsänen J, Downs JB, Stock MC: Cardiovascular effects of conventional positive pressure ventilation and airway pressure release ventilation. Chest 1988; 93:911.
64. Räsänen J, Cane RD, Downs JB, et al: Airway pressure release ventilation during acute lung injury: A prospective multicenter trial. Crit Care Med 1991; 19:1234.
65. Cane RD, Peruzzi WT, Shapiro BA: Airway pressure release ventilation in severe acute respiratory failure. Chest 1991; 100:460.
66. Valentine DD, Hammond MD, Downs JB, et al: Distribution of ventilation and perfusion with different modes of mechanical ventilation. Am Rev Respir Dis 1991; 143:1262.
67. Jousela IT, Nikki P, Tahvanainen J: Airway pressure release ventilation by mask. Crit Care Med 1988; 16:1250.
68. Rouby J-J: Pressure release ventilation. *In:* Update in Intensive Care Medicine. Vol 10. Vincent JL (Ed). Berlin, Springer-Verlag, 1990, pp 185–195.
69. Räsänen J: IMPRV: Synchronized APRV, or more? Intensive Care Med 1992; 18:65.
70. Rouby J-J, Ben Ameur M, Jawish D, et al: Continuous positive airway pressure vs. intermittent mandatory pressure release ventilation (IMPRV) in patients with acute respiratory failure. Intensive Care Med 1992; 18:69.

CHAPTER 99

High-Frequency Ventilation and Oscillation

Sid M. Viner, MD • Keith L. Stein, MD, FCCP, FCCM

In contrast to modes of conventional mechanical ventilation (CMV) in which tidal volume exceeds dead space and respiratory frequency is maintained in the normal physiologic range, *high-frequency ventilation* (HFV) refers to modes of assisted mechanical ventilation using rapid rates and small tidal volumes.[1–3] HFV is defined as ventilation occurring at frequencies greater than 60 breaths per minute. Rates range from 60 to 3000 breaths per minute (1–50 Hz) with tidal volumes that are near or less than anatomic dead space.

In recent years, the therapeutic limitations associated with conventional modes of mechanical ventilation have spurred efforts to develop new approaches to ventilatory support. HFV techniques have been developed with the goals of improving carbon dioxide (CO_2) elimination and oxygenation while minimizing lung injury in patients with respiratory failure, minimizing potential adverse hemodynamic effects related to mechanical ventilation, and facilitating ventilation during certain procedures, such as laryngoscopy or bronchoscopy.[1]

The three modes of HFV in clinical use today vary in their rates, tidal volumes, and the systems used to deliver gas flow (see Table 99–1). The three distinct modes are high-frequency positive-pressure ventilation (HFPPV), high-frequency jet ventilation (HFJV), and high-frequency oscillation (HFO). HFO is quite different from the other modes in that tidal volumes are routinely smaller than dead space, both inspiratory and expiratory phases are active, and HFO may be applied to the airways, chest wall, or body surface.

TYPES OF HIGH-FREQUENCY VENTILATION

High-Frequency Positive-Pressure Ventilation

HFPPV was first developed by Sjostrand and coworkers in 1967.[4] While studying the carotid sinus reflex in dogs, they sought to eliminate respiration synchronous fluctuations in blood pressure by ventilating the animals with small tidal volume, high-frequency breaths at rates between 60 and 100 breaths per minute. They found that HFPPV provided adequate ventilation with low transpulmonary pressures and minimal circulatory effects. Clinical studies soon thereafter demonstrated the usefulness of the technique during general anesthesia in humans[5] and during procedures such as bronchoscopy and laryngoscopy.[6]

HFPPV is best delivered by a ventilator with low internal and circuit compliance and negligible compressible volume.[4] Breaths may be pressure or volume controlled with gas flow directed through an insufflation catheter placed in the airway or more commonly directed through the side arm of a pneumatic valve attached to an endotracheal tube or bronchoscope (Fig. 99–1). The main channel of the connector may remain open and be used for insertion of bronchoscopic or laryngoscopic equipment. Although an open system exists, gas entrainment does not occur. HFPPV uses frequencies of 60 to 100 breaths per minute, tidal volumes of 3 to 5 mL/kg, and inspiratory-expiratory ratios of less than 0.3. Expiration is passive.[2]

Although HFPPV is basically intermittent positive-pressure ventilation at increased rates and small tidal volumes, ventilators used to provide CMV often will not effectively provide HFPPV because of high internal and circuit compliances.[4] Nonetheless, conventional ventilators with external circuits using low-compliance tubing have been used successfully to deliver HFPPV.[7,8]

High-Frequency Jet Ventilation

In 1977 Klain and Smith[9] described the technique of HFJV in which small tidal volumes of gas were delivered as high-velocity jets via a catheter placed in the trachea. Because of entrainment of additional ambient gas by a Venturi effect, the actual delivered tidal volume was significantly greater

TABLE 99–1. Modes of High-Frequency Ventilation

Mode	*Rate (breaths per min)*	*Tidal Volume (mL/kg)*	*Exhalation*	*Gas Entrainment*
HFPPV	60–100	3–5	Passive	None
HFJV	100–150	2–5	Passive	Yes
HFO	Up to 2400	<3	Active	Yes

Abbreviations: HFPPV = high-frequency positive-pressure ventilation; HFJV = high-frequency jet ventilation; HFO = high-frequency oscillation.

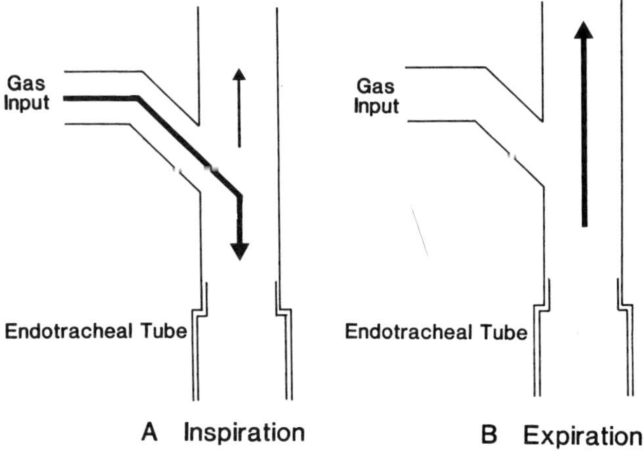

Figure 99–1. Schematic diagram of the pneumatic valve system for HFPPV.

than the volume of gas delivered from the jet catheter. Modern ventilators providing HFJV deliver gas under high pressure (10–50 psi) through a small cannula (14–16 gauge) placed within an endotracheal tube, incorporated within the wall of a specially designed endotracheal tube (NCC Hi-Lo Jet Tube, Argyle, NY), or less commonly via a catheter placed directly into the trachea. Ventilation is provided as gas flow is intermittently interrupted by a fluidic, pneumatic, or solenoid valve regulated by a timer. An ancillary circuit providing a continuous flow of humidified gas is directed through a side port into the endotracheal tube (Fig. 99–2). The jet stream entrains this gas by a Venturi effect, thus augmenting the tidal volume delivered. The tidal volume delivered by the jet ventilator is proportional to the size of the jet catheter, driving pressure, and inspiratory time. Entrained volume is a function of the velocity of jet flow, the jet velocity profile, position of the jet cannula in the airway, and resistance and compliance characteristics of the patient's lungs.[10, 11] Generally, frequencies of 100 to 150 breaths per minute are used with driving pressures of 10 to 40 psi with resultant tidal volumes in the range of 2 to 5 mL/kg. Inspiratory-expiratory ratio ranges from 0.1 to 0.5. Exhalation is passive.[12] Humidification of the high-velocity jet flow presents a difficult problem and is generally accomplished by directing a coaxial flow of saline in front of the jet cannula. The saline is nebulized by the jet flow and humidification occurs. Entrained gas may be humidified with a cascade-type or any other humidifier used with a conventional ventilator.[13]

A variation on HFJV is high-frequency flow interruption. As in HFJV, a high-pressure source of gas is interrupted by a valve such that pulsatile flow is delivered to the patient's airway. A rotating cam or Emerson rotating ball is often used to interrupt flow. In contrast to HFJV, gas is delivered well back from the patient's airway, and a source of bias gas flow is often used to magnify delivered tidal volume. Compared with HFJV, clinical and experimental data on HFFI are limited.

Initiation of High-Frequency Jet Ventilation

When switching a patient from CMV to HFJV, initial ventilator settings are somewhat empiric, but typical settings would dictate a frequency of 100 to 150, inspiratory time of 0.3, fraction of inspired oxygen (F_{IO_2}) and positive end-expiratory pressure (PEEP) equal to prejet level, and driving pressure adjusted to produce a mean airway pressure equal to that present when the patient was ventilated on CMV. If possible, mean airway pressure should be measured at a site 5 to 10 cm distal to the jet cannula because monitoring more proximally will result in underestimation of mean airway and alveolar pressure as a result of the presence of dynamic hyperinflation and auto-PEEP.[14] Arterial oxygenation is determined by F_{IO_2}, mean airway pressure, and functional residual capacity. Thus, an increase in partial pressure of oxygen (P_{O_2}) may be achieved by increasing F_{IO_2}, PEEP, driving pressure, or inspiratory time.[11, 15, 16] Determinants of partial pressure of arterial CO_2 (Pa_{CO_2}) are more complex. Although Pa_{CO_2} is inversely proportional to the product of frequency and tidal volume, changes in ventilatory frequency above 100 to 150 per minute have little effect on alveolar ventilation. Increases in frequency above 150 per minute may actually result in an increase in partial pressure of CO_2 (P_{CO_2}) because of a decrease in both the volume

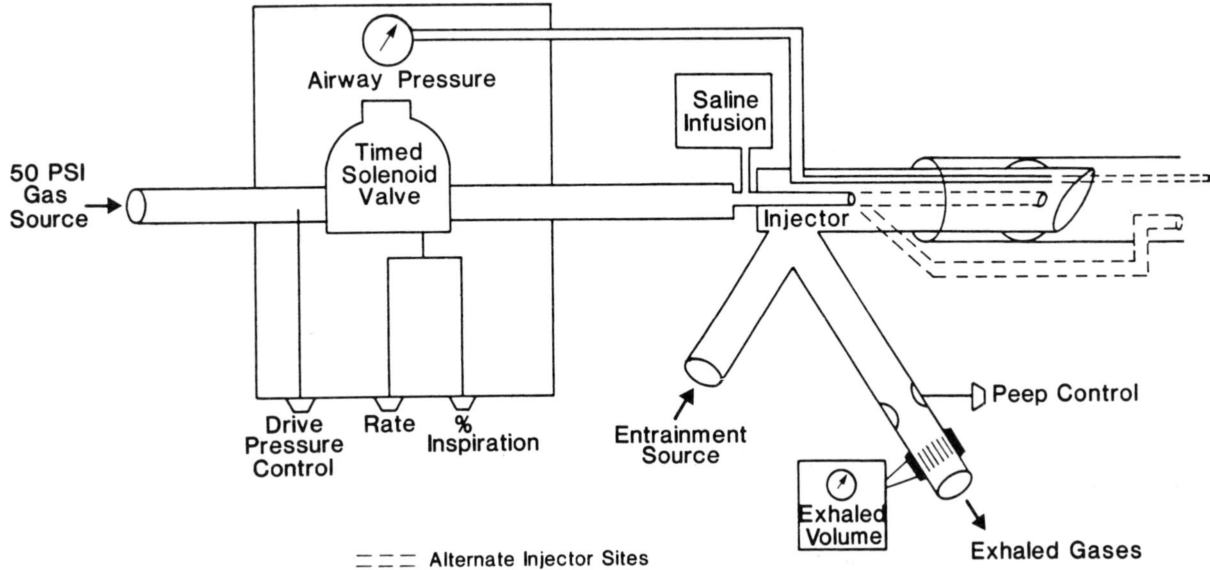

Figure 99–2. Schematic diagram of an HFJV system. (From MacIntyre NR: New forms of mechanical ventilation in the adult. Clin Chest Med 1988; 9:49.)

delivered through the jet and the entrained volume and increased gas trapping. At frequencies of 100 to 150 per minute, increases in alveolar ventilation are best accomplished by increasing driving pressure or inspiratory time, thus increasing tidal volume.[17]

High-Frequency Oscillation

In 1972, while performing studies of cardiac physiology in apneic dogs, Lukenheimer and colleagues[18] discovered that normocapnia was maintained when small volumes of air were oscillated in the animals' airways at rapid frequencies of up to 40 Hz. Over the ensuing years, an increasing number of studies have examined the role of HFO in adults, children, and particularly neonatal patients with respiratory failure. HFO differs from the other modes of HFV in that both the inspiratory and expiratory phases are active, tidal volumes are smaller, and frequencies are higher. The various devices used to generate high-frequency, sinusoidal, oscillatory flows at the airway opening have included piston pumps, loudspeakers, and linear magnetic motors. Reciprocating flows have also been generated using high-pressure impulses of gas directed 180° out of phase. A nozzle directed toward the lung acts as an injector, the other as an ejector.[19] A microprocessor-controlled, hybrid flow interrupter is now commercially available. All HFO ventilators incorporate a bias flow of fresh humidified gas delivered across the tubing connecting the oscillator to the patient (Fig. 99–3).

Arterial P_{CO_2} is affected by tidal volume and frequency at oscillatory frequencies less than 4 Hz (240 breaths per minute), with frequency becoming less important above this rate.[20] Typically, frequencies of 4 to 15 Hz are used with the oscillatory amplitude and rate of bias flow adjusted as needed to correct hypocapnia or hypercapnia. Oxygenation is determined by lung volume and F_{IO_2}; thus, arterial P_{O_2} may be improved by increasing PEEP, oscillatory amplitude (driving pressure), frequency, or the F_{IO_2} of the bias flow.[21] Lung volume history also has an important effect on oxygenation. If a sustained high-pressure inflation is provided to maximize alveolar recruitment before initiation of HFO, subsequent lung volume will be higher at any given mean airway pressure and oxygenation will be improved.[22] In an animal model, Bond and Froese showed that volume recruitment maneuvers not only improved oxygenation at any given mean airway pressure but also decreased progression of lung injury.[23]

In contrast to the other modes of HFV, HFO may be applied to the chest wall or body surface rather than to the airway opening.[24] Methods used to provide mechanical coupling between the ventilator and the patient have included an inflatable vest placed around the chest[25] and a cuirass apparatus designed to fit around the chest.[26] Pressure changes in the thorax are produced when a reciprocating pump moves air in and out of the vest or cuirass. Pressure is oscillated around a mean value, which may be positive, atmospheric, or subatmospheric.

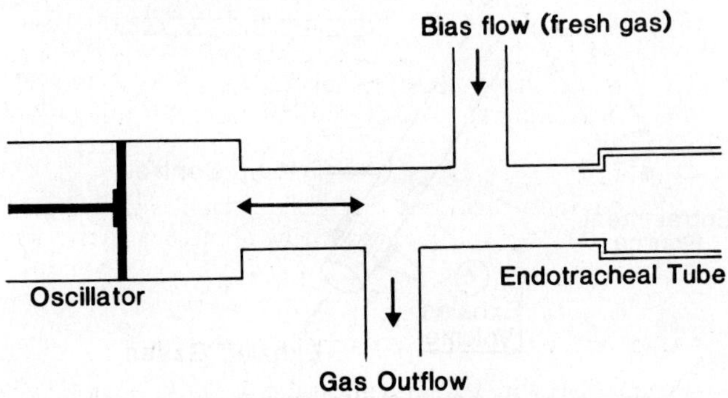

Figure 99–3. Schematic diagram of a high-frequency oscillator.

MECHANISMS OF GAS TRANSPORT

Mechanisms of gas transport during HFV are not well understood, and the importance of different mechanisms varies depending on the mode of HFV used. As in CMV, bulk (convective) flow is important, particularily in HFPPV and HFJV. As detailed in reviews by Chang[27] and Froese and Bryan,[1] the following mechanisms of gas transport are believed to be of most importance in HFV.

1. Direct alveolar ventilation: Alveoli with short path lengths from the conducting airways receive direct alveolar ventilation.
2. Pendelluft: Within the lung there are regional differences in resistance and compliance (time constants) with the effect that lung units fill and empty at varying rates and gas movement may occur between fast and slow units. *Pendelluft* refers to this movement of gas that occurs between adjacent regions of lung, resulting in intraregional gas mixing and homogenization of peripheral gas concentrations.
3. Asymmetric velocity profiles: In the distal small airways, where gas flow is predominantly laminar, viscous shear is created by the airway walls producing inspiratory velocity profiles that are asymmetric and parabolic, with molecules in the center of the airway moving more rapidly than those in the periphery. Expiratory velocity profiles are flatter; thus, in the center of the airway, there is net convective gas transport toward the alveoli, whereas along the periphery of the airway alveolar gas moves away from the alveoli.
4. Augmented (Taylor) dispersion: Axial convection, resulting from asymmetric velocity profiles, and oscillatory flows produce very turbulent gas movement, with resultant eddies and swirling gas flows leading to increased dispersion and mixing of gases.
5. Cardiogenic oscillations: Airway oscillations produced by the beating heart act to improve peripheral gas mixing. Cardiogenic oscillations have been shown to be of minor importance as a mechanism of gas transport in HFV.[28]
6. Molecular diffusion: This is the major gas transport mechanism operative once gas moves through the conducting airways and into the alveoli.

CLINICAL USES OF HIGH-FREQUENCY VENTILATION

Although HFV offers potential advantages in certain clinical situations (see Table 99–2), there is no situation in which HFV would be absolutely indicated over other modes of ventilatory support. Furthermore, the different modes of HFV have been found to be of varying benefit in different age groups. Although HFJV has been applied successfully

TABLE 99–2. Potential Clinical Applications of High-Frequency Ventilation

Difficult airway management	Bronchopleural fistula
Procedures involving upper airway	Hemodynamic instability
Lithotripsy	Enhanced secretion clearance
Tracheal and thoracic surgery	Weaning from ventilator support
Respiratory distress syndromes	

in pediatric and adult patients, the utility of HFO has been largely limited to the neonatal age group.

Management of the Difficult Airway

Percutaneous transtracheal HFJV may be used emergently in patients who can neither be intubated nor ventilated adequately by mask ventilation.[29] For instance, in patients with facial trauma, airway access may be a particularly difficult problem. In such patients, transtracheal HFJV may be a faster and simpler alternative to emergent cricothyroidotomy or tracheostomy. Transtracheal HFJV has been used extensively in the operating room to ventilate patients with difficult airways while fiberoptic intubation was accomplished.[29, 30] HFJV is achieved by puncturing the cricothyroid membrane with a 14- to 16-gauge catheter, which is then connected via noncompliant tubing to a jet injector connected to a high-pressure gas source. Complete upper airway obstruction is a contraindication to transtracheal HFJV as a result of the attendant risk of hyperinflation and barotrauma because instilled gas has no egress.

Ventilation During Diagnostic or Surgical Procedures

Both HFJV and HFPPV have been used extensively to support ventilation during laryngoscopy, bronchoscopy, endoscopic laser surgery, and upper airway and tracheal surgery.[6, 31–33] For procedures involving the upper airway, the advantages offered by HFV compared with CMV include maximization of surgical access to the airway, decreased motion of the surgical field, and the achievement of adequate ventilation without the need for a closed (gas-tight) system. HFV may be delivered through a nasotracheal or orotracheal catheter, through a catheter placed percutaneously into the trachea below the level of the vocal cords, or through the side port of a rigid bronchoscope (as first described by Sanders in 1967).[34]

HFV may be of greater benefit than CMV for any procedure in which it is advantageous to minimize lung or diaphragmatic movement. It has been demonstrated that HFJV during extracorporeal shock wave lithotripsy minimizes stone movement, reducing the number and intensity of required shock waves.[35] Speiss and associates[36] reported on the use of HFPPV during anterior thoracic spinal fusion to prevent incursion of the lung into the surgical field. Perera and colleagues[32] reported on the use of HFJV delivered via two separate catheters during tracheal resection. During surgery, the HFJV technique provided minimum obstruction to the surgical field, minimum lung movement, and adequate gas exchange in the presence of surgically disrupted airways.

Infant and Adult Respiratory Distress Syndrome

Because HFV maintains higher mean lung volumes with lower peak airway pressures than CMV, HFV is theoretically of particular benefit in patients with diffuse lung damage and poor lung compliance. Expected benefits include an improvement in oxygenation and minimization of lung injury and barotrauma.

A direct reduction in lung injury itself might be expected from the work of Kolobow's group,[37] who demonstrated that cyclic tidal ventilation as used in CMV may initiate and perpetuate lung injury. Related experimental evidence suggests that if early phasic pressure swings are reduced or eliminated, pulmonary injury will be reduced.[38, 39]

Studies of the respiratory distress syndrome have failed to clearly show any benefits. The HiFi study group[40] randomly assigned 673 preterm neonates with infant respiratory distress syndrome (IRDS) to either CMV or HFO. There was no difference between the groups in mortality, incidence of bronchopulmonary dysplasia, or level of ventilatory support required in the first 28 days. In fact, the number of treatment failures was higher with HFV, as was the occurence of pulmonary air leaks, intracranial hemorrhage, and periventricular leukomalacia. However, several experienced investigators criticized the design of this study, commenting that there was often a delay in institution of HFO during which time infants were maintained on CMV and that volume recruitment maneuvers and mean airway pressures were inadequate.[41] In a more recent study, Clark and colleagues[42] randomized 83 neonates to CMV or HFO using a high lung volume strategy to recruit and maintain alveolar volume. Although mortality and nonpulmonary morbidity were the same for the two groups, there was a reduction in chronic lung disease in the HFO group. Several other studies[43, 44] have shown HFO to be efficacious in supporting critically ill neonates with respiratory failure caused by IRDS. In contemporary neonatal critical care, HFO using a high lung volume strategy is now common, and in many instances, infants successfully treated with HFV would otherwise require treatment with extracorporeal membrane oxygenation, a much more invasive and labor-intensive modality.[42, 45]

In considering patients with adult respiratory distress syndrome (ARDS), published randomized trials have again failed to show any significant advantage of HFV over CMV. In a large prospective trial, Carlon and colleagues[12] compared 309 patients randomly assigned to HFJV or CMV at the onset of ARDS. There was no difference in the number of days in the intensive care unit or overall survival between groups. Schuster and associates[46] compared HFJV with CMV and found no difference in oxygenation at comparable levels of PEEP and mean airway pressure in eight patients with respiratory failure. Holzapfel and coworkers[47] studied 16 patients with ARDS and found no improvement in gas exchange on HFJV. In fact, some of the patients on HFJV required higher levels of PEEP, which produced higher mean airway pressures and lower cardiac indexes.

Because HFJV is accomplished at lower peak airway pressures than CMV, it was expected that the incidence of barotrauma would be lower in patients with ARDS ventilated on HFV. However, presumably because mean airway pressures are comparable and a significant level of auto-PEEP is present,[48, 49] clinical studies have also not shown any decrease in the incidence of barotrauma with HFV.[12]

Thus, despite theoretic advantages of HFV over CMV, in adults with diffuse lung disease and respiratory failure, group data from prospective randomized trials comparing CMV to HFV show that if comparable mean airway pressures are maintained, HFV does not appear to offer any significant advantages. However, the total number of patients studied in these trials is relatively small and further trials are needed, focusing particularly on new approaches such as combined HFV superimposed on low-frequency CMV and HFV used with adjunctive therapies such as exogenous surfactant. In individual patients with ARDS, HFJV offers an alternative to CMV that may occasionally be lifesaving. Borg and associates[50] reported on 35 patients with ARDS refractory to support on CMV. This group had an extremely high predicted mortality. On initiation of HFV, there was both an improvement in oxygenation and survival of 23%.

Bronchopleural Fistula and Airway Disruption

During CMV, in the presence of a large bronchopleural fistula (BPF), much of the tidal volume may be lost through the fistula, resulting in decreased alveolar ventilation and inadequate gas exchange. If ventilation is provided at high frequency, gas flow patterns are dictated preferentially by airway, not parenchymal properties, and overall alveolar ventilation is increased despite the presence of an air leak. Although the amount of gas lost through the fistula generally does not decrease,[51] animal[52] and human studies[53, 54] have shown HFV to provide superior oxygenation and CO_2 elimination in the presence of a BPF with a large pulmonary air leak. Patients with unilateral lung disease, with and without a BPF, have been successfully ventilated with independent lung ventilation and unilateral HFJV after failing on CMV.[55] However, an improvement in gas exchange may be realized only if higher mean airway pressures are generated. Bishop and associates[56] reported on seven patients with combined ARDS and BPF. They found that when patients were changed from CMV to HFJV at equal mean airway pressures, there was a deterioration in oxygenation and CO_2 elimination. Thus, in patients with underlying lung disease and BPF, HFV may be efficacious only if one uses higher mean airway pressures and accepts the accompanying increase in the pulmonary air leak volume.

Hemodynamic Instability

Because HFV is accomplished with smaller swings in intrathoracic pressure, HFV may cause less hemodynamic compromise in unstable patients. Matuschak and colleagues[57] ventilated acutely hypovolemic dogs with jet ventilation synchronized to late diastole and found stroke volume to be improved. In an experimental model of cardiac tamponade, HFJV was compared with CMV in animals ventilated to achieve equivalent levels of $Paco_2$. The study showed that adequate levels of ventilation were achieved at lower peak and mean airway pressures on HFJV with a higher stroke volume index and cardiac output.[58] In an animal model of acute mitral regurgitation, Stein and colleagues[59] compared the effect of cardiac cycle-specific (synchronized) HFJV, asynchronous HFJV, and CMV on left ventricular stroke volume and left ventricular filling pressure. Compared with CMV or apnea, both asynchronous and synchronous HFJV increased left ventricular stroke volume and reduced left ventricular filling pressure. HFJV synchronized to cardiac systole was most effective in augmenting forward flow. In a study on patients with left ventricular failure, Pinsky and coworkers[60] used HFJV synchronized to cardiac systole and demonstrated an augmentation of cardiac output. Fusciardi and others[61] studied patients with distributive shock ventilated on CMV and HFJV at equal mean airway pressures. They found no difference in hemodynamics in patients without circulatory shock, but in patients with distributive shock cardiac output and oxygen delivery were higher on HFJV. Other studies found that hemodynamic compromise occurs to a similar extent with either HFV or CMV and is largely related to mean airway pressure.[8, 46, 62–64] Similarly, Traverse and coworkers[65] compared the hemodynamic effects of HFJV and HFO and found that hemodynamic changes were independent of ventilator frequency or type of HFV but were determined by mean airway pressure and lung compliance. Thus, although HFV offers no major advantage over CMV in terms of hemodynamic effects, there may be subsets of patients with hemodynamic instability who will benefit from HFV.

Enhanced Mucus Clearance

Freitag and coworkers[66] studied five patients with bronchiectasis, superimposing HFO on spontaneous breathing using a mouthpiece. Asymmetric HFO (15 Hz) was used in which expiratory peak flows exceeded inspiratory peak flows. They demonstrated enhanced clearance of sputum, with an increased volume of sputum appearing in the central airways. Although HFO provided at the airway may prove useful as an adjunct to physiotherapy, HFO with asymmetric flow oscillations is needed, and currently available commercial HFO ventilators generate sinusoidal flows that have not been found to be efficacious.[67] A noninvasive alternative may be high-frequency chest wall oscillation, which has also been shown to enhance clearance of secretions from the lung.[68]

Weaning/Assist to Spontaneous Ventilation

Calverley and colleagues[69] studied high-frequency chest wall oscillation in five spontaneously breathing normal subjects. Although minute ventilation decreased up to 40%, there was no change in Pco_2 and either no change or an improvement in Po_2. Harf and coworkers[70] also demonstrated that high-frequency chest wall oscillation superimposed on spontaneous breathing produced an improvement in alveolar ventilation presumably as a result of enhanced intrapulmonary gas mixing.

The ability of HFV to suppress respiratory drive[71] may be of value in some patients to decrease their subjective sense of dyspnea during weaning. Klain and coworkers[72] described nine patients who failed attempts at weaning from CMV but were successfully weaned from mechanical ventilation when HFJV was instituted. They attributed their success to less asynchrony between patient and ventilator on HFV, with greater patient comfort and a decreased need for sedation.

Although preliminary studies suggest that HFO applied to the chest wall or airway may be an adjunct to weaning and assist spontaneous ventilation, further studies are needed to determine whether clinically significant improvements in gas exchange will occur when HFV is used for longer time intervals in patients with underlying lung disease. The use of HFV, or HFV superimposed on CMV, during weaning also warrants further investigation.

POTENTIAL COMPLICATIONS AND LIMITATIONS

Although certain complications and limitations are common to all types of mechanical ventilation, others are relatively unique to HFV. Necrotizing tracheobronchitis is a severe form of airway damage that is often fatal and has been linked with the use of HFPPV and HFJV.[73, 74] Development of necrotizing tracheobronchitis is believed to be related to high-velocity gas flows impacting on airways (jackhammer effect) and difficulty in humidifying inspired gas adequately during HFJV. Inadequate humidification during HFJV has also been shown to lead to problems with airway obstruction by desiccated, inspissated airway secretions and epithelium.[75] Various new approaches to humidification have been developed and may help circumvent the aforementioned problems.[76]

Dynamic hyperinflation occurs not only with HFPPV and HFJV, in which the expiratory phase is passive,[48, 49] but also with HFO, in which the expiratory phase is active.[77] Although sometimes of benefit in improving oxygenation, dynamic hyperinflation may lead to barotrauma and have deleterious hemodynamic consequences. HFV, particularly HFJV, should probably be avoided in patients with airflow obstruction because of the risk of generating very high levels of intrinsic PEEP.

Another significant limitation to the use of HFV is the lack of familiarity with the technique itself by medical personnel. Ventilator parameters are very different from CMV, monitoring of standard variables such as tidal volume or minute ventilation is often less precise, and initial ventilator settings as well as further adjustments are largely empiric based on patients' clinical responses and frequent arterial blood gas analyses. Improvements in ventilator design, with greater sophistication in monitoring and alarm functions, are helping to circumvent some of these drawbacks.

FUTURE APPLICATIONS

With diffuse parenchymal lung injury as seen in ARDS, lung compliance is low and much of the lung is atelectatic. During exhalation on CMV, as airway pressure falls there is a progressive collapse of lung units. During the subsequent inspiratory phase of the respiratory cycle, a pressure in excess of alveolar opening pressure must be generated to open alveoli and achieve gas exchange. This repetitive opening and closing of lung units under high pressure may induce further lung injury in the already damaged lung. In HFV, mean airway pressure is similar to that seen with CMV, but fluctuations about the mean are much smaller. Thus, during exhalation, there is less tendency for alveolar collapse, and during inspiration, the small tidal volumes used avoid the large increases in peak airway pressure seen with CMV. Thus, there is the possibility that HFV may yet prove to be of value in patients with ARDS. Further investigation is needed in the use of HFV in combination with other therapy such as exogenous surfactant or combined HFV with CMV at low tidal volumes.[78] Another area in which HFV may prove to be of benefit is as an adjunct to other types of noninvasive ventilation in patients with respiratory failure. When combined with noninvasive ventilation, HFO applied to the chest wall or airway may help avoid the need for tracheal intubation. Although initial enthusiasm for HFV in adult critical care has waned, in current practice, HFV is of particular value on an individual basis and may prove to be of greater value when combined with other newly evolving therapies.

References

1. Froese AB, Bryan AC: High frequency ventilation. Am Rev Respir Dis 1987; 135:1363.
2. Standiford T, Morganroth ML: High-frequency ventilation. Chest 1989; 96:1380.
3. Slutsky AS: Nonconventional modes of ventilation. Am Rev Respir Dis 1988; 138:175.
4. Sjostrand U: High-frequency positive pressure ventilation (HFPPV): A review. Crit Care Med 1980; 8:345.
5. Heijman K, Heijman L, Jonzon A, et al: High frequency positive pressure ventilation during anesthesia and routine surgery in man. Acta Anaesthesiol Scand 1972; 16:176.
6. Borg U, Eriksson I, Sjostrand U: High frequency positive pressure ventilation (HFPPV): A review based upon its use during bronchoscopy and for laryngoscopy and microlaryngeal surgery under general anesthesia. Anesth Analg 1980; 59:594.
7. Abu-Dbai J, Flatau E, Lev A, et al: The use of conventional ventilators for high frequency positive pressure ventilation. Crit Care Med 1983; 11:356.
8. Nakatsuka M, Colquhoun A, Gehr L: Right ventricular function and high-frequency positive-pressure ventilation during coronary artery bypass grafting. Ann Thorac Surg 1989; 48:263.
9. Klain M, Smith RB: High frequency percutaneous transtracheal jet ventilation. Crit Care Med 1977; 5:280.
10. Carlon GC, Ray C, Griffin J, et al: Tidal volume and airway pressure on high frequency jet ventilation. Crit Care Med 1983; 11:83.
11. Guntapalli KK, Pinsky MR, Marquez J, et al: Determinants of ventilation during high frequency ventilation. J Crit Care 1987; 2:93.
12. Carlon G, Howland W, Ray C Jr, et al: High frequency jet ventilation: A prospective randomized evaluation. Chest 1983; 84:551.
13. Carlon GC, Barker RL, Benua RS, et al: Airway humidification with high-frequency jet ventilation. Crit Care Med 1985; 13:114.
14. Sutton JE Jr, Glass DD: Airway pressure gradient during high-frequency ventilation. Crit Care Med 1984; 12:774.
15. Jonson B, Lachmann B: Setting and monitoring of high-frequency jet ventilation in severe respiratory distress syndrome. Crit Care Med 1989; 17:1020.
16. Rouby JJ, Fusciardi J, Bourgain JL, et al: High frequency jet ventilation in postoperative respiratory failure: Determinants of oxygenation. Anesthesiology 1983; 59:281.
17. Rouby JJ, Simonneau G, Benhamou D, et al: Factors influencing pulmonary volumes and CO_2 elimination during high frequency jet ventilation. Anesthesiology 1985; 63:473.
18. Lukenheimer PP, Rafenbeul W, Keller H, et al: Application of transtracheal pressure oscillations as a modification of diffusion respiration (Letter to the editor). Br J Anaesth 1972; 44:627.
19. Mutz N, Baum M, Benzer H, et al: Clinical experience with several types of high frequency ventilation. Acta Anaesthesiol Scand Suppl 1989; 90:140.
20. Rossing T, Slutsky AS, Lehr J, et al: Tidal volume and frequency dependence of carbon dioxide elimination by high frequency ventilation. N Engl J Med 1981; 305:1375.
21. McEvoy RD: High frequency oscillatory ventilation: Technical development and experimental evaluation. *In*: High Frequency Ventilation in Intensive Care and During Surgery. Carlon GC, Howland WS (Eds). New York, Marcel Dekker, 1985, p 217.
22. Walsh M, Waldemar A: Sustained inflation during HFOV improves pulmonary mechanics and oxygenation. J Appl Physiol 1988; 65:368.
23. Bond DM, Froese AB: Volume recruitment maneuvers are less deleterious than persistent low lung volumes in the atelectasis-prone rabbit during high-frequency oscillation. Crit Care Med 1993; 21:402.
24. Chang HK: Transthoracically-induced high frequency ventilation. Br J Anaesth 1989; 63:24S.
25. Zidulka A, Gross D, Minami H, et al: Ventilation by high frequency chest wall compression in dogs with normal lungs. Am Rev Respir Dis 1983; 127:709.
26. Dolmage TE, Hayek Z, De Rosie A, et al: Effects of high frequency chest wall oscillation (HFCWO) at 1.5 Hz on gas exchange in normal lungs. Am Rev Respir Dis 1992; 145:A528.
27. Chang HK: Mechanisms of gas transport during ventilation by high frequency oscillation. J Appl Physiol 1984; 56:553.
28. Meyer M, Calzia E, Mohr M, et al: Cardiogenic mixing: Mechanisms and experimental evidence in dogs. Br J Anaesth 1989; 63:95S.
29. Benumof JL, Scheller MS: The importance of transtracheal jet ventilation in the management of the difficult airway. Anesthesiology 1989; 71:769.
30. Nakatsuka M, MacLeod AD: Hemodynamic and respiratory effects of transtracheal high-frequency jet ventilation during difficult intubation. J Clin Anesth 1992; 4:321.
31. MacIntyre NR, Ramage JE, Follett JV: Jet ventilation in support of fiberoptic bronchoscopy. Crit Care Med 1987; 15:303.
32. Perera ER, Vidic DM, Zivot J: Carinal resection with two high-frequency jet ventilation delivery systems. Can J Anaesth 1993; 40:59.
33. Giunta F, Chiaranda M, Manani G: Clinical uses of high frequency jet ventilation in anaesthesia. Br J Anaesth 1989; 63:102S.
34. Sanders RD: Two ventilating attachments for bronchoscopes. Del Med J 1967; 39:170.
35. Warner MA, Warner ME, Buck CF, et al: Clinical efficacy of high frequency jet ventilation during extracorporeal shock wave lithotripsy of renal and ureteral calculi: A comparison with conventional mechanical ventilation. J Urol 1988; 139:486.
36. Speiss BD, Wong CA, Tuman KJ, et al: High frequency positive pressure ventilation for anterior thoracic spine fusion after a previous pneumonectomy. Anesth Analg 1988; 67:411.
37. Tsuno K, Prato P, Kolobow T: Acute lung injury from mechanical ventilation at moderately high airway pressures. J Appl Physiol 1990; 69:956.
38. Pesenti A, Kolobow T, Buckhold D, et al: Prevention of hyaline membrane disease in premature lambs by apneic oxygenation

and extracorporeal carbon dioxide removal. Intensive Care Med 1982; 8:11.
39. Meredith KS, deLemos RA, Coalson JJ, et al: Role of lung injury in the pathogenesis of hyaline membrane disease in premature baboons. J Appl Physiol 1989; 66:2150.
40. HiFi Study Group: High-frequency oscillatory ventilation compared with conventional mechanical ventilation in the treatment of respiratory failure in preterm infants. N Engl J Med 1989; 320:88.
41. Froese AB, Bryan AC: Reflections on the HiFi trial. Pediatrics 1991; 87:565.
42. Clark RH, Gerstmann DR, Null DM Jr, et al: Prospective randomized comparison of high frequency oscillatory and conventional ventilation in respiratory distress syndrome. Pediatrics 1992; 89:5.
43. Froese A, Butler P, Fletcher W, et al: High frequency oscillatory ventilation in premature infants with respiratory failure: A preliminary report. Anesth Analg 1987; 66:814.
44. Kocis KC, Meliones JN, Dekeon MK, et al: High-frequency jet ventilation for respiratory failure after congenital heart surgery. Circulation 1992; 86(Suppl II): II–127.
45. deLemos R, Yoder B, McCurnin D, et al: The use of high frequency oscillatory ventilation (HFOV) and extracorporeal membrane oxygenation (ECMO) in the management of the term/near term infant with respiratory failure. Early Hum Dev 1992; 29:299.
46. Schuster D, Klain M, Snyder J: Comparison of high frequency jet ventilation to conventional mechanical ventilation during severe acute respiratory failure in humans. Crit Care Med 1982; 10:625.
47. Holzapfel L, Perrin RF, Gaussorgues P, et al: Comparison of high-frequency jet ventilation to conventional ventilation in adults with respiratory distress syndrome. Intensive Care Med 1987; 13:100.
48. Benhamou D, Ecoffey C, Rouby JJ, et al: Impact of changes in operating pressure during high frequency jet ventilation. Anesth Analg 1984; 63:19.
49. Beamer WC, Prough DS, Royster RL, et al: High-frequency jet ventilation produces auto-PEEP. Crit Care Med 1984; 12:734.
50. Borg U, Stoklosa JC, Siegel JH, et al: Prospective evaluation of combined high-frequency ventilation in post-traumatic patients with adult respiratory distress syndrome refractory to optimized conventional ventilatory management. Crit Care Med 1989; 17:1129.
51. Roth MD, Wright JW, Bellamy PF: Gas flow through a bronchopleural fistula: Measuring the effects of high frequency jet ventilation and chest tube suction. Chest 1988; 93:210.
52. Mayers I, Long R, Breen P, et al: Artificial ventilation of a canine model of bronchopleural fistula. Anesthesiology 1986; 64:739.
53. Carlon GC, Ray C Jr, Klain M, et al: High-frequency positive pressure ventilation in management of a patient with bronchopleural fistula. Anesthesiology 1980; 50:160.
54. Turnbull AD, Carlon G, Howland WS, et al: High frequency jet ventilation in major airway or pulmonary disruption. Ann Thorac Surg 1981; 32:468.
55. Crimi G, Candiani A, Conti G: Clinical applications of independent lung ventilation with unilateral high-frequency jet ventilation (ILV-UHFJV). Intensive Care Med 1986; 12:90.
56. Bishop MJ, Benson MS, Satyo P, et al: Comparison of high frequency ventilation with conventional ventilation for bronchopleural fistula. Anesth Analg 1987; 66:833.
57. Matuschak G, Pinsky M, Klain M: Hemodynamic effects of synchronous high-frequency jet ventilation during acute hypovolemia. J Appl Physiol 1986; 61:44.
58. Goto K, Goto H, Benson KT, et al: Efficacy of high-frequency jet ventilation in cardiac tamponade. Anesth Analg 1990; 70:375.
59. Stein KL, Kramer DJ, Killian A, et al: Hemodynamic effects of synchronous high-frequency jet ventilation in mitral regurgitation. J Appl Physiol 1990; 69:2120.
60. Pinsky M, Marquez J, Martin D, et al: Ventricular assist by cardiac cycle-specific increases in intrathoracic pressure. Chest 1987; 91:709.
61. Fusciardi J, Rouby JJ, Barakat T, et al: Hemodynamic effects of high-frequency jet ventilation in patients with and without circulatory shock. Anesthesiology 1986; 65:485.
62. Fusciardi J, Rouby JJ, Benhamou D, et al: Hemodynamic consequences of increasing mean airway pressure during high frequency jet ventilation. Chest 1984; 86:30.
63. Otto C, Quan S, Conahan T, et al: Hemodynamic effects of high frequency jet ventilation. Anesth Analg 1983; 62:298.
64. Mayers I, Mink J: Cardiac output effects of high-frequency oscillatory ventilation in normal dogs. Respir Physiol 1989; 75:247.
65. Traverse JH, Korvenranta H, Adams EM, et al: Cardiovascular effects of high-frequency oscillatory and jet ventilation. Chest 1989; 96:1400.
66. Freitag L, Kim WM, Long J, et al: Mobilization of mucous by airway oscillations. Acta Anaesthesiol Scand Suppl 1989; 90:93.
67. McEvoy RD, Davies NJH, Hedenstierna G, et al: Lung mucociliary transport during high frequency ventilation. Am Rev Respir Dis 1982; 126:452.
68. Gross D, O'Brien C, Wight D, et al: Enhanced peripheral mucus clearance with high frequency chest wall compression. J Appl Physiol 1985; 58:1157.
69. Calverley PMA, Chang HK, Vartian V, et al: High-frequency chest wall oscillation: Assistance to ventilation in spontaneously breathing subjects. Chest 1986; 89:218.
70. Harf A, Zidulka A, Chang HK: Nitrogen washout during tidal breathing with superimposed high-frequency chest wall oscillation. Am Rev Respir Dis 1985; 132:350.
71. Butler WJ, Bohn DJ, Bryan AC, et al: Ventilation by high frequency oscillation in humans. Anesth Analg 1980; 59:577.
72. Klain M, Kalla R, Sladen A, et al: High-frequency ventilation in weaning the ventilator dependent patient. Crit Care Med 1984; 12:780.
73. Wiswell TE, Clark RH, Null DM, et al: Tracheal and bronchial injury in high-frequency oscillatory ventilation and high-frequency flow interruption compared with conventional positive-pressure ventilation. J Pediatr 1988; 112:249.
74. Boros S, Mammel M, Lewallen P, et al: Necrotizing tracheobronchitis: A complication of high frequency ventilation. J Pediatr 1986; 109:95.
75. Boros SJ, Mammel M, Coleman JM, et al: Neonatal high frequency jet ventilation: Four years' experience. Pediatrics 1985; 75:657.
76. Fuchs W: Humidification techniques in high-frequency ventilation: A review. Acta Anesthesiol Scand Suppl 1989; 90:120.
77. Hoskyns EW, Milner AD, Hopkin IE: Dynamic lung inflation during high frequency oscillation in neonates. Eur J Pediatr 1992; 151:846.
78. Barzilay E, Kessler D, Raz R: Superimposed high frequency ventilation with conventional mechanical ventilation. Chest 1989; 95:681.

CHAPTER 100

Independent Lung Ventilation*

John M. Chandler, MD • Morris I. Bierman, MD
Keith L. Stein, MD, FCCP, FCCM

Independent lung ventilation (ILV) has revolutionized the approach to mechanical ventilatory support of patients with refractory hypoxemia. This diverse but select group with pathologic, asymmetric lung function[1] has demonstrated a failure to improve, or a further deterioration in oxygenation, as a result of the maldistribution of pulmonary perfusion and ventilatory mismatching, particularly in the presence of positive end-expiratory pressure (PEEP). Conventional techniques, when applied to asymmetric lung diseases, have often failed to achieve an acceptable arterial oxygen tension

*The views expressed in this chapter are those of the authors alone and do not reflect the views or position of the National Naval Medical Center, the United States Naval Medical Corps, or the United States Navy.

(PaO_2) with less toxic levels of inspired oxygen (FIO_2) and are complicated by problems of inadequate or wasted alveolar ventilation ($\dot{V}A$). Radiographic evidence of improvement is seen after insertion of a double-lumen endobronchial (DLEB) tube when conventional single-lumen tube ventilation has failed (Figs. 100–1 and 100–2). The advent of ILV in the critical care setting has allowed patients with refractory hypoxemia to be salvaged through the lessons learned from intraoperative management[2, 3] and through experimental models[4, 5] of one-lung ventilation. ILV is derived from the design concept introduced in 1949 by Carlens for bronchospirometry,[6] which was subsequently employed to differentially deliver positive-pressure mechanical ventilation to one lung while intraoperative soiling of the contralateral lung was avoided.[7]

Over the past 50 years, technologic advances in DLEB tube composition[8, 9] and design[10] have resulted in effective isolation of the left or right mainstem bronchus.[11, 12] Maintenance of alveolar oxygenation (PAO_2) and $\dot{V}A$ in critically ill patients with unilateral lung disease has been applied to other patient populations outside the operating room.[13, 14] Previously employed for relatively brief intervals during the operative event (lasting for only minutes to hours), this technique of gas exchange is now used in intensive care units for periods of days to weeks.[15] The appealing intraoperative advantages of modern short-term ILV include the relative ease of placement and maintenance of DLEB tubes, a low incidence of complications, and the ability to alternate between conventional ventilation to single-lung ventilation. During extended long-term maintenance of ILV, these advantages are not easily translated to the critical care setting. A wide range of personnel are needed to accomplish ILV outside the operating room, including physicians, nurses, and respiratory therapists. Expertise is required not only in maintaining ILV but also in promptly discerning when malpositioning of the DLEB tube has led to hypoxemia, hemodynamic instability, and ventilatory compromise in patients with complex cardiopulmonary interactions. Simply stabilizing the DLEB tube and neck during positioning for a chest radiograph[16] can cause major cardiopulmonary instability and loss of the benefits afforded by differential ventilation. Complicating matters further, extended ventilatory support often requires combined sedation and paralysis of a patient. As with conventional ventilation for respiratory failure,[17] immobility during ILV may contribute to the development of significant complications, such as prolonged paralysis[18] and myopathy.[19, 20] Hence, the risks of using ILV with its potential morbidity must be weighed along with the difficulties in maintaining optimal tube positioning within the mainstem bronchus (which may mean a distance of only a few millimeters in either proximal or distal movement).[12] In this context of prolonged mechanical ventilation, the applicability of ILV in critical care has expanded to fill the void left by traditional and conventional methods that have failed to maintain adequate cardiopulmonary support in unstable patients.

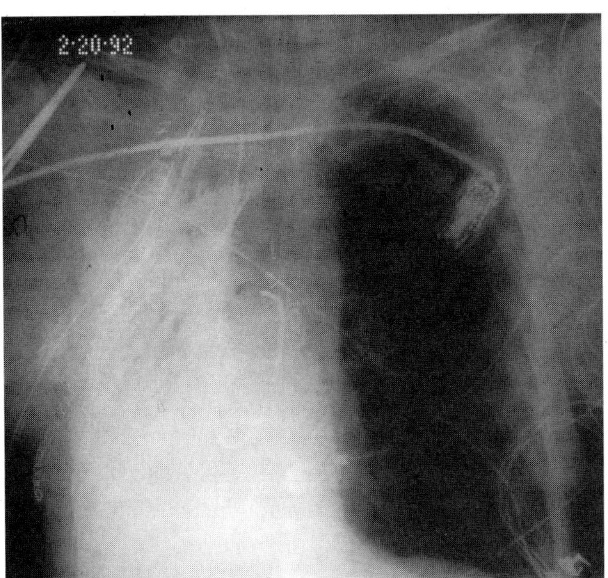

Figure 100–1. Single-lumen ventilation after preservation injury following single-lung transplantation.

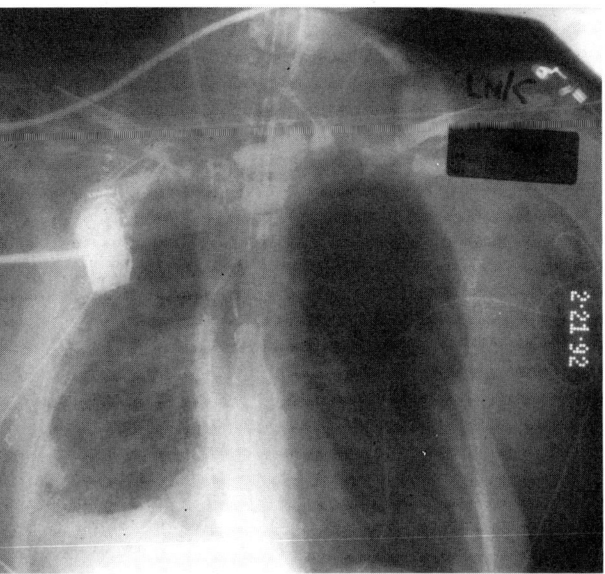

Figure 100–2. Double-lumen ventilation after preservation injury following single-lung transplantation.

CLINICAL INDICATIONS

ILV is justified when conventional pulmonary support fails in the patient with any kind of acute lung injury that results in asymmetry on the basis of radiographic and physiologic findings. Many anecdotal case reports and observations attest to the clinical utility of ILV outside the operating room, but as of yet few studies have addressed large numbers of prospectively randomized patients who require long-term ILV. Conditions for which ILV have been most commonly used can be summarized broadly into the following categories:

1. Selective airway protection: lavage for pulmonary alveolar proteinosis,[21–23] aspiration of purulent secretions,[7] and massive hemoptysis[24]
2. Correction of severe, life-threatening hypoxemia due to ventilation-perfusion ($\dot{V}/\dot{Q}$) mismatching: pneumonia,[14, 25] pulmonary contusion,[26] pulmonary hemorrhage,[27] and refractory atelectasis[13, 28]
3. Management of bronchopleural fistula[29, 30]
4. Single-lung and double-lung transplantation[31–33]

When ILV is contemplated in the intensive care setting, dependent lung factors (such as gravitational redistribution of pulmonary blood flow [$\dot{Q}pa$]), independent lung factors (such as optimization of the components that affect hypoxic pulmonary vasoconstriction [HPV]), and augmentation of cardiac performance have already been considered.

CRITERIA AND METHODS FOR INSTITUTION OF INDEPENDENT LUNG VENTILATION

Although a minority of patients exhibiting arterial hypoxemia present with asymmetric lung disease, proper management of this subset of candidates[34] necessitates an orderly sequence in the application of mechanical ventilation. This sequence ordinarily begins with the spontaneous ventilation of a patient before intubation. A trial of combined gravitational maneuvers (i.e., positioning), noninvasive mechanical ventilation administered via facemask (e.g., continuous positive airway pressure [CPAP],[35,36] and aggressive respiratory therapy are initiated to reverse the primary disorder. If hypoxemia persists, intubation with an ordinary single-lumen endotracheal tube is appropriate.

During mechanical ventilation with a conventional single-lumen endotracheal tube, the gravitational effect on $\dot{Q}pa$ as well as differential pleural pressures (Ppl) on lung tissue (which allow for greater amounts of transpulmonary pressure to be applied to areas that are uppermost) are evaluated in concert with radiologic abnormalities.[36a] Specific maneuvers designed to recruit collapsed and underventilated alveoli include lateral decubitus positioning,[37] with the affected lung uppermost, combined with periodic hyperoxic hyperinflations (i.e., the raising of airway pressure [Paw] to 40 cm H_2O in a sustained fashion for 15–30 seconds).[38] Although it has proved successful in improving acute lobar collapse due to atelectasis in intubated and nonintubated patients,[39] the results of directed recruitment are disappointing in patients with hypoxemic respiratory failure. Patients with established collapse of greater than 24 hours' duration who are on mechanical ventilation and are unresponsive to conventional bag suctioning techniques show no improvement in oxygenation, physiologic deadspace ($\dot{V}DS$), shunt fraction, or static compliance (Cst).[38] Unless other therapies (e.g., bronchoscopy) are effective at removing tenacious secretions, alveolar collapse is inevitable. Hence, patients with alveolar instability leading to $\dot{V}/\dot{Q}$ mismatching that is not acute (<24 hours' duration) may require ILV.

Clinical and experimental findings have demonstrated that patients with asymmetric lung disease have a striking maldistribution of both PEEP, tidal volume (VT), and $\dot{Q}pa$. The distribution of ventilation to both lungs is defined by the regional time constant (τ) of each lung.[40] The τ is the product of the airway resistance (Raw) and the compliance of a given system. During negative-pressure ventilation, as occurs with spontaneous ventilation, the disbursement of VT is influenced by regional τ, whereas $\dot{Q}pa$ is conditional, being dependent on gravitational forces[41] and on vascular tone.[42] Pathologic lung conditions that are amenable to the benefits of ILV are those diseases in which bulk gas flow is affected because of either unilateral differences in Raw or compliance, or in both. These differences are accounted for by the dyshomogeneity and parallel inequality that exist within diseased airways. As numerous studies[43, 44] have reported a substantial improvement in oxygenation in the presence of acute lung injury, a predictable deterioration in PaO_2 was observed in some individuals who had progressive amounts of PEEP added.[58] PaO_2 paradoxically increased as PEEP was removed, indicating a lessening shunt fraction and a consequent reduction of pulmonary venous admixture ($\dot{Q}sp/\dot{Q}t$). A scenario of a paradoxical response to PEEP in the absence of an intracardiac shunt strongly implies inhomogeneous lung disease. This finding is noteworthy, regardless of the lag in radiographic change that is sometimes seen in early asymmetric lung disease. Acute lung injury has been clearly shown with dynamic computed tomography to be inhomogeneous, as revealed by aerated, poorly aerated, and nonaerated lung tissue and regional overdistention of alveoli.[45, 46] Unless clear asymmetry exists in a right-to-left distribution, ILV has no theoretic or practical benefit. Nevertheless, ILV has been studied in patients with symmetric but inhomogeneous acute lung injury with the use of the inert gases technique.[47] Although titration and restoration of $\dot{V}/\dot{Q}$ matching is attained more effectively than with conventional means,[47] it is doubtful that such a small improvement in supportive care alone would gain favor in the management of acute lung injury. Of greater practical relevance is the avoidance of ventilator-associated pulmonary barotrauma. The matching of VT, gas flow, and PEEP to the specific dynamic compliance (Cdyn) in unilateral lung disease may avoid the high Paw associated with ventilator-induced pulmonary barotrauma.[48, 49]

To document the failure of whole-lung ventilation, some authors have suggested that the redistribution of $\dot{Q}pa$ and the increase in $\dot{Q}sp/\dot{Q}t$ that occur as whole PEEP is applied be illustrated as a function of elevated Cst, with concomitant overdistention of alveoli and loss in functional residual capacity,[34] before a shift to ILV is made. Furthermore, elevations in mean Paw attained through alternative means, such as pressure control–inverse ratio ventilation[50] or high-frequency jet ventilation,[51] in an effort to recruit and to maintain diseased but functioning alveoli that are able to participate in gas exchange[52, 53] may obviate the need for ILV. Unfortunately, as mean Paw increases, cardiac instability may ensue because of a reduction in right ventricular performance, which is usually due to alteration in preload or afterload, or both. Since the heart is an intrathoracic structure dependent on systemic venous return to fill the right atrium, right atrial pressure varies with changes in intrathoracic pressure (ITP). It follows that positive-pressure ventilation limits venous return during lung inflation to such a degree that ITP changes are relayed to the right atrium, increasing right atrial pressure and, in turn, lowering the pressure gradient for venous return to fill the right atrium and, hence, the right ventricle.[54] Thus, a deceleration in venous return decreases cardiac output by reducing right ventricular stroke volume. Right ventricular function can also be affected by resistance to right ventricular ejection (i.e., increased afterload). Again, as ITP varies with systolic right ventricular performance, the pressure gradient is defined as the mean pulmonary artery pressure (Ppa) relative to the ITP that is transmitted to the pulmonary circulation. The importance of lung volumes, as they relate to positive-pressure ventilation and to transmitted ITP, has been long recognized.[55] As usually occurs with positive-pressure ventilation, pulmonary vascular resistance increases as lung volumes are raised above functional residual capacity owing to alveolar vessel compression. Alternatively, if resting lung volumes fall below functional residual capacity, as in hypoxemia secondary to atelectasis, and if pulmonary vascular resistance increases because of compression of extra-alveolar vessels, restoration of lung volumes may actually decrease pulmonary vascular resistance.[56] Moreover, HPV and thus PVR may be reduced if collapsed alveoli are opened and reoxygenated.[57] This beneficial effect is minimized or reversed altogether should overinflation of alveoli occur because of heterogeneous lung involvement in acute lung injury. Since few clinicians routinely utilize serial pulmonary contrast or nuclear angiography[58] or computed tomography studies to detect subtle variations in $\dot{V}/\dot{Q}$ inequalities, ILV is most commonly reserved for patients with radiographic intraparenchymal asymmetry and some reduction in $\dot{Q}sp/\dot{Q}t$ with positional changes and variations in PEEP during standard, single-lumen, whole-lung ventilation.

Parallel inequality as it relates to lung inflation and deflation during whole-lung mechanical ventilation varies the bulk distribution of gas within the lung itself. Variability in bronchial diameters, turbulence, and airway plugging as well as the specific dynamic compliance of individual lung units can affect the dispersion of the individual components of mechanical ventilation. PEEP, VT, inspiratory-expiratory flow rate and duration, and respiratory frequency are the parameters that show the greatest variability. These parameters, which alter ITP during ventilation, have an important role in cardiopulmonary interactions whether they are delivered synchronously or asynchronously.

As ILV is begun, equal VTs are usually delivered to each lung and are adjusted while Paw is monitored. If differential pressures are elevated with maintenance of a routine VT of 5 to 7.5 mL/kg to each lung, the lowering of VT, which is inversely proportional to the degree of compliance of each lung, reduces airway pressures. Usually, the more compliant lung receives the larger proportion of VT in an attempt to reduce pulmonary barotrauma. Constructing a pressure-volume curve for each lung is helpful when the duration of flow and the shape of the inspiratory flow curve are recorded in relation to the inspiratory time. Initially, the combined minute ventilation ($\dot{V}E$) is maintained, if possible, at the same level as was used for whole-lung ventilation. PEEP is applied to maintain the same mean Paw as occurs with whole-lung ventilation. Ultimately, the amount of PEEP applied to each lung is modified in relation to the air trapping that occurs as a function of its dependence on differential flow rates and on inspiratory-expiratory ratios to adjust $\dot{V}E$ while both peak Paw and mean Paw are optimized.

Ordinarily, most people can sustain an acceptable level of PaO_2 by means of an autoregulatory reduction in flow through a small region of hypoxic lung due to an intact hypoxic pulmonary vasoconstrictor response. However, during one-lung anesthesia, moderate to severe hypoxemia with PaO_2 less than 80 mm Hg occurs in 15% to 35% of patients.[59, 60] HPV occurs in response to alveolar hypoxia, raising the pressure gradient across pulmonary arterioles and capillaries and, in turn, diverting $\dot{Q}pa$ to regions that have better oxygenation.[61] This appears to affect directly pulmonary arterioles with diameters less than 500 μm.[62, 63] The reactivity of HPV depends on many factors that may be present to varying degrees (Table 100–1). Factors shown to

TABLE 100–1. Differential Diagnosis of Altered Hypoxic Pulmonary Vascular Tone During Independent Lung Ventilation

Decreased Reactivity
Elevated Ppa
Hypothermia
Hypocarbia
Metabolic alkalosis
High mixed venous PO_2
Sepsis/pneumonia
Surgical manipulation of lungs
Drugs: nitroprusside, nitroglycerin, calcium channel antagonists, β_2-adrenergic agonists, inhaled anesthetics, prostaglandin I_2
Increased Reactivity
Hyperthermia
Hypercarbia
Metabolic acidosis
Low mixed venous PO_2
Almitrine bismesylate

TABLE 100–2. Differential Diagnosis of Arterial Hypoxemia During Independent Lung Ventilation

Mechanical Tube Obstruction
Distal migration of either right or left DLEB, which impairs ventilation
Distal migration of the tracheal cuff into the unintubated mainstem bronchus
Proximal migration of the DLEB cuff with herniation into the trachea or opposing mainstem bronchus
Inadvertent intubation of the opposing mainstem bronchus
Intraluminal obstruction caused by secretions or blood
Extraluminal obstruction caused by kinking, mediastinal mass, or cuff overinflation
Nondependent Lung Factors (Shunt Physiology)
Pulmonary: altered HPV
Cardiac: pulmonary hypertension with a patent foramen ovale or atrial septal defect
Dependent Lung Factors (Gravitational Effects of $\dot{Q}pa$)
Worsening of $\dot{V}/\dot{Q}$ matching due to mediastinal and diaphragmatic shifts in decubitus positions
Cardiac Output–Related Factors (Cardiopulmonary Interactions)
Auto-PEEP limiting venous return with elevation in right ventricular afterload and reduced cardiac output
DLEB cuff inflation obstructing pulmonary artery outflow and limiting cardiac output

decrease pulmonary vascular reactivity include elevation of Ppa that results from pulmonary hypertension of any cause, including chronic obstructive pulmonary disease, pulmonary embolism, hypothermia, mitral or aortic valvular diseases, and volume overload. In the case of chronic obstructive pulmonary disease, responsiveness to hypoxia may be lost if arteriole hyperplasia produces a fixed pulmonary vascular resistance.[64] Other conditions that produce decreased reactivity include hypocarbia,[65] metabolic alkalosis, elevated oxygen tension of mixed venous blood,[4] sepsis, pneumonia, and those produced by drugs such as nitroprusside,[66] nitroglycerin,[67] calcium channel antagonists,[68, 69] β_2-adrenergic agonists,[70] inhaled anesthetics,[71] and prostaglandin I_2.[72] Factors shown to increase pulmonary vascular reactivity are hyperthermia, hypercarbia,[65] metabolic acidosis, low oxygen tension of mixed venous blood,[4] and almitrine bismesylate.[73]

Thus, the differential diagnosis of arterial hypoxemia during ILV must include assessment not only of physical and mechanical factors related to the patency of the airway and the tube lumina themselves but also of nondependent factors in the loss of HPV or intracardiac shunt, of dependent (gravitational) factors, and of a diminished cardiopulmonary interaction that leads to right ventricular dysfunction (Table 100–2). Besides fulfilling the need of physically separating either lung to prevent contamination by blood, purulent matter, or fluid, ILV is primarily useful in redistributing the delivery of positive-pressure ventilation to efficiently match $\dot{Q}pa$, thereby enhancing oxygenation and carbon dioxide elimination.

In addition to matching variations in regional Raw and compliance, ILV is useful in the management of bronchopleural fistulas, which are frequently associated with lung disorders and cause an increase in $\dot{Q}sp/\dot{Q}t$, a reduction in functional residual capacity, and a decrease in Cst. Measures to reduce the air leak in the presence of bronchopleural fistulas should not only address the mechanical problem of volume loss but also the functional derangements in ventilation and oxygenation. Most important, the components of mechanical ventilation responsible for keeping the fistula open must be limited (Table 100–3). Above a critical opening pressure of the fistula, both mean Paw and peak Paw

TABLE 100–3. Goals for Management of Bronchopleural Fistula During Independent Lung Ventilation

- Keep Paw throughout the respiratory cycle below the opening pressure of the fistula
- Lowest effective differential VT
- Least number of mechanical positive pressure breaths (f)
- Lowest PEEP (avoid auto-PEEP)
- Shorten inspiratory time

must be considered. Ensuring ventilation to the healthier lung, the affected lung can be managed with ILV that combines hypoventilation and reduced PEEP; this lowers mean Paw and peak Paw to below the critical opening pressure. Both inspiratory time and inspiratory flow rates can be similarly used to lower Paw. Potential advantages of this technique include a decrease in $\dot{V}_E$ through the anatomic defect, which promotes closure; and a reduction in mean Paw and peak Paw to the unaffected lung while ventilation is maintained and lowering of F_{IO_2} is permitted owing to better matching of $\dot{V}/\dot{Q}$. Although combinations of PEEP versus no PEEP,[29] synchronous versus asynchronous ILV,[30] and high-frequency jet ventilation[74] have been used, no one strategy is clearly superior, as all have met with success. ILV suffers from a lack of clinically controlled and randomized trials to delineate those attributes of patients that lead to improvement in outcome and to reduction in associated morbidity when compared with conventional single-lumen tube ventilation and other modes of mechanical ventilation; however, it may be effective nonetheless.

SYNCHRONOUS VERSUS ASYNCHRONOUS INDEPENDENT LUNG VENTILATION

A number of ventilatory techniques that involve dual ventilation patterns have been combined to administer ILV and selective PEEP. Whether or not the two ventilators are synchronized with each other during inflation and deflation, the goal remains the maximization of gas exchange and oxygenation as well as preservation or augmentation of cardiac output. To the extent that cardiac output varies with changes in ITP, inspiration and expiration can either impede or augment cardiac output.[75] These effects of ventilation on cardiac function depend on lung inflation pressure[76, 77] and intravascular volume and can be further augmented if phasic high ITP during ventilation is linked to the cardiac cycle.[78] Unilateral high-frequency jet ventilation and conventional contralateral positive-pressure ventilation have been used with success during ILV without synchrony between the phasic ITP changes and the cardiac cycle.[79] The importance of synchrony between the cardiac cycle and ITP changes has been only preliminarily studied as it relates to either synchronous or asynchronous differential lung inflation. However, during thoracic surgery in patients in the lateral decubitus position, cardiac output changes minimally when two-lung and one-lung ventilation are alternated[80] in patients with normal pulmonary compliance. In this situation, with synchronous versus asynchronous lung inflation[5] (with asynchrony of 180° between the right lung and left lung inflation), only minor alterations in circulatory function occur—namely in heart rate, systemic blood pressure, cardiac output, and intracardiac pressures. In addition, $\dot{Q}sp/\dot{Q}t$ and systemic blood gas parameters do not change significantly between these ventilation patterns despite significant changes in lung mechanics, Paw, and lung compliance. Further studies of the effect of differential lung ventilation on cardiac performance are needed.

Synchronous ILV was initially accomplished with a single ventilator and a selective distribution circuit that split the flow to each lung.[81] Currently, two ventilators are most commonly used to split flow in a synchronous (right and left lung)[1] or an asynchronous[82] mode, with the latter being easier to perform. The choice between synchrony and asynchrony remains empiric at present. Synchronization both between the two ventilators and with the cardiac cycle is an interesting but unexplored concept.

INTUBATING TECHNIQUE

Intubation may be accomplished with many types of DLEB tubes (Fig. 100–3). The DLEB tubes supplied for clinical use currently include the Mallinckrodt Broncho-Cath (Mallinckrodt Critical Care, Glen Falls, NY), the Rüsch endobronchial tube (Rüsch, Duluth, GA), and the Sheridan Broncho-Trach (Sheridan, Argyle, NY). Left-sided DLEB tubes are indicated for most clinical situations except those in which left bronchial mainstem stenosis or obstruction or thoracic aortic aneurysms preclude placement. In general, given the short length of the right mainstem bronchus before the origin of the right upper-lobe orifice compared with the longer mainstem bronchus to left upper-lobe interval, left-sided endobronchial intubation is more practical and safer than right-sided intubation. With right-sided tubes, occlusion of the right upper lobe can follow in as many as 89% of patients.[11] For most cases, a rigid stylet positions the DLEB tube's distal curved angle anteriorly as it moves between the vocal cords. After negotiating the cords, the stylet is removed, and the DLEB tube is advanced toward the intended mainstem bronchus after it has been rotated 90°. With the placement of left-sided DLEB tubes, the average depth of inser-

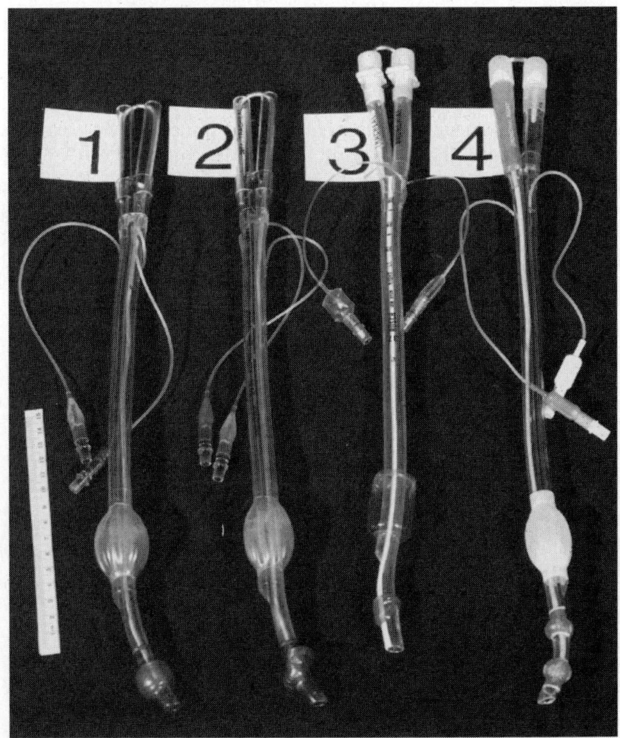

Figure 100–3. Types of double-lumen endobronchial tubes. 1 and 2 = Mallinckrodt left-sided and right-sided* Broncho-cath (Mallinckrodt Critical Care, Glen Falls, NY); 3 = right-sided* Rüsch endobronchial tube (Rüsch, Duluth, GA); 4 = right-sided* Sheridan Broncho-Trach (Sheridan, Argyle, NY). (*Variable distal lumens designed to ventilate the right upper lobe.)

tion from the teeth for both men and women 170 cm in height is 29 cm and varies for every ±10 cm in height by an average of ±1 cm.[83] In determining an average placement depth, it has been noted that the insertion depth for a patient of any given height is normally distributed, and thus proper confirmatory techniques are still required. In practice, the DLEB tube is advanced gently until slight resistance is encountered.

Proper positioning is necessary owing to the small margin of safety involved in the placement of both left-sided and right-sided DLEB tubes. The most proximal and distal positions acceptable are defined with regard to the patency of all bronchi and tube lumens (Fig. 100–4).[12] For all manufactured left-sided DLEB tubes, the average margin of safety in positioning, defined as the length of the left mainstem bronchus minus the distance from the proximal margin of the endobronchial cuff to the lumen tip, ranges from 16 to 19 mm. Right-sided DLEB positioning presents a particularly difficult problem, as right upper-lobe obstruction is frequently observed[11] owing to a narrow margin of safety that ranges from 1 to 4 mm or from 1 to 8 mm, depending on the particular manufacturer.[12] Confirmation of DLEB tube position may take place either "blindly" or with fiberoptic visualization. Currently, no consensus exists regarding the routine use of fiberoptic bronchoscopy in the placement of DLEB tubes.[84, 85] Intubating airway experience, interpatient variability, degree of difficulty, and access to fiberoptic bronchoscopy are all factors that affect use of the technique

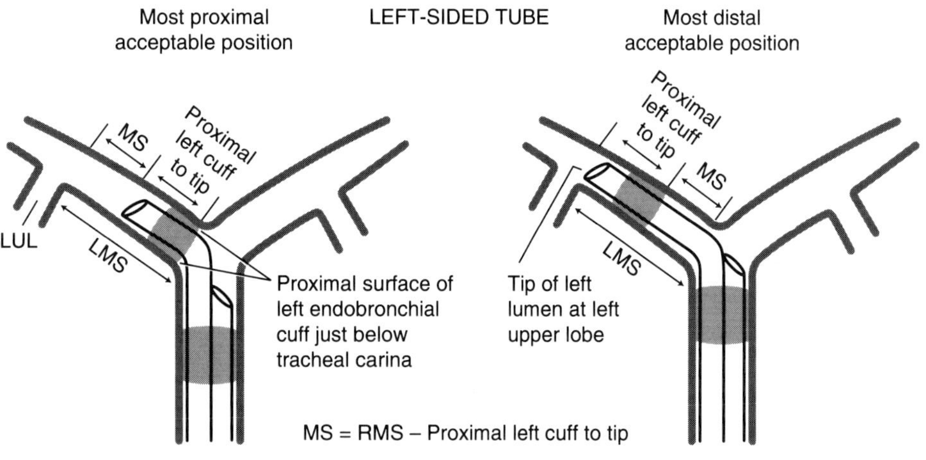

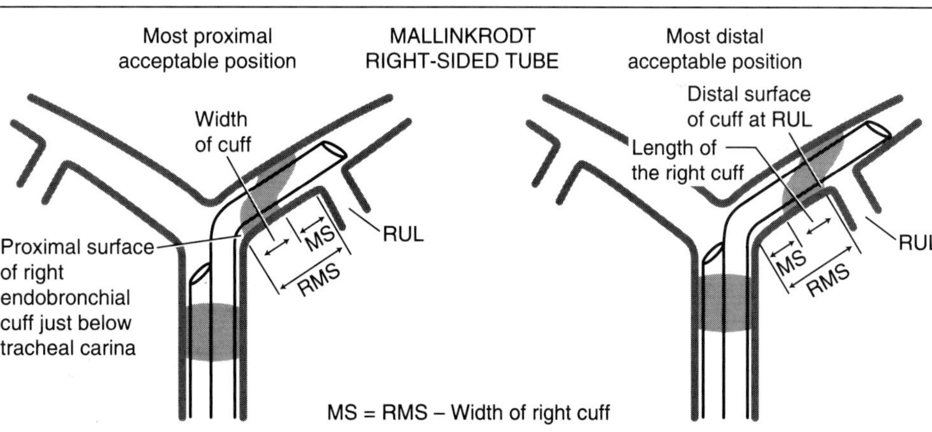

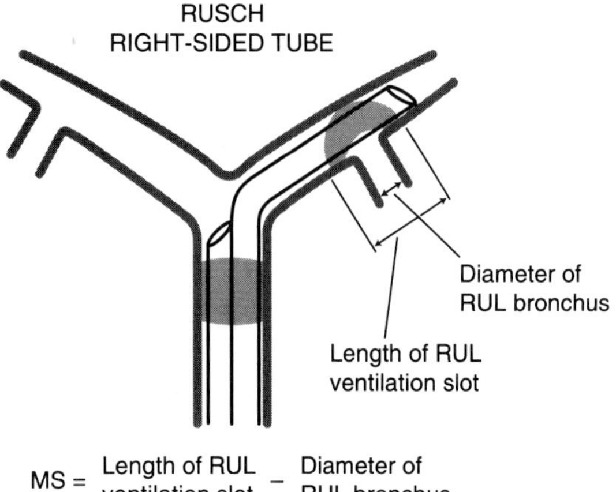

Figure 100–4. Margin of safety (MS) in the most distal and the most proximal positioning of left-sided and right-sided double-lumen endotracheal tubes. *Abbreviations*: LUL = left upper lobe; LMS = left mainstem bronchus; RUL = right upper lobe; RMS = right mainstem bronchus. (From Benumoff JL, Partridge BL, Salvatierra C, et al: Margin of safety in positioning modern double-lumen endotracheal tubes. Anesthesiology 1987; 67:729–738.)

for DLEB tube positioning. Fiberoptic bronchoscopy is the standard confirmatory method used if any question regarding optimal placement exists.

A method for secure fixation of the DLEB tube is required for long-term use of ILV. Physical factors that mitigate against proper tube placement include tubing weight, which causes gravitational pull and displacement during mechanical ventilation; slippery contact with oral secretions; and inflation of the DLEB cuff in a bronchus that in itself is fluted in configuration. All of these factors also may contribute to cuff herniation above the carina. Short of physically securing the DLEB tube to the upper teeth,[29] an acceptable and reliable technique has been to combine neck stabilization with DLEB tube fixation. Optimal tube positioning can vary by as much as 15 to 35 mm owing to a shorter radius in the posterior pharynx during neck flexion.[16] Although soft collars permit up to 75% of normal neck movement[86] and are not acceptable to prevent DLEB tube migration, a rigid collar, such as the Philadelphia collar, reduces flexion and extension to about 30% of normal and rotation and lateral movement to about 50% of normal.[87] Limitation of neck movement combined with the use of fixation devices, such as the SecureEasy oral endotracheal tube holder (IPI Medical Products, Chicago, IL) helps ensure proper tube placement. DLEB tubes have also been used successfully in patients with tracheostomies who require one-lung anesthesia;[88] however, suitable fixation during prolonged ILV in such patients is less likely to be maintained. Newer double-lumen tracheostomy tubes may improve fixation.

Currently, five sizes of DLEB tubes are available in clinical practice. The tubes range in odd-number sizes from 35 to 41 French to allow appropriate sizing for each adult patient (Table 100–4).

MONITORING DURING INDEPENDENT LUNG VENTILATION

Once ILV has been chosen as the method of ventilation, compulsive monitoring should be undertaken to ensure proper separation of ventilation (Table 100–5). Instead of bronchoscopically visualizing the position of each mainstem bronchus and carina through the tracheal lumen, the blue endobronchial cuff, and the segmental bronchi to ensure patency (described in detail elsewhere),[89] less invasive serial evaluation comparing differential pulmonary physiology can be used. Each tool has its own limitations, but when used in concert, correct DLEB tube positioning can be accomplished and maintained. Although alternating axillary chest auscultation may be useful when left and right lungs are sequentially ventilated immediately after intubation, transmission of breath sounds across the midline limits its usefulness during maintenance of ILV. More helpful are serial recordings of exhaled VT and peak Paw and volume-time and pressure-time curves for each lung. If asynchronous dual ventilation is used, auto-PEEP may be reflected either by the end-expiratory occlusion method[90] or qualitatively expressed by the flow-time curve as passive exhalation flow that does not return to zero flow prior to inspiration.

Although end-tidal carbon dioxide pressure (P_{ETCO_2}) monitoring may not detect malplacement of DLEB tubes,[91] individual capnographic waveform analysis in each lung is sufficiently sensitive to detect communication or obstruction during ILV. With carbon dioxide exhalation, inflection of the capnographs during synchronous or asynchronous ventilation unmistakably identifies either tube displacement or obstruction.[92] Some clinicians have even used monitoring of differential carbon dioxide elimination ($\dot{V}CO_2$) as a means to calculate VDS over time as an indirect assessment of individual $\dot{Q}pa$.[26] P_{ETCO_2} ratios that compare contused and noncontused lungs should be used with caution, as their use as a method of analysis may lead to underestimation of differential perfusion ratios.[93]

TABLE 100–4. Comparison of Double-Lumen Endobronchial Tube Sizes/Applications

Tube Size (French)	*Maximum Circumference (mm)*	*Lumenal Diameters (mm)*	*Usual Patient Applications*
35	38	5.0	Children > 40 kg
37	40	5.5	Small adults, usually women
39	44	6.0	Medium-sized adults
41	45	6.5	Large adults, usually men

(Data adapted from Burton NA, Watson DC, Brodsky JB, et al: Advantages of a new polyvinyl chloride double-lumen tube in thoracic surgery. Ann Thorac Surg 1983; 36:78–84.)

TABLE 100–5. Monitoring of Effective Lung Separation During Independent Lung Ventilation*

Chest Auscultation
Clamping and declamping of tracheal and endobronchial lumens sequentially

Serial Analysis of Differential Pulmonary Parameters
Exhaled VT
Peak Paw
Auto-PEEP
Varying FIO_2
Comparison of dual-capnograms
Pressure-volume loop hysteresis loops

Chest Radiographs

Flexible Fiberoptic Bronchoscopy

*Serial documentation in establishing a baseline for comparison is more helpful than any one parameter alone.

COMPLICATIONS ASSOCIATED WITH DOUBLE-LUMEN ENDOBRONCHIAL TUBES

Although several generations of DLEB tubes have been manufactured, the clinical applicability of these tubes continues to be limited by their design.[10] The airway injuries seen with the use of the antiquated, nondisposable Carlens tube and the red rubber Robertshaw tubes (Leyland) resulted from their size, shape (carinal hook, which can cause tracheal trauma), stiffness, and cuff design (low-volume, high-pressure) as well as from the materials used to construct the tubes. A rare and disastrous complication of the use of DLEB tubes is tracheal rupture following insertion.[94] Risk factors described along with tracheobronchial rupture include placement by an inexperienced laryngoscopist, use of an intubating stylet, multiple vigorous attempts at placement, tracheal abnormalities, overdistention of either the tracheal or bronchial cuffs, and advanced patient age.[95, 96] Moving the patient into the lateral decubitus position while the endobronchial cuff is inflated may result in bronchial laceration.[96] Signs of injury may become manifest for hours and can present as hemorrhage, air leak, pneumothorax, subcutaneous emphysema, or compliance changes. Airway trauma leading to ischemic injury and airway rupture may result from cuff overinflation, even with cuffs designed to have low pressures and high volumes. Insidious pressure changes may occur with the diffusion of anesthetic gases (e.g., nitrous oxide) and cause elevation in cuff pressures.[8]

The pressure-volume relationships for the endobronchial cuffs of tubes manufactured by Mallinckrodt, Rüsch, Sheridan, and Leyland are similar. Only 2 mL of air produced pressures greater than 80 mm Hg. However, when endobronchial tube cuffs were inflated to occlusion, only the Mallinckrodt and Rüsch cuffs had pressures lower than 20 mm Hg.[97] Given that the measurement of pressures within endotracheal tube cuffs is prone to error related to the equilibration of pressures within the manometer and pilot tubing, falsely low cuff pressures[98] may be obtained as a result of the added dead space. This error in measurement would only be exaggerated by the longer pilot tubing of DLEB tubes. Cuff inflation with the minimum occluding volume to minimize leak may be better than attempting to attain any particular minimum volume or pressure. If more than 3 mL is required for occlusion, cuff herniation above the carina usually exists.

WEANING FROM INDEPENDENT LUNG VENTILATION

Weaning from ILV should commence when the physiologic differences between the two lungs have either resolved or diminished to the point at which conventional pulmonary support is not only possible but avoids barotrauma.[99] The criteria that are used to predict success in converting from ILV back to single-lumen tube ventilation require equilibration of lung perfusion and lung ventilation (Table 100–6). The indicators that were used for instituting ILV must show continuous improvement such that differential PEEP, lung volumes, flow rates, minute ventilations, and nontoxic levels of oxygenation can all be accomplished with the single-lumen endotracheal tube. To examine whether compliance and Raw have improved in response to supportive therapy, separate pressure-volume curves can be used to test both Cst and Cdyn, as was originally described for acute respiratory distress during whole-lung ventilation.[100] To test the feasibility of whole-lung ventilation and the termination of ILV, the endobronchial cuff may be deflated and a Y-adapter inserted to allow single ventilatory support through the DLEB tube. If hemodynamic and gas exchange parameters remain stable after a period of time (usually 2–4 hours), successful exchange of endotracheal tubes is permitted. Occasionally, radiographs may be used as an indicator of success or failure: the return of atelectasis and derecruitment of alveoli indicate the need for continued ILV.

SUMMARY

ILV is a unique ventilatory modality owing to its ability to segregate the lungs from one another. It is a potentially lifesaving intervention in patients with asymmetric pulmonary pathophysiology, and it should be considered when conventional whole-lung ventilation fails. Further research addressing the indications for and the physiologic consequences of ILV are necessary.

TABLE 100–6. Weaning Criteria to Single-Lumen Ventilation from Independent Lung Ventilation

- PEEP differential < 5 cm H_2O
- Compliance differential < 10 mL/cm H_2O
- Raw < 3 cm $H_2O \cdot L^{-1} \cdot S^{-1}$
- Stability of PaO_2 on equalizing selective PEEP*
- Stability of left-sided and right-sided heart function on equalizing selective PEEP*
- Chest radiographic resolution of asymmetry after equalizing selective PEEP*
- Combined differential minute ventilation ($\dot{V}_E$) < 12 L/min
- Bronchopleural fistula closure

*Deflation of endobronchial cuff with Y-adapter linking the tube to a single mechanical ventilator.

References

1. Carlon GC, Ray C, Klein R, et al: Criteria for selective positive end-expiratory pressure and independent synchronized ventilation of each lung. Chest 1978; 74:501–507.
2. Cohen E, Eisenkraft JB, Thys DM, et al: Oxygenation and hemodynamic changes during one-lung ventilation: Effects of $CPAP_{10}$, $PEEP_{10}$, and $CPAP_{10}/PEEP_{10}$. J Cardiothorac Anesth 1988; 2:34–40.
3. Benumof JL: One-Lung ventilation and hypoxic pulmonary vasoconstriction: Implications for anesthetic management. Anesth Analg 1985; 64:821–833.
4. Benumof JL, Pirlo AF, Johanson I, et al: Interaction of $P\bar{v}O_2$ with PAO_2 on hypoxic pulmonary vasoconstriction. J Appl Physiol 1981; 51:871–874.
5. Muneyuki M, Konishi K, Horiguchi R, et al: Effects of alternating lung ventilation on cardiopulmonary function in dogs. Anesthesiology 1983; 58:353–356.
6. Carlens E: A new double-lumen catheter for bronchospirometry. J Thorac Surg 1949; 18:742.
7. Björk VO, Carlens E: The prevention of spread during pulmonary resection by the use of a double-lumen catheter. J Thorac Surg 1950; 20:151–157.
8. Neto PPR: Bronchial cuff pressure: Comparison of Carlens and polyvinylchloride (PVC) double-lumen tubes. Anesthesiology 1987; 66:255–256.
9. Burton NA, Watson DC, Brodsky JB, et al: Advantages of a new polyvinyl chloride double-lumen tube in thoracic surgery. Ann Thorac Surg 1983; 36:78–84.
10. Benumof JL: Improving the design and function of double-lumen tubes. J Cardiothorac Anesth 1988; 2:729–733.
11. McKenna MJ, Wilson RS, Botelho RJ: Right upper lobe obstruction with right-sided double-lumen endobronchial tubes: A comparison of two tube type. J Cardiothorac Anesth 1988; 2:734–740.
12. Benumof JL, Partridge BL, Salvatierra C, et al: Margin of safety in positioning modern double-lumen endotracheal tubes. Anesthesiology 1987; 67:729–738.
13. Glass DD, Tonnesen AS, Gabel JC, et al: Therapy of unilateral pulmonary insufficiency with a double-lumen endotracheal tube. Crit Care Med 1976; 4:323–326.
14. Powner DJ, Eross B, Grenvik A: Differential lung ventilation with PEEP in the treatment of unilateral pneumonia. Crit Care Med 1977; 5:170–172.
15. Zandstra DF, Stoutenbeek CP, Bams JL: Monitoring lung mechanics and airway pressures during differential lung ventilation (DLV) with emphasis on weaning from DLV. Intensive Care Med 1989; 15:458–463.
16. Saito S, Dohi S, Naito H: Alteration of double-lumen endobronchial tube position by flexion and extension of the neck. Anesthesiology 1985; 62:696–697.
17. Hansen-Flaschen JH, Brazinsky S, Basile C, et al: Use of sedating drugs and neuromuscular blocking agents in patients requiring mechanical ventilation for respiratory failure: A national survey. JAMA 1991; 266:2870–2875.
18. Segredo V, Caldwell JE, Matthay MA: Persistent paralysis in critically ill patients after long-term administration of vecuronium. N Engl J Med 1992; 327:524–528.
19. Danon MJ, Carpenter S: Myopathy with thick filament (myosin) loss following prolonged paralysis with vecuronium during steroid treatment. Muscle Nerve 1991; 99:176–184.
20. Subramony SH, Carpenter DE, Raju S, et al: Myopathy and prolonged neuromuscular blockade after lung transplant. Crit Care Med 1991; 19:1580–1582.
21. Smith JD, Millen JE, Safar P, et al: Intrathoracic pressure, pulmonary vascular pressures and gas exchange during pulmonary lavage. Anesthesiology 1970; 33:401–405.
22. Lippman M, Mok MS: Anesthetic management of pulmonary lavage. Anesthesiology 1978; 33:401.
23. Claypool WD, Rogers RM, Matuschak GM: Update on the

clinical diagnosis, management, and pathophysiology of pulmonary alveolar proteinosis (phospholipidosis). Chest 1984; 85:550.
24. Shivaram U, Finch P, Nowak P: Plastic endobronchial tubes in the management of life-threatening hemoptysis. Chest 1987; 92:1108–1110.
25. Zandstra DF, Stoutenbeek CP: Treatment of massive unilateral pulmonary embolism by differential lung ventilation. Intensive Care Med 1987; 13:422–424.
26. Zandstra DF, Stoutenbeek CP: Monitoring differential CO_2 excretion during differential lung ventilation in asymmetric pulmonary contusion: Clinical implications. Intensive Care Med 1988; 14:106–109.
27. Carlon GC, Kahn R, Howland WS, et al: Acute life-threatening ventilation-perfusion inequality: An indication for independent lung ventilation. Crit Care Med 1978; 6:380–383.
28. Sachdeva SP: Treatment of post-operative pulmonary atelectasis by active inflation of the atelectatic lobe(s) through an endobronchial tube. Acta Anaesthesiol Scand 1974; 18:65.
29. Rafferty TD, Palma J, Motoyama EK, et al: Management of a bronchopleural fistula with differential lung ventilation and positive end-expiratory pressure. Respir Care 1980; 25:654–657.
30. Benjaminsson E, Klain M: Intraoperative dual-mode independent lung ventilation of a patient with bronchopleural fistula. Anesth Analg 1981; 60:118–119.
31. Conacher ID: Isolated lung transplantation: A review of problems and guide to anaesthesia. Br J Anaesth 1988; 61:468–474.
32. Smiley RM, Navedo AT, Kirby T, et al: Postoperative independent lung ventilation in a single-lung transplant recipient. Anesthesiology 1991; 74:1144–1148.
33. Heerdt PM, Triantafillou A: Perioperative management of patients receiving a lung transplant. Anesthesiology 1991; 75:922–923.
34. Kvetan V, Carlon GC, Howland WS: Acute pulmonary failure in asymmetric lung disease: Approach to management. Crit Care Med 1982; 10:114–118.
35. Brochard L, Isabey D, Piquet J: Reversal of acute exacerbations of chronic obstructive lung disease by inspiratory assistance with a face mask. N Engl J Med 1990; 323:1523–1530.
36. Farias E, Rudski L, Zidulka A: Delivery of high inspired oxygen by face mask. J Crit Care 1991; 6:119–124.
36a. Lamm WJE, Graham MM, Albert RK: Mechanism by which the prone position improves oxygenation in acute lung injury. Am J Respir Crit Care Med 1994; 150:184–193.
37. Syracuse DC, Hyman AI, King TC: Postural influences on arterial blood gases in patients with unilateral pulmonary consolidation. Surg Forum 1979; 30:173.
38. Novak RA, Shumaker L, Snyder JV, et al: Do periodic hyperinflations improve gas exchange in patients with hypoxemic respiratory failure? Crit Care Med 1987; 15:1081–1085.
39. Scholten DJ, Novak RA, Snyder JV: Directed manual recruitment of collapsed lung in intubated and nonintubated patients. Ann Surg 1985; 51:530.
40. Otis AB, McKerrow CB, Bartlett RA, et al: Mechanical factors in the distribution of pulmonary ventilation. J Appl Physiol 1956; 8:427–443.
41. Remolina C, Kahn AU, Santiago TV, et al: Positional hypoxemia in unilateral lung disease. N Engl J Med 1981; 304:523.
42. Pirlo AF, Benumof JL, Trousdale FR: Atelectatic lung lobe blood flow: open vs closed chest, positive pressure vs spontaneous ventilation. J Appl Physiol 1981; 50:1022–1026.
43. Kumar A, Falke KJ, Geffin B, et al: Continuous positive-pressure ventilation in acute respiratory failure. N Engl J Med 1970; 283:1430.
44. Leftwich IE, Witorsch RJ, Witorsch P: Positive end-expiratory pressure in refractory hypoxemia. Ann Intern Med 1973; 79:187.
45. Gattinoni L, Pesenti A, Bombino M, et al: Relationships between lung computed tomographic density, gas exchange, and PEEP in acute respiratory failure. Anesthesiology 1988; 69:824–832.
46. Gattinoni L, D'Andrea L, Pelosi P, et al: Regional effects and mechanisms of positive end-expiratory pressure in early adult respiratory distress syndrome. JAMA 1993; 269:2122–2127.
47. Hedenstierna G, Baehrendtz S, Klingstedt C, et al: Ventilation and perfusion of each lung during differential ventilation with selective PEEP. Anesthesiology 1984; 61:369–376.
48. Parker JC, Hernandez LA, Longenecker GL, et al: Lung edema caused by high peak inspiratory pressures in dogs. Am Rev Respir Dis 1990; 142:321–328.
49. Kolobow T, Moretti MP, Fumagalli R, et al: Severe impairment in lung function induced by high peak airway pressures during mechanical ventilation. Am Rev Respir Dis 1987; 135:312–315.
50. Lain DC, DiBenedetto R, Morris SL, et al: Pressure control inverse ratio ventilation as a method to reduce peak inspiratory pressure and provide adequate ventilation and oxygenation. Chest 1989; 95:1081–1088.
51. Rouby JJ, Fusciardi J, Bourgain JL, et al: High-frequency jet ventilation in postoperative respiratory failure: Determinants of oxygenation. Anesthesiology 1983; 59:281.
52. Marini JJ, Ravenscraft SA: Mean airway pressure: Physiologic determinants and clinical importance: Part 1. Physiologic determinants and measurements. Crit Care Med 1992; 20:1461–1472.
53. Marini JJ, Ravenscraft SA: Mean airway pressure: Physiologic determinants and clinical importance: Part 2. Clinical implications. Crit Care Med 1992; 20:1604–1616.
54. Morgan BC, Abel FL, Mullins GL, et al: Flow-patterns in cavae, pulmonary artery, pulmonary vein and aorta in intact dogs. Am J Physiol 1966; 210:903.
55. Permutt S, Howell JBL, Proctor DF, et al: Effect of lung inflation on static pressure-volume characteristics of pulmonary vessels. J Appl Physiol 1961; 16:64.
56. Canada E, Benumof JL, Tousdale FR: Pulmonary vascular resistance correlated in intact normal and abnormal canine lungs. Crit Care Med 1982; 10:719.
57. Marshall BE, Marshall C: Continuity of response to hypoxic pulmonary vasoconstriction. J Appl Physiol 1980; 49:189.
58. Kanarek DJ, Shannon DC: Adverse effect of PEEP on pulmonary perfusion and arterial oxygenation. Am Rev Respir Dis 1975; 112:457.
59. Flacke JW, Thompson DS, Read RC: Influence of tidal volume and pulmonary artery occlusion on arterial oxygenation during endobronchial anesthesia. South Med J 1976; 69:619–626.
60. Tarhan S, Lundborg RO: Effects of increased expiratory pressure on blood gas tensions and pulmonary shunting during thoracotomy with use of the Carlens catheter. Can Anaesth Soc J 1970; 17:4–11.
61. Siegal LC, Pearl RG, Shafer SL, et al: The longitudinal distribution of pulmonary resistance during unilateral hypoxia. Anesthesiology 1989; 70:527–532.
62. Hales CA: The site and mechanism of oxygen sensing for pulmonary vessels. Chest 1985; 88 (Suppl):235S–240S.
63. Staub NC: Site of hypoxic pulmonary vasoconstriction. Chest 1985; 88 (Suppl):240S–245S.
64. Bergman NA: Hypoxic pulmonary vasoconstriction. Semin Anesth 1987; 6:188–195.
65. Benumof JL, Mathers JM, Wahrenbrock EA: Cyclic hypoxic pulmonary vasoconstriction induced by concomitant carbon dioxide changes. J Appl Physiol 1976; 41:466–499.
66. Colley PS, Cheney FW: Sodium nitroprusside increases $\dot{Q}s/\dot{Q}t$ in dogs with regional atelectasis. Anesthesiology 1977; 47:338–341.
67. Casthely PA, Lear S, Cotterell JE, et al: Intrapulmonary shunting during induced hypotension. Anesth Analg 1982; 61:231–235.
68. Nakazawa K, Amaha K: Effect of nicardipine hydrochloride on regional hypoxic pulmonary vasoconstriction. Br J Anaesth 1988; 60:547–554.
69. Tucker A, McMurtry IF, Grover RF, et al: Attenuation of hypoxic pulmonary vasoconstriction by verapamil in intact dogs. Proc Exp Biol Med 1976; 151:611–614.
70. Conover WB, Benumof JL, Key TC: Ritodrine inhibition of hypoxic pulmonary vasoconstriction. Am J Obstet Gynecol 1983; 146:652.
71. Domino KB, Borowec L, Alexander CM, et al: Influence of isoflurane on hypoxic pulmonary vasoconstriction in dogs. Anesthesiology 1986; 64:423–429.

72. Mayers I, Hurst T, To T, et al: Vasodilators or vasoconstrictors prevent hypoxic pulmonary vasoconstriction. J Crit Care 1991; 6:125–135.
73. Takasaki M, Oh-Oka T, Saito Y, et al: Low dose almitrine bismesylate improves pulmonary gas exchange during canine one-lung hypoxia. Crit Care Med 1989; 17:661–665.
74. Feely TW, Keating D, Nishimura T: Independent lung ventilation using high-frequency ventilation in the management of a bronchopleural fistula. Anesthesiology 1988; 69:420–422.
75. Snyder JV, Powner DJ: Effects of mechanical ventilation on the measurement of cardiac output by thermodilution. Crit Care Med 1982; 10:677–682.
76. Hakim TS, Michel RP, Minami H, et al: Site of pulmonary hypoxic vasoconstriction studied with arterial and venous occlusion. J Appl Physiol 1983; 54:1298–1302.
77. Brower H, Gottlieb J, Wise RA, et al: Locus of hypoxic vasoconstriction in isolated ferret lungs. J Appl Physiol 1987; 63:59–65.
78. Pinsky MR, Summer WR: Cardiac augmentation by phasic high intrathoracic support (PHIPS) in man. Chest 1983; 84:370–375.
79. Crimi G, Candiani A, Conti G, et al: Clinical applications of independent lung ventilation with unilateral high-frequency jet ventilation (ILV-UHFJV). Intensive Care Med 1986; 12:90–94.
80. Aalto-Setälä M, Heinonen J, Salorinne Y: Cardiorespiratory function during thoracic anaesthesia: A comparison of two-lung ventilation and one-lung ventilation with and without $PEEP_5$. Acta Anaesth Scand 1975; 19:287.
81. Gallagher TJ, Banner MJ, Smith RA: A simplified method of independent lung function. Crit Care Med 1980; 8:390.
82. Hillman KM, Barber JD: Asynchronous independent lung ventilation (AILV). Crit Care Med 1980; 8:390.
83. Brodsky JB, Benumof JL, Ehrenwerth J: Depth of placement of left double-lumen endobronchial tubes. Anesth Analg 1991; 73:570–572.
84. Ehrenwerth J: Pro: Proper positioning of a double-lumen endobronchial tube can only be accomplished with endoscopy. J Cardiothorac Anesth 1988; 2:101–104.
85. Brodsky JB: Con: Proper positioning of a double-lumen endobronchial tube can only be accomplished with endoscopy. J Cardiothorac Anesth 1988; 2:105–109.
86. Colachis SC, Strohm BR, Ganter EL: Cervical spine motion in normal women: Radiographic study of effect of cervical collars. Arch Phys Med Rehabil 1973; 54:161–169.
87. Johnson RM, Hart DL, Simmons EF, et al: Cervical orthoses. J Bone Joint Surg 1977; 59A:332–339.
88. Coe VL, Brodsky JB, Mark JBD: Double-lumen endobronchial tubes for patients with tracheostomies. Anesth Analg 1984; 63:882.
89. Slinger PD: Fiberoptic bronchoscopic positioning of double-lumen tubes. J Cardiothorac Anesth 1989; 3:486–496.
90. Bates JHT, Milic-Emili J: The flow interruption technique for measuring respiratory resistance. J Crit Care 1991; 6:227–238.
91. deVries JW, Haanschoten MC: Capnography does not reliably detect double-lumen endotracheal tube malplacement. J Clin Monit 1992; 8:236–237.
92. Shafieha MJ, Sit J, Kartha R, et al: End-tidal CO_2 analyzers in proper positioning of the double-lumen tubes. Anesthesiology 1986; 64:844–845.
93. Zandstra DF, Stoutenbeek CP: Reflection of differential pulmonary perfusion in polytrauma patients on differential lung ventilation (DLV). Intensive Care Med 1989; 15:151–154.
94. Wagner DL, Gammage GW, Wong ML: Tracheal rupture following the insertion of a disposable double-lumen endotracheal tube. Anesthesiology 1985; 63:698–700.
95. Blanc FV, Tremblay NAG: Complications of tracheal intubation: A new classification with a review of the literature. Anesth Analg 1974; 53:202–213.
96. Tornvall SS, Jackson KH, Oyanedel ET: Tracheal rupture, complication of cuff endotracheal tube. Chest 1971; 59:237–239.
97. Brodsky JB, Adkins MO, Gaba DM: Bronchial cuff pressures of double-lumen tubes. Anesth Analg 1989; 69:608–610.
98. Cox PM, Schatz ME: Pressure measurements in endotracheal cuffs: A common error. Chest 1974; 65:84–87.
99. Hurst JM, DeHaven CB, Branson RD: Comparison of conventional mechanical ventilation and synchronous independent lung ventilation (SILV) in the treatment of unilateral lung injury. J Trauma 1985; 25:766–770.
100. Bone RC: Diagnosis of causes for acute respiratory distress by pressure volume curves. Chest 1976; 70:740–746.

CHAPTER 101

Computerized Management of Mechanical Ventilation

Thomas D. East, PhD • Alan H. Morris, MD
Reed M. Gardner, PhD

It is ironic that the man whose name was chosen for the international unit of pressure, Blaise Pascal, was also the 17th century inventor of the first calculating machine.[1, 2] In a sense, the link between mechanical positive-pressure ventilation and computers has existed from the beginnings of these two technologies. The introduction of the minicomputer and the microcomputer in the 1970s dramatically increased the availability of computers. It was during this era that computers first began to be routinely used in hospitals and intensive care units (ICUs). The initial systems typically used teletypewriters and primitive video terminals as user interfaces. The proliferation of the early personal computer and its clones in the early 1980s greatly enhanced the spread of computers in medicine in general. The evolution of the computer industry in the mid- to late 1980s blurred many of the previous distinctions between minicomputers, microcomputers, and mainframe computers. It rapidly became possible to provide what used to be considered mainframe computing power with a single microchip the size of a postage stamp.

Why would anyone use a computer to manage mechanical ventilation? If the history of computers is examined, it becomes clear that computers were created to help the human mind deal with large amounts of information, complex mathematics, and complex data manipulation as well as to automatically perform well-defined, repetitive tasks. There are few devices in medicine that are as complex, data intensive, and associated with well-defined repetitive tasks (e.g., delivering breaths repeatedly) as a modern mechanical ventilator. Since the late 1970s, the fundamental operation of the mechanical ventilator has been increasingly turned over to microprocessor control.[3] In addition to their computing capabilities, microprocessor systems provide an excellent platform on which to build devices that can easily be modified and updated. Microprocessor-controlled systems make it easy (with software changes) to modify ventilators without the need to change expensive physical components. As a result, an explosion of new modes and monitoring techniques occurred during the 1980s. Automation of the routine management of mechanical ventilation has been attempted since 1953,[4] only 10 years after the first electronic digital computer was constructed. Automation of mechanical ventilation management has continued to evolve, with increasing success and areas of clinical application, over the last 40 years.[5] The purpose of this chapter is to review the use of computers in the management of mechanical ventilation. The primary areas of computer application in management of mechanical ventilation are operation of mechanical ventilators, charting and information systems, and decision support.

COMPUTERS IN THE OPERATION OF MECHANICAL VENTILATORS

A fundamental part of a mechanical ventilator is that component that controls the timing and delivery of a gas under positive pressure to a patient. The early mechanical ventilators either used a mechanical system or a pneumatic system to control both the timing and delivery of the gas.[3] A good example of the mechanical system was the piston pump system. The piston pump was driven by a motor that turned a camshaft. The speed of the motor and the mechanical linkage between the camshaft and the piston determined the timing and volume of a breath. The bellows (or "bag-in-box") ventilator (still in use in anesthesiology) is a good example of the pneumatic system, in which gas under pressure is used to compress a bellows and to deliver a volume of gas to a patient. The timing of the ventilator was controlled by pneumatic valves that switched on or off as pressure in the circuit crossed certain thresholds. As ventilators became more sophisticated, a merging of mechanical, pneumatic, and electric systems occurred. One significant advance was the use of proportional gas delivery valves that used a high-pressure gas source to produce whatever flow or pressure profile was desired. Siemens (Cupertino, CA) was the first manufacturer to introduce electronic feedback control of these proportional valves (Servo 900B) to produce a variety of different flow and pressure waveforms. These "Servo"-controlled proportional valves were really the key to the birth of the variety of ventilator modes that are now available. Even though many of the modern ventilators introduced in the 1960s and 1970s included electronic control of the ventilator, it was not until the late 1970s that a digital computer was used to control the valves in the ventilator.

It was inevitable that digital computers would be used to operate ventilators, and it is not surprising that it was only a few years after the initial design of a microcomputer when the first Food and Drug Administration 510 K approval was given for a microprocessor-controlled ventilator, the Rodder ventilator (Rodder Instruments, Los Altos, CA).[5] The Rodder ventilator was followed by the manufacturer of a couple of microprocessor-controlled infant ventilators and then by the introduction of the Bear 5 (Bear Medical, Riverside, CA) and the Puritan Bennett 7200 (Puritan Bennett Corporation, Carlsbad, CA) adult ventilators. The previous analog systems were excellent; however, they lacked the ability to be easily changed and adapted. With the electronic ventilators of the 1970s and early 1980s, addition of a new mode of mechanical ventilation required the addition of all new analog control circuits. Typically, these analog systems were not designed for such expansion. The microprocessor offers the unique ability of providing rapid and precise control of gas delivery and of simultaneously running the user interface, collecting data, and monitoring ventilator performance. In addition, the computer could easily be reprogrammed to add new modes and other features. The control and operation of mechanical ventilators seemed an ideal application for the digital microcomputer.

Figure 101–1 is an illustration of how microcomputers are used in a modern ventilator. The primary function of the microprocessor is to regulate the proportional function of the valves delivering air and oxygen to the patient. Typically, these valves are closed-loop controlled. For example, to produce pressure support ventilation, the ventilator monitors airway pressure and opens or closes a valve as needed to maintain a desired pressure level. These fast closed-loop control systems are good; however, they are not perfect and do exhibit undesired control behavior, such as overshoot and ringing (Fig. 101–2). The same concept applies for volume control with a constant inspiratory flow profile. The only difference is that the proportional valve is feedback-controlled to maintain a desired flow rate. Typically, the computer in the ventilator is updating the position of the proportional valve at least every 1/100 of a second. In the new Siemens Servo 300, the valve is adjusted every 1/1000 of a second.[6] The advantage of such a closed-loop controller is that the valve does not need to be linear or necessarily stable over time. What is critical is that the input to the controller—flow or pressure—must be accurate and precise, otherwise the function of the entire system will be inaccurate. In addition, the control algorithm must be carefully adjusted to provide optimal performance over the operating range of the system. This adjustment is not an easy task when one considers that a ventilator such as the Siemens Servo 300 must ventilate with tidal volumes ranging from 2 mL to 4 L with only one valve. As can be seen in Figure 101–1, it is easy for manufacturers to provide a variety of modes, such as pressure support, pressure control, and volume control. Several new modes of ventilation include a second feedback loop that is superimposed on the existing ones for pressure support or pressure control. Figure 101–3 illustrates the new modes of volume support and pressure-regulated volume control that were introduced with the Siemens Servo 300. These include an outer feedback loop that adjusts, over several breaths, the set point of the faster inner feedback loop. This concept has been in use since the mid-1980s in modes such as mandatory minute ventilation, in which the support level is adjusted slowly over several breaths to maintain a desired minute ventilation range. It is unclear what impact the new ventilator modes have on patient outcome; however, the new modes represent a new level of sophistication and complexity in the control of gas delivery.

The concepts of feedback control also can be applied to the expiratory valve. The Siemens 900C ventilator uses the pressure measured in the inspiratory limb of the patient circuit as feedback control to adjust the expiratory pinch valve to maintain a desired positive end-expiratory pressure (PEEP) value (Fig. 101–4). The inspiratory limb has zero flow during expiration, ensuring measurement of pressure at the patient manifold, even though the pressure transducer is within the ventilator. The advantage of using a feedback-controlled valve is that a relatively simple valve and pressure sensor can be made to behave like a threshold resistor (zero resistance until pressure reaches the PEEP value, and thereafter resistance is infinite). An additional advantage is that it is easy for the microprocessor to control this expiratory valve for measurements, such as of intrinsic PEEP, whose determination requires an end-expiratory hold. Not all microprocessor-based ventilators use a computer-controlled expiratory valve. For example, the Puritan Bennett 7200 uses a pneumatically controlled expiratory valve that depends only on pressures in the breathing circuit, and it has no computer control.

Charting and Information Systems

Despite the large amount of clinical respiratory care data and the obvious difficulty in their management with handwritten records, respiratory care information systems have not had widespread acceptance as modalities for recording information during mechanical ventilation. Much of the reason probably lies in cost justification of such systems. Such systems are typically cost justified based on the extent to

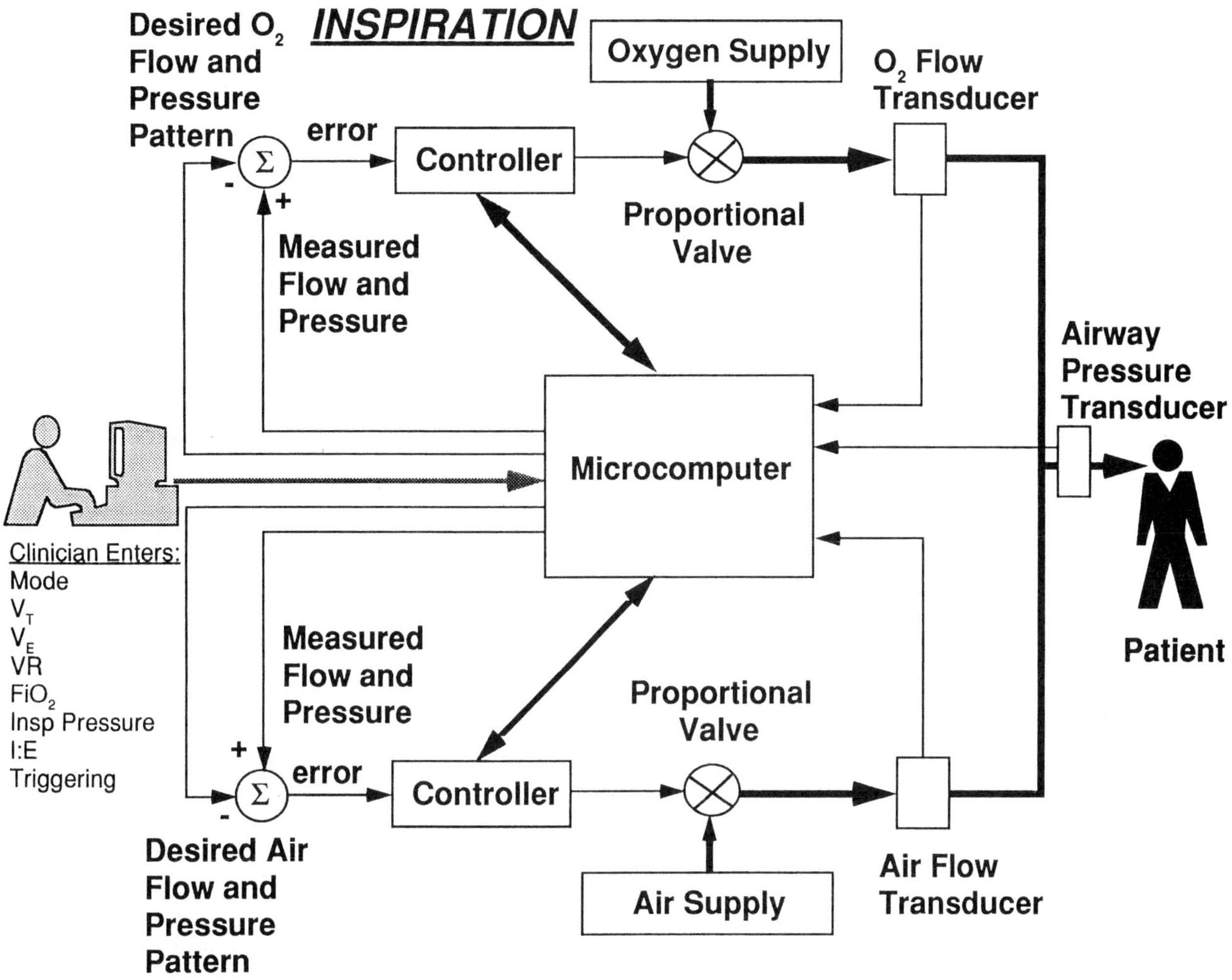

INSPIRATION

Desired O_2 Flow and Pressure Pattern
Oxygen Supply
O_2 Flow Transducer
error
Controller
Proportional Valve
Measured Flow and Pressure
Airway Pressure Transducer
Microcomputer
Patient
Clinician Enters:
Mode
V_T
V_E
VR
FiO_2
Insp Pressure
I:E
Triggering
Measured Flow and Pressure
Proportional Valve
error
Controller
Desired Air Flow and Pressure Pattern
Air Supply
Air Flow Transducer

Figure 101–1. Microprocessor-controlled mechanical ventilator. The microprocessor uses data from the flow and pressure sensors as well as input from the user to determine the correct positioning of the proportional gas supply valve. Separate control systems for air and oxygen provide the desired fraction of inspired oxygen. *Abbreviations*: V_T = tidal volume; V_E = expired minute volume; VR = respiratory rate; FiO_2 = fraction of inspired oxygen; Insp = inspiratory; I:E = ratio of inspiratory time to expiratory time.

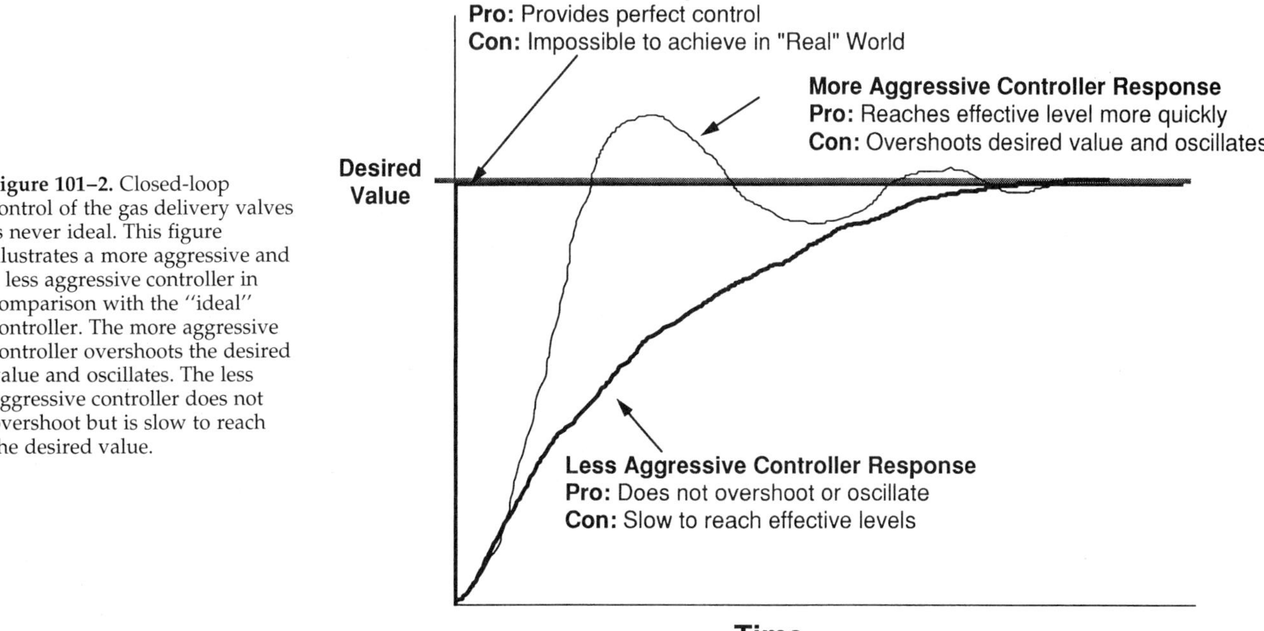

Figure 101–2. Closed-loop control of the gas delivery valves is never ideal. This figure illustrates a more aggressive and a less aggressive controller in comparison with the "ideal" controller. The more aggressive controller overshoots the desired value and oscillates. The less aggressive controller does not overshoot but is slow to reach the desired value.

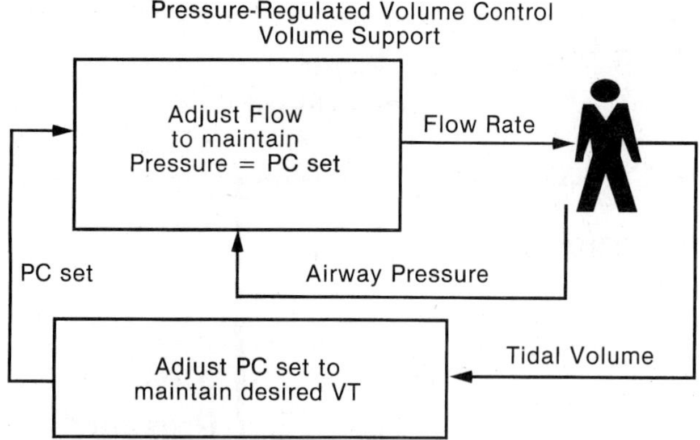

Figure 101–3. Volume support and pressure-regulated volume control are examples of double-feedback systems. The standard inner feedback loop adjusts the gas delivery valve to provide the desired pressure. An outer feedback loop adjusts the desired pressure level of the inner loop to deliver the desired tidal volume.

which the reduced time spent on charting and performing record audits, the implication being that money would be saved if such systems could decrease staffing requirements. Andrews and coworkers reported that the respiratory care charting portion of the HELP system at LDS Hospital (Salt Lake City, UT) was associated with an 18.2% increase in productivity and a 20.9% increase in work volume.[7] Full-time equivalent staffing requirements did not change. An average of 2.6 minutes was spent on each documentation in 1984 compared with 1.37 minutes in 1992.[8] Some have claimed that information systems are cost justified based on the reduction in full-time equivalents that they provide; however, this is controversial. Hammond and associates have demonstrated that an ICU patient data management system can significantly reduce the number of errors found in paper flow charts[9] and improve the quality, accuracy, and timely capture and retrieval of data. They did not show a reduction in the required nursing full-time equivalents.[10] Bradshaw and colleagues showed a reduction in nursing time spent on direct patient care (from 49.1% to 43.2%) and an increase in time spent on clinical data entry (from 18.2% to 24.2%).[11] Many anecdotal reports exist describing the impact of such systems on the quality of patient care; however, few conclusive studies clearly demonstrate improvement in the quality of patient care. One would assume that the improvements in the quality of a patient's charting would impact on the quality of the patient's care; however, some have estimated that at least 6000 patients would be required to be able to statistically detect any impact on patient outcome[12] (assuming a reduction in mortality from 16% to 14.4%). It may be possible to observe an impact on the quality of patient care by looking at other intermediate indicators, such as the length of hospital stay and the incidence of mistakes. It is essential that carefully designed studies be performed to evaluate the impact of these systems.

The main problem with demonstrating efficacy of information systems for mechanical ventilation may be that the current systems that focus on automating the charting process do not really address the needs of the clinician in the ICU environment. What are the real needs of the clinician (physician, nurse, and respiratory therapist) at the bedside? Not long ago, the author (AHM) went to the bedside of one critically ill patient and counted the current information categories (not repeated measures) that were reviewed one morning during ICU rounds and found that the total number of variable categories exceeded 236.[13] Eddy summarized the problem best: "It is simply unrealistic to think that individuals can synthesize in their head scores of pieces of evidence, accurately estimate the outcomes of different options, and accurately judge the desirability of those outcomes for patients. . . . All confirm what would be expected from common sense: the complexity of modern medicine exceeds the inherent limitations of the unaided human mind."[14] The next generation of computers for mechanical ventilation *must* help the clinician to assimilate the myriad data and to quickly make effective decisions. It is not enough to merely display data in a large spreadsheet or on a complex colorful graph. New data display concepts and

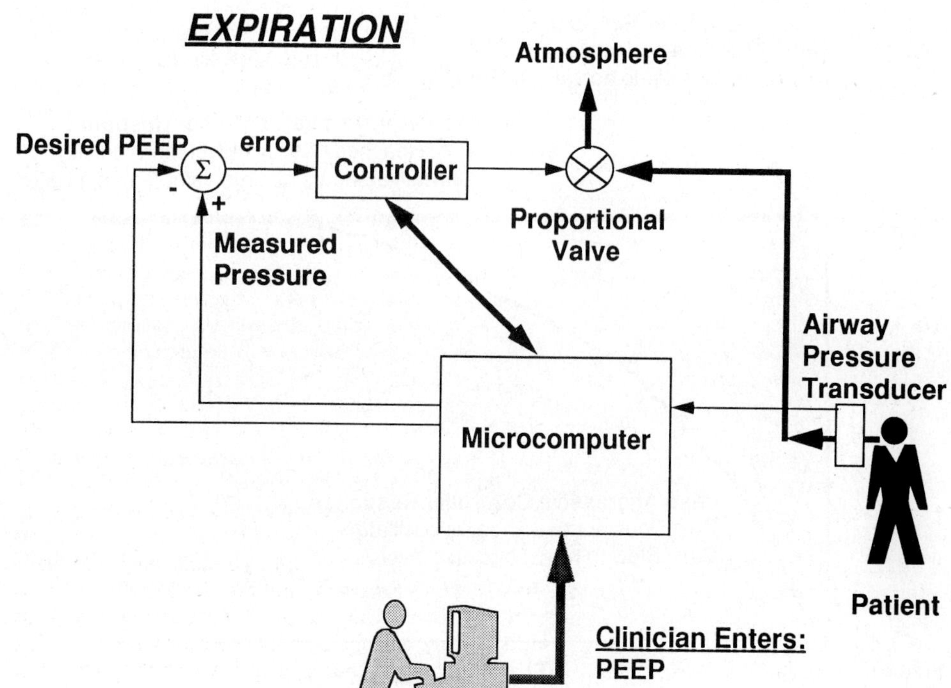

Figure 101–4. Many microprocessor-based ventilators use an active exhalation valve that is under computer control. The computer uses a feedback control system to adjust the expiratory valve to maintain the desired PEEP level.

expert systems need to be included in commercial ventilator products. Very few computer systems for the ICU currently provide any tools for decision support. If the next generation of ICU computer systems is to have a significant impact on the quality of patient care, they must include a fully integrated data base, automated charting of data from mechanical ventilators, and tools for decision-making support.

Fully Integrated Data Base

An effective system needs to interface with or already include sources of data from more than just the ICU. These sources include the admission, discharge, and transfer department, laboratories, radiology department, operating rooms, and outpatient clinics. The introduction of prospective reimbursement has resulted in the performance of as many tests as possible on an outpatient basis before hospitalization. It is essential that the data from the outpatient visits be available and integrated with the ICU data.[15, 16] If data base integration is handled by an interface with other systems, the interface must guarantee accurate and timely data collection (response time delay < 1 minute) and avoid the pitfalls of duplicating a copy of a remote data base. The risk is that some interface techniques might download data periodically from a remote system. This does not guarantee "timely" access to data, and it may not guarantee that changes are communicated to the ICU computer system if the data are edited at the original laboratory. There is a movement toward the establishment of local, regional, national, and international data bases that would track all medical information on a patient from birth to death.[16] It is obvious that access to such systems would facilitate medical care in our highly mobile society. The integrated data base must not only be available in the ICU but also made accessible to other departments and divisions that need to complete their own integration. This includes the billing and accounting departments, where all procedures charted in the ICU can be billed separately, thus improving charge capture and reducing lost charges to third-party payers.

Automated Charting of Data from Mechanical Ventilators

Several commercially available systems interface with selected ventilators. The Puritan Bennett Clinivision (Puritan Bennett, Carlsbad, CA) interfaces directly with the manufacturer's 7200 ventilator. Various ICU computer systems have developed interfaces for the Puritan Bennett 7200, Siemens 900C (Siemens-Elema, Solna, Sweden) with the 990 Servo computer module, Hamilton Amadeus (Hamilton Ventilators, Reno, CA), Hamilton Alveolar, Bear 5 (Bear Medical, Riverside, CA), and other ventilators that have digital communication ports. These interfaces are usually custom interfaces that are specifically matched to a particular ventilator. These custom interfaces can be expensive and difficult to maintain. This means that if an existing computer system in a hospital is to be connected the ventilators, most likely a great deal of time and money will have to be spent to accomplish the task. The vast majority of ventilators have digital communication ports that remain unused.

Several successful research systems have interfaced ventilators with computers. Shabot and Gardner at Cedar-Sinai Hospital (Los Angeles, CA) have interfaced their Hewlett-Packard (Palo Alto, CA) ICU computer system with the Puritan Bennett 7200 ventilator.[17, 18] In this system, data is only sent from the ventilator when the clinician at the bedside pushes a button or when a setting is changed. The authors have developed individual research systems that interface with the Siemens 900C and 900i ventilators[19–22] as well as with the Hamilton Amadeus[23] and the Puritan Bennett 7200.[24]

To facilitate automatic data acquisition from a wide variety of medical devices, a standardized Medical Information Bus (MIB) has been proposed.[17] The MIB provides a local area network around a patient. The MIB can be interfaced with all bedside devices and allows data from each of the devices to be stored in a central data base in a standard format.[25–28] The MIB is being standardized by the Institute of Electrical and Electronics Engineers (IEEE, New York, NY) so that all hospitals and vendors can use a common data format and easily communicate with multiple bedside devices.[17] The MIB addresses issues unique to the medical data communications environment, such as the need for automatic recognition of new devices placed at a bedside, automatic reconfiguration of a network, and logical association of a device to a particular patient.[17] Unfortunately, the currently proposed MIB does not include standards for artifact rejection and significant event identification.[29, 30] It is ironic that the largest amount of effort in developing the MIB standard has been spent on the standardization of digital communication and that this feature is the least important to medical decision making.

A preliminary version of the MIB was installed at the 520-bed LDS Hospital and connected to the HELP system[29–32] (Fig. 101–5). An MIB interface for ventilators has been constructed at the LDS Hospital.[24, 33] The authors have completed studies investigating techniques for identifying artifacts and significant events.[34] Data were collected for 617 hours from 10 patients ventilated using the Puritan Bennett 7200 ventilator. Data from the ventilator was sampled at 10-second intervals and stored in a research data base. This large research data base was then used to examine six different filters designed to eliminate artifact: moving average, moving median, two different moving exponentially weighted averages, LOWESS (a robust locally weighted regression technique)[35], and a moving LOWESS. Significant events were identified as values that were above a defined threshold for a period of time (intervals of both 1 and 3 minutes were tested). The output from each of these algorithms was compared with the concurrent data in the HELP system that had been entered by the respiratory therapist with a bedside keyboard. Some differences between the ventilator settings charted by the registered technician and by the MIB were found. The "error" rate for manual charting of ventilator settings was 3%. From careful screening, most of the difference was found to come from technician "back-charting" with the wrong time-stamp and from the "time delay" of the automated charting algorithms. Respiratory care therapists tended to enter data and stamp the chart with the time that they "thought" was the time of the events' occurrence. Occasionally, this time stamping was in error. The error rate for manual charting was reduced to 1% if all the errors caused by back-charting were neglected.[34]

Figure 101–6 is an example of the tidal volume data collected during this study.[24] The raw data contained a lot of "noise" and "artifact." In general, all the filtering algorithms helped to reduce artifact; however, the moving LOWESS filter performed best. The disadvantage of the moving LOWESS filter is that it requires much more computer time than does a simple moving median filter. The moving median seemed to be the best choice because it did not follow transient events (i.e., suctioning, cough) and was relatively simple to implement. Large differences between the number of events found by the filtering algorithms to be "significant" and the number of those charted manually were found. Two main differences were observed: (1) the therapists did not chart what occurred when they were not

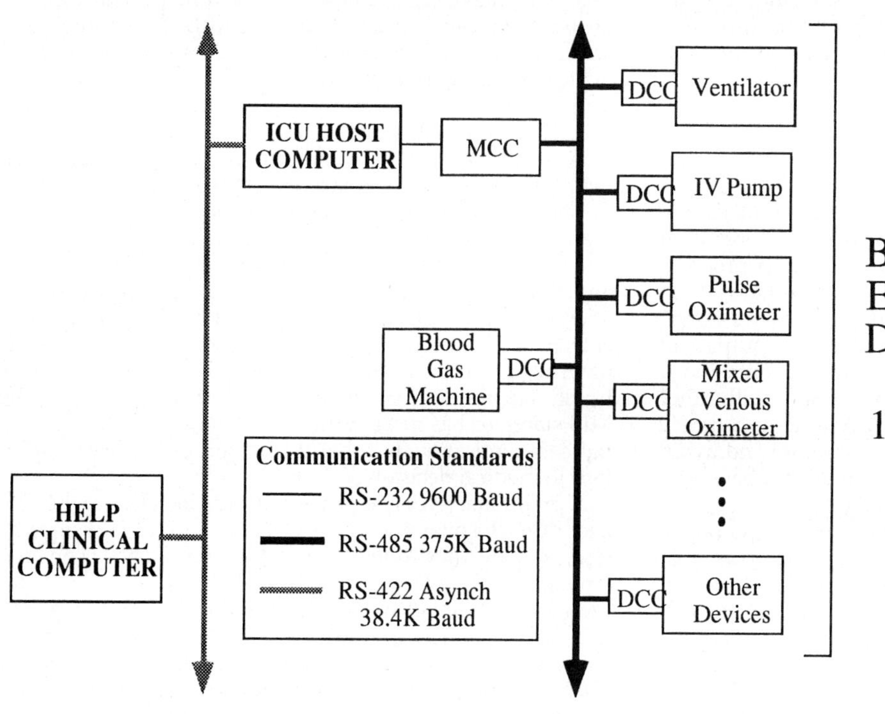

Figure 101–5. MIB on HELP system. *Abbreviations*: DCC = device communications controller; MCC = master communications controller. (From East TD, Young WH, Gardner RM: Digital electronic communication between ventilators and computers and printers. Respir Care 1992; 1113–1123.)

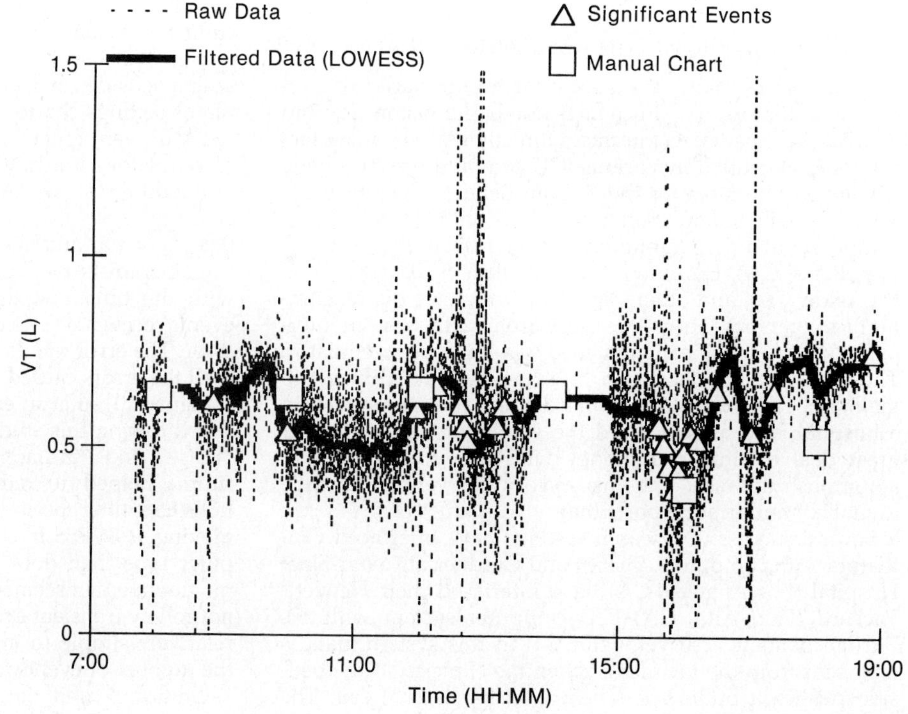

Figure 101–6. An example of tidal volume data collected from a ventilator at 10-second intervals. The effect of filtering the data with a LOWESS filter is shown, and only the significant events indicated are actually stored in the patient's record. The points actually recorded in the manual chart are included for comparison. (From East TD, Young WH, Gardner RM: Digital electronic communication between ventilators and computers and printers. Respir Care 1992; 1113–1123.)

at the bedside; and (2) when they charted, they typically recorded a "snapshot" of data for the few seconds that they were working on a ventilator, and this record was not really representative of a patient's overall status. Our recommendation for an optimal algorithm for automated respiratory care charting is as follows:[24, 30, 34]

Sampling frequency: Sample data from the ventilator every 10 seconds

Ventilator settings: Report every ventilator setting change that lasts longer than 3 minutes

Measurement of respiratory care data: Filter raw MIB-collected data with a 3-minute moving median; report one filtered value every hour; use a threshold table[24] for defining significant events; report changes that are above threshold for over 3 minutes; and report all measured respiratory care data values 1 minute following any setting change

Few or no data are available on how automated charting of mechanical ventilation data may impact patient outcome. In their study, the authors found that ventilator setting charting errors could be reduced from about 3% to near 0% with the institution of automated charting. For measured parameters, the automated charting found significant events that had previously gone undetected. However, no studies have been performed to determine what impact these results might have on patient care. Automation of other areas of the patient record keeping has been shown to improve the quality of the data and to reduce the amount of time spent on charting.[9] If electronic communication with mechanical ventilation is to become an effective and routine part of clinical care, then the standardization of digital communication with these devices must move forward. A standard that simplifies the physical connection of the devices (such as the MIB) must be adopted. In addition, much more research into the elusive definitions of "artifact" and "significant events" is needed. In the next 10 years, the respiratory care community must actively take part in this standardization process. Without clinical input the standardization process is doomed to failure from the beginning. We anticipate that one day connection of a ventilator to a computer will be as simple as plugging in a telephone and that the quality of collected data will be relied upon to be valid and representative of a patient's true condition.

Tools for Decision-Making Support

These tools must provide decision-making support that includes the following: (1) seamless access to information systems, such as bibliographies (e.g., MEDLINE and BRS Colleague); on-line access to reference and training materials; (2) alarms and alerts; (3) expert systems; and (4) closed-loop control.

On-Line Access to Reference and Training Materials

The National Library of Medicine[36] as well as several other integrated advanced information system research sites have been working on integrating the availability of reference material—such as that contained in MEDLINE (which is accessed through tools such as GRATEFUL MED) and even full text references—into the everyday work environment of the hospital. It has been suggested that eventually context-sensitive searches will be issued automatically by information systems. For example, if a clinician is currently examining data on mechanical ventilation, the computer could issue a query for current references explaining the interpretation of the data and for potential therapies. If the clinician needed help at any point, he or she could push a button and obtain both textual and graphic information. Furthermore, integration of the training and teaching process could occur at the bedside. For example, if a clinician is reviewing a flow-volume loop on the computer and wants more information on the interpretation, the computer could retrieve the latest journal articles for review and then enter into a hypermedia training program that would describe, at the user's discretion, many different problems of pulmonary function measurement and interpretation. The hypermedia might include color images of devices and of anatomy, recordings of typical auscultation sounds, graphic representations, and text. This type of computer-based learning is not new.[37] The advantages of computer-based learning as an independent learning modality were highlighted in the recommendations of the Association of American Medical Colleges' 1984 report of the Project Panel on the General Professional Education of the Physician and College Preparation for Medicine.[38, 39] In fact, such systems have already been designed for teaching pulmonary auscultation,[39] blood gas and acid-base interpretation,[40] diagnosis of chest pain,[41] diagnosis of acute respiratory failure,[42] airway management,[43] and a general model of the pulmonary system known as MacPuf.[44] Although assessments of whether computer-based learning is better than traditional training are inconclusive, the field of computer-based learning is still in its infancy, and it is commonly believed that "point-of-care" learning will be far more valuable than traditional lecture- and book-based learning formats.

Integrated Alarms and Alerts

Both the HELP system at the LDS Hospital[11, 45–49] and the patient data management system at Cedar-Sinai Hospital provide alarms and alerts.[46] Automated alarms and alerts that are generated on a wide variety of data types can help to direct decision making. At the LDS Hospital, alarms and alerts are generated for drug allergies, drug-drug interactions, drug selection and dosing,[50, 51] blood ordering,[52, 53] infectious disease surveillance, and organ dysfunction or critical changes in laboratory or physiologic parameters.[11, 47–49, 54] The alerts are automatically generated every time a new piece of information that meets the alert criteria is entered into the system. An integrated data base that includes more than ICU data is essential if these functions are to be adequately performed. For example, a respiratory care manager's alert is generated when nosocomial infections are observed in different patients who are served by the same respiratory therapist.[55, 56] The respiratory care department manager can then review proper policy and procedures with the therapist in an effort to reduce the incidence of nosocomial infections in the future. This particular example requires data from respiratory care charting as well as data from the microbiology laboratory. Other respiratory care alerts are triggered in response to elevated endotracheal tube cuff pressures, high PEEP exposure, high fraction of inspired oxygen (FIO_2) exposure, and the presence of carboxyhemoglobin in a patient receiving oxygen (which indicates that he or she is smoking while receiving oxygen). Such alerting systems have a high benefit-to-cost ratio.[50, 52, 53]

Expert Systems

Expert systems are collections of knowledge that are represented in the computer in a variety of different ways. The knowledge may be represented as a set of rules, such as "if A is greater than 2, then do B," or it may be represented as a Bayesian probability, such as "if A is greater than 2, then there is a 60% probability of B." The concept of expert systems is not new. Expert systems for medical applications have been developed for over 20 years. Figure 101–7 illus-

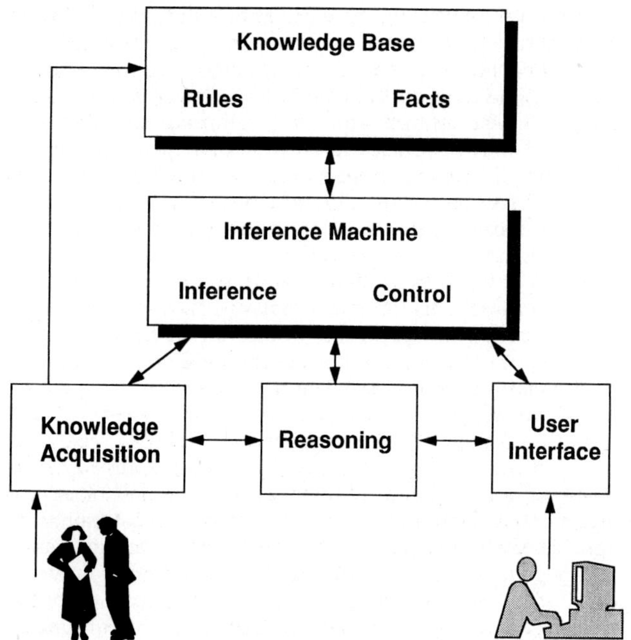

Figure 101–7. The function of an expert system. (From Klar R, Zaiss A: Medical expert systems: Design and applications in pulmonary medicine. Lung 1990; 168:1201–1209.)

trates the function of an expert system.[57] The heart of the system is the inference engine (machine shown in Fig. 101–7). This engine takes the data from the data base and takes rules from the knowledge base and delivers the inferences. The knowledge base contains medical rules, heuristics (rules of thumb), and facts. For the system to acquire knowledge, there must be a knowledge acquisition process. In general, expert systems fall into two categories: those for diagnostic purposes, and those for therapeutic purposes.

Pulmonary diagnostic expert systems have been developed for interpretation of blood gas data.[58–63] Hingston and coworkers[61] performed an interesting study illustrating that although 61% of the participants at medical grand rounds believed that they knew how to interpret blood gas data, 71% believed that an expert system was unnecessary. The audience was able to answer only 39% of the questions correctly. This type of study indicates that despite their perceptions, clinicians are not capable of remembering everything in infinite detail and that bedside decision support may be an important asset. Other diagnostic support systems include a system for community-acquired pneumonia,[64] occupational lung disease,[65] interstitial lung diseases,[66] and the detection of breaths from flow and capnography data.[67]

Several different expert systems have been developed for ventilator management.[68–80] These expert systems can be divided into those that are designed for general management of the mechanical ventilator[68–76, 80] and those that are designed specifically for weaning.[77–79]

The systems designed for the management of mechanical ventilation have been constructed in a variety of different ways. The majority are traditional rule-based expert systems.[68, 70–72, 74–76, 80] Two examples are the VQ-Attending system and KUSIVAR system. The VQ-Attending system, developed by Miller,[70] was designed as a critiquing system. Physicians enter the current ventilator settings, blood gas data, and their suggestions for new settings. The VQ-Attending system implements rules, frames, and semantic nets in the LISP programming language. The expert system interprets the manually entered current data, infers the appropriate treatment goals, and then compares the findings with the physicians' suggested settings. It then provides a printed critique. VQ-Attending system was used as a teaching tool in anesthesiology; however, it was never put into routine clinical practice. The KUSIVAR system[80] is an expert system designed to aid in management of adults with respiratory distress. KUSIVAR was implemented in the LISP

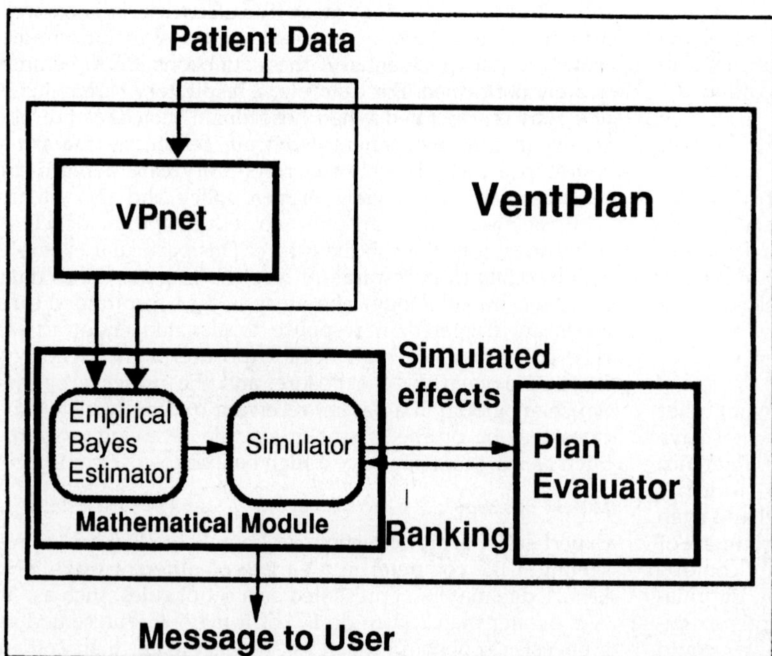

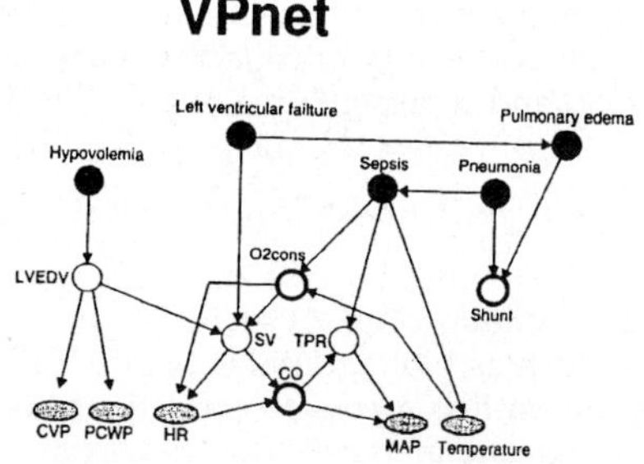

The belief network represents causal relationships with diagnostic nodes (black circles), intermediate nodes (open circles), and subnetworks containing time, report, and measured-variable nodes (grey circles)

Figure 101–8. The VentPlan expert system for managing mechanical ventilation. This system was designed at Stanford University by Rutledge and coworkers.[69, 73, 81] (From Rutledge G, Thompson G, Farr B, et al: VentPlan: A ventilator-management advisor. 15th Annual Symposium on Computer Applications in Medical Care. Washington, DC, IEEE Computer Soc Press, 1991, pp 869–871.)

programming language on a high-powered, expert system workstation (Explorer Workstation, Unisys, Detroit, MI). Knowledge was represented in the KUSIVAR system as a set of rules. A mathematic model was used to predict patient responses to a proposed therapy change. Because KUSIVAR has not been used in an extensive clinical trial, it is unclear what impact it would have on patient outcome.

The VentPlan system designed at Stanford University (Stanford, CA)[69, 73, 81] (Fig. 101–8) is different from most rule-based systems in that it uses a Bayesian network and a physiologically based mathematic model to predict the impact of a recommended therapy plan. The mathematic model, which is at the core of the system, consists of equations that describe a three-compartment model of the cardiopulmonary circulation. An empirical Bayesian estimator calculates the best fit for the parameters of its equations using parameter estimates and current laboratory test values. The system fit represents the VentPlan system's understanding of a patient's current physiologic state. A simulator then works in conjunction with the plan evaluator to determine the appropriate recommendation for the ventilator settings. The simulator uses the fitted parameters to calculate the effects of certain ventilator settings. The plan evaluator ranks the plans based on results from the simulations. A belief network, known as the "VP-net," is used to calculate the prior parameter estimates for the model. Without this network, only population estimates could be used. The belief network (see Fig. 101–8) collects hemodynamic, gas exchange, and other diagnostic information as it becomes available from the patient and updates the estimates of the model parameters. This system has been evaluated using data collected from 14 patients at the Palo Alto Veterans Administration Medical Center (Palo Alto, CA). The results show that the concept is sound and that the estimates from the model agree well with actual data. The VentPlan system has yet to be placed into routine clinical use at the bedside.

The WEANPRO system developed by Tong[77, 78] is a good example of an expert system designed particularly for weaning patients from mechanical ventilation (Fig. 101–9). The knowledge for the system was obtained from four domain experts (physicians who were "experts" at weaning). The knowledge base consists of 406 general and 133 global rules. The system runs on any personal computer. Approximately 6 man-months of work were required to establish the system. Fifty-four patients were studied in a prospective trial; 16 of these patients were weaned using the WEANPRO system. However, only 13 patients were successfully weaned. The remaining three exhibited conditions that were not adequately addressed by WEANPRO's knowledge base. WEANPRO required fewer blood gas determinations than did clinicians (3.4 ± 0.5 versus 6.2 ± 1.9) and made more ventilator adjustments per blood gas determination than did clinicians (1.17 ± 0.2 versus 0.8 ± 0.3). A review of the WEANPRO system's therapy suggestions by experts showed 96% acceptance. The WEANPRO system has been rewritten in the MUMPS computer language and is currently in clinical use at Baptist Memorial Hospital in Memphis, Tennessee.

At the LDS Hospital, the development of expert systems for the management of mechanical ventilation was originally stimulated by the investigative needs of a clinical trial of extracorporeal carbon dioxide removal in patients with adult respiratory distress syndrome (ARDS).[82–84] The intent was to develop protocols to standardize therapy[13, 22] that could be used by the routine clinical staff. It was reasoned that standardization of therapy would increase the interpretability and credibility of clinical trial results.[84] The protocol control goals were to ensure uniformity of care, equal intensity and frequency of monitoring, consistent decision-making logic, and common therapeutic goals (e.g., maintenance of arterial oxygen tension [PaO_2]). Protocols were developed for volume control (in continuous positive-pressure ventilation [CPPV]), pressure control–inverse ratio ventilation, low-frequency positive-pressure ventilation–extracorporeal carbon dioxide removal, intermittent mandatory ventilation, and continuous positive airway pressure for application in patients with ARDS. A special protocol was developed for the management of ventilation and intrinsic PEEP for pressure control–inverse ratio ventilation.[22] After completion of the clinical trial in 1991, new protocols were written for ventilation and arterial pH control.

The protocols were developed using an iterative approach that used the clinical environment as an integral part of the development process.[85, 86] It was believed that this was the only way to generate a successful protocol that could handle the majority of circumstances encountered and be acceptable to the clinical care staff. A therapy consensus committee initially consisting of 14 physicians, 3 nurses, 1 respiratory therapist, and 1 doctor of philosophy in medical informatics developed and refined protocol logic.[22] The committee members had appointments in the Pulmonary Division, the Critical Care Department, and the Respiratory Care at the LDS Hospital and in the Anesthesiology Department at the University of Utah and included two research associate physicians from Dr. Gattinoni's group at the University of

WEANPRO Expert System For Weaning

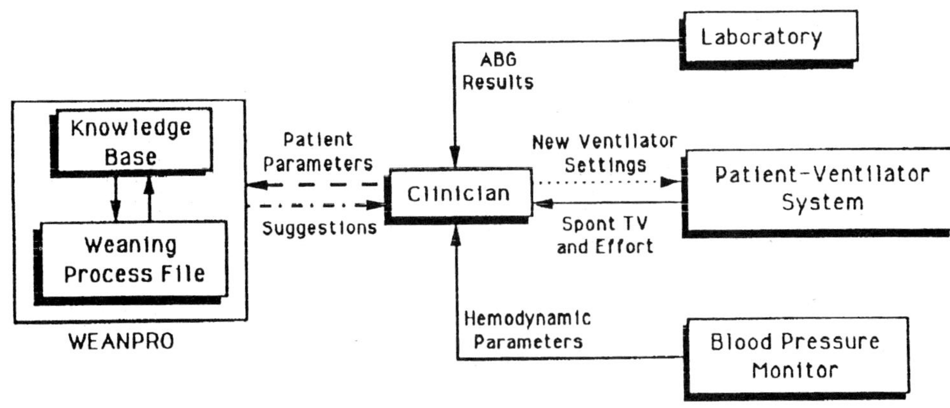

Figure 101–9. The WEANPRO system developed by Tong and coworkers[77, 78] is an expert system designed particularly for weaning patients from mechanical ventilation. (From Tong DA: Weaning patients from mechanical ventilation: A knowledge based approach. 14th Annual Symposium on Computer Applications in Medical Care. Washington, DC, IEEE Computer Soc Press, 1990, pp 79–85.)

Milan. The composition of this group has changed over time as a result of personnel changes and because of the evolution of new areas for protocol development. All physicians agreed to forego personal treatment style and to accept the consensus recommendations that were incorporated into the protocol logic.

The operation of the protocols is demonstrated in Figure 101–10. The protocols are automatically started whenever a new pulse oximeter saturation ($Sp{O_2}$) or a new $Pa{O_2}$ is entered into the computer. The protocol first classifies the arterial oxygenation into one of five categories: "threatening hypoxemia," "marginal hypoxemia," "acceptable," "satisfactory," and "supersatisfactory." This protocol also determines the appropriateness of using the $Sp{O_2}$ to perform this classification. In the "gray" areas (between $Sp{O_2}$'s of 82% and 92%), specific rules dictate whether a $Pa{O_2}$ must be measured to accurately classify the arterial oxygenation. The protocols are automatically activated by the new arterial oxygen classification. The protocol determines whether the patient needs a therapy increase, requires a therapy reduction, or needs to wait without a therapy change.

These protocols were computerized using the HELP system at the LDS Hospital[13, 19, 22, 74–76, 86, 87] As shown in Figure 101–10, the computer displays instructions on the terminal at the bedside. A member of the clinical care team, typically the respiratory therapist, reads the instructions and makes the indicated ventilator setting change. This is *not* a closed-loop system. The computer never makes any adjustments of therapy directly. The clinical care team members always have the option of refusing to execute an instruction. However, if they refuse to implement an instruction, they must provide a reason. The record of reasons for refusal provides critical feedback that permits protocol refinement.

The ability of the CPPV oxygenation protocols to control care during around-the-clock application in the ICU was evaluated. The study was approved by the LDS Hospital's Research and Human Rights Committee. A total of 111 patients with ARDS were enrolled in the trial. The diagnosis of ARDS was defined by the following criteria:

1. A $Pa{O_2}$ to alveolar $P{O_2}$ ratio ≤ 0.2
2. Total static thoracic compliance $\leq$ 50 mL/cm H_2O
3. No evidence of heart failure or fluid overload (pulmonary artery occlusion pressure $\leq$ 15 mm Hg)
4. Acute onset of illness accompanied by an ARDS risk factor
5. Radiographic evidence of bilateral diffuse infiltrates

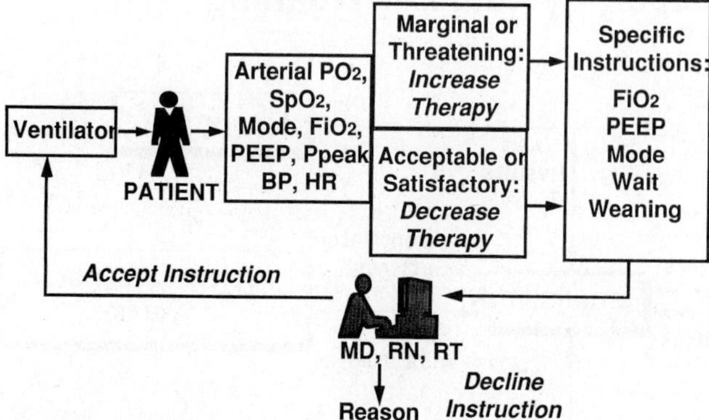

Figure 101–10. Diagram illustrating the function of the oxygenation portion of the decision support system developed at LDS Hospital, Salt Lake City, Utah.[74, 84] *Abbreviations*: $Sp{O_2}$ = pulse oximeter saturation; Ppeak = peak pressure; BP = mean arterial blood pressure; HR = heart rate.

Detailed data about patient demographics, the use of protocols, and patient physiology during protocol use were collected for the first 45 patients. Only outcome data were measured on the remaining 66 patients. Outcome was compared, using a chi-squared test, with that of two historical controls: one from the Massachusetts General Hospital (Boston, MA) between 1978 and 1988,[88] and the other from the European Collaborative Study.[89] The CPPV oxygenation protocols were applied until patients were weaned to continuous positive airway pressure or died. In the first 45 patients, all instructions generated by the computerized CPPV oxygenation protocol were logged, as was the acceptance or rejection of an instruction by the clinical staff. If an instruction was not followed, the clinical staff member was asked to identify a reason from a menu.[85, 90]

Figure 101–11 summarizes the results of the CPPV oxygenation protocol used in 111 ARDS patients. In the first 45 patients, the CPPV oxygenation protocol was applied for 19 ± 18 days (mean $\pm$SD, range: 0.2–78 days). The protocols controlled care 95% of the time (22.8 hours of a 24-hour day). The protocol was suspended when the patient required transportation to other hospital sites for procedures such as surgery or chest tube placement, for diagnostic procedures such as computed tomography scanning, or for intense therapy for nonprotocol problems such as septic shock.

The specific reasons for why the clinical staff did not follow instructions are described in Figure 101–12. The most frequent reason given by the staff was that instructions were incorrect because of incorrect or inappropriate respiratory care data (typographic errors or neglected charting) or blood gas data (resulting from inappropriate sample handling or sample collection during a nonsteady state); such incorrect instructions occurred with a frequency of 3.1% (358 out of 11,708 total instructions). Only 110 instructions (1%) of the total number of instructions were not followed because the clinical staff challenged the medical logic of the protocols.

The success of these CPPV oxygenation protocols clearly indicates the feasibility of using expert systems for the direct management of care for critically ill patients. The data of interest for clinical decision making were integrated effectively. Specific instructions that could be followed by nursing or respiratory therapy personnel were generated. Many of the "out of protocol" hours were explained by the clinical circumstances of the ARDS patient: hemodynamic instability as well as the need for the placement of chest tubes, diagnostic or therapeutic procedures, and other surgical and nursing interventions. Traditional ventilator therapy titration would also generally have been stopped during these periods. The physicians, respiratory therapists, and nurses commented that the computerized protocol, which produced "standing orders," simplified the management of mechanical ventilation. The CPPV oxygenation protocol is now in routine clinical use for ARDS patients.

The survival of patients cared for with the CPPV oxygenation protocol is shown in Figure 101–13. The survival of the whole group was greater than that of similar patients at the Massachusetts General Hospital[88] and from the collaborative European ARDS Study.[89] This difference was statistically significant (CPPV Protocol versus Massachusetts General Hospital: $\chi^2_{1df} = 26.5$, $P < .001$; CPPV Protocol versus European ARDS Study: $\chi^2_{1df} = 40.0$, $P < .001$). The survival of the subsets of the 111 patients who met or did not meet extracorporeal membrane oxygenation (ECMO) entry criteria was also higher than that published previously[88] (ECMO entry criteria: $\chi^2_{1df} = 10.2$, $P < .001$, non-ECMO entry criteria: $\chi^2_{1df} = 4.9$, $P = .034$).

The reported mortality associated with ARDS varies

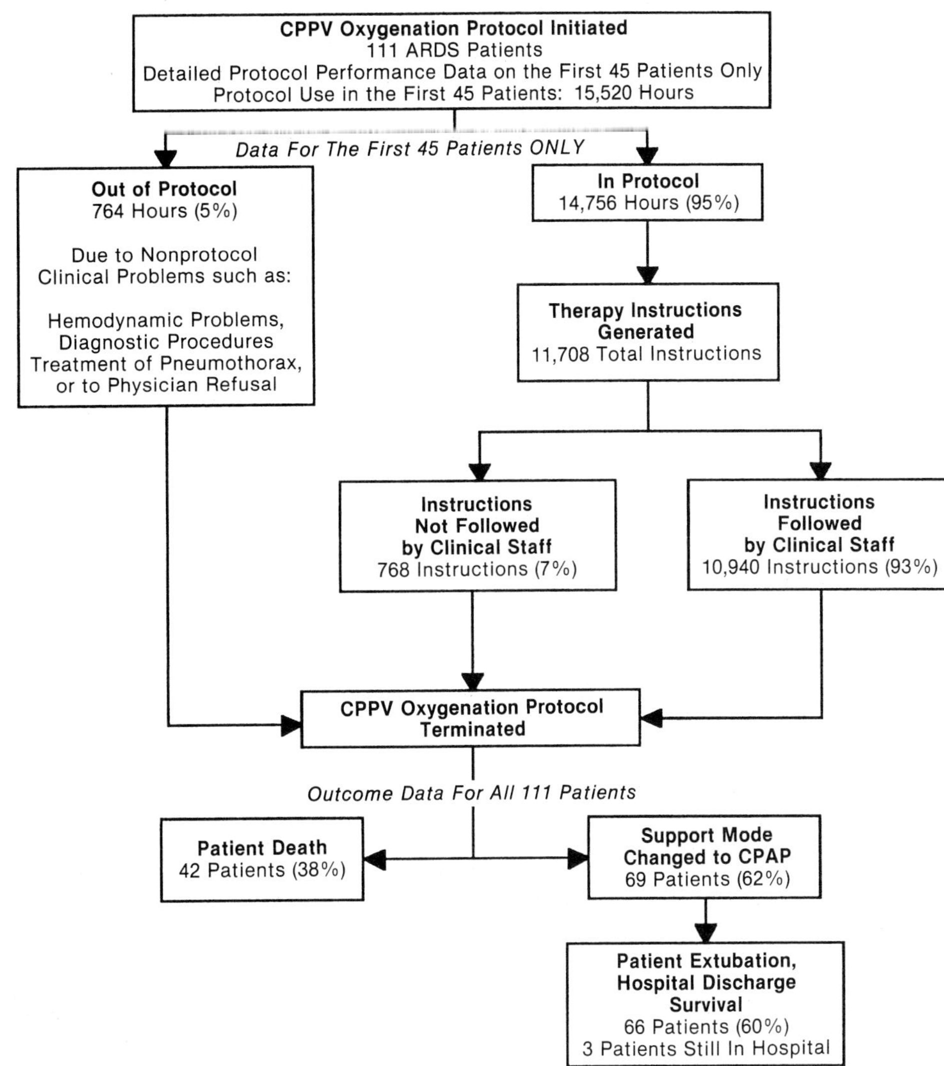

Figure 101–11. This figure summarizes the results of the CPPV oxygenation protocol use in 111 ARDS patients in the shock trauma ICU at LDS Hospital, Salt Lake City, Utah.[74, 84]

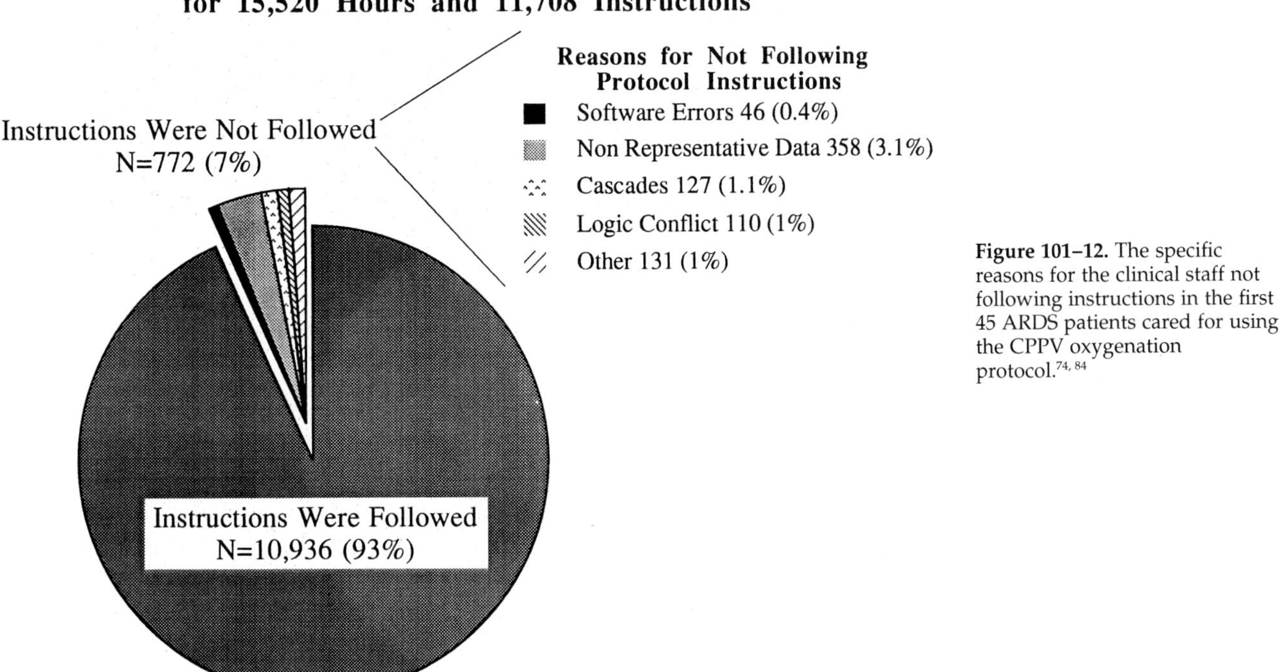

Figure 101–12. The specific reasons for the clinical staff not following instructions in the first 45 ARDS patients cared for using the CPPV oxygenation protocol.[74, 84]

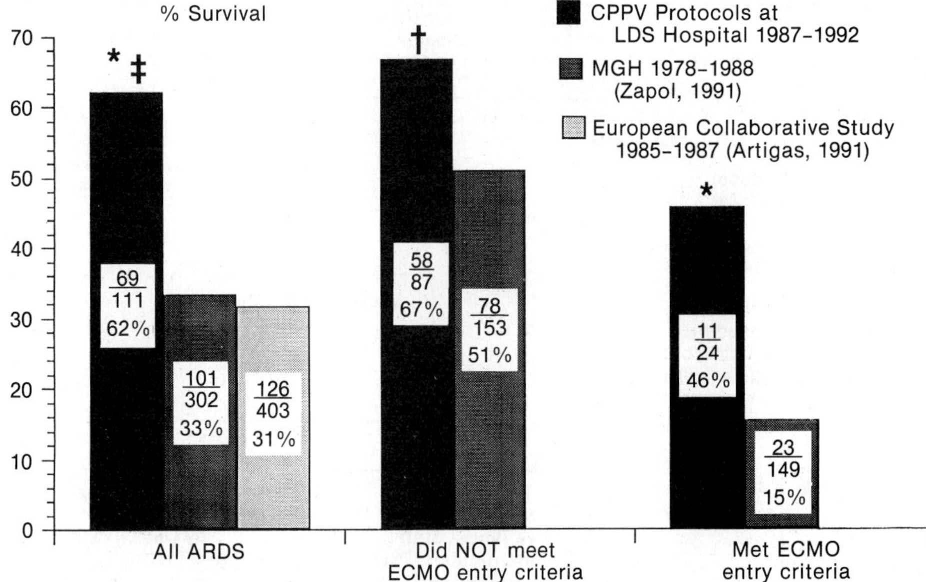

Figure 101–13. Survival results of CPPV oxygenation protocol use in 111 ARDS patients in the shock trauma ICU at LDS Hospital, Salt Lake City, Utah.[74, 84] *Key:* * = $P<.001$ versus MGH; † = $P<.05$ versus MGH; ‡ = $P<.001$ versus European Collaborative Study.

widely in the literature. We have chosen two of the largest studies as historical controls. The data from the Massachusetts General Hospital[88] and from the European Collaborative ARDS Study[89] are a good summary of the experience in both the United States and Europe in the late 1980s. In addition, the data from the Massachusetts General Hospital provided outcome data on patients meeting the ECMO entry criteria, making it possible to compare outcome in the subgroups of severe ARDS patients (meeting ECMO entry criteria) and less severe ARDS patients (not meeting ECMO entry criteria). As shown in Figure 101–13, the survival of patients cared for with the protocols was significantly higher than that of either of these historical control groups. This was true for all ARDS patients as well as the two subgroups of patients with severe and less severe ARDS. Without randomized clinical trials with concurrent controls, no definitive conclusion can be drawn concerning the impact of protocol control on patient survival. Nevertheless, the outcome of patients cared for with these protocols appears to be at least as good as the published outcomes. This suggests that computerized protocols can be used successfully and safely to manage mechanical ventilation in critically ill patients. To the authors' knowledge, this is the first demonstration that a computerized decision support system can be used effectively in the critical care environment. Similar protocols could be used in several different arenas (1) to control future clinical trials as part of the ongoing nationwide effort to determine the efficacy of existing and new therapies; (2) to standardize the management of mechanical ventilation, an essential part of the continuous quality improvement process; and (3) to provide decision support in the management of mechanical ventilation for patients with ARDS who are in a variety of settings in which a clinical expert in the management of ARDS is unavailable.

A randomized, controlled, prospective clinical trial is underway to objectively compare this protocol control with physician-directed care. This study will answer two questions: (1) Can a computerized decision support system be exported to other centers and be used by clinicians uninvolved with its development? and (2) Does the protocol control of mechanical ventilation have an impact on ARDS patient outcome? During year 1, the knowledge base (protocol logic rules) was transferred from the HELP system at LDS Hospital to a personal computer–based ICU system known as ARGUS Windows. The ARGUS Windows system has been installed at all 12 beds of the surgical ICU at King Drew Medical Center (Los Angeles, CA). This system is now in routine use for respiratory care charting, and the decision-making support system has been used successfully to care for five ARDS patients in a pilot study of feasibility. The authors have started a prospective, randomized clinical trial to test the efficacy of computerized protocols. Four hundred patients with ARDS are to be enrolled. This study will be conducted at a minimum of two different clinical sites: King Drew Medical Center, a county hospital in the Watts district of Los Angeles; and Hermann Hospital, a private hospital in Houston affiliated with the University of Texas Medical School. The null hypothesis (HØ) is defined as follows: there is no difference in efficacy between protocol and non-protocol controlled critical care. Efficacy is defined using a hierarchical, four-level approach: efficacy → (1) survival, (2) length of ICU stay, (3) morbidity, and (4) incidence and severity of barotrauma. Generalizability of the computerized decision-making support system will be determined by examining (1) the percentage of total time in the trial during which protocols controlled patient care, (2) the number of protocol instructions that were not followed, (3) the number of objections to protocol logic that, based on medical evidence, forced a change in the logic. As of August 1993, 11 patients were randomized into this study at King Drew Medical Center (6 controls, and 5 protocol-controlled care patients).

Closed-Loop Control

Closed-loop control is similar to an expert system except that the computer directly adjusts the mechanical ventilator. Figure 101–14 is a typical diagram of a closed-loop controller.[91] The heart of many of the simple controllers is a proportional, integral, and differential (PID) controller. PID controllers are used frequently throughout industry for controlling many different processes. A home thermostat and the furnace it controls are an example of a simple closed-loop control. The thermostat is either on (when the temperature is too cold) or off (when the temperature is too hot). It might be possible to have a more comfortable home that is heated more efficiently if the furnace were hotter when it was very cold in the home and became cooler as it approached the desired temperature. This is the concept of *proportional control.* The disadvantage of proportional control is that it will typically reach a steady state at a value that differs from the desired set point. To force the system to reach exactly the desired set point, one can integrate the error—that is, the difference between the desired value and the actual value. Even a small error eventually integrates into a large error over time, and such an error forces the system to the exact set point. This is the concept of the *integral control. Derivative control* attempts to anticipate what is going to happen within the system. If your house was heating up very rapidly, then it would be good if the thermostat could recognize this and slow down the heating process so that the set point is not overshot. This can be accomplished by adding some control that is dependent on the time rate of change of the error signal (the derivative). Although many other types of closed-loop controller have been used, the PID controller remains a central element in most of them. In computerized systems, the PID controller can be represented in a recursive form that can be easily programmed.[91, 92]

An analog closed-loop control system for mechanical ventilation was first introduced in 1953 by Frumin.[4, 5] This sophisticated system included oxygen and carbon dioxide analyzers and adjusted the FIO_2 and tidal volume during anesthesia. Several other analog closed-loop control systems were reported between 1953 and 1973.[5] Coles and coworkers introduced the first computerized, closed-loop controller for mechanical ventilation.[93] This system controlled FIO_2 and tidal volume during anesthesia. Several other different systems were designed since the early 1970s for closed-loop control of tidal volume and ventilatory rate based on monitoring of expired carbon dioxide.[5, 91, 94–98] Most systems were designed to maintain a desired end-tidal carbon dioxide fraction or percentage. Although all of these systems worked well, they did not enjoy widespread clinical use because of the differences between end-tidal carbon dioxide tension and $PaCO_2$ in patients who have a large physiologic dead space. Some closed-loop controllers have been designed for managing oxygenation. Most of these systems are simple and were designed to adjust FIO_2 to produce a desired PaO_2 or SpO_2.[99–101] Morozoff and Evans demonstrated in neonates that computer control was able to maintain a desired SpO_2 with an accuracy greater than that afforded by manual control.[99] East and colleagues designed a system for control of PEEP based on the normalization of functional residual capacity.[20] Strickland and Hasson have developed a closed-loop controller for weaning from synchronized intermittent mandatory ventilation with pressure support in postoperative cardiac patients.[79, 102] This controller decreased the SIMV rate by 2 breaths per minute every 5 minutes until a rate of 2 breaths per minute was reached; it then decreased pressure support by 4 cm H_2O every 5 minutes as long as the patient met the following criteria: respiratory rate from 8 to 25 breaths per minute; minute ventilation from 6 to 14 L/min; and $SpO_2 \geq 90\%$. This rule-based controller automatically adjusted a Puritan Bennett 7200 ventilator. This system was used in a prospective, randomized trial of 15 patients (9 had computer control, and 6 manual control). The results showed that the group with computer-controlled ventilation used significantly fewer blood gases than that with manually controlled ventilation (1.4 ± 0.7 versus 7.2 ± 4.3), had shorter weaning times (18.7 ± 5.9 versus 25.6 ± 5.6 hours) and less time spent outside acceptable respiratory rate and tidal volume bounds (3.2 ± 2.8 versus 6.6 ± 4.1 minutes).[102] The system examined in this study is an interesting contrast to the WEANPRO expert system developed by Tong.[77, 78] WEANPRO is a far more complex system that requires hemodynamics and a variety of other sources of data not required by the LDS Hospital protocols. The simple weaning system developed at the LDS Hospital[74] focuses on spontaneous ventilatory rate as a primary variable and on PaO_2 or SpO_2 as a secondary variable. The LDS Hospital protocols have been used to successfully wean 68 patients. Despite the simplicity of Strickland's and our expert system, it appears to work as well or better than the more sophisticated WEANPRO system. This reaffirms our belief in the "KIS" principle: Keep It Simple.

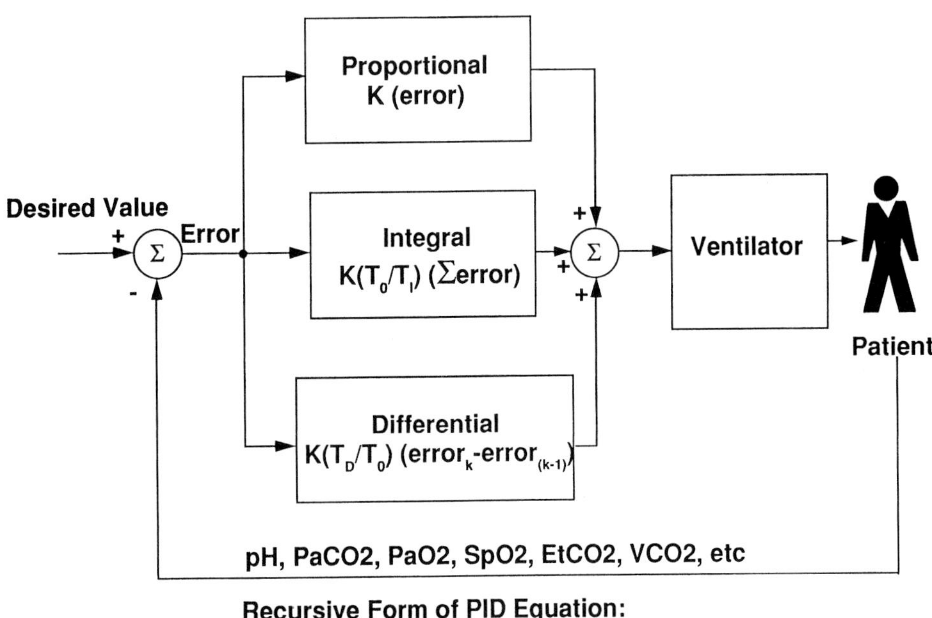

Figure 101–14. A typical diagram of a closed-loop controller. The heart of many of the simple controllers is a proportional, integral, and differential (PID) equation. This equation can be easily written in a recursive form that is amenable to processing by computer. K is the overall gain of the controller, T_0 is the sample interval, T_I is the integration time (essentially, the integral gain constant), and T_D is the differential time (essentially, the differential gain constant). The values of K, T_0, T_I, and T_D are adjusted so that the controller can provide the best performance. When the PID equation is written in the recursive form, new gain constants q_0, q_1, and q_2 are introduced to simplify the equation. These new constants are mathematically related to the original gain constants (K, T_0, T_I, and T_D) by the equations shown.

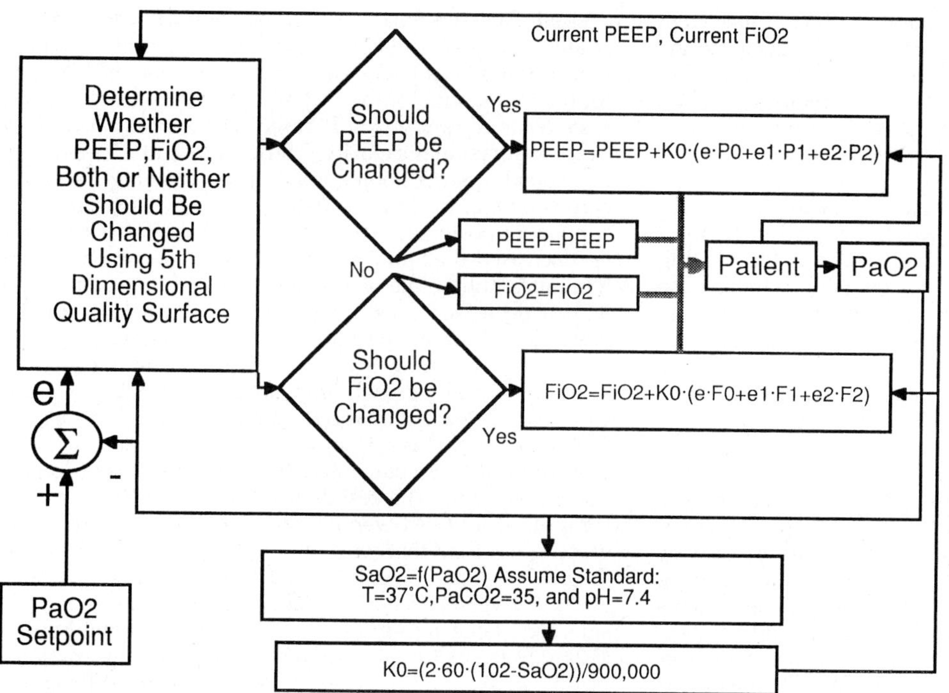

Figure 101–15. A nonlinear closed-loop controller for adjusting PEEP and FIO_2. PEEP and FIO_2 are automatically adjusted to maintain PaO_2 at a desired setpoint. The size and direction of a therapy change are determined by the PaO_2 error "e" (difference between measured and desired PaO_2). A record of the previous two values for the error (e1 and e2) is kept. The decision regarding which variable to change—PEEP or FIO_2, or both—was determined from a fifth dimensional quality surface that described the tradeoff between PEEP and FIO_2 changes for a specific combination of current PEEP, FIO_2, and PaO_2 values. The quality surface is generated from the clinically proven protocols. Once it is decided which variables are to be changed, the amount of change is calculated by a PID controller. The controller uses the current (e) and previous values (e1 and e2) to calculate the actual change in PEEP or FIO_2. The PID gain constants (P0, P1, P2, F0, F1, and F2) are adjusted to provide the best controller performance. The overall gain of the controller (K0) is a function of the arterial oxygen saturation (SaO_2). This provides an aggressive response to hypoxemia and a more conservative response to hyperoxia. Arterial oxygen saturation was calculated from the PaO_2 (assuming pH = 7.4, $PaCO_2$ = 35 mm Hg, and temperature = 37°C), using standard equations. (From East TD: The magic bullets in the war on ARDS: Aggressive therapy for oxygenation failure. Respir Care 1993; 38:690–704.)

Despite the development of several very clever and sophisticated systems, none of the discussed closed-loop controllers for mechanical ventilation have had a major impact on clinical care. There are two primary reasons for this: (1) these systems all rely on input data from sensors (e.g., for PaO_2, end-tidal carbon dioxide tension, transcutaneous PO_2, and SaO_2) that are too unreliable to trust in a closed-loop control; and (2) most of these systems were designed by engineers in the laboratory, and although they are excellent engineering exercises, they do not closely reflect the realities of clinical practice.

The authors have addressed this problem by designing a system based on well-established protocols for the management of mechanical ventilation[22, 75, 76] that provides continuous closed-loop control of oxygenation (Fig. 101–15).[23] A Hamilton Amadeus ventilator was controlled by an Apple Macintosh SE-30 computer (Apple Computer, Inc., Cupertino, CA). A Shiley Continucath intra-arterial electrode (Shiley, Inc., Irvine, CA) was used to provide continuous measurement of PaO_2. Arterial oxygen saturation was calculated from the PaO_2, pH, $PaCO_2$, and temperature with standard equations. The magnitude and direction of a therapy change were determined by the PaO_2 error (difference between the measured and the desired PaO_2). The overall gain of the controller was a function of the arterial oxygen saturation. This control strategy provided an aggressive response to hypoxemia and a more conservative response to hyperoxia. The content of the therapy change was determined from a fifth dimensional quality surface that described the tradeoff between PEEP and FIO_2 changes for a specific combination of current PEEP, FIO_2, and PaO_2 values. The quality surface was generated from our extensively used protocols applied clinically in an open-loop manner[22, 75, 76] (see earlier discussion of expert systems). The controller was tested in five mongrel dogs with oleic acid lung injury. After injury, the controller was activated, and the animals were monitored at 30-minute intervals for 6 hours. The controller performed as designed for all five animals, and no hazardous or failure conditions were noted. A small clinical trial of this closed-loop controller has been started at the LDS Hospital to evaluate its safety and effectiveness in patients with ARDS. Hopefully, this careful management of potentially toxic therapies will improve the outcome of patients with hypoxic respiratory failure.

SUMMARY

Computers have been a part of mechanical ventilation therapy for over two decades. Are we much better off than we were when we had the pneumatic ventilators that delivered pressure-limited ventilation? In many ways, we have gone full circle, moving from pressure- to volume-controlled ventilators and back to pressure-controlled ventilators. The big difference is that now the devices are elaborate computerized systems that cost between $15,000 and $30,000. The newer systems certainly have better alarms and monitoring packages; however, little evidence is available to prove that these systems have made a dramatic impact on patient outcome. The next generation of computers for mechanical ventilation *must* help clinicians to assimilate the myriad data from mechanical ventilators and to make fast and effective decisions. It is not enough to merely display the data in a large spreadsheet or on a complex colorful graphic display versus time. New data display concepts and expert systems need to be incorporated into the commercial products. The next generation of computer systems for the management of mechanical ventilation will have to include a fully integrated data base, automation charting of data from mechanical ventilation, and tools for decision-making support if they are to have a significant positive impact on the quality and cost of patient care.

ACKNOWLEDGMENTS

Dr. East would like to thank his wife Katherine and his children Thomas, Rosemary, and Patrick; without their support and understanding that "Dad" had to work long hours at night and on weekends, this work would have not been possible.

Research on the development of the MIB for respiratory care was initially supported by Siemens Life Support Systems (Solna, Sweden) and was continued by Puritan Bennett Corporation (Carlsbad, CA).

Research on the closed-loop control of oxygenation was supported by Hamilton Ventilators (Bonaduz, Switzerland).

Research on expert systems was supported in part by grants from the Deseret Foundation (LDS Hospital), the National Institutes of Health (NHLBI grant HL36787), the Agency for Health Care Policy and Research (AHCPR grant HS06594), and the Respiratory Distress Syndrome Foundation. The ACT/PC Corporation (Madison, WI) is an active supporter of the ongoing clinical trial of our expert systems for mechanical ventilation. The Siemens 900C ventilators, carts, and supplies were loaned by Siemens Life Support Systems.

References

1. Bernstein J: The Analytical Engine: Past, Present, and Future. New York, William Morrow & Co, 1981.
2. Heebink DM: Computers in pulmonary medicine. Respir Care 1982; 27:793–794.
3. Sanborn WG: Microprocessor-based mechanical ventilation. Respir Care 1993; 38:72–109.
4. Frumin JR: Clinical use of a physiological respirator producing N_2O amnesia-analgesia. Anesthesiology 1957; 18:290–299.
5. Thompson JD: Computerized control of mechanical ventilation: Closing the loop. Respir Care 1987; 32:440.
6. Siemens: Servo Ventilator 300 Reference Manual. Solna, Sweden, Siemens Life Support Systems, 1992.
7. Andrews RD, Gardner RM, Metcalf SM, et al: Computer charting: An evaluation of a respiratory care computer system. Respir Care 1985; 30:695–707.
8. Greenway L, Jeffs M, Turner K: Computerized management of respiratory care. Respir Care 1993; 38:42–53.
9. Hammond J, Johnson HM, Varas R, et al: A qualitative comparison of paper flowsheets vs a computer-based clinical information system. Chest 1991; 99:155–157.
10. Hammond J, Johnson MH, Ward CG, et al: Clinical evaluation of a computer-based patient monitoring and data management system. Heart Lung 1991; 20:119–124.
11. Bradshaw KE, Sittig DF, Gardner RM, et al: Computer-based data entry for nurses in the ICU. MD Comput 1989; 6:274–280.
12. Hilberman M, Kamm B, Tarter M, et al: An evaluation of computer-based patient monitoring at Pacific Medical Center. Comput Biomed Res 1975; 8:447–460.
13. East T: Computers in the ICU: Panacea or plague? Respir Care 1992; 37:170–180.
14. Eddy DM: Clinical decision making. JAMA 1990; 263:1265–1275.
15. Dick RS, Steen EB (Eds): The Computer-Based Patient Record: An Essential Technology for Health Care. Washington, DC, National Academy Press, 1991.
16. Stead WW: Systems for the year 2000: The case for an integrated database. MD Comput 1991; 8:103–110.
17. Shabot MM: Standardized acquisition of bedside data: The IEEE P1073 medical information bus. Int J Clin Monit Comput 1989; 6:197–204.
18. Gardner RM, Shabot MM: Computerized ICU data management: Pitfalls and promises. Int J Clin Monit Comput 1990; 7:99–105.
19. East TD, Andriano KP, Pace NL: Automated measurement of functional residual capacity by sulfur hexafluoride washout. J Clin Monit 1987; 3:14–21.
20. East TD, in't Veen JCCM, Jonker TA, et al: Computer-controlled positive end-expiratory pressure (PEEP) titration for effective oxygenation without frequent blood gases. Crit Care Med 1988; 16:252–257.
21. East TD, Wortelboer PJ, van Ark E, et al: Automated sulfur hexafluoride washout functional residual capacity measurement system for any mode of mechanical ventilation as well as spontaneous respiration. Crit Care Med 1990; 18:84–91.
22. East TD, Böhm SH, Wallace CJ, et al: A successful computerized protocol for clinical management of pressure control–inverse ratio ventilation in ARDS patients. Chest 1992; 101:697–710.
23. East TD: The magic bullets in the war on ARDS: Aggressive therapy for oxygenation failure. Respir Care 1993; 38:690–704.
24. East TD, Young WH, Gardner RM: Digital electronic communication between ventilators and computers and printers. Respir Care 1992; 37:1113–1123.
25. Furst E: Cardiovascular technology. J Cardiovasc Nurs 1989; 4:68–78.
26. Gardner RM, Bradshaw KE, Hollingsworth KW: Computerizing the intensive care unit: Current status and future directions. J Cardiovasc Nurs 1989; 4:68–78.
27. Shabot MM, LoBue M, Leyerle B: An automatic PDMS interface for the Urotrack Plus 220 urimeter. Int J Clin Monit Comput 1988; 5:125–131.
28. McDonald CJ, Hammond WF: Standard formats for electronic transfer of clinical data (Editorial). Ann Intern Med 1989; 110:333–335.
29. Gardner RM, Hawley WL, East TD, et al: Real time data acquisition: Experience with the Medical Information Bus (MIB). Proc Annu Symp Comput Appl Med Care 1991; 15:813–817.
30. Gardner RM, Hawley WL, East TD, et al: Real time data acquisition: Recommendations for the Medical Information Bus (MIB). Int J Clin Monit Comput 1991; 8:251–258.
31. Gardner RM: Computerized management of intensive care patients. MD Comput 1986; 3:36–51.
32. Hawley WL, Tariq H, Gardner RM: Clinical implementation of an automated medical information bus in an intensive care unit. Proc Annu Symp Comput Appl Med Care 1988; 12:621–624.
33. East TD, Yang W, Tariq H, et al: The IEEE medical information bus for respiratory care. Crit Care Med 1989; 17:S80.
34. Young W: Automated respiratory care charting: Artifact rejection and data reduction [Doctoral dissertation]. Salt Lake City, UT, University of Utah, 1993.
35. Cleveland WS, Devlin SJ: Locally weighted regression: An approach to regression analysis by local fitting. J Am Stat Assoc 1988; 9:596–609.
36. Lindberg DAB, Schoolian HM: The National Library of Medicine and medical informatics. West J Med 1986; 145:786–790.
37. Jones A: Interactive Videodisc Technology: An overview for respiratory care education. Respir Care 1989; 34:890.
38. Muller S: Physicians for the twenty-first century: Report of the project panel on the general professional education of the physician and college preparation for medicine. J Med Educ 1984; 59:Part 2.
39. Muller WJ, Hess GD, Scherer PW: A model of cigarette smoke particle deposition. Am Ind Hyg Assoc J 1990; 51:245–256.
40. Hess D: The hand-held computer as a teaching tool for acid-base interpretation. Respir Care 1984; 29:375–379.
41. Pincetl P, Hoffer E, Barnett O: Chest pain, an exercise in problem solving. Baltimore, Williams & Wilkins Electronic Media, 1988.
42. Cyberlog: Acute Respiratory Failure. Munich, CMS–Biomedical Verlag, 1989.
43. Rubens AJ: Testing airway management skills: Interactive video courseware vs ACLS instructor. Respir Care 1991; 36:849.
44. Ingram J, Dickison P, Ahmed M. MacPuf. Oxford, Oxford University Press, 1988.
45. Gardner RM, Cannon GH, Morris AH, et al: Computerized blood gas interpretation and reporting system. Proc Annu Symp Comput Appl Med Care 1975; 8:39–45.
46. Shabot MM, LoBue M, Leyerle BJ, et al: Decision support alerts

for clinical laboratory and blood gas data. Int J Clin Monit Comput 1990; 7:27–31.
47. Evans RS, Gardner RM, Bush AR, et al: Development of a computerized infectious disease monitor (CIDM). Comput Biomed Res 1985; 18:103–113.
48. Tate K, Gardner R, Weaver L: A computerized laboratory alerting system. MD Comput 1990; 7:296–301.
49. Bradshaw KE, Gardner RM, Pryor TA: Development of a computerized laboratory alerting system. Comput Biomed Res 1989; 22:575–587.
50. Evans RS, Pestotnik SL, Burke JP, et al: Reducing the duration of prophylactic antibiotics use through computer monitoring of surgical patients. DICP 1990; 24:351–360.
51. Classen DC, Pestotnik SL, Evans RS, et al: Computerized surveillance of adverse drug events in hospital patients. JAMA 1991; 266:2847–2851.
52. Lepage ER, Gardner RM, Laub RM, et al: Assessing the effectiveness of a computerized blood order "consultation" system. Proc Annu Symp Comput Appl Med Care 1991; 15:33–37.
53. Gardner RM, Laub RM, Golubjatnikov OK, et al: Computer-critiqued blood ordering using the HELP system. Comput Biomed Res 1990; 23:514–528.
54. Kuperman GJ, Garder RM, Pryor TA: HELP: A Dynamic Hospital Information System. *In*: Computers and Medicine. Orthner HF (Ed). New York, Springer-Verlag, 1991.
55. Morris AH: Use of monitoring information in decision making. *In*: Respiratory Monitoring. Tobin MJ (Ed). New York, Churchill Livingstone, 1991.
56. Elliot CG: Computer-assisted quality assurance: Development and performance of a respiratory care program. QRB Qual Rev Bul 1991; 17:84–90.
57. Klar R, Zaiss A: Medical expert systems: Design and applications in pulmonary medicine. Lung 1990; 168:1201–1209.
58. Silage DA, Maxwell C: An acid-base map/arterial blood-gas interpretation program for hand-held computers. Respir Care 1984; 29:833–838.
59. Hess D, Eitel D: A portable and inexpensive computer system to interpret arterial blood gases. Respir Care 1985; 31:797.
60. Hess D, Silage D, Maxwell C: An arterial blood gas interpretation program for hand-held computers. Respir Care 1984; 29:756–759.
61. Hingston DM, Irwin RS, Pratter MR, et al: A computerized interpretation of arterial pH and blood gas data: Do physicians need it? Respir Care 1982; 27:809–815.
62. Gardner RM, Clemmer TP, Morris AH: Computerized medical decision-making, an evaluation in acute care. *In*: Computers in Critical Care and Pulmonary Medicine. Vol 2. Prakash O (Ed). New York, Plenum Press, 1982, pp 147–150.
63. Moore MJ, Bleich HL: Consulting the computer about acid-base disorders. Respir Care 1982; 7:834–838.
64. Verdaguer A, Patak A, Sancho JJ, et al: Validation of the medical expert system PNEUMON-IA. Comput Biomed Res 1992; 25:511–526.
65. Harber P, McCoy JM, Howard K, et al: Artificial intelligence–assisted occupational lung disease diagnosis. Chest 1991; 100:340–346.
66. Asada N, Doi K, MacMahon H, et al: Potential usefulness of an artificial neural network for differential diagnosis of interstitial lung diseases: Pilot study. Radiology 1990; 177:857–860.
67. Govindarajan N, Prakash O: Breath detection algorithm in digital computers. Int J Clin Monit Comput 1990; 7:59–64.
68. Shahsavar N, Gill H, Wigertz O, et al: Kave: A tool for knowledge acquisition to support artificial ventilation. Comput Methods Programs Biomed 1991; 34:115–123.
69. Polaschek J, Rutledge G, Andersen S, et al: Using belief networks to interpret qualitative data in the ICU. Respir Care 1993; 38:60–72.
70. Miller PL: Goal oriented critiquing by computer for ventilatory management. Comput Biomed Res 1985; 18:422–438.
71. Menn SJ, Barnett GO, Schnechel D, et al: A computer program to assist in the care of acute respiratory failure. JAMA 1973; 223:308–312.
72. Grossman R, Hew E, Aberman A: Assessment of the ability to manage patients on mechanical ventilators using a computer model. Acute Care 1984; 10:95–102.
73. Fagan L, Kunz J, Feigenbaum E, et al: Representing time-dependent relations in a medical setting [Doctoral dissertation]. Stanford, CA, Stanford University, 1980.
74. East TD, Morris AH, Wallace CJ, et al: A strategy for development of computerized critical care decision support systems. Int J Clin Monit Comput 1991; 8:263–269.
75. Henderson S, Crapo RO, Wallace CJ, et al: Performance of computerized protocols for the management of arterial oxygenation in an intensive care unit. Int J Clin Monit Comput 1991; 8:271–280.
76. Henderson S, Crapo RO, East TD, et al: Computerized clinical protocols in an intensive care unit: How well are they followed? Proc Annu Symp Comput Appl Med Care 1990; 14:284–288.
77. Tong DA: Weaning patients from mechanical ventilation: A knowledge-based system approach. Comput Methods Programs Biomed 1991; 35:267–278.
78. Tong DA: Weaning patients from mechanical ventilation: A knowledge-based approach. Proc Annu Symp Comput Appl Med Care 1990; 14:79–85.
79. Strickland JH Jr, Hasson JH: A computer-controlled ventilator weaning system. Chest 1991; 100:1096–1099.
80. Rudowski R, Frostell C, Gill H: A knowledge-based support system for mechanical ventilation of the lungs: The KUSIVAR concept and prototype. Comput Methods Programs Biomed 1989; 30:59–70.
81. Rutledge G, Thomsen G, Farr B, et al: VentPlan: A ventilator-management advisor. Proc Annu Symp Comput Appl Med Care 1991; 15:869–871.
82. Morris AH, Wallace CJ, Clemmer TP, et al: Extracorporeal CO_2 removal therapy for adult respiratory distress syndrome patients. Respir Care 1990; 35:224–231.
83. Morris AH, Wallace CJ, Clemmer TP, et al: Extracorporeal CO_2 removal therapy for adult respiratory distress syndrome patients: A computerized protocol–controlled trial. Rean Soins Intens Med Urg 1990; 6:485–490.
84. Morris AH, Wallace CJ, Clemmer TP, et al: Final Report: Computerized protocol controlled clinical trial of new therapy which includes ECCO2R for ARDS. Am Rev Respir Dis 1992; 145:A184.
85. Gardner RM, West BJ, Pryor TA, et al: Computer-based ICU data acquisition as an aid to clinical decision-making. Crit Care Med 1982; 10:823–830.
86. Sittig DF, Pace NL, Gardner RM, et al: Implementation of a computerized patient advice system using the HELP clinical information system. Comput Biomed Res 1989; 22:474–487.
87. Sittig DF, Gardner RM, Morris AH, et al: Clinical evaluation of computer-based respiratory care algorithms. Int J Clin Monit Comput 1990; 7:177–185.
88. Zapol WM, Frikker MJ, Pontoppidan H, et al: The adult respiratory distress syndrome at Massachusetts General Hospital: Etiology, progression and survival rates, 1978–1988. *In*: Adult Respiratory Distress Syndrome. Walz F (Ed). New York, Marcel Dekker, 1991, pp 367–380.
89. Artigas A, Carlet J, Le Gall JR, et al: Clinical presentation, prognostic factors, and outcome of ARDS in the European Collaborative Study (1985–1987). *In*: Adult Respiratory Distress Syndrome. Zapol WM, Lemaire F (Eds). New York, Marcel Dekker, 1991, pp 37–63.
90. Gardner RM, Hawley WL: Standardizing Communications & Networks in the ICU: Patient Monitoring and Data Management Conference. Arlington, VA, American Association of Medical Instrumentation, 1985, pp 59–63.
91. East TD: Real-time data acquisition and control. *In*: Diagnostic Methods in Critical Care: Automated Data Collection and Interpretation. Shoemaker WC, Abraham E (Eds). New York, Marcel Dekker, 1987, pp 285–310.
92. Isermann R: Digital Control Systems. Heidelberg, Germany, Springer-Verlag, 1981.
93. Coles JR, Brown WA, Lampard DG: Computer control of respiration and anesthesia. Med Biol Eng 1973; 11:262–267.
94. Rudowski R, Skreta L, Baehrendtz S, et al: Lung function analysis and optimization during artificial ventilation: A personal computer–based system. Comput Methods Programs Biomed 1990; 31:33–42.

95. East TD, Westenskow DR, Pace NL, et al: A microcomputer-based differential lung ventilation system. IEEE Trans Biomed Eng 1982; 29:736–740.
96. Chapman FW, Newell JC, Roy RJ: A feedback controller for ventilatory therapy. Ann Biomed Eng 1985; 13:359–372.
97. Verkaaik AP, van Dijk G, Westerkamp B, et al: Gas exchange in the lung, computer feed back–controlled physiological matching of artificial ventilation. Adv Exp Med Biol 1992; 317:325–330.
98. Ohlson KB, Westenskow DR, Jordan WS: A microprocessor-based feedback controller for mechanical ventilation. Ann Biomed Eng 1982; 10:3548–3555.
99. Morozoff PE, Evans RW: Closed-loop control of Sa_{O_2} in the neonate. Biomed Instrum Technol 1992; 26:117–123.
100. Verkaaik AP, Erdmann W, van Dijk G, et al: On-line oxygen uptake measurement (VO_2): A computer feed-back–controlled rebreathing circuit for long-term oxygen uptake registration. Adv Exp Med Biol 1992; 316:195–202.
101. Tehrani FT: A microcomputer oxygen control system for ventilatory therapy. Ann Biomed Eng 1992; 20:547–558.
102. Strickland JH Jr, Hasson JH: A computer-controlled ventilator weaning system: A clinical trial. Chest 1993; 103:1220–1226.

CHAPTER 102

Hemodynamic Effects of Artificial Ventilation

Michael R. Pinsky, MD

The use of artificial ventilation has significantly improved our ability to support critically ill patients in the intensive care unit. With the widespread application of positive-pressure ventilation has come the realization that complex cardiopulmonary interactions can occur that may significantly alter cardiac output and thus oxygen delivery to the tissues.[1, 2] For example, if positive-pressure ventilation decreases cardiac output to a greater degree than it increases arterial oxygen content, then oxygen delivery to the tissues decreases. Because a major therapeutic goal in the critically ill patient is to maximize oxygen delivery to the tissues,[3] any ventilatory therapy aimed at improving arterial oxygenation that simultaneously decreases cardiac output is counterproductive to good patient care. Accordingly, the critical care physician must understand the hemodynamic effects of artificial ventilation to optimize cardiorespiratory therapy.

EFFECTS OF VENTILATION ON LUNG VOLUME AND INTRATHORACIC PRESSURE

Ventilation directly affects cardiovascular performance by changing either lung volume or intrathoracic pressure (ITP). Although most studies have demonstrated that mechanical factors are primarily responsible for hemodynamic alterations,[1, 4, 5] neuroreflex mechanisms (autonomic tone)[6, 7] and humoral cardiac depressant substances have also been implicated.[8, 9] Lung inflation at normal tidal volumes induces cardioacceleration, which is caused primarily by withdrawal of vagal tone. This phenomenon is called *respiratory sinus arrhythmia.* A residual respiratory sinus arrhythmia persists in humans even after total denervation of the heart;[10] this suggests that mechanical stretch receptors may also influence chronotropism. The implication of these findings is that the demonstration of respiratory sinus arrhythmia is an inadequate criterion with which to validate normal sympathetic innervation of the heart. Because the absence of respiratory sinus arrhythmia is often used to assess autonomic dysfunction, this limitation in such an assessment is important.

Large tidal volumes (>15 mL/kg) induce a reflex vasodilation, bradycardia, and a negative inotropic response. This vasodepressor response is directly proportional to ventilatory frequency and tidal volume. The bradycardia is affected by tidal volume. The receptors for this response, whose fibers travel in the vagus nerve, tonically inhibit the vasomotor center.[7] Lung inflation may also produce humoral substances that depress myocardial performance.[8, 9] These nonmechanical factors may induce transient cardiovascular changes, but their effect is not great enough to explain most of the hemodynamic changes. These reflex interactions appear to be most pronounced in neonates, in whom sympathetic tone is high, and with the use of high-frequency ventilation.

As lung volume changes during a breath, pulmonary vascular capacitance[11] and resistance[12] may vary. If the pulmonary vasculature is engorged with blood and pulmonary capillary pressure is subsequently increased, then lung distention squeezes blood out of the alveolar vessels, increasing pulmonary venous blood flow and augmenting left ventricular (LV) filling. Conversely, if intrathoracic blood volume is low and pulmonary capillary pressure reduced, lung distention has a minimum effect on pulmonary capillary blood volume. However, extra-alveolar vessels do dilate, and this causes blood to pool in large pulmonary arterial and venous vessels and blood flow to decelerate in the pulmonary veins, thus limiting LV filling. Furthermore, as lung volume increases, alveolar pressure increases relative to ITP, which is the extramural pressure for extra-alveolar pulmonary vessels, whereas alveolar pressure is the extramural pressure for alveolar vessels. Thus, increasing lung volume causes the pressure gradient between the outside of the extra-alveolar and alveolar vessels to increase. This extravascular pressure gradient, referred to as *transpulmonary pressure,* not only distends the lungs but also constricts the alveolar vessels, increasing their resistance to flow as these vessels pass from extra-alveolar to alveolar loci. This phenomenon is usually seen with increases in lung volume above functional residual capacity (FRC). If lung volumes increase excessively, as with hyperinflation or a deep inspiration, mechanical heart-lung interactions in which the inflated lungs compress the heart and limit diastolic ventricular filling can also occur.[13–15] Decreases in lung volume below FRC can also increase pulmonary vascular resistance (PVR). In this case, the mechanism is thought to be vasoconstriction of the large extra-alveolar vessels as alveoli collapse[16] with decreasing lung volume. These mechanical factors can affect cardiac performance; whereas some increase the work necessary to pump blood from the right ventricle (RV) across the pulmonary vasculature, others inhibit diastolic filling of both ventricles.

Changes in ITP can also affect cardiovascular function independent of changes in lung volume. The heart within the thorax is a pressure chamber within another pressure chamber. Thus, changes in ITP affect the pressure gradient both for systemic venous return[17–19] and for LV output independent of the pressures generated by the heart itself.[20] Because the pressure gradient for venous return is small compared with that for LV ejection, small changes in ITP have a greater effect on the pressure gradient for systemic venous drainage than on LV ejection. Only in conditions in which cardiac function is reduced and intravascular volume is expanded or when changes in ITP are excessive do changes in ITP have a significant primary effect on LV systolic performance.[21–24]

Because ITP increases during positive-pressure inspiration and decreases during spontaneous inspiration (whereas lung volume increases during both types of breathing), the effects of positive-pressure ventilation on cardiovascular performance may not be the same as those of spontaneous respiration, despite similar changes in lung volume. Any cardiovascular differences between spontaneous breathing and positive-pressure ventilation relate primarily to differences in the changes in ITP with tidal breathing and to differences in the work of breathing.

RIGHT VENTRICULAR PERFORMANCE

RV systolic performance is determined by diastolic (preload) and systolic (afterload) components as well as by the level of cardiac contractility. The exact determinants of RV function are unknown but appear to vary from those defining LV function. However, Sibbald and coworkers[25] found that RV end-diastolic volume correlates with RV stroke volume. The RV end-diastolic volume (preload), in turn, is determined by both ventricular diastolic compliance and distending pressure. Diastolic compliance of the RV may decrease in response to acute chamber dilation, ischemia, neurohumoral stimulation, or overdistention of the LV (reverse interdependence).[26] Distending pressure in the RV can be defined as the intracavity pressure minus the extracavity (pericardial) pressure, both of which are measured relative to atmospheric pressure. Pericardial pressure rarely equals atmospheric pressure and during respiration may fluctuate widely. Therefore, to estimate accurately RV distending pressure, extracavity pressure must be measured. If the pericardium does not limit diastolic filling, ITP can be used to approximate extracavity (pericardial) pressure. Esophageal pressure is often used as an estimate of pleural pressure.[27] Although in upright humans esophageal pressure parallels negative fluctuations in pleural pressure, it may underestimate the positive fluctuations[28] because of the stenting effect of the mediastinum and of the esophagus on intraluminal esophageal pressure. During the application of positive end-expiratory pressure (PEEP), differences between pericardial pressure or ITP and esophageal pressure can be large.[29] Because the RV receives its blood from contiguous intrathoracic structures such as the right atrium and vena cavae, which are easily deformed by ITP, RV distending pressure can be estimated as right atrial pressure (Pra) minus ITP (transmural Pra). With this formula, if esophageal pressure underestimates the increase in ITP, the observer calculates incorrectly a greater RV distending pressure than actually exists; this may lead to the assumption that RV preload is adequate when in fact it is low. With this in mind, Pinsky and associates[30] measured pericardial pressure, Pra, and RV volumes as PEEP was varied from 0 to 15 cm H_2O in patients who had undergone cardiac surgery. They demonstrated that RV end-diastolic volume may vary greatly without measurable changes in transmural Pra. The explanation of these findings was that under most physiologic conditions, RV filling occurs below the unstressed volume of the RV such that conformational changes in the RV occur without changes in RV wall stress. Accordingly, measurements of Pra either alone or relative to pericardial pressure are insensitive determinants of RV volumes when RV volumes are either normal or reduced. Presumably, when the RV dilates beyond some limiting volume, distending pressure varies with volume. However, the degree to which these findings are applicable clinically is unknown. It is sufficient to state that unless one measures RV volumes by some means, it is difficult to assess the adequacy of RV preload with measures of RV filling pressures.

Unlike RV filling pressure, the driving pressure for systemic venous return is determined by the pressure gradient between the small systemic veins and Pra, both of which are measured relative to atmospheric pressure.[18] Because the right atrium is an intrathoracic structure, changes in ITP directly affect Pra. During spontaneous inspiration, as ITP becomes more negative, Pra also decreases; this creates an increased pressure gradient between the systemic veins and the right atrium that accelerates venous blood flow.[17] Accordingly, spontaneous inspiration is usually associated with an increase in systemic venous return, which is manifested as an increase in RV end-diastolic volume (preload); thus, RV stroke volume is augmented. Conversely, positive-pressure inspiration increases ITP and, thus, Pra, which decreases the pressure gradient for venous return and decelerates venous blood flow.[19] This decrease in venous return during positive-pressure inspiration is associated with a decrease in RV end-diastolic volume, which decreases RV stroke volume[31] and, ultimately, cardiac output. The reciprocal change in Pra and transmural Pra (RV filling pressure) during both spontaneous (intermittent negative-pressure) breathing and intermittent positive-pressure breathing (IPPB) is depicted in Figure 102–1. Note that Pra tends to follow ITP. The resultant reciprocal change in venous blood flow into the RV induces a parallel change in transmural Pra; however, as noted previously, the transmural Pra does not faithfully reflect RV volume. These ventilation-induced fluctuations in Pra should not be confused with the steady-state effect of intravascular volume loading on Pra. With volume loading, mean Pra (often referred to as *central venous pressure*) increases, although phasic changes in Pra still persist (see Fig. 102–1). During positive-pressure ventilation with a small tidal volume, when Pra increases, RV stroke volume decreases proportionally. When data—such as

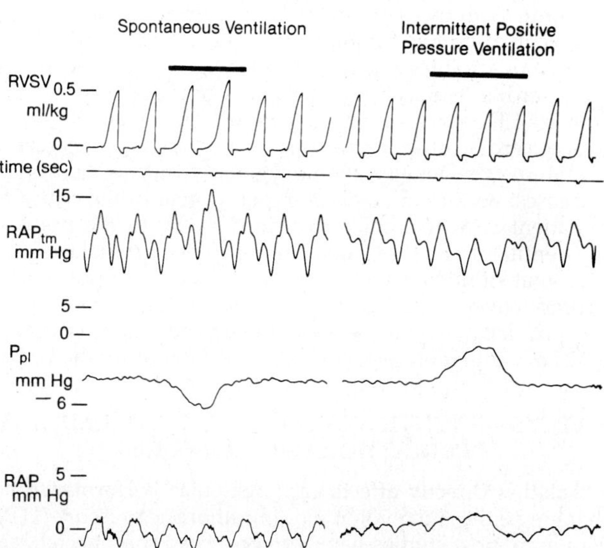

Figure 102–1. From *bottom* to *top*, Trend records of right atrial pressure (RAP), juxtacardiac pleural pressure (P_{pl}), and RAP measured relative to P_{pl} (called transmural RAP [RAP_{tm}]), and RV stroke volume (RVSV) during spontaneous *(left)* and positive-pressure *(right)* breathing in an intact, anesthetized canine model. *Solid bars* represent inspiration. Note that right atrial pressure and pleural pressure follow each other but that transmural right atrial pressure (RV filling pressure) moves in the opposite direction. As transmural right atrial pressure varies, so does RV stroke volume on the subsequent beat. (From Snyder JV, Pinsky MR [Eds]. Oxygen Transport in the Critically Ill. Chicago, Year Book Medical Publishers, 1987, p 321.)

those described for positive-pressure breaths shown in Figure 102–1—are plotted as RV stroke volume versus Pra, an "instantaneous venous return curve" similar to one created with right-sided heart bypass techniques is generated[31] (Fig. 102–2). Such analyses can be used to assess cardiovascular status.[32]

Because the pressure gradient for systemic venous blood flow can be defined as Pra minus the hydrostatic pressure in the small venules,[18] a decrease in the driving pressure for venous return can occur owing to an increase in Pra, to a decrease in peripheral venous pressure, or to both. Thus, the obligatory decrease in the pressure gradient for venous return during positive-pressure ventilation is exacerbated by hypovolemia, sepsis, or spinal shock, each of which may decrease systemic venous pressure. This decrease in the pressure gradient for venous return can be minimized either by reducing mean ITP to lower mean Pra (decreasing inspiratory time, increasing inspiratory flow rate for a fixed tidal volume)[4] or by increasing systemic venous pressure by volume infusion or the use of vasotonic agents.[33] Either maneuver maintains cardiac output. When pulmonary parenchymal compliance is low, however, increases in airway pressure do not increase ITP to the same degree as when lung compliance is normal.[34] Thus, in patients with stiff lungs, artificial ventilation may have less effect on venous return and overall cardiovascular hemostasis than would be expected based on the changes in airway pressure observed in persons with healthy lungs. However, as lung volume increases during the positive-pressure breath, ITP also increases proportionally, independent of the compliance of the lungs. Thus, even when lung compliance is low (as occurs in states of acute lung injury), if tidal volume is kept constant, then the changes in ITP during breathing are also constant, despite markedly increasing airway pressures. Because the hemodynamic effects of positive-pressure ventilation are due to changes in both lung volume and ITP, keeping both constant results in a constant hemodynamic state, regardless of changes in lung compliance.

The detrimental effects of positive-pressure ventilation are primarily due to an inspiration-associated decrease in systemic venous return. These effects may not be as pronounced as was originally thought.[33] When inspiration is associated with an increase in lung volume, then diaphragmatic descent also increases abdominal pressure. Because abdominal pressure is the surrounding pressure for intra-abdominal blood vessels, increasing abdominal pressure increases the intra-abdominal vascular pressure relative to atmospheric pressure just as increases in ITP increase Pra relative to atmospheric pressure. This increase in abdominal pressure minimizes the resultant decrease in the pressure gradient for venous return. Takata and Robotham[35] demonstrated that this effect functionally resulted in a parallel shift of the venous return curve to the right with pressure on the *x*-axis in a fashion analogous to that with volume resuscitation. Thus, to the extent that inspiration also increases intra-abdominal pressure, venous return is not reduced by positive-pressure ventilation. Accordingly, one would predict that in the presence of tense ascites, venous return would not be reduced during positive-pressure ventilation, whereas if abdominal pressure were to decrease to atmospheric pressure (as occurs with an open abdomen, e.g., with laparotomy), the deleterious effects of positive-pressure ventilation on venous return would be maximum. This loss of the abdominal pressure stenting of mean systemic pressure may account for the hemodynamic instability seen in patients with portal hypertension and ascites in whom a pericentesis removes large quantities of fluid.

RV afterload can be defined as stress to the RV wall during systole, which is a function of end-diastolic volume and systolic RV pressure.[36] Because the RV and pulmonary circulation are surrounded by an ITP that may not equal atmospheric pressure, functional systolic RV pressure is defined more accurately as pulmonary artery pressure (Ppa) minus ITP (transmural Ppa). If transmural Ppa increases, RV ejection is impeded. However, under most clinical conditions, transmural Ppa does not increase greatly because the pulmonary arteries can dilate easily. If, however, transmural Ppa increases by a large amount, then the RV also dilates. Because the RV cannot empty as well against an increased transmural Ppa, RV end-systolic volume increases, and stroke volume initially decreases. For cardiac output to remain unchanged by the Frank-Starling mechanism, RV filling pressures must increase to augment RV end-diastolic volume. This increase in RV filling pressure

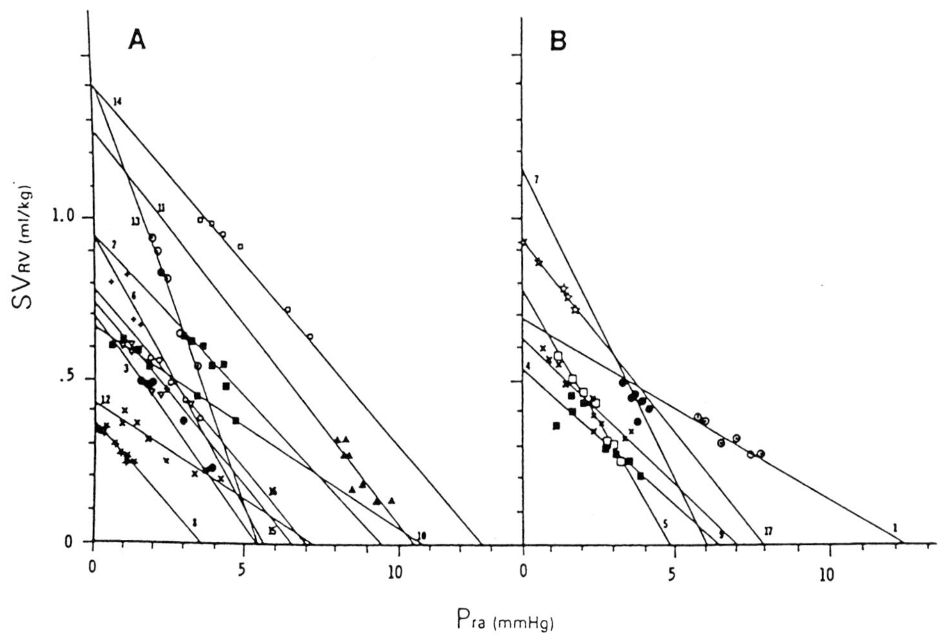

Figure 102–2. Relationship between RV stroke volume (SVrv) and right atrial pressure (Pra) during nonvolemic intermittent positive-pressure ventilation for all animals is shown on 2 separate graphs for clarity *(A and B)*. Each data point represents the SVrv-Pra relationship of one cardiac cycle, and all data points represent sequential beats throughout inspiration. (From Pinsky MR: Instantaneous venous return curves in an intact canine preparation. J Appl Phys 1984; 56:765–771.)

causes Pra to increase. Although in the chronic state increased sympathetic tone and fluid retention return the pressure gradient for venous return toward normal, thereby allowing normal cardiac output despite increased transmural Ppa and Pra,[25] acute increases in transmural Ppa may induce profound hemodynamic compromise owing to a decrease in the pressure gradient for systemic venous return.

Transmural Ppa may increase either owing to a passive back-up of pressure from the LV or as a result of increased PVR. Pulmonary hypertension resulting from LV pump failure may precipitate cardiogenic pulmonary edema and respiratory failure, necessitating artificial ventilation; however, this condition is not usually in itself a consequence of artificial ventilation. Most increases in transmural Ppa during artificial ventilation result from increased PVR. As lung volume increases above FRC, alveolar vessels are compressed, and PVR increases because the extravascular transpulmonary pressure increases.[12] Overdistention of the lungs, as occurs with obstructive airway disease, ventilation with large tidal volumes, and excessively high levels of PEEP, increases PVR. Normal resting tidal volume is less than 10 mL/kg[37]; this increases PVR at end-inspiration in healthy lungs by no more than 12%.[38] Accordingly, Piene and Sund[39] have noted that RV systolic performance changes minimally during normal ventilation. In further support of this concept, Pinsky[31] showed that during normal tidal breathing, changes in RV end-diastolic volume are the only determinants of changes in RV stroke volume.

Therefore, small changes in lung volume that occur during normal ventilation in patients without pulmonary hypertension do not affect RV systolic performance. Artificial ventilation may actually decrease PVR in certain conditions. In acute respiratory failure, resting lung volumes are often below FRC, and alveolar hypoxia may be present owing to collapse of terminal airways and absorption atelectasis.[3] When the lung volume falls below FRC, compression of extra-alveolar vessels causes PVR to increase. In addition, hypoxia can increase PVR by inducing hypoxic pulmonary vasoconstriction.[40] If artificial ventilation increases the concentration of oxygen in the alveoli or returns lung volume to its normal end-expiratory level, then PVR may decrease. Canada and coworkers[41] recently demonstrated in a dog model with healthy lungs that increasing end-expiratory volumes from the use of 10 cm H_2O of PEEP increases PVR, whereas after the induction of acute respiratory failure by oleic acid, the same amount of PEEP decreases PVR. Regarding the interaction of RV preload and afterload, one can readily see that if the RV is highly compliant during diastole and that, relative to the LV; it has a lesser end-systolic elastance, increases in RV end-diastolic volume should also increase RV end-systolic volume, even if RV stroke volume increases as well. Studies by Reuse and coworkers[42] and by Pinsky and associates[30] support the concept and underscore the dissimilarities between RV and LV function.[16] That the relation of RV end-systolic volume to end-diastolic volume is highly linear suggests that RV contractility does not vary with changes in RV end-diastolic volume, a concept foreign to the assessment of LV function.

Thus, the effects of positive-pressure ventilation on RV performance depend on the degree to which venous return (preload) is compromised and PVR (afterload) is affected. In almost all patients, however, positive-pressure ventilation increases Pra, owing to either passive transmission of ITP to intrathoracic venous structures or to RV dilation caused by increases in PVR. If increased airway pressure is sustained, RV performance is impaired only in those patients with preexisting RV dysfunction.[42a] Increasing Pra decreases the pressure gradient for venous return;[18, 43] this decelerates venous blood flow and thus decreases cardiac output compared with that seen during spontaneous breathing.[4, 31] The most common and important hemodynamic effect of artificial ventilation is to decrease cardiac output by decreasing the pressure gradient for systemic venous return.

LEFT VENTRICULAR PERFORMANCE

Left ventricular performance is determined by its preload (end-diastolic volume), contractility, afterload (systolic wall stress), and the heart rate.[44] By the Frank-Starling mechanism,[45] when LV contractility is not reduced, LV stroke volume depends primarily on LV end-diastolic volume, and small changes in the heart rate or LV afterload, as may occur during positive-pressure ventilation, do not significantly affect it.[1]

Artificial ventilation can significantly alter LV end-diastolic volume (preload) in several ways. First, if Pra increases because of an increase in either ITP or RV afterload, venous return decreases. This must eventually decrease pulmonary venous blood flow and LV end-diastolic volume. Second, because LV end-diastolic volume is a function of LV diastolic compliance and distending pressure, it is altered by a change in either. Because lung inflation increases PVR and, thus, RV systolic pressure load, if the RV dilates during artificial ventilation, LV diastolic volume may be compromised by one of two mechanisms: (1) a leftward shift of the intraventricular septum,[46] which decreases LV diastolic compliance (ventricular interdependence); or (2) the limitation imposed by the semirigid pericardium on absolute biventricular end-diastolic volume (tamponade).[26, 47] Sudden increases in airway pressure caused by increasing lung volume may dilate the RV owing to the increase in RV afterload.[48] However, such increases in lung volume also immediately decrease venous return; this in turn decreases RV end-diastolic volume[49] and minimizes ventricular interaction. Robotham and colleagues[50] demonstrated minimal septal shift during positive-pressure ventilation that was abolished by the application of PEEP. Similarly, LV end-systolic volume is unaffected by septal shift.[49, 50] Therefore, ventricular interdependence is probably not a significant factor in depressing steady-state LV performance during positive-pressure ventilation, unless marked cardiomegaly and large increases in transmural Ppa occur. Independent of ventricular interdependence, as lung volume increases, the space within the thorax where the heart resides (the cardiac fossa) becomes more constricting because of the mechanical compressive effects of the expanding lungs.[15, 51] Wallis and coworkers[14] and Lloyd[13] demonstrated that this form of mechanical heart-lung interaction decreases LV end-diastolic volume by increasing juxtacardiac pleural pressure. This effect of inflation-induced cardiac compression becomes more important as lung volume or heart size increases. Because the compliance of the LV measured relative to juxtacardiac pleural pressure is unchanged,[52] increasing LV filling pressure by volume infusion usually overcomes the decrease in end-diastolic volume and restores cardiac output to normal.[53] Although septal shift, pericardial volume limitations, and mechanical heart-lung interactions function by different means, they all create conditions in which LV filling pressure, when measured as either left atrial pressure or pulmonary artery occlusion pressure relative to atmospheric pressure, overestimates actual LV end-diastolic volume. Thus, all three mechanisms can be considered to decrease the "effective" LV diastolic compliance. Similarly, all three mechanisms respond to intravascular volume challenge by increasing cardiac output. Therefore, positive-pressure ventilation may decrease LV preload by decreasing either systemic venous return to the RV or effective LV diastolic compliance.

Because the LV delivers its stroke volume into the aorta, a vascular structure with free extrathoracic drainage, changes in ITP may affect the ejecting LV independent of aortic pressure measured relative to atmospheric pressure. Buda and colleagues[20] have shown that the LV systolic pressure load is represented more accurately by LV pressure relative to ITP (transmural LV pressure) than by LV pressure alone when ITP varies widely. If aortic pressure remains constant, positive fluctuations in ITP decrease the transmural LV pressures, thus decreasing LV afterload, whereas negative fluctuations in ITP increase LV afterload (Fig. 102–3). Spontaneous inspiratory efforts in the setting of upper airway obstruction,[54] bronchospasm,[55] or decreased lung compliance[56] significantly decrease ITP and thus increase LV afterload by increasing transmural LV pressure; this may precipitate or worsen cardiogenic pulmonary edema. Giving patients with these conditions positive-pressure ventilation may improve LV performance by abolishing the negative fluctuations in ITP seen during spontaneous inspiration and by adding positive ITP during the positive-pressure breaths. Calvin and coworkers[21] showed that increasing ITP with the addition of PEEP in patients with severe LV dysfunction did not depress LV function and, in some patients, improved LV performance. Mathru and associates[22] demonstrated in patients with high LV filling pressures (>15 mm Hg) and presumably decreased myocardial performance that increasing ITP with the application of 10 cm H_2O of PEEP improved cardiac output, whereas in patients with low LV filling pressures (<15 mm Hg), the same amount of PEEP decreased cardiac output. Similar results were obtained by Räsänen.[57] Artificial ventilation may improve LV performance for a given LV preload by eliminating the negative fluctuations in ITP seen during spontaneous ventilation. Thus, changes in ITP may directly affect LV performance by altering either LV end-diastolic compliance or LV afterload. To the extent that cardiac performance depends on venous return and LV end-diastolic volume, positive-pressure ventilation decreases cardiac output. If LV end-diastolic volume can be maintained, increases in ITP do not depress LV performance[58] and may even improve it when contractility is depressed by decreasing LV afterload.[59] A commonly accepted method of assessing LV function is to plot LV pressure versus volume for a cardiac cycle. If sudden changes in either preload or afterload can be induced, one can generate a series of cardiac cycles with varying end-systolic pressure-volume data pairs. The slope of the end-systolic pressure-volume relation so created is believed to be a measure of LV contractility.[60] If this slope increases, contractility is better, whereas if the slope decreases, contractility is worse. Similarly, if the end-systolic pressure-volume point moves upward and to the left of the end-systolic pressure-volume relation, then contractility must be improved (Fig. 102–4). When the LV pressure-volume history during positive-pressure ventilation is examined in an intact dog preparation using this analysis (Fig. 102–5), it can be seen that the LV pressure-volume relation during a positive-pressure breath moves upward as if contractility were improved relative to a reference value of apneic end-systolic pressure-volume relation. As can be seen in this example, positive-pressure ventilation reduces both LV end-diastolic volume and end-systolic volume. The decrease in LV end-diastolic volume presumably occurs because of the compression of the heart in the cardiac fossa by the expanding lungs. However, the LV end-systolic volume decreases as well, and it decreases to a pressure-volume

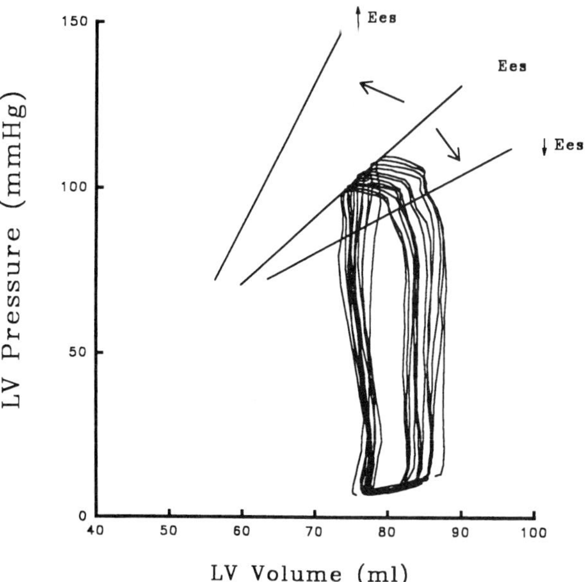

Figure 102–4. Relationship between LV pressure and volume as LV preload is rapidly reduced in a closed-chest canine model in which LV volume is measured with a conductance catheter. The maximum ratio of pressure to volume defines maximum or end-systolic elastance (Ees) in this model. Changes in Ees reflect concomitant changes in cardiac contractility. Drawn onto these pressure volume loops are two other Ees lines that reflect increased contractility (↑ Ees) and decreased contractility (↓ Ees).

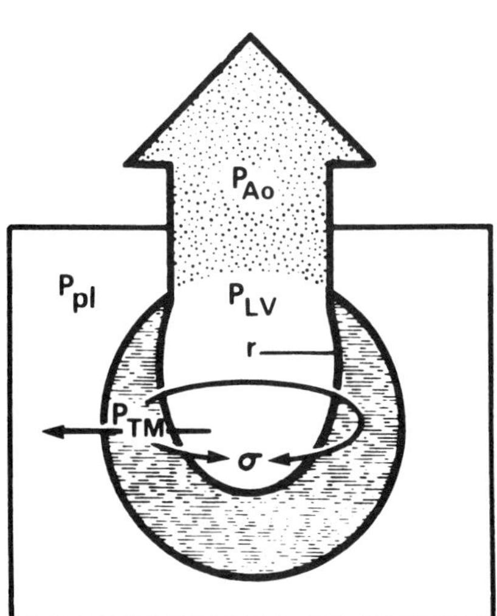

$$\text{MYOCARDIAL WALL TENSION} = f(P_{TM}) = f(\sigma, \text{GEOMETRY})$$

$$P_{TM} = P_{LV} - P_{pl}$$

Figure 102–3. Schematic representation of the LV wall, thoracic cavity, and aorta. According to the Laplace relationship, myocardial wall tension is a function of LV transmural pressure (P_{TM}) and of the geometry of the left ventricle (r). (From Dantzker D [Ed]. Cardiopulmonary Critical Care. Philadelphia, WB Saunders, 1991, p 102.)

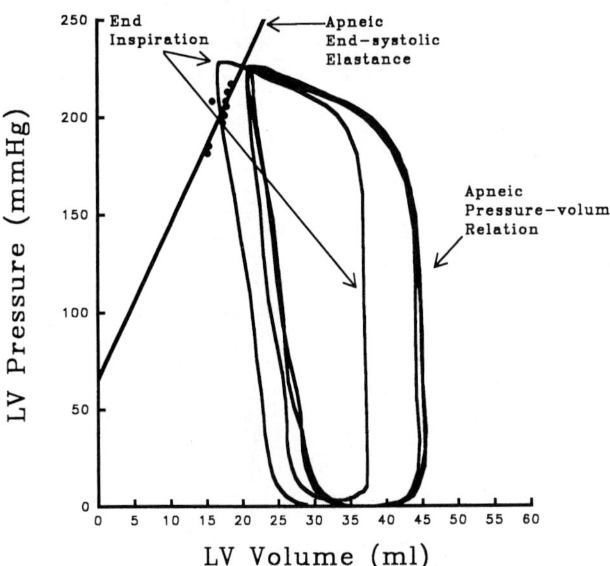

Figure 102–5. The LV pressure-volume relationship during apnea and inspiration of a single breath. The apneic end-systolic elastance curve and its corresponding end-systolic pressure-volume points during an acute interior vena cava occlusion are included for reference. Note that inspiration decreases both end-diastolic and end-systolic volume and shifts the end-systolic pressure-volume relation to the left of the apneic end-elastance domain.

location to the left of the apneic value of the end-systolic pressure-volume relationship. This shift can be explained by the increase in ITP decreasing the LV ejection pressure (transmural LV pressure), which, when plotted as LV pressure alone, cannot be accounted for. Thus, positive-pressure ventilation dynamically alters both LV preload and afterload. The net hemodynamic effect is determined by the balance between preload and afterload.

CARDIAC PERFORMANCE DURING THE VENTILATORY CYCLE

Throughout the ventilatory cycle, phasic and continuous changes occur in autonomic tone, lung volume, transpulmonary pressure, and ITP, all of which affect instantaneous blood flow. Similarly, the degree to which blood flow is affected depends on the functional state of the heart, lungs, and vasculature. Thus, the effect of any ventilatory mode on cardiovascular performance is not uniform for all clinical conditions. However, under normal conditions with tidal volume ventilation in the range of 5 to 15 mL/kg, the hemodynamic effects of either spontaneous or positive-pressure ventilation are reasonably predictable (Table 102–1). The cardiovascular system never exists in a circulatory steady state, with LV and RV output equal and constant from one beat to the next.[5, 19, 61] Thus, measurements averaged throughout the respiratory cycle may not accurately represent the hemodynamic interactions present during specific phases of the respiratory cycle or predict the response of the system to sudden changes in preload or afterload.

The instantaneous changes in intrathoracic vascular pressures on ventricular output during spontaneous and positive-pressure ventilation in a dog model are illustrated in Figures 102–6 and 102–7, respectively. Spontaneous respiratory efforts, by decreasing ITP, decrease Pra (see Fig. 102–6). During spontaneous inspiration, a decrease in Pra increases the pressure gradient for venous return; this, in turn, increases RV filling pressure and results in an increase in RV stroke volume and transmural Ppa on the following systole. Intrathoracic blood volume increases; within two to three cardiac cycles, as the increased pulmonary blood flow reaches the LV, LV filling pressure (transmural left atrial pressure) and LV stroke volume increase as well. This phase lag in the outputs of the two ventricles in response to respiration-induced changes in venous return to the RV can cause the peak output of each ventricle to be completely out of phase with that of the other and may complicate an analysis of the effects of ventilation on LV performance[61] unless LV volume and transmural pressure during the breath are continuously known. Because this criterion is unreasonable under most clinical conditions, our assessment of the hemodynamic effects of ventilation is based primarily on inferential data. Advances in cardiac imaging methodologies, however, are markedly reducing the information gap.

TABLE 102–1. Factors That Determine Heart-Lung Interactions

Lung volume
PVR
Ventricular interdependence
Mechanical heart-lung interactions
Pressure gradient for systemic venous return, modified by:
Circulating blood volume
Peripheral vasomotor tone
Intra-abdominal pressure
Pressure gradient for LV ejection, modified by:
Ventricular contractility
Mitral valve function

In general, the phasic variations in RV stroke volume during the ventilatory cycle are greater than those in LV stroke volume. This is because ventilation has a greater effect on the pressure gradient for systemic venous return than does LV filling, as both the pulmonary circulation and the LV undergo a similar increase in ITP. However, transmural left atrial pressure may increase either during one phase of ventilation or during another by (1) direct transmission of the pressure pulse from the pulmonary artery (no change in preload),[62] (2) acceleration of pulmonary venous blood flow during inspiration via the squeezing of alveolar vessels (increase in preload),[11, 19] (3) decreased LV diastolic compliance from the suddenly dilated RV through the mechanism of ventricular interdependence (decrease in preload),[26, 46, 47] or (4) decreased LV ejection due to negative ITP that increases the LV systolic pressure load or vice versa (change in afterload).[20] Ventilation-associated changes in aortic pressure and flow are usually less than those in the pulmonary circulation because systemic venous return is affected more by small changes in Pra[17] than LV ejection is by similar changes in transmural aortic pressure.[20, 63] However, to the extent that spontaneous respiratory efforts alter ITP and lung volume, affecting venous return and LV diastolic compliance, LV output may also be affected. In the setting of decreased lung compliance or increased resistance to inspiration, spontaneous inspiratory efforts may be associated with profound negative fluctuations in ITP that increase venous return and reduce LV output,[43] resulting in a tendency for blood to pool in the chest. This promotes pulmonary edema and further decreases lung compliance. Such a negative feedback process has been postulated as a cause of pulmonary edema in patients with asthma[55] and upper airway obstruction[54] and may be important in the progression of pulmonary edema associated with acute myocardial

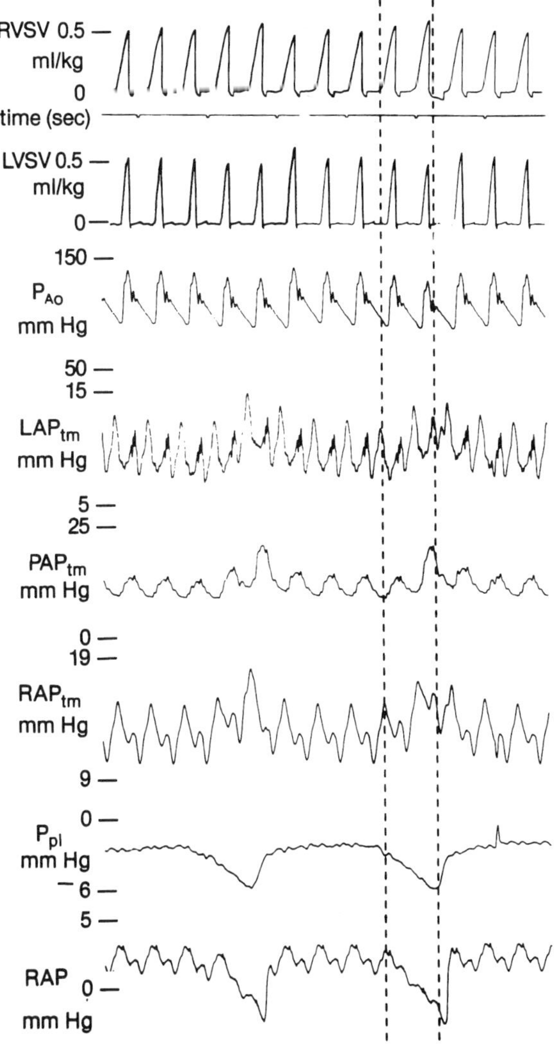

Figure 102–6. Trend records of various hemodynamic variables during spontaneous ventilation for an intact anesthetized canine model. RV stroke volume (RVSV) and LV stroke volume (LVSV) are displayed with the corresponding pressures for the aorta (P_{AO}), pleural space (P_{pl}), and right atrium (RAP) as well as for the transmural (relative to Ppl) left atrial (LAP_{tm}), pulmonary arterial (PAP_{tm}), and right atrial (RAP_{tm}) pressures. The two vertical *dotted lines* serve as reference points for end-inspiration for two breaths. (From Snyder JV, Pinsky MR [Eds]. Oxygen Transport in the Critically Ill. Chicago, Year Book Medical Publishers, 1987, p 325.)

infarction. The use of artificial ventilation to treat patients with cardiogenic pulmonary edema alleviates these exaggerated negative fluctuations in ITP;[57] this in turn decreases intrathoracic blood volume and possibly allows a more rapid resolution of pulmonary edema than would otherwise occur.[64] Similarly, spontaneous expiratory grunting, which increases ITP, may relieve pulmonary vascular congestion in the presence of pulmonary edema.[23, 65] The cost of the work of breathing is minimal under normal resting conditions, accounting for approximately 8% of basal oxygen consumption. However, with increasing elastic loads (pulmonary edema, fibrosis) or resistive loads (bronchospasm, airway collapse), the respiratory muscles may use more than 80% of the total oxygen delivery.[66] This stress may overtax a failing cardiovascular system, even if the blood oxygen-carrying capacity and blood volume are within an acceptable range for resting conditions.[67] As the cost of the work of breathing increases, blood flow to the respiratory muscles also increases, and this may compromise flow to other organs.[60] For example, if cardiac output is limited, this increased oxygen consumption in the respiratory muscles may limit exercise capacity. If ventilation-perfusion imbalance exists, the decreasing mixed venous oxygen content associated with an increase in oxygen consumption may cause arterial oxygen content and oxygen delivery to decrease, as deoxygenated mixed venous blood flows through intrapulmonary shunts. To the extent that artificial ventilation minimizes the cost of the work of breathing, oxygen consumption decreases, and this in turn increases the mixed venous oxygen content. Under these conditions, artificial ventilation may increase the arterial oxygen content without primarily affecting either gas exchange or cardiac output.

By increasing airway pressure, positive-pressure inspira-

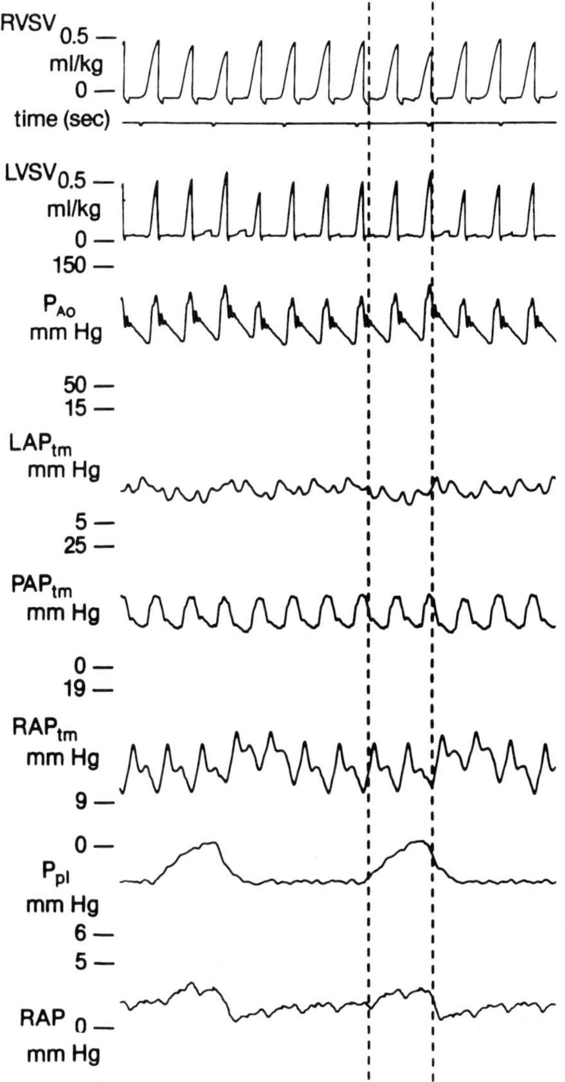

Figure 102–7. Trend records of the hemodynamic variables shown in Figure 102–6 during positive-pressure ventilation at approximately the same tidal volume and frequency. (From Snyder JV, Pinsky MR [Eds]. Oxygen Transport in the Critically Ill. Chicago, Year Book Medical Publishers, 1987, p 325.)

tion (see Fig. 102–7) distends the lungs and causes ITP to increase. This increased ITP passively increases Pra, which in turn decreases venous return, RV filling pressure, and RV stroke volume. Because the pulmonary circulation is intrathoracic and has a high capacitance relative to the right side of the heart, transmural left atrial pressure (LV filling pressure) and LV stroke volume do not vary as much as RV stroke volume does during ventilation, despite similar changes in venous return and pulmonary arterial blood flow. During positive-pressure ventilation, the decrease in LV stroke volume (see Fig. 102–7) is delayed by two to three beats from that in RV stroke volume and represents the decreases in venous return that subsequently affect the LV. Such decreases in LV stroke volume are accentuated in the setting of hypovolemia,[69] decreased vasomotor tone,[69] large tidal volume breathing,[4] or prolonged inspiratory time.[4, 24] The first two factors decrease the upstream pressure for venous return, and the last two increase the back pressure to venous return. Inspiratory increases in LV stroke volume may also occur during positive-pressure ventilation (reverse pulsus paradoxus) in the presence of heart failure and are manifest as an increase in aortic pulse pressure over end-expiratory levels.[70] Such matched changes in inspiration to pulse pressure usually do not represent relative hypovolemia but rather states of decreased LV contractility or volume overload. Thus, it is not enough to ascertain whether the pulse and systolic pressures in the aorta vary with artificial ventilation; the timing of such changes and their direction relative to the cardiac cycle are also important.

The importance of matching when the change in aortic pulse pressure or systolic arterial pressure occurs relative to both positive-pressure ventilation and LV volume changes is exemplified by the studies of Perel and coworkers,[71] Jardin and associates,[72] and others who, by not matching these changes in time, assumed the presence of heart-lung interactions that may be invalid. Perel and coworkers[71] observed that systolic arterial pressure decreased in a cyclic fashion relative to apneic values during positive-pressure ventilation in dogs. This decrease was accentuated by hemorrhage and minimized by fluid resuscitation. Because these variations in systolic arterial pressure had the same frequency as did respiratory rate, these workers hypothesized that the decrease in systolic arterial pressure reflected decreases in LV end-diastolic volume caused by positive-pressure ventilation. In support of this hypothesis, Jardin et al.[72] demonstrated that this decrease in systolic arterial pressure correlated with echocardiographic estimates of mean LV end-diastolic area made a few minutes before the measurement of the pressure changes. Furthermore, Pizov and colleagues[73] demonstrated that increases in systolic arterial pressure occurred in dogs with heart failure after fluid resuscitation; this is consistent with the "reverse pulsus paradoxus" described earlier.[70] They hypothesized that this increase in systolic arterial pressure reflected increased LV stroke volume due to an increase in LV afterload that decreased ITP. However, the relation between the phase of the ventilatory cycle or dynamic changes in LV volumes and the observed changes in systolic arterial pressure was not made. It has become possible to assess LV area on-line with the use of echocardiographic techniques.[74] When such techniques are used to measure arterial pressure, airway pressure, and LV area during positive-pressure ventilation in humans, preliminary reports have shown that the changes in arterial pressure correspond to changes in airway pressure, not to those in LV volumes.[75] These data suggest that although the clinical observation of cardiovascular instability correlates with respiration-induced changes in systolic arterial pressure, the mechanism is not one of in-phase changes in preload or afterload. Thus, the changes in systolic arterial pressure cannot be used to infer changes in LV preload or afterload; however, they do reflect a more complex interaction between the heart and lungs. An example of this phenomenon in one subject is shown in Figure 102–8. Note that systolic arterial pressure increases and decreases in phase with airway pressure changes, whereas LV areas vary in a direction opposite to that hypothesized earlier. This example serves to underscore the importance of considering the timing of specific hemodynamic changes within the ventilatory cycle before making inferences as to the mechanism for such effects.

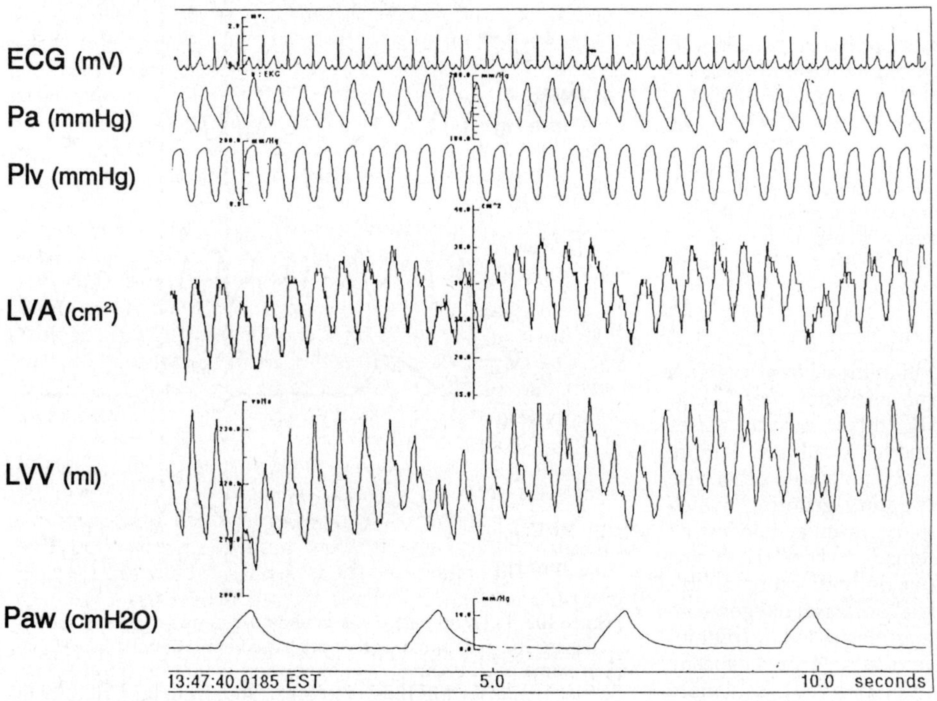

Figure 102–8. Effect of positive-pressure inspiration on arterial pressure (Pa), LV pressure (Plv), LV area (LVA), LV volume (LVV), and airway pressure (Paw) in a closed-chest patient prior to cardiac surgery. Note the phase relation and magnitude of the Pa and LVA signals compared with the Paw signal.

EFFECT OF CARDIOVASCULAR STATUS ON THE HEMODYNAMIC RESPONSE TO ARTIFICIAL VENTILATION

Cardiac output depends primarily on the level of cardiac performance, circulating blood volume, and peripheral vasomotor tone. Because ventilation and ventilatory maneuvers alter all of these cardiovascular variables by changing lung volume and ITP, the hemodynamic effect of any specific mode of ventilation is clearly the result of interactions among many factors. Given these complex, interrelated forces, the hemodynamic effect of ventilation under all conditions is impossible to define accurately.

Two warnings, however, may allow the physician to predict with some certainty the hemodynamic response that a specific mode of ventilation might induce. First, under normal conditions, venous return is the dominant force determining cardiac output.[45] Second, intrathoracic blood volume varies inversely with ITP,[24, 33] and measurements of intrathoracic blood volume estimate LV preload better than do values of pulmonary artery occlusion pressure (Ppao).[4, 76] Thus, ventilatory maneuvers that decrease ITP, such as spontaneous ventilation and spontaneous breathing during intermittent mandatory ventilation and continuous positive airway pressure, are associated with greater intrathoracic blood volume, ventricular preload, and, therefore, cardiac output than is the case during ventilatory conditions that increase ITP, such as IPPB and PEEP.

The previous approach to predicting the hemodynamic effects of artificial ventilation is unfortunately simplistic. ITP is also a component of the ejection pressure for LV emptying (afterload), such that decreases in ITP increase LV afterload, whereas increases in ITP decrease the LV afterload.[20] If the increase in afterload exceeds the ability of the LV to empty, then LV failure worsens. This further increases intrathoracic blood volume, thus potentially causing or worsening pulmonary edema.[64] These points have been discussed earlier but not in the context of specific cardiovascular conditions. Because most physicians approach patient care—and, specifically, cardiovascular response—from the standpoint of baseline physiologic status, the hemodynamic effects of artificial ventilation in regard to particular cardiovascular states are worth re-examining. Normal cardiovascular status is addressed first, and reduced ventricular performance, altered vasomotor tone, and low blood volume are then considered. In each condition, the impact of conditions in which the lungs are either normal, stiff, or overly compliant (with and without increases in bronchomotor tone) are discussed.

Normally, venous return is sensitive to changes in the driving pressure for venous blood flow (mean systemic pressure minus Pra).[18, 43] Any process that increases Pra decreases cardiac output. Ventilation-associated increases in Pra can occur during both spontaneous and positive-pressure ventilation by one of two mechanisms: (1) ITP can increase during positive-pressure breathing, thus increasing Pra directly; or (2) PVR can increase with lung overdistention, thus impeding RV ejection and increasing Pra secondarily. During spontaneous breathing, air trapping due to inadequate expiratory time (auto-PEEP or occult PEEP)[77] or premature airway closure (chronic obstructive airway disease) also increases lung volume.[78] Similarly, externally applied PEEP increases lung volume. As the lungs increase in volume, they expand against the rib cage, diaphragm, and mediastinum, increasing ITP. As the right atrium and intrathoracic vena cavae are compliant and easily affected by ITP, Pra also increases. Thus, in patients with normal cardiovascular status, mean ITP should be kept at the lowest level that ensures adequate ventilation to minimize the deleterious effect of increasing ITP on venous return. Increases in lung volume above FRC (hyperinflation) increase PVR.[12] If spontaneous or positive-pressure ventilation results in hyperinflation, as may occur in patients with obstructive lung disease, PVR increases; this in turn impedes RV ejection. This impediment must eventually increase RV filling pressure, as the RV, unable to empty, dilates. As the RV dilates, Pra increases as well, thus decreasing venous return.[19] Thus, a primary cardiovascular goal of ventilatory therapy for all patients should be to maintain resting lung volume at or near FRC, although this goal may seem at cross-purposes with the use of PEEP in the ventilator-dependent patient. When used properly, PEEP usually returns abnormally low lung volumes back to FRC,[3] which decreases PVR.[41] In fact, many respiratory therapies used to improve oxygenation, such as suctioning and periodic hyperinflation, are performed to reopen collapsed air spaces and to allow resting lung volume to increase to FRC.

In conditions involving heart failure, ventricular pump function is impaired. Normal compensatory physiologic processes and routine therapeutic interventions usually produce adequate cardiac output but also result in a greatly expanded blood volume. Although intrathoracic blood volume and LV filling pressures are increased in conditions involving heart failure, most of the increased blood volume resides in the peripheral vasculature owing to its vastly greater capacitance.[79] Under these conditions, spontaneous ventilatory efforts may worsen gas exchange and cardiac output by further increasing both intrathoracic blood volume and LV afterload, promoting pulmonary edema. If cardiac output is fixed, then the increased oxygen consumption by the respiratory muscles may significantly limit oxygen availability for other tissues; this results in venous desaturation, increased anaerobic metabolism,[67] and, in the setting of intrapulmonary shunts, arterial desaturation. The management of congestive heart failure usually includes administration of diuretics to reduce systemic and pulmonary venous pressures and that of vasodilators to reduce LV afterload. Thus, by increasing ITP, positive-pressure ventilation reduces intrathoracic blood volume and decreases LV afterload, resulting in a similar therapeutic effect. Accordingly, positive-pressure ventilation should not impair cardiovascular function. In patients with congestive heart failure, positive-pressure ventilation usually does not decrease cardiac output,[34] whereas in severely impaired patients it may actually augment blood flow.[21, 22] If patients with heart failure also have decreased lung compliance, the hemodynamic benefits of positive-pressure ventilation are greater as will be the hemodynamic stress of weaning from mechanical ventilation.[57]

Critically ill patients may have impaired venous return before ventilatory support is initiated. Intravascular volume depletion (hemorrhage, dehydration, and third-space volume loss) and loss of vasomotor tone (vasomotor shock, anaphylaxis, and septic shock) often occur. These patients are sensitive to increases in Pra, as the driving pressure of venous blood flow is already reduced[18, 69] and sympathetic tone is already near maximum and cannot increase mean systemic pressure further. Although the function of the cardiac pump often decreases in these conditions, the hemodynamic effects are usually exceeded by the preload dependence of the heart (Frank-Starling mechanism). Because intravascular volume is often inadequate when positive-pressure ventilation is begun, care must be taken to apply the minimum positive airway pressure necessary to provide adequate ventilation as well as to give intravascular fluid resuscitation promptly if cardiovascular status deteriorates upon initiation of mechanical ventilation. Likewise, when intravascular volume loss is ongoing, increases in ITP that may once have been acceptable may now induce hypotension and inadequate cardiac output owing to decreasing venous return. To the extent that positive-pressure ventilation can be avoided through the use of intermittent mandatory ventilation, pressure support, or continuous positive airway pressure or by adjustments in the fraction of inspired oxygen, a patient's cardiovascular status will benefit. However, care should be taken when leaving the nonsupported patient with respiratory distress to breathe spontaneously. In an animal model of low cardiac output, failure of the primary respiratory bellows occurred and caused subsequent cardiac arrest.[80] Similarly, respiratory arrest in humans may precede cardiac arrest, especially in patients with lung disease. Thus, all hemodynamically unstable patients who are breathing spontaneously must undergo adequate respiratory monitoring to detect potential respiratory arrest. Furthermore, it may be preferable clinically to intubate and ventilate hemodynamically unstable patients who have an increased cost of the work of breathing to stabilize their cardiovascular states quickly.

HEMODYNAMIC EFFECT OF SPECIFIC MODES OF ARTIFICIAL VENTILATION

Modes of artificial ventilation can be classified as those that generate a tidal breath through the application of positive pressure to the airway (IPPB, high-frequency jet ventilation [HFJV]) and those that increase end-expiratory lung volume through the maintenance of positive pressure at end-expiration, during either IPPB (PEEP) or spontaneous breathing (continuous positive airway pressure). This classification can be refined further by the inclusion of positive-pressure breathing interspersed with spontaneous breathing (intermittent mandatory ventilation) and minimum supplemental positive airway pressure to ensure an adequate spontaneous tidal volume (pressure support) (Table 102–2).

TABLE 102–2. Artificial Ventilation Modes

Intermittent positive-pressure breathing
IPPB
HFJV
Partial ventilatory support
Intermittent mandatory ventilation
Pressure support
Positive end-expiratory pressure
PEEP
Continuous positive airway pressure
Apneic ventilation
Constant tracheal insufflation

Positive-Pressure Breathing

Positive-pressure breathing (IPPB and HFJV) proportionally increases ITP and lung volume.[24] The hemodynamics are similar for IPPB and HFJV for the same mean airway pressure or ITP.[24, 81] Under certain conditions, however, HFJV may result in a higher ITP than would be predicted from the mean airway pressure because the short expiratory time of the HFJV breath precludes complete exhalation of one delivered breath before the next is delivered (occult PEEP).[77, 78] With any form of positive-pressure breathing, adequate expiratory time is necessary to minimize the possibility of inadvertent hyperinflation.[77] Hyperinflation occurs most commonly in patients with airflow obstruction[78] and when large tidal volumes and rapid ventilatory frequencies[77] are both used. Because hyperinflation also increases PVR, acute cor pulmonale and cardiovascular collapse may occur in patients who already have compromised RV function.

The pressure gradient for venous return decreases in proportion to the increase in ITP owing to an increase in Pra independent of the level of ventricular pump function. As venous blood flow decreases, intrathoracic blood volume decreases as well. This decrease in intrathoracic blood volume can be reversed by increasing venous pressure (through volume infusion or by increasing vasomotor tone)[33] or by minimizing the increase in Pra (small tidal volume, minimum inspiratory time).[4] The increase in ITP may also decrease LV afterload.[20, 64] Of greater clinical importance, however, is the ability of IPPB to abolish the negative fluctuations in ITP associated with spontaneous ventilation and, thus, remove the preexisting increased LV afterload that the negative swings in ITP created. Numerous case reports of patients with normal cardiac function have documented the beneficial effects of IPPB in reversing pulmonary edema induced by profound negative swings in ITP, such as may occur during forceful spontaneous inspiration against an occluded airway (laryngospasm),[54] when increased airway resistance is present (asthma),[55] or when pulmonary compliance is decreased (pulmonary fibrosis, pulmonary edema).[56] Thus, under most conditions, IPPB reduces cardiac output by reducing LV preload through the mechanism of a reduced pressure gradient for venous return. This reduction in venous return is minimized in those patients with already increased intravascular volume who can tolerate the decrease in LV filling pressure without a decrease in output, and in patients whose respiratory pathology results in a predominant hemodynamic increase in LV afterload during spontaneous breathing.

Positive End-Expiratory Pressure

PEEP is used routinely in the treatment of acute hypoxemic respiratory failure. Although the mechanism by which PEEP improves arterial oxygenation is still a subject of controversy,[82] most investigators[83] have demonstrated that improvement does not occur unless PEEP increases lung volume. Thus, it presumably functions by opening collapsed or partially collapsed airspaces. The effect of PEEP on cardiovascular function is slightly more complex than that of IPPB if only because of the greater increase in lung volume and ITP that it creates. The increase in lung volume has three primary effects. As with IPPB, when lung volume increases, ITP increases as well; this decreases the pressure gradient for venous return. Similarly, PVR may also increase; this impedes RV ejection. Finally, by increasing lung volume, PEEP may squeeze the heart within the cardiac fossa,[13–15] thus mechanically limiting diastolic filling. This process is similar to the lung-induced limitation of diastolic filling seen in patients with chronic airway obstruction who have hyperinflation during exercise.[84] To the extent that PEEP returns lung volume to the original FRC, neither ITP nor PVR increase above normal levels,[2] and no significant hemodynamic effects occur.

By increasing lung volume, PEEP depresses the diaphragm, and this increases intra-abdominal pressure. This increase in intra-abdominal pressure is minimized when the abdomen is open (e.g., during laparotomy) and is accentuated when intra-abdominal pressure is already increased (e.g., in the presence of tense ascites or abdominal binding). Because intra-abdominal pressure surrounds the intra-abdominal vasculature (where a large proportion of the ve-

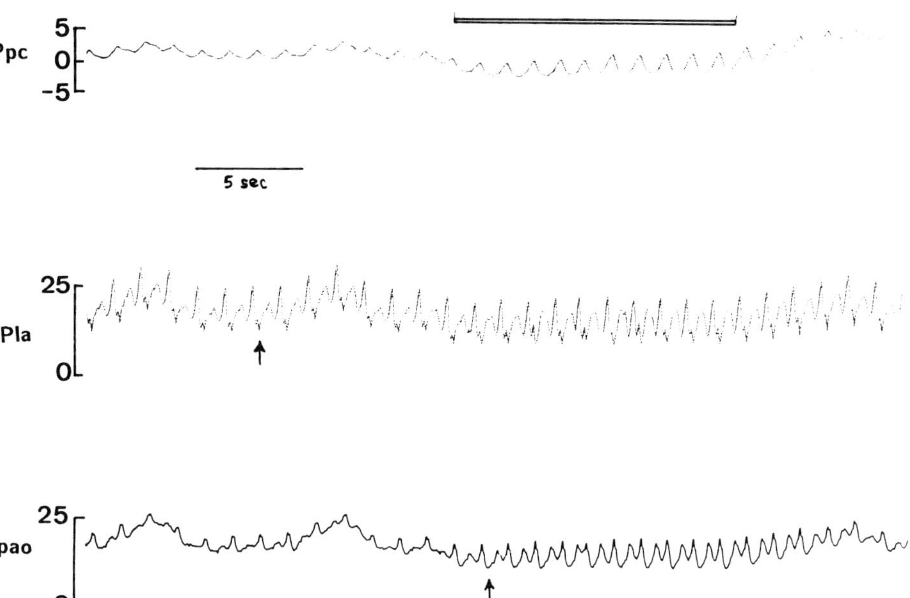

Figure 102–9. Strip chart recording of pericardial pressure (Ppc), pulmonary artery occlusion pressure (Ppao), and left atrial pressure (Pla) during both 15 cm H_2O PEEP *(left side)* and immediately after airway disconnection (off-PEEP, indicated by *bar* above strip chart). Measurements of on-PEEP Pla and Ppao are timed at the first *arrow* (showing Pla), whereas the nadir Ppao is timed at the second *arrow*. (From Pinsky MR, Vincent JL, DeSmet JM: Estimating left ventricular filling pressure during positive end-expiratory pressure in humans. Am Rev Respir Dis 1991; 143:25–31.)

nous blood volume resides), the increase in intra-abdominal pressure mechanically increases mean systemic pressure. Operationally, this would be represented by a shift in the venous return curve to the right. However, maximum venous return would still be depressed because of the obligatory increase in Pra. Thus, PEEP may not decrease cardiac output as much as originally predicted because mean systemic pressure is also increased, and this minimizes the decrease in the pressure gradient for venous return.

Considerable controversy exists regarding the hemodynamic effects of PEEP.[84–86] The issues raised include whether PEEP depresses contractility,[8] induces increased ventricular interdependence,[49] or augments cardiac output.[21, 22, 57, 64] The notion that PEEP depresses LV performance stemmed from technical inaccuracies involved in the measurement of LV filling pressure and end-diastolic volume. LV filling pressure is intracavitary pressure relative to surrounding pressure. Although intracavitary pressure can usually be measured (LV end-diastolic pressure), surrounding pressure (pericardial pressure) cannot. Pericardial pressure can increase with the application of PEEP either because absolute biventricular end-diastolic volume exceeds pericardial unstressed volume[14] and the pericardium becomes a limiting membrane, or because the expanding lungs compress the pericardium and heart, limiting absolute biventricular volume to less than pericardial unstressed volume.[13, 15] In either case, measuring LV filling pressure as LV end-diastolic pressure or determining its bedside estimate (Ppao) overestimates true LV filling pressure.[87] This overestimation of LV end-diastolic pressure can be minimized if the Ppao is meas-

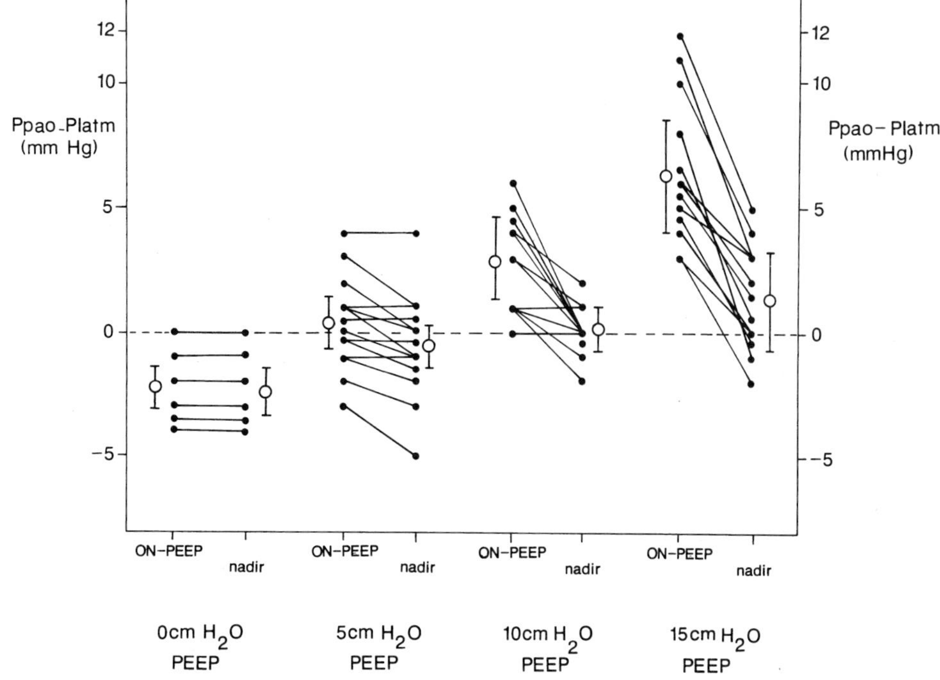

Figure 102–10. Difference between on-PEEP pulmonary artery occlusion pressure (Ppao) and nadir Ppao after airway disconnection (nadir Ppao) and transmural left atrial pressure (Platm) for all patients. Separate panels for 0, 5, 10, and 15 cm H_2O PEEP are presented. *Open circles* and *bars* represent means ±SD. The difference between on-PEEP Ppao and nadir Ppao increased with increasing levels of PEEP. On-PEEP Ppao overestimated on-PEEP Platm at ≥10 cm H_2O PEEP, whereas nadir Ppao was not affected. (From Pinsky MR, Vincent SL, DeSmet JM: Estimating left ventricular filling pressure during positive end-expiratory pressure in humans. Am Rev Respir Dis 1991; 143:25–31.)

ured at its nadir immediately after airway disconnection. As shown in Figure 102–9, this event occurs within 1 to 2 seconds after airway disconnection (arrow) and need not impair gas exchange. Using this technique, Pinsky and colleagues[88] demonstrated that nadir Ppao reflected LV filling pressure with PEEP faithfully up to the PEEP limit of 15 cm H_2O; Ppao consistently overestimated LV filling pressure (Fig. 102–10). Numerous studies have demonstrated that when either LV end-diastolic volume[49] or transmural LV filling pressure[53, 58] is kept constant, LV performance is unimpaired by PEEP. Similarly, LV performance may actually improve[20, 22, 23] owing to the decrease in LV afterload. As a first approximation, some have suggested that about one third of the increase in airway pressure is transmitted to the pleural space. Thus, subtracting one third of the airway pressure (in mm Hg) from Ppao should give an accurate estimate of transmural Ppao. Unfortunately, lung compliance varies widely from patient to patient and within individual patients over time. Pinsky and colleagues[88] demonstrated that the simplification routine was often inaccurate, and they recommended that it not be used.

References

1. Grenvik A: Respiratory, circulatory and metabolic effects of respiratory treatment. Acta Anaesthesiol Scand Suppl 1966; 19:1.
2. Vuori A, Jalonen J, Laaksonen V: Continuous positive airway pressure during mechanical and spontaneous ventilation. Effects on central hemodynamic and oxygen transport. Acta Anaesthesiol Scand 1979; 23:453.
3. Pontoppidan H, Green B, Lowenstein E: Acute respiratory failure in the adult. N Engl J Med 1972; 87:690.
4. Cournaud A, Motley HL, Werko L, et al: Physiological studies of the effect of intermittent positive pressure breathing on cardiac output in man. Am J Physiol 1948; 152:162.
5. Conway CM: Haemodynamic effects of pulmonary ventilation. Br J Anaesth 1975; 47:761.
6. Vatner SF, Rutherford JD: Control of the myocardial contractile state by carotid chemo- and baroreceptors and pulmonary inflation reflexes in conscious dogs. J Clin Invest 1978; 63:1539.
7. Glick C, Wechsler AS, Epstein SE: Reflex cardiovascular depression produced by stimulation of pulmonary stretch receptors in the dog. J Clin Invest 1969; 48:467.
8. Patten MT, Liebman PR, Hectmann HB: Humorally mediated decreases in cardiac output associated with positive end-expiratory pressure. Microvasc Res 1977; 13:137.
9. Berend N, Christopher KL, Voelkel NF: Effect of positive end-expiratory pressure on functional residual capacity: Role of prostaglandin production. Am Rev Respir Dis 1982; 126:641.
10. Bernardi L, Keller F, Saunders M, et al: Respiratory sinus arrhythmia in the denervated human heart. J Appl Physiol 1989; 67:1447.
11. Bower R, Wise RA, Hassapoyannes C, et al: Effect of lung inflation on lung blood volume and pulmonary venous flow. J Appl Physiol 1961; 58:754.
12. Permutt S, Howell JBL, Proctor DF, et al: Effect of lung inflation on static pressure-volume characteristics of pulmonary vessels. J Appl Physiol 1961; 16:64.
13. Lloyd TC Jr: Mechanical cardiopulmonary interdependence. J Appl Physiol 1982; 52:333.
14. Wallis TW, Robotham JL, Compean R, et al: Mechanical heart-lung interaction with positive end-expiratory pressure. J Appl Physiol 1983; 54:1039.
15. Butler J: The heart is in good hands. Circulation 1983; 67:1163.
16. Hakim TS, Michel MP, Minami H, et al: Site of pulmonary hypoxic pulmonary vasoconstriction studied with arterial and venous occlusion. J Appl Physiol 1983; 54:1298.
17. Brecher GA, Hubay CA: Pulmonary blood flow and venous return during spontaneous respiration. Circ Res 1955; 3:210.
18. Guyton AC, Lindsey AW, Abernathy B, et al: Venous return at various right atrial pressure and the normal venous return curve. Am J Physiol 1957; 189:690.
19. Morgan BC, Abel FL, Mullins GL, et al: Flow patterns in cavae, pulmonary artery, pulmonary vein, and aorta in intact dogs. Am J Physiol 1966; 210:903.
20. Buda AJ, Pinsky MR, Ingels NB, et al: Effect of intrathoracic pressure on left ventricular performance. N Engl J Med 1979; 301:453.
21. Calvin JE, Driedger AA, Sibbald WJ: Positive ventricular function in patients with pulmonary edema. Am Rev Respir Dis 1981; 124:121.
22. Mathru M, Rao TLK, El-Etr AA, et al: Hemodynamic response to changes in ventilatory patterns in patients with normal and poor left ventricular reserve. Crit Care Med 1982; 10:423.
23. Pinsky MR, Matuschak GM, Itzkoff JM: Respiratory augmentation of left ventricular function during spontaneous ventilation in severe left ventricular failure by grunting: An auto-PEEP effect. Chest 1983; 84:370.
24. Pinsky MR, Matuschak GM, Klain M: Determinants of cardiac augmentation by elevations in intrathoracic pressure. J Appl Physiol 1985; 58:1189.
25. Sibbald WJ, Driedger AA, Myers ML, et al: Biventricular function in the adult respiratory distress syndrome: Hemodynamic and radionuclide assessment with special emphasis on right ventricular function. Chest 1983; 84:126.
26. Taylor RR, Corell JW, Sonnenblick EH, et al: Dependence of ventricular distensibility on filling of the opposite ventricle. Am J Physiol 1967; 213:711.
27. Milic-Emili J, Mean J, Turner JM, et al: Improved technique for estimating pleural pressure from esophageal balloons. J Appl Physiol 1964; 19:207.
28. Agostoni E: Mechanics of the pleural space. Physiol Rev 1972; 52:57.
29. Dhainaut JF, Devaux JY, Monsallier JF, et al: Mechanisms of decreased left ventricular preload during continuous positive-pressure ventilation in ARDS. Chest 1986; 90:74.
30. Pinsky MR, Vincent JL, DeSmet JM: Effect of positive end-expiratory pressure on right ventricular function in man. Am Rev Respir Dis 1992; 146:681.
31. Pinsky MR: Determinants of pulmonary artery flow variation during respiration. J Appl Physiol 1984; 56:1237.
32. Pinsky MR, Matuschak GM: Cardiovascular determinants of the hemodynamic response to acute endotoxemia in the dog. J Crit Care 1986; 1:18.
33. Braunwald E, Binion JT, Morgan WL, et al: Alterations in central blood volume and cardiac output induced by positive breathing and counteracted by metaraminol (Aramine). Circ Res 1987; 5:670.
34. Ellman H, Denbin H: Lack of a diverse hemodynamic effect of PEEP in patients with acute respiratory failure. Crit Care Med 1982; 10:711.
35. Takata M, Robotham JL: Effects of inspiratory diaphragmatic descent on inferior vena caval venous return. J Appl Physiol 1992; 72:597.
36. Mathay RA, Berger HJ: Non-invasive assessment of right and left ventricular function in acute and chronic respiratory failure. Crit Care Med 1983; 11:329.
37. Tobin MH, Dhadha TS, Jenouri G, et al: Breathing patterns: I. Normal subjects. Chest 1983; 84:202.
38. Shuler RH, Ensor C, Gunning RE, et al: The differential effects of respiration on the left and right ventricles. Am J Physiol 1942; 137:620.
39. Piene H, Sund T: Does normal pulmonary impedence constitute the optimal load for the right ventricle? Am J Physiol 1982; 242:H154.
40. Ahmed T, Oliver W Jr: Does slow-reacting substance of anaphylaxis mediate hypoxic pulmonary vasoconstriction? Am Rev Respir Dis 1983; 127:566.
41. Canada E, Benumof JL, Tousdale FR: Pulmonary vascular resistance correlated in intact normal and abnormal canine lungs. Crit Care Med 1982; 10:719.
42. Reuse C, Vincent JL, Pinsky MR: Measurements of right ventricular volumes during fluid challenge. Chest 1990; 98:1450–1454.

42a. Imai T, Uchiyama N, Marayama N, et al: Influence of constant sustained positive airway pressure on right ventricular performance. Intensive Care Med 1993; 19:8.

43. Pinsky MR: Instantaneous venous return curves in an intact canine preparation. J Appl Physiol 1984; 56:756.

44. Sarnoff SJ: Myocardial contractility as described by the ventricular function curves: Observations on Starling's law of the heart. Physiol Rev 1955; 35:756.
45. Patterson SW, Piper H, Starling EH: The regulation of the heart beat. J Physiol 1914; 48:465.
46. Brinker JA, Weiss I, Lappe DL, et al: Leftward septal displacement during right ventricular loading in man. Circulation 1980; 61:626.
47. Janiki JS, Weber KT: The pericardium and ventricular interaction distensibility and function. Am J Physiol 1980; 238:H494.
48. Jardin F, Fercot J-C, Gueret P, et al: Echocardiographic evaluation of ventricles during continuous positive airway pressure breathing. J Appl Physiol 1984; 56:619.
49. Rankin JS, Olsen CO, Arentzen CE, et al: The effects of airway pressure on cardiac function in intact dogs and man. Circulation 1982; 66:108.
50. Robotham JL, Bell RC, Badke FR, et al: Left ventricular geometry during positive end-expiratory pressure. Crit Care Med 1985; 13:617.
51. Brookhart JM, Boyd TE: Local differences in intrathoracic pressure and their relationship to cardiac filling pressure in the dog. Am J Physiol 1947; 148:434.
52. Marini JJ, Culver BN, Butler J: Mechanical effect of lung distension with positive pressure in cardiac function. Am Rev Respir Dis 1981; 124:382.
53. Prewitt RM, Wood LDH: Effects of positive end-expiratory pressure on ventricular function in dogs. Am J Physiol 1979; 236:H534.
54. Lee KWT, Downes JJ: Pulmonary edema secondary to laryngospasm in children. Anesthesiology 1983; 59:347.
55. Stalcup SA, Mellins RB: Mechanical forces producing pulmonary edema in acute asthma. N Engl J Med 1977; 297:592.
56. Milic-Emili J, Rubb F: Effects of pulmonary congestion and edema on the small airways. Bull Physiol Pathol Respir 1977; 7:1181.
57. Räsänen J: Ventilatory support in respiratory failure following acute myocardial infarction. Intensive Crit Care Digest 1985; 4:29.
58. Qvist J, Pontoppidan H, Wilson RS, et al: Hemodynamic response to mechanical ventilation with PEEP: The effect of hypervolemia. Anesthesiology 1975; 42:45.
59. Pinsky MR, Summer WR: Cardiac augmentation by phasic high intrathoracic pressure support. Chest 1983; 84:370.
60. Suga H, Sagawa K: Instantaneous pressure-volume relationships and their ratio in the excised supported canine left ventricle. Circ Res 1974; 35:117.
61. Scharf SM, Brown R, Saunders N, et al: Hemodynamic effects of positive-pressure inflation. J Appl Physiol 1980; 49:124.
62. Maloney JE, Bergel DH, Blazier JB, et al: Transmission of pulsatile blood pressure and flow through the isolated lung. Circ Res 1968; 23:11.
63. Suga H, Sagawa K: Instantaneous pressure-volume relationships and their ratio in the excised, supported canine left ventricle. Circ Res 1974; 35:117.
64. Rasanen J, Nikki P, Heikkila J: Acute myocardial infarction complicated by respiratory failure, the effect of mechanical ventilation. Chest 1984; 85:21.
65. Harrison VC, DeV Heese H, Klein M: The significance of grunting in hyaline membrane disease. Pediatrics 1968; 41:549.
66. Roussos C, Macklem PT: The respiratory muscles. N Engl J Med 1982; 126:648.
67. Aubier M, Viires N, Syllie G, et al: Respiratory muscle contribution to lactic acidosis in low cardiac output. Am Rev Respir Dis 1982; 126:648.
68. Viires N, Sillye G, Aubier M, et al: Regional blood flow distribution in dog during induced hypotension and low cardiac output. Spontaneous breathing versus artificial ventilation. J Clin Invest 1983; 72:935.
69. Matuschak GM, Pinsky MR, Klain M: Hemodynamic effects of synchronous high-frequency jet ventilation during acute hypovolemia. J Appl Physiol 1986; 61:44.
70. Massumi RA, Mason DT, Vera Z, et al: Reversed pulsus paradoxus. N Engl J Med 1973; 289:1272.
71. Perel A, Pizov R, Cotev S: Systolic blood pressure variation is a sensitive indicator of hypovolemia in ventilated dogs subjected to graded hemorrhage. Anesthesiology 1987; 67:498.
72. Jardin F, Farcot JC, Gueret P, et al: Echocardiographic evaluation of ventricles during continuous positive airway pressure. J Appl Physiol 1984; 56:619.
73. Pizov R, Ya'ari Y, Perel A: The arterial pressure wave form during acute ventricular failure and synchronized external chest compression. Anesth Analg 1989; 68:150.
74. Gorcsan J 3rd, Gasior TA, Mandarino WA, et al: On-line estimation of changes in left ventricular stroke volume by transesophageal echocardiographic automated border detection in patients undergoing coronary artery bypass grafting. Am J Cardiol 1993; 72:721.
75. Denault AY, Ondulick B, Pinsky MR: Effect of positive-pressure ventilation in left ventricular pressure-volume relationships (Abstract). Am Rev Respir Dis 1993; 147:A610.
76. Pinsky MR, Matuschak GM, Klain M: Determinants of cardiac augmentation by increases in intrathoracic pressure. J Appl Physiol 1985; 58:1189.
77. Bergman NA: Intrapulmonary gas trapping during mechanical ventilation at rapid frequencies. Anesthesiology 1972; 37:626.
78. Pepe JE, Marini JJ: Occult positive end-expiratory pressure in mechanically ventilated patients with airflow obstruction: The auto-PEEP effect. Am Rev Respir Dis 1982; 126:166.
79. Rothe C: Physiology of venous return, an unappreciated boost to the heart. Arch Intern Med 1986; 146:977.
80. Aubier M, Trippenbach T, Roussos CL: Respiratory muscles fatigue during cardiogenic shock. J Appl Physiol 1981; 51:499.
81. Shinozaki T, Deane RS, Perkins FM, et al: Comparison of high-frequency jet ventilation with conventional mechanical ventilation. J Thorac Cardiovasc Surg 1985; 89:269.
82. Ralph DD, Robertson HT, Weaver LJ, et al: Distribution of ventilation and perfusion during positive end-expiratory pressure in the adult respiratory distress syndrome. Am Rev Respir Dis 1985; 131:54.
83. Richardson P, Carlstrom JR: Effects of end-expiratory lung volume on lung mechanics in normal and edematous lungs. Respiration 1985; 47:90.
84. Albert RK, Muramoto A, Caldwell J, et al: Increases in intrathoracic pressure that occur during exercise in patients with chronic obstructive pulmonary disease. Am Rev Respir Dis 1985; 132:623.
85. Dorinsky PM, Whitcomb ME: The effect of PEEP on cardiac output. Chest 1983; 84:210.
86. Wood LDH, Prewitt RM: Cardiovascular management in acute hypoxemic respiratory failure. Am J Cardiol 1981; 47:963.
87. Carter RS, Snyder JV, Pinsky MR: LV filling pressure during PEEP measured by nadir wedge pressure after airway disconnection. Am J Physiol 1985; 249:H770.
88. Pinsky MR, Vincent JL, DeSmet JM: Estimating left ventricular filling pressure during positive end-expiratory pressure in humans. Am Rev Respir Dis 1991; 143:25.

CHAPTER 103

Weaning from Mechanical Ventilation

Edward R. Garrity, Jr., MD • Martin J. Tobin, MD

Mechanical ventilation has been identified with the development of critical care units more than any other technologic advance. Although it is frequently lifesaving, mechanical ventilation poses a risk of serious complications[1, 1a] while markedly increasing the cost of care for ventilator-dependent patients.[2] Consequently, every effort should be made to discontinue mechanical ventilation as soon as a patient can sustain spontaneous ventilation. In the majority of patients, ventilator support can be discontinued without any difficulty. However, as many as 20% of patients experience difficulty during the time of ventilator discontinuation,[3,4] and this group of patients requires a gradual approach to the transition between mechanical ventilation and spontaneous breathing—the process referred to as *weaning*.

DETERMINANTS OF WEANING OUTCOME

The pathophysiologic determinants of weaning outcome are adequacy of pulmonary gas exchange, performance of the respiratory muscle pump, and psychologic factors. Although cardiac dysfunction can certainly affect gas exchange and the respiratory muscle pump, it is not addressed in this chapter, but rather in Chapter 102.

Adequacy of Pulmonary Gas Exchange

Attempts to restore spontaneous respiration after a period of mechanical ventilation may result in hypoxemia as a consequence of impaired pulmonary gas exchange, hypoventilation, or decreased oxygen (O_2) content of venous blood. A detailed investigation of gas exchange abnormalities at the time of weaning from mechanical ventilation was undertaken by Torres and colleagues[5] using the multiple inert gas technique. Discontinuation of ventilator support and resumption of spontaneous breathing was associated with a decrease in tidal volume (VT), an increase in frequency, and no change in minute ventilation. Significant changes included an increase in arterial carbon dioxide tension ($Paco_2$), a decrease in pH, and increases in mixed venous oxygen tension ($P\bar{v}o_2$) and cardiac output. Despite the abnormalities in alveolar ventilation-perfusion ratio, a fall in Pao_2 was prevented by the associated increase in cardiac output. Unfortunately, comparable detailed investigations of gas exchange in patients failing a weaning trial have not been conducted.

Respiratory Muscle Performance

Failure of the respiratory muscle pump is probably the most common cause of failure to wean from mechanical ventilation. This may result from decreased neuromuscular capacity, increased respiratory muscle pump load, or a combination of both factors (Table 103–1).

TABLE 103–1. Causes of Respiratory Muscle Pump Failure

Decreased Neuromuscular Capacity
Decreased respiratory center output
Phrenic nerve dysfunction
Neuromuscular disorders
Decreased respiratory muscle strength or endurance
Hyperinflation
Malnutrition
Decreased oxygen supply
Respiratory acidosis
Mineral and electrolyte abnormalities
Endocrinopathy
Disuse muscle atrophy
Respiratory muscle fatigue
Increased Respiratory Muscle Pump Load
Increased ventilatory requirements
Increased CO_2 production
Increased dead space ventilation
Inappropriately increased respiratory drive
Increased work of breathing

Decreased Neuromuscular Capacity

Respiratory Center Output

Patients who fail a weaning trial commonly develop respiratory acidosis, raising the possibility that respiratory center drive may be decreased. However, indexes of drive, such as airway occlusion pressure at 0.1 second ($P_{0.1}$) or mean inspiratory flow (VT/TI), are usually above the normal range in such patients.[6–9] Furthermore, an increase in VT/TI has been observed in patients who developed severe alveolar hypoventilation during an unsuccessful weaning trial (Fig. 103–1).[6]

Phrenic Nerve Function

Phrenic nerve dysfunction should be suspected in patients who have undergone coronary artery bypass surgery if weaning proves difficult in the postoperative period. Estenne and colleagues[10] and others have found hemidiaphragmatic paralysis in 10% of these patients, especially after internal mammary grafting.[11] Most injuries are due to hypothermia from the topical cooling and are more common when a pericardial insulating pad is not used during surgery. Unilateral diaphragmatic paralysis is rarely life threatening but may make weaning difficult in the first several days after surgery. A small number of patients develop bilateral diaphragmatic paralysis resulting in prolonged ventilator dependency.

Respiratory Muscle Function

Respiratory muscle function may be impaired by various conditions commonly observed in critically ill patients (see Table 103–1).[12] These conditions are discussed in detail throughout this book, and the following review focuses on their role during the weaning process.

Of the clinical conditions that cause a decrease in respiratory muscle strength or endurance, *hyperinflation* is one of the most important.[6] Dynamic hyperinflation often results from altered patterns of breathing during weaning.[6] Adverse effects are numerous[12] and are illustrated in Figure 103–2.

Malnutrition is particularly common in critically ill patients[13] because a large percentage of ventilated patients receive inadequate nutrition. Malnutrition has a number of adverse effects on respiratory function related to weaning, including decreased ventilatory response to hypoxia,[14] a decrease in muscle mass and thickness,[15] and a reduction in respiratory muscle strength and endurance.[16] In addition, altered host defenses predispose to nosocomial pneumonia, which can increase the load on the respiratory system.[13]

The *O_2 supply* to a muscle is decreased if cardiac output falls, the O_2 content of arterial blood decreases (hypoxemia, anemia),[17] or O_2 extraction is impaired (sepsis).[18] A helpful study illustrates hemodynamic compromise during weaning: Substantial hemodynamic changes occurred during failed weaning trials in 15 patients with chronic obstructive pulmonary disease and cardiovascular disease.[19] After 10 minutes of spontaneous breathing, the patients showed an increase in transmural pulmonary artery wedge pressure, cardiac index, and left and right ventricular end-diastolic volume indexes, with subsequently successful weaning in nine patients after diuresis.

Several other issues may affect muscle function as well. Information about hypoxic harm to respiratory muscle function is accumulating,[17] but controversy still exists. Acute respiratory acidosis may decrease contractility and endurance time of the diaphragm in healthy subjects.[20] Several *metabolic abnormalities* including abnormalities of phosphate,[21] potassium, calcium,[22] or magnesium[23] may adversely affect respiratory muscle function. *Endocrine disturbances* such as hyperthyroidism or hypothyroidism may also

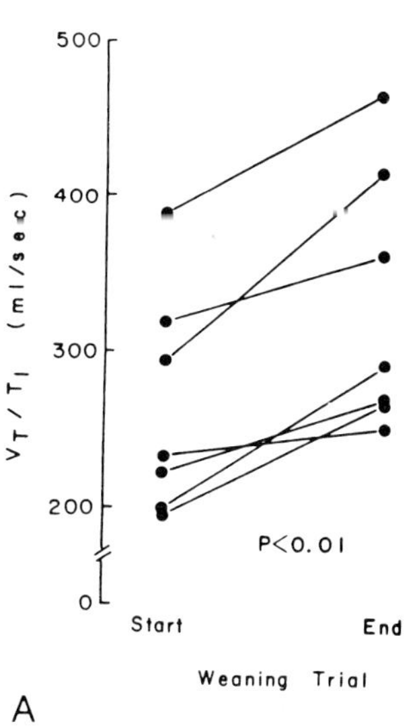

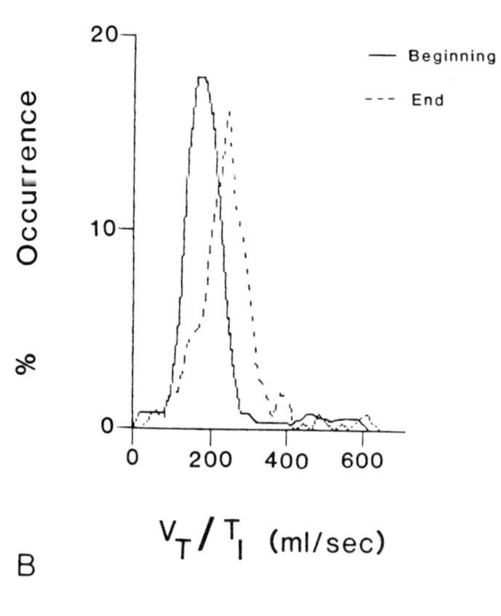

Figure 103–1. *A*, Measurements of VT/TI in seven patients who failed a trial of weaning from mechanical ventilation. *B*, The increase in the frequency histogram distribution of VT/TI from the beginning to the end of the weaning trial in a single, representative patient with an unsuccessful weaning outcome ($P < .002$, Mann-Whitney U tests of medians and variability). An increase in VT/TI of this magnitude was individually observed in all but one of the patients in the failure group. (From Tobin MJ, Perez W, Guenther SM, et al: The pattern of breathing during successful and unsuccessful trials of weaning from mechanical ventilation. Am Rev Respir Dis 1986; 134:1111.)

impair respiratory muscle function. Probably more relevant to the weaning situation is the use of corticosteroid therapy, potentially leading to steroid myopathy.[24]

Respiratory muscle atrophy and decreased performance due to prolonged mechanical ventilation have been demonstrated in baboons,[25] but animal data may not translate well to the human condition. The respiratory muscles are not completely immobilized with mechanical ventilation, and as little as one diaphragmatic contraction daily may be enough to prevent atrophy.[26]

The question of whether *respiratory muscle fatigue* occurs during the weaning process is of major importance. On one hand, patients failing a weaning trial often display marked abnormalities in respiratory mechanics, inefficient respiratory muscle function, and marked increase in the O_2 cost of breathing, all of which predispose to respiratory muscle fatigue. On the other hand, rest via mechanical ventilation is the major therapy for fatigue, but prolonged rest may produce atrophy (discussed earlier). Consequently, the optimal timing and pace of weaning are particularly problematic in these patients, but very few data have been obtained in patients with respiratory failure. In one influential study, Cohen and colleagues[27] suggested that respiratory muscle fatigue may be a major cause of weaning failure. During weaning, they found that 7 of 12 difficult-to-wean patients developed electromyographic (EMG) changes representative of fatigue. Six who displayed EMG changes also exhibited paradoxical motion of the abdomen (inward displacement during inspiration), accompanied by "respiratory alternans" (phasic alternation in the contribution of the rib cage and abdomen to VT) in four patients and an increase in respiratory frequency in six. None of these signs were observed in the patients who did not develop EMG changes. The researchers considered that these changes in breathing pattern permit a diagnosis of respiratory muscle fatigue to be made with reasonable certainty. However, all of the patients were returned to mechanical ventilation within 40 minutes, thus limiting the clinical significance of these findings. Also, the EMG changes may not be shown to be related to the form of fatigue that is physiologically important (i.e., low-frequency fatigue, whose physiologic basis remains unknown),[28] and factors other than fatigue may affect the EMG power spectrum.[29] In addition, no attempt was made to distinguish the effect of work of breathing from fatigue in these patients.

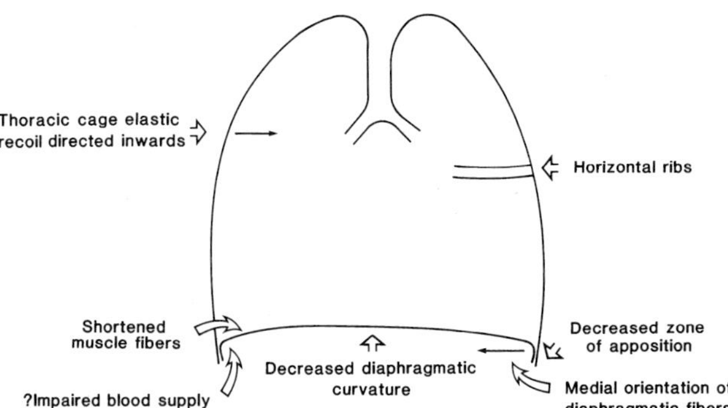

Figure 103–2. The detrimental effects of hyperinflation on respiratory muscle function. (From Tobin MJ. Respiratory muscles in disease. Clin Chest Med 1988; 9:263–286.)

In a series of detailed studies of breathing pattern during weaning, Tobin and coworkers[6, 30, 31] found that patients who could not be weaned displayed rapid, shallow breathing and abnormal rib cage–abdominal motion immediately on discontinuation of ventilator support, with no further progression during the period of the weaning trial (Fig. 103–3). Conceptually, it is difficult to reconcile this response of immediate alteration in the breathing pattern without subsequent progression to respiratory muscle fatigue. In another study of healthy volunteers breathing against inspiratory resistive loads,[31] respiratory muscle fatigue was found to be neither a sufficient nor a necessary condition for the development of rib cage–abdominal asynchrony or paradox, and the abnormal motion was found to be primarily determined by load rather than muscle fatigue per se (Fig. 103–4).

Increased Respiratory Load

An increase in the load on the respiratory muscle pump may result from increased ventilatory requirements or increased work of breathing.

INCREASED VENTILATORY REQUIREMENTS. Factors causing an increase in ventilatory requirements include increased CO_2 production ($\dot{V}CO_2$), increased dead space ventilation, and an inappropriately elevated respiratory drive. Although an increase in $\dot{V}CO_2$ predisposes to the development of CO_2 retention, it is never the sole cause of hypercapnia. There has

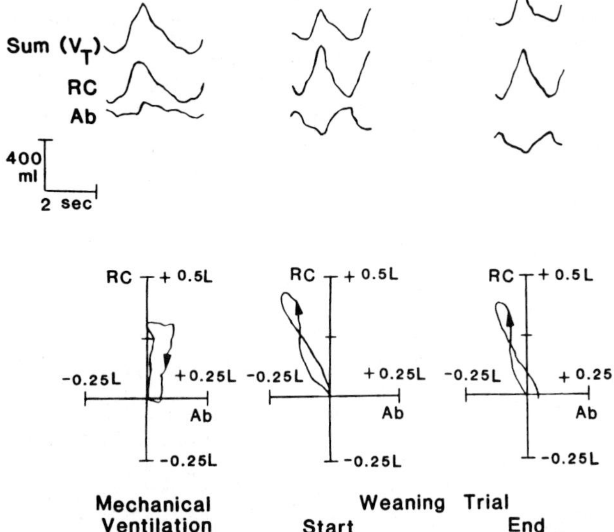

Figure 103–3. Analog tracing of the sum (V_T), rib cage (RC), and abdominal (Ab) signals during mechanical ventilation and at the beginning and end of a weaning trial in a patient with an unsuccessful weaning outcome. The respective Konno-Mead plots of the RC-Ab relationship are displayed below each of the breaths. During mechanical ventilation, some Ab paradox occurs; this increases immediately on discontinuation of the ventilator, with no further progression during weaning. (From Tobin MJ, Guenther SM, Perez W, et al: Konno-Mead analysis of rib cage–abdominal motion during successful and unsuccessful trials of weaning from mechanical ventilation. Am Rev Respir Dis 1987; 135:1320.)

been little in the way of systematic investigation of $\dot{V}CO_2$ in patients undergoing a weaning trial.

DEAD SPACE VENTILATION. Physiologic dead space is usually related to VT (i.e., VDS/VT), and in healthy subjects the VDS/VT ratio is between 0.33 and 0.45. High regional alveolar ventilation-perfusion ratios and thus increased dead space occur in a number of disease states and require increased minute ventilation to avoid hypercapnia. If $\dot{V}CO_2$ is high, an increase in VDS/VT to 0.60 or greater is generally considered to be a poor indicator of weaning success because the increase in minute ventilation needed to maintain adequate gas exchange encroaches on ventilatory reserve. In addition, patients with increased dead space often have decreased lung compliance and increased airway resistance, causing further increases in the work of breathing. The importance of VDS/VT as a determinant of weaning outcome has not been systematically studied in a large group of patients, but in a small group, VDS/VT could not predict success or failure of weaning.[32]

INCREASED RESPIRATORY DRIVE. Although inadequate respiratory drive causes hypoventilation and respiratory acidosis, an inappropriately heightened drive places excessive stress on the respiratory muscle pump and predisposes to fatigue. Possible sources of excessive drive include stimulation of pulmonary irritant or J receptors, neurologic lesions, or psychologic stress. Several studies have shown high levels of drive in patients who could not be weaned,[6–8] but the level of drive does not appear to be inappropriate in relation to chemical stimulation.[6, 32]

WORK OF BREATHING. To achieve normal ventilation, work is performed to overcome the elastic and frictional impedances of the lungs and chest wall. In the presence of increased resistance or decreased compliance, a greater swing in pleural pressure is required to achieve a given VT, thus increasing the work of breathing. Although several investigators have measured work of breathing in patients being weaned from mechanical ventilation (Table 103–2), there is considerable overlap of the groups able to be weaned with those who remained ventilator dependent, and threshold values differed among the studies. When assessing work of breathing, it is important to consider it in terms of both work per liter of ventilation (reflecting respiratory mechanics) and work per minute (taking into account ventilatory requirements).[33] Unfortunately, because the thresholds tabulated were determined on a post hoc basis, the predictive value of respiratory work as an index of successful weaning remains unclear.

Respiratory work load can be assessed also in terms of the O_2 cost of breathing. This is usually taken as the difference in total body O_2 consumption between spontaneous breathing and O_2 consumption per unit time ($\dot{V}O_2$) when a patient is relaxed and ventilated mechanically.[34] In healthy subjects at rest, the O_2 cost of breathing is less than 5% of the total body O_2 consumption,[35] whereas it can exceed 50% in patients being weaned from mechanical ventilation.[34] Although a number of investigators[34, 36, 37] have found O_2 cost of breathing to be higher in patients who could not be weaned, this index does not provide a clear distinction between weaning success and weaning failure. Last but very importantly, Oh and colleagues[38] dispel the notion that O_2 cost is due solely to the work of breathing; rather, it is at least partly due to elevated catecholamine levels during weaning.

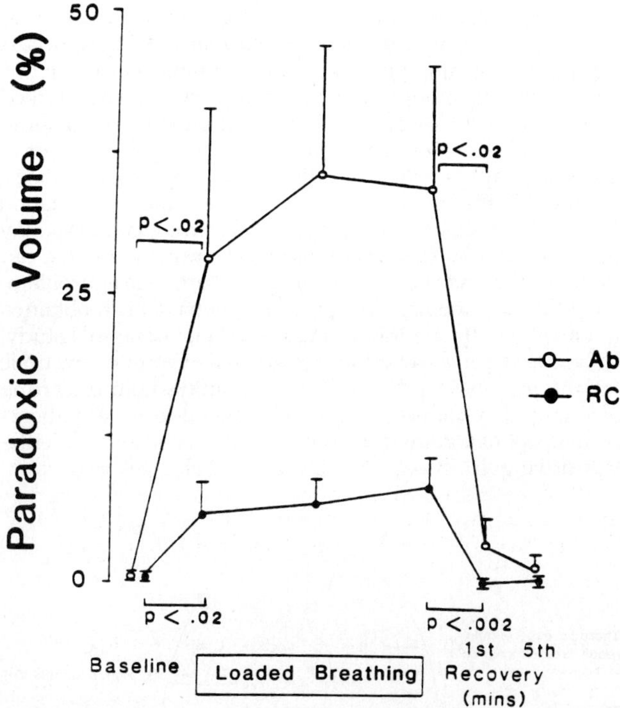

Figure 103–4. Effect of breathing against a fatiguing resistive load on the volume of inspiratory paradoxic volume of the rib cage (RC) and abdomen (Ab). Values depicted are those at baseline, at the first, middle, and penultimate minutes of the "fatigue run," and at the first and fifth minute of recovery. Values are mean ±SE for six subjects. Paradoxic volumes increased during the first minute of loaded breathing, did not progress during the loaded breathing run, and returned to baseline immediately following discontinuation of the load. (From Tobin MJ, Perez W, Guenther SM, et al: Does rib cage–abdominal motion signify respiratory muscle fatigue? J Appl Physiol 1987; 63:851–860.)

TABLE 103–2. Work of Breathing as a Determinant of Weaning Outcome

	Ventilator Dependent		*Ventilator Independent*	
	Work/L (kg · m/L)	*Work/min (kg · m/min)*	*Work/L (kg · m/L)*	*Work/min (kg · m/min)*
Peters et al[64]	≥ 0.10	≥ 1.00	< 0.10	< 1.00
Proctor and Woolson[65]	—	> 1.34	—	< 1.34
Henning et al[66]	—	> 1.70	—	< 1.00
Fiastro et al[67]	—	≥ 1.62	< 0.13	≥ 1.60

Psychologic Factors

Psychologic factors may contribute to weaning difficulties in some patients, because feelings of insecurity, anxiety, fear, agony, and panic have been associated with dependence on mechanical ventilation.[39] Apart from a few isolated reports, there is little information on the prevalence or nature of psychologic disturbances in ventilator-dependent patients or the degree to which they contribute to ventilator dependency.

PREDICTING WEANING OUTCOME

Determining the optimal time to discontinue ventilator support can be difficult. Although experience may allow a physician to predict weaning success in an individual patient, predictive indexes that can be easily measured and widely applied are desirable. The uses of such indexes are to identify the earliest time that a patient is able to resume and sustain spontaneous breathing and to identify patients who are likely to fail weaning, thus sparing them additional distress. In addition, these indexes may provide insight into the reasons for ventilator dependency in an individual and suggest an alteration in management. The commonly used indexes are listed in Table 103–3.

Gas Exchange

No single index of oxygenation is universally accepted to prohibit weaning, and a number of different criteria derived from arterial blood gas measurements have been proposed. The oxygenation criteria in Table 103–3 have been passed from one review article to another without systematic studies. Krieger and Ershowsky[40] examined retrospectively the predictive power of the arterial to inspired O_2 ratio ($Pa{O_2}/F{IO_2}$), and found in 269 patients that a ratio of 238 (equivalent to a PaO_2 of 50 mm Hg with an FIO_2 of 0.21) had a positive preditive value of 90% but a negative predictive value of only 10%. This ratio also cannot account for fluctuations in $PaCO_2$. Of the indexes of gas exchange calculated from conventional arterial blood gases, the arterial-alveolar O_2 tension ratio (PaO_2/PAO_2) is preferred because it is more stable with changing levels of FIO_2 than the alveolar-arterial PO_2 gradient (PAO_2–PaO_2).[41] In a study of predictors of weaning outcome, Yang and Tobin[42] found that a PaO_2/PAO_2 ratio of 0.35 was the value that provided the best prediction of weaning success versus weaning failure in a preliminary "training data set" of 36 patients. However, prospective evaluation of 64 patients undergoing weaning yielded a positive predictive value for this ratio of only 0.59 but a negative predictive value of only 0.53.

TABLE 103–3. Variables Used to Predict Weaning Success

Gas Exchange
PaO_2 of ≥ 60 mm Hg with FIO_2 of ≤ 0.35
Alveolar-arterial PO_2 gradient of < 350 mm Hg
PaO_2/FIO_2 ratio of > 200

Ventilator Pump
Vital capacity of > 10–15 mL/kg body weight
Maximum negative inspiratory pressure < −30 cm H_2O
Minute ventilation < 10L/min
Maximum voluntary ventilation more than twice resting minute ventilation

Maximum Inspiratory Pressure

Respiratory muscle function is probably the single most important factor in determining weaning outcome. A global assessment of respiratory muscle strength can be obtained by measuring maximum inspiratory pressure (PImax)[43] using an aneroid manometer at the opening of an endotracheal tube, during a maximum inspiratory effort. Sahn and Lakshminarayan[3] popularized the test with their excellent results in 100 patients, who were successfully weaned if PImax was −30 cm H_2O or less and unsuccessfully weaned if PI was −20 cm H_2O or greater. Since then, however, other investigators, especially Tahvanainen and coworkers,[4] found prospectively that a PImax value of −30 cm H_2O was falsely negative in 100% of patients (predicted failure but actual success) and falsely positive in 26%.

Lack of patient cooperation has been cited for the poor predictive power of PImax, and thus Marini and associates[44] modified the PImax technique. A one-way valve ensured that inspiratory efforts were made at a low lung volume while occlusion was maintained for 20 seconds. PImax gradually improved during the 20 seconds of occlusion, and values with the one-way valve were approximately one third more negative than values without it. Prospectively, however, Yang and Tobin[42] showed continued poor performance of PImax of −30 cm H_2O as a predictor of weaning outcome: positive predictive value of only 0.58.

Vital Capacity

A normal vital capacity is between 65 and 75 mL/kg, and a value of 10 mL/kg or more[45] has been suggested as essential to sustain spontaneous ventilation. This value is approximately twice the predicted tidal volume. Although vital capacity exceeding 10 to 15 mL/kg has been used as a standard predictor of weaning outcome,[45] Tahvanainen and colleagues[4] found that a vital capacity of 10 mL/kg was falsely positive in 18% and falsely negative in 50% of patients. Similarly, in a prospective study of 33 postoperative patients, when weaning success was defined as sustained spontaneous respiration with a pH of greater than 7.35, Milbern and associates[46] found that a vital capacity of 15 mL/kg was falsely positive in 15% and falsely negative in 63% of patients.

Respiratory System Compliance

Static compliance of the respiratory system is a direct determinant of respiratory work and has been suggested as a useful predictor of weaning outcome, with the added attraction that it is not highly dependent on patient's cooperation.[47] Noting the VT and the airway pressure plateau during "inspiratory hold" permits calculation of static thoracic compliance: Static compliance = tidal volume/ (plateau pressure–positive end-expiratory pressure) The normal range for adult patients receiving mechanical ventilation is generally accepted to be 60 to 100 mL/cm H_2O,[41] but in their prospective study, Yang and Tobin[42] found that a static thoracic compliance of 33 mL/cm H_2O had a positive predictive value of only 0.60 and a negative predictive value of 0.53.

Minute Ventilation and Maximum Voluntary Ventilation

The relationship between resting minute ventilation and maximum voluntary ventilation indicates the proportion of a patient's ventilatory capacity required to maintain a given level of $PaCO_2$ and identifies the degree of reserve available for further respiratory demands. In the study by Sahn and Lakshminarayan,[3] the combination of a minute ventilation of less than 10 L/min and the ability to double this value during a maximum voluntary ventilation maneuver identified all patients who could be weaned, whereas 71% of those who could not meet both criteria required continued support. However, Tahvanainen and colleagues[4] found a minute ventilation of 10 L/min to be falsely positive in 11% and falsely negative in 25% of patients. The ability to double minute ventilation during a maximum voluntary ventilation maneuver was falsely positive in 5% of patients and falsely negative in 76%. Similarly, a minute ventilation of 10 L/min proved to be quite a misleading predictor for Yang and Tobin:[42] Positive and negative predictive values were only 0.50 and 0.40, respectively.

Airway Occlusion Pressure

The use of airway occlusion pressure as a predictor of weaning outcome has been evaluated by a number of investigations. Pressures generated are negative, but $P_{0.1}$ values are generally reported in positive units, and the values are usually less than 2 cm H_2O in healthy subjects.[7] Herrera and colleagues[7] and Sassoon and associates[8] reported that $P_{0.1}$ was elevated in all of their patients with respiratory failure and that successful weaning could be predicted by threshold values of $P_{0.1}$ less than or equal to 4.2 cm H_2O[7] and less than 6 cm H_2O,[8] respectively. Similarly, Murciano and coworkers[9] studied 16 patients with chronic obstructive pulmonary disease and found that the $P_{0.1}$ values for successfully weaned patients decreased substantially from the start of ventilation support to extubation. In the weaning failure group, no decrease was evident.

Using a different approach, Montgomery and colleagues[32] first observed little difference of $P_{0.1}$ values between their successfully and unsuccesfully weaned patients, and then they found that they could not predict success or failure using a threshold. The investigators then performed hypercapnic challenges and found that the ratio of CO_2 stimulated $P_{0.1}$/baseline $P_{0.1}$ was higher in successfully than in unsuccessfully weaned patients. Further studies may clarify the role of $P_{0.1}$ as a predictor of weaning outcome.

Rapid Shallow Breathing

Although the conventional approach to predicting weaning outcome has focused on gas exchange indexes and measurements of maximum inspiratory pressure, vital capacity, and maximum voluntary ventilation (see Table 103–3), simple bedside measurements such as respiratory frequency have received less emphasis despite ease and potential utility.[48] Using respiratory inductive plethysmography to obtain breath-by-breath measurements, Tobin and colleagues[6] demonstrated an immediate increase to at least 25 breaths per minute in 7 patients who could not be weaned, whereas only 3 of 10 successfully weaned patients breathed as rapidly. Tachypnea was associated with a fall in VT, and all of the patients who failed to be weaned had a VT of less than 300 mL, whereas higher values were observed in eight (80%) of the successfully weaned patients.

Subsequently, Yang and Tobin[42] measured VT and respiratory frequency with a simple bedside spirometer attached to a patient's endotracheal tube while the patient spontaneously breathed room air for 1 minute. Measurements of frequency (f) and VT were combined into an index of rapid shallow breathing—the f/VT ratio. In an initial training data set obtained in 36 patients, they found that an f/VT value of 105 breaths per minute per liter best differentiated patients who were successfully weaned from those in whom weaning failed. The predictive power of this value was then assessed in 64 patients who constituted the "prospective-validation data set" (Fig. 103–5). The positive and negative predictive values were 0.78 and 0.95, respectively, which were the highest values noted for any of the predictive indexes in the study. As a predictive index, the f/VT ratio has a number of attractive features: It is easy to measure, it

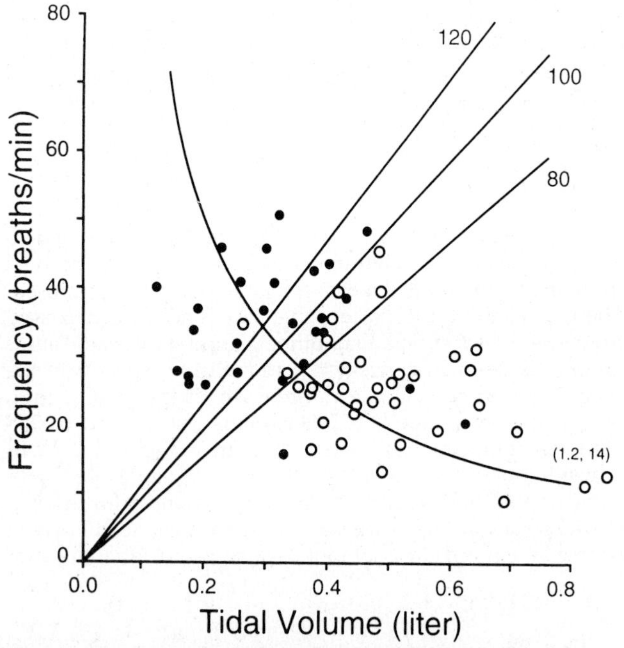

Figure 103–5. Isopleths for the ratio of frequency to tidal volume (f/VT). Different degrees of rapid shallow breathing are represented. Patients who fell to the left of the 100 breaths per minute per liter isopleth had a 95% likelihood of failing a weaning trial, whereas patients who fell to the right of this isopleth had an 80% likelihood of a successful weaning outcome. The *hyperbola* represents a minute ventilation of 10 L/min, a criterion commonly used to predict weaning outcome. It is apparent that this criterion was of little value in discriminating between weaning success patients *(open circles)* and weaning failure patients *(solid circles)*. Values for one patient (VT = 1.2 L, f = 14 breaths per minute) lay outside the graph. (From Yang KL, Tobin MJ: A prospective study of indexes predicting the outcome of trials of weaning from mechanical ventilation. N Engl J Med 1991; 324:1445–1450. Reproduced by permission of *The New England Journal of Medicine*.)

is independent of a patient's effort and cooperation, it appears to be quite accurate in predicting the ability to sustain ventilation, and fortuitously, it has a "rounded off" threshold value (100) that is easy to remember. The mechanism of rapid shallow breathing remains unknown.

Rib Cage–Abdominal Motion

The potential importance of abnormal rib cage–abdominal motion as a guide to weaning was first emphasized by Cohen and colleagues[27] and discussed earlier (see *Respiratory Muscle Function*). Tobin and colleagues[30] used respiratory inductive plethysmography to obtain breath-to-breath measurements of rib cage–abdominal motion in 17 patients being weaned from mechanical ventilation and to quantify indexes of asynchrony and paradox from Konno-Mead plots of rib cage–abdominal motion. It was found that marked asynchrony and paradoxical motion of both the rib cage and abdomen distinguished weaning success from failure. Likewise, marked variability in breath-by-breath contribution of the rib cage to V_T distinguished patients who failed to be weaned from successfully weaned patients, who showed much less variability in breaths.

Integrative Indexes

Weaning failure is commonly multifactorial in origin, and thus it is not very surprising that an index that assesses a single function, such as respiratory muscle strength, is not a powerful predictor of outcome.[49] Accordingly, an index that integrates a number of physiologic functions should have greater predictive accuracy. Such an index is the CROP index (an acronym for compliance, rate, oxygenation, and pressure), which incorporates a measure of pulmonary gas exchange and an assessment of the demands placed on the respiratory system and the capacity of the respiratory muscles to handle them.[42] The rationale for this index and its derivation are detailed elsewhere.[42] The index equation is displayed here:

$$\text{CROP index} = \frac{C_{dyn} \times PImax \times (PaO_2/PAO_2)}{\text{Rate}}$$

In their study of patients being weaned from ventilator support, Yang and Tobin[42] found that a CROP index value of 13 mL per breath per minute was the best discriminator between weaning success and weaning failure in the training data set obtained in 36 patients. When evaluated in the prospective-validation data set in 64 patients, its positive and negative predictive values were 0.71 and 0.70, respectively.

METHODS OF DISCONTINUING MECHANICAL VENTILATION

Abrupt Discontinuation

Patients who receive ventilator support for short periods, especially postoperative patients, can commonly be extubated without prolonged weaning trials. Quasha and coworkers[50] undertook a prospective randomized study of 38 patients undergoing coronary artery bypass surgery and observed no differences in cardiorespiratory morbidity in patients who were extubated within 2 hours of bypass versus those who were extubated 18 hours after bypass.

Spontaneous Breathing Trials

Before extubation, patients are usually observed during spontaneous breathing trials without ventilator support. Such a trial may be conducted while a patient breathes spontaneously through a T-tube system or through the ventilator circuit, but careful efforts to minimize respiratory work are important. When a T-tube system is used, the gas source flow to the inspiratory limb should be at least twice that of the patient's spontaneous minute ventilation in order to meet the patient's peak inspiratory flow rate,[51] and an extension piece should be added to the expiratory limb to prevent entrainment of room air. Although construction of the circuitry is now reasonable, the conduct of the trials remains unclear. Full ventilatory support can frequently give way to a T-tube trial and extubation in short order. If deterioration occurs, however, more gradual weaning is needed. A reasonable approach is to begin with relatively brief T-tube trials (lasting about 5 min) and gradually increase their duration according to a patient's respiratory performance. Trials are commonly performed every 1 to 3 hours, without knowing the optimal period of rest. If muscle fatigue is likely to have developed, preliminary studies suggest 24 hours or more may be necessary for recovery.[52] In the authors' opinion, extubation can usually be safely performed if a patient can undertake a T-tube trial for 30 to 60 consecutive minutes without undue respiratory distress or significant deterioration in gas exchange.

During a trial of spontaneous breathing, a patient's clinical status should be closely monitored by a physician, nurse, or therapist. The degree of change in breathing pattern during the transition from mechanical ventilation to spontaneous breathing depends on the ventilator settings. In a group of 10 patients who were successfully weaned and extubated, the transition from mechanical ventilation to the first 15 minutes of spontaneous breathing (while still intubated) was associated with no change in the volume and time components of the breathing pattern,[6] but slight increases occurred in the amount of asynchronous and paradoxical motion of the rib cage and abdomen.[30] As the trial of spontaneous breathing continued for 1 hour, these patients developed slight increases in minute ventilation (of 1 L/min) and respiratory frequency (of 3 breaths per minute)[6] but no significant changes in arterial blood gases. In the authors' opinion, spontaneous breathing trials constitute the preferred method of weaning.

Intermittent Mandatory Ventilation

Patients receiving intermittent mandatory ventilation (IMV) can breathe spontaneously and receive periodic positive-pressure breaths at a preset volume and rate from the ventilator.[53] When used as a weaning technique, IMV can be initiated after a period of mechanical ventilation delivered in the assist-control mode or in the IMV mode. When a patient is ready for weaning, the IMV rate is reduced in steps, usually one to three breaths per minute at each step, and arterial blood gases are measured after 30 minutes or more at that setting. If the pH remains greater than 7.30[54] or 7.35,[55] the IMV rate is reduced in further steps until a rate of zero or close to zero is reached. Thus, weaning is guided by monitoring the pH response to stepwise reductions in the number of mechanically delivered breaths, and predictions based on physiologic measurements are not used.

Proponents suggest several advantages of IMV such as preventing patients from "fighting" the ventilator, reducing the need for sedation and muscle paralysis, decreasing respiratory alkalemia, achieving more normal matching of ventilation and perfusion and more rapid weaning[54] and other benefits. Data to support these claims are few and are largely based on comparison between IMV and controlled mechanical ventilation.

A major disadvantage of IMV is the fact that it produces a marked increase in the work of breathing when IMV demand-valve circuits are incorporated. The excessive reduction in airway pressure necessary to activate the demand valve, combined with the inadequate delivery of instantaneous gas flow, may cause a twofold or more increase in the work of breathing[55] and O_2 consumption.[56] Incorporation of a reservoir bag into the system provides both a volume and a pressure reservoir to match more closely a patient's peak inspiratory flow rate and thus minimize the work of breathing.

In patients receiving IMV, it has been generally assumed a patient's effort is spared in proportion to the number of breaths delivered by the ventilator, but Marini and others[57, 57a] showed that as the synchronized IMV rate was decreased, inspiratory work and pressure-time product increased progressively for both the spontaneous and assisted breaths. These findings indicate that patients display little breath-to-breath adaptation to machine assistance during synchronized IMV. Of particular concern is the observation that tension-time index is commonly above the fatigue threshold for both the assisted and spontaneous breaths, suggesting that the common practice of using low levels of IMV may hinder satisfactory recovery from respiratory muscle fatigue.

The efficacy of IMV as a weaning technique has been evaluated prospectively in two studies. Hastings and coworkers[58] studied 18 stable patients after cardiac surgery. The patients were randomized to a T-tube trial or IMV at four breaths per minute, after meeting a number of weaning criteria. The duration of weaning to the time of extubation was similar for each group. Tomlinson and associates[59] undertook a prospective randomized comparison of IMV and T-tube weaning techniques in 165 patients who received ventilator support for an average of 3.6 days and who met several typical weaning criteria. The weaning time again was similar for the two patient groups. Unfortunately, this latter study[59] enrolled patients receiving short-term ventilator support; two thirds of the patients who were weaned in 2 hours were postoperative patients who had been ventilated for less than 72 hours. In the former study,[58] little difficulty with weaning would have been anticipated owing to the short period of support and the patients' good pulmonary function.

Pressure Support Ventilation

Pressure support ventilation (PSV) is available on most of the new generation of mechanical ventilators[60, 61] and is described in detail elsewhere in this text (see Chapter 98). PSV is considered to be more comfortable than conventional ventilatory modes because patients can control the depth, length, and flow profile of each breath[60] while the PSV counteracts the resistive load due to endotracheal tubes and ventilator circuits and simultaneously decreases the elastic work of breathing.[62] Controversy exists regarding patient comfort with the use of any form of mechanical ventilatory support.[62a]

The level of PSV is set on an empirical basis, with or without continuous positive airway pressure, and titrated to a patient's respiratory frequency and clinical status. Pressures of 5 to 15 cm H_2O are used most commonly, but higher levels have been used.[60, 61, 61a] Brochard and colleagues[63] reported that monitoring of sternocleidomastoid muscle EMG activity is useful in deciding the optimal level of PSV. Weaning from PSV can be performed by gradually decreasing the level of PSV in 3- to 6-cm H_2O decrements according to tolerance by a patient, and extubation can be performed at a PSV level of 5 cm H_2O. No study has demonstrated the superiority of PSV over other techniques of weaning.

SUMMARY

Although most patients can be easily weaned from mechanical ventilation, a substantial minority pose considerable difficulty. The major respiratory determinants of weaning outcome include respiratory muscle performance, adequacy of gas exchange, and psychologic factors. In addition, cardiac dysfunction may affect both muscle performance and gas exchange. Because weaning failure is usually multifactorial, indexes that assess a single physiologic function are frequently inaccurate in predicting weaning outcome. An index of rapid shallow breathing, the f/VT ratio, appears to be more accurate in predicting weaning outcome than traditional indexes, such as maximum inspiratory pressure or minute ventilation. Although a number of different weaning techniques exist, no data support the superiority of one technique over another. Indeed, too much attention has been focused on techniques of weaning, and instead, management should be directed at the underlying pathophysiology.

References

1. Pierson DJ: Complications associated with mechanical ventilation. 1990; 6:711–724.
1a. Tobin MJ: Mechanical ventilation [Review]. N Engl J Med 1994; 330:1056–1061.
2. Rosen RL, Bone RC: Financial implications of ventilator care. 1990; 6:785–805.
3. Sahn SA, Lakshminarayan S: Bedside criteria for discontinuation of mechanical ventilation. Chest 1973; 63:1002–1005.
4. Tahvanainen J, Salenpera M, Nikki P: Extubation criteria after weaning from intermittent mandatory ventilatory and continuous positive airway pressure. Crit Care Med 1983; 11:702–707.
5. Torres A, Reyes A, Roca J, et al: Ventilation-perfusion mismatching in chronic obstructive pulmonary disease during ventilator weaning. Am Rev Respir Dis 1989; 140:1246–1250.
6. Tobin MJ, Perez W, Guenther SM, et al: The pattern of breathing during successful and unsuccessful trials of weaning from mechanical ventilation. Am Rev Respir Dis 1986; 134:1111–1118.
7. Herrera M, Blasco J, Venegas J, et al: Mouth occlusion pressure ($P_{0.1}$) in acute respiratory failure. Intensive Care Med 1985; 11:134–139.
8. Sassoon CSH, Te TT, Mahutte CK, et al: Airway occlusion pressure: An important indicator for successful weaning in patients with chronic obstructive pulmonary disease. Am Rev Respir Dis 1987; 135:107–113.
9. Murciano D, Boczkowski J, Lecocguic Y, et al: Tracheal occlusion pressure: A simple index to monitor respiratory muscle fatigue during acute respiratory failure in patients with chronic obstructive pulmonary disease. Ann Intern Med 1988; 108:800–805.
10. Estenne M, Yernault JC, De Smet JM, et al: Phrenic and diaphragm function after coronary artery bypass grafting. Thorax 1985; 40:293–299.
11. Wilcox PG, Paré PD, Pardy RL: Recovery after unilateral phrenic injury associated with coronary artery revascularization. Chest 1990; 98:661–666.
12. Tobin MJ: Respiratory muscles in disease. Clin Chest Med 1988; 9:263–286.
13. Pingleton SK, Harmon GS: Nutritional management in acute respiratory failure. JAMA 1987; 257:2094–2099.
14. Doekel RC, Zwillich CW, Scoggin CH, et al: Clinical semistarvation: Depression of hypoxic ventilatory response. N Engl J Med 1976; 295:358–361.
15. Arora NS, Rochester DF: Effect of body weight and muscularity on human diaphragm muscle mass, thickness, and area. J Appl Physiol 1982; 52:64–70.
16. Arora NS, Rochester DF: Respiratory muscle strength and maximal voluntary ventilation in undernourished patients. Am Rev Respir Dis 1982; 126:5–8.

17. Jardim J, Farkas G, Prefaut C, et al: The failing inspiratory muscles under normoxic and hypoxic conditions. Am Rev Respir Dis 1982; 124:274–279.
18. Hussain SNA, Simkus G, Roussos C: Respiratory muscle fatigue: A cause of ventilatory failure in septic shock. J Appl Physiol 1985; 58:2033–2040.
19. Lemaire F, Teboul JL, Cinotti L, et al: Acute left ventricular dysfunction during unsuccessful weaning from mechanical ventilation. Anesthesiology 1988; 69:171–179.
20. Juan G, Calverley P, Talamo C, et al: Effect of carbon dioxide on diaphragmatic function in human beings. N Engl J Med 1984; 310:874–979.
21. Fisher J, Magrid M, Kallman C, et al: Respiratory illness and hypophosphatemia. Chest 1983; 83:504–508.
22. Aubier M, Viires N, Piquet J, et al: Effects of hypocalcemia on diaphragmatic strength generation. J Appl Physiol 1985; 58:2054–2061.
23. Molloy DW, Dhingra S, Solven F, et al: Hypomagnesemia and respiratory muscle power. Am Rev Respir Dis 1984; 129:497–498.
24. Knox AJ, Mascie-Taylor BH, Muers MF: Acute hydrocortisone myopathy in acute severe asthma. Thorax 1986; 41:411–412.
25. Anzueto A, Tobin MJ, Moore G, et al: Effect of prolonged mechanical ventilation on diaphragmatic function: A preliminary study of a baboon model (Abstract). Am Rev Respir Dis 1987; 135:A201.
26. Muller EA: Influence of training and of inactivity on muscle strength. Arch Phys Med Rehabil 1970; 51:449–462.
27. Cohen C, Zagelbaum G, Gross D, et al: Clinical manifestations of inspiratory muscle fatigue. Am J Med 1982; 73:308–316.
28. Moxham J, Edwards RHT, Aubier M, et al: Changes in the EMG power spectrum (high-to-low) with force fatigue in humans. J Appl Physiol 1982; 53:1094–1099.
29. Walsh JM, Romano S, Grassino A: The effect of diaphragm length on the EMG power spectrum. Clin Res 1990; 38:847A.
30. Tobin MJ, Guenther SM, Perez W, et al: Konno-Mead analysis of ribcage-abdominal motion during successful and unsuccessful trials of weaning from mechanical ventilation. Am Rev Respir Dis 1987; 135:1320–1328.
31. Tobin MJ, Perez W, Guenther SM, et al: Does ribcage abdominal paradox signify respiratory muscle fatigue? J Appl Physiol 1987; 63:851–860.
32. Montgomery AB, Holle RHO, Neagley SR, et al: Prediction of successful ventilator weaning using airway occlusion pressure and hypercapnic challenge. Chest 1987; 91:496–499.
33. Fleury B, Murciano D, Talamo C, et al: Work of breathing in patients with chronic obstructive pulmonary disease in acute respiratory failure. Am Rev Respir Dis 1985; 131:822–827.
34. Lewis WD, Chwals W, Benotti PN, et al: Bedside assessment of the work of breathing. Crit Care Med 1988; 16:117–122.
35. Campbell EJM, Westlake EK, Cherniack RM: Simple methods of estimating oxygen consumption and efficiency of the muscles of breathing. J Appl Physiol 1957; 11:303–308.
36. Kemper M, Weissman C, Askanazi J, et al: Metabolic and respiratory changes during weaning from mechanical ventilation. Chest 1987; 92:979–983.
37. Hubmayr RD, Loosbrock LM, Gillespie DJ, et al: Oxygen uptake during weaning from mechanical ventilation. Chest 1988; 94:1148–1155.
38. Oh TE, Bhatts, Lin ES, et al: Plasma catecholamines and oxygen consumption during weaning from mechanical ventilation. Intensive Care Med 1991; 4:199.
39. Bergbom-Engberg I, Haljamäe H: Assessment of patients' experience of discomforts during respiratory therapy. Crit Care Med 1989; 17:1068–1072.
40. Krieger BP, Ershowsky P: Noninvasive detection of respiratory failure in the intensive care unit. Chest 1988; 94:254–261.
41. Tobin MJ: State of the art: Respiratory monitoring in the intensive care unit. Am Rev Respir Dis 1988; 138:1625–1642.
42. Yang K, Tobin MJ: A prospective study of indexes predicting outcome of trials of weaning from mechanical ventilation. N Engl J Med 1991; 324:1445–1450.
43. Black LF, Hyatt RE: Maximal respiratory pressures: Normal values and relationship to age and sex. Am Rev Respir Dis 1968; 99:696–702.
44. Marini JJ, Smith TC, Lamb V: Estimation of inspiratory muscle strength in mechanically ventilated patients: The measurement of maximal inspiratory pressure. J Crit Care 1986; 1:32–38.
45. Feeley TW, Hedley-White J: Weaning from controlled ventilation and supplemental oxygen. N Engl J Med 1975; 292:903–906.
46. Milbern SM, Downs JB, Jumper LC, et al: Evaluation of criteria for discontinuing mechanical ventilation support. Arch Surg 1978; 113:1441–1443.
47. Fallat RJ: Bedside pulmonary function and ICU monitoring: Indications and interpretation. In: Pulmonary Function Testing: Indications and Interpretations. Wilson AF (Ed). Orlando, Grune & Stratton, 1985, pp 293–309.
48. Gravelyn TR, Weg JR: Respiratory rate as an indicator of acute respiratory dysfunction. JAMA 1980; 244:1123–1125.
49. Tobin MJ. Predicting weaning outcome (Editorial). Chest 1988; 94:227–228.
50. Quasha AC, Loeber N, Feeley TW, et al: Postoperative respiratory care: A controlled trial of early and late extubation following coronary care artery bypass grafting. Anesthesiology 1980; 52:135–141.
51. Dean SE, Keenan RL: Spontaneous breathing with a T-piece circuit: Minimum fresh gas/minute volume ratio which prevents rebreathing. Anesthesiology 1982; 56:449–452.
52. Laghi F, D'Alfonso N, Doud J, et al: Time course of recovery from diaphgragmatic fatigue assessed by magnetic stimulation of the phrenic nerves. Am Rev Respir Dis 1993; 147:A956.
53. Kirby RR, Robison EJ, Schulz J, et al: A new pediatric volume ventilator. Anesth Analg 1971; 50:533–537.
54. Downs JB, Block AJ, Vennum KG. Intermittent mandatory ventilation in the treatment of patients with chronic obstructive pulmonary disease. Anesth Analg 1974; 53:437–443.
55. Gherini S, Peters RM, Virgilio RW: Mechanical work on the lungs and work of breathing with positive end-expiratory pressure and continuous positive airway pressure. Chest 1979; 76:251–255.
56. Henry WC, West GA, Wilson RS: A comparison of the oxygen cost of breathing between a continuous-flow CPAP system and a demand-flow CPAP system. Respir Care 1983; 28:1273–1281.
57. Marini JJ, Smith TC, Lamb VJ: External work output and force generation during synchronized intermittent mandatory ventilation: Effect of machine assistance on breathing effort. Am Rev Respir Dis 1988; 138:1169–1179.
57a. Imsand C, Feihl F, Perret C, Fitting JW: Regulation of inspiratory neuromuscular output during synchronized intermittent mechanical ventilation. Anesthesiology 1994; 80:13–22.
58. Hastings PR, Bushnell LS, Skillman JJ, et al: Cardiorespiratory dynamics during weaning with IMV versus spontaneous ventilation in good-risk cardiac-surgery patients. Anesthesiology 1980; 53:429–431.
59. Tomlinson JR, Miller KS, Lorch DG, et al: A prospective comparison of IMV and T-piece weaning from mechanical ventilation. Chest 1989; 96:348–352.
60. MacIntyre NR: Respiratory function during pressure support ventilation. Chest 1986; 89:677–683.
61. Kacmarek RM: The role of pressure support ventilation in reducing work of breathing. Respir Care 1988; 33:99–120.
61a. Nathan SD, Ishaaya AM, Koerner SK, Belman MJ: Prediction of minimal pressure support during weaning from mechanical ventilation. Chest 1993; 103:1215–1219.
62. Van de Graaff WB, Gordey K, Dornseif SE, et al: Pressure support: Changes in ventilatory pattern and components of the work of breathing. Chest 1991; 100:1082–1089.
62a. Knebel AR, Janson-Bjerklie SL, Malley JD, et al: Comparison of breathing comfort during weaning with two ventilatory modes. Am J Respir Crit Care Med 1994; 149:14–18.
63. Brochard L, Harf A, Lorino H, et al: Inspiratory pressure support prevents diaphragmatic fatigue during weaning from mechanical ventilation. Am Rev Respir Dis 1989; 139:513–521.
64. Peters RM, Hilberman M, Hogan JS, et al: Objective indications for respiratory therapy in post-trauma and postoperative patients. Am J Surg 1972; 124:262–269.
65. Proctor HJ, Woolson R: Prediction of respiratory muscle fatigue by measurements of the work of breathing. Surg Gynecol Obstet 1973; 136:367–370.
66. Henning RJ, Shubin H, Weil MH: The measurement of the work of breathing for the clinical assessment of ventilator dependence. Crit Care Med 1977; 5:264–268.
67. Fiastro JF, Habib MP, Shon BY, et al: Comparison of standard weaning parameters and mechanical work of breathing in mechanically ventilated patients. Chest 1988; 94:232–238.

CHAPTER 104

Positive-Pressure Ventilation Without Tracheal Intubation

Mark H. Sanders, MD, FCCP • Ronald A. Stiller, MD, PhD, FCCP
Patrick J. Strollo, MD, FCCP

Although unquestionably a clinical milestone, endotracheal intubation is not without its complications. These may be divided into four loosely defined groups: (1) those associated with the act of placing the tube within the airway, (2) those associated with compromising the integrity of the glottic aperture, (3) those occurring during extubation, and (4) those that affect a patient at a time remote from intubation (Table 104–1).[1,2] These problems are discussed in detail in Chapters 78, 79, and 80. Because of such adverse consequences, some of which may be magnified by administering positive pressure via endotracheal tube, significant benefit may be conferred by successful noninvasive approaches to mechanical ventilatory support.

In this chapter, various aspects of positive-pressure ventilation without tracheal intubation are described. The discussion initially addresses noninvasive interfaces that have been used to administer positive pressure to patients during acute resuscitative efforts in the field and emergency department, in the operating room, and for sustained ventilatory support. Subsequently, the utility of various techniques of noninvasive positive-pressure ventilation used in an intensive care setting are also addressed.

INTERFACES FOR DELIVERY OF POSITIVE-PRESSURE VENTILATION THAT DO NOT REQUIRE TRACHEAL INTUBATION

During cardiopulmonary resuscitative efforts in the field and in the operating room, the primary focus of medical attention is to rapidly establish a secure airway through which positive-pressure ventilatory assistance can be applied. Under these circumstances, the nature of the airway is a more critical issue than the method or modality of positive pressure that is applied through it. In the prehospital setting, remote from sophisticated equipment and medical expertise, it is desirable to have techniques that can be used by paramedical personnel with various levels of training and experience to facilitate rapid stabilization of the airway with minimum risk of medical misadventure.

The noninvasive interfaces used to allow ventilatory support during resuscitative efforts in the field are generally intended to provide access to the airway for the finite period required for successful resuscitation or transport to an acute-care facility. Although a mask covering the nose and mouth with a bag-and-valve system has historically been used for this purpose, the high risk of inadequate ventilation owing to poor sealing at the mask-skin interface as well as the need for two hands to secure the mask has led clinicians to seek alternative interfaces. Three such alternatives include the esophageal obturator airway (EOA) the pharyngotracheal lumen airway (PTL), and the laryngeal mask airway (LMA).

Esophageal Obturator Airway

Although the EOA was initially described more than two decades ago,[3,4] its application in the acute setting has remained controversial. Designed to facilitate establishing a patent airway by personnel with diverse levels of skill and experience in resuscitation techniques and to permit maintenance of satisfactory arterial blood gases and acid-base balance with minimum complications, the superiority of the EOA to endotracheal intubation in the prehospital environment remains to be demonstrated.

Although an exhaustive review of the literature addressing the EOA is beyond the scope of this chapter, several investigations have demonstrated that this device can be a useful tool for delivering short-term positive-pressure ventilatory support to patients in the field and in the emergency department. In one of the earliest studies, Schofferman and coworkers[5] reported no significant difference in arterial blood gas values between periods of support with the EOA and after endotracheal intubation. No statistical analyses were performed, however, and examination of the data reveals that the EOA was associated with substantially worse arterial oxygen tension (Pa_{O_2}) and carbon dioxide tension (Pa_{CO_2}) in some patients when compared with ventilation via endotracheal tube, specifically in those patients requiring continued chest compression. The researchers suggested that because of difficulty predicting the adequacy of ventilation with respect to Pa_{CO_2} using the EOA, efforts should

TABLE 104–1. Complications of Tracheal Intubation

During the Intubation Procedure	*While the Airway Is Being Intubated*	*During Extubation of the Airway*	*Late Complications Remote from Extubation*
Epistaxis	Tracheal damage	Glottic trauma	Odynophagia, dysphagia
Dental trauma	Pneumothorax	Laryngospasm	Vocal cord paralysis/paresis
Retropharyngeal dissection	Aspiration	Bronchospasm	Lingual nerve damage
Laryngeal dissection, trauma	Infectious complications	Aspiration	Stricture of nostril, vocal cords, trachea
Esophageal intubation	Inability to speak		Tracheomalacia
Bronchial intubation			
Pneumothorax			
Aspiration			
Laryngospasm			
Bronchospasm			
Cardiac arrhythmias			
Arterial hypotension			

(Adapted from Applebaum EL, Bruce DL: Tracheal Intubation. Philadelphia, WB Saunders, 1976, pp 78–79.)

be made to "overventilate" patients pending measured blood gas results. The data reported by Meislin[6] were similar to those of Schofferman and demonstrated that on average, ventilation via the EOA was as good as that delivered via endotracheal tube in patients undergoing resuscitation from cardiac arrest, albeit with substantial patient-to-patient variability. Donen and Tweed[7] observed comparable PaO_2 values during ventilation with the EOA and a conventional facemask–oral airway system, although neither was as effective as ventilation via endotracheal tube, which provided significantly better oxygenation. Hammargren and coworkers[8] also reported comparable arterial blood gas values during ventilation using either the EOA or endotracheal tube, although the study population was highly selected. In this study, patients who appeared to be responding poorly with the EOA were subsequently intubated and excluded from the analysis.

A common but perhaps unavoidable criticism of all the foregoing studies is that arterial blood gas values obtained during ventilation with either the EOA or endotracheal tube were sampled and analyzed in the controlled setting of an emergency department and may not reflect conditions in the field. Furthermore, arterial blood gases during ventilation via endotracheal tube were invariably taken *after* those obtained during EOA use. It is therefore possible that the improvement seen after tracheal intubation reflected improvement in the patient's physiologic status rather than benefit derived specifically from changing the route by which ventilatory assistance was delivered.

The ease and rapidity of establishing a stable airway using the EOA have also been evaluated with variable but generally favorable results. Goldenberg and colleagues[9] reported a significantly greater success rate in securing the airway using the EOA (98.3%) than endotracheal intubation (79.6%) in patients undergoing prehospital resuscitation. Along similar lines, Donen and Tweed[7] reported satisfactory EOA passage in 96% of patients. Other investigators have reported inability to pass either the EOA or an endotracheal tube in 2% to 20% of attempts.[7, 10, 11] The rapidity with which a stable airway can be established is of obvious importance. Michael[11] reported that after training, house staff required approximately 5 seconds for EOA insertion and 30 seconds for tracheal intubation. This difference is of arguable clinical significance, however.

When using the EOA, potential adverse consequences should be kept in mind. Unrecognized tracheal intubation with the EOA is often if not invariably associated with a fatal outcome.[12] Bryson and colleagues[10] noted significantly reduced tidal volumes when using the EOA compared with a facemask–oropharyngeal airway and attributed this to poor fit and mouth leakage with the former device. In addition, supraglottic obstruction frequently occurred during use of the EOA, prompting these investigators to comment that successful passage of the EOA does not guarantee a patent airway. Another complication that may be associated with EOA use is gastric rupture.[13] To minimize this possibility, the device has been modified to permit passage of a nasogastric tube via the esophageal obturator in order to avoid overdistention of the stomach. Another untoward consequence of attempted EOA insertion is esophageal trauma. As evidenced by mucosal lacerations, this complication has been reported in 8% to 10% of patients evaluated at autopsy after EOA use.[7, 9] Esophageal rupture may occur in approximately 2% of patients.[14, 15]

Contraindications to the use of the EOA are listed in Table 104–2. In addition, careful consideration should be given before using this device in edentulous patients and individuals with unusual facial morphology because of reported difficulty in achieving an adequate mask seal.[8, 15] Because adequate ventilation with the EOA may require at least two operators, attempted insertion by a single rescuer may be imprudent. It is, of course, recognized that under such circumstances, ventilation with a standard bag and facemask might be equally difficult.

TABLE 104–2. Contraindications for Use of the Esophageal Obturator Airway

Known esophageal or gastric disease or trauma
Corrosive poisoning
Known supraglottic or tracheal disease or trauma
Trauma to facial anatomy
Conscious or semi-conscious patients

In summary, although most investigators agree that tracheal intubation is the optimal technique for establishing a secure airway either in the field or in a hospital setting,[15, 16] it appears that satisfactory arterial blood gas values can usually be achieved with positive-pressure ventilation using the EOA. Successful insertion of the EOA is likely to be highly dependent on the training and expertise of the responsible healthcare personnel as well as the clinical condition of patients selected to undergo this procedure. If the EOA is used, the operator must accept an additional degree of uncertainty about the integrity of the airway in comparison with airway patency after placement of an endotracheal tube.

Pharyngeal Tracheal Lumen Airway

The EOA can be simply described as a facemask with an esophageal obturator to divert gas flow into the trachea and prevent gastric insufflation. As described earlier, inadvertent tracheal intubation with the EOA, recognized by absence of chest wall movement with inspiratory positive pressure, mandates immediate removal of the device and either another attempt at insertion or abandonment of the technique. The PTL takes the EOA concept one further step in an attempt to avoid potentially lethal esophageal intubation and consequent failure to ventilate a patient. The PTL has two tubes, one longer than the other and each with an inflatable cuff. The large low-pressure cuff located proximally on the shorter tube inflates in the pharynx (Fig. 104–1) and seals it from above. This arrangement allows delivery of gas via the tubes without the need for a facemask, as required by the EOA. During PTL insertion, a semi-rigid stylet remains in the longer tube. After the PTL is inserted into the airway, both cuffs are inflated and gas is administered under positive pressure through the shorter tube while the operator observes the chest wall for motion. If the chest wall is noted to rise, the esophagus has been intubated with the longer tube and subsequent efforts to ventilate the patient are made via the shorter one. The inflated pharygeal cuff prevents loss of delivered gas through the mouth. The stylet should remain in the longer tube to prevent aspiration of gastric contents. On the other hand, if the chest wall does not rise with positive-pressure gas insufflation through the shorter tube, the operator should assume that the trachea has been intubated by the longer tube and the route of positive-pressure delivery should be changed accordingly. Under these circumstances, the cuff around the longer tube should remain inflated to facilitate ventilation and as a precaution against aspiration pneumonia.

Only limited studies have investigated the utility and safety of the PTL. In anesthetized volunteers, comparable arterial blood gas values were obtained using positive pres-

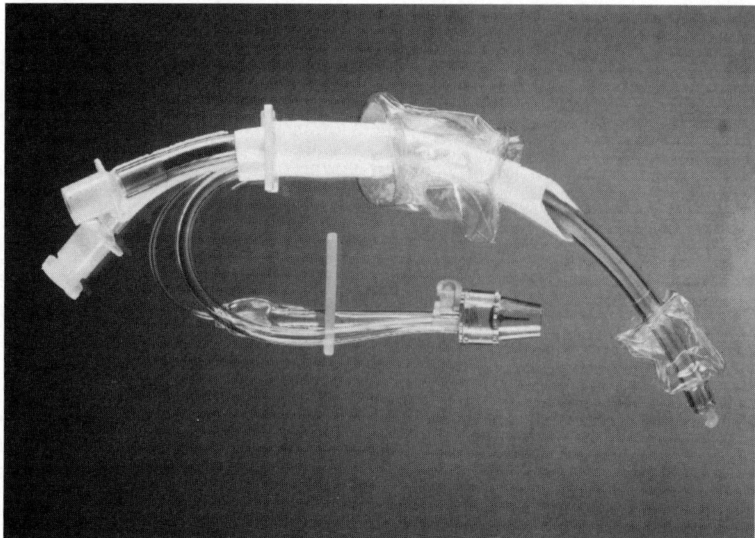

Figure 104–1. A PTL device. (Courtesy of Respironics, Murrysville, PA.)

sure with both the PTL and an endotracheal tube.[17, 18] Other studies[15, 19] have shown no difference in the average arterial blood gas values in patients ventilated via these two routes, as reflected by similar average arterial blood gas values in patients undergoing unsuccessful resuscitation from cardiac arrest. Nonetheless, despite the absence of significantly different Pa_{CO_2} values using the two devices, Neiman and coworkers observed that some patients had a considerably greater degree of respiratory acidosis during ventilation with the PTL.[19] Because minute ventilation was not specifically measured in this study, however, differences in Pa_{CO_2} during PTL and endotracheal tube use may be not be related to the interface per se but may possibly be due to differences in ventilation for other reasons. Bartlett and coworkers[20] compared the PTL and endotracheal tube in the prehospital setting, where the devices were inserted by paramedical personnel in patients requiring resuscitation in the field. No significant difference between the two airways was noted with respect to the number of attempts needed for successful passage. In addition, the time required for successful insertion of the PTL was statistically less than that for the endotracheal tube, although the difference was probably not clinically significant. Comparable levels of ventilation were maintained regardless of the tube interface. These observations are generally similar to those by McMahan and coworkers,[21] except that the latter investigators found that patients with head and facial injuries were inadequately ventilated using the PTL. McMahan and associates also reported that the PTL was more difficult to insert.[21]

The importance of maintaining adequate pressure in the pharyngeal cuff during ventilation should be emphasized. Neiman and colleagues[19] emphasized the need to maintain pressure in the pharyngeal cuff of the PTL at levels that are at least as great as those used for ventilation. In this regard, both McMahan and colleagues and Barlett and coworkers[20, 21] used either a bag-valve-mask or a manually triggered oxygen powered system rather than a conventional positive-pressure ventilator. The latter could generate higher peak airway pressure and increase the risk of air leakage through the mouth.

Although the PTL does not specifically use positive pressure, Kern and colleagues reported an interesting and unique application of the PTL during cardiopulmonary resuscitation.[22] In anesthetized, paralyzed, and apneic dogs, insufflation of 10 L/min of oxygen via the PTL during chest compression maintained adequate oxygenation and Pa_{CO_2}. If the oxygen insufflation catheter can be stabilized within the PTL, this technique could enhance the efficiency of resuscitative efforts when only one rescuer is available. Importantly, Kern and coworkers observed that sufficient ventilation could be achieved only when the pharyngeal cuff of the PTL was deflated, allowing for adequate "expiratory" gas flow. Clearly, however, more studies are required before this technique can be introduced into routine clinical use.

The limited available data suggest that the PTL can usually be used to establish a secure airway and to deliver adequate ventilation. In light of these findings, the device has been approved by the Food and Drug Administration for use in the prehospital setting. Nonetheless, more information from randomized controlled studies that examine its utility in the field and in the emergency department is needed before the efficacy of the PTL and its role relative to the gold standard, endotracheal intubation, are defined.

Laryngeal Mask Airway

The LMA was described by Brain in the early 1980s.[23–25] The device is a modified endotracheal tube that has been obliquely cut anteriorly with fixation of an inflatable, low-pressure cuff around the oblique lumen opening (Fig. 104–2). During insertion, the LMA is blindly advanced over the tongue until resistance is met. The cuff is then inflated, theoretically isolating the glottic aperture from the rest of the pharynx. The patient may then be ventilated via the tube. Tracheal or esophageal cannulation during insertion is unlikely owing to the size of the device.

Several studies have found that passage of the LMA may be accomplished by trained medical or paramedical personnel as rapidly as placement of a conventional endotracheal tube.[26, 27] After a brief training period, paramedical personnel successfully placed the LMA in 94% of attempts, whereas an endotracheal tube was successfully inserted in 51% of attempts.[27] In a study of 100 spontaneously breathing patients, physicians with various levels of medical experience were reported to have an 80% success rate in placing the LMA on the first attempt.[28] Including all attempts, the success rate was 98%.[28] However, the latter studies were conducted in the controlled environment of an operating room and once again may not accurately reflect conditions in the field. In a single case report, Calder and colleagues

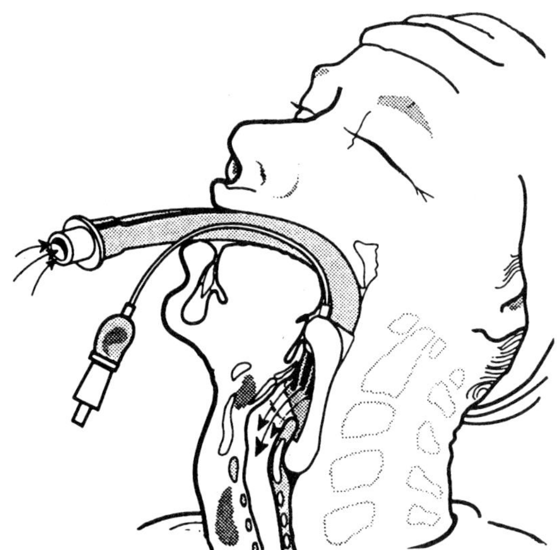

Figure 104–2. An LMA device. (From Davies PRF, Tighe SQM, Greenslade GL, et al: Laryngeal mask airway and tracheal tube insertion by unskilled personnel. Lancet 1990; 336:977–979. © by the Lancet Ltd., 1990.)

described successful use of the LMA in an emergent situation when endotracheal intubation was not possible.[29]

Studies addressing the utility of the LMA have been very limited in scope. There are no comparative data, using $Paco_2$ as a criterion, with respect to the efficacy of ventilation via LMA versus a conventional endotracheal tube. Brodrick and coworkers[28] reported that applying 17 cm H_2O pressure via the LMA resulted in substantial mouth leakage in 10% of patients. In a number of these individuals, the leak was sufficiently large to preclude delivery of adequate ventilation. Another limitation of the LMA is the need to anesthetize patients during its insertion and subsequent removal. Not only is this necessary to minimize patients' discomfort, but inadequate anesthesia with LMA use has been associated with coughing or laryngospasm.[28] Other factors that may reduce enthusiasm for the LMA, particularly outside an operating room setting, include its inability to protect the airway against aspiration of gastric contents, gastric insufflation if the LMA is improperly placed, down-folding of the epiglottis, and laryngospasm.[26, 28] Brodrick and associates suggested that using an introducer during insertion may facilitate proper placement of the LMA.[28]

In summary, there are too few data to suggest that the LMA is a viable alternative to tracheal intubation in the field by either skilled or unskilled personnel. Furthermore, there is no conclusive information demonstrating that adequate ventilation may be delivered through the LMA for the period of time likely to be required during field resuscitation or during short periods outside the operating room. Finally, the utility of the LMA in conjunction with standard positive-pressure ventilators, rather than with manual resuscitation bags as described in the literature, remains to be established.

Positive-Pressure Ventilation Via Mouthpiece

Administration of positive-pressure ventilation via mouthpiece was described by Garay and colleagues in 1981[30] in patients with chronic ventilatory failure. Although this interface does not appear to lend itself to use in the setting of cardiopulmonary resuscitation or in the long-term management of patients with acute respiratory failure (ARF) in the intensive care unit (ICU), it merits discussion because of its successful use in providing ventilatory support to patients with chronic hypercapnia.[31–33] Bach and coworkers have demonstrated that a lip-seal mouthpiece, held in place with a head harness, can be successfully used for nocturnal positive-pressure ventilatory support in patients with neuromuscular and chest wall diseases. These investigators acknowledge that among the problems with this interface are the potential risk of aspiration pneumonia, the development or worsening of dental malocclusion, temporomandibular joint problems, and leakage of delivered tidal volume via the nose or mouth (particularly in edentulous patients and those with buccopharyngeal muscle weakness). Despite the many potential difficulties, however, Bach and his colleagues have indicated that these have neither been frequent nor major factors affecting patients' care.

It is conceivable that ventilatory assistance via the mouth could also be considered for postoperative patients who experience short-term difficulty after extubation. This application would be limited by the anticipated duration of continuous use, the ability to maintain a tight mouth seal, and the risk of aspiration. In general, however, because of concerns about its efficacy and safety and because there are no data describing its application in acutely ill patients, the use of a mouthpiece for noninvasive ventilation in this patient population is not considered to be a routine therapeutic option.

Nasal or Facemask Interfaces for Positive-Pressure Ventilation

The utility of positive-pressure ventilation via mask has been long recognized in the form of continuous positive airway pressure (CPAP) (discussed later). The application of CPAP via nasal interface in adult patients with obstructive sleep apnea was initially described by Sullivan and associates.[34, 35] In this report, CPAP was administered via nasal prongs that were sealed within the patients' nares with silicon rubber. Other researchers subsequently described various self-sealing nasal masks and prongs through which positive pressure could be applied.[36–40]

Several years after the utility of nasal CPAP for the treatment of obstructive sleep apnea was recognized, the nasal route was also used to deliver nocturnal positive-pressure ventilatory support to patients with chronic and acute ventilatory failure, due to various causes.[2, 41–56] The nasal route of delivery offered the safety of an unencumbered oral airway through which a patient could breathe in the event of mechanical ventilator failure and reduced the likelihood of aspiration of gastric contents. A significant potential problem with the nasal interface, however, is leakage of delivered gas through the mouth. This may prevent administration of adequate tidal volumes when using a volume-cycled ventilator or may cause dysfunctional cycling of pressure-limited ventilators. Mouth leakage may be a particularly troublesome issue in patients who are unable to keep their mouth closed secondary to neuromuscular disease or air hunger or during sleep. Chin straps have been used in an effort to enforce mouth closure, although the authors have frequently found them to be ineffective because of leakage between the teeth.[57] Consequently, oronasal interfaces have been found to be useful in selected patients[57] (Fig. 104–3.)

No conclusive data support mandatory insertion of a nasogastric tube when using an oronasal mask. Clearly, a nasogastric tube should be used in patients who are at risk for vomiting or in those who cannot remove the mask themselves, unless close, continuous observation of the patient is feasible, as in an ICU. During positive-pressure ventilatory assistance via oronasal mask, consideration also should be

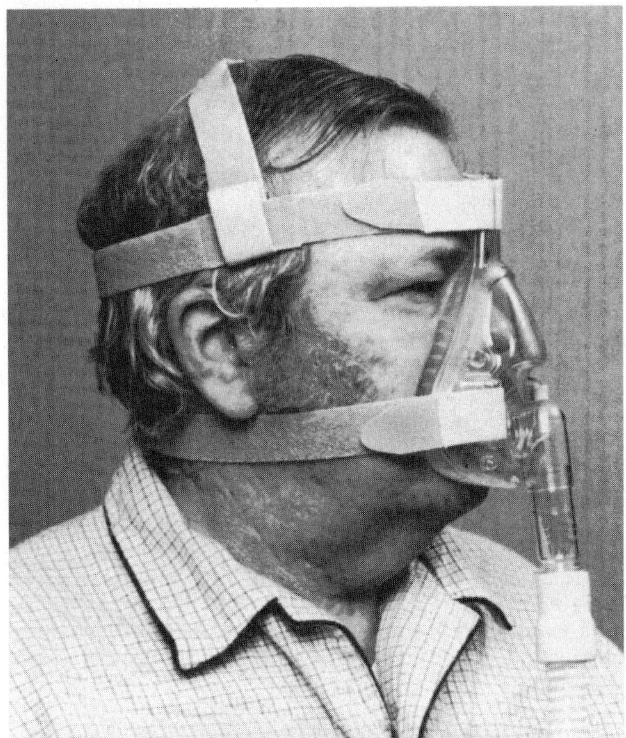

Figure 104–3. Oronasal interface. (Courtesy of Respironics, Murrysville, PA.)

given to incorporating a safety valve in the positive-pressure circuit through which a patient may entrain room air with minimal dead space, in the event of mechanical failure. As described later, nasal and oronasal masks have become the mainstay for delivering noninvasive positive-pressure ventilatory support.

NONINVASIVE POSITIVE-PRESSURE VENTILATION TO PREVENT TRACHEAL INTUBATION IN ACUTELY ILL PATIENTS

Continuous Positive Airway Pressure for Patients with Acute Respiratory Failure

Positive-pressure therapy via mask is not a new concept, having been described in the early 20th century by Bunnell to deliver nitrous oxide and oxygen anesthesia as well as to enhance intraoperative lung inflation[58] (Fig. 104–4). During subsequent decades, the beneficial impact of CPAP by mask in the treatment of patients with cardiogenic pulmonary edema and other forms of ARF has been reported. Barach and coworkers, as well as other investigators, reported successful treatment of patients in acute pulmonary edema with positive pressure delivered via either mask or hood.[59, 60] These investigators hypothesized that application of positive pressure minimized the magnitude of negative pleural pressure swings and prevented fluid shifts into the alveoli.[61] The findings of these early studies have been reinforced by others who demonstrated successful application of mask CPAP in the treatment of patients with cardiogenic pulmonary edema.[62–64] In two separate but similar studies, Rasanen and colleagues[63] and Bersten and coworkers[64] observed that patients in acute pulmonary edema who were treated with mask CPAP, supplemental oxygen, and conventional pharmacologic intervention had more rapid reduction in respiratory rate and $Pa{CO_2}$ than did a control population who were treated conventionally without CPAP. Patients treated with mask CPAP also experienced more rapid improvement in $Pa{O_2}$ and normalization of pH (Fig. 104–5). Despite these differences, however, neither in-hospital mortality nor the duration of hospitalization was influenced by the use of mask CPAP.

Possibly on the basis of its reported success in the treatment of both infant respiratory distress syndrome and cardiogenic pulmonary edema, CPAP has also been administered to treat patients with ARF. Greenbaum and colleagues[65] examined the impact of positive-pressure administration by mask in 14 patients with ARF due to various causes (Fig. 104–6). This therapy was deemed successful in preventing endotracheal intubation in eight patients, five of whom may have had at least some component of cardiogenic pulmonary edema. Two of the 14 patients experienced significant carbon dioxide retention during positive-pressure administration. It is important to note that the positive pressure provided to patients in this study, which the authors labeled as CPAP, actually reflected expiratory pressures that exceeded inspiratory pressures by 2 to 12 cm H_2O. Indeed, five patients received positive pressure *exclusively* during expiration. The work of breathing may have been substantially increased under these circumstances compared with CPAP defined in more contemporary terms (in which airway pressure is maintained at a constant level throughout both phases of the ventilatory cycle),[66, 67] and this may have adversely affected the study results.

In 44 patients with mild to moderate ARF due to unspecified causes, Smith and colleagues[68] observed improvement in $Pa{O_2}$ after applying an average of 9 cm H_2O CPAP by facemask. One patient required endotracheal intubation after developing respiratory acidemia during mask therapy.

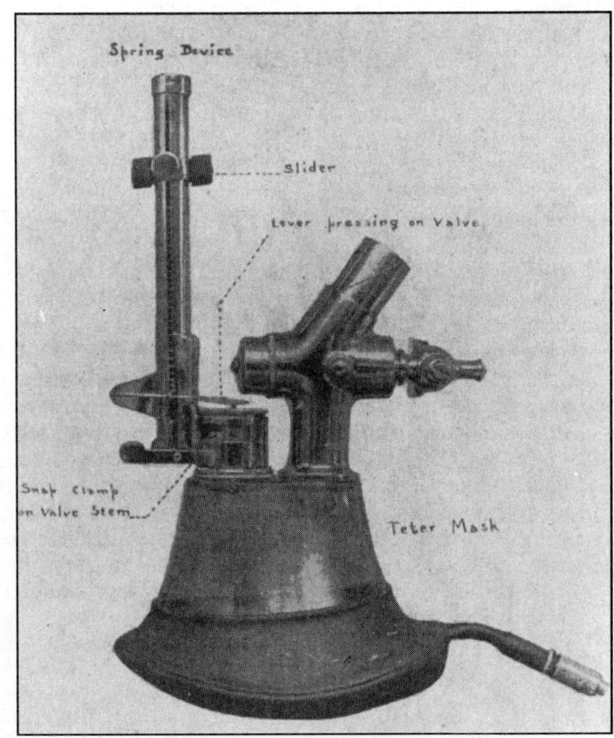

Figure 104–4. Attachment of a valve system to a Teter mask for delivery of intraoperative positive pressure. (From Bunnel SJ: The use of nitrous oxide and oxygen to maintain anesthesia and positive pressure for thoracic surgery. Am Med Assoc 1912; 58:835–838.)

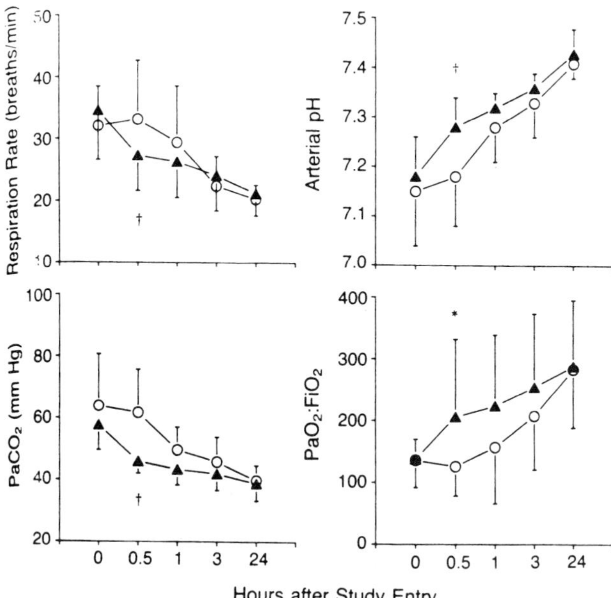

Figure 104–5. Comparison of ventilatory parameters in patients with cardiogenic pulmonary edema treated with oxygen at ambient pressure *(open circles)* and in patients who were treated with mask CPAP and supplemental oxygen. The *asterisk* indicates $P = .01$, and the daggers indicate $P < .01$ for comparison between the two groups. (From Bersten AD, Holt AW, Vedig AE, et al: Treatment of severe cardiogenic pulmonary edema with continuous positive airway pressure delivered by face mask. N Engl J Med 1991; 325:1825–1830. Reproduced by permission of *The New England Journal of Medicine.*)

Covelli and coworkers[62] applied at least 10 cm H_2O mask CPAP to 35 patients with adult respiratory distress syndrome due to various causes. Two patients had cardiogenic pulmonary edema, and three patients had what was described as noncardiogenic pulmonary edema of unknown cause. Patients were selected on the basis of having adequate alveolar ventilation before CPAP therapy and sufficient cognitive function to follow commands. Five of the 35 individuals who were treated with mask CPAP required tracheal intubation. Although Covelli and associates observed no change in the average Pa_{CO_2} of the study group after initiation of mask CPAP, the development of hypercapnia was reported by Meduri and colleagues in two patients with adult respiratory distress syndrome treated with this therapy at 10 and 18 cm H_2O, respectively.[69] These data extend the earlier experience of Smith and coworkers.[68]

Interpreting studies addressing the application of mask CPAP for treatment of ARF is confounded by the virtual absence of randomly selected control populations. It is therefore difficult to make definite conclusions about the impact of this treatment intervention on patients' outcome. In the absence of controlled trials, it is also impossible to assess the likelihood that mask CPAP will precipitate or exacerbate hypercapnia and ventilatory failure. Although many authorities have suggested that inability to maintain adequate spontaneous ventilation is a contraindication for the use of mask CPAP,[62, 70, 71] the variable experience in this regard mandates further research before definitive recommendations can be made. For the present, important questions remain about whether mask CPAP is an appropriate modality for noninvasive management of patients with ARF.

Continuous Positive Airway Pressure by Mask for Patients with Lower Airways Obstruction

In 1973, Barach and associates[72] first described the impact of CPAP, then termed continuous positive pressure breathing, on patients with emphysema, bronchitis, and asthma. Patients with emphysema had a significant reduction in minute ventilation with maintenance of Pa_{CO_2} while breathing with CPAP delivered via mouthpiece at 6.5 cm H_2O. The investigators speculated that CPAP reduced inspiratory effort and improved alveolar ventilation owing to reduced expiratory bronchiolar collapse. Patients with mixed emphysema and bronchitis, chronic bronchitis, and chronic asthma, however, were observed to have augmented minute ventilation while receiving 6.5 cm H_2O CPAP.

In eight asthmatic patients with histamine-induced bronchospasm, Martin and colleagues[73] examined the effect of CPAP applied via mouthpiece at a level of 12 cm H_2O over an interval of approximately 1 minute. CPAP was associated with a significant increase in mean inspiratory and expiratory airflow as well as decreased airway resistance. Furthermore, application of CPAP during bronchoconstriction increased minute ventilation by increasing both tidal volume and breathing frequency, reduced the pressure-time product (a measure of work) of the inspiratory muscles, decreased inspiratory swings in transdiaphragmatic pressure, and reduced the peak diaphragmatic electromyogram activity in two of the three individuals in whom this variable was measured. These data suggested decreased inspiratory work per liter ventilation and reduced diaphragm energy expenditure during inspiration. Because of the patients' increased breathing frequency, however, no change oc-

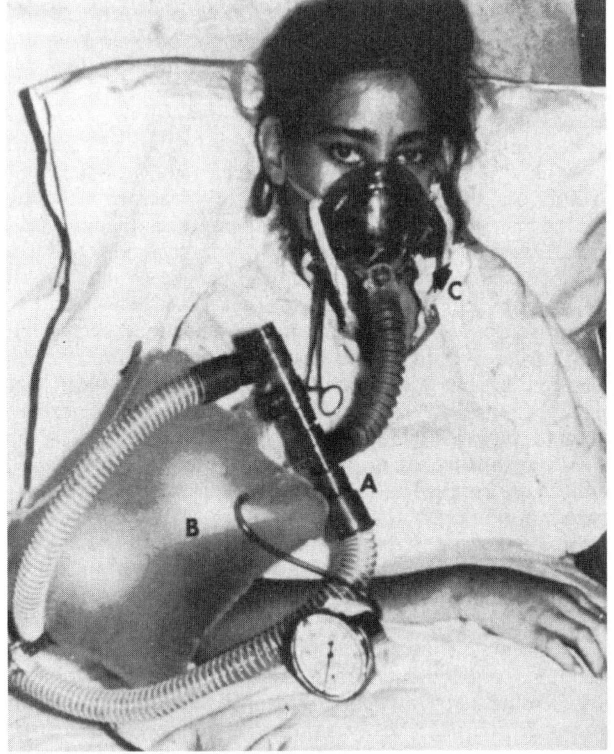

Figure 104–6. System used to administer CPAP or expiratory positive airway pressure by facemask. (From Greenbaum DM, Millen JE, Eross B, et al: Continuous positive airway pressure without tracheal intubation in spontaneously breathing patients. Chest 1976; 69:615–620.)

curred in the work performed by the inspiratory muscles per minute during CPAP administration.

The reduced airway resistance that was observed by Martin and coworkers[73] during CPAP administration may in part be related to increased lung volume, but it may also be attributable to reflex dilatation of the airways associated with stimulation of stretch receptors in the trachea or widening of the glottic aperture.[74] If these latter mechanisms are important, noninvasive application of CPAP may present a theoretic advantage over ventilatory support via endotracheal tube because it provides positive airway pressure without the untoward effects of an endotracheal tube. The reduced inspiratory work per liter ventilation during CPAP may occur at the expense of increased expiratory work to defend functional residual capacity (FRC) and prevent hyperinflation, which may tend to occur during CPAP therapy. Evidence for increased expiratory work during CPAP administration includes a smaller than expected increase in end-expiratory lung volume during positive-pressure breathing, increased expiratory gastric pressure, and increased expiratory airflow that cannot be explained by the reduced airway resistance. Maintaining FRC during CPAP therapy may confer the advantage of increasing inspiratory muscle efficiency. Changes in Pa_{CO_2} and dead space ventilation were not examined by Martin and colleagues. Although their findings are of substantial interest, the uncertain impact of increased expiratory work and unchanged inspiratory work over time during CPAP administration limits extrapolation of the data to the clinical setting, where bronchoconstriction may be more prolonged than during the brief experimental period of data collection.

Limited data have been collected *under clinical conditions* that systematically address the utility of noninvasively applied CPAP to patients with lower airways obstruction. Shivaram and coworkers reported in abstract form[75] on the impact of CPAP by mask in 20 patients who were hospitalized with acute bronchospasm. These investigators observed a progressive increase in end-expiratory flow with increasing levels of CPAP, whereas breathing frequency increased only after CPAP levels exceeded 6 cm H_2O. In part, these observations may be explained by the beneficial impact of low levels of positive expiratory pressure on reducing intrinsic positive end-expiratory pressure, together with recruitment of expiratory muscles, as suggested by Martin and coworkers.[73] In another study, Shivaram and associates[76] observed that 5 to 6 cm H_2O CPAP by mask reduced the duty cycle (ratio of inspiratory time to total cycle time) and increased the comfort of patients with acute bronchoconstriction. These data reinforced the previous work suggesting that CPAP reduces the inspiratory work of breathing under clinical circumstances.

Data regarding the impact of CPAP therapy on nocturnal asthma are conflicting. Chan and coworkers[77] reported that application of nasal CPAP successfully ameliorated nocturnal asthma in patients who also snored. It was speculated that stabilization of the upper airway prevented snoring-induced, reflex-mediated bronchoconstriction. This theory is supported by the observations by Guilleminault and coworkers, who evaluated the effect of nasal CPAP on the frequency of nocturnal asthma attacks in patients with narrow posterior airway spaces and obstructive apneas, hypopneas, or snoring.[78] As expected, the frequency of obstructive apneas and hypopneas was substantially reduced after initiating nocturnal nasal CPAP therapy. In addition, however, no episodes of nocturnal asthma were reported during the subsequent 6 to 14 months. Although CPAP may have been of benefit owing to elimination of snoring-induced reflex activation, an alternative explanation for the apparent relief of nocturnal asthma during CPAP therapy in these patients is prevention of snoring or apnea-related increases in vagal tone[79] and parasympathetic activity, which may promote bronchoconstriction. Finally, the excessively negative pleural pressures generated during obstructive sleep apnea may predispose patients to gastroesophageal reflux, which in turn may induce bronchospasm.[80] Minimizing the negative pleural pressure swings during sleep in these patients with CPAP may reduce the degree of reflux and have a beneficial effect on nocturnal asthma.[81]

In contrast to the foregoing observations of patients who have sleep-related upper-airway obstruction as well as nocturnal asthma, Martin and Pak[82] reported that in general, nasal CPAP administered during sleep had no beneficial effect on nocturnal asthma in patients without sleep apnea, hypopnea, or snoring. In fact, application of CPAP impaired the patients' sleep quality. The difference between the experiences of Martin and coworkers and those of others may be explained by differences in the study populations. The pathogenesis of nocturnal bronchospasm in those individuals with snoring and upper-airway obstruction during sleep may differ from that of individuals with nocturnal asthma alone. Therefore, it is plausible that the impact of CPAP on the two patient groups may also differ.

Although the literature suggests that application of CPAP by mask may be of benefit to patients with acute bronchospasm, no large, randomly controlled trials have tested the hypothesis that this modality offers a clinical or cost advantage over current, conventional treatment regimens. In addition, the effect of potentially increased expiratory work remains to be explored. For these reasons, judgment regarding the routine use of CPAP for the treatment of acute asthmatic attacks must await further investigation. Similarly, there are too few data defining the utility and risks associated with CPAP therapy for nocturnal asthma. Further studies are necessary to define which patient populations are likely to derive benefit from mask CPAP and to determine if it has advantages over existing treatment protocols.

Continuous Positive Airway Pressure by Mask for Patients Suffering Chest Wall Trauma or Lung Contusion

In the past decade, mask CPAP has been used to provide chest wall stabilization and maintain FRC in trauma victims with flail chest or lung contusion. Linton and Potgeiter[83] reported that application of CPAP by mask at pressures of at least 5 cm H_2O was associated with fewer complications and shorter length of stay in an ICU compared with administration of intermittent mandatory ventilation (IMV) via endotracheal tube. Assignment of patients to the mask CPAP or IMV groups was not random in this study, and although the two populations appeared to be clinically equivalent, physician bias cannot be precluded as an influential factor in the results of this study. This concern notwithstanding, more recent experience has also suggested that mask CPAP is a viable therapeutic alternative in patients with flail chest or pulmonary contusion. Branson and coworkers reported successful noninvasive therapy in 94% of these patients.[71] It would therefore appear that although published data are limited and prospective randomized control trials have not been performed, mask CPAP is a reasonable approach to the treatment of those patients with chest trauma who are capable of maintaining adequate ventilation in conjunction with administration of adequate analgesia. Care must be taken, however, to monitor the Pa_{CO_2} carefully during therapy because of the potential for unacceptable hypoventilation due to patient's underlying disease and the possible effects of CPAP per se. Caution in this regard is particularly warranted if analgesics that may suppress ventilatory chemosensitivity and load compensation are used.

Continuous Positive Airway Pressure by Mask for Patients with Atelectasis

Using an experimental model of atelectasis, Anderson and coworkers observed that lung re-expansion could be achieved with lower peak transpulmonary pressure and attenuated swings in transpulmonary pressure when CPAP was applied, compared with "deep breathing" and mechanical ventilation using ambient end-expiratory pressure.[84] In a subsequent prospective, randomized controlled study of postoperative patients, Andersen and colleagues[85] observed that approximately 15 cm H_2O CPAP by mask, applied once per hour, provided better resolution of atelectasis than physical therapy with postural drainage, deep breathing, and endotracheal suction. In separate case reports, Williamson and Modell[86] described successful treatment of refractory atelectasis after application of CPAP in a trauma victim, whereas Duncan and colleagues[87] used CPAP via nasal mask in postoperative patients.

Although the foregoing studies suggest that CPAP via mask may facilitate resolution of atelectasis, several studies have demonstrated that prophylactic intervention with this modality does not prevent the development of postoperative pulmonary complications. Stock and coworkers[88] compared the incidence of pneumonia, deterioration of spirometric parameters of pulmonary function, gas exchange, and FRC, as well as the radiographic incidence of atelectasis after median sternotomy, in 38 patients who were randomly assigned to receive "cough and deep-breathing," incentive spirometry, or mask CPAP. No difference was noted among the three postoperative regimens with respect to any outcome variable, except that 72 hours after surgery the incidence of atelectasis was lower in those patents who received CPAP. It should be noted, however, that the overall incidence of pneumonia for the entire study population was only 3%, which may be too low to detect treatment differences. The observations by Stock and associates[88] were consistent with those by Good and coworkers,[89] who found no reduction in the incidence of postoperative radiographic complications between ventilation using positive end-expiratory pressure and ambient end-expiratory pressure. The unimpressive performance of intermittent mask CPAP therapy relative to other, conventional efforts to reduce postoperative pulmonary complications may in part be attributable to the very transient nature of CPAP-related improvement in pulmonary function. Deterioration in FRC and forced vital capacity to pre-CPAP levels has been reported to occur within 10 minutes after termination of CPAP application.[90] Nonetheless, Stock and colleagues[88] concluded that although intermittent mask CPAP therapy does not confer substantial benefit over other postoperative protocols, efforts to prevent pulmonary complications may have value in avoiding pulmonary function deterioration and complications. They further suggested that CPAP by mask may be a preferable approach to this aspect of postoperative care because of its non–effort-dependent nature and because it is not associated with as much discomfort as incentive spirometry or coughing with deep breathing. In contrast, Bartlett[91] suggested that postoperative prophylaxis for pulmonary complications can be satisfactorily provided by having patients spontaneously inhale to maximum lung volume several times per hour. He added, however, that intermittent positive pressure using any modality via mouthpiece may be useful in those patients who cannot sustain a sufficient inspiratory volume. This suggestion is based on the concept that development of an adequate transpulmonary pressure is instrumental in preventing decrement of lung volume and consequent intrapulmonary shunting. Bartlett speculated that using a mouthpiece to administer CPAP in patients who are predisposed to losing consciousness (perhaps facilitated by administration of sedating analgesics) would reduce the risk of gastric distention or aspiration of gastric contents compared with using a tight-fitting oronasal mask.[91] Under these circumstances, in contrast to an oronasal mask held in place with straps, the mouthpiece would most likely fall out of a patient's mouth if consciousness were lost.

Continuous Positive Airway Pressure by Mask for Patients with Tracheobronchomalacia

Although tracheobronchomalacia is a relatively uncommon problem, it represents a therapeutic challenge in patients with difficulty clearing airway secretions, atelectasis, and dyspnea. Application of CPAP via mask may improve sputum clearance by moving the equal-pressure point peripherally. In addition, pneumatic stenting of the airway by CPAP may relieve dyspnea and facilitate re-expansion of collapsed lung parenchyma.[92] Ferguson and Benoist[92] described three patients with tracheobronchomalacia who obtained symptomatic relief and resolution of lobar atelectasis with CPAP by nasal mask at 10 cm H_2O during sleep as well as during chest physical therapy. One patient used nasal CPAP during both stationary bicycle exercise and at night, with improved exertional tolerance even without CPAP. Although there are no systematic studies addressing the utility of CPAP in patients with tracheobronchomalacia, the available evidence suggests that it may be therapeutically useful in at least some patients.

Noninvasive Positive-Pressure Ventilation

During the past decade, numerous investigators have described noteworthy success using nasal CPAP in the treatment of obstructive sleep apnea and using noninvasive, nocturnal positive pressure in the treatment of patients with chronic respiratory failure due to neuromuscular diseases and chest wall deformities.[34, 35, 37, 41–44, 46–50, 93–95, 95a] In light of these experiences, interest has been renewed in administering various positive-pressure modalities via mask to patients who do not require endotracheal intubation to facilitate clearance of airway secretions.

In 1989, Meduri and colleagues[69] evaluated the efficacy of mechanical ventilation via facemask in 10 patients with ARF. Six patients had acute hypercapnia and respiratory acidosis, and four patients had acute hypoxemic failure (defined by Pa_{O_2}/F_{IO_2} less than 200 with or without hypercapnia). Those patients with acute hypercapnic failure had chronic obstructive pulmonary disease (COPD) in conjunction with either congestive heart failure or evidence of a respiratory tract infection. Those with hypoxemic failure had ARDS (secondary to sepsis or pneumonia) or cardiogenic pulmonary edema. Within hours of initiating therapy with either pressure support or pressure control modes of ventilation via mask, the patients with hypercapnic ventilatory failure had a reduction in Pa_{CO_2} and improvement in arterial pH. Before application of noninvasive mechanical ventilation, the patients with hypoxemic failure had signs of ventilatory fatigue with respiratory acidosis on CPAP. After initiation of noninvasive ventilatory support, all four patients showed substantial improvement in oxygenation. One patient eventually became intolerant of the facemask and required endotracheal intubation. For the entire patient population, the mean duration of ventilatory support via facemask was 33 hours. The only complication from noninvasive ventilation was skin abrasion at the bridge of the nose. It should be noted that a nasogastric tube was placed before beginning ventilation via facemask as a precaution against pulmonary aspiration of gastric contents and aerophagia.

Meduri and coworkers subsequently extended their findings in an additional 18 patients with various degrees of acute respiratory acidosis.[96] Twelve patients had COPD either alone (nine patients) or in combination with congestive heart failure (two patients) or pneumonia (one patient). Of the remaining patients, two had pulmonary edema, two had asthma, one had pneumonia, and one had fibrothorax. Patients were initially placed on pressure support ventilation via facemask using a conventional life-support ventilator, although mask leak occasionally necessitated a change to the IMV mode of ventilatory support. Of the 18 patients included in the study, noninvasive ventilatory support failed in 6 patients, who required endotracheal intubation. One of these patients required intubation to facilitate secretion clearance and presumed aspiration pneumonia during noninvasive therapy. Two other patients became intolerant of the mask but required no further ventilatory support. Thus, if a successful outcome is defined as avoidance of endotracheal intubation and tolerance of the technique, noninvasive support was successful in 56% of patients. Of interest, the investigators observed that the rapidity of improvement on noninvasive ventilatory support predicted the outcome. Those patients who exhibited an increase in arterial pH from a value less than 7.30 to a value greater than 7.30, 2 to 6 hours after the institution of therapy, were more likely to have a successful outcome (positive predictive value = 92%). Similarly, more than a 15% decrease in Pa_{CO_2} during this period also predicted a successful outcome. Similarly, Bott and colleagues[96a] found nasal ventilation via a volume-cycled ventilator to be effective in reducing Pa_{CO_2}, increasing pH, and reducing breathlessness in patients with COPD and ARF.

To further identify those factors associated with a successful outcome with noninvasive ventilation, Wysocki and colleagues[97] treated 17 patients with ARF using a conventional life-support ventilator to deliver pressure support ventilation via facemask. The study group were highly selected, however, with exclusion of patients with neurologic disease, multisystem organ failure, otolaryngologic or gastric surgery, facial trauma, asthma, or postcardiopulmonary resuscitation. Four patients who were included in the study developed ARF after postoperative extubation, and two patients developed ARF after extubation from a resolving episode of ARF. Of the 17 patients, 8 (47%) had successful noninvasive ventilation (defined as not requiring intubation and surviving until discharge from the ICU). There was no difference between the patients with successful and unsuccessful noninvasive ventilation with respect to the cause of ARF, although those individuals with postextubation ARF appeared to fare better. In addition, patients with hypercapnia but lower overall physiologic derangement scores also appeared to have better outcomes. Only two patients were considered treatment failures on the basis of inability to tolerate the mask or an inadequate mask fit.

Brochard and coworkers examined the physiologic impact of pressure support ventilation via facemask using a customized system in 11 patients with COPD.[98] All but one of these patients were hypercapnic. After 45 minutes of intervention, the study group had exhibited a statistically significant reduction in breathing rate and an increase in minute ventilation, with consequent reduction in Pa_{CO_2}. Transdiaphragmatic pressure was significantly reduced, and diaphragm electromyogram activity was decreased during pressure support therapy, suggesting a decrease in the work of breathing despite augmented minute ventilation. These investigators subsequently described the clinical outcome of 13 patients hospitalized for exacerbations of COPD and treated intermittently with pressure support via facemask for periods ranging from 3 to 12 hours.[98] Outcome data were compared with 13 matched historical control patients who had not been treated with noninvasive ventilatory assistance. None of the patients treated with pressure support via mask required endotracheal intubation, compared with 11 of the 13 historical control patients. Although there was no difference in hospital mortality between the two groups, the duration of stay in the ICU was shorter in the pressure support–treated patients. No complications from mask ventilatory support were reported, although in this context, it may be significant to note that mask pressure was kept below 25 cm H_2O.

In a study of noninvasive positive-pressure ventilation in a group composed largely of postoperative patients experiencing ARF after extubation, Pennock and colleagues examined the efficacy of noninvasive bilevel positive airway pressure ventilation in avoiding reintubation.[56, 56a] Bilevel positive airway pressure permits independent adjustment and delivery of inspiratory positive airway pressure (IPAP) and expiratory positive airway pressure (EPAP). This means of ventilatory support has been shown to provide effective noninvasive ventilatory assistance both to patients with chronic ventilatory failure and to patients with obstructive sleep apnea.[41, 43, 44, 48, 94] Pennock and coworkers selected patients who had undergone surgery at least 36 hours earlier and who had clinical evidence of ventilatory muscle fatigue including use of accessory muscles of ventilation, tachypnea, chest wall paradox, or Pa_{CO_2} greater than 50 mm Hg. Patients were also included in the study if they had Pa_{O_2} less than 60 mm Hg despite an F_{IO_2} of 0.55. Bilevel positive airway pressure was initially applied at 10 cm H_2O IPAP and 5 cm H_2O EPAP to patients with hypoxemic respiratory failure and 10 cm H_2O IPAP and 2 cm H_2O EPAP to patients with hypercapnic ventilatory failure. Pressure settings were subsequently adjusted for patients' comfort. If oxygenation remained at unacceptable levels, IPAP and EPAP were concomitantly raised such that the gradient between the two pressures was kept constant. For persistently unacceptable hypercapnia, IPAP was progressively raised in 2-cm H_2O increments to augment tidal volume. After successful institution of therapy, patients had a rapid decrease in respiratory rate, relief of dyspnea, and generally improved arterial blood gas values. Twenty-two of 29 patients (76%) successfully recovered without requiring endotracheal intubation. Despite the fact that a nasogastric tube was placed in only one patient, no instances of aspiration, gastric distention, or other complications, with the exception of minor abrasions on the bridge of the nose, were reported.

The results of the foregoing studies, which suggest that noninvasive positive-pressure therapy can be effectively used to treat acutely ill patients with COPD, are to be contrasted with the results reported by Foglio and colleagues.[99] In a retrospective study, these investigators examined the outcome of 49 patients who were hospitalized because of acute ventilatory failure secondary to exacerbation of COPD. All patients underwent a daily trial of positive-pressure ventilation via nasal interface using a volume-cycled ventilator in the control mode. The outcomes of those individuals who were both tolerant of and compliant with ventilator support were compared with those who received a standard treatment regimen without noninvasive ventilatory assistance. Patients who received noninvasive ventilation were treated with four 1-hour sessions per day. Despite initial identification as candidates for noninvasive therapy, 10 of the 49 patients refused nasal noninvasive ventilation and 14 additional patients were unable to tolerate it after beginning the therapeutic regimen. After 10 days, no significant difference in arterial blood gas values was noted between those patients who ultimately used noninvasive ventilation as directed and those who did not. Although of interest because of its discordant findings, this study may be biased by the fact that patients were not randomly assigned to the mask ventilation group and control group. Rather, patients who were intolerant of noninvasive ventilation were selected as controls, thus possibly obscuring differences between groups. It is also possible that the limited duration of positive-pressure application to the patients contributed to the similar outcomes of the two study groups. Foglio and coworkers also observed various side effects resulting from noninvasive positive-pressure ventilatory assistance, including air leakage at the mask-skin interface, skin/eye irritation, mask discomfort, nasal dryness, and gastric distention (despite the use of the nasal interface).

Chevrolet and colleagues[100] examined noninvasive positive-pressure therapy in acutely ill patients from the very important perspective of its implications on nursing care. These investigators reported their experience in six consecutive patients who were hospitalized in an ICU with ARF. Nasal ventilation with a volume-cycled ventilator in the assist-control mode was used in all six individuals. Three patients had a restrictive pulmonary process, and three had COPD. A significant reduction in Pa_{CO_2} was observed in all patients during nasal ventilation. The researchers' enthusiasm for this form of therapy was diminished by the observation that nursing attendance at the bedside was required during virtually the entire period of noninvasive ventilation in the three individuals with COPD (average of about 90% across the three patients). In contrast, nurses were required at the bedside of the patients with restrictive pulmonary processes for less than 50% of the treatment period (average of about 40% across the three patients). The greater demand for nursing time during noninvasive ventilation by patients with COPD was not explained by differences in the severity of illness, and the reason for this observation remains uncertain. Chevrolet and coworkers did note that the nasal mask was poorly tolerated by patients with COPD and that nursing time was often devoted to alleviating fear and anxiety. They also speculated that the assist-control mode may not be optimally tolerated by some patients and suggested that pressure support ventilation may be preferable.

In summary, a review of the literature suggests that noninvasive ventilation may be effectively used to avoid endotracheal intubation in a substantial proportion of patients with ARF. Although it is clear that this treatment technique is useful in certain individuals, it is also noteworthy that none of the published studies reviewed here included contemporary, randomly selected control populations, thus precluding precise data interpretation. Similarly, there are no published, controlled trials examining the relative impact of various noninvasive modes of positive-pressure ventilation on the outcome and cost of care in acutely ill patients. More work is needed to identify the patient populations most likely to benefit from noninvasive positive-pressure ventilation, to clarify the most efficacious manner in which it should be administered, and to define what risks, if any, are associated with it.

It is clear that positive-pressure ventilatory support has evolved considerably since the 19th century, when surgical cannulation of the trachea was the state of the art. Healthcare delivery is progressing to make obsolete those previous, revolutionary advances that proved lifesaving at the time and in some cases continue to do so. It is our task to continue to refine our therapeutic approaches in a manner that preserves the positive aspects of existing medical interventions and eliminates or at least modifies those features that are risky and undesirable. Toward this end, maintenance of a stable airway and administration of adequate alveolar ventilation are inherently laudable objectives. Achieving these goals without placing a foreign body into the airway would represent progress.

References

1. Applebaum EL, Bruce DL: Tracheal Intubation. Philadelphia, WB Saunders, Co. 1976; pp 1–5.
2. Heironimus TWI, Bageant RA: Artificial airways uses and complications. *In*: Mechanical Artificial Ventilation. Adriani J (Ed). Springfield, IL, Charles C Thomas, 1977; pp 402–428.
3. Michael DTA: Mouth to lung airway for cardiac resuscitation. Lancet 1968; 2:1329.
4. Michael DTA: Esophageal obturator airway. Med Instrum 1977; 11:331–333.
5. Schofferman J, Oill P, Lewis AJ: The esophageal obturator airway. A clinical evaluation. Chest 1976; 69:67–71.
6. Meislin HW: The esophageal obturator airway: A study of respiratory effectiveness. Ann Emerg Med 1980; 9:54–59.
7. Donen N, Tweed A: The esophageal obturator airway: An appraisal. Can Anaesth Soc J 1983; 30:194–200.
8. Hammargren Y, Clinton JE, Ruiz E: A standard comparison of esophageal obturator airway and endotracheal tube ventilation in cardiac arrest. Ann Emerg Med 1985; 14:953–958.
9. Goldenberg IF, Campion BC, Siebold CM, et al: Morbidity and mortality in patients receiving the esophageal obturator airway and the endotracheal tube in prehospital cardiopulmonary arrest. Minn Med 1986; 69:707–713.
10. Bryson TK, Benumof JL, Ward CF: The esophageal obturator airway. A clinical comparison to ventilation with a mask and oropharyngeal airway. Chest 1978; 74:537–539.
11. Michael DTA: The role of the esophageal obturator airway in cardiopulmonary resuscitation. Circulation 1986; 74:IV134–IV137.
12. Gertler JP, Cameron DE, Shea K, et al: The esophageal obturator airway: Obturator or obtundator? J Trauma 1985; 25:424–426.
13. Crippen D, Olvey S, Graffis R: Gastric rupture: An esophageal obturator airway complication. Ann Emerg Med 1981; 10:370–373.
14. Kassels SJ, Robinson WA, O'Bara KJ: Esophageal perforation associated with the esophageal obturator airway. Crit Care Med 1980; 8:386–389.
15. McCabe CJ, Browne BJ: Esophageal obturator airway, ET tube, and pharyngeal-tracheal lumen airway. Am J Emerg Med 1986; 4:64–71.
16. Pons PT: Esophageal obturator airway. Emerg Med Clin North Am 1988; 6:693–698.
17. Merrifield AJ, Waldmann C, Blundell MD: Ventilation through a new emergency airway in an anesthetized man. Proceedings of the Anesthetic Research Society, 1983.
18. Hooks PJ, Scarberry EN, Bryan-Brown C: The pharyngeal tracheal airway lumen (PTL) airway: A single handed emergency resuscitation tube. Society of Critical Care Medicine, 1983.
19. Nieman JT, Rosborough JP, Meyers R, et al: The pharyngeotracheal lumen airway: Preliminary investigation of a new adjunct. Ann Emerg Med 1984; 13:591–596.
20. Bartlett RL, Martin SD, McMahon JMJ, et al: A field comparison of the pharyngeotracheal lumen airway and the endotracheal tube. J Trauma 1992; 32:280–284.
21. McMahan S, Ornato JP, Racht EM, et al: Multi-agency, prehospital evaluation of the pharyngeo-tracheal lumen (PTL) airway. Prehospital and Disaster Medicine 1992; 7:13–18.
22. Kern KB, Nelson JR, Norman SA, et al: Oxygenation and ventilation during cardiopulmonary resuscitation utilizing contin-

uous oxygen delivery via a modified pharyngeal-tracheal lumened airway. Chest 1992; 101:522–529.
23. Brain AIJ: The laryngeal mask airway—a possible new solution to airway problems in the emergency situation. Arch Emerg Med 1984; 1:229–232.
24. Brain AIJ: The laryngeal mask—a new concept in airway management. Br J Anaesth 1983; 55:801–805.
25. Brain AIJ: Three cases of difficult intubation overcome by the laryngeal mask airway. Anaesthesia 1985; 40:353–355.
26. Sarma VJ: The use of a laryngeal mask airway in spontaneously breathing patients. Acta Anaesthesiol Scand 1990; 34:669–672.
27. Davies PRF, Tighe SQM, Greenslade GL, et al: Laryngeal mask airway and tracheal tube insertion by unskilled personnel. Lancet 1990; 336:977–979.
28. Brodrick PM, Webster NR, Nunn JF: The laryngeal mask airway. A study in 100 patients during spontaneous breathing. Anesthesia 1989; 44:238–241.
29. Calder I, Ordman AJ, Jackowski A, et al: The brain laryngeal airway. Anesthesia 1990; 45:137–139.
30. Garay SM, Turino GM, Goldring RM: Sustained reversal of chronic hypercapnia in patients with alveolar hypoventilation syndromes. Long-term maintenance with noninvasive nocturnal mechanical ventilation. Am J Med 1981; 70:269–274.
31. Bach JR, Alba AS, Bohatiuk G, et al: Mouth intermittent positive pressure ventilation in the management of postpolio respiratory insufficiency. Chest 1987; 91:859–864.
32. Bach JR, Alba A, Mosher R, et al: Intermittent positive pressure ventilation via nasal access in the management of respiratory insufficiency. Chest 1987; 92:168–170.
33. Bach JR, Alba AS, Saporito LR: Intermittent positive pressure ventilation via the mouth as an alternative to tracheostomy for 257 ventilator users. Chest 1993; 103:174–182.
34. Sullivan CE, Berthon-Jones M, Issa FG, et al: Reversal of obstructive sleep apnoea by continuous positive airway pressure applied through the nares. Lancet 1981; 1:862–865.
35. Sullivan CE, Issa FG, Berthon-Jones M, et al: Home treatment of obstructive sleep apnoea with continuous positive airway pressure applied through a nose mask. Bull Eur Physiopathol Respir 1984; 20:49–54.
36. Rapoport DM, Sorkin B, Garay SM, et al: Reversal of the "pickwickian syndrome" by long-term use of nocturnal nasal airway pressure. N Engl J Med 1982; 307:931–933.
37. Sanders MH: CPAP via nasal mask: A treatment for sleep apnea. Chest 1983; 83:144–145.
38. Mayer LS, Kerby GR, Whitman RA: Evaluation of a new nasal device for administration of continuous positive airway pressure for obstructive sleep apnea. Am Rev Respir Dis 1989; 139:A114.
39. Mayer LS, Kerby GR, Whitman RA, et al: Continued evaluation of a new nasal device for administration of continuous positive airway pressure. Am Rev Respir Dis 1990; 141:A684.
40. Harris C, Daniels B, Peterson R, et al: Comparison of cannula and mask systems for administration of nasal continuous positive airway pressure for treatment of obstructive sleep apnea. Sleep Res 1990; 19:233.
41. Waldhorn R: Nocturnal nasal intermittent positive pressure ventilation with bi-level positive airway pressure (BiPAP) in respiratory failure. Chest 1992; 101:516–521.
42. Segall D: Noninvasive nasal mask-assisted ventilation in respiratory failure of Duchenne muscular dystrophy. Chest 1988; 93:1298–1300.
43. Sanders MH, Kern NB: Long-term experience with BiPAP in neuromuscular disease patients: Clinical and physiologic implications. Presented at the Third World Congress for Sleep Apnea and Rhonchopathy. Tokyo, Japan, 1991, p 22.
44. Sanders MH, Black J, Stiller RA, et al: Nocturnal ventilatory assistance with bi-level positive airway pressure. Operative technique. Otolaryngol Head Neck Surg 1991; 2:56–62.
45. Rodenstein DO, Stanescu DC, Delguste P, et al: Adaptation to intermittent positive pressure ventilation applied through the nose during day and night. Eur Respir J 1989; 2:473–478.
46. Leger P, Jennequin J, Gerard M, et al: Home positive pressure ventilation via nasal mask for patients with neuromuscular weakness or restrictive lung or chest-wall disease. Respir Care 1989; 34:73–79.
47. Kerby GR, Mayer LS, Pingleton SK: Nocturnal positive pressure ventilation via nasal mask. Am Rev Respir Dis 1987; 135:738–740.
48. Hill N, Eveloff S, Carlisle C, et al: Efficacy of nocturnal ventilation in patients with restrictive thoracic disease. Am Rev Respir Dis 1992; 145:365–371.
49. Hill NS, Eveloff SE, Carlisle CC, et al: Efficacy of nocturnal nasal ventilation administered by the BiPAP ventilator in restrictive pulmonary diseases. Am Rev Respir Dis 1991; 143:A602.
50. Goldstein RS, De Rosie JA, Avendano MA, et al: Influence of noninvasive positive pressure ventilation on inspiratory muscles. Chest 1991; 99:408–415.
51. Gay P, Patel A, Viggiano R, et al: Nocturnal nasal ventilation for treatment of patients with hypercapnic respiratory failure. Mayo Clin Proc 1991; 66:695–703.
52. Ellis ER, Grunstein RR, Chan S, et al: Noninvasive ventilatory support during sleep improves respiratory failure in kyphoscoliosis. Chest 1988; 94:811–815.
53. Ellis ER, Bye PTP, Bruderer JW, et al: Treatment of respiratory failure during sleep in patients with neuromuscular disease. Positive-pressure ventilation through a nose mask. Am Rev Respir Dis 1987; 135:148–152.
54. Carroll N, Branthwaite MA: Control of nocturnal hypoventilation by nasal intermittent positive pressure ventilation. Thorax 1988; 43:349–353.
55. Branthwaite MA: Home mechanical ventilation. Eur Respir J 1990; 3:743–745.
56. Pennock BE, Kaplan PD, Carlin BW, et al: Pressure support ventilation with a simplified support system administered with a nasal mask in patients with respiratory failure. Chest 1991; 100:1371–1376.
56a. Pennock BE, Cranshaw L, Kaplan PD: Noninvasive nasal mask ventilation for acute respiratory failure: Institution of a new therapeutic technology for routine use. Chest 1994; 105:441–444.
57. Sanders MH, Kern NB, Costantino JP, et al: Use of oro-nasal interfaces for positive pressure ventilation. Chest (in press).
58. Bunnell S: The use of nitrous oxide and oxygen to maintain anesthesia and positive pressure for thoracic surgery. JAMA 1912; 58:835–838.
59. Barach AL, Martin J, Eckman M: Positive pressure respiration and its application to the treatment of acute pulmonary edema. Ann Intern Med 1938; 12:754.
60. Ansbro PF: Positive pressure respiration in the treatment of acute pulmonary edema. Am J Surg 1945; 118:185–194.
61. Barach AL, Martin J, Eckman L: Positive pressure respiration and its application to the treatment of acute pulmonary edema and respiratory obstruction. J Clin Invest 1937; 16:664.
62. Covelli HD, Weled BJ, Beekman JF: Efficacy of continuous positive airway pressure administered by face mask. Chest 1982; 81:147–150.
63. Räsänen J, Heikkilä J, Downs J, et al: Continuous positive airway pressure by face mask in acute cardiogenic pulmonary edema. Am J Cardiol 1985; 55:296–300.
64. Bersten AD, Holt AW, Vedig AE, et al: Treatment of severe cardiogenic pulmonary edema with continuous positive airway pressure delivered by face mask. N Engl J Med 1991; 325:1825–1830.
65. Greenbaum DM, Millen JE, Eross B, et al: Continuous positive airway pressure without tracheal intubation in spontaneously breathing patients. Chest 1976; 69:615–620.
66. Schlobohm RM, Falltrick RT, Quan SF, et al: Lung volumes, mechanics, and oxygenation during spontaneous positive-pressure ventilation: The advantage of CPAP over EPAP. Anesthesiology 1981; 55:416–422.
67. Gherini S, Peters RM, Virgilo RW: Mechanical work on the lungs and work of breathing with positive end-expiratory pressure and continuous positive airway pressure. Chest 1979; 76:251–256.
68. Smith RA, Kirby RR, Gooding JM, et al: Continuous positive airway pressure (CPAP) by face mask. Crit Care Med 1980; 8:483–485.
69. Meduri GU, Conoscenti CC, Menashe P, et al: Noninvasive face mask ventilation in patients with acute respiratory failure. Chest 1989; 95:865–870.

70. Hoff BH, Flemming DC, Sasse F: Use of positive airway pressure without endotracheal intubation. Crit Care Med 1979; 7:559–561.
71. Branson RD, Hurst JM, DeHaven CBJ: Mask CPAP: State of the art. Respir Care 1985; 30:846–857.
72. Barach AL, Bickerman HA, Rodgers J: Continuous positive pressure breathing in chronic obstructive lung disease: Effect on minute ventilation and blood gases. Ann Allergy 1973; 31:72–78.
73. Martin JG, Shore S, Engel LA: Effect of continuous positive airway pressure on respiratory mechanics and pattern of breathing in induced asthma. Am Rev Respir Dis 1982; 126:812–817.
74. Widdicombe JG: Reflex effects of lung inflation in tracheal volume. J Appl Physiol 1963; 18:681–686.
75. Shivaram U, Donath J, Khan F, et al: Continuous positive airway pressure (CPAP) in the treatment of acute bronchial asthma: clinical study of 20 patients. Am Rev Respir Dis 1984; 29:A41.
76. Shivaram U, Donath J, Khan FA, et al: Effects of continuous positive airway pressure in acute asthma. Respiration 1987; 52:157–162.
77. Chan CS, Woolcock AJ, Sullivan CE: Nocturnal asthma: Role of snoring and obstructive sleep apnea. Am Rev Respir Dis 1988; 137:1502–1504.
78. Guilleminault C, Quera-Salva MA, Powell N, et al: Nocturnal asthma: Snoring, small pharynx and nasal CPAP. Eur Respir J 1988; 1:902–907.
79. Guilleminault C, Tilkian A, Lehrman K, et al: Sleep apnea syndrome: States of sleep and autonomic dysfunction. J Neurol Neurosurg Psychiatry 1977; 40:718–725.
80. Harper PC, Bergner A, Kaye MD: Antireflux treatment for asthma. Improvement in patients with associated gastroesophageal reflux. Arch Intern Med 1987; 147:56–60.
81. Kerr P, Shoenut JP, Millar T, et al: Nasal CPAP reduces gastroesophageal reflux in obstructive sleep apnea syndrome. Chest 1992; 101:1539–1544.
82. Martin RJ, Pak J: Nasal CPAP in nonapneic nocturnal asthma. Chest 1991; 100:1024–1027.
83. Linton DM, Potgeiter PD: Conservative management of blunt chest trauma. S Afr Med J 1982; 61:917–919.
84. Andersen JB, Qvist J, Kann T: Recruiting collapsed lung through collateral channels with positive end-expiratory pressure. Scand J Respir Dis 1979; 60:260–266.
85. Andersen JB, Olesen KP, Eikard B, et al: Periodic continuous positive airway pressure, CPAP, by mask in the treatment of atelectasis. Eur J Respir Dis 1980; 61:20–25.
86. Williamson DC, Modell JH: Intermittent continuous positive airway pressure by mask. Its use in the treatment of atelectasis. Arch Surg 1982; 117:970–972.
87. Duncan SR, Negrin RS, Mihm FG, et al: Nasal continuous positive airway pressure in atelectasis. Chest 1987; 92:621–624.
88. Stock MC, Downs JB, Cooper RB, et al: Comparison of continuous positive airway pressure, incentive spirometry, and conservative therapy after cardiac operations. Crit Care Med 1984; 12:969–972.
89. Good JT Jr, Wolz JF, Anderson JT, et al: The routine use of positive end-expiratory pressure after open heart surgery. Chest 1979; 76:397–400.
90. Stock CM, Downs JB, Corkran ML: Pulmonary function before and after prolonged continuous positive airway pressure by mask. Crit Care Med 1984; 12:973–974.
91. Bartlett RH: Respiratory therapy to prevent pulmonary complications of surgery. Respir Care 1984; 29:667–679.
92. Ferguson GT, Benoist J: Nasal continuous positive airway pressure in the treatment of tracheomalacia. Am Rev Respir Dis 1993; 147:457–461.
93. Sanders MH: Nasal CPAP effect on patterns of sleep apnea. Chest 1984; 86:839–844.
94. Sanders MH, Kern N: Treatment of obstructive sleep apnea by using independently adjusted inspiratory and expiratory positive pressure via nasal mask. Physiologic and clinical implications. Chest 1990; 98:317–324.
95. Heckmatt J, Loh L, Dubowitz V: Night-time nasal ventilation in neuromuscular disease. Lancet 1990; 335:579–582.
95a. Hill NS: Noninvasive ventilation: Does it work? Am Rev Respir Dis 1993; 147:1050–1055.
96. Meduri GU, Abou-Shala N, Fox RC, et al: Noninvasive face mask mechanical ventilation in patients with acute hypercapnic respiratory failure. Chest 1991; 100:445–454.
96a. Bott J, Carroll MP, Conway JH, et al: Randomised controlled trial of nasal ventilation in acute ventilatory failure due to chronic obstructive airway disease. Lancet 1993; 341:1555–1557.
97. Wysocki M, Tric L, Wolff MA, et al: Noninvasive pressure support ventilation in patients with acute respiratory failure. Chest 1993; 103:907–913.
98. Brochard L, Isabey D, Piquet J, et al: Reversal of acute exacerbations of chronic obstructive lung disease by inspiratory assistance with a face mask. N Engl J Med 1990; 323:1523–1530.
99. Foglio C, Vitacca M, Quadri A, et al: Acute exacerbations in severe COLD patients. Treatment using positive pressure ventilation by nasal mask. Chest 1992; 101:1533–1538.
100. Chevrolet J-C, Jolliet P, Abajo B, et al: Nasal positive pressure ventilation in patients with acute respiratory failure. Difficult and time-consuming procedure for nurses. Chest 1991; 100:775–782.

CHAPTER 105

Extracorporeal and Intravascular Gas Exchange Devices

Harry L. Anderson, III, MD • Robert H. Bartlett, MD

Extracorporeal perfusion was first used successfully as therapy for respiratory failure in 1972, when Hill reported the recovery of a patient with the adult respiratory distress syndrome (ARDS) using prolonged extracorporeal support.[1] Since then, this type of bedside cardioperfusion technology has found use in selected neonatal, pediatric, and adult patients and is used for treatment of both respiratory and cardiac dysfunction. *Extracorporeal life support* (ECLS), a new term that replaces the term *extracorporeal membrane oxygenation* (ECMO), has many other names (Table 105–1). Most designations refer to extracorporeal passage of blood through a gas exchange device, or oxygenator, and then return of blood to a major vein or artery, thus providing a unique means of assisting respiration or blood pressure—hence the term *extracorporeal life support*. In this chapter, after the evolution of ECLS is described, the current technology and management of patients is discussed, as are worldwide results of ECLS for selected patient populations. The intravascular oxygenator (IVOX) is discussed at the conclusion of this chapter.

BACKGROUND

The first description of cardiopulmonary bypass dates back to 1937, when Gibbon described a system that consisted of a roller pump and a vertically mounted cylinder over which blood was pumped, allowing gas exchange of the blood with ambient gas.[2] This system was able to provide complete support of blood pressure and respiration when the pulmonary artery was occluded at the time of operation within the chest. It was with this system that cardiopulmonary bypass was born. Refinements in this technology as applied to cardiac surgery have led to more efficient membrane oxygenators and pumping systems and a better un-

TABLE 105–1. Common Acronyms for Types of Artificial Cardiac or Pulmonary Support

ECLS	Extracorporeal life support
ECMO	Extracorporeal membrane oxygenation
ECCOR or $ECCO_2R$	Extracorporeal CO_2 removal
$PECCO_2R$	Partial extracorporeal CO_2 removal
ECLA	Extracorporeal lung assist
CPS	Cardiopulmonary support
CPB	Cardiopulmonary bypass
LVAD	Left ventricular assist device
RVAD	Right ventricular assist device
IVOX	Intravascular oxygenator

derstanding of the interaction of blood with polymeric surfaces. Through these same avenues, ECLS was conceived, and this spinoff of cardiopulmonary bypass was modified for prolonged support of reversible heart or lung dysfunction at the bedside.

TECHNIQUE OF EXTRACORPOREAL LIFE SUPPORT

The ECLS perfusion circuit is depicted in Figure 105–1. In a manner similar to cardiopulmonary bypass, blood is drained from the vena cava, pumped through an oxygenator device (where exchange of oxygen [O_2] and carbon dioxide [CO_2] with blood takes place), warmed by a water-jacketed heat exchanger, and then returned to a major artery (carotid, femoral, aortic arch) in the case of venoarterial bypass or to a major vein (internal jugular, femoral) in the case of venovenous bypass. *Venoarterial bypass* provides both cardiac (i.e., blood pressure) and respiratory support (i.e., oxygenation and ventilation), whereas *venovenous bypass* provides respiratory support only (cardiac function and blood pressure must be normal or nearly normal). With venovenous bypass, the venous blood is oxygenated and CO_2 removed before reentering the venous system and mixing with venous blood from systemic circulation, raising the already low O_2 content of venous blood returning to the heart.

Bypass pump flow is limited by the rate at which venous blood is siphoned from a patient; therefore, the lowest-resistance configuration is selected for the drainage portion of the circuit. Large-bore, high-flow catheters are usually selected, and the internal jugular vein is usually chosen because it is the largest extrathoracic vein available by simple cutdown or by percutaneous access. Other veins that can be used for venous drainage (in order of decreasing preference) are the femoral vein or iliac vein (exposed by infraperitoneal dissection), as well as direct cannulation of the right atrium via thoracotomy.

Warmed, oxygenated blood is usually returned to (in decreasing order of preference) the common carotid artery, femoral artery, aortic arch, or axillary artery, in the case of venoarterial perfusion. In collateral-poor arterial beds (i.e., the leg supplied by the femoral artery, the arm supplied by the axillary artery), perfusion must also be supplied distal to the site of cannulation to prevent ischemia of the limb. With cannulation of the aortic arch through the right common carotid artery, the distal vessel is usually ligated; collateral perfusion from the external carotid, the circle of Willis, and the vertebrobasilar system prevent unilateral hemispheric cerebral ischemia. When venovenous perfusion is selected, the oxygenated blood is usually returned to the internal jugular, femoral, or iliac vein.

Vessel cannulation is usually carried out at the patient's bedside, with the assistance of an operating room team. Patients are first systemically heparinized before insertion of catheters. For arterial cannulation, it is necessary to expose the vessels surgically; Pesenti and colleagues have described venous cannulation for $ECCO_2R$ (see Respiratory Failure) by the percutaneous route,[3] and we have found this to be the preferred method of cannulation for patients with pure respiratory failure. Single-catheter venovenous systems can use a continuous-flow, double-lumen catheter or tidal flow (so-called push-pull, or to-and-fro) to propel oxygenated blood into the right atrium.[4–7] These modifications allow cannulation using a single site and in neonates can provide total respiratory support.

Pumping systems are of several varieties, the most common and simple of which is the servocontrolled roller pump.[8] Alternatively, the centrifugal (vortex) pump has been the mainstay of many cardiac perfusion teams and can be selected for ECLS perfusion. The centrifugal pump has the advantage of a lesser requirement of regulating the pump speed by the rate of venous blood drainage from the patient, but this advantage is somewhat offset by a higher device cost, potential cavitation, and hemolysis of blood. Cavitation (creating air bubbles) and hemolysis are of particular concern during periods of occlusion of the drainage inlet line supplying blood to the centrifugal pump head. A passively filling, servoregulated pump has been described,[9] and a version of this pump is currently used in Europe.[6]

Oxygenators are usually of the coil membrane type (Kolobow membrane lung) or the hollow fiber type. Both types of oxygenators have undergone extensive clinical use, both

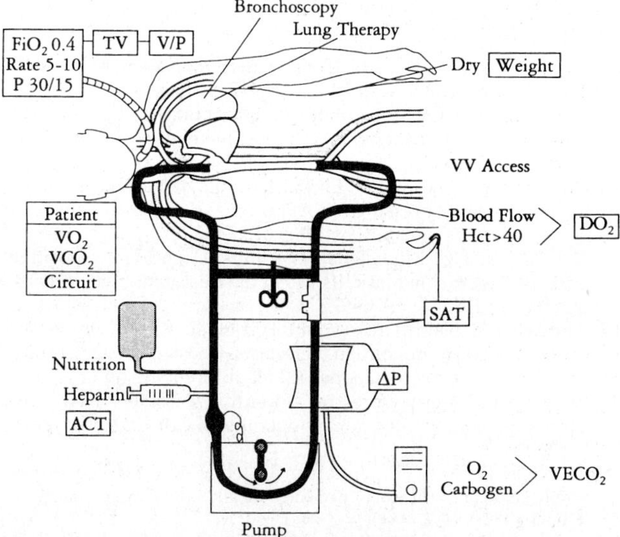

Figure 105–1. Diagram of venovenous ECLS perfusion circuit. Blood is drained from the right atrium by a catheter placed through the right jugular vein. Warmed and oxygenated blood is finally returned to the vena cava through a catheter placed in the right femoral vein. Parameters contained within boxes are those that are continuously monitored during ECLS. *Abbreviations*: FiO_2 = inspired oxygen fraction; P = pressure; TV = tidal volume; V/P = volume/pressure, or compliance; VV = venovenous; Hct = hematocrit; DO_2 = oxygen delivery; SAT = hemoglobin saturation by oxygen; ΔP = pressure drop across membrane oxygenator; $VECO_2$ = percentage of carbon dioxide in outlet sweep gas; ACT = activated clotting time; VO_2 = oxygen consumption; VCO_2 = carbon dioxide production. (From Anderson HL III, Steimle CM, Shapiro MB, et al: Extracorporeal life support for adult cardiorespiratory failure. Surgery 114:162, 1993.)

short term in the operating room and for long-term perfusion. Because the need for systemic heparinization is predicated by the extensive contact of blood with foreign surfaces of the perfusion circuit, particularly in the oxygenator, significant effort is under way to perfect nonthrombogenic coating of bypass components. Heparin-bonded circuitry has enjoyed acceptance for short-term perfusion in the operating room; however, when this existing technology of heparin coating is used for long-term perfusion, leakage of plasma from the blood phase to the gas phase in the oxygenator results and limits its attractiveness.

The blood leaving the oxygenator, now oxygenated, is warmed to body temperature by a water-jacketed heat exchanger before returning to the patient. A "bridge" connects the venous drainage limb and return limb of the ECLS circuit together, near the patient, and is occluded by a clamp during the bypass run. The bridge is opened every 15 to 20 minutes to "flash" the transiently stagnant blood within this section of tubing. This bridge has particular importance just before connecting the ECLS circuit to the patient: It allows continuous flow of blood within the circuit and avoids stagnation (and thrombus formation) of the blood prime. The bridge is also used during a "trial off" of ECLS, when heart or lung recovery has occurred and a patient is temporarily taken off extracorporeal support. Blood can continue to flow within the circuit without actually disconnecting the patient and cannulas from the circuit.

Anticoagulation during the ECLS run is accomplished by continuous systemic heparinization and is monitored by the activated clotting time (ACT). Because ACT is a measure of the heparin effect on whole blood, it is preferred over the partial thromboplastin time or other measures of heparin activity. Normal ACT is 100 to 120 seconds, and systemic heparinization is maintained to an ACT range of 160 to 200 seconds, usually in the range of 160 to 180 seconds. At higher ACTs, bleeding (e.g., from endobronchial, cannulation, or chest tube sites) and gross blood loss are greater, whereas at ACT levels less than 160 seconds, the likelihood of clot formation in circuit components (especially the membrane oxygenator) increases. Perfusion of patients without systemic heparin for short periods has been described. One must plan for the eventual loss of the circuit to thrombosis and the need to replace it quickly with a new one.

Blood product administration is usually performed through the perfusion circuit and it is usually necessary to replace the red blood cells, platelets, and clotting factors, which are normally consumed, sequestered, or lost in bulk amount (e.g., bleeding, laboratory sampling). Packed red blood cells are transfused to achieve a hematocrit of 45% to 50%, to maximize O_2 delivery from the perfusion circuit. Platelets are slowly consumed by the perfusion circuit (particularly the membrane oxygenator) during an ECLS run, and any circulating platelets that remain are rendered dysfunctional by the extensive blood-foreign surface contact and by activation of the many inflammatory cascades within blood. A platelet level exceeding $100{,}000/mm^3$ usually results in satisfactory hemostasis during a bypass run and a lesser likelihood of bleeding. Fresh frozen plasma or cryoprecipitate is used to replace factors consumed during extracorporeal perfusion, particularly Factor II (fibrinogen), antithrombin III, and so on.

Fluids other than blood products (parenteral nutrition, intravenous fluids, intravenous medications, and others) can be similarly administered through the perfusion circuit and are concentrated as much as possible to minimize the fluid given to a patient in each 24 hours. Exquisite control of daily fluid balance can also be achieved through ultrafiltration using a minidialyzer membrane, taking advantage of the pressurized portion of the bypass circuit between the roller pump and the membrane oxygenator as the driving force for ultrafiltration through a dialyzer membrane. Slow continuous ultrafiltration (SCUF) for simple serum/fluid removal can be used, or dialysis can be added (SCUF-D),[10] a simple modification of techniques patterned after continuous arteriovenous hemofiltration (CAVH or CAVH-D).

A patient's typical course is depicted in Figure 105–2. ECLS, when used for respiratory failure, allows "lung rest" from the high fraction of inspired O_2 (FIO_2) and high ventilatory pressures required to oxygenate and ventilate these patients adequately. Thus, the ventilator support is turned down to more moderate O_2 fraction, pressures, and rate. As pulmonary function improves, bypass pump flow (venoarterial or venovenous) is slowly weaned in response to increasing arterial partial pressure of oxygen (PaO_2) (or decreasing arterial partial pressure of CO_2 [$PaCO_2$]), until support is considered to be less than 10% of the patient's metabolic needs. The ventilator is then increased to modest settings (e.g., FIO_2 of 0.5, moderate inflating pressures and minute ventilation), and the patient is "tried off" of bypass by clamping drainage and return catheters and opening the bridge, again allowing blood within the circuit to continue to circulate. If recovery of pulmonary function has been sufficient and adequate blood gases and hemodynamic parameters remain after 2 to 4 hours of a trial off, decannulation from bypass is usually considered. If not, the patient is returned to bypass support until the next trial off, usually 24 to 48 hours later. In cases of cardiac failure treated by ECLS, a trial off of venoarterial bypass is considered after cardiac function improves and blood pressure, O_2 delivery, and perfusion also improve and are sustained when pump flow is weaned. Again, a trial off of bypass is performed, after ensuring adequate cardiac preload and using only minimum or moderate levels of inotropes.

When the decision to decannulate has been made, catheters placed percutaneously in veins are removed and the skin puncture sites closed with a simple pursestring or mattress suture. Cannulas placed operatively in vessels are removed after operative exposure of the cannulas and vessels. Veins are usually ligated after removal of surgically placed cannulas but can be repaired. Cannulated arteries supplying areas of poor collateral circulation (e.g., end-arterial beds of the femoral or axillary arteries) require primary repair (end-to-end anastomosis) or are repaired using autogenous vessel as a patch or interposition graft. Ligation of the common carotid artery is usually performed after carotid artery decannulation. Several centers have successfully performed repair of the common carotid artery in neonates after decannulation, with good results,[11, 12] although a small risk of distal embolization, pseudoaneurysm formation, or stenosis at the site of the arterial repair still remains. Unilateral carotid artery ligation has been safely performed in thousands of neonatal, pediatric, and adult patients with virtually minimum or no morbidity, and any alternative techniques beyond simple carotid decannulation and ligation must be compared with this standard. The long-term effect of unilateral carotid ligation after treatment with ECLS is not known. The oldest surviving patient who underwent therapy with venoarterial ECLS and subsequently underwent carotid artery ligation is neurologically and developmentally normal at age 18 years. Long-term follow-up of these patients is important to discern whether (if at all) neurologic or developmental sequelae arise from unilateral carotid artery ligation.

An alternative to immediate decannulation after a trial off of bypass is heparinization of the indwelling bypass cannulas after removal of the bypass circuit. A continuous infu-

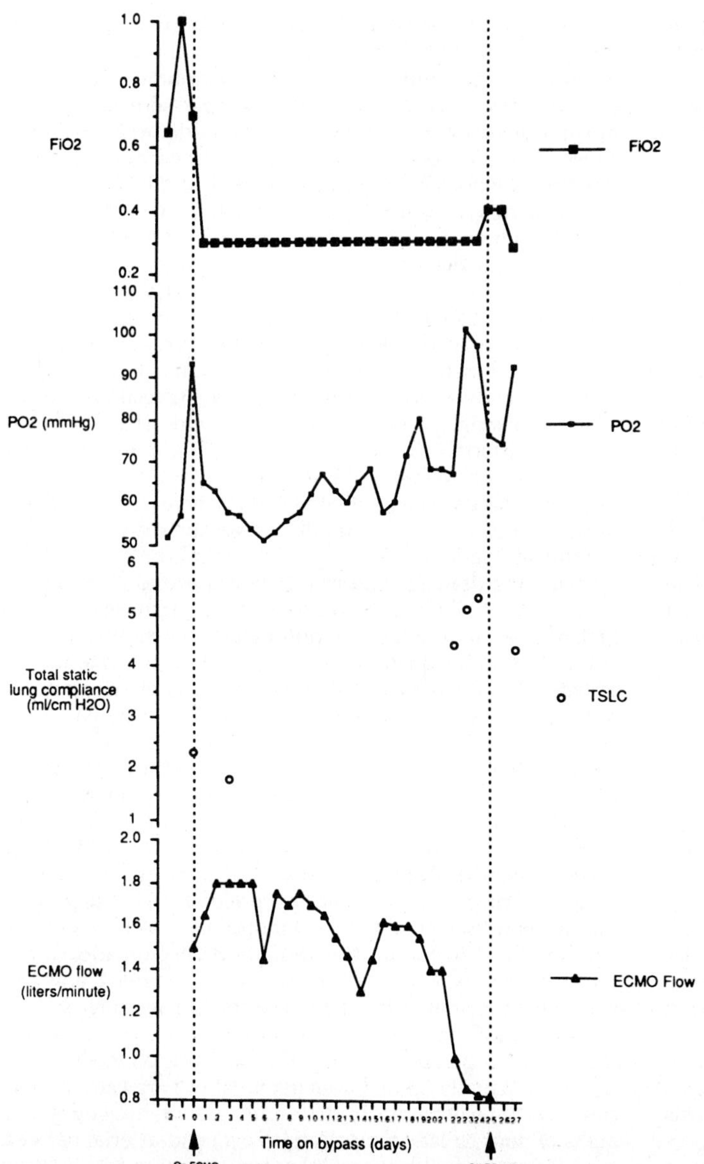

Figure 105–2. ECLS course of 2-year-old infant with respiratory failure from varicella pneumonia. Inspired oxygen fraction (FiO_2), arterial oxygen pressure (pO_2), total static lung compliance (TSLC), and ECLS pump flow are plotted against time. At day 25, the patient successfully weaned from bypass and was decannulated. This patient was subsequently discharged. (From Anderson HL III, Attorri RJ, Custer JR, et al: Extracorporeal membrane oxygenation [ECMO] for pediatric cardiorespiratory failure. J Thorac Cardiovasc Surg 1990; 99:1015.)

sion of a heparin-containing solution is attached to the cannulas until 12 to 24 hours have passed and the patient's condition continues to merit the removal of catheters. Should a patient's condition deteriorate before catheters are removed, with this technique, a new bypass circuit can be primed and the patient again placed back on ECLS.

PATIENT SELECTION

Selection of Neonates

Much attention has been given to the topic of patient selection, particularly in the pediatric and adult patient population, when ECLS is considered for primary respiratory or cardiac failure. ECLS for neonates became standard therapy for neonatal respiratory failure by 1984,[13] and indications have become relatively standardized from medical center to medical center. Minimum differences exist in individual entry criteria of each center, because mortality for a given level of illness in any patient varies from center to center.

Five pathophysiologic conditions (excluding congenital cardiac anomaly) of the newborn period are typically responsible for respiratory failure within the first 2 weeks of life: meconium aspiration syndrome, respiratory distress syndrome, persistent pulmonary hypertension of the newborn/persistent fetal circulation, pneumonia/sepsis, and congenital diaphragmatic hernia. All these conditions have some component of persistent fetal circulation due to elevated pulmonary vascular resistance (and pulmonary hypertension), with right-to-left shunt.[8] Conventional therapy calls for higher FIO_2 and higher mean airway pressures by mechanical ventilation to improve oxygenation. Oxygen toxicity and barotrauma are the usual result.

Most neonatal centers select a 90% mortality threshold, as defined by physiologic and ventilatory parameters, as criteria for placement on ECLS. The oxygenation index (OI), defined as

$$\text{OI} = \text{mean airway pressure (cm } H_2O) \times \frac{FIO_2 \times 100}{PaO_2 \text{ (mm Hg)}}$$

was developed as one predictor of mortality. In the authors' neonatal intensive care unit, an OI of 25 predicts a mortality of 50% and an OI of 40 predicts a mortality of 80%. Some centers use postductal alveolar-arterial O_2 gradient as a predictor of mortality. Krummel reported a predicted mortality of 94% with an alveolar-arterial O_2 gradient consistently at 600 mm Hg or greater despite 12 hours of maximum conventional therapy.[8, 14]

The authors have used an OI consistently greater than 25 despite maximum conventional management for 12 hours (50% predicted mortality) or attainment of an OI of 40 (80% predicted mortality) as indications for ECLS in neonates. For neonates between 2.5 and 4.5 kg, without severe cardiac dysfunction, an attempt is made at placement of the double-lumen venovenous catheter, thereby sparing ligation of the carotid.

In most cases, time permits early ultrasonographic evaluation of a patient's head to rule out intracranial bleeding. Also as part of the evaluation routine, major congenital cardiac anomalies are excluded by echocardiography. Neonates with respiratory failure identified early in the disease course are usually evaluated by cranial ultrasonography and echocardiogram; in the event that urgent cannulation becomes necessary late at night, all the preparatory screening studies will have been done. Conditions that might exclude a patient from consideration for ECLS are major chromosomal aberration, major cardiac anomaly, bleeding (particularly *any* evidence of intraventricular hemorrhage), and estimated gestational age less than 32 weeks.

Selection of Pediatric and Adult Patients

Respiratory Failure

The pathophysiology of respiratory or cardiac failure in an older child or adult patient is much more complex when compared with the reversibility of respiratory failure in a neonate. Criteria used in the National Institutes of Health–sponsored ECMO trial of the 1970s have been modified for use today. It is clear that with advancement in the technology of ventilators and advances in the field of respiratory care, ARDS still caries a high mortality.[15] Indications and exclusionary criteria for older and adult patients are listed in Table 105–2. Physiologic criteria of low static lung compliance and high transpulmonary shunt as predictors of mortality have been reverified during the years; the authors currently use a 90% mortality threshold as an indicator for ECLS.

Gattinoni and colleagues, in Milan, Italy, have used similar entry criteria but use a different approach to ECLS (termed $ECCO_2R$), emphasizing CO_2 removal by a low-flow system (1–2 L/min blood flow in the circuit) and apneic oxygenation by the native lungs.[16] They have placed no limitation on the time of mechanical ventilation before institution of $ECCO_2R$, although our series would suggest that the optimal time period for institution of ECLS is within 10 days of intubation.

TABLE 105–2. Indications and Contraindications for the Institution of Extracorporeal Life Support for Pediatric and Adult Patients

Indications
Total static lung compliance <0.5 mL · cm H_2O^{-1} · kg^{-1}
Transpulmonary shunt >30% on inspired oxygen fraction of 0.6 or greater
Reversible respiratory failure
Time on mechanical ventilation ≤ 5 days (10 days absolute maximum)
Exclusions
Potential for severe bleeding
Time on mechanical ventilation 11 days or greater
Necrotizing pneumonia
Poor quality of life (those patients with metastatic malignancy, major central nervous system injury, or quadriplegia)
Age over 60 years

Once a patient has successfully been placed on ECLS, the ventilator settings can be turned down, affording true lung rest. Typical rest settings include an FIO_2 of 0.5 or less, peak pressures limited at 40 cm H_2O, positive end-expiratory pressure of 10 to 15 cm H_2O, and respiratory rate of 10 per minute. The inspiratory period is often increased, reversing the inspiratory-expiratory ratio and providing prolonged alveolar "inflation."

Cardiac Failure

The use of venoarterial ECLS for support of a failing heart is an area that has only recently received renewed attention, particularly in children. Selected pathologic conditions include preoperative support of the failing heart ("bridge to transplant") or postoperative support after cardiac operation or cardiac transplantation, when cardiac index is less than 2 L/min · m^2. Typical reversible medical conditions treated with ECLS are myocarditis and cardiomyopathy.[10, 17, 18]

One advantage of ECLS over the use of the right ventricular assist device or the left ventricular assist device is the fact that major operation with median sternotomy is not required for cannulation, allowing rapid institution of bypass support for these patients in the intensive care unit or emergency room. Later thoracic operation is not compromised should cardiac surgery or cardiac transplantation be necessary.

Although it would seem that recent sternotomy or thoracotomy would prove to be a contraindication to institution of ECLS, because of the potential for severe bleeding, the authors usually approach this by placing the patient on bypass, leaving the sternum open, and closing the skin over the open sternum, or by closing the skin defect with a Gore-Tex or Silastic patch. This method allows bedside evacuation of hematoma, minimizes the potential for cardiac tamponade, and allows easy access for correction of hemorrhage and hemothorax within the chest. For postoperative cardiac surgery patients placed on ECLS, ACT levels are maintained low (150–170 s) and platelets and fresh frozen plasma are transfused to keep platelet count greater than 150,000/mm^3 and fibrinogen level greater than 200 mg/dL.

Major and irreversible organ failure (e.g., kidney, hepatic, global neurologic insult), often associated with hypotension and low-flow states in any patient, must be carefully ruled out before consideration for ECLS.

RESULTS

To facilitate collection and exchange of information and data with regard to ECLS and ECMO, an organization of health-care professionals interested in ECLS was founded in 1989.[8] The Extracorporeal Life Support Organization (ELSO) and the ELSO Registry are based at the University of Michigan and coordinate education of and multicenter studies for their member institutions. Data with respect to number of active centers, numbers of patients treated, survival, complications, and so forth are summarized each quarter for centers within the United States, in Canada, and overseas. A summary can be found in Table 105–3.

The largest patient experience with ECLS is for the treatment of neonatal respiratory failure, with an overall survival of 81%.[19] Patient survival at each new center improves over time as the center becomes more experienced and more patients are accrued, thereby giving support to the concept of a learning curve with this specialized technology. Survival is highest in patients with the meconium aspiration syndrome (93% survival) and lowest in neonates treated for

TABLE 105–3. Neonatal and Pediatric ECLS Results Compiled by the ELSO Registry (Ann Arbor, Michigan) as of May 1994

Group	*Patients Reported*	*Number Survived*	*% Survival*
Neonatal respiratory	8913	7213	81%
Pediatric respiratory	672	336	50%
Pediatric cardiac	1109	493	44%
Totals	10,694	8042	75%

congenital diaphragmatic hernia (58% survival). This disparity reflects the complexity of treating patients with congenital diaphragmatic hernia, whether ECLS is used as rescue therapy for deterioration in the immediate postpartum period or is used for respiratory deterioration after surgical repair of the diaphragmatic defect. Controversy still exists about the optimal timing for operative repair of congenital diaphragmatic hernia and the institution of ECLS for the respiratory decompensation that can precede or follow operation.

The most common physiologic complication of ECLS is bleeding, owing to the use of systemic heparinization; it occurs in as many as 20% of cases. Bleeding can be minor and easily corrected when occurring in a cannulation site or may be serious if it occurs intracranially—often mandating immediate discontinuance of ECLS. Mechanical complications with the ECLS circuit happen less frequently (e.g., failure of a membrane oxygenator or rupture of tubing) and often can be corrected with minimum disruption in the ECLS run.

Follow-up of neonates treated with ECLS has shown normal neurologic development in about three fourths of patients, with the remaining one quarter sustaining either minor or major neurologic handicap. Analysis of risk factors for intracranial bleeding or intraventricular hemorrhage implicated prematurity or younger gestational age.[20]

Since 1990, the use of ECLS for the treatment of pediatric respiratory or cardiac failure has increased markedly. As more and more neonatal centers join the current list of ECLS centers, a natural transition is from neonatal ECLS to pediatric ECLS. This trend involves larger circuits with greater membrane surface area (to accommodate greater gas exchange), larger catheters, and obviously larger patients. What is not readily appreciated is the fact that the time course for non-neonatal patients on ECLS is typically 1 to 3 weeks in duration instead of only 4 to 7 days for a neonate. This longer period can involve a significant investment in hospital and medical personnel resources, with particular use of more laboratory studies and blood products and often requiring the frequent replacement of oxygenators or complete bypass circuits during these longer runs.

Typical respiratory diseases treated in pediatric patients include bacterial or viral pneumonia, aspiration, ARDS, and near-drowning. As in neonates, both venoarterial access (using the carotid artery) and venovenous access (usually with a two-catheter system) are used. Cardiac diseases treated by ECLS can include cardiac failure before or after cardiac operation (particularly from congenital cardiac disease or before or after cardiac transplantation), viral myocarditis, and cardiomyopathy. Approximately 25% of pediatric patients with cardiac failure are placed on ECLS in the operating room owing to the inability to wean from cardiopulmonary bypass.[19] Results of ECLS for the treatment of pulmonary and cardiac failure in pediatric patients are also summarized in Table 105–3.

As the experience with ECLS for pediatric patients has continued to expand, with the more experienced centers accepting and treating non-neonatal patients, the next level of difficulty is ECLS support of adult patients. After the results of the National Institutes of Health–sponsored multicenter adult ECMO trial were reported in 1977, ECMO for adults was abandoned as therapy for respiratory failure because no benefit was found over conventional medical management. It was not until 1986 that Gattinoni reported 48.8% survival (21 patients surviving of 43 patients total) using a low-flow $ECCO_2R$ and apneic oxygenation.[16] Renewed interest in the treatment of adults, in both Europe and the United States, using 1990s technology and critical care techniques, currently results in a 50% survival rather than the dismal 10% survival of the 1970s trial (Table 105–4). Several centers now use an 80% to 90% mortality threshold (by current physiologic parameters) as the decision point for the institution of ECLS, similar to what was used in the 1970s National Institutes of Health trial. It would appear that ECLS as practiced in 1994, with newer perfusion technology and attention to lung rest (as opposed to the high FIO_2 and high ventilatory pressures used *with* ECMO in the 1970s trial) has made significant advances in treating respiratory failure in adults.

Clemmer and colleagues, of Salt Lake City, tested the hypothesis that conventional mangement ("control therapy") was as good as or better than pressure-controlled, inverse-ratio ventilation plus $ECCO_2R$ ("new therapy"). They used a computer-driven ventilatory protocol for each group, randomizing patients with ARDS to treatment with either standard positive-pressure ventilation or the new

TABLE 105–4. International and United States Centers Performing ECLS for Adult Patients

Center	*n*	*Survivors (% Survival)*
Milan-Monza, Italy	93	41 (44%)
Marburg, Germany	150	86 (57%)
Berlin, Germany	41	22 (55%)
Paris, France	64	27 (42%)
Stockholm, Sweden	26	9 (35%)
Freiburg, Germany	19	11 (58%)
Lund, Sweden	3	2 (67%)
University of Michigan (Ann Arbor, MI)	46	25 (54%)
LDS Hospital, University of Utah (Salt Lake City, UT)	21	7 (33%)
Hershey Medical Center (Hershey, PA)	—*	—*
Sharpe Memorial Hospital (San Diego, CA)	9	3 (33%)
University of Pittsburgh (Pittsburgh, PA)	11	7 (64%)
Totals	483	240 (50%)

*Information not available.

therapy group, with $ECCO_2R$.[21] No difference in survival was found between the two groups in this study, which incorporated phase I use of $ECCO_2R$.[22] They did, however, find that with the use of computer monitoring and standardizing of ventilator changes with previously agreed-on and programmed algorithm, an improvement in survival (42% overall survival) in treating ARDS was greater than what would have been expected with the nonprotocol, individual judgment approach to mechanical ventilation (10% expected survival) practiced in critical care units today. Consistency in ventilator changes mandated by such computer-directed protocols may have appeal for clinical studies, in that confounding variables in a clinical study of two techniques can be held to a minimum.

The authors' experience with ECLS for treating respiratory failure[23] has mirrored the experience of the Milan group[24] and that of Lennartz and Müller of Marburg, Germany, approaching 50% survival. As we have left the learning curve of our first 10 patients[25] and are now completing a phase I trial of ECLS for adults, several key points are worth summarizing: (1) ECLS is reasonable therapy for adult patients with respiratory failure, particularly that due to ARDS. This technology is expensive in both resources of equipment and personnel and cannot be considered standard therapy, yet its safety and efficacy have shown that it might be more properly categorized as extraordinary therapy. (2) Early intervention in the disease process (within the first 10 days of intubation and mechanical ventilation) is probably key to improved outcome. (3) A phase II comparison of conventional therapy versus ECLS, involving centers experienced in the technique of ECLS, still needs to be conducted to answer the question, Is ECLS better than conventional medical management for the treatment of *severe* respiratory failure?

NEW INNOVATIONS FOR EXTRACORPOREAL LIFE SUPPORT

As clinical application of ECLS has grown and as the indications and age groups have expanded beyond the neonate, new problems have surfaced with extracorporeal technology and support. Much attention has been directed to the question, How can we perform ECLS more safely and better? As one would expect, advances in perfusion technology for cardiac surgery cross over to many areas of ECLS, particularly with regard to the actual propulsion of blood through the bypass circuit.

Automation or servoregulation of the ECLS system will be one such advance. The ability to place a patient on ECLS and have the system wean pump flow automatically based on multiplexed physiologic information, directly input by hard-wired technology that can include arterial blood gases, mixed venous oxygen saturation, and pulmonary mechanics from the ventilator, would simplify the process tremendously. Such a servoregulated system could be attached to the patient and be supervised by the one intensive care unit nurse caring for the patient, rather than having a round-the-clock ECLS specialist (which is the current practice) also at the bedside. Servo-regulation has been implemented successfully in the laboratory[26] and should soon find an active role for ECLS in the critical care unit.

Catheter technology, geared toward thin-wall, wire-reinforced designs (e.g., those marketed by the Bio-Medicus Corporation, a division of Medtronic, Inc., Minneapolis, MN), have simplified cannulation by percutaneous technique, as previously described by Pesenti and colleagues.[3] These small-diameter catheters allow higher blood flow without collapse of the catheters, owing to lower intrinsic resistance and to wire reinforcing of the catheter wall. Montoya and associates described the *M number*, a numeric system by which catheters can be categorized according to their flow/pressure characteristics.[27] Sinard and coworkers tested perfusion catheters currently in use for ECLS today and determined the M number for each.[28] Knowing the required flow to support a given patient, the appropriate size and type catheter can be selected, using the working pressure of the system and calculating the M number necessary for those constraints.

Single-site cannulation using a double-lumen catheter for venovenous bypass has been successfully used for neonatal ECLS[4, 6, 29] and in a multicenter comparison was found to be at least as safe as venoarterial bypass.[5] Double-lumen catheters of sufficient size are currently not available for use in larger pediatric and adult patients. Single-site cannulation with these catheters would allow quick and easy cannulation and decannulation and would decrease bleeding from the cannulation site.[24]

Gas exchange surface technology and development of oxygenators have been primarily driven by their use in clinical cardiopulmonary bypass. Heparin coating of perfusion components has been accomplished by two manufacturing groups, Medtronic/Carmeda (Carmeda BioActive Surface; Stockholm, Sweden)[30, 31] and Baxter-Bentley Laboratories (DuraFlo II, Irvine, CA).[32] Although heparin coating of the hollow-fiber lung has shown the greatest promise for ECLS, it is still handicapped by plasma leakage from blood to the gas phase, resulting in profuse production of soapsudslike foam from the gas port of the oxygenator. A system that does not require full systemic heparinization would ultimately be ideal, decreasing bleeding from the patient (and reducing the need for blood transfusion).

The ideal pumping system for long-term perfusion is a continuous topic of controversy. The classic roller pump has had decades of clinical use, with advantages of relative inexpense, minimum hemolysis, and the fact that it has no spinning impeller to propel blood through the circuit. Regulation of pump speed based on venous drainage from the patient is a method of servo-regulation by which the pump is stopped when venous drainage stops (i.e., a venous return line is kinked), preventing cavitation of the stationary blood within the pump raceway. The centrifugal pump, of which the Bio-Medicus Bio-Pump is a popular model, is found in many cardiac operating rooms today. No discrete servo-control, based on venous drainage, is necessary for the centrifugal pump, obviating the need for the distensible "bladder" in the venous drainage line often used with roller pump systems. Cavitation of blood and creation of air bubbles in the blood path during inflow occlusion of the centrifugal pump pose a potential hazard. The centrifugal pump is a more expensive system owing to the magnetically coupled impeller chamber that propels the blood and must be replaced every few days. Again, neither of the pumping systems can be referred to as the perfect system.

Several European centers currently use a passively filling, roller-type pump known as the Rhone-Poulenc pump (Collin Cardio, Paris, France).[6] This pump system combines advantages of both the roller pump and the centrifugal pump: As venous drainage decreases or when a venous return line is occluded, the distensible pump raceway tubing collapses, and no blood is moved through the pump (thus, there is no cavitation). Should a high-pressure return line become kinked or occluded, the pump raceway tubing becomes circular rather than ovoid, overcoming the occlusion of the rollers and halting propulsion of blood through the tubing. High pressures are therefore avoided, preventing tubing rupture due to high pressure within the blood return portion of the circuit. Thus, the Rhone-Poulenc system incorporates the benefits of the previously mentioned pumping systems without the expensive hardware that either of the two systems requires. This system is not available in the United States, although a prototype for manufacture within the United States is currently in development in our laboratory.[9]

Pharmacologic modulation of the inflammatory and coagulation cascade has shown some promise in preserving platelet number and function and in decreasing overall blood loss in patients undergoing cardiopulmonary support. Tranexamic acid, a plasmin inhibitor, has both clinically and experimentally been demonstrated to decrease blood loss and preserve platelet number and function during cardiac operation.[33, 34] Aprotinin, an inhibitor of fibrinolysis, has been shown to decrease postoperative bleeding when administered before cardiopulmonary bypass.[35] As more is learned about the coagulation and inflammatory cascades, agents that prevent their activation in blood when in contact with foreign surfaces and agents that preserve platelet number and function during bypass will make long-term ECLS perfusion safer, with less bleeding and less need for blood product transfusion.

The Intravascular Oxygenator

The IVOX represents a different approach to extrapulmonary augmentation of gas exchange in patients with respiratory failure. A multicenter phase I trial of this device has been under way in 31 centers across the United States and overseas. Although the IVOX was not designed to completely take over all respiratory function, it functions best at augmenting CO_2 removal, thereby allowing a decrease in minute ventilation (and a decrease in ventilatory pressures), reducing barotrauma.

The IVOX (CardioPulmonics, Inc., Salt Lake City, UT) was introduced in 1987 as an implantable device,[36] which in application should be more correctly referred to as an *intracorporeal* respiratory support device. It is inserted transvenously through the right femoral or jugular vein after surgical exposure of the vessel and resides in the vena cava (Figs. 105–3 and 105–4). Before insertion, it is wound tightly (similar to an intra-aortic balloon pump catheter) to decrease the diameter of the device. Once it is placed and its position is confirmed fluoroscopically, the IVOX is unwound or "unfurled," the fibers expanding to occupy the lumen of the vena cava.

The small-diameter, hollow fibers are composed of siloxane-coated microporous polypropylene and carry O_2 gas from the distal end of the device to the proximal end, where a negative pressure (vacuum) is applied. As bulk movement of the O_2 through the fibers is achieved with subatmospheric pressure, gas embolization to the patient is unlikely should any fiber break—blood instead enters the broken fiber and clots, occluding it. Gas exchange between blood in the vena cava and the O_2 within the fiber occurs through diffusion

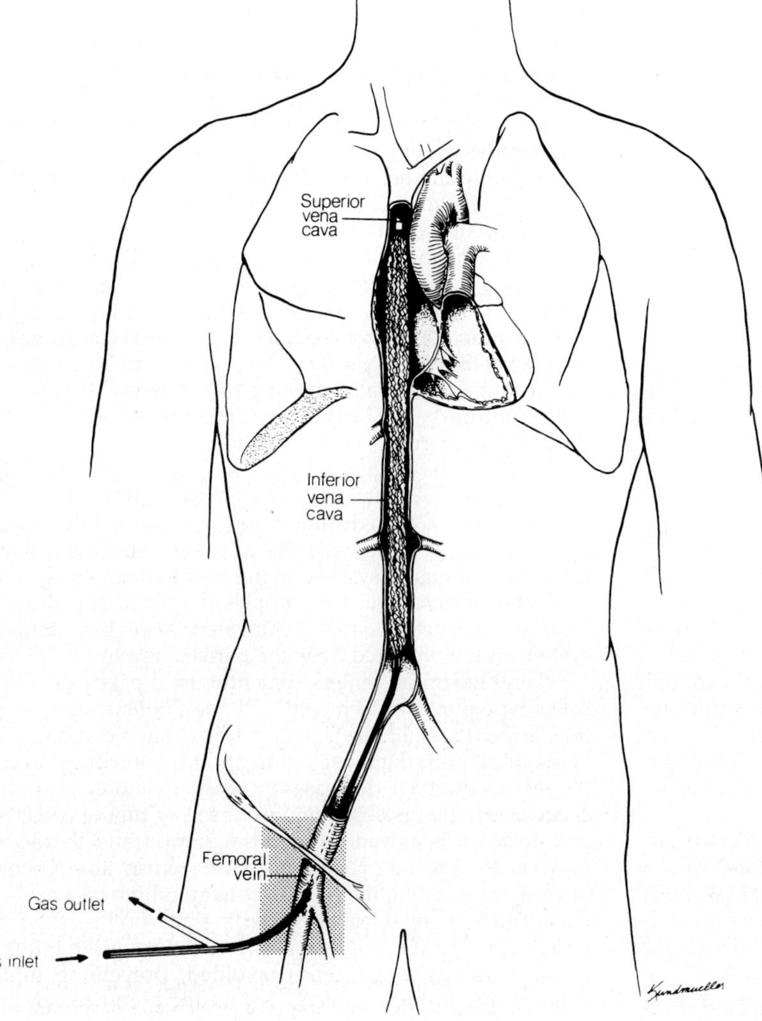

Figure 105–3. The IVOX intravascular oxygenator. This device is inserted through surgical exposure of the right femoral or right internal jugular vein. Venous blood flowing past the device exchanges oxygen and carbon dioxide with the oxygen sweep gas flowing through the individual hollow fibers. (Courtesy of CardioPulmonics, Salt Lake City, UT.)

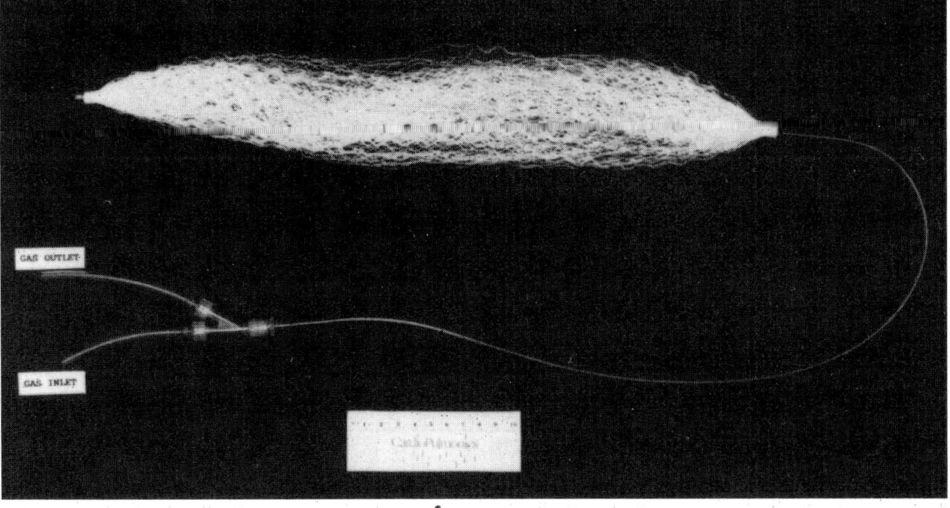

Figure 103–4. The IVOX intravascular oxygenator unfurled, prior to insertion. The device is first twisted on its axis; this spirally compacts the fibers and creates a smaller diameter for insertion. Once in place in the vena cava, the device is unfurled. (Courtesy of CardioPulmonics, Salt Lake City, UT.)

across the fiber wall. Effluent gas can be measured for CO_2 concentration, and thus CO_2 extraction from a patient can be calculated by multiplying by the effluent gas flow rate.

Several groups have reported safety and efficacy of the IVOX device.[37–39] The device is manufactured in four sizes, and maximum CO_2 removal capability is approximately one third of the metabolically produced CO_2. The device is less efficient at O_2 transfer to venous blood. Cox and colleagues described a conceptual mathematic model of the use of the IVOX, based on laboratory and clinical data.[37] They too confirmed the observations by Hickling and coworkers[40] of the benefit of permissive hypercapnia to the augmentation of CO_2 removal. Using their mathematic model, a $Pa{CO_2}$ of 75 to 80 mm Hg was required to achieve CO_2 removal rates of 90 to 100 mL of CO_2 per minute.

Although the IVOX cannot achieve the same gas exchange capabilities of extracorporeal circulation, it nonetheless may provide critical care physicians with a means to supplement the ventilator when treating patients with moderately severe respiratory failure.

CONCLUSION

ECLS is a critical care technique that has gained popularity in recent years, particularly after its acceptance as *standard therapy* for neonatal respiratory failure. As the technology of ECLS has made significant advances in recent years, more complete respiratory and cardiac support and safety are now provided to patients. It is clear that in pediatric and adult patients with respiratory failure, *early* intervention is key to a successful outcome. ECLS technology can be expensive in terms of medical resources and personnel; however, improved results in recent years, owing to better patient selection and better understanding of pulmonary pathophysiology, make ECLS another lifesaving technique in the armamentarium of critical care physicians.

References

1. Hill JD, O'Brien TG, Murray JJ, et al: Extracorporeal oxygenation for acute post-traumatic respiratory failure (shock-lung syndrome): Use of the Bramson membrane lung. N Engl J Med 1972; 286:629–634.
2. Gibbon JH Jr: Artificial maintenance circulation during experimental occlusion of the pulmonary artery. Arch Surg 1937; 34:1105.
3. Pesenti A, Gattinoni L, Kolobow T, et al: Extracorporeal circulation in adult respiratory failure. ASAIO Trans 1988; 34:43–47.
4. Anderson HL III, Otsu T, Chapman RA, et al: Venovenous extracorporeal life support in neonates using a double lumen catheter. ASAIO Trans 1989; 35:650–653.
5. Anderson HL III, Snedecor SM, Otsu T, et al: Multicenter comparison of conventional venoarterial access versus venovenous double lumen catheter access in newborn infants undergoing extracorporeal membrane oxygenation. J Pediatr Surg 1993; 28:530–535.
6. Durandy Y, Chevalier JY, Lecompte Y: Single cannula venovenous bypass for respiratory membrane lung support. J Thorac Cardiovasc Surg 1990; 99:404–409.
7. Tsuno K, Terasaki H, Tsutsumi R, et al: To-and-fro veno-venous extracorporeal lung assist for newborns with severe respiratory distress. Intensive Care Med 1989; 15:269–271.
8. Bartlett RH: Extracorporeal life support for cardiopulmonary failure. Curr Probl Surg 1990; 27:621–705.
9. Montoya JP, Merz SI, Bartlett RH: Laboratory experience with a novel, nonocclusive, pressure-regulated peristaltic pump. ASAIO J 1992; 38:M406–M411.
10. Anderson HL III, Attorri RJ, Custer JR, et al: Extracorporeal membrane oxygenation (ECMO) for pediatric cardiopulmonary failure. J Thorac Cardiovasc Surg 1990; 99:1011–1019.
11. Spector ML, Wiznitzer M, Walsh-Sukys MC, et al: Carotid reconstruction in the neonate following ECMO. J Pediatr Surg 1991; 26:357–359.
12. Taylor BJ, Seibert JJ, Glasier CM, et al: Evaluation of the reconstructed carotid artery following extracorporeal membrane oxygenation. Pediatrics 1992; 90:568–572.
13. Andrew AF, Roloff DN, Bartlett RH: Use of extracorporeal membrane oxygenation in persistent pulmonary hypertension of the newborn. Clin Perinatol 1984; 11:729–735.
14. Krummel TM, Greenfield LJ, Kirkpatrick BV, et al: Alveolar-arterial oxygen gradients versus the neonatal pulmonary insufficiency index for prediction of mortality in ECMO candidates. J Pediatr Surg 1984; 19:380–384.
15. Sloane PJ, Gee MH, Gottlieb JE, et al: A multicenter registry of patients with acute respiratory distress syndrome: Physiology and outcome. Am Rev Respir Dis 1992; 146:419–426.
16. Gattinoni L, Pesenti A, Mascheroni D, et al: Low-frequency positive-pressure ventilation with extracorporeal CO_2 removal in severe acute respiratory failure. JAMA 1986; 256:881–886.
17. Pennington GD, Swartz MT: Circulatory support in infants and children. Ann Thorac Surg 1993; 55:233–237.
18. Klein MD, Shaheen KW, Whittlesey GC, et al: Extracorporeal membrane oxygenation for the circulatory support of children after repair of congenital heart disease. J Thorac Cardiovasc Surg 1990; 100:498–505.
19. ECMO Quarterly Report (May 1994). Ann Arbor, MI, ECMO Registry of the Extracorporeal Life Support Organization (ELSO), 1994.
20. Cilley RE, Zwischenberger JB, Andrews AF, et al: Intracranial hemorrhage during extracorporeal membrane oxygenation in neonates. Pediatrics 1986; 78:699–704.

21. Clemmer T, Morris A, Suchyta M, et al: Extracorporeal support does not improve ARDS survival (Abstract). Crit Care Med 1992; 20:S61.
22. Morris AH, Menlove RL, Rollins RJ, et al: A controlled clinical trial of a new 3-step therapy that includes extracorporeal CO_2 removal for ARDS. ASAIO Trans 1988; 34:48–53.
23. Anderson HL III, Steimle CN, Shapiro MB, et al: Extracorporeal life support for adult cardiorespiratory failure. Surgery 1993; 114:161–173.
24. Pesenti A, Gattinoni L, Bombino M: Long term extracorporeal respiratory support: 20 years of progress. Intensive Crit Care Dig 1993; 12:15–18.
25. Anderson HL III, Delius RE, Sinard JM, et al: Early experience with adult extracorporeal membrane oxygenation in the modern era. Ann Thor Surg 1992; 53:553–563.
26. Merz S, Montoya PJ, Shanley CJ, et al: Implementation of a controller for extracorporeal life support (Abstract). ASAIO Trans 1993; 22:69.
27. Montoya JP, Merz SI, Bartlett RH: A standardized system for describing flow/pressure relationships in vascular access devices. ASAIO Trans 1991; 37:4–8.
28. Sinard JM, Merz SI, Hatcher MD, et al: Evaluation of extracorporeal perfusion catheters using a standardized measurement technique—the M-number. ASAIO Trans 1991; 37:60–64.
29. Delius RE, Anderson HL III, Schumacher RE, et al: Venovenous compares favorably to venoarterial access for extracorporeal membrane oxygenation in neonatal respiratory failure. J Thorac Cardiovasc Surg 1993; 106:329–338.
30. Bindslev L: Adult ECMO performed with surface-heparinized equipment. ASAIO Trans 1988; 34:1009–1013.
31. Shanley CJ, Hultquist KA, Rosenberg DM, et al: Prolonged extracorporeal circulation without heparin: Evaluation of the Medtronic Minimax oxygenator. ASAIO Trans 1992; 38:M311–M316.
32. Toomasian JM, Hsu L-C, Hirschl RB, et al: Evaluation of Duraflo II heparin coating in prolonged extracorporeal membrane oxygenation. ASAIO Trans 1988; 34:410–414.
33. Plotz FB, van Oeveren W, Aloe LS, et al: Prophylactic administration of tranexamic acid preserves platelet numbers during extracorporeal circulation in rabbits. ASAIO Trans 1987; 37:M416–M417.
34. Nakashima A, Matsuzaki K, Hisahara M, et al: Tranexamic acid decreases blood loss after cardiopulmonary bypass (Abstract). ASAIO Trans 1993; 22:64.
35. Lavee J, Raviv Z, Smolinsky A, et al: Platelet protection by low-dose aprotonin in cardiopulmonary bypass: Electron microscopic study. Ann Thorac Surg 1993; 55:114–119.
36. Mortensen JD: An intravenacaval blood gas exchange (IVCBGE) device—preliminary report. ASAIO Trans 1987; 33:570–573.
37. Cox CS Jr, Zwischenberger JB, Grave DF, et al: Intracorporeal CO_2 removal and permissive hypercapnia to reduce airway pressure in acute respiratory failure: The theoretical basis for permissive hypercapnia with IVOX. ASAIO J 1993; 39:97–102.
38. Jurmann JM, Demertzis S, Schaefers H-J, et al: Intravascular oxygenation for advanced respiratory failure. ASAIO J 1992; 38:120–124.
39. Conrad SA, Eggerstedt JM, Morris VF, et al: Prolonged intracorporeal support of gas exchange with an intravenacaval oxygenator. Chest 1993; 103:158–161.
40. Hickling KG, Henderson SJ, Jackson R: Low mortality associated with low volume pressure limited ventilation with permissive hypercapnia in severe adult respiratory distress syndrome. Intensive Care Med 1990; 16:372–377.

CHAPTER 106

Hyperbaric Oxygen in Critical Care

Richard E. Moon, MD, FACP, FCCP, FRCP(C)
Guy de Lisle Dear, MB, FRCA • *Bryant W. Stolp, MD, PhD*

The value of supplemental oxygen (O_2) to avert the danger of hypoxia in high-altitude balloon flights was first recognized by Bert more than 100 years ago.[1] In later years, others described the value of supplemental O_2 to treat hypoxemia caused by lung pathology. Within the past 40 years, the physiologic and pharmacologic effects of breathing O_2 at increased ambient pressure have been recognized. Several of these effects—namely, to increase O_2 partial pressure (Po_2) and content in the arterial blood—have been exploited clinically.

Patients with carbon monoxide (CO) poisoning, acute decompression illness, and necrotizing infection are often critically ill, requiring the modern techniques of invasive monitoring, mechanical ventilation, and hemodynamic support. This chapter provides the background information, rationale, and practical aspects of the use of hyperbaric O_2 (HBO) treatment in critically ill patients (Table 106–1).

PHYSIOLOGY OF HYPEROXIA

At normal atmospheric pressure, the O_2 in arterial blood is almost entirely bound to hemoglobin. At an arterial Po_2 of 90 mm Hg and hemoglobin concentration of 12 g/dL, less than 2% of the total arterial O_2 content is dissolved in the

TABLE 106–1. Range of Pressures Used in Clinical Hyperbaric Oxygen Therapy

	Equivalent Depth		
Ambient Pressure (Atmospheres Absolute [ATA])	*Feet of Seawater (fsw)*	*Meters of Seawater (msw)*	
1	0	0	Sea level
2	33	10	Commonly used treatment pressure range for chronic indications
2.5	45	14	
2.8	60	18	Most commonly used initial treatment pressure for decompression illness
3.04	68	21	Duke treatment pressure for clostridial myonecrosis
6	165	50	Occasionally used for arterial gas embolism, using 21–50% O_2 in patient breathing gas. Significant nitrogen narcosis in caregivers breathing air.

TABLE 106–2. Mean Blood Oxygen, Acid-Base, and Cardiovascular Responses to Hyperbaric Oxygenation

		Arterial Blood								*Venous Blood†*						
Atmospheric Pressure (ATA)	*Inspired Gas*	*Inspired* P_{O_2} *(mm Hg)*	P_{AO_2} *(mm Hg)*	P_{O_2} *(mm Hg)*	*pH**	P_{CO_2}* *(mm Hg)*	Ca_{O_2}‡ *(Total) (mL/dL)*	Ca_{O_2} *(Dissolved) (mL/dL)*	*% Dissolved*	P_{O_2} *(mm Hg)*	*pH**	P_{CO_2}* *(mm Hg)*	*Cardiac Output* (L/min)*	*Heart Rate (bpm)*	*Stroke Volume (mL/beat)*	*Mean Blood Pressure (mm Hg)*
1	Air	150	102	89	7.45	37	16.3	0.3	2	41	7.42	41	6.1	75	81	89
1	O_2	713	673	507	7.46	37	18.2	1.5	8	57	7.42	42	5.8	71	82	90
3.04	Air	475	427	402	7.45	39	17.9	1.2	7	68	7.41	44	5.7	68	85	88
3.04	O_2	2263	2223	1721	7.47	37	21.8	5.2	24	424	7.40	45	5.3	63	92	92

*Data from Whalen RE, Saltzman HA, Holloway DH, et al: Cardiovascular and blood gas responses to hyperbaric oxygenation. Am J Cardiol 1965; 15:638–646.

†Obtained from a catheter with tip at the junction of the superior vena cava and right atrium.

‡Arterial oxygen concentration (Ca_{O_2}) calculated from measured arterial P_{O_2}, assuring hemoglobin = 12 g/dL.

plasma (0.3 mL/dL out of 16.6 mL/dL). However, while breathing 100% O_2 at 3 atmospheres absolute (ATA), 24% of arterial O_2 is in the dissolved form (5.2 mL/dL out of 21.8 mL/dL; Table 106–2).

At a constant metabolic rate, this increase in arterial O_2 content would be expected to result in a rise in P_{O_2}. Indeed such an increase in tissue oxygenation can be observed from direct measurements of mixed venous, transcutaneous and tissue P_{O_2}, and cytochrome redox using near-infrared spectroscopy (see Table 106–2).

Hyperoxia results in peripheral vasoconstriction and a reduction in tissue blood flow. At 3.04 ATA (inspired O_2 = 100%), cardiac output is reduced by 13%,[2] as shown in Table 106–2. While breathing 100% O_2, cerebral blood flow is reduced around by 15% at 1 ATA and 25% at 3.5 ATA. This reduction in regional blood flow without reduction of P_{O_2} has been used therapeutically for the treatment of cerebral edema (discussed later), edema due to crush injury,[3] and burns (discussed later). Physiologic effects of hyperbaric hyperoxia have been summarized by Fife and Camporesi.[4]

PHARMACOLOGY OF HYPEROXIA

Antibacterial Effects

Hypoxia in ischemic tissue can support the growth of anaerobic bacteria. These organisms lack antioxidant defense mechanisms. Therefore, HBO therapy, which can increase the production of O_2 free radicals, is directly toxic to anaerobic bacteria. The increased P_{O_2} that results from HBO therapy would therefore be expected to be bactericidal to these organisms. Indeed, ample experimental and clinical evidence shows that HBO is useful in the treatment of anaerobic infection (discussed later).

In addition, killing of aerobic bacteria by leukocytes is dependent on generation of reactive O_2 species within the lysosomes,[5] which is P_{O_2} dependent. Mader and colleagues[6] have shown in vitro that phagocytic killing of *Staphylococcus aureus* by polymorphonuclear leukocytes becomes progressively impaired as ambient P_{O_2} is decreased from 100 to 23 mm Hg. This mechanism appears also to be important in vivo when tissue P_{O_2} is low—for example, in bone infections.[6] In an animal model of osteomyelitis, tobramycin had increased killing power against *Pseudomonas* when HBO was added.[7]

Cellular Effects

In addition to the physiologic effects of hyperoxia related to O_2 transport, some tissue effects that are noted are presumably due to cellular or subcellular mechanisms. Zamboni and colleagues[8] have described a delayed decrease in blood flow after reperfusion of myocutaneous tissue flaps. This flow reduction appears to be due to adherence of leukocytes to the endothelium of the microcirculation. HBO administration minimizes this effect. A similar flow reduction observed in the microcirculation of the brain after arterial gas embolism (AGE)[9] has also been attributed to leukocyte accumulation in the capillaries.[10] It has been speculated that part of the beneficial effect of HBO in AGE might be due to prevention of such leukocyte adherence. The mechanism for this effect of HBO is unknown but may involve migration of leukocytes to the pulmonary circulation in response to alveolar hyperoxia.

HBO administration after CO exposure can reduce the lipid peroxidation in the brain that occurs during or after removal of CO.[11]

Oxygen Toxicity

Pharmacology

Exposure of an animal to increased P_{O_2} results in higher rates of endogenous production of reactive O_2 species, including superoxide anion, hydroxyl radical, hydrogen peroxide, and singlet O_2. It is believed that these reactive species underlie the mechanisms of tissue O_2 toxicity.[12, 13] Toxic effects of these species depend on both dose and duration of O_2 exposure and include lipid peroxidation, sulfhydryl group inactivation, oxidation of pyridine nucleotides, inactivation of Na^+-K^+ adenosine triphosphatase, and inhibition of deoxyribonucleic acid and protein synthesis.

Organ Effects

BRAIN. Oxygen toxicity affects the central nervous system (CNS) producing a wide variety of symptoms (Table 106–3). The most dramatic effect is generalized convulsions, which most commonly occur during clinical HBO therapy when the inspired P_{O_2} exceeds 3 ATA. These are usually self-limited and without evidence of lasting side effects when the inspired O_2 fraction (F_{IO_2}) is decreased to normal levels.[14] Factors that increase the risk of CNS O_2 toxicity include hypercapnia, exertion, and (in divers) water immersion. Although in-water convulsions in divers have been recorded at an inspired P_{O_2} of 1.3 ATA, convulsions during clinical HBO therapy are rare at an inspired P_{O_2} less than 3 ATA. In the authors' clinical experience, the risk of convulsions is approximately 0.02% at an inspired P_{O_2} of 2 ATA and around 4% at 3 ATA. Mild symptoms of CNS toxicity can be managed by discontinuing the supplementary O_2. Common symptoms such as nausea or facial paresthesias then resolve spontaneously and will not usually recur if the O_2 is restarted.

Prophylactic anticonvulsant therapy probably reduces the

TABLE 106–3. Symptoms and Signs of Central Nervous System Oxygen Toxicity

Facial pallor	Unpleasant olfactory sensations
Sweating	Unpleasant gustatory sensations
Bradycardia	Respiratory changes
Choking sensation	Panting
Sleepiness	Grunting
Depression	Hiccups
Euphoria	Inspiratory predominance
Apprehension	Diaphragmatic spasms
Changes of behavior	Severe nausea
Fidgeting	Spasmodic vomiting
Disinterest	Vertigo
Clumsiness	Fibrillation of lips
Visual symptoms	Lip twitching
Loss of acuity	Twitching of cheek and nose
Dazzle	Palpitations
Lateral movement	Epigastric tensions
Decrease of intensity	Syncope
Constriction of visual field	Convulsions
Acoustic symptoms	
Music	
Bell ringing	
Knocking	

(From Clark JM: Oxygen toxicity. *In*: The Physiology and Medicine of Diving. Bennett PB, Elliott DH [Eds]. Philadelphia, WB Saunders, 1993, pp 121–169.)

risk of convulsions when using clinical treatment schedules with significant risk of CNS O_2 toxicity (e.g., treatment pressure ~3 ATA). The authors' practice is to load patients with phenobarbital before HBO treatment and maintain the serum concentration within the anticonvulsive range during the entire period of treatment at this pressure. Phenytoin and benzodiazepines have also been used for this purpose. When using inspired P_{O_2} of 2.8 ATA or less, the risk of convulsions is sufficiently low that prophylactic anticonvulsant therapy is unnecessary.

LUNGS. Pulmonary O_2 toxicity is manifested initially as tracheobronchitis. Symptoms include burning substernal chest pain, cough, and ultimately dyspnea. Functional abnormalities include a reduction in forced vital capacity and CO transfer factor. Continued exposure to O_2 results in hyaline membrane formation, proliferation of type II pneumocytes,[15] and fibrosis. Pulmonary O_2 toxicity symptoms may not be evident in patients who are sedated and mechanically ventilated. Moreover, such patients often have pulmonary infiltrates for various reasons, and it may be impossible to distinguish the possible additive effects of pulmonary O_2 toxicity.

One method of qualifying pulmonary O_2 toxicity is to measure the resulting change in vital capacity. Reduction in vital capacity is related to both P_{O_2} and duration of exposure in a fashion described by Lambertsen[16] as shown in Figure 106–1. Mild symptoms of pulmonary O_2 toxicity may occur after a prolonged HBO treatment (e.g., extended United States Navy [USN] Table 6—see Fig. 106–6*B*), although greater exposures are necessary to cause measurable changes in pulmonary mechanics.

At present, reduction of the risk of pulmonary O_2 toxicity to a minimum is based on limiting exposure. Although the *maximum* safe inspired P_{O_2} during clinical HBO therapy is largely based on CNS O_2 toxicity limits, the *duration* is limited by pulmonary effects. Although the UPTD system (discussed next) can be used as an approximate guide to pulmonary O_2 toxicity risk, in awake patients the presence of burning of retrosternal chest pain is often more useful as an endpoint. Intermittent O_2 exposure reduces the rate of onset of toxic manifestations (Fig. 106–2). For this reason, many HBO treatment schedules include periods of air breathing ("air breaks") interspersed between the therapeutic periods of 100% O_2 breathing.

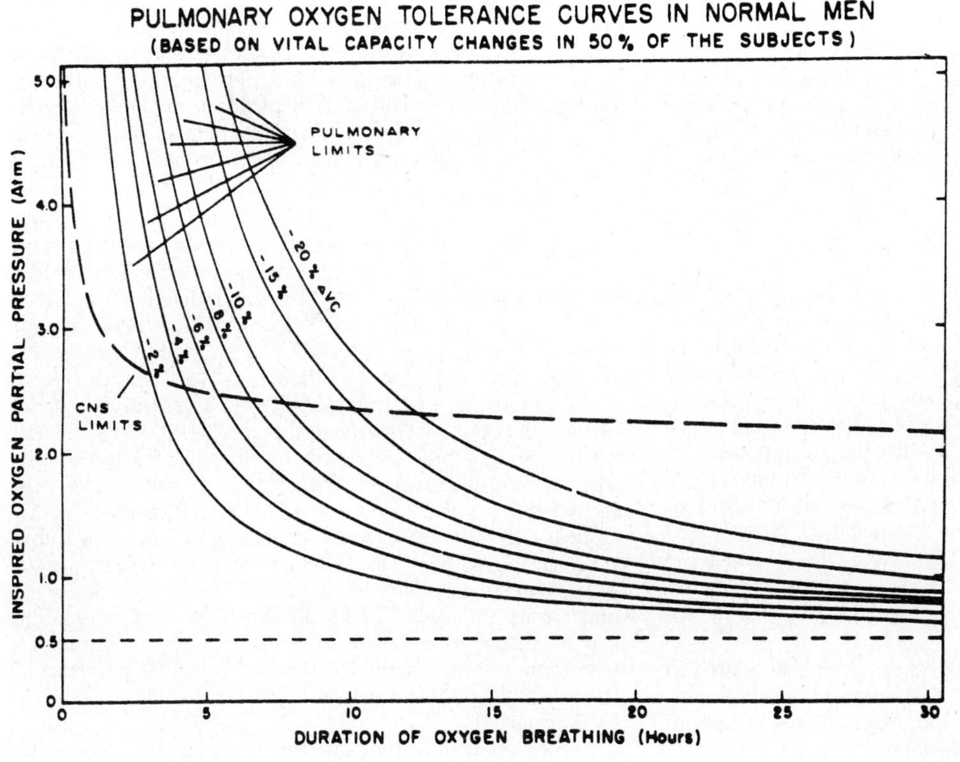

Figure 106–1. Dose-response curves for O_2 tolerance in humans. (From Clark JM: Oxygen toxicity. *In*: The Physiology and Medicine of Diving. Bennett PB, Elliott DH [Eds]. Philadelphia, WB Saunders, 1993, pp 121–169.)

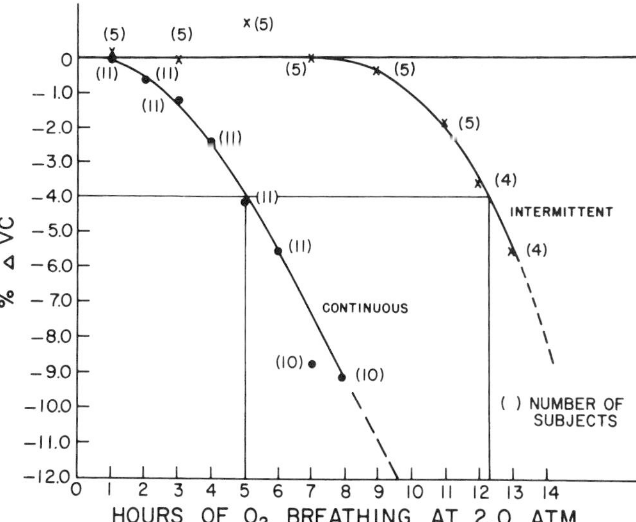

Figure 106–2. Rate of decrease of vital capacity (VC) during O_2 exposure in normal volunteers—continuous versus intermittent exposure. Insertion of air breaks into periods of 100% O_2 breathing during HBO therapy reduces the rate of development of pulmonary O_2 toxicity. (From Clark JM: Oxygen toxicity. *In*: The Physiology and Medicine of Diving. Bennett PB, Elliott DH [Eds]. Philadelphia, WB Saunders, 1993, pp 121–169.)

The following equation has been used to define the unit pulmonary toxic dose (UPTD):

$$\text{UPTD} = t \cdot m \sqrt{\frac{0.5}{P_{O_2} - 0.5}} \quad \text{[Equation 1]}$$

where P is inspired P_{O_2} in ATA, m is an empirically derived slope constant with a value of −1.2, and t is exposure time in minutes.[17] The UPTD calculated is related to a certain reduction in vital capacity. For example, 1425 UPTD units results in approximately a 10% reduction in vital capacity, whereas 2190 UPTD units results in around a 20% reduction. A simpler representation of the data is shown in the following equation, in which the per cent reduction in vital capacity is related to P_{O_2} and minutes of exposure (t):[18]

$$\%\Delta VC = -0.009 \cdot (P_{O_2} - 0.38) \cdot t \quad \text{[Equation 2]}$$

The UPTD concept has proved useful in generating approximate guidelines for O_2 exposure. However, interindividual variability in O_2 susceptibility is considerable. Moreover, other factors such as intermittent exposure, O_2 administration before HBO exposure, sepsis, tissue leukocytes, and probably a number of unknown modifiers may limit the accuracy of prediction.

Supplemental O_2 administration at 1 ATA between treatments may promote the development of pulmonary O_2 toxicity. Therefore, it is prudent to use the lowest safe F_{IO_2} between HBO treatments. However, the effects of mild or even moderate pulmonary O_2 toxicity are usually reversible. Therefore, in life-threatening situations requiring aggressive HBO therapy, some degree of pulmonary O_2 toxicity may be acceptable (Fig. 106–3).

The risk of pulmonary O_2 toxicity due to HBO therapy in patients with previous exposure to agents suspected of pro-

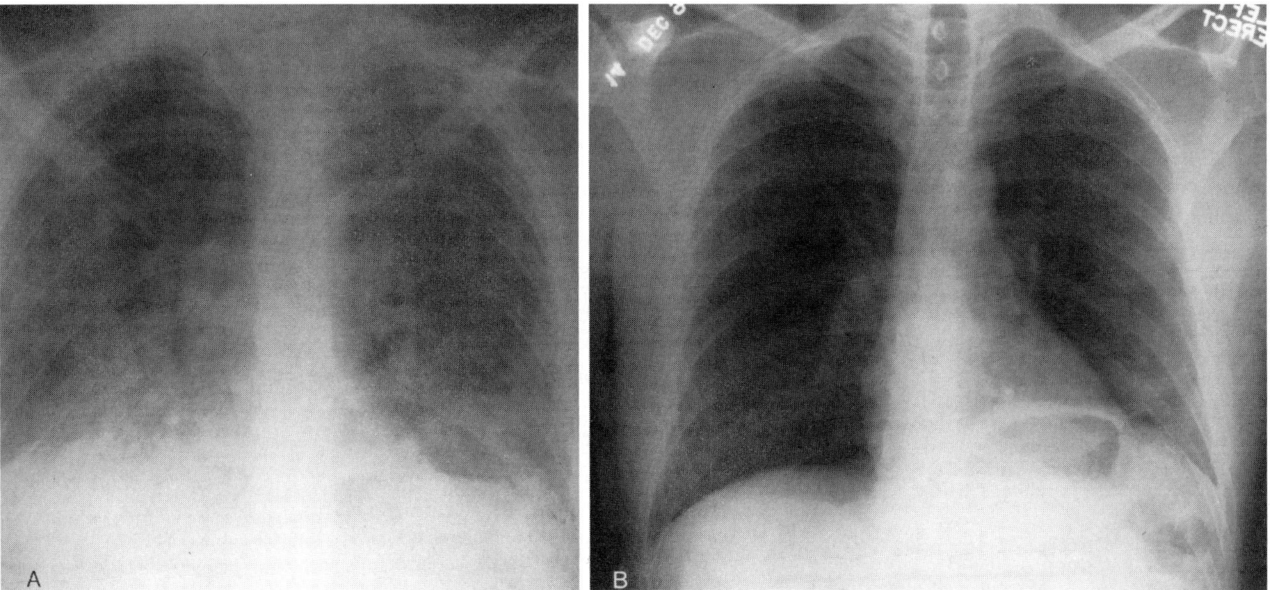

Figure 106–3. Severe pulmonary O_2 toxicity. The patient is a 40-year-old diver who developed dense paraplegia after exceeding safe depth-time limits during a scuba dive. *A*, Bilateral pulmonary edema due to O_2 toxicity after the patient had been exposed to around 3000 UPTD, and simultaneous significant neurologic improvement. Over the 2 to 3 days after discontinuation of supplemental O_2, his pulmonary symptoms resolved. *B*, Radiograph of the patient in *A* taken 2 weeks after initial radiography shows an almost complete return to normal.

moting O_2 toxicity, such as bleomycin or mitomycin C, is unknown, although the authors have treated several such individuals with HBO. Some of these individuals seem to have an enhanced propensity to develop mild pulmonary O_2 toxicity symptoms such as retrosternal burning chest pain, but life-threatening manifestations have not been reported.

EYE. Repetitive HBO therapy can result in myopia, which is probably caused by a change in the lens.[19] Twenty or more exposures are usually required to observe any change in visual acuity, although acute deterioration can sometimes occur after only one prolonged treatment. The myopia usually resolves at a rate approximately equal to that of onset but may occasionally only partially reverse.

Palmquist and colleagues[20] have suggested that HBO treatment may predispose to nuclear cataract formation. Although this possibility cannot be discounted, many of the patients in Palmquist's study received hundreds of hours of HBO treatment, considerably more than is customary. In addition, nuclear cataracts are associated with diabetes, which is often present in patients requiring prolonged, repetitive HBO therapy.

PERIPHERAL NERVE. After HBO exposure, some patients experience paresthesias, usually in their fingers and toes. These symptoms generally occur after repetitive HBO exposures but occasionally are noted after only a single (usually prolonged) HBO treatment. They normally resolve within a day or two, have no known clinical significance, and are not a reason to discontinue HBO therapy.

USE OF HYPERBARIC OXYGEN FOR SPECIFIC DISEASES

Gas Bubble Disease

The Spectrum of Gas Bubble Disease

ACCIDENTAL BUBBLE INJECTION. Intra-arterial injection of only small quantities of gas can result in acute stroke, myocardial infarction, or cardiac arrest. Iatrogenic AGE is usually caused by accidental arterial injection of air during diagnostic procedures or cardiopulmonary bypass. AGE can also be caused by pulmonary overpressurization from mechanical ventilation and penetrating lung trauma.

On the other hand, similar volumes of gas can be injected intravenously without clinical consequence because it is usually filtered by the pulmonary circulation. However, injection of greater than 0.35 mL/kg of gas can cross the pulmonary circulation directly or traverse the interatrial septum via a patent foramen ovale. Larger mounts of intravenous gas can also totally fill the right side of the heart and the pulmonary arteries, resulting in "vapor lock." Such a situation has been most commonly described during craniotomy in the sitting position, in which air may enter the vascular system via the intraosseous sinuses. In animal studies, the fatal bolus dose of intravenous gas injection is 4 to 5 mL/kg. Lower doses are often tolerated, although in dogs, constant infusions at 0.6 $mL \cdot kg^{-1} \cdot min^{-1}$ can cause electrocardiographic changes and 2 $mL \cdot kg^{-1} \cdot min^{-1}$ can result in severe hypotension.[21] In humans, fatalities have been recorded after intravenous injection of as little as 100 mL.[22, 23]

In addition to obstructing the flow of blood, gas can damage the vascular endothelium, causing changes in permeability. Intravenous air injection can thus cause pulmonary edema, which in divers is termed *cardiorespiratory decompression illness* ("chokes," discussed later). Similarly, AGE can cause cerebral edema.

GAS EMBOLISM IN DIVERS. Pulmonary overpressurization is the mechanism by which AGE occurs in scuba divers. During a dive, gas is delivered to the diver from the scuba regulator at a pressure equal to the ambient hydrostatic pressure. During ascent from the dive, gas-containing spaces within the body must be vented or they expand. Such spaces include bubbles within the gastrointestinal tract, paranasal sinuses, middle ear cavities, and lungs. During ascent, gas trapped within the lungs either by breath holding or by regional gas trapping (e.g., mucus plugging, bronchospasm, bullae, or blebs) therefore results in an increase in alveolar pressure. If intra-alveolar pressure exceeds tissue elastic pressure, gas may enter pulmonary capillaries. This can occur at a pressure between 80 and 100 mm Hg.[24] Hence, a breath-hold ascent from a scuba dive as shallow as 4 to 5 ft may result in AGE. Gas may also enter the pulmonary interstitium, from where it may track into the mediastinum or the pleural space, causing pneumomediastinum or pneumothorax.

Once bubbles have entered the arterial tree, they may cause symptoms or signs due to infarction of any end-organ, including the heart. However, the most common syndromes involve the brain:

CASE HISTORY

A 21-year-old diver trainee breathed from a scuba tank in a swimming pool at a depth of 10 ft. He made a panic ascent, and when he reached the surface had a generalized convulsion. A few minutes later, he regained consciousness but was hemiplegic.

IN SITU BUBBLE FORMATION. When a gas is dissolved in a liquid, an acute reduction in ambient pressure may allow the gas to come out of solution and form bubbles in a fashion analagous to carbon dioxide (CO_2) bubbling out of a carbonated beverage when the bottle cap is removed. Symptoms due to this phenomenon were first described in the 19th century in workers who were engaged in construction of bridge abutments, tunnels, or mines in an environment in which the pressure had been raised in order to prevent water from entering the workplace (caisson). On decompressing from the work environment, many of these men developed limb pain and neurologic symptoms, and death sometimes ensued. These events were subsequently described in divers. Similar effects can also occur in aviators who decompress during high-altitude flight (usually > 18,000 ft), and even moderate altitude exposure can cause decompression illness, particularly in a person who has been scuba diving within the past 24 hours.[25]

Bubbles can form in any tissue but appear to have a predilection for the areas around the joints, spinal cord, brain, and skin. Symptoms commonly consist of joint pain, paresthesias, limb weakness, and occasionally ataxia and loss of consciousness. A list of common presenting symptoms is shown in Table 106–4. A more detailed discussion can be found in Elliott and Moon.[26]

Traditionally, in situ gas formation has been called *decompression sickness,* to differentiate it from *arterial gas embolism.* This differentiation at one time had therapeutic significance because different recompression schedules were used for the two disorders. Decompression sickness has been classified as *type I* (musculoskeletal, skin, lymphatic, fatigue) and *type II* (neurologic, cardiorespiratory, inner ear, shock). Decompression sickness has been treated using USN Tables 5 or 6 (discussed later), whereas AGE has been treated using USN Table 6A (see Figs. 106–5 and 106–6). It has increasingly been recognized that the two syndromes often occur simultaneously. In addition, there is evidence that USN Table 6 is as effective as Table 6A for the treatment of AGE (discussed later). AGE (in divers) and both subclassifications of decompression sickness are now most commonly referred to using the umbrella term *decompression illness.*

TABLE 106–4. Distribution of Symptoms in 1249 Cases of Decompression Illness in Recreational Divers Reported to the Divers Alert Network

Initial Symptom	%	*Symptom at Any Time*	%
Pain	40.7	Pain	56.7
Altered skin sensation	19.2	Altered skin sensation	52.1
Dizziness	7.8	Weakness	22.4
Extreme headache	5.7	Dizziness	18.6
Headache	5.7	Extreme fatigue	17.1
Weakness	4.8	Headache	16.1
Nausea	2.9	Nausea	13.9
Difficulty breathing	2.5	Difficulty walking	10.2
Altered level of consciousness	2.1	Difficulty breathing	8.7
Itching	1.6	Altered level of consciousness	6.9
Visual disturbance	1.5	Visual disturbance	6.4
Rash	1.1	Paralysis	6.3
Paralysis	1.0	Itching	5.0
Personality change	0.8	Restlessness	4.6
Difficulty walking	0.7	Muscle twitching	4.0
Restlessness	0.4	Rash	3.5
Muscle twitching	0.4	Urethral/anal sphincter dysfunction	3.5
Urethral/anal sphincter dysfunction	0.4	Personality change	3.0
Tinnitus	0.2	Speech disturbance	2.8
Speech disturbance	0.2	Tinnitus	1.7
Convulsions	0.2	Hearing loss	1.1
Hearing loss	0.1	Convulsions	1.0
		Hemoptysis	0.7
Total	100.0		

(From Elliot DH, Moon RE: Manifestations of the decompression disorders. *In*: The Physiology and Medicine of Diving. Bennet PB, Elliot DH [Eds]. Philadelphia, WB Saunders, 1993, pp 481–505.)

CASE HISTORY

A 39-year-old man made three dives over 2 days, to depths of 104 ft, 97 ft, and 147 ft, respectively. During ascent from the third dive, he noted discomfort in the area of the distal biceps tendon in one arm. The pain gradually increased in intensity, and 12 hours after surfacing he experienced paresthesias in his ipsilateral hand. Physical examination revealed no abnormality. Twenty-four hours after surfacing from his last dive, he was recompressed using USN Table 6. The paresthesias resolved, and the pain was reduced in intensity. The following morning, the discomfort in his arm was almost imperceptible.

CASE HISTORY

A 42-year-old dive instructor made six dives during the course of 3 days, each dive to a depth of 77 ft for around 30 minutes. During decompression from his last dive, he noticed weakness in his legs. When he reached the surface, he was disoriented and had profound weakness in his legs and his left arm. He received treatment with USN Table 6A approximately 1 hour after injury, but the abnormalities only partially resolved. After being transferred to a tertiary referral center, he was found to have cortical blindness, paraplegia, urinary retention, and profound left arm weakness. Computed tomography of his brain showed hypodensity at the gray-white junction of both occipital lobes and in the thalamus. He received three USN Table 6 treatments and then nine more treatments at 2 ATA for 2 hours each. After treatment, he was able to walk with a cane and managed his bladder with intermittent self-catheterization.

Treatment

PREHOSPITAL TREATMENT. In addition to the standard principles of resuscitation, patients should be well hydrated with either oral or intravenous fluid and administered as high an FIO_2 as possible. Supplemental O_2 washes out blood and tissue nitrogen stores and therefore increases the partial pressure gradient for nitrogen to diffuse from bubbles into tissue or blood. Tissue hypoxia may result from vascular occlusion or pulmonary abnormalities such as aspiration, pneumothorax, or pulmonary edema due to venous gas embolism. Supplemental O_2 therefore hastens bubble shrinkage and ameliorates hypoxia. Oxygen is best administered with a tightly fitting facemask and demand valve or, if necessary, an endotracheal tube. Oxygen administered by nasal cannulas or a loose-fitting facemask, although undoubtedly beneficial, is probably less effective.

The head-down position was previously recommended for the treatment of AGE on the basis that because of buoyancy effects, residual gas in the pulmonary veins or left side of the heart might be less likely to "float to the head" and result in cerebral infarction. In addition, it was hypothesized that dilatation of the cerebral vessels secondary to hydrostatic loading would promote distal migration of bubbles and hence less cerebral ischemia. Indeed, Van Allen and colleagues[27] observed a higher mortality in dogs when they were embolized in the head-up position. Furthermore, Atkinson[28] demonstrated that placing embolized cats in a head-down position caused redistribution of bubbles in the direction of arterial flow. However, Butler and coworkers[29] demonstrated that buoyancy has minimum importance for the distribution of arterial gas. In addition, Atkinson observed a tendency for the development of cerebral edema in his cat preparation, an observation that has been confirmed by Dutka.[30] The supine position is therefore recommended by most practitioners for conscious victims with intact airway reflexes, and the lateral decubitus position for patients at increased risk of pulmonary aspiration or vomiting.

Intravenous fluid administration can reverse, at least for a short period of time, signs of decompression illness in dogs.* In severe cases of human decompression illness, hemoconcentration has been observed,[31] for which isotonic

*Hallenbeck JM: Personal communication.

crystalloid or colloid solutions are recommended. As in other CNS diseases, it is probably advisable to avoid glucose-containing fluids.

PHYSICAL REMOVAL OF GAS. Aspiration of gas from the superior vena cava or right atrium from an appropriately placed catheter has been lifesaving in some instances of massive venous gas embolism.[32] Removal of arterial bubbles caused by accidental injection during cardiopulmonary bypass has been performed using reversal of pump flow.[33] In most instances, however, physical removal of gas bubbles from the vascular tree is not feasible and is unlikely to be complete.

COMPRESSION. An increase in the ambient pressure results in a reduction in volume of tissue gas bubbles. For instance, recompression from 1 ATA to 6 ATA reduces a gas bubble to one sixth of its original volume.

Recompression therapy remains the mainstay of treatment for tissue gas. Originally, air was used as the breathing gas during treatment. This has the disadvantage that it results in additional inert gas (N_2) uptake, which might then promote bubble formation during the subsequent decompression.

Bert[1] demonstrated more than 100 years ago that the signs of decompression illness could be resolved in experimental animals by administering supplemental O_2. Yarbrough and Behnke[34] suggested that breathing 100% O_2 during recompression therapy would result in increased efficacy of treatment. In addition to eliminating excess inert gas uptake, O_2 breathing results in a significantly greater partial pressure gradient for nitrogen to diffuse out of bubbles (Fig. 106–4). Increased arterial O_2 content could also result in normalization of tissue O_2 in the event of low blood flow due to bubble fibrin or platelet accumulation.

Initial recommendations for the recompression pressure were based on the empirical tradeoff between the greatest bubble size reduction versus the risk of CNS system O_2 toxicity. A recompression "depth" of 60 ft of seawater (2.82 ATA) was initially suggested and remains the most commonly used recompression pressure for decompression illness.

Although no controlled studies have compared the outcomes of patients treated with HBO versus untreated, the preponderance of evidence supports the use of recompression therapy in gas bubble disease. In the 19th century and the early part of this century, large numbers of untreated cases of decompression illness due to caisson work were reported. Although the majority of cases of pain-only decompression illness resolved spontaneously, as did some cases of neurologic decompression illness, many other patients remained symptomatic or died. Keays[35] retrospectively reviewed decompression illness in caisson workers treated versus not treated. Around 14% of patients who did not receive recompression therapy had residual symptoms, compared with fewer than 1% of patients who were treated with recompression therapy. Evidence from the Diver's Alert Network (Durham, NC) indicates that in recreational divers with decompression illness, those who are treated early are less likely to have residual long-term symptoms than those treated after significant delay.[36] Similarly, a retrospective review of patients with AGE, both iatrogenic and dive related, strongly supports the use of hyperbaric treatment.[37]

Individuals with gas bubble disease treated early are more likely to have complete relief of symptoms than those treated after a delay. However, delays up to several days do not preclude significant clinical improvement after recompression therapy.[38–40]

SPECIFIC TREATMENT PROTOCOLS

The most commonly used treatment schedules were developed by the U.S. Navy[41] and are shown in Figures 106–5

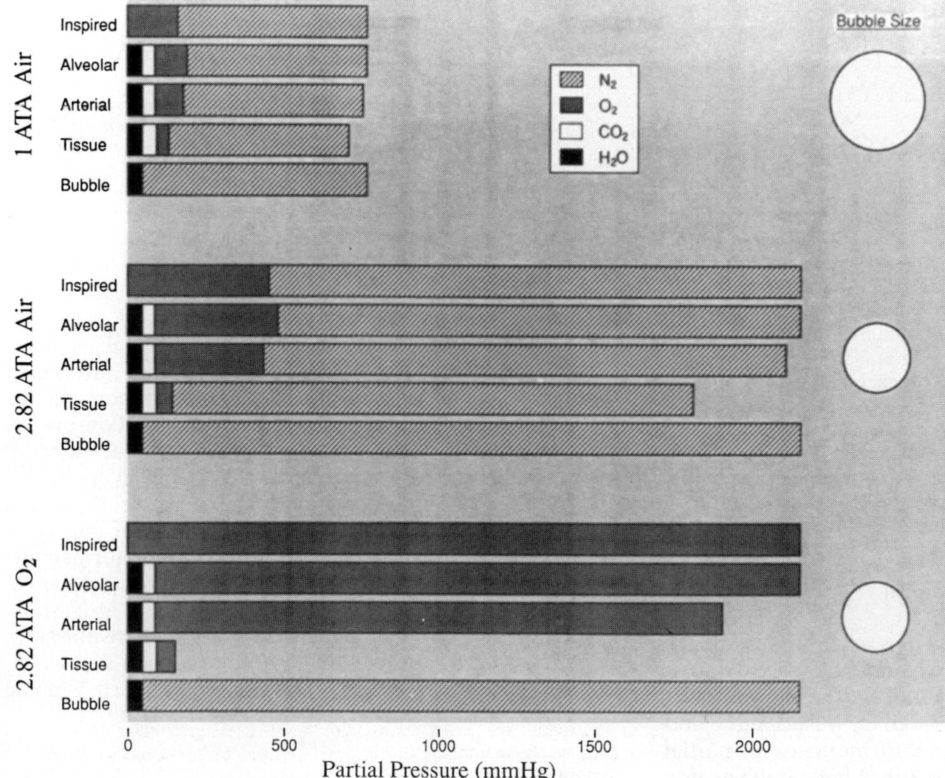

Figure 106–4. Partial pressures of gases within a bubble under various conditions. The *top panel* shows a bubble at 1 ATA while the patient breathes air. P_{N_2} in the bubble is slightly greater than that in the surrounding tissue; this tends to favor resorption of the gas. Compression to 2.82 ATA increases this gradient somewhat, as shown in the *middle panel*. Breathing 100% O_2 at 2.82 ATA *(bottom panel)* washes out nitrogen from the tissue surrounding the bubble, substantially increasing the gradient for diffusion of nitrogen and, hence, the rate of resolution of the bubble. (From Moon RE: Treatment of gas bubble disease. Probl Respir Care 1991; 4:232–252.)

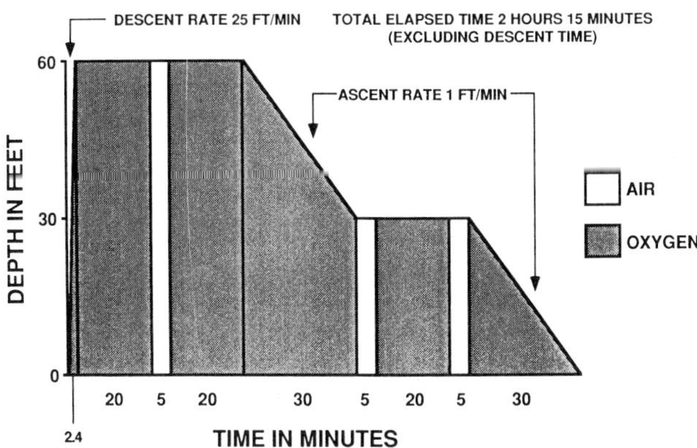

Figure 106–5. US Navy Table 5. This treatment table is designed for the management of patients with pain-only or skin bends, in which complete relief of symptoms occurs within 10 minutes of reaching the equivalent depth of 60 feet (2.82 ATA). (From Moon RE, Gorman DF: Treatment of decompression disorders. *In*: The Physiology and Medicine of Diving. Bennett PB, Elliott DH [Eds]. Philadelphia, WB Saunders, 1993, pp 121–169.)

and 106–6. Each treatment table includes periods of 100% O_2 breathing with air breaks interspersed to reduce the probability of O_2 toxicity. The initial treatment pressure is 2.82 ATA (60 ft of seawater, fsw). After a period at that pressure, the chamber is slowly decompressed to a pressure of 1.9 ATA (30 fsw). USN Table 5 is reserved for decompression illness in which pain is the only symptom and in which symptoms are completely resolved within 10 minutes of beginning recompression.

USN treatment Table 6 (Fig. 106–6*B*) is a longer version, using the same basic two-step paradigm. Additional O_2 cycles can be administered at both 60 and 30 fsw. Maximum duration at each pressure level is determined by pulmonary O_2 toxicity limits. Further details of specific treatment protocols can be found in USN Diving Manual[41] and in Moon and Gorman.[36]

USN Table 6A was designed for the treatment of AGE (see Fig. 106–6*A*). It consists of a Table 6 protocol preceded by a 30-minute period at 6 ATA (165 fsw), in an attempt to "crush" arterial bubbles. Because increasing the ambient pressure from 2.8 to 6 ATA results in only a small additional bubble diameter reduction, the utility of recompression to pressures greater than 2.82 ATA (60 fsw equivalent depth) has been questioned. The majority of animal studies do not support the use of higher pressures.[42–45] Use of 47% O_2 as the breathing gas at 6 ATA provided no measurable benefit using cortical evoked potentials as the endpoint in anesthetized cats.[46] In a retrospective review of human cases of decompression illness, Leitch and Green[47] concluded that clinical benefit could rarely be obtained by recompressing to a higher pressure than 2.82 ATA. On the other hand, Lee and colleagues,[48] using 40% O_2 during a 1-hour period at 6 ATA, presented clinical evidence in favor of using compression to 6 ATA in unresponsive or severe cases.

In the event that a patient has serious neurologic symptoms and shows ongoing improvement during the initial period of recompression, or deteriorates during decompression, then *saturation* treatment can be instituted. Saturation treatment consists of an indefinite period of O_2 and air breathing at a specified treatment pressure. Once the patient's clinical condition has stabilized, then decompression may be commenced. All tissues in both the patient and the individual caring for the patient are assumed to be fully saturated with inert gas at the increased ambient pressure. Therefore, in order to avoid inducing decompression illness in the caregiver or worsening of symptoms in the patient, decompression must be carried out at a significantly lower rate than for standard short recompression tables. An example of a saturation table (USN treatment Table 7) is shown in Figure 106–7.

If a single HBO treatment does not resolve all symptoms, repetitive treatments may produce additional improvement. Follow-up treatments are recommended until a patient is asymptomatic or improvement stops.

Adjunctive Measures

CORTICOSTEROIDS. Corticosteroids have been used both experimentally and clinically in decompression illness. In a retrospective review of 132 divers with AGE,[49] use of dexamethasone was associated with a reduced relapse rate: 10.8% in treated versus 29.5% in untreated individuals.

However, in a model of canine spinal decompression illness, using somatosensory evoked responses as an endpoint, Frances and Dutka[50] reported no additional benefit when methylprednisolone (20 mg/kg) was administered in addition to recompression treatment. In a canine study,[51]

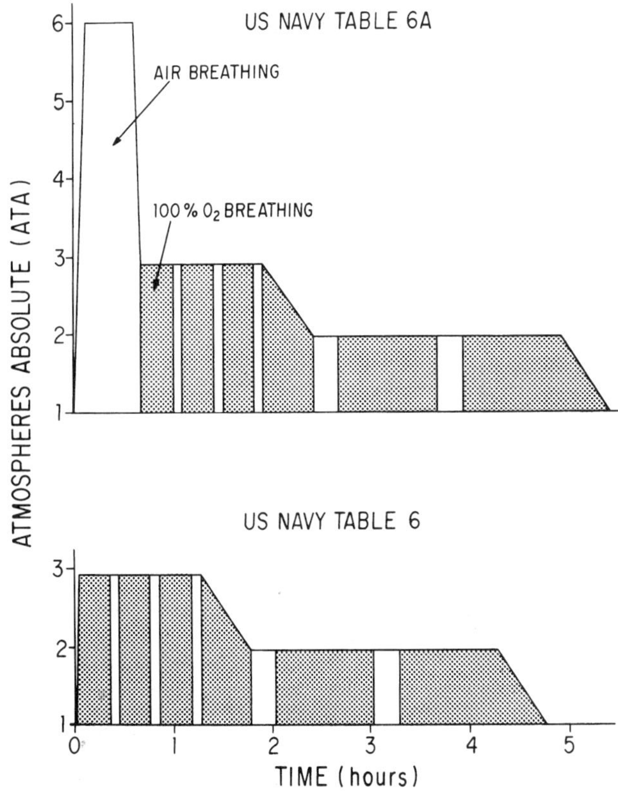

Figure 106–6. US Navy treatment tables for serious decompression illness. The *top panel* shows Table 6A, which was designed originally for the treatment of arterial gas embolism. Although originally designed to have the patient breathe air during the 30-minute exposure at 6 ATA, many diving physicians administer 40% to 50% O_2 during this phase. The *bottom panel* shows US Navy Table 6. Additional periods of O_2 breathing can be administered at both 2.82 and 1.9 ATA during use of these treatment tables. The majority of recompression treatments in patients with decompression illness use US Navy Table 6. If a patient fails to respond completely to an initial treatment, then repetitive treatments are given until no further stepwise improvement occurs. (From Moon RE: Treatment of gas bubble disease. Probl Respir Care 1991; 4:232–252.)

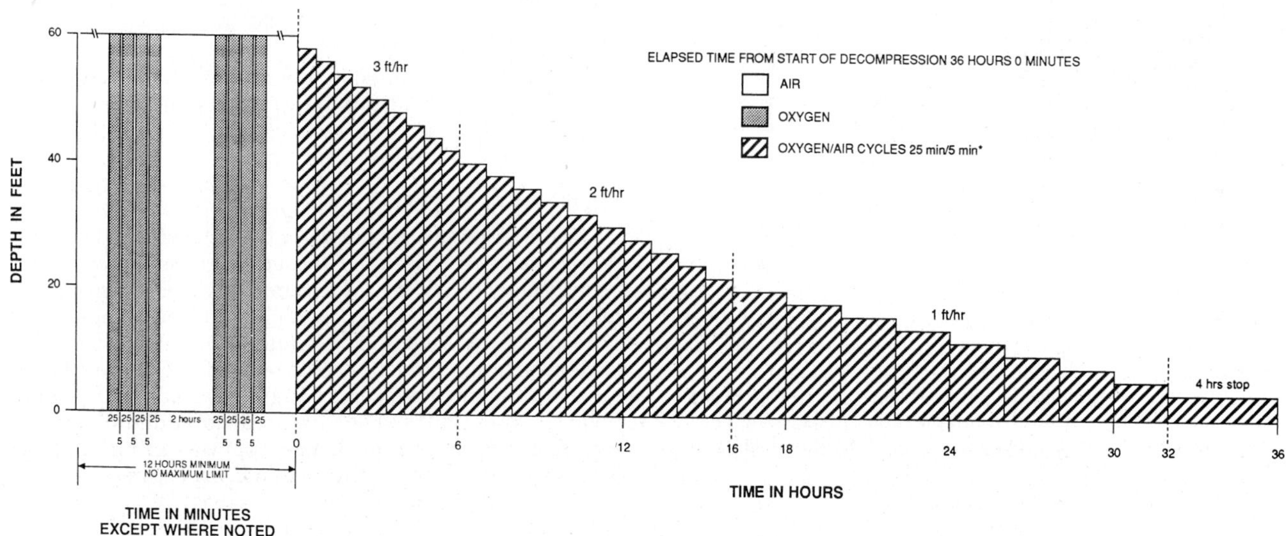

Figure 106–7. US Navy Table 7 (saturation table). The patient may spend an indefinite period of time at 60 feet (2.82 ATA), receiving intermittent periods of O_2 exposure. For details on administration, see the *USN Diving Manual* published by the US Navy.[51] This treatment may last several days. Therefore, in order to administer this treatment, the chamber facility must employ personnel who can work around-the-clock. Two on-duty "tenders" are preferable. Control of the chamber atmosphere must be carefully maintained to prevent fluctuations of the levels of O_2 and CO_2. (From Moon RE: Treatment of gas bubble disease. Probl Respir Care 1991; 4:232–252.)

dexamethasone was administered in addition to recompression therapy after experimental embolism of anesthetized animals. A slight benefit was noted with administration of dexamethasone, 1 mg/kg, 3 to 4 hours before and immediately after carotid artery embolization, but no effect when 2 mg/kg was administered after injection of air. Dexamethasone treatment did not prevent cerebral edema. On the other hand, the Second National Acute Spinal Cord Injury Study[52] showed that when methylprednisolone was given in a dose of 30 mg/kg bolus within 8 hours after acute mechanical spinal cord injury followed by a continuous infusion of 5.4 $mg \cdot kg^{-1} \cdot h^{-1}$ for 23 hours, significant benefit was observed 6 months after injury. The potential value of corticosteroids administered in these high doses to patients with decompression illness is unknown.

ANTICOAGULANTS. Intravascular bubble formation induces accumulation of platelets and fibrin at the blood-bubble interface, suggesting that anticoagulant therapy may be beneficial in the treatment of decompression illness. Diving physicians have been cautious about using therapeutic anticoagulation because of the tissue hemorrhage that may accompany spinal cord and inner ear decompression illness. However, various anticoagulants have been administered to patients with neurologic decompression illness in an attempt to minimize the secondary coagulation effects. Reeves and Workman[53] did not demonstrate a beneficial effect of using intravenous heparin in experimental decompression illness in dogs. A single case report of neurologic decompression illness treated with heparin[54] described neither adverse nor beneficial effect.

Nonsteroidal anti-inflammatory drugs also have antiplatelet activity and are commonly administered to patients who receive HBO therapy for pain-only decompression illness. It is not known whether this class of drugs has any benefit other than analgesia.

Despite the unknown value of anticoagulants in the treatment of decompression illness, they may have an important role in prophylaxis against deep vein thrombosis. Patients with paraplegia due to decompression illness are probably at high risk for this complication. Low-dose subcutaneous heparin or other prophylaxis for deep vein thrombosis may therefore be beneficial.

LIDOCAINE. Evans and colleagues showed both a prophylactic[55] and therapeutic[56] effect when lidocaine was used in experimental AGE in anesthetized cats. McDermott and associates,[57] using embolized, anesthetized cats, were unable to demonstrate a significant additive effect of lidocaine when added to HBO. However, using a more realistic model, which included a period of transient hypertension at the time of embolization of anesthetized dogs, Dutka and coworkers[58] reported that when intravenous lidocaine was used in addition to recompression, recovery of cortical evoked potential amplitude was twice as great as with recompression alone. No controlled human data exist at the time of this writing; however, in a case report of a diver with neurologic decompression illness poorly responsive to recompression therapy, significant clinical improvement occurred after an intravenous infusion of lidocaine was begun.[59] The mechanism of action of lidocaine in this setting has been speculated to be reduction in intracranial pressure and increased cerebral blood flow.[58]

FLUOROCARBONS. Fluorocarbons have a higher solubility for inert gases than plasma. One might therefore expect that intravenous administration of fluorocarbons could result in faster bubble resolution by virtue of providing a greater sink into which tissue and bubble nitrogen can diffuse. Indeed, Menasché and colleagues[60] have shown that infusion of the fluorocarbon FC-43 intravenously into rats allows more than 3 times the volume of air to be injected into the carotid artery before irreversible flattening of the electroencephalogram occurs. Decompression illness in experimental animals has also been treated with FC-43 and 100% O_2, resulting in a significantly improved survival.[60a]

Poisonings

Carbon Monoxide

CO binds to hemoproteins, resulting in impaired O_2 transport and utilization. CO binds to hemoglobin about 200 times as avidly as does O_2. The result is decreased amounts of hemoglobin available for O_2 transport and increased avidity of hemoglobin for O_2 (shift of the hemoglobin-O_2 dissociation curve to the left). Although these are important mechanisms for CO toxicity, the binding of CO to intracellular proteins (e.g., myoglobin, cytochrome c oxidase) may also be important.[61] Piantadosi and associates[62] demonstrated evidence for CO toxicity in rats in which blood was exchanged for fluorocarbon. During reoxygenation, after exposure to CO, O_2 free radical–mediated damage may occur.[63]

Acute toxicity can result in dysfunction of multiple organ systems, particularly the CNS. Commonly reported symptoms and signs include headache, nausea, vomiting, confusion, and loss of consciousness. A cursory neurologic examination may fail to detect cortical dysfunction caused by CO poisoning, which can often be demonstrated by simple bedside neuropsychologic testing.[64] Late neurologic sequelae can occur, sometimes after a lucid interval of a few days. The most useful clinical information in CO poisoning is a history of exposure and the degree of functional impairment at or shortly after exposure. Although carboxyhemoglobin (COHb) level is a useful marker of exposure, it does not correlate well with clinical outcome.

Pace and coworkers[65] demonstrated the relationship between COHb elimination half-life and inspired P_{O_2}. While breathing air at 1 ATA, the half-life of COHb degradation was 214 minutes. The half-life decreased to 42 minutes when breathing 100% O_2 at the same ambient pressure and to 18 minutes while breathing 100% O_2 at 2.5 ATA. In addition to this accelerated rate of elimination of CO from hemoglobin, removal from intracellular binding sites is probably enhanced by HBO treatment,[66] allowing more rapid recovery of energy metabolism.[67] During HBO treatment, the increased dissolved O_2 in the plasma can support tissue oxygenation pending elimination of CO. This is also evidence that HBO treatment can minimize damage due to lipid peroxidation, which occurs after clearance of CO.[11]

A prospective study compared normobaric O_2 with HBO therapy in a series of CO-poisoned patients and found no apparent benefit of HBO.[68] Unfortunately, this conclusion is not well supported by the published data, because the patients selected for this comparison were only mildly poisoned and would not have been expected a priori to have derived major benefit. Moreover, several patients were treated after significant delay (up to 12 h), during which time they were usually receiving supplemental O_2, therefore minimizing a possible favorable effect of subsequent HBO.

Clinical evidence exists suggesting that use of HBO in moderate to severe CO poisoning offers significant clinical benefits. Two comparable series of patients with CO poisoning were treated, respectively, with 100% O_2 at atmospheric pressure[69] and HBO.[70] Considering those patients who lost consciousness, in the HBO treated group, mortality was 50% lower and neurologic sequelae 80% lower than in the patients treated with 100% O_2 at 1 ATA. In a prospective, randomized study of HBO versus normobaric O_2 in moderately severe CO poisoning, Thom and associates[71] reported a significant reduction in late neurologic sequelae in patients treated with HBO.

Reasonable indications for the use of HBO in CO poisoning are as follows:[72]

- COHb level 25% or greater
- History of neurologic impairment including loss of consciousness
- Evidence of cardiac abnormalities (ischemia, arrhythmias, ventricular failure)

Another reasonable indication is significant CO exposure while pregnant. Although theoretic concern about the risk of HBO in pregnancy might cause hesitancy in using it, individual case reports and a published series provide evidence that the risk to the fetus of HBO treatment in CO poisoning is low.[73–76]

The window of opportunity for HBO in the treatment of CO poisoning is likely to be within the first few hours. Occasional cases of CO poisoning treated after 6 to 8 hours have improved after HBO, although no current evidence shows that hyperbaric treatment administered to patients after this length of time improves the ultimate outcome.

Carbon monoxide–poisoned patients with unremitting nausea, vomiting, or headache despite normobaric O_2 therapy are also occasionally considered for treatment.

Treatment of CO poisoning with HBO is customarily administered at 2 to 3 ATA for 90 to 150 minutes. Definitive studies comparing different treatment pressures and durations have not been published. A single treatment is almost always sufficient to reduce the COHb to baseline levels. However, CO binding to other sites cannot currently be measured, and patients who are still symptomatic after a single treatment are often treated one to three more times. In addition to eliminating CO from hemoproteins, HBO may produce additional benefit by reducing cerebral edema and possibly also pulmonary edema associated with concomitant smoke inhalation.[76a]

CASE HISTORY

A 35-year-old woman was found unconscious in her bed 48 hours after going to sleep. She was taken to an emergency room. On arrival she was stuporous and had several small peripheral retinal hemorrhages. COHb level was 41%. After breathing O_2 she began to awaken and remembered waking up several times at home with headache, nausea, and vomiting. On examination, she was unable to walk without assistance. Computed tomography of her brain showed normal findings. She was treated with O_2 at 2.5 ATA for 90 minutes with improvement. After three additional HBO treatments, she was asymptomatic and had normal findings on neurologic examination.

Cyanide

The major mode of toxicity of cyanide is interference with O_2 transport at cytochrome c oxidase; however, unlike CO, cyanide binding with cytochrome oxidase is not dependent on P_{O_2}. Therefore, the rationale for the use of HBO in acute cyanide poisoning is not as strong as it is for CO poisoning, particularly given the efficacy of conventional chemical treatment using sodium nitrate and thiosulfate.

Chemical treatment of cyanide poisoning with nitrite causes formation of methemoglobin, which then binds cyanide to produce cyanmethemoglobin. Neither hemoglobin variant binds O_2. Therefore, patients may have some degree of functional anemia in cyanide poisoning. If this is of sufficient magnitude to impair tissue O_2, then HBO administration could be of benefit, by augmenting the quantity of O_2

dissolved in plasma. Indeed, anecdotal reports suggest efficacy of HBO when standard chemical measures have failed.[77]

It should be noted that in addition to other toxic products such as CO, cyanide is frequently produced from combustion of building materials such as plastics. Patients exposed to products of combustion frequently have significant exposure to both CO and cyanide.

Hydrogen Sulfide

Hydrogen sulfide inhibits respiration at the level of the cell by virtue of reaction with cytochrome c oxidase. Sulfide binding to this enzyme is also not PO_2 dependent. Sulfide can also combine with hemoglobin to form sulfhemoglobin, which does not transport O_2. Clinical manifestations include pulmonary edema and loss of consciousness.

As with cyanide poisoning, the main rationale for use of HBO in hydrogen sulfide poisoning is to overcome the reduction in O_2 transport due to sulfhemoglobin. Anecdotal case reports suggest a beneficial effect of HBO in this toxicity.[78,79]

Carbon Tetrachloride

Poisoning with carbon tetrachloride typically results in CNS and hepatic toxicity. The possible value of HBO in this condition is exemplified by a report of a patient with circumstantial evidence of CO poisoning who appeared to respond to treatment with HBO. There was no definitive evidence of CO exposure, and after regaining consciousness, the patient admitted to having ingested approximately 250 mL of carbon tetrachloride (a lethal dose) 4 hours before HBO administration.[80]

Carbon tetrachloride is believed to exert its toxic effects by virtue of free radical generation[81] ($CCl_3^{\cdot}$ and $CCl_3OO^{\cdot}$), which may then cause lipid peroxidation. High hepatic PO_2 has been shown to reduce the conversion of carbon tetrachloride to its reactive metabolites, and evidence suggests that lipid peroxidation is reduced when experimental animals poisoned with carbon tetrachloride are treated with HBO.[82]

Necrotizing Infection

Clostridial Infections

Because anaerobic bacteria lack antioxidant defenses such as superoxide dismutase, the growth of these organisms in tissue tends to be inversely related to tissue PO_2. In vitro studies show that HBO can inhibit the growth of clostridia and alpha-toxin production. Another possible mechanism is a generalized increase in O_2 delivery to both infected and noninfected tissues.[83] Using animal models of clostridial myonecrosis,[84–86] an independent beneficial effect of HBO has been demonstrated when added to surgical débridement and antibiotics. Bakker[87] demonstrated that early HBO treatment and antibiotics provide adequate time for demarcation of necrotic tissue, which can then be removed surgically.

HBO treatment is typically administered between 2.5 and 3 ATA for around 90 minutes. Two to three treatments are usually given within the first 24 hours, and then two treatments daily until a patient is clinically stable and the infection is under control (usually 5–10 treatments).

A review of the literature examining the outcome of clostridial infection demonstrates a lower mortality when adjunctive HBO therapy is used (Table 106–5).

Nonclostridial Bacterial Infections

Necrotizing infections due to organisms other than clostridia are often mixed aerobic and anaerobic infections. Although the same rationale can be used to suggest that HBO can be beneficial, many of these infections are indolent, and an immediate clinical benefit of HBO may be difficult to discern.

Nevertheless, the benefit of HBO in nonclostridial necrotizing infection is supported by a controlled trial reported by Riseman and coworkers.[113] Additionally, a similar meta-analysis suggests a significant beneficial effect of HBO on clinical outcome (Table 106–6).

HBO schedules in this disease are usually similar to those advocated for the treatment of clostridial infections. Empirical endpoints of treatment include resolution of the acute infection and reduction in "toxicity." In view of the indolence of many of these infections and the lack of a well-defined endpoint, patients often receive a more protracted HBO therapy, sometimes lasting 2 weeks or more.

Mucormycosis

Rhinocerebral mucormycosis is due to infection with fungi from the family *Mucoraceae.* These fungi grow well in an environment with low PO_2, invade blood vessels, and cause infarction. Impaired leukocyte function in the hypoxic tissue allows greater proliferation of the organism. This disease usually occurs in diabetic patients and often is associated with ketoacidosis. The rationale for HBO treatment in this disease is to increase tissue PO_2 and enhance killing of the organism. Several case reports[122–126] and a retrospective re-

TABLE 106–5. Mortality in Gas Gangrene

Without Hyperbaric Oxygen				*With Hyperbaric Oxygen*			
Reference	*Number of Patients*	*Died*	*Mortality (%)*	*Reference*	*Number of Patients*	*Died*	*Mortality (%)*
DeLalande et al[88]	22	9	40.9	Bakker[96]	409	48	11.7
Freischlag et al[89]	21	11	52.0	Caplan and Kluge[97]	34	11	32.4
Gibson and Davis[90]	17	12	70.6	Gibson and Davis[90]	29	9	31.0
Hitchcock and Bubrick[91]	33	14	42.4	Gurtner[99]	73	23	31.5
Kaiser and Cerra[92]	20	8	40.0	Hart and Lamb[100]	139	27	19.4
Katlic and Derkac[93]	7	5	71.4	Heimbach[101]	58	3	5.2
Pailler and Labeeu[94]	20	8	41.0	Hirn and Niinikoski[102]	32	9	8.1
Vo and Watson[95]	77	31	40.0	Holland et al[86]	49	13	26.5
Total	**217**	**98**	**45.2**	Nier and Kremer[103]	78	30	38.5
				Shupak et al[104]	4	1	25.0
				Unsworth and Sharp[105]	73	15	20.5
				Total	**978**	**189**	**19.3**

TABLE 106–6. Mortality in Nonclostrdial Fasciitis

Without Hyperbaric Oxygen				*With Hyperbaric Oxygen*			
Reference	*Number of Patients*	*Died*	*Mortality (%)*	*Reference*	*Number of Patients*	*Died*	*Mortality (%)*
Brown et al[121a]*	24	10	41.7	Aasen et al[118]	9	1	11.1
Farrell et al[106]	11	5	45.5	Bakker[87]	27	5	18.5
Ledingham[107]	3	0	0	Brown et al[121a]*	30	9	30.0
Mader[108]	12	6	50.0	Chevallier et al[119]	13	4	30.8
Majeski[109]	20	10	50.0	Gozal et al[120]	16	2	12.5
Oh et al[110]	28	10	35.7	Hirn and Niinikoski[102]	11	1	9.1
Pessa and Howard[111]	33	13	39.4	Krasova et al[121]	11	3	27.3
Reigels-Nielsen et al[112]	5	1	20.0	Ledingham[107]	9	8	88.9
Riseman et al[113]	12	8	66.7	Mader[108]	10	2	20.0
Rouse and Malangoni[114]	27	20	74.1	Riseman et al[113]	17	4	23.5
Spirnak et al[115]	20	9	45.0	**Total**	**153**	**39**	**25.5**
Wang and Shih[116]	18	6	33.3				
Woodburn and Ramsay[117]	19	7	36.8				
Total	**232**	**105**	**45.3**				

*9 patients with clostridial myonecrosis included, in whom the breakdown between HBO and no HBO was not reported.

view comparing the outcomes of patients treated with or without adjunctive HBO[127] suggest a beneficial effect of HBO in this disease.

Head Injury

The reduction of cerebral blood flow that occurs during HBO therapy has previously been shown to be associated with a reduction in intracranial pressure.[128] This decrease in intracranial pressure in response to hyperoxia has been reported to be transient[129] and does not occur when cerebral autoregulation is absent.

Because of this ameliorative effect of HBO on intracranial hypertension, it has been suggested that HBO may also have a long-term beneficial effect on acute head injury. Indeed, Holbach and colleagues[130] treated 99 patients with severe head injuries using HBO. The mortality rate in the treated individuals was significantly lower than in the controls (33% vs. 74%), and the percentage of patients who made a good recovery was significantly greater in the HBO-treated individuals (33% vs. 6%). Rockswold and associates[131] studied 168 patients who suffered head injuries and who had a Glasgow Coma Scale score of 9 or less for 6 hours or more. All patients were treated with standard techniques for management of head injuries. Eighty-four patients were randomly selected to receive HBO, which was administered at 1.5 ATA for 1 hour every 8 hours for 2 weeks or until the patient was either brain dead or awake. Mortality rate was significantly lower in the HBO-treated patients (17% vs. 32% in controls). Despite this improvement in acute mortality, the outcome at 12 months was not significantly different in the two groups.

Thermal Injury

Ikeda and colleagues[132] reported on a series of patients who experienced CO poisoning due to coal mine explosions and fire. Patients who were treated for CO poisoning with HBO and who also had burns showed more rapid healing and less infection than other burned patients who did not receive HBO. Although some studies have failed to demonstrate a beneficial effect of HBO,[133] many others support its use. Korn and associates[134] studied the effect of twice-daily HBO treatment at 2 ATA for 90 minutes on burn healing in guinea pigs. HBO resulted in more rapid epithelialization and return of vascularity to the burn wound. Hammarlund and coworkers[135] inflicted 5-mm-diameter ultraviolet-irradiated blister wounds on normal volunteers. Three HBO treatments within 24 hours at 2.8 ATA for 60 minutes each resulted in a significant reduction in burn diameter and fluid exudation rate. In a randomized prospective study, Hart and colleagues[136] demonstrated that HBO treatment of patients with burns was associated with a significant reduction in healing time. Niu and associates[137] reported a comparative study of 266 patients with burns (mean 34% of body surface area) treated with HBO and a control group of 609 patients who did not receive HBO (mean 36% of body surface area). Although overall mortality did not differ between the groups, among patients aged 15 to 45 years with burns covering 35% to 75% of body surface area, mortality in the HBO-treated group was significantly reduced (6.8% vs. 14.8%). Cianci and coworkers[138] reported a controlled trial of HBO in which patients treated with HBO at 2 ATA for 90 minutes twice daily were in the hospital for a mean of 20.8 days versus 33 days in controls. In another report, in addition to shorter hospital stay, HBO-treated patients had lower average hospital costs ($60,350) than did controls ($91,960).[139]

As recent information has demonstrated a benefit of adjunctive O_2 therapy for the treatment of burns,[139a] clinical utilization of this modality has grown. In addition to any beneficial effects of HBO on the burn itself, many individuals with severe burns also have CO poisoning, which can be detected by measurement of blood COHb and appropriately treated with HBO.

Other Indications

HBO has been used to support tissue oxygenation transiently in patients with severe anemia when their blood cannot readily be crossmatched or in patients who refuse transfusion.[140] HBO has also been used to maintain arterial P_{O_2} during therapeutic lung lavage, during which gas exchange must be maintained on a single lung.[141]

HBO is also used for various nonacute conditions (Table 106–7). The common theme that underlies the rationale for treatment of these conditions is insufficient tissue oxygenation. A complete review of accepted indications can be found in a biannual publication of the Undersea and Hyperbaric Medical Society.[142] Additional reference sources are listed in Greenbaum and Mathias.[143]

TABLE 106–7. A Partial List of Conditions for Which Hyperbaric Oxygen Has Been Successfully Used

Gas bubble disease
- Air embolism[144, 145]
- Decompression sickness[36]

Poisoning
- Carbon monoxide[72]
- Cyanide[77]

Infections
- Clostridial myonecrosis[87]
- Other soft-tissue necrotizing infections[113]
- Refractory chronic osteomyelitis[146]
- Mucormycosis[126]

Acute ischemia
- Crush injury[3]
- Compromised skin flaps[8]

Chronic ischemia
- Radiation necrosis (soft tissue, radiation cystitis, and osteoradionecrosis)[147, 148, 148a,b]
- Ischemic ulcers, including diabetic ulcers[149, 149a]

Central nervous system edema[128]

Acute hypoxia
- Support of oxygenation during therapeutic lung lavage[141]
- Exceptional blood loss anemia (when transfusion delayed or unavailable)[140]

Thermal injury (burns)[137, 139, 139a]

MECHANICS

Chambers

Hyperbaric chambers are commonly classified according to the number of individuals inside. A multiplace chamber can accommodate one or more patients along with a caregiver (tender). The caregiver is typically a nurse who can provide assistance to the patient and manage intravascular monitoring catheters, obtain blood samples, administer medications, and evaluate patients. Multiplace chambers (Fig. 106–8) are usually compressed using air. Oxygen is administered to patients with either a tightly fitting facemask, head tent, or endotracheal tube. Medications, food, and blood samples can be moved into or out of the chamber using transfer locks. Prolonged treatment up to several days for patients with decompression illness (saturation treatment) can be accomplished using multiplace chambers. Additional personnel can also move into and out of the chamber using personnel locks. Multiplace chambers can typically be compressed to at least 6 ATA.

Monoplace chambers (Fig. 106–9), usually constructed of Plexiglas, can accommodate a single patient. They are generally compressed with 100% O_2, to a maximum operating pressure of around 3 ATA. Some practitioners have compressed these chambers with air, providing 100% O_2 to a patient via a tight-fitting mask. Patient monitoring connections can be made via through-hull penetrators adjacent to a patient's head. Although hands-on treatment of patients in monoplace chambers is not possible, intravenous fluid administration, intravascular monitoring, mechanical ventilation, and chest tube management all can be accomplished in these units.[151] If prolonged treatments are required (e.g., USN Table 6) air breaks can be administered to patients via a tight-fitting mask equipped with a demand valve.

Critically ill patients can more easily be cared for in multiplace chambers. Patients can easily be fed, and urine and stool elimination can also be managed. On the other hand, installation of a multiplace chamber requires a specially designed and engineered room. Multiplace chambers are costly and require a chamber operator in addition to inside and outside caregivers. Monoplace chambers, despite some practical shortcomings, are inexpensive, can be connected to standard hospital O_2 supplies, and require only one operator, who can also be a nurse.

Ventilatory Care

Important considerations in the choice of a ventilator for use in a hyperbaric environment include fire safety, simplicity, and small size. Fire hazard increases substantially when combustible materials are in contact with O_2 at high ambient pressure (discussed later). Therefore, it is preferable that ventilators not require electrical power but rather be fluidically or pneumatically controlled. Flammable lubricants

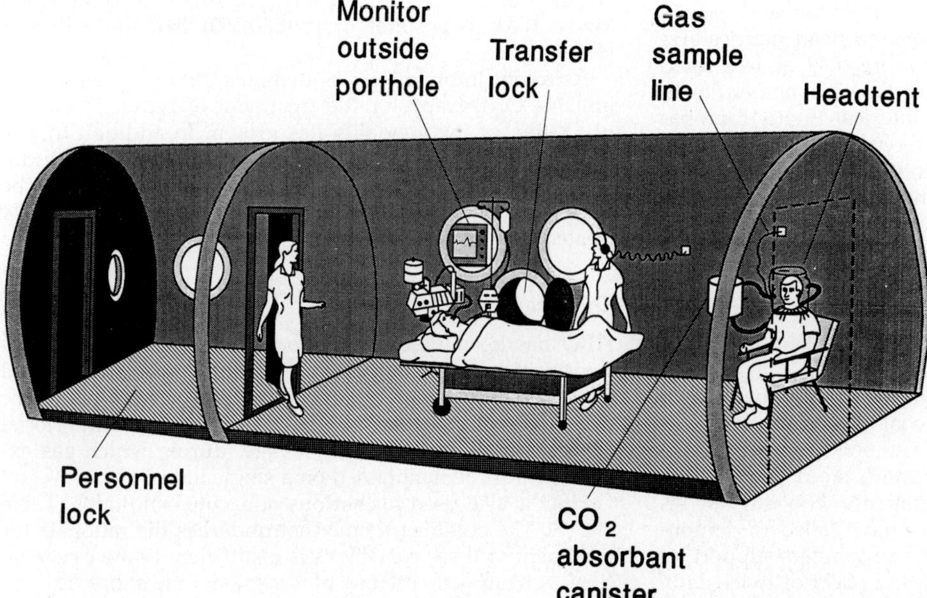

Figure 106–8. A multiplace chamber. Oxygen can be administered to the patient with a headtent (shown), endotracheal tube (shown), or a tight-fitting facemask (not shown). Many patients can be treated simultaneously. Medical personnel (tenders) accompany the patient during treatment. Additional personnel can enter the chamber using the personnel lock. Supplies can also be transferred via the transfer lock. Monitor displays are most conveniently kept outside the chamber to minimize electrical hazards and to prevent implosion of cathode ray tubes. Maximum pressure for multiplace chambers is usually at least 6 ATA (165 feet). The chamber atmosphere in hospital-based chambers and in most other multiplace chambers is composed of compressed air. Helium-oxygen is occasionally used in the chamber for the treatment of divers with decompression illness sustained while diving and breathing He–O_2. (From Moon RE, Camporesi EM: Operational use and patient monitoring in a multiplace hyperbaric chamber. Probl Respir Care 1991; 4:172–188.)

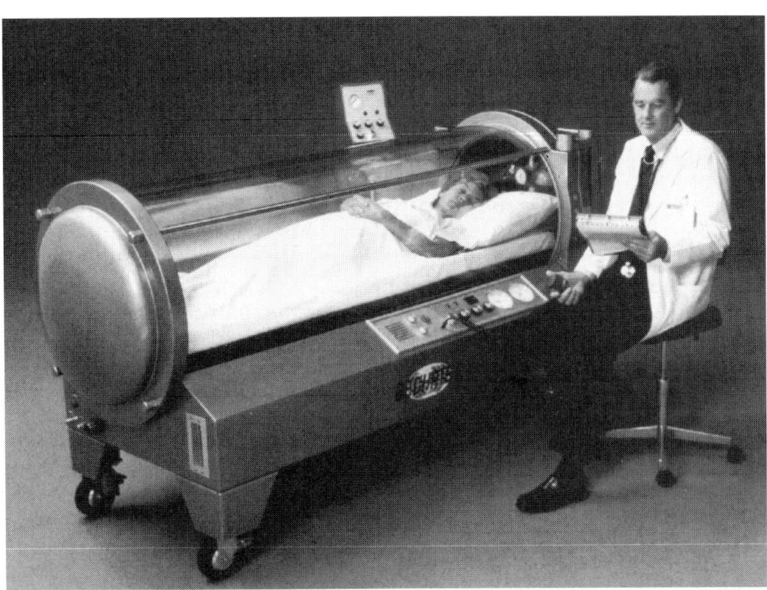

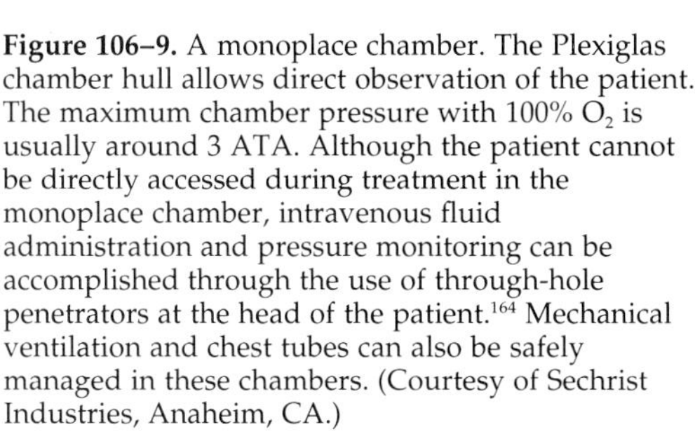

Figure 106–9. A monoplace chamber. The Plexiglas chamber hull allows direct observation of the patient. The maximum chamber pressure with 100% O_2 is usually around 3 ATA. Although the patient cannot be directly accessed during treatment in the monoplace chamber, intravenous fluid administration and pressure monitoring can be accomplished through the use of through-hole penetrators at the head of the patient.[164] Mechanical ventilation and chest tubes can also be safely managed in these chambers. (Courtesy of Sechrist Industries, Anaheim, CA.)

should be avoided if possible: Hydrocarbons spontaneously ignite when in contact with aluminum at increased ambient Po_2. In addition, gas density increases in proportion to ambient pressure, resulting in a net rise in airways resistance. Therefore, volume-cycled ventilators are preferable. Table 106–8 summarizes the characteristics of a number of ventilators that have been used in hyperbaric environments.

Compression of the chamber results in a reduction in volume of any enclosed gas-containing space, including endotracheal tube cuffs. This can be managed by continuous addition of air during chamber compression. However, gas must be removed during decompression in order to avoid hyperinflation of the balloon. It is safer and easier to remove all air from an endotracheal tube cuff before compression and to replace it with an appropriate volume of water.

Intravenous Infusion Devices

Intravenous infusion of fluids contained in flexible plastic bags poses no major difficulty. The only minor adjustment is of the amount of air within the drip chamber. The air volume tends to decrease with compression and expand with decompression. Nonvented glass intravenous fluid

TABLE 106–8. Ventilators Used in Hyperbaric Chambers

Ventilators	*Comments*	*References*
Bennett PR-2	Controlling circuitry can be separated from the actuator and kept outside the chamber.	Weaver[151]
Bird	Pressure-cycled ventilators, operating characteristics vary significantly as ambient pressure is changed.	Gallagher et al[153]
Dräager Oxylog	Extremely compact fluidically controlled ventilator.	
Dräager Hyperlog	Extremely compact fluidically controlled ventilator designed specifically for hyperbaric use.	Pelaia et al[154]
LAMA RCH (Laboratories de Mechanique Appliqué, Egly, France)	Designed for use up to 6 ATA.	Le Masson et al[155]
Logic 03		Degauque et al[156]
Monaghan 225	Fluidically controlled ventilator. Satisfactory performance at least to 7 ATA, with some slowing of rate at increasing ambient pressure. Modification possible to allow compressed air actuation.	Moon et al[157]
Ohio 550	Fluidically controlled ventilator; preliminary tests at Duke revealed satisfactory operation to 4 ATA.	
Penlon Nuffield 200		Lewis et al[158]
Penlon Oxford	Successfully tested at 31 ATA.	Saywood et al[159]
Pneumatic Emerson	Controller; intermittent mandatory ventilation circuit added separately if needed. Originally designed using leather bellows and mineral oil lubricant, which would require modification for safe hyperbaric use.	Gallagher et al[153]
PneuPAC Variant HB	Compact ventilator designed for use in monoplace chambers.	Spittal et al[160]
Sechrist 500A	Compact fluidically controlled ventilator designed for monoplace chamber use. Some alteration of performance with changes in supply pressure, thoracic compliance, and at ambient pressure higher than 2.2 ATA.	Weaver[151, 152]
Siemens 900C	Sophisticated, compact, electronically controlled ventilator. High O_2 levels near electric components. Expired volume monitor may not be accurate except at 1 ATA.	Holcomb et al[161]

containers can potentially be extremely dangerous, however. Implosion during compression and explosion during decompression are risks.

Accurate fluid administration using flow-controlled pumps is possible. IVAC 260 Volumetric Controllers and Variable Pressure Volumetric Pumps (San Diego, CA) work satisfactorily under steady-state conditions in a hyperbaric chamber. Because they use drop counting to measure the flow rate, inaccuracy may result during compression and decompression as the gas within the drip chamber compresses and expands. IMED pumps (IMED Corp., San Diego, CA) do not require a drip chamber for monitoring of flow. The IMED 208 and 905 pumps have been tested satisfactorily to 6.75 ATA. Abbott Life Care 5000 Infusion Pumps (Abbott Laboratories, North Chicago, IL) work extremely well without any significant changes in flow during compression and decompression.

In order to minimize fire hazard due to electric sparks, many hyperbaric facilities purge the cowling of electrically powered instruments with 100% nitrogen (discussed later).

Arterial Blood Gas

Measurement

While arterial PO_2 increases along with inspired PO_2 during hyperbaric exposure, arterial pH and PCO_2 continue to be regulated by the body to near 7.4 and 40 mm Hg, respectively (see Table 106–2). Blood gas electrodes cannot be calibrated accurately at PO_2 values higher than around 700 mm Hg unless the electrodes or the blood gas machine is pressurized. Therefore, extremely precise PO_2 measurements are best performed on a blood gas machine inside the chamber. A modified blood gas instrument and analysis protocols are required, as well as a technician specially trained in this technique.

It is much more convenient, therefore, to measure blood gases on samples decompressed to 1 ATA. Indeed, pH and PCO_2 can accurately be measured on such samples. However, because the PO_2 is usually higher than 700 mm Hg, supersaturation of O_2 occurs during decompression, and there is a tendency for bubble formation and hence a tendency for the PO_2 in the sample to decrease. Weaver and colleagues[162] have shown that despite this theoretic objection, PO_2 values can be reasonably accurate if the sample is measured immediately after decompression. Furthermore, for clinical purposes it may not be necessary to have more than 10% to 20% accuracy under hyperbaric conditions.

PO_2 attained during hyperbaric treatment can be estimated reasonably accurately from blood gas measurements obtained at 1 ATA. Gilbert and Keighley[163] showed that the ratio of arterial to alveolar PO_2 (PaO_2/PAO_2) is reasonably constant over a range of FIO_2 from 0.21 to 1.0. The PaO_2/PAO_2 ratio is in fact reasonably constant up to an inspired PO_2 of 3 ATA. Therefore, 1 ATA blood gas measurement can be used to predict the PO_2 under hyperbaric conditions, according to the following equation:

$$PO_2\ (\text{predicted}) = PaO_2/PAO_2 \cdot [760 \cdot P_{ATA} - 47 - PCO_2] \quad \text{[Equation 3]}$$

where P_{ATA} is the chamber pressure in atmospheres absolute. Alveolar PO_2 is calculated from the following equation:

$$PAO_2 = (P_b - PH_2O) \cdot FIO_2 - PACO_2 \cdot \left[FIO_2 + \frac{(1 - FIO_2)}{R} \right] \quad \text{[Equation 4]}$$

where P_b is the ambient pressure (usually 760 mm Hg) and PH_2O the saturated vapor pressure of water at body temperature (usually 47 mm Hg); $PACO_2$ is alveolar PCO_2 (usually assumed equal to arterial PCO_2); and R is respiratory quotient (usually 0.8).

In the presence of lung disease, Equation 3 tends to underestimate the actual PO_2 under hyperbaric conditions, for two reasons. First, PaO_2 while breathing an inspired O_2 mixture less than 1.0 is affected by both alveolar ventilation-perfusion ($\dot{V}A/\dot{Q}$) mismatch and intrapulmonary shunt; while breathing 100% O_2, $\dot{V}A/\dot{Q}$ mismatch has no influence on arterial PO_2. Second, under hyperbaric conditions, mixed venous blood may be almost fully saturated, and thus right-to-left shunt has quantitatively less of an effect on arterial PO_2.

Hypercapnia results in cerebral vasodilatation, which may increase the risk of hyperoxic convulsions. In ventilated patients it is often helpful, therefore, to measure arterial PCO_2 shortly after compression in order to ensure adequacy of ventilation. Individuals with hypercapnia under 1 ATA conditions are likely to experience an acute rise in PCO_2 when administered HBO. This is because of both a reduced respiratory drive induced by hyperoxia and relative hypoventilation because of the increased respiratory effort associated with breathing dense gas. Therefore, if HBO treatment of such individuals is considered necessary, mechanical ventilation may be required.

Patient Monitoring

Patient monitoring in a multiplace chamber should ideally include a display that is visible to the caregivers inside the chamber as well as to the outside chamber operator, nurse, or physician. Cathode ray tubes are likely to implode at high ambient pressure. If such devices are used, it is safest to place the monitor outside the chamber facing one of the view ports. Liquid crystal display units can be used in hyperbaric chambers.

Electrical monitoring is easily accomplished using cables plumbed through the chamber hull. In order to isolate preamplifiers from the chamber wall, it is best to use individual shielded wires for each electrode.

Standard sphygmomanometers with stethoscope can be used inside hyperbaric chambers. However, spillage of mercury inside a hyperbaric chamber can produce a dangerously high mercury vapor pressure. It is therefore recommended that aneroid pressure gauges be used rather than mercury-filled ones. Automatic noninvasive blood pressure monitors can be used in the hyperbaric environment.

Strain gauge pressure transducers used for invasive pressure monitoring require no modification when used under hyperbaric conditions. Whereas older Statham-type transducers tend to vary their zero offset during chamber compression and decompression, the newer disposable type are acceptably stable. Pressure transducers can be readily zeroed to chamber pressure. If pneumatically inflated pressure bags are used in conjunction with continuous-flow systems, they must be further inflated on compression in order to maintain a constant 300 mm Hg pressure and subsequently deflated before decompression. An alternative is to use a spring-loaded rather than a pneumatically pressurized device.

During compression and decompression of the chamber, pulmonary artery catheter balloon ports must be vented to the chamber atmosphere. In other words, the balloon inflation syringe must be disconnected from the inflation port. If this is not done, the balloon may be forcefully pressed against the internal port during compression, causing tearing; during decompression, the balloon may explode or rupture a pulmonary vessel.

Fire Hazard

The extremely high Po_2 that may be present in the chamber atmosphere or in isolated instruments (e.g., ventilators) can result in a significant increase in fire risk. A child undergoing hyperbaric treatment was incinerated when fire was started by a spark from a toy that had been allowed inside the chamber. In another instance, a preheated bed sheet caught fire when compressed to 2 ATA.[164a]

Minimization of fire hazard may require a number of modifications of standard intensive care unit practice. First, the inevitable increase in chamber Po_2 in multiplace facilities should be minimized. This increase in Po_2 occurs because of leakage from headtents, masks, or ventilators. Continuous monitoring of the chamber Po_2 can provide guidance as to when the chamber should be vented with air to reduce O_2 concentration to an acceptable level (typically 23%). Sources of spark and heat should be eliminated if possible. An additional safety measure is purging of electric instruments with 100% nitrogen at a flow rate sufficient to maintain the Po_2 within the instrument at a level that would not support combustion.

Patients must be forbidden from carrying sources of combustion into the chamber. These restrictions include matches, cigarette lighters, or battery-operated devices. Static electricity can result in a fire; therefore, cotton garments are safer than ones manufactured out of synthetic material. Hair grease should be removed, and hydrocarbon lubricants should be avoided. Fluorocarbon lubricants that are nonflammable are preferred. Humidification of the breathing gas within headtent systems further reduces fire hazard.

Sparking that might occur when electric instruments are plugged in or unplugged should be minimized. High-voltage (120 V) instruments can be plugged into hard-wired extension cords before compression of the chamber, and the connection securely taped. An alternative to hard wiring is to use explosion-proof plugs, such as Arktite Series (Crouse-Hinds, Division of Cooper Industries, Syracuse, NY).

Defibrillation is another source of sparking. Low-resistance electrode gel or use of preapplied disposable defibrillator pads is likely to minimize this risk.

Atmosphere Control

Trace gases exert their toxic effects according to partial pressure. Because partial pressure increases directly with ambient pressure, trace contaminants may become toxic under hyperbaric conditions. It is important to ensure periodically that gases that can be produced by the compressors (e.g., hydrocarbons and CO) are at a safe level. Other trace contaminants include alcohol from skin disinfectant solutions, mercury vapor from sphygmomanometers and glass thermometers, and other gases such as hydrogen and sulfur dioxide, which can be released from batteries.

Many hyperbaric chamber facilities use non–alcohol-based skin disinfectant solutions. Lithium and mercury batteries are best avoided. The Gates lead acid, gelled electrolyte battery has been specifically tested to 8 ATA. Alkaline cells are also usually considered to be safe.

It is important that the gas delivered to a patient contains an appropriate concentration of O_2 and a safe concentration of CO_2. Use of a semi-closed partially recirculating gas circuit to deliver O_2 to a headtent can be associated with CO_2 accumulation. It is the practice of many facilities to monitor both inspired O_2 and CO_2. Inspired CO_2 should probably be kept less than 3.8 mm Hg (0.5% "surface equivalent" concentration); Fio_2 should be 0.98 or higher.

Evaluation of Patients for Hyperbaric Oxygen Therapy

Evaluation of patients must take into consideration both the efficacy of HBO for each patient and the risk of complications.

A patient's disease must be amenable to HBO therapy. Guidelines for acceptable indications are published by the Undersea and Hyperbaric Medical Society.[142] It is important that a therapeutic arterial Po_2 be attained, which might be precluded in the presence of severe pulmonary disease or cyanotic heart disease.

The most common side effect of HBO therapy is otic barotrauma. Patients with middle ear disease, respiratory tract infections, allergic rhinitis, or swallowing disorders and intubated or unconscious patients may be unable to equilibrate middle ear pressure as ambient pressure is raised. Pain, middle ear hemorrhage, tympanic membrane rupture, or labyrinthine (round or oval) window rupture can result.[164] It is the practice of many physicians to perform prophylactic myringotomies on these patients before HBO therapy.

The risk of pulmonary barotrauma should be assessed before instituting HBO therapy. Patients with a pneumothorax may require thoracostomy. Bullous lung disease and severe airways obstruction are risk factors for pulmonary barotrauma. If possible, airways obstruction should be treated pharmacologically before HBO treatment.

Commonly used treatment schedules are designed to minimize both cerebral and pulmonary O_2 toxicity. However, pulmonary O_2 toxicity can still occur, particularly if supplemental O_2 is required between treatments. Myopia is a risk, usually after a prolonged series of treatments, although it rarely influences the decision to undertake HBO therapy. However, this possibility should always be discussed with patients, who may be unwilling to accept this risk if they have preexisting visual impairment.

SUMMARY

In the past 20 years, HBO therapy has been increasingly used in patients with conditions amenable to this type of treatment. With this wider use has followed a demand for more sophisticated care in this unusual environment. Although new pharmacologic therapies may obviate the need for HBO in some conditions, for the foreseeable future the need to deliver high-pressure O_2 to a select group of patients will continue. Ongoing update of hyperbaric technology will ensure that standards of intensive care will be available in the hyperbaric environment.

References

1. Bert P: Barometric Pressure (La Pression Barometrique). Hitchcock M, Hitchcock FA (Translators). Bethesda, MD, Undersea and Hyperbaric Medical Society, 1978, pp 961–971.
2. Whalen RE, Saltzman HA, Holloway DH, et al: Cardiovascular and blood gas responses to hyperbaric oxygenation. Am J Cardiol 1965; 15:638–646.
3. Nylander G, Lewis D, Nordstrom H, et al: Reduction of postischemic edema with hyperbaric oxygen. Plast Reconstr Surg 1985; 76:596–603.
4. Fife CE, Camporesi EM: Physiologic effects of hyperbaric hyperoxia. Probl Respir Care 1991; 4:142.
5. Klebanoff SJ: Oxygen-dependent cytotoxic mechanisms of phagocytes. *In*: Advances in Host Defence Mechanisms. Gallin JI, Fauci AS (Eds). New York, Raven Press, 1982, pp 111–162.
6. Mader JT, Brown GL, Guckian JC, et al: A mechanism for the amelioration by hyperbaric oxygen of experimental staphylococcal osteomyelitis in rabbits. J Infect Dis 1980; 142:915–922.

7. Mader JT, Adams KR, Sutton TE: Infectious diseases: Pathophysiology and mechanisms of hyperbaric oxygen. J Hyperbaric Med 1987; 2:133–140.
8. Zamboni WA, Roth AC, Russell RC, et al: Morphologic analysis of the microcirculation during reperfusion of ischemic skeletal muscle and the effect of hyperbaric oxygen. Plastic Reconstruct Surg 1993; 91:1110–1123.
9. Helps SC, Parsons DW, Reilly PL, et al: The effect of gas emboli on rabbit cerebral blood flow. Stroke 1990; 21:94–99.
10. Helps SC, Gorman DF: Air embolism of the brain in rabbits pretreated with mechlorethamine. Stroke 1991; 22:351–354.
11. Thom SR: Antagonism of carbon monoxide-mediated brain lipid peroxidation by hyperbaric oxygen. Toxicol Appl Pharmacol 1990; 105:340–344.
12. Gerschman R, Gilbert DL, Nye SW, et al: Oxygen poisoning and x-irradiation: A mechanism in common. Science 1954; 119:623–626.
13. Freeman BA, Crapo JD: Biology of disease: Free radicals and tissue injury. Lab Invest 1982; 47:412–426.
14. Donald K: Oxygen and the Diver. Hanley Swan, The SPA, 1992, pp 27–79.
15. Crapo JD: Morphologic changes in pulmonary oxygen toxicity. Annu Rev Physiol 1986; 48:721–731.
16. Lambertsen CJ: Effects of hyperoxia on organs and their tissues. *In*: Extrapulmonary Manifestations of Respiratory Disease. Robin ED (Ed). Vol 8 of Lung Biology in Health and Disease. Leufent C (Ed). New York, Marcel Dekker, 1978, pp 239–303.
17. Clark JM: Oxygen toxicity. *In*: The Physiology and Medicine of Diving. Bennett PB, Elliott DH (Eds). Philadelphia, WB Saunders, 1993, pp 121–169.
18. Harabin AL, Homer LD, Weathersby PK, et al: An analysis of decrements in vital capacity as an index of pulmonary oxygen toxicity. J Appl Physiol 1987; 63:1130–1135.
19. Anderson B Jr, Shelton DL: Axial length in hyperoxic myopia. *In*: Proceedings of the 9th International Symposium on Underwater and Hyperbaric Physiology. Bove AA, Bachrach AJ, Greenbaum LJ, (Eds). Bethesda, MD, Undersea and Hyperbaric Medical Society, 1987, pp 607–611.
20. Palmquist BM, Philipson B, Barr PO: Nuclear cataract and myopia during hyperbaric oxygen therapy. Br J Ophthalmol 1984; 68:113–117.
21. Adornato DC, Gildenberg PL, Ferrano CM, et al: The pathophysiology of intravenous air embolism in dogs. Anesthesiology 1978; 49:120–127.
22. Yeakel A: Lethal air embolism from plastic blood storage container. JAMA 1968; 204:267–269.
23. Seidelin PH, Stolarek IH, Thompson AM: Central venous catheterization and fatal air embolism. Br J Hosp Med 1987; 38:438–439.
24. Malhotra MS, Wright HC: The effects of a raised intrapulmonary pressure on the lungs of fresh unchilled cadavers. J Pathol Bacterial 1961; 82:198–202.
25. Vann RD, Denoble P, Emmerman MN, et al: Flying after diving and decompression sickness. Aviat Space Environ Med 1993; 64:801–807.
26. Elliott DH, Moon RE: Manifestations of the decompression disorders. *In*: The Physiology and Medicine of Diving. Bennett PB, Elliott DH (Eds). Philadelphia, WB Saunders, 1993, pp 481–505.
27. Van Allen CM, Hydrina LS, Clark J: Air embolism from the pulmonary vein. Arch Surg 1929; 19:567–599.
28. Atkinson JR: Experimental air embolism. Northwest Med 1963; 62:699–703.
29. Butler BD, Laine GA, Leiman BC, et al: Effect of the Trendelenburg position on the distribution of arterial air emboli in dogs. Ann Thorac Surg 1988; 45:198–202.
30. Dutka AJ: Therapy for dysbaric central nervous system ischemia: Adjuncts to recompression. *In*: Diving Accident Management. Bennett PB, Moon RE (Eds). Bethesda, Undersea and Hyperbaric Medical Society, 1990, pp 222–234.
31. Brunner FP, Frick PG, Bühlmann AA: Post decompression shock due to extravasation of plasma. Lancet 1964; 1:1071–1073.
32. Michenfelder JD, Martin JT, Altenburg BM, et al: Air embolism during neurosurgery. An evaluation of right atrial catheters for diagnosis and treatment. JAMA 1969; 208:1353–1358.
33. Stark J, Hough J: Air in the aorta: Treatment by reversed perfusion. Ann Thorac Surg 1986; 41:337–338.
34. Yarbrough OD, Behnke AR: The treatment of compressed air illness using oxygen. J Ind Hyg Toxicol 1939; 21:213–218.
35. Keays FL: Compressed Air Illness with a Report of 3,692 Cases. Vol. 2, Ithaca, NY, Department of Medical Publications, Cornell University Medical College 1909, pp 1–55.
36. Moon RE, Gorman DF: Treatment of the decompression disorders. *In*: The Physiology and Medicine of Diving. Bennett PB, Elliott DH (Eds). Philadelphia, WB Saunders, 1993, pp 506–541.
37. Dutka AJ: Air or gas embolism. *In*: Hyperbaric Oxygen Therapy: A Critical Review. Camporesi EM, Barker AC (Eds). Bethesda, Undersea and Hyperbaric Medical Society, 1991, pp 1–10.
38. Meyers RAM, Bray P: Delayed treatment of serious decompression sickness. Ann Emerg Med 1985; 14:254–257.
39. Rudge FW, Shafer MR: The effect of delay on treatment outcome in altitude-induced decompression sickness. Aviat Space Environ Med 1991; 62:687–690.
40. Ball R: Effect of severity, time to recompression with oxygen, and re-treatment on outcome in forty-nine cases of spinal cord decompression sickness. Undersea Hyperbaric Med 1993; 20:133–145.
41. US Navy Department: US Navy Diving Manual. Vol 1: Air Diving. NAVSEA 0994-LP-001-9010. San Pedro, Best, 1993.
42. Leitch DR, Greenbaum LJ Jr, Hallenbeck JM: Cerebral arterial embolism: I. Is there benefit in beginning HBO treatment at 6 bar? Undersea Biomed Res 1984; 11:221–235.
43. Leitch DR, Greenbaum LJ Jr, Hallenbeck JM: Cerebral arterial embolism: II. Effect of pressure and time on cortical evoked potential recovery. Undersea Biomed Res 1984; 11:237–248.
44. Leitch DR, Hallenbeck JM: Pressure in the treatment of spinal cord decompression sickness. Undersea Biomed Res 1985; 12:291–305.
45. McDermott JJ, Dutka AJ, Koller WA, et al: Comparison of two recompression profiles in treating experimental cerebral air embolism. Undersea Biomed Res 1992; 19:171–185.
46. McDermott JJ, Dutka AJ, Koller WA, et al: Effects of an increased Po_2 during recompression therapy for the treatment of experimental cerebral arterial gas embolism. Undersea Biomed Res 1992; 19:403–413.
47. Leitch DR, Green RD: Additional pressurization for treating nonresponding cases of serious air decompression sickness. Aviat Space Environ Med 1985; 56:1139–1143.
48. Lee HC, Niu KC, Chen SH, et al: Therapeutic effects of different tables on type II decompression sickness. J Hyperbaric Med 1991; 6:11–17.
49. Pearson RR, Goad RF: Delayed cerebral edema complicating cerebral arterial gas embolism: Case histories. Undersea Biomed Res 1982; 9:283–296.
50. Frances TJR, Dutka AJ: Methylprednisolone in the treatment of acute spinal cord decompression sickness. Undersea Biomed Res 1989; 16:165–174.
51. Dutka AJ, Mink RB, Pearson RR, et al: Effects of treatment with dexamethasone on recovery from experimental cerebral arterial gas embolism. Undersea Biomed Res 1992; 19:131–141.
52. Bracken MB, Shephard MJ, Collins WF, et al: A randomized, controlled trial of methylprednisolone or naloxone in the treatment of acute spinal-cord injury study. N Engl J Med 1990; 322:1405–1411.
53. Reeves E, Workman RD: Use of heparin for the therapeutic-prophylactic treatment of decompression sickness. Aerospace Med 1971; 42:20–23.
54. Kindwall EP, Margolis I: Management of severe decompression sickness with treatment ancillary to recompression: Case report. Aviat Space Environ Med 1975; 46:1065–1068.
55. Evans DE, Kobrine AI, LeGrys DC, et al: Protective effect of lidocaine in acute cerebral ischemia induced by air embolism. J Neurosurg 1984; 60:257–263.
56. Evans DE, Catron PW, McDermott JJ, et al: Therapeutic effect of lidocaine in experimental cerebral ischemia induced by air embolism. J Neurosurg 1989; 70:97–102.

57. McDermott JJ, Dutka AJ, Evans DE, et al: Treatment of experimental cerebral air embolism with lidocaine and hyperbaric oxygen. Undersea Biomed Res 1990; 17:525–534.
58. Dutka AJ, Mink R, McDermott J, et al: Effect of lidocaine on somatosensory evoked response and cerebral blood flow after canine cerebral air embolism. Stroke 1992; 23:1515–1520.
59. Drewry A, Gorman DF: Lidocaine as an adjunct to hyperbaric therapy in decompression illness: A case report. Undersea Biomed Res 1992; 19:187–190.
60. Menasché P, Pinard E, Desroches A-M, et al: Fluorocarbons: A potential treatment of cerebral air embolism in open heart surgery. Ann Thorac Surg 1985; 40:494–497.
60a. Spiess BD, McCarthy RJ, Tuman KJ, et al: Treatment of decompression sickness with a perfluorocarbon emulsion (FC-43). Undersea Biomed Res 1988; 15:31–37.
61. Brown SD, Piantadosi CA: In vivo binding of carbon monoxide to cytochrome c oxidase in rat brain. J Appl Physiol 1990; 68:604–610.
62. Piantadosi CA, Lee PA, Sylvia AL: Direct effects of CO on cerebral energy metabolism in bloodless rats. J Appl Physiol 1988; 65:878–887.
63. Zhang J, Piantadosi CA: Mitochondrial oxidative stress after carbon monoxide hypoxia in the rat brain. J Clin Invest 1992; 90:1193–1199.
64. Messier LD, Myers RA: A neuropsychological screening battery for emergency assessment of carbon monoxide poisoned patients. J Clin Psychol 1991; 47:675–684.
65. Pace N, Strajman E, Walker EL: Acceleration of carbon monoxide elimination in man by high pressure oxygen. Science 1950; 111:652.
66. Brown SD, Piantadosi CA: Reversal of carbon monoxide-cytochrome c oxidase binding by hyperbaric oxygen in vivo. Adv Exp Med Biol 1989; 248:747–754.
67. Brown SD, Piantadosi CA: Recovery of energy metabolism in rat brain after carbon monoxide hypoxia. J Clin Invest 1992; 89:666–672.
68. Rafphael J-C, Elkharrat D, Jars-Guincestre M-C, et al: Trial of normobaric and hyperbaric oxygen for acute carbon monoxide intoxication. Lancet 1989; 2:414–419.
69. Krantz T, Thisted B, Strom J, et al: Acute carbon monoxide poisoning. Acta Anaesthesiol Scand 1988; 32:278–282.
70. Norkool DM, Kirkpatrick JN: Treatment of acute carbon monoxide poisoning with hyperbaric oxygen: A review of 115 cases. Ann Emerg Med 1985; 14:1168–1171.
71. Thom SR, Taber RL, Mendiguren I, et al: Delayed neuropsychiatric sequelae following CO poisoning and the role of treatment with 100% O_2 or hyperbaric oxygen—a prospective, randomized, clinical study. Undersea Biomed Res 1992; 19(Suppl):47.
72. Piantadosi CA: The role of hyperbaric oxygen in carbon monoxide, cyanide and sulfide intoxication. Probl Respir Care 1991; 4:215–231.
73. Hollander DI, Nagey DA, Welch R, et al: Hyperbaric oxygen therapy for the treatment of acute carbon monoxide poisoning in pregnancy. A case report. J Reprod Med 1987; 32:615–617.
74. Van Hoesen KB, Camporesi EM, Moon RE, et al: Should hyperbaric oxygen be used to treat the pregnant patient for carbon monoxide poisoning? A case report and literature review [published erratum in JAMA 1990; 273:2750]. JAMA 1990; 261:1039–1043.
75. Koren G, Sharav T, Pastuszak A, et al: A multicenter, prospective study of fetal outcome following accidental carbon monoxide poisoning in pregnancy. Reprod Toxicol 1991; 5:397–403.
76. Brown DB, Mueller GL, Golich FC: Hyperbaric oxygen treatment for carbon monoxide poisoning in pregnancy; A case report. Aviat Space Environ Med 1992; 63:1011–1014.
76a. Stewart RJ, Mason SW, Taira MT, et al: Effect of radical scavengers and hyperbaric oxygen on smoke-induced pulmonary edema. Undersea Hyperb Med 1994; 21:21–30.
77. Litovitz TL, Larkin RF, Myers RAM: Cyanide poisoning treated with hyperbaric oxygen. Am J Emerg Med 1983; 1:94–101.
78. Whitcraft DD, Bailey TD, Hart GB: Hydrogen sulfide poisoning treated with hyperbaric oxygen. J Emerg Med 1985; 3:23–25.
79. Smilkstein MJ, Bronstein AC, Pickett HM, et al: Hyperbaric oxygen therapy for severe hydrogen sulfide poisoning. J Emerg Med 1985; 3:27–30.
80. Truss CD, Killenberg PG: Treatment of carbon tetrachloride with hyperbaric oxygen. Gastroenterology 1982; 82:767–769.
81. Burkhart KK, Hall AH, Gerace R, et al: Hyperbaric oxygen treatment for carbon tetrachloride poisoning. Drug Saf 1992; 6:332–338.
82. Berk RF, Lane JM, Patel K: Relationship of oxygen and glutathione in protection against carbon tetrachloride-induced hepatic microsomal lipid peroxidation and covalent binding in the rat. Rationale for the use of hyperbaric oxygen to treat carbon tetrachloride ingestion. J Clin Invest 1984; 74:1996–2001.
83. Shoemaker WC, Appel PL, Kram HB: Role of oxygen debt in the development of organ failure, sepsis and death in high risk surgical patients. Chest 1992; 102:208–215.
84. Hill GB, Osterhout S: Experimental effects of hyperbaric oxygen on selected clostridial species. II. In vivo studies in mice. J Infect Dis 1972; 125:26–35.
85. Demello FJ, Haglin JJ, Hitchcock CR: Comparative study of experimental *Clostridium perfringens* infection in dogs treated with antibiotics, surgery and hyperbaric oxygen. Surgery 1973; 73:936–941.
86. Holland JA, Hill GB, Wolfe WG, et al: Experimental and clinical experience with hyperbaric oxygen in the treatment of clostridial myonecrosis. Surgery 1975; 77:75–85.
87. Bakker DJ: The use of hyperbaric oxygen in the treatment of certain infectious diseases especially gas gangrene and acute dermal gangrene. Wageningen, Netherlands, Drukkerij Veenman BV, 1984.
88. DeLalande JP, Perramant M, Tanguy RL: Postoperative gas gangrene. Apropos of 22 cases. Ann Anesthesiol Fr 1981; 22:351–358.
89. Freischlag JA, Ajalat G, Busuttil RW: Treatment of necrotizing soft tissue infections. The need for a new approach. Am J Surg 1985; 149:751–755.
90. Gibson A, Davis FM: Hyperbaric oxygen therapy in the management of *Clostridium perfringens* infections. N Z Med J 1986; 99:617–620.
91. Hitchcock CR, Bubrick MP: Gas gangrene infections of the small intestine, colon and rectum. Dis Colon Rectum. 1976; 19:112–119.
92. Kaiser RE, Cerra FB: Progressive necrotizing surgical infections—a unified approach. J Trauma 1981; 21:349–355.
93. Katlic MR, Derkac WM: *Clostridium septicum* infection and malignancy. Ann Surg 1981; 193:361–364.
94. Pailler JL, Labeeu F: Gas gangrene: A military disease? Acta Chir Bel 1986; 86:63–71.
95. Vo NM, Watson S, Bryant LR: Infections of the lower extremities due to gas forming and non-gas forming organisms. South Med J 1986; 79:1493–1495.
96. Bakker DJ: Clostridial myonecrosis. *In*: Problem Wounds: The Role of Oxygen. Davis JC (Ed). New York, Elsevier, 1988, pp 153–172.
97. Caplan ES, Kluge RM: Gas gangrene: A review of 34 cases. Arch Intern Med 1976; 136:788–791.
98. Gibson A, Davis FM: Hyperbaric oxygen therapy in the management of *Clostridium perfringens* infections. N Z Med J 1986; 99:617–620.
99. Gurtner T: Gas gangrene. Unfallchirurgie 1983; 9:172–174.
100. Hart GB, Lamb RC: Gas gangrene. J Trauma 1983; 23:991–1000.
101. Heimbach RD: Gas gangrene: Review and update. HBO Rev 1980; 1:41–46.
102. Hirn M, Niinikoski J: Hyperbaric oxygen in the treatment of clostridial gas gangrene. Ann Chir Gynaecol 1988; 77:37–40.
103. Nier H, Kremer K: Gas gangrene—still a diagnostic and therapeutic problem. Zentralbl Chir 1984; 109:402–417.
104. Shupak A, Halpern P, Ziser A, et al: Hyperbaric oxygen therapy for gas gangrene casualties in the Lebanon War, 1982. Isr J Med Sci 1984; 20:323–326.
105. Unsworth IP, Sharp PA: Gas gangrene. An 11-year review of 73 cases managed with hyperbaric oxygen. Med J Aust 1984; 140:256–260.

106. Farrell LD, Karl SR, Davis PK, et al: Postoperative necrotizing fasciitis in children. Pediatrics 1988; 82:874–879.
107. Ledingham IM, Tehrani MA: Diagnosis, clinical course and treatment of acute dermal gangrene. Br J Surg 1975; 62:364–372.
108. Mader JT: Mixed anaerobic and aerobic soft tissue infection. *In*: Problem Wounds: The Role of Oxygen. Davis JC (Ed): New York, Elsevier, 1988, pp 173–186.
109. Majeski JA: Necrotizing fasciitis. Am Fam Physician 1984; 30:221–223.
110. Oh C, Lee C, Jacobson JH: Necrotizing fasciitis of perineum. Surgery 1982; 91:49–51.
111. Pessa ME, Howard RJ: Necrotizing fasciitis. Surg Gynecol Obstet 1985; 161:357–361.
112. Reigels-Neilsen P, Hesselfeldt-Neilsen J, Bang-Jesen E, et al: Fournier's gangrene: 5 patients treated with hyperbaric oxygen. J Urol 1984; 132:918–920.
113. Riseman JA, Zamboni WA, Curtis A, et al: Hyperbaric oxygen therapy for necrotizing fasciitis reduces mortality and the need for debridements. Surgery 1990; 108:847–850.
114. Rouse TM, Malangoni MA: Necrotizing fasciitis: A preventable disaster. Surgery 1982; 92:765–770.
115. Spirnak JP, Resnick MI, Hampel N, et al: Fournier's gangrene: A report of 20 patients. J Urol 1984; 131:289–291.
116. Wang KC, Shih CH: Necrotizing fasciitis of the extremities. J Trauma 1992; 32:179–182.
117. Woodburn KR, Ramsay G: Retroperitoneal necrotizing fasciitis. Br J Surg 1992; 79:342–344.
118. Aasen AO, Ruud TE, Haffner J, et al: Surgical treatment of necrotizing fasciitis. Tidsskr Nor Laegeforen 1989; 109:2768–2772.
119. Chevallier D, Amiel J, Michetti C, et al: Gangrenous states of the perineum and genital region. J Urol (Paris) 1987; 93:145–150.
120. Gozal D, Ziser A, Shupak A, et al: Necrotizing fasciitis. Arch Surg 1986; 121:233–235.
121. Krasova Z, Matusek A, Chmelar D: Hyperbaric oxygenation in the treatment of necrotizing fasciitis. Vnitr Lek 1992; 38:640–644.
121a. Brown DR, Davis NL, Lepawsky M, et al: A multicenter review of the treatment of major truncal necrotizing infections with and without hyperbaric oxygen therapy. Am J Surg 1994; 167:485–489.
122. Price JC, Stevens DL: Hyperbaric oxygen in the treatment of rhinocerebral mucormycosis. Laryngoscope 1980; 90:737–747.
123. Nathan MD, Keller AP, Lerner CJ, et al: Entomophthorales infection of the maxillofacial region. Laryngoscope 1982; 92:767–769.
124. Couch L, Theilen F, Mader JT: Rhinocerebral mucormycosis with cerebral extension successfully treated with adjunctive hyperbaric therapy. Arch Otolaryngol Head Neck Surg 1988; 114:791–794.
125. Anand VK, Alemar G, Griswold JA Jr: Intracranial complications of mucormycosis: An experimental model and clinical review. Laryngoscope 1992; 102:656–662.
126. Kemper J, Kuijper EJ, Mirck PGB, et al: Recovery from rhinocerebral mucormycosis in a ketoacidotic diabetic: A case report. J Laryngol Otol 1993; 107:233–235.
127. Ferguson BJ, Mitchell TG, Moon R, et al: Adjunctive hyperbaric oxygen for treatment of rhinocerebral mucormycosis. Rev Infect Dis 1988; 10:551–559.
128. Sukoff MH, Ragatz RE: Hyperbaric oxygenation for the treatment of acute cerebral edema. Neurosurgery 1982; 10:29–38.
129. Ohta H, Hadeishi H, Nemoto M, et al: Transient effect of hyperbaric oxygen on cerebral blood flow and intracranial pressure. J Hyperbaric Med 1990; 5:3–13.
130. Holbach KH, Wassmann H, Kolberg T: Verbesserte Reversibilität des traumatischen Mittelhirnsyndroms bei Anwendung der hyperbaren Oxygenierung. Acta Neurochir 1974; 30:247–256.
131. Rockswold GL, Ford SE, Anderson DC, et al: Results of a prospective randomized trial for treatment of severely brain injured patients with hyperbaric oxygen. J Neurol Surg 1992; 76:929–934.
132. Ikeda K, Ajiki H, Nagao H, et al: Experimental and clinical use of hyperbaric oxygen in burns. *In*: Proceedings of the 4th International Congress on Hyperbaric Medicine. Wada J, Iwa T (Eds). Baltimore, Williams & Wilkins, 1970, pp 377–380.
133. Perrins DJD: A failed attempt to limit tissue destruction in scalds of pig skins with hyperbaric oxygen. Proceedings of the 4th International Congress on Hyperbaric Medicine. Baltimore, Williams & Wilkins, 1970, pp 381–387.
134. Korn HN, Wheeler ES, Miller TA: Effect of hyperbaric oxygen on second-degree burn wound healing. Arch Surg 1977; 112:732–737.
135. Hammarlund C, Svedman C, Scedman P: Hyperbaric oxygen treatment of healthy volunteers with UV-irradiated blister wounds. Burns 1991; 17:296–301.
136. Hart GB, O'Reilly RR, Broussard ND, et al: Treatment of burns with hyperbaric oxygen. Surg Gynecol Obstet 1974; 139:693–696.
137. Niu AKC, Yang C, Lee HC, et al: Burns treated with adjunctive hyperbaric oxygen therapy: A comparative study in humans. J Hyperbaric Med 1987; 2:75–85.
138. Cianci P, Lueders HW, Lee H, et al: Adjunctive hyperbaric oxygen therapy reduces length of hospitalization in thermal burns. J Burn Care Rehabil 1989; 10:432–435.
139. Cianci P, Williams C, Lueders HW, et al: Adjunctive hyperbaric oxygen in the treatment of thermal burns: An economic analysis. J Burn Care Rehabil 1990; 11:140–143.
139a. Cianci P, Sato R: Adjunctive hyperbaric oxygen therapy in the treatment of thermal burns: A review. Burns 1994; 20:5–14.
140. Hart GB, Lennon PA, Strauss MD: Hyperbaric oxygen in exceptional acute blood-loss anemia. J Hyperbaric Med 1987; 2:205.
141. Camporesi EM, Moon RE: Hyperbaric oxygen as an adjunct to therapeutic lung lavage in pulmonary alveolar proteinosis. *In*: Underwater and Hyperbaric Physiology IX: Ninth International Symposium on Underwater and Hyperbaric Physiology. Bove AA, Bachrach AJ, Greenbaum LJ (Eds). Bethesda, MD, Underwater Hyperbaric Medical Society, 1987, p 955.
142. Undersea & Hyperbaric Medical Society: Hyperbaric Oxygen Therapy: A Committee Report. Bethesda, MD, Undersea & Hyperbaric Medical Society, 1992.
143. Greenbaum LJ Jr, Mathias RA: Information sources in the hyperbaric field. Probl Respir Care 1991; 4:269–272.
144. Leitch DR, Green RD: Pulmonary barotrauma in divers and the treatment of cerebral arterial gas embolism. Aviat Space Environ Med 1986; 57:931–938.
145. Kizer KW: Management of dysbaric diving casualties. Emerg Med Clin North Am 1983; 1:659–670.
146. Davis JC, Heckman JD, DeLee JC, et al: Chronic non-hematogenous osteomyelitis treated with adjuvant hyperbaric oxygen. J Bone Joint Surg [Am] 1986; 68:1210–1217.
147. Farmer JC, Shelton DL, Angelillo JD, et al: Treatment of radiation-induced tissue injury with hyperbaric oxygen. Ann Otol Rhinol Laryngol 1978; 87:707–715.
148. Norkool DM, Hampson NB, Gibbons RP, et al: Hyperbaric oxygen therapy for radiation-induced hemorrhagic cystitis. J Urol 1993; 150:332–334.
148a. Weiss JP, Mattei DM, Neville EC, et al: Primary treatment of radiation-induced hemorrhagic cystitis with hyperbaric oxygen: 10-year experience. J Urol 1994; 151:1514–1517.
148b. Feldmeier JJ, Heimbach RD, Davolt DA, et al: Hyperbaric oxygen as an adjunctive treatment for severe laryngeal necrosis: A report of nine consecutive cases. Undersea Hyperb Med 1993; 20:329–335.
149. Baroni G, Porro T, Faglia E, et al: Hyperbaric oxygen in diabetic gangrene treatment. Diabetes Care 1987; 10:81–86.
149a. Hammarlund C, Sundberg T: Hyperbaric oxygen reduced size of chronic leg ulcers: A randomized double-blind study. Plast Reconstr Surg 1994; 93:829–833.
150. Moon RE, Camporesi EM: Operational use and patient monitoring in a multiplace hyperbaric chamber. Probl Respir Care 1991; 4:172–188.
151. Weaver LK: Clinical applications of hyperbaric oxygen-monoplace chamber use. Probl Respir Care 1991; 4:189–214.
152. Weaver LK: Air breaks with the Sechrist 500A monoplace hyperbaric ventilator. J Hyperbaric Med 1988; 3:179–186.
153. Gallagher TJ, Smith RA, Bell GC: Evaluation of mechanical ventilators in a hyperbaric environment. Aviat Space Environ Med 1978; 49:375–376.
154. Pelaia P, Volturo P, Rocco M, et al: Mechanical ventilation in hyperbaric environment: Experimental evaluation of the Drager Hyperlog. Minerva Anestesiol 1990; 56:1371.

155. Le Masson Y, Le Pechon J Cl, Barratt M, et al: Ventilator for Space Station Freedom. *In*: Proceedings of the Joint Meeting on Diving and Hyperbaric Medicine. Schmutz J, Wendling J (Eds). Basel, Foundation for Hyperbaric Medicine, 1992, pp 78–82.
156. Degauque C, Lamy M, Stas M: Use of the Logic 03 for controlled ventilation in hyperbaric oxygen therapy. Acta Anaesthesiol Belg 1977; 28:251–259.
157. Moon RE, Bergquist LV, Conklin B, et al: Monaghan 225 ventilator use under hyperbaric conditions. Chest 1986; 89:846–851.
158. Lewis RP, Szafranski J, Bradford RH, et al: The use of the Penlon Nuffield 200 in a monoplace hyperbaric oxygen chamber. An evaluation of its use and a clinical report in two patients requiring ventilation for carbon monoxide poisoning. Anaesthesia 1991; 46:767–770.
159. Saywood AM, Howard R, Goad RF, et al: Function of the Oxford Ventilator at high pressure. Anaesthesia 1982; 37:740–744.
160. Spittal MJ, Hunter SJ, Jones L: The pneuPAC hyperbaric variant HB: A ventilator suitable for use within a one-man hyperbaric chamber. Br J Anaesth 1991; 67:488–491.
161. Holcomb JR, Matos-Navarro AY, Goldmann RW: Critical care in the hyperbaric chamber. *In*: Problem Wounds: The Role of Oxygen. Davis JC, Hunt TK (Eds). New York, Elsevier, 1988, pp 187–209.
162. Weaver LK, Howe S, Berlin SL: Normobaric measurement of O_2 tension of blood and saline tonometered under hyperbaric O_2 conditions. J Hyperbaric Med 1990; 5:29–38.
163. Gilbert R, Keighley JF: The arterial/alveolar oxygen tension ratio. An index of gas exchange applicable to varying inspired oxygen concentrations. Am Rev Respir Dis 1974; 109:142–145.
164. Farmer JC Jr: Otological and paranasal sinus problems in diving. *In*: The Physiology and Medicine of Diving. Bennett PB, Elliott DH (Eds). Philadelphia, WB Saunders, 1993, pp 267–300.
164a. Youn BA, Gordon D, Moran C, et al: Fire in the multiplace hyperbaric chamber. J Hyperb Med 1989; 4:63–67.

SECTION VIII

ABDOMINAL ORGAN DYSFUNCTION

William C. Shoemaker • Ake Grenvik

CHAPTER 107

The Acute Abdomen

Kenneth Waxman, MD, FACS

Sir Zachary Cope, in his 1921 monograph "The Early Diagnosis of the Acute Abdomen," eloquently outlined the importance of a carefully taken history and physical examination.[1] Despite all technologic advances, the history and physical examination remain the most important tools in the initial assessment of a patient who complains of abdominal pain. Although critically ill patients may be more difficult to evaluate, the data from their history and physical examination are, nonetheless, paramount, as this information obtained allows either definitive diagnosis or direct further evaluation. During an initial assessment, the physician should obtain a thorough understanding of a patient's underlying medical problems, of the precise nature and chronicity of the abdominal pain, of its association with related symptoms such as vomiting, diarrhea, and dysuria. In the course of a complete physical examination, the physician evaluates a patient for signs of shock, infection, cardiopulmonary disease, neurologic disorders, rectal masses or occult blood, and pelvic or genital masses or tenderness as well as for abdominal tenderness and peritoneal irritation. Following this initial assessment, the following questions can be addressed:

1. Does the patient require immediate resuscitation?
2. Does the patient require invasive cardiorespiratory monitoring?
3. Are additional diagnostic tests necessary?
4. Does the patient require urgent operation?

DOES THE PATIENT REQUIRE IMMEDIATE RESUSCITATION?

Patients with acute abdominal pain often have hypovolemia due to gastrointestinal losses from vomiting or diarrhea as well as the extravascular sequestration of fluid and electrolytes in the intestinal, peritoneal, retroperitoneal, and interstitial spaces. Thus, patients with acute abdominal conditions frequently require aggressive fluid and electrolyte infusion.

Altered pulmonary function is also common in patients with acute abdominal pain. Abdominal pain and distention often limit tidal volume; this results in increased respiratory rate and sometimes ventilatory failure. Furthermore, atelectasis and pneumonia can ensue, and this in turn can lead to hypoxia.[2] Certain acute abdominal diseases, such as pancreatitis, are particularly likely to cause hypoxia. Also, the abdominal pain itself can be caused by primary pulmonary pathology, especially lower lobe pneumonia, pleuritis, or pulmonary infarction. Oxygenation and ventilation must therefore always be assessed and often supported in patients with abdominal pain.

Antibiotic therapy is important during the resuscitation of patients with intra-abdominal bacterial contamination or infection. Antibiotic therapy may be definitive therapy, such as in uncomplicated diverticulitis and pelvic inflammatory disease. In addition, the early preoperative initiation of presumptive antibiotic therapy, which is effective against suspected bacterial flora, is indicated prior to emergency laparotomy in the setting of acute abdominal pain. One important caution, however, is that the initiation of such antibiotic therapy should generally be delayed until a definite decision to operate has been made. If the decision to operate itself is delayed owing to observation for progression of disease, then antibiotic therapy is contraindicated because antibiotics may mask the signs and symptoms upon which such observation is based.

Other physiologic alterations (including temperature elevation, anemia, and clotting abnormalities) also frequently require correction in the preoperative resuscitation period.

DOES THE PATIENT REQUIRE INVASIVE CARDIORESPIRATORY MONITORING?

The majority of patients with acute abdominal disease can be effectively resuscitated with the use of physical examination data, vital signs, and urine output as guidelines. In selected patients, however, the early utilization of invasive monitoring may be useful both for titrating preoperative resuscitation and for determining when the patients are best able to undergo anesthesia and operation. Patients in whom such invasive preoperative monitoring should be considered include those with severe cardiac, pulmonary, or renal disease; these patients may require precise regulation of fluid therapy and are also more likely to require afterload and contractility agents than are patients with less severe disease. Invasive preoperative monitoring is also indicated for patients with severe preoperative shock, sepsis, or blood loss because optimal titration of preoperative resuscitation may be very important in determining these patients' ability to tolerate the ensuing anesthesia and operation. In each case, the time necessary to institute invasive monitoring as well as any additional time required for resuscitation must be weighed against the benefits of early operation.

The nature of preoperative monitoring should be individualized to particular situations. Monitoring of clinical signs and symptoms, vital signs, and urine output is sufficient to monitor resuscitation in the great majority of patients. When central venous catheterization is initiated in the emergency setting, central venous pressure is most often measured. Monitoring of central venous pressure has the advantages of simple institution and a minimal equipment requirements. However, both the absolute value of central venous pressure as well as the response of this parameter to therapy may be misleading if used as a guide of cardiac function; thus, central venous pressure values must be interpreted with caution.[3] In selected instances, monitoring of pulmonary artery and wedge pressures and measurement of cardiac output provide critical information and are thus justified. Again, however, in all instances care must be taken not to unduly delay an urgent operation in order to institute such monitoring. The use of noninvasive monitoring devices, which rapidly provide monitoring information with minimum risk, is extremely attractive in this setting and deserves wider application and study.[4]

ARE DIAGNOSTIC TESTS NECESSARY?

Diagnostic tests should be reserved for those patients in whom indications for surgery are unclear. For patients with clear-cut signs of peritonitis requiring laparotomy, further diagnostic tests to define the precise etiology prior to operation are not necessary. In fact, the extra time taken to perform such diagnostic tests may delay both resuscitation and operation and thus may be harmful. Diagnostic tests should therefore be performed selectively.

Laboratory Testing

Several blood tests are of frequent importance in evaluating patients with abdominal pain. The white blood cell count is often of diagnostic value. A mild leukocytosis (white blood cell count: 12,000–20,000) is most frequently seen in patients with peritonitis; however, early in the course of disease, no leukocytosis may be present. White blood cell counts of greater than 20,000 are seen uncommonly in peritonitis, usually only in patients with severe intra-abdominal infection or bowel infarction.[5] Peritonitis may also be present in patients with a normal white blood cell count but also a "left shift" or increase in the number of polymorphonuclear leukocytes; this is most often seen in elderly and debilitated patients. Finally, in patients with severe sepsis, leukopenia may supervene. Thus, although leukocytosis is characteristic of peritonitis that requires operation, a great number of exceptions exist. Although an elevated white blood cell count is supportive of a diagnosis of peritonitis, a normal count should not delay operation if history data and physical examination findings are clear.

Tests of the coagulation system are sometimes diagnostically useful. Increased prothrombin and partial thromboplastin times and decreased platelet counts are often seen in patients with severe intra-abdominal infections.

Serum amylase determination is a useful test in patients with abdominal pain because pancreatitis, which is best treated medically, can easily be confused with other causes of peritonitis. Detection of hyperamylasemia may suggest the correct diagnosis and thus help to avoid unnecessary laparotomy. It is important to recognize, however, that serum amylase values may be increased in other surgical conditions. Furthermore, serum amylase may not be increased in pancreatis, even in the presence of severe disease.[6]

Urinalysis may also be helpful in patients with abdominal pain. Pyuria may indicate the presence of a urinary tract infection, and hematuria may indicate a ureteral stone. However, it is also possible that inflammatory processes adjacent to the kidney, ureter, or bladder may be responsible for abnormal urinalysis results. Thus, abnormal urinalysis results do not rule out the need for laparotomy in patients with signs of peritonitis.

Radiologic Evaluation

If a diagnosis of peritonitis requiring operation is clear, then radiologic evaluation is not necessary and may in fact delay resuscitation and operation. On the other hand, if diagnosis is unclear—particularly if conditions not requiring immediate operation are in the differential diagnosis—then radiologic evaluation may prove very helpful. Examples of situations in which plain abdominal and chest radiographs may be useful include the diagnosis of intestinal obstruction, the diagnosis of ureteral stone, and the finding of free intraperitoneal air. Gastrointestinal contrast studies may be useful to confirm a diagnosis of intestinal perforation or obstruction. However, care must be taken in the emergency situation to avoid the introduction of barium into a perforated intestinal tract; water-soluble contrast agents should be utilized. Intravenous pyelogram may be indicated to differentiate ureteral obstruction as the cause of abdominal pain and to define genitourinary involvement in intra-abdominal infections.

Abdominal ultrasound may also be useful during the evaluation of acute abdominal pain. Ultrasound may indicate the presence of intra-abdominal fluid, blood, or abscess; help evaluate solid organs; detect abnormalities of the biliary system; may detect abdominal aortic aneurysm. Ultrasound has the advantage of portability; that is, it may be performed at the bedside. However, in many critically ill patients, ultrasound may be technically difficult to perform, often because of ileus. Ultrasound evaluation of patients with acute abdominal pain is best utilized to answer specific questions, such as Are gallstones present? Are the bile ducts dilated? and Is there a pancreatic abscess?

Computed tomography (CT) is currently the most specific diagnostic test for the diagnosis of the acute abdominal conditions. CT has the ability to detect intra-abdominal fluid or blood, to determine the presence and location of intra-abdominal and retroperitoneal abscesses, and to detect abnormalities of the abdominal wall, pancreas, liver, spleen, gallbladder, genitourinary system, retroperitoneum, and, in some cases, intestine. A positive finding on CT is usually quite specific and allows a high degree of diagnostic certainty.[7] However, CT does have disadvantages that should be considered when the decision to perform this test is being made. First, the patient must be transported to the scanner; if the patient is critically ill and requires intensive monitoring and resuscitation, this may be difficult. Second, CT is not extremely sensitive in detecting abnormalities of the gastrointestinal tract, and thus important causes of peritonitis may not be detected. Third, CT scans are expensive. For these reasons, diagnostic CT scanning should be carefully considered and selectively performed.

Nuclear medicine imaging techniques may be useful in some instances. Iminodiacetic acid scans are useful in confirming the diagnosis of acute cholecystitis in questionable cases. Ventilation-perfusion lung scans may be helpful in differentiating pulmonary embolism as the source of abdominal pain. Other nuclear imaging techniques, such as gallium scans or labeled leukocyte scans, have been of only limited value in the evaluation of acute abdominal pain.

Angiography is uncommonly necessary for evaluation of acute abdominal pain but may be occasionally indicated to evaluate for the presence of mesenteric arterial occlusion.

Peritoneal Lavage and Laparoscopy

Diagnostic peritoneal lavage is an important diagnostic tool in patients with blunt abdominal trauma. The usefulness of diagnostic peritoneal lavage in other patients with abdominal pain is less well established. In selected patients, it may be quite useful, particularly in those whose abdominal examinations may be difficult to perform because of altered mental status or critical illness.

Peritoneal lavage may be performed in several ways. In

all cases, the bladder should be emptied by a Foley catheter and the stomach decompressed by nasogastric suction. A peritoneal dialysis catheter is then introduced. In patients with nondistended abdomens and who have not had previous abdominal surgery, a percutaneous technique may be used. Following local anesthesia, an 18-gauge catheter is introduced through the midline 1 to 2 cm below the umbilicus; entry into the peritoneal cavity can be appreciated by a palpable decrease in resistance. A metal guide wire can then be passed through the catheter, over which the peritoneal dialysis catheter is introduced. Alternatively, in patients with intestinal distention or with possible intraabdominal adhesions, it is safer to place the peritoneal catheter with the direct cut down technique through a 2- to 4-cm incision made below the umbilicus. The linea alba is divided, and the dialysis catheter is introduced directly through an incision in the peritoneum.

Following placement of the peritoneal catheter, aspiration may yield fluid for analysis. If it does not, 1000 mL of warm sterile isotonic saline solution is introduced (40 mL/kg in children). When infusion is complete, the saline bag is placed on the floor, and lavage fluid, returned by gravity, is then sent for analysis. In particular, the presence of significant numbers of red blood cells, white blood cells, or bacteria indicates the need for laparotomy.

Laparoscopy may also be useful in evaluating acute abdominal pain.[8] Laparoscopy may be performed with either local or general anesthesia and may allow both diagnosis and treatment. The possibility of bedside diagnostic laparoscopy in the emergency department or intensive care unit makes this procedure particularly appealing for critically ill patients.

DOES THE PATIENT REQUIRE URGENT OPERATION?

Early operation is essential for a patient with acute abdominal pain who requires laparotomy. However, for many patients, a preoperative period of resuscitation is beneficial. The optimal period of time to continue this resuscitation and delay operation is to a great extent dependent on an individual patient's physiologic response to illness and to resuscitation. Although benefit is gained by correcting preoperative deficits with resuscitation, undue operative delay may result in continued hemorrhage, obstruction, and infection and, thus, may contribute to a net worsening of the patient's physiologic status.

In general, acute abdominal disorders fall into three categories: (1) those that require early surgery with resuscitation performed as quickly as possible; (2) those that benefit from a definitive period of medical therapy before operation; and (3) those that are best treated nonoperatively.

Examples of conditions requiring rapid resuscitation and urgent surgery include abdominal trauma, ruptured aortic aneurysm, intestinal necrosis, ruptured ectopic pregnancy, large intestinal obstruction, appendicitis, and perforated ulcer. Although early operation is clearly important in each of these disorders, resuscitation may need to be prolonged under certain circumstances. For example, patients with appendicitis usually require little preoperative care and are best served with early operation. However, a subgroup of patients with appendicitis have severe generalized peritonitis, intestinal obstruction, or intra-abdominal abscess and may be critically ill on presentation. Children, the elderly, and patients with underlying medical diseases often fall into this category. These patients may benefit from a period of preoperative resuscitation lasting several hours. As another example, patients with perforated peptic ulcer may have a significant peritonitis and may benefit from aggressive preoperative resuscitation. In selected patients with perforated ulcer and severe underlying illness for whom emergency operation is very high-risk intervention, water-soluble contrast radiography may be performed; if no intraperitoneal extravasation of contrast medium is observed, the patients can be treated nonoperatively with nasogastric suction, antibiotics, and intensive supportive care.[9, 9a]

Other conditions are best treated medically before operation. One example is gallstone pancreatitis. When pancreatitis is due to gallstones, patients should undergo cholecystectomy and, possibly, common bile duct exploration. The timing of operation remains controversial, but most studies recommend a period of medical therapy to allow resolution of pancreatitis before operation.[10] Although such improvement occurs in most patients, a minority develops progressive pancreatitis; these patients require urgent surgery. An additional example is small bowel obstruction. Patients with small bowel obstruction may benefit greatly from intravenous hydration and nasogastric suction. If improvement of pain, abdominal examination, and abdominal x-ray occurs within 8 to 12 hours, nonoperative management may be continued and, in some patients, operation may be avoided. However, if at any time signs of peritonitis, fever, or leukocytosis occur, patients must undergo prompt laparotomy. Furthermore, if progressive improvement does not occur, then immediate operation is necessary.[11]

Finally, patients with abdominal pain may also have conditions that cause severe illness for which intensive nonoperative care may be definitive therapy. Examples of such illnesses include acute pancreatitis, pelvic inflammatory disease, and severe gastroenteritis. Aggressive medical therapy and supportive intensive care are often mandatory in such patients if a successful outcome is to be achieved. It is also important to recognize that these nonoperative conditions are easily confused with conditions for which operative therapy is necessary. It is often good medical practice to perform laparotomy under these circumstances to establish a definitive diagnosis.

INTRAOPERATIVE MANAGEMENT

Intraoperative management of patients undergoing emergency abdominal surgery presents special problems for both the anesthesiologist and the surgeon.

The anesthesiologist is often disadvantaged by having little or no time for perioperative assessment of a patient who may be very seriously ill and who may also have a chronic disease that increases the risk of anesthesia. The emergency nature of the illness also increases the risk of anesthesia, for on presentation to the operating room the patient may be dehydrated and hypovolemic, may have electrolyte and acid-base disturbances, and may have acute pulmonary compromise. Of special concern in such a patient is that he or she may have recently eaten or have bowel obstruction or ileus; thus, the risk of vomiting and aspiration of gastric contents may be greatly increased. This risk of vomiting may be even greater if the patient has been given preoperative narcotics or sedatives (which should preferentially be avoided for this reason). In the face of these problems, a careful anesthetic approach is essential.

Of major concern during induction of anesthesia is the prevention of vomiting and aspiration. A common technique that is useful to minimize this risk is rapid-sequence intubation, in which the patient is rapidly anesthetized, paralyzed, and intubated with a cuffed endotracheal tube. During this process, an assistant exerts cricoid pressure by pressing firmly against the anterior portion of the neck over the cricoid cartilage in order to compress the esophagus; this helps to prevent aspiration of gastric contents before inflation of the endotracheal cuff.

Avoidance of cardiac decompensation and hypotension during anesthesia for these emergency surgery patients may also be difficult because they may have sepsis, vasodilatation, and unrecognized hypovolemia. The appropriate choices of anesthetic agents, monitoring techniques, intraoperative fluid management modalities, and cardiotonic or vasopressor drugs demand expert care by the anesthesiologist.

Sound surgical technique and judgment are also critical in the treatment of patients undergoing emergency laparotomy. Often, a number of options exists regarding the specific procedure to perform; the surgeon must choose one of these options. Optimally, these decisions are based not solely on the specific intra-abdominal pathology but also on a patient's physiologic condition. Although specific surgical approaches to the various intra-abdominal diseases cannot be here discussed, several general decisions that often effect postoperative management deserve special mention.

BOWEL ANASTOMOSIS VERSUS EXTERIORIZATION. Although primary bowel anastomosis obviates the need for stomal care as well as that for subsequent surgery for ostomy closure, the risks accompanying anastomosis must always be considered. In particular, patients with preoperative shock or sepsis, or both, may have decreased mesenteric blood flow, and thus their anastomotic blood supply may be marginal. Furthermore, patients who are severely ill and particularly those with compromised cardiorespiratory reserve would be less able to tolerate the sepsis resulting from possible anastomotic leak. Thus, when these factors are present, it is good judgment to create intestinal stomas rather than to perform intestinal anastomosis.

WOUND CLOSURE TECHNIQUE. A number of factors contribute to increased incidence of abdominal wound dehiscence and evisceration, which are often disastrous postoperative complications. These factors include shock, malnutrition, respiratory failure, recent laparotomy, steroid therapy, and intra-abdominal infection. When these factors are present, particular care should be utilized in fascial wound closure, and the use of retention suture techniques should be considered.

The risks of postoperative subcutaneous wound infection should also be considered during operation. When factors such as shock, bowel obstruction, intraperitoneal contamination, and infection are present, the risk of subcutaneous wound infection is considerable. In these conditions, wound infection can be avoided by leaving the skin and subcutaneous tissues open for subsequent secondary or delayed primary closure. Again, this should especially be considered for those patients who would not tolerate the sepsis of postoperative wound infection.

INTRA-ABDOMINAL DRAINAGE. The specifics of intraabdominal drainage remain controversial, as a number of approaches have their own advocates.[12] However, several general concepts are accepted.

First, use of drains has negative aspects. Drains not only drain infection from the peritoneum to the outside, but they also act as conduits for bacteria to enter the peritoneal cavity. In addition, drains can erode intra-abdominal structures, causing bleeding, abscesses, or fistulas. Finally, the presence of a foreign body within the abdominal cavity may decrease the intrinsic immunologic resistance of the peritoneal cavity to infection and may impair wound healing.

Second, the entire peritoneal cavity cannot be effectively drained, as any drainage tube is relatively quickly isolated by intraperitoneal reaction. Drainage should therefore be reserved for management of localized intra-abdominal abscesses or for attempts to control fistula output through a defined outflow tract.

Third, dependent drainage is preferable. Drains should be placed in as dependent a position as possible, optimally through the flank or retroperitoneum.

Fourth, closed drainage systems may have advantages over open systems but are often prone to occlusion. The use of sump drains may help to some extent. All drainage systems, and particularly open ones, need be cared for in the postoperative period with sterile technique.

Fifth, percutaneous drains may be very effective at draining selected intra-abdominal abscesses and may obviate the need for formal anesthesia and operation. When an intra-abdominal abscess is diagnosed preoperatively, it is appropriate to consider the possibility of percutaneous drainage. When such drainage is technically feasible and when a patient does not require laparotomy to treat underlying problems, percutaneous drainage may be advantageous.

Finally, peritoneal lavage has been advocated in certain situations, such as generalized peritonitis and pancreatitis, but its application remains controversial. Although the advantages of continuously "cleansing" the peritoneal cavity seem appealing, lavage may also decrease the effectiveness of the peritoneal defense mechanisms. Net benefit of therapeutic peritoneal lavage remains to be proved.[12]

POSTOPERATIVE CARE

It is important to recognize that many determinants of why postoperative complications occur are already present before the postoperative period. The metabolic stress of the underlying illness, the deficits resulting from preoperative shock and sepsis, and the superimposed stress of anesthesia and operation have all occurred prior to the postoperative period. The patient who has undergone emergency abdominal surgery has thus already undergone such significant stress that his or her needs for survival are no longer the same as those of normal individuals. Bland and coworkers have emphasized these differing physiologic needs of such patients and have described "optimal" therapeutic goals that are significantly different from "normal" physiologic states.[13] These optimal therapeutic goals reflect the requirements of postoperative emergency patients to compensate physiologically for the combined stresses of preoperative illness, shock, sepsis, anesthesia, and surgery.

Several other aspects of postoperative care deserve emphasis. Expectant physiologic monitoring should be initiated early in the postoperative period in patients at high risk for the development of complications. Rather than waiting for complications to occur, early monitoring of patients at risk allows titration of postoperative therapy to achieve optimal physiologic goals. In particular, increased cardiac output, increased oxygen delivery, and increased oxygen consumption are necessary in the early postoperative period. Titration of therapy to optimize tissue oxygenation improves both cellular and organ recovery from shock and resistance to infection.[14]

Every effort must be made to prevent septic complications. Compulsive maintenance of sterile technique during insertion of indwelling catheters cannot be overemphasized. Furthermore, intravascular as well as urinary monitoring catheters should be removed as soon as possible—that is, as soon as the information they provide is no longer essential to patient care.

Aggressive pulmonary care helps prevent pulmonary complications that lead to sepsis. This care should include administration of positive end-expiratory pressure and frequent suctioning with sterile technique for intubated patients and early ambulation and incentive spirometry for extubated patients.

Wound care should be meticulous. Of particular importance is avoidance of the spread of bacteria from drainage sites or wounds to other patients. Hand washing is critical in this regard.

Surgical drains placed into the peritoneal cavity have the potential to introduce contamination as well as act as conduits for drainage. Thus, they should be removed as early as feasible. Drains placed to remove blood (for example, splenic bed drains placed following splenectomy) may be removed after one day if bleeding is not evident. Drains placed to remove secretions (e.g., drains placed following cholecystectomy) should be removed when fluid drainage ceases. Drains placed into established abscess cavities are removed by advancing them slowly as the cavity size decreases or a drainage tract becomes well established. Drains placed to control fistula output should be left in place until the fistula has closed or until a very well-established tract has been formed.

Despite excellent postoperative care, an incidence of postoperative septic complications is inevitable following emergency abdominal surgery. The key to the successful management of these complications is continuing suspicion and early diagnosis.

Careful daily physical examination, with particular attention devoted to the chest, abdomen, and wounds, is essential. The diagnosis of sepsis in the postoperative period can often be made prior to definitive culture identification on the basis of signs such as fever, hyperventilation, worsening mental status, decreased systemic vascular resistance, or deterioration of organ function. Therapy of suspected sepsis should be instituted as early as possible, and great emphasis should be placed on signs of physiologic decompensation. Antibiotic therapy appropriate to the suspected bacteriologic flora is indicated, sometimes even before specific culture results are available. Suspected intra-abdominal sources of sepsis must be vigorously pursued.

ACUTE ABDOMINAL COMPLICATIONS THAT DEVELOP IN THE INTENSIVE CARE UNIT

The critical illness caused by acute abdominal disease has been discussed in this chapter. Conversely, acute abdominal disease can also be caused by critical illness. The diagnosis and treatment of acute abdominal complications occurring in patients who are already critically ill can be difficult and deserves particular emphasis. Several such complications occur with such a frequency and have such a significant impact (particularly if unrecognized) that they deserve special mention.

Ileus

Ileus is a frequent occurrence in critically ill patients. It is particularly prevalent in patients who have had shock or sepsis, possibly because of the decrease in mesenteric blood flow that results from these conditions. Patients with respiratory failure also frequently develop ileus, again perhaps due to a decrease in oxygen delivery to the gut. In addition, ileus may be an early sign of unrecognized intra-abdominal infection.[15]

Ileus in critically ill patients leads to several very serious problems. First, the inability to tolerate oral or enteral feedings interferes with nutritional support. Second, the abdominal distention resulting from ileus can significantly impair pulmonary function. Third, large volumes of fluid can be sequestered in the intestinal lumen, causing hypovolemia and electrolyte disturbances. Finally, massive colonic ileus (so-called *Ogilvie's syndrome*) can result in perforation of the colon, a disastrous complication.

The diagnosis of ileus is usually apparent. Abdominal distention and vomiting occur in a patient with a serious underlying illness. Bowel sounds are hypoactive or absent. Abdominal radiographs show distention of the small and large intestine. At times, however, it may prove difficult to differentiate ileus from mechanical small bowel obstruction; gastrointestinal contrast studies may be useful in this differentiation.

Early recognition and treatment of ileus is essential, because the more distended the intestine becomes, the less effective peristalsis becomes and the more prolonged the bowel dysfunction will be. To some extent, ileus can be prevented or minimized with optimal hemodynamic support. Electrolyte disturbances should be corrected. In particular, hypokalemia and hypomagnesemia commonly intensify bowel dysfunction. An active search for intra-abdominal infection must be undertaken. Of great importance is the early cessation of oral fluid and food intake and the initiation of nasogastric suction. Nasogastric tubes are of two types: simple tubes (e.g., Levine tubes), which require intermittent suction; or sump tubes (e.g., Salem tubes), which require constant suction. Nasogastric suction can effectively prevent intestinal distention, but tube patency must be frequently checked. Consideration should always be given to the initiation of intravenous nutritional support, since it is frequently many days before a patient is able to tolerate oral or enteral feedings. Finally, if massive or progressive colonic distention is present, it can be effectively reversed by colonoscopic decompression, and cecal perforation can be prevented.[16] If colonoscopy is not available, operative or percutaneous decompression with cecostomy may be necessary.

Stress Ulcer

The occurrence of stress ulceration of the stomach or duodenum was previously a frequent cause of morbidity in critically ill patients owing to bleeding or perforation. Although endoscopy reveals significant mucosal injury in most intensive care unit patients, bleeding and perforation are now uncommon because of widespread use of prophylactic antacid therapy.[17] These complications do, however, continue to occur in very severely stressed and septic patients, particularly if antacid therapy is inadequate. The optimal regimen in preventing bleeding from stress ulcers appears to be hourly titration of antacid therapy to maintain a gastric pH of 4.0 or greater.

When upper gastrointestinal bleeding does occur in intensive care unit patients, endoscopy is indicated to differentiate possible causes. If bleeding from diffuse gastric stress ulceration is identified, then medical management consisting of hemodynamic resuscitation, saline lavage, and antacids is usually successful. Continued bleeding may respond to intravenous administration of vasopressin. Further bleeding that does not respond to these measures has a poor prognosis. Attempts at arteriographic embolization may be undertaken. Surgery therapy consisting of subtotal gastrectomy or vagotomy and pyloroplasty with oversewing of gastric ulcers has a high risk of mortality but may be successful.

Perforated peptic ulcer in critically ill intensive care unit patients also carries a very high risk of mortality. Early diagnosis and prompt laparotomy are mandatory.

Acalculous Cholecystitis

This entity is due to acute biliary stasis without stone formation and is most common in the critically ill patient with prolonged illness who has been on long-term intravenous hyperalimentation without oral intake and who often has had shock or sepsis. Stasis of the gallbladder can be due to absent gastrointestinal stimulation, sepsis, or ischemia.

A high degree of suspicion is necessary for diagnosis of this condition because many patients are too ill to communicate their symptoms. Unexplained abdominal tenderness, ileus, and fever as well as possible abnormal liver function test results suggest the diagnosis. Bedside ultrasound may show a distended gallbladder with thickened wall. The gallbladder does not contract despite cholecystokinin administration. The gallbladder does not appear to fill on iminodiacetic acid scan, even after morphine administration.[18]

Therapy should be initiated as soon as possible following diagnosis. Options for therapy include laparotomy and cholecystectomy, cholecystostomy performed under local anesthesia, laparoscopic cholecystostomy, and percutaneous drainage of the gallbladder with ultrasound guidance.

Intestinal Necrosis

Ischemic intestinal necrosis may occur in critically ill patients for a variety of reasons. It may be associated with occlusive disease of the mesenteric arteries that is either due to an acute embolic event (usually associated with cardiac arrhythmias) or due to a low flow state superimposed upon arteriosclerotic mesenteric disease. Advanced pseudomembranous colitis may also progress to intestinal necrosis. It may also occur without occlusion of the arterial inflow, usually in association with severe or prolonged low flow states and, sometimes, with mesenteric venous thrombosis. Intestinal necrosis often represents a very difficult diagnostic dilemma because patients in whom it occurs may be too ill to communicate any of their symptoms. Ileus and abdominal distention may be the only signs present. Stool may contain occult blood. Plain abdominal x-rays may have "thumbprinting." It is often associated with severe systemic toxicity, fever, and very significant leukocytosis. Acidosis and thrombocytopenia also are often present. When such signs occur in critically ill patients, especially in patients who have had recent arrhythmias or low flow states, a diagnosis of intestinal necrosis should be considered. Diagnostic peritoneal lavage is a useful diagnostic test as it can rapidly be performed at the bedside and is quite sensitive. Arteriography may be useful in diagnosing occlusive mesenteric infarction but may not exclude nonocclusive disease. The only successful therapeutic modalities are laparotomy and bowel resection.

Pancreatitis

Hyperamylasemia is relatively common in critically ill patients. Serious pancreatitis, however, is unusual. When pancreatitis is severe, it manifests as abdominal pain, ileus, hypovolemia, pulmonary failure, hypocalcemia, and multiple organ failure. Among other possible etiologic factors, inadequate blood flow may both cause and potentiate acute pancreatitis. Thus, patients with severe pancreatitis occurring in the postoperative period or superimposed upon critical illness benefit from aggressive hemodynamic resuscitation to optimize cardiac output. Fluid requirements may be enormous, hemodynamic instability is common, and respiratory failure is often severe. Intensive cardiopulmonary monitoring, optimal fluid therapy, and aggressive supportive care are essential for maximizing a patient's chances for survival.

Intra-Abdominal Abscess

Intra-abdominal abscesses are a common cause of sepsis in critically ill patients. They most commonly occur following previous intra-abdominal trauma, infection, and operation. On occasion, however, intra-abdominal abscess, such as hepatic or splenic abscess, may occur without prior abdominal disease and secondary to hematogenous spread from distant infection.

The diagnosis of intra-abdominal abscesses in critically ill patients may be difficult, as symptoms and signs are often difficult to elicit and to interpret. A high index of suspicion is necessary in patients who are at high risk because of prior abdominal disease and operation and in those who have occult sepsis. The presence of fever, leukocytosis, and coagulopathy are additional clues. The best diagnostic test is CT, which has high sensitivity and specificity for the diagnosis of intra-abdominal abscess. Localization of abscesses with CT is also of great value in planning either percutaneous or operative drainage. If a patient is too unstable for transfer to the CT suite, bedside ultrasound imaging, if technically possible, may localize abscesses.

References

1. Cope SZ: The Early Diagnosis of the Acute Abdomen. 14th ed. London, Oxford University Press, 1972.
2. Lindberg P, Gunnarsson L, Tokics L, et al: Atelectasis and lung function in the postoperative period. Acta Anaesthesiol Scand 1992; 36:546–553.
3. Mark JB: Central venous pressure monitoring: Clinical insights beyond the numbers. J Clin Vasc Anesthesia 1991; 5:163–173.
4. Moore FA, Haenel JB, Moore EE: Alternatives to Swan-Ganz cardiac output monitoring. Surg Clin North Am 1991; 71:699–721.
5. Chang R, Wong GY: Prognostic significance of marked leukocytosis in hospitalized patients. J Gen Intern Med 1991; 6:199–203.
6. Winslet M, Hall C, London NJ, et al: Relation of diagnostic serum amylase levels to aetiology and severity of acute pancreatitis. Gut 1992; 33:982–986.
7. Taourel P, Baron MP, Pradel J, et al: Acute abdomen of unknown origin: Impact of CT on diagnosis and management. Gastrointest Radiol 1992; 17:287–291.
8. Easter DW, Cuschieri A, Nathonson LK, et al: The utility of diagnostic laparoscopy for abdominal disorders: Audit of 120 patients. Arch Surg 1992; 127:379–383.
9. Donovan AJ, Vinson TL, Maulsby GO, et al: Selective treatment of duodenal ulcer with perforation. Ann Surg 1979; 189:627–636.
9a. Hamby LS, Zweng TN, Stroedel WE: Perforated gastric and duodenal ulcer: An analysis of prognostic factors. Am Surg 1993; 59:319–324.
10. Patti MG, Pelligrini CA: Gallstone pancreatitis. Surg Clin North Am 1990; 70:1277–1295.
11. Bizer LS, Liebling RW, Delay HM, et al: Small bowel obstruction: The role of nonoperative treatment in simple intestinal obstruction and predictive criteria for strangulation obstruction. Surgery 1981; 89:407–413.
12. Dougherty SH, Simmons RL: The biology and practice of surgical drains. Curr Probl Surg 1992; 24:561–685.
13. Bland R, Shoemaker WC, Shabot MM: Physiologic monitoring goals for the critically ill patient. Surg Gynecol Obstet 1978; 147:833–841.
14. Sawyer RG, Pruett TL: Wound infections. Surg Clin North Am 1994; 74:519–536.
15. Dark DS, Pingleton SK: Nonhemorrhagic gastrointestinal complications in acute respiratory failure. Crit Care Med 1989; 17:755–758.

16. Jetmore AM, Timmcke AE, Gathright JB, et al: Ogilvie's syndrome: Colonoscopic decompression and analysis of predisposing factors. Dis Colon Rectum 1992; 35:1135–1142.
17. Marrone GC, Silen W: Pathogenesis, diagnosis and treatment of acute gastric mucosal lesions. Clin Gastroenterol 1984; 13:635–650.
18. Cornwall EE, Rodriguez A, Merves SE, et al: Acute acalculous cholecystitis in critically injured patients: Preoperative diagnostic imaging. Ann Surg 1989; 210:52–55.

CHAPTER 108

Failure of the Gastrointestinal Tract Barrier

Mitchell P. Fink, MD

As Wilmore and coworkers have pointed out, clinicians have tended to view the gut in critically ill patients as a quiescent organ.[1] This notion has been fostered by the frequent presence of ileus and the availability of means for providing completely parenteral nutritional support. Furthermore, acute failure of other organs, in particular the heart and lungs, can be immediately life-threatening, whereas the consequences of gastrointestinal (GI) dysfunction typically are subtle and difficult to discern.

In the past few years, however, this view of the gut in critical illness has changed considerably. Indeed, it has been proposed that the GI tract is not only a "central organ" after surgical stress[1] but also may be the very "motor" of multiple organ system dysfunction.[2] These notions, of course, are not really new at all.[3] Early in this century, Metchnikoff suggested that the systemic absorption of microorganisms or their toxins from the GI tract could lead to mortality.[4] Later, the great physiologist Walter B. Cannon suggested that a toxic factor originating from the gut was responsible for the development of irreversibility in patients with prolonged, profound shock.[5] This hypothesis was extended and subjected to extensive experimental testing by Fine and associates, who proposed that Cannon's toxic factor was endotoxin derived from intraluminal, gram-negative bacteria.[6] The ideas of Fine and associates were not widely accepted, in part because of the publication of contradictory findings by other workers.[7, 8] Currently, however, an updated version of Fine's hypothesis has found a receptive audience among clinicians and investigators who are studying the problem of multiple organ system dysfunction in critical illness.

The premise for the idea that the GI tract may play a pivotal role in the pathogenesis of multiple organ system dysfunction is that the gut serves not only as physiologic portal for the entry of water and nutrients into the body but also as a barrier that limits the systemic absorbtion of intraluminal microbes or microbial products (e.g., endotoxin). In its barest outline, the current incarnation of the "gut hypothesis for multiple organ dysfunction" proposes that trauma, sepsis, and various critical illnesses lead to derangements in this barrier's function that permit dissemination of intraluminal bacteria, yeast, and associated substances to mesenteric lymph nodes or other organs (especially the liver) that are "downstream" from the GI tract. The pathologic absorbtion of gut-derived proinflammatory substances activates Kupffer's cells, macrophages, and other immune cells and results in the release of various mediators (cytokines, nitric oxide, eicosanoids, platelet activating factor) implicated as being important in the pathogenesis of organ system dysfunction. Although supported only by circumstantial evidence, this "gut hypothesis" is attractive because it might explain why signs and symptoms of sepsis, such as fever, leukocytosis, hypermetabolism and organ system dysfunction, frequently are present in critically ill patients, even in the absence of a well-defined focus of infection.[9, 10]

MICROBIAL TRANSLOCATION

Translocation is the transepithelial passage of microbes, microbial fragments, or even inert particles such as latex beads from the lumen of the gut to extraluminal sites.[11] In experimental studies, the extent of microbial translocation usually is quantified by enumerating viable colony-forming units in various extraintestinal organs. This approach probably underestimates the number of organisms that traverse the epithelium because most are killed by phagocytic cells in the lamina propria of the gut, mesenteric lymph nodes, liver, lung, or spleen.[12] This is an issue of importance, since nonviable microbes or microbial products may be as capable as living cells in eliciting the release of inflammatory mediators. Because only viable organisms are detected in most experimental studies of translocation using animal models, pathologic increases in the extent of translocation may be caused by an increase in the penetration of the epithelium of the gut by microbes, a decrease in the capacity of the host to kill microbes in extraluminal sites, or a combination of both of these phenomena.

The mechanisms responsible for penetration of the epithelium by translocating microbes remain to be completely elucidated. Whereas some data suggest that microbes traverse the mucosal barrier through microscopic discontinuities in the epithelial sheet,[13, 14] other findings indicate that macromolecules and even intact microorganisms are ingested by enterocytes and are transported across the mucosa via a transcellular pathway.[15–17] The uptake of antigens by the gut ("antigen sampling") is a key event in the development of immunoglobulin A (IgA)–mediated mucosal immunity.[18] Although the transepithelial passage of certain macromolecules (e.g., maternally derived immunoglobulins) is a receptor-dependent process,[19] other macromolecular substances are bound and transported across the epithelium by a nonspecific, nonsaturable mechanism.[20] The uptake and transport of microbes and macromolecules across the epithelium occurs by endocytosis[15, 16, 21] and appears to be energy-dependent.[17] Although macromolecules are absorbed by the epithelium of the gut under normal conditions, recent data suggest that this process is accelerated under conditions of stress such as thermal injury.[21]

GASTROINTESTINAL MUCOSAL PERMEABILITY

Permeability refers to the passage of hydrophilic compounds or ions across the epithelial barrier. Were it not for the presence of various ion channels and transporters, the plasma membrane of enterocytes would be impermeable to hydrophilic compounds. Nevertheless, highly hydrophilic compounds can permeate the intestinal epithelium by traversing the paracellular channels between adjacent enterocytes.[22] Permeation via this pathway, however, is not unrestricted because of the presence of tight junctions (zonula occludens) between the cells that make up the epithelial monolayer. Formerly, it was believed that permeation was restricted to relatively small molecules and ions (i.e., with a Stokes radius < 11.5 Å), but recent observations indicate that even molecules as large as inulin (Stokes radius = 14–20 Å) can traverse the paracellular pathway in the normal rat intestine.[23]

Paracellular permeability to hydrophilic molecules is dynamically regulated by the size of the pores created by the tight junctions.[22] Under physiologic conditions, intestinal permeability is increased by activation of sodium ion–coupled cotransporters on the apical membrane of the cell by intraluminal substrates, such as glucose or amino acids.[24] Certain drugs, such as L-tryptophan[25] and cyclooxygenase inhibitors (in pharmacologic doses),[23, 26] increase gut epithelial permeability, whereas other agents, such as prostaglandin E analogs,[23] decrease paracellular conductance of water-soluble probes. It is noteworthy that prolonged exposure of certain model epithelia (T84 and MDCK monolayers) to cytokines, such as interferon-γ or tumor necrosis factor–α, also increases paracellular permeability.[27, 28]

Recently, Kubes showed that pharmacologic inhibition of nitric oxide synthase markedly increases small intestinal mucosal permeability in the cat.[29] Nitric oxide synthetase inhibitors have been used experimentally to treat sepsis or endotoxemic shock,[30, 31] but Kubes's data suggest that this therapeutic strategy might worsen sepsis-induced derangements in mucosal permeability.

FACTORS CONTRIBUTING TO INCREASED TRANSLOCATION OR MUCOSAL HYPERPERMEABILITY, OR BOTH

In experimental animals, the incidence and extent of microbial translocation is enhanced by a wide variety of pathologic insults, including obstructive jaundice,[32] thermal trauma,[33] endotoxemia,[34, 35] hemorrhage,[14] immunosuppression,[36] alterations in diet,[37] and sterile inflammation.[38] Similarly, a large number of pathologic conditions, including intestinal ischemia-reperfusion,[39–42] total parenteral nutrition,[43] cutaneous thermal injury,[44] endotoxemia,[35, 45–47] and pancreatitis,[48] have been shown to increase intestinal permeability in experimental animals. At present, it is not clear how these various insults promote translocation or mucosal hyperpermeability, or both.

Ischemia

One factor that may be important in the promotion of translocation or hyperpermeability, or both—at least in certain models—is mucosal ischemia. Because of the architecture of microvasculature of the intestinal mucosa, this tissue is very susceptible to ischemic damage. Blood is supplied to the intestinal villus by a central nutrient arteriole and is drained by an arbor of venules surrounding the inflow vessel. This anatomic arrangement causes the tip of the villus to be relatively hypoxic, even under normal conditions.[49] The most important reason for this is that tissue oxygen tension decreases along the length of the villus from base to tip because of consumption of oxygen by cells along this axis.[49] In addition, the arrangement of the nutrient arteriole and draining venules constitutes a countercurrent exchange network. Thus, the base-to-tip oxygen tension gradient induced by oxygen consumption is exaggerated by diffusional arteriovenous shunting. Although Lundgren and others have proposed that the base-to-tip oxygen tension gradient is exaggerated under conditions of low flow due to increased arteriovenous shunting within the villous microvasculature,[50, 51] recent theoretic calculations suggest that shunting actually decreases when flow is diminished.[49] Nevertheless, because of the effect of oxygen consumption along the axis of the villus, tissue oxygen tension at the tip decreases dramatically during hypoperfusion. This accounts for the characteristic tip-to-base pattern of necrosis induced by increasing periods of mucosal ischemia.[52]

Mucosal hypoperfusion can result from anatomic occlusion of the superior or inferior mesenteric arteries due to atherosclerotic vascular disease or thromboembolism. However, a more common mechanism responsible for mucosal hypoperfusion in critical illness is excessive vasoconstriction in the splanchnic arterial supply during periods of low cardiac output that result from hypovolemia or myocardial dysfunction. Reilly and coworkers have shown that inflow impedance in the splanchnic network increases out of proportion to the increase in that of the arterial system as a whole when cardiac output is diminished.[53] This effect is mediated by excessive release of the potent vasoconstrictor angiotensin II.[53]

Mesenteric arteriolar vasoconstriction also occurs in certain experimental models of sepsis, endotoxemia, and sterile peritonitis, even when cardiac output is maintained at normal or supranormal levels.[54–58] Mesenteric hypoperfusion due to sepsis probably results from the release of vasoconstricting mediators, such as thromboxane A_2 and leukotriene D_4,[47, 59, 60] as well as from functional alterations in the capacity of resistance vessels in the mesenteric bed to respond appropriately to vasodilatory agonists.[61] Sepsis also may lead to alterations in the density of perfused capillaries in the intestinal microvascular network.[62]

The notion that mesenteric ischemia promotes translocation and increases mucosal permeability is supported by several observations. Morris and coworkers and Saydjari and colleagues have documented that mesenteric perfusion decreases and bacterial translocation increases in ovine and porcine models of cutaneous thermal injury.[63–65] Moreover, these authors have documented that bacterial translocation can be prevented in burned sheep if mesenteric hypoperfusion is prevented with the infusion of a vasodilator (sodium nitroprusside) directly into the mesenteric artery.[63] Using a similar experimental design, Jones and associates showed that thermal injury in rats is associated with a 46% decrease in small intestinal blood flow and a significant increase in bacterial translocation.[33] Pretreatment with an angiotensin-converting enzyme inhibitor (enalapril) prevented intestinal hypoperfusion and decreased the incidence of bacterial translocation after thermal injury.[33] The author has shown that administration of lipopolysaccharide to pigs markedly increases intestinal permeability to a medium-size hydrophilic probe (chromium 51–labeled ethylenediaminetetraacetic acid), an effect that can be abrogated if lipopolysaccharide-induced mesenteric hypoperfusion is prevented with infusion of a colloid solution (hetastarch) and an inotropic agent (dobutamine).[46] Using a guinea pig model of cutaneous thermal injury, Gianotti and colleagues showed that the incidence of translocation of *Candida albicans* is inversely related to villous blood flow measured using colored microspheres.[66]

Mucosal ischemia might promote translocation or hyperpermeability directly. In addition, by promoting the conversion of xanthine dehydrogenase to xanthine oxidase, ischemia *followed by reperfusion* might promote the production of reactive oxygen metabolites,[67] thus leading to cellular damage and altered barrier function. Xu and colleagues and Deitch and coworkers have obtained considerable data over the past few years to support the idea that ischemia-induced activation of xanthine oxidase plays a key role in the derangement of gut barrier dysfunction that is induced by hemorrhage or endotoxemia.[35, 58, 68–70] In contrast, recent data from these groups suggest that xanthine oxidase is relatively unimportant in the pathogenesis of translocation that is induced with a sterile proinflammatory stimulus.[71]

Not all data support the notion that ischemia is a major factor contributing to derangements in gut barrier function. The author found that administration of lipopolysaccharide to pigs reduces mesenteric blood flow to about 50% of the normal value and increases ileal mucosal permeability to chromium 51–labeled ethylenediaminetetra-acetic acid.[45] When mesenteric perfusion was reduced to a similar extent in normal animals with the application of a mechanical occluder, no derangement in barrier function was demonstrated.[45] In several recent studies, the ability of hemorrhagic shock to induce bacterial translocation has been questioned. Using rats, LaRocco and associates found that hemorrhage to a blood pressure of 30 mm Hg for as long as 90 minutes did not lead to bacterial translocation when methoxyflurane (instead of pentobarbital) was employed as the anesthetic agent.[72] Similar findings have been reported in halothane-anesthetized swine subjected to hemorrhage.[73, 74]

Microbiologic Factors

Experiments in animals have provided clear evidence that bacterial translocation is modulated by the microbiologic ecology of the gut lumen. Not all microorganisms penetrate the epithelial barrier equally well—that is, some microbes are "good" translocators, whereas others are not.[75, 76] Obligate anaerobes tend not to translocate.[77] Moreover, obligate anaerobes in the gut lumen suppress the growth of more pathogenic organisms (enteric gram-negative bacilli and aerobic gram-positive cocci) that are more likely to translocate; this phenomenon, originally described by van der Waaij and colleagues, has been termed "colonization resistance."[78–80] When animals are treated with antibiotics that suppress the growth of obligate anaerobes, the extent of translocation is enhanced.[81, 82]

Nutritional, Hormonal, and Immunologic Considerations

Results obtained by Cappellar and coworkers suggest that derangements in IgA-mediated mucosal immunity may be an important factor contributing to increased bacterial translocation in many experimental models.[83] The major source of intraluminal IgA is secretory IgA in bile,[83] and the amount of IgA secreted into bile is markedly diminished in a variety of conditions associated with enhanced translocation, including total parenteral nutrition (TPN) (with glutamine-deficient formulas),[84] thermal injury,[83] glucocorticoid administration,[36] and endotoxemia.[85] Bile duct ligation also increases bacterial translocation,[32] possibly by interupting the delivery of secretory IgA into the intestinal lumen.

Dietary composition has been shown by numerous investigators to be a key factor influencing the degree of translocation in experimental animals. With a few exceptions,[43, 86] most studies have found that translocation is increased after prolonged TPN.[37, 87–89] Since enteral administration of a TPN formula or an elemental diet also is associated with increased translocation,[37, 88, 90] it seems likely that the deleterious effect of TPN is due to the lack of one or more key nutrients rather than to the parenteral route of administration.

One key substrate that is lacking from conventional TPN formulas is glutamine. Glutamine supplementation has been shown to diminish the incidence of bacterial translocation in several different systems.[84, 87, 91] Glutamine has numerous biologic effects that might account for the salutary action of this amino acid on the degree of translocation observed in experimental studies. Glutamine is a key nutrient for enterocytes[92] and immune cells,[93] and it also is one of the amino acids that make up glutathione, an important endogenous antioxidant.[94]

Fiber is another factor that may contribute to an increase in translocation in animals fed parenterally or enterally with an elemental diet. In 1990, Spaeth and associates in Shreveport reported that enteral administration of cellulose powder abrogated the increased incidence of translocation induced by TPN or enteral feeding of an elemental diet.[37] The mechanism or mechanisms underlying this phenomenon remain to be established. Deitch and associates have hypothesized that administration of fiber may modulate the production of hormones trophic for the intestinal mucosa. Accordingly, these investigators examined the effect that two key gut hormones, bombesin and somatostatin, have on bacterial translocation.[90] Bombesin, which promotes the release of several trophic hormones, was shown to prevent increased translocation induced by an elemental diet without fiber. In contrast, somatostatin, which blocks the release of trophic gut hormones, induced translocation in animals fed a normal enteral diet. Cellulose-like compounds also may influence translocation by other mechanisms, such as interference with adherence of bacteria to the mucosa, as evidenced by the work of Wang and colleagues.[95]

Hormones and autocoids other than bombesin have been shown to ameliorate bacterial translocation in certain animal models. Gianotti and coworkers[96] and Fukushima and associates[97] at the University of Cincinnati have shown that oral administration of analogs of prostaglandin E_1 decreases translocation and improves survival in mice subjected to thermal injury. Interestingly, other investigators have reported that treatment with prostaglandin E_2 maintains the structural integrity of the mucosa in TPN-fed rats but that this therapy fails to prevent increased translocation in this model.[98] Huang and colleagues have shown that treatment with insulin-like growth factor 1 reduces gut atrophy and bacterial translocation after burn trauma in rats.[99] Zapata-Sirvent and coworkers have reported similar findings from a study of epidermal growth factor in burned mice.[100] Gianotti and associates have reported that another hormone, fibroblast growth factor, diminishes translocation in thermally injured mice.[101]

TRANSLOCATION OR HYPERPERMEABILITY AS FACTORS CONTRIBUTING TO MORTALITY IN ANIMAL MODELS

Accumulating data suggest that microbial translocation or gut-derived endotoxemia, or both, contribute to mortality in several animal models of critical illness; however, interpretation of some findings is difficult because observations among studies are discordant. For example, Bruce and colleagues have found that survival is significantly greater in germ-free rats compared with conventional rats subjected to hemorrhagic shock.[102] In contrast, in studies performed more than 30 years ago, neither Zweifach and colleagues[8] nor McNulty and Linares[103] found that hemorrhage was better tolerated by germ-free animals than by normal animals.

Gathiram and colleagues[104, 105] and Gaffin and coworkers[106] have documented elevated circulating endotoxin levels in experimental animals subjected to superior mesenteric arterial ischemia and reperfusion, heat stroke, and arterial hypoxemia. In their studies, circulating endotoxin levels were lower than the limit of detection in appropriate controls. Endotoxemia associated with mesenteric ischemia is abrogated by prior treatment with nonabsorbable antibiotics to eradicate gram-negative aerobic enteric bacteria[104]; this indicates that the gut is the source of the endotoxin in plasma in this model. Zanotti and associates,[107] Gaffin and associates,[108] and Gathiram and coworkers[109] also have shown that administration of a polyvalent antiendotoxin antibody preparation improves survival in rabbits subjected to mesenteric ischemia, cats subjected to hemorrhagic shock, and monkeys subjected to heat stroke. Thus, in these models, convincing evidence exists to support the idea that mortality is caused at least in part by leakage of gut-derived endotoxins into the systemic circulation.

Bacterial translocation also has been studied in an animal model of the "systemic inflammatory response syndrome."[110] In this model, developed by Goris and coworkers,[111] rats are injected intraperitoneally with sterile zymosan. Bacterial translocation has been documented in this model.[112, 113] In this model, early deaths, which normally occur in about one third of animals, are not observed in germ-free animals,[111] rats treated with oral antibiotics to "decontaminate" the GI tract,[113, 114] or rats treated with systemic antibiotics (cefoxitin or streptomycin).[38] Thus, it seems likely that translocation is an important determinant of early mortality in this paradigm of critical illness, although delayed deaths (later than 5 days) appear to result from other factors.

Using a thermal injury model in mice, Fukushima and associates obtained further evidence that the extent of translocation is a key determinant of mortality.[97] These authors showed that duration of survival was inversely correlated ($r = .4$, $P < .05$) with the degree of translocation, as quantified by measurement of radioactivity in blood after loading (by gavage) of the GI tract with radioactively labeled bacteria. Thus, at least in various animal models of acute illness, gut-derived bacteria or endotoxins, or both, appear to play a key role in the pathogenesis of mortality.

EVIDENCE FOR TRANSLOCATION OR MUCOSAL HYPERPERMEABILITY IN MAN

Solid evidence supports the view that mucosal permeability is increased in humans with a variety of pathologic conditions. For example, O'Dwyer and coworkers reported that intestinal permeability to a hydrophilic probe (lactulose) was increased in volunteers injected with a very small dose of endotoxin.[115] Mucosal permeability also has been shown to be increased in critically ill patients, including those with burns,[116, 117] trauma,[118] sepsis,[119] or other conditions.[120]

Although limited, some data exist to support the idea that microbial translocation also occurs in humans. For example, Deitch showed that cultures of mesenteric lymph nodes were positive for enteric gram-negative bacilli in 10 (59%) of 17 patients undergoing laparotomy for nonstrangulated intestinal obstruction, whereas positive culture results were obtained in only 1 (4%) of 25 patients who underwent surgery for other reasons.[121] Krause and associates reported that oral ingestion of a suspension containing numerous viable *C. albicans* resulted in fungemia and funguria in a human volunteer,[122] Soriano and colleagues found that the incidence of spontaneous bacterial peritonitis in hospital patients with cirrhosis was significantly decreased by selective digestive decontamination—that is, oral administration of an antibiotic active against the aerobic gram-negative but not against the strictly anaerobic microflora of the GI tract.[123] Finally, in a study of 50 trauma patients, Rush and colleagues reported that blood culture results obtained within 3 hours of admission were positive in 56% of the patients with a systolic blood pressure less than 80 mm Hg, whereas the results of only 4% were positive in the patients without hemorrhagic shock.[124]

Other clinical investigators, however, have questioned the importance of both translocation and hyperpermeability as phenomena that contribute to morbidity or mortality in critical illnesses. Perhaps the most important study in this regard was performed by Moore and coworkers,[125] who, at the time of laparotomy, placed portal venous catheters in 20 patients with major injuries. Using this indwelling portal catheter as well as more conventional arterial and central venous catheters, these investigators assayed portal and systemic blood samples for the presence of bacteria and endotoxin over the first 5 days of hospitalization. The results of only 9 (2%) of 424 blood cultures were positive; moreover, most of the organisms isolated were probably contaminants. Endotoxin levels were below the lower limit of detection for all samples assayed. Despite the minimal evidence for leakage of gut-derived bacteria or endotoxin into the portal or systemic circulations, six of the patients developed evidence of multiple organ dysfunction syndrome. In a related study by a different group of investigators, mesenteric lymph node biopsies were obtained at the time of laparotomy from 25 trauma patients and 4 patients with primary GI problems. None of the trauma patients had positive results on mesenteric lymph node cultures, whereas culture results were positive for samples from three of the four patients with GI problems. Despite the lack of evidence for translocation, 40% of the trauma patients had major complications, including pneumonia and adult respiratory distress syndrome. Further casting doubt on the "gut hypothesis" are two other studies that have failed to detect any relationship between gut mucosal permeability to a hydrophilic probe (lactulose) and outcome in critically ill patients.[118, 120]

Despite the "negative" studies just cited, the notion that the gut is somehow a pivotal organ in critical illness remains viable because of other circumstantial evidence from clinical studies. Certainly, it is now well established that septic complications are diminished by provision of early enteral nutrition to trauma patients.[126, 127] Furthermore, several studies have shown that tonometric evidence of gastric mucosal acidosis, especially if persistent, portends a bad outcome in critically ill patients.[128–131] Although tonometrically estimated mucosal acidosis might simply be an early warning sign of tissue hypoperfusion, it is worth noting that in animal experiments, the presence of mucosal acidosis has been associated with intestinal hyperpermeability.[45] Thus, the association of mucosal acidosis with mortality in critically ill patients might reflect a relationship between derangements in gut barrier function and outcome.

SUMMARY AND RECOMMENDATIONS

Despite a large body of data from both laboratory and clinical studies, the precise role of gut barrier dysfunction as a mechanism for disease in humans remains to be established. Although hard evidence to support the "gut hypothesis" is lacking, certain conclusions appear to be warranted. First, patients should be fed enterally unless overwhelming contraindications to providing nutritional support via this route are present. Second, antibiotics that deplete the gut of obligate anaerobes should be eschewed unless the use of such agents is clearly indicated. Because these agents interfere with the phenomenon of "colonization resistance," their use may promote the overgrowth of microorganisms (aerobic gram-negative enteric bacilli, enterococci, yeast) that are much more prone to translocation than are obligately anaerobic species. Third, although further studies are clearly needed, GI mucosal tonometry appears to be a useful means for titrating resuscitation (i.e., intravascular volume loading, inotropic support) to ensure the adequacy of splanchnic perfusion.

References

1. Wilmore DW, Smith RJ, O'Dwyer ST, et al: The gut: A central organ after surgical stress. Surgery 1988; 104:917.
2. Carrico CJ, Meakins JL, Marshall JC, et al: Multiple-organ-failure syndrome. Arch Surg 1985; 121:196.
3. Fink MP: The leaky gut hypothesis: A historical perspective. Crit Care Med 1990; 18:579.
4. Metchnikoff E: The nature of man. *In:* Studies in Opportunistic Philosophy. Mitchell PC (Ed). New York, G.P. Putnam's Sons, 1908, p 309.
5. Cannon WB: Traumatic Shock. New York, Appleton, 1923.
6. Fine J, Frank ED, Rutenberg SH, et al: The bacterial factor in traumatic shock. N Engl J Med 1959; 260:214.
7. Nadler AL, Zweifach BW: Pathogenesis of experimental shock: II. Absence of endotoxic activity in blood of rabbits subjected to graded hemorrhage. J Exp Med 1961; 114:195.
8. Zweifach BW, Gordon HA, Wagner M, et al: Irreversible hemorrhagic shock in germ-free rats. J Exp Med 1958; 107:437.
9. Goris RJ, Beokhorst PA, Nuytinck KS: Multiple organ failure: Generalized autodestructive inflammation. Arch Surg 1986; 120:1109.
10. Marshall JC, Christou NV, Horn R, et al: The microbiology of multiple organ failure: The proximal gastrointestinal tract as an occult resevoir of pathogens. Arch Surg 1988; 123:309.
11. Mora EM, Cardona MA, Simmons RL: Enteric bacteria and ingested inert particles translocate to intraperitoneal prosthetic materials. Arch Surg 1991; 126:157.
12. Alexander JW, Gianotti L, Pyles T, et al: Distribution and survival of *Escherichia coli* translocating from the intestine after thermal injury. Ann Surg 1991; 213:558.
13. Deitch EA, Morrison J, Berg R, et al: Effect of hemorrhagic shock on bacterial translocation, intestinal morphology, and intestinal permeability in conventional and antibiotic-decontaminated rats. Crit Care Med 1990; 18:529.
14. Deitch EA, Bridges W, Baker J, et al: Hemorrhagic shock–induced bacterial translocation is reduced by xanthine oxidase inhibition or inactivation. Surgery 1988; 104:191.
15. Wells CL, Jechorek RP, Erlandsen SL: Evidence for the translocation of *Enterococcus faecalis* across the mouse intestinal tract. J Infect Dis 1990; 162:82.
16. Alexander JW, Boyce ST, Babcock GF, et al: The process of microbial translocation. Ann Surg 1990; 212:496.
17. Walker WA, Cornell R, Davenport LM, et al: Macromolecular absorption: Mechanism of horseradish peroxidase uptake and transport in adult and neonatal rat intestine. J Cell Biol 1972; 54:195.
18. Bienstock J, Befus AD: Mucosal immunology. Immunology 1980; 41:249.
19. Casanova JE: Transepithelial transport of macromolecules. Chest 1992; 101:55S.
20. Sterns M, Walker WA: Food proteins and gut mucosal barrier: I. Binding and uptake of cow's milk proteins by adult rat jejunum in vitro. Am J Physiol 1984; 246:556.
21. Carter EA, Gonnell A, Tompkins RG: Increased transcellular permeability of rat small intestine after thermal injury. Burns 1992; 18:117.
22. Madara JL: Loosening tight junctions: Lessons from the intestine. J Clin Invest 1989; 83:1089.
23. Ma TY, Hollander D, Erickson RA, et al: Is the small intestinal epithelium truly "tight" to inulin permeation? Am J Physiol 1991; 260:G669.
24. Pappenheimer JR, Volpp K: Transmucosal impedance of small intestine: Correlation with transport of sugars and amino acids. Am J Physiol 1992; 263:C480.
25. Madara JL, Carlson S: Supraphysiologic L-tryptophan elicits cytoskeletal and macromolecular permeability alterations in hamster small intestinal epithelium in vitro. J Clin Invest 1991; 87:454.
26. Bjaranson I, Williams P, Smethurst P, et al: Effect of nonsteroidal anti-inflammatory drugs and prostaglandins on the permeability of the human small intestine. Gut 1986; 27:1292.
27. Madara JL, Stafford J: Interferon-gamma directly affects barrier function of cultured intestinal epithelial monolayers. J Clin Invest 1989; 83:724.
28. Mullin JM, Snock KV: Effect of tumor necrosis factor on epithelial tight junctions and transepithelial permeability. Cancer Res 1990; 50:2172.
29. Kubes P: Nitric oxide modulates epithelial permeability in the feline small intestine. Am J Physiol 1992; 262:G1138.
30. Lubbe AS, Garrison RN, Cryer HM, et al: EDRF as a possible mediator of sepsis-induced arteriolar dilation in skeletal muscle. Am J Physiol 1992; 262:H880.
31. Petros A, Bennett D, Vallance P: Effect of nitric oxide synthase inhibitors on hypotension in patients with septic shock. Lancet 1991; 338:1557.
32. Deitch EA, Sittig K, Li M, et al: Obstructive jaundice promotes bacterial translocation from the gut. Am J Surg 1990; 159:79.
33. Jones WG II, Minei JP, Barber AE, et al: Splanchnic vasoconstriction and bacterial translocation after thermal injury. Am J Physiol 1991; 261:H1190.
34. Deitch EA, Berg RD, Specian RD: Endotoxin promotes the translocation of bacteria from the gut. Arch Surg 1987; 122:185.
35. Deitch EA, Specian RD, Berg RD: Endotoxin-induced bacterial translocation and mucosal permeability: Role of xanthine oxidase, complement activation, and macrophage products. Crit Care Med 1991; 19:785.
36. Alverdy J: The effect of glucocorticoid administration on bacterial translocation: Evidence for an acquired mucosal immunodeficient state. Ann Surg 1991; 214:719.
37. Spaeth G, Berg RD, Specian RD, et al: Food without fiber promotes bacterial translocation from the gut. Surgery 1990; 108:240.
38. Deitch EA, Kemper AC, Specian RD, et al: A study of the relationships among survival, gut-origin sepsis, and bacterial translocation in a model of systemic inflammation. J Trauma 1992; 32:141.
39. Bulkley GB, Kvietys PR, Parks DA, et al: Relationship of blood flow and oxygen consumption to ischemic injury in the canine small intestine. Gastroenterology 1985; 89:852.
40. Langer JC, Sohal SS: Increased mucosal permeability after intestinal ischemia-reperfusion injury is mediated by local tissue factors. J Pediatr Surg 1992; 27:329.
41. Horton JW: Alterations in intestinal permeability and blood flow in a new model of mesenteric ischemia. Circ Shock 1992; 36:134.
42. Salzman AL, Wollert PS, Wang H, et al: Intraluminal oxygenation ameliorates ischemia/reperfusion-induced gut mucosal hyperpermeability in pigs. Circ Shock 1993; 40:37.
43. Illig KA, Ryan CK, Hardy DJ, et al: Total parenteral nutrition–induced changes in gut mucosal function: Atrophy alone is not the issue. Surgery 1992; 112:631.
44. Epstein MD, Tchervenkov JI, Alexander JW, et al: Increased gut permeability following burn trauma. Arch Surg 1991; 126:198.
45. Fink MP, Antonsson JB, Wang H, et al: Increased intestinal permeability in endotoxic pigs: Mesenteric hypoperfusion as an etiologic factor. Arch Surg 1991; 126:211.
46. Fink MP, Kaups KL, Wang H, et al: Maintenance of superior mesenteric arterial perfusion prevents increased intestinal mucosal permeability in endotoxic pigs. Surgery 1991; 110:154.
47. Fink MP, Kaups KL, Wang H, et al: Ibuprofen improves survival but does not ameliorate increased gut mucosal permeability in endotoxic pigs. Arch Surg 1992; 127:49.
48. Ryan CM, Schmidt J, Lewandrowski K, et al: Gut macromolecular permeability in pancreatitis correlates with severity of disease in rats. Gastroenterology 1993; 104:890.
49. Shepherd AP, Kiel JW: A model of countercurrent shunting of oxygen in the intestinal villus. Am J Physiol 1992; 262:H1136.
50. Lundgren O: Studies on blood flow distribution and countercurrent exchange in the small intestine. Acta Physiol Scand Suppl 1967; 303:1.
51. Lundgren O: Microcirculation of the gastrointestinal tract and pancreas. *In:* Handbook of Physiology: The Cardiovascular System: Microcirculation. Bethesda, MD, American Physiological Society, 1984, p 799.

52. Marston A: Vascular occlusion. *In:* Splanchnic Ischemia and Multiple Organ Failure. Marston A, Bulkley GB, Fiddian-Green RG, et al (Eds). London, Edward Arnold, 1989, p 51.
53. Reilly PM, MacGowan S, Miyachi M, et al: Mesenteric vasoconstriction in cardiogenic shock in pigs. Gastroenterology 1992; 102:1968.
54. Fink MP, Cohn SM, Lee PC, et al: Effect of lipopolysaccharide on intestinal intramucosal hydrogen ion concentration in pigs: Evidence of gut ischemia in a normodynamic model of septic shock. Crit Care Med 1989; 17:641.
55. Whitworth PW, Cryer HM, Garrison RN, et al: Hypoperfusion of the intestinal microcirculation with decreased cardiac output during live *Escherichia coli* sepsis in rats. Circ Shock 1989; 27:111.
56. Steeb GD, Wilson MA, Garrison RN: Pentoxyfylline preserves small-intestine microvascular blood flow during bacteremia. Surgery 1992; 112:756.
57. Scalia S, Sharma P, Rodriguez J, et al: Decreased mesenteric blood flow in experimental multiple organ failure. J Surg Res 1992; 52:1.
58. Xu D, Lu Q, Guillory D, et al: Mechanisms of endotoxin-induced intestinal injury in a hyperdynamic model of sepsis. J Trauma 1993; 34:676.
59. Fink MP, Rothschild HR, Deniz YF, et al: Systemic and mesenteric O_2 metabolism in endotoxic pigs: Effect of ibuprofen and meclofenamate. J Appl Physiol 1989; 67:1950.
60. Fink MP, Kruithoff KL, Antonsson JB, et al: Delayed treatment with an LTD_4/E_4 antagonist limits pulmonary edema in endotoxic pigs. Am J Physiol 1991; 260:R1007.
61. Wylam ME, Samsel RW, Umans JG, et al: Endotoxin *in vivo* impairs endothelium-dependent relaxation of canine arteries *in vitro.* Am Rev Respir Dis 1990; 142:1263.
62. Drazenovic R, Samsel RW, Wylam ME, et al: Regulation of perfused capillary density in canine intestinal mucosa during endotoxemia. J Appl Physiol 1992; 72:259.
63. Morris SE, Navaratnam N, Townsend CM Jr, et al: Decreased mesenteric blood flow independently promotes bacterial translocation in chronically instrumented sheep. Surg Forum 1989; 40:88.
64. Morris SE, Navaratnam N, Townsend CM Jr, et al: Bacterial translocation and mesenteric blood flow in a large animal model after cutaneous thermal smoke inhalation injury. Surg Forum 1988; 39:189.
65. Saydjari R, Beerthuizen GIJM, Townsend CM Jr, et al: Bacterial translocation and its relationship to visceral blood flow, gut mucosal ornithine decarboxylase activity, and DNA in pigs. J Trauma 1991; 31:639.
66. Gianotti L, Alexander JW, Fukushima R, et al: Translocation of *Candida albicans* is related to blood flow of individual intestinal villi. Circ Shock 1993; 40:250.
67. Bulkley GB: Free radicals and other reactive oxygen metabolites: Clinical relevance and the therapeutic efficacy of antioxidant therapy. Surgery 1993; 113:479.
68. Deitch EA, Ma L, Ma JW, et al: Inhibition of endotoxin-induced bacterial translocation in mice. J Clin Invest 1989; 84:36.
69. Deitch EA, Specian RD, Berg RD: Induction of early-phase tolerance to endotoxin-induced mucosal injury, xanthine oxidase activation, and bacterial translocation by pretreatment with endotoxin. Circ Shock 1992; 36:208.
70. Deitch EA, Bridges W, Baker J, et al: Hemorrhagic shock–induced bacterial translocation is reduced by xanthine oxidase inhibition or inactivation. Surgery 1988; 104:191.
71. Mainous MR, Xu D, Deitch EA: Role of xanthine oxidase and prostaglandins in inflammatory-induced bacterial translocation. Circ Shock 1993; 40:99.
72. LaRocco MT, Rodriguez LF, Chen CY, et al: Reevaluation of the linkage between acute hemorrhagic shock and bacterial translocation in the rat. Circ Shock 1993; 40:212.
73. Gelfand GAJ, Morales J, Jones RL, et al: Hemorrhagic shock and bacterial translocation in a swine model. J Trauma 1991; 31:867.
74. Morales J, Kibsey P, Thomas PD, et al: The effects of ischemia and ischemia-reperfusion on bacterial translocation, lipid peroxidation, and gut histology: Studies on hemorrhagic shock in pigs. J Trauma 1992; 33:221.
75. Steffen EK, Berg RD, Deitch EA: Comparison of translocation rates of various indigenous bacteria from the gastrointestinal tract to the mesenteric lymph node. J Infect Dis 1988; 157:1032.
76. Wells CL, Jechorek RP, Olmsted SB, et al: Effect of LPS on epithelial integrity and bacterial uptake in polarized human enterocyte-like cell line Caco-2. Circ Shock 1993; 40:276.
77. Wells CL, Maddaus MA, Reynolds CM, et al: Role of the anaerobic flora in the translocation of aerobic and facultatively anaerobic intestinal bacteria. Infect Immun 1987; 55:2689.
78. van der Waaij D, Berghuis-deVries JM, Lekkerkerk–van der Wees JEC: Colonization resistance of the digestive tract in conventional and antibiotic treated mice. J Hygiene 1971; 69:405.
79. van der Waaij D, Berghuis-deVries JM, Lekkerkerk–van der Wees JEC: Colonization resistance of the digestive tracts and the spread of bacteria to the lymphatic organs in mice. J Hygiene 1972; 70:335.
80. van der Waaij D, Berghuis-deVries JM, Lekkerkerk–van der Wees JEC: Colonization resistance of the digestive tract of mice during systemic antibiotic treatment. J Hygiene 1972; 70:605.
81. Berg RD: Promotion of the translocation of enteric bacteria from the gastrointestinal tract of mice by oral treatment with penicillin, clindamycin, or metronidazole. Infect Immun 1981; 33:854.
82. Deitch EA, Maejima K, Berg RD: Effect of oral antibiotics and bacterial overgrowth on the translocation of the GI tract microflora in burned rats. J Trauma 1985; 25:385.
83. Cappellar WA, Bloch KJ, Hatz RA, et al: Reduction in biliary IgA after burn injury: Role of diminished delivery via the thoracic duct and of enhanced loss from the systemic circulation. Ann Surg 1992; 215:338.
84. Alverdy JC, Aoys E, Weiss-Carrington P, et al: The effect of glutamine-enriched TPN on gut immune cellularity. J Surg Res 1992; 52:34.
85. Alverdy JC, Aoys E: The effect of dexamethasone and endotoxin administration on biliary IgA and bacterial adherence. J Surg Res 1992; 53:450.
86. Kueppers PM, Miller TA, Chen C-YK, et al: Effect of total parenteral nutrition plus morphine on bacterial translocation in rats. Ann Surg 1993; 217:286.
87. Burke DJ, Alverdy JC, Aoys E, et al: Glutamine-supplemented total parenteral nutrition improves gut immune function. Arch Surg 1989; 124:1396.
88. Alverdy JC, Moss GS: Total parenteral nutrition promotes bacterial translocation from the gut. Surgery 1988; 104:185.
89. Zaloga GP, Roberts P, Black KW, et al: Gut bacterial translocation/dissemination explains the increased mortality produced by parenteral nutrition following methotrexate. Circ Shock 1993; 39:263.
90. Haskel Y, Xu D, Deitch E: Elemental diet-induced bacterial translocation can be hormonally modulated. Ann Surg 1993; 217:634.
91. Fox AD, Kripke SA, de Paula J, et al: Effect of glutamine-supplemented enteral diet on methotrexate-induced enterocolitis. JPEN J Parenter Enter Nutr 1988; 12:325.
92. Souba WW, Klimberg VS, Plumley DA, et al: Current research review: The role of glutamine in maintaining a healthy gut and supporting the metabolic response to injury and infection. J Surg Res 1990; 48:383.
93. Newsholme EA: Nutrition of immune cells: The implications for whole-body metabolism. *In:* Yearbook of Intensive Care Medicine. Vincent J-L (Ed). Berlin, Springer-Verlag, 1993, p 187.
94. Hong RW, Helton WS, Rounds JD: Glutamine-supplemented TPN preserves hepatic glutathione and improves survival following chemotherapy. Surg Forum 1990; 41:9.
95. Wang X, Andersson R, Soltesz V, et al: Water-soluble ethylhydroxyethyl cellulose prevents bacterial translocation induced by major liver resection in the rat. Ann Surg 1993; 217:155.
96. Gianotti L, Alexander JW, Pyles T, et al: Prostaglandin E_1 analogues misoprostol and enisoprost decrease microbial translocation and modulate the immune response. Circ Shock 1993; 40:243.
97. Fukushima R, Gianotti L, Alexander JW, et al: The degree of bacterial translocation is a determinant factor for mortality after burn injury and is improved by prostaglandin analogs. Ann Surg 1992; 216:438.

98. Helton WS, Garcia R: Oral prostaglandin E_2 prevents gut atrophy during intravenous feeding but not bacterial translocation. Arch Surg 1993; 128:178.
99. Huang KF, Chung DH, Herndon DN: Insulin-like growth factor 1 (IGF-1) reduces gut atrophy and bacterial translocation after severe burn injury. Arch Surg 1993; 128:47.
100. Zapata-Sirvent RL, Hansbrough JF, Wolf P, et al: Epidermal growth factor limits structural alterations in gastrointestinal tissues and decreases bacterial translocation in burned mice. Surgery 1993; 113:564.
101. Gianotti L, Alexander JW, Fukushima R, et al: Reduction of bacterial translocation with oral fibroblast growth factor and sucralfate. Am J Surg 1993; 165:195.
102. Bruce CJ, Rush BF Jr, Ferraro FJ, et al: The effect of the germ-free state on survival following hemorrhagic shock: A study in germ-free and germ-bearing rats. Surg Forum 1992; 53:47.
103. McNulty WP Jr, Linares R: Hemorrhagic shock of germfree rats. Am J Physiol 1960; 198:141.
104. Gathiram P, Wells MT, Brock-Utne JG, et al: Oral administered non-absorbable antibiotics prevent endotoxemia in primates following intestinal ischemia. J Surg Res 1988; 45:187.
105. Gathiram P, Gaffin SL, Brock-Utne JG, et al: Time course of endotoxemia and cardiovascular changes in heat-stressed primates. Aviat Space Environ Med 1987; 58:1071.
106. Gaffin SL, Brock-Utne JG, Zanotti A, et al: Hypoxia-induced endotoxemia in primates: Role of reticuloendothelial system function and anti-lipopolysaccharide plasma. Aviat Space Environ Med 1986; 57:1044.
107. Zanotti AM, Gaffin SL: Prophylaxis of superior mesenteric artery occlusion shock in rabbits by antilipopolysaccharide (anti-LPS) antibodies. J Surg Res 1985; 38:113.
108. Gaffin SL, Grinberg Z, Abraham C, et al: Protection against hemorrhagic shock in the cat by human plasma containing endotoxin-specific antibodies. J Surg Res 1981; 31:18.
109. Gathiram P, Wells MT, Brock-Utne JG, et al: Antilipopolysaccharide improves survival in primates subjected to heat stroke. Circ Shock 1987; 23:157.
110. Members of the American College of Chest Physicians/Society of Critical Care Medicine Consensus Conference Committee: Definitions for sepsis and organ failure and guidelines for the use of innovative therapies in sepsis. Crit Care Med 1992; 20:864.
111. Goris RJA, Boekholtz WKF, van Bebber IPT, et al: Multiple-organ failure and sepsis without bacteria. Arch Surg 1986; 121:897.
112. Mainous MR, Tso P, Berg RD, et al: Studies of the route, magnitude, and time course of bacterial translocation in a model of systemic inflammation. Arch Surg 1991; 126:33.
113. Goris RJA, van Beeber IPT, Mollen RMH, et al: Does selective decontamination of the gastrointestinal tract prevent multiple organ failure? An experimental study. Arch Surg 1991; 126:561.
114. Rosman C, Wubbels GH, Manson WL, et al: Selective decontamination of the digestive tract prevents secondary infection of abdominal cavity, and endotoxemia and mortality in sterile peritonitis in laboratory rats. Crit Care Med 1992; 20:1699.
115. O'Dwyer ST, Michie HR, Ziegler TR, et al: A single dose of endotoxin increases intestinal permeability in healthy humans. Arch Surg 1988; 123:1459.
116. Deitch EA: Intestinal permeability is increased in burn patients shortly after injury. Surgery 1990; 107:411.
117. Ryan CM, Yarmush ML, Burke JF, et al: Increased gut permeability early after burns correlates with the extent of burn injury. Crit Care Med 1992; 20:1508.
118. Roumen RMH, Hendriks T, Wevers RA, et al: Intestinal permeability after severe trauma and hemorrhagic shock is increased without relation to septic complications. Arch Surg 1993; 128:453.
119. Ziegler TR, Smith RJ, O'Dwyer ST, et al: Increased intestinal permeability associated with infection in burn patients. Arch Surg 1988; 123:1313.
120. Harris CE, Griffiths RD, Freestone N, et al: Intestinal permeability in the critically ill. Intensive Care Med 1992; 18:38.
121. Deitch EA: Simple intestinal obstruction causes bacterial translocation in man. Arch Surg 1989; 124:699.
122. Krause W, Matheis H, Wulf K: Fungaemia and funguria after oral administration of *Candida albicans.* Lancet 1969; i:598.
123. Soriano G, Guarner C, Teixido M, et al: Selective intestinal decontamination prevents spontaneous bacterial peritonitis. Gastroenterology 1991; 100:477.
124. Rush BF, Sori AJ, Murphy TF, et al: Endotoxemia and bacteremia during hemorrhagic shock. Ann Surg 1988; 207:549.
125. Moore FA, Moore EE, Poggetti R, et al: Gut bacterial translocation via the portal vein: A clinical perspective with major torso trauma. J Trauma 1991; 31:629.
126. Kudsk KA, Croce MA, Fabian TC, et al: Enteral versus parenteral feeding: Effects on septic morbidity after blunt and penetrating abdominal trauma. Ann Surg 1992; 215:503.
127. Moore FA, Moore EE, Jones TN, et al: TEN versus TPN following major abdominal trauma—reduced septic morbidity. J Trauma 1989; 29:916.
128. Maynard N, Bihari D, Beale R, et al: Assessment of splanchnic oxygenation by gastric tonometry in patients with acute circulatory failure. J Am Med Assoc 1993; 270:1203.
129. Gutierrez G, Palizas F, Doglio G, et al: Gastric intramucosal pH as a therapeutic index of tissue oxygenation in critically ill patients. Lancet 1992; 339:195.
130. Gys T, Hubens A, Neels H, et al: Prognostic value of gastric intramural pH in surgical intensive care patients. Crit Care Med 1988; 16:122.
131. Doglio GR, Pusajo JF, Egurrola MA, et al: Gastric mucosal pH as a prognostic index of mortality in critically ill patients. Crit Care Med 1991; 19:1037.

CHAPTER 109

Acute Pancreatitis

Michael L. Steer, MD

CLASSIFICATION, PATHOLOGIC FACTORS, AND CAUSE

Pancreatitis is an inflammatory disease of the pancreas that is frequently associated with a number of other processes referred to as the causes of pancreatitis. By convention, the term *acute pancreatitis* refers to an attack involving a pancreas that was normal, both functionally and morphologically, before the onset of symptoms and that returns to normal after resolution of the attack. In contrast, the term *chronic pancreatitis* refers to a disease process in which functional and/or morphologic changes in the pancreas precede or follow the attack. In practice, however, the distinction between an attack of either acute or chronic pancreatitis is often difficult because, in each, the symptoms and clinical findings are frequently sudden in onset and the functional as well as the morphologic status of the gland before and after the attack is unknown. As a result, sudden-onset attacks are usually considered symptomatic of acute pancreatitis, whereas attacks characterized by long periods of waxing and waning symptoms are commonly considered symptomatic of chronic pancreatitis.

The pathologic changes of pancreatitis include interstitial edema, infiltration of inflammatory cells into the pancreas, and evidence of fat necrosis. In chronic pancreatitis, areas of fibrosis as well as atrophy of acinar tissue can also be seen. To a great extent, the morphologic changes of pancreatitis parallel the clinical severity of an attack, and, in severe cases, focal or diffuse areas of glandular necrosis are usually present. In addition, there may be thrombosis of intra- or

TABLE 109–1. Causes of Pancreatitis

Biliary tract stones	Trauma
Ethanol abuse	Postoperative
Obstructive lesions	Drugs
Infections	Miscellaneous
Parasites	Idiopathic
Metabolic abnormalities	

peripancreatic vessels with intraparenchymal hemorrhage and abscess formation.

The so-called causes[1] of acute pancreatitis are listed in Table 109–1. In any given population, roughly 80% of the cases are associated with either biliary tract stone disease or alcohol abuse, and 10% to 15% of the cases have no identified cause. These latter cases are identified as "idiopathic" acute pancreatitis. In the remaining 5% to 10% of cases, patients have an attack that is associated with a variety of other processes, including periampullar tumors or other obstructing lesions, infections such as mumps or coxsackievirus, parasites such as Clonorchis sinensis and Ascaris lumbricoides, or metabolic abnormalities such as hyperlipoproteinemia or hyperparathyroidism. Trauma to the pancreas can cause a diffuse form of acute pancreatitis as a result of pancreatic contusion or, more commonly, can lead to ductal disruption and an obstructive form of chronic pancreatitis. In such cases, the ductal disruption usually occurs near the junction between the body and tail of the pancreas, where the gland passes over the spine and can be cracked by blunt abdominal injury. Acute pancreatitis can also follow a variety of operative procedures including distal gastrectomy, sphincteroplasty, and common bile duct exploration. Endoscopic retrograde cholangiopancreatography is a relatively common iatrogenic cause of pancreatitis. Pancreatitis has also been noted to occur with increased frequency after either cardiac or renal transplantation and after cardiopulmonary bypass. Acute pancreatitis can also be precipitated by a variety of drugs including the thiazide diuretics, furosemide, ethacrynic acid, azathioprine, tetracycline, estrogens, and valproic acid. Certain drugs used to treat acquired immunodeficiency syndrome such as pentamidine and dideoxyinosine can also cause acute pancreatitis.

PATHOGENESIS

The mechanism by which ethanol abuse leads to pancreatitis is not known. For the most part, the symptoms of pancreatitis appear only after many years of ethanol abuse, and, in these cases, fibrosis and atrophy of the gland are already established. Evidence of exocrine and/or endocrine insufficiency may be present, and, as a result, these patients are usually given the diagnosis of chronic pancreatitis.[2] On occasion, however, an attack of pancreatitis may occur after only a brief period of ethanol abuse, and there may be no evidence of chronic morphologic and/or functional abnormality.

In contrast to the paucity of information concerning the events that relate ethanol abuse to pancreatitis, our knowledge concerning the pathogenesis of gallstone-related pancreatitis is much further developed. The studies of Acosta and Ledesma,[3,4] as well as others, clearly showed that pancreatitis is triggered by stone passage into or through the terminal biliopancreatic duct.

Three theories have been advanced to explain the mechanism by which stone passage might precipitate pancreatitis. The so-called common-channel theory proposed by Opie in 1901 suggested that a stone might occlude the biliopancreatic duct, creating behind it a common channel through which bile might reflux into the pancreatic duct and, presumably, injure the pancreas.[5] Objections to this theory include the observation that because pancreatic duct pressure exceeds bile duct pressure,[6] bile reflux into the pancreatic duct is unlikely. In addition, it is known that perfusion of the pancreatic duct with bile under physiologic pressures does not induce pancreatitis.[7]

The second theory, frequently referred to as the *duodenal reflux theory*, suggests that stone passage through Oddi's sphincter renders that sphincter incompetent, and, as a result, duodenal juices containing activated digestive enzymes can reflux through the incompetent sphincter into the pancreatic duct.[8] The currently recognized fact that the sphincter can be surgically or endoscopically divided (i.e., sphincterotomy or sphincteroplasty) without causing repeated episodes of pancreatitis certainly indicates that the duodenal reflux theory is an unlikely explanation for the development of gallstone-related pancreatitis.

The third theory and, by exclusion, the most likely explanation for the events relating stone passage to pancreatitis involves pancreatic duct obstruction. Presumably, either the offending stone or the edema and inflammation of the distal pancreatic duct that follows stone passage causes obstruction of the pancreatic duct. With continued secretion into the obstructed duct system, pancreatic duct hypertension would be expected. Experimental studies using various animal models of pancreatitis suggest that this could lead to intra-acinar cell activation of digestive enzyme precursors (zymogens) by the lysosomal hydrolase cathepsin-B and that this phenomenon could result in acinar cell injury and pancreatitis.[9–12]

CLINICAL PRESENTATION

History and Physical Examination

A history and physical examination[13] reveal the classic symptoms of acute pancreatitis, including abdominal pain, nausea, and vomiting. The pain typically begins abruptly and precedes the onset of nausea. It slowly increases in severity over several hours and thereafter remains constant. It is usually most severe in the epigastrium and radiates through to the midback. Frequently, the degree of discomfort is lessened by either leaning forward or assuming the knee-chest position. Patients frequently describe the pain as having a knifelike or boring character. The nausea and vomiting of an attack of pancreatitis usually persist even after the stomach has been emptied and the vomiting has become unproductive.

Patients with acute pancreatitis usually appear anxious as they constantly move about in search of a comfortable position. They may have mild, or sometimes severe, mental status alterations as a result of ethanol or drug exposure, hypotension, or hypoxemia. Jaundice is common, even in the absence of bile duct obstruction. Patients with gallstone-related pancreatitis also may have evidence of cholangitis, but, even in the absence of cholangitis, fever is often noted. Abdominal examination usually reveals areas of tenderness as well as both voluntary and involuntary guarding. Although these changes are usually most pronounced in the epigastrium, where a mass may be felt, tenderness and guarding can also be observed elsewhere or even diffusely in the abdomen. Abdominal distension is common, and bowel sounds are frequently diminished or absent. As a result of hypovolemia and dehydration, the skin and mucous membranes may be dry, neck veins may be collapsed, and hypotension as well as tachycardia may be present.

Evidence of retroperitoneal bleeding (Grey Turner's sign, Cullen's sign) is sometimes observed. Examination of the chest may reveal diminished breath sounds, especially at the bases, and evidence of pleural effusions.

Laboratory Tests

The routine laboratory tests usually show a number of nonspecific changes including leukocytosis with a leftward shift of the differential, an elevated hematocrit, hyperglycemia, hypoalbuminemia, and an increase in the creatinine and blood urea nitrogen. Hypocalcemia, sometimes out of proportion to the degree of hypoalbuminemia, can occur. Mild elevations of the alkaline phosphatase, transaminases, and bilirubin level are common even in those without gallstone-related pancreatitis. Hypertriglyceridemia may be present in those with alcohol-related pancreatitis or pancreatitis caused by hyperlipoproteinemia.[14, 15]

Patients with acute pancreatitis usually have elevated serum and urine levels of amylase.[16, 17] Unfortunately, hyperamylasemia is not a finding that is specific to pancreatitis. Other causes of hyperamylasemia are listed in Table 109–2. Hyperamylasemia caused by perforated viscus, mesenteric infarction, bowel obstruction, or cholangitis may be particularly difficult to distinguish from hyperamylasemia caused by pancreatitis. Attempts have been made to improve the diagnostic accuracy in pancreatitis by measuring the amylase–creatinine clearance ratio, serum pancreatic amylase isoenzymes, and serum level of other pancreas-derived digestive enzymes such as trypsinogen.[16] Unfortunately, these tests have not proven useful, and, for the most part, they are not widely used. Measurement of serum lipase and/or urine amylase levels may be useful in identifying those patients who are first seen several days after the onset of pancreatitis, because, in those patients, hyperlipasemia and hyperamylasuria may persist even after serum amylase levels have returned to normal.[16] Measurement of urine amylase levels may also aid in identifying those patients whose hyperamylasemia is caused by macroamylasemia rather than pancreatitis. In macroamylasemia, amylase is bound to an abnormal circulating protein, and, as a result, urine amylase levels are very low.[18]

Routine radiographic examinations of the chest may reveal basal atelectasis and pleural effusions, which are more common on the left than on the right side. Abdominal radiographs may demonstrate pancreatic calcifications in patients with chronic pancreatitis. The gaseous pattern of a paralytic ileus is frequently noted. Routine abdominal x-ray films may also suggest displacement of various organs by an inflammatory pancreatic mass, and in patients with pancreatic abscess, retroperitoneal gas can, on occasion, be noted. In general, however, these routine radiographic studies are not of great value in the diagnosis of acute pancreatitis. Similarly, ultrasonography is of only limited value because the gaseous distention of bowel during the early stages of pancreatitis usually precludes a complete ultrasonographic examination.[19] Even in such cases, however, ultrasonographic evidence of gallbladder stones and/or dilated bile ducts may aid in identifying those patients whose pancreatitis is caused by gallstones.

In contrast to routine radiography and ultrasonography, computed tomography (CT) may be extremely valuable in the diagnosis and management of pancreatitis.[20] The CT is not limited by the presence of gas-filled loops in the upper abdomen, and it can detect the presence of relatively mild as well as severe pancreatitis. As noted later, routine CT, along with dynamic contrast-enhanced CT, may be of value in predicting the severity of an attack of pancreatitis. Finally, CT may be of value in identifying those patients mistakenly diagnosed with pancreatitis, because, in such individuals, the pancreas will appear normal on CT.

TABLE 109–2. Causes of Hyperamylasemia

Pancreatic	*Malignant Tumors*
Pancreatitis, pseudocyst, ascites	Lung
Pancreatic duct obstruction	Prostate
Secretagogue stimulation	Ovary
Pancreatic trauma	Pancreas
Endoscopic retrograde cholangiopancreatography	Breast
Pancreatic tumor	*Genitourinary*
Nonpancreatic Intra-Abdominal	Ovarian cyst
Bowel obstruction	Ruptured ectopic pregnancy
Perforated ulcer or viscus	Renal failure
Appendicitis	Pregnancy
Bowel infarction	Prostatic disease
Salivary	*Miscellaneous*
Mumps	Burns
Trauma	Diabetic ketoacidosis
Duct obstruction	
Radiation	
Pulmonary	
Pneumonia	
Cancer	

Differential Diagnosis

Acute pancreatitis must be distinguished from the large number of other processes that can cause upper abdominal pain, nausea, and vomiting.[21] Pancreatitis frequently causes hyperamylasemia and hyperlipasemia, whereas many of the other diseases in the differential diagnosis do not cause these changes. Some diseases such as perforated viscus, bowel obstruction, cholangitis, and mesenteric ischemia can have modest rises in circulating amylase and lipase levels, and distinguishing these processes from pancreatitis may be quite difficult. Factors that favor the diagnosis of pancreatitis include (1) a markedly elevated amylase level rather than the elevation of one to one and one half times, which is seen in nonpancreatic diseases, (2) CT changes of pancreatitis, and (3) improvement after institution of aggressive nonoperative treatment. When doubt about the diagnosis persists, however, exploratory laparotomy for diagnostic purposes may be indicated, particularly if the patient's condition is deteriorating in spite of aggressive treatment.

Prognosis

Although only 10% to 15% of patients with pancreatitis have a severe attack, the mortality and serious morbidity among this group may exceed 50%. Identifying those individuals most likely to experience a severe attack would be helpful in allowing for comparison of various treatment strategies in prospective trials as well as in selecting those individuals who are in need of intensive care. A number of clinical, radiographic, and the biochemical methods of identifying such individuals are currently available (Table 109–3).[22] The most widely used clinical prognostic system is that developed by Ranson and colleagues[23] (Table 109–4). Those with fewer than three Ranson signs have a mortality rate of less than 1%, whereas those with seven to eight prognostic signs have a mortality rate of 90%. Because of its greater flexibility, the APACHE-II system may replace the Ranson or Imrie systems for predicting the severity of an attack on clinical

TABLE 109–3. Prognostic Markers

Clinical
Ranson's scoring system
Imrie's scoring system
APACHE-II scoring system

Radiographic
Non–contrast-enhanced computed tomography
Dynamic contrast-enhanced computed tomography

Biochemical
Polymorphonuclear elastase
C-reactive protein
Trypsinogen activation peptide
Antiprotease levels

grounds.[24] From a radiologic standpoint, the dynamic contrast-enhanced CT can also predict the severity of an attack. As noted by Balthazar and associates,[25] the presence of one or more pancreatic or peripancreatic fluid collections and lack of contrast enhancement of 50% of the pancreas is associated with a high probability of septic complications and/or death. A number of serum markers for severity have been evaluated (see Table 109–3), but the ultimate value of these tests in the management of patients with pancreatitis remains to be established. The most widely used are the C-reactive protein and polymorphonuclear elastase measurements. The ultimate value of these tests may be in the fact that low levels of these markers indicate a benign course and that, in this setting, particularly if the clinical scoring system also suggests a benign course, the contrast-enhanced dynamic CT may not be needed.[22]

TREATMENT OF ACUTE PANCREATITIS

The goals of initial management in pancreatitis include establishing the diagnosis, relieving pain, and supporting fluid as well as electrolyte needs. Usually, the diagnosis can be securely established when the clinical presentation and findings are appropriate, the amylase level is markedly elevated, the CT scan is convincing, and/or the patient improves with appropriate treatment. On occasion, however, exploratory laparotomy may be required to establish the diagnosis when uncertainty persists, particularly if the patient fails to improve with aggressive treatment.

The pain of pancreatitis may be severe, and, for the most part, narcotic medications are needed. In gallstone pancreatitis, meperidine (Demerol) rather than morphine should be used because the former relaxes Oddi's sphincter whereas morphine causes contraction of the sphincter.[26]

The early stages of acute pancreatitis are frequently characterized by marked intravascular volume contraction and hypovolemia. Injury caused by release of agents from the inflamed pancreas leads to exudation of fluid into the retroperitoneum. In addition, there is repeated vomiting and nasogastric aspiration of fluid. Overall, the lost fluid in pancreatitis usually has a plasmalike content of electrolytes and protein. Thus, although serum electrolyte concentrations may not change dramatically, a rise in hematocrit can be expected, and the magnitude of this rise may be useful in calculating fluid replacement needs. If vomiting and/or nasogastric fluid aspiration volumes are large, a hypochloremic alkalosis may result. On the other hand, poor tissue perfusion can favor development of a metabolic acidosis. Hypocalcemia and/or hypomagnesemia can occur either as a result of preexisting malnutrition, especially in alcoholics, or as a result of the pancreatitis itself. Usually, the hypocalcemia is merely a reflection of hypoalbuminemia, and ionized calcium levels remain normal. In severe cases of pancreatitis, however, the degree of hypocalcemia may be out of proportion to the hypoalbuminemia and reflect a decline in ionized calcium levels. Tetany and carpopedal spasm can be seen, and, when noted, aggressive calcium and magnesium replacement should be instituted.

During the early stages of pancreatitis, the heart rate, cardiac output, and cardiac index may rise and total peripheral resistance may decline. The degree of intrapulmonary shunting may rise and hypoxemia can develop. These changes are, most likely, caused by hypovolemia, atelectasis, and the release of vasoactive agents and cytokines from the inflamed pancreas.

Treatment of the early stages of a severe attack of acute pancreatitis requires meticulous management of fluid, electrolyte, and respiratory needs. Central filling pressures and volume needs can be monitored using a Swan-Ganz catheter. The hematocrit can be used to quantitate extracellular fluid losses. An indwelling arterial catheter, used to track arterial blood gasses and pH, may identify those individuals in need of endotracheal intubation and ventilatory support. Renal function can be monitored by placement of a urethral catheter. A fluid-balance flow sheet may be particularly useful in managing these complicated and seriously ill patients.

The role of peritoneal lavage in the management of patients with severe attacks of pancreatitis remains controversial. A number of uncontrolled or anecdotal reports suggested that lavage, by removing harmful agents released from the inflamed pancreas, might be beneficial. More recently, however, a randomized, multicenter study suggested that lavage does not alter the outcome of an attack.[27] The issue probably warrants further study because the randomized study used only short-term lavage, and the possibility that longer periods of lavage might be of benefit has not been adequately evaluated.[28] The potential value of prophylactic antibiotics in the treatment of severe pancreatitis is also controversial; some studies suggested a benefit,[29] whereas others concluded that antibiotics are not beneficial. Given these uncertainties, my practice is to not administer peritoneal lavage and to confine the use of prophylactic antibiotics to patients with gallstone pancreatitis.

Many additional therapies for pancreatitis have been proposed, but the benefit of most of them remains unproven.[21, 30] These include attempts to (1) reduce pancreatic function using atropine, somatostatin, glucagon, or calcitonin; (2) inhibit the activity of pancreatic digestive enzymes using aprotinin, chlorophyll-a, procainamide, or gabexate; and (3) inhibit inflammation and cytotoxicity using indomethacin

TABLE 109–4. Ranson's Criteria

On Admission
Age greater than 55 years
White blood cell count greater than 16,000/mm^3
Blood glucose level greater than 200 mg/dL
Lactate dehydrogenase level greater than 350 IU/L
Glutamic-oxaloacetic transaminase level greater than 250 SFU/dL

During Initial 48 Hours
Hematocrit decrease greater than 10%
Blood urea nitrogen rise greater than 5 mg/dL
Serum Ca^{2+} less than 8 mg/dL
PaO_2 less than 60 mm Hg
Base deficit greater than 4 mEq/L
Fluid sequestration greater than 6 L

Abbreviations: Ca^{2+} = calcium ion; PaO_2 = partial pressure of arterial oxygen.

or prostaglandins. Nasogastric decompression appears to improve patient comfort, but it does not alter the course or severity of pancreatitis. Antacids and histamine$_2$ receptor antagonists do not appear to alter the severity of an attack, but these agents may be of value in preventing stress ulcer bleeding.

TREATMENT OF BILIARY TRACT STONE DISEASE

Most patients with gallstone pancreatitis experience only a relatively mild attack that resolves as the offending stone is either passed into the duodenum or becomes disimpacted by moving more proximally in the biliary tree. These individuals need no immediate treatment for their biliary tract stones but should eventually have a ductal stone–clearance procedure with or without cholecystectomy to prevent repeated attacks of gallstone pancreatitis. The method of ductal stone clearance in the management of such patients could be either surgical (common duct exploration, sphincteroplasty, bilioenteric anastomosis) or endoscopic (sphincterotomy with stone extraction, lithotripsy, or stone dissolution) depending on the locally available expertise and/or individual preference. Currently, most patients are now managed endoscopically. Removal of the gallbladder can usually be accomplished laparoscopically. Some evidence suggests that cholecystectomy is not mandatory, especially in high-risk patients who have only a cholangitis/pancreatitis clinical picture and who lack symptoms of acute or chronic cholecystitis.[31] Most of these individuals, if treated for their ductal disease, will not require a later cholecystectomy.

Approximately 10% to 15% of patients with gallstone pancreatitis suffer from a severe attack. Acosta and coworkers[32] reported that the incidence of these severe attacks could be reduced by subjecting all patients with gallstone pancreatitis to early surgical duct clearance, but Kelly and Wagner[33] later reported that early surgical intervention in such patients resulted in an increased mortality rate. More recent attention has been directed to the role of early endoscopic approaches to duct clearance in such patients. Two reports[34, 35] indicated that early endoscopy with sphincterotomy and ductal clearance of stones for patients with severe gallstone pancreatitis is both safe and beneficial. It is not entirely clear whether the benefit of this approach results from the reduction in the ultimate severity of pancreatitis or, alternatively, from the relief of cholangitis. On the basis of currently available evidence, however, early endoscopic attempts at clearing the ductal stones seems to be the treatment of choice for individuals with severe gallstone pancreatitis.

TREATMENT OF THE SYSTEMIC COMPLICATIONS OF ACUTE PANCREATITIS

The systemic complications of acute pancreatitis, for the most part, occur during the early stages of an attack. They include renal failure, respiratory failure, cardiovascular collapse, disseminated intravascular coagulopathy, and gastrointestinal bleeding. During the early stages of an attack, severe hypovolemia may result from extensive fluid losses. Vasoactive agents and activated digestive enzymes may be released into the circulation, and, in a setting of hypovolemia, these agents can have profound effects on cardiac, pulmonary, and renal function. Treatment should be directed at supporting cardiac, pulmonary, and renal function while aggressively replacing fluid losses. Close monitoring of venous filling pressure, cardiac output, urinary output, blood oxygenation, and hematocrit is critical. Endotracheal intubation and/or hemodialysis may be required. Theoretically, peritoneal dialysis might allow for removal of toxic agents released from the inflamed pancreas, but the value of peritoneal lavage in this setting remains controversial. Plasmapheresis may be another method of achieving the same goal. The value of these modalities is currently under investigation at several centers.

Gastrointestinal bleeding during acute pancreatitis may occur by several mechanisms, including bleeding from stress-induced gastroduodenal ulcers. In addition, there may be erosion of the peripancreatic inflammatory process into major vessels and/or a hollow viscus. Depletion of coagulation factors as a result of disseminated intravascular coagulation can occur. Finally, portal hypertension caused by splenic and/or portal vein thrombosis can occur. The management of these complications of pancreatitis should be dictated by the nature of the lesion present but, for the most part, is similar to that used when bleeding is caused by these processes in the absence of pancreatitis.

TREATMENT OF THE LATE LOCAL COMPLICATIONS OF ACUTE PANCREATITIS

The local complications of acute pancreatitis can be separated into two groups based on the presence of abscess or infection.[36] Sterile complications include areas of pancreatic and peripancreatic necrosis, pancreatic pseudocysts, and pancreatic ascites. These lesions usually appear several days to weeks after the onset of an attack and can be identified using ultrasonography (Fig. 109–1) and CT (Fig. 109–2). The latter technique is especially useful when performed using dynamic contrast enhancement to identify areas of necrosis (Fig. 109–3). Paracentesis and/or thoracentesis for measurement of the amylase level in the removed fluid can identify patients with pancreatic ascites or pancreaticopleural fistulas, and ERCP in such patients can be used to localize the site of pancreatic duct disruption (Fig. 109–4).

Each of these sterile complications of pancreatitis can become secondarily infected, usually as a result of transmigration of organisms into the inflamed area from adjacent segments of the gastrointestinal tract. When infection is

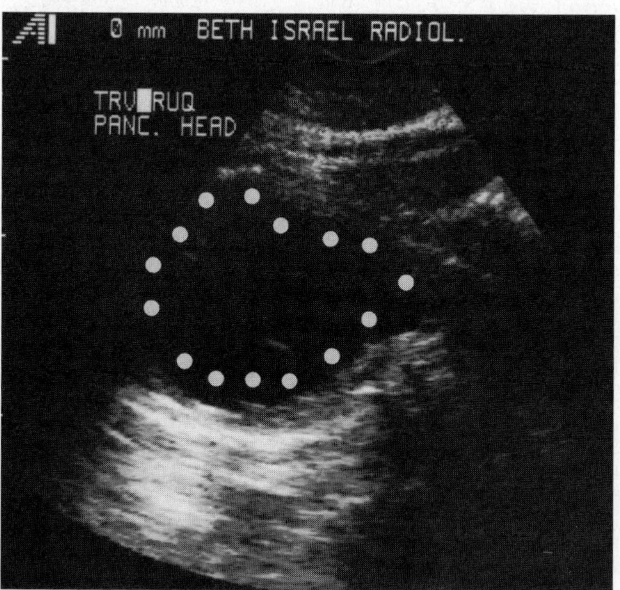

Figure 109–1. Ultrasound examination of pancreas reveals a pseudocyst (the nonechogenic area identified by the *white dots*).

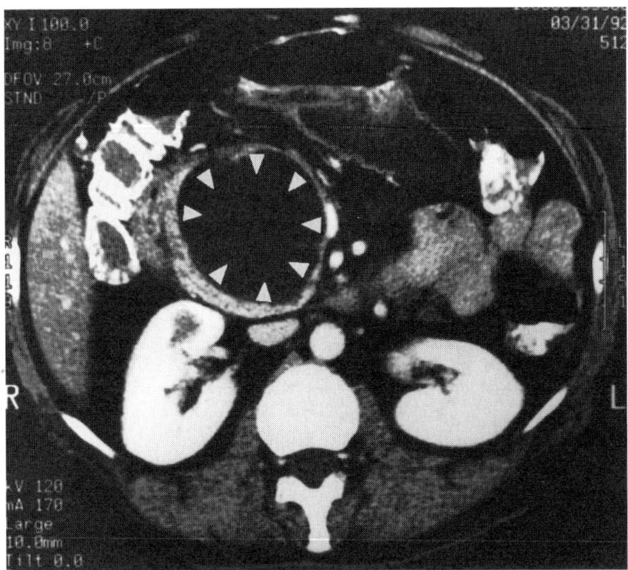

Figure 109–2. CT of pancreas reveals a pseudocyst (the low-density area outlined by *arrowheads*).

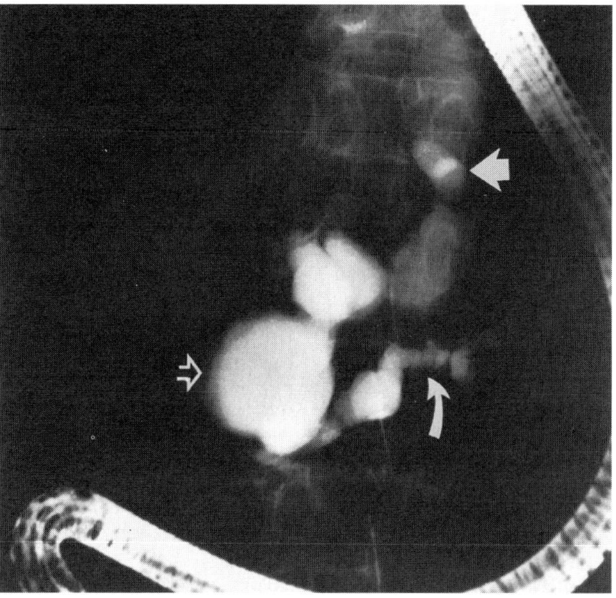

Figure 109–4. Pancreaticopleural fistula. Endoscopic retrograde cholangiopancreatography reveals a dialated pancreatic duct *(curved arrow)* filling a pseudocyst *(open arrow)* that communicates to the pleural space via a fistulous tract *(solid arrow)*.

present, the terms *infected pancreatic/peripancreatic necrosis* and *infected pseudocyst* are usually used. The latter lesion is also frequently referred to as a *pancreatic abscess*. When in doubt, the presence of infection can be documented using the technique of CT-guided fine-needle aspiration.[37]

At present, the treatment of these sterile complications of pancreatitis is the subject of considerable controversy. Most surgeons prefer to avoid operation for sterile pancreatic necrosis, although some, particularly the group in Ulm, Germany, have advocated necrosectomy in such cases and claimed that that procedure can lessen the overall morbidity and mortality of pancreatitis.[38] Until recently, it was generally believed that pancreatic pseudocysts greater than 6 cm in diameter and persisting longer than 6 weeks after an attack of pancreatitis should be treated by either internal or percutaneous drainage.[39] However, two reports indicated that asymptomatic pseudocysts, even if persistent and quite large, can be left untreated with little or no long-term morbidity.[40, 41] In contrast to these areas of controversy, there is general agreement regarding the treatment of pancreatic ascites and pancreaticopleural fistulas. These lesions result from major pancreatic duct disruptions. In general, initial attempts to treat these lesions should include nutritional support and reduction of pancreatic secretion by the use of parenteral nutrition and administration of somatostatin.[42–44] Pancreatic duct stents, placed endoscopically across the point of duct disruption, may reduce the fluid leak.[45] If these efforts fail, treatment should include either resection of the pancreas proximal (i.e., to the left) to the ductal injury or internal drainage using a Roux-en-Y anastomosis of a jejunal limb to the site of duct disruption.

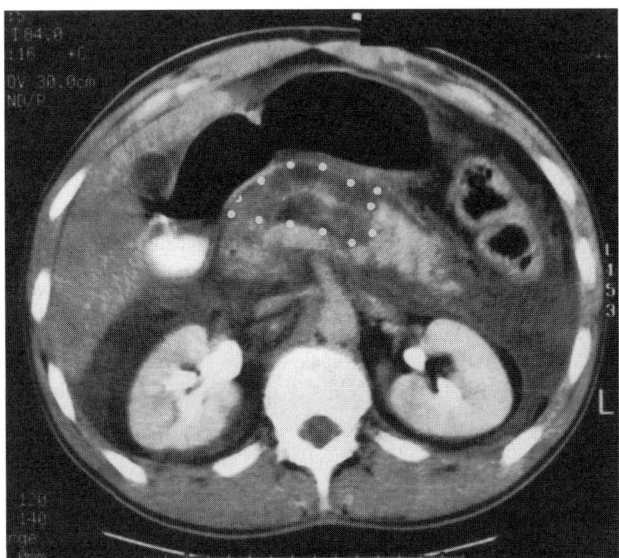

Figure 109–3. Necrosis of pancreas. Contrast-enhanced, dynamic CT reveals area of pancreatic underperfusion (outlined by the *white dots*) around a central core of remaining, perfused pancreatic tissue.

When areas of peripancreatic or pancreatic necrosis become infected, surgical intervention with debridement is almost always required.[46] The organisms recovered from such lesions include *Escherichia coli, Klebsiella, Proteus, Enterococcus, Pseudomonas,* and *Candida*.[47] Antibiotic therapy is never sufficient for treating such lesions. In addition, attempts to drain such areas nonoperatively usually fail because the infected material is puttylike and not amenable to drainage through catheters. Frequently, repeated operations for debridement are required.[46] In contrast to infected necrosis, infected pseudocysts (also referred to as pancreatic abscesses) can frequently be treated using percutaneously placed drainage catheters because, for the most part, the infected fluid in these lesions is liquid pus, which can pass through the drainage catheters. On occasion, however, surgical intervention for debridement, drainage, or resection may be required for the treatment of pancreatic abscesses also.

References

1. Steer ML: Etiology and pathophysiology of acute pancreatitis. *In*: The Exocrine Pancreas: Biology, Pathobiology, and Diseases. Go VLW, DiMagno EP, Gardner JD, et al (Eds). New York, Raven Press, 1993, pp 581–592.
2. Sarles H: Chronic pancreatitis: Etiology and pathophysiology. *In*: The Exocrine Pancreas: Biology, Pathobiology, and Diseases. Go VLW, Brooks F, DiMagno E, et al (Eds). New York, Raven Press, 1986, p 37.
3. Acosta JL, Ledesma CL: Gallstone migration as a cause for acute pancreatitis. N Engl J Med 1974; 290:484.
4. Acosta JL, Ross R, Ledesma CL: The usefulness of stool screening for diagnosing cholelithiasis in acute pancreatitis: A description of the technique. Am J Dig Dis 1977; 22:168.
5. Opie EL: The relationship of cholelithiasis to disease of the pancreas and fat necrosis. Am J Med Surg 1901; 12:27.
6. Menguy RB, Hallenbeck GA, Bollman JL, et al: Intraductal pressures and sphincteric resistance in canine pancreatic and biliary ducts after various stimuli. Surg Gynecol Obstet 1958; 106:306.
7. Robinson TM, Dunphy JE: Continuous perfusion of bile protease activators through the pancreas. JAMA 1963; 183:530.
8. McCutheon AD: Reflux of duodenal contents in the pathogenesis of pancreatitis. Gut 1964; 5:260–265.
9. Steer ML, Meldolesi J: The cell biology of experimental pancreatitis. N Engl J Med 1987; 316:144–150.
10. Steer ML: How and where does acute pancreatitis begin? Arch Surg 1992; 127:1350–1353.
11. Lerch MM, Saluja AK, Runzi M, et al: Pancreatic duct obstruction triggers acute necrotizing pancreatitis in the opossum. Gastroenterology 1993; 104:853–861.
12. Steer ML, Saluja AK: Experimental acute pancreatitis: Studies of the early events that lead to cell injury. *In*: The Exocrine Pancreas: Biology, Pathobiology, and Diseases. Go VLW, DiMagno EP, Gardner JR, et al (Eds). New York, Raven Press, 1993, pp 489–500.
13. Silen W: Cope's Early Diagnosis of the Acute Abdomen. 15th ed. New York, Oxford University Press, 1979.
14. Fredrickson DS, Lees RS: Familial hyperlipoproteinemia. *In*: The Metabolic Basis of Inherited Disease. 1st ed. Stanbury JB, Wyngaarden LB, Fredrickson DS (Eds). New York, McGraw-Hill, 1966, pp 429–485.
15. Cameron JL, Crisler C, Margolis S, et al: Acute pancreatitis with hyperlipemia. Surgery 1971; 70:53.
16. Leavitt MD, Edkfeldt JH: Diagnosis of acute pancreatitis. *In*: The Exocrine Pancreas: Biology, Pathobiology, and Disease. Go VLW, Brooks F, DiMagno E, et al (Eds). New York, Raven Press, 1986, p 481.
17. Salt WB, Schenker S: Amylase: Its clinical significance: A review of the literature. Medicine (Baltimore) 1976; 55:269–289.
18. Berk JE, Kizu H, Wilding P: A newly recognized cause for elevated serum amylase activity. J Engl J Med 1967; 277:941.
19. McKay AJ, Imrie CW, O'Neill J, et al: Is an early ultrasound scan of value in acute pancreatitis. Br J Surg 1982; 69:369–372.
20. Freeny PC: Incremental dynamic bolus computed tomography of acute pancreatitis. Int J Pancreatol 1993; 13:147–158.
21. Steer ML: Acute pancreatitis. *In*: Textbook of Gastroenterology. Yamada T, et al (Eds). Philadelphia, JB Lippincott, 1991, pp 1854–1874.
22. Malfertheiner P, Dominguez-Munoz JE: Prognostic factors in acute pancreatitis. Int J Pancreatol 1993; 14:1–8.
23. Ranson JHC, Rifkind KM, Roses DF, et al: Prognostic signs and the role of operative management in acute pancreatitis. Surg Gynecol Obstet 1974; 139:69–81.
24. Larvin M, McMahon MJ: Apache-2 score for assessment and monitoring of acute pancreatitis. Lancet 1989; 2:201–205.
25. Balthazar EJ, Robinson DL, Megibow AJ, et al: Acute pancreatitis: Value of CT in establishing prognosis. Radiology 1990; 174:331–336.
26. Thune A, Baker RA, Saccone GT, et al: Differing effects of pethidine and morphine on human sphincter of Oddi motility. Br J Surg 1990; 77:992–995.
27. Mayer AD, McMahon MJ, Corfield AP, et al: Controlled clinical trial of peritoneal lavage for the treatment of severe acute pancreatitis. N Engl J Med 1985; 312:399–404.
28. Ranson JH, Berman RS: Long peritoneal lavage decreases pancreatic sepsis in acute pancreatitis. Ann Surg 1990; 211:708–716.
29. Pederzole P, Bassi C, Vesentini S, et al: A randomized multicenter trial of antibiotic prophylaxis of septic complications in acute necrotizing pancreatitis with imipenem. Surg Gynecol Obstet 1993; 176:480–483.
30. Steer ML: Acute pancreatitis. *In*: Gastrointestinal Emergencies. Taylor MW, Gollan J, Peppercorn MA, et al (Eds). Baltimore, Williams & Wilkins, 1992, pp 171–179.
31. Davidson BR, Neoptolemos JP, Carr-Locke DL: Endoscopic sphincterotomy for common bile duct calculi in patients with gall bladder in situ considered unfit for surgery. Gut 1988; 29:114–120.
32. Acosta JM, Rossi R, Galli OMR, et al: Early surgery for acute gallstone pancreatitis: Evaluation of a systematic approach. Surgery 1978; 83:367.
33. Kelly TR, Wagner DS: Gallstone pancreatitis: A prospective randomized trial of the timing of surgery. Surgery 1988; 104:600.
34. Neoptolemos JP, Carr-Locke DL, London NJ, et al: Controlled trial of urgent endoscopic retrograde cholangiopancreatography and endoscopic sphincterotomy versus conservative treatment for acute pancreatitis due to gallstones. Lancet 1988; 2:979.
35. Fan ST, Lai ECS, Mok FPT, et al: Early treatment of acute biliary pancreatitis by endoscopic papillotomy. N Engl J Med 1993; 328:228–232.
36. Bradley EL: A clinically based classification system for acute pancreatitis. Arch Surg 1993; 128:586–590.
37. Gerzoff SG, Banks PA, Robbins AH, et al: Early diagnosis of pancreatic infection by computed tomography-guided aspiration. Gastroenterology 1987; 93:1315.
38. Beger HG, Krautzberger W, Bittner R, et al: Results of surgical treatment of necrotizing pancreatitis. World J Surg 1985; 9:972–979.
39. Bradley EL, Clements JL, Gonzales AC: The natural history of pancreatic pseudocysts: A unified coincept of management. Am J Surg 1979; 137:135.
40. Yeo CJ, Bastidas JA, Lynch-Nyhan A, et al: The natural history of pancreatic pseudocysts documented by computed tomography. Surg Gynecol Obstet 1990; 170:411–417.
41. Vitas GJ, Sarr MG: Selected management of pancreatic pseudocysts: Operative versus expectant management. Surgery 1992; 111:123–130.
42. Sankaren S, Walt AJ: Pancreatic ascites: Recognition and management. Arch Surg 1976; 111:430.
43. Cameron JL, Kieffer RS, Anderson WJ, et al: Internal pancreatic fistulas: Pancreatic ascites and pleural effusions. Ann Surg 1976; 184:587.
44. Gislason H, Growbech JE, Soreide O: Pancreatic ascites: Treatment by continuous somatostatin infusion. Am J Gastroenterol 1991; 86:519–521.
45. Kozarek RA, Ball TH, Paterson DJ, et al: Endoscopic transpapillary therapy for disrupted pancreatic duct and peripancreatic fluid collections. Gastroenterology 1991; 100:1362–1370.
46. Bradley EL: A fifteen year experience with open drainage for infected pancreatic necrosis. Surg Gynecol Obstet 1993; 177:215–222.
47. Ranson JHC: Complications of pancreatitis. *In*: Gastrointestinal Emergencies. Taylor MW, Gollan J, Peppercorn MA, et al (Eds). Baltimore, Williams & Wilkins, 1992, pp 180–192.

CHAPTER 110

Severe Liver Disease

Mary McDonald, MD • David D. Ralph, MD
Robert L. Carithers, Jr., MD

The care of patients with liver disease is difficult because of the multitude of possible complications suffered by these patients, the limited forms of therapy available, and the high rate of recurrent complications if the underlying hepatic function does not improve. The development of hepatic transplantation has, however, dramatically changed the prognosis for patients with severe liver disease. In addition, it has provided new challenges for the critical care physician, namely, patient management before and after transplantation. Because some forms of therapy that may be useful in patients who are not candidates for transplantation such as portocaval shunt procedures are contraindicated in patients being considered for transplantation, it has become important to determine promptly whether patients are appropriate candidates for transplantation and to tailor the therapy based on such eligibility.

Three conditions account for most intensive care unit (ICU) admissions of patients with liver disease: decompensated cirrhosis, fulminant hepatitis, and liver transplantation. The specific complications of each are described to illustrate the important principles of critical care for patients with severe liver disease.

CIRRHOSIS

Cirrhosis is the end-stage of all severe chronic liver diseases. The most common causes of cirrhosis include alcoholic liver disease, chronic autoimmune hepatitis, chronic hepatitis caused by either hepatitis B or hepatitis C virus infections, metabolic disorders such as Wilson's disease, alpha$_1$-antitrypsin deficiency, and idiopathic hemochromatosis, hepatotoxic drugs such as methydopa (Aldomet) and isoniazid, biliary disorders such as primary biliary cirrhosis and sclerosing cholangitis, and vascular disorders including longstanding chronic heart failure and hepatic vein occlusion. A variety of complications, many of which require optimal care for survival, may occur because of the various profound physiologic alterations that can occur in patients with cirrhosis.

Physiologic Changes in Cirrhosis

Physiologic alterations in hemodynamics, renal function, blood gases, acid-base status, coagulation, and drug metabolism are seen in patients with cirrhosis. Some of these alterations are similar to those seen with other causes of multiple organ system failure (MOSF), but several are different from those seen in other critically ill patients.

Hemodynamic Alterations

Blood volume is increased in patients with cirrhosis; nevertheless, effective circulating volume often seems to be decreased. Patients with severe liver disease typically have a hyperdynamic circulatory state. Cardiac output is increased and systemic vascular resistance (SVR) is decreased. Typical mean values for cardiac index (CI) range from 4.5 to 5.25 L/min · m^2. SVR is decreased by a third to 800 to 900 dyne · s/cm^5 · m^2. Some patients will have an SVR as low as 400 dyne · s/cm^5 · m^2.[1] The relationship between CI and SVR is well documented, but it is not clear which occurs first. Systemic blood pressure (BP) often is mildly reduced, although the degree of reduction is small and variable. Despite the increase in blood volume, pulmonary artery wedge pressures are usually normal (4–6 mm Hg). Pulmonary artery pressures are usually normal (mean PAP = 12 mm Hg). Significant elevations of pulmonary pressures have been demonstrated by heart catheterization in 2% of patients with portal hypertension.[2] Such pulmonary hypertension seems to be related to the duration of portal hypertension and portends a poor survival rate.[3]

Renal Function

Avid renal sodium retention is the rule in patients with decompensated cirrhosis. A state of hyper-responsiveness to mineralocorticoid effect may be present. Sodium retention, hypokalemia from poor nutrition, and reduced bicarbonate excretion often lead to metabolic alkalosis. Potassium and chloride replacement as well as restoration of an effective circulating volume is required to correct the acid-base balance.

Blood Gases

Mild hyperventilation is usually present in clinically significant cirrhosis. Respiratory rate and tidal volume are increased and partial pressure of arterial carbon dioxide ($Pa{CO_2}$) is reduced to the range of 30 to 35 mm Hg. Although respiratory alkalosis worsens with increasing degrees of hepatic encephalopathy, it can be found at all levels of consciousness. The cause of respiratory alkalosis is uncertain; it is not explained by the concomitant mild degree of hypoxemia and probably reflects instead respiratory stimulation from altered chemoreceptor function as a result of the disordered metabolism of liver failure.

Mild arterial blood gas abnormalities are very common in patients with cirrhosis. Mild hypoxemia (partial pressure of arterial oxygen [$Pa{O_2}$] of 65 to 85 mm Hg) and increased alveolar-arterial oxygen differences (20–30 mm Hg) are almost universal. A minority of patients will have severe hypoxemia ($Pa{O_2}$ = 30–65 mm Hg) in spite of clear chest radiographs.[4] Several mechanisms for hypoxemia have been documented. The distribution of ventilation is disturbed in cirrhotic patients. Basal lung units close prematurely; in some cases, closing capacity exceeds functional residual capacity, indicating gas trapping even during resting ventiiation. Although ascites and elevated diaphragms may contribute to these abnormalities,[5] even patients without clinical ascites often have elevated closing capacities. Hypoxemia is worsened in these poorly ventilated units because there may also be inadequate hypoxic pulmonary vasoconstriction caused by circulating vasoactive substances. A variety of intrapulmonary vascular dilatations have been demonstrated in cirrhotic patients, including intrapulmonary, portopulmonary, and pleural arteriovenous connections.[6] These shunts are more common in patients with severe hypoxemia and may be demonstrated by contrast echocardiography[7] with delayed detection of bubbles in the left atrium or by transpulmonary transit of injected labeled macroaggregated albumin. Finally, some studies suggest that a diffusion limitation for oxygen transfer can result from the high pulmonary blood flow through vascular dilatations.[8] Multiple inert gas studies show that individual patients have varying combinations of low ventilation-perfusion regions and of physiologic shunt.[9] Fortunately, the elevated cardiac output and ventilation that usually accompany liver failure also blunt the degree of hypoxemia caused by the ventilation-perfusion mismatching in these patients.[4]

Several points relative to the hypoxemia of liver disease are clinically important. First, the degree of hypoxemia and shunting is poorly related to the results of liver function tests, the presence of ascites, enlargement of the spleen, portal or pulmonary hypertension, or specific type of liver disease but may be associated with the presence of vascular spider angiomata.[9] Second, 50% of nonsmokers and 70% of smokers with cirrhosis have reduced diffusing capacities, and 25% have reduced lung volumes;[10] however, most of these patients have no evidence of fibrosis on biopsy or autopsy and so should not be rejected as transplantation candidates. Third, in some patients hypoxemia worsens (15–25 mm Hg) in the upright position, a condition known as orthodeoxia. These patients may also have dyspnea when sitting or standing (platypnea). Finally, bilirubin accumulation in the skin can cause erroneous values for oxygen saturation measured by ear oximetry; measured oxyhemoglobin saturations are 5% to 15% lower than values determined by direct arterial blood gas measurements.

Drug Metabolism

The metabolism of a number of drugs commonly used in the ICU is altered in patients with cirrhosis. Drug metabolism may be altered by decreased drug delivery to the liver because of decreased hepatic blood flow, by decreased hepatic metabolic capacity caused by hepatocyte destruction, or by changes in volume of distribution of individual drugs. Affected drugs include bronchodilators, antibiotics, corticosteroids, and histamine blockers.

Theophylline is metabolized in the liver via hydroxylation and demethylation. Although cholestasis and compensated cirrhosis have little effect on the metabolism of theophylline, passive congestion and decompensated cirrhosis have major effects on its clearance. Serum albumin levels have been suggested as a good indicator of impaired theophylline clearance; however, the correlation is not sufficiently precise to obviate the need for frequent determinations of serum theophylline levels.

Two frequently used analgesics, morphine and meperidine, are eliminated by the liver. The elimination rate of morphine is normal in patients with stable cirrhosis. Although morphine intolerance is sometimes identified, it is probably due to increased cerebral sensitivity rather than altered hepatic metabolism of the drug. In contrast, meperidine metabolism is decreased in cirrhotic patients. If the drug is used, smaller doses and longer intervals between doses are necessary to prevent accumulation of toxic levels of its metabolites.

Complications of Cirrhosis

Gastrointestinal (GI) hemorrhage, hepatic encephalopathy, ascites, renal failure, and life-threatening infections are major complications for which ICU admission is required in cirrhotic patients.

Gastrointestinal Hemorrhage

GI hemorrhage is the most dramatic complication encountered in patients with cirrhosis. Exsanguination, aspiration pneumonia, adult respiratory distress syndrome (ARDS), acute renal failure, myocardial ischemia, and other potentially fatal complications can develop. In addition, bleeding can precipitate hepatic encephalopathy and coma, which, although rarely fatal, complicate the clinical care of the patient. Timely and adroit management of any episode of GI hemorrhage is essential if these complications are to be avoided.

GI bleeding from any cause should be diagnosed and treated systematically. Rapid assessment of hemodynamic stability (pulse, BP, and orthostatic changes) and hematocrit determination guide the need for intravascular volume expansion through large-bore peripheral or central catheters. Blood volume must be maintained to ensure adequate circulation and oxygen delivery to the liver and other vital organs. Any existing coagulopathy should be partially corrected with fresh-frozen plasma, and severe thrombocytopenia should be corrected with platelet infusions. Desmopressin acetate (DDAVP) may improve platelet function altered by the liver disease or concomitant uremia.[11]

Early intubation of the airway should be considered because aspiration and pneumonia are common and often fatal pulmonary complications of upper GI bleeding. When bleeding is brisk, upper airway reflexes may be overwhelmed by the large volume of blood. In addition, premedication of patients for endoscopy may result in respiratory depression and may precipitate encephalopathy in patients with marginal hepatic function, further reducing the efficiency of normal airway defenses.

In the rapid-sequence intubation technique, the patient is given high concentrations of supplemental oxygen and then an analgesic, sedative, and muscle relaxant in rapid sequence. Compression of the esophagus with pressure on the cricoid cartilage (Sellick's maneuver) is used to prevent aspiration until intubation is accomplished under direct visualization. Failure to intubate on the first attempt is the major risk with this technique. Cirrhotic patients can experience hypotension and prolonged effects from the administered drugs. Atracurium is a good choice as a paralytic agent for intubation or other procedures because it undergoes spontaneous degradation with a short half-life and is not dependent on liver or kidney function for its elimination. Etomidate, a barbiturate sedative, has a short action duration and low frequency of cardiac depression. In contrast, thiopental can cause a sudden drop in BP. Morphine has a normal half-life in patients with cirrhosis; nevertheless, it can cause hypotension through venodilation and histamine release. Fentanyl has a more rapid onset and shorter duration of action and causes less hypotension.

Hemorrhage from duodenal or gastric ulcers, Mallory-Weiss tears, portal gastropathy, and esophageal varices is common in patients with cirrhosis. Because upper GI bleeding often is from a source other than varices and because the management of variceal bleeding differs so dramatically from that used for other causes of hemorrhage, early identification of the bleeding site by endoscopy is essential.

Ulcers

Peptic ulcer disease is the cause in 40% to 50% of patients with upper GI bleeding. Urgent flexible fiberoptic upper endoscopy within 12 hours of hospitalization yields a greater chance of identifying the bleeding lesion. Early endoscopy also can help identify predictors of persistent or recurrent bleeding in patients with ulcer disease.

Medical treatment should be used alone only for uncomplicated ulcer bleeding.[12] Approved drugs for the acute treatment of duodenal ulcer include histamine$_2$ (H_2) blockers, sucralfate, and antacids. When used appropriately, their ability to heal ulcers is comparable. The newest agents for the treatment of acid-peptic disorders are the proton-pump inhibitors. These drugs suppress gastric acid secretion by noncompetitively and irreversibly inhibiting acid secretion. Omeprazole is the first drug available in this class and seems to be more effective than prior agents in the rate of ulcer healing.[12] Currently, omeprazole is approved for short-term use in the treatment of erosive esophagitis, resistant gastroesophageal reflux disease, Zollinger-Ellison syndrome, and resistant peptic ulcer disease.

Patients with active bleeding as evidenced by pulsatile arterial bleeding and those with a visible vessel or clot in the ulcer base are at risk for ongoing bleeding or significant rebleeding.[13] These patients should be considered for endoscopic hemostatic therapy. Multipolar electrocoagulation and heater probes are comparable in their efficacy in treating bleeding ulcers. The yttrium-aluminum-garnet laser is similarly effective but expensive, and the greater technical expertise required makes it a secondary choice of treatment. Injection therapy with agents such as epinephrine and absolute alcohol is comparable in efficacy to thermal methods.[14] If these endoscopic hemostatic methods are unsuccessful in stemming hemorrhage from a peptic ulcer, surgical intervention is required.[15]

Mallory-Weiss Tear

A Mallory-Weiss tear is a nonpenetrating mucosal laceration in the distal esophagus or proximal stomach. These lacerations have been noted after sudden increases in intra-abdominal pressure and have been seen with increased frequency in patients with portal hypertension.[16] Most Mallory-Weiss tears stop bleeding spontaneously. Endoscopic hemostasis can be achieved with either injection treatment or multipolar electrocautery. If bleeding cannot be controlled endoscopically, surgery is necessary.

Portal Hypertensive Gastropathy

Portal hypertensive gastropathy is a well-recognized complication of cirrhosis. Severe gastropathy is associated with increased portal venous pressure and impaired metabolic activity of the liver, both of which have important therapeutic implications.[17] Bleeding occurs in a significant proportion of patients with severe portal hypertensive gastropathy. The severity of portal hypertensive gastropathy correlates with the severity of the liver disease.[18] Propranolol can significantly reduce bleeding by altering local gastric hemodynamics in addition to reducing portal pressure.[19] Suggested doses to achieve control of bleeding are 80 to 160 mg, with long-term treatment to prevent rebleeding. Surgical portal-systemic shunts can be used to arrest bleeding in severe portal hypertensive gastropathy. Little information is available on transjugular intrahepatic portolsystemic shunts (TIPS) in controlling bleeding from portal hypertensive gastropathy, but theoretically this technique should be effective.

Esophageal Varices

One of the most challenging complications of end-stage liver disease is variceal hemorrhage. The mortality associated with variceal bleeding averages 50% in the United States. A number of splanchnic vasoconstrictors reduce portal blood flow and portal pressure. The most commonly used are β-blockers, vasopressin, and somatostatin.

Propranolol, a nonselective β-blocker, is effective for prophylaxis of variceal bleeding.[20] By using a dose that reduces the resting heart rate by 25%, patients also have a reduced rebleeding rate.[21] However, there is no role for the use of β-blockers in acute variceal hemorrhage.

Vasopressin produces an increase in mesenteric vascular resistance and a reciprocal fall in portal venous flow and pressure.[22] Unfortunately, it also increases peripheral vascular resistance and arterial pressure and reduces cardiac output. As a consequence, cardiovascular side effects such as transient ischemia, myocardial infarction, and cardiac arrhythmias are often seen. The addition of nitroglycerin not only reduces portal pressure further than vasopressin alone but also significantly reduces systemic complications.[23]

Somatostatin has been used to treat variceal hemorrhage because of its ability to decrease splanchnic blood flow. In cirrhotic patients, there are varying effects on hepatic blood flow, wedged hepatic venous pressure, and intravariceal pressure.[24, 25] Equally varying results have been observed in clinical trials of acute variceal hemorrhage.[26]

BALLOON TAMPONADE. Balloon tamponade has been used for emergency treatment of bleeding esophageal varices since the 1950s. Three types of balloons are available. The Linton device has a single gastric balloon with both gastric and esophageal aspiration ports. The Sengstaken-Blakemore tube has both gastric and esophageal balloons but only a single gastric aspiration lumen. The Minnesota balloon has gastric and esophageal balloons, with both a gastric and an esophageal lumen, which allows suctioning of the esophagus above the esophageal balloon, theoretically lowering the possibility of aspiration.[27]

Airway protection with an endotracheal tube is recommended to prevent aspiration and to provide airway control. The major acute complication of balloon placement is esophageal perforation. Accordingly, these balloons should be placed only by experienced physicians. The gastric balloon should be partially inflated and checked for position with a radiograph before full inflation and traction tamponade. Traction on the inflated gastric balloon often stops variceal hemorrhage; inflation of the esophageal balloon is infrequently required. If inflated, the pressure in the esophageal balloon should be carefully determined to reduce the risk of mucosal necrosis. Gastric balloon tamponade can be continued safely for 48 to 72 hours; however, esophageal tamponade should not be used for more than 24 hours because of esophageal susceptibility to pressure necrosis.[27] The effectiveness of balloon tamponade in arresting acute bleeding varies from 44% to 92%.[28] Complications include pulmonary aspiration, mucosal pressure necrosis, and esophageal rupture.

ENDOSCOPIC SCLEROTHERAPY. Endoscopic sclerotherapy is effective in controlling acute variceal bleeding in 75% to 90% of patients and is more effective than pharmacologic agents alone.[29] Although sclerotherapy has not been shown to be more effective than balloon tamponade in arresting acute variceal bleeding,[30] it is certainly equally as effective.

Serious complications are seen in 10% to 30% of patients after sclerotherapy; the procedure has a 0.5% to 2% mortality.[31] Minor complications include fever, retrosternal chest pain, and transient dysphagia. Major complications include deep esophageal ulcerations with bleeding, mediastinitis, pleural effusions, esophageal strictures, bronchoesophageal fistulas, ARDS, pneumothorax, and portal venous thrombosis. Because of the risk of postoperative bleeding from esophageal ulcerations, most surgeons are opposed to sclerotherapy immediately before liver transplantation. Bacteremia has been demonstrated after the procedure, but the incidence is too low to warrant the routine use of prophylactic antibiotics.

ENDOSCOPIC VARICEAL BAND LIGATION. Variceal ligation is performed using a modified endoscope equipped with a preloaded elastic rubber band. The endoscope is repeatedly passed through an overtube into the esophagus. Suction is used to draw the variceal mucosa into the cylinder affixed to the endoscope tip; a trip wire is used to release a rubber band around the base of the suctioned varix. The variceal tissue eventually sloughs, leaving a superficial ulcer in the esophagus. Variceal ligation compares favorably with sclerotherapy for treatment of bleeding esophageal varices. Control of active bleeding is equally effective; however, there are fewer complications and treatment sessions required for eradication using band ligation. Furthermore, patients treated with band ligation have a better survival compared with patients treated with sclerotherapy.[32]

TRANSJUGULAR INTRAHEPATIC PORTOSYSTEMIC SHUNT. The TIPS procedure provides a nonoperative approach to variceal bleeding. Portal decompression is achieved via a percutaneous route by creating a communication between the hepatic and portal veins. A transjugular approach is used to manipulate a guide wire through the superior vena cava, right atrium, and inferior vena cava into the middle or right hepatic vein using fluoroscopic guidance.[33] A needle is used to advance the guiding sheath through the liver parenchyma into the right portal vein. Using a guide wire, an angioplasty balloon is used to dilate the tract between the hepatic and portal veins, allowing placement of a self-expanding metallic stent.[34]

Percutaneous shunt placement requires considerable technical expertise. In experienced hands, the procedure can be performed in 2 to 3 hours. An appealing advantage of the procedure is that it does not require general anesthesia. Complications include capsular perforation, intra-abdominal bleeding, stent migration, stent occlusion, hematobilia arteriovenous, fistulas, and hepatic encephalopathy.[35, 36] The long-term benefits of TIPS remain to be demonstrated. Currently, it is a practical option for patients who have failed standard techniques to stem variceal hemorrhage and for patients with bleeding gastric varices. It also provides an effective bridge to orthotopic liver transplantation.

SURGERY. When used for the emergent control of variceal hemorrhage, portosystemic shunts are associated with high morbidity and mortality.[37] Although effective in controlling variceal hemorrhage, operative mortality for emergency shunts is 46% versus 9% for elective procedures.[38] Although some surgeons advocate earlier consideration of emergency surgical shunting, portocaval shunts are being used less and less frequently because of the increased risk of subsequent liver transplantation.[38, 39]

Hepatic Encephalopathy

Hepatic encephalopathy is a diffuse disturbance in cerebral function that commonly complicates the clinical management of patients with cirrhosis. Alterations in cerebral function range from subtle disturbances in thought processes to deep coma. Although the pathogenesis of the condition remains controversial, effective treatment is available.

Pathogenesis

The encephalopathy associated with severe liver disease is believed to be caused by inadequate hepatic degradation of metabolic toxins that, when present in sufficient concentrations, interfere with the cellular function of the brain. Impaired degradation of these toxins presumably occurs because either the mass of functioning hepatocytes is too small or uptake of toxins into hepatocytes is compromised by shunting of blood around or through the liver.

Potential toxins include ammonia, methionine, and fatty acids. Reversible hepatic encephalopathy can be produced experimentally by administration of either ammonium salts or ammonium cation resins. Oral administration of either methionine or fatty acids also causes reversible encephalopathy in patients with cirrhosis. If antibiotics are given before administration, no alteration in mental status is seen, suggesting that metabolites produced by intestinal bacteria, rather than the parent compounds, are responsible for the encephalopathy. There also is evidence for a synergistic action between mercaptans and ammonia and between fatty acids and ammonia. Although the pathogenesis of hepatic encephalopathy is clearly more complex than simple accumulation of ammonia, therapeutic maneuvers that decrease ammonia levels within the body are effective in preventing and treating the disorder.

Ammonia is a key intermediate in the excretion of nitrogenous residues from the body. Major sites of ammonia production are the intestine and the kidney. Within the intestine, nitrogenous substances, including blood and dietary protein, are the major substrates for ammonia production. It is estimated that 4 g of ammonia are absorbed daily into the portal vein under normal physiologic conditions. Ammonia produced in the renal tubular cell by deamidization of glutamine can combine with excess hydrogen ions to form ammonium ions and facilitate urinary hydrogen ion excretion or may be released into the renal vein. When carbonic anhydrase inhibitors such as acetazolamide (Diamox) are used, ammonia concentration in the renal veins increases, adding an additional source of ammonia to the blood.

The liver contains unique urea cycle enzymes that convert ammonia into urea. These enzymes are reduced significantly in patients with cirrhosis and portal hypertension. Reduced capacity for urea synthesis in addition to shunting of portal blood around and through the liver combine to diminish urea production and cause systemic accumulation of ammonia.

The brain normally removes small amounts of ammonia from the blood; however, when blood ammonia levels rise, the brain rapidly responds by removing larger amounts. The concentration of ammonia is always higher in the brain than in the blood. Because the brain is devoid of a urea cycle, ammonia is converted exclusively to glutamine.[40] When brain levels of ammonia rise, glutamine increases and α-ketoglutarate decreases. Rapid accumulation of glutamine can result in osmotic attraction of water, cell swelling, and cerebral edema.[41] Cerebrospinal fluid (CSF) glutamine concentrations correlate better than any other biochemical parameter with the severity of neurologic impairment in patients with hepatic encephalopathy.[42] It also has been postulated that depression in α-ketoglutarate, a key intermediate in Krebs' cycle, impairs cerebral oxidative metabolism. Another proposed mechanism for depressed cortical function in patients with hepatic encephalopathy is accumulation of "false neurotransmitters" as a result of absorption of biogenic amines from the gut. Much recent interest has centered on excessive activity of central nervous system gamma-aminobutyric acid (GABA) receptors (the receptors for benzodiazepines and other sedatives) in states of high brain ammonia concentration. Increased levels of substances that bind to benzodiazepine receptors have been seen in patients with hepatic encephalopathy.[43] However, more evidence is needed before the importance of GABA receptors in the pathogenesis of hepatic encephalopathy can be determined.

Diagnostic Evaluation

The diagnosis of hepatic encephalopathy is based on a constellation of clinical features and supportive laboratory studies. Many patients with cirrhosis have subtle brain dysfunction, which may be difficult to detect clinically. A close family member often is the best source for identifying these early changes. In addition, a variety of simple bedside tests including the digit-symbol, Reitan trail-making block design, and Purdue peg board tests are effective in detecting subclinical encephalopathy.[44]

Once hepatic encephalopathy is diagnosed, it is useful to grade the degree of impairment on a clinical scale. The most widely used grading system separates patients into four stages of encephalopathy based on alterations in mentation, reflexes, and the electroencephalogram (EEG).

STAGE I ENCEPHALOPATHY. This is characterized by subtle alterations in thought processes and personality. Patients may note difficulty in performing calculations, may become sloppy in their personal habits, and may have difficulty writing legibly. However, they may be able to conceal the condition from family and physicians for some time. Asterixis is not seen at this stage of encephalopathy, and the EEG usually shows only subtle, if any, alterations. A rigorous mental status examination may be necessary to detect any abnormalities. Often, however, the patient will have difficulty constructing simple figures and may be unable to connect a series of numbers; one of the most helpful clinical exercises for detection of this stage of encephalopathy is the number connection test. An elevated arterial ammonia level may be a clue to the presence of encephalopathy, although a normal value does not exclude the diagnosis.[45]

STAGE II ENCEPHALOPATHY. This stage is associated with overt alterations in cerebral function characterized by confusion, abnormal sleep patterns, inappropriate behavior, loss of attention span, and drowsiness. Asterixis is present and the reflexes are brisk; clonus can usually be elicited, and extensor plantar reflexes are often present. The EEG is usually abnormal with obvious slowing and appearance of theta waves.

STAGE III ENCEPHALOPATHY. This stage is marked by accentuated disturbance in thought processes. The patient usually is quite confused, has a short attention span, sleeps most of the time, and cannot perform fine motor movements such as writing; however, the patient does respond to noxious stimuli. If the patient can cooperate, asterixis can be elicited without difficulty. In those who cannot cooperate with dorsiflexion of the hands, asterixis can be demonstrated by having the patient squeeze the physician's hand or a blood pressure cuff and finding rhythmic contraction and relaxation of the grip. The EEG is usually grossly abnormal with triphasic waves.

STAGE IV ENCEPHALOPATHY. These patients are comatose. As the degree of coma deepens, they become less responsive to noxious stimuli. Decerebrate movements of the extremities often are seen, but oculocephalic reflexes remain intact until the deepest stages of coma are reached. Deep-tendon reflexes are depressed rather than exaggerated. The EEG shows bilateral slowing with replacement of the triphasic waves by delta waves.

Any patient suspected of having hepatic encephalopathy should receive a complete neurologic evaluation. It is particularly important to rule out subdural hematomas if there is any history of head trauma. Lumbar puncture should be performed with caution if there is a coagulopathy or if there is any question of increased intracranial pressure (ICP).

No laboratory tests are sensitive or specific for hepatic encephalopathy. The ammonia level is elevated in most, but not all, patients and may be useful in observing the course of an individual patient. If ordered, a fasting arterial sample should be obtained, placed on ice, and tested by a laboratory experienced in its measurement. CSF glutamine levels are elevated in most patients with hepatic encephalopathy. The EEG is helpful in staging the degree of encephalopathy; however, the changes seen are not specific for hepatic encephalopathy.

Treatment

The major goal of therapy is to decrease further accumulation of ammonia and other toxins in the circulation and brain by reversing any precipitating factors. It is important to search for factors such as the use of sedatives or narcotics, increased ammonia absorption from the intestine resulting from dietary indiscretion, GI bleeding or constipation, uremia, acid-base disturbances, and infections. All sedatives and narcotics should be discontinued and infections treated. GI bleeding must be stopped, and the gut should be cleansed with purgatives. Good renal function should be maintained to prevent urea accumulation, and acid-base balance should be normalized to prevent exaggerated movements of ammonia and other toxins into the brain.

Acid-base balance has a profound effect on the movement of ammonia into and out of cells. Both gaseous nonionized ammonia and ammonium ions are normally found in the blood and tissues. Gaseous ammonia freely diffuses across lipid membranes. In contrast, these membranes are impermeable to the ionized ammonium ion. If there is a pH gradient across a membrane, ammonium ions will accumulate on the side with the higher hydrogen ion concentration as they are trapped by ionization. As a consequence, there is always a movement of ammonia from areas of relative alkalinity to those of relative acidity. For example, the normal pH in brain is 6.95 versus blood pH of 7.40; this promotes the movement of ammonia into the brain. Systemic alkalosis enhances ammonia accumulation in the brain by increasing the pH gradient across the blood-brain barrier.

The amount of ammonia and other toxins absorbed from the gut can be decreased by lactulose, a nondigestible disaccharide that is metabolized by the intestinal flora into a variety of small organic acids. Acidification of the colon results in catharsis, diminished bacterial production of ammonia, and trapping of ammonia within the gut because of lowered colonic pH.[46] Oral neomycin also is effective in diminishing ammonia absorption from the intestine by interfering with the conversion of urea to ammonia by colonic bacteria.[47] Vancomycin and metronidazole can be used in resistant cases, although the latter should be used with caution because it is metabolized by the liver.[48]

Although a great deal has been written on the use of branched-chain amino acids, there is no good evidence that they reduce hepatic encephalopathy or affect mortality.[49] Flumazenil treatment has resulted in dramatic improvement in mental status in some patients; however, until a well-controlled clinical trial is conducted to test its safety and efficacy, it cannot be considered appropriate treatment for patients with hepatic encephalopathy.[50]

Ascites

Ascites is a serious complication in patients with cirrhosis. Early satiety makes it difficult for patients with ascites to maintain adequate nutrition. Massive ascites also may impair respiratory function by elevating the diaphragm and causing both basilar lung atelectasis and less effective diaphragmatic contraction. Umbilical hernias, which may potentially rupture, can develop. Finally, the presence of ascitic fluid continuously exposes the patient to the possibility of peritonitis.

The treatment of ascites has undergone radical revision over the past few years. Cautious diuresis has been replaced by vigorous paracentesis. The remarkable safety and efficacy of large-volume paracentesis also have led to a reexamination of the pathogenesis of ascites.

Pathogenesis

The mechanisms of ascites formation are complex and controversial; however, it is generally agreed that three areas are important: local factors, the systemic hemodynamic milieu, and renal response to the altered hemodynamic state.

Ascites presumably develops as a result of perturbation of Starling forces throughout the hepatic sinusoids and splanchnic capillary bed. The hepatic sinusoids have a discontinuous membrane that permits free egress of plasma proteins. As a consequence, there is minimal oncotic pressure to oppose any increase in hydrostatic pressure within this large vascular bed. Occlusion of the inferior vena cava above the liver results in a massive outpouring of lymph into the abdominal cavity. When the capacity of the thoracic duct to drain the abdomen is overwhelmed, ascites develops.

Significant ascites would not accumulate were it not for avid renal retention of sodium; however, the factors that initiate this process remain highly controversial. The classic "underfill" theory presumes that ascites formation causes a progressive depletion of intravascular volume and that sodium is retained by the kidney as a normal compensatory mechanism. Saline, mannitol, albumin infusions, and head-out water immersion each result in a brisk diuresis in patients with cirrhosis and ascites, providing support for this theory.

However, most investigators have found increased, rather than decreased, plasma volume in patients with cirrhosis and ascites. In dogs with chemically induced cirrhosis, avid renal sodium retention occurs before any ascites accumulates. These observations support the "overflow" theory of ascites formation, which proposes that renal retention of sodium is the primary event in initiation of ascites formation and that expansion of the intravascular volume and intra-abdominal fluid accumulation are secondary events.

A third hypothesis for ascites formation recently has been proposed in which it is presumed that the arterial circulation is the primary fluid compartment responsible for modulating renal sodium and water excretion. The two primary determinants of overfilling or underfilling of the arterial circulation are cardiac output and peripheral vascular resistance. Peripheral arterial dilatation is thought to be the primary event that leads to renal sodium retention and ascites formation. Thus, sodium and water retention occur as a response to arterial underfilling.[51] The specific causes of peripheral arterial vasodilatation remain to be defined. Prostaglandins, substance P, endotoxins, calcitonin gene-related peptide, and endorphins are a few candidates.

Treatment

Bed rest and dietary sodium restriction have been the cornerstones of ascites therapy. Recumbence decreases activation of renin, angiotensin, and aldosterone; decreases sympathetic output; and increases glomerular filtration rate (GFR) and sodium excretion.[52] Reduction of sodium intake is the other major component of ascites management. In the ICU it is particularly important to avoid excessive sodium administration in intravenous fluids. Because 20% of cirrhotics with ascites excrete relatively high amounts of sodium in the urine, reducing the sodium content in the diet to 40 to 60 mEq per day is effective.[53] In the remaining cirrhotics with ascites, in whom urinary sodium excretion is often less than 10 mEq per day, diets containing as little as 10 to 20 mEq of sodium are required. However, a negative sodium balance often cannot be obtained in these patients without the aid of diuretics.

The goal of diuretic therapy is to promote a safe and sustained diuresis. Loop diuretics give a good natriuresis in only 50% of nonazotemic cirrhotics with ascites. In contrast, spironolactone is followed by a good natriuretic response in most patients.[54] Spironolactone is usually started at a dose of 100 to 400 mg per day. If no response is seen in 3 to 5 days, furosemide can be added to enhance the natriuretic effect. Doses can be increased stepwise to 160 mg per day of furosemide and 400 to 600 mg per day of spironolactone.[53] Patients who do not respond to salt restriction and this type of diuretic regimen are considered diuretic resistant. However, it is important to search for overlooked sources of sodium intake such as sodium-rich antacids and intravenous antibiotics. In addition, drugs such as nonsteroidal anti-inflammatory drugs and β-blockers that interfere with renal sodium excretion should be avoided.[55, 56]

Azotemia secondary to intravascular volume depletion is a common complication of diuretic therapy. Fortunately, this is usually reversible with diuretic withdrawal. Diuretic-induced azotemia is less common in patients with both ascites and peripheral edema. Other complications of diuretic therapy include hyponatremia, muscle cramps, decreased libido, gynecomastia, and hepatic encephalopathy.

Therapeutic paracenteses and peritoneovenous shunts can be used in patients in whom diuresis cannot be achieved safely with sodium restriction and diuretics. Repeated large-volume paracenteses are more effective than diuretics in removing ascites.[53, 57] Hyponatremia, azotemia, and hepatic encephalopathy also are less frequent in patients treated with paracentesis than in those treated with diuretics.[58] Furthermore, complete removal of ascites with a single paracentesis has a complication rate similar to that seen with repeated large-volume paracenteses.[59]

The peritoneovenous shunt produces sustained blood volume expansion by continuously shunting ascites to the central circulation. Either a Le Veen or Denver shunt can be used. Unfortunately, peritoneovenous shunts are associated with many complications including bacterial infection, diffuse intravascular coagulation, pulmonary edema, esophageal variceal hemorrhage, and congestive heart failure. Shunt obstruction occurs in more than 30% of patients. Vascular thrombosis also occurs and can result in pulmonary embolism. Nevertheless, a recently reported clinical trial revealed that peritoneovenous shunts were as effective as paracentesis.[60] TIPS also can be very effective in patients with diuretic-resistant ascites.

Renal Failure

Oliguria occurs frequently in patients with cirrhosis. The major causes are prerenal azotemia from volume depletion, acute tubular necrosis (ATN), and the hepatorenal syndrome. If treated aggressively, many patients with prerenal azotemia and ATN survive. In contrast, the mortality without transplantation in patients with the hepatorenal syndrome is 90%.

Acute Tubular Necrosis

ATN is the most common cause of renal failure in patients with cirrhosis. Excessive diuresis with volume depletion, use of nephrotoxic antibiotics, and sepsis secondary to indwelling catheters all too commonly result in acute renal failure. Patients with ATN usually have a history of shock, nephrotoxic drug use, and deep jaundice. Although shock can be corrected and toxic agents removed, tubular necrosis and severe liver disease often are a deadly combination. Patients with liver disease are unusually sensitive to the nephrotoxic effects of aminoglycosides.[61] As a consequence, these agents should be used with trepidation in patients with cirrhosis. Plasma levels should be monitored daily; a rising trough level should prompt discontinuation of the drug.

Hepatorenal Syndrome

The hepatorenal syndrome is characterized by progressive oliguria, normal intravascular volume, and highly concentrated urine essentially free of sodium. The renal failure in patients with the hepatorenal syndrome is functional in origin. Kidneys removed from patients with the syndrome function normally after kidney transplantation. In addition, the hepatorenal syndrome has been reversed by liver transplantation.[62] It has been proposed that renal deterioration is mediated by a signal or reflex from the liver.[63] Infusion of glutamine into the superior mesenteric vein leads to a marked reduction in renal plasma flow, GFR, and urinary flow rate, an effect abolished by spinal transection and hepatic or renal denervation.[64]

Diagnosis and Treatment

When a patient with cirrhosis experiences oliguria or a rise in serum creatinine, it is important to exclude any potentially treatable form of renal dysfunction such as urinary tract infections and volume depletion with prerenal azotemia. Plasma and urine sodium concentrations, osmolality, and creatinine should be obtained before any diuretics are administered and the urine sediment should be examined. Prerenal azotemia and the hepatorenal syndrome are characterized by normal urinary sediment and preservation of renal concentrating ability with urine sodium concentration of less than 10 mEq/L, urine-plasma creatinine ratio greater than 30:1, and urine osmolality greater than 100 mOsm. In contrast, the urine of patients with ATN often is rich in casts and cellular debris. Urine sodium is greater than 30 mEq/L, the urine–plasma creatinine ratio is less than 20:1, and the urine osmolality is equal to the plasma osmolality.

If the urine examination is consistent with prerenal azotemia or the hepatorenal syndrome, it is essential to assess the patient's volume status with a pulmonary artery catheter. About 10% to 15% of patients initially thought to have the hepatorenal syndrome are merely volume depleted and respond promptly to volume replacement;[65] other patients may respond more slowly to volume replacement. Thus, lack of response should be considered only after acute and chronic volume expansion. Patients with the hepatorenal syndrome usually die of complications of liver disease within a short time without hepatic transplantation.

Infections

Spontaneous bacterial peritonitis (SBP) accounts for 60% to 70% of all serious infections in patients with cirrhosis.[66] The organisms most frequently cultured are aerobic gram-negative bacteria. *Escherichia coli* and *Klebsiella* are the most frequently isolated gram-negative species. Streptococci and enterococci are less frequently isolated. Anaerobes rarely cause SBP. The mortality associated with SBP is 30%; moreover, those who recover have a 70% chance of a recurrent episode within a year.[66] It is important to differentiate spontaneous peritonitis from intestinal perforation and secondary peritonitis. The clinical features of each may be quite similar; however, patients with intestinal perforation usually have lower ascitic fluid glucose levels, higher lactate dehydrogenase (LDH) levels, and higher total protein concentrations than patients with spontaneous peritonitis.[67] In addition, patients with perforation often grow multiple organisms in contrast to the single organism usually cultured in patients with spontaneous peritonitis.

Most patients with infected ascites have neither fever nor abdominal tenderness; a diagnostic paracentesis is required for diagnosis. Placing ascitic fluid in blood culture bottles at the bedside significantly improves the yield of bacteria.[68] The number of polymorphonuclear leukocytes (PMNs) in the ascites is the main laboratory indicator of SBP.[69] A PMN count greater than 500/mm^3 is indicative of SBP. Glucose, LDH, protein, pH, and lactate concentrations are not as useful in differentiating infected from sterile ascites.[69] Early institution of antibiotics in suspected SBP can improve survival.[70] Empirical therapy often includes ampicillin and an aminoglycoside; however, the high risk of aminoglycoside nephrotoxicity limits their usefulness. Cefotaxime is more effective than ampicillin and aminoglycosides in the treatment of SBP and is not nephrotoxic.[71] Ceftriaxone and ampicillin-clavulanic acid also have been shown to be effective.[72] Once culture results are available, antibiotic therapy can be tailored to the organism recovered. Aztreonam is effective for most gram-negative organisms.[73] Cefotaxime administered for 5 days is as efficacious as 10- to 14-day courses of therapy and is significantly less expensive.[74] There is a high risk of recurrent infections, which can be reduced with norfloxacin prophylaxis.[75]

Pneumonia, septicemia, and endocarditis also are common in patients with liver failure. Almost a quarter of patients admitted with GI bleeding acquire bacterial infections. Selective bowel decontamination with oral norfloxacin significantly reduces the incidence of infections in these patients.[76]

FULMINANT HEPATIC FAILURE

Fulminant hepatic failure (FHF) is the sudden onset of hepatic failure in a patient without preexisting liver disease, characterized by marked prolongation of prothrombin time and development of hepatic encephalopathy within 8 weeks of symptom onset. The mortality rate for FHF ranges from 40% to 85%. Medical treatments attempted for patients with FHF have included corticosteroids, exchange transfusions, plasmapheresis, charcoal hemoperfusion, and prostaglandins; none have been shown to be useful. In the United States, the most common cause of FHF is viral hepatitis, usually hepatitis B or non-A, non-B hepatitis. Other common causes of FHF include acetaminophen hepatotoxicity and drug-induced hepatitis from halothane, methyldopa, or isoniazid. Less common causes include hepatitis A infection, Wilson's disease, Budd-Chiari syndrome, and Amanita mushroom poisoning.

Several independent factors influence survival in FHF, including cause and patient age. Cause is a particularly important prognostic factor. Most patients with FHF resulting from hepatitis A and acetaminophen hepatotoxicity recover. In contrast, the possibility of recovery is less than 20% for patients with FHF resulting from non-A, non-B hepatitis or drug-induced hepatitis. Patients with hepatitis B have a 40% chance of spontaneous recovery, whereas patients with FHF caused by Wilson's disease almost never recover.[77] Approximately one third of patients between the ages of 10 and 40 years recover from FHF. In contrast, very few patients older than 40 years survive without transplantation.

A variety of dynamic variables also are useful in predicting the outcome of patients with FHF. These include the degree of hepatic encephalopathy, prothrombin time, factor V level, serum bilirubin, serum creatinine, α-fetoprotein level, and arterial pH.[78] The degree of hepatic encephalopathy has a profound influence on the outcome of patients with FHF. Patients who reach only stage II encephalopathy have a recovery rate of 65% to 70%. In contrast, patients who reach stage IV encephalopathy have less than a 20% chance of recovery.

Because no specific form of treatment has been proven beneficial in FHF, the goal of critical care management is to temporize until hepatic regeneration occurs or until urgent transplantation can be performed. Prevention and timely recognition and management of major complications is crucial. These include hepatic encephalopathy, respiratory failure, infections, profound coagulopathy, bleeding, renal failure, and cerebral edema.

The timing of transplantation in patients with FHF is critical. Complete recovery occurs after surgery in most patients who undergo transplantation with stage III or early stage IV encephalopathy; however, major neurologic complications can occur because of cerebral edema in patients who have prolonged stage IV hepatic encephalopathy before transplantation.

Hepatic Encephalopathy

Hepatic encephalopathy can develop with amazing rapidity in FHF. Patients can pass through the various stages of encephalopathy within a few hours and can recover with equal rapidity. With early encephalopathy, young patients may exhibit bizarre, combative behavior with profanity, violent movements, and even seizures. Sedatives, which unfortunately are often given to these patients, can cause rapid deterioration of mental status. Because decisions concerning transplantation rely so heavily on the progression of encephalopathy, any type of sedative should be avoided.

Respiratory Failure

Patients should be considered for intubation for airway protection when they reach stage II or certainly stage III encephalopathy. Intubation and ventilation also decrease the excessive oxygen consumption caused by the increased work of breathing in hyperventilating patients. In spite of adequate PaO_2 values, tissue oxygenation may be inadequate because of the MOSF that occurs with FHF. It has been postulated that an altered balance between vasodilator and vasoconstrictor substances is present. Acetylcysteine administration increases cardiac output, with a resultant increase in oxygen extraction ratio and total oxygen consumption.[79] However, prostacyclin administration does not reproduce these beneficial results, so the role of these alterations in tissue oxygenation remains unclear.

Infections

Bacterial infection can be documented in 80% of patients with FHF.[80] Pulmonary and urinary tract infections are most common. One third of patients also acquire fungal infections.[81] Very few patients have fever or elevated white blood cell counts. These features and the preponderance of infections suggest that patients with FHF are severely immunosuppressed. Spontaneous bacterial peritonitis also is common in patients with FHF, occurring in almost one third of patients.[82] Patients with SBP or bacteremia are more likely to experience renal failure and GI bleeding and have a significantly higher mortality than noninfected patients. Because of the high risk of infections in patients with FHF, some centers routinely place these patients on an oral selective bowel decontamination preparation, including polymyxin, gentamicin, and nystatin plus low-dose amphotericin before transplantation. Although infections can be significantly reduced with selective enteral and parenteral antibiotic prophylaxis, survival is not enhanced.[83]

Coagulopathy

The coagulopathy of FHF is a complex disorder consisting of reduction in coagulation factors normally produced by the liver, enhanced fibrinolysis with intravascular coagulation, and reduction in the number and function of platelets.

Factors I (fibrinogen), II (prothrombin), V, VII, IX, and X are synthesized exclusively by the liver. The rapid changes in prothrombin time values that occur during the course of FHF probably reflect changes in Factor VII, which has a half-life of only 2 hours. Although individual factor levels can be measured, the prothrombin time continues to be the most useful test for monitoring the relative synthesis of coagulation factors during the course of the disease.

Patients with FHF also can have depressed levels of plasminogen activator and plasminogen, increased levels of fibrin and fibrinogen–split products, and deficiency of antithrombin III, which can lead to intravascular clotting. However, despite the plethora of laboratory abnormalities, diffuse intravascular coagulation is rarely an important clinical problem unless there is a precipitating event such as sepsis. Platelet counts less than $80,000/mm^3$ are seen in approximately half of patients. A variety of abnormalities in platelet function also can be measured, each of which resolves with recovery of hepatic function.

The most effective management of coagulopathy is conservative and consists of parenteral vitamin K replacement, administration of fresh frozen plasma to maintain a reasonable prothrombin time level, platelet transfusions when necessary, and possibly desmopressin administration.[11] Despite the profound coagulopathy, overt bleeding from sources other than the GI tract is surprisingly uncommon. The most common cause of GI bleeding is stress ulceration, which can be dramatically reduced by prophylactic administration of antacids or H_2 blockers.

Renal Failure

Renal failure is an ominous development in patients with FHF. Many patients are oliguric on ICU admission because of volume depletion from poor fluid intake. Volume expansion usually results in rapid improvement in urine output and may prevent the development of ATN, which usually appears later in the clinical course. The hepatorenal syndrome is uncommon and, when seen, is usually a preterminal event. As in patients with cirrhosis, the most important clinical measurement is a good assessment of the intravascular volume status, which usually requires the insertion of a pulmonary artery catheter. Despite the potential hazards of catheter placement in patients with a severe coagulopathy, maintenance of adequate blood volume is crucial.

Cerebral Edema

The primary cause of death in patients with FHF is cerebral edema, which is found in 60% to 70% of patients who die with this disease. Proposed pathogenetic mechanisms include disruption of the blood-brain barrier with leakage of plasma into the CSF and cellular mechanisms that allow increased uptake of water into brain cells. The clinical observation that mannitol is effective and corticosteroids are ineffective in reducing ICP in patients with FHF strongly supports the latter mechanism. Cellular swelling may be due to the osmotic effects of glutamine, which is generated from the deamidization of ammonia by glutamine synthetase in cortical astrocytes. Rats given infusions of ammonium acetate acquire brain edema; however, prior administration of glutamine synthetase inhibitors prevents the increase in brain water.[41] These findings suggest that there is nothing unique about FHF but that brain edema and increased CSF pressure may develop in any patient with markedly increased cerebral ammonia levels.

Classic signs of elevated ICP often are absent in patients with FHF. Computed tomographic (CT) scans of the head are an insensitive method of detecting cerebral edema in these patients.[84] However, a CT scan should be performed to exclude subdural and intraparenchymal hematomas. ICP monitoring has been increasingly used in patients with FHF. Despite the coagulopathy usually present in these patients, ICP monitors can be used safely. Epidural monitors are commonly used. Although they are safer to place, they are somewhat less accurate than subdural bolts. However, the latter have a higher incidence of hemorrhagic complications.[85] Monitoring of ICP may be valuable in the management of patients with FHF in stage III to stage IV coma by not only providing a guide for therapy but also allowing the exclusion of patients from emergency liver transplantation who have sustained elevations of ICP.[86]

Mannitol and hyperventilation are effective in reducing ICP; however, their use can occasionally be counterproductive. Hyperventilation can transiently decrease ICP; however, not all patients with stage IV coma are hyperemic. In these patients, hyperventilation can decrease cerebral blood flow inappropriately and result in cerebral ischemia. Likewise, mannitol can be very useful in transiently decreasing elevated ICP but can be dangerous in patients with renal failure.

Despite aggressive medical management and supportive care, the mortality rate in FHF remains high. Orthotopic liver transplantation is quickly becoming the treatment of choice in patients who have little chance of spontaneous recovery. Survival after liver transplantation has ranged from 50% to 90%.[86]

LIVER TRANSPLANT PATIENTS

Liver transplantation has become an accepted therapeutic procedure for selected patients with severe acute and chronic liver disease. Technical improvements in surgery, improved patient selection, the availability of cyclosporine for immunosuppression, and improved methods for organ procurement and preservation have resulted in dramatic improvements in survival rates.[87] One-year survival rates in many centers approach 90%. As a result, liver transplantation is now performed at more than 75 centers throughout the United States.

The primary indications for liver transplantation in adults include chronic active hepatitis, cryptogenic cirrhosis, primary biliary cirrhosis, and primary sclerosing cholangitis. The major indications for transplantation in children include biliary atresia, with in-born errors of metabolism and chronic hepatitis less often. Other less frequent indications include hepatic vein thrombosis, fulminant hepatitis, and primary malignancy of the liver and bile ducts. It has been shown that in properly selected patients the results of transplantation in alcoholic cirrhosis are as good as those for other diseases;[88] this has now become one of the major indications for transplantation. More controversy surrounds transplantation for patients with cirrhosis resulting from chronic hepatitis B virus infection because of recurrence of viral infection in the graft. Recipients older than 50 years have a 5-year survival after transplantation, similar to that of younger patients.[89] Contraindications to transplantation include malignancy, systemic infection, and advanced cardiopulmonary disease. Severe hypoxemia with right-to-left shunts, previously believed to be an absolute contraindication to liver transplantation, may improve substantially after the operation and should be reviewed only as a relative contraindication.[6, 90] Thrombosis of mesenteric, splenic, or portal veins previously made transplantation virtually impossible. This obstacle has been overcome in many patients with the use of vein grafts. Most complications of portal vein reconstruction have been in patients with prior shunt operations. Mesocaval and distal splenorenal shunts have been less deleterious because they do not involve dissection of the portal hilum.[91]

Preoperative Complications and Management

The most common causes of death in patients awaiting transplantation are GI bleeding and infection. Most patients have severe portal hypertension and varices. Although management of variceal hemorrhage is generally the same as with any cirrhotic patient, sclerotherapy ulcers can delay transplantation. Overly vigorous sclerotherapy also occasionally can result in portal vein thrombosis. Banding and TIPS are other therapeutic options that can be used to temporize variceal hemorrhage and provide an effective bridge to transplantation. Placement of a Minnesota tube followed by a TIPS procedure is one of the best methods of controlling variceal bleeding without interfering with subsequent transplantation.

Life-threatening infections commonly occur in these critically ill patients. A simple urinary tract infection can trigger overwhelming sepsis within a period of hours. As a consequence, any fever must be addressed aggressively with blood, urine, and peritoneal fluid cultures combined with a search for identification of any other potential source of infection. Infections should be treated with the narrowest spectrum of antibiotics possible because of the risk of fungal infections after liver transplantation.

Transplant Operation

The transplant operation consists of removal of the recipient liver, anastomosis of the vena cava above and below the liver, anastomoses of the portal vein and hepatic artery, and biliary reconstruction. Biliary reconstruction is usually performed with an end-to-end anastomosis of the common bile duct over a T tube or, if this is not possible, anastomosis of the donor common duct to a Roux-en-Y loop of jejunum. Because many adults requiring transplantation have a coagulopathy and severe portal hypertension, blood loss during the operation can be significant. The average adult requires 10 to 20 units of packed cells; however, this can be far exceeded during difficult operations. At the time of reperfusion of the newly inserted donor liver, a number of active substances are released with sequelae including hypotension, increased ICP, intravascular coagulation, and pulmonary hypertension. It is important to be aware of intraoperative events because they can have a bearing on early postoperative care.

Postoperative Complications

Postoperative complications are now the major obstacle to prolonged survival after hepatic transplantation. The frequency of postoperative complications correlates well with the duration of surgery. A variety of unique complications can occur. These complications can be surgical, immunologic, or medical in nature, which adds to the complexity of postoperative management.

The most prominent surgical complications include nonfunction of the graft, intra-abdominal bleeding, hepatic artery thrombosis, and biliary obstruction or leak. In a patient with a functioning graft, there is rapid production of bile, spontaneous correction of coagulation deficiencies, and metabolic alkalosis from conversion of citrate in infused blood into citrate by the liver. Patients usually are alert and can be extubated within 12 to 24 hours after surgery. A marked rise in aminotransferases in the first 24 to 48 hours after surgery, absence of bile flow, coagulopathy, and stupor all suggest the presence of primary graft nonfunction, which occurs in 5% to 20% of liver transplants. These patients usually become profoundly cholestatic and require urgent retransplantation.

Intra-abdominal bleeding, which usually occurs within the first 24 hours after transplantation, can be recognized clinically by a rapidly rising pulse and decreasing BP associated with a rapid drop in hemoglobin. Patients tolerate reoperation well if the bleeding is recognized promptly and the patient can be stabilized with transfusions and returned quickly to the operating room. In contrast, a delay in diagnosis can result in irreversible hypotensive damage to the kidneys and liver. Hepatic artery thrombosis can result in a marked rise in hepatic transaminases because of ischemia to the graft; however, many cases are very subtle. Doppler ultrasonography is an extremely useful screening examination of the vascular anastomoses. The diagnosis of hepatic artery thrombosis can be confirmed with angiography. Prompt repair is essential if the graft is to be salvaged.[87, 92]

Biliary tract obstruction and bile leak typically present with a sustained and steady rise in the bilirubin level with or without elevation of the alkaline phosphatase level. However, myriad other conditions including allograft rejection, infection, hemolysis, and renal insufficiency also can elevate serum bilirubin in these patients. Differentiating biliary tract complications from these disorders usually requires cholangiography. In patients with a T tube, cholangiography can be performed without difficulty. However, in patients with an internal biliary anastomosis to a Roux-en-Y loop of bowel, a transhepatic cholangiogram is required.

The major immunologic complications seen after liver transplantation include rejection of the allograft and a limited graft-versus-host disease with hemolytic anemia and renal failure. Allograft rejection, which occurs in 30% to 70% of patients, often begins with an insidious but sustained elevation of the serum bilirubin with little or no change in transaminase and alkaline phosphatase values; however, transaminase elevations typically occur as rejection progresses. Differentiation from biliary tract disorders, hepatic artery thrombosis, systemic infection, and other forms of hepatocellular injury including viral hepatitis can be difficult. The most accurate diagnostic approach is to exclude other possibilities through cholangiography, arteriography, and cultures followed by liver biopsy. The biopsy allows exclusion of other forms of hepatocellular injury and often shows the typical histologic picture of rejection, which includes periportal inflammation with mononuclear cells, cholestasis, and invasion of the vascular endothelium and biliary epithelium by mononuclear cells.[93] If recognized promptly, episodes of acute rejection usually respond favorably to bolus injections of corticosteroids. In selected patients, antilymphocyte preparations such as OKT3 are required. With currently available immunosuppressive agents, most episodes of rejection can be controlled; however, delay in diagnosis may result in irreversible, fatal rejection.[94] Patients who receive ABO-incompatible grafts can experience a limited graft-versus-host reaction characterized by hemolytic anemia. Lymphocytes carried over with the donor organ survive for 6 to 8 weeks after transplantation and can react against recipient red cells, producing anti-A or anti-B antibodies and triggering an acute hemolytic anemia, which usually occurs 10 to 14 days after transplantation.[95] Massive hemolysis can result in renal failure requiring dialysis. However, with appropriate support, most patients survive with spontaneous resolution of hemolysis and recovery of renal function.

A number of medical complications also may occur in liver transplant recipients. Metabolic alkalosis, sodium retention, and a right-sided pleural effusion are the rule in the immediate postoperative period. Several factors may be responsible for the metabolic alkalosis. Renal adaptations to cirrhosis include avid renal sodium retention and bicarbonate resorption. This adaptation persists for a variable length of time after transplantation. Sodium citrate, used as a preservative in red blood cells and fresh frozen plasma, is metabolized to bicarbonate by the functioning liver. Because each unit of fresh frozen plasma contains approximately 20 g of citrate, the added alkali load is quite sizable in patients who require large numbers of transfusions during surgery. Chloride depletion is also often a significant part of alkalosis. This may be in part secondary to pretransplant chloride deficits. In addition, many blood products are deficient in chloride. The natural consequence of metabolic alkalosis is respiratory compensation with hypercarbia. Excessive mechanical ventilation worsens the alkalemia, whereas failure to treat the alkalosis can result in atelectasis and difficulty weaning the patient from assisted ventilation. Correction of intravascular volume deficits and provision of adequate chloride are helpful; however, intravenous acetazolamide or hydrochloric acid occasionally may be required.

In cirrhotic patients with ascites, increased tubular resorption of sodium persists for an indefinite period of time after transplantation. Excessive use of crystalloid during the operation and postoperatively in the ICU can lead to massive weight gain and expansion of the extracellular fluid volume. In extreme circumstances, this can increase the work of breathing and prolong the need for assisted ventilation.

The hyperdynamic changes after liver transplantation are quite complex. Before surgery, many patients have a hyperdynamic circulation with increased cardiac output and diminished peripheral vascular resistance as well as increased splanchnic blood flow and evidence for portosystemic shunting. The splanchnic hemodynamics and portosystemic shunts do not change in the early postoperative period.[96] There is an increase toward normal in SVR, and many patients become hypertensive as a result of volume expansion and the effects of cyclosporine.[97] However, changes in cardiac output have been more variable; some studies have shown a return toward normal,[1, 98] whereas in others no change has been seen for as long as 2 years after transplantation.[99]

A variety of pulmonary abnormalities are present in the immediate postoperative period. Right lower lobe atelectasis secondary to poor excursion of the right hemidiaphragm either from damage during prolonged traction in the intraoperative period or because of generalized diaphragmatic dysfunction as a result of the wide surgical incisions is a frequent postoperative finding. Right-sided pleural effusions, which appear to be a sympathetic response to manipulation of the diaphragm during the transplant procedure, are often seen in the week after surgery. These have the characteristic features of a transudate. They do not require thoracentesis unless they become large enough to impair ventilation and oxygenation or unless occult infection is being sought. Weaning from mechanical ventilation can proceed in spite of this abnormality; many patients are weaned successfully with $PaCO_2$ in the range of 48 to 52 mm Hg. High levels of positive end-expiratory pressure should be avoided because they may decrease cardiac output or create excessive venous pressures in the transplanted liver. One patient has been described in whom pulmonary hypertension partially normalized after transplantation.[100] The severe hypoxia associated with cirrhosis can reverse after transplantation; however, these patients often require prolonged assisted ventilation and rehabilitation.

Much more ominous are the complications of acute renal failure and infection. In the first 24 to 48 hours after transplantation, urinary output often must be supported with large volumes of intravenous fluid and small amounts of potent diuretics, even though clinical signs and measurement of intravascular pressures indicate satisfactory intravascular volume. Frequently, the blood urea nitrogen increases as a result of operative trauma; therefore, the serum creatinine is a more reliable indicator of renal function.

Renal failure poses a significant hazard to patients in the immediate postoperative period because it restricts the choice of immunosuppressive agents and may eventually lead to the need for dialysis with its potential complications. Renal failure may develop for many reasons, including acute intraoperative of postoperative hypotension secondary to hemorrhage, arrhythmias, or sepsis; the use of nephrotoxic antibiotics; inadequate volume replacement; and the use of cyclosporin A. Although maintenance of stable hemodynamics with good renal blood flow may prevent renal failure, acute renal failure may occur even with meticulous management. For this reason, the support of an experienced hemodialysis team is essential to any liver transplantation program. With sustained dialysis, patients often recover from the acute episode with normal or near-normal renal function.

Infection is the leading cause of death in liver transplant recipients. Preoperative malnutrition, the invasive nature and extent of the operation, the catabolic postoperative state, the need for indwelling catheters and ventilators, and immunosuppression all expose the patient to an inordinate risk of infection with a wide variety of organisms. Early infectious complications include pneumonias, catheter-related sepsis, intra-abdominal abscesses, and peritonitis. Gram-negative enteric organisms are frequently encountered in the situation, although catheter-related infections are most frequently caused by coagulase-negative staphylococci. Systemic candidiasis and aspergillosis as well as herpesvirus and cytomegalovirus infections more often develop later during the postoperative course.[92]

SUMMARY

The preoperative management of patients with acute and chronic liver failure and the management of patients after liver transplantation have become exciting new areas of clinical experience for the critical care physician. It is becoming more apparent that optimum management in the ICU for many of these patients can make the difference between death and survival with excellent quality of life after liver transplantation.

References

1. Glauser F: Systemic hemodynamic and cardiac function changes in patients undergoing orthotopic liver transplantation. Chest 1990; 98:1210–1215.
2. Hadengue A, Benahyoun M, Lebrec D, et al: Pulmonary hypertension complicating portal hypertension: Prevalence and relation to splanchnic hemodynamics. Gastroenterology 1991; 100:520–528.
3. Robalino B, Moodie D: Association between primary pulmonary hypertension and portal hypertension: Analysis of its pathophysiology and clinical, laboratory, and hemodynamic manifestations. J Am Coll Cardiol 1991; 17:492–498.
4. Agust'i AG, Roca J, Bosch J, et al: The lung in patients with cirrhosis. J Hepatol 1990; 10:251–257.
5. Hanson C, Ritter A, Duran W, et al: Ascites: Its effect upon static inflation of the respiratory system. Am Rev Respir Dis 1990; 142:39–42.
6. Krowka M, Cortese D: Hepatopulmonary syndrome: An evolving perspective in the era of liver transplantation. Chest 1990; 98:1053–1054.
7. Krowka MJ, Tajik AJ, Dickson ER, et al: Intrapulmonary vascular dilatations (IPVD) in liver transplant candidates: Screening by two-dimensional contrast-enhanced echocardiography. Chest 1990; 97:1165–1170.
8. Hedenstierna G, Soederman C, Eriksson LS, et al: Ventilation-perfusion inequality in patients with non-alcoholic liver cirrhosis. Eur Respir J 1991; 4:711–717.
9. Rodriguez-Roisin R, Roca J, Agusti AG, et al: Gas exchange and pulmonary vascular reactivity in patients with liver cirrhosis. Am Rev Respir Dis 1987; 135:1085–1092.
10. Hourani J, Bellamy P, Tashkin D, et al: Pulmonary dysfunction in advanced liver disease: Frequent occurrence of an abnormal diffusing capacity. Am J Med 1991; 90:693–700.
11. Cattaneo M, Tenconi PM, Alberca I, et al: Subcutaneous desmopressin (DDAVP) shortens the prolonged bleeding time in patients with liver cirrhosis. Thromb Haemost 1990; 64:358–360.
12. Rubin W: Medical treatment of peptic ulcer disease. Med Clin North Am 1991; 75:981–998.
13. Wara P: Endoscopic prediction of major rebleeding: A prospective study of stigmata of hemorrhage in bleeding ulcer. Gastroenterology 1985; 88:1209–1214.
14. Laine L: Multipolar electrocoagulation versus injection therapy in the treatment of bleeding peptic ulcers. Gastroenterology 1990; 99:1303–1306.
15. Sachdeva AK, Zaren HA, Sigel B: Surgical treatment of peptic ulcer disease. Med Clin North Am 1991; 75:999–1012.
16. Paquet K-J, Mercado MA, Kalk J-F: Frequency, significance and therapy of the Mallory-Weiss syndrome in patients with portal hypertension. Hepatology 1990; 11:879–883.
17. Iwao T, Toyonaga A, Sumino M, et al: Portal hypertensive gastropathy in patients with cirrhosis. Gastroenterology 1992; 102:2060–2065.
18. Sarin SK, Sreenivas DV, Lahoti D, et al: Factors influencing development of portal hypertensive gastropathy in patients with portal hypertension. Gastroenterology 1992; 102:994–999.
19. Lebrec D, Poynard T, Hillon P, et al: Propranolol for prevention of recurrent gastrointestinal bleeding in patients with cirrhosis. N Engl J Med 1981; 305:1371–1374.
20. Conn HO, Grace ND, Bosch J, et al: Propanolol in the prevention of the first hemorrhage from esophagogastric varices: A multicenter, randomized clinical trial. Hepatology 1991; 13:902–912.
21. Vinel J-P, Lamouliatte H, Cales P, et al: Propranolol reduces the rebleeding rate during endoscopic sclerotherapy before variceal obliteration. Gastroenterology 1992; 102:1760–1763.
22. Rodriguez-Perez F, Groszmann RJ: Pharmacologic treatment of portal hypertension. Gastroenterol Clin North Am 1992; 21:15–40.
23. Tsai YT, Lay CS, Lai KH, et al: Controlled trial of vasopressin plus nitroglycerin vs vasopressin alone in the treatment of bleeding esophageal varices. Hepatology 1986; 6:406–409.
24. Bosch J, Karvetz D, Rodes J: Effects of somatostatin on hepatic and systemic haemodynamics in patients with cirrhosis of the liver: Comparison with vasopressin. Gastroenterology 1981; 80:518–525.
25. Kleber G, Sauerbruck T, Fischer G, et al: Somatostatin does not reduce oesophageal variceal pressure in liver cirrhotics. Gut 1988; 29:153–156.
26. Silvain C, Fort E, Beauchant M: Somatostatin and acute variceal hemorrhage. Gastroenterology 1991; 101:874–875.
27. Matloff DS: Treatment of acute variceal bleeding. Gastroenterol Clin North Am 1992; 21:103–118.
28. Panes J, Teres J, Bosch J, et al: Efficacy of balloon tamponade in treatment of bleeding gastric and esophageal varices. Dig Dis Sci 1988; 33:454–459.
29. Larson A, Cohen H, Zweiban B, et al: Acute esophageal variceal sclerotherapy: Results of a prospective randomized controlled trial. Hepatology 1986; 255:447–500.
30. Teres J: Balloon tamponade vs. endoscopic sclerotherapy: In the management of active variceal hemorrhage. Hepatology 1990; 11:898–899.
31. Schuman BM, Berkman JW, Tedesco FJ, et al: Complications of endoscopic injection sclerotherapy: A review. Am J Gastroenterol 1987; 82:823–829.
32. Stiegmann GV, Goff JS, Michaletz-Onody PA, et al: Endoscopic sclerotherapy as compared with endoscopic ligation for bleeding esophageal varices. N Engl J Med 1992; 326:1527–1532.
33. Richter GM, Noeldge G, Roessle M, et al: Transjugular intrahepatic portosystemic shunt (TIPSS). Radiology 1990; 174:1027–1030.

34. Ring EJ, Lake JR, Roberts JP, et al: Using transjugular intrahepatic portosystemic shunts to control variceal bleeding before liver transplantation. Ann Intern Med 1992; 116:304–309.
35. Zemel G, Katzen BT, Becker GJ, et al: Percutaneous transjugular portosystemic shunt. JAMA 1991; 266:390–393.
36. Gordon JD, Colapinto RF, Abecassis M, et al: Transjugular intrahepatic portosystemic shunt: A nonoperative approach to life-threatening variceal bleeding. Can J Surg 1987; 30:45–49.
37. Terblanche J, Burroughs AK, Hobbs KEF: Controversies in the management of bleeding esophageal varices. N Engl J Med 1989; 320:1393–1398.
38. Lacaine F, LaMuraglia GM, Malt RA: Prognostic factors in survival after portasystemic shunts: Multivariate analysis. Ann Surg 1985; 202:729–734.
39. Terblanche J, Burroughs AK, Hobbs KEF: Controversies in the management of bleeding esophageal varices (second of two parts). N Engl J Med 1989; 320:1469–1475.
40. Lockwood AH, Yap EWH, Wong WH: Cerebral ammonia metabolism in patients with severe liver disease and minimal hepatic encephalopathy. J Cereb Blood Flow Metab 1991; 11:337–347.
41. Swain M, Butterworth RF, Blei AT: Ammonia and related amino acids in the pathogenesis of brain edema in acute ischemic liver failure in rats. Hepatology 1992; 15:449–453.
42. Lavoie J, Giguere JF, Pomier LG, et al: Amino acid changes in autopsied brain tissue from cirrhotic patients with hepatic encephalopathy. J Neurochem 1987; 49:692–697.
43. Mullen KD, Mendelson WB, Martin JV, et al: Could an endogenous benzodiazepine ligand contribute to hepatic encephalopathy? Lancet 1988; 1:457–459.
44. Gitlin N: Subclinical portal-systemic encephalopathy. Am J Gastroenterol 1988; 83:8–11.
45. Butterworth RF, Giguere JF, Michaud J, et al: Ammonia: Key factor in the pathogenesis of hepatic encephalopathy. J Cereb Blood Flow Metab 1987; 6:1–12.
46. Uribe M, Campollo O, Cote C: Effect of lactulose on the metabolism of short chain fatty acids (comment). Hepatology 1990; 12:1251–1252.
47. Weber FL Jr, Fresard KM, Lally BR: Effects of lactulose and neomycin on urea metabolism in cirrhotic subjects. Gastroenterology 1982; 82:415–420.
48. Tarao K, Ikeda T, Hayashi K, et al: Successful use of vancomycin hydrochloride in the treatment of lactulose resistant chronic hepatic encephalopathy. Gut 1990; 31:702–706.
49. Munoz SJ: Nutritional therapies in liver disease. Semin Liver Dis 1991; 11:278–281.
50. Jones EA, Basile AS, Mullen KD, et al: Flumazenil: Potential implications for hepatic encephalopathy. Pharmacol Ther 1990; 43:331–343.
51. Schrier RW: Body fluid volume regulation in health and disease: A unifying hypothesis. Ann Intern Med 1990; 113:155–159.
52. Ring-Larsen H, Henrilsen JH, Wilken C, et al: Diuretic treatment in decompensated cirrhosis and congestive heart failure: Effects of posture. Br Med J 1986; 292:1351.
53. Arroyo V, Gines P, Planas R: Treatment of ascites in cirrhosis: Diuretics, peritoneovenous shunt, and large-volume paracentesis. Gastroenterol Clin North Am 1992; 21:237–255.
54. Perez ARM, Arroyo V, Planas R, et al: Randomized comparative study of efficacy of furosemide versus spironolactone in nonazotemic cirrhosis with ascites. Gastroenterology 1984; 84:961.
55. Mirouze D, Zipser RD, Reynolds TB: Effect of inhibitors of prostaglandin synthesis on induced diuresis in cirrhosis. Hepatology 1983; 3:50–55.
56. Rector WG Jr, Reynolds TB: Propranolol in the treatment of cirrhotic ascites. Hepatology 1982; 2:678.
57. Gines P, Tito LI, Arroyo V, et al: Randomized comparative study of therapeutic paracentesis with and without intravenous albumin in cirrhosis. Gastroenterology 1988; 94:1493.
58. Gines P, Arroyo V, Quintero E, et al: Comparison of paracentesis and diuretics in the treatment of cirrhotics with tense ascites: Results of a randomized study. Gastroenterology 1987; 93:234.
59. Tito L, Gines P, Arroyo V, et al: Total paracentesis with intravenous albumin management of patients with cirrhosis and ascites. Gastroenterology 1990; 98:146–151.
60. Gines P, Arroyo V, Vargas V, et al: Paracentesis with intravenous infusion of albumin as compared with peritoneovenous shunting in cirrhosis with refractory ascites. N Engl J Med 1991; 325:829–835.
61. Moore RD, Smith CR, Leitman PS: Increased risk of renal dysfunction due to interaction of liver disease and aminoglycosides. Am J Med 1986; 80:1093–1097.
62. Wilkinson SP, Moore KP, Arroyo V: Pathogenesis of ascites and hepatorenal syndrome. Gut 1992; Sep; Suppl:S12–S17.
63. Safirstein R, Levitt MF: A hepatorenal depressor reflex: A possible clue to the pathogenesis of the hepatorenal syndrome. Hepatology 1991; 14:734–735.
64. Lang F, Tschernko E, Schulze E, et al: Hepatorenal reflex regulating kidney function. Hepatology 1991; 14:590–594.
65. Tristani FE, Cohn JN: Systemic and renal hemodynamics in oliguric renal failure: Effect of volume expansion. J Clin Invest 1967; 46:1894.
66. Hoefs JC: Spontaneous bacterial peritonitis: Prevention and therapy. Hepatology 1990; 12:776.
67. Runyon BA, Hoefs JC: Ascitic fluid analysis in the differentiation of spontaneous bacterial peritonitis from gastrointestinal tract perforation into ascitic fluid. Hepatology 1984; 4:447.
68. Bobadilla M, Sifuentes J, Garcia-Tsao G: Improved method for bacteriological diagnosis of spontaneous bacterial peritonitis. J Clin Microbiol 1989; 27:2145–2147.
69. Abillos A, Cuervas-Mons V, Millan I, et al: Ascitic fluid polymorphonuclear cell count and serum to ascites albumin gradient in the diagnosis of bacterial peritonitis. Gastroenterology 1990; 98:134–140.
70. Hoefs JC, Canawatai HN, Sapico FL, et al: Spontaneous bacterial peritonitis. Hepatology 1982; 2:399–407.
71. Felisart J, Rimola A, Arroyo V, et al: Cefotaxime is more effective than is ampicillin-tobramycin in cirrhotics with severe infections. Hepatology 1985; 5:457–462.
72. Grange JD, Amiot X, Grange V, et al: Amoxicillin-clavulanic acid therapy of spontaneous bacterial peritonitis: A prospective study of twenty-seven cases in cirrhotic patients. Hepatology 1990; 11:360–364.
73. Ariza J, Xiol X, Esteve M, et al: Aztreonam vs. cefotaxime in the treatment of gram-negative spontaneous peritonitis in cirrhotic patients. Hepatology 1991; 14:91–98.
74. Runyon BA, McHutchison JG, Antillon MR, et al: Short-course versus long-course antibiotic treatment of spontaneous bacterial peritonitis: A randomized controlled study of 100 patients. Gastroenterology 1991; 100:1737–1742.
75. Gines P, Rimola A, Planas R, et al: Norfloxacin prevents spontaneous bacterial peritonitis recurrence in cirrhosis: Results of a double-blind, placebo-controlled trial. Hepatology 1990; 12:716–724.
76. Soriano G, Guarner C, Tomas A, et al: Norfloxacin prevents bacterial infection in cirrhotics with gastrointestinal hemorrhage. Gastroenterology 1992; 103:1267–1272.
77. O'Grady JG, Gimson AES, O'Brien CJ, et al: Controlled trials of charcoal hemoperfusion and prognostic factors in fulminant hepatic failure. Gastroenterology 1988; 94:1186–1192.
78. O'Grady JG, Alexander GJM, Hayllar KM, et al: Early indicators of prognosis in fulminant hepatic failure. Gastroenterology 1989; 97:439–445.
79. Harrison PM, Wendon JA, Gimson AES, et al: Improvement by acetylcysteine of hemodynamics and oxygen transport in fulminant hepatic failure. N Engl J Med 1991; 324:1852–1857.
80. Rolando N, Harvey F, Brahm J, et al: Prospective study of bacterial infection in acute liver failure: An analysis of 50 patients. Hepatology 1990; 11:49–53.
81. Rolando N, Harvey F, Brahm J, et al: Fungal infection: A common, unrecognized complication of acute liver failure. J Hepatology 1991; 12:1–9.
82. Chu C-M, Chiu K-W, Liaw Y-F: The prevalence and prognostic significance of spontaneous bacterial peritonitis in severe acute hepatitis with ascites. Hepatology 1992; 15:799–803.
83. Rolando N, Gimson A, Wade J, et al: Prospective controlled trial of selective parenteral and enteral antimicrobial regimen in fulminant liver failure. Hepatology 1993; 17:196–201.

84. Munoz SJ, Robinson M, Northrup B, et al: Elevated intracranial pressure and computed tomography of the brain in fulminant hepatocellular failure. Hepatology 1991; 13:209–212.
85. Keays R, Potter D, O'Grady J, et al: Intracranial and cerebral perfusion changes before, during, and immediately after orthotopic liver transplantation for fulminant hepatic failure. Q J Med 1991; 79:425–433.
86. Lidofsky SD, Bass NM, Prager MC, et al: Intracranial pressure monitoring and liver transplantation for fulminant hepatic failure. Hepatology 1992; 16:1–7.
87. Starzl TE, Demetris AJ, Van Thiel DH: Medical progress: Liver transplantation. N Engl J Med 1989; 321:1014–1022.
88. Starzl TE, Van Thiel DH, Tzakis AG, et al: Orthotopic liver transplantation for alcoholic cirrhosis. JAMA 1988; 260:2542–2544.
89. Starzl TE, Todo S, Gordon R, et al: Liver transplantation in older patients. N Engl J Med 1987; 316:484–485.
90. Erickson L, Soderman C, Ericzon BG, et al: Normalization of ventilation/perfusion relationships after liver transplantation. Hepatology 1990; 12:1350–1357.
91. Lerut J, Tzakis AG, Bron K, et al: Complications of venous reconstruction in human orthotopic liver transplantation. Ann Surg 1987; 205:404–414.
92. Starzl TE, Demetris AJ, Van Thiel DH: Medical progress: Liver transplantation. N Engl J Med 1989; 321:1092–1099.
93. Williams JW, Foster PF, Sankary HN: Role of liver allograft biopsy in patient management. Semin Liver Dis 1992; 12:60–72.
94. Williams JW, Peters TG, Vera SR, et al: Biopsy-directed immunosuppression following hepatic transplantation in man. Transplantation 1985; 39:589–596.
95. Ramsey G, Nusbacher J, Starzl TE, et al: Isohemagglutinins of graft origin after ABO-unmatched liver transplantation. N Engl J Med 1984; 311:1167–1170.
96. Henderson JM, Gilmore GT, Mackay GJ, et al: Hemodynamics during liver transplantation: The interactions between cardiac output and portal venous and hepatic arterial flows. Hepatology 1992; 16:715–718.
97. Curtis J: Distinguishing the causes of post-transplantation hypertension. Pediatr Nephrol 1991; 5:108–111.
98. Navasa M, Feu F, Garcai-Pagan JC, et al: Hemodynamic and humoral changes after liver transplantation in patients with cirrhosis. Hepatology 1993; 17:355–360.
99. Hadengue A, Lebrec D, Moreau R: Persistence of systemic and splanchnic hyperkinetic circulation in liver transplant recipients. Hepatology 1993; 17:175–178.
100. Ettinger N, Trulock E: Pulmonary considerations of organ transplantation. Am Rev Respir Dis 1991; 1386–1405.

CHAPTER 111

Severe Gastrointestinal Hemorrhage

Thomas J. Savides, MD • Dennis M. Jensen, MD

Severe gastrointestinal (GI) bleeding is defined as documented GI bleeding (i.e., hematemesis, melena, hematochezia, or positive nasogastric lavage) accompanied by either shock or orthostatic hypotension, decrease of hematocrit by 6% to 8%, or transfusion of at least two units of packed red blood cells. Most of these patients are admitted to intensive care units (ICUs) for resuscitation. Acute management of these patients is conducted by a team of physicians including gastroenterologists, surgeons, and critical care specialists. Improvement in patient outcomes will occur as a result of successful medical resuscitation, precise endoscopic diagnosis, and appropriate use of therapeutic endoscopy and surgery.

INITIAL APPROACH TO THE PATIENT WITH SEVERE GASTROINTESTINAL BLEEDING

Initial Assessment

Initial patient assessment includes history, vital signs with orthostatic blood pressure determination, physical and rectal examinations, and nasogastric lavage. One or two large-bore (14- or 16-gauge) intravenous catheters should be placed. Blood should be sent for hematocrit, platelets, prothrombin time, partial thromboplastin time, chemistry panel, and type and crossmatch for packed red blood cells. Resuscitation should be initiated simultaneously with assessment. Normal saline is infused as fast as needed to keep systolic blood pressure greater than 100 mm Hg and pulse lower than 100 beats per minute. Patients are transfused with packed red blood cells, platelets, and fresh-frozen plasma as necessary to keep the hematocrit greater than 24%, platelet count greater than 50,000/mm,[3] and prothrombin time less than 15 seconds. A gastroenterologist and a surgeon should be notified as soon as possible to expedite patient diagnosis and possible therapy.

Intensive Care Unit Management

Patients with severe GI bleeding should be admitted to an ICU-monitored intermediate care unit. Patients should have automatic blood pressure monitoring every 5 minutes if unstable and hourly if stable. Each patient should receive cardiac rhythm monitoring to observe for arrhythmias as well as to follow the heart rate as a sign of continued or recurrent bleeding. Laboratory-determined hematocrits (not finger-stick hematocrits, which are less reliable) should be obtained every 4 to 6 hours until the patient has a stable hematocrit. In cases of active bleeding, an indwelling bladder catheter should be placed to help monitor fluid status. Swan-Ganz catheter monitoring is unnecessary except for patients with a history of congestive heart failure or unstable cardiac disease. Patients older than 60 years should also be evaluated for myocardial infarction with electrocardiograms and creatinine kinase measurements.

Localization of the Site of Hemorrhage

Hematemesis, coffee-ground emesis, or a nasogastric lavage with blood or large amounts of coffee-ground emesis indicates an upper GI source. A small amount of coffee-ground emesis that clears easily may represent an upper GI source of bleed or only mucosal trauma from the nasogastric tube. A clear nasogastric aspirate does not necessarily indicate a more distal GI source; 16% of patients with actively bleeding lesions have had clear nasogastric aspirates.[1] Guaiac tests of nasogastric aspirates are not helpful because of high rates of false-positive and false-negative test results.[2] The presence of bile in the nasogastric tube makes upper GI bleeding less likely but may be consistent with an upper GI source that bleeds intermittently.

Use, Timing, and Complications of Endoscopy

Experienced endoscopists diagnose a source of upper GI bleeding in greater than 90% of cases, and this facilitates simultaneous treatment via endoscopy.[1,3] Endoscopy should be done only when safe and if the information will influence patient care. Patients should be hemodynamically stable, with a heart rate of less than 100 beats per minute and systolic blood pressure greater than 100 mm Hg. Respiratory insufficiency, altered mental status, or ongoing hematemesis may indicate the need for endotracheal intubation before emergency endoscopy for patient stabilization and protection of the airway. Coagulopathy and thrombocytopenia should be corrected with transfusions.

Patients with active hemorrhage (i.e., bloody nasogastric lavage) should undergo urgent endoscopy after medical resuscitation. In patients with massive bleeding and shock, endoscopy can be performed in the operating room. Patients who have acute self-limited blood loss with no evidence of ongoing bleeding can undergo endoscopy within 24 hours, with the exception of patients with cirrhosis, possible aortoenteric fistula, or evidence of rebleeding. Middle-of-the-night endoscopy should be avoided, if possible, because well-trained endoscopy nurses, endoscopy equipment, and surgical back-up may not be available.

Complications related to emergency endoscopy occur in up to 1% of patients.[1, 4] The most common complications include perforation, aspiration, induced hemorrhage, medication reaction, hypotension, and hypoxia.[1, 4] Because of the risk of aspiration, especially in encephalopathic or massively bleeding patients, prophylactic intubation for airway protection before endoscopy is often advisable.

In severe upper GI bleeding, gastric lavage with a large (34-French) orogastric tube is performed to evacuate blood from the stomach to prevent aspiration and to clear the stomach before endoscopy. There is no value in using iced-saline lavage to prevent or decrease upper GI bleeding.[5] Gastric lavage with lukewarm tap water is as safe as that with saline and significantly less expensive.[6]

In cases of suspected lower GI bleeding, patients should undergo urgent colonoscopy after rapid sulfate purge.[3] In the ICU, patients receive 4 to 6 L of polyethylene glycol (i.e., GoLYTELY) either orally or via nasogastric tube over 3 to 5 hours until the rectal effluent is clear of stool, blood, and clots. Metoclopramide, 10 mg, may be given intravenously before the purge and repeated every 3 to 4 hours to facilitate gastric emptying and reduce nausea.

Use and Timing of Angiography and Surgery in Severe Gastrointestinal Bleeding

Most patients with severe GI bleeding are admitted to medical ICUs and have surgical consultation. Patients who have massive hemorrhage and cannot be stabilized with ICU resuscitation should undergo urgent surgical exploration either without prior endoscopy or with emergency endoscopy in the operating room. Emergency angiography may also be used to diagnose severe bleeding of obscure origin and possible hemostasis in patients with massive bleeding who can be resuscitated.

UPPER GASTROINTESTINAL BLEEDING

Upper GI bleeding is a common medical emergency that accounts for more than 300,000 hospital admissions each year or approximately 150 patients with severe upper GI bleeds per 100,000 population per year.[7] Despite advances in medical therapy, ICU care, endoscopy, and surgery, the mortality rate of 10% for severe upper GI bleeding has not changed over the past 30 years.[8, 9] The lack of decline of mortality may be explained by an increase in the proportion of elderly patients with GI bleeding who usually die from worsening of other medical problems and not from exsanguination.[8, 9]

The most common causes of severe upper GI bleeding among patients admitted to University of California, Los Angeles (UCLA) Medical Center and the West Los Angeles Veterans Affairs Hospital are shown in Table 111–1. The frequency of causes of bleeding reflects the population served by the hospital. For example, fewer patients with bleeding ulcers and more bleeding varices and Mallory-Weiss tears are admitted to hospitals caring for greater numbers of alcoholic patients.

TABLE 111–1. Causes of Severe Upper Gastrointestinal Bleeding in 948 Consecutive Patients at University of California, Los Angeles Medical Center and the West Los Angeles Veterans Administration Medical Center

Diagnosis	%
Peptic ulcer	55
Gastric or esophageal varix	14
Angioma	6
Mallory-Weiss tear	5
Tumor	4
Erosions	4
Esophagitis	4
Other	8

Bleeding is self-limited in 80% to 85% of patients with upper GI hemorrhage, even without specific therapy.[8, 10] Of the remaining 15% to 20% who continue to bleed or rebleed, the mortality rate is 30% to 40%.[1, 10] Patients at high risk for continuous bleeding or rebleeding potentially can benefit the most from acute medical, endoscopic, and surgical therapy; this is discussed in more detail later in this chapter.

PEPTIC ULCER HEMORRHAGE

Peptic ulcers are the leading cause of severe upper GI bleeding in the United States and account for 50% of bleeds and approximately 100,000 hospitalizations per year.[11, 12] Poor prognostic factors in peptic ulcer bleeding are shown in Table 111–2. These factors are associated with increased morbidity and mortality. Knowledge of these risk factors can identify patients at high risk for rebleeding and assist in ICU utilization and timing of endoscopy.

Medical Therapy for Severe Peptic Ulcer Hemorrhage

No medical therapy has been found significantly to decrease transfusions, rebleed rates, surgery rates, or mortality in patients with severe peptic ulcer hemorrhage.[13] Although most patients with upper GI bleeding are treated with histamine$_2$ (H_2) receptor antagonists before endoscopy, there are no conclusive results from randomized, placebo-controlled trials or meta-analysis that H_2 blockers stop active bleeding or prevent acute rebleeding. Likewise, studies of omeprazole, sucralfate, somatostatin, vasopressin, prostaglandin E_1, estrogens, and tranexamic acid have not been

TABLE 111–2. Adverse Prognostic Factors in Peptic Ulcer Hemorrhage

Age greater than 60 years
Comorbid medical illness
Shock or orthostatic hypotension
Coagulopathy
Bleeding onset in hospital
Multiple transfusions required
Fresh blood in nasogastric tube
Higher lesser curve gastric ulcer (adjacent to left gastric artery)
Posterior duodenal bulb ulcer (adjacent to gastroduodenal artery)
Endoscopic finding of arterial bleeding or visible vessel

shown to improve patient outcome in acute peptic ulcer bleeding.

Helicobacter pylori has been implicated as a possible pathogen in the cause of peptic ulcers. Although there may be a role for *H. pylori* eradication to reduce ulcer recurrence or rebleeding, there is no role for acute *H. pylori* eradication in the management of severe upper GI bleeding.[14]

Endoscopic Therapy for Severe Peptic Ulcer Hemorrhage

The endoscopic appearance (stigmas of hemorrhage) of peptic ulcer bases and the associated risks of rebleeding are shown in Table 111–3. The patients at highest risk for rebleeding are those with active arterial bleeding, a visible vessel, or an adherent clot.[15] These are the patients who may benefit from endoscopic hemostasis. Patients with clean-based ulcers or flat spots have very low rates of rebleeding and can leave the ICU soon after endoscopy and immediately begin a regular diet.[16] Patients with oozing bleeding in the absence of a visible vessel or adherent clot have an intermediate rebleeding rate of less than 20%. Treatment of these lesions is controversial; some endoscopists elect to treat these lesions.

The goal of endoscopic hemostasis is to coagulate or thrombose the underlying artery. This can be done with various thermal devices including contact probes (monopolar electrocoagulation, bipolar electrocoagulation, heater probe) or laser devices (neodymium–yittrium-aluminum-garnet [YAG] or argon). Animal studies have shown that these thermal devices are effective in coagulating arteries up to 2 mm in diameter, which is the size of arteries in resected bleeding human peptic ulcers.[17, 18] Monopolar electrocoagulation is generally not used because of concern for excessive tissue damage. Laser is not used for acute GI bleeding because of lack of portability to the ICU and expense of the equipment. A 1989 National Institutes of Health consensus conference concluded that the two "most promising techniques" of endoscopic hemostasis for bleeding ulcers were multipolar electrocoagulation and heater probe.[19] In addition, injection therapies using epinephrine, polidocanol, or alcohol have been introduced as effective but less expensive alternatives.

Randomized, controlled studies have shown that multipolar electrocoagulation probe, bipolar electrocoagulation probe, and injection therapy are all better than medical therapy alone for treating peptic ulcers with active bleeding or visible vessels in terms of reducing transfusions, length of hospital stay, and need for emergency surgery.[20–23] Table 111–4 shows the results of one such large, randomized University of California, Los Angeles Medical Center/Center for Ulcer Research and Education study of multipolar electrocoagulation and heater probe compared with medical therapy alone in the treatment of peptic ulcers with active bleeding or nonbleeding visible vessels. The results of several randomized studies comparing the different thermal modalities versus the injection therapy suggest that both methods have similar efficacy and safety[24, 25] (see Table 111–5). The results of ongoing, randomized, controlled trials will help determine the optimal treatment techniques.

Bleeding stress ulcers that occur in either the duodenum or stomach in severely ill inpatients in ICUs, do not seem to respond as well to endoscopic therapy as do peptic ulcers that start to bleed before hospitalization.[26] The cause of these in-hospital ulcers is unknown, but the poor prognosis and high rebleeding rates are often related to impaired wound healing and multiple organ failure. Generally, patients with these lesions should be supported medically, and these ulcers will heal as the patient's overall medical status improves. We treat actively bleeding ulcers in these inpatients twice with endoscopic hemostasis. If the patient continues to have severe bleeding, then surgery is recommended.

Surgery for Bleeding Peptic Ulcers

Acute surgical intervention is indicated when there is an exsanguinating bleeding and the patient cannot be medically resuscitated. Patients with recurrent bleeding despite two sessions of endoscopic hemostasis should receive surgical therapy. Patients should also be referred for surgery if the endoscopist does not feel comfortable treating a very large or pulsating visible vessel (e.g., one in a deep, posterior duodenal ulcer, which may represent the gastroduodenal artery).

VARICEAL HEMORRHAGE

Esophageal variceal bleeding related to portal hypertension is the second most common cause of severe upper GI bleed-

TABLE 111–3. Endoscopic Appearance of Peptic Ulcer Bases After Recent Hemorrhage: Prevalence and Rate of Rebleeding*

Endoscopic Appearance (Stigmas of Hemorrhage)	*Prevalence (%)*	*Rebleeding Rate (%)*
Active arterial bleeding	10	90
Nonbleeding visible vessel	25	50
Nonbleeding adherent clot	10	25
Oozing without visible vessel	5	<20
Flat spot	15	<10
Clean ulcer base	35	<5

*Data are compiled from Freeman.[15]

TABLE 111–4. Comparison of Multipolar Electrocoagulation, Heater Probe, and Medical Therapy for Peptic Ulcers with Active Bleeding or Nonbleeding Visible Vessels*

Variable	*Medical Therapy (n = 32)*	*Electro-coagulation (n = 30)*	*Heater Probe (n = 32)*
Initial hemostasis (%)	20.0	90.0†	93.0†
Rebleeding (%)	72.0	44.0	22.0†
Blood transfusions (units)	3.5	3.7	1.3
Emergency surgery (%)	41.0	33.0	3.0
Mortality	9.0	3.0	3.0

*Data compiled from Jensen and colleagues.[20]
†$P < .05$ versus medical therapy.

TABLE 111–5. Comparison of Multipolar Electrocoagulation Versus Alcohol Injection for Peptic Ulcers with Active Bleeding or Nonbleeding Visible Vessels*

Variable	*Electro-coagulation (n = 31)*	*Injection (n = 29)*	P
Further bleeding (%)	6.0	10.0	NS
Blood transfusions (units)	1.8	1.3	NS
Emergency surgery (%)	6.0	7.0	NS
Hospital stay (days)	5.8	7.2	NS
Mortality (%)	3.0	3.0	NS

*Data compiled from Laine.[24]
Abbreviation: NS = not significant.

ing after peptic ulcers. The acute mortality is approximately 30% with each bleed, and the long-term survival rate is less than 40% after 1 year with medical management in one large Veterans Administration series.[27] Despite advances in medical therapy, endoscopic hemostasis, and portosystemic shunt surgery, survival rates have not improved for variceal bleeding. The exception is with liver transplantation, which can improve survival in selected patients. Survival in nontransplanted patients is heavily influenced by the extent of underlying liver disease, with much worse survival rates for Child's class C patients than class A or B patients.

Bleeding gastric varices are a difficult therapeutic problem because, unlike with bleeding esophageal varices, most nonsurgical treatments are not effective. An exception is when isolated gastric varices are found without accompanying esophageal varices. This raises the possibility of splenic vein thrombosis, which often occurs in association with pancreatitis or pancreatic cancer. The diagnosis of splenic vein thrombosis can be made with Doppler ultrasound or angiography. The best treatment of bleeding gastric varices secondary to splenic vein thrombosis is splenectomy.

Medical Management of Acute Variceal Bleeding

Vasopressin can lower portal pressure by vasoconstriction of the splanchnic arteriolar bed. Although widely used for variceal bleeding, clinical trials have not shown intravenous vasopressin to be significantly better than placebo for hemostasis or survival.[28] Vasopressin has a high incidence of cardiac complications as a result of nonspecific vasoconstriction, which can be reduced with the simultaneous use of intravenous or sublingual nitroglycerin.[29, 30] Somatostatin infusion may cause selective splanchnic vasoconstriction without cardiac complications. Studies have shown mixed results as to whether somatostatin is more effective than placebo in managing variceal bleeding, but it seems to be as effective as vasopressin and much safer.[31–33] No studies have shown any survival benefit to patients with variceal bleeding using vasopressin or somatostatin.

Balloon Tamponade of Varices

Because varices lie in the esophageal and gastric submucosa, they are amenable to physical tamponade. There are three types of tamponade balloons. The Sengstaken-Blakemore tube has gastric and esophageal balloons, with a single aspirating port in the stomach. The Minnesota tube also has gastric and esophageal balloons but has aspiration ports in the esophagus and in the stomach. The Linton-Nicholas tube has a single large gastric balloon and aspiration ports in the stomach and esophagus. Most reports suggest that balloon tamponade provides initial tamponade in 85% to 98%, but variceal rebleeding recurs soon after deflating the balloon in 21% to 60% of patients.[34, 35] The major problem with tamponade balloons is a 30% rate of serious complications such as aspiration pneumonia, esophageal rupture, and airway obstruction.[36] Patients should be intubated before placement of tamponade balloons to minimize the pulmonary complications. Clinical studies have not shown any significant difference in efficacy between vasopressin and balloon tamponade.

Endoscopic Variceal Sclerotherapy

Endoscopic variceal sclerotherapy involves injecting sclerosants into or adjacent to esophageal varices. The most commonly used sclerosants are ethanolamine oleate, sodium tetradecyl sulfate, sodium morrhuate, and ethanol. Cyanoacrylate is a glue that is very effective for both esophageal and gastric varices, but it is difficult to use and not available in the United States. Various techniques are used, with the common goal being initial hemostasis and then weekly sclerotherapy until obliteration of all varices. Esophageal varices are much more amenable to endoscopic therapy than gastric varices.

Prospective, randomized trials show mixed results but suggest improved immediate hemostasis and a reduction in acute rebleeding with sclerotherapy compared with medical therapy for treatment of bleeding esophageal varices.[37–40] The complications of endoscopic variceal sclerotherapy include esophageal ulcers, which can bleed or perforate, esophageal strictures, mediastinitis, pleural effusions, aspiration pneumonia, adult respiratory distress syndrome, chest pain, fever, and bacteremia.

Endoscopic Variceal Band Ligation

Endoscopic band ligation is a technique similar to that used in band ligation of internal hemorrhoids. A rubber band is placed over a varix with subsequent thrombosis, sloughing, and fibrosis. Prospective, randomized, controlled trials show that endoscopic band ligation is equally effective as sclerotherapy in initial hemostasis and in reducing rebleeding rates for bleeding esophageal varices.[41, 42] Banding seems to have fewer local complications, especially in terms of esophageal strictures. Banding may be more technically difficult to perform than endoscopic sclerotherapy during active variceal bleeding. Banding also requires the use of an endoscopic overtube, which has been reported to cause proximal esophageal perforations during placement.

Surgical Portosystemic Shunts

Various surgical portosystemic shunts can be performed to reduce portal venous pressure. When compared with sclerotherapy, surgical shunts significantly decrease the rebleed rate but result in no survival difference.[43–47] Some groups suggest that survival can be improved by using the combination of endoscopic sclerotherapy and surgical shunt rescue for those who rebleed despite sclerotherapy.[44] Surgical shunts may be associated with increased hepatic encephalopathy. Surgical shunts do have an advantage over endoscopic techniques in terms of reducing portal hypertension to treat gastric variceal bleeding.

Radiologic Transjugular Intrahepatic Portosystemic Shunt (TIPS)

Transjugular intrahepatic portosystemic shunt (TIPS) is an interventional radiology procedure in which a percutaneously placed expandable metal stent is placed between the hepatic and portal veins, thereby creating an intrahepatic portosystemic shunt. TIPS seems to be effective in the short-term control of bleeding gastroesophageal varices.[48, 48a,b] Initially envisioned to be a bridge to transplant, it is becoming used more frequently in nontransplant settings. The actual utility of TIPS will depend on efficacy and safety results of future randomized, controlled trials comparing it with endoscopic or surgical therapy. As more long-term data become available, it appears that shunt obstruction or stenosis (and therefore the risk of recurrent variceal hemorrhage) occurs in up to 59% of patients after 2 years.[49] In addition, TIPS seems to induce hepatic encephalopathy in approximately 35% of patients.[50] Given the expense of this procedure, further trials will be needed to identify which patients will benefit most from this procedure.

OTHER BLEEDING UPPER GASTROINTESTINAL LESIONS

Esophagitis

In the acute setting, severe bleeding from esophagitis is treated medically with H_2 receptor antagonists followed by omeprazole when the patient is eating. There is generally no role for therapeutic endoscopy or surgery in the management of bleeding esophagitis.

Mallory-Weiss Tear

Mallory-Weiss tears are lacerations of mucosa at the gastroesophageal junction related to vomiting. These usually stop bleeding without therapy, but in cases of active bleeding, endoscopic therapy with bipolar electrocoagulation, heater probe, and injection therapy has been successful.[51–53] Rebleeding is uncommon after endoscopic therapy unless patients have portal hypertension.[52, 53]

Dieulafoy's Lesion

Dieulafoy's lesion is an aberrant, large submucosal artery that ruptures into the gastric lumen and causes massive bleeding. It usually occurs within 6 cm of the gastroesophageal junction. It is characterized by recurrent gastric hemorrhage with no source found unless active bleeding or visible vessel is noted. By definition, there is no surrounding ulceration. Endoscopic therapy has been reported to be successful. However, at least 50% of patients rebleed after endoscopic therapy.[54] The definitive treatment is surgical resection if patients rebleed after endoscopic therapy. The cause of this lesion is unknown.

Upper Gastrointestinal Angiodysplasia

Angiodysplasia are ectatic submucosal vessels that appear as cherry-red spiderlike lesions on endoscopy. The cause is unknown, but some patients have Osler-Weber-Rendu disease, chronic renal failure, and aortic stenosis. They can occur in the upper and lower GI tracts and small intestine. Patients usually present with self-limited or occult bleeding, but some may have massive bleeding. Endoscopic therapy can be used to stop bleeding and decrease transfusion rates.[55]

Upper Gastrointestinal Tumors

Upper GI tumors represent approximately 1% of severe upper GI bleeds. Bleeding usually occurs from large, ulcerated, malignant esophageal or gastric tumors.[56] Endoscopic hemostasis with heater probe, bipolar electrocoagulation, or injection can be used to control active bleeding and allow for medical stabilization of the patient before palliative surgical resection. The 1-year mortality rate is 90% for UCLA/CURE patients who have had a severe upper GI bleed resulting from bleeding tumor despite endoscopic or surgical treatment.[56]

Aortoenteric Fistulas

Aortoenteric fistulas generally occur in patients who have undergone abdominal aortic artery reconstructive surgery for aneurysms. The upper portion of the aortic graft often lies in direct contact with the second portion of the duodenum and results in fistulous communication. Aortic graft infection appears to be important in the pathogenesis of the fistula. Patients usually present with an initial self-limited bleed ("herald bleed") followed by an exsanguinating hemorrhage. Patients with an abdominal aortic artery graft and GI bleed should have urgent upper endoscopy to attempt to identify the graft or localize the blood in the duodenum. Because the level of the fistula varies, a colonoscope introduced orally may be necessary to examine further down the small bowel rather than the proximal duodenum. A computed tomographic scan rather than an angiogram may also help localize the fistula. Surgery is indicated in patients with suspected aortoenteric fistulas. The surgery consists of bypassing the fistula (or removing the graft and fistula) and performing axillary femoral bypass.

SEVERE LOWER GASTROINTESTINAL BLEEDING

Severe lower GI hemorrhage usually manifests itself as hematochezia. Diagnosis is generally by colonoscopy after urgent sulfate purge.[3] When internal hemorrhoids are excluded in adults, the most common causes of severe hematochezia are colonic angiomas and diverticulosis (Table 111–6). Rarely, technetium 99m red blood cell scanning or visceral angiography is necessary to diagnose a bleeding site.

Seventy per cent to 90% of ambulatory patients with acute lower GI bleeding will stop bleeding spontaneously. This allows for elective diagnosis and treatment in most cases. For the 10% to 30% of patients with ongoing or recurrent hematochezia, urgent diagnosis and treatment are required to control the bleeding. In a large series of patients at UCLA Medical Center and Wadsworth Veterans Administration Hospital, 64% of patients with severe hematochezia required some therapeutic intervention for control of continued bleeding or rebleeding.[3] Among these patients, 39% underwent endoscopic hemostasis, 1% had angiographic embolization, and 24% underwent surgery.

Colonic Angiomas

Colonic angiomas are often found in the right colon and can be missed unless patients are resuscitated and careful colonoscopic examination is performed. As with angiomas in other parts of the GI tract, they may be associated with chronic renal failure, aortic stenosis, or Osler-Weber-Rendu disease. Individual angiomas can be coagulated endoscopically with bipolar electrocoagulation, heater probe, or YAG laser.[57] In our experience, endoscopic coagulation can con-

TABLE 111–6. Cause of Severe Hematochezia in 80 Patients*

Lesion Site	*Percentage of Patients*
Colonic	74
Angiomas	30
Diverticulosis	16
Polyps or cancer	11
Colitis	9
Rectal lesions	4
Bleeding polyp stalk	3
Endometriosis	1
Upper Gastrointestinal	11
Small Bowel†	9
No Site Found	6

*Data taken from Jensen and Machicado.[3]
†Diagnosis of small bowel made when upper endoscopy and colonoscopy were negative but fresh blood or clots seen coming through the ileocecal valve.

trol colonic angioma bleeding in 80% of patients, although 20% of these patients will have rebleeding. With repeated treatments, patients successfully treated endoscopically have a significant decrease in the frequency of bleeding episodes and the number of units of packed red blood cells transfused per year and an increase in mean hematocrit.[57] Complications of colonoscopic coagulation of angiomas occur in less than 5% of patients and include perforation, postcoagulation syndrome (pain, fever, leukocytosis), and secondary bleeding from the ulcers induced by coagulation.

Colonic Diverticular Bleeding

Colonic diverticular bleeding is usually self-limited but may be severe. When barium enema was used for diagnosis of diverticular hemorrhage in 50 patients with hematochezia requiring transfusions, 58% of patients stopped bleeding during hospitalization and had no further bleeding, 20% had recurrent bleeding in the hospital, and 22% had ongoing bleeding requiring surgery.[58] Overall, in 70% of patients bleeding stopped with conservative management; of those patients, 22% experienced recurrent bleeding events.

Colonoscopic treatment of bleeding diverticula has been successfully performed with heater probe and bipolar electrocoagulation.[59, 60] These techniques are experimental, should be reserved for experienced therapeutic endoscopists, and need to be compared with surgical resection with long-term follow-up. However, they offer a promising new nonsurgical approach to management of diverticular bleeding in elderly patients who may have higher morbidity or mortality from surgery.

Colon Cancer

Focal ulceration of colonic tumors can occasionally present with severe lower GI bleeding. Diagnosis and initial hemostasis can be performed with a colonoscope. Subsequent therapy may be surgical resection or palliative endoscopic laser treatment.

Ischemic Bowel Disease

Ischemic bowel disease usually is secondary to a hypotensive event with decreased perfusion of the watershed area of the colon near the splenic flexure. However, ischemia may cause acute or chronic damage anywhere in the colon depending on the patient's collateral circulation. Patients generally present with acute hematochezia and, on urgent colonoscopy, have normal rectal mucosa with a sharp demarcation of swollen, friable tissue near the ischemic area. Ischemic lesions of the colon may resolve with medical therapy, may perforate, or may cause colonic strictures. The latter two complications require surgery.

Inflammatory Bowel Disease

Rarely, ulcerative colitis or Crohn's disease will present with massive hematochezia. Patients with a history of ulcerative colitis that has been quiescent but suddenly becomes more active should have stool studies to exclude an infectious cause. Colonoscopy with biopsies will assist in diagnosing inflammatory bowel disease. Acute medical therapy generally involves bowel rest, steroids, and possibly cyclosporine. Urgent colectomy is reserved for those patients refractory to several days of aggressive medical management.

ACKNOWLEDGMENT

The clinical and laboratory research reported in this chapter was supported in part by a National Institutes of Health (NIH) Core Grant NIDDK 41301 (Human Subjects Core) to the Center for Ulcer Research and Education, NIH RO1 Grant NIDDK 33273, and Veterans Administration Research Funds (merit review to Dennis M. Jensen).

References

1. Gilbert DA, Silverstein FE, Tedesco FJ, et al: The national ASGE survey on upper gastrointestinal bleeding: III. Endoscopy in upper gastrointestinal bleeding. Gastrointest Endosc 1981; 27:94–102.
2. Layne EA, Mellow MH, Lipman TO: Insensitivity of guaiac slide tests for the detection of blood in gastric juice. Ann Intern Med 1981; 94:774–776.
3. Jensen DM, Machicado GA: Diagnosis and treatment of severe hematochezia. Gastroenterology 1988; 95:1569–1574.
4. Katon RM: Complications of upper gastrointestinal endoscopy in the gastrointestinal bleeder. Dig Dis Sci 1981; 26(Suppl):47S–54S.
5. Andrus CH, Ponsky JL: The effects of irrigant temperature on upper gastrointestinal hemorrhage: A requiem for iced saline lavage (Editorial). Am J Gastroenterol 1987; 82:1062–1063.
6. Rudolph JP: Automated gastric lavage and a comparison of 0.9% normal saline solution and tap water irrigant. Ann Emerg Med 1985; 14:1156–1159.
7. Cutler JA, Mendeloff AI: Upper gastrointestinal bleeding: Nature and magnitude of this problem in the U.S. Dig Dis Sci 1981; 26(Suppl):90S–96S.
8. Allan R, Dykes P: A study on the factors influencing mortality rates from gastrointestinal hemorrhage. Q J Med 1976; 45:533–550.
9. Silverstein FE, Gilbert DA, Tedesco FJ, et al: The national ASGE survey of upper gastrointestinal bleeding: Part II. Clinical prognostic factors. Gastrointest Endosc 1981; 27:80–93.
10. Fleischer D: Etiology and prevalence of severe persistent upper gastrointestinal bleeding. Gastroenterology 1983; 84:538–543.
11. Silverstein FE, Gilbert DA, Tedesco FJ, et al: The national ASGE survey on upper gastrointestinal bleeding: Part I. Study design and baseline data. Gastrointest Endosc 1981; 27:73–79.
12. Kurata JH, Corboy ED: Current peptic ulcer time trends: An epidemiologic profile. J Clin Gastroenterol 1988; 10:259–268.
13. Zuckerman GR, Buse PE: Current medical and surgical management of nonvariceal upper gastrointestinal bleeding. Gastrointest Endosc Clin North Am 1991; 1:263–289.
14. Graham DY, Lew GM, Klein PD, et al: Effect of treatment of *Helicobacter pylori* infection on the recurrence of gastric ulcers or duodenal ulcers: A randomized controlled study. Ann Intern Med 1992; 116:705–708.
15. Freeman ML: The current endoscopic diagnosis and intensive care unit management of severe ulcer and other nonvariceal upper gastrointestinal hemorrhage. Gastrointest Endosc Clin North Am 1991; 1:209–239.
16. Laine L, Cohen H, Brodhead J, et al: Prospective evaluation of immediate versus delayed refeeding and prognostic value of endoscopy in patients with upper gastrointestinal hemorrhage. Gastroenterology 1992; 102:314–316.
17. Swain CP, Storey DW, Bown GS, et al: Nature of the bleeding vessel in recurrently bleeding gastric ulcers. Gastroenterology 1986; 90:595–608.
18. Johnston JH, Jensen DM, Auth D: Experimental comparison of endoscopic yttrium-aluminum-garnet laser, electrosurgery, and heater probe for canine gut arterial coagulation: Importance of compression and avoidance of erosion. Gastroenterology 1987; 92:1101–1108.
19. NIH Consensus Development Conference: Therapeutic endoscopy and bleeding ulcers. JAMA 1989; 262:1369–1372.
20. Jensen DM, Machicado GA, Kovacs TOG, et al: Controlled randomized study of heater probe and BICAP for hemostasis of severe ulcer bleeding (Abstract). Gastroenterology 1988; 94:A208.
21. Laine L: Multipolar electrocoagulation in the treatment of active upper gastrointestinal hemorrhage: A prospective controlled trial. N Engl J Med 1987; 316:1613–1617.
22. Laine L: Multipolar electrocoagulation in the treatment of peptic ulcers with nonbleeding visible vessels. Ann Intern Med 1989; 110:510–514.

23. Chung SC, Leung JW, Steel RJ, et al: Endoscopic injection of adrenaline for actively bleeding ulcers: A randomized trial. Br Med J 1988; 296:1631–1633.
24. Laine L: Multipolar electrocoagulation versus injection therapy in the treatment of bleeding peptic ulcers. Gastroenterology 1990; 99:1303–1306.
25. Chung SC, Leung JW, Sung JY, et al: Injection or heat probe for bleeding ulcers. Gastroenterology 1991; 100:33–37.
26. Jensen DM, Machicado GA, Kovacs TOG, et al: Current treatment and outcome of patients with bleeding "stress ulcers" (Abstract). Gastroenterology 1988; 94:A208.
27. Grahm DY, Smith JL: The course of patients after variceal hemorrhage. Gastroenterology 1981; 80:800–809.
28. Fogel MR, Knauer M, Andres LL, et al: Continuous intravenous vasopressin in active upper gastrointestinal bleeding: A placebo-controlled trial. Ann Intern Med 1982; 96:565–569.
29. Tsai YT, Lay CS, Lai KH, et al: Controlled trial of vasopressin plus nitroglycerin vs. vasopressin alone in the treatment of bleeding esophageal varices. Hepatology 1986; 6:406–409.
30. Gimson AES, Westaby D, Hegarty J, et al: A randomized trial of vasopressin and vasopressin plus nitroglycerin in the control of acute variceal hemorrhage. Hepatology 1986; 6:410–413.
31. Kravetz D, Bosch J, Teres J, et al: Comparison of intravenous somatostatin and vasopressin infusions in treatment of acute variceal hemorrhage. Hepatology 1984; 4:442–446.
32. Valenzuela JE, Schubert T, Fogel MR, et al: A multicenter, randomized, double-blind trial of somatostatin in the management of acute hemorrhage from esophageal varices. Hepatology 1989; 10:958–961.
33. Burroughs AK, McCormick PA, Hughes MD, et al: Randomized, double-blind, placebo-controlled trial of somatostatin for variceal bleeding: Emergency control and prevention of early variceal rebleeding. Gastroenterology 1990; 99:1388–1395.
34. Pitcher J: Safety and effectiveness of the modified Sengstaken-Blakemore tube: A prospective study. Gastroenterology 1971; 61:291–298.
35. Novis GH, Duys GO, Barbezat O, et al: Fibreoptic endoscopy and the use of the Sengstaken tube in acute gastrointestinal hemorrhage with portal hypertension and varices. Gut 1976; 17:258–263.
36. Conn HO, Simpson JA: Excessive mortality associated with balloon tamponade of bleeding varices: A critical reappraisal. JAMA 1967; 202:587–591.
37. Larson AW, Cohen J, Zweiban B, et al: Acute esophageal variceal sclerotherapy: Results of a prospective randomized controlled trial. JAMA 1986; 255:497–500.
38. Paquet KJ, Feussner H: Endoscopic sclerosis and esophageal balloon tamponade in acute hemorrhage from esophagogastric varices: A prospective controlled randomized trial. Hepatology 1985; 5:580–583.
39. The Copenhagen Esophageal Varices Sclerotherapy Project: Sclerotherapy after first variceal hemorrhage in cirrhosis: A randomized multicenter trial. N Engl J Med 1984; 311:1594–6000.
40. Westaby D, Hayes PC, Gimson AES, et al: Controlled clinical trial of injection sclerotherapy for active variceal bleeding. Hepatology 1989; 9:274–277.
41. Stiegmann GV, Goff JS, Michaletz-Ondey PA, et al: Endoscopic sclerotherapy as compared with endoscopic ligation for bleeding esophageal varices. N Engl J Med 1992; 326:1527–1532.
42. Laine L, El-Newihi HM, Migikovsky B, et al: Endoscopic ligation compared with sclerotherapy for the treatment of bleeding esophageal varices. Ann Intern Med 1993; 119:1–7.
43. Cello JP, Grendell JH, Crass RA, et al: Endoscopic sclerotherapy versus portacaval shunt in patients with severe cirrhosis and acute variceal hemorrhage: Long-term follow-up. N Engl J Med 1987; 316:11–15.
44. Henderson JM, Kutner MH, Millikan WJ, et al: Endoscopic variceal sclerosis compared with distal splenorenal shunt to prevent recurrent variceal bleeding in cirrhosis: A prospective, randomized trial. Ann Intern Med 1990; 112:262–269.
45. Teres J, Bordas JM, Bravo D, et al: Sclerotherapy vs. distal splenorenal shunt in the elective treatment of variceal hemorrhage: A randomized controlled trial. Hepatology 1987; 7:430–436.
46. Planas R, Boix J, Broggi M, et al: Portacaval shunt versus endoscopic sclerotherapy in the elective treatment of variceal hemorrhage. Gastroenterology 1991; 100:1078–1086.
47. Spina GP, Stantabrogio R, Opocher E, et al: Distal splenorenal shunt versus endoscopic sclerotherapy in the prevention of variceal rebleeding. Ann Surg 1990; 211:178–186.
48. Ring EJ, Lake JR, Roberts JP: Using transjugular intrahepatic portosystemic shunts to control variceal bleeding before liver transplantation. Ann Intern Med 1992; 116:304–309.
48a. LaBerge JM, Ring EJ, Gordon RL, et al: Creation of transjugular intrahepatic portosystemic shunts with the Wallstent endoprosthesis: Results in 100 patients. Radiology 1993; 187:413–420.
48b. Rossle M, Haag K, Ochs A, et al: The transjugular intrahepatic portosystemic stent-shunt procedure for variceal bleeding. N Engl J Med 1994; 330:165–171.
49. Peron JM, Rousseau H, Vinel JP, et al: Long term follow up study of transjugular intrahepatic portasystemic shunts (TIPS) (Abstract). Hepatology 1993; 18:102A.
50. Shonk T, Moats R, Lee JH, et al: Increased incidence of subclinical hepatic encephalopathy associated with TIPS procedures (Abstract). Gastroenterology 1993; 104:A994.
51. Laine L: Multipolar electrocoagulation in the treatment of active upper gastrointestinal tract hemorrhage: A prospective controlled trial. N Engl J Med 1987; 316:1613–1617.
52. Kovacs TOG, Jensen DM: Endoscopic diagnosis and treatment of bleeding Mallory-Weiss tears. Gastrointest Endosc Clin North Am 1991; 1:387–400.
53. Paquet KJ, Mercado-Diaz M, Kalk JF: Frequency, significance and therapy of the Mallory-Weiss syndrome in patients with portal hypertension. Hepatology 1990; 11:879–883.
54. Narayan S, Jensen DM, Randall GA, et al: Gastric bleeding from Dieulafoy's lesion versus peptic ulcer (Abstract). Gastrointest Endosc 1992; 38:239.
55. Machicado GA, Jensen DM: Upper gastrointestinal angiomata: Diagnosis and treatment. Gastrointest Endosc Clin North Am 1991; 1:241–262.
56. Savides TJ, Jensen DM, Randall GM, et al: The role of endoscopy in the diagnosis and treatment of severe UGI bleeding from tumors compared to peptic ulcers (Abstract). Gastrointest Endosc 1993; 39:288.
57. Jensen DM, Machicado GA: Endoscopic diagnosis and treatment of bleeding colonic angiomas and radiation telangiectasia. *In*: Prospectives in Colon and Rectal Surgery. Vol. 2. Schrock T (Ed). St. Louis, Quality Medical Publishing, 1989, pp 99–113.
58. McGuire HH, Haynes BW: Massive hemorrhage from diverticulosis of the colon: Guidelines for therapy based on bleeding patterns observed in fifty cases. Ann Surg 1972; 175:847–853.
59. Johnston J, Sones J: Endoscopic heart probe coagulation of the bleeding colonic diverticulum (Abstract). Gastrointest Endosc 1986; 32:160.
60. Savides TJ, Jensen DM: Colonoscopic hemostasis for recurrent diverticular hemorrhage associated with a visible vessel: A report of three cases. Gastrointest Endosc 1994; 40:70–73.

CHAPTER 112

Acute Gastrointestinal Disorders

Kenneth K. W. Lee, MD • Wolfgang H. Schraut, MD, PhD

Acutely evolving, life-threatening conditions may arise in the gastrointestinal tract anywhere along its length. Although quite varied in their clinical presentation and course, these emergencies can be described in several broad categories. Bleeding, the most common emergency, is discussed in Chapter 111; obstruction, perforation, vascular compromise, and fulminant infection or inflammation are subjects of this section. In the intensive care setting, management of these problems does not, in general, differ from that in other settings. In particular, therapeutic options and indications for surgical intervention are largely unchanged. However, recognition and diagnosis of these problems may be challenging. The patient's underlying condition and concurrent medications may render the patient's history and physical examination unreliable. Accordingly, a high index of suspicion must be maintained so that the problems are promptly recognized. Appropriate therapy for these emergencies can then be instituted in a timely manner, thereby minimizing morbidity and mortality.

OBSTRUCTION

Advancement of ingested food and endogenous secretions is one of the physiologic tasks of the gastrointestinal tract. At any site along the course of the gastrointestinal tract, impediment by a number of mechanisms may occur: obstruction by obturation (tumor, foreign body, food bolus), external compression (adhesion, volvulus, compression), and peristaltic paralysis (toxic or metabolic ileus). This halts or impairs the main task of the gastrointestinal tract (i.e., absorption) and may lead to fluid losses, electrolyte disturbances, loss of barrier function, vascular compromise, rupture of the bowel, and other life-threatening complications such as aspiration. The cause, presentation, evaluation, and treatment vary with the site of obstruction, and the outcome is influenced by an array of factors such as the patient's age and medical or surgical history.

Acute *esophageal obstruction* usually is precipitated by the ingestion and impaction of a foreign body. In adults, such obstruction is commonly associated with underlying esophageal disease such as a stricture or web, a tumor, or a motility disorder and may be caused by a poorly chewed food bolus or foreign objects such as coins and dentures. Poor dentition may also be a contributory factor in this setting. The obstructive event may be associated with a choking sensation and retrosternal discomfort that may mimic cardiac symptoms; dysphagia or odynophagia and profuse salivation may be noted.

When acute esophageal obstruction by a foreign body is suspected, radiologic evaluation, including lateral views, may be helpful to confirm, localize, and characterize the obstruction, if uncertain. Barium contrast studies may be used to evaluate obstruction by a foreign body, but caution must be exercised to avoid aspiration during the study; also, barium administration may obscure subsequent endoscopic procedures. Radiologic studies confirm esophageal perforation if this is suspected to have occurred in association with the obstruction.

Endoscopic examination is diagnostic and can be therapeutic for acute esophageal obstruction caused by a foreign body. Impacted foreign bodies can be readily identified and usually removed under direct vision; the instrumentation and techniques for these procedures are well described in appropriate reference sources. Particular note, however, should be made of the risks of aspiration and perforation during these procedures, and general anesthesia with endotracheal intubation and mechanical ventilation is a prudent choice for airway protection in children and in adults who are unable to tolerate or cooperate with the procedure. Perforation of the esophagus is the main concern during the procedure, particularly if a rigid instrument is used, or during manipulation and withdrawal of the foreign body if it is sharp or pointed, such as an open safety pin. Use of an overtube reduces the risk of perforation and decreases trauma and patient discomfort if multiple insertions of the endoscope are necessary. If perforation is suspected, an aggressive diagnostic stance is imperative (see later discussion). Finally, enzymatic digestion of impacted food material has also been widely used but should be avoided because esophageal perforation and aspiration have been reported with its use.

Obstruction from intrinsic esophageal disease is typically more gradual than obstruction from foreign body ingestion. Common causes include esophageal neoplasms, benign strictures, and congenital abnormalities such as webs. Motility disorders such as achalasia may also result in functional esophageal obstruction. Obstruction caused by intrinsic esophageal disease typically presents as progressive dysphagia; as the degree of obstruction worsens, liquids and finally the patient's own saliva cannot be swallowed, often leading to recurrent episodes of aspiration. Accompanying complaints may include odynophagia, hematemesis, and weight loss.

Evaluation in these patients is directed at identifying the underlying abnormality of the esophagus and is centered on endoscopic and radiographic evaluation. The specific nature of the abnormality then guides further studies; for example, a computed tomographic (CT) scan is the most informative test for esophageal malignancies, whereas esophageal manometry studies are indicated if a motility disorder such as achalasia is suspected.

Treatment or prevention of aspiration and maintenance of the patient's nutritional state are of primary importance in patients with any form of esophageal obstruction. Antibiotic therapy should be initiated if aspiration pneumonia exists. Placement of the patient in an upright position and drainage of the esophagus proximal to the level of obstruction may help to reduce the risk of subsequent aspiration. When the obstruction is not complete, oral nutrition may be possible or passage of a feeding tube beyond the site of obstruction will permit enteral feeding; otherwise, parenteral nutrition becomes necessary. Ultimately, however, prevention of aspiration and restoration of adequate enteral nutrition are best accomplished by treatment of the specific underlying esophageal problem.

Intraluminal *obstruction of the stomach* by mass lesions or bezoars is rarely an acute event and is readily diagnosed by endoscopic and radiologic means; therapies follow established guidelines. Obstruction of the gastric outlet may result from bulky intraluminal or intramural tumors arising in the antrum or prepyloric region or, more commonly, from chronic peptic ulcer disease with pyloric or duodenal scarring; less commonly, obstruction may result from anastomotic tumor recurrences or ulcers. Obstruction of the gastric outlet presents as nonbilious emesis, and often a history of peptic ulcer disease is elicited. Upper endoscopy readily confirms the diagnosis of gastric outlet obstruction and permits biopsies to determine the cause of the obstruction.

Urgent intervention to relieve the obstruction is unwarranted because there is no risk of infarction. Instead, initial treatment should consist of gradual correction of fluid and electrolyte abnormalities that have resulted from frequent emesis, and gastric decompression to prevent further emesis and aspiration. Decompression by a nasogastric tube in conjunction with suppression of gastric acid secretion reduces the edema, which is usually superimposed on the chronic irreversible partial obstruction of the outlet channel. Once evaluation of the obstruction has been completed, definitive treatment can be performed electively.

Volvulus of the stomach may occur acutely with complete obstruction or chronically with partial or intermittent obstruction of the stomach. Laxity, disruption, or absence of the suspensory attachments of the stomach permits rotation of the greater curvature toward the lesser curvature along the longitudinal axis of the stomach (organoaxial volvulus) or of the pylorus toward the cardia (mesenteroaxial volvulus). Abnormalities of adjacent organs may predispose to volvulus of the stomach; among these, hiatal or paraesophageal hernias, congenital diaphragmatic hernias, and eventration or rupture of the diaphragm are particularly common.

Acute volvulus typically produces epigastric pain and is associated with nonbilious vomiting followed by retching, gastric distention, and inability to pass a nasogastric tube. This triad (Borchardt's triad) is pathognomonic for gastric volvulus, and little further diagnostic evaluation is necessary. An electrocardiogram should be obtained to rule out myocardial ischemia as the cause of the patient's epigastric pain. Plain abdominal x-ray films will demonstrate a markedly dilated stomach in which a double air-fluid level is seen. Barium studies are usually not warranted, because there is significant risk of regurgitation and aspiration, and little barium is able to pass through the obstruction at the cardia. In contrast, the presentation of chronic gastric volvulus may be quite varied. Pain may be absent or variable in intensity; the severity of obstructive symptoms may also be quite variable. Early satiety, epigastric fullness, and epigastric pressure are frequent complaints. With chronic volvulus, barium studies are often undertaken to evaluate chronic upper abdominal complaints, and inasmuch as obstruction is incomplete, the volvulus is often defined.

Acute gastric volvulus results in a closed-loop obstruction and may lead to ischemia and infarction of the stomach and consequently requires prompt correction. Vigorous fluid resuscitation and correction of electrolyte abnormalities should be initiated; persistent efforts to pass a nasogastric tube should be avoided to prevent perforation of the stomach or esophagus. Urgent laparotomy must be performed. At operation, the gastric volvulus should be reduced and gangrenous segments resected; the stomach should be transfixed and coexistent abnormalities such as a diaphragmatic hernia repaired to minimize the risk of recurrence. With chronic volvulus, the absence of complete obstruction and risk of infarction permits more deliberate evaluation of the situation and the overall health and operative risk of the patient and less urgent operative intervention if the patient's condition allows such delay.

Acute mechanical *small-bowel obstruction* may arise from a wide range of causes that vary with age; for example, obstruction caused by intussusception is common in infancy and early childhood, whereas obstruction from adhesions or malignancy is more common in adulthood. Although the specific cause and site of the obstruction bear on the clinical presentation, in general, small-bowel obstruction presents as nausea, vomiting, crampy abdominal pain, abdominal distention, and absent or decreased passage of flatus or stool. On auscultation, the typical alterations of bowel sounds support the diagnosis of small-bowel obstruction. Plain abdominal x-ray examination demonstrates the telltale air-fluid levels or fluid-filled bowel loops. Paralytic ileus, in contrast, also presents with abdominal distention but is less likely to be associated with crampy abdominal pain or hyperactive bowel sounds, and plain abdominal radiographs typically demonstrate generalized bowel distention.

Regardless of the cause, the initial management of a small-bowel obstruction is uniform and should consist of fluid resuscitation, correction of electrolyte abnormalities, and decompression of the gastrointestinal tract. Placement of central venous and Foley catheters may be useful for monitoring the adequacy of the fluid resuscitation. Nasogastric and intestinal (e.g., Cantor or Miller-Abbott) tubes each have their advocates for the treatment of small-bowel obstruction. In our own practice, we use nasogastric tubes for decompression, although we occasionally use intestinal tubes for treatment of partial obstructions. Serial examinations and radiographic studies should demonstrate whether the obstruction is resolving.

Despite numerous reports, to date no single test or any combination has proven reliable for determining whether a complete mechanical obstruction is associated with strangulation of the bowel. Surgical intervention to relieve the bowel obstruction and to correct the underlying abnormality (e.g., lysis of adhesions, hernia repair, reduction or resection of an intussusception) is, therefore, indicated for the complete mechanical bowel obstruction that fails to resolve within a relatively short interval.

Certain exceptions to this policy deserve mention. Treatment of obstruction secondary to active Crohn's disease should be directed against the underlying inflammatory process. Although this approach will frequently lead to resolution of the obstruction, the possibility that the obstruction is not caused by inflammation but rather by a mechanical process must be borne in mind because it will dictate earlier operative intervention. Obstruction caused by malignancy should be treated similarly to obstruction from other causes unless carcinomatosis is known to be present; in this case, continued nonoperative management may be appropriate. Finally, more extended nonoperative management may also be warranted in the setting of an early postoperative bowel obstruction or of radiation injury to the intestinal tract.

Colonic obstruction usually presents as abdominal distention and obstipation and most commonly results from primary tumors, inflammation caused by diverticular disease, or colonic volvulus; differentiation among these causes is generally straightforward because the clinical presentations and x-ray findings are distinctive. Obstruction associated with acute diverticulitis can initially be managed by nonoperative means (bowel rest and antibiotics). In this setting, strangulation is rare, and the obstruction may resolve as the acute inflammation subsides. In contrast, obstruction secondary to a colonic tumor will not regress and requires surgical treatment; the timing of surgery is dependent on the completeness of the obstruction. If the obstruction is incomplete, preparation of the bowel may be possible, thereby permitting resection followed by a primary anastomosis; otherwise, resection and exteriorization may be necessary. Occasionally, the condition of the patient precludes definitive treatment of a primary tumor. Instead, proximal diversion of the fecal stream by means of an ileostomy or colostomy is first undertaken, and resection of the obstructing tumor is deferred to a subsequent operation.

Volvulus of the colon may affect the cecum or sigmoid colon and rarely the transverse colon or splenic flexure. As with volvulus elsewhere along the gastrointestinal tract, volvulus of the colon carries a risk of vascular compromise; consequently, prompt recognition and treatment are mandatory. The presentation of a sigmoid volvulus resembles that of a distal colonic obstruction secondary to carcinoma or diverticulitis: crampy abdominal pain, obstipation and absence of flatus associated with abdominal distention, and eventually nausea and vomiting. Tenderness, tympany, and in some instances a tender mass are found on physical examination. Plain radiographs are frequently diagnostic and demonstrate a markedly dilated sigmoid loop, often appearing as the bent inner tube or upside-down U sign. Contrast enema studies may aid in the diagnosis of a sigmoid volvulus but must be avoided if gangrene of the colon is suspected.

Once sigmoid volvulus is diagnosed, endoscopic reduction and decompression should be attempted using a rigid or flexible sigmoidoscope. If the volvulus can be successfully reduced, a rectal tube should be placed into the sigmoid colon to decrease the risk of early recurrent volvulus. Unless the operative risk of the patient is prohibitive, elective sigmoid resection with primary anastomosis should then be undertaken because the risk of recurrent volvulus after decompression is 35% to 90%, and the mortality after decompression alone is 14%. Urgent operation must be undertaken if the volvulus cannot be reduced endoscopically, if after reduction the colonic mucosa does not appear viable, or if clinical signs develop suggestive of colonic ischemia. At operation, the volvulus, if still present, is reduced; to prevent recurrence of the volvulus, the redundant sigmoid colon is resected irrespective of its viability. Because the colon is unprepared, creation of a colostomy rather than primary anastomosis is a prudent choice. Fixation of the sigmoid colon may be considered as an alternative to resection because it avoids the need for a colostomy, but this approach has been associated with an increased risk of recurrent volvulus. The recent advances in laparoscopic surgery may provide less extensive, better tolerated approaches to this problem. If viability of the colon is confirmed during laparoscopy, preparation of the bowel followed by resection with primary anastomosis may be considered. If endoscopic reduction of the volvulus has been unsuccessful, a laparoscopic approach may be considered; however, manipulation of the distended sigmoid volvulus may be a formidable undertaking.

Cecal volvulus may involve the terminal ileum and cecum or a fold of the cecum alone, referred to as a cecal bascule. In contrast to a sigmoid volvulus, a cecal volvulus typically presents with the signs and symptoms of a distal small-bowel obstruction. Plain radiographs characteristically demonstrate the markedly dilated cecum, which, because of a lengthy mobile mesentery, may be displaced into the left upper abdomen. Contrast studies may confirm the presence of the volvulus but again must be used with caution to avoid perforation of the colon.

Whereas endoscopic reduction and evaluation of the colon are often successful with sigmoid volvulus, treatment of a cecal volvulus is primarily surgical. After appropriate resuscitation of the patient, urgent laparotomy should be undertaken. The volvulus is reduced, and if the bowel is not viable, resection is performed. Otherwise, measures to prevent a recurrent volvulus should be considered. These include creation of a cecostomy (a less favored option because it is associated with a significant recurrence rate as well as frequent local complications directly related to the cecostomy), resection of the redundant cecum (which prevents recurrent volvulus but risks anastomotic complications), and wide fixation of the cecum to the parietal peritoneum.

Massive acute colonic distention without mechanical obstruction may mimic true mechanical obstruction of the colon. This condition, referred to as pseudo-obstruction of the colon or Ogilvie's syndrome, is particularly likely among hospitalized patients and must be recognized and distinguished from mechanical obstruction of the colon because surgical intervention is usually not necessary. Many precipitating or associated conditions have been identified. As with obstruction of the colon, pseudo-obstruction presents with marked abdominal distention; however, other features such as colicky abdominal pain, nausea and vomiting, and fever and leukocytosis are frequently absent. Physical examination commonly reveals a soft abdomen with minimal tenderness, absence of peritoneal irritation, and absence of obstructive bowel sounds.

The diagnosis of pseudo-obstruction of the colon can usually be confirmed with plain abdominal radiographs; these demonstrate marked colonic dilatation, often predominantly present in the ascending and transverse colon. Small-bowel dilatation is absent unless the ileocecal valve is incompetent. If mechanical obstruction cannot be confidently excluded (e.g., sigmoid volvulus), radiographic study with water-soluble contrast may confirm the suspected diagnosis of pseudo-obstruction.

In the absence of peritoneal irritation or other signs questioning the viability of the bowel, nonoperative therapy is indicated and involves nasogastric decompression, intravenous fluids, and withdrawal of medications that may predispose to impaired intestinal motility and heighten distention, such as narcotics, neuroleptics, and anticholinergics. Placement of a rectal tube may be helpful, particularly if colonic distention involves the rectosigmoid colon. Resolution of the pseudo-obstruction should be followed by serial physical examinations and radiographs. If the dilatation fails to respond to these measures, then decompression of the colon should be performed by means of colonoscopy.

If peritoneal irritation is present or the viability of the colon is in question, prompt laparotomy and resection of questionable bowel segments should be undertaken after appropriate resuscitation. If the colon is viable, intraoperative decompression of the colon should be performed. Placement of a cecostomy tube can accomplish this and be used to prevent subsequent colonic distention, but local complications may result. In a patient with a history of recurrent pseudo-obstruction, consideration should be given to performing an abdominal colectomy with ileosigmoid or ileorectal anastomosis.

PERFORATION

Perforations may occur along the length of the gastrointestinal tract. With the exception of anastomotic fistulas, perforation of the esophagus is most frequently caused by instrumentation of the esophagus. Although perforation may rarely result from passage of nasogastric tubes and other catheters, most commonly it occurs during diagnostic endoscopic procedures or during dilatation of esophageal strictures. Technical difficulties, unsuspected esophageal disease, prior surgery on or in the vicinity of the esophagus, general anesthesia, and an uncooperative patient all heighten the risk of perforation during passage of an instrument. When dilating esophageal strictures, failure to pass a guide wire or the initial dilator under direct vision or fluoroscopic guidance and failure to dilate strictures progressively also increase the risk of esophageal disruption. Pneumatic dilatation for achalasia is also associated with perforation of the esophagus.

Spontaneous perforation of the esophagus may occur in the absence of underlying esophageal disease (Boerhaave's syndrome). Conditions usually associated with such an event are a full stomach, forceful spontaneous or induced vomiting and retching, and transient obstruction of a segment of the esophagus leading to generation of high intraesophageal pressures. Typically, such spontaneous perforations occur in the distal third of the esophagus. Spontaneous perforation of the esophagus may also occur in the absence of such factors; the physiologic basis for such perforations is unclear. Perforation may occur as a result of underlying esophageal disease (e.g., tumors or infections), although penetration into adjacent structures with fistula formation is more common. Carcinomas of the esophagus, for example, may erode into the tracheobronchial tree, and Barrett's ulcers arising in the setting of chronic gastroesophageal reflux may penetrate into surrounding tissues. On rare occasions, such ulcers may penetrate into the pericardium or even the heart or aorta, with catastrophic consequences. Finally, perforation of the esophagus may occur in association with ingested foreign bodies or corrosive substances or as a result of trauma; as is predictable, esophageal perforation is more common with external penetrating rather than blunt trauma.

With acute intrapleural perforation, the clinical course is typically one of rapidly progressive sepsis, whereas mediastinal perforations may initially follow a more gradual course. Intra-abdominal perforation of the distal esophagus presents in the usual manner of an intraperitoneal perforation and peritonitis (see later discussion). Pain, the most common symptom associated with esophageal perforation, is usually severe and substernal or upper abdominal; later the pain may radiate to the back between the scapulae. Signs of progressive sepsis and shock, dyspnea, dysphagia or odynophagia, cervical crepitus, and a mediastinal crunch are frequently found. Plain radiographs usually demonstrate a pleural effusion, which may increase rapidly with intrapleural perforation. The aspirate is typically brown, foul smelling, and rich in amylase, and, if perforation has occurred in the setting of violent postprandial vomiting, it may contain food materials. Plain radiographs may also demonstrate mediastinal widening and air (Fig. 112–1). The diagnosis and localization of an esophageal perforation can best be made by means of a barium swallow examination; if the study is nondiagnostic but clinical suspicion remains high, a repeat examination should be considered. Esophagoscopy is less sensitive and may result in further disruption of the esophagus.

The differential diagnosis of esophageal perforation is broad and includes acute myocardial infarction, dissecting or ruptured thoracic aortic aneurysm, perforated duodenal or gastric ulcer, acute pancreatitis, and acute pericarditis. However, because the outcome and management of esophageal perforations are strongly influenced by the timeliness of diagnosis and institution of therapy, a rapid diagnosis is imperative. Any patient in whom unexplained pain, fever, or other signs of possible perforation develop after esophageal instrumentation or surgery or after forceful vomiting must be evaluated promptly. Penetrating trauma in proximity to the esophagus (e.g., injuries to the midchest or that cross the mediastinum) mandates evaluation to rule out esophageal injury.

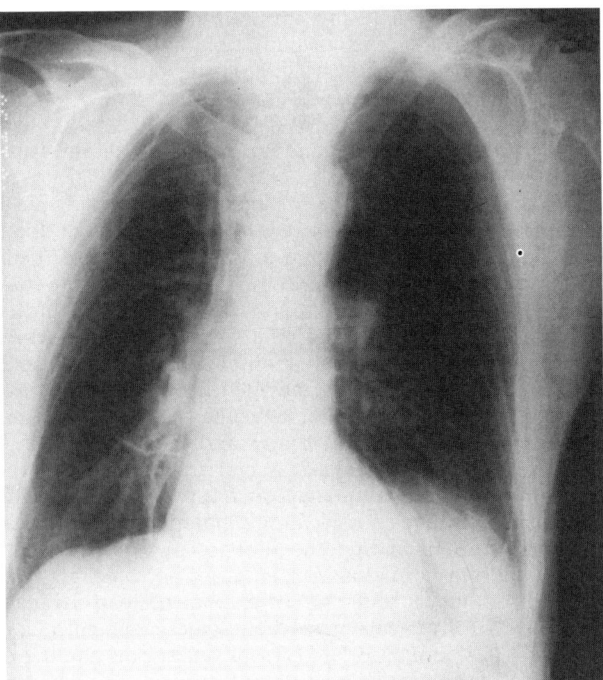

Figure 112–1. Mediastinal air resulting from perforation of the esophagus during attempted esophageal dilatation for achalasia.

With few exceptions, esophageal perforations require surgical treatment. The goals of treatment are to prevent further soilage from the perforation, to treat soilage that has already occurred, and, if possible, to re-establish gastrointestinal continuity for enteral alimentation. When the perforation is recognized before extensive local inflammation and infection have evolved and there is no underlying esophageal disease, primary closure of the defect can often be performed; techniques that buttress the repair such as mobilization of pleural or pericardial flaps may be useful. An esophagectomy is a rarely chosen option but may be appropriate to treat underlying esophageal disease (e.g., perforated esophageal cancer) when the perforation is promptly recognized. However, when the diagnosis of esophageal perforation is delayed, attempts at definitive repair or treatment carry increased risks of failure, morbidity, and mortality. In this setting, diversion of oral secretions by means of a cervical esophagostomy and extensive mediastinal and/or pleural drainage combined with antibiotic therapy is most appropriate. In instances in which reflux of gastric contents into the perforated esophagus is a concern, the gastroesophageal junction should be closed. To provide a route for long-term enteral alimentation, a feeding tube should also be placed. If esophageal reconstruction by a gastric pull-up is anticipated, then a jejunostomy tube rather than a gastrostomy tube is preferable.

Intraperitoneal perforation, whether originating from the stomach, duodenum, or intestine, results in soilage and irritation of the peritoneal cavity (i.e., peritonitis); the clinical picture ranging from localized discomfort to overwhelming sepsis in a moribund patient obviously depends on the extent to which the process is localized or generalized. A free intraperitoneal rupture gives rise to diffuse peritonitis; the onset of symptoms is characteristically quite abrupt, and in many instances the patient can relate the exact onset of symptoms. In contrast, contained perforation, such as a posterior perforation of a gastric ulcer into the lesser sac or perforation of the appendix localized to the right lower quadrant of the abdomen, frequently evolves into an abscess with much more limited symptoms and findings. Sudden worsening of the patient's condition and complaints occurs if the walled-off process suddenly disrupts.

The diagnosis of intraperitoneal perforation, primarily a clinical diagnosis, is often confirmed by plain radiographs. Upright or decubitus radiographs are most useful for demonstrating free intraperitoneal air. With perforation into the lesser sac, haziness in the midabdomen ("football" sign) may be evident. With retroperitoneal perforations, air may outline the kidneys or other retroperitoneal structures and may dissect into the mediastinum and subcutaneous tissues (Fig. 112–2). If perforation is suspected but cannot be verified with plain radiographs, then contrast studies using water-soluble contrast may be helpful; these studies should also be obtained if expectant nonoperative management of a perforation is being considered (see later discussion). CT scan is also a sensitive means of detecting small amounts of free air or extravasated contrast and is particularly useful in the evaluation of acute abdominal complaints when history, physical examination, and plain radiographs are not diagnostic.

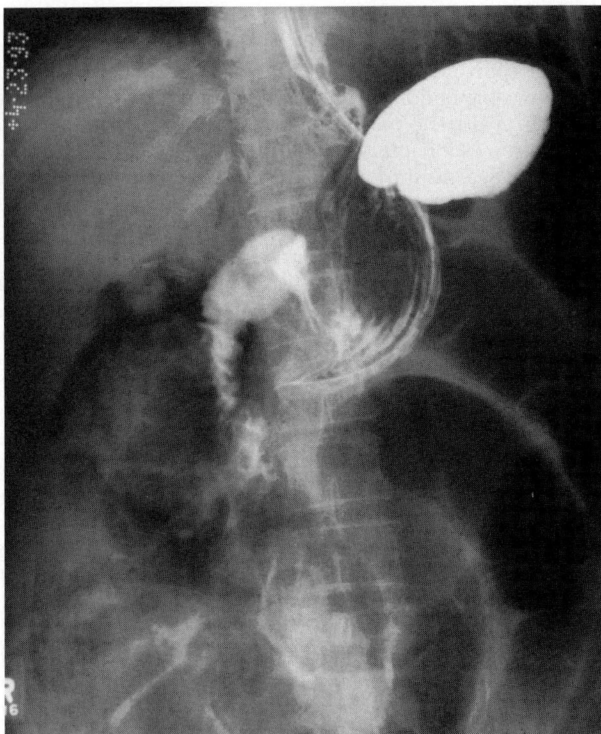

Figure 112–2. Extensive retroperitoneal air in the subhepatic region resulting from perforation of the duodenum secondary to endoscopic sphincterotomy.

Once intraperitoneal perforation of a hollow viscus is suspected or confirmed, prompt fluid resuscitation and antibiotic therapy are instituted to prepare the patient for urgent laparotomy if diffuse peritonitis is a threat. In most instances, precise preoperative localization of the site of perforation is unnecessary because the site can be readily determined intraoperatively. Operative management is aimed at stopping further leakage and clearing the peritoneal cavity of contaminants as much as possible. Relaparotomy, open packing, and continued lavage are subsequent measures that may aid in this effort. The site of perforation, the extent of peritonitis, and the general health of the patient will determine the specific measures to be taken and ultimately the final outcome. A prolonged course of care in the intensive care unit leading to multiple organ system failure and death is still not uncommon.

CT- or ultrasound-guided percutaneous drainage techniques have become the standard approach for perforations associated with contained collections in the absence of diffuse peritonitis. Management by percutaneous drainage may result in a cutaneous fistula, which can be dealt with later in an elective surgical procedure; if resection is required, this approach often avoids the need for a staged procedure and creation of an enterostoma. Failure of percutaneous drainage to control the focus of sepsis adequately will require operative intervention.

Nonoperative management of perforated peptic ulcers has been successful in carefully selected patients in whom the perforation has spontaneously sealed. This approach has generally been limited to patients judged to be poor operative risks in whom diffuse peritonitis is absent and sealing of the perforation site has been verified by water-soluble contrast studies. Careful selection and monitoring of patients managed in this manner are mandatory.

Acute perforation of the rectum has customarily been treated by abdominal exploration, diversion of the fecal stream, and wide drainage of the presacral space. However, with a limited injury and minimal contamination, primary repair may be undertaken. Should the perforation be below the peritoneal reflection and a rectal contrast study fail to demonstrate free extravasation, then antibiotic therapy and expectant management may be pursued in the otherwise healthy individual. If a low pelvic or perineal abscess should develop, then this can be drained percutaneously or by incision. Rarely, a previously unrecognized colonic or rectal perforation presents as an infection of the upper leg as a result of the process dissecting downward into the leg (Fig. 112–3). In these instances, identification and treatment of the perforation must be combined with aggressive treatment of the soft-tissue infection. History and physical examination supplemented by CT scan, transrectal or transvaginal ultrasound, or proctosigmoidoscopy will detect and delineate these and other rectal perforations.

VASCULAR COMPROMISE

Ischemia of the gastrointestinal tract may result from arterial embolization or arterial or venous thrombosis. As the numbers of critically ill patients increase and because critical illness is often accompanied by hemodynamic instability requiring the use of vasoactive medications, nonocclusive ischemia has become an increasingly common cause of visceral ischemia. Although all parts of the gastrointestinal tract may be subject to ischemia, ischemia in the distribution of the superior mesenteric artery (i.e., affecting the small and large intestine), is clinically most important; ischemia of the esophagus or stomach is uncommon and usually reflects global ischemia occurring as a preterminal event.

Acute small intestine ischemia typically presents with abdominal pain that is most often centrally located. Increased peristaltic activity may be present and be associated with vomiting and diarrhea. Bleeding per rectum is usually not an initial event but may develop later once mucosal necrosis has occurred. Physical examination is often unimpressive, giving rise to the classic axiom that the patient's complaints are out of proportion to the physical findings; the presence of peritoneal irritation may signify full-thickness necrosis of the bowel. If untreated, systemic signs of a catastrophe gradually evolve: progressive tachycardia, hypotension, hypovolemia resulting from massive fluid sequestration, respiratory decompensation, and eventually multiple organ system failure.

The diagnosis of mesenteric ischemia may be difficult to confirm without laparotomy, and the clinician must maintain a high degree of suspicion for this diagnosis. Plain radiographs are of little help in the diagnosis of acute mesenteric ischemia. Intramural or intraportal air is a diagnostic but late finding of intestinal infarction. A CT scan, which may be obtained in the evaluation of the patient's abdominal pain, may demonstrate bowel wall thickening; intramural or intravascular air may also be seen. If prompt exploration after resuscitation is not mandated by the patient's physical findings, immediate visceral angiography may be helpful in establishing the diagnosis. If an embolus is demonstrated, operative embolectomy should be undertaken. In the absence of this finding, the utility of angiography is less clear because a normal angiogram does not preclude nonocclusive ischemia, and the presence of occlusive disease does not confirm the diagnosis of mesenteric ischemia. Nevertheless, in the appropriate clinical setting, the finding of severe occlusive disease may sway the clinician in favor of this diagnosis. In advanced ischemic states, leukocytosis and metabolic acidosis commonly are present, as are elevations

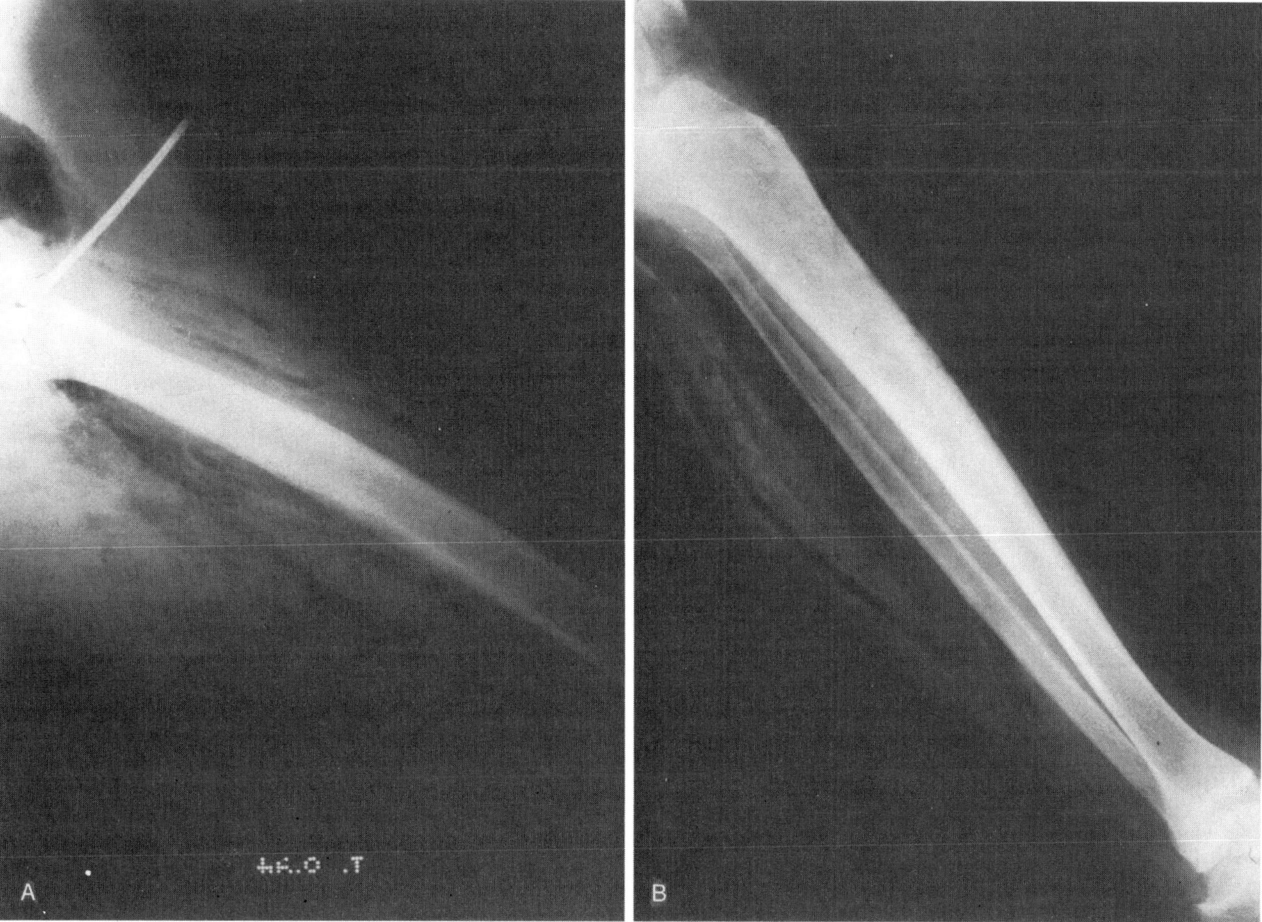

Figure 112–3. Gas in the soft tissues of the upper (*A*) and lower (*B*) leg resulting from perforation of the sigmoid colon with dissection into the leg and subsequent infection by gas-producing organisms.

of the serum amylase, lactate dehydrogenase, alkaline phosphatase, and phosphate levels. However, neither these tests separately nor collectively nor other laboratory tests have proven sufficiently reliable to diagnose timely and accurately the presence of intestinal ischemia when the bowel is still salvageable.

The initial management of the patient with acute mesenteric ischemia consists of fluid resuscitation, correction of electrolyte and other metabolic abnormalities, and initiation of antibiotic therapy. A decision regarding surgical exploration must then be made. Some investigators advocate that, in the absence of physical findings dictating operative intervention, initial trials of intra-arterial infusion of vasodilators such as papaverine, particularly if nonocclusive mesenteric ischemia is suspected, or of thrombolytic agents can be attempted. With this approach, prompt exploration is warranted if the patient's condition worsens. A limitation of this approach is that focal areas of bowel necrosis may go undetected until perforation and peritonitis ensue. Others advocate early operation in all patients in whom the diagnosis of acute mesenteric ischemia has been made. With this approach, angiography may not be necessary because it delays operative intervention; if obtained, it serves primarily as a guide should embolectomy or revascularization through a bypass procedure of the mesenteric circulation be performed.

With the increasing effectiveness of both parenteral and enteral nutrition, the short-gut syndrome, the consequence of loss of a major portion of the intestinal tract, has become a manageable problem. Thus, an aggressive surgical approach should be considered for most patients with intestinal ischemia. At operation, intestine that is obviously not viable is resected. If additional compromised but potentially salvageable segments of intestine are encountered, occluded vessels that can be thrombectomized or bypassed should be sought. If the viability of the remaining intestine cannot be determined with confidence using such methods as fluorescein dye injection and Doppler ultrasound or if the patient exhibits continuing signs of hemodynamic instability or mesenteric ischemia, a second-look laparotomy should be performed 24 hours later to re-evaluate the intestinal segments in question. Postoperative care is directed toward control of infection, maintenance of fluid and electrolyte balance, and nutritional support.

Colonic ischemia may result from outright thrombotic or embolic vascular occlusion or from low-flow states that may occur perioperatively or in the course of severe illnesses. Additionally, colonic ischemia may result from interruption of the arterial blood supply as a consequence of aortic, and less commonly colonic or gastric, surgery. Most commonly, ischemic colitis affects the left colon; the splenic flexure and sigmoid colon, which are watershed areas between the distributions of the superior and inferior mesenteric arteries and the inferior mesenteric and iliac arteries, are particularly susceptible to injury. Ischemic colitis associated with aortic surgery usually results from occlusion or ligation of the inferior mesenteric artery in the absence of adequate collateral flow, and accordingly, the sigmoid colon is particularly at risk; rectal ischemia is quite uncommon but may occur with coexisting disease or interruption of the internal iliac arteries. With prolonged periods of hypotension and hypoperfusion, as may be seen in the intensive care setting, ischemia of the right colon or entire colon is more frequent.

Ischemic colitis usually presents as lower, often left-sided, cramping abdominal pain associated with diarrhea. The diarrhea is usually bloody, and this particular finding after aortic surgery strongly suggests the possibility of colonic ischemia. However, substantial blood loss is uncommon and diarrhea without bleeding may also occur. Abdominal tenderness and distention, ileus, fever, and leukocytosis are other common findings.

Endoscopic evaluation is particularly useful as a means of confirming the diagnosis of ischemic colitis. Moreover, it provides an assessment of the severity of the ischemic changes and may aid in the identification or exclusion of other diagnoses such as infectious colitis. Endoscopic findings may range from mucosal edema to frank mucosal necrosis. Plain radiographs may show characteristic thumbprinting of the colon resulting from submucosal hemorrhage; with severe ischemia, intramural or intraportal air may be seen. Contrast radiographs may more readily detect mucosal thumbprinting but add little beyond endoscopy to the diagnostic evaluation. In the chronic setting, barium contrast studies may demonstrate colonic strictures. However, such strictures generally require endoscopic evaluation to exclude an underlying malignancy despite an antecedent history of colonic ischemia. CT scan findings of colonic ischemia are similar to those observed for mesenteric ischemia. Angiography generally is not useful for the evaluation of colonic ischemia because patency of the major vessels does not exclude ischemia, whereas vessel occlusion is often inconsequential.

Immediate operative intervention is indicated when frank gangrene or peritonitis is present. In the absence of these findings, initial management should be supportive. Low-flow states that may induce or worsen colonic ischemia must be corrected. Intravenous fluids and antibiotics should be administered and bowel rest instituted while careful observation is continued. If the mucosal abnormalities are severe on the initial endoscopic examination, early repeat endoscopy is warranted. In most instances, the ischemia reverses without sequelae. However, deterioration of the patient's condition warrants prompt surgical intervention. Resection of the ischemic colon segment with creation of a temporary stoma is a prudent choice. Intervention before colonic perforation has occurred will substantially reduce overall morbidity and mortality.

INFLAMMATION

A broad range of inflammatory processes may affect the gastrointestinal tract. Although the condition and treatment of the patient in the intensive care setting may obscure diagnosis of these processes, their treatment, in general, follows standard guidelines and, with few exceptions, is initially nonoperative.

Uncomplicated peptic esophagitis, gastritis, duodenitis, and frank ulceration present as pain and are treated with acid-reducing (histamine receptor antagonists, antacids, proton-pump inhibitors) or cytoprotective medications. In the intensive care setting, prophylaxis against these conditions should be routinely used. When complications such as bleeding, perforation, or obstruction arise, specific interventions, often surgical, are required.

Several conditions may cause focal inflammation of the intestine. Although most common in the first two decades of life, acute appendicitis may occur at any age. Particularly among the elderly or when the appendix lies in a retrocecal position, its presentation is often atypical, and it should be considered as a possible source of unexplained sepsis. Treatment is primarily surgical. Focal small-bowel inflammation or bleeding may result from a Meckel's diverticulum with associated ectopic, acid-producing gastric mucosa. Although radionuclide studies may aid in the diagnosis of this condition, the diagnosis is frequently made at the time of operation performed for suspected acute appendicitis, perforation, or bleeding. Diverticular inflammation may occur throughout the intestine but most often affects the sigmoid or descending colon, presenting as left lower abdominal pain and tenderness; however, right-sided abdominal pain and tenderness may result from right-sided diverticular disease or from a redundant diseased sigmoid colon. In the absence of complications, initial treatment of acute diverticulitis consists of bowel rest and antibiotic therapy. If the acute process fails to resolve on such therapy or if complications such as free perforation, abscess formation, or fistulization (e.g., colovesical) develop, then operative intervention is warranted.

Perianal processes such as perirectal abscesses, fistulas in ano, hemorrhoids, and anal fissures are readily diagnosed by direct inspection, palpation, or anoscopic examination. These processes can be managed by the standard means of bowel regulation, local symptomatic treatments, and operative intervention. These seemingly trivial perineal problems merit mention because they are often overlooked sources of sepsis, bleeding, or pain among critically ill patients.

Crohn's disease may affect the entire digestive tract. Standard medical treatment (e.g., corticosteroids, sulfasalazine, 5-ASA preparations, 6-MP) is indicated for active disease but may obscure recognition of acute surgical processes related or unrelated to Crohn's disease. Surgical treatment is reserved for specific acute complications such as perforation, obstruction, and less commonly bleeding and for chronic disease unresponsive to medical treatment. Localized perforations presenting as abscesses are common and, if possible, should be drained percutaneously. An enterocutaneous fistula may develop, which can be treated subsequently by a definitive procedure. Obstruction often results from acute inflammation superimposed on fixed narrowing of the bowel and may resolve with aggressive medical management. However, one must keep in mind that a simple mechanical obstruction unrelated to Crohn's disease may be the cause of the patient's complaints, in which case operative intervention may be warranted sooner rather than later.

The presentation of ulcerative colitis may vary from mild diarrhea to fulminant colitis associated with sepsis and severe hemorrhage. In most instances, an initial trial of medical therapy is warranted. However, when fulminant colitis fails to respond promptly or if severe colitis with colonic dilatation (toxic megacolon) is suspected, total abdominal colectomy with end-ileostomy should be performed promptly.

INFECTION

With increasing numbers of debilitated or immunocompromised patients and wider use of antibiotics, infectious problems and superinfections of the gastrointestinal tract have assumed increasing importance. Although most gastrointestinal tract infections cause only mild self-limited symptoms and require supportive but no specific therapy, some lead to illness of such severity as to require aggressive antimicrobial therapy and, in some instances, prompt surgical therapy.

Debilitated or immunocompromised patients are particularly susceptible to infections of the esophagus, most commonly of viral or fungal, rather than bacterial, cause. Viral ulcerations of the esophagus typically appear as discrete, well-rounded, punched-out ulcerations with raised edges. The diagnosis can, in most instances, be established by typical changes seen at light microscopic evaluation of biopsy specimens (ballooning degeneration, eosinophilic nuclear inclusions, and multinucleated giant cells). Acyclovir and dihydroxy-2 proproxymethyl guanine (DHPG) are usually effective treatments even in the face of continuing immunosuppressive therapy.

Candida esophagitis usually causes dysphagia, which may be accompanied by retrosternal pain, nausea, vomiting, and gastrointestinal bleeding. Upper endoscopy reveals typical *Candida* lesions consisting of white plaques overlying friable erythematous mucosa; biopsy of the lesions is warranted to determine whether tissue infiltration by yeast hyphae is present. *Candida* esophagitis should be treated promptly to relieve symptoms, to prevent dissemination in the setting of chronic immunosuppression, and to avert local complications such as stricture formation or perforation. Topical (oral) therapy may be effective and may also be useful prophylaxis. Systemic therapy consisting of ketoconazole or amphotericin B is instituted when topical therapy fails, for extensive or disseminated infection, and for chronic esophagitis.

Suppurative gastritis is a rare but potentially fatal infection that occurs in immunocompromised patients and in those with chronic gastritis, gastric cancer, or hypochlorhydria or achlorhydria. Most of these infections are caused by α-hemolytic streptococci; *Staphylococcus, Escherichia coli, Proteus,* and *Clostridium perfringens* have also been implicated. Patients so afflicted present with sudden onset of abdominal pain, nausea, and vomiting. Purulent emesis is a rare but pathognomonic sign. Radiologic evaluation is often nonspecific but may demonstrate gastric pneumatosis. Treatment of suppurative gastritis consists of broad-spectrum antibiotic therapy and urgent total or subtotal gastrectomy.

Although enteric infection by many species of bacteria may cause diarrheal syndromes, surgically important infections result primarily from *Salmonella, Yersinia,* and *Shigella* infections. Stool cultures are diagnostic for these infections; blood cultures may also be positive, particularly in *Salmonella* infection. Antibiotic treatment using fluoroquinolones, trimethoprim-sulfamethoxazole, ampicillin, or chloramphenicol is usually effective, but in a small percentage of patients bleeding or intestinal perforation, most commonly occurring in the terminal ileum, necessitates operative intervention. Rarely, necrotizing enteritis, a rapidly progressive form of gas gangrene of the bowel, may result from ingestion of food heavily contaminated with *C. perfringens* type C. Patients experience nausea, vomiting, crampy abdominal pain, and diarrhea; peritonitis and shock rapidly ensue. Resuscitation is followed by an emergency operation to resect necrotic bowel. The diagnosis is confirmed by intraoperative Gram's stains demonstrating gram-positive rods.

Use of antibiotics and immunosuppressive agents has led to the emergence of several clinically important forms of colitis. Infection by toxin-producing *C. difficile* depends on alterations in colonic flora and has become increasingly common with the growing use of antibiotics. Although administration of any antibiotic can predispose to *C. difficile* infections, treatment with ampicillin, cephalosporins, and clindamycin has most commonly been associated with the development of these infections. Clinical presentation ranges from an asymptomatic carrier state to pseudomembranous colitis, which can culminate in fulminant life-threatening colitis requiring surgical intervention. Most often, patients present with diarrhea, although obstipation may also occur. With more severe colitis, abdominal pain, distention, tenderness, fever, and leukocytosis are likely and hematochezia may occur. The pathogenesis of the colitis derives from toxins produced by the bacteria; accordingly, strains of *C. difficile* that do not produce the toxins are not pathogenic, and the detection of the toxins, rather than bacteria, in stool specimens confirms the diagnosis. With advanced disease, pseudomembranes consisting of leukocytes, fibrin, and debris may be found on colonoscopy, which is a strong diagnostic clue. Plain radiographs are not helpful, and a CT scan, although demonstrating colonic thickening consistent with colitis, is usually unnecessary for purposes of diagnosis.

Management of *C. difficile* colitis consists of discontinuation of ongoing antibiotic therapy and treatment with oral vancomycin or metronidazole; intravenous metronidazole can be given if oral delivery is not possible or unreliable. In most instances, this treatment is sufficient, although relapse may occur in 5% to 20% of patients. In rare but increasingly frequent instances, *C. difficile* infection may present as fulminant colitis associated with signs of systemic sepsis and multiple organ system impairment. Unless an immediate response to vancomycin and metronidazole therapy occurs, these patients should undergo emergency total abdominal colectomy.

Chronic immunosuppressive therapy and immunodeficiency states predispose to unusual infections in the gastrointestinal tract. Among transplant patients, intestinal infection by *Aspergillus, Histoplasma,* and *Mycobacterium* species presenting as gastrointestinal bleeding or perforation has been reported (see Chapter 187); cytomegalovirus (CMV) infection of the gastrointestinal tract is also common in this patient population. In the colon, CMV infection may cause ulceration, especially of the cecum, and present as bleeding or perforation. In the absence of such complications that require more specific intervention, treatment consists of reduction of immunosuppressive therapy as allowed and administration of antiviral therapy (DHPG).

Finally, mucosal damage coupled with profound neutropenia, usually resulting from chemotherapy, may lead to invasive infection of the intestinal wall by enteric organisms. In this disorder, referred to as neutropenic colitis, the terminal ileum and cecum are most often affected, and pathologic changes range from mucosal inflammation to transmural necrosis. The typical presentation includes fever, abdominal pain and distention, and right lower quadrant tenderness. Abdominal radiographs and CT scan may demonstrate bowel wall thickening and detect evidence of bowel perforation or compromise. In the absence of clear indications for operative intervention, bowel rest, decompression, nutritional support, antibiotics, and possibly the administration of granulocyte–colony-stimulating factors should be used rather than surgery because the risks of a nontherapeutic laparotomy in a profoundly neutropenic patient are substantial. Close monitoring of the patient with frequent examinations and radiographs is essential so that surgical intervention can be undertaken before perforation occurs.

Suggested Readings

Bondestam S: Ultrasound-guided drainage of abdominal abscesses and fluid collections. Ann Chir Gynaecol 1993; 82:131–133.

Cameron JL (Ed): Current Surgical Therapy: 4. Philadelphia, BC Decker, 1992.

DeLaurier GA, Ivey RK, Johnson RH: Peritoneal fluid lactic acid and diagnostic dilemmas in acute abdominal disease. Am J Surg 1994; 167:302–305.
Goletti O, Lippolis PV, Chiarugi M, et al: Percutaneous ultrasound-guided drainage of intra-abdominal abscesses. Br J Surg 1993; 80:336–339.
Greenfield LJ, Mulholland MW, Oldham KT, et al (Eds): Surgery: Scientific Principles and Practice. Philadelphia, JB Lippincott, 1993.
Heys SD, Brittenden J, Crofts TJ: Acute mesenteric ischemia: The continuing difficulty in early diagnosis. Postgrad Med J 1993; 69:48–51.
Kelly CB, Pothoulakis C, LaMont JT: *Clostridium difficile* colitis. N Engl J Med 1994; 330:257–262.
Larson FA, Haller C, Delcore R, et al: Diagnostic peritoneal lavage in acute peritonitis. Am J Surg 1992; 164:449–452.
Lee YC, Luh SP, Wu RM, et al: A rational surgical approach for intra-thoracic esophageal perforation. Int Surg 1993; 78:307–310.
Levinson MA: Percutaneous versus open operative drainage of intra-abdominal abscesses. Infect Dis Clin North Am 1992; 6:525–544.
Medich DS, Lee KKW, Simmons RL, et al: Laparotomy for fulminant pseudomembranous colitis. Arch Surg 1992; 127:847–853.
Menzies D: Postoperative adhesions: Their treatment and relevance in clinical practice. Ann R Coll Surg Engl 1993; 75:147–153.
Ripamonti C, De Conno F, Ventafridda V, et al: Management of bowel obstruction in advanced and terminal cancer patients. Ann Oncol 1993; 4:15–21.
Salo JA, Isolauri JO, Heikkila LJ, et al: Management of delayed esophageal perforation with mediastinal sepsis. J Thorac Cardiovasc Surg 1993; 106:1088–1091.
Simmons RL, Howard RJ: Surgical Infectious Diseases. Norwalk, CT, Appleton & Lange, 1988.
Sleisenger MH, Fordtran JS (Eds): Gastrointestinal Disease: Pathophysiology, Diagnosis, Management. Philadelphia, WB Saunders, 1989.
Steinberg W, Tenner S: Acute pancreatitis. N Engl J Med 1994; 330:1198–1210.
Stoney RJ, Cunningham CG: Acute mesenteric ischemia. Surgery 1993; 114:489–490.
Svanes C, Lie RT, Svanes K, et al: Adverse effects of delayed treatment for perforated peptic ulcer. Ann Surg 1994; 220:168–175.
van Ooijen B, van der Burg ME, Planting AS, et al: Surgical treatment or gastric drainage only for intestinal obstruction in patients with carcinoma of the ovary or peritoneal carcinomatosis of other origin. Surg Gynecol Obstet 1993; 176:469–474.
Wade DS, Nava HR, Douglass HO: Neutropenic colitis. Cancer 1992; 69:17–23.
Zuidema GD (Ed): Shackelford's Surgery of the Alimentary Tract. Philadelphia, WB Saunders, 1991.

CHAPTER 113

Clinical Assessment of Renal Function

Anton C. Schoolwerth, MD • *Todd W. B. Gehr, MD*

Abnormalities in renal function constitute a major problem in critical care units. It has been estimated that from 5% to 15% of intensive care unit (ICU) patients experience acute deterioration in renal function.[1,2] Conversely, renal dysfunction adds substantially to the morbidity and mortality of these patients. Moreover, changes in renal function directly affect drug disposition. Thus, a means to assess renal function is essential for optimal management. In this chapter, we review selected aspects of renal physiology with an emphasis on measurement of renal function, consequences of altered function, and approaches to improving renal function. The focus is on measurement and optimization of glomerular filtration rate (GFR) and renal blood flow (RBF) and sodium and water homeostasis.

RENAL BLOOD FLOW

Under physiologic conditions, blood flow to the kidneys is 20% of cardiac output. This is a high rate of blood flow, approximately 1 to 1.2 L per minute, a particularly remarkable value considering that the kidneys make up only 0.5% of total body weight. The high blood flow rate is due, at least in part, to the unique anatomic arrangement of the renal vasculature in that the interlobar and arcuate vessels offer little resistance to flow. This, in turn, is due to the fact that the interlobular arteries originate from the arcuates in a parallel arrangement and that the afferent arterioles also arise in a parallel arrangement from the interlobular vessels. It is this parallel arrangement that accounts for the low resistance because the total resistance of n equal parallel paths, each with a resistance R, is R/n.[3] Major resistance vessels in the kidney are the afferent and efferent arterioles, which bind the glomerular capillary network. As will be discussed later, although total resistance is a function of resistance across each of these vessels, it is a unique feature of the kidney that variations in the individual resistances across the afferent and efferent arteriole, respectively, may lead to alterations in glomerular capillary pressure and, hence, in GFR.

Despite a wide range of perfusion pressures, RBF and GFR are maintained relatively constant, a process described as *autoregulation*. Although in the kidney autoregulation has generally been used to refer to the relative constancy of GFR over a range of perfusion pressures, studies have also addressed the regulation of RBF. Emphasis has been placed on the preglomerular vasculature, mainly the afferent arterioles, as the major site by which renal perfusion is regulated. However, some studies also suggest that the larger vessels, such as the interlobulars, may respond to a variety of vasoactive stimuli and participate in an autoregulatory phenomenon. A variety of hypotheses have been generated to explain the autoregulatory response of the kidney with respect to RBF. There is evidence to suggest mediation by neural, humoral, or intrarenal factors that regulate the renal circulation.[4] Although the list of neurohumoral factors that may potentially regulate renal hemodynamics is growing rapidly, emphasis has been placed on several known mediators of this process.

The renin-angiotensin pathway has been shown to have a significant effect on renal hemodynamics. Renin, elaborated in the juxtaglomerular cells, may be released in response to a decrease in renal perfusion pressure and to altered sodium chloride delivery to the ascending limb and macula densa cells. Increased renin secretion, in turn, leads to increased formation of angiotensin II (AII) at the local nephron level. AII, in turn, influences renal vascular resistance by affecting both the afferent and efferent arterioles, predominantly the latter.

Renal eicosanoids are also known to affect renal hemodynamics.[5] Eicosanoids are biologically active fatty acid products of arachidonic acid and are synthesized in the kidney in response to a variety of stimuli, with local release and effect on the renal vasculature. Stimulation of the cyclooxygenase pathway and prostaglandin synthetases leads to the formation of endoperoxides (PGG_2, PGH_2), prostaglandins (PGD_2 and prostaglandins E_2, $F_{2\alpha}$, I_2), and thromboxane (TXA_2). Leukotrienes are synthesized by another major pathway involving the enzyme lipoxygenase. In the kidney, the major products of arachidonic acid metabolism are PGE_2, PGI_2, and, to a lesser extent, $PGI_{2\alpha}$. These compounds have a predominant effect to relax renal vascular smooth muscle and lead to vasodilatation, whereas TXA_2 is a vasoconstrictor prostanoid. It is believed that in disease states endogenous vasodilator prostaglandins serve a protective function to maintain renal perfusion and GFR in response to vasoconstrictor stimuli, including AII and enhanced sympathetic nervous system activity. In contrast, release is inhibited by nonsteroidal anti-inflammatory drugs.

Other vasoactive compounds that affect the renal circulation include the plasma and glandular kallikreins and kinins and endothelium-derived vasoactive factors such as nitric oxide and endothelin.[4, 6] Among the catecholamines, α- and β-adrenergic agonists are known to affect renal vascular tone by causing vasoconstriction and vasodilatation, respectively. In addition, dopamine in low doses leads to renal vasodilatation. Emphasis has been placed on atrial natriuretic peptide and purinergic agents such as adenosine.[7, 8] The effect is likely to be influenced by changes in salt intake and extracellular fluid volume as well as hydration status. For example, the influence of AII on renal hemodynamics is greater in sodium depletion, which also activates the sympathetic nervous system.[9] In response to mild nonhypotensive hemorrhage, renal hemodynamics are relatively well maintained. However, with further reductions in volume associated with a more severe hemorrhage, renal ischemia, mediated by activation of the renin-angiotensin system, renal efferent adrenergic nerves, and circulating catecholamines, may occur (see Arendshorst and Navar[4]). Finally, modification of dietary protein and amino acid intake may affect renal hemodynamics. Dietary protein intake in excess of 1 g/kg per day has been associated with renal vasodilatation, as have infusions of casein hydrolysates and amino acids.[10, 11] Conversely, chronic consumption of a low-protein diet may be associated with renal vasoconstriction.

Measurement of Renal Blood Flow

RBF is measured conventionally by the clearance of infused para-aminohippurate (PAH), which is cleared almost totally from the arterial plasma by both filtration and secretion. Thus, its clearance approximates the rate of renal plasma flow (RPF):

$$RPF = UPAH \cdot V/PPAH$$

where UPAH and PPAH refer to urine and plasma PAH concentrations, respectively and V is urine flow rate (milliliters per minute). RBF can be estimated by correction for the hematocrit (Hct):

$$RBF = RPF/[1 - Hct]$$

Although available, this test is rarely used in clinical practice. In fact, direct quantitation of RPF and RBF is rarely indicated outside of research studies. However, there are situations in which it is necessary to document that the kidneys are being perfused. In this case, one of three additional methods may be used: selective arteriography, Doppler ultrasound, and external radionuclide scanning (see Oken and Schoolwerth[3]). Because the latter two methods are noninvasive, they are preferred. With respect to the nuclide study, scanning is usually performed using iodine 131 iodohippurate.

Clinical Correlates

Although a significant body of data has been obtained to indicate a complex relationship between neurocirculatory factors and renal hemodynamics, several points can be made from a clinical perspective. Optimization of cardiac output and extracellular fluid (ECF) volume, including the intravascular space, is essential for the maintenance of renal perfusion. Particularly because the effects of vasoactive compounds such as AII and catecholamines are accentuated in the face of renal hypoperfusion and volume contraction, attention should be directed to assessing ECF volume, with correction of any deficits, and to optimizing cardiac function. Frequently, pharmacologic agents have been used to maintain renal perfusion in situations in which this may be compromised. Specifically, there has been widespread use of so-called low-dose or renal dose dopamine infusions. This is based on the observation that in low doses (<3 μg/kg per min) dopamine leads to a renal vasodilatation.[12] At higher doses, renal vasoconstriction may occur. As emphasized,[13] beneficial effects of dopamine infusion have not been documented in patients who are sodium chloride and volume depleted; nor has the use of dopamine been shown to be effective beyond a short period of infusion.[14] That is, infusions of renal dose dopamine for 24 to 36 hours may be beneficial in the appropriate circumstance, but there is no evidence supporting the long-term use of this agent. Thus, justification for prolongation of its use beyond several days is currently not supported by available data. Additionally, beyond anecdotes, there are no compelling data to support the use of other potential vasodilator substances such as prostaglandins. Although high-protein feeding and amino acid infusions may increase renal hemodynamics[10, 11] by an undefined mechanism, there is no justification for using these therapies solely from a hemodynamic point of view.

GLOMERULAR FILTRATION RATE

Of the 500 to 700 mL of plasma delivered per minute to the kidneys (corresponding to a renal blood flow of 1 to 1.2 L/min), approximately 20% to 25% is filtered. Glomerular filtration is a major function of the kidney and averages approximately 130 mL/min/1.73 m^2 in normal males and 120 mL/min/1.73 m^2 in females.[15] Because each kidney normally contains approximately 1 million nephrons, the GFR of the two kidneys is determined by the sum of individual nephron GFRs (SNGFR). SNGFR is determined by the glomerular capillary hydraulic pressure (P_{GL}) and opposed by the sum of the hydrostatic pressure in Bowman's space (P_{BS}) and the mean colloid osmotic pressure (COP) of the plasma flowing through the glomerulus. The ultrafiltration coefficient (K_f) determines the rate of filtration at any given filtration pressure, ΔP, so that

$$SNGFR = K_f[P_{GL} - (P_{BS} + COP)] = Kn_f \cdot \Delta P$$

P_{GL} is one of the major determinants of GFR and in turn is affected by RPF and the preglomerular and/or postglomerular vascular resistance across the glomerulus. The extent to which alteration of K_f produced by various physiologic and pathophysiologic states may affect changes in GFR is, at present, not settled. Nevertheless, estimation or direct measurement of GFR remains one of the most important measurements of renal function and is widely used in clinical practice.

Measurement of Glomerular Filtration Rate

GFR is classically measured as the clearance (Cl_{in}) of inulin, a fructose polymer with a mean molecular weight of approximately 5 kd. Because this substance is not present endogenously, it must be given by constant infusion after a loading dose. The amount filtered is the product of the GFR and plasma inulin (P_{in}) concentration. The amounts filtered and excreted are equal such that:

$$GFR \cdot P_{in} = U_{in} \cdot V$$

where U_{in} is urine inulin. By rearrangement,

$$GFR = U_{in} \cdot V/P_{in}$$

Thus, the GFR can be measured from the amount of inulin excreted over a given time period divided by the plasma inulin concentration. Inulin is available commercially but is expensive, often difficult to obtain, and cumbersome to use. As a result, Cl_{in} is rarely used in clinical practice except for research protocols. Although inulin is generally measured chemically, tritium- and carbon 14–labeled inulin are also available but are expensive. Other radiolabeled nuclides have been found to be satisfactory substitutes for inulin and have advantages in the measurement of GFR. Particularly, technetium 99m–labeled diethylene triamine penta-acetic acid (DTPA) and ^{125}I- or ^{131}I-labeled iothalamate clearances closely approximate Cl_{in}.[16, 17] Technetium 99m DTPA has been used and found to give measurements that correlated closely with Cl_{in} in ICU patients.[18, 19] In addition, the clearance of gentamicin has been used in a limited fashion to measure GFR.[20] At present, it is not common that GFR is measured directly. Rather, the GFR is estimated by the endogenous creatinine clearance or serum creatinine determination (see later discussion).

The normal values for GFR given previously apply for individuals ranging in age from the teens to approximately 35 years. Thereafter, GFR declines in most individuals at a relatively constant rate of approximately 10 mL/min per decade.[21–23] In addition, a circadian rhythm for GFR has been described.[24, 25] The GFR is maximal in daytime, whereas a minimum value during the night has been found in normal individuals. Whether this circadian pattern of GFR occurs in critically ill hospitalized patients is not known.

CREATININE CLEARANCE AND SERUM CREATININE

The endogenous creatinine clearance (Cl_{cr}) enjoys widespread use as a reasonable gauge of GFR when great precision is not demanded; it rarely is in clinical practice. The use of creatinine as a marker of GFR has the advantage that creatinine is endogenously produced and is easily measured by inexpensive methods. Creatinine, like inulin, is freely filtered and absorbed not at all or to a minimum extent. However, creatinine is secreted, the contribution of secretion to total excretion increasing as the GFR decreases and serum creatinine rises. At GFRs below 40 mL/min, Cl_{cr} exceeds Cl_{in} by 50% to 100%.[16, 26] When the GFR is significantly depressed and it is deemed important to obtain a more precise measurement of GFR, one of the previously mentioned methods to estimate GFR directly might be used. Additionally, because Cl_{cr} overestimates GFR and the clearance of urea underestimates GFR (see later), the mean value of simultaneously obtained creatinine and urea clearances has been shown to provide a close estimation of Cl_{in}[27] when the latter is less than 20 mL/min. Volume expansion in humans causes a small rise in GFR, whereas volume depletion, severe heart failure, hypotension, anesthesia, surgery, trauma, sepsis, and even mild intestinal bleeding without frank hypotension may depress the GFR substantially.

Various methods are available to measure creatinine. Creatinine is frequently measured using the Jaffé alkaline picric reaction. Although widely used, it should be recognized that this reaction also measures other chromogens, which may lead to a false elevation in the estimated serum creatinine measurement. Substances such as acetoacetate (in ketoacidosis), pyruvate, ascorbate, 5-flucytosine, certain (but not all) cephalosporin antibiotics, and very high urate artifactually raise serum creatinine (S_{cr}) in normal subjects by 0.5 to 2 mg/dL.[28–34] These substances are excreted into the urine but contribute trivially compared with overall urine creatinine. Thus, noncreatinine chromogens affect the S_{cr} but have little effect on the urine creatinine (U_{cr}). In individuals with normal renal function, the contribution of serum noncreatinine chromogens to raising the S_{cr} is approximately equal to the contribution of secretion to creatinine excretion such that the Cl_{cr} closely approximates the GFR. As GFR decreases, the contribution of noncreatinine chromogens to the total measured serum creatinine becomes less than the secreted moiety, and the Cl_{cr} overestimates GFR to a greater extent. Direct enzymatic creatinine measurements are not affected by noncreatinine chromogens. Very high serum glucose (>1000 mg/dL) and 5-flucytosine may interfere with the enzymatic reaction, whereas high bilirubin (>5 mg/dL) levels affect the autoanalyzer method[32] and lead to falsely low S_{cr} values. It is, therefore, important to know the method by which a given laboratory measures serum creatinine. Competing for the same proximal tubular organic base secretory site as creatinine, certain pharmacologic agents may suppress this process and lead to a rise in S_{cr}. Trimethoprim, probenecid, and cimetidine but not ranitidine are organic bases that inhibit creatinine secretion competitively and can result in a mild elevation in S_{cr}, usually 0.5 mg/dL or less.[35–38] This effect has been used to obtain a more accurate estimate of GFR. Specifically, Cl_{cr} obtained in the presence of cimetidine (400 mg as a priming dose followed by 200 mg every 3 hours) yielded values that closely approximated Cl_{in}.[39, 40]

As with all clearance methods, the Cl_{cr} is subject to errors that may amount to as much as 10% to 15% or more. In addition to potential problems in estimating serum and urine creatinine, errors in timing of urine collection, incomplete collection, and inaccurate measurement of urine volume are other factors that contribute to errors.[41] Although 24-hour urine Cl_{cr} has been widely used, there is no specified time period required for the clearance to be obtained. In fact, in patients passing adequate amounts of urine (not oliguric), shorter collection periods of several hours may be more accurate, particularly if the patient is not in a steady state (see later). To reduce errors in volume measurement, a water diuresis can be induced in stable subjects before beginning the test. However, this is rarely practical in the ICU setting. Nevertheless, because many ICU patients have indwelling Foley catheters, it should be possible for accurately timed urine collections to be obtained and for Cl_{cr} to be measured with reasonable accuracy.

Because of the practical and technical problems in obtaining estimates of GFR by clearance methods, renal function is most commonly estimated by monitoring the serum creatinine in hospitalized patients. Creatinine is formed nonenzymatically from creatine and phosphocreatine in muscle cells and is normally present in the serum at a concentration of 0.8 to 1.4 mg/dL in adults and 0.3 to 0.6 mg/dL in children and pregnant subjects. The actually measured S_{cr} depends on the method of measurement as discussed previously, the GFR, rate of creatinine production and volume of distribution (e.g., S_{cr} is lower in anasarca), and the extent of its tubular secretion and intestinal degradation.[3] Because creatinine production is closely related to muscle mass, S_{cr} is generally less in females than in males and decreases as muscle mass is lost with aging or with debilitating illnesses. The relationship between S_{cr} and Cl_{cr} (and hence GFR) can

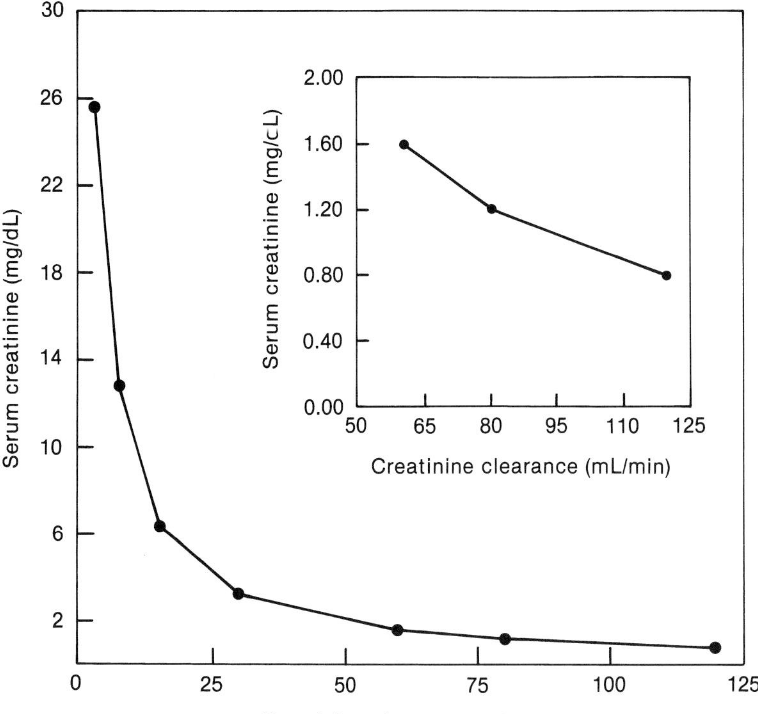

Figure 113–1. Relationship between C_{cr} and S_{cr}. In the steady state, the S_{cr} should increase twofold for each 50% reduction in C_{cr}. The *inset* represents an enlarged view of the changes in S_{cr} as C_{cr} decreases from 120 to 60 mL/min. Note that if S_{cr} is 0.8 mg/dL when the C_{cr} is 120 mL/min, C_{cr} can decrease by 33% such that the increased S_{cr} is still within the normal range.

be described by a rectangular hyperbola.[41] However, it must be emphasized that this relationship applies in the steady state and assumes a constant rate of creatinine production (Fig. 113–1). Thus, a doubling of the serum creatinine reflects a 50% decrease in Cl_{cr}, a fourfold increase in S_{cr}, a 75% drop in GFR, and so on. Because creatinine production may not remain constant, serum creatinine may underestimate the decrease in GFR in critically ill patients who have a decrease in muscle mass secondary to an ongoing catabolic state. Moreover, it should be appreciated that S_{cr} is an insensitive marker of change early in the course of renal disease. Thus, a 33% fall in GFR may raise the S_{cr} from 0.8 to 1.2 mg/dL, a value that is still within the normal range. If the prior value is not known, this fall in GFR may go unrecognized. S_{cr} provides a close estimate of GFR only in the steady state. With an abrupt decrease in GFR, as may occur in acute renal failure, creatinine production would be expected to continue unchanged, but, because of the decrease in GFR, creatinine excretion will be impaired. As a result, the S_{cr} will increase until a new steady state is obtained, at which time the amount of creatinine produced equals the amount filtered ($GFR \cdot S_{cr}$) and excreted ($U_{cr} \cdot V$). Depending on the extent of damage and decrease in GFR, it may take several days for a new steady state to be achieved (Fig. 113–2). Therefore, after an insult leading to an abrupt decrease in GFR, the serum creatinine will rise progressively over the next several days. This should not be interpreted as a new insult each day but rather that a steady state has not yet been obtained. While the S_{cr} is changing, its absolute value cannot be used as an accurate measure of the decrease in GFR. Should an accurate measurement of GFR be needed during this period of time, a short Cl_{cr} can be obtained.

A variety of equations have been developed to estimate Cl_{cr} based on the S_{cr} without collecting urine. These equations generally take into consideration muscle mass (estimated as body weight), sex (males having a higher GFR than females), and age. Aging, hepatic diseases, excessive muscle wasting, severe muscular atrophy or dystrophy, hyperthyroidism, paralysis, and chronic glucocorticoid therapy have been associated with reduced creatinine generation.[19] In addition, particularly at low levels of GFR, correction for nonrenal creatinine metabolism is also recommended.[42, 43] One of the most commonly used equations is that developed by Cockcroft and Gault:[44]

$$Cl_{cr} = \frac{(140 - \text{age}) \cdot \text{lean weight}}{72 \cdot S_{cr}}$$

where age is expressed in years and weight in kilograms. This expression is multiplied by 0.85 for females. These equations have been adapted as follows:

$$Cl_{cr} = (28 - 0.2\text{age}) \cdot S_{cr}^{-1} - 0.04 \text{ L/kg per day in men}$$

$$Cl_{cr} = (23.8 - 0.17\text{age}) \cdot S_{cr}^{-1} - 0.04 \text{ L/kg per day in women}$$

where Cl_{cr} is expressed in liters per kilogram per day; the added expression (−0.04 L/kg per day) accounts for creatinine degradation, which, when used, reduces the error of estimating Cl_{cr} from S_{cr}.[42, 45]

Serum Urea Nitrogen

Although less accurate as a marker of GFR than the S_{cr}, serum urea nitrogen (SUN) (or blood urea nitrogen) is still used extensively in clinical practice to estimate renal function. Although this was the earliest available indicator of renal function, several other factors should be appreciated in the use of this substance. Like creatinine, urea is freely filtered and is retained in the blood as GFR falls. However, in contrast to creatinine, urea may be reabsorbed to a significant extent, its excretion tending to be increased with increasing urine flow rates, whereas its excretion is reduced when tubular fluid reabsorption is enhanced. More important, urea production is more variable than is creatinine. Produced in the liver, urea will increase with high protein

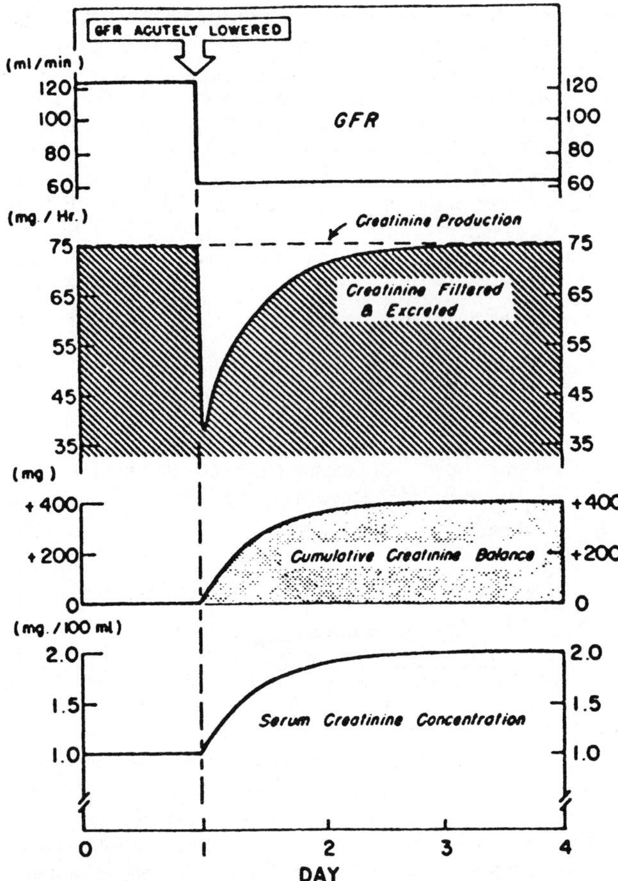

Figure 113–2. Expected changes in S_{cr} resulting from an acute decrease in the GFR level and the attainment of a new steady state. Between days 0 and 1, the patient excretes all the creatinine that is produced, and S_{cr} remains stable at 1.0 mg/dL. A 50% reduction in GFR level on day 1 results in an abrupt decrease in filtered (and, therefore, excreted) creatinine. Release of creatinine from muscle remains constant; as a result, creatinine is retained, and its serum concentration is increased. As creatinine concentration rises progressively, the filtered (and excreted) creatinine concentration also increases until the excreted creatinine concentration returns to control levels and matches creatinine production. This new steady state (days 3 to 4) is achieved by the doubling of S_{cr} concentration; this maintains the filtered creatinine load at control levels in the face of the halving of the GFR. A greater decrease in GFR concentration would lead to a greater increase in the steady state (e.g., a 90% reduction in GFR concentration would lead to a 10-fold increase in S_{cr}) and would take a longer period of time to achieve. (From Kassirer JP: Clinical evaluation of kidney function–glomerular function. N Engl J Med 1971; 285:385. Reprinted with permission from *The New England Journal of Medicine*.)

intake, amino acid infusions, and hypercatabolic states. In addition, endogenous sources of protein such as absorbed hemoglobin from gastrointestinal bleeding may contribute to increased urea synthesis. Even at a constant GFR, SUN may rise in subjects on high-protein intake and fall with protein restriction or on refeeding of previously starved, nonhypercatabolic subjects. In addition, several pharmacologic agents may affect urea nitrogen (UN) formation. Tetracyclines may lead to an increase in SUN by an antianabolic effect without any detectable change in GFR, whereas glucocorticoids and severe illnesses or trauma do the same by inducing endogenous protein hypercatabolism. Because of the widespread use of hyperalimentation in ICU patients, an impairment in renal function is often associated with a marked disproportion in the elevation of SUN compared with S_{cr}. For this reason, the issue is raised as to whether SUN elevation itself poses an important threat to the patient if the GFR is in a range that should not lead to enhanced morbidity by itself. In those circumstances, it is useful to measure the rate of urea appearance (or generation) to estimate whether other factors such as gastrointestinal bleeding, excessive amino acid infusions, and protein administration are contributing to the increase in SUN over and above that expected by the decrease in GFR.[42, 43] UN appearance can be determined from urine UN, SUN, and body weight as follows:

$$UN = U_{UN} \cdot V + \Delta \text{body pool UN}$$

where $U_{UN} \cdot V$ is 24-hour UN excretion and

$$\Delta \text{body pool UN} = 0.6 \cdot \text{nonedematous weight (kilograms)} \cdot \Delta SUN/\text{day}$$

or if the weight is changing[43, 44]

$$\Delta \text{body pool UN} = (0.6 \cdot \text{nonedematous weight} \cdot \Delta SUN) + (\Delta \text{weight} \cdot \text{final SUN}).$$

Nitrogen balance (B_N) is calculated as:

$$B_N = I_{UN} - UN - NUN$$

where I_{UN} is UN intake and NUN is nonurea nitrogen excretion.[43] The latter, which includes fecal nitrogen, urinary creatinine, uric acid, and unmeasured nitrogen, averages 0.031 g nitrogen/kg per day.[43] The data obtained from these measurements may be quite useful in evaluating the cause of disproportionate elevations in SUN. If the patient is in a steady state (with a stable weight and SUN), B_N is 0, and I_{UN} can be estimated from UN plus NUN.[43] Also, because catabolism, except in cases of severe trauma and burns, is usually 2 to 4 g of nitrogen per day, additional conclusions can be drawn if the patient is not in the steady state. For example, if it is known that I_{UN} is less than UN plus NUN, gastrointestinal bleeding plus or minus excess catabolism would be suggested. Similarly, one can evaluate if the increase in SUN is a reflection of excessive exogenous protein and amino acid administration (usually >1.5 g/kg per day; grams of UN ÷ 0.16 = grams of protein or amino acids). If I_{UN} is greater than UN, such as in severe liver disease, the clinician might more carefully evaluate changes in weight and SUN as well as clearances because the latter may be more severely depressed than initially suspected.

SODIUM BALANCE AND EXTRACELLULAR FLUID VOLUME

Sodium is the primary cation of the extracellular fluid volume (ECF), present in a concentration of 140 to 142 mmol. The volume of the ECF is approximately 20% of total body weight and represents one third of total body water. Regulation of ECF volume is governed by factors regulating sodium balance and sodium excretion. Readers are referred to several excellent reviews on this topic.[46, 47] For the purposes of this discussion, several factors are emphasized. Under physiologic conditions and in the steady state, sodium balance pertains, and the amount of sodium excreted equals that which enters the body by oral and intravenous routes. Sodium excretion and the fraction of filtered sodium that is excreted (FE_{Na}) can be readily determined. Absolute sodium excretion is measured as the product of the urine sodium concentration (U_{Na}) and the urine volume,

$$Na^+ \text{ excretion} = (U_{Na} \cdot V)$$

FE_{Na} can be determined as follows:

$$FE_{Na} = U_{Na} \cdot V/GFR \cdot S_{Na}$$

where S_{Na} is the serum sodium concentration. For practical reasons, the Cl_{cr} ($U_{cr} \cdot V/S_{cr}$) is used to estimate GFR, such that

$$FE_{Na} = U_{Na} \cdot V/U_{cr} \cdot V/S_{cr} \cdot S_{Na}$$

Because the V term in the numerator and denominator cancels out,

$$FE_{Na} = U_{Na}/S_{Na} \cdot S_{cr}/U_{cr}$$

Thus, FE_{Na} can be calculated from the sodium and creatinine determined in a random urine sample and serum (or plasma) simultaneously. The resulting calculation is expressed as a percentage by multiplying by 100. This test is of value in the setting of acute renal failure to aid in distinguishing a prerenal from a renal parenchymal cause.[48] It is not usually helpful in aiding in the diagnosis of urinary tract obstruction or in patients with underlying chronic renal insufficiency (CRI). The reason for the difficulty in interpreting CRI can be illustrated by the following considerations. At a GFR of 130 mL/min and a dietary sodium intake of 3 g of sodium (130 mmol), an individual in sodium balance will excrete 0.5% of the filtered load (FE_{Na} = 0.5%). For sodium balance to be maintained at lower levels of GFR with the same sodium intake, FE_{Na} must be increased progressively. Successive decreases in GFR by one half from 130 would result in an FE_{Na} of 1%, 2%, 4%, and 8%, respectively. Thus, interpretation of the FE_{Na} in a patient with acute renal failure superimposed on CRI will be problematic unless the prior steady-state FE_{Na} is known; this is rarely the case.

The fractional excretion of chloride (FE_{Cl}) has been suggested to be more accurate than that of sodium in aiding in distinguishing prerenal from parenchymal causes of acute renal failure.[49] This is particularly so when acute renal failure occurs with simultaneous metabolic alkalosis. If the urine contains substantial amounts of bicarbonate (HCO_3) ($U_{pH} > 7$), sodium excretion will increase to maintain electroneutrality. Under these circumstances, the FE_{Na} may give misleading information, but the FE_{Cl} can be used to obtain the same information.

Although urinary sodium excretion can be used to help make determinations with respect to ECF volume under certain circumstances, this may be fraught with potential errors. There is no laboratory test available that will provide this information. Rather, the astute clinician must rely on bedside evaluation complemented, when appropriate, with measurements of central venous pressure and pulmonary capillary wedge pressure to assist in making determinations with respect to ECF volume status. For example, a low FE_{Na} (<1%) in the setting of acute renal failure usually indicates a decrease in renal perfusion but does not provide information on the status of the patient's ECF volume. Because a low FE_{Na} can be seen with either ECF volume contraction or severe congestive heart failure, these conditions must be distinguished at the bedside. Moreover, there are circumstances, (enumerated in Chapter 114) in which a low FE_{Na} exists despite parenchymal renal disease, such as acute glomerulonephritis, severe burn, and radiocontrast nephropathy. Finally, it must be appreciated that administration of potent diuretic agents can alter the FE_{Na} and lead to misleading interpretations. For this reason, urine samples should be obtained before diuretics are administered (avoid the "furosemide [Lasix] reflex").

A few additional points are worthy of note with respect to diuretic use. There is now ample evidence to support the notion that in a patient in positive sodium balance diuretic therapy should not be used without simultaneously restricting sodium intake if negative sodium balance and reduction in edema fluid are desired.[50] In general, this requires restriction of dietary sodium intake, usually to less than 2 g of sodium per day (≈88 mmol) if the patient has an edema-forming state. Although diuresis can be affected even with liberal sodium intake, this requires higher doses of diuretics and more frequent administration of these agents.[51] The coexistence of hyponatremia should not deter the clinician from restricting sodium intake but rather should also lead to a restriction in solute-free water intake. Of course, it is recognized that, under certain circumstances, obligatory intakes make it difficult to achieve optimal restriction to assist diuresis. That is, with various pharmacologic drips, blood products, and feeding regimens necessary in acutely ill patients in the ICU, this may become a difficult problem. Under those circumstances, increasing doses of diuretics, including continuous infusions of loop diuretics,[51] may be required.

SELECTED ASPECTS OF WATER BALANCE

Water balance is achieved through a variety of factors including water intake, excretion, and insensible fluid losses.[52, 53] Contributing to the maintenance of water balance is the sensation of thirst, elaboration by osmoreceptors in the hypothalamus of antidiuretic hormone (ADH) with its release into the circulation from the posterior pituitary, and ADH action on the kidney. ADH increases renal water permeability by opening water channels in the collecting tubule, leading to osmotic equilibrium between the medullary interstitium of the kidney and tubular fluid. As a consequence, increased water reabsorption with reduced excretion occurs and urine concentration increases. A variety of abnormalities in urine concentration and dilution are encountered in clinical practice. A detailed discussion is beyond the scope of this chapter, and selected aspects only are reviewed.

Under physiologic conditions, urine flow rate is determined by water intake and by the need to achieve osmotic balance. That is, water ingested in excess of the needs of the organism will be excreted, but the urine volume will also be affected by the osmotic load ingested or infused. It has been estimated that a typical North American diet contains approximately 600 mOsm of solute, which must be excreted to maintain osmotic balance. In fact, it is this estimate, plus the knowledge that the human kidney can concentrate urine maximally to a value of 1200 to 1400 mOsm/kg of water (H_2O), that has led to the definition of oliguria as a urine volume below 400 to 500 mL per day. It should also be appreciated that, under physiologic conditions, a diurnal variation in urine flow rate has been documented; urine flow is lowest and urine concentration maximal at night, with rising flow and decreasing concentration during the first hours after awakening.[54] Although it is possible that diurnal variation is lost in the critically ill patient in the ICU setting, there is little documentation of the needs for a minimum urine flow rate per hour. Thus, the view that urine flow should exceed 30 to 40 mL/h appears to have little justification. As discussed in Chapter 114 on renal failure, when urine flow rate is clearly reduced (very low urine flow rate for several hours or more) leading to positive osmotic balance, one should address the cause for the low urine flow rate rather than treat the symptom (low urine flow rate) alone (the "*Lasix* reflex" revisited).

The primary constituents of urine contributing to osmolality are sodium, potassium, chloride, and other particles

TABLE 113–1. Relationship Between Creatinine Urine/Plasma (U/P) Ratios and Percentage of Water Excreted and Reabsorbed

*Creatinine U/P Ratio**	*% Filtered Water Excreted ([P/U] × 100)†*	*% Filtered Water Reabsorbed (1 − [P/U] × 100)†*
2	50.0	50.0
5	20.0	80.0
10	10.0	90.0
20	5.0	95.0
50	2.0	98.0
100	1.0	99.0
200	0.5	99.5

*Creatinine U/P ratio = ratio of creatinine measured in urine and plasma (or serum), both in units of milligrams per deciliter.

†The percentages of filtered water excreted and reabsorbed are calculated assuming that creatinine is freely filtered and neither reabsorbed nor secreted. Because creatinine is known to be secreted, these calculations will overestimate the percentage excreted and underestimate the percentage reabsorbed, especially when the serum creatinine is elevated.

of which urea is a major component. Although osmolality can be readily determined in the laboratory by use of an osmometer, in the setting of acute renal failure renal water handling is more usefully assessed from the urine–plasma creatinine ratio (U/P_{cr}).[55, 56] The basis for this is as follows: creatinine is freely filtered at the glomerulus and is reabsorbed to a negligible extent; creatinine secretion can be ignored for these purposes. One can interpret a rise in urine creatinine concentration, relative to the plasma or serum, as a measure of water reabsorption. Thus, as indicated in Table 113–1, plasma–urine creatinine ratios (P/U_{cr}) provide a rough estimate of fractional water excretion, and [1 − (P/U_{cr})] provides a measure of fractional water reabsorption. Together with FE_{Na}, these indexes may be used to determine that the kidney is responding to decreased perfusion or, in the face of a decrease in GFR, exhibiting a decrease in tubular sodium and water reabsorption.[55]

Serum compositional changes generally denote alterations in water balance. Specifically, hypernatremia and hyponatremia represent problems with hyperosmolality and hypo-osmolality, respectively. Hypernatremia and hyperosmolality commonly occur in the setting of dehydration with loss of water in excess of sodium. This can usually be confirmed by history and physical examination, the latter involving findings compatible with a decrease in ECF volume and total body water. The response of the kidney is expected to mirror the decrease in ECF volume: a low urine sodium concentration (<20 mmol), FE_{Na} (<1%), and an increased U/P_{cr} ratio (>20) and urine osmolality (>400). Uncommonly, hypernatremia occurs with an increased ECF volume and total body sodium. Circumstances in which this may pertain include aggressive treatment with sodium bicarbonate after cardiopulmonary resuscitation; administration of large amounts of blood products, such as plasma or albumin in addition to isotonic saline, in a febrile patient; or administration of these agents in patients with acute or chronic renal insufficiency. In these situations, efforts should be made to induce enhanced sodium removal from the body by use of diuresis and, where appropriate, dialysis.

With respect to hyponatremia and hypo-osmolality, several points can be made. Hyponatremia represents an increase in body water relative to sodium; this can occur in the setting of a reduced, normal, or increased total body sodium as determined by estimation of the ECF volume.[57] It is important to make this distinction early because it will have a major impact on therapy. In addition to physical examination, a urine sodium concentration should be obtained, with values less than 20 mmol suggesting a decrease in ECF volume, if supported by bedside examination. Volume expansion should be more easily determined by the presence of expanded interstitial edema, pulmonary vascular congestion, and elevated filling pressures, as might occur in the patient with congestive cardiac failure, cirrhosis, or nephrotic syndrome. The urine sodium is usually low in these conditions, reflecting the edema-forming state.

Patients who appear to be neither volume contracted nor volume expanded are the most difficult to assess. Under all circumstances, it is advisable to measure urine osmolality because this provides information with regard to the bioactivity of ADH. A urine osmolality of less than 100 mOsm/kg suggests little or no ADH activity, such as might occur with psychogenic polydipsia. A urine osmolality (U_{Osm}) of greater than 100 mOsm/kg indicates ADH activity. It is not necessary for the U_{Osm} to exceed the simultaneously obtained serum osmolality, although the latter circumstance may be encountered frequently in clinical practice.[58] The majority of patients with hyponatremia will have evidence of increased ADH activity. It is essential to recall that there are both osmotic and nonosmotic stimuli to the release of ADH.[53] In response to an increase in serum osmolality, ADH is released. This is a sensitive response and usually begins when serum osmolality exceeds a value of 280 mOsm/kg H_2O.[59] From the point of osmotic balance, ADH release is not appropriate in the hypo-osmolar patient. However, under these circumstances, one may often find that ADH is being released in response to nonosmotic stimuli. As shown in Table 113–2 and Figure 113–3, a variety of factors may lead to nonosmotic release of ADH. These include ECF volume depletion, pain, surgery, anesthesia, and pharmacologic agents. Hyponatremia as a result of nonosmotic stimuli for ADH release with ongoing fluid intake commonly occurs perioperatively related to anesthesia and surgery, after diuretic therapy, and after excessive extrarenal fluid losses such as diarrhea. It is only when these are not present that the diagnosis of inappropriate secretion of ADH becomes probable. In one review, 97% of hospitalized patients with hyponatremia were found to have evidence for nonosmotic ADH release.[60] For the patient who is hyponatremic in the setting of decreased ECF volume, administration of isotonic saline to replete ECF volume is appropriate. A comprehensive discussion of the physiologic basis and treatment of hyponatremia is available.[61]

ACID-BASE BALANCE

Arterial hydrogen ion (H^+) is maintained by buffering and the several organ systems that regulate the components of the primary buffer system in the body: the bicarbonate carbonic acid buffer system. Specifically, H^+ is determined by

TABLE 113–2. Osmotic and Nonosmotic Stimuli for Antidiuretic Hormone Secretion

Osmotic
- *Hyperosmolality*

Nonosmotic
- *Hypovolemia*
- *Pain*
- *Anesthesia*
- *Hypoxemia*
- *Hypoglycemia*
- *Drugs*
  - Nicotine
  - Morphine
  - Other

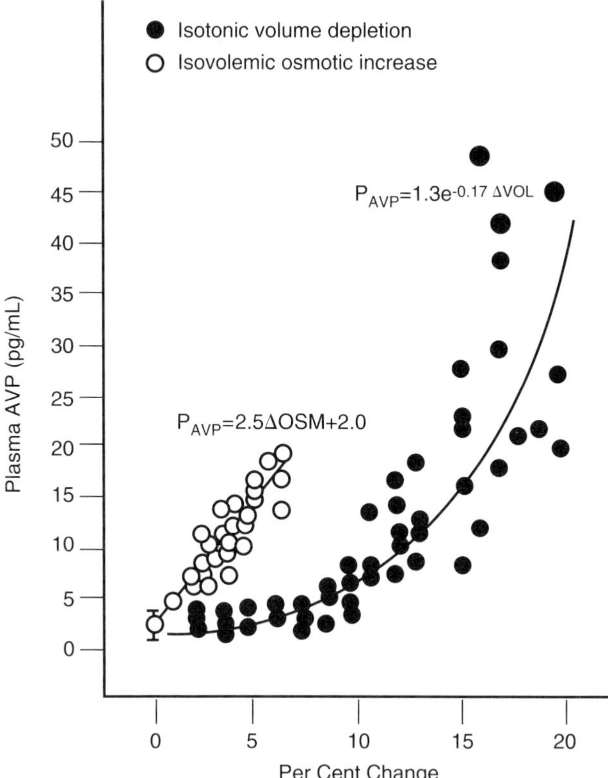

Figure 113–3. Plasma arginine vasopressin (AVP) response to changes in blood osmolality *(open circles)* or volume *(closed circles)*, expressed as per cent change from normal. (Reproduced from Dunn FL, Brennan TJ, Nelson AE, et al: The role of blood osmolality and volume in regulating vasopressin in renal medulla in situ. J Clin Invest 1973; 52:3212, by copyright permission of the American Society for Clinical Investigation.)

the ratio of carbonic acid to bicarbonate (HCO_3) as described in the Henderson equation:

$$H^+ = 24 \cdot \frac{PCO_2}{HCO_3}$$

where PCO_2 is the partial pressure of carbon dioxide. In recent years the Henderson equation has been used more widely than the Henderson-Hasselbalch equation.[62] Although the Henderson-Hasselbalch equation has the advantage that one need not deal with small numbers (nmoles of H^+), one must deal with logarithmic expressions. The Henderson equation obviates the latter and requires only the measurement of pH and PCO_2 in the blood with conversion of pH to H^+. This can be done by any use of simple conversion factors listed in Figure 113–4.

PCO_2 is regulated by pulmonary ventilation, whereas the HCO_3 concentration is regulated by the kidneys. Although it has been suggested that other organ systems, particularly the liver, may play a major role in HCO_3 homeostasis, this remains a controversial area.[63–66] For the purposes of this discussion, we still use the conventional view. Renal regulation of HCO_3 concentration requires that the kidneys reabsorb all filtered HCO_3 (approximately 4500 mmol daily under physiologic conditions) to prevent depletion of HCO_3 stores. In addition, new HCO_3 must be formed to replace that consumed by nonvolatile acids. As with HCO_3 reabsorption, this process occurs primarily in the proximal tubule in association with ammonium synthesis and excretion.[67] The formation of new HCO_3 by the kidney can be estimated by measurements of urinary ammonium excretion.

Urine Net Charge

Because the measurement of urinary ammonium is not available in most clinical laboratories, it has been suggested that urinary ammonium can be estimated, under appropriate circumstances, by measurements of the urine net charge (UNC) or anion gap, defined as urine $Na^+ + K^+ - Cl^-$.[68]

$$UNC = Na^+ + K^+ - Cl^-$$

Ammonium (NH_4^+) must be excreted with an anion, usually chloride. The urine pH should be less than 6.5 to exclude the presence of HCO_3^-. It has been stated that on a regular diet other anions and divalent cations do not change markedly, with the former exceeding the latter by approximately 80 mmol/d.[68]

$$Na^+ + K^+ + NH_4^+ = Cl^- + 80$$

Estimation of UNC is useful in dissecting the cause of normal anion gap or hyperchloremic metabolic acidosis (HCMA).[68, 69] If urine Cl^- is greater than Na^+ plus K^+, urine NH_4^+ exceeds 80 mmol/d; this indicates that the kidney is responding to metabolic acidosis with enhanced ammonium excretion and is not the cause for the acidosis. Excess urinary ammonium in this setting points to an extrarenal cause for the acidosis such as diarrhea. If urine Cl^- is less than Na^+ plus K^+, a major defect in NH_4^+ excretion (e.g., renal tubular acidosis) is suggested. Furthermore, if the U_{pH} is less than 5.5, a defect in NH_4^+ synthesis is likely; if the U_{pH} is ≈6 or higher, a defect in H^+ secretion is suggested. There are certain situations in which NH_4^+ will be underestimated

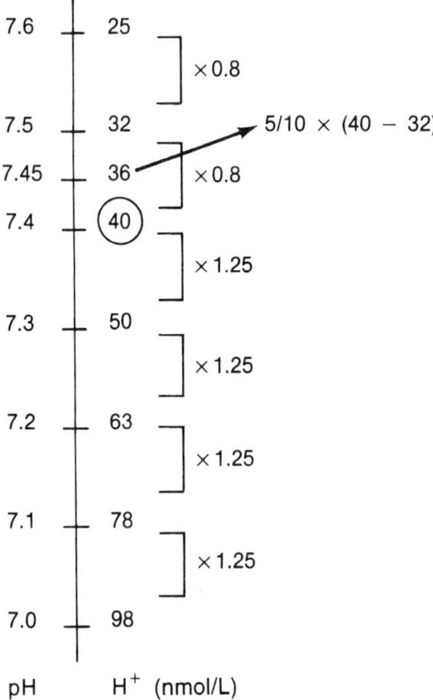

Figure 113–4. Conversion of pH to H^+. At a pH of 7.40, H^+ is 40 nmol/L. For each 0.1-unit decrease in pH, H^+ is obtained by multiplying H^+ by 1.25; for each 0.1-unit increase in pH above 7.40, H^+ is obtained by multiplying the previous H^+ value by 0.8. H^+ is estimated from intermediate pH values by interpolation: 7.45 is 5/10 between 7.40 and 7.50; H^+ is equal to 5/10 × 40 nmol/L (pH 7.40) minus 32 nmol/L (pH 7.50) = 36 nmol/L.

using the UNC: ketonuria and the excretion of certain drugs such as penicillins or salicylates.[70, 71]

Serum Anion Gap

In metabolic acidosis associated with an increase in serum anion gap ($Na^+ - [Cl^- + CO_2]$), it is useful to evaluate whether the change in anion gap and serum HCO_3 (or total CO_2) are approximately the same.[72] That is, in a situation in which metabolic acidosis occurs with an increased anion gap, such as lactic acidosis, the decrease in HCO_3 from normal should be approximately the same as the increase in anion gap from the normal value of 12 ± 2 mmol. If the changes are not closely related, the presence of another superimposed acid-base disturbance is likely. For example, if the increase in anion gap is greater than the decrease in HCO_3, metabolic alkalosis likely is present as well. Conversely, if the increase in anion gap is substantially less than the decrease in HCO_3, this indicates the presence of an additional cause for metabolic acidosis, viz. a normal anion gap metabolic acidosis. Readers are referred to several excellent reviews on this topic.[72–74]

Metabolic alkalosis is usually due to loss of acid with excess generation of HCO_3 by the gastrointestinal tract or kidneys.[75] Less commonly, it may occur as a result of excess administration of sodium HCO_3. The latter circumstance is relatively uncommon because of the capacity of normal kidneys to excrete HCO_3. However, in states in which urinary HCO_3 excretion is impaired, such as with severe renal failure, metabolic alkalosis may occur from excess HCO_3 administration. For example, administration of high doses of sodium HCO_3 after cardiac resuscitation in a patient with end-stage renal disease or transfusion of many units of citrated blood may lead to metabolic alkalosis. For the most part, other causes of metabolic alkalosis can be subdivided into those that are sodium chloride responsive or sodium chloride resistant. Under the first category (Table 113–3), metabolic alkalosis occurs in the setting of a sodium (and hence ECF volume) deficit with activation of the renin-angiotensin-aldosterone system. This commonly occurs with protracted vomiting or nasogastric suction and in patients treated aggressively with diuretics. Sodium chloride–resistant metabolic alkalosis occurs generally in situations associated with increased mineralocorticoid activity, such as primary aldosteronism or administration of high doses of corticosteroids without sodium restriction. Under these circumstances, metabolic alkalosis is generated by the kidneys and is sustained by ongoing potassium depletion.

In general, the factors leading to the generation and maintenance of metabolic alkalosis need to be considered separately. The causes explaining the generation of alkalosis are usually readily apparent, whereas those for maintenance are often less clear. HCO_3 reabsorption may be maintained despite an elevation in plasma HCO_3 by such factors as a decrease in GFR, hypokalemia, hypochloremia, and ECF volume contraction.[76, 77] In the situation of a decreased GFR or volume contraction, one would anticipate finding a low urinary chloride concentration, whereas in settings in which the alkalosis is maintained by excess mineralocorticoid activity directly related to hypokalemia, urine chloride is usually in excess of 20 mmol. Repletion of ECF volume with sodium chloride often improves the sodium chloride–responsive alkalosis appreciably but is not effective in patients with sodium chloride–resistant conditions; in the latter states, efforts should be made to replete decreased potassium stores, usually with potassium chloride. Ultimately, full correction of the alkalemic state is possible only when the underlying condition is corrected.

TABLE 113–3. Causes of Metabolic Alkalosis

Chloride Responsive	*Chloride Resistant*
Gastric Fluid Loss	*Primary Hyperaldosteronism*
Vomiting	*Secondary Hyperaldosteronism*
Nasogastric suction	Malignant hypertension
Stool Chloride Loss	Renal artery stenosis
Chloride-wasting diarrhea	Renin-secreting tumor
Villous adenoma	*Glucocorticoid Hormone Excess*
Posthypercapnia	Cushing's syndrome
Nonreabsorbable Anion Delivery	Exogenous glucocorticoids
Carbenicillin	*Bartter's syndrome*
Penicillin	*Alkali Ingestion*

TABLE 113–4. Expected Compensatory Responses in Simple Acid-Base Disturbances

Metabolic acidosis	P_{CO_2} should fall 1.0 to 1.5 mm Hg for each mmol/L fall in HCO_3^-
Metabolic alkalosis	P_{CO_2} should increase 0.7 mm Hg for each mmol/L rise in HCO_3^-; P_{CO_2} rarely >55 mm Hg as compensation
Respiratory acidosis	
Acute	HCO_3^- should increase 0.1 mmol/L for each mm Hg rise in P_{CO_2}; HCO_3^- rarely >30 mmol/L as compensation
Chronic	HCO_3^- should increase 0.4 mmol/L for each mm Hg rise in P_{CO_2}
Respiratory alkalosis	
Acute	HCO_3^- should decrease 0.2 mmol/L for each mm Hg fall in P_{CO_2}; usually not <18 mmol/L
Chronic	HCO_3^- should decrease 0.4 mmol/L for each mm Hg fall in P_{CO_2}, usually not <14 mmol/L

Abbreviations: P_{CO_2} = partial pressure of carbon dioxide; HCO_3^- = bicarbonate

Compensation

Acid-base disturbances are frequently encountered in the ICU setting. Aid in recognition and approach to these problems is facilitated by an understanding of the compensation or response to each simple acid-base disturbance. As shown in Table 113–4, consideration of rules of thumb for compensation is useful.[78] To address them, it is necessary to have a pH, P_{CO_2}, and HCO_3 obtained from an arterial blood sample and to correlate these with the anion gap determined from serum electrolyte measurements. It is frequently stated clinically that the calculated HCO_3 from arterial blood gases is less accurate than the directly measured CO_2. This statement is misleading and subject to frequent confusion among students and staff. Although it is a calculated value, there is only one correct HCO_3 concentration assuming accurate measurement of pH and P_{CO_2}. Thus, the calculation of HCO_3 is as accurate as the two direct measurements from which it is determined. It is important to use the HCO_3 from the same sample because it represents an HCO_3 from the same vascular location (arterial versus venous) and at the same time as the pH and P_{CO_2}. All too frequently, efforts to interpret acid-base balance are based on electrolytes and arterial blood gases obtained at widely disparate points in time (often hours); this leads to the potential for erroneous conclusions if the clinical status of the patient has changed in the intervening time.

POTASSIUM BALANCE

The kidneys play a major role in the maintenance of potassium homeostasis. On a daily basis, approximately 60 to 100 mmol of potassium are ingested and must be excreted for balance to be maintained. Excretion occurs almost entirely by the kidneys. Potassium is filtered freely at the glomerulus and is largely reabsorbed by nephron segments before the collecting tubule. The excreted potassium represents potassium secreted into the tubular lumen in the collecting tubule.[79] Under steady-state conditions, the amount excreted balances exactly the amount ingested in the diet.

Potassium is the major intracellular cation, present at approximately 150 mmol in intracellular fluid (ICF). The ECF potassium concentration is between 3.5 and 5.0 mmol, indicating that only 2% of total body potassium is located within this space. Alterations in potassium balance are encountered frequently in ICU patients. To understand these disorders, which manifest as hyperkalemia and hypokalemia, it is important to evaluate both external balance (excretion) as well as internal balance (changes in distribution of potassium between ECF and ICF). Various factors can alter the normal distribution of potassium between these two fluid compartments. Hormones, particularly insulin, catecholamines (specifically beta$_2$ agonists), possibly mineralocorticoids, and HCO_3 result in increased potassium uptake by cells from the ECF.[80, 81] Conversely, potassium movement into cells may be retarded in insulin deficiency (uncontrolled diabetes), reduced beta$_2$-agonist activity (caused by administration of β-blocking agents), possibly by hypertonicity (e.g., hyperglycemia), and in hyperchloremic metabolic acidosis. In hyperchloremic metabolic acidosis, but not increased anion gap metabolic acidosis, potassium efflux from cells into the ECF occurs in exchange for H^+ that enters cells and is buffered.[82, 83] Although hyperkalemia is seen frequently (e.g., diabetic ketoacidosis), this is not due to the acidosis directly because the organic anions (ketones) accompany H^+ into cells, obviating a need for cation efflux as potassium; rather, in ketoacidosis, insulin lack is the primary mechanism that accounts for hyperkalemia. The factors affecting internal potassium balance should be considered as part of the evaluation and treatment of patients with altered serum potassium concentration.

As part of the evaluation of hyperkalemia, possible sources of potassium should also be considered. Excess potassium could result from increased exogenous administration and/or from increased endogenous release of potassium, as might occur with tissue damage. Hyperkalemia can also result from decreased excretory capacity in the face of a normal potassium load. In most situations with significant hyperkalemia, renal function is decreased to some extent. In hypokalemia, increased cellular uptake and enhanced loss of potassium from the body, either by the gastrointestinal tract or kidneys, should be considered.

As part of the assessment of alterations in potassium concentration, the cause for the abnormality should be identified. With regard to hyperkalemia, sources of increased K^+ entry into the ECF (endogenous and exogenous loads as well as internal shifts) and renal function should be evaluated. When serum K^+ is elevated, the expected renal response is an increase in potassium excretion. Conversely, potassium depletion caused by extrarenal potassium loss should lead to renal conservation of potassium. Under each circumstance, the renal response can be evaluated by measurement of the urine K^+. For example, increased urinary K^+ excretion would be expected in hyperkalemia if it is not directly due to defective renal excretory function. On the other hand, extrarenal potassium loss should lead to renal potassium conservation and a low (10–15 mmol if hypokalemia is chronic) urinary potassium concentration. Estimation of urinary K^+ may also provide evidence suggesting an inappropriate renal response to potassium depletion and thus might implicate the kidneys in the genesis of the potassium abnormality.

Calculation of the transtubular potassium concentration gradient has been introduced as a semiquantitative tool to assist in the evaluation of alterations of potassium balance.[84–86] The rationale for this test is to permit separate evaluation of the urine K^+ and the urine flow rate, the two major determinants of total potassium excretion ($U_{K+} \cdot V$ = total K^+ excretion). The concentration of potassium in the cortical collecting tubule lumen is affected largely by aldosterone and nonabsorbable anions.[84, 86] Beyond the cortical collecting tubule, urine osmolality rises from iso-osmolar values as a result of water reabsorption in the medullary collecting duct. The luminal K^+ in the cortical collecting duct can be deduced by correcting for this more distal water abstraction by factoring the urine K^+ by the urine to plasma osmolality. This can be done as follows:

$$K^+\text{urine}/(\text{Osm})\text{urine}/(\text{Osm})\text{plasma}$$

The transtubular potassium gradient (TTKG) can be calculated as follows:

$$\text{TTKG} = K^+\text{urine}/(U/P)\text{osm}/K^+\text{plasma}$$

where osm is osmolality. In normal subjects, during hypokalemia of nonrenal origin, the TTKG was approximately 1.[86] In hypokalemia resulting from hyperaldosteronism, this value rose to 7 and was 12 in normal subjects receiving the potent mineralocorticoid 9-α-fludrocortisone.[86] In hyperkalemic individuals, the TTKG was in excess of 10.[86] This test can provide information with respect to the renal response to changes in serum potassium and may aid in therapeutic maneuvers. For example, if a low TTKG is found in a hyperkalemic patient, confirmation of a deficiency in aldosterone state could be supported if the TTKG rises above 7 in response to 9-α-fludrocortisone (3 hours after 50 μg).[86]

References

1. Jochimsen F, Schafer JH, Maurer A, et al: Impairment of renal function in medical intensive care: Predictability of acute renal failure. Crit Care Med 1990; 18:480.
2. Menashe PI, Ross SA, Tottlieb JE: Acquired renal insufficiency in critically ill patients. Crit Care Med 1988; 16:1106.
3. Oken DE, Schoolwerth AC: The kidney. *In*: Laboratory Medicine: The Selection and Interpretation of Clinical Laboratory Studies. Noe DA, Rock RC (Eds). Baltimore, Williams & Wilkins, 1994, pp 401–461.
4. Arendshorst WJ, Navar LG: Renal circulation and glomerular hemodynamics. *In*: Diseases of the Kidney. 5th ed. Vol 1. Schrier RW, Gottschalk CW (Eds). Boston, Little, Brown and Co, 1993, pp 65–117.
5. Baer PG, McGiff JC: Hormonal systems and renal hemodynamics. Annu Rev Physiol 1980; 42:582.
6. Palmer RMJ, Ashton DS, Moncada S: Vascular endothelial cells synthesize nitric oxide from L-arginine. Nature 1988; 333:664.
7. Cogan MG: Renal effects of atrial natriuretic factor. Annu Rev Physiol 1990; 52:699.
8. Osswald H, Nabakowski G, Hermes H: Adenosine as a possible mediator of metabolic control of glomerular filtration rate. Int J Biochem 1978; 12:263.
9. Navar LG, Marsh DJ, Blantz RC, et al: Intrinsic control of renal hemodynamics. (symposium report). Fed Proc 1982; 41:3022.
10. Bergstrom J, Ahlberg M, Alvestrand A: Influence of protein intake on renal hemodynamics and plasma hormone concentrations in normal subjects. Acta Med Scand 1985; 217:189.
11. Bosch JP, Saccaggi A, Lauer A, et al: Renal functional reserve in humans. Am J Med 1983; 75:943.
12. McDonald RH Jr, Goldberg LI, McNay JL, et al: Effects of dopamine in man: Augmentation of sodium excretion, glomerular

filtration rate, and renal plasma flow. J Clin Invest 1964; 43:1116.
13. Szerlip HM: Renal-dose dopamine: Fact and fiction. Ann Intern Med 1991; 115:153.
14. Orme ML, Breckenridge A, Dollery CT: The effects of long term administration of dopamine on renal function in hypertensive patients. Eur J Clin Pharmacol 1973; 6:150.
15. Wesson LG Jr: The Physiology of the Kidney. New York, Grune & Stratton, 1969, pp 640–642.
16. Shemesh O, Golbetz H, Riss JP, et al: Limitations of creatinine as a filtration marker in glomerulopathic patients. Kidney Int 1985; 28:830.
17. Blaufox MD: Radionuclide techniques for the diagnosis of urinary tract disease. *In*: Contemporary Issues in Nephrology: 25. Diagnostic Techniques in Renal Disease. Narins RG, Stein JH (Eds). New York, Churchill Livingstone, 1992, pp 305–329.
18. Wharton WW, Sondeen JL, McBiles M, et al: Measurement of glomerular filtration rate in ICU patients using ^{99m}Tc-DTPA and inulin. Kidney Int 1992; 42:174.
19. Robert S, Zarowitz BJ: Is there a reliable index of glomerular filtration rate in critically ill patients? DICP Ann Pharmacother 1991; 25:169.
20. Salazar DE, Corcoran GB: Predicting creatinine clearance and renal drug clearance in obese patients from estimated fat-free body mass. Am J Med 1988; 84:1053.
21. Davies DF, Shock NW: Age changes in glomerular filtration rate, effective renal plasma flow and tubular excretory capacity in adult males. J Clin Invest 1950; 29:496.
22. Rowe JW, Andres R, Tobin JD, et al: The effect of age on creatinine clearance in men: A cross-sectional and longitudinal study. J Gerontology 1976; 31:155.
23. Kafetz K: Renal impairment in the elderly: A review. J Roy Soc Med 1983; 76:398.
24. Koopman MG, Koomen GCM, Krediet RT, et al: Circadian rhythm of glomerular filtration rate in normal individuals. Clin Sci 1989; 77:105.
25. Van Acker BAC, Koomen GCM, Koopman MG, et al: Discrepancy between circadian rhythms of inulin and creatinine clearance. J Lab Clin Med 1992; 120:400.
26. Bauer JH, Brooks CS, Burch RN: Clinical appraisal of creatinine clearance as a measurement of glomerular filtration rate. Am J Kidney Dis 1982; 2:337.
27. Lubowitz H, Slatopolsky E, Shankel S, et al: Glomerular filtration rate: Determination in patients with chronic renal disease. JAMA 1967; 199:252.
28. Gerard SK, Khayam-Bashi H: Characterization of creatinine error in ketotic patients: A prospective comparison of alkaline picrate methods with an enzymatic method. Am J Clin Pathol 1985; 84:659.
29. Molitch ME, Rodman E, Hirsch CA, et al: Spurious serum creatinine elevations in ketoacidosis. Ann Intern Med 1980; 93:280.
30. Cruickshank AM, Shenkin A: A comparison of the effect of acetoacetate concentration on the measurement of serum creatinine using Technicon SMAC II, Beckman Astra and enzymatic techniques. Ann Clin Biochem 1987; 24:317.
31. Mascioli SR, Bantle JP, Freier EF, et al: Artifactual elevation of serum creatinine level due to fasting. Arch Intern Med 1984; 144:1575.
32. Levey AS, Perrone RD, Madias NE: Serum creatinine and renal function. Annu Rev Med 1988; 39:465.
33. Kroll MH, Elin RJ: Mechanism of cefoxitin and cephalothin interference with the Jaffe method for creatinine. Clin Chem 1983; 29:2044.
34. Kroll MH, Koch TR, Drusano GL, et al: Lack of interference with creatinine assays by four cephalosporin-like antibiotics. Am J Clin Pathol 1984; 82:214.
35. Berglund F, Killander J, Pompeius R: Effect of trimethoprim-sulfamethoxazole on the renal excretion of creatinine in man. J Urol 1975; 114:802.
36. Odlind B, Hällgren R, Sohtell M, et al: Is ^{125}I iothalamate an ideal marker for glomerular filtration? Kidney Int 1985; 27:9.
37. Dubb JW, Stote RM, Familiar R, et al: Effect of cimetidine on renal function in normal man. Clin Pharmacol Ther 1978; 24:76.
38. Rocci ML Jr, Vlasses PH, Ferguson RK: Creatinine serum concentrations and H_2-receptor antagonists. Clin Nephrol 1984; 22:214.
39. Hilbrands LB, Artz MA, Wetzels JFM, et al: Cimetidine improves the reliability of creatinine as a marker of glomerular filtration. Kidney Int 1991; 40:1171.
40. Van Acker BAC, Koomen GCM, Koopman MG, et al: Creatinine clearance during cimetidine administration for measurement of glomerular filtration rate. Lancet 1992; 340:1326.
41. Kassirer JP: Clinical evaluation of kidney function–glomerular function. N Engl J Med 1971; 285:385.
42. Maroni BJ, Steinman TI, Mitch WE: A method for estimating nitrogen intake of patients with chronic renal failure. Kidney Int 1985; 27:58.
43. Mitch WE: Nutritional therapy and the progression of renal insufficiency. *In*: Nutrition and the Kidney. Mitch WE, Klahr S (Eds). Boston, Little, Brown and Co, 1988, pp 154–179.
44. Cockcroft DW, Gault MH: Prediction of creatinine clearance from serum creatinine. Nephron 1976; 16:31.
45. Mitch WE: Measuring the rate of progression of renal insufficiency. *In*: Contemporary Issues in Nephrology: 26. The Progressive Nature of Renal Disease. Mitch WE, Stein JH (Eds). New York, Churchill Livingstone, 1992, pp 203–221.
46. Moe GW, Legault L, Skorecki KL: Control of extracellular fluid volume and pathophysiology of edema formation. *In*: Breener BM, Rector FC Jr (Eds). The Kidney. 4th ed. Vol 1. Philadelphia, WB Saunders, 1991, pp 623–676.
47. Reeves WB, Andreoli TE: Tubular sodium transport. *In*: Diseases of the Kidney. 5th ed. Vol 1. Schrier RW, Gottschalk CW (Eds). Boston, Little, Brown and Co, 1993, pp 139–179.
48. Espinel CH: The FE_{Na} test: Use in the differential diagnosis of acute renal failure. JAMA 1976; 236:579.
49. Anderson RJ, Gross PA, Gabow P: Urinary chloride concentration in acute renal failure. Miner Electrolyte Metab 1984; 10:92.
50. Wilcox CS, Mitch WE, Kelly RA, et al: Response of the kidney to furosemide: I. Effects of salt intake and renal compensation. J Lab Clin Med 1983; 102:450.
51. Rudy D, Sica DA, Nunley J, et al: Continuous intravenous infusion of furosemide in diuretic resistant critical care patients. Manuscript submitted for publication.
52. Lassiter WE, Gottschalk CW: Regulation of water balance: Urine concentration and dilution. *In*: Diseases of the Kidney. 5th Ed. Vol 1. Schrier RW, Gottschalk CW (Eds). Boston, Little, Brown and Co, 1993, pp 119–138.
53. Dunn FL, Brennan TJ, Nelson AE, et al: The role of blood osmolality and volume in regulating vasopressin in renal medulla in situ. J Clin Invest 1973; 52:3212.
54. Wesson LG Jr: Physiology of the Human Kidney. New York, Grune & Stratton, 1969, p 433.
55. Bastl CP, Rudnick MR, Narins RG: Diagnostic approaches to acute renal failure. *In*: Contemporary Issues in Nephrology: 6. Acute Renal Failure. Brenner BM, Stein JH (Eds). New York, Churchill Livingstone, 1980, pp 17–51.
56. Anderson RJ, Linas SL, Berns AS, et al: Nonoliguric acute renal failure. N Engl J Med 1977; 296:1134.
57. Berl T, Schrier RW: Disorders of water metabolism. *In*: Renal and Electrolyte Disorders. 3rd ed. Schrier RW (Ed). Boston, Little, Brown and Co, 1986, pp 1–78.
58. Bartter FC, Schwartz WB: The syndrome of inappropriate secretion of antidiuretic hormone. Am J Med 1967; 42:790.
59. Robertson GL, Shelton RL, Athar S: The osmoregulation of vasopressin. Kidney Int 1976; 10:25.
60. Anderson RJ, Chung H-M, Kluge R, et al: Hyponatremia: A prospective analysis of its epidemiology and the pathogenetic role of vasopressin. Ann Intern Med 1985; 102:164–168.
61. Berl T: Treating hyponatremia: Damned if we do and damned if we don't. Kidney Int 1990; 37:1006.
62. Narins RG, Emmett M: Simple and mixed acid-base disorders: A practical approach. Medicine 1980; 59:161.
63. Atkinson DE, Bourke E: Metabolic aspects of the regulation of systemic pH. Am J Physiol 1987; 252:F947.
64. Halperin ML, Jungas RL, Cheema-Dhadli S, et al: Disposal of the daily acid load: An integrated function of the liver. Trends Biochem Sci 1987; 12:197.
65. Guder WG, Haussinger D, Gerok W: Renal and hepatic nitrogen metabolism in systemic acid base regulation. J Clin Chem Biochem 1987; 25:457.
66. Cohen RD: Roles of the liver and kidney in acid-base regulation and its disorders. Br J Anaesth 1991; 67:154.

67. Halperin ML, Kamel KS, Ethier JH, et al: Biochemistry and physiology of ammonium excretion. *In*: The Kidney. 2nd ed. Vol 2. Seldin DW, Giebisch G (Eds). New York, Raven Press, 1992, p 2645.
68. Goldstein MB, Bear R, Richardson RMA, et al: The urine anion gap: A clinically useful index of ammonium excretion. Am J Med Sci 1986; 292:198.
69. Batlle DC, Hizon M, Cohen E, et al: The use of the urinary anion gap in the diagnosis of hyperchloremic metabolic acidosis. N Engl J Med 1988; 318:594.
70. Halperin ML, Kamel KS, Narins RG: Use of urine electrolytes and osmolality: Bringing physiology to the bedside. *In*: Diagnostic Techniques in Renal Disease. Narins RG, Stein JH (Eds). New York, Churchill Livingstone, 1992, p 1.
71. Kamel KS, Ethier JH, Richardson RMA: Urine electrolytes and osmolality: When and how to use them. Am J Nephrol 1990; 10:89.
72. Narins RG: Acid-base disorders: Definitions and introductory concepts. *In*: Clinical Disorders of Fluid and Electrolyte Metabolism. 4th ed. Maxwell MH, Kleeman CR, Narins RG (Eds). New York, McGraw-Hill, 1987, pp 585–595.
73. Emmett M, Narins RG: Clinical use of the anion gap. Medicine 1977; 56:38.
74. Gabow PA: Disorders associated with an altered anion gap. Kidney Int 1985; 27:472.
75. Harrington JT: Metabolic alkalosis. Kidney Int 1984; 26:88.
76. Alpern RJ, Emmett M, Seldin DW: Metabolic alkalosis. *In*: The Kidney. 2nd ed. Vol 2. Seldin DW, Giebisch G (Eds). New York, Raven Press, 1992, pp 2733–2758.
77. Sabatini S, Kurtzman NA: The maintenance of metabolic alkalosis: Factors which decrease bicarbonate excretion. Kidney Int 1984; 25:357.
78. Halperin ML, Goldstein MB: Fluid, Electrolyte, and Acid-Base Emergencies. Philadelphia, WB Saunders, 1988, p 33.
79. Wright FS, Giebisch G: Regulation of potassium excretion. *In*: The Kidney. 2nd ed. Vol 2. Seldin DW, Giebisch G (Eds). New York, Raven Press, 1992, pp 2209–2247.
80. Sterns RH, Cox M, Feig PU, et al: Internal potassium balance and the control of the plasma potassium concentration. Medicine 1981; 60:339.
81. Ponce SP, Jennings AE, Madias NE, et al: Drug-induced hyperkalemia. Medicine 1985; 64:357.
82. Adrogue HJ, Madias NE: Changes in plasma potassium concentration during acute acid-base disturbances. Am J Med 1981; 71:456.
83. Halperin ML, Goldstein MB: Fluid, Electrolyte, and Acid-Base Emergencies. Philadelphia, WB Saunders, 1988, pp 216–219.
84. West ML, Bendz O, Chen CB, et al: Development of a test to evaluate the transtubular potassium concentration gradient in the cortical collecting duct in vivo. Miner Electrolyte Metab 1986; 12:226.
85. West ML, Marsden PA, Richardson RMA, et al: New clinical approach to evaluate disorders of potassium excretion. Miner Electrolyte Metab 1986; 12:234.
86. Ethier JH, Kamel KS, Magner PO, et al: The transtubular potassium concentration in patients with hypokalemia and hyperkalemia. Am J Kidney Dis 1990; 15:309.

CHAPTER 114

Adult Acute and Chronic Renal Failure

Todd W. B. Gehr, MD • Anton C. Schoolwerth, MD

The term *acute renal failure* (ARF) is used to describe any abrupt and almost complete cessation of renal function. *Chronic renal insufficiency* refers to an irreversible reduction in renal function that is usually progressive in nature and ultimately leads to chronic renal failure. The term *end-stage renal disease* is applied to the patient with chronic renal failure who also requires some type of renal replacement therapy, such as dialysis or kidney transplantation. Although ARF is more relevant to critical care, patients with renal insufficiency, dialysis patients, and kidney transplantation patients all have unique critical care requirements.

Renal hypoperfusion that results in functional or prerenal renal failure, urinary tract obstruction, and acute renal parenchymal damage that leads to a reduction in renal function produce characteristic responses that form the basis for diagnostic and therapeutic approaches. It is customary to refer to acute renal parenchymal failure in mechanistic terms (e.g., acute tubular necrosis, vasomotor nephropathy), even though these terms are not entirely accurate.[1] Some of the confusion in terminology is a result of the fact that ARF has a variety of causes, the most common of which are listed in Table 114–1. Whereas ARF and chronic renal failure are addressed in this chapter in general terms, five specific causes of ARF that are particularly important in critical care are discussed in detail: ARF associated with cardiac failure and sepsis; interstitial nephritis; hepatorenal syndrome; myoglobinuric ARF (rhabdomyolysis); and pulmonary-renal syndromes.

ACUTE RENAL FAILURE

Clinical Presentation

ARF is commonly induced by shock, sepsis, or trauma and is characterized by an abrupt decrease in the glomerular filtration rate (GFR). Oliguria (defined as a urine output <400 mL/d) is typical,[2] although nonoliguric ARF is becoming increasingly common.[3] Whether or not oliguria is present, the urine volume is quite constant from day to day and, once renal failure has fully developed, usually does not increase significantly even when large doses of furosemide or ethacrynic acid are administered.[3,4] However, the urinary output may decrease in parallel with decreases in blood pressure and cardiac output if a patient is intermittently hypotensive.

The GFR remains fixed at a very low level until recovery. As a result, the serum creatinine concentration rises steadily by 1 to 4 mg/dL per day. It would be quite atypical for the serum creatinine concentration to increase by 2 mg/dL on the first day, fall slightly on the next, and then rise by 0.5 mg/dL during the third day. However, such a pattern is common in ARF secondary to functional (pre) renal failure and in urinary outflow obstruction.

Although renal failure may last 3 or 4 weeks in some patients, renal function usually begins to improve 10 to 12 days after onset of the disease.[2] In general, nonoliguric renal failure is of significantly shorter duration than oliguric renal failure and often lasts only 5 to 6 days.[5] In both, recovery is heralded by initially small increases in urine volume on successive days (1–2 L/d or more). Massive diuresis (increases of 3–5 L/d) during the recovery period is no longer common, probably because the aggressive application of dialysis now prevents the severe fluid overload and high blood urea nitrogen (BUN) level that were commonplace in the predialysis era.

Total anuria is so atypical of uncomplicated ARF that its presence for longer than 2 or 3 days in a hemodynamically stable patient should prompt suspicion of urinary outflow obstruction, compromise of the major renal vessels, renal cortical necrosis, glomerular or small-vessel disease, or a ruptured bladder as a possible cause.

Causes

ARF occurs most commonly in a setting of surgery, trauma, sepsis, hypotension, hemolytic reaction, or poisoning. Un-

TABLE 114–1. Causes of Renal Failure

Glomerulopathy (Especially Necrotizing, Proliferative, Membranoproliferative, and Rapidly Progressive)
Streptococcal or other bacterial infection
Viral infection
Lupus erythematosus
Goodpasture's syndrome
Eclampsia
Mixed cryoglobulinemia

Vascular and Thrombotic Disease
Malignant hypertension
Wegener's granulomatosis
Hypersensitivity angiitis
Periarteritis nodosa
Thrombotic thrombocytopenic purpura
Hemolytic uremic syndrome
Postpartum acute renal failure
Disseminated intravascular coagulation (cortical necrosis)
Scleroderma
Acute allograft rejection
Fat or cholesterol embolism
Renal venous–vena caval thrombosis
Post-traumatic renal arterial thrombosis or avulsion
Aortic coarctation, dissection, or thrombosis
Renal artery dysplasia

Interstitial Disease
Allergic, postinfectious, or idiosyncratic interstitial nephritis
Fulminating pyelonephritis (in infants)
Papillary necrosis

Functional (Pre)renal Failure
Severe volume depletion
Shock
Sepsis
Trauma
Heart failure

Acute Renal Parenchymal Failure (Acute Tubular Necrosis, Vasomotor Nephropathy)
All causes of functional renal failure (e.g., nephrotic syndrome, sepsis, hemorrhage, vomiting, diarrhea, and hypotension) if not adequately treated
Blunt trauma
Burns
Surgery
Bone fractures
Intravascular hemolysis
Heat stroke
Malaria
Snake bite
Electric shock
Dissecting aneurysm (e.g., Marfan's syndrome, homocystinuria)
Septicemia
Rhabdomyolysis
Antibiotics
Poisoning with mercury, bismuth, phosphorus, lead, carbon tetrachloride, ethylene glycol, methanol, poisonous mushrooms, and Lysol household spray
Methoxyflurane
Cyclosporin
Chemotherapeutic agents
Uric acid

Hepatorenal Syndrome

Urinary Obstruction
Ureter, bladder, or urethra (due to inflammation, calculus, blood clot, urate crystallization, tumor, retroperitoneal mass, hemorrhage, or fibrosis

Bladder Rupture

fortunately, a number of these predisposing factors may be concomitantly present in critically ill patients.

Once common, obstetric complications such as intra- and postpartum hemorrhage, placenta previa, and abruptio placentae still produce ARF in a small but significant number of patients.[6] Septic abortion, especially when attended by clostridial endometritis, is the leading cause of ARF in areas of the world where contraception and medically supervised abortion are not readily available.[7] Transfusion accidents, formerly a major contribution to the syndrome, also have become quite uncommon as blood bank techniques for the detection of ABO and Rh blood group mismatch have improved.[8] Hemolytic crises due to glucose-6-phosphate dehydrogenase deficiency[9] and paroxysmal nocturnal hemoglobinuria[10] are rare potential causes of the syndrome. Other uncommon causes associated with hemolysis include intra-amniotic infusions of hypertonic saline,[11] intracervical instillation of various solutions for self-induced abortion,[12] intravenous glycerol therapy for cerebral edema,[13] snake bite,[14] malarial blackwater fever,[15] and acute arsine poisoning.[16]

A variety of industrial and household chemicals may produce both severe acute illness and ARF. Carbon tetrachloride, ethylene glycol (found in antifreeze), methanol, trichlorethylene (solvent), toluene, paraquat, and chlordane have been among the most commonly identified causative agents in the past but appear to have become less common offenders since their attendant dangers have become widely known. Industrial exposure to these compounds and to certain heavy metals (especially mercury and lead) is still a problem. Some poisons exert a direct nephrotoxic effect, whereas others, such as *Amanita* species mushrooms and carbon tetrachloride, cause ARF by inducing severe volume depletion and cardiovascular collapse.[17, 18] Certain other poisons produce ARF secondary to myoglobinuria,[19] hemolysis,[20] or fulminating hepatic failure.[16]

Antibiotics, particularly aminoglycoside antibiotics, continue to be a frequent cause of ARF. With the exception of streptomycin, aminoglycoside antibiotics are universally nephrotoxic when given in sufficiently large doses for extended periods of time.[21] These agents are excreted almost exclusively via the kidney (predominantly through glomerular filtration) and have a relatively low therapeutic index. Their dosage must be carefully adjusted in the setting of renal insufficiency. The half-life of gentamicin in the serum of normal patients is approximately 2 hours, whereas in renal tissue of the same individuals it is about 4 days.[22] Thus, the concentration of the drug in renal tissue increases inexorably with each injection. With careful dosing, the tissue concentration usually does not reach a frankly toxic level during a typical 5- to 7-day course of treatment, although small changes in renal function may be seen even when the peak and trough concentrations of these antibiotics have been consistently within the acceptable range.[23] The potential for nephrotoxicity seems to be about the same for gentamicin and amikacin but may be lower for tobramicin, which has a distinctly lower rate of tissue accumulation.[24] Nevertheless, tobramicin is still a potent nephrotoxin and must be administered with the same dosing precautions as for gentamicin and amikacin.

The degree of renal functional impairment produced by the aminoglycoside antibiotics ranges from mild renal insufficiency, with a maximum serum creatinine concentration of approximately 1.5 to 3 mg/dL, to frank renal failure, which is indistinguishable from typical ARF. Even if it is uncertain whether mild renal insufficiency in hemodynamically unstable patients is caused by aminoglycoside toxicity, further use of these agents before the full return of renal function should be avoided if possible. On the other hand, dialysis is by far preferable to fatal sepsis. In general, the incidence or severity of aminoglycoside nephrotoxicity can be minimized by careful limitation of the duration of antibiotic therapy, adjustment of dosage according to a patient's renal function, and maintenance of adequate volume status throughout the treatment period. In most patients, alternative antibiotics can be safely employed.

Amphotericin, another commonly used antibiotic, also inevitably causes renal damage. As with aminoglycosides, the occurrence of renal dysfunction is dosage dependent, with cumulative doses of 2 to 3 g being necessary before important toxicity occurs.[25] Hypokalemia and renal acidification and concentrating defects commonly precede reductions in GFR.[26–29]

ARF severity following the intravenous administration of radiographic contrast agents ranges from mild nonoliguric reductions in GFR to irreversible renal failure. In normal patients, the incidence is probably less than 2%.[30, 31] Predisposing risk factors lead to a much higher incidence, particularly in the ICU setting. Preexisting renal insufficiency is probably the most important of these risk factors,[32–34] but diabetes mellitus,[35, 36] multiple myeloma,[37] intravascular volume depletion,[38] and congestive heart failure[40] as well as the amount of contrast material used[34] and a patient's age,[39] are additional important risk factors. The use of noniodinated contrast materials may reduce the incidence of this serious complication, although the results of studies to date do not suggest that this is the case.

Pathogenesis

The pathogenic mechanisms responsible for ARF have been the subject of debate ever since the syndrome first became widely recognized about 50 years ago.[42] A number of mechanisms have been proposed to explain the cessation of glomerular filtration characteristic of this syndrome. These mechanisms are based on a variety of animal models of ARF, four of which are intratubular obstruction,[43] tubular backleak of filtrate,[44] filtration failure related to disturbed renal hemodynamics,[45] and reduction in glomerular permeability.[46] It is likely that no one mechanism explains this syndrome because measures aimed at preventing it (e.g., diuresis, use of vasodilators) invariably fail. In addition, the type of renal injury may be an important determinant of a particular mechanism. Combinations of mechanisms are probably necessary to explain the pathogenesis of this complex syndrome, although the susceptibility of the epithelial cells in the renal tubule to ischemic injury may be central to our understanding.[47, 47a]

Differential Diagnosis

The diagnostic approach to a patient with reduced renal function is outlined in Figure 114–1. This approach should be utilized for all patients so that potentially reversible diagnoses are not missed. Determining the time course of the reduction in renal function and whether the dysfunction is acute or chronic and subsequent categorization of the cause of the failure as either functional (prerenal), renal parenchymal, or related to urinary tract obstruction are useful.

ACUTE VERSUS CHRONIC RENAL FAILURE

On admission to the hospital, a severely ill renal dysfunction patient often has an elevated serum creatinine concentration, which may be either recent (ARF) or long-standing (chronic renal insufficiency). In the latter case, the patient may have been unaware of a kidney problem because chronic renal disease usually does not have obvious symptoms except when it is associated with renal colic, dysuria, gross hematuria, or anuria. Instead, renal disease may be discovered when the patient seeks medical care either for unrelated reasons or because of the dramatic and life-threatening complications that develop during end-stage renal failure.

Since ARF usually causes serum creatinine concentration to increase by about 1 to 3 mg/dL per day, a patient admitted for an acute illness of 1 or 2 days' duration who has a serum creatinine level of 10 to 12 mg/dL or greater, either has had ARF considerably longer than the history would suggest or has chronic renal disease that may have gone unrecognized. A carefully taken history may be very helpful in distinguishing between these possibilities. Most forms of ARF are associated with a sudden and marked reduction in urine volume that patients may not report unless they are specifically asked. By contrast, nocturia is an almost universal hallmark of chronic renal disease, and its absence or very recent development strongly suggests a relatively acute process. A long history of difficulties with micturition (e.g., hesitancy, urgency, dribbling, or incontinence in particular) suggests chronic bladder outflow obstruction as the cause of renal dysfunction. A history of any form of renal disease, proteinuria, or abnormal urinary sediment; repeated bouts of dysuria and other symptoms of pyelonephritis; long-standing and severe hypertension; prior abdominal or pelvic irradiation for the treatment of malignancy; diabetes of many years' duration or other systemic diseases that commonly cause chronic renal failure; repeated passage of renal stones; chronic analgesic ingestion; or a family history of polycystic kidney disease, Alport's syndrome, or other hereditary renal disease suggests chronic renal involvement.

On physical examination, a patient with chronic renal failure frequently displays a highly characteristic, yellow-tan, sallow coloration of the skin that is not found in the acutely uremic patient. Although pruritus is often an extremely bothersome symptom in acute as well as chronic renal failure, the association of both old and new pruritic excoriations of the skin is an unmistakable sign of chronicity. Symptomatic renal osteodystrophy with pain and difficulty in walking are hallmarks of chronic (but not acute) renal failure. Nerve deafness or keratoconus may indicate chronic renal failure due to Alport's syndrome, and detection of large cystic kidneys on abdominal palpation provide almost prima facie evidence of polycystic kidney disease. A lax rectal sphincter and perianal anesthesia are hallmarks of a neurogenic bladder, whereas a palpable bladder or an impaired ability to initiate or sustain urination suggests bladder outflow problems. Marked prostatic enlargement in men, cervical or pelvic malignancies in women, and a rectal mass in patients of either sex may suggest the existence and cause of chronic obstructive uropathy.

Very few laboratory determinations are helpful in distinguishing ARF from chronic renal failure; however, the detection of normocytic, normochromic anemia in a patient whose serum creatinine concentration has not yet reached 6 mg/dL favors a chronic process. The serum electrolyte profile can be equally abnormal in the two conditions. ARF frequently causes a rapid depression of calcium level and an increase in phosphorus concentration comparable with that found in chronic renal failure, and acidosis may be severe in acutely ill hypercatabolic patients very early in the course of ARF. Urinary sodium, potassium, and creatinine concentrations are usually comparable in the two conditions; urine concentrating capacity is also equally affected, and the excreted fraction of filtered sodium are elevated.

An abdominal radiograph or ultrasound examination can be very helpful in diagnosis. At 2 or more days after the onset of ARF, the kidney typically is notably enlarged and usually has normal echogenicity; in contrast, most forms of chronic renal failure result in small, abnormally echogenic kidneys. Both radiography and ultrasound can detect nephrocalcinosis and stag-horn calculi found in some forms of chronic renal failure as well as ureteral stones that might be the cause of acute obstructive renal failure. The ultrasonic examination is now used routinely to rule out acute upper

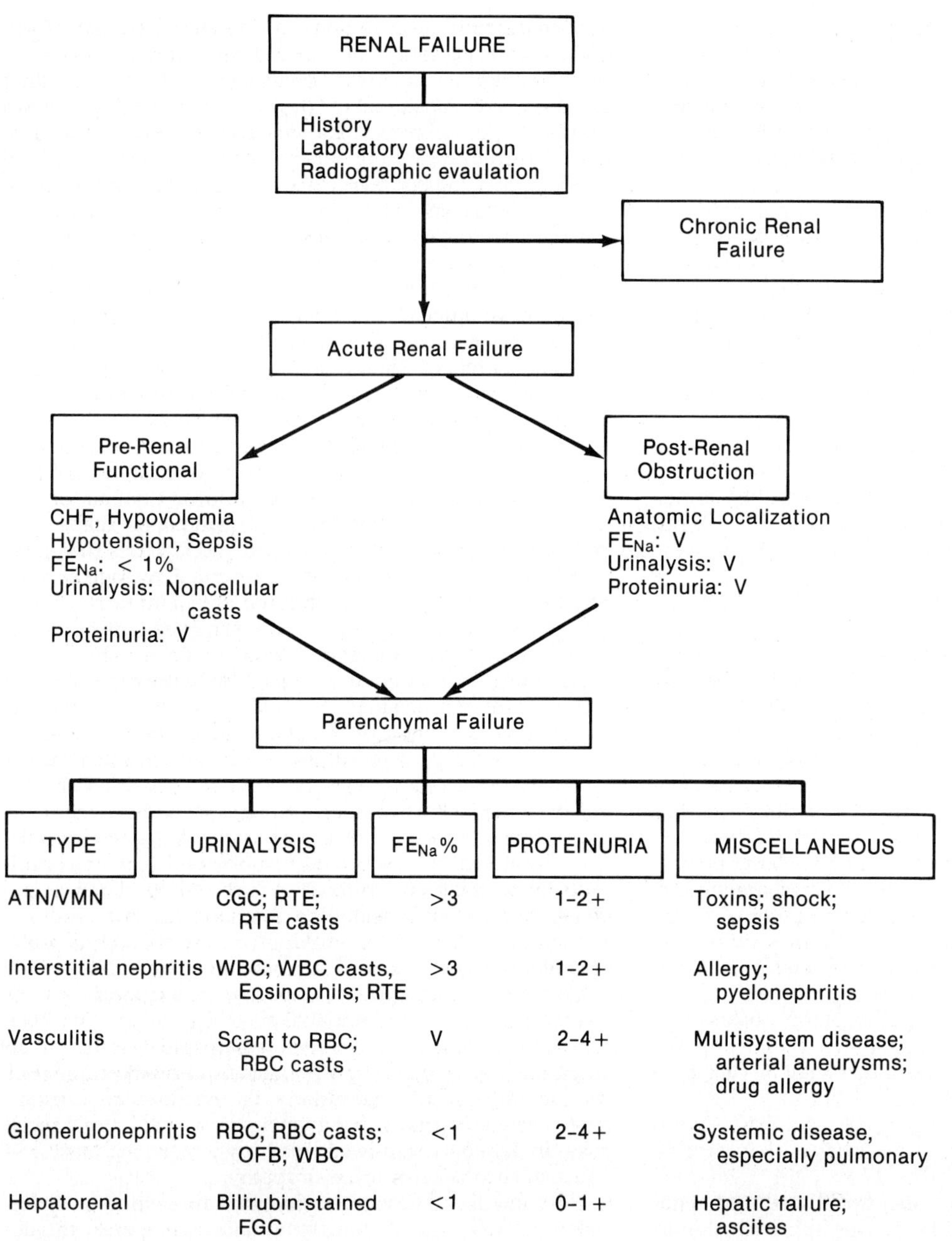

Figure 114–1. Diagnostic approach to renal failure. *Abbreviations*: CHF = congestive heart failure; ATN = acute tubular necrosis; VMN = vasomotor nephropathy; CGC = coarsely granular casts; FGC = finely granular casts; RBC = red blood cell; WBC = white blood cell; RTE = renal tubular epithelium; FE_{Na} = fractional excretion of sodium; V = variable; OFB = oval fat bodies. (Adapted from Rudnick MR, Bastl CP, Elfinbein IB, et al: The differential diagnosis of acute renal failure. *In*: Acute Renal Failure. Brenner BM, Lazarus MJ [Eds]. New York, Churchill Livingstone, 1983, p 177.)

urinary tract obstruction.[48] However, the typical hydronephrotic dilatation of the renal pelvis is not invariably found in patients with proven acute upper tract obstruction.[49] Therefore, the ultrasound procedure should be followed by direct urologic assessment (cystoscopy and retrograde pyelography) when obstruction is strongly suspected in a patient with no obvious other cause for renal failure. Radiographic studies of the outer clavicle and hands can document the presence of osteomalacia and other changes of long-standing hyperparathyroidism that are not seen in ARF.

ACUTE RENAL FAILURE DUE TO RENAL PARENCHYMAL FAILURE VERSUS FUNCTIONAL (PRERENAL) RENAL FAILURE

Severe volume depletion reduces both GFR and renal blood flow. In young and otherwise healthy individuals, the serum creatinine concentration usually does not exceed 3 mg/dL unless the volume deficit is severe enough to cause hypotension. However, severe volume depletion in subjects with even mild chronic renal disease, in elderly patients, and in patients with diabetes and hypertension may lead to a far more serious reduction in GFR with oliguria and a progressive rise in the serum creatinine concentration sufficiently great to suggest ARF. Unlike functional renal failure, ARF cannot be reversed by normalizing a patient's hemodynamic status, and no other presently available treatment appears to significantly alter its course. Thus, prevention is more practical than is the attempt to find a cure.

ASSESSING VOLUME STATUS

The clinical assessment of a patient's volume status is often inexact. Skin turgor, axillary moistness, and the moistness of the mucous membranes of the mouth are often examined to judge the degree of dehydration, but these indicators are not always reliable. Orthostatic hypotension is probably the most reliable physical indicator of serious volume depletion. Changes of 15 to 20 mm Hg and of 10 mm Hg in systolic and diastolic pressures, respectively, suggest the loss of about 20% or more of body water. However, orthostatic changes also are found in seemingly euvolemic patients after prolonged bed rest, in some patients taking antihypertensive medications, phenothiazines, narcotics, or antidepressants; in subjects with severe diabetic neuropathy; and in others with certain rare forms of neurogenic dysautonomia. It should be stressed that the absence of an orthostatic change in blood pressure or of a change in heart rate does not rule out a degree of volume depletion that can be especially harmful to renal function in elderly subjects or in patients with relatively mild chronic renal insufficiency.

The pulmonary artery wedge pressure is a valuable and widely used indicator of the adequacy of a patient's plasma volume. However, a high wedge pressure does not necessarily signify a normal or supernormal plasma volume. The wedge pressure reflects both the effective blood volume and the competence of the heart to accommodate the volume presented to it. Thus, severe plasma volume depletion is partly offset by an increase in capacitance vessel tone that may help sustain normal central venous and wedge pressures. In this case, rapid intravenous infusions may produce a significant central pressure increase, even when the volume deficit is still significant. Slowing or temporarily stopping the infusion does not uncommonly cause the return of pressure to or even below the preinfusion value; slow and careful continuation of the infusion can then be reinstituted. However, when cardiac failure is determined to be the primary cause of reduced renal perfusion, as in a patient with pulmonary edema following an acute myocardial infarction, attempts to restore renal function by further volume expansion obviously are contraindicated until the cardiac problem has been adequately treated. The determination of other central hemodynamic parameters such as cardiac index and systemic vascular resistance often further assists in both volume assessment and therapeutic maneuvers.

The fluid balance, calculated by comparing fluid intake with loss through both renal and extrarenal routes, is an important indicator of the adequacy of hydration when it is accurately recorded. Fluid balance calculated only from fluid intake and measurable output ignores insensible fluid loss through the skin and lungs, which can be substantial. Basal insensible water loss averages 0.5 to 0.6 mL per kilogram of body weight per hour (840–1000 mL/d in an individual weighing 70 kg); this loss increases by about 300 mL/d for each 1°C change in body temperature.[50] Additional fluid is lost as the relative humidity of the environment falls and the ambient temperature rises; thus, insensible losses of 2 L or more per day are not unusual in febrile patients who live in hot, dry environments. This insensible water loss is offset to some extent by the amount of water formed through metabolism, which may be as much as 500 mL/d in the catabolic patient. Fortunately, close monitoring of body weight can help identify any error in fluid balance estimates made because of insensible fluid loss. Except in individuals whose intravascular compartment is depleted by concealed bleeding or extravascular sequestration of fluid, change in body weight is among the most important and reliable indicators of an acute change in fluid volume. In fact, in patients with rapidly changing statuses, determining body weight more than once per day may be necessary.

The accurate assessment of urine volume is of obvious importance in the evaluation of ARF. The term *anuria* refers to the most severe reduction of urine volume (100 mL/d or less). *Oliguria* is a reduction of excreted urine volume to 100 to 400 mL/d. Whereas in the past the term *polyuria* was used to describe the excretion of urine volumes greater than 400 mL/d in the setting of ARF, the term *nonoliguria* is now often applied in its place to the ARF patient with excreted urine volumes of between 400 mL/d and 2 L/d. *Polyuria* now is applied to the patient with urine excretion of greater than 3 L/d.

Anuria may result from complete urinary tract obstruction, bilateral cortical necrosis, acute glomerulonephritis or vasculitis, or bilateral renal arterial or venous occlusion. The presence of alternating anuria and polyuria is strongly suggestive of intermittent urinary tract obstruction. Although most cases of ARF result in oliguria, anuria is more common than was once thought.[51] Whereas transient episodes of reversible anuria lasting up to 6 hours can occur with hypotension and dehydration, sustained anuria argues against the presence of functional renal failure.

Oliguria may occur with functional renal failure, ARF, or urinary tract obstruction. When oliguria accompanies functional renal failure, the urine is concentrated and has a low sodium content. With usual solute loads of 500 to 600 mOsm/d and a normal urinary concentrating ability of 1200 mOsm/L, a urine volume of 400 to 500 mL is necessary to maintain solute balance. Therefore, a urine volume of less than 400 to 500 mL/d results in the accumulation of excess solutes (e.g., BUN, creatinine). In critically ill patients, the usual solute load may be increased dramatically owing to increased catabolism and parenteral nutrition. This large solute load may increase the obligatory urine volume to greater than 1 L/d, so that even with nonoliguric or polyuric volumes, accumulation of excess solute may occur.

Otherwise normal subjects with purely functional renal failure excrete a concentrated urine that has a vanishingly low urine sodium concentration, a urine-plasma creatinine ratio far greater than 20, a high urine osmolality, and a benign urinary sediment. The fractional excretion of sodium, which was defined in the preceding chapter, is probably the best single indicator of renal function and is usually below 1%. No difficulty is encountered in separating such individuals from those with ARF on this basis alone (see Fig. 114–1). However, the situation often becomes rather blurred in volume-depleted patients with preexisting renal disease as well as in the elderly, whose capacity to maximally conserve sodium and to concentrate the urine appropriately may be severely blunted by benign nephrosclerosis.[52] In these patients, urine sodium concentration and the urine-plasma creatinine and osmolality ratios may approach those expected in ARF despite the presence of marked volume depletion, significant hypotension, or cardiac failure. Prompt return of renal function following correction of volume abnormalities or a salutary response to diuretic therapy often proves the functional origin of renal failure that otherwise might be mistaken for atypical ARF.

Assessment of the urinary composition may be complicated if the patient has received potent diuretics within the preceding 12 hours or is undergoing an osmotic diuresis maintained by glycosuria or mannitol infusions; even in the presence of serious volume depletion, the urine sodium concentration is apt to be much higher than it would otherwise be, whereas the osmolality and urine-plasma creatinine ratio may be reduced. Recently administered infusions of radiologic contrast medium exert the same osmotic effect, and irrigation of the bladder with either a glucose or saline solution grossly distorts the composition of urine obtained soon thereafter. These considerations must be kept in mind when interpreting the pathophysiologic connotations of urine composition. Furthermore, urine sodium, osmolality, and urine-plasma creatinine values that typify functional renal failure may be encountered with any parenchymal renal disease that greatly reduces renal perfusion while largely sparing tubular function (e.g., hepatorenal syndrome,[53] vasculitis, or glomerulonephritis), despite evidence of euvolemia or even plasma volume expansion.

Chemical and microscopic examination of the urine can offer valuable diagnostic clues in the evaluation of ARF. A positive reaction for blood on an orthotoluidine-impregnated dipstick test indicates the presence of heme pigment, either in the form of myoglobin (seen in rhabdomyolysis) or free hemoglobin (seen in transfusion reaction and hemolytic anemia), of red blood cells, or of both. A positive result and the absence of red blood cells on microscopic examination support the former two diagnoses, which can be confirmed by more specific laboratory methods. Knowledge of the quantity and quality of protein is also helpful. Minimal proteinuria characterizes functional renal failure and urinary tract obstruction. Glomerular disease leads to selective albuminuria, whereas ARF and acute interstitial nephritis lead to nonselective proteinuria.[54] Light-chain proteinuria, as seen in multiple myeloma, causes ARF and can be determined with urinary immunoelectrophoresis.

The urinary sediment in functional renal failure and urinary tract obstruction tends to be unimpressive and often consists of increased numbers of hyaline and finely granular casts. The presence of a large number of tubular epithelial cells, both free and in casts, and of many coarsely granular casts characterizes the urinary sediment in ARF due to parenchymal failure. Inflammatory diseases of the kidney (glomerulonephritis, vasculitis, or interstitial nephritis) result in the presence of red blood cells and white blood cells, both free and in casts, in the urine. The importance of identifying these cellular elements in the urine cannot be overstated.

IMPORTANT ETIOLOGIES FOR ACUTE RENAL FAILURE IN THE CRITICAL CARE SETTING

Acute Renal Failure Associated with Cardiac Failure, Hypoxia, or Sepsis

Hemodynamic instability due to cardiac failure, hypoxia, or sepsis occurs commonly in the intensive care setting, and its incidence has increased since the advent of sophisticated life-support systems. Indeed, sepsis has been identified as an important predisposing factor in up to one third of patients who develop ARF.[55] The normal kidney responds to heart failure in much the same way as it does to uncomplicated volume depletion: the GFR and renal blood flow decrease modestly, urinary sodium excretion is reduced, and the urine osmolality is high. The urinary sediment should be relatively benign in the absence of chronic renal disease, but, in contrast to in the volume-depleted state, the elevated central venous pressure and decreased renal perfusion in heart failure may cause a significant degree of proteinuria.

Despite normal or hyperdynamic cardiac function, sepsis is often associated with reductions in renal function. Like the kidney in heart failure, the urinary characteristics suggest functional or prerenal renal failure. The etiology of this renal vasoconstriction remains unknown but may be related to the stimulation of a number of vasoconstrictor substances such as endothelin and arachidonic acid derivatives.[56]

As blood pressure is reduced, glomerular filtration is maintained through autoregulatory mechanisms. Autoregulation is apparently blunted in many elderly patients and in those with underlying renal disease, especially after severe surgical trauma or during sepsis. In this population, systemic hypotension or compromised cardiac output, or both, may cause large reductions in renal perfusion and glomerular filtration that suggest the development of ARF. The true cause becomes apparent if the patient retains the capacity to conserve sodium appropriately and to concentrate the urine; exhibits either spontaneous fluctuations in urine volume or an increased urine output in response to therapy with diuretic agents or to an improvement in blood pressure; and rapidly recovers renal function after hemodynamic instability is reversed. As in volume depletion, patients with preexisting renal disease may not show the expected urinary characteristics, making differentiation from ARF rather difficult. This sequence of events is common after cardiovascular surgery, especially in patients who require vasopressor and inotropic agents for several days postoperatively.

Unlike simple volume depletion in which the underlying basis for renal dysfunction usually can be easily corrected, heart failure, sepsis, and hypoxia often do not immediately respond to treatment. Additional synergistic factors, such as the use of aminoglycoside antibiotics, may also be important.[57] It is not unusual for patients to present a rather baffling clinical picture that suggests ARF and that may last for many days. However, the rate of increase in serum creatinine concentration may be inconstant, a clear improvement in urine volume or a smaller rise in serum creatinine may occur on days when the hemodynamic status is ameliorated, some modest response to diuretics may be observed, and the urine volume may fluctuate significantly from day to day. All these features are highly atypical of acute renal parenchymal failure. Nevertheless, dialytic therapy may be required either for treatment of progressive volume overload, hyperkalemia, acidosis, or worsening azotemia. The true basis for renal failure in such patients may be confirmed only retrospectively when hemodynamic abnormalities are finally corrected.

Acute Interstitial Nephritis

Patients in an intensive care unit receive a variety of medications, often over an extended period. Some of these, the penicillin-related β-lactam antibiotics in particular,[58] cause ARF that differs both clinically and mechanistically from that associated with ischemia or aminoglycoside antibiotics. Methicillin, ampicillin, nafcillin, oxacillin, amoxicillin, carbenicillin, cephradine, and cephalexin are not nephrotoxic per se and produce renal failure only in certain susceptible individuals, usually after at least 10 days of treatment.[59] Such individuals usually have no prior history of penicillin allergy.[60]

ARF caused by acute interstitial nephritis has a distinct clinical presentation that is typified by a patient's exposure to methicillin.[61] Fever is almost invariably present but, unfortunately, is often considered as part of the infectious process for which the antibiotic was originally prescribed. Microscopic hematuria is also characteristic; only about one third of all patients have gross hematuria. Morbilliform or maculopapular rash, with or without arthralgias, can suggest a possible immune basis for renal failure, but rashes are found in no more than one half of all patients. A blood smear reveals peripheral eosinophilia in perhaps three quarters of patients; however, eosinophilia often does not persist beyond 1 to 3 days and as a result may be missed.[62] However, sterile pyuria, which can be frequently profuse, and eosinophiluria remain evident as long as mononuclear and eosinophilic cell infiltration exists in the renal interstitium.[63] Proteinuria is often present but usually not massive, and erythrocyte casts are more suggestive of an allergic vasculitis or other causes of renal failure. Bilateral flank pain is a common complaint; when coupled with fever and pyuria, it not infrequently leads to an erroneous initial diagnosis of acute pyelonephritis. However, acute pyelonephritis per se almost never causes ARF unless complicated by urinary obstruction, septic shock, severe volume depletion, or acute papillary necrosis.

Although hematuria, fever, rash, eosinophilia, and eosinophiluria are hallmarks of allergic interstitial nephritis due to any of the β-lactam antibiotics, the variability of these findings in individual patients makes the recognition of the entity somewhat difficult unless it is routinely considered in the differential diagnosis of ARF. A patient's past and present drug intake would be carefully scrutinized, each of the classic presenting features looked for, and further work-up initiated if necessary. Skin biopsy can often definitively identify the origin of even relatively innocent-looking skin rashes, and a Wright's or Hansel's stain of the urinary sediment can establish the presence of eosinophiluria. Most commonly, 30% or more of the leukocytes in urine are eosinophils,[58] but any degree of eosinophiluria in a patient with unexplained renal failure is worthy of note. An intensely positive result on gallium scanning can be very helpful to separate this entity from ARF,[58] but renal biopsy may still be required for a definitive diagnosis.

A host of other agents also causes an acute interstitial nephritis but without all of the characteristic clinical manifestations of the penicillin-related drugs. Cimetidine, rifampin, virtually any of the nonsteroidal anti-inflammatory agents, allopurinol, trimethoprim-sulfamethoxazole, furosemide, thiazide diuretics, phenytoin, and barbiturates are but a few of the many medications that have been implicated.[58, 62] Although a skin rash, fever, pyuria, or flank pain may signal a reaction to these agents, peripheral eosinophilia and eosinophiluria generally are absent when interstitial nephritis is caused by these drugs.

Once the diagnosis of interstitial nephritis is made, the patient's entire medication list should be carefully scrutinized. No penicillin-related drug should be continued or prescribed, especially since it is rarely essential and because there is no easy way to identify which drug among several is the actual causative agent. The same is true of the thiazide and loop diuretics. Of course, decisions must be individualized in patients who are receiving essential anticonvulsive and antiarrhythmic medications. No consensus on the necessity of corticosteroid therapy exists; however, since treatment usually lasts only a few days, many nephrologists prescribe steroids.

Hepatorenal Syndrome

Although the pathogenesis of the hepatorenal syndrome remains unknown, the combination of systemic vasodilatation and renal vasoconstriction results in a dramatic reduction in renal function that often portends a grave prognosis.[64, 65] The term *hepatorenal syndrome* was originally applied to patients who developed ARF following hepatobiliary surgery[66] but now is reserved for those patients who have ARF associated with hepatic failure from any cause and with portal hypertension.[67] If patients have chronic liver failure, they often have the physical signs of their disease: ascites, spider angiomata, palmar erythema, splenomegaly, hypothermia, and cachexia. Jaundice is usually present, although its severity bears no relationship to the degree of renal insufficiency.[68] Hypotension is a late development in most instances. Oliguria is a characteristic feature. Cardiac dysfunction may be an important concomitant disorder that is usually secondary to alcohol-induced cardiomyopathy. The fact that many cases occur in hospitalized patients points to iatrogenic initiators of the syndrome. These include volume depletion induced by diuretics, paracentesis, or gastrointestinal bleeding; drugs, the most important of which are nonsteroidal anti-inflammatory drugs; and infection of any kind.

Laboratory studies confirm the presence of advanced liver dysfunction with elevations of prothrombin time, reduction of the serum albumin and cholesterol concentrations, and an increased bilirubin concentration.[69] BUN concentrations and creatinine levels are sometimes difficult to interpret in the patient with liver failure. BUN levels tend to be low in cirrhotic patients because of both reduced protein intake and hepatic urea synthesis. Creatinine also is low owing to reduced muscle mass characteristic of this patient population. Falsely low serum creatinine values may result from assay interference by high bilirubin concentrations. Normal or high normal concentrations of BUN or creatinine may in fact indicate a significant reduction in renal function.

Specific urinary electrolyte changes are suggestive of functional renal failure (e.g., urinary sodium <10 mEq/L; urine-plasma creatinine level of >20; excreted fraction of filtered sodium <1%; and urinary osmolarity >450 mOsm/L). Even in patients who develop typical ARF, urinary electrolytes continue to indicate a prerenal state.[70] Microscopic examination of the urine reveals many bilirubin-stained hyaline and granular casts; the sediment is typically acellular.

Exclusion of reversible causes of ARF is essential when treating the patient with liver and renal failure. Once obstruction is ruled out, differentiating hepatorenal syndrome from functional renal failure is difficult. Central hemodynamic monitoring may be useful, but often the parameters are difficult to interpret because of tense ascites. A low pulmonary capillary wedge pressure and cardiac output should prompt efforts to bring about volume repletion. An empirical trial of colloid infusion is often indicated to exclude functional renal failure, although such an infusion is not without risks.[71] Systemic vasoconstrictors have been employed to counter the systemic vasodilatation that is characteristic of this syndrome, but they are only of transient or negligible benefit.[72, 73] On the other hand, renal vasodilator agents have also been used to counter the intense renal vasoconstriction seen in hepatorenal syndrome. Dopamine, prostaglandins, saralasin, phentolamine, isoproterenol, acetylcholine, and thromboxane synthetase inhibitors are but a few of these agents that have been used unsuccessfully to restore renal function.[74–76]

A number of other therapies have also been tried, but all either have little or transient benefit (e.g., paracentesis with or without colloid infusion) or exchange "renal death" for another form of complication such as hemorrhage or sepsis (e.g., portosystemic shunt).[77] Dialysis has been employed in hepatorenal syndrome patients[78] but should be reserved for those patients who are expected to demonstrate recovery of their liver failure, for those who have other causes of ARF, or for those who are awaiting liver transplantation. Cadaveric liver transplantation offers the best chance of curing both the hepatorenal syndrome and the liver failure.[79]

Since the therapy for hepatorenal syndrome is usually ineffective, prevention is the key when caring for patients with decompensated liver disease. Avoiding vigorous diuresis (0.5 kg/d in those patients without peripheral edema), treating hemorrhage early and aggressively, removing ascitic fluid cautiously with hemodynamic monitoring (large-volume paracentesis with albumin replacement is often more effective than the administration of large doses of diuretics[80]), using lactulose wisely to avoid heavy diarrhea, and, finally, avoiding the use of nephrotoxic drugs such as aminoglycosides (even neomycin) and nonsteroidal anti-inflammatory drugs are all measures that should be employed.

Myoglobin-Induced Acute Renal Failure (Rhabdomyolysis)

Myoglobinuric ARF remains an important cause of ARF in the critical care setting. Although its course is typical of other forms of ARF, several distinctive clinical features and therapeutic interventions make this cause of ARF unique. The causes of myoglobinuric ARF are summarized in Table 114–2 and are divided into traumatic and nontraumatic causes. Although "crush" injury and ischemia constitute the majority of these cases, important causes include sustained strenuous exercise,[81] drug overdose,[82] carbon monoxide poisoning,[83] inherited glycogen storage diseases,[84, 85] and electrolyte abnormalities.[86, 87] Ethanol intoxication is, in fact, a frequent forerunner of rhabdomyolysis and myoglobinuric ARF, even in the absence of overt muscle injury;[88] the attendant hypomagnesemia, hypokalemia, and hypophosphatemia found so commonly in chronic alcoholics are likely contributing factors.

The characteristic clinical presentation results from the large quantity of muscle necrosis with its attendant delivery of intracellular contents into the extracellular space. Hyperkalemia, hyperuricemia, and hyperphosphatemia are much more pronounced than in typical ARF.[89, 90] Hypocalcemia is also common and is most likely related to the deposition of calcium salts within necrotic muscle[91]; however, skeletal resistance to parathyroid hormone[92] and altered vitamin D metabolism[93] have also been implicated. Creatinine level is often elevated out of proportion to the BUN concentration and may increase by more than the usual 1 mg/dL per day.[90] A BUN:creatinine ratio less than the usual 10 may suggest the presence of rhabdomyolysis. Examination of the urine reveals darkly pigmented, coarsely granular casts and tubular cell casts. As mentioned previously, a positive result on a dipstick test for blood in the face of a negative microscopic examination for blood is evidence to support that myoglobin is present in the urine. Evidence of muscle necrosis is invariably present with elevation of creatine phosphokinase, aldolase, lactate dehydrogenase, and alkaline phosphatase concentrations. Concomitant volume depletion or hypotension, or both, are important factors that contribute to the development of the ARF.

Therapy is first directed toward prevention. Mannitol and furosemide have been employed in this regard, although evidence to support their effectiveness is scant. Alkalinization of the urine with volume repletion is probably the most useful maneuver.[94] Care must be exercised if oliguric ARF develops, since mannitol or sodium bicarbonate therapy can precipitate pulmonary edema. Dialysis is often necessary for the treatment of hyperkalemia well before there are other indications for dialysis. As renal recovery occurs, hypercalcemia may become a problem as calcium is mobilized from muscle.

TABLE 114–2. Causes of Myoglobinuric Acute Renal Failure

Traumatic

Crush injury, seizures, strenuous exercise, ischemia, status asthmaticus, delirium tremens, air embolism

Nontraumatic

Myopathic: phosphorylase deficiency, phosphofructokinase deficiency, myxedema, dermatomyositis/polymyositis

Drug: alcohol, narcotics, sedatives, amphetamines, lysergic acid diethylamide, salicylate, clofibrate, lovastatin

Metabolic: hyperpyrexia, hyperosmolarity, hypokalemia, hypophosphatemia, carbon monoxide poisoning, idiopathic paroxysmal myoglobinuria

Pulmonary-Renal Syndrome

A diverse number of systemic immunologic diseases may present with both ARF and acute pulmonary disease. Although Goodpasture's syndrome[95] is the best known of these, systemic lupus erythematosus,[96] Wegener's granulomatosis,[97] polyarteritis nodosa (both classic and microvascular),[98, 99] sarcoidosis,[100] and right-sided endocarditis[101] may all present with similar characteristics. Although a detailed description of each of these diseases is beyond the scope of this chapter, recognition of this group of diseases is important to direct often life-saving therapy.

The presentation of patients with this syndrome may be dominated by either the pulmonary disease or the renal disease. The pulmonary disease may vary, ranging from mild, patchy infiltrates to life-threatening diffuse hemorrhage. ARF is frequently accompanied by hypertension and evidence of volume expansion. Examination of the urine often reveals albuminuria, red blood cells, and red blood cell casts. Since the renal tubules are often unaffected early in the course of the disease, the urine is concentrated, and urine sodium level is low. The excreted fraction of filtered sodium is often less than 1%. Later in the course of the disease, renal ischemia results in tubular dysfunction and the usually observed values for urinary indices.

Serologic evaluation may be helpful in establishing a diagnosis. Antiglomerular basement membrane antibody in Goodpasture's syndrome,[102] antineutrophil cytoplasmic antibody in Wegener's granulomatosis and polyarteritis,[103] and antinuclear antibodies in systemic lupus erythematosus[104] are sensitive and specific markers for these diseases. Less specific but still helpful in diagnosis are hepatitis B antigen status,[105] complement activity,[106] and cryoglobulin level.[107] Assessment of these serologic markers is also helpful in following patients once treatment has begun. Although serologic evaluation is often helpful, obtaining results may be somewhat delayed because specialized laboratories are often used. Therefore, correct pathologic diagnosis is imperative owing to the diversity of diseases that can present in this dramatic manner. Percutaneous renal biopsy may be too hazardous, and open biopsy of the kidney is often necessary. Angiography is very helpful in establishing the diagnosis of polyarteritis nodosa, precluding the need for renal biopsy.

Therapy, if initiated before oliguria develops or before dialysis is necessary, is often effective in reversing the renal and pulmonary disease. "Pulse" intravenous administration of methylprednisolone, cytotoxic drugs such as cyclophosphamide or azathioprine, and plasma exchange constitute the treatment of choice for Goodpasture's syndrome,[108] whereas the use of steroids and cyclophosphamide is the preferred therapy for Wegener's granulomatosis, polyarteritis nodosa, and systemic lupus erythematosus.[109–112] Pulse steroid administration may be particularly effective in controlling the diffuse pulmonary hemorrhage that occurs in all of these diseases of this syndrome. Because of the potential for reversibility of the disease process, rapid diagnosis and treatment is imperative.

PROGNOSIS OF RECOVERY AND SURVIVAL

The major determinant of survival in the patient with ARF is the number and severity of concomitant illnesses.[113–115] Intensive supportive care in the intensive care unit make death that occurs directly owing to the complications of renal failure a rarity; death occurs primarily as a result of infectious,[116, 117] cardiovascular,[114] or respiratory complications.[118] Mortality rates, unfortunately, remain high in patients with ARF, ranging from approximately 20% in obstetric patients to 50% to 60% in postoperative and trauma patients. Although some improvement in survival may occur in postsurgical and traumatic ARF, it is generally acknowledged that survival has reached a plateau.[118] This lack of improvement is most likely related to both an increase in the age of the population and the occurrence of multiorgan failure.[116, 119–122] When ARF is a part of multiorgan failure, mortality approaches 100%.[114] Urine volume in patients with ARF also impacts on survival. Patients with nonoliguric ARF have a significantly lower mortality rate than those patients with either oliguric or anuric ARF.[114, 123, 124] This difference is related to a reduction in the number of complications in the nonoliguric patients.[125]

PREVENTION AND TREATMENT OF ACUTE RENAL FAILURE

Since ARF is usually not immediately reversible, prevention remains the most effective tool. When a patient is at risk for developing ARF because of disordered hemodynamics rather than the presence of nephrotoxins, prompt and full restoration of blood volume and adequate cardiovascular support are the key prophylactic measures. The dramatic reduction in post-traumatic ARF that occurred in the wounded during the Vietnam War compared with that during the Korean War is mainly attributed to rapid volume resuscitation delivered in the field.[126] Reliance on mannitol, loop diuretics, or vasopressor agents without consideration of the underlying abnormality is not wise. Careful monitoring of both serum creatinine and serum antibiotic concentrations and maintaining optimal renal function whenever aminoglycoside agents are given may limit the incidence and severity of renal toxicity.

The use of diuretics, particularly furosemide, to prevent, ameliorate, or speed recovery in ARF continues to be a controversial subject. Although few controlled studies have addressed the effects of furosemide on human ARF, these studies show that furosemide increases urine volume[127] and occasionally reduces the need for dialysis,[128] but that it has no effect on clinical outcome.[127] The detrimental effects of furosemide or ethacrynic acid, such as permanent deafness and volume depletion, should be weighed against the small and inconsistent benefit of their use.

Mannitol, dopamine, calcium channel blockers, angiotensin-converting enzyme inhibitors, atrial natriuretic peptide, adenosine triphosphate, magnesium chloride, prostaglandins, heparin, and thyroxine have also been employed in human ARF, but whether they are of benefit continues to be speculated.

Once ARF becomes established, therapy should be directed toward the prevention of complications (Table 114–3). Complications may arise quite rapidly in the hypercatabolic patient or may arise more subtly in the nonoliguric patient with significant residual renal function. Meticulous attention to fluid and electrolyte balance, drug use, and nutritional support prevents many of these complications. Unfortunately, even with meticulous attention, patients with sepsis, multiorgan failure, or trauma often develop life-threatening complications such as hyperkalemia, acidosis, and volume overload.

Without aggressive nutritional support, loss of body mass can be extreme in such catabolic patients. Few controlled studies concerning the role of parenteral nutrition in ARF are available. The ones performed have generally shown a beneficial effect of amino acid infusions on ARF recovery but have failed to show a significant benefit in terms of overall patient survival.[129, 130] Although enteral nutrition is the preferred route of administration, parenteral nutrition is often necessary because many critically ill patients have a poorly functioning gastrointestinal tract. The prescription for calories and protein is dependent on the severity of the illness as well as on whether dialysis is required. In the situation in which oliguria is expected to be brief (1–3 days), the goal should be to minimize tissue breakdown through the supply of the minimum nutritional requirements. In this case, restriction of fluid and protein may avoid the need for dialysis. In prolonged oliguric ARF, the administration of calories and protein can be more generous because dialysis is invariably required. Even with dialysis, though, the overzealous administration of amino acids, fluid, and glucose may overwhelm the capacity of routine hemodialysis and lead to fluid overload or uremia.

Because recovery from ARF may be delayed, dialysis therapy is often necessary to both prevent and treat complications as they arise. Indications for dialysis are listed in Table 114–4, but dialysis is often initiated well before the development of these complications. Clearly, dialysis therapy has had a significant impact on improving survival in some patients with ARF.[131] Although the appropriate "intensity" of dialysis is a subject of debate, most studies support the early use of aggressive dialysis.[132] However, one study showed little benefit of intensive dialysis with respect to a patient's survival.[133]

Dialysis therapy should be modified to fit the particular needs of each patient. Currently, five modalities may be

TABLE 114–3. Complications of Acute Renal Failure

Metabolic	*Gastrointestinal*
Hyperkalemia	Nausea
Acidosis	Vomiting
Hypocalcemia	Gastritis/duodenitis
Hyperphosphatemia	Anorexia
Hyperuricemia	Ileus
Hypermagnesemia	*Hematologic*
Insulin resistance	Platelet dysfunction
Malnutrition	Factor VII dysfunction
Cardiovascular	Anemia
Pulmonary edema	*Infectious*
Arrhythmias	Pneumonia
Hypertension	Septicemia
Pericarditis	Urinary tract infection
Neurologic	Indwelling catheter–related infection
Asterixis	
Myoclonus	
Confusion	
Somnolence	
Coma	
Seizures	
Nonspecific electroencephalographic changes	

TABLE 114–4. Indications for Dialysis

Uremia*	Hypercalcemia/hyperphosphatemia
Fluid overload	Platelet dysfunction
Pericarditis	Metabolic acidosis or alkalosis
Hyperkalemia	Neurologic symptoms (confusion, seizures)
Hyponatremia†	

Rough guidelines:
*BUN >100 mg/dL or serum creatinine level >10 mg/dL.
†The rapid correction of serum sodium concentrations may be harmful owing to osmolality shifts.

TABLE 114–5. Advantages and Disadvantages of Renal Replacement Therapy in Acute Renal Failure Patients

Modality	*Advantages*	*Disadvantages*
Hemodialysis	Efficient and rapid; preferred for hyperkalemic and catabolic patients; citrate/sodium chloride flush; anticoagulation	Hemodynamically stressful; technically complicated; special personnel required
Peritoneal dialysis	Simple; no vascular access needed; no anticoagulation; preferred for hemodynamically unstable patients	Inefficient and slow; glucose load; not for patients with previous abdominal surgery
Continuous arteriovenous hemo(dia)filtration	Simple; no specialized personnel needed; preferred for hypotensive patients; large fluid intake possible	Arterial access; anticoagulation; blood pressure–dependent
Continuous venovenous hemo(dia)filtration	No arterial access needed; preferred for hypotensive patients; large fluid intake possible; more dependable blood flow	Anticoagulation; specialized equipment needed; intensive care unit nurses with specialized training needed
Slow continuous ultrafiltration	Fluid removal only; preferred for hypotensive patients	Poor clearance; anticoagulation

utilized, each of which offers certain advantages to the particular patient. *Intermittent hemodialysis* is the most widely used form of dialysis but may be difficult to perform in the hemodynamically unstable intensive care unit patient. Continuous renal replacement therapies such as *peritoneal dialysis, continuous arteriovenous hemo(dia)filtration, continuous venovenous hemo(dia)filtration,* and *slow continuous ultrafiltration* all offer unique advantages to unstable ARF patients. Specific advantages and disadvantages are summarized in Table 114–5. Technologic advances in dialysis equipment have made dialysis safer, although meticulous attention is necessary if dialysis complications are to be avoided. Dialysis-induced hypotension, a complication that may prolong the course of ARF,[134] excessive or inappropriate systemic anticoagulation, and dialysis-induced electrolyte disturbances such as hypokalemia and alkalosis all can worsen an intensive care unit patient's condition.

SPECIAL CONSIDERATIONS IN PATIENTS WITH CHRONIC RENAL INSUFFICIENCY/FAILURE

The intensive care unit patients with chronic, stable renal insufficiency present special clinical problems. Not only are these patients more prone to develop acute deterioration in their renal function, but all aspects of their care, nutritional and fluid support, drug therapy, and diagnostic testing are affected by the presence of renal dysfunction.

The first consideration in these patients is preservation of renal function. To this end, maintenance of extracellular volume status is of primary importance to ensure adequate renal perfusion. However, because of the kidney's reduced ability to excrete salt and water, care should be exercised in administering fluid to these patients. Central pressure monitoring may be helpful, if not necessary, to direct this fluid administration. In patients who are volume depleted, the indiscriminate use of vasopressor drugs may also depress renal perfusion and worsen renal function.

Hypertension is a common feature in chronic renal insufficiency, and the incidence increases as renal function worsens.[135] Stage 4 hypertension (blood pressure >210/120 mm Hg) may cause rapid deterioration of renal function, particularly when chronic renal insufficiency exists and should be treated aggressively. Since orally administered drugs are often not practical in the intensive care unit, the use of parenteral antihypertensive medications is often necessary. Sodium nitroprusside is the most potent of these agents and has the advantages of rapid onset of action and short half-life.[136] Unfortunately, the metabolic byproducts cyanide and thiocyanate have long half-lives and accumulate in renal insufficiency. Toxicity may occur within 48 hours and leads to metabolic acidosis, confusion, hyperreflexia, and seizures. Other parenteral antihypertensive medications can be used as alternatives, including methyldopa, labetalol, esmolol, hydralazine, and enalaprilat. The hypotensive effects of these drugs can be extreme and must be avoided, particularly in chronic renal insufficiency patients.

Finally, the prevention of renal deterioration in the intensive care unit setting depends on the judicious use of drugs and diagnostic tests. Drug toxicity is often enhanced in chronic renal insufficiency patients owing to altered drug disposition as well as to increased susceptibility. Some drugs, such as aminoglycoside antibiotics, amphotericin, and cyclosporin A, may cause predictable decreases in renal function that should be monitored carefully. Avoiding these drugs may not be possible so the determination of blood concentrations is essential if toxicity is to be prevented. Radiocontrast agents should be avoided, if possible, since preexisting renal insufficiency is a predisposing factor for the development of ARF.

Many of the drugs utilized in the intensive care unit are excreted in the urine as intact drug or drug metabolites; with diminished function, these drugs or metabolites often accumulate. Vigilance is therefore necessary to prevent serious toxicity. Most intensive care units rely on hospital pharmacy services to help in supporting this vigilance, although the daily review and prudent use of medications by the physicians caring for a patient are essential to good intensive care.

References

1. Oken DE: Nosologic considerations in the nomenclature of acute renal failure. Nephron 1971; 8:505.
2. Swan RC, Merrill JP: The clinical course of acute renal failure. Medicine 1953; 32:215.
3. Epstein M, Schneider NS, Befeler B: Effect of intrarenal furosemide on renal function and intrarenal hemodynamics in acute renal failure. Am J Med 1975; 58:510.
4. Muth RG: Furosemide in acute renal failure. *In*: Conference on Acute Renal Failure. Friedman EA, Eliahou HE (Eds). Washington, DC. US Department of Health, Education and Welfare publication (NIH) 74–608, 1973, pp 245–263.
5. Anderson RJ, Linas SL, Berns AS, et al: Nonoliguric acute renal failure. N Engl J Med 1977; 296:1134.
6. Smith K, Browne JC, Shackman R, et al: Acute renal failure of obstetric origin: An analysis of 70 patients. Lancet 1968; ii:351.
7. Chugh KS, Singhal PC, Sharma BK, et al: Acute renal failure of obstetric origin. Obstet Gynecol 1976; 48:642.
8. Solanki D, McCurdy PR: Delayed hemolytic transfusion reactions: An often-missed entity. JAMA 1978; 239:729.
9. Guluti PD, Rizva SNA: Acute reversible renal failure in G-6-PD deficient siblings. Postgrad Med J 1976; 52:83.

10. Hartmann RC, Auditore JV: Paroxysmal nocturnal hemoglobinuria: 1. Clinical studies. Am J Med 1959; 27:389.
11. Eisner GM, Piver JS: Acute renal failure after therapeutic abortion by intra-amniotic saline administration. N Engl J Med 1968; 279:360.
12. Thomas TA, Galizia FJ, Wensley RT: Termination of pregnancy with Utus paste: Report of a fatal case. Br Med J 1975; 1:375.
13. Hagvenik K, Gordon E, Lins LE, et al: Glycerol-induced haemolysis with haemoglobinuria and acute renal failure: Report of three cases. Lancet 1974; i:78.
14. Warrell DA, Ormerod LD, Davidson NM: Bites by puff-adder *(Bitis arietans)* in Nigeria, and value of antivenom. Br Med J 1975; 4:697.
15. Rosen S, Hano JE, Inman MM, et al: The kidney in blackwater fever: Light and electron microscopic studies. Am J Clin Pathol 1968; 49:358.
16. Muehrcke RC, Pirani CL: Arsine-induced anuria: A correlative clinicopathological study with electron microscopic observations. Ann Intern Med 1968; 68:853.
17. Grossman CM, Malbin B: Mushroom poisoning: A review of the literature and report of two cases caused by a previously undescribed species. Ann Intern Med 1954; 40:249.
18. Sinicrope RA, Gordon JA, Little JR, et al: Carbon tetrachloride nephrotoxicity: A reassessment of pathophysiology based upon urinary diagnostic indices. Am J Kidney Dis 1984; 3:362.
19. Carlton BE, Tufts E, Girard DE: Water hemlock poisoning complicated by rhabdomyolysis and renal failure. Clin Toxicol 1979; 14:87.
20. Sitprija V, Benyajati C, Boonpucknavig V: Further reservations of renal insufficiency in snakebite. Nephron 1974; 13:396.
21. Zager RA: Gentamicin effects on renal ischemia/reperfusion injury. Circ Res 1992; 70:20.
22. Schentag JJ, Cumbo TJ, Jusko WJ, et al: Gentamicin tissue accumulation and nephrotoxic reactions. JAMA 1978; 240: 2067.
23. Plaut ME, Schentag JJ, Jusko WJ: Aminoglycoside nephrotoxicity: Comparative assessment in critically ill patients. J Med 1979; 10:257.
24. de Rosa F, Buoncristiani U, Capitanucci P, et al: Tobramycin: Toxicological and pharmacological studies in animals and pharmacokinetic research in patients with varying degrees of renal impairment. J Intern Med Res 1974; 2:100.
25. Butler WT, Bennett JE, Alling DW, et al: Nephrotoxicity of amphotericin B: Early and late effects in 81 patients. Ann Intern Med 1964; 61:175.
26. Eknoyan G, Roberts AD: Nephrotoxicity of amphotericin B: Observations in the mechanism of hypokalemia. Antimicrob Agents Chemother 1962; 2:497.
27. Holeman CW Jr, Einstein H: The toxic effects of amphotericin in man. Calif Med 1963; 99:90.
28. McCurdy DK, Frederic M, Elkinton JR: Renal tubular acidosis due to amphotericin B. N Engl J Med 1968; 278:124.
29. Barbour GL, Straub KD, O'Neal BL, et al: Vasopressin-resistant nephrogenic diabetes insipidus: A result of amphotericin B therapy. Arch Intern Med 1979; 139:86.
30. D'Elia J, Alday M, Gleason R, et al: Acute renal failure following angiography: Prospective study of 150 patients, preliminary results. Proc Clin Dial Transplant Forum 1978; 8:123.
31. Port FK, Wagoner RD, Fulton RE: Acute renal failure after angiography. AJR 1974; 121:544.
32. Taliercio CP, Vlietstra RE, Fisher LD, et al: Risks for renal dysfunction with cardiac angiography. Ann Intern Med 1986; 104:501.
33. Martin-Paredero V, Dixon SM, Baker JD: Risk of renal failure after major angiography. Arch Surg 1983; 118:1417.
34. Gomes AS, Baker JD, Martin-Paredero V, et al: Acute renal dysfunction after major arteriography. AJR 1985; 145:1249.
35. Harkonen S, Kjellstrand C: Intravenous pyelography in nonuremic diabetic patients. Nephron 1979; 24:268.
36. Weisberg LS, Kurnik PB, Kurnik BRC: Risk of radiocontrast nephropathy in patients with and without diabetes mellitus. Kidney Int 1994; 45:259.
37. Holland MD, Galla JH, Sanders PW, et al: Effect of urinary pH and diatrizoate on Bence Jones protein nephrotoxicity in the rat. Kidney Int 1985; 27:46.
38. Swartz RD, Rubin JE, Leeming BW, et al: Renal failure following major angiography. Am J Med 1978; 65:31.
39. Byrd L, Sherman RL: Radiocontrast-induced acute renal failure: A clinical and pathophysiologic review. Medicine (Baltimore) 1979; 58:270.
40. Older RA, Korobkin M, Cleeve DM, et al: Contrast-induced acute renal failure: Persistent nephrogram as clue to early detection. AJR 1980; 134:339.
41. Schwab SJ, Hlatky MA, Pieper KS, et al: Contrast nephrotoxicity: A randomized controlled trial of a nonionic and an ionic radiographic contrast agent. N Engl J Med 1989; 320:149.
42. Bywaters EGL, Beall D: Crush injuries with impairment of renal function. Br Med J 1941; 1:427.
43. Minami S: Über Nierenveränderungen nach Verschüttung. Arch Pathol Anat 1923; 245:247.
44. Richard AN: Direct observations of changes in function of the renal tubule caused by certain poisons. Trans Assoc Am Phys 1929; 44:64.
45. Oken DE: An analysis of glomerular dynamics in rat, dog and man. Kidney Int 1982; 22:136.
46. Blantz RC: The mechanism of acute renal failure after uranyl nitrate. J Clin Invest 1975; 55:621.
47. Brezis M, Rosen S, Epstein FH: Acute renal failure. *In*: Brenner BM, Rector FC Jr (Eds). The Kidney. 4th ed. Philadelphia, WB Saunders, 1991, pp 1011–1015.
47a. Bonventre JV: Mechanisms of ischemic acute renal failure. Kidney Int 1993; 43:1160.
48. Ellenbogen PH, Scheible FW, Talner LB, et al: Sensitivity of gray scale ultrasound in detecting urinary tract obstruction. Am J Roentgenol 1978; 130:731.
49. Rascoff JH, Golden RA, Spinowitz BS, et al: Non-dilated obstructive uropathy. Arch Intern Med 1983; 143:696.
50. Merrill JP: The Treatment of Renal Failure. 2nd ed. New York, Grune & Stratton, 1965, p 147.
51. Schrier RW, Henderson HS, Fisher CS, et al: Nephropathy associated with heat stress and exercise. Ann Intern Med 1967; 67:56.
52. Sporn IN, Lancestremere RG, Papper S: Differential diagnosis of oliguria in aged patients. N Engl J Med 1962; 267:130.
53. Papper S: Hepatorenal syndrome. Contrib Nephrol 1980; 23:55.
54. MacLean PR, Robson JS: Unselective proteinuria in acute ischaemic renal failure. Clin Sci 1966; 30:91.
55. Werb R, Linton AL: Aetiology, diagnosis, treatment and prognosis of acute renal failure in an intensive care unit. Resuscitation 1979; 29:95.
56. Badr KF: Sepsis-associated renal vasoconstriction: Potential targets for future therapy. Am J Kidney Dis 1992; 20:207.
57. Zager RA: Endotoxemia, renal hypoperfusion, and fever: Interactive risk factors for aminoglycoside and sepsis-associated acute renal failure. Am J Kidney Dis 1992; 20:223.
58. Linton AL, Clark WF, Dridger AA, et al: Acute interstitial nephritis due to drugs. Ann Intern Med 1980; 93:735.
59. Van Ypersele de Strihou C: Acute oliguric interstitial nephritis. Kidney Int 1979; 16:751.
60. Braulinger AE, Remington JS: Nephropathy associated with methicillin allergy. JAMA 1968; 203:125.
61. Baldwin DW, Levine BB, McCluskey RT, et al: Renal failure and interstitial nephritis due to penicillin and methicillin. N Engl J Med 1968; 29:1245.
62. Levin ML: Patterns of tubulo-interstitial damage associated with nonsteroidal antiinflammatory drugs. Semin Nephrol 1984; 4:1.
63. Zollinger HU, Mihatsch MJ: Morphology of acute interstitial nephropathy. Contrib Nephrol 1979; 16:118.
64. Shear L, Kleinerman J, Gabuzda GJ: Renal failure in patients with cirrhosis of the liver: I. Clinical and pathological characteristics. Am J Med 1965; 39:184.
65. Levy M: Hepatorenal syndrome. Kidney Int 1993; 43:737.
66. Flint A: Clinical report on hydro-peritoneum, based on an analysis of forty-six cases. Am J Med Sci 1963; 45:306–339.
67. Papper S: The role of the kidney in Laënnec's cirrhosis of the liver. Medicine 1958; 37:299–316.
68. Baldus WP, Feichter RN, Summerskill WHJ, et al: The kidney in cirrhosis: II. Disorders of renal function. Ann Intern Med 1964; 60:366.
69. Baldus WP, Feichter RN, Summerskill WHJ, et al: The kidney

in cirrhosis: I. Clinical and biochemical features of azotemia in hepatic failure. Ann Intern Med 1964; 60:353.
70. Diamond JR, Yoburn DC: Nonoliguric acute renal failure associated with a low fractional excretion of sodium. Ann Intern Med 1982; 96:597–600.
71. Reynolds TB, Lieberman FL, Redeker AF: Functional renal failure with cirrhosis. Medicine 1967; 46:191.
72. Cohn JN, Tristani FE, Khatri M: Renal vasodilator therapy in the hepatorenal syndrome. Med Ann DC 1970; 39:154.
73. Sugarman HJ, Berkowitz HD, Miller KD: Metaraminol in "hepatorenal syndrome." N Engl J Med 1971; 285:180.
74. Barnardo DE, Baldus WP, Maher FT: Effects of dopamine on renal function in patients with cirrhosis. Gastroenterology 1970; 58:524.
75. Zusman RM, Axelrod L, Tolkoff-Rubin N: The treatment of the hepatorenal syndrome (HRS) with intrarenal administration of prostaglandin E. Prostaglandins 1977; 13:814.
76. Zipser RD, Kronborg I, Rector W, et al: Therapeutic trial of thromboxane synthesis inhibition in the hepatorenal syndrome. Gastroenterology 1984; 87:1228–1232.
77. Moskovits M: The peritoneovenous shunt: Expectations and reality. Am J Gastroenterol 1990; 85:917–929.
78. Davenport A, Will EJ, Davison AM: Effect of renal replacement therapy on patients with combined acute renal and fulminant hepatic failure. Kidney Int 1993; 43(Suppl 41):S245.
79. Iwatsuki S, Popovtzer MM, Corman JL, et al: Recovery from "hepatorenal syndrome" after orthotopic liver transplantation. N Engl J Med 1973; 289:1155.
80. Gines P, Arroyo V, Quintero E, et al: Comparison of paracentesis and diuretics in the treatment of cirrhotics with tense ascites. Gastroenterology 1987; 93:234–241.
81. Jackson RC: Exercise-induced renal failure and muscle damage. Proc R Soc Med 1970; 63:566.
82. Cadnapaphornchai P, Taher S, McDonald FD: Acute drug-associated rhabdomyolysis: An examination of its diverse renal manifestations and complications. Am J Med Sci 1980; 280:66.
83. Bessoundo R, Gray J: Carbon monoxide poisoning and nonoliguric acute renal failure. Can Med Assoc J 1978; 119:41.
84. Nixon JC, Hobbs WK, Greenblat J: Myoglobinuria and skeletal muscle phosphorylase deficiency: Report of a case of McArdle's disease. Can Med Assoc J 1966; 94:977.
85. Reza MI, Kar NC, Pearson CM, et al: Recurrent myoglobinuria due to muscle carnitine palmityl transferase deficiency. Ann Intern Med 1978; 88:610.
86. Anchor RWP, Smith LA: Nutritional deficiency syndrome and diarrhea resulting in hypopotassemia, muscle degeneration and renal insufficiency: Report of a case with recovery. Mayo J Clin Proc 1955; 49:185.
87. Knochel JP, Bablenas C, Cotton JR, et al: Hypophosphatemia and rhabdomyolysis. J Clin Invest 1978; 62:1240.
88. Rubin E, Kantz AM, Lieber CS, et al: Muscle damage produced by chronic alcohol consumption. Am J Pathol 1976; 83:499.
89. Grossman RA, Hamilton RW, Morse BM, et al: Nontraumatic rhabdomyolysis and acute renal failure. N Engl J Med 1974; 291:807.
90. Chugh KS, Nath IV, Ubroi HS, et al: Acute renal failure due to non-traumatic rhabdomyolysis. Postgrad Med J 1979; 55:386.
91. Akmal M, Goldstein DA, Telfer N, et al: Resolution of muscle calcification in rhabdomyolysis and acute renal failure. Ann Intern Med 1978; 89:928.
92. Massry SG, Arieff AI, Coburn JW, et al: Divalent ion metabolism in patients with acute renal failure: Studies on the mechanism of hypocalcemia. Kidney Int 1974; 5:437.
93. Pietrek J, Kokot F, Jadwiga K: Serum 25-hydroxyvitamin D and parathyroid hormone in patients with acute renal failure. Kidney Int 1978; 13:178.
94. Ron D, Taitelman U, Michaelson MD, et al: Prevention of acute renal failure in traumatic rhabdomyolysis. Arch Intern Med 1984; 144:277.
95. Duncan DA, Drummond KN, Michael AF, et al: Pulmonary hemorrhage and glomerulonephritis. Ann Intern Med 1964; 62:920.
96. Eagen JW, Memoli VA, Roberts JL, et al: Pulmonary hemorrhage in systemic lupus erythematosus. Medicine 1978; 57:545.
97. Appel GB, Gee B, Kashgarian M, et al: Wegener's granulomatosis: Clinical pathologic correlations and long-term course. Am J Kidney Dis 1981; 1:27.
98. Nuzum JW Jr, Nuzum JW Sr: Polyarteritis nodosa: Statistical review of 175 cases from the literature and report of a "typical" case. Arch Intern Med 1954; 94:789.
99. Parkin TW, Rusted IE, Burchell HB, et al: Hemorrhagic and interstitial pneumonitis with nephritis. Am J Med 1955; 18:220.
100. Allegri L, Olivetti G, David S, et al: Sarcoid granulomatous nephritis with isolated and reversible renal failure. Nephron 1980; 25:207.
101. Schwartz EE, Teplick JG, Onesti G, et al: Pulmonary hemorrhage in renal disease: Goodpasture's syndrome and other causes. Radiology 1977; 122:39.
102. Wilson CB, Dixon FJ: Anti-glomerular basement membrane antibody–induced glomerulonephritis. Kidney Int 1973; 3:74.
103. Jennette JC, Falk RJ: Diagnostic classification of antineutrophil cytoplasmic autoantibody–associated vasculitides. Am J Kidney Dis 1991; 18:184.
104. Emlen W, Pisetsky D, Taylor R: Antibodies to DNA: A perspective. Arthritis Rheum 1986; 29:1417.
105. Ronco P, Verroust P, Mignon F, et al: Immunopathological studies of polyarteritis nodosa and Wegener's granulomatosis: A report of 43 patients with 51 renal biopsies. Q J Med 1983; 52:212.
106. Lloyd W, Schur PH: Immune complexes, complement and anti-DNA in exacerbations of systemic lupus erythematosus (SLE). Medicine 1981; 60:208.
107. Gamble CN, Ruggles SW: The immunopathogenesis of glomerulonephritis associated with mixed cryoglobulinemia. N Engl J Med 1978; 299:81.
108. Lockwood C, Boulton-Jones J, Lowenthal R, et al: Recovery from Goodpasture's syndrome after immunosuppressive treatment and plasmapheresis. Br Med J 1975; 2:252.
109. Salant DJ, Adler S, Bernard DB, et al: Acute renal failure associated with renal vascular disease, vasculitis, glomerulonephritis, and nephrotic syndrome. *In*: Acute Renal Failure. 2nd ed. Brenner BM, Lazarus JM (Eds). New York, Churchill Livingstone, 1988, p 398.
110. Aldo MA, Benson MD, Comerford FR, et al: Treatment of Wegener's granulomatosis with immunosuppressive agents. Arch Intern Med 1970; 126:298.
111. Kimberly RD, Lockshin MD, Sherman RL, et al: High-dose intravenous methylprednisolone pulse therapy in systemic lupus erythematosus. Am J Med 1981; 70:817.
112. Barron KS, Person DA, Brewer EJ Jr, et al: Pulse methylprednisolone therapy in diffuse lupus nephritis. J Pediatr 1982; 101:137.
113. Kennedy AC, Burton JA, Luke RG, et al: Factors affecting the prognosis in acute renal failure. Q J Med 1973; 42:73.
114. Bullock ML, Umen AJ, Finkelstein M, et al: The assessment of risk factors in 462 patients with acute renal failure. Am J Kidney Dis 1985; 5:97.
115. McMurray SD, Luft FC, Maxwell DR, et al: Prevailing patterns and predictor variables in patients with acute tubular necrosis. Arch Intern Med 1978; 138:950.
116. Fry DE, Pearlstein L, Fulton RL, et al: Multiple system organ failure: The role of uncontrolled infection. Arch Surg 1980; 115:136.
117. Montgomerie JZ, Kalmanson GM, Guze LB: Renal failure and infection. Medicine 1968; 47:1.
118. Cameron JS: Acute renal failure: The continuing challenge. Q J Med 1986; 228:337.
119. Stott RB, Cameron JS, Ogg CS, et al: Why the persistently high mortality in acute renal failure? Lancet 1972; ii:75.
120. Butkus DE: Persistent high mortality in acute renal failure: Are we asking the right questions? Arch Intern Med 1983; 143:209.
121. Balslow JT, Jorgensen HE: A survey of 499 patients with acute anuric renal insufficiency: Causes, treatment, complications, and mortality. Am J Med 1963; 34:75.
122. Eisman B, Beart R, Norton L: Multiple organ failure. Surg Gynecol Obstet 1977; 144:323.
123. Baek SM, Makabali GG, Shoemaker WC: Clinical determinants of survival from postoperative renal failure. Surgery 1975; 140:685.
124. Rasmussen H, Ibels LS: Acute renal failure: Multivariate analysis of causes and risk factors. Am J Med 1982; 73:211.

125. Anderson RJ, Linas SL, Berns AS, et al: Nonoliguric acute renal failure. N Engl J Med 1977; 296:1134.
126. Whelton A, Donadio JV: Post-traumatic acute renal failure in Vietnam. Johns Hopkins Med J 1969; 124:95.
127. Minuth AN, Terrell JB, Suki WN: Acute renal failure: A study of the course and prognosis of 104 patients and of the role of furosemide. Am J Med Sci 1976; 271:317.
128. Fries D, Pozet N, Dubois N, et al: The use of large doses of furosemide in acute renal failure. Postgrad Med J 1971; 47:18.
129. Abel RM, Beck CH Jr, Abbott WM, et al: Improved survival from acute renal failure after treatment with intravenous essential L-amino acids and glucose: Results of a prospective double-blind study. N Engl J Med 1973; 288:695.
130. Baek SM, Makabali GG, Bryan-Brown CW, et al: The influence of parenteral nutrition on the course of acute renal failure. Surg Gynecol Obstet 1975; 141:405.
131. Kleinknecht D, Jungers P, Chanard J, et al: Uremic and nonuremic complications in acute renal failure: Evaluation of early and frequent dialysis on prognosis. Kidney Int 1972; 1:190.
132. Conger JD: A controlled evaluation of prophylactic dialysis in post-traumatic acute renal failure. J Trauma 1975; 15:1056.
133. Gillum DM, Dixon BS, Yanover MJ, et al: The role of intensive dialysis in acute renal failure. Clin Nephrol 1986; 25:249.
134. Kelleher SP, Robinette JB, Miller F, et al: Effect of hemorrhagic reduction in blood pressure on recovery from acute renal failure. Kidney Int 1987; 31:725.
135. Blythe WB: Natural history of hypertension in renal parenchymal disease. Am J Kidney Dis 1985; 5:A50.
136. Tuzel IH: Sodium nitroprusside: A review of its clinical effectiveness as a hypotensive agent. J Clin Pharmacol 1974; 14:494.

CHAPTER 115

Hemofiltration

Rinaldo Bellomo, MBBS, MD, FRACP

The management of acute renal failure (ARF) has changed over the last two decades. ARF is now most frequently seen in critically ill patients with hemodynamic instability and multiple organ failure.[1–4] In these patients, conventional forms of renal replacement therapy (intermittent hemodialysis and peritoneal dialysis) are associated with clinically important undesirable side effects. In an attempt to circumvent the shortcomings of conventional treatment, novel modalities of renal replacement therapy have been developed over the last decade. They all, in essence, rely on the continuous application of hemofiltration with various technical modifications. Over the last few years, their clinical application has markedly increased. In many circumstances, continuous dialytic techniques have all but replaced conventional dialysis.

HISTORICAL BACKGROUND

Continuous arteriovenous (AV) hemofiltration (CAVH) was first used by Peter Kramer and colleagues for the treatment of refractory edema.[5] Only later did its potential as a form of renal replacement become widely appreciated.[6–8] After initial clinical experience, modifications were developed to augment its otherwise limited solute clearances. Initially, this was achieved by increasing convective solute clearances by either ultrafiltrate suction or blood predilution.[9, 10] In 1984, Geronemus and Schneider combined hemofiltration with countercurrent dialysate flow in a technique they named *CAVHD*.[11] This slow dialytic technique doubled the solute clearances achieved during continuous hemofiltration. Further, clinicians were able to avoid the need for arterial vascular access by using double-lumen venous catheters and peristaltic blood pumps (continuous venovenous hemofiltration).[12] This technique was further refined by the addition of a diffusive component (continuous venovenous hemodiafiltration) that ensured urea clearances greater than 30 L/d, low invasiveness, and minimal morbidity.[13] Hemofiltration has rapidly evolved over a decade to become a more adaptable, safe, and efficacious technique. Its clinical application in the critically ill with acute renal failure has increased accordingly.

THE TECHNIQUES

Continuous Arteriovenous Hemofiltration

CAVH is the original and technically simplest hemofiltration technique. Arterial blood is typically obtained either by femoral artery cannulation or by surgical construction of a Scribner shunt. Blood then passes through the hemofilter driven by the patient's own blood pressure and returns to either a femoral venous cannula or the venous limb of the AV shunt (Fig. 115–1). The patient's blood pressure sustains ultrafiltration through the highly porous filter membrane.

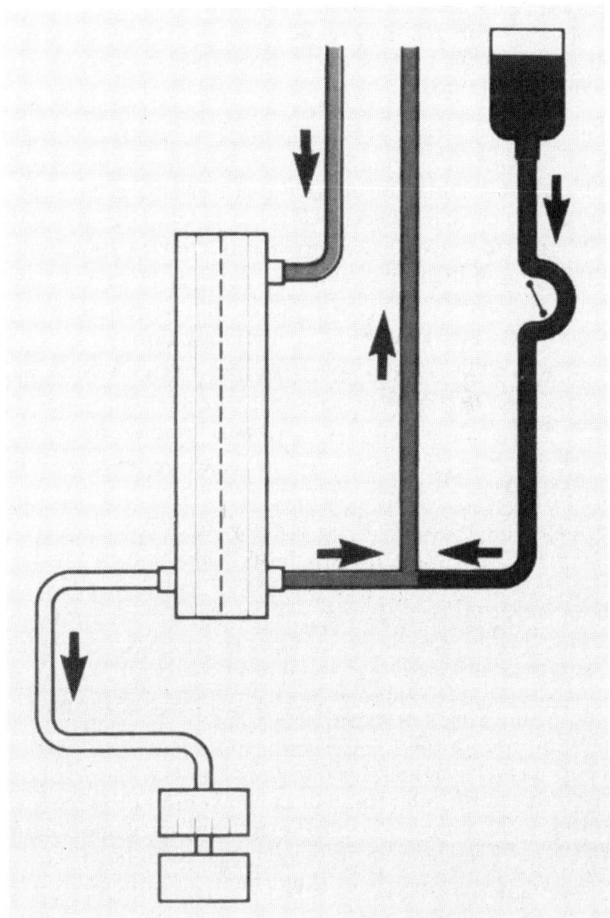

Figure 115–1. Representation of a continuous arteriovenous hemofiltration (CAVH) circuit. The *gray line* represents arterial blood, which, as indicated by the *arrows,* enters and then exits the filter (*white rectangle*) to return to the venous circulation (*gray line, continued*). The ultrafiltrate formed is collected in a volumetric device placed in a dependent position (*white line* and *white rectangles* in lower left). Replacement fluid (*black line*) is pumped into the venous limb of the circuit. (Courtesy of Hospal International Marketing, Lyon, France.)

The ultrafiltrate formed is collected in a volumetric container. Typically, although affected by multiple variables (type of membrane, type of vascular access, patient's mean blood pressure, serum albumin concentration, and so on), approximately 10 to 14 L of ultrafiltrate are produced daily. Urea clearances are in the range of 10 to 12 mL/min. Solute clearances are convective; transmembrane pressure drives ultrafiltration and the greater the ultrafiltrate volume produced, the greater the solute clearance achieved. To augment convective clearances, suction can be applied to the ultrafiltrate port of the hemofilter. Ultrafiltrate production can be increased if isotonic replacement fluids are administered before the filter (predilution). These modifications can increase total urea and creatinine clearances to 15 to 17 mL/min.

A major advantage of CAVH over intermittent hemodialysis is that large fluid volumes are easily and safely removed. This allows prompt treatment of pulmonary edema and markedly facilitates the safe administration of blood, blood products, nutritional fluids, and antibiotics. Very importantly, this is achieved with an outstanding degree of hemodynamic stability. Another advantage is simplicity. It allows the immediate implementation of renal replacement therapy in the intensive care unit (ICU) without the need for trained hemodialysis nurses and hemodialysis machines. Centers in which hemodialysis facilities are not available need not expose a critically ill patient to the dangers associated with interhospital transfer merely because of a need for dialytic support.

The major shortcomings of CAVH relate to the need for arterial access, the possible immobilization associated with femoral vascular cannulation, the need for extracorporeal circuit anticoagulation, and the relatively low solute clearances achieved. If solute clearances obtained with CAVH are low, adjunctive hemodialysis is often needed to control azotemia adequately.

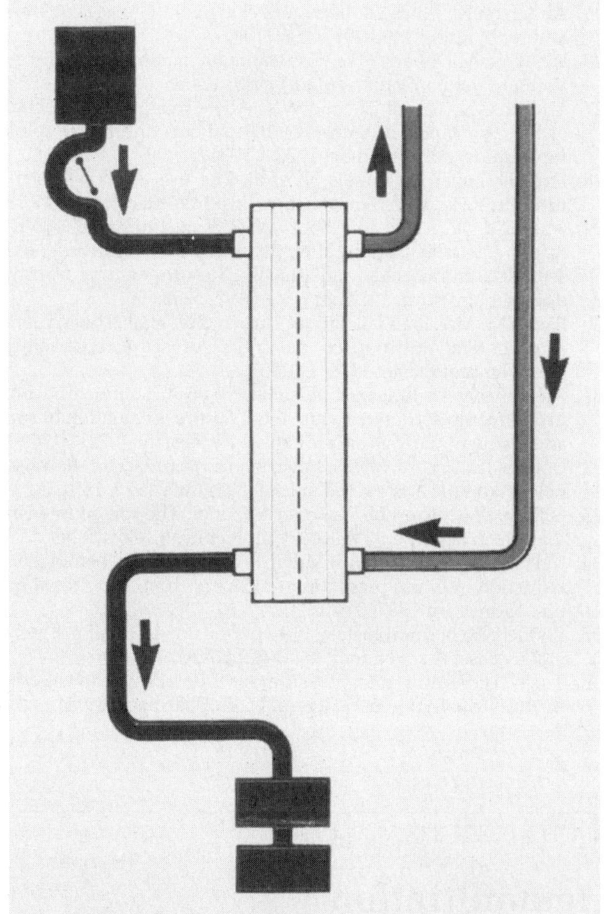

Figure 115–2. Representation of a continuous arteriovenous hemodiafiltration (CAVHD) circuit. The *gray line* represents arterial blood entering the filter (*white rectangle*). The blood returns to the venous circulation (*gray line*) after traversing the blood compartment of the filter. Simultaneously, dialysate (*black*) is pumped (the thin diagonal line with dots at each end represents a pump) into the nonblood compartment of the filter in a direction countercurrent to blood flow. The resultant ultradiafiltrate is collected in a volumetric collecting device placed in a dependent position (*black rectangles*). The replacement fluid (not represented) is delivered to the venous limb of the circuit. (Courtesy of Hospal International Marketing, Lyon, France.)

Continuous Arteriovenous Hemodiafiltration

Continuous AV hemodiafiltration (CAVHD) is a modification of CAVH. It increases urea and creatinine clearances by adding a diffusive (dialytic) solute clearance component (solute movement is driven by chemical gradients) to the convective process used in hemofiltration. For this reason, terms such as *CAVH with dialysis* have also been used. Whatever the expression, blood flows through the filter as in CAVH, while countercurrent dialysate solution is simultaneously delivered to the nonblood compartment of the filter (Fig. 115–2). Typically, dialysate flow rates are 1 L/h, although this can easily be increased to augment solute clearances further. Large volumes of fluids can still be removed, as in CAVH, and urea and creatinine clearances reach values of 23 to 25 mL/min.[14]

With this approach, even septic and highly catabolic patients receiving aggressive nutritional protein supplementation can achieve full control of azotemia (urea blood concentration <30 mL/L). CAVHD, therefore, overcomes one of the major shortcomings of CAVH. It retains, however, the need for arterial access with its attendant increase in morbidity.[14]

Continuous Venovenous Hemofiltration

Continuous venovenous hemofiltration (CVVH) was developed to circumvent the need for arterial access. Vascular access is usually obtained by means of a double-lumen, large-bore venous catheter. Blood is then pumped at a preset flow rate (150–200 mL/min or more) by a peristaltic pump. It flows from the "outlet" lumen of the catheter into the filter and returns to the venous circulation via the "inlet" lumen of the catheter (Fig. 115–3).[12] Ultrafiltrate is collected as for CAVH, but, because of the high blood flows with higher transmembrane pressures, larger ultrafiltrate volumes can be achieved (>35 L/d) with increased convective solute clearances. The technique of predilution can be applied to increase the effectiveness of CVVH further. This approach is attractive because venous access can usually be easily obtained with little morbidity, and treatment can be initiated rapidly. Its application, however, adds the complexity and cost of operating a peristaltic pump. This change mandates adequate nursing staff education. It also requires very close supervision of fluid replacement management, given the particularly large volumes being removed. The possibility of air embolism in association with pump use also requires continuous vigilance. All modern pumps are equipped with an air trap and other safety features. Finally, the morbidity associated with gaining venous access with a

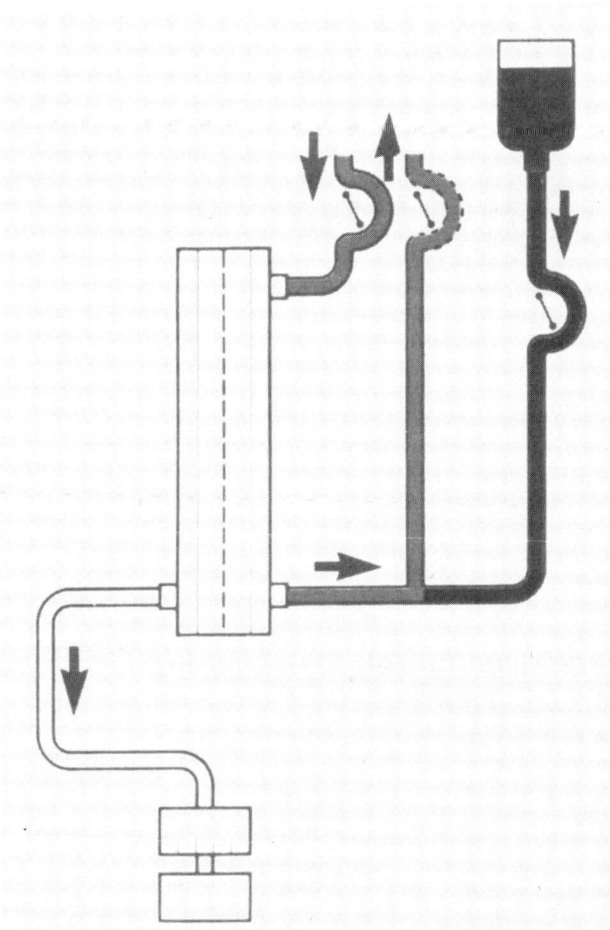

Figure 115–3. Representation of a continuous venovenous hemofiltration (CVVH) circuit. Venous blood is pumped into and out of (*large white rectangle*) the filter by means of peristaltic pumps (symbolized by diagonal lines with dots at each end). Replacement fluid (*black line*) is delivered by volumetric pump (postfiltration, in this case). Ultrafiltrate is collected in a volumetric collecting device (*white rectangles at bottom*).

double-lumen venous catheter should not be underestimated.

Continuous Venovenous Hemodiafiltration

Continuous venovenous hemodiafiltration (CVVHD) seeks to combine the advantages of double-lumen venous access with those of diffusive solute clearance. Blood is pumped by a peristaltic pump (as in CVVH) and dialysate is delivered countercurrent to blood flow in the nonblood compartment of the hemofilter (as in CAVHD) (Fig. 115–4). The combination of high blood flow, high convective clearances, and the additional diffusive solute clearance component results in average urea and creatinine clearances of approximately 25 mL/min (at 1 L/h of dialysate flow rates).[15] This approach adds the complexity of a peristaltic blood pump and of a volumetric pump for dialysate delivery. It nonetheless remains substantially less complex than intermittent hemodialysis. Trained hemodialysis nurses are not needed for the application of CVVHD. Further, CVVHD has the advantage over CVVH of being associated with smaller net filtrate volumes (600–700 mL/h) while maintaining high solute clearances. The use of dialysate at a given sodium concentration also allows serum tonicity to be essentially "servo-controlled;" the serum sodium concentration is kept within a narrow range by continuous equilibration with the concentration of sodium in the dialysate. This increases the ease and safety of overall fluid management.

BIOCHEMICAL PRINCIPLES OF HEMOFILTRATION AND HEMODIAFILTRATION

In CAVH, the major determinant of urea clearance is the ultrafiltration rate. This is determined to a major degree by the transmembrane pressure (TMP), which is the net pressure gradient driving fluid across the membrane as defined by Starling law:

$$\text{TMP} = \text{hydrostatic pressure} - \text{oncotic pressure}$$

The hydrostatic pressure is the sum of the positive pressure generated by the patient's blood pressure and the negative pressure in the filtrate compartment (PF), which is due to the gravity effect of the lower position of the collecting bag in relation to the filter.[16] The magnitude of PF depends on

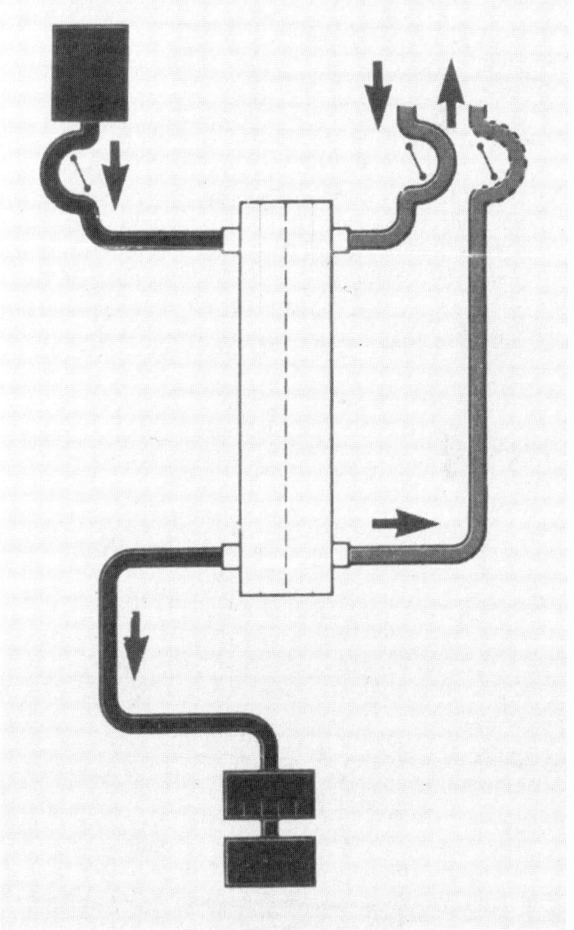

Figure 115–4. Representation of a continuous venovenous hemodiafiltration (CVVHD) circuit. Venous blood is pumped from one limb of the double-lumen intravenous catheter into the filter inlet (*gray line leading to the white rectangle*). It later exits the filter outlet to return to the venous circulation via the other limb of the catheter (*gray line leading from the white rectangle*). Simultaneously, dialysate is pumped into the nonblood compartment of the filter (*black line leading to the white rectangle*). The ultradiafiltrate is collected in a volumetric collection device (*black rectangles at bottom*). (Courtesy of Hospal International Marketing, Lyon, France.)

the length of the filtrate column between filter and collecting device:

PF = height (centimeter) × 0.74 mm Hg (conversion factor for cm H_2O to mm Hg)

The mean hydrostatic pressure (MHP) in the filter will, therefore, be given by the equation

$$\text{MHP} = \frac{\text{prefilter blood pressure} + \text{postfilter blood pressure}}{2} + \text{PF}$$

Equally, the mean oncotic pressure (MOP) can be easily calculated by the following:

$$\text{MOP} = \frac{\text{oncotic pressure inlet} + \text{oncotic pressure outlet}}{2}$$

The gradient between MHP and MOP will determine the filtration fraction (FF)

$$\text{FF (\%)} = \text{Qf/QPi}$$

where Qf is the ultrafiltration rate and QPi is the plasma flow at the filter inlet (both in milliliters per minute). The total amount of ultrafiltrate is, therefore, a function of filter plasma flow at a given stable FF (Fig. 115–5). Plasma flow at the inlet is a fraction of total blood flow (Qbi). This can be calculated using the equation:

$$\frac{\text{Qbi} = \text{Qf} \times \text{Hct outlet}}{\text{Hct outlet} - \text{Nct inlet}}$$

where Qf is the ultrafiltration rate measured from the ultrafiltration collection device (milliliters per minute). The hematocrit (Hct) values are obtained by sampling blood along the arterial and venous catheters. Plasma flow is then calculated as

$$\text{QPi} = \text{Qbi} - \text{erythrocyte mass}$$

where inlet erythrocyte mass is equal to

$$\frac{\text{Qbi} \times \text{Hct inlet}}{100}$$

From these observations, it is clear that the total ultrafiltrate at a given state of membrane function and resistance will depend on blood flow, arterial inlet pressure, venous outlet pressure, Hct, and oncotic pressure. Dynamically, filtration will be greater in the proximal segments of the filter and will then progressively diminish distally as oncotic pressure rises because of the loss of plasma water. Present evidence suggests that equilibrium between hydrostatic and oncotic pressure (zero filtration rate) is not reached in most currently used filters.

If a dialytic component is added to convection-based clearances, the total solute clearance achieved is the sum of each separate clearance; that is,

$$\text{Kt} = \text{Kc} + \text{Kd}$$

where Kt is the total clearance achieved, Kc is the clearance achieved in the absence of dialysate flow, and Kd is that obtained at zero ultrafiltration. Kc is easily calculated from the equation

$$\text{Kc} = \frac{\text{Cuf} \times \text{Vuf}}{\text{Cpl}}$$

where Cuf and Cpl are solute concentrations in ultrafiltrate and plasma and Vuf is the volume of ultrafiltrate produced per unit of time. Equally, Kt is easily calculated according to the same principle:

$$\text{Kt} = \frac{\text{Cudf} \times \text{Vudf}}{\text{Cpl}}$$

where Cudf refers to the solute concentration in the ultradiafiltrate when dialysis is added to filtration and Vudf is the volume of ultradiafiltrate. The difference between Kt and Kc is the solute clearance added by diffusion. In CAVHD, where dialysate flow rate is much less than blood flow at inlet (Qbi), full diffusion equilibrium is achieved, and, in the absence of filter clotting, for molecules the size of urea, the concentration at dialysate outflow approximates plasma concentration.[17, 18] In a patient with a plasma urea concentration of 40 mmol/L, a similar ultradiafiltrate concentration is achieved in a new filter in vivo at 1 L/h of

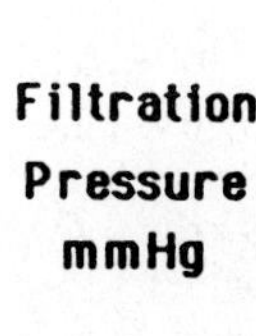

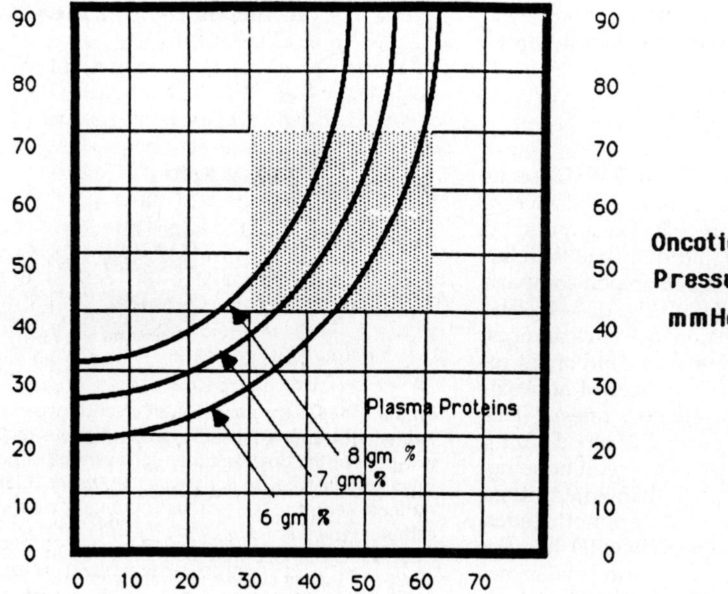

Figure 115–5. Diagram showing the relationship that links filtration pressure, oncotic pressure, and filtration fraction. The *shaded area* represents the usual range of filtration pressure. The *curved lines* show oncotic pressures for different filter inlet protein concentrations. (From Bosch JP, Ronco C: Continuous arteriovenous hemofiltration (CAVH) and other continuous replacement therapies: Operational characteristics and clinical use. *In*: Replacement of Renal Function by Dialysis. Maher JF [Ed]. Dordrecht, Kluwer Academic Publishers, 1989, p 351.)

TABLE 115–1. Features of Some Available Hemofilters (Continuous Arteriovenous Hemodiafiltration Data)

Maker	*Name*	*Material*	*Configuration*	*Cl_{cr} (mL/min)*
Hospal	AN 69S	Polyacrylonitrile	Parallel plate	~17
ASAHI	PAN 50	Polyacrylonitrile	Hollow fiber	~14
Gambro	FH 66	Polyamide	Hollow fiber	~9
Amicon	Diafilter 30	Polysulphone	Hollow fiber	~10
Fresenius AG	AV 400	Polysulphone	Hollow fiber	~10
Renal Systems	Renaflo 0.5	Polysulphone	Hollow fiber	~11

Abbreviation: Cl_{cr} = creatinine clearance.

dialysate flow. With a typical daily ultradiafiltrate production of 35 L a day, slightly more than a mole of urea is removed each day (6×10^{23} molecules of urea). This means that approximately 7×10^{18} molecules of urea cross the filtering membrane each second and that, for each square millimeter of membrane, billions of urea molecules move across in the same time span!

THE HEMOFILTERS

The filters now available for continuous hemofiltration are highly biocompatible. These membranes are polyacrylonitrile, polysulphone, or polyamide (Table 115–1). These types of membranes are not associated with many of the hematologic consequences seen with cuprophane-based membranes commonly used for intermittent hemodialysis (e.g., leukopenia, complement activation, increased pyrogen production). Filter membranes are highly porous with pore size up to 50,000 ds.[19] This allows the removal of many molecules (drugs, hormones, microglobulin) that are retained within the circulation during hemodialysis. It also allows the extraction or absorption of potentially noxious cytokines such as tumor necrosis factor-α and interleukin (IL)-1β.[20] In this regard, polyacrylonitrile membranes may be superior to others.[21] Polyacrylonitrile may also be superior in terms of urea and creatinine clearance. It is now apparent that fiber configuration may be an important variable determining filtration efficiency. High-flux membranes are available in both parallel plate (i.e., flat layers of membrane overlapping each other as in a sandwich) and hollow fiber (i.e., tubular structures with a hollow core) configurations. The parallel plate configuration has been shown to offer less resistance to blood flow, higher diffusive clearances, and higher ultrafiltrate volumes (Table 115–2).[22] The decreased resistance to blood flow may have clinically important implications with regard to the requirements for filter anticoagulation. Their better overall performance would lead one to consider flat plate (parallel) fiber polyacrylonitrile membranes to be the filter membranes of choice for continuous hemofiltration therapies.

TABLE 115–2. Filter Performance During CAVHD*

Filter	*Kt (mL/min)*	*Kd (mL/min)*	*Qf (mL/min)*	*Cdo/Cbi*
Parallel plate	17.9 ± 0.6	12.6 ± 0.4	7.2 ± 0.5	0.76 ± 0.03
Hollow fiber				
Gambro FH 66	8.8 ± 1.0	6.3 ± 0.5	5.6 ± 1.0	0.38 ± 0.03
Cobe PAN	9.2 ± 3.2	7.0 ± 2.1	3.9 ± 1.3	0.41 ± 0.12
Combined	9.0 ± 1.2†	6.5 ± 0.6†	5.0 ± 0.6†	0.39 ± 0.03†

(Modified from Yohay D, Butterly DW, Schwat SJ, et al: Continuous arteriovenous hemodialysis: Effect of dialyzer geometry. Kidney Int 1992; 42:448–451.)

*All values represent mean ± standard error of the mean.

†Significant difference from parallel plate at $P < .05$.

Abbreviations: CAVHD = continuous arteriovenous hemodiafiltration; Kt = total urea clearance; Kd = diffusive clearance; Qf = ultrafiltration rate; Cdo/Cbi = ratio between urea concentration at dialysate outlet (Cdo) and at blood inlet (Cbi); combined = data from both hollow fiber dialyzers.

Fluid Replacement

Continuous hemofiltration leads to the removal of large amounts of isotonic fluids. Depending on the technique, up to 35 L of fluid can be removed each day. Most of this fluid must be replaced, which poses a number of challenges to the clinician. The first challenge is determining the volume of isotonic fluid that should be infused. A 1:1 replacement regimen is simple but ignores administered nutritional fluids (often 2 to 2.5 L/d), blood or blood products, and fluids associated with antibiotics or other intravenous drugs. The volume of the therapeutic fluids administered can be subtracted from the estimate of daily losses, and the difference can be infused as replacement fluids. This approach, however, would lead to an even fluid balance and would not address the treatment of pulmonary and peripheral edema. A clinical assessment of such therapeutic needs, therefore, must be added to any equation so that more or less total volume is administered as replacement fluid to maintain desired intravascular or extravascular volumes. For example, it may be decided that under-replacement by 150 or 200 mL/h is an appropriate therapeutic goal in a mildly volume overloaded patient receiving approximately 3 L a day in "additional" fluids. Volumetric pumps and precision weighing scales have been introduced in some ICUs to regulate administered volume automatically on the basis of ongoing losses.[23]

Another approach is to control ultrafiltration rates by means of a pump that is set at a rate 100 to 200 mL greater than that of the volumetric pump administering dialysate. These strategies are, generally speaking, effective. They rely, however, on the precision and accuracy of these pumps, which, unfortunately, are limited.[24]

Another simple strategy is to measure the ultrafiltrate produced hourly and then change the setting of the volumetric pump each hour to administer the desired volume. This approach is time consuming and labor intensive. The problem ideally lends itself to closed-loop control strategies. Initial work indicates that an adaptable intravascular volume-responsive, computer-driven, closed-loop control system for the administration of replacement fluids is feasible and effective. It allows for rapid modifications (every 5 seconds) in fluid infusion rates to meet the ever-changing hemodynamic needs of these critically ill patients.[25]

Once the issue of fluid replacement has been addressed, the quality of fluids to be administered needs to be considered. Commercial replacement fluids with the appropriate electrolyte composition are now available. Simple saline-based replacement schedules have also been described (Table 115–3).[14] Whatever the choice, one needs to be aware of

TABLE 115–3. Fluid Replacement During CAVHD/CVVHD

Liter No.	*Constitution*	*Additives*
1	Normal saline	None
2	Normal saline	10 mL of 10% calcium gluconate
3	Normal saline	5 mmol of magnesium sulfate
4	5% dextrose	150 mL of 8.4% sodium bicarbonate

(Modified with permission from Bellomo R, Ernest D, Love J, et al: Continuous arteriovenous hemodiafiltration: Optimal therapy for acute renal failure in an intensive care setting? Aust N Z J Med 1990; 20:237–242.)

Abbreviations: CAVHD = continuous arteriovenous hemodiafiltration; CVVHD = continuous venovenous hemodiafiltration.

and responsive to the electrolyte and acid-base requirements of the individual patient.

During CAVH or CVVH, the ultrafiltrate electrolyte composition mirrors that of plasma. With countercurrent dialysate (CAVHD or CVVHD), ultradiafiltrate composition is modified, particularly if, as is usually the case, potassium is added to standard dialysate at 4 to 5 mmol/L concentrations. Under these conditions, potassium, calcium, and magnesium requirements are altered in a clinically important way, and overall electrolyte replacement schedules must take this into account.[17]

Finally, one has to decide where in the circuit replacement fluid should be administered. There is good evidence that prefilter fluid delivery increases clearance in techniques that use convective clearance (CAVH or CVVH). It possibly also prolongs filter life by a flushing effect. When diffusive clearance is in use (CAVHD or CVVHD), prefilter dilution may actually result in a net fall in urea clearance. With dialytic techniques, therefore, fluid replacement is usually administered after the filter.

VASCULAR CATHETERS AND CIRCUIT

When AV hemofiltration is used (CAVH or CAVHD), vascular access can be achieved by either the insertion of femoral arterial and venous cannulas (10 to 14 French) or the construction of a Scribner shunt. The former approach (percutaneous insertion by sterile Seldinger technique) seems to offer higher blood flows, the potential for better filtration and dialysis, and the possibility of prolonged filter life with diminished anticoagulation. One disadvantage lies in a greater degree of patient immobilization. Further, femoral cannulation is relatively contraindicated in grossly obese patients, in those with groin intertrigo, and in patients with severe peripheral vascular disease.

The use of a Scribner shunt may provide greater patient comfort but is usually associated with lower blood flows. In hypotensive patients, this results in diminished filter perfusion and increased risk of filter clotting. The choice of AV access devices should take into account the hemodynamic and clinical features of the individual patient.

The surface area of the vascular tubing of the circuit contributes to increased blood coagulation. Tubing should, therefore, be as short as possible. The filtrate collection device can be placed at different levels in relation to the filter. At higher levels, ultrafiltrate flow is diminished. This step is taken by some clinicians to control ultrafiltrate production, even though solute clearance is diminished. If large amounts of ultrafiltrate (>1.5 L/h) are being produced, as is often the case in the first 2 to 3 hours of filter life, it seems wiser to simply provide adequate and rapid fluid replacement as necessary.

The use of a double-lumen dialysis catheter (percutaneous insertion by sterile Seldinger technique usually either in the femoral or subclavian vein position) and a peristaltic pump (CVVH or CVVHD) simplifies vascular access and significantly reduces complications[26] but requires a longer extracorporeal circuit. In theory, this should result in an increased chance of extracorporeal formation of clot. Clinical experience so far does not bear out this concern perhaps because higher blood flows achieved with a pump (150–200 mL/min) are protective.

EXTRACORPOREAL CIRCUIT ANTICOAGULATION

All continuous filtration techniques require the avoidance of blood clotting in the extracorporeal circuit (catheters, tubing, and filters) because all the components provide a clinically important thrombogenic stimulus through contact activation of the coagulation cascade. It is generally believed that some form of anticoagulation is needed to maintain filtering function for an acceptable period of time (>24 hours).[27]

Various approaches have been described, most of which are based on the use of intravenous heparin.[24] Heparin can be given to achieve systemic anticoagulation. This is effective prophylaxis against filter clotting but is often contraindicated in critically ill patients. Heparin can also be given before the filter at low dose, thus achieving a degree of filter protection without a major systemic anticoagulant effect. Various low-dose regimens have been described that range from prefilter heparin at 10 IU/h to the fixed administration of 250 to 500 IU/h. These follow the priming of the filter with heparin-containing saline (2000–5000 IU in 2 L). The regimen chosen for a given patient usually follows a clinical and laboratory assessment of risk of bleeding.

An alternative approach is to anticoagulate the membrane aggressively with prefilter heparin and then reverse its effect with postfilter protamine, typically at a ratio of 100 IU:1 mg (regional anticoagulation).[28] This strategy results in prolongation of filter life compared with low-dose heparin (500 IU/h before the filter) in patients receiving CAVHD via a Scribner shunt without an increase in bleeding complications.[29] When blood flow is high (e.g., CAVHD with femoral cannulas), low-dose heparin was not superior to "no anticoagulation." One may, therefore, wish to avoid using heparin altogether in patients thought to be at very high risk of bleeding. In fact, even during CVVHD in high-risk patients, one can achieve acceptable mean filter lives (>24 h) without anticoagulation.[29] When no anticoagulation is used, some clinicians seek to prevent filter clotting by administering regular saline flushes (100 mL each hour) to the filter. No evidence exists to support this clinical practice.[29a]

If anticoagulation is desired but one wishes to avoid the specific complications associated with the use of heparin (especially thrombocytopenia), other modes of anticoagulation are available. The chelation of calcium with prefilter citrate has been shown to be effective. The local anticoagulant effect is reversed by the postfilter administration of calcium. This approach is associated with a 25% incidence of transient metabolic alkalosis and requires the use of an especially prepared low-sodium, calcium- and alkali-free dialysate solution. It has so far only been described by a single group of investigators.[29a, 30]

Low-molecular-weight heparin appears to be associated with fewer side effects than standard heparin with possibly a better overall safety profile. It has been used effectively in small numbers of patients so far, but it has been compared with unfractionated heparin in only one small study.[31–33] More information is needed to determine whether there are clinically important advantages in its use over its less expensive unfractionated counterpart.

TABLE 115–4. Anticoagulation During Continuous Hemofiltration

Method	*Advantages*	*Disadvantages*	*Dosage*	*Monitoring*
No anticoagulant	Safest	Early filter clotting if no evidence of coagulopathy	None	None
Low-dose heparin	Safe, simple, and inexpensive	Thrombocytopenia	500 IU/h	APTT
Heparin	Very effective	Increased risk of bleeding, thrombocytopenia	Full dose	APTT>1.5–<2.5 times control
LMW heparin	Effective, fall in bleeding risk?	Expensive, monitoring not readily available	10–40 mg every 6 h	anti-Xa activity >0.25–<0.5 IU/mL
Regional heparin	Very effective	Complex, cumbersome, preserved risk of bleeding	100 IU/1 mg heparin to protamine	Filter APTT >2 and patient APTT <1.5 control values
Regional citrate	Effective	Complex, alkalosis, Ca^{++} monitoring needed	4% citrate 150 mL/h	APTT 1.5–2.5 × controls; free Ca^{++} 0.96–1.2 mmol/L
Prostacyclin	Less heparin	Hypotension, not easily reversed	4–6 ng · kg^{-1} · min^{-1}	Skin bleeding time APTT
Nafamostat mesylate	No heparin Less bleeding	Little clinical experience Efficacy?	0.1 mg · kg^{-1} · h^{-1}	ACT
Gabexate mesylate	No heparin Less bleeding	Little clinical experience Efficacy?	10–15 mg · kg^{-1} · h^{-1}	ACT
Saline flush	No bleeding	No proven efficacy	100 mL/h	None

Abbreviations: APTT = activated partial thromboplastin time; LMW = low molecular weight; Xa = activated factor X; Ca^{++} = calcium ion; ACT = activated clotting time.

Prostacyclin infusion has also been used as a means of filter anticoagulation.[34–36] It acts by inhibiting platelet aggregation and adhesion. It has been used in combination with heparin and low-molecular-weight heparin or alone. Experience, however, is limited, cost is high, immediate reversibility is unavailable, and evidence of clinically important advantages is absent.

Finally, protease inhibitors such as gabexate or nafamostat mesylate have also been used.[37] Experience with these new drugs is encouraging, but reports have included only small numbers of patients, and no comparative data are yet available.

The approaches to extracorporeal anticoagulation are summarized in Table 115–4.

CLINICAL CONSEQUENCES OF HEMOFILTRATION

Extensive experience has now accumulated on the use of hemofiltration in its various forms.[38–49] All techniques have been found to be generally safe and effective. A number of important issues, however, require separate discussion because of their clinical relevance.

Hemorrhage and Vascular Access–Related Complications

The initial experience with CAVH and CAVHD indicates that there is a 10% to 15% combined incidence of hemorrhagic, infectious, and/or vascular-related complications with the use of these techniques.[42, 42a, 43] Most of these complications are of limited clinical importance, but their occurrence highlights the problems associated with continuous anticoagulation and vascular cannulation in critically ill patients. These complications must also be viewed in comparison to those seen with alternate therapies such as intermittent hemodialysis and peritoneal dialysis. A retrospective review suggested that the overall number of complications is less during continuous hemodiafiltration. Further, the introduction of CVVH and CVVHD, with the need for a single venous puncture, diminishes vascular and hemorrhagic complications.[44] Venous access also potentially allows full mobility to the patient, circumventing another potential problem associated with earlier versions of these continuous dialytic techniques.

Hemodynamic Consequences

There is ample reported and anecdotal evidence to indicate that continuous hemofiltration is associated with an excellent degree of hemodynamic stability.[39–44] Fluid can be readily and rapidly removed from edematous patients without associated hypotension.[41, 42] Initiation of continuous hemofiltration therapy is not associated with any of the fluctuations in blood pressure and heart rate often seen with intermittent hemodialysis schedules; in fact, improvements in cardiopulmonary variables have been reported in critically ill patients after initiation of therapy.[47]

Control of Azotemia

Whereas initial forms of therapy such as CAVH had limited urea and creatinine clearances and required additional intermittent hemodialysis in up to 20% of patients to achieve control of azotemia, newer techniques (CAVHD/CVVHD) can achieve steady and excellent degrees of azotemia control even in catabolic patients weighing more than 100 kg who are receiving aggressive parenteral nitrogen supplementation (Fig. 115–6). In these patients, plasma urea can be kept below 30 mmol/L throughout the entire course of treatment. This contrasts with the fluctuations in plasma solute concentrations seen during conventional intermittent hemodialysis and may translate into clinically important gains.

Nutrition

A major problem in patients with ARF is protein catabolism. This often occurs in patients in whom it is problematic to

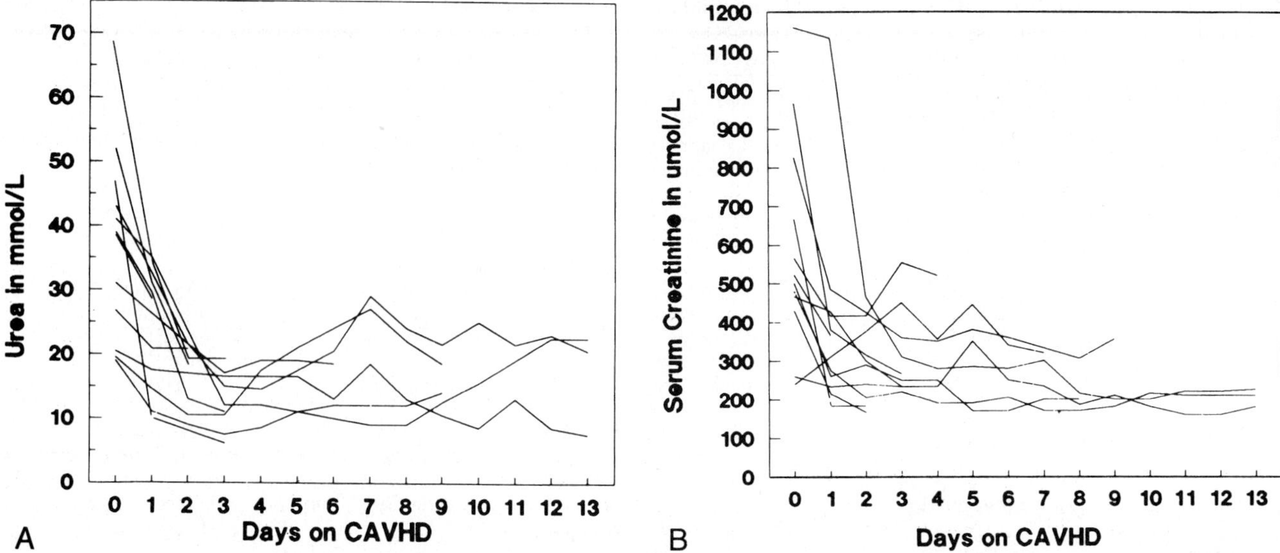

Figure 115–6. Graphs illustrating the impact of CAVHD on urea (*A*) and creatinine (*B*) blood concentrations. Each line represents one patient's concentration throughout the duration of therapy. Note how urea and creatinine levels are rapidly brought under control and kept below 30 mmol/L. (From Bellomo R, Ernest D, Love J, et al: Continuous arteriovenous hemodiafiltration: Optimal therapy for acute renal failure in an intensive care setting? Aust N Z J Med 1990; 20:237–242.)

administer adequate nutritional fluids because of issues associated with volume overload or when adequate protein nitrogen administration exacerbates azotemia. In this respect alone, continuous hemofiltration has truly represented a major step forward.[48, 49] The issue of volume overload has been effectively eliminated. With high urea clearance techniques (especially CAVHD and CVVHD), a high-protein diet (2 g or more of protein per kilogram per day) can be administered without unacceptable azotemia (plasma urea >35 mmol/L). The impact of CAVHD on major nutrient balances has been investigated.[50] It has been shown that, even in septic ARF, a near-neutral nitrogen balance can be achieved despite the obligatory loss of 10% of infused amino acids into the ultradiafiltrate (Table 115–5).[50–52] This is a major improvement on previous results[53] and may ultimately translate into a better prognosis.[54, 55] With techniques that use glucose-containing dialysates, glucose transfer to the blood compartment takes place in clinically important quantities. Using a 1.5% dextrose-containing solution, approximately 150 g of carbohydrate enter the circulation each day.[50, 56] These 600 kcal/d should be taken into account in the prescription of parenteral nutrition. The amount of glucose transferred to blood increases linearly with increasing dialysate dextrose concentrations and with dialysate flow rates. Blood lipids are not directly affected by hemofiltration. No lipid losses into the ultradiafiltrate can be documented in vivo.

There are few data on trace elements and their extraction during continuous hemofiltration. Preliminary findings indicate that zinc, copper, manganese, selenium, and iron are ultrafiltered in negligible amounts.[57] No data are available on vitamin losses during hemofiltration, and it seems wise to provide regular vitamin supplementation during therapy.

Drugs

The clearance of many drugs used in the ICU is significantly affected by hemofiltration techniques. This aspect of renal failure management is discussed in detail in a separate chapter dealing with drug-kidney interactions (Chapter 116).

Hormones

Few data have so far been published on the effects of continuous hemofiltration on hormones. Catecholamine clearance

TABLE 115–5. Impact of Continuous Arteriovenous Hemodiafiltration on Nitrogen Balance

Measured Variables	*Mean Value*	*95% Confidence Interval*
Nitrogen mass transfer per day	24.1 g	20.9–27.3 g
Urea nitrogen mass transfer per day	15.1 g	14.6–15.6 g
Urea nitrogen production per day	14.7 g	13.4–16.1 g
Blood urea concentration	18 mmol/L	15.3–20.8 mmol/L
Ultradiafiltrate urea concentration	15.1 mmol/L	13.8–17.6 mmol/L
Urea clearance	32.7 L/d	29.8–35.6 mmol/L
Intravenous nitrogen given per day	20.5 g	17.9–23.1 g/d
Nitrogen balance per day	−0.045 g/kg	−0.024–0.056 g

(Modified with permission from Bellomo R, Martin H, Parkin G, et al: Continuous arteriovenous hemodiafiltration in the critically ill: Influence on major nutrient balances. Intensive Care Med 1991; 17:399–402.)

has been formally studied during CAVHD and CVVHD. The findings indicate that the loss of dopamine, epinephrine, and norepinephrine over a period of 24 hours is clinically and pharmacologically negligible, even in patients receiving high-dose intravenous infusions and achieving high plasma catecholamine concentrations.[58] Hemodiafiltration clearance accounts for less than 1% of the total administered dose and is not associated with any increase in drug requirements. Insulin clearances are also minimal.[59] Other hormones such as aldosterone, parathyroid hormone, testosterone, cortisol, triiodothyronine, thyroxine, and thyroid-stimulating hormone are also only removed in minute quantities by continuous hemodiafiltration.[57] This suggests that continuous hemodiafiltration does not significantly modify the hormonal response to critical illness.

Blood Purification During Sepsis

Strong evidence indicates that many of the adverse physiologic consequences of sepsis are due to humoral "mediators of injury." Many molecules have been shown in vivo to be produced in the presence of sepsis and to be capable of triggering pathophysiologic changes that mimic sepsis. Their molecular size allows their potential extraction from the circulation during hemofiltration. A number of studies now suggest that continuous hemofiltration may offer a degree of "blood purification" over and above the removal of urea and creatinine.[59a] Hemofiltration lowers pulmonary artery pressures and pulmonary resistance in a model of endotoxic shock.[60] It reverses left ventricular dysfunction during experimental endotoxemia in dogs.[61] This may be due to the extraction of tumor necrosis factor-α which is a known myocardial depressant.[62–64] High-volume venovenous hemofiltration increases cardiac output, left ventricular stroke volume, mean arterial pressure, and right ventricular ejection fraction in a pig model of endotoxic shock (Figs. 115–7 and 115–8).[65, 66]

Hemofiltration also decreases extravascular lung water,[67] removes thromboxane, bradykinin, β-endorphin,[68] and IL-1β.[69] Finally, there is suggestive evidence that more intensive hemofiltration or hemodiafiltration may be associated with a better overall clinical outcome.[69, 70] Although these data require confirmation and their clinical significance needs further clarification, they also suggest that hemofiltration offers the additional advantage of down-regulating the potentially noxious inflammatory response associated with sepsis.

Continuous Hemofiltration or Conventional Dialysis

It remains unclear whether the many practical and theoretical advantages of continuous hemofiltration can translate into improved overall survival in ARF compared with treatment by conventional dialytic techniques (intermittent hemodialysis and peritoneal dialysis). The reasons for this are many. Studies of ARF outcome with conventional dialysis offer variable patient population mixes and widely variable outcome figures. They also rarely give an illness severity score for the population under study. This makes retrospective, meaningful comparisons impossible. Detection of falls in mortality of 20% to 25% with the use of hemofiltration techniques will require the study of large numbers of patients. Single institutions need many years to achieve sufficient numbers. Multicenter studies are difficult because of large diversities in expertise, techniques used, and regional philosophic commitments to a given dialytic approach. Despite these limitations, there are some retrospective comparative data that suggest that the use of continuous hemodiafiltration may translate into diminishing morbidity and mortality for patients with ARF in the setting of critical illness (Table 115–6).[43, 43a, 44, 48, 71, 72] The present view is that more information is necessary before continuous hemofiltration techniques become completely established as *the only* renal replacement therapy to be used in intensive care.[73]

THE FUTURE

It is likely that the use of hemofiltration will increase. Further technical refinements will take place. They will provide more precise peristaltic and volumetric pumps, heparin

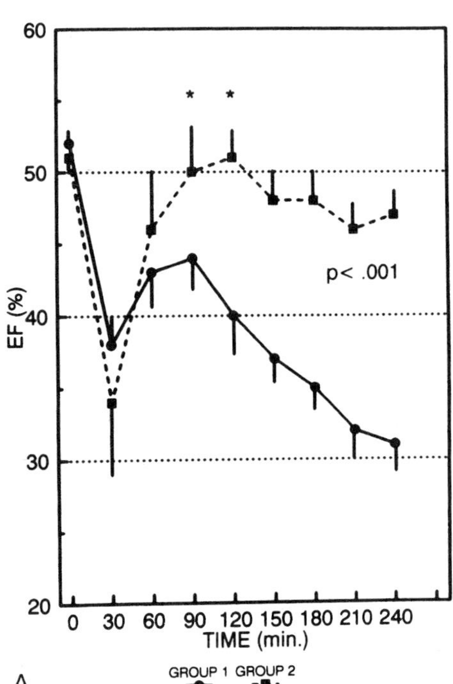

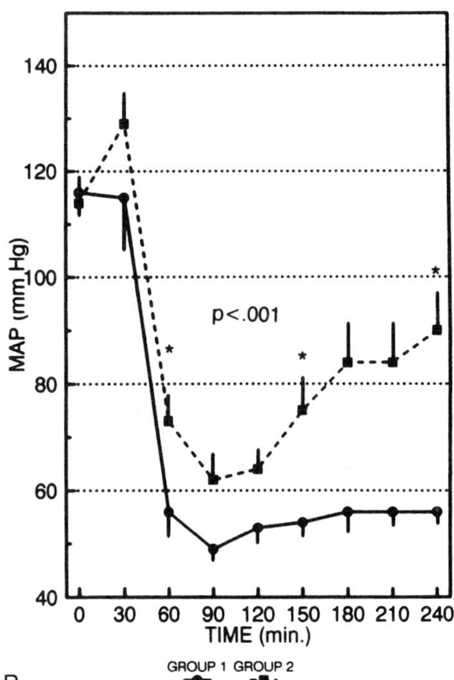

Figure 115–7. Diagrams showing the effect of high-volume CVVH on right ventricular ejection fraction (EF, *A*) and mean arterial pressure (MAP, *B*) in a porcine model of endotoxic shock. The *squares* and *dashed lines* identify the treated animals, and the *circles* and *continuous lines* identify the control animals. Right ventricular ejection fraction and mean arterial blood pressure are positively affected in a significant way. (From Grootendorst AF, van Bonnell EFH, van der Hoven B, et al: High volume hemofiltration improves right ventricular function in endotoxin-induced shock in the pig. Intensive Care Med 1992; 18:235–240.)

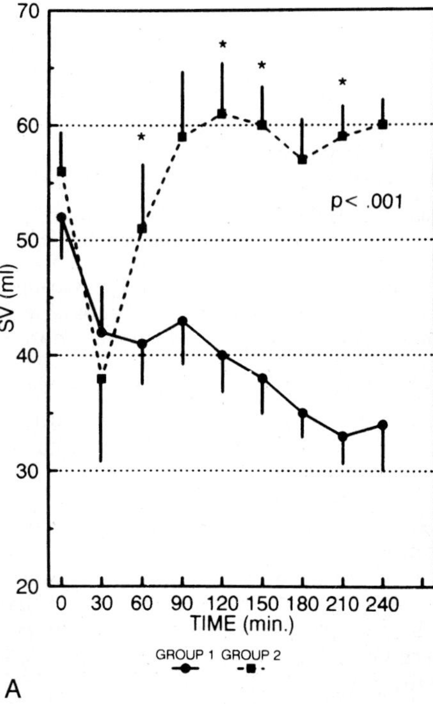

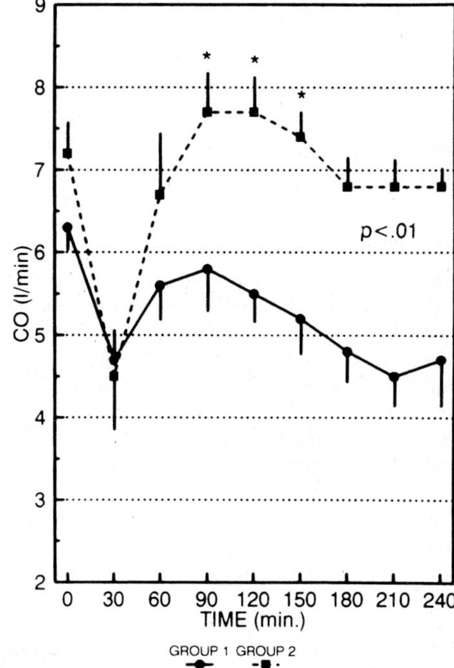

Figure 115–8. *A* and *B,* Diagrams showing the impact of high-volume CVVH on cardiac output (CO) and left ventricular stroke volume (SV) in a porcine model of endotoxic shock. The *squares* and *dashed lines* indicate the treated animals, and the *circles* and *continuous lines* the control animals. Cardiac output and stroke volume are maintained at pre-endotoxemia levels if hemofiltration is applied. Their levels fall significantly in the control animals. (From Grootendorst AF, van Bonnell EFH, van der Hoven B, et al: High volume hemofiltration improves right ventricular function in endotoxin-induced shock in the pig. Intensive Care Med 1992; 18:235–240.)

TABLE 115–6. Comparison of Acute Continuous Hemodiafiltration (ACHD) with Conventional Dialytic Therapy (CDT)

Clinical Effects	*CDT*	*ACHD*	*P*
Overall survival	25/84 (29.8%)	34/83 (41%)	NS
Survival with two or fewer failing organs	6 of 12	14 of 16	NS
Survival with two to four failing organs	17 of 58	26 of 50	<.025
Survival with more than four failing organs	6 of 23	6 of 31	NS
APACHE II score <24	17 of 37	14 of 26	NS
APACHE II score 24 to 29	3 of 24	13 of 28	<.025
Full-dose total parenteral nutrition	28 of 52	42 of 47	<.025
Median duration of hospital stay (days)	45 (range = 7–176)	29 (range = 14–123)	NS

(Modified with permission from Bellomo R, Mansfield D, Rumble S, et al: Acute renal failure in critical illness: Conventional dialysis [CD] vs. acute continuous hemodiafiltration [ACHD]. ASAIO J 1992; 38:M654–M657.)

bonding of filtering membranes,[74, 75] vascular catheters with protection from bacterial biofilm formation, and the binding to filtering membranes of molecules that may allow the removal of endotoxin.[76] Technical advances will make fluid replacement simpler, diminish or abrogate the need for extracorporeal anticoagulation, decrease the risk of catheter-associated infection, and possibly help influence the pathophysiology of septic shock while continuing to offer excellent and consistent control of azotemia.

ACKNOWLEDGMENTS

My thanks go to my wife, Debrah, for her continuing and patient support during the preparation of this chapter. My gratitude goes to Neil Boyce, MD, Daniel Martich, MD, Derek Angus, MD, and Morris Bierman, MD, for their friendly and useful advice.

GLOSSARY

Renal replacement therapy: any dialytic technique (intermittent hemodialysis, peritoneal dialysis, hemofiltration) that replaces kidney function in patients with renal failure.

Conventional dialysis: the kind of dialytic therapy typically offered to renal failure patients before the advent of hemofiltration. The expression includes intermittent hemodialysis with cuprophane membranes and peritoneal dialysis.

Continuous arteriovenous hemofiltration (CAVH): a technique that provides renal replacement therapy by allowing blood to run from an artery through a highly porous filter before returning to the venous circulation. Arterial blood pressure drives blood flow through the filter and induces ultrafiltrate production. The filter acts as an artificial glomerulus, and, by allowing the production of ultrafiltrate, it provides a degree of urea clearance (convective clearance). The fluid loss associated with CAVH requires isotonic fluid replacement.

Slow, continuous ultrafiltration (SCUF): a technique for the removal of fluid that is essentially the same as CAVH without fluid replacement. The term is often loosely used to mean CAVH, especially in the United States.

Predilution: a technique of isotonic fluid replacement during hemofiltration whereby the fluid is administered via an infusion port situated just before the inflow side of the hemofilter. It results in blood dilution, diminished oncotic pressure, increased ultrafiltrate production, and higher solute clearances.

Suction: a technique whereby negative pressure is applied to the ultrafiltrate collection chamber to augment transmembrane pressure, ultrafiltrate production, and solute clearances.

Continuous arteriovenous hemodiafiltration (CAVHD): a modification of CAVH in which dialysate (usually peritoneal dialysate) is pumped into the nonblood compartment of the filter countercurrent to blood flow to add diffusive (dialytic) solute clearance to convective clearance. Urea clearance doubles with CAVHD if dialysate flow is 1 L/h and can be further increased by increasing dialysate flow rates. CAVHD has also been called *continuous arteriovenous hemodialysis* (even though it is hemofiltration that is taking place) or *continuous arteriovenous hemofiltration with dialysis.*

Continuous venovenous hemofiltration: a filtration technique whereby blood is pumped through the filter by a peristaltic pump using a double-lumen intravenous catheter for vascular access. Blood flow is kept at rates that ensure the production of large amounts of ultrafiltrate with associated high solute clearances.

Continuous venovenous hemodiafiltration (CVVHD): this technique adds a dialytic component to CVVHD just as CAVHD does for CAVH. It increases solute clearances considerably. It has also been called *continuous venovenous hemodialysis, continuous venovenous hemofiltration with dialysis,* and even SCUF with dialysis (in the absence of fluid replacement).

References

1. Woodrow J, Turney JH: Cause of death in acute renal failure. Nephrol Dial Transplant 1992; 7:230–234.
2. Maher ER, Robinson KN, Scoble JE, et al: Prognosis of critically ill patients with acute renal failure. Q J Med 1989; 269:857–866.
3. Wheeler DC, Feehally J, Walls J: High risk acute renal failure. Q J Med 1986; 61:977–984.
4. Spiegel DM, Ullian ME, Zerbe GO, et al: Determinants of survival and recovery in acute renal failure patients dialyzed in intensive care units. Am J Nephrol 1992; 11:44–47.
5. Kramer P, Wegger W, Rieger J, et al: Arteriovenous hemofiltration: A new and simple method for treatment of overhydrated patients resistant to diuretics. Klin Wochenschr 1977; 55:1121–1122.
6. Kramer P, Seegers J, Bohnsack E, et al: Therapeutic potential of hemofiltration. Clin Nephrol 1979; 11:145–147.
7. Kramer P, Schraeder J, Bohnsack E, et al: Continuous arteriovenous hemofiltration (CAVH): A new kidney replacement therapy. Proc Eur Dial Transplant Assoc 1981; 18:743.
8. Mault JR, Dechert RE, Lees P, et al: Continuous arteriovenous filtration: An effective treatment for surgical acute renal failure. Surgery 1987; 101:478–484.
9. Kaplan AA: Enhanced efficiency during CAVH: Clinical trials with predilution and vacuum suction. *In*: International Symposium on CAVH. La Greca G, Fabris A, Ronco C (Eds). Milano: Wichtig Editore, 1986, pp 49–52.
10. Kaplan AA, Longnecker RE, Folkert VW: Suction-assisted continuous arteriovenous hemofiltration. Trans Am Soc Artif Intern Organs 1983; 29:412.
11. Geronemus R, Schneider N: Continuous arteriovenous hemodialysis: A new modality for the treatment of acute renal failure. Trans Am Soc Artif Intern Organs 1984; 30:610–613.
12. Wendon J, Smithies M, Sheppard M, et al: Continuous high volume veno-venous hemofiltration in acute renal failure. Intensive Care Med 1989; 15:358–363.
13. Bellomo R, Parkin G, Love J, et al: Use of continuous hemodiafiltration: An approach to the management of acute renal failure in the critically ill. Am J Nephrol 1992; 12:240–245.
14. Bellomo R, Ernest D, Love J, et al: Continuous arteriovenous hemodiafiltration: Optimal therapy for acute renal failure in an intensive care setting? Aust N Z J Med 1990; 20:237–242.
15. Bellomo R, Parkin G, Love J, et al: Management of acute renal failure in the critically ill with continuous veno-venous hemodiafiltration. Ren Fail 1992; 14:183–186.
16. Olbricht CJ, Haubitz M, Habel U, et al: Continuous arteriovenous hemofiltration: In-vivo functional characteristics and its dependence on vascular access and filter design. Nephron 1990; 55:49–57.
17. Sigler MH, Teehan BP: Solute transport in continuous hemodialysis: A new treatment for acute renal failure. Kidney Int 1987; 32:562–571.
18. Pallone T, Hyver S, Peterson J: The simulation of continuous arteriovenous hemodialysis with a mathematical model. Kidney Int 1989; 35:125–133.
19. Bosch JP, Ronco C: Continuous arteriovenous hemofiltration (CAVH) and other continuous replacement therapies: Operational characteristics and clinical use. *In*: Replacement of Renal Function by Dialysis. Maher JF (Ed). Dordrecht, Holland, Kluwer Academic Publishers, 1989.
20. Kierdorf H, Melzer D, WeiBen D, et al: Elimination of tumor necrosis factor-alpha by continuous veno-venous hemofiltration (Abstract). Ren Fail 1992; 14:98.
21. Brown A, Mehta R: Effect of CAVH membranes on transmembrane flux of TNF-alpha (Abstract). *In*: Proceedings of the Annual Scientific Meeting of the American Society of Nephrology, Washington, DC, 1992, p 316.

22. Yohay D, Butterly DW, Schwat SJ, et al: Continuous arteriovenous hemodialysis: Effect of dialyzer geometry. Kidney Int 1992; 42:448–451.
23. Sodemann K, Niedenthal A, Russ A, et al: Automated fluid balance in continuous hemodialysis with blood safety module BSM22/VPM. Contrib Nephrol 1991; 93:184–192.
24. Roberts M, Winney RJ: Errors in fluid balance with pump control of continuous hemodialysis. Int J Artif Organs 1992; 15:99–102.
25. Parkin G, Wright C, Bellomo R, et al: Computerized closed loop control of fluid replacement during acute continuous hemodiafiltration (ACHD) (Abstract). *In*: Proceedings of the 38th Annual Meeting of American Society of Artificial Internal Organs, p 92.
26. Bellomo R, Parkin G, Love J, et al: A prospective comparative study of continuous arteriovenous hemodiafiltration and continuous veno-venous hemodiafiltration in critically ill patients. Am J Kidney Dis 1993; 21:400–404.
27. Mehta R, Dobow GJ, Ward DM: Anticoagulation in continuous renal replacement procedures. Semin Dial 1992; 5:61–68.
28. Kaplan AA, Petrillo R: Regional heparinization for continuous arteriovenous hemofiltration. Trans Am Soc Artif Intern Organs 1987; 33:312–315.
29. Bellomo R, Teede H, Boyce N: Anticoagulant regimens in acute continuous hemodiafiltration: A comparative study. Intensive Care Med 1993; 19:329–332.
29a. Ward DM, Mehta RL: Extracorporeal management of acute renal failure patients at high risk of bleeding. Kidney Int 1993; 41:S237–244.
30. Mehta RL, McDonald BR, Aguilar MM, et al: Regional citrate anticoagulation for continuous arteriovenous hemodialysis in critically ill patients. Kidney Int 1990; 38:976–981.
31. Schrader J, Stibbe W, Kandt M, et al: Low molecular weight heparin versus standard heparin: A long term study in hemodialysis and hemofiltration patients. Trans Am Soc Artif Intern Organs 1990; 36:28–32.
32. Hory B, Cachaux A, Toulemonde F: Continuous arteriovenous hemofiltration with low-molecular-weight heparin. Nephron 1985; 42:125.
33. Wynckel A, Bernieh B, Toupance O, et al: Guidelines to the use of enoxaparin in slow continuous hemodialysis. Contrib Nephrol 1991; 93:221–224.
34. Journois D, Chanu D, Pouard P, et al: Assessment of standardized ultrafiltrate production rate using prostacyclin in continuous veno-venous hemofiltration. Contrib Nephrol 1991; 93:202–204.
35. Maurin N: Antithrombotic management with a stable prostacyclin analogue during extracorporeal circulation. Contrib Nephrol 1991; 93:205–209.
36. Ponikvar R, Kandus A, Buturovic J, et al: Use of prostacyclin as the only anticoagulant during continuous veno-venous hemofiltration. Contrib Nephrol 1991; 93:218–220.
37. Ohtake Y, Hirasawa H, Sugai AT: Nafamostat mesylate as anticoagulant in continuous hemofiltration and continuous hemodiafiltration. Contrib Nephrol 1991; 93:215–217.
38. Tam PYW, Huraib S, Mahan B, et al: Slow continuous hemodialysis for the management of complicated acute renal failure in an intensive care unit. Clin Nephrol 1988; 30:79–85.
39. Reynolds HN, Borg U, Belzberg H, et al: Efficacy of continuous arteriovenous hemofiltration with dialysis in patients with renal failure. Crit Care Med 1991; 19:1387–1394.
40. Pattison ME, Lee SM, Ogden D: Continuous arteriovenous hemodiafiltration: An aggressive approach to the management of acute renal failure. Am J Kidney Dis 1988; 11:43–48.
41. Macias WL, Mueller BA, Scarim SK, et al: Continuous venovenous hemofiltration: An alternative to continuous arteriovenous hemofiltration and continuous arteriovenous hemodiafiltration in acute renal failure. Am J Kidney Dis 1991; 18:451–458.
42. Kaplan AA, Longnecker RE, Folkert VW: Continuous arteriovenous hemofiltration: A report of six months' experience. Ann Intern Med 1984; 100:358–367.
42a. Tominaga GT, Ingegno M, Ceraldi C, et al: Vascular complications of continuous arteriovenous hemofiltration in trauma patients. J Trauma 1993; 35:285–288.
43. Bellomo R, Mansfield D, Rumble S, et al: Acute renal failure in critical illness: Conventional dialysis (CD) vs. acute continuous hemodiafiltration (ACHD). ASAIO J 1992; 38:M654–M657.
43a. Kruczynski K, Irvine-Bird K, Toffelmire EB, et al: A comparison of continuous arteriovenous hemofiltration and intermittent hemodialysis in acute renal failure patients in the intensive care unit. ASAIO J 1993; 39:M778–M781.
44. Bellomo R, Boyce N: Continuous veno-venous hemodiafiltration vs. conventional dialysis in critically ill patients with acute renal failure. ASAIO J 1993; 39:M794–M797.
45. Olbricht C, Mueller C, Schurek HJ, et al: Treatment of acute renal failure by continuous spontaneous hemofiltration. Trans Am Soc Artif Intern Organs 1982; 28:33–39.
46. Lauer A, Saccaggi A, Ronco C, et al: Continuous arteriovenous hemofiltration in the critically ill patient. Ann Intern Med 1983; 99:455–460.
47. DiCarlo JV, Dudley TE, Sherbotie JR, et al: Continuous arteriovenous hemofiltration/dialysis improves pulmonary gas exchange in children with multiple system failure. Crit Care Med 1990; 18:822–826.
48. Bartlett RH, Mault JR, Dechert RE, et al: Continuous arteriovenous hemofiltration: Improved survival in surgical acute renal failure? Surgery 1986; 2:400–408.
49. Weiss L, Danielson BG, Wilkstrom B, et al: Continuous arteriovenous hemofiltration in the treatment of 100 critically ill patients with acute renal failure: Report on clinical outcome and nutritional aspects. Clin Nephrol 1989; 31:184–189.
50. Bellomo R, Martin H, Parkin G, et al: Continuous arteriovenous hemodiafiltration in the critically ill: Influence on major nutrient balances. Intensive Care Med 1991; 17:399–402.
51. Davies SP, Reaveley DA, Brown EA, et al: Amino acid clearances in patients with acute renal failure treated by continuous arteriovenous hemodialysis. Crit Care Med 1991; 19:1510–1515.
52. Davenport A, Roberts NB: Amino acid losses during continuous high-flux hemofiltration in critically ill patients. Crit Care Med 1989; 17:1010–1014.
53. Bouffard Y, Viale JP, Annat G, et al: Energy expenditure in the acute renal failure patient mechanically ventilated. Intensive Care Med 1987; 13:401–404.
54. Abel RM, Shih UE, Abbott WM, et al: Amino acid metabolism in acute renal failure: Influence of intravenous essential L-amino acid hyperalimentation therapy. Ann Surg 1974; 180:350–356.
55. Abel RM, Beck CH, Abbott WM, et al: Improved survival from acute renal failure after treatment with intravenous essential L-amino acids and glucose: Results of a prospective, double blind study. N Engl J Med 1973; 288:659–665.
56. Bonnardeaux A, Pichette V, Quimer I, et al: Solute clearances with high dialysate flow rates and glucose absorption from the dialysate in continuous arteriovenous hemodialysis. Am J Kidney Dis 1992; 10:31–38.
57. Bellomo R, Daskalakis M, Martin H, et al: Nutritional and biochemical consequences of continuous arteriovenous hemodiafiltration (Abstract). *In*: Proceedings of the 15th Australian and New Zealand Scientific Meeting on Intensive Care, Adelaide, Australia, 1990, p 59.
58. Bellomo R, McGrath B, Boyce N: The impact of continuous veno-venous hemodiafiltration on hormone and catecholamine clearance in critically ill patients with acute renal failure. Crit Care Med 1994; 22:833–837.
59. Bellomo R, Colman P, Caudwell J, et al: Acute continuous hemodiafiltration: Its impact on insulin levels and glycemic control in the critically ill. Crit Care Med 1992; 20:1672–1676.
59a. Lee PA, Matson JR, Pryor RW, et al: Continuous arteriovenous hemofiltration therapy for *Staphylococcus aureus*-induced septicemia in immature swine. Crit Care Med 1993; 21:914–924.
60. Stein B, Pfenninger E, Grunert A, et al: Influence of continuous hemofiltration on hemodynamics and central blood volume in experimental endotoxic shock. Intensive Care Med 190; 16:494–499.
61. Gomez A, Wang R, Unruh H, et al: Hemofiltration reverses left ventricular dysfunction during sepsis in dogs. Anesthesiology 1990; 73:671–685.
62. Bellomo R, Tipping P, Boyce N: Tumor necrosis factor clearances during veno-venous hemodiafiltration in the critically ill. Trans Am Soc Artif Intern Organs 1991; 37:M324–M325.
63. Bellomo R, Tipping P, Boyce N: Continuous veno-venous hemofiltration with dialysis removes cytokines from the circulation in septic patients. Crit Care Med 1993; 21:508–513.
64. Heard SO, Perkins MW, Fink MP: Tumor necrosis factor-alpha causes myocardial depression in guinea pigs. Crit Care Med 1992; 20:523–527.
65. Grootendorst AF, van Bonnell EFH, van der Hoven B, et al:

High volume hemofiltration improves hemodynamics of endotoxin-induced shock in the pig. J Crit Care 1992; 7:67–75.
66. Grootendorst AF, van Bonnell EFH, van der Hoven B, et al: High volume hemofiltration improves right ventricular function in endotoxin induced shock in the pig. Intensive Care Med 1992; 18:235–240.
67. Stein B, Pfenninger E, Grunert A, et al: The consequences of continuous hemofiltration on lung mechanics and extravascular lung water in a porcine endotoxic shock model. Intensive Care Med 1990; 17:239–248.
68. Gotloib J, Barzilay E, Shustak A, et al: Hemofiltration in septic ARDS: The artificial kidney as an artificial endocrine lung. Resuscitation 1986; 13:123–132.
69. Storck M, Hart WH, Zimmerer E, et al: Comparison of pump-driven and spontaneous continuous hemofiltration in postoperative acute renal failure. Lancet 1991; 337:452–455.
70. Barzilay E, Kessler D, Berlot G, et al: Use of extracorporeal supportive techniques as additional treatment for septic induced multiple organ failure patients. Crit Care Med 1989; 17:634–637.
71. Kierdorf H: Continuous versus intermittent treatment: Clinical results in acute renal failure. Contrib Nephrol 1991; 93:1–12.
72. McDonald B, Mehta R: Decreased mortality in patients with acute renal failure undergoing continuous arteriovenous hemodialysis. Contrib Nephrol 1991; 93:51–56.
73. Bellomo R, Boyce N: Does continuous hemodiafiltration improve survival in acute renal failure. Semin Dial 1993; 6:16–19.
74. DeTong S, Chien Hsu L: Non-thrombogenic hemofiltration system for acute renal failure treatment. ASAIO J 1992; 38:M702–M706.
75. Arakawa M, Nagao M, Gejyo F, et al: Development of a new antithrombogenic continuous ultrafiltration system. Artif Organs 1991; 15:171–179.
76. Sato T, Orlowski J, Shahin A, et al: The experimental study of extracorporeal endotoxin removal against endotoxin shock (Abstract). *In*: Proceedings of the 39th Annual Scientific Meeting of the American Society of Artificial Internal Organs, 1993, p 94.

CHAPTER 116

Drug-Kidney Interactions

Rinaldo Bellomo, MBBS, MD, FRACP

The subject of drug-kidney interactions is extremely broad. A detailed description of how each drug affects kidney function or is affected by renal disease is beyond the scope of this chapter. The focus of the following pages is on a number of specific drug-kidney interactions as they relate to pharmacologic agents commonly used in the intensive care unit.

This chapter discusses the following topics in detail:

1. General principles of drug disposition and dosage in renal failure.
2. The effect of renal failure on drug use and dosage.
3. The effect of conventional dialytic therapy on drug clearance and use.
4. The effect of novel techniques of continuous renal replacement therapy on drug clearance and use.
5. The pathophysiology, consequences, and prevention of drug-induced nephrotoxicity.

PHARMACOLOGIC PRINCIPLES OF DRUG USE IN PATIENTS WITH RENAL DYSFUNCTION

The effect of renal failure on drug pharmacokinetics is pervasive. First, if a drug is administered to a patient with renal failure via the gastrointestinal tract, its bioavailability may be altered by the presence of uremia. This may be due to edema of the gut wall or to changes in the rate of gastric emptying.[1] Second, no matter what the drug's absorption may be, the presence of uremia may affect the fluid volume in which the drug is distributed at equilibrium. This volume is referred to as the *volume of distribution* (Vd). Vd is calculated according to the equation:

$$Vd = Dt/Dpl \qquad \text{[Equation 1]}$$

where Dt is the total amount of drug administered, and Dpl is the concentration of drug in plasma water at equilibrium (the concept of Vd is useful from a therapeutic point of view because it helps in calculating the expected plasma concentration of a drug from a given dosage). Uremia, as previously stated, affects the Vd of a number of drugs. For example, Vd for digoxin is diminished by renal failure, so that its loading dose must be decreased by approximately 50%.[2]

Most drugs bind to plasma proteins, and the extent of this binding influences a drug's distribution and elimination rate. As a rule, polar drugs are more significantly affected by protein binding. Decreased protein binding of drugs, particularly for acidic drugs,[4] has been described[3] in the presence of uremia. These drugs are displaced from binding sites by accumulated endogenous organic acids.[5] The consequence of this phenomenon is an increase in the proportion of unbound drug. This may lead to misinterpretation of serum concentrations of a drug like phenytoin,[6] for which total concentrations fall, whereas unbound concentrations remain unchanged. If a laboratory only measures total concentration, the result may mislead a clinician to increase the dose of phenytoin, and this could result in the possible development of toxicity.[7] The therapeutic range for this drug, therefore, needs to be redefined for uremic patients.[8] Uremia also affects the biotransformation of drugs by the liver. Notably, drugs like phenytoin and propranolol are more rapidly oxidized by the liver in patients with renal failure,[9] whereas quinidine is oxidized more slowly in the same patients.[10]

In summary, renal failure affects the bioavailability, distribution, protein binding, and metabolism of several drugs beyond any considerations related to drug clearance and excretion. However, other pharmacologic issues are also of importance in renal failure. Electrolyte and acid-base derangements seen in uremia can predispose patients to changes in drug sensitivity. Hyperkalemia potentiates the effects of quinidine and procainamide on the conduction system; alkalosis, hypokalemia, and hypomagnesemia predispose to digoxin-induced arrhythmias. The presence of renal insufficiency makes it difficult to achieve therapeutic antibiotic levels in the urine of patients with urinary tract infection; thus, the eradication of infection is particularly difficult, especially if aminoglycosides are used (these reach the urine through glomerular filtration).[11] Drugs frequently contain accompanying substances (e.g., sodium, potassium, water, and magnesium) and thus impose a degree of "solute load" that failing kidneys cannot adequately excrete (Table 116–1). Uremia may also modify the effect of certain drugs on laboratory tests (e.g., those for determination of creatinine, bilirubin, and urate), leading to incorrect measurement.[12, 13]

By far the most important pharmacologic effect of renal failure relates to diminished extraction of drugs and their metabolites. The concept of *clearance* is fundamental in this regard. Clearance is defined as the rate of elimination of a solute (by all routes) relative to its plasma concentration. Clinically, clearance is used to indicate the volume of

TABLE 116–1. Intensive Care Unit Drugs That Impose Additional Metabolic Loads in Renal Failure

Imposed Load	*Drug*
Sodium/volume	Ampicillin, carbenicillin, ticarcillin, piperacillin, moxalactam, cephalothin, amphotericin, sulphamethoxazole, trimethoprim
Urea	Corticosteroids
Acid	Acetazolamide
Alkali	Antacids, plasma protein fraction solutions, carbenicillin
Magnesium	Antacids
Potassium	Spironolactone, potassium salt of penicillin, neuromuscular blocking drugs

plasma from which a drug has been completely eliminated per time unit. In the case of the kidney,

$$\text{Renal clearance} = \frac{\text{Uex/t}}{\text{C}} \qquad \text{[Equation 2]}$$

where Uex is the amount of drug being excreted in the urine during time t, and C is the plasma concentration of the drug.

Equation 2, however, refers to a specific time—a value that cannot be directly measured. The amount excreted over a designated time interval, in practice, is measured and is related to the mean solute plasma concentration (Cmean) during that period of time:

$$\text{Renal clearance} = \frac{\text{Uex/t}}{\text{Cmean}} \qquad \text{[Equation 3]}$$

The units of clearance thus become those of volume over time (e.g., mL/min), and the expression clinically used in renal physiology becomes

$$\text{Renal clearance (mL/min)} = \frac{\text{Uc} \times \text{V}}{\text{PC}} \qquad \text{[Equation 4]}$$

where Uc is the urinary concentration of the substance under study, V is the urine volume produced during a given period of time, and PC is the plasma concentration of the substance at the time of measurement. Drug clearance by the kidney reflects the usual renal excretory processes: filtration, secretion, and reabsorption. Most drugs are renally cleared by first-order kinetics, in which the plasma concentration of the drug diminishes exponentially with time from its initial level at time zero all the way to zero at time infinity. The disappearance of these drugs is usually expressed in terms of *biologic half-life* ($t\frac{1}{2}$), which is the time needed for their concentrations to decrease to one half of the equilibration value.

A useful approximate relationship between half-life, clearance (Cl), and volume of distribution is given by the following equation:

$$t_{1/2} = 0.693 \times \text{Vd/Cl} \qquad \text{[Equation 5]}$$

It follows that a diminution in a drug's clearance or an increase in its volume of distribution (Vd) prolongs the half-life of the drug, according to first-order kinetics (the constant $k = 0.693$, a value derived using the natural logarithm of 2). The half-life concept is useful in estimating drug-dosing intervals and the approximate time needed for the removal of a drug from the body.

It is clear from the previous discussion that a clinically sound and practical approach to drug prescription in renal failure requires knowledge of

1. the degree of renal dysfunction,
2. the effect of renal dysfunction on the pharmacokinetics of the chosen drug,
3. the appropriate changes in dose or dosage intervals required to achieve drug levels that are both nontoxic and efficacious, and
4. the effect of any dialytic procedure on drug removal.

Excretory renal function can be estimated by measuring 24-hour creatinine (Cr) clearance. However, this method is often too cumbersome and time consuming. A practical formula commonly used for estimating clearance from the serum creatinine[14] is as follows:

$$\text{CrCl} = \frac{(140 - \text{Age in years}) \times (\text{Ideal body weight in kilograms})}{72 \times (\text{Serum creatinine in mg/dL})} \qquad \text{[Equation 6]}$$

For estimating creatinine clearance in women, the value obtained with this equation is multiplied by 0.85.

Dosing of drugs depends on whether an infusion is being administered or whether multiple doses are given. For constant infusions,

$$\text{Dosing rate} = \text{Cl} \times \text{Css} \qquad \text{[Equation 7]}$$

where Cl is the total drug clearance by all routes, and Css is the steady-state drug concentration in plasma.

For multiple doses, the equation can be expressed as

$$\text{Cl} \times \text{Cp ave} = \text{Dose/I} \qquad \text{[Equation 8]}$$

where Cp ave is the average plasma drug concentration during the dosing interval (I).

In general, drug dosage adjustments may be made as follows:

1. By changing dose and maintaining interval
2. By changing interval and maintaining dose
3. By changing both dose and interval

For toxic antibiotics like gentamicin, these approaches may still result in either a loss of peak levels or exposure to relatively high drug levels for long periods of time. Clearly, all of the previous observations are altered by the application of dialytic techniques such as intermittent hemodialysis, peritoneal dialysis, and continuous hemofiltration.

Since clearances are additive, the total clearance of a drug by the body during dialysis can be expressed as

$$\text{Cl total} = \text{Cl} + \text{Cl d} \qquad \text{[Equation 9]}$$

where Cl d is the additional clearance provided by dialysis. Of course, the increased clearance provided by dialysis shortens the $t_{1/2}$ of the drug. Many factors affect drug clearance during dialysis: molecular weight, water solubility, degree of protein binding, and type of membrane used. Drugs with a molecular weight greater than 500 are poorly cleared by conventional membranes as are drugs with large volumes of distribution, high lipid solubility, or a high degree of protein binding.

Important changes in clearance, however, are seen with new more permeable and more biocompatible membranes that are sometimes used for intermittent high-flux dialysis and that are always used for continuous hemofiltration (polysulfone, polyamide, and polyacrylonitrile). For example, larger molecules such as vancomycin (molecular weight >1000), which are not cleared by conventional dialysis, are removed in significant amounts during hemofiltration; thus, they must be administered either once per day or even twice per day.[15] To further complicate the situation, the evolution of continuous hemofiltration, from the arteriovenous to the pumped venovenous technique with the addition of a dialytic component (continuous arteriovenous hemodiafiltration and continuous venovenous hemodiafiltration), means that drug clearance during hemofiltration does not only depend on the type of membrane used, on the degree of protein binding, or on the lipophilic or hydrophilic nature of the drug, but also on the type of technique.[16, 17]

IMPACT OF RENAL FAILURE ON DRUG USE

Many patients in the intensive care unit have significant renal dysfunction but do not require dialytic therapy. However, their degree of renal failure requires considerable modifications of drug dosage aimed at minimizing adverse effects.[17a]

A number of drugs are primarily cleared by nonrenal mechanisms, and their dosage does not require modifications (Table 116–2). Most drugs, however, require a decrease in the dose administered or a longer interval between doses, or both (Table 116–3). Importantly, the presence of renal insufficiency increases the likelihood of adverse effects due to antibiotics.[18] For example, renal insufficiency predisposes to the development of seizures induced by penicillin and its derivatives; such is also the case with imipenem. Ototoxicity may be seen with erythromycin as well as with vancomycin and the aminoglycosides. The risk of coagulopathy due to penicillins and cephalosporins is increased by the platelet dysfunction seen in uremia, the frequent vitamin K deficiency, and the use of heparin with dialysis. Hypoglycemia may be induced by sulfonamides, which stimulate

TABLE 116–2. Intensive Care Unit Drugs That Typically Do Not Require Dosage Changes During Renal Failure

Drug Type	*Drug Name*
Sedatives	Clonazepam, lorazepam, midazolam, temazepam, haloperidol, chlorpromazine, ketamine, tricyclic antidepressants
Anticonvulsants	Carbamazepine, phenytoin
Antibiotics, antifungals, antivirals	Chloramphenicol, clindamycin, doxycycline, nafcillin, rifampin, erythromycin, ketoconazole, amphotericin, zidovudine
Cardiovascular drugs	Nifedipine, nimodipine, verapamil, diltiazem, propranolol, labetalol, metoprolol, clonidine, isosorbide, nitroglycerin
Antiarrhythmic drugs	Lidocaine, amiodarone, quinidine, propafenone
Miscellaneous drugs	Theophylline, corticosteroids, cyclosporine, FK-506, methimazole, propylthiouracil, acetaminophen

TABLE 116–3. Drugs Commonly Used in the Intensive Care Unit: General Dosage Guidelines During Renal Failure*

		Approximate Dose Based on the Degree of Renal Failure as Measured by Creatinine Clearance (mL/min)		
Drug Name	*Volume of Distribution (L/kg)*	*>60*	*10 to 60*	*<10*
Acyclovir	0.7	5 mg/kg every 8 h	5 mg/kg every 12–24 h	5 mg/kg every 48 h
Ganciclovir	0.5	5 mg/kg every 8 h	2 mg/kg every 24 h	1.2 mg/kg every 24 h
Amikacin	0.4	7 mg/kg every 12 h	5 mg/kg every 24 h	4 mg/kg every 48 h
Gentamicin	0.45	2 mg/kg every 12 h	1.5 mg/kg every 16 h	1.5 mg/kg every 72 h
Tobramycin	0.45	2 mg/kg every 12 h	1.5 mg/kg every 16 h	1.5 mg/kg every 72 h
Cefamandole	0.25	2 g every 6 h	1 g every 8 h	1 g every 12 h
Cefotaxime	0.35	2 g every 8 h	2 g every 12 h	1 g every 12 h
Cefotetan	0.15	2 g every 12 h	2 g every 24 h	1 g every 24 h
Ceftazidime	0.3	1 g every 8 h	1 g every 12 h	0.5 g every 24 h
Ceftriaxone	0.1	2 g every 24 h	1 g every 24 h	1 g every 24 h
Penicillin G	2.0†	2 MU every 4 h	1 MU every 4 h	1 MU every 6 h
Amoxicillin	0.5	1 g every 6 h	1 g every 8 h	1 g every 12 h
Ampicillin	0.3	1 g every 6 h	1 g every 8 h	1 g every 12 h
Aztreonam	0.4	2 g every 8 h	2 g every 12 h	1 g every 24 h
Carbenicillin	0.2	5 g every 4 h	3 g every 8 h	3 g every 24 h
Cloxacillin	0.2	500 mg every 6 h	250 mg every 6 h	250 mg every 6 h
Imipenem	0.4	1 g every 8 h	1 g every 12 h	0.5 g every 12 h
Piperacillin	0.5	4 g every 6 h	3 g every 6 h	2 g every 8 h
Ticarcillin	0.2	3 g every 4 h	2 g every 6 h	1.5 g every 12 h
Ciprofloxacin	2.1†	500 mg every 12 h	250 mg q 12 h	500 mg every 24 h
Norfloxacin	3.0†	400 mg every 12 h	400 mg q 16 h	400 mg every 24 h
Trimethoprim sulfate	2.0†	Usually every 12 h	50% dose q 12 h	50% dose every 24 h
Metronidazole	0.9	500 mg every 8 h	500 mg q 8 h	500 mg every 12 h
Vancomycin	0.7	750 mg every 12 h	750 mg q 24 h	1 g every 6–7 d
Fluconazole	0.8	200 mg every 24 h	100 mg q 24 h	100 mg every 24 h
Flucytosine	0.7	2 g every 6 h	2 g q 12 h	1.5 g every 24 h
Ranitidine	1.0	300 mg/d	150–300 mg/d	150 mg/d
Famotidine	1.3†	40 mg every 24 h	20 mg q 24 h	20 mg every 48 h
Cimetidine	1.0	300 mg every 8 h	300 mg q 12 h	300 mg every 24 h
Codeine	4.0†	No change	25% less	50% less
Cyclophosphamide	0.7	Usual dose	Usual dose	25–50% less
Digoxin	4.0†	25% less	50% less	75% less
Allopurinol	0.6	300 mg every 24 h	300 mg q 48 h	100 mg every 24 h

*See Table References for further information.
†Drugs with a Vd greater than body weight.

insulin secretion in a clinical setting of usually decreased insulin catabolism. Furthermore, aminoglycosides may be inactivated by high serum concentrations of unexcreted penicillins,[19] resulting in persistently subtherapeutic aminoglycoside levels despite administration of seemingly adequate dosages. This phenomenon may compound the effect of the increased volume of distribution for aminoglycosides seen in critically ill patients, which makes routine loading dosage inadequate.[20]

Monitoring of serum concentrations for toxic antibiotics such as the aminoglycosides and vancomycin is strongly indicated in critically ill patients with renal insufficiency because the degree of renal dysfunction is rarely constant during the treatment period; this makes underdosage or overdosage a likely occurrence. In this context, disagreement exists concerning which aminoglycoside concentrations are "toxic" and which are "therapeutic." This is not surprising, as toxicity is most likely related to tissue accumulation, which in turn is probably related to the integral of the area under the serum concentration–over–time curve[21] and not to episodically measured "peak" and "trough" drug levels. Despite such limitations in our understanding of therapeutic gains versus toxic side effects, peak concentrations of greater than 5 mg/L for gentamicin and tobramycin and of >15 mg/L and >8 mg/L for amikacin and netilmicin as a minimum are considered advisable.[22] In order to minimize toxicity, "trough" concentrations <2 mg/L are considered advisable. Similarly "peak" levels of 30 to 40 mg/L and "trough" levels of 5 to 10 mg/L appear appropriate for vancomycin.

Another important issue in renal insufficiency relates to the accumulation of drug metabolites with pharmacological effects. N-acetylprocainamide, for example, accumulates in renal failure and shows a degree of potency and toxicity similar to that of its parent compound.[23] A number of other active and/or toxic metabolites of drugs used in the ICU may accumulate with deleterious consequences (Table 116–4). Of particular importance is the accumulation of morphine glucuronides. Their accumulation may result in a prolonged period of sedation (days) despite the cessation of morphine administration. The 3-hydroxy metabolites of vecuronium and pancuronium[24] also accumulate in patients with renal failure. They may induce prolonged (days) neuromuscular blockade and trigger the development of a myopathy.[25]

TABLE 116–4. Active or Toxic Metabolites That Accumulate During Renal Failure

Drug Type	*Drug Name (Reaction)*
Narcotics/analgesics	3- and 6-Glucuronides of morphine (prolonged sedation)
	Norpethidine from pethidine (seizures, prolonged sedation)
	Norpropoxyphene from propoxyphene (depressed cardiac conduction)
Cardiovascular drugs	*N*-Acetylprocainamide from procainamide (cardiac toxicity)
	Thiocyanate from sodium nitroprusside (anoxia, muscle spasms, psychosis)
	Methyldopa-*O*-sulfate from methyldopa (marked hypotension)
Miscellaneous drugs	Oxypurinol from allopurinol (fever, eosinophilia, rash)
	Desmethyldiazepam from diazepam (prolonged sedation)
	3-Hydroxypancuronium from pancuronium (prolonged paralysis, myopathy)
	3-Hydroxyvecuronium from vecuronium (prolonged paralysis, myopathy)

DRUG USE IN PATIENTS RECEIVING CONVENTIONAL DIALYSIS

During conventional dialysis, solute removal is almost entirely via diffusion. This solute removal is expressed as its dialysance (D) in milliliters per minute, according to the following formula:

$$D = Qb\,\frac{Bi - Bo}{Bi - Di} \quad \text{or} \quad = Qd\,\frac{Do - Di}{Bi - Di} \qquad \text{[Equation 10]}$$

where Qb and Qd are blood and dialysate flow rates, respectively; Bi and Bo are the dialyzer inflow and outflow blood concentrations of solute, respectively; and Di and Do are the comparable dialysate solute concentrations, respectively. As drug concentration in the dialysate is zero at the inlet (i.e., Di = 0), dialysance in the case of drugs is equivalent to the drugs' clearance. This dialysis-induced clearance depends on many factors. First, a drug must not be bound to proteins or cells (i.e., it is only the free drug that is dialyzed). Second, the total amount of the drug in the body that is found in blood must be substantial for clearance to be significant. Some drugs are in such rapid equilibrium with plasma water that this effect may be overcome. Third, the drug must be water soluble. Fourth, the drug's molecules must be small enough to move through a dialyzing membrane. With conventional dialyzing membranes, solutes with a molecular weight greater than 500 are either poorly dialyzed or not dialyzed at all. Finally, as is clear from Equation 10, blood and dialysate flow rates are important determinants of drug clearance.

Peritoneal dialysis typically leads to lower drug clearances than does intermittent hemodialysis, even when peritoneal dialysate flow rates are kept high.[26] In general, peritoneal dialysis is not an effective method of removing drugs, and its impact on drug therapy in the intensive care unit is minor. Furthermore, the intrinsic properties of the peritoneal membrane vary significantly with infection, blood flow changes, abdominal scarring, and fluid loculation, making it almost impossible to accurately predict drug extraction.

Table 116–5 summarizes dialytic clearance for drugs commonly used in the intensive care unit.

CONTINUOUS HEMOFILTRATION-BASED DIALYTIC THERAPIES

Continuous hemofiltration removes solutes by convection, and, because highly porous membranes are used, drug movement across the filtering membrane is not limited by molecular weight. Theoretically, therefore, the concentration of unbound drug in plasma should closely approximate the concentration in the ultrafiltrate. Knowledge of the degree of drug-protein binding then should provide enough information to calculate clearance over a given time period:

$$Cl = \frac{UFc \times VUF}{PLc} \qquad \text{[Equation 11]}$$

where clearance is equal to the concentration of the drug in the ultrafiltrate (UFc) multiplied by the volume of the ultrafiltrate (VUF) produced over that given time period and divided by the concentration of the drug in plasma (PLc). In vivo, however, the observed drug sieving coefficient (ratio of arterial plasma drug concentration to ultrafiltrate drug concentration) may not always be as easily predicted be-

TABLE 116–5. Dialytic Clearance for Drugs Commonly Used in the Intensive Care Unit

Clearance	*Drug Type*	*Drug Name*
Negligible	*Antibiotics*	Cefotetan, clindamycin, cloxacillin, nafcillin, doxycycline, vancomycin, amphotericin B, itraconazole, ketoconazole, zidovudine, erythromycin, ciprofloxacin
	Cardiovascular drugs	Amiodarone, disopyramide, propafenone, esmolol, labetalol, metoprolol, digoxin, diltiazem
	Miscellaneous drugs	Morphine, propoxyphene, benzodiazepines, phenytoin, cimetidine, famotidine, omeprazole, cyclosporine, prednisone
Significant (Postdialysis Redosing Recommended)	*Antibiotics*	Aminoglycosides, most cephalosporins, imipenem, aztreonam, ampicillin, piperacillin, sulfamethoxazole/trimethoprim, flucytosine, metronidazole, isoniazid, acyclovir, ganciclovir
	Other drugs	Ranitidine, cyclophosphamide, sotalol, captopril, allopurinol, atenolol, N-acetylprocainamide

cause of protein-membrane and drug-membrane interaction as well as the significant variability in the degree of protein binding. Likewise, ultrafiltrate production depends on many variables (e.g., oncotic pressure, blood flow, hydrostatic pressure, and membrane age) and is neither constant nor predictable. Despite these caveats, useful approximations can be reached and used as guidelines for drug administration in these patients (Amount removed = Arterial steady state drug concentration × Unbound fraction × Ultrafiltrate produced).

Hemofiltration has been combined with a dialytic component[27, 28] to augment clearance. Drug removal during continuous arteriovenous or venovenous hemodiafiltration is thus predictably different and usually greater than with filtration alone because with the former diffusion is combined with convection. Once again, the membrane, protein binding factors, the drug's volume of distribution, and its water solubility have an important role in determining the drug's overall extraction. Because these techniques are new, only limited data on them are available (Table 116–6).

DRUG-INDUCED NEPHROTOXICITY

The renal parenchyma is particularly vulnerable to drugs and toxins. The ability of the kidneys to concentrate urine allows drugs to reach luminal concentrations in individual nephrons that are much higher than their concentrations in blood. The high perfusion rate also results in the delivery of large amounts of drug per time unit, and mechanisms of solute transport facilitate drug entry into cells, where toxic metabolites may develop. In critically ill patients, other mechanisms of renal injury may be at work (e.g., hypovolemia, endotoxemia, ischemia), and these mechanisms can augment the injurious effects of nephrotoxic drugs.[29–31] A number of drugs administered to critically ill patients are known to be potential nephrotoxins and a common cause of in-hospital–acquired renal failure.[32]

TABLE 116–6. Dosage of Drugs Removed During Continuous Hemofiltration/Hemodiafiltration*

Drug Name	*Drug Dosage*
Cefuroxime	750 mg every 12 h
Tobramycin	120 mg every 24 h
Amikacin	250–500 mg every 24 h
Imipenem	500 mg every 12 h
Metronidazole	500 mg every 8 h
Ceftazidime	500 mg every 12 h
Gentamicin	80–100 mg every 24 h
Vancomycin	500–1000 mg every 24 h
Ciprofloxacin	500 mg every 24 h
Piperacillin	4 g every 8 h

*These values are approximate and depend on the technique in use.

Aminoglycosides and Antibiotics

Aminoglycosides are a common cause of in-hospital–acquired renal failure,[33, 34] having an overall incidence of between 5% and 15% during treatment courses.[35, 36] These epidemiologic data, however, are based on a drug-induced increase in serum creatinine and underestimate the true incidence of nephrotoxicity.[37] A number of pathogenetic mechanisms appear to mediate aminoglycoside nephrotoxicity: accumulation and binding to anionic phospholipids (especially phosphoinositol) in the brush border membrane[38, 39]; translocation to the lysosomes[40] and other cell constituents[41, 42]; inhibition of action of phospholipases and of renal protein kinase C[43]; and severe damage to the phosphoinositol second messenger pathway.[44] Furthermore, by altering membrane phospholipids, aminoglycosides alter tubular cell transport functions; in mitochondria, they inhibit oxidative phosphorylation while enhancing the generation of free oxygen radicals.[44, 44a] These mechanisms of renal dysfunction are all rapidly operative after drug administration, suggesting that a degree of aminoglycoside nephrotoxicity may be inevitable. Only in rather severe cases is damage diagnosed with the use of our relatively insensitive measures of renal function.

The clinical pattern of aminoglycoside nephrotoxicity is characterized by the initial appearance of lysosomal enzymes in the urine followed by polyuria and then by a decrease in glomerular filtration rate. Typically, the urinary sodium concentration is greater than 40 mEq/L, and renal failure is nonoliguric, occurring 7 to 10 days after initiation of treatment. Oliguria may be seen in combination with sepsis and hypotension.

A number of risk factors have been reported to predispose to nephrotoxicity (Table 116–7). Worthy of particular note is vancomycin, which may potentiate the nephrotoxic effect of aminoglycosides.[45, 46] The issue of comparative nephrotoxicity among various aminoglycosides remains strongly debated.[47] Gentamicin has been found to be more nephrotoxic than tobramycin and netilmicin in animal studies[48, 49]; it may also be more nephrotoxic than amikacin.[50] The clinical significance of such potential or real differences in nephrotoxicity is unclear. It appears prudent to use those agents that have the least nephrotoxicity in high-risk patients. In critically ill patients, careful monitoring of renal function and of peak and trough levels is needed if the incidence of nephrotoxicity is to be diminished. More re-

TABLE 116–7. Risk Factors for Aminoglycoside Toxicity

High dosage and prolonged administration
High peak and trough levels
Concurrent nephrotoxins
  Vancomycin, amphotericin, cisplatin, cyclosporine, FK-506, radiocontrast media, nonsteroidal anti-inflammatory agents
Concurrent renal insults
  Intravascular volume depletion, hepatic disease, sepsis, hypotension
Acid-base/electrolyte disorders
  Hypercalcemia, hypomagnesemia, hypokalemia, metabolic acidosis
Factors related to patient status
  Old age, chronic renal impairment, prior treatment with aminoglycosides

cently, experimental and clinical data[51, 52] suggest that once-daily aminoglycoside dosing may reduce nephrotoxicity while maintaining efficacy.[53, 54] Finally, third-generation cephalosporins, aztreonam, or imipenem may represent a safer and cheaper[55] therapeutic alternative in critically ill patients unless aminoglycoside therapy is mandated by the particular antibiotic sensitivity of the microbial isolate.

Penicillin, penicillin-derived antibiotics, and sulfonamides can induce cell-mediated acute interstitial nephropathy. This condition causes renal failure, typically between the first week and the first month of antibiotic exposure. Most affected patients (85%) have nonoliguric renal failure.[56] Removal of the offending agent is necessary for recovery. In severe cases, a short course of high-dose steroid administration may speed recovery.

Vancomycin is nephrotoxic in animals; however, when used alone in clinically correct doses and in a suitably purified preparation, it may not be nephrotoxic to humans.[45] It is probably best avoided when aminoglycosides are being administered.

Rifampin has been associated with the development of acute interstitial nephropathy, especially when reinstituted after a pause in therapy.

Pentamidine has been reported to be associated with azotemia.[57] The significance of this association is unclear because many of the affected patients were also receiving other potential nephrotoxins.

Acyclovir has been associated with dose-dependent nephrotoxicity owing to its intraluminal precipitation.[58] Acute renal failure may develop and can be prevented by prehydration and infusion of the drug over a longer period of time (e.g., 1 hour).

Amphotericin B affects renal function in a number of ways. It induces an increase in hydrogen ion– and potassium ion–permeable tubular cells, causing distal tubular acidosis and potassium wasting.[59] Its infusion induces a decrease in renal blood flow and glomerular filtration rate that persists for hours.[60] Over time, dose-related, nonoliguric renal failure develops, following earlier proteinuria and abnormal urinary sedimentation. Typically, hyperkalemia and hypomagnesemia accompany this type of drug-induced azotemia.

Radiologic Contrast Media

Contrast media are the most common cause of in-hospital drug-induced renal failure,[32] exceeding aminoglycosides in frequency. Critically ill patients with previous renal disease, diabetes, and fluid depletion who require large doses of contrast medium are at particularly high risk (Table 116–8). Depending on the presence of one or more of these risk factors and on their severity, the probability of radiocontrast-induced renal failure may be as high as 55%.[61, 62] Particularly important in this regard is the presence of a baseline serum creatinine level greater than 2 mg/dL or of diabetes mellitus.[62a] Most patients develop oliguric renal failure, the duration of which depends on their previous renal function. In some patients with previous serious renal impairment, hemodialysis may become temporarily or permanently necessary.[63] Typically, however, the serum creatinine begins to rise within 24 hours of contrast administration, peaks within 96 hours, and returns to baseline values within 7 to 10 days. The damaging effects appear to be mediated by renal ischemia and hypoxia possibly combined with a direct nephrotoxic effect of the iodinated contrast agent.[63a] Prevention strategies are based on rehydration, avoidance of other nephrotoxins, and maintenance of diuresis (Table 116–9). Newer nonionic contrast agents have been promoted as being significantly less nephrotoxic than the usual media. However, scientific evidence shows a similar degree of nephrotoxicity[63, 64] and a much higher cost.

Other Drugs

A number of drugs used in oncologic intensive care units are nephrotoxic. Cisplatin can induce nonoliguric renal failure and severe hypomagnesemia. This toxicity is reduced by slow infusion, rehydration, and maintenance of diuresis. Nitrosoureas are associated with dose-dependent, diffuse tubulointerstitial nephropathy and the development of slow, progressive renal dysfunction. Methotrexate and one of its metabolites appear to induce renal failure through their precipitation in the distal nephron. Fluid administration and alkalinization of urine may be protective. Finally, mitomycin C is associated with a microangiopathic hemolytic anemia that can cause renal failure.

Drugs used to induce immunosuppression in patients who are to undergo organ transplantation are also associated with renal failure. Cyclosporin A is a powerful nephrotoxin that deleteriously affects renal function in a number of ways. The major mechanism of injury, particularly in patients with episodes of acute renal dysfunction, appears to be severe vasoconstriction and ischemia.[65] The diagnosis of nephrotoxicity can be particularly difficult in renal transplant recipients because its clinical and histologic features may mimic those of rejection.[66] A number of strategies are available to minimize its nephrotoxicity, such as low-dose therapy, avoidance in the early treatment of renal grafts with primary nonfunction, and adjunctive pharmacotherapy directed at minimization of vasospasm. In this regard, calcium channel blockers show considerable promise.[67, 68] Other powerful newer immunosuppressive agents such as FK-506 also appear to have considerable nephrotoxicity.[69]

Angiotensin-converting enzyme inhibitors are frequently used in cardiac intensive care units. They have been shown to induce reversible acute renal failure in patients in whom

TABLE 116–8. Risk Factors for Radiocontrast Medium–Induced Renal Failure

Chronic renal failure (creatinine >1.5 mg/dL)	Dehydration
Diabetes	Hyperuricemia
Age > 60 y	Liver disease
Hypertension	Cardiac failure
Exposure to nephrotoxins	Solitary kidney
Radiocontrast dose >2 mL/kg	Multiple myeloma
Multiple studies	Proteinuria

TABLE 116–9. Approach to the Prevention of Radiocontrast Medium–Induced Renal Failure

General Steps

Remove other nephrotoxins, minimize volume of contrast administered, space performance of radiologic procedures, avoid dehydration

Specific Steps

Infuse 500 mL of 5% mannitol at 100 mL/h beginning 1 h before procedure

or

Infuse 1500 mL of 0.45% saline beginning a few hours before procedure and 250 mL of 20% mannitol within 1 h of contrast exposure

or

Infuse 500 mL of 20% mannitol with 100 mg furosemide for each 1 mg/dL of serum creatinine at an infusion rate of 20 mL/h beginning 1 h before procedure and continuing for at least 6 h; replace urinary output in 1-to-1 ratio with intravenous fluids

or

Infuse 1500 mL of 5% dextrose in 0.45 saline before the procedure and 125 mL/h for 4 h thereafter

glomerular filtration pressure is dependent on angiotensin II–induced efferent arteriolar vasoconstriction, as in bilateral renal artery stenosis.[70] However, the presence of nonrenovascular kidney dysfunction before treatment does not increase the likelihood that renal deterioration will occur in these patients.[71, 72] Nonsteroidal anti-inflammatory drugs such as ibuprofen, which may be used in an attempt to modulate chemical mediators or septic organ injury, can induce acute renal failure,[73] particularly when glomerular filtration is dependent on afferent arteriolar vasodilation.[74] Their combination with converting enzyme inhibitors is particularly dangerous. Finally, if given repeatedly and in excessive amounts (total dose >300 g), as sometimes occurs in neurosurgical patients with elevated intracranial pressure, mannitol may induce acute renal failure. In fact, at such high levels, mannitol can produce severe vasoconstriction and a major degree of renal ischemia.[75]

CONCLUSION

Renal failure and dialysis profoundly affect all aspects of pharmacotherapy. Safe and efficacious drug use depends on a working knowledge of the basic principles of pharmacokinetics during renal failure and dialysis before administration of any drug to affected patients. Furthermore, newer techniques of continuous hemofiltration, with their own separate drug clearance effects, make it impossible for individuals to correctly remember and predict appropriate drug dosage. Monitoring drug levels and obtaining all pertinent pharmacologic information before drug use are vital to the correct management of patients with renal failure. Many drugs used in the intensive care unit are significantly nephrotoxic. Their use should be cautious and guided by careful monitoring of serum concentrations, particularly in patients in whom other nephrotoxic insults may significantly aggravate drug effects.

ACKNOWLEDGEMENTS

My deep gratitude goes to my wife Debrah for helping with the typing of the manuscript and for offering her constant and patient support.

References

1. Bennett WM, Blythe WB: Use of drugs in patients with renal failure. *In*: Diseases of the Kidney. 4th ed. Schreier RW, Gottschalk CW (Eds). Boston, Little, Brown, and Co, 1988, pp 3441–3442.
2. Scheiner LB, Rosenberg BG, Marathe VV: Estimation of population characteristics of pharmacokinetic parameters from routine clinical data. J Pharmacokinet Biopharm 1977; 5:445–479.
3. Brater DC, Sokol PP, Hall SD, et al: Disposition and dose requirements of drugs in renal insufficiency. *In*: The Kidney: Physiology and Pathophysiology. 2nd ed. Seldin DW, Giebisch G (Eds). New York, Raven Press, 1992, pp 3672–3675.
4. Reidenberg MM, Drayer DE: Alteration of drug-protein binding in renal disease. Clin Pharmacokinet 1984; 9(Suppl 1):18–26.
5. Depner TA, Gulyassay PF, Stanfel LA, et al: Plasma protein binding in uremia: Extraction and characterization of an inhibitor. Kidney Int 1980; 18:86–94.
6. Greenblatt DJ, Sellers EM, Koch-Wester J: Importance of protein binding for the interpretation of serum and plasma drug concentrations. J Clin Pharmacol 1982; 22:259–263.
7. McKichan JJ: Protein binding drug displacement interactions: Fact or fiction? Clin Pharmacokinet 1989; 16:65–73.
8. Reidenberg MM, Affrime M: Influence of disease on binding of drugs to plasma proteins. Ann N Y Acad Sci 1973; 226:115–126.
9. Bianchetti G, Graziani G, Brancaccio D, et al: Pharmacokinetics and effects of propranolol in terminal uremic patients and in patients undergoing regular dialysis treatment. Clin Pharmacokinet 1976; 1:373–379.
10. Drayer DE, Lowenthal DT, Restivo KM, et al: Steady-state serum levels of quinidine and active metabolites in cardiac patients with varying degrees of renal function. Clin Pharmacol Ther 1978; 24:31–36.
11. Bennett WM, Hartnett MN, Craven R, et al: Gentamicin concentrations in blood, urine and renal tissue of patients with end-stage renal disease. J Lab Clin Med 1977; 90:389–393.
12. Burgess E, Blair A, Krichman K, et al: Inhibition of renal creatinine secretion by cimetidine in humans. Renal Physiol 1982; 5:27–30.
13. Rainer G, Rosenberg AR: Effect of co-trimoxazole on the glomerular filtration rate of healthy adults. Chemotherapy 1981; 27:229–232.
14. Cockroft DW, Gault MH: Prediction of creatinine clearance from serum creatinine. Nephron 1976; 15:31–36.
15. Bellomo R, Ernest D, Parkin G, et al: Clearance of vancomycin during continuous arteriovenous hemodiafiltration. Crit Care Med 1990; 18:181–183.
16. Kronfol NO, Lau AH, Colon-Rivera J, et al: Effect of CAVH membrane types on drug-sieving coefficients and clearances. Trans Am Soc Artif Intern Organs 1986; 32:85–87.
17. Golper TA, Wendel SK, Kaplan AA, et al: Drug removal during continuous arteriovenous hemofiltration: Theory and clinical observations. Intern Artif Organs 1985; 8:307–312.

17a. Talbert RL: Drug dosing in renal insufficiency. J Clin Pharmacol 1994; 34:99–110.

18. Manian FA, Stone WJ, Alford RH: Adverse antibiotic effects associated with renal insufficiency. Rev Infect Dis 1990; 12:236–249.
19. Ervin FR, Bullock WE Jr, Nuttal CE: Inactivation of gentamicin by penicillins in patients with renal failure. Antimicrob Agents Chemother 1976; 9:1004–1011.
20. Triginer G, Izquierdo I, Fernandez R, et al: Gentamicin volume of distribution in critically ill septic patients. Intensive Care Med 1990; 16:303–306.
21. Follath F, Wenk M, Vozeh S: Plasma concentration monitoring of aminoglycosides. J Antimicrob Chemother 1981; 8(Suppl A):37–43.
22. Moore RD, Smith CR, Lietman PS: The association of aminoglycoside plasma levels with mortality in patients with gram-negative bacteremia. J Infect Dis 1984; 149:443–448.
23. Drayer DE: Active drug metabolites and renal failure. Am J Med 1977; 62:486–489.
24. Segredo V, Caldwell JE, Matthay MA: Persistent paralysis in critically ill patients after long-term administration of vecuronium. N Engl J Med 1992; 327:524–528.
25. Hansen-Flaschen J, Cowen J, Raps EC: Neuromuscular blockade in the intensive care unit: More than we bargained for. Am Rev Respir Dis 1993; 147:234–236.
26. Manuel MA, Paton TW, Cornish WR: Drugs and peritoneal dialysis. Perit Dial Bull 1983; 3:117–125.

27. Bellomo R, Parkin G, Love J, et al: The use of continuous hemodiafiltration: An approach to the management of acute renal failure in the critically ill. Am J Nephrol 1992; 12:240–245.
28. Bellomo R, Parkin G, Love J, et al: Management of acute renal failure in the critically ill with continuous veno-venous hemodiafiltration. Ren Fail 1992; 14:183–186.
29. Zager RA: Endotoxemia, renal hypoperfusion, and fever: Interactive risk factors for aminoglycoside and sepsis-associated acute renal failure. Am J Kidney Dis 1992; 20:223–230.
30. Spiegel DM, Shanley PF, Molitoris BA: Mild ischemia predisposes the S3 segment to gentamicin toxicity. Kidney Int 1990; 38:459–464.
31. Badr KF, Kelley VE, Brenner BM: Selective antagonism of thromboxane A2 and sulfidopeptide leukotrienes ameliorates endotoxin-induced renal ischemia. Kidney Int 1986; 30:474–480.
32. Hou S, Bushinsky DA, Wish JB, et al: Hospital-acquired renal insufficiency: A prospective study. Am J Med 1983; 74:243–248.
33. Tablan OC, Reyes MD, Rintelman WF, et al: Renal and auditory toxicity of high dose, prolonged therapy with gentamicin and tobramycin in *Pseudomonas* endocarditis. J Infect Dis 1984; 149:257–263.
34. Keys TF, Kurtz SB, Jones JD, et al: Renal toxicity during therapy with gentamicin or tobramycin. Mayo Clin Proc 1981; 56:556–598.
35. Appel GB: Aminoglycoside nephrotoxicity. Am J Med 1990; 88(Suppl 3C):16S–20S.
36. Kahlmeter G, Dahlager JI: Aminoglycoside toxicity: A review of clinical studies published between 1975 and 1982. J Antimicrob Chemother 1984; 13(Suppl A):9–22.
37. Walker RJ, Duggin GG: Cellular mechanisms of drug nephrotoxicity. *In*: The Kidney: Physiology and Pathophysiology. 2nd ed. Seldin DW, Giebisch G (Eds). New York, Raven Press, 1992, p 3581.
38. Morin JP, Viotte G, Vandewalle A, et al: Gentamicin-induced nephrotoxicity: A cell biology approach. Kidney Int 1980; 18:583–590.
39. Sastrasinh M, Knauss TC, Weinberg JM, et al: Identification of the aminoglycoside binding site in rat renal brush border membrane. J Pharmacol Exp Ther 1982; 222:350–358.
40. Feldman S, Wang MY, Kaloyanides GJ: Aminoglycosides induce a phospholiposis in the renal cortex of the rat: An early manifestation of nephrotoxicity. J Pharmacol Exp Ther 1982; 220:514–520.
41. Kaloyanides GJ: Renal pharmacology of aminoglycoside antibiotics. Contrib Nephrol 1984; 42:148–167.
42. Ramsammy LS, Josepovitz C, Lane B, et al: Effect of gentamicin on phospholipid metabolism in cultured rabbit proximal tubular cells. Am J Physiol 1989; 256:C204–C213.
43. Hagiwara M, Inagaki M, Kanamura K, et al: Inhibitory effects of aminoglycosides on renal protein phosphorylation by protein kinase C. J Pharmacol Exp Ther 1988; 244:355–360.
44. Bennett WM: Mechanisms of aminoglycoside nephrotoxicity. Clin Exp Pharmacol Physiol 1989; 16:1–6.
44a. Hishida A, Nakajima T, Yamada M, et al: Roles of hemodynamic and tubular factors in gentamicin-medicated nephropathy. Ren Fail 1994; 16:109–116.
45. Appel GB, Given DB, Levine LR, et al: Vancomycin and the kidney. Am J Kidney Dis 1986; 8:75–80.
46. Wold TJ, Turnipseed SA: Toxicology of vancomycin in laboratory animals. Rev Infect Dis 1981; 3:224–235.
47. Evans DA, Buring J, Mayrent S, et al: Qualitative overview of randomized trials of aminoglycosides. Am J Med 1986; 80(Suppl 6B):39–43.
48. Cone LA: A survey of prospective controlled clinical trials of gentamicin, tobramycin, amikacin and netilmicin. Clin Ther 1982; 5:155–162.
49. Soberon L, Bowman RL, Pastoriza-Munoz E, et al: Comparative nephrotoxicities of gentamicin, netilmicin, and tobramycin in the rat. J Pharmacol Exp Ther 1979; 210:334–343.
50. Smith CR, Boughman KL, Edwards CQ, et al: Controlled comparison of amikacin and gentamicin. N Engl J Med 1977; 296:349–354.
51. Kapusnik JE, Hackbarth CJ, Chambers HF, et al: Single large daily dosing versus intermittent dosing of tobramycin for treating experimental *Pseudomonas* pneumonia. J Infect Dis 1988; 158:7–12.
52. Prins JM, Bueller HR, Kuijper EJ, et al: Once versus thrice daily gentamicin in patients with serious infections. Lancet 1993; 341:335–339.
53. Kapusnik JE, Sande MA: Challenging conventional aminoglycoside dosing regimens: The value of experimental models. Am J Med 1986; 80(Suppl 6B):179–181.
54. Zahnel GG, Ariano RE: Once daily aminoglycoside dosing: Maintained efficacy with reduced nephrotoxicity? Ren Fail 1992; 14:1–9.
55. Eisenberg JM, Koffer H, Glick HA, et al: What is the cost of nephrotoxicity associated with aminoglycosides? Ann Intern Med 1987; 107:900–909.
56. Galpin JE, Shinaberg JH, Stanley TM, et al: Acute interstitial nephritis due to methicillin. Am J Med 1978; 65:756–761.
57. Anderson R, Boedecher M, Ma M, et al: Adverse reactions associated with pentamidine isothionate in AIDS patients: Recommendations for monitoring therapy. Drug Intell Clin Pharmacol 1986; 20:862–866.
58. Sawyer MA, Webb PE, Balow JE, et al: Acyclovir-induced renal failure. Am J Med 1988; 84:1067–1071.
59. Finn JT, Cohen LH, Steinmetz PR: Acidifying defect induced by amphotericin B: Comparison of bicarbonate and hydrogen ion permeabilities. Kidney Int 1977; 11:261–266.
60. Cheng JT, Witty T, Robinson RR, et al: Amphotericin B nephrotoxicity: Increased renal resistance and tubular permeability. Kidney Int 1982; 22:626–633.
61. Berns A: Nephrotoxicity of contrast media. Kidney Int 1989; 36:730–740.
62. Teruel JL, Marcer R, Onaindia JM, et al: Renal function impairment caused by intravenous urography. Arch Intern Med 1981; 141:1271–1274.
62a. Weisberg LS, Kurnik PB, Kurnik BR: Risk of radiocontrast nephropathy in patients with and without diabetes mellitus. Kidney Int 1994; 45:259–265.
63. Cronin RE: Southwestern Internal Medicine Conference: Renal failure following radiologic procedures. Am J Med Sci 1989; 298:342–356.
63a. Porter GA: Effects of contrast agents on renal function. Invest Radiol 1993; 28:S1–5.
64. Schwab SJ, Hlatky MA, Pieper KS, et al: Contrast nephrotoxicity: A randomized controlled trial of a nonionic and an ionic radiographic contrast agent. N Engl J Med 1989; 320:149–153.
65. Greenberg A, Holley J, McCauley J: The spectrum of ciclosporin nephrotoxicity. Am J Nephrol 1990; 10:296–309.
66. Bellomo R, Berlangieri S, Wong C, et al: Renal allograft scintigraphy with Tc-99m-DTPA: Its role during cyclosporin A therapy. Transplantation 1992; 53:143–145.
67. Finn WF: Prevention of ischemic injury in renal transplantation. Kidney Int 1990; 37:171–180.
68. Alvanis P, Grekas D, Bougioukas G, et al: Reduction of Cy A nephrotoxicity by nifedipine during and after experimental in-situ renal preservation. Ren Fail 1992; 14:485–491.
69. Armitage JM, Kormos RL, Morita S, et al: Clinical trial of FK-506 immunosuppression in adult cardiac transplantation. Ann Thorac Surg 1992; 54:205–211.
70. Coulie P, De Plaen JF, van Y Persele de Strihou C: Captopril-induced acute reversible renal failure. Nephron 1983; 108:35–40.
71. Bauer JH, Gaddy P: Effects of enalapril alone and in combination with hydrochlorothiazide, on renin-angiotensin-aldosterone, renal function, salt and water excretion, and body fluid composition. Am J Kidney Dis 1985; 6:222–232.
72. Gottlieb SS, Weir MR: Renal effects of angiotensin-converting enzyme inhibition in congestive heart failure. Am J Cardiol 1990; 66:14D–21D.
73. Whelton A, Hamilton CW: Nonsteroidal anti-inflammatory drugs: Effects on kidney function. J Clin Pharmacol 1991; 31:588–598.
74. Tan SY, Shapiro R, Franco R, et al: Indomethacin-induced prostaglandin inhibition with hyperkalemia. Ann Intern Med 1979; 90:783–785.
75. Dorman HR, Sondheimer JH, Cadnapaphornchai P: Mannitol-induced acute renal failure. Medicine 1990; 69:153–159.

Table References

Note: As drug-specific references are too numerous to permit their citation in the tables themselves, only major papers are listed here. Each of these papers provides a review of the area mentioned in its title and of various tables in this chapter. The data presented in the tables found in this chapter are the result of the cross-checking of multiple tables and references.

1. Brater DG, Sokol PP, Hall SD, et al: Disposition and dose requirements of drugs in renal insufficiency. *In*: The Kidney: Physiology and Pathophysiology. 2nd ed. Vol 3. Seldin DW, Giebish G (Eds). New York, Raven Press, 1992, pp 3671–3695.
2. Bennett WM, Blythe WB: Use of drugs in patients with renal failure. *In*: Diseases of the Kidney. 4th ed. Vol. 3. Schrier RW, Gottschalk CW (Eds). Boston, Little, Brown and Co, 1988, pp 3437–3506.
3. Bennett WM: Guide to drug dosage in renal failure. Clin Pharmacokinet 1988; 15:326–354.
4. Gambertoglio JG, Aweeka FT, Blythe WB: Use of drugs in patients with renal failure. *In*: Diseases of the Kidney. 5th ed. Vol 3. Schrier RW, Gottschalk CW (Eds). Boston, Little, Brown, and Co, 1993, pp 3211–3268.
5. Bernstein JM, Erk SD: Choice of antibiotics, pharmacokinetics, and dose adjustment in acute renal failure. Med Clin North Am 1990; 74:1059–1076.
6. Shuler CL, Bennett WM: Principles of drug usage in dialysis patients. *In*: Dialysis Therapy. 2nd ed. Niessenson AR, Fine RN (Eds). Philadelphia, Hanley and Belfus, 1993, pp 327–332.
7. Golper TA: Drug dosage adjustment in dialysis patients including continuous ambulatory peritoneal dialysis, the treatment of peritonitis, and continuous arteriovenous hemofiltration. Contemp Issues Nephrol 1987; 17:21–48.
8. Verbeek RG, Branch RA, Wilkinson GR: Drug metabolites in renal failure: Pharmacokinetics and clinical implications. Clin Pharmacokinet 1981; 6:329–345.
9. Golper TA, Wedel SK, Kaplan AA, et al: Drug removal during continuous arteriovenous hemodiafiltration: Theory and clinical observations. Int J Artif Organs 1985; 8:307–312.
10. Davies SP, Kox WJ, Brown EA: Clearance studies in patients with acute renal failure treated by continuous arteriovenous hemodialysis. Contrib Nephrol 1991; 93:117–119.
11. Kroh UF, Dehne M, El Abed K, et al: Drug dosage during continuous hemofiltration: Pharmacokinetics and practical implications. Contrib Nephrol 1991; 93:127–130.
12. Bodenham A, Shelly MP, Park GR: The altered pharmacokinetics and pharmacodynamics of drugs commonly used in critically ill patients. Clin Pharmacokinet 1988; 14:347–373.
13. Kroh UF, Holl T, Feussner KD: Pharmacokinetics and dosage adjustment of antibiotics during continuous extracorporeal lung assistance and hemofiltration. Artif Organs 1992; 16:457–460.
14. Vos MC, Vincent HH, Yzerman EPF: Clearance of imipenem/cilastatin in acute renal failure patients treated by continuous hemodiafiltration (CAVHD). Intensive Care Med 1992; 18:282–285.
15. Davies SP, Lacey LF, Kox WJ, et al: Pharmacokinetics of cefuroxime and ceftazidime in patients with acute renal failure treated by continuous arteriovenous hemodialysis. Nephrol Dial Transplant 1991; 6:971–976.
16. Davies SP, Azadian BS, Kox WJ, et al: Pharmacokinetics of ciprofloxacin and vancomycin in patients with acute renal failure treated by continuous hemodialysis. Nephrol Dial Transplant 1992; 7:848–854.
17. Old CW, Lehrner LM: Prevention of radiocontrast-induced acute renal failure with mannitol. Lancet 1980; i:1980.
18. Anto HR, Chou SY, Porush JG, et al: Infusion intravenous pyelography and renal function: Effect of hypertonic mannitol in patients with chronic renal insufficiency. Arch Intern Med 1981; 141:1652–1656.
19. Berkseth RO, Kjellstrand CM: Radiologic contrast–induced nephropathy. Med Clin North Am 1984; 68:351–371.

CHAPTER 117

Acute Renal Failure in Infants and Children

Edward J. Ruley, MD • *Glenn H. Bock, MD*

Acute renal failure (ARF) is defined as the sudden impairment of homeostatic renal function that is characterized by the retention of nitrogenous metabolites. ARF occurs frequently in critical care patients, usually with conditions associated with high mortality rates.[1–3] Often, however, ARF is a reversible process providing that an early diagnosis is made, the cause correctly discerned, and appropriate treatment measures instituted. The incidence of ARF in industrialized nations is lower than in underdeveloped countries. Surgery (particularly cardiac surgery), the hemolytic-uremic syndrome, drug toxicity, and trauma constitute the major pediatric causes in industrialized countries, whereas infectious illnesses (with or without dehydration) are the predominant cause of ARF in underdeveloped areas.[1–6] Regardless, the reported incidence of ARF in any population is usually underestimated, since nonoliguric forms often go undetected.

ETIOLOGY AND PATHOGENESIS

In normal individuals, renal function can be maintained, despite significant homeostatic alterations, through the interplay of intrarenal and extrarenal mechanisms. The intrarenal mechanisms, usually termed *autoregulation,* include alterations in renal blood flow, glomerular arteriolar tone, renin release, and tubular reabsorption of solutes. Extrarenal compensatory mechanisms include changes in systemic blood distribution, systemic vascular tone, cardiac output, and blood pressure. The importance of the interplay of intrarenal and extrarenal factors is made evident by a consideration of the physiologic response to acute volume depletion. With a sudden reduction in renal perfusion pressure, stimuli to increase the release of renin from the macula densa are intrinsically generated. Renin acts extrarenally to increase systemic vascular tone, thereby raising blood pressure. In addition, renin stimulates aldosterone release by the adrenal cortex, which then acts intrarenally to increase tubular sodium reabsorption through a direct effect on the distal nephron. These responses serve to normalize renal perfusion, thereby maintaining the glomerular filtration rate (GFR).

Traditionally, ARF has been classified as prerenal, intrinsic-renal, or postrenal, implying the principal site of the pathologic process. Prerenal azotemia, which can be considered a form of functional renal failure (FRF), occurs when there is a reduction in renal perfusion that exceeds the regulatory capacity of the intrarenal and extrarenal mechanisms. In the critically ill patient with FRF, the renal ischemia is usually but one component of generalized inadequate tissue perfusion. Selective renal ischemia can occur in such conditions as bilateral renal artery stenosis and hepatorenal syndrome. Intrinsic renal failure, also termed *parenchymal renal failure* (PRF), may result from pathology that is essentially limited to the kidney (e.g., kidney transplant rejection, glomerulonephritis, specific nephrotoxins) or a process that involves the kidney as part of a systemic disease (e.g., ARF due to hemolytic-uremic syndrome). Postrenal causes of ARF include those in which the egress of urine from the kidney is impaired because of acquired or congenital obstruction of the urinary tract.

Although such a compartmentalized concept facilitates an approach to etiologic mechanisms, the boundaries between these groupings are indistinct—that is, more than one type of ARF may be operative in a patient at the same time. For example, severe physiologic derangements that result in FRF may persist long enough to produce renal injury, thereby creating an aspect of PRF. Such interactions are very important clinically, since it is the responsibility of the caretakers to rapidly distinguish FRF from PRF so that intervention can minimize the subsequent development of parenchymal renal injury. Although the clinical syndrome of PRF may arise from many different types of primary injuries, the ultimate expression of these injuries may be quite similar. The patient must therefore be carefully scrutinized for subtle clues so that timely therapeutic intervention may be facilitated.

The following discussion of the causes and pathogenesis of human ARF is organized by cause rather than by site of injury, since any given renal insult may have variable manifestations that depend on the degree, duration, and timing of the injury.

TABLE 117–1. Immunologic Disorders Associated with Acute Renal Failure

Specifically Directed Autoimmunity
Goodpasture's syndrome*
Antiglomerular basement membrane disease*
Renal transplant rejection
Immunity-Related
Postinfectious glomerulonephritis (including poststreptococcal)†
Systemic lupus erythematosus
Henoch-Schönlein purpura
Immunoglobulin A–immunoglobulin G (Berger's) nephropathy†
Membranous nephropathy*†
Idiopathic crescentic glomerulonephritis
Hypersensitivity tubulointerstitial nephritis
Immune Mechanism Unknown
Membranoproliferative glomerulonephritis Type I†
Membranoproliferative glomerulonephritis Type II
Wegener's granulomatosis*

*Rare in childhood.
†ARF in a very small percentage of patients.

Cardiovascular Causes

Effective renal blood flow may be impaired by a reduction in cardiac output or inadequate intravascular volume. The former may result from decreased venous return, heart rate, or myocardial contractility as seen in congenital heart disease, conduction disturbances, and cardiomyopathies. Inadequate vascular volume can be on a true depletion basis as in severe dehydration or hemorrhagic shock, or a functional volume depletion as in septicemia or gram-negative shock. Regardless, as effective renal blood flow decreases, autoregulation attempts to maintain the GFR by avid sodium and water reabsorption, which results in decreased urine production. Generally, creatinine excretion is less changed than urea, since filtered creatinine is not significantly reabsorbed in the tubules, whereas urea is freely reabsorbed. This disparity in the tubular handling of urea and creatinine accounts for the elevated plasma urea–creatinine ratio that frequently accompanies FRF. If renal hypoprofusion is severe and prolonged, renal parenchymal damage may result.

Immunologic and Infectious Causes

A large number of suspected or proven immune disorders may cause ARF (Table 117–1). The most common causes in children are the postinfectious glomerulopathies. Although the specific pathogenetic mechanisms of these immune disorders remain incompletely understood, the development of ARF is primarily due to extensive injury to the glomerular capillary wall, which results in a decreased GFR. The clinical syndrome of rapidly progressive glomerulonephritis, in which a rapid relentless progression of renal failure occurs, is produced by proliferation of the parietal epithelium of Bowman's capsule and fibrin deposition; this results in glomerular crescents that compress the glomerular capillary tuft. Its presence is determined by renal biopsy.

Fulminating pyelonephritis as a cause or complication of ARF is most common in infants, although older children may also be affected.[7, 8] Histologically, a massive polymorphonuclear leukocytic interstitial infiltrate produces widespread tubular injury. Recovery of normal renal function may be incomplete even after appropriate antibiotic therapy.

Acute tubulointerstitial nephritis is generally considered an uncommon cause of ARF. However, recent data suggest that this entity may be underdiagnosed.[7] It may be secondary to a toxic or acute hypersensitivity reaction to a drug or associated with an infectious illness. The mechanism of injury in such cases appears to be inflammation of the renal tubules, which causes a secondary decrease in GFR.

Toxic Causes

The kidneys are uniquely sensitive to a number of chemical compounds and biologic agents. The reasons for this sensitivity include the high proportion of cardiac output delivered to the kidney, the countercurrent concentrating gradient in the renal medulla, and the relatively high oxygen requirement necessary for normal kidney function.

Chemical nephrotoxins may directly impair renal cell function, participate in immune or inflammatory reactions, and/or aggravate an underlying renal disorder.[8] Those toxins most commonly seen in children, as well as their clinical manifestations and specific therapies, are outlined in Table 117–2. Consideration of nephrotoxins is important, since recognition of their role in a child with ARF and their prompt withdrawal alone or in combination with the provision of specific therapy, may dramatically influence outcome.

Renovascular Causes

Primary or secondary vascular disease of the renal blood vessels may result in ARF. Bilateral renal artery thrombosis, although a rare entity, is most frequently a complication of injury to the renovascular pedicle or is associated with umbilical artery catheterization in the newborn. Renal artery stenosis may lead to ARF, particularly when accompanied by accelerated hypertension. Patients with hypertension and bilateral renal artery stenoses may develop ARF when treated with angiotensin II–converting enzyme inhibitors.[11, 12] The immediate consequence of sudden partial or complete renal arterial occlusion is ischemic renal failure, which may lead to a decrease in the size of the kidney. The extent of the diminished blood flow determines the extent and reversibility of the cortical ischemic renal lesion. Similarly, in the early stages of accelerated hypertension, the unprotected renal arterial microvasculature may undergo intimal proliferation and luminal narrowing, resulting in

TABLE 117–2. Drugs and Toxins Most Commonly Associated with Acute Renal Failure in Childhood

	Associated Manifestations	*Therapy*
Immune Reaction or Hypersensitivity		
Penicillins Sulfonamides Cephalosporins	Fever, rash, serum sickness, eosinophilia, eosinophiluria, exfoliative dermatitis (sulfonamides)	Supportive corticosteroids, dialysis
Direct Toxicity		
Heavy metals (mercurials, lead, bismuth, gold, iron, copper)	CNS, GI, circulatory collapse (iron), hemolytic anemia (copper)	Emesis, albumin, charcoal chelation, supportive, dialysis
Glycols	CNS, cardiac failure, pulmonary edema	Immediate hemodialysis, gastric lavage
Organic solvents (carbon tetrachloride, turpentine)	CNS, hepatic, GI	Gastric lavage, catharsis, supportive
Aminoglycosides	Ototoxicity, exacerbated by poor hydration	Hydration
Amphotericin B	Hypokalemia, nonoliguric renal failure Toxicity dose-related; exacerbated by poor hydration	Hydration
Mushroom (especially *Amanita phalloides*)	GI, shock, severe liver dysfunction	Dialysis, hemoperfusion (within 24 to 36 h), supportive
Salicylates	Tinnitus, hyperpnea, acidosis, GI, hemorrhage, CNS depression	Alkalinization of urine, hydration, gastric lavage, dialysis
Methoxyflurane, enflurane	ARF frequently nonoliguric; toxicity may be accentuated by aminoglycosides, tetracycline, and obesity	Supportive, possibly early dialysis to remove fluoride
Uricosuric or hyperuricemic agents (pancreatic enzymes, furosemide, salicylates, radiographic contrast media, antineoplastic agents)		Supportive, diuresis, alkalinization, hemodialysis

Abbreviations: CNS = central nervous system; GI = gastrointestinal.

further activation of the renin-angiotensin-aldosterone axis and distal renal ischemia. Successful therapy depends on the interruption of this cycle through the control of blood pressure. However, overly aggressive treatment of the hypertension may produce or exacerbate renal ischemia, further impairing renal function.

Bilateral renal vein occlusion is a more common major vascular lesion, particularly in newborn infants. It is frequently associated with maternal diabetes mellitus, birth asphyxia, and cyanotic congenital heart disease (especially after angiocardiography or other intravascular uses of contrast material). In older infants, bilateral renal vein thrombosis may be associated with hyperosmolar dehydration, accidental or surgical trauma to the major renal veins, or the nephrotic syndrome. In nephrotic syndrome, thrombosis is presumed to be a multifactorial event resulting from elevated levels of coagulation Factors V and VIII, thrombocytosis, and extremely low plasma levels of antithrombin III and plasminogen.[13] Although marked swelling of the kidneys may produce compression of the collecting systems, this process is often nonhomogeneous, thus allowing recovery of a significant amount of renal function. Emboli, particularly pulmonary emboli, may complicate the early course, whereas severe hypertension due to irreversible fibrosis of the parenchyma may be a late complication.

Cortical or medullary renal parenchymal necrosis, or both, may be associated with major renovascular lesions or microvascular disease. Medullary necrosis may result from sickle cell disease or acute pyelonephritis. The two most common causes for microvascular thrombosis in childhood are disseminated intravascular coagulation and the hemolytic-uremic syndrome. The former may progress to renal arteriolar thrombosis and cortical necrosis, whereas the latter, which is characterized by glomerular endocapillary thrombosis, is the most common cause of oliguric ARF in young children.[4] The sudden appearance of azotemia and oliguria accompanied by microangiopathic hemolytic anemia suggests hemolytic-uremic syndrome. This disorder is often preceded by a prodrome of symptoms that suggests a gastrointestinal infectious cause. This fact and the histologic similarity to the Shwartzman reaction are compatible with endotoxin-mediated capillary endothelial injury. Some investigators have proposed that imbalance of the normal microvascular proaggregants and antiaggregants may be an important aspect of its pathophysiology.[15] Evidence also supports the role of a Shiga-like enterotoxin ("verotoxin") in the pathogenesis of the hemolytic-uremic syndrome. These cytotoxic products of certain bacteria (including some enteric *Escherichia coli* serotypes) can cause the watery diarrhea and hemorrhagic colitis often seen during the prodrome and may play a role in the glomerular capillary endothelial damage that occurs.[16] The severity of the acute hemolytic-uremic syndrome appears to be unrelated to outcome, since more than 95% of patients survive with appropriate therapy. Chronic renal insufficiency and hypertension can be late complications.

Obstructive Uropathy

Urinary tract obstruction can produce FRF or PRF, or both. Acute obstruction increases intratubular pressure, leading to a reduction in GFR that may be associated with decreased urinary flow and increased sodium and water reabsorption.[17] A concentrated urine with little sodium may erroneously suggest a defect in effective renal blood flow. Prolonged partial obstruction in which the GFR is maintained while tubular function is impaired is usually associated with isotonic or hypotonic urine with a relatively high sodium content. These findings, as well as defective hydrogen and potassium elimination, resemble the abnormalities seen in parenchymal nonoliguric renal failure.

Acute PRF may arise as a complication of obstructed urinary outflow. Bilateral anatomic obstruction occurs most often in male infants and is due to congenital posterior urethral valves. Oliguric ARF may occur in older infants who have an undiagnosed solitary kidney that becomes acutely obstructed. This obstruction may be due to an anatomic abnormality or to an acquired intraluminal lesion such as a renal calculus or ureteral debris. Extrinsic compression of the urethral outflow tract by lesions such as a periurethral abscess, pelvic hematoma, or neoplasm is rare but must be suspected in any patient with acute bilateral obstruction.

The infrequent onset of acute obstructive uropathy after the newborn period does not diminish its importance, since early diagnosis and correction may avert permanent parenchymal damage. Total anuria strongly suggests a major renovascular accident or total obstruction. An acute partial or intermittent obstruction may be more difficult to clinically diagnose.

CLINICAL MANIFESTATIONS

In the child presenting with ARF, the initial history and physical examination can be very useful in discerning the cause. Acutely decompensated underlying chronic renal failure should be suspected in the child with a prior history of urinary tract infections, preexisting anorexia or fatigue, poor growth, abnormal voiding habits, rachitic bone abnormalities, or unexplained anemia. A prodrome of diarrhea or vomiting associated with physical signs of severe volume depletion suggests the possibility of PRF with acute tubular necrosis or renal vein thrombosis. When accompanied by bloody stools, these same findings suggest hemolytic-uremic syndrome. The presence of anuria or palpable flank masses raises the possibility of acute bilateral urinary obstruction. Vasculitic rashes, arthritis, lymphadenopathy, or other organ involvement should raise suspicion of an underlying multisystemic disorder. The ingestion of nephrotoxic drugs or poisons should be routinely considered in children with unexplained ARF.

ARF that occurs in the critically ill patient usually has a discernible cause with a definite time of onset. The signs and symptoms in this setting usually result from interactions of the underlying disease with the consequent renal dysfunction and treatment. The predominant findings vary with the type and severity of the disease. Since the symptoms of ARF may have more than one cause, the clinician must keep in mind the relative contribution of multiple factors when considering the physical findings in each individual patient.

Oliguria (urine output <250 mL/m^2 per day) is not considered a necessary condition for ARF, since ARF can be associated with any volume of urine excretion. The term *nonoliguric ARF* describes renal dysfunction associated with a normal or even excessive urine volume. Clinical findings directly ascribable to renal failure or to the homeostatic adjustments that occur in response to renal failure are uncommon early in its course. As the metabolic disturbances of ARF become more severe, the chance that the symptoms of renal dysfunction will become manifest also increases. Lethargy, disorientation, vomiting, and diarrhea usually do not occur until the blood urea nitrogen (BUN) values exceed 120 mg/dL.

Patients with ARF and hyperkalemia are usually asymptomatic. Neuromuscular findings such as paresthesias, weakness, and ascending paralysis rarely occur. More importantly, hyperkalemia may produce sudden life-threatening cardiac conduction abnormalities. Acidosis, hypocalcemia, and hyperphosphatemia rarely cause symptoms unless exacerbated by overaggressive or ill-advised therapy.

BIOCHEMICAL ABNORMALITIES

ARF produces a wide spectrum of biochemical abnormalities that may reflect the duration and severity of renal dysfunction. Hypervolemia in oliguric ARF may dilute serum sodium, hemoglobin, and protein concentrations. Conversely, diuresis during the recovery phase of oliguric renal failure may produce abnormally high serum concentrations if fluid is not adequately replaced.

Hyperkalemia is common in oliguric ARF and can be quite severe when extensive tissue injury, large hematomas, infection, metabolic acidosis, hypoxemia, or hemolysis is present. The adverse effects of hyperkalemia are potentiated by concomitant hyponatremia, hypocalcemia, hypomagnesemia, and digitalis use. Hyperkalemia in an ARF patient should be monitored with serial electrocardiography. Increasingly severe hyperkalemia causes peaking of the T waves with shortening of the QT interval, followed by prolongation of the QRS complex, atrioventricular block, flattening and then disappearance of the P wave, the appearance of a sine wave,[18] and finally ventricular fibrillation or asystole. Factitious hyperkalemia may occur in patients with thrombocytosis when intracellular potassium is released into the serum as the blood clots in the collection tube.[19] This artifact can be confirmed by comparing potassium concentrations in serum and plasma specimens obtained simultaneously; factitious hyperkalemia corresponds to a serum potassium value that is more than 0.5 mEq/L greater than the plasma value. The electrocardiogram is also helpful in the diagnosis of factitious hyperkalemia. Hyperkalemia is uncommon in nonoliguric ARF.

Metabolic acidosis may appear early in ARF and can be particularly intractable in children with reduced tissue perfusion or with a hypermetabolic state that increases organic acid production in the presence of a reduced capacity for acid excretion. Metabolic acidosis in the critically ill child may be complicated by respiratory acidosis due to concomitant pulmonary injury, infection, or edema.

Hypocalcemia associated with elevated levels of immunoreactive parathyroid hormone may develop as early as 2 days after the onset of ARF.[20] Although calcium values are commonly reduced to a range of 6.3 to 8.3 mg/dL, the ratio of ionized to nonionized calcium is generally normal. The mechanisms that produce hypocalcemia remain incompletely understood. Hyperphosphatemia is common but does not usually occur as early as hypocalcemia, and phosphate levels rarely exceed 8 mg/dL. Hypermagnesemia is also common in ARF, but corresponding symptoms are rare unless magnesium-containing compounds such as antacids or laxatives are administered to the patient with oliguric ARF.

Hematologic abnormalities are common in children with ARF. Anemia usually occurs at some time during the illness. Factors contributing to anemia include vascular volume overexpansion, blood loss, and diminished erythrocyte production. Thrombocytopenia is common following cardiopulmonary bypass or in association with renal vein thrombosis, disseminated intravascular coagulation, and the hemolytic-uremic syndrome. Abnormalities of clotting factors are most striking in children with disseminated intravascular coagulation.

DIAGNOSIS

The first consideration of a diagnostic algorithm (Fig. 117–1) is differentiation of ARF from occult chronic renal failure that has suddenly become symptomatic. Chronic renal failure may be insidious in onset and progression, so that its

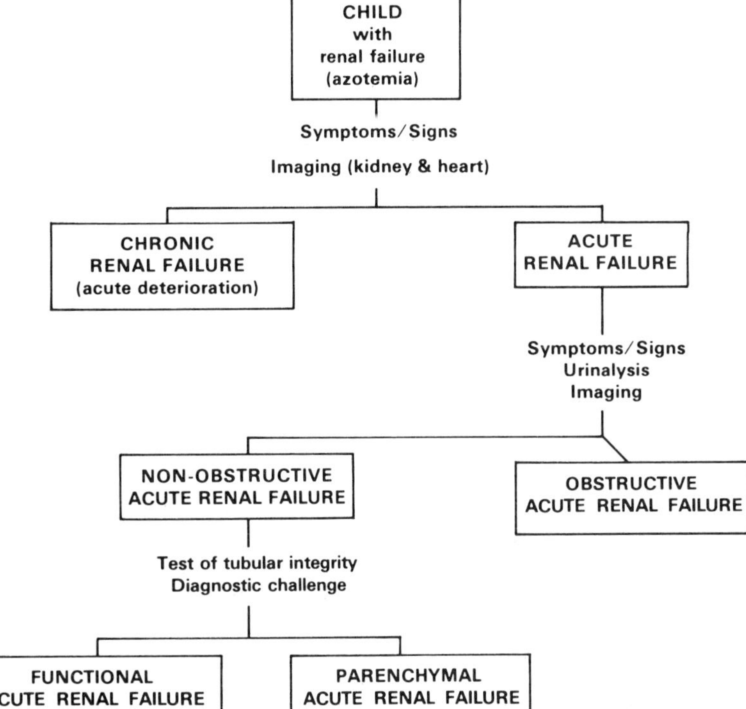

Figure 117–1. A systematic approach to the child with renal failure.

subtle symptoms are not appreciated by the parents or child. An intercurrent illness such as gastroenteritis with dehydration can make the patient suddenly symptomatic. A careful history and physical and laboratory examination usually distinguish acute from chronic renal failure. A history of vague symptoms, including polyuria, polydipsia, episodic fever, anorexia, vomiting, diarrhea, or easy fatigue, all of which antedate the onset of acute illness, may be elicited from a child with undiagnosed chronic renal failure. Physical examination may demonstrate poor growth or rachitic bone changes. Laboratory evaluation may demonstrate electrocardiographic or echocardiograhic evidence of long-standing hypertension, and ultrasonography may reveal small or cystic kidneys.

If symptoms and signs suggest ARF, the next step in the algorithm is differentiation of obstructive from nonobstructive causes. Children with obstructive ARF often have abdominal or flank pain referable to the obstructed systems. Palpable renal masses suggest an obstructed urinary system, although masses may be associated with other causes of ARF such as renal vein thrombosis or polycystic kidneys. Renal masses associated with a palpable bladder in a male strongly suggest urinary tract obstruction from posterior urethral valves. The urinary sediment associated with obstruction is usually normal unless coexisting infection is present.

Imaging techniques should be used in ARF of undetermined cause to rule out obstruction. A simple radiograph of the abdomen may determine kidney size or demonstrate calcifications. When compared with other imaging techniques, excretory urography may carry some risk of further renal parenchymal injury[21–23] in the oliguric or anuric patient and usually provides incomplete information owing to poor visualization of the urinary system in children with high BUN levels. Visualization is also usually poor in young infants. Ultrasonography accurately assesses renal size and identifies urinary obstructions and thus is the imaging technique of choice. Radionuclide studies help to delineate functional, parenchymal, and obstructive causes of ARF.[24]

Once obstructive causes of renal failure have been ruled out, PRF must be differentiated from FRF. Such a differentiation should not begin until clinical evidence indicates that the patient is well hydrated. If the child remains oliguric after hydration, the clinician may then choose among the battery of laboratory urinary diagnostic tests (Table 117–3) described below or conduct clinical challenges of renal function (Table 117–4) to make this differentiation. The clinical challenge may include intravenous or oral administration of 2 mg/kg furosemide, accompanied by intravenous mannitol (0.5 g/kg given over 5 minutes or an infusion of 20 mL/kg over 4 hours). In FRF, the output increases to at least 12 mL/m^2 per hour, whereas in PRF it does not. However, this diagnostic challenge may be unreliable in children who are malnourished, and false-negative responses can occur in those who are markedly dehydrated. Moreover, mannitol is contraindicated in patients with vascular volume expansion. Bladder catheterization is required to accurately measure the response to clinical challenge, but the catheter should be removed at the end of the test to prevent infection. Urine specimens for sodium, osmolality, and urea should always be obtained prior to the administration of fluid, mannitol, or diuretics.

Laboratory Tests

By definition, the diagnosis of renal failure is based on the presence of azotemia. The nitrogenous compounds most commonly measured in clinical practice are BUN and serum creatinine. However, since the BUN is affected by factors other than nitrogen excretion by the kidney (Table 117–5), it is an unreliable single indicator of renal function. Serum creatinine is relatively unaffected by extrarenal factors and therefore is a better indicator of glomerular function. Serum creatinine is a function of muscle mass, which is affected by

TABLE 117–3. Laboratory Tests to Discriminate Functional from Parenchymal Acute Renal Failure

Test	Calculation	*Expected Results* Functional ARF	Parenchymal ARF	Discrimination	References
Tests of Tubular Sodium Reabsorption					
Urine sodium concentration	Direct measurement	<20 mEq/L	>40 mEq/L	Poor	27–29
Fractional excretion of sodium (Fe_{Na})	$U/S_{Na} \div U/S_{cr} \times 100$	< 1	> 1*	Good	
Tests of Tubular Water Reabsorption					31, 39
Urine specific gravity	Direct measurement	>1.020	<1.010	Poor	
Urine osmolality	Direct measurement	>500 mOsm/kg	<350 mOsm/kg	Poor	
Urine-serum osmolality ratio	Direct measurement	>2	<1.1	Fair	4, 43
Free water clearance (CH_2O)	Urine vol − C osm [C osm = (U osm × U volume) ÷ S osm]	Negative values	Positive values	Good	45
Urine-serum creatinine	Direct measurement	>40	<20	Fair	48
Urine-serum urea ratio	Direct measurement	>20	<10	Fair	32, 33
Renal excretory index	U/S urea × (24-h urine vol ÷ 100)	>200	<84		49

*Some investigators use 3 on the cutoff value.
Abbreviations: U = urine; S = serum; Na = sodium; cr = creatinine; vol = volume; osm = osmolality; C = clearance.

age, gender, and body build.[25] The observation that the serum creatinine concentration is related to height and that creatinine clearance is proportional to body surface area has led to the development of a formula for estimating GFR without a timed urine collection[26, 27]:

$$Ccr = \frac{f \times (\text{Height, in centimeters})}{Cr}$$

where Ccr is the creatinine clearance (mL/min · 1.73 m^2) and Cr is the serum creatinine (mg/dL). The derived factor, f, equals 0.55 if creatinine is measured by the total chromogen method,[26] or 0.43 if measured by the true creatinine method.[27] Estimates of GFR by this formula correlate well with calculations using the classic endogenous creatinine clearance method[26, 27] or the inulin clearance method[26] but are less accurate in children under 3 years of age and at higher GFR levels.[28] None of these techniques is as precise as measuring the clearance of intravenously injected edetic acid labeled with chromium 51[27, 28]; however, for practical reasons, the endogenous creatinine clearance remains the most commonly used clinical method to estimate GFR.

Although changes in serum creatinine level reflect alterations in GFR, the significance of these changes depends on the initial level of renal function. For example, although a 50% decrease in creatinine clearance in a child with normal function produces only a slight increase in serum creatinine level (Fig. 117–2), a 10% decrease in clearance in the child with established renal failure produces a large increase in serum creatinine level. Furthermore, a sudden marked change in GFR causes only a gradual adjustment in the creatinine level, which often takes several days to reach a new steady state that reflects the reduced filtration. The use of a formula based on the difference in serum creatinine values obtained several hours apart circumvents this lag problem and accurately estimates creatinine clearance in adults and children with unstable renal function.[29]

The most common clinical problem in the child with oliguric ARF is the differentiation of FRF from PRF once obstructive causes of renal failure have been ruled out. Prompt diagnosis of FRF is critical, since it is reversible if renal perfusion is restored promptly; otherwise, long-standing renal hypoperfusion can result in PRF that is not readily reversible. Conversely, vigorous volume therapy in the child with established PRF can lead to fluid overload, which may adversely affect other organ systems, particularly the central nervous system and the lungs. Laboratory determinations purported to differentiate FRF from PRF (see Table 117–3) assess the functional integrity of the renal tubule by measuring tubular reabsorption of sodium or water, or tubular damage.

TABLE 117–4. A Clinical Approach to the Differentiation of Functional from Parenchymal Acute Renal Failure

1. Catheterize bladder—urinalysis on residual urine.
2. Collect urine for 1 h. Measure volume, osmolality, urea, creatinine, sodium.
3. At the end of 1 h, obtain serum for measurements of osmolality, urea, creatinine, and sodium.
4. Administer furosemide and fluid/mannitol challenge.
5. Collect urine for 3 h for volume determination.
6. Differentiate functional from parenchymal renal failure by:
   a. Calculation of U/S osm, U/S urea, U/S_{cr}, CH_2O, and FeNa (see laboratory tests).
   b. Urinary output response to the furosemide and fluid/mannitol challenge.

TABLE 117–5. Extrarenal Factors That Affect Blood Urea Nitrogen and Creatinine Concentrations

Blood Urea Nitrogen	
Increased By:	*Decreased By:*
High-protein diet	Low-protein diet
Starvation	High-caloric diet
GI hemorrhage	Liver disease
Dehydration	Hypometabolism
Corticosteroid administration	Hyperlipidemia
Hypercatabolic states (fever, sepsis, etc.)	
Creatinine	
Increased By:	*Decreased By:*
Rhabdomyolysis	Loss of muscle mass (amputations, dystrophy, atrophy)
Dehydration	Burns
	Hyperlipidemia

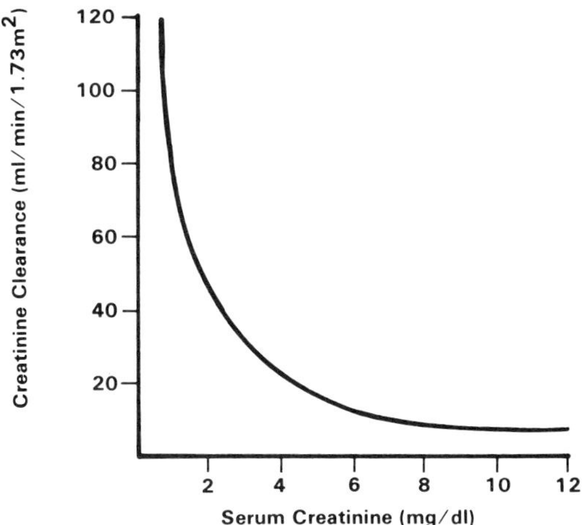

Figure 117–2. The relationship between creatinine clearance and serum creatinine level.

Tests of Tubular Reabsorption of Sodium

An underperfused but functionally intact kidney (as in FRF) actively reabsorbs sodium as a compensatory response to volume depletion, whereas a kidney with parenchymal damage is relatively unable to perform this function. Thus, a urinary sodium (U_{Na}) concentration less than 20 mEq/L is often consistent with FRF, whereas a U_{Na} of greater than 40 mEg/L is more often found in PRF.[30–32] Although these differences often reach statistical significance in groups of patients, U_{Na} is of limited value in individual cases,[33–37] particularly postoperative patients,[38] those who have undergone cardiopulmonary bypass,[39] and infants with hypernatremic dehydration.[40]

To improve the sensitivity of urinary sodium measurements, the urine/serum creatinine ratio (U/S_{cr}) may be combined with the urine/serum sodium ratio (U/S_{Na}) to calculate the fractional excretion of sodium (Fe_{Na}).[34] Using the criteria given in Table 117–3, several investigators have found these tests to be highly reliable in the differentiation of FRF from oliguric PRF.[41, 42] However, as the Fe_{Na} has been more widely applied in clinical practice, an increasing number of reports of low reabsorption (i.e., >1%) in patients with PRF have appeared.[43] This has led several investigators to suggest that tests of sodium excretion are not as useful as free water clearance or 2-hour creatinine clearance measurements.[43, 44] All tests of urinary sodium excretion are of limited value in children who have received large sodium loads or diuretics[45] or who have nonoliguric ARF.[46] Use of tests of tubular sodium reabsorption in neonates must take maturational factors into account. The Fe_{Na} has been shown to be inversely proportional to gestational age.[47] and to decrease with increasing postnatal age.[48] Several studies have shown that an Fe_{Na} of 2.5% or greater differentiates PRF in infants greater than 32 weeks' gestation provided that the other limitations (e.g., diuretic use) are observed.[45, 49, 50]

Tests of Tubular Reabsorption of Water

Reabsorption of water also requires a functionally intact tubule. Urinary specific gravity measurement has the advantage of being a simple and readily available test in which values over 1.020 strongly suggest FRF. However, falsely high values occur in the presence of albumin, dextran, glucose, bilirubin, radiographic dyes, or other high-molecular-weight substances in the urine. Urine osmolality measurements are not significantly affected by these substances. Although groups of patients with FRF usually have an average urine osmolality greater than 500 mOsm/L and PRF groups have an average urine osmolality less than 350 mOsm/L, considerable overlap exists among individuals. The urine-serum osmolality ratio has been proposed as a more sensitive test.[51] A ratio of greater than 2.0 suggests FRF, whereas a ratio that approaches 1.0 is consistent with PRF.[4] However, this ratio can be unreliable in children who have received hypotonic fluids or are malnourished.

Free water clearance (C_{H_2O}) is a test of urinary concentrating capacity. C_{H_2O} represents the *volume* of pure water that would have to be added *to* or removed *from the* urine to make it isosmotic to plasma. Thus, the C_{H_2O} should be negative (−25 to −100 mL/h) in patients with FRF but approaches or exceeds zero in PRF patients (see Table 117–3). Some investigators have found that the C_{H_2O} accurately differentiates FRF from PRF in patients with ARF after cardiopulmonary bypass.[39, 43, 44, 52–54] C_{H_2O} may be factitiously altered by diuretics, hyperosmolar agents, vigorous fluid infusion, and head injuries.[55] Others have suggested that the combination of C_{H_2O} and creatinine clearance improves diagnostic accuracy.[44, 55]

U/S_{cr} has been suggested as a measure of the ability of the kidney to reabsorb water.[33, 41, 56] A ratio above 40 correlates with FRF, and one below 20 indicates PRF (see Table 117–3).[41] In adults with ARF, this test distinguishes FRF from PRF in 75% of the cases,[42] although individual values frequently overlap.[41]

Use of the urine-serum urea ratio to differentiate FRF from PRF assumes a properly functioning medullary countercurrent system (see Table 117–3).[35, 36] Urine-serum urea ratio is of value in children with ARF,[40] including those who are malnourished[4]; it has been used in combination with the renal excretory index (see Table 117–3).[57]

Evidence of Tubular Damage

Careful microscopic examination of the centrifuged urinary sediment can help differentiate FRF from PRF.[58] FRF is characterized by hyaline and finely granular casts, whereas PRF is evidenced by the presence of tubular epithelial cell casts, degenerating tubular cell casts, and free tubular cells. However, the rather subjective nature of the urine sediment examination and its inability to differentiate between complete and partial PRF limit the value of this test.

Renal biopsy is rarely helpful in differentiating FRF from PRF because biopsy findings correlate poorly with renal dysfunction.[30, 33, 56, 59] However, for selected patients who demonstrate inconclusive evidence of tubular necrosis or whose course is not typical, renal biopsy may be useful in arriving at the correct diagnosis.[60]

Attempts to detect the urinary excretion of various intracellular enzymes[61] or tubular antigens[62] in patients with acute tubular injury are interesting but not generally available or of proven clinical value at the present time.

TREATMENT

Treatment of PRF should address the underlying disorder while maintaining homeostasis and preventing complications from reduced renal function or therapy, or both. Generally, the faster the underlying disorder is corrected, the more rapidly renal function is restored. Certain causes such as acute glomerulonephritis or acute tubular necrosis are self-limited and do not require specific therapy.

Homeostasis is maintained by correcting the biophysiologic abnormalities with medical therapy and dialysis. This requires surveillance and treatment of fluid and electrolyte imbalances, acidosis, calcium-phosphorus abnormalities, anemia, blood pressure abnormalities, and nutritional deficits.

Water and Sodium Imbalances

After initial deficits have been corrected, the goal of water and sodium replacement is to maintain a zero balance. Fluid balance is most often estimated from measurements of intake and output and confirmed by observation of daily body weight changes. It must be kept in mind that the fluid-balanced acutely ill child may lose as much as 0.5% of lean body weight per day. The design of a fluid and sodium replacement regimen must be individualized for each patient. The fluid and sodium replacement prescription should be estimated from calculated or measured insensible losses and urine volume as well as from losses from the gastrointestinal tract or cavity drainage. The presence of fever, the need for mechanical ventilation, and metabolic disturbances must also be considered in the estimate of fluid needs. In the absence of appreciable gastrointestinal or cavity fluid losses, the markedly oliguric patient should receive replacement solutions that are relatively free of sodium. By contrast, patients with nonoliguric renal failure or those with large amounts of drainage should receive fluid and sodium at a rate that is based on their measured losses.

Hyperkalemia

Hyperkalemia is a potentially fatal complication of ARF requiring continuous monitoring of both the serum potassium level and the electrocardiogram. The treatment of hyperkalemia depends on its severity. Patients with mildly elevated serum potassium concentrations between 5.0 and 6.5 mEq/L often require no treatment; however, these patients should be observed closely for a continued rise in potassium concentration. Moderate (6.5–8.0 mEq/L) and severe (>8.0 mEq/L) potassium elevations and neuromuscular or electrocardiographic abnormalities should always be treated.

Treatment of hyperkalemia may be considered to have four aspects: reversal of membrane abnormalities, shifting of potassium into the intracellular space, removal of potassium from the body, and reduction of future potassium loads. Intravenous administration of calcium gluconate (Table 117–6) is a temporizing measure that decreases membrane excitability by reducing the membrane threshold potential. Although it quickly reduces the chance of neuromuscular or cardiac conduction abnormalities, its effect is only transient because the serum concentration of potassium is unchanged. The administration of calcium allows the clinician time to institute other, more definitive measures. Hypertonic sodium solutions, including isotonic sodium chloride to which sodium bicarbonate has been added, have been used in place of calcium gluconate for patients who have hyponatremia associated with hyperkalemia.[63]

Intravenous glucose, glucose and insulin, beta agonists such as albuterol,[64] and sodium bicarbonate cause extracellular potassium to move into the intracellular space, reducing the serum potassium level (see Table 117–6). The effect is rapid and may last several hours.

Potassium can be removed by cation exchange resins (see Table 117–6) or by dialysis. Sodium polystyrene sulfonate, which exchanges sodium for potassium in the colon,[65] may be administered orally or rectally in combination with sorbitol. Sorbitol acts as an osmotic cathartic, which prevents constipation and consequent resin retention. In addition, it may provide the secondary benefit by inducing diarrhea in the oliguric patient, thereby increasing potassium and water losses from the gut. Occasionally, the diarrhea and the resin-sorbitol mixture may irritate the rectum and cause rectal bleeding, in which case the resin must be discontinued. Since these resins exchange sodium for potassium, they may produce significant sodium and fluid retention. Intractable or imminently life-threatening hyperkalemia is an indication for dialysis.

Reduction of the potassium burden is important to maximize the effect of therapy and to prevent the recurrence of hyperkalemia. This can be accomplished by (1) eliminating

TABLE 117–6. Treatment of Hyperkalemia

Agent	*Action*	*Dose*	*Onset/Duration*	*Remarks*
Calcium gluconate (10%)	Stabilization of membrane potential	0.5 mg elemental Ca^{+2}/kg IV over 2–4 min	Rapid (min)/transient (h)	Monitor electrocardiograph for bradycardia during administration May be repeated once; further repetition not recommended
Glucose (50%)	Promotes cellular uptake of K^+	1 mL/kg IV by slow push	1–2 h/transient (h)	Do not use in diabetics
Glucose (50%) and insulin	Promotes cellular uptake of K^+	1 mL/kg of glucose with 0.1 U regular insulin/kg IV by slow push or rapid drip	Rapid (30 min)/ transient (h)	*Never* give insulin alone
Sodium bicarbonate (7.5%)	Promotes cellular uptake of K^+	2.5 mEq/kg (~ 3 mL/kg) by slow push or rapid drip	Rapid (30 min)/ transient (h)	May be repeated with caution, although often ineffective
Albuterol	Promotes cellular uptake of K^+	0.1 mg/kg by aerosol	Rapid (30–45 min)/ transient	May repeat every 30–60 min. Can synergize with glucose/ insulin
Sodium polystyrene sulfonate (Kayexalate, Breon Labs, NY)	Cation exchange resin	1 g/kg PO (with 3–4 mL of 70% sorbitol/g of resin) or PR (with 10 mL of 70% sorbitol/g of resin)	Hours/days	Unpalatable Enemas should be retained at least 30 min Oral administration more effective/effect delayed Rectal administration less effective/effect rapid Also chelates Ca^{+2} and Mg^{+2}

Abbreviations: k^+ = potassium; Ca^{+2} = calcium; IV = intravenous; PO = perioral; PR = perirectal Mg^{+2} = magnesium.

sources of potassium intake, including medications; (2) promptly treating infections; (3) débriding devitalized tissues; (4) removing blood accumulations; and (5) providing enough exogenous calories to prevent tissue breakdown. Should all of the above treatment methods fail, dialysis becomes the treatment of choice.

Acidosis

Mild metabolic acidosis (serum bicarbonate level of greater than or equal to 15 mEq/L) need not be treated. Moderate acidosis (serum bicarbonate level of 10 to 15 mEq/L) may be ameliorated by use of a 7.5% solution of intravenous sodium bicarbonate, although this therapy is limited by the amount of sodium and fluid that can be tolerated by the patient. Adequate caloric intake minimizes acidosis in most patients. Severe or intractable acidosis is best treated by dialysis.

Hypocalcemia and Hyperphosphatemia

The problems of hypocalcemia and hyperphosphatemia are best treated by reducing the serum phosphorus level with orally administered aluminum hydroxide or calcium carbonate, which render gastrointestinal phosphate less resorbable. Usually, the serum calcium level rises as the phosphorus level falls. After the phosphorus level is reduced, additional elemental calcium can be administered. It is not advisable to administer supplemental calcium before controlling phosphorus concentration because metastatic calcification may occur when there is a high serum calcium-phosphorus product.

Anemia

The anemia of ARF is usually not severe enough to require treatment. If transfusion does become necessary, it should be done with great caution because children with ARF are very sensitive to the volume-expanding effects of transfusion and may develop severe hypertension or congestive heart failure. Blood transfusions may also exacerbate hypocalcemia or hyperkalemia. Transfusions should be given as packed red blood cells unless persistent bleeding is present. Administration of blood as an exchange transfusion or during dialysis often minimizes the adverse effects of the transfusion volume.

Blood Pressure Abnormalities

Hypotension may be associated with ARF as a result of diminished intravascular volume (i.e., dehydration or bleeding), as a manifestation of cardiac failure (i.e., after open-heart surgery), or with underlying systemic illnesses (e.g., septic shock and capillary leak). The treatment of hypotension depends on its pathophysiology. The rapidity with which normal blood pressure is restored affects the severity and duration of ARF.

Hypertension in ARF patients is most often associated with glomerulonephritis or excessive intravenous fluid and sodium administration. Treatment includes the use of parenteral or oral antihypertensive drugs in the former instance, and the reduction of intravascular volume by dialysis in the latter. Hypertension is uncommon in nonoliguric ARF.

Nutritional Deficits

Nutritional support is a very important part of the treatment plan that should be implemented early. Provision of adequate calories and high–biologic value protein prevents complications due to catabolism and speeds the recovery from ARF. The degree of caloric support varies with the age of the patient and associated injuries (e.g., burns), which may pose additional nutritional burdens. To maintain a positive nitrogen balance, the child should be provided with 80 to 120 mg of nitrogen per kilogram per day, depending on the degree of catabolism. The provision of nutritional support is limited by whether the GI tract is functional, what vascular access is available, and whether the patient has oliguric or nonoliguric ARF. If the gut is functional, it should be used as the vehicle for caloric and protein provision. The caloric content of ingested foods and fluids should be increased as much as possible without causing osmotic diarrhea. Hard candy is an excellent caloric source for children and contributes minimally to the volume. All intravenously administered fluids should have their caloric content maximized to help meet the daily caloric requirements. Whether the patient can tolerate hypertonic glucose solutions is limited by the location of vascular access (peripheral or central sites). If adequate nutritional support cannot be administered using a combined oral and peripheral intravenous regimen, parenteral alimentation should be considered.

Preliminary studies of parenteral nutrition in ARF patients suggest that infusion of essential amino acids or a combination of essential and nonessential amino acids can decrease urea nitrogen production and improve nitrogen balance.[66–69] These regimens appear to significantly improve the overall recovery of renal function and survival in high-risk ARF patients with underlying septic or surgical disorders. Provision of increased calories and protein can usually be achieved in children with nonoliguric ARF who have minimal or no volume limitation.

Use of Drugs in Acute Renal Failure

It is appropriate to review, at regular intervals, the drug regimens of patients with ARF. The use of drugs in patients with ARF, particularly those primarily excreted by the kidneys, must be done cautiously to avoid overdosing or underdosing. Many aspects of drug metabolism also can be altered during ARF, including biotransformation, plasma protein binding, and distribution volumes. When using a drug whose elimination is altered during renal failure, reasonable estimates of dose adjustments can be made using dose and dose-interval prescription changes.[70] These dose-modifications are generally based on stratifications from creatinine clearances. Creatinine clearance can usually be adequately estimated using the formula presented earlier in this chapter. In addition, the concomitant use of dialysis or hemofiltration may generate the need for supplemental drug doses if significant amounts of the drug are removed by these procedures.[70]

Use of Dialysis

Dialysis is indicated for volume-overloaded ARF patients who are unresponsive to conservative therapy or are developing congestive heart failure or pulmonary edema. It may also be used to treat patients with symptoms of uremia; intractable or life-threatening electrolyte disturbances, especially hyperkalemia and acidosis; uncontrolled hypertension, particularly if on a volume basis; and to create vascular volume deficits so that parenteral nutrition or high volume parenteral infusion therapy,[71] can be employed. Hemodialysis, hemofiltration, and peritoneal dialysis for infants and children with ARF should be available in pediatric centers.

Hemodialysis is more effective in the treatment of poisoning with dialyzable compounds[72] and in general offers more efficient dialysis and ultrafiltration. However, peritoneal dialysis is less destabilizing and therefore less likely to produce the disequilibrium syndrome or hemodynamic instability. Furthermore, it has been shown to be sufficient for the treatment of ARF in a variety of settings.[73, 74] Moreover, it is simpler to perform. Peritoneal dialysis is relatively contraindicated in patients who have undergone recent abdominal surgery, especially bowel procedures, and it may compromise respiratory function. Other complications include the considerable amount of protein that is lost in the peritoneal dialysate and the high frequency of infection.

Continuous arteriovenous hemofiltration and slow, continuous ultrafiltration are being used with increasing frequency for patients with ARF.[75, 76] These procedures are better tolerated by the more unstable patients than is hemodialysis[77] and can be used when a coexistent contraindication to peritoneal dialysis exists. They are particularly valuable for treatment vascular overload or for creating a vascular deficit in the oliguric patient so that hyperalimentation and medications can be administered intravenously and that hemofiltration can be effectively utilized in infants.[78, 79, 80]

Despite these facts, the arteriovenous extracorporeal circulatory route of continuous arteriovenous hemofiltration in general may be limiting in infants, children, and critically ill patients. The efficiency of these procedures can be limited by arterial cannula core size, actual blood flow, and blood pressure through the extracorporeal circuit. For these reasons, pump-assisted continuous hemofiltration and, particularly, pump-assisted venovenous hemofiltration techniques have evolved. These have been demonstrated to be at least as effective as continuous arteriovenous hemofiltration in both adult and pediatric patients.[81–83] Nonetheless, continuous venovenous hemofiltration remains a technically more difficult procedure and its performance requires specially trained personnel.

COMPLICATIONS

The most common complications of ARF are infection and gastrointestinal hemorrhage. The incidence of infection varies from 11% to 88% and is more common in trauma or surgical patients.[1, 3, 84, 85] Infection is also the leading cause of death in ARF, accounting for one third to two thirds of all mortalities.[1, 85] The most common site of infection is the urinary tract. Reduced urine output and prolonged urinary bladder catheterization are important predisposing factors, followed by septicemia and respiratory infection.[84] The risk of infection can be reduced by the early removal of urinary catheters, meticulous care of intravenous catheters, vigorous respiratory therapy, and avoidance of prophylactic antibiotics.[84] Although bladder catheterization is useful in the early evaluation of the child with ARF, its convenience and diagnostic value must be weighed against the higher risk of infection, particularly when the catheter is kept in place for longer than 3 days. Regular surveillance cultures should be routine for all ARF patients, and proven infections should be treated vigorously, with adjustment of the dose of antibiotics to the state of renal function.

Gastrointestinal hemorrhage occurs in over 20% of adults with ARF and is a leading cause of death.[85] Gastritis and ulcer formation are frequent, occurring most commonly following surgery, major trauma, or head injury. Prophylaxis is difficult owing to the danger of magnesium toxicity from magnesium-containing antacids and to the adverse effects of cimetidine on cerebral function in patients with renal failure.[86]

OUTCOME

Outcome is largely dependent on the underlying condition that produced renal failure. Death is most often attributed to the underlying illness or the major complications of ARF, that is, gastrointestinal hemorrhage and infection. Despite the availability of dialysis and parenteral nutrition, the mortality rate in children developing ARF after surgery ranges from 25% to 70%. Mortality is particularly high when renal perfusion remains markedly reduced by persistently poor cardiac function following open-heart surgery or when prolonged periods of hypotension accompany multiple trauma. Other factors associated with high mortality include young age and a poor nutritional state before development of ARF.[4] Also, the oliguric forms of ARF have a higher morbidity and mortality than do the nonoliguric forms. However, specific definitive predictors of survival in ARF children have not emerged; prompt recognition and differentiation of the various pathophysiologic types of ARF and expeditious therapeutic intervention are therefore vital to reduce mortality and minimize residual renal dysfunction.

The actual long-term adverse consequences of ARF on renal function in patients who do survive ARF are relatively small. Adult patients have been noted to have persistent mild decreases of creatinine clearances.[87, 88] Children recovering from ARF have evidence for some loss of the overall nephron population but generally maintain normal glomerular filtration rates and tubular function.[89]

PREVENTION

The high morbidity and mortality of ARF, particularly after surgery, severe medical illness, or trauma, increase the importance of prophylactic measures. Certain clinical conditions are associated with a relatively high risk of ARF in the pediatric patient. These include preexisting renal insufficiency, diabetes mellitus, and severe dehydration. In these high-risk patients, avoidance of prolonged hypotension and the judicious use of radiographic contrast media, nephrotoxic antibiotics, and other agents known to be associated with nephrotoxicity (i.e., uricosuric agents) minimize the occurrence of ARF.

Considerable controversy exists with respect to therapeutic agents that avert or ameliorate impending ARF. Intravenous mannitol has been purported to reduce the incidence of ARF in high-risk patients and in patients with impending oliguric renal failure. The theoretic benefit of mannitol is based on its actions as a pharmacologically inert osmotic diuretic that can cause a solute diuresis, maintain high urine flow, diminish renin secretion, and reduce endothelial cell swelling. Experimental data suggest that mannitol may maintain the GFR above control values in the hypoperfused kidney, presumably by acting as an intratubular osmotic agent.[90] High-risk clinical conditions such as rhabdomyolysis and myoglobinuria may respond to mannitol administration.[91] Similarly, mannitol has been advocated for patients undergoing cardiac surgery, patients with high serum uric acid levels, and patients receiving nephrotoxic drugs or undergoing radiographic contrast studies. Care must be used in the administration of mannitol to potentially oliguric patients because, in the absence of urinary excretion, mannitol acts as an intravascular volume expander.

Many studies examining the efficacy of high-dose furosemide in the prevention of ARF have demonstrated improved urine flow and decreased duration of dialysis.[92–94] However, care must be taken with its use, since high doses may be ototoxic. Alternatively, low doses of dopamine hydrochloride (5–10 $\mu g \cdot kg^{-1} \cdot min^{-1}$), either alone or combined with furosemide, markedly increase renal blood flow.[95–98]

Thus, although the prevention of high-risk clinical situations is the optimal form of prophylaxis for ARF, the use of furosemide in combination with a low-dose dopamine infusion may be an effective adjunct therapy in the patient with early renal failure. Although the presence of renal failure may not be affected, the conversion of the patient's status from oliguric ARF to nonoliguric ARF simplifies therapy and improves the overall prognosis.

References

1. Hodson EM, Kjellstrand CM, Mauer SM: Acute renal failure in infants and children: Outcome of 53 patients requiring hemodialysis treatment. J Pediatr 1978; 93:756.
2. Griffin NK, McElnea J, Barratt TM: Acute renal failure early in life. Arch Dis Child 1976; 51:459.
3. Chesney RW, Kaplan BS, Freedom RM, et al: Acute renal failure: An important complication of cardiac surgery in infants. J Pediatr 1975; 87:381.
4. Gordillo-Paniagua G, Velasquez-Jones L: Acute renal failure. Pediatr Clin North Am 1976; 23:817.
5. Gokcay G, Emre S, Tanman F, et al: An epidemiological approach to acute renal failure in children. J Trop Pediatr 1991; 37:191.
6. Gokalp AS, Oguz A, Gultekin A: Acute renal failure related to infectious disease in infancy and childhood. Ann Trop Paediatr 1991; 11:119.
7. Greenhill AH, Norman ME, Cornfeld D, et al: Acute renal failure secondary to acute pyelonephritis. Clin Nephrol 1977; 8:400.
8. Lorentz WB, Iskandar S, Browning MC, et al: Acute renal failure due to pyelonephritis. Nephron 1990; 54:256.
9. Ellis D, Fried WA, Yunis EJ: Acute interstitial nephritis in children: A report of 13 cases and review of the literature. Pediatrics 1981; 67:862.
10. Schreiner SE, Maher JF: Toxic nephropathy. Am J Med 1965; 38:409.
11. Coulie P, De Plaen JF, van Ypersele de Strihou C: Captopril-induced acute reversible renal failure. Nephron 1983; 35:108.
12. Dominiczak A, Isles C, Gillen G, et al: Angiotensin-converting enzyme inhibition and renal insuficiency in patients with bilateral renovascular disease. J Hum Hypertens 1988; 2:53.
13. Lau SO, Tkachuck JY, Hasegawa DK, et al: Plasminogen and antithrombin III deficiencies in the childhood nephrotic syndrome associated with plasminogenuria and antithrombinuria. J Pediatr 1980; 96:390.
14. Goldstein MH, Churg J, Strauss L, et al: Hemolytic-uremic syndrome. Nephron 1974; 23:263.
15. Remizzi G, Marchesi D, Mecca G, et al: Hemolytic uremic syndrome: Deficiency of plasma factors regulating prostacyclin activity. Lancet 1978; ii:871.
16. Kaplan BS, Cleary TG, Obrig TG: Recent advances in understanding the pathogenesis of the hemolytic uremic syndrome. Pediatr Nephrol 1990; 4:276.
17. Suki W, Eknoyan G, Rector PC, et al: Patterns of nephron perfusion in acute and chronic hydronephrosis. J Clin Invest 1966; 45:122.
18. Weidner NJ, Guam WE, Chou T-C, et al: Hyperkalemia-electrocardiographic abnormalities. J Pediatr 1978; 93:462.
19. Hartman RC, Mellinkoff SN: The relationship of platelets to the serum potassium concentration. J Clin Invest 1958; 37:699.
20. Massry SG, Arieff AI, Coburn JW, et al: Divalent ion metabolism in patients with acute renal failure: Studies on the mechanism of hypocalcemia. Kidney Int 1974; 5:437.
21. Long S, Gaudio KM, Siegel NJ: Nondialytic treatment of acute renal failure. *In*: Pediatric Kidney Disease. 2nd ed. Edelmann CM Jr (Ed). Boston, Little, Brown and Co, 1992, pp 806.
22. Sanders RC, Menon S, Sanders AD: The complementary uses of nuclear medicine and ultrasound in the kidney. J Urol 1978; 120:521.
23. Schleigel JV, Lang EK: Computed radionuclide urogram for assessing acute renal failure. AJR 1980; 134:129.
24. Mattern W, Staab EV: Imaging studies in renal failure: Emphasis on selection and sequencing in the clinical setting. CRC Rad Nuc Med 1975; 6:459.
25. Schwartz GJ, Haycock GB, Spitzer A: Plasma creatinine and urea concentration in children: Normal values for age and sex. J Pediatr 1976; 88:828.
26. Schwartz GJ, Haycock GB, Edelmann CM, et al: A simple estimate of glomerular filtration rate in children derived from body length and plasma creatinine. Pediatrics 1976; 58:259.
27. Counahan CC, Ghazali S, Kirkwood B, et al: Estimation of glomerular filtration rate from plasma creatinine concentration in children. Arch Dis Child 1976; 51:875.
28. Evans GO, Griffiths PD: Limitations concerning the use in children of the relationship between plasma creatinine and body height to derive glomerular filtration rate. Ann Clin Biochem 1981; 18:295.
29. Hallynck T, Soep HH, Thomas J, et al: Prediction of creatinine clearance from serum creatinine concentration based on lean body mass. Clin Pharmacol Ther 1981; 30:414.
30. Orecklin JR, Brosman SA: Current concepts in the diagnosis of acute renal failure. J Urol 1972; 107:892.
31. Joekes AM, Mowbray JF, Dormandy K: Oliguria with urine of fixed specific gravity. Lancet 1957; ii:864.
32. Swann RC, Merrill JP: The clinical course of acute renal failure. Medicine 1953; 32:215.
33. Handa SP, Morrin PA: Diagnostic indices in acute renal failure. Can Med Assoc J 1967; 96:78.
34. Espinal CH: The FE Na test: Use in the differential diagnosis of acute renal failure. JAMA 1976; 236:579.
35. Kennedy AC: Acute renal failure and the anesthetist. Proc Soc Med 1968; 6:1165.
36. Perlmutter M, Grossman SL, Rothenberg S, et al: Urine-serum urea nitrogen ratio: Simple test of renal function in acute azotemia and oliguria. JAMA 1959; 170:1533.
37. Werb R, Linton AL: Aetiology, diagnosis, treatment and prognosis of acute renal failure in an intensive care unit. Resuscitation 1979; 7:95.
38. Figdor PP, Holtl G, Zinnbauer B: Diagnostic differentiation between advanced functional and acute organic renal failure. Int Urol Nephrol 1972; 4:71.
39. Heimann T, Brau S, Sakurai H, et al: Urinary osmolal changes in renal dysfunction following open heart operations. Ann Thorac Surg 1976; 22:44.
40. Banister A, Hatcher GW: Renal tubular and papillary necrosis after dehydration in infancy. Arch Dis Child 1973; 48:36.
41. Miller TR, Anderson RJ, Linas SL, et al: Urinary diagnostic indices in acute renal failure. A prospective study. Ann Intern Med 1978; 89:47.
42. Espinal CH, Gregory AW: Differential diagnosis of acute renal failure. Clin Nephrol 1980; 13:73.
43. Zarich S, Fang LST, Diamond JR: Fractional excretion of sodium: Exceptions to its diagnostic value. Arch Intern Med 1985; 145:108.
44. Brown R, Babcock R, Talbert J, et al: Renal function in critically ill postoperative patients: Sequential assessments of creatinine, osmolar, and free water clearance. Crit Care Med 1980; 8:68.
45. Mathew OP, Jones AS, James E, et al: Neonatal renal failure: Usefulness of diagnostic indices. Pediatrics 1980; 65:57.
46. Anderson RJ, Linas SL, Berna AS, et al: Non-oliguric acute renal failure. N Engl J Med 1977; 296:1134.
47. Siegel SR, Oh W: Renal function as a marker of human fetal maturation. Acta Pediatr Scand 1976; 65:481.
48. Engelke SC, Shah BL, Vasan U, et al: Sodium balance in very low-birth-weight infants. J Pediatr 1978; 93:837.
49. Anand SK: Acute renal failure in the neonate. Pediatr Clin North Am 1982; 29:791.
50. Ellis EN, Arnold WC: Use of urinary indexes in renal failure in the newborn. Am J Dis Child 1982; 136:615.
51. Eliahou HE, Bata A: The diagnosis of acute renal failure. Nephron 1965; 2:287.
52. Baek SM, Brown RS, Shoemaker WC: Early prediction of acute renal failure and recovery: I. Sequential measurements of free water clearance. Ann Surg 1973; 177:253.
53. Landes RG, Lillehei RC, Lindsay WG, et al: Free-water clearance and the early recognition of acute renal insufficiency after cardiopulmonary bypass. Ann Thorac Surg 1976; 22:41.
54. Baek SM, Makabali GG, Brown RS, et al: Free-water clearance patterns as predictors and therapeutic guides in acute renal failure. Surgery 1975; 77:632.
55. Shin B, Isenhower NM, McAslan TC, et al: Early recognition of

renal insufficiency in post-anesthetic trauma victims. Anesthesiology 1979; 50:262.
56. Stokes JM: Diagnostic indices and postoperative renal failure. Arch Surg 1968; 97:291.
57. Lindsay RM, Linton AL, Longland CJ: Assessment of postoperative renal function. Lancet 1965; 8:978.
58. Levinsky NG: The interpretation of proteinuria and the urinary sediment. DM 1967; 3:40.
59. Finckh ES, Jeremy D, Whyte HM: Structural renal damage and its relation to clinical features in acute oliguric renal failure. Q J Med 1962; 31:429.
60. Wilson DM, Turner DR, Cameron JS, et al: Value of renal biopsy in acute intrinsic renal failure. Br Med J 1976; 2:459.
61. Nobel RE, Brainerd HD: Urine and serum lysozyme alterations in a case of acute renal failure. J Urol 1966; 96:852.
62. Zager RA, Carpenter CB: Radioimmunoassay for urinary renal tubular antigen: A potential marker of tubular injury. Kidney Int 1978; 13:505.
63. Garcia-Palmieri MR: Reversal of hyperkalemic cardiotoxicity with hypertonic saline. Am Heart J 1962; 64:483.
64. Allon M, Copkney C: Albuterol and insulin for treatment of hyperkalemia in hemodialysis patients. Kidney Int 1990; 38:869.
65. Fleisher DS: Cation exchange resin therapy for hyperkalemia in infants and children. J Pediatr 1961; 58:486.
66. Feinstein EI, Blumenkrantz MJ, Healy M, et al: Clinical and metabolic responses to parenteral nutrition in acute renal failure. Medicine 1981; 60:124.
67. Leonard CD, Luke G, Siegel RR: Parenteral essential amino acids in acute renal failure. Urology 1975; 6:154.
68. Baek S, Makabali GG, Bryan-Brown CW, et al: The influence of parenteral nutrition on the course of acute renal failure. Surg Gynecol Obstet 1975; 141:405.
69. Abel RM, Beck CH, Abbott WM, et al: Improved survival from acute renal failure after treatment with intravenous essential L-amino acids and glucose. N Engl J Med 1973; 288:695.
70. Schrier RW, Gambertoglio JG: Handbook of Drug Therapy in Liver and Kidney Disease. Boston, Little, Brown and Co, 1991.
71. Kuttnig M, Zobel G, Ring E, et al: Nitrogen and amino acid balance during total parenteral nutrition and continuous arteriovenous hemofiltration in critically ill anuric children. Child Nephrol Urol 1991; 11:74.
72. Winchester JF: Active methods for detoxification. *In*: Clinical Management of Poisoning and Drug Overdosage. 2nd ed. Haddad LM, Winchester JF (Eds). Philadelphia, WB Saunders, 1990, p 148.
73. Reznik VM, Griswold WR, Peterson BM, et al: Peritoneal dialysis for acute renal failure in children. Pediatr Nephrol 1991; 5:715.
74. Giuffre RM, Tam KH, Williams WW, et al: Acute renal failure complicating pediatric cardiac surgery: A comparison of survivors and nonsurvivors following acute peritoneal dialysis. Pediatr Cardiol 1992; 13:208.
75. Golper TA: Continuous arteriovenous hemofiltration in acute renal failure. Am J Kid Dis 1985; 6:373.
76. Paganini EP, Nakamoto S: Continuous slow ultrafiltration in oliguric acute renal failure. Trans Am Soc Artif Intern Organs 1980; 26:201.
77. Bellomo R, Mansfield D, Rumble S, et al: Acute renal failure in critical illness: Conventional dialysis versus acute continuous hemodiafiltration. ASAIO J 1992; 38:M654.
78. Lieberman KV, Nardi L, Bosch JP: Treatment of acute renal failure in an infant using continuous arteriovenous hemofiltration. J Pediatr 1985; 106:646.
79. Zobel G, Kuttnig M, Ring E: Continuous arteriovenous hemodialysis in critically ill infants. Child Nephrol Urol 1990; 10:196.
80. Continuous arteriovenous hemofiltration after cardiac operations in infants and children. J Thorac Cardiovasc Surg 1992; 104:1225.
81. Zobel G, Ring E, Kuttnig M, et al: Five years' experience with continuous extracorporeal renal support in paediatric intensive care. Intensive Care Med 1991; 17:315.
82. Macias WL, Mueller BA, Scarim SK, et al: Continuous venovenous hemofiltration: An alternative to continuous arteriovenous hemofiltration and hemodiafiltration in acute renal failure. Am J Kidney Dis 1991; 18:451.
83. Storck M, Hartl WH, Zimmerer E, et al: Comparison of pump-driven and spontaneous continuous haemofiltration in postoperative acute renal failure. Lancet 1991; 337:452.
84. Zech P, Bouletreau R, Moskoutchenko JR, et al: Infection in acute renal failure. Adv Nephrol 1971; 1:231.
85. Kleinknecht D, Junges P, Chanard J, et al: Factors influencing immediate prognosis in acute renal failure, with special reference to prophylactic hemodialysis. Adv Nephrol 1971; 1:207.
86. Schentag JJ, Cerra FB, Calleri G, et al: Pharmacokinetic and clinical studies in patients with cimetidine-associated mental confusion. Lancet 1979; i:177.
87. Finkenstaedt JT, Merrill JP: Renal functional studies in acute tubular necrosis. Clin Sci 1950; 9:379.
88. Fox M: Progressive renal fibrosis following acute tubular necrosis: An experimental study. J Urol 1967; 97:196.
89. Georgaki-Angelaki HN, Steed DB, Chantler C, et al: Renal function following acute renal failure in childhood: A long-term follow-up study. Kidney Int 1989; 35:84.
90. Morris CR, Alexander EA, Bruns SJ, et al: Restoration and maintenance of glomerular filtration by mannitol during hypoperfusion of the kidney. J Clin Invest 1972; 51:1555.
91. Eneas JF, Schoenfeld PY, Humphreys MH: The effect of infusion of mannitol-sodium bicarbonate on the clinical course of myoglobinuria. Arch Intern Med 1979; 139:801.
92. Borirakchanyavat D, Dongsthongsri M, Sitprija D: Furosemide and acute renal failure. Postgrad Med J 1978; 54:30.
93. Cantarovich F, Galli C, Benedetti L, et al: High dose furosemide in established acute renal failure. Br Med J 1973; 4:449.
94. Prandota J: High doses of furosemide in children with acute renal failure: A preliminary retrospective study. Int Urol Nephrol 1991; 23:383.
95. Henderson IS, Beattie TJ, Kennedy AC: Dopamine hydrochloride in oliguric states. Lancet 1980; ii:827.
96. Lindner A, Cutler RE, Goodman WG, et al: Synergism of dopamine plus furosemide in preventing acute renal failure in the dog. Kidney Int 1979; 16:158.
97. Davis RF, Lappas DG, Kirklin JK, et al: Acute oliguria after cardiopulmonary bypass: Renal functional improvement with low-dose dopamine infusion. Crit Care Med 1982; 10:852.
98. Graziani G, Cantaluppi A, Casati S, et al: Dopamine and furosemide in oliguric acute renal failure. Nephron 1984; 37:39.

METABOLISM AND PHARMACOLOGY

Bart Chernow

CHAPTER 118

Thyroid Emergencies*

Robert C. Smallridge, MD, FACP

Patients with hyperthyroidism and hypothyroidism are usually treated as outpatients. However, when hyperthyroidism is severe, is associated with other medical illnesses, or reaches a state of decompensation (thyroid storm), then intensive inpatient management is indicated. Similarly, patients who develop profound hypothyroidism or myxedema coma benefit from being treated in the critical care environment. Furthermore, patients may be euthyroid but need specialized care because they have an anatomic enlargement of the thyroid gland that has created an emergency.

Aside from the bona fide conditions of thyroid hormone excess and deficiency, a common problem encountered in acutely ill patients is a constellation of thyroid blood test abnormalities. This condition is referred to as *nonthyroidal illness* or *euthyroid sick syndrome*,[1, 2] and hormone replacement therapy for it is not generally recommended.[3] However, the literature suggests that in certain circumstances thyroid hormone therapy may be beneficial; the current status of this controversy is described in this chapter.

THYROID PHYSIOLOGY

An overview of the brain-hypothalamic-pituitary-thyroid axis is depicted in Figure 118–1. The dominant influence controlling thyroid hormone secretion is the pituitary hormone thyrotropin (TSH), a glycoprotein that is under both positive and negative feedback regulation. Thyrotropin-releasing hormone is principally responsible for stimulating the secretion of TSH, whereas estrogen has a minor positive effect, enhancing the TSH response to thyrotropin-releasing hormone. The thyroid hormones thyroxine (T_4) and triiodothyronine (T_3) play an essential role in the negative feedback inhibition of TSH secretion. In addition, several other hormones, including cortisol (and other glucocorticoids), dopamine, and somatostatin, all inhibit TSH release.

TSH, by acting through a plasma membrane receptor on thyroid follicular cells, stimulates iodide uptake and thyroid hormone synthesis and secretion. Under certain conditions, patients with autoimmune thyroid disease develop circulating immunoglobulins that can affect thyroid function by binding to the TSH receptor. These proteins (TSH-receptor antibodies) can produce hyperthyroidism (Graves' disease). Alternatively, some antibodies bind to the TSH receptor without causing stimulation, and these may produce hypothyroidism.

Under normal circumstances, TSH maintains circulating levels of T_4 and T_3 within a narrow physiologic range. All of the T_4 is produced and secreted by the thyroid gland. This amounts to about 90 μg per day. However, only approximately 20% of circulating T_3 is manufactured by the thyroid gland; the rest is derived from deiodination by the enzyme 5′-deiodinase. This process occurs in many peripheral tissues, especially those of the liver and kidney. Other pathways of metabolic degradation of thyroxine exist,[4] and it has been suggested that sulfation may play a prominent role in critically ill individuals.[5]

Thyroid hormones circulate bound to three proteins (T_4-binding globulin, transthyretin, and albumin). The amount of T_4 circulating in its unbound form is only 0.03%, and that

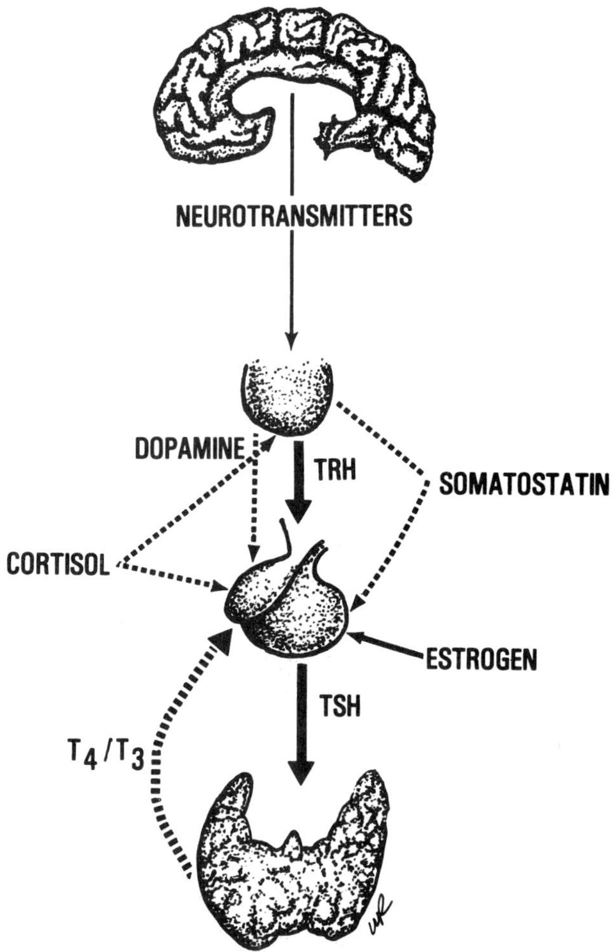

Figure 118–1. Schematic drawing of the hypothalamic-pituitary-thyroid axis and its hormonal control. *Solid lines* indicate a positive influence, and *dashed lines* represent a negative influence. The width of a line represents the relative importance of the effect. *Abbreviations:* TRH = thyrotropin (TSH)–releasing hormone; T_4 = thyroxine; T_3 = triiodothyronine. (From Smallridge RC: Thyrotropin-secreting pituitary tumors. Endocrinol Metab Clin North Am 1987; 16:766.)

*The opinions or assertions contained in this chapter are the private views of the author and are not to be construed as official or as reflecting the views of the Department of the Army or of the Department of Defense.

of T_3 is but 0.3%. Nevertheless, it is only this extremely small fraction of hormone (especially of T_3) that is transported into cells and is responsible for the myriad biologic responses influenced by thyroid hormones.

THYROID FUNCTION TESTS

Thyroid hormones affect virtually every tissue and organ system in the body, and the symptoms and signs elicited by their excess or deficiency are numerous. Unfortunately, none of the symptoms or signs is specific for thyroid disease; thus, clinical examination, although an important element of any evaluation, is not diagnostic of thyroid dysfunction. In the setting of severe illness, the accurate diagnosis of thyroid disease can be difficult. Thyroid function tests, especially measurements of serum hormones, are an essential element in the decision-making process.

The selection of appropriate available tests, in conjunction with an appreciation of the multiple variables that can confound their interpretation in hospitalized patients, can simplify the testing procedure. Even so, pitfalls await the skilled clinician. An overview of commonly ordered tests and of the directional changes observed in various diseases is given in Table 118–1. The total T_4 level has been used for more than two decades. Since almost all of the T_4 measured in this assay is protein bound, factors altering the quantity, affinity, or capacity of these proteins elevate or lower the T_4 value and mislead the physician into thinking that a patient is either hyperthyroid or hypothyroid. This difficulty has been avoided by simultaneously performing an in vitro test (the T_3 uptake test) and then by deriving a free T_4 index. The latter correlates well with the "gold standard" thyroid test, the measurement of free T_4 (measured by equilibrium dialysis). Measurement of free T_4 traditionally has not been readily available because of its involved cost and time factors. Unfortunately, the free T_4 index is not always reliable in the setting of critical illness, and in response diagnostic products companies have produced many kit assays designed to measure free T_4 levels. Several assays that appear to be reliable in measuring thyroid function in critically ill patients have been reported in the literature.[6] Additional experience with these kits is eagerly awaited.

A serum T_3 determination is not helpful in evaluating hospitalized patients suspected of being hypothyroid, because inhibition of 5′-deiodinase activity results in low T_3 levels in euthyroid persons afflicted with a variety of medical or surgical disorders.[1, 2] Documentation of an increased total or free T_4 level is usually sufficient to support a diagnosis of hyperthyroidism. In some cases, T_4 level is normal, and one must demonstrate a high T_3 level (a condition known as *T_3 toxicosis*). A reverse T_3 level may be helpful—this hormone's level is low in patients with hypothyroidism but elevated in those with nonthyroidal illness. The reason for the increase in reverse T_3 is that the enzyme that converts T_4 to T_3 also is responsible for the degradation of reverse T_3.

Measurements of serum TSH also are valuable. TSH is suppressed in all patients with hyperthyroidism except for those with the rare disorders of thyroid hormone resistance and TSH-secreting pituitary tumors. An elevation of TSH is diagnostic of primary hypothyroidism. However, in critical illness, TSH levels may be partially suppressed, and some patients with hypothyroidism have values within the normal range. The mechanism may include the effects of increased endogenous cortisol or of the administration of steroids or dopamine, or both, to such patients.

THYROTOXICOSIS AND THYROID STORM

Thyrotoxicosis is present whenever excess amounts of thyroid hormones are circulating in the bloodstream. When the underlying process is overproduction and secretion of hormone by the thyroid gland, then hyperthyroidism exists.

Pathophysiology

Numerous organ systems are affected. The cardiovascular system is subject to many changes, including an increase in heart rate, stroke volume, cardiac output, and cardiac contractility. Peripheral vascular resistance is reduced.[7, 8] Changes in the respiratory system include tachypnea, a reduction in vital capacity, diffusing capacity, and lung compliance in combination with an increase in the ventilatory responses to hypercapnia and hypoxia.[9] Muscle weakness accounts at least in part for these disturbances.[10] Gastrointestinal function is enhanced,[11, 12] with a shortening of intestinal transit time, an increase in duodenal basal electrical activity, and, at times, a secretory diarrhea. The central nervous system is subject to an increase in catecholamine turnover and an increase in receptor sensitivity to neurotransmitters.

Clinical Presentation

The symptoms and signs of the typical case of hyperthyroidism reflect the enhancing influence of excessive amounts of thyroid hormone on the function of many organs (Table 118–2). At times, one system may predominate; that is, a patient may be referred to a cardiologist because of tachyarrhythmias, to a pulmonologist because of dyspnea, to a rheumatologist because of myopathy, to a gastroenterologist because of diarrhea, or to a dermatologist because of severe pruritus. Older patients may have a paucity of symptoms and signs, with thyroid enlargement frequently being absent.[13, 14]

A patient may require hospitalization because of compli-

TABLE 118–1. Serum Thyroid Hormone Tests in Health and Disease

	Total T_4	*T_3U*	*FT_4 Index*	*Free T_4*	*T_3*	*rT_3*	*TSH*
Euthyroid	N	N	N	N	N	N	N
Hyperthyroid	↑	↑	↑	↑	↑	↑	↓
Hypothyroid	↓	↓	↓	↓	N, ↓	↓	↑
TBG excess	↑	↓	N	N	↑	↑	N
TBG deficiency	↓	↑	N	N, ↓	↓	↓	N
Nonthyroidal illness	N, ↓	↑	N, ↓	↑,N, ↓	↓	↑	N, ↓
FDH	↑	N	↑	N	N	N	N

(Reprinted with permission from Smallridge RC: Metabolic and anatomic thyroid emergencies: A review. Crit Care Med 1992; 20:276. © Williams & Wilkins, 1992.)

Abbreviations: TBG = Thyroxine-binding globulin; FDH = familial dysalbuminemic hyperthyroxinemia; T_3U = T_3 uptake; FT_4 = free T_4; rT_3 = reverse T_3; N = normal; ↑ = increased; ↓ = decreased.

TABLE 118–2. Symptoms and Signs of Thyrotoxicosis and Thyrotoxic Crisis

Thyrotoxicosis	*Crisis*
Neuromuscular	*Neuromuscular*
Emotional lability	Agitation
Short attention span	Emotional lability
Tremor	Apathy
Weakness	Delirium
Periodic paralysis	Seizures
	Coma
Cardiovascular	*Cardiovascular*
Tachycardia	Congestive heart failure
Systolic hypertension	Arrhythmias
Atrial fibrillation	
Thermoregulation	*Thermoregulation*
Warm, moist skin	Fever
Heat intolerance	
Gastrointestinal	*Gastrointestinal*
Hyperdefecation	Vomiting
	Diarrhea
	Jaundice
Nutritional	*Nutritional*
Increased appetite	Severe weight loss
Weight loss	Vitamin deficiencies

cations arising from his or her hyperthyroid state. Older patients frequently develop atrial fibrillation, with incidences of approximately 30% to 40%.[13, 14] Significant cardiovascular events include congestive heart failure, unstable angina, and myocardial infarction (even in patients with normal coronary arteries). Other less common arrhythmias include complete heart block and ventricular arrhythmias, which can be lethal. A variety of neurologic conditions such as stroke, myasthenia gravis, periodic paralysis, seizures, and myopathies may also prompt hospital admission.[15] Pregnant women with hyperemesis gravidarum may develop increases of both total and free T_4 and T_3 levels; interestingly, these abnormalities usually resolve spontaneously.[16]

The most dangerous complication of hyperthyroidism is a state of systemic decompensation known as *thyroid storm.*[16a] The hallmarks of this life-threatening disorder include fever, cardiac dysfunction (arrhythmias, congestive heart failure), and neurologic changes ranging from agitation and restlessness to confusion, disorientation, delirium, seizures, and coma. Thyroid storm develops in the setting of untreated or undertreated hyperthyroidism and is associated with some precipitating event. Situations known to trigger this critical condition include surgery; infections and other acute medical illnesses; trauma; labor and delivery; and emotional stress. It is imperative that an initiating factor be carefully sought for and corrected.

Differential Diagnosis

Thyrotoxicosis is suspected when blood tests show an elevated free T_4 index or free T_4. An assortment of conditions collectively referred to as *euthyroid hyperthyroxinemia*[17] must be distinguished from thyrotoxicosis (Table 118–3). Individuals with euthyroid hyperthyroxinemia are clinically euthyroid, and a carefully taken history and observations on physical examination should suggest the correct diagnosis. Occasionally, thyrotoxicosis is suspected clinically, but the serum T_4 level is normal. When this scenario arises, a determination of serum T_3 level should be ordered, as T_3-toxicosis may be present.

TABLE 118–3. Differential Diagnosis of Euthyroid Hyperthyroxinemia

- Alterations in thyroid hormone/plasma protein binding
  - Inherited
    - TBG excess
    - TBPA excess
    - Familial dysalbuminemic hyperthyroxinemia
  - Acquired
    - Nonthyroidal illness
      - Liver disease
      - Acute intermittent porphyria
      - Estrogen secreting tumors
    - Drugs
      - Narcotics (e.g., methadone, heroin)
      - Oral contraceptives
      - Perphenazine
      - 5-Fluorouracil
      - Clofibrate
    - Physiologic (pregnancy)
    - T_4 autoantibodies
- Transient hyperthyroxinemia
  - Acute medical illness
  - Acute psychiatric disease
  - Hyperemesis gravidarum
- Drug-induced hyperthyroxinemia
  - Amiodarone
  - Iodinated contrast agents (e.g., ipodate, iopanoate)
  - Heparin
- Thyroid hormone resistance (generalized)

(Reprinted with permission from Smallridge RC: Metabolic and anatomic thyroid emergencies: A review. Crit Care Med 1992; 20:276. © Williams & Wilkins, 1992.)
Abbreviation: TBPA = Thyroxine-binding prealbumin.

The most reliable test for distinguishing between hyperthyroidism and all other causes of thyrotoxicosis is the radioactive iodine uptake test. Table 118–4 indicates how this test can narrow the differential diagnosis. Graves' disease is the most common cause of hyperthyroidism and is associated with an undetectable serum TSH level. Toxic multinodular goiter is less common in the United States than in other countries. Although symptoms are often less pronounced than in Graves' disease, older patients are susceptible to the development of complications (especially if they receive an

TABLE 118–4. Differential Diagnosis of Thyrotoxicosis

- Increased RAIU
  - Diffuse hyperplasia (Graves' disease)
  - Toxic multinodular goiter
  - Solitary autonomous nodule
  - Neonatal thyrotoxicosis
  - Syndromes of inappropriate TSH secretion
    - TSH tumors
    - Thyroid hormone resistance (central)
  - Trophoblastic tumor
- Decreased RAIU
  - Destructive thyroiditis
    - Subacute (viral)
    - Postpartum (autoimmune)
    - Painless, nonpostpartum
  - Iodine-induced (e.g., amiodarone)
  - Thyrotoxicosis factitia
  - Metastatic thyroid carcinoma
  - Struma ovarii

(Reprinted with permission from Smallridge RC: Metabolic and anatomic thyroid emergencies: A review. Crit Care Med 1992; 20:276. © Williams & Wilkins, 1992.)
Abbreviation: RAIU = radioactive iodine uptake.

iodine load, as may occur when diagnostic radiographic dye studies are performed). Inappropriate TSH secreting disorders,[18–20] although uncommon, are being recognized much more often than in the past owing to the advent of sensitive TSH assays. Patients with these disorders usually do not present with such acute disease that hospitalization is likely. Neonatal thyrotoxicosis, due to transplacental transfer of maternal thyroid-stimulating immunoglobulins, occurs in the offspring of fewer than 1% of women with a history of Graves' disease. It should be suspected in any pregnant woman with such a history, even if her hyperthyroidism had been treated years previously. Newborns with this illness may develop heart failure and thus require careful observation until the condition resolves over several weeks to months after birth.

Most causes of low radioactive iodine uptake thyrotoxicosis do not produce illness of such severity that hospitalization is necessary. However, accidental or suicidal ingestion of large amounts of thyroid hormone can be quite serious.[21] Similarly, patients who develop drug-induced thyrotoxicosis (e.g., that caused by iodine or amiodarone) may have life-threatening disease.[22]

Therapy

Management of patients with uncomplicated hyperthyroidism of mild to moderate severity can be accomplished on an outpatient basis. Patients are usually rendered euthyroid with antithyroid drugs (either methimazole or propylthiouracil). Adrenergic symptoms can be controlled initially with β-blocker therapy. Approximately one third of patients with Graves' disease may go into long-term remission after a year of antithyroid drug treatment. Individuals with small goiters (<40 g) and a short duration of symptoms (<6 months) are more likely to respond. Thyroid ablation, preferably with iodine-131 but occasionally with surgical thyroidectomy, is quite effective not only for patients with Graves' disease but also for those with nodular diseases. Thyroid ablation is *not* recommended for the syndromes of TSH secretion; proper therapy should focus on decreasing TSH secretion.

Patients with severe hyperthyroidism may benefit from a period of hospitalization. Restricted activity, ensurance of compliance with medications, and education may promote recovery. Certainly, anyone who manifests confounding medical problems may need to be admitted to a hospital. It is important to remember that the metabolism of some drugs is enhanced by hyperthyroidism. Specifically, digoxin[23] and adrenergic blockers[24] may be required in larger than usual doses, and patients should be carefully monitored for side effects.

Once euthyroidism is attained, atrial fibrillation often spontaneously converts to sinus rhythm. Nakazawa and coworkers[25] found this to be true in 62% of 163 patients. In most individuals, conversion occurred within 3 weeks of euthyroidism, and never after 4 months. Therefore, elective cardioversion is recommended if atrial fibrillation persists for more than 16 weeks. Some studies have recommended anticoagulation for patients with thyrotoxic atrial fibrillation to reduce the likelihood of a cerebrovascular accident. However, Petersen and Hansen[26] retrospectively evaluated 610 patients with untreated thyrotoxicosis, of whom 91 had atrial fibrillation; they found that age, but not atrial fibrillation, was a significant risk factor for the development of stroke.

The most severe form of hyperthyroidism, thyroid storm, should always be managed in the intensive care unit. Table 118–5 outlines the recommended approach. General supportive measures are essential in the overall scheme. Fever reduction decreases metabolic demands and also the per cent of free T_4. Since salicylates may affect the binding of thyroid hormones to plasma proteins, acetaminophen is the preferred antipyretic. Nicoloff[27] has advocated the use of chlorpromazine and meperidine to prevent the shivering response.

Large fluid losses due to sweating, vomiting, and diarrhea need to be aggressively replaced with fluids and electrolyte solutions. Glucose and vitamins are also important, as these patients have been catabolic for a prolonged period of time. Hemodynamic monitoring may be required, since heart failure (including high output) may be present. As noted above, higher doses of digoxin may be needed, and β-blockers should be used with caution.

Pharmacologic intervention is essential and should be approached in several ways. Antithyroid drugs should be given initially and frequently to prevent further thyroid hormone synthesis. Either propylthiouracil or methimazole can be given orally or crushed and delivered by nasogastric tube. Rectal delivery of methimazole has also been reported.[28]

Inhibition of the release of T_4 and T_3 acutely from the thyroid gland is of utmost importance and has traditionally been accomplished with either a saturated solution of potassium iodide or sodium iodide. This therapy works immediately and is effective for several weeks. It must be remembered that an initial dose of antithyroid drug must be given *before* the first dose of iodide because administration of iodide to an unblocked thyroid gland can worsen a patient's status. Lithium can also be used, but this drug's side effects limit its popularity. If lithium is used, its blood levels must be monitored and maintained within a range of 0.5 to 1.5 mmol/L.

A third means of improving the clinical condition in thyroid storm is to inhibit conversion of T_4 to T_3. The most effective agent, and one which has been studied extensively, is ipodate sodium (Oragrafin). In one study, patients' serum T_3 levels fell by 73% within 1 day and remained at this level for almost 6 months with continued daily ipodate sodium therapy.[29] Caution in its long-term use is advised, since escape from its beneficial effects has been reported.[30] An additional acute effect of this drug is inhibition of hormone secretion, since it contains large amounts of iodide. Propylthiouracil and glucocorticoids may block conversion of T_4 to T_3 and have an additive effect when combined.[31]

Reduction of the hyperadrenergic state is desired, and β-blocker therapy is quite effective in this regard. Propranolol has been favored for many years, in part because it has been shown to inhibit conversion of T_4 to T_3 in hyperthyroid patients. It should be noted that some severely hyperthyroid individuals with cardiac disease maintain their cardiac output by increasing their heart rate. Injudicious use of a β-blocker could precipitate heart failure.[32] The short-acting β_1-blocker esmolol has been used in several patients with thyrotoxic crisis[33] and may offer some advantage over propranolol for two reasons: (1) it is a more cardioselective antagonist and (2) its biologic effects dissipate more rapidly. Two loading doses may be needed, and maintenance doses of up to 350 $\mu g \cdot kg^{-1} \cdot min^{-1}$ have been used.

The last management option involves T_4 removal. Occasional reports have demonstrated the efficacy of plasmapheresis and hemoperfusion.[34, 35] In a few Graves' disease patients who developed thyrotoxic crisis while receiving medical therapy, immediate surgical thyroidectomy has been shown to be successful.[36] Hopefully, with aggressive management as outlined above, these latter approaches need be entertained only rarely.

TABLE 118–5. Management of Decompensated Hyperthyroidism (Thyroid Crisis)

Management	*Route of Administration*
General measures	
Antipyresis	
Acetaminophen	PO
Cooling blankets	
Blockade of central nervous system thermoregulatory centers	IV
Hydration: fluids, electrolytes	IV
Nutrition: glucose, vitamins	IV
Antibiotics	IV
Cardiac therapy	IV, PO
Specific measures	
Inhibition of T_4 synthesis	
PTU: 200–400 mg PO every 6 h	PO, NG
MMI: 20–40 mg PO every 6 h	PO, NG, rectal
Inhibition of T_4 release	
Iodides	
SSKI: 5 drops every 6 h	PO
NaI 1–2 g	IV
Lithium: 300–900 mg/d	PO
Sodium ipodate (see below)	PO
Inhibition of conversion of T_4 to T_3	
PTU	PO, NG
Sodium ipodate: 0.5–1.0 g/d	PO
Glucocorticoids (dexamethasone, 2 mg every 6 h)	IV, PO
Propranolol (see below)	IV, PO
Inhibition of adrenergic effects	
Propranolol: 1.0 mg (IV); 40–120 mg every 6 h (PO)	IV, PO
Esmolol: 500-μg/kg loading dose over 1 min; then, 50–200 μg/kg per minute	IV
T_4 removal	
Plasmapheresis	
Dialysis	
Hemoperfusion	
Bile salt–binding resins	

(Reprinted with permission from Smallridge RC: Metabolic and anatomic thyroid emergencies: A review. Crit Care Med 1992; 20:276. © Williams & Wilkins, 1992.)

Abbreviations: PO = oral; IV = intravenous; NG = nasogastric; PTU = propylthiouracil; MMI = methimazole; SSKI = saturated solution of potassium iodide; NaI = sodium iodide.

Most forms of thyrotoxicosis associated with a low radioactive iodine uptake do not pose a medical emergency. Two that do are thyrotoxicosis factitia and iodine-induced thyrotoxicosis. Factitious disease is usually brought on accidentally in children and as the result of suicide attempt in adults. Emesis and gastric lavage should be instituted acutely. Beta-blockers and barbiturates have been recommended for management of tachycardia and for sedation. Other reported therapies have included plasmapheresis, steroid therapy, and treatment with iopanoic acid.[21] Bile acid sequestrants have also been employed.[37]

Patients receiving large doses of iodine-containing compounds chronically, such as asthmatics or cardiac patients (of the latter, those taking amiodarone), may develop severe hyperthyroidism up to the point of thyroid storm. This can pose difficult management problems because the body stores of iodine may remain elevated for months. Surgery has been used successfully when medical therapy does not control the disease.[38]

HYPOTHYROIDISM AND MYXEDEMA COMA

Hypothyroidism can be either primary (thyroid gland failure) or secondary (due to pituitary insufficiency). Primary hypothyroidism is most commonly the result of an autoimmune destruction of the thyroid gland (autoimmune thyroiditis, or Hashimoto's disease). Thyroid disease is 5- to 10-fold more common in women than in men, and the incidence of symptomatic disease increases with age. Above the age of 60 years, approximately 5% of women become hypothyroid. Because hypothyroidism develops gradually and because many of the symptoms are attributed to advancing age, the diagnosis is frequently delayed. Other causes of primary thyroid insufficiency include ablation (with iodine ^{131}I or surgery) and the use of certain drugs (e.g., lithium and diphenylhydantoin). Amiodarone can produce hypothyroidism as well as hyperthyroidism.

Secondary hypothyroidism is much less common than primary hypothyroidism. The most likely cause would be a pituitary tumor, but hypothalamic injury (meningiomas, infiltrative diseases such as sarcoidosis or tuberculosis) or carotid artery aneurysms occasionally produce hypothyroidism. In all of these situations, careful attention should be devoted to determination of the possible existence of other pituitary hormone deficiencies.

Pathophysiology

Hypothyroidism alters the function of many organs, generally in a fashion opposite to that of hyperthyroidism.[15] The cardiovascular system responds with bradycardia and a reduction in stroke volume, cardiac index and contractility, and oxygen consumption as well as with an increase in peripheral vascular resistance.[7] Pulmonary changes include hypoventilation and an impaired hypoxemic and hypercapnic ventilatory drive as well as muscle weakness and obstructive sleep apnea.[39, 40] These abnormalities may lead to acute hypercapnic respiratory failure. Central nervous system changes involve a decrease in oxygen and glucose utilization, a reduction in cerebral blood flow, and an increase in cerebrovascular resistance. The kidneys may have impaired renal water excretion, and the intestinal tract may manifest impaired motility. Anemia—both physiologic (from reduced oxygen demands) and secondary (both iron deficiency and megaloblastic) is common. Myopathic changes are frequent, and peripheral and cranial nerve neuropathies have been reported.

Clinical Presentation

Symptoms and signs commonly observed in hypothyroidism are listed in Table 118–6. Additionally, hypothyroidism may present as other common illnesses such as heart failure, intestinal pseudo-obstruction, bleeding disorder (an acquired von Willebrand's abnormality), anemia, or cerebrovascular disease.[41, 42]

The most severe presentation of hypothyroidism is myxedema coma, with or without respiratory failure.[42a] This condition usually follows exposure to an external stress. Precipitating events include infections, surgery, trauma, injudicious use of oxygen, or a variety of acute medical illnesses. Use of medications, especially sedatives and hypnotics, can produce a decompensated state in older hypothyroid patients. The condition is more likely to occur in the winter, since hypothermia is also a triggering factor.

Differential Diagnosis

The diagnosis of primary hypothyroidism is readily made when a patient's serum TSH concentration is elevated and his or her T_4 level is low or low normal. Difficulty arises when a total T_4 value is below normal, but the TSH is within the normal range. In the outpatient setting, the possibilities include a protein binding abnormality and secondary or central hypothyroidism. A normal free T_4 index or free T_4 concentration would be expected with the former possibility. If pituitary or hypothalamic disease is suspected, then a careful history and physical examination should be performed to seek evidence of the presence of other hormone deficiencies. Measurement of other anterior pituitary hormones confirms the diagnosis and characterizes the extent of pituitary insufficiency.

TABLE 118–6. Symptoms and Signs of Hypothyroidism and Myxedema Coma

Hypothyroidism	*Myxedema (Coma)*
Neuromuscular	*Neuromuscular*
Fatigue	
Weakness	
Slowed mentation	Psychosis
Delayed deep tendon reflexes	Obtundation/coma
Muscle cramps	
Cardiovascular	*Cardiovascular*
Bradycardia	Bradycardia
Hypertension	Pericardial effusion
Gastrointestinal	*Gastrointestinal*
Constipation	Ileus
	Megacolon
Thermoregulation	*Thermoregulation*
Cold intolerance	Hypothermia
Cool dry skin	

When a hospitalized patient with a systemic illness is found to have a low T_4 level and a normal TSH concentration, then one must consider several possibilities. Most commonly, nonthyroidal illness is responsible. Although one would expect the free T_4 level to be normal, when measured with some commercial assays it is found to be either increased or reduced. The results of several commercial assays have compared well with equilibrium dialysis measurements in hospitalized patients.[6] Confounding the situation is the occurrence of normal TSH levels in some ill patients with primary hypothyroidism; once the acute illness resolves, TSH increases. Finally, secondary hypothyroidism must also be entertained. Although not readily available, serum reverse T_3 assay may clarify the problem, as this hormone's level is low in hypothyroidism but elevated in nonthyroidal illness. A more readily available test—that for the measurement of the resin T_3 uptake—may provide similar information: resin T_3 uptake is low in hypothyroidism and increased (often markedly) in nonthyroidal illness.

Management

Uncomplicated hypothyroidism is treated on an outpatient basis.[42b] Young patients with mild to moderate disease can be started on L-thyroxine (L-T_4), 50 to 100 μg/d, and their serum TSH levels measured at 4 to 6 weeks later. Upward adjustment of hormone dosage should be performed until the TSH value is suppressed to within the normal range. The full replacement dose is approximately 1.7 $\mu g \cdot kg^{-1} \cdot d^{-1}$.[43] Older individuals or any patients with known coronary artery disease should be managed more conservatively. L-T_4 can initiate or exacerbate angina,[44] so treatment should proceed slowly. An initial dose of L-T_4 should be no greater than 12.5 to 25 μg/d. Patients should be questioned about the development of any cardiac symptoms, and serum TSH level should be measured before any increase in dosage is made. Changes in dosage should be small (12.5–25 μg) and be made no more frequently than every 6 weeks. Although central hypothyroidism is much less common than primary disease, it is important to recognize. Patients with concomitant secondary adrenal insufficiency should receive replacement hydrocortisone therapy before initiation of thyroid hormone treatment, since an increase in metabolic rate caused by the latter might induce acute adrenal insufficiency.

Profound hypothyroidism/myxedema coma is an endocrine emergency with a high mortality rate. The diagnosis should be considered in any obtunded or comatose patient for whom no obvious cause can be identified. Hypothermia or the absence of fever in a patient with a known infection is possible.

Management of myxedema coma should be conducted in the intensive care unit. A variety of general supportive measures are essential (Table 118–7). If hypothermia is present, covering the patient with blankets is helpful. Active warming with heating devices should be avoided, however, because doing so may produce vasodilation and a lowering of blood pressure. An adequate blood volume should be restored. Hypothyroidism impairs free water clearance; monitoring of electrolytes is important to avoid hyponatremia. Adequate glucose maintenance is required to prevent the development of hypoglycemia. Dilated cardiomyopathy has been reported[45]; thus, careful hemodynamic monitoring is essential. Drug metabolism is prolonged, so care must be taken to avoid toxicity if digoxin is used.[46] Stress doses of steroids are often recommended because the integrity of the pituitary-adrenal axis is usually unknown. Formal testing can be done at a later time. A careful search for an underly-

TABLE 118–7. Management of Decompensated Hypothyroidism (Myxedema Crisis)

General measures
- Hypothermia
  - Use blankets only—no heating devices
- Hydration
  - Maintain adequate blood volume
  - Avoid water intoxication
- Nutrition: glucose, vitamins
- Antibiotics
- Cardiac therapy
  - Correct hypotension
  - Glucocorticoids (stress doses)
  - Anticipate and treat heart failure
  - Correct anemia
- Pulmonary therapy
  - Monitor arterial blood gases
  - Ventilatory support
  - Treat infection
- Intestinal atony

Specific measures
- Thyroid hormone
  - Initial dose: 200–300 μg L-T_4 IV
  - Maintenance: 50–100 μg L-T_4 per day IV

(Reprinted with permission from Smallridge RC: Metabolic and anatomic thyroid emergencies: A review. Crit Care Med 1992; 20:276. © Williams & Wilkins, 1992.)

ing infection is a must, and broad-spectrum antibiotic coverage is advised pending the receipt of culture results.

Close monitoring of pulmonary status is vital. Patients with hypothyroidism may hypoventilate, and they are sensitive to drugs that can depress respiration. They may require therapy for acute respiratory failure. Gastrointestinal tract abnormalities may also complicate the management plan, as hypotonia, ileus, or megacolon may occur.

Ideally, therapy for hypothyroidism in comatose patients should be restricted to only those persons identified as unequivocally hypothyroid. Unfortunately, this is not always possible, because laboratory values available at the time of decision making do not always distinguish between this disorder and nonthyroidal illness. Since delay in therapy can be fatal, early treatment with thyroid hormone has been advocated,[27, 42a] even though this approach may mean that some individuals may be treated unnecessarily. Thyroid therapy can be discontinued as a patient's situation becomes more clear.

Because absorption may be impaired, thyroid hormone should be given intravenously. A loading dose of 500 μg followed 4 to 7 days later by daily doses of 50 to 100 μg has been recommended.[27, 47] The rationale for a large initial dose is that endogenous stores of thyroid hormone are depleted. Kaptein and coworkers[48] have reported that large doses of L-T_4 may not cause cardiovascular complications in critically ill patients. However, Hylander and Rosenqvist[49] reported a greater mortality rate in patients who had high serum T_3 levels when treated for myxedema coma. In the absence of definitive guidelines for management of this disorder, an intermediate approach of giving 200 to 300 μg L-T_4 followed by daily doses of 50 to 100 μg might lessen the possibility of the occurrence of cardiac complications.

Therapy in Surgical Patients

Some patients are recognized to be hypothyroid shortly before surgery is needed. In the past, it was believed that anesthetic and surgical complications were more common in such patients.[50] Three studies performed in the 1980s have provided more complete information on this subject. In two of the reports,[51, 52] mild to moderate hypothyroidism had little influence on surgical complications. Ladenson and associates[53] reported the occurrence of intraoperative hypotension, heart failure, and some postoperative gastrointestinal and neuropsychiatric problems that were managed without sequelae. Importantly, they observed no increased occurrence of cardiopulmonary difficulties, infections, impaired wound healing, or blood loss nor any increase in the number of days spent in the hospital or in the incidence of death. Whether these observations can be extrapolated to all patients with hypothyroidism, including those with longstanding and severe disease, is unknown.

When surgery is elective, it seems reasonable to delay the procedure until the hypothyroid state has been reversed. However, these studies suggest that if surgery is more urgent, then a patient has a reasonably good chance of tolerating the operation successfully. One special situation is surgery for the cardiac patient who presents with severe angina pectoris.[50] In individuals undergoing cardiac bypass, surgery was found to be more successful if thyroid replacement was begun after the operation (presumably because of the impact of thyroid hormone on myocardial oxygen consumption). At the time of this writing, cardiac patients should be at even less of a risk because the introduction of better antianginal drugs and balloon angioplasty has eliminated the potential risk of general anesthesia in the hypothyroid patient.

Neurosurgeons must be familiar with the issues involved in managing hypothyroidism, particularly as it relates to hypothalamic and pituitary disorders. Before surgery, patients must be screened for the possibility of deficiencies of multiple pituitary hormones. Most critical is the recognition of adrenocorticotropic hormone deficiency because administration of stress doses of glucocorticoids are required perioperatively. Should surgery be indicated for a benign tumor, such as a pituitary adenoma, the decision to correct the hypothyroidism before surgery depends on whether resection is urgent because the tumor impinges on vital structures, such as the optic chiasm. It should be noted that, in hypothyroid patients, not all pituitary masses require surgery. Some persons with primary hypothyroidism develop generalized compensatory pituitary enlargement from prolonged TSH production. These individuals may present with visual field changes, and computed tomography and magnetic resonance imaging scans show a pituitary mass with suprasellar extension. Surgery is *not* the appropriate treatment; thyroid hormone use will decrease the size of the pituitary gland back to normal.[18] Thus, it is essential to measure serum TSH concentration in any patient before surgical exploration is performed.

THYROID HORMONE AND CRITICAL ILLNESS

Numerous studies have shown that serum T_3 and, in some patients, T_4 levels are reduced in critical illness. Serum free T_4, measured by equilibrium dialysis, is usually normal or elevated, and TSH level is not increased. This reduction in T_3 level is reproduced in fasted subjects. In the latter, physiologic supplements of oral T_3 have increased skeletal muscle breakdown, and it is believed that the impairment of conversion of T_4 to T_3 in such situations protects a patient from excessive catabolism. Therefore, administering thyroid hormone to patients with nonthyroidal illness has been discouraged.[3] Two controlled studies have addressed this issue. Becker and colleagues[54] gave L-T_3 to patients with extensive burns and found neither beneficial nor detrimental effect. Brent and Hershman[55] gave L-T_4 to a small group of patients with severe medical or surgical disease and also found no benefit. The tissue concentrations of thyroid hormones in patients with nonthyroidal illness have not been well studied. Recently, Arem and coworkers[56] measured cell contents of T_4 and T_3 in 12 patients dying from nonthyroidal illness and in another 10 healthy persons killed suddenly by trauma. Tissue concentrations of T_3 were reduced in the liver, lung, kidney, pituitary, hypothalamus, and cerebral cortex of patients with nonthyroidal illness; T_4 levels were lower in liver. The crucial question raised by these findings is whether they indicate the presence of tissue hypothyroidism.

Since the mid-1980s, several bodies of literature have provided evidence—albeit preliminary or controversial—for a beneficial role of thyroid hormone in selected circumstances related to critical illness. The most numerous works are found in the literature on organ transplantation. Several investigators have claimed that giving small doses of thyroid hormone to donors before organ removal improves organ survival.[57, 58] Animal studies indicate that the effect may be due to improvement in cellular metabolic function. Not all reports are favorable and worsening of metabolic acidosis with T_3 therapy has been reported.[59]

In one study, it was claimed that T_3, given in sufficient quantity to raise serum free T_3 levels to normal, acts as an inotropic agent in patients undergoing myocardial revascularization.[60] T_3 also enhances left ventricular function after myocardial ischemia in pigs.[60a] Finally, evidence from studies in experimental animals demonstrates that pharmacologic doses of T_4 protect against the development of acute renal failure.[61] This result may be because of an effect of the hormone on plasma membrane functions. Several clinical trials evaluating the possible benefits of this therapy in acute renal failure are in progress.

At this time, thyroid hormone use cannot be recommended in any of the conditions described in this section. The results do raise the possibility that thyroid hormone use may be warranted under specific circumstances but that its clinical application, if any, requires additional carefully designed clinical trials.

OBSTRUCTIVE THYROID EMERGENCIES

Thyroid enlargement, in the absence of biochemical abnormalities, can create a surgical emergency.[15] Although the thyroid gland usually can expand when located in its normal cervical location, a substernally located thyroid gland can cause obstruction within the thoracic inlet. Frequent symptoms include dyspnea, dysphagia, and a sense of fullness or choking. Less common but more serious is the occurrence of acute respiratory failure, respiratory arrest, or the superior vena cava syndrome. The most useful diagnostic tool for detecting upper airway obstruction is the flow-volume loop,[62] which should be obtained for every patient with a substernal or intrathoracic goiter. Although the superior vena cava syndrome is most often caused by a malignancy, this disorder occasionally may be due to a benign goiter.[63] It can be cured by surgery.

Rarely, massive upper gastrointestinal hemorrhage that results from downhill varices produced by goiter has been reported.[64] Although most goiters are benign, sudden thyroid enlargement should suggest the presence of malignancy, such as a thyroid lymphoma or an anaplastic carcinoma. The former is amenable to therapy,[65] whereas the latter carries a dismal prognosis.[66]

CONCLUSIONS

Thyroid emergencies are not common. When they do occur, they may be attributed to either biochemical or anatomic abnormalities. The management of patients with these disorders is multidisciplinary and may require the expertise of a critical care physician and nurse, an endocrinologist, a pulmonologist, a cardiologist, and a surgeon.

References

1. Wartofsky L, Burman KD: Alterations in thyroid function in patients with systemic illness: The "euthyroid sick syndrome." Endocr Rev 1982; 3:164.
2. Zaloga GP, Smallridge RC: Thyroidal alterations in acute illness. Semin Respir Med 1985; 7:95.
3. Utiger RD: Decreased extrathyroidal triiodothyronine production in nonthyroidal illness: Benefit or harm? Am J Med 1980; 69:807.
4. Engler D, Burger AG: The deiodination of the iodothyronines and of their derivatives in man. Endocr Rev 1984; 5:151.
5. LoPresti JS, Mizuno L, Nimalysuria A, et al: Characteristics of 3,5,3′-triiodothyronine sulfate metabolism in euthyroid man. J Clin Endocrinol Metab 1991; 73:703.
6. Wong TK, Pekary AE, Hoo GS, et al: Comparison of methods for measuring free thyroxin in nonthyroidal illness. Clin Chem 1992; 38:720.
7. Klein I: Thyroid hormone and the cardiovascular system. Am J Med 1990; 88:631.
8. Woeber KA: Thyrotoxicosis and the heart. N Engl J Med 1992; 327:94.
9. Kendrick AH, O'Reilly JF, Laszlo G: Lung function and exercise performance in hyperthyroidism before and after treatment. Q J Med 1988; 256:615.
10. Siafakas NM, Milona I, Salesiotou V, et al: Respiratory muscle strength in hyperthyroidism before and after treatment. Am Rev Respir Dis 1992; 146:1025.
11. Shafer RB, Prentiss RA, Bond JH: Gastrointestinal transit in thyroid disease. Gastroenterology 1984; 86:852.
12. Culp KS, Piziak VK: Thyrotoxicosis presenting with secretory diarrhea. Ann Intern Med 1986; 105:216.
13. Davis PJ, Davis FB: Hyperthyroidism in patients over the age of 60 years. Medicine 1974; 53:161.
14. Tibaldi JM, Barzel US, Albin J, et al: Thyrotoxicosis in the very old. Am J Med 1986; 81:619.
15. Smallridge RC: Metabolic and anatomic thyroid emergencies: A review. Crit Care Med 1992; 20:276.
16. Swaminathan R, Chin RK, Lao TTH, et al: Thyroid function in hyperemesis gravidarum. Acta Endocrinol 1989; 120:155.
16a. Burch HB, Wartofsky L: Life-threatening thyrotoxicosis: Thyroid storm. Endocrinol Metab Clin North Am 1993; 22:263.
17. Borst GC, Eil C, Burman KD: Euthyroid hyperthyroxinemia. Ann Intern Med 1983; 98:366.
18. Smallridge RC: Thyrotropin-secreting pituitary tumors. Endocrinol Metab Clin North Am 1987; 16:765.
19. Smallridge RC: Thyrotropin-secreting tumors. *In*: Endocrine Tumors. Mazzaferri E, Samaan NA (Eds). Oxford, Blackwell Scientific Publications, 1993, p 136.
20. Refetoff S, Weiss RE, Usala SJ: The syndromes of resistance to thyroid hormone. Endocr Rev 1993; 14:348.
21. Cohen JH III, Ingbar SH, Braverman LE: Thyrotoxicosis due to ingestion of excess thyroid hormone. Endocr Rev 1989; 10:113.
22. Georges J-L, Normand J-P, Lenormand M-E, et al: Life-threatening thyrotoxicosis induced by amiodarone in patients with benign heart disease. Eur Heart J 1992; 13:129.
23. Bonelli J, Haydl H, Hruby K, et al: The pharmacokinetics of digoxin in patients with manifest hyperthyroidism and after normalization of thyroid function. Int J Clin Pharmacol 1978; 16:302.
24. Feely J, Stevenson IH, Crooks J: Increased clearance of propranolol in thyrotoxicosis. Ann Intern Med 1981; 94:472.
25. Nakazawa HK, Sakurai K, Hamada N, et al: Management of atrial fibrillation in the post-thyrotoxic state. Am J Med 1982; 72:903.

26. Petersen P, Hansen JM: Stroke in thyrotoxicosis with atrial fibrillation. Stroke 1988; 19:15.
27. Nicoloff JT: Thyroid storm and myxedema coma. Med Clin North Am 1985; 69:1005.
28. Nabil N, Miner DJ, Amatruda JM: Methimazole: An alternative route of administration. J Clin Endocrinol Metab 1982; 54:180.
29. Shen D-C, Wu S-Y, Chopra IJ, et al: Long-term treatment of Graves' hyperthyroidism with sodium ipodate. J Clin Endocrinol Metab 1985; 61:723.
30. Roti E, Gardini E, Minelli R, et al: Sodium ipodate and methimazole in the long-term treatment of hyperthyroid Graves' disease. Metabolism 1993; 42:403.
31. Croxson MS, Hall TD, Nicoloff JT: Combination drug therapy for treatment of hyperthyroid Graves' disease. J Clin Endocrinol Metab 1977; 45:623.
32. Ikram H: The nature and prognosis of thyrotoxic heart disease. Q J Med 1985; 213:19.
33. Brunette DD, Rothong C: Emergency department management of thyrotoxic crisis with esmolol. Am J Emerg Med 1991; 9:232.
34. Tajiri J, Katsuya H, Kiyokawa T, et al: Successful treatment of thyrotoxic crisis with plasma exchange. Crit Care Med 1984; 12:536.
35. Preuschof L, Keller F, Bogner U, et al: Plasma exchange and hemoperfusion in iodine-induced thyrotoxicosis. Blood Purif 1991; 9:164.
36. Schaaf L, Greschner M, Paschke R, et al: Thyrotoxic crisis in Graves' disease: Indication for immediate surgery. Klin Wochenschr 1990; 68:1037.
37. Shakir KMM, Michaels RD, Hays JH, et al: The use of bile acid sequestrants to lower serum thyroid hormones in iatrogenic hyperthyroidism. Ann Intern Med 1993; 118:112.
38. Köbberling J, Hintze G, Becker H-D: Iodine-induced thyrotoxicosis—A case for subtotal thyroidectomy in severely ill patients. Klin Wochenschr 1985; 63:1.
39. Ambrosino N, Pacini F, Paggiaro PL, et al: Impaired ventilatory drive in short-term primary hypothyroidism and its reversal by 1-triiodothyronine. J Endocrinol Invest 1985; 8:533.
40. Rajagopal KR, Abbrecht PH, Derderian SS, et al: Obstructive sleep apnea in hypothyroidism. Ann Intern Med 1984; 101:491.
41. Robuschi G, Safran M, Braverman LE, et al: Hypothyroidism in the elderly. Endocr Rev 1987; 8:142.
42. Tachman ML, Guthrie GP Jr: Hypothyroidism: Diversity of presentation. Endocr Rev 1984; 5:456.
42a. Nicoloff JT, LoPresti JS: Myxedema coma: A form of decompensated hypothyroidism. Endocrinol Metab Clin North Am 1993; 22:279.
42b. Mandel SJ, Brent GA, Larsen PR: Levothyroxine therapy in patients with thyroid disease. Ann Intern Med 1993; 119:492.
43. Hennessey JV, Evaul JE, Tseng Y-C, et al: L-Thyroxine dosage: A reevaluation of therapy with contemporary preparations. Ann Intern Med 1986; 105:11.
44. Levine HD: Compromise therapy in the patient with angina pectoris and hypothyroidism. Am J Med 1980; 69:411.
45. Ladenson PW, Sherman SI, Baughman KL, et al: Reversible alterations in myocardial gene expression in a young man with dilated cardiomyopathy and hypothyroidism. Proc Natl Acad Sci 1992; 89:5251.
46. Croxson MS, Ibbertson HK: Serum digoxin in patients with thyroid disease. Br Med J 1975; 3:566.
47. McConahey WM: Diagnosing and treating myxedema and myxedema coma. Geriatrics 1978; 33:61.
48. Kaptein EM, Quion-Verde H, Swinney RS, et al: Acute hemodynamic effects of levothyroxine loading in critically ill hypothyroid patients. Arch Intern Med 1986; 146:662.
49. Hylander B, Rosenqvist U: Treatment of myxoedema coma-factors associated with fatal outcome. Acta Endocrinol 1985; 108:65.
50. Becker C: Hypothyroidism and atherosclerotic heart disease: Pathogenesis, medical management, and the role of coronary artery bypass surgery. Endocr Rev 1985; 6:432.
51. Weinberg AD, Brennan MD, Gorman CA, et al: Outcome of anesthesia and surgery in hypothyroid patients. Arch Intern Med 1983; 143:893.
52. Drucker DJ, Burrow GN: Cardiovascular surgery in the hypothyroid patient. Arch Intern Med 1985; 145:1585.
53. Ladenson PW, Levin AA, Ridgway EC, et al: Complications of surgery in hypothyroid patients. Am J Med 1984; 77:261.
54. Becker RA, Vaughan GM, Ziegler MG, et al: Hypermetabolic low triiodothyronine syndrome of burn injury. Crit Care Med 1982; 10:870.
55. Brent GA, Hershman JM: Thyroxine therapy in patients with severe nonthyroidal illnesses and low serum thyroxine concentration. J Clin Endocrinol Metab 1986; 63:1.
56. Arem R, Wiener GJ, Kaplan SG, et al: Reduced tissue thyroid hormone levels in fatal illness. Metabolism 1993; 42:1102.
57. Novitsky D, Cooper DKC, Chaffin JS, et al: Improved cardiac allograft function following triiodothyronine therapy to both donor and recipient. Transplantation 1990; 49:311.
58. Orlowski JP, Spees EK: Improved cardiac transplant survival with thyroxine treatment of hemodynamically unstable donors: 95.2% graft survival at 6 and 30 months. Transplantation Proc 1993; 25:1535.
59. Randell TT, Höckerstedt KAV: Triiodothyronine treatment is not indicated in brain-dead multiorgan donors: A controlled study. Transplantation Proc 1993; 25:1552.
60. Novitsky D, Cooper DKC, Barton CI, et al: Triiodothyronine as an inotropic agent after open heart surgery. J Thorac Cardiovasc Surg 1989; 98:972.
60a. Dyke CM, Ding M, Abd-Elfattah AS, et al: Effects of triiodothyronine supplementation after myocardial ischemia. Ann Thorac Surg 1993; 56:215.
61. Cronin RE, Brown DM, Simonsen R: Protection by thyroxine in nephrotoxic acute renal failure. Am J Physiol 1986; 251:F408.
62. Miller MR, Pincock AC, Oates GD, et al: Upper airway obstruction due to goitre: Detection, prevalence and results of surgical management. Q J Med 1990; 274:177.
63. Aasted A, Bertelsen S: Superior vena caval syndrome in benign mediastinal goitre. Acta Chir Scand 1981; 147:405.
64. Fleig WE, Stange EF, Ditschuneit H: Upper gastrointestinal hemorrhage from downhill esophageal varices. Dig Dis Sci 1982; 27:23.
65. Butler JS Jr, Brady LW, Amendola BE: Lymphoma of the thyroid: Report of five cases and review. Am J Clin Oncol 1990; 13:64.
66. Nel CJC, van Heerden JA, Goellner JR, et al: Anaplastic carcinoma of the thyroid: A clinicopathologic study of 82 cases. Mayo Clin Proc 1985; 60:51.

CHAPTER 119

The Critically Ill Diabetic

Christine R. Schneyer, MD • Gary J. Kerkvliet, MD

Disorders of glucose metabolism are common endocrine problems, with diabetes mellitus alone afflicting at least 5% of the United States population. Diabetes affects an even greater proportion of hospitalized patients because of the high frequency of its complications, such as heart disease, stroke, peripheral vascular disease, retinopathy, and nephropathy. The association of hyperglycemia with stress renders the critically ill patient particularly susceptible to glucoregulatory derangements. Life-threatening sequelae to disturbances of glucose regulation are diabetic ketoacidosis, hyperosmolar hyperglycemic nonketotic coma (HHNC), and hypoglycemia. This chapter reviews the pathophysiology, diagnosis, and treatment of these major disorders of glucose regulation, which are encountered in the critical care setting both in adults and in children.

CLASSIFICATION OF DIABETES MELLITUS

Diabetes mellitus is a metabolic disorder characterized by hyperglycemia. As shown in Table 119–1, it is broadly subdivided into three major subclasses.[1] Flexibility is required

TABLE 119–1. Major Clinical Subclasses of Diabetes Mellitus

Type	*Clinical Features*
Insulin-dependent diabetes mellitus	Comprises ~10% of diabetic patients. They are usually <30 years old, thin, severely insulinopenic, and ketosis prone. They depend absolutely on exogenous insulin for survival.
Non–insulin-dependent diabetes mellitus	Comprises ~90% of diabetic patients. Patients are typically >30 years old, obese, insulin resistant, and not ketosis prone except during stress. They do not require insulin to sustain life, but it is often prescribed to control hyperglycemia.
Other types of diabetes mellitus	Secondary to pancreatic disease, e.g., chronic pancreatitis, pancreatectomy, hemochromatosis, and cystic fibrosis.
	Secondary to endocrine disease, e.g., Cushing's syndrome, acromegaly, primary hyperaldosteronism, and pheochromocytoma.
	Drug or chemical induced, e.g., by thiazide diuretics, furosemide, glucocorticoids, catecholamines, or estrogen-containing drugs.
	Insulin-receptor abnormalities and genetic syndromes, e.g., autoimmune disorders, hyperlipidemia, muscular dystrophy, and acute intermittent porphyria.

in the use of these classifications; for example, some patients with type I, or insulin-dependent, diabetes mellitus may be overweight, and some individuals with type II, or non–insulin-dependent, diabetes mellitus may develop ketoacidosis, especially during periods of severe stress, such as sepsis, surgery, or myocardial infarction.

Insulin-dependent diabetes mellitus is caused by destruction of insulin-secreting beta cells in the pancreas in a genetically susceptible host.[2] Presumably, external factors (e.g., viral infections, environmental toxins) incite immune-mediated beta cell damage, which is manifested by the presence of islet cell and, less often, insulin autoantibodies in most newly diagnosed patients. The pathogenesis of non–insulin-dependent diabetes mellitus is less well characterized. One important hypothesis (syndrome X) suggests that the primary disturbance is insulin resistance, which is genetically determined and exacerbated by obesity, inactivity, and aging. The resultant hyperinsulinism produces non–insulin-dependent diabetes mellitus as well as hypertension, dyslipidemia, and atherosclerotic vascular disease.[3]

NORMAL PHYSIOLOGY

Insulin has a crucial role in maintaining normal metabolism by facilitating utilization and storage of energy derived from ingested nutrients. Insulin exerts both anabolic and anticatabolic actions on adipose tissue, liver, and skeletal muscle. In adipose tissue, insulin stimulates triglyceride synthesis from glycerol and free fatty acids and prevents lipolysis. In the liver, it increases glycolysis as well as synthesis of glycogen and fatty acids; it prevents glycogenolysis (breakdown of glycogen into glucose), gluconeogenesis (conversion of noncarbohydrate precursors to glucose), and ketogenesis (formation of ketone bodies from fatty acids). In muscle, insulin stimulates amino acid and glucose uptake and protein and glycogen synthesis; it inhibits glycogenolysis and breakdown of protein.

STRESS HYPERGLYCEMIA

Metabolic Effects of Stress

Severe illness is often associated with deterioration of glycemic control in formerly well-controlled diabetics and with precipitation of hyperglycemia in patients not previously diagnosed as diabetic. This phenomenon of "stress hyperglycemia" is attributed to hypersecretion of the counterregulatory hormones, catecholamines, glucagon, cortisol, and growth hormone. These hormones induce a state of marked catabolism in direct opposition to the anabolic and anticatabolic effects of insulin, hence the term *counterregulatory*. The sympathetic branch of the autonomic nervous system plays a key role in the stress-mediated glycemic response. Catecholamines exert an overall inhibitory effect on insulin secretion by activation of α_2-adrenergic receptors in pancreatic beta cells.[4] Activation chiefly of β-adrenergic receptors raises plasma insulin levels.[5]

The net effect of counterregulatory hormone hypersecretion is a surge in circulating glucose derived from glycogenolysis, gluconeogenesis, and impaired peripheral utilization of glucose. The substrates for gluconeogenesis are glycerol and amino acids (which are derived from counterregulatory hormone-induced breakdown of fat and protein, respectively) and lactate (a product of muscle metabolism). Hyperglycemia itself impairs peripheral glucose utilization[6] and residual insulin secretion.[7] Insulinopenic individuals taking fixed doses of insulin, or those with borderline insulin secretory reserve, are unable to increase insulin secretion adequately to counteract these intense catabolic effects. Ketoacidosis may develop in patients with the most severe insulin deficits because of unrestrained lipolysis and ketogenesis.

Rationale for Treatment of Hyperglycemia

The goals of therapy for hyperglycemia in a critical care unit are to minimize morbidity and mortality and to hasten recovery. Avoidance of excessive hyperglycemia prevents ketoacidosis as well as dehydration and electrolyte imbalance secondary to the accompanying osmotic diuresis. Good glycemic control may also be desirable for reducing susceptibility to infection,[8] normalizing wound healing,[9, 10] and improving outlook after myocardial infarction and stroke.[11]

A large body of evidence suggests that serious infection is more likely to develop in the setting of hyperglycemia and ketosis than in nondiabetic individuals. For example, patients with diabetes may be at greater risk for staphylococcal and gram-negative pneumonia and reactivation of tuberculosis.[12] Defects in neutrophil phagocytic function and other host defense mechanisms are associated with diabetes, and they may increase the risk of infection.[13, 13a] Wound healing in patients with diabetes is possibly also impaired. In diabetic animals, repair of deep wounds requiring collagen formation is reduced, but it is correctable by insulin administration and improved glycemic control.[10]

Finally, hyperglycemia per se, even in previously nondiabetic patients, is associated with increased mortality after acute myocardial infarction and stroke.[11] One group has reported a marked reduction in this excess mortality (from 42–17%) when glycemic control was maintained by insulin infusion techniques,[14] whereas others have found no significant differences.[15, 16] In hyperglycemic animals with induced cerebral ischemia, the extent of functional damage is decreased when the blood glucose level is corrected.[17] Comparable trials in humans have been inconclusive.[18]

Management of Hyperglycemia in the Critical Care Setting

Considering both the established and theoretic advantages of adequate glycemic control, it is prudent to restore normoglycemia and to maintain glucose concentrations within a range of about 90 to 180 mg/dL. Glycemic control in critically ill patients is best accomplished with a continuous intravenous infusion of insulin, which provides smoother control than intermittent subcutaneous insulin administration. Adjustments in the insulin infusion rate are based on bedside determination of capillary blood glucose levels obtained with a glucose monitor. Oral hypoglycemic therapy is not recommended, because it is generally ineffective in critically ill individuals.[15]

Patients with significant hyperglycemia should have glucose-containing solutions withheld and regular insulin (prepared for adults as described in Table 119–2; the pediatric dose is 50 U of regular insulin per 50 mL of isotonic saline) infused at a rate of about 0.05 $U \cdot kg^{-1} \cdot h^{-1}$. Insulin sensitivity varies with the patient and the associated illness, and modification of doses, based on hourly glucose readings, is often required.

Once the blood glucose level drops to about 250 mg/dL, glucose control may be maintained by simultaneous infusion of insulin, glucose, and potassium. This regimen was originally proposed for the perioperative treatment of patients with diabetes but has since been found to be of general utility in acute care units. Infusion of 0.25 to 0.35 U of insulin per gram of glucose usually produces acceptable glycemic control in patients with uncomplicated diabetes who undergo the stress of surgery and anesthesia.[19] Based on these studies in surgical patients, suggested guidelines for the maintenance of glycemic control in adults in intensive care are outlined in Table 119–2. Sufficient glucose, approximately 10 g/h, should be provided to meet basal energy requirements and to prevent catabolism and negative nitrogen balance. In children, the corresponding starting dose of insulin is 0.05 $U \cdot kg^{-1} \cdot h^{-1}$, accompanied by adequate amounts of dextrose and potassium.[20] This methodology may also be readily adapted to facilitate glycemic control in patients receiving total parenteral nutrition or continuous tube feedings.[21] The insulin infusion should be administered separately from the replacement fluids to permit flexibility in adjustment of the insulin dosage.

Certain caveats exist in the care of hyperglycemic patients. One is the potential for errors in bedside capillary blood glucose level monitoring[22, 23]; therefore, laboratory plasma or serum glucose testing should be performed intermittently to confirm the accuracy of bedside monitoring. Another is the predictable rapid decline in metabolic control following more than a brief discontinuation of intravenous insulin administration (which has about a 5-minute plasma half-life and an approximately 20-minute biologic effect).[24] If the insulin infusion is stopped because of concern about hypoglycemia, hourly glucose monitoring must be continued; then, the infusion may be quickly restarted at a new rate to prevent excessive swings in glucose concentration.

DIABETIC KETOACIDOSIS

Diabetic ketoacidosis is a life-threatening complication of diabetes. In its pure form, it is manifested by ketoacidosis and modest hyperglycemia without significant hyperosmolality. More often, however, ketoacidosis and hyperosmolality occur together. Interestingly, the severity of the hyperosmolality correlates more closely with mortality than does the acidosis. Diabetic ketoacidosis has been the subject of numerous reviews.[20, 25–29a]

TABLE 119–2. Maintenance of Glucose Control in Adults

Treatment Element	*Action*
Insulin	• Prepare insulin* and piggy back insulin line to maintenance fluid line. • Infuse insulin at rate of 30 mL/h (to provide 3 U/h)†
Fluids	• Add 20 mEq of potassium chloride to 1000 mL of 10% dextrose and normal saline.‡ • Infuse at 100 mL/h (to provide 10 g of glucose and 2 mEq of potassium chloride/h).
Glucose	• Measure blood glucose level with test strips every hour.§ • If glucose level is 90–180 mg/dL, continue ongoing rate of insulin infusion. • If glucose level is > 180 mg/dL, increase the hourly insulin infusion rate by 0.5 U/h until glucose level is < 180 mg/dL. • If glucose level is < 90 mg/dL, decrease hourly insulin infusion rate by 0.5 U/h until glucose level stabilizes at 90–180 mg/dL.
Potassium	• Measure serum potassium level every 1–2 h. • If potassium level is < 3.5 mEq/L, double rate of potassium infusion by adding extra potassium chloride to the fluids. If potassium level is > 5.5 mEq/L, discontinue potassium infusion by administering fluids containing only glucose.

(Data from Gavin LA: Perioperative management of the diabetic patient. Endocrinol Metab Clin North Am 1991; 21:457, and Alberti KGMM, Marshall SM: Diabetes and Surgery. *In*: The Diabetes Annual/4. Alberti KGMM, Krall LP [Eds]. New York, Elsevier, 1988.)

*Insulin solutions are 0.1 U/mL (50 U regular insulin/500 mL isotonic saline). Flush 50 mL through the line before connecting it to the patient to saturate insulin binding sites on the tubing.

†Insulin dose adjustments:

1. For obesity, hepatic disease, increase 1.5×.
2. For severe infection, steroid therapy, or renal transplant surgery, increase 2.0×.
3. For coronary artery bypass surgery, increase 3.0–5.0×.

‡If 5% dextrose is used, decrease insulin infusion rate by 50%.

§Monitoring frequency can be reduced when glucose level stabilizes.

Mortality rates for diabetic ketoacidosis are high; this complication accounts for about 10% of diabetic deaths in the United States. In contrast to popular belief, diabetic ketoacidosis is more common in adults than in children.[30] Mortality increases substantially with aging, with those patients over 65 years at greatest risk.[31, 32] Most deaths are due to coexistent illnesses, such as cardiovascular or renal disease. Unfortunately, up to one third of deaths, particularly in patients under 45 years of age, are due to potentially reversible metabolic complications.[31]

Pathogenesis

Hyperglycemia, hyperketonemia, and acidosis are the hallmarks of diabetic ketoacidosis, developing in patients with either an absolute or a relative insulin deficiency (Fig. 119–1). Diabetic ketoacidosis occurs when insulin levels are too low to oppose the effects of excessive concentrations of the counterregulatory hormones (glucagon, catecholamines, cortisol, and growth hormone) that are secreted in response

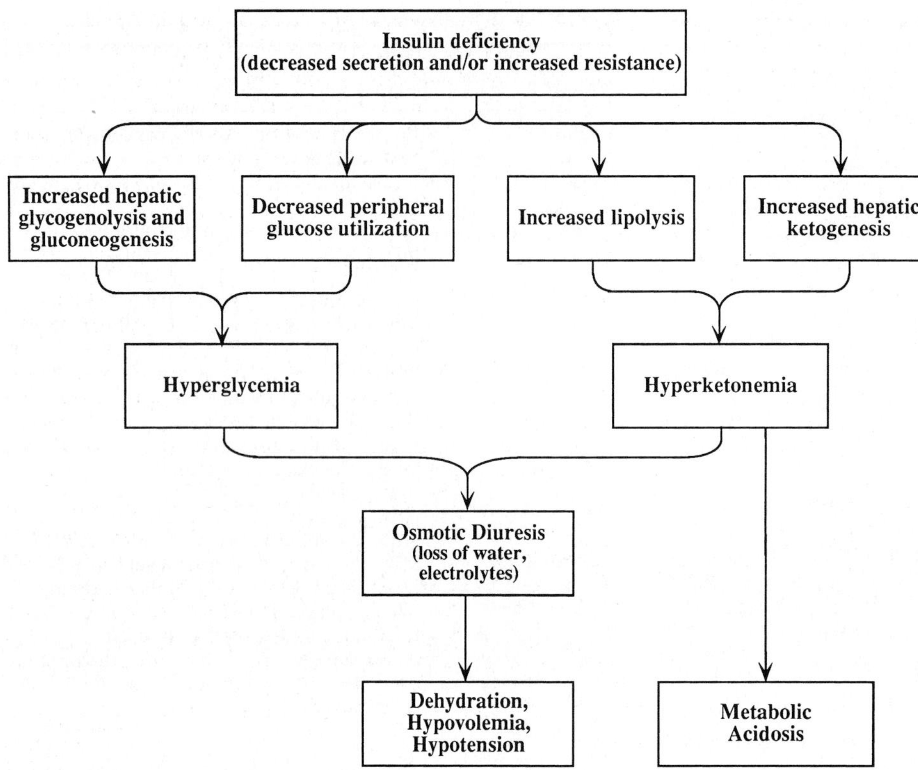

Figure 119–1. Pathophysiology of diabetic ketoacidosis. (Adapted from Barrett EJ, DeFronzo RA: Diabetic ketoacidosis: Diagnosis and treatment. Hosp Pract [Off Ed] 1984; 19:91. Illustration by Albert Miller.)

to such stress as trauma, sepsis, or shock. The constellation of metabolic derangements is similar to that described for stress hyperglycemia in that an outpouring of glucose into the circulation occurs. However, a major difference between the two clinical syndromes is related to the exquisite sensitivity of adipose tissue to the antilipolytic properties of insulin. Inhibition of lipolysis is mediated by much lower concentrations of insulin than are required for the hormone's glucoregulatory effects.[33] Thus, only in the setting of profound insulin deficiency, or insulin resistance, or both, does significant lipolysis occur. Free fatty acids released during lipolysis serve as substrates for the hepatic synthesis of ketoacids, a process in which glucagon plays a central stimulatory role. Levels of circulating ketone bodies increase, as a result of both increased production and decreased utilization. The ketones acetoacetate and β-hydroxybutyrate are moderately strong acids, and their accumulation in large amounts produces metabolic acidosis. High plasma concentrations of glucose and ketones evoke an osmotic diuresis, in which loss of free water and electrolytes, and consequently dehydration and hypovolemia, occur. The negative charge of ketones necessitates the excretion of such cations as sodium and potassium. Phosphorus, calcium, and magnesium are also excreted in large amounts.

Precipitating Factors

Infection is the most common precipitant of diabetic ketoacidosis, causing over half of the cases in some series.[30, 32] Other conditions that can cause this disorder include abdominal disorders, myocardial infarction, hyperthyroidism, and trauma. Treatment errors, including noncompliance with diet or medications, inadequate insulin therapy, and mechanical dysfunction of insulin infusion pumps, account for about one fourth of cases.[30, 32] Drugs that affect carbohydrate metabolism may also cause diabetic ketoacidosis. A classic example is glucocorticoid therapy, which stimulates gluconeogenesis and increases peripheral resistance to insulin. Other agents, such as β-blockers, phenytoin, and thiazides (by inducing hypokalemia) impair insulin secretion. Additional offending drugs include β-sympathomimetic agents (e.g., dobutamine[34] and terbutaline[35]) and pentamidine.[36] In the 20% of patients in whom no precipitating cause is identified, physical or emotional stress is the presumed cause.

Symptoms and Signs

Patients with advanced diabetic ketoacidosis present with a characteristic set of symptoms and signs that usually develop rapidly over fewer than 24 hours (Table 119–3). Abdominal pain, sometimes mimicking an acute abdomen, is especially common in children, but the precise cause has not been elucidated; the usual explanation is ileus induced by electrolyte disturbances. Acidosis causes peripheral vasodilatation, resulting in exacerbation of hypotension, mild hypothermia (~36°C), and warm skin. Therefore, if fever is present, infection is likely.

Laboratory Values

GLUCOSE. Glucose concentration is typically greater than 250 mg/dL in patients with diabetic ketoacidosis (see Table 119–3). However, some patients have significantly lower levels, occasionally less than 100 mg/dL.[37] This situation may occur when a patient with diabetes is stressed because of an intercurrent illness but nonetheless is able to maintain sufficient hydration to promote renal glucose excretion. Likewise, in pregnant women, the increased glomerular filtration rate lowers the renal threshold for glucose, resulting in enhanced urinary excretion of glucose and the development of ketoacidosis at lower glucose values than those customarily observed.

ACID-BASE BALANCE. Plasma ketone bodies may be de-

TABLE 119–3. Clinical Features of Diabetic Ketoacidosis

Symptoms	*Signs*	*Laboratory Test Results*
Polyuria	Dehydration	Glucose level > 250 mg/dL
Polydipsia	Hypotension	Positive serum ketones
Oliguria	Tachycardia	High anion gap
Dyspnea	Hypothermia	$HCO_3^- < 15$ mEq/L
Fatigue	Warm skin	pH < 7.3
Anorexia	Hyperventilation	Serum Na^+ level variable
Nausea and vomiting	Acetone breath	Serum K^+ level variable
Abdominal pain	Stupor, coma	Leukocytosis
Muscle cramps		Increased hematocrit value
		Hyperamylasemia

tected at the patient's bedside by test strips or tablets. If test strips are employed, a result of 1+ or greater is significant. If tablets are used (with diluted plasma), a positive result at a greater than eightfold dilution is considered significant. The three ketone bodies formed in diabetic ketoacidosis are β-hydroxybutyrate and acetoacetate (usually in a ratio of about 3:1 to 5:1), and acetone, which is not a ketoacid. An elevation in the ratio of reduced to nonreduced hepatic mitochondrial nicotinamide-adenine dinucleotide ($NADH:NAD^+$) favors synthesis of β-hydroxybutyrate from acetoacetate. In patients with severe tissue hypoxemia (e.g., that resulting from sepsis and shock), the ratio of β-hydroxybutyrate:acetoacetate may be as high as 20:1. Under these conditions, a false-negative result for ketones may be obtained from bedside ketone body measurements because in these tests, the nitroprusside reaction measures primarily acetoacetate, less so acetone, and β-hydroxybutyrate not at all. The key to this diagnostic dilemma is the anion gap, which is elevated in ketoacidosis in proportion to accumulation of either ketoacid.

The anion gap is calculated by subtracting the measured anions (chloride and bicarbonate) from the measured cations (sodium and potassium). If potassium is omitted (as it often is), the normal anion gap is 8 to 12 mEq/L and consists of negatively charged albumin and phosphates, sulfates, and organic acids (chiefly lactate). In diabetic ketoacidosis, the anion gap is characteristically increased as a result of accumulation of β-hydroxybutyrate and acetoacetate. Increased blood lactate levels often accompany diabetic ketoacidosis and should be suspected particularly in a diabetic patient with a high–anion-gap acidosis and an unimpressive reaction on the nitroprusside test.

ELECTROLYTES. Patients with diabetic ketoacidosis are usually markedly dehydrated, with total body deficits of water of 100 mL/kg and sodium (Na^+) of up to 7 to 10 mEq/kg of body weight.[38] The Na^+ concentration is usually low, presumably because glucose is an osmotically active substance; hyperglycemia draws cellular water into the intravascular space, causing dilution of serum Na^+. To more accurately assess the severity of dehydration, serum Na^+ may be "corrected" by adding 1.6 mEq/L to the measured serum Na^+ for each 100 mg/dL that the measured serum glucose level is above 100 mg/dL.[39] A high corrected serum Na^+ level implies a greater free water deficit and more severe intracellular dehydration. Confusing laboratory values may be caused by lipemic serum, which can cause a spurious lowering of the serum Na^+ (pseudohyponatremia), as well as of other measured plasma constituents.

The serum potassium level is usually normal or high in patients presenting with diabetic ketoacidosis, despite estimated total body deficits of 3 to 5 mEq/kg of body weight[38] that result from kaliuresis, vomiting, and decreased intake. These high levels occur because K^+, chiefly an intracellular cation under physiologic conditions, rises extracellularly because of the combined derangements of ketoacidemia and hyperglycemia. Reduced K^+ excretion due to renal dysfunction may also contribute to hyperkalemia.[40]

Blood urea nitrogen (BUN) is usually elevated out of proportion to the creatinine level because of dehydration and prerenal azotemia. The serum creatinine level may be falsely increased (by about 1.4 mg/dL) if it is measured using the alkaline picrate method because of interference by acetoacetate with this automated method of creatinine determination.[41] The serum phosphate level may be normal or slightly increased at presentation, although total body phosphate is diminished by 1 mmol/kg of body weight.[38] Like K^+, phosphate is largely an intracellular ion that is driven out of the cell in patients with diabetic ketoacidosis and is excreted in large amounts in the urine. Hypomagnesemia is also common with decreases of 0.5 to 1.0 mEq/kg of body weight,[38] but its clinical significance is unclear.

SERUM OSMOLALITY. A strong correlation exists between serum osmolality and depression of consciousness, and coma is observed in some patients whose total serum osmolality is greater than 340 mOsm/kg of water.[42, 43] In contrast, neither hyperglycemia nor acidosis causes coma. Therefore, serum osmolality should be calculated to determine if hypertonicity can account for the observed mental status changes or if another etiology, such as meningitis or stroke, should be considered. Total serum osmolality is easily calculated by the following equation:

$$2\ (Na^+ + K^+ \text{ in mEq/L}) + (\text{glucose in mg/dL} \div 18) + (\text{BUN in mg/dL} \div 2.8)$$

The so-called "effective" serum osmolality is determined by deleting the BUN from this equation. This is a more accurate assessment of body fluid tonicity because urea passes freely across cell plasma membranes and is osmotically inactive.[44] Patients with an effective osmolality of greater than 320 mOsm/kg are often comatose.[45]

Treatment

The fundamentals of diabetic ketoacidosis therapy may be divided into the following categories: general therapeutic measures, fluids, insulin, K^+, and alkali. A flow sheet is invaluable for recording vital signs, weight, composition and volume of fluid administered, insulin dosage, hourly urine output, electrolyte levels, and acid-base status. During the course of treatment, blood glucose levels are determined hourly, and electrolyte levels every 2 hours until the serum bicarbonate (HCO_3^-) level rises to about 15 mEq/L. Subsequently, these blood tests may be performed every 4 to 6 hours until acidosis is completely resolved and the patient is able to tolerate adequate oral intake without vomiting. Initially, BUN, creatinine, calcium, and phosphate values are monitored every 4 to 8 hours, depending on baseline values and choice of fluid therapy.

GENERAL THERAPEUTIC MEASURES. Measurement of central venous or pulmonary artery occlusion pressure may be needed to guide fluid replacement, especially in patients who are in shock, in the elderly, or in individuals with heart disease. (To reduce the risk of iatrogenic infection, deep catheterization should be discontinued as soon as it is no longer necessary.) Assessment of urine output is essential to establish that the patient is not in renal failure and to assess responsiveness to therapy. Bladder catheterization should be performed in patients who do not urinate spontaneously. In comatose patients, a nasogastric tube should be inserted to prevent pulmonary aspiration. Oxygen should be administered to maintain the Po_2 at greater than 80 mm Hg. An assiduous search for the precipitating cause of diabetic ketoacidosis must be conducted. If there is any suggestion of infection, broad-spectrum antibiotic therapy should be begun after the requisite cultures have been obtained. Because hypercoagulability is a feature of diabetic ketoacidosis, prophylactic therapy with subcutaneous heparin may be beneficial, especially in elderly patients and in those with severe hyperosmolality.

FLUIDS. Hydration is the mainstay of therapy for diabetic ketoacidosis and may independently cause a 20% or greater reduction in the glucose level by improving renal perfusion and augmenting urinary glucose losses. Table 119–4 provides guidelines for fluid administration. As shown in this table, slightly different guidelines exist for children and adults, not only for fluid therapy but also for other aspects of diabetic ketoacidosis treatment. These differences are based more on convention than on rigorous investigation. The choice of fluids used in therapy has been controversial, although in hypotensive patients, normal saline is usually recommended to rapidly replenish intravascular volume. Lactated Ringer's solution is favored by some clinicians for initial hydration. However, because of possible concomitant lactic acidosis, we prefer not to use lactate-containing solutions. Rarely, colloid (albumin) may be necessary to resolve persistent hypotension. Severely dehydrated patients require rapid infusion rates. In patients with very mild volume depletion, reducing the rate of fluid administration by about 50% appears to speed recovery from acidosis.[46]

The fluid and electrolyte requirements of a child with diabetic ketoacidosis must be calculated with extreme care because of the greater risk for developing potentially fatal cerebral edema, as is discussed later. After initial rehydration, the fluid deficit (based on an assumed 10% dehydration) is replaced over at least 36 to 48 hours. Daily maintenance fluids (~1500 mL/m^2) are provided in conjunction with ongoing correction of the deficit. Unusual fluid losses due to vomiting or diarrhea should be replaced. Many clinicians also add the amount of urine output (osmotic diuresis) in the first few hours to the parenteral fluids as ½ normal saline. Some investigators have suggested that the overall rate of fluid administration should not exceed 4 L/m^2 per day, so as to diminish the risk of cerebral edema (see *Cerebral Edema*).[47]

TABLE 119–4. Therapy for Diabetic Ketoacidosis

	Adults	*Children*
Fluid		
Type	NS if hypotensive *or* if Na level < 130 mEq/L. ½ NS if not hypotensive *or* if Na level > 150 mEq/L. Add 5% or 10% dextrose to IV fluids when serum glucose level reaches ~ 250–300 mg/dL. NS (rather than ½ NS) if necessary to prevent hypo-osmolality.	NS until hypotension and perfusion improved. Then ½ NS. Add 5% or 10% dextrose to IV fluids when serum glucose level reaches ~ 250–300 mg/dL. NS (rather than ½ NS) if necessary to prevent hypo-osmolality.
Rate	1 L/h for ~2 h (longer if hypotension persists). Then 500 mL/h for ~4 h. Then 250 mL/h for ~4 h.	10–20 mL/kg boluses as quickly as possible and as frequently as necessary until hypotension and perfusion improve. Calculate fluid requirements as sum of estimated deficit (administered over 36–48 hr) + maintenance fluids (~ 1500 mL/m^2) = ~ 1.5 × maintenance. Amount of ongoing fluid losses (urinary output) may be added to IV fluids as ½ NS for first few h.
Insulin*	10 U IV bolus optional. 0.1 U/kg/h continuous IV infusion. Double infusion rate every 2 h that glucose level does not fall by ~ 50–100 mg/dL. If blood glucose level falls too low despite addition of dextrose, decrease rate of insulin infusion by ~ 50%. When serum bicarbonate level reaches 18–20 mEq/L and patient is tolerating oral fluids and food, begin intermediate-acting SC insulin.	0.1 U/kg IV bolus optional. 0.1 U/kg/h continuous IV infusion. If no improvement in acidosis after ~ 2 h, increase IV insulin infusion rate to 0.15–0.20 U/kg/h. If blood glucose level falls too low despite addition of dextrose, decrease rate of insulin infusion by ~ 50%. When the acidosis is cleared and the patient is tolerating oral fluids and food, begin intermediate-acting SC insulin.
Potassium	40 mEq/h if serum K^+ <3 mEq/L. 30 mEq/h if serum K^+ level is 3–4 mEq/L. 20 mEq/h if serum K^+ level is 4–5 mEq/L.	40 mEq/L of IV fluids if serum K^+ level is normal or low. 60–80 mEq/L of IV fluids for severe hypokalemia (not to exceed 0.5 mEq/kg/h).

(Data from Weigle CGM: Metabolic and endocrine disease in pediatric intensive care. *In*: Textbook of Pediatric Intensive Care. Rogers MC [Ed]. Baltimore, Williams & Wilkins, 1987, pp 1057–1109; Siperstein MD: Diabetic ketoacidosis and hyperosmolar coma. Endocrinol Metab Clin North Am 1992; 21:415; Fleckman AM: Diabetic ketoacidosis. Endocrinol Metab Clin North Am 1993; 22:181; Kecskes SA: Diabetic ketoacidosis. Pediatr Clin North Am 1993; 40:355; Plotnick LP: Insulin-dependent diabetes mellitus. *In*: Principles and Practice of Pediatrics Update. Oski FA, McMillan JA [Eds]. Philadelphia, JB Lippincott, 1993, pp 1–13; Kitabchi AE, Fisher JN, Murphy MB, et al: Diabetic ketoacidosis and the hyperglycemic, hyperosmolar nonketotic state. *In*: Joslin's Diabetes Mellitus. 13th ed. Kahn CR, Weir GC [Eds]. Philadelphia, Lea & Febiger, 1994, pp 738–770; and Davidson MB: Ketoacidosis and hyperosmolar nonketotic syndrome. *In*: Diabetes Mellitus: Diagnosis and Treatment. 3rd ed. New York, Churchill Livingstone, 1991, pp 175–212.)

*Prepare insulin infusion for adults as in Table 119–2; pediatric dose is 50 U of regular insulin/50 mL of isotonic saline. Concentration and rate of insulin infusion may require changes for patients with renal insufficiency or heart disease.

NS = normal saline.

Resolution of acidosis usually requires a more extended period of treatment than does lowering of the blood glucose level. Therefore, when glucose concentrations have decreased to about 250 to 300 mg/dL, 5% or 10% dextrose should be added to prevent hypoglycemia during ongoing insulin therapy for acidosis.

INSULIN. A well-accepted protocol consists of administering a continuous IV infusion of regular insulin at a rate of $0.1\ U \cdot kg^{-1} \cdot h^{-1}$ (see Table 119–4). An initial bolus of intravenous insulin is optional because no convincing evidence exists that it offers additional therapeutic benefit. The intravenous route of insulin delivery is preferred because absorption from intramuscular or subcutaneous sites may be impaired in a dehydrated patient. As in other situations in which an intravenous insulin infusion is used, the insulin and rehydration solutions should be administered separately to allow flexibility in their individual delivery rates.

Within 12 to 24 hours of therapy, the acidosis is usually resolved, and patients are ready to begin receiving subcutaneous insulin. In patients with preestablished insulin requirements, subcutaneous administration of intermediate-acting insulin (e.g., neutral protamine Hagedorn [NPH] or insulin zinc suspension [Lente]) may then be resumed. Generally, adults with new-onset insulin-dependent diabetes mellitus may be started on a dose of intermediate-acting insulin in the range of 0.2 to $0.3\ U \cdot kg^{-1} \cdot d^{-1}$ (two-thirds of the total amount in the morning, and one-third in the evening); a reasonable starting dose in children is also about $0.3\ U \cdot kg^{-1} \cdot d^{-1}$. The first injection of intermediate acting insulin should be given at a routine time (before breakfast or dinner). Intravenous insulin should be continued at a low dose for 1 to 2 hours after the first injection of intermediate-acting insulin to provide insulin coverage of the meal during the 2- to 4-hour interval preceding the onset of action of the longer-acting insulin.

POTASSIUM. Although the serum K^+ level is usually normal or high at the onset, it invariably falls with treatment. Rehydration lowers the serum K^+ level by exerting a dilutional effect and by increasing urinary K^+ excretion. Both insulin therapy and correction of acidosis lower the serum K^+ level by stimulating intracellular K^+ uptake.

Because of profound adverse effects of severe hypokalemia and hyperkalemia on the cardiovascular and respiratory systems, recommendations for K^+ replacement are directed toward maintaining a normal serum K^+ level (see Table 119–4). If serum electrolyte levels are not immediately available, hyperkalemia or hypokalemia can be rapidly detected by observing peaked or flattened T waves, respectively, on an electrocardiogram. Many clinicians recommend waiting to begin K^+ therapy until urine flow is established. However, because hypokalemia is potentially life threatening, K^+ repletion, if necessary, may be initiated cautiously before urine output is confirmed. K^+ is usually replaced as potassium chloride, either alone or alternating with potassium phosphate (K_3PO_4) (see *Other Electrolytes*). Some clinicians prefer to use potassium acetate in severely acidotic patients because of possible endogenous conversion of acetate to HCO_3^-.

BICARBONATE. Acidosis may cause severe adverse effects, including hypotension, myocardial depression, arrhythmias, central nervous system depression, and insulin resistance. Nevertheless, several studies have been unable to demonstrate any substantial benefits from administering HCO_3^- to patients with diabetic ketoacidosis whose arterial pH was as low as 6.9.[48] In addition, HCO_3^- therapy has potential adverse consequences, including hypokalemia, Na^+ overload and hyperosmolality, late alkalemia due to additional endogenous generation of HCO_3^- from ketoacids, and worsening of paradoxical cerebral acidosis. This last condition develops because HCO_3^- combines with a hydrogen ion and dissociates to carbon dioxide and water. Whereas HCO_3^- passes slowly across the blood-brain barrier, carbon dioxide diffuses freely, further decreasing cerebral pH.

HCO_3^- administration in diabetic ketoacidosis remains controversial, and indications for its use have not been well delineated. A currently accepted practice is to administer HCO_3^- only if the pH is below 7.0. Other indications for alkali therapy are coexistent lactic acidosis and severe hyperkalemia. HCO_3^- should never be given as an intravenous bolus, because of the danger of precipitating hypokalemia and fatal arrhythmias. In addition, it should not be given to hypokalemic patients until K^+ therapy has been started. For adults, one ampule of $NaHCO_3$ (containing 44 mEq each of Na^+ and HCO_3^-) should be added to ½ normal saline and given over 1 to 2 hours. The corresponding pediatric dose is 1 to 2 mEq/kg of $NaHCO_3$ administered in a similar manner. The pH should be checked about 30 minutes after the infusion. The goal of therapy is a small increase in pH, to a maximum of about 7.2.

OTHER ELECTROLYTES. Deficits of phosphate occur in diabetic ketoacidosis, but their clinical relevance is unclear, as are the benefits of replacement therapy. Although serum phosphate may fall to undetectable levels during therapy for diabetic ketoacidosis, several studies have failed to show any beneficial effect of phosphate replacement on clinical outcome.[49] Furthermore, phosphate therapy is potentially hazardous, as was documented in case reports of children with diabetic ketoacidosis who developed hypocalcemia and tetany secondary to phosphate supplementation.[50] However, theoretic advantages to phosphate therapy include prevention of respiratory depression and neurologic dysfunction and accelerated regeneration of erythrocyte 2,3-diphosphoglycerate, thereby causing a shift of the oxygen dissociation curve to the right and improved oxygen delivery to tissues. Because of these potential benefits, many diabetologists recommend phosphate therapy when the serum level is low, less than about 2 mEq/L. Phosphate may be administered as a potassium salt, by giving half the potassium as potassium chloride and half as potassium phosphate. This therapy may also help to avoid subsequent development of hyperchloremic acidosis, as is discussed later. Potassium phosphate contains 90 mg (3 mmol) of elemental phosphorus and 4.4 mEq of potassium per milliliter. Replacement doses should be administered cautiously in normal saline or ½ normal saline over 6 or more hours, and serum calcium and phosphate levels should be frequently monitored.

Magnesium (Mg^{2+}) deficiency is associated with diminished parathyroid hormone secretion and impaired tissue sensitivity to this hormone. Therefore, Mg^{2+} supplementation should be considered in hypomagnesemic patients to prevent hypocalcemia, especially in patients receiving phosphate replacement.

Complications of Treatment

CEREBRAL EDEMA. Cerebral edema is a potentially fatal complication of diabetic ketoacidosis. It occurs most commonly in children under 5 years of age and in new-onset insulin-dependent diabetes mellitus patients, and it accounts for over 30% of deaths in diabetic ketoacidosis patients under 20 years of age.[51] Subclinical brain swelling may be detectable at the time of presentation and often worsens with therapy. Typically, clinical and biochemical indices are improving when a sudden deterioration in mental status occurs.

Conditions that have been investigated but not definitively linked to the development of cerebral edema are the osmolality of administered fluids, the rate of fall of the blood glucose or Na^+ level, and the use of HCO_3^-.[51] A possible correlation has been found by some[47] but not all[51] investigators between fluid administration of greater than 4 L/m^2 per day and development of brain herniation. A lack of serum Na^+ level increase in association with falling glucose levels may be an indicator of excess free water and may help distinguish patients who will subsequently develop cerebral edema.[47] Despite the uncertain pathogenesis of this disorder, it is prudent to avoid rapid and extreme decreases in serum osmolality. Blood glucose concentration should be lowered gradually. Serum osmolality should be calculated intermittently (especially if the serum Na^+ level remains low or decreases); if the osmolality drops below normal or falls precipitously, normal saline rather than ½ normal saline should be administered.[29]

Warning signs of cerebral dysfunction occur in about half of patients and include severe headache, blood pressure changes, abnormal temperature regulation, decreased arousability, and seizures. If cerebral edema is suspected, aggressive measures to decrease intracranial pressure should be initiated. Such measures include intubation and hyperventilation, fluid restriction, and mannitol administration (0.25–1.0 g/kg IV over 20 minutes). Mannitol should be kept at the bedside during the first 24 hours of therapy.[47] Unfortunately, even when treatment is introduced early, nearly 50% of patients suffer disabling or fatal cerebral damage.[51]

PULMONARY EDEMA. Pulmonary edema secondary to adult respiratory distress syndrome is a rare complication of severe diabetic ketoacidosis.[52] It afflicts predominantly young patients (less than 50 years of age) with severe acidosis and has a striking mortality of about 90%. The diagnosis should be suspected in any patient who develops dyspnea, hypoxia, rales, or infiltrates. The etiology is not understood, but like cerebral edema, its development may be related to rapid decreases in serum osmolality during treatment with large volumes of hypotonic fluids. Increased pulmonary capillary permeability induced by acidosis and hyperventilation may also play a role.[53]

Special Problems in Diagnosis and Management

GASTROINTESTINAL DISTURBANCES. Abdominal pain, nausea, and vomiting are common presenting symptoms in diabetic ketoacidosis and are usually metabolic in origin. However, diabetic ketoacidosis may be precipitated by an intra-abdominal emergency. Complicating this differential diagnosis is the common occurrence of hyperamylasemia (with or without abdominal pain) and occasional unexplained elevations in hepatic transaminase, creatine phosphokinase, and 5′-nucleotidase levels.[54] A reasonable approach is to initiate therapy for diabetic ketoacidosis and to evaluate the patient frequently for progression of symptoms. If gastrointestinal symptoms do not improve after several hours, the possibility of true intra-abdominal pathology should be considered. If significant pancreatitis is suspected, the serum lipase level should be measured.

ELECTROCARDIOGRAPHIC ABNORMALITIES. Electrolyte derangements of diabetic ketoacidosis may produce ST-segment abnormalities simulating those seen in acute myocardial infarction. However, these electrocardiographic changes occur in the absence of other indicators of cardiac disease, and they resolve with treatment of the diabetic ketoacidosis.[55]

NONCLASSIC ACID-BASE DISTURBANCES. A broad spectrum of acid-base patterns may be encountered in patients with diabetic ketoacidosis. A normal–anion-gap hyperchloremic acidosis may be present at the onset of therapy, or more commonly, is observed during the recovery period.[56] One explanation for this phenomenon is enhanced chloride (Cl^-) reabsorption in the proximal tubule in conjunction with ketonuria that occurs with vigorous hydration. Loss of ketoacids reduces available reserves of this important substrate for HCO_3^- synthesis. Importantly, this metabolic disorder is self-limited and spontaneously resolves over several days with restoration of normal dietary intake and insulin therapy.

A less common condition is diabetic ketoacidosis with alkalemia, which is the coexistence of a primary high–anion-gap metabolic acidosis due to diabetic ketoacidosis, with a primary metabolic alkalosis, possibly secondary to vomiting, diuretic use, or alkali ingestion. In the case of vomiting, Cl^- loss through emesis combined with HCO_3^- loss through buffering of ketoacids markedly elevates the anion gap, but the pH is higher than expected from the PCO_2 measurement.[57]

FAILURE OF KETOSIS TO RESOLVE WITH THERAPY. During recovery from diabetic ketoacidosis, spontaneous generation of acetone may increase the nitroprusside reaction and give a spurious impression of worsening ketoacidosis. Evidence of resolving ketosis, however, can be found in the anion gap, which decreases despite an increase in acetone because the latter is not an anion.

RENAL FAILURE. Patients with diabetic ketoacidosis and concomitant renal failure pose special management problems. Administered K^+ and fluid are retained in the body. Furthermore, ketoacids are not excreted and are available as substrates for HCO_3^- regeneration. Fluid should be administered in much lower volumes than those previously outlined for patients who are not in renal failure; it may be delivered as repetitive fluid challenges, 10 mL/min over 10 to 20 minutes, and the patient should be carefully monitored for evidence of volume overload.[26] Hyperkalemia may be unresponsive to insulin therapy and may require dialysis for management.

HYPEROSMOLAR HYPERGLYCEMIC NONKETOTIC COMA

Hyperosmolar hyperglycemic nonketotic coma (HHNC) and diabetic ketoacidosis should be considered as syndromes at opposite ends of a continuum of hyperglycemic states. Patients with classic HHNC have marked hyperosmolality secondary to hyperglycemia and little if any ketosis. Several reviews have been published on this topic.[20, 25, 28, 29a, 54, 58–60] Most patients with HHNC have non–insulin-dependent diabetes mellitus, and in about one third of cases, HHNC is the first indication of the presence of diabetes.[61] The syndrome is rare in children[20] and typically strikes the elderly, especially nursing home residents.[61] Mortality rates of 40% to 70% are attributed to associated illnesses.[59, 60]

Pathogenesis

The pathogenesis of HHNC is unclear. It has been theorized that a combination of insulin resistance and relative insulin deficiency result in insulin levels sufficient to inhibit lipolysis and ketogenesis. However, the level is inadequate to suppress hepatic glucose production and to stimulate peripheral glucose utilization in the presence of counter-regulatory hormone hypersecretion. Another potential mechanism involves dehydration and hyperosmolality, themselves inhibitory to lipolysis and ketogenesis.[58, 60]

Hyperglycemia induces an osmotic diuresis and early volume depletion, which in the elderly may not necessarily stimulate thirst.[58] Some patients, especially those who are very young or very old, may sense thirst but have limited access to fluid intake. A decreasing glomerular filtration rate secondary to extracellular volume depletion worsens glucose retention; this phenomenon results in a vicious spiral of accelerated hyperglycemia, hyperosmolality, and dehydration.

Precipitating Causes

As with diabetic ketoacidosis, infection is the major precipitating factor for HHNC.[59–61] Myocardial infarction, cerebrovascular accident, burns, and intravenous hyperalimentation are also associated with HHNC. In nondiabetic children, this syndrome has been observed with gastroenteritis, improper dilution of infant formula, epinephrine treatment for asthma, and suprasellar surgery.[20] Many of the same drugs that cause diabetic ketoacidosis may also precipitate HHNC, including glucocorticoids, thiazides, β-blockers, and phenytoin. Death from this disorder has been described in at least two nondiabetic young adults after only a few weeks of glucocorticoid therapy.[62]

Symptoms and Signs

Patients with HHNC experience most of the same symptoms described for diabetic ketoacidosis (see Table 119–3), with the exception of dyspnea, which is not present because of the absence of severe acidosis. In contrast to the rapid course of diabetic ketoacidosis, symptoms of HHNC are usually slowly progressive over a period of days to weeks, and patients are brought to medical attention because of altered consciousness.

With the exception of severe dehydration, the physical signs of patients with HHNC differ considerably from those with diabetic ketoacidosis. Fever due to infection is common, and signs of acidosis (e.g., hyperventilation, acetone breath, and warm skin) are often absent. Unlike diabetic ketoacidosis, focal neurologic signs and seizures may be dominant clinical features, resulting in a common misdiagnosis of stroke.

Laboratory Values

The major chemical features of classic HHNC are marked hyperglycemia (the blood glucose level is usually greater than 500 mg/dL) and minimal ketosis, with a normal serum HCO_3^- level and arterial pH. In mixed diabetic ketoacidosis–hyperosmolar syndromes, serum ketone and lactate levels may both be elevated and should be measured if the anion gap is increased. The serum Na^+ level tends to be high, and calculated total osmolality is typically greater than 340 mOsm/kg of water and often exceeds 400 mOsm/kg. As previously discussed, depression of sensorium is closely correlated with hyperosmolality of greater than 340 mOsm/kg but is not correlated with hyperglycemia or acidosis. Therefore, alternative causes for coma must be investigated if the total serum osmolality is below 340 mOsm/kg.

Treatment

General therapeutic measures are similar to those recommended for patients with diabetic ketoacidosis. Precipitating causes of HHNC should be carefully sought and treated. Patients are at high risk of thrombosis because of dehydration and immobilization. Therefore, in the absence of contraindications, anticoagulation therapy with low-dose heparin should be administered.

Fluid therapy for patients with HHNC is similar to that for patients with diabetic ketoacidosis (see Table 119–4). In elderly patients with a fragile cardiovascular status, reasonable guidelines are to correct about half of the fluid deficit during the first 12 to 24 hours and the remainder over the ensuing 24 to 48 hours. Monitoring of central venous pressure or pulmonary wedge pressure is extremely helpful.

Hypertonic dehydration is the major disturbance in HHNC, and insulin assumes a lesser role than in diabetic ketoacidosis. Nevertheless, because of the central role of insulin in restoring and maintaining normal glucose metabolism, we advocate treating patients with a continuous intravenous insulin infusion in the same manner as for diabetic ketoacidosis (see Table 119–4). Some clinicians prefer to use lower doses of insulin, for example, 0.05 $U \cdot kg^{-1} \cdot h^{-1}$, particularly in children.[20] Dextrose should be added to the rehydration fluids when the glucose level approaches 250 mg/dL. At this time, the insulin drip may also require reduction. K^+ deficits and other electrolyte disturbances should be corrected as for diabetic ketoacidosis. Full recovery may take several days. In contrast to diabetic ketoacidosis patients, many individuals with HHNC can be successfully treated with oral hypoglycemic agents or with diet alone after recovery.

HYPOGLYCEMIA

Hypoglycemia defines a laboratory value and a clinical syndrome. Although the normal lower limit of the fasting plasma glucose level is 60 mg/dL, development of symptoms is highly variable at a wide range of values below this limit. Criteria for the diagnosis of clinical hypoglycemia are based on modifications of Whipple's triad set forth in 1938: a blood glucose level lower than 50 mg/dL (<45 mg/dL in children); simultaneous neuroglycopenic symptoms, such as confusion and coma; and relief of these symptoms with correction of the low blood glucose level.[63, 64]

The physiologic response to hypoglycemia is a decrease in insulin levels and an increase in counterregulatory hormone secretion to augment glucose production. The critical physiologic goal is to supply glucose to the brain, which via insulin-independent mechanisms is absolutely dependent on glucose and ketones as metabolic fuels. Providing an immediate supply of glucose is vital because it may take several days for the brain to adapt to ketone utilization. Glucagon and catecholamines (especially epinephrine) are the major hormonal defense against hypoglycemia, with glucagon playing the dominant role. Cortisol and growth hormone appear to be less important, exerting mainly permissive effects on key enzymes required for glycogenolysis and gluconeogenesis. Hepatic glycogenolysis is the primary source of glucose during the initial hours of hypoglycemia. Gluconeogenesis becomes progressively more important as glycogen stores are depleted.

Differential Diagnosis

Hypoglycemia can be broadly classified as either drug induced, fasting (unrelated to food and usually occurring more than 4 hours after the last meal), postprandial (within 4 hours of a meal), or artifactual (Table 119–5). The most common cause of hypoglycemia in hospitalized adults is excessive insulin administration for the treatment of diabetes.[65] The risk of hypoglycemia in diabetic subjects with

TABLE 119–5. Causes of Hypoglycemia

Type	*In Adults*	*Additional Causes in Children*
Drug-induced (insulin-dependent)	Insulin	
	Sulfonylureas	
	Other sulfa compounds	
	Pentamidine	
	Quinine	
	Selegiline	
	Pyriminil (Vacor)	
Drug-induced (non–insulin-dependent)	Ethanol	Salicylates
	Nonselective β-blockers	
Fasting (insulin-dependent)	Autonomous insulin production (insulinoma)	Autonomous insulin production (nesidioblastosis)
	Humoral tumor–induced (IGF II)	Leucine-sensitive hypoglycemia
	Autoimmunity (antibodies to insulin receptor or insulin)	
	Abrupt cessation of total parenteral nutrition	
Fasting (non–insulin-dependent)	Decreased glucose production	Decreased glucose production
	Liver dysfunction	Liver dysfunction
	Congestive heart failure	Enzymatic defects in carbohydrate, fat, and amino acid metabolism (e.g., glycogen storage diseases, carnitine deficiency)
	Cirrhosis	
	Septic shock	
	Substrate deficiency	
	Uremia	
	Malnutrition	Reye's syndrome
	Hormone deficiency states	Cyanotic heart disease
	Adrenal insufficiency	Substrate deficiency
	Hypothyroidism	Ketotic hypoglycemia
	Increased glucose utilization	Growth hormone deficiency
	Advanced pregnancy	
	Seizures	
	Tumors (sarcomas, hepatomas)	
Postprandial	Idiopathic	
	Alimentary hyperinsulinism (rapid gastric emptying)	
	Prediabetic functional hypoglycemia	
Artifactual	Leukocytosis (infection, leukemia)	
	Polycythemia	

IGF II = Insulin-like growth factor II.

(Data from Comi RJ: Approach to acute hypoglycemia. Endocrinol Metab Clin North Am 1993; 22:247; Rowland MJ, Bransome Ed Jr, Hendry LB: Hypoglycemia caused by selegiline, an antiparkinsonian drug: Can such side effects be predicted? J Clin Pharmacol 1994; 34:80; Haymond MW: Hypoglycemia in infants and children. Endocrinol Metab Clin North Am 1989; 18:211; Miller JA, Hallenbeck JM: Pharmacologic approach to acute seizures. *In*: Essentials of Critical Care Pharmacology. 2nd ed. Chernow B, Holaday JW, Zaloga GP, et al [Eds]. Baltimore, Williams & Wilkins, 1989, pp 222–235; and Field JB: Exercise and deficient carbohydrate storage and intake as causes of hypoglycemia. Endocrinol Metab Clin North Am 1989; 18:155.)

associated renal insufficiency is even greater because of decreased renal insulin degradation and clearance. Hypoglycemia may also occur during insulin treatment of hyperkalemia in patients with renal insufficiency or hyperglycemia related to total parenteral nutrition. Numerous other drugs may cause hypoglycemia, particularly in patients with decreased carbohydrate intake. Sulfonylureas account for most cases, especially the long-acting agents chlorpropamide and glyburide. In children as well as adults, ethanol ingestion is perhaps the most common cause of debilitating and lethal hypoglycemic coma.[66] Increased reduction in nicotinamide-adenine dinucleotide (NADH) production and an increase in the ratio of NADH to NAD associated with ethanol metabolism impairs hepatic gluconeogenesis. Many other agents can cause hypoglycemia,[66a] and this subject has been the topic of a comprehensive review.[66]

In the critical care setting, hypoglycemia may follow abrupt cessation of total parenteral nutrition (TPN). Hypoglycemia is attributed to a sudden lack of circulating glucose in the presence of persistent hyperinsulinemia induced by previous infusion of concentrated dextrose solutions. Interestingly, abrupt discontinuation of TPN does not appear to cause hypoglycemia in children older than 2 years of age.[66b]

Hypoglycemia occurs in end-stage liver disease because of diminished glycogen stores and impaired gluconeogenesis. Liver dysfunction due to passive venous congestion associated with congestive heart failure can cause hypoglycemia, which usually resolves with improvement of the congestion. Hypoglycemia is common in children who have accelerated glucose demands caused by medical or surgical stress, depleted glycogen stores due to chronic disease, and an inadequate caloric supply secondary to fasting and insufficient dextrose administration.[20,67]

Artifactual hypoglycemia refers to blood glucose levels that are depressed because of mishandling of blood samples. Both leukocytes and erythrocytes metabolize glucose via glycolysis for cellular energy. If blood is drawn and allowed to stand, the blood glucose level can fall from 10 to $20\ mg \cdot dL^{-1} \cdot h^{-1}$. An increase in blood cells, especially leukocytes, exacerbates the condition because of augmented glycolysis. Artifactual hypoglycemia has been observed in patients with leukemia and leukemoid reactions as well as polycythemia vera. Fluoride and oxalate inhibit glycolysis and are contained in gray-topped tubes, which should therefore be used for blood collection should the question of artifactual hypoglycemia arise.[23]

Presentation and Evaluation

Symptoms and signs of hypoglycemia are of two types: adrenergic and neuroglycopenic. Increased catecholamines cause adrenergic manifestations of sweating, weakness, nervousness, and tachycardia. If hypoglycemia continues, signs and symptoms of neuroglycopenia ensue. These signs represent the direct effect of hypoglycemia on neurologic function and include headache, confusion, focal neurologic deficits, seizures, and coma. The most dreaded complications of hypoglycemic coma are irreversible neurologic dysfunction and death.

The diagnosis of hypoglycemia in a symptomatic patient may be instantly established at the patient's bedside with a glucose monitor reading. If hypoglycemia is detected, blood samples should be drawn before therapeutic intervention for the measurement of glucose, cortisol, plasma insulin, and connecting peptide (C peptide, the cleaved portion of the proinsulin molecule). Extra serum should be stored in case additional tests are required.

Nonketotic hypoglycemia suggests insulin-induced hypoglycemia. Hyperinsulinemia is diagnosed when an inappropriately high plasma insulin level (>5 μU/mL) occurs in conjunction with a glucose level of less than 40 mg/dL.[63] If a concomitant measurement of C peptide is similarly elevated (>0.6 mg/dL), endogenous insulin overproduction is confirmed. On the other hand, hyperinsulinemia in association with a suppressed C peptide level implicates exogenous (presumably surreptitious) insulin administration. Sulfonylureas stimulate endogenous insulin secretion, and their occult use may be detected by measurement of drug levels in serum or urine.

Treatment

A favorable clinical outcome is dependent on the speed of restoration of normoglycemia. Adult patients should receive 25 g of glucose intravenously (50 mL of 50% dextrose). If malnutrition is suspected, thiamine should be administered before the glucose to prevent acute neurologic injury. Subsequent therapy should be geared to maintain mild hyperglycemia. One suggested protocol in adults[66] is to infuse 10% glucose at a rate sufficient to sustain the blood glucose level at greater than 100 mg/dL. If hyperglycemia cannot be achieved despite 200 mL/h infusion of 10% dextrose, then 100 mg of hydrocortisone and 1 mg of glucagon are added to each liter of 10% dextrose. Diazoxide, an inhibitor of insulin secretion, may also be useful. It is added to 5% dextrose and administered in dosages of 3 to 8 $mg \cdot kg^{-1} \cdot d^{-1}$ until the blood glucose level stabilizes at greater than 100 mg/dL. When the patient awakens, a high carbohydrate diet of greater than 300 g/d is started. Increasing hyperglycemia is the sign to slowly withdraw therapy over a period of 24 hours. Throughout the treatment period, glucose levels should be monitored frequently to prevent a relapse of severe hypoglycemia.

Comparable therapeutic measures are recommended in children.[20] A bolus of 25% dextrose (0.5 g/kg) is administered, followed by a constant infusion of 10% dextrose. Glucagon, 0.1 to 0.3 mg/kg (up to a maximum of 1 mg), may be given either IV or IM. Hydrocortisone (5 $mg \cdot kg^{-1} \cdot d^{-1}$) is used in children with persistent hypoglycemia. Diazoxide may also be employed, but the enteral route (10 $mg \cdot kg^{-1} \cdot d^{-1}$ in two to three doses) is preferred because of its potent hypotensive effect. The IV dose of diazoxide is about 1 mg/kg by slow infusion, and blood pressure is carefully monitored. Other useful agents include octreotide (a long-acting analogue of somatostatin), which has proved to be efficacious in the treatment of children with hyperinsulinemia secondary to nesidioblastosis when surgery has been unsuccessful.[63]

Prevention

In the critically ill patient, blood glucose levels should be checked at least daily (more frequently in infants). Liver enzyme, BUN, and creatinine levels should also be monitored to detect worsening hepatic or renal function, which may disturb gluconeogenesis, glycogenolysis, and insulin metabolism. Diabetic patients who receive less than the usual caloric intake should have their insulin doses adjusted.

The critically ill patient has increased metabolic demands and must not be deprived of a source of calories. Children in particular should never be deprived of oral intake without a constant adequate supply of intravenous dextrose. Enteral or parenteral hyperalimentation should be initiated promptly as necessary to maintain adequate nutrition. To prevent possible hypoglycemia when total parenteral nutrition is discontinued, the infusion rate of the solution should be gradually tapered. In adults, this goal may be accomplished by decreasing the caloric intake 1000 kcal/d until the patient's daily intake is 2000 kcal. The infusion may then be changed to 5% dextrose (2 to 3 L/d) and subsequently stopped when the patient is able to ingest adequate amounts of food. A comparable tapering regimen may be used in children, although it may not be necessary.[66b]

References

1. National Diabetes Data Group: Classification and diagnosis of diabetes mellitus and other categories of glucose intolerance. Diabetes 1979; 28:1039.
2. Muir A, Schatz DA, Maclaren NK: The pathogenesis, prediction, and prevention of insulin-dependent diabetes mellitus. Endocrinol Metab Clin North Am 1992; 21:199.
3. Karam JH: Type II diabetes and syndrome X. Endocrinol Metab Clin North Am 1992; 21:329.
4. Nakaki T, Nakadate T, Kato R: α_2-Adrenoreceptors modulating insulin release from isolated pancreatic islets. Naunyn-Schmiedebergs Arch Pharmacol 1980; 313:151.
5. Ahren B, Taborsky GJ Jr, Porte D Jr: Neuropeptidergic versus cholinergic and adrenergic regulation of islet hormone secretion. Diabetologia 1986; 29:827.
6. Yki-Jarvinen H, Helve E, Koivisto VA: Hyperglycemia decreases glucose uptake in type I diabetes. Diabetes 1987; 36:892.
7. Imamura T, Koffler M, Helderman JH, et al: Severe diabetes induced in subtotally depancreatized dogs by sustained hyperglycemia. Diabetes 1988; 37:600.
8. Rayfield EJ, Ault MJ, Keusch GT, et al: Infection and diabetes: The case for glucose control. Am J Med 1982; 72:439.
9. Rubenstein A, Pierce CE, Bloomgarden Z: Rapid healing of diabetic foot ulcers with continuous subcutaneous insulin infusion. Am J Med 1983; 75:161.
10. McMurry JF Jr: Wound healing with diabetes mellitus. Surg Clin North Am 1984; 64:769.
11. Yudkin JS, Hendra TJ: Vascular events and diabetes: Acute myocardial infarction and stroke. *In*: International Textbook of Diabetes Mellitus. Alberti KGMM, DeFronzo RA, Keen H, et al (Eds). New York, John Wiley & Sons, 1992, pp 1185–1210.
12. Wheat LJ: Infection and diabetes mellitus. Diabetes Care 1980; 3:187.
13. Reeves WG, Wilson RM: Infection, immunity, and diabetes. *In*: International Textbook of Diabetes Mellitus. Alberti KGMM, DeFronzo RA, Keen H, et al (Eds). New York, John Wiley & Sons, 1992, p 1165.

13a. Sentochnik DE, Eliopoulos GM: Infection and diabetes. *In*: Joslin's Diabetes Mellitus. 13th ed. Kahn CR, Weir GC (Eds). Philadelphia, Lea & Febiger, 1994, pp 867–888.

14. Clark RS, English M, McNeill GP, et al: Effect of intravenous infusion of insulin in diabetics with acute myocardial infarction. Br Med J 1985; 291:303.

15. Husband DJ, Alberti KGMM, Julian DG: Methods for the control of diabetes after acute myocardial infarction. Diabetes Care 1985; 8:261.
16. Gwilt DJ, Nattrass M, Pentecost BL: Use of low-dose insulin infusions in diabetics after myocardial infarction. Br Med J 1982; 285:1402.
17. Siemkowicz E: Hyperglycemia in the reperfusion period hampers recovery from cerebral ischemia. Acta Neurol Scand 1981; 64:207.
18. Toni D, Sacchetti ML, Argentino C, et al: Does hyperglycaemia play a role in the outcome of acute ischaemic stroke patients? J Neurol 1992; 239:382.
19. Husband DJ, Thai AC, Alberti KGMM: Management of diabetes during surgery with glucose-insulin-potassium infusion. Diabet Med 1986; 3:69.
20. Weigle CGM: Metabolic and endocrine disease in pediatric intensive care. *In*: Textbook of Pediatric Intensive Care. Rogers MC (Ed). Baltimore, Williams & Wilkins, 1987, pp 1057–1109.
21. Gavin LA: Perioperative management of the diabetic patient. Endocrinol Metab Clin North Am 1991; 21:457.
22. Presti B, Kircher T, Reed C: Capillary blood glucose monitor: Evaluation in a newborn nursery. Clin Pediatr (Phila) 1989; 28:412.
23. Horwitz DL: Factitious and artifactual hypoglycemia. Endocrinol Metab Clin North Am 1989; 18:203.
24. Home PD, Massi-Benedetti M, Shepard GA, et al: A comparison of the activity and disposal of semi-synthetic human insulin and porcine insulin in man by the glucose clamp technique. Diabetologia 1982; 22:41.
25. Siperstein MD: Diabetic ketoacidosis and hyperosmolar coma. Endocrinol Metab Clin North Am 1992; 21:415.
26. Fleckman AM: Diabetic ketoacidosis. Endocrinol Metab Clin North Am 1993; 22:181.
27. Kecskes SA: Diabetic ketoacidosis. Pediatr Clin North Am 1993; 40:355.
28. Marshall SM, Alberti KGMM: Diabetic ketoacidosis and hyperglycaemic non-ketotic coma. *In*: International Textbook of Diabetes Mellitus. Alberti KGMM, DeFronzo RA, Keen H, et al (Eds). New York, John Wiley & Sons, 1992, pp 1151–1164.
29. Plotnick LP: Insulin-dependent diabetes mellitus. *In*: Principles and Practice of Pediatrics Updates. Oski FA, McMillan JA (Eds). Philadelphia, JB Lippincott, 1993, pp 1–13.
29a. Kitabchi AE, Fisher JN, Murphy MB, et al: Diabetic ketoacidosis and the hyperglycemic, hyperosmolar nonketotic state. *In*: Joslin's Diabetes Mellitus. 13th ed. Kahn CR, Weir GC (Eds). Philadelphia, Lea & Febiger, 1994, pp 738–770.
30. Faich GA, Fishbein HA, Ellis SE: The epidemiology of diabetic acidosis: A population-based study. Am J Epidemiol 1983; 117:551.
31. Connell FA, Louden JM: Diabetes mortality in persons under 45 years of age. Am J Public Health 1983; 73:1174.
32. Snorgaard O, Eskildsen PC, Vadstrup S, et al: Diabetic ketoacidosis in Denmark: Epidemiology, incidence rates, precipitating factors and mortality rates. J Int Med 1989; 226:223.
33. Jensen MD, Caruso M, Heiling V, et al: Insulin regulation of lipolysis in nondiabetic and IDDM subjects. Diabetes 1989; 38:1595.
34. Wood SM, Milne JR, Evans SF, et al: Effect of dobutamine on insulin requirement in diabetic ketoacidosis. Br J Surg 1981; 282:946.
35. Tibaldi JM, Lorber DL, Nerenberg MD: Diabetic ketoacidosis and insulin resistance with subcutaneous terbutaline infusion: A case report. Am J Obstet Gynecol 1990; 163:509.
36. Lambertus MW, Murthy AR, Nagami P, et al: Diabetic ketoacidosis following pentamidine therapy in a patient with the acquired immunodeficiency syndrome. West J Med 1988; 149:602.
37. Brandt KR, Miles JM: Relationship between severity of hyperglycemia and metabolic acidosis in diabetic ketoacidosis. Mayo Clin Proc 1988; 63:1071.
38. Martin HE, Smith K, Wilson ML: The fluid and electrolyte therapy of severe diabetic acidosis and ketosis. Am J Med 1958; 24:376.
39. Katz MA: Hyperglycemia-induced hyponatremia: Calculation of expected serum sodium depression. N Engl J Med 1973; 289:843.
40. Adrogue HJ, Lederer ED, Suki WN, et al: Determinants of plasma potassium levels in diabetic ketoacidosis. Medicine (Baltimore) 1986; 65:163.
41. Assadi FK, John EG, Fornell L, et al: Falsely elevated serum creatinine concentration in ketoacidosis. J Pediatr 1985; 107:562.
42. Arieff AI, Carroll HJ: Cerebral edema and depression of sensorium in nonketotic hyperosmolar coma. Diabetes 1974; 23:525.
43. Fulop M, Tannenbaum H, Dreyer N: Ketotic hyperosmolar coma. Lancet 1973; ii:635.
44. Gennari FJ: Serum osmolality: Uses and limitations. N Engl J Med 1984; 310:102.
45. Daugirdas JT, Kronfol NO, Tzamaloukas AH, et al: Hyperosmolar coma: Cellular dehydration and the serum sodium concentration. Ann Intern Med 1989; 110:855.
46. Adrogue HJ, Barrero J, Eknoyan G: Salutary effects of modest fluid replacement in the treatment of adults with diabetic ketoacidosis. JAMA 1989; 262:2108.
47. Duck SC, Wyatt DT: Factors associated with brain herniation in the treatment of diabetic ketoacidosis. J Pediatr 1988; 113:10.
48. Morris LR, Murphy MB, Kitabchi AE: Bicarbonate therapy in severe diabetic ketoacidosis. Ann Intern Med 1986; 105:836.
49. Fisher JN, Kitabchi AE: A randomized study of phosphate therapy in the treatment of diabetic ketoacidosis. J Clin Endocrinol Metab 1983; 57:177.
50. Zipf WB, Bacon GE, Spencer ML, et al: Hypocalcemia, hypomagnesemia, and transient hypoparathyroidism during therapy with potassium phosphate in diabetic ketoacidosis. Diabetes Care 1979; 2:265.
51. Rosenbloom AL: Intracerebral crises during treatment of diabetic ketoacidosis. Diabetes Care 1990; 13:22.
52. Carroll P, Matz R: Adult respiratory distress syndrome complicating severely uncontrolled diabetes mellitus: Report of nine cases and a review of the literature. Diabetes Care 1982; 5:574.
53. Brun-Buisson CJL, Bonnet F, Bergeret S, et al: Recurrent high-permeability pulmonary edema associated with diabetic ketoacidosis. Crit Care Med 1985; 13:55.
54. Davidson MB: Ketoacidosis and hyperosmolar nonketotic syndrome. *In*: Diabetes Mellitus: Diagnosis and Treatment. 3rd ed. New York, Churchill Livingstone, 1991, pp 175–212.
55. Khardori R, Cohen B, Taylor D, et al: Electrocardiographic finding simulating acute myocardial infarction in a compound metabolic aberration. Am J Med 1985; 78:529.
56. Adrogue HJ, Wilson H, Boyd AE, et al: Plasma acid-base patterns in diabetic ketoacidosis. N Engl J Med 1982; 307:1603.
57. Zonszein J, Baylor P: Diabetic ketoacidosis with alkalemia—A review. West J Med 1988; 149:217.
58. Wachtel TJ: The diabetic hyperosmolar state. Clin Geriatr Med 1990; 6:797.
59. Arieff AI, Carroll HJ: Nonketotic hyperosmolar coma with hyperglycemia: Clinical features, pathophysiology, renal function, acid base balance, plasma cerebrospinal fluid equilibria and the effects of therapy in 37 cases. Medicine (Baltimore) 1972; 51:73.
60. Khardori R, Soler NG: Hyperosmolar hyperglycemic nonketotic syndrome: Report of 22 cases and brief review. Am J Med 1984; 77:899.
61. Wachtel TJ, Silliman RA, Lamberton P: Predisposing factors for the diabetic hyperosmolar state. Arch Intern Med 1987; 147:499.
62. Fujikawa LS, Meisler DM, Nozik RA: Hyperosmolar hyperglycemic nonketotic coma: A complication of short-term systemic corticosteroid use. J Ophthalmol 1983; 90:1239.
63. Comi RJ: Approach to acute hypoglycemia. Endocrinol Metab Clin North Am 1993; 22:247.
64. Whipple AO: The surgical therapy of hyperinsulinism. J Int Chir 1938; 3:237.
65. Fischer KF, Lees JA, Newman JH: Hypoglycemia in hospitalized patients. N Engl J Med 1986; 315:1245.
66. Seltzer HS: Drug-induced hypoglycemia. Endocrinol Metab Clin North Am 1989; 18:163.
66a. Rowland MJ, Bransome ED Jr, Hendry LB: Hypoglycemia caused by selegiline, an antiparkinsonian drug: Can such side effects be predicted? J Clin Pharmacol 1994; 34:80.
66b. Werlin SL, Wyatt D, Camitta B: Effect of abrupt discontinuation of high glucose infusion rates during parenteral nutrition. J Pediatr 1994; 124:441.

67. Haymond MW: Hypoglycemia in infants and children. Endocrinol Metab Clin North Am 1989; 18:211.
68. Barrett EJ, DeFronzo RA: Diabetic ketoacidosis: Diagnosis and treatment. Hosp Pract (Off Ed) 1984; 19:89.
69. Alberti KGMM, Marshall SM: Diabetes and surgery. *In*: The Diabetes Annual/4. Alberti KGMM, Krall LP (Eds). New York, Elsevier, 1988.
70. Miller JA, Hallenbeck JM: Pharmacologic approach to acute seizures. *In*: Essentials of Critical Care Pharmacology. 2nd ed. Chernow B, Holaday JW, Zaloga GP, et al (Eds). Baltimore, Williams & Wilkins, 1989, pp 222–235.
71. Field JB: Exercise and deficient carbohydrate storage and intake as causes of hypoglycemia. Endocrinol Metab Clin North Am 1989; 18:155.

CHAPTER 120

Adrenal Dysfunction in the Intensive Care Unit

Michael Salem, MD • Anthony H. Guarino, MD
Bart Chernow, MD, FACP

The adrenal glands play a vital role in the body's endogenous response to numerous physical stressors.[1-4] The biologically active products of the adrenal cortex (glucocorticoids, mineralocorticoids) and the adrenal medulla (catecholamines) are requisite for normal development and cellular function (e.g., blood flow, heart rate, food and water intake, thermoregulation, and sexual behavior). Further, these secretory products are the peripheral components of many complex neuroendocrine systems, such as the hypothalamic-pituitary-adrenal (HPA) axis, the reproductive axis, growth axis, and the autonomic nervous system axis, which serve an adaptive role in responding to behavioral and physical stressors.[5] As our knowledge of intercellular communications and cell signal transduction increases, considerable experimental evidence supports the concept of a regulatory circuit between the neuroendocrine and immune systems.[6-11] Glucocorticoids secreted as a consequence of immunologic or inflammatory challenge serve as effectors to modulate the immune response.

Although adrenal dysfunction is not common, nor is it commonly recognized among critically ill patients, intensive care physicians may treat disease states that affect the adrenal glands. These states include adrenal hyperfunction (Cushing's syndrome, pheochromocytoma, and primary aldosteronism) and adrenal insufficiency (primary or secondary). In addition, critically ill patients face many clinically important physical stressors (major trauma, hypotension, infection, or hypoxia). Therefore, this chapter includes a discussion both of disorders of the adrenal gland and of stress-associated adrenal gland regulation and dysfunction. The remainder of this chapter details (1) adrenal physiology and regulation, (2) adrenal function in critical illness, (3) adrenal insufficiency, and (4) conditions of adrenal hormonal excess.

ADRENAL FUNCTION AND PHYSIOLOGY

Structure

The paired adrenal glands (average individual weight, 4–6 g at autopsy) are situated retroperitoneally at the upper poles of the kidneys. They are structurally divided into a head, body, and tail from inferomedial to superior aspects. The yellow adrenal cortex, which accounts for 90% of the weight of the gland, surrounds the gray medulla. Histologically, the mesodermally derived cortex is divided both functionally and by light microscopic characteristics into three zones. Aldosterone is the main mineralocorticoid secreted by the outer zona glomerulosa. Both the zona fasciculata and the zona reticularis contain the appropriate enzymes for the biosynthesis of cortisol and androgens, although it has been generally thought that the major byproducts of the zona reticularis are the adrenal androgens. The ectodermally derived adrenal medulla predominantly consists of chromaffin cells that produce and release catecholamines into the circulation in response to central nervous system–mediated activation of cholinergic preganglion neurons.

Neural Innervation and Adrenal Blood Flow

The neural innervation of the adrenal gland was first described about 100 years ago.[12] Now, morphologic evidence indicates that the adrenal glands are richly innervated.[13] Traditionally, sympathetic preganglionic and cholinergic nerve fibers were thought to pass through the cortex to the chromaffin cells of the medulla where catecholamines stored in granules are secreted in response to central nervous system–mediated signals. More recent work,[13-15] however, supports the concept of direct postganglionic adrenergic and peptinergic adrenal cortical innervation. In addition to increasing medullary secretory activity, neural control has been implicated as one of several regulatory mechanisms that modulate adrenal blood flow.[16]

The blood supply to the adrenal glands, although somewhat variable, originates from branches of the abdominal aorta, the renal arteries, and the inferior phrenic arteries. The major arteries branch in the outer cortex into a capillary plexus and sinusoids, and some arteries pass directly into the medulla.[17] The main venous drainage of the left adrenal gland is into the left renal vein, and the right adrenal gland drains directly into the inferior vena cava.

Although the adrenal glands receive only 0.14% of the cardiac output,[18] their blood supply is considerably in excess of that required for routine metabolism,[19] and is highly conserved under many life-threatening conditions. Regulation of adrenal gland blood flow is complex and incompletely understood. Further, marked differences exist between blood flow regulatory mechanisms between the vascular beds of the cortex and the medulla. The reader is referred to an excellent subject review,[16] although several general statements concerning regulation of adrenal blood flow can be made:

1. Blood flow to the adrenal glands increases significantly in response to such physical stressors as hemorrhage[20] and hypoxia.[16]
2. Neural stimulation of the medulla causes vasodilatation and a concomitant increase in catecholamine secretion rates. Neurally induced stimulation of cortical vasodilation has been postulated but not yet conclusively demonstrated.
3. Regional adrenal blood flow is modulated by many pharmacologic agents, including catecholamines,[21] nitric oxide,[22] adenosine,[23] acetylcholine,[24] histamine, and serotonin,[25] either by direct vascular action or through their action as neurotransmitters.
4. Adrenocorticotropic hormone (ACTH), at least in large doses, increases the rate of adrenal cortical blood flow through mast cell–mediated cortical vasodilation.[25-27]

Regulation of Glucocorticoid Release

Corticotropin-releasing hormone (CRH) is the principal regulatory peptide of the HPA axis.[28] Released at multiple central nervous system sites (predominantly from neurons of the hypothalamus that are probably under tonic opioid inhibition), CRH is transported via its portal circulation to the anterior pituitary, where it stimulates cellular ACTH release.[29] Although other hormones (catecholamines, vasopressin, oxytocin, vasoactive intestinal peptide, and naloxone), induce ACTH release, CRH is the principal mediator of ACTH release.

ACTH, a 39-amino-acid peptide derived from the cleavage of pro-opiomelanocortin, acutely and chronically stimulates steroidogenesis (including cortisol, corticosterone, aldosterone, and androgens) in adrenal cortical cells.[25] Acutely, ACTH engages the adrenal cortical cell membrane adenylate cyclase second-messenger system, which results in increased cytosolic cyclic adenosine monophosphate (cAMP) concentrations.[30] Increases in adrenal cellular cAMP concentrations result in enzymatic cleavage of a cholesterol side chain and rapid mobilization of intracellular cholesterol,[30] the rate limiting step in steroidogenesis. Chronically, ACTH has trophic effects (hypertrophy and hyperplasia) on the adrenal glands, which subsequently increase steroidogenesis. In addition to the neural input mentioned earlier, at least three other major mechanisms modulate ACTH release:

1. Pulsatile and *circadian rhythm* of ACTH and cortisol release. Circulating concentrations of ACTH and cortisol rise to a peak at about 8 AM, with subsequent declination in levels throughout the day, reaching a nadir at about 12 AM in subjects with a normal sleep-wake cycle. The ACTH secretory episodes probably result from pulsatile CRH release.[31]
2. Long and short *negative feedback loops* of glucocorticoids on CRH and ACTH release.[32] Increases in circulating glucocorticoid concentrations suppress the release of CRH and ACTH. Decreases in circulating glucocorticoid levels lead to increases in ACTH release. In addition, increasing concentrations of ACTH in a short feedback loop inhibit CRH release.
3. *Stress-associated activation* of the HPA axis. The release of CRH, ACTH, and glucocorticoids are modulated by physical and emotional stressors that lead to sustained activation of the HPA axis (see *Immune-HPA Axis*).

Glucocorticoid Actions

The normal daily production rates of cortisol in healthy subjects are estimated to be 12 to 15 mg/m^2 per day,[30] although recent work[33] suggests this may be an overestimate. The diverse biologic actions of glucocorticoids can generally be characterized as maintenance of normal and stress-associated cellular and tissue function. Most glucocorticoid effects are produced by tissue-specific induction or suppression of protein synthesis. Cytoplasmic glucocorticoid receptors contain both glucocorticoid and DNA binding sites.[34] Glucocorticoid-receptor binding results in an uncovering of the DNA binding site. When activated, the complex migrates into the nucleus and binds specific DNA sequences, activating or suppressing transcription and subsequent protein synthesis.

By increasing circulating glucose concentrations, glucocorticoids protect glucose-dependent tissue functions.[30] Glucocorticoids promote hepatic gluconeogenesis and glycogen storage, diminish the peripheral utilization of glucose in select tissues, and promote protein catabolism from which amino acid substrates are utilized for glucose production. Lipid metabolism is affected by glucocorticoid- and catecholamine-induced mobilization of lipids from peripheral stores, and by the subsequent provision of increased circulating concentrations of free fatty acids and glycerol as fuel substrates. Increases in circulating glucose concentrations result in increases in insulin release, which counter-regulates several glucocorticoid effects.

The fact that glucocorticoids are important for normal β-adrenergic receptor function[35, 36] may partly explain their importance in the cardiovascular system. Animal[37, 38] and human tissue studies[39] suggest that glucocorticoids increase synthesis of new β-adrenergic receptors, reverse β-adrenergic receptor dysfunction, and increase coupling between cell membrane β-adrenergic receptors and second-messenger systems. The mineralocorticoid properties (sodium ion and water retention) of some glucocorticoids also contribute to their effects on the maintenance of intravascular volume, and hence to cardiovascular stability.

The central nervous system effects of glucocorticoids have been described in relation to both the therapeutic use of glucocorticoids and the disease states associated with hormone excess or insufficiency. Glucocorticoids stimulate appetite and have profound effects on mood and behavior. Patients with adrenal insufficiency may manifest apathy, depression, or psychoses.[30] Central nervous system changes associated with glucocorticoid excess include euphoria, increased psychomotor activity, and psychoses.[39]

Regulation of Mineralocorticoid Release and Actions

The synthesis and secretion of the principal mineralocorticoid aldosterone is a complex and highly regulated process. Several secretagogues, such as potassium ions, angiotensin II, ACTH, serotonin, and β-endorphin, increase adrenal glomerulosa cellular synthesis of aldosterone, whereas others, such as atrial natriuretic peptide, dopamine, and somatostatin, appear to inhibit aldosterone synthesis. The stimulatory secretagogues, through different adrenal cortical cell second-messenger systems or voltage-activated calcium ion channels (in the case of potassium), increase intracellular free calcium concentrations. Increases in cellular free calcium concentrations correlate with increases in aldosterone production.[40–41] Cellular free calcium ions activate several protein kinases, resulting in an increased conversion of cholesterol to aldosterone.

The renin-angiotensin system is an important control mechanism of extracellular fluid volume. Renin is secreted by the kidney juxtaglomerular apparatus and enzymatically converts the hepatically derived angiotensinogen to angiotensin I. Enzymatic activation of angiotensin I to angiotensin II occurs in several tissue beds, but the primary site is the lungs. Angiotensin II modulates aldosterone synthesis and increases peripheral vascular resistance. Renin release is regulated by the integrated effects of many factors: volume-sensitive stretch receptors in the juxtaglomerular cells in afferent renal arterioles, chemoreceptors in the macula densa of the distal tubule that are sensitive to lumen sodium ion concentrations, neural innervation, and circulating factors (e.g., potassium ions, angiotensin II, and atrial natriuretic peptide).

Aldosterone increases sodium ion reabsorption in the renal distal tubule and collecting ducts. Increases in sodium ion reabsorption are linked to increased excretion of potassium and hydrogen ions. The net result of this activity is sodium and water retention and intravascular expansion.

Cytosolic mineralocorticoid receptors,[42] located primarily in the kidney but also found in the heart and brain, may encode for proteins that increase sodium reabsorption and increase the sodium-dependent adenosine triphosphatase.

ADRENAL FUNCTION IN CRITICAL ILLNESS

Immune-HPA Axis

Although the HPA axis response to physical stressors has been well described, little has been known regarding the purpose of the sustained increases in circulating concentrations of the products of the HPA axis in meeting the demands of stress (other than the provision of glucose substrate). Recent work details extensive bidirectional communication between the neuroendocrine (e.g., the HPA axis) and the immune systems. Increasing experimental and clinically based evidence supports the concept that the illness- or stress-associated systemic immune (inflammatory) response is a potent stimulus for sustained activation of the HPA axis. Further, secretory products of the HPA axis counter-regulate (dampen) the inflammatory response. Our emerging understanding of this "stress system" may provide an explanation for the spectrum of HPA responses described in critically ill patients and may stimulate investigation in this rapidly expanding field of immune-endocrine research in critically ill patients.

Woloski and colleagues[6] provided some of the first experimental in vitro evidence that interleukin-1 (IL-1) stimulated the release of ACTH and glucocorticoids. This work was supported by that of Besedovsky and coworkers,[8] who showed that infusions of IL-1 in vivo were associated with increases in circulating concentrations of ACTH and glucocorticoids. The results of numerous studies[7–9] now support the concept of immune (IL-1, IL-2, IL-6, and tumor necrosis factor) activation of the HPA axis. This activation may be mediated by CRH,[43–45] although there is also experimental evidence for direct cytokine-induced pituitary activation.

Several cytokines directly stimulate adrenal steroidogenesis. Tominaga and his colleagues[46] recently described in vitro increases in glucocorticoid production rates in response to the administration of several interleukins. Other investigators[47, 48] have shown that infusions of tumor necrosis factor cause sustained increases in circulating glucocorticoid concentrations in animal models. However, not all immune-system modulators are stimulatory. Transforming growth factor-β has been shown to inhibit the actions of ACTH on adrenal cortical cells.[49, 50] Similarly, certain macrophage and neutrophil secretagogues may inhibit steroidogenesis.[44, 51]

Glucocorticoids and, potentially, ACTH serve a reciprocal role in modulating the immune-inflammatory response through several negative-feedback loops. Snyder and Unanue[52] reported that cortisol decreased the in vitro production of IL-1 by macrophages. Staruch and Wood[53] showed that pretreatment of mice with dexamethasone was associated with significant decreases in circulating concentrations of IL-1 in an endotoxic shock model. Other investigators[54] showed that pretreatment of animals with dexamethasone was associated with a decrease in tumor necrosis factor release. In human patients with severe burn injury, Marano and his colleagues[55] described higher circulating cortisol concentrations in patients whose circulating tumor necrosis factor levels were not detectable.

Glucocorticoids' diverse immunomodulatory effects[44, 45] also include (1) induction of lymphocytopenia and monocytopenia, (2) interference with T cell antigen processing, (3) decreases in B cell antibody production, (4) inhibition of some cytotoxic T cell functions, (5) stimulation of neutrophil release from bone marrow, and (6) decrease in natural killer cell activity.

Other anti-inflammatory effects of glucocorticoids may be mediated by glucocorticoid-induced production of a family of proteins, lipocortins. Experimental evidence[56] suggests that lipocortins inhibit the enzyme phospholipase A_2, and hence eicosanoid release. The gene for the protein lipocortin-1 has been cloned and is inducible by glucocorticoids. Experimental evidence[56] suggests that in animal models, lipocortin-1 inhibits the release of prostacyclin, thromboxane A_2, and leukotriene C_4. Further work should elucidate the precise role of lipocortins and other modulators of the anti-inflammatory actions of glucocorticoids.

HPA Axis in Critical Illness

Our emerging understanding of the complex role of the secretory products of the adrenal gland in the immune-HPA axis may provide a plausible explanation for the variability reported in the adrenocortical responses to critical illness. The hormonal responses to surgery, trauma, and critical illness have been extensively studied over the past 15 to 20 years. ACTH, circulating cortisol, and urinary free cortisol concentrations all increase in response to acute medical illness,[57, 58] surgery,[1–4, 59–63] critical illness,[64–68] and trauma and burn injury.[5, 55, 69] Considerable interindividual variation exists in these responses. There also appear to be critical illness–induced shifts in steroidogenesis from androgens[70, 71] and aldosterone[72] toward the production of glucocorticoids. Illness- or stress-associated increases in circulating ACTH and glucocorticoid concentrations may modulate the systemic inflammatory response associated with illness or injury.

Span and his coworkers[67] described higher plasma cortisol concentrations among nonsurvivors in a population of 159 critically ill patients compared with survivors. Only one patient had biochemical evidence of adrenal insufficiency. They[67] and others[73, 74] suggest using circulating glucocorticoid concentrations or evaluation of HPA axis function as a potential marker for severity of illness. Schein and his colleagues[75] reported similar very high circulating glucocorticoid concentrations in patients who met criteria for sepsis. Plasma cortisol concentrations, however, *did not* correlate with survival and they suggest that cortisol values could not be used as an outcome predictor.

Rothwell and his colleagues[74] administered a short ACTH stimulation test to 32 patients who met criteria for sepsis associated with shock. In findings similar to those of others, they reported that baseline cortisol values were high (greater than 300 nmol/L in all but one patient), and that survivors had an increased response to ACTH stimulation (>250 nmol/L increase in cortisol values compared with baseline values) compared with that of nonsurvivors. In a recent study,[76] Reincke and his colleagues evaluated the HPA axis in 53 medical intensive care patients by performing an overnight dexamethasone suppression test or a CRH stimulation test. They report increased mean baseline ACTH and cortisol values in critically ill patients compared with control patients. Further, despite high baseline ACTH and glucocorticoid values, mean ACTH and cortisol concentrations decreased but were not entirely suppressed by dexamethasone administration and were increased in response to the administration of CRH.[76] The authors speculated that the illness-associated immune-HPA activation may be responsible for the altered HPA responses to dexamethasone and CRH.[76] Similarly, other investigators[77] showed that cortisol levels were not suppressible by dexamethasone administration in a group of critically ill patients who had a diagnosis of sepsis. In light of multiple stress system interactions operative in the setting of critical illness, the evaluation of adrenal function and the diagnosis of adrenal dysfunction, like other forms of organ dysfunction, may be complex. Further longitudinal studies relating critical illness–associated neuroendocrine and immune function may be important.

Stress-Associated and Perioperative Glucocorticoid Administration

Perioperative adrenal insufficiency is an excellent model for studying stress-associated adrenal crisis. In 1952, Fraser and his colleagues[78] reported the first case of surgery-associated adrenal insufficiency as a consequence of preoperative withdrawal of glucocorticoid therapy. A similar case was reported by Lewis and coworkers[79] later that year, and in both cases, only autopsy findings of adrenal hemorrhage (no biochemical evidence) supported the diagnosis of adrenal insufficiency. The Lewis case report concluded with a list of recommendations for glucocorticoid-dependent patients who require anesthesia and surgery. They suggested that patients receive their normal dose of glucocorticoid and 300 mg of cortisol preoperatively and "30 to 50 mL of aqueous adrenal cortical extract" during surgery.[79] The recommendations from this case report became the standard for perioperative care. Glucocorticoid-dependent patients who require anesthesia and surgery routinely receive 300 to 400 mg of cortisol daily in the perioperative period.[79] Our knowledge of the adrenal cortical responses to varying degrees of surgical stress has been refined over the past 10 to 15 years; however, recommendations for perioperative or stress-associated glucocorticoid administration have not been altered.[79a]

Although perioperative adrenal insufficiency is an uncommon complication of surgery, a review[2] of all the reported surgery-associated instances of death or hypotension in glucocorticoid-treated patients supports the concept that adrenal insufficiency may be a consequence of lack of perioperative glucocorticoid coverage. Glucocorticoid-dependent patients who manifest HPA axis suppression as a result of glucocorticoid administration for their disease process require perioperative glucocorticoid supplementation. Patients whose HPA axis is intact (i.e., a normal result from a 30-minute ACTH stimulation test) do not require supplemental glucocorticoid administration in the perioperative period beyond what they require for their baseline disease process. For elective surgical cases, we recommend a preoperative 30-minute ACTH stimulation test to evaluate HPA integrity. In urgent or emergent situations, the clinician must rely on vague clinical signs and laboratory information suggestive of adrenal dysfunction.

We believe that stress-associated glucocorticoid coverage should be provided based on the patient's preoperative glucocorticoid dosing regimen and the known stress-associated glucocorticoid production rate. After the provision of local analgesia, the HPA response to minor surgery is minimal in that replacement therapy beyond the patient's baseline dose is unnecessary. For minor surgical stress (e.g., inguinal herniorraphy, excisional biopsy), daily cortisol secretion rates suggest that the glucocorticoid target is 25 mg of hydrocortisone equivalent. Therefore, a patient should probably take his or her normal glucocorticoid dose 2 hours before surgery. If no complications occur, the patient can return to his or her normal dosing regimen the next day.

For moderate surgical stress, such as that resulting from abdominal hysterectomy, joint replacement, lower extremity revascularization, or segmental colon resection, cortisol production rates suggest that the daily glucocorticoid target is 50 to 75 mg of hydrocortisone equivalent for 2 days. These equivalents can be administered enterally or parenterally, depending on the nature of surgery.

Kehlet and Binder[80] used ^{3}H-cortisol to evaluate glucocorticoid production rates in major surgical stress and estimated that patients produced 75 to 150 mg of cortisol during the operative day. For major surgical stress (e.g., esophagogastrectomy, total abdominal colectomy, or cardiac surgery involving cardiopulmonary bypass), the glucocorticoid target is 100 to 150 mg of hydrocortisone equivalent per day for 2 to 3 days. In the absence of complications, cortisol secretion rates return rapidly (24–48 hours) to baseline values. Many clinicians use return of bowel function as an indicator to resume patients' normal glucocorticoid dosing regimen. No data indicate that these recommended glucocorticoid targets should be exceeded. Therefore, if a patient's baseline glucocorticoid dose exceeds the glucocorticoid targets, the patient should not require supplemental dosing.

ADRENOCORTICAL INSUFFICIENCY

Adrenocortical insufficiency, although an uncommon diagnosis in the intensive care unit, is an important one to consider because of potential life-threatening consequences. Primary adrenocortical insufficiency, first described in detail by Sir Thomas Addison,[81] is characterized by decreased adrenal gland production of glucocorticoids and mineralocorticoids. The incidence of Addison's disease, which has a marked female predilection and usually occurs in the third to fifth decades of life, is 20 to 60 cases per million in North America.[82] Secondary adrenal insufficiency is defined as adrenocortical hypofunction in response to decreased CRH- or ACTH-induced adrenal gland stimulation. Once recognized, adrenal insufficiency is relatively easy to treat.

Etiology and Pathogenesis

Autoimmune Addison's disease accounts for 65% to 80% of the currently recorded cases of primary adrenal insufficiency.[82] The disease process includes a combined antibody- and cell-mediated immune reaction against adrenocortical cells. Pathologic examination of adrenal gland specimens from patients with this diagnosis shows fibrous cortical replacement and relative medullary sparing. Before the advent of antituberculosis medication regimens, tuberculosis, which now accounts for 30% of recorded cases, accounted for most cases of primary adrenal insufficiency. How the frequency of tuberculosis-induced Addison's disease will change in light of the recent resurgence in strains of therapy-resistant tuberculosis remains to be elucidated. Other less frequent etiologies of primary adrenal insufficiency include adrenal hemorrhage resulting from injury, sepsis, coagulation disorders, ischemia, connective tissue disorders, or traumatic shock; neoplasia; amyloidosis; drug use; and familial disorders.

Acquired immunodeficiency syndrome (AIDS) has been associated with adrenal dysfunction and insufficiency, based both on clinical findings in AIDS patients (symptoms of weight loss, weakness, anorexia, myalgias, diarrhea) and on numerous autopsy reports of adrenocortical necrosis and infection.[83, 84] Glasgow and his colleagues[83] examined adrenal pathology specimens in 41 patients who died of AIDS. They[83] and others[84] reported frequent adrenal cortical necrosis (50–70%) and associated glandular infection (*Mycobacterium avium-intracellulare*, cytomegalovirus, cryptococcus), or glandular involvement with Kaposi's sarcoma, or both. These observations led some investigators to hypothesize a human immunodeficiency virus (HIV)-induced adrenal dysfunction in AIDS patients. Hilton and colleagues[85] in a prospective study of 11 patients with AIDS, found a normal response to a rapid ACTH stimulation test in all patients. One potential explanation for the paradox of biochemical evidence of normal HPA axis function and clinical symptoms of adrenal insufficiency in AIDS patients may be peripheral resistance to glucocorticoids induced by AIDS-associated functionally abnormal lymphocyte glucocorticoid receptors.[86] Causes of adrenal insufficiency are detailed in Table 120–1.

Secondary adrenocortical insufficiency occurs most frequently as a result of HPA axis suppression from the withdrawal of exogenous glucocorticoid therapy. Axelrod[87] states that anyone receiving the equivalent of 20 to 30 mg of prednisone per day for more than a week should be evaluated for HPA axis suppression. Functionally, the HPA axis suppression observed in exogenous glucocorticoid administration is primarily mediated by glucocorticoid-induced decreases in CRH secretion.

Diseases of the pituitary that cause hypopituitarism (ACTH deficiency and subsequent secondary adrenal insufficiency) include infarction (from traumatic injury or Sheehan's syndrome), neoplasia (e.g., craniopharyngiomas, adenomas, or metastatic lesions from lung or breast), lymphoproliferative malignancies, granulomatous disease (e.g., tuberculosis, sarcoidosis), previous pituitary surgery or transient adrenocortical insufficiency secondary to successful pituitary surgery, infection, or autoimmune disease.

Clinical Manifestations

Table 120–2 details the clinical manifestations associated with adrenal insufficiency. The clinical presentation of adrenal insufficiency is variable, ranging from vague nonspecific symptoms developing over several days in the unstressed patient to sudden cardiovascular collapse (addisonian crisis) in the patient undergoing clinically important physical stressors. In patients with chronic adrenal insufficiency, the most common general presenting symptoms are typically vague and nonspecific (e.g., weight loss, fatigue, anorexia, weakness, myalgias, and dehydration).[88] The fact that only extensive glandular destruction (>90%) is associated with decreases in basal glucocorticoid production rates may explain why many patients remain minimally symptomatic until faced with physical stressors, such as illness or injury.

Other clinical features of adrenal insufficiency may include:

1. *Hyperpigmentation* (secondary to increased melanocyte stimulating factor activity), which may be evident over extremity extensor surfaces, palmar creases, previous scars, on the lips and buccal mucosa, and on the gingiva of the mouth.

TABLE 120–1. Causes of Adrenal Insufficiency

Primary Adrenal Insufficiency	
Autoimmune	Malignancy
Infections	Primary
Tuberculosis	Metastatic disease
HIV associated	Lung
Cytomegalovirus	Gastrointestinal
Mycobacterium avium–intracellulare	Breast
Cryptococcus	Lymphoma
Toxoplasmosis	Melanoma
Kaposi's sarcoma	Adrenal Hemorrhage
Fibrosis	Sepsis
Infarction	Anticoagulant therapy
Histoplasmosis	Heparin
Blastomycosis	Warfarin
Coccidioidomycosis	Infarction
Meningococcus	ITP
Pneumococcus	Lupus anticoagulant
Medications	Familial
Metyrapone	Familial glucocorticoid deficiency
Aminoglutethimide	Infiltrating Diseases
Ketoconazole	Amyloidosis
Rifampin	Sarcoidosis
Phenytoin	Hemochromatosis
Etomidate	
Mitotane	
Phenobarbital	
Secondary Adrenal Insufficiency	
Exogenous glucocorticoid withdrawal	Surgery-induced
Hypothalamic or pituitary disease	Post-transsphenoidal pituitary surgery
Tumor	Removal of a functional adrenal lesion
Adenoma	Isolated ACTH deficiency
Sarcoidosis	
Hemorrhage	
Autoimmune	

Abbreviations: ACTH = adrenocorticotropic hormone; HIV = human immunodeficiency virus; ITP = idiopathic thrombocytopenic purpura.

TABLE 120–2. Clinical Manifestations of Adrenal Insufficiency

Glucocorticoid Deficiency Manifestations	
Cardiovascular	Renal
Hypotension	Impaired free water excretion
Impaired hemodynamic response to catecholamine administration	Metabolic
Orthostatic hypotension	Impaired gluconeogenesis
Gastrointestinal	Impaired lipogenesis
Nausea	Hypoglycemia
Vomiting	Hyponatremia
Anorexia	Muscular
Weight loss	Weakness
Abdominal pain	Fatigue
Change in bowel habits	Myalgias
Diarrhea	Arthralgias
Constipation	Neurologic
Cutaneous	Confusion
Hyperpigmentation	Apathy
Extensor surfaces	Lethargy
Palmar creases	Sensory deficits
Areolae	Psychoses
Scar tissue	Miscellaneous
Mucous membranes	Hematologic
Gingiva	Lymphocytosis
Respiratory	Eosinophilia
Reactive airways	Anemia
	Fever
Mineralocorticoid Deficiency Manifestations	
Cardiovascular	Metabolic
Hypotension	Electrolyte abnormalities
Hypovolemia	Hyponatremia
Shock	Hyperkalemia
Decreased cardiac output	Acidosis
Impaired hemodynamic response to catecholamine administration	Renal
	Azotemia

2. *Gastrointestinal symptoms* including nausea and vomiting (90% of cases), diarrhea (20%), and chronic abdominal pain (12–30%).

3. *Hemodynamic effects*, including orthostatic or frank hypotension.

4. *Behavioral abnormalities*, including depression, apathy, confusion, and various psychoses.

5. *Electrolyte abnormalities*, including hyponatremia, hyperkalemia, elevated blood urea nitrogen level, mild acidosis, and hypercalcemia. In primary adrenal insufficiency, electrolyte abnormalities are common and are related to glucocorticoid and mineralocorticoid deficiencies. In secondary adrenal insufficiency, isolated glucocorticoid deficiencies are typically observed, and electrolyte abnormalities are usually isolated to mild hyponatremia. Circulating glucose concentrations are usually in the low-normal range unless patients are not being nourished, which may occur in the inpatient hospital setting.

6. *Hematologic abnormalities*, including eosinophilia (10–20% of patients), normochromic normocytic anemia, and lymphocytosis.

7. *Androgen deficiency*, which may be associated with body hair loss in female patients.

Diagnostic Modalities

The diagnosis of adrenal insufficiency can be suspected, but not confirmed, by patient medication histories, physical examination, and electrolyte abnormalities. The accurate diagnostic assessment of the HPA axis is based on laboratory determinations. A random plasma cortisol concentration of greater than 500 nmol/L (18.1 μg/dL) argues strongly against a diagnosis of adrenal insufficiency; however, in most patients, random cortisol concentrations are less than 500 nmol/L. The episodic, pulsatile, and variable nature of the HPA response to physical stressors strongly suggests that a provocative test is important in evaluating HPA axis function, particularly in critically ill patients.

A very good initial diagnostic study to confirm a suspected diagnosis of primary adrenocortical insufficiency is a 30-minute ACTH stimulation test. A baseline blood sample is obtained for subsequent cortisol determination, followed by intravenous administration of 250 μg of synthetic ACTH (Cortrosyn, cosyntropin). A second blood sample for plasma cortisol is collected 30 minutes later. A plasma cortisol concentration of greater than 500 nmol/L (18–20 μg/dL) after the administration of ACTH excludes the diagnosis of primary adrenocortical insufficiency, but not secondary adrenal insufficiency. The 30-minute ACTH stimulation test has been criticized as not reflecting HPA axis function because of its peripheral stimulation of the HPA axis.[89] Other available provocative tests that centrally stimulate the HPA axis are the insulin-induced hypoglycemia, metyrapone, and CRH stimulation tests. Kehlet and his colleagues have repeatedly shown[90–92] a close correlation between results of the 30-minute ACTH stimulation test and the insulin tolerance tests, although they note that discordant results may be obtained in the first 1 to 2 weeks after pituitary surgery.

In the intensive care setting, the 30-minute ACTH stimulation test is an accurate and safe diagnostic tool for assessing HPA axis function and hence adrenal insufficiency. If the ACTH stimulation test results are abnormal or equivocal, then a plasma ACTH determination should be performed. A blood sample for subsequent ACTH determination should be obtained at the same time as the baseline blood sample for the 30-minute ACTH stimulation test. In primary adrenocortical insufficiency, cortisol concentrations remain low after ACTH administration, whereas the plasma ACTH concentration is high.

A 3-day ACTH stimulation test may be helpful in distinguishing primary from secondary adrenal insufficiency in patients for whom the diagnosis is equivocal. Synthetic ACTH (250 μg) is administered intravenously on 3 consecutive days. Daily cortisol determinations and 24-hour urine collections for subsequent 17-hydroxycorticosteroid determinations are performed. A normal test result includes a rise in circulating cortisol concentrations to 1000 nmol/L and an increase in urinary 17-hydroxycorticosteroid concentrations of greater than 15 mg/24 h. If circulating cortisol concentrations are not greater than 500 nmol/L, then primary adrenal insufficiency is present. A diagnosis of secondary adrenal insufficiency is suggested by progressive increases in circulating cortisol concentrations and urinary 17-hydroxycorticosteroid concentrations over the 3-day testing period in response to daily ACTH administration.

In addition to laboratory data, results of diagnostic imaging modalities, such as computed tomography (CT) and magnetic resonance imaging (MRI) can be quite useful in the diagnosis of adrenal insufficiency. Both modalities are sensitive and specific in diagnosing anatomic lesions of the HPA axis. CT images can precisely identify small atrophic glands (autoimmune adrenal insufficiency, calcifications, granulomatous disease), bilateral glandular enlargement (hemorrhage, neoplasia), and central nervous system lesions. Magnetic resonance technology provides excellent cortical and medullary resolution as well as potentially enhanced resolution of vascular invasion compared with that imaged by CT.[93]

Therapeutic Strategies and Prognosis

Treatment of adrenal insufficiency in the intensive care unit includes hormone replacement therapy and elimination or treatment of potential causative factors, such as neoplasia or infection. In the case of addisonian crisis, prompt recognition and treatment is critical. Immediate therapeutic intervention in acute adrenal insufficiency includes obtaining blood samples for subsequent cortisol and ACTH determinations and simultaneously administering 2 mg of intravenous dexamethasone daily or 100 mg of hydrocortisone (every 6 to 8 hours) until the results of diagnostic evaluation of the HPA axis are complete. Dexamethasone is the traditional glucocorticoid preparation used in this circumstance because it reportedly does not cross-react with cortisol assays. In our experience, however, all glucocorticoid preparations may cross-react with current cortisol assays, and this factor should be taken into account when results of HPA axis function tests are interpreted. Patients with acute adrenal insufficiency are treated aggressively with intravascular volume resuscitation, using isotonic crystalloid solutions that contain dextrose, and hemodynamic monitoring. A 30-minute ACTH stimulation test should be performed to establish the diagnosis when the patient is hemodynamically stable.

Once the patient has stabilized, maintenance hormonal therapy can be instituted. Replacement doses consist of 30 mg of hydrocortisone equivalent, administered daily; typically, 20 mg is administered in the morning and 10 mg at night. Alternatively, 5 mg of prednisone can be administered in the morning and 2.5 mg at night. This dosing regimen can be titrated to the patient's symptomatic improvement. Relative potencies of commonly used steroids are detailed in Table 120–3.

Chronic adrenocortical insufficiency requires both glucocorticoid and mineralocorticoid replacement. Glucocorticoids are administered in a dosing regimen (see earlier discussion) to simulate the daily cortisol secretion rates (12–15 mg/m^2). Care should be taken to avoid excessive administration of glucocorticoids, which may result in features of Cushing's syndrome and other potential negative effects of glucocorticoid administration. Mineralocorticoid replacement is administered to patients with primary adrenal insufficiency. The dosage range for fludrocortisone (Florinef) is 0.05 to 0.2 mg/d, and the usual starting dose is 0.1 mg/d. The dosing may be altered in patients with hypertension. Excessive mineralocorticoid dosing may cause congestive heart failure, metabolic alkalosis, hypokalemia, or hypertension. Patients requiring chronic adrenal replacement therapy should be informed of their need for lifetime medication and should wear a "Medical Alert" identification.

Implications in the Intensive Care Unit

The reported frequency of adrenocortical insufficiency in the critical care setting is extremely variable, ranging from less than 1%[57, 94] to 35%,[58, 65] depending on the study. Jurney and his colleagues[66] reported only one case (based on a rapid ACTH stimulation test) of primary adrenal insufficiency in 70 intensive care unit patients. Sibbald and coworkers[64] reported sepsis-associated adrenal insufficiency in 5 of 26 (19%) patients. Other investigators,[75] however, have described very high circulating cortisol concentrations associated with sepsis. Large prospective studies are not available that define the frequency of critical illness–associated adrenal insufficiency. Similarly, the potential issues related to *relative* adrenal insufficiency in addressing the HPA axis response to critical illness have not been sufficiently answered. Increasing recognition of the varied potential causes of adrenal insufficiency in the intensive care unit should lead the critical care practitioner to consider this diagnosis because of the high morbidity and mortality associated with unrecognized disease progression.

ISOLATED HYPOALDOSTERONISM

Isolated hypoaldosteronism is a syndrome characterized by a hypoaldosterone state accompanied by normal adrenocortical cell glucocorticoid production. It is commonly associ-

TABLE 120–3. Relative Potencies of Steroids

			Potency	
Agent	*Dose (mg)*	*Duration (h)*	*Mineralo-corticoid*	*Gluco-corticoid*
Dexamethasone	0.75	72	0	25
Methylprednisolone	4.0	36	0.5	5
Prednisolone	5.0	24	0.8	4
Prednisone	5.0	24	0.8	4
Cortisol	20.0	8	1.0	1
Cortisone	25.0	8	1.0	0.8
Hydrocortisone	25.0	8	1.0	0.8

ated with hyporeninemia. In patients with decreased or absent aldosterone secretion, potassium clearance is severely diminished, and clinically important hyperkalemia can result.

Etiology and Pathogenesis

Isolated hypoaldosteronism may be associated with any of the following: (1) decreased circulating concentrations of angiotensin, (2) decreased renal renin production, (3) decreased or absent angiotensin-converting enzyme, (4) decreased or abnormal angiotensin II adrenal cortical cell receptors, and (5) inability of the adrenal gland to produce aldosterone (primary hypoaldosteronism). The most common causes of isolated hypoaldosteronism are related to defective renal renin secretion (hyporeninemic hypoaldosteronism). These disorders include diabetes mellitus,[95] chronic renal disease,[96] systemic lupus erythematosus,[97] AIDS,[98] interstitial nephritis,[99] some medications, and congenital familial defect in renin production. A congenital form exists that is due to inborn errors (an enzymatic deficiency in corticosterone methyl oxidase) in aldosterone synthesis or peripheral mineralocorticoid resistance.

Other causes of isolated hypoaldosteronism are associated with increases in circulating concentrations of renin and include transient postoperative deficiency after removal of an adrenal lesion, autoimmune disease,[100] heparin administration,[101] hemochromatosis,[102] and hypoparathyroidism.[103]

Clinical Manifestations

One important clinical feature associated with hypoaldosteronism is hyperkalemia. Increases in circulating potassium ion concentrations may be asymptomatic; however, hyperkalemia can induce clinically important derangements in cardiac conduction and rhythm, syncope, weakness, and potentially sudden death. Sodium ion depletion and significant renal sodium losses are not usually clinically apparent.[88] Patients may manifest a mild hyperchloremic metabolic acidosis in conjunction with impaired ammonia excretion.

Diagnostic Modalities

Typically, hyperkalemia does not occur as a result of diminished renal function until glomerular filtration rates decrease to less than 10 mL/min; therefore, the presence of hyperkalemia in patients who manifest mild renal dysfunction should alert the clinician to the potential diagnosis of isolated hypoaldosteronism. The diagnosis can be established by plasma aldosterone and renin determinations; if both values are diminished, the diagnosis is established. Frequently, provocative tests of the HPA axis are performed to eliminate the possibility of global adrenal insufficiency.

Therapeutic Strategies and Prognosis

In many patients with mild, isolated hypoaldosteronism, no therapy is required. Performing disease-specific interventions, such as diabetic control, may improve the function of the renin-angiotensin system, and recognizing and treating interstitial nephritis may prevent hypoaldosteronism. Medications that cause renin-angiotensin suppression (β-adrenergic receptor blockers, prostaglandin-synthesis inhibitors, heparin, and potassium-sparing diuretics) should be avoided in patients who manifest hypoaldosteronism. Correction of chronic volume expansion and reduction in the potassium intake can have beneficial effects on the degree of hypoaldosteronism.

In cases in which mineralocorticoid replacement therapy is necessary, fludrocortisone acetate is administered in doses of 0.1 to 0.2 mg/d. The hyperkalemia and acidosis observed may respond to diuretic therapy by reducing chronic volume expansion and inducing kaliuresis. The use of diuretic agents may be more appropriate in older patients because of potential concomitant hypertension, renal insufficiency, or cardiac insufficiency, whereas salt and mineralocorticoid replacement may be more appropriate in younger patients.[104] In the intensive care unit, commonly administered medications, such as heparin, some antibiotics, β-adrenergic receptor blockers, and nonsteroidal anti-inflammatory agents, may induce hypoaldosteronism. When the syndrome is recognized, particularly when hyperkalemia is present, the offending agents should be discontinued.

ADRENAL HORMONAL EXCESS

Cushing's Syndrome

Cushing's syndrome is characterized by abnormally high circulating concentrations of glucocorticoids. Cushing's disease is defined as bilateral adrenocortical hyperplasia resulting from excessive stimulation by CRH or ACTH. The constellation of symptoms is related to chronic excess glucocorticoid secretion.

Etiology and Pathogenesis

About 40% to 60% of patients with adrenocortical hyperplasia have lesions of the pituitary gland that secrete ACTH (ACTH-dependent Cushing's syndrome). The tumors are typically microadenomas (50–80% of cases); however, some adenomas can grow larger and become locally invasive. *Ectopic ACTH syndrome* refers to a group of nonpituitary lesions that produce ACTH with resulting bilateral adrenal hyperplasia. In these lesions (e.g., small-cell lung carcinoma), ACTH is produced by tumor-associated amine precursor uptake and decarboxylate cells.[105] Several tumor lines have now been described that produce CRH[106] and subsequently cause bilateral adrenal hyperplasia. Cushing's syndrome may be caused by some functional adrenal adenomas and adrenal carcinomas (non–ACTH-dependent Cushing's syndrome). Another common source of excess circulating glucocorticoids that causes Cushing's syndrome is iatrogenically administered glucocorticoids. Table 120–4 details causes of Cushing's syndrome.

Clinical Manifestations

The clinical syndrome first described by Harvey Cushing[107] and others[108] is characterized by truncal obesity, hypertension, fatigue, weakness, hirsuitism, amenorrhea, abdominal striae, decrease in subcutaneous tissue mass, tissue edema, diabetes mellitus, and osteoporosis. Lipid distribution is altered so that fat is mobilized from the lower part of the body and deposited in (1) the posterior thoracic region (buffalo hump), (2) the supraclavicular regions, and (3) the face (moon facies). Extremity muscle wasting is a prominent feature. Generalized arteriosclerosis and nephrosclerosis may also be noted. Chronic excess circulating concentrations of glucocorticoids may have deleterious effects on the immune system. For example, glucocorticoids permit viral (e.g.,

TABLE 120–4. Causes of Cushing's Syndrome

Pituitary
Microadenoma
Macroadenoma
Hyperplasia
Adrenal
Adenoma
Carcinoma
Nodular dysplasia
Ectopic ACTH
Small cell carcinoma
Pancreatic tumor
Carcinoid tumor
Thymoma
Other bronchial tumors
Medullary thyroid carcinoma
Pheochromocytoma
Ganglioneuroma
Breast carcinoma
Ovarian carcinoma
Prostate carcinoma

Abbreviation: ACTH = adrenocorticotropic hormone.

herpes virus) dissemination and may reactivate pulmonary tuberculosis, histoplasmosis, and other fungal infections.

Glucocorticoid-induced osteoporosis can contribute to fracture development. Bone density loss results from both the osteolytic effects of glucocorticoids and the glucocorticoid-associated antagonism of vitamin D–induced calcium absorption. Avascular necrosis can also occur. Muscle wasting, negative nitrogen balance, reduced tissue repair rates, and resultant myopathy are caused by glucocorticoid-induced protein breakdown. Glucocorticoids stimulate hepatic gluconeogenesis, and increases in circulating glucose concentrations lead to glucose intolerance and potentially diabetes mellitus. Central nervous system effects include agitation, sleep disorders, depression, euphoria, and psychoses.

In terms of biochemical derangements, circulating cortisol concentrations are markedly increased. Normal diurnal variation is absent, and urinary levels of free cortisol, 17-hydroxycorticosteroids, and 17-ketosteroids are elevated. Electrolytes and other analyte values are typically normal (with the exception of glucose); however, with marked excess cortisol secretion, a hypokalemic metabolic alkalosis may be observed. Lymphocytopenia, monocytopenia, and leukocytosis may be seen in the peripheral blood smear.

Diagnostic Modalities

Patients with Cushing's disease uniformly manifest elevations in circulating cortisol and urinary free cortisol concentrations. Cushing's syndrome is also associated with increased cortisol production, but occurs as a consequence of adrenal adenoma or carcinoma, ectopic ACTH or CRH production, and nodular adrenal dysplasia. The differentiation of these conditions is important so that disease-specific treatment can be instituted.

A good screening test for Cushing's syndrome is the dexamethasone suppression test.[109] Dexamethasone suppression tests are useful in differentiating pituitary from ectopic causes of Cushing's syndrome. One milligram of dexamethasone is administered at the hour of sleep initiation, and a blood sample for subsequent cortisol determination is obtained the next morning. The administered dexamethasone should suppress cortisol production, leading to a morning plasma cortisol concentration of less than 138 nmol/L. If the morning cortisol level is greater than 138 nmol/L, then ACTH secretion is probably autonomous, and the patient likely has Cushing's disease. Pituitary or hypothalamic lesions are "reset" at a higher level of ACTH or CRH secretion and *do suppress* cortisol and 24-hour urinary free cortisol values with *high* doses of dexamethasone (2 mg of dexamethasone administered every 6 hours for 2 days). Failure to suppress cortisol production at high doses of dexamethasone suggests an adrenal or ectopic cause of Cushing's syndrome. A plasma ACTH determination should also be performed. The CRH stimulation test performed in combination with the dexamethasone suppression test may improve the accuracy in the differentiation of causes of Cushing's syndrome.[110]

After biochemical testing, localization and characterization studies of tumors are performed. Contrast-enhanced CT scanning, although not a particularly sensitive test for small pituitary tumors, provides important information to the surgeon. Gadolinium-enhanced MRI of the pituitary may be more sensitive than CT scanning[111]; however, further investigations should determine which modality is more specific for pituitary lesions. If the adrenal gland, and not the pituitary, is determined to be the primary cause of Cushing's syndrome, abdominal CT scanning is very sensitive and specific for adrenal gland lesions. Inferior petrosal sinus sampling may provide important localizing information that confirms a pituitary source of ACTH overproduction.[109] If ectopic ACTH production is deemed the cause of Cushing's syndrome after routine testing (chest radiograph, hematologic and biologic screening, tumor marker evaluation), a CT scan of both the chest and the abdomen is performed.

Therapeutic Strategies and Prognosis

The treatment of Cushing's syndrome is directed at the source of hypersecretion. The preferred therapy for Cushing's disease is transsphenoidal surgery performed at a large referral center. Cure rates in patients with documented microadenomas are about 90%.[112] The transsphenoidal approach is associated with a prompt response, low morbidity, and rarely hypopituitarism. Recovery of postoperative endocrine function (mean recovery time, 11 months) is dependent on the amount of tissue removed. Postoperatively, patients are treated for secondary adrenal insufficiency until HPA axis competence is assured. Some recent reports[113, 114] suggest that urinary free cortisol determinations may help to predict outcome of transsphenoidal pituitary surgery.

External-beam radiation of the pituitary as primary therapy for Cushing's disease is associated with relatively low remission rates in adults (15–25%) but may be more successful in children.[115] The onset of effectiveness is slow, and if this treatment modality is selected, combined medical therapy is usually required. Radiation therapy may be considered as an adjunct if surgery fails. Surgical abdominal exploration and removal of adrenal adenomas is curative, and removal, or debulking, or both, of carcinomas is useful. Ten per cent of adenomas are bilateral, and both glands should be examined if preoperative testing suggests bilateral disease.

Medical therapy may be used in candidates who are poor operative risks or in those with disseminated disease. Several agents, such as aminoglutethimide, metyrapone, and *o,p'*-DDD (mitotane), are available that inhibit cortisol synthesis. Other potential agents, such as ketoconazole, somatostatin, low-dose etomidate, or cortisol receptor antagonists (RU-38486) are being investigated.[109] Patients are closely monitored when taking these agents to avoid potential adrenal insufficiency.

Implications in Critical Care

Cushing's syndrome is difficult to diagnose in the setting of critical illness (sustained stress–associated HPA axis activation). No accurate tests can be performed in this setting to differentiate the two conditions. After pituitary microsurgery, the patient should be closely monitored for diabetes insipidus and potential adrenal insufficiency. Other complications after pituitary surgery include hemorrhage, meningitis, or cerebrospinal fluid leak that requires repair. Most neurosurgeons provide patients with glucocorticoids during the perioperative period. Glucocorticoid dosing is then decreased postoperatively until standard replacement dosing is achieved.

PRIMARY ALDOSTERONISM

Primary aldosteronism refers to the disorder of increased aldosterone production that is independent of the renin-angiotensin axis. The clinical manifestations include hypertension, hypokalemia, and hypernatremia.

Etiology and Pathogenesis

Originally described by Conn in 1955, the classic cause (60–90% of cases) of primary aldosteronism is a solitary, aldosterone-producing adrenocortical adenoma (Conn's syndrome). Bilateral adrenal hyperplasia (idiopathic hyperaldosteronism) accounts for 20% to 30% of cases of primary aldosteronism. Idiopathic hyperaldosteronism is characterized by diffuse nodular changes of the adrenal glands and zona glomerulosa hyperplasia. Other, rare (<1%), causes are aldosterone-producing adrenal carcinoma, glucocorticoid-suppressible aldosteronism, and congenital aldosteronism. In each case, the common defect is excess production of aldosterone, resulting in increases in renal sodium reabsorption and concomitant potassium and hydrogen ion excretion, as well as suppression of plasma renin activity.

Clinical Manifestations

The most common clinical abnormalities observed are longstanding hypertension and hypokalemia.[116] The incidence of primary hyperaldosteronism in hypertensive patients is 0.5 to 2.0%. The peak age is between the third and fifth decade, and there is a 3:1 female predominance. Signs and symptoms related to potassium wasting include neuromuscular weakness, cardiac dysrhythmias, polyuria, polydipsia, cramps, paresthesias, tetany, paralysis, visual disturbances, and sudden death.[117] Carbohydrate intolerance due to the interference with the release and peripheral actions of insulin as a result of hypokalemia are present in 50% of patients. In many cases, mild-to-moderate hypertension may be the only symptom, and malignant hypertension is rare.

Biochemical abnormalities include hypokalemic alkalosis, hypernatremia, and hypomagnesemia.[117] Urinary abnormalities may include increased ammonium excretion, impaired urine concentrating function secondary to hypokalemia, mild proteinuria, and an increased frequency of bacteriuria and pyelonephritis.

Diagnostic Modalities

Because this disorder is a reversible cause of hypertension, the diagnosis should be considered in any hypertensive patient who has concomitant hypokalemia. Diuretic therapy, if administered as part of the antihypertensive regimen, should be discontinued for 3 to 6 weeks before evaluation. A normal circulating potassium ion concentration obtained on three separate occasions (when the patient is consuming >120 mEq/d of sodium) eliminates the possibility of primary aldosteronism. In patients with persistent hypokalemia, without other attributable causes, a plasma renin concentration should be determined. Primary aldosteronism is unlikely to be present in patients with normal or elevated plasma renin concentrations. If circulating concentrations of renin are low, the definitive diagnosis rests on the following criteria: (1) plasma or urinary aldosterone levels that do not suppress when the patient is salt loaded, (2) plasma renin activity that cannot be stimulated with salt restriction and upright posture, (3) persistent hypokalemia when the patient is salt loaded, and (4) normalization of circulating potassium concentrations with sodium restriction.

Once the diagnosis of primary aldosteronism has been biochemically established, localization studies (CT or MRI) are performed.[116] The differentiation between adrenal adenoma and bilateral hyperplasia causing aldosteronism is established in most cases by current imaging modalities. In difficult cases, selective adrenal vein blood sampling is both sensitive and specific in localizing the site of increased aldosterone production.[117]

Therapeutic Strategies and Prognosis

During the diagnostic evaluations, the major goals are to control hypertension and reverse potassium depletion. Unfortunately, therapy aimed at these abnormalities interferes with the diagnostic process. Blood pressure can be controlled with calcium channel antagonists or α-methyldopa without interfering with test results. Medical treatment of mineralocorticoid hypertension can be accomplished with aldosterone antagonists and potassium-sparing diuretics, such as spironolactone (200–400 mg) or amiloride (20–60 mg).

The treatment of choice for adenoma is unilateral adrenalectomy. Preoperative correction of potassium depletion with potassium supplements, low-sodium diet, and spironolactone therapy is important. Successful antihypertensive treatment with spironolactone may be predictive of a successful surgical result.[118] After an adrenalectomy is performed for an adenoma, all patients show improvement in their hypertension; however, 1 year later, only 70% of patients will be normotensive, and at 5 years, 40% to 50% will develop hypertension, but not hyperaldosteronism.

Medical therapy (spironolactone or amiloride, low-sodium diet) is used in patients with bilateral hyperplasia. Surgery is no longer advised, because adrenalectomy in these cases provides poor control of hypertension.[119] At times, additional antihypertensive agents (calcium channel antagonists) or potassium supplementation may be required to provide maximal medical therapy.

Implications in Critical Care

Preoperative control of hypokalemia and hypertension is requisite. Intraoperative blood pressure and electrolyte monitoring is performed, particularly when adrenal gland manipulation is in progress. Because the remaining adrenal gland may take several months to recover, stress-associated glucocorticoid coverage may be provided. Postoperatively, patients may develop hyperkalemia due to the hypoaldosterone state, and blood pressure may require therapeutic intervention.

PHEOCHROMOCYTOMA

A pheochromocytoma is a catecholamine-secreting chromaffin tumor most commonly found in the adrenal gland.[120]

Etiology and Pathogenesis

The hallmark of a pheochromocytoma is its ability to produce catecholamines (dopamine, epinephrine, and norepinephrine). Although it is a rare entity, occurring in fewer than 1% of hypertensive patients, it has clinical importance as a potentially curable cause of hypertension. Alternatively, if it is not treated, the clinical consequences include paroxysmal and potentially lethal hypertension. Pheochromocytomas are located in the adrenal gland in 80% to 90% of patients.[120] Extra-adrenal tumors are typically found in the sympathetic ganglia in the abdomen and thorax and in the organs of Zuckerkandl at the abdominal aortic bifurcation. Other rare locations include the neck, brain, or bladder. Five per cent to 10% of lesions are malignant. Most pheochromocytomas secrete norepinephrine as well as epinephrine in lesser amounts; rarely, a tumor secretes epinephrine predominantly or exclusively.[121]

Pheochromocytomas, along with medullary carcinoma of the thyroid and primary hyperparathyroidism, make up the multiple endocrine neoplasia (MEN II) syndrome. This syndrome is inherited as an autosomal dominant trait. Pheochromocytoma is also associated with neurofibromatosis (von Recklinghausen's disease) and hemangiomas (von Hippel–Lindau disease).

Clinical Manifestations

Pheochromocytomas have been reported to occur over a wide age range (5 months–82 years), but the highest frequency is reported in the third to fifth decades. The usual presenting symptom is sustained (50%) or paroxysmal hypertension (50%). Occasionally, hypertension is absent. Hypertension results from increases in baseline circulating catecholamine concentrations or episodic, tumor-associated catecholamine release. Signs and symptoms of pheochromocytoma most commonly include diaphoresis, headache, and palpitations.[122] Other, less frequent symptoms include tachycardia, dyspnea, postural hypotension, tachypnea, flushing, tremor, angina, vertigo, a sense of impending doom, weight loss, wasting of fat stores, diarrhea, and nausea.[122] Patients may develop clinically important supraventricular and ventricular dysrhythmias or cardiac arrest. There is no unifying pattern to the onset, duration, precipitating factors, or the frequency of attacks.

Unless patients are having an acute exacerbation, physical examination may reveal only hypertension, orthostatic hypotension, tremor, or weight loss. In patients with MEN II, a thyroid nodule may be palpable, or neurofibromas may be evident. Occasionally, an abdominal mass may be palpable. Routine biochemical determinations are normal in patients with pheochromocytoma but may demonstrate hyperglycemia, glycosuria, hypertriglyceridemia, or frank diabetes mellitus.

Diagnostic Modalities

Similar to that for other diseases of the adrenal gland, the diagnosis of pheochromocytoma requires a high index of suspicion. The triad of diaphoresis, headache, and tachycardia occurring in a hypertensive patient should suggest the disease. Once suspected, a 24-hour urine collection should be performed for determinations of subsequent free catecholamines and their metabolites. Total metanephrines, unconjugated catecholamines, and vanillylmandelic acid are all excreted in significant quantities in the urine. If the tumor secretes dopamine exclusively, urinary homovanillic acid and dopamine concentrations are elevated. Before urinary tests are performed, patients should avoid alcohol, tobacco, caffeine, food containing vanillylmandelic acid, and certain medications (e.g., methyldopa and exogenous catecholamines). Under standardized conditions, plasma catecholamine determinations can then be performed to establish the diagnosis. These conditions include a fasting patient who is currently taking none of the above-mentioned substances and who has remained supine for 30 minutes or longer.

Anatomic localization studies such as CT or MRI are performed. CT scanning localizes most tumors; however, MRI may be more effective in localizing extra-adrenal tumors.[123] Scintigraphy using iodine 131–metaiodobenzylguanidine (MIBG) measures and localizes the functional capability of the tumor.[123] The test may be particularly useful in cases of recurrent pheochromocytoma, or in cases in which the lesion is particularly difficult to detect. The differential diagnosis of pheochromocytoma includes hyperadrenergic essential hypertension, medications (e.g., monoamine oxidase inhibitors, clonidine withdrawal), and anxiety attacks.

Therapeutic Strategies

The treatment of a patient with pheochromocytoma is surgical excision. Most tumors are benign, which facilitates this process. Preoperative α-adrenergic blockade (phenoxybenzamine, 10 mg orally twice daily, with increasing doses in the week before surgery, or prazosin, 2 to 5 mg twice daily) in addition to intravascular expansion consisting of preoperative hydration may mitigate intraoperative paroxysmal hypertension.[124] A β-adrenergic receptor antagonist is added, after α-adrenergic blockade, to this regimen if tachycardia or dysrhythmias are observed. Propranolol or another β-adrenergic receptor antagonist can be administered preoperatively (10 mg orally 3 to 4 times daily) or intraoperatively (1–2 mg IV).

Intraoperative hemodynamic monitoring through an indwelling arterial catheter, a pulmonary artery flotation catheter, and an indwelling Foley catheter, is essential for patient management. It has been suggested that atropine-like agents and halogenated hydrocarbons should be avoided. For the management of intraoperative hypertension, sodium nitroprusside or phentolamine are the rapidly acting agents of choice. Postoperative plasma and urinary catecholamine concentrations can remain increased for about 1 week. Operative mortality is reported to be less than 1%.[125] Hypertension is cured in 75% of patients, and in the remaining 25%, the hypertension is usually amenable to antihypertensive therapy. After successful surgical resection, recurrence rates are about 10% and life expectancy approaches the age-adjusted norms.

Malignant pheochromocytomas are characterized by functional metastases to sites that are not typical for chromaffin tissue. Management may include debulking procedures and prolonged medical therapy with α- and β-adrenergic blockade to control symptoms. Malignant lesions are generally chemoresistant and radioresistant, although a few reports indicate responses to either therapeutic modality.[126] Reported 5-year survival rates from malignant pheochromocytomas are less than 50%.[125]

Implications in Critical Care

The intensive care specialist commonly sees the pheochromocytoma patient postoperatively; however, occasionally these patients are brought to the intensive care unit for preoperative hemodynamic monitoring and optimization before surgery. Cardiovascular complications may be reduced by adrenergic receptor blockade and judicious intravenous hydration.

References

1. Chernow B, Alexander HR, Thompson WR, et al: The hormonal responses to surgical stress. Arch Intern Med 1987; 147:1273–1278.
2. Kehlet H: Clinical Course and Hypothalamic-Pituitary-Adrenocortical Function in Glucocorticoid-Treated Surgical Patients. Copenhagen, FADL's Forlag, 1976.
3. Udelsman R, Ramp J, Gallucci WT, et al: Adaptation during surgical stress—A re-evaluation of the role of glucocorticoids. J Clin Invest 1986; 44:1377–1381.
4. Meguid MM, Brennan MF, Aoki TT, et al: Hormone-substrate interrelationship following trauma. Arch Surg 1974; 109:776–783.
5. Chrousos GP, Gold PW: The concepts of stress and stress system disorders. JAMA 1992; 267:1244–1252.
6. Woloski BM, Smith EM, Meyer WJ, et al: Corticotropin-releasing activity of monokines. Science 1985; 230:1035–1037.
7. Bernton EW, Beach JE, Holaday JW, et al: Release of multiple hormones by a direct action of interleukin-1 on pituitary cells. Science 1987; 238:519–521.
8. Besedovsky H, Del Rey A, Sorkin E, et al: Immunoregulatory feedback between interleukin-1 and glucocorticoid hormones. Science 1986; 233:652–654.
9. Naitoh Y, Fukata J, Tominaga T, et al: Interleukin-6 stimulates the secretion of adrenocorticotropic hormone in conscious, freely-moving rats. Biochem Biophys Res Commun 1988; 155:1459–1463.
10. Breder CD, Dinarello CA, Saper CB: Interleukin-1 immunoreactive innervation of the human hypothalamus. Science 1988; 240:321–323.
11. Spangelo BL, MacLeod RM, Isakson PC: Production of interleukin-6 by anterior pituitary cells in vitro. Endocrinology 1990; 126:582–586.
12. Dogiel JW: Die Nervenendingungen in den Nebennieren der Saugethiere. Arch Anat Physiol 1894; S90:104.
13. McNicol AM: The human adrenal gland, aspects of structure, function, and pathology. *In*: The Adrenal Gland. 2nd ed. James VHT (Ed). New York, Raven Press, 1992, pp 1–42.
14. Rundle SE, Canny BJ, Robinson PM, et al: Innervation of the sheep adrenal cortex: An immunohistochemical study with rat corticotropin releasing factor and anti-serum. Neuroendocrinology 1988; 48:8–15.
15. Holzwarth MA, Cunningham LA, Kleitman N: The role of adrenal nerves in the regulation of adrenocortical functions. Ann N Y Acad Sci 1987; 512:449–464.
16. Breslow MJ: Regulation of adrenal medullary and cortical blood flow. Am J Physiol 1992; 262:H1317–H1330.
17. Sasano N, Sasano H: The adrenal cortex. *In*: Functional Endocrine Pathology. Kovacs K, Asa SL (Eds). Boston, Blackwell Scientific Publications, 1990, pp 546–584.
18. Sapirstein LA, Goldman H: Adrenal blood flow in the albino rat. Am J Physiol 1959; 196:159–162.
19. Sakima NT, Breslow MJ, Raff H, et al: Lack of coupling between adrenal cortical metabolic activity and blood flow in dogs. Am J Physiol 1991; 261:H410–H415.
20. Houck PC, Lutherer LO: Regulation of adrenal blood flow: Response to hemorrhagic hypotension. Am J Physiol 1981; 241:H872–H877.
21. Valenta LJ, Elias AN, Eisenberg H: ACTH stimulation of adrenal epinephrine and norepinephrine release. Horm Res 1986; 23:16–20.
22. Breslow MJ, Tobin JR, Bredt DS, et al: Nitric oxide as a regulator of adrenal blood flow. Am J Physiol 1993; 264:H464–H469.
23. Hinson JP, Vinson GP, Kapas S, et al: The relationship between perfusion medium flow rate and steroid secretion in the isolated perfused rat adrenal gland in situ. J Endocrinol 1986; 111:391–396.
24. Kennedy JG, Breslow MJ, Tobin JR, et al: Cholinergic regulation of adrenal medullary blood flow. Am J Physiol 1991; 261:H1836–H1841.
25. Vinson GP, Hinson JP: Blood flow and hormone secretion in the adrenal gland. *In*: The Adrenal Gland. 2nd ed. James VHT (Ed). New York, Raven Press, 1992, pp 71–86.
26. Hartman FA, Brownell KA, Liu TY: Blood flow through the dog adrenal. Am J Physiol 1955; 180:375–377.
27. Hinson JP, Vinson GP, Pundney J, et al: Adrenal mast cells modulate vascular and secretory responses in the intact adrenal gland of the rat. J Endocrinol 1989; 121:253–260.
28. Orth DN: Corticotropin-releasing hormone in humans. Endocr Rev 1992; 13:164–191.
29. Wynn PC, Aguilera G, Morrell J, et al: Properties and regulation of high affinity pituitary receptors for corticotropin-releasing factor. Biochem Biophys Res Commun 1983; 110:602–608.
30. Haynes RC: Adrenocorticotropic hormone; adrenocortical steroids and their synthetic analogs; inhibitors of the synthesis and actions of adrenocortical steroid hormones. *In*: The Pharmacological Basis of Therapeutics. 8th ed. Gilman AG, Goodman LS, Rall TW, et al (Eds). New York, Macmillan, 1990, pp 1431–1462.
31. Avgerinos PC, Schurmeyer TH, Gold PW, et al: Pulsatile administration of human corticotropin-releasing hormone in patients with secondary adrenal insufficiency—Restoration of the normal cortisol secretory pattern. J Clin Endocrinol Metab 1986; 62:816–821.
32. Keller-Wood ME, Dallman MF: Corticosteroid inhibition of ACTH secretion. Endocr Rev 1984; 5:1–24.
33. Esteban N, Loughlin T, Yergey A, et al: Daily cortisol production rate in man determined by stable isotope dilution, mass spectrometry. J Clin Endocrinol Metab 1991; 71:39–45.
34. Munck A, Mendel DB, Smith LI, et al: Glucocorticoid receptors and actions. Am Rev Respir Dis 1990; 141:S2–S10.
35. Brodie BB, Davies JI, Hynie S, et al: Interrelationships of catecholamines with other endocrine systems. Pharmacol Rev 1966; 18:273–289.
36. Svedmyr N: Action of corticosteroids on beta-adrenergic receptors. Am Rev Respir Dis 1990; 141:S31–38.
37. Mackenzie CW: Dexamethasone inhibits isoproterenol desensitization of bovine tracheal trips. Fed Proc 1982; 42:1048.
38. Stephan WC, Chick TW, Avner BP, et al: Tachyphylaxis to inhaled isoproterenol and the effect of methylprednisolone in dogs. J Allergy Clin Immunol 1980; 65:105–109.
39. Varney NR, Alexander B, MacIndoe JH: Reversible steroid dementia in patients without steroid psychosis. Am J Psychiatry 1982; 100:660–665.
40. Braley LM, Menarchery AM, Brown EM, et al: Comparative effect of angiotensin II, potassium adrenocorticotropin and cyclic adenosine 3′, 5′-monophosphate on cytosolic calcium in rat adrenals. Endocrinology 1986; 119:1010–1019.
41. Capponi AM, Lew PD, Jornot L, et al: Correlation between cytosolic free Ca^{++} and aldosterone production in bovine glomerulosa cells. J Biol Chem 1984; 259:8863–8869.
42. Quinn SJ, Williams GH: Regulation of aldosterone secretion. *In*: The Adrenal Gland. 2nd ed. James VHT (Ed). New York, Raven Press, 1992, pp 159–189.
43. Berkenbosch F, Van Oers J, Del Rey A, et al: Corticotropin releasing factor-producing neurons in the rat activated by interleukin-1. Science 1987; 238:524–526.

44. Bateman A, Singh A, Dral T, et al: The immune-hypothalamic-pituitary-adrenal axis. Endocr Rev 1989; 10:92–112.
45. Imura H, Fakata J, Mori T: Cytokines and endocrine function: An interaction between the immune and neuroendocrine systems. Clin Endocrinol 1991; 35:107–115.
46. Tominaga T, Fukata J, Naito Y, et al: Prostaglandin-dependent in vitro stimulation of adrenocortical steroidogenesis by interleukins. Endocrinology 1991; 128:526–531.
47. Tracey KJ, Lowry SF, Fahey TJ, et al: Cachectin/tumor necrosis factor induces lethal shock and stress hormone responses in the dog. Surg Gynecol Obstet 1987; 164:415–422.
48. Bertini R, Bianchi M, Ghezzi P: Adrenalectomy sensitizes mice to the lethal effects of interleukin-1 and tumor necrosis factor. J Exp Med 1988; 167:1708–1712.
49. Feige JJ, Cochet C, Rainey WE, et al: Type β transforming growth factor affects adrenocortical cell differentiation functions. J Biol Chem 1987; 262:13491.
50. Hotta M, Baird A: Differential effects of transforming growth factor type β on the growth and function of adrenocortical cells in vitro. Proc Natl Acad Sci U S A 1986; 83:7795–7796.
51. Mathison JC, Schrieber RD, Laforest AC, et al: Suppression of ACTH induced steroidogenesis by supernatants from LPS treated peritoneal exudate macrophages. J Immunol 1983; 130:2757–2760.
52. Snyder DS, Unanue ER: Corticosteroids inhibit murine macrophage Ia expression and interleukin 1 production. J Immunol 1982; 129:1803–1806.
53. Staruch MJ, Wood DD: Reduction of serum interleukin 1 line activity after treatment with dexamethasone. J Leukoc Biol 1985; 37:193.
54. Malcolm D, Hinson D, Chia J: Dexamethasone inhibits endotoxin-induced tumor necrosis factor release in vivo (Abstract). Circ Shock 1988; 24:296.
55. Marano MA, Fong Y, Moldawer LL, et al: Serum cachectin/tumor necrosis factor in critically ill patients with burns correlates with infection and mortality. Surg Gynecol Obstet 1990; 170:32–38.
56. Peers SH, Flower RJ: The role of lipocortin in corticosteroid actions. Am Rev Respir Dis 1991; 141:S18–21.
57. Drucker D, Shandling M: Variable adrenocortical function in acute medical illness. Crit Care Med 1985; 13:477.
58. Tapper ML, Rotterdam HZ, Lerner CW, et al: Adrenal necrosis in the acquired immunodeficiency syndrome. Ann Intern Med 1984; 100:239–241.
59. Mattingly D, Tyler C: Plasma 11-hydroxycorticoid levels in surgical stress. Proc R Soc Med 1965; 58:24–26.
60. Khilnani P, Munoz R, Salem M, et al: The hormonal responses to surgical stress in children. J Pediatr Surg 1993; 28:1–4.
61. Alford WC Jr, Meador CK, Mihalevich J, et al: Acute adrenal insufficiency following cardiac surgical procedures. J Thorac Cardiovasc Surg 1979; 78:478–493.
62. Hume DM, Bell CC, Bartter F: Direct measurement of adrenal secretion during operative trauma and convalescence. Surgery 1962; 52:174–187.
63. Naito Y, Tamai S, Shingu K, et al: Responses of plasma adrenocorticotropic hormone, cortisol, and cytokines during and after upper abdominal surgery. Anesthesiology 1992; 77:426–431.
64. Sibbald WJ, Short A, Cohen MP, et al: Variations in adrenocortical responsiveness during severe bacterial infection. Ann Surg 1977; 186:29.
65. Finlay WE, McKee JI: Serum cortisol levels in severely stressed patients. Lancet 1982; i:1414.
66. Jurney TH, Cockrell JL, Lindberg JS, et al: Spectrum of serum cortisol response to ACTH in ICU patients. Chest 1987; 92(2):292–295.
67. Span LFR, Hermus ARMM, Bartelink AKM, et al: Adrenocortical function: An indicator of severity of disease and survival in chronic critically ill patients. Intensive Care Med 1992; 18:93–96.
68. Catalano RD, Parameswaran V, Ramachandran J, et al: Mechanisms of adrenocortical depression during *Escherichia coli* shock. Arch Surg 1984; 119:145.
69. Hume DM, Nelson DH, Miller DW: Blood and urinary 17-hydroxycorticosteroids in patients with severe burns. Ann Surg 1956; 143:316–329.
70. Wade CE, Lindberg JS, Lamiell JM, et al: Upon admission adrenal steroidogenesis is adapted to the degree of illness in intensive care unit patients. J Clin Endocrinol Metab 1988; 67:223–227.
71. Parker LN, Levin ER, Lifrak ET: Evidence for adrenocortical adaptation to severe illness. J Clin Endocrinol Metab 1985; 60:947–952.
72. Zipser RD, Davenport MW, Martin KL, et al: Hyperreninemic hypoaldosteronism in the critically ill: A new entity. J Clin Endocrinol Metab 1981; 53:867–873.
73. Barton RN, Stoner HB, Watson SM: Relationships among plasma cortisol, adrenocorticotrophin, and severity of injury in recently injured patients. J Trauma 1987; 27:384–392.
74. Rothwell PM, Udwadia ZF, Lawler PG: Cortisol response to corticotropin and survival in septic shock. Lancet 1991; 337:582–583.
75. Schein RMH, Sprung CL, Marcial E, et al: Plasma cortisol levels in patients with septic shock. Crit Care Med 1990; 18:259–263.
76. Reincke M, Allolio B, Wurth G, et al: The hypothalamic-pituitary-adrenal axis in critical illness: Response to dexamethasone and corticotropin-releasing hormone. J Clin Endocrinol Metab 1993; 77:151–156.
77. Perrot D, Bonneton A, Dechaud H, et al: Hypercortisolism in septic shock is not suppressible by dexamethasone infusion. Crit Care Med 1993; 21:396–401.
78. Fraser CG, Preuss FS, Bigford WD: Adrenal atrophy and irreversible shock associated with cortisone therapy. JAMA 1952; 149:1542–1543.
79. Lewis L, Robinson RF, Yee J, et al: Fatal adrenal cortical insufficiency precipitated by surgery during prolonged continuous cortisone infusion. Ann Intern Med 1953; 39:116–125.
79a. Chernow B, Salem M, Tainsh R, et al: Perioperative glucocorticoid coverage: A reassessment 41 years after emergence of a problem. Ann Surg 1994; 219:416–425.
80. Kehlet K, Binder C: Value of an ACTH test in assessing hypothalamic-pituitary-adrenocortical function in glucocorticoid-treated patients. Br Med J 1973; 2:147–149.
81. Addison T: On the Constitutional and Local Effects of Diseases of the Suprarenal Capsules. London, Samuel Highley, 1855.
82. Wulffraat NM, Drexhage HA, Bottazzo GF: Autoimmune aspects of Addison's disease. *In*: The Adrenal Gland. 2nd ed. James VHT (Ed). New York, Raven Press, 1992, pp 263–288.
83. Glasgow BJ, Steinsapir KD, Anders K, et al: Adrenal pathology in acquired immunodeficiency syndrome. Am J Clin Pathol 1985; 84:594–597.
84. Welch K, Finkbeiner W, Alpers CE, et al: Autopsy findings in the acquired immune deficiency syndrome. JAMA 1984; 252:1152–1159.
85. Hilton CW, Harrington PT, Prasad C, et al: Adrenal insufficiency in the acquired immunodeficiency syndrome. South Med J 1988; 81:1493–1495.
86. Norbiato G, Bevilacqua M, Vago T, et al: Cortisol resistance in acquired immunodeficiency syndrome. J Clin Endocrinol Metab 1992; 74:608–613.
87. Axelrod L: Glucocorticoid therapy. Medicine 1976; 55:39–63.
88. Tyrrell JB, Baxter JB: Disorders of the adrenal cortex. *In*: Cecil Textbook of Medicine. 17th ed. Wyngaarder JB, Smith LH (Eds). Philadelphia, WB Saunders, 1985, pp 1300–1320.
89. Reschini E, Catania A, Giustina G: Plasma cortisol response to ACTH does not accurately indicate the state of hypothalamic-pituitary-adrenal axis. J Endocrinol Invest 1982; 5:259–261.
90. Lindholm J, Kehlet H, Blichert-Toft M, et al: Reliability of the 30-minute ACTH test in assessing hypothalamic-pituitary-adrenal function. J Clin Endocrinol Metab 1978; 47:272–274.
91. Hjortrup A, Kehlet J, Lindholm L, et al: Value of the 30-minute ACTH test in demonstrating hypothalamic-pituitary-adrenocortical insufficiency after acute ACTH deprivation. J Clin Endocrinol Metab 1983; 57:668–670.
92. Lindholm L, Kehlet H: Re-evaluation of the clinical value of the 30-minute ACTH test in assessing the hypothalamic-pituitary-adrenocortical function. Clin Endocrinol 1987; 26:53–59.

93. Rafal RB, Kosovsky PA, Markisz JA: Magnetic resonance imaging of the adrenal glands—A subject review. Clin Imaging 1990; 14:1–10.
94. Sarnsbury JR, Stoddart JC, Watson MJ: Plasma cortisol levels—A comparison between sick patients and volunteers given intravenous cortisol. Anesthesia 1981; 36:16.
95. Perez G, Siegel L, Schreiner GE: Selective hypoaldosteronism with hyperkalemia. Ann Intern Med 1972; 76:757–763.
96. Schambelan M, Sebastian A, Biglieri EG: Prevalence, pathogenesis and functional significance of aldosterone deficiency in hyperkalemic patients with renal insufficiency. Kidney Int 1980; 17:89–101.
97. deFronzo RA, Cooke CR, Goldberg M, et al: Impaired renal tubular potassium secretion in systemic lupus erythematosus. Ann Intern Med 1977; 86:268–271.
98. Kalin MF, Poretsky L, Seres DS, et al: Hyporeninemic hypoaldosteronism associated with acquired immune deficiency syndrome. Am J Med 1987; 82:1035–1038.
99. Don BR, Schambelan M: Hyperkalemia in acute glomerulonephritis due to transient hyporeninemic hypoaldosteronism. Kidney Int 1990; 38:1159–1163.
100. Saenger P, Levine LS, Irvine WJ, et al: Progressive adrenal failure in polyglandular autoimmune disease. J Clin Endocrinol Metab 1982; 54:863–868.
101. O'Kelly R, Magee F, McKenna TJ: Routine heparin therapy inhibits adrenal aldosterone production. J Clin Endocrinol Metab 1983; 56:108–112.
102. Thomas JP: Aldosterone deficiency in a patient with idiopathic haemochromatosis. Clin Endocrinol 1984; 21:271–277.
103. Marieb NJ, Melby JC, Lyall SS: Isolated hypoaldosteronism associated with idiopathic hypoparathyroidism. Arch Intern Med 1974; 134:424–429.
104. Melby JC, Griffing GT: Isolated hypoaldosteronism. *In*: Current Therapy in Endocrinology. Krieger DT, Bardin CW (Eds). Philadelphia, BC Decker, 1983, pp 131–134.
105. Loriaux DLL: The treatment of Cushing's syndrome and adrenal cancer. Endocrinol Metab Clin 1991; 20:767–771.
106. Upton GV, Amatruda TT: Evidence for the presence of tumor peptides with corticotrophin-releasing-factor like activity in the ectopic ACTH syndrome. N Engl J Med 1971; 285:419–424.
107. Cushing H: The Pituitary Body and its Disorders. Philadelphia, JB Lippincott, 1912.
108. Osler W: An acute myxoedematous condition, with tachycardia, glycosuria, melena, mania, and death. J Nerv Ment Dis 1899; 26:65–71.
109. Klibanski A, Zervas NT: Diagnosis and management of hormone secreting pituitary adenomas. N Engl J Med 1991; 324:822–831.
110. Flack MR, Oldfield EH, Cutler GB, et al: Urine free cortisol in the high-dose dexamethasone suppression test for the differential diagnosis of the Cushing syndrome. Ann Intern Med 1992; 116:211–217.
111. Kaye TB, Crapo L: The Cushing syndrome: An update on diagnostic tests. Ann Intern Med 1990; 112:434–444.
112. Mamjpalam TJ, Tyrrell JC, Wilson CB: Transsphenoidal microsurgery for Cushing's disease. A report of 216 cases. Ann Intern Med 1988; 109:487–493.
113. Tahir AH, Sheeler LR: Recurrent Cushing's disease after transsphenoidal surgery. Arch Intern Med 1992; 152:977–981.
114. Arnott RD, Pestell RG, McKelvie PA, et al: A critical evaluation of transsphenoidal pituitary surgery in the treatment of Cushing's disease: Prediction of outcome. Acta Endocrinol (Copenh) 1990; 123:423–430.
115. Littley MD, Shalet SM, Beardfwell CG, et al: Long-term follow-up of low-dose external pituitary irradiation for Cushing's disease. Clin Endocrinol 1990; 33:445–455.
116. Semple PF: Mineralocorticoid excess. *In*: The Adrenal Gland. 2nd ed. James VHT (Ed). New York, Raven Press, 1992, pp 373–389.
117. Melby JC, Griffing GT: Primary aldosteronism: *In* Current Diagnosis. Conn RB (Ed). Philadelphia WB Saunders, 1985, pp 867–871.
118. Saruta I, Suzuke H, Takita T, et al: Pre-operative evaluation of the prognosis of primary aldosteronism owing to adenoma. Acta Endocrinol (Copenh) 1987; 116:229–234.
119. Ferriss JB, Brown JJ, Freser R, et al: Hypertension with aldosterone excess and low plasma renin: Pre-operative distinction between patients with and without tumor. Clin Endocrinol Metab 1981; 10:419–452.
120. Cryer PE: Pheochromocytoma. Clin Endocrinol Metab 1985; 14:203–220.
121. Page LB, Raker JW, Beberich FR: Pheochromocytoma with predominant epinephrine secretion. Am J Med 1969; 48:648–652.
122. Bravo EL, Gifford RW Jr: Pheochromocytoma: Diagnosis, localization, and management. N Engl J Med 1984; 311:1298–1303.
123. Quint LE, Glazer GM, Francis IR, et al: Pheochromocytoma and paraganglioma: Comparison of MR imaging with CT and I-131 MIBG scintigraphy. Radiology 1987; 165:89–93.
124. Sjoerdsma A, Engleman K, Waldman TA, et al: Pheochromocytoma: Current concepts and diagnosis and treatment. Ann Intern Med 1966; 65:1302–1326.
125. Sheps SG, Jiang NS, Klee GG, et al: Recent developments in the diagnosis and treatment of pheochromocytoma. Mayo Clin Proc 1990; 65:88–95.
126. Averbuch SD, Steakley CS, Young RC, et al: Malignant pheochromocytoma: Effective treatment with a combination of cyclophosphamide, vincristine and dicarbazine. Ann Intern Med 1988; 109:267–276.

CHAPTER 121

Nutrition in Critical Illness

Khursheed N. Jeejeebhoy, MB, BS, PhD, FRCP(C)

METABOLIC EFFECTS OF STARVATION, INJURY, ILLNESS, AND SEPSIS

The human body is in a constant state of flux. Tissue constituents are continuously being synthesized and broken down, or catabolized. These processes need energy, as do the functions of several vital organs, such as the brain, liver, kidneys, and intestine. Consequently, humans have to ingest nutrients to meet energy needs and to repair tissues that are being catabolized. In the normal adult human, food intake equals energy needs and losses that result from catabolism. Many factors disturb this equilibrium in critical illness, including anorexia and inability to eat, possible associated gastrointestinal disease, increased or altered requirements, and altered utilization.

The imbalance between reduced intake and augmented or altered requirements results in effects that are similar to those of starvation. In addition, altered utilization imposes additional derangement, which may result in loss of body tissue and altered function. Hence, the provision of adequate nutritional support in such patients requires an understanding of the metabolic effects of starvation and hypocaloric intake, acute injury, and sepsis.

Starvation and Hypocaloric Intake

Whenever a deficit between needs and intake occurs, the balance must come from body stores. The predominant aim of adaptation is to supply glucose or ketones to the brain. These nutrients are mandatory for brain functioning; in their absence, the brain is rapidly injured. The secondary aim of adaptation is to preserve the structural elements of the body, namely protein. To understand the availability of

TABLE 121–1. Sources of Energy and Protein in a 75-kg Man

Source	*Amount (kg)*	*Energy (kcal)*
Triglycerides	12	110,000
Protein	12	50,000
Carbohydrates	0.62	2480

TABLE 121–2. Basal Energy Consumption of a 75-kg Man*

Organ	*% of Basal Energy*	*Energy Consumed (kcal/d)*
Brain	20	288
Heart	5	72
Kidneys	10	144
Viscera	30	480
Muscle and other organs	45	648

*Basal energy consumption of 1 kcal/min = 1440 kcal/d.

these stores, it is necessary to understand the nature of the available stores and the basal energy requirements.

Carbohydrates, presenting mainly as glycogen, are not present in sufficient quantities to meet requirements for more than 24 hours (Tables 121–1 and 121–2). Theoretically, protein stores can supply energy for about 30 days; however, the resultant wasting would cause death long before the end of this interval. Therefore, body proteins cannot provide energy without destroying the structure of organs. The only remaining source of proteins is body fat, which is an expendable source of substrate and is energy dense. However, fat cannot supply glucose, an essential substrate for the brain, which requires 72 g/d of this carbohydrate. In early starvation, this requirement is met by gluconeogenesis from protein catabolism and from glycerol derived from lipolysis. However, with prolonged energy deficit, fatty acids transported to the liver are converted to ketones, which the brain progressively uses for energy; thus, body protein is spared.

The energy density of storage determines how much weight loss occurs when these stores are being utilized. Fat manifesting as triglyceride is stored in adipose tissues as an oil with little water, protein, and electrolytes. Pure triglyceride has an energy density of 9 kcal/g, which is only slightly higher than that of adipose tissue, which has an energy density of 8 kcal/g. In contrast, carbohydrate (manifesting as glycogen) and proteins are stored in cytosol along with water and potassium at an energy density of 1 kcal/g, instead of the 4 kcal/g for pure glycogen or protein.

Early Starvation

ENERGY METABOLISM. A fall in insulin level and a rise in glucagon level occur in early starvation. These hormonal changes result in a breakdown of glycogen and a release of glucose for the brain. Unfortunately, total glycogen stores can provide energy for a maximum of 24 hours (see Table 121–1). Therefore, alternative sources of energy must be mobilized and used. The most important such sources are free fatty acids (FFA) from triglyceride and glucose synthesized by gluconeogenesis from lactate, amino acids, and glycerol. The lower insulin levels activate hormone-sensitive lipase in adipose tissue, the lipase then hydrolyzes triglyceride in adipose tissue to FFA and glycerol. FFA becomes a source of energy to muscle and liver, and glycerol is available for glucose synthesis.

PROTEIN METABOLISM. The decrease in insulin levels results in protein hydrolysis in muscle and transamination of nitrogen from amino acids to pyruvate and α-ketoglutarate. This action causes the formation of alanine and glutamine. Alanine is a precursor for gluconeogenesis by the liver, and glutamine also carries nitrogen to the liver and is an energy substrate for the gut and lymphocytes and a substrate for ammonia synthesis by the kidney. Thus, this flow of amino acids from the muscle to the viscera maintains visceral and plasma protein synthesis despite wasting of muscle. Ultimately, nitrogen not incorporated into visceral proteins is converted to urea and is excreted. The nitrogen lost as urea is initially equal to the nitrogen intake before the start of starvation or the start of reduced protein intake. In Figure 121–1, the nitrogen intake was reduced from 16 to 5 g/d. The nitrogen loss continued, and a negative balance of about 50 g of nitrogen occurred before equilibrium was restored. Hence, at the start of protein-calorie malnutrition, nitrogen losses are high, but they rapidly fall until losses equal intake.

WEIGHT LOSS. As mentioned earlier, glycogen and protein are stored with water in a state of low-energy density. Therefore, during early starvation, weight loss is rapid, but as protein loss is reduced and body fat is used, the weight loss slows.

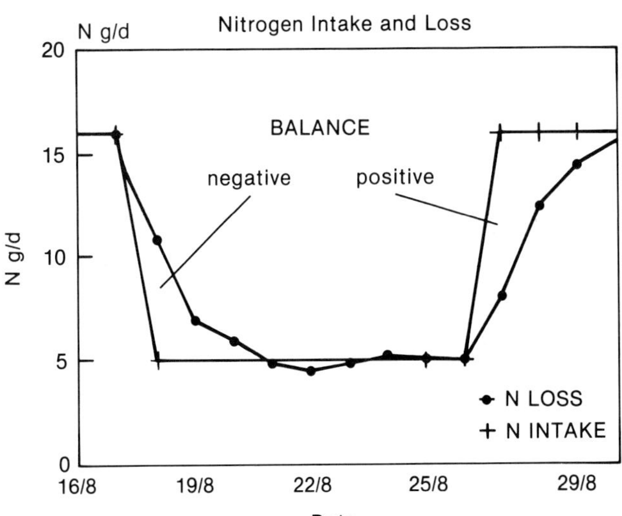

Figure 121–1. Nitrogen loss with reduced changes in intake.

Prolonged Starvation

In this state, the FFA level rises, and the acids are converted to ketones by the liver. In Figure 121–2, the control points are numbered 1 to 3. The reasons for the development of ketosis are (1) increased availability of FFA to the liver because low insulin levels promote lipolysis (2, 1), (2) reduced glucose to form glycerol for re-esterification to triglyceride (2, 2), and (3) reduced fat oxidation in the liver because the liver needs oxaloacetate for trichloroacetate cycle function, and oxaloacetate is used by increased gluconeogenesis because of low insulin levels (2, 3). These ketones are used instead of glucose as a source of energy by the brain and other tissues. The body conserves protein and uses fat as a source of energy, thus sparing body protein.

ENDOCRINE CHANGES. Endocrine changes occurring in protein-calorie malnutrition and their effects are given in Table 121–3. Reduced insulin and increased cortisol levels occurring during protein deficit cause increased catabolism and wasting. Despite increased growth hormone production, insulin-like growth factor I is reduced, and growth stops. In protein deficiency in patients with adequate energy intake, the renin-aldosterone level increases, and edema occurs. Reduced thyroid hormones and gonadotropins cause menstrual abnormalities and reduced basal metabolic rate.

HEMATOLOGY. Anemia is common and does not respond to iron or vitamin supplementation until protein intake is increased. However, iron deficiency due to blood loss or vitamin B_{12} or folate deficiency may occur concurrently as a result of the condition that caused the protein-calorie malnutrition, and this condition may aggravate the anemia.

ELECTROLYTES. A change in membrane potential and abnormalities of the Na-K adenosine triphosphatase pump results in a decrease in cell potassium level and an increase in cell sodium level. These factors may cause muscle abnormalities and fatigue.

CARDIOVASCULAR SYSTEM. Cardiac output and blood pressure are reduced and renal function is impaired in prolonged starvation. In severe cases, shock may occur.

IMMUNE SYSTEM AND CYTOKINES. Major defects of the T lymphocytes and complement systems occur. Although circulating B lymphocyte levels are normal, as are circulating immunoglobulins, secretory immunoglobulin production may be reduced. Gram-negative bacterial sepsis is common. Cytokine interleukin-1 production by macrophages is reduced, resulting in reduced leukocyte response to infections.

KWASHIORKOR AND MARASMUS SYNDROMES. The response to protein-calorie malnutrition in children may be wasting or wasting with edema. The former is called *marasmus* and the latter, *kwashiorkor*. These terms have been inappropriately used to describe adult clinical states not resulting from reduced nutrient intake but from diseases that cause wasting and hypoalbuminemia due to increased catabolism and protein loss. The protein loss can be through ulcerated bowel or through the kidneys. A pertinent clinical question is why do some individuals have edema and reduced plasma albumin levels and others have wasting and normal plasma albumin levels? The exact cause is unclear, but it is recognized that administration of carbohydrates with a low protein intake results in edema and hypoproteinemia. The likeliest explanation is that carbohydrate causes sodium retention when it is fed to malnourished individuals, resulting in "refeeding edema." The provision of carbohydrate energy increases insulin levels and prevents the mobilization of muscle protein (manifesting as amino acids) to supply nitrogen to the viscera. This phenomenon causes reduced liver and plasma protein synthesis.

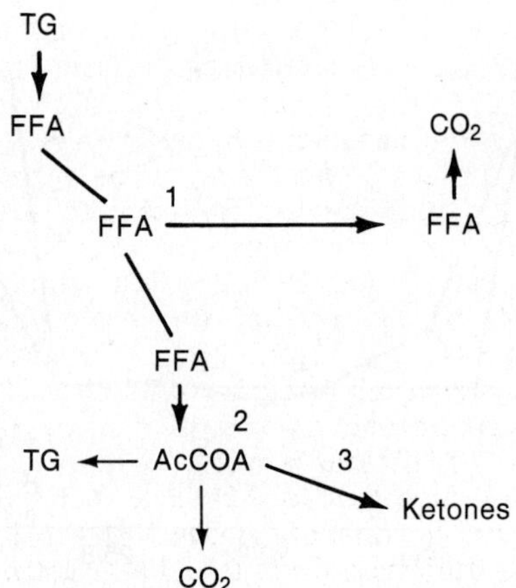

Figure 121–2. Pathways of ketosis. See text for explanation.

TABLE 121–3. Hormonal Effects of Protein-Calorie Malnutrition

Hormone	*Energy Deficit*	*Protein Deficit*	*Effect*
Insulin	–	–	↑ Catabolism
Growth hormone	±	+ +	↓ Urea synthesis
IGF-I	±	–	↓ Growth
Cortisol	+ +	+	↑ Catabolism
Aldosterone	None	+ +	Edema
Thyroid	–	–	↓ Metabolism
Gonadotropin	–	–	↓ Menstruation

IGF-I = insulin-like growth factor.

Effect of Injury and Sepsis

Injury and sepsis have similar effects on the metabolism of nutrients and often occur together. Therefore, the metabolic effects of trauma and sepsis may also be considered together. For example, a person suffering from a fractured pelvis and rupture of the bowel often develops peritonitis, and burn patients have burn wound sepsis.

PROTEIN AND ENERGY. Sir David Cuthbertson is credited with the first comprehensive observations of the effect of trauma on metabolism. He described patients after bone fracture and rats subjected to experimental fracture. In humans, increased protein catabolism, mainly from muscle, occurred. The nitrogen present in the chemical form of urea, sulfate, and phosphorus excretion increased to a maximum between the third and eighth day after injury and then declined. Associated with the increase in protein catabolism was an increase in metabolic rate. However, if the animal or human was malnourished, the excess catabolism was not seen. It is believed that the increased catabolism is related to mobilization of the labile nitrogen pool (see section on Obligatory Nitrogen Losses and Nitrogen Balance). Similarly, in rats, the increased metabolic rate is not seen if they are protein depleted. Therefore, hypercatabolism appears to be related to the protein nutrition of the animal or human in pure trauma.

GLUCOSE AND LIPID METABOLISM. Gluconeogenesis, the production of glucose from lactate and alanine in the liver, is markedly enhanced and is not sensitive to insulin infusion. In normal individuals, the administration of small amounts of insulin results in complete suppression of gluconeogenesis. In trauma-septic patients, gluconeogenesis is not suppressed by insulin, a phenomenon called *insulin re-*

sistance. In addition, increased lipolysis occurs because insulin resistance prevents insulin from suppressing lipolysis. FFA output rises, and fat oxidation is increased, resulting in hyperglycemia and mild acidosis.

HORMONAL AND NEUROENDOCRINE RESPONSE. A marked rise occurs in the counter-regulatory hormones, that is, the hormones that oppose the action of insulin. These hormones are glucagon, catecholamines, and cortisol (see Table 121–3). Note that total parenteral nutrition (TPN) increases the levels of these hormones and that despite high insulin levels, glucose levels are high, and FFA production is not shut off. The rise in glucagon level increases glucose output from the liver. The increase in catecholamine level increases the metabolic rate, increases liver glucose output, and increases lipolysis. Cortisol increases protein catabolism, mobilizes amino acids from muscle, and increases hepatic glucose production. The increases in cortisol and catecholamines are probably mediated by the central nervous system through the hypothalamic activation of the sympathetic nervous system and the release of corticotropin-releasing factor. Corticotropin-releasing factor in turn increases adrenocorticotropic hormone, which stimulates the adrenal glands to secrete cortisol.

CYTOKINES. Cytokines are peptides secreted by macrophages, lymphocytes, and endothelial cells in response to endotoxin and injury. They act on other organs to alter metabolism. The cytokines that are associated with trauma-sepsis are tumor necrosis factor α, interleukin-1, and interleukin-6. These cytokines cause anorexia and weight loss due to reduced intake. However, if attempts are made to feed tumor necrosis factor–infused animals to promote weight gain, they develop multisystem organ failure,[1a] a phenomenon seen in septic human patients. They have severe hyperglycemia, azotemia, and liver failure. Therefore, feeding trauma-sepsis patients is not a simple matter of giving many nutrients to meet the patient's metabolic requirement.

SUMMARY OF METABOLIC EFFECTS OF TRAUMA AND SEPSIS. The effects of trauma-sepsis are increased metabolic rate and increased mobilization of amino acids from muscle to viscera under the influence of hormones and cytokines. The hormonal effects are partly caused by activation of the central nervous system. Insulin resistance and tendency to glucose intolerance also occur.

Changes in Body Composition in Acutely Ill Patients

Clinically, the trauma-sepsis patient suffers wasting, despite receiving what appears to be an adequate caloric intake. How does this happen? In the past, the metabolic rate in these patients was believed to be excessive; therefore, the only way of preventing weight loss was presumed to be through the administration of massive amounts of calories. As is discussed later, the measured metabolic rate is not substantially increased in these patients. Reflection about the metabolic reaction to injury provides the answer. In this reaction, specific breakdown of muscle and release of energy substrates occurs. These substrates can be oxidized or stored as fat. Muscle is 80% water and 20% solid matter. Assuming that most of the solid matter is protein and carbohydrate, 1 kg of muscle = 800 kcal. In contrast, 1 kg of fat = 7000 kcal. Thus, specific muscle catabolism results in substantial weight loss because of the weight-calorie ratio of muscle to fat. For instance, a metabolic rate of 2000 kcal/d requires catabolism of 2.5 kg of muscle per day or only 0.3 kg of fat per day. As a result, in pure starvation, weight loss is minimized because body fat is the main source of energy. In contrast, in trauma-sepsis patients, in whom muscle provides much energy, weight loss and wasting are greater. Thus, muscle catabolism may cause dramatic wasting without hypermetabolism.

MACRONUTRIENTS

Proteins

Obligatory Nitrogen Losses and Nitrogen Balance

The fasting animal and human excrete nitrogen at rates that are proportional to their metabolic rates. Munro[1] indicated that endogenous nitrogen excretion is 230, 77, and 45 mg · kg^{-1} · d^{-1} in rats, dogs, and humans in relation to their basal metabolic rates of 108, 38, and 23 kcal · kg^{-1} · d^{-1}, making the endogenous nitrogen loss about 2 mg · kg^{-1} · d^{-1}. This value, called the *obligatory nitrogen loss,* varies between 41 to 69 mg · kg^{-1} · d^{-1}.[2] On the other hand, when a person who has had no oral intake is re-fed protein, nitrogen excretion does not rise in proportion to the intake, so that a gain of body nitrogen occurs. This gain in early refeeding has been found to be due to a rapid accumulation of nitrogen in the liver, to a lesser extent in the kidneys, and even less in muscle.[1] Thus, the early benefit of refeeding of protein appears to be an increase in liver protein. However, this early and spectacular nitrogen retention is not sustained, and nitrogen retention slows rapidly within 4 to 7 days. This phenomenon should be considered when short-term nitrogen balance data are interpreted, as is discussed later. Recent papers have emphasized the role of nitrogen balance for the determination of nutrient needs during parenteral nutritional therapy. Hence, it is appropriate to analyze the value and interpretation of nitrogen balance data. The human adult has finite cellularity of muscle and viscera, which determines the body nitrogen content. Hence, a well-nourished adult cannot have a positive nitrogen balance unless there is hypertrophy of existing muscle and viscera or an increase in tissue that is a part neither of muscle nor of viscera. Such an increase has been shown to occur mainly with deposition of adipose tissue; the added nitrogen is believed to be required to permit the development of supporting structures, such as connective tissue and blood vessels, and the increase in muscle fiber size required to support the additional weight of the adiposity. Experimentally, this concept has been supported by the studies of Keys and coworkers[3] in volunteers, and by Elwyn[4] in patients receiving parenteral nutrition.

Munro[1] noted that the nitrogen excretion in urine is partly dependent on the preceding nitrogen intake. Hence, the amount of nitrogen required to maintain balance in any individual depends on the previous intake of dietary nitrogen. When an individual receiving a high-protein diet starves or reduces his or her protein intake, the previously high urinary nitrogen loss continues for a few days, despite the reduced intake, resulting in a negative nitrogen balance, the magnitude of which is directly proportional to the previous intake level. The higher the preceding nitrogen intake, the greater the negative balance following subsequent starvation and vice versa. Interestingly, in rats, Munro[1] showed that the catabolic reaction to injury was greatest in well-nourished animals. The reaction was not clearly seen in malnourished rats. In addition, nitrogen loss after injury is greatest in healthy males and is lowest in malnourished subjects. However, within a few days of injury, the urinary nitrogen excretion falls until it is equal to the level of protein intake or is equivalent to at least 2 mg/kcal of the metabolic rate. Hence, protein catabolism rises with an increase in metabolic rate. However, the high initial negative nitrogen balance referred to earlier results in a limited loss of about

50 to 60 g (of a total of about 1800 to 2000 g of total body nitrogen), after which excretion falls to the low value of about 2 mg/kcal of the metabolic rate. These data indicate that short-term nitrogen balances reflect changes in the labile nitrogen pool of between 50 and 60 g only.

Protein-Energy Interrelationships

Years ago investigators showed in humans that increasing energy intake either as fat or carbohydrate increased nitrogen retention by 4 and 2 mg, respectively, of nitrogen per extra kilocalorie fed.[1] Calloway and Spector[5] showed that nitrogen retention increased when either nitrogen or energy intake was increased. However, the effect of each alone was restricted if given in insufficient amounts to meet requirements.

In injured subjects, nitrogen excretion rises in proportion to the rise in metabolic rate.[6] Thus, protein appears to become an important source of energy in injured subjects. Greenberg and colleagues[7, 8] noticed that the quantity of nitrogen given was an important determinant of nitrogen balance; when 2 g/kg of amino acids were given per day to such patients, a positive nitrogen balance was seen, even when total calories were less than metabolic requirements. Hoffer and coworkers[9] showed that in obese patients on a protein-modified fast, feeding a high nitrogen intake of 1.4 g/kg maintained nitrogen balance, whereas a lower nitrogen intake of 0.8 g/kg was associated with a negative nitrogen balance. Hence, giving amino acids alone made possible the induction of nitrogen balance in depleted adults. The ability of proteins to modulate nitrogen retention, independent of other factors, has been named *anabolic drive* by Millward.[10]

The ability of protein intake to modulate nitrogen retention, independent of the amount of energy or its source, explains three other observations. Yeung and associates[11] showed that patients receiving TPN gained a lot of weight, compared with those patients receiving an elemental diet. However, weight gain was due to an increase in body water and fat, but nitrogen retention was equivalent in the two groups. Even in patients with burns, who are traditionally regarded as having high caloric needs, Burke and coworkers[12] showed that when the protein intake was as high as 2.78 $g \cdot kg^{-1} \cdot d^{-1}$, the effect of additional glucose calories on protein synthesis or catabolism was minimal. In studies by Collins and colleagues,[13] total body nitrogen level after major surgery was as well maintained with an infusion of amino acids as with amino acids and glucose. Thus, based purely on total body nitrogen level, amino acid infusions by themselves apparently meet the previously held goal of a positive nitrogen balance. However, in functional terms, it is of interest that Young and Hill[14] showed that even though body nitrogen was as well maintained with amino acids alone as with amino acids plus "energy," the group of patients receiving supplemental calories recovered earlier and had fewer complications. This observation underscores the need for alteration of our views concerning nitrogen balance and body nitrogen as the best measurement of the effects of nutritional therapy. We have shown that the effect of nutrition on muscle function may be rapid and may occur even when little or no detectable change occurs in overall body composition.[15]

Protein Requirements

From the foregoing discussion of protein metabolism, it is clear that protein requirements are dependent on numerous metabolic factors, such as previous nutritional status, degree of nutritional depletion, provision of nonprotein energy, and rate of desired repletion. The more protein given, the less the effect of nonprotein energy intake and the greater the degree of nitrogen retention in the protein-depleted patient.

Protein requirements have been estimated by observing the amount of protein and energy needed to achieve nitrogen balance; that is, the observed difference between intake and measured losses should be zero or mildly positive. The tacit assumption is that when losses exceed intake, the patient is losing body protein, and vice versa. Another way of estimating requirements is by determining the amount of protein required to meet the requirements of essential amino acids. In addition, because cystine and tyrosine can replace approximately 30% and 50% of their essential precursors, the requirements of these amino acids also should be considered.

YOUNG ADULTS. On the basis of nitrogen balance data, the mean protein requirement for young males is an estimated 0.6 $g \cdot kg^{-1} \cdot d^{-1}$, with a standard deviation of 12.5%. Thus, 0.75 g/kg would encompass 2 standard deviations above the mean and be estimated to meet the requirements of 97% of young males. However, this amount is based on a reference protein of the composition of egg protein, which has a high proportion of essential amino acids. For mixed diets, the amount must be adjusted to meet essential amino acid requirements. The data are also applicable to young females. Are the data applicable for elderly patients as well? In theory, the amino acid needs for the elderly should be less. Unfortunately, the data on this topic are sparse, but available data suggest that amino acid requirements *do not* change with age.

CHILDREN AND ADOLESCENTS. The requirements of protein for children and adolescents have been estimated by adding the incremental protein requirements for growth to the intake necessary for balance. Based on these calculations, protein requirements at different ages are given in Figure 121–1. In this figure, the safe requirement is 2 standard deviations above the mean and is represented by the upper limits of the error bars.

PARENTERAL NUTRITION. The questions of whether intravenous amino acids are as effective in promoting nitrogen retention as oral proteins, and whether all amino acid preparations are comparable in their ability to promote nitrogen retention, are often asked. Patel and coworkers[16] compared the nitrogen balance achieved by intravenous administration of graded amounts of casein hydrolysate with that achieved by oral administration of casein and its hydrolysate. This study demonstrated that the amino acid composition of the hydrolysate given intravenously was not optimal and resulted in a lower balance than when the same casein, as intact protein, was administered orally. The finding that the nitrogen balance during the intravenous administration of casein hydrolysate was the same as that observed when it was given orally, keeping all other parameters constant, indicated that oral and intravenous amino acids were utilized identically as far as gross nitrogen economy was concerned. The authors surmised that the difference between the hydrolysate and the whole casein was due to a loss of sulfur-containing and aromatic amino acids during the process of hydrolysis. Anderson and colleagues[17] devised and infused an amino acid mixture enriched in these two groups of amino acids. Using a similar study design, they showed that with this more suitable amino acid composition, the intravenously administered amino acids were as effective in promoting nitrogen balance as was oral protein, and about 1 g/kg of ideal body weight was sufficient to promote positive nitrogen balance in patients.

Several interacting factors determine how much protein should be given. The nitrogen requirement for balance in normal adults is only 0.4 g · kg^{-1} · d^{-1}, and this was also found to be true for intravenously administered amino acids in the study by Anderson and colleagues.[17] However, increased nitrogen retention occurs with increasing intake, and this gain is linear over a range of 0.25 to 2 g · kg^{-1} · d^{-1}. Also, an increase in metabolic rate increases nitrogen loss, raising the basal needs for balance. Finally, the higher the nitrogen intake, the less dependent the balance on energy intake in depleted patients. On the other hand, poor renal and hepatic function reduces tolerance to amino acid loads. Taking all these factors into account, it seems desirable to give, as a first approximation, 1 to 1.5 g of a balanced amino acid mixture per kilogram of ideal body weight per day and to monitor the response of plasma proteins and urea nitrogen excretion in patients receiving parenteral nutrition.

Energy

General Concepts

CARBOHYDRATES. About 400 g of carbohydrate is eaten per day in a normal diet: 60% as starch, 30% as sucrose, and 10% as lactose. Starch is made up of 80% amylopectin and 20% amylose. Amylose is a straight-chain molecule with alpha (1–4) linkages. In contrast, amylopectin, in addition to these linkages, has branch points with alpha (1–6) linkages. Sucrose and lactose are disaccharides composed of glucose and fructose (sucrose) and glucose and galactose (lactose), respectively.

FATS. Dietary fat is composed of triglyceride of mainly four long-chain fatty acids; two saturated fatty acids, palmitic (C_{16}) and stearic (C_{18}) acids; and two unsaturated fatty acids, oleic (C_{18} with one double bond) and linoleic (C_{18} with two double bonds) acids. In addition, smaller amounts of linoleic acid (C_{18} with three double bonds) and medium-chain fatty acids (C_6 to C_{10}) are contained in the diet. Linoleic acid and its derivatives eicosapentaenoic and docosahexanoic acids are derived from fish. They have special anti-inflammatory and cholesterol-lowering properties.

Two unsaturated fatty acids, linoleic and linolenic acids, are called essential fatty acids because they cannot be synthesized in vivo from nondietary sources. Both fatty acids have 18 carbon atoms, but the position of the first double bond, called the omega (ω) number, is between the sixth and seventh carbons for linoleic acid and between the third and fourth carbons for linolenic acid. Linoleic acid is converted by chain elongation to arachidonic acid, which is the precursor of prostaglandins of the E^2 series, whereas linolenic acid is chain elongated to eicosapentaenoic acid and docosahexenoic acid and is a precursor of prostaglandins of the E^3 series.

Energy Requirements

The intake of energy is expressed as kilocalories or kilojoules (kilocalories × 4.18) per day of available energy. The availability depends on the amount of energy present in food that can be absorbed. This is close to the theoretic value for foods that do not contain fiber. The output of energy is due to basal metabolism (defined as the energy expenditure 12 hours after eating and soon after awakening from sleep in the morning), to physical activity, to the thermogenic effect of eating, and to anabolic processes such as growth, pregnancy, and lactation. In turn, these components are dependent on factors that include the body surface area (derived from height and weight), age, sex, and trauma-sepsis.

RESTING ENERGY EXPENDITURE. Resting requirements are most commonly predicted for normal humans by the Harris-Benedict equations. The equations for calculating the resting energy expenditure are as follows:[18]

Men:

$$\text{kcal/24 h} = 66.473 + 13.7516 \times \text{weight (kg)} + 5.0033 \times \text{height (cm)} - 6.7550 \times \text{age (year)}$$

Women:

$$\text{kcal/24 h} = 655.0955 + 9.5634 \times \text{weight (kg)} + 1.8496 \times \text{height (cm)} - 4.6756 \times \text{age (y)}$$

ACTIVITY FACTOR. The activity factor depends on the person's occupation and leisure activities. The activity factor is expressed as the multiple of the resting energy expenditure as given in Table 121–2. The total energy expenditure for a day can be estimated by multiplying the factor by the number of hours during which this factor is applicable and then summing the values for 24 hours (Table 121–2).

THERMIC EFFECT OF FEEDING. Eating or infusing nutrients increases the metabolic rate within an hour of eating, depending on the nutrient fed. The thermic effect is higher for glucose (6–8% of intake) and lower for lipids (2–3% of intake).[19] The thermic effect of carbohydrate administration is partly due to increased catecholamine secretion, which does not occur when lipids are infused. In patients with burns, the thermic effect is increased to 23% of the calories fed.[20]

PREGNANCY AND LACTATION. Pregnancy increases energy requirements by 300 kcal/d during the second and third trimester. Lactation increases energy requirements by 500 kcal/d.

GROWTH. The energy requirement for growth has been computed to be 5 kcal/g of tissue.[21] Because the weight gain in adolescence is about 5 kg/y, with an increase in height of between 4 to 6 cm/y from the ages of 12.5 to 16.5 years of age, the excess energy requirement will be 25,000 kcal/y, or 5000 kcal/cm. Clearly, any energy deficit will impair growth.

MALNUTRITION AND TRAUMA-SEPSIS. Malnutrition reduces the resting energy expenditure to an extent that exceeds that expected simply on the basis of weight loss. Injury, sepsis, and especially burns were believed to increase energy requirements by approximately 30%, 60%, and 100%, respectively.[6] However, recently, the degree of hypermetabolism in injured and septic patients has come into question. This matter is not only of theoretic but also of practical importance. If it is held that such patients lose weight because of hypermetabolism, then the logical treatment is to give a large excess of calories. Such excess feeding, however, increases the risk of metabolic complications.

Three studies, two of them based on controlled protocols, failed to find that septic patients are markedly hypermetabolic. Roulet and associates[22] found a metabolic rate increase of only 12.9% in critically ill patients in respiratory failure. Baker and colleagues[23] came to the same conclusion. In any case, an increase in metabolic rate of 60% in a 70-kg man, when referred to the basal energy expenditure (which is about 25 kcal · kg^{-1} · d^{-1}), requires only 40 kcal · kg^{-1} · d^{-1}, or 2800 kcal. Hence, little evidence exists of a need for 4000 to 6000 kcal, as has been claimed in the past.

Sources of Energy

Gamble,[24] in his classic studies, showed that feeding a modest amount (100 g) of glucose reduced the urinary excretion of nitrogen in normal, fasting subjects, demonstrating the protein-sparing effect of glucose. Based on the known protein-sparing effects of glucose and the increased metabolic rate and nitrogen loss observed in trauma-sepsis patients, TPN using very large amounts of glucose was advocated, in the belief that this therapy would promote nitrogen retention or reduce catabolism. This concept received support from the studies of Woolfson and coworkers[25] and Long and coworkers,[26] who showed that in burned patients, glucose was the only substrate capable of reducing nitrogen excretion and improving nitrogen balance. Recently, the paramount importance of glucose has come into question.

We[27] showed that in contrast to the observation of Long and coworkers in burned subjects,[26] patients with gastrointestinal disease utilize glucose and fat equally well, and both glucose and fat promote nitrogen retention to a similar extent. Askanazi and associates[28] showed that injured and septic patients, including those with burns, have an obligatory need for fat energy and continue to oxidize significant amounts of fat, despite being provided with all nonprotein calories as glucose. Furthermore, when a substantial amount of glucose is administered, not all the infused glucose is utilized directly for energy. The excess glucose calories must be stored. Once liver glycogen is repleted, the excess is converted to fat, which is deposited in the liver, resulting in hepatic steatosis.[29] Hence, it is now clear that the injured or septic patient needs a mixed substrate of glucose and fat to meet energy needs.

Essential Fatty Acid Deficiency

Certain fatty acids, principally linoleic acid, are essential for humans. Linoleic acid (18 carbon atoms, two double bonds) is converted to a longer-chain fatty acid (20 carbon atoms, four double bonds, i.e., a tetraene) called *arachidonic acid.* When linoleate is deficient, the same system that elongates the chain of linoleate apparently uses oleate (18 carbon atoms, one double bond) as a substrate and elongates it to a 20-carbon fatty acid with three double bonds (i.e., a triene) called *eicosatrienoic acid.* Because oleate can be synthesized from carbohydrates, an alteration in the plasma fatty acid pattern occurs during essential fatty acid deficiency. Linoleic acid and its daughter product arachidonic acid are both reduced, and, in place of the latter, eicosatrienoic acid appears in the circulation. The ratio of eicosatrienoic to arachidonic acid is called the triene:tetraene ratio, which is elevated in essential fatty acid deficiency.

During fat-free TPN, essential fatty acid deficiency occurs in adults. Clinically, essential fatty acid deficiency in patients receiving TPN is characterized by skin rash, reduced plasma levels of linoleate, and elevated triene:tetraene ratio. These changes were corrected by infusion of an intravenous lipid emulsion containing linoleate. Wene and colleagues[30] showed that the plasma pattern of essential fatty acid deficiency can be observed as early as 10 days after starting fat-free parenteral nutrition, before the onset of any clinically observable features. The reason for the early occurrence of essential fatty acid deficiency in adults receiving TPN is that when glucose is infused continuously, high insulin levels prevent the release of free fatty acids from adipose tissue stores. Hence, plasma fatty acids can originate only from either exogenously infused lipids or, in the case of fat-free parenteral nutrition, from endogenously synthesized lipids derived from carbohydrates. Because the endogenously synthesized lipids do not include linoleate, the pattern of fatty acids alters rapidly to that seen with essential fatty acid deficiency. Hence, during continuous glucose infusion, the only way to maintain plasma essential fatty acid levels is to infuse continuously lipids that contain them. Because intravenous lipid can reverse and prevent essential fatty acid deficiency, various regimens have been suggested in which variable amounts of lipid are given either once a week, twice a week, or three times a week, but none of these regimens has been tested rigorously. However, the more recent indication that lipid would be advantageous as a calorie source has made superfluous the concept of giving lipids only as a source of essential fatty acid.

Recommendations for Energy Intake

The energy requirements in normal persons depend on the mean activity factor of the individual and the resting energy expenditure. On the other hand, patients with malnutrition and trauma-sepsis have different requirements. In stable or malnourished individuals receiving either parenteral or enteral diets, the caloric requirements can be roughly computed from the relationships that about 30 kcal/kg (0.13 MJ/kg) maintains body weight and 40 kcal/kg (0.17 MJ/kg) induces weight gain. What should the energy intake be for the critically ill patient? Hitherto, based on the concept that these patients are grossly hypercatabolic, 4000 to 5000 kcal was often given to sick patients. In experiments using graded inputs of calories, we found that the most striking increase in nitrogen balance, with an increase in caloric intake, occurred when the intake increased from 0 to 40 kcal/kg of ideal body weight, and that increasing the intake of calories above this level did not appreciably increase nitrogen balance (see Fig. 121–2). This figure corresponds to the theoretic maximum calculated on the basis of a 60% increase in the metabolic rate referred to earlier and amounts to an intake of 2800 kcal/d in the 70-kg man. This caloric intake also comfortably exceeds the energy requirements noted for injured and septic patients by Askanazi and colleagues,[28] Roulet and colleagues,[22] and Baker and colleagues.[23]

Electrolytes

General Aspects

The importance of fluid and electrolyte replacement for the promotion of tissue perfusion and ionic equilibrium is self-evident. In addition, the processes of malnutrition and refeeding are both associated with major changes in electrolyte balance. With protein-calorie malnutrition, loss of the intracellular ions potassium (K^+)[31] and magnesium (Mg^{2+}) occurs,[32] together with a gain in sodium (Na^+)[33] and water.[34] On refeeding, potassium,[35] magnesium,[36] phosphorus (as monovalent or divalent phosphate),[35] and zinc (Zn^{2+})[37] must be given to ensure optimum nitrogen retention. Initially, the sodium balance may become markedly positive and may cause water retention during refeeding, particularly with carbohydrate.[38] This rapid weight gain, seen during the early phases of resumption of food intake, has been noted clinically—the so-called refeeding edema. Diuresis occurs as the nutritional status improves, and the edema disappears. In emaciated patients, refeeding must be undertaken with caution because pulmonary edema may occur if attempts are too vigorous. Furthermore, these patients may have hyponatremia[39] due to an inability to excrete free water, perhaps as a result of Mg^{2+} and K^+ deficiencies.[40]

Sodium and Chloride

SOURCE. Milk, cheese, bread, and cereals are rich sources of sodium. Fruits and potatoes are relatively low in sodium. Foods high in sodium are often high in chloride; however, chloride is also high in foods that are low in sodium and high in potassium, such as bananas, tomatoes, and sweet potatoes. Processing and preserving foods introduce large amounts of sodium and chloride in the form of sodium chloride.

ABSORPTION. Sodium is actively transported in association with carbohydrate. The absorption of sodium is enhanced by the ingestion of glucose. Chloride absorption occurs by various mechanisms. Chloride is absorbed as a passive process that follows the potential difference created by sodium absorption across the mucosa. In the ileum and colon, it is coupled to bicarbonate secretion. In addition, a transcellular neutral sodium chloride absorption may occur in the intestine.

DISTRIBUTION. Sodium and chloride are the most abundant extracellular ions and are responsible for maintaining the osmolality of the extracellular fluid. When intake is restricted, sodium is avidly reabsorbed by the kidneys under the influence of aldosterone. Normally, most of the bodily sodium and chloride is in the extracellular fluid, where these elements are present in concentrations of about 140 and 100 mmol/L, respectively. Because extracellular fluid amounts to about 20% of body weight, the total amounts of sodium and chloride in the extracellular fluid are about 1960 and 1400 mmol, respectively. In contrast, the sodium and chloride concentrations in the intracellular fluid are only about 5 and 2 mmol/L, respectively. Because intracellular fluid amounts to 50% of body weight, total intracellular sodium and chloride levels are therefore only 175 and 70 mmol, respectively. Thus, total body sodium level in the 70-kg adult averages 30 mmol/kg of body weight. In malnourished children, total body sodium level is increased. In surgical patients, most of whom were below 85% of ideal body weight, Hill and associates[41] found that total body sodium level was 2789 mmol (53.9 mmol/kg, nearly double the expected normal value of 30 mmol/kg) in patients whose average weight was 51.7 kg. After TPN administration, total body sodium level rose to a mean of 3038 mmol and was accompanied by an average weight gain of 2.6 kg. Thus, total body sodium level of these surgical patients increased to 56 mmol/kg, although the authors did not find this elevation to be statistically significant. In another study, in which oral diets were used, Veverbrants and Arky[38] indicated that carbohydrate feeding induces sodium retention, which is not seen when isocaloric amounts of fat or protein are fed. Hence, in malnourished patients great care should be taken to prevent salt and water overload, especially in elderly subjects and in those patients with cardiopulmonary disease. The more malnourished the patient, the greater the danger, especially when large amounts of carbohydrate are being infused. The obvious clinical manifestation of fluid overload is the appearance of refeeding edema.

RECOMMENDATIONS. The recommendations for sodium and chloride are similar. The minimum amount of sodium lost is about 5 mmol/d. However, sweating during physical activity and temperature changes result in an increased requirement, estimated to be about 20 mmol/d in the normal individual. No known advantages exist to taking more sodium, and the disadvantage is the development of hypertension in susceptible individuals. In most patients with gastrointestinal disease, about 100 to 200 mmol/d of sodium can be given. This amount should be supplemented with extra sodium to cover abnormal losses via the gastrointestinal tract. In severely malnourished patients and in those with cardiopulmonary disease, the sodium intake should be restricted to 50 to 60 mmol/d, and the amount infused should be gradually increased as the patient tolerates the fluid load. In this context, potassium and magnesium deficiency has been shown to hinder the excretion of free water, resulting in hyponatremia, because even though total body sodium is increased, total body water is increased even more. Under these circumstances, replacement of these two ions and the use of diuretics may be necessary.

Potassium

SOURCE. Potassium is present in many foods and is especially abundant in milk, meat, potatoes, and fruits. Traditionally, orange juice and bananas are considered rich sources of potassium.

ABSORPTION. Potassium absorption in the ileum is a passive process and depends on the concentration gradient. Potassium is secreted by the colon, and in patients with diarrhea, this loss may be aggravated, as it may be also by the long-term use of laxatives.

DISTRIBUTION. Potassium is the main intracellular cation, and its concentration in cells amounts to about 140 mmol/L. Based on water distribution in different body compartments, a 70-kg man has 4900 mmol of intracellular potassium. Based on an average extracellular potassium of 4 mmol/L, the extracellular content of potassium amounts to a total of only 56 mmol, giving a total body potassium level of 71 mmol/kg. In children with protein-calorie malnutrition, the total body potassium level is markedly reduced, but this deficiency is not reflected in lower plasma levels. In malnourished surgical patients, recalculation of the data by Hill and coworkers[41] for the total body showed that potassium level was only 39 mmol/kg and that TPN increased it to 43 mmol/kg without an increase in total body nitrogen level. We[42, 43] also noted that body potassium level was disproportionately reduced in malnourished patients when compared with nitrogen and was replenished by short-term (30-day) TPN[42] and oral refeeding[43] without alteration in total body nitrogen level. In contrast, long-term TPN increased both nitrogen and potassium levels.[42] Accordingly, potassium deficiency is an integral part of malnutrition and needs repletion apart from nitrogen. Rudman and colleagues[35] showed that a positive nitrogen balance during glucose-based TPN did not occur unless potassium was also given.

RECOMMENDATIONS. The range of normal dietary intake is determined by the fact that potassium is not as well conserved as sodium and that significant fecal and renal losses occur. To maintain body stores and normal plasma levels, 40 to 50 mmol/d of potassium must be given. In children, growth results in the deposition of 60 to 80 mmol of potassium per kilogram of weight gain. In growing children, an estimated 2 mmol per 100 kcal of energy intake should be given. Calculations of potassium requirements during parenteral nutrition must take into consideration that (1) glucose infusions increase the need for potassium, (2) about 3 mEq of K^+ are retained with each gram of nitrogen, and (3) based on the data of both Hill and colleagues[41] and Jeejeebhoy and colleagues,[42] the total deficit of potassium may be between 800 to 900 mmol in the 50- to 70-kg adult. Hence, during TPN, relatively larger amounts of potassium should be infused. The infusion of about 80 to 120 mEq/d aids in replenishing stores and in meeting daily needs.

Magnesium

SOURCE. Milk, meat, cheese, and leafy vegetables are rich in magnesium.

ABSORPTION. Only about 30% of oral intake of magnesium is absorbed. Most of the absorption takes place in the ileum because of slow transit in that area and the fact that uptake is passive. Absorption is linearly related to intake, without obligatory losses.

DISTRIBUTION. Apart from potassium, magnesium is the most abundant intracellular cation. Intracellularly, it is bound to protein and is necessary for numerous vital cellular functions, including membrane and mitochondrial integrity and enzyme activation (including that of adenosine triphosphatase and adenylate cyclase), and also for the synthesis and stability of nuclear DNA. It is also necessary for control of neuromuscular excitability. The average concentration of magnesium in plasma is 1.0 mmol/L, or 2.0 mEq/L. Based on a normal extracellular volume, a 70-kg man has about 14 mmol of magnesium extracellularly, constituting only about 3% of the total because intracellular magnesium is about 500 mmol in the average 70-kg man.

RECOMMENDATIONS. The amount of magnesium required to maintain balance in normal individuals has been estimated to vary between 0.125 to 0.187 mmol · kg^{-1} · d^{-1}. The upper limit of this dose is the recommended daily allowance.[44] To accommodate requirements for growth, 0.25 mmol · kg^{-1} · d^{-1} has been recommended for children. During pregnancy and lactation, the requirements can be met by incorporating the recommendations for children.

In patients with protein-calorie malnutrition, magnesium deficiency has been documented, and in surgical patients, increasing the magnesium intake to about 15 mmol/d improved nitrogen balance. In malnourished patients receiving home TPN, we have documented a markedly positive magnesium balance and noted that 15 to 17 mmol/d was required to maintain balance and normal serum levels over the long term. Furthermore, in patients with a short bowel, the needs were especially high, owing to losses from diarrhea and stomal drainage. In these patients, we have documented that the absorption of orally fed magnesium is only 30%. Therefore, to meet nutritional needs, oral magnesium must be given at a dosage of 0.5 to 0.6 mmol · kg^{-1} · d^{-1}. This dosage causes diarrhea or intensifies diarrhea if it is fed in a bolus. Also, the sulfate ion of magnesium sulfate is not absorbed and adds to the problem. To avoid this difficulty, we recommend that magnesium as the heptogluconate be diluted in oral rehydration solution and be consumed gradually during the day.

Calcium

SOURCE. The major source of calcium is milk and milk products. Calcium in vegetables is less available because it complexes with phytates and oxalates.

ABSORPTION. The luminal contents of the intestine influence the availability of calcium. Gastric acid converts calcium to an ionized absorbable chloride salt. In contrast, high intraluminal phosphate, fatty acid, oxalate, and phytate levels bind calcium and prevent absorption. Hence, most calcium is absorbed proximally. Bile acids, amino acids, and monosaccharides and disaccharides enhance absorption. The mucosal cell binds and pumps calcium, aided by a vitamin D–dependent system of calcium-binding protein and a Ca^{2+}-Mg^{2+} adenosine triphosphatase complex. The 1,25-dihydroxy derivative of vitamin D (1,25-dihydroxycholecalciferol) is the most potent facilitator of calcium absorption.

DISTRIBUTION. About 98% of the total body calcium is in the skeleton. Intracellular concentration of calcium is extremely low because it is toxic to the cell. However, a small amount of calcium residing in the sarcoplasmic reticulum of muscle cells and calcium entering through the cell membrane plays a very important part in cell contraction and relaxation. The remaining calcium is distributed in the extracellular space and is closely regulated by parathormone and 1,25-dihydroxycholecalciferol levels. The concentration of extracellular calcium plays a very important part in nerve and muscle cell excitability.

RECOMMENDATIONS. In recent years, much pressure has been exerted in the lay press to recommend a large intake of calcium in an effort to prevent osteoporosis in later life. The evidence for the benefits accruing from these high intakes is not convincing, and recent controlled trials have not shown that calcium supplements benefit patients with osteoporosis unless previous intake has been below 20 mmol/d. The recommended daily allowance[44] for calcium has been set at 60 mmol/d during adolescence and up to the age of 24, during which time maximal calcium retention occurs, and it is reduced to 40 mmol/d for older persons. During pregnancy and lactation, 60 mmol/d is considered a prudent intake.

This intake must be augmented in patients with a short bowel because of increased losses. In patients with a short bowel, we noted that the mean absorption of calcium was 32% of intake, with a range of 18% to 46%. The recommended daily allowance for normal individuals has been computed based on an absorption of 40%; therefore, a prudent intake for patients with a short bowel based on a lower absorption should be 90 mmol/d in older adults and up to 120 mmol/d in adolescents. Calcium should always be added to parenteral nutrition regimens: at least 12 to 15 mmol/d should be given, and additional calcium should be added to cover losses in gastrointestinal secretions.

Phosphorus

SOURCE. Milk, meat, and cereals are rich sources of phosphorus.

ABSORPTION. The absorption of phosphorus is remarkably efficient, and 70% to 90% of dietary intake is absorbed. Hence, dietary hypophosphatemia is rare.

DISTRIBUTION. Phosphorus is the major intracellular anion. In the cell, among other functions, it is a part of buffer systems of energy-storing nucleotides (adenosine triphosphate), of membranes (as phospholipids), and of oxygen-transfer systems in the form of erythrocyte 2,3-diphosphoglycerate. The total body extraskeletal phosphorus level amounts to 600 mmol in the 70-kg man.

Because serum levels are only about 1.2 mmol/L, total extracellular phosphorus level is only 17 mmol in the 70-kg man. Thus, most of this element is in bone or is intracellular. Data recalculated from Hill and colleagues[41] show that the total body phosphorus level in malnourished surgical patients was only 281 mmol/kg, compared with their normal level of 374 mmol/kg. If in acute malnutrition skeletal phosphorus is presumably unchanged, the lower total body phosphorus level would suggest that intracellular phosphorus is proportionately even more depleted.

The serum phosphorus decreases rapidly during TPN, and the literature is full of reports about the serious effects of hypophosphatemia, which in some cases has proved to be lethal. Silvis and Paragas[45] showed that during parenteral nutrition in which all nonprotein calories were given as glucose, serum phosphorus level may drop precipitously, followed by the development of tremors, impaired mentation, paresthesias, muscular weakness, convulsions, and coma. These symptoms usually occur only when glucose is used to provide all caloric needs for a malnourished patient, such as in a system of parenteral nutrition not using fat. However, in our experience, this syndrome has not been seen in any patient infused with a mixed fuel (glucose-lipid)–based nutrient regimen, and hence, such a dual substrate system is safer in severely malnourished patients. In addition, Rudman and associates[35] showed that a positive nitrogen balance was associated with phosphorus retention; therefore, this element is important in the promotion of anabolism.

RECOMMENDATION. The recommended daily allowance[44] for phosphorus is set at a 1:1 ratio with calcium. Therefore, in normal and orally fed patients, the phosphorus intake should approximate the calcium intake. In patients receiving TPN, the total needs for phosphorus amount to about 14 to 16 mmol/d when a glucose-lipid source of nonprotein energy is being given as a source of energy. This recommended dose is due partly to the fact that lipid emulsions have phospholipids, which themselves act as an additional source of phosphorus in the dual-energy system. It is also partly due to the high insulin level associated with the glucose-only system, which increases the cellular uptake of phosphorus.

References

1. Munro HN: General aspects of the regulation of protein metabolism by diet and by hormones. *In:* Mammalian Protein Metabolism. Vol 1. Munro HN, Allison JB (Eds). New York, Academic Press, 1964, pp 381–481.
1a. Matsui J, Cameron RG, Kurian R, et al: Nutritional, hepatic, and metabolic effects of cachectin/tumor necrosis factor in rats receiving total parenteral nutrition. Gastroenterology 1993; 104:235–243.
2. WHO (World Health Organization): Energy and protein requirements. Report of a joint FAO/WHO/UNU expert consultation. Technical Report Series 724. Geneva, World Health Organization, 1985, p 206.
3. Keys A, Brozek J, Hanschel A, et al: The Biology of Human Starvation. Minneapolis, University of Minnesota Press, 1950.
4. Elwyn DH: Nutritional requirements of adult surgical patients. Crit Care Med 1980; 8:9–20.
5. Calloway DH, Spector H: Nitrogen balance as related to calorie and protein intake in active young men. Am J Clin Nutr 1954; 2:405–415.
6. Kinney JM, Long CL, Duke JH: Carbohydrate and nitrogen metabolism after injury. Ciba Found Symp 1970; 103–126.
7. Greenberg GR, Marliss EB, Anderson GH, et al: Protein-sparing therapy in the postoperative patient: Effects of added hypocaloric glucose or lipid. N Engl J Med 1976; 194:1411–1416.
8. Greenberg GR, Jeejeebhoy KN: Intravenous protein-sparing therapy in patients with gastrointestinal disease. JPEN J Parenter Enteral Nutr 1979; 3:427–432.
9. Hoffer LJ, Bistrian BR, Young VR, et al: Metabolic effects of very low calorie weight reduction diets. J Clin Invest 1984; 73:750–758.
10. Millward DJ: The hormonal control of protein turnover. Clin Nutr 1990; 9:115–126.
11. Yeung CK, Smith RC, Hill GL: Effect of an elemental diet on body composition. Comparison with intravenous nutrition. Gastroenterology 1979; 77:652–657.
12. Burke JF, Wolfe RR, Mullany CJ, et al: Glucose requirements following burn injury. Ann Surg 1979; 190:274–285.
13. Collins JP, Oxby CB, Hill GL: Intravenous amino acids and intravenous hyperalimentation as protein-sparing therapy after major surgery: A controlled clinical trial. Lancet 1978; i:788–791.
14. Young GA, Hill GL: A controlled study of protein-sparing therapy after excision of the rectum. Ann Surg 1980; 192:183–190.
15. Pichard C, Jeejeebhoy KN: Muscle dysfunction in malnourished patients. Q J Med 1988; 69:1021–1045.
16. Patel D, Anderson GH, Jeejeebhoy KN: Amino acid adequacy of parenteral casein hydrolysate and oral cottage cheese in patients with gastrointestinal disease as measured by nitrogen balance and blood aminogram. Gastroenterology 1973; 65:427–437.
17. Anderson GH, Patel DG, Jeejeebhoy KN: Design and evaluation by nitrogen balance and blood aminograms of an amino acid mixture for total parenteral nutrition of adults with gastrointestinal disease. J Clin Invest 1974; 53:904–912.
18. Harris JA, Benedict FG: Standard basal metabolism constants for physiologists and clinicians. *In:* A Biometric Study of Basal Metabolism in Man. Publication 279, The Carnegie Institute of Washington. Philadelphia, JB Lippincott, 1919, pp 223–250.
19. Jequier E, Tiebaud D: Effects of glucose and lipid infusions on energy expenditure in man. *In:* New Aspects of Clinical Nutrition. Kleinberger G, Deutch E (Eds). Basel, Karger, 1983, pp 25–30.
20. Allard JP, Jeejeebhoy KN, Whitwell J, et al: Factors influencing energy expenditure in patients with burns. J Trauma 1988; 28(2):199–202.
21. Roberts SB, Young VR: Energy costs of fat and protein deposition in the human infant. Am J Clin Nutr 1988; 48:951–955.
22. Roulet M, Detsky AS, Marliss EB, et al: A controlled trial of the effect of parenteral nutritional support on patients with respiratory failure and sepsis. Clin Nutr 1983; 2:97–105.
23. Baker JP, Detsky AS, Stewart S, et al: A randomized trial of total parenteral nutrition in critically ill patients: Metabolic effects of varying glucose-lipid ratios as the energy source. Gastroenterology 1984; 87:53–59.
24. Gamble JL: Physiological information gained from studies on the life raft ration. Harvey Lect 1946–1947; 247–273.
25. Woolfson AMJ, Heatley RV, Allison SP: Insulin to inhibit protein catabolism after injury. N Engl J Med 1979; 300:14–17.
26. Long JM, Wilmore DW, Mason AD Jr, et al: Fat-carbohydrate interaction: Nitrogen-sparing effect of varying caloric sources for total intravenous feeding. Surg Forum 1974; 25:61–63.
27. Jeejeebhoy KN, Anderson GH, Nakhooda AF, et al: Metabolic studies in total parenteral nutrition with lipid in man: Comparison with glucose. J Clin Invest 1976; 57:125–136.
28. Askanazi J, Carpentier YA, Elwyn DH, et al: Influence of total parenteral nutrition on fuel utilization in injury and sepsis. Ann Surg 1980; 191:40–46.
29. Messing B, Bitoun A, Galian A, et al: La steatose hepatique au cours de la nutrition parenterale depend-elle de l'apport calorique glucidique? Gastroenterol Clin Biol 1977; 1:1015–1025.
30. Wene JD, Connor WE, DenBesten L: The development of essential fatty acid deficiency in healthy men fed fat-free diets intravenously and orally. J Clin Invest 1975; 56:127–134.
31. Garrow JS: Total body potassium in kwashiorkor and marasmus. Lancet 1965; ii:455–458.
32. Montgomery RD: Magnesium metabolism in infantile protein malnutrition. Lancet 1960; ii:74–76.
33. Garrow JS, Smith R, Ward EE: Electrolyte Metabolism in Severe Infantile Malnutrition. Oxford, Pergamon Press, 1968, p 56.
34. Brinkman GL, Bowie MD, Frus-Hansen B, et al: Body water composition in kwashiorkor before and after loss of edema. Pediatrics 1965; 36:94–103.
35. Rudman D, Millikan WJ, Richardson TJ, et al: Elemental balances during intravenous hyperalimentation of underweight adult subjects. J Clin Invest 1975; 33:94–104.
36. Freeman JB: Magnesium requirements are increased during total parenteral nutrition. Surg Forum 1977; 28:61–62.
37. Wolman SL, Anderson GH, Marliss EB, et al: Zinc in total parenteral nutrition. Requirements and metabolic effects. Gastroenterology 1979; 76:458–467.
38. Veverbrants E, Arky PA: Effects of fasting and refeeding: I. Studies on sodium, potassium and water excretion on a constant electrolyte and fluid intake. J Clin Endocrinol 1969; 29:55–62.
39. Waterlow JC, Golden MHN, Patrick J: Protein-energy malnutrition: Treatment. *In:* Nutrition in the Clinical Management of Disease. Dickerson JWT, Lee HA (Eds). London, Edward Arnold Ltd., 1978, pp 49–71.
40. Manitius A, Epstein FH: Some observations on the influence of a magnesium-deficient diet on rats, with special reference to renal concentrating ability. J Clin Invest 1963; 42:208–215.
41. Hill GL, King RFGJ, Smith RC, et al: Multi-element analysis of the living body by neutron activation analysis—Application to critically ill patients receiving intravenous nutrition. Br J Surg 1979; 66:868–872.
42. Jeejeebhoy KN, Baker JP, Wolman SL, et al: Critical evaluation of the role of clinical assessment and body composition studies in patients with malnutrition and after total parenteral nutrition. Am J Clin Nutr 1982; 35:1117–1127.
43. Russell DMcR, Prendergast PJ, Darby PL, et al: A comparison between muscle function and body composition in anorexia nervosa: The effect of refeeding. Am J Clin Nutr 1983; 38:229–237.
44. Recommended Dietary Allowances. 10th ed. Washington, DC, National Academy Press, 1989.
45. Silvis SE, Paragas PD: Paresthesias, weakness, seizures and hypophosphatemia in patients receiving hyperalimentation. Gastroenterology 1972; 62:513–520.

CHAPTER 122

Total Parenteral Nutrition: Priorities and Practice

Andrew S. Kenler, MD • George L. Blackburn, MD, PhD
Timothy J. Babineau, MD

Total parenteral nutrition (TPN) got its start by saving patients with gastrointestinal disorders from starvation and now ranks as one of the most important medical discoveries of the 20th century. During the past 25 years, the administration of TPN has progressed from the provision of excess calories and protein, in a futile attempt to promote a "positive" nitrogen balance in the critically ill, to more appropriate metabolic and nutritional support, in which calories and protein are supplied to meet energy requirements. This change has resulted in improved nutritional support and in avoidance of the problems associated with overfeeding critically ill patients.

The metabolic response to injury and the goals of nutritional support have become linked in our understanding of critical illness. In the starved-stressed state, most patients are hypermetabolic, as reflected by their increased resting energy expenditure. If it is allowed to progress unopposed, the unchecked catabolism that characterizes the inflammatory state can lead to nitrogen losses of up to 40 g/d[1] and to rapid depletion of energy reserves (10,000 kcal). This metabolic response is in contrast to the malnutrition of the nonstressed semistarved state (e.g., that resulting from anorexia nervosa), in which the metabolic rate is often decreased. In the absence of a superimposed infection or stress, this type of malnutrition may be tolerated for longer periods than that type developing during critical illness.

The usual metabolic response to injury is mediated by the counter-regulatory hormones (growth hormone, glucagon, cortisol, and catecholamines), the monokines interleukin-1 and tumor necrosis factor, and other immunologic mediators that lead to a redistribution of macronutrients (protein, fat, and glycogen) from skeletal muscle and adipose tissue to more metabolically active structures (liver, bone, and visceral organs) (Fig. 122–1).[2,3] Initially, this hypermetabolic response is beneficial, providing energy and amino acids for protein synthesis during the stressed state.[4] Although this response is adaptive for the first 5 to 7 days of an illness, if it proceeds unopposed, multisystem organ failure may be initiated.

The injury response, which is characterized by tachycardia, increased oxygen consumption, increased respiratory rate, increased core body temperature, and a negative nitrogen balance, is dynamic.[5,6] Cuthbertson divided this shock state into ebb and flow phases.[7] The ebb phase occurs during the first hours after injury and is characterized by the body's attempt to restore normal tissue perfusion. The flow phase, which begins once the shock state has been reversed, can last for days, weeks, or months and is the dynamic state of acute injury that is exemplified by catabolism and a negative nitrogen balance. A third phase (not described by Cuthbertson) is the anabolic phase, which is characterized by the slow reaccumulation of protein and body fat once the metabolic response to injury has subsided (Fig. 122–2). During the flow phase, TPN can be particularly efficacious by providing the stressed host with calories and a protein substrate that can be used to promote a positive nitrogen balance. Parenteral nutritional support potentially can offset the endogenous catabolism that occurs during the flow phase of injury, thereby helping to minimize the loss of lean body tissue, preserve vital organ function, and maintain immunocompetence. Failure to provide such nutritional support to the critically ill patient may lead to an unopposed loss of lean tissue and vital organ structure (with subsequent dysfunction) and immunosuppression. Multisystem organ failure often becomes the final common pathway of these adverse results. The critically ill patient is characterized by a redistribution of macronutrients from la-

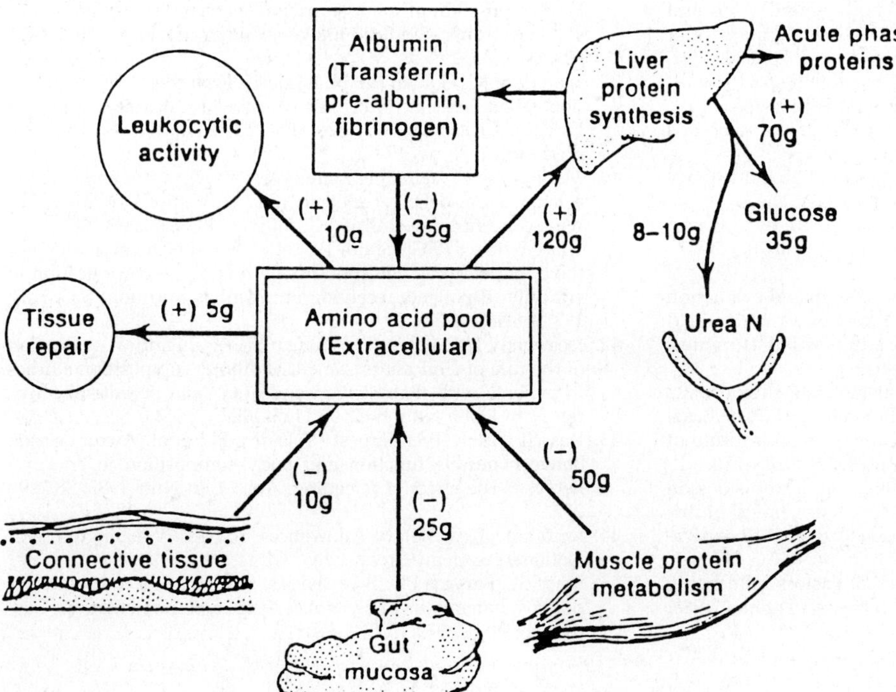

Figure 122–1. Functional redistribution of body cell mass after injury or surgery provides nitrogen for protein synthesis. *Arrows* reflect the net release (−) in grams from connective tissue, gut mucosa, and muscle, as well as uptake (+) of amino acids into tissues whose net anabolism is associated with survival. The conversion of protein into glucose and urea is a minor source of energy but is an important part of the role of the liver to produce the heat necessary to maintain core temperature. Approximately 120 g of protein per day is redistributed by day 3 to day 5 of acute stress. (From Blackburn GL: Nutrition in surgical patients. *In*: Hardy's Textbook of Surgery. Hardy JD, Kukora JS, Pass HI [Eds]. Philadelphia, JB Lippincott, 1988, pp 86–105.)

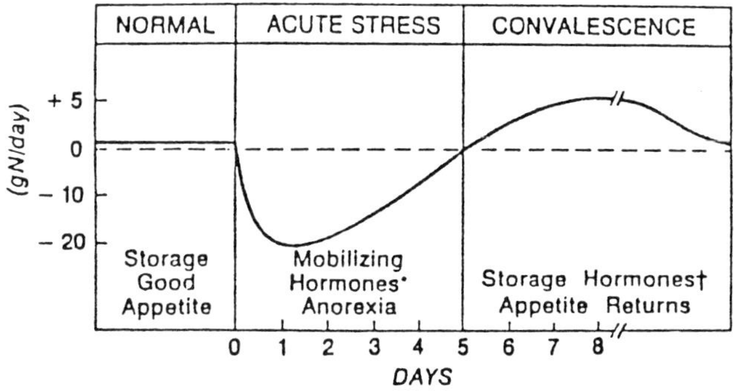

Figure 122–2. Biphasic hormonal response to injury in the normal postoperative patient. *Abbreviation*: gN = grams of nutrition. (From Blackburn GL: Nutrition in surgical patients. *In*: Hardy's Textbook of Surgery. Hardy JD, Kukora JS, Pass HI [Eds]. Philadelphia, JB Lippincott, 1988, pp 86–105.)

bile reserves (fat, muscle, and glycogen) to more metabolically active tissues for the purpose of host defense, thermogenesis, and protein synthesis. The net redistribution of protein is approximately 120 g/d. If the expendable labile protein pool is 600 to 700 g, these stores can be depleted within 5 to 7 days of ongoing injury. In addition, studies have demonstrated a mortality of 86% in intensive care unit (ICU) patients who accumulate a 10,000-cal deficit.[8] For these reasons, nutritional support should be started as early as possible in the course of a patient's critical illness. Once the resuscitation period has ended and the "shock" state reversed, which usually occurs between 48 and 72 hours into the ICU stay, exogenous calories and protein should be supplied. The exogenous calories and protein help limit the catabolic response to stress and maintain the metabolic response to injury by providing substrates that are utilized by the liver, bone marrow, and healing wound. In this fashion, the metabolically active tissues are supported without an increase in the catabolism of muscle protein, connective tissue, and gut mucosa. As long as the patient remains in a stressed state, however, nutritional support can, at best, only prevent further protein wasting and maintain organ structure and function.

ASSESSMENT OF PATIENTS

Multiple measurements and assessments are required for the adequate assessment of the nutritional status of the critically ill patient. Two major types of protein-calorie malnutrition have been identified: a stress-induced hypoalbuminemic form and a marasmic form that is generated by uncomplicated or adaptive starvation.[9] The latter, rarely seen in the ICU setting, is typified by the semistarved patient with anorexia nervosa or cancer cachexia. Patients with the marasmic form appear obviously malnourished and wasted. In contradistinction, hypoalbuminemic malnutrition results from the injury response and is thought to be mediated primarily by monokines in association with the counter-regulatory hormones. This form of malnutrition is more typically encountered in the ICU than is the marasmic form. Patients with stress-induced hypoalbuminemic malnutrition may not appear grossly malnourished and may be difficult for the untrained eye to recognize because of the fluid overload that often accompanies the postresuscitative state. The diagnosis of hypoalbuminemic malnutrition, however, is suggested by decreased serum levels of visceral proteins, such as albumin and transferrin.[10, 11] Importantly, these patients are at the same increased risk as patients with marasmic type malnutrition for malnutritionally associated infectious complications, sepsis, and eventually, multisystem organ failure and death.[9, 12]

TABLE 122–1. Evaluation of Weight Change in Critically Ill Patients

Time	*Significant Weight Loss (%)*	*Severe Weight Loss (%)*
1 wk	1–2	>2
1 mo	5	>5
3 mo	7.5	>7.5
6 mo	10	>10

(From Blackburn GL, Bistrian BR, Maini BS, et al: Nutritional and metabolic support of the hospitalized patient. JPEN J Parenter Enteral Nutr 1977; 1:17.)

The nutritional assessment should begin with a history and physical examination. Important questions in the history include recent unintentional weight loss (> 10%) (Table 122–1), recent surgical stress, protracted nausea or vomiting, diarrhea, and the presence of comorbid illnesses. During the physical examination, the clinician should look for signs of chronic wasting (e.g., temporal muscle wasting) and decreased fat stores. Anthropometrics also provide a valuable adjunct to the nutritional assessment (Table 122–2). Upper-arm anthropometry reveals information about lean body mass and fat that is based on available standards for American men and women.[13, 14] However, like weight, anthropometrics in the critically ill may be inaccurate because of the effects of excess fluid. A 24-hour urine collection for creatinine is another method of obtaining information about lean body mass. The amount of creatinine produced over a 24-hour period is proportional to the total body skeletal muscle mass, and this level decreases with worsening malnutrition.[15–17] The creatinine height index, as described by Bistrian and coworkers, is the ratio of measured creatinine excreted to the expected excreted creatinine based on that of control subjects matched by age, sex, and ideal body weight (Table 122–3). Values below 60% of expected creatinine excretion signify severe loss of lean body mass.[13]

Numerous laboratory values can be used to quantify the visceral protein stores of a patient. These measurements differ from morphologic techniques of nutritional assessment, which seek to determine the somatic protein mass. These laboratory values, however, are often a reflection of the stressed state and are not a true marker for malnutrition. Historically, the serum albumin level has been used as the primary marker of malnutrition. In the absence of a metabolic stress, protein deprivation causes decreased catabolism and decreased production of albumin.[18] Despite the

TABLE 122–2. Standards for Arm Muscle Circumference and Triceps Skinfold

	Standard (mm)	*Lower Fifth Percentile (mm)*	*Percent of Standard Represented by Fifth Percentile*
Upper-Arm Muscle Circumference			
Male	270	220	81
Female	213	177	83
Triceps Skinfold			
Male	11	4	36
Female	19	9	47

(From Bistrian BR: Anthropometric norms used in assessment of hospitalized patients. Am J Clin Nutr 1980; 30:2212. © American Society for Clinical Nutrition.)

TABLE 122–3. Ideal Urinary Creatinine Values

*Men**		*Women*†	
Height (cm)	*Ideal Creatinine Value (mg)*	*Height (cm)*	*Ideal Creatinine Value (mg)*
157.5	1288	147.3	830
160.0	1325	149.9	851
162.6	1359	152.4	875
165.1	1386	154.9	900
167.6	1426	157.5	925
170.2	1467	160.0	949
172.7	1513	162.6	977
175.3	1555	165.1	1006
177.8	1596	167.6	1044
180.3	1642	170.2	1076
182.9	1691	172.7	1109
185.4	1739	175.3	1141
188.0	1785	177.8	1174
190.5	1831	180.3	1206
193.0	1891	182.9	1240

(From Blackburn GL, Bistrian BK, Maini BS, et al: Nutritional and metabolic support of the hospitalized patient. JPEN J Parenter Enteral Nutr 1977; 1:15.)
*Creatinine coefficient for men = 23 mg/kg of ideal body weight.
†Creatinine coefficient for women = 18 mg/kg of ideal body weight.

decrease in synthesis, the large body pool (3–5 g/kg) and long half-life (18–21 days) of albumin lead to only modest changes in serum albumin concentration during unstressed starvation. In the stressed or injured state, three major events take place that cause a decrease in serum albumin: (1) increased degradation of albumin, (2) decreased synthesis of albumin, and (3) redistribution of albumin secondary to extravascular sequestration.[19, 20] Serum albumin levels in the critically ill reflect more the disease state and the concomitant inflammatory response than the nutritional status of the stressed patient. The finding of a low serum albumin level, however, is predictive of an increased morbidity and mortality in hospitalized patients.[21, 22] Exogenous albumin administration may raise serum albumin levels in the injured patient but does not decrease morbidity or mortality.[23, 24] Its addition to the TPN admixture is probably not efficacious and is not recommended. When used to transiently increase intravascular oncotic pressure to aid in diuresis, albumin is best administered in bolus fashion, followed immediately by diuretic therapy.

Protein-calorie malnutrition can lead to depression of both humoral- and cell-mediated immunity and can cause a subsequent increase in morbidity and mortality.[25, 26] Restoration of adequate nutritional status has been shown to reverse the immunosuppressive effect of malnutrition.[27–29] The total lymphocyte count, which is equal to the total white blood cell count multiplied by the percentage of lymphocytes in the differential, may be useful in the nutritional assessment of the ICU patient. Although not specific, a total lymphocyte count of less than 1000/mm^3 is associated with decreased immunocompetence and malnutrition. Delayed hypersensitivity skin testing, which evaluates cell-mediated immunity, can also be used to help assess the nutritional status of a patient. However, many conditions (e.g., uremia, infections, surgery, and liver disease) can affect cell-mediated immunity and can reduce the value of delayed hypersensitivity testing, making it a less valuable marker of malnutrition during acute illness.[30–32]

Twenty-four-hour urine collections for urea nitrogen provide further information on the metabolic state of the critically ill patient. Nitrogen balance is calculated by the following equation:[33]

$$\text{Nitrogen balance} = \text{nitrogen intake} - (\text{urine urea nitrogen level} + 4)$$

where nitrogen intake = protein intake in grams/6.25 and 4 represents the presumed nitrogen losses from stool, skin, and nonurea nitrogen losses in the urine (note: 6.25 g of protein ≈ 1 g of nitrogen). Placing a critically ill patient into a positive nitrogen balance is not often possible and should not necessarily be the goal of TPN in the ICU. Rather, nutritional support should attempt to limit the catabolism of lean body mass and prevent severe negative balance. Exogenous calories and protein delivered to meet the energy expenditure of the stressed patient should be reflected in a reduction of the net negative nitrogen balance seen in the stressed patient.[34, 35] A nitrogen balance between 0 and −5 g/d represents a moderate stress, whereas a nitrogen balance of greater than −5 g/d represents a severe stress (Figs. 122–3 and 122–4).[36] Hence, nitrogen balance can be used to help assess and guide the nutritional support of critically ill patients.

PROTEIN AND ENERGY REQUIREMENTS

Historically, the resting energy expenditure of a patient has been estimated by the Harris-Benedict equation.[37] Moreover, the Harris-Benedict equation has usually been multiplied by a "stress" factor to further estimate the energy expenditure of the critically ill.[38] These values have frequently proved to be inaccurate; they either overestimate or underestimate the true energy expenditure of the critically ill patient.[39, 40] Such errors can cause underfeeding or overfeeding. Overfeeding critically ill patients may produce numerous deleterious effects, including hyperglycemia, depressed white blood cell

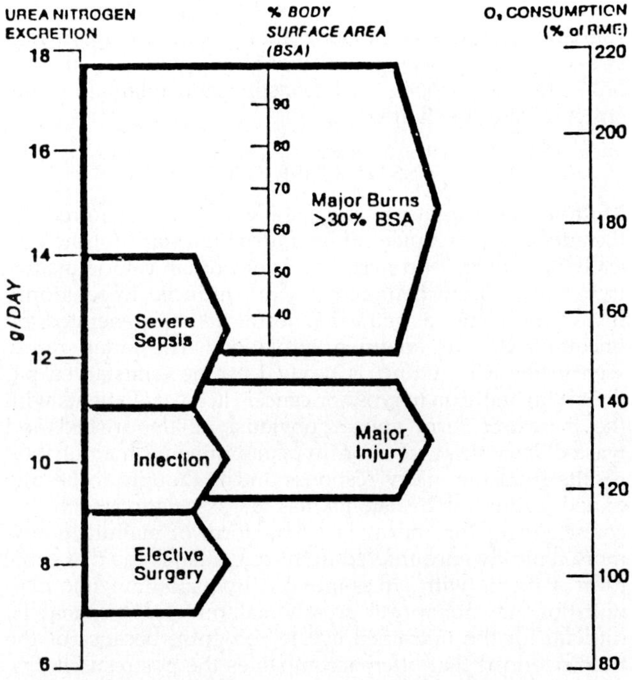

Figure 122–3. Rates of hypermetabolism estimated from urinary urea nitrogen excretion. (From Blackburn GL, Bistrian BR, Maini BS, et al: Nutritional and metabolic support of the hospitalized patient. J Parenter Enteral Nutr 1977; 1:21.)

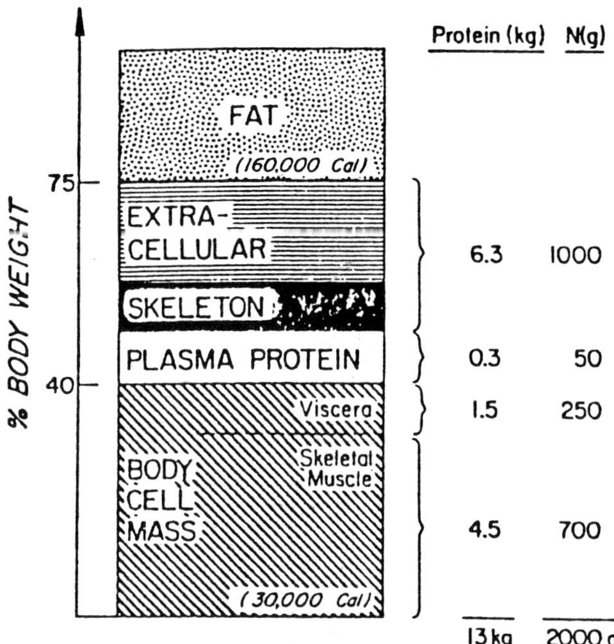

Figure 122–4. Relative size and protein content of the four major body compartments. (From Blackburn GL, Bistrian BR, Maini BS, et al: Nutritional and metabolic support of the hospitalized patient. J Parenter Enteral Nutr 1977; 1:12.)

function and chemotaxis, decreased immunoglobulin and macrophage function, respiratory decompensation, and liver steatosis.[41, 42] A more reasonable approach to determining the caloric needs of the critically ill appears to be the administration of approximately 25 to 30 kcal · kg^{-1} · d^{-1}.[43, 44] This calculation is not appropriate for use in burned, head-injured, or trauma patients, who may require 40 to 45 kcal · kg^{-1} · d^{-1}. The weight used to determine caloric need in these calculations should be the weight that is halfway between the ideal body weight and the current weight, for the obese or morbidly obese patient; the ideal weight, for the patient who has not undergone significant weight loss; and the usual weight, for the patient who has undergone significant weight loss.[45]

The most accurate way to determine energy expenditure in the critically ill patient is through the use of the metabolic cart and indirect calorimetry.[46] The metabolic cart uses the modified Wier formula to measure oxygen and carbon dioxide gas exchange as a determinant of energy expenditure.[47] Furthermore, the metabolic cart can be used to calculate the respiratory quotient, which is defined as the ratio of moles of carbon dioxide produced to moles of oxygen consumed. Metabolism of a mixed fuel results in a respiratory quotient of approximately 0.82 to 0.83, whereas excessive carbohydrate feeding, lipogenesis, and increased carbon dioxide production result in respiratory quotients of greater than 1. A poor correlation between measured energy expenditure determined by the metabolic cart and estimated energy expenditure calculated by the Harris-Benedict equation has been demonstrated.[48] The advantage of the metabolic cart is that it allows specific determination of patients' energy requirements. Subsequently, a tailored feeding regimen can be employed in which energy delivery matches energy expenditure. Patients who are TBW overloaded, morbidly obese, very small, or ventilator dependent for a prolonged period are ideal candidates for the metabolic cart.

Determining the protein requirements of the critically ill patient is more straightforward than determining energy expenditure. In the absence of renal or liver disease, most critically ill patients should receive 1.5 g of protein per kilogram per day. The weight used to calculate protein needs is the ideal body weight for the morbidly obese patient; the present weight, for the patient who has not had significant weight loss; and the usual weight, for the patient who has had significant weight loss.[45] Protein intake of greater than 2 g · k^{-1} · d^{-1} is poorly utilized and increases ureagenesis.[49, 50]

TOTAL PARENTERAL NUTRITION IN THE INTENSIVE CARE UNIT

The evolution of TPN has included the realization that TPN is more than a vehicle for the delivery of calories and protein; the TPN admixture can also be used to help regulate fluid, electrolyte, and acid-base homeostasis. When TPN is initiated in the critical care setting, the *volume status* of the patient is of primary concern. As discussed earlier, many critically ill patients have volume overload. Furthermore, the multitude of drugs that a critically ill patient receives may exacerbate the fluid-overloaded state.[51] In these cases, the patient may be able to tolerate only an additional 1000 mL of nutritional fluid. Initially, this volume restriction often precludes meeting the caloric and protein requirements of most critically ill patients. Once the volume status has improved, however, increased amounts of protein and calories can be delivered. Overzealous attempts to meet the energy needs of the critically ill patient who has fluid overload can lead to a worsening of this state and an increased tissue oxygen debt and may increase morbidity and mortality.[52, 53]

Electrolyte abnormalities are common in the critically ill patient and need to be monitored and corrected on a daily basis. Manipulation of serum electrolyte levels can be safely accomplished via the TPN solution. All fluid and electrolyte losses (e.g., those occurring through a nasogastric tube, stool, fistulas, and urine) should be quantified when possible to accurately guide replacement therapy.

Sodium homeostasis requires replacement based on need. Serum sodium concentration is a measure of tonicity, not necessarily volume status. Hyponatremia and hypernatremia may be seen in patients with hypovolemia, isovolemia, or hypervolemia. Many antibiotics are supplied in the sodium salt form, which can lead to hypernatremia. Hypernatremia can also be seen in patients undergoing exogenous steroid administration, as a result of the mineralocorticoid effect of these drugs on the kidney. Conversely, hyponatremia is commonly seen in cirrhosis and in renal failure patients as a result of excess free water. Furthermore, the ubiquitous use of $histamine_2$-blocking agents can lead to excess sodium loss from the stomach.[54] Correction of serum sodium concentration that is greater than 10 mEq/L within a 24-hour period should be avoided because it may cause potentially lethal accompanying osmotic changes in the brain.[55]

Potassium replacement should be guided by quantifying losses as well. Excessive potassium losses can be seen with diuretic, amphotericin B, and corticosteroid administration. Conversely, hyperkalemia may be seen with potassium-sparing diuretics, overzealous potassium replacement, and renal dysfunction. In addition, acid-base homeostasis affects potassium homeostasis.[56] Potassium shifts intracellularly with elevations of arterial pH; however, decreasing serum pH causes potassium to shift out of the cell. Chloride replacement usually parallels sodium and potassium replacement.

Maintenance of serum pH within a narrow range is also important. Optimal oxygen delivery, enzymatic processes, and renal and respiratory dynamics are all affected by changes in pH. Manipulation of serum pH can be accomplished via the TPN admixture with the addition of acetate (as sodium or potassium salts) or hydrochloric acid. Importantly, TPN alone causes neither acidosis nor alkalosis.

The five most common etiologies of metabolic alkaloses in the ICU patient are (1) increased nasogastric tube losses or protracted emesis, (2) diuretic therapy, (3) steroid administration, (4) large-bowel diarrhea, and (5) citrate toxicity from excessive blood product administration. All of these alkaloses can initially be treated with chloride repletion in the form of sodium and potassium chloride, except the alkalosis produced by steroid administration. In this case, sodium chloride may worsen the alkalosis by promoting exchange at the distal renal tubule for potassium and hydrogen ions. In such cases and in cases of more severe alkalosis, the use of hydrochloric acid (HCl) in the TPN bag can be a quite effective treatment.[57] The easiest and most accurate method to calculate HCl requirement is the *base excess method*:[58]

$$\text{Dose of HCl (mEq/L)} = [\text{body weight (kg)} \times 0.6] \times [\text{observed serum bicarbonate} - 24].$$

The 0.6 should become 0.5 for female patients because women typically have less total body water.

Two restrictions concerning HCl administration in the TPN admixture are noteworthy:

1. The maximum recommended dose of HCl in the TPN bag is 100 mEq/L; higher doses have resulted in central venous line (CVL) damage.[58]
2. HCl cannot be added to lipid-containing TPN admixtures. The fat emulsion (which is negatively charged) can potentially coalesce and "crack" with the addition of HCl (which is positively charged), thereby liberating free lipid particles and potentially lethal fat emboli.[59]

Serial arterial or venous blood gases should be employed to monitor therapy. Venous blood gases obtained from central venous lines can be used in patients receiving TPN to monitor acid-base status by employing conversion factors for venous pH and $P\text{CO}_2$. To determine arterial pH, 0.04 pH units are added to venous pH, and 6 mm Hg are subtracted from the venous $P\text{CO}_2$ to calculate arterial $P\text{CO}_2$.[60] These conversion constants may obviate arterial blood gases in the monitoring of acid-base status of patients on TPN.

Metabolic acidoses are also observed in the critically ill patient. Amphotericin B and the aminoglycoside antibiotics are commonly associated with non–anion-gap metabolic acidoses. Both agents can induce renal tubular acidosis[61] because of their nephrotoxic effect on the kidney. Small-bowel diarrhea, losses from gastrointestinal fistulas, and ureteral diversions can also lead to metabolic acidosis secondary to bicarbonate losses. Anion-gap acidoses are commonly secondary to renal failure or lactic acidosis. Treatment involves calculating the base deficit and replacing the bicarbonate loss with the addition of sodium and potassium acetate to the TPN bag. Sodium bicarbonate is not employed in the TPN admixture because of its reactive nature with the divalent cations (Ca^{2+}, Mg^{2+}) and the possibility of it forming insoluble coprecipitates.

Blood glucose homeostasis is of paramount importance in the management of the critically ill patient. Glucose, because it is an obligate energy source for the renal medulla, brain, and erythrocytes, is administered as dextrose in the TPN bag.[62] Glucose is then metabolized via oxidative pathways (aerobic or anaerobic glycolysis) and produces adenosine triphosphate or undergoes nonoxidative disposal (glycogen formation or lipogenesis). During the stress of critical illness, glucose metabolism is altered; cortisol, glucagon, and catecholamines may produce a state of abnormal glucose tolerance and regulation.[63] These hormones increase glycogenolysis and gluconeogenesis, inhibit insulin secretion, produce hepatic and peripheral insulin resistance, and decrease glucose utilization and clearance, all of which lead to hyperglycemia.[64] Blood glucose levels of greater than 220 mg/dL have been associated with an increased incidence of infection, perhaps related to depressed phagocytosis, decreased chemotaxis, and glycosylation of immunoglobulins.[65–67] Baxter and colleagues[68] demonstrated an increased incidence of nosocomial infections in diabetics during the immediate postoperative period, when serum blood glucose levels were greater than 220 mg/dL. The potential benefit of TPN is negated if hyperglycemia is allowed to persist.

MACRONUTRIENTS

GLUCOSE. Glucose, or dextrose, is the macronutrient that provides most of the calories in the TPN admixture (between 50–75%). Its caloric value in the hydrated form is 3.4 kcal/g. Nondiabetics typically receive 200 g of dextrose per day in their TPN admixture, to mimic endogenous glucose production by the liver (i.e., 2 mg · kg^{-1} · min^{-1} in the 70-kg patient).[64] In patients with diabetes mellitus, 1 mg · kg^{-1} · min^{-1} (approximately 100 g in the 70-kg patient) of dextrose is a reasonable amount for the initiation of carbohydrate feeding. Once euglycemia has been achieved, the dextrose load can be increased by 50 g/d. Most critically ill patients do not require, nor do they tolerate, more than 400 g of glucose per day. This rate of dextrose infusion (4 mg · kg^{-1} · min^{-1}) is optimal and should be considered the upper limit of exogenous glucose infusion.[69] Increasing rates of infusion can lead to nonoxidative disposal of glucose (increased hepatic lipogenesis), and subsequent liver steatosis, which is characterized by increased aspartate aminotransferase, alkaline phosphatase, and total serum bilirubin levels. Furthermore, excessive carbohydrate administration can lead to increased carbon dioxide production (reflected in a respiratory quotient > 1), and a subsequent increased minute ventilation and work of breathing.[70] Inability to wean a patient from mechanical ventilation may be due to overfeeding. Finally, hyperglycemia and its associated deleterious effects on immune function can predominate as a result of excessive carbohydrate administration.

PROTEIN. Endogenous protein catabolism mobilizes amino acids for energy production and for the hepatic synthesis of acute phase proteins. This accelerated protein catabolism, and the subsequent amino acid oxidation, leads to the increased urinary nitrogen excretion and negative nitrogen balance that is characteristic of the stress response to injury. Protein (caloric value = 4 kcal/g), in the form of crystalline amino acids, is administered in the amount of 1.5 to 2.0 g · kg^{-1} · d^{-1} (patients with nitrogen retention disorders may receive less exogenous protein). Most of the exogenously delivered protein is oxidized; hence, the total calories delivered in the TPN solution should be calculated to include the contribution from protein.

LIPID. Lipid metabolism during stress is a complex and incompletely understood process. Initially, lipolysis occurs from the release of free fatty acids. Subsequent oxidation provides energy for the host during the initial acute inflammatory response to injury. Once exogenous nutritional support is provided, free fatty acid levels and subsequent oxidation depend on glucose metabolism and the accompanying insulin level (increased insulin levels inhibit lipolysis). During stress, lipids are incorporated into the feeding regimen for several reasons. Lipid emulsions added to TPN can help alleviate some of the problems related to excessive carbohydrate feeding. In addition, fat is protein sparing for the critically ill patient, and delivery of exogenous fat may decrease or inhibit de novo hepatic lipogenesis. Intravenous lipid emulsions currently available in the United States are derived from safflower or soybean oils and are composed solely of long-chain triglycerides (LCTs). Fat calories should make up no more than 30% of the total calories delivered or no more than approximately $1\ g \cdot kg^{-1} \cdot d^{-1}$. Fat should be given continuously over a 24-hour period to help prevent the reticuloendothelial system dysfunction that has been observed when lipids are given in a discontinuous, or bolus, fashion.[71] This potentially deleterious effect on immune function has led to the use of other fat substrates, namely medium-chain triglycerides (MCTs), or "physical" mixtures of MCTs and LCTs, and "structured" lipids, which consist of both medium- and long-chain fatty acids attached to the same glycerol backbone.[72] These alternative fat sources, although studied primarily in enteral products, have been shown in animal models to have less interference from the reticuloendothelial system than occurs with LCTs.[73] Also, MCTs are cleared more rapidly from the bloodstream. The rapidity and completeness of the B-oxidation of MCTs may relate to their direct and independent transportation into mitochondria. LCTs are primarily dependent on the "carnitine shuttle" to enter mitochondria. Of note, investigators have shown that the stress of critical illness is associated with decreased carnitine levels, perhaps related to decreased hepatic production.[74] This carnitine deficiency could decrease oxidation of LCTs during the stressed state and therefore make MCTs a more efficient energy source.

MICRONUTRIENTS

Calcium, magnesium, phosphate, and trace elements are typically added to the TPN admixture on a daily basis, although the exact requirements have not been well studied. A maintenance dose of 0.2 to 0.3 $mEq \cdot k^{-1} \cdot d^{-1}$ for calcium and 0.35 to 0.45 $mEq \cdot k^{-1} \cdot d^{-1}$ for magnesium should maintain normal serum concentrations in the absence of excessive losses. Approximately half of serum calcium is bound to albumin, and stressed, hypoalbuminemic patients have falsely depressed serum calcium concentrations. The ionized (physiologically active) calcium measurement is often more useful in this setting. The usual parenteral daily supplementation of phosphate is 30 to 40 mmol/d. Many clinical states (e.g., renal failure) and medications (e.g., steroids and diuretics) affect serum calcium, magnesium, and phosphorous concentrations. Daily administration should be based on serum concentrations.

Trace elements are added on a daily basis to replenish lost elements and meet daily requirements. Serum zinc and iron levels can be decreased during stress as part of the metabolic response to injury. Therefore, replacement is at times largely empirical. Zinc is an important cofactor in numerous enzymatic reactions and plays an important role in wound healing. Large zinc losses can be expected with high gastrointestinal outputs (e.g., those resulting from ileostomies and fistulas). Approximately 10 mg of zinc are lost per liter of diarrhea. Three to 10 mg of zinc can be added to the TPN admixture each day. Supplemental iron is added to the TPN admixture only when an iron deficiency anemia is diagnosed.

Finally, although rarely seen in the stressed hospitalized patient, vitamin deficiencies do occur when supplementation is not provided. A multivitamin containing the 12 essential vitamins is added on a daily basis to the TPN admixture. Vitamin K (10 mg) is given separately, once per week by intramuscular or subcutaneous injection, unless contraindicated.

CENTRAL VENOUS LINES: INSERTION, MAINTENANCE, AND COMPLICATIONS

By definition, TPN requires dedicated central venous access. CVLs are most commonly placed in the subclavian or internal jugular veins. The preferred location of central access for TPN is in the subclavian vein because improved dressing care may decrease infectious complications. In the ICU, patients may already have central access. Although a new, dedicated noncontaminated catheter is preferred, TPN may be infused through any available central line until clinical stability allows for catheter exchange.

The maintenance of the CVL dedicated to TPN requires skilled personnel so as to decrease the incidence of the two most common problems that arise once access has been established: infection and thrombosis. The incidence of CVL infection is usually reduced by a nutrition support service, in which improved dressing and line care is provided by dedicated and highly skilled nurses.[75] Appropriately administered TPN does not lead to an increased incidence of line infections. Line infections are prevented by a strict aseptic insertion technique and proper dressing and line care. Patients receiving TPN who develop a fever, increased white blood cell count or hyperglycemia may have a CVL infection. Blood cultures should be obtained from the CVL and peripherally. Although beyond the scope of this chapter, specific algorithms exist to aid in the diagnosis and treatment of CVL infections (Table 122–4).[76] Finally, routine catheter exchange is not performed unless specific clinical indications exist for this procedure.

A second major complication associated with CVLs is thrombosis, either catheter or central vein related. Strategies have been devised to help decrease the incidence of this complication. Heparin is added to the TPN admixture on a daily basis to reduce the incidence of thrombosis.[77] Six thousand units per day are added initially, with the goal of keeping the partial thromboplastin time in the high-normal range (28 to 30 seconds). We have found that doses less than 3000 U may not prevent thrombosis. Doses greater than 12,000 U have been associated with partial thromboplastin time prolongation and may cause bleeding. Thrombocytopenia (platelet counts $< 100{,}000$) may require that the amount of heparin administered be decreased. Certain patient populations have been found to have an accelerated partial thromboplastin time (i.e., < 25 seconds). Risk factors associated with a shortened partial thromboplastin time include inflammatory bowel disease, obesity, pancreatitis, certain cancers, and a history of smoking. These patients are at particularly high risk for catheter and central vein thrombosis, and maintenance of their partial thromboplastin times at greater than 25 seconds is optimal.

TOTAL PARENTERAL NUTRITION ADDITIVES

Use of the TPN admixture for drug delivery can be advantageous. First, this practice can be cost effective because materials as well as personnel time can be eliminated when drugs are added to the TPN admixture. Second, the addition of drugs to the TPN solution can eliminate extraneous volume that the patient may receive from piggybacked intravenous solutions. Third, violations of the central ports of the

TABLE 122–4. Interpretation of Qualitative Cultures and Treatment of Catheter-Related Sepsis

Culture Result				*Treatment*	
Catheter Tip	*Peripheral Blood Count*	*Aspiration Blood Culture*	***Interpretation***	*Temporary Catheter*	*Long-term Catheter**
Negative	Negative	Negative	No infection	None	None
Negative	Positive	Positive	Sepsis, not related to catheter	Systemic antibiotics; catheter change over guide wire	Systemic antibiotics
Negative	Positive	Negative			
Positive	Negative	Negative	Catheter colonization or infection†	Catheter change over guide wire	Culture-specific antibiotic administration through catheter; catheter removal or exchange over guide wire
Negative	Negative	Positive			
Positive	Negative	Positive			
Positive	Positive	Positive	Catheter sepsis	Catheter removal, culture-specific antibiotics, and re-site catheter	Catheter removal, culture-specific antibiotics, re-site catheter; culture-specific antibiotics through catheter and catheter exchange over guide wire (only for patients with severe limitations in central venous access)
Positive	Positive	Negative			

(From Lowell JA, Bothe AJ: Venous access: Preoperative, operative, and postoperative dilemmas. Surg Clin North Am 1991; 71:1238.)
*Tunneled catheter or implantable venous infusion port.
†Colonization or infection with virulent bacteria (e.g., *Staphylococcus aureus*) or fungi warrants treatment as catheter sepsis.

CVL can be decreased, which may decrease the incidence of catheter infections. Last, the continuous administration of certain medications (e.g., histamine$_2$ antagonists) can produce a steady-state drug level, which may enhance drug efficacy.

Histamine$_2$ antagonists are routinely used in the care of the critically ill ICU patient. Benefits include prevention and treatment of stress-related gastritis, reduction of nasogastric tube losses, and decrease in small-bowel and ostomy losses.[78] Histamine$_2$ antagonists can be added directly to the TPN admixture. From a clinical perspective, continuous administration of histamine$_2$ antagonists may minimize fluctuations in serum drug concentration, potentially leading to enhanced drug efficacy and reduced drug-drug interactions and drug toxicity.[78] Finally, metoclopramide, aminophylline, and steroids are also commonly added to the TPN admixture.

TOTAL PARENTERAL NUTRITION AND THE CRITICALLY ILL

Preoperative Total Parenteral Nutrition

Certain malnourished patients may benefit from preoperative nutritional support. Although enteral nutrition is the preferred route of nutrient administration, many disease states preclude its use. Furthermore, when a short, defined period of time for feeding exists, TPN may offer a more reliable method of nutrient delivery than enteral nutrition.[79] Decreased morbidity and mortality from preoperative TPN has been demonstrated in severely malnourished patients[79, 80]; this improvement in outcome is thought to be secondary to protein repletion in the liver and bone marrow, as well as other tissues with rapid turnover. Furthermore, glycogen stores can be replenished. Approximately 1 week of preoperative TPN is necessary for a decrease in morbidity and mortality to occur. Appropriately administered TPN (e.g., correct estimation of energy expenditure with proper caloric and protein delivery, maintenance of normal serum blood glucose levels, proper CVL catheter care, and maintenance of metabolic homeostasis) is mandated. Overfeeding, hyperglycemia, and iatrogenic catheter complications militate against the beneficial effects of TPN. Emergent surgery should never be delayed to allow for TPN administration.

Diabetes Mellitus

Diabetes is not a contraindication to TPN. However, special considerations are required when TPN is delivered to the diabetic patient. Parenteral insulin may be added to the TPN admixture in most acutely ill diabetic patients. The amount of insulin required can be estimated from the patient's routine insulin requirement. The ratio of the preadmission insulin needs to the basal energy expenditure of the patient is approximately equal to the ratio of the initial in-hospital insulin needs to the initial exogenously delivered protein and carbohydrate calories.[81] For example, a patient receiving an 1800-calorie-per-day American Diabetes Association diet who usually takes 20 U of insulin would receive 10 U of insulin in the TPN admixture for 900 calories delivered exogenously. Most patients receiving this regimen require greater than 100% of their insulin needs once they receive their estimated energy requirements. If the preadmission insulin requirement is not known, an estimation of initial insulin needs is approximately 0.1 U of insulin per gram of dextrose delivered. Capillary blood glucose levels should be monitored, at least initially, every 6 hours to ensure adequate blood glucose control. A sliding-scale insulin regimen via subcutaneous delivery can simultaneously be employed. Approximately two thirds of the 24-hour sliding-scale insulin requirement can be added to the TPN admixture the following day to help achieve euglycemia. Because a variable amount (10–90%) of the intravenous insulin is metabolically active as a result of loss by adherence to the infusate material, insulin requirements are almost always safely underestimated.

The route of insulin administration should follow the route of dextrose delivery. Parenterally administered hypertonic dextrose is best managed with intravenous insulin, whereas enterally administered dextrose is best managed with subcutaneous, long-acting (i.e., neutral protamine Hagedorn) insulin. A potentially overlooked source of dextrose administration is via glucose-containing dialysate solutions in peritoneal dialysis. Peritoneal dialysis patients may absorb as much as 300 g of dextrose per day from the dialysate, and the insulin needed to metabolize this glucose load should be added directly to the dialysate solution.

Finally, once established, the dose of insulin for a given dextrose load should remain stable unless a metabolic stress (e.g., new infection) occurs. Hyperglycemia in a patient who was previously euglycemic may be an early sign of infection. As demonstrated by Hongsermeir and Bistrian,[81] infection increases insulin resistance and leads to higher insulin:dextrose ratios in the TPN admixture.

Pulmonary Dysfunction

Protein-calorie malnutrition can lead to respiratory dysfunction. Furthermore, baseline respiratory dysfunction (e.g., chronic obstructive pulmonary disease) is associated with malnutrition.[82] TPN provides calories and protein that are necessary to limit the loss of pulmonary musculature, function, and respiratory defense mechanisms that occur with starvation. Appropriate caloric delivery is critical in the ventilator-dependent patient. Inadequate energy delivery can lead to increased catabolism of the diaphragm and accessory muscles of respiration, and to continued respiratory failure. Overfeeding increases carbon dioxide production and minute ventilation, both of which increase the work of breathing and may prolong ventilator dependence. Strategies that may help prevent respiratory dysfunction during the injury state include (1) use of the metabolic cart to determine resting energy expenditure to ensure accurate energy delivery; (2) delivery of no more than 4 $mg \cdot kg^{-1} \cdot min^{-1}$ of carbohydrate to prevent hepatic lipogenesis and subsequent increased carbon dioxide production; and (3) use of mixed fuel systems that incorporate fat, which can be beneficial by limiting the amount of dextrose provided and decreasing hepatic lipogenesis.[83] Lipids, however, should be delivered with caution in patients with adult respiratory distress syndrome because pulmonary function may be worsened when patients receive lipid-containing TPN.[84] Unless contraindicated by liver or renal failure, 1.5 $g \cdot kg^{-1} \cdot d^{-1}$ of protein should be provided to limit the catabolism (loss of skeletal muscle mass) associated with the stress response.

Cardiac Dysfunction

The term *cardiac cachexia* is used to describe the wasting that is seen in patients with heart failure secondary to valvular heart disease, coronary heart disease, or cardiomyopathy. The cause of cachexia is thought to be multifactorial; decreased dietary intake and a decreased cardiac output can lead to wasting of lean body mass and body fat stores. First, these patients have limited reserve, and their volume status is critical to their metabolic management. Second, the hypermetabolism seen during acute injury may put an additional burden on the patients' stressed heart. Initiation of TPN can cause water retention secondary to the antinatriuretic effect of insulin, and this increased intravascular volume may exacerbate preexisting heart failure. Furthermore, fluxes in potassium and phosphorus levels may occur with TPN initiation. These electrolyte abnormalities, which can be associated with cardiac arrhythmias, should be avoided. TPN in the stressed patient with cardiac dysfunction should be administered cautiously and should provide calories to meet, not exceed, energy expenditure.

Renal Dysfunction

The mortality rate for acute renal failure is at least 25%,[85] and although nutritional support has not been shown to affect recovery of renal function, the associated catabolism of stress that accompanies acute renal failure mandates nutritional support. TPN is employed if enteral support is not possible. Protein is provided at 1.5 $g \cdot kg^{-1} \cdot d^{-1}$, and dialysis is employed to control nitrogen retention and the potential deleterious sequelae of uremia. No difference in survival has been conclusively shown either with essential amino acids alone or with a mixture of essential and nonessential amino acids.[86] Most TPN solutions have approximately a 1:1 ratio of essential and nonessential amino acids. At present, the standard crystalline amino acid formulation with a full complement of essential amino acids (i.e., the solution has high biologic value) is employed. Branched-chain amino acids, however, when combined with the usual complement of amino acids, improve protein utilization. Branched-chain amino acids (leucine, isoleucine, valine) are essential for protein synthesis and are an energy source for peripheral skeletal muscle. Finally, the inability of the liver to oxidize branched-chain amino acids decreases the formation of blood urea nitrogen. We advocate the use of a branched-chain amino acid–enriched formulation when a patient's blood urea nitrogen level is greater than 100 mg/dL or when uremic complications exist. In these cases, protein delivery is usually decreased to 1 $g \cdot kg^{-1} \cdot d^{-1}$.

Liver Dysfunction

Hepatic dysfunction, acute or chronic, is associated with increased catabolism. Most liver failure patients have total body water and sodium overload; hence, the volume of parenteral nutrition may need to be restricted in many cases. Diuretic therapy may be necessary to allow the delivery of adequate protein and calories. Incorporation of fat can help alleviate glucose intolerance. Furthermore, endogenous hepatic lipogenesis may be reduced when exogenous fat is employed. This effect may be beneficial to the dysfunctional liver by providing energy stores that would have been consumed during de novo hepatic lipogenesis and would now be used for more important metabolic activities in the injured liver. Protein is provided at 1.5 $g \cdot kg^{-1} \cdot d^{-1}$ to help reduce the catabolism and the subsequent loss of lean tissue that accompanies liver failure. Restriction to 1 $g \cdot kg^{-1} \cdot d^{-1}$ of protein is necessary only when severe hepatic encephalopathy is present. Branched-chain amino acids have been used in liver failure, although controversy exists concerning their efficacy in decreasing encephalopathy and mortality. Branched-chain amino acids are preferentially utilized by skeletal muscle during injury and promote muscle and visceral protein synthesis and inhibit proteolysis.[87,88] Their oxidation occurs primarily in skeletal muscle, not in the liver; hence, branched-chain amino acids may be beneficial with respect to blood urea nitrogen production and subsequent hepatic encephalopathy.

Liver Transplantation

Nutritional support is often employed before and after liver transplantation. The pretransplantation time period may be of varied duration, depending on the condition of the potential recipient and the availability of a suitable donor. Short-duration TPN can help correct metabolic abnormalities and achieve homeostasis before transplantation. If a longer period of time exists before transplantation (5–7 days) and the patient is in the ICU, TPN can also provide calories (25 to 30 $kcal \cdot kg^{-1} \cdot d^{-1}$) and protein (1 $g \cdot kg^{-1} \cdot d^{-1}$) to help the recipient initiate and maintain an effective metabolic response to injury. Standard amino acid formulas are employed unless the blood urea nitrogen level is greater than

100 g/dL or encephalopathy or hepatic coma is present. In these situations, the standard amino acid formula is enriched with branched-chain amino acids to achieve a final branched-chain amino acid concentration of approximately 50%. This specialized formula delivers a full complement of amino acids (i.e., it has high biologic value), while providing protein that may be better utilized.

After transplantation, metabolic support may initially take precedence over delivery of adequate calories and protein. Liver transplantation operations are lengthy, and patients may receive large amounts of fluid in the form of crystalloid, colloid, and blood products. Their total body water overloaded state may initially limit the amount of fluid that can be allocated for TPN, and a maximally concentrated admixture can be particularly efficacious. One of the most common metabolic abnormalities seen in the liver transplant patient is metabolic alkalosis. The cause of this acid-base disorder is multifactorial but relates primarily to blood product replacement. Fresh frozen plasma has the most citrate per unit of blood product, approximately 14 mEq/U of fresh frozen plasma, and as little as 10 U of fresh frozen plasma can lead to a significant base excess. A functioning liver is needed to convert citrate to bicarbonate, and the presence of metabolic alkalosis may be an early sign of allograft function. Metabolic support provided by TPN may decrease morbidity and shorten ICU length of stay in liver transplant patients.[89]

Obesity with Stress

Obesity (weight that is 130% above ideal body weight) and morbid obesity (weight that is 100 pounds above ideal body weight) are associated with increased morbidity and mortality.[90] Although difficult to determine by prospective analysis, obesity may increase ICU length of stay as well as morbidity and mortality during critical illness. Stressed obese patients lose lean body mass and fat stores, which can lead to protein-calorie malnutrition. In the nonstressed obese patient, a protein-sparing modified diet has been employed for weight loss. A modification of this approach (moderately hypocaloric TPN) has been developed in which protein is supplied in normal stress amounts ($1.5 \text{ g} \cdot \text{kg}^{-1} \cdot \text{d}^{-1}$ based on ideal body weight), and total calories are provided at approximately 500 kcal less than the expected resting energy expenditure.[91] In females, this amount is approximately 3.6 to 4.5 kcal/kg and in males, 4.5 to 5.5 kcal/kg. This feeding approach offers both long- and short-term advantages for the critically ill obese patient. First, this lipolytic regimen promotes loss of fat stores and long-term reduction in cardiovascular risk.[92] Second, only a small quantity (200 g/d) of dextrose is provided, which may improve blood glucose regulation. Nonoxidative disposal of glucose in the form of hepatic lipogenesis is decreased with this smaller dextrose load. Finally, lipids are not usually administered unless hyperglycemia supervenes.

AIDS

Before acute secondary infection occurs, many acquired immunodeficiency syndrome (AIDS) patients suffer from protein-calorie malnutrition of the marasmic form. They have typically lost lean body mass, and they have diminished fat stores. In similar fashion to the patient with anorexia nervosa, their energy and protein reserves are limited. The injury response characterized by hypermetabolism (increased energy expenditure) and hypercatabolism can rapidly deplete these already marginal protein and energy stores. TPN in the critically ill acquired immunodeficiency syndrome patient is initiated similarly to that for any patient with protein-calorie malnutrition who cannot receive enteral nutrition. Calories are provided to meet energy expenditure based on lean body mass. Protein is provided ($1.5 \text{ g} \cdot \text{kg}^{-1} \cdot \text{d}^{-1}$) based on the patient's usual weight. Metabolic support is provided by correcting electrolyte, fluid, and acid-base disturbances.

Many patients with acquired immunodeficiency syndrome have abnormal lipid metabolism[93]; and an increase in plasma triglyceride and very low-density lipoprotein levels can be seen. The cause of the abnormal lipid metabolism is multifactorial, and tumor necrosis factor, interleukin-1, and interferon-α have all been implicated.[92,94] Serum triglyceride levels should be determined before TPN containing lipids is initiated. Currently, we withhold lipids from patients with serum triglyceride levels greater than 400 mg/dL to prevent the potential deleterious sequelae of hypertriglyceridemia (mental status changes, pancreatitis, and lipemic serum and respiratory dysfunction).

SUMMARY

TPN can provide nutritional as well as metabolic support for the critically ill patient when the enteral route is not available. Through the provision of calories and protein, the net catabolism that accompanies the metabolic response to stress can be reduced. Furthermore, exogenous delivery of protein and calories helps to maintain immunocompetence, lean body mass, and visceral organ function. TPN also acts as a vehicle for metabolic homeostasis. TPN should be delivered with emphasis on two main objectives: (1) the *appropriate* feeding of the critically ill patient, in which energy delivery meets energy expenditure, and (2) the maintenance of metabolic homeostasis via the TPN admixture. Aggressive nutritional support as part of the ICU strategy for the critically ill patient may lead to a shortened length of stay in the ICU and to decreased morbidity, with the ultimate goal being improved patient survival.

CASE STUDY

To highlight the important issues of TPN delivery in the critically ill patient, a common clinical scenario is presented.

The patient is a 60-year-old, 70-kg male with type II diabetes mellitus, who has undergone subtotal gastrectomy for carcinoma of the stomach. The patient had a 5% weight loss from his usual weight over the previous 3 months. Preadmission insulin needs for a 2000-kcal diet are approximately 20 U of insulin per day.

Nutritional Goals:
25 kcals × 70 kg = 1750 kcal/d

Postoperative Day One:
1.5 g of protein × 70 kg = 105 g of protein per day
Patient has volume overload—TPN is restricted to 1 L.

Stock Pharmacy Solutions. 15% amino acids, 70% dextrose, 20% fat

Amino Acids. 105 g = 700 mL = 10.5% amino acids = 420 kcal
Dextrose. 210 g = 300 mL = 21% dextrose = 714 kcal fat.

Electrolytes, micronutrients, and vitamins are administered as required; approximately half of preadmission insulin (for half the calories) is included in TPN admixture. Sliding scale insulin coverage is used.

Postoperative Day Three:
Mobilization of excess water–increased volume for TPN occurs (1500 mL); triglyceride level is normal. Blood glucose level is between 100 and 200 mg/dL.

Amino Acid. 105 g = 700 mL = 7% amino acids = 420 kcal
Dextrose. 250 g = 285 mL = 16.6% dextrose = 850 kcal
Fat. 45 g = 225 mL = 3% fat = 405 kcal (~ 25% of total

kilocalories)

Totals: 1675 kcal and 105 g of protein per day
Additional insulin is added to TPN.

Postoperative Day Six:

The patient is at preoperative weight; no fluid restriction is necessary. Patient is started on sips of clear liquids. TPN maintenance fluids, approximately 30 mL/kg or approximately 2000 mL/d.

Amino Acids. 105 g = 700 mL = 5.25% amino acids = 420 kcal
Dextrose. 250 g = 285 mL = 12.5% dextrose = 850 kcal
Fat. 50 g = 250 mL = 2.5% fat = 450 kcal
Totals: 1720 kcal and 105 g of protein per day

References

1. Kudsk KA, Stone JM, Sheldon FGF: Nutrition in trauma and burns. Surg Clin North Am 1983; 62:183.
2. Schwartz JH, Bistrian BR: The role of cytokines in intermediary metabolism. *In*: Cellular and Molecular Aspects of Endotoxin Reactions. Nowotny JJ, Spitzer EJ, Ziegler (Eds). New York, Elsevier Science Publishing B.V. (Biomedical Division), 1990, pp 427–445.
3. Blackburn GL: Nutrition in Surgical Patients. 2nd ed. Philadelphia, JB Lippincott, 1988.
4. Johnston IDA: The endocrine response to trauma. *In*: Scientific Basis of Medicine Annual Reviews. London, Oxford University Press, 1968, pp 224–241.
5. Grant JP: Handbook of Total Parenteral Nutrition. 2nd ed. Philadelphia, WB Saunders, 1992, pp 215–233.
6. Bessey PQ, Warrens JM, Brooks DR, et al: Combined hormonal infusion stimulates the metabolic response to injury. Ann Surg 1984; 200:264.
7. Cuthbertson DP: Post-shock metabolic response. Lancet 1942; i:433.
8. Bartlett RH, Dechert RE, Mault JR, et al: Measurement of metabolism in multiple organ failure. Surgery 1982; 4:771.
9. McClave SA, Mitoraj TE, Thielmeier KA, et al: Differentiating subtypes (hypoalbuminemic vs. marasmic) of protein-calorie malnutrition: Incidence and clinical significance in a university hospital setting. JPEN J Parenter Enteral Nutr 1992; 4:337.
10. Torosian MH, Mullen JL: Nutritional assessment. *In*: Hyperalimentation—A Guide for Clinicians. Kaminski MV (Ed). New York, Marcel Dekker, 1985.
11. Dudrick SJ, O'Donnell JJ, Weinmann-Winiker S, et al: Nutritional assessment: Indications for nutritional support. *In*: Nutrition in Clinical Surgery. Deitel M (Ed). Baltimore, Williams & Wilkins, 1985.
12. Bistrian BR: Nutritional assessment of the hospitalized patient: A practical approach. *In*: Nutritional Assessment. Wright RA, Heymsfield J (Eds). Boston, Blackwell Scientific Publications, 1984, p 183.
13. Frisancho AR: Triceps skinfold and upper arm muscle size norms for assessment of nutritional status. Am J Clin Nutr 1974; 27:1052.
14. Frisancho AR: New norms of upper limb fat and muscle areas for assessment of nutritional status. Am J Clin Nutr 1981; 34:2540.
15. Turner WJ, Cohn S: Total body potassium and 24 hour creatinine excretion in healthy males. Clin Pharmacol Ther 1975; 18:405.
16. Muldowney FP, Crooks J, Bluhm MM: The relationship of total exchangeable potassium and chloride to lean body mass, red cell mass and creatinine excretion in man. J Clin Invest 1957; 36:1375.
17. Boileau RA, Horstman DH, Buskirk ER: The usefulness of urinary creatinine excretion in estimating body composition. Med Sci Sports Exerc 1972; 4:85.
18. James WPT, Hay AM: Albumin metabolism: Effect of the nutritional state and the dietary protein intake. J Clin Invest 1968; 47:1958.
19. Rothschild MA, Oratz M, Schreiber SS: Albumin synthesis: Part II. N Engl J Med 1972; 286:816.
20. Gray GE, Meguid MM: Can total parenteral nutrition reverse hypoalbuminemia in oncology patients? Nutrition 1990; 6:225.
21. Harvey KB, Moldawer LL, Bistrian BR, et al: Biological measures for the formulation of a hospital prognostic index. Am J Clin Nutr 1981; 34:2013.
22. Muller JL, Buzby GP, Matthews DC, et al: Reduction of operative morbidity and mortality by combined preoperative and postoperative support. Ann Surg 1980; 142:604.
23. Foley EF, Borlase BC, Benotti PN, et al: Albumin therapy in the critically ill. Arch Surg 1990; 125:739.
24. Strong FM, Shah S, Pollak A, et al: Total albumin replacement during parenteral nutrition: Is it helpful (Abstract)? JPEN J Parenter Enteral Nutr 1990; 14(Suppl 1):15.
25. Bistrian BR, Sherman M, Blackburn GL: Cellular immunity in adult marasmus. Arch Intern Med 1977; 137:1408.
26. Bistrian BR, Blackburn GL, Scrimshaw MS: Cellular immunity in semistarved states in hospitalized patients. Am J Clin Nutr 1975; 28:1148.
27. Meakins JL, Pietsch JB, Bubenick D, et al: Delayed hypersensitivity: Indicator of acquired failure of host defenses in sepsis and trauma. Ann Surg 1977; 186:241.
28. Dionffi R, Zonta A, Dominioni Z, et al: The affects of TPN on immunodepression due to malnutrition. Ann Surg 1977; 185:467.
29. Van Buren CT, Rudolph FB, Kulkarni A, et al: Reversal of immunosuppression induced by a protein free diet: Comparison of nucleotides, fish oil, and arginine. Crit Care Med 1990; 18:S114.
30. Rhoads JE: Diuretics as an adjuvant in disposing of extra water employed as a vehicle in parenteral hyperalimentation. Fed Proc 1962; 21:389.
31. Griffin RE, Champagne C, Bistrian BR, et al: Delayed cutaneous hypersensitivity testing in patients receiving nutritional support for protein-calorie malnutrition. Clin Pharm 1983; 2:43.
32. Twomey P, Ziegler D, Rombeau J: Utility of skin testing in nutrition assessment: A critical review. JPEN J Parenter Enteral Nutr 1982; 6:50.
33. Mackenzie T, Blackburn GL, Flatt JP, et al: Clinical assessment of nutrition status using nitrogen balance. Fed Proc 1974; 33:653.
34. Streat SJ, Bleddoe AH, Hill GL: Aggressive nutrition support does not prevent protein loss despite fat gain in septic intensive care patients. J Trauma 1987; 27:262.
35. Shaw JHF, Wolfe RR: An integrated analysis of glucose, fat, and protein metabolism in severely traumatized patients. Ann Surg 1989; 209(1):63.
36. Bistrian BR: A simple technique to estimate severity of stress. Surg Gynecol Obstet 1979; 148:675.
37. Harris JA, Benedict FG: Biometric Study of Basal Metabolism (Publication #279). Washington, DC, Carnegie Institute of Washington, 1919.
38. Rutten P, Blackburn GL, Flatt JP, et al: Determination of optimal hyperalimentation infusion rate. J Surg 1975; 18:477.
39. Quebbeman EJ, Autman RK, Schneider TC: A reevaluation of energy expenditure during parenteral nutrition. Ann Surg 1982; 195:282.
40. Hunter DC, Jaksic T, Lewis D, et al: Resting energy expenditure in the critically ill: Estimations versus measurement. Br J Surg 1988; 75:875.
41. Daly JM, Heymsfield SB, Head CA, et al: Human energy requirements: Overestimation by widely used prediction equations. Am J Clin Nutr 1985; 42:1170.
42. Foster GD, Knox LT, Dempsey DT, et al: Caloric requirements in TPN. J Am Coll Nutr 1987; 6:231.
43. Paauw JP, McCamish MA, Dean RE, et al: Assessment of caloric needs in stressed patients. J Am Coll Nutr 1984; 3:51.
44. Mann S, Westenskow DR, Houtchens BA: Measured and predicted caloric expenditure in the acutely ill. Crit Care Med 1985; 13:173.
45. McMahon MM, Bistrian BR: The physiology of nutrition assessment and therapy in protein-calorie malnutrition. Dis Mon 1990; 36:375.
46. Feurer I, Muller JL: Bedside measurement of resting energy expenditure and respiratory quotient via indirect calorimetry. Nutr Clin Prac 1986; 1:43.
47. Wier JB: New methods for calculating metabolic rate with special reference to protein metabolism. J Physiol 1949; 109:1.
48. Makk LJ, McClave SA, Creech PW, et al: Clinical application of

the metabolic cart to the delivery of TPN. Crit Care Med 1990; 18:1320.
49. Shaw JHF, Widbore M, Wolfe RR: Whole body protein kinetics in severely septic patients: The response to glucose infusion in TPN. Ann Surg 1987; 205:66.
50. Shaw JHF, Wolfe RR: Whole body protein kinetics in patients with early and advanced gastrointestinal cancer: The response to glucose infusion in TPN. Surgery 1988; 103:148.
51. McCarthy ET, Baptista RJ: Fluid status and central venous access in ICU patients receiving intravenous antibiotics: Pharmacy implications. Infusion 1984; 8:187.
52. Nuytinck HK, Kubar K: Whole-body inflammation in trauma patients. Arch Surg 1988; 123:1519.
53. Shoemaker WC, Appel PL, Kram HB: Tissue oxygen debt as a determinant of lethal and nonlethal postoperative organ failure. Crit Care Med 1988; 16:1117.
54. Driscoll DF: Drug-induced metabolic disorder and parenteral nutrition in the ICU: A pharmaceutical and metabolic perspective. Ann Pharmacother 1989; 23:363.
55. Illowsky BP, Laureno R: Encephalopathy and myelinolysis after rapid correction of hyponatremia. Brain 1987; 110:855.
56. Adrogué HJ, Madiar NE: Changes in plasma potassium concentration during acute acid-base disturbances. Am J Med 1981; 71:456.
57. Martin WJ, Matzke GR: Treating severe metabolic alkalosis. Clin Pharm 1982; 1:42.
58. Lopel PF, Durbin CG: Pulmonary artery catheter deterioration during hydrochloric acid infusion for the treatment of metabolic alkalosis. Crit Care Med 1989; 17:688.
59. Driscoll DF: Clinical issues regarding the use of total nutrient admixtures. Ann Pharmacother 1990; 24:296.
60. Kenler AS, Campbell K, Driscoll DF, et al: Venous blood gas analysis can be used to monitor acid/base homeostasis in surgical ICU patients (Abstract). Crit Care Med 1993; 21:S203.
61. Bistrian BR, Bothe A, Blackburn GL: Complications of TPN. Clin Anesthesiol 1983; 1:693.
62. Blackburn GL, Wolfe RR: Clinical biochemistry and intravenous hyperalimentation. *In*: Recent Advances in Clinical Biochemistry. Alberti, KGMM, Price CP (Eds). Edinburgh, Churchill Livingstone, 1981, pp 197–228.
63. Long C, Smith O, Fri E: Actions of cortisol and related compounds on carbohydrate and protein metabolism. *In*: Metabolic Effects of Adrenal Hormones. Wolstenhom O, Connor M (Eds). London, 1960.
64. McMahon M, Manji N, Driscoll DF, et al: Parenteral nutrition in patients with diabetes mellitus: Theoretical and practical considerations. JPEN J Parenter Enteral Nutr 1989; 13:545.
65. Rayfield E, Ault M, Deusch G, et al: Infection and diabetes: The case for glucose control. Am J Med 1982; 72:439.
66. Davidson M, Sowder J, Fletcher J: Defective phagocytosis in insulin controlled diabetes: Evidence for a reaction between glucose and opsonising proteins. J Clin Pathol 1984; 37:783.
67. Washibi M, Smith R, Baltch A, et al: The effect of diabetes mellitus on chemotactic and bactericidal activity of human polymorphonuclear leukocytes. Diabetes Res Clin Pract 1987; 4:27.
68. Baxter JK, Babineau TJ, Apovian CM, et al: Perioperative glucose control predicts increased nosocomial infections in diabetics (Abstract). Crit Care Med 1990; 18:S207.
69. Wolfe R, O'Donnell T, Stone M, et al: Investigation of factors determining the optimal glucose infusion rate in TPN. Metabolism 1980; 29:892.
70. Askanazi J, Weissman C, Rosenbaum SH, et al: Nutrition and the respiratory system. Crit Care Med 1982; 10:163.
71. Seidner DL, Mascioli EA, Istan NW, et al: The effects of long chain triglyceride emulsions on reticuloendothelial system function in humans. JPEN J Parenter Enteral Nutr 1989; 13:614.
72. Mascioli EA, Bistrian BR, Babayan VK, et al: Medium chain triglycerides and structured lipids as unique nonglucose energy sources in hyperalimentation. Lipids 1987; 22:421.
73. Hamaway KJ, Moldawer LL, Georgieff M, et al: The effect of lipid emulsions on reticuloendothelial system function in the injured animal. JPEN J Parenter Enteral Nutr 1985; 9:559.
74. Tao RC, Yoshimura NN: Carnitine metabolism and its application in parenteral nutrition. JPEN J Parenter Enteral Nutr 1980; 4:469.
75. Nelson DB, Kien CL, Mohr B, et al: Dressing changes by specialized personnel reduce infection rates in patients receiving central venous parenteral nutrition. JPEN J Parenter Enteral Nutr 1986; 10:220.
76. Lowell JA, Bothe AJ: Venous access: Preoperative, operative, and postoperative dilemmas. Surg Clin North Am 1991; 71:1231.
77. Imperial J, Bistrian BR, Bothe A, et al: Limitation of central vein thrombosis in parenteral nutrition by continuous infusion of low dose heparin. J Am Coll Nutr 1983; 2:263.
78. Driscoll DF, Lowell JA, Nompleggi D, et al: Continuous versus intermittent cimetidine infusion in critically ill hospitalized patients: Role of TPN admixture as drug vehicle. Nutrition 1990; 6:383.
79. Muller JM, Keller HW, Brenner U, et al: Indications and effects of preoperative parenteral nutrition. World J Surg 1986; 10:53.
80. The Veterans Affairs Total Parenteral Nutrition Cooperative Study Group: Perioperative total parenteral nutrition in surgical patients. N Engl J Med 1991; 325:525.
81. Hongsermeir T, Bistrian BR: Evaluation of a practical technique for determining insulin requirements in diabetic patients receiving TPN. JPEN J Parenter Enteral Nutr 1993; 17:11.
82. Suchner U, Rothkopf MM, Stanislaus G, et al: Growth hormone and pulmonary disease: Metabolic effects in patients receiving parenteral nutrition. Arch Intern Med 1990; 150:1225.
83. Abbott WC, Grakauskas AM, Bistrian BR, et al: Metabolic and respiratory effects of continuous and discontinuous lipid infusions. Arch Surg 1984; 119:1367–1371.
84. Hwang TS, Huang SL, Chen MF: Effects of intravenous fat emulsions on respiratory failure. Chest 1990; 97:934.
85. Hou SH, Bushinsky DA, Wish JB, et al: Hospital-acquired renal insufficiency: A prospective study. Am J Med 1983; 74:243.
86. Feinstein EI, Blumenkrantz MJ, Healy M, et al: Clinical and metabolic responses to parenteral nutrition in acute renal failure: A controlled double-blind study. Medicine (Baltimore) 1981; 60:124.
87. Cerra FB, Upson D, Angelico R, et al: Branched chains support postoperative protein synthesis. Surgery 1982; 92:192.
88. Kern KA, Bower RH, Atamian S, et al: The effect of a new branched chain–enriched amino acid solution on postoperative catabolism. Surgery 1982; 92:780.
89. Reilly J, Mehta R, Teperman L, et al: Nutritional support after liver transplantation: A randomized prospective study. JPEN J Parenter Enteral Nutr 1990; 14:386.
90. Hubert HB, Feinleib M, McNamara PM, et al: Obesity as an independent risk factor for cardiovascular disease: 26 year followup of participants in the Framingham Heart Study. Circulation 1983; 67:968.
91. Baxter JK, Bistrian BR: Moderate hypocaloric parenteral nutrition in the critically ill, obese patient. Nutr Clin Pract 1989; 4:133.
92. Bistrian BR: Clinical use of a protein-sparing modified fast. JAMA 1972; 240:2299.
93. Grunfeld C, Pang M, Doerrler W, et al: Lipids, lipoproteins, triglyceride clearance and cytokines in human immunodeficiency virus infection and the acquired immunodeficiency syndrome. J Clin Endocrinol Metab 1992; 74:1045.
94. Grunfeld C, Feingold KR: The metabolic effects of tumor necrosis factor and other cytokines. Biotherapy 1991; 3:143.

CHAPTER 123

Enteral Feeding

M. H. Parsa, MD • William C. Shoemaker, MD

Nutritional requirements should be satisfied daily to prevent reduced body function and vitality. After only a 24-hour fast, an otherwise healthy person feels weak and apathetic. These early functional effects of starvation are aggra-

TABLE 123–1. Conditions That May Limit or Preclude Peroral or Enteral Feedings

- Poor appetite, nausea, and vomiting
- Inability to swallow in spite of a patent gastrointestinal tract
- Inability to swallow because of tumors, strictures, or inflammation of the mouth, pharynx, and esophagus secondary to infections, trauma, or operations
- Tumors and ulcers of stomach, complicated peptic ulcer, or pyloric obstruction
- Acute and chronic relapsing pancreatitis
- Perforated viscus, generalized peritonitis, paralytic ileus, abdominal wound dehiscence, and immediately after intra-abdominal operations
- Small-bowel fistula, gastrocolic fistula, or enterourinary fistula
- Intestinal obstruction
- Sepsis, severe stress and/or trauma after major intra-abdominal operations
- Severe malnutrition
- Short-bowel and malabsorption syndromes
- Inflammatory bowel disease
- Severe brain injury[1]

TABLE 123–3. Sequential Steps for the Insertion of Nasoenteral Tubes

1. Place the patient in an upright or semiupright position.
2. If the patient is conscious, spray his or her nasopharyngeal passage with a topical anesthetic.
3. Lubricate the tube well.
4. Have the conscious patient swallow water while you pass the tube through the opening of the esophagus.
5. Check for correct placement in the stomach by auscultation during insufflation of air, by aspiration of gastric contents, and, if necessary, by irrigation with 10–50 mL of water.
6. Tape the tube to the nose without exerting pressure on the nasal alae; check security of the fixation frequently.
7. Confirm the tube's position by taking an abdominal radiographic film.
8. Keep the head of the bed elevated about 45° to reduce the chance of gastric contents reflux and aspiration into the tracheobronchial tree.
9. Repeat steps 5 through 7 whenever the tube is manipulated or repositioned.

vated and yet masked by the disease. Thus, timely, sufficient, and appropriate nutritional support is a major component of critical care for patients recovering from severe illnesses.

Feeding natural foods by the gastrointestinal route is the best and safest method for providing nutrition in health or illness. Alternative routes and foods are used only when feeding natural foods perorally or enterally is not possible or is inadequate, such as occurs in severely ill patients who cannot ingest some or all of their increased nutritional requirements[1] (Table 123–1). Such patients should receive enteral feeding supplemental to their oral intake (Table 123–2); those patients who do not tolerate sufficient oral or enteral feeding should receive supplemental intravenous feeding; those who cannot tolerate any enteral feeding should receive parenteral nutrition only. Those patients who do not tolerate or cannot utilize sufficient parenteral feeding and remain in negative nitrogen and energy balance may not survive if their utilization of nutrients is not augmented to meet their daily needs. In general, the feeding techniques used for critically ill patients, in order of frequency are: total parenteral, combined enteral and parenteral, combined oral and parenteral, combined oral and enteral, and oral feeding.

ENTERAL TUBES: INSERTION TECHNIQUES

Nasogastric and Nasoduodenal Tubes, Gastrostomy and Jejunostomy Buttons

Insertion, maintenance, and use of gastrointestinal tubes and buttons for feeding require expertise. Following the insertion steps described in Table 123–3 produces the best results, using a 12-French tube; smaller-sized tubes have rigid stylets and tend to pierce the pharynx or esophagus during insertion. Nasogastric tubes can be passed into the duodenum blindly in about 15% of cases; fluoroscopic guidance increases this figure to 95%.[4, 5] When necessary, the tip of the tube can be advanced from the stomach into the duodenum with the help of fluoroscopy or gastroscopy.[4–7]

TABLE 123–2. Alternative Enteral Routes to Oral Feeding

- Nasogastric and nasoduodenal tubes
- Simultaneous decompression of stomach and intraduodenal feeding
- Pharyngostomy gastric or duodenal tubes
- Gastrostomy tube and gastrostomy duodenal tube
- Jejunostomy tube or catheter
- Gastrostomy and jejunostomy buttons[2, 3]

Moss Nasoduodenal and Gastrostomy Duodenal Tubes

The Moss nasoduodenal tube[8] has an inflatable balloon to block the cardia by a ball-valve mechanism. One of its other three lumens opens in the esophagus above the balloon, in the stomach, and in the duodenum consecutively. The nasoduodenal tube is placed during or at the end of intra-abdominal operations for immediate low-power esophageal and gastric suction and for simultaneous feeding into the duodenum. For correct Moss nasoduodenal tube placement, the pylorus should be visualized and held manually while the tube's tip is guided into the duodenum. Decompression of the esophagus and stomach combined with immediate postoperative feeding into the duodenum make this tube uniquely effective.[9, 10] Using this method of immediate postoperative tube feeding, vigorous ambulation, and coughing followed by early postoperative oral feeding, Moss was able to discharge patients from the hospital within 48 hours after cholecystectomy and partial colectomy. Other investigators have indicated that intraduodenal feeding and gastric decompression following elective cholecystectomy are not necessary.[11]

Pharyngostomy Tubes

Small nasogastric catheters can be inserted percutaneously via a needle through the lateral wall of the pharynx.[12] Larger tubes can be first inserted via nasogastric route, and then their nasal ends can be brought out through a small lateral pharyngotomy.

Gastrostomy Tubes

Gastrostomy tubes are placed through the anterior stomach wall at a high cephalad point. When the head of the bed is elevated 30° to 45°, the gastric contents gravitate down to the antrum. The tube is sutured to the gastric and abdominal walls, leaving a slack in the peritoneal space as a safeguard against the pull of distention and traction exerted against the tube accidentally. Feeding via gastrostomy tubes should be delayed a few days after their insertion until gastric emptying is effective. When this tube is removed, the tract heals shortly afterward, especially if the patient is kept in a Fowler's position and given oral feedings in frequent but small increments.

Immediately after insertion of a Moss gastrostomy-duodenal tube, the stomach is continuously decompressed via the gastric port, and an elemental diet is administered through the duodenal port. If the head of the bed is elevated to about 30° to 45°, the feedings rarely back up alongside the tube or into the esophagus.

Percutaneous insertion of gastrostomy tubes under the control of fluoroscopy[13] and gastroscopy are alternatives that avoid surgery. Gastrostomy can also be performed laparoscopically.

Jejunostomy Tubes and Catheters

Jejunostomy using a 16-gauge catheter was popularized by Delany and coworkers.[14] However, the narrow lumen of this catheter is vulnerable to frequent clogging so that only elemental diets can be administered. Use of 13-gauge catheters eliminates this problem,[15] but limitations still exist.[16] Nonsterile tap water with added salt, sugar, broth, and milk can be administered through jejunostomy catheters after major intra-abdominal operations,[17] thus eliminating the need for intravenous fluids except as a vehicle for antibiotics. We have kept jejunostomy catheters in place for up to 120 days.[17] When long-term jejunostomy tubes are accidentally or intentionally pulled out, they usually can be replaced through the tract if this action is performed promptly.

Intraoperative Insertion of Jejunal Tubes and Catheters

The junction of jejunum and duodenum at the ligament of Treitz is identified, and a segment of jejunum about 12 inches from its origin is selected for the insertion site. The catheter is introduced into the lumen of jejunum via a needle tangentially inserted through the jejunal wall at the antimesenteric border. After the catheter is advanced, the needle is withdrawn while the tip of the catheter is held inside the jejunum by pinching it. The catheter's exit site is then checked for leakage of gas or fluid by trapping gas, or fluid, or both, in that segment and squeezing toward the catheter site from both sides.[17, 18] If a leak exists, a circular (pursestring) suture is placed around the exit site, tied firmly, and tested again for leakage.

The catheter is directed out through the abdominal wall via a needle inserted from the outside. A piece of intact omentum is sutured at jejunal catheter exit site. The jejunum near the catheter site is sutured to the abdominal wall as far laterally as possible with three or four linear longitudinal interrupted sutures to provide a broad fixation base to the abdominal wall. This method avoids sharp kinking of the jejunum, which may cause an obstruction that mimics superior mesenteric syndrome. Intraluminal placement of the catheter tip is checked by injection of air and fluid with a syringe via the catheter into the bowel, which results in distention of the jejunal loop and no crepitus or edema in the bowel wall. This condition indicates that the catheter is within the lumen of the jejunum. The catheter is then fixed externally to the abdominal wall by a suture, and the abdomen is closed. Before feeding is started, radiopaque material is injected via the catheter, and a radiograph of the abdomen is taken to confirm that the catheter tip is within the bowel lumen and that peristalsis and bowel motility are present.

This technique is usually performed at the end of major intra-abdominal operations. However, in patients who otherwise do not need intra-abdominal operations, the catheter can be inserted by a small midline or transverse upper abdominal incision. We recommend that the segment of jejunum between the ligament of Treitz and the catheter site be attached to the parietal peritoneum by continuous or interrupted sutures.[18] Catheter jejunostomy has also been performed percutaneously and laparoscopically.[19–21]

COMPOSITION OF ENTERAL DIETS

Enteral liquid feedings can be prepared from fresh foods, with all essential nutrients,[21a] according to a patient's needs; however, many hospitals prefer to use commercially prepared diets (Table 123–4). Usually, 1500 to 3000 mL of these formulas meet the United States recommended daily allowance of necessary nutrients. The non–renal failure formulas contain 53 to 211 nonprotein calories per gram of nitrogen.

In patients with normal blood urea nitrogen (BUN) and serum creatinine levels, higher protein intakes with low calorie to nitrogen ratios are preferred.[22] Patients with a normal BUN level should receive about 1.5 to 2.5 g of protein per kg of body weight per day.

If BUN and serum creatinine levels remain lower than 40 mg/dL and 2 mg/dL, respectively, giving larger amounts of nitrogen is appropriate. However, protein intake should be decreased if BUN and serum creatinine levels increase to 80 mg/dL and 3 mg/dL, respectively. Protein/nitrogen intake should also be limited in patients with renal insufficiency, who generally need higher nonprotein calorie to nitrogen ratios to prevent BUN elevations. When about 25 to 50 g of protein per 24 h given simultaneously with sufficient nonprotein calories do not stop BUN and creatinine levels from increasing, dialysis should be considered to ensure that adequate amounts of protein are administered before these patients become irreversibly catabolic.

Formulas enriched with branched-chain amino acids and immunoenhancement formulas[22a] may be beneficial in patients with sepsis, severe trauma, and hepatic failure.[23, 24] However, their cost and questionable long-term benefit limit their use.[25] Provision of essential amino acids as the source of nitrogen in patients with renal failure is generally no more effective in controlling the level of BUN than the nitrogen equivalent as all amino acids or whole protein provided over 24 hours a day simultaneously with non-nitrogenous calories.

Carbohydrates

Adults should receive at least 100 g but no more than 500 g of carbohydrates per day; amounts larger than 500 g can significantly increase serum hepatic enzyme levels and can sometimes cause hepatomegaly.[17] Blood glucose levels should be maintained at between 100 and 200 mg/dL; higher blood glucose levels may lead to metabolic complications. Patients with mild renal insufficiency may develop metabolic acidosis and blood lactate accumulation from prolonged hyperglycemia. In these patients, carbohydrate intake should be decreased and sodium chloride intake should be replaced with acetate salt[17] to alleviate metabolic acidosis.

Fat

Fat can be given in amounts of 1 to 3 g/kg of body weight per day. The serum should be visually checked for clarity; triglyceride and serum cholesterol concentrations should be determined weekly or more often, if necessary. In patients who tolerate carbohydrate and fat well, the nonprotein calories are provided by both. When the patient is intolerant to fat or carbohydrate, the nonprotein calories are provided mostly by the one that is better tolerated. We recommend giving fat and carbohydrate separately: fat during the day

TABLE 123–4. Commercially Available Enteral Diets

*Product**	*Manufacturer*	*Nonprotein Calories/g Nitrogen†*
Whole-Protein Diets		
Sustacal High Protein	Mead Johnson	79
Sustacal 8.8	Mead Johnson	153
Sustacal HC	Mead Johnson	134
Isocal	Mead Johnson	167
Isocal HN	Mead Johnson	125
Isocal HCN	Mead Johnson	145
Sustacal with fiber	Mead Johnson	120
Ensure	Ross Laboratories	153
Ensure HN	Ross Laboratories	125
Ensure plus	Ross Laboratories	146
Ensure plus HN	Ross Laboratories	125
Ensure with fiber	Ross Laboratories	148
Osmolite	Ross Laboratories	153
Osmolite HN	Ross Laboratories	125
Two-Cal HN	Ross Laboratories	125
Promote	Ross Laboratories	75
Isosource	Sandoz Nutrition	148
Isosource HN	Sandoz Nutrition	116
Isotein HN	Sandoz Nutrition	86
Citrotein	Sandoz Nutrition	76
Replete	Clintec Nutrition Company	75
Replete with fiber	Clintec Nutrition Company	75
Elemental Diets		
Vivonex TEN	Sandoz Nutrition	149
Vivonex HN	Sandoz Nutrition	127
Vital HN	Ross Laboratories	125
Criticare HN	Mead Johnson	148
Peptamen	Clintec Nutrition Company	131
Diets Specialized for Disease		
Immun-Aid	Kendall McGaw	53
Hepatic-Aid II	Kendall McGaw	148
Amin-Aid	Kendall McGaw	800
Stresstein	Sandoz Nutrition	97
Impact	Sandoz Nutrition	71
Impact with fiber	Sandoz Nutrition	71
TraumaCal	Mead Johnson	91
Pulmocare	Ross Laboratories	125
NutriVent	Clintec Nutrition Company	116
Travasorb hepatic diet	Clintec Nutrition Company	211
Travasorb renal diet	Clintec Nutrition Company	339

*Preparations contain a range of 53 to 211 nonprotein calories per gram of nitrogen in non–renal failure formulas. They consist of protein, fat, carbohydrate, minerals, and vitamins sufficient to satisfy 100% United States recommended daily allowance in liquid or powder forms. In patients with normal renal function, formulas with lower nonprotein calorie:nitrogen ratio have proportionately higher nutritional values.

†Total calories can be calculated by adding 25 calories for 1 g of nitrogen to the nonprotein calories.

Supplemental Components

ProMod protein supplement powder (Ross Laboratories) per one scoop (6.6 g) contains protein (5 g), fat (0.60 g), carbohydrate (0.67 g), calcium (44 mg), sodium (15 mg), potassium (65 mg), and phosphorus (33 mg). MCT oil (Mead Johnson) contains 933 g of medium-chain triglycerides per liter, 7.7 calories per mL. For short-bowel and malabsorption syndromes.

Vegetable oils (corn oil, safflower oil, soybean oil, soybean-cottonseed blend) can be used as a calorie supplement in diabetics and renal insufficiency/failure patients.

Poly-Vi-Sol multivitamin supplement (Mead Johnson) contains (in 1 mL) vitamin A (1500 IU), vitamin D (400 IU), vitamin E (5 IU), vitamin C (35 mg), thiamine (0.5 mg), riboflavin (0.6 mg), niacin (8 mg), vitamin B_6 (0.4 mg), and vitamin B_{12} (2 μg).

The most important factor in nutritional value of these formulas is the appropriateness of calorie to nitrogen ratio for individual patients; patients who have a blood glucose level of 100 to 150 mg/dL can be given formulas containing carbohydrate and fat. Patients who have a blood glucose level of 180 to 200 mg/dL before starting the nutrition support and without receiving large amounts of carbohydrates should receive formulas that contain mainly fat and amino acids. If a suitable formula cannot be found among commercially available formulas, the desirable composition should be prepared by mixing components or alternating the formulas. The detailed composition of each product can be found in the manufacturer's brochure.

(6 AM to 6 PM) and carbohydrate during the night (6 PM to 6 AM), each given simultaneously with nitrogen-containing food.

Vitamins and Minerals

To ensure adequate replacement of trace elements and other minerals, particularly in patients receiving dilute-strength formulas, serum levels should be determined at least once weekly until they have stabilized. The normal serum values of minerals are listed in Table 123–5. Selenium deficiency may occur, especially in burn[26] and cancer patients, because the amounts of selenium in commercially available diets are often not sufficient.

The vitamin content of liquid feedings may decrease if shelf life is prolonged. Clinical assessment (Table 123–6) may help provide appropriate amounts of vitamins for each patient; a general recommendation is the inclusion of an additional 1 mL (for children) and 5 mL (for adults) of a multivitamin preparation in daily feedings to meet requirements (Table 123–7).

TABLE 123–5. Clinical Assessment of Minerals

Mineral	*Clinical Manifestations of Deficiency*	*Normal Serum Values*	*Deficient Serum Values*
Calcium	Osteomalacia; tetany	2.2–2.7 mM 8.6–10.6 mg/dL	<2.2 mM <8.6 mg/dL
Chloride	Metabolic alkalosis	95–105 mEq/L	<85 mEq/L
Chromium	Glucose intolerance	2–4 ng/mL	<1 ng/mL
Cobalt	Unknown	2–5 ng/mL	<2 ng/mL
Copper	Anemia; neutropenia	90–130 μg/dL	<50 μg/dL
Iodine	Cretinism; myxedema	4–11 μg/dL	<4 μg/dL if binding protein normal
Iron	Hypochromic; microcytic anemia	Serum iron >60 μg/dL TIBC <250 μg/dL Ferritin >30 μg/dL	<50 mg/dL >250 μg/dL <12 μg/dL
Magnesium	Tetany; muscle weakness	1.2–2.5 mg/dL	<1 mg/dL
Manganese	Abnormal clotting	6–10 ng/dL	<5 ng/dL
Molybdenum	Confusional state	0.5–2 ng/dL	<0.5 ng/dL
Phosphorus	Osteomalacia; tetany	2.5–4.5 mg/dL	<2.5 mg/dL
Potassium	Muscular weakness; cardiac irritability; alkalosis	3.5–5.5 mEq/L	<3.5 mEq/L
Selenium	Muscle weakness; anemia	0.02 ng/mL	<0.02 ng/mL
Sodium	Hypovolemia; hypotension; reduced urinary volume	135–142 mEq/L	<135 mEq/L
Sulfur	Unknown	Unknown	Unknown
Zinc	Retarded growth; delayed wound healing; coagulopathies	70–120 μg/dL	<1 μg/dL

Abbreviation: TIBC = total iron-binding capacity.

Precautions and Monitoring

Listed in Tables 123–8 and 123–9 are precautions and steps for monitoring for the care of enteral tubes and feeding. When a patient has 2 g/dL of urine glucose, he or she should receive 20 U of crystalline insulin every 2 hours until the urine glucose level is less than 2 g/dL. If 2 g/dL spillage does not stop by this insulin coverage in 4 hours, the feeding should be stopped until the patient is rehydrated and the blood glucose level is returned to normal limits with the administration of adequate amounts of exogenous insulin. The feeding may then be resumed with lesser amounts of intake or lower amounts of carbohydrate.

Patients whose glucose utilization is limited should receive mostly protein and fat, with only minimal carbohydrate. Patients whose blood glucose level is higher than 200 mg/dL and whose BUN level is higher than 80 mg/dL should receive mainly fat by the enteral route and concentrated albumin intravenously. If they cannot tolerate sufficient fat, glucose clearance from the blood should be in-

TABLE 123–6. Clinical Assessment of Vitamins

Vitamin	*Clinical Manifestations of Deficiency*	*Normal Values*	*Deficient Values*
Ascorbic acid	Scurvy; bleeding of gums, hair follicles, and subperiosteum; delayed wound healing	0.5–1 mg/dL	<0.1 mg/dL
Biotin	Alopecia; dermatitis; neuritis	200–500 pg/mL	<200 pg/mL
Cobalamin	Megaloblastic anemia; neuropathy	200–900 pg/mL	<150 pg/mL
Folic acid	Megaloblastic defect of red cells and mucous membranes	Serum: 3–9 ng/mL Cells: 150–600 ng/mL	<3 ng/mL <100 ng/mL
Niacin	Pellagra; dermatitis; mucous membrane ulceration; CNS depression	4–9 μg/mL	<3 μg/mL
Pantothenic acid	Irritability; paresthesia	150–400 ng/mL	<150 ng/mL
Pyridoxine	Glossitis; neuritis; microcytic hypochromic anemia	Red cell GOT index >1.5	Red cell GOT index <1.5
Riboflavin	Cheilosis; glossitis; dermatitis	<1.2 erythrocyte glutathione reductase activity	>1.2 erythrocyte glutathione reductase activity
Thiamine	Polyneuritis; high-output cardiac failure	8–15 IU transketolase activity	<8 IU transketolase activity
Vitamin A	Night blindness; xerophthalmia; keratosis	20–60 μg/dL	<20 μg/dL
Vitamin D	Osteomalacia; rickets; muscle weakness	10–80 ng/mL	<10 ng/mL
Vitamin E	Hemolytic anemia in neonate; CNS and retinal changes	0.8–1.2 mg/dL	<0.5 mg/dL
Vitamin K	Bleeding tendency	Prothrombin time <1 s over control	Prothrombin time >2 s over control

Abbreviations: CNS = central nervous system; GOT = glutamic-oxaloacetic transaminase.

TABLE 123–7. Recommended Daily Amounts of Vitamins and Trace Elements for Enteral Administration to Adult Patients

Supplement	*Daily Amounts**
Vitamins	
Ascorbic acid	250–500 mg
Riboflavin	25 mg
Thiamine	25–50 mg
Niacin	50–200 mg
Pantothenic acid	50 mg
Pyridoxine	50–100 mg
Folic acid	1–5 mg
Cyanocobalamin	5–10 μg
Phytonadione	5–10 mg
α-Tocopherol	50–200 IU
Ergocalciferol	200–500 IU
Retinoic acid	2000–5000 IU
Elements	
Zinc	20 mg
Iron	25 mg
Copper	0.5–2 mg
Selenium	50–150 μg
Chromium	30 μg
Manganese	0.7–2.5 mg

*Depending on the degree of intestinal absorption, these amounts may have to be adjusted to each patient's need. Parenteral daily requirements are less than these amounts.

creased by the administration of adequate crystalline insulin. Protein intake can be increased by dialysis. Protein/nitrogen intake in renal failure patients should be constant and uninterrupted during 24 hours by frequent oral feedings or by constant enteral tube feeding to maximize nitrogen efficiency.

TABLE 123–8. Precautions for the Care of Gastrointestinal Tubes Used for Feeding

- Prevent retraction or progression of the tube by taping it securely to the skin around the exit/entry site and frequently checking its adequate and appropriate fixation.
- Do not allow the nasoenteral tube to press against the nostril and create soreness or sore.
- Be sure that the outer end of the nasoenteral tube is larger than the nostril to prevent intranasal migration.
- Flush the feeding tube daily with 10–50 mL of sterile water at least every 8 hours and
  After administration of viscous medications and crushed tablets
  After intragastric or intrajejunal increment feedings to clear the food from the lumen of the tube
- Clamp the tube to prevent reflux of food material into the tube between incremental feedings.
- Aspirate for gastric residual before each intragastric feeding (or every 4 hours during drip feeding) and withhold the next increment (or slow down or stop the drip) if more than 100 mL of material is retrieved from the stomach in adults.
- Administer the contents of each feeding bag or container no longer than 12, but preferably within 4, hours.
- Replace connection tubings and the feeding bag or container every 24 hours.
- Prepare feedings with sterile technique, and culture the last 5–10 mL of the feeding material before changing bag or container and tubings, especially when the patient has diarrhea.
- Encourage oral intake when the patient can swallow so that tube and tube feeding can be discontinued as soon as possible.
- Alternate nostrils if the nasoenteral tube must be replaced; replace nasoenteral tube weekly when possible.
- Cleanse the jejunostomy and gastrostomy tube skin sites every day.

TABLE 123–9. Monitoring of Patients Receiving Enteral Feeding

Clinical
- Examine the abdomen for distention and bowel sounds.
- Record the frequency and consistency of stools, and their color, odor, and estimated weight or volume.
- Note patient's complaints of fullness, nausea, vomiting, abdominal pain, or tenderness.

Blood
- Measure blood glucose, blood urea nitrogen, and serum electrolyte levels at least twice a week or more frequently if they are abnormal.
- Measure SGOT, SGPT, LDH, serum protein, serum albumin, bilirubin, calcium, magnesium, and phosphate levels once a week.
- Measure serum triglyceride and cholesterol levels at least once a week in patients receiving fat in their diets.

Urine
- Test for glucose every 6 hours and cover with crystalline insulin as follows: 5U for 0.25 g/dL, 10U for 0.5 g/dL, 15 U for 1 g/dL, and 20U for 2 g/dL.
- Repeat the test hourly for 2 g/dL and cover with 20U for 2 g/dL every 2 hours. Draw blood to obtain glucose level when urine glucose level is 2 g/dL two consecutive times, and inform physician if 2 g/dL glycosuria lasts for 4 consecutive hours. Depending on the blood glucose level, feeding must be diminished (blood glucose level, 200–450 mg/dL) or stopped (blood glucose level >450 mg/dL) until the blood glucose level is <200 mg/dL. Then resume feeding with a lesser rate or with a formula containing less carbohydrate.

Abbreviations: LDH = lactate dehydrogenese; SGOT = serum glutamic-oxaloacetic transaminase; SGPT = serum glutamic-pyruvic transaminase.

BOLUS AND CONTINUOUS-DRIP ENTERAL FEEDING

Bolus feeding in the stomach is more physiologic; because the formulas are not administered by drip methods at room temperature, less chance of bacterial contamination and growth exists. However, problems with bolus feeding in the stomach include (1) more frequent intolerance in patients with short-bowel and malabsorption syndromes; (2) greater chance of pulmonary aspiration in semiconscious or unconscious patients; (3) physiologic intolerance to the bolus of carbohydrate, protein, or fat; and (4) a more time-consuming feeding schedule. Incremental feeding in the normal stomach every 4 to 6 hours is usually well tolerated; however, if the serum albumin level is less than 2.5 g/dL, gastric emptying and intestinal motility may be sluggish, especially immediately following intra-abdominal operations. In such patients, serum albumin level should be raised to at least 3.5, or preferably, to 4 g/dL for optimal gastrointestinal tract function.

Drip feeding may be easier, but a danger of bacterial overgrowth exists when feeding material bags hang at room temperature for long periods.[27–30] Therefore, the formulas should not remain at room temperature for longer than 12 hours, especially in warm environments. The bags and connection tubing should be changed once a day or more frequently if contamination occurs.

Feeding into the small bowel should be given by continuous drip; however, jejunal feeding also may be given by smaller but more frequent feeding increments than those given into the stomach.[31] Also, small increments of feeding are usually a more reliable way to deliver the heavy viscous foods than drip feeding when large fluid volumes are not tolerated.

ELEMENTAL VERSUS NONELEMENTAL DIETS

The usefulness of elemental diets is limited by their high cost and limited nutritional values compared with natural foods. In general, these diets are appropriate only when nutrition cannot be attained with nonelemental diets. Specific indications include: (1) short bowel and malabsorption syndromes[31a]; (2) reduction of fecal matter and the enteric stream in patients with gastrointestinal fistula, perineal wounds and burns, or perioperative colon operations; and (3) feeding via a gastrointestinal feeding tube that is too small to allow easy flow of nonelemental formulas.

ENTERAL VERSUS PARENTERAL NUTRITION

Parenteral nutrition should not be used unless provision of nutrients by the enteral route is impossible or limited.[31b, 31c, 31d] Conditions such as gastrointestinal fistulae can be treated initially by parenteral feeding, then by the combination of parenteral and enteral feeding, and eventually by enteral feeding alone.

The daily output through the fistula is quantitated while the patient is given parenteral nutrition only. After this initial assessment, enteral nutrition is initiated in the forms and quantities that do not increase the daily fistula output. When the quantity of enteral nutrition meets the estimated metabolic needs of the patient, then parenteral nutrition can be stopped. The gastrointestinal tracts of patients who receive adequate parenteral nutrition to maintain their well nourished state, unlike malnourished patients, tolerate enteral feeding well, and the gastrointestinal readjustments promptly occur.[32] Patients with serum albumin levels of less than 2.5 g/dL may not tolerate enteral feedings well in sufficient quantities. However, if the rate of administration of nutrients is adjusted to the tolerance of the patients, even in those patients with low serum albumin levels, they may tolerate enteral feeding proportionately.[33] Feedings enriched with glutamine are considered to preserve gut structure and function and to promote nitrogen balance.[34, 35, 35a] Addition of fiber to enteral feeding products is considered necessary to maintain the integrity of the intestinal mucosa.[36] Nevertheless, a reported formation of bezoar in the cecum that caused intestinal obstruction was believed to have formed as a result of the fiber-enriched enteral feedings.[37] With the refinements of enteral diets and the variety of means of delivery of these nutrients, patients with pancreatitis, pancreatic fistula,[38, 39] short-bowel syndrome, and inflammatory bowel disease[40, 41, 41a] may be given enteral instead of parenteral feeding at a certain point; this method may reduce the need for long-term parenteral nutrition, along with its inevitable consequent venous thrombosis and intravenous catheter–related sepsis. Branched-chain amino acid–enriched feedings in patients with hepatic failure may be effective temporarily, but the ultimate outcome cannot be altered unless the pathologic condition is reversed.[42] In patients with renal failure who do not have sepsis, it may be possible to reduce to or maintain the BUN level at an acceptable range. However, frequently the tolerated essential amino acids or the limited amounts of all amino acids or proteins may fall short of their daily nitrogen requirements. These patients should receive dialysis to provide their basic nitrogen needs for anabolism and energy production.[43] In enteral feeding, patients may have liquid stools because of the lack of formed material in their diets. If the loose but limited amounts of stools are not to be categorically called diarrhea, the daily stools should be quantitated.[44] Providing nutrition in presence of sepsis, or multiple organ failure, or both, by the safest effective means possible is fundamental to the prevention of metabolic failure.[45] Metabolic death is the consequence of irreversible catabolism; when this stage is reached, death occurs rapidly.

The most effective means of providing nutritional requirements in the critically ill is a combination of parenteral and enteral feedings. Whenever possible, in this combined feeding, we recommend giving fats parenterally and proteins and carbohydrates enterally, which is closer to the physiologic assimilation pathways of these nutrients. In infection-prone and in septic patients, parenteral nutrition should be given intermittently in alternate periods of 7 to 10 days on and 7 to 10 days off. In this method of periodic intravenous feeding, as days of intravenous nutrition accumulate, it may be necessary to limit the number of days of parenteral feeding periods and increase the number of days off of parenteral feeding to prevent catheter-related sepsis or to eradicate the existing sepsis.

NUTRIENT UTILIZATION AND NUTRITIONAL ASSESSMENT IN PREDICTION OF OUTCOME

A patient's daily needs for calories, nitrogen, electrolytes, vitamins, and minerals can be estimated and supplied by the most physiologic route when malnutrition is not present. Preexisting malnutrition can be assessed by the patient's appearance; vigor; nutritional history; drinking and smoking habits; ethnic, cultural, and religious backgrounds, socioeconomic history; present illness; body weight; clinical presence of edema; serum albumin level; and lymphocyte count. Many of these variables, particularly the patient's vigor and sense of well-being, can be reassessed daily to follow up the nutritional status.

Nutrient utilization and serum chemistries can be used to index a patient's nutritional status and predict nutritional outcome. Thus, a metabolically good risk is an adult utilizing 2.5 g of protein, 8 g of carbohydrate, and 3 g of fat per kg of ideal body weight per day without evidence of abnormally high blood glucose, BUN, and triglyceride levels. On the other hand, the adult patient with a BUN level above 40 mg/dL, blood glucose level of greater than 250 mg/dL, and high serum triglyceride level while receiving only about half of the aforementioned amounts of protein, carbohydrate, and fat is a metabolically poor risk. The risk is proportional to the degree of elevation of these serum values and is inversely related to the tolerated amounts of daily intake or utilization of nutrients. The extent of physical activity in the past and present is also directly related to a patient's ability to metabolize food substrates.

COMPLICATIONS OF FEEDING CONDUITS AND ENTERAL FEEDING

Complication of tubes and feeding are listed in Tables 123–10 and 123–11. Perforation of the esophagus, trachea, bronchi, or lungs during blind insertion of small-bore feeding tubes with rigid stylets is a relatively common problem.[46–57] These tubes must be inserted with caution and without undue force. Placement of the tip in the stomach or duodenum must be checked clinically and radiographically before the feedings are administered.[57a]

Tracheoesophageal fistula is a serious complication that may occur if the endotracheal or tracheostomy tube cuffs press against the nasogastric tube, causing necrosis of the opposing tracheal and esophageal walls. The use of small diameter, soft nasogastric tubes and low-pressure tracheostomy or endotracheal tube cuffs may prevent this complication.[18]

Inadvertent connection of an enteral feeding administration set to an intravenous catheter can easily be avoided by using clearly distinguishable and non–cross-fitting infusion adapters for the enteral tubes.[58, 59]

Intended percutaneous gastrostomy tubes have been misplaced into the jejunum and transverse colon.[60] Pneumatosis intestinalis has been reported after insertion of a feeding catheter jejunostomy;[61] this complication resolved by removal of the catheter and administration of systemic antibiotics. Reports have also been published of poor results with percutaneous endoscopic jejunostomies.[62, 63]

Malfunction and obstruction of enteral feeding tubes are common. To prevent feeding tube obstruction, the team caring for the patient must ensure uninterrupted inflow of fluids during drip feedings. We recommend forcefully flushing these tubes with at least 10 to 50 mL of sterile water three times a day to prevent accumulation of deposits and debris within the tube. Clogging can occur most commonly with feeding materials that contain milk products,[64] which can also obstruct the esophagus in the event of reflux or leakage from the tube into the esophagus.[65] Even large-bore tubes have become occluded by overgrowth of yeast colonies.[66] We believe that these kinds of blocking can be avoided by frequent daily flushing. Enteral tubes can become a reservoir of microorganisms once contaminants gain access to the inside of the feeding tube. Microorganisms can gain access to the inside of tubes by contaminated nutrient solutions or by ascending contamination from the gut. Frequent and forceful flushing of these tubes several times a day can diminish the number of contaminant microorganisms. Feeding tubes that are intermittently clamped should be frequently flushed and filled with sterile water to diminish growth of microorganisms.

TABLE 123–10. Potential Complications of Enteral Feeding Tubes

Nasoenteric Tubes
- Misplacement of the tube into trachea, bronchi, and pleural space by perforation through the bronchus and lung tissue.
- Perforation of pharynx, esophagus, trachea, and bronchus.
- Retraction of the tip of the tube from the stomach into the esophagus and from the duodenum upward and displacement to outside.
- Erosion of nostril, pharynx, and esophageal, gastric, and duodenal mucosa.
- Disappearance of the outer end of the tube into the nasal passage.
- Tracheoesophageal fistula in patients with simultaneous nasoenteral tube and endotracheal or tracheostomy tube with high-pressure cuff.
- Inability to pass the tube into the stomach or duodenum.
- Knotting and blockage.

Gastrostomy Tubes
- Dislodgement of the tip into the peritoneal cavity or to the outside.
- Inability to guide the tip of the tube into the duodenum transpylorically.
- Leakage of gastric contents from around the tube aggravated by retching, coughing, and straining.
- Nonhealing of the gastrostomy fistula tract requiring operative closure after removal of the gastrostomy tube.

Jejunostomy Tubes or Catheters
- Leakage of feeding from around the tube or catheter.
- Inadvertent intravenous infusion of jejunostomy feeding material.
- Dislodgement of the tip of the tube into the peritoneal cavity or to outside.
- Intestinal obstruction due to adhesion bands or volvulus of the jejunum affixed to the abdominal wall.

All Tubes
- Clogging.
- Mucosal erosions.
- Downward/caudad progression of the tip of the tube.
- Outward/cephalad regression of the tip of the tube.

TABLE 123–11. Complications of Enteral Tube Feeding

- Extraenteral administration of feedings by failing to recognize the misplaced tips of the tubes.
- Diarrhea due to
  - High osmolality
  - Rapid feeding of large volumes
  - Low serum albumin level, <2.5 g/dL
  - Sensitivity and allergy to the feeding
  - Contamination and overgrowth of organisms in the food
- Distention*
- Abdominal pain and cramps secondary to rapid administration of hypertonic feeding
- Dumping
- Fullness*
- Vomiting*
- Dehydration
- Hypermagnesemia or hypomagnesemia
- Azotemia
- Hyperphosphatemia or hypophosphatemia
- Hyperglycemia
- Hyperkalemia or hypokalemia
- Metabolic acidosis
- Elevation of serum hepatic enzymes, hepatomegaly, and excessive glycogen or fat storage in the liver.

*In patients with abnormally high gastric residual volume, the intragastric feeding must be reduced or stopped until gastric emptying is effective.

Pulmonary aspiration in all patients with enteral tubes and feeding is a common problem. Patients with feeding tubes aspirate more frequently than when they do not have enteral tube feeding. Even patients with jejunostomy feedings can develop pulmonary aspiration.[67] Constant attendance to the patient and elevation of the head of the bed about 35° help reduce the frequency and amounts of aspiration, but aspiration cannot be completely prevented, because some of the patients tend to regurgitate and aspirate even without enteral feeding tubes and feeding.

References

1. Norton JA, Ott LG, McClain C, et al: Intolerance to enteral feeding in the brain-injured patient. J Neurosurg 1988; 68:62.
2. Al Malki T, Langer JC, Thompson V, et al: A prospective evaluation of the button gastrostomy in children. Can J Surg 1991; 34:247.
3. Stellato TA, Gauderer MW: Jejunostomy button as a new method for long term jejunostomy feeding. Surg Gynecol Obstet 1989; 168:552.
4. Marian M, Rappaport W, Cunningham D, et al: The failure of conventional methods to promote spontaneous transpyloric feeding tube passage and the safety of intragastric feeding in the critically ill ventilated patient. Surg Gynecol Obstet 1993; 176:475.
5. Prager R, Laboy V, Venus B, et al: Value of fluoroscopic assistance during transpyloric intubation. Crit Care Med 1986; 14:151.
6. Mann NS, Nair PK, Mann SK, et al: Nasoenteral feeding tube insertion via fiberoptic endoscope for enteral hyperalimentation. J Am Coll Nutr 1984; 3:333.
7. Kim IG: Endoscopic guided intubation of long nasointestinal decompression tube. Surg Gynecol Obstet 1985; 161:282.
8. Moss G: Efficient gastroduodenal decompression with simultaneous full enteral nutrition: A new gastrostomy catheter technique. JPEN J Parenter Enteral Nutr 1984; 8:203.
9. Takala J, Havia T, Heinonen R, et al: Immediate enteral feeding after abdominal surgery. Acta Chir Scand 1985; 151:143.
10. Seidmon EJ, Pizzimenti KV, Blumenstock FA, et al: Immediate postoperative feeding in urological surgery. J Urol 1984; 131:1113.
11. Elmore MF, Gallagher SC, Jones JG, et al: Esophagogastric decompression and enteral feeding following cholecystectomy: A

controlled randomized prospective trial. JPEN J Parenter Enteral Nutr 1989; 13:377.
12. Bucklin DL, Gilsdorf RB: Percutaneous needle pharyngostomy. JPEN J Parenter Enteral Nutr 1985; 9:68.
13. Ho CS, Gray RR, Goldfinger M, et al: Percutaneous gastrostomy for enteral feeding. Radiology 1985; 156:349.
14. Delany HM, Carnevale N, Garvey J, et al: Postoperative nutritional support using needle catheter feeding jejunostomy. Ann Surg 1977; 186:165.
15. Delany HM: An improved technique for needle catheter jejunostomy. Arch Surg 1980; 115:1235.
16. Hayashi JT, Wolfe BM, Calvert CC: Limited efficacy of early postoperative jejunal feeding. Am J Surg 1985; 150:52.
17. Parsa MH, Shoemaker WC: Nutritional failure. *In*: Textbook of Critical Care. 1st ed. Shoemaker WC, Thompson WL, Holbrook PR (Eds). Philadelphia, WB Saunders, 1984, pp 664–694.
18. Parsa MH, Tabora F, Al-Sawwaf M, et al: Enteral feeding. *In*: Textbook of Critical Care. 2nd ed. Shoemaker WC, Ayres S, Grenvik A, et al (Eds). Philadelphia, WB Saunders, 1989, pp 1073–1080.
19. Rosenblum J, Taylor FC, Lu CT, et al: A new technique for direct percutaneous jejunostomy tube placement. Am J Gastroenterol 1990; 85:1165.
20. Duh QY, Way LW: Laparoscopic jejunostomy using T-fasteners as retractors and anchors. Arch Surg 1993; 128:105.
21. O'Regan PJ, Scarrow GD: Laparoscopic jejunostomy. Endoscopy 1990; 22:39.
21a. Grimble GK: Dietary nucleotides and gut mucosal defence. Gut 1994; 35(Suppl 1):46S.
22. Cerra FB, Shronts EP, Raup S, et al: Enteral nutrition in hypermetabolic surgical patients. Crit Care Med 1989; 17:619.
22a. Alexander JW: Immunoenhancement via enteral nutrition. Arch Surg 1993; 128:1242.
23. Cerra FB, Shronts EP, Konstantinides NN, et al: Enteral feeding in sepsis: A prospective, randomized double-blind trial. Surgery 1985; 98:632.
24. Barber JR, Teasley KM: Nutritional support of patients with severe hepatic failure. Clin Pharmacol 1984; 3:245.
25. Yu YM, Wagner DA, Walesreswski JC, et al: A kinetic study of leucine metabolism in severely burned patients. Comparison between a conventional and branched-chain amino acid-enriched nutritional therapy. Ann Surg 1988; 207:421.
26. Hunt DR, Lane HW, Beesinger D, et al: Selenium depletion in burn patients. JPEN J Parenter Enteral Nutr 1984; 8:695.
27. Anderson KR, Norris DJ, Godfrey LB, et al: Bacterial contamination of tube-feeding formulas. JPEN J Parenter Enteral Nutr 1984; 8:673.
28. Anderton A: The potential of *Escherichia coli* in enteral feeds to cause food poisoning: A study under simulated ward conditions. J Hosp Infect 1984; 5:155.
29. Bussy V, Marechal F, Nasca S: Microbial contamination of enteral feeding tubes occurring during nutritional treatment. JPEN J Parenter Enteral Nutr 1992; 16:552.
30. Payne-James JJ, Rana SK, Bray MJ, et al: Retrograde (ascending) bacterial contamination of enteral diet administration systems. JPEN J Parenter Enteral Nutr 1992; 16:369.
31. Rumley TO, Lineaweaver W, Goff K, et al: Self-administered bolus jejunostomy feeding and gastric fluid reinfusion in patients with gastric atony. JPEN J Parenter Enteral Nutr 1985; 9:626.
31a. McArdle AH: Protection from radiation injury by elemental diet: Does added glutamine change the effect? Gut 1994; 35(Suppl 1):60S.
31b. Bell SJ, Borlase BC, Swails W, et al: Experience with enteral nutrition in a hospital population of acutely ill patients. J Am Diet Assoc 1994; 94:414.
31c. Sax HC, Souba WW: Enteral and parenteral feedings: Guidelines and recommendations. Med Clin North Am 1993; 77:863.
31d. Haglund U: Gut ischaemia. Gut 1994; 35(Suppl 1):73S.
32. Jackson WD, Grand RJ: The human intestinal response to enteral nutrients: A review. J Am Coll Nutr 1991; 10:500.
33. Patterson ML, Dominguez JM, Lyman B, et al: Enteral feeding in hypoalbuminemic patient. JPEN J Parenter Enteral Nutr 1990; 14:362.
34. Brown MG, Campbell GR, Rowlands BJ: Glutamine-enhanced enteral diet improves nitrogen balance without increasing portal ammonia. Br J Surg 1991; 78:1305.
35. Swails WS, Bell SJ, Borlase BC, et al: Glutamine content of whole proteins: Implication for enteral formulas. Nutr Clin Pract 1992; 7:77.
35a. Booth IW: Enteral nutrition as primary therapy in short bowel syndrome. Gut 1994; 35(Suppl 1):69S.
36. Shankardass K, Chuchmach S, Chelswick K, et al: Bowel function of long-term tube-fed patients consuming formulae with and without dietary fiber. JPEN J Parenter Enteral Nutr 1990; 14:508.
37. McIvor AC, Meguid MM, Curtas S, et al: Intestinal obstruction from cecal bezoar: A complication of fiber-containing tube feedings. Nutrition 1990; 6:115.
38. Pisters PW, Ranson JH: Nutritional support for acute pancreatitis. Surg Gynecol Obstet 1992; 175:275.
39. Kellum JM, Holland GF, McNeill P: Traumatic pancreatic cutaneous fistula: Comparison of enteral and parenteral feedings. J Trauma 1988; 28:700.
40. Dudrick SJ, Latifi R, Fosnocht DE: Management of short-bowel syndrome. Surg Clin North Am 1991; 71:625.
41. Dudrick SJ, Latifi R, Schrager R: Nutritional management of inflammatory bowel disease. Surg Clin North Am 1991; 71:609.
41a. Fernandez-Banares F, Cabre E, Gonzalez-Huix F, et al: Enteral nutrition as primary therapy in Crohn's disease. Gut 1994; 35(Suppl 1):55S.
42. Latifi R, Killam RW, Dudrick SJ: Nutritional support in liver failure. Surg Clin North Am 1991; 71:567.
43. Compher C, Mullen JL, Barker CF: Nutritional support in renal failure. Surg Clin North Am 1991; 71:597.
44. Benya R, Layden TJ, Mobarhan S: Diarrhea associated with tube feeding: The importance of using objective criteria. J Clin Gastroenterol 1991; 13:167.
45. Baue AE: Nutrition and metabolism in sepsis and multisystem organ failure. Surg Clin North Am 1991; 71:549.
46. Bell MD, Tate LG, Hensley GT: Esophageal-atrial fistula resulting in systemic "meat and vegetable" emboli. Am J Forensic Med Pathol 1992; 13:137.
47. Wendell GD, Lenchner GS, Promisloff RA: Pneumothorax complicating small-bore feeding tube placement. Arch Intern Med 1991; 151:599.
48. McWey RE, Curry NS, Schabel SI, et al: Complications of nasoenteric feeding tubes. Am J Surg 1988; 155:253.
49. Lipman TO, Kessler T, Arabian A: Nasopulmonary intubation with feeding tubes: Case report and review of the literature. JPEN J Parenter Enteral Nutr 1985; 9:618.
50. Valentine RJ, Turner WW Jr: Pleural complications of nasoenteric feeding tubes. JPEN J Parenter Enteral Nutr 1985; 9:605.
51. Olbrantz KR, Gelfand D, Choplin R, et al: Pneumothorax complicating enteral feeding tube placement. JPEN J Parenter Enterol Nutr 1985; 9:210.
52. Saltzberg DM, Goldstein M, Levine GM: Feeding tube-induced pneumothorax. JPEN J Parenter Enteral Nutr 1984; 8:714.
53. Eldar S, Meguid MM: Pneumothorax following attempted nasogastric intubation for nutritional support. JPEN J Parenter Enteral Nutr 1984; 8:450.
54. Miller KS, Tomlinson JR, Sahn SA: Pleuropulmonary complications of enteral tube feedings. Two reports, review of the literature and recommendations. Chest 1985; 88:230.
55. Dorsey JS, Cogordan J: Nasotracheal intubation and pulmonary parenchymal perforation. An unusual complication of naso-enteral feeding with small-diameter feeding tubes. Chest 1985; 87:131.
56. Hand RW, Kempster M, Levy JH, et al: Inadvertent transbronchial insertion of narrow-bore feeding tubes into the pleural space. JAMA 1984; 251:2396.
57. Schorlemmer GR, Battaglini JW: An unusual complication of naso-enteral feeding with small-diameter feeding tubes. Ann Surg 1984; 199:104.
57a. Metheny N: Minimizing respiratory complications of nasoenteric tube feedings: State of the science. Heart Lung 1993; 22:213.
58. Stellato TA, Donziger LH, Nearman HS, et al: Inadvertent intravenous administration of enteral diet. JPEN J Parenter Enteral Nutr 1984; 8:453.
59. Stapleton GN, Symmonds KL, Immelman EJ: Septicemia result-

ing from inadvertent intravenous administration of enteral nutrient solution. A case report. S Afr Med J 1988; 73:542.
60. Bul HD, Dang CV, Schlater T, et al: A new complication of percutaneous endoscopic gastrostomy. Am J Gastroenterol 1988; 83:448.
61. Smith CD, Sarr MG: Clinically significant pneumatosis intestinalis with postoperative enteral feedings by needle catheter jejunostomy: An unusual complication. JPEN J Parenter Enteral Nutr 1991; 15:328.
62. DiSario JA, Poutch PG, Sanowski RA: Poor results with percutaneous endoscopic jejunostomy. Gastrointest Endosc 1990; 36:257.
63. Smith-Choban P, Max MH: Feeding jejunostomy: A small bowel stress test? Am J Surg 1988; 155:112.
64. Marcuard SP, Stegall KS: Unclogging feeding tubes with pancreatic enzymes. JPEN J Parenter Enteral Nutr 1990; 14:198.
65. Turner JS, Fyfe AR, Kaplan DK, et al: Oesophageal obstruction during nasogastric feeding. Intensive Care Med 1991; 17:302.
66. Marcuard SP, Finley JL, McDonald KG: Large-bore feeding tube occlusion by yeast colonies. JPEN J Parenter Enteral Nutr 1993; 17:187.
67. Weltz CR, Morris JB, Mullen JL: Surgical jejunostomy in aspiration risk patients. Ann Surg 1992; 215:140.

CHAPTER 124

Nutritional Failure

M. H. Parsa, MD • William C. Shoemaker, MD

All Deaths Are Hateful to Miserable Mortals, But the Most Pitiable Death of All Is to Starve

HOMER, XII, p 341

Nutritional failure follows hypercatabolic states, starvation, severe infections, parasitic infestations, and chronic wasting diseases. It is likely to occur in patients with severe illnesses, insufficient intake of nutrients, and inadequate nutritional reserves. The onset of nutritional failure is insidious, and its manifestations are subtle, but the end stage may be lethal. The nutritionally debilitated patient usually dies from sepsis and organ failure associated with amino acid and nitrogen deficiencies, inadequate protein synthesis, and failed immune mechanisms. Therapy of nutritional failure is time consuming and not dramatic, but its timely and effective correction may reverse the course of this life-threatening condition.

NUTRITIONAL RESERVES AND THEIR DEPLETION

Calorie Depletion

The average healthy adult male with a body weight of 75 kg stores only 200 to 300 g of carbohydrate, equivalent to about 800 to 1200 kcal, mostly as glycogen. The normal body is made of about 15% to 30% fat, or 11 to 22 kg, and 14% to 20% protein, or 10 to 15 kg; the average total caloric value is about 200,000 kcal, 75% of which is fat. Women have 5% to 10% more fat than men and slightly less protein.[1–4] Although an individual's normal total dispensable caloric storage could potentially sustain life for about 3 to 5 months, functionally most individuals would die after burning about 140,000 kcal, or about 75% of body fat and 50% of body protein.[1, 2, 5] Thus, in the complete absence of food intake, an otherwise healthy person would catabolize 1 to 2 g/kg of protein and 2 to 3 g/kg of fat per day, which provide 1650 to 2200 kcal; at death, about 5% of body weight would be unexpended fat.

Protein Depletion

Reduced or absent dietary protein does not completely stop endogenous protein catabolism and in some instances may increase protein turnover. Normally, the dietary nitrogen intake of 10 to 30 g per day closely approximates the excretion of nitrogen. Fasting gradually decreases nitrogen excretion to 6 to 8 g per day, which is equivalent to about half a pound of lean protein. Prolonged fasting subsequently reduces nitrogen excretion to about 3 to 4 g per day.[1, 4, 5] Inadequate protein food intake initially accompanies urinary losses of 10 to 15 g of nitrogen per day, which decreases within a week to 6 to 8 g per day. The administration of 100 g of carbohydrates further reduces the nitrogen losses 3 to 4 g per day, which represents the well-known nitrogen-sparing effect of carbohydrates.[2] However, a nitrogen-free diet reduces liver and plasma proteins, interferes with fat transport, elevates serum hepatic enzymes, and may lead to fatty liver.

Although the healthy subject with suddenly reduced nitrogen intake will adapt over 5 to 10 days to excrete less nitrogen, the critically ill patient's adaptation may be more than offset by the increased nitrogen requirements associated with wound healing, sepsis, hyperthermia, and increased functional needs.[1, 6] Moreover, critically ill patients are also more vulnerable to extrarenal nitrogen losses from transudates and exudates; burn surfaces; biliary, pancreatic, and enteric fistulas; gastrointestinal fluids in ulcerative colitis or chronic diarrhea; direct tissue injury resulting from trauma; and hemorrhage.

Although protein depletion affects the protein content of all organs, the brain is less affected. Most tissues catabolize fat for most of their energy requirements, whereas the brain normally consumes glucose because free fatty acids do not cross the blood-brain barrier. In the absence of carbohydrate/glucose intake, the brain catabolizes acetoacetate, β-hydroxybutyrate, and acetone, all of which are water-soluble keto acids; this reduces cerebral glucose requirements and spares the need for gluconeogenesis from endogenous amino acids.

In contrast to the brain, the liver and gut are rapidly affected by inadequate protein intake. In severe protein depletion states, the gut may be unable to tolerate or digest food. This condition may be corrected by intravenous amino acid administration; presumably, protein is needed to produce gastrointestinal secretions and enzymes necessary for digestion. The most severely depleted organ in starved patients is skeletal muscle, which may lose as much as 70% of its protein. Moreover, because collagen losses are smaller than intracellular protein losses, the loss from active protoplasmic muscle mass may be considerably greater than what appearance suggests.

The plasma albumin synthesis rate responds rapidly to dietary changes; it is high on high-protein diets and low on low-protein diets.[7] However, responses in albumin catabolism are delayed by 1 to 2 weeks. Decreased albumin catabolism may be mediated by growth hormone because plasma growth hormone levels are elevated in protein depletion.[8]

Protein-Calorie Depletion

Severe protein-calorie depletion is an important problem in critically ill patients. The incidence of various degrees of depletion is unknown, but severe depletion frequently occurs in hospitalized patients because their nutritional deficits are often unsuspected and the relationship of nutritional failure to morbidity may not always be recognized. For example, the patient with carcinoma of the esophagus who has lost 30 pounds before an extensive ablative operation may receive nothing by mouth for 10 days postoperatively while being maintained on intravenous solutions of 5% glucose and electrolytes. Such a regimen is equivalent to major starvation, which further increases the patient's vulnerability to infection, failure of wound healing, wound dehiscence, and organ failure.

Response to Trauma and Sepsis

Trauma and sepsis are associated with hypercatabolic states that decrease protein synthesis and increase nitrogen excretion in proportion to the severity of the trauma, sepsis, associated medical conditions, and immune deficiencies.

After uncomplicated surgical procedures of moderate severity, such as internal fixation of femoral fractures, nitrogen balance remains negative for about a week. During this time, urinary nitrogen losses parallel increases in oxygen consumption.[9] In otherwise healthy subjects, mild and transient nitrogen losses are well tolerated for 1 to 7 days and are readily replaced by subsequent oral feeding; prophylactic nutritional therapy usually is not necessary.

By contrast, the fasting patient recovering from major trauma catabolizes considerable lean tissue and fat. Patients with severe body surface burns may expend as much as 5000 to 6000 kcal/day.[1, 4, 5, 10] Endogenous peripheral amino acids are mobilized and gluconeogenesis increases, mediated in part by glucocorticoids. Severe trauma with sepsis is characterized by increased body metabolism with fever and increased oxygen consumption;[6] accelerated glucose turnover;[10] reduced insulin release; increased adrenal glucocorticoid, glucagon, and catecholamine release; early hyperglycemia followed by late hypoglycemia; and high circulating free fatty acid levels. Muscle proteins are broken down to amino acids, which are used as substrates for gluconeogenesis to supply glucose for glucose-dependent tissues such as the brain.[1] The greater the stress of trauma and sepsis relative to the patient's state of well-being and immune competence, the greater is the catabolic response. In these patients, preoperative reversal of malnutrition more effectively reduces mortality and morbidity than does nutritional therapy limited to the postoperative period.

CLINICAL AND LABORATORY DIAGNOSIS OF NUTRITIONAL FAILURE

Evaluation of nutritional status in seriously ill patients is made difficult by the lack of specific tests for protein-calorie malnutrition.

Nutritional History

A history of nausea, anorexia, diarrhea, weight loss, or nutritional deficiency is important. The medical history should also assess the possible influence of the current illness and its therapy on appetite, taste sensation, chewing, swallowing, and absorption. Dietary intake may be estimated from careful inquiry into the patient's eating patterns and weight changes. If possible, a food diary or hospital calorie count may be used to confirm the dietary intake. Evaluation of energy expenditure is a rough-value judgment[10a, 10b, 10c] that may be affected by increased work of breathing, high fever, and hypercatabolism[10d] (particularly in postoperative septic states), major body surface burns, and severe trauma. Social factors including alcohol intake, drug use, ethnic and cultural influences, socioeconomic status, dietary supplements,[10e] dietary nonnutrients,[10f] and degree of independence and mobility may also directly or indirectly influence the patient's nutritional status.

Physical Examination

The routine physical examination should note signs suggesting possible nutritional deficiencies,[10g] including muscle wasting or weakness, dermatitis, keratosis and scaling of skin, ulceration of mucous membranes, osteomalacia, metabolic alkalosis, tetany, growth retardation, delayed wound healing, central nervous system depression, paresthesias, glossitis, night blindness, ecchymosis, epistaxis, congestive heart failure, goiter, thyrotoxicosis, bleeding tendency, and diabetes mellitus. Height should be verified because of possible loss with age or bone disease; weight may be expressed as a percentage of change over a given time interval.

The normal weight for healthy males is about 106 pounds for 5 feet plus 6 pounds for every inch thereafter (plus 10% of the calculated weight over 50 years of age);[11] the normal for females is 100 pounds for 5 feet plus 5 lb for every inch thereafter (plus 10% of the calculated weight over 50 years of age). Table 124–1 lists ideal body weights in relation to height. A decreasing ratio of actual weight to ideal weight, expressed as a percentage, may roughly reflect a degree of malnutrition: mild (>90%), moderate (50–90%), or severe (<50%).

The nutritional history and physical examination provide only a gross qualitative picture of nutritional status that is limited by the patient's recall and by the accuracy of hospital records, which often neglect the potential effects of malabsorption, drug use, or lifestyle. Even the assessment of weight change has limitations because the pre-illness weight obtained by history may be unreliable, and current weight may be hard to obtain in the critically ill, bedridden subject. Moreover, weight losses of fat have quite different implications for the nutritional status than losses of lean body mass.

Laboratory Tests

Laboratory tests should include complete blood count, total lymphocyte count, blood smear, reticulocyte count, plasma osmolality, blood glucose and electrolytes (sodium, potassium, chloride, bicarbonate, calcium, phosphate, magnesium, and iron), albumin and total protein concentrations, and measurements of blood urea nitrogen (BUN), serum creatinine, triglycerides, and cholesterol. Less commonly available tests include serum transferrin (TFN), retinol-binding protein, fibronectin, plasma ferritin, various vitamins,

TABLE 124–1. Ideal Weight for Height

Height (cm)	*Weight (kg)*	
	Males	*Females*
145	51.8	47.5
150	54.5	50.4
155	57.2	53.1
160	60.5	56.2
165	63.5	59.5
175	70.1	66.3
180	74.2	
185	78.1	

(Adapted from the Metropolitan Life Insurance Statistics Bulletin 1981; 40:1.)

trace elements, and essential fatty acids. Many of these measurements are affected by the bulk movements of fluids and electrolytes between plasma and interstitial water; these provide only a rough index of nutritional status.

Anthropometric Measurements

Table 124-2 lists measurements that are increasingly used to estimate the proportions of body fat and muscle mass assumed to reflect caloric and protein intakes, respectively.[11, 12] Individually, these are only gross estimates; however, they may be used in combination to derive useful indexes.[12a] For example, preoperative values of serum albumin, triceps skin-fold thickness (TSF), TFN, and delayed cutaneous hypersensitivity (DCH) have been compiled to derive an empiric prognostic nutritional index (PNI) that is directly related to the risk of complications in postoperative patients.[13] The PNI is calculated as follows:

$$\text{PNI (\%)} = 158 - 16.6\,(\text{albumin, g/dL}) - 0.78\,(\text{TSF, mm}) - 0.2\,(\text{TFN, mg/dL}) - 5.8\,(\text{DCH, graded as 0, 1, or 2})$$

For example, one study found that, of 100 patients scheduled for gastrointestinal operations, those whose index was less than 40% had an 8.3% postoperative complication rate and 2.8% mortality, whereas those patients whose index was greater than 50% had a 46% postoperative complication rate and 33% mortality.[13] Mortality and morbidity in the high-risk group (index above 50%) were significantly reduced by preoperative nutritional support.

Creatinine-Height Index

The creatinine-height index uses the 24-hour urinary creatinine output to relate body muscle mass to height.[14] This measure assumes that protein deficiency depletes muscle protein and thus lowers the daily creatine excretion. This index is not useful in patients with diseases, trauma, or myolysis.

DCH testing, a nonspecific method for evaluating immune function, also may reflect protein nutritional status. T cell suppressor function can be reduced by protein-calorie malnutrition[15, 16]; depleted children and adults have proportionate degrees of lymphopenia. In our experience, patients on intravenous feeding for 2 to 4 weeks without catheter-related sepsis are clinically assumed to be immune competent.

BODY FLUID DISTRIBUTIONS IN NUTRITIONAL FAILURE

Nutritional deficiencies as well as severe acute accidental and surgical trauma are associated with major fluid shifts between intracellular water (ICW), extracellular water (ECW), and interstitial water. Frequently, patients with chronic diseases or nutritional depletion appear to be dehydrated when, in fact, maldistribution of body water has produced intracellular dehydration and increased the ECW despite associated hypovolemia.[17] Patients successfully resuscitated from severe shock often experience some degree of peripheral or dependent edema; pitting edema of the ankles, in particular, is commonly associated with weight gain. These water dislocations reflect an energy deficit caused by metabolic needs that exceed nutritional intake and reserves.

TABLE 124–2. Anthropometric Measures

Body weight
Current body weight to ideal body weight = % ideal weight
Triceps skin fold
Subscapular skin fold
Midarm muscle circumference
Urinary creatinine excretion
Serum albumin concentration
Serum transferrin concentration
Skin tests of immune function

Understanding the changes in the distribution of body water may be crucial in the care of the critically ill patient because fluid imbalances may be exacerbated by overadministration of electrolyte solutions or corrected by adequate administration of nutrients.[17, 18] However, fluid maldistributions often cannot be inferred from clinical observations; direct quantitative measurements are needed. Most body composition studies are done in special study areas where serial measurements are only infrequently repeated to monitor relatively long-term changes. They are, therefore, usually limited to only a few patients with specific problems.

Hemodynamic and oxygen transport monitoring may be useful in acutely very ill or unstable patients with suspected fluid problems. Suboptimal oxygen delivery ($D\text{O}_2$) and oxygen consumption ($V\text{O}_2$) suggest that there may be inadequate blood volume, left ventricular preload, or cardiac performance in addition to inadequate nutrition. Body metabolism requires the supply of both oxygen and oxidative substances.[6]

Plasma Volume and Blood Volume

Iodine 125–radioiodinated human serum albumin (RIHSA) is used to measure plasma volume.[2, 17, 19] Three to 5 μCi of RIHSA are injected intravenously after obtaining duplicate 1-mL aliquots of plasma for control measurements. Blood is sampled after 5, 10, 20, and 30 minutes; samples are counted in a well-type gamma-scintillation counter and compared with standard dilutions of the injected RIHSA. Counts are plotted on a semilog scale; the radioactivity corresponding to instantaneous mixing of RIHSA and plasma is obtained by extrapolating these values back to the time of injection.

Blood volume (BV) may be calculated as the plasma volume divided by whole-body hematocrit. The latter is assumed to be 0.874 times the large-vessel hematocrit measured by standard microcapillary centrifugation.[2, 17] Normal BVs are approximately 2.74 L/m^2 for men and 2.35 L/m^2 for women.[20, 21]

Total Body Water and Extracellar Water

The total body water (TBW) is determined by dilution technique with tritiated water, and ECW is measured by a variety of tracers including inulin, sucrose, thiocyanate, and isotopically labeled sodium ($^{22}Na^+$, $^{24}Na^+$), chloride, sulfate, and bromide ($^{82}Br^-$); of these, $^{82}Br^-$, $^{22}Na^+$, and $^{24}Na^+$ have been used clinically, and they reach a stable plasma concentration within 4 to 5 hours, even in sick patients.[2, 22-28] In normal subjects, measurements of both ^3H_2O and $^{82}Br^-$ are highly reproducible;[28] however, severe illness may increase the permeability of cells to bromide, increasing the bromide space and causing overestimation of ECW and underestimation of ICW. The extent of this discrepancy can be determined by measuring exchangeable potassium,[19, 29] as described next.

Intracellular Water and Exchangeable Potassium

The ICW may be calculated as the difference between TBW and ECW or directly measured as the exchangeable radiopotassium (^{42}K). However, although ICW may be accurately measured by ^{42}K, equilibration time is 3 days in normal subjects and probably longer in seriously ill patients,[29] and results are not available until 4 days after the test has been completed. Also, loss of potassium may be proportionately greater than loss of body cell mass in patients with heart failure, hyperadrenalism, acute stress, trauma, and other diseases.[30, 31] Thus, exchangeable ^{42}K is not practical for clinical estimation of body cell mass.

Potassium 40 is a naturally occurring isotope that represents 0.012% of all naturally occurring potassium. Total body counting of ^{40}K is an alternative to isotope dilution for measurement of total body potassium. This method closely correlates with exchangeable potassium measured by ^{42}K.[32]

Measurements of Fluid Distribution

Because ICW content fluctuates only within narrow limits, a change in the ICW reflects changes in the total body cell mass and therefore is a more accurate index of protein-calorie depletion than is weight loss,[17, 19] except in dehydrated patients. In one series, weight losses averaged only 16%, whereas ICW decreased 22% (Table 124–3).[19] The loss of more than 50% of the body cell mass (measured as ICW) usually is irreversible, but lesser losses can be restored with adequate parenteral and enteral alimentation.[18, 19]

The major source of error in the use of ICW to evaluate the nutritional status is the approximately 12% variation in the expected normal value used to calculate gains or losses. This error limits the usefulness of ICW in patients with mild depletion.[19] However, ICW remains the most relevant index of moderate or severe nutritional depletion. The major errors are technical and reflect variations of about 5% to 10% errors expected in serial body composition measurements.

Because the ECW-TBW ratio is largely independent of body weight or fat content, it is a more reliable index of nutritional depletion than ICW measurements. Expected ratios of ECW to TBW are affected by age and sex; normal values range from 0.40 for a 16-year-old boy to 0.50 for an 80-year-old man or woman.[2] Illness increases the ECW-TBW ratio by increasing ECW and decreasing ICW. Increases of 0.05 greater than the expected normal value suggest significant dislocations of body water.

Body Composition Patterns in Acute and Chronic Illness

In their extreme forms, protein deficiency and combined protein-calorie deficiency correspond to the clinical syndromes of kwashiorkor and marasmus, respectively.[8, 33, 34] Both syndromes, which most frequently occur in children with severe malnutrition, consist of weight loss and failure to grow and reductions in organ size, protein content, and plasma proteins; the latter is more pronounced in kwashiorkor. Patients with marasmus have a relatively normal body composition, but kwashiorkor is characterized by markedly increased ECW, pitting edema, ascites, and anasarca as well as decreased lean body mass, decreased plasma albumin, changes in plasma amino acid and enzyme patterns, fatty liver, muscle wasting, lethargy, and loss of hair pigment. One week of carbohydrate feeding to an already undernourished child with marasmus can produce the fully developed kwashiorkor syndrome.[33]

Increased ECW has been reported in chronic wasting diseases,[2] in German soldiers on repatriation from Russian prison camps after World War II,[35] after weight loss and surgery,[2, 17, 19, 22, 26, 36, 37] and after resuscitation from trauma and hemorrhage.[38] These ECW increases are relative as well as absolute, despite considerable weight loss and an even greater loss of body cell mass.[19] Thus, ECW is greatly expanded compared with ICW or TBW, particularly in patients who are chronically depleted (see Table 124–3). Combined depletion-dehydration may be accompanied by relatively normal TBW; the increased ECW may be offset by dehydration.

THERAPY

The interactions of therapy in the nutritionally depleted patient are now briefly reviewed.

Effects of Crystalloids in Depleted Patients

Fluid retention in critically ill patients may be partly due to the administration of saline or carbohydrate as the sole caloric intake, particularly in those who are chronically depleted. Intravenous glucose administration can produce acute fluid retention in fasting but otherwise healthy young men by reducing sodium excretion. This effect is increased when sodium chloride is given simultaneously. Because an expanded ECW may contribute to respiratory failure in critically ill patients, the routine administration of 5% glucose and electrolyte solutions should be replaced with adequate parenteral nutrition mainly composed of amino acids, fat, vitamins, minerals, and carbohydrates only in quantities that maintain the blood glucose between 100 and 200 mg/dL.[39]

Clinically, when glucose administration exceeds the clearance or utilization rates and continues, there will be a gradual increase in serum alkaline phosphatase, hepatic enzymes, and bilirubin[40–43] before the patient manifests stupor

TABLE 124–3. Observed Body Composition Values Expressed as Percentage of Deviation from Predicted Values Based on Current and Normal Expected Weights

		Current Weight			*Normal Weight*			
Variable	*No. of Subjects*	*ECW*	*TBW*	*ICW*	*Wt.**	*ECW*	*TBW*	*ICW*
Postoperative	16	+25	+7	−7	−10	+11	−4	−18
Depleted	11	+39	+13	−12	−22	+15	−7	−28
Depleted-dehydrated	4	−8	−6	−6	−24	−27	−24	−22
All patients	31	+25	+7	−9	−16	+7	−8	−22
Controls	3	−1	+5	+9	−3	−3	+2	+7

(Reprinted with permission from Elwyn DH, Bryan-Brown CW, Shoemaker WC: Nutritional aspects of body water dislocations in postoperative and depleted patients. Ann Surg 1975; 182:76.)

*Decreases in body weight given as % of normal: − = decrease; + = increase.

Abbreviations: Wt. = weight; ECW = extracellular water; TBW = total body water; ICW = intracellular water.

and hepatic coma. Administration of glucose in excess of clearance and utilization rates in patients with unrecognized or clinically inapparent renal insufficiency causes the development of metabolic acidosis, which can be alleviated by reducing the daily intake of glucose.[42] In fact, this metabolic acidosis may be the first early sign of renal insufficiency in patients with borderline renal function. Thus, glucose administration must be adjusted to avoid blood glucose levels of greater than 200 mg/dL to prevent continuing increase of serum hepatic enzymes and augmentation of metabolic acidosis from either renal insufficiency or the overwhelming of the renal compensatory functions.

At the early phase of our experience with intravenous hyperalimentation, exogenous crystalline insulin was used to augment glucose clearance in patients who manifested hyperglycemia greater than 200 mg/dL despite inadequate amounts of glucose administration.[39, 42, 43] However, now we rarely use exogenous insulin except in diabetics requiring exogenous insulin and in post total pancreatectomy patients. The liberal use of the exogenous insulin in the nondiabetic to augment glucose clearance and utilization is not recommended.

Amino Acid and Protein Feeding

Indirect calorimetry[44] may serve as a guide to determine the daily energy needs, but it may not reflect the actual daily nutritional deficits, especially in patients with metabolic acidosis from nutritional deficiency. A number of special amino acid formulations are commercially available. Branched-chain amino acid–enriched formulas have been used in the management of hepatic coma and in severely stressed patients[45, 46] with favorable results. Other investigators recommend using special amino acid formulations with caution and skepticism about the final outcome.[47]

We use the BUN level as an indicator for administration/intake of amino acids/nitrogen similar to using the blood sugar as a guide for carbohydrate intake. In patients with the BUN within normal limits, the highest rate of nitrogen intake should not increase BUN levels to greater than 30 mg/dL. In patients with BUN values of greater than 30 mg/dL, the highest rate of intake should not raise the BUN to greater than 40 mg/dL; in patients with BUN values of 40 mg/dL, the highest rate of intake should not raise the BUN to greater than 60 mg/dL; in patients with BUN of 60 mg/dL, the highest rate of nitrogen intake should not raise the BUN to greater than 80 mg/dL. Patients with a BUN of 80 mg/dL or higher can be given protein or amino acid solutions evenly over each 24-hour period only at a rate that does not cause the BUN level to increase above the preinfusion preintake level.

In patients receiving hemodialysis, intravenous nutrition composed of amino acids, glucose, and fat can be administered during the dialysis cycle to provide for the metabolic needs and to offset some of the losses of the nutrients in the dialysate.[48] Administration of concentrated human albumin (25%) in patients with renal insufficiency or renal failure is the most effective means of rapidly restoring serum albumin levels to normal limits.

We believe that a steady rate of amino acids or protein administration simultaneously with non-nitrogenous sources of calories provides the highest nitrogen metabolic efficiency. Additionally, active or passive exercises, or a combination, prescribed several times daily as tolerated by the patient help further increase the nitrogen efficiency.

Fat emulsion provides some of the needed calories in patients with sharply limited tolerance to carbohydrates and amino acids or proteins; fat intake can help provide some of the needed calories. Fat can be given to patients with carbohydrate intolerance or diabetes mellitus. However, administration of long-chain and even medium-chain triglycerides in excess of utilization rate may result in fat uptake by the reticuloendothelial system[49–52]; this result may make the immunodeficient patient vulnerable to intravenous catheter infection.

Continuous and steady administration of fat emulsions with amino acids or proteins provides the most efficient utilization of fat. We prefer not to administer fat and carbohydrates simultaneously. Diabetic patients with hyperglycemia greater than 200 mg/dL and a BUN level greater than 40 mg/dL are largely dependent on the intake of fat as the main source of calories.

Patients with metabolic derangements are at high risk for intravenous catheter infection. Therefore, the period of intravenous nutrition must be effectively and efficiently curtailed to avoid catheter infection. Oral/enteral feeding must be started as soon as possible and by any possible means. When intravenous feeding in patients at high risk for infection is essential for a long time, we recommend removing the catheter once a week with another week interval free of intravenous catheters. This intermittent venous cannulation may help prevent the almost inevitable catheter infection resulting from prolonged continuous indwelling venous catheters.

SUMMARY OF THERAPEUTIC ASPECTS

Patients in whom nutritional failure has developed must be slowly resuscitated nutritionally and metabolically. The administration of nutrients must be constantly readjusted to the clearance from blood and utilization rates until a normal nutritional status is reached. The key to patient survival is to feed only what can be utilized at the time to keep the metabolic fire aflame but not extinguish it; this adjusted nutritional rehabilitation is particularly crucial in the elderly,[53] in cancer patients,[54] and in patients with acquired immunodeficiency syndrome.[55] When malnourished patients reach close to the normal nutritional status, the daily amounts of nutrient intakes may have to be reduced to avoid overdose of nutrients. However, some patients with severe stress, trauma, sepsis, advanced cancer, and acquired immunodeficiency syndrome may never utilize their nutritional intakes. In such patients, the use of growth factors may enhance metabolism and recovery.[56–58]

Patients who continue to remain in a deficient nitrogen and calorie balance because of starvation or insufficient calorie-nitrogen utilization eventually will experience an irreversible catabolic state and metabolic failure, which is the end-stage in all dying patients. When the irreversible catabolic state is reached, death is imminent, and, in fact, intake of nutrients may accelerate the inevitable demise because of the effects of unutilized nutrients. Philosophically, we believe in providing nutritional support for patients in preterminal disease stages because even in the preterminal stage nutrients help maintain some physical vigor and strength necessary for the critically ill patient to cope with dying. This approach, we believe, can be as comforting to the otherwise listless and apathetic patient as analgesics are in alleviating the pain. However, when irreversible metabolic failure sets in, the intake of unutilizable nutrients should be withheld.

References

1. Vanamee P, Shils M, Meng HC, et al: Symposium on Total Parenteral Nutrition. Chicago, American Medical Association, 1972.

2. Moore FD, Olesen KH, McMurrey JD, et al: Body Cell Mass and Its Supporting Environment. Philadelphia, WB Saunders, 1963.
3. Brozek JD (Ed): Human Body Compositions: Approaches and Applications. New York, Pergamon Press, 1965.
4. Cahill GF Jr, Owen OE: Some observations on carbohydrate metabolism in man. *In*: Carbohydrate Metabolism and Its Disorders. Dickens F, Randle PJ, Whelan WJ (Eds). London, Academic Press, 1968.
5. Meng HC, Law DH: Parenteral Nutrition. Springfield, IL, Charles C Thomas, 1968.
6. Shoemaker WC: Cardiorespiratory patterns in complicated and uncomplicated septic shock. Ann Surg 1971; 174:119.
7. Elwyn DH: Role of the liver in regulation of amino acid and protein metabolism. *In*: Mammalian Protein Metabolism. Vol 4. Munro HN (Ed). New York, Academic Press, 1970, p 523.
8. Waterlow JC: Assessment of protein nutrition and metabolism in the whole animal with special reference to man. *In*: Mammalian Protein Metabolism. Vol 3. Munro HN (Ed). New York, Academic Press, 1969, p 325.
9. Cuthbertson DP: Observations on the disturbance of metabolism produced by injury of the limbs. Q J Med 1932; 25:233.
10. Long CL, Spencer JL, Kinney JM, et al: Carbohydrate metabolism in man: Effect of elective operations and major injury. J Appl Physiol 1971; 31:110.
10a. Beaton GH: Approaches to analysis of dietary data: Relationship between planned analyses and choice of methodology. Am J Clin Nutr 1994; 59(Suppl 1):253S.
10b. Bingham SA: The use of 24-h urine samples and energy expenditure to validate dietary assessments. Am J Clin Nutr 59(Suppl 1): 227S.
10c. Foltz MB, Schiller MR, Ryan AS: Nutrition screening and assessment: Current practices and dietitians' leadership roles. J Am Diet Assoc 1993; 93:1388.
10d. Kelly KG: Advances in perioperative nutritional support. Med Clin North Am 1993; 77:465.
10e. Block G, Sinha R, Gridley G: Collection of dietary-supplement data and implications for analysis. Am J Clin Nutr 1994; 59(Suppl 1):232S.
10f. Petersen BJ, Chaisson CF, Douglass JS: Use of food-intake surveys to estimate exposures to nonnutrients. Am J Clin Nutr 1994; 59(Suppl 1):240S.
10g. Lupo L, Pannarale O, Altomare D, et al: Reliability of clinical judgement in evaluation of the nutritional status of surgical patients. Br J Surg 1993; 80:1553.
11. Keys A: Overweight, obesity, coronary heart disease and mortality. Nutr Rev 1980; 38:297.
12. Howard L, Meguid MM: Nutritional assessment in total parenteral nutrition. Clin Lab Med 1981; 4:611.
12a. Dwyer JT, Gallo JJ, Reichel W: Assessing nutritional status in elderly patients. Am Fam Physician 1993; 47:613.
13. Buzgy GP, Mullen JL, Matthews DC, et al: Prognostic nutritional index in gastrointestinal surgery. Am J Surg 1979; 139:160.
14. Forbes GB, Bruining GJ: Urinary creatinine excretion and lean body mass. Am J Clin Nutr 1976; 29:1359.
15. Chandra RK: Immunodeficiency in undernutrition and overnutrition. Nutr Rev 1981; 39:225.
16. Chandra RK: Immunocompetence. Clin Lab Med 1981; 1:631.
17. Shoemaker WC, Bryan-Brown CW, Quigley L, et al: Body fluid shifts in depletion and poststress states and their correction with adequate nutrition. Surg Gynecol Obstet 1973; 136:371.
18. Shoemaker WC, Bryan-Brown CW, Elwyn DH: Therapy of nutritional failure. Semin Drug Treatment 1973; 3:301.
19. Elwyn DH, Bryan-Brown CW, Shoemaker WC: Nutritional aspects of body water dislocations in postoperative and depleted patients. Ann Surg 1975; 182:76.
20. Davis HA: Blood Volume Dynamics. Springfield, IL, Charles C Thomas, 1962.
21. Nadler SB, Hidalgo JV, Bloch T: Prediction of blood volume in normal human adults. Surgery 1962; 52:224.
22. Cleland MB, Pluth JR, Tauxe WN, et al: Blood volume and body fluid compartment changes soon after closed and open intracardiac surgery. J Thorac Surg 1960; 52:698.
23. Barratt TM, Walser M: Extracellular fluid in individual tissues and in whole animals: The distribution of radiosulfate and radiobromide. J Clin Invest 1969; 48:56.
24. Berson SA, Yalow RS: Critique of extracellular space measurements with small ions. Science 1955; 121:34.
25. Dyrbye MO, Kragelund E: Simultaneous determination of the apparent ^{3}HOH, ^{82}Br, ^{125}I human albumin and ^{51}Cr red cell volumes in human subjects. Scand J Clin Lab Invest 1970; 26:61.
26. Kragelund E: Changes of the apparent ^{3}HOH, ^{82}Br, ^{125}I human albumin and ^{51}Cr red blood cell dilution volumes before, during and after operation in human subjects. Ann Surg 1970; 172:116.
27. Leth A, Binder C: The distribution volume of ^{82}Br as a measurement of the extracellular fluid volume in normal persons. Scand J Clin Lab Invest 1970; 25:291.
28. Nicholson JP, Zilva JF: Estimation of extracellular fluid volume using radiobromide. Clin Sci 1960; 10:391.
29. Zollinger RM, Van DeWater JM, Maletskos CJ, et al: Exchangeable potassium in man using a new radioisotope ^{42}K. Surg Forum 1970; 21:213.
30. Flear CTG: Significance of potassium and sodium masses in cardiac diseases. *In*: Compartments, Pools, and Spaces in Medical Physiology. Bergner PE, Lushbaugh EE (Eds). Springfield, IL, US Atomic Energy Commission, 1967, pp 53–93.
31. Muldowney FP, Healy JJ: Lean body mass and total body potassium. *In*: Compartments, Pools, and Spaces in Medical Physiology. Bergner PE, Lushbaugh EE (Eds). Springfield, IL, US Atomic Energy Commission, 1967, pp 95–109.
32. Novak LP: Aging, total body potassium, fat-free mass, and cell mass in males and females between ages 18 and 85 years. J Gerontol 1972; 27:438.
33. Viteri F, Behar M, Arroyave G, et al: Clinical aspects of protein malnutrition. *In*: Mammalian Protein Metabolism. Vol 1. Munro HN, Allison JB (Eds). New York, Academic Press, 1964, p 523.
34. Elwyn DH: A kwashiorkor-like syndrome in hospitalized patients. Surg Gynecol Obstet 1973; 137:837.
35. McCance RA, Widdowson EM: A method of breaking down the weights of living persons into terms of extracellular fluid, cell mass, and fat, and some applications of it to physiology and medicine. Proc R Soc Lond (Biol) 1951; 138:115.
36. Pluth JR, Cleland J, Meador C, et al: Effect of surgery on the volume distribution of ECF determined by sulfate and bromide methods. *In*: Compartments, Pools, and Spaces in Medical Physiology. Bergner PE, Lushbaugh EE (Eds). Springfield, IL, US Atomic Energy Commission, 1967, p 217.
37. Bryan-Brown CW, Savitz MH, Elwyn DH, et al: Cerebral edema unresponsive to conventional therapy in neurosurgical patients with unsuspected nutritional failure. Crit Care Med 1973; 1:125.
38. Doty DB, Hufnagle HV, Mosely RV: The distribution of body fluids following hemorrhage and resuscitation in combat casualties. Surg Gynecol Obstet 1970; 130:453.
39. Parsa MH, Shoemaker WC: Nutritional failure. *In*: Textbook of Critical Care Medicine. 1st ed. Shoemaker WC, Thompson WL, Holbrook PR (Eds). Philadelphia, WB Saunders, 1984, p 681.
40. Leaseburge LA, Winn NJ, Schloerb PR: Liver test alterations with total parenteral nutrition and nutritional status. JPEN J Parenter Enteral Nutr 1992; 16:348.
41. Messing B, Colombel JF, Heresbach D, et al: Chronic cholestasis and macro nutrient excess in patients treated with prolonged parenteral nutrition. Nutrition 1992; 8:30.
42. Parsa MH, Habif DV, Ferrer JM, et al: Intravenous hyperalimentation: Indications, technique and complications. Bull NY Acad Med 1972; 48:920.
43. Parsa MH, Ferrer JM, Habif DV: Safe Central Venous Nutrition: Guidelines for Prevention and Management of Complications. Springfield, IL, Charles C Thomas, 1974, p 234.
44. Driscoll DF, Blackburn GL: Total parenteral nutrition 1990: A review of its current status in hospitalised patients, and the need for patient-specific feeding. Drugs 1990; 40:346.
45. Fischer JE: Branched-chain enriched amino acid solutions in patients with liver failure: An early example of nutritional pharmacology. JPEN J Parenter Enteral Nutr 1990; 14(Suppl):249S.
46. Kawamura I, Yamazaki K, Tsuchiya H, et al: Optimum branched-chain amino acids concentration for improving protein catabolism in severely stressed rats. JPEN J Parenter Enteral Nutr 1990; 14:398.
47. Heyman MB: General and specialized parenteral amino acid formulations for nutrition support. J Am Diet Assoc 1990; 90:401.
48. Cano N, Labastie-Coeyrehourq J, Lacombe P, et al: Peridialytic

parenteral nutrition with lipids and amino acids in malnourished hemodialysis patients. Am J Clin Nutr 1990; 52:726.
49. Hirschberg Y, Pomposelli EA, Bistrian BR, et al: Effect of tracer and intravenous fat emulsion on the measurement of reticulo endothelial system function. JPEN J Parenter Enteral Nutr 1990; 14:463.
50. Jensen GL, Mascioli EA, Seidner DL, et al: Parenteral infusion of long- and medium chain triglycerides and reticuloendothelial system function in man. JPEN J Parenter Enteral Nutr 1990; 14:467.
51. Macfie J, Courtney DF, Brennan TG: Continuous versus intermittent infusion of fat emulsion during total parenteral nutrition: Clinical trial. Nutrition 1991; 7:99.
52. Rosenthal E, Weissman B, Kyllonen K: Use of parenteral medium-chain triglyceride emulsion for maintaining seizure control in a 5-year-old girl with intractable diarrhea. JPEN J Parenter Enteral Nutr 1990; 14:538.
53. Driscoll DF, Bistarian BR: Special considerations required for the formulation and administration of total parenteral nutrition therapy in the elderly patient. Drugs Aging 1992; 2:395.
54. Daly JM, Redmond HP, Gallagher H: Perioperative nutrition in cancer patients. JPEN J Parenter Enteral Nutr 1992; 16(Suppl):100S.
55. Kofler DP, Tierney AR, Culpepper-Morgan JA, et al: Effect of home total parenteral nutrition on body composition in patients with acquired immunodeficiency syndrome. JPEN J Parenter Enteral Nutr 1990; 14:454.
56. Wilmore DW: Catabolic illness: Strategies for enhancing recovery. N Engl J Med 1991; 325:695.
57. Ziegler TR, Rombeau JL, Young LS, et al: Recombinant growth hormone enhances the metabolic efficacy of parenteral nutrition: A double-blind, randomized controlled study. J Clin Endocrinol Metab 1992; 74:865.
58. Ponting GA, Ward HC, Halliday D, et al: Protein and energy metabolism with biosynthetic human growth hormone in patients on full intravenous nutrition support. JPEN J Parenter Enteral Nutr 1990; 14:437.

CHAPTER 125

Pharmacologic Principles

Barbara J. Zarowitz, PharmD, FCCP

Comprehension of pharmacologic principles is essential for optimizing drug therapy in critically ill patients. Variability in pharmacologic response may be a function of alterations in drug disposition (pharmacokinetics) or drug effects (pharmacodynamics) resulting from organ system impairment, instrumentation, concurrent drug therapy, metabolic aberration, or altered receptor number or sensitivity. Vast new knowledge has allowed for the provision of individualized pharmacotherapeutics. Advanced pharmacy practitioners are at the bedside in many intensive care units (ICUs) as a part of the patient care team providing comprehensive pharmacokinetically based dosing services, identifying and preventing adverse drug reactions and drug interactions, individualizing medication delivery systems, ensuring intravenous compatibility and nutritional support, selecting pharmacologic regimens, and participating in clinical research.[1, 2] This chapter reviews ICU-associated alterations in pharmacokinetics, and pharmacodynamics, reviews drug interactions, and provides recommendations for optimizing the pharmacologic aspects of care for critically ill patients.

PHARMACOKINETIC PRINCIPLES

Clinical pharmacokinetics is defined as the study and characterization of the time course of drug absorption, distribution, metabolism, and excretion and the relationship of these processes to the intensity and time course of therapeutic and adverse effects of drugs in humans.[3] Multiple system organ dysfunction in critically ill patients predisposes to large interindividual variability in each phase of drug disposition.

Absorption

The pharmacokinetic description of the extent of drug absorption is termed *bioavailability*.[3] When a drug is administered intravenously, it is completely available systemically or 100% bioavailable (bioavailability [F] = 1) as opposed to orally administered drugs, which pass through the gastrointestinal tract or liver before entering the general circulation. Impaired oral bioavailability may result from incomplete disintegration or dissolution, resulting in poor absorption or significant biotransformation and extraction of the drug by the liver before reaching the general circulation.[4] Gut wall edema, stasis, and alterations in gastric or intestinal blood flow as well as concurrent therapy with anticholinergics and narcotic analgesics account for delayed or incomplete drug absorption and altered gastrointestinal transit time in the critically ill. Gut wall absorptive capacity is diminished after hemorrhagic shock.[5] Bioavailability may be decreased by 70% to 80% for drugs such as phenytoin when coadministered with antacids or enteral feeding products.[6] Coadministration of enteral feedings may speed or delay the rate or extent of absorption of various drugs (Table 125–1).[7, 8] Individual absorption characteristics of each drug must be examined before relying on the adequacy of this route of administration.

Bioavailability considerations also exist with intravenous, intramuscular, subcutaneous, rectal, and aerosolized drug delivery routes. A decrease in bioavailability of as much as 50% can occur when intravenously administered nitroglycerin and diazepam bind to the polyvinylchloride constituent of intravenous tubing and containers.[9] Subcutaneous, intramuscular, and rectal routes of administration are not recommended, except for subcutaneous heparin, in the ICU because the absorption time may be dramatically delayed and absolute bioavailability limited by alterations in blood flow to the injection site or rectal mucosa. Aerosolization of drugs such as epinephrine, β_2 receptor agonists, lidocaine, anticholinergics, and corticosteroids has been shown to be reliable in the critically ill because of the extensive alveolocapillary membrane surface area.[10–12] Bronchodilation associated with aerosolized β_2 receptor agonists exceeds that achieved orally and is similar to that attained after intravenous administration.[11, 12]

The intravenous route is the primary medication delivery mode in the ICU. Access for multiple, concurrently administered intravenous medications has been facilitated by the use of multilumen central venous catheters in which high blood flow rates alleviate most concerns of drug incompati-

TABLE 125–1. Absorption Alterations in Critically Ill Patients

Drugs Well Absorbed Orally	*Drugs with Documented Absorption Difficulties*
Cimetidine	Cyclosporine
Fluconazole	Digoxin
Quinolone antibiotics*	Famotidine
Rifampin	Ketoconazole
Theophylline elixir	Omeprazole
	Phenytoin
	Theophylline (sustained release)

*Avoid concurrent antacid administration.

bility and volume restriction requirements for fluid-overloaded patients. In spite of accurate high-technology infusion control devices, delays in drug response may occur when drug concentrations are changed without priming the intravenous tubing.

Distribution

The relationship between the amount of drug in the body and the plasma concentration after absorption and distribution is expressed by a proportionality constant called the *apparent volume of distribution* (V). It reflects a nonphysiologic compartment into which the drug disperses and may be affected by body size, physicochemical characteristics of the drug, tissue binding, plasma protein binding, and regional blood flow.[3] The early part of the serum concentration–time curve (Fig. 125–1) is the distributive phase and primarily represents drug diffusion from the intravascular space into extravascular fluids and tissue. Knowledge of drug volumes of distribution is helpful in choosing adequate loading doses to achieve rapid therapeutic effects, particularly for drugs such as theophylline, anticonvulsants, antiarrhythmics, and many antibiotics.

The concentration of plasma proteins, which changes dramatically in response to critical illness, may also affect drug distribution.[13, 14] Albumin, prealbumin, and transferrin concentrations decrease in patients with burns, cancer, chronic bronchitis, diabetes mellitus, heart failure, liver disease, malnutrition or sepsis, and uremia. Albumin concentration decreases significantly after trauma.[13] Acidic drugs, which bind to albumin, exhibit a larger, unbound fraction in hypoalbuminemic patients, potentially producing a greater pharmacologic effect. The concentration of acute phase–reactant proteins, including α_1–acid glycoprotein, increases in patients with burns, cancer, epilepsy, infection, myocardial infarction, surgery, and trauma. Alpha$_1$–acid glycoprotein increases three- to fourfold after severe multiple trauma, reaching peak concentrations by the sixth day after injury, and remains elevated for 15 to 21 days.[14] In this situation, increased binding of basic drugs (e.g., lidocaine)

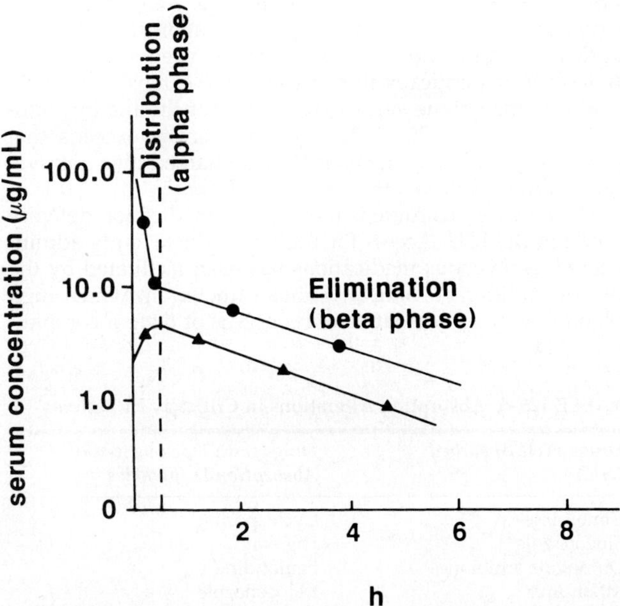

Figure 125–1. Serum concentration-time curve of a drug showing the distribution and elimination phases after rapid intravenous injection *(black circles)* and oral administration *(black triangles)*.

TABLE 125–2. Protein Binding of Drugs to Albumin or α_1-Acid Glycoprotein

Drugs Bound Primarily to Albumin (Acidic Drugs)	*Drugs Bound Primarily to α_1–Acid Glycoprotein (Basic Drugs)*
Cephalosporins	Clindamycin
Penicillins	Disopyramide
Phenobarbital	Imipramine
Phenytoin	Lidocaine
Theophylline	Meperidine
Valproic acid	Quinidine
Warfarin	Propranolol
	Verapamil

may lead to decreased effect, necessitating greater than usual doses. This effect reverses with recovery from the acute injury phase (Table 125–2).

Alterations in drug binding status may be responsible for changes in the pharmacologic effect because only unbound drug is available to equilibrate with receptor sites in tissues.[15] Drugs with a narrow therapeutic range are most likely to produce important increases in pharmacologic effect with binding alterations. For these medications serum concentrations producing the desired pharmacologic effect and those that produce toxicity may overlap. Clinically important binding changes occur in hypoalbuminemic or uremic patients. For example, hypoalbuminemic patients receiving phenytoin may have total phenytoin concentrations that are normal or low and yet the unbound concentrations are adequate.[13, 15] Alternately, postmyocardial infarction patients with increases in α_1–acid glycoprotein tolerate total lidocaine concentrations that are normally associated with toxicity.[16, 17] Careful patient and pharmacokinetic assessment of both unbound and total drug concentrations is recommended before dosage adjustment.

Large interindividual variability in the volume of distribution of water-soluble drugs, such as aminoglycoside antibiotics, has been reported in critically ill, surgical, acutely ill, malnourished, medical, burn, and spinal cord injury patients.[18–23] Increased extracellular and total body water and decreased body cell mass can occur, even in the face of central volume contraction in hypoalbuminemic patients. Assessment of the distribution of fluids is essential to ensure that adequate loading doses are administered.

Clearance

Clearance is a term based on the concept of the whole body acting as a drug-eliminating system. Clearance is the sum of the individual clearance rates of the various drug-eliminating organs.[3] Many drugs are metabolized by the liver or excreted unchanged in the urine. Decreased glomerular filtration (GFR), as may be seen in low cardiac output states, decreases renal elimination and drug clearance.[24]

Generally, a linear relationship exists between renal drug clearance and creatinine clearance (Cl_{cr}), which is often used as a marker for GFR. Patients may demonstrate low-normal serum creatinine values because of immobility, age, or malnutrition and yet have significantly impaired GFR and drug clearance.[24–26] Although limitations in accuracy exist, Cl_{cr} can be calculated by several equations, such as the Cockcroft and Gault method.[27]

$$Cl_{cr}(\text{ml/min}) = \left(\frac{(140 - \text{age}) \times \text{weight}}{72 \times \text{serum creatinine}}\right) \times 0.85 \text{ for female patients}$$

where weight is measured in kilograms.

Because aminoglycoside antibiotics are filtered but minimally secreted and reabsorbed, aminoglycoside clearance has been shown to be a more accurate predictor of GFR than Cl_{cr} in critically ill medical patients.[26] Doses of other filtered drugs can be altered on the basis of aminoglycoside clearance. Linear regression equations and empirical recommendations are available to modify dosage regimens before characterization by serum concentration monitoring.[21-28] The effects of dialysis, ultrafiltration, hemodiafiltration, and peritoneal removal techniques on drug elimination have been well documented.[29, 30] Water-soluble drugs with small distribution volumes, low protein binding, and a substantial renal component to total body clearance demonstrate greater dialytic removal, requiring dosage replacement after dialysis.

Drugs eliminated primarily by the liver may demonstrate decreased or increased clearance in critically ill patients. High intrinsic clearance drugs, whose elimination from the body is dependent primarily on liver blood flow, may show reduced clearance with splanchnic and hepatic hypoperfusion. Hepatic hypoperfusion can occur directly as a function of penetrating injury, through decreased cardiac output and thus liver blood flow, or by flow redistribution in shock states. Hepatic blood flow is decreased within the first 24 hours of multiple severe trauma and returns to normal values by the sixth day after injury. Studies using indocyanine green clearance as a marker of liver blood flow have yielded conflicting results in animal models of hemorrhagic shock and neurotrauma.[31-34] Increases in serum bilirubin and transient, nonspecific increases in ammonia and transaminases follow hypoperfusion injury. Drugs that rely on liver blood flow for clearance (Table 125–3) may require dosage adjustment and careful monitoring.

Decreases in liver functional capacity consistent with hypoalbuminemia, hyperbilirubinemia, and prolongation in partial thromboplastin time are seen in alcoholic cirrhosis

TABLE 125–3. Characterization of Drugs Eliminated Primarily by the Liver

	Approximate Extraction (E)	*Protein Binding (%)*	*Comments on Effects of Liver Disease*
Flow-limited drugs			
Chlormethiazole	0.70	99	Changes in liver blood flow and intrinsic clearance associated with liver disease affect these drugs. The shunting of blood around the liver has important effects on the bioavailability of these drugs.
Labetalol	0.85	40	
Lidocaine	0.60	65	
Lorcainide	0.65	70	
Morphine	0.75	35	
Pentazocine	0.60	65	
Propoxyphene	>0.90	75	
Propranolol	0.65	95	
Verapamil	0.80	92	
Flow/enzyme-sensitive drugs			
Acetaminophen	0.30	20	Changes in liver blood flow, free intrinsic clearance, and free fraction of drug in blood may be important for this class of drugs.
Chloramphenicol	0.28	70	
Chlorpromazine	0.30	95	
Erythromycin	0.30	80	
Isoniazid	0.27	10	
Meperidine	0.50	70	
Methohexital	0.53	—	
Metoprolol	0.56	10	
Nafcillin	0.27	90	
Nortriptyline	0.50	95	
Quinidine	0.27	85	
Ranitidine	0.28	15	
Enzyme-limited, binding-insensitive drugs			
Antipyrine	0.05	10	This class of drugs is most sensitive to changes occurring in the free intrinsic drug clearance with liver disease.
Amylobarbital	0.03	60	
Caffeine	0.04	31	
Cyclophosphamide	0.08	14	
Hexobarbital	0.15	47	
Theophylline	0.05	62	
Enzyme-limited, binding-sensitive drugs			
Cefoperazone	0.04	90	This class of drugs will be influenced by changes in free fraction of drug in blood and free intrinsic drug clearance. The overall change in drug clearance will be governed by which one of these factors changes the most as a result of the disease process.
Chlordiazepoxide	0.02	96	
Diazepam	0.02	97	
Diphenylhydantoin	0.03	92	
Fenprofen	0.13	>99	
Indomethacin	0.08	90	
Naproxen	0.005	>99	
Phenylbutazone	0.01	99	
Rifampin	0.11	85	
Tolbutamide	0.02	98	
Valproic acid	0.02	89	
Warfarin	0.005	99	

(Used with permission from Arns PA, Wedland PJ, Branch RA: Adjustment of medications in liver failure. *In*: The Pharmacologic Approach to the Critically Ill Patient. 2nd ed. Chernow B (Ed). Baltimore, Williams & Wilkins, 1988.)

and biliary stasis. Animal models of traumatic injury have demonstrated differential decreases in both phase I (nonsynthetic functionalization reactions: oxidation, reduction, hydrolysis) and phase II (synthetic conjugation reactions: glucuronidation, sulfation, acetylation, and methylation) biotransformation, although phase II reactions appear to be less affected than phase I reactions.[35–37] Antipyrine, a marker of oxidative capacity, and lorazepam, a marker of glucuronidation, have been used to demonstrate decreased enzymatic function in head trauma patients and experimental models of hemorrhagic shock.[33, 34] On the other hand, glucuronidation is preserved in burn trauma patients.[38] Drugs dependent primarily on enzymatic function rather than liver blood flow for clearance are considered low-extraction drugs and may require dosage adjustment in patients with liver dysfunction. An exception to this is phenytoin, a low-extraction drug whose dosage requirements may continue to increase in neurotrauma patients with either induction of metabolism as a result of influences of stress on hepatic metabolic activity or decreases in protein binding.[34] Specific recommendations for dosage adjustment of hepatically cleared drugs are available.[39] Further study is needed to elaborate on the interrelationships of organ dysfunction and drug clearance. Preliminary information suggests a decrease in hepatic clearance of drugs metabolized through oxidation by the P45OIID6 isozyme in patients with renal failure.[40]

Enzyme functional capacity can be altered by concurrent drug therapy with enzyme-inducing agents such as phenobarbital, phenytoin, cigarette smoke, rifampin, carbamazepine, or inhibiting agents such as cimetidine, omeprazole, and quinolone antibiotics.[41] The effect may be small or significant depending on the potency of the offending agent, fraction of total clearance accounted for by metabolism, isozyme family affected, route of administration, and dosage selected. The time course of induction varies from 2 to 10 days depending on the inducing agents and reverses at a similar rate upon drug discontinuation. Direct metabolic inhibition can occur more immediately and produce clinically important toxicity. Selected examples of induction and inhibition interactions are provided in Table 125–4.

Microsomal enzyme function is decreased by interleukin-1, interleukin-6, tumor necrosis factor, interferon, and endotoxin, whereas no effect of these cytokines has been demonstrated on glucuronidation.[42, 43] The cytokines appear to bind to receptors on the surface of the hepatocytes during the acute phase response. Cytokine suppression of hepatocyte mixed-function oxidation and subsequent reduction in drug clearance may have significant clinical importance warranting further investigation.

The influence of mechanical ventilation and positive end-expiratory pressure (PEEP) on drug clearance is a consideration in critically ill patients. Mechanical ventilation and PEEP additively decrease cardiac output, hepatic and renal blood flow, GFR, and urine flow.[44] A 22% decrease in lidocaine clearance, consistent with a reduction in hepatic blood flow, has been demonstrated after initiation of mechanical ventilation.[45] The role of invasive mechanical assist devices, such as balloon counterpulsation, in altering drug disposition needs elaboration.

Half-Life

Half-life ($t_{1/2}$) represents the time required for a drug concentration to decrease by 50% after absorption and distribution.[3] The elimination rate constant (k) is the fraction of drug eliminated per unit of time, usually per hour, and is inversely related to half-life ($t_{1/2} = \ln 2/k$). Figure 125–2 depicts the relationship between half-life and elimination rate constant. Half-life is dependent on both V and clearance but nevertheless represents a useful parameter to estimate the time to steady state and time necessary for drug removal in situations of overdose.

Dosage regimens are usually designed to provide minimum fluctuation around a therapeutically effective concentration. Four to five half-lives are required before the full effects of the dosage regimen can be evaluated by serum concentration measures. At steady state, the drug reaches an equilibrium in the body wherein the amount of drug entering is equal to the amount of drug being eliminated. Subsequent peak and trough concentrations will be equal unless drug clearance changes (Fig. 125–3).

Summary of Pharmacokinetic Considerations

In critically ill patients, irrespective of the primary pathophysiology, standard approaches to drug therapy individualization can be used if consequences of physiologic sequelae are accounted for in the interpretation of functional markers. Individualization of drug doses with carefully timed serum concentrations of total and, where applicable, unbound drug is recommended whenever possible. Figure 125–4 summarizes hypoperfusion-related changes in drug disposition in the critically ill.

DRUG INTERACTIONS

Adverse reactions of drugs are a potentially lethal complication of therapy in hospitalized patients. Approximately 6.5% of all drug reactions have been attributed to drug interactions.[46] Because critically ill patients usually require complex drug combinations and exhibit impaired organ function, they are believed to be at higher risk for adverse pharmacotherapy events. Recognition that interindividual differences of drug action may be exaggerated in critically ill patients should prompt anticipation of resultant variability in the pharmacologic effect of the drug interaction. Table 125–4 summarizes representative drug interactions in critically ill patients.

PHARMACODYNAMIC ALTERATIONS IN CRITICAL ILLNESS

Pharmacodynamics has been defined as the study of the biologic effects resulting from the interaction between drugs and biologic systems.[47] Whereas pharmacokinetics describes drug disposition, pharmacodynamics pertains to drug effects. Numerous mechanisms are responsible for altered pharmacodynamics in critically ill patients (Fig. 125–5). Pharmacologic intensity of effect can be altered both by pharmacokinetic factors (inadequate drug concentration at the receptor site from altered absorption, distribution, or elimination) and parameters associated with the receptor such as occupancy, number, and translocation of the receptor within the membrane.[47] Competing drugs, active metabolites, or endogenous inhibitors may occupy receptors. Regional receptor distribution, number, and affinity may be altered in response to drug treatment and various disease states (Table 125–5).[48] Secondary messengers or cofactors may be depleted, impairing the drug-receptor interface. The range of doses of inotropes, catecholamines, opioids, and sedative drugs required to produce the desired clinical response is so varied that it is futile to define average doses.[48] Clinical endpoints must be chosen and doses titrated cautiously to the desired clinical endpoint.

Text continued on page 1149

TABLE 125–4. Selected Drug Interactions in Critically Ill Patients

Drug	*Drug*	*Effect*	*Mechanism*	*Comments*
Aminoglycosides	Loop diuretics	Increased risk of ototoxicity	Additive	Transient or permanent hearing loss
	Neuromuscular blocking agents	Increased neuromuscular blockade	Additive	Reversible with calcium
	Penicillins	Inactivation of both antibiotics	Formation of inactive conjugates	Separate administration times by 1–2 hours
Amphotericin B	Digitalis	Increased risk of digitalis toxicity	Amphotericin-induced renal potassium wasting	Monitor serum potassium
	Neuromuscular blocking agents	Increased curariform effect	Amphotericin-induced renal potassium wasting	Monitor serum potassium
Antacids	Angiotensin-converting enzyme inhibitors Histamine$_2$ antagonists Ketoconazole Quinolone antibiotics (norfloxacin, ciprofloxacin)	Decreased effect	Decreased absorption	Separate administration times, avoid combination
	Quinidine	Increased quinidine effect	Decreased renal clearance	Monitor quinidine serum concentration, and adjust dose
Barbiturates (phenobarbital)	Beta-blockers	Decreased β-blockade	Induction of microsomal enzymes	Increase dose as required
	Corticosteroids	Increased barbiturate effect	Induction of microsomal enzymes	Increase steroid dose as required
	Quinidine	Decreased quinidine effect	Induction of microsomal enzymes	Increase quinidine dose as required
	Rifampin	Decreased barbiturate effect	Induction of microsomal enzymes	Increase barbiturate dose as required
	Valproic acid	Increased barbiturate effect	Inhibition of microsomal enzymes	Monitor barbiturate levels
Beta-blockers	Anesthetics, general	Hypotension	Potentially additive	Monitor blood pressure
	Barbiturates	Decreased β-blockade	Induction of microsomal enzymes	Increase β-blocker dose as required
	Cimetidine	Increased β-blocker effect	Decreased hepatic clearance	Observe closely
	Lidocaine	Increased lidocaine effect	Decreased hepatic clearance	Observe closely
	Neuromuscular blocking agents	Prolonged blockade	Potentially synergistic	Monitor closely
	Theophylline	Increased theophylline effect	Decreased theophylline clearance	Monitor theophylline serum concentrations
	Verapamil	Increased negative chronotropic and inotropic effects	Additive	Caution using this combination
Calcium channel blockers	Beta-blockers	Increased negative chronotropic and inotropic effects	Additive	Caution using this combination
Cimetidine	Alprazolam Diazepam Narcotic analgesics Phenytoin Theophylline Warfarin	Increased effect	Inhibition of microsomal enzymes	Monitor and adjust dose as required
	Beta-blockers Lidocaine	Increased effect	Decreased hepatic clearance	Monitor and adjust dose as required
	Procainamide	Increased PA/NAPA effect	Decreased renal clearance	Monitor PA/NAPA serum concentrations
	Ketoconazole	Decreased antifungal effect	Decreased absorption	Avoid combination

Table continued on following page

TABLE 125–4. Selected Drug Interactions in Critically Ill Patients *(Continued)*

Drug	*Drug*	*Effect*	*Mechanism*	*Comments*
Cyclosporin	Cimetidine Diltiazem Erythromycin Fluconazole Ketoconazole Metoclopramide Nicardipine Norfloxacin Steroid hormones Sulindac Verapamil	Increased cyclosporine effect	Inhibition of metabolism	Monitor cyclosporine serum concentrations and lower dose as required
	Carbamazepine Nafcillin Phenobarbital Phenytoin Octreotide Rifampin Sulfonamides	Decreased cyclosporine effect, risk of rejection	Induction of microsomal enzymes	Avoid concurrent use
Digoxin	Cholestyramine Kaolin pectin Metoclopramide Neomycin Sulfasalazine	Decreased digoxin effect	Reduced oral absorption	Separate administration times by 4–6 hours
	Amiodarone Quinidine Verapamil	Increased digoxin effect	Reduced renal or nonrenal clearance	Decrease dose by half, monitor closely
	Erythromycin and other oral antibiotics	Increased digoxin effect	Inactivation of gut flora by antibiotic, increased oral absorption	May occur in 10–20% of patients; monitor and reduce dose as required
	Amphotericin B Diuretics	Increased digoxin effect	Hypokalemia	Monitor serum potassium and replace as required
	Vasodilators (hydralazine, nitroprusside)	Decreased digoxin effect	Increased renal clearance	Monitor, may require dosage increase
Neuromuscular blocking agents (pancuronium, vecuronium, atracurium)	Aminoglycoside antibiotics	Neuromuscular blockade	Additive	Reversible with calcium
	Amphotericin B	Increased curariform effect	Renal potassium wasting	Monitor serum potassium and replace as required
	Clindamycin	Neuromuscular blockade	Additive	Monitor patient closely
	Diuretics	Increased curariform effect	Hypokalemia	Monitor serum potassium and replace as required
	Lidocaine	Increased curariform effect	Potentiation	Monitor patient closely
	Narcotic analgesics	Respiratory depression	Additive	Monitor patient closely
	Procainamide	Increased curariform effect	Additive	Monitor patient closely
	Quinidine	Increased curariform effect	Additive	Monitor patient closely
Omeprazole	Diazepam Phenytoin	Omeprazole causes increased drug effect	Inhibition of metabolism	Monitor patient and decrease dose as required
Phenytoin	Cimetidine Fluconazole Isoniazid Valproic acid	Increased phenytoin effect	Inhibition of metabolism	Monitor phenytoin serum concentrations and decrease dose as required
	Folic acid Rifampin	Decreased phenytoin effect	Induction of phenytoin metabolism	Monitor serum phenytoin concentrations and increase dose as required
	Corticosteroids Quinidine Theophylline	Decreased drug effect	Phenytoin induces metabolism of other drug	Monitor drug therapy and increase dose as required
	Enteral feeds Sucralfate	Decreased phenytoin effect	Decreased phenytoin absorption	Monitor serum phenytoin concentrations and increase dose as required

TABLE 125–4. Selected Drug Interactions in Critically Ill Patients *(Continued)*

Drug	*Drug*	*Effect*	*Mechanism*	*Comments*
Sucralfate	Cimetidine Digoxin Phenytoin Quinidine Quinolone antibiotics	Decreased effect	Decreased absorption	Separate administration times
Theophylline	Adenosine	Theophylline impairs adenosine effect, adenosine reverses theophylline hemodynamic instability and neurologic toxicity	Receptor sensitivity	Avoid theophylline use in patients requiring adenosine
	Allopurinol Cimetidine Erythromycin Propranolol Quinolone antibiotics	Increased theophylline effect	Decreased theophylline clearance	Monitor theophylline serum concentrations and decrease dose as required
	Phenobarbital Phenytoin Rifampin	Decreased theophylline effect	Induction of microsomal enzymes and clearance	Monitor theophylline serum concentrations and increase dose as required

Abbreviations: PA = procainamide; NAPA = *N*-acetyl procainamide.

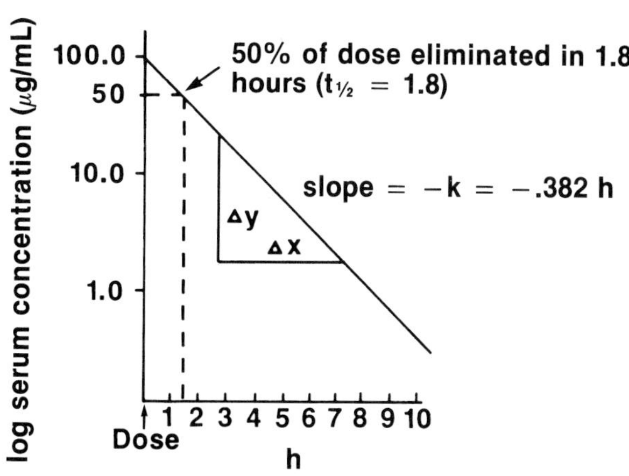

Figure 125–2. Mathematical derivation of half-life ($t_{1/2}$) and elimination rate constant (k). The slope is calculated as follows:

$$\frac{\Delta y}{\Delta x} = (\ln 32 - \ln 5) = -.382$$

$$t_{1/2} = .693/k = \frac{.693}{.382} = 1.8 \text{ h.}$$

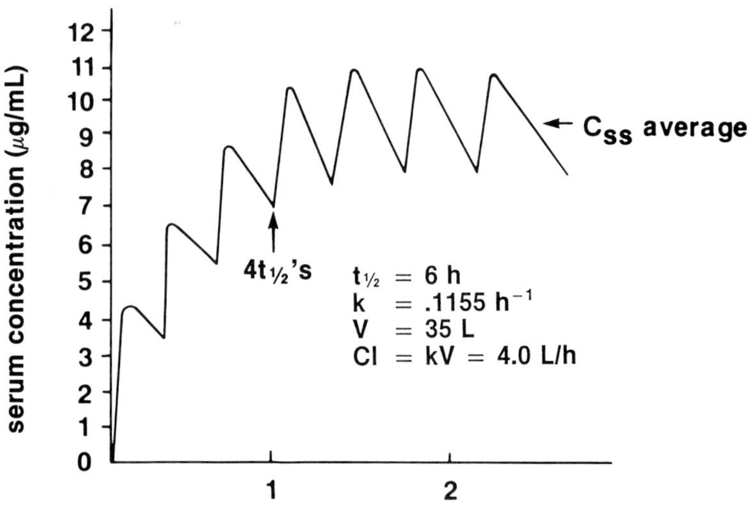

Figure 125–3. Serum concentration-time profile of a drug during multiple dosing. The time required to reach 90% of steady-state is four $t_{1/2}$'s. If this patient received 300 mg of theophylline elixir every 8 hours, the average steady-state concentration (C_{ss}) would be

$$C_{ss} = \frac{F \times \text{dose}}{Cl \times \text{dosing interval}}$$

$$= \frac{(1.0)\ (300)}{(4.0)\ (8.0)} = 9.3\ \mu g/mL$$

where F = 1.0 (100% bioavailability).

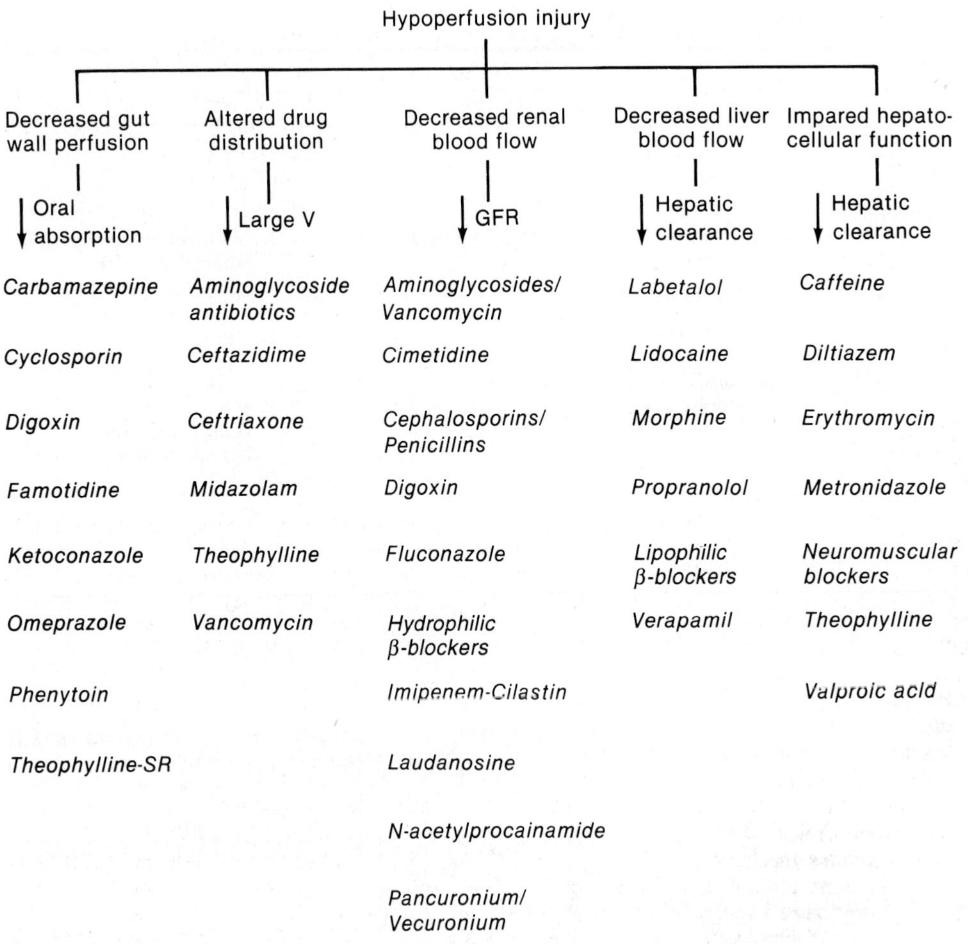

Figure 125–4. Hypoperfusion-induced changes in blood flow and organ system function may result in decreased absorption, altered distribution, impaired renal excretion, and decreased hepatic metabolism of clinically important drugs.

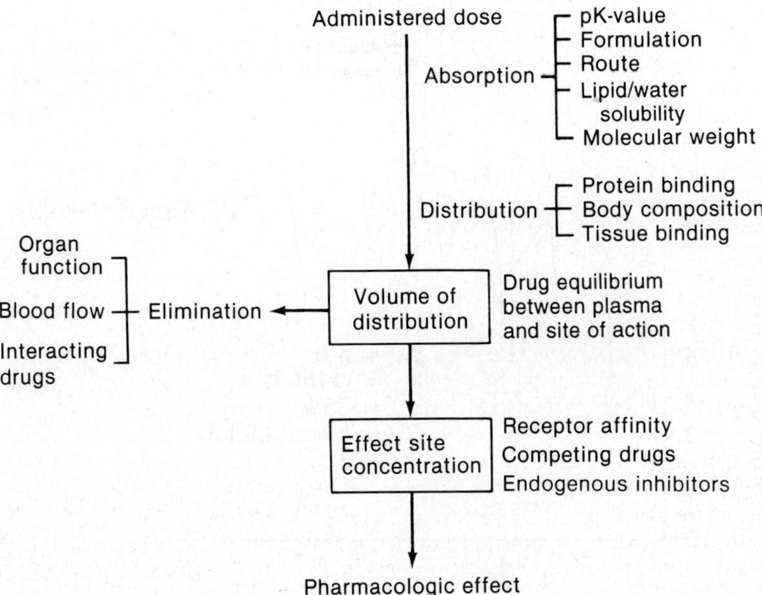

Figure 125–5. Drug pharmacokinetic and pharmacodynamic factors can alter the intensity of the pharmacologic effect. Factors that affect absorption, distribution, effect site concentration, and elimination are schematically represented.

TABLE 125–5. Selected Examples of Pharmacodynamic Variability in Critically Ill Patients[48–50]

Drug	*Variability/Cause*	*Recommendations*
Opioids	Greater than 10-fold range of daily requirements for adequate pain relief; μ-receptor sensitivity	Doses should be titrated to pain relief Decrease morphine dose in renal failure, avoid meperidine (active normeperidine accumulates)
Diazepam	$t_{1/2}$ of 24–72 hours Accumulation of active metabolites Wide range of required doses and duration of effect	Choice of shorter acting agents (e.g., midazolam) or agent without active metabolites (e.g., lorazepam)
Theophylline	Toxicity within the usual therapeutic range	Careful monitoring, cautious dosage titration
	Underlying cardiovascular disease predisposes to toxicity Clearance is also impaired	Choose desired concentrations at the lower end of the therapeutic range
Nondepolarizing neuromuscular blockers	Varying dosage requirements Prolonged paralysis after discontinuation Altered clearance Metabolite accumulation Acid-base, temperature, and concurrent drug interaction effects	Reduce dosage in elderly, organ system–compromised patients; lighten paralysis daily, and monitor with peripheral nerve stimulation Consider shorter acting agents in susceptible patients
Dobutamine	Impaired β-receptor function	Doses must be titrated to response
Catecholamines	Reduced myocardial performance in septic shock Hypersensitization and up-regulation early, followed by desensitization and down-regulation Circulating catecholamines and mediators of inflammation	More evident with β_1 than α_2 receptors
Furosemide	Wide range of dosing requirements Renal sodium threshold varies with renal function and underlying disease	Titrate dose to achieve adequate diuresis, then repeat effective dose as needed to achieve clinical endpoints

(Modified with permission from Runciman WB, Myburgh JA, Upton RN: Pharmacokinetics and pharmacodynamics in the critically ill. Baillieres Clin Anaesth 1990; 4:271.)

Abbreviation: $t_{1/2}$ = half-life.

Recommendations for Optimizing Pharmacotherapy

It is difficult to establish meaningful outcome parameters in critically ill patients because many clinically desirable responses do not have easily monitored markers of activity. Reductions in mortality and morbidity are global outcome goals, yet neither assists the clinician in managing the patient at the bedside. Clinicians are left with monitoring available parameters and setting intermediate endpoints.

Specific pharmacologic endpoints should be set to provide optimal therapeutic effect with minimum toxicity. Knowledge of the alterations in both pharmacokinetic and pharmacodynamic behavior of drugs in critically ill patients is fundamental to setting appropriate endpoints and individualizing pharmacotherapy regimens. Physiologic modifications resulting from acute illness change not only the drug effects but also the monitoring endpoints. Patient assessment and pharmacotherapeutic individualization become very dynamic processes.

Common problems encountered in optimizing drug therapy regimens include (1) underestimating the time required for a regimen to reach steady state, (2) misinterpreting the physiologic parameters chosen as therapy endpoints, and (3) failing to anticipate the altered response resulting from either pharmacokinetic or pharmacodynamic changes. Assessment of the time required to reach steady state is a function of the estimated change in drug half-life. Clinicians must have knowledge of customary drug half-lives and then estimate the likely prolongation in half-life resulting from concurrent organ dysfunction. For most drugs, blood for serum concentration monitoring can be drawn after four half-lives have elapsed. Drugs with a narrow therapeutic range given intermittently may warrant assessment of both peak and trough concentrations for dosage individualization. If doses have been appropriately spaced (i.e., one to two half-lives apart), steady state can be assumed after the third dose in most cases. Administration of a loading dose, large enough to account for the potentially enlarged volume of distribution for water-soluble drugs, is recommended when immediate drug effects are desired. Steady state may not be attained in patients with rapidly changing organ function, necessitating clinical reassessment with each administered dose.

Misinterpretation of physiologic parameters can lead to grossly inaccurate assessment of organ function. Low or normal serum creatinine values should not imply unaffected GFR or drug clearance. Hyperbilirubinemia, hypoprothrombinemia, and hypoalbuminemia correlate better with decreased hepatic function than elevated transaminase values for most drugs.

Failure to recognize that critical illness may be responsible for exaggerated drug effects can lead to significant overdosing of drugs. Centrally acting agents, neuromuscular blockers, opioids, theophylline, and histamine$_2$ receptor antagonists are examples of medications with the potential to alter response and disposition in the critically ill. Dosage titration to minimally effective concentrations or pharmacologic response is recommended to avoid prolonged, unwanted effects or toxicity. The prolonged half-life portends delayed elimination and continued effect beyond that expected in non-ICU patients. There are also many situations in which drug elimination and effect may be enhanced.

CONCLUSIONS

Extensive information describing the pharmacologic idiosyncrasies of critically ill patients has become available and yet the challenges of management continue. Clinicians are often forced to extrapolate from knowledge of drug behavior in non-ICU patients to fashion individualized therapy in this special population.

References

1. Ellinoy BR, Clarke JE, Wagers PW, et al: Comprehensive pharmaceutical services in a medical intensive-care unit. Am J Hosp Pharm 1984; 41:2335.
2. Dasta JF, Angaran DM: Evolving role of the pharmacist in critical care. Crit Care Med 1992; 20:563.
3. Gibaldi M, Levy G: Pharmacokinetics in clinical practice: Concepts. JAMA 1976; 235:1864.
4. Pond SM, Tozer TN: First-pass elimination: Basic concepts and clinical consequences. Clin Pharmacokinet 1984; 9:1.
5. Singh G, Chaudry KI, Chudler LC, et al: Depressed gut absorptive capacity after trauma-hemorrhagic shock. Ann Surg 1991; 214:712.
6. Hooks MA, Longe RL, Taylor AT, et al: Recovery of phenytoin from an enteral nutrient formula. Am J Hosp Pharm 1986; 43:685.
7. Holtz L, Milton J, Sturek JK: Compatibility of medications with enteral feedings. JPEN J Parenter Enteral Nutr 1987; 11:183.
8. Cutie AJ, Altman E, Lenkel L: Compatibility of enteral products with commonly employed drug additives. JPEN J Parenter Enteral Nutr 1983; 7:186.
9. Martens HJ, DeGoede PN, VanLoenen AC: Sorption of various drugs in polyvinyl chloride glass, and polyethylene-lined infusion containers. Am J Hosp Pharm 1990; 47:369.
10. Emergency Cardiac Care Committee and Subcommittees, American Heart Association: Guidelines for cardiopulmonary resuscitation and emergency cardiac care. JAMA 1992; 268:2199.
11. Louridas G, Kakoura M, Galenis N, et al: Bronchodilatory effects of inhaled versus oral salbutamol in bronchial asthma. Respiration 1983; 44:439.
12. Lawford P, Jones BJ, Milledge JS: Comparison of intravenous and nebulised salbutamol in initial treatment of severe asthma. Br Med J 1978; 1:84.
13. Boucher BA, Rodman JH, Fabian TC, et al: Disposition of phenytoin in critically ill trauma patients. Clin Pharm 1987; 6:881.
14. Edwards DJ, Lalka D, Cerra F, Slaughter RL: Alpha$_1$-acid glycoprotein concentration and protein binding in trauma. Clin Pharmacol Ther 1982; 31:62.
15. Perucca E, Grimaldi R, Crema A: Interpretation of drug levels in acute and chronic disease states. Clin Pharmacokinet 1985; 10:498.
16. Levy RH, Moreland TA: Rationale for monitoring free drug levels. Clin Pharmacokinet 1984; 9:1.
17. Routledge PA, Barchowsky BS, Bjornsson TD, et al: Lidocaine plasma protein binding. Clin Pharmacol Ther 1980; 27:347.
18. Fuhs DW, Mann HJ, Kubajak CA, et al: Intrapatient variation of aminoglycoside pharmacokinetics in critically ill surgical patients. Clin Pharm 1988; 7:207.
19. Dasta JF, Armstrong DK: Variability in aminoglycoside pharmacokinetics in critically ill surgical patients. Crit Care Med 1988; 16:327.
20. Zarowitz BJ, Pilla AM, Popovich J: Expanded gentamicin volume of distribution in patients with indicators of malnutrition. Clin Pharm 1990; 9:40.
21. Sawchuk RJ, Zaske DE: Pharmacokinetics of dosing regimens which utilize multiple intravenous infusions: Gentamicin in burn patients. J Pharmacokinet Biopharm 1976; 4:183.
22. Friedrich LV, White RL, Kays MB, et al: Aztreonam pharmacokinetics in burn patients. Antimicrob Agents Chemother 1991; 35:57.
23. Segal JL, Brunnemann SR: Clinical pharmacokinetics in patients with spinal cord injuries. Clin Pharmacokinet 1989; 17:109.
24. Robert S, Zarowitz BJ: Is there a reliable index of glomerular filtration rate in critically ill patients? DICP, Ann Pharmacother 1991; 25:169.
25. Hickling KG, Berry EJ, Perry RE, et al: Serum aminoglycoside clearance is predicted as poorly by renal aminoglycoside clearance as by creatinine clearance in critically ill patients. Crit Care Med 1991; 19:1041.
26. Zarowitz BJ, Robert S, Peterson EL: Prediction of glomerular filtration rate using aminoglycoside clearance in critically ill medical patients. Ann Pharmacother 1992; 26:1205.
27. Cockcroft DW, Gault MH: Prediction of creatinine clearance from serum creatinine. Nephron 1976; 16:31.
28. Bennett WM, Aronoff GR, Golper TA, et al: Drug prescribing in renal failure. 2nd ed. Philadelphia, American College of Physicians, 1991.
29. Matzke GR, Millikin SP: Influence of renal function and dialysis on drug disposition. *In*: Applied Pharmacokinetics: Principles of Therapeutic Drug Monitoring. 3rd ed. Evans WE, Schentag JJ, Jusko WJ (Eds). Vancouver, WA, Applied Therapeutics Inc, 1991, pp 8-1–8-49.
30. Golper TA: Continuous arteriovenous hemofiltration in acute renal failure. Am J Kidney Dis 1985; 6:373.
31. Gottlieb ME, Sarfeh IJ, Stratton H, et al: Hepatic perfusion and splanchnic oxygen consumption in patients postinjury. J Trauma 1983; 23:836.
32. Minard G, Fabian TC, Croce M, et al: Effect of isolated hepatic ischemia on organic anion clearance and oxidative metabolism. J Trauma 1992; 32:514.
33. DiPiro JT, Hooker KD, Sherman JC, et al: Effect of experimental hemorrhagic shock on hepatic drug elimination. Crit Care Med 1992; 29:810.
34. Boucher BA, Kuhl DA, Fabina TC, et al: Effect of neurotrauma on hepatic drug clearance. Clin Pharmacol Ther 1991; 50:487.
35. Griffeth LK, Rosen GM, Tschanz C, et al: Effect of model traumatic injury on hepatic drug metabolism in the rat: 1. In vivo antipyrine metabolism. Drug Metab Dispos 1983; 11:517.
36. Griffeth LK, Rosen GM, Rauckman EJ: Effects of model traumatic injury on hepatic drug metabolism in the rat: IV. Glucuronidation. Drug Metab Dispos 1988; 13:391.
37. Griffeth LK, Rosen GM, Rauckman EJ: Effects of model injury on hepatic drug metabolism in the rat: V. Sulfation and acetylation. Drug Metab Dispos 1985; 13:398.
38. Martyn J, Greenblatt DJ: Lorazepam conjugation is unimpaired in burn trauma. Clin Pharmacol Ther 1987; 43:250.
39. Kubisty CA, Arns PA, Wedland PJ, Branch RA: Adjustment of medications in liver failure. *In*: Pharmacologic Approach to the Critically Ill Patient. 3rd ed. Chernow B (Ed). Baltimore, Williams & Wilkins, 1994, pp 95–113.
40. Touchette MA, Slaughter RL: The effect of renal failure on hepatic drug clearance. DICP, Ann Pharmacother 1991; 25:1214.
41. Brouwer KCR, Dukes GE, Powell JR: Influence of liver function on drug disposition. *In*: Applied Pharmacokinetics: Principles of Therapeutic Drug Monitoring. 3rd ed. Evans WE, Schentag JJ, Jusko J (Eds). Vancouver, WA, Applied Therapeutics Inc, 1992, pp 6-1–6-59.
42. Sujita K, Okuno F, Tanaka Y, et al: Effect of interleukin 1 (IL-1) on the levels of cytochrome P-450 involving IL-1 receptor on the isolate hepatocytes of rat. Biochem Biophys Res Comm 1990; 168:1217.
43. Chen YL, Florentin I, Batt AM, et al: Effects of interleukin-6 on cytochrome P450-dependent mixed function oxidases in the rat. Biochem Pharmacol 1992; 44:137.
44. Perkins MW, Dasta JF, DeHaven B: Physiologic implications of mechanical ventilation on pharmacokinetics. DICP, Ann Pharmacother 1989; 23:316.
45. Richard C, Berdeaux A, Delion F, et al: Effect of mechanical ventilation on hepatic drug pharmacokinetics. Chest 1986; 90:837.
46. Greenlaw CW, Zellers DD: Computerized drug-drug interaction screening. Am J Hosp Pharm 1978; 35:567.
47. Lalonde RL: Pharmacodynamics. *In*: Applied Pharmacokinetics: Principles of Therapeutic Drug Monitoring. 3rd ed. Evans WE, Schentag JJ, Jusko WJ (Eds). Vancouver, WA, Applied Therapeutics Inc, 1992, pp 4-1–4-33.
48. Runciman WB, Myburgh JA, Upton RN: Pharmacokinetics and pharmacodynamics in the critically ill. Baillieres Clin Anaesth 1990; 4:271.
49. Silverman HJ, Penaranda R, Orens JB, et al: Impaired β-adrenergic receptor stimulation of cyclic adenosine monophosphate in human septic shock: Association with myocardial hyporesponsiveness to catecholamines. Crit Care Med 1993; 21:31.
50. Forse RA, Saint-Vil D, Gagner M, et al: Intra-abdominal sepsis and adrenergic receptor response. J Trauma 1992; 32:564.

CHAPTER 126

Providing Pharmaceutical Services in Critical Care Areas

Deborah K. Armstrong, PharmD, FCCM • Judith Jacobi, PharmD, FCCM • Joseph F. Dasta, MSc (Pharm), FCCM, FCCP

Provision of optimal pharmaceutical services is essential to the care of the critically ill patient. As with that of other specialists in critical care medicine, the role of critical care pharmacists is evolving into an integral component of healthcare. Pharmacists, using their unique training and skills, are making important contributions to the optimization of pharmacotherapy of the critically ill patient.[1, 2, 2a] The goal of this chapter is to provide information on the expanding role of the critical care pharmacist and to describe methods to implement cost-effective pharmaceutical services to the critically ill patient.

REVIEW OF PHARMACEUTICAL SERVICES

Pharmacists are taking an increasingly active role in drug therapy. As such, their focus is changing from the traditional drug product orientation to the optimal care of the patient from the bedside. To consolidate the varied aspects of pharmacy, a new paradigm, *pharmaceutical care,* has arisen.[3] This concept highlights the pharmacist's direct responsibility to the patient to provide optimal drug therapy with the intent of improving quality of life. It focuses on pharmacists' joint responsibility with physicians, nurses, and other healthcare professionals to ensure the safe preparation, timely delivery, and appropriateness of drug therapy to achieve the desired pharmacotherapeutic outcome for the patient. To effectuate these outcomes, pharmacists have become active participants in the drug therapy decision-making process. Interactions with physicians and other healthcare personnel on drug-related matters occur during patient care rounds, while monitoring prescribed drug therapy for a patient, and by providing in-service lectures on pharmacotherapy issues. Efficient use of information technology and technical support are key elements in the expansion of these patient-focused services.

Adverse drug effects, however, continue to occur. One study reported more than three prescribing errors for every 1000 drug orders.[4] These authors also found that up to 43% of hospitalized patients experience an adverse drug reaction. Implementing pharmaceutical care, and its associated active pharmacist participation in drug therapy, is a potential solution to this problem. Sophisticated drug delivery systems in hospitals have increased the efficiency and accuracy of medications administered to the patient. Unit-dose and intravenous admixture services exist in more than 70% of hospitals in the United States.[5] These developments have been paralleled by the increased use of the pharmacist's cognitive skills in drug therapy selection and monitoring for efficacy and toxicity and expansion of clinical pharmacy services.[5a] For example, nearly 80% of hospitals surveyed have pharmacists actively involved in drug therapy monitoring, and 90% have adverse drug reaction and drug use evaluation programs.[5] More than 40% of hospitals have formalized pharmacokinetic consult services, with most recommendations being accepted by the physician. In a detailed report of data on patient-focused pharmacy services summarized from studies published during an 11-year period, the outcomes of optimal drug use were described: reduced numbers of unnecessary drug levels, more appropriate interpretation of drug levels, lower drug costs, and improved quality of care.[6] Furthermore, one yearlong study conducted at Walter Reed Army Medical Center revealed a shorter length of hospital stay and reduced drug costs when a pharmacist attended rounds in general medicine and general surgery services. Cost savings in this study were estimated at $377 per patient or an annual savings of $150,000.[7]

In response to the increased sophistication of modern healthcare, pharmaceutical education has expanded the training of pharmacists. Many schools currently offer the doctor of pharmacy degree, which provides advanced clinical training in various aspects of physiology, pharmacology, and pharmacokinetics.[8] Many of these doctorate-possessing pharmacists subsequently pursue clinical residencies and fellowships to specialize in several areas, including critical care. Clinical pharmacists are sometimes referred to as *clinical pharmacologists.* They should be differentiated because the training of a clinical pharmacist differs from that of a physician or doctorate-possessing clinical pharmacologist. Dr. George Lundberg, editor of *Journal of the American Medical Association,* concluded that clinical pharmacy has emerged from a need for an interface between drugs and people, and the most qualified individual at this interface is the pharmacist.[9]

CRITICAL CARE PHARMACEUTICAL SERVICES

In the last 10 years, pharmacists have increasingly specialized in critical care practice.[1, 2, 8] Pharmacy services have been reported in virtually all types of intensive care units (ICUs) (pediatric, neonatal, adult medical, surgical, and trauma), the operating room, and the emergency department.[1, 9a] Critically ill patients, by their disease acuteness, require a rapid response time for drug preparation and delivery. Accuracy and sterility of drugs for parenteral administration are especially crucial for the patient with a tenuous physiologic status. Pharmaceutical care services provided include drug distribution systems tailored to the critically ill patient coupled with prospective drug therapy evaluation and monitoring.

A national survey of critical care pharmaceutical services revealed that unit-dose services were provided to 85% of ICU patients; however, only about 50% of these hospitals reported complete intravenous admixture services to these patients.[10] Whereas only 13% of hospitals reported that nurses prepared nearly all intravenous products, this number increased to 20% in hospitals without an ICU satellite pharmacy. The increased time required by nurses to prepare intravenous medications detracts from their direct patient care responsibilities, which is particularly problematic during periods of nursing shortages. Critical care pharmacists responding to the survey were involved in a variety of patient-focused activities such as monitoring efficacy of antibiotics, total parenteral nutrition solutions, vasoactive or inotropic agents, and antiarrhythmics. These pharmacists also conducted concurrent reviews of drug orders, provided pharmacokinetic consultations, participated in resuscitative attempts, and developed cost-containment programs.

The stimuli for the growth of this area of practice are composed, in part, of the unique and complex drug-related issues surrounding the critically ill patient. Approximately 6% to 20% of ICU admissions are drug related, and more than 50% of iatrogenic cardiac arrests are caused by medications.[11–13] The ICU patient receives, on average, 6 to 9 drugs per day and 8 to 12 different drugs during an ICU stay.[8] Examples of commonly prescribed drugs include antibiotics, analgesics/sedatives, agents for stress ulcer prophylaxis, antiarrhythmics, and antianginal drugs. In one study, drugs administered to patients admitted to the surgical ICU (SICU) accounted for 14% of hospital charges, and these admissions produced a net deficit of nearly $18,000 per patient under prospective reimbursement plans.[14] Pharmacy costs were significantly decreased in another study after implementing a satellite pharmacy in the SICU for a group of patients with similar severity of illness.[15]

It is well recognized that ICU patients have altered pharmacokinetics and pharmacodynamics.[16] Changes in organ blood flow, changes in fluid status, dysfunction of drug-eliminating organs, and altered plasma proteins account for many of these changes. Examples of drugs with known pharmacokinetic alterations in critically ill patients include aminoglycosides, β-lactam antibiotics, lidocaine, vancomycin, phenytoin, theophylline, and midazolam. Many other drugs are probably affected by these pharmacokinetic changes but have yet to be studied. The critical care pharmacist applies principles of pharmacology and physiology to design regimens to achieve and maintain therapeutic serum concentrations of many drugs rapidly and to optimize monitoring. A pharmacist-coordinated theophylline dosing system in a medical ICU (MICU), for example, resulted in fewer serum theophylline concentrations and less inappropriately obtained serum levels (15 versus 40%).[17] Another study demonstrated cost savings when the clinical pharmacist intervened in the scheduling and interpretation of serum drug concentrations compared with cost savings of $2128 for unjustifiable serum drug concentrations.[18] Much attention has been focused on the increased distribution volume of the aminoglycosides in critically ill patients and the subsequent need for large loading doses to achieve therapeutic concentrations.[19] Furthermore, pharmacist-managed aminoglycoside therapy achieved a significantly lower mortality rate.[20] For drugs with readily available serum concentrations, one study revealed that a large percentage of levels were incorrectly drawn or inappropriately ordered.[21] The potential for suboptimal decisions increases when drug concentrations are not appropriately obtained or incorrectly interpreted. Thus, an important function of the critical care pharmacist involves dosing and monitoring of drugs using pharmacokinetic principles. However, more studies are needed to continue to document the impact of therapeutic drug monitoring on outcome and associated costs.

Critical care pharmacists have organized their efforts in professional societies. In addition to specialty critical care sections in two professional pharmacy associations, the Clinical Pharmacology and Pharmacy section of the Society of Critical Care Medicine, formed in 1989, had more than 300 members as of February 1993. Pharmacists have also collaborated with physician colleagues on research. For example, a review of *Critical Care Medicine* articles from 1989 to 1993 revealed 77 studies with pharmacist authors; in 30 of these articles, the pharmacist was the primary author. Since 1982, the *Annals of Pharmacotherapy* has published a column in the pharmacy literature entitled "Critical Care," which focuses on pharmacotherapeutic issues of this specialized population.

IMPLEMENTING CRITICAL CARE PHARMACY SERVICES

The pharmacy of the future may be realized sooner than expected. With the focus on the provision of optimal drug therapy, monitoring, and outcomes, the satellite pharmacy will also change. The need for the provision of 24-hour, 7-day a week services has not been eliminated because the patients will continue to be dynamic and have acute needs.[22] However, with pharmaceutical care, the emphasis has shifted toward the pharmacists' responsibility for ensuring that the therapy chosen is optimal for the patient before it is dispensed. Pharmacists must be patient advocates for drug therapy selection and screen for potential adverse reactions or interactions from the bedside. Well-trained technicians are needed to support the dispensing functions and facilitate efficient drug availability. Ideally, the drugs should be dispensed in a patient-specific, ready-to-use form to minimize the amount of nursing time spent in drug preparation.

Another change may be in the physical characteristics of the satellite. With automated dispensing technology (Pyxis, Meditrol, Sure-Med, ATC 212, Medispence), the physical size of the satellite may decrease.[23] However, a pharmacy facility is still needed preferably within close proximity to the critical care patient area. A laminar flow hood should be used for aseptic preparation of all intravenous products.[24] Standard procedures for preparation and dilution will produce a more consistent product that has the flexibility to be relabeled for another patient, thereby minimizing waste.[25, 26] However, individualized formulation will still be needed for many patients to minimize fluid overload.[27, 28] Pharmacists have demonstrated successful improvements in the fluid status of ICU patients by individualizing preparation techniques.[29] Critical care pharmacists will use other resources that include a library or drug information center to supplement the critical care and drug therapy literature in the satellite. References such as a pharmacotherapy/therapeutics text (adult and pediatric), a critical care text, a pharmacology text,[16] a pharmacokinetic text, current Advanced Cardiac Life Support/Pediatric Advanced Life Support (ACLS/PALS) guidelines, and a toxicology data base should be standard. Also, sources for current information on intravenous drug compatibility and drug interactions need to be available.

Additionally, the pharmacist must have a strong knowledge base in critical care to anticipate and initiate therapy recommendations when the order is written. This will require good communication skills and an effective working relationship with the critical care team. The drug dose should be evaluated on the basis of renal-hepatic function estimates and the appropriate therapeutic drug monitoring initiated. Other important roles of the critical care pharmacist are nutritional support, pharmacokinetic dosing, profile review for elimination of unnecessary drug therapy, and report of adverse drug reactions. The pharmacist must provide education to other health professionals on the team and may be called on to obtain a medication history.[2, 30] These patient-focused services have been projected to require 13 hours per day in one 20-bed surgical ICU.[31] Productivity measurements must include the time spent in patient-focused activities.

Critical care pharmacists must document their contributions to patient care. The record of pharmacist drug therapy evaluations should be a part of the medical record just as is standard for other personnel. Optimally, pharmaceutical care plans will be developed around the problem-oriented analysis of drug therapy selection, dosing, monitoring, and follow-up for desired outcome. To facilitate efficient service, the members of the critical care team should develop practice guidelines and algorithms for selection and use of drugs in their ICU population. These guidelines (or critical paths) must consider optimal drug therapy outcome and the potential costs of the therapy.[32, 33]

An important challenge for critical care pharmacists is to assess the impact of the pharmaceutical care services on patient outcome. Reports of outcome assessment should be used by committees such as critical care, pharmacy and therapeutics, and infection control as evidence of continuous drug use improvement or continuous quality improvement.[34–36] The objective evaluation of outcome will also be needed to determine the role of new and more expensive therapies.

Justification of new critical care pharmacy services has been demonstrated in several ways.[37–39] Generally, a pilot study is conducted over a short period of time, collecting prospective data on prescribing trends, adverse drug reactions, and usage of serum drug concentrations, and dispensing response time (from the time the order is written to when the drug is administered to the patient). These data are then presented to a committee of hospital administrators, key physicians, and nurses as evidence for expanded pharmacy services. The impact of established critical care pharmaceutical services on the cost of patient care has been described,[1, 40–42] with savings demonstrated in a variety of units; more than seven abstracts were presented at the 1992 American Society of Hospital Pharmacists Midyear Clinical Meeting. Savings are primarily the result of cost avoidance measures and have generally been significant enough to justify pharmacist positions to hospital administration. Cost avoidance estimates from direct pharmacist involvement in drug therapy have been calculated to range from $72,000 for a 14-bed MICU to $96,000 for a 12-bed MICU per year.[43, 44, 44a] Other methods to justify development of a satellite pharmacy have included pharmacist scheduling of therapeutic drug monitoring serum concentrations, with the potential to avoid nearly $40,000 in unnecessary/poorly scheduled laboratory tests in a SICU.[21] Economic and patient care benefits were confirmed after satellite implementation in another study.[45] Justification of a pediatric ICU/neonatal ICU satellite was accomplished through analysis of medication administration errors.[46] After observing frequent errors related to dose preparation and timing and rate of administration, the authors established the need for more effective pharmacy services.

The potential expense of expanded pharmacy services to the ICU must also be considered, but through cost avoidance, charge capture, and improved drug delivery, a satellite was justified for 28 ICU beds.[47] A combination of many of these approaches and an estimate of the value of avoiding potential adverse drug reactions also produced a significant savings for a satellite serving 20 ICU beds (critical care unit/SICU).[48] A satellite may be successfully implemented with fewer than 24 hours of coverage.[47–49a] This allows pharmacists to document their impact and plan for expanded coverage. A study of total pharmacy costs for postoperative cardiac patients after the initiation of a satellite in a SICU showed a significant decrease when compared with presatellite costs for the first week postoperative.[15]

SUMMARY

Nursing and physician shortages—human resource issues—require efficient use of the healthcare team. Critical care pharmacists have become recognized as important contributors to the pharmaceutical care of critically ill patients. As healthcare dollars decrease, it is imperative to provide cost-effective care that improves outcomes. Critical care pharmacy services using a satellite with a critical care specialist active on the healthcare team is the preferred model for the provision of optimal pharmaceutical care for the critically ill patient.

Critical care pharmacy specialists have demonstrated benefit for the patient and documented cost savings. As healthcare reform focuses on optimal therapy and monitoring outcomes with minimal costs, the expertise of clinical pharmacists will be in greater demand. Pharmacists need to continue to document their contributions to pharmaceutical care in the literature and solicit support from critical care physicians and nurses to expand current services or establish new services.

References

1. Majerus TC, Dasta JF (Eds): Practice of Critical Care Pharmacy. Rockville, MD, Aspen Systems, 1985, pp 1–315.
2. Dasta JF, Angaran DM: Evolving role of the pharmacist in critical care. Crit Care Med 1992; 20:563–565.

2a. Dasta JF, Jacobi J: The critical care pharmacist: What you get is more than what you see. Crit Care Med 1994; 22:906–909.

3. Hepler CD, Strand LM: Opportunities and responsibilities in pharmaceutical care. Am J Hosp Pharm 1990; 47:533–543.
4. Lesar TS, Briceland LL, Delcoure K, et al: Medication prescribing errors in a teaching hospital. JAMA 1990; 263:2329–2334.
5. Crawford SY, Myers CE: ASHP national survey of hospital-based pharmaceutical services—1993. Am J Hosp Pharm 1993; 50:1371–1404.

5a. Bond CA, Raehl CL, Pitterle ME: 1992 National Clinical Pharmacy Services Study. Pharmacotherapy 1994; 14:282–304.

6. Hatoum HT, Catizone C, Hutchinson RA, et al: An eleven-year review of the pharmacy literature: Documentation of the value and acceptance of clinical pharmacy. Drug Intell Clin Pharm 1986; 20:33–48.
7. Bjornson DC, Hiner WO, Potyk RP, et al: Effect of pharmacists on healthcare outcomes in hospitalized patients. Am J Hosp Pharm 1993; 50:1875–1884.
8. Dasta JF, Jacobi J, Armstrong DK: Role of the pharmacist in caring for the critically ill patient. *In*: The Pharmacologic Approach to the Critically Ill Patient. 3rd ed. Chernow B (Ed). Baltimore, Williams & Wilkins, 1994, pp 156–166.
9. Lundberg GD: The clinical pharmacist. JAMA 1983; 249:1193.

9a. Levy DB: Documentation of clinical and cost-saving pharmacy interventions in the emergency room. Hosp Pharm 1993; 28:624–653.

10. Dasta JF, Segal R, Cunningham A: National survey of critical-care pharmaceutical services. Am J Hosp Pharm 1989; 46:2308–2312.
11. Bedell SE, Dietz DC, Leeman D, et al: Incidence and characteristics of preventable iatrogenic cardiac arrests. JAMA 1991; 265:2815–2820.
12. Trunet P, Borda IT, Rouget AV, et al: The role of drug-induced illness in admissions to an intensive care unit. Intensive Care Med 1986; 12:43–46.
13. Tietze KJ, Wittbrodt ET, Lanken PN: The frequency of drug-related MICU/IMCU admissions (Abstract). Clin Pharmacol Ther 1992; 53:214.
14. Dasta JF, Armstrong DK: Pharmacoeconomic impact of critically ill surgical patients. Drug Intell Clin Pharm 1988; 22:994–998.
15. Wilt JL, Johnson RF, Melby MS, et al: The cost effectiveness of a satellite pharmacy in the surgical intensive care unit (Abstract). Chest 1992; 102:192S.
16. Chernow B (Ed): The Pharmacologic Approach to the Critically Ill Patient. 3rd ed. Baltimore, Williams & Wilkins, 1994.
17. Dager WE, Albertson TE: Impact of therapeutic drug monitoring of intravenous theophylline regimens on serum theophylline concentrations in the medical intensive care unit. Ann Pharmacother 1992; 26:1287–1291.
18. Wragge T, Angaran D, Kilroy R: Evaluation of serum drug concentration ordering and appropriateness of subsequent actions in two intensive care units (Abstract). Crit Care Med 1993; 21:S179.
19. Watling SM, Dasta JF: Aminoglycoside dosing considerations in intensive care unit patients. Ann Pharmacother 1993; 27:351–357.
20. Whipple JK, Ausman RK, Franson R, et al: Effect of individualized pharmacokinetic dosing on patient outcome. Crit Care Med 1991; 19:1480–1485.
21. Crisp CB, Lane JR, Murray W: Audit of serum drug concentra-

tion analysis for patients in the surgical intensive care unit. Crit Care Med 1990; 18:734–737.
22. Task Force on Guidelines: Recommendations for services and personnel for delivery of care in a critical care setting. Crit Care Med 1989; 16:810–811.
23. Dasta JF: Computers in critical care: Opportunities and challenges. DICP Ann Pharmacother 1990; 24:1084–1092.
24. Quercia RA, Hills SW, Klimek JJ, et al: Bacteriologic contamination of intravenous infusion delivery systems in an intensive care unit. Am J Med 1986; 80:364–367.
25. Gonzalez ER, Sojka PA, Clapham CE, et al: Cost containment in the intensive care unit: Standardized regimens of dopamine and dobutamine. Parenterals 1988; 6:1–8.
26. Sulzbach LM, Munro BH: Survey of nursing practice related to decanting intravenous solutions. Heart Lung 1991; 20:624–630.
27. Hall K, Guay M, Armstrong G, et al: Development of an intravenous drug manual for a critical care satellite pharmacy. Can J Hosp Pharm 1982; 35:189–191.
28. Robinson DC, Cookson TL, Grisafe JA: Concentration guidelines for parenteral antibiotics in fluid-restricted patients. Drug Intell Clin Pharm 1987; 21:985–989.
29. Broyles JE, Brown RO, Vehe KL, et al: Pharmacist interventions improve fluid balance in fluid-restricted patients requiring parenteral nutrition. DICP Ann Pharmacother 1991; 25:119–122.
30. Ellinoy BR, Clarke JE, Wagers PW, et al: Comprehensive pharmaceutical services in a medical intensive-care unit. Am J Hosp Pharm 1984; 41:2335–2342.
31. Ferris NH, Crisp CB, Hoyt DB, et al: Analysis of workload and staffing requirements for a critical-care satellite pharmacy. Am J Hosp Pharm 1990; 47:2473–2478.
32. Hadbavny AM, Hoyt JW: Promotion of cost-effective benzodiazepine sedation (Letter to the editor). Am J Hosp Pharm 1993; 50:660–661.
33. Dobson K, Holt P, Falkowski M, et al: The establishment of a critical care pharmacy: A nursing perspective. Crit Care Nurs 1984; 4:20–22.
34. Blissenbach H: The justification of critical care pharmacy positions in hospitals. *In*: Practice of Critical Care Pharmacy. Majerus TC, Dasta JF (Eds). Rockville, MD, Aspen Systems Corp, 1985, pp 13–27.
35. Strand LM, Cipolle RJ, Morley PC: Documenting the clinical pharmacist's activities: Back to basics. Drug Intell Clin Pharm 1988; 22:63–67.
36. Hynniman CE: Drug product distribution systems and departmental operations. Am J Hosp Pharm 1991; 48:S24–S35.
37. Hawlins VA, Powell MF: Justification for a pediatric satellite pharmacy at a tertiary-care institution. Am J Hosp Pharm 1992; 49:2192–2197.
38. Stroup JW, Iglar AM: Implementation and financial analysis of an operating room satellite pharmacy. Am J Hosp Pharm 1992; 49:2198–2202.
39. Ullman HD, Rivalsky EJ, Oliver AM: Validating the need for a satellite pharmacy within a surgical intensive care unit (Abstract P-232E). Presented at the ASHP Midyear Clinical Meeting, Las Vegas, NV, December 1990.
40. McCulloch LM, Wong AF, Brethauer B: Cost impact of an intensive care nursery satellite pharmacy (Abstract P-571E). Presented at the ASHP Midyear Clinical Meeting, Orlando, FL, December 1992.
41. Dove KS, Nosal BL: Impact of a pharmacy satellite in a level I trauma center (Abstract P-320). Presented at the ASHP Midyear Clinical Meeting, Orlando, FL, December 1992.
42. Orynchak I, Hoying M, Powell MF: Evaluation of a critical care/OR satellite at a tertiary care institution (Abstract MCS-101). Presented at the ASHP Midyear Clinical Meeting, Orlando, FL, December 1992.
43. Miyagawa CI, Rivera JO: Effect of pharmacist interventions on drug therapy costs in a surgical intensive-care unit. Am J Hosp Pharm 1986; 43:3008–3013.
44. Katona BG, Ayd PR, Walters JK, et al: Effect of a pharmacist's and nurse's interventions on cost of drug therapy in a medical intensive-care unit. Am J Hosp Pharm 1989; 46:1179–1182.
44a. Montazeri M, Cook DJ: Impact of a clinical pharmacist in a multidisciplinary intensive care unit. Crit Care Med 1994; 22:1044–1048.
45. Ferris NH: Justification of a critical care satellite pharmacy. Calif J Hosp Pharm 1990; 2:35–37.
46. Tisdale JE: Justifying a pediatric critical-care pharmacy by medication-error reporting. Am J Hosp Pharm 1986; 43:368–371.
47. Caldwell RD, Tuck B: Justification and operation of a critical-care satellite pharmacy. Am J Hosp Pharm 1983; 40:2141–2145.
48. Bearce WC, Willey GA, Coleman LT: Documentation of clinical interactions: Quality of care issues and economic considerations in critical care pharmacy. Hosp Pharm 1988; 23:883–890.
49. Kelly WN, Meyer JD, Flatley CJ: Cost analysis of a satellite pharmacy. Am J Hosp Pharm 1986; 43:1927–1930.
49a. Chuang LC, Sutton JD, Henderson GT: Impact of a clinical pharmacist on cost saving and cost avoidance in drug therapy in an intensive care unit. Hosp Pharm 1994; 29:215–221.

CHAPTER 127

Drug Monitoring

Bertil K. J. Wagner, PharmD

Patients in the intensive care unit (ICU) receive more drugs than other hospitalized patients, and the ICU drug cost ranges from 15% to 40% of total hospital stay drug cost.[1] Adverse effects from drugs may be difficult to detect and have exaggerated consequences in unstable patients with multiple organ failure. Therefore, it is essential from a cost-effective and therapeutic standpoint that drug therapy be monitored carefully in the ICU and tailored to the patient's individual needs. Studies show that therapeutic drug monitoring (TDM) improves the therapeutic response and decreases the length of hospital stay, number of adverse reactions, and number of inappropriate serum drug concentrations in the general hospital patient population.[2, 3]

Only a few studies have examined the effects of TDM in the critical care population. TDM of aminoglycoside antibiotics in ICU patients has been shown to decrease patient mortality.[4, 5] Other studies indicated that TDM of theophylline in the ICU can decrease the number of adverse reactions and improve the likelihood that plasma theophylline concentrations will be in the therapeutic range.[6, 7] Patient survival in the ICU is not solely influenced by TDM, but an increasing body of literature suggests that individualized drug dosing may improve patient response and decrease drug toxicity for certain medications.

TDM focuses generally on maintaining serum drug concentrations in the therapeutic range. This range of concentrations between minimum effective and subtoxic concentrations is not absolute for all patients and may change in an individual patient over time as a result of concurrent disease and drug therapy. Serum drug concentration monitoring should be performed only with medications that show a consistent relationship between drug effect and concentration. An expanded focus of TDM includes pharmacodynamic (drug effect) monitoring of medications that exhibit variable dose-response or concentration-response relationships. Optimal results of TDM are achieved with a multidisciplinary group of healthcare professionals, including physicians, pharmacists, nurses, and medical technologists. This approach improves professional communication, team spirit, data gathering and analysis, and implementation of recommended changes as well as opportunities for related research.

PHARMACOKINETIC ANALYSIS

Pharmacokinetic drug monitoring uses the concept of the therapeutic range. The therapeutic range is the range of drug concentrations between minimum effective and minimum toxic concentrations. Approximately 20 drugs have established therapeutic ranges.[8] However, the ranges show significant inter- and intrapatient variability, and therapeutic ranges obtained in the general patient population may not apply to critically ill patients. The therapeutic range is, therefore, only a guide, the specific patient pharmacodynamic response is the primary endpoint. Frequent sampling of blood may be detrimental to the patient, and drug concentration data may not be necessary if pharmacodynamic data provide similar information. Drug concentrations should generally be obtained during early therapy to document concentration and response relationships or when dosing changes are planned because of suboptimal therapy or toxicity. Drug concentrations are also useful to determine compliance and to establish a diagnosis after overdoses.

To use pharmacokinetic forecasting methods and maximize the benefit of serum drug concentration monitoring, timing of drug samples is essential. Serum drug concentrations are obtained once steady-state conditions have been achieved. The time required to achieve greater than 90% of the pharmacokinetic steady state, when the rate of drug input is equal to the rate of drug elimination, is at least 3.5 elimination half-lives. Drug concentration samples should be obtained 2 to 4 hours after the administration (peak) of rapid-release medications, immediately before the next dose (trough) for slow-release or anticonvulsant and antiarrhythmic medications, and at any time after steady state has been attained during a constant-rate intravenous infusion. Distributional characteristics of drugs also need to be considered. Serum samples for drugs should be obtained after distribution between plasma and tissues has taken place to avoid misinterpretation of increased predistributional serum concentrations. Alternatively, plasma concentrations of many drugs a few hours after hemodialysis are low because of slow redistribution from tissues and should, therefore, not be used for dosage predictions.[9]

Several factors may adversely influence drug assay results. Active metabolites and endogenous substances may cross-react with the parent compound, producing falsely elevated measured concentrations. The clinician may, therefore, lower the dose when, in reality, no change in volume of distribution or drug clearance exists. Resultant inadequate therapy may, therefore, ensue. Most laboratories use automated enzyme multiplied immunoassay techniques and fluorescence immunoassays, or fluorescence polarization immunoassay (FPIA), instead of the older and more time-consuming methods, such as gas-liquid chromatography, high-performance liquid chromatography (HPLC), radioimmunoassay (RIA), and bioassays. RIAs are extremely sensitive, but their clinical usefulness is limited by poor specificity and precision, expensive equipment, and concerns over the disposal of radioactive wastes. The HPLC assays are useful in the analysis of drugs with active metabolites that may cross-react with the parent compound if other assays are used. The immunoassays determine the amount of drug in the serum by antibody displacement reactions and are used in hospital, commercial, and office laboratories to assay aminoglycoside, anticonvulsant, chloramphenicol, digoxin, tricyclic antidepressant, antiarrhythmic, and theophylline serum concentrations. More recently, extremely rapid, disposable enzyme immunochromatography methods that use finger-stick blood samples have been developed for monitoring of theophylline and anticonvulsant medications.[10, 11]

Dosing nomograms are generally useful to estimate initial drug dosing but usually perform poorly in comparison to individualized pharmacokinetic monitoring. The majority of dosing nomograms do not use a critical care data base and may lead to erroneous dosing because both the pharmacokinetic and pharmacodynamic differences of these patients are ignored. Bayesian forecasting, a method in which population data are combined with individualized pharmacokinetic or dynamic parameters, offers significant improvement of drug dosing,[12a] even during non–steady-state conditions, but requires use of powerful computers.[12–13]

ANTIMICROBIALS

Antibiotics and antifungals are the most commonly used drugs in the critical care setting and are also the most likely to produce significant adverse effects.[1, 14] Optimal dosing of aminoglycosides improves patient survival.[4, 5] Antimicrobial pharmacokinetics are often drastically altered in critically ill patients.[15, 16] Monitoring of antimicrobial therapy is, therefore, paramount to optimize patient care. Pharmacodynamic factors, such as minimum inhibitory concentration (MIC) and serum bactericidal concentrations, and synergistic or antagonistic drug combinations should also be considered for antibiotic selection in prophylaxis or treatment of established infections.

High peak-dose concentrations of gentamicin and tobramycin in the range of 5 to 10 μg/mL produce an optimum response.[17] This translates into a desirable peak-dose concentration of 20 to 40 μg/mL for amikacin. Early achievement of gentamicin therapeutic concentrations increases the cure rate in patients with sepsis, pneumonia, wound, and urinary tract infections.[18] However, renal toxicity may occur in up to 25% of patients and is more common with gentamicin and amikacin peak levels of greater than 10 and 38.5 μg/mL, respectively, as well as with increased trough levels (>2 or 8 μg/mL, respectively). Other predisposing factors for renal toxicity are prolonged therapy (>11 days), use of diuretics and nephrotoxic agents, increased initial serum creatinine, female gender, liver disease, old age, shock, and congestive heart failure (CHF).[19–21] Risk factors for ototoxicity are the same as for renal toxicity.[22] Aminoglycoside-induced ototoxicity is not reversible, is usually difficult to detect, and occurs in 2% to 10% of patients receiving aminoglycosides.

Published nomograms of aminoglycoside dosing are generally of little use in critically ill patients and may predispose the patient to toxicity or suboptimal dosing.[23, 24] Individualized dosing with peak and trough serum drug concentrations should be used to maximize efficacy and minimize toxicity. Aminoglycoside concentrations can be obtained in all patients; however, aminoglycosides are inactivated *in vitro* by semisynthetic penicillins, and samples that contain high concentrations of these drugs should be placed on ice and analyzed immediately or frozen before analysis.[25] Besides optimization of serum drug concentrations, the clinician should avoid factors that increase the risk for nephrotoxicity and monitor for changes in renal function. However, serum creatinine concentrations are affected by many drugs and diseases, and the levels do not increase until after renal damage has occurred.[26]

The need for vancomycin serum concentration monitoring is controversial. The individualized aminoglycoside model more accurately predicts peak and trough concentrations than published nomograms.[27, 28] However, the relationship between drug concentrations and efficacy or toxicity has not been well-defined. Serum vancomycin concentration monitoring is most useful in patients who exhibit decreased renal function, receive concurrent nephrotoxic drugs, or suffer from life-threatening methicillin-resistant staphylococcal or enterococcal sepsis. Peak concentrations of 20 to 40 μg/mL and trough concentrations of 5 to 10 μg/mL are generally sufficient, and serum drug concentrations should not be obtained more frequently than once weekly.

Integration of pharmacokinetics with MIC data results in optimal dosing of other antibiotics. The time of plasma concentrations of β-lactam antibiotics above the MIC correlates best with eradication of gram-negative bacteria.[29, 30] Serum bactericidal titers have been shown to be useful in patients with endocarditis or immunocompromised states.[31] The postantibiotic effect[32] of the aminoglycosides and vancomycin for gram-negative and gram-positive organisms, respectively, would allow use of lower and less toxic trough concentrations. Synergistic combinations of antibiotics (combinations of β-lactamase antibiotics with aminoglycosides, fluoroquinolones, or β-lactamase inhibitors) are useful to treat less susceptible organisms, prevent resistance, and decrease drug-induced toxicity.[33]

Amphotericin B, a nephrotoxic antifungal agent, is often used in patients who receive concurrent aminoglycoside or vancomycin therapy. The risk for amphotericin B–induced nephrotoxicity with potassium and magnesium wasting is decreased by administering sodium supplements, avoiding dehydration, and limiting the cumulative dose to less than 4 to 5 g.[34] Although some clinicians advocate the use of alternate-day amphotericin B dosing to decrease nephrotoxicity, little evidence supports this practice. Monitoring for amphotericin-induced nephrotoxicity includes serum concentrations of creatinine, magnesium, and potassium.

ANTICOAGULANTS

Warfarin inhibits vitamin K epoxide reductase and the regeneration of vitamin KH_2 in the liver, which is a cofactor for the carboxylation (activation) of Factors II, VII, IX, and X and proteins C and S. The onset of full anticoagulant effect is delayed by 3 to 4 days because of the long half-life (>24 hours) of Factors II, IX, and X. Initial depletion of the natural anticoagulant proteins C and S may predispose the patient to embolization. Therefore, heparin is usually given concurrently during early warfarin therapy to prevent the formation of emboli. Heparin binds to antithrombin III and catalyzes the inactivation of Factors IXa, Xa, XIa, XIIa, kallikrein, and thrombin.[35]

The prothrombin time (PT) is sensitive to decreases in Factors II, VII, and X and is used to measure warfarin anticoagulation. The test is performed by adding calcium and thromboplastin to citrated plasma. Because commercial thromboplastins have different sensitivities to the reduction of vitamin K–dependent factors, variable PT ratios (patient-laboratory control value) may be reported for the same level of anticoagulation. The international normalized ratios (INRs) standardize the PT ratios according to the World Health Organization's reference thromboplastin and should be used to monitor warfarin anticoagulant response:

$$\text{INR} = (\text{observed PT ratio})^{\text{ISI}}$$

where ISI is the international sensitivity index based on the type of thromboplastin used.[36] The recommended INRs are listed in Table 127–1. The INR should be monitored daily until it has stabilized over a 2- to 3-day period. Abnormal responses should be investigated for drug interactions, altered vitamin K intake, concurrent disease states, and, rarely, genetic warfarin resistance.[37]

The activated partial thromboplastin time (APTT) is sensitive to the inhibition of Factors IIa, IXa, and Xa and is the standard parameter of heparin anticoagulation monitoring. Prolongation of the APTT versus laboratory control of one and one half to two and one half times provides adequate anticoagulation and minimizes the risk for bleeding. The APTT should be measured before and 6 hours after the initiation of the heparin infusion, with subsequent measurements taken once daily. Therapeutic drug monitoring using APTT is described in Table 127–2. The rapidly performed activated clotting time (ACT) test is used during cardiac surgery. The ACT shows a linear relationship to heparin doses up to 400 seconds. The therapeutic range of ACT is 150 to 190 seconds or 400 to 600 seconds for patients receiving extracorporeal circulation.[38, 39]

The primary adverse effect of warfarin and heparin is bleeding, which can be reversed with fresh frozen plasma, factor concentrates, vitamin K (warfarin), and protamine (heparin). Elderly patients, those with comorbid conditions, and those who receive more intensive anticoagulation are at greater risk for major bleeding episodes when receiving warfarin or heparin.[40] Small intravenous doses of vitamin K (0.5–1.0 mg) after a warfarin overdose may be advantageous in patients who need to be restarted on warfarin.[41] Heparin may cause a bimodal incidence of thrombocytopenia, requiring monitoring of the platelet count every 2 to 3 days. The early thrombocytopenia occurs within 2 to 4 days and reverses with continued heparin treatment. The delayed thrombocytopenia, an autoimmune reaction, occurs after 7

TABLE 127–1. Recommended INR for Warfarin Therapy

	Minimum Effective INR	*Recommended INR*
Prevention of subclavian venous thrombosis	1.2	N/A
Prevention of deep venous thrombosis	1.5–2.5	2.0–3.0
Treatment of deep venous thrombosis	2.0–2.5	2.0–3.0
Acute myocardial infarction (MI)		
Prevention of stroke	2.0	2.0–3.0
Prevention of recurrent MI	2.7–4.5	3.0–4.5
Reduction of mortality	2.7–4.5	3.0–4.5
Peripheral arterial disease		
Prevention of death	2.6–4.5	N/A
Atrial fibrillation		
Prevention of systemic thromboembolism	2.0–3.0	2.0–3.0
Cardiac valve replacement		
Tissue valves	2.0–2.25	2.0–3.0
Mechanical valves	1.9–3.6	2.5–3.5

(Used with permission from Hirsh J, Dalen DE, Deykin D, et al: Oral anticoagulants. Chest 1992; 102:312S.)

Abbreviations: INR = international normalized ratio; N/A = not applicable.

TABLE 127–2. Therapeutic Monitoring of Heparin Anticoagulation Using Activated Partial Thromboplastin Time (APTT)*

Measurement Result	*Intervention*
APTT 1.0–1.2 × control	Loading dose of 25–50 U/kg and increase infusion by 200 U/h (3–4 U · kg^{-1} · h^{-1})
APTT 1.2–1.3 × control	Loading dose of 15–25 U/kg and increase infusion by 100 U/h (1–2 U · kg^{-1} · h^{-1})
APTT 1.3–1.5 × control	Increase infusion by 100 U/h (1–2 U · kg^{-1} · h^{-1})
APTT 1.5–2.0 × control	No change necessary
APTT 2.0–2.5 × control	Decrease infusion by 100 U/h (1–2 U · kg^{-1} · h^{-1})
APTT 2.5–3.5 × control	Stop infusion for 1–2 hours and decrease infusion by 200 U/h (3–4 U · kg^{-1} · h^{-1})
APTT >3.5 × control	Stop infusion for 2–4 hours and decrease infusion by 300 U/h (4–5 U · kg^{-1} · h^{-1})

(Data compiled from Carter BL: Therapy of acute thromboembolism with heparin and warfarin. Clin Pharm 1991; 10:503.)

*The APTT should be determined within 6 to 8 hours after changing the heparin infusion.

TABLE 127–3. Drug Interactions That Alter Warfarin Drug Action

Pharmacokinetic	*Pharmacodynamic*	*Mechanism Unknown*
Prolonges Prothrombin Time	*Prolongs Prothrombin Time*	*Prolongs Prothrombin Time*
Decreased clearance of warfarin	Blocks vitamin K regeneration	Relationship clearly established
Phenylbutazone*	2nd- and 3rd-generation cephalosporins	Erythromycin
Metronidazole*	Other mechanisms	Anabolic steroids
Sulfa antibiotics*	Clofibrate	Relationship less clearly established
Disulfiram*	Inhibition of blood coagulation	Ketoconazole
Cimetidine†	Heparin	Fluconazole
Omeprazole†	Increased factor metabolism	Isoniazid
Amiodarone*†	Thyroid hormones	Piroxicam
		Tamoxifen
		Quinidine
		Vitamin E (megadose)
		Phenytoin
		Fluoroquinolones
Reduces Prothrombin Time	*Inhibits Platelet Function*	*Reduces Prothrombin Time*
Reduced warfarin absorption	Aspirin	Penicillins
Cholestyramine	Other NSAIDs	Griseofulvin
Increased clearance of warfarin	Ticlopidine	
Barbiturates	Moxalactam	
Rifampin	Carbenicillin and high doses of other penicillins	
Griseofulvin		
Carbamazepine		

(Adapted from Hirsh J: Oral anticoagulant drugs. N Engl J Med 1991; 324:1865, by permission of the New England Journal of Medicine.)
*Decreased clearance of S isomer.
†Decreased clearance of R isomer.
Abbreviation: NSAIDs = nonsteroidal anti-inflammatory drugs.

to 10 days in less than 5% of patients but requires discontinuation of the drug.[42, 43] Warfarin, a strongly protein-bound (>97%) and hepatically metabolized agent, is susceptible to many drug interactions. Table 127–3 lists drug interactions with warfarin. Drugs that inhibit platelet function will enhance the anticoagulant action of heparin.[44]

ANTICONVULSANTS

Phenytoin, valproic acid, and phenobarbital are used in the prevention and treatment of generalized and focal seizures in the ICU. Table 127–4 lists the therapeutic concentration ranges and adverse effects for these agents. Phenytoin undergoes zero-order (saturable) hepatic elimination and is a low hepatic extraction ratio drug. The drug is 90% bound to albumin, and decreases in protein binding in hypoalbuminemia, renal failure, and jaundice, and following displacement reactions with other drugs can significantly increase drug clearance with resultant decreases in total but not free drug concentrations. The total phenytoin concentration is usually a good indicator of clinical response, but free serum phenytoin concentrations show a better correlation with clinical response in patients with altered serum protein binding.[45] Therefore, free serum drug concentrations should be measured when the potential for altered protein binding exists. Alternatively, the total phenytoin concentration corrected for protein binding can be estimated:

$$\text{C normal binding} = \frac{\text{C observed}}{(\delta \cdot \text{albumin}) + 0.1}$$

where C normal binding is the phenytoin concentration observed if protein binding is normal, C observed is the measured total phenytoin concentration, albumin is the albumin concentration (grams per deciliter), and δ is the adjustment factor for protein binding (0.2 in normal patients, 0.1 in uremic patients).

Although the bioavailability of high-quality preparations approaches 100%, changes in dosage form or brand should be avoided to prevent the risk of subtherapeutic effect or toxicity. Phenytoin absorption is significantly decreased by enteral feedings, and the intravenous route is preferred in these patients. When using the oral suspension or parenteral phenytoin sodium, the daily dose should be split into two or three doses to avoid peak concentration toxicity. Pheny-

TABLE 127–4. Therapeutic Ranges and Adverse Effects of Anticonvulsant Agents

Agent	*Therapeutic Range*	*Adverse Effects*
Phenytoin	Total: 10–20 μg/mL Free: 1–2 μg/mL	Far-lateral nystagmus or seizures (>20 μg/mL total concentration) Ataxia (>30 μg/mL total concentration) Altered mental status (>40 μg/mL total concentration)
Valproic acid	Total: 40–100 μg/mL Free: 3–10 μg/mL	Gastrointestinal complaints (tolerance observed with continued use) Transient elevation of LFTs in 40% of patients Dose-dependent weight gain (>4 kg) in 50% of patients Hepatotoxicity in 0.01% of patients (mostly in children <2 years old) Tremor, confusion (≥80 μg/mL total concentration)
Phenobarbital	Total: 10–25 μg/mL	Sedation and ataxia (35–80 μg/mL) Coma with intact reflexes (65–117 μg/mL) Coma without DTR (>100 μg/mL)

Abbreviations: LFT = liver function tests; DTR = deep tendon reflexes.

toin trough serum concentrations should be measured approximately 24 hours after a loading dose and once every 5 to 10 days thereafter until the patient has been stabilized. Phenytoin oral and intravenous loading doses can be estimated by the following equation:

$$\text{Dose (mg/kg)} = 0.7\ \text{L/kg} \cdot (\text{C desired} - \text{C observed})$$

The phenytoin maintenance dose is usually estimated by the Michaelis-Menten equation:

$$\text{Dose (mg/d)} = \frac{\text{Vmax} \cdot \text{Css}}{\text{S} \cdot \text{F} \cdot (\text{Km} + \text{Css})}$$

where Vmax is the maximum rate of metabolism, Css is the steady-state concentration, S is the sodium salt form factor (0.92), F is the bioavailability (0.95 for oral preparations), Km is a constant equal to the plasma concentration at which the rate of metabolism is 50% of Vmax, Vmax is 7 $\text{mg} \cdot \text{kg}^{-1} \cdot \text{d}^{-1}$ and Km is 4 mg/L.[46] These values have been shown to be different in head trauma patients (Vmax is 17.5 $\text{mg} \cdot \text{kg}^{-1} \cdot \text{d}^{-1}$, Km is 4.8 mg/L).[47] Vmax and Km can be estimated and adjusted from clinical data. A simpler, more conservative method can also be used:[48]

$$\text{New dose} = \text{current dose} \cdot \text{Css (desired)}^{0.2} \cdot \text{Css (achieved)}^{-0.2}$$

Valproic acid has a relatively short half-life (9–18 hours) and is administered several times daily. Longer dosing intervals with higher doses may be equally effective but increase the risk for gastrointestinal side effects. Unlike the other anticonvulsants, valproic acid decreases hepatic enzyme drug metabolizing capacity, and the dose of other anticonvulsants may need to be reduced during polytherapy. Valproic acid is a low-extraction ratio drug that also exhibits dose-dependent protein binding with resultant wide fluctuations in both total and free drug concentrations. Serum drug concentrations may also vary significantly if different oral preparations are used. Peak plasma concentrations are usually reached after 3 to 8 hours with the enteric-coated preparation and within 2 hours with other oral dosage forms. Valproic acid trough concentrations should be obtained every 2 to 3 days after the initial loading dose until the patient is stable.[49]

Phenobarbital undergoes rapid and complete absorption from oral and intramuscular sites. The drug is 50% bound to albumin, and an increased therapeutic effect or risk for toxicity is expected in patients with severe hypoalbuminemia. Phenobarbital is metabolized by the liver and induces hepatic enzyme metabolism of other drugs. The renal clearance accounts for 40% of total clearance and is increased 5- to 10-fold with urinary alkalinization.[50] Phenobarbital exhibits a linear dose-concentration relationship, making dosage adjustments easy. The drug has a very long half-life (96 hours), and frequent sampling for serum concentrations is useful only in patients in whom toxicity or inadequate therapy is suspected.

CARDIOVASCULAR AGENTS

Antiarrhythmics

TDM of antiarrhythmic agents is complicated by variable concentration-effect relationships, changing drug pharmacokinetics, and variable treatment endpoints. Drug selection is often based on adverse-effect profiles of individual drugs that can range from mild gastrointestinal discomfort to proarrhythmia and death. In general, patients with complicated, preexisting, sustained ventricular arrhythmias and left ventricular dysfunction appear to be most at risk for drug-induced arrhythmias.[51, 52] Class Ia, Ic, and III agents and certain antidepressants and neuroleptic drugs prolong both QRS and QT_c and can, in addition to low potassium, magnesium, and calcium levels, cause torsades de pointes.[53] QT prolongation is also a risk factor for sudden death.[54] Drug combinations that increase the risk for torsades de pointes should be avoided and underlying electrolyte abnormalities corrected, especially in the high-risk, critically ill population. Prolongation of the QT_c interval greater than 0.6 seconds (normal <0.45 seconds) during antiarrhythmic therapy without control of arrhythmia warrants a trial with another agent. Assessment of antiarrhythmic therapy includes long-term electrocardiogram (ECG) monitoring, exercise testing, electrophysiologic-pharmacologic testing, and drug concentrations. Table 127–5 lists the therapeutic concentration ranges of commonly used antiarrhythmics and the relationship between serum concentrations and adverse effects.

Quinidine and Procainamide

Quinidine and procainamide are class Ia antiarrhythmics and are used extensively for both ventricular and supraventricular arrhythmias. Quinidine is strongly bound to both albumin and α_1–acid glycoprotein; protein binding is decreased in liver disease and increased after trauma and surgery and during myocardial infarction due to increases in α_1-acid/glycoprotein levels. Because quinidine is a high-extraction ratio drug, changes in plasma protein binding directly alter free drug concentrations, and drug toxicity would most likely occur in patients with poor hepatic blood flow and decreased protein binding. Increased oral bioavailability resulting from decreased first-pass metabolism would also be expected in heart failure patients. Quinidine

TABLE 127–5. Therapeutic Ranges and Adverse Effects of Antiarrhythmic Agents

Agent	*Therapeutic Range*	*Adverse Effects*
Quinidine	2–5 μg/mL	12% of patients with myocardial toxicity at Q = 6–8 μg/mL Q >10 μg/mL increases risk for toxicity to >30%
Procainamide NAPA	4–12 μg/mL 10–30 μg/mL	27% of patients with minor toxicity (GI disturbances, 10–30% prolongation of PR, QRS, and QT interval) at PA = 12.1–16.0 μg/mL 16% of patients with serious toxicity (hypotension, >30% prolongation of PR, QRS, and QT intervals) at PA = 12.1–16 μg/mL PA >16.0 μg/mL increased incidence of minor and serious toxicity to 62% and 35%, respectively Risk for toxicity is increased with PA + NAPA >25 μg/mL
Lidocaine	Total: 3–6 μg/mL Free: 0.5–2.0 μg/mL	Drowsiness, dizziness, paresthesias, and euphoria at L = 3–6 μg/mL Fasciculations, visual disturbances, and tinnitus at L = 6–8 μg/mL Seizures and obtundation at L >8 μg/mL

Abbreviations: Q = quinidine; PA = procainamide; NAPA = *N*-acetyl procainamide; GI = gastrointestinal; L = lidocaine.

is metabolized to several active metabolites of which 3-OH quinidine is the most important.[55]

Procainamide is 50% renally eliminated; the remainder is metabolized to active *N*-acetyl procainamide (NAPA), which is 85% renally eliminated.[56] Procainamide is only 15% bound to albumin, and clearance and plasma concentrations are not altered by protein-binding changes. Liver, renal, and cardiac insufficiency decrease procainamide clearance. Procainamide concentrations should be obtained in patients with these conditions, and dosing should be adjusted accordingly. Treatment of certain ventricular arrhythmias may require procainamide serum concentrations greater than 10 μg/mL. The significance of NAPA as a contributor to antiarrhythmic activity and drug-induced torsades de pointes is controversial, and NAPA concentrations should be obtained only in patients with renal insufficiency or in patients who show signs of drug toxicity.

Lidocaine

Lidocaine (class Ib) is frequently chosen in the treatment of ventricular arrhythmias because of its low incidence of hemodynamic complications. However, the drug has a narrow therapeutic concentration range and clinically important central nervous system toxicity. Lidocaine is a high-extraction ratio drug, and its clearance is dependent on cardiac function and hepatic blood flow. Approximately 70% of lidocaine is bound to albumin and α_1–acid glycoprotein, and drug toxicity is correlated with increasing amounts of total and free drug. Lidocaine protein binding is decreased in patients with hypoalbuminemia and is increased after myocardial infarction. The renally eliminated metabolites monoethylglycinexylidide and glycinexylidide possess 80% to 90% and 10% to 26%, respectively, of the antiarrhythmic potency of lidocaine but have not been correlated to adverse events during lidocaine therapy. Lidocaine clearance is decreased by CHF and other low-flow states and liver disease.[57] Monitoring of lidocaine toxicity is difficult because of the initial subtle signs of toxicity and the significant number of patients who may require lidocaine concentrations greater than 6 μg/mL for arrhythmia control.

Digoxin

Digoxin is currently used in the control of supraventricular arrhythmias and severe CHF. Therapy with digoxin should be monitored carefully because the agent is known to cause practically any type of arrhythmia but primarily atrioventricular (AV) junctional tachycardia. The absorption of digoxin is dependent on the preparation used, with tablets being the least (70–80%) and the liquid-filled capsules the most (90–100%) bioavailable. Digoxin is primarily renally excreted, and the dose can be adjusted during renal insufficiency using the following formula:

$$\text{Maintenance dose} = \frac{\text{Cl digoxin} \cdot \text{Css} \cdot \tau}{\text{F}}$$

where Cl digoxin is digoxin clearance (liters per day), Css is steady-state concentration (nanogram per milliliter), τ is dosing interval (days), and F is bioavailability (ranging from 0.7 for tablets to 0.9 for liquid-filled capsules). The digoxin clearance can be estimated by using the patient's creatinine clearance (Cl_{cr}):

$$\text{Cl digoxin} = 1.02(Cl_{cr}) + 57 \text{ mL/min (CHF not present)}$$
$$\text{Cl digoxin} = 0.88(Cl_{cr} + 23 \text{ mL/min (CHF present)}$$

The currently accepted therapeutic range of digoxin is 0.8 to 2.0 ng/mL, but treatment of atrial fibrillation may require concentrations of 1.6 ng/mL or greater. The risk for digoxin toxicity is increased by hypokalemia, hypercalcemia, hypothyroidism, and drug interactions (quinidine, verapamil, and spironolactone). Nonspecific ECG changes (ST depression, T wave abnormalities, and QT shortening) do not correlate with drug effects. Serum digoxin concentration monitoring is further complicated by RIA interference by digoxin-like immunoreactive substance (DLIS), an endogenous compound, which produces falsely elevated serum digoxin concentrations in neonates and patients with liver or renal impairment.[58] The FPIA is less influenced by DLIS and is preferred when the presence of DLIS is suspected.[59] The response to digoxin therapy is best evaluated by improvement in the patient's clinical status or reversal of the arrhythmia. Patients with atrial fibrillation not controlled with digoxin despite "adequate" serum concentrations may benefit from the addition of another AV node suppressant medication, such as a β-adrenergic or calcium channel blocking agent.

Calcium Channel and β-Blocking Agents

Calcium channel and β-blocking agents are often used to control supraventricular arrhythmias. Verapamil and diltiazem are given as single-bolus doses or continuous infusions. Hypotension is the most common adverse effect with these agents but can be prevented with intravenous administration of calcium.[60] Most of the β-blockers (propranolol, metoprolol, atenolol, labetalol) used in the ICU block the sinoatrial and AV node for up to several hours as a result of nonlinearity of the plasma concentration-response relationship.[61] Continuous infusions of esmolol, an ultra short-acting β-blocker, have become popular because of easier modulation of drug effect. However, like all β- and calcium channel blocking agents, esmolol can cause profound hypotension in patients with limited cardiovascular reserve capacity and in patients who are dehydrated. Close monitoring of heart rate and blood pressure is warranted when these agents are used.

Antihypertensives

Severely injured patients often present with hyperadrenergic crisis, manifested by persistent systemic hypertension and tachycardia. Because of the loss of cerebral autoregulation, cerebral edema and increased intracranial pressure may occur.[62] The use of vasodilators in these patients requires careful monitoring of intracranial pressure as well as systemic blood pressure. Hydralazine, nitroprusside, and nitroglycerin decrease mean arterial pressure and cerebral perfusion pressure but increase intracranial pressure secondary to an increase in cerebral blood volume. Beta-blocking agents do not increase intracranial pressure.[63]

The metabolism of nitroprusside may lead to life-threatening cyanide or thiocyanate toxicity in patients with end-organ dysfunction.[64] Most cyanide from nitroprusside reacts with thiosulfate to form renally eliminated thiocyanate. Normal hepatic clearance of cyanide by conversion to thiocyanate corresponds to a nitroprusside infusion of less than 2 $\mu g \cdot kg^{-1} \cdot min^{-1}$. Unmetabolized cyanide binds to cytochrome oxidase and blocks cellular respiration. Nitroprusside infusions in excess of 4 $\mu g \cdot kg^{-1} \cdot min^{-1}$ can produce toxic cyanide levels in 5 to 10 hours. The acute clinical manifestations of cyanide toxicity can range from headache, dizziness, tachypnea, and tachycardia to apnea, convulsions, and lactic acidosis. Patients with renal insufficiency are also at risk for the development of thiocyanate toxicity, which may manifest as confusion, hyperreflexia, hallucinations, convulsions, coma, and death. Nitroprusside should be dosed carefully in patients with hepatic dysfunction, and prolonged infusions exceeding 2 $\mu g \cdot kg^{-1} \cdot min^{-1}$ should be

TABLE 127–6. Hemodynamic Effects of Catecholamines

Drug	*Dose* ($\mu g \cdot kg^{-1} \cdot min^{-1}$)	*Predominant Receptor Activity*	*Effect*
Dopamine	1–3	Dopaminergic	Diuresis
	2.5–6	Beta	Increased CO and vasodilation
	>6	Alpha	Vasoconstriction
Epinephrine	<0.03	Beta	Increased CO and vasodilation
	0.03–0.15	Beta and alpha	Mixed
	>0.15	Alpha	Vasoconstriction
Norepinephrine	0.01–0.05	Beta and alpha	Mixed
	>0.05	Alpha	Vasoconstriction
Isoproterenol	0.02–0.1	Beta	Increased CO and vasodilation
Dobutamine	5–15	Beta	Increased CO and vasodilation
Phenylephrine	0.2–0.9	Alpha	Vasoconstriction

Abbreviation: CO = cardiac output.

avoided. Serum thiocyanate concentrations should be measured in patients who receive nitroprusside infusions at rates exceeding 10 $\mu g \cdot kg^{-1} \cdot min^{-1}$ for more than 48 hours or who have renal insufficiency.

Vasopressor and Inotropic Agents

Dopamine, epinephrine, and norepinephrine are the only naturally occurring catecholamines used in the ICU. Isoproterenol, dobutamine, and phenylephrine are synthetic catecholamines with special pharmacologic properties. The effects of catecholamines are mediated by β- and α-adrenergic and dopaminergic (DA) receptors. Both β_1 and β_2 receptors increase cardiac inotropy and vasodilation. Stimulation of β_2 receptors promotes peripheral vasodilation, glycogenolysis, and hypokalemia, whereas α_1 and α_2 receptor stimulation causes vasoconstriction and vasodilation, respectively. Other effects mediated by α receptors include glycogenolysis and decreased insulin secretion. DA receptors increase coronary, renal, and mesenteric blood flow.[65] The synthetic catecholamine inotropes, isoproterenol and dobutamine, stimulate both β_1 and β_2 receptors. Although both agents will increase cardiac output, isoproterenol is more potent and will greatly increase heart rate, myocardial oxygen consumption, and the potential for arrhythmias. Phenylephrine is an α-adrenergic agonist with predominant pressor activity and low potential for cardiac stimulation and arrhythmias. The hemodynamic effects of the catecholamines are shown in Table 127–6. Selection and monitoring of catecholamines are dependent on the hemodynamic effects desired and the potential for arrhythmias and renal insufficiency. Low-dose dopamine plays a particular role in maintaining renal perfusion if used together with α-adrenergic vasopressor agents.[66]

Amrinone, milrinone, and related agents produce inotropy and vasodilation independently of β receptor activity by blocking the phosphodiesterase F-III enzyme, which degrades cyclic adenosene monophosphate. Phosphodiesterase inhibitors are hepatically cleared, and the half-life of amrinone is significantly increased in patients with congestive heart failure and in those who exhibit slow acetylator phenotype status. After an intravenous bolus dose, a maximum hemodynamic effect is seen within 10 minutes, and a continuous infusion is needed to prolong the effect beyond 60 to 90 minutes. Amrinone may cause excessive hypotension in fluid-depleted patients, and short-term intravenous administration has been associated with a 2.4% incidence of dose-related, reversible thrombocytopenia and an incidence of elevated hepatic enzyme levels of less than 2%.[67] Milrinone use has not been associated with changes in platelet count or hepatic enzyme levels.[68] Many approaches to monitoring and optimization of vasoactive therapy have been proposed.[66a] Much controversy surrounds the methods and goals of inotropic therapy optimization.[66b] However, therapy should be adjusted individually for each patient in order to optimize tissue perfusion without causing undue risk to the patient. The selection of multiple hemodynamic and laboratory monitoring parameters to achieve this goal is recommended.

SEDATIVES

Sedatives, hypnotics, and anxiolytics are used to provide sedation, sleep, and adjunct pain control. These potent drugs require specialized monitoring to avoid oversedation and cardiorespiratory depression. Decreased metabolic clearance pathways often prolong drug action, and the presence of long-acting, active metabolites further complicates patient management.[69] Misconception of drug action further confuses the treatment approach.[70] Limited trials with short-acting agents show improved sedation control and a decreased risk of adverse events.[71, 72]

The level of sedation is dependent on several factors. Concurrent illness, lack of communication, invasive catheters, noise, interruption of day-night cycles, and drugs promote agitated behavior. Monitoring of sedation is complicated by a lack of well-defined objective parameters. Several subjective rating scales for clinical assessment of sedation have been developed. However, these methods require patient cooperation and cannot be used in paralyzed or otherwise immobile patients. Indirect measurements of blood pressure and heart rate may also be influenced by concurrent illness. Electroencephalogram (EEG) monitoring is a promising development, but the equipment is expensive and requires

TABLE 127–7. Factors That Affect Neuromuscular Blockade

Drugs	*Disease States*
Factors Increasing Neuromuscular Blockade	
Calcium channel blockers	Hypermagnesemia
Procainamide	Myasthenia gravis
Quinidine	Muscular dystrophies
Antibiotics	Myopathies
Steroids	Neuropathies
Dantrolene	Acidosis
Local anesthetics	Renal disease
Lithium	Hepatic disease
Trimethaphan	Hypothermia
Factors Decreasing Neuromuscular Blockade	
Azathioprine	Alkalosis
Furosemide	Burns
Phenytoin	
Calcium	

technical expertise, and EEG distribution patterns vary with medications or concurrent disease states.[73]

PARALYTIC AGENTS

Neuromuscular blocking agents are used in critically ill patients to facilitate respiratory management; to reduce skeletal muscle activity and oxygen consumption during tetanus, status epilepticus, and severe shivering; and to decrease the potential for injury in patients with uncontrolled agitation and hyperactivity. Prolonged skeletal muscle blockade is primarily accomplished with continuous intravenous infusions of the nondepolarizing agents pancuronium, vecuronium, and atracurium. Both pancuronium and vecuronium have active metabolites that have been implicated in cases of prolonged paralysis.[74, 75] Laudanosine, the metabolite of atracurium, produces seizures in dogs and can accumulate in patients with biliary obstruction or cirrhosis.[76] Therefore, patients with head trauma, uremia, cerebral hypoxia, or hepatic dysfunction who receive large or prolonged infusions of atracurium should receive EEG monitoring.[77, 78] Other potential complications of neuromuscular blockade are muscle weakness and development of decubitus ulcers and infections.[79] Patients who receive paralytics can also become profoundly agitated and require concurrent sedative and anxiolytic therapy.

Many drugs and disease states alter the paralytic response to neuromuscular blocking agents (Table 127–7). Monitoring for paralysis is often accomplished by using clinical signs, such as voluntary movements (opening of eyes, swallowing, head lift) and respiratory parameters (negative inspiratory force, vital capacity). However, these parameters may be inappropriate in unconscious patients or in patients who receive large doses of medications with respiratory depressant properties. Peripheral nerve stimulation is a more applicable and accurate method of estimating neuromuscular blockade. It can be performed using electromyography (most sensitive) or stimulation with visualization (least sensitive) of muscle twitches. The train-of-four (TOF) is the most commonly used estimate of neuromuscular blockade. The test consists of four impulses 0.5 seconds apart applied to the ulnar nerve with measurement of the response (adduction of thumb). The posterior tibial nerve (plantar flexion of the foot), lateral popliteal nerve (dorsiflexion of the foot), and facial nerve (facial and orbicularis oculi muscle contraction) can also be used. The number of twitches indicates the degree of paralysis (0 = 100% blockade, 1 = 90% blockade, 2 = 80% blockade, 3 = 75% blockade, 4 = <75% blockade). Clinical paralysis is achieved at 80% to 90% blockade, and a patient can safely be extubated at less than 50% blockade. The TOF cannot adequately define blockade less than 75%, and clinical signs (head lift >5 seconds, open eyes widely, cough effectively, and generate a negative inspiratory force >20 cm H_2O) should be used in conjunction with an overall assessment of the patient's status to determine the appropriate time of extubation after paralysis.[80]

THEOPHYLLINE

Theophylline is commonly used for the treatment of respiratory disorders in the ICU and is one of the few drugs with a relatively well-defined dose-response relationship.[81] Although the onset of activity with theophylline is delayed, pulmonary function (forced expiratory volume in 1 second or forced vital capacity) will improve 2% for each microgram per milliliter increase in serum theophylline concentration from 5 to 20 μg/mL. However, the risk for toxicity will increase from 0% to 7% over the same concentration range and may exceed 80% for concentrations greater than 25 μg/mL in some patients. Theophylline-induced seizures and arrhythmias (primarily sinus tachycardia, paroxysmal supraventricular tachycardia, or ectopic beats) may occur at 20 to 25 μg/mL, especially in older patients and in those with underlying neurologic and cardiovascular disorders.

TABLE 127–8. Factors Affecting Theophylline Elimination*

Decreased Clearance	*Increased Clearance*
Disease States	
Cirrhosis (65%)	Cystic fibrosis (100%)
Congestive heart failure (50%)	Smoking (40%)
Hypothyroidism (20%)	Hyperthyroidism (35%)
Drugs	
Enoxacin (60%)	Phenytoin (50%)
Propranolol (30%)	Phenobarbital (30%)
Cimetidine (30%)	Rifampin (20%)
Ciprofloxacin (30%)	
Pefloxacin (30%)	
Oral contraceptives (30%)	
Erythromycin (25%)	
Verapamil (20%)	

*Values in parentheses indicate magnitude of clearance changes.

The drug is moderately protein bound (40%) and undergoes hepatic metabolism (low-extraction ratio). Several drugs and disease states have been shown to alter theophylline clearance (Table 127–8). Dosing of theophylline is easily adjusted because the dose-plasma concentration relationship is linear up to a dose of approximately 1500 mg per day. The steady-state concentration clearance equation (clearance = infusion rate/Cp_{ss}) provides the most accurate estimate of the patient's theophylline clearance. However, the Chiou equation provides an estimate of theophylline clearance before the achievement of steady-state conditions:

$$\text{Clearance} = \frac{2K_0(t_2 - t_1)}{(Cp_1 + Cp_2)} + \frac{2Vd(Cp_1 - Cp_2)}{(Cp_1 + Cp_2)(t_2 - t_1)}$$

where K_0 is the infusion rate, t_1 is time of first sample, t_2 is time of second sample, Cp_1 is the first serum concentration, Cp_2 is the second serum concentration, and Vd is volume of distribution (0.45 L/kg lean body weight). However, to use this equation, the infusion rate must be constant and the concentrations must be spaced by at least one half-life.

CONCLUSIONS

TDM should be routinely performed in the ICU because these patients receive many drugs and are prone to exaggerated drug responses. The focus of TDM has changed from serum concentration monitoring to drug effect monitoring as the ultimate outcome parameter, with drug concentrations playing an ancillary role. Patient mortality and morbidity associated with drug therapy can be decreased using TDM, but additional studies are needed to define the role of TDM adequately in the process of healthcare provision. A multidisciplinary healthcare team should provide TDM for maximum impact on patient care, teaching, and research.

References

1. Dasta JF, Armstrong DK: Pharmacoeconomic impact of critically ill surgical patients. Drug Intell Clin Pharm 1988; 22:994.
2. Reents S, Hatton RC: Influence of methods on the evaluation of therapeutic drug-monitoring services. Am J Hosp Pharm 1991; 48:1553.
3. Ried LD, McKenna DA, Horn JR: Meta-analysis of research on the effect of clinical pharmacokinetics services on therapeutic drug monitoring. Am J Hosp Pharm 1989; 46:945.
4. Zaske DE, Bootman JL, Solem LB, et al: Increased burn patient

survival with individualized dosages of gentamicin. Surgery 1982; 91:142.

5. Whipple JK, Ausman RK, Franson T, et al: Effect of individualized pharmacokinetic dosing on patient outcome. Crit Care Med 1991; 19:1480.
6. Mungall D, Marshall J, Penn D, et al: Individualizing theophylline therapy: The impact of clinical pharmacokinetics on patient outcomes. Ther Drug Monit 1983; 5:95.
7. Dager WE, Albertson TE: Impact of therapeutic drug monitoring of intravenous theophylline regimens on serum theophylline concentrations in the medical intensive care unit. Ann Pharmacother 1992; 26:1287.
8. Brown GR, Miyata M, McCormack JP: Drug concentration monitoring: An approach to rational use. Clin Pharmacokinet 1993; 24:187.
9. Lee CS, Marbury TC: Drug therapy in patients undergoing haemodialysis. Clin Pharmacokinet 1984; 9:42.
10. Vaughan LM, Milavetz G, Ellis E, et al: Multicentre evaluation of disposable visual measuring device to assay theophylline from capillary blood sample. Lancet 1986; 1:184.
11. Monaco F, Gianelli M, Dimanico U, et al: A simple and disposable visual measuring device to assay antiepileptic drugs from whole blood samples. Ther Drug Monit 1990; 12:359.
12. Sheiner LB, Beal SL: Bayesian individualization of pharmacokinetics: Simple implementation and comparison with non-Bayesian methods. J Pharm Sci 1982; 71:1344.
12a. Rodvold KA, Pryka RD, Kuehl PG, et al: Bayesian forecasting of serum gentamicin concentrations in intensive care patients Clin Pharmacokinet 1990; 18:409.
13. Yuen GJ, Taylor JW, Ludden TM, et al: Predicting phenytoin dosages using Bayesian feedback: A comparison with other methods. Ther Drug Monit 1983; 5:437.
14. Leape LL, Brennan TA, Laird N, et al: The nature of adverse events in hospitalized patients. N Engl J Med 1991; 324:337.
15. Shikuma LR, Ackerman BH, Weaver RH, et al: Effects of treatment and the metabolic response to injury on drug clearance: A prospective study with piperacillin. Crit Care Med 1990; 18:37.
16. Fuhs DW, Mann HJ, Kubajak CAM, et al: Intrapatient variation of aminoglycoside pharmacokinetics in critically ill surgery patients. Clin Pharm 1988; 7:207.
17. Moore RE, Lietman PS, Smith CR: Clinical response to aminoglycoside therapy: Importance of the ratio of peak concentration to minimal inhibitory concentration. J Infect Dis 1987; 155:93.
18. Noone P, Parsons TMC, Pattison JR, et al: Experience in monitoring gentamicin therapy during treatment of serious gram-negative sepsis. Br Med J 1974; 1:477.
19. Meyer RD: Risk factors and comparisons of clinical nephrotoxicity of aminoglycosides. Am J Med 1986; 80(Suppl 6B):119.
20. Leehy DJ, Braun BI, Tholl DA, et al: Can pharmacokinetic dosing decrease nephrotoxicity associated with aminoglycoside therapy? J Am Soc Nephrol 1993; 4:81.
21. Smith CR, Lipsky JJ, Laskin OL, et al: Double-blind comparison of the nephrotoxicity and auditory toxicity of gentamicin and tobramycin. N Engl J Med 1980; 302:1106.
22. Jackson GG, Arcieri G: Ototoxicity of gentamicin in man: A survey and controlled analysis of clinical experience in the United States. J Infect Dis 1971; 124(Suppl):S130.
23. Lesar TS, Rotschafer JC, Strand LM, et al: Gentamicin dosage errors with four commonly used nomograms. JAMA 1982; 248:1190.
24. Hickling K, Begg E, Moore ML: A prospective, randomized trial comparing individualized pharmacokinetic dosage prediction for aminoglycosides with prediction based on estimated creatinine clearance in critically ill patients. Intensive Care Med 1989; 15:233.
25. Pickering LK, Rutherford I: Effect of concentration and time upon inactivation of tobramycin, gentamicin, netilmicin, and amikacin by azlocillin, carbenicillin, mecillinam, mezlocillin, and piperacillin. J Pharmacol Exp Ther 1981; 217:345.
26. Smith CL, Hampton EM: Using estimated creatinine clearance for individualized drug therapy: A reassessment. DICP, Ann Pharmacother 1990; 24:1185.
27. Sawchuk RJ, Zaske DE: Pharmacokinetics of dosing regimens which utilize multiple intravenous infusions: Gentamicin in burn patients. J Pharmacokinet Biopharm 1976; 4:183.
28. Rybak MJ, Boike SC: Individualized adjustment of vancomycin dosage: Comparison with two dosage nomograms. Drug Intell Clin Pharm 1986; 20:64.
29. Vogelman B, Gudmundsson S, Leggett J, et al: Correlation of antimicrobial pharmacokinetic parameters with therapeutic efficacy in an animal model. J Infect Dis 1988; 158:831.
30. Schentag JJ, Smith IL, Swanson DJ, et al: Role of dual individualization with cefmenoxime. Am J Med 1984; 77(Suppl 6A):43.
31. Wolfson JS, Swartz MN: Serum bactericidal activity as a monitor of antibiotic therapy. N Engl J Med 1985; 312:968.
32. Zhanel GG, Hoban DJ, Harding GKM: The postantibiotic effect: A review of in vitro and in vivo data. DICP, Ann Pharmacother 1991; 25:153.
33. Eliopoulos GM, Eliopoulos CT: Antibiotic combinations: Should they be tested? Clin Microbiol Rev 1988; 1:139.
34. Branch RA: Prevention of amphotericin B–induced renal impairment: A review on the use of sodium supplementation. Arch Intern Med 1988; 148:2389.
35. Majerus PW, Broze GJ, Miletich JP, et al: Anticoagulant, thrombolytic, and antiplatelet drugs. *In*: The Pharmacological Basis of Therapeutics. Gilman AG, Rall TW, Nies AS, Taylor P (Eds). New York, Pergamon Press, 1990, pp 1311–1331.
36. Hirsh J, Dalen JE, Deykin D, et al: Oral anticoagulants. Chest 1992; 103:312S.
37. Bentley DP, Backhouse G, Hutchings A, et al: Investigation of patients with abnormal response to warfarin. Br J Clin Pharmacol 1986; 22:37.
38. Cipolle RJ, Rodvold KA: Heparin. *In*: Applied Pharmacokinetics: Principles of Therapeutic Drug Monitoring. 3rd ed. Evans WE, Schentag JJ, Jusko WG (Eds). Spokane, WA, Applied Therapeutics Inc, 1992.
39. Tinker JH, Roberts SL: Management of cardiopulmonary bypass. *In*: Cardiac Anesthesia. 2nd ed. Kaplan JA (Ed). Philadelphia, WB Saunders, 1987.
40. Landefeld CS, Cook EF, Flatley M, et al: Identification and preliminary validation of predictors of major bleeding in hospitalized patients starting anticoagulant therapy. Am J Med 1987; 82:703.
41. Shetty HGM, Bentley DP, Routledge PA: Effective reversal of warfarin-induced excessive anticoagulation with low dose vitamin K_1. Thromb Haemost 1992; 67:13.
42. Ramierez-Lassepas M, Cipolle RJ, Rodvold KA, et al: Heparin-induced thrombocytopenia in patients with cerebrovascular ischemic disease. Neurology 1984; 34:736.
43. Cola C, Ansell J: Heparin-induced thrombocytopenia and arterial thrombosis: Alternative therapies. Am Heart J 1990; 119:368.
44. Sethi GK, Copeland JG, Goldman S, et al: Implications of preoperative administration of aspirin in patients undergoing coronary artery bypass grafting. J Am Coll Cardiol 1990; 15:15.
45. Peterson GM, Khoo BHC, von Witt RJ: Clinical response in epilepsy in relation to total and free serum levels of phenytoin. Ther Drug Monit 1991; 13:415.
46. Tozer TN, Winter ME: Phenytoin. *In*: Applied Pharmacokinetics: Principles of Therapeutic Drug Monitoring. 3rd ed. Evans WE, Schentag JJ, Jusko WG (Eds). Spokane, WA, Applied Therapeutics Inc, 1992.
47. Boucher BA, Rodman JH, Jaresko GS, et al: Phenytoin pharmacokinetics in critically ill trauma patients. Clin Pharmacol Ther 1988; 44:675.
48. Graves NM, Leppik IE, Termond E, et al: Phenytoin clearances in a compliant population: Description and application. Ther Drug Monit 1986; 8:427.
49. Levy RH, Wilensky AJ, Anderson GD: Carbamazepine, valproic acid, phenobarbital, and ethosuximide. *In*: Applied Pharmacokinetics: Principles of Therapeutic Drug Monitoring. 3rd ed. Evans WE, Schentag JJ, Jusko WG (Eds). Spokane, WA, Applied Therapeutics Inc, 1992.
50. Skoutakis VA, Acchiardo SR: Barbiturates. *In*: Clinical Toxicology of Drugs: Principles and Practice. Skoutakis VA (Ed). Philadelphia, Lea & Febiger, 1982.
51. Podrid PJ, Lampert J, Graboys TB, et al: Aggravation of arrhythmia by antiarrhythmic drugs: Incidence and predictors. Am J Cardiol 1987; 59:38E.
52. Morganroth J: Risk factors for the development of proarrhythmic events. Am J Cardiol 1987; 59:32E.
53. Stratman HG, Kennedy HL: Torsades de pointes associated with drugs and toxins. Am Heart J 1987; 113:1470.

54. Moss AJ, Schwartz PJ: Sudden death and the idiopathic long Q-T syndrome. Am J Med 1979; 66:4.
55. Ueda CT. Quinidine. *In*: Applied Pharmacokinetics: Principles of Therapeutic Drug Monitoring. 3rd ed. Evans WE, Schentag JJ, Jusko WG (Eds). Spokane, WA, Applied Therapeutics Inc, 1992.
56. Coyle JD, Lima JJ: Procainamide. *In*: Applied Pharmacokinetics: Principles of Therapeutic Drug Monitoring. 3rd ed. Evans WE, Schentag JJ, Jusko WG (Eds). Spokane, WA, Applied Therapeutics Inc, 1992.
57. Pieper JA, Johnson KE: Lidocaine. *In*: Applied Pharmacokinetics: Principles of Therapeutic Drug Monitoring. 3rd ed. Evans WE, Schentag JJ, Jusko WG (Eds). Spokane, WA, Applied Therapeutics Inc, 1992.
58. Reuning RH, Geraets DR, Rocci ML, et al: Digoxin. *In*: Applied Pharmacokinetics: Principles of Therapeutic Drug Monitoring. 3rd ed. Evans WE, Schentag JJ, Jusko WG (Eds). Spokane, WA, Applied Therapeutics Inc, 1992.
59. Pleasants RA, Gadsden RH, McCormack JP, et al: Interference of digoxin-like immunoreactive substances with three digoxin immunoassays in patients with various degrees of renal function. Clin Pharm 1986; 5:810.
60. Salerno DM, Anderson B, Sharkey PJ, et al: Intravenous verapamil for treatment of multifocal atrial tachycardia with and without calcium pretreatment. Ann Intern Med 1987; 107:623.
61. Kazierad DJ, Schlanz KD, Bottorf MB: Beta Blockers. *In*: Applied Pharmacokinetics: Principles of Therapeutic Drug Monitoring. 3rd ed. Evans WE, Schentag JJ, Jusko WG (Eds). Spokane, WA, Applied Therapeutics Inc, 1992.
62. Simard J, Bellefleur M: Systemic arterial hypertension in head trauma. Am J Cardiol 1989; 63:32C.
63. Bertel O, Marx BE, Conen D: Effects of antihypertensive treatment on cerebral perfusion. Am J Med 1987; 82(Suppl 3B):29.
64. Zerbe BA, Wagner BKJ: Use of vitamin B_{12} in the treatment and prevention of nitroprusside-induced cyanide toxicity. Crit Care Med 1993; 21:465.
65. Lefkowitz RJ, Hoffman BB, Taylor P: Neurohumoral transmission: The autonomic and somatic motor nervous system. *In*: The Pharmacological Basis of Therapeutics. 8th ed. Gilman AG, Rall TW, Nies AS, Taylor P (Eds). New York, Pergamon Press, 1990, pp 84–121.
66. Schaer GL, Fink MP, Parillo JE: Norepinephrine alone versus norepinephrine plus low-dose dopamine: Enhanced renal blood flow with combination pressor therapy. Crit Care Med 1985; 13:492.
66a. Schlichtig R, Tønnesen TI, Nemoto EM: Detecting dysoxia in "silent" organs. *In*: Critical Care: State of the Art. Vol. 14. Prough DS, Traystman RJ (Eds). Anaheim, CA, Society of Critical Care Medicine, 1993.
66b. Hayes MA, Timmins AC, Yau EHS, et al: Elevation of systemic oxygen delivery in the treatment of critically ill patients. N Engl J Med 1994; 330:1717.
67. Wood MA, Hess ML: Amrinone. *In*: Cardiovascular Drug Therapy. Messerli FH (Ed). Philadelphia, WB Saunders, 1990.
68. DiBianco R: Milrinone. *In*: Cardiovascular Drug Therapy. Messerli FH (Ed). Philadelphia, WB Saunders, 1990.
69. Bodenham A, Shelly MP, Park GR: The altered pharmacokinetics and pharmacodynamics of drugs commonly used in critically ill patients. Clin Pharmacokinet 1988; 14:347.
70. Loper KA, Butler S, Nessly M, et al: Paralyzed with pain: The need for education. Pain 1989; 37:315.
71. Aitkenhead AR, Willatts SM, Park GP, et al: Comparison of propofol and midazolam for sedation in critically ill patients. Lancet 1989; 2:704.
72. Kong KL, Willatts SM, Prys-Roberts C: Isoflurane compared with midazolam for sedation in the intensive care unit. Br Med J 1989; 298:1277.
73. Shelly MP: The assessment of sedation. Br J Intensive Care 1992; 2:195.
74. Segredo V, Caldwell JE, Matthay MA, et al: Persistent paralysis in critically ill patients after long-term administration of vecuronium. N Engl J Med 1992; 327:524.
75. Vanderbrom RHG, Wierda JMKH: Pancuronium bromide in the intensive care unit: A case of overdose. Anesthesiology 1988; 69:996.
76. Agoston S, Vanderbrom RHG, Wierda JMKH: Clinical pharmacokinetics of neuromuscular blocking drugs. Clin Pharmacokinet 1992; 22:94.
77. Shearer ES, O'Sullivan EP, Hunter JM: An assessment of the Cerebrotrac 2500 for continuous monitoring of cerebral function in the intensive care unit. Anaesthesia 1991; 46:750.
78. Wadon AJ, Dogra S, Anand S: Atracurium infusion in the intensive care unit. Br J Anaesth 1986; 58:64S.
79. OpdeCoul A, Lambregts P, Koeman J: Neuromuscular complications in patients given Pavulon® (pancuronium bromide) during mechanical ventilation. Clin Neurol Neurosurg 1985; 87:17.
80. Ali HH: Monitoring of neuromuscular function. Semin Anesth 1989; 9:158.
81. Edwards DJ, Zarowitz BJ, Slaughter RL: Theophylline. *In*: Applied Pharmacokinetics: Principles of Therapeutic Drug Monitoring. 3rd ed. Evans WE, Schentag JJ, Jusko WG (Eds). Spokane, WA, Applied Therapeutics Inc, 1992.

CHAPTER 128

Sedatives and Muscle Relaxants in the Intensive Care Unit

Phillip D. Lumb, MBBS, FCCM
T. James Gallagher, MD, FCCP, FCCM

Although healthcare providers recognize a responsibility to provide appropriate analgesia after trauma, the requirement to modify stress and mental discomfort is more controversial, and available therapies are difficult to titrate because of a lack of clear-cut therapeutic goals. Patients in intensive care units (ICUs) with a variety of illnesses including severe respiratory insufficiency, trauma, and multiple organ system failure receive muscle relaxants to help manage mechanical ventilation. Uniform indications for use and clinical endpoints against which dosage can be titrated do not exist, and prescription of these drugs is difficult and confusing. The triad of hypnosis, analgesia, and muscle relaxation provides an important framework on which to base the prescription of agents capable of producing specific effects. Inhalation anesthetic agents in increasing concentrations can produce these effects, but the concentrations required depress circulatory function disproportionately. In the past, muscle relaxation of appropriate degree for surgical manipulation became synonymous with anesthetic overdose and resultant toxicity. Recognition that animals were killed with darts and arrows coated with a poison that obviously did not poison the meat led to the discovery that the animals died of asphyxia secondary to respiratory muscle paralysis. Subsequently it was demonstrated that if the animal was ventilated during paralysis, it recovered fully. These observations led to the preparation and introduction of *d*-tubocurarine as the first muscle relaxant used in clinical practice and initiated research into the motor end-plate and neuromuscular transmission.

Anesthesiologists have become familiar with the use of muscle relaxants for the specific purposes of facilitating intubation after anesthetic induction, providing muscle relaxation to enable surgical exposure and manipulation, and providing a means to isolate one of the three required anesthetic components. Further uses have been described in critical care medicine (CCM) and other environments, and one of the purposes of this discussion is to specify indications, dosing, and adjuvant therapy for their appropriate use.

NEUROMUSCULAR JUNCTION

Acetylcholine is the chemical neurotransmitter manufactured and stored in the nerve and released into the space between the nerve terminal and the muscle: the synaptic cleft. The acetylcholine reacts with an area of the underlying muscle (motor end-plate), causing conformational changes in specialized acetylcholine receptors. The receptors are composed of several protein subunits manufactured in the muscle and inserted into the cell membrane. They are arranged to provide a passage between the muscle cell surface and the cytoplasm. Normally, they are impermeable to ionic traffic. When two α subunits are stimulated by acetylcholine, the tube opens and sodium and calcium ions flow into the cytoplasm while potassium ions move in the opposite direction. This ionic movement produces an end-plate potential (EPP) that can be measured electrically. When adequate numbers of EPPs occur simultaneously, the motor unit is stimulated and the muscle membrane contracts.

Acetylcholine is synthesized in the nerve terminal and stored in small, round structures called *vesicles*. The acetylcholine stored in the synaptic vesicles is released as a single bolus or quantum, and the release of many quanta simultaneously leads to the production of an EPP and stimulates subsequent events leading to muscle contraction. The action of acetylcholine is transient because it is destroyed by acetylcholinesterase, found in high concentration in the synaptic cleft. The synaptic cleft is a complex, circumscribed structure with multiple invaginations into the muscle mass and is suited ideally for the rapid destruction of acetylcholine, which terminates the muscle activity.

Two basic mechanisms of neuromuscular blockade can be inferred from this discussion. Drugs can either mimic the action of acetylcholine or compete with it for the motor end-plate binding sites. The former mechanism is characteristic of the neuromuscular blocking agent succinylcholine and, because an initial end-plate depolarization occurs after injection, it is called a *depolarizing agent*. Succinylcholine is not deactivated by pseudocholinesterase; therefore, its action is prolonged, causing flaccid paralysis by blocking transmembrane ion flux.

When drugs that compete with acetylcholine for the end-plate receptors are used, no initial depolarization occurs because the agents block conformational subunit change. This nondepolarizing blockade is representative of the most common class of muscle relaxants used in CCM. The major difference between the actions of acetylcholine and the synthetic muscle relaxants is one of degree and the rapidity of their clearance from the synaptic cleft. Normally, the release of acetylcholine from the nerve terminal occurs as a small, rapid pulse, the effects of which are disseminated long before another nerve impulse arrives to activate the muscle.

In the case of the depolarizing relaxants, the drug binds to the receptor initially, as does acetylcholine. It remains in the synaptic cleft, and as it dissociates from one receptor it is available to attach to another one immediately. Ionic fluxes persist across the motor end-plate, and the muscle achieves a state of relaxation, in contrast to the case with nondepolarizing relaxants. Because of muscular activity before the onset of blockade, the drug may be associated with potassium release.

Many drugs can compete with the neuromuscular receptor and alter neuromuscular transmission. These drugs are involved in two important reactions: desensitization and channel blockade.[1] Desensitization blockade describes the condition in which a receptor is capable of binding acetylcholine molecules appropriately but is incapable of then undergoing the conformational changes necessary to promote ionic transfer and subsequent depolarization. The receptor population is finite, and the number of desensitized receptors will affect the efficiency of neuromuscular transmission. The appropriate dosing of neuromuscular blocking agents will depend on the overall relationship between the number of normal receptors and the number of desensitized receptors, and drug titration can be carried out only if appropriate neuromuscular transmission monitoring is performed. Many drugs causing these changes are used in the perioperative period and in the ICU (Table 128–1). These interactions are important in the immediate postoperative period because receptors may become desensitized, thereby reducing the number of effective receptors in the active pool. This reduces the usual margin of safety inherent in the large total number. The desensitized receptor can be trapped in this state by the use of conventional neuromuscular reversal agents, which act by increasing the effective concentration of acetylcholine in the synaptic cleft.

TABLE 128–1. Drugs That May Alter Desensitization of Nicotinic Cholinergic Receptors and Be Administered in the Postoperative or ICU Patient Population*

Volatile Anesthetics	***Local Anesthetics***
Halothane	Lidocaine
Barbiturates	***Phenothiazines***
Thiopental	Chlorpromazine
Pentobarbital	
Alcohol	***Calcium Channel Blockers***
Ethanol	Verapamil
Acetylcholinesterase Inhibitors	
Neostigmine	
Pyridostigmine	

(Adapted from Standaert FG: Basic physiology and pharmacology of the neuromuscular junction. *In*: Anesthesia. 2nd ed. Vol 2. Miller RD [Ed]. New York, Churchill Livingstone, 1986, p 853.)

*All of these agents may act to weaken neuromuscular transmission or diminish the margin of safety that usually exists with motor function.

Pharmacologic interference of ionic flow through a transmembrane channel can occur in two ways.[1] Either a drug blocks the channel before it opens by occupying a position at the mouth of the channel, similar to a bath plug in a drain, or it enters an open channel and sticks somewhere in the path. In either case, transmembrane ion flux is impeded and neuromuscular transmission is altered. These changes are well recognized in non-neuromuscular settings (e.g., the effects of calcium entry channel blockade on the heart and vessels or the action of local anesthetics on sodium channels). These observations emphasize the importance of appropriate dosing and monitoring of all patients receiving neuromuscular blocking agents in the operating room, post-anesthesia care unit, and ICU.

MONITORING NEUROMUSCULAR BLOCKADE

Physiologic monitoring is an integral component of CCM, and patient management using hemodynamic parameters has become commonplace. Increasingly, the use of pharmacokinetic principles is guiding the administration of antibiotics and antiarrhythmics. Therefore, it is surprising that monitoring neuromuscular function is seldom routine, especially in those units that receive patients directly from the operating room. This attitude may be reinforced by the perception that a residual degree of paralysis results in easier patient management during transport from the operating room and easier initial stabilization in the ICU. The ready availability of mechanical ventilators capable of synchronizing with and assisting spontaneous respiratory efforts allows easy weaning and extubation over a few hours. This exceeds the pharmacologic half-life of the relaxant in most cases. The clinician's prime concern is to select the appropriate time for extubation, and the possibility that residual paralysis may be a complicating factor is seldom germane. However, pulmonary mechanics measurements associated with the other clinical tests performed before extubation are tests of muscle function more so than of pulmonary performance. Assessment of muscle strength should be a component of all clinical examinations in patients who have received muscle relaxants. Costly errors may be avoided and patients spared unnecessary suffering. The following cases illustrate the importance of neuromuscular monitoring and an appreciation of the actions of muscle relaxants.

CASE HISTORY 1

A 48-year-old man was admitted to the surgical ICU (SICU) after emergency evacuation of a hematoma surrounding a newly transplanted kidney. Pancuronium bromide (Pavulon) was used as the relaxant in both the transplant and re-exploration, and there was some concern that the patient could have suffered a cerebral ischemic insult secondary to severe hypotension before re-exploration. Thirty-six hours after readmission to the ICU, the patient was unresponsive to all stimuli and exhibited no respiratory efforts. A neurology consultation was obtained, and physical examination revealed flaccid paralysis with normal pupillary signs. During the examination the patient became tachycardic and hypertensive. The patient was scheduled for a computed tomographic scan, but on discussion with the ICU attending physician, peripheral nerve stimulation studies were performed and the patient demonstrated signs of a residual, nondepolarizing motor block. After administration of routine pharmacologic reversal agents, the patient "awoke" and was extubated without difficulty. However, on questioning, the patient had extremely unpleasant memories of this experience and recounted the discussions surrounding his possible diagnoses in great detail.

CASE HISTORY 2

A 7-year-old male near-drowning victim was admitted to the pediatric ICU after resuscitation in the field. Initial stabilization was successful, and the patient remained hemodynamically stable with acceptable blood gases and chemistries for the 12 hours after admission. Then generalized seizures developed, and the patient became increasingly difficult to ventilate. Phenytoin sodium (Dilantin) was started, but the seizures continued and a continuous muscle relaxant infusion was initiated to prevent the patient from "fighting" the ventilator. After several days, the patient was believed to be improving, and the nurses noted that occasionally he grimaced to painful stimuli and on turning. Unfortunately, the patient did not "recover" fully until the muscle relaxant infusion was discontinued. Subsequently, his vivid and unpleasant recollections of this experience became the subject of a videotaped interview.

These examples underscore the need to assess continuously the requirement for relaxant therapy and to monitor the blockade obtained. Muscle relaxants that are prescribed chronically mask the symptom that stimulated prescription and may exacerbate an underlying problem. The addition of analgesic and hypnotic medications is extremely important in these patients.

Clinical assessment of appropriate muscle strength before extubation is easier than regulating a chronic dosing regimen to an appropriate level. Table 128–2 presents a list of common clinical criteria for a successful extubation.

In contrast to this relatively simple task is the choice of the correct dose of muscle relaxant to administer to a patient who has been paralyzed electively to facilitate chronic management. In this setting, ancillary medication use cannot be ignored, and the use of appropriate sedatives and analgesics becomes of paramount importance. Muscle relaxants have neither sedative nor analgesic properties. Appropriate treatment of patients receiving these agents mandates inclusion of other sedative and analgesic agents. Paralysis without

TABLE 128–2. Common Clinical Criteria Used to Determine Appropriate Conditions for a Successful Extubation

An awake patient responding appropriately to command should be able to
- Open the eyes widely
- Cough effectively
- Sustain tongue protrusion
- Sustain hand grip
- Sustain head lift for 5 s or greater
- Produce a vital capacity of 15–20 mL/kg
- Generate an inspiratory force of at least 25 cm H_2O negative pressure
- Sustain a tetanic stimulation of 50 Hz for 5 s
- Have a respiratory rate less than 25–30 breaths per minute
- Produce a voluntary end-inspiratory hold on command before exhalation

A patient who is unable to respond to command should be able to
- Produce a normal tidal volume
- Sustain a tetanic stimulation of 50 Hz for 5 s
- Generate an inspiratory force of at least 25 cm H_2O negative pressure
- Have a respiratory rate less than 25–30 breaths per minute
- Have a minimal requirement for endotracheal suctioning to control secretions

(Adapted from Ali HH, Miller RD: Monitoring of neuromuscular function. *In*: Anesthesia. 2nd ed. Vol 2. Miller RD [Ed]. New York, Churchill Livingstone, 1986, p 882.)

adjuvant hypnosis and analgesia is inappropriate and inhumane. The degree of relaxation required to provide an appropriate clinical response will depend, in part, on the degree to which the patient has been sedated with other agents. After paralysis, the patient's motor response is unavailable as a guide to the degree to which the patient perceives pain or is anxious. Muscle relaxation rather than paralysis is an appropriate endpoint to which these drugs should be titrated. If appropriate guidelines are used, the patient will retain the ability to indicate discomfort in a conventional fashion, and the physiologic condition necessitating pharmacologic control can be monitored routinely.

The practical assessment of the presence, type, and degree of muscle paralysis in the operating room and ICU depends on the fact that, if a peripheral nerve is stimulated electrically, the motor unit supplied by the nerve will respond by contracting. To make the measurement of muscle contraction reproducible within and comparable among patients, specific criteria have been developed for research preparations. However, a clinically oriented approach will suffice for the purposes of this discussion and ICU practice. The electrical nerve stimulators available for use in the operating room and ICU control the following four variables:

1. Stimulus frequency: with a constant dose of nondepolarizing muscle relaxant, paralysis will appear greater at higher stimulus frequency. In the presence of a competitive blockade, a relatively greater amount of transmitter will be required to produce an equivalent contraction.
2. Stimulus duration: the duration of the electrical pulse should be as short as possible. It must be shorter than the muscle's refractory period to avoid restimulation of the muscle during the decay phase of the stimulus itself. Duration is usually less than 0.2 milliseconds.[2]
3. Stimulus waveform: Ideally, the stimulus waveform should be a square wave pulse to avoid repetitive nerve firing caused by the stimulus and provoking a tetany-like response.[2]
4. Stimulus intensity: A stimulation greater than necessary to provoke muscle contraction (supramaximal) ensures full recruitment of the nerve fibers and, therefore, full activation of the muscle fibers.[2] Most nerve stimulators produce currents in the range of 0 to 75 mA.

The pattern of a muscle's response to stimulation of its motor nerve in the presence of neuromuscular blocking drugs depends on the pattern of the stimulus applied to the nerve and the degree and type of blockade present. The ulnar nerve supplies the adductor pollicis brevis, which causes adduction of the thumb. The muscle is positioned at some distance from the stimulating nerve, and this diminishes the likelihood that the muscle will contract by direct electrical stimulation. Clinically, much useful information can be gained by careful observation of finger flexion and thumb adduction in response to ulnar nerve stimulation. The most common locations to stimulate the ulnar nerve are the elbow and wrist. If the hand is inaccessible, many clinicians observe the reaction of the orbicularis muscles of the eye after stimulation of the facial and supraorbital nerves. By monitoring these reactions, an appreciation of the appropriateness of muscle relaxant administration is gained. Stimuli are administered in four distinct patterns: single-twitch stimuli, tetanic stimuli, train-of-four (TOF) stimuli, and post-tetanic facilitation (PTF).

In single-twitch stimuli, a supramaximal stimulus is administered every 1 to 10 seconds. Shortly after administration of a muscle relaxant, the single-twitch response will diminish and, dose-dependently, disappear. The measurement provides a quantitative measurement of relaxation in that, at the depression of twitch, approximately 70% of the receptors are blocked. If the twitch response is abolished, the dose of relaxant is reduced, and return of some twitch activity should be awaited before repeat dosing. Single-twitch response can return to normal appearance in the presence of a significant proportion of receptor blockade. Therefore, appearance of a single twitch after stimulation should never be considered an indication of returned motor strength.

Regarding tetanic stimuli, when the single-twitch response returns to normal, approximately 20% of the receptor pool is free of relaxant. Diaphragmatic activity may be almost normal, and the return of spontaneous respiratory efforts is one of the first signs of emergence. Although the diaphragm is active, the patient is at risk because an 80% receptor blockade may remain. Therefore, it is important to document the full return of neuromuscular transmission before extubation. The application of a stimulus at either 50 or 100 Hz to a normally active neuromuscular unit results in a profound muscle contraction for the duration of the stimulus application. In the presence of a nondepolarizing blockade, the contraction will begin to lose strength before 5 seconds has passed, and the hand will relax. This phenomenon is described as *fade*. Fade can be detected at 100 Hz when as few as 50% of the receptors are occupied. At 50 Hz the discrimination falls to a receptor blockade of as much as 70%. However, the response evoked by a 50-Hz stimulus equals that of a voluntary maximal effort, and the higher frequency stimulus may not be necessary or physiologic.[2] Tetanic stimuli are painful and not useful in the awake, unanesthetized patient. Sustained tetanus at 100 Hz is presumptive that neuromuscular transmission is adequate for normal respiratory function.

In TOF stimuli, the nerve unit is stimulated with four supramaximal stimuli occurring 0.5 second apart. The ratio of the height of the fourth twitch to the first twitch is used to quantitate the degree of blockade. This test is not as painful as tetanic stimulation, and it provides a built-in control. The twitch height ratio is a useful and reproducible indicator of the degree of receptor blockade. Even if there has been a change in the electrode resistance or in the positioning of the electrodes, the ratio of the first and fourth twitches is still valuable. The degree of block may be estimated by noting the number of twitches present after the four stimulus pulses. When only one twitch is present, there is a 90% block. All four twitches return when there is a 75% depression of the single-twitch response. Recovery from neuromuscular blockade occurs when all four twitches have returned to the same height. This indicates approximately 25% freedom of the receptor population. The TOF is a more discriminating test than the single twitch.

In PTF, after the application of a supramaximal tetanus, the next set of contractions produced by either a TOF or single-twitch pulse will be enhanced in the presence of a nondepolarizing muscle relaxant. This result is explained by the increased synthesis and mobilization of acetylcholine, which occurs during the tetanic stimulation. In the poststimulus period, more transmitter is available to compete with the receptors occupied by the nondepolarizing agent for a brief period. PTF is not observed in the presence of a depolarizing relaxant.

CLINICALLY USEFUL MUSCLE RELAXANTS

In the ICU, nondepolarizing muscle relaxants are used almost exclusively. Succinylcholine is the primary depolarizing relaxant in clinical use, and in most instances its use is confined to facilitating intubation after induction of anesthesia. Succinylcholine causes fasciculations of skeletal muscles before causing relaxation, and this reaction may lead to significant potassium release and cardiac arrest, especially in patients who have suffered spinal cord injuries, closed head injury, intra-abdominal infections, renal failure, and burns.[3] Although the duration of succinylcholine's action after injection is short, these and other undesirable characteristics minimize its use in the ICU.

A new addition to the muscle relaxant armamentarium, rocuronium bromide (Zemuron), may prove useful in facilitating emergency ICU intubation. Rocuronium is a nondepolarizing neuromuscular blocking agent with a rapid-to-intermediate onset of action, depending on the initial dose. Intubating conditions were assessed in 230 patients in 6 clinical trials in which anesthesia was induced with either thiopental (3–6 mg/kg) or propofol (1.5–2.5 mg/kg) in combination with either fentanyl (2–5 μg/kg) or alfentanil (1 mg). Most of the patients also received a premedication such as midazolam or temazepam. Most patients had intubation attempted within 60 to 90 seconds of administration of rocuronium bromide injection, 0.6 mg/kg, or succinylcholine, 1 to 1.5 mg/kg. Excellent or good intubating conditions were achieved in 119 of 120 of those (99% [95% confidence interval 95–99.9%]) receiving rocuronium bromide and in 108 of 110 of those patients (98% [94–99.8%]) receiving succinylcholine. The duration of action of rocuronium bromide, 0.6 mg/kg, is longer than that of succinylcholine and at this dose is approximately equivalent to the duration of other intermediate-acting neuromuscular blocking drugs.[4a] Clinical experience with this compound in the ICU is lacking, and usage patterns have yet to be determined.

Until recently, perhaps the most common muscle relaxant used in CCM was pancuronium bromide. However, the introduction of newer agents with cleaner pharmacologic profiles has increased therapeutic options in CCM. This discussion focuses on three long-acting and two intermediate muscle relaxants: pancuronium, doxacurium (Nuromax), pipercuronium (Arduan), atracurium (Tracrium), and vecuronium (Norcuron). Although other nondepolarizing agents are available in the United States (metocurine, gallamine, *d*-tubocurarine), their use in the ICU is limited by undesirable side effects and custom. Indications for the use of muscle relaxants in CCM are discussed separately.

Pancuronium Bromide

Pancuronium is a nondepolarizing muscle relaxant with a relatively long elimination half-life reported from 89 to 161 minutes, a volume of distribution of 241 to 280 mL/kg, and plasma clearance of 1.1 to 1.9 mL · kg^{-1} · min^{-1}. Pancuronium is excreted primarily by the kidneys, with 40% of the total dose administered recovered from the urine. In addition, 11% of the dose has been recovered from the bile.[4] Dosage must be adjusted in patients with liver or renal disease. The major side effect of importance to the ICU clinician is tachycardia, which may be severe. Concomitantly, an expected increase in blood pressure and cardiac output has been noted. Because of its long half-life, pancuronium is usually administered in intermittent boluses, and dosage should be individualized with peripheral nerve stimulator titration. For endotracheal intubation, pancuronium should be administered in a bolus dose of 0.06 to 0.15 mg/kg.[4] All ICUs should prepare protocols for failed intubation, and the availability of emergency airway and tracheostomy sets should be immediate and ensured.

After intravenous injection, appropriate intubating conditions are present in approximately 4 minutes, and the patient will remain paralyzed for 45 to 90 minutes on average. Subsequent dosing of pancuronium should be from 0.01 to 0.05 mg/kg approximately each hour.[4] If appropriate neuromuscular monitoring is used, the likelihood of inappropriate overdose will be minimized. The major disadvantages of overdose are prolongation of the neuromuscular block and prolonged ventilator dependence. Careful dosing is important in patients who have received or are receiving intravenously or intraperitoneally large doses of certain antibiotics that may themselves intensify an existing neuromuscular block or cause one independently. Antibiotics implicated are aminoglycosides (neomycin, streptomycin, kanamycin, gentamicin, and dihydrostreptomycin), tetracyclines, bacitracin, polymyxin B, colistin, and sodium colistimethate.[4] (These caveats are equally applicable to the use of all nondepolarizing muscle relaxants.)

Atracurium Besylate

Atracurium is a nondepolarizing skeletal muscle relaxant with a duration of action of approximately one half to one third of that seen with pancuronium at initially equipotent doses.[5] Time to onset decreases and duration increases with increasing dose. The dose required to produce 95% twitch height depression with a balanced anesthetic is 0.23 mg/kg, and initial doses of 0.4 to 0.5 mg/kg produce maximum dose effect within 3 to 5 minutes of injection and good intubating conditions within 2 to 2½ minutes in most patients.[5] Under balanced anesthesia, recovery of twitch can be anticipated within 20 to 35 minutes after injection, and recovery to 25% of control is achieved at approximately 35 to 45 minutes after injection and is 95% complete at 60 to 70 minutes.[5] Unlike with most other relaxants, repeat doses have no cumulative effect, and recovery from atracurium blockade is predictable in all clinical settings. The pharmacokinetics of atracurium are linear within the 0.3- to 0.6-mg/kg dose range, and the elimination half-life is approximately 20 minutes.[5] The duration of blockade does not correlate with plasma pseudocholinesterase levels and is unaffected by renal or hepatic compromise. Atracurium is inactivated in plasma by two nonoxidative mechanisms: ester hydrolysis catalyzed by nonspecific esterases and Hoffman elimination, a nonenzymatic chemical process that occurs at physiologic pH.[5] Atracurium injection may cause histamine release, although in most instances reactions are mild and easily controlled. The possibility of a significant histamine reaction must be anticipated if an initial dose is 0.6 mg/kg or greater. Side effects may be minimized if the drug is given in divided doses over 1 to 2 minutes or if an infusion technique is used.

Appropriate dosing for intubation and initial muscle relaxation is 0.4 to 0.5 mg/kg.[5] Dosage ranges of 0.005 to 0.01 mg · kg^{-1} · min^{-1} have been successful in maintaining adequate operating conditions in most situations, although individual variation is possible.[5] Of concern has been the fact that laudanosine is the primary metabolite of Hoffman elimination.[6] Potential for neurologic toxicity has been raised with this compound, but to date no significant damage has been reported after either single-bolus injections or intermittent dosing or continuous infusion therapies that have been maintained for prolonged periods. The degradation characteristics of atracurium may make it the most predictable in geriatric patients, who demonstrate variable organ perfusion and decreased capacity to metabolize some compounds by conventional methods.

Vecuronium Bromide

Vecuronium is a nondepolarizing skeletal muscle relaxant of intermediate duration and is reportedly about one-third more potent than pancuronium.[7] The duration of effect is significantly less than that of pancuronium. When the drug is used in a continuous infusion for prolonged periods, the duration of effect is seldom increased beyond that expected from a single dose after cessation of the infusion. A dose of 0.08 to 0.15 mg/kg produces first depression of twitch within 1 minute and appropriate intubating conditions within 2½ to 3 minutes. Subsequently, maintenance doses of 0.01 to 0.04 mg/kg may be administered every 20 to 30 minutes with minimal cumulative effect.[7] After an intravenous dose, 60% to 80% of vecuronium is protein bound at normal clinical doses, with a distribution half-life of 4 minutes. The elimination half-life is 65 to 75 minutes in both healthy surgical patients and in renal failure patients who are candidates for transplant surgery. In late pregnancy, the elimination half-life may be decreased to 35 to 40 minutes.[7] The steady-state volume of distribution is approximately 300 to 400 mL/kg, with a systemic clearance rate of 3 to 4.5 mL · kg^{-1} · min^{-1}. In humans, urine recovery varies from 3% to 35% within 24 hours; however, information derived after cholecystectomy with T-tube drainage of the common bile duct suggests that 25% to 50% of the total injected dose may be excreted in the bile within 42 hours.[7] Data obtained from multiple preparations and from humans suggest that the duration of paralysis from a single dose in patients with liver failure is prolonged.[7] No clinically detectable changes in elimination characteristics are noted in renal failure.

Because of its elimination characteristics and lack of cumulative drug effects, vecuronium may be used successfully as a continuous infusion in the operating room and ICU. After an initial loading dose, an infusion of 0.075 to 0.10 mg · kg^{-1} · h^{-1} has been used successfully for prolonged periods. In some series, recovery to 10% to 25% of control has occurred within 7 minutes of stopping the infusion,[8] although longer times to recovery have been noted.

Doxacurium Chloride

Doxacurium is a recently released, long-acting, nondepolarizing muscle relaxant. As with all agents of this class, it binds competitively and reversibly to cholinergic receptors on the motor end-plate to antagonize the action of acetylcholine and block neuromuscular transmission. Pharmacodynamically, it is two and one-half to three times more potent than pancuronium and has a duration of action that is similar when administered in equipotent doses. The average effective dose (ED_{95}) is 0.025 mg/kg in adults receiving balanced anesthesia.[9] When the drug is administered at this dose, time to maximum block is approximately 9.3 minutes, with an average duration to 25% recovery of 55 minutes. At a dose three times ED_{95}, the time to onset of maximum block is reduced to 3.5 minutes, with a duration of 160 minutes.[9] As with other agents of this class, clinical response to recommended dose exhibits considerable interpatient variability, and it is important to individualize doses carefully and follow recommendations for monitoring depth of neuromuscular blockade, as previously described. The pharmacokinetics of doxacurium are similar in both young and elderly patients. Although there appears to be little or no accumulation with repeat administration, to avoid prolonged action, careful determination of appropriate patient-specific dosing intervals must be performed. The manufacturer recommends a dosing schedule based on ideal body weight (IBW) calculated from the following formulas: men, IBW (in kilograms) = [106 + (6 × inches in height >5 feet)]/2.2; women, IBW (in kilograms) = [100 + (5 × inches in height >5 feet)]/2.2.[9] An anesthetic relaxant dose associated with appropriate intubating conditions in approximately 5 minutes is 0.05 mg/kg with a duration of approximately 100 minutes. More rapid onset and longer duration are anticipated with doses in the 0.08-mg/kg range. Maintenance doses in the 0.005-mg/kg range are advised.[9] Recommendations for use in the ICU are not available because of the newness of the agent.

The major difference between doxacurium and pancuronium is the absence of cardiovascular side effects in the former. Injection of doses up to and including 0.08 mg/kg (~3 × ED_{95}) over 5 to 15 seconds in healthy adult patients during stable-state, balanced anesthesia and in patients with serious cardiovascular disease undergoing coronary artery bypass grafting, cardiac valvular repair, or vascular repair produced no dose-related effects on mean arterial blood pressure (MAP) or heart rate (HR). No dose-related changes in MAP or HR were observed after administration of up to 0.05 mg/kg over 5 to 15 seconds in 2- to 12-year-old children receiving halothane anesthesia. Doses of 0.03 to 0.08 mg/kg (1.2–3 × ED_{95}) were not associated with dose-dependent changes in mean plasma histamine concentration.[9]

In summary, doxacurium chloride is a new, hemodynamically stable, long-acting, nondepolarizing muscle relaxant that can be used safely in the operating room and ICU if precautions are taken to ensure appropriate dose titration and provide other safeguards necessary for the management of any paralyzed patient.

Pipercuronium Bromide

Pipercuronium is a new long-acting, nondepolarizing neuromuscular blocking agent that acts by competing for cholinergic receptors at the motor end-plate, and, as is the case with drugs of this class, the action is antagonized by acetylcholinesterase inhibitors, such as neostigmine.[10] Pipercuronium was shown to have an onset time and clinical duration (range and variability) similar to those of pancuronium bromide at comparable doses (historical data and limited comparisons).[10] As with doxacurium, the potential benefit of pipercuronium is its lack of cardiovascular side effects after injection. According to the product literature, clinically significant bradycardia, hypotension, and hypertension, reasonably associated with the administration of pipercuronium, have been reported in approximately 3% of 592 patients.[10] However, these are not unexpected side effects when it is recognized that muscle relaxants are never used in isolation and are always accompanied by adjuvant drugs, the combination of which would be expected to produce these side effects. However, unlike with pancuronium and its associated tachycardia and rate-related increase in MAP, use of the newer relaxants should be carefully controlled until familiarity is gained by all potential users. Paralysis and associated mechanical ventilation will have deranging effects on any patient's hemodynamic stability, and use must be tempered by experience and ability to control hemodynamic responses.

Pipercuronium is no different from other drugs in its class in demonstrating variability in duration from doses based on patient weight. Therefore, care must be taken to individualize doses, and careful attention must be paid to the patient's underlying renal function. Studies of distribution, metabolism, and excretion in animals indicate that pipercuronium is eliminated primarily by the kidneys (more than 75% of the drug is recovered in the urine, primarily as the unchanged drug).[10] The package insert lists several formulas to adjust drug dose based on renal function, and the user is advised to review these recommendations before use. They are similar to those seen with other muscle relaxants, and, as is the case with all agents in this class, all doses should be individualized and titrated to the desired effect.

The primary advantage of pipercuronium over pancuronium and other available relaxants (with the exception of doxacurium) is its absence of hemodynamic side effects after injection and its prolonged duration of action. Its use in CCM is being researched and established currently.

Summary

Popular muscle relaxants used in the critical care unit today are doxacurium, pancuronium, and pipercuronium (long action) and atracurium and vecuronium (intermediate action). With the exception of pancuronium, these pharmacologically clean drugs are a powerful armamentarium that can be titrated appropriately in all patients irrespective of diagnosis or severity of illness. However, this recognition places increased responsibility on the clinician to understand the pharmacology of the drug as well as the physiology attendant with its use.

INDICATIONS FOR THE USE OF MUSCLE RELAXANTS IN THE INTENSIVE CARE UNIT

No specific indications exist that make paralysis a sine qua non of pharmacologic care in CCM. For purposes of discussion, indications are divided into the areas of perioperative care, specific disease states, and postoperative considerations and potential beneficial effects. Inappropriate use of a muscle relaxant to control agitation and movement in the absence of adequate analgesia and hypnosis may lead to lasting psychologic trauma in those patients who survive the experience. Critical care personnel should always be conscious of the possibility of cognitive function in all patients no matter how ill or advanced in their disease.

Perioperative Use of Muscle Relaxants

Stable Transport from Operating Room to Intensive Care Unit

After complex or lengthy surgical procedures, the anesthesiologist is faced with managing a prolonged, complicated patient transport from the operating room to an ICU. Transport may be easier to manage if the patient is kept sedated and paralyzed. Certainly, the situation in which a patient becomes agitated and combative in a constricted elevator between floors is one to be avoided at all costs, and muscle relaxation provides a practical approach to avoiding this problem. This practice will have significant implications for the receiving ICU team, and communication between the transport and care teams must be detailed and precise. The ICU team must be familiar with the effects and anticipated duration of all drugs administered in the operating room and must be prepared to treat the patient appropriately based on clinical evaluation and pharmacologic expectation.

Rewarming/Suppression of Postoperative Shivering

General anesthetics abolish shivering. After emergence from prolonged surgical procedures during which the patient's core temperature may fall to 32°C or lower in spite of fluid and inspired gas warming, shivering occurs often. Although this is a normal response to cold in health, the metabolic consequences in postoperative and critically ill patients with unknown oxygen deficits may be excessive. Shivering is associated with increases in heart rate and blood pressure, which, in turn, increases rate pressure product and myocardial oxygen consumption. Total body oxygen consumption and carbon dioxide production are raised secondary to increased muscle work, and rewarming leads to peripheral vasodilation and hypotension, which place further demands on the myocardium. Abolition of shivering during external rewarming may be beneficial, allowing for more controlled rewarming. Provision for mechanical ventilatory assistance must be made and prolongation of the recovery period anticipated, although appropriate management may actually minimize the delay in emergence and subsequent extubation.

Specific Wounds

No specific recommendations exist for prolonging muscle relaxation in the postoperative period in the event of a difficult or technically complex surgical wound closure. Some patients appear to benefit from postoperative paralysis and mechanical ventilation. It should not be anticipated that surgical healing will occur during the period of relaxant use. Rather, a stable period after the end of the surgical procedure may encourage early perfusion of the wound with benefit to the recently traumatized tissues. Other patients who were thought to benefit from prolonged postoperative ventilation (e.g., those with severe chronic lung disease) now may receive regional or combination general and regional techniques to control postoperative pain to attempt the earliest possible extubation. Vigorous encouragement of normal ventilatory effort and its associated beneficial effects on cardiac output and hemodynamic stability has proven beneficial for many.

Intubated, ventilated patients are at increased risk for the development of nosocomial pneumonias, especially when gastrointestinal bleeding prophylaxis with antacids and histamine$_2$ blockers is used.[11] The decision to paralyze a patient postoperatively, specifically to help wound management, must not supplant the use of more conventional and successful methods. Finally, the absolute dependence of a paralyzed patient on the nursing staff and ancillary personnel must be emphasized. Of paramount importance is the recognition that a healthcare provider must be in attendance at all times, and a 1:1 patient-nurse ratio is mandatory if private rooms are used. A ventilator disconnect is fatal in this situation, and appropriate alarms must be set at all times. Therefore, the decision to paralyze a patient under any circumstances must not be taken lightly, and the practical, financial, and medical problems associated with long-term maintenance cannot be underestimated.

Clinical Indications for Prolonged Muscle Relaxant Use

Although specific indications for prolonged muscle relaxant use are difficult to determine, the following conditions have been managed using paralysis as an adjunct to care:

Bronchopleural fistula
Certain diagnostic tests[12]
Control of intracranial pressure[13]
Decerebrate rigidity after anoxic injury[14]
Diaphragmatic hernia
Extensive mouth care
Hyaline membrane disease[15]
Increased peak inflation pressures[16, 17]
Mechanical ventilation/respiratory failure[16, 17]
Multiple system organ failure[18]
Postoperative neuroleptic malignant syndrome[19]
Reye's syndrome[13]
Tetanus[20]
Tracheal disruption

This list is not intended to be either exhaustive or exclusive. Rather, it provides a sample of the multiple situations in which muscle relaxants have been used. Careful attention should be paid to those comments that indicate that, although a muscle relaxant may have appeared to be appropriate initially, subsequent patient outcome indicated that paralysis may not have been of primary importance in altering respiratory function.

For example, in one reported series, "improvement in oxygenation was unrelated to changes in ventilation in most infants,"[21] and the authors "expected paralysis to improve oxygenation in infants who were struggling. However, few of our patients were actually resisting the respirator, and most were given pancuronium as a 'last resort' for severely impaired gas exchange. Most patients did not change their oxygenation immediately after paralysis, and few worsened, while respirator settings and inspired oxygen concentration remained stable. . . . As lung compliance improves, spontaneous respiratory efforts would be expected to contribute a greater portion of total ventilation. Thus, paralysis of a patient with less severe disease or who is recovering might result in deteriorating blood gas values unless compensating respirator adjustments are made."[21]

Another author recommends the use of muscle relaxants "when the patient is first placed on artificial ventilation, whilst monitoring lines are being inserted, or when lung compliance is poor, making artificial ventilation difficult."[18]

The common themes supporting the use of relaxants in the critically ill population relate to the perceived benefits of immobility and decreased muscular work. The following case illustrates this point.

CASE HISTORY 3

A 23-year-old female victim of a high-speed automobile accident was transported to the emergency department via helicopter transport in a pneumatic antishock garment. Intravenous resuscitation had been pursued vigorously, and initial assessment revealed a hemodynamically unstable patient with severe supraventricular tachycardia (rate = 160) and respiratory distress in a neck collar and on a long back board immobilizer. Abdominal paracentesis was markedly positive, and the patient was transported directly to the operating room. At laparotomy, a ruptured spleen was removed, and a fractured liver, mesenteric avulsions, and a gastric perforation with associated diaphragmatic disruption were repaired. An arch aortogram performed in the operating room showed the presence of an aortic disruption at the level of the ligamentum arteriosum, but a severe coagulopathy made further surgical exploration of the chest and repair of the transection impossible. Several hours after return to the SICU, the patient remained in unstable condition with marginal renal function, decreased pulmonary compliance, and worsening arterial oxygen saturation. Peak inflation pressures were approximately 95 cm H_2O, and the patient was hemodynamically unstable with systolic blood pressure in the 85-mm Hg range on high-dose dopamine. Arterial oxygenation was poor, with a saturation of 89%, a fraction of inspired oxygen (FIO_2) of 1.0, positive end-expiratory pressure (PEEP) of 10 cm H_2O, and a tidal volume of 750 mL. Any alteration in tidal volume, PEEP, or ventilator rate caused significant increase in peak ventilator pressures and worsening hypotension. During this time, the patient (admitted with a core temperature of 32.7°C) began to shiver, and arterial and mixed venous oxygen saturations fell precipitously. Clinical evaluation confirmed bilateral small pupils reactive to light with no other significant findings. Reinstitution of neuromuscular blockade was felt to be advantageous, and 6 mg of vecuronium was given in two divided doses. Shortly after the second dose, the shivering was arrested, peak inflation pressure decreased, and arterial and venous saturations rose. PEEP was increased to 30 cm H_2O without a significant increase in ventilator pressures, and over the course of the next few hours, FIO_2 was successfully reduced to 50%. Initial hypotension after paralysis was managed with crystalloid volume infusions to maintain adequate pulmonary artery occluded pressure and cardiac output, and, overall the patient made significant improvement acutely.

Improvement in oxygenation could have resulted from a decrease in abdominal and chest wall rigidity, thereby increasing pulmonary compliance, as reflected in a decreased peak ventilatory inflation pressure. Sequentially, this would be expected to improve venous return to the right side of the heart and increase cardiac output. In addition, the improvements in compliance permitted an increase in PEEP without unacceptable increases in peak inflation pressure, which recruited alveoli into the functional lung volume available for alveolar gas exchange. Also, decreased inflation pressures may diminish the risks of developing pulmonary barotrauma, which may be associated with increased ventilatory pressures acutely or for prolonged periods. Finally, the abolition of shivering diminished overall oxygen consumption and decreased the venous desaturation necessary to maintain oxygen delivery in an already compromised system. Muscle relaxation was assessed with a peripheral nerve stimulator, and dosage was adjusted to preserve one to two twitches on TOF testing. Hypnosis and analgesia were accomplished with infusions of midazolam (Versed) and morphine sulfate.

Detrimental effects of paralysis in an underresuscitated patient are detailed in the following example.

CASE HISTORY 4

An 18-year-old woman with toxemia secondary to a hydatidiform molar pregnancy was admitted to the SICU in extremis. She was incoherent, combative, and noticeably cyanotic on 100% face mask oxygen, with a respiratory rate of 58 breaths per minute. Initial blood gas determination revealed a partial pressure of arterial oxygen (PaO_2) of 45 mm Hg, partial pressure of carbon dioxide ($PaCO_2$) of 24 mm Hg, and pH of 7.46. Pulse rate was 164 and blood pressure was 95 mm Hg by palpation. Initial attempts to control the airway were unsuccessful, and the patient's condition continued to deteriorate. Endotracheal intubation without paralysis was impossible, and the patient received 8 mg of pancuronium to facilitate intubation and mechanical ventilation. Shortly after administration, the patient became more hypotensive and hemodynamically unstable ventricular tachycardia developed. The airway was secured, and massive amounts of frothy sputum were suctioned from the endotracheal tube. The patient was cardioverted successfully and volume resuscitated with a combination of balanced salt solution in addition to packed cells, platelets, and fresh frozen plasma. Postintubation blood gas determination showed a PaO_2 of 56 mm Hg on 100% oxygen and a $PaCO_2$ of 74 mm Hg. Volume resuscitation was continued, and the patient was placed on 20 cm H_2O PEEP with controlled mechanical ventilation. The patient was taken to the operating room for a hysterectomy. Ventilatory support was tapered over the next several days and the patient was extubated with reasonable pulmonary function 10 days after the initial event.

In this situation, the negative impact of muscle relaxants and mechanical ventilation can be seen in the early phases of management. The physiologic implications in paralyzing a critically ill patient to control mechanical ventilation are significant and must be understood. The patient who is struggling to breathe without an endotracheal tube is seldom paralyzed to make him or her look better; the same logic should apply to mechanically ventilated patients, and the first approach to a struggling patient should be to ensure appropriate ventilatory support, a subject beyond the scope of this chapter.

CLINICAL IMPLICATIONS OF MUSCLE RELAXANT USE IN THE INTENSIVE CARE UNIT

There are few specific situations in which paralysis is recognized as a mandatory adjunct to patient care, although in cases of tetanus and some specialized pulmonary management problems, most practitioners would be able to reach a consensus on the appropriateness of use. The remaining situations in which paralysis is used are likely to depend on the the unit physicians' and nursing staff's familiarity with the physiologic effects of paralysis and the perceived and measured benefits of therapy. Measurement of effect is especially important with the use of these agents, as is the use of a peripheral nerve stimulator to adjust dosage. Therefore, appropriate measurement of oxygen transport and other metabolic data will help adjudicate overall requirement. Also, improvement in ventilatory parameters will predict accurately the patient's ability to be weaned from the drugs. Too often, drug use is continued beyond the time required to correct the initial clinical problem, and it is in situations such as these that adjuvant therapies become confused, and inappropriately the patient is left awake and paralyzed.

Prescription and titration of drug use to anticipated outcome should enable appropriate use and accurate dosing of these agents. Anticipated physiologic effects by system are discussed next.

Central Nervous System Effects

Muscle relaxants have no known sedative or analgesic properties. They do not alter the perception of pain, and they act only at the neuromuscular junction of skeletal muscles. Normal pupil reactivity is preserved in patients receiving nondepolarizing muscle relaxants. Severe agitation is masked by these agents, and dosing of routinely prescribed sedatives and analgesics is difficult. Careful titration of muscle relaxant dose is important so that the patient will be able to respond visibly to noxious stimuli. Variations in pulse rate and blood pressure may be related to inadequate pharmacologic blunting of affect as much as to an acute hemodynamic insult.

Metabolic Effects

Muscle relaxants may be valuable in controlling hypermetabolic states associated with increased skeletal muscle activity such as shivering. The use of these agents in postoperative neuroleptic malignant syndrome and in postanoxic convulsive states has been reported.[14, 19] In all instances, the patient must be monitored to ensure adequate oxygen delivery to meet metabolic demand. If muscle relaxants are continued, an improvement in oxygen transport should be demonstrated. The patient's physiologic needs must be met appropriately, and successful management will provide adequate monitoring sophistication to ensure that the prescribed drugs are correct in both dose and anticipated activity.

Respiratory Effects

One of the most common uses of muscle relaxants in the ICU is to ensure adequate ventilation in the face of decreased pulmonary performance. A common use is to control the patient who is "fighting" the ventilator. Early patient assessment should recognize that, in many instances, the patient is reacting to inadequate ventilatory support to meet physiologic demands. Often, adjustment of PEEP, tidal volume, pressure support level, or ventilator rate will cause a dramatic improvement in the patient's sense of well-being, and agitation will decrease markedly. Dyspnea may have a physiologic basis because of inappropriate lung expansion secondary to the erosion of functional residual capacity common to the postoperative period and associated particularly with thoracic, upper abdominal, and some retroperitoneal procedures. In a number of patients, even the most careful ventilator adjustments have a minimal effect in controlling ventilator disharmony, which leads to an increased work of breathing, ventilation-perfusion mismatch, and possibly increases the risks of pulmonary barotrauma secondary to increased ventilator pressures. In these situations, muscle relaxants may be beneficial and increase the efficiency of ventilator support to the patient's benefit.

If paralysis is initiated, the resultant cardiorespiratory consequences must be managed. Paralysis will eliminate spontaneous respiratory effort, and accordingly the normal negative intrathoracic pressure generated during inspiration will be replaced with positive-pressure breaths delivered at constant tidal volume and pressure. The diaphragm becomes a passive demarcation between the thorax and abdomen, and instead of the creation of optimal areas of lung expansion during active inspiration, movement is controlled by pressure relationships that depend on intra-abdominal factors as well as thoracic compliance. The normal matching of ventilation to perfusion is absent, and ventilation-perfusion mismatch occurs to the detriment of blood exchange. Detailed discussion of these changes is beyond the scope of this chapter, but when administering any muscle relaxants, one must consider the possibility of detrimental effects that may worsen the clinical situation and require corrective action.

Hemodynamic Effects

Any physiologic manipulation of the pulmonary system will have significant effects on cardiovascular performance. Venous return is affected adversely by positive intrathoracic pressure. Cardiac output is compromised because of an overall decrease in stroke volume secondary to a decreased preload. Intravascular volume expansion to counteract cardiac depression is mandatory during mechanical ventilation. Adequate sedative and analgesic medications must be administered before and during administration of relaxants. Narcotics and hypnotics are cardiac depressants and peripheral vasodilators, and an unfortunate synergy with the decrease in preload may cause severe hemodynamic instability after relaxant administration. This response is predictable, and adequate preload supplementation before paralysis prevents significant problems. However, rapid corrective action is mandatory if the patient experiences severe cardiorespiratory embarrassment after paralysis. Paralysis alters mechanical cardiorespiratory function, whereas sedatives and analgesics depress cardiac function and alter autonomic responsiveness to stress.

SEDATION AND THE USE OF MUSCLE RELAXANTS

Although paralyzed patients do not complain visibly, there is no doubt that their pain perception and anxiety are not controlled or altered. There is an absolute indication to provide adequate sedative and analgesic medication if muscle relaxants are used in the ICU. There is no particular regimen for sedation, analgesia, or relaxation, and individual practitioners will find a variety of available agents with distinct pharmacologic properties for use in these situations. The goal is to provide adequate levels of analgesia and hypnosis to minimize patient discomfort while preserving or improving hemodynamic and respiratory function.

Sedative-Hypnotic Drugs

Benzodiazepines are used frequently in the ICU, and midazolam has become the sedative of choice in some units because of its short elimination half-life, water solubility, and lack of adverse hemodynamic side effects if carefully titrated.[22, 23] However, more recent reports indicate that dosage variability among patients may be high, and prolonged effects after continuous infusion have been noted.[24] Patients acquire acute tolerance early during infusion, and if abrupt weaning is attempted, withdrawal is noted. This includes acute restlessness, tachycardia, marked blood pressure lability, hypermetabolism, and other symptoms that usually require reinstitution of the infusion. These effects may be predictable based on work presented by Persson and colleagues,[25] who noted that the sedative actions of midazolam may be modified by coadministration of opioids and that dosages may need to be modified. Midazolam remains a useful drug in ICU practice. Continuous infusion has become an increasingly accepted method of administration, and most patients tolerate the drug well.

Two other benzodiazepines, diazepam (Valium) and lorazepam (Ativan), are also popular. In contrast to diazepam, lorazepam and midazolam lack active metabolites and have more predictable elimination half-lives. This may be a disadvantage in situations in which weaning from a continuous infusion of any of the drugs is accompanied by agitation. Administration of a hypnotic with a longer duration of action may provide an opportunity to discontinue the short-acting agent without complication. It is important to provide adequate sedation in all situations in which a patient requires mechanical ventilation and associated administration of muscle relaxants. Monitoring adequacy of sedation in this patient population is extremely difficult because of vast changes in volumes of drug distribution, hemodynamic parameters, nutritional and protein concentration imbalances, and altered drug metabolic processes.

Narcotic Analgesics

Drug prescription in the ICU should be guided specifically to the effects desired. The availability of new delivery systems and specific, short-acting narcotics such as fentanyl (Sublimaze), sufentanil (Sufenta), and alfentanil (Alfenta) may alter the more routine prescriptions for morphine sulfate and meperidine hydrochloride (Demerol). Indeed, complicated surgical dressing changes may be facilitated by appropriate use of these agents in combination with short-acting hypnotic agents. In some instances, adequate and safe procedural conditions can be created in the ICU that may obviate the need to return repeatedly to the operating room for many of these activities.

Appropriate narcotic prescription will promote increased patient cooperation, and, occasionally, some discussion will be held regarding appropriate prescriptions for weaning patients from mechanical ventilation if narcotics are not discontinued. Normally, $Pa{CO_2}$ is maintained at levels approximating 40 mm Hg in a wide variety of conditions. Narcotic analgesics should be titrated appropriately to control pain, especially during the resumption of normal ventilatory effort. Although narcotics diminish the set point at which the respiratory center perceives the necessity to ventilate in response to carbon dioxide, once the threshold is reached, increasing concentrations provoke a relatively normal and effective ventilatory response.

Correct narcotic prescription is an essential component of ICU patient management, especially in those instances in which the patient's normal responses have been eliminated pharmacologically.

Reversal Agents

Agents used to reverse the effects of nondepolarizing muscle relaxants increase the availability of acetylcholine at the motor end-plate by inhibiting the action of acetylcholinesterase. Because nondepolarizing neuromuscular blockade is competitive, the subsequent increase in concentration of acetylcholine in the synaptic cleft leads to appropriate transmission of the neurologic stimulus at the postjunctional motor end-plate. Unopposed use of these drugs may cause unwanted muscarinic side effects of increased secretions and severe bradycardia. Common practice dictates the use of either atropine or glycopyrrolate (Robinul) whenever acetylcholinesterase inhibitors are used. The three drugs in common use, and recommended dosing ranges, are as follows: (1) neostigmine bromide (Prostigmin), 2.5 to 5.0 mg/70 kg; (2) pyridostigmine bromide (Regonol), 0.1 to 0.20 mg/kg with a 25-mg maximum in a 70-kg patient; and (3) edrophonium chloride (Tensilon, Enlon, Reversol), 10 to 40 mg/70 kg. Use of atropine, 0.6 to 1.5 mg/70 kg, or glycopyrrolate, 0.5 to 1.0 mg/70 kg, provides an appropriate antimuscarinic dose and will promote the desired nicotinic effects. Of major importance in the ICU is that the effectiveness of these agents be documented before extubation, and restoration of neuromuscular transmission must be demonstrated with a peripheral nerve stimulator.[26]

Some of the factors that determine effectiveness of reversal agents are as follows:

1. Has adequate time elapsed between the administration of the antagonist and the anticipated response? In most situations, this will take at least 15 to 30 minutes.
2. Is the neuromuscular blockade too intense to be reversed? These agents work by competitive inhibition, and even in the presence of an acetylcholinesterase inhibitor, the blocking agent may be present in greater concentration than transmitter at the neuromuscular junction.
3. The acid-base status of the patient may affect reversal in that respiratory acidosis and metabolic alkalosis augment nondepolarizing muscle blockade. This result may reflect the fact that extracellular potassium and calcium concentrations may be more important to the success or failure of reversal than the pH itself.
4. Has the patient received any of the antibiotics mentioned previously that may depress neuromuscular transmission? In this situation, administration of calcium may improve strength, but antibiotic metabolism will permit normal restoration of neuromuscular function as long as the airway is protected and appropriate ventilation ensured.
5. A delay in reversal may occur in cases of renal failure for the relaxants pancuronium and *d*-tubocurare. Newer relaxants that are excreted nonrenally are not affected.[3]

CONCLUSIONS

Appropriate pharmacotherapy in the critically ill patient is a therapeutic challenge, and the prescribing physician should have a clear understanding of the pharmacologic vagaries of the drugs used and of the anticipated clinical goals of therapy. In using muscle relaxants, disagreement surrounds not only appropriate indications but also the choice of obligatory hypnotic and analgesic therapy. The preceding discussion has not provided specific recommendations for a particular combination of agents. Rather, information has been presented that should enable clinicians to make rational choices from the selections available. Because the drug synthesis breakthroughs of recent years have provided increasingly "clean" drugs with absence of major side effects, the tendency is to minimize the dangers associated with inappropriate use. Unfortunately, the opportunities for untoward reactions are great with muscle relaxants, and the penalties may be divided equally between psychologic damage and hemodynamic instability associated with initiation of muscle relaxant–controlled mechanical ventilation. Certainly, when used with care, these agents may prove to be extremely beneficial in the management of acute hemodynamic and respiratory compromise.

Therapeutic goals must be defined before administration, especially in critically ill patients, whose tolerance for prescription error is low. Newer agents have relatively short durations of action with few pharmacologic side effects or associated drug interactions. The physiologic consequences of paralyzing a hypovolemic patient whose respiratory effort is the prime mechanism supporting adequate oxygen transport to hypoxic tissues may be catastrophic. A useful way to determine the correct mix of drugs is to consider the needs of muscle relaxation, analgesia, and hypnosis separately. Dosing specifically targeted agents is easier, and all members of the healthcare team should be educated in the desired effects of each of the components used so that patients' responses can be judged. This approach provides positive feedback to the management team and may prevent inappropriate patient management.

Muscle relaxant prescription is not a benign intervention. However, when used for specific indications, muscle relaxants can provide benefit by decreasing work of breathing and associated excessive oxygen consumption, improving ventilation-perfusion relationships in carefully selected patients, and minimizing peak inflation pressures in patients with poorly compliant lungs who require ventilatory support. All paralyzed patients, in spite of apparently appropriate sedation, should be treated as though they were alert. Paralysis is no substitute for careful medical care. Most patients do not "fight" the ventilator; rather, the clinician prescribes inappropriate settings to which the patient reacts appropriately. This point must be recognized for the valuable clinical information given and not hidden by the reflex use of muscle relaxants.

Noncautious use of these agents may lead to clinical and emotional disaster. It is hoped that this brief discussion will have provoked clinical questions and provided some insight into the appropriate use of muscle relaxants and sedatives in critical care practice.

ANALGESIA

There are a number of reasons for ensuring that the critically ill patient receives adequate analgesia.[27] Pain in the postoperative patient stimulates catechol release, and the high circulating levels increase the overall as well as individual organ metabolic demands and contribute to clinically important increases in blood pressure and heart rate. Those patients with compromised myocardial function may be especially vulnerable to the associated hypertension or tachycardia. Additionally, pain increases overall oxygen demands.

Reduction of pain awareness contributes to patient ambulation and ultimate recovery. Early activity minimizes the risk of other complications such as pulmonary embolism. The ability to cough, turn, and deep breathe adequately enhances mobilization of secretions and reduces the incidence of pulmonary complications such as atelectasis and pneumonia.

Finally, patient well-being and humaneness both imply the provision of adequate analgesia. Today, our strategy has been completely revised from earlier plans, which minimized medication, particularly narcotics, for fear of habituation. Today, we recognize that adequate pain relief during critical illness does not lead to drug dependency and is a vital and integral part of the recovery process.

Several different routes are available for analgesic delivery. These include intermittent intravenous and intramuscular injection, continuous intravenous infusion, epidural and intrathecal administration, and patient-controlled analgesia (PCA) pump. For the critically ill patient in an ICU, intramuscular use of narcotics seems totally unwarranted given the fact that almost every patient will have adequate intravenous access. Intermittent medication taken as occasion requires provided by the nurse on patient request today seems ancient and out of place within modern critical care practice. Perhaps for non-narcotic analgesics such as ketorolac, intermittent intravenous or intramuscular administration may be justified.

Ketorolac represents one of the few non-narcotic analgesics that actually works. Ketorolac can ordinarily be given in 30- to 60-mg dosages either intravenously or intramuscularly.[28] The agent can interfere with platelet aggregation. Therefore, the dosages may need to be adjusted or the drug entirely eliminated when thrombocytopenia develops or when an increased risk to bleeding exists.

Continuous or basal narcotic infusion has continued to gain favor in the critical care environment. This method provides excellent ongoing pain relief. It requires less direct nursing involvement except observation for complications. Basal infusions can be used to supplement PCA or epidural analgesia. This is a particularly desirable route of administration for the patient maintained on mechanical ventilation. Because of the back-up from the mechanical ventilator, the clinician may have less concern about cumulative dosage and resultant respiratory depression.

The two different agents most commonly used for continuous infusion are morphine and fentanyl or derivatives such as alfentanil or sufentanil. In our opinion, morphine remains a mainstay of intravenous therapy because of its reliable analgesic properties. Ordinarily, in the average-sized individual, dosages may range from 0.5 mg per hour to as high as 4 to 6 mg per hour. In our practice, the dosages are usually between 2 and 4 mg per hour. Because of its reliable respiratory depressant effects, mainly centering on reduction of rate, morphine can be used to aid in the mechanical ventilatory support of the patient in respiratory failure. The reduction in spontaneous rate during mechanical ventilation may promote better distribution of gases and overall enhancement of gas exchange.

The fat solubility of fentanyl implies its rapid uptake and usage. Therefore, as opposed to the water-soluble morphine, it is less likely to accumulate and fewer problems will potentially develop. In general, during continuous infusion, rates up to 1.25 μg per hour of fentanyl can provide good to excellent analgesia and not result in any significant respiratory depression.

Epidural analgesia can provide excellent pain relief. This is particularly so after various operative procedures or blunt trauma to the chest. Analgesia is usually maintained by continuous or intermittent infusion depending on the specific agent. However, some clinicians have had success with patient control of the drug injection. Patient control of dosages is much like that with intravenous PCA.

The epidural catheter is usually placed at the lumbar level L2–4 or the thoracic level T6–10. Lumbar administration will provide adequate pain relief for most abdominal and thoracic surgical procedures.[29–31] Thoracic area pain relief may require somewhat larger dosages than does abdominal pain relief.

The uptake and distribution of epidural narcotics help explain the analgesia at a site distant from placement of the agent.[32] Mechanisms of action include interaction directly on the μ receptors present in the spinal cord. Migration of the analgesic along nerve routes of the central nervous system offers another explanation. Once into the cerebrospinal fluid (CSF), migration continues to the brain. Sufficient evidence exists to support intravenous uptake of the agents at the site of the epidural injection. Thoracic epidural analgesia at the T6–10 level can provide adequate pain relief after chest surgery or blunt injuries to the chest, resulting in either fractured ribs or a flail chest. The method can also be beneficial for some patients requiring tube thoracostomy.[33–36]

The narcotics used for epidural analgesia include morphine, fentanyl, and derivatives such as alfentanil and sufentanil.[37, 38] The fat solubility of fentanyl favors continuous infusion. The water solubility of morphine better lends itself to intermittent administration. However, in small dosages, the drug can be administered by continuous infusion. Ordinarily, fentanyl dosages up to 1 μ/kg per hour will provide adequate analgesia without significant respiratory depression. When morphine is chosen, bolus administration of preservative-free drug of 4 to 6 mg every 8 to 24 hours usually proves to be adequate. For continuous infusion, most adults of average size will tolerate dosages of 0.1 to 0.5 mg per hour. Because of the large potential volume of the epidural space, the drugs must be mixed in sufficient volume to have effective action. Ordinarily, morphine is in 1 mg/mL and fentanyl in 5.0 μ/mL concentrations.

Supplements such as local anesthetics are often added to the epidural infusion, particularly with fentanyl. Such additives reduce the overall drug requirements while still providing excellent analgesia. The most often used local anesthetic is bupivacaine. It is usually delivered in concentrations of ⅛% to 1⁄16%. At such dosages, the local anesthetics are able to block the smaller sensory pain fibers and yet have little effect on the much larger motor fibers. Patients so treated are still able to maintain ambulation and not experience the paralysis common when local anesthetics are used to provide operative analgesia.

Epidural catheters can be left in place for variable amounts of time. In general, most clinicians advise removal between 3 and 7 days. However, there are a number of reports of catheters being left in place for at least 2 weeks. Furthermore, patients on home infusion analgesia may have catheters in place for substantially longer periods of time. The risk of infection at the wound site can be minimized by treating such catheters in the manner similar to that for intravenous hyperalimentation catheters. This approach includes dressing changes on a regular basis by teams well versed in sterile technique.

Common complications of epidural analgesia include nausea, vomiting, pruritus, and urinary retention. The incidence varies between 20% and 50% in most series and relates to the actual drug dosage.[39] Although most concerns are related to respiratory depression, the overall incidence is extremely low (approximately 1%).[40–42] Other concerns include inadvertent penetration of the dura at the time of catheter placement. Drug introduction into the epidural space at the same level can migrate through the hole and into the CSF. When inserted via the needle, the epidural catheter can penetrate the dura, resulting in drug administration into the subarachnoid space. Catheters can also be inadvertently placed in a vessel in the epidural space; consequently, unwanted intravenous infusion may occur. Both problems can be best detected by intermittent aspiration of the catheter to ensure that neither the clear CSF nor blood is present in the catheter. If so, usage of the catheter should be immediately discontinued.

Anticoagulation is a contraindication to epidural catheter placement. There is considerable variation of opinion regarding the removal of catheters in patients who are subsequently anticoagulated after placement of the catheter. Several large patient series suggest that this is a minimal problem.[43–45] However, many clinicians who anticipate anticoagulation after catheter placement will refrain from such therapy.

Patients should be monitored for levels of sedation during analgesic treatment with epidural narcotics. Dosages should be adjusted accordingly. Because pain relief remains a major goal, the patient needs to be evaluated for both subjective pain relief and the response of such vital signs as HR and blood pressure to pain. Although the incidence of respiratory depression remains low, its development can have serious ramifications. Respiratory rate will be depressed. However, most monitors, other than direct observation, may provide only a false sense of security. Pulse oximetry may be used to detect respiratory depression, but this technique requires a continuously low baseline oxygen saturation. The modality relies on the accumulation of carbon dioxide to displace oxygen further in the alveoli, resulting in greater decrease in the oxygen saturation. Accordingly, the patient must be maintained at a level of oxygenation close to the shoulder of the oxyhemoglobin dissociation curve. Apnea monitors may also be used. However, an obstructed patient may have substantial chest movements that the apnea monitor may confirm as respiratory efforts but which, in fact, underlie upper airway obstruction. Nasal cannula may be used to monitor expired carbon dioxide. However, most patients seem to have major difficulties maintaining the nasal cannula in the appropriate location.

Recently, interest has developed in non-narcotic agents for epidural administration pain relief. Clonidine has been advocated most often. This α_2-adrenergic agonist can provide pain relief and can probably reduce overall narcotic requirements.[46]

Intrathecal drug administration has had limited use as a means of providing pain relief in the critically ill. However, the technique works quite well and requires smaller dosages and volumes than in epidural delivery.[47] Almost always, placement is via the lumbar approach. Placement below L2–3 avoids any inadvertent damage to the spinal cord, which ends at L1–2. The majority of experience has been obtained with the use of morphine in dosages of 0.25 to 1.25 mg in single-dose administration. Infection of the subarachnoid space may result in severe complications. Therefore, the duration of catheter placement, if used at all, is usually less than that described for epidural catheters.

Other complications of intrathecal administration include respiratory depression secondary to rapid movement of agents into the brain CSF. Monitoring techniques are similar to those described for the use of epidural narcotics. Ordinarily, local anesthetics are not added to intrathecal infusions of morphine.

PCA is another major mainstay of analgesic administration in critically ill patients.[48, 49] The technique appeals to most patients. It is obviously less invasive than epidural or intrathecal administration of agents. However, it does require that the patient be able to at least grasp the concept. Perhaps one of the greatest problems involves patients not attempting to push the button at the first sign of discomfort but rather waiting too long. This waiting results in uneven drug levels and can contribute to some of the problems such as hypertension and tachycardia that the analgesia is intended to prevent.

Because of the intermittent nature of the technique, morphine best lends itself to such therapy. Patients can obviously be maintained for indefinite periods of time. Overdosage is a potential complication. At times, this has developed because of overzealous friends or family members who activate the pump while visiting. Pump failure could result in a runaway pump and overdosage or failure to deliver any drug at all. Drug accumulation can occur and, as a result, respiratory depression may also develop.

When ordering a PCA pump, the clinician usually specifies the dosage and the interval between dosages (lockout time) during which, despite repeated activation of the pump button, no drug will be received by the patient. The orders usually include a cumulative dose that the patient will receive over an extended period of time, usually 4 to 6 hours. In general, for most adults, morphine can be administered in 1.0- to 1.5-mg doses, with a 6-minute lockout time. This would result in a dosage schedule of 10 to 15 mg per hour. It is rare that patients, after the first hour or two, use anywhere near the upper limits of the drug allowed by the ordering methods.

Clinicians should be regularly apprised of both the amounts of drug that the patient has received and the frequency of pump utilization. Multiple attempted activations of the pump may indicate inadequate analgesia by the current prescription or patient misunderstanding of the entire concept.

Intrapleural analgesia has been used to a limited extent. Local anesthesia such as 0.5% bupivacaine can be instilled through either a chest tube or a catheter placed for such a purpose. It appears to have a direct effect on pain fibers in the chest wall and ultimately on the neural sheath below each rib. Up to 20 mL may be required to provide analgesia. The adequacy of pain relief can be affected by position as the fluid moves in the chest. The response tends to remain unpredictable.[50]

SEDATION

There are several indications for sedation of critically ill patients. Overall, sedation can reduce stress, resulting in decreased individual organ and total body oxygen requirements. This result will promote return of vital signs to normal ranges with a concomitant reduction in myocardial oxygen requirements. Appropriate sedation can better enable the patient to tolerate the critical care environment, particularly mechanical ventilation, invasive procedures, and the overall milieu. Sedation is also a mainstay of the therapy for withdrawal syndrome, which may be part of the ongoing patient care. Finally, the judicious use of sedatives will generally result in amnesia for most of the patient's stay in the ICU. Those patients who require paralysis during mechanical ventilation also should be sedated if there is any indication of awareness of the situation. A judicious use of sedatives will also reduce the overall amount of analgesics given because clinicians often order dosages large enough to also provide sedation along with pain relief.

When sedatives are ordered, both the physician and the nurse should be clear on the desired end points. To that end, sedation scales have been introduced.[51] These scales provide a range of levels from relatively deep sedation to extreme agitation. Various clinical situations will require different levels of sedation. Because the defined levels can be interpreted differently, the definitions should be understandable to all who care for the patient.

As with analgesics, it seems that there are few if any indications for the use of intramuscular administration for the critically ill patient having multiple sources of intravenous access. Some patients may require only an intermittent, irregular administration of a sedative. An example might be for a specific invasive procedure. Other patients, because of the nature of their underlying illness or during a recovery phase from anesthesia, may require sedation only at a specific time, such as manipulation of the patient while in the bed, chest physiotherapy, bathing, or the like. The unsteady state of other patients may lend themselves only to intermittent administration.

For those patients anticipated to require long-term sedation, continuous infusion may be the preferred method. This will allow maintenance of a steady state. However, deep sedation may mask the onset of neurologic changes. Therefore, in such patients, short-acting agents may enhance rapid return to the individual baseline state. Long-term administration may result in accumulation of either the primary agent or its metabolites, again prolonging the recovery phase.

Today, benzodiazepines remain a mainstay of sedation therapy for critically ill patients. The most commonly used drugs are lorazepam and midazolam.[52, 53] These drugs can be administered by either continuous or intermittent infusion. Dosages range from 0.01 to 1.0 mg/kg per hour for midazolam to 0.1 to 2.0 mg per hour for lorazepam. To date, most data suggest minimal impact on cardiovascular function with both lorazepam and midazolam. In higher concentrations both drugs can suppress respiration, blood pressure, and cardiac output. Discontinuation of continuous infusions of midazolam generally allows return to baseline states within 30 to 40 minutes. Lorazepam has a half-life of 4 to 8 hours, and discontinuation may not result in rapid recovery.

Recently, a benzodiazepine-competitive antagonist (flumazenil) has become available. The agent may be administered as a single dose or by continuous infusion.[54, 55] Major benefits appear to be reversal of benzodiazepine overdose and a return to baseline state for other clinical reasons. Compared with the agents it is intended to reverse, flumazenil has a relatively short duration of action. Therefore, it may require either continuous infusion or frequent readministration of a single-bolus dose. It is recommended that flumazenil not be administered to patients on long-term benzodiazepine therapy for fear of untoward reactions.

Propofol is a nonbenzodiazepine sedative. The drug is also used in the operating room for induction technique as part of the administration of anesthesia. Because of its water insolubility, the drug is prepared in a lipid emulsion. Propofol elimination relies on liver blood flow and the ability to be rapidly conjugated by the liver.[56–59] Only in severe liver disease would any accumulation be expected. The drug can have significant vasodilating properties of which the clinician should be aware. However, once a steady state is reached, this is no longer a problem. The usual dosage is between 0.2 and 0.4 mg/kg per hour.

Thiopental sodium (Pentothal) and etomidate are also anesthetic induction agents that can be used to provide short-term sedation.[60] These agents are generally used for various procedures such as an intubation. Their effects are rapidly dissipated within 3 to 5 minutes. In the case of thiopental sodium, this involves redistribution in the fatty tissues. Etomidate has primarily hepatic clearance. Whereas thiopental sodium can result in hypotension, etomidate has minimal effects on blood pressure or the cardiovascular system.[61] Sodium thiopental is usually administered in dosages of 50- to 75-mg increments. Etomidate can be administered in 10-mg increments. Large dosages (>80 mg) or prolonged administration can result in significant clonus. These agents are not intended for long-term continuous infusion.

Haloperidol decanoate (Haldol), a butyrophenone, has been used for sedation in the elderly. After several days in the ICU, elderly patients may experience a disorientation syndrome, particularly in the evening. This effect often results in severe agitation, including attempts to remove catheters, and, if not intubated, loud vocalization. Intermittent dosages of haloperidol decanoate, 1 to 2 mg every 4 to 6 hours, seem to work quite well in this group to relieve the agitation.

References

1. Standaert FG: Basic Physiology and pharmacology of the neuromuscular junction. *In*: Anesthesia. 2nd ed. Vol 2. Miller RD (Ed). New York, Churchill Livingstone, 1986.
2. Ali HH, Miller RD: Monitoring of neuromuscular function. *In*: Anesthesia. 2nd ed. Vol 2. Miller RD (Ed). New York, Churchill Livingstone, 1986.
3. Miller RD, Savarese JJ: Pharmacology of muscle relaxants and their antagonists. *In*: Anesthesia. 2nd ed. Vol 2. Miller RD (Ed.). New York, Churchill Livingstone, 1986.
4. Physicians' Desk Reference. 42nd ed. Oradell, NJ, Medical Economics Company, 1988, p 1491.

4a. Zemuron (rocuronium bromide) package insert. West Orange, NJ, Oraganon, Incorporated, March 1994.

5. Physicians' Desk Reference. 45th ed. Oradell, NJ, Medical Economics Company, 1991, p 803.
6. Merrett RA, Thompson CW, Webb FW: In vitro degradation of atracurium in human plasma. Br J Anaesth 1983; 55:61–66.
7. Physicians' Desk Reference. 45th ed. Oradell, NJ, Medical Economics Company, 1991, p 1585.
8. Mirakhur RK: Muscle relaxation with an infusion of vecuronium. Anesthesiology 1984; 61:A293.
9. Nuromax (doxacurium chloride) package insert. Research Triangle Park, NC, Burroughs Wellcome Company, March 1991.
10. Arduan (pipercuronium bromide) package insert. West Orange, NJ, Organon Incorporated, June 1990.
11. Driks MR, Craven DE, Celli BR, et al: Nosocomial pneumonia in intubated patients given sucralfate as compared with antacids or histamine type H-2 blockers: The role of gastric colonization. N Eng J Med 1987; 317:1376–1382.
12. Hutchins WW, Vogelzang RL, Fuld IL, et al: Utilization of temporary muscle paralysis to eliminate CT motion artifact in the critically ill patient. J Comput Assist Tomogr 1984; 8:181–183.
13. Trauner DA: What is the best treatment for Reye's syndrome? Arch Neurol 1986; 43:729–731.
14. Penn F, Shalhoub R, Lisby-Sutch S, et al: Continuous vecuronium infusions for sustained skeletal muscle relaxation in two pediatric patients. Presented at the 45th Annual Meeting of the American Society of Hospital Pharmacists, San Francisco, June 1988.
15. Hamza J, Macquin I, Wood C, et al: Cardiovascular effects of vecuronium vs. pancuronium in preemies with hyaline membrane disease. Anesthesiology 1984; 67:A515.
16. Smith CL, Hunter JM, Jones RS: Vecuronium infusions in patients with renal failure in an ITU. Anaesthesia 1987; 42:387–393.
17. Griffiths RB, Hunter JM, Jones RS: Atracurium infusions in patients with renal failure in an ITU. Anaesthesia 1986; 41:375–381.
18. Hunter JM: Infusions of atracurium and vecuronium in patients with multisystem organ failure in the intensive therapy unit. Insights Anaesthesiol 1987; 1:23–27.
19. Patel P, Bristow G: Postoperative neuroleptic malignant syndrome: A case report. Can J Anaesth 1987; 34:515–518.
20. Powles AB, Ganta R: Use of vecuronium in the management of tetanus. Anaesthesia 1985; 40:879–881.
21. Stark AR, Bascom R, Frantz ID III: Muscle relaxation in mechanically ventilated infants. J Pediatr 1979; 94:439–443.
22. Heizmann P, Eckert M, Ziegler WH: Pharmacokinetics and bioavailability of midazolam in man. Br J Clin Pharmacol 1983; 16:9S–43S.
23. Dundee JW, Halliday NJ, Harper KW, et al: Midazolam: A review of its pharmacological properties and therapeutic use. Drugs 1984; 28:519–543.
24. Oldenhof H, deJong M, Steenhoek A, et al: Clinical pharmacokinetics of midazolam in intensive care patients: A wide interpatient variability? Clin Pharmacol Ther 1988; 43:263–269.
25. Persson MP, Nilsson A, Hartvig P: Relation of sedation and

amnesia to plasma concentrations of midazolam in surgical patients. Clin Pharmacol Ther 1988; 43:324–331.
26. Physicians' Desk Reference. 45th ed. Oradell, NJ, Medical Economics Company, 1991, pp 1090, 1094.
27. Coleman DL: Control of postoperative pain: Nonnarcotic and narcotic alternatives and their effect on pulmonary function. Chest 1987; 92:520–528.
28. Grass JA, Sakima NT, Valley M, et al: Assessment of ketorolac as an adjuvant to fentanyl patient-controlled epidural analgesia after radical retropubic prostatectomy. Anesthesiology 1993; 78:642–648.
29. Chaplan SR, Duncan SR, Brodsky JB, et al: Morphine and hydromorphone epidural analgesia: A prospective, randomized comparison. Anesthesiology 1992; 77:1090–1094.
30. Glass PAS, Estok P, Ginsberg B, et al: Use of patient-controlled analgesia to compare the efficacy of epidural to intravenous fentanyl administration. Anesth Analg 1992; 74:345–351.
31. Fischer RL, Lubenow TR, Liceaga A, et al: Comparison of continuous epidural infusion of fentanyl-bupivacaine and morphine-bupivacaine in management of postoperative pain. Anesth Analg 1988; 67:559–563.
32. Dahl JB, Rosenberg J, Hansen BL, et al: Differential analgesic effects of low-dose epidural morphine and morphine-bupivacaine at rest and during mobilization after major abdominal surgery. Anesth Analg 1992; 75:362–365.
33. Guinard JP, Mavrocordatos P, Chiolero R, et al: A randomized comparison of intravenous versus lumbar and thoracic epidural fentanyl for analgesia after thoracotomy. Anesthesiology 1992; 77:1108–1115.
34. Cicala RS, Voeller GR, Fox T, et al: Epidural analgesia in thoracic trauma: Effects of lumbar morphine and thoracic bupivacaine on pulmonary function. Crit Care Med 1990; 18:229–231.
35. Whiting WC, Sandler AN, Lau LC, et al: Analgesic and respiratory effects of epidural sufentanil in patients following thoracotomy. Anesthesiology 1988; 69:36–43.
36. Benzon HT, Wong HY, Belavic AM Jr, et al: A randomized double-blind comparison of epidural fentanyl infusion versus patient-controlled analgesia with morphine for postthoracotomy pain. Anesth Analg 1993; 76:316–322.
37. Geller E, Chrubasik J, Graf R, et al: A randomized double-blind comparison of epidural sufentanil versus intravenous sufentanil or epidural fentanyl analgesia after major abdominal surgery. Anesth Analg 1993; 76:1243–1250.
38. Chauvin M, Hongnat JM, Mourgeon E, et al: Equivalence of postoperative analgesia with patient-controlled intravenous or epidural alfentanil. Anesth Analg 1993; 76:1251–1258.
39. Bronage PR, Camporesi EM, Durant PAC, et al: Nonrespiratory side effects of epidural morphine. Anesth Analg 1982; 61:490–495.
40. Jayr C, Thomas H, Rey A, et al: Postoperative pulmonary complications: Epidural analgesia using bupivacaine and opioids versus parenteral opioids. Anesthesiology 1993; 78:666–676.
41. Renaud B, Brichant JF, Clergue F, et al: Ventilatory effects of continuous epidural infusion of fentanyl. Anesth Analg 1988; 67:971–975.
42. Ready LB, Loper KA, Nessly M, et al: Postoperative epidural morphine is safe on surgical wards. Anesthesiology 1991; 75:452–456.
43. Odoom JA, SIH IL: Epidural analgesia and anticoagulant therapy. Anaesthesia 1983; 38:254–259.
44. Baron HC, LaRaja RD, Rossi G, et al: Continuous epidural analgesia in the heparinized vascular surgical patient: A retrospective review of 912 patients. J Vasc Surg 1987; 6:144–146.
45. Rao TLK, El-Etr AA: Anticoagulation following placement of epidural and subarachnoid catheters: An evaluation of neurologic sequelae. Anesthesiology 1981; 55:618–620.
46. Bonnet F, Boico O, Rostaing S, et al: Clonidine-induced analgesia in postoperative patients: Epidural versus intramuscular administration. Anesthesiology 1990; 72:423–427.
47. Neustein SM, Cohen E: Intrathecal morphine during thoracotomy: Part II. Effect on postoperative meperidine requirements and pulmonary function tests. J Cardiothorac Vasc Anesth 1993; 7:157–159.
48. Sechzer PH: Patient-controlled analgesia (PCA): A retrospective. Anesthesiology 1990; 72:735–736.
49. Parker RK, Holtmann B, White PF: Patient-controlled analgesia: Does a concurrent opioid infusion improve pain management after surgery? JAMA 1991; 266:1947–1952.
50. Reistad F, Stromskag KE: Intrapleural catheter in the management of postoperative pain. Reg Anesth 1986; 11:89–90.
51. Ramsey MAE, Savage TM, Simpson BRJ, et al: Controlled sedation with alphaxolone/alphadolone. Br Med J 1974; 2:656–659.
52. Reves JG, Fragen RJ, Vinik HR, et al: Midazolam: Pharmacology and uses. Anesthesiology 1985; 62:310–324.
53. Bailey PL, Pace NL, Ashburn MA, et al: Frequent hypoxemia and apnea after sedation with midazolam and fentanyl. Anesthesiology 1990; 73:826–830.
54. Winkler E, Almog S, Kriger D, et al: Use of flumazenil in the diagnosis and treatment of patient with coma of unknown etiology. Crit Care Med 1993; 21:538–542.
55. Blouin RT, Conard PF, Perreault S, et al: The effect of flumazenil on midazolam-induced depression of the ventilatory response to hypoxia during isohypercarbia. Anesthesiology 1993; 78:635–641.
56. Carrasco G, Molin R, Costa J, et al: Propofol vs midazolam in short-, medium- and long-term sedation of critically ill patients: A cost-benefit analysis. Chest 1993; 103:557–564.
57. Harris CE, Grounds RM, Murray AM, et al: Propofol for long-term sedation in the intensive care unit: A comparison with papaveretum and midazolam. Anaesthesia 1990; 45:366–372.
58. McMurray TJ, Collier PS, Carson IW, et al: Propofol sedation after open heart surgery: A clinical and pharmacokinetic study. Anaesthesia 1990; 45:322–326.
59. Cooks P: Propofol as a sole agent for prolonged infusion in intensive care. J Drug Dev 1989; 2:65–67.
60. Mayer N, Legat K, Weinstabl C, et al: Effects of propofol on the function of normal, collateral-dependent and ischemic myocardium. Anesth Analg 1993; 76:33–39.
61. White PF: What's new in intravenous anesthetics? Anesth Clin North Am 1988; 6:297–318.

CHAPTER 129

Drug Abuse, Overdose, and Withdrawal Syndromes

Sidney H. Schnoll, MD, PhD

Drug abuse poses a significant problem for society and the healthcare system. Although it is recognized as a medical problem, drug abuse retains the stigma of a moral problem or lack of will by the abuser. The misconceptions about drug abuse persist despite mounting evidence from both animal and human studies that genetics play a significant role in the cause of addiction.[1]

Healthcare professionals, especially physicians, tend to ignore the problem because of the lack of medical education regarding treatment of drug abuse. This lack of education has led to an inordinate fear of addiction and more comfort dealing with the acute medical sequelae associated with addiction rather than the addiction itself. It is currently estimated that drug abuse, including alcoholism, costs our society more than $140 billion a year, with some of that cost related to admission to critical care facilities.[2] These costs are exclusive of the costs associated with tobacco use. A recent study of intensive care unit admissions found that 28% were related to substance abuse, and these admissions accounted for more than 39% of the costs. The substance abuse–related admissions also had significantly longer lengths of stay.[3]

This chapter addresses the medical sequelae of drug ad-

TABLE 129–1. Definitions

Addiction: a chronic disorder characterized by compulsive use of drugs (craving) resulting in physical, psychologic, and social harm and continued use despite evidence of that harm (denial).
Dependence: an adaptation at the cellular level to drugs such that when the drug is removed there is a characteristic set of signs and symptoms called the *withdrawal syndrome.*
Cross-dependence: the development of dependence to a drug to which the patient has never been exposed because of exposure to a drug to which dependence developed.
Abuse: the use of an illicit drug or the use of a licit drug outside of legitimate medical practice.
Tolerance: an adaptation at the cellular level to the presence of a drug such that more drug is needed to achieve the desired effect.
Cross-tolerance: the development of tolerance to a drug to which the patient has never been exposed because it contains similar characteristics to a drug for which tolerance has developed.
Withdrawal: the gradual reduction in the amount of drug given to an individual who is dependent to reduce the severity of the withdrawal syndrome (abstinence syndrome).
Detoxification: the clearance of a drug from the body through metabolic and excretory mechanisms.
Multiple drug use: the use or abuse of more than one drug simultaneously, sequentially, or inadvertently.
Recovery program: the steps taken by an individual in the treatment of the addiction; this may include formal treatment such as individual or group therapy and informal treatment such as 12-step programs

diction and abuse, with emphasis on the acute problems of intoxication and withdrawal and how they should be treated in the critical care setting. Despite this focus on the acute issues, it must be stressed that, although the acute care problems are being treated, it is time to begin to address the long-term treatment of addiction.

Several definitions are important to comprehend the scope of the problem (Table 129–1). The critical issues to remember regarding addiction are the chronicity, the consequences, and the failure to recognize the severity of those consequences. Dependence occurs with and without addiction and is not a problem, except that the patient must be gradually withdrawn from the drugs to reduce the possibility of producing a withdrawal syndrome. Abuse of drugs can exist independently from both addiction and dependence and is more common than addiction and dependence.

When treating patients who are suffering the consequences of addiction or abuse, as in any other medical condition, the patient must be treated in a nonjudgmental and confidential atmosphere. Because of the understanding by the federal government that confidentiality must be maintained for patients to seek treatment, very stringent laws have been developed regarding confidentiality with drug abusers. It is impossible in this chapter to discuss in detail these laws, but it is strongly recommended that, should questions arise, one should contact the hospital attorney or a drug abuse program to learn more about these laws. Concern about legal issues should never deter one from adequately treating the patient. Because of the patient's fears of legal reprisals, it is often necessary to bring in significant others who can provide you with important information. It is vital, however, to make sure that releases are signed, if possible, to gather the information.

Despite all the problems associated with drug abuse and the concerns about treating it, it is a highly treatable disorder. As a chronic disease, there is no cure, but effective treatment can significantly alter the course of addiction and result in changes in the person's lifestyle. However, like any other chronic disorder, addiction is characterized by remissions and exacerbations; when an exacerbation occurs, rather than blame the patient for recurrence of the illness, treatment should be intensified.

Early intervention into the problems of addiction results in better outcome. Failure to initiate treatment for the addiction results in progression of the illness, which is often fatal. It is erroneously assumed by many physicians that simply withdrawing the patient from the drugs of abuse is sufficient treatment. This is treatment for the dependence and not treatment for the addiction. Treatment for the addiction is a long-term process, often being quite intense in the first few weeks or months with lesser intensity over time depending on the progress that the patient makes.

EPIDEMIOLOGY

Although the exact prevalence of addiction in the population is not known, a study of nearly 20,000 adults found a lifetime prevalence of alcoholism of 13.5% and a lifetime prevalence of other drug abuse of 6.1%.[4] These prevalence rates are exclusive of nicotine dependence. In hospitalized patients, it is estimated that, at any time, between 25% and 40% are suffering from problems of alcohol and other drug addiction and are hospitalized because of medical sequelae of the addiction.[5] These percentages may be even higher in inner-city and in Veterans Administration hospitals.

All segments of the population are at risk, and addiction is surely an equal opportunity disorder. However, use of drugs is most prevalent in the 18- to 25-year age group and then tapers off.[6] Recent evidence indicates that women are also at high risk for addiction.[7] Because genetics plays an important role in the risk for addiction, certain ethnic groups may be at higher risk than others. Individuals from Scandinavian and Irish backgrounds have been shown to be at higher risk for alcoholism as have some tribes of Native Americans. Therefore, a history of alcohol or drug abuse in the family places the patient at high risk.

Because of the intoxicating nature of the drugs, individuals who use them are at high risk for trauma. This fact frequently brings them into hospitals, where they may wind up in critical care settings. In some institutions, as many as 70% of the patients presenting with trauma are intoxicated at the time of the traumatic event.[8] More than 60% of spinal cord injuries occur in persons who have ingested intoxicating substances.[9] Drug use is a major risk factor in human immunodeficiency (HIV) infection, and currently in some cities more than 50% of new HIV infections are in individuals who are injection drug users (IDUs) or have had sexual relations with IDUs. This group is also at higher risk for tuberculosis and other infectious diseases.[10]

The most common pattern of drug use is multiple drug use. This creates significant problems for the clinician because of the mixed picture of intoxications and the need to handle multiple withdrawals. Therefore, it is important to define to the greatest extent possible all the drugs that an individual has been using, including licit, illicit, and over-the-counter substances. Table 129–2 lists the most common patterns of drug use presenting in emergency departments.[11]

CLASSES OF DRUGS INVOLVED

Almost any drug can be abused by an individual. However, the classes of drugs that cause medical or legal problems

TABLE 129–2. Distributions of Drug Mentions (%)

Drug Groups	*None*	*One*	*Two*	*Three or More*
Benzodiazepines	22.6	38.0	23.7	15.7
Narcotic analgesics	35.2	35.4	18.8	10.7
Sedative-hypnotics	34.9	35.2	15.6	14.3
Amphetamines	41.8	28.2	21.1	9.0
Hallucinogens and PCP	40.8	30.1	16.9	12.2
Alcohol in combination	—	69.2	21.2	9.6
Cocaine	42.3	42.2	11.8	3.7
Marijuana	20.0	38.1	30.8	10.7

(Based on data from National Institute of Drug Abuse.[11])
Abbreviation: PCP = phencyclidine.

TABLE 129–3. Narcotic Analgesics

Agonists	*Antagonists*	*Partial Agonists*
Morphine	Pentazocine	Buprenorphine
Methadone	Butorphanol	Dezocine
Hydromorphone	Nalbuphine	
Meperidine		
Oxycodone		
Levorphanol		
Fentanyl		

most frequently are opioids, alcohol and other sedative-hypnotics, cocaine and other psychostimulants, phencyclidine (PCP) and other arylcyclohexylamines, hallucinogens, marijuana, and volatile inhalants.

Opioids can be divided into three groups: agonists, agonist/antagonists, and partial agonists. The agonists have primary action at the μ receptor, which is the main opioid receptor involved in analgesia and are best characterized by morphine. Agonist/antagonist drugs have agonist actions and, as the dose increases, they also display antagonist actions. The prototype drug in this category is pentazocine (Talwin). Recently, partial agonist drugs have been developed that display agonist activity at lower doses but have a ceiling effect whereby increasing doses does not produce increasing levels of analgesia. This drug type is in distinction to the pure agonists that have no ceiling effect.[12] Examples of the three classes of opioid drugs are listed in Table 129–3.

Sedative-hypnotics are among the most widely prescribed drugs in the world, and all sedative-hypnotics have a very close relationship with alcohol with which they display both cross-tolerance and cross-dependence. The oldest group of prescribed sedative-hypnotic drugs is the barbiturates. Barbiturates fall into ultrashort-acting, short-acting, intermediate-acting, and long-acting groups. The ultrashort-acting, short-acting, and intermediate-acting barbiturates have a very low therapeutic index, resulting in a significant chance for overdose. An important characteristic of the barbiturates is that, as tolerance develops to the therapeutic effects of the drug, tolerance does not develop to the lethal effect of the drug at the same rate; therefore, over time with continued use, the therapeutic index decreases.[13]

Barbiturates have been replaced to a large extent with the benzodiazepines. The benzodiazepines and their characteristics are listed in Table 129–4. As with the barbiturates, the benzodiazepines now are available in ultrashort-acting, short-acting, and longer acting preparations. This provides greater flexibility in their use. For the most part, the benzodiazepines have an extremely high therapeutic index and, therefore, are safer to use than the barbiturates and other nonbarbiturate sedative-hypnotics.[14]

Alcohol is the most widely used of all the sedative-hypnotics. Alcohol shows cross-tolerance and cross-dependence with all the other sedative-hypnotic drugs and has an extremely low therapeutic index. Other nonbarbiturate and nonbenzodiazepine sleeping pills are available but are not used widely. They all show cross-tolerance and dependence with the other sedative-hypnotic drugs.

Both the opioids and the sedative-hypnotics produce intoxication, dependence, and tolerance, and when stopped abruptly they can produce withdrawal syndromes. Of significance is the fact that the opioid withdrawal syndrome, although uncomfortable, rarely produces discomfort beyond that of a bad case of flu. However, the sedative-hypnotic withdrawal syndrome can result in status epilepticus and a major withdrawal syndrome (delirium tremens, or DTs) that can produce severe autonomic dysfunction leading to death if not adequately treated.[15]

Epidemics of amphetamine and other psychostimulant use have occurred periodically in the United States. The most recent epidemic has been related to the use of cocaine in the smokable form, known as free base or crack. Psychostimulants cause marked excitation of the central nervous system, resulting in hyperactivity, seizures, and increased blood pressure. Cocaine is unique among the psychostimulants in that, besides its stimulant activity, it has properties of a local anesthetic. All of the psychostimulants show cross-tolerance and cross-dependence with one another and, when administered in a blind fashion to users, are indistinguishable.[16]

PCP is the prototypic arylcyclohexylamine. It was devel-

TABLE 129–4. Benzodiazepines

Drug	*Latency*	*Active Metabolite*	*Half-Life (Hours)*
Alprazolam	Intermediate	Yes	12–15
Chlordiazepoxide	Intermediate	Yes	5–30
Clonazepam	Fast	No	18–50
Clorazepate	Fast	Yes	36–200
Diazepam*	Fast	Yes	20–50
Flurazepam	Intermediate	Yes	40–150
Halazepam	Intermediate	Yes	50–100
Lorazepam*	Intermediate	No	10–14
Midazolam*	Ultrafast	No	1–2
Oxazepam	Slow	No	5–10
Prazepam	Slow	Yes	36–200
Temazepam	Intermediate	Yes	8–12
Triazolam	Intermediate	No	2–5

*Available in parenteral form.

oped as a general anesthetic but, because of its epileptogenic properties and psychotic-like sequelae, was withdrawn from the market. Although the popularity of these drugs waxes and wanes, there are still pockets of significant use, particularly in the Los Angeles area and in Washington, D.C. PCP is often a contaminant found in other street drugs, and, because of the ease with which it is manufactured, numerous analogs have been produced and are also found on the street. Because of PCP's binding to the *N*-methyl-D-aspartate receptor, it has recently become an important tool in the study of that receptor's actions.[17]

The hallucinogens and marijuana and its derivatives, although popular drugs of abuse, do not cause problems that would be important in the critical care setting.

It was previously believed that volatile inhalants were primarily used by preadolescents before they had access to other drugs. However, these ubiquitous compounds are used not only by preadolescents but also by adults who have become exposed to them in industrial settings. When used chronically, because of their toxic nature, damage to the liver, kidneys, and other organs can occur. The volatile inhalants are closely related to general anesthetics and show properties similar to the sedative-hypnotics.[18]

Because many abused drugs are sold on the illicit market, even those that may have legitimate medical use, it is not always possible to use our knowledge of the pharmacology of the pure drug when it comes to treating problems associated with street drugs. The street drug market is highly volatile and often creates its own set of problems. When purchasing a street drug, one is not always sure what is being purchased. Over the years, analyses of street drugs have demonstrated that, in more than 50% of cases, individuals may not get the drug they thought they were purchasing. Besides the problem of deception, there is no consistency in dose or purity. To increase their profits, drug dealers often cut their drugs with other substances. These can be other drugs that produce effects similar to or different than those of the drug the person was buying or inert substances that are added to bulk up the material. These contaminants, both drugs and nondrugs, can have their own side effects. If insoluble materials are used to bulk up drugs that are used intravenously, showers of emboli can go to the lungs and other organs. In addition, there can be significant interactions between the various drugs used to cut street drugs.[19]

The most significant factor increasing morbidity and mortality associated with drug use is route of administration. Infectious diseases are frequently associated with intravenous administration of drugs, and the threat of acquired immunodeficiency syndrome has resulted in a move away from intravenous use to smoking or snorting drugs. It is important to keep these problems associated with street drugs in mind when treating overdose or withdrawal problems in a street drug user.

Besides the pharmacology of the abused drugs, it is important to understand the pharmacology of the drugs used in the treatment of withdrawal or overdose syndromes. Usually when treating withdrawal syndromes in noncritical care settings, long-acting drugs are used that show cross-tolerance to the drugs on which the patient is dependent. Long-acting drugs are used because they provide more consistent blood levels, and it has been demonstrated that the withdrawal syndrome associated with long-acting drugs is less severe than that seen with short-acting drugs. However, in the critical care setting, where conditions are changing rapidly, the use of a long-acting drug may prove to be detrimental if it is necessary to adjust dosages very rapidly. Therefore, it may be more appropriate to use continuous intravenous infusions of short-acting drugs so rapid changes in drug levels can be achieved by changing the infusion rate. In addition, the first-pass effects in the liver are avoided, eliminating the development of metabolites that may be problematic. Also, by bypassing the liver, hepatic function is not altered. Finally, it is most important to use a drug that has few interactions with other drugs, thereby reducing interactions with other therapies. In discussing the treatment of overdose and withdrawal syndromes, these pharmacologic principles are used extensively.

RECOGNITION AND DIAGNOSIS

Substance abuse is frequently overlooked in healthcare settings because clinicians are not taught how to make the diagnosis. As with any disorder, it is important to take a careful history, stressing areas that will assist in making the diagnosis, or to recognize patients who potentially will have a problem with drug use.

One of the best indicators of substance abuse problems is a history of drug abuse. As a chronic disorder, it is not uncommon to return to drug use during stressful situations. A family history of drug use is significant because genetics play an important role in addictive behavior. It is vital to go back at least two generations because the problem will often skip a generation. Individuals who associate with known drug abusers also are at high risk and frequently are involved with addicts because of their own use. There is no stereotypic addict. Addiction involves patients from all racial, ethnic, and socioeconomic backgrounds.

The physical examination is also critical in making the diagnosis. We have all been taught the stigmas of cirrhosis such as spider angiomas, rhinophyma, palmar erythema, and so on that can be helpful in recognizing the alcoholic. IDUs may have tracks over sites of intravenous injection. When injection drug use is suspected, it is important to look not only in the antecubital fossa but at other sites as well because drug users will try to hide their use and may inject in the axilla, under the tongue, in breast veins, and in the dorsal vein of the penis. In individuals who have been unable to maintain good venous access, scars and ulcers may be present from subcutaneous injection, known as *skin-popping*. To disguise track marks, drug users will often draw elaborate tattoos that incorporate the tracks. These tattoos will look homemade, but at times professional tattoos will be used to disguise the track marks.

Other signs of heavy drug use include cigarette burns on the fingers and on the chest from "nodding off" while high from the drug use. Those who snort drugs will show inflammation of the nasal mucosa, and heavy chronic users may even show perforation of the nasal septum. However, this is rare. Hepatomegaly is common from alcohol use as well as from hepatitis and other problems associated with injection drug use. Murmurs also may be found from endocarditis that develops from injecting drugs.

Alterations in consciousness may also be present from drug use. Opioids and sedative-hypnotics can cause effects from sedation to coma. They will also decrease vital signs with decreased respirations, pulse, and blood pressure. Stimulants like cocaine or amphetamines cause hyperactivity and paranoia. Physically, they produce hyperthermia, agitation, tachycardia, and hypertension. Ocular manifestations of drug use include nystagmus with sedatives and alcohol. PCP will cause both horizontal and vertical nystagmus. Opioids cause myosis and mydriasis in withdrawal except for meperidine, which produces mydriasis during intoxication. On fundoscopic examination, microemboli have been seen occluding retinal vessels. Despite good studies describing the physical findings associated with drug

TABLE 129–5. Duration of Drug Detection in Urine and Limits of Sensitivity*

Drug	*Approximate Duration of Detectability*	*Limits of Sensitivity*
Amphetamine	48 h	100 ng/mL
Methamphetamine	48 h	100 ng/mL
Barbiturates		
Short-acting		
Hexobarbital		1.0 μg/mL
Pentobarbital	24 h	100 ng/mL
Secobarbital		100 ng/mL
Intermediate-acting		
Amobarbital		1.0 μg/mL
Butabarbital	48–72 h	0.5 μg/mL
Butalbital		1.5 μg/mL
Long-acting		
Phenobarbital	7+ d	1.0 μg/mL
Benzodiazepines	3+ d†	100 ng/mL
Cocaine		
Benzoyl ecgonine	2–3 d	50 ng/mL
Ecgonine methyl ester	2–3 d	50 ng/mL
Methadone	3+ d	0.5 μg/mL
Codeine	48 h	0.5 μg/mL
Morphine (heroin)	48 h	100 ng/mL
Propoxyphene	6–48 h	0.5 μg/mL
Cannabinoids	3–21 d‡	10 ng/mL
Phencyclidine	±8 d§	10 ng/mL

(Adapted from Schnoll SH, Lewis DE: Drug screening in the workplace: Pros and cons. Semin Occupat Med 1986; 243–251, by permission of Thieme Medical Publishers.)

*Interpretation of detectability must take into account many factors: metabolism, physical condition, state of hydration, route and frequency of administration, and method of detection used.

†Therapeutic doses.

‡Dependent on frequency and chronicity of use.

§Poorly excreted in alkaline urine.

use, the presenting signs are often difficult to interpret because of the use of multiple substances that have numerous interactions. This problem makes the performance of toxicologic screens critical.

One of the best ways to confirm suspicions about drug use is through laboratory findings. Because of the high rates of trauma associated with drug use, urine toxicologic screens should be performed on all patients who present for critical care from trauma. It is wise to collect a urine toxicology on all patients presenting for critical care to anticipate patients who may later show withdrawal syndromes. If there is concern about alcohol use, blood alcohol levels can be sent or breath alcohol levels obtained. Elevations of liver enzymes, HIV infection, tuberculosis, and increased mean corpuscular volume could all be indicators of alcohol and other drug use.

For toxicology, urine screens are superior to plasma levels because the drugs are concentrated in the urine and may be present in urine when not present in the blood. With urine toxicology, there is a window of opportunity, and a negative screen does not totally rule out that the person has not used those drugs in the recent past. Table 129–5 gives information about the time after use that urine tests might remain positive for various drugs.[20]

TREATMENT OF ACUTE INTOXICATION

General Considerations

In recent years, there has been the fortunate development of specific antagonists for some of the common drugs with abuse potential. The presence of these pure antagonists has not only provided rapid reversal of intoxication but also diagnosis of the intoxicating agent. In cases of coma of unknown origin, in addition to infusion of 50% glucose, naloxone (Narcan) and flumazenil (Mazicon) should be administered intravenously to determine whether the coma is secondary to hypoglycemia or opioid or benzodiazepine intoxication.

Although intoxicated patients can become extremely agitated and at times violent, physical restraints should be avoided unless all other measures fail. Placing an intoxicated patient in restraints will only precipitate more agitation and aggressive behavior. When possible, chemical restraints should be used to control agitation and aggressive behavior.

Treatment of Opioid Intoxication

Opioid intoxication is a problem that, fortunately, can now be rapidly treated through the use of a narcotic antagonist. Naloxone has been available for close to 20 years and is an extremely safe drug that can be administered intramuscularly, subcutaneously, and intravenously in large quantities without any significant adverse effects. The signs and symptoms of opioid intoxication are listed in Table 129–6.

When administering naloxone, two important points must be kept in mind. First, naloxone is extremely short acting, its effects lasting 60 to 90 minutes. This duration of action is significantly shorter than almost all opioids except the ultrashort-acting drugs such as fentanyl and its analogs. Because of this, naloxone must be administered repeatedly or through continuous intravenous infusion to avoid relapse into coma. Second, naloxone can precipitate withdrawal in an individual who is dependent on opioids. However, this problem can be alleviated by titrating the amount of naloxone that relieves respiratory depression without precipitating withdrawal. All opioids are antagonized by naloxone including the agonist/antagonists and the partial agonists.

Treatment of Sedative-Hypnotic Intoxication

Intoxication with sedative-hypnotics in conjunction with alcohol is one of the most frequent combinations seen in the emergency department. Table 129–7 lists the signs and symptoms of overdose with sedative-hypnotic medication. The recent release of flumazenil has been an important addition for the treatment of benzodiazepine intoxication and

TABLE 129–6. Opioid Intoxication and Overdose

Signs	Depressed respirations Miotic pupils (meperidine intoxication produces mydriasis) Bradycardia Hypotension Pulmonary edema Coma
Treatment	Step 1: Secure adequate airway, maintain cardiovascular system, draw appropriate blood studies, and do not administer stimulants. Step 2: Administer naloxone, 2–4 mg IV or SC, administer 50% glucose IV, and administer flumazenil 0.2–3 mg IV or SC. This administration of multiple drugs is necessary because of the frequency of multiple drug intoxications. Step 3: Once symptoms are relieved, give the patient naloxone every 60–90 minutes or add naloxone to intravenous fluids (4 mg/L), titrating a small dose over time to a desired level of consciousness. Naloxone is short-acting, requiring repeated doses to prevent the patient from slipping back into coma.

TABLE 129–7. Sedative-Hypnotic/Alcohol Intoxication and Overdose

Signs	Loss of coordination Respiratory depression Nystagmus Depressed deep-tendon reflexes Hypotension Dysarthria Coma
Treatment	Step 1: Secure adequate airway, maintain cardiovascular system, draw appropriate blood studies, and do not administer stimulants. Step 2: Administer flumazenil, 0.2–3.0 mg IV or SC, administer 50% glucose intravenously and administer naloxone, 2–4 mg IV or SC. This administration of multiple drugs is necessary because of multiple drug intoxications. Step 3: If the patient responds to flumazenil, give repeated doses every 30–60 minutes because most benzodiazepines are longer acting than flumazenil. Flumazenil can be added to intravenous fluids to titrate level of consciousness. Step 4: Because most sedative-hypnotics are taken orally, give activated charcoal orally to prevent absorption of drug still in the gut and reduce reabsorption of active metabolites in the enterohepatic circulation. Step 5: For patients who do not respond to the above steps, dialysis or hemoperfusion may be necessary to reduce coma. Most sedative-hypnotic medications are extremely lipophilic and are, therefore, removed slowly by these methods.

overdose.[21] However, like naloxone, flumazenil is a short-acting preparation and, therefore, requires either repeated dosing every 30 minutes or intravenous infusion over time to cover the longer acting effects of most benzodiazepines. Also, like naloxone, flumazenil can precipitate a withdrawal syndrome in an individual who is dependent on benzodiazepines. This effect can result in seizures and a major withdrawal syndrome with severe autonomic dysfunction similar to that seen in DTs.

Although flumazenil reverses most of the effects of a benzodiazepine overdose, it does not always reliably reverse respiratory depression. This may be due to the high frequency of intoxication with other drugs in conjunction with benzodiazepines. Flumazenil does not antagonize the effects of other sedative-hypnotics, including alcohol, barbiturates, and the nonbenzodiazepine, nonbarbiturate sleeping pills. Treatment of overdose with these drugs may require dialysis to clear the drug from the system because no antagonists of these drugs are currently available. When the drug has been taken orally, administration of activated charcoal can be important in reducing absorption of more drug into the body and preventing reabsorption of drug through the enterohepatic circulation.

With both the opioids and the sedative-hypnotics, as the intoxication clears, a withdrawal syndrome may develop. Therefore, it is important to monitor for withdrawal and treat it appropriately, as is described later. Failure to do this will result in more severe problems and, with sedative-hypnotics, the potential for status epilepticus and delirium.

Treatment of Psychostimulant Intoxication

The most common psychostimulant intoxication seen at this time occurs with cocaine. Cocaine overdoses are very common in the emergency department because, as with other street drugs, individuals taking cocaine are never aware of the purity of the drug they are buying. The signs and symptoms of the psychostimulant overdose syndrome and treatment are listed in Table 129–8. Unlike the opioids and benzodiazepines, there is no specific antagonist available for the effects of cocaine or other psychostimulants; therefore, depending on the presenting problems, other drugs may be needed to treat specific effects of the overdose. Although cocaine itself is relatively short acting, there is evidence that some of its metabolites, particularly benzoyl ecgonine, may produce long-acting effects after cocaine has cleared the system.[21] In addition, some of the cardiac effects of cocaine can occur a week to 10 days after the individual has stopped using the cocaine. Individuals who use alcohol with cocaine can synthesize coca ethylene, which may be more toxic than cocaine.[22]

One of the most difficult problems associated with severe cocaine and other psychostimulant intoxication is the psychosis, which may be indistinguishable from a naturally occurring psychosis. This problem is best treated with high-potency antipsychotic medications, such as haloperidol. It is best to give haloperidol intravenously because the absorption intramuscularly may be erratic and not rapid enough to give the desired effect. Haloperidol may lower the seizure threshold. Therefore, care should be taken when it is administered.[23] For excessive stimulation, an intravenously administered benzodiazepine can be very useful.[24] Benzodiazepines should not be administered intramuscularly because of erratic absorption from the intramuscular injection site. Depending on the nature of the problem, several choices can be used. Lorazepam intravenously has a duration of action of approximately 2 hours. Diazepam has a duration of action, when given intravenously, of about 30 to 40 minutes, and if an ultrashort-acting drug is necessary, midazolam could be used. The choice of drug will depend on the circumstances, and the availability of this range of drugs

TABLE 129–8. Psychostimulant Intoxication and Overdose

Signs	Hyperactivity Diaphoresis Mydriasis Tremor Tachycardia and arrhythmias Hypertension Hyperpyrexia Stereotypic behavior (picking at skin) Seizures Paranoia
Treatment	Step 1: Administer lorazepam, 2 mg, by slow intravenous infusion to reduce agitation and seizure potential. Give repeated doses as needed to control stimulant effects. Lorazepam has a duration of action of 90–120 minutes IV. A shorter acting parenteral benzodiazepine such as diazepam or midazolam can be used if the long duration of action of lorazepam is clinically contraindicated. Step 2: Beta-blockers may be used to treat ventricular arrythmias. When there is evidence of ischemic injury, calcium channel blockers should be used. Step 3: In patients who are paranoid or violent, administer haloperidol, 5 mg IV and repeat the dose every 30 min until symptoms subside or side effects are seen. Haloperidol and other antipsychotics may lower the seizure threshold and, therefore, should be used judiciously. Step 4: Administer ascorbic acid, 500 mg three or four times daily, to enhance excretion of amphetamine and its derivatives. Administer a diuretic when urinary pH is below 6.0.

certainly is a therapeutic advantage. Because respiratory depression can occur with the use of intravenous benzodiazepines, in particular midazolam, it is best to start with a low dose and titrate up on the basis of the clinical picture.

Arrhythmia is associated with cocaine use and can be treated with β-blockers and, if associated with myocardial ischemia, calcium channel blockers can also be used. Again, the choice of drug will depend on the circumstance, and intravenous administration provides more precise control of medication. All of the psychostimulants can cause hypertension, and it may be necessary to administer antihypertensive medications should the blood pressure be at a problematic level. Hypertensive effects usually ameliorate as the drug clears the system.[25]

Cocaine is a short-acting drug with a duration of action of several hours. However, some of the amphetamines are long acting and, if taken in high doses, effects can persist for several days. To reduce the duration of these effects, acidification of the urine will enhance excretion of amphetamines. Acidification can be accomplished through the use of ascorbic acid, 500 mg three or four times a day, or ammonium chloride. However, the latter may produce hepatic toxicity. Once the urinary pH is less than 6.0, a diuretic should be administered to enhance drug excretion.[26]

Treatment of Phencyclidine Intoxication

Overdoses with PCP and other arylcyclohexylamines, although not common in all parts of the country, can present very challenging clinical problems. The signs and symptoms of PCP overdose and its treatment are presented in Table 129–9. PCP is a weak acid with a pK of 8.5. Because of this, the nonionized drug is frequently taken up by cells where it cannot be excreted, resulting in a prolonged effect.

One of the most severe problems with PCP is hypertensive crisis, which needs to be addressed vigorously with potent antihypertensive medications such as nitroprusside. Psychoses and catatonia can also occur with PCP intoxication. Individuals on PCP have also been known to become violent. There have been reports of individuals exhibiting superhuman strength while intoxicated with PCP. However, these are anecdotal. The acute psychosis and agitation with PCP can be treated in a similar manner to that associated with amphetamines through the use of intravenous haloperidol and benzodiazepines. The doses used are similar to those used for psychostimulants.[27]

PCP, like the amphetamines, is best excreted in an acid urine, which will significantly decrease the duration of effects from the drug. Ascorbic acid, 500 mg three or four times a day, or ammonium chloride can be used to acidify the urine, and it is important to try to reduce the urinary pH to 5.5 or below to enhance the excretion of the drug. There is a 100-fold difference in the rate of excretion between pH 5.5 and pH 6. Once the pH is down to the 5.5 level, a diuretic should be administered to facilitate excretion of the drug. This will significantly decrease the duration over which PCP effects persist.[27]

Treatment of Hallucinogen Intoxication

With the recent increased use of hallucinogens, particularly on college campuses, once again acute reactions to hallucinogens are appearing in the emergency department. Of particular concern are seizures that can occur with high doses and the acute disorientation resulting in confusion and severe anxiety known as a "bad trip." In severe cases, antipsychotics such as haloperidol have been shown to be effective in reducing some of these problems and sedation can be effected with benzodiazepines. Problems with hallucinogens are rarely seen in the critical care setting unless the person is severely injured while intoxicated. The effects of these drugs can last up to 12 hours.[28]

In the past, hallucinogens were frequently contaminated with other drugs, resulting in unusual reactions when attempts were made to medicate these patients. When there is concern about administering drugs to these individuals, placing the person in a softly lighted room with minimal stimulation can be helpful in reducing the anxiety, and having someone there to talk to the patient—a procedure known as a *talk down*—can calm the person down rapidly.

TABLE 129–9. Arylcyclohexylamine (PCP) Intoxication and Overdose

Signs	**Low-Dose Effects**	
	Tachycardia	Distorted perception
	Numbness	Agitation
	Hypertension	Sensory isolation
	High-Dose Effects	
	Incoordination	Loss of sensation
	Catatonia	Loss of corneal and gag reflexes
	Nystagmus (vertical and horizontal)	Estrangement
	Hyperacusis	Diaphoresis
	Hypersalivation	Apathy
	Convulsions	Aggressive behavior
		Coma
Treatment	Step 1: Secure adequate airway, maintain cardiovascular system, draw appropriate blood studies.	
	Step 2: Administer flumazenil; 0.2–3.0 mg IV or SC, administer 50% glucose IV and administer naloxone, 2–4 mg IV or SC. This administration of multiple drugs is necessary because PCP is often mixed with other drugs.	
	Step 3: Administer lorazepam, 2 mg by slow intravenous infusion, to reduce agitation and seizure potential. Give repeated doses as needed to control stimulant effects. Lorazepam has a duration of action of 90–120 min IV. Repeated doses may be necessary because PCP is a long-acting drug. In patients who are paranoid or violent, administer haloperidol, 5 mg IV and repeat the dose every 30 min until symptoms subside or side effects are seen. Haloperidol and other antipsychotics may lower the seizure threshold and, therefore, should be used judiciously.	
	Step 4: For patients with severe hypertension, administer nitroprusside or other rapidly acting antihypertensive drugs to avoid a hypertensive crisis.	
	Step 5: Administer ascorbic acid, 500 mg three or four times daily, to enhance excretion of PCP and its derivatives. Administer a diuretic when urinary pH is below 5.5. This procedure may have to be repeated for several days until the urine is clear of PCP.	

Abbreviation: PCP = phencyclidine.

Treatment of Solvent Intoxication

Acute problems with volatile inhalants are rare; however, they can be quite serious. The most significant is arrhythmias, which develop from the hydrofluorocarbons and other volatile substances that resemble some of the older general anesthetics. These arrhythmias occur from sensitization of the heart to catecholamines and have been fatal at times. Fortunately, the effects of these drugs are short lived, and these problems reverse themselves very rapidly. However, in patients in whom arrhythmias may persist, β-blockers may be effective in reducing the problems.

TREATMENT OF WITHDRAWAL SYNDROMES

For the patient in the critical care unit, withdrawal may significantly complicate care and produce new but potentially avoidable problems. Therefore, it is critical to anticipate when a withdrawal syndrome may occur and treat it vigorously to prevent new problems. Withdrawal syndromes should not be treated as occasion requires because, once the withdrawal syndrome occurs, it is more difficult to stop it than to maintain the patient in a state free of withdrawal signs.

When withdrawing patients from dependency-producing drugs, it is important to reduce gradually the amount of drug the individual is taking. This can be safely done by reducing the dose of the drug at a rate of approximately 10% of the initial dose per day, resulting in a gradual withdrawal over approximately 10 days. In an individual who is more stable and if a long-acting drug is being used to effect the withdrawal, then a 20% per day taper can be used, completing the withdrawal in 5 days.

When developing a withdrawal schedule, the most common mistake is to increase the interval between doses of medication, often going beyond the duration of action of the drug. This error results in repeated withdrawal symptoms throughout the day that may be partially relieved when the next dose of drug is administered. The more appropriate way to effect the withdrawal is to maintain a dosing interval within the duration of action of the drug and reduce the amount of drug given at each dose to achieve the 10% to 20% reduction a day. In most instances, because of their reduced severity of withdrawal, long-acting medications are used to provide a smooth withdrawal for the individual. Therefore, drugs like methadone for opioid withdrawal and phenobarbital for sedative-hypnotic withdrawals are used in the noncritical care setting. However, in the critical care setting, to obtain a more precise control over the medication without accumulation and other unanticipated side effects, shorter acting drugs may be more appropriate.

Because tolerance develops to most of the drug classes, which can cause dependence, it is impossible from historic information to determine how much drug may be needed to control the withdrawal syndrome. Therefore, it is necessary to titrate the amount of drug to the withdrawal signs of the patient. This technique can be most effectively and rapidly performed through intravenous administration of medication. In a tolerant individual, very high doses of medication may be necessary to accomplish the reduction in withdrawal signs. Short-acting drugs can be rapidly titrated to achieve maximum benefit without under- or overmedication, which may compromise the patient's care.

When selecting a drug to treat the withdrawal syndrome, the first choice should be a drug that shows cross-dependence and cross-tolerance with the drugs causing the withdrawal syndrome. Adjunctive medications described later can also be used, if necessary, to facilitate a smooth withdrawal.

Treatment of Opioid Withdrawal

Although street addicts are inordinately concerned about opioid withdrawal, rarely has anyone died from its effects. In most cases, opioid withdrawal is no more severe than a bad case of the flu with lacrimation, rhinorrhea, nausea, vomiting, diarrhea, and piloerection. It is from the piloerection that the term *cold turkey* was originated. The signs and symptoms of opioid withdrawal and its treatment are listed in Table 129–10. Although opioid withdrawal is not life threatening, the patient can be extremely disruptive and uncomfortable. Therefore, it is important to treat withdrawal vigorously to avoid other problems that can be very disruptive to the unit and the patient.

Traditionally, opioid withdrawal has been treated with methadone, a long-acting narcotic, or more recently in combination with the α_2 agonist clonidine.[29] Methadone can cause problems because of its extremely long half-life and because it can accumulate over time in cases of hepatic or renal impairment. If the patient's condition is rapidly changing and there is a need to alter the dose of the withdrawal medication quickly, methadone may be inappropriate. However, if a long-acting narcotic is desired and will not interfere with the patient's condition or treatment, methadone should be the treatment of choice. Unlike many narcotics, methadone does not have significant first-pass metabolism and, therefore, is a good drug to use orally. However, if parenteral administration is necessary, it is preferable to use morphine intravenously because there can be erratic absorption from subcutaneous or intramuscular injection sites.

The easiest way to deal with opioid withdrawal is to treat the signs and symptoms as they appear. A simple scoring system for determining the dose of methadone necessary is described in Table 129–10.[28] An alternative approach is to use intravenous morphine. Although very short acting, intravenous morphine can be titrated precisely to the dose necessary to maintain the patient in a withdrawal-free state. Morphine should be increased at a minimum of 1 mg per hour or as rapidly as 1 mg every 5 minutes until signs and symptoms of withdrawal are relieved. The scoring system described in Table 129–10 can be used to determine how close the dose of morphine is to the dose necessary to relieve withdrawal. Once stabilized on morphine, the patient can either be maintained on that amount of morphine or withdrawn at a rate of 10% of the total daily dose each day. As the patient begins to recover and can be switched to oral medication, it is important to remember that the oral dose of morphine is six times the parenteral dose because of significant first-pass metabolism. If there is going to be a switch from parenteral to oral medication, it may be more satisfactory to switch the patient to methadone, as described in Table 129–10. The methadone can then be reduced to 5 mg per day in a fixed volume of liquid.

Treatment of Sedative-Hypnotic and Alcohol Withdrawal

The withdrawal from alcohol and other sedative-hypnotics is the only life-threatening withdrawal. Patients in whom major withdrawal (DTs) develops can have mortality rates as high as 5%, even in treated cases. Therefore, it is important to treat major withdrawal vigorously, and, more importantly, unless the patient arrives in the hospital in major withdrawal, it should not be permitted to occur in the hospital setting. There is no way to predict who will experience major withdrawal, except that those patients who have had major withdrawal in the past are more likely to experience it in the future. There is no correlation with the amount of drug or alcohol ingested or other medical conditions. Pa-

TABLE 129–10. Opioid Withdrawal

Signs	Insomnia	Anxiety
	Lacrimation	Mydriasis
	Rhinorrhea	Spontaneous orgasms
	Diarrhea	Cramps
	Nausea and vomiting	Tachycardia
	Yawning	Piloerection
Treatment	**If Oral Medications Are to Be Used** Step 1: Score patient on the above signs, rating "0" if absent, "1" if present mildly, and "2" if strongly present. Step 2: If score is 5 or less, give no medication. If score is greater than 5, give 1 mg of methadone for each point. Repeat steps 1 and 2 every 6 hours for 24 h. Each scoring period is independent of the previous scoring period. Patient will agitate for more medication. Scoring should be based on objective signs, not patient's subjective complaints. Step 3: Add up the amount of methadone given in the 24-h period. This is the amount of methadone necessary to prevent withdrawal in the patient. This can be given as a single daily dose or in a divided dose every 12 h. Step 4: Reduce the dose of methadone 5 mg per day. Do not tell the patient the dose or the withdrawal schedule. Give the medication in a fixed volume of liquid to disguise the withdrawal schedule. Step 5: If patient shows signs of breakthrough withdrawal, either slow the withdrawal rate or start clonidine, 0.1 mg twice daily, and increase dose until breakthrough signs are treated. It may be necessary to give more than 1 mg of clonidine a day. Gradually reduce the clonidine dose after the withdrawal is completed to avoid rebound hypertension. **If Parenteral Medications Are to Be Used** Step 1: Score patient on the above signs, rating "0" if absent, "1" if present mildly, and "2" if strongly present. Step 2: Administer morphine sulfate intravenously until withdrawal score is 0–5. Morphine can be increased rapidly in 1-mg increments every 5 min to reduce withdrawal signs. Step 3: Once patient's withdrawal is stabilized, reduce total daily dose of morphine 10% a day. If patient is to be converted to oral medication, give oral methadone in fixed volume at a morphine-methadone conversion of 1:10. (If the patient is receiving morphine 3 mg/h, then give methadone 30 mg/d or 15 mg every 12 h.) Then follow steps 3 and 4 above.	

tients with a history of chronic alcohol dependence are often vitamin depleted; therefore, it is imperative to give thiamine and multivitamins before glucose to prevent the precipitation of Wernicke's and Korsakoff's syndromes.

Withdrawal from alcohol and other sedative-hypnotics is divided into minor and major withdrawal. Minor withdrawal precedes major withdrawal and is more common than major withdrawal. It is during minor withdrawal that seizures occur. The signs and symptoms of major and minor withdrawal and their treatment are listed in Table 129–11. With alcohol, an extremely short-acting drug, minor withdrawal occurs in the first 48 hours, and major withdrawal occurs 48 to 72 hours after drinking has stopped. Patients taking other sedative-hypnotic medications that are longer acting than alcohol will show a significant time shift, with minor withdrawal not appearing for 2 to 3 days after drug use has stopped and major withdrawal appearing 8 to 10 days after drug use has ceased.

In a patient with a history of alcohol or other sedative-hypnotic use, it is critical to begin prophylactic treatment to prevent the patient from going into sedative-hypnotic withdrawal because this can be severely disruptive to any other conditions with which the patient is presenting. In most cases, a long-acting benzodiazepine or long-acting barbiturate such as phenobarbital can be used as treatment or prophylaxis for sedative-hypnotic and alcohol withdrawal. However, both of these drugs, given orally, can create significant problems in the critical care setting.

Phenobarbital is extremely long acting, with a half-life of more than 72 hours and also is an enzyme inducer that could result in interference with the metabolism of other medications. However, if it can be used, phenobarbital is the treatment of choice because of its long duration of action and the fact that 30% is excreted unchanged in the urine. It is also available in many different dosage and delivery forms, allowing very precise dosage adjustments. Phenobarbital also has a long latency, which reduces its abuse potential. Long-acting benzodiazepines are converted to the long-acting form only on passage through the liver. Therefore, parenteral administration bypasses the liver, and the long-acting metabolites will not be generated. Only three benzodiazepines can be given parenterally: midazolam, diazepam, and lorazepam. Midazolam is an ultrashort-acting benzodiazepine, and unless there is specific need for an ultrashort-acting medication, it should not be used. Diazepam intravenously has a half-life of about 30 minutes, and lorazepam intravenously has a half-life of about 2 hours. Therefore, the choice of medication will be based on specific need. Because the latency of intravenous benzodiazepines is very short (minutes), the drug can be titrated very rapidly to relieve withdrawal symptoms.

Lorazepam has a specific advantage over diazepam in that there is less protein binding, and it is excreted with only glucuronidation, which is preserved even in severe liver damage. On the other hand, diazepam has to go through multiple metabolic steps using mixed oxidase systems, which can be compromised in a patient with severe liver damage.

In a patient in major withdrawal, massive doses of intravenous medication may be needed. The simplest sign to monitor is tachycardia; in this case, the heart rate should be brought down below 120 beats per minute. The other autonomic signs and the hallucinations will respond more slowly once the patient's withdrawal state is brought under control. It is necessary to maintain a level of sedative-hypnotic drug in the system and gradually reduce the level 10% per day from the total daily dose. If the withdrawal condition is brought under control and medication is stopped, the patient will very rapidly go back into the withdrawal state.

There are instances in which patients with extremely high blood alcohol levels begin to show signs of withdrawal before total clearance of alcohol from the system. Patients with high blood alcohol levels should be monitored closely for the development of withdrawal, and medications should be initiated when the withdrawal signs and symptoms appear. If phenobarbital is to be used, the patient should be given 30 mg of phenobarbital for each .05 mg per cent drop in blood alcohol level. If intravenous lorazepam is going to be used, 1 mg should be given for each .05 mg per cent drop in blood alcohol level. At this point, the total amount of medication needed can be rapidly calculated because alcohol is metabolized by first-order kinetics. Therefore, if two

TABLE 129–11. Alcohol and Other Sedative-Hypnotic Withdrawal

MINOR WITHDRAWAL	
Signs	Tremors Mild diaphoresis Hallucinations Seizures Minimal disorientation Mild temperature increases Mild tachycardia Mild increases of blood pressure
Treatment	**If Oral Medications Are to Be Used** Step 1: To determine level of tolerance, give pentobarbital, 200 mg PO and wait 1 h. Look for signs of nystagmus, ataxia, drowsiness, dysarthria, decreased blood pressure, and decreased pulse. If two or more signs are present, stop the procedure; if not, give pentobarbital, 100 mg PO, every hour until two or more signs are present or a total of pentobarbital, 600 mg, has been given. Step 2: Convert to phenobarbital, 30 mg for every 100 mg of pentobarbital given. Then decrease phenobarbital 10% of the initial dose per day in a fixed volume of liquid. **If Parenteral Medications Are to Be Used** Step 1: If a long-acting medication can be used, infuse phenobarbital intravenously until patient shows signs of mild intoxication as described in step 1 above. Once that dose is determined, it is the daily dose required to block withdrawal. If a short-acting medication is to be used, choose among midazolam, diazepam, or lorazepam, depending on rapidity of reversal of effects required. Infuse medication intravenously until signs of intoxication or reduction of withdrawal signs occurs, as in step 1 above. Step 2: Reduce dose 10% a day. Because phenobarbital is long acting even when administered intravenously, it can be given as a single daily dose. For the short-acting intravenous medications, adjust frequency of administration to duration of action of the medication and reduce the total daily dose 10% a day.
MAJOR WITHDRAWAL	
Signs	Tremors Increased psychomotor activity Increased autonomic activity Marked diaphoresis Tachycardia (usually > 120 beats per minute) Rapid blood pressure changes Disorientation Hallucinations No seizures
Treatment	Step 1: Administer lorazepam 4 mg IV every 5–10 min until tachycardia is reduced to less than 120/min. Step 2: For sustained effect, continue to administer lorazepam at required dose every 2 h and reduce total dose 10% a day or administer phenobarbital, 120 mg PO twice a day or 60 mg parenterally twice a day, and reduce at 10% a day.

blood alcohol levels are drawn at least an hour apart, the drop in blood alcohol level is linear, and medications can then be appropriately timed.

Treatment of Other Drug Withdrawals

The withdrawal from psychostimulants, including cocaine, is not life threatening. During the first 24 to 48 hours after stimulant medication is discontinued, the patient may be hypersomnolant for 16 to 24 hours, at which point hyperactivity and insomnia can develop. There is debate in the literature over whether or not a stimulant withdrawal syndrome actually exists. Some individuals will experience depression secondary to withdrawal from psychostimulants, and this can persist for a week to 10 days after the person has discontinued use of the stimulant. Should the depression persist beyond this point, a psychiatric evaluation to determine whether or not an underlying depression exists is warranted. Numerous medications, including antidepressants and dopamine agonists, have been tried to treat the stimulant withdrawal syndrome. Many of these medications have looked positive in open trials, but few have shown any significant benefit when studied in a double-blind fashion. Therefore, at this time, no medication is recommended.

The same lack of specific withdrawal treatment exists for PCP and the other arylcyclohexylamines, hallucinogens, marijuana, and the volatile inhalants. None of these drugs shows clear-cut withdrawal syndromes, and there is little concern over any severe conditions developing during the withdrawal period. If medications are warranted, they should be for symptomatic treatments if at all.

SUMMARY

The problems of addiction and drug abuse have become prominent in our society and can severely affect healthcare. Most important, they can have profound effects on patients who are being treated for other medical conditions, and it is often the sequelae of drug use that bring the patient to the hospital. Intoxication and withdrawal can severely complicate the treatment of a patient in the critical care setting. Therefore, it is important that physicians be aware of the signs and symptoms of both intoxication and withdrawal syndromes and the most appropriate methods to treat them. These conditions are treatable and can reduce complications that develop. However, it is critical to recognize that the treatment of intoxication and withdrawal is not the treatment of addiction, and all of these patients should be referred for long-term treatment of their addiction. Otherwise, they become part of the revolving-door syndrome that plagues many healthcare systems.

References

1. Anthenelli RM, Schuckit MA: Genetics. *In*: Substance Abuse: A Comprehensive Textbook. 2nd ed. Lowinson JH, Ruiz P, Millman RB (Eds). Baltimore, Williams & Wilkins, 1985, pp 39–50.
2. Rice DP, Kelman S, Miller LS, et al: Economic costs of alcohol and drug abuse and mental illness: 1985. Rockville, MD, U.S. Dept. of Health and Human Services, Public Health Service, Alcohol Drug Abuse, and Mental Health Administration, 1990, p 296.
3. Baldwin WA, Rosenfeld BA, Breslow MJ, et al: Substance abuse–related admissions to adult intensive care. Chest 1993; 103:21.
4. Regier DA, Farmer FE, Rae DS, et al: Cormorbidity of mental disorders with alcohol and other drug abuse: results from the Epidemiologic Catchment Area (ECA) Study. JAMA 1990; 264:2511–2518.
5. Moore RD, Bone LR, Geller G, et al: Prevalence, detection and treatment of alcoholism in hospitalized patients. JAMA 1989; 261:403–407.
6. National Institute on Drug Abuse: National Household Survey on Drug Abuse Main Findings: 1990. Rockville, MD, National Institute on Drug Abuse, 1992.
7. Ray BA, Braude MC (Eds): Women and Drugs: A New Era for Research. Rockville, MD, National Institute on Drug Abuse, 1986.
8. Clark RF, Harchelroad F: Toxicology screening of the trauma patient: A changing profile. Ann Emerg Med 1991; 20:151–153.
9. Heinemann AW, Mamott BD, Schnoll SH: Substance use by persons with recent spinal cord injuries. Rehabil Psychol 1990; 35:4.

10. Selwyn PA, O'Connor PG: Diagnosis and treatment of substance abusers with HIV infection. Prim Care 1992; 19:119–159.
11. National Institute on Drug Abuse: Drug Abuse Warning Network. Rockville, MD, National Institute on Drug Abuse, 1992.
12. Jaffee JH, Martin WR: Opioid analgesics and antagonists. *In*: Goodman and Gelman's The Pharmacological Basis of Therapeutics. 8th ed. Gilman AG, Rall TW, Nies AS, et al (Eds). New York, Pergamon Press, 1990, pp 485–521.
13. Harvey SC: Hypnotics and sedatives. *In*: Goodman and Gelman's The Pharmacological Basis of Therapeutics. 7th ed. Gilman AG, Goodman LS, Rall TW, et al (Eds). New York, MacMillan Publishing Co, 1985, pp 339–371.
14. Roy-Byrne PP, Cowley DS (Eds): Benzodiazepines in Clinical Practice: Risks and Benefits. Washington, DC, American Psychiatric Association Press, 1991.
15. Wesson DR, Smith DE, Seymour RA: Sedative-hypnotics and tricyclics. *In*: Substance Abuse: A Comprehensive Textbook. 2nd ed. Lowinson JH, Ruiz P, Millman RB (Eds). Baltimore, Williams & Wilkins, 1985, pp 271–279.
16. Gawin FH, Ellinwood EH Jr: Cocaine and other stimulants. N Engl J Med 1988; 318:1173–1182.
17. Johnson KM, Jones SM: Neuropharmacology of phencyclidine: Basic mechanisms and therapeutic potential. Ann Rev Pharmacol Toxicol 1990; 30:707–750.
18. Sharp CW, Rosenberg NL: Volatile substances. *In*: Substance Abuse: A Comprehensive Textbook. 2nd ed. Lowinson JH, Ruiz P, Millman RB (Eds). Baltimore, Williams & Wilkins, 1985, pp 303–327.
19. Schnoll SH: Pharmacological aspects of youth drug abuse. *In*: Youth Drug Abuse—Problems, Issues, and Treatment. Beschner GM, Friedman AS (Eds). Lexington, MA, Lexington Books, 1979, pp 255–275.
20. Schnoll SH, Lewis DE: Drug screening in the workplace: Pros and cons. Semin Occupat Med 1986; 1:243.
21. Weinbroun A, Halpern P, Geller E: The use of flumazenil in the management of acute drug poisoning: A review. Intensive Care Med 1991; 17:S32–S38.
22. Brogan WC III, Lange RA, Glaman DB: Recurrent, coronary vasoconstriction caused by intranasal cocaine: Possible role for metabolites. Ann Intern Med 1992; 116:556–561.
23. Baily DN: Plasma cocaethylene concentrations in patients treated in the emergency room or trauma unit. Am J Clin Pathol 1993; 99:123–127.
24. Ungar JR: Current drugs of abuse. *In*: Schwartz GR, Bucker N, Hanke BK, et al (Eds). Emergency Medicine: The Essential Update. Philadelphia, WB Saunders, 1989, pp 210–224.
25. Weiss RD, Mirin SM: Intoxication and withdrawal syndromes. *In*: Manual of Psychiatric Emergencies. Hyman SE (Ed). Boston, Little, Brown, and Co, 1988, pp 233–244.
26. Om A, Ellaham S, DiSciascio A: Management of cocaine-induced cardiovascular complications. Am Heart J 1993; 125:469–475.
26. Caldwell J: The metabolism of amphetamines and related stimulants in animals and man. *In*: Amphetamines and Related Stimulants: Chemical, Biological, Clinical, and Social Aspects. Caldwell J (Ed). Boca Raton, FL, CRC Press, 1980.
27. Daghestani AN, Schnoll SH: Phencyclidine abuse and dependence. Treat Psychiatr Disord 1989; 2:1209–1218.
28. Schnoll SH: Aiding the drug abuser. Hosp Med 1983; 19:116–155.
29. Jasinski DR, Johnson RE, Kocher TE: Clonidine in morphine withdrawal: Differential effects on signs and symptoms. Arch Gen Psychiatry 1985; 42:1066–1076.

CHAPTER 130

Poisoning

Cathleen Clancy, MD • Toby L. Litovitz, MD

Poisoning remains a serious public health problem despite regulatory intervention and medical advances. In 1993, over 1.7 million exposures to potential poisons were reported to poison centers participating in the American Association of Poison Control Centers Toxic Exposure Surveillance System (AAPCC TESS). Only 0.48% of the poisoned individuals suffered life-threatening effects or major disability or died. The site of exposure was a residence in 90.3% of cases. Although most reported poison exposures were managed at home with the advice of a poison control center, a significant proportion (24.4%) were managed in healthcare facilities. Children younger than 6 years were involved in 56% of the exposures but were among only 4.3% (27) of the fatalities. Suicide was the reported reason in 54% of the fatal poisonings.[1a]

Poison control centers serve as an invaluable but underutilized resource for physicians managing poisoned patients. Because these centers are able to guide the management of most poisoned patients at home, thus preventing unnecessary emergency department visits, poison control centers provide a highly cost-effective means of managing poisonings. There are currently 36 certified regional poison control centers in the United States, each meeting minimum quality standards set by the AAPCC. Certified regional poison control centers offer:

1. 24-hour staffing by specialists in poison information, each of whom has met rigorous training requirements leading to required certification as a specialist in poison information after 1 year of experience in the center,
2. Extensive on-site and computerized resources, often including hundreds of texts, tens of thousands of journal articles, and Poisindex, a CD-ROM database of computerized product and protocol information,
3. 24-hour back-up by clinical and medical toxicologists,
4. Extensive public education programs in poison prevention as well as professional education in poisoning management at all levels, including education for first responders; paramedics; students in nursing, pharmacy, and medical schools; intensive care unit and emergency department nurses and physicians, and
5. Participation in the nationwide poisoning surveillance program through submission of data on each reported poisoning to the AAPCC TESS.

Poisoning surveillance allows detection of hazards of new products before needless injuries occur, leading to repackaging, reformulation, product recall, or product ban. Every physician can aid in this nationwide surveillance effort by reporting each and every poisoning to a regional poison control center.

This chapter provides a brief overview of poisonings that are frequently managed (or mismanaged) in the critical care setting. It is not intended to be comprehensive or to replace consultation with a certified regional poison control center, as therapeutic strategies in toxicology are rapidly evolving. Seventeen specific drugs or chemicals are discussed in depth; these substances were chosen because they involve new, controversial, or unusual therapies or because they have been associated with high morbidity and mortality.

TREATMENT MODALITIES

Decontamination

Decontamination of the eyes, skin, and gastrointestinal tract is the first and foremost task to perform in any poisoning emergency. Gastrointestinal decontamination involves the use of emetics, gastric lavage, oral sorbents, cathartics, and whole-bowel irrigation.

Emetics

Ipecac is currently the emetic of choice. The ipecacuanha alkaloids, emetine and cephaeline, act by local activation of peripheral sensory receptors in the gastrointestinal tract and by central stimulation of the chemoreceptor trigger zone in the medulla. Vomiting begins 20 to 30 minutes after administration of ipecac and lasts from 30 minutes to 2 hours. The type and amount of liquid (e.g., milk, water) given after ipecac administration may be unimportant.[2–4] Antiemetics do not seem to inhibit effectiveness. Stored ipecac syrup has been shown to be effective in inducing emesis without delay for up to 4 years after the expiration date.[5]

Contraindications to the use of ipecac include the potentially imminent onset or presence of a decreased level of consciousness or seizures, uncontrolled hypertension, and prior ingestion of acid or alkali. Ipecac is generally not indicated for low-viscosity petroleum distillate ingestions unless a toxic coingestant is implicated. The incidence of diarrhea and lethargy is 13% and 11.6%, respectively.[6] Uncommon complications include aspiration, Mallory-Weiss tears, diaphragmatic rupture, pneumomediastinum, intracerebral hemorrhage, and foreign body aspiration.

Gastric Lavage

Orogastric lavage is frequently used for gastric decontamination in the emergency department. Tracheal intubation should precede lavage in patients with seizures, depressed mental status, or an absent gag reflex. Lavage is contraindicated in patients with caustic ingestions. The complications include aspiration; airway obstruction; esophageal, gastric, or laryngeal damage; water intoxication in children when tap water is used; and gastrointestinal hemorrhage. Orogastric lavage is indicated in patients with life-threatening ingestions who reach medical attention within 1 to 2 hours postingestion, and possibly longer with substances associated with delayed gastric emptying such as anticholinergics.

Activated Charcoal

The maximum binding capacity of activated charcoal is dependent on its surface area, which ranges from 950 m^2/g to 2000 m^2/g. Activated charcoal adsorbs most drugs but is *not* very effective for alcohols, hydrocarbons, organophosphates, carbamates, cyanide, acids, alkali, lithium, and iron. The dosage should reflect an activated charcoal-to-drug ratio of 10:1. However, because the amount ingested is rarely accurately known, it is common practice to dose activated charcoal based on a patient's body weight (1–2 g/kg).

Activated charcoal appears to be very effective in the treatment of a wide range of poisonings. Complications from the use of activated charcoal are infrequent. Activated charcoal aspiration does occur, although aspiration of gastric contents is more problematic. Intestinal obstruction and bezoars have been reported. Endoscopic visualization of the mucosa is obscured following activated charcoal administration.

Cathartics and Whole Bowel Irrigation

Activated charcoal is often mixed with a cathartic to speed gastrointestinal transit time. Magnesium citrate or sorbitol is commonly mixed or given with activated charcoal and may decrease drug absorption by decreasing gastrointestinal transit time. Despite the routine use of cathartics with activated charcoal, only one study has demonstrated efficacy. Keller and Schwab showed that sorbitol leads to a 28% decrease in the absorption of salicylates in a crossover study of activated charcoal with sorbitol compared with activated charcoal alone.[7] In contrast, another study found no difference in acetaminophen levels over 8 hours between groups treated with activated charcoal and activated charcoal with sorbitol.[8] Relative contraindications include ingestion of corrosives, recent bowel surgery, or absence of bowel sounds. Contraindications for use of magnesium-containing cathartics include renal disease, nephrotoxic ingestion, and potential for myoglobinuria (i.e., the presence of seizures, or poisoning with cocaine or phencyclidine hydrochloride).

Whole-bowel irrigation involves the use of a polyethylene glycol electrolyte lavage solution—a nonabsorbable, osmotically active compound—that is given continuously for about 4 to 6 hours until the rectal effluent is clear. Whole-bowel irrigation may be useful in patients who have ingested large quantities of substances that are difficult to remove, such as sustained-release capsules, iron tablets, lead pellets, lithium tablets, cocaine packets, and crack vials. The dose is 0.5 L/h for small children and 2.0 L/h for adolescents and adults. Rosenberg and coworkers showed that activated charcoal alone was more effective than whole-bowel irrigation in three volunteers given 650 mg of salicylate.[9] In a crossover study, Tenenbein and associates described a 67% reduction in serum ampicillin concentrations following whole-bowel irrigation in nine volunteers compared with controls.[10] Anecdotal reports suggest efficacy following overdoses with iron[11] and sustained-release preparations.

Enhanced Elimination

Alkalinization

Sodium bicarbonate therapy enhances the elimination of certain toxic drugs by altering drug ionization and also decreases toxicity by changing sodium gradients or receptor binding or by buffering acidemia.

Ionization of weak acids like salicylate occurs whenever the pH of the serum or urine is greater than the acid dissociation constant (pK_a). Ionized substances do not readily cross cell membranes. Urinary alkalization can significantly increase the elimination of some renally excreted drugs. Weakly acidic drugs cannot be reabsorbed after glomerular filtration into alkaline urine because a large proportion of the drug will have become ionized in the alkaline medium. In the same manner, ionization of a drug in the plasma prevents tissue penetration. The drugs that respond to urine and serum alkalization in this fashion include salicylic acid ($pK_a = 3.0$), phenobarbital ($pK_a = 7.24$), chlorpropamide ($pK_a = 4.8$), and the chlorophenoxy herbicide 2,4-dichlorophenoxyacetic acid ($pK_a = 2.6$).

The cyclic antidepressants are weak bases with a high pK_a; thus, alkalinization does not promote elimination. Nonetheless, sodium bicarbonate therapy is efficacious in the management of cyclic antidepressant overdoses. One postulated mechanism for the observed clinical effect is an increase in protein binding with an increase in pH, resulting in a lesser amount of free (active) drug.[12] Variable results following the administration of α_1–acid glycoprotein (a binding protein) have raised doubts that this is the true mechanism.[13, 14] Sodium channel blockade, a major mechanism of cyclic antidepressant toxicity, is sensitive to pH, and alkalinization prevents this blockade. In addition, sodium administration alone may overcome sodium channel blockade and enhance the efficacy of sodium bicarbonate.[15]

Sodium bicarbonate may also be useful in the treatment of overdose of other cardiotoxic drugs that produce a widened QT interval, including carbamazepine, procainamide, quinidine, and quinine; however, poisoning with these drugs has been less well studied. Sodium bicarbonate therapy for ethylene glycol, methanol, and isoniazid, as well as other drugs, is based on the buffering capability of bicarbonate and does not enhance elimination.

Multidose Activated Charcoal

Multidose activated charcoal has been shown to increase systemic clearance of many drugs, including carbamazepine, cyclosporin, dapsone, diazepam, digoxin, disopyramide, meprobamate, methotrexate, nadolol, phenobarbital, phenylbutazone, phenytoin, and theophylline. Although clinical efficacy has been confirmed with only a relatively small number of drugs, the risk of complications from therapy is minimal.

The model drug for successful use of multidose activated charcoal is one that is actively secreted by or diffuses across the gastrointestinal mucosa, has a low volume of distribution, and is effectively adsorbed by activated charcoal. Theophylline and phenobarbital suit this model well. Multidose activated charcoal has been shown to double the clearance of intravenous aminophylline in adult volunteers[16] and has been used successfully in infants.[17] In six volunteers given 2.85 mg/kg of phenobarbital intravenously and multidose activated charcoal, Berg and colleagues demonstrated a decrease in serum half-life from 110 to 45 hours.[18] The data on cyclic antidepressant and salicylate poisonings is controversial, but multidose activated charcoal is generally recommended.

The dosage of activated charcoal is approximately 50 to 100 g in adults for the first dose, given with a cathartic, and then about 20 to 50 g given at 2- to 4-hour intervals *without* a cathartic. Adverse reactions include vomiting, aspiration, and bowel obstruction. Diarrhea with dehydration may be seen when repeated doses of cathartic are mistakenly included with the multiple doses of activated charcoal. When activated charcoal is required in a patient with drug-induced vomiting, as in theophylline toxicity, ranitidine has been recommended as an antiemetic agent.[19] Metoclopramide, ondansetron, or droperidol may also be used. Therapy should be discontinued if bowel sounds are absent, vomiting is persistent, or the level of the drug (and metabolites, when applicable) decreases to the therapeutic range.

Extracorporeal Modalities

Hemodialysis involves arterial to venous blood flow with diffusion of substances through a semipermeable membrane. The blood flows by the semipermeable membrane, and soluble chemicals diffuse into the dialysate down a steep concentration gradient. Electrolytes can diffuse back into the plasma. Drugs and chemicals that are well dialyzed have low molecular weights, high water solubility, low lipid solubility, low plasma protein binding, low volume of distribution (low tissue binding), and a short distribution phase. Hemodialysis is routinely used in severe ethylene glycol, lithium, methanol, and salicylate poisonings. Many other drugs and toxic substances reportedly have increased clearance with the application of hemodialysis. Although theophylline is cleared by hemodialysis, charcoal hemoperfusion is more effective than dialysis and is the procedure of choice. In some overdose patients, dialysis may also be indicated to manage refractory hyperkalemia, acidosis, renal failure, or volume overload.

Hemoperfusion removes toxic substances by directing blood from an arterial source, through a cartridge filled with an adsorbent material, then back to the patient intravenously. This method is more effective than hemodialysis for removing substances with high protein binding but cannot correct electrolyte or fluid balance abnormalities. The adsorbent materials in use are coated activated charcoal or synthetic resin, although the latter has limited availability. Charcoal hemoperfusion is commonly used for theophylline overdose patients and may be indicated for the removal of amatoxins (from mushrooms), methotrexate, phenobarbital, paraquat, and other poisons. In some cases, charcoal hemoperfusion and hemodialysis have been used in series to increase clearance and correct fluid and electrolyte abnormalities.

The complications of hemodialysis and hemoperfusion include bleeding from the anticoagulation required for these procedures, hypotension, thrombocytopenia, and metabolic abnormalities.

Other Modalities

Exchange transfusion involves the removal of circulating blood and the infusion of red blood cells and plasma products. This method has limited utility in the removal of toxic substances but can be used in life-threatening cases of methemoglobinemia (chlorates, aniline) or in severe hemolysis (arsine).

Plasmapheresis has a similar technique of blood removal, but the cellular elements removed are separated and resuspended in fresh plasma or colloid and returned to the patient. Plasmapheresis has little utility in the management of intoxications, although theoretically it might be useful for treatment of poisoning with substances that are highly toxic and tightly bound to proteins.

Peritoneal dialysis is very similar to hemodialysis in that a semipermeable membrane, the peritoneum, separates the blood from the dialysate. The concentrations equilibrate in both compartments before removal of the dialysate. Although peritoneal dialysis is much less efficient than hemodialysis, it can be performed on a continuous, 24-hour basis and does not produce the complications of arterial and venous access and anticoagulation.

Continuous arteriovenous hemofiltration (see Chapter 115) can be used to remove non–protein-bound drugs and to manage fluid overload and electrolyte imbalances in a continuous fashion. Drugs with high volumes of distribution may be removed by this method. Little data is currently available on the efficacy of continuous arteriovenous hemofiltration in specific intoxications.

Antidotes and Chelators: Controversies and New Issues

Antidotes can be virtually miraculous when used appropriately, but their misuse can cause more severe toxicity than that of the offending agent. Controversies abound, and new drugs are constantly being made available. Table 130–1 outlines currently used antidotes and chelators.

N-*Acetylcysteine*

N-Acetylcysteine (NAC) use has been widely accepted as antidotal therapy for acetaminophen overdose. A remarkable hepatoprotective effect was demonstrated in a multicenter trial[20] with 2540 patients who were treated with the oral NAC regimen (a 140-mg/kg load, followed by 70 mg/kg every 4 hours for 17 doses). Only 2.4% of patients had an aspartate aminotransferase level greater than 1000 IU/L when NAC was started within 8 hours of the ingestion. Hepatotoxicity increased in a stepwise fashion when treatment initiation was delayed for 8 to 12 hours or for 12 to 16 hours after acetaminophen ingestion. However, those patients treated 16 to 20 hours and 20 to 24 hours after ingestion were also found to have a lower incidence (42%) of severe hepatotoxicity than was expected. Thus, therapy is unquestionably indicated for up to 24 hours following ingestion. Therapy initiated later than 24 hours after ingestion—even in the absence of persistent acetaminophen levels in the blood—has been recommended by some authors. These authors' recommendations are supported by a recent study in which 50 consecutive patients with fulminant hepatic failure induced by acetaminophen were randomized to receive NAC or supportive care. Forty-eight per cent of patients in the NAC-treated group survived, whereas only 20% of those in the control group survived.[21]

TABLE 130–1. Antidotes and Chelators

Antidote	*Trade/Common Name*	*Toxin*	*Indications*	*Complications*
Antivenin (Crotalidae) polyvalent	Snakebite antivenin	Venom from Crotalidae family members (e.g., rattlesnake, copperhead, cotton mouth)	Symptomatic envenomation within 12–24 h of bite (e.g., coagulopathy, severe extremity swelling, hemodynamic compromise)	Serum sickness, anaphylaxis
Antivenin (*Latrodectus mactans*)	Black widow spider antivenin	Venom of all American widow spiders (*Latrodectus* species)	Failure of conservative management (e.g., muscle cramps, hypertension)	Serum sickness, anaphylaxis
Atropine sulfate	Atropine sulfate	Acetylcholinesterase-inhibiting pesticides, physostigmine excess, synthetic choline esters (e.g., urecholine), *Clitocybe* and *Inocybe* mushrooms	Symptoms of muscarinic cholinergic excess (salivation, lacrimation, urination, defecation, vomiting)	Anticholinergic symptoms
Benztropine mesylate	Cogentin	Phenothiazines and related compounds	Acute dystonia, extrapyramidal symptoms	Anticholinergic side effects (drowsiness, urinary retention, dry mouth)
Botulism antitoxin	Trivalent A,B, and E antitoxins supplied by the CDC&P	*Clostridium botulinum* toxin	Suspected botulism	Hypersensitivity, anaphylaxis
Edetate calcium disodium, EDTA	Calcium Disodium Versenate	1. Lead 2. Manganese, cadmium, copper, zinc, and other heavy metals	1. Symptomatic lead poisoning or laboratory evidence of significant lead accumulation	Renal tubular necrosis, decrease in iron, zinc, and other trace metal stores, dermatitis
1. Calcium gluconate 2. Calcium chloride	1. Calcium gluconate 2. Calcium chloride	1., 2. Hydrofluoric acid, black widow venom, calcium channel blockers, β-blockers	Symptomatic exposure, envenomation, overdose	1., 2. Hypercalcemia 2. Local necrosis at infusion site if extravasation occurs
Cyanide antidote kit: 1. amyl nitrite inhalant 2. sodium nitrite 3. sodium thiosulfate	Lilly Cyanide Antidote Kit	1., 2., 3. Cyanide 1., 2. Hydrogen sulfide	Suspected cyanide or hydrogen sulfide intoxication	Methemoglobinemia, hypotension
Deferoxamine mesylate	Desferal Mesylate	1. Iron 2. Aluminum	1. Serum iron >350 μg/dL with symptoms 2. Related encephalopathy, osteomalacia with renal failure	Hypotension, shock, anaphylaxis, ocular and auditory toxicity, adult respiratory distress syndrome with greater than 24-h infusion
2,3-Dimercaptosuccinic acid (DMSA)	Chemet, Succimer	1. Lead 2. Arsenic, mercury	1. Oral therapy for blood lead over 45 μg/dL in children; may also be indicated at lower levels	Transient liver enzyme elevation, nausea, vomiting, diarrhea
Diphenhydramine	Benadryl	Phenothiazines and related compounds	Acute dystonia, extrapyramidal symptoms	Anticholinergic side effects (drowsiness, urinary retention, dry mouth)
Ethanol	Ethanol	Methanol, ethylene glycol	Methanol or ethylene glycol ingestion, level >20 mg/dL	Central nervous system depression, hypoglycemia (primarily in pediatric patients)
Flumazenil	Mazicon	Benzodiazepines	Suspected benzodiazepine overdose without proconvulsant coingestants or past history of seizures	Seizures, benzodiazepine withdrawal
Folic acid/leucovorin	B complex vitamin 1. Folic acid 2. Leucovorin (active form of folic acid)	1. Methanol (adjunct) 2. Folic acid antagonists (e.g., methotrexate, trimethoprim, pyrimethamine)	1. Methanol intoxication 2. Symptomatic methanol intoxication, folic acid antagonist overdose	Allergic reactions
Glucagon	Glucagon	Beta-blockers, calcium channel blockers, hypoglycemic agents	Symptomatic overdose	Nausea, vomiting, hypersensitivity, hyperglycemia, hypokalemia

Table continued on following page

TABLE 130–1. Antidotes and Chelators *Continued*

Antidote	*Trade/Common Name*	*Toxin*	*Indications*	*Complications*
Methylene blue (methylthioninium chloride)	Methylene blue	Methemoglobinemia (e.g., dapsone, benzocaine, aniline, nitrites)	Methemoglobin level >20–30% with symptoms	Ineffective and causes hemolysis in glucose-6-phosphate dehydrogenase–deficient patients; releases cyanide if given after nitrite antidote in cyanide intoxication
N-Acetylcysteine	Mucomyst, Mucosol	Acetaminophen	Serum level above lower line on Rumack-Matthew nomogram longer than 4 h after ingestion	Vomiting from hypertonicity, foul odor
Naloxone hydrochloride	Narcan	Opiates	Respiratory depression	Acute opioid withdrawal
Niacinamide	Niacinamide, nicotinamide, nicotinic acid amide, 3-pyridine-carboxamide	Vacor (PNU), Alloxan, streptozotocin	Suspected exposure	Postural hypotension
D-Penicillamine	Cuprimine	1. Lead 2. Copper, arsenic, mercury, bismuth	1. Second line as oral therapy for mild lead intoxication	Fever, rash, bone marrow depression, cross-reactivity in patients with penicillin allergy
Physostigmine salicylate	Antilirium	Anticholinergics (e.g., diphenhydramine, jimson weed)	Severe anticholinergic poisoning (e.g., hallucinations, seizures, hypertension, arrhythmias)	Seizures, cholinergic crisis
Phytonadione (vitamin K)	AquaMEPHYTON, Konakion, Mephyton	Long-acting coumarins (e.g., brodifacoum, diphacinone)	Severe bleeding diathesis, hemorrhage	Shock, anaphylaxis
Pralidoxime chloride (2-PAM)	Protopam chloride	Acetylcholinesterase-inhibiting pesticides (organophosphates, possibly some carbamates)	Symptomatic poisoning (e.g., bradycardia, bronchorrhea, hypotension)	Overdoses with the carbamate carbaryl may worsen
Protamine sulfate	Protamine	Heparin	Coagulopathy with bleeding, or preoperative	Hypotension, bradycardia, hypersensitivity
Pyridoxine hydrochloride	Vitamin B_6	Isoniazid, ethylene glycol, monomethyl-hydrazine–containing mushrooms	Suspected intoxication	Peripheral neuropathy (only in high doses [10 g] or chronic overdosage)
Thiamine hydrochloride	Vitamin B_1	Ethylene glycol, ethanol	Suspected intoxication, acute Wernicke's encephalopathy	Hypersensitivity
Sodium polystyrene sulfonate	Kayexalate	Potassium	Symptomatic hyperkalemia	Hypokalemia

Abbreviation: CDC&P = Centers for Disease Control and Prevention.

The concurrent administration of NAC and activated charcoal may be problematic. Activated charcoal has been shown in vitro to bind to NAC.[21a] In contrast, several studies on humans have shown no statistically significant decrease in serum NAC levels with concurrent use of activated charcoal.[22, 23] However, one study in 12 volunteers did show a 39% decrease in the area under the curve for serum NAC levels and a 29% reduction in the peak NAC level when activated charcoal was administered concurrently.[24] No studies demonstrate that the liver or serum NAC levels obtained with current dosing protocols are required for NAC efficacy, yet the studies suggesting avoidance of concurrent activated charcoal and NAC are based on this assumption. The initial studies on which the current NAC dosage regimens are based were done in mice. The overwhelming hepatoprotective effect shown in the multicenter trials,[20] regardless of concurrent activated charcoal use and the presence of coingestants, suggests that the current NAC dose is greater than required. Thus, current recommendations are to administer both activated charcoal and NAC in their usual doses. If a patient presents well within the 8-hour window for maximum NAC efficacy, activated charcoal should be administered first, and NAC about 1 hour later in the usual doses. The use of intravenous NAC conveniently prevents an interaction between NAC and activated charcoal.

Intravenous NAC is widely used in Europe and Canada. Its efficacy has clearly been demonstrated in comparison with that of the oral form.[25] Unfortunately, no pyrogen-free preparation is commercially available in the United States because NAC has not been approved by the Food and Drug Administration for intravenous use. The complications of intravenous NAC are limited to local irritation at the infusion site and allergic reactions. Also, cases of anaphylaxis have been reported. Because intravenous NAC is given over a shorter time-course (20–48 hours) than the oral form, the length and cost of hospitalization are decreased.

Flumazenil

Flumazenil is a 1,4-imidazobenzodiazepine that competitively inhibits benzodiazepines at the central receptors, effectively blocking their clinical effect. It was approved for use in the United States in 1991. Double-blind, placebo-controlled trials have shown significant improvement in central nervous system depression following flumazenil administration in benzodiazepine-intoxicated patients.[26–28] The median interval for resedation was 60 to 90 minutes. Mild adverse reactions were noted in 27% of the 162 patients treated with flumazenil, whereas the placebo group (164 patients) had adverse reactions in only 14%. The adverse reactions included agitation, crying, nausea, and vomiting. More serious reactions (predominantly seizures) were seen in four patients. Two of the three patients with seizures had also ingested cyclic antidepressants.[27, 29]

Contrary to popular belief, benzodiazepine overdose alone can cause death or serious morbidity. Coingestants often potentiate toxicity.[30] In 1993, more than 32,000 benzodiazepine exposures were reported to the AAPCC, and 1 of the 33 deaths involving benzodiazepines was not associated with coingestants.[1a, 31]

Animal studies have confirmed a relationship between cyclic antidepressant intoxication and flumazenil-induced seizures that may be related to the unmasking of a proconvulsant effect. In one study, 24 mongrel dogs were randomized to receive amitriptyline and placebo or amitriptyline and midazolam. Then, six dogs in each group received flumazenil, whereas the other six were treated with a placebo. The number of dogs with seizures induced by amitriptyline (4 of 6) was identical in both the amitriptyline-plus-placebo and the amitriptyline-plus-midazolam-and-flumazenil groups. Midazolam administration alone was shown to have a reversible, protective anticonvulsant effect.[32] Acute benzodiazepine withdrawal has also been reported following flumazenil administration, although this effect is not life threatening.[26, 33, 34]

Flumazenil is an effective benzodiazepine antagonist that may decrease morbidity, complications, and therapeutic intervention required in patients with benzodiazepine overdose. The risk of precipitating convulsions in tricyclic antidepressant overdoses dictates that caution be taken when flumazenil is administered in patients with mixed drug overdoses with undetermined agents.

Physostigmine

Physostigmine, a reversible acetylcholinesterase inhibitor, is an alkaloid extract from the Calabar or (ordeal) bean of the West African climbing vine *Physostigma venenosum.* As an uncharged, lipophilic, tertiary ammonium compound, physostigmine easily crosses the blood-brain barrier. The other reversible acetylcholinesterase inhibitors are quaternary ammonium compounds (edrophonium, neostigmine, pyridostigmine) and do not penetrate the blood-brain barrier.

Although physostigmine is effective in reversing both central and peripheral manifestations of anticholinergic drug overdose, adverse reactions are common. Symptoms of a cholinergic crisis, including salivation, lacrimation, urination, defecation, and bronchorrhea, may occur if physostigmine is administered in the absence of true anticholinergic poisoning. Even when given in the setting of pure anticholinergic overdose, physostigmine may cause seizures. Physostigmine use in anticholinergic poisonings should be limited to patients with life-threatening manifestations who are unresponsive to other therapy.

Complications are particularly frequent in the treatment of cyclic antidepressant overdose, in which the use of physostigmine is strongly discouraged. Physostigmine is not recommended in the treatment of cyclic antidepressant overdose because cardiac abnormalities unrelated to anticholinergic effects usually predominate as the cause of mortality.

A REVIEW OF SELECTED TOXIC AGENTS

Acetaminophen

Acetaminophen (*N*-acetyl-*p*-aminophenol, APAP, paracetamol) is the most prevalent analgesic implicated in overdose today. Twenty-seven deaths caused by acetaminophen alone were reported to the AAPCC in 1993. This figure represents 0.04% of all acetaminophen exposures reported to the AAPCC and is considerably less than the 0.13% fatality rate seen in aspirin exposures (only acetaminophen and aspirin formulated without other active ingredients are considered in this analysis).[1a]

Acetaminophen is rapidly absorbed from the gastrointestinal tract, reaching peak plasma concentrations within 40 to 60 minutes. The metabolism of acetaminophen is complex (Fig. 130–1) and varies as the blood levels and cumulative dosage change. Therapeutic doses of acetaminophen are metabolized (with an elimination half-life of 2–4 hours) to nontoxic glucuronide (42%) and sulfate conjugates (52%). Both routes can be saturated in the overdose setting. About 5% of the remaining metabolite is converted to a very toxic metabolite, *N*-acetyl-*p*-benzoquinonimine (NAPQI) by the cytochrome P_{450} mixed-function oxidase system. In small quantities, NAPQI is rapidly detoxified by conjugation with glutathione and excreted in the urine as mercapturic acid and cysteine conjugates. Pretreatment with a P_{450} inducer like phenobarbital increases the formation of NAPQI.[35] In the overdose state, the production of NAPQI outstrips the available amount of glutathione. When the supply of glutathione drops by 70%, the unconjugated NAPQI binds covalently to various hepatocellular macromolecules, producing massive centrilobular hepatocyte necrosis with periportal sparing. The half-life of acetaminophen in this setting can increase from 3 hours, as seen with therapeutic dosing, to 15 hours (or even longer) as the hepatic necrosis progresses.

Potential for a clinically significant overdose can be seen with acute acetaminophen ingestions of 150 mg/kg or of 7.5 to 10 g in an adult. The clinical presentation, primarily hepatotoxicity, is often delayed. Three general stages occur[36]:

- *Stage I* can begin within hours, with symptoms of nausea, vomiting, and diaphoresis; however, many patients remain asymptomatic. The symptoms gradually subside over 24 hours.
- *Stage II* occurs 24 to 48 hours after the ingestion, when gastrointestinal symptoms are minimal but hepatic injury is progressing. Right upper quadrant abdominal pain and early liver function abnormalities are noted (e.g., elevations in levels of alanine aminotransferase, aspartate aminotransferase, total bilirubin, and prothrombin time). Alkaline phosphatase and amylase levels remain near normal. The disproportionate rise in transaminase levels compared with the small increases in bilirubin concentration can help in the differentiation among acetaminophen-induced hepatic injury, viral hepatitis, and biliary obstruction.
- In *Stage III,* which occurs 3 to 4 days after ingestion, is when hepatic necrosis and liver function abnormalities peak. Hepatic encephalopathy, bleeding diatheses, and hypoglycemia may be present. By 7 to 9 days, most patients recover full hepatic function without evidence of cirrhosis.

Young children seem somewhat protected from the hepatotoxicity of acetaminophen. In a study of 417 children younger than 5 years who ingested more than 150 mg/kg of acetaminophen, only 55 had toxic serum levels, 43 received NAC, and only 3 had hepatotoxic reactions. All of these last three children had received a full course of NAC,

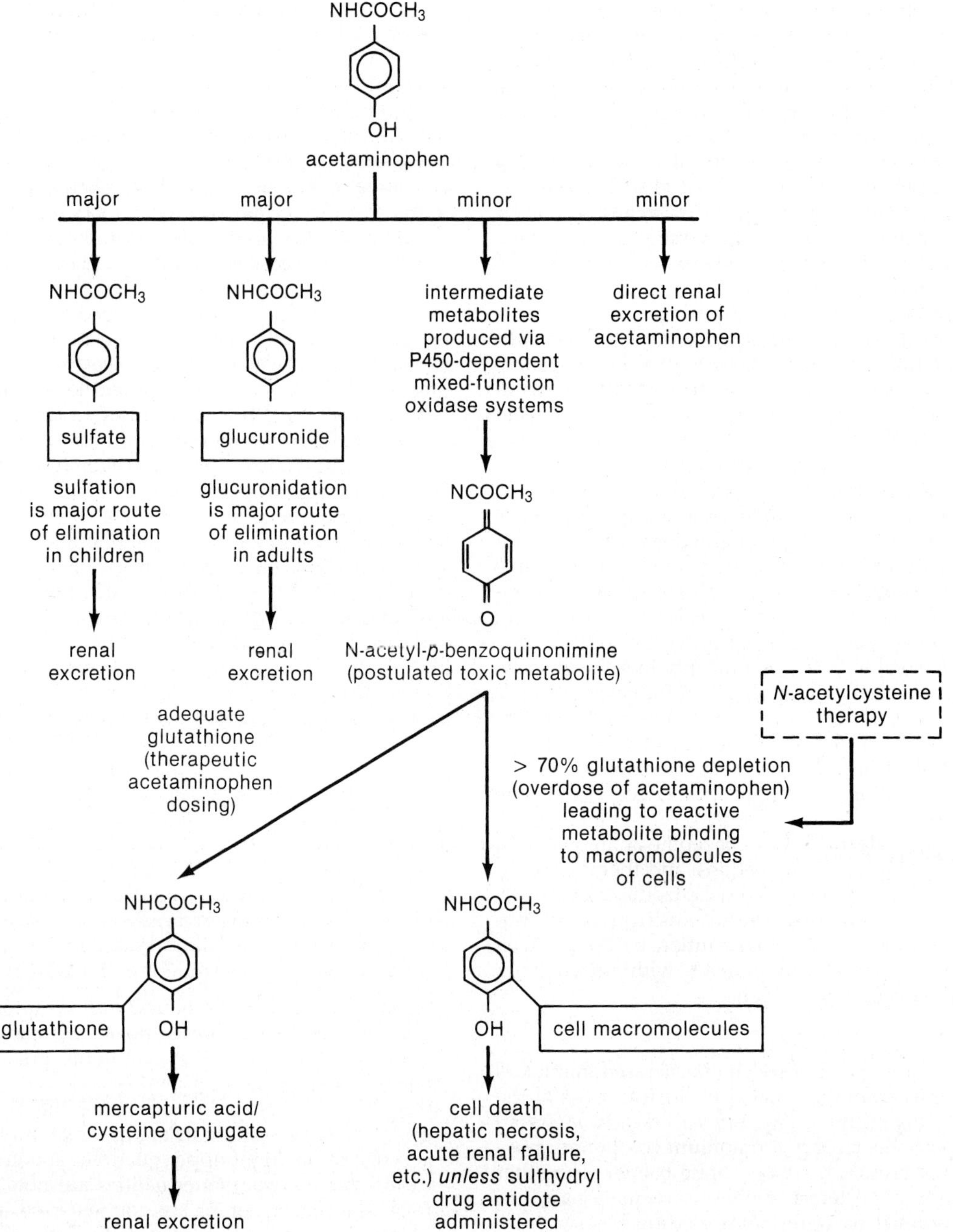

Figure 130–1. Metabolism of acetaminophen. (Adapted from Kunkle DB: Updating acetaminophen toxicity. Emerg Med 1985; 17:121.)

although this therapy was begun more than 16 hours after ingestion. No child died. The reason for the relative hepatic sparing seen in young children is unknown. Postulated mechanisms include an increased rate of glutathione turnover and disproportionate sulfonation compared with glucaronidation seen in children younger than 9 years of age.[37] Fetal acetaminophen levels and hepatic metabolism are similar to those observed in the pregnant mother who has been poisoned by acetaminophen, putting the fetus at risk of hepatotoxicity.[38]

Other organ systems can manifest acetaminophen toxicity. Acute renal failure with or without hepatic involvement may occur. The cardiac effects of acetaminophen toxicity are not common, but cases of pericarditis, myocardial necrosis, and diffuse electrocardiogram changes have been reported. Pancreatitis also has been reported but is uncommon.

Treatment of acetaminophen overdose is based on identification of potential victims, decontamination, assessment of risk based on serum concentration and a nomogram, early therapy with NAC, intensive supportive care, and early consultation for liver transplantation in refractory patients. The often overlooked presence of acetaminophen in medicinal products mandates evaluation of all overdose patients for possible acetaminophen exposure. In a prospective study of 486 overdose patients, 365 patients had a negative history of acetaminophen ingestion; however, 1.9% of these tested positive for the drug, and one patient had potential hepatotoxicity.[39]

The Rumack-Matthew nomogram used for the assessment of risk (Fig. 130–2[40]) is based on the serum acetaminophen level and the time since ingestion as correlated with hepatotoxicity data obtained from 30 overdose patients. A second line has been added below the original Rumack-Matthew nomogram line to allow for 25% laboratory-related inconsistency and for inaccuracies of the medical history regarding the time of ingestion.[20] The nomogram is valid only for an acute ingestion that occurred 4 hours or more before the first serum level was determined. The nomogram cannot be used for chronic ingestions. Any patient with a serum concentration above the lower nomogram line should receive a full 18-dose course of NAC, which is most effective if begun within 8 hours of drug ingestion.

With the advent of liver transplantation, early assessment of prognosis in overdose has become more important. Bilirubin and prothrombin time were shown in one study to be the most reliable prognostic indicators of fulminant hepatic failure and death.[40a] Other studies have shown that a serum pH less than 7.3 in combination with a serum creatinine concentration greater than 3.4 mg/dL, a prothrombin time greater than 100 milliseconds, or grade III or IV encephalopathy could identify over three quarters of potentially fatal cases.[41, 42] A rising prothrombin time on the fourth day after paracetamol ingestion and a peak prothrombin time of greater than 180 seconds has also been shown to identify patients with a less than 8% chance of survival.[43]

Pearls and Perils

- If initially indicated, oral NAC administration *must* be continued for the entire 18-dose course (loading dose and 17 maintenance doses) even if the serum acetaminophen level falls below the nomogram line during therapy.
- An acetaminophen level can only be plotted on the nomogram if (1) the ingestion is acute and (2) the level was determined 4 or more hours after ingestion.

Alcohols

Isopropanol, ethylene glycol, and methanol are the toxic alcohols that are commonly implicated in poisonings. More than 7000 exposures to isopropanol were reported to the AAPCC in 1993; however, no fatalities occurred. In contrast, about 2000 and 4000 exposures were reported for methanol and ethylene glycol, with 14 and 12 related deaths, respectively.[1a] The diagnosis and management of methanol and

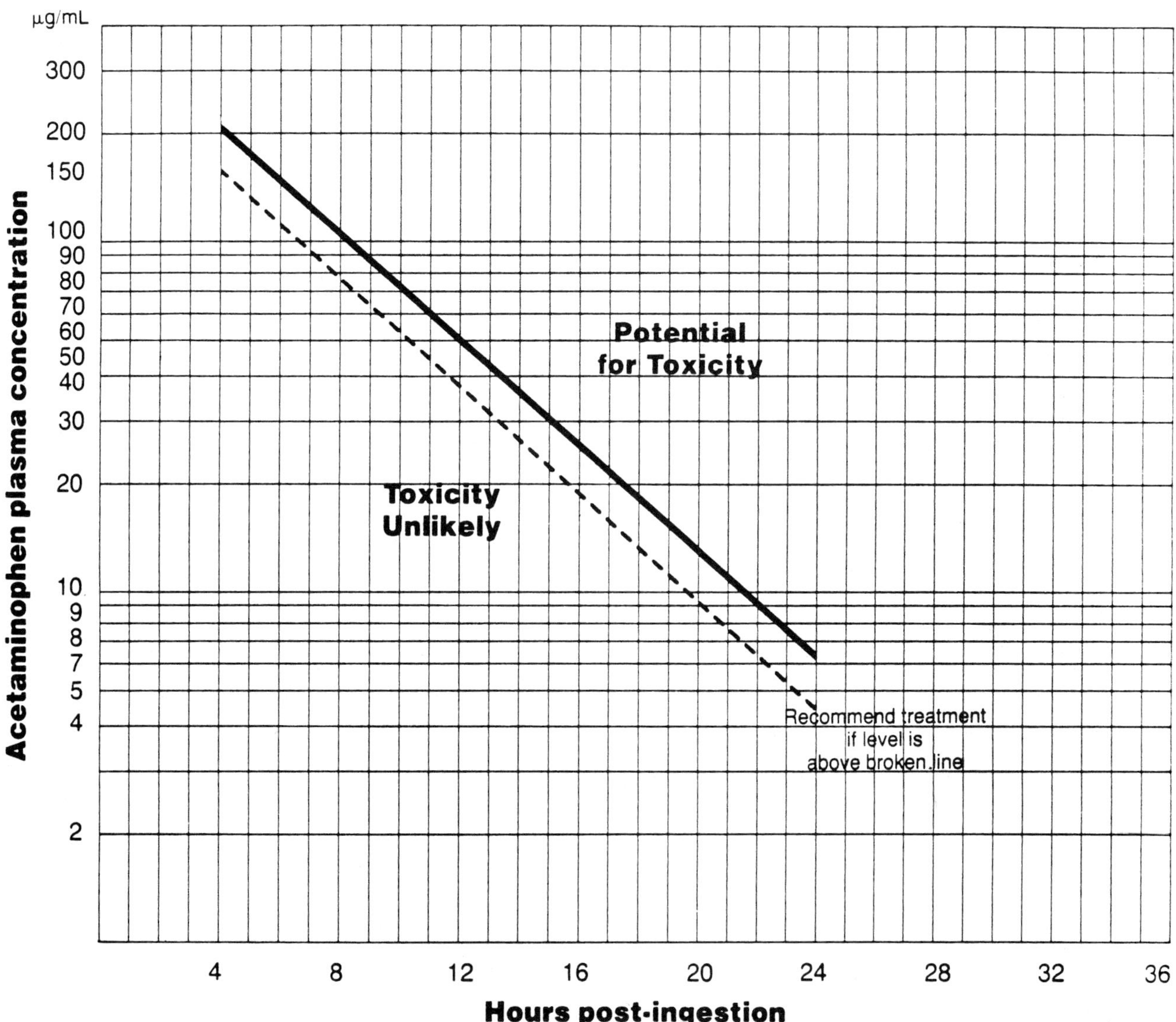

Figure 130–2. Nomogram: plasma or serum acetaminophen concentration as it relates to the time after acetaminophen ingestion. (Adapted from Rumack BH, Matthew H: Acetaminophen poisoning and toxicity. Pediatrics 1975; 55:871–876. Adapted by permission of Pediatrics.)

ethylene glycol overdose can be quite difficult, and morbidity and mortality are significant. Inappropriate management, especially early in the course of treatment, is common.

Ethylene glycol is found in antifreeze, de-icers, and industrial solvents. Methanol is referred to as "wood alcohol," whereas ethanol is known as "grain alcohol." Methanol can be found in paint remover, duplicator fluid, gas-line antifreeze, windshield washing fluid, solid canned fuel (4%), alternative fuels, denatured ethanol (added to ethanol to make it unfit to drink), and bootlegged whiskey (as a contaminant). Isopropanol is found in rubbing alcohol (although some rubbing alcohols contain ethanol), skin lotions, hair tonics, after-shave, and glass cleaners.

Alcohols are absorbed to varying degrees cutaneously, by inhalation, or by ingestion and can reach toxic blood levels within 1 hour (ethylene glycol can take up to 4 hours to reach these levels). They have low protein binding and a volume of distribution that is close to the amount of total body water (0.6 L/kg).

The metabolism of ethylene glycol and methanol produces the actual toxic metabolites. Ethylene glycol toxicity does not result from the glycol itself, but rather from the accumulation of four major metabolites: glycoaldehyde (which causes central nervous system depression), glycolate (which causes acidosis), formic acid (which causes acidosis), and oxalate (which causes calcium oxalate crystal formation and deposition in tissues). The oxidation of methanol proceeds at a rate that is one seventh that of ethanol and is independent of dose. Toxicity is related to the breakdown products formic acid and formaldehyde, and not to the methanol itself. The rate-limiting step in metabolism is the breakdown of methanol to formaldehyde by alcohol dehydrogenase. The formaldehyde is rapidly converted to formic acid and then, with folate as a cofactor, to carbon monoxide and water. As methanol is oxidized to formaldehyde, nicotinamide-adenine dinucleotide (oxidized form) (NAD^+) is converted to nicotinamide-adenine dinucleotide (reduced form) (NADH), favoring the reduction of pyruvate to lactate and causing additional acid formation. Isopropanol is metabolized by alcohol dehydrogenase more slowly than is ethanol. The major metabolite is acetone, which causes inebriation and central nervous system depression.

Ethylene glycol is odorless and sweet tasting, characteristics that make the clear liquid palatable to children. Blue or green fluorescent dye is added to most ethylene glycol–containing antifreeze products. Intoxication is similar to inebriation from ethanol. Four stages of clinical toxicity have been delineated:

- *Stage I* of ethylene glycol toxicity occurs over the first 30 minutes to 12 hours after ingestion, and is predominantly characterized by central nervous system effects and acidosis. The poisoned patient has nystagmus and depressed reflexes and appears intoxicated with Kussmaul's respirations owing to pronounced metabolic acidosis. Coma with focal seizures may develop, and tetany from hypocalcemia, although unusual, may ensue.
- *Stage II* occurs within the first 24 hours, when deposition of calcium oxalate crystals in the myocardium, lung, and vasculature causes multisystem complications, including hypertension, tachycardia, and pulmonary edema.
- At *Stage III* (24–72 hours), oliguric renal failure develops.
- *Stage IV* is characterized by delayed neurologic sequelae that occur 6 to 15 days after the original insult. Patients present with hyperreflexia, ataxia, facial nerve paralysis, and other cranial nerve abnormalities.[44, 45]

Methanol, like ethylene glycol, is also clear and odorless; however, in its crude form, it is bitter tasting, and this in part explains its use as an additive in denatured ethanol. Early central nervous system signs reflect inebriation, which may be followed by an asymptomatic period. The delayed effects begin after 6 to 36 hours, with vertigo, motor restlessness, delirium, blurred or whitened vision, hyperemia of optic disk, dilated pupils, and, occasionally, blindness. The classic description of visual changes is "seeing as if through a blizzard." Pulmonary findings include Kussmaul's respirations owing to the severe acidosis caused by formate and lactate. Bradycardia is uncommon, and its presence confers a grave prognosis. Abdominal pain, vomiting, and diarrhea are common.

Isopropanol is clear, colorless and bitter tasting and leaves the smell of acetone or "alcohol" on the breath. The neurologic symptoms of intoxication are similar to those of ethanol; however, isopropanol is twice as potent as ethanol, and this causes marked central nervous system depression, ataxia, headache, and depression of deep tendon reflexes. Gastrointestinal irritation, nausea, vomiting, abdominal pain, and hematemesis are common. Respiratory depression with progression to respiratory arrest and myocardial depression that causes hypotension can be seen in severe overdose.

The laboratory diagnosis is based on determination of the presence of an osmolar gap, an anion gap, and serum levels. The calculated osmolality (measured in milliosmoles per kilogram of water or in milliosmoles per liter) can be estimated with the following equation:

$$\text{Calculated osmolality} = 2 \times \text{Sodium (in mEq/L)} + \text{BUN (in mg/dL)}/2.8 + \text{Glucose (in mg/dL)}/18 + \text{Ethanol (in mg/dL)}/4.6,$$

where BUN is blood urea nitrogen level. Some authors suggest multiplying the sodium level by 1.86 rather than by 2 or multiplying the entire sum by 0.93 because serum is 93% water. Freezing point osmometry must be used to measure osmolality when volatile solutes such as alcohols are present. The use of vapor pressure osmometry can lead to a falsely low measured serum osmolality. The following relationship can be used to estimate the serum concentration:

$$\text{Serum concentration (in mg/dL)} = \text{Osmolar gap (in mOsm/L)} \times \text{MW (in mg/mOsm)}/10.8$$

A marked osmolar gap (0.2 mOsm/L for every 1 mg/dL of ethylene glycol) and an anion gap acidosis are present with ethylene glycol ingestions. However, the serum level of ethylene glycol may be low despite a persistent anion gap, suggesting that much of the ethylene glycol has been metabolized to glycolate. Ethylene glycol toxicity can be suggested by the presence of dihydrate or monohydrate calcium oxalate crystals in the urine. Although it has been said that Wood's lamp causes urine to fluoresce if certain dye additives were present in the formulation of antifreeze and were ingested within 2 to 4 hours, this is neither a sensitive nor a specific finding.[46] Hematuria and proteinuria associated with oliguria can be seen. The electrocardiogram may show evidence of QT_c prolongation from hypocalcemia that is induced by the formation of calcium oxalate crystals.

Methanol poisoned patients also have an osmolar gap (0.34 mOsm/L for every 1 mg/dL of methanol) and a marked anion gap acidosis from the metabolite formate. No crystals are seen in the urine. Computed tomography scans may show a hemorrhagic or nonhemorrhagic focal necrosis of the putamen.

Isopropanol produces an osmolar gap (0.17 mOsm/L for every 1 mg/dL of isopropanol) and ketonuria because 15% of it is metabolized to acetone. The ketonuria is accompanied by only minimal acidosis and no glycosuria. Determination of serum acetone levels can be helpful.

The treatment of ethylene glycol and methanol poisoning

is based on prevention of the formation of toxic metabolites. Gastric emptying may be effective early. Activated charcoal use is ineffective. Ethanol administration should be started *early* to prevent the metabolism of ethylene glycol to glycoaldehyde and that of methanol to formaldehyde by competitively inhibiting the hepatic enzyme alcohol dehydrogenase. Ethanol can be administered orally or intravenously. The oral ethanol should be in solution of 20% or greater, and intravenous ethanol should be in solution of 5% to 10%. A product's "proof" is twice the per cent ethanol by volume. Begin treatment with an intravenous bolus of 7.9 to 10 mL/kg of 10% ethanol in 5% dextrose in water over 30 minutes. A maintenance infusion can be estimated at 1 to 2 $mL \cdot kg^{-1} \cdot h^{-1}$ of 10% ethanol in 5% dextrose in water; the higher end of the range should be chosen for the chronic drinker. A serum level of just over 100 mg/dL should be maintained. Acidosis should be aggressively treated with sodium bicarbonate. Hemodialysis should be instituted early for ethylene glycol intoxication if the level is greater than 50 mg/dL or if a patient has metabolic or hemodynamic evidence of toxicity; for methanol intoxication, hemodialysis should be instituted if the methanol level is greater than 50 mg/dL or if a patient has clinical manifestations of toxicity, such as visual changes or acidosis. Glycolate, the major contributor to acidosis in ethylene glycol overdose, is well dialyzed. During hemodialysis, ethanol can be added to the dialysate bath to achieve a concentration of 100 mg/dL in the dialysate.

Specific additional therapies for an ethylene glycol overdose patient include administration of thiamine (100 mg intravenously per day) and pyridoxine (100 mg intravenously per day) to enhance the metabolism of glyoxylate. Experimental therapies include the use of 4-methylpyrazole, which is a potent inhibitor of alcohol dehydrogenase. The benefits of this agent are oral bioavailability and no central nervous system depression as seen with ethanol. Case reports of 4-methylpyrazole treatment show success.[47] This drug is currently for experimental use only in the United States.

Specific therapies for methanol intoxication include administration of folic acid and its metabolite leucovorin (folinic acid), which is a cofactor in the metabolism of formate. The dose is 1 to 2 mg/kg intravenously every 4 hours for six doses. Leucovorin, the active form, is preferred in patients who are already symptomatic. Experimentally, 4-methylpyrazole also has been proposed as an alternative to ethanol as initial therapy for methanol intoxication.

Isopropanol therapy is predominantly supportive; hemodialysis is reserved for patients with hypotension that is unresponsive to fluid administration. Isopropanol and acetone are effectively dialyzed, but the procedure is infrequently needed.

Pearls and Perils

- Patients are often asymptomatic early, and the history of ingestion may be in doubt; meanwhile, toxic metabolites are being formed. The metabolism should be blocked with ethanol until determination of the level is made.
- Look for methanol or ethylene glycol poisoning in any patient with an anion gap acidosis or an osmolar gap, or with both. Toxicologic screens do not routinely test for methanol or ethylene glycol.

Alkalis, Acids, and Hydrofluoric Acid

Liquid, granular, and solid forms of alkali (usually sodium or potassium hydroxide) are present in many households. Liquid and granular forms can be found mostly in drain openers, oven cleaners, automatic dishwasher detergents, and other household cleaning products. Automotive airbags can also release a sodium hydroxide powder if they burst on impact. The tablets used to test urine for sugar (e.g., Clinitest) and tablets to clean dentures also contain alkali. Acids are usually liquid or granular and are found in toilet bowl cleaners, battery acids, antirust compounds, and some drain cleaners. Hydrofluoric acid can be found in rust removal agents, automobile tire cleaners, and glass-etching solutions.

Injury occurs on contact with the caustic agents through inhalation, ingestion, dermal contact, or ocular exposure. The severity of the injury associated with exposure to the caustics is variable and depends on the pH (and molarity), concentration, viscosity, ingested volume, form of compound, current stomach contents, heat of reaction, and associated toxic substances. In general, tissue exposure to a pH of greater than 12 or less than 2 is associated with damage. The measurement of titratable acid-alkaline reserve, a concept similar to normality, has been suggested as a better predictor of caustic potential than pH. Titratable acid-alkaline reserve is defined as the number of milliliters of a 0.1 molar solution of hydrochloric acid or sodium hydroxide required to titrate 100 mL of a 1% solution of test product to pH 8.0.[48] As the concentration, viscosity, and volume increase, the amount and duration of tissue exposure also increase. Cement, for example, liberates calcium hydroxide with a pH of 11 to 13 when it is mixed with water. The thick, tenacious material causes third-degree burns only after hours of contact, usually in individuals who have been kneeling in wet cement.[49] The form of the ingestant is important, in that granular products are rarely swallowed completely. The heat of neutralization becomes important if prehospital neutralization has erroneously been attempted. The heat of neutralization describes an exothermic reaction caused by contact of an acid with a base. Clinitest tablets contain citric acid and sodium hydroxide, and when dissolved in 1.5 mL of water, temperatures of up to 69.5°C are generated.[50]

The mechanism of injury for acids and alkali differ. Alkali cause liquefaction necrosis during contact with and penetration of tissues. Destruction of protein and collagen, saponification of fat, and thrombosis of blood vessels occurs within minutes after exposure. Acids, however, tend to cause coagulation necrosis and have more limited penetration. Destruction begins with the columnar epithelium and progresses through the submucosa and muscularis mucosa to the loose connective tissue and blood vessels in which thrombosis and coagulation occur. A protective hard eschar is formed, limiting further penetration. Hydrofluoric acid is actually a weak acid that dissociates poorly in solution. This property actually enhances the toxicity of the fluoride component. Although the free proton may contribute to tissue damage, as with other acids, it is the uncharged hydrogen fluoride complex that penetrates deeply into tissues. In the tissues, dissociation takes place, slowly releasing the strongly negative fluoride ions that bind avidly to calcium and magnesium.

Symptoms may be deceptively mild as compared with the mucosal damage and long-term sequelae following alkaline burns. For example, within minutes alkali can begin to penetrate the corneal stroma, interfering with sensory nerves and producing anesthesia. Penetration then continues, sometimes without pain, to involve the structures of the anterior chamber and retina, causing total blindness. In contrast, acid injuries are usually painful, are limited to the cornea, and only rarely cause blindness. Inhalation of either acids or alkali can produce coughing, stridor, and severe damage to the respiratory mucosa, leading to pulmonary edema and respiratory failure. Dermal exposure can produce first- to third-degree burns. Acids, however, infrequently cause third-degree burns but do cause significant pain. Low concentrations (<20%) of hydrofluoric acid can cause pain, erythema, and necrosis, which may be delayed for up to 24 hours after contact. Gastrointestinal symptoms with significant injury are usually present. Dysphagia, odynophagia, drooling, vomiting, hematemesis, and oropharyngeal, substernal, and abdominal pain may be observed. Evidence of pneumomediastinum or intra-abdominal perforation may also be present. Alkali causes oral and circumferential esophageal burns with subsequent scarring and stricture formation. The stomach and small bowel are less frequently involved. Long-term follow-up of serious alkaline burns often reveals esophageal obstruction and stricture formation. The incidence of esophageal carcinoma may be increased 100-fold in patients with prior alkaline injuries. Acids, however, tend to traverse the esophagus quickly and cause more damage at the gastric antrum and pylorus. Relaxation of the pyloric sphincter allows passage of the acid into the small bowel, where perforation occurs.

Endoscopists have categorized mucosal burns into three degrees of severity. First-degree burns have visible erythema and edema but are without the blistering, superficial ulceration, or fibrinous exudate that characterize second-degree burns. Third-degree burns are characterized by erythema, deep ulceration, friability, eschar formation, and possibly perforation.

Three studies have attempted to clarify which symptoms suggest severe—grade 2 or grade 3—gastrointestinal pathology. Gaudreault and coworkers retrospectively evaluated signs and symptoms in 378 children who had endoscopy following acid or alkaline ingestion. None of the individual signs—vomiting, dysphagia, drooling, abdominal pain, refusal to drink, or oropharyngeal burns—was found to reliably predict injury. In fact, 10 patients without symptoms had second-degree burns, and 1 of these developed a stricture.[51] Another retrospective study evaluated 79 children for signs of drooling, vomiting, or stridor and found that the presence of two or more of these signs accurately identified those patients with severe burns.[52] A prospective study of 63 patients with alkaline ingestion who underwent endoscopy showed that no completely asymptomatic patient had a grade 2 or grade 3 lesion and that there was no particular symptom that identified all the patients with severe injury. Incidentally, suicidal patients were more likely to have significant lesions, as determined by endoscopy (53%).[53] In summary, symptomatic patients with a history of caustic ingestion should be examined with endoscopy to assess the extent of their injury. Suicidal patients may be less cooperative and are at increased risk for serious lesions; thus, a lower threshold for endoscopy may be warranted.

Systemic symptoms following alkali exposure are usually secondary to perforation, tissue damage, and edema. Patients who have ingested significant amounts of acid can develop metabolic acidosis, hemolysis, and shock directly from acid absorption. Dermal, pulmonary, or gastrointestinal exposure to hydrofluoric acid can cause systemic fluoride poisoning. Patients with burns of more than 1% of body surface area with a more than 50% solution are at risk, as are patients with inhalation or ingestion exposures. Signs of fluoride poisoning include marked hypocalcemia, tetany, muscle spasms, hyperkalemia, metabolic acidosis, seizures, and lethal arrhythmias.

The treatment of all dermal and ocular exposures begins with copious irrigation and removal of contaminated clothing. Neutralization is not recommended. Ocular irrigation should continue until the ocular pH has returned to the neutral range and all particulate material has been removed. Alkaline burns require irrigation for at least 1 hour and sometimes for up to 12 hours. Lid retractors and topical anesthetics are important adjuncts. The skin exposed to alkali should be washed until the soapy feeling has been removed. Ophthalmology consultation is merited for all severe alkaline eye burns, and prolonged irrigation as well as use of topical mydriatics, cycloplegics, antibiotics, steroids, and collagenase inhibitors may be required.

The airway and ventilatory status of patients with pulmonary inhalation is of the utmost importance. Rapid progression of pharyngeal and laryngeal edema may necessitate early intubation or cricothyroidotomy with subsequent tracheostomy.

Emesis and lavage are usually contraindicated for acid and alkali ingestions, and use of activated charcoal is ineffective. Dilution (not neutralization) with milk or water is routinely advised. Although the efficacy of this measure remains unproven in humans, rat studies suggest a beneficial effect.[53a] Early endoscopy in symptomatic patients may reveal necrosis or esophageal lesions that are prone to stricture formation. The use of corticosteroids or antibiotics, or both, has been a controversial issue for decades. A prospective, randomized study of 60 children showed no correlation between treatment with methylprednisolone and ampicillin and stricture formation.[54] Antibiotics are often used in conjunction with steroids in an effort to decrease infectious complications but are not indicated prophylactically in the absence of symptoms in patients who are not receiving steroids.[55] Esophageal replacement or repeated esophageal dilation may eventually be required.

Hydrofluoric acid burns are treated with similar attention to decontamination and respiratory status, but calcium is used as an adjunct. Superficial skin burns can be treated with a topical gel of 2.5% calcium gluconate mixed as 3.5 g of USP calcium gluconate powder in 5 oz of surgical lubricant.[56a] This can be repeated as often as necessary to relieve pain. If pain is not relieved or if the burns are deep, subcutaneous calcium gluconate infiltration may be required. A 5% to 10% calcium gluconate solution is injected with a 30-gauge needle in a dose of 0.5 mL/cm^2 of affected tissue. Calcium chloride should never be infiltrated in place of calcium gluconate because it is very irritating. Intra-arterial infusions of calcium gluconate are less painful and may be more effective than subcutaneous injections for digital burns.[57, 58] Administration of large amounts of intravenous calcium chloride or gluconate may be required to prevent hypocalcemia in patients with systemic fluoride toxicity.

Pearls and Perils

- Gastric lavage with a soft tube may be indicated in patients who have ingested substantial amounts to decrease the risk of severe, potentially lethal fluoride toxicity.
- Watch for systemic toxicity, as it may become fatal rapidly.
- Monitor all patients with hydrofluoric acid ingestion for hypocalcemia. Urgent treatment with large doses of intravenous calcium may be required.

Beta-Blockers

Beta-blockers are competitive antagonists and block endogenous catecholamine activity. Beta$_1$ receptors are located in the heart, and β_2 receptors are located primarily in the bronchial tree and in blood vessel walls. The more selective a drug is for the β_1 receptors, which are located primarily in the heart, the fewer peripheral effects that are observed (e.g., bronchospasm, hypoglycemia). The more cardioselective agents include acebutolol, atenolol, betaxolol, esmolol, and metoprolol. The membrane-stabilizing effect (or quinidine-like effect) refers to interference with depolarization brought about by an interaction with the sodium channels; this produces depression of the myocardium that can manifest as widening of the QRS complex and depression of cardiac output. Examples of the β-blockers commonly associated with this effect are acebutolol, betaxolol, penbutolol, pindolol, and propranolol. Intrinsic sympathomimetic effects of partial agonist activity is present with acebutolol, carteolol, penbutolol, and pindolol. Weak α-adrenergic blocking properties are present with labetalol. Lipid solubility varies with different drugs; propranolol is the most soluble and thus has the greatest blood-brain penetration and the most profound effect on the central nervous system. The elimination half-life of individual β-blockers also varies tremendously and is increased in the overdose patient.

The clinical manifestations following a β-blocker overdose vary in severity with the type and the amount of drug ingested. Some patients become symptomatic following ocular exposure to β-blocker–containing ophthalmic products. The cardiovascular manifestations are the major cause of morbidity and mortality. They include bradycardia, atrioventricular blocks, arrhythmias, and hypotension; with the partial agonists, especially pindolol, tachycardia and hypertension can occur. Other effects include bronchospasm, wheezing, dyspnea, delirium, lethargy, decreased level of consciousness, and seizures. Hypoglycemia may occur, especially in children, due to inadequate glycogen mobilization in response to epinephrine. Hyperglycemia has also been reported in chronic poisoning.

The treatment of β-blocker overdoses begins with immediate decontamination. Administration of activated charcoal and gastric lavage are the methods of choice for substantial ingestions because the possibility for rapid cardiovascular collapse renders emesis unsafe. Multidose activated charcoal has been shown to enhance the elimination of several β-blockers. With sustained-release preparations, whole-bowel irrigation may be indicated. Cardiovascular effects predominate and should be treated aggressively with intravenous glucagon administration and a combination of fluid resuscitation, vasopressor agents and atropine therapy, and transvenous pacing. Glucagon is a polypeptide hormone with positive inotropic and chronotropic action that is mediated by adenyl cyclase. It causes an increase in cyclic adenosine monophosphate formation, an increase in intracellular calcium flux, and an increase in catecholamines without utilization of the β receptors.[59] Experience with the use of glucagon in human overdose patients has been limited to case studies, but improvement in hemodynamic status has been documented.[60, 61] An initial bolus of 5 to 10 mg in adults given intravenously over 1 minute is followed by an infusion of 1 to 10 mg/h titrated to response. Sterile saline or 5% dextrose in water should be used in place of the manufacturer's diluent (Eli Lilly and Company, Indianapolis, IN), which contains phenol (0.2%). Reversal of the negative inotropic and chronotropic effects should be observed within 1 to 3 minutes and last 15 to 30 minutes. Isoproterenol, epinephrine, and norepinephrine can be useful in reversing hypotension.[62] A Swan-Ganz catheter, transvenous pacer, intra-aortic balloon pump, and cardiopulmonary bypass are sometimes required to maintain adequate perfusion during an acute overdose. Bronchospasm can be treated with aminophylline and nebulized beta$_2$ agonists. When pharmacotherapy fails, hemodialysis or hemoperfusion may be considered for the more water-soluble agents with low volumes of distribution (specifically, atenolol and acebutolol); however, glucagon and other drug therapy should be used preferentially.

Pearls and Perils

- Hypoglycemia, especially in children, can be the occult cause of severe complications.
- The administration of high doses of glucagon required for some patients can rapidly deplete hospital stores, so check with the pharmacy early.

Calcium Channel Blockers

Death from overdose of calcium channel blockers has increased dramatically in frequency over the past decade. During the 5-year period from 1985 through 1989, 10,432 calcium channel blocker exposures were reported to the AAPCC, including 165 patients who suffered a major effect (life-threatening effect or permanent disability) and 61 fatalities.[63–67] The number of reports continued to increase gradually, and in 1993 alone, there were 6730 reports of calcium channel blocker exposure, including 182 patients with a major effect and 35 fatalities.[1a]

Immediate-release and sustained-release products are now available, and these products have a wide variety of pharmacologic effects. The immediate-release products include diltiazem, nicardipine, nifedipine, nimodipine, and verapamil. Three calcium antagonists are currently available in sustained-release form: diltiazem, nifedipine, and verapamil.

The pharmacokinetics of the various immediate-release products are similar. These drugs reach peak serum levels within 0.5 to 3 hours, are 90% to 99% protein bound, and have high first-pass metabolism that limits their bioavailability to between 10% and 60%. Their half-lives are more variable, ranging from 1 to 12 hours, and even longer if they are taken in overdose. The slow-release preparations (which tend to aggregate and thus slow dissolution) have even longer and less predictable half-lives.

The primary action of this class of agents is to oppose calcium flux at cell membranes. Calcium flux plays an integral role in cardiac contractility, intrinsic cardiac conduction, pacemaker function, and the regulation of systemic vascular tone. The electrical activity of the sinoatrial node and the atrioventricular node is dependent on the "slow inward current" that is provided by calcium entry. Calcium is also required for skeletal and myocardial muscle contraction.

Cardiac toxicity usually predominates as the major cause of morbidity and mortality. Hypotension and cardiac arrhythmias, including sinus bradycardia, junctional rhythms, second- and third-degree heart block, and asystole are commonly reported. Nifedipine acts primarily on the peripheral vasculature as a vasodilator and thus manifests fewer conduction delays and less myocardial depression when taken in overdose. Verapamil overdose more commonly causes arrhythmias, conduction blockade, and decreased myocardial contractility. Diltiazem overdose results in impairment of conduction and contractility to a greater extent than does nifedipine but to a lesser extent than does verapamil.[68] Central nervous system effects include dizziness, lethargy, confusion, slurred speech, and rarely seizures. Hyperglycemia and lactic acidosis are not infrequent.[69]

The treatment of calcium antagonist overdose patients involves decontamination, calcium and glucagon administration, and specific management of arrhythmias and hypotension that may involve multiple invasive techniques (e.g., Swan-Ganz catheterization, external or internal pacemaker placement, intra-aortic balloon pump, or cardiopulmonary bypass). Decontamination is primary and should begin with gastric emptying and administration of activated charcoal and a cathartic. Ipecac is contraindicated in patients who have ingested substantial quantities because rapid deterioration of mental and cardiovascular status can occur. In patients with large ingested amounts or who have taken sustained-release products, multidose activated charcoal and whole-bowel irrigation may be indicated, although data confirming the efficacy of this measure is unavailable. Whole-bowel irrigation can be instituted with a polyethylene glycol–electrolyte lavage solution (GoLYTELY; Colyte) as a slow infusion via nasogastric tube or orally (0.5 L/h for children, and 2 L/h in adults) until the rectal effluent is clear. Exogenous calcium salts (chloride or gluconate) function by increasing extracellular calcium and enhancing intracellular calcium flux. Calcium chloride is 27% elemental calcium, whereas calcium gluconate is only 9% elemental calcium; this partially explains the preferential use of the chloride salt in patients with good intravenous access and a reasonable acid-base status. Also, some evidence indicates that calcium chloride, even in equimolar amounts, produces a more reliable increase in extracellular serum calcium and greater inotropic action than does calcium gluconate.

Glucagon is a polypeptide hormone having positive inotropic and chronotropic actions that seem to be mediated by adenyl cyclase, which increases cyclic adenosine monophosphate formation.[59, 70, 71] Experience in human overdose patients is limited to case reports, but improvement in hemodynamic status has been documented.[72, 73] Cardiopulmonary bypass, transvenous pacing, and intra-aortic balloon pumps have all been used effectively as supportive care. Hemoperfusion and hemodialysis have not been used extensively because the high volume of distribution and high protein binding of the calcium antagonists suggest that these measures would have limited efficacy.

Pearls and Perils

- The high doses of glucagon required in some patients can rapidly deplete hospital stores. Check with the hospital pharmacy early.
- Intravenous access should be rechecked for patency before each dose of calcium chloride is administered because extravasation into the local tissues can cause severe tissue necrosis.

Carbon Monoxide

Carbon monoxide is ubiquitous. It is the leading single agent implicated in suicide-related deaths.[74] The odorless gas causes permanent disability and death, not only of suicide victims, but also of many unsuspecting individuals as well. Almost all exogenous carbon monoxide is man-made. Its source can vary but is primarily the incomplete combustion of carbonaceous materials. Natural gas does not contain carbon monoxide, but carbon monoxide is generated if natural gas is incompletely burned. Heavy traffic can cause carbon monoxide levels of 115 parts per million (ppm; 0.1% = 1000 ppm). The Office of Safety and Health Administration recommended that 8-hour, time-weighted average exposure limit is 50 ppm.[75] Other sources include furnaces, hot water heaters with malfunctioning exhaust mechanisms, and all internal combustion engines. Sterno, kerosene heaters, butane, charcoal, and gas cooking stoves can all release carbon monoxide. One study showed that selecting patients who used a stove for household heating and who had symptoms of headache or dizziness correctly predicted all patients with random carboxyhemoglobin levels greater than 10%.[76] Fire fighters and smokers are at increased risk for carbon monoxide poisoning. During a fire, the normal minute ventilation can rise from 6 L/min to 30 L/min, and because ambient carbon monoxide level may be 2000 ppm, carboxyhemoglobin levels can increase to 25% within 4 minutes.[77] Methylene chloride (a paint stripper) and methylene iodide (used to analyze gem quality) are metabolized within hours to clinically significant amounts of carbon monoxide.

Inhaled carbon monoxide rapidly diffuses across the alveolocapillary membrane and becomes bound to the four binding sites of hemoglobin. The relative affinity of carbon monoxide for hemoglobin is 200 times that of oxygen, and carbon monoxide adherence to one of these binding sites inhibits oxygen release at the other three. In addition, 10% to 15% of carbon monoxide stores are bound to extravascular tissues and interfere with cellular respiration through different mechanisms. There has been some controversy regarding carbon monoxide's mechanism of toxicity. In the past, the hypoxia and clinical manifestations of carbon monoxide poisoning were attributed to the decreased oxygen-carrying capacity of hemoglobin and to the leftward shift of the oxyhemoglobin dissociation curve. More recent studies have shown that carbon monoxide binding to myoglobin and cytochrome oxidase also interferes with intracellular respiration.[78]

The half-life of carboxyhemoglobin in room air is 3 to 5 hours, and in 100% oxygen it is 30 to 80 minutes; binding to myoglobin and cytochrome oxidases cannot be directly measured. In the hyperbaric oxygen chamber, the half-life of carboxyhemoglobin is reduced to 20 to 30 minutes. Those at high risk for carbon monoxide poisoning include fetuses, pregnant women, children younger than 15 to 16 years of age, and the elderly. Often, infants, children, and pets are the first to manifest symptoms of increased ambient carbon monoxide because they have increased metabolic demands.

The symptoms of mild to moderate carbon monoxide poisoning are usually seen at carboxyhemoglobin levels of 10% to 30% and may include headache, dizziness, weakness, nausea, dyspnea, visual disturbances, irritability, and decreased concentration. The signs are mild tachycardia, tachypnea, mild systolic hypotension, vomiting, and confusion. In severe carbon monoxide poisoning, the carboxyhemoglobin level is usually over 30% to 50%, and findings include visual field defects, blindness, papilledema, retinal hemorrhages, adult respiratory distress syndrome, arrhythmias, hypotension, syncope, and angina. Neurologic features include intense headaches, subtle confusion that progresses to coma, seizures, agitation, cranial nerve deficits, increased deep tendon reflexes, hyperventilation, muscular rigidity, and ataxia.

The subacute and chronic manifestations can resolve over years or be permanent. Although three types of cortical lesions were described in a pathologic review of 22 cases with delayed neurologic deterioration, bilateral necrosis of the globus pallidus was the most common, reflecting selective hypoperfusion.[79] The clinical findings in the delayed neurologic syndrome are widespread and include cortical blindness, psychosis, extrapyramidal rigidity, akinesia, aphasia, dementia, and choreoathetosis. More subtle findings include memory impairment, personality alterations, and parietal lobe dysfunction with visual agnosia, dyspraxia, dysnomia, and dysgraphia.[80] Neurologic sequelae were documented in 2.7% of a group of 2360 patients with clinical carbon monoxide intoxication. At 2-year follow-up, 11.8% of the admitted patients in this series were found to have permanent neurologic sequelae.[81]

Common laboratory tests, including complete blood count and chemistry determinations, are not of value in the diagnosis of carbon monoxide poisoning. In a study of 114 cases of carbon monoxide intoxication, 40 patients (35%) had electrocardiographic abnormalities, but none of the abnormalities was specific for carbon monoxide toxicity.[82] Arterial blood gas determinations are notoriously unreliable for assessing oxyhemoglobin level because PO_2 is a measurement of the partial pressure of oxygen in millimeters of mercury, *not* of the oxygen saturation of hemoglobin. Furthermore, oxygen saturation determined by pulse oximetry is unreliable in the setting of carbon monoxide poisoning. Urine that tests positive for myoglobin suggests rhabdomyolysis. Computed tomography scanning is useful in determining prognosis. Lesions involving the globus pallidus are associated with a poor medical outcome.

Specific laboratory tests can be helpful if used correctly. Spot tests, such as those involving the addition of ammonia or sodium bicarbonate to dilute serum, are very unreliable.[83] Carboxyhemoglobin spectrophotometry has been the standard for many years and is accurate for assessing current carboxyhemoglobin content; however, extrapolation back to the initial carboxyhemoglobin level (using the half-life) may be important in determining the need for hyperbaric oxygen therapy. Carboxyhemoglobin saturations of 0.5% to 3% can be found in nonsmoking adults. Smokers have levels of up to 7%, and in those with hemolytic anemia, levels up to 6% have been reported. Carbon monoxide breath analyzers have been shown to produce results that correlate with those of spectrophotometric testing.[84] Early psychometric testing has been recommended as a more reliable indicator of the severity of carbon monoxide intoxication. A carbon monoxide neuropsychologic screening battery has been developed for this purpose.[85]

The therapy of mild to moderate carbon monoxide poisoning is controversial.[85a] Mild to moderate acidosis should not be aggressively treated because hydrogen ions shift the hemoglobin dissociation curve to the right, thus enhancing oxygen delivery to tissues. The only currently accepted treatment of carbon monoxide poisoning is administration of oxygen. Hyperbaric oxygen therapy can oxygenate tissues much more effectively than normobaric oxygen therapy, yet no controlled studies support that superior clinical outcomes occur with hyperbaric oxygen treatment.

The indications for hyperbaric oxygen therapy are unknown, but guidelines have been proposed by various centers that offer hyperbaric oxygen therapy. Generally, candidates for this therapy include all patients with a known carbon monoxide exposure and at least one of the following:

Coma or a history of coma at some point after the exposure
Neurologic impairment as determined by psychometric testing or other means
Cardiovascular involvement, including chest pain, ischemic electrocardiographic findings, or cardiac arrhythmias
Symptoms that do not resolve after 6 hours of continuous 100% normobaric oxygen therapy
A carboxyhemoglobin level greater than 40%
Pregnancy, with a carboxyhemoglobin level greater than 15% to 20% or signs of fetal distress[86]
Recurrent symptoms up to 3 weeks after treatment with normobaric oxygen
A history of ischemic heart disease and levels of carbon monoxide greater than 20%

The complications of hyperbaric oxygen therapy include vomiting, sinus barotrauma, claustrophobia, pneumothorax, air embolism, corneal injury under contact lenses, odontalgia, and tympanic membrane rupture.

Pearls and Perils

- Any patient with injuries associated with smoke inhalation should be evaluated for carbon monoxide toxicity.
- Historical information concerning family and pets should be obtained from patients with the protean manifestations of carbon monoxide toxicity.
- Normal arterial blood gas values do not rule out the possibility of carbon monoxide toxicity.

Cyanide

Throughout the ages, cyanide has been used for suicide, murder, and mass executions. In the 1940s, Nazi extermination camps used the gas hydrogen cyanide (Zyklon B) for execution, and to this day it is still used for judicial executions in the United States. In 1978 in Jonestown, Guyana, 913 people died after drinking cyanide-laced Kool-Aid in a mass suicide. In 1982, seven unrelated people in the Chicago area died after accidentally ingesting potassium cyanide–contaminated Extra Strength Tylenol capsules.[87, 88]

Cyanide is used in industry for electroplating, refining precious metals, and hardening steel. Hydrogen cyanide gas can be liberated during a fire; by pyrolysis of wool, silk, nylons, polyurethanes, and polyacrylonitriles; from cyanide salts that have been mixed with acid in a laboratory; or when cyanide powders are used as pesticide fumigants in horticulture. Cyanogenic glycosides are found in over 1000 plants (e.g., sorghum, flax, lima beans, cassava roots) and in the kernels of fruit pits (e.g., apple, peach, plum, apricot [Laetrile], bitter almond). Nitrile compounds (acetonitrile, propiononitrile) and sodium nitroprusside also contain cyanide that can be liberated by metabolism.

Cyanide can be inhaled as cyanide gas, injected, ingested, or absorbed through mucosal membranes and intact skin. Absorption is rapid (within seconds to minutes) by almost any route. Some compounds appear to have delayed absorption (30 minutes to 2 hours or longer) because cyanide is released as a product of metabolism. For example, the seeds and pits of some fruits contain the cyanogenic glycoside amygdalin, which is converted to hydrogen cyanide by a reaction catalyzed by the enzyme β-glucosidase. This enzyme is present in the moistened, crushed pit and in the human gastrointestinal tract. This reaction takes place faster at an alkaline pH; this partially explains the delay in onset of symptoms because the seed must reach the alkaline environment of the duodenum.

After absorption, cyanide is transported to the liver where, metabolism by an endogenous enzyme, rhodanese, takes place. Thiocyanate is produced by this rhodanese catalyzed reaction as long as a sulfur substrate, thiosulfate, is available. Although thiocyanate is much less toxic than cyanide, high serum levels can cause symptoms. The usual half-life of this reaction for a nonlethal dose is from 20 minutes to 1 hour; however, in the overdose state, the half-life can extend to 19 hours.[89]

The mechanism of toxicity is based on the binding of cyanide to the ferric ion (Fe^{3+}) in the cytochrome oxidase enzymes and on interruption of electron transport and, thus, oxidative phosphorylation. Pyruvate can no longer be metabolized in the Krebs' cycle and is converted to lactate by anaerobic metabolism, resulting in metabolic acidosis.

Clinically, patients with cyanide poisoning present in extremis without signs that are specific for cyanide intoxication. The odor of bitter almonds is detectable for a genetically predetermined 65% of the population.[88] Early symptoms include anxiety, agitation, flushing, tachycardia, tachypnea, and dizziness. These early symptoms are followed rapidly by the progressive onset of metabolic acidosis, seizures, coma, and cardiovascular collapse. The cellular extraction of oxygen from the blood decreases so profoundly that arterial and venous Po_2 and retinal artery and vein color are similar. Individual organ systems manifest the symptoms of hypoxemia.

Therapy is effective if instituted early in the course. Oxygen, decontamination, nitrites, and sodium thiosulfate are the mainstays of therapy. Initially, oxygen given by facemask or endotracheal tube should be employed to deliver as close to 100% inspired oxygen as possible. Administration of nitrites should not be delayed by decontamination procedures or by prolonged resuscitation in the field. Amyl nitrite, the immediately available part of the cyanide antidote regimen, has a high abuse potential and has been removed from the formulary of many ambulance units, making immediate transport to a hospital even more imperative. Lavage is only helpful in patients with recent ingestions, and cyanide binds poorly to activated charcoal. Inhalation of amyl nitrite pearls produces a 5% methemoglobinemia, and one "ampule" of sodium nitrite (300 mg in 10 mL of a 3% solution) in an adult produces a methemoglobin level of approximately 20%. Methemoglobinemia should not be treated with methylene blue, as this measure causes the liberation of free cyanide. Methemoglobin can bind to free cyanide to form cyanmethemoglobin and thus prevent binding to the cytochrome oxidase enzymes in cells. As cyanide is slowly released from the cyanmethemoglobin compound, thiocyanate is formed and excreted in the urine. Intravenous administration of sodium nitrite should follow amyl nitrite therapy as soon as possible. Amyl nitrite therapy may be omitted if an intravenous route is already established. Following the nitrite therapy, sodium thiosulfate should be given intravenously to provide additional substrate to allow formation of thiocyanate. In patients who do not respond to antidotal therapy, hyperbaric oxygen therapy has no proven efficacy.[90, 91]

Pearls and Perils

- The course of cyanide intoxication is fulminant. Treat the patient immediately if cyanide intoxication is suspected.
- Methemoglobinemia is expected in the course of treatment. Treatment of the methemoglobinemia with methylene blue *liberates* cyanide and causes increased cyanide toxicity.
- Vomitus and other body fluids can contain significant amounts of cyanide. Healthcare providers should protect themselves.

Cyclic Antidepressants

Antidepressant exposures were responsible for the largest absolute number of fatalities (115) and largest fatality/exposure rate (0.66%) of all exposure categories reported to the AAPCC in 1993.[1a] Approximately 70% of individuals who have taken fatal overdoses of cyclic antidepressants are pronounced dead before medical assistance can be provided.

The cyclic antidepressants include the tertiary amines (amitriptyline, imipramine, doxepin, trimipramine) and the secondary amines (nortriptyline, protriptyline, desipramine). Several of the tertiary amines are metabolized to secondary amines before excretion. For example, imipramine is metabolized to desipramine, and amitriptyline is metabolized to nortriptyline. Other cyclic antidepressants with significant toxicity include amoxapine, bupropion, and maprotiline. Other antidepressants, such as fluoxetine, sertraline, and trazodone, are not similar in structure to the cyclic antidepressants and are substantially less toxic.

The oral absorption of the cyclic antidepressants is delayed in patients with overdose because of the delayed gastric emptying and ileus caused by these drugs' anticholinergic effects. These drugs are extensively protein bound (≥90%) and highly lipophilic. Protein binding is enhanced by increases in pH. Their volume of distribution is very large, ranging from 10 L/kg for amitriptyline to 59 L/kg for desipramine, with rapid distribution to tissues. The half-lives of the parent compounds and their active metabolites are very long (8–52 hours). Toxicity is likely if more than 20 mg/kg is ingested.

The clinical manifestations of cyclic antidepressant overdose are based on the four toxic mechanisms: direct muscarinic receptor blockade (anticholinergic), neurotransmitter reuptake blockade (adrenergic excess), α-adrenergic receptor blockade, and type I antiarrhythmic action.

The direct anticholinergic effects include sinus tachycardia, ileus, urinary retention, pupillary dilation, mental status changes, coma, impaired sweating with hyperthermia, and possibly seizures.[92] Norepinephrine, dopamine, and serotonin reuptake blockade causes sinus tachycardia through the elevation of intracardiac catecholamine levels, transient early hypertension, and arrhythmias. Alpha-adrenergic receptor blockade contributes to hypotension by causing vasodilation and arteriolar dilation, and it can cause pupillary constriction. The type I antiarrhythmic action seen with cyclic antidepressants stems from sodium channel blockade, similar in mechanism to that of quinidine. These agents inhibit fast sodium channels and slow phase 0 depolarization in His-Purkinje tissue and ventricular myocardium, causing direct myocardial depression, QRS prolongation, and ventricular arrhythmias.

Clinical manifestations stem directly from the drugs' mechanisms. The pupillary size is unreliable, but dry skin, ileus, urinary retention, and hyperthermia are common. The cardiovascular signs often include hypotension, which can be refractory, arrhythmias (sinus tachycardia, supraventricular tachycardia, ventricular tachycardia), and conduction disturbances. Neurologic findings commonly include central nervous system depression. Myoclonus, hallucinations, and choreoathetosis are less common. Seizures are especially frequent with amoxapine, bupropion, and maprotiline poisonings. In a review of 29 patients with cyclic antidepressant–induced seizures, most seizures were short and self-limited, and 23% occurred when patients were alert. All but two patients had seizures within 3 hours of drug ingestion. Four patients' cardiovascular status deteriorated immediately following seizure.[93]

The overdose profiles of amoxapine, maprotiline, and bupropion are different from those of typical cyclic antidepressants in that cardiovascular abnormalities are greatly diminished as are anticholinergic effects. Central nervous system depression and seizures predominate.[94, 94a]

The laboratory studies that may aid therapy and predict outcome include electrocardiography, serum drug level determinations, and the arterial blood gas analysis. Electrocardiographic abnormalities—such as a prolonged PR interval, a QRS duration greater than 100 to 160 ms, QT_c prolongation, a terminal 40 ms QRS axis between 120° and 270°, and a rightward deviation of the QRS axis—suggest a significant ingestion. The arterial pH should be maintained at approximately 7.45 to 7.55.

The treatment of cyclic antidepressant overdose patients can be very challenging. The mainstays of decontamination, multidose activated charcoal administration, and lavage are important in the early stages. The anticholinergic properties of cyclic antidepressants make lavage for up to 3 to 5 hours after ingestion worthwhile. Ipecac has no role in treatment of the cyclic antidepressant overdose. Repeated doses of activated charcoal over the first 24 hours shortens the elimination half-life of active metabolites.[95]

Alkalinization of the serum is essential and can be accomplished by sodium bicarbonate infusion or bolus therapy, or by hyperventilation. Bicarbonate is effective in reversing QRS prolongation, ventricular arrhythmias, and hypotension but has no effect on cyclic antidepressant–induced seizures. However, the use of bicarbonate to correct any acidosis that develops with seizure activity is essential to prevent cardiotoxicity precipitated by acidosis. More clinical data support the use of sodium bicarbonate alkalinization than support hyperventilation therapy. Sodium bicarbonate offers the additional theoretic advantage of providing excess sodium to minimize sodium channel inhibition.

Multiple measures can be undertaken to control the variety of arrhythmias seen in these overdose patients, including serum alkalinization, antiarrhythmic therapy, administration of magnesium and rarely β-blockers, isoproterenol use, and overdrive pacing. Use of the type Ia and Ic antiarrhythmic agents (procainamide, quinidine, flecainide, encainide, amiodarone, and disopyramide) is absolutely contraindicated. Phenytoin has been suggested as a prophylactic agent because it increases conduction velocity and improves membrane responsiveness, thus opposing the quinidine-like effects of these drugs. However, Mayron and Ruiz used a crossover rabbit study to show that prophylactic phenytoin (17 mg/kg) is not useful in preventing cardiotoxicity.[96] Callaham and coworkers used a dog model to show that pretreatment with phenytoin (19 mg/kg) actually increases the frequency of ventricular tachycardia without other positive effects.[97]

Hypotension can be managed initially by fluid resuscitation; then, α-adrenergic agonists such as norepinephrine should be used instead of dopamine. In the presence of α-blockade, dopamine can have unopposed beta effects and may theoretically worsen hypotension. However, animal studies have failed to substantiate this theoretic effect.

Although physostigmine is effective in reversing the anticholinergic effects in cyclic antidepressant overdose, it is not indicated because the cardiotoxic effects seen in cyclic antidepressant overdose can worsen. Therefore, physostigmine is not recommended in the routine treatment of cyclic antidepressant overdose because cardiac abnormalities usually predominate as the cause of mortality.

Seizures should be treated sequentially with benzodiazepines (diazepam, lorazepam), phenytoin, and phenobarbital. If these modalities are ineffective, paralysis (vecuronium, pancuronium) and barbiturate coma should be considered early in the course. Ineffective treatments include forced diuresis, hemodialysis, and hemoperfusion.

Patients should be monitored for 24 hours after resolution of all signs and symptoms, assuming that they have been passing charcoal stools and have bowel sounds.[98] Late complications usually are the result of aspiration, prolonged seizures, or anoxia during the acute illness. Delayed sudden death is rare, but cases of sudden death after apparent recovery from severe cyclic antidepressant overdose have been reported.[99]

Pearls and Perils

- Serum, not urine, alkalization is the mainstay of early therapy because only very small amounts of cyclic antidepressants are excreted in the urine.
- Initiate alkalization at the earliest sign of electrocardiographic abnormality.

Hypoglycemic Agents

Oral hypoglycemic agents are more commonly implicated in poison exposures (2272 reported to AAPCC in 1993) than is insulin (868 reported).[1a] The sulfonylureas are the only oral hypoglycemic agents available in the United States today. They can be divided into the first-generation compounds acetohexamide, chlorpropamide, tolazamide, and tolbutamide and into the more potent second-generation compounds glyburide and glipizide. The sulfonylureas stimulate the pancreatic islet tissue to secrete insulin, increase the conversion of glucose to glycogen, and may increase the binding of insulin to receptors or increase the number of the receptors. Phenformin, a biguanide compound unrelated to the sulfonylureas, is still used as an oral hypoglycemic agent in Europe; however, it was taken off the market in the United States in 1977 because of the severe lactic acidosis that it can cause. Other agents that can cause hypoglycemia include β-blockers, ethanol, salicylates, and the unripe akee fruit (grown in Jamaica).

Prolonged absorption from massive subcutaneous administration of insulin is common in intentional overdose patients.[100] In one case report of a 2500-U overdose of NPH insulin, intravenous glucose therapy was required for 6 days.[101] The absorption of the oral agents varies tremendously, with peak levels ranging from 1 to 2 hours for glipizide to 6 hours for glyburide and tolbutamide. They are more than 90% protein bound and have low volumes of distribution. Chlorpropamide has the longest half-life, averaging 36 hours or even longer in the overdose state. In one review of 40 sulfonylurea overdoses, the longest reported recurrence of hypoglycemia was 82 hours.[102]

The clinical presentation can be delayed up to 24 hours (and possibly even 48 hours) after ingestion. Symptoms are the same as those seen in hypoglycemia, including diaphoresis, confusion, agitation, nausea, and tachycardia, which can progress to seizures, coma, bradycardia, and asystole if treatment is not instituted in a timely manner. Cutaneous examination of patients with large parenteral insulin exposures can reveal an erythematous, boggy injection site. Patients concurrently taking β-blockers may be at increased risk for accidental overdose and delayed diagnosis because the early signs of hypoglycemia in the presence of such therapy are masked. A disulfiram-like reaction has occurred in patients maintained on chlorpropamide following ingestion of ethanol. Sulfonylurea abuse can mimic an insulinoma.

Assays for determination of blood levels of the sulfonylureas are available in some laboratories; however, their results do not correlate well with clinical effect and are rarely helpful in acute management. Elevated serum free insulin measurements, in the presence of low or normal C-peptide levels, can confirm the persistence of insulin following a parenteral insulin overdose.[101]

Treatment is primarily supportive. Decontamination with emesis or lavage can be helpful when an acute ingestion of an oral agent is involved. Some authors advocate surgical debulking at the site of a massive insulin overdose.[103] Activated charcoal has been shown to reduce absorption of chlorpropamide by 90%, although multidose activated charcoal was ineffective in reducing the plasma half-life.[104] Urinary alkalization to a pH of 8 can increase the urinary clearance of chlorpropamide fourfold.[104] Although it has not been studied, alkalization also may be useful with overdose of other oral hypoglycemic agents.

Intravenous glucose administration is the mainstay of therapy. Administration of 25 g of dextrose solution is appropriate initial therapy, but an infusion of 5% to 10% dextrose must follow. Oral glucose administration alone is insufficient, and recurrent hypoglycemia is common with oral therapy.[105] Glucagon also has been used in the prehospital setting and in refractory cases but not as a substitute for glucose. Glucagon is a polypeptide hormone that stimulates gluconeogenesis and glycogenolysis. Adequate liver glycogen stores must be present for an adequate response to be obtained with this therapy.

Diazoxide administration has been proposed as an adjunct to traditional therapy. Diazoxide is a benzothiadiazine antihypertensive agent that relaxes smooth muscles in the peripheral arterioles and directly inhibits insulin release from the pancreas; thus, it commonly causes hyperglycemia when used as an antihypertensive agent. Anecdotal success in treating refractory hypoglycemia due to the sulfonylureas with diazoxide has been reported.[102, 106] Hypotension does not seem to be a frequent complication. Dialysis is unlikely to be effective for oral hypoglycemic agents because of the high degree of protein binding. Hemoperfusion was effective in a single reported case of chlorpropamide poisoning.[107]

Pearls and Perils

- The onset of hypoglycemia may be delayed 24 to 48 hours following a sulfonylurea ingestion.
- Patients receiving chronic insulin therapy can have prolonged effects following massive subcutaneous overdosage.
- Rebound hypoglycemia commonly occurs following the discontinuation of intravenous glucose therapy.

Iron

Iron poisoning is the leading cause of pediatric accidental ingestion fatalities in the United States. In 1991, 11 iron-related pediatric deaths were reported to the AAPCC, accounting for 65% of all unintentional pharmaceutical ingestion fatalities in children younger than 6 years of age.[108] Iron salts formulated as attractively colored dietary iron supplements and prenatal multivitamins are implicated in these poisonings.

Absorption of environmental iron, found primarily as ferric oxide or hydroxide, is minimal. Ferrous iron (Fe^{2+}), however, is absorbed from the gastrointestinal mucosa, oxidized to ferric iron (Fe^{3+}), and binds to ferritin or transferrin. Ascorbic acid (vitamin C) reduces ferric to ferrous iron and facilitates absorption. Ferrous salts (sulfate, gluconate, fumarate) are much better absorbed than are ferric compounds (ferric chloride, ferric ammonium citrate). There is no route for the excretion of iron other than cell turnover and bleeding, which eliminate approximately 1 mg/d in men and 2 mg/d in women.

Iron has a direct irritant effect on the gastrointestinal mucosa. Additionally, when the iron binding sites on the transferrin, hemosiderin, and ferritin molecules become saturated, the serum free iron levels rise and systemic toxicity develops. Clinical toxicity is likely following ingestion of 40 to 60 mg/kg of elemental iron, although serious complications usually require ingestion greater than 100 mg/kg. To estimate the severity of an ingestion, the amount of elemental iron must be calculated. For example, the sulfate salt of iron (ferrous sulfate) is 20% elemental iron, the gluconate salt—12%, and the fumarate salt—33%. Four stages of clinical toxicity occur:

- *Stage I* occurs within 30 minutes to 2 hours after ingestion. The findings include nausea, vomiting with hematemesis (and hypotension in massive overdoses), abdominal pain, and lethargy.
- *Stage II,* occurring 6 to 12 hours after ingestion, is also called *the quiescent period* because the patient may become asymptomatic.
- In *Stage III,* which takes place between 12 and 48 hours after ingestion, life-threatening complications occur, including metabolic acidosis, increased lethargy, coma, vasomotor collapse, gastrointestinal bleeding, and perforation.
- In *Stage IV,* which occurs 2 to 4 days after the ingestion, liver failure develops as a direct effect of iron on mitochondria in the liver.

Some authors describe a fifth, late stage of toxicity in which systemic symptoms have resolved but in which gastric obstruction occurs as a result of scar formation at the sites of earlier iron-induced mucosal damage.[109]

The laboratory studies that have been used to assist in the clinical evaluation of iron overdose patients include determination of serum iron, total iron-binding capacity, complete blood count, and serum glucose as well as abdominal radiography. Routine laboratory analyses, including arterial blood gas testing, electrocardiography, serum electrolyte measurement, coagulation parameter assessment, liver and renal function studies, and chest radiography also are warranted. Although serum iron levels are imprecise clinical indicators, a serum iron level of greater than 350 mg/dL is often associated with moderate manifestations of toxicity. However, the total iron-binding capacity was found to be falsely elevated following a 20-mg/kg iron ingestion in volunteers; thus, the traditional concept of using chelation therapy for patients with a serum iron level that is greater than the measured total iron binding capacity has come into question.[110, 111] Treatment should be based on a history of the amount ingested, symptoms, and the peak serum iron level (usually observed 3–6 hours after the ingestion). The presence of deferoxamine in the serum may cause the measured iron level to be falsely low, by chelating iron liberated during the laboratory test. The iron in the deferoxamine-iron complex (ferrioxamine) may also be liberated, further affecting the results. Atomic absorption spectrophotometry can accurately measure the serum iron in the presence of deferoxamine. Thus, this laboratory method should be used, or the serum iron level should be determined before deferoxamine is given. In cases in which serum iron levels are not immediately available, elevated glucose level (>150 mg/dL), leukocytosis (≥15,000 per cubic millimeter), vomiting, diarrhea, and the visualization of radiopaque material on a radiograph suggest a serum iron concentration of greater than 300 μg/dL. However, the absence of these individual findings does not ensure that the serum iron level is less than 300 μg/dL.[112]

Treatment for iron intoxication relies heavily on gastrointestinal decontamination and emptying. Activated charcoal is ineffective. Emesis may be induced when the estimated ingestion is 20 to 60 mg/kg and the patient is asymptomatic; however, following massive ingestions or in the symptomatic patient, lethargy may complicate emetic therapy with ipecac syrup. The safety and efficacy of oral lavage solutions (sodium bicarbonate, phosphate solutions) is questionable. Whole-bowel irrigation with polyethylene glycol electrolyte solutions has been used effectively in both adult and pediatric patients, with evidence of large amounts of undissolved iron remaining in the gastrointestinal tract.[113]

The indications for deferoxamine chelation are not well defined. Intravenous or intramuscular therapy is generally recommended when the serum iron concentration exceeds 350 μg/dL or if a serum iron concentration cannot be obtained in a timely manner and the patient is symptomatic. In patients who present with hypotension or severe poisoning, the intravenous form of deferoxamine should be used. As chelated iron is excreted, the urine turns a pink to orange color. The resolution of this "vin rose" urine in patients has been used as a clinical endpoint for deferoxamine therapy. Not all patients exhibit a visible urinary color change; thus, this finding cannot be used as a reliable confirmation of suspected toxicity.

Pearls and Perils

- Activated charcoal does not adsorb iron.
- Beware of stage II, the quiescent period, and do not underestimate the potential for serious complications to follow.

- Do not forget to calculate the percentage of elemental iron when calculating the milligrams per kilogram of iron ingested.

Isoniazid

Isoniazid (isonicotinic acid hydrazide [INH]) was introduced into clinical practice in 1952 for the chemotherapy of tuberculosis. The resurgence of mycobacterial disease has led to an increase in the intentional and accidental ingestion of acutely toxic amounts of INH. From 1991 to 1993, nine INH-related deaths were reported to the AAPCC, whereas from 1983 to 1990 only two fatal cases were reported.[1, 1a, 63–67, 108, 114–116] The acute toxicity of INH has clinical manifestations and therapy that are very different from the side effects seen with INH chronic therapy and their management.

Oral absorption of INH is rapid, reaching peak serum levels within 1 to 2 hours after ingestion. Distribution throughout the plasma occurs quickly, with very little protein binding (volume of distribution: 0.6 L/kg). In patients receiving chronic therapy, metabolism by the enzyme *N*-acetyltransferase to inactive metabolites (e.g., acetylhydrazine) occurs by acetylation in the liver and intestinal mucosa. Acetylhydrazine can be hepatotoxic. The rate of acetylation is genetically determined. In patients who are slow acetylators, the mean half-life is about 3 hours, whereas in those who are fast acetylators, the half-life is 80 minutes. Fast acetylators seem to be at increased risk for hepatotoxicity. In contrast, slow acetylators are at greater risk of INH-induced peripheral neuropathy, which is thought to be caused by unmetabolized INH.

Pyridoxine phosphokinase, which converts pyridoxine to its active form, pyridoxal phosphate, is inhibited by INH. The resultant acute pyridoxal phosphate deficiency can decrease the formation of γ-aminobutyric acid from glutamic acid, leading to the onset of convulsions in the acute overdose. Numerous enzymes are affected, and this causes other metabolic changes.

Clinical intoxication can occur with INH overdoses of 10 to 30 mg/kg and death with doses greater than 50 mg/kg. Early signs and symptoms may include nausea, vomiting, abdominal pain, slurred speech, dizziness, and visual changes (mydriasis, blurring, nystagmus), although seizures may be the presenting symptom. Characteristically, severe intoxication produces seizures that may progress to status epilepticus, coma, and a refractory anion gap metabolic acidosis.

Treatment involves early gastric decontamination, activated charcoal administration, and aggressive management of the seizures and acidosis. Seizure activity, acidosis, and coma should be treated with pyridoxine. One gram of pyridoxine is administered for every gram of INH ingested, or 5 g are given initially if the amount of INH is unknown.[117, 118] Benzodiazepines, paralysis, and barbiturate coma may also be required to control refractory seizures.[119] Peripheral neuropathy from pyridoxine is seen only with chronic administration of large doses. Acidosis results primarily from production of lactic acid during seizures, although ketone formation and interference with conversion of lactate to pyruvate also contribute. Hemodialysis, peritoneal dialysis, and exchange transfusion effectively clear INH but are not indicated in view of the efficacy of pyridoxine.

Pearls and Perils

- Large quantities of pyridoxine may be required, exhausting the hospital supplies. Check with the pharmacy early.

Lithium

Lithium is a metallic ion in group IA on the periodic table of the elements (like sodium and potassium) and was prescribed in Europe as early as 1897 as a treatment of periodic depression. In the United States, lithium was originally used as an over-the-counter salt substitute and in the soft drink 7-Up in the 1940s. A number of deaths were attributed to the use of these products. The Food and Drug Administration finally approved the drug in 1970 for the treatment of manic-depressive disorders. Overdose frequency has risen over the years in parallel with the drug's increasing availability.

Lithium is available primarily as a carbonate salt formulated in immediate and slow-release carbonate tablets and capsules. Liquid citrate preparations are also available in slow and immediate-release forms. Lithium is used industrially in nuclear reactors, lubricants, alloy manufacture, porcelain enamels, and disk batteries. Lithium toxicity from the ingestion or explosion of batteries has not occurred, and other occupational exposure is rare.

Lithium ions are completely absorbed from the gastrointestinal tract, with peak serum concentrations achieved within 3 to 5 hours after therapeutic dosing. Its binding to protein is minimal (volume of distribution: 0.79 L/kg); however, its distribution into and out of the tissue compartment can take as long as 25 to 30 hours with therapeutic doses of the sustained-release preparations and longer when the drug is taken in overdose. Lithium is not metabolized but is eliminated almost entirely by the kidneys. The initial half-life is 6 to 12 hours; thereafter, as the tissue compartment releases bound drug, the half-life extends to 24 hours or longer. The proximal and distal tubules reabsorb about 80% of the filtered lithium, and the reabsorption is markedly increased in low sodium states. The mechanism of clinical efficacy and toxicity is thought to relate to cationic substitution at the cellular level; however, all of the specific mechanisms are as yet unclear.

Lithium has a very narrow therapeutic index, and serum levels above the therapeutic range (0.8 to 1.2 mEq/L) result in toxicity. The clinical manifestations of lithium intoxication vary tremendously, depending on a patient's serum drug levels, underlying illnesses, concurrent drug therapy, coingestants, hydration status, and overdose chronicity. The main clinical effects are on the central nervous system, the kidneys, and the heart. Early nervous system findings are confusion, tremor, and hyperreflexia. Symptoms may progress to delirium, choreiform movements, spasticity, hallucinations, coma, and seizures. Long-term memory impairment and neurologic deficits have been documented following lithium toxicity.[120] Renal damage with a gradual decline in glomerular filtration rate and a reversible vasopressin-resistant renal concentrating defect are seen in patients receiving chronic therapy. These changes result in dehydration and in the worsening of toxicity. Hypotension, arrhythmias, and electrocardiographic abnormalities that include diffuse T wave flattening, QT prolongation, and U waves are common.[121] Symptoms of nausea, vomiting, and diarrhea may also be present. Other effects are blurred vision, nystagmus, dry mouth, hyperthermia or hypothermia, and profound weakness. Chronically overmedicated patients have a greater risk of complications.[122]

An ingestion of 40 mg/kg of a lithium salt can raise the serum level to more than 2 mEq/L and cause symptoms. The treatment of the acute lithium overdose patient begins with gastric emptying. Activated charcoal does not adsorb lithium well, and it is not indicated unless coingestants are present. Preliminary evidence does show that the exchange resin sodium polystyrene sulfonate binds lithium and prevents some absorption.[123] The complications of sodium polystyrene sulfonate use include sodium overload, hypokalemia, hypocalcemia, nausea, vomiting, and constipation. Lithium carbonate is a poorly soluble lithium salt and can form bezoars. Whole-bowel irrigation with a polyethylene glycol electrolyte lavage solution has been shown to decrease the absorption of a sustained-release lithium preparation by 67% when compared with control therapy.[124]

Once lithium has been absorbed, enhancing its elimination becomes important because the drug is not metabolized. In the past, treatment with saline diuresis and forced alkaline diuresis were used but have since been found to be dangerous and ineffective.[125] Diuretics act on the ascending limb of the loop of Henle or on the distal tubule and have little effect on the reabsorption of lithium, which occurs primarily in the proximal tubules. Intravenous normal saline or 0.45% saline should be infused to maintain a normal urine output and to correct dehydration and sodium depletion. Hemodialysis is the treatment of choice, although the indications for its use are poorly defined. Peritoneal dialysis is less effective than hemodialysis. Serum lithium levels are an inaccurate reflection of tissue levels. Mild toxicity occurs in acute overdose patients with serum levels of 1.5 to 2.5 mEq/L; however, in an overdose patient already receiving therapeutic lithium, this level could have severe complications. Hemodialysis should be considered when the peak serum level (at least 6 hours after ingestion) is greater than 3.5 mEq/L, or when it is greater than 2.5 mEq/L *with* symptoms in a chronic overdose patient. However, patients often require dialysis at lower levels, especially symptomatic patients with chronic overmedication. Patients with renal insufficiency or renal failure cannot excrete lithium normally and should also undergo dialysis at lower serum levels. Following dialysis, a drug rebound occurs as the drug redistributes, and repeat hemodialysis may be required.

Pearls and Perils

- Patients chronically maintained on lithium therapy require dialysis to prevent permanent renal and neurologic damage.
- Hydration to normovolemia, not saline diuresis, is required to assist the excretion of lithium.

Monoamine Oxidase Inhibitors

In 1954, when the drug iproniazid, a monoamine oxidase (MAO) inhibitor, was undergoing clinical trials for the treatment of tuberculosis, mood elevation was noted in trial subjects. The use of MAO inhibitors as well as their misuse in accidental and suicidal overdose has increased since the mid-1980s. In 1993, 556 exposures to MAO inhibitors, including 3 deaths, were reported to the AAPCC.[1, 1a]

The MAO inhibitors bind irreversibly to MAO, resulting in the latter's permanent inactivation and thus preventing degradation of biogenic amines by this route. Although reversible agents are under investigation, none has been approved for use in the United States. MAOs of subtypes A and B are flavoprotein enzymes located on the outer mitochondrial membrane of mammalian tissues. In the brain, liver, and gastrointestinal tract, MAO inactivates neurotransmitters (e.g., serotonin, epinephrine, norepinephrine, and dopamine) and other monoamines (e.g., tyramine) through oxidative deamination. MAO-A preferentially deaminates serotonin and norepinephrine and is likely related to the antidepressant effects seen when the drug is given in therapeutic doses.[126] MAO-B preferentially deaminates phenylethylamines such as dopamine. Some of the newer investigational agents, when given in therapeutic doses, selectively bind to MAO-A (clorgyline, moclobemide) or MAO-B (selegiline). Most of the older agents (phenelzine, tranylcypromine, pargyline, isocarboxazid, nialamide) are not selective.

Although the MAO inhibitors are rapidly absorbed from the gastrointestinal tract, reaching peak serum levels within 1 to 2 hours, after an overdose, reaching the peak toxicity can take 6 to 24 hours. These compounds are highly protein bound and are rapidly metabolized by acetylation in the liver, with a half-life of 1.5 to 3.5 hours. The irreversible nature of MAO binding causes a delay in the resolution of clinical effects, pending the resynthesis of MAO.

The clinical manifestations of overdose do not necessarily mimic the clinical effects of MAO inhibitor interactions with drugs and foods. The onset of symptoms in overdose patients is often delayed for 6 to 24 hours. A wide range of symptoms has been described. One review of 12 overdose cases found one or more of the following in more than 50% of patients: excitement or agitation, sinus tachycardia, mydriasis, muscle rigidity, coma, or hyperthermia. Hypertension was present in only 17% of patients. Other symptoms included sweating, hyperreflexia, nystagmus, writhing or grimacing, tachypnea, seizures, hypotension, cardiac arrest, hallucinations, papilledema, and peaked T waves on electrocardiography.[127] Recovery can be delayed for 3 to 7 days as MAO is synthesized.

Coingestants are of particular concern in patients taking MAO inhibitors. The interaction of MAO inhibitors with food products and indirectly acting sympathomimetic agents can result in toxicity even when therapeutic doses are given. The food products known to cause toxicity (e.g., aged cheeses, wines [especially chianti], fava beans, and pickled herring) often contain monoamines, such as tyramine, that are usually degraded in the gastrointestinal tract and liver by MAO. With MAO inhibition, undegraded monoamines enter the circulation and precipitate the release of large quantities of stored norepinephrine. This results in hypertension, tachycardia, headache, hyperthermia, and other hyperadrenergic symptoms. Similar symptoms occur with indirectly acting sympathomimetic amines (e.g., amphetamines, phenylpropanolamine, and pseudoephedrine), opioids (e.g., meperidine), and cocaine. Many indirectly acting sympathomimetic amines are available over the counter.[128] The directly acting sympathomimetic amines (e.g., epinephrine, norepinephrine, and isoproterenol) are not potentiated by MAO inhibitors. Drug interaction occurs with numerous preparations, including some anticholinergic drugs, antihypertensive agents, asthma medications, hypoglycemic agents, and barbiturates.

The treatment of MAO inhibitor overdose begins with aggressive decontamination. Use of activated charcoal with a cathartic is indicated, and gastric emptying may be valuable if the patient presents early. Urinary acidification is not recommended because excretion is only minimally enhanced and because the risk of renal failure secondary to rhabdomyolysis and myoglobinemia would increase. Supportive treatment is the mainstay of therapy. Hyperthermia must be treated immediately with external cooling and control of muscular activity. Administration of dantrolene sodium, a lipid-soluble hydantoin analog that directly relaxes skeletal muscle, has been shown to be effective in some case reports, although the drug's mechanism is unclear.[129, 130] Seizures and agitation may be controlled initially with benzodiazepines or phenytoin. Potentiation of the sedative effects of barbiturates is possible; however, barbiturates may be used for the management of refractory seizures. Neuromuscular paralysis may be required if convulsions persist. Hypotension that is unresponsive to fluid therapy may be controlled through the cautious use of directly acting sympathomimetic agents, which include epinephrine, norepinephrine, and isoproterenol. Hypertension may be treated with nitroprusside or phentolamine. Beta-blocker use is contraindicated because the unopposed α effects can lead to hypertension. The safety of calcium channel blockers in this setting has not been determined.

A hyperserotonergic state has been postulated as the cause of some clinical manifestations in animal studies.[131] In one case report, the neuromuscular effects of therapeutic doses of phenelzine (possible coingestant, tryptophan) were relieved by the administration of cyproheptadine, a serotonin antagonist.[132] The high degree of protein binding and the rapid metabolism of the MAO inhibitors suggest that hemodialysis and hemoperfusion are not likely to be useful. Charcoal hemoperfusion was found to decrease the serum level of phenelzine in one patient from 19.5 to 6.5 ng/mL; however, the status of this patient did not change.[129]

Pearls and Perils

- The onset of clinical manifestations of an MAO inhibitor overdose can be delayed for 6 to 24 hours, and no laboratory tests are available to help make the diagnosis.
- A patient with a mixed overdose may develop severe toxicity from drug-drug or food-drug interactions without having an actual overdosage of an MAO inhibitor.

Salicylates

The incidence of acute salicylism has declined over the past two decades since acetaminophen and ibuprofen have entered the market for analgesics. Nonetheless, acute and chronic salicylism remains a major but often unrecognized cause of poisoning morbidity and mortality. Over 15,000 exposures and 20 fatalities (0.13%) related to salicylates alone were reported to the AAPCC in 1993. From the same data base, it was learned that the fatality rate was 0.04% for acetaminophen and 0.009% for ibuprofen.[1a]

The salicylates commonly encountered as ingredients in pharmaceutical products include aspirin (acetylsalicylic acid), sodium salicylate, salicylic acid (keratolytic), and methyl salicylate. Methyl salicylate (oil of wintergreen, a common component of liniments) is the most concentrated of these: one teaspoon contains 7000 mg of salicylate, the equivalent of approximately 21 regular-strength aspirin tablets. Using grains as a measure of acetylsalicylic acid adds to the confusion. One grain is equivalent to 65 mg of aspirin (5 grains = 325 mg). Also, enteric-coated aspirin tablets are available, and these may delay attainment of peak serum concentrations.[133, 134] Salsalate (salicylsalicylic acid) yields two molecules of acetylsalicylic acid after metabolism and results in typical salicylate toxicity. Salicylamide, however, is an amide derivative of acetylsalicylic acid and has only mild toxicity, unrelated to salicylism.

Acetylsalicylic acid is a weak acid and very well absorbed from the acid environment of the stomach and the small bowel. Large doses of aspirin can delay gastric emptying and are poorly soluble in gastric acid; this can lead to bezoar formation. When given therapeutically, peak levels are usually seen within 2 hours, but in overdose, the peak may be delayed for 6 hours or longer. The small volume of distribution (2.1 L/kg) increases in the presence of acidosis, as the nonionized (uncharged) salicylate molecules cross cell membranes, including those of the blood-brain barrier. Protein binding usually ranges from 50% to 80%, but with overdoses or the presence of hypoalbuminemia, or in the elderly, binding sites are saturated and more drug remains unbound, and this increases toxicity. Once acetylsalicylic acid is absorbed, metabolism to the active compound salicylic acid is rapid (20 minutes). Further metabolism to salicyluric acid (75%) and phenolic glucuronide (10%) occurs through pathways that become saturated in overdose. Thus, the half-life with therapeutic dosages of 2 to 4.5 hours can increase to 20 hours or more[135] in overdose. When the urinary pH is greater than 8.0, most of the unmetabolized drug passing through the tubules is ionized and not reabsorbed; this decreases the half-life to less than 8 hours.

Clinical manifestations of acute salicylism may include mild confusion, tinnitus, and decreased auditory acuity. As the salicylate level in the serum and central nervous system increases, other symptoms begin to appear, including agitation or lethargy, vertigo, convulsions, hyperventilation, metabolic acidosis, coagulation abnormalities, nausea, and vomiting. Although fever is a hallmark of pediatric salicylism, its presence in adults is less frequent and a poor prognostic sign. If the serum salicylate levels increase, noncardiogenic pulmonary edema (rarely seen in pediatric salicylism), refractory seizures, and death are common. Chronic salicylism produces similar symptoms, although at much lower serum levels; however, chronic salicylism is often occult, and delays in diagnosis can result in increased mortality.

The metabolic derangements seen with salicylate overdose deserve special mention. Salicylates directly stimulate the medulla to increase the rate and depth of respirations, causing respiratory alkalosis. Concurrent direct effects on intracellular metabolism cause an increased metabolic rate and result in formation of lactate, pyruvate, and other organic acids that, in turn, produce an anion gap metabolic acidosis. The combination of respiratory alkalosis and metabolic acidosis usually produces alkalemia in adults unless central nervous system depressants were also ingested or the overdose is severe. An overriding metabolic acidosis is more common in children. Fluid and electrolyte disorders are common and include dehydration, hypokalemia, hypocalcemia, and hyperglycemia or hypoglycemia. Therapy with intravenous bicarbonate can worsen hypokalemia. A paradoxic aciduria is also common because hydrogen ions are excreted in an attempt to retain potassium ions. The central nervous system is the site of the lethal effects of salicylates.

Salicylate levels in cerebrospinal fluid correlate more closely with incidence of death than do serum levels. A critical cerebrospinal fluid salicylate level is achieved over a wide range of serum levels because of equilibration, protein binding, and acid-base status. In chronic overdoses, equilibration has a lesser role, and toxicity is increased.

Treatment of patients with suspected salicylate overdose includes recognition of the diagnosis, early gastric decontamination followed by multidose activated charcoal, urinary alkalization, monitoring of serial serum salicylate levels (until a decline is confirmed), a close monitoring of fluid and electrolyte balance, and possibly hemodialysis. The effectiveness of urinary alkalization without forced diuresis is based on the marked increase in urinary excretion of salicylate that occurs at a urinary pH of 7.5 to 8.0. Although rehydration is important, forced diuresis does not increase the efficacy of urinary alkalization and is fraught with complications because salicylate-intoxicated patients are at risk for noncardiogenic pulmonary edema and cerebral edema.

The Done nomogram was developed to assess and predict the clinical severity of acute salicylism based on the study of 38 acutely poisoned children in 1960 (Fig. 130–3).[135] Although the nomogram was based on pediatric data alone and although complex statistic kinetic analysis was not yet available, the nomogram, if used properly, is still clinically useful as a *rough* guide of severity in *acute* overdose patients. A critical review has shown that the nomogram is not as reliable a predictor as was once thought.[134]

The indications for hemodialysis are primarily clinical. Dialysis should be considered and is often necessary in patients with a serum level of 100 to 120 mg/dL or with

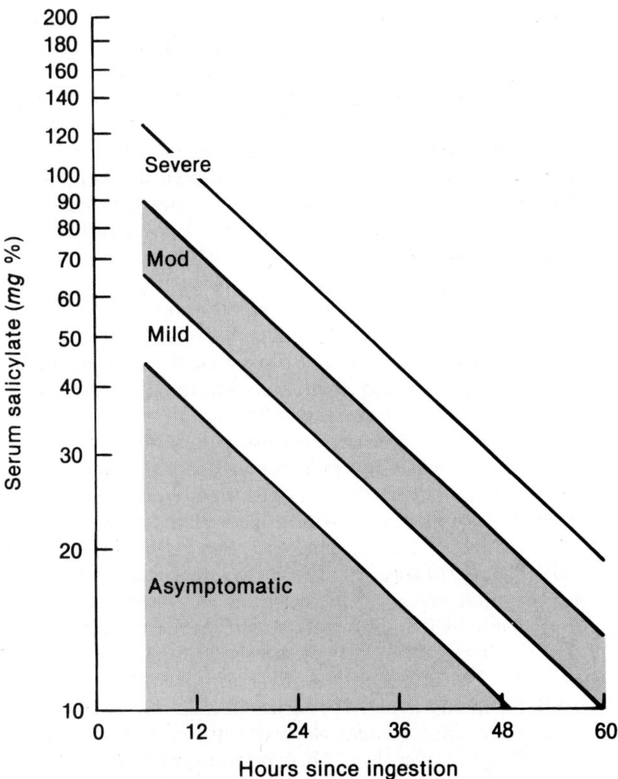

Figure 130–3. Nomogram relating salicylate concentration and expected severity of intoxication at varying intervals following the ingestion of a single dose of salicylate. (From Done AK: Salicylate intoxication. Pediatrics 1960; 26:800. Reproduced by permission of Pediatrics.)

deteriorating clinical status (worsening acidosis, decline in mental status, seizures, noncardiogenic pulmonary edema). In chronic overdose, dialysis may be necessary for symptomatic patients with a salicylate level greater than 60 mg/dL.

Pearls and Perils

- Be aware of the proper unit of measure when using the Done nomogram (mg/dL, *not* mg/L, μg/L, or mmol/L).
- Start potassium supplementation early (in the absence of renal insufficiency) because hypokalemia makes urinary alkalization impossible.
- The nomogram is only useful for *acute* overdoses with serum levels determined at least 6 hours after ingestion.

Strychnine

Medicinal use of strychnine dates back to 1540. Early in the 20th century, it became widely available in the United States in tonics, bitters, and cathartics. Strychnine, 0.5 to 1.0 mg, was mixed in various combinations with belladonna, cascara, quinine, and iron. Strychnine was finally removed from nonprescription medicines in 1962, although it is still found in some homeopathic preparations. Ten strychnine-related deaths have been reported to the AAPCC since 1988.[1, 1a, 66, 67, 108, 116]

Although the dried gray-green seeds of the vinelike *Strychnos nux-vomica* (the strychnine tree) are the main source of strychnine extracts, powders, and tinctures, all parts of the plant contain strychnine. Currently, strychnine is available in veterinary products, homeopathic medications, and rodenticides, avicides, and other pesticides in concentrations from 0.3% to 0.5%. Licensed exterminators have access to products containing up to 5% strychnine. Strychnine is a bitter tasting, white, crystalline material that is sometimes used as an adulterant mixed into illegal street heroin and cocaine.

Absorption of strychnine is rapid via the nasal and gastrointestinal mucosa. Peak serum levels are observed within 5 minutes in nasal exposures, and clinical symptoms usually occur within 15 to 30 minutes after ingestion. Metabolism occurs primarily in the liver by microsomal enzymes, and the half-life of strychnine is about 10 hours.[136]

Strychnine acts as a competitive antagonist of the inhibitory neurotransmitter glycine at the postsynaptic receptor. Some evidence suggests that strychnine acts on an allosterically separate binding site on the receptor but lowers the affinity for glycine.[137] Tetanus toxin also blocks the effect of glycine, but it does so by inhibiting its release from the nerve ending. The interference with the negative feedback provided by glycine results in a marked increase in motor neuron activity. Although glycine receptors are found primarily on the motor neurons of the ventral horn of the spinal cord, other receptor sites have been identified in the brain stem and the dorsal horn of the spinal cord.[138]

The clinical manifestations of strychnine poisoning occur rapidly. A prodromal phase of agitation, anxiety, and increased sensory awareness may precede the diffuse, painful muscle spasms that resemble seizures and characterize poisoning with this agent. These muscle spasms are tetanic and last 1 to 2 minutes; during this time, the patient often remains alert and without a postictal period, in contrast to that which occurs with true generalized seizures. All the muscles of the body are affected. Spasms of the strongest groups of muscles predominate and lead to opisthotonos, trismus, and the grin of risus sardonicus. The arms are flexed, the legs are in extension, and nystagmus can be seen. The increased sensory awareness continues, and loud noises, physical stimuli, or bright lights can precipitate diffuse spasms. The excessive muscular activity causes severe lactic acidosis, hyperthermia, rhabdomyolysis, and compartment syndromes. Diaphragmatic and chest wall spasms can lead to respiratory arrest. Long-term complications are usually a result of anoxia, hyperthermia, and renal failure, with resultant cerebral injury or multisystem organ failure. Primary renal, hepatic, pulmonary, or gastrointestinal effects do not seem to occur.

The lethal dose of strychnine is estimated to be 1.5 to 2 mg/kg. Fatal serum levels range from 0.5 to 90 mg/L and do not accurately reflect toxicity. The therapy starts with decontamination with administration of activated charcoal and gastric lavage. The affinity of activated charcoal for strychnine was graphically demonstrated in 1830 by Touéry, who survived the ingestion of a lethal amount of strychnine with 15 g of activated charcoal taken as a demonstration during a meeting of the French Academy of Medicine.[139] Repeated doses of activated charcoal may be of value. Emesis is contraindicated, and lavage should be limited to patients with recent ingestions because the stimulation may induce muscle spasms. Beyond the initial decontamination, care is largely supportive. The tetanic muscle spasms and convulsions can be treated initially with benzodiazepines, which may raise the threshold for convulsions and actually displace some of the strychnine bound to receptor sites.[140] For refractory convulsions, intubation and neuromuscular blockade, general anesthesia, or barbiturate-induced coma are recommended. Phenobarbital has been recommended as the anticonvulsant of choice because of its longer duration of action and effect on the other inhibitory neurotransmitter, γ-aminobutyric acid.[141] Aggressive treatment of hyperthermia and rhabdomyolysis with cooling, hydration, urinary alkalization, and neuromuscular blockade (to block persistent muscular hyperactivity) should be undertaken. Urinary acidification theoretically increases the excretion of strychnine but is not used because it increases the risk of myoglobinuric renal failure. Hemodialysis is not likely to have a role in enhancing elimination but may be required to control a patient's acidosis.

Pearls and Perils

- Supportive care is the mainstay of therapy.
- Induction of paralysis and sedation is probably required to control muscular activity and to prevent hyperthermia, acidosis, rhabdomyolysis, and renal failure.

Superwarfarins

The so-called "sweet clover disease" was a hemorrhagic disorder of cattle that ingested spoiled sweet clover silage earlier this century. In 1939, the causative agent was identified in a laboratory as bishydroxycoumarin (dicoumarol). In 1944, the congener warfarin was developed in the same laboratory and became widely used as a rodenticide. Although these compounds are relatively nontoxic to humans following a single ingestion, the "superwarfarins" developed in the mid-1980s to combat warfarin-resistant rodent populations are considerably more toxic.

The superwarfarins are a number of agents within the two main groups of rodenticide anticoagulants. The hydroxycoumarin group, which contains warfarin, also contains the 4-hydroxycoumarins brodifacoum, difenacoum, bromadiolone, and coumatetralyl, which are considerably more potent and longer acting than warfarin. The indandione group contains diphacinone, chlorphacinone, valone, and pindone, which also are potent, longer-acting analogs of warfarin. These products are often packaged as round, green-blue pellets, cakes, or powders and are sometimes left in areas accessible to toddlers and are thus the cause of significant morbidity. Rodent feces have been shown to contain clinically significant amounts of brodifacoum.[142]

The superwarfarins are effectively absorbed through the skin, by inhalation, and from the gastrointestinal tract. Their hematologic effects may not be seen for 24 to 48 hours after exposure.[143] The half-life of brodifacoum in dogs has been estimated to be 120 days.[144] Hematologic effects in humans have been reported to last for 2 to 3 months and, in some cases, for 8 or 13 months.[142, 145] Metabolism occurs in the liver, where warfarin and its analogs are hydroxylated to inactive compounds by the mixed-function oxidase system. They are then renally excreted. The superwarfarins produce more potent inhibition of vitamin K_1 epoxide reductase and bind irreversibly to the epoxide reductase with 100-fold greater affinity when compared with warfarin.[144, 146] The reductase converts 2,3-epoxy-vitamin K_1 to vitamin K_1. Vitamin K_1 catalyzes the carboxylation of the glutamic acid residues on the vitamin K-dependant clotting Factors II, VII, IX, and X, allowing them to function. During this reaction, vitamin K_1 is oxidized to become 2,3-epoxy-vitamin K_1, and the cycle begins again.

The clinical effects of these rodenticides relate directly to their anticoagulant properties. In children, these effects can manifest after ingestion of "only a mouthful." Anticoagulation can present with epistaxis, cutaneous ecchymoses, bleeding gums, hemoptysis, melena, hematuria, or menorrhagia. Bleeding may begin within 24 to 48 hours of ingestion, and hematologic abnormalities can last for months or longer, especially in cases of chronic ingestion. Although the indandiones have produced some cardiovascular and neurologic effects in rats when given in large doses, these effects have not been reported in humans.[147]

Laboratory evaluations can assist in uncovering the covert abuse of these substances. Elevations in prothrombin and partial thromboplastin times with normal mixing studies in the absence of malnutrition or liver disease should suggest the diagnosis. Techniques to measure warfarin levels do not detect the long-acting vitamin K antagonists. However, assays for vitamin K_1, urinary γ-carboxylglutamic acid, and 2,3-epoxy-vitamin K_1 are available. In the absence of vitamin K_1, there are measurable decreases in the levels of urinary γ-carboxylglutamic acid, elevated levels of the precursor 2,3-epoxy-vitamin K_1 in serum, and an abnormally high ratio of 2,3-epoxy-vitamin K_1 to vitamin K_1 (normal ratio: 0.1 to 0.2). In a 7-month-old girl with brodifacoum poisoning, the determined ratio was 20:1.[142] Brodifacoum serum levels can be measured with the use of high-pressure liquid chromatography.

Therapy involves early decontamination with emesis or gastric lavage in addition to the administration of activated charcoal. If prolongation of the prothrombin time is already present, emesis and gastric lavage are contraindicated. Decontamination is indicated even when visible evidence of ingestion is lacking. Green-blue oral discoloration from the water-soluble dyes added to some products does not appear to be useful in predicting which children have an elevated prothrombin time.[143] The specific antidote for symptomatic patients is intravenous phytonadione (vitamin K_1). In adults, a minimum dose of 10 mg is given intravenously diluted in saline or in 5% dextrose in water and infused over 20 minutes. Initial doses of 25 to 400 mg have been required in patients with active bleeding. Neither vitamin K_4 (menadiol) nor vitamin K_3 (menadione) can reverse the effects of coumadin derivatives. The effects of intravenous vitamin K_1 may take 4 to 6 hours to manifest, so patients with hemodynamic compromise or active bleeding should receive fresh frozen plasma. Because of the increased risk of blood-borne pathogens, preparations of pooled clotting factors should be reserved for those patients with uncontrolled bleeding or for patients unable to tolerate the volume load of fresh frozen plasma. Oral and intramuscular phytonadione therapy may be used for the milder cases or as long-term maintenance. Patients on therapeutic anticoagulation merit special attention and may need heparin therapy to safely maintain anticoagulation while their drug-induced vitamin K deficiency is reversed. Anecdotal evidence seems to support the use of phenobarbital to induce the hepatic microsomal enzyme system and to increase the metabolism of the superwarfarin compounds.[142, 148]

Pearls and Perils

- Recognize surreptitious superwarfarin use in patients with unusually high vitamin K requirements.
- Use fresh frozen plasma in patients with acute bleeding because production of vitamin K–dependent clotting factors may take 6 hours.
- Phytonadione is the only vitamin K preparation that should be used to reverse anticoagulation from coumadin-related poisonings.

References

1. Litovitz TL, Holm KC, Clancy C, et al: 1992 Annual Report of the American Association of Poison Control Centers Toxic Exposure Surveillance System. Am J Emerg Med 1993; 11:495.

1a. Litovitz TL, Clark LR, Soloway RA: 1993 Annual Report of the American Association of Poison Control Centers Toxic Exposure Surveillance System. Am J Emerg Med (in press).

2. Grbcich PA, Lacouture PG, Lewander WJ, et al: Effect of milk on ipecac-induced emesis. J Pediatrics 1987; 110:973.

3. Grbcich PA, Lacouture PG, Lovejoy FH: Effect of fluid volume on ipecac-induced emesis. J Pediatrics 1987; 110:970.

4. Klein-Schwartz W, Litovitz T, Oderda GM: The effect of milk on ipecac-induced emesis. J Toxicol Clin Toxicol 1991; 29:505.
5. Grbcich PA, Lacouture PG, Kreses JJ, et al: Expired ipecac syrup efficacy. Pediatrics 1986; 78:1085.
6. Czajka PA, Russell SL: Non-emetic effects of ipecac syrup. Pediatrics 1985; 75:1101.
7. Keller RE, Schwab RA: Contribution of sorbitol combined with activated charcoal in prevention of salicylate absorption. Ann Emerg Med 1990; 19:654.
8. McNamara RM, Aaron CK, Gemborys M, et al: Sorbitol catharsis does not enhance efficacy of charcoal in a simulated acetaminophen overdose. Ann Emerg Med 1988; 17:243.
9. Rosenberg PJ, Livingstone DJ, McLellan BA: Effect of whole-bowel irrigation on the antidotal efficacy of oral activated charcoal. Ann Emerg Med 1988; 17:681.
10. Tenenbein M, Cohen S, Sitar DS: Whole bowel irrigation as decontamination procedure after acute drug overdose. Arch Intern Med 1987; 147:905.
11. Everson GW, Bertaccini EJ, O'Leary J: Use of whole bowel irrigation in an infant following iron overdose. Am J Emerg Med 1991; 9:369.
12. Levitt MA, Sullivan JB, Owens SM, et al: Amitriptyline plasma protein binding: Effect of plasma pH and relevance to clinical medicine. Am J Emerg Med 1986; 4:121.
13. Seaberg DC, Weiss LD, Yealy DM, et al: Effects of alpha-1-acid glycoprotein on the cardiovascular toxicity of nortriptyline in a swine model. Vet Hum Toxicol 1991; 33:226.
14. Pentel PR, Keyler DE: Effects of alpha-1-acid glycoprotein on desipramine toxicity in rats. J Pharmacol Exp Ther 1988; 246:1061.
15. Pentel PR, Benowitz N: Efficacy and mechanism of action of sodium bicarbonate in the treatment of desipramine toxicity in rats. J Pharmacol Exp Ther 1984; 231:387.
16. Berlinger WG, Spector R, Goldberg MJ, et al: Theophylline clearance by oral activated charcoal. Clin Pharmacol Ther 1983; 33:35.
17. Shannon M, Amitai Y, Lovejoy FH: Multiple dose activated charcoal for theophylline poisoning in young infants. Pediatrics 1987; 80:368.
18. Berg MJ, Berlinger WG, Goldberg MJ, et al: Acceleration of the body clearance of phenobarbital by oral activated charcoal. N Engl J Med 1982; 307:642.
19. Amitai Y, Yeung AS, Moye J, et al: Repetitive oral activated charcoal and control of emesis in severe theophylline toxicity. Ann Emerg Med 1986; 105:386.
20. Smilkstein MJ, Knapp GL Kulig KW, et al: Efficacy of oral *N*-acetylcysteine in the treatment of acetaminophen overdose. N Engl J Med 1988; 319:1557.
21. Keays R, Harrison PM, Wendon JA, et al: Intravenous acetylcysteine in paracetamol-induced fulminant hepatic failure: A prospective controlled trial. Br Med J 1991; 303:1026.
21a. Klein-Schwartz W, Oderta GM: Absorption of oral antidotes for acetaminophen poisoning (methionine and *N*-acetylcysteine). Clin Toxicol 1981; 18:283.
22. Renzi FP, Donovan JW, Martin TG, et al: Concomitant use of activated charcoal and *N*-acetylcysteine. Ann Emerg Med 1985; 14:568.
23. North DS, Peterson RG, Krenzelok EP: Effect of activated charcoal administration on *N*-acetylcysteine serum levels in humans. Am J Hosp Pharm 1981; 38:1022–1024.
24. Ekins BR, Ford DC, Thompson MI, et al: The effect of activated charcoal on *N*-acetylcysteine absorption in normal subjects. Am J Emerg Med 1987; 5:483.
25. Prescott LF: Treatment of severe acetaminophen poisoning with intravenous acetylcysteine. Arch Intern Med 1981; 141:386.
26. O'Sullivan GF, Wade DN: Flumazenil in the management of acute drug overdosage with benzodiazepines and other agents. Clin Pharm Ther 1987; 42:254.
27. Bayer MJ, Danzl D, Gibler B, et al: Treatment of benzodiazepine overdose with flumazenil: The flumazenil in benzodiazepine intoxication multicenter study group. Clin Ther 1992; 14:859.
28. Aarseth HP, Bredesen JE, Grynne B, et al: Benzodiazepine-receptor antagonist: A clinical double-blind study. J Toxicol Clin Toxicol 1988; 26:283.
29. Roche Laboratories: Mazicon (flumazenil) product monograph. Nutley, NJ, Hoffman–La Roche Inc, 1992.
30. Litovitz T: Fatal benzodiazepine toxicity? Am J Emerg Med 1987; 5:472.
31. Höjer J, Behrendtz S, Gustafsson L: Benzodiazepine poisoning: Experience of 702 admissions to an intensive care unit during a 14-year period. J Intern Med 1989; 226:117.
32. Lheureux P, Vranckx M, Leduc D, et al: Flumazenil in mixed benzodiazepine/tricyclic antidepressant overdose: A placebo-controlled study in the dog. Am J Emerg Med 1992; 10:184.
33. Amrein R, Leishman B, Bentzinger C, et al: Flumazenil in benzodiazepine antagonism: Actions and clinical use in intoxications and anesthesiology. Med Toxicol 1987; 2:411.
34. Hruby K, Prischl F, Donner A, et al: Value of flumazenil in benzodiazepine self-poisoning. Eur J Anaesthesiol Suppl 1988; 2:309.
35. Douidar SM, Ahmed AE: A novel mechanism for the enhancement of acetaminophen hepatoxicity by phenobarbital. J Pharmacol Exp Ther 1987; 240:578.
36. Rumack BH: Acetaminophen overdose. Am J Med 1983; 75:104.
37. Rumack BH: Acetaminophen overdose in young children. Am J Dis Child 1984; 138:428.
38. Kumar A, Goel KM, Rae MD: Paracetamol overdose in children. Scott Med J 1990; 35:106.
39. Ashbourne JF, Olson KR, Khayam-Bashi H, et al: Value of rapid screening for acetaminophen in all patients with intentional drug overdose. Ann Emerg Med 1989; 18:1035.
40. Rumack BH, Matthew H: Acetaminophen poisoning and toxicity. Pediatrics 1975; 55:871.
40a. Clark R, Borirakchanyavat V, Davidson AR, et al: Hepatic damage and death from overdose of paracetamol. Lancet 1973; i:66.
41. O'Grady J, Alexander GM, Hayller KM, et al: Early indicators of prognosis in fulminant hepatic failure. Gastroenterology 1989; 97:439.
42. Schafer DF, Shaw BW: Fulminant hepatic failure and orthotopic liver transplantation. Semin Liver Dis 1989; 9:189.
43. Harrison PM, O'Grady JG, Keays RT, et al: Serial prothrombin time as prognostic indicator in paracetamol-induced fulminant hepatic failure. Br Med J 1990; 301:964.
44. Palmer BF, Eigenbrodt EH, Henrich WL: Cranial nerve deficit: A clue to the diagnosis of ethylene glycol poisoning. Am J Med 1989; 87:91.
45. Mallya KB, Mendis T, Guberman A: Bilateral facial paralysis following ethylene glycol ingestion. Can J Neurol Sci 1986; 13:340.
46. Locke KD, Ellis JH, Dart RC, et al: A randomized, double-blind, placebo-controlled study of fluorescein detection in human urine. Ann Emerg Med 1993; 22:891.
47. Galliot M, Astier A, Vu Bien D, et al: Treatment of ethylene glycol poisoning with intravenous 4-methylpyrazole. N Engl J Med 1986; 319:97.
48. Hoffman RS, Howland MA, Kamerow HN, et al: Comparison of titratable acid/alkaline reserve and pH in potentially caustic household products. Clin Toxicol 1989; 27:241.
49. Early SH, Simpson RL: Caustic burns from contact with wet cement. JAMA 1985; 254:528.
50. Rumack BH, Burrington JD: Caustic ingestions: A rational look at diluents. Clin Toxicol 1977; 11:27.
51. Gaudreault P, Parent M, McGuigan MA, et al: Predictability of esophageal injury from signs and symptoms: A study of caustic ingestion in 378 children. Pediatrics 1983; 71:767.
52. Crain EF, Gershel JC, Mezey AP: Caustic ingestions: Symptoms as predictors of esophageal injury. Am J Dis Child 1984; 138:863.
53. Gorman RL, Khin-Maung-Gyi MT, Klein-Schwartz W, et al: Initial symptoms as predictors of esophageal injury in alkaline corrosive ingestions. Am J Emerg Med 1992; 10:189.
53a. Homan CS, Maitra SR, Lane BP, et al: Therapeutic effects of water and milk for alkali injury of the esophagus. Ann Emerg Med 1994; 24:14.
54. Anderson KD, Rouse TM, Randolph JG: A controlled trial of corticosteroids in children with corrosive injury of the esophagus. N Engl J Med 1990; 323:637.
55. Howell JM: Alkaline ingestions. Ann Emerg Med 1987; 15:820.

56. Bracken WM, Cuppage F, McLaury RL, et al: Comparative effectiveness of topical treatments for hydrofluoric acid burns. J Occup Med 1985; 27:733.
56a. Burkhart KK, Brent J, Kirk MA, et al: Comparison of topical magnesium and calcium treatment for dermal hydrofluoric acid burns. Ann Emerg Med 1994; 24:9.
57. Henry JA, Hla KK: Intravenous regional calcium gluconate perfusion for hydrofluoric acid burns. Clin Toxicol 1992; 30:203.
58. Vance MV, Curry SC, Kunkel DB, et al: Digital hydrofluoric acid burns: Treatment with intra-arterial calcium infusion. Ann Emerg Med 1986; 15:890.
59. Chernow B, Zaloga GP, Malcolm D, et al: Glucagon's chronotropic action is calcium dependent. J Pharmacol Exp Ther 1987; 241:833.
60. Smith RC, Wilkinson F, Hall RL: Glucagon for propranolol overdose. JAMA 1985; 254:2412.
61. Peterson CD, Leeder S, Sterner S: Glucagon therapy for β-blocker overdose. Drug Intell Clin Pharm 1984; 18:398.
62. Weinstein RS: Recognition and management of poisoning with beta-adrenergic blocking agents. Ann Emerg Med 1984; 13:1123.
63. Litovitz TL, Normann SA, Veltri JC: 1985 Annual Report of the American Association of Poison Control Centers National Data Collection System. Am J Emerg Med 1986; 4:427.
64. Litovitz TL, Martin TG, Schmitz B: 1986 Annual Report of the American Association of Poison Control Centers National Data Collection System. Am J Emerg Med 1987; 5:427.
65. Litovitz TL, Schmitz B, Matyunas N, et al: 1987 Annual Report of the American Association of Poison Control Centers National Data Collection System. Am J Emerg Med 1988; 6:479.
66. Litovitz TL, Schmitz B, Holm KC: 1988 Annual Report of the American Association of Poison Control Centers National Data Collection System. Am J Emerg Med 1989; 7:495.
67. Litovitz TL, Schmitz B, Bailey KM: 1989 Annual Report of the American Association of Poison Control Centers National Data Collection System. Am J Emerg Med 1990; 8:394.
68. Ramoska EA, Spiller HA, Winter M, et al: A one-year evaluation of calcium channel blocker overdoses: Toxicity and treatment. Ann Emerg Med 1993; 22:196.
69. Pearigen PD, Benowitz NL: Poisoning due to calcium antagonists: Experience with verapamil, diltiazem, and nifedipine. Drug Saf 1991; 6:408.
70. Zaritsky AL, Horwitz M, Chernow B: Glucagon antagonism of calcium channel blocker–induced myocardial dysfunction. Crit Care Med 1988; 16:246.
71. Chernow B, Reed L, Geelhoed GD, et al: Glucagon: Endocrine effects and calcium involvement in cardiovascular actions in dogs. Circ Shock 1986; 19:393.
72. Kuo MJ, Tseng YZ, Chen TF, et al: Verapamil overdose and severe hypocalcemia. Clin Toxicol 1992; 30:309.
73. Wolf LR, Spadafora MP, Otten EJ: The use of amrinone and glucagon in a case of calcium channel blocker overdose (abstract). Vet Hum Toxicol 1991; 33:35.
74. Cobb N, Etzel RA: Unintentional carbon monoxide–related deaths in the United States, 1979 through 1988. JAMA 1991; 266:659.
75. Llano AL, Raffin TA: Management of carbon monoxide poisoning. Crit Care Med 1990; 97:165.
76. Heckerling PS, Leikin JB, Maturen A: Occult carbon monoxide poisoning: Validation of a prediction model. Am J Med 1988; 84:251.
77. Heimbach DM, Waeckerle JF: Inhalation injuries. Ann Emerg Med 1988; 17:1316.
78. Halebian P, Robinson N, Barie P, et al: Whole-body utilization during acute carbon monoxide poisoning and isocapneic nitrogen hypoxia. J Trauma 1986; 26:110.
79. Ginsberg MD: Carbon monoxide intoxication: Clinical features, neuropathology, and mechanisms of injury. Clin Toxicol 1985; 23:281.
80. Schwartz A, Hennerici M, Wegener OH: Delayed choreoathetosis following acute carbon monoxide poisoning. Neurology 1985; 35:98.
81. Choi IS: Delayed neurologic sequelae in carbon monoxide intoxication. Arch Neurol 1983; 40:433.
82. Lustman F: Letter. Am J Med 1985; 85:462.
83. Otten EJ, Rosen JM, Tasset JT: An evaluation of carboxyhemoglobin spot tests. Ann Emerg Med 1985; 14:850.
84. Kurt TL, Anderson RJ, Reed WG: Rapid estimation of carboxyhemoglobin by breath sampling in an emergency setting. Vet Hum Toxicol 1990; 32:227.
85. Myers RA, Britten JS: Are arterial blood gases of value in treatment decisions for carbon monoxide poisoning? Crit Care Med 1989; 17:139.
85a. Seger D, Welch L: Carbon monoxide controversies: Neuropsychologic testing, mechanism of toxicity, and hyperbaric oxygen. Ann Emerg Med 1994; 24:242.
86. Van Hoesen KB, Camporesi EM, Moon RE, et al: Should hyperbaric oxygen be used to treat the pregnant patient for acute carbon monoxide poisoning? JAMA 1989; 261:1039.
87. Gee DJ: Cyanides in murder, suicide and accident. *In*: Clinical and Experimental Toxicology of Cyanides. Ballantyne B, Marrs TC (Eds). Bristol, England, IOP Publishing, 1987, pp 209–216.
88. Hall AH, Rumack BH, Schaffer MI, et al: Clinical toxicology of cyanide: North American clinical experience. *In*: Clinical and Experimental Toxicology of Cyanides. Ballantyne B, Marrs TC (Eds). Bristol, England, IOP Publishing, 1987, pp 312–333.
89. Hall AH, Doutre WH, Ludden T, et al: Nitrate/thiosulfate treated acute cyanide poisoning: Estimated kinetics after antidote. Clin Toxicol 1987; 25:121.
90. Myers RA, Schnitzer BM: Hyperbaric oxygen use, update 1984. Postgrad Med 1984; 76:83.
91. Litovitz TL, Larkin RF, Myers RA: Cyanide poisoning treated with hyperbaric oxygen. Am J Emerg Med 1983; 1:94.
92. Malatynska E, Knapp RJ, Masaaki I, et al: Antidepressants and seizure interactions at the GABA-receptor chloride-ionophore complex. Life Sci 1988; 43:303.
93. Ellison DW, Pentrel PR: Clinical features and consequences of seizures due to cyclic antidepressant overdose. Am J Emerg Med 1989; 7:5.
94. Litovitz TL, Troutman WG: Amoxapine overdose seizures and fatalities. JAMA 1983; 250:1069.
94a. Spiller HA, Ramoska EA, Krenzelok EP: Bupropion overdose: A 3-year multi-center retrospective analysis. Am J Emerg Med; 12:43.
95. Scheinin M, Virtanen R, Lisalo E: Effect of single and repeated doses of activated charcoal on the pharmacokinetics of doxepin. Int J Clin Pharmacol Ther Toxicol 1985; 1:38.
96. Mayron R, Ruiz E: Phenytoin: Does it reverse tricyclic antidepressant–induced cardiac conduction abnormalities? Ann Emerg Med 1986; 15:876.
97. Callaham M, Schumaker H, Pentel P: Phenytoin prophylaxis of cardiotoxicity in experimental amitriptyline poisoning. J Pharmacol Exp Ther 1988; 248:216.
98. Goldberg RJ, Capone RJ, Hunt JD: Cardiac complications following tricyclic antidepressant overdose. JAMA 1985; 254:1772.
99. McAlpine SB, Calabro JJ, Robinson MD, et al: Late death in tricyclic antidepressant overdose revisited. Ann Emerg Med 1986; 11:1349.
100. Roberge RJ, Martin TG, Delbridge TR: Intentional massive insulin overdose: Recognition and management. Ann Emerg Med 1993; 22:228.
101. Samuels MH, Eckel RH: Massive insulin overdose: Detailed studies of free insulin levels and glucose requirements. Clin Toxicol 1989; 27:157.
102. Palatnick W, Meatherall RC, Tenenbein M: Clinical spectrum of sulfonylurea overdose and experience with diazoxide therapy. Arch Intern Med 1991; 151:1859.
103. McIntyre AS, Woolf VJ, Burnham WR: Local excision of subcutaneous fat in the management of insulin overdose. Br J Surg 1986; 73:157.
104. Neuvonen PJ, Karkkainen S: Effects of charcoal, sodium bicarbonate, and ammonium chloride on chlorpropamide kinetics. Clin Pharmacol Ther 1983; 33:386.
105. Stapczynski SJ, Haskell RJ: Duration of hypoglycemia and need for intravenous glucose following intentional overdoses of insulin. Ann Emerg Med 1984; 13:505.
106. Jeffrey WH, Graham EM: Treatment of chlorpropamide overdose with diazoxide. Drug Intell Clin Pharm 1983; 17:372.

107. Ludwig S, McKenzie J, Faiman C: Chlorpropamide overdose in renal failure: Management with charcoal hemoperfusion. Am J Kidney Dis 1987; 10:457.
108. Litovitz TL, Holm KC, Bailey KM, et al: 1991 Annual Report of the American Association of Poison Control Centers National Data Collection System. Am J Emerg Med 1992; 10:452.
109. Tenenbein M, Littman C, Stimpson RE, et al: Gastrointestinal pathology in adult iron overdose. Clin Toxicol 1990; 28:311.
110. Tenenbein M: The total iron-binding capacity in iron poisoning: Is it useful? Am J Dis Child 1991; 145:437.
111. Burkhart KK, Kulig KW, Hammond KB, et al: The rise in the total iron-binding capacity after iron overdose. Ann Emerg Med 1991; 20:532.
112. Lacoutre PG, Wason S, Temple AR, et al: Emergency assessment of severity in iron overdose by clinical and laboratory methods. J Pediatr 1981; 99:89.
113. Tenenbein M: Whole-bowel irrigation in iron poisoning. J Pediatr 1987; 111:142.
114. Veltri JC, Litovitz TL: 1983 Annual Report of the American Association of Poison Control Centers National Data Collection System. Am J Emerg Med 1984; 2:420.
115. Litovitz T, Veltri JC: 1984 Annual Report of the American Association of Poison Control Centers National Data Collection System. Am J Emerg Med 1985; 3:423.
116. Litovitz TL, Bailey KM, Schmitz BF, et al: 1990 Annual Report of the American Association of Poison Control Centers National Data Collection System. Am J Emerg Med 1991; 9:461.
117. Brent J, Vo N, Kulig K, et al: Reversal of prolonged isoniazid-induced coma by pyridoxine. Arch Intern Med 1990; 150:1751.
118. Cash JM, Zawada ET: Isoniazid overdose: Successful treatment with pyridoxine and hemodialysis. West J Med 1991; 155:644.
119. Bredemann JA, Krechel SW, Eggers GN: Treatment of refractory seizures in massive isoniazid overdose. Anesth Analg 1990; 71:554.
120. Saxena S, Mallikarjuna P: Severe memory impairment with acute overdose lithium toxicity: A case report. Br J Psychiatry 1988; 152:853.
121. Brady HR, Horgan JH: Lithium and the heart, unanswered questions. Chest 1988; 93:166.
122. Shannon MW, Eisen T, Linakis J, et al: Clinical features of acute versus chronic lithium intoxication. Vet Hum Toxicol 1989; 31:370.
123. Tomaszewski C, Musso C, Pearson RJ: Lithium absorption prevented by sodium polystyrene sulfonate in volunteers. Ann Emerg Med 1992; 21:1308.
124. Smith SW, Ling LJ, Halstenson CE: Whole-bowel irrigation as a treatment for acute lithium overdose. Ann Emerg Med 1991; 20:536.
125. Jacobson D, Aasen G, Friedericksen P, et al: Lithium intoxication: Pharmacokinetics during and after terminated hemodialysis in acute intoxications. J Toxicol Clin Toxicol 1987; 25:81.
126. Brown C, Taniguchi G, Yip K: The monoamine oxidase inhibitor–tyramine interaction. J Clin Pharmacol 1989; 29:529.
127. Meredith TJ, Vale JA: Poisoning due to psychotropic agents. Adverse Drug React Acute Poisoning Rev 1985; 4:83.
128. Harrison WM, McGrath PJ, Stewart JW, et al: MAOIs and hypertensive crises: The role of OTC drugs. J Clin Psychiatry 1989; 50:2.
129. Kaplan RF, Feinglass NG, Webster W, et al: Phenelzine overdose treated with dantrolene sodium. JAMA 1986; 255:642.
130. Verrilli MR, Salanga VD, Kozachuk WE, et al: Phenelzine toxicity responsive to dantrolene. Neurology 1987; 37:865.
131. Marley E, Wozniak KM: Interactions of a nonselective monoamine oxidase inhibitor, phenelzine, with inhibitors of 5-hydroxytryptamine, dopamine or noradrenaline. 1984; 18:173.
132. Lieberman JA, Kane JM, Reife R: Neuromuscular effects of monoamine oxidase inhibitors. J Clin Psychopharmacol 1985; 5:221.
133. Wortzman DJ: Delayed absorption following enteric-coated aspirin overdose. Ann Emerg Med 1987; 16:434.
134. Dugandzic RM, Tierney MG, Dickenson GE, et al: Evaluation of the validity of the Done nomogram in the management of acute salicylate intoxication. Ann Emerg Med 1989; 18:1186.
135. Done AK: Salicylate intoxication. Pediatrics 1960; 26:800.
136. Heiser JM, Daya MR, Magnussen RA: Massive strychnine intoxication: Serial blood levels in a fatal case. Clin Toxicol 1992; 30:269.
137. Marvizon JG, Vazquez J, Calvo MG, et al: The glycine receptor: Pharmacological studies and mathematical modeling of the allosteric interaction between the glycine- and strychnine-binding sites. Mol Pharmacol 1986; 30:590.
138. Probst A, Cortés R, Palacio JM: The distribution of glycine receptors in the human brain: A light microscopic autoradiographic study using (3H) strychnine. Neurosci 1986; 17:11.
139. Anderson AH: Experimental studies on the pharmacology of activated charcoal. Acta Pharmacol 1946; 2:69.
140. Sangiah S: Effects of glycine and other inhibitory amino acid transmitters on strychnine convulsive threshold in mice. Vet Hum Toxicol 1972; 27:747.
141. Boyd RE, Spyker DA: Strychnine poisoning: Recovery from profound lactic acidosis, hyperthermia, and rhabdomyolysis. Am J Med 1983; 74:507.
142. Watts RG, Castleberry RP, Sadowski JA: Accidental poisoning with a superwarfarin compound (brodifacoum) in a child. Pediatrics 1990; 86:883.
143. Smolinske SC, Scherger DL, Kearns PS, et al: Superwarfarin poisoning in children: A prospective study. Pediatrics 1989; 84:490.
144. Lipton RA, Klass EM: Human ingestion of a "super warfarin" rodenticide resulting in a prolonged anticoagulant effect. JAMA 1984; 252:3004.
145. Exner DV, Brien WF, Murphy MJ: Superwarfarin ingestion. Can Med Assoc J 1992; 146:34.
146. Bachmann RA, Sullivan TJ: Dispositional and pharmacodynamic characteristic of brodifacoum in warfarin-sensitive rats. Pharmacology 1983; 27:281.
147. Murdoch DA: Prolonged anticoagulation in chlorphacinone poisoning. Lancet 1983; i:355.
148. Barucoa CH, Mura P, Rovert R, et al: Chlorphacinone intoxication: A biological and toxicological study. Clin Toxicol 1989; 27:79.

SECTION X

INFECTIOUS DISEASE

Stephen M. Ayres • Peter Linden

CHAPTER 131

Prevention and Management of Infections in Critically Ill Trauma Victims and Patients with Hematologic Malignancies

Wayne N. Campbell, MD • Stephen C. Schimpff, MD

Physicians involved in critical care medicine encounter a wide variety of serious problems regarding infections that require immediate attention. This includes recognition of the factors that predispose a patient to infection, the development of an approach to diagnosis even when normal inflammatory responses are muted, appreciation of the approach to empiric therapy, and, equally important, attention to infection prevention.

The critically ill person who has sustained multiple trauma or the leukemic patient undergoing chemotherapy has an exceedingly high incidence of infection that is related to tissue or mucous membrane damage, iatrogenic bypass of normal anatomic barriers, and impaired host immune defense mechanisms. The higher risk of infection, especially nosocomial infection, is reflected in increased costs of hospitalization and, more important, by increased morbidity and mortality. Important factors that may predispose the critical care patient to infection are outlined in Table 131–1. These factors differ among patient groups, but their presence can suggest appropriate diagnostic procedures, empiric antibiotic therapy, and prevention measures. Physicians must recognize these predisposing factors as quickly as possible because the type of infection that occurs in each setting is distinctly different and, as a result, the proper approach to early therapy varies widely. Infections in these populations of critically ill patients are to a certain extent preventable with the proper use of routine methods. Seldom do we devote adequate attention to this fact. Appropriately, measures to prevent the most common nosocomial infections are discussed first.

PREVENTING IATROGENIC INFECTIONS

Handwashing Techniques

A century ago, Semmelweis pointed out the importance of handwashing to prevent transmission of infections from patient to patient in an obstetric ward. Because a great percentage of nosocomial infections are caused by pathogens acquired during hospitalization, often through contact with medical personnel, it is surprising that handwashing is practiced so infrequently. For example, at a major cancer center, where the physicians were well acquainted with the problems of organism transmission and where handwashing had been emphasized, observation of physician behavior during routine morning work rounds during a 1-month period indicated that only one clinician on one occasion washed his or her hands. This is not an uncommon observation in the medical and surgical wards of the hospital, yet no surgeon would consider entering the operating room without adhering precisely to the routine of handwashing before surgery. In essence, the problem is psychologic: the preparation for surgery is a fixed procedure demanding a particular approach, whereas the preparation for routine patient contact has no specific protocol.

Nevertheless, handwashing is thought by many to be the single most important procedure for reducing the frequency of nosocomial infections. Even in the absence of overt contamination, all medical personnel should wash their hands before and after any physical contact with patients. Good mechanical friction with soap and running water eliminates the vast majority of the transiently acquired organisms likely to be transmitted to another patient. This is not to denigrate the added value of antiseptic agents but rather to emphasize that the most important potential pathogens are not part of the individual's resident hand flora and usually can be easily removed with mechanical handwashing. Nevertheless, in a critical care setting, in which the risk of infection is exceedingly high and close physical proximity increases the risk of transmission, use of an antiseptic is

TABLE 131–1. Factors Predisposing Patients to Infection

Iatrogenic Procedures
Urinary catheters
Intravenous catheter and infusions
Respiratory assist devices
Implantation of prosthetic materials
Lack of handwashing
Failure to follow infection control guidelines
Damage of Anatomic Barriers to Microbe Entry
Skin (e.g., trauma, venipuncture, surgical wounds, drainage tubes)
Alimentary canal mucosa (e.g., surgery, cancer chemotherapy, radiation therapy)
Obstruction of Natural Passages
Bronchus (e.g., tumor, hemothorax, pneumothorax)
Urinary tract (e.g., stone, tumor)
Humoral Immune Deficiency
Congenital immune deficits
Tumors (e.g., multiple myeloma)
Splenectomy
Cellular Immune Deficiency
Transplantation (e.g., renal, cardiac)
Acquired immunodeficiency syndrome
Lymphomas (i.e., Hodgkin's disease)
Therapy with immunosuppressive drugs or radiation therapy
Extensive soft tissue injury
Granulocytopenia
Bone marrow failure states (e.g., aplastic anemia, leukemia)
Intensive cancer chemotherapy (e.g., small-cell lung cancer, testicular cancer)

appropriate.[1] A 2% solution of chlorhexidine is nonirritating to the skin and has a sudsing action similar to that of soap, yet it has an extremely high activity against most gram-positive and gram-negative bacteria, yeasts, and many viruses. In addition, if used regularly, chlorhexidine accumulates on the skin to maintain an antimicrobial effect for prolonged periods.

Body Substance Isolation Precautions

In 1985, Universal Blood-Borne Disease precautions were created as a strategy to minimize the risk of transmitting blood-borne pathogens in the workplace.[2] This policy applied its Blood and Body Fluid Precautions to the blood or blood-stained body fluids of all patients. The use of gloves and gowns and the proper handling of sharps were intended to protect hospital personnel from infectious agents in patients' blood. Many aspects of universal precautions have been endorsed and enforced by the Occupational Safety and Health Administration (OSHA) of the Department of Labor.

Resulting from concerns that all moist body substances should be considered potentially infectious for hospital personnel and that these personnel are unrecognized sources of potentially transmissible nosocomial pathogens led to the formulation of the Body Substance Isolation policy in 1987. This included the use of barrier precautions for the moist body substances of all patients, regardless of their diagnosis. These policies incur added costs to patient care; however, if properly implemented, they should result in dual benefit by preventing (1) the transmission of infection to healthcare providers and (2) the transmission of nosocomial pathogens among patients. Prospective evidence for the latter effect is not convincingly evident at the present time. Body substance isolation is outlined in Table 131–2.[3]

PREVENTING BACTERIAL COLONIZATION OF INFUSION AND DRAINAGE DEVICES

Urinary Catheters

The placement of indwelling urinary catheters is the most common procedure that predisposes patients to hospital infection. The Centers for Disease Control and Prevention (CDCP) estimates that nearly 40% of nosocomial infections originate from the urinary tract and that urinary catheters are responsible for 80% of these. Bacteriuria (the presence of bacteria in the urine) occurs in 10% to 20% of patients catheterized for at least 1 day. The risk of developing bacteriuria increases 5% to 10% per day for each day that the catheter remains in place.[4] Bacteriuria is not synonymous with the term *urinary tract infection* (UTI). In general, 20% to 30% of catheterized bacteriuric patients develop a UTI. UTI is best distinguished from bacteriuria by the presence of associated symptoms such as fever, abdominal or flank pain, dysuria, frequency, or evidence of bladder inflammation (e.g., pyuria).

TABLE 131–2. Body Substance Isolation

1. Gloves are worn for anticipated contact with blood, secretions, mucous membranes, nonintact skin, and moist body substances of all patients. (Handwashing is not necessary when gloves are worn unless the hands become visibly soiled.) Gloves are changed before another patient is treated.
2. After other types of patient contact, hands are washed.
3. Gowns, plastic aprons, masks, or goggles are worn when secretions, blood, or body fluids are likely to soil or splash on clothing, skin, or the face.
4. Soiled reusable items, linen, and trash are contained to prevent leaking. Double-bagging is not necessary unless the outside of the bag is visibly soiled.
5. Needles (without recapping them) and sharp items are placed in puncture-resistant, rigid containers.
6. Private rooms are indicated for patients with some diseases transmitted exclusively or in part by the airborne route, such as pulmonary tuberculosis and other diseases listed in the Strict Isolation category of the CDC Guidelines for Isolation Precautions in Hospitals.[4] Private rooms are also indicated for patients who soil articles in the environment with body substances.

(Data from Lynch P, Jackson MM, Cummings J, et al: Rethinking the role of isolation precautions in the prevention of nosocomial infections. Ann Intern Med 1987; 107:243.)

Reducing the frequency of bacteriuria, and consequently UTI, is important. Although these infections are generally local and easily treated, they increase hospital costs and can culminate in bacteremia, particularly with multiresistant organisms. Because of their frequency, the expense of their treatment, and a small, but important, incidence of serious complications, they are a major concern for epidemiologists and clinicians. The urinary catheterization predisposes to bacteriuria by (1) perturbing the protective mucopolysaccharide coating of the bladder and promoting inflammation; (2) providing a conduit for endogenous periurethral bacteria to enter the bladder; and (3) serving as a nidus for bacterial attachment, protected growth, and persistence. The infecting organisms are frequently identical to those found on a patient's perineal skin surfaces. These organisms may derive either from the patient's own enteric flora or were acquired during hospitalization.[5] Exogenous direct contamination of the catheter system by other catheterized patients via crossinfecton may also result in nosocomial UTI epidemics.

The CDCP has developed a set of recommendations for the prevention of catheter-associated UTIs.[6] Adherence to these guidelines substantially reduces catheter-associated bacteriuria and their sequelae. Catheters should be used only when essential and not as a simple convenience for the medical staff, and they must be inserted with aseptic technique and sterile equipment. The drainage system must be of the closed type and should never be opened. Urine samples for culture should be aspirated with a syringe and needle from the rubber catheter tubing after cleansing with alcohol. The collecting bag must always be lower than the patient's bladder to prevent retrograde flow of potentially contaminated urine.

A number of other measures have been evaluated in addition to the simple procedures outlined. The majority either have failed to reduce bacteriuria, have done so inconsistently, or have not proved to be worth their expense. In all but the most immunocompromised of patients, selective decontamination of the bowel with oral or systemic antibiotics has not been found to be cost effective and may even increase the risk of infection with antibiotic-resistant organisms. Likewise, bladder irrigations with antibiotics or disinfectants predispose to infection with resistant organisms. Regular cleansing of the urethral meatus with soap and water or povidone-iodine solution has failed to show any protective value. A water-soluble polyantimicrobial ointment applied three times a day to the catheter-meatal junction did reduce the incidence of bacteriuria but was not clearly cost effective.[7] Use of antibacterial silver- or chlorhexidine-impregnated catheters has been inconsistent in reducing bacteriuria; considering their expense, more obvious benefit will need to be demonstrated to warrant their regular use in all but selected cases.

Central and Peripheral Vascular Catheters (see also Chapter 138)

The importance of intravenous catheters as a source of septic thrombophlebitis and systemic infection has been emphasized since the mid-1960s and must always be considered in patients with unexplained fever. Most catheter-associated infections occur as a result of improper insertion or maintenance practices, or of prolonged use.

Several factors increase the likelihood of catheter colonization. These include (1) improper sterile insertion technique; (2) placement or maintenance of the catheter by inexperienced personnel; (3) the number of catheter lumens; (4) the frequency of catheter manipulation; (5) the type of catheter material; (6) the use of occlusive catheter dressings; and (7) the duration for which the catheter is in place.[8] Reducing the incidence of catheter colonization and subsequent catheter-related infections begins with the adherence of an experienced operator to aseptic techniques during placement. With central catheters, this includes the use of sterile gowns, gloves, and drapes. Handwashing by all personnel inserting or maintaining the catheter is mandatory. The patient's skin must be cleansed before insertion with povidone-iodine and then with 70% alcohol or a chlorhexidine gluconate scrub. Daily inspection of the catheter site and removal of the catheter if signs of inflammation are present are mandatory, as are dressing changes every 48 hours with dry, nonocclusive dressings.[9] Topically applied polymyxin-neomycin-bacitracin ointment may be used at the insertion site. This reduces the bacterial colonization of peripheral and central catheters but may be associated with an increased risk of fungal colonization.[10]

Considerable debate and numerous opinions focus on the regularly scheduled changing of central catheters. Clearly, the risk of catheter colonization increases with the length of time it is in place. Changing the site of peripheral catheters every 48 hours is generally not difficult or risky, but changing central catheters does pose some risk to the patient (e.g., pneumothorax or bleeding). Changing a catheter-over-wire should reduce these mechanical complications, but evidence supports that it may increase the risk of bacterial colonization of the catheter.[11] In critically ill surgical patients with adequate vascular access sites, we believe routine changing of the catheter has merit. For patients who are ill but do not appear acutely infected, we permit one routine guidewire catheter change. If a patient is stable and afebrile and if the catheter site is clean, it is not clear that any manipulation of the catheter is warranted.[11] Anytime a patient appears acutely infected and demonstrates a clinical picture consistent with sepsis syndrome and no source for infection is obvious, we either remove all catheters or change them over a wire. The intradermal catheter segments are cultured semiquantitatively.[12] If blood culture results are positive or if a catheter is heavily colonized, then any line changed over a wire is removed. It is absolutely imperative that any unused or unnecessary catheter be removed. The idle catheter is not uncommon and poses an unacceptable risk.[13] A well-presented set of recommendations for central vascular catheter care is available.[14]

PREVENTING INFECTIONS RELATED TO RESPIRATORY ASSIST DEVICES

Inhalation therapy equipment and mechanical ventilators, much like indwelling intravascular catheters, have had a major impact on medical care but have also created the potential for contamination of the respiratory tract with hospital-associated microbes. Moreover, patients who require inhalation therapy or ventilatory assistance may have significant preexisting pulmonary pathology predisposing them to respiratory tract contamination that can lead to bronchitis or pneumonia.

Pneumonia accounts for 10% to 15% of nosocomial infections. The incidence of pneumonia in mechanically ventilated patients may be as high as 40%, with the risk depending on the degree of acute or chronic pulmonary disease and on the duration of ventilatory assistance. Nosocomial pneumonia in ventilated patients does contribute to hospital stay and cost and to patient mortality, particularly if the infecting organisms are *Pseudomonas* or *Acinetobacter*.[15] Colonization of the oropharynx with hospital-acquired gram-negative bacteria is believed to precede infection of the respiratory tract. This colonization occurs rapidly in patients admitted to the intensive care unit, particularly if they are intubated and receive systemic antibiotics. Bacteria from the oropharynx may enter the respiratory tract (1) by leakage of pooled secretions around the endotracheal tube cuff; (2) by the dislodging of aggregates of bacteria that colonize the endotracheal tube during suctioning; (3) by inhalation of infected aerosolized droplets of water from the ventilator tubing condensate or from contaminated humidification devices or medication nebulizers; or (4) from the hands of hospital personnel during suctioning or manipulation of the endotracheal tube if appropriate aseptic techniques are not followed. Strategies to reduce respiratory infections might be divided into two categories: those designed to reduce aspiration or aerosolization of infectious water droplets, and those designed to reduce colonization of the oropharynx with pathogenic bacteria. Examples of the former include reducing unnecessary manipulation or suctioning of the endotracheal tube, strict use of aseptic technique (use of gloves, sterile tubing, and sterile water), using humidifiers that do not produce aerosols, using heated circuits or traps to collect condensate within ventilator tubing, using clean medication nebulizers, and implementing hospital infection control programs to monitor pulmonary infections associated with inhalation therapy or mechanical ventilation.[16]

Measures to reduce oropharyngeal colonization with pathogenic bacteria include early enteral feeding to maintain gastrointestinal epithelial integrity and resistance to bacterial translocation.[17] The use of sucralfate for stress ulcer prophylaxis may be superior to histamine$_2$ receptor antagonists because sucralfate does not interfere with the ability of gastric acid to limit colonization of the stomach with gram-negative bacteria. More well-controlled studies are needed to resolve this issue. A recent meta-analysis supported an association of sucralfate use with a reduction in respiratory infections when compared with the use of histamine$_2$ receptor antagonists.[18] Selective decontamination of the oropharynx and gastrointestinal tract with nonabsorbed oral and topical suspensions of antibiotics remains a controversial modality for reducing the incidence of nosocomial pneumonia. The large number of studies that employ this approach are very different and therefore difficult to assess and compare. Some are not randomized or blinded. Some include different definitions of pneumonia, different patient populations, different antibiotic regimens (some include systemically administered antibiotics), and incomplete explanations of methodology. It may be that selective decontamination reduces the frequency of pneumonia, but whether this reduction is significant and cost effective, leads to reduction in mortality, and occurs without leading to the development of antimicrobial resistance is not sufficiently answered. A fine review of this difficult topic has been published.[19]

ANTIBIOTIC PROPHYLAXIS

Appropriate use of prophylactic antibiotics significantly reduces the incidence of certain nosocomial infections. Prophylaxis in the neutropenic host is addressed later in this chapter.

The blunt or penetrating trauma victim often requires

multiple surgical interventions. For the trauma patient, antibiotic prophylaxis is as important to reducing infection as are the previously described measures for reducing site-specific nosocomial infection. Indications for prophylaxis and specific antibiotic regimens are beyond the scope of this chapter, but an excellent review of these subjects is available.[20] An understanding of and adherence to the fundamentals of prophylaxis are essential. These fundamentals are as follows: (1) the antibiotic selected should kill the endogenous or acquired *pathogenic* organisms that colonize the site where the invasive procedure is to be performed; (2) the antibiotic should be bactericidal; (3) attention to the timing of administration is important, so that adequate levels of the antibiotic are in the tissue at the time contamination is most likely; (4) the antibiotic should ideally have a long half-life and should be redosed during lengthy surgical procedures; (5) the antibiotic should be of low potential toxicity; and (6) the duration of prophylaxis should be as short as possible. The trend in surgical antibiotic prophylaxis regimens is decidedly toward the use of antibiotics only during the intraoperative period. Exceptions to this might include orthopedic trauma with high-grade open fractures or penetrating large bowel injuries with peritoneal soiling. In these situations, the use of the term "prophylaxis" is incorrect.

INFECTIONS IN CRITICALLY ILL TRAUMA VICTIMS

Altered Host Immunity

The victim of acute blunt or penetrating trauma is not immunologically normal. The cause of immunosuppression in the trauma patient is multifactorial. During the first few days, altered immunity correlates with the extent and severity of soft tissue injury. Hence, blunt trauma patients may be somewhat more compromised than victims of penetrating trauma. Later, host immunity may be adversely influenced by multiple blood transfusions, infections, nutritional deficiency, and medications.

Specific immunologic changes secondary to trauma have been comprehensively reviewed by Stillwell and Caplan.[21] Total lymphocyte counts drop quickly following injury, and the proliferation of stimulated lymphocytes is suppressed. The reduction of T lymphocyte number and function may persist for many days after injury and is correlated with injury severity. Anergy (the inability to respond with a delayed-type hypersensitivity reaction to a previously known antigen) is a common manifestation of this lymphocyte impairment and may occur in up to 75% of trauma patients. Severity of injury and patient age also correlate with the presence of anergy. Outcome measures that are associated with anergy include length of hospital stay, incidence of infection, and overall mortality. B lymphocyte counts may also decrease after injury, burn, or hemorrhage, with small declines in serum concentrations of immunoglobulin (Ig)G and IgM protein.

Neutrophils generally undergo a substantial increase in number after the trauma period. Very often, their chemotaxis is impaired. Chemiluminescence, an indirect assessment of enzyme-mediated bactericidal neutrophil function, is also reduced. In addition, reticuloendothelial cell phagocytic function is impaired after trauma. These defects in phagocyte function may increase the risk of bacterial infection.

Trauma-induced activation of inflammatory pathways may also impair normal immune defense. In the case of severe blunt trauma, single or multiple organ failure can occur very early—less than 72 hours after injury. Although infection is often considered to be the most likely cause for multiple organ failure in the trauma patient, early-onset organ failure clearly occurs before infection is expected or can be identified in up to 50% of the patients.[22] The early development of multiorgan failure is an accurate indication that activation of the inflammatory cascade has occurred. The magnitude of activation may correlate with the extent of soft tissue injury, circulatory shock or tissue hypoxia.[22] The inflammatory mediator cascade may adversely affect cell-mediated, humoral, or neutrophil-related defenses. Inflammatory mediators with immune-altering effects following trauma may include interleukin (IL)-1, IL-2, IL-6, IL-8, tumor necrosis factor-α, interferon-γ, and prostaglandins. Furthermore, the development of single or multiple organ failure further compromises the patient by necessitating longer intensive care unit stay and more invasive interventions.

As described, multiple impairments of normal immunologic defenses occur following trauma. It is likely that they increase the risk of developing infection. These abnormalities work in concert with the major predisposition to infection in the trauma patient—the breech of normal anatomic barriers. When evaluating the febrile, critically ill trauma patient for infection, the vast majority of infections are found where the host has been invaded or where normal defenses have been bypassed—that is, traumatic and surgical wounds, fractured bones, crushed tissue, the lungs, pleural and peritoneal spaces, the urinary tract, and bloodstream. These sites should be the focus of the clinician. Fever certainly does arise from noninfectious causes such as venous thrombosis, pancreatitis, large tissue hematomas, and intracranial injuries; infrequently, some febrile episodes are related to infectious complications such as hepatitis, acute acalculous cholecystitis, or *Clostridium difficile* colitis. However, as a group, all of these are much less common than infection at the site of iatrogenic or traumatic invasion.

Approach to the Critically Ill Trauma Patient

When evaluating a trauma patient for infection, the search should begin where the patient has been invaded. However, fever and leukocytosis, the classic hallmarks of infection, are both very nonspecific and are not always indicative of infection in trauma patients. Often, fever is secondary to activation of the acute inflammatory cascade by extensive soft tissue and bone injury, head injury, surgical manipulation of ischemic tissue, large soft tissue hematoma, transient atelectasis, or reaction to some specific administered medication or blood product. Therefore, whereas the presence of fever should institute a search for infection, it does not mean that an infection is definitely present or that antibiotics are necessarily indicated. Leukocytosis, the cardinal sign of infection, is also very nonspecific in the postsurgical or acutely traumatized patient. Acute inflammatory response, significant blood loss, stress, and the use of many drugs may cause an increase in the count of the peripheral circulating leukocytes. Therefore, it is not uncommon for the acutely traumatized patient to have both fever and leukocytosis without infection.

Limiting antibiotic use as much as possible lessens the incidence of superinfection with resistant organisms. In the majority of instances, we do not begin administration of antibiotics for fever and leukocytosis until a site of infection has been clearly established or is strongly suspected. However, any time a patient manifests cardiovascular instability, exhibiting parameters of cardiac index and systemic vascular resistance consistent with sepsis, and there is no other adequate explanation, then empiric antibiotics should be instituted. Specific recommendations for empiric antibiotic therapy require knowledge of two critical pieces of information: (1) the organisms that normally reside and typically cause infection at the suspected site of infection (i.e., wound infections with *Staphylococcus aureus* or *Streptococcus* species, or abdominal infections with gram-negative rods and anaerobic organisms); and (2) the pathogens resident in the specific intensive care unit and the pattern of their antibiotic susceptibility. In our trauma intensive care unit, for example, *Enterobacter cloacae,* which is often resistant to both β-lactam and third-generation cephalosporin antibiotics, is a concern.

The close association between antibiotic use patterns and the prevalence of multiple drug–resistant bacteria and fungal pathogens cannot be overemphasized. Broad-spectrum empiric antibiotic regimens must be used judiciously, and once the site or organism causing infection is identified, the empiric regimens must be appropriately narrowed. The careful and selective use of antibiotics at our institution has resulted in significantly fewer infections with nosocomial multiple drug–resistant pathogens, such as *Xanthomonas maltophilia* or *Pseudomonas* species, and systemic fungal infections. Since 1992, we have found only 7 documented blood-borne fungal infections among more than 2500 patients admitted to our trauma intensive care units.

Surgical Wound Infections

Surgical wounds account for only 10% of all infections in our postsurgical trauma patients. Most wound infections become evident approximately 48 hours or more after the surgical event. However, infections due to group A β-hemolytic streptococci or *Clostridium* species may occur within 24 hours and are usually fulminant. They must be identified and treated aggressively with débridement and antibiotics. Of the wound infections that occur more than 48 hours after surgery, staphylococcal ones are by far the most common. Gram-negative rods do cause wound infections, and along with enterococci and anaerobes are often present in necrotizing infections or abdominal-perineal wounds. Purulent material obtained from the wound should be examined immediately with a Gram's stain, and if the patient has systemic signs and symptoms of infection, use of appropriate antibiotics should accompany proper surgical management of the wound. If the wound infection is superficial, above the fascia, and not accompanied by cellulitis, simple opening of the wound may be adequate therapy.

Daily inspection of all surgical wounds for swelling, heat, erythema, and purulent or copious serous discharge is mandatory.

Intra-abdominal Infection

In the blunt trauma victim whose initial results on abdominal computed tomography or diagnostic peritoneal lavage, or both, are negative, the development of intra-abdominal infection is unusual. Infrequent exceptions include acute acalculous cholecystitis[23] or, even more unusual, post-traumatic appendicitis.[24] Even patients who have required celiotomy on admission for nonintestinal intra-abdominal injury have a less than 5% likelihood of developing an intra-abdominal infection.[25]

Occasionally, a blunt trauma victim has bowel injury with intra-abdominal soiling that is often associated with injury to the liver, spleen, or pancreas. The risk of postoperative infection in these patients seems to be similar to that of those with penetrating bowel injuries and is increased if the victim is older, has left-sided colon injury necessitating colectomy, has a larger number of injured organs, and requires a lot of blood products.[26] The time elapsed between peritoneal soiling and surgical débridement may also be a factor.

The risk of intra-abdominal infection is much greater for the victims of penetrating abdominal injuries. The vast majority of these are gunshot or stab wounds. During surgery, the abdominal cavity is vigorously lavaged, and perforated bowel injuries receive 24 to 48 hours of an antibiotic regimen with anaerobic and gram-negative aerobe activity. The majority of patients do not develop infections; however, the cases of infection that do occur can be extremely complicated. Such cases are closely followed with abdominal computed tomography and surgical or percutaneous catheter drainage of collections, when indicated. The difficult patients are the ones who have free abdominal fluid or blood or multiple small collections in the pelvis or between loops of bowel. It is often impossible to determine which if any of these fluid collections are infected. Often, following a course of empiric antibiotic therapy, we must simply observe the patient closely for systemic indications of intra-abdominal abscess. Close cooperation among the surgical team, critical care physicians, and the infectious disease consultants is the optimal way to manage these patients.[26a]

Pneumonia

Respiratory tract infection in the intensive care unit population carries the highest fatality rate among all nosocomial infections. When a patient is placed on a respirator, all airway defense mechanisms are circumvented, and the alveoli are exposed directly to the outside environment. Clearly, prevention is better than treatment, and early treatment is better than late treatment.

Pneumonia is diagnosed based on the identification of signs and symptoms of infection: a new pulmonary infiltrate that does not change with aggressive physical therapy, and a Gram's stain of tracheal secretions that shows many polymorphonuclear cells and many organisms. The diagnosis is not solely dependent on culture results, in particular because patients on mechanical ventilation often have nosocomial pathogens that do not in themselves signify infection. Physical examination alone is not an adequate screening procedure. All patients on respirators should undergo portable upright chest radiography on a daily basis so that pulmonary infection can be identified as early as possible. A patient who has fever, leukocytosis, pulmonary infiltrate on chest radiographs, and growth of a potential pathogen should receive aggressive mechanical physical therapy directed at the area of the infiltrate. Therapeutic bronchoscopy may be employed in those patients who do not respond to conventional chest physiotherapy or in patients whose chest films show the absence of proximal air bronchograms; however, this technique's benefit remains unproven. If a subsequent radiograph obtained 3 to 6 hours later shows no change in the infiltrate and if the results of Gram's staining are as described earlier, the patient is treated for a bacterial pneumonia. Frequently, however, aggressive physical therapy resolves the infiltrate appreciably; if this is the case, the patient probably has atelectasis rather than pneumonia. Also, if the results of Gram's staining are not consistent with bacterial pneumonia (i.e., polymorphonuclear leukocytes are not seen or few organisms are noted), then a diagnosis of bacterial pneumonia is in doubt, and other possible causes for the infiltrate should be sought. Blood gas analyses are quite helpful in determining whether a new infectious process exists, as patients with improving blood gas values rarely have an active pulmonary infection.

The diagnosis of pneumonia becomes very difficult in febrile patients who have diffuse parenchymal abnormalities on radiography that are consistent with adult respiratory distress syndrome, lung contusion, or aspiration pneumonitis. These patients often have been intubated for several days or weeks, their sputum is colonized with nosocomial gram-negative rods, and they have abnormal gas exchange. Whether to attribute the fever to pneumonia or to continue the search for more remote causes requires careful clinical discrimination. Furthermore, if pneumonia is believed to be present, the determination of the specific inciting pathogen based only on sputum culture results is quite problematic. Diagnostic bronchoscopy that is directed at the radiographically consolidated area may be helpful in discriminating the true pathogen or pathogens from colonizing flora. Either protected specimen brushings or bronchoalveolar lavage methods may be employed. These specimens may be sent for Gram's staining of the cytospin pellet and quantitative culture. Accepted diagnostic thresholds are $\geq 10^3$ bacteria/mL for protected specimen brushing and $\geq 10^4$ bacteria/mL for bronchoalveolar lavage.[26b, 27] Chest computed tomography in the critically ill, recumbent patient can contribute valuable information about unidentified areas of consolidation, pleural effusion, abscess, pneumatocele, or pericardial effusion that are not seen on the recumbent portable chest radiograph.[28]

One subset of patients in whom the early institution of antibiotics for possible pulmonary infection is warranted are those with pulmonary contusions. Pneumonia may develop rapidly in these patients and often is caused by *Haemophilus influenzae* or *St. aureus,* or both. Blood in the pulmonary parenchyma supports the proliferation of these pathogens, which can evolve into serious necrotizing pneumonias. We perform Gram's staining and cultures of daily sputum samples in these patients. If the sputum becomes purulent and has many bacteria, and if the chest radiograph fails to show the expected early resolution of simple contusion, we begin antibiotic therapy for the isolated pathogen or pathogens.

Sinusitis

Nosocomial sinusitis is a complication that results from the use of nasotracheal or nasogastric tubes.[29] The frequency of this infection has decreased dramatically as our use of nasal tubes has decreased. Nevertheless, we still consider nosocomial sinusitis in our differential diagnosis of fever in the trauma intensive care unit patient if he or she has or has had a nasal tube and, importantly, facial trauma. In the intubated, sedated, recumbent patient, sinusitis is often unrecognized because it is cryptic, represented only by fever and a mild leukocytosis with very few physical findings on examination. Fewer than half of patients have purulent nasal drainage.

Sinusitis can occur as early as 2 days after nasal intubation but usually occurs somewhat later. The diagnosis is often assisted by examination of portable sinus radiographs. In the absence of previous facial trauma, we look for complete opacification or an air-fluid level in the sinus. Portable films, however, may be of poor technical quality if the intensive care unit patient is uncooperative. If our suspicion for sinusitis is strong and the portable films are unsatisfactory, computed tomography is an excellent means to evaluate all of the paranasal sinuses. If the plain radiography or computed tomography findings are compatible with sinusitis, aspiration of the maxillary sinus is performed. In patients who have had facial trauma, often only blood is obtained. If purulent material is obtained, Gram's staining is performed, and antibiotics are instituted based on the morphology of the organisms observed. The nasal tube is removed, and if a tube is still required, it is placed in the oral cavity. Most patients respond well, only a few require a temporary drain to be left in place.

Post-traumatic Central Nervous System Infections

Hospital-acquired infections of the central nervous system are uncommon in most intensive care unit patients; thus, lumbar puncture is not part of the routine work-up in the critically ill patient who appears to have sepsis. However, patients who have undergone neurosurgical procedures or patients with open central nervous system trauma are at risk for developing meningitis and, less commonly, brain abscess. Patients with evidence on physical examination or computed tomography of a basilar skull fracture, or patients who have significant severe midface bone fractures may have an unrecognized cerebrospinal fluid fistula. As many as 40% of patients with fractures of the middle third of the facial skeleton have cerebrospinal fluid leaks. Rhinorrhea and otorrhea are often not evident. Remarkably, very few of these patients develop meningitis, and the cerebrospinal fluid fistulas spontaneously close.[30] Despite the low incidence of meningitis, in patients with head and face injuries associated with cerebrospinal fluid leaks, any fever, leukocytosis, or a change in mental status must be assessed immediately. If there is any suspicion of meningitis, administration of antibiotics should be begun, and computed tomography of the head should be performed. Head trauma is one situation in which computed tomography is indicated before lumbar puncture is performed to avoid complications of the procedure. If lumbar puncture is not neurologically contraindicated, it should be performed. If results of Gram's staining, culture, cell counts, or latex agglutination studies of the cerebrospinal fluid are remarkable, a therapeutic course of antibiotics should be completed. An excellent review of post-traumatic central nervous system infections is available.[31]

Urinary Tract Infection

Since most intensive care unit patients have a Foley catheter in place, it is not surprising that the urinary tract accounts for a substantial portion of the infections encountered in this group. The true difficulty with catheter-associated urinary tract infections is differentiating colonization of the catheter from infection of the urinary tract. It is common for patients to have bacteria colonizing their urinary tracts, depending on the duration that the catheter has been indwelling. The presence of symptoms is useful to separate the colonized from the infected patient; however, in the trauma patient, critical illness, sedation, confusion, head trauma, or spinal cord trauma all obviate the ability to assess symptoms. Noting the presence of pyuria can be quite useful. The febrile patient with persistent bacteriuria and pyuria probably has a UTI, and therapy should be instituted. Pyuria, however, is not an absolute indication of infection and may be absent or present without infection.[32] There is also a misconception about the critical number of organisms (colony forming units [CFU]/mL) required to diagnose a UTI. Urine colony counts of less than 10^5 CFU/mL have clinical significance for catheterized patients. Low-level colonization of catheter urine progresses to high level bacteriuria ($>10^5$ CFU/mL) in 95% of patients who are not treated with catheter removal or antibiotics. Therefore, clinicians should consider colony counts of 10^2 to 10^3 organisms as representing "significant" bacteriuria.[33] The microbiology laboratory should identify organisms that are recovered in colony counts of 10^3 CFU/mL or greater in catheterized patients.

Another misconception is that the presence of polymicrobial urine isolates is always an indication of specimen contamination. Up to 15% of hospitalized patients with catheters may have polymicrobial UTIs.[34]

The diagnosis of UTI in the catheterized patient is difficult and requires the clinician to assess and weigh the results of the urinalysis and urine culture within the context of the physical examination and the patient's clinical status.

Primary Bacteremia

Ten per cent of our bacteremic patients have no definite site of infection. A primary bacteremia is the occurrence of two positive blood cultures in a patient with systemic signs of infection and from whom the same organism is not isolated from any other site. Primary bacteremias are often due to coagulase-negative staphylococci, *St. aureus,* enterococci, or one of the gram-negative rods (Table 131–3). Since this infection can only be defined based on positive blood cultures, the culturing of blood from two separate venipunctures should be routine for all intensive care unit patients who demonstrate signs of infection. If the patient is stable and no primary site of infection can be found, antibiotics may be withheld. If, on the other hand, a patient shows signs of cardiovascular instability or manifests sepsis syndrome, then antibiotics are instituted on the basis of the most resistant organisms residing within the particular intensive care unit. Persistence of the same organism in the bloodstream without an identifiable primary focus should prompt a search for an endovascular focus (e.g., endocarditis, suppurative thrombophlebitis, arteritis or mycotic aneurysm, infected prosthetic material).

INFECTIONS IN PATIENTS WITH HEMATOLOGIC MALIGNANCIES

Patients with hematologic malignancies experience profound compromise of their host defenses owing to either their native oncologic condition or therapeutic interventions (e.g., chemotherapy, radiation, splenectomy). The type and severity of infectious complications in such patients are a function of which host defense mechanisms (humoral, granulocyte, cell-mediated) are affected in addition to elements of nosocomial exposure and previous exposure. The combination of all these factors has been appropriately termed the "net state of immunosuppression."[35]

Humoral Immune Defect

Common examples of hematologic malignancies characterized by humoral dysfunction include chronic lymphocytic leukemia and multiple myeloma. Both disorders are associated with hypogammaglobulinemia and an impaired de novo antibody response to important antigenic challenges, which result in the lack of opsonizing antibodies to a variety of common pyogenic bacteria. Such patients thus have a fairly predictable spectrum of infections caused by the encapsulated pathogens, *S. pneumoniae, H. influenzae,* and, rarely, *Neisseria meningitidis.*

Patients who undergo bone marrow transplantation for hematologic malignancy have an increased risk of pneumococcal infection when antibody production against *S. pneumoniae* is depressed before full marrow engraftment. This risk is decreased in older individuals who have come in contact with and formed antibody against most pneumococcal serotypes.

Because the spleen is essential for initial recognition and antibody formation against each serotype of pneumococci, patients who have undergone splenectomy are also at increased risk of infection. The risk of *S. pneumoniae* or *H. influenzae* bacteremia is very low but nevertheless should be considered in any splenectomized patient who experiences sudden fever and shaking chills. Such patients should have immediate medical attention; hospitalization for treatment with intravenous ampicillin is appropriate, except in settings where penicillin-resistant pneumococcus or ampicillin-resistant *H. influenzae* is prevalent (in this case, a third-generation cephalosporin should be effective). Splenectomized children should receive both the polyvalent pneumococcal vaccine and the new *H. influenzae* type b vaccine, preferably before splenectomy. *N. meningitidis* vaccine should also be considered. Adults should at least receive the pneumococcal vaccine.

TABLE 131–3. Shock Trauma Center, January–December 1992: Microbes Causing Nosocomial Bloodstream Infections

Organism	*Primary Bacteremia*	*Secondary Bacteremia*	*Total*
Coagulase-negative staphylococci	26	6	32
Enterococci	12	4	16
Staphylococcus aureus	11	6	17
Methicillin-resistant *Staphylococcus aureus*	6	7	13
Pseudomonas aeruginosa	6	7	13
Enterobacter species	2	7	9
Klebsiella species	2	4	6
Candida species	3	2	5
Acinetobacter species	3	2	5
Group A streptococci	2	1	3

Cellular Immune Dysfunction

Intact cell-mediated immunity depends on a qualitative and quantitative intact line of T helper (CD4), T suppressor (CD8), other effector lymphocytes, and cell-derived lymphokines that function as nonspecific and specific activators to lymphocyte proliferation. Common examples of hematologic malignancy with cell-mediated immunity defects include Hodgkin's disease, lymphoma, and the lymphocytic leukemias. In addition, drugs such as azathioprine, cyclosporin, corticosteroids, and cytotoxic agents as well as antilymphocyte antibodies and irradiation all have variable deleterious effects on cellular immunity. An extraordinarily wide spectrum of pathogens may cause infection owing to cell-mediated immunity defects. These include (1) intracellular bacteria (*Mycobacterium tuberculosis,* atypical mycobacteria, *Listeria, Legionella, Nocardia,* and nontyphoidal *Salmonella*); (2) fungi (*Aspergillus* species, *Cryptococcus neoformans, Histoplasma capsulatum, Coccidioides immitis*); (3) protozoa (*Pneumocystis carinii, Toxoplasma gondii*; (4) *Herpesvirus* species (herpes simplex, varicella-zoster, cytomegalovirus); and (5) helminths (*Strongyloides stercoralis*).

Granulocytopenia

Granulocytopenia is associated with hematologic malignancies, therapy with myelosuppressive agents, and bone marrow transplantation. It is probably the most important predisposing factor to infection in the immunocompromised patient. The granulocyte count is inversely correlated with the incidence of infection, particularly at granulocyte counts below 100/μL (Fig. 131–1).[36]

The granulocytopenic patient does not usually have the classic signs of inflammation; severe infection may be present with minimal or no physical findings. Thus, patients with pharyngitis often have fever and sore throat, but only a few develop an exudate or even erythema. Similarly, ano-

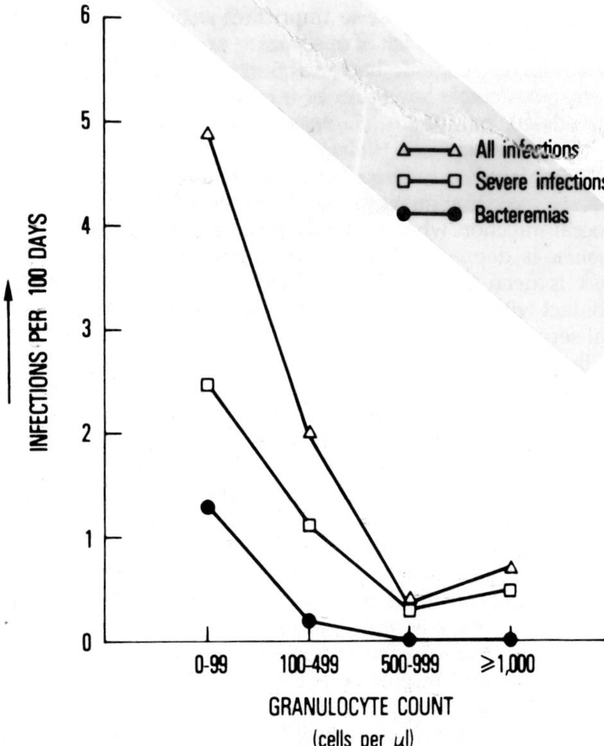

Figure 131–1. Granulocytopenia. Incidence of infection in acute nonlymphocytic leukemia during induction therapy. Infection incidence rises as the granulocyte count falls; almost all bacteremias occur when there are essentially no circulating granulocytes. (From Schimpff SC: Infections in the compromised host: an overview. *In*: Principles and Practice of Infectious Diseases. 3rd ed. Mandell GL, Douglas RG Jr, Bennett JE [Eds]. New York, Churchill Livingstone, 1989, pp 2258–2265.)

rectal lesions may be suggested by fever, local pain, and occasionally induration, but true formation of an abscess is rare and usually occurs only after partial recovery of marrow function.

Patients with pneumonia and profound granulocytopenia usually have fever and dry cough, but sputum production is minimal and, because of the impaired inflammatory response, physical or radiologic findings of consolidation may not be present for the first few days. By the same token, patients with urinary tract infections usually fail to show dysuria, urinary frequency, or flank pain, and very seldom demonstrate pyuria. For these reasons, fever, which is almost invariably present during infection, is considered the early primary sign, and its recognition has substantial therapeutic implications.

Infections in granulocytopenic patients frequently occur at only five or six sites and are usually caused by a small number of pathogens.[37] Major sites of infection are the upper alimentary canal (periodontium, oropharynx, and lower third of the esophagus), lower colon and perianum, lungs, skin, and, to a lesser degree, urinary tract. Infection usually follows mucosal damage produced by chemotherapeutic agents and occasionally is exacerbated by repeated episodes of vomiting or diarrhea, suppression of pulmonary clearance mechanisms (e.g., the mucociliary function of the tracheobronchial tree), or damage to the integuments at sites of venipuncture or bone-marrow aspiration, as well as moist, warm areas such as the axillae or groin, where replication of the organism is unimpeded. Urinary infections are uncommon except in patients with predisposing anatomic defects or bladder instrumentation.

The major pathogens (Table 131–4) are enteric gram-negative bacilli such as *Escherichia coli*, *Klebsiella pneumoniae*, and *P. aeruginosa* as well as some gram-positive organisms such as α-hemolytic streptococci and *S. epidermidis*. Yeasts (*Candida albicans* and *C. tropicalis*) and filamentous fungi (*A. flavus* and *A. fumigatus*) are rarely involved in the first infectious episode but are prominent pathogens after prolonged use of broad-spectrum antibiotics during persistent granulocytopenia.

Routine surveillance cultures of samples from the nose, gingiva, skin, and rectum reveal that gram-negative infections tend to occur at sites where the organisms were already colonizing; more than half of the infections are caused by hospital-acquired bacteria, which often have a more resistant pattern of antibiotic susceptibility.[38] Not all colonizing organisms, however, cause infection, and the relative virulence of the organism is important in determining pathogenicity. For example, antecedent colonization by *P. aeruginosa* has a higher predictive value for subsequent infection during granulocytopenia than prior colonization by *Proteus* species, *Citrobacter* species, or other less virulent *Pseudomonas* species. Colonization by *Klebsiella* and *Serratia* species appears to be of intermediate virulence in this setting.

Diagnostic Process

Evaluating infection in the patient with hematologic malignancy should include an overall assessment of which host defense mechanisms are actively compromised; this may provide diagnostic insight to both the site of infection and to pathogen or pathogens involved.

The diagnostic process begins by looking for obvious predisposing factors, such as peripheral or central intravenous lines, arterial catheters, and bladder catheters. A meticulously recorded history and emphasis on apparently minor complaints such as minimal cough or slight dyspnea, pain on defecation, or substernal discomfort with dysphagia may suggest pneumonitis, perianal cellulitis, or esophagitis, respectively; a careful physical examination must follow to detect even minimal inflammatory changes. A urine specimen should always be obtained and examined for bacteriuria by the physician.

Infection of the oral cavity is commonly associated with granulocytopenia and is usually clinically difficult to distinguish from mucosal damage caused by cytotoxic drugs. Sudden onset of pain and difficulty in swallowing in combination with fever, chills, and tenderness in the submandibular area are usually suggestive of bacterial or fungal infection. A significant portion of these patients have concurrent bacteremia. Esophagitis is a much more frequent infection than is commonly recognized, and the lower third

TABLE 131–4. Common Pathogens During Neutropenia*

Gram-Positive Bacteria
Staphylococcus epidermidis
α-Hemolytic streptococci
Gram-Negative Bacteria
Escherichia coli
Klebsiella pneumoniae
Pseudomonas aeruginosa
Yeasts and Fungi
Candida albicans and *C. tropicalis*
Aspergillus flavus and *A. fumigatus*

*As a general rule, about 85% of bacterial infections are caused by these five bacteria, and 85% of fungal infections are caused by these yeasts and filamentous fungi.

of the esophagus is the most vulnerable area, probably because of a combination of mucosal damage and gastric acid reflux. *Candida* species, herpes simplex virus, and cytomegalovirus are the three most common pathogens. The characteristic symptoms of esophagitis are substernal pain on swallowing and occasional dysphagia, symptoms often overlooked by the patient and the physician. Barium swallow may demonstrate mucosal damage but does not define the causative agent. Upper endoscopy is the preferred diagnostic procedure. Since therapeutic approaches vary with the causative pathogen, a definitive diagnosis depends on direct visualization, brushing, and biopsy of the affected mucosa. Samples obtained on esophagoscopy should be sent for bacterial, fungal, and viral culturing as well as for cytologic and histopathologic analysis.

Pneumonitis may initially cause minimal or no symptoms and few, if any, physical findings. The initial chest radiograph may yield a negative result even with severe infection and bacteremia, probably because too few cells are present to mount an inflammatory response; repeated radiologic studies, however, eventually demonstrate an infiltrate. The development of pneumonia is one of the most common and serious complications among immunocompromised patients and is associated with a mortality of 40% to 50% or greater. It requires prompt diagnosis and specific treatment. Because of the diverse spectrum of opportunistic pathogens in these immunocompromised hosts, the evaluation of pneumonia may require both semi-invasive and invasive procedures to determine the cause and to guide appropriate therapy. Common bacterial organisms include the aerobic gram-negative bacilli and *St. aureus*. The filamentous fungi (*Aspergillus* species, *Mucor* species) or yeasts (*Candida* species, Torulopsis glabrata) may be responsible for later infections in patients who have received prolonged antibiotic therapy or had prolonged nosocomial exposure. Other opportunistic pathogens such as *Nocardia* species, *Cryptococcus* species, *P. carinii,* and cytomegalovirus are usually associated with concomitant deficits in cell-mediated immunity. Several causes of noninfectious pulmonary infiltrates must also be considered; these include tumor, radiation pneumonitis, drug-induced pulmonary toxicity, hemorrhage, and nonspecific interstitial pneumonitis. The different causes of lung infiltrates in the compromised host have been detailed in excellent reviews.[39, 40]

In most instances, the patient with early pneumonitis should receive empiric therapy after appropriate cultures have been performed. If significant doubt still exists with regard to the inciting pathogen or if the patient fails to show an early favorable clinical response, then further invasive diagnostic procedures become necessary. The decision frequently depends on the ability of the physician to recognize the most likely pathogen in a given epidemiologic setting (neutropenia, immunosuppressive therapy, previous antibiotic therapy) and to assign probabilities on an individual basis. The initial clinical evaluation must be followed by chest radiography; sputum examination is usually unhelpful because during granulocytopenia its production is minimal and always nonpurulent. In addition, expectorated material is contaminated by oropharyngeal microorganisms.

Blood cultures and surveillance cultures of samples from the nose and gingiva may be of value. Nose sample cultures positive for *Aspergillus* in the granulocytopenic patient suggest that the same pathogen is responsible for the pulmonary infiltrate. Transtracheal aspiration, transtracheal brushing, percutaneous needle aspiration, transbronchial lung biopsy, and open lung biopsy have been employed with different degrees of success. Numerous reports have appeared in the literature about the diagnostic yield of fiberoptic bronchoscopy in immunocompromised patients with pulmonary infiltrates; the procedure is relatively simple, can be done without general anesthesia, and can provide samples for histologic examination as well as brushings and alveolar washings from which specimens can be sent for culture, cytologic analysis, and direct antibody staining. The use of protected catheters minimizes specimen contamination by oropharyngeal flora. We favor fiberoptic bronchoscopy as a first invasive procedure after initial clinical and microbiologic evaluations have failed to provide etiologic information. In patients with a rapidly progressing process or with contraindications to bronchoscopic biopsy, tissue diagnosis from open-lung biopsy has a diagnostic accuracy of greater than 80% and a low operative mortality.

Lower colon infections are the origin of many bacteremias in the granulocytopenic patient and usually occur in the setting of extensive and severe mucosal damage by cytotoxic agents, which allows easy passage of potentially pathogenic organisms from the intestinal lumen to the bloodstream. These infections are difficult to diagnose accurately because of the difficulty in accessing the affected area to obtain samples for culture or pathologic analysis; however, patients usually complain of diarrhea, abdominal cramps, and, occasionally, distention. Anorectal lesions are particularly common in patients with acute monocytic and myelocytic leukemia, especially those with preexisting hemorrhoidal disease or bowel dysfunction. Easily overlooked in their early stage because of the minimal inflammatory response, these lesions may progress rapidly to widespread cellulitis and overwhelming sepsis. Meticulous examination usually reveals small mucosal tears with erythema and tenderness. Anorectal lesions are frequently associated with bacteremia, especially with *P. aeruginosa* and Enterobacteriaceae. It is unclear why anaerobes such as *Bacteroides fragilis* are rarely involved.

Skin lesions are frequently found in the axillae or groin or are associated with areas of trauma from venipuncture or bone marrow aspiration. The high incidence of infections in axillae and inguinal regions probably reflects the combination of moisture, temperature, local trauma (axillary shaving), and obstruction of hair follicles and sweat glands by the use of occlusive antiperspirants. Unlike infections at these sites in noncompromised patients, gram-negative bacilli are responsible for over half of these lesions. In addition, cutaneous lesions may be secondary to disseminated bacterial (*Pseudomonas, Staphylococcus, Nocardia*), fungal (*Candida, Aspergillus*), or viral (herpes simplex, varicella-zoster) infections.

Although granulocytopenia does not predispose patients to urinary tract infections, it obscures the usual signs and symptoms, making diagnosis somewhat difficult. Use of catheters and other invasive instruments or obstructive lesions are important antecedents of infectious episodes that usually carry a high incidence of bacteremia. Early recognition usually depends on prompt examination of the urine for bacteriuria.

Approach to Therapy

Because infections in granulocytopenic patients have a high early fatality rate, antibiotic therapy is often given empirically—that is, before culture and susceptibility results are available. In a large population of granulocytopenic patients who develop fever, 60% have microbiologically or clinically documented infection, 20% have equivocal signs of infection, and another 20% in retrospect prove not to have an infection. Fever is therefore usually a sign of infection in these patients, and empiric antibiotic therapy is necessary

TABLE 131–5. Available Antibiotics for Initial Empirical Therapy of Febrile, Neutropenic Patients

Beta-Lactams	*Aminoglycosides*
Penicillins	Gentamicin
Piperacillin	Tobramycin
Mezlocillin	Amikacin
Azlocillin	
Cephalosporins	
Ceftazidime	
Cefoperazone	
Carbapenem	
Imipenem (with cilastatin)	
Ticarcillin (with clavulanic acid)	

Note: Whether to add vancomycin to the initial regimen is discussed in the text.

because other signs of inflammation are muted and because mortality is high.

Empiric antibiotics administered to the granulocytopenic patient must be selected according to the following considerations:

1. The antimicrobial spectrum must include the most common pathogenic gram-negative bacilli and gram-positive cocci, since infections with these agents usually cannot be distinguished on clinical grounds alone (Table 131–5).
2. The antibiotics must be bactericidal in the face of granulocytopenia. Antibiotic combinations should preferably be synergistic.
3. Adequate dosages by intravenous administration are used to ensure reliable and sufficient drug concentrations.
4. Toxicities should be minimized, since 20% or more of patients treated do not have an infection.
5. Duration of therapy must be long enough to allow complete resolution of the infection but be short enough to avoid unnecessary toxicity or propensity for superinfection.

The semisynthetic penicillins have good spectra of action but when used alone predispose to the rapid development of bacterial resistance. Aminoglycosides are inadequate when used as single agents in profoundly neutropenic patients; this is probably because the serum aminoglycoside level corresponding to minimum bactericidal concentration is maintained for only a short period of time.

Combinations of antibiotics expand the antibacterial spectrum and may have a synergistic effect against common pathogens. Although the concept of antimicrobial synergy is intriguing, models for synergism have been described only for the following combinations: penicillin and an aminoglycoside against enterococcal endocarditis; ticarcillin and gentamicin against *P. aerguinosa;* and cephalothin and an aminoglycoside against *K. pneumoniae.* However, the use of synergistic combinations is associated with an improved response rate in immunocompromised patients with documented infections,[41, 42] and numerous antibiotic combinations have been evaluated as empiric therapy for the febrile, granulocytopenic patient. The combination of an acylampicillin (azlocillin, mezlocillin, or piperacillin) and an aminoglycoside (gentamicin, tobramycin, or amikacin) depends largely on the resistance patterns of gram-negative bacilli in a given institution; when used to treat susceptible bacteria, the efficacy among aminoglycosides has been shown to be similar.

Although ticarcillin is not sufficiently active to be useful against *K. pneumoniae,* the addition of the β-lactamase inhibitor clavulanic acid enhances its gram-negative coverage against most β-lactamase–producing gram-negative flora except for *P. aeruginosa,* for which piperacillin remains the ideal agent.

The third-generation cephalosporins include those with a spectrum of activity that covers *P. aeruginosa* (e.g., cefotaxime, cefoperazone, and ceftazidime). These compounds are active against most pathogens that affect the granulocytopenic patient, and they display in vitro synergistic activity against most gram-negative bacilli when combined with an aminoglycoside. Moreover, their low level of antibiotic-related side effects makes the combination of one of these agents with an aminoglycoside a very reasonable choice for empiric therapy.[42a]

Another therapeutic option, termed *double β-lactam therapy,* employs an acylampicillin in combination with either a third-generation cephalosporin or the monobactam aztreonam. Such a combination would provide double coverage against most pathogens and avoid aminoglycoside-related nephrotoxicity and ototoxicity. Laboratory and clinical trials have demonstrated such combinations to be clinically effective in this patient population and to reduce nephrotoxicity and ototoxicity. However, combinations of a β-lactamase inducer (cefoxitin, ceftazidime) and a susceptible β-lactam antibiotic (piperacillin) should be avoided to prevent the emergence of inducible, multiresistant gram-negative bacteria (e.g., *Enterobacter* and *Pseudomonas* species).

The clinical response of infected granulocytopenic patients to antibiotic therapy depends on both the return of the granulocyte count and whether the infecting pathogen or pathogens are susceptible to the chosen antibiotic therapy. Even a minimal increase in the granulocyte count (to >100 cells/μL) can significantly improve response rates (Fig. 131–2)[42]; however, in patients with no rise in granulocyte count, susceptibility of the infecting pathogen to both antibiotics in a combination has been associated with higher improvement rates than if the pathogen is susceptible to only one of the antibiotics used. We therefore recommend antibiotic combinations both to broaden the spectrum of coverage and to provide synergistic bactericidal activity.

During the 1980s, a number of new antibiotics, such as ceftazidime and imipenem-cilastatin have become available;

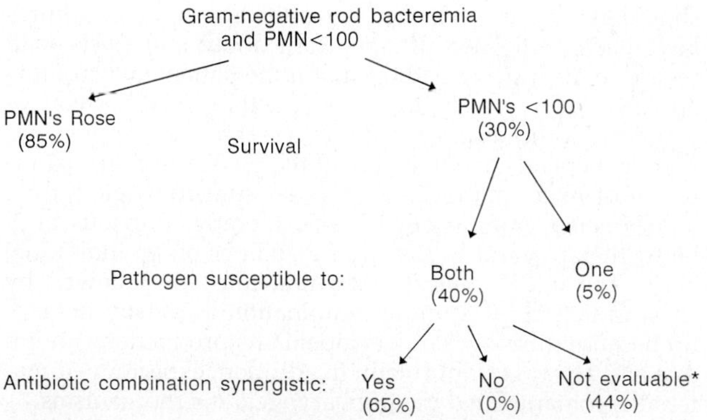

Figure 131–2. Response (survival) of 75 consecutive patients who developed gram-negative bacteremia when their absolute granulocyte count was less than 100 per microliter. Response was much worse for those with aplastic marrow and persistence of neutropenia; in this subgroup, combination therapy was superior, and synergy appears to be useful. *Abbreviation:* PMN = Polymorphonuclear cells. (From Schimpff SC, Scott DA, Wade JC: Infections in cancer patients: Some controversial issues. Support Care Cancer 1994; 2:94–104.)

these antibiotics have such a broad spectrum of coverage that they essentially "cover" most of the major bacterial pathogens (excluding methicillin-resistant *St. aureus,* some enterococci, and certain gram-negative bacilli) that commonly infect the neutropenic patient. As a result, a number of trials have demonstrated that empiric monotherapy with these agents is both safe and effective compared with standard combination therapy.[42b] However, we offer two caveats with respect to empiric monotherapy. First, prescribing physicians need to have a firm understanding of the susceptibility patterns of recent isolates from their institution and, preferably, knowledge of the recent isolate susceptibilities from the area of the institution where cancer patients are treated. The risk of empiric monotherapy is unwarranted in the setting in which the prevalence of multiresistant organisms is high. The rapid emergence of resistance acquired during therapy of *E. cloacae* to the third-generation cephalosporins reduces the efficacy of ceftazidime monotherapy if this organism is part of the nosocomial flora. Second, patients with an aplastic bone marrow and profound granulocytopenia with gram-negative bacteremia should receive a synergistic combination of antibiotics, even though the survival rate in this setting is quite low (Table 131–6).[43] The rationale for this recommendation derives from studies that demonstrate a higher survival rate with synergistic therapy and the relative lack of available efficacy data for monotherapy in this setting. An excellent review of antibiotic therapy for neutropenic patients is available.[44]

Duration of Therapy

The optimal duration of empiric antibiotic therapy during granulocytopenia remains controversial. Superinfection or subsequent infection, or both, occur among 10% to 20% of neutropenic patients treated with empiric, broad-spectrum antibiotic regimens. Although the major predisposing factor to further infection is persistent granulocytopenia, prolonged antibiotic therapy also contributes to superinfection with multiresistant bacteria or fungi. Therefore, it is important to discontinue the use of empiric antibiotics when both the clinical and microbiologic findings permit. More studies are necessary to define the optimal length of therapy in patients with documented infections; a general guideline is 10 to 14 days of therapy for patients with gram-positive or gram-negative bacteremia, provided that their progress is favorable and that the source of infection has resolved within this period. Serious nonbacteremic infections, either microbiologically or clinically documented, are treated for a similar period; less severe infections are treated for 7 to 10 days. In all cases, therapy is continued until the infection has resolved and the patient has been afebrile for 4 to 5 days. Patients with equivocal signs of infection who have an apparent clinical response to antibiotic administration are also treated until they have remained afebrile for 4 to 5 days (usually a total of 7 to 9 days of therapy). Patients receiving empiric antibiotic therapy should have their antibiotic treatment discontinued as soon as tests confirm an elevation in temperature related to a noninfectious cause (e.g., red blood cell or platelet transfusions, chemotherapy, or other drugs). This is usually possible within 4 days.

Perhaps the most difficult therapeutic decision relates to the patient without definitive signs of infection or positive culture results who still has persistent fever and granulocytopenia. Most infected patients, although severely granulocytopenic, show specific symptoms or signs of infection in addition to fever after 72 to 96 hours, provided that careful clinical evaluation has been performed on a daily basis from the moment of the initial febrile episode. For that reason, antibiotic therapy can usually be discontinued in the febrile patient after 4 days if repeated history, physical examination, and laboratory and radiographic evaluations are unrevealing and if the patient is not systemically ill with negative cultures. However, the patient must be watched closely and re-evaluated if fever continues; if necessary, antibiotic therapy can be restarted.

If, on the other hand, a patient presents with conflicting evidence of infection, another antimicrobial agent may be added to cover the possibility of a resistant organism; alternatively, amphotericin B may be administered for possible occult fungal infection.[45,46] Modification of the initial empiric antibiotic regimen should be made after careful review of the particular epidemiologic setting. Examples of common modifications include the addition of vancomycin for suspected catheter-related infection caused by coagulase-negative staphylococci or methicillin-resistant *St. aureus,* clindamycin for suspected anaerobes (perirectal cellulitis, oral infection, or typhlitis) or the addition of an appropriate antibiotic to cover the isolation of a multiresistant organism from oropharyngeal or rectal surveillance cultures. Patients with prolongation of fever and granulocytopenia beyond 7 days or with the presence of *Candida* species or filamentous fungi are candidates for amphotericin B therapy.

TABLE 131–6. Response of Patients with Gram-Negative Bacteremia and Less Than 100 Polymorphonuclear Neutrophil Leukocytes per Microliter

	*Number Responding/Number with Bacteremia (%)**
Persistent granulocytopenia	12/53 (23%)
Recovery of granulocytes	62/76 (82%)

(Data from EORTC International Antimicrobial Therapy Cooperative Group: Ceftazidime combined with a short or long course of amikacin for empirical therapy of gram-negative bacteremia in cancer patients with granulocytopenia. N Engl J Med 1987; 317:1692–1698.)
*$P < .001$.

Treatment of Fungal Infections

Overall, 85% of fungal infections are caused by *Candida* and *Aspergillus* species. Fungi may be of either endogenous origin (*Candida* species, *T. glabrata*), with colonization of the upper and lower alimentary canal, or exogenous origin (*Aspergillus* and *Mucor* species) via the deposition of airborne fungal spores in the lungs and paranasal sinuses. Suppression of local and systemic defense mechanisms may result in their dissemination to contiguous and distant tissues.

The drugs currently available for the therapy of these infections include amphotericin B, 5-flucytosine, the imidazole derivatives miconazole and ketoconazole, and the newer triazoles fluconazole and itraconazole. Amphotericin B is still the most effective agent; however, it is associated with significant morbidity, largely owing to its nephrotoxicity. The drug is given intravenously in doses of 0.3 to 0.6 $mg \cdot kg^{-1} \cdot d^{-1}$ for most *C. albicans* infections. For more resistant *Candida* strains or for neutropenic patients with invasive aspergillosis, doses of 0.7 to 1.5 $mg \cdot kg^{-1} \cdot d^{-1}$ may be required. No clear guidelines exist for determining the total dose of amphotericin B required to achieve cure in patients with serious fungal infection and granulocytopenia.

Flucytosine has been used as an adjunct to amphotericin B for the therapy of candidiasis and cryptococcosis. There are limited data to recommend its use for disseminated candidiasis, and it has no activity against filamentous fungal infections. Its main advantage may be its relatively rapid onset of action and its excellent penetration of the central nervous system. Bone marrow suppression is the principal limiting side effect; however, maintaining serum peak levels at less than 80 μg/mL reduces its occurrence.

Fluconazole holds some promise for infections due to sensitive strains of *Candida* species. Whether or not it is equivalent to amphotericin B is the subject of an ongoing study conducted by the National Institutes of Health. Fluconazole may be adequate for esophagitis, cystitis, or skin infections with *C. albicans* in the non-neutropenic host. Itraconazole has good in vitro activity against *Aspergillus* species. Several case reports demonstrate apparent clinical improvement or cure of patients with aspergillosis following failure of amphotericin B therapy. However, evidence to suggest its efficacy over amphotericin B in the neutropenic host with invasive aspergillosis is insufficient. The main advantage of the triazoles is their good absorption with oral administration and their relative lack of important toxicity when compared with amphotericin.

Most granulocytopenic patients develop fungal infections during or after several prolonged courses of antibacterial therapy and after the infecting organism has been found colonizing one or more sites. For these reasons, empiric therapy with amphotericin B has been recommended for patients with fever of unknown origin who have not responded to antimicrobial therapy, especially if granulocytopenia has been prolonged and if multiple broad-spectrum antibiotic treatments have been given during the past weeks or days. A more recently described fungal infection in the neutropenic patient is chronic disseminated candidiasis, also known as "hepatosplenic candidiasis." This is a *Candida* infection of liver, spleen, lungs, and kidneys that presents with persistent fever and abnormal hepatic chemistries in a patient who is recovering from neutropenia. This is a serious infection that is best treated with amphotericin B, with or without flucytosine.

The high mortality associated with fungal infections in the patient with hematologic malignancy has led to numerous investigations of prophylaxis against fungal infections. The efficacy of fungal prophylaxis has been shown in other immunocompromised populations, including acquired immunodeficiency syndrome patients (fluconazole) and bone marrow recipients (fluconazole, low-dose amphotericin).[47,48] Oral administration of nonabsorbable polyene antibiotics such as nystatin and amphotericin B have failed to show a significant and consistent decrease in the incidence of serious fungal infection during granulocytopenia.[49,50] For patients who are expected to have prolonged neutropenia, fluconazole use may reduce the risk of fungal infection, but this approach still requires prospective investigation to assess efficacy. A major concern is that the systematic use of fluconazole may lead to the emergence of resistant species of fungus such as *C. krusei* or *T. glabrata*.[51]

Prevention of Infection

Most infections are caused by organisms that already colonize the patient, especially along the alimentary canal. About 50% of these organisms are acquired during hospitalization. Thus, a rational plan for the prevention of infection should be to reduce the incidence of colonization with nosocomial pathogens before the period of profound granulocytopenia, when the host is most vulnerable.[52]

The principal sources of new organisms are food, hands, water, and air, probably in that order. Unfortunately, little attention is usually paid to food. Green, leafy vegetables are naturally colonized by gram-negative bacilli, including large numbers of *Klebsiella* species and *E. coli.* Similarly, the pulp of tomatoes is frequently heavily colonized by *P. aeruginosa.* Because fruit juices are prepared in bulk, they usually contain large numbers of yeasts such as *C. tropicalis.* However, most cooked foods and commercially canned products are sterile or nearly sterile, and pasteurized products rarely contain pathogenic organisms. Therefore, eliminating salads and other uncooked vegetables along with fresh fruit juices substantially reduces the number of organisms reaching the patient. The second major area of prophylaxis is proper handwashing by both staff and patients. Observation indicates that most physicians are lax about handwashing. Particular attention also needs to be given to paramedical personnel who may have substantial daily patient contact, such as blood-drawing personnel and respiratory therapists. Water supplies, especially ice machines, are frequently contaminated with water-loving gram-negative rods such as *P. aeruginosa* and *Serratia marcescens.* Finally, air is a source of spore-forming organisms, such as *Aspergillus* species, and of organisms that are carried on particles.

Standard reverse isolation does not address three of the major sources of new organism acquisition—food, water, and air—whereas it overemphasizes reducing direct contact with the use of gowns, gloves, masks, booties, and caps in lieu of handwashing. A practical alternative that can be used in any hospital setting and substantially reduces the acquisition of important pathogens is to ensure that the patients are placed in single-bed rooms, are given a diet with low microbe content and water from tested sources, and are attended by medical personnel who are careful about personal hygiene, including handwashing. A program of sensible housekeeping is also desirable.

Complete reverse isolation with laminar airflow and high-efficiency particulate air filtration may be required for a few specific high-risk patient groups such as bone marrow recipients or aplastic anemia patients who will have a period of prolonged granulocytopenia. Although the maintenance of rooms with such features is both costly and labor intensive, certain airborne pathogens such as *Aspergillus* species can be eliminated.

For patients who will have periods of profound granulocytopenia (cell count <100/μL for longer than 2 weeks), suppression of potentially pathogenic intestinal flora (aerobic/facultative gram-negative organisms) may be beneficial. Oral nonabsorbable antibiotics, such as the combination of gentamicin, polymyxin, and nystatin, administered as a liquid formulation reduce colonization and may reduce infections arising from these sites. Unfortunately, these drugs' high cost and poor taste limit the usefulness of this approach in a setting other than complete reverse isolation. Also, on discontinuation of such therapy, aerobic gram-negative bacilli may rapidly repopulate the alimentary canal in large numbers, leading to gram-negative bacteremia if the patient is still profoundly granulocytopenic. Alternative approaches include the use of trimethoprim-sulfamethoxazole, ciprofloxacin, or norfloxacin; these relatively low-cost compounds suppress many aerobes but leave the anaerobic flora intact. A number of prospective controlled trials indicate that these agents reduce infections in the granulocytopenic patient. However, colonization resistance does not usually remain completely intact, and patients may subsequently become colonized by either a trimethoprim-sulfamethoxazole–resistant or quinolone-resistant form of *E. coli,* which ultimately leads to bacteremia. Although the number of febrile episodes is not always reduced, some studies have shown a reduced need for parenteral broad-spectrum antibiotics.[53]

References

1. Steere AC, Mallison GF: Handwashing practices for the prevention of nosocomial infections. Ann Intern Med 1975; 83:683.
2. Centers for Disease Control: Update: Universal precautions for prevention and transmission of human immunodeficiency vi-

rus, hepatitis B virus, and other blood-borne pathogens in health care settings. MMWR 1988; 37:377.
3. Lynch P, Jackson MM, Cummings J, et al: Rethinking the role of isolation precautions in the prevention of nosocomial infection. Ann Intern Med 1987; 107:243.
4. Garner JS, Simmons BP: CDC guidelines for isolation precautions in hospitals. Am J Infect Control 1984; 12:103.
5. Garibaldi RA, Burke JP, Dickman ML, et al: Factors predisposing to bacteriuria during indwelling urethral catheterization. N Engl J Med 1974; 291:213.
6. Wong ES, Hooton TM: Guidelines for prevention of catheter-associated urinary tract infections. Infect Control 1981; 2:126.
7. Classen DC, Larsen RA, Burke JP, et al: Daily mental care for prevention of catheter-associated bacteriuria: Results using frequent applications of polyantibiotic cream. Infect Control Hosp Epidemiol 1991; 12:157.
8. Hampton AA, Sherertz RJ: Vascular-access infections in hospitalized patients. Surg Clin North Am 1988; 66:57.
9. Conly JM, Grieves K, Peters B: A prospective, randomized study comparing transparent and dry gauze dressing for central venous catheters. J Infect Dis 1989; 159:310.
10. Maki DG, Band JD: A comparative study of polyantibiotic and iodophor ointments in prevention of vascular catheter-related infection. Am J Med 1991; 70:739.
11. Cobb DK, High KP, Snyder RG, et al: A controlled trial of scheduled replacement of central venous and pulmonary-artery catheters. N Engl J Med 1992; 327:1062.
12. Maki DG, Weise CE, Sarafin HW: A semiquantitative culture method for identifying intravenous-catheter–related infection. N Engl J Med 1977; 296:1305.
13. Lederle FA, Parenti CM, Berskow LC, et al: The idle intravenous catheter. Ann Intern Med 1992; 116:737.
14. Corona ML, Peters SG, Narr BJ, et al: Infections related to central venous catheters. Mayo Clin Proc 1990; 65:979.
15. Fason JY, Chastre J, Hance AJ, et al: Nosocomial pneumonia in ventilated patients: A cohort study evaluating attributable mortality and hospital stay. Am J Med 1993; 94:281.
16. Craven DE, Steger KA, Duncan RA: Prevention and control of nosocomial pneumonia. *In*: Prevention and Control of Nosocomial Infections. Wenzel RP (Ed). Baltimore, Williams & Wilkins, 1993, pp 580–600.
17. Deitch EA, Berg R: Bacterial translocation from the gut: A mechanism of infection. J Burn Care Rehabil 1987; 8:475.
18. Tryba M: Sucralfate versus antacids or H_2-antagonists for stress ulcer prophylaxis: A meta-analysis on efficacy and pneumonia rate. Crit Care Med 1991; 19:942.
19. Hamer DH, Barsa M: Prevention of hospital-acquired pneumonia in critically ill patients. Antimicrob Agents Chemother 1993; 37:931.
20. Page CP, Bohmen JMA, Fletcher JR, et al: Antimicrobial prophylaxis for surgical wounds. Arch Surg 1993; 128:79.
21. Stillwell M, Caplan ES: The septic multiple-trauma patient. Crit Care Clin 1988; 4:345.
22. Waydhas C, Nast-Kolb D, Jochum M, et al: Inflammatory mediators, infection, sepsis, and multiple organ failure after severe trauma. Arch Surg 1992; 127:460.
23. Frazee RC, Nagorney DM, Mucha P: Acute acalculous cholecystitis. Mayo Clin Proc 1989; 64:163.
24. Hennington MH, Tinsley EA, Proctor HJ, et al: Acute appendicitis following blunt trauma. Ann Surg 1991; 214:61.
25. Goins WA, Rodriguez A, Joshi M, et al: Intra-abdominal abscess after blunt abdominal trauma. Ann Surg 1990; 212:60.
26. Nichols RL, Smith JW, Klein DB, et al: Risk of infection after penetrating abdominal trauma. N Engl J Med 1984; 311:1065.
26a. McClean RL, Sheehan GJ, Harding GKM: Intraabdominal infection: A review. Clin Infect Dis 1994; 19:100.
26b. Niederman MJ, Torres A, Summer W: Invasive diagnostic testing is not needed routinely to manage suspected ventilator-associated pneumonia. Am J Respir Crit Care Med 1994; 150:565.
27. Meduri GU: Ventilator-associated pneumonia in patients with respiratory failure. Chest 1990; 97:1208.
28. Mirvis SE, Tobin KD, Kostrubiak I, et al: Thoracic CT in detecting occult disease in critically ill patients. Am J Radiol 1987; 148:685.
29. Caplan ES, Hoyt NJ: Nosocomial sinusitis. JAMA 1982; 647:639.
30. O'Brien MD, Rende PC: The management of dural tear from mid-face fracture. Head Neck Surg 1984; 6:810.
31. Clark RA, Hyslop NE Jr: Posttraumatic meningitis. *In*: Infections of the Nervous System. Schlossberg D (Ed). New York, Springer-Verlag, 1990, pp 50–63.
32. Steward DK, Wood GL, Cohen RL, et al: Failure of the urinalysis and quantitative urine culture in diagnosing symptomatic urinary tract infections in patients with long-term urinary catheters. Am J Infect Control 1985; 13:154.
33. Stark RP, Maki D: Bacteriuria in the catheterized patient: What quantitative level of bacteriuria is relevant? N Engl J Med 1984; 311:560.
34. Asher EF, Oliver BG, Fry DE: Urinary tract infections in the surgical patient. Ann Surg 1988; 54:466.
35. Schimpff SC, Young VM: Epidemiology and prevention of infection in the compromised host. *In*: Clinical Approach to Infection in the Compromised Host. Rubin RH, Young LS (Eds). New York, Plenum Publishing, 1981, pp 5–33.
36. Schimpff SC: Infections in the compromised host: An overview. *In*: Principles and Practice of Infectious Diseases. 3rd ed. Mandell GL, Douglas RG Jr, Bennett JE (Eds). New York, Churchill Livingstone, 1989, pp 2258–2265.
37. EORTC International Antimicrobial Therapy Project Group: Three antibiotic regimens in the treatment of infection in febrile granulocytopenic patients with cancer. J Infect Dis 1978; 137:14.
38. Schimpff SC, Young VM, Greene WH, et al: Origin of infection in acute nonlymphocytic leukemia: Significance of hospital acquisition of potential pathogens. Ann Intern Med 1972; 77:707.
39. Fanta CH, Pennington FE: Fever and new lung infiltrates in the immuno-compromised host. Clin Chest Med 1981; 2:19.
40. Shelhamer JH: Respiratory diseases in the immunosuppressed patient. Ann Intern Med 1992; 117:415.
41. Anderson EJ, Young LS, Hewitt WL: Antimicrobial synergism in the therapy of gram-negative bacteremias. Chemotherapy 1978; 24:45.
42. de Jongh CA, Schimpff SC, Joshi JH, et al: Antibiotic synergism and response in gram-negative bacteremias among granulocytopenic cancer patients. Am J Med 1986; 80:96.
42a. International Antimicrobial Therapy Cooperative Group of the European Organization for Research and Treatment of Cancer: Efficacy and toxicity of single daily doses of amikacin and ceftriaxone versus multiple daily doses of amikacin and ceftazidine for infection in patients with cancer and granulocytopenia. Ann Intern Med 1993; 119:584.
42b. DePauw BE, Derensinski SC, Feld R, et al: Ceftazidine compared with pipericillin and tobramycin for the empiric treatment of fever in neutropenic patients with cancer. Ann Intern Med 1994; 120:834.
43. EORTC International Antimicrobial Therapy Cooperative Group: Ceftazidime combined with a short or long course of amikacin for empirical therapy of gram-negative bacteremia in cancer patients with granulocytopenia. N Engl J Med 1987; 317:1692–1698.
44. Pizzo PA: Management of fever in patients with cancer and treatment-induced neutropenia. N Engl J Med 1993; 328:1323.
45. Pizzo PA, Robichaud KJ, Gill FA, et al: Empiric antibiotic and antifungal therapy for cancer patients with prolonged fever and granulocytopenia. Am J Med 1982; 72:101–111.
46. EORTC International Antimicrobial Therapy Cooperative Group: Empiric antifungal therapy in febrile granulocytopenic patients. Rev Infect Dis 1991; 13:496–503.
47. Nightingale SD, Cal SX, Peterson DM, et al: Primary prophylaxis with fluconazole against systemic fungal infections in HIV-positive patients. AIDS 1992; 6:191.
48. Goodman JL, Winston DJ, Greenfield RA, et al: A controlled trial of fluconazole to prevent fungal infections in patients undergoing bone marrow transplantation. N Engl J Med 1992; 326:845.
49. DeGregoria MW, Lee WMF, Ries CA: *Candida* infections in patients with acute leukemia: Ineffectiveness of nystatin prophylaxis and relationship between oropharyngeal and systemic candidiasis. Cancer 1982; 50:2780–2784.
50. Dekker AW, Rozenberg-Arska MK, Sixma JJ, et al: Prevention of infection by trimethoprim-sulfamethoxasole plus amphotericin B in patients with acute nonlymphocytic leukemia. Ann Intern Med 1981; 95:555–559.
51. Wingard JR, Merz WG, Rinaldi MG, et al: Association of Toru-

lopsis glabrata infections with fluconazole prophylaxis in neutropenic bone marrow transplant patients. Antimicrob Agents Chemother 1993; 37:1847–1849.
52. Scott DA, Schimpff SC: Prevention of infection in cancer patients. *In*: Handbook of Medical Supportive Care in Cancer. Klastersky J, Schimpff SC (Eds). New York, Marcel Dekker (in press).
53. The GIMEMA Infection Program: Prevention of bacterial infection in neutropenic patients with hematologic malignancies: A randomized multicenter trial comparing norfloxacin and ciprofloxacin. Ann Intern Med 1991; 115:7.

CHAPTER 132

Infections in the Surgical Critical Care Unit

Steven M. Steinberg, MD • Ronald Lee Nichols, MD, MS, FACS

Postoperative infectious complications are a frequent cause of morbidity and mortality in the surgical intensive care unit (ICU). These infections most commonly involve the urinary or respiratory tract, invasive catheters, or the operative wound. Patients in ICUs are, by the nature of their clinical status, much more likely to develop nosocomial infections than is the general hospital population. Although the rate of hospital-acquired infection in the general hospital population is approximately 5%,[1] it has been estimated that the rate of nosocomial infection in surgical ICU patients is two- to fivefold higher.[2] Many factors that seem to be associated with this increased risk of infection have been described. Craven and colleagues[3] found that ICU confinement of longer than 3 days, the presence of shock, the use of arterial catheters, and the use of urinary catheterization for longer than 10 days were all linked to significant increases in the incidence of nosocomial infection. Many clinical risk characteristics seem to be related to the development of infection in ICU patients (Table 132–1). Additionally, the association between nosocomial infection and outcome appears to be clear. Both Fry and coworkers[4] and Pin and associates[5] have reported that infection is related to the development of the multiple system organ failure syndrome and to increased mortality.

The evaluation of the critically ill patient in the ICU to determine the focus of infection is often difficult and frequently provides conflicting data. Furthermore, we have come to realize that clinical signs of sepsis such as fever, leukocytosis, high cardiac output, and low peripheral vascular resistance may result from other noninfectious causes. Shock resulting from any cause, severe multiple trauma, acute pancreatitis, the presence of nonviable tissue, and reperfusion injury may all result in the clinical picture of sepsis. Such underlying conditions should be vigorously sought and treated. Patients with these conditions should be supported by all hemodynamic, ventilatory, nutritional, and other means available. However, we often search for a "treatable" source of a patient's sepsis, which is most frequently a nosocomial infection. We have found that a systematic, head-to-toe search for the site of infection in the critically ill surgical patient with sepsis is of utmost importance. However, first and foremost, any search for infection in a surgical patient must take into account the prior condition of the patient. This includes not only the patient's preexisting diseases but also any history of invasive procedures that have been performed. Frequently, the occurrence of infectious complications or organ failure in a surgical ICU patient is closely associated with complications of the operations previously performed. Any investigation for the site of infection in a critically ill patient must start at that patient's known site of disease or operation. For example, in the patient who has undergone a gastrointestinal tract operative procedure, the clinician's index of suspicion must be extremely high for complications of that operation, including anastomotic dehiscence, peritonitis, and intra-abdominal abscess. Before the sepsis can be attributed to an infection at a distant site, the patient must be evaluated for complications of the original disease process or operation that may have resulted in infection. Investigation for other hospital-acquired infections should be carried out either concomitantly or after the original disease site has been examined.

In this chapter, those infections acquired in the hospital setting that may result in sepsis in the critically ill surgical patient are reviewed (Table 132–2).

TABLE 132–1. Risk Factors for the Development of Intensive Care Unit Infections

Age >70 y	Mechanical ventilation
Shock	Invasive monitoring
Coma	Urinary catheter use >10 d
Steroids	Acute renal failure
Chemotherapy	Head or multiple trauma
ICU stay >3 d	Surgical versus medical patient
Previous antibiotic therapy	

TABLE 132–2. Nosocomial Infections Common to the Intensive Care Unit Patient

Surgical Site	*Abdomen*
Wound infection	Peritonitis
Head and Neck	Abscess
Sinusitis	*Clostridium difficile* enterocolitis
Meningitis	Urinary tract infection
Ventriculitis	*Catheter-Related Infections*
Parotitis	Arterial catheters
Chest	Central venous catheters
Pneumonia	Swan-Ganz catheters
Lung abscess	
Empyema	

WOUND INFECTION

The overall incidence of postoperative wound infection was reported to be 7.5% in a frequently cited national study published in 1964.[6] The incidence varied from surgeon to surgeon, from hospital to hospital, and from one surgical procedure to another. The lowest infection rate (2%) followed "clean" operations, such as elective orthopedic procedures and herniorrhaphy, in which the possible sources of wound contamination were solely airborne or exogenous. "Clean-contaminated" operations that resulted in the additional exposure of the operative site to the endogenous microflora had higher rates or infection (>5%). Green and Wenzel[7] reported that the average hospital stay doubled and that hospitalization costs were thus increased when postoperative wound infection developed after any of six common elective operations were performed.

The economic, physical, and psychologic impact of postoperative wound sepsis and other serious infections mandates the use of preventive methods. The most critical of these are proper operative technique and sound judgment (i.e., in the choice of operation, on the part of a responsible surgeon and his team). In addition, well-controlled prospective, blinded clinical studies have defined the circumstances in which antibiotic prophylaxis is of benefit as well as the situations in which the risks of prophylaxis outweigh the expected benefits.

Classification of Surgical Wounds

Surgical wounds are generally classified as *clean, clean-contaminated, contaminated,* or *dirty.*[8] Clean wounds are those in which the gastrointestinal (GI), genitourinary, or respiratory tracts has not been entered during the course of operation. The usual cause for postoperative infections in this case is the aerobic exogenous bacteria, such as staphylococci, that enter the wound during the course of operation. The overall infection rate in clean surgical procedures is often quoted to be in the range of 2% to 3%.

Clean-contaminated wounds include elective operations in which the GI, genitourinary, or respiratory tract has been entered during the course of elective surgery. The risk of infection in this case is higher than in clean surgical procedures and is generally between 5% and 10%. The primary cause of infection in these patients is the endogenous microflora of the organ that has been surgically resected.

Contaminated wounds include those in which acute inflammation (without pus formation) or gross spillage of GI contents is encountered at the time of operation. Infections in this case again are primarily due to endogenous bacteria, and the infection rate is about 20%.

Dirty wounds include those in which gross pus is encountered at operation. Once again, the infections are primarily related to the involved organ's endogenous microflora and have incidence rates approaching 40%.

Non–Antibiotic-Associated Factors That Influence Wound Infection Rates

Many factors have been considered, without convincing evidence, as influencing the incidence of postoperative wound infection in clean operations: preoperative scrub technique, surgical glove damage, barrier materials, and "laminar" flow air systems in the operating room (Table 132–3).[8] Several, however, are clearly associated with increased risk of wound infection.

The longer the preoperative period of hospitalization, the greater the infection rate.[8] Northey observed that virtually every patient is colonized with nosocomial bacteria within 2 weeks of admission to a critical care unit.[9] These colonizations are usually by hospital-acquired, antibiotic-resistant organisms.

Preoperative showering with hexachlorophene-containing antiseptics on the evening before surgery is associated with a significantly decreased postoperative wound infection rate.[8] The decrease in infection rate was not observed when regular soap was used in the preoperative shower.

Razor shaving of the operative site on the day before surgery has been demonstrated to increase the postoperative infection rate.[8] This increase is due to the growth and multiplication of skin microorganisms in the damaged epithelium after the razor shave. For this reason, when razor shaving is to be employed, it should be confined to the immediate preoperative period. However, studies have shown that the lowest postoperative infection rate occurs if no shaving is performed; clipping with a barber's shears or using a depilatory cream before surgery has been associated with a low wound infection rate.[8, 10]

Generally speaking, each added hour of operation results in a doubling of the infection rate.[8] Shapiro and coworkers have reported on a prospective study of risk factors for infection after hysterectomy.[11] They observed that the statistically significant benefit of antibiotic prophylaxis in decreasing wound sepsis in operations lasting 1 hour was lost in operations lasting over 3.3 hours. This finding undoubtedly relates to the pharmacokinetics of antibiotic prophylaxis as well as to increased bacterial wound colonization in lengthy, complicated operative procedures. Repeat doses of prophylactic antibiotics given during the operation may be necessary for procedures lasting over 3 hours, especially when agents with short half-lives are used.

Nora and colleagues reported on the dangers of using prophylactic drains in abdominal surgery. Based on their frequent findings of skin bacteria at the interior of the abdominal drains, these authors have stressed the "two-way street" concept in that bacteria may just as easily enter the body along the drain tract as be removed.[12] Magee demonstrated that the presence of either Silastic or latex Penrose drains in an experimental wound dramatically enhanced the wound's infection rate, even in the presence of subinfective doses of bacteria.[13] Based on these experimental and clinical studies, it appears safe to conclude that the prophylactic use of abdominal drains is unwarranted and may indeed be a dangerous practice. When drains are required to empty localized collections, they should be placed through sites other than the primary surgical incision to decrease the incidence of subsequent wound infection.

Significant increases in postoperative wound infection occur when an elective procedure is done in the presence of an active remote infection.[8] It is therefore prudent to initiate treatment for urinary, pulmonary, or skin infections at least 48 hours before elective operative procedures are attempted.

TABLE 132–3. Factors Influencing the Development of Postoperative Wound Infections in Clean Surgical Procedures: Degree of Importance

Very Important (Infection Rate Doubled)
Period of preoperative hospitalization prolonged
Shaving of the operative site on the day before surgery
Duration of the operation prolonged
Use of prophylactic abdominal drains
Operation done in the presence of an active remote infection
Important (Infection Rate Less Than Doubled but Significantly Increased)
Preoperative showering with antiseptic not done
Probably Not Important (No Significant Increase in Infection Rate)
Surgeon's hand scrub: iodophor versus hexachlorophene
Patient skin preparation: iodophor versus hexachlorophene
Use of plastic skin drapes
Use of "laminar" flow air systems

Types of Clinical Wound Sepsis

The majority of postoperative wound infections are uncomplicated, involving only the skin and subcutaneous tissues. Infrequently, they progress to become necrotizing infections, which may involve the fascia and muscle. The usual clinical presentation of uncomplicated wound infection includes local incisional pain (dolor), tenderness, swelling (tumor), redness (rubor), increased warmth (calor), and elevated body temperature, all of which often begin between the 4th and 8th postoperative days. When infection occurs during the first 48 hours after operation, it is characteristically caused by either clostridia or β-hemolytic streptococci. In such a case, the dramatic clinical presentation of gangrenous infections may include profound systemic toxicity and rapid local advance of the infection, which often involves all layers of the body wall. A high mortality rate (60%–80%) can be expected unless a rapid diagnosis is made on the basis of clinical presentation as well as the results of Gram's staining of wound fluid. Treatment includes parenteral administration of antimicrobial agents (usually penicillin G alone) and aggressive, prompt surgical débridement of all infected tissue. Additionally, hyperbaric oxygen treatments should be employed if they are locally available.

In clean operations in which the GI, genitourinary, and respiratory tracts have not been entered, exogenous *Staphylococcus aureus* is the usual cause of infection; in contrast, infection by a polymicrobial aerobic-anaerobic flora that closely resembles the normal endogenous microflora of the surgically resected organ occurs in clean-contaminated operations. The cardinal features of treatment of an uncomplicated wound infection are operative drainage and local wound care.

Prevention of Wound Infection

Great progress has been made since the mid-1980s in the appropriate use of antibiotic prophylaxis in the patient undergoing surgery. Well-controlled, prospective, blinded studies have outlined many areas in which antibiotic prophylaxis is of benefit as well as those clinical settings in which the risks of antibiotic prophylaxis outweighed the expected value.[14]

Historically, the most common errors included the widespread use of antibiotic prophylaxis in clean surgical procedures as well as the faulty timing of the initial administration of the selected agents. Currently, the most common error is the practice of continuing use of the antibiotic agents beyond the time necessary for maximum benefit (>72 hours).[15]

In order to obtain the greatest effect with the use of prophylactic antibiotics, one must be aware of the following factors: the timing of administration should offer maximum benefit while minimizing adverse effects; the route of administration must be appropriate; the choice of antibiotic agent should be based on the types of organisms that usually cause infection; and a dosage necessary to attain efficacious tissue or serum levels must be administered.

Timing of Antibiotic Prophylaxis

The effective use of prophylactic antibiotics depends to a great extent on the appropriate timing of their administration.[16] Intravenously administered antibiotics in effective doses should first be given 30 minutes before the operative incision is made. This is accomplished by having the anesthesiologist start the antibiotic infusion when he or she establishes intravenous access in the operating room just before the induction of anesthesia. Such timing of administration results in the presence of therapeutic drug levels in the wound and related tissues during the operation, but it does not allow for the development of bacterial resistance. Administration of the drugs should be continued for less than 24 hours, a period during which the concentration of bacteria in the wound may exceed the capacity of the tissues to destroy them. Continuation of prophylactic drug therapy beyond 24 hours increases the risk of drug toxicity or bacterial superinfection and does not reduce the incidence of subsequent infection. One to three doses of antimicrobial agents, with the first dose beginning just before operative incision, are sufficient for prophylaxis.

When prophylaxis is accomplished with orally administered antibiotics, as is frequently practiced in elective colon resection, the agents should be given only during the 24 hours before operation. Longer periods of preoperative preparation are not necessary and have been associated with the isolation of resistant organisms within the colonic lumen at the time of resection.[17]

Route of Administration of Prophylactic Antibiotics

Intravenous administration is preferred in most surgical patients. Administering antibiotics intravenously in a relatively small volume of diluent over a short period of time results in high serum concentrations that are reflected in more rapid entry and greater early concentrations of antibiotics in wound fluid. Administration of equivalent doses of antibiotics by either continuous intravenous infusion or intermittent intramuscular injection produces lower blood concentrations and retarded entry of the antibiotics into wound fluid. Oral administration of poorly absorbed antibiotics has a major role only in the elective preparation of patients before colon operations.[18]

Choice of Antibiotics

No single antibiotic agent or combination of agents can be relied on for effective prophylaxis in the various clinical settings of the surgical critical care unit. The agent or agents employed should be chosen primarily on the basis of their efficacy against the microorganisms that usually cause the infectious complications in each clinical setting.[8] For example, in uncomplicated cardiovascular or orthopedic operations, the usual cause of postoperative infections is aerobic

TABLE 132–4. Microorganisms Most Commonly Isolated from Sites of Postoperative Infection

Infection Site	*Aerobes*	*Anaerobes*
Gastrointestinal		
Mouth	Streptococci	Bacteroides (other than *Bacteroides fragilis*), peptostreptococci, fusobacteria
Esophagus	Same as for mouth	Same as for mouth
Stomach	Enteric gram-negative bacilli, streptococci	Same as for mouth
Biliary	Enteric gram-negative bacilli, group D streptococci	Clostridia
Distal ileum	Enteric gram-negative bacilli	*B. fragilis*, peptostreptococci, clostridia
Colon	Same as for distal ileum	Same as for distal ileum
Gynecologic	Same as for distal ileum	Same as for distal ileum
Orthopedic	Staphylocci, streptococci	
Thoracic	Streptococci, pneumococci	Bacteroides (other than *B. fragilis*), peptostreptococci
Cardiovascular	Staphylococci, streptococci	
Urologic	Enteric gram-negative bacilli, group D streptococci	

streptococci or staphylococci. The organisms responsible for infection after GI or gynecologic surgery are more complex, and selecting appropriate prophylactic antibiotics requires an understanding of the polymicrobial nature of the endogenous microflora at each site. The microorganisms usually responsible for infection in different surgical disciplines are listed in Table 132–4.

Antibiotic Prophylaxis in Clean Surgical Procedures

In the past, the use of prophylactic antibiotics in clean surgical cases has been limited to procedures in which a prosthetic foreign body has been implanted.[14] Operations in which prophylactic antibiotics are not frequently used are listed in Table 132–5. The general attitude has been that any benefit from the use of antibiotic prophylaxis in clean surgical cases is outweighed by its potentially harmful effects, which include toxic and allergic drug reactions as well as bacterial or fungal superinfections. Low infection rates in clean cases are best obtained through strict adherence to the principles of good surgical technique. However, the presence of any foreign body disables wound healing. Even a single suture in a wound is sufficient to cause suppuration with a bacterial inoculum that by itself does not result in infection.[19] Foreign material disables normal wound defense mechanisms, so that fewer bacteria are necessary to cause infection. However, a large, multicenter, prospective randomized study of antibiotic prophylaxis in clean surgery, such as inguinal hernia repair or breast procedures, has demonstrated the apparent value of antibiotic prophylaxis in reducing wound infection.[20]

The risk of infections in patients undergoing clean surgical procedures with prosthetic devices, such as total hip replacement or implantation of cardiac valves or vascular grafts, is low. However, when infection does occur in these patients, the result most often is catastrophic. Prophylaxis with antistaphylococcal drugs may reduce the incidence of postoperative infection in such procedures and is therefore recommended.[14] Penicillinase-resistant penicillins, such as methicillin, oxacillin, and nafcillin, have commonly been employed for prophylaxis in this clinical setting. Recently, increased numbers of infections have been reported to be due to *S. epidermidis,* an organism that has a degree of resistance to this group of semisynthetic penicillins. It is for this

TABLE 132–5. Operations in Which Prophylactic Antibiotics Are Frequently Not Employed*

Operative Procedure	*Exceptions*
General Surgery	
Breast surgery	
Cholecystectomy	Clinical risk factors are present Positive intraoperative Gram stain of bile
Head and neck surgery	Anticipate cutting across contaminated area (oropharynx, hypopharynx, nasopharynx) Enter dura during such procedures as ethmoidectomy
Inguinal hernia repair	
Incisional hernia repair	
Mastectomy (modified or radical)	
Parathyroidectomy	
Soft tissue surgery	Human bite Major soft tissue injury
Stripping of varicose veins	
Splenectomy	
Thyroidectomy	
Gastrectomy	Gastric ulcer or complications of duodenal ulcer
Pyloroplasty	Same as for gastrectomy
Gastrectomy	As above and gastric malignancy
Gynecologic Surgery	
Cesarean section	Membranes have been ruptured
Oophorectomy	
Tubal ligation	
Neurosurgery	
All procedures	Large area of dead space or devitalized bone Insertion of ventricular shunt or other foreign body
Neurosurgery	
All procedures	Large area of dead space or devitalized bone Insertion of ventricular shunt or other foreign body
Orthopedic Surgery	
All procedures	Open fracture Foreign body implanted Amputation in presence of gangrene
Thoracic Surgery	
All procedures	Penetrating wounds with extensive soft tissue damage Perforation or transection of esophagus Transection of bronchial tree
Urologic Surgery	
All procedures	Patient with positive urine culture results Obstructive uropathy
Cardiovascular Surgery	
All procedures	Presence of foreign body Cardiac bypass employed

*Some authorities advise the prophylactic use of antibiotics in all procedures if evidence for the existence of patient risk factors is present.[8]

reason that first-generation cephalosporins, which frequently exhibit good activity against many of the organisms that commonly cause postoperative sepsis, continue to be the drugs of choice. If significant antibiotic resistance is suspected or proven, the use of vancomycin may be desirable.

PERITONITIS AND INTRA-ABDOMINAL ABSCESS

Significant improvement in the survival of patients with intra-abdominal infection occurred early in this century, with mortality rates falling from 90% to 40 to 50% primarily because of the realization that surgical intervention was necessary to cure most intra-abdominal infections. However, the mortality rate has only minimally decreased over the past 50 years, despite the discovery and use of effective antibiotics and the advent of modern critical care. Secondary bacterial peritonitis primarily occurs following the leakage of the endogenous microflora from a diseased or traumatized intraperitoneal hollow viscus. The extent of dissemination and the severity of the infection within the peritoneal cavity depend on a number of factors, including the source of contamination, the duration of contamination, the presence of adjuvant substances, bacterial synergy, and the adequacy of the host defense response. Hemoglobin, ascitic fluid, fibrin clots, necrotic tissue, bile, and barium sulfate have all been demonstrated to promote the establishment of intra-abdominal bacterial infection.[21]

The polymicrobial nature of intra-abdominal infections and the pathogenic characteristics of anaerobes were first recognized by Altemeier in patients with perforated appendicitis.[22, 23] The conclusions of his studies were that (1) the majority of the bacteria do not produce a fatal peritonitis when injected in pure culture; (2) many avirulent strains of bacteria, particularly *Escherichia coli,* become highly virulent in the presence of dead tissue; (3) in mixed culture, these bacteria show a synergistic action, producing a high degree of pathogenicity; and (4) peritonitis appears to be an infection resulting from the synergistic activities of the various bacterial symbionts present. These studies were not elaborated on for nearly three decades until modern anaerobic microbiologic techniques were introduced and allowed for the better classification of these organisms in both normal flora and postoperative infection studies.[24]

Experimental models of intra-abdominal sepsis have provided much insight with regard to bacterial synergy and also the need to treat such infection with antibiotics active against both aerobes and anaerobes. Intra-abdominal sepsis is, at times, a two-phase disease process, with acute peritonitis and bacteremia occurring early, and with survivors developing intra-abdominal abscesses later on. Aerobes seem to be responsible for the high mortality in acute peritonitis, whereas anaerobes are necessary for the development of intra-abdominal abscesses in the survivors. The use of antibiotics directed against both aerobes and anaerobes is important in decreasing the mortality rate associated with early peritonitis and late abscess formation in experimental intra-abdominal sepsis.[25, 26] Subsequent studies have demonstrated that the most important virulence factor for *Bacteroides fragilis* is its polysaccharide capsule, which is found only in *B. fragilis* subspecies *fragilis.*[27, 28]

Clinical Presentation

The diagnosis of intra-abdominal infection is usually suggested on the basis of a patient's history and the typical physical findings. Abdominal pain is present in almost all patients with peritonitis or abscess. In patients with abscesses, the physical findings of involuntary guarding and tenderness are localized; in contrast, these findings are diffuse in patients with generalized peritonitis. The pain and tenderness are worsened by any movement, including coughing or jarring of the hospital bed. Absence of bowel sounds and abdominal distention occur owing to paralytic ileus. Patients with intra-abdominal infection also have fever, and they may have other symptoms and signs related to hypovolemia due to fluid sequestration within the peritoneal cavity. With adequate fluid resuscitation, the patients manifest the typical hyperdynamic state associated with sepsis. Increases in the peripheral leukocyte count frequently exceed 15,000 cells per cubic millimeter, with a shift to the left often observed.

Plain or contrast radiologic examinations of the abdomen and chest may be helpful in demonstrating perforations, ileus, space-occupying lesions, and free fluid. Specialized radiologic tests such as ultrasound and computed tomography are most helpful in searching for localized intra-abdominal fluid collections. In patients with ascites, paracentesis may be helpful. In patients without ascites and borderline findings on physical examination, peritoneal lavage may be extremely helpful. The technique was first described in this clinical setting by Richardson and colleagues in 1983.[29] This procedure requires the placement of a catheter intraperitoneally, either by cutdown or by the percutaneous route, followed by the instillation of 1 L of saline. The fluid is then drained off, and an aliquot is examined. If gross pus, bile, or feces is present in the fluid, the cell count is greater than 500 polymorphonuclear leukocytes per cubic millimeter, or bacteria or food fibers are seen on microscopic examination, the diagnosis of peritonitis is made. It is important to culture both the fluid from peritoneal lavage and that from paracentesis for both aerobes and anaerobes.

Therapy

The most critical aspect of the treatment of secondary peritonitis is early diagnosis and prompt intervention. Pitcher and Musher found a strong correlation between the interval from presentation to treatment and the subsequent perioperative morbidity and mortality. Antibiotic use, ICU care, and other adjunctive modalities do not compensate for delays in definitive treatment.[30]

Frequently, the exact cause of the peritonitis is not ascertained until abdominal exploration is performed. For therapeutic purposes, it is helpful to classify intra-abdominal infections as either diffuse or localized. Those which are localized are most frequently amenable to operative resection, surgical drainage, or percutaneous catheter drainage. Diffuse suppurative peritonitis is not particularly responsive to these types of treatment alone, and other approaches such as open abdominal packing, radical peritoneal débridement, peritoneal lavage, and planned repeated abdominal explorations have been recommended as additional therapeutic options.

Treatment Methods for Localized Infection

RESECTION. Resectional therapy for diseases such as gangrenous appendicitis or cholecystitis, bowel infarction, or perforated diverticulitis is the standard of care. In the past, the operative treatment for perforated diverticulitis was conducted in three stages: (1) drainage of abscess with diverting colostomy, (2) resection of the involved colon, and finally (3) closure of the colostomy. Most surgeons today combine the first and second stages. However, with the ability to drain abscesses percutaneously, another potential approach is to first drain the peridiverticular abscess percutaneously, allowing the patient's symptoms and signs of infection to resolve. This is followed by mechanical and antibiotic colon preparation and then by resection of the involved portion of colon with primary anastomosis. It remains to be seen whether this approach will become widely applicable.

DRAINAGE. The optimal method of treating abscesses continues to be incision and drainage, and there are many techniques available to accomplish this. Percutaneous drainage of intra-abdominal abscesses was first reported by Grønvall and colleagues in 1977.[31] Comparisons of percutaneous and surgical drainage of abdominal abscesses are extremely variable and suffer from the lack of evidence from prospective, randomized studies comparing the two drainage approaches. Based on currently available data, we believe that percutaneous drainage of intra-abdominal abscesses is not advisable in the presence of the following: (1) complex abscesses, which are defined as those with more than two septations, that are in continuity with the gastrointestinal tract, that are filled with thick debris, or that contain primarily fungi; (2) more than two abscesses; (3) pancreatic abscesses; or (4) drainage pathways that necessitate traversing bowel or uncontaminated body cavities. The success rate for percutaneous drainage of favorable abscesses should range from 80% to 90%.

Treatment Methods for Diffuse Intra-Abdominal Infections

Although the overriding principle in the management of localized purulent collections (incision and drainage) is accepted and the major controversies concerning management are over differences in technique, the same cannot be said about the treatment principles for diffuse suppurative peritonitis. Several different approaches to this condition are available.

SIMPLE DRAINAGE. Simple drainage of the peritoneal cavity in the setting of diffuse suppurative peritonitis is totally ineffective. This is possibly because drains are rapidly walled off by fibrin deposition along the drain tract.

CONTINUOUS POSTOPERATIVE PERITONEAL LAVAGE. Continuous peritoneal lavage refers to the placement of irrigation catheters in the peritoneal cavity *at the time of operation* to irrigate the peritoneal cavity with fluid in an effort to dilute or wash away bacteria and other toxic substances during the postoperative period. It is extremely important to note that the use of this technique has been proposed only as a therapeutic adjunct after exploratory laparotomy has been used to control the inciting factors in the development of peritonitis and that it is of no use by itself. The technique usually involves instilling 1 L of fluid over 5 to 10 minutes, allowing it to remain in the peritoneal cavity for approximately 30 minutes, and then draining it out over another 20 to 25 minutes.[32] This process is repeated until either the effluent becomes totally clear or an arbitrary point in time has been reached. The choice of fluid and of any additives to it, such as antibiotics and heparin, varies widely among the proponents of this technique. Although many nonrandomized studies have shown a survival advantage with the use of continuous postoperative peritoneal lavage, of the six prospective studies reported in the literature, five show no improvement with lavage.[33] Because this technique has not convincingly been demonstrated to improve survival, we believe it should be used only in selected patients, such as those with peritonitis and renal failure who require peritoneal dialysis for their renal failure.

INTRAOPERATIVE IRRIGATION. Although intraoperative irrigation with crystalloid solutions has not been shown to decrease either mortality or the recurrence of abscesses, virtually all studies have supported the use of intraoperative peritoneal irrigation with or without antibiotic-containing solutions in patients with diffuse bacterial peritonitis. Schumer and colleagues demonstrated that crystalloid irrigation reduced the number of bacteria remaining in the peritoneal cavity.[34] Although Rosato and coworkers also demonstrated a reduction in the concentration of adjuvant substances following irrigation, they were unable to show any reduction in either mortality or subsequent abscess formation.[35] Various antibiotics, including cephalothin (1 g/L), kanamycin (1 g/L), and bacitracin (50,000 U/L), chloramphenicol, and other aminoglycosides have all been used enthusiastically but have rarely been shown to decrease the incidence of recurrent intra-abdominal infection. Attention should be devoted to possible antibiotic toxicities that may occur owing to rapid absorption and the presence of high systemic serum levels.

RADICAL PERITONEAL DÉBRIDEMENT. In 1975, Hudspeth introduced the concept of radical peritoneal débridement for the treatment of generalized peritonitis.[36] The technique involves the complete exposure of the entire peritoneal cavity. Initially, all free peritoneal fluid and pus are suctioned out of the abdomen. Then, the entire peritoneal cavity is meticulously débrided. All fibrin peels are removed from the serosal surfaces of the bowel. In the only study comparing radical peritoneal débridement with standard therapy, Polk and Fry reported no difference in outcome.[37]

LEAVING THE PERITONEAL CAVITY OPEN. The concept of treating the peritoneal cavity as a large abscess cavity and of managing generalized peritonitis by packing it open was revived in 1979.[38] Since that time, several reports on the use of this technique or modifications of it have been published. The combination of the use of polypropylene mesh to avoid evisceration and of planned repeated returns to the operating room has been widely adopted and practiced in the specific group of patients having severe generalized bacterial peritonitis. The decision is made at the initial operation, based on the operative findings, to return the patient to the operating room daily to break up loculations and débride dead tissue. The abdomen is closed when no further fluid collections or necrotic debris can be found. No prospective, randomized clinical studies comparing the packing of the abdomen open or any of its variations with any other form of treatment have been published. This open type of treatment has been proposed to have several advantages over standard therapy: (1) a decrease in intra-abdominal pressure, which improves blood flow to the abdominal viscera; (2) daily elimination of purulent and necrotic material to maintain control over infection by lessening the bacterial burden; and (3) the prompt recognition of intra-abdominal complications. An increased risk of bowel perforation and fistula formation may exist with this procedure.

Antibiotic Selection

Unlike patients with superficial wound abscesses in whom surgical drainage alone suffices, those with intra-abdominal infections are best managed by a combination of surgical repair, excision, diversion, or drainage along with therapy with appropriately chosen, parenterally administered antibiotics. The antibiotic therapy should be initiated as soon as the diagnosis is made preoperatively, and it should be continued during the operation and into the postoperative period. The choice of the ideal agent or agents and of the necessary length of the therapeutic course remains controversial. Based on experimental and clinical studies, the chosen antibiotics must have activity against both colonic aerobes and anaerobes, including *B. fragilis*.[26, 39] Conventional antibiotic regimens for peritonitis have included an aminoglycoside and either clindamycin or metronidazole;

TABLE 132–6. Parenteral Antibiotic Agents Currently Used For Therapy of Intra-Abdominal Infection

Combination Therapy	
*Aerobic Coverage**	
Amikacin	Ciprofloxacin
Aztreonam	Gentamicin
Cefotaxime	Tobramycin
Ceftriaxone	
Anaerobic Coverage†	
Chloramphenicol	
Clindamycin	
Metronidazole	
Single-Drug Therapy	
Aerobic/Anaerobic Coverage: Single Agents	
Ampicillin/sulbactam	Imipenem/cilastatin
Cefotetan	Piperacillin/tazobactam
Cefoxitin	Ticarcillin/clavulanic acid
Ceftizoxime	

*To be combined with a drug having anaerobic activity.
†To be combined with a drug having aerobic activity.

however, the use of single-antibiotic therapy effective against both aerobic and anaerobic organisms has been espoused. The antibiotics that are commonly used singly or in combination are listed in Table 132–6. The appropriate duration of antibiotic therapy in patients with established peritonitis is controversial. The data of Lennard and coworkers indicate that if a patient still has leukocytosis without fever at the conclusion of the antibiotic course, the risk of his or her having ongoing or recurrent intra-abdominal infection is 33%.[40] Seventy-nine per cent of patients who were still febrile at the conclusion of their antibiotic course developed recurrent infection. No patient who was both afebrile and had a normal white blood cell count developed recurrent intra-abdominal infection. We believe that, in patients with established intra-abdominal infections, antibiotic use should be continued for a minimum of 5 to 7 days; however, it may be appropriate to continue antibiotic therapy until both fever and leukocytosis have resolved.

In summary, the successful treatment of intra-abdominal infection depends primarily on early appropriate operative intervention combined with the use of efficacious parenteral antibiotic agents. The use of human monoclonal antibody against endotoxin in this clinical setting may be of value only in those patients with associated gram-negative bacteremia and shock.[41] Its use at the present time remains investigational, and its efficacy unproven.

HEAD AND NECK INFECTIONS

The most common hospital-acquired infections of the head and neck are sinusitis and central nervous system infections, including meningitis and ventriculitis.

Sinusitis

Sinusitis is a frequently overlooked source of sepsis and should be suspected in patients who have sustained facial trauma or who have any type of tube passing through the nares. Since Arens and coworkers first described this problem and reported a 2% incidence in an ICU population, several other reports have appeared that indicate that sinusitis is an even more common occurrence in ICU patients than was previously thought.[42] O'Reilly and colleagues reported a 27% incidence of sinusitis; reviews of the subject describe occurrence rates that range between the two values just discussed.[43]

Sinusitis is most commonly associated with nasotracheal intubation, but its occurrence with the use of nasogastric tubes has also been reported. Facial trauma is also a predisposing factor. The maxillary sinuses are involved in one half to three fourths of all cases of facial trauma, and the involved sinus is almost always on the same side as the nasal tube. The mechanism by which sinusitis occurs is assumed to be obstruction of the sinus ostia that results in the accumulation of fluid in the sinus and then in secondary infection. Diagnosis is difficult because most patients do not exhibit the typical symptoms of sinusitis or, because of depressed mental status, cannot relate their symptoms to their physicians. The diagnosis is most easily made with computed tomography of the face and sinuses. Plain sinus radiographs are not particularly helpful, probably because of the difficulty in properly positioning these critically ill patients to obtain adequate radiographic images. Unlike in primary sinusitis, the bacteria involved are usually gram-negative bacilli, *S. aureus,* or anaerobes. Treatment includes removal of the nasal tube, use of decongestant sprays and antibiotics appropriate for the implicated organism, and, most important, drainage of the sinus.

Parotitis

Parotitis is rarely seen in the critically ill surgical patient. It is probably caused by inspissation of saliva in Stensen's duct in dehydrated patients that results in ductal obstruction. With a better understanding of fluid therapy in these patients, postoperative parotitis seems to be a disease of the past. Early reports of the disease tended to stress the importance of *S. aureus;* however, several reports of parotitis due to gram-negative bacilli have appeared in the literature.

THORACIC INFECTIONS

The intrathoracic infections most commonly seen in the ICU include pneumonia, lung abscess, and empyema. Additionally, because of the great number of cardiac surgical procedures performed in this country, mediastinitis is not infrequently seen in surgical ICUs in the United States.

Pneumonia

The incidence of pneumonia is related to underlying lung injury (e.g., that caused by adult respiratory distress syndrome or pulmonary contusion), mechanical ventilation for longer than 48 hours, prolonged preoperative hospitalization, thoracic or upper abdominal incision, and possibly the use of certain types of stress ulcer prophylactic agents.[44] The mechanism by which pneumonia occurs in ICU patients is thought to be aspiration, inhalation, or hematogenous spread. Aspiration of upper airway and oropharyngeal secretions seems to be the most common mode. The bacteriology of ICU-acquired pneumonias tends to confirm this assertion. Approximately 70% to 75% of ICU-related pneumonias are caused by aerobic gram-negative bacilli, whereas 15% to 20% are caused by *S. aureus* and 5% to 15% are caused by *Candida* species.[45] Only 2% to 15% of normal humans have gram-negative bacilli colonizing their upper airways; however, in critically ill patients, the colonization of the upper airway occurs within the first few days of the ICU stay in 55% to 75% of patients. Driks and colleagues have demonstrated an association between the colonization of the stomach by gram-negative bacilli and the subsequent development of pneumonia in the presence of the same organisms.[46]

A number of factors, both related to the primary illness

TABLE 132–7. Risk Factors for Intensive Care Unit–Related Pneumonia

Age	Prior use of antibiotics
Aspiration	Prolonged preoperative hospitalization
Head trauma	Pulmonary edema
History of smoking	Stress ulcer prophylaxis with antacids or histamine$_2$ blockers
Intubation/mechanical ventilation	Upper abdominal or chest incision
Lung injury–adult respiratory distress syndrome, pulmonary contusion	

and iatrogenic in nature, contribute to the increased risk of pneumonia in ICU patients (Table 132–7). Normal barriers to infection are breached, including the mucociliary clearance mechanism in the tracheobronchial tree and the normally acidic nature of the stomach. Endotracheal tubes prevent the normal mucociliary mechanism from functioning and from clearing secretions. In order to minimize the risk of stress-related GI ulceration, we alkalize the stomach; this allows for overgrowth of lower GI tract bacteria in the stomach, which then colonize the upper aerodigestive tract. The patient's mental status may be depressed because of head trauma, narcotics, sedatives, or central nervous system failure from sepsis; the presence of these factors leads to a decreased ability to cough.

Diagnosis

The diagnosis of pneumonia in otherwise critically ill patients can be very difficult to establish. Patients often have other reasons to account for their fever and leukocytosis. Chest radiography is frequently not helpful, as many pneumonia patients already have infiltrates secondary to other pulmonary pathology such as adult respiratory distress syndrome or pulmonary contusion. Because of these difficulties, a number of diagnostic techniques that involve sputum analysis have been developed. Determination of the quantity and quality of the sputum, Gram's staining of sputum, and sputum culture can suggest a diagnosis but are not diagnostic tests. We have found examination of the quantity and quality of sputum to be a good guide to the diagnosis of pneumonia. The presence of copious amounts of purulent sputum is consistent with the pneumonia process, and the diagnosis can usually be confirmed by Gram's staining of the sputum. The absence of white blood cells in a sputum sample obtained through an endotracheal tube almost completely precludes the diagnosis of pneumonia, whereas the presence of white blood cells in combination with intracellular bacteria ensures the diagnosis. However, many times, Gram's staining of sputum demonstrates white blood cells and one or more morphologic types of bacteria, none of which is intracellular. In this instance, the findings of sputum analysis should guide the choice of antibiotics; once the sputum culture and sensitivities return, the choice of antibiotics used may be altered if necessary. However, in patients without endotracheal tubes, 25% to 50% of routine sputum cultures show a discrepancy with respect to the organisms they contain compared with cultures of sputum collected more distally in the tracheobronchial tree. This finding almost certainly represents either colonization of the upper airways with organisms different from those causing the pneumonia or contamination by the oral flora. Various techniques have been described to improve the specificity of sputum culture in these patients, including transtracheal aspiration and bronchoscopic protected brush sampling of the lower respiratory tract. Transtracheal aspiration is performed by passing a small angiocatheter through the cricothyroid membrane and obtaining a sputum sample via the angiocatheter. This collection method has the advantage of bypassing the mouth and thus avoiding contamination by oral flora. Analysis of a sample obtained in this manner to identify the true pathogen is much more reliable than analysis of an expectorated sputum sample. However, this technique cannot be performed when an endotracheal tube is in place, and it is associated with a small risk of pneumothorax, subcutaneous emphysema, and hemorrhage. Bronchoscopy has also been utilized to obtain sputum samples. Some contamination by oral flora always occurs because the bronchoscope must pass through the upper aerodigestive tract. Two recently described techniques include protected brush and protected bronchoalveolar lavage techniques of sputum sampling. With the first, a sterile brush protected within a plastic tube is passed through the bronchoscope. When the area to be sampled is reached, the brush is pushed out of the end of the plastic tube, the sample is obtained, and the brush is withdrawn back into the plastic tubing. Protected specimen bronchoalveolar lavage is similar except that, in place of a brush, sterile saline is introduced through the sterile plastic tubing, aspirated, and cultured. Both methods of sputum sampling have significantly improved accuracy when compared with other techniques of sputum sampling. We suggest using this technique if a patient does not seem to respond clinically to treatment directed by standard sputum sampling techniques.

Most ICU-acquired pneumonias reflect the ICU's bacterial flora. Within a short time of arriving in an ICU, a patient's own normal bacterial flora is replaced by the ICU flora. This process is exacerbated by the use of broad-spectrum antibiotics, which decimate the patient's more antibiotic-sensitive normal bacterial flora and allow for overgrowth of the resistant ICU bacteria.

Prevention of Intensive Care Unit–Acquired Pneumonia

Several concepts and techniques that seem to decrease the incidence of ICU-related pneumonia have been developed since the mid-1980s. These include the use of enteral (as opposed to parenteral) nutrition, alteration of the type of stress ulcer prophylaxis, selective gut decontamination, and early fixation of pelvic and long bone fractures.

Enteral Versus Parenteral Nutrition

Since the initial discovery that it is possible to maintain patients' nutrition with total parenteral nutrition (TPN), it has become clear that this modality represents a great advance and that it has saved many patients' lives. However, its use in critically ill patients has not met with total success. Since the concepts of the "gut origin septic state" and the role of the gastrointestinal tract in sepsis and multiple organ failure have become fashionable, studies comparing TPN and enteral nutrition have repeatedly demonstrated the superiority of enteral feedings in decreasing infectious complications as well as the intensity of the sepsis syndrome.[47] At least two prospective studies comparing enteral nutrition with parenteral nutrition in critically ill trauma patients have shown a lower incidence of ICU-related pneumonia in patients who receive enteral nutrition. In a study by Moore and coworkers, 59 patients who sustained severe abdominal trauma were randomized to receive equal amounts of calories and protein by either the enteral ($n = 29$) or parenteral ($n = 30$) route.[48] No patients who received enteral nutrition developed pneumonia, whereas 20% (6 of 30) in the group receiving TPN developed pneumonia ($P < .03$ between groups). In the second study by Kudsk and colleagues, 68 patients who sustained blunt and penetrating abdominal trauma were randomized to receive enteral nutrition or TPN.[49] In this report, 6% of patients who received enteral feedings developed pneumonia, whereas 29% of patients who received TPN did. These authors recommend placing feeding tubes in the small bowel using either surgically placed jejunostomy tubes or nasoduodenal tubes (which may be placed either intraoperatively or under fluoroscopic guidance). We generally begin enteral feedings on the first postoperative day as soon as the patient is hemodynamically stable. Feeding into the stomach of a critically ill patient is poorly tolerated and is linked to an increase in aspiration.

Stress Ulcer Prophylaxis

One of the great advances in modern critical care has been the recognition that the incidence of significant GI stress hemorrhage can be decreased from approximately 15% to 5% through the use of antacids, histamine$_2$ blockers (e.g., cimetidine, ranitidine, famotidine), sucralfate, or misoprostol. Because of the association among increased gastric pH, gastric colonization with enteric organisms, and the development of ICU-related pneumonia with these same organisms, the relationship between the type of stress ulcer prophylaxis and pneumonia has been the subject of several investigations. In 1987, Driks and associates[46] and Tryba[50] both reported that the use of sucralfate as opposed to antacids seemed to be related to a lower incidence of ICU-acquired pneumonia.[46, 50] More recently, Kappstein and coworkers found the same to be true when they compared sucralfate and cimetidine.[51] They reported a 46% incidence of nosocomial pneumonia in the cimetidine group and a 27% incidence of pneumonia in the sucralfate group. All of these researchers suggested that the increase in gastric pH, which is associated with the use of antacids or histamine$_2$ blockers and with the subsequent colonization of the stomach with enteric organisms, is the primary factor related to the increased incidence of pneumonia. However, several reports have concluded that no relationship exists between stress ulcer prophylaxis regimen and ICU-acquired pneumonia. Simms and colleagues found no difference in the incidence of pneumonia in their subjects who received antacids (30%), cimetidine (28%), or sucralfate (27%).[52] Additionally, Cook and associates, using meta-analysis techniques, found no compelling evidence to support the concept that one form of stress ulcer prophylaxis is superior to any other form in minimizing the risk of nosocomial pneumonia.[53] They concluded that most of the prior studies suffered from methodologic deficiencies, including small sample size and the failure to separate antacids and histamine$_2$ receptor blockers in the study groups.

In our own unpublished prospective, randomized study comparing antacids, cimetidine, and sucralfate, we found no difference in the incidences of ICU-acquired pneumonia. We did find, as others have reported, a relation among bacteria cultured from the stomach, oropharynx, and sputum.

Early Fracture Fixation

Until recently, fractures in multiple trauma patients were fixed almost as an afterthought: the other serious injuries would be dealt with at the time of presentation, and the patient would then be taken to the ICU, where the fractures would be treated with bedrest and traction. Through the insight of such traumatologists as John Border and Thomas Rüedi, the recognition that multiple trauma patients "did better" with early fracture fixation piqued the interest of a number of trauma groups. Seibel and coworkers demonstrated a reduction in the rate of occurrence of acute respiratory failure in patients who had early fixation (within 24–48 hours of injury) of femur fractures compared with those who had late fixation.[54] Bone and coworkers[55] and Behrman and associates[56] demonstrated a decrease in the incidence of pneumonia and noted shorter requirements for mechanical ventilation, lower incidence of adult respiratory distress syndrome, fewer ICU and hospital days, lower mortality rate, and lower care costs in the groups that had immediate stabilization of femur fractures compared with the groups treated initially with traction followed by late fixation. These authors have theorized that early fracture fixation accomplishes a number of positive results: (1) it allows for the early mobilization of the patient, so that he or she may be transferred from the bed and into the upright position early postoperatively; (2) it decreases ongoing blood loss with the resultant possibility of shock; and (3) it helps to minimize ongoing soft tissue injury.

Selective Gut Decontamination

The concept of selective gut decontamination grew out of the belief that some pneumonias are due to the aspiration of gastric contents colonized by enteric organisms. It was thought that if the cycle could be interrupted before the aspiration stage, then the incidence of ICU-acquired pneumonia might decrease. It had previously been noted that this technique, in which nonabsorbable antibiotics effective against aerobic gram-negative bacteria and *Candida* species were swabbed in the oropharynx and given via a nasogastric tube, is effective in preventing infections in patients with leukemia.[57] Stoutenbeek and colleagues were the first to demonstrate the efficacy of this approach in trauma patients.[58] They used a regimen that included the application of a sticky paste containing 2% each of polymyxin E, tobramycin, and amphotericin B four times daily along with the administration of the same antibiotics via the nasogastric tube and the intravenous administration of a third-generation cephalosporin. In a nonrandomized trial against historical controls from their own ICU, they found that selective gut decontamination decreased the incidence of pneumonia, urinary tract infection, bacteremia, and wound infection.

Three other prospective, randomized studies have confirmed the findings of Stoutenbeek's group. Kerver and coworkers used the exact antibiotic regimen used by Stoutenbeek and colleagues in a patient population that included both trauma and nontrauma surgical patients and found a significant decrease in pneumonia and intra-abdominal infections but no alteration in the mortality rate of the group receiving the selective gut decontamination regimen.[59] Using only polymyxin E, tobramycin, and amphotericin B by capsule or nasogastric tube (no oropharyngeal paste or systemic antibiotics), Godard and associates were also able to verify the previous findings: a reduction in the overall number of gram-negative infections and a decreased incidence of ICU-acquired pneumonia.[60] A 12% mortality rate was found in the selective decontamination group compared with an 18% rate in the control group (not a significant difference). This study had the advantage of studying all patients admitted to the ICU and included trauma, nontrauma surgical, and medical patients. Also, Flaherty and coworkers found that selective gut decontamination (with polymyxin, gentamicin, and nystatin) and stress ulcer prophylaxis with antacids or histamine$_2$ receptor blockers, or both, significantly decreased the incidence of all infections, including pneumonia, when compared with sucralfate therapy for stress ulcer prophylaxis and no selective gut decontamination.[61] Overall, the rate of all infections was 12% in the selective decontamination group compared with 27% in the sucralfate group; the incidence of pneumonia was similarly less in the former group (2% and 9%, respectively).

A recent study by Cerra and colleagues, who used nystatin and norfloxacin in 94 critically ill patients via nasogastric tube (no oropharyngeal application), demonstrated a decrease in the incidence of pneumonia and other nosocomial infections in the group receiving selective gut decontamination.[62] However, no reduction in mortality or in the incidence of multiple organ failure or adult respiratory distress syndrome was reported. Similarly, Gastinne and coworkers were not able to demonstrate any difference in either the incidence of pneumonia or mortality with selective gut decontamination compared with placebo.[63] Although the use of nonabsorbable antibiotics in the oropharynx and GI tract may reduce the incidence of nosocomial pneumonia, the intravenous use of antibiotics to prevent ICU-related pneumonia has not been successful. In a large, multicenter study carried out in Europe, approximately 1300 patients were randomized to receive either cefoxitin, penicillin G, or no antibiotic.[64] The incidence of pneumonia was 6% in both the cefoxitin and penicillin groups and 7% in the group not receiving prophylactic antibiotics.

Empyema

Empyema is a complication of pneumonia, trauma, or chest tube placement. After trauma, empyema most commonly follows the incomplete evacuation of blood from the pleural space. It has been recommended that hemothoraces that are not completely drained by tube thoracostomy should be operatively evacuated within 3 to 7 days of injury.

Controversy surrounds the use of prophylactic antibiotics for the duration of chest tube placement.[14] Since the mid-1980s, several retrospective and prospective reviews on this subject have appeared in the literature. The reporting authors' conclusions are divided with regard to whether antibiotics are helpful in preventing empyema in patients with chest trauma who require tube thoracostomy. In these reports, the risk of empyema ranged from 1.2% to 7%. The authors who reported the higher rate of empyema found that antibiotics lowered the empyema rate, whereas those who observed a lower rate of empyema found no benefit attributable to prophylactic antibiotics. It seems likely that factors such as emergency placement of a chest tube, hemothorax (as opposed to pneumothorax), and manipulation of the chest tube are all associated with an increased incidence of empyema.

Lung Abscess

Lung abscess most commonly is a complication of pneumonia, and its bacteriology is dependent on the cause and microbiology of the pneumonia. For example, pneumonias secondary to aspiration cause abscesses that harbor anaerobes. Regardless of the pathogen, the treatment of lung abscesses involves their drainage. In the majority of patients, this involves repeated bronchoscopy to break into the abscess cavity and to drain the abscess internally into the tracheobronchial tree. We recommend at least daily bedside flexible bronchoscopy until the amount of purulence is significantly decreased and the patient's systemic signs of infection begin to resolve. External drainage or resection of pulmonary abscesses is infrequently necessary and fraught with complications. The most common and most devastating complication is bronchopleural fistula.

CATHETER-RELATED INFECTIONS

(see also Chapter 138)

It is estimated that 2.5 million central venous catheters and 100,000 arterial catheters are placed in patients in the United States each year. Because catheter-related sepsis occurs in 3% to 5% of all intravascular catheter placements, the magnitude of the problem is clear. Catheter-related sepsis has been defined as either bacteremia associated with intravascular catheters or sepsis (fever, leukocytosis) that resolves with removal of the catheter. The diagnosis is strengthened when the organism cultured from the blood is the same as that obtained from the catheter tip. Catheter contamination from the skin is the most common mode of infection, followed by seeding of the catheter from a remote site, catheter/tubing contamination at the connecting hub, and infusate colonization. The most frequently encountered organisms associated with catheter-related infection are staphylococci (*S. aureus* and *S. epidermidis*), *C. albicans*, and gram-negative bacilli. Each accounts for approximately 25% of catheter-related infections.

Risk factors related to the development of catheter-related infection include the nature of the underlying disease, the duration of catheterization, the location of the catheter, the expertise of the physician who places the catheter, catheter care, the material of which the catheter is constructed, and the use of multiple catheter lumens. Those patients who are in critical care units are more likely to develop catheter-related sepsis than are patients on hospital wards. However, it is not clear whether this finding is a result of patients' underlying illnesses or of the fact that intravascular catheters used in ICU patients tend to be manipulated more, are in place longer, and are more often placed under emergency circumstances than are catheters used in hospital ward patients. A duration of catheterization of longer than 3 days has been shown to be linked with an increased rate of catheter sepsis.[65] The site of cannulation is an important determinant in that femoral venous cannulas are the most likely to be colonized, followed by internal jugular catheters, with subclavian catheters having the lowest risk. Although results of studies comparing single- and multiple-lumen catheters are mixed, triple-lumen catheters tend to present a higher risk of colonization than do single-lumen catheters.

The development of catheter-related bacteremia is closely related to the number of colony-forming units cultured off the catheter tip on semiquantitative culture.[66] When fewer than 15 colony-forming units are cultured from the catheter tip, catheter-related bacteremia is rare. This fact is the basis for many of the suggested plans of catheter maintenance. The most controversial aspect of catheter maintenance concerns the routine changing of catheters in the nonseptic patient. Recommendations to change the catheter to a different site every 3 to 7 days, to change the catheter-over-guide wire every 3 to 7 days, and to leave the catheter in place without routine replacement have all been made. Recently, Eyer and associates reported a study in which 112 consecutive surgical ICU patients were randomized to three catheter management protocols.[67] The regimens consisted of changing the catheter to an entirely new site every 7 days, changing the catheter-over-guide wire every 7 days, or no weekly change at all. The study evaluated central venous, pulmonary artery, and arterial catheters. All catheters were changed if a positive blood culture result was obtained since the most recent catheter change, if evidence of exit site infec-

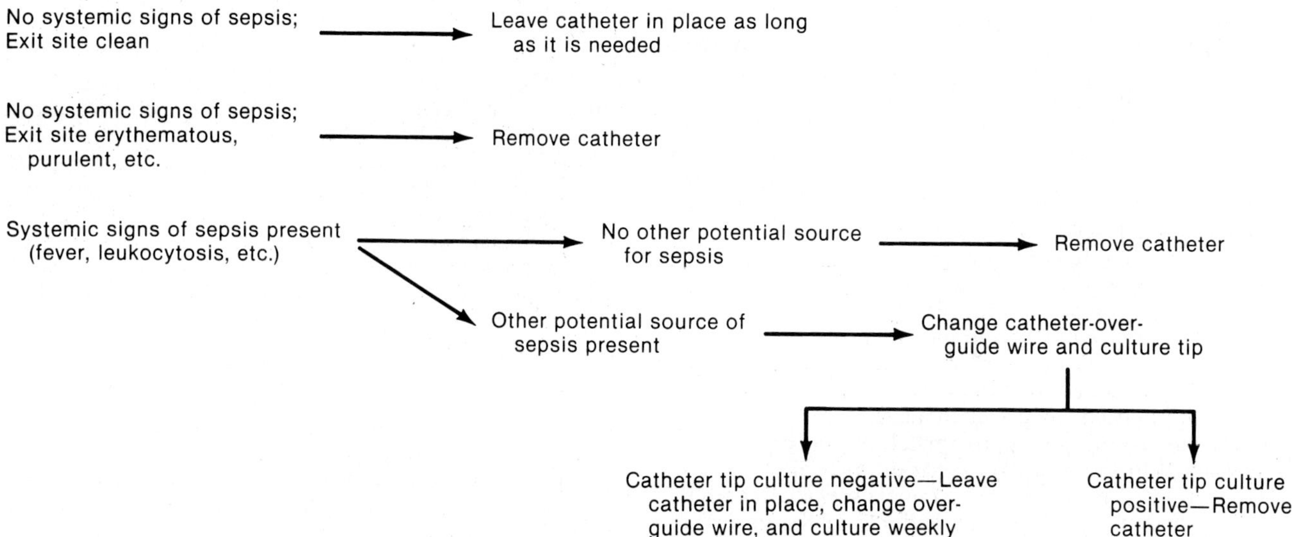

Figure 132–1. Algorithm for managing arterial, central venous, and pulmonary artery catheters.

tion was present, or if the patient manifested sepsis without any other obvious source. The incidence of catheter-related sepsis episodes per patient was similar for all groups (0.17 for guide wire changes, 0.22 for complete changes, and 0.16 for no changes). The algorithm for catheter changes that we follow is detailed in Figure 132–1.

The treatment of catheter-related infection involves removal of the catheter and the administration of antibiotics. The appropriate duration of antibiotic therapy is a subject of controversy. Most clinicians continue antibiotic therapy only as long as a patient manifests systemic signs of infection (e.g., fever, leukocytosis). However, longer courses of antibiotic therapy (up to 10–14 days) may be necessary to prevent complications of staphylococci-related bacteremias. In retrospective studies, both Raad and Sabbagh[68] and Mylotte and McDermott[69] suggested that continuing antibiotic therapy for 10 to 14 days may be associated with a lower incidence of recurrent bacteremia or of endocarditis.

The most important means of decreasing the incidence of catheter-related sepsis is the strict adherence to aseptic technique during catheter placement and care. Caps, masks, gowns, and gloves should certainly be used during placement of pulmonary artery and central venous catheters and possibly even arterial catheters. A number of other adjunctive techniques have been developed to minimize the incidence of catheter-related sepsis. These include the bonding of antibiotics and silver compounds to the catheter, the use of a sterile, protective plastic sleeve over pulmonary artery catheters, and utilization of a silver ion–impregnated cuff. The silver ion–impregnated cuff fits over the catheter at the time of placement. It is made of collagen and allows for a firm anchoring of the catheter in the subcutaneous tissue. It acts as both a mechanical and chemical barrier to bacteria and has been shown to minimize the incidence of skin site infections as well as catheter-related sepsis.

The incidence of subacute bacterial endocarditis and suppurative thrombophlebitis of the great veins is an uncommon but deadly complication of the placement of central venous and pulmonary artery catheters and of transvenous pacemakers. It has been demonstrated that, within 1 to 2 days after placement of a central venous or pulmonary artery catheter, damage to the endothelium occurs; this damage is hypothesized to be responsible for the increased risk of endocarditis and phlebitis.

ABDOMINAL INFECTIONS

Most intra-abdominal infections that occur in critically ill surgical patients are secondary to the patients' underlying disease or represent a complication of a surgical procedure. However, several "abdominal" infections do not fall into these categories.

Clostridium difficile–Related Enterocolitis

Clostridium difficile–related enterocolitis is not uncommon in the critically ill patient treated with antibiotics. It tends to cluster in "mini-epidemics" and almost always follows the use of antibiotics. There may be a substantial lag between the withdrawal of antibiotics and the development of colitis. It is our experience that *C. difficile*–related enterocolitis can present with a full spectrum of features, from mild diarrhea and other nonspecific symptoms to a necrotizing enterocolitis with bowel perforation. Diagnosis is made on the basis of results from assay of a stool specimen for *C. difficile* toxin. The disease commonly (but not always) affects the distal sigmoid colon and rectum and can be diagnosed on sigmoidoscopic examination by detection of the classic pseudomembranes. However, presence of the disease cannot be excluded if pseudomembranes are not seen. The first line of treatment is generally oral administration of vancomycin. Metronidazole, administered either orally or intravenously, has also been used, but a higher relapse rate appears to occur when it rather than vancomycin is used. Occasionally, patients develop a fulminant form of enterocolitis, and systemic signs of sepsis result from their *C. difficile* infection. If bowel perforation occurs, if signs of peritoneal irritation are present, or if sepsis becomes increasingly more severe, the patient should undergo exploratory laparotomy and resection of the involved colon.

Urinary Tract Infection

Urinary tract infection is the most common hospital-acquired infection; however, it seems to be a less important problem in critically ill patients than in hospital ward patients. The development of urinary tract infection is directly related to the duration of urinary bladder catheterization. In one study, only 2.6% of urine specimens cultured were positive in patients whose catheters had been in for fewer than 4 days.[70] The rate of positive urine culture results increases dramatically after 5 days of catheterization.

The diagnosis is usually easily made on the basis of urinalysis and culture results. The combination of white blood cells on microscopic examination and the growth of an organism (usually >100,000 colony-forming units per milliliter) confirms the diagnosis. The most common organisms isolated are gram-negative aerobes and *Candida* species. Urinary tract infection seems to be declining in incidence. This may be because of the use of closed drainage systems and improvement in nursing protocols for catheter care. Performance of routine catheter culture in patients without sepsis, use of prophylactic antibiotics, and frequent catheter changes are not necessary and do not seem to reduce the incidence of urinary tract infection.

SUMMARY

A multitude of infections can result in sepsis in critically ill patients. We believe that the best way to evaluate these patients is to develop a list of diagnostic possibilities based on whether they have risk factors for specific infections, and not to simply perform "pan-culturing." We believe that this type of evaluation yields useful diagnostic information and that it avoids inadequate, ineffective, and unnecessary treatment, whether it be with antibiotics or with any other therapeutic modalities.

References

1. Pories SE, Gamelli RL, Mead PB, et al: The epidemiologic features of nosocomial infections in patients with trauma. Arch Surg 1991; 126:97.
2. Maki DG: Risk factors for nosocomial infection in intensive care. Arch Intern Med 1989; 149:30–35.
3. Craven DE, Kunches LM, Lichtenberg DA, et al: Noscomial infection and fatality in medical surgical intensive care unit patients. Arch Intern Med 1988; 148:1161.
4. Fry DE, Pearlstein L, Fulton RL, et al: Multiple system organ failure: The role of uncontrolled infection. Arch Surg 1980; 115:136.
5. Pin RW, Wertz MJ, Lennard ES, et al: Determinants of organ malfunction or death in patients with intra-abdominal sepsis: A discriminant analysis. Arch Surg 1983; 118:242.
6. Ad Hoc Committee of the Committee on Trauma, National Research Council Division of Medical Sciences: Factors influencing the incidence of wound infection. Ann Surg 1964; 160(Suppl):32.
7. Green JW, Wenzel RP: Postoperative wound infection: A controlled study of the increased duration of hospital stay and direct cost of hospitalization. Ann Surg 1977; 185:264.
8. Nichols RL: Surgical wound infection. Am J Med 1991; 91(Suppl 3B):54S.
9. Northey D: Microbial surveillance in a surgical intensive care unit. Surg Gynecol Obstet 1974; 139:321.
10. Balthazar ER, Colt J, Nichols RL: Preoperative hair removal: A random, prospective study. South Med J 1982; 75:799.
11. Shapiro M, Munoz A, Tager IB, et al: Risk factors for infection at the operative site after abdominal or vaginal hysterectomy. N Engl J Med 1982; 307:1661.
12. Nora PF, Vanecko RM, Bransfield JJ: Prophylactic abdominal drains. Arch Surg 1972; 105:173.
13. Magee C: Potentiation of wound infection by surgical drains. Am J Surg 1976; 131:547.
14. Antimicrobial prophylaxis for surgery. Med Lett 1993; 35:91.
15. Shapiro M, Townsend TR, Rosner B, et al: Use of antimicrobial drugs in general hospitals: Patterns of prophylaxis. N Engl J Med 1979; 301:351.
16. Burke JF: The effective period of preventive antibiotic action in experimental incisions and dermal lesions. Surgery 1961; 50:161.

16a. Nichols RL: Current approaches to antibiotic prophylaxis in surgery. Infect Dis Clin Pract 1993; 2:149.

17. Nichols RL: Bowel preparation. *In:* Surgical Infections: Diagnosis and Treatment. Meakins JL (Ed). New York, Scientific American, 1994, p 151.
18. Nichols RL, Condon RE, Grobach SL, et al: Efficacy of preoperative antimicrobial preparation of the bowel. Ann Surg 1972; 176:227.
19. Howe CW: Experimental studies on determinants of wound infection. Surg Gynecol Obstet 1966; 123:507.
20. Platt R, Zaleznik DF, Hopkins CC, et al: Perioperative antibiotic prophylaxis for herniorrhaphy and breast surgery. N Engl J Med 1990; 322:153.

20a. Platt R, Zucker JR, Zalenik DF, et al: Perioperative antibiotic prophylaxis and wound infection following breast surgery. J Antimicrob Chemother 1993; 31(Suppl B):43.

21. Dunn D, Rotstein O, Simmons R: Fibrin in peritonitis: IV. Synergistic intraperitoneal infection caused by *Escherichia coli* and *Bacteroides fragilis* within fibrin clots. Arch Surg 1984; 119:139.
22. Altemeier W: The bacterial flora of acute perforated appendicitis: A bacteriologic study based upon one hundred cases. Ann Surg 1938; 107:517.
23. Altemeier W: The pathogenicity of the bacteria of appendicitis peritonitis: An experimental study. Surgery 1942; 11:374.
24. Nichols RL, Smith JW: Anaerobes from a surgical perspective. Clin Infect Dis 1994; 18(Suppl 4):S280.

24a. Nichols RL, Smith JW: Wound and intraabdominal infections: Microbiological considerations and approaches to treatment. Clin Infect Dis 1993; 16(Suppl 4):266.

25. Weinstein WM, Onderdonk AB, Bartlett JG, et al: Experimental intra-abdominal abscesses in rats: Development of an experimental model. Infect Immun 1974; 10:1250.
26. Nichols RL, Smith JW, Fossedal EN, et al: Efficacy of parenteral antibiotics in the treatment of experimentally induced intra-abdominal sepsis. Rev Infect Dis 1979; 1:302.
27. Kasper DL: The polysaccharide capsule of *Bacteroides fragilis* subspecies *fragilis*: Immunochemical and morphologic definition. J Infect Dis 1976; 133:79.
28. Onderdonk AB, Kasper DL, Cisneros RL, et al: The capsular polysaccharide of *Bacteroides fragilis* as a virulence factor: Comparison of the pathogenic potential of encapsulated and unencapsulated strains. J Infect Dis 1977; 136:82.
29. Richardson J, Flint L, Polk H: Peritoneal lavage: A useful diagnostic adjunct for peritonitis. Surgery 1983; 94:826.
30. Pitcher W, Musher D: Critical importance of early diagnosis and treatment of intra-abdominal infection. Arch Surg 1982; 117:328.
31. Grønvall J, Grønvall S, Hegedüs V: Ultrasound-guided drainage of fluid-containing masses using angiographic catheterization techniques. AJR 1977; 131:323.
32. Stephen M, Loewenthal J: Continuing peritoneal lavage in high-risk peritonitis. Surgery 1979; 85:603.
33. Leiboff AR, Soroff HS: The treatment of generalized peritonitis by closed postoperative peritoneal lavage: A critical review of the literature. Arch Surg 1987; 122:1005.
34. Schumer W, Lee D, Jones B: Peritoneal lavage in postoperative therapy of late peritoneal sepsis. Surgery 1964; 55:841.
35. Rosato E, Oram-Smith J, Mullis W, et al: Peritoneal lavage treatment in experimental peritonitis. Ann Surg 1972; 175:384.
36. Hudspeth A: Radical surgical débridement in the treatment of advanced generalized bacterial peritonitis. Arch Surg 1975; 110:1233.
37. Polk H, Fry D: Radical peritoneal débridement for established peritonitis: The results of a prospective randomized clinical trial. Ann Surg 1980; 192:350.
38. Steinberg D: On leaving the peritoneal cavity open in acute generalized suppurative peritonitis. Am J Surg 1970; 137:216.
39. Walker AP, Nichols RL, Wilson RF, et al: Efficacy of a β-lactamase inhibitor combination for serious intra-abdominal infections. Ann Surg 1993; 217:115.

39a. Nichols RL, Smith JW, Robertson GD, et al: Prospective alterations in therapy for penetrating abdominal trauma. Arch Surg 1993; 128:55.
40. Lennard E, Dellinger E, Wertz M, et al: Implications of leukocytosis and fever at conclusion of antibiotic therapy for intra-abdominal sepsis. Ann Surg 1982; 195:19.
41. Ziegler EJ, Fisher CJ, Sprung CL, et al: Treatment of gram-negative bacteremia and septic shock with HA-1A human monoclonal antibody against endotoxin. N Engl J Med 1991; 324:429.
42. Arens JF, LeJeune FE, Webre DR: Maxillary sinusitis, a complication of nasotracheal intubation. Anesthesiology 1974; 40:415.
43. O'Reilly MJ, Reddick EJ, Black W, et al: Sepsis from sinusitis in nasotracheally intubated patients: A diagnostic dilemma. Am J Surg 1984; 147:601.
44. Craven DE, Kunches LM, Kilinsky V, et al: Risk factors for pneumonia and fatality in patients receiving continuous mechanical ventilation. Am Rev Respir Dis 1986; 133:729–736.
45. Burchard K: Diagnosis and treatment of pneumonia in the surgical intensive care unit. Surg Gynecol Obstet 1989; 171(Suppl):35–40.
46. Driks MR, Craven DE, Celli BR, et al: Nosocomial pneumonia in intubated patients given sucralfate as compared with antacids or histamine type 2 blockers. N Engl J Med 1987; 317:1376–1382.
47. Border JR, Hassett J, LaDuca J, et al: The gut origin septic states in blunt multiple trauma (ISS = 40) in the ICU. Ann Surg 1987; 206:427.
48. Moore FA, Moore EE, Jones TN, et al: TEN versus TPN following major abdominal trauma: Reduced septic morbidity. J Trauma 1989; 29:916.
49. Kudsk KA, Croce MA, Fabian TC, et al: Enteral vs. parenteral feeding: Effects on septic morbidity following blunt and penetrating abdominal trauma. Ann Surg 1992; 215:503.
50. Tryba M: Risk of acute stress bleeding and nosocomial pneumonia in ventilated intensive care unit patients: Sucralfate versus antacids. Am J Med 1987; 83(Suppl 3B):117.
51. Kappstein I, Schulgen G, Friedrich T, et al: Incidence of pneumonia in mechanically ventilated patients treated with sucralfate or cimetidine as prophylaxis for stress bleeding: Bacterial colonization of the stomach. Am J Med 1991; 91(Suppl 2A):125S.
52. Simms HH, DeMaria E, McDonald L, et al: Role of gastric colonization in the development of pneumonia in critically ill trauma patients: Results of a prospective randomized trial. J Trauma 1991; 31:531.
53. Cook DJ, Laine LA, Guyatt GH, et al: Nosocomial pneumonia and the role of gastric pH: A meta-analysis. Chest 1991; 100:7.
54. Seibel R, LaDuca J, Hassett J, et al: Blunt multiple trauma (ISS 36), femur traction, and the pulmonary failure-septic state. Ann Surg 1985; 202:283.
55. Bone LB, Johnson KD, Weigelt J, et al: Early versus delayed stabilization of femoral fractures: A prospective randomized study. J Bone Joint Surg [Am] 1989; 71:336.
56. Behrman SW, Fabian TC, Kudsk KA, et al: Improved outcome with femur fractures: Early vs. delayed fixation. J Trauma 1990; 30:792.
57. Sleyfer DT, Mulder NH, de Vries-Hospers HG, et al: Infection prevention in granulocytopenic patients by selective decontamination of the digestive tract. Eur J Cancer 1980; 16:859.
58. Stoutenbeek CP, van Saene HK, Miranda DR, et al: The effect of selective decontamination of the digestive tract on colonization and infection rate in multiple trauma patients. Intensive Care Med 1984; 10:185.
59. Kerver AJ, Rommes JH, Mevissen-Verhage EA, et al: Prevention of colonization and infection in critically ill patients: A prospective randomized study. Crit Care Med 1988; 16:1087.
60. Godard J, Guillaume C, Reverdy ME, et al: Intestinal decontamination in a polyvalent ICU: A double-blind study. Intensive Care Med 1990; 16:307.
61. Flaherty J, Nathan C, Kabins S, et al: Pilot trial of selective decontamination for prevention of bacterial infection in an intensive care unit. J Infect Dis 1990; 162:1393.
62. Cerra FB, Maddaus MA, Dunn DL, et al: Selective gut decontamination reduces nosocomial infections and length of stay but not mortality or organ failure in surgical intensive care unit patients. Arch Surg 1992; 127:163.
63. Gastinne H, Wolff M, Delatour F, et al: A controlled trial in intensive care units of selective decontamination of the digestive tract with nonabsorbable antibiotics. N Engl J Med 1992; 326:594.
64. Mandelli M, Mosconi P, Langer M, et al: Prevention of pneumonia in an intensive care unit: A randomized multicenter clinical trial. Crit Care Med 1989; 17:501.
65. Gil RT, Kruse JA, Thill-Baharozian MC, et al: Triple- vs. single-lumen central venous catheters: A prospective study in a critically ill population. Arch Intern Med 1989; 149:1139.
66. Maki DG, Weise CE, Sarafin HW: A semiquantitative method for identifying intravenous catheter–related infection. N Engl J Med 1977; 296:1305.
67. Eyer S, Brummitt C, Crossley K, et al: Catheter-related sepsis: Prospective, randomized study of three methods of long-term catheter maintenance. Crit Care Med 1990; 18:1073.
68. Raad II, Sabbagh MF: Optimal duration of therapy for catheter-related *Staphylococcus aureus* bacteremia: A study of 55 cases and review. Clin Infect Dis 1992; 14:75.
69. Mylotte JM, McDermott C: *Staphylococcus aureus* bacteremia caused by infected intravenous catheters. Am J Infect Control 1987; 15:1.
70. Martinez OV, Civetta JM, Anderson K, et al: Bacteriuria in the catheterized surgical intensive care patient: A prospective survey of 100 patients. Crit Care Med 1986; 14:188.

CHAPTER 133

Antimicrobial Therapy in the Critical Care Setting

Joan E. Kapusnik-Uner, PharmD • *David Woods, PharmD*
Merle A. Sande, MD

The diagnosis and therapy of infections represent a major function of the critical care physician. Intensive care unit (ICU) infections are often severe and are encountered either as a cause for admission to an ICU or as a complication of other severe illnesses. Also, bacterial sepsis remains the most common cause of late death in trauma victims.[1] The diagnosis of infection in the ICU patient may be obvious or extremely difficult. Infection may have a dramatic presentation with high temperatures, leukocytosis with left shift, hypotension, disseminated intravascular coagulopathy, renal insufficiency, and respiratory failure. On the other hand, patients admitted to the ICU for presumed shock, respiratory insufficiency, or coma may ultimately not have infection as an underlying diagnosis despite the presence of classic signs and symptoms. The patient presenting with respiratory insufficiency is an excellent example of the dilemma faced by the ICU physician, who must try to distinguish between infectious and noninfectious causes. In this chapter, we discuss a rational approach to the diagnosis and treatment of infections encountered by the ICU physician. Diagnostic tests and a general approach to selecting empiric antibiotic treatments are described. A summary of the pertinent pharmacology data for the individual antibiotics is given, with an emphasis on spectrum of activity, pharmacokinetics, toxicity, and dosing guidelines.[2] Infections commonly found in the ICU patient are also described, along with a rationale approach to their antimicrobial treatment.

DIAGNOSIS OF INFECTION

Once infection is suspected in the ICU patient, the physician's goal is to identify the infecting pathogen. Currently, a specific bacteriologic diagnosis is made only through isolation of the pathogen by culture or identification by staining techniques. Before the availability of culture data in a particular patient, clues as to the identity of the pathogen may be obtained by performing a Gram's stain of material from the suspected site of infection. When the Gram's stain reveals only a single morphologic type of bacteria, such as gram-positive cocci or gram negative bacilli, this organism should be treated empirically as the etiologic pathogen. Morphologic characteristics cannot indicate whether the pathogen is anaerobic or aerobic, but certain clues can help to identify the organism. For example, gram-positive cocci in clusters are likely to be staphylococci, encapsulated gram-positive diplococci are probably *Streptococcus pneumoniae*, small gram-negative cocci are *Neisseria* species, and coccobacillary organisms are consistent with *Haemophilus* species. When the Gram's stain reveals multiple morphologic types of bacteria, this may represent contamination during the process of obtaining the specimen (e.g., the normal skin flora contaminating a wound swab specimen), or the presence of multiple morphologic types of bacteria can be an accurate reflection of a polymicrobial, or mixed, infection. Note that the specificity and usefulness of the Gram's stain/culture specimens are related directly to the care with which the specimen is obtained. Compulsive care must be used to minimize contamination. This is obviously difficult when obtaining samples from nonsterile body sites (e.g., respiratory secretions obtained from a patient on a ventilator, because the endotracheal tube/upper airway is colonized by large numbers of bacteria).

SELECTION OF ANTIBIOTICS

A number of historic and clinical factors must be taken into account before selecting an empiric antibiotic regimen.[3] For example, several aspects of the patient's history must be considered. First, is the infection community acquired or hospital acquired? Community-acquired infections are, in general, caused by bacteria that are more susceptible to a wide range of antimicrobials and may be treated with "standard," less toxic, and less expensive agents. Hospital-acquired (nosocomial) infections, however, may be caused by pathogens with complex antimicrobial resistance patterns and may require potentially more toxic and expensive drugs. Second, what is the patient's underlying illness? Certain diseases predispose patients to infections caused by specific pathogens. For example, multiple myeloma is associated with infections caused by encapsulated bacteria, such as *S. pneumoniae* and *Haemophilus influenzae*, patients with leukemia and leukopenia and burn victims are predisposed to infections with *Pseudomonas aeruginosa*, and diabetes mellitus is associated with polymicrobial infections caused by *Staphylococcus aureus* and anaerobic organisms. Thus, if a patient with such an underlying illness is suspected to have an infection, the empiric antibiotic regimen is tailored to cover these organisms. Third, what is the suspected primary focus of infection? Different anatomic sites are characteristically infected by specific microorganisms. For example, the urinary tract and biliary tree are usually infected by enteric (aerobic) gram-negative bacilli, whereas endocarditis is caused by aerobic gram-positive cocci, such as *S. aureus* and viridans streptococci, and meningitis is caused by encapsulated organisms, such as *S. pneumoniae, Neisseria meningitidis,* and *H. influenzae.* Fourth, has the patient been treated with antibiotics recently? If the patient has acquired a new infection during or shortly after treatment with antibiotics, the new infection or superinfection is likely to be caused by a more resistant pathogen. Last, in patients receiving antibiotics, bacterial growth in cultures obtained may be suppressed owing to the presence of antibiotic in the actual culture specimen, thus culture results may be unhelpful for pathogen identification.

The appropriate selection of antimicrobials for empiric therapy also requires a reasonable understanding of pharmacology, including the mechanism of action (bactericidal versus bacteriostatic), antimicrobial spectrum of activity, pharmacokinetics, potential toxicities, and appropriate dose/dosing interval for a given clinical scenario. There are several important considerations. First, when should a bactericidal versus a bacteriostatic antibiotic be selected? Bactericidal antibiotics kill bacteria without the assistance of host defenses and thus are important for the cure of infections when the host immune response is not adequate. Three clinical settings require bactericidal therapy for cure: meningitis, because there are decreased antibodies and complement (C3b) in cerebrospinal fluid (CSF) as well as the lack of surface phagocytosis; infectious endocarditis, in which a dense fibrin-platelet meshwork encases a large bacterial inoculum (vegetation) and is impermeable to the effects of circulating white blood cells (WBCs); and infections in neutropenic patients. Bacteriostatic drugs, in contrast, inhibit the normal growth cycle of bacteria but do not lyse or kill the organisms. Bacteriostatic agents such as tetracyclines, macrolides, and clindamycin generally provide adequate therapy when host defenses are intact. Second, the general spectrum of activity for an antimicrobial agent must be understood. The usefulness of a specific agent in an institution may be monitored by the microbiology department or the infection control department. An antibiogram, which outlines an institution's susceptibility pattern to specific microorganisms, is helpful for the empiric antimicrobial selection process. The ICU physician must be informed of susceptibilities of common ICU pathogens because they may vary among institutions and also within a given institution (e.g., *Enterobacter* species, *Pseudomonas* species, and *Xanthomonas* species).

Third, pharmacokinetics are important because the physician must understand the distribution and elimination characteristics of an antimicrobial agent. For example, infections occurring in the CSF (i.e., meningitis), biliary tract, or urinary tract may be difficult to treat because certain drugs may not adequately distribute to those sites. The routes of elimination for each agent are important for the drug selection process to ensure adequate urine and bile concentrations for the treatment of infection at these sites. Also, toxicities may occur when elimination routes are impaired. Fourth, dose/dosing intervals are selected with the following factors in mind: the pathogen's minimum inhibitory concentration (MIC), the severity of infection, the size of the patient, and the ease of drug elimination. Inadequate drug regimens can result in treatment failure and the emergence of antimicrobial resistance, whereas excessive drug administration may result in toxicity and unnecessary expense. Fifth, the toxicity profile of antimicrobial agents is important for the overall clinical outcome. Factors that contribute to potential toxicities may be avoided or carefully monitored (i.e., excessive serum drug concentrations, renal dysfunction, concomitant administration of drugs with similar toxicities).

During the first 48 to 72 hours of empiric antimicrobial therapy, the patient must be watched closely for signs of clinical deterioration or improvement. If the patient's status deteriorates, the following possibilities should be considered: the presence of an undrained or undebrided focus of infection; too-narrow spectrum of antimicrobial coverage; inadequate penetration of drug to the focus of infection;

subtherapeutic dose/interval for the severity of infection or size of the patient.

When culture and sensitivity results are available, the antimicrobial regimen should be reassessed and tailored to the narrowest spectrum, least toxic, and least expensive agents. It is critical to tailor antimicrobials, even when patients have "responded" to therapy. This is done to minimize the alterations in the patient's bacterial flora, which occur with prolonged use of broad-spectrum antibiotics. Shortened courses of therapy and narrow-spectrum coverage both help to minimize the "antibiotic pressure" that promotes antimicrobial resistance[4] and reduces the incidence of bacterial superinfections caused by resistant pathogens (e.g., fungi and *Enterococcus* species). Drug toxicities and expense may also be reduced by decreasing the duration of therapy.

ANTIMICROBIALS

Beta-Lactam Antimicrobials

Penicillin G

Penicillin G remains clinically useful for a variety of serious infections. Penicillin G potassium is acid labile and, therefore, is not used widely as an oral agent. Phenoxypenicillin, penicillin VK, is more acid stable and is the preferred oral penicillin salt formulation. Aqueous crystalline penicillin G potassium is administered parenterally (intramuscular or intravenous), as are the procaine and benzathine salts for intramuscular injection. These latter preparations are less useful for ICU infections because relatively low serum concentrations result after drug administration. The mechanism of action of β-lactam antimicrobials (penicillins, cephalosporins, monobactams, and carbapenems) is related to their ability to inhibit bacterial cell wall synthesis and in some organisms trigger lysis of the cell wall. Beta-lactams bind to various intracellular proteins called penicillin-binding proteins (PBPs) and exert their effects at several stages of cell wall synthesis. The affinity and specificity of different β-lactams for different PBPs may help explain why the various agents have differing spectrums of activity. Alterations in binding to certain PBPs also have been associated with antimicrobial resistance.

Bacteria may become resistant to the penicillins by several mechanisms. The most important mechanism is through the production of enzymes called β-lactamases. These enzymes act irreversibly on the β-lactam drug molecule itself, causing hydrolysis of the β-lactam ring. Gram-positive bacteria produce, for the most part, plasmid-mediated β-lactamases, which are secreted extracellularly (ie., out of the bacteria) into the environment. Conversely, gram-negative organisms uniformly produce β-lactamases (chromosome mediated or plasmid mediated; constitutive or inducible), but concentrate these enzymes intracellularly in the periplasmic space. Other mechanisms of resistance include decreased antibiotic penetration through the outer cell wall membrane and changes in binding to PBPs.

Aerobic and anaerobic gram-positive cocci, including group A streptococci *(Streptococcus pyogenes)*, group B streptococci *(Streptococcus agalactiae)*, group C streptococci, viridans streptococci, *S. pneumoniae, (Streptococcus bovis), Peptostreptococcus* species, and *Peptococcus* species, for the most part have remained highly sensitive to penicillin G. *Listeria monocytogenes* is also susceptible. Routine sensitivity testing may not be performed for these organisms because resistance is rare. However, recent reports of *S. pneumoniae* resistance to penicillin makes screening of these organisms necessary.[5] The majority of strains of *S. aureus* and *S. epidermidis* do produce β-lactamases and are, therefore, resistant to penicillin G and ampicillin. Additionally, most strains of *S. epidermidis* are also methicillin resistant (MRSE), a resistance mechanism mediated by elaboration of a unique enzyme, PBP-2A.[6] There is an increasing incidence of methicillin-resistant *S. aureus* (MRSA) such that an ICU physician should be aware of the MRSA incidence in their institution. The susceptibility testing of cephalosporins against MRSE and MRSA may give misleading information because standard sensitivity tests do not detect small numbers of these resistant organisms. *Therefore, no cephalosporin is recommended in the treatment of infection caused by MRSE or MRSA.*

Penicillin G is eliminated from the body primarily by renal tubular secretion and glomerular filtration. Therefore, dosage adjustments must be made in patients with significant renal insufficiency (<40 mL/min). The serum elimination half-life of penicillin is approximately 30 minutes in patients with normal renal function. Penicillin distributes widely into body fluids, except for CSF, although in patients with meningitis (inflamed meninges) penicillin enters the CSF more easily and achieves therapeutic concentrations against susceptible bacteria when high-dose penicillin is administered (12–20 MU/d). Intravenous aqueous crystalline penicillin G is usually administered by intermittent infusion. One to 2 MU every 2 to 6 hours will adequately treat moderate to severe infections caused by susceptible organisms (Table 133–1). For meningitis and endocarditis, the higher doses (12–20 MU/d) are usually recommended.

The major adverse reactions from penicillin G are hypersensitivity reactions. Several chemical entities have been implicated in penicillin-induced hypersensitivity reaction. Antigenic determinants (metabolites) of penicillin hypersensitivity are formed by in vivo hydrolysis of the β-lactam ring and are classified as major and minor determinants, depending on how frequently they are involved in hypersensitivity reactions. The major antigenic determinant, the penicilloyl metabolite, elicits an IgE antibody response but results in accelerated urticarial reactions and maculopapular rashes. The various minor determinants elicit an IgE antibody response, which mediates most of the anaphylactic reactions. Skin testing with the single, commercially available preparation penicilloyl-polylysine (Pre-Pen) will not routinely predict which patient will have the more important anaphylactic reaction. It is, therefore, inadequate and is not routinely recommended. Skin testing with extemporaneously prepared penicillin solutions is also inadequate.

TABLE 133–1. Miscellaneous Penicillins

Variable	*Aqueous Penicillin G (Potassium Salt)*	*Ampicillin*	*Nafcillin*
Elimination half-life (hours)	0.5	1.0	1.0
Route(s) of elimination	Renal	Renal and biliary	Hepatic, biliary, and renal
Average peak concentration (dose)	10 μg/mL (1 MU)	47 μg/mL (2 g)	40 μg/mL (1 g)
Dosage regimen	1–2 MU every 2–6 h	1–3 g every 4–6 h	1–2 g every 4–6 h
Sodium (Na^+) content/dose	0.3 mEq/MU	3.0 mEq/g	2.9 mEq/g

Other than hypersensitivity reactions, penicillin G rarely causes toxicity. Drug accumulation in renal failure may predispose patients to generalized seizures, which are less responsive to anticonvulsant therapy. Central nervous system (CNS) toxicity may also manifest as lethargy, confusion, and multifocal myoclonus. Cation intoxication may occur during high-dose penicillin therapy because of the large potassium load and also because of excessive obligate anion excretion of the penicillin molecules. In patients with renal failure, serum potassium should be monitored during high-dose therapy with the potassium penicillin salt preparation, or, alternatively, penicillin G sodium may be specially ordered.

Clinically, penicillin G is still the single agent of choice for therapy of most streptococcal infections. Because *Enterococcus* species are tolerant to penicillin's action (i.e., results in only a bacteriostatic effect), penicillin should be combined with gentamicin to achieve bactericidal activity for therapy of enterococcal endocarditis. The "synergistic" effect achieved with penicillin and gentamicin against Enterococcus species is also produced by the combination of penicillin and gentamicin against viridans streptococci, a combination again only used in special circumstances (i.e., short-course therapy for endocarditis).

Ampicillin

Ampicillin, a semisynthetic derivative of penicillin, is active against most strains of bacteria sensitive to penicillin G and against some aerobic gram-negative bacilli. Susceptible Enterobacteriaceae include some strains of *Escherichia coli, Proteus* species, and *Salmonella* species. Ampicillin distributes throughout body tissues and fluids and is eliminated by renal and biliary mechanisms. The normal serum elimination half-life in adults is 1.1 to 1.3 hours, and dosage adjustments may be necessary only in severe renal impairment. Ampicillin cannot be detected in CSF with uninflamed meninges, but therapeutic concentrations for susceptible organisms are achieved in meningitis with large doses of drug. Dosages range from 1 to 2 g every 4 to 6 hours (see Table 133–1). Amoxicillin, a close chemical and pharmacologic relative of ampicillin, is more acid stable and is, therefore, more effectively absorbed from the gastrointestinal tract. Amoxicillin is available only as an oral preparation in the United States. Its spectrum of activity is identical to that of ampicillin, although it is not recommended in the treatment of infectious diarrhea because of low bile/stool concentrations achieved. Ampicillin and amoxicillin are more likely to cause rashes than do other penicillins, but these are usually benign, macular rashes and are *unrelated* to "true penicillin allergy."

Nafcillin

The emergence of staphylococcal resistance to penicillin G made necessary the development of β-lactamase–stable drugs. Nafcillin, methicillin, and oxacillin, so-called penicillinase-resistant penicillins, are parenteral semisynthetic agents. The use of nafcillin is restricted appropriately to the treatment of suspected or documented *S. aureus* infections. Nafcillin is less active than penicillin G against the other "penicillin-sensitive" organisms, such as streptococci, and is not an acceptable alternative in the treatment of enterococcal infections. Nafcillin is excreted unchanged in the urine (30%) to a lesser extent than other penicillins. Most of the drug is metabolized in the liver or eliminated in bile. The serum elimination half-life of nafcillin is approximately 1 hour, and penetration into CSF is usually adequate for the treatment of staphylococcal meningitis. Dosing ranges from 1 to 2 g every 4 to 6 hours (see Table 133–1).

Adverse reactions associated with nafcillin are similar to those observed with other penicillins. Additionally, dose-related neutropenia is reported to occur with high-dose (>10 g/d), long-term (>10 days) therapy. Interstitial nephritis associated with methicillin and hepatotoxicity associated with oxacillin have somewhat reduced the clinical usefulness of these two drugs, making nafcillin the parenteral penicillinase-resistant penicillin of choice.

Antipseudomonal Penicillins

TICARCILLIN, MEZLOCILLIN, PIPERACILLIN. Carbenicillin, introduced in 1967, was the first β-lactam antibiotic with reliable antipseudomonal activity and represented a dramatic improvement in the prognosis of pseudomonal infections. Unfortunately, larger carbenicillin dosages needed to be given (30 g/d), which meant a large salt load as well. Ticarcillin has a spectrum of activity similar to that of carbenicillin but is more active by weight and is active against more strains of *Pseudomonas* species. This increased activity by weight meant that patients could be administered smaller dosages and, therefore, a lower salt load. The main mechanism of resistance against these drugs is inactivation by β-lactamases, although decreased cell wall permeability has also been documented. Mezlocillin and piperacillin have greater activity against gram-negative anaerobes, anaerobic/aerobic streptococci, and *Enterococcus* species compared with ticarcillin. They have activity that is equal to (mezlocillin) or better (piperacillin) against *P. aeruginosa*. These compounds owe their increased activity against *Pseudomonas* species to increased cell wall permeability and increased binding to PBP-3 (responsible for bacterial septation).

The elimination half-life of these agents varies from approximately 1 hour for ticarcillin to 1.3 hours for both piperacillin and mezlocillin. These latter two agents may have an even longer half-life with higher doses because of dose-dependent rates of elimination. Thus, higher doses (4 g) that are given less frequently (every 6–8 hours) are used to take advantage of this pharmacokinetic feature. The dosing schedule for ticarcillin is usually 3 g every 4 to 6 hours for a serious infection (every 4 hours for pseudomonal infections).

The distribution and penetration of these penicillins into CSF, even with inflamed meninges, are negligible. Thus, they should not be relied on in the treatment of meningitis. Their primary route of elimination is the kidney, but biliary elimination also plays a major role for mezlocillin and piperacillin (Table 133–2).

TABLE 133–2. Extended-Spectrum, Antipseudomonal Penicillins

Variable	*Ticarcillin*	*Mezlocillin*	*Piperacillin*
Elimination half-life (hours)	1.0	1.0–1.3 (dose dependent)	1.0–1.3 (dose dependent)
Route(s) of elimination	Renal	Renal and biliary	Renal and biliary
Average peak concentration (dose)	218 μg/mL (3 g)	217 μg/mL (3 g)	227 μg/mL (4 g)
Dosage regimen	3 g every 4–6 h	2–4 g every 6 h	4 g every 6 h
Sodium (Na^+) content/dose	5.2–6.5 mEq/g	1.75–1.85 mEq/g	1.85 mEq/g

Adverse reactions include those seen with other penicillins. Additionally, they can cause a qualitative platelet defect in which the antibiotic blocks platelet aggregation. Another problem resulting from administering large daily doses of these penicillins is the concomitant salt load. Each antibiotic molecule is dibasic and, if excreted, acts as an obligate anion when eliminated, leading to potassium wasting. The large amount of sodium administered with these antibiotics may also lead to fluid retention.

Beta-Lactamase Inhibitor Combination Antimicrobials

AMPICILLIN PLUS SULBACTAM (UNASYN), TICARCILLIN PLUS CLAVULANATE (TIMENTIN), PIPERACILLIN PLUS TAZOBACTAM (ZOSYN). Sulbactam, clavulanate (clavulanic acid), and tazobactam are unique compounds that will irreversibly bind to and inactivate β-lactamase enzymes. When combined with ampicillin, ticarcillin, and piperacillin, respectively, they prevent destruction by β-lactamases and have increased our utilization of these "older" drugs.[7] These combination drugs are active against previously susceptible organisms but have an expanded spectrum of activity, which notably includes *S. aureus* (not MRSA) and *Bacteroides fragilis*. Some aerobic gram-negative bacilli also are included in the expanded spectrum, although the chromosome-mediated β-lactamases found in *Citrobacter* species, *Enterobacter* species, indole-positive *Proteus* species, *Providencia* species, and *Serratia* species may not be uniformly inhibited.

The development of ampicillin plus sulbactam became of interest because β-lactamase enzymes elaborated from gram-positive and gram-negative bacteria had diminished the usefulness of ampicillin monotherapy. Sulbactam, when combined with ampicillin in the commercially available 2:1 ratio, has been shown to inhibit important plasmid-mediated β-lactamases, thus increasing the spectrum of activity of ampicillin to include β-lactamase–producing strains of *Neisseria* species, *Moraxella catarrhalis, S. aureus, E. coli, Proteus* species, *Klebsiella* species, *Acinetobacter* species, and *Bacteroides* species, including *B. fragilis*. Organisms that are ampicillin susceptible remain so with the combination and include *Enterococcus* species, aerobic and anerobic streptococci, and *L. monocytogenes*. It is important to note that *P. aeruginosa* and other nosocomial gram-negative bacilli remain resistant to ampicillin plus sulbactam, as does MRSA and MRSE. Because the spectrum of activity is so broad for this combination agent, it has been effective monotherapy for many community-acquired mixed infections, such as pelvic inflammatory disease and other intra-abdominal infections, as well as in polymicrobial skin/soft-tissue infections, including diabetes-related infections. The addition of sulbactam to ampicillin does not change the biodisposition of ampicillin. Both drugs have a serum elimination half-life of approximately 1 hour, with renal elimination being the primary route (see Table 133–1). Biliary excretion of sulbactam appears to be less than that of ampicillin, which may impact the adequate treatment of certain infections caused by β-lactamase–producing organism. Although ampicillin and sulbactam have been reported to penetrate into CSF in patients with meningitis, there is a lack of clinical efficacy studies for this indication. The toxicity profile of ampicillin plus sulbactam is essentially the same as that observed for ampicillin, with the most common adverse reactions being diarrhea, skin reactions, and nausea/vomiting.

The addition of clavulanic acid to ticarcillin has broadened its spectrum of activity in the same way as ampicillin plus sulbactam. Organisms that were susceptible to ticarcillin remain so with the combination; however, *S. aureus* and *B. fragilis* (major producers of β-lactamases) are now also susceptible. Elimination is not altered with the clavulanic acid/ticarcillin product. Ticarcillin, 3 g, is combined with clavulanic acid, 100 mg, in the commercially available preparation. Dosages of 3.1 g every 4 to 6 hours are recommended. Piperacillin/tazobactam has been approved by the U.S. Food and Drug Administration (FDA) and is given in a dose of 3.375 g every 6 hours (Table 133–3). Adverse reactions to these β-lactamase inhibitor combinations are similar to those observed with the individual antibiotics; however, the incidence of diarrhea is reported to be higher.

First- and Second-Generation Cephalosporins

CEFAZOLIN. *Cephalosporium* is a fungus that produces cephalosporin C. Most of the presently available cephalosporin antibiotics are semisynthetic derivatives of this compound. The cephalosporin nucleus is very similar to that of the penicillins with the same β-lactam ring; and their mechanism of action is similar. Cefazolin is a first-generation cephalosporin that has proved to be safe and effective against many pathogenic aerobic gram-positive cocci and gram-negative bacilli. It became a popular substitute in patients who gave a history of penicillin allergy. Approximately 5% to 10% of patients who demonstrate allergy to penicillin will, however, experience a cross-reaction to the cephalosporins. Although this may be an acceptable risk in patients reporting non–life-threatening reaction from penicillin (e.g., hives, rash), greater caution must be used if the patient gives a history of anaphylaxis. There is no skin test that will predict which penicillin-allergic patient will experience cross-reaction. When antimicrobial therapy is indicated in a patient with a history of penicillin anaphylaxis, most authorities recommend a non–β-lactam antibiotic if available.[8]

Gram-positive cocci that are not inhibited by cefazolin (or any other cephalosporin) include *Enterococcus* species, MRSE, even though in vitro tests may sometimes give contrary data. The aerobic gram-negative bacilli that are usually sensitive include *E. coli, Klebsiella* species, and *Proteus mirabilis*, although nosocomial strains are often resistant. Oral gram-positive anaerobic streptococci are sensitive, but gram-negative anaerobes are resistant (e.g., *Bacteroides* species).

Cefazolin offers some advantages over cephalothin, which was the first available parenteral cephalosporin. It has the same spectrum of activity, although in vitro cephalothin may be more stable against β-lactamase enzymes.

TABLE 133–3. Beta-Lactamase Inhibitor Combination Antimicrobials

Variable	*Ampicillin Plus Sulbactam*	*Ticarcillin Plus Clavulanic Acid*	*Piperacillin Plus Tazobactam*
Elimination half-life (hours)	1.0	1.0	1.0
Route(s) of elimination	Renal and biliary	Renal	Renal and biliary
Average peak concentration (dose)	47 μg/mL (2 g)	324/8 μg/mL (3.1 g)	247/19.8 μg/L (3.375 g)
Dosage regimen	1.5–3.0 g every 6 h	3.1 g every 4–6 h	3.375/g every 6 h
Sodium (Na^+) content/dose	5 mEq/1.5 g	4.75 mEq/g	N/A

TABLE 133–4. First- and Second-Generation Cephalosporins

Variable	*Cefazolin*	*Cefuroxime*	*Cefoxitin*	*Cefotetan*
Elimination half-life (hours)	1.2–2.2	1.0–2.0	0.7–1.1	2.8–4.6
Route(s) of elimination	Renal	Renal	Renal	Renal and biliary
Average peak concentration (dose)	140 μg/mL (1 g)	51.1 μg/mL (750 mg)	75 μg/mL (1 g)	140 μg/mL (1 g)
Dosage regimen	1–2 g every 8 h	0.75 or 1.5 g every 8 h	1–2 g every 4–8 h	1–2 g every 12 h
Sodium (Na^+) content/dose	2 mEq/g	2.4 mEq/g	2.3 mEq/g	3.5 mEq/g

However, cefazolin is used more often because of its favorable pharmacokinetic profile, with a more prolonged serum half-life (0.5 hour for cephalothin versus 1.5–2 hours for cefazolin), thus allowing less frequent administration. Cefazolin is also better tolerated as an intramuscular injection. Cefazolin is excreted primarily by glomerular filtration, so dosage adjustments must be made in patients with decreased renal function. The therapeutic dose range is 0.5 to 2 g every 8 hours. Only small quantities of the drug are excreted into the bile, and unreliable drug concentrations are found in CSF, even with inflamed meninges (Table 133–4).

Local reactions (e.g., phlebitis) related to intravenous administration of cefazolin are the most frequently observed adverse effects. Hypersensitivity (allergic) reactions may occur but to a lesser degree than with penicillins. They may manifest as anaphylaxis, immediate reaction with shortness of breath and urticarial rash, Serum Sickness, a positive Coombs' reaction with or without hemolytic anemia, morbilliform rash, fever, pruritus, and eosinophilia. There is a significant rate of cross-reaction in patients allergic to penicillin who will then have an allergic reaction to cephalosporins. This is why a complete allergy history is important, in that, if anaphylaxis is reported from the penicillin, cephalosporins should be avoided when possible.

CEFUROXIME. This drug is active against cefazolin-sensitive organisms, but importantly it is also active against *H. influenzae*, even β-lactamase producing strains. Nosocomial strains of *E. coli*, *Proteus* species, and *Klebsiella* species may be more sensitive to cefuroxime than to cefazolin. However, *S. aureus* is less susceptible. Drug distribution occurs widely throughout the body, including penetration into CSF. Cefuroxime, however, has been shown to be less effective in the treatment of *H. influenzae* meningitis compared with ceftriaxone and is, therefore, not routinely recommended.[9] The main route of elimination is the kidneys with a serum elimination half-life of approximately 80 minutes. This prolonged half-life allows for dosing 750 mg or 1.5 g every 8 hours. Most infections require only the 750-mg dose. Side effects from cefuroxime include those described for cefazolin.

CEFOXITIN, CEFOTETAN. These agents are predominantly active against the same bacteria as cefuroxime. Important additions to their spectrum of activity are anaerobic gram-negative organisms especially *B. fragilis*, as well as *Neiserria gonorrhoeae*, and aerobic gram-negative bacilli such as *Serratia* species. A unique characteristic of cefoxitin is its increased resistance to hydrolysis by various β-lactamases. Cefoxitin and cefotetan are, on the other hand, less active against some gram-positive organisms, including staphylococci and streptococci. Cefoxitin and cefotetan are eliminated mainly by the kidneys; therefore, dosage adjustments must be made in patients with decreased renal function. A peak serum concentration of 75 μg/mL is achieved after a 1-g intravenous dose of cefoxitin, and the elimination half-life is approximately 45 minutes, compared with cefotetan with a half-life of 3 to 4.6 hours and a peak serum concentration of 158 μg/mL of cefoxitin. Dosage regimens for treatment of infections (as opposed to lower doses for surgical prophylaxis) range from 0.5 to 2 g every 4 to 6 hours, whereas the regimen for cefotetan is 1 to 2 grams every 12 hours (see Table 133–4). Potential adverse reactions from these agents are similar to those from other cephalosporins, with the exception that cefotetan can cause a disulfiram (Antabuse)-like reaction and bleeding from inhibition of the synthesis of vitamin K–dependent coagulation factors. These reactions have rarely been reported at the currently recommended dosing range of 1 to 2 g every 12 hours.

Third-Generation Cephalosporins

The third-generation cephalosporins represented a significant advance in spectrum of activity and pharmacokinetics over older cephalosporins. Important features include greater β-lactamase stability, increased affinity for gram-negative bacilli PBP-1 and PBP-3, longer serum elimination half-lives, and better penetration into CSF. These compounds show enhanced activity against *H. influenzae* and *Neisseria* species as well as most strains of Enterobacteriaceae, including nosocomial strains. Like other cephalosporins, they are not active against *Enterococcus* species, *L. monocytogenes*, MRSA, and MRSE and have variable activity against *B. fragilis* and *P. aeruginosa*. The chromosome-mediated β-lactamases of aerobic gram-negative bacilli hydrolyze most third-generation cephalosporins to some degree. All show an inoculum effect (i.e., an increase in MIC when an increased inoculum of bacteria is present), indicating their unique sensitivity to β-lactamases. Ceftazidime is the most β-lactamase stable, showing an inoculum effect only with some *Enterobacter* species. The resistance of various organisms to third-generation cephalosporins must be evaluated on an individual basis because the susceptibility of various bacteria to these new drugs is variable. In general, higher, more predictable CSF concentrations, greater than 10% of the simultaneous serum concentrations, are achievable, making these cephalosporins useful for the treatment of meningitis caused by susceptible organisms.

CEFOTAXIME. Cefotaxime and its desacetyl-cefotaxime metabolite are active against most Enterobacteriaceae except for *Enterobacter* species. The metabolite may be less active by weight than cefotaxime. Some evidence suggests that cefotaxime and desacetyl-cefotaxime may act synergistically against some bacteria. A significant inoculum effect is seen with the chromosome-mediated β-lactamases of *Serratia* species, indicating that, for certain infections, a high concentration of β-lactamase enzymes may destroy the drug's activity. Cefotaxime is unfortunately readily hydrolyzed by the plasmid-mediated β-lactamases of *Pseudomonas* species and by the β-lactamases from *B. fragilis*. The gram-positive activity of cefotaxime is comparable to that of cefuroxime.

The pharmacokinetics of both cefotaxime parent compound and its active metabolite should be considered when making decisions concerning dosing. Cefotaxime is eliminated by liver metabolism to desacetyl-cefotaxime as well as eliminated by the kidneys and bile. After a 2-g intravenous dose of cefotaxime, serum levels of 80 to 90 μg/mL are achieved but cefotaxime has a relatively short half-life of 0.9 to 1.7 hours. The desacetyl metabolite, on the other hand, is eliminated more slowly (half-life of 1.4–1.9 hours), mainly by further liver metabolism and renal excretion. In renal failure, the clearance of cefotaxime and metabolite is minimally affected, and thus dosage adjustments do not need to be made, except in cases of severe insufficiency (<20 mL/min). The "usual" dosing schedule varies widely for cefotaxime, from 1 to 2 g every 4 to 8 hours. Complications of cefotaxime therapy are similar to those of other β-lactam antibiotics (Table 133–5).

CEFTAZIDIME. The aerobic gram-negative spectrum for ceftazidime is exceptionally broad. Ceftazidime appears to be the most β-lactamase stable of the third-generation cephalosporins. It alone is stable with respect to the chromosomal β-lactamase of *Serratia* species and is the most stable against the β-lactamase of *Pseudomonas* species. Ceftazidime is also the most active against *Proteus* species because of its stability with respect to its chromosomal β-lactamases. However, ceftazidime is readily hydrolyzed by β-lactamases from *B. fragilis* and, therefore, should not be used as a single agent when infection with this organism is suspected. Gram-positive activity is adequate for nonenterococcal streptococci but is marginal for most nafcillin-sensitive *S. aureus*.

A peak serum concentration of 200 μg/mL is obtained from a 2-g intravenous dose with a serum elimination half-life of approximately 1.4 to 2 hours. The dosing range is 1 to 2 g every 6 to 12 hours. Ceftazidime is cleared predominantly by the kidneys and some in the bile; thus, in renal insufficiency dosage adjustments should be made (see Table 133–5).

Ceftazidime has been used as a single agent and in combination with an aminoglycoside to treat a variety of infections including pneumonia, osteomyelitis, sepsis, abscesses, cellulitis, urinary tract infections, and especially infection caused by *P. aeruginosa*, including those infections complicating cystic fibrosis. Febrile neutropenic cancer patients (WBC <500/mm^3) are often empirically given ceftazidime monotherapy.[10] Adverse reactions reported with ceftazidime include those ordinarily found with other β-lactam antibiotics.

CEFTIZOXIME. The spectrum of antimicrobial activity for ceftizoxime is similar to that of cefotaxime. The drug is hydrolyzed by chromosomal β-lactamase of *Enterobacter* species and is not usually active against *P. aeruginosa*. A potential difference between this third-generation cephalosporin and the others is its improved activity against *B. fragilis*, which is comparable to that of cefoxitin and cefotetan. The gram-positive spectrum of activity and patterns of resistance are similar to those of cefotaxime.

Approximately 85% to 88% of the drug is excreted by the kidneys, with a serum elimination half-life ranging between 1.4 to 1.9 hours, thus allowing a dosing interval of 6 to 8 hours. Ceftizoxime is concentrated in the bile in the absence of biliary obstruction. Dosage must be adjusted for patients with renal failure (see Table 133–5).

CEFTRIAXONE. This has a number of unique properties. Ceftriaxone is quite active against gram-negative bacteria and is stable against their chromosomal and plasmid-mediated β-lactamases. The gram-negative antibacterial spectrum for ceftriaxone is similar to that of cefotaxime and ceftizoxime, except for *P. mirabilis* and *Morganella morganii*, which are more sensitive to ceftriaxone, and it is less active against *Pseudomonas* species. The gram-positive antibacterial spectrum is also similar to that of cefotaxime. Like ceftazidime, ceftriaxone should not be relied on for coverage of *B. fragilis*. Ceftriaxone's pharmacokinetics are unique among the third-generation cephalosporins, with both very high serum drug concentrations and a very long serum elimination half-life. This is in part due to the high protein binding of this agent. A 1-g intravenous dose yields a peak serum concentration of approximately 150 μg/mL, and the serum elimination half-life ranges from 5.4 to 10.9 hours. Thus, ceftriaxone may be given once every 24 hours for most infections. Penetration into the CSF is impressive in patients with inflamed meninges with concentrations of 7% to 11% of the simultaneous serum levels. Dosing in meningitis should be more frequent (1–2 g every 12 hours) to maintain an adequate CSF drug concentration. Sixty per cent of drug is excreted by the kidneys and 40% is metabolized by the liver or excreted in bile; therefore, dosage adjustments are not necessary in patients with renal insufficiency (see Table 133–5). Adverse reactions reported are similar to those of other β-lactam agents. Additionally, there are several reports of ceftriaxone causing biliary sludging, stone formation, and biliary obstruction thought to be due to drug chelation with calcium.[11]

Monobactam and Carbapenem Agents

AZTREONAM. This synthetic monobactam antibiotic is truly "a narrow-spectrum" antimicrobial agent with activity only against aerobic gram-negative bacilli. Although stable with respect to most of the plasmid- and chromosome-mediated β-lactamases produced by these organisms, an inoculum effect is seen with *Serratia marcescens, Enterobacter* species, *Klebsiella* species, and *Pseudomonas* species. This compound is hydrolyzed by the β-lactamase of *B. fragilis. H. influenzae, Neisseria* species, many Enterobacteriaceae (*E. coli, Enterobacter aerogenes, Klebsiella* species, *Proteus* species), *Salmonella*, and *Shigella* have very low MICs, ranging from 0.05 to 0.25 μg/mL. The nosocomial gram-negative bacteria such as *Enterobacter cloacae, Citrobacter freundii,* and *Serratia* species have higher MICs from 2 to 4 μg/mL, whereas *Acinetobacter* species have an MIC of 6 μg/mL and *P. aeruginosa* has an MIC of greater than or equal to 8 μg/mL.

The average peak serum drug concentration after a 1-g intravenous infusion ranges from 90 to 164 μg/mL. The half-life is reported to be 1.3 to 2.2 hours, with the kidney being the primary excretion route, although the half-life is increased with renal or liver disease (Table 133–6). Usual dosing ranges from 1 to 2 g every 8 hours. Significant CSF penetration has been reported in patients with inflamed meninges, although this drug is not routinely recommended in meningitis. Aztreonam penetrates into other tissues, fluids, and urine at concentrations many times the MIC of most sensitive pathogens.

TABLE 133–5. Third-Generation Cephalosporins

Variable	*Cefotaxime*	*Ceftizoxime*	*Ceftriaxone*	*Ceftazidime*
Elimination half-life (hours)	0.9–1.7	1.4–1.9	5.4–10.9	1.4–2.0
Route(s) of elimination	Liver, renal, biliary	Renal	Renal and biliary	Renal
Average peak concentration (dose)	45 μg/mL (1 g)	84.4 μg/mL (1 g)	137 μg/mL (1 g)	69 μg/mL (1 g)
Dosage regimen	1–2 g every 4–8 h	1–2 g every 8 h	1–2 g every 12–24 h	1–2 g every 6–12 h
Sodium (Na^+) content/dose	2.2 mEq/g	2.6 mEq/g	3.6 mEq/g	2.3 mEq/g

Adverse reactions to aztreonam are similar to those reported for other β-lactam antimicrobials. Aztreonam appears to display very low immunologic cross-reactivity with other β-lactam antibiotics and may be useful in patients with non–life-threatening allergies to β-lactams. Its safety in patients with a β-lactam anaphylaxis history has not been sufficiently proven. A potential benefit of aztreonam's narrow spectrum of activity (ie, not active against anaerobic bacteria or gram-positive aerobes) is that it may have minimal effect on normal gastrointestinal flora, thus decreasing the incidence of diarrhea and superinfections.

IMIPENEM/CILASTATIN. Imipenem is the first carbapenem β-lactam to be FDA approved in the United States. This drug is highly resistant to degradation by the β-lactamase enzymes produced by gram-negative and gram-positive organisms, particularly those that are plasmid mediated. This broad-spectrum drug is very potent against community-acquired gram-positive organisms as well as the more resistant nosocomial gram-negative bacilli. Imipenem does not have reliable activity against *Enterococcus* species, *Mycoplasma pneumoniae, Chlamydia* species, *Legionella* species, and *L. monocytogenes.*

A 500-mg intravenous infusion of imipenem results in a peak serum concentration of 33 μg/mL and has a serum elimination half-life of approximately 0.85 to 1.3 hours. This serum concentration is low; however, imipenem is a very potent drug, with most gram-negative bacilli having low MICs. Imipenem is primarily excreted by the kidneys (70–80%). However, high urine concentrations are not observed because of significant drug hydrolysis (metabolism) by proximal tubule brush border dehydropeptidase enzymes. Unfortunately, the resulting metabolites are nephrotoxic. Therefore, the currently marketed imipenem product also contains cilastatin, a dipeptidase inhibitor. The addition of cilastatin results in higher urine imipenem concentrations and decreased formation of the potentially nephrotoxic metabolites. Imipenem dosages must be adjusted in renal failure because drug accumulation may lead to neurotoxicity (e.g., seizures). CSF penetration of simultaneous serum concentrations is excellent (20–30%); however, because of the potential for CNS toxicity, imipenem is used rarely in the treatment of meningitis (see Table 133–6).

Adverse reactions for imipenem are similar to those reported for other β-lactam antimicrobials. However, because of its broad spectrum of activity, superinfections are reported to occur with enterococci and fungi. Mild renal failure has been seen along with elevated liver enzymes. Of some concern is the association of this drug with seizures. The reported incidence is less than 1% and occurs in patients with renal failure or with preexisting seizure disorders.[12] Imipenem does cross-react in patients who are allergic to penicillins or cephalosporins and thus should be avoided if possible in patients with a history of anaphylaxis from other β-lactams.

TABLE 133–6. Monobactam and Carbapenem Agents

Variable	*Aztreonam*	*Imipenem*
Elimination half-life (hours)	1.3–2.2	0.85–1.3
Route(s) of elimination	Renal and liver	Renal and metabolism ?
Average peak concentration (dose)	90–164 μg/mL (1 g)	33 μg/mL (500 mg)
Dosage regimen	1–2 g every 8 h	0.5–1.0 g every 6–8 h
Sodium (Na^+) content/dose	None	2.8–3.2 mEq/g

Aminoglycosides

The most commonly used parenteral aminoglycoside antibiotics are gentamicin, tobramycin, and amikacin. Streptomycin usefulness has declined for the treatment of bacterial infections but has increased in the therapy of *Mycobacterium tuberculosis*, especially for multidrug-resistant strains. Aminoglycosides are rapidly bactericidal, although their exact mechanism of action is not completely understood. Drug easily passes via aqueous porin channels through the outer cell wall membranes of gram-negative bacilli entering into the periplasmic space. Aminoglycosides are not able to pass easily through the thicker outer cell wall membrane of gram-positive bacteria and thus have higher MICs to these organisms. Drug molecules are then transported across the cytoplasmic membrane, which appears to be an active process closely linked to electron transport, oxidative phosphorylation, and cellular respiration. This transport mechanism is shown to be impaired under conditions of low pH, high osmolality, and reduced oxygen tension. Thus, in certain clinical settings, aminoglycoside antimicrobials may not be maximally effective (e.g., acidic fluids, such as ascites; anaerobic environments, such as poorly diffused tissue or abscesses). Aminoglycosides are known to bind irreversibly to the 30s ribosomal subunit and to alter protein synthesis.

There are three well-described mechanisms by which bacteria develop resistance to the aminoglycosides. First, ribosomal mutation alters the site of aminoglycoside attachment. This phenomenon has been rare except for some strains of enterococci. Second, bacteria may become resistant to aminoglycosides by preventing penetration of the drug through the outer bacterial cell membrane or by preventing active transport through the cytoplasmic membrane. Anaerobic organisms are thought to be resistant because of the latter mechanism (the absence of the oxygen-dependent active transport system). Finally, the most important mechanism of bacterial resistance for aerobic gram-negative bacilli is plasmid-mediated enzyme production, which occurs within the periplasmic space.

Aminoglycosides have exposed hydroxyl and amino groups that are the potential sites of enzymatic modification. These enzymes inactivate aminoglycosides by adenylation, acetylation, or hosphorylation. Amikacin is the most stable aminoglycoside to these enzymatic effects because it has fewer sites for enzymatic attack. The antibacterial activity of aminoglycosides is directed primarily against aerobic gram-negative bacilli. Most are active against strains of Enterobacteriaceae, such as *E. coli, Klebsiella* species, *Enterobacter* species, *Proteus* species, and *Serratia* species. Strains of *P. aeruginosa, Citrobacter* species, *Acinetobacter* species, and *Providencia stuartii* usually are more resistant. When performing in vitro testing, tobramycin appears to be the most active aminoglycoside against the various *Pseudomonas* species, including *P. aeruginosa.* Other pseudomonal strains, such as *P. cepacia* are more resistant to all aminoglycosides. Their synergistic activity with penicillins or vancomycin against aerobic gram-positive bacteria is primarily limited to viridans streptococci, *Enterococcus* species, and *Staphylococcus* species.

Aminoglycoside concentrations are generally low in various infected secretions and tissues, such as respiratory secretions, pleural fluid, CSF, and aqueous humor. These low concentrations are predictable because of the simultaneously low serum concentrations, high molecular polarity, and the relatively short serum elimination half-life. Very high drug concentrations are, however, found in the renal tubular cells of the cortex, which is thought to correlate with the nephrotoxic potential of aminoglycosides.[13] Careful drug dosing is needed for aminoglycosides because of their narrow therapeutic window. An aminoglycoside loading dose is usually given to achieve the desired peak serum concentration immediately (5–10 μg/mL for gentamicin and tobramycin and 15–30 μg/mL for amikacin). Maintenance doses and dosing intervals are adjusted based on the patient's estimated creatinine clearance because glomerular filtration is the major route of elimination. Empiric maintenance doses for gentamicin and tobramycin range from 1.2 to 1.5 mg/kg every 8 hours and 7.5 mg/kg every 8 hours for amikacin. Clinical scenerios when dosage reductions may be necessary include advanced age, decreased renal blood flow, intrinsic renal disease, and azotemia. Higher drug dosages may be required in neonates or in patients with burns or with cystic fibrosis.

Serum drug concentration monitoring is necessary for all patients with life-threatening gram-negative infections.[14] Peak serum concentrations (30 minutes after a 30-minute infusion) are measured to ensure the adequacy of antimicrobial activity against a specific pathogen. Therefore, the desired peak concentration may be different among patients, ranging from 5 to 10 μg/mL. Measuring the trough serum concentration (just before receiving a dose) allows assessment of whether or not drug accumulation is occurring, which is a risk factor for nephrotoxicity and ototoxicity. Most clinicians adjust dosing to achieve a trough concentration of less than 2 μg/mL. The frequency of monitoring serum drug concentrations will vary among patients (usually once weekly throughout therapy) but should be more frequent in patients with changing renal function or in those with more resistant pathogens (Table 133–7).

Life-threatening adverse reactions from aminoglycosides are rare but may include neuromuscular blockade, similar to that seen with d-tubocurarine, which may result in muscular weakness and respiratory depression with apnea, especially when administered by rapid intravenous bolus dosing. Patients at increased risk include those who have myasthenia gravis and severe hypocalcemia and patients who have been concurrently receiving a neuromuscular blocking agent. All aminoglycosides can cause irreversible or reversible damage to the hair cells of the inner ear. Auditory and vestibular toxicity has been reported with equal frequency for amikacin, tobramycin, and gentamicin, whereas streptomycin appears to cause predominantly vestibular toxicity. The ototoxic effects of aminoglycosides may be potentiated by concurrent administration of other ototoxic agents (e.g., loop diuretics). It is postulated that all persons receiving an aminoglycoside will incur some damage to the hair cells, an effect that will accumulate over time with subsequent use of aminoglycosides, other ototoxic drugs, or auditory insults.

Nephrotoxicity is the most common complication of aminoglycoside therapy. It appears to be most common in elderly, debilitated patients and in those with preexisting renal disease. Additionally, ICU patients with hypotension or contracted intravascular volume from volume depletion, diuretic therapy, or contrast dyes are at specific risk. Nephrotoxicity is also incurred in patients who have had previous aminoglycoside therapy or who are receiving concurrent drugs known to be nephrotoxic (e.g., amphotericin). Nephrotoxicity is usually mild and reversible. Because aminoglycosides are useful in the treatment of serious infections, their use should not be avoided just because of the potential risk of nephrotoxicity. Close monitoring of serum drug concentrations will help to minimize this toxicity.

A new strategy for dosing aminoglycosides is being used by some clinicians. A single large daily dose of aminoglycosides may be more effective (or at least as effective) and less toxic than the traditional divided daily doses.[15] This new regimen takes advantage of the concentration-dependent killing power of aminoglycosides (i.e., the higher the drug serum concentration, the faster the rate of bacterial killing).[16] Additionally, this new dosing regimen provides a prolonged period of time at the end of the dosing interval when the serum drug concentration is low (or undetectable). This allows drug to eflux out of the cells (hair cells of the ear and proximal tubular cells of the kidney) and results in reduced ototoxicity and nephrotoxicity.

Antianaerobe Antimicrobials

CLINDAMYCIN. This semisynthetic derivative of lincomycin is a bacteriostatic antimicrobial agent. The exact mechanism by which clindamycin inhibits bacterial protein synthesis is not known but is eventually accomplished by binding to the 50s ribosomal subunit. Aerobic gram-positive organisms other than enterococci are susceptible, whereas aerobic gram-negative bacilli are completely resistant. Clindamycin is effective against most clinically important anaerobes (gram-positive cocci and gram-negative bacilli), including *B. fragilis*, although rates of resistance from *B. fragilis* of 15% and higher have been reported in specific institutions. Clindamycin is available as oral and intravenous-intramuscular formulations. After a 600-mg intravenous infusion, the peak serum concentration achieved is approximately 10 μg/mL, many times the MICs of susceptible organisms. The drug is well distributed into most body tissues and fluids but does not penetrate the blood-brain barrier to any reliable extent. Therefore, this drug would not be appropriate for the treatment of meningitis. In addition, it only exerts a bacteriostatic effect. Adequate parenteral therapy ranges from 300 to 900 mg every 8 hours. Clindamycin is predominantly metabolized by the liver to inactive compounds (90%), but a small amount of unchanged drug is also eliminated by the kidneys. Thus, no adjustments need to be made for renal insufficiency, but they may be necessary in severe liver disease. The normal serum elimination half-life is 2 to 4 hours (Table 133–8).

Pseudomembranous colitis (diarrhea, abdominal pain, fever, mucus and blood in the stool), a highly publicized complication of clindamycin therapy, is due to the production of exotoxin by resistant strains of *Clostridium difficile*.

TABLE 133–7. Aminoglycosides

Variable	*Gentamicin*	*Tobramycin*	*Amikacin*
Elimination half-life (hours)	2–3	2–3	2–3
Route(s) of elimination	Renal	Renal	Renal
Target trough concentration (μg/mL)	<2.0	<2.0	5–10
Target peak concentration (μg/mL)	5–10 (for GNR) 3–4 (for GPC)	5–10 (for GNR)	15–30 (for GNR)
Dosage regimen (for GNR)	1.2–1.5 mg/kg every 8 h	1.2–1.5 mg/kg every 8 h	7.5 mg/kg every 12 h

Abbreviations: GNR = gram-negative rods; GPC = gram-positive cocci.

TABLE 133–8. Antianaerobe Antimicrobials

Variable	*Clindamycin*	*Metronidazole*
Elimination half-life (hours)	2–4	6–8
Route(s) of elimination	Liver	Liver and renal
Average peak concentration (dose)	10 μg/mL (600 mg)	26 μg/mL (7.5 mg/kg)
Dosage regimen	600 or 900 mg every 8 h	500 or 750 mg every 8–12 h

Treatment consists first of discontinuing clindamycin and then administering oral metronidazole or vancomycin if symptoms persist.[17] This adverse effect has also been associated with most other antibiotics and is not specific for clindamycin. Other reported adverse effects from clindamycin include nausea, vomiting, diarrhea, rash, local thrombophlebitis, and increased liver enzymes.

METRONIDAZOLE. This is a nitroimidazole drug that is highly active against obligative anaerobes but does not have clinically significant activity against facultative anaerobic and aerobic organisms. Its mechanism of action has not been fully elucidated but probably has to do with its nitro group being reduced within anaerobes by low-redox-potential electron transport proteins. It is also effective in the treatment of trichomoniasis, amebiasis, and giardiasis. Metronidazole is a rapidly bactericidal agent that is active against gram-negative anaerobic bacilli such as the various *Bacteroides* species including *B. fragilis*. Gram-positive bacilli, such as *Clostridium* species, are nearly all sensitive as well. Unfortunately, anaerobic gram-positive cocci are less susceptible (*Peptococcus* and *Peptostreptococcus*) but are inhibited, whereas other anaerobic streptococci are resistant. Until recently, acquired resistance to metronidazole was not described; however, reports of resistant *B. fragilis* isolates and treatment failures of trichomonal infections have now been reported.

The peak serum concentration achieved after a 7.5-mg/kg intravenous dose of metronidazole is approximately 26 μg/mL and the serum elimination half-life is 6 to 8 hours. Usual dosing varies widely depending on the site and severity of infection. The most frequently administered dose of metronidazole for bacterial infections is 500 mg because it is available in a premixed minibag. Higher dosages (7.5 mg/kg) may be necessary in large patients or for the treatment of CNS infections. A dosing interval of every 8 to 12 hours should be used because this agent has a very long half-life. Most of an intravenous dose of metronidazole is metabolized by the liver to inactive metabolites, which are then eliminated by the kidney. No dosage adjustments need be made in renal failure. However, with significant hepatic dysfunction, therapy should be monitored for toxicities and dosage reductions should be made. Metronidazole penetrates well into body tissues and fluids, including penetration into CSF where concentrations have been reported to be 43% of simultaneous serum concentrations in patients with meningitis (see Table 133–8).

Adverse reactions specific to metronidazole have been reported to include metallic taste, anorexia, and nausea. The urine may turn dark or reddish brown, causing some unnecessary concern. Neurologic side effects include peripheral neuropathy, manifesting as tingling and paresthesias, as well as CNS effects including vertigo, seizures, and ataxia. A disulfiram-like reaction may also occur during concurrent drug therapy with an alcohol-containing product or ingestion of alcoholic beverages. Symptoms of a disulfiram reaction are hypotension, nausea, flushing, and tachycardia. Metronidazole may be responsible for clinically significant drug-drug interactions with warfarin. Metronidazole is thought to decrease warfarin metabolic clearance (increasing the half-life) and thus increase or prolong warfarin's hypoprothrombinemic effects.

Miscellaneous Agents

VANCOMYCIN. This was the agent of choice in the 1950s for penicillin-resistant staphylococci; however, after the introduction of penicillinase-resistant penicillins (e.g., nafcillin) and later cephalosporins, it relinquished this status. When first introduced in 1956, preparations contained approximately 80% vancomycin and 20% impurities with unknown microbiologic activity and toxicity. A high incidence of adverse reactions including nephrotoxicity, ototoxicity, fever, and phlebitis was initially reported. Current preparations are more pure and thus cause fewer reactions.

Vancomycin is a narrow-spectrum drug that exerts its bactericidal effect by irreversibly binding to the cell wall of susceptible gram-positive bacteria and inhibits synthesis. Vancomycin has unique antimicrobial activity against MRSA and MRSE.[18] It is also active against gram-positive bacilli, streptococci, and *Enterococcus* species. Like the penicillins, vancomycin is not bactericidal against enterococci. When a bactericidal effect is necessary to treat enterococcal endocarditis, it may be attained with the synergistic combination of vancomycin plus an aminoglycoside (usually gentamicin). *Clostridium* species and *Corynebacterium* species are gram-positive bacilli and are usually susceptible to vancomycin; however, gram-negative aerobes and anaerobes are all resistant.

Vancomycin is not absorbed from the gastrointestinal tract; thus, the oral route of administration has been reserved for the treatment of pseudomembranous colitis. Intramuscular administration of vancomycin is contraindicated because of adverse reactions (e.g., pain, tenderness, or muscle necrosis). Intravenous drug should only be administered over a period of at least 60 minutes because rapid infusions may cause the "red neck" or "red man's" syndrome with nausea, chills, hypotension, urticaria, and macular rashes.[19] Also, thrombophlebitis can be minimized by administering vancomycin in at least 200 mL of fluid and by reducing the infusion rate.

There is conflict in the literature regarding appropriate monitoring of peak and trough vancomycin concentrations.[20] The peak concentration should be monitored in patients if there is concern over drug accumulation (e.g., in acute renal failure) and should be kept below 60 μg/mL to minimize ototoxicity. The trough concentration should be monitored for efficacy and should remain in the 5- to 10-μg/mL range (above the MIC of the pathogen being treated). To achieve these desired steady-state serum concentrations quickly, it is recommended to give an initial loading dose of approximately 17.5 mg/kg (use total body weight in the calculation). The maintenance dose regimen is based on the patient's renal function. Patients with normal renal function may require a total daily maintenance dose of 20 to 30 mg/kg divided every 12 hours. Adjustments for decreased renal function can be estimated by monitoring serum drug concentrations (Table 133–9). Vancomycin penetrates well into various body fluids except the CSF. Penetration of vancomycin, even in patients with meningitis, may be erratic, and thus intrathecal drug administration may be required. Vancomycin is not significantly concentrated, specifically in the bile or aqueous humor.

ERYTHROMYCIN. This is currently the only available parenteral macrolide antibiotic. It is a bacteriostatic agent mostly active against gram-positive organisms such as streptococci (nonenterococcal). *S. aureus* may also be suscep-

TABLE 133–9. Miscellaneous Agents

Variable	*Vancomycin*	*Erythromycin (Lactobionate)*	*Trimethoprim-Sulfamethoxazole*	*Ciprofloxacin*	*Ofloxacin*
Elimination half-life (hours)	4–6	0.8–3.0	8–11/10–13	3–5	4–8
Route(s) of elimination	Renal	Liver and biliary	Metabolism and renal	Renal and liver	Renal
Average peak concentration (dose)	20 μg/mL (1 g)	10 μg/mL (500 mg)	9.0/105 μg/mL (160/800 mg)	4.6 μg/mL (400 mg)	5.5 μg/mL (400 mg)
Dosage regimen	1 g every 12 h (adjust for renal function)	0.5–1.0 g every 6 h	5–10 $mg \cdot kg^{-1} \cdot d^{-1}$ of (trimethoprim) divided every 8–12 h	400 mg every 8–12 h	400 mg every 12 h

tible, but resistance may develop to erythromycin during therapy. This may be exclusively erythromycin resistance or may also include resistance to clindamycin. Erythromycin is also clinically useful for the treatment of infections resulting from *Treponema pallidum* (syphilis) as well as atypical organisms such as *M. pneumoniae, Chlamydia* species, and *Legionella pneumophila.* Erythromycin inhibits bacterial protein synthesis by reversibly binding to the 50s ribosomal subunit. Erythromycin more rapidly penetrates bacterial cell walls when in the nonionic drug state (pKa 8.8) and thus is most effective in an alkaline environment; and activity decreases in acidic surroundings such as abscesses or urine.

Erythromycin lactobionate and erythromycin gluceptate are the available intravenous preparations. Intramuscular injection is avoided because of pain. These two erythromycin esters are inactive, and in vivo hydrolysis must occur to free active erythromycin base. Peak serum concentrations after 500 mg of the lactobionate salt are approximately 10 μg/mL. Erythromycin is mostly metabolized by the liver but is eliminated to a small degree as unchanged drug in the urine and bile. The serum elimination half-life of erythromycin ranges from 0.8 to 3.0 hours. Erythromycin penetrates fairly well into body tissues and fluids, except CSF, even in patients with inflamed meninges. For serious infections, 0.5 to 1.0 g should be administered every 6 hours (see Table 133–9).

Thrombophlebitis associated with drug infusion is a frequent problem; however, severe adverse reactions (i.e., tinnitus and transient deafness) have rarely been reported with intravenous administration. The oral formulations have all been known to cause an exceptionally high incidence of gastrointestinal side effects, and erythromycin estolate has been associated with reversible jaundice.

TRIMETHOPRIM-SULFAMETHOXAZOLE. This broad-spectrum combination product is available as a fixed 1:5 ratio of trimethoprim-sulfamethoxazole (TMP-SMX). Both drugs are folate synthesis antagonists and act synergistically to inhibit or kill susceptible bacteria. Aerobic streptococci and staphylococci are susceptible as are aerobic enteric gram-negative bacilli. *Enterococcus* species and anaerobic gram-negative bacilli, such as *B. fragilis,* are resistant. Most strains of *P. aeruginosa* are resistant; however, *Xanthomonas maltophilia,* a multiresistant nosocomial pathogen, is usually very susceptible.

TMP-SMX is well absorbed from the gastrointestinal tract and is also tolerated after intravenous infusion (except for some thrombophlebitis). Therapeutic ratio concentrations of 1:20 result in most body fluids, which appears to be an optimal ratio for synergistic activity. Both drugs are metabolized by the liver and also eliminated renally. Serum elimination half-lives are 8 to 11 hours and 10 to 13 hours, respectively. Drug accumulation can occur in severe renal insufficiency, as well as toxic metabolite accumulation, such that dosage reduction is recommended. TMP-SMX does penetrate into CSF (40–50%) in meningitis; however, this drug is mostly bacteriostatic and is, therefore, not acceptable for the routine treatment of bacterial meningitis. Drug dosages are calculated as total daily dose of TMP, 5 to 10 mg/kg per day; serious gram-negative bacillary infections require the higher dosage. The total daily dose is divided every 12 hours so that no more than 400 mg of TMP will be given at one time. The dose-limiting toxicity of intravenous TMP-SMX is usually gastrointestinal intolerance. For the treatment of *Pneumocystis carinii* pneumonia, dosing is higher (15 to 20 mg/kg per day TMP) (see Table 133–9).

Other adverse reactions to TMP-SMX include, most notably, hypersensitivity reactions such as rash, fever, epidermal necrolysis, and Stevens-Johnson syndrome. Hematologic toxicities (anemia, neutropenia, and thrombocytopenia) may be treatable with concomitant administration of folinic acid. Hepatitis and CNS reactions are also reported, but most patients tolerate this drug well. The incidence, however, of TMP-SMX–induced adverse reactions has been reported to be extremely high in patients with acquired immunodeficiency syndrome. The mechanism for this increased risk of toxicity is not well understood but is thought to be related to altered drug metabolism. A clinically significant drug-drug interaction is reported with TMP-SMX and warfarin, which results in increased prothrombin time and possible bleeding.

CIPROFLOXACIN AND OFLOXACIN. These are the currently available parenteral quinolone antimicrobials. The bactericidal mechanism of action for these agents is unique and involves inhibition of deoxyribonucleic acid gyrase (topoisomerase) enzymes. Their spectrum of activity is similar; most aerobic gram-negative bacilli are susceptible, including *P. aeruginosa.* All anaerobic organisms are resistant, whereas aerobic gram-positive cocci have variable susceptibility. Specifically for respiratory tract infections, great care should be taken to rule out the possibility of *S. pneumoniae* infection before selecting a quinolone because these antimicrobials are not recommended even though in vitro tests results may show this organism to be marginally susceptible.[21] *S. aureus* and *S. epidermidis,* including MRSA and MRSE, have been susceptible. With regards to most gram-positive bacteria, quinolones have a "narrow therapeutic window;" that is, the achievable (nontoxic) peak concentrations are very close to the organisms' MICs. However, the uncontrolled use of ciprofloxacin has quickly promoted the rapid emergence of ciprofloxacin resistance both for *S. aureus* and *P. aeruginosa* (with cross-resistance conferred to other quinolones).[22] The addition of rifampin to a ciprofloxacin regimen is believed to help prevent this emergence of resistance. Quinolones also have activity against atypical organisms including *Chla-*

mydia species and *Legionella* species, as well as various strains of *Mycobacterium*, including *M. tuberculosis.*

Ciprofloxacin is eliminated by the kidneys and by liver metabolism, whereas ofloxacin is mostly excreted by the kidney. Their approximate serum elimination half-lives are 3 to 5 hours and 4 to 8 hours, respectively. Drug accumulation will occur to a significant extent in renal insufficiency; thus, dosage adjustment will be necessary. Drug distribution occurs widely throughout body tissues and fluids, with concentrations in many fluids exceeding serum drug concentrations. Penetration into CSF (11–46%) is reported to occur in patients with meningitis. However, because these drugs have a narrow therapeutic window, they are not routinely recommended in the treatment of meningitis. Dosing recommendations are 200 to 400 mg every 12 hours; however, every 8 hours has been used in severe infections or with *P. aeruginosa* infections (see Table 133–9).

Adverse reactions have limited quinolone dosing to the extent that it is not recommended that peak serum drug concentrations exceed 6.0 μg/mL because of the risks of CNS toxicities. Headache and restlessness, as well as seizures and psychosis, have been reported in 1% to 2% of patients. Other adverse reactions include gastrointestinal side effects, rash, arthralgias, and increased liver enzymes. The arthropathy observed in children is severe enough that the drugs are contraindicated except in life-threatening infections (e.g., resistant pseudomonal infection in cystic fibrosis patients). A clinically significant drug-drug interaction is reported with ciprofloxacin and warfarin, which results in increased prothrombin time and possible bleeding.[23]

COMMONLY ENCOUNTERED INTENSIVE CARE UNIT INFECTIONS[24]

Pneumonias

Community-Acquired Pneumonias

Community-acquired pneumonias in relatively healthy people rarely result in illness severe enough to require ICU admission. However, in persons with significant underlying medical disease (alcoholism, malignancies, malnutrition, diabetes, sickle cell disease, congestive heart failure, or chronic obstructive lung disease [COPD]), pneumonia can have severe consequences.

S. pneumoniae is a common cause of adult (>40 years old) pneumonia in the community, whereas pneumonia in younger adults and children may be caused by viruses, *M. pneumoniae, Chlamydia pneumoniae*, and *Legionella* species as well. Community-acquired bacterial pneumonia is usually characterized by respiratory symptoms, cough, shortness of breath, purulent sputum, and occasionally pleuritic chest pain. The diagnosis requires signs of infection such as fever, chills, leukocytosis, and an abnormal chest x-ray film. The sputum Gram's stain should show polymorphonuclear cells and a predominant microorganism with rare epithelial cells. The diagnosis may be confirmed by sputum culture and occasionally by positive blood cultures.

Because *S. pneumoniae* is the most common cause of community-acquired pneumonia, a penicillin will be the treatment of choice in most cases. However, the respiratory tract of patients with chronic obstructive pulmonary disease or smokers is frequently colonized by *H. influenzae*; therefore, multiple organisms may be seen on sputum Gram's stain or culture. Consequently, the true pneumonic pathogen may not be distinguishable, so empiric treatment with ampicillin, which covers both organisms, may be initiated. Unfortunately, in some communities, the prevalence of β-lactamase–producing *H. influenzae* may be significant; thus, TMP-SMX and cefuroxime serve as alternatives. Atypical pneumonias must be treated with erythromycin and in the rare case of *Klebsiella pneumoniae,* which is reported to occur in elderly, debilitated patients and alcoholics, an extended-spectrum penicillin or cephalosporin plus gentamicin should be added. When aspiration is believed to be a contributing factor in the pathogenesis of pneumonia, oral anaerobe coverage including *Bacteroides* species needs to be added. This can be achieved by administering clindamycin, cefoxitin, or β-lactamase inhibitor combination agents. *P. carinii* pneumonia must always be considered in a patient with human immunodeficiency virus infection and is treated with TMP-SMX.

Hospital-Acquired Pneumonias

Hospitalized patients, especially those with endotracheal tubes or tracheostomies undergoing mechanical ventilation, are at increased risk for pneumonia. Hospital-acquired pneumonia develops in 5 to 10 patients per 1000 hospital admissions and has a mortality rate of 20% to 50%.[25] They are most commonly caused by aerobic gram-negative bacilli including *K. pneumoniae, Proteus* species, *S. marcescens, E. coli, E. cloacae,* and *P. aeruginosa*. Additionally, *S. aureus* is reported to be responsible for some nosocomial pneumonias and appears to be more common in patients on ventilators. Other organisms, such as anaerobes and fungi, are infrequently responsible for nosocomial pneumonias. Fungal pneumonia may especially occur in immunocompromised patients (e.g., transplant patients) or in patients who have been taking broad-spectrum antibiotics for prolonged periods of time.

The gram-negative bacilli encountered in nosocomial pneumonias may be resistant to many standard antibiotics such as ampicillin, cefazolin, gentamicin, and TMP-SMX. Consequently, the extended-spectrum penicillins and third-generation cephalosporins are required. If the extended-spectrum penicillins are selected, the addition of gentamicin or tobramycin is recommended because of their lack of stability against some β-lactamases and for synergy. Again, because of the high morbidity and mortality for gram-negative pneumonia (i.e., *Pseudomonas* pneumonia), synergistic combination therapy is frequently recommended, especially in the septic patient. The specific choice of drugs may depend on the unique sensitivity pattern of an ICU.

If gram-positive cocci are seen on the Gram's stain, *S. aureus* must be considered as a potential pathogen. Vancomycin is the drug of choice for MRSA, which may be common in the ICU setting. As previously described, cephalosporins should not be considered a substitute for vancomycin in the treatment of infections resulting from MRSA or MRSE, even if in vitro tests show the organism to be susceptible.

Urinary Tract Infections

Community-acquired urinary tract infections rarely cause urosepsis unless there is a structural abnormality of the genitourinary (GU) tract. Patients may occasionally appear with sepsis from pyelonephritis and have normal GU anatomy; however, usually the patients may have ignored symptoms for prolonged periods or are debilitated. In hospitalized patients, instrumentation or the presence of a urinary catheter will predispose the patient to urinary tract infection. Community-acquired urinary tract infections are usually caused by enteric gram-negative bacilli, which are increasingly resistant to ampicillin and TMP-SMX but remain susceptible to most first-generation cephalosporins, quinolones, and aminoglycosides. The organisms causing hospital-acquired urinary tract infections are those nosocomial gram-negative bacilli that colonize the patient and may include more resistant organisms such as *P. aeruginosa*. Extended-spectrum penicillins, third-generation cephalosporins, or β-lactamase inhibitor combination agents may be used as monotherapy. Alternatively, in cases of septic shock, the addition of an aminoglycoside is recommended. There are theoretical reasons why aminoglycosides may be less effective when used alone in the treatment of complicated urosepsis. Within renal abscess cavities or the renal medulla, aminoglycosides may be relatively inactive owing to low pH or anaerobic environment.

Urosepsis should be suspected in the patient who has signs of systemic infection (e.g., chills, fever, leukocytosis, and hypotension) in addition to flank pain and lower abdominal pain. Confirmatory laboratory findings include pyuria with or without WBC casts and Gram's stain of urine with many bacteria of a single morphologic type. The diagnosis is confirmed by isolation of the infecting organism from blood or urine cultures. Treatment must include assessment (with sonogram, intravenous pyelogram, or computed tomographic scan) and removal of the urinary tract obstruction because antibiotic therapy alone is not adequate. Nevertheless, antibiotics are essential for treating bacteria in the bloodstream and the GU tract.

Meningitis

Patients with bacterial meningitis may be admitted to an ICU because of lethargy, obtundation and need for airway protection, treatment of seizures and hemodynamic instability, or other systemic consequences of infection (see Chapter 139). Cure of meningitis requires the administration of adequate doses of bactericidal antibiotic and early institution of adjuvant steroid therapy (dexamethasone), which has been shown to reduce meningitis-induced morbidity in children.[26] *S. pneumoniae* is the most common cause of community-acquired meningitis in adults, followed by *N. meningitidis*, *L. monocytogenes*, and rarely *H. influenzae*. Postneurosurgical meningitis may be caused by varied pathogens including nosocomial gram-negative bacilli as well as staphylococci.

The diagnosis of meningitis should be suspected on the basis of the appropriate clinical syndrome but is established by Gram's stain and culture of CSF and blood. When a primary site of pneumococcal or *H. influenzae* infection, such as the lung or sinus, is identified, meningitis is probably due to the same organism. Meningitis associated with CSF leaks or rhinorrhea (post-traumatic) is usually caused by *S. pneumoniae*. The CSF findings characteristic of bacterial meningitis are high WBC count with a predominance of polymorphonuclear cells, a decrease in CSF glucose concentrations (less than 50% that of serum glucose), and elevated protein. If the infecting agent is not isolated by cultures, a bacteriologic diagnosis can sometimes be made by detecting the capsular antigens in the CSF or blood by counterimmunoelectrophoresis.

Thus, empiric therapy of bacterial meningitis in most patients consists of ampicillin or high-dose penicillin G (20 MU per day adjusted for renal insufficiency). Patients at risk for enteric gram-negative bacilli or *H. influenzae* infection should be administered ceftriaxone. None of the cephalosporins are active against *L. monocytogenes*, so penicillin or ampicillin needs to be included in a patient's regimen if this organism is suspected (i.e., elderly, immunocompromised, neonates). Vancomycin should be administered if MRSA or MRSE is suspected in postneurosurgical patients. It is recommended for the treatment of pneumococcal meningitis because of the rising incidence of penicillin-resistant *S. pneumoniae*. Adjuvant therapy with dexamethasone is important for children with *H. influenzae* meningitis. Its use in adults is controversial (see Chapter 139) but may be used to reduce cerebral edema in patients with increased intracranial pressure or CNS dysfunction such as an altered mental status or a focal neurologic deficit.

Endocarditis and Endovascular Infections

Endocarditis is an infection in which the host defense has limited ability to control bacterial growth. Vegetations on heart valves are avascular masses of fibrin, platelets, and bacteria that do not contain WBCs. Consequently, the choice of bactericidal antibiotics is crucial for cure.

Left-sided native valve endocarditis may have a wide variety of presentations that require ICU admission or complicate a patient's hospital course. Patients may be admitted with a stroke, cerebral hemorrhage, bowel infarct, myocardial infarction, limb ischemia, or renal failure. These manifestations are consequences of systemic embolization or congestive heart failure resulting from valve dysfunction. Patients with right-sided endocarditis (particularly common in intravenous drug users) may develop septic pulmonary emboli. The diagnosis is based on recognition of the appropriate clinical syndrome, as described previously, and documentation of sustained bacteremia. At least two blood cultures taken 30 minutes apart should be positive for a single organism; an echocardiogram may be helpful if valve vegetations are seen but is negative in a significant number of the cases.

Left-sided native valve endocarditis is most commonly caused by streptococci (Viridans streptococci 30–40%; *Enterococcus* species, 5–18%; others, 15–25%), staphylococci cause 20% to 35% of cases mostly from *S. aureus*, with few cases of *S. epidermidis*; and aerobic gram-negative bacilli causes 1.5% to 13%. Intravenous drug users are particularly susceptible to *S. aureus* infection of the tricuspid valve.

Empiric therapy for community-acquired native valve endocarditis must include an antimicrobial active against viridans streptococci; therefore, penicillin plus gentamicin (low-dose 1 mg/kg every 8 hours) is administered. Coverage for *S. aureus* with nafcillin may be added depending on the clinical presentation and risk factors. First-generation cephalosporins can be substituted for nafcillin/penicillin combination in the penicillin-allergic patient. Vancomycin should be reserved for MRSA and for patients who have anaphylaxis hypersensitivity reactions to β-lactams. The duration of therapy is usually 4 to 6 weeks. The addition of low-dose gentamicin is to achieve synergy with nafcillin against *S. aureus* and may decrease the period of fever and positive blood cultures. The synergistic combination of nafcillin/gentamicin may also decrease the total duration of therapy in select patients with right-sided endocarditis from 4 weeks to 2 weeks. For streptococcal endocarditis (nonenterococcal), penicillin plus gentamicin is the regimen of choice. The addition of gentamicin may decrease required treatment duration to 2 weeks, whereas enterococcal endocarditis treatment is always prolonged (4–6 weeks) because it is difficult to cure. Therapy must continue with the combination of penicillin or ampicillin (or vancomycin in penicillin-allergic patients) plus gentamicin because the penicillin alone is not bactericidal against the enterococcus. Gentamicin is the aminoglycoside of choice; however, increasing resistance to gentamicin is being observed, such that all strains causing endocarditis should have susceptibility testing.

Prosthetic valve endocarditis is usually subdivided into two stages: early (less than 2 months postoperative) and late. Staging this infection is important because the bacteriology is different in these two groups. In early prosthetic valve endocarditis, *S. epidermidis* (27%), *S. aureus* (20%), aerobic gram-negative bacilli (19%), and fungi (13%) are the most common organisms. Empiric therapy must include vancomycin for MRSA and MRSE as well as an aminoglycoside. If *S. epidermidis* is isolated, rifampin, 300 mg orally twice a day; may be added. Unfortunately, valve replacement is frequently required, with streptococcal infections having the best prognosis. Late endocarditis is usually caused by streptococci, but staphylococci and gram-negative bacilli are not uncommon. Therefore, empiric therapy for late prosthetic valve endocarditis needs to include coverage for all of these organisms.

References

1. Morgan AS: Risk factors for infection in the trauma patient. J Natl Med Assoc 1992; 84:1019.
2. The American Hospital Formulary Service: Drug Information '92. McEvoy GK (Ed). Bethesda, MD, American Hospital Pharmacists, Inc, 1992.
3. Sande MA, Kapusnik-Uner JE, Mandell GL: Chemotherapy of microbial diseases. *In*: Goodman and Gilman's The Pharmacological Basis of Therapeutics. 8th ed. Gilman AG, Rall TW, Nies AS, et al (Eds). New York, Pergamon Press, 1990, p 1018.
4. Kunin CM: Resistance to antimicrobial drugs: A worldwide calamity. Ann Intern Med 1993; 118:557.
5. Appelbaum PC: Antimicrobial resistance in *Streptococcus pneumoniae*: An overview. Clin Infect Dis 1992; 15:77.
6. Hackbarth CJ, Chaambers HF: Methicillin-resistant staphylococci: Genetics and mechanisms of resistance. Antimicrob Agents Chemother 1989; 33:991.
7. Livermore DM: Determinants of activity of beta-lactamase inhibitor combinations. J Antimicrob Chemother 1993; 31(Suppl A):9.
8. Mandell GL, Sande MA: Antimicrobial agents: Penicillins, cephalosporins, and other beta-lactam antibiotics. *In*: Goodman and Gilman's The Pharmacological Basis of Therapeutics. 8th ed. Gilman AG, Rall TW, Nies AS, et al (Eds). New York, Pergamon Press, 1990, p 1065.
9. Lebel MH, Hoyt MJ, McCracken GH Jr: Comparative efficacy of ceftriaxone and cefuroxime for treatment of bacterial meningitis. J Pediatr 1989; 114:1049.
10. Pizzo PA, Hathorn JW, Hiemenz J, et al: A randomized trial comparing ceftazidime alone with combination antibiotic therapy in cancer patients with fever and neutropenia. N Engl J Med 1986; 315:552.
11. Park HZ, Lee SP, Schy AL: Ceftriaxone-associated gallbladder sludge. Gastroenterol 1991; 100:1665.
12. Pestotnik SL, Classen DC, Evans RS, et al: Prospective surveillance of imipenem/cilastatin use and associated seizures using a hospital information system. Ann Pharmacother 1993; 27:497.
13. Aronoff GR, Pottratz ST, Brier ME, et al: Aminoglycoside accumulation kinetics in rat renal parenchyema. Antimicrob Agents Chemother 1983; 23:74.
14. Watling SM, Dasta JF: Aminoglycoside dosing considerations in intensive care unit patients. Ann Pharmacother 1993; 27:351.
15. Prins JM, Buller HR, Kuiijpeer EJ, et al: Once versus thrice daily gentamicin in patients with serious infections. Lancet 1993; 341:335.
16. Kapusnik JE, Hackbarth CJ, Chambers HF, et al: Single, large, daily dosing versus intermittent dosing of tobramycin for treating experimental pseudomonas pneumonia. J Infect Dis 1988; 158:7.
17. Fekety R, Shah AB: Diagnosis and treatment of *Clostridium difficile* colitis. JAMA 1993; 269:71.
18. Hackbarth CJ, Chambers HF: Methicillin-resistant staphylococci: Detection methods and treatment of infections. Antimicrob Agents Chemother 1989; 33:995.
19. Newfield P, Roizen MF: Hazards of rapid administration of vancomycin. Ann Intern Med 1979; 91:581.
20. Freeman CD, Quintiliani R, Nightingale CH: Vancomycin therapeutic drug monitoring: Is it necessary? Ann Pharmacother 1993; 27:594.
21. Lee BL, Padula AM, Kimbrough RC, et al: Infectious complications with respiratory pathogens despite ciprofloxacin therapy. N Engl J Med 1991; 325:520.
22. Ball P: Emergent resistance to ciprofloxacin amongst *Pseudomonas aeruginosa* and *Staphylococcus aureus*. Clinical significance and therapeutic approaches. J Antimicrob Chemother 1990; 26(Suppl F):165.
23. Marchbanks CR: Drug-drug interactions with fluoroquinolones. Pharmacother 1993; 13:23S.
24. Sanford JP: Guide to Antimicrobial Therapy 1993. Dallas, TX, Antimicrobial Therapy, Inc, 1994.
25. Scheld WM, Mandell GL: Nosocomial pneumonia: Pathogenesis and recent advances in diagnosis and therapy. Rev Infect Dis 1991; 9:743S.
26. Schaad UB, Lips U, Gnehm HE, et al: Dexamethasone therapy for bacterial meningitis in children: Swiss Meningitis Study Group. Lancet. 1993; 342:457.

CHAPTER 134

Infections After Solid Organ Transplantation

Peter Linden, MD, DMD

Infections occurring after allograft transplantation are still generally acknowledged to be a major variable contributing to organ recipient morbidity and mortality.[1, 2] A reciprocal relationship between allograft viability and infection is often apparent; allograft dysfunction caused by technical errors often manifests as infection (e.g., cholangitis resulting from hepatic allograft vascular compromise or urosepsis complicating a ureteral anastomotic leak in a kidney recipient). Alternatively, infectious complications may adversely affect the allograft either directly (cytomegalovirus [CMV] hepatitis in hepatic grafts) or indirectly, as in the case of rejection that ensues after the withdrawal or tapering of immunosuppression in the face of overwhelming nonopportunistic or opportunistic infection. Superimposed on a 20-year trend of decreasing overall 1- and 5-year post-transplant mortality rates, infection remains the leading primary or associated cause of mortality for all categories of organ transplantation.[1] Nevertheless, there have been enormous advances made over the past 15 years that have created a more favorable standard of care. These have included, in part, the chemoprophylaxis of viral (herpes simplex, CMV) disease and protozoa *(Pneumocystis carinii)* infection, improved surgical techniques, and the more refined utilization of conventional cyclosporine-based immunosuppression plus the introduction of alternative agents, including FK-506.[3] The development of large tertiary care centers with coordinated organ transplantation programs has also accelerated the "learning curve" of knowledge, thus favoring the early diagnosis and treatment of post-transplant infection. The net effect of these interventions has, to a certain extent, diminished the incidence of life-threatening infection in allograft recipients. In addition, these innovations have also altered the frequency, timing, clinical presentation, and outcome of certain post-transplant infections.

One should, however, not underestimate the continuing challenges that include evolving drug-resistant bacteria, fungi, and viruses; a progressively sicker candidate population; and the undertaking of more prolonged, contaminated surgery with the intestinal and multivisceral transplants. A contemporaneous discussion of this dynamic and complicated aspect of the post-transplant period must consider these relevant features and the new trends they are establishing.

TABLE 134–1. Rates of Serious Infection Based on the Category of Solid Organ Transplant*

Transplant Category	*Institution*	*Years*	*Infections (%)*⁺	*Associated Mortality (%)*
Liver	Pittsburgh	1985–1987	83	23
Liver	Mayo Clinic	1984–1985	53	9
Liver	Baylor	1988–1989	47	8
Kidney	Minnesota	1987–1990	65	8
Kidney	Netherlands	1985–1986	26	NA
Heart	Loyola	1986	67	0
Heart	Multicenter	1980–1987	57	5

*Cyclosporine-treated recipients only.
⁺Major infections.
Abbreviation: NA = not available.

EPIDEMIOLOGY OF POST-TRANSPLANT INFECTION

The rate of occurrence of serious infection in organ recipients is illustrated in Table 134–1, which summarizes infection rates from several major series of organ recipients within the past 10 years.[4–10] The frequency and severity of infections are clearly a function of the type of transplanted organ, with both heart-lung and liver recipients experiencing higher overall rates of infection and infection-related mortality. The extensive nature of both the liver and heart-lung transplant surgical procedure and its required immunosuppressive intensity contribute significantly to their higher rates of serious infection when compared with kidney transplants. Early limited aggregate data on intestinal transplants also demonstrate a very high rate of infection-related mortality. Variance among medical centers is, in part, secondary to both candidate selection policies and the intensity and quality of immunosuppression regimens.

TEMPORAL PATTERN OF POST-TRANSPLANT INFECTION

The time course of infections in the post-transplant period is conveniently grouped into three consecutive but overlapping periods: (1) early infections within the first post-transplant month, (2) a middle period between the second and sixth months, and (3) late infections that may occur sporadically during the lifetime of the recipient. This stereotypic pattern was conveniently fabricated into a timetable for kidney recipients 15 years ago[11] and remains applicable today for all solid organ recipient groups. Early, middle, and late infections are summarized in Table 134–2. The most severe and life-threatening infections also tend to cluster within the first 4 months of transplantation. Biologic and iatrogenic factors act together to establish this temporal pattern of infection. The disruption of anatomic barriers, establishment of artificial vascular and excretory (urine, bile) anastomoses, and the sheer duration of surgery are major predisposing factors for early postoperative infection.[5] Pretransplant host conditions (diabetes, uremia, alcoholism, liver failure, malnutrition, and immunosuppression) whose effects are carried through into the postoperative period may impair wound healing and further compromise local host defenses. Infections present or incubating before the transplantation may become manifest clinically only after the transplant procedure. Allograft immunotolerance is lowest during the early months, thus requiring both higher baseline and supplemental immunosuppression to prevent and treat rejection. Early primary dysfunction of the allograft, especially in liver and heart-lung recipients, may culminate in either single or multiple system organ failure and enhance the risk for infection.

Early infections within the first month are most commonly postoperative superficial or deep wound infections. Bacterial pathogens derived from the host's endogenous or antibiotic-modified flora predominate. However, fungal infections, particularly *Candida* species and *Torulopsis,* also pose a serious threat. Reactivated mucocutaneous herpes simplex infections are classically associated with this early period as well. However, the utilization of acyclovir prophylaxis has reduced the frequency of this complication.

During the intermediate period (months 2–6), there are several major categories of infection that classically have their onset, most important of which is the presentation of serious viral infection and disease. CMV is, by far, the most

TABLE 134–2. Common Infections After Solid Organ Transplantation Based on the Time of Presentation

Early (Weeks 1–4)
All Solid Organ Recipients
Superficial wound infection
Bacterial pneumonia
Urinary tract infection
Catheter infection
Kidney Recipients
Pyelonephritis
Perinephric/parenchymal abscess
Liver Recipients
Cholangitis
Intra-abdominal abscess
Peritonitis
Hepatic abscess
Heart and Heart-Lung Recipients
Sternal wound infection
Mediastinitis
Empyema
Middle (Months 2–6)
Cytomegalovirus
Epstein-Barr Virus (PTLD)
Legionellosis
Tuberculosis
Nocardia
Aspergillus
Pneumocystis
Late (After 6 Months)
Pneumocystis
Cryptococcosis
Herpes Zoster Virus
CMV Retinitis
Community-Acquired Pathogens
Streptococcus pneumonia
Influenza

Abbreviations: PTLD = post-transplant lymphoproliferative disorder; CMV = cytomegalovirus.

common viral pathogen in organ recipients, with a wide range of presentations including febrile syndrome, focal invasive disease (pneumonia, hepatitis, or enteritis), and disseminated disease. Serious short-term sequelae of CMV disease include allograft rejection mediated either by CMV-induced up-regulation of allograft class II human lympocyte antigen (HLA) expression compounded by the iatrogenic tapering of immunosuppression. In addition, CMV disease appears to potentiate the subsequent risk for the development of other opportunistic infections (fungi, protozoa) probably mediated by viral-induced, cell-mediated dysfunction.[12, 13] The cumulative effects of iatrogenic immunosuppression, nosocomial epidemiologic exposure, and perhaps antibiotic pressure may culminate in serious, life-threatening infection as a result of certain bacteria (*Mycobacterium tuberculosis, Legionella, Listeria, Nocardia*), fungi (*Aspergillus, Cryptococcus*), and protozoa (*Pneumocystis, Toxoplasma gondii*).

Late infections are composed of a diverse spectrum of pathogens. The frequency and severity of infection in this period may be partially related to the intensity and duration of antecedent immunosuppressive therapy. Patients with chronic rejection and a high immunosuppressive requirement maintain a higher risk for late infections. Relapsing forms of infection such as bronchitis in lung recipients, cholangitis in patients undergoing liver grafts with biliary duct disease, and chronic urinary tract infections in kidney recipients are not uncommon. Endogenous reactivation of viruses (herpes zoster varicella, hepatitis B and C, Epstein-Barr virus [EBV]), and bacteria (*Mycobacterium tuberculosis*) are most common in this category. CMV chorioretinitis is well described in this late period[14] as is a more recent trend of late CMV infection in graft recipients treated with an intense CMV prophylaxis regimen.[15] Exogenous infections with community-acquired pathogens (influenza, *Streptococcus pneumoniae, Staphylococcus aureus*) also occur but potentially with a more fulminant course or atypical clinical presentation. *P. carinii* pneumonia was the most frequent protozoal pathogen with the highest attack rates in heart and heart-lung recipients. Trimethoprim-sulfamethoxasole (TMP-SMX) prophylaxis has significantly diminished this threat, but pneumocystosis sporadically occurs as a result of either physician withdrawal of TMP-SMX or patient noncompliance. Rarely, late technical complications such as hepatic artery thrombosis in a liver recipient may also occur and present as sepsis with enteric bacteremia or candidemia.

SOURCES OF PATHOGENS CAUSING CLINICAL DISEASE IN ORGAN RECIPIENTS

The organ recipient is susceptible to an enormously broad range of potential pathogens in large part because of the compromise of anatomic barriers and iatrogenic immunosuppression principally directed toward cell-mediated immunity. Placed in simple perspective, these pathogens are either endogenous (i.e., originating from within the host) or exogenous (i.e., newly acquired from the physical environment [human contacts or inanimate surroundings], allograft, or transfused blood products). A more subtle distinction is required, however, because certain organisms may either be exogenously acquired and cause early clinical disease (primary tuberculosis, CMV-positive allograft causing infection in a CMV-seronegative recipient) or endogenously acquired as a tissue-latent phase that is reactivated in the setting of host immunosuppression (reactivated pulmonary tuberculosis or CMV disease in a CMV-seropositive recipient).

Endogenous bacterial flora colonizes the mucosal surfaces of the upper respiratory, gastrointestinal, and genitourinary tracts as well as the skin surface (predominantly gram-positive flora). The composition of this "normal" flora is usually modified by exposure to the physical nosocomial environment (other patients via the healthcare worker vector). In addition, prior antibiotic usage favors the proliferation of multiresistant bacterial flora and overgrowth of *Candida* and *Aspergillus* species. This "modified endogenous flora" is a real concern because many allograft recipients have had an extended period of intensive care unit (ICU) or non-ICU nosocomial exposure during the donor search before their transplant procedure. This more virulent flora may be resistant to the routine antibacterial prophylaxis administered for the transplant procedure and may be more difficult to treat when causing active local or systemic infection. Examples include vancomycin-resistant *Enterococcus*, methicillin-resistant *S. aureus*, and multiresistant *Enterobacter* and *Pseudomonas* species.

Latent endogenous organisms are characteristically contained within certain organ tissues by an intact host cell–mediated immune system. After a variable period of cell-mediated immunosuppression, these organisms reactivate to cause clinical disease in the allograft recipient. Organisms with reactivation potential are represented in all the major categories including bacteria (*M. tuberculosis*), the herpesviruses (herpes simplex, varicella-zoster, CMV, and EBV), fungi (*histoplasmosis, Coccidioides*), protozoa (*Toxoplasma gondii*), and parasites (*Strongyloides stercoralis*). The probability of harboring these organisms is dependent on specific variables for each. For instance, geographic origin is the major determinant for having latent infection with *Coccidioides immitis* (southwestern United States) and *Strongyloides* (southeastern United States, Caribbean). However, seroprevalence studies demonstrate a uniformly high rate of latent infection for type I herpes simplex, varicella-zoster, and EBV, with greater than 95% of adults demonstrating seropositivity. CMV is an important exception, with a variable range of 40% to 100% of adults possessing serum immunoglobulin G antibodies indicative of a prior primary infection.[16] Laboratory evidence that confirms the presence of a tissue-latent phase for a particular organism before transplantation is crucial because it can prospectively guide prophylactic and diagnostic management in the post-transplant period. These may include isoniazid prophylaxis for candidates with positive purified protein derivative of tuberculin (PPD) skin tests and CMV hyperimmune globulin for CMV-seronegative recipients of seropositive allografts. In contrast to bone marrow transplantation, the shortage of donor solid organs prevents the prospective matching of CMV-seronegative allografts exclusively for CMV-seronegative recipients.

Exogenous organisms may be transmitted to the organ recipient via the physical inanimate environment (air, water, bed linens, food), by direct contact with healthcare personnel, and from the donor allograft or transfused blood products. Outbreaks of infections with certain exogenous organisms among cohorted transplant patients can be the sentinel that a contaminated environmental source exists.[17] Airborne spread of *Aspergillus* spores from hospital construction and recirculated ventilation patterns has been associated with well-documented cluster epidemics of invasive aspergillosis.[18, 19] *Cryptococcus, Mucorales, Histoplasma*, and many other less common fungi (*Dactylaria, Fusaria, Pseudoallescheria boydii*) invade via airborne lung entry. However, the precise environmental contact source is usually unknown. Exogenous bacterial pathogens to which transplant recipients are particularly vulnerable include *Legionella, Listeria monocytogenes*, and *Nocardia* species. Best described are nosocomial outbreaks of pneumonia caused by

Legionella pneumophila, L. micdadei, and several other species from a contaminated hospital hot-water supply.[20, 21] However, because *Legionella* bacteria are fairly ubiquitous community pathogens, sporadic cases of legionellosis may affect the organ recipient any time in the post-transplant period. Nocardiasis remains an uncommon infection, although prior series reported a somewhat higher incidence among cardiac and lung recipients. *Listeria* most commonly is transmitted via contaminated food sources and is still the most common bacterial central nervous system (CNS) pathogen among organ recipients. It has been speculated that the common use of TMP-SMX for the prophylaxis of pneumocystosis may afford incidental protection from these bacterial pathogens.[22]

The donor allograft represents a proven source of potential pathogens that is unique to the organ recipient population. Over the past 30 years, this route of transmission has generally been narrowed to either undetectable organisms or pathogens for which there is no prospective indication to eliminate the potential donor from consideration. Clinician knowledge of organisms in this latter group may still be significant for guiding subsequent prophylaxis in the recipient. Examples include CMV, toxoplasmosis, and the tracheal bacterial cultures of lung donors. Before the availability of screening methods, there were numerous reports of transmission of hepatitis B and C and human immunodeficiency virus-1 (HIV-1) with serious or fatal sequelae. Before the availability of HIV-1 screening in 1985, cases of donor-to-recipient HIV-1 transmission with rapid progression to full-blown acquired immunodeficiency syndrome (AIDS) were reported for all major solid organ transplant groups.[23, 24] HIV transmission has also rarely occurred since the use of systematic HIV antibody screening as a result of false-negative tests occurring in the "window" period of HIV seroconversion.[25] Further sophistication of HIV screening has largely eliminated HIV as a transmissible agent in the transplant setting. Serologic screening has drastically diminished the threat of donor transmission of this agent; however, hepatitis C transmission may still occur because of the significant window period when there is no detectable C antibody. Some transplant centers continue to use donor organs from hepatitis C–seropositive donors for recipients who are already seropositive for this virus. Rare but well-documented cases of proven donor-to-recipient transmission are reported for herpes simplex and tuberculosis.[26, 27]

ROLE OF IATROGENIC IMMUNOSUPPRESSION

The multicomponent immunosuppressive regimens required by all solid organ recipients for the prevention and treatment of allograft rejection are a key determinant for the development of post-transplant infection. The major immunosuppressants can be categorized as corticosteroids, cytotoxic/antiproliferative drugs including azathioprine and cyclophosphamide, and agents directed either at the CD4 lymphocyte (OKT3, antilymphocyte globulin or rabbit antithymocyte globulin) or at its lymphokine production (cyclosporine, FK-506). The "infection-potentiating" effect of any immunosuppressive drug has some specificity based on its immunologic targets. It is difficult, however, to attribute any given infection to one specific immunosuppressive agent because most regimens contain multiple immunosuppressants, and there are multiple other immunosuppressive and nonimmunosuppressive risk factors for the development of infection.

Corticosteroids cause a broad impairment of host defenses with effects on the neutrophil inflammatory response, macrophage antigen processing, antibody production, and cell-mediated immunity. These effects are, to some extent, both dose and duration dependent. This association is best illustrated by the fall in the incidence of both infections and infection-related mortality in kidney, liver, and heart recipients coincident with the introduction of cyclosporine, which allowed a relative reduction of the corticosteroid requirement.[28–30] Recent data from the University of Pittsburgh liver transplant program demonstrate a further decline in mortality caused by infections to only 7% for recipients administered FK-506–based immunosuppression, which appears primarily because of the corticosteroid-sparing effect.[3] Notably, steroids are not potent inducers of CMV disease or other invasive viral illnesses. Other relevant effects of steroid therapy in organ recipients include the impairment of wound healing and an altered clinical presentation that may result in a delayed diagnosis of serious infection.

Both cyclosporine and FK-506 appear to lower the risk-benefit ratio as it pertains to the risk of infectious complications. This effect is basically mediated by the diminished need for other immunosuppressants to prevent or treat rejection. Both agents selectively depress helper T lymphocyte interleukin-2 synthesis without depressing neutrophil, macrophage, or antibody-mediated defense.[31, 32] After the introduction of cyclosporine in 1980, multiple prospective or historically controlled trials consistently demonstrated a fall in the rates of serious bacterial and viral infection (although not fungal infection) compared with steroid/azathioprine/antilymphocyte regimen–treated recipient groups.[33] The availability of serum or blood cyclosporine level monitoring was a further refinement that allowed the individualization of dosing. The excellent therapeutic profile is further illustrated by the improvement in both allograft and actuarial organ recipient survival.[28–30] Moreover, the low rates of infection in cyclosporine-treated nonorgan recipients (i.e., autoimmune disease) are additional evidence of its favorable infection risk profile.[34]

Antilymphocyte therapy with either polyclonal (antilymphocyte globulin [ALG]) or monoclonal (murine OKT3) antibody is used at many transplant centers for either induction in the early post-transplant period or for treatment of steroid-refractory acute rejection. Several reports suggested higher rates of invasive CMV disease in kidney, liver, and heart recipients when compared either with historic or contemporaneous controls.[35, 36] EBV-mediated post-transplant lymphoproliferative disorder (PTLD) was also highly associated with a prior course of OKT3 or sequential use of Minnesota ALG and OKT3 in kidney recipients.[37, 38]

Recent evidence from the Birmingham liver transplant program demonstrates that complete withdrawal of corticosteroids could be accomplished after 3 months in 85% of recipients without excess rejection or allograft loss.[39] O'Connell and colleagues reported successful steroid-free maintenance in cardiac recipients receiving cyclosporine-based immunosuppression.[40] The ability to detect a state of host-donor chimerism in liver recipients lays the groundwork for further studies that investigate achieving host immunotolerance without incurring the infection-producing risks of iatrogenic immunosuppression.[41]

INFECTIONS RELATED TO THE TRANSPLANT PROCEDURE

The category of organ transplantation is a major determinant for the sites of infection, particularly in the early post-transplant period. Both the allograft organ and the contiguous tissue structures are especially vulnerable to infection for a variety of reasons relating to retained fluid collections, foreign bodies, and technical complications. Such infections merit separate discussion based on the type of transplant. In contrast, certain opportunistic infections occur in all types of transplant recipients because all are exposed to exogenous organisms from similar sources (donor graft, blood products, nosocomial, and community physical environments), and all uniformly require varying degrees of T cell–directed immunosuppression. Therefore, a separate pathogen-based discussion for these infections with an emphasis on notable differences between organ transplant types is also presented subsequently.

Kidney Transplantation

The most common infectious problems are urinary tract infections (UTIs), with some series demonstrating rates exceeding 40% within the first year of transplantation. Independent risk factors include prolonged bladder catheterization, degree of organ mismatch, patient age, and presence of prior urologic complications. The spectrum of infecting organisms does not differ from that causing native UTI with aerobic gram-negative bacilli and enterococci predominating. UTI occurring earlier are characteristically more refractory to conventional therapy and associated with more severe sequelae (pyelonephritis, bacteremia, and sepsis) than those occurring after the third post-transplant month. Both symptomatic and asymptomatic infections merit aggressive therapy. Appropriate management includes 4 to 6 weeks of antibiotic therapy, removal of the bladder drainage catheter if possible, and post-therapy follow-up urine cultures. Tapering of immunosuppression is rarely indicated except in the settings of superimposed sepsis. Recurrent infections or relapse with the same organism should prompt a search for structural sources (parenchymal abscess) and functional abnormalities (ureterovesical reflux, urethral stricture, neurogenic bladder). Rarely, graft nephrectomy is indicated for complicated upper tract infection. Prophylaxis with TMP-SMX or ciprofloxacin has shown a clear reduction in the rate of early UTI.[42]

Wound infection rates in most series are generally within the expected range for clean contaminated surgery (5–10%) with appropriate antibiotic prophylaxis. Preoperative host risk factors include poorly controlled uremia, diabetes, and malnutrition. The majority of wound infections are superficial and easily treatable with antibiotics and drainage. Postoperative hematomas, lymphoceles, and urinomas resulting from technical errors greatly potentiate the risk for deep perinephric wound infection. These may have devastating consequences, including mycotic aneurysm formation of the vascular pedicle, sepsis, and graft failure. Transplant nephrectomy is often the only life-saving measure for deep perinephric space infections. Rare causes of early infections in kidney recipients are also described, including direct transmission of infectious agents via the donor kidney such as tuberculosis and herpes simplex,[26, 27] primary or reactivated papovavirus infection manifesting as a ureteral stenosis,[43] hemorrhagic pyelonephritis caused by adenovirus,[44] and deep wound infection with *Mycoplasma hominis*.[45]

Liver Transplantation

Serious infectious complications after liver transplantation are most likely to occur within the first 4 to 6 postoperative weeks. Surgical entry into the biliary tree and proximal gastrointestinal tract is a necessary but predisposing cause of the high infection rates postoperatively. Such infections are principally intra-abdominal and closely related to a number of factors, including duration of surgery, type and viability of the biliary anastomosis, and adequacy of vascular supply via a reconstructed recipient to host the hepatic arterial system.

Duration of Surgery

A prospective analysis from the University of Pittsburgh demonstrated a significant correlation between the number of operative hours (composed of the transplant operation alone or subsequent surgery, or both) with the number of episodes of infection and the probability of deep-seated fungal infection.[5] Such a relationship probably captures multiple inherent risk factors for which operative time is an easily measurable marker, including hemorrhage, technical difficulties, and the risk of intra-abdominal contamination with endogenous flora.

Type and Viability of the Biliary Anastomosis

A second operation (retransplantation or duct revision) requiring a choledochojejunostomy anastomosis is also associated with a significantly higher infection rate than choledochocholedochostomy.[5] Serious intra-abdominal infection may occur secondary to a bile leak or biliary obstruction. Leakage of bile may manifest as fever or sepsis with or without enteric bacteremia and usually presents within the first 2 weeks after transplantation. An elevated serum bilirubin is characteristic and occasionally mistaken for acute rejection. Underlying reasons for a bile leak are usually either vascular insufficiency or are purely technical in nature. Management includes early surgical correction or temporary external biliary drainage along with appropriate antibiotic therapy.[46] Biliary obstruction usually presents later and is most commonly due to anastomotic stenosis or intrahepatic strictures.

Adequacy of Vascular Supply Via a Reconstructed Recipient to Host Hepatic Arterial System

Thrombosis of the hepatic artery may present as relapsing enteric bacteremias, hepatic abscess, fulminant hepatic necrosis, or indolent breakdown of the extrahepatic biliary anastomosis or intrahepatic biliary tree.[47] The quality and intensity of immunosuppression probably are not major inciting risk factors for these infections; however, continued immunosuppression may contribute to poor healing and impair recovery from a serious pyogenic infection.

Heart and Lung Transplantation

The most significant sites of infection after heart, lung, or heart-lung transplantation involve the lung parenchyma and other compartments of the chest cavity (pleural space, mediastinum). Independent risk factors for early infection include prolonged cardiopulmonary bypass time, prior implantation of an artificial heart device, and the presence of oral flora in the donor tracheal culture in lung recipients.[48–50] Mediastinitis is an uncommon but potentially devastating complication in heart recipients, with an incidence ranging from 2.5% to 2.8% in two recent series[48, 49] and a higher incidence of attributable mortality. Risk factors include prior sternotomy, early post-transplant hemorrhage, staphylococcal pneumonitis, diabetes, and early rejection. The inciting origins are either primary contamination at transplantation, a sternal wound infection, or leakage of secretions from the tracheal anastomosis into the peritracheal tissue in lung recipients. *S. aureus* or *S. epidermidis* are predominant; however, gram-negative bacteria and other less common causes, including *M. hominis*[51] and *Nocardia*,[52] have been reported. Presenting local signs include incisional erythema or purulent drainage and an unstable sternum.

Computed tomographic (CT) scanning provides confirmatory evidence in most cases. Successful management can be achieved in the majority of cases with a combination of systemic antibiotics and open debridement with irrigation or closure using muscle flaps. Lung and heart-lung recipients have a high disposition to bacterial pneumonia as a result of, for example, compromised secretion clearance, anastomotic breakdown, the loss of lymphatic drainage, donor inoculum of organisms, and pretransplant conditions predisposing to chronic lung infection such as cystic fibrosis or obstructive lung disease. Pneumonia may occur as early as the second post-transplant day. Diagnostic confusion with early acute graft rejection is not uncommon. However, this distinction is best made by careful clinical and laboratory examination. Therapy is guided by knowledge of donor trachea cultures and cultures obtained from the distal airways via bronchoscopic lavage or brushing.

Pancreas Transplantation

Cumulative early experience with pancreatic transplantation has shown a high rate of serious intra-abdominal infections with significant associated mortality.[53] The majority of such complications are deep wound infections arising in the retroperitoneum or frank peritonitis. Both allograft pancreatitis secondary to ischemic preservation injury or operative trauma and bowel contamination are the principal mechanisms. For these reasons, the donor pancreatic ampulla is now commonly anastomosed to the recipient bladder to reduce the degree of abdominal contamination. Pancreaticocystostomy has resulted in significantly lower rates of serious infection and improved allograft survival.

Bowel and Multivisceral Transplantation

Transplantation of the small intestines with or without other intra-abdominal viscera is associated with the highest rates of early infection among all categories of solid organ transplantation.[54] This association results from the extensive and prolonged nature of the surgery and the heavy immunosuppression required to control the strong tendency for allograft rejection. There is a high incidence of apparent intestinal translocation of enteric bacteria and fungi as a result of intraluminal overgrowth and loss of mucosal integrity caused by concomitant graft rejection. Paradoxically, immunosuppression must be intensified during these episodes to restore intestinal integrity.[55]

OPPORTUNISTIC INFECTIONS IN THE SOLID ORGAN RECIPIENT

Opportunistic Bacteria

Infections with opportunistic bacteria may occur either in an epidemic fashion, usually in the nosocomial setting, or as sporadic cases, usually in the late post-transplant period. Many opportunistic bacteria are pathogenic, even in those with normal host defense. However, the immunocompromised organ recipient is notable for several aspects including a higher attack rate after exposure, a more virulent and therapy-refractory course, and an altered clinical presentation in comparison to immunocompetent hosts. This enhanced virulence is partially due to the inherent property of facultative intracellular growth, which, in the setting of cell-mediated immunosuppression, results in overwhelming infection.

Legionellosis

Within several years after the 1976 Philadelphia legionnaires' disease epidemic, there came several reports of nosocomial legionellosis in renal transplant units with significant morbidity and mortality figures.[21, 56] Since that time, there has been a rapid growth of knowledge pertaining to the prevention of legionellosis with hyperchlorination of the hospital water supply, better diagnostic techniques, and emphasis on early effective treatment. Nevertheless, *Legionella* remains a low-frequency pathogen that is more often a late community-acquired infection, although nosocomial epidemics resulting from undetected failure of the water eradication system are still described. Thus, any case of *Legionella* in a transplant unit should prompt a search for nosocomial sources. *L. pneumophila*, serogroup 1, causes the vast majority (80–90%) of cases, with other *L. pneumophila* serogroups and *L. micdadei* accounting for most others. Direct aerosolization into the distal airways and aspiration of contaminated water are believed to be the principal modes of acquisition.[57] Early reports emphasized a high prevalence of nonspecific clinical and laboratory signs (nonproduction of sputum, diarrhea, hyponatremia, elevated transaminase levels, and de novo renal insufficiency); however, current opinion derived from aggregate experience has diminished their prospective diagnostic value.[57] The overwhelming majority of transplant recipients with legionellosis will still manifest a high-grade fever even in the presence of corticosteroid administration. Chest radiographic findings in the transplant recipient are typically uni- or multilobar alveolar infiltrates that do not differ much from normal hosts, although early cavitation appears to be more frequently described among immunosuppressed patients.[58] In recent years, extrapulmonary *Legionella* infection, including cellulitis, sternal wound infection, prosthetic endocarditis, and peritonitis, have been reported. Such evidence demonstrates the true systemic nature and possible extrapulmonary portals of entry for this organism.

Diagnosis necessitates a high index of suspicion because special microbiologic stains and culture methods are required. Rapidly available tests are most valuable because they may prompt early therapeutic intervention. Direct fluorescent antibody examination of respiratory secretions was the most frequently used rapid method, but it has only 50% sensitivity. Both the legionella gene probe, which detects all *Legionella* species with excellent sensitivity and specificity, and the urine radioimmunoassay for the detection of antigenuria, have superior sensitivity and even remain positive during early therapy. *Legionella* culture still remains the "gold standard." However, growth requires special media (buffered charcoal yeast agar) and may not be positive until the fifth day. *Legionella* bacteremia is detectable in up to 20% of documented pneumonia cases but also requires specific communication with the microbiology laboratory because special subplating methods are required. Treatment delay is poorly tolerated in transplant recipients and should be started on an empiric basis for clinically suspected cases. Intravenous erythromycin (4 g/d) has the longest cumulative record of success, although no prospective comparative trials against other in vitro effective agents are available. Coadministration of rifampin is recommended for severe cases or refractory disease. Interference with cyclosporine or FK-506 metabolism is well described for both erythromycin and rifampin, which presents a unique problem for the organ recipient. Close monitoring of drug levels is recommended for guiding appropriate immunosuppressive dosage. Agents with less or no drug interference that appear promising for the treatment of *Legionella* include the quinolones (ciprofloxacin, ofloxacin) and the new generation macrolide antibiotic, clarithromycin.[59, 60] Duration of treatment should be a minimum of 21 days because relapses are described with shorter courses. Cavitary disease or slow responders may require longer periods of therapy.

Tuberculosis

The incidence of *M. tuberculosis* disease among solid organ recipients is higher than in the general population but still relatively low. Two large series of renal recipients from Denver and Minnesota showed an occurrence of only three cases each of a total recipient population of 400 and 845, respectively.[61, 62] A study over a 9-year period of liver transplantation at the University of Pittsburgh revealed only five documented cases from a total of 2380 recipients.[63] These observations are somewhat unexpected because of the number of risk factors favoring a higher incidence of reactivated tuberculosis (TB). These include pretransplant chronic conditions associated with TB (alcoholism, uremia, cirrhosis, and steroid therapy), organ recipients from endemic countries, and post-transplant immunosuppression. The actual incidence is probably higher because of missed diagnosis ante mortem and a falling postmortem exam rate at many transplant centers. Moreover, the rising incidence of TB over the past decade in both the general population and other immunocompromised groups, such as the HIV infected, may favor higher rates of TB in the organ recipient population in the future. The majority of tuberculous disease in transplant recipients is due to the reactivation of latent endogenous foci. However, systematic cohorting of hospitalized transplant patients and a poor primary T cell containment response resulting from immunosuppression make the organ recipient extremely susceptible to primary disease after exposure to an active case of pulmonary disease.

Nosocomial outbreaks are described with fulminant progressive primary disease and high mortality rates.[64] The spectrum of clinical presentation is more diverse, with the incidence of disseminated disease in one study of kidney recipients[65] as high as 38.7% with a 59.8% rate of extrapulmonary disease compared with 17.5% of cases in the overall U.S. population.[66] Other atypical features in transplant recipients include middle and lower lobe reactivated pulmonary disease, poorly visible or absent tissue granulomas, a high rate of bone and joint disease, and transmission to the recipient via reactivation in the donor organ.[67] Diagnostic methodology is no different than that for TB in the general population. However, the value of the PPD skin test is significantly diminished because of the high prevalence of cutaneous anergy. Prior bacille Calmette-Guérin vaccination may cause a positive PPD reaction; however, this does not necessarily confer immunity among adult organ recipients. Preliminary data from two new diagnostic modalities, gene probe and polymerase chain reaction, appear promising.

No data from prospective trials of antituberculous therapy among organ recipients are available. Standard treatment with a minimum of three first-line agents (isoniazid [INH], rifampin, ethambutol, pyrazinamide) is generally used, with excellent treatment success even with continued immunosuppression. The efficacy of 6-month regimens for transplant recipients is unknown and thus cannot be recommended at present. It is imperative to implement full respiratory isolation measures (negative-pressure, closed room, and proper mask wearing) for suspected or documented pulmonary disease with positive acid-fast bacilli smears. Infectivity should rapidly wane within 1 to 2 weeks of initiating appropriate antituberculous therapy. Recipients with risk factors for isoniazid resistance or multidrug resistance such as isoniazid prophylaxis failure, prior incomplete therapy, or foreign natives will require broader empiric regimens until definitive susceptibility results are available. Treatment may be problematic because of isoniazid and rifampin hepatotoxicity, particularly in the liver recipient, and the potentiation of cyclosporine and FK-506 metabolism by rifampin.

Atypical mycobacteria are less common opportunistic bacterial pathogens in solid organ recipients. The most common organism in this category is *Mycobacterium kansasii* for which there are numerous reports of both focal and disseminated invasive disease. Others include *M. haemophilum, M. chelonei, M. marianum,* and *M. avium-intracellulare.* In contrast to tuberculosis, these organisms are not capable of person-to-person spread, and thus cases with pulmonic involvement do not require respiratory isolation measures. Treatment is multifaceted with both multidrug chemotherapy directed by susceptibility testing and surgical debridement in some instances.

Nocardiasis

Nocardia asteroides is a gram-positive or modified acid-fast–positive, rod-shaped structure with characteristic beading and branching morphology. Despite its ubiquitous environmental presence, the documented incidence of infection in the transplant population has always been quite low. Over the past decade, speculation has existed that the widespread use of sulfa prophylaxis for *P. carinii* may have further diminished the incidence of nocardiasis; however, this remains unproven. Qualitative improvements in immunosuppression may also be instrumental, because a recent series of nocardiosis in renal transplant recipients demonstrated a 0.7% incidence in the postcyclosporine era compared with a rate of 2.6% in precyclosporine era controls.[68] *Nocardia* bacteria usually gain entry via inhalation of aerosolized organisms with secondary hematogenous spread most commonly to the CNS, skin, and subcutaneous tissues, although involvement in any viscera is described. Initial clinical presentation is most frequently a subacute febrile illness with clinical and radiographic pulmonic disease. In the minority of patients, the pulmonary focus is silent and only a skin, CNS, or other visceral manifestation is present. *Nocardia* species grow aerobically on routine blood agar, but their growth properties are slower than most bacteria. Thus, early notification of the microbiology laboratory that there is clinical suspicion of nocardiasis may be instrumental in detecting the organism. Because of its low rate of occurrence, there are no prospective trials comparing the therapeutic efficacy of agents with in vitro activity against species of *Nocardia.* Sulfa drugs (TMP-SMX, sulfisoxazole, or sulfadiazine) have the longest track record of success when used for an optimal duration of at least 3 to 6 months.[69, 70] Sulfa-intolerant individuals have responded to alternative agents including minocycline and amoxicillin/clavulanic acid.

Opportunistic Fungal Infection

Infection secondary to opportunistic fungi continues to have the highest associated case fatality rates among all the categories of infectious agents in the solid organ recipient. Despite improved survival in the cyclosporine era, there was no measured decrease in the incidence of fungal infection in a recent combined series of kidney and heart recipients.[33] The incidence of fungal infections is highest among liver recipients and is progressively lower among heart-lung, heart, and kidney recipients, respectively.[71] *Candida, Aspergillus,* and *Cryptococcus* constitute greater than 90% of all fungal infection. *Candida* species bacteria are the predominant cause in all organ transplant groups with the exception of heart recipients, who have a higher incidence of *Aspergillus* infection.[72] Other less common fungal species that have become increasingly recognized pathogens include *Mucorales* and other filamentous, nonpigmented fungi *(Fusarium, Curvularia, Trichosporon beigleii)* and pigmented fungi *(Dactylaria).* Finally, fungi with a strong geographic concentration, termed *endemic,* such as *Coccidioides, Histoplasma,* and *Blastomyces,* may occasionally cause either reactivated disease in organ recipients native to these regions or progressive primary infection after initial exposure. The discussion is limited to post-transplant infection resulting from the major fungal pathogens *Candida*, *Aspergillus*, and *Cryptococcus*.

Candida Infection

Invasive disease secondary to *Candida* species remains the most common type of fungal infection in the organ transplant population. Such infection is most often diagnosed within the first 2 to 3 post-transplant months when recent surgery and other fungal selection factors have their strongest influence. The majority of *Candida* infections are believed to arise from the host's endogenous intestinal flora. However, cluster outbreaks of non–*Candida albicans* infections suggest that transmission from exogenous sources may occur as well. Risk factors for candidiasis have been most extensively studied in the liver transplant population. A multivariate analysis of 91 fungal infections among 355 liver recipients demonstrated the following as statistically significant risk factors: retransplantation, reintubation, severe illness at time of transplant, higher intraoperative transfusion requirements, choledochojejunostomy biliary reconstruction, and post-transplant course complicated by bacterial infection, antibiotic use, and vascular problems related to the graft.[73]

The spectrum of infectious disease caused by *Candida* species ranges from mucosal involvement only (stomatitis, esophagitis, cystitis) to bloodstream infection indicative usually of either a catheter-related source or true multivisceral invasion. The crude mortality rates associated with candidemia in immunocompromised patients still range upward of 50%.[74, 75] However, the sensitivity of candidemia as an indicator of deep-seated disease is notoriously poor, with only 30% to 40% of patients with postmortem invasive disease having a demonstrable candidemia. Conversely, candidemia should never be managed presumptively as either a transient event or as a catheter-related source for which only simple catheter removal is performed. There are few other specific signs of candidiasis in the organ recipient population; nodular skin lesions and retinal infiltrates are occasionally seen in the oncologic population but only rarely observed in the transplant recipient. The presence of *Candida* at multiple sites (urine, respiratory, stool) has poor positive predictive value for the presence of a deep-seated *Candida* infection because many organ recipients have either preexisting colonization or experience de novo colonization in the post-transplant period.[76] However, the predictive value of non–*C. albicans* species *(Candida tropicalis)* in surveillance cultures for invasive disease has been shown to be higher than *C. albicans*.[77] Other reliable diagnostic tests include the histopathologic demonstration of yeast or pseudohyphae in deep tissue specimens or positive cultures from a sterile body site (e.g., ascites, pericardial fluid, joint fluid).

Superficial *Candida* infections (stomatitis, esophagitis) are usually responsive to nystatin or fluconazole, whereas severe cases may be treated with systemic amphotericin. The prognosis of invasive candidiasis infection still remains poor even in the setting of aggressive therapy. Amphotericin B at dose ranges of 0.5 to 1.0 $mg \cdot kg^{-1} \cdot d^{-1}$ remains the primary treatment modality. Improved outcome with the addition of 5-flucytosine has been reported. A recent clinical trial comparing fluconazole to amphotericin B for candidemia demonstrated equal efficacy.[78] Several species *(Candida krusei, Torulopsis glabrata)*, however, are fluconazole resistant. In addition, fluconazole may cause a rise in either cyclosporine or FK-506 levels because of the down-regulation of hepatic metabolism. The value of liposomal amphotericin preparations is currently undergoing prospective evaluation.

Aspergillus Infection

Aspergillus are filamentous fungi that are ubiquitous in the environment (soil, dust) and are capable of causing contamination of laboratory specimens, true colonization, or invasive disease. Conditions that favor the airborne release and spread of spores (hospital construction or heavy dust contamination in air conduits) clearly enhance the risk of aspergillosis in the post-transplant period. The vast majority of infections are secondary to two species: *Aspergillus fumigatus* and *Aspergillus flavus*. The primary host defense against aspergillosis consists of the alveolar macrophage, which contains the spore phase and the neutrophil, which has activity against the hyphal form.[79] Organ recipients are rendered vulnerable to invasive disease primarily because of the depression of the pulmonary mononuclear cell line (alveolar macrophage) and perhaps qualitative suppression of the neutrophil. The first 3 post-transplant months have the highest incidence because of the combined effects of high immunosuppression, antibiotic pressure, and nosocomial exposure. Invasive disease most commonly begins in the lungs as a febrile focal pneumonitis. The radiographic picture may also include solitary or multiple nodules with or without cavitation. Hemoptysis, although nonspecific, may be a clinical manifestation of angioinvasive pulmonary disease. Less common sites of primary inoculation include the sinuses, open surgical wounds, and the skin. Not uncommonly, the primary site of infection is either subclinical or undiagnosed, with the subsequent diagnosis established in distant organs as endocarditis, a cerebral abscess, or disseminated disease.

Establishing a definitive diagnosis of invasive aspergillosis can be difficult. The histopathologic demonstration of tissue-invasive hyphal forms with dichotomous 45°-angle branching remains the accepted gold standard. However, because less common pathogenic fungi may also have a similar morphologic appearance on tissue stains (e.g., *Pseudoallescheria boydii, Dactylaria, Alternaria, Fusaria*), concomitant growth of an *Aspergillus* species in the specimen confirms the diagnosis. The sole presence of an *Aspergillus* isolate in a respiratory specimen in the organ recipient still carries a fairly high positive predictive value for ongoing or incipient invasive aspergillosis.[80] Conversely, invasive aspergillosis may evolve without antecedent positive cultures in at least 20% of cases in one series.[81] Despite its well-known ability for hematogenous dissemination, *Aspergillus* rarely grows in routine or fungal blood cultures. Innovative methods for detecting aspergillosis including tests for metabolites and polymerase chain reaction are promising but still not widely available.

The prognosis for invasive aspergillosis in all organ recipient groups has remained uniformly grim, with attributable mortality in excess of 90% in several series. Responsible factors include difficulties in establishing an early diagnosis when disease is localized, a poor in vivo response to amphotericin B, and fatal relapse after the completion of amphotericin B. Recent reports demonstrate favorable experience with oral itraconazole and liposome formulations of amphotericin; however, the overall numbers are small.[82, 82a, 83] In addition to high-dose amphotericin (1 $mg \cdot kg^{-1} \cdot d^{-1}$), aggressive surgical measures should be considered in those patients in whom only local disease is suspected, such as a single-lung abscess or primary skin lesion.[84, 85] A respiratory *Aspergillus* isolate in the early and middle post-transplant periods should be interpreted with the bias that ongoing or incipient invasive disease is present, especially with a compatible clinical picture of unexplained radiographic infiltrates, fever, or sepsis. Measures to prevent aspergillosis have included preventing patient contact with the airborne spores with high-efficiency particulate air (HEPA) filtration, which has reduced both aspergillus colonization and disease in kidney recipients.[86] Localized prophylaxis with nebulized or intranasal amphotericin B appears promising in bone marrow and cancer patients but is untested in organ recipients. Finally, systemic prophylaxis with oral itraconazole is also undergoing clinical trials at present.

Cryptococcus Infection

Cryptococcus neoformans is a ubiquitous yeast pathogen that causes a sporadic low frequency of infection in all categories of solid organ recipients. Unlike *Candida* and *Aspergillus* infections, cryptococcosis may occur in the very late post-transplant period. No specific environmental or host risk factors have been discovered that favor the development of cryptococcal disease. Pretransplant harboring of the organism has been rarely demonstrated; however, routine screening with cryptococcal serology is not regarded as either cost-effective or clinically efficacious. The organism usually gains entry via inhalation of airborne yeast forms. Pulmonary manifestations are usually subclinical. However, on occasion, a febrile pneumonitis is evident. Early diagnosis and treatment of the infection at this stage may abort the development of the two most common sequelae; meningitis and disseminated disease. Other uncommon primary manifestations have included skin nodules, cellulitis, and retinitis. The meningeal syndrome is usually characterized by a subacute (weeks) progressive fever, headache, and visual disturbances with or without true meningism.

Cerebrospinal fluid (CSF) findings include a mononuclear pleocytosis of fewer than 500 cells, moderate elevation in protein, and a normal or mildly depressed glucose level. CSF cryptococcal antigen (latex agglutination) is invariably positive, whereas a positive India ink stain is present in 40% to 50% of patients. Head CT findings are variable. Findings may include noncommunicating hydrocephalus, meningeal enhancement, and rarely discrete lesions (cryptococcoma). Poor prognostic factors include a positive blood culture, high CSF cryptococcal antigen titer, and an attenuated CSF inflammatory response.[87] Combination therapy with amphotericin B ($0.5\ mg \cdot kg^{-1} \cdot d^{-1}$) and flucytosine ($150\ mg \cdot kg^{-1} \cdot d^{-1}$ divided every 6 hours) for a minimum of 6 weeks is recommended.[88] Intrathecal or intraventricular amphotericin B (0.1–0.5 mg/d) has been reported to enhance the clinical response in severe cases[89]; however, its independent contribution has not been rigorously studied. Fluconazole has shown equivalent efficacy in the AIDS population, and early noncomparative results in transplant patients are promising.[90, 91] Despite in vitro susceptibility of *Cryptococcus* to either amphotericin or fluconazole, clinical failures are not infrequent principally because of late presentation, mechanical CNS complications such as hydrocephalus, and late clinical relapse.

Viral Infections

The herpesvirus family constitutes the dominant group of viral pathogens in solid organ recipients largely because of their widespread prevalence as latent organisms in the general population and their capability for reactivation. Thus, both the donor organ and certain recipient tissues may harbor these potentially pathogenic viruses. All viruses in this family are implicated as important causes of post-transplant morbidity and mortality. These include herpes simplex virus (HSV), CMV, varicella-zoster virus (VZV), and EBV. A more recently identified virus, human herpesvirus-6, is recognized to cause reactivation infection in organ recipients; however, whether it produces a tissue invasive disease is still unknown.[92] Other significant viral pathogens include hepatitis B, hepatitis C, papovavirus, adenovirus, and papillomavirus. Our discussion focuses on infectious and other sequelae of the herpesviruses only.

Herpes Simplex Virus

Localized reactivated herpes simplex infections may occur in seropositive recipients usually during the early post-transplant period. Common sites include the oropharynx and genital mucocutaneous areas. Classically, lesions are painful vesicles; however, traumatized or unroofed lesions may appear as coalesced ulcers. Localized mucocutaneous HSV usually is responsive to intravenous or oral acyclovir therapy, which hastens healing, shortens the period of viral shedding, and may prevent progression to more serious disease.[93] Less commonly, disseminated cutaneous infection or visceral involvement (esophagitis, hepatitis, pneumonitis) may cause life-threatening sequelae. The more severe spectrum of HSV disease may represent a true primary infection in a seronegative recipient via HSV transmission from the donor organ. These infections may have a fulminant course with high mortality despite acyclovir therapy. Definitive diagnosis for any HSV infection requires the demonstration of typical multinucleated giant cells on either cytologic or histologic specimens, cytopathologic effect in viral cell culture, or immunofluorescent staining for HSV antigens. Low-dose oral acyclovir (200 mg twice daily) appears to offer HSV chemoprophylaxis.[94] Notably, not all solid organ transplant programs use this approach because of the relatively low frequency of serious HSV disease.

Varicella-Zoster Infection

The vast majority of adult solid organ recipients are VZV seropositive as a result of childhood chickenpox and are thus considered immune to an exogenous reinfection with varicella. Rare instances of primary varicella may occur in VZV-seronegative recipients after exposure to an incubating case of chickenpox. Such cases can be severe with interstitial pneumonitis–induced respiratory failure and multiple organ dissemination. Postexposure prophylaxis with varicella zoster immune globulin (administered within 72 hours of exposure) may abort or modify the primary varicella syndrome. Reactivated disease, commonly termed *herpes zoster* or *shingles*, occurs in organ recipients at a constant low frequency of 10% to 15%. The time of occurrence may be months or even years after transplantation. Single- or multidermatomal, painful vesicular eruption is the most common clinical manifestation. Although usually self-limited, some may progress from cutaneous disease to visceral dissemination. Early intervention with high-dose intravenous acyclovir ($30\ mg \cdot kg^{-1} \cdot d^{-1}$) may shorten the clinical syndrome, promote healing, and prevent progression to visceral dissemination in immunosuppressed patients.[95]

Cytomegalovirus Infection

CMV remains the most common single infectious agent in all categories of organ transplantation, with both early direct and delayed adverse effects on the host and graft function. McCarthy and colleagues demonstrated its significant economic impact as a result of extended hospitalization in a kidney recipient population.[96] The extended biologic effects of CMV infection and disease are many and include potentiation of the risk of subsequent fungal and protozoal infection, enhanced graft rejection as a result of increased class II HLA expression, and tapered immunosuppression.[97, 98] In addition, many have speculated that late graft dysfunction (vanishing bile duct syndrome in liver recipients, glomerulotubular damage in renal recipients, and atherosclerotic disease in cardiac grafts) are late sequelae of CMV disease.[99–101] The virus is either transmitted via the donor organ, and less frequently blood products or latent virus is reactivated. Seropositive recipients may have either a reactivation of the latent strain or superinfection with the donor strain. CMV infection may be defined as either asymptomatic, which only denotes evidence of either prior acquisition of the virus (positive serology) or viral shedding without symptoms, or symptomatic, also termed *disease*, in which the host has clinical, biochemical, virologic, or histopathologic findings of an active CMV process. The status of the recipient's native CMV immunity is a major determinant of the frequency and severity of CMV disease after transplantation;[102] CMV-seronegative recipients who sustain a primary CMV infection have a rate of symptomatic CMV infection as high as 70% in some series, more serious morbidity, and more frequent relapses than seropositive recipients with either reactivation or superinfection.

Immunosuppression with antilymphocyte therapy also potentiates the risk of CMV disease.[103] Symptomatic CMV disease tends to cluster between the second and sixth posttransplant months with or without CMV-directed chemoprophylaxis. Clinical presentation is diverse, ranging from a simple CMV syndrome of fever, malaise, and atypical lymphocytosis to serious focal or disseminated invasive disease. Thus, CMV pneumonitis in heart-lung and lung recipients tends to dominate the clinical picture, whereas CMV hepatitis is a more frequent problem in the liver recipient. The attributable mortality is variable in many series because of differences in the definition of disease and organ transplant category. CMV pneumonia has a mortality as high as 64% among solid organ recipients even with antiviral therapy.[103]

The common and rare acute manifestations of CMV disease are shown in Table 134–3. Diagnosis of invasive disease requires at least the demonstration of typical CMV inclusions in tissue or cytology (e.g., pneumonitis) or virologic evidence of CMV along with a compatible clinical picture. The rapid shell vial centrifugation method allows for the fast detection (24–48 hours) of CMV early antigens in a buffy coat, urine, respiratory, and tissue specimens and has enhanced the clinician's ability to direct antiviral therapy earlier and in nonempiric fashion.[104] There is no utility for CMV serologic testing in organ recipients.

Several treatment options have become available over the past 5 years for the management of symptomatic CMV infections. Ganciclovir, a guanosine analog, is virucidal against most CMV strains, although resistance has been described.[105] Numerous noncomparative series in solid organ recipients perceived acute clinical benefit with ganciclovir therapy, but there are no placebo-controlled trials available.[106, 107] Ganciclovir therapy may, however, permit continued immunosuppression for concomitant graft rejection and thus ameliorate the risk of worsening the CMV disease.[108] The principal limiting toxicity is bone marrow suppression, resulting in leukopenia and thrombocytopenia. Foscarnet is a recently approved antiviral agent with in vitro CMV activity, but cumulative experience in solid organ recipients is currently limited. Finally, CMV specific hyperimmune globulin has demonstrated clear survival benefit in bone marrow recipients with CMV pneumonia; however, its adjunctive therapeutic benefit in solid organ recipients is undergoing investigation at present.[108a]

There has been a flurry of clinical investigations examining several different CMV-directed chemoprophylaxis strategies. Balfour and colleagues showed a significant decrease in the rates of CMV disease from 29% in placebo recipients to 7.5% with the use of high-dose oral acyclovir (3200 mg/d) after kidney transplantation.[109] Early 14-day courses of ganciclovir in both heart and liver recipients have shown similar results in the seropositive recipients.[15, 110] Singh and colleagues demonstrated superior prophylactic efficacy with a 7-day, pre-emptive ganciclovir course started at the onset of CMV shedding when compared with high-dose oral acyclovir in liver transplant recipients.[110a]

TABLE 134–3. Acute and Delayed Manifestations of Cytomegalovirus Disease

Organ Invasive Disease
Mononucleosis syndrome
Hepatitis
Pneumonitis
Gastroesophagitis
Enteritis
Colitis
Encephalitis
Retinitis
Adrenalitis
Cutaneous vasculitis
Immunologic
Allograft rejection
Superinfection with nonviral pathogens
Allograft dysfunction
Glomerulonephritis
Vanishing bile duct syndrome
Accelerated coronary atherosclerosis

Epstein-Barr Virus Infection

Serologic evidence of prior EBV infection is present in greater than 95% of adult solid organ recipients; thus, symptomatic primary EBV infection is commonly manifested in seronegative pediatric recipients and rarely in adults. The major sequelae of either primary or reactivated EBV infection are due to its oncogenic potential. Strong evidence linking EBV with the PTLD includes the isolation of EBV deoxyribonucleic acid sequences and viral proteins in both hyperplastic and frank lymphatic and visceral tumor tissue.[111] High EBV IgG viral capsid antibody titer may be present. The histologic appearance of such tumors ranges from polymorphous hyperplasia to frank lymphoma with monomorphic cells.[112] The incidence and severity of PTLD appear greatest in those recipients with primary EBV infection and possibly the prior use of OKT3.[37, 38] The median time from transplantation to presentation is 3 to 5 months in most solid organ groups, with the highest incidence in the heart and heart-lung groups. A favorable clinical response may occur with judicious tapering of immunosuppression alone.[113] Antiviral therapy with acyclovir is often added; however, its true clinical benefit is unknown. Occasionally, both surgical excision and antineoplastic chemotherapy are required for aggressive visceral disease with monoclonal cell surface markers and autonomous tumor behavior that is unresponsive to recovery of the host's immune system.

CHEMOPROPHYLAXIS AND OTHER PREVENTIVE MEASURES

Measures to prevent certain types of infectious complications in organ recipients may vary depending on the transplant category or transplant center. There is a poor consensus on many of these interventions because of inherent difficulties in performing comparative prospective trials. Some are well supported in nontransplant populations such as AIDS or cancer patients and have been adapted for use in the solid organ recipients. Table 134–4 summarizes some preventive and chemoprophylactic strategies based on the mechanisms discussed next.

TABLE 134–4. Chemoprophylaxis and Other Preventive Measures After Solid Organ Transplantation

Pathogen(s)	*Chemoprophylaxis*	*Other Measures*
Herpes simplex	Acyclovir	
CMV	High-dose acyclovir	Vaccination*
	Ganciclovir*	CMV (−) products
	Hyperimmune CMV globulin*, +	
Varicella	VZIG*	
Pneumocystis	Trimethoprim-sulfamethoxasole	
	Aerosolized pentamidine	
Toxoplasmosis	Pyrimethamine*	
Aspergillus	Itraconazole+	HEPA
	Aerosolized amphotericin B+	
Candida	Systemic amphotericin B	
	Nystatin	
Bacteria	Antibiotic (wound prophylaxis)	Gut decontamination
Mycobacterium tuberculosis	Isoniazid†	
Streptococcus pneumoniae		Pneumovax

*In seronegative recipient.
+Investigational.
† (+) purified protein derivative or high-risk exposure.
Abbreviations: CMV = cytomegalovirus; VZIG = varicella zoster immune globulin; HEPA = high-efficiency particulate air filtration.

1. Serologic screening of donor organs and blood products for CMV, toxoplasmosis, HIV-1, hepatitis B and C, and syphilis: On the basis of this information, management options may include complete avoidance (HIV, hepatitis B) or postexposure prophylaxis (CMV, toxoplasmosis).
2. Environmental controls to abolish contact with the organism: HEPA filtration is capable of dramatically decreasing the quantity of airspace pathogens, including *Aspergillus* spores, although its cost and impracticality for wide implementation limit its usefulness. Other interventions such as hyperchlorination or superheating of the hot-water supply in hospital facilities and respiratory isolation of known patients with active TB are routine protection measures. Protective or "reverse" isolation does not provide any extra protection from post-transplant infection than do conventional measures.[114]
3. Vaccination with killed or inactivated preparations before transplantation (pneumococcal vaccine [Pneumovax]) or before a high-risk seasonal period (influenza vaccine): The efficacy of such vaccination in organ recipients remains unproven because of a variable immune response.
4. Suppression of pathogenic colonization (aerobic gram-negative bacteria, *Candida*) of the gastrointestinal tract and oropharynx with nonabsorbable antibiotics (e.g., colistin, gentamicin, nystatin).
5. Systemic chemoprophylaxis directed at specific pathogens: This is a broad category that includes bacterial wound prophylaxis at transplantation, prophylaxis against organisms that either have a latent existence in the host (CMV, HSV, *P. carinii, M. tuberculosis*) or to which the host has de novo exposure and is thus considered a very high risk (CMV-positive graft transplanted to CMV-negative recipient, TB exposure, or chickenpox exposure in a VZV-seronegative recipient). Prophylactic intervention in the latter situations is termed *postexposure prophylaxis.*

The majority of solid organ transplant programs are now using oral TMP-SMX for *Pneumocystis* prophylaxis and some form of CMV prophylaxis. Selective decontamination of the gut resulted in a decreased infection rate with aerobic gram-negative bacteria in one study of liver recipients, although a reciprocal increase in gram-positive infections was noted.[115] There still is a wide disparity of opinion regarding whether to use isoniazid prophylaxis in PPD-positive organ recipients and the duration of prophylaxis. Other areas of controversy include low-dose systemic amphotericin B for organ recipients with a high risk for invasive candidiasis, aerosolized amphotericin or itraconazole for the prevention of aspergillosis, and the efficacy of CMV vaccination for CMV seronegative recipients. As such, this is a ripe area for future investigation of both the clinical and cost efficacy of novel prophylactic interventions.

References

1. Dummer JS: Infections after transplantation: Past, present and future. Transplant Sci 1992; 2:93–99.
2. Rubin RH: Infection in the renal and liver transplant patient. *In*: Clinical Approach to Infection in the Compromised Host. 2nd ed. Rubin RH, Young LS (Eds). New York, Plenum Press, 1988.
3. Kusne S, Fung J, Alessiana M, et al: Infections during a randomized trial comparing cyclosporine to FK 506 immunosuppression in liver transplantation. Trans Proc 1992; 24:429–430.
4. Mora NP, Gonwa TA, Goldstein RM, et al: Risk of postoperative infection after liver transplantation: A univariate and stepwise logistic regression analysis of risk factors in 150 consecutive patients. Clin Trans 1992; 46:443–449.
5. Kusne S, Dummer JS, Ho M, et al: Infections after liver transplantation: An analysis of 101 consecutive cases. Medicine 1988; 67:132–143.
6. Paya CV, Hermans PE, Washington JA, et al: Incidence, distribution, and outcome of episodes of infection in 100 orthotopic liver transplantations. Mayo Clin Proc 1989; 64:555–564.
7. O'Connell JB, Pirarre R, Sullivan HJ, et al: Heart transplantation at Loyola University Medical Center: The first two years. J Heart Transplant 1986; 5:54.
8. Linder J: Infection as a complication of heart transplantation. J Heart Transplant 1988; 7:390–394.
9. van Dorp WT, Kootte AM, van Gemerrt GW, et al: Infections in renal transplant patients treated with cyclosporine or azathioprine. Scand J Infect Dis 1989; 21:75–80.
10. Brayman KL, Stephanian E, Matas A, et al: Analysis of infectious complications occurring after solid organ transplantation. Arch Surg 1992; 127:38–47.
11. Rubin RH, Wolfson JS, Cosimi AB, et al: Infection in the renal transplant recipient. Am J Med 1981; 70:405.
12. Rubin RH: The indirect effects of cytomegalovirus infection on the outcome of organ transplantation. JAMA 1989; 261:3607.
13. Rand KH, Pollard RB, Merigan TC, et al: Increased pulmonary superinfection in cardiac transplant patients undergoing primary cytomegalovirus infection. N Engl J Med 1978; 298:951.
14. Egbert PR, Pillard RB, Gallagher JB, et al: Cytomegalovirus retinitis in immunosuppressed hosts. Ann Intern Med 1980; 93:664–670.

15. Martin M, Manez R, Linden PK, et al: A prospective randomized trial comparing sequential ganciclovir-high dose acyclovir to high dose acyclovir for the prevention of cytomegalovirus disease in adult liver transplant recipients. Transplantation (in press).
16. Krech U: Complement-fixing antibodies against cytomegalovirus in different parts of the world. Bull WHO 1973; 49:103–106.
17. Rubin RH: The compromised host as sentinel chicken (Editorial). N Engl J Med 1987; 317:1151.
18. Sarubbi FA, Kopt HB, Wilson MB, et al: Increased recovery of Aspergillus from respiratory specimens during hospital construction. Am Rev Respir Dis 1982; 125:33.
19. Lentino JR, Rosenkranz MA, Michaels JA, et al: Nosocomial aspergillosis: A retrospective review of airborne disease secondary to road construction and contaminated air conditioners. Am J Epidemiol 1982; 116:430.
20. Doebbbeling BN, Ishak MA, Wade BH, et al: Nosocomial *Legionella micdadei* pneumonia: 10 years experience and a case-control study. J Hosp Infect 1989; 13:289–298.
21. Tobin JO, Beare J, Dunnill MS, et al: Legionnaire's disease in a transplant unit: Isolation of the causative agent from shower baths. Lancet 1980; 2:118–121.
22. Andreone PA, Olivari MT, Elick B, et al: Reduction of infectious complications following heart transplantation with triple-drug immunotherapy. J Heart Transplant 1986; 5:13–19.
23. Prompt CA, Reiss MM, Grillo FM, et al: Transmission of AIDS virus at renal transplantation. Lancet 1985; 2:672.
24. Rubin RH, Jenkins RL, Shaw BW, et al: The acquired immunodeficiency syndrome and transplantation. Transplantation 1987; 44:1–4.
25. Simonds RJ, Holmberg SD, Hurwitz RL, et al: Transmission of human immunodeficiency virus type 1 from a seronegative organ and tissue donor. N Engl J Med 1992; 326:726–732.
26. Dummer JS, Armstrong J, Ho M, et al: Transmission of infection with herpes simplex virus by renal transplantation. J Infect Dis 1987; 155:202–206.
27. Peters TG, Reiter CG, Boswell RL: Transmission of tuberculosis by kidney transplantation. Transplantation 1984; 38:514–516.
28. Dummer JS, Hardy A, Poorsattar A, et al: Early infections in kidney, heart, and liver transplant recipients on cyclosporine. Transplantation 1983; 36:259–267.
29. Hofflin JM, Potasman I, Baldwin JC, et al: Infectious complications in heart transplant recipients receiving cyclosporine and corticosteroids. Ann Intern Med 1987; 106:209–216.
30. The Canadian Multicentre Transplant Study Group: A randomized clinical trial of cyclosporine in cadaveric renal transplantation. N Engl J Med 1986; 314:1219–1225.
31. Borel JF, Feurer C, Gubler GU, et al: Biological effects of cyclosporine A: A new antilymphocytic agent. Agents Actions 1976; 6:468–475.
32. Sawada S, Suzuki G, Kawase Y, et al: Novel immunosuppression agent, FK 506 in vitro effects on the cloned T cell activation. J Immunol 1987; 139:1797–1803.
33. Kim JH, Perfect JR: Infection and cyclosporine. Rev Infect Dis 1989; 11:677–690.
34. Palestine AG, Nussenblatt RB, Chan CC: Side effects of systemic cyclosporine in patients not undergoing transplantation. Am J Med 1984; 77:652–656.
35. Singh N, Dummer JS, Ho M, et al: Infections with cytomegalovirus and other herpes viruses in 121 liver transplant recipients: Transmission by donated organ and the effect of OKT3 antibodies. J Infect Dis 1988; 154:124–131.
36. Nicol DL, MacDonald AS, Beliltsky P, et al: Reduction by combination prophylactic therapy with CMV hyperimmune globulin and acyclovir of the risk of primary CMV disease in renal transplant recipients. Transplantation 1993; 55:841.
37. Swinnen LJ, Costanzo-Nordin MR, Fisher SG, et al: Increased incidence of lymphoproliferative disorder after immunosuppression with the monoclonal antibody OKT3 in cardiac transplant recipients. N Engl J Med 1990; 323:1723.
38. Cockfield SM, Preiksaitis J, Harvey E, et al: Is sequential use of ALG and OKT3 in renal transplants associated with an increased incidence of fulminant post-transplant lymphoproliferative disorder? Tran Proc 1991; 23:1106.
39. Padbury RT, Gunson BK, Dousset B, et al: Steroid withdrawal from long term immunosuppression in liver allograft recipients. Transplantation 1993; 55:789–794.
40. O'Connell JB, Bristow MR, Rasmussen LG, et al: Cardiac allograft function with corticosteroid-free maintenance immunosuppression. Circulation 1990; 82(Suppl IV):318–321.
41. Starzl TE, Demetris AJ, Trucco M, et al: Systemic chimerism in human female recipients of male livers. Lancet 1992; 340:876–877.
42. Fox BC, Sollinger HW, Belzer FO, et al: A prospective, randomized, double-blind study of trimethoprim-sulfamethoxazole for prophylaxis of infection in renal transplantation: Clinical efficacy, absorption of trimethoprim-sulfamethoxazole, effects on the microflora, and the cost-benefit of prophylaxis. Am J Med 1990; 89:255–274.
43. Gardner SD, Mackenzie EFD, Smith C, et al: Prospective study of the human polyomarviruses BK and JC and cytomegalovirus in renal transplant recipients. J Clin Pathol 1984; 37:578–586.
44. Shinohara Y, Hashimoto K, Ikegami M, et al: Hemorrhagic kidney graft pyelonephritis caused by type 37 adenovirus infection. Transplant Proc 1992; 24:1565–1566.
45. Miranda C, Carazo C, Banon R, et al: Mycoplasma hominis infection in three renal transplant recipients. Diagn Microbiol Infect Dis 1990; 13:329–331.
46. Lerut J, Gjordon RD, Iwatsuki S, et al: Biliary tract complications in human orthotopic liver transplantation. Transplantation 1987; 43:47–50.
47. Tzakis AG, Gordon RD, Shaw BW, et al: Clinical presentation of hepatic artery thrombosis after liver transplantation in the cyclosporine era. Transplantation 1987; 40:667–671.
48. Baldwin RT, Radovanevic B, Sweeny MS, et al: Bacterial mediastinitis after heart transplantation. J Heart Lung Transplant 1992; 1:545–549.
49. Karwande SV, Renlund DG, Olsen SL, et al: Mediastinitis in heart transplantation. Ann Thorac Surg 1992; 54:1039–1045.
50. Zenati M, Dowling RD, Dummer JS, et al: Influence of the donor lung on development of early infections in lung transplant recipients. J Heart Transplant 1990; 9:508–509.
51. Boyle EM, Burdine J, Bolman RM: Successful treatment of *Mycoplasma* mediastinitis after heart-lung transplantation. J Heart Lung Transplant 1993; 12:508–512.
52. Thaler F, Gotainer B, Teodori G, et al: Mediastinitis due to *Nocardia asteroides* after cardiac transplantation. Intensive Care Med 1992; 18:127–128.
53. Hesse UJ, Sutherland DER, Najarian JS, et al: Intra-abdominal infections in pancreas transplantation recipients. Ann Surg 1985; 203:153–162.
54. Reyes J, Abu-Elmagd K, Tzakis A, et al: Infectious complications after human small bowel transplantation. Transplant Proc 1992; 24:1249–1250.
55. Starzl TE, Todo S, Tzakis A, et al: Multivisceral and intestinal transplantation. Transplant Proc 1992; 24:1217–1223.
56. Haley CE, Cjohen ML, Halter J, et al: Nosocomial Legionnaire's disease: A continuing common-source epidemic at Wadsworth Medical Center. Ann Intern Med 1979; 90:583–586.
57. Edelstien PH: Legionnaire's disease. Clin Infect Dis 1993; 16:741–749.
58. Gombert ME, Josephson A, Goldstein EJC, et al: Cavitary Legionnaire's pneumonia: Nosocomial infection in renal transplant recipients. Am J Surg 1984; 147:402–405.
59. Meyer RD: Role of the quinolones in the treatment of legionellosis. J Antimicrob Chemother 1991; 28:623–625.
60. Hamedani P, Juzar A, Hafeez S, et al: The safety and efficacy of clarithromycin in patients with legionella pneumonia. Chest 1991; 100:1503–1506.
61. Neff TA, Hudgel DW: Miliary tuberculosis in a renal transplant recipient. Am Rev Respir Dis 1973; 108:677.
62. Ascher NL, Simmons RL, Marker S, et al: Tuberculous joint disease in transplant patients. Am J Surg 1978; 135:853.
63. Higgins RD, Kusne S, Reyes J, et al: Mycobacterium tuberculosis after liver transplantation: Management and guidelines for prevention. Clin Transplant 1992; 6:81–90.
64. Sundberg R, Shapiro RR, Darras F, et al: A tuberculosis outbreak in a renal transplant program. Transplant Proc 1991; 23:3091–3092.

65. Quinibi WY, Al-Sibai B, Taher S, et al: Mycobacterial infection after renal transplantation: Report of 14 cases and review of the literature. Q J Med 1990; 77:1039–1060.
66. Rieder HL, Snider DE, Cauthen GM: Extrapulmonary tuberculosis in the United States. Am Rev Respir Dis 1990; 141:347–351.
67. Wong LL, Levin BS, Collins GM, et al: Unusual manifestations of tuberculosis in cyclosporine-treated renal transplant recipients. Clin Transplant 1993; 7:18–24.
68. Arduino RC, Johnson PC, Miranda AG: Nocardiosis in renal transplant recipients undergoing immunosuppression with cyclosporine. Clin Infect Dis 1993; 16:505–512.
69. Simpson GL, Stinson EB, Egger MJ, et al: Nocardial infections in the immunocompromised host: A detailed study in a defined population. Rev Infect Dis 1981; 3:492–507.
70. Wallace RJ, Septimus EJ, Williams TW, et al: Use of trimethoprim-sulfamethoxazole for treatment of infections due to Nocardia. Rev Infect Dis 1982; 4:312–325.
71. Paya CV: Fungal infections in solid-organ transplantation. Clin Infect Dis 1993; 16:677–689.
72. Linder J: Infection as a complication of heart transplantation. J Heart Transplant 1988; 7:390–394.
73. Castaldo P, Stratta RJ, Wood RP, et al: Clinical spectrum of fungal infections after orthotopic liver transplantation. Arch Surg 1991; 126:149–156.
74. Rantala A, Niinikoski J, Lehtonen O-P: Yeasts in blood cultures: Impact of early therapy. Scand J Infect Dis 1989; 21:557–561.
75. Komshian SV, Uwaydah AK, Sobel JD, et al: Fungemia caused by *Candida* species and *Torulopsis glabrata* in the hospitalized patient: Frequency, characteristics, and evaluation of factors influencing outcome. Rev Infect Dis 1989; 11:379–390.
76. Tollemar J, Ericzon BG, Holmberg K, et al: The incidence and diagnosis of invasive fungal infections in liver transplant recipients. Transplant Proc 1990; 22:242–244.
77. Tollemar JU, Holmberg K, Ringden O, et al: Surveillance tests for the diagnosis of invasive fungal infections in bone marrow transplant recipients. Scand J Infect Dis 1989; 21:205–212.
78. Rex JH, Bennett JE, Sugar AM, et al: Fluconazole vs amphotericin B for treatment of candidemia: Results of a randomized multicenter trial (Abstract 805). In Proceedings of the 33rd ICAAC, October 1993.
79. Khardori N: Host-parasite interaction in fungal infections. Eur J Clin Microbiol Infect Dis 1989; 8:331–351.
80. Yu VL, Muder RR, Poorsatar A: Significance of isolation of *Aspergillus* from the respiratory tract in diagnosis of invasive pulmonary aspergillosis. Am J Med 1986; 81:249–254.
81. Kusne S, Torre-Cisneros J, Manez R, et al: Factors associated with invasive lung aspergillosis and the significance of positive *Aspergillus* culture after liver transplantation. J Infect Dis 1992; 166:1379–1383.
82. Denning DW, Tucker RM, Hanson LH, et al: Treatment of invasive aspergillosis with itraconazole. Am J Med 1989; 86:791–800.
82a. Denning DW, Lee JY, Hostetler JS, et al: NIAID Mycoses Study Group multicenter trial of oral itraconazole therapy for invasive aspergillosis. Am J Med 1994; 97:135–144.
83. Katz NM, Pierce PF, Anzeck RA, et al: Liposomal amphotericin B for treatment of pulmonary aspergillosis in a heart transplant patient. J Heart Transplant 1990; 9:14.
84. Mayer JM, Nimer L, Carroll K: Isolated pulmonary aspergillus infection in cardiac transplant recipient: Case report and review. Clin Infect Dis 1992; 15:698–700.
85. Loria KM, Salinger MH, Frohlich TG, et al: Primary cutaneous aspergillosis in a heart transplant recipient treated with surgical excision and oral itraconazole. J Heart Lung Transplant 1992; 11:156–159.
86. Bodey GP, Vartivarian S: Aspergillosis. Eur J Clin Microbiol Infect Dis 1989; 8:413–437.
87. Diamond RD, Bennett JE: Prognostic factors in cryptococcal meningitis: A study of 111 cases. Ann Intern Med 1974; 80:181.
88. Bennett JE, Dismukes WE, Duma RJ, et al: A comparison of amphotericin B alone and combined with flucytosine in the treatment of cryptococcal meningitis. N Engl J Med 1979; 301:126–131.
89. Polsky B, Depman MR, Gold JWM, et al: Intraventricular therapy of cryptococcal meningitis via a subcutaneous reservoir. Am J Med 1986; 81:24–28.
90. Robinson PA, Knirsch AK, Joseph JA: Fluconazole for life-threatening fungal infections in patients who cannot be treated with conventional antifungal agents. Rev Infect Dis 1990; 12(Suppl 3):S349–S363.
91. Conti DJ, Tolkoff-Rubin, Baker GP, et al: Successful treatment of invasive fungal infection with fluconazole in organ transplant recipients. Transplantation 1989; 48:692–695.
92. Morris DJ, Littler E, Arrand JR, et al: Human herpesvirus 6 infection in renal transplant recipients. N Engl J Med 1989; 320:1560.
93. Chou S, Gallagher JC, Merigan TC: Controlled clinical trial of intravenous acyclovir to treat mucocutaneous herpes simplex after marrow transplantation. Lancet 1981; 1:1392–1394.
94. Pettersson E, Hovi T, Ahonen T, et al: Prophylactic oral acyclovir after renal transplantation. Transplantation 1985; 39:279.
95. Shepp DH, Dandliker PS, Meyers JD: Treatment of varicella-zoster virus infection in severely immunocompromised patients. N Engl J Med 1986; 314:208–212.
96. McCarthy JM, Karim MA, Krueger H, et al: The cost impact of cytomegalovirus disease in renal transplant recipients. Transplantation 1993; 555:1277–1282.
97. Schooley RT, Hirsch MS, Colvin RB, et al: Association of herpesgroup virus infections with T-lymphocyte subset alterations, glomerulopathy and opportunistic infections following renal transplantation. N Engl J Med 1983; 308:307–313.
98. Pouteil-Noble C, Ecochard R, Landrivon G, et al: Cytomegalovirus infection: An etiological factor for rejection? Transplantation 1993; 55:851–857.
99. O'Grady JG, Alexander GJM, Sutherland S, et al: Cytomegalovirus infection and donor/recipient HLA antigens: Interdependent cofactors in pathogenesis of vanishing bile duct syndrome after liver transplantation. Lancet 1988; 2:302.
100. Richardson WP, Colvin RB, Cheeseman SH, et al: Glomerulopathy associated with cytomegalovirus viremia in renal allografts. N Engl J Med 1981; 305:57.
101. Grattan MT, Moreno-Cabral CE, Stames VA, et al: Cytomegalovirus infection is associated with cardiac allograft rejection and atherosclerosis. JAMA 1989; 261:3561.
102. Weir MR, Irwin BC, Maters AW, et al: Incidence of cytomegalovirus disease in cyclosporine-treated renal transplant recipients based on donor/recipient pretransplant immunity. Transplantation 1987; 43:187.
103. Snydman DR: Treatment of cytomegalovirus pneumonia in solid organ recipients. *In*: Ganciclovir Therapy for Cytomegalovirus Infection. Spector S (Ed). New York, Marcel Dekker, 1991, p 145.
104. Paya CV, Smith TF, Ludwig J, et al: Rapid shell viral culture and tissue histology compared with serology for the rapid diagnosis of cytomegalovirus infection in liver transplantation. May Clin Proc 1989; 64:670.
105. Erice A, Chou S, Biron KK, et al: Progressive disease due to ganciclovir-resistant cytomegalovirus in immunocompromised patients. N Engl J Med 1989; 320:289–293.
106. Dunn DL, Mayoral JL, Gillingham KT, et al: Treatment of invasive cytomegalovirus disease in solid organ transplant recipients with ganciclovir. Transplantation 1991; 51:98.
107. Snydman DR: Ganciclovir therapy for cytomegalovirus disease associated with renal transplants. Rev Infect Dis 1988; 10:S554.
108. Dunn DL, Mayoral JL, Gillingham KT, et al: Simultaneous treatment of concurrent rejection and tissue invasive cytomegalovirus disease without detrimental effects upon patient or allograft survival. Clin Transplant 1992; 46:413–420.
108a. Zaia JA: Prevention and treatment of cytomegalovirus pneumonia in transplant recipients. Clin Infect Dis 1993; 17(Suppl 2):S392–S399.
109. Balfour HH Jr, Chace BA, Stapleton JT, et al: A randomized placebo-controlled trial of oral acyclovir for the prevention of cytomegalovirus disease in recipients of renal allografts. N Engl J Med 1989; 320:1381.
110. Merigan TC, Renlund DG, Keay S, et al: A controlled trial of ganciclovir to prevent cytomegalovirus disease after heart transplantation. N Engl J Med 1992; 326:1182–1186.
110a. Singh N, Yu VL, Mieles L, et al: High-dose acyclovir compared with short-course preemptive ganciclovir therapy to

prevent cytomegalovirus disease in liver transplant recipients. Ann Intern Med 1994; 120:375–381.
111. Ho M, Jaffe R, Miller G, et al: The frequency of Epstein-Barr virus infection and associated lymphoproliferative syndrome after transplantation and its manifestations in children. Transplantation 1988; 45:719–727.
112. Starzl T: The diagnosis and treatment of posttransplant lymphoproliferative disorders. Curr Probl Surg 1988; 25:371–465.
113. Starzl TE, Nalesnik MA, Porter KA, et al: Reversibility of lymphomas and lymphoproliferative lesions developing under cyclosporine-steroid therapy. Lancet 1984; 1:583.
114. Walsh TR, Guttendorf J, Dummer JS, et al: The value of protective isolation procedures in cardiac allograft recipients. Ann Thorac Surg 1989; 47:539–545.
115. Wiesner RH, Hermans PE, Rakela J, et al: Selective bowel decontamination to decrease gram negative aerobic bacterial cand candida colonization and prevent infection after orthotopic liver transplantation. Transplantation 1988; 45:570.

CHAPTER 135

Laboratory Diagnosis of Infection

Michael R. Jacobs, MB, BCh, PhD, MRC Path

Infections in critically ill patients, either as primary diseases or as complications of other conditions, carry a high mortality and require prompt and appropriate diagnosis and therapy. The laboratory diagnosis of infection in critical care medicine includes collection and direct examination of specimens; culture for bacterial, viral, and fungal pathogens; antimicrobial susceptibility testing; and serologic diagnosis of infection.

SPECIMEN COLLECTION

Collection of adequate, appropriate, and representative samples is crucial to successful laboratory examination,[1] particularly in critical care medicine, in which basic antiseptic precautions can easily be omitted in the flurry of activity surrounding a critically ill patient and diagnostic material may be unavailable or obtained only after institution of antimicrobial therapy. Results of investigations performed on a specimen are valid only if the specimen is correctly collected, transported, and processed.

Ideal specimens are collected from normally sterile body sites and should not contaminated by indigenous organisms of the skin or mucous membranes.[2, 3] They should be adequate in quantity, particularly if examined for low numbers of multiple groups of organisms. Tissue rather than swabs should be submitted whenever possible.

Specimens should be promptly transported to the laboratory under conditions designed to protect fastidious organisms and prevent overgrowth of any contaminants. Each specimen is accompanied by relevant information about the patient, including clinical diagnosis and examinations required, and each should be promptly examined and cultured on appropriate media.

If possible, specimens are collected before the institution of antimicrobial therapy, and use of topical anesthetics or preservative-containing solutions should be avoided.[2] Procedure guides for collecting and transporting of specimens and information about facilities available, routine laboratory practices, and interpretation of results should be obtained from laboratory staff.

Respiratory Specimens

Important respiratory tract infections in critically ill patients include acute primary pneumonias as well as pneumonias secondary to endotracheal intubation, impaired host defenses (resulting from malignancies, immunosuppressive drugs, or chemotherapy), diabetes, alcoholism, and congestive heart failure. Because expectorated sputum is often difficult or impossible to obtain from these patients, material for examination can be sampled by bronchoscopy, transtracheal aspiration, or open lung biopsy.[4] Bronchoscopy with double-lumen catheters minimizes oropharyngeal contamination of specimens; however, the local anesthetic agents that are used during bronchoscopy possess antibacterial properties, and results of bronchoscopically obtained specimens should be interpreted with caution. Protected brush or alveolar lavage sampling permits the use of quantitative culture techniques.

Transtracheal aspiration is indicated when sputum cannot be obtained, when Gram's stain or culture of sputum does not yield a clear pathogen, when a patient has responded poorly to antimicrobial therapy, and when there is a possibility of superinfection.[4] The technique is used less commonly than before because of the ease of bronchoscopic sampling. Transtracheal aspiration is carried out by hyperextending the patient's neck, injecting a local anesthetic agent over the cricothyroid membrane, and entering the trachea through the membrane with a large-bore needle containing an indwelling catheter. The needle is angled downward toward the patient's coccyx. After the needle has entered the trachea, the catheter is advanced several inches and the needle is withdrawn. Sputum is then aspirated from the catheter with a syringe; if no material is obtained, 1 to 2 mL of preservative-free sterile saline can be injected and aspirated. Transtracheal aspirates bypass the oropharynx and can, therefore, be cultured in both anaerobic and aerobic media. Significant complications of transtracheal aspiration are hemoptysis, subcutaneous emphysema, aspiration, and cellulitis. The procedure can have false-positive results because of oropharyngeal aspiration or tracheal colonization and false-negative results caused by prior antimicrobial therapy or bronchial obstruction.

Open lung biopsy is an alternative to bronchoscopy but is usually necessary only in immunocompromised hosts. The procedure has a low mortality and morbidity but is contraindicated in patients with hypoxia and thrombocytopenia.[4]

Blood Specimens

Patients with septicemia are often in septic shock and, therefore, critically ill. Prompt, adequate, and aseptic collection of blood for culture is essential to confirm the diagnosis and identify the causative pathogen and its antimicrobial susceptibility before starting antimicrobial therapy.[2]

Blood is best collected by direct venipuncture with a needle and syringe or a sterile transfer set; to avoid contamination, vacuum tubes should be used with sterile, prepackaged needle holders. Additional specimens can be collected from arterial or venous access catheters, but such specimens may only demonstrate colonization of the line and not septicemia and should not be the only blood specimens submitted for culture.

The venipuncture site is first disinfected with 70% alcohol, followed by 2% iodine or an iodophor, which should remain in contact with the skin for at least a minute. Residual iodine is then removed with an alcohol pad, and 10 to 20 mL of blood is collected in a syringe by venipuncture. The syringe needle is changed and the blood is injected into two broth bottles, one aerobic and one anaerobic. The optimal volume ratio of blood to broth is 1:10; commercial broth bottles usually contain 30 to 100 mL of broth, requiring 3 to 10 mL of blood per bottle.[1]

Bacteremia is best demonstrated by detecting the same organism in multiple blood cultures collected over several hours from different venipuncture sites. In critical care medicine, it is often not possible to delay antimicrobial therapy beyond the initial set of cultures; the alternative is to collect two culture sets from different venipuncture sites with a delay as short as a few minutes or to collect a second set of cultures in commercially available resin-containing antimicrobial removal systems shortly after beginning antimicrobial therapy. Because multiple specimens should be collected in all patients with suspected septicemia, the collection time should be clearly noted on each requisition to assess the relationship among clinical condition, antimicrobial therapy, procedures performed, and culture results.

Vascular catheter tips should be submitted for culture when removed.[2] Blood to culture for viruses and *Leptospira* can be collected in sterile, heparinized tubes.[3]

Urine Specimens

Urine is best collected as a clean-catch, midstream specimen after appropriate cleansing of the external genitalia.[1] This is usually not possible in critically ill patients, and the laboratory should be notified about specimens not optimally collected. Should urine culture be particularly important, suprapubic aspiration can be used to obtain a specimen. Suprapubic aspirates should be clearly identified because any growth from these specimens is significant.

In catheterized patients, urine should be collected with a needle and syringe directly from the clamped catheter. Such specimens should be clearly identified because conventional quantitation is not used. Urinary catheter tips should not be submitted for culture because they reflect only what is colonizing the catheter and not necessarily the patient.

Urine specimens should be transported to the laboratory as soon as possible and should be cultured within an hour of collection. Specimens can be refrigerated if any delay is anticipated.

Other Specimens

Body fluids and exudates, pus, and swabs of mucous membranes should be submitted to the laboratory as rapidly as possible.[1, 2] If anaerobic culture is required, anaerobic transport medium should be used.

DIRECT EXAMINATION OF SPECIMENS

Direct microscopic examination of specimens, either as wet mounts or stained smears, is extremely important in the diagnosis of many infections.[1, 2] Specimens can be examined for various microbial antigens and other products as well as for inflammatory cells and chemical composition.

Wet Mounts

Direct examination of a fluid specimen on a slide and under a coverslip can be extremely useful for demonstrating protozoa and inflammatory cells. Dark-ground or phase-contrast illumination reveals bacteria, including spirochetes, and other organisms. *Cryptococcus neoformans* can be demonstrated by mixing a drop of India ink with a drop of cerebrospinal fluid (CSF) or other body fluid; the India ink is a negative stain that outlines the capsule of the organism. Potassium-hydroxide wet mounts are useful for detecting fungi, particularly in sputum.

Stained Smears

Gram's Stains

Stained smears are commonly performed on a wide variety of specimens and often provide diagnostic information in infectious conditions. Gram's-stained smears of body fluids and exudates can show inflammatory cells as well as bacteria. Clumps of gram-positive cocci suggest staphylococci or peptococci; chains of gram-positive cocci suggest streptococci or peptostreptococci; large gram-positive bacilli suggest clostridia; large gram-negative bacilli suggest Enterobacteriaceae; and small gram-negative bacilli suggest *Pseudomonas, Haemophilus,* or *Bacteroides* species. However, bacterial morphology can be highly variable, particularly in material from abscesses or from patients on antimicrobial therapy, and overinterpretation of smears must be avoided.

Gram's stains of sputum are helpful when inflammatory cells suggest pneumonia; however, if there are oral squamous epithelial cells and a wide variety of organisms, the specimen includes saliva and should be discarded.[1] Pneumonia caused by *Streptococcus pneumoniae, Haemophilus influenzae, Staphylococcus aureus,* and Enterobacteriaceae can often be diagnosed with a high degree of accuracy from a sputum Gram's stain.[4]

Gram's stains of urine are highly suggestive of significant bacteriuria if two or more bacteria are seen per oil-immersion field of well-mixed, uncentrifuged urine.[1] Gram-negative bacilli suggest Enterobacteriaceae, and gram-positive cocci suggest enterococci or staphylococci.

A Gram's stain can be easily and rapidly performed by the physician attending the patient. Good results, however, require considerable experience and expertise because decolorization time depends on the nature of the material being stained. Again, overinterpretation of smears should be avoided. Because many organisms have similar appearances, those in Gram's-stained smears should be described by their morphology as well as their degree of staining. Finally, the preparation of Gram's stain reagents should be checked, and a supply of smears containing a mixture of gram-positive cocci and gram-negative bacilli should be provided as quality control slides to be stained by anyone using the reagents.

Acid-Fast and Fluorescent Stains

Mycobacteria do not stain readily with Gram's method, but they resist acid decolorization and can, therefore, be identified by various acid-fast stains of sputum and other specimens.[2] Both Ziehl-Neelsen stain using hot carbolfuchsin and Kinyoun stain using cold, concentrated carbolfuchsin will stain mycobacteria red. Auramine will stain mycobacteria a bright yellow under suitable fluorescent illumination.

Fluorescein-tagged fluorescent antibody stains are useful in demonstrating various pathogens, such as *Legionella pneumophila, Pneumocystis carinii, Francisella tularensis,* and common respiratory viruses.[1, 5] Fluorescein appears bright green under suitable fluorescent illumination. Other staining methods include silver stains of biopsies for fungi and *P. carinii* and Giemsa stains of blood smears for malarial parasites. All staining procedures, particularly fluorescent stains, require adequate controls.

DETECTION OF MICROBIAL PRODUCTS

The only commonly available techniques for detecting microbial products directly in specimens are various immunologic methods used to identify microbial antigens and direct gene probes to detect *Neisseria gonorrhoeae* and *Chlamydia trachomatis*.[5,6] Considerable advances have been made in the development of amplified gene probes, for example by the polymerase chain reaction.[6] Ready availability of commercial products has, however, not been attained.[6]

In patients with meningitis, capsular polysaccharide antigens of *H. influenzae, Streptococcus pneumoniae, Neisseria meningitidis*, or *C. neoformans* can be detected in CSF and sometimes in serum, sputum, urine, and effusion fluids. Antigens can be demonstrated by counterimmunoelectrophoresis (CIE), latex agglutination, or staphylococcal coagglutination,[5] but false-positive and false-negative results limit the application of these procedures. CIE of CSF is best for the diagnosis of bacterial meningitis, and latex agglutination of CSF or serum is best for the diagnosis of cryptococcal infection. CIE of serum, sputum, and urine detects up to 75% of bacteremic pneumococcal pneumonias but only 45% of nonbacteremic cases. Moreover, antigen can persist in urine for up to 6 weeks after onset of illness and may not accurately reflect a patient's current disease.[6]

Enzyme-linked immunosorbent assays (ELISAs) are being developed for the detection of bacterial and viral antigens, using enzyme-labeled antibodies. Examples of infections that can be diagnosed by the ELISA technique include rotavirus infection, gonorrhea, and legionnaires' disease.

CULTURE METHODS

The wide variety of bacteria, fungi, viruses, and protozoa that can cause infections requires different isolation techniques. Most laboratories choose techniques based on ease of use, local prevalence of various infectious diseases, clinical usefulness, and availability of equipment and facilities.[1] Physicians should be aware of which procedures are routine and which are available on request, either on site or at a referral laboratory. To ensure its optimal laboratory handling, each specimen should be identified by the patient's age, clinical presentation and diagnosis, travel history, known exposure to specific pathogens, and any antimicrobial therapy.[1,2] Laboratory tests should be specifically requested, particularly when unusual infections are suspected.

Specimens are usually processed for groups of organisms, such as rapidly growing bacteria (aerobic and anaerobic), mycobacteria, fungi, chlamydia, and viruses. Rapidly growing bacteria are generally isolated from specimens that are streaked onto a variety of agar media and incubated aerobically (supplemented with 5% to 10% carbon dioxide (CO_2), if necessary) or anaerobically. Selective and enrichment media are used to select pathogens from normal flora. Blood agar allows the growth of many common bacteria in 24 to 48 hours, whereas chocolate agar encourages the growth of more fastidious organisms such as *Haemophilus* and *Neisseria* species and MacConkey agar is specific for growth and differentiation of enteric gram-negative bacilli.

Mycobacteria can be isolated on various solid media, such as Lowenstein-Jensen agar, in 2 to 3 weeks. Detection within a week is possible using liquid media containing carbon 14–labeled substrates.[7]

Fungi can be readily isolated on most bacteriologic media after prolonged incubation if antibacterial agents are added to inhibit bacterial growth. Incubation for several weeks at 30°C and 37°C may be required for growth of systemic fungi.[1] Special techniques are required for the isolation of molds from blood, such as the lysis-centrifugation method.

Viruses and chlamydia can be isolated by animal inoculation or by inoculation of hens' eggs or mammalian cell cultures.[3,8] Cell cultures are commonly used but will not grow all viruses.

Respiratory Specimens

Bacterial pneumonia can be diagnosed by culturing sputum, transtracheal aspirates, or biopsy material on blood agar under CO_2 for pneumococci and staphylococci, on chocolate agar under CO_2 for *Haemophilus*, on MacConkey agar for enteric gram-negative bacilli, and on enriched blood agar incubated anaerobically for anaerobes (only for suitable specimens such as transtracheal aspirates or material from open lung biopsies).[1,2] *Mycoplasma pneumoniae* can be isolated on special media, but isolation is rarely attempted owing to the slow growth of this organism and inadequate material for culture.[8] Mycobacteria and many fungi require prolonged aerobic incubation. *Legionella pneumophila* and other *Legionella* species can be cultured from respiratory specimens on charcoal-yeast extract agar under CO_2; sputum is the least suitable specimen for isolating these organisms. Viral isolation can be attempted from all respiratory specimens.[3]

Blood Specimens

The diagnosis of septicemia is best made by demonstrating sustained bacteremia. After direct inoculation of blood into liquid culture media, culture broths are incubated at 35°C and examined several times daily. Growth is detected by macroscopic turbidity, blind subculture, measurement of CO_2 released from ^{14}C-labeled substrates or other indicators of bacterial metabolic activity.[1,2]

Most bacteria and yeasts will grow in common commercial blood culture media, but prolonged incubation is often required to isolate yeasts and *Brucella* species. Biphasic broth/agar media can also be used for prolonged incubation. Antimicrobial-removing resin media or lysis-centrifugation systems may be used in addition to these media when patients are receiving antimicrobial therapy or are suspected of having a fungal infection.

Urine Specimens

Quantitation of organisms in voided urine is used to differentiate infection (more than 100,000 organisms per milliliter) from urethral and perineal contamination (less than 10,000 mixed organisms per millilter).[1] Urine is cultured quantitatively on blood and MacConkey agar, using a calibrated 1-μL loop. Any growth may be significant in catheter and suprapubic specimens, and culture results in patients on antimicrobial therapy need to be interpreted with caution.

Other Specimens

Specimens from normally sterile sites are usually cultured for bacteria aerobically and anaerobically on blood agar; chocolate agar is used if fastidious organisms are suspected.[1,2] Specimens from mucous membranes or the gastrointestinal tract often require selective and enrichment media to allow isolation of specific pathogens (e.g., *Salmonella* species from feces and *Neisseria gonorrhoeae* from cervix, urethra, throat, or rectum).[1,2]

Identification of Isolates

Most common bacteria, fungi, and mycobacteria are identified by their ability to grow on cell-free media, their colonial morphology on solid media, their rate of growth, temperature requirements and stained microscopic morphology, and a variety of tests to differentiate biochemical or antigenic properties. Atypical isolates, unusual organisms, and differentiation of phage types of serotypes of an organism are generally referred to a reference laboratory for investigation. Identification of epidemic strains can be achieved by many molecular methods such as deoxyribonucleic fingerprinting, plasmid profiles, and multilocus enzyme electrophoresis.[9]

Growth of viruses and chlamydia can be detected in cell cultures by cytopathic effects such as cell rounding, cell clustering, syncytial formation, and intranuclear or intracytoplasmic inclusions.[8] Hemadsorption, direct immunofluorescence, and interference can also indicate viral growth. Final identification of a virus requires specific neutralization of viral activity by homologous antiserum.

ANTIMICROBIAL SUSCEPTIBILITY TESTS

Determining the susceptibility of isolated pathogens to appropriate antimicrobial agents is an important function of clinical microbiology laboratories. The development and spread of resistant bacteria such as nosocomial pathogens, as well as the increasing numbers of immunocompromised patients and new antimicrobial agents, emphasize the importance of rapid and accurate susceptibility testing of isolates from critically ill patients.

In vivo susceptibility is influenced by several factors: host defense mechanisms; the concentrations of antimicrobial agents at the site of infection; the natural course, nature, and severity of the infection; any delay in starting therapy; and effects of other therapeutic measures such as surgery. In vitro susceptibility depends on organism, growth medium, atmosphere, inoculum size, and length and temperature of incubation; because these factors have been standardized for common rapidly growing bacteria,[10] the outcome of infection is mainly affected by in vivo factors.

Organisms are regarded as susceptible to an antimicrobial agent if they are inhibited in vitro by a concentration of the agent that is lower than serum concentrations achievable with the usual drug dosage.[11] Resistant organisms are not inhibited or are inhibited only at concentrations above those attainable. Susceptibility and resistance are expressed as the minimal inhibitory concentration (MIC) of an antimicrobial agent required to inhibit growth of a defined population of organisms or as categories based on antimicrobial levels in various body sites. Most susceptibility tests are based directly or indirectly on MIC determination[10] and require strict standardization and quality control.

Minimal Inhibitory Concentration Determination

Serial twofold dilutions of antimicrobial agents in a suitable growth medium, such as Mueller-Hinton broth, are prepared in test tubes (macrodilution method) or in microdilution wells (microdilution method), with an inoculum of 10^5 to 10^6 organisms per milliliter.[10, 11] MICs can also be performed by the agar dilution method; multiple inocula of 10^4 organisms are placed on antimicrobial-containing plates with a replicating device. After overnight incubation at 35°C, the lowest antimicrobial concentration completely inhibiting growth is the MIC. Minimal bactericidal concentrations (MBCs) can be determined by quantitative subculture; the MBC is the lowest concentration of antimicrobial producing at least a 99.9% reduction in the original inoculum.[10] However, MBCs are now rarely performed because of a lack of reproducibility of results and absence of quality-control strains.

The macrodilution method produces reproducible MIC results, but it is time consuming and expensive. The microdilution method produces results identical to those obtained with macrodilution for gram-positive bacteria and results one dilution lower for enteric gram-negative bacteria;[12] this method is commercially available in the form of frozen or lyophilized trays. Agar dilution is the most reproducible MIC determination method and allows testing of up to 36 organisms simultaneously on a standard agar plate.[10] A new method for MIC determination is the E test, which is performed with a plastic carrier strip that releases an antimicrobial gradient when placed on an agar plate and combines the simplicity of disk diffusion with the accuracy of MIC determination. The E test is particularly useful for susceptibility testing of fastidious organisms such as *S. pneumoniae, H. influenzae*, and anaerobes.

MICs are expressed in micrograms per milliliter and should be at least twofold to fourfold lower than mean achievable drug levels to produce an adequate therapeutic response. MICs can also be qualitatively expressed by predetermined resistance categories based on achievable serum drug concentrations.[10] A susceptible organism is inhibited by antimicrobial levels readily attained in the blood on usual dosage, including oral when applicable; a moderately susceptible organism is inhibited only by blood levels achieved with fairly high dosage or when the drug is concentrated (e.g., in urine); and a resistant organism is resistant to commonly achievable levels (Table 135–1). These general categories are influenced by the patient's condition, drug pharmacokinetics, renal and hepatic disease, patient's age, presence of shock, and effects of other drugs. They may need to be modified for infections in sites of poor drug penetration, such as CSF.

Disk-Diffusion Tests

The zone of growth inhibition around an antimicrobial-containing disk is inversely proportional to the MIC of the antimicrobial.[13, 14] Up to 12 different disks can be placed on a 15-cm diameter Petri dish containing Mueller-Hinton agar seeded with a test organism. Zones of inhibition are recorded after overnight incubation at 35°C. The degree of microbial growth inhibition is categorized as susceptible, intermediate (moderately susceptible), or resistant on the basis of the diameter of the zone of inhibition around each disk. The disk-diffusion method usually used is the Kirby-Bauer procedure, which is limited by the range of drugs and organisms that can be tested. Anaerobes should not be tested by disk diffusion.[13]

Automated Tests

The MIC and disk-diffusion methods require overnight incubation in addition to the 24 hours usually required to isolate the organism. The obvious need for faster turnaround times in the care of critically ill patients led to commercial systems that produce susceptibility results in 3 to 7 hours.[15] Staphylococci, enterococci, and enteric gram-negative bacilli can be tested by any of several commercially available systems that read and interpret results photometrically.[16] These automated systems perform adequately in comparison with MIC results and can test between 9 and 20 drugs at one time. However, they should be used with caution, and results for important isolates should be confirmed by conventional methods. Manufacturers' recommendations must be strictly adhered to with these systems to avoid erroneous results.

TABLE 135–1. MIC Interpretative Standards (in μg/mL) for Enteric Gram-Negatives, Staphylococci, and Enterococci

Antimicrobial Agent	*Susceptible*	*Intermediate**	*Resistant*
β-Lactams			
Penicillins			
Ampicillin, ampicillin-sulbactam, and amoxicillin-clavulanate			
When testing Enterobacteriaceae	≤8.00	16	>16.00
When testing staphylococci	≤0.25	—	>0.25
When testing enterococci	≤8.00	—	>8.00
When testing other gram positives	≤0.12	0.25–2	>2.00
Penicillin G			
When testing staphylococci	≤0.12	—	>0.12
When testing enterococci	≤8.00	—	>8.00
When testing pneumococci	≤0.06	0.12–1	>1.00
When testing other gram positives	≤0.12	0.25–2	>2.00
Oxacillin and nafcillin†			
When testing staphylococci	≤2.00	—	>2.00
Mezlocillin, ticarcillin, ticarcillin-clavulanate, piperacillin			
When testing Enterobacteriaceae	≤16.00	32–64	>64.00
When testing *Pseudomonas aeruginosa*	≤64.00	—	>64.00
Cephalosporins			
Cephalothin, cefazolin, cefoxitin, cefuroxime, ceftazidime	≤8.00	16	>16.00
Cefotaxime, ceftriaxone, ceftizoxime	≤8.00	16–32	>32.00
Cefotetan, cefoperazone	≤16.00	32	>32.00
Carbapenems			
Imipenem	≤4.00	8	>8.00
Monobactams			
Aztreonam	≤8.00	16	>16.00
Aminoglycosides			
Gentamicin, tobramycin	≤4.00	8	>8.00
Amikacin	≤16.00	32	>32.00
Glycopeptides			
Vancomycin	≤4.00	8–16	>16.00
Macrolides			
Erythromycin, clindamycin	≤0.50	1–4	>4.00
Azithromycin, clarithromycin	≤2.00	4	>4.00
Quinolones			
Ciprofloxacin	≤1.00	2	>2.00

*Intermediate MICs approach achievable blood and tissue levels, and response rates may be lower than for strains with susceptible MICs. Strains with intermediate MICs can be treated at body sites where drugs are concentrated, such as in urine, or when high dosage of drugs such as β-lactams are used. This category also indicates a buffer zone to allow for minor technical errors with toxic agents.

†Oxacillin- or nafcillin-resistant staphylococci are resistant to all β-lactams.

Abbreviation: MIC = minimal inhibitory concentration.

Beta-Lactamase Production

Penicillin and ampicillin-resistant strains of *H. influenzae* and *S. aureus* produce β-lactamases that can be demonstrated by various methods. Beta-lactamase production by *H. influenzae* can be rapidly detected by the acidimetric or chromogenic cephalosporin methods.[17] Demonstration of β-lactamase production by *S. aureus* is more difficult and may require induction by oxacillin or methicillin.

Choosing Susceptibility Tests and Agents

Choice of method depends on the organism to be tested, the techniques available, and the need for speed or accuracy. The choice of antimicrobial agents to be tested depends on the organism to be tested, its site of isolation, and local patterns of susceptibility and antimicrobial usage.[18] Some antimicrobials, such as amikacin and the newer β-lactams, are tested or reported only if resistance to older aminoglycosides or β-lactams is detected. Susceptibility to groups of antimicrobial agents can be determined by testing one of the group (Table 135–2).

Because critically ill patients are often treated with combinations of antimicrobial agents, the interaction of these agents is important.[17,19] Effective antimicrobial combinations are either synergistic or additive. These effects can be assessed in vitro by testing the rate of killing of an organism with drugs alone and in combined drugs in a checkerboard titration. Many drug combinations are known to be synergistic in vivo, particularly β-lactams with aminoglycosides, and do not need to be tested in combination.[19] Combinations known to be antagonistic in vivo include penicillin G with tetracycline in pneumococcal meningitis and chloramphenicol with a β-lactam agent in meningitis caused by enteric gram-negative bacilli.

Severe mycobacterial infections such as miliary tuberculosis are rare but are increasingly being encountered in critically ill patients. Conventional mycobacterial susceptibility tests take 2 to 3 weeks but can be performed within a week on isolates of *Mycobacterium tuberculosis* using a radiometric method.[7,20]

Susceptibility of yeasts and molds to amphotericin B and imidazoles can be determined using techniques similar to MIC determinations for bacteria.[21] These techniques, however, are difficult to perform and are best done by specialist reference laboratories.

DETERMINING BACTERICIDAL ACTIVITY OF BODY FLUIDS

The bactericidal activity of serum and other body fluids reflects the adequacy of antimicrobial therapy.[17,22] The best

TABLE 135–2. Recommended Antimicrobial Agents to be Tested According to Organism and Site of Isolation*

Enteric Gram-Negative Isolates from Urine	
Ampicillin†	Gentamicin
Amoxicillin-clavulanate	Tobramycin
Ampicillin-sulbactam	Amikacin
Trimethoprim	Cephalothin†
Tetracycline†	Cefoxitin
Nitrofurantoin	Cefuroxime
Sulfisoxazole†	Third-generation cephalosporins‡
Nalidixic acid	Imipenem
Mezlocillin, piperacillin, or ticarcillin	Ciprofloxacin
Enteric Gram-Negative Isolates from Other Sites	
Ampicillin†	Imipenem
Amoxicillin-clavulanate	Cephalothin†
Ampicillin-sulbactam	Cefoxitin
Trimethoprim	Cefuroxime
Chloramphenicol	Mezlocillin, piperacillin, or ticarcillin
Aztreonam	Third-generation cephalosporins‡
Gentamicin	Ciprofloxacin
Tobramycin	
Amikacin	
Pseudomonas, Xanthomonas, and Acinetobacter	
Azlocillin or piperacillin	Gentamicin
Aztreonam	Tobramycin
Mezlocillin or ticarcillin	Netilmicin
Ceftazidime	Amikacin
Trimethoprim-sulfamethoxazole	Imipenem
Staphylococci	
Penicillin G	Imipenem
Amoxicillin-clavulanate	Vancomycin
Ampicillin-sulbactam	Gentamicin
Oxacillin or nafcillin	Amikacin
Cephalothin	Clarithromycin or azithromycin
Erythromycin	Ciprofloxacin
Clindamycin	Trimethoprim-sulfamethoxazole
Enterococci	
Ampicillin†	Gentamicin (high-level resistance)
Pencillin G	Nitrofurantoin§
Ciprofloxacin	Vancomycin
Nonenterococcal Streptococci	
Penicillin G	Clarithromycin or azithromycin
Erythromycin	Vancomycin
Clindamycin	
Streptococcus pneumoniae	
Penicillin G‖	Erythromycin
Cefotaxime or ceftriaxone	Vancomycin
Haemophilus influenzae	
Ampicillin†	Tetracycline
Amoxicillin-clavulanate or ampicillin-sulbactam	Trimethoprim
Cefotaxime or ceftriaxone	Sulfisoxazole†
Clarithromycin or azithromycin	Ciprofloxacin
Anaerobes	
Penicillin G	Clindamycin
Ampicillin	Imipenem
Ampicillin-clavulanate or ampicillin-sulbactam	Metronidazole
Ticarcillin, mezlocillin or piperacillin	Cefoxitin
Ticarcillin-clavulanate	

*The most appropriate antimicrobials to test are best determined by the clinical laboratory in consultation with medical staff, infectious disease practitioners, and pharmacy. Antimicrobials in this table have proven clinical efficacy for that organism group and acceptable *in vitro* test performance.

†These agents represent similar agents (e.g., ampicillin represents amoxicillin, cephalothin represents cephaloridine, cephalexin, cefazolin, cephradine, and so on).

‡Cefotaxime, ceftazidime, ceftizoxime, ceftriaxone, or moxalactam.

§For urinary isolates only.

‖For disk-diffusion testing, oxacillin or methicillin disks reflect penicillin G susceptibility more accurately than penicillin G disks.

assessment is made by drawing peak and trough serum samples; peak samples are drawn 15 to 30 minutes after intravenous infusion or 1 hour after intramuscular injection; trough samples are drawn just before the next drug dose.

Serum bactericidal activity, often referred to as the Schlichter test, is performed by preparing serial twofold dilutions of the patient's serum in tubes of Mueller-Hinton broth and inoculating each tube with a suspension of 5×10^5 organisms per milliliter.[17] After overnight incubation, bacteriostatic levels are read and tubes are subcultured to determine bactericidal dilutions. Results are expressed as endpoint serum dilutions. Criteria for acceptable bactericidal levels have not been clearly defined, except in endocarditis in which peak serum bactericidal dilutions of 1:8 or greater correlate with a favorable outcome.

MONITORING ANTIMICROBIAL LEVELS

Measurement of concentrations of antimicrobial agents in serum and other body fluids can confirm that therapeutic drug levels (i.e., above in vitro MIC values) have been attained while avoiding levels approaching toxicity.[23, 24] Although most drugs do not usually require monitoring, aminoglycosides,[23, 24] chloramphenicol,[25, 26] and vancomycin[24] produce dose-related toxicity. Gentamicin and tobramycin trough values greater than 2 μg/mL and amikacin values greater than 10 μg/mL are associated with nephrotoxicity.[23, 27] Reversible hematopoietic toxicity of chloramphenicol occurs with serum concentrations greater than 25 μg/mL, particularly in patients with liver and renal disease.[25, 26] Renal disease, obesity, dehydration, edema, major burns, and fever can all alter aminoglycoside distribution, resulting in potentially toxic drug levels.[24]

Peak and trough serum samples for antimicrobial assay should be drawn as discussed previously. All specimens must be labeled with sampling time, times of drug administration, drug dosage and route of administration, and other drugs being administered, particularly antimicrobial agents. This is necessary to minimize drug interactions, such as the inactivation of aminoglycosides by high concentrations of carbenicillin, and to ensure that the assay procedure is appropriate.[28, 29]

Drugs can be assayed by microbiologic, biochemical, and chromatographic methods.[1] Microbiologic methods require at least 24 hours and are difficult to perform if patients are receiving multiple antimicrobial agents. Biochemical methods using antibodies with radioactive, enzyme, or fluorescent labels are widely used for aminoglycosides. Chloramphenicol, which is now rarely used, is best assayed by high-pressure liquid chromatography.[30]

SEROLOGIC DIAGNOSIS OF INFECTIONS

Although antibody detection is rarely useful for the management of critically ill patients, serology can be important in providing a diagnosis during convalescence.[31] Acute-phase sera should be collected whenever possible in patients with febrile illnesses, and convalescent samples should be drawn 1 to 6 weeks later. There are many techniques to detect antibodies, and commercial reagents are increasingly available. Examples of infections causing severe illness that can be diagnosed serologically include typhoid fever, brucellosis, tularemia, legionnaires' disease, all acute viral diseases, histoplasmosis, rickettsial typhus and spotted fevers, toxoplasmosis, and amebiasis.[31]

VALUE OF DIAGNOSTIC MICROBIOLOGY IN CRITICAL CARE MEDICINE

Diagnostic microbiologic procedures can identify the infectious cause of a disease and determine its optimal therapy. Rapid determination of these results is vital in critical care medicine, particularly for patients with septicemia, pneumonia, meningitis, or neutropenia. Faster bacterial isolation, identification, and susceptibility tests now allow results on the day after specimen collection rather than 2 days after. For results to be of value for the initial management of critically ill patients, however, this time delay needs to be shortened to 1 or 2 hours; only antigen-detection procedures currently fulfill this requirement, and their usefulness is limited. Direct microscopic examination of specimens remains the only rapid diagnostic procedure that is always available and can be performed with simple reagents and microscopes.

In critically ill patients with suspected infections, broad-spectrum therapy can be guided by Gram's stain results until culture and susceptibility results are known. Adequate collection of appropriate specimens is crucial for the generation of meaningful laboratory results and should not be neglected in the rush to initiate antimicrobial therapy in a critically ill patient.

Microbiology laboratories can provide valuable information about the antimicrobial susceptibility of pathogens, serum bactericidal activity, serum drug levels, and activity of drugs in combination. However, corresponding antimicrobial therapy may still fail owing to failure of drug absorption or distribution, accelerated drug inactivation, inadequate dosage, inactivation of drugs when mixed in infusion fluids before administration, failure of drugs to reach organisms in abscesses or the central nervous system, development of pathogen resistance during therapy, drug antagonism, superinfection, or impairment of local or general host defenses.[18] Consultation among physicians and clinical microbiology personnel will do much to identify many of these factors and to optimize patient care. Improvements in rapid diagnostic procedures will be a major advance in the diagnosis and management of the critically ill patient.

References

1. Washington JA (Ed): Laboratory Procedures in Clinical Microbiology. 2nd ed. New York, Springer-Verlag, 1985.
2. Isenberg HD, Washington JA, Doern GV, et al: Specimen collection and handling. *In*: Manual of Clinical Microbiology. 5th ed. Balows A, Hausler JR, Herrmann KL, et al (Eds). Washington, DC, American Society for Microbiology, 1991, p 15.
3. Lennette DA: Preparation of specimens for virological examination. *In*: Manual of Clinical Microbiology. 5th ed. Balows A, Hausler JR, Herrmann KL, et al (Eds). Washington, DC, American Society for Microbiology, 1991, p 818.
4. Donowitz GR, Mandell GL: Acute pneumonia. *In*: Principles and Practices of Infectious Diseases. 2nd ed. Mandell GL, Douglas RG, Bennett JE (Eds). New York, John Wiley & Sons, 1985, p 394.
5. Fung JC, Tilton RC: Detection of bacterial antigens by counterimmunoelectrophoresis, coagglutination and latex agglutination. *In*: Manual of Clinical Microbiology. 4th ed. Lennette EH, Balows A, Hausler JR, et al (Eds). Washington, DC, American Society for Microbiology, 1985, p 883.
6. Tenover FC: Molecular methods for the clinical microbiology laboratory. *In*: Manual of Clinical Microbiology. 5th ed. Balows A, Hausler JR, Herrmann KL, et al (Eds). Washington, DC, American Society for Microbiology, 1991, p 119.
7. Horstmeier CD, DeYoung DR, Doerr KA, et al: A comparison of a radiometric method and conventional media for recovery of mycobacteria in clinical specimens (Abstract no. C187). *In*: Abstracts of the 82nd Annual Meeting of the American Society for Microbiology, 1982.
8. Menegus MA, Douglas RG: Viruses, rickettsia, chlamydia and mycoplasmas. *In*: Principles and Practices of Infectious Diseases. 2nd ed. Mandell GL, Douglas RG, Bennett JE (Eds). New York, John Wiley and Sons, 1985, p 138.
9. Pfaller MA: Typing methods for epidemiological investigation. *In*: Manual of Clinical Microbiology. 5th Edition. Balows A, Hausler JR, Herrmann KL, et al (Eds). Washington, DC, American Society for Microbiology, 1991, p 171.
10. National Committee for Clinical Laboratory Standards: Methods for Dilution Antimicrobial Susceptibility Tests for Bacteria Which Grow Aerobically. 3rd ed. Villanova, PA, NCCLS, 1993.
11. Barry AL: The Antimicrobial Susceptibility Test: Principles and Practices. Philadelphia, Lea & Febiger, 1976.
12. Barry AL, Jones RN, Gavan TL: Evaluation of the Micro-Media system for quantitative antimicrobial susceptibility testing: A collaborative study. Antimicrob Agents Chemother 1978; 13:61.
13. National Committee for Clinical Laboratory Standards: Performance Standards for Antimicrobic Disk Susceptibility Tests. 5th edition. Villanova, PA, NCCLS, 1993.
14. National Committee for Clinical Laboratory Standards: Per-

formance Standard for Antimicrobial Susceptibility Testing: Fourth Informational Supplement. Villanova, PA, NCCLS, 1992.
15. Randall EL: State of the art susceptibility testing with the Autobac MTS. *In*: Rapid Methods and Automation in Microbiology. Tilton RC (Ed). Washington, DC, American Society for Microbiology, 1982, p 295.
16. Kelly MT, Latimer JM, Balfour LC: Comparison of three automated systems for antimicrobial susceptibility testing of Gram-negative bacilli. *In*: Rapid Methods and Automation in Microbiology. Tilton RC (Ed). Washington, DC, American Society for Microbiology, 1982, p 302.
17. Schoenknecht FD, Sabath LD, Thornsberry C: Special tests. *In*: Manual of Clinical Microbiology. 4th ed. Lenette EH, Balows A, Hausler JR, et al (Eds). Washington, DC, American Society for Microbiology, 1985, p 1000.
18. Sanders WG, Sanders CC: Significance of *in vitro* antimicrobial susceptibility tests in care of the infected patient. *In*: Significance of Medical Microbiology in the Care of Patients. Lorain V (Ed). Baltimore, Williams & Wilkins, 1977, p 186.
19. Krogstad DJ, Moellering RC: Antimicrobial combinations. *In*: Antibiotics in Laboratory Medicine. 2nd ed. Lorain V (Ed). Baltimore, Williams & Wilkins, 1986, p 537.
20. McClatchy JK: Antimycobacterial drugs: Mechanisms of action, drug resistance, susceptibility testing, and assays of activity in biological fluids. *In*: Antibiotics in Laboratory Medicine. 2nd ed. Lorain V (Ed). Baltimore, Williams & Wilkins, 1986, p 181.
21. Shadomy S, Pfaller MA; Laboratory studies with antifungal agents: Susceptibility tests and quantitation in body fluids. *In*: Manual of Clinical Microbiology. 5th ed. Balows A, Hausler JR, Herrmann KL, et al (Eds). Washington, DC, American Society for Microbiology, 1991, p 1173.
22. Stratton CW, Weinstein MP, Reller LB: Correlation of serum bactericidal activity with antimicrobial agent level and minimal bactericidal concentration. J Infect Dis 1982; 145:160.
23. Appel GB, Neu HC: The nephrotoxicity of antimicrobial agents. N Engl J Med 1977; 296:722.
24. Pechere JC, Dugal R: Clinical pharmacokinetics of aminoglycoside antibiotics. Clin Pharmacokin 1979; 4:170.
25. Scott JL, Finegold SM, Belkin GA, et al: A controlled double-blind study of the hematologic toxicity of chloramphenicol. N Engl J Med 1965; 272:1137.
26. Suhrland LG, Weisberger AS: Chloramphenicol toxicity in liver and renal disease. Arch Intern Med 1963; 112:747.
27. Dahlgren JG, Anderson ET, Hewitt WL: Gentamicin blood levels: A guide to nephrotoxicity. Antimicrob Agents Chemother 1975; 8:58.
28. Henderson JL, Polk RE, Kline BJ: *In vitro* inactivation of gentamicin, tobramycin, and netilmicin by carbenicillin, azlocillin, or mezlocillin. Am J Hosp Pharm 1981; 38:1167.
29. Pickering LK, Gearhart P: Effect of time and concentration upon interaction between gentamicin, tobramycin, netilmicin, or amikacin and carbenicillin or ticarcillin. Antimicrob Agents Chemother 1979; 15:592.
30. Pickering LK, Hoecker JL, Kramer WG, et al: Assays for chloramphenicol compared: Radioenzymatic, gas chromatographic with electron capture and gas chromatographic-mass spectrophotometric. Clin Chem 1979; 25:300.
31. White A: Serologic diagnosis. *In*: Principles and Practices of Infectious Diseases. Mandell GL, Douglas RG, Bennett JE (Eds). New York, John Wiley and Sons, 1979, p 192.

CHAPTER 136

Pneumonia in the Immunosuppressed Patient

Henry Masur, MD

Over the past two decades, considerable progress has been made in managing pneumonia in all patient populations. First, the natural history of many infectious processes has been clarified. Second, the relationship of infection to specific forms of immunosuppression is better delineated, allowing clinicians to predict when certain infectious processes are likely to occur. Third, diagnostic procedures are more sensitive, more specific, and more available, allowing more accurate diagnoses to be made. Fourth, therapy is more successful because of improved methods of respiratory support and a vastly expanded armamentarium of drugs. These advances provide the intensivist with the tools to reduce the morbidity and mortality associated with pneumonia. Successful management depends on utilization of these tools in an organized and expeditious manner.[1]

SPECTRUM OF CAUSATIVE PROCESSES

When patients present with respiratory symptoms, respiratory signs, or chest radiographic abnormalities, a wide variety of infectious, neoplastic, toxic, embolic, and cardiogenic processes may be responsible (Table 136–1). This chapter focuses on pneumonia, but it is important to assess whether an infection is the causative process or whether pulmonary dysfunction is, in fact, due to one of the noninfectious processes listed in Table 136–1.

Pneumonia can be caused by organisms that were acquired recently (primary infection) or by reactivation of latent organisms that were previously acquired. Influenza A and legionellosis are examples of primary processes. Alternatively, tuberculosis, cryptococcosis, pneumocystosis, or cytomegalovirus (CMV) disease may represent reactivation of previously acquired infection that has remained latent, even in immunologically normal individuals.

Pneumonia may be acquired in the community, especially by aerosolization, suggesting a certain spectrum of pathogens based on the season, geographic location, and other factors unique to an individual patient's environment. The organisms may, alternatively, be acquired in a healthcare facility, suggesting a very different spectrum of organisms. The causative organisms for a nosocomial process are a reflection of the microbial flora of a particular hospital or clinic and the defects in the patient's pulmonary defense mechanisms brought about by iatrogenic procedures as well as the underlying disease and immunosuppressive therapies.

Table 136–2 provides an overview of microorganisms that cause pneumonia. Table 136–3 summarizes pulmonary defense mechanisms, including nonimmunologic as well as immunologic components of host defense. Table 136–4 provides examples of which causative organisms are more likely when specific defenses are compromised.

When approaching the diagnosis of pneumonia in immunosuppressed patients, it is important to keep in mind that common, community-acquired pneumonia as well as opportunistic processes can develop in these patients. Thus, a patient with human immunodeficiency virus (HIV) infection and a CD4+ T lymphocyte count of 50/mm^3 is highly predisposed to *Pneumocystis carinii* pneumonia (Fig. 136–1), but when influenza or respiratory syncytia virus (RSV) is prevalent in the community, these latter pathogens need to be a

TABLE 136–1. Causes of Diffuse Pulmonary Infiltrates

Pneumonia	Radiation pneumonitis
Aspiration pneumonia	Leukoagglutinin reactions
Congestive heart failure	Hematologic malignancy
Adult respiratory distress syndrome	Lymphangitic spread of carcinoma
Pulmonary emboli with infarction	Alveolar hemorrhage
Drug-induced pneumonitis	Oxygen toxicity

TABLE 136–2. Potential Causes of Pulmonary Infection in Immunosuppressed Patients

Community-Acquired Bacterial Pneumonia	***Viral Pneumonia***
Streptococcus pneumoniae	Cytomegalovirus
Haemophilus influenzae	Influenza, parainfluenza
Branhamella catarrhalis	Adenovirus
Staphylococcus aureus	Herpes simplex, varicella zoster
Escherichia coli	***Fungal Pneumonia***
Klebsiella pneumoniae	*Aspergillus fumigatus*
Mycoplasma pneumoniae	*Histoplasma capsulatum*
Chlamydia pneumoniae	*Cryptococcus neoformans*
Legionella pneumophila	*Blastomyces dermatitidis*
Nosocomial Bacterial Pneumonia	*Coccidioides immitis*
Enteric gram-negative bacilli	*Candida* species
Pseudomonas aeruginosa	*Mucor-Rhizopus-Absidia*
Pseudomonas species (other)	*Pneumocystis carinii*
Xanthomonas maltophilia	***Parasitic Pneumonia***
Other Bacterial Pneumonia	*Strongyloides stercoralis*
Nocardia species	*Toxoplasma gondii*
Mycobacterium tuberculosis	
Atypical mycobacteria (*M. avium* complex, *M. Kansasii,* and others)	
Aspiration Pneumonia	
Anaerobic rods and cocci	
Staphylococcus aureus	
Steptococcus species	
Enteric gram-negative bacilli	

prime concern in planning the diagnostic approach and the initial empirical therapeutic regimen. It is important for the clinician not to focus exclusively on opportunistic processes.

When assessing the cause of pneumonia, it is important to appreciate the relationship of host defense mechanisms, both nonimmunologic and immunologic, to the likelihood that a specific pathogen is involved.[1–7] Nonimmunologic mechanisms, as listed in Table 136–3, include physical barriers like the epiglottis; if, for example, the epiglottis is compromised by drugs that impair neurologic function or by an endotracheal tube, then microorganisms from the oropharynx or the gastrointestinal tract can gain access to the lower respiratory tract, which they ordinarily could not do. Similarly, chemical barriers are important. Gastric acidity, for example, reduces the population of bacteria in the stomach.[8, 8a, 9] Achlorhydria, produced by disease or by drugs such as histamine$_2$ blockers or antacids, allows gram-negative bacilli to populate the upper gastrointestinal tract.[8] Thus, when organisms are aspirated into the lungs from gastric or oropharyngeal material, the organisms are more likely to be gram-negative bacilli rather than exclusively aerobic and anaerobic cocci, thus changing the microbiology of aspiration pneumonia.[8a]

The relationship of causative processes to defects in inflammatory and immunologic mechanisms is also important. The organisms that cause pneumonia in patients with diminished number or diminished function of neutrophils are quite distinct from those that cause pneumonia in patients with deficient immunoglobulin G, complement, or CD4 + T lymphocytes, as shown in Table 136–4.[3–6, 10–16] The degree of deficiency in inflammatory and immunologic mechanisms is important to measure; clinical relationships have been established that show the degree of deficiency that is required before the likelihood of infection is enhanced. For instance, neutrophil counts can fall to the 750 to 1000/mm^3 range before there is predisposition to infection.[10–16] Similarly, life-threatening opportunistic infections rarely occur until the CD4 + T lymphocyte falls from a normal range of 800 to 1200/mm^3 to 200 to 300/mm^3 (see Fig. 136–1).[3]

TABLE 136–3. Defects in Respiratory Host Defenses That May Lead to Infection

Host Mechanism	*Defect*	*Potential Impact of Defects on Respiratory Host Defenses*
Conducting Airways		
Mechanical barriers (upper airway structures)	Intubation of the trachea	Aspiration or direct aerosol entry of organisms into the airway
Mucociliary clearance	Intrinsic structural defects	Stasis of secretions, bronchiectasis
Bronchoconstriction	Hyperactive airways	Poor clearance of secretions, excessive secretions
Local immunoglobulin coating	IgA deficiency, functional deficiency from breakdown by bacterial proteases	Sinopulmonary infections
Iron-containing proteins	Iron deficiency	Lack of killing of certain bacteria
Alveolar Milieu		
Other immunoglobulins	Acquired hypogammaglobulinemia Selective IgG$_4$ and IgG$_2$ deficiency	Sinopulmonary infections, pneumonia with encapsulated bacteria
Alternative complement pathway	C3 and C5 deficiency	Recurrent infections
Surfactant	Decreased synthesis Acute lung injury	Loss of opsonization activity, alveolar collapse
Alveolar macrophages	Intracellular killing	Propensity of *Legionella* infections; poor containment of mycobacteria
Polymorphonuclear leukocytes	Decreased numbers Intrinsic defects Absence of chemotactic stimulus	Poor inflammatory response; bacterial and fungal infections
Augmenting Mechanisms		
Initiation of immune responses	Immunosuppression	Inadequate S-IgA or IgG antibody available; susceptible to viral, mycoplasmal, and bacterial infections
Generation of inflammatory response (influx of inflammatory cells and mediators)	Usually reflects supply of PMN leukocytes; impaired adherence	Same as for PMN leukocytes; C5 deficiency might decrease inflammatory reaction

(From Reynolds HY: Pulmonary host defenses. *In:* Respiratory Disease in the Immunosuppressed Host. Shelhamer J, Pizzo PA, Parrillo JE, et al [Eds]. Philadelphia, JB Lippincott, 1991, p 4.)

Abbreviations: Ig = immunoglobulin; PMN = polymorphonuclear.

TABLE 136–4. Infections Associated with Common Defects in Inflammatory or Immunologic Response

Host Defect	*Diseases/Therapies Associated with Defects*	*Common Causes of Infections*
Inflammatory Response		
Neutropenia	Hematologic malignancies, cytotoxic chemotherapy, aplastic anemia	Gram-negative bacilli, *Staphylococcus aureus, Candida* species, *Aspergillus* species
Chemotaxis	Chédiak-Higashi disease	*Staphyloccus aureus, Streptococcus pyogenes*
Phagocytosis (cellular)	Systemic lupus erythematosus, chronic myelogenous leukemia, megaloblastic anemia	*Streptococcus pneumoniae, Haemophilus influenzae*
Splenectomy	Trauma, therapy for thrombocytopenia	*Haemophilus influenzae, Streptococcus pneumoniae,* other streptococci, DF-2, *Babesia microti*
Microbicidal defect	Chronic granulomatous disease	Catalase-positive bacteria and fungi: staphylococci, *Escherichia coli, Klebsiella* species, *Pseudomonas aeruginosa, Candida* species, *Aspergillus* species, *Nocardia* species
	Chédiak-Higashi disease	*Staphylococcus aureus, Streptococci pyogenes*
Complement System		
C3	Congenital, liver disease	*Staphylococcus aureus, Streptococcus pneumoniae*
	Systemic lupus erythematosus	*Pseudomonas* species, *Proteus* species
C5	Congenital	*Neisseria* species, gram-negative rods
C6, C7, C8	Congenital, systemic lupus erythematosus	*Neisseria meningitidis, Neisseria gonorrhoeae*
Alternative complement pathway	Sickle cell disease	*Streptococcus pneumoniae, Salmonella* species
Immune Response		
T lymphocyte deficiency/dysfunction	Thymic aplasia, thymic hypoplasia, Hodgkin's disease, sarcoid, lepromatous leprosy	*Listeria monocytogenes, Mycobacterium* species, *Candida* species, *Aspergillus* species, *Cryptococcus neoformans,* herpes simplex, herpes zoster
	Human immunodeficiency virus	*Pneumocystis carinii,* cytomegalovirus, herpes simplex, *Mycobacterium avium-intracellulare, Cryptococcus neoformans, Candida* species
	Mucocutaneous candidiasis	*Candida* species
	Purine nucleoside phosphorylase deficiency	Fungi, viruses
B cell deficiency/dysfunction	Bruton's X-linked agammaglobulinemia, hypogammaglobulinemia, chronic lymphocytic leukemia, multiple myeloma, dysglobulinemia	*Streptococcus pneumoniae,* other streptococci, *Haemophilus influenzae, Neisseria meningitidis, Staphylococcus aureus, Klebsiella pneumoniae, Escherichia coli, Giardia lamblia, Pneumocystis carinii,* enteroviruses
	Selective IgM deficiency	*Streptococcus pneumoniae, Haemophilus influenzae, Escherichia coli*
	Selective IgA deficiency	*Giardia lamblia,* viral hepatitis, *Streptococcus pneumoniae, Haemophilus influenzae*
Mixed T and B cell deficiency/dysfunction	Common variable hypogammaglobulinemia	*Pneumocystis carinii,* cytomegalovirus, *Streptococcus pneumoniae, Haemophilus influenzae,* varicella, other bacteria
	Ataxia-telangiectasia	*Streptococcus pneumoniae, Haemophilus influenzae, Staphylococcus aureus,* rubella, *Gardia lamblia*
	Severe combined immunodeficiency	*Candida albicans, Pneumocystis carinii,* varicella, rubella, cytomegalovirus
	Wiskott-Aldrich syndrome	Infections seen in T and B cell abnormalities

Abbreviations: Ig = immunoglobulin.

Anticipating infectious complications in terms of when they are likely to occur also facilitates the diagnostic and therapeutic approach. Many immunodeficiencies are produced by immunosuppressive drugs or procedures. Clinical experience permits the infectious complications to be predicted, for instance, during discrete time periods after institution of immunosuppressive drugs for organ transplantation.[17, 18] Figure 136–2 shows the viral complications that typically follow allogeneic bone marrow transplantation. The precise pattern may be modified by the underlying disease and the particular immunosuppressive regimen being used. However, it is very useful to know when CMV pneumonia, for example, is most likely to occur after allogeneic bone marrow transplantation.

DIAGNOSIS

It is particularly important for immunosuppressed patients to have an expeditious diagnostic evaluation when they present with an apparent pneumonia. First, the differential diagnosis in the population is very broad, making it unlikely that any reasonable empirical regimen could cover all the common pathogens. Second, clinical presentations are particularly likely to be misleading. Atypical presentations and mixed processes (e.g., tumor plus infection), as well as mixed infections (e.g., *Pneumocystis carinii* plus CMV), make clinical presentations diagnostically confusing. Third, progressive infection can develop in immunosuppressed patients very rapidly. A rapid deterioration can preclude performing diagnostic procedures such as bronchoscopy or open lung biopsy if the patient becomes too unstable to tolerate the procedure. Fourth, failure to institute appropriate therapy promptly has obvious negative implications for survival. Last, immunosuppressed patients often have compromised function of multiple organs because of underlying disease or previous therapy, and they are often receiving multiple drugs. Thus, the administration of antimicrobial agents may cause toxicities and drug interactions that might be avoided if a specific diagnosis was quickly established.

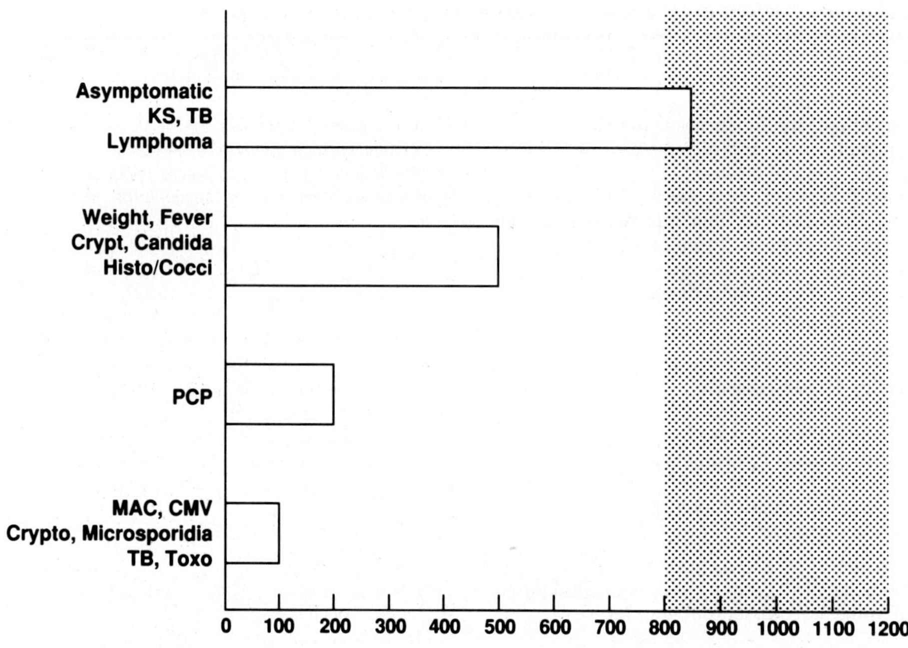

Figure 136–1. The relationships of circulating CD4+ T lymphocyte count and the causative organisms for opportunistic processes in patients with HIV infection. *Abbreviations*: KS = Kaposi's sarcoma; TB = tuberculosis; PCP = *Pneumocystis carinii* pneumonia; MAC = *Mycobacterium avium* complex.

Chest radiographs present useful information about the location and extent of pulmonary involvement. The pattern of radiologic abnormality can be useful for suggesting specific causes because the differential diagnosis for a diffuse interstitial infiltrate is quite different from that for a lobar infiltrate, for cavitating nodules, or for wedge-shaped, pleural-based lesions. These clues are helpful diagnostically, but they should not be relied on for individual patients. As mentioned, pathogens can manifest atypically or unusual pathogens can mimic the classic presentations of common organisms. Thus, "pattern recognition" should not be a substitute for establishing a specific diagnosis. It is also appropriate to emphasize that a normal chest radiograph does not exclude the possibility of pneumonia. There can be substantial pulmonary dysfunction before any abnormality is apparent on chest radiograph. Thus, there may be instances when a diagnostic work-up, including invasive procedures, may be warranted despite an apparently normal chest radiograph.

Other chest imaging studies may be useful. Computed tomographic scans and magnetic resonance imaging may reveal pulmonary disease not apparent on routine chest radiograph. This may be useful for directing diagnostic procedures or assessing the extent or change of disease over time.

Examination of respiratory secretions continues to be the mainstay for diagnosis (Table 136–5).[19–25a] Examination of sputum by Gram's stain, wet mount, or a mycobacterial technique can often establish a diagnosis expeditiously (Table 136–6). Better sputum specimens in terms of quality and quantity can often be obtained by induction techniques that emphasize high-flow nebulized saline to produce an adequate specimen. When appropriate techniques are used by the laboratory to process and stain the specimen, the diagnostic yield can be substantial. For pneumocystis pneumonia, for example, induced sputum can establish a diagnosis in 80% to 95% of patients with HIV infection.[26–28] There are fewer data for other pathogens.

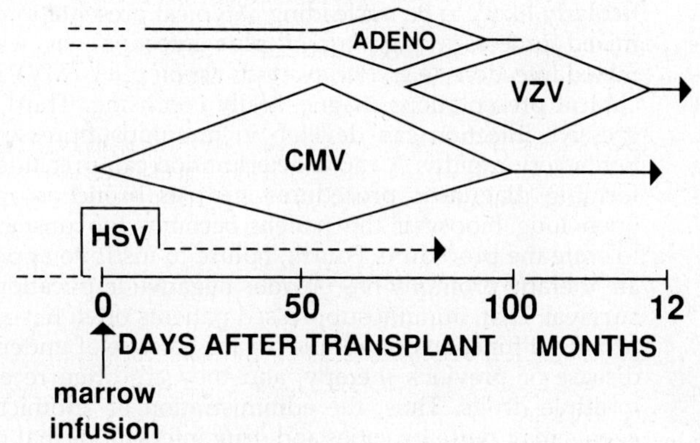

Figure 136–2. The temporal pattern of opportunistic infections among patients who have undergone allogeneic bone marrow transplantation. *Abbreviations*: ADENO = adenovirus; VZV = varicella-zoster virus; HSV = herpes simplex virus. (From Myers JD: Infection in bone marrow transplant recipients. *In:* Principles and Practice of Infectious Disease. 3rd ed. Mandell GL, Douglas RG, Bennett J [Eds]. New York, Churchill Livingstone, 1990.)

TABLE 136–5. Sequence of Diagnostic Pulmonary Procedures and Characterization of Pathogenic Processes Yielded in Immunosuppressed Hosts

Procedure	*Pathogenic Process*
Induced sputum with hypertonic sodium chloride	*Pneumocystis carinii*
Sputum specimen for Gram's stain, culture, and cytology	Bacterial, fungal, and mycobacterial pneumonias or neoplasia
Bronchoalveolar lavage for microbiologic stains, cultures, and cytology	Bacterial, fungal, mycobacterial, viral, and *Pneumocystis* pneumonias; neoplasia; alveolar hemorrhage
Transbronchial biopsy	Bacterial, fungal, mycobacterial, viral, and *Pneumocystis* pneumonias; neoplasia; diffuse alveolar damage; hemorrhage; fibrosis
Open lung biopsy	Bacterial, fungal, mycobacterial, viral, and *Pneumocystis* pneumonias; neoplasia; diffuse alveolar damage; hemorrhage; fibrosis

(From Ognibene FP: An approach to the management of respiratory disease in the immunosuppressed adult. *In:* Respiratory Disease in the Immunosuppressed Hosts. Shelhamer J, Pizzo PA, Parrillo JE, Masur H [Eds]. Philadelphia, JB Lippincott, 1991, p 731.)

If examination of a sputum sample does not establish a definitive diagnosis, bronchoscopy is usually warranted. Bronchoalveolar lavage has replaced bronchial washings or brushings as the procedure of choice for most infectious processes.[21–26] The repertoire of stains for a bronchoalveolar lavage is similar to that outlined for sputum (Fig. 136–3). If the lavage is nondiagnostic, a repeat bronchoscopy with a second lavage plus a transbronchial biopsy should be considered. Histopathology of a biopsy specimen may reveal organisms that were not apparent in the lavage (Fig. 136–4). Moreover, some causes of pneumonitis, such as CMV, can be established definitively only by visualization of typical inclusion bodies, at least in some patient populations such as those with acquired immunodeficiency syndrome.[29] Culture of sputum, bronchoalveolar lavage, or lung biopsy may reveal the causative organism if a definitive pathogen such as *Cryptococcus, Histoplasma,* or tuberculosis is grown. However, in immunosuppressed patients, these culture results are not available rapidly (they may take days or weeks), and a definitive diagnosis must be sought by direct examination of secretions or tissue so that appropriate therapy can be initiated promptly. Bronchoscopy can be performed safely in almost any patient as long as the patient can be ventilated and oxygenated with the bronchoscope in the airway. Transbronchial biopsy can be performed in many patients, but not in those with thrombocytopenia, coagulopathy, severe hypoxemia, or unilateral lung function. In situ-

TABLE 136–6. Evaluation of the Utility of Sputum Diagnosis of Respiratory Disease Caused by Various Pathogens in Immunocompromised Patients

Pathogen	*Utility of Sputum Diagnosis*	*Comment*
Bacteria		
Streptococcus pneumoniae	Useful	Few squamous cells, sheets of PMNs (except in neutropenia), plus characteristic organisms are highly suggestive.
Staphylococcus aureus	Useful	Cellular features as above but less reliable. High colonization rate in immunocompromised patients.
Enterobacteriaceae and *Pseudomonas aeruginosa*	Useful	As above.
Legionella pneumophila	Useful	Direct fluorescent antibody supplemented by culture is diagnostic.
Chlamydia trachomatis	Probably useful	Immunofluorescent stain appears helpful. Conventional stains and culture are difficult.
Mycobacterium tuberculosis	Useful	Acid-fast stains and culture are diagnostic. Induced sputum helpful if necessary.
Nocardia asteroides	Often not useful	0–50% sensitivity.
Fungi		
Blastomyces dermatitidis	Useful	Characteristic morphology in KOH preparations. Culture is confirmatory.
Histoplasma capsulatum	Useful	As above.
Coccidioides immitis	Useful	As above.
Cryptococcus neoformans	Useful	As above.
Candida species	Not useful	Diagnosis requires demonstration of organism in lung tissue. High colonization rate in immunocompromised patients.
Aspergillus sp.	Possibly useful	Sputum culture has low sensitivity for invasive disease, but specificity appears good in patients with neutropenia and/or leukemia.
Pneumocystis carinii	Useful	Induced sputum with conventional stains has high sensitivity; improves to >90% when combined with immunofluorescent testing.
Viruses		
Cytomegalovirus	Possibly useful	Histopathology necessary to diagnose invasive disease. Sputum cytology may be helpful. In bone marrow transplant recipients and probably other transplant recipients, positive CMV cultures often warrant therapy.
Herpes simplex virus	Not useful	As above.
Adenoviruses	Not useful	As above.
Influenza virus	Useful	Nasopharyngeal swabs or washings are preferred. Culture is diagnostic.
Parainfluenza virus	Useful	As above.
Respiratory syncytial virus	Useful	As above.

(Adapted with permission from Lipschik GY, Kovacs JA: Sputum evaluation and nonbronchoscopic lavage. *In:* Respiratory Disease in the Immunosuppressed Host. Shelhamer J, Pizzo PA, Parrillo JE, Masur H [Eds]. Philadelphia, JB Lippincott, 1991, p 65.)

Abbreviations: PMNs = polymorphonuclear leukocytes; KOH = potassium hydroxide; CMV = cytomegalovirus.

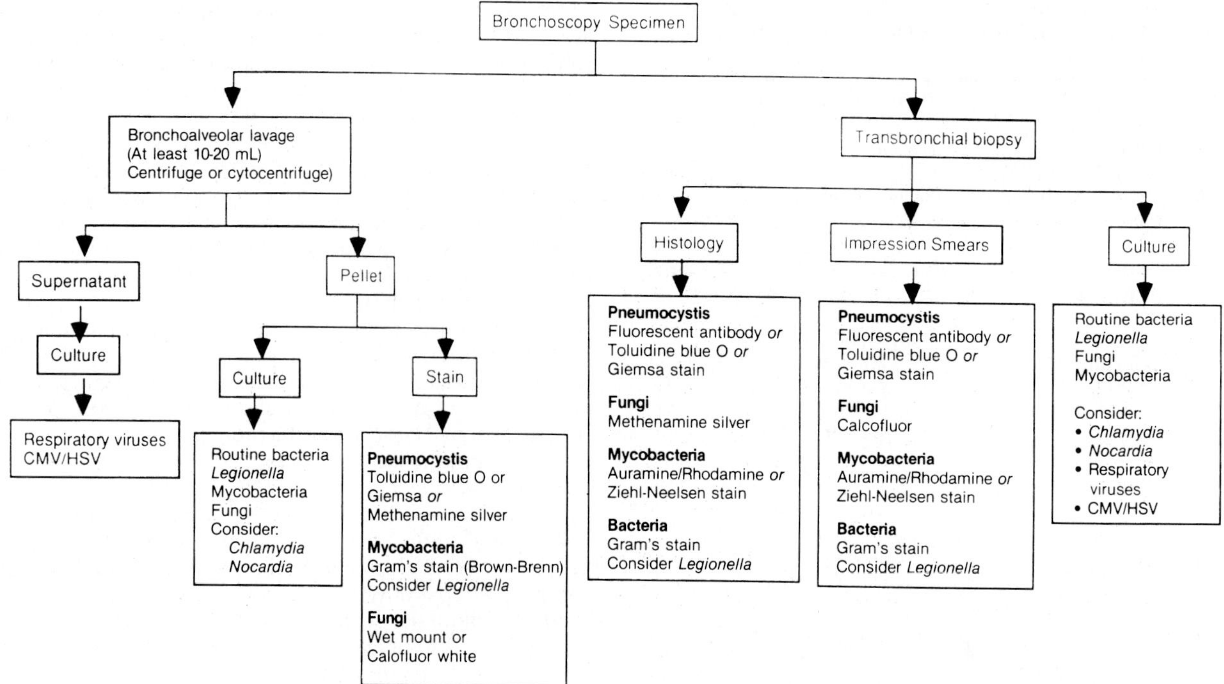

Figure 136–3. Schematic representation of laboratory evaluation of bronchoalveolar lavage in immunosuppressed patients.

ations in which no diagnosis is established by bronchoscopic approaches, an open lung biopsy should be considered (see Fig. 136–4).[30–32] However, in many situations, empirical therapy may be preferable to the morbidity associated with open lung biopsy. Many studies suggest that, with current bronchoscopic techniques, open lung biopsy will only rarely reveal a treatable process. If it is to be useful, open lung biopsy should probably be performed early before empirical therapy refuses the diagnostic yield and before the patient is so sick that morbidity is excessive.

If there is evidence of pleural fluid, examination of a sample by direct microscopy and by culture can be useful for establishing a diagnosis and should be attempted. Similarly, blood cultures can be useful if a pathogen such as *Streptococcus pneumoniae, Cryptococcus,* or even *Mycobacterium tuberculosis* grows. Serum antigen detection approaches are useful in a few situations, such as for *Cryptococcus* or *Histoplasma.*

A variety of techniques to establish a diagnosis by detecting ribonucleic acid or deoxyribonucleic acid sequences in blood, respiratory secretions, urine, or even stool hold considerable promise because of their high degree of sensitivity.

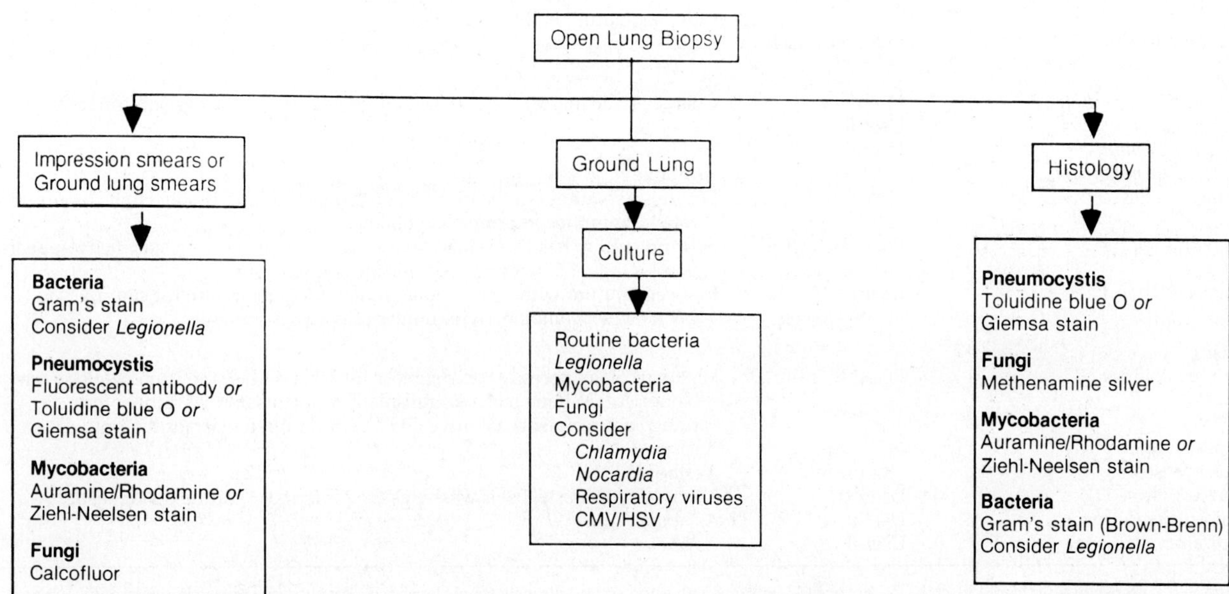

Figure 136–4. Schematic representation of laboratory evaluation of lung biopsy in immunosuppressed patients.

The specificity of these techniques, or their accuracy and reproducibility in a routine laboratory setting, have yet to be determined.

EMPIRICAL THERAPY

In most immunosuppressed patients, it is reasonable and appropriate to institute empirical therapy while the diagnostic evaluation is being initiated. The choice of agents depends on the patient's immunologic status as well as epidemiologic considerations such as recent patient exposures and community-wide trends and outbreaks. Generally, an empirical regimen needs to treat likely community-acquired pathogens such as *Streptococcus pneumoniae, Haemophilus influenzae,*[33] and perhaps *Legionella,*[35] *Chlamydia pneumoniae,* and *Mycoplasma pneumoniae.*[25, 36] In addition, the likely opportunistic pathogens, chosen with knowledge of the immunologic lesion, must be treated.

Some reasonable empirical regimens are outlined in Table 136–7. A frequent concern about empirical regimens is that they will reduce the likelihood that the diagnostic procedures will be useful or that they will introduce unneeded toxicity. Although each of these concerns has some validity, the need to try to reverse the disease may require precedence depending on the severity of the pneumonia. In terms of toxicity, it is important to recognize that a few days of empirical therapy can usually be tolerated without major difficulty.

PREVENTING NOSOCOMIAL SPREAD OF PATHOGENS

Whenever a patient presents in an intensive care unit with pulmonary disease, immediate attention needs to be given to reducing the likelihood of transmitting air- or blood-borne pathogens to the healthcare staff, other patients, and visitors.[37–41] For airborne pathogens, tuberculosis is the major concern.[38–40] In immunosuppressed patients and especially in patients with HIV infection, tuberculosis can present with essentially any radiologic pattern; the typical presentations of primary or reactivated disease are not necessarily seen.[40, 42]

In the 1990s, there are increasing numbers of reports of nosocomial transmission of tuberculosis.[38–40] Some of these have involved more than a dozen patients. Most of these outbreaks have occurred because tuberculosis was overlooked as a possible causative agent. Thus, a high index of suspicion is necessary when evaluating any patient, particularly in areas where tuberculosis is endemic. The epidemic of tuberculosis is spreading rapidly in the United States, however, and is not restricted to large urban areas. Thus, all clinicians need to consider *M. tuberculosis* in the differential diagnosis of pulmonary disease.

Respiratory precautions need to be considered for all patients.[43, 44] The patients at highest risk are probably those with HIV infection who live in areas with high tuberculosis rates. Other immunosuppressed patients, especially those with defective cell-mediated immunity, are also at risk. Precautions include the use of some type of mask by all healthcare practitioners and support personnel (as well as others) who come into contact with the patient. The type of mask that provides optimal protection has not been scientifically determined. It is currently uncertain what type of mask will be mandated by regulatory organizations.[44] The use of isolation rooms with negative airflow and adequate air exchange dynamics is desirable but is not attainable for economic and logistic reasons at many facilities. Whether ultraviolet lights add to protection is controversial. The patients who pose the highest risk are those with high quantities of organisms. In the past, these patients were classically those with laryngeal or cavitary tuberculosis. Now immunosuppressed patients without these types of disease can also have large quantities of organisms. Particular caution is appropriate during procedures likely to aerosolize secretions or induce coughing such as bronchoscopy, intubation, sputum induction, or aerosol drug treatments such as aerosol pentamidine.

At some institutions, all patients with HIV infection and apparent pulmonary disease are placed in respiratory isolation until three sputum smears or a bronchoalveolar lavage specimen are demonstrated to be negative by direct microscopy for mycobacteria. On the basis of local epidemiologic patterns, hospitals need to individualize their isolation policies while trying to establish the causative process. If tuberculosis is documented, careful attention to isolation precautions is mandatory until it is clear that the patient is no longer contagious.

Respiratory transmission can occur with other pathogens such as varicella, influenza, RSV, *Neisseria meningitidis,* or *Pasteurella,* for example. Tuberculosis is the major concern

TABLE 136–7. Typical Empirical Antimicrobial Regimens for Severe Pneumonias for Patients with Different Types of Immunodeficiency

Type of Immunodeficiency	*Initial Empirical Antimicrobial Regimen*	*Pathogens Treated*
Deficiency in cell-mediated immunity (i.e., Hodgkin's disease, corticosteroid therapy)	TMP-SMX and erythromycin; may also consider cephalosporin (e.g., ceftriaxone) and aminoglycoside	*Pneumocystis carinii, Nocardia, Legionella, Mycoplasma* Aerobic gram-positive and gram-negative bacteria (not usually *Pseudomonas*)
Deficiency in neutrophils (i.e., neutropenia, chronic granulomatous disease)	Third-generation cephalosporins (e.g., ceftriaxone) plus aminoglycoside plus vancomycin plus erythromycin; may also consider TMP-SMX and amphotericin B	Gram-negative bacteria (including *Pseudomonas*) Gram-positive bacteria *Legionella, Mycoplasma* *Pneumocystis carinii* Fungi (primarily *Mucor* and *Aspergillus*)
HIV infection	TMP-SMX or pentamidine and erythromycin; consider third-generation cephalosporin such as ceftriaxone	*Pneumocystis carinii* *Legionella* species, *Chlamydia, Mycoplasma* Pyogenic bacteria (*Haemophilus, Streptococcus pneumoniae*)
Deficiency in immunoglobulin	Ceftriaxone alone or vancomycin plus aztreonam	*Streptococcus pneumoniae* *Haemophilus influenzae*

Abbreviations: TMP-SMX = trimethoprim-sulfamethoxazole; HIV = human immunodeficiency virus.

in most patient populations and geographic areas, but outbreaks of influenza or RSV, for example, can cause fatalities in debilitated patients and can cause major staff shortages among hospital personnel.

Prevention of transmission of blood-borne pathogens such as HIV and hepatitis B needs attention as well, as is appropriate for any hospital patient, by emphasizing techniques to use universal precautions and to reduce the likelihood of injuries with sharp instruments.

PNEUMONIA IN CANCER PATIENTS WITH NEUTROPENIA

Patients with neutrophil counts less than 500/mm^3 or neutrophil counts that are falling rapidly toward 500/mm^3 or less, are a special high-risk population for the development of life-threatening pulmonary infections.[10–16] As emphasized previously, the approach to management must include an initial assessment to determine whether the process might be noninfectious. For cancer patients who have received chemotherapy, drug-related pulmonary disease must be considered, such as that caused by methotrexate, busulfan, cyclophosphamide (Cytoxan), vinblastine, melphalan, or mitomycin C. Cardiogenic pulmonary edema, caused by adriamycin-related cardiomyopathy, for example, also deserves consideration.

In this population, the differential diagnosis is extremely broad. Community-acquired processes such as pneumonia caused by *Pneumococcus, Haemophilus, Mycoplasma, Legionella,* or *Chlamydia* are possibilities that need to be treated empirically until a definite cause is established.[25, 30] Bacterial processes, in addition to those caused by *Pneumococcus* and *Haemophilus,* include less common community-acquired pneumonias such as those caused by enteric gram-negative bacilli and *Staphylococcus aureus.* Those processes cause pneumonia as a result of immunosuppression and the altered flora in patients who have often received multiple courses of antibiotics. Cancer patients have also frequently been hospitalized regularly, allowing acquisition of nosocomial pathogens including gram-positive cocci (e.g., enterococci, *S. aureus,* and *S. pneumoniae*) and gram-negative bacilli (e.g., *Pseudomonas* species, *Enterobacter,* and *Klebsiella*), which may be resistant to the antimicrobial agents that might initially be chosen. Patients who have been neutropenic for prolonged periods are predisposed to fungal pneumonias caused by *Aspergillus,* Rhizopus-Mucor-Absidia, endemic fungi *(Cryptococcus, Histoplasma, Blastomyces,* and *Coccidioides),* and perhaps to *Candida.* Finally, if their underlying disease or their chemotherapy has affected their cell-mediated immunity, pneumocystis, CMV, and *Nocardia* become considerations.

Thus, it is clear that an expeditious effort to establish a specific diagnosis is especially important in this population. Table 136–7 provides some possible empirical regimens while the diagnostic process is underway. Table 136–8 provides regimens for specific pathogens once they are identified as the causative organism.

The prognosis in this patient population depends on how long they remain neutropenic, how sensitive the pathogen is to specific therapy, and how severe the process has become at the time optimal therapy is initiated. Granulocyte colony–stimulating factor (G-CSF) can be very useful in accelerating granulocyte proliferation in some patients.[45, 46] Neutrophil transfusion has never been proven useful in adults with cancer.

PATIENTS WITH HIV INFECTION

The CD4+T lymphocyte count is a useful indicator of the degree of immunosuppression in patients with HIV infection.[3] For patients with CD4+T lymphocyte counts greater than 300 to 400/mm^3, the approach to management is similar to that for immunologically normal individuals with several notable exceptions. First, patients with HIV infection have an extraordinary susceptibility to tuberculosis at all ranges of CD4+T lymphocyte counts. Thus, respiratory iso-

TABLE 136–8. Suggested Antimicrobial Therapy for Pulmonary Infections in Immunosuppressed Patients

Infective Agent	*Primary*	*Alternative/Substitute*
Bacteria		
Streptococcus pneumoniae	Penicillin G	First-generation cephalosporin, vancomycin
Staphylococcus aureus	Oxacillin or nafcillin	First-generation cephalosporin, vancomycin
Haemophilus influenzae	Ampicillin-sulbactam	Ceftriaxone, aztreonam
Enteric gram-negative bacilli	Ceftazidime + aminoglycoside	Piperacillin + aztreonam or ciprofloxacin + aztreonam
Pseudomonas aeruginosa	Piperacillin + aminoglycoside	Ciprofloxacin + aminoglycoside
Legionella	Erythromycin ± rifampin	Ciprofloxacin
Mycobacterium tuberculosis	Isoniazid + rifampin + ethambutal + pyrazinamide	Isoniazid + ethambutol + pyrazinamide + streptomycin
Nocardia	Trimethoprim-sulfamethoxazole	Minocycline
Viruses		
Cytomegalovirus	Ganciclovir ± immune globulin	Foscarnet ± immune globulin
Herpes simplex	Acyclovir	Foscarnet
Adenovirus	None effective	—
Influenza A	Rimantadine	Amantadine
Fungi		
Aspergillus	Amphotericin B	Itraconazole
Cryptococcus neoformans	Amphotericin B ± flucytosine	Fluconazole
Histoplasma capsulatum	Amphotericin B	Itraconazole
Coccidioides immitis	Amphotericin B	Itraconazole
Candida species	Amphotericin B ± flucytosine	Fluconazole
Pneumocystis carinii	Trimethoprim-sulfamethoxazole	Pentamidine (intravenous) or trimetrexate-leucovorin
Parasites		
Strongyloides stercoralis	Thiabendazole	—
Toxoplasma gondii	Sulfadiazine + pyrimethamine	Clindamycin + pyrimethamine

lation needs to be considered in any patient with HIV infection and pulmonary disease until one or more smears of respiratory secretions has been examined for mycobacteria.[44, 45] This may be unnecessary in certain geographic areas or for patients who have an extremely low risk of lifetime exposure. Second, certain endemic mycoses such as cryptococcus, histoplasmosis, coccidiodomycosis, or blastomycosis can be common in certain geographic areas. For example, in Indianapolis, *Histoplasma* is as common as pneumocystis as a cause of pulmonary disease in this patient population.[47–49] Third, neoplastic processes such as Kaposi's sarcoma and lymphoma occur with increased frequency.

At lower CD4 + T lymphocyte counts, opportunistic processes must be added to the differential diagnosis (see Fig. 136–3). Pneumocystis pneumonia is the most common of the treatable processes, but fungal disease and CMV are also considerations. If an induced sputum examination does not reveal pneumocystis or any other pathogen, bronchoalveolar lavage is indicated. Transbronchial and open lung biopsy are appropriate, sequentially, if no diagnosis is established and the patient's condition is not improved on empirical therapy. Lung biopsy is rarely needed to establish a diagnosis of pneumocystis pneumonia because essentially all cases should be evident by bronchoalveolar lavage. Lung biopsy may be necessary to document CMV, fungus, mycobacteria, or tumor as the causative process.

When respiratory failure develops in patients with HIV infection, the appropriateness of ventilatory support is often questioned.[50–55] Most intensivists approach this issue no differently in patients with HIV infection than in other immunosuppressed populations. A realistic assessment of the patient's prognosis and the patient's wishes in terms of intensity of support are the major issues. Retrospective reviews indicate that, for most HIV-infected patients, pneumocystis pneumonia is the cause of respiratory failure. Thirty per cent to 50% of patients will survive to leave the hospital.[50–52] Patients need to be selected carefully for support; those who were active and functional before their illness, who do not have immediately life-threatening concurrent problems, and who have received only a few days of antipneumocystis therapy at the time of respiratory failure probably have the best prospects for survival.

PNEUMONIA IN TRANSPLANT RECIPIENTS

Pneumonia is a frequent complication of all transplantation procedures that involve immunosuppression.[17, 18, 29, 56] The frequency of infectious complications varies tremendously among transplant recipients depending on the organ being transplanted and the immunosuppressive regimen being used. When recipients are neutropenic for long periods of time or are treated with a more potent immunosuppressive like antithymocyte globulin, mucocutaneous barriers are damaged by surgery, foreign bodies are implanted (e.g., chest tubes, urinary catheters, or stints), or immunosuppressive infections such as CMV develop, patients acquire particular predispositions to infection. Infections posttransplantation occur with a characteristic timing that is dependent on a variety of factors, particularly the organ being transplanted and the immunosuppressive regimen being used. An example is shown in Fig. 136–2.

Immunosuppression after transplantation is largely time limited. Neutropenia will resolve if the patient can survive long enough for the drug effect to wane or for CMV disease to be treated. G-CSF may be helpful in such circumstances. The immunosuppressive effects of antilymphocyte serum, prednisone, azathioprine (Imuran), cyclophosphamide, or other agents diminish as the doses of these agents are reduced and as time passes since those agents were administered. Classically, infectious complications fit into three periods: the initial several weeks when the infection is related to surgical complications or neutropenia; the following 4 to 6 months when opportunistic infections, especially CMV, are common; and the period more than 6 months after transplant when, if the graft is functioning well, immunosuppressive therapy is minimal. In this situation, opportunistic complications other than chronic CMV or hepatitis B virus are minimal.

ADDENDUM

Adult respiratory distress syndrome resulting from a newly recognized hantavirus has received considerable attention since recognition of this syndrome in June 1993 (see Chapter 142B). Sporadic cases have been recognized in the western United States; through December 31, 1993, 53 persons meeting the case definition had been reported. Thirty-two of these 53 patients have died. There is no evidence yet that this illness occurs more commonly in immunosuppressed patients.

Because the reservoir for this virus (the deer mouse, *Peromyscus maniculatus*, as well as numerous other small rodent species) can be found throughout most of the United States except the southeast and Atlantic seaboard, this disease may not remain geographically circumscribed. Diagnosis can be established by polymerase chain reaction or culture at reference laboratories. The infection does not appear to be transmissible from person to person. Therapy is supportive.

This hantavirus is likely to be named *Muerto Canyon virus*. Why this clinical entity appears to be occurring in the United States now is not entirely clear, but a temporary increase in the deer mouse population may be relevant.

References

1. Shelhamer J, Pizzo PA, Parrillo JE, Masur H (Eds): Respiratory Disease in the Immunosuppressed Host. Philadelphia, JB Lippincott, 1991.
2. Tramont EC: General or nonspecific host defense mechanisms. *In*: Principles and Practice of Infectious Disease. 3rd ed. Mandell GL, Douglas RG, Bennett JE (Eds). New York, Churchill Livingstone, 1990.
3. Masur H, Ognibene FP, Yarchoan R, et al: CD4 counts as predictors of pneumonias in human immunodeficiency virus infected individuals. Ann Intern Med 1989; 111:223.
4. Dwyer JM: Manipulating the immune system with immune globulin. N Engl J Med 1992; 326:107.
5. Frank MM: Complement in the pathophysiology of human disease. N Engl J Med 1987; 316:1525.
6. Figueroa JE, Densen P: Infectious diseases associated with complement deficiencies. Clin Microbiol Rev 1991; 4:359.
7. Tolkoff-Rubin NE, Rubin RH: Infection in organ transplant recipients. *In*: Infectious Diseases. Gorbach SL, Bartlett JG, Blacklow NR (Eds). Philadelphia, WB Saunders, 1992.
8. Driks MR, Craven DE, Celli BR, et al: Nosocomial pneumonia in intubated patients given sucralfate as compared with antacids or histamine type 2 blockers. N Engl J Med 1987; 317:1376.

8a. Prod'hom G, Leuenberger P, Koerfer J, et al: Nosocomial pneumonia in mechanically ventilated patients receiving antacid, ranitidine, or sucralfate as prophylaxis for stress ulcer: A randomized controlled trial. Ann Intern Med 1994; 120:653–662.

9. Torres A, Aznar R, Gatell JM, et al: Incidence, risk, and prognosis factors of nosocomial pneumonia in mechanically ventilated patients. Am Rev Respir Dis 1990; 142:523.
10. Pizzo PA: Management of fever in patients with cancer and treatment induced neutropenia. N Engl J Med 1993; 328:1323–1332.
11. Hughes WT, Armstrong D, Bodey GP, et al: Guidelines for the use of antimicrobial agents in neutropenic patients with unexplained fever. J Infect Dis 1990; 161:381.

12. Pizzo PA, Hathorn JW, Hiemenz J, et al: A randomized trial comparing ceftazidine alone with combination antibiotic therapy in cancer patients with fever and neutropenia. N Engl J Med 1986; 315:552.
13. Winston DJ, Ho WG, Bruckner DA, et al: Beta-lactam antibiotic therapy in febrile granulocytopenic patients: A randomized trial comparing cefoperazone plus piperacillin, ceftazidime plus piperacillin, and imipenem alone. Ann Intern Med 1991; 115:849.
14. Pizzo PA, Rubin M, Freifeld A, et al: The child with cancer and infection: I. Empiric therapy for fever and neutropenia, and preventive strategies. J Pediatr 1991; 119:679–694.
15. Pizzo PA, Rubin M, Freifeld A, et al: The child with cancer and infection: II. Nonbacterial infections. J Pediatr 1991; 119:845–857.
16. Pizzo PA, Robichaud KJ, Wesley R, et al: Fever in the pediatric and young adult patient with cancer: A prospective study of 1001 episodes. Medicine (Baltimore) 1982; 61:153–165.
17. Rubin RH: Infectious disease complications of renal transplantation. Kidney Int 1993; 44:221–236.
18. Cunningham I: Pulmonary infections after bone marrow transplant. Semin Respir Infect 1992; 7:132–138.
19. Thorpe J, Baugham R, Frame PT, et al: Bronchoalveolar lavage for diagnosing acute bacterial pneumonia. J Infect Dis 1987; 155:855.
20. Khan FW, Jones JM: Diagnosing bacterial respiratory infections by bronchoalveolar lavage. J Infect Dis 1987; 155:862.
21. Fagon JY, Chastre J, Hance AJ, et al: Detection of nosocomial lung infection in ventilated patients: Use of a protected specimen brush and quantitative culture techniques in 147 patients. Am Rev Respir Dis 1988; 138:110.
22. Torres A, De La Bellacasa JP, Xaubet A, et al: Diagnostic value of quantitative cultures of bronchoalveolar lavage and telescoping plugged catheters in mechanically ventilated patients with bacterial pneumonia. Am Rev Respir Dis 1989; 140:306.
23. Williams DE, Yungbluth M, Adams G, et al: The role of fiberoptic bronchoscopy in the evaluation of immunocompromised hosts with diffuse pulmonary infiltrates. Am Rev Respir Dis 1985; 131:880.
24. Baselski V: Microbiologic diagnosis of ventilator associated pneumonia. Infect Dis Clin North Am 1993; 7:331.
25. Marrie TJ, Durant H, Yates L: Community-acquired pneumonia requiring hospitalization: 5-year prospective study. Rev Infect Dis 1989; 11:586.
25a. Marrie TJ: Community-acquired pneumonia. Clin Infect Dis 1994; 18:501–515.
26. Kovacs JA, Ng V, Masur H, et al: Diagnosis of *Pneumocystis carinii* pneumonia: Improved detection in sputum with use of monoclonal antibodies. N Engl J Med 1988; 318:589.
27. Lode H, Schaberg T: Rational approach to the diagnosis of pneumocystis pneumonia. Eur Respir J 1993; 6:166.
28. Glenny RW, Pierson DG: Cost reduction in diagnosing *Pneumocystis carinii* pneumonia-sputum induction versus bronchoalveolar lavage as the initial diagnostic procedure. Am Rev Respir Dis 1992; 145:1425.
29. Meyers JD, Flournoy N, Thomas ED: Risk factors for cytomegalovirus infection after human marrow transplantation. J Infect Dis 1986; 153:478.
30. Pachon J, Prados MD, Capote F, et al: Severe community-acquired pneumonia: Etiology, prognosis and treatment. Am Rev Respir Dis 1990; 142:369.
31. Warner DO, Warner MA, Divertie MB: Open lung biopsy in patients with diffuse pulmonary infiltrates and acute respiratory failure. Am Rev Respir Dis 1988; 137:90.
32. Potter DP, Pass HI, Brower S, et al: Prospective randomized study of open lung biopsy versus empirical antibiotic therapy for acute pneumonitis in non-neutropenic cancer patients. Am Thorac Surg 1985; 40:422.
33. Simon HB, Southwick FS, Moellering RC, et al: *Haemophilus influenzae* in hospitalized adults: Current perspectives. Am J Med 1980; 69:219.
34. Hager H, Verghese A, Alvarez S, et al: *Branhamella catarrhalis* respiratory infections. Rev Infect Dis 1987; 9:1140.
35. Woodhead MA, MacFarlane JT: Legionnaires' disease: A review of 79 community-acquired cases in Nottingham. Thorax 1986; 41:635.
36. Grayston JT: Infections caused by *Chlamydia pneumoniae* strain TWAR. Clin Infect Dis 1992; 15:757.
37. Hamer DH, Barza M: Prevention of hospital acquired pneumonia in critically ill patients. Antimicrob Agents Chemother 1993; 37:931.
38. Pearson ML, Jereb JA, Frieden TR, et al: Nosocomial transmission of multidrug-resistant *Mycobacterium tuberculosis*: A risk to patients and health care workers. Ann Intern Med 1992; 117:191.
39. Daley CL, Small PM, Schecter GF, et al: An outbreak of tuberculosis with accelerated progression among persons infected with the human immunodeficiency virus: An analysis using restriction-fragment-length polymorphisms. N Engl J Med 1992; 326:231.
40. Barnes PF, Bloch AB, Davidson PT, et al: Tuberculosis in patients with human immunodeficiency virus infection. N Engl J Med 1991; 324:1644.
41. Gerberding JL, Henderson DK: Management of occupational exposures to bloodborne pathogens: Hepatitis B virus, hepatitis C virus, and HIV. Clin Infect Dis 1992; 14:1179.
42. Barnes PF, Steele MA, Young SMM, et al: Tuberculosis in patients with human immunodeficiency virus infection: How often does it mimic *Pneumocystis carinii* pneumonia? Chest 1992; 102:428.
43. Centers for Disease Control: Tuberculosis and human immunodeficiency virus infection: Recommendations of the advisory committee for the elimination of tuberculosis. MMWR 1989; 38:236.
44. Centers for Disease Control: The use of preventive therapy for tuberculosis infection in the United States: Recommendations of the advisory committee for the elimination of tuberculosis. MMWR 1990; 39:9.
45. Vadhan-Raj S, Broxmeyer HE, Hittelman WN, et al: Abrogating chemotherapy-induced myelosuppression by recombinant granulocyte-macrophage colony-stimulating factor in patients with sarcoma: Protection at the progenitor cell level. J Clin Oncol 1992; 10:1266.
46. Lieschke GJ, Burgess AW: Granulocyte colony-stimulating factor and granulocyte-macrophage colony-stimulating factor. N Engl J Med 1992; 327:28.
47. Wheat LJ, Connolly-Stringfield PA, et al: Disseminated histoplasmosis in the acquired immunodeficiency syndrome: Clinical findings, diagnosis, and treatment and review of the literature. Medicine (Baltimore) 1990; 69:361–374.
48. Galgiani JN, Catanzaro A, Cloud GA, et al: Fluconazole therapy for coccidioidal meningitis: The NIAID Mycosis Study Group. Ann Intern Med 1993; 119:28–35.
49. Vincent T, Galgiani JN, Huppert M, et al: The natural history of coccidiodal meningitis: VA-Armed Forces Cooperative studies. Clin Infect Dis 1993; 16:247.
50. Wachter RM, Luce JM, Hopewell PC: Critical care of patients with AIDS. JAMA 1992; 267:541.
51. Wachter RM, Russi MB, Bloch DA, et al: *Pneumocystis carinii* pneumonia and respiratory failure in AIDS: Improved outcomes and increased use of intensive care units. Am Rev Respir Dis 1991; 143:251.
52. Wachter RM, Luce JM, Hearst N, et al: Decisions about resuscitation: Inequities among patients with different diseases but similar prognoses. Ann Intern Med 1989; 111:525.
53. Masur H: Approach to the patient with human immunodeficiency virus infection: Clinical features. *In*: Infectious Diseases. Gorbach SL, Bartlett JG, Blacklow NR (Eds). Philadelphia, WB Saunders, 1992.
54. Montaner JSG, Lawson LM, Levitt N, et al: Corticosteroids prevent early deterioration in patients with moderately severe *Pneumocystis carinii* pneumonia and the acquired immunodificiency syndrome (AIDS). Ann Intern Med 1990; 113:14.
55. Emanuel EJ: Do physicians have an obligation to treat patients with AIDS? N Engl J Med 1988; 318:1686.
56. Cooper DKC, Novitsky D, Schlegel V, et al: Successful management of symptomatic cytomegalovirus disease with ganciclovir after heart transplantation. J Heart Lung Transplant 1991; 10:656.
57. Nichol ST, Spiropoulon CF, Morzunov S, et al: Genetic identification of a hantavirus associated with an outbreak of acute respiratory illness. Science 1993; 262:914–917.

CHAPTER 137

Infection with HIV, AIDS, and the Intensive Care Unit

Stephen M. Ayres, MD

The Centers for Disease Control, in 1981, became aware of 26 cases of Kaposi's sarcoma and 15 cases of *Pneumocystis carinii* pneumonia (PCP) in previously healthy homosexual men from San Francisco and New York. The report raised the curtain on a tragic global epidemic that has not yet reached its peak and shows little evidence for early control. By December 1982, 878 cases had been reported and by December 1986, the cumulative number of acquired immunodeficiency syndrome (AIDS) cases had increased to 28,098.[1] In June 1991, at the end of the first decade of the worldwide human immunodeficiency virus (HIV) epidemic, 182,834 cases had been reported in the United States.[2]

The epidemic rapidly became a major challenge to intensivists because patients with AIDS commonly presented with PCP and acute respiratory failure. Although patients exhibited acute hypoxemic failure, it was not the same as the syndrome of capillary leak that had just been christened the acute adult respiratory distress syndrome. It soon became apparent that this new disease was unique and extremely difficult to treat. HIV-1 was identified as the causal agent and was found to have an affinity for mononuclear cells, which led to widespread destruction of both macrophages and T lymphocytes. Macrophage infection with virus particles explained the not uncommon involvement of the brain, but the primary target of the virus was the helper T lymphocyte. This widespread defect in cellular immunity placed patients at risk for the development of a group of unusual opportunistic infections such as PCP pneumonia, toxoplasmosis, cryptococcosis, atypical mycobacterial infection, cytomegalovirus infection, and other "exotic" infectious diseases that were only briefly discussed in medical school and were not readily treatable by commonly available antimicrobial agents.

The rapid appearance of a specific and hitherto undescribed critical illness raised treatment and other ethical issues that had lain dormant in the early years of critical care medicine. Should individuals with almost untreatable infectious diseases and no chance of ultimate survival be treated with life-support systems in intensive care units (ICUs)? Was active euthanasia an option for young individuals who clearly had but a short time left to live? How could health-care workers be protected against what appeared to be a highly communicable disease? Should the development of new drugs be hastened by sidestepping the carefully designed double-blind statistical trials, used for less fatal chronic illnesses, and replaced by single-patient studies of whatever agents appeared capable of prolonging life? How could molecular research find the Achilles' heel of the AIDS virus and kill it the way that penicillin long ago had been able to eliminate the pneumococcus from patients with pneumococcal pneumonia?

PNEUMOCYSTIS CARINII PNEUMONIA

At one time, 75% of AIDS patients acquired PCP.[3] The parasite, *Pneumocystis carinii*, produces an acute interstitial pneumonitis that impairs the diffusion of oxygen and leads to decreased pulmonary compliance. Unlike many other acute lung injury processes, repair is associated with rapid fibrogenesis so that interstitial fibrosis may limit gas exchange and alveolar ventilation even if the acute process is controlled. DeVita and Greenbaum[4] described the first 69 patients admitted with PCP to Saint Vincent's Hospital in New York City before December 31, 1985. Severe dyspnea and hypoxemia with arterial oxygen tensions below 40 mm Hg were common. The chest radiograph could be normal or could demonstrate interstitial infiltration. Bacterial superinfection, pulmonary embolism, pneumothorax, and subcutaneous emphysema attributable to high-pressure mechanical ventilation, low cardiac output, and elevated serum lactic dehydrogenase were observed. Diarrhea was found in 78% of patients, hypoalbuminemia in 70%, creatinine concentrations above 2.5 in 37%, and pancreatitis in 4%. Hyponatremia and hypotension were common.

A hyperdynamic syndrome similar to that seen in bacterial pneumonia with sepsis was reported by Parker and colleagues.[5] They studied 31 consecutive patients with bacterial pneumonia and 41 with PCP. The diagnosis of PCP was based on the finding of at least two clumps of cysts on toluidine blue O or Gomori's methenamine silver stains in appropriate specimens. Both groups of patients exhibited a hyperdynamic syndrome with increased cardiac index and decreased systemic vascular resistance. More patients with bacterial sepsis required vasopressors than did those with PCP; in contrast, more of the patients with PCP required mechanical ventilation. Parker and coworkers pointed out the unusual finding that patients with PCP became more hypoxemic within 40 to 72 hours of beginning therapy. The cause of this deterioration has not been identified but may be associated with parasite necrosis and an exacerbation of the immunologic process.

The incidence of PCP in patients with AIDS began to decline in 1988 when primary and secondary prophylaxis with pentamidine or trimethoprim-sulfamethazole was initiated. This preventive regimen delays the incidence of the first AIDS-related illness by 6 to 12 months. Hoover and associates[3] compared the incidence of opportunistic infection in individuals receiving PCP prophylaxis. The incidence of PCP dropped from 46.3% to 14.5% in the treated group. In contrast, the incidence of *Mycobacterium avium* complex disease, wasting syndrome, cytomegalovirus disease, and esophageal candidiasis was significantly increased. The incidence of cryptosporidiosis, progressive multifocal leukoencephalopathy, HIV-1–related dementia, cryptococcal disease, toxoplasmosis, lymphoma, Kaposi's sarcoma, disseminated herpes simplex, and other opportunistic infections was not increased. Chemoprophylaxis changed the mode but not the likelihood of death.

The wasting syndrome, a unique but uncommon constellation of metabolic disturbances, was increased from less than 1% in patients not receiving prophylactic treatment to 10.9% in those receiving such therapy.[3] The syndrome[6] is reminiscent of the autocannibalism seen in prolonged sepsis and emphasizes the important role of cytokines like cachectin (tumor necrosis factor) in the evolution of the septic syndrome. It is difficult to understand how suppression of *P. carinii* can somehow activate the cascade of mediators leading to the wasting syndrome.

EPIDEMIOLOGY/NATURAL HISTORY OF AIDS

The Centers for Disease Control estimated, in 1990, that about 1 million Americans were HIV-positive. In the early years, homosexual and bisexual men and intravenous drug users accounted for most of the cases of AIDS. More recently, increases in homosexual AIDS have been blunted, and the number of cases among heterosexuals and intravenous drug users has increased dramatically. Minority populations are disproportionately represented; 44% of cases have occurred among African Americans and Hispanics.[7] Of all AIDS cases among women, 34% were attributed to heterosexual transmission.[7] Sixty-eight per cent of reported patients were dead by 1991,[8] and, in 1992, HIV infection became the leading cause of death among people between the ages of 25 and 44 years.[9]

HIV infection was the leading cause of death among black men aged 25 to 44 years during 1991 and 1992, accounting for 21.4% and 25.3% of deaths, respectively. It was second, behind unintentional injury, among white men in that age group in 1991, accounting for 17.8% of deaths in 1991 and 18.5% in 1992. HIV was the second most common cause of death in black women during that time period, behind unintentional injuries, accounting for 12.1% of deaths in 1991 and 16.5% in 1992. It was the sixth leading cause of death in white women. The death rate from HIV infection in 1982 for persons aged 25 to 44 years was three times as high for black men as for white men and 12 times as high for black women as for white women. HIV infection was the leading cause of death among Hispanic men and the third leading cause of death among Hispanic women in that same age group.

The pathogenesis of HIV infection is now reasonably well understood.[10] The HIV viral particles penetrate CD4 (helper) T cells and become uncoated as they are incorporated into genomic ribonucleic acid and then, aided by the enzyme reverse transcriptase, integrate their unique coded sequences into proviral deoxyribonucleic acid (DNA). The DNA sequences of HIV are then replicated and infect other CD4 cells in the body. There is a gradual reduction of CD4 cells as they are progressively infected by the replicating virus. At some point, the number of CD4 T cells falls below a critical level, and an opportunistic infection announces the presence of clinical AIDS. The time from infection to expression averages 6 to 10 years but may be longer than 10 years or less than 1 year.

The understanding of the pathogenesis of HIV infection was enhanced by parallel discoveries in the field of immunology. The ability to identify and measure subsets of T and B lymphocytes made it possible to learn that the helper, or CD4, lymphocyte was the target cell for HIV infection. Measurement of peripheral CD4 cells has become a marker of severity and has led to a new definition of AIDS by the Centers for Disease Control. The long asymptomatic or latent period makes it difficult to assign a consistent definition for the onset of the disease AIDS. In the past, AIDS was diagnosed when an opportunistic infection revealed immunodeficiency and the diagnosis was confirmed by the identification of the HIV virus. The Centers for Disease Control have extended the diagnosis to include HIV-positive individuals with CD4 counts less than 200/mm^3 as well as HIV patients with cervical cancer, tuberculosis, and recurrent pneumonia.[11]

Although quantifying CD4 cells has been useful in staging HIV infection and measuring the effectiveness of prophylactic and therapeutic drugs, recent observations have suggested that simple counting alone may be insufficient. It is now known that CD4 depletion is a late occurrence and may be influenced by a variety of cofactors. Schechter and colleagues[12] studied 473 patients with combined HIV and human T cell lymphotrophic infection type I (HTLV-I). HTLV-I is a newly identified retrovirus associated with neurologic disease and lymphomas. Coinfection is particularly common in intravenous drug users. They observed that those infected with both viruses had evidence of more severe disease than patients with only one virus but that they had a higher CD4 count than those infected with HIV only. Because patients infected with both viruses had more serious disease and higher counts of CD4 cells than expected, many new questions arise. What has altered the usual relationship between HIV disease stage and CD4 cell count? Are factors other than CD4 cell depletion playing a pathogenetic role? Are the CD4 cells less functional with combined infection? These concerns are important for intensivists treating patients with opportunistic infections and emphasize that interpretations of CD4 cell counts be made with some caution.

TREATMENT OF HIV INFECTION

Information about the replication of the human immunodeficiency has provided leverage points for the development of chemotherapeutic agents. A concerned and frightened American public has endorsed the race for effective agents, although reports of large-scale health expenditures for such agents has led to some backlash among supporters of other health problems who have lamented what they consider to be the disproportionate amount spent on AIDS research. Hirsch and D'Aquila provided a comprehensive review of the currently available therapeutic agents.[13] Most attention thus far has been directed at inhibitors of reverse transcriptase, protease, and a regulatory protein, Tat.

Zidovudine (AZT) was originally developed as an anticancer drug in 1964. It undergoes glucuronidation during the first pass through the liver and then enters the cells. Reverse transcriptase catalyzes the incorporation of the drug into nucleic acid and leads to competitive inhibition of the enzyme. Thymidine-5′-triphosphate is a cofactor in this competitive inhibition. Early randomized trials at a dose of 1500 mg daily showed substantial increases in survival compared with placebo, but significant side effects such as macrocytic anemia and granulocytopenia were observed. Lower doses were soon found to be as effective as higher ones and to produce fewer side effects. The current recommended dose is 500 to 600 mg daily. Two hundred mg every 8 hours is a common dose schedule.

Therapy initiated before the development of symptoms delays the onset of AIDS, but survival appears to be similar whether it is begun in the asymptomatic state or later in the course of the illness.[14] The present recommendations in the United States are to begin therapy at 500 to 600 mg/d in all HIV-infected people with CD4 counts below 500/mm^3.

Side effects such as anemia and leukopenia have been reduced with the introduction of lower doses and can be further reduced with the use of bone marrow–stimulating factors. Prolonged therapy may produce a myopathy that can be distinguished from the myopathy of HIV itself only by discontinuing the drug. Therapy with zidovudine increases life expectancy modestly, but median survival is still less than 3 years from the diagnosis of AIDS because of the development of resistance, decreased cellular activation to the active triphosphate form, increased virulence of the virus, and increased virus burden resulting from further loss of immune control.

Didanosine, another reverse transcriptase inhibitor, was the second drug approved by the U.S. Food and Drug Administration to treat HIV infection.[13] Although the outcomes are relatively similar, there are some differences that may be important. There is some evidence that switching patients from zidovudine to didanosine may be beneficial after a certain period of zidovudine therapy, although the optimal time for switching is not clear.[15] Side effects of didanosine are quite different from those of zidovudine and include a dose-limiting peripheral neuropathy, which has been found in 13% to 34% of patients. Pancreatitis, elevation of uric acid, headache, and diarrhea have also been observed. Another reverse transcriptase inhibitor, zalcitabine, has been approved for combination therapy with zidovudine for patients who exhibit continued deterioration.

The Tat protein is a regulator of gene expression that has no cellular homologue. It appears to stabilize and increase the initiation of the stabilization process. Two benzodiazepine derivatives appear to antagonize Tat function and are presently under investigation. Other agents under development are an HIV protease, which may prevent processing of the viral core, and agents designed to attack the CD4 membrane receptors. Combination therapy with different antiretroviral agents, interferons, interleukins, and specific drugs aimed at different opportunistic infections show promise and could lead to increased longevity if not cure.[16]

Vaccination against HIV would be an important element in any AIDS prevention program. Efforts to develop vaccines that either prevent the acquisition of HIV (prophylactic vaccines) or delay or prevent progression of disease in already infected individuals are under vigorous development. By April 15, 1993, 15 possible vaccines had been proposed and at least 10 therapeutic vaccines had been evaluated in a phase I or phase II trial. Because HIV infection in many developing countries occurs in more than 10% of the population, many vaccine trials will be implemented in those areas. Lurie and colleagues[17] described the great promise of such vaccines for the entire world. They discussed important ethical, social, and behavioral issues that surround vaccine trials in developing countries.

ETHICAL CONSIDERATIONS ASSOCIATED WITH CARE OF THE PATIENT WITH AIDS

The impact of HIV on medicine in general and critical care in specific is more far reaching than almost anyone could imagine. Critical care can be said to have come of age in the mid-1970s as it shifted its attention from what could be done to what should be done. The Karen Quinlan case focused attention on the persistent vegetative state; physicians, ethicists, and others began to focus on life and death issues as the concepts of autonomy, burden, beneficence, hospice care, and passive euthanasia became the focus of intensive study. The HIV epidemic magnified and raised the stakes on such ethical decision making as young adults turned to their physicians and nurses for advice about whether they should attempt to keep on living. (See Chapters 201 and 205.)

At first, patients with severe PCP were routinely intubated and ventilated just like any other patient with acute hypoxemic failure. DeVita and Greenbaum reported that 84% of the first 69 patients admitted to Saint Vincent's Hospital in New York City were cared for in the ICU. Most required ventilatory support, and 60% of the patients required a minute ventilation of more than 30 L/min. Peak airway pressure frequently exceeded 65 cm H_2O.[4] In contrast, only 15% of 111 patients admitted to the San Francisco General Hospital with AIDS, during the second quarter of 1984, were admitted to the ICU.[18] By 1985 only 3% of patients were admitted to the ICU and the hospital death rate was 87%.

Because there are no known long-term survivors from AIDS, the ethical implications of admission to the ICU become important. Forty of the 45 patients who were intubated and mechanically ventilated at the San Francisco General Hospital died. The median survival for those who left the unit was 7 months, and the median survival for all hospitalized patients with PCP was 8 months.

The San Francisco General Hospital group supported the right of competent patients to decide whether they wished to undergo potentially painful and probably futile treatment. A study of 188 patients with AIDS by Steinbrook and colleagues[19] revealed that 45% would not want intubation and mechanical ventilation, even though their answers to a questionnaire indicated they were unrealistically optimistic over the outcome of such care; they believed that 53% survived hospital care compared with the actual 13%. Physicians expressed similar views. Most of the residents (82%) and attending medical staff (62%) stated they would not wish to be intubated if they had PCP and AIDS themselves. They also admitted that their views had changed remarkably over the preceding 2 years, because 80% of the physicians would have recommended intubation if queried at an earlier date. These attitudes on the part of both physicians and patients in San Francisco explains why the ratio of ICU to hospital admissions for PCP declined from 21% to 4% between 1984 and 1985. The presence of a large homosexual population, with its strong relationships with one another, certainly enhanced the exchange of information and, ultimately, the change of behavior.

PROGNOSIS OF THE PATIENT WITH AIDS

A study of two large cohorts of homosexual men between 1983 and 1993 provides instructive information about prognosis and is probably relevant to individuals with AIDS in other risk groups.[20] These two cohorts were initiated in San Francisco in 1983 and 1984 and contain 462 and 796 homosexual and bisexual men. Median time from a clinical AIDS diagnosis to death did not change significantly over three time periods and averaged 15.9 months. The relative frequency of *P. carinii* as a presenting diagnosis decreased from 57% to 31%, and patients had a decline in the median CD4 count at diagnosis compared with earlier years.

There was a significant increase of about 1 year in survival time from the time of a CD4 count of 200/mm^3 to death. Most of the improved time after observation of a low CD4 count was due to improved survival after the diagnosis of PCP. Improved survival was due to the combined use of PCP prophylaxis and an antiretroviral drug but not to the antiretroviral drug alone. It was also found that the median 3-year survival between identification of a 200 CD4 count and death was independent of the clinical diagnosis, underscoring the importance of the immunosuppressed state rather than the opportunistic infection or malignancy in determining outcomes.

COST OF THE AIDS EPIDEMIC IN THE UNITED STATES

DeVita and Greenbaum[4] emphasized the enormous impact that the AIDS epidemic had on "hospitals, ICUs, the homosexual community, and society at large." Data for 1984 from their large urban hospital in Greenwich Village indicated that 30 of 240 medical beds (13%) were occupied by AIDS patients. Close to one third of all medical ICU beds were used for patients with AIDS. By 1987, AIDS patients filled 21% of all medical beds.

As AIDS patients become more numerous and live longer, the cost of their care becomes a major burden on the U.S. healthcare system. Hellinger estimated that the average cost of treating a patient with AIDS is $32,000 per year, with an average lifetime cost of $85,000.[21] The total cost of all persons with HIV in the United States for 1991 is estimated to be $5.8 billion. These costs represent somewhat less than 2% of all national health expenditures and are substantially greater than the amount currently invested in research into the eradication of the disease.

PROTECTION OF HEALTH WORKERS

Epidemiologic studies performed early in the AIDS epidemic identified that the virus was transmitted by sexual, blood-borne, and perinatal routes. The risk for transmission in the healthcare setting is bidirectional; healthcare personnel may contract HIV from patients and patients can contract the virus from healthcare providers.

Several prospective studies in the healthcare setting demonstrate that the risk of transmission to a health worker from a single percutaneous exposure is 0.3% to 0.4%.[22] The risk for mucous membrane or skin exposure to blood from HIV-positive individuals is substantially less. Only one seroconversion was noted after mucous membrane exposure in 1100 instances in institutional and home settings. The estimated transmission rate was 0.006% to 0.5%.[23] The risk of transmission after cutaneous exposure to HIV-infected blood is probably much smaller because no instances were observed after more than 2700 reported exposures, and the transmission rate was estimated to be 0% to 0.11%.[24] Recently, a case of child-to-child transmission in the family setting was documented by genetic sequencing of the virus from each child. The sick child had open skin lesions that may have facilitated transmission.[25]

Transmission of HIV from provider to patient is rare. In 1990, the Centers for Disease Control reported the first case of apparent transmission from a health provider—a Florida dentist—to a patient. Four additional cases were subsequently identified from the same source. The dentist was HIV-positive, had Kaposi's sarcoma in the mouth, was intermittently taking zidovudine, and was a patient of the dental hygienist in his office.[26] Other cases of HIV-infected healthcare providers have been identified, but retrospective studies have failed to reveal transmission to others. The numbers studied have been small, however, and examples of transmission may well be uncovered as the number of retrospective studies increases.

Health workers in ICUs are at great risk of exposure to HIV-infected blood and must assiduously follow published guidelines designed to protect themselves from such infection. The incidence of infection HIV in some inner-city ICUs is as high as 60%.[27] The Centers for Disease Control included a section titled "Blood and Body Fluid Precautions" in their 1983 document *Guidelines for Isolation Precautions in Hospitals*.[28] In August 1987,[29] the Centers for Disease Control expanded their concept to what was called "Universal Precautions,"[24] based on the belief that the HIV status of all patients under care could not be known with certainty and that it was vital to consider that all patients could be infected with HIV. The inability to test all patients because of autonomy issues and the realization that the antibodies take a number of weeks to develop before a test becomes positive has justified the importance of their judgment. The details of universal precautions were further modified in June 1988[30] and began:

Universal precautions apply to blood and other body fluids containing visible blood. Occupational transmission of HIV and HBV [hepatitis B virus] to health-workers by blood is documented. Blood is the single most important source of HIV, HBV and other blood borne pathogens in the occupational setting. Infection control efforts and other blood borne pathogens must focus on preventing exposures to blood as well as on delivery of HBV immunization . . . Universal precautions are intended to supplement rather than replace recommendations for routine infection control, such as hand washing and using gloves to prevent gross microbial contamination of hands. Because specifying the types of barriers necessary for every possible clinical situation is impractical, some judgment must be exercised.

CENTERS FOR DISEASE CONTROL RECOMMENDATIONS FOR UNIVERSAL PRECAUTIONS

1. Hands should be washed immediately before and after contact with HIV-infected patients, their blood, and secretions.
2. Gloves should be worn when contact with body fluids is anticipated. They should be used for routine phlebotomy. They cannot prevent penetrating injuries caused by needles or other sharp instruments. Take care to prevent injuries when using sharp instruments by using care when cleaning or disposing of used instruments. Do not recap needles by hand; do not remove needles from disposable syringes by hand and do not bend, break, or otherwise manipulate used needles by hand. Place all sharp items in puncture-resistant containers as close to the use area as possible. Gloves should be sterile when used for procedures involving normally sterile areas of the body. There are no reported differences between intact latex and intact vinyl gloves.
3. Other protective barriers reduce the risk of exposure of the healthcare worker's skin or mucous membranes to infective materials. A gown should be worn when there is a possibility of contamination of clothing. Gowns are not necessary for routine patient care.
4. A mask should be worn if the patient is suspected of having pulmonary tuberculosis or other infections spread by aerosol or when there is a risk of blood contamination to the face.
5. Protective eye wear should be used to avoid conjunctival exposure when aerosols are likely to be generated.
6. Resuscitation equipment, including airways, ventilation bags, and masks, should be readily available.
7. Laboratory specimens should be identified with an easily recognized biohazard warning and placed in waterproof bags or containers for transport to the laboratory. A similar sign should be posted near the patient to alert personnel.
8. Disposable food trays are unnecessary. Glassware and utensils may be handled according to routine hospital procedure.
9. Private rooms are unnecessary for patients with AIDS unless they have transmissible infections such as tuberculosis. These patients should not share a room with other immunosuppressed persons, including those with AIDS.

In July 1991, the Centers for Disease Control published recommendations for the prevention of HIV and hepatitis B virus to patients during exposure-prone invasive procedures. These recommendations underscored the importance of continued use of universal precautions and indicated that health professionals who carry out invasive procedures defined as *exposure prone* should know their HIV and hepatitis B serologic status. Additionally, the guidelines recommend that if the infected provider continues to perform exposure-prone invasive procedures, patients should be notified of their HIV or hepatitis B status.

CONCLUSIONS

Infection with HIV has dramatically changed the practice of medicine. Even if appropriate antiviral agents and vaccines are developed, other new and more contagious infectious agents may enter the environment. Many issues surrounding the treatment of patients with HIV are philosophic as well as biomedical. In their 1994 position paper, the American College of Physicians[22] recommended important approaches to the many complex problems that involve the patient with HIV; this paper should be read by all providers whether or not they anticipate caring for such individuals.

In particular, the position paper dealt with the moral imperative for physicians to treat all patients, including those with HIV infection. Because the diagnosis of HIV carries with it an enormous number of psychosocial and economic issues, physicians must recommend the routine testing for its presence with great care. Confidentiality concerns are critical because the knowledge of HIV infection could lead to loss of income and family status. Equally important is the conflict faced by the diagnosis of HIV infection in a health provider for whom the protection of others may be as important as confidentiality of his or her own status.

The country is both alarmed and shocked at the proportions of the HIV epidemic. Moralists declaim the presumed decay of public conduct, public health officials seek to prevent transmission of the virus, and scientists search for biologic solutions to control the virus. The general public wonders whether the resources expended are appropriate to the number of people infected, not realizing that the next retrovirus to become epidemic could be transmitted by less selective methods and that a better understanding of the retrovirus could assist in the treatment of other viral illnesses as well as cancer.

Intensivists face the risk of infected arterial, venous, and pulmonary artery blood on a regular basis and must learn how to protect themselves and their colleagues from serious disease. At the same time, they must be certain that they do not treat those infected with HIV in a manner different from those who are uninfected.

All physicians must help their patients understand the transmission of AIDS and other sexually transmitted diseases. History provides tales of general panic in the face of epidemics of plague, leprosy, influenza, tuberculosis, and poliomyelitis. Only solid information, presented without emotion or ideologic bias, can help the general public understand the truth about this important disease and those that follow.

References

1. Centers for Disease Control: Update: Acquired immunodeficiency syndrome: United States. MMWR 1986; 35:757.
2. Centers for Disease Control: HIV/AIDS Surveillance: U.S. AIDS Cases Reported Through June 1991. Atlanta GA, Centers for Disease Control, 1991.
3. Hoover DR, Saah AJ, Bacellar MA, et al: Clinical manifestations of AIDS in the era of pneumocystis prophylaxis. N Engl J Med 1993; 329:1922.
4. DeVita ME, Greenbaum DM: The critically ill patient with the acquired immunodeficiency syndrome. In: Textbook of Critical Care. 2nd ed. Shoemaker WC, Ayres S, Grenvik A, et al (Eds). Philadelphia, WB Saunders, 1989.
5. Parker MM, Ognibene FP, Rogers P, et al: Severe *Pneumocystis carinii* pneumonia produces a hyperdynamic profile similar to bacterial pneumonia with sepsis. Crit Care Med 1994; 22:50.
6. Grunfeld C, Feingold KR: Metabolic disturbances and wasting in the acquired immunodeficiency syndrome. N Engl J Med 1992; 327:329.
7. The second 100,000 cases of acquired immunodeficiency syndrome: United States, June 1981–1991. MMWR 1992; 41:28.
8. Centers for Disease Control and Prevention: HIV/AIDS Surveillance Year-End Edition. Atlanta, GA, Centers for Disease Control, 1993.
9. Update: Mortality attributable to HIV infection among persons 25–44 years: United States, 1991 and 1992. MMWR 1993; 42:869.
10. Fauci AS, Schmittman SM, Poli G: Immuno-pathogenic mechanisms in human immunodeficiency virus (HIV) infection. Ann Intern Med 1991; 114:678.
11. Revised classification system for HIV infection and expanded surveillance case definition for AIDS among adolescents and adults. MMWR 1992; 41:1.
12. Schechter M, Harrison LH, Halsey NA, et al: Co-infection with human T-cell lymphotrophic virus type I and HIV in Brazil: Impact on markers of HIV disease progression. JAMA 1994; 271:353.
13. Hirsch MS, D'Aquila: Therapy for human immunodeficiency virus infection. N Engl J Med 1993; 328:1686.
14. Aboulker J-P, Swart AM: Preliminary analysis of the Concorde trial. Lancet 1993; 34:889.
15. Kahn JO, Lagakos SW, Richman DD, et al: A controlled trial comparing continued zidovudine with didanosine in human immunodeficiency virus infection. N Engl J Med 1992; 327:581.
16. Johnson VA, Merrill DP, Videler JA, et al: Two-drug combinations of zidovudine, didanosine, and recombinant interferon-alpha A inhibit replication of zidovudine-resistant human immunodeficiency virus type I synergistically in vitro. J Infect Dis 1991; 164:43.
17. Lurie P, Bishaw M, Chesney MA, et al: Ethical, behavioral, and social aspects of HIV vaccine trials in developing countries. JAMA 1994; 271:295.
18. Wachter RM, Luce JM, Turner J, et al: Intensive care of patients with the acquired immunodeficiency syndrome: Outcome and changing patterns of utilization. Am Rev Respir Dis 1986; 134:891.
19. Steinbrook R, Lo B, Moulton J, et al: Preferences of homosexual men with AIDS for life-sustaining treatment. N Engl J Med 1986; 314:457–460.
20. Osmond D, Charlebois E, Lang W: Changes in AIDS survival time in two San Francisco cohorts of homosexual men, 1983 to 1993. JAMA 1994; 271:1083.
21. Hellinger FJ: Forecasting the medical care costs of the HIV epidemic: 1991–1994. Inquiry 1991; 28:213.
22. Human immunodeficiency virus (HIV) infection. (Position Paper, American College of Physicans). Ann Intern Med 1994; 120:310.
23. Ippolito G, Puro V, DeCarli G: Italian study on occupational risk of HIV infection: The risk of occupational immunodeficiency infection in health care workers: Italian Multicenter Study. Arch Intern Med 1993; 153:1451.
24. Henderson DK, Fahey BJ, Willy M, et al: Risk for occupational transmission of human immunodeficiency virus type 1 (HIV-1) associated with clinical exposure: A prospective evaluation. Ann Intern Med 1990; 113:740.
25. Fitzgibbon JE, Gaur S, Frenkel LD, et al: Transmission from one child to another of human immunodeficiency virus type I with a zidovudine-resistance mutation. N Engl J Med 1993; 329:1835.
26. Update: Transmission of HIV infection during invasive dental procedures—Florida. MMWR 1991; 40:377.
27. Parsa M: Personal Communication, 1994.
28. Garner JS, Simmons BP: Guideline for isolation precautions in hospitals. Infect Control 1983; 4:245.
29. Conte JE: Infection with human immunodeficiency virus in the hospital. Ann Intern Med 1986; 105:730.
30. Update: Universal precautions for prevention of transmission of human immunodeficiency virus, hepatitis B virus, and other bloodborne pathogens in health-care settings. MMWR 1988; 37:377.

CHAPTER 138

Catheter-Related Infections and Associated Bacteremia

Scott Norwood, MD, FACS, FCCM

Despite their ubiquitous presence and an abundance of literature on the subject, the prevention, diagnosis, and treatment of catheter-related infections remain controversial. The principal life-threatening complication in patients with catheter-associated infections is bacteremia or fungemia, occurring in 3% to 7% of patients with central venous catheters and in about 1% of patients with arterial catheters. Catheter-related bacteremia develops in approximately 50,000 patients yearly in the United States.[1] More than 90% of these infections are associated with central venous or arterial catheters.[2] The incidence of bacteremia may be considered relatively low, but the problem is significant because it is estimated that more than 850,000 device-related infections occur annually in hospitalized patients; up to 45% of these infections occur in the intensive care unit (ICU) population.[3]

In this chapter, clarification of commonly used terms associated with catheter-related infections is presented along with the present theories of pathogenesis, risk factors for infection, diagnostic techniques, and a synopsis of the existing data on infections associated with specific types of vascular catheters.

DEFINITIONS

Catheter infection is an imprecise term. Although it is clear that inanimate objects do not become "infected," there is strong evidence to suggest that bacteria may be able to live and multiply on catheter surfaces, deriving nutrients from catheter polymers, the deposited glycocalix of certain bacterial species, and other nonviable bacteria.[4] Erroneous delineation of contamination, colonization, and actual infection has lead to confusion and incorrect interpretation of many clinical investigations.[5] The following definitions are generally accepted and used in most studies addressing the problem of catheter infection.

Catheter-related infection: Frequently used for a positive catheter segment culture. If semiquantitative cultures are used, the presence of at least 15 colonies on a blood-agar plate is considered positive.[6] Although a true infection should be defined by more than just a specific number of organisms recovered from a catheter segment, the objective finding of a positive catheter segment culture is frequently used to define a catheter-related infection. The term *catheter-related infection* does *not* necessarily imply that a locally invasive infection is present and certainly does not justify antibiotic therapy. Many studies have also used the term *catheter colonization* for the presence of at least 15 colonies of bacteria in the absence of associated bacteremia or obvious clinical signs of local infection such as gross purulence or severe inflammation.

Catheter-related bacteremia (or septicemia): A diagnosis based on simultaneous isolation of the same organism from a catheter-segment quantitative or semiquantitative culture and a peripheral blood culture. The presence of the same organisms on the catheter and in peripheral blood is considered by most investigators to be positive proof that the catheter is the source for bacteremia.

PATHOGENESIS

Bacterial colonization within or around a catheter probably begins almost immediately after insertion,[4] and the final determinant of whether such colonization causes clinical infection is multifactorial. Multiple sites are incriminated as potential sources for microbial entry into an intravenous or intra-arterial delivery system (Fig. 138–1).

Three pathogenic theories for catheter-related bacteremia have been proposed. The prevailing hypothesis is that bacterial colonization and subsequent bacteremia begin at the interface of the catheter and the skin insertion site.[7, 7a, 7b] Bacteria either advance or multiply distally along the external catheter surface within the subcutaneous tract, gaining access to the venous or arterial circulation. The skin is the most common source for organisms causing catheter-related infection and bacteremia.[8, 9] The majority of catheter-related infections and bacteremias are caused by 21 different species of coagulase-negative staphylococci[10] or *Staphylococcus aureus*. At least half of all fungal infections also develop from skin colonization.[9, 10]

In vitro electron microscopy identifies coagulase-negative staphylococci adherent to irregularities in catheter surfaces within 30 minutes.[4] Within 1 hour, microcolonies develop, with heavy colonization occurring within 6 to 12 hours.[11] These colonies eventually become covered with a glycocalix coating, serving as a barrier against antibiotics, phagocytic neutrophils, and macrophages.[4, 11–14] In vitro studies show that bacteria can grow on catheter surfaces, even when externally supplied nutrients are absent.[4, 14a, 14b] This seems possible only if bacteria are capable of using catheter components or other bacterial cells as nutrient sources. Catheter surface erosion does occur, suggesting that catheter components or added antithrombogenic layers are possible nutritional sources.

A second theory suggests that the catheter hub may be a source for catheter-related bacteremia.[15] Bacteria are introduced via the hub from frequent manipulations, migrating down the inner luminal surface and gaining access to the venous circulation. One study evaluating the pathogenesis and epidemiology of pulmonary artery (PA) catheter-related infections showed that approximately 17% occurred from hub contamination.[16] However, species antibiograms and plasmid profiles of bacterial isolates confirmed that 80% of catheter-related infections still developed from skin entry sites.[16]

Although it is possible that remote infections may produce bacteremia and catheter seeding and may be considered a third mechanism, hematogenous catheter seeding is probably uncommon.[3] It is suggested that many fungal catheter-related infections and enteric organisms such as enterococci, *Escherichia coli*, and *Klebsiella* may infect catheters by hematogenous spread.[9]

Infusate contamination has also been implicated in the past as a possible fourth mechanism.[17–19] Parenteral nutrition solutions[20] and lipid emulsions[21] can both support bacterial and fungal growth,[3] but the present risk from infusate contamination is considered very low.

RISK FACTORS

Risk factors for catheter-related infection and associated bacteremia can be grouped into patient-related and hospital-related factors.[3] Age (i.e., younger than 1 year, older than 60 years), altered host defense mechanisms, severity of underlying disease, remote infections, and the "systemic inflammatory response syndrome" may all be considered patient-related risk factors. Patient-related factors usually cannot be altered but should be considered when developing catheter maintenance protocols.

Many hospital-related factors can be altered, and prevention should focus on these risks.[13, 22, 23] Although the number of catheter manipulations and the experience of the individual performing the insertion procedure may also be risk factors, these cannot necessarily be changed or controlled. Cut downs should be avoided if possible because the incidence of catheter-related complications is higher than with the percutaneous technique.[24] The most common risk factors that can potentially be altered or controlled are discussed separately.

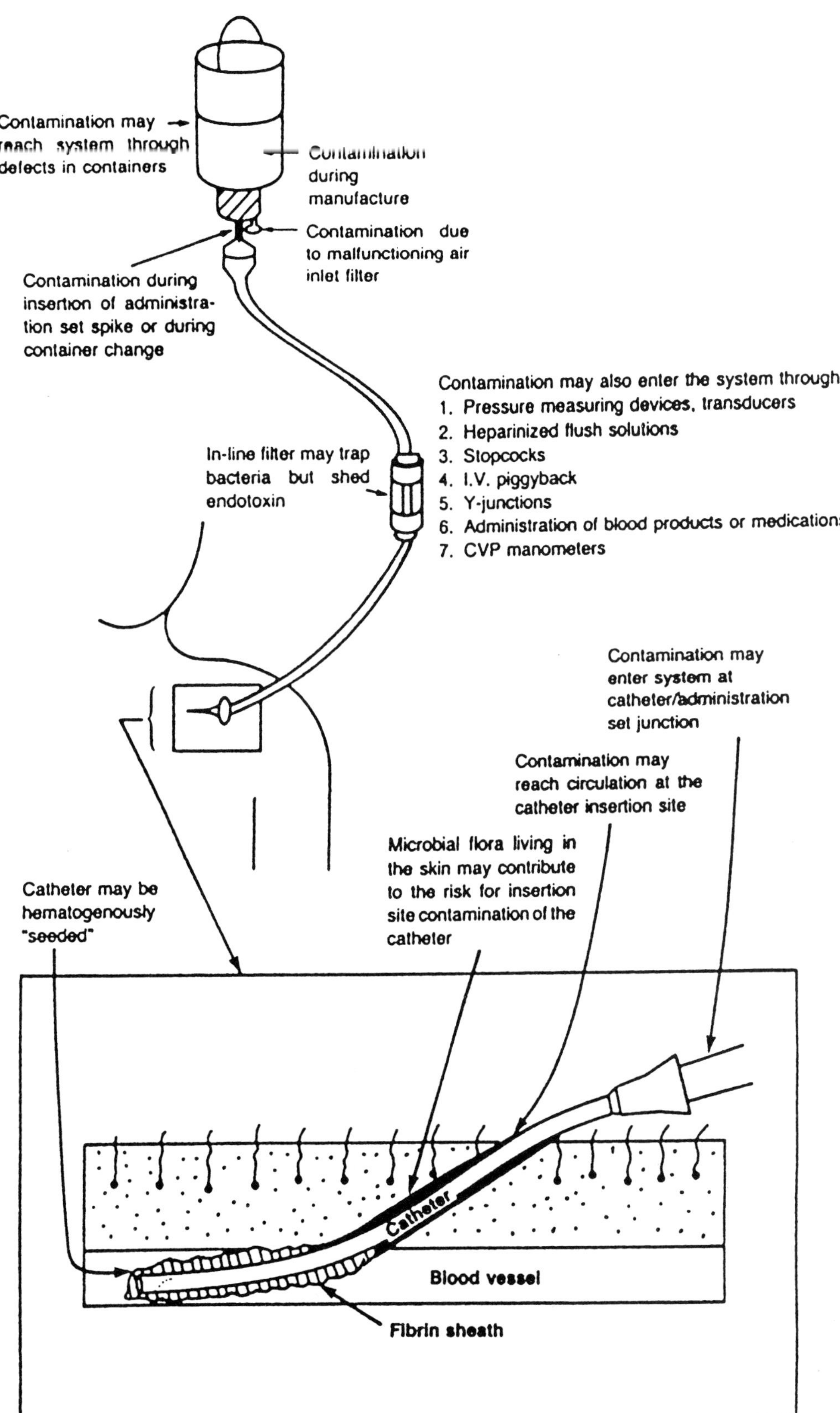

Figure 138–1. Potential sites of microbial entry, colonization, and catheter-related infection for intravenous delivery systems. (From Henderson DK: Intravascular device–associated infection: Current concepts and controversies. Infect Surg 1988; 7:366.)

Anatomic Site of Insertion

Early studies showed no difference between subclavian and internal jugular insertion-site PA catheter infections.[25] More recent studies, however, strongly suggest that the internal jugular site is associated with a higher risk for infection.[16, 26, 27] Possible explanations include the close proximity to oropharyngeal secretions, increased catheter motion as a result of neck movement, and difficulty with maintaining a sterile occlusive dressing.[16]

It is commonly believed that femoral artery and vein catheters are also at higher risk for infection. One recent study supports this belief.[27a] It is my experience that properly placed femoral catheters, placed under sterile conditions and appropriately managed, are at no higher risk for infection than those placed at other sites, especially in predominantly supine, critically ill patients. Recent studies support this experience.[28, 28a]

Duration of Catheter Site Use

The incidence of catheter-related infection and bacteremia is directly proportional to the duration of catheter site use. The optimal time for catheter removal, however, is unknown. The risk of any catheter site becoming infected is low if the catheter is removed within 3 days. Critically ill patients frequently need venous access for prolonged periods, and it is not clear when a catheter should be removed to prevent infection and yet optimize time of use. Two studies suggested that central venous and PA catheters should not have a predetermined life span.[29, 30] Because risk factors are multifactorial, global recommendations for duration of catheter usage are not applicable to all patients. Individual hospitals, ICUs, and, in certain situations, individual practitioners should study their catheter infection rates to develop guidelines that are appropriate for their practice or environment. Recommendations and guidelines for catheter exchange may be used to optimize prevention of catheter-related infection and to prolong site use based on existing published data.

Generally, catheters should be removed when they are no longer needed or if a catheter-related infection is suspected based on examination of the catheter entry site and appropriate cultures (see discussion of diagnostic techniques) to confirm clinical suspicions.

Critically Ill Versus Noncritically Ill Patients

A review of all prospective studies using quantitative culture techniques reported data that varied from a low risk of 0.7% per day in catheters used only for total parenteral nutrition to 3.3% per day for central venous catheters.[31] Many of these studies did not distinguish critically ill patients from other hospitalized patients or septic from nonseptic patients. One study examining multilumen catheter infection rates in critically ill patients reported no infections in critically ill, nonseptic patients compared with a 26.3% incidence of catheter-related infection and a 9.6% incidence of associated bacteremia in critically ill, septic patients.[32] This study also suggested that the number of days hospitalized before catheter insertion may contribute to a higher incidence of catheter-related infection.

Catheter Composition

Earlier, stiffer catheters were associated with a higher risk for thrombosis and infection.[33, 34] Although it has been suggested that the more flexible silicone and polyurethane catheters are less thrombogenic with less in vitro bacterial adherence,[35] more recent studies have questioned the validity of these findings. Gilsdorf and colleagues studied four different intravenous catheter materials and concluded that the decreased in vitro bacterial adherence and thrombogenicity attributed to newer catheter materials did not improve resistance to catheter-related infection and bacteremia.[13] This study demonstrated that *Staphylococcus epidermidis* was adherent to Silastic, Teflon, and two types of polyurethane. The authors speculated that bacterial adherence to these catheter materials in the absence of nutrients probably reflects organism resistance to nutritional inadequacy, the ability to use catheter materials as nutrients, or the expression of adherence factors that are not dependent on either growth or nutrition.[13]

DIAGNOSTIC TECHNIQUES

Catheter-related infection is associated with positive skin site cultures, especially quantitative cultures yielding at least 50 colonies of organisms, and erythema at the insertion site measuring more than 4 mm in diameter.[36] A skin site infection is considered the most common precursor to catheter-related bacteremia. Routine broth cultures are too sensitive for diagnosing catheter-related infection,[31] giving rates of false-positive results up to 50%.[6] Routine swab cultures may also be too sensitive, although some investigators suggested that periodic semiquantitative swab cultures of central venous catheter skin sites may have a negative predictive value of at least 95%.[37]

Various quantitative culture techniques have been developed to better delineate infection risk from colonization.[31] The semiquantitative technique developed by Maki and colleagues[6] is used extensively and provides reliable results. This culture is performed by rolling a 5-cm catheter segment (tip or intracutaneous) across a blood-agar plate in a reproducible, defined manner. In the original study, a positive culture was defined as at least 15 colonies per plate,[6] although the majority of culture-positive catheters yielded confluent growth. A positive catheter segment culture resulted in a 16% risk of catheter-related bacteremia. It is customary to culture the tip of most central venous and PA catheters, although the intracutaneous segment will usually provide more information because the majority of infections begin at the skin site. One study of infections in PA catheters showed that only 61% of semiquantitative tip cultures were positive in catheters known to be infected. Intracutaneous segment cultures were positive in 83%, and culturing both the tip and intracutaneous segment (of the catheter introducer) resulted in a 94% positive rate.[38] Other more complex techniques have been used, including Gram's staining techniques,[39] broth quantitative cultures,[40] and "sonicated" quantitative catheter cultures.[41] Moyer and associates compared various culture techniques for diagnosing catheter-related infection and bacteremia.[42] They considered semiquantitative culture the best test for diagnosing catheter-related infection, but quantitative blood cultures withdrawn through the catheter may also be an acceptable approach in those patients with very difficult venous access or permanent indwelling catheters.[42, 43]

One study suggested that central venous catheters removed within 5 days of placement may not require culture because the information usually has no clinical impact on therapy.[44] This should not be extrapolated to imply that catheters left in place for longer periods should not be cultured. It is generally recognized that the risk of infection is very low if catheters are placed under sterile conditions, cared for appropriately, and removed after only a few days of use. Therefore, routinely culturing such catheters is not indicated. Bedside plating for semiquantitative culture immediately on catheter removal may also increase sensitivity and specificity.[45]

A recurring question concerns the value of broth blood cultures obtained through the catheter (TTC) to diagnose bacteremia or catheter-related infection. TTC cultures have been advocated for diagnosing bacteremia but not specifically for catheter-related bacteremia.[46] This practice should be considered only when catheters have been in place for relatively short periods of time (fewer than 4 days) and when strict disinfection of the hubs is mandatory to prevent false-positive cultures.[46] Catheter microbial colonization may contaminate TTC blood specimens, and more data are needed before this practice can be routinely recommended. Generally, TTC cultures should be avoided unless the physician knows precisely how such cultures are obtained and the length of catheter use. TTC cultures are indicated only if it is impossible to obtain blood cultures from peripheral venipuncture. TTC cultures should not be used to diagnose catheter-related infection unless some form of quantitative culture technique is used.

CATHETER AND SITE MAINTENANCE

The initial preparation of the skin site and subsequent maintenance after insertion is a crucial factor in preventing catheter-related bacteremia. Long-term maintenance of catheters and insertion sites has been studied extensively, including the type and frequency of dressing changes, intravenous tubing changes, type of skin antiseptic, antimicrobial ointment use, and guide wire exchange to diagnose or prevent infection. Great care should be taken in preparing the site for catheter insertion, including careful antiseptic preparation of the skin and wide, sterile draping of the area. In addition, sterile gowns, gloves, surgical head covers, and masks ideally should be worn during nonurgent situations and when time permits.

Antiseptics, Ointments, and Dressing Materials

A study assessing the efficacy of cutaneous antiseptics evaluated 668 catheters randomized to skin preparation with 10% povidone-iodine, 70% alcohol, or 2% aqueous chlorhexidine.[47] Chlorhexidine provided the best protection against catheter-related infection with an incidence of 2.3% versus 7.1% and 9.3% for alcohol and povidone-iodine, respectively ($P = .02$). The rate of bacteremia was also lower, with a rate of 0.5% versus 2.3% and 2.6%, respectively. Another study evaluating epidural catheter colonization also strongly supported the use of chlorhexidine as the first-line skin antiseptic.[48]

Chlorhexidine, a cationic biguanide, is a potent germicide against nearly all nosocomial bacteria and yeasts.[47] Unlike povidone-iodine or alcohol, chlorhexidine provides residual cutaneous antibacterial activity that persists for several hours after application, and its germicidal activity is not neutralized by blood, serum, and other protein-rich biomaterials.[47]

Various ointments are also routinely used. The authors of one large prospective study[49] concluded that topical antimicrobial ointments conferred only modest protection, primarily for peripheral venous catheters remaining in place for more than 4 days. If ointments are used at all, the authors recommended topical polymyxin-neomycin-bacitracin ointment for peripheral catheters and iodophor ointment for central parenteral nutrition and arterial catheters.[49]

The frequency of dressing changes and the type of dressing material have also been extensively studied. It is recommended that peripheral intravenous catheters be removed at 72 hours with one interim dressing change at 48 hours.[50] A large study of more than 2000 Teflon peripheral catheters showed no difference in skin site colonization, catheter-related infection, or bacteremia when comparing dry gauze with transparent polyurethane and iodophor-transparent dressings.[51] The authors recommended that in peripheral catheters placed under sterile conditions either sterile dry gauze or a transparent dressing could be left in place until the catheter was removed.[51] Other investigators showed that bacterial colonization with peripheral catheters is increased, correlating transparent dressings with increased catheter-tip colonization and hospital costs.[52]

Two studies implicated transparent dressings for central venous catheters with a higher incidence of catheter-related infection and associated bacteremia when compared with dry gauze dressings.[53, 54] A meta-analysis of all studies published in the English literature evaluating the use of transparent polyurethane dressings concluded that there is a significantly increased risk of catheter-related infection associated with transparent dressings compared with dry gauze dressings.[55] This study reported a 53% increased risk of catheter-related infection for peripheral catheters and a 63% to 78% increased risk for central venous catheters.[55] Transparent dressings probably impede moisture evaporation from the insertion site and may, therefore, enhance bacterial colonization, especially in critically ill or diaphoretic patients.[52–54] Transparent dressings should probably be avoided in these patients.

Replacement Schedules and Guide Wire Exchange

Two schools of thought exist regarding prophylaxis for catheter-related infection and bacteremia. The first suggests that routine exchange to a new site or by guide wire at a predetermined interval confers protection; the second allows for central venous catheters to be left in place until clinical suspicion or signs of catheter-related infection develop. Both of these practices have inherent risks. With routine catheter exchange, the patient is exposed to the potential risk of pneumothorax or injury to major vessels.[5] Recontamination and subcutaneous tract infection may occur during guide wire exchange.[5] Also, the risk of infection increases with time if catheters remain in place indefinitely.

Most studies evaluating guide wire exchange show that the technique is safe and effective for diagnosing catheter-related infection and for prolonging catheter site use.[32, 56, 57] Guide wire exchange is effective in diagnosing catheter-related infection as long as every attempt is made to "sterilize" the entire external portion of the catheter and the surrounding skin before exchange. This not only prevents contamination of the new catheter during exchange but also yields more accurate semiquantitative cultures because the catheters are removed through a "sterile field."[18] If bacteria are truly capable of growing and multiplying on catheter surfaces without external nutrient sources, as suggested by in vitro studies,[4, 11–13] then guide wire exchange may assist in preventing infection by removing significant numbers of externally and internally adherent bacteria before developing a number sufficient to cause bacteremia and local infection. One criticism of guide wire exchange is that intracutaneous tract colonization or contamination while performing the guide wire exchange may perpetuate local infection or allow for subsequent infection of the new catheter. One study proved this to be unlikely, because 12 culture-positive catheters were replaced with new catheters by guide wire exchange, and subsequent catheters removed from the same sites showed no growth in 8, probable contamination in 1, and positive cultures in only 3.[29] This suggests, as previously hypothesized by Bozzetti and colleagues,[58] that guide wire exchange may confer some protection against catheter-related infection. However, because there is an increased risk of bacteremia when catheters are positive (≥15 colonies), it is generally suggested to remove the new catheter from the potentially infected site and to replace it with another catheter at a different site. If culture of the removed segment demonstrates only colonization (<15 colonies) by semiquantitative culture, then the new catheter placed via guide wire into the old site may be left in place.

Two studies investigated the infection risk of different methods for managing long-term vascular catheters in critically ill patients.[29, 30] Cobb and associates[30] studied four different methods of replacing central venous and PA catheters. Patients were randomized to receive (1) a new catheter at a new site every 3 days, (2) a guide wire exchange at the existing site every 3 days, (3) a new catheter and new site only when clinically indicated, or (4) a guide wire exchange only when infection was suspected. Of the 160 patients studied, 5% had catheter-related bacteremia, 16% had catheter-related infections (which the authors termed *colonization*), and 9% had major mechanical complications. Insertions at new sites were associated with more mechanical complications (5% versus 1%, $P = .005$). Although not statistically significant, patients who were randomly assigned to guide wire exchange were considered more likely to have bacteremia after the first 3 days of catheterization (6% versus 0%, $P = .06$). The authors concluded that routine replacement of central vascular catheters every 3 days does not prevent infection and that exchanging catheters by a guide wire technique may increase the risk of bacteremia (although not statistically significant). However, insertion of catheters at new sites was associated with an increased risk of mechanical complications.[30]

Eyer and associates[29] evaluated three different methods of site management for multilumen, single-lumen central, PA, and arterial catheters used for 7 or more days: (1) catheter exchange to a new site every 7 days; (2) no scheduled change at any particular time but exchange to a new site when clinically indicated; and (3) guide wire exchange every 7 days. In all groups, a catheter change was mandatory for a positive blood culture, skin site infection (defined as purulent drainage, expanding erythema or cellulitis, or a positive qualitative swab culture), or clinical signs of sepsis without a definite source. These authors found no difference in infection risk among the three methods of long-term catheter care, recommending that the method with the fewest complications and least expense should be used. These two studies support the general guideline of not routinely changing catheters at a specific time interval. The study by Eyer and coworkers[29] suggested that guide wire exchange is appropriate when a new catheter is needed or when catheter-associated bacteremia is suspected (because it is safer). If there is evidence of skin site infection, then removing the old catheter and placing a new catheter at a new site would be most appropriate. Other studies also suggested that catheters should not have a predetermined life span and that routine exchange either to a new site or by guide wire does not provide added protection from catheter-related infection or bacteremia.[5]

Suggested Method for Guide Wire Exchange

The method of guide wire exchange that I have found most acceptable involves a complete sterilization of the external portion of the existing catheter before placing the guide wire. All intravenous tubing, including parenteral nutrition tubing, is carefully separated from the catheter hubs and replaced with Luer-Lok adapter plugs. The intravenous tubing tips are also protected with either a sterile, capped needle or the sterile covering from the Luer lock adapter plug.

Sterile disposable gowns and gloves are worn along with surgical hats and masks, and a sterile field for the necessary equipment is prepared on a bedside table. The distal ports of the catheter to be exchanged are placed on a sterile paper barrier, and the insertion site, along with a 10-cm circumferential area of skin, and the entire external portion of the catheter from insertion site to capped hubs, is scrubbed for 5 minutes with 10-cm × 10-cm gauze pads soaked in 4% chlorhexidine skin cleanser. After this scrub, the soap is carefully removed from the area with dry 10-cm × 10-cm gauze pads, and the skin sutures securing the catheter are removed with a No. 11 disposal scalpel. The 10-cm area and the catheter are then cleansed four times with 70% alcohol, and the entry site and catheter are allowed to dry completely.

At this point, the operator should change sterile surgical gloves, and the entire area is draped with six sterile cloth surgical towels, with the distal hubs being carefully removed from the previously sterile paper barrier to the new sterile cloth barrier. A sterile guide wire is then carefully inserted through the distal port of the catheter after removing the heparin lock, ensuring that the wire does not contact the external surface of the hub. The old catheter is carefully removed, taking care to avoid contact with the surrounding skin. Appropriate cultures are then obtained by amputating the 5-cm intracutaneous segment of the catheter and the 5-cm distal tip of the catheter. This can be done with sterile disposable suture removal kits (Johnson & Johnson Products, Inc., Skillman, NJ).

The segments are then placed into two separate culturettes (Baxter Health Care Corporation, McGaw Park, IL) and transported immediately to the microbiology laboratory for semiquantitative cultures. The portion of the guide wire protruding from the skin is cleansed with a 4% chlorhexidine and alcohol solution, and the new catheter is then placed over the guide wire into the proper anatomic position. All catheters are sutured into place after the guide wire is removed. Chest x-ray film is generally not required after guide wire exchange.

INFECTION RISKS OF SPECIFIC CATHETER TYPES

Pulmonary Artery Catheters

Mermel and colleagues[16] published their extensive study on the pathogenesis and epidemiology of PA infections. Overall, they found a 22% incidence of catheter-related infection and a 0.7% incidence of bacteremia. In another study of 69 pulmonary artery catheters, a 21.7% incidence of catheter-related infection was reported.[38] The duration of catheterization for more than 5 days was significantly associated with a higher risk of catheter-related infection. This study reported a 13.3% risk of bacteremia if a catheter-related infection developed. The risk of a catheter-related infection was 41.2% if the catheter remained in place for more than 5 days and only 15.4% if used for no more than 5 days. These two studies and other previous studies[59–61] demonstrated that the risk of catheter-related bacteremia from PA catheters is relatively low when used for no more than 5 days and when reasonable site care is given. Clearly, the risk increases when PA catheters are used for prolonged periods.

Multilumen Central Venous Catheters

The risk of catheter-related infection for multilumen central venous pressure catheters ranges from 6.9% to 11.5%, with an associated bacteremia rate of 1.3% to 13.1% in several studies.[62–65] Some authors condemned their use, showing much higher infection rates when compared with single-lumen catheters.[64] Many of these studies used total parenteral nutrition as the entry criterion for patient selection; others combined PA catheter data. Such criteria and comparisons may bias these studies because patients with multilumen or PA catheters are usually more critically ill than those patients with single-lumen catheters. Therefore, the perceived higher infection rate may not be related to the type of catheter but rather to difficulty in maintaining sterility, more frequent catheter manipulations, and the patient's own immune status. One such study examined the rate of catheter-related bacteremia in 78 patients receiving single-lumen catheters and 99 patients who received triple-lumen catheters.[64] These patients were considered high risk for catheter-related infection. The authors concluded that more frequent catheter manipulations with triple-lumen catheters caused a higher rate of infection and, therefore, should not be used routinely for total parenteral nutrition.[64] Eyer and colleagues[29] reported a 3.4% incidence of catheter-related infection with an associated 2.1% incidence of catheter-related bacteremia in triple-lumen catheters used for an average of 22.6 days. Several other studies also demonstrated no increased risk of catheter-related bacteremia associated with triple-lumen catheters.[27a, 32, 56, 62, 63, 65]

Another study separated multilumen catheter infections in septic and nonseptic critically ill surgical patients.[32] There were no catheter-related infections or bacteremic episodes in the nonseptic critically ill patients, but the incidence of catheter-related infection in the septic group was 26.3%, with a 9.6% incidence of bacteremia.[32] The catheter infection rate per 100 days, however, was only 0.9 for both septic and nonseptic patients combined, which is very similar to rates previously published for single-lumen catheters.[32] The authors concluded that the risk of multilumen catheter infection is no higher than for single-lumen catheters, but septic patients are probably at higher risk regardless of the type of catheter used.[32]

Arterial Catheters

In 1979 Band and Maki studied arterial catheter-related infections and determined that the predominant variables for infection risk at that time were percutaneous versus cut down insertion (ninefold increase in catheter-related bacteremia with cut downs) and extended arterial cannulation time.[66] The overall incidence of catheter-related infection was 18%, with 70% of the catheter-related infections occurring in catheters used for longer than 96 hours. All five episodes of catheter-related bacteremia occurred in patients with catheter sites used for more than 96 hours.[66] A more recent study[67] also supported extended cannulation time as an important factor and re-emphasized that the risk of infection for catheter sites used for fewer than 96 hours is virtually nonexistent. In the latter study,[67] 27% of sites used for more than 96 hours became colonized, as evidenced by positive swab culture of the entry site. Catheter-related infection developed in 9.5% of radial and femoral artery sites used for up to 14 days (mean = 6.4 days), although there were no documented episodes of catheter-related bacteremia. Forty-four percent of axillary sites became infected after 96 hours of use.[67] The authors concluded that radial and femoral artery sites could be used for prolonged periods if skin site colonization were controlled with strict local site care.[67] Further, guide wire exchange could also be used to confirm the presence of catheter-related infection for arterial catheters.[67] This relatively low risk of arterial catheter-related infection and bacteremia has been reconfirmed in other studies.[68]

NOVEL TECHNOLOGIES

An attachable subcutaneous cuff made of an inner silicone sleeve and an outer layer of bovine collagen impregnated with silver ions (Vitacuff, Vitaphore Corporation, Plainsboro, NJ) is one of the first significant technological advances specifically designed for preventing catheter-related infection. The results of two prospective, randomized studies suggested that the cuff may substantially reduce the risk of catheter-related infection.[2, 69] These studies reported reductions in rates of catheter-related infection from 28.9% to 9.1% (P = .002)[2] and 34.5% to 7.7%.[69] No significant differences in the rates of bacteremia were identified with the use of the cuff in either study.[2, 69] Other studies failed to demonstrate any benefit of the collagen cuff in critically ill and septic patients.[5, 56] One of these studies[56] showed a higher rate of catheter-related infection with *Candida* species (31%), with 20% of all the associated bloodstream infections caused by *Candida* fungemia.

Recently, a multilumen catheter coated with silver sulfadiazine and chlorhexidine antiseptic has become commercially available. A prospective, randomized study compared this new catheter to a standard polyurethane multilumen central venous catheter.[70] The results of 405 catheters studied showed that the antiseptic-coated catheters were twofold less likely to be colonized with bacteria than control catheters (24.6% vs. 13.6%, P = .003) and were fourfold less likely to cause bacteremia (4.7% vs. 1.0%, P = .02).[70] I also recently concluded a study of the efficacy of these antiseptic-coated catheters in 101 different catheter sites in 87 critically ill trauma patients. The catheter-related infection rate in this study was only 7.0%, with a 4% rate of bacteremia. All four cases of bacteremia were from gram-negative organisms: three from *Enterobacter* species, and one from a *Pseudomonas* species (unpublished data). Because the silver sulfadiazine and chlorhexidine coating protects the inner as well as the outer surfaces of the catheter, luminal bacterial contaminants as well as skin bacterial contaminants may be inhibited.[70] These antiseptics also appear to be more protective against the more virulent organisms that cause catheter-related bacteremia such as *S. aureus* and *Candida* species.[70]

Other authors[71, 72] demonstrated that coating central venous catheters with various antibiotics will also significantly reduce the rate of catheter-related infection and associated bacteremia. Such technology is presently available. Clearly, the successful strategy for future reductions in infection rates appears to be in developing catheter surfaces that are resistant to colonization either by developing new catheter materials or by coating catheter surfaces with antiseptics and antibiotics. Currently, coating catheter surfaces seems to be the area of greatest promise.[70, 73]

RECOMMENDATIONS

The following recommendations are based on the studies previously reviewed in this chapter and, to some extent, on my personal experience. Physicians in critical care units should be encouraged to study their own patient populations to determine the incidence of catheter-related infection and to develop appropriate guidelines for catheter exchange and site maintenance. On the basis of currently available information, peripheral arterial, central venous, and PA catheters do not require routine exchange. Although the risk of colonization and bacteremia increases with time, the optimal time for catheter removal is not known. Routine central, PA, and peripheral arterial catheter exchange in critically ill patients does not seem to alter infection risk significantly. Axillary arterial catheters may be associated with higher rates of catheter-related infection after 96 hours and should not be used for longer periods.

Catheters that are placed under less than ideal conditions should be treated as potential sources for infection. Generally, these catheters should be removed and a new catheter inserted at a different site if the need for catheterization is longer than 48 hours. Ideal conditions for catheter insertion include the use of sterile, disposable surgical gowns, surgical masks, hats and sterile gloves, careful preparation of the skin site with an antiseptic solution (preferably 4% chlorhexadine), and wide draping of the area to create an adequate sterile field. The subclavian site is preferred over the internal jugular site for long-term (>72 hours) catheter use because of the higher infection rates associated with neck insertions.

The absolute indication for either removal of a catheter or for guide wire exchange is the presence of an unexplained bacteremia. I prefer guide wire exchange using the strict protocol previously described in this chapter because only about 20% to 25% of catheters removed for suspected infection will have positive semiquantitative cultures and less than 10% will be associated with bacteremia.

I prefer daily site cleansing with 4% chlorhexidine followed by placement of dry sterile gauze and tape dressings. Antibiotic ointments do not seem to provide any added benefit, and clear plastic dressings should be avoided. It is my opinion that strict daily site care is crucial in critically ill patients if catheters are to remain in place for prolonged periods without increasing the risk for infection.

References

1. Maki DG: Pathogenesis, prevention, and management of infections due to intravascular devices used for infusion therapy. *In*: Infections Associated with Indwelling Medical Devices. Bisno A, Waldvogel F (Eds). Washington, DC, American Society for Microbiology, 1989, pp 161–177.
2. Maki DG, Cobb I, Carman JK, et al: An attachable silver-impregnated cuff for prevention of infection with central venous catheters: A prospective, randomized multi-center trial. Am J Med 1988; 85:307.
3. Henderson DK: Intravascular device-associated infection: Current concepts and controversies. Infect Surg 1988; 7:365.
4. Peters G, Loui R, Pulverer G: Adherence and growth of coagulase-negative staphylococci on surfaces of intravenous catheters. J Infect Dis 1982; 146:479.
5. Bonawitz SC, Hammell EJ, Kirkpatrick JR: Prevention of central venous catheter sepsis: A prospective randomized trial. Am Surg 1991; 57:618.
6. Maki DG, Weise CE, Sarafin HW: A semiquantitative culture method for identifying intravenous catheter-related infection. N Engl J Med 1977; 296:1305.
7. Beam TR: Vascular access catheters and infections. Infect Surg 1989; 5:156.

7a. Kruse JA, Shah NJ: Detection and prevention of central venous catheter-related infections. Nutr Clin Pract 1993; 8:163.

7b. Bjornson HS: Pathogenesis, prevention, and management of catheter-associated infections. New Horizons 1993; 1:271.

8. Syndman DR, Pober BR, Murray SA, et al: Predictive value of surveillance skin cultures in total-parenteral-nutrition-related infections. Lancet 1982; 2:1385.
9. Bjornson HS, Colley R, Bower RH, et al: Association between microorganism growth at the catheter insertion site and colonization of the catheter in patients receiving total parenteral nutrition. Surgery 1982; 92:720.
10. Martin MA, Pfaller MA, Wenzel RP: Coagulase-negative staphylococcal bacteremia. Ann Intern Med 1989; 110:9.
11. Passerini L, Lam K, Costerton JW, et al: Biofilms on indwelling vascular catheters. Crit Care Med 1992; 20:665.
12. Gristina AG: Biomaterial-centered infection: Microbial adhesion versus tissue integration. Science 1987; 237:1588.
13. Gilsdorf JR, Wilson K, Beals TF: Bacterial colonization of intravenous catheter materials in vitro and in vivo. Surgery 1989; 106:37.
14. Franceschi D, Gerding RL, Phillips G, et al: Risk factors associated with intravascular catheter infections in burned patients: A prospective randomized study. J Trauma 1989; 29:811.

14a. Herrmann M, Lai QJ, Albrecht RM, et al: Adhesion of staphylococcus aureus to surface-bound platelets: Role of fibrinogen, fibrin, and platelet integrins. J Infect Dis 1993; 167:312.

14b. Wang I-W, Anderson JM, Marchant RE: Staphylococcus epidermidis adhesion to hydrophobic biomedical polymer is mediated by platelets. J Infect Dis 1993; 167:329.

15. Linares J, Sitges-Serra A, Garan J, et al: Pathogenesis of catheter sepsis: A prospective study with quantitative and semiquantitative cultures of catheter hub and segments. J Clin Microbiol 1985; 21:357.
16. Mermel LA, McCormick RD, Springman SR, et al: The pathogenesis and epidemiology of catheter-related infection with pulmonary artery Swan-Ganz catheters: A prospective study utilizing molecular subtyping. Am J Med 1991; 91(Suppl 3B):197S.
17. Kovacevich DS, Faubion WC, Bender JM, et al: Association of parenteral nutrition catheter sepsis with urinary tract infections. JPEN J Parenter Enteral Nutr 1986; 10:639.
18. Pettigrew RA, Lang SDR, Haydock DA, et al: Catheter-related sepsis in patients on intravenous nutrition: A prospective study of quantitative catheter cultures and guidewire changes for suspected sepsis. Br J Surg 1985; 72:52.
19. Maki DG, Rhame FS, Mackel DC, et al: Nationwide epidemic of septicemia caused by contaminated intravenous products: I. Epidemiologic and clinical features. Am J Med 1976; 60:471.
20. Goldman DG, Martin WT, Worthington JW: Growth of bacteria and fungi in total parenteral nutrition solutions. Am J Surg 1973; 126:314.
21. Crocker KS, Noga R, Filibeck DG, et al: Microbial growth comparisons of five commercial parenteral lipid emulsions. JPEN J Parenter Enteral Nutr 1984; 8:391.
22. Rotrosen D, Gibson TR, Edwards JE Jr: Adherence of *Candida* species to intravenous catheters. J Infect Dis 1982; 147:594.
23. Sheth NK, Franson TR, Rose HD, et al: Colonization of bacteria on polyvinyl chloride and Teflon intravascular catheters in hospitalized patients. J Clin Microbiol 1983; 18:1061.
24. Moran JM, Atwood RP, Rowe MI: A clinical and bacteriologic study of infections associated with venous cutdowns. N Engl J Med 1965; 272:554.
25. Senagore A, Waller JD, Bonell BW, et al: Pulmonary artery catheterization: A prospective study of internal jugular and subclavian approaches. Crit Care Med 1987; 15:35.
26. Richet H, Hubert B, Nitemberg G, et al: Prospective multicenter study of vascular-catheter-related complications and risk factors for positive central-catheter cultures in intensive care unit patients. J Clin Microbiol 1990; 28:2520.
27. Hagley MT, Martin B, Gast P, et al: Infections and mechanical complications of central venous catheters placed by percutaneous venipuncture and over guidewires. Crit Care Med 1992; 20:1426.

27a. Kemp L, Burge J, Choban P, et al: The effect of catheter type and site on infection rates in total parenteral nutrition patients. JPEN J Parenter Enteral Nutr 1994; 18:71.

28. Murr MM, Rosenquist MD, Lewis RW, et al: A prospective study of femoral vein versus nonfemoral vein catheterization in patients with burns. J Burn Care Rehabil 1991; 12:576.

28a. Friedman B, Kanter G, Titus D: Femoral venous catheters: A safe alternative for delivering parenteral nutrition. Nutr Clin Pract 1994; 9:69.

29. Eyer S, Brummitt C, Crossley K, et al: Catheter-related sepsis: Prospective, randomized study of three methods of long-term catheter maintenance. Crit Care Med 1990; 18:1073.
30. Cobb DK, High KP, Sawyer RG, et al: A controlled trial of scheduled replacement of central venous and pulmonary-artery catheters. N Engl J Med 1992; 327:1062.

31. Hampton AA, Sheretz RJ: Vascular access infections in hospitalized patients. Surg Clin North Am 1988; 68:57.
32. Norwood SH, Jenkins G: An evaluation of triple-lumen catheter infections using a guidewire exchange technique. J Trauma 1990; 30:706.
33. Welch GW, McKeel DW, Silverstein P, et al: The role of catheter composition in the development of thrombophlebitis. Surg Gynecol Obstet 1974; 138:421.
34. Stillman RM, Soliman F, Garcia L, et al: Etiology of catheter-associated sepsis. Arch Surg 1977; 112:1497.
35. Linder LE, Curelaru I, Gustavsson B, et al: Material thrombogenicity in central venous catheterization: A comparison between soft, antebrachial catheters of silicone elastomer and polyurethane. JPEN J Parenter Enteral Nutr 1984; 8:399.
36. Armstrong CW, Mayhall CG, Miller KB, et al: Clinical predictors of infection of central venous catheters used for total parenteral nutrition. Infect Control Hosp Epidemiol 1990; 11:71.
37. Cercenado E, Ena J, Rodriguez-Creixems M, et al: A conservative procedure for the diagnosis of catheter-related infections. Arch Intern Med 1990; 150:1417.
38. Rello J, Coll P, Net A, et al: Infection of pulmonary artery catheters: Epidemiologic characteristics and multivariate analysis of risk factors. Chest 1993; 103:132.
39. Cooper GL, Hopkins GC: Rapid diagnosis of intravascular catheter-associated infection by direct gram staining of catheter segments. N Engl J Med 1985; 312:1142.
40. Cleri DJ, Corrado ML, Seligman SJ: Quantitative culture of intravenous catheters and other intravascular inserts. J Infect Dis 1980; 141:781.
41. Raad II, Sabbagh MF, Rand KH, et al: Quantitative tip culture methods and the diagnosis of central venous catheter-related infections. Diagn Microbiol Infect Dis 1992; 15:13.
42. Moyer MA, Edwards LD, Farley L: Comparative culture methods on 101 intravenous catheters. Arch Intern Med 1983; 143:66.
43. Wing EF, Norden CW, Shadduck RK, et al: Use of quantitative bacteriologic techniques to diagnose catheter-related sepsis. Arch Intern Med 1979; 287:482.
44. Widmer AF, Nettleman M, Flint K, et al: The clinical impact of culturing central venous catheters. Arch Intern Med 1992; 152:1299.
45. Hnatiuk OW, Pike J, Stoltzfus D, et al: Value of bedside plating of semiquantitative cultures for diagnosis of central venous catheter-related infections in ICU patients. Chest 1993; 103:896.
46. Wormser GP, Onorato IM, Preminger TJ, et al: Sensitivity and specificity of blood cultures obtained through intravascular catheters. Crit Care Med 1990; 18:152.
47. Maki DG, Ringer M, Alvarado CJ: Prospective randomized trial of povidone-iodine, alcohol, and chlorhexidine for prevention of infection associated with central venous and arterial catheters. Lancet 1991; 338:339.
48. Shapiro JM, Bond EL, Garman JK: Use of a chlorhexidine dressing to reduce microbial colonization of epidural catheters. Anesthesiology 1990; 73:625.
49. Maki DG, Band JD: A comparative study of polyantibiotic and iodophor ointments in prevention of vascular catheter-related infection. Am J Med 1981; 70:739.
50. Center for Disease Control: Guidelines for Prevention of Intravascular Infections. Washington, DC, U.S. Department of Health and Human Services, 1982.
51. Maki DG, Ringer M: Evaluation of dressing regimens for prevention of infection with peripheral intravenous catheters. JAMA 1987; 258:2396.
52. Craven DE, Lichtenberg DA, Kunches LM, et al: A randomized study comparing a transparent polyurethane dressing to a dry gauze dressing for peripheral intravenous catheter sites. Infect Control 1985; 6:361.
53. Conly JM, Grieves K, Peters B: A prospective randomized study comparing transparent and dry gauze dressings for central venous catheters. J Infect Dis 1989; 159:310.
54. Dickerson N, Horton P, Smith S, et al: Clinically significant central venous catheter infections in a community hospital: Association with type of dressing. J Infect Dis 1989; 160:720.
55. Hoffman KK, Weber DJ, Samsa GP, et al: Transparent polyurethane film as an intravenous catheter dressing: A meta-analysis of the infection risks. JAMA 1992; 267:2072.
56. Norwood S, Hajjar G, Jenkins L: The influence of an attachable subcutaneous cuff for preventing catheter infections in critically ill surgical and trauma patients. Surg Gynecol Obstet 1992; 175:33.
57. Civetta JM, Hudson-Civetta JA, Nelson LD, et al: Utility and efficacy of guidewire changes (Abstract). Crit Care Med 1987; 15:380.
58. Bozzetti F, Terno G, Bonfanti G, et al: Prevention and treatment of central venous catheter sepsis by exchange via a guidewire. Ann Surg 1983; 198:48.
59. Myers ML, Austin TW, Sibbald WJ: Pulmonary artery catheter infections. Ann Surg 1985; 201:237.
60. Hudson-Civetta JA, Civetta JM, Martinez OV, et al: Risk and detection of pulmonary artery catheter-related infection in septic surgical patients. Crit Care Med 1987; 15:29.
61. Civetta JM, Hudson-Civetta JA, Dion L: Duration of illness affects catheter-related infection and bacteremia (Abstract). Presented at the 27th Interscience Conference on Antimicrobial Agents and Chemotherapy, Atlanta, October 11–12, 1988.
62. Manglano R, Martin M: Safety of triple lumen catheters in the critically-ill. Am Surg 1991; 57:370.
63. Farkas JC, Liu N, Bleriot JP, et al: Single-versus triple-lumen central catheter-related sepsis: A prospective randomized study in a critically-ill population. Am J Med 1992; 93:277.
64. Clark-Christoff N, Watters VA, Sparks W, et al: Use of triple-lumen subclavian catheters for administration of total parenteral nutrition. JPEN J Parenter Enteral Nutr 1992; 16:403.
65. Lee RB, Buckner M, Sharp KW: Do multi-lumen catheters increase central venous catheter sepsis compared to single-lumen catheters? J Trauma 1988; 28:1472.
66. Band JD, Maki DG: Infections caused by arterial catheters used for hemodynamic monitoring. Am J Med 1979; 67:735.
67. Norwood SH, Cormier B, McMahan NG, et al: Prospective study of catheter-related infection during prolonged arterial catheterization. Crit Care Med 1988; 16:836.
68. Leroy O, Beuscart C, Santre C, et al: Nosocomial infections associated with long-term artery cannulation. Intensive Care Med 1989; 15:241.
69. Flowers RH, Schwenzer KJ, Kopel RF, et al: Efficacy of an attachable subcutaneous cuff for the prevention of intravascular catheter-related infection. JAMA 1989; 261:878.
70. Carlson R: Antiseptic-releasing catheter reduces infections: An interview with Dennis Maki, M.D. Oncology Times 1992; 14:23.
71. Trooskin SZ, Donetz AP, Harvey RA, et al: Prevention of catheter sepsis by antibiotic bonding. Surgery 1985; 97:547.
72. Kamal GD, Pfaller MA, Rempe LE, et al: Reduced intravascular catheter infection by antibiotic bonding. JAMA 1991; 265:2364.
73. Sherertz RJ, Carruth WA, Hampton AA, et al: Efficacy of antibiotic-coated catheters in preventing subcutaneous staphylococcus aureus infection in rabbits. J Infect Dis 1993; 167:98.

CHAPTER 139

Central Nervous System Infections

David W. Haas, MD • Allen B. Kaiser, MD

Physiologic and anatomic barriers make direct medical and surgical intervention difficult in critically ill patients with central nervous system (CNS) infection. Physiologically, the blood-brain barrier impairs delivery of many antimicrobials, and anatomic barriers are created by the bony calvarium and the central location of the ventricular system.

In addition, noninfectious conditions may mimic CNS infection. For example, a necrotic brain tumor may be clinically indistinguishable from a brain abscess. In general, it is prudent to address the infectious possibilities immediately in such situations.

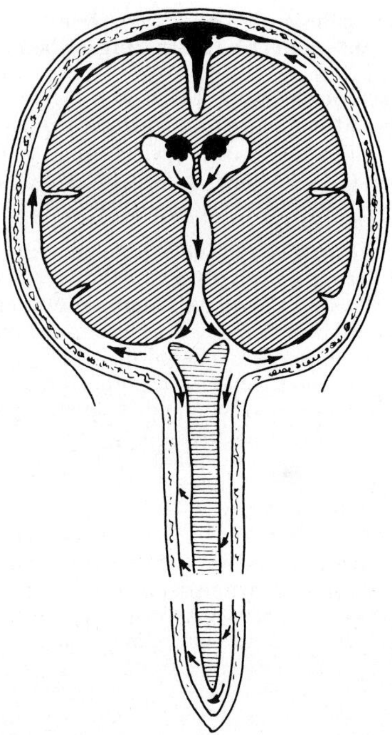

Figure 139–1. CSF flow within the CNS. CSF formed at the choroid plexus of the cerebral ventricles rapidly enters the subarachnoid space at the foramina of Luschka and Magendie. From the cisterna magna, an organized flow of CSF occurs around the convexities of the brain to the arachnoid villi. There are multiple pathways of bidirectional flow around the spinal cord.

A final problem is that many pathogens produce identical clinical syndromes. Timely identification of the specific etiologic agent is crucial. Fortunately, most pathogens can be identified from early laboratory tests, such as Gram's stains of cerebrospinal fluid (CSF) or of pus aspirated from a brain abscess. Epidemiologic clues may also suggest specific microorganisms; pathogens associated with community-acquired infections differ from those acquired in a hospital. In short, proper therapy of CNS infection demands an understanding of the anatomy and physiology of the CNS, the pharmacokinetics of antimicrobial agents, and the epidemiology of infecting pathogens.

BACTERIAL MENINGITIS

Anatomy

Bacterial meningitis is a pyogenic infection of the cerebral ventricles and the subarachnoid space, with bacteria usually confined to the nutrient-rich CSF. Most CSF is formed in the choroid plexus of the ventricles, flows into the subarachnoid space at the cisterna magna and around the cerebral hemispheres, and is reabsorbed by the arachnoid villi (Fig. 139–1). In adults, CSF is produced at approximately 500 mL/day but the CSF space averages 140 mL in volume. The cerebral subarachnoid space joins the spinal subarachnoid space at the cisterna magna. Flow through the spinal subarachnoid space is of variable velocity and direction.

There are numerous potential and actual spaces among the layers of the meninges (Fig. 139–2). Meningitis involves the actual space (i.e., the subarachnoid space). The brain parenchyma is usually not infected in uncomplicated bacterial meningitis, even when the illness follows a fulminant course. Exceptions occur in neonates, in whom *Citrobacter freundii* and *Haemophilus influenzae* may cause focal cerebritis or microabscesses adjacent to the pia. In adults, *Listeria monocytogenes* meningitis may be complicated by cerebritis, brain abscess, or both.

How does bacterial meningitis cause such profound CNS dysfunction when neural tissues are not directly infected or involved in the associated inflammatory response? Likely factors may include (1) bacterial toxins that affect underlying neural structures; (2) occlusion of cortical blood vessels that traverse the subarachnoid space (see Fig. 139–2); (3) damage to nerve roots that traverse the subarachnoid space, causing cranial or spinal nerve dysfunction; (4) impairment of CSF flow (see Fig. 139–1), leading to hydrocephalus; (5) bacterial products that stimulate release of cytokines, which cause capillary leakage and cerebral edema.

The CSF-filled space should not be viewed as a single compartment. The small size of the foramina of Luschka and Magendie probably ensures unidirectional caudal flow.

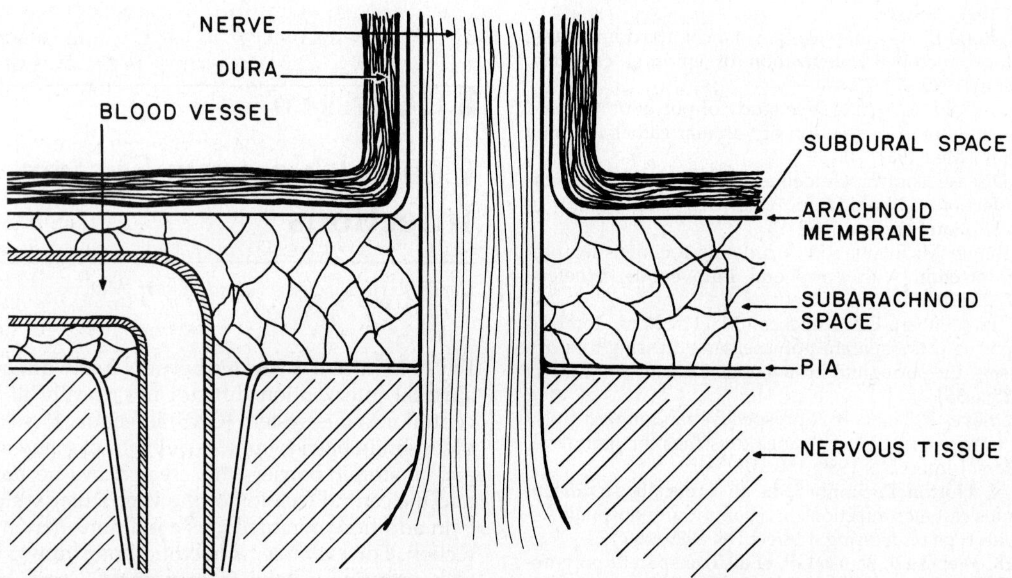

Figure 139–2. This diagram of the potential and actual spaces between the layers of the meninges shows the relationship of blood vessels and nerve roots to the subarachnoid space.

This intraventricular flow, the cephalad flow within the cerebral subarachnoid space, and the imprecise flow within the lumbar area suggest three distinct compartments. This compartmentalization has implications for therapy, because movement of medications and infectious agents between compartments depends on rates and directions of CSF flow.

Infectious agents may invade the CSF by at least three routes (Table 139–1). First, the vascular structures of the choroid plexus and pia and the vessels that traverse the subarachnoid space may serve as conduits during systemic bacteremia. The frequency of ventriculitis during meningitis suggests that the choroid plexus is an important route.

A second, less common route is direct invasion across the protective meninges. Disruption of the dura by trauma or surgery may allow direct invasion of the CSF, and CSF drainage from sites of surgery and trauma indicates a break in dural continuity. Emissary veins provide another pathway for bacteria to spread from contiguous foci into the subarachnoid space. These veins traverse the skull and dura, directly connecting the soft tissues of the head and neck with the venous system of the brain and meninges, including the arachnoid villi. Although blood in the emissary veins usually flows away from the brain, the CNS veins and dural sinuses do not contain valves, and retrograde flow of bacteria is possible. Congenital defects may occur at any point from the glabrata to the cauda equina, offering additional direct communication with the subarachnoid space.[1]

Finally, organisms may reach the ventricles or subarachnoid space from within the neural tissue. For example, rupture of a brain abscess into the CSF may cause a disastrous complication.

Pathophysiology

The unique anatomy and composition of the CSF-filled compartments create an environment that, relative to other tissues, encourages persistence of microorganisms. Phagocytosis is most effective when polymorphonuclear leukocytes can trap a bacterium against a host tissue surface; the large fluid-filled spaces of the ventricles and subarachnoid space deny such phagocytic surfaces. Mobilization of polymorphonuclear leukocytes is delayed during the early stages of infection. Additionally, CSF contains little immunoglobulin.[2] Most importantly, complement, which rapidly kills many bacteria and assists in chemotaxis, phagocytosis, and intracellular killing, is absent from normal CSF. These features dictate that once the CSF is inoculated with pathogens, a self-limited illness is virtually impossible.[2a]

These limited local defense mechanisms may explain the importance of using bactericidal antibiotics in bacterial meningitis. Lepper and Dowling showed that treatment of pneumococcal meningitis with penicillin was associated with lower mortality than the combination of penicillin and tetracycline.[3] Tetracycline neutralizes the bactericidal activity of penicillin. Although tetracycline may be as effective as penicillin for many extra-CNS infections and produces acceptable CSF levels, its inferior performance suggests that host defenses cannot compensate for its lack of bacterial killing. Similarly, chloramphenicol is bactericidal against most *H. influenzae* and pneumococci and may be as effective as ampicillin for meningitis caused by susceptible strains of these organisms. (Chloramphenicol may not be optimal therapy for pneumococci that are highly resistant to penicillin, as discussed later). However, it is rarely bactericidal against gram-negative enteric bacilli, and failures are common when gram-negative bacillary meningitis is treated with chloramphenicol.[4]

TABLE 139–1. Routes by Which Bacteria May Enter the Subarachnoid Space

Bloodstream

Most likely pathogens: pneumococci, meningococci, *H. influenzae, E. coli* (neonates), group B streptococci (neonates)

- *Choroid plexus:* may be most common site of invasion
- *Meningeal blood vessels:* located throughout the subarachnoid space
- *Arachnoid villi:* a possible route of invasion, located between the sagittal sinus and subarachnoid space

Transdural

Most likely pathogens: pneumococci, gram-negative enteric bacilli, staphylococci (especially coagulase-negative) and *H. influenzae*

- *Surgery:* including ventriculoatrial and ventriculoperitoneal shunts
- *Trauma:* especially when cribriformplate or petrous bone is fractured
- *Parameningeal infective focus:* including sinusitis, otitis, osteomyelitis; emissary veins may serve as conduit
- *Congenital defects:* including myelomeningocele and spinal dermal sinus

Transparenchymal

Most likely pathogens: anaerobic bacteria

Occurs when brain abscess ruptures into ventricles or subarachnoid space

CLINICAL COURSE OF PYOGENIC MENINGITIS

Most patients with bacterial meningitis exhibit only modest impairment of higher integrative functions on presentation. Several days of malaise, fever, and headache are typical, and meningismus is usually present.[4a] The CSF indices are almost always abnormal, and Gram's stain or culture of the fluid usually reveals the infecting pathogen unless antibiotics were administered beforehand. Despite the availability of antibiotics active against all common causes of acute bacterial meningitis in adults, the overall mortality remains approximately 25%.[5]

For unclear reasons, in some patients, pyogenic meningitis follows a different course. Such patients experience a fulminant illness that rapidly (<48 h) produces signs and symptoms of both systemic and CNS infections. In addition to having fever, headache, and meningismus, such patients exhibit early impairment of sensorium, ranging from lethargy to coma. Despite appropriate antimicrobial therapy, mortality rates of approximately 50% have been reported for such patients.[6]

A successful outcome is inversely related to the degree of impairment of higher integrative functions when therapy is initiated. At some point, progression to morbidity or mortality becomes irreversible. In herpes simplex encephalitis, mortality is 50% to 65% in patients who present with severe cognitive impairment versus 10% to 30% without such impairment.[7,8] Adults who are obtunded on admission with community-acquired bacterial meningitis may be three times more likely to die of the infection than more alert patients.[5]

Syndromes of Central Nervous System Infection

Definitive diagnosis of bacterial meningitis requires laboratory confirmation. Involvement of the CNS by other pathogens (e.g., viruses, fungi, mycobacteria) and noninfectious processes (e.g., subarachnoid hemorrhage) may produce identical syndromes. *Subacute CNS infection syndrome* is a slowly evolving syndrome characterized by fever, headache,

TABLE 139–2. Etiology of Acute and Subacute Syndromes of Central Nervous System Infection

Acute meningitis syndrome (rapid onset [<24–48 h] of fever, headache, and/or meningismus, with early impairment of higher integrative functions)	
Common:	Pyogenic meningitis (pneumococcal, meningococcal, *Haemophilus*, other)
Uncommon:	Viral encephalitis (especially herpes simplex), subarachnoid bleed, and brain tumor (with rupture)
Rare:	Viral meningitis, granulomatous meningitis (cryptococcal, mycobacterial), carcinomatous meningitis, and brain tumor
Subacute CNS infection syndrome (subacute onset [>24–48 h] of fever, headache, and/or meningismus, with no or gradual impairment of higher integrative functions)	
Common:	Viral meningitis, viral encephalitis, pyogenic meningitis
Uncommon:	Brain abscess, brain tumor, granulomatous meningitis
Rare:	Cerebrovascular accident, carcinomatous meningitis

and meningismus. These features plus an acute onset (<24–48 h) and early impairment of higher integrative functions represent *acute meningitis syndrome* (Table 139–2).

The following sections outline approaches to acute meningitis and subacute CNS infection syndromes. These approaches prioritize the competing needs of obtaining a precise etiologic diagnosis versus instituting early antimicrobial therapy.

Acute Meningitis Syndrome

Early recognition and therapy of acute meningitis syndrome are essential to prevent mortality. The initial manifestation may be subtle, with a low-grade headache or upper respiratory tract infection. However, once meningeal symptoms (vomiting, severe headache, and stiff neck) develop, the clinical course is dramatic. Patients appear "toxic," and higher integrative functions may deteriorate rapidly. In the elderly, the signs and symptoms may be indistinct, consisting only of fever, irritability, confusion, poor appetite, or seizures. Nonetheless, such cases may progress to coma within hours. Therapy should begin within 30 minutes of encountering a patient with acute meningitis syndrome; therapy should not be withheld while awaiting CSF Gram's stain results (Fig. 139–3). A brief history should elicit antibiotic (especially penicillin) allergy and identify risk factors such as immunosuppression, recent surgery, or trauma. A brief physical examination should preclude papilledema or focal neurologic defects. Papilledema or focal defects (excluding Todd's paralysis) are rare in acute meningitis and are indications for immediate empirical antimicrobial therapy with a third-generation cephalosporin (cefotaxime or ceftriaxone) combined with either metronidazole or chloramphenicol because of the possibility of an abscess caused by anerobic organisms. A computed tomography (CT) or magnetic resonance imaging (MRI) scan should follow immediately in order to rule out a mass lesion, which might produce uncal herniation if a lumbar puncture were performed.

Antibiotics must be administered in the first 30 minutes to patients with the acute meningitis syndrome even if diagnostic results are incomplete (see the later section on therapy). Therapy is often delayed in practice because physicians make the mistake of waiting for the results of a scan or lumbar puncture before starting therapy.[9] The importance of administering antibiotics to patients with the acute meningitis syndrome within 30 minutes, *regardless of how far the diagnostic process has progressed*, cannot be overemphasized. Therapy can be modified later based on Gram's stain or culture results. Rarely does a noninfectious process, such as a subarachnoid hemorrhage, produce this syndrome.

Subacute Central Nervous System Infection Syndrome

Febrile illness associated with a somewhat more gradual progression of signs and symptoms of CNS involvement represents the subacute CNS infection syndrome. Headache can be mild or severe, and neck stiffness can be minimum or marked. However, patients should be oriented and clinically stable, as evidenced by a gradual (>24–48 h) progression of symptoms. Although pyogenic organisms are frequently implicated, many cases are caused by nonpyogenic pathogens and noninfectious factors.

Herpes simplex encephalitis, brain abscess, and meningitis due to fungi, mycobacteria, or viruses all may produce moderate fever, worsening headache, and progressive impairment of higher integrative functions. On occasion, carcinomatous meningitis, brain tumor, and subarachnoid bleeding cause similar findings (see Table 139–2). To avoid inappropriate therapy and unnecessary hospitalization, the decision to institute antimicrobials should be carefully weighed. However, if pyogenic meningitis is still a possibility after evaluation, antimicrobial therapy should be given as outlined later.

The first priority when managing subacute CNS infection syndrome is "rapid diagnosis" versus the "rapid therapy" approach to acute meningitis syndrome. A physician should take 1 to 2 hours to carefully evaluate a patient and relevant laboratory data (Fig. 139–4). Peripheral blood granulocytosis (>10,000/mm^3), CSF pleocytosis (cell counts >1000/mm^3), elevated CSF protein (>100 mg/dL), or decreased CSF glucose (<40 mg/dL) favor a bacterial cause.

If the history and examination findings suggest a space-occupying lesion, lumbar puncture and even antimicrobial therapy can be safely delayed for 1 to 2 hours pending results of emergency CT or MRI scan. However, if longer delays are likely, empirical therapy before lumbar puncture may be preferred if a space-occupying lesion is a possibility. Other causes of subacute CNS infection syndrome are discussed later (see *Brain Abscess* and *Viral Infections of the Central Nervous System*).

Therapy of Pyogenic Meningitis

Pneumococci, meningococci, and rarely *H. influenzae* cause most community-acquired bacterial meningitis in previously healthy adults.[10] Intravenous penicillin (18–24 million units/d) traditionally was the treatment of choice. However, β-lactamase-positive *H. influenzae* and, more importantly, pneumococci, which are intermediately (minimum inhibitory concentration ≥0.1 μg/mL) or highly (minimum inhibitory concentration >1 μg/mL) resistant to penicillin, have altered this approach. The extent to which penicillin-resistant pneumococci are resistant to cephalosporins, chloramphenicol, sulfonamides, and tetracyclines is highly variable. To date, vancomycin is active against virtually all pneumococci. Initial therapy for most patients with bacterial meningitis should include a third-generation cephalosporin such as cefotaxime or ceftriaxone. These drugs are strongly bactericidal against the common pathogens of acute meningitis and are adequate for most penicillin-resistant pneumococci. If resistance to cephalosporins is a concern, vancomycin should be added. Vancomycin should not be used alone as initial therapy because of its marginal CNS penetration and poor activity against *H. influenzae*. Chloramphenicol for

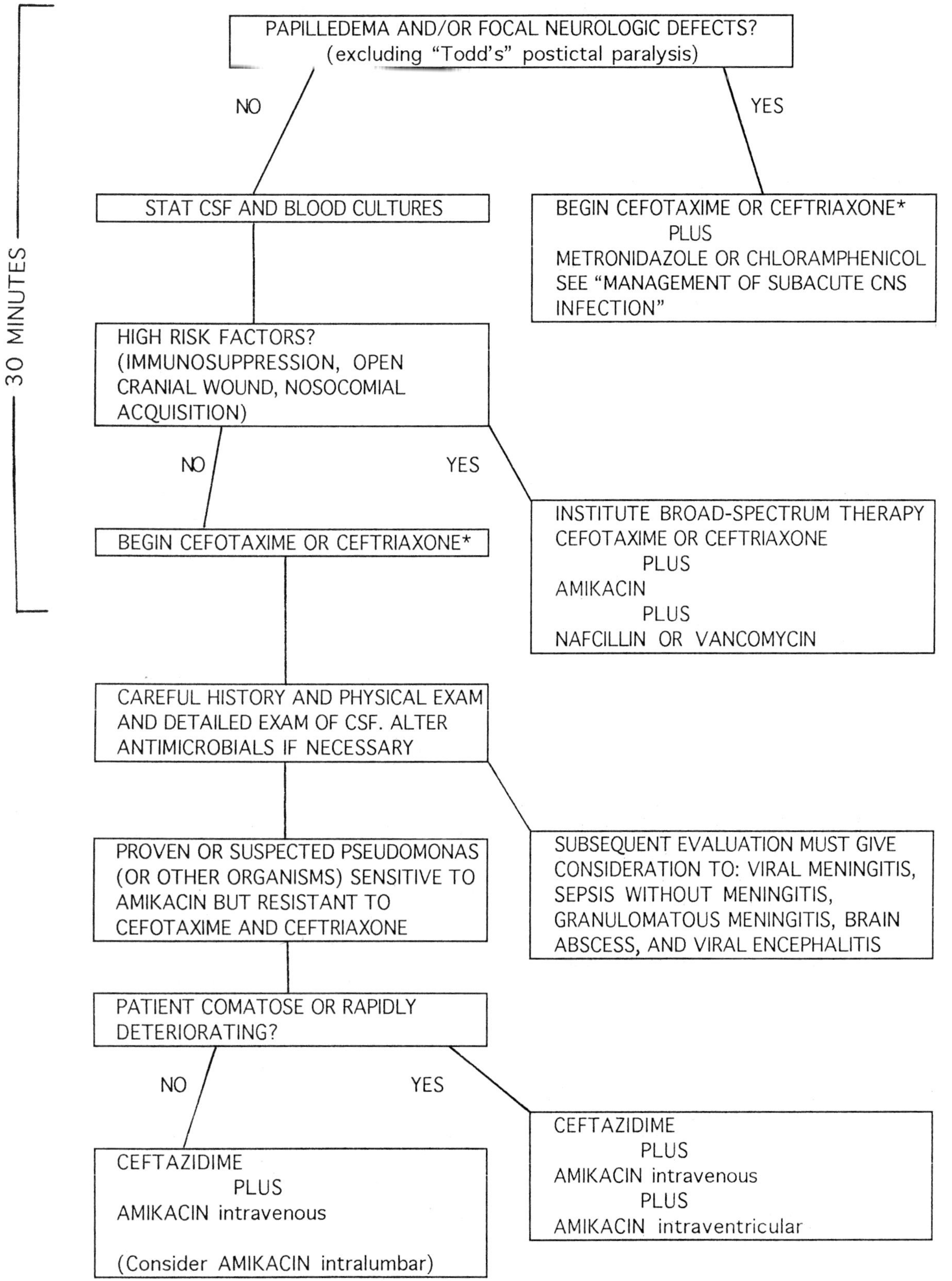

Figure 139–3. Algorithm for the management of patients with the acute meningitis syndrome. (*Consider adding vancomycin as empiric coverage against high-level penicillin-resistant pneumococci that may also be resistant to cephalosporins. See Table 139–3 for specific antimicrobial doses.)

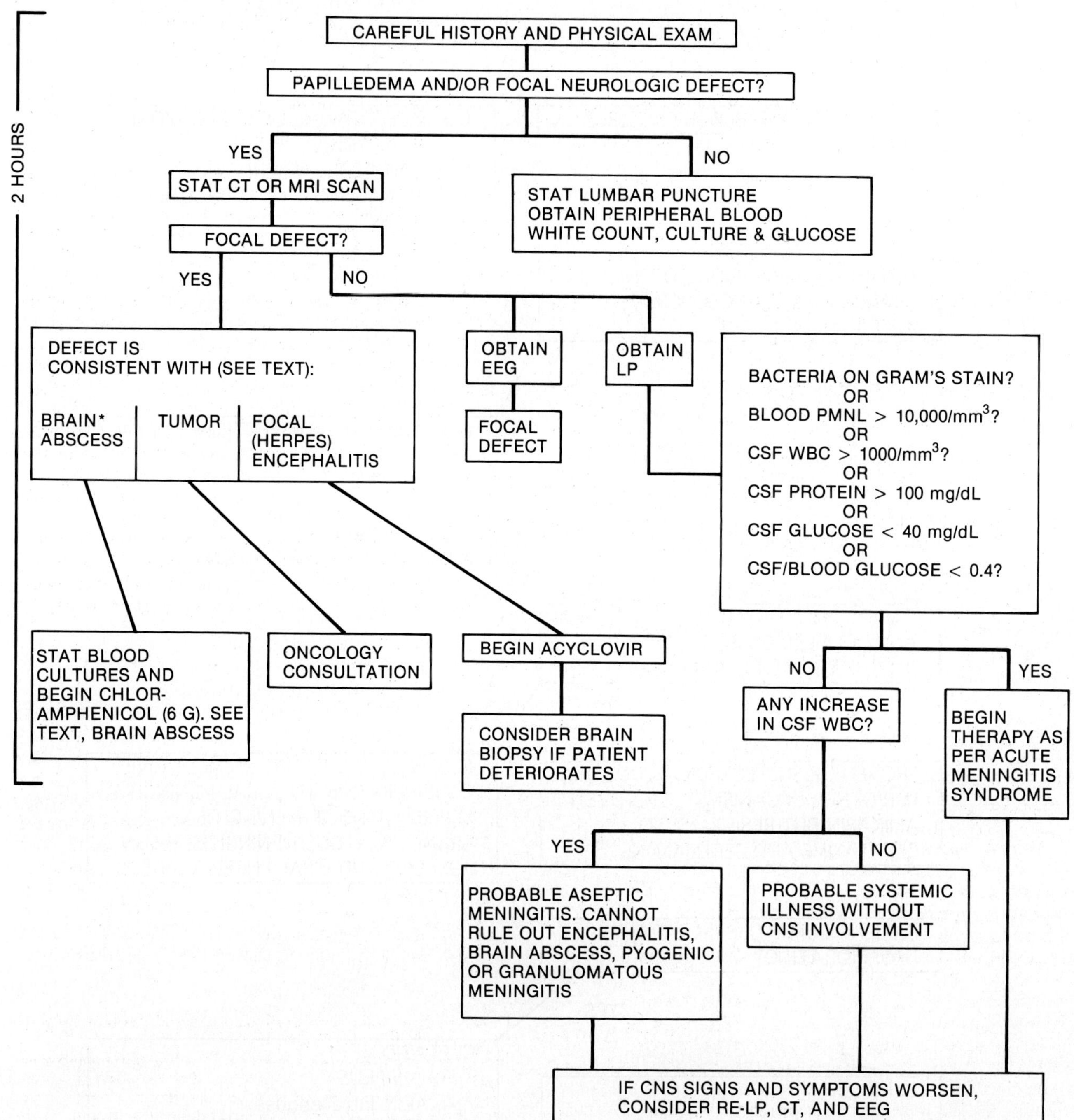

Figure 139–4. Algorithm for the management of patients with the subacute CNS infection syndrome. (*If CT not diagnostic, multiple antimicrobial therapy may be indicated pending further evaluation.)

TABLE 139–3. Dosages of Antimicrobials for Therapy of Central Nervous System Infection

Drug	*Dosage (by Total Body Weight)*	*Usual Dosage (for 70-kg Adult)*
Acyclovir	10 mg/kg IV every 8 h	700 mg IV every 8 h
Amikacin	15 mg/kg IV load, then 7.5 mg/kg every 12 h*	1050 mg IV load, then 525 mg IV every 12 h*
Intrathecal	$0.1\ mg \cdot lb^{-1} \cdot d^{-1}$	15 mg/d
Intraventricular	$0.1\ mg \cdot lb^{-1} \cdot d^{-1}$	15 mg/d
Ampicillin	30 mg/kg IV every 4 h	2 g IV every 4 h
Cefotaxime	30 mg/kg IV every 4 h	2 g IV every 4 h
Ceftazidime	30 mg/kg IV every 6 h	2 g IV every 6 h
Ceftriaxone	30 mg/kg IV every 12 h	2 g IV every 12 h
Chloramphenicol	15 mg/kg IV every 6 h	1 g IV every 6 h
Metronidazole	7.5 mg/kg IV every 6 h	500 mg IV every 6 h
Nafcillin	30 mg/kg IV every 4 h	2 g IV every 4 h
Penicillin G	60,000–70,000 units/kg IV every 4 h	4–5 million units IV every 4 h
Trimethoprim-sulfamethoxazole	5 mg/kg IV every 6 h	350 mg IV every 6 h†
Vancomycin	15–30 mg/kg IV every 12 h	1–2 g IV every 12 h*

*Adjust dose based on serum levels.
†Dose indicates trimethoprim component.

high-level penicillin-resistant pneumococcal meningitis has been associated with a high failure rate, even when the organism is susceptible to chloramphenicol in vitro.[11] Pneumococci are the most common cause of bacterial meningitis in the elderly, and these same considerations apply. However, gram-negative bacilli and *L. monocytogenes* are commonly implicated in elderly patients.[10] A wide spectrum of pathogens causes meningitis in immunosuppressed patients. On rare occasions, in patients with no immunologic defects, fungi, protozoa, and unusual bacteria may cause acute or subacute meningitis. After initiating therapy, every effort should be made to identify the infecting pathogen.

Large systemic doses of third-generation cephalosporins (e.g., cefotaxime and ceftriaxone) are bactericidal against the common pathogens of bacterial meningitis (pneumococci, meningococci, and all *H. influenzae*).[12] The third-generation cephalosporins are also effective in enteric gram-negative meningitis. *Escherichia coli, Klebsiella*, and other susceptible bacilli can be treated with these agents. A third-generation cephalosporin is indicated for patients who are relatively stable and infected with an enteric gram-negative pathogen presumed to be sensitive to the cephalosporins (see Fig. 139–3). Successful therapy of enteric gram-negative meningitis is associated with trough CSF antibiotic levels 5 to 10 times the minimum inhibitory concentration of the organism.[13] Third-generation cephalosporins are not indicated for every case of bacterial meningitis. Moribund patients, patients with resistant organisms, or patients who do not respond to cephalosporin therapy may require intraventricular aminoglycoside therapy (see Fig. 139–3). The doses of antimicrobials used for CNS infections are presented in Table 139–3. Some CNS pathogens cannot be reliably treated with cefotaxime or ceftriaxone, and alternative therapy is presented in Table 139–4.

The duration of therapy in bacterial meningitis varies with the pathogen and the clinical response. A normal host with pneumococcal or meningococcal meningitis is unlikely to suffer relapse after clinical improvement, and appropriate antibiotics should be given for 7 days.[14] Relapses occasionally occur with *H. influenzae* meningitis, and in such cases 10 to 14 days of therapy are recommended. Because antibiotic penetration into CSF falls as meningeal inflammation subsides, parenteral antibiotics are recommended for the entire course.

Abnormalities of the CSF (high protein and cell count and low glucose) persist for days to weeks. Resolution of symptoms should serve as adequate evidences of success. In patients who respond poorly to 48 hours of therapy, repeat lumbar puncture and head CT or MRI are indicated. Neither scans nor repeat lumbar puncture is indicated for patients with pneumococcal or meningococcal meningitis that steadily improves with therapy. In contrast, the response to therapy in gram-negative enteric meningitis is less consistent. Results of CSF cultures and Gram's stain should be monitored daily. After the CSF becomes sterile, an additional 7 days of aggressive antimicrobial therapy is warranted.

Adults with acute bacterial meningitis commonly have predisposing infections, including pneumonia, sinusitis, otitis, or endocarditis.[5] Therapy for meningitis usually treats the primary cause. Exceptions include endocarditis, which requires prolonged therapy with bactericidal antibiotics, and brain abscess, which may require surgical drainage.

Use of Corticosteroids

Much of the morbidity of bacterial meningitis is caused by the vigorous inflammatory response. Corticosteroids block inflammation, and animal studies clearly show that the addition of corticosteroids to antibacterial regimens improves survival. However, the role of corticosteroids for patients with pyogenic meningitis is controversial. Four double-blind placebo-controlled studies of dexamethasone adjuvant therapy for children with acute bacterial meningitis showed benefits, including decreased neurologic sequelae (mostly in terms of hearing loss) and in one study improved survival.[15–17] However, most patients were infected with *H. influenzae*, now an unusual cause of meningitis in developed countries. Nevertheless, dexamethasone administration

TABLE 139–4. Bacterial Meningitis Pathogens Not Adequately Treated with Cefotaxime or Ceftriaxone

Organism	*Antimicrobial*
P. aeruginosa	Ceftazidime plus amikacin
L. monocytogenes	Trimethoprim-sulfamethoxazole or ampicillin
S. aureus (methicillin susceptible)	Nafcillin
S. aureus (methicillin resistant)	Vancomycin
Enterobacter species (β-lactam resistant strains)	Trimethoprim-sulfamethoxazole
Pneumococci (some high-level penicillin-resistant strains)	Vancomycin or imipenem

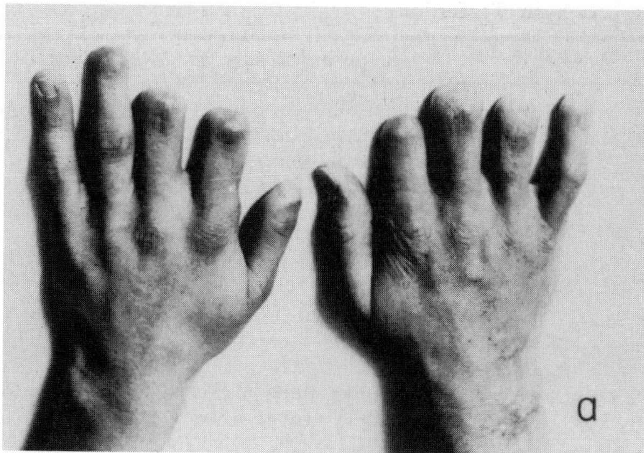

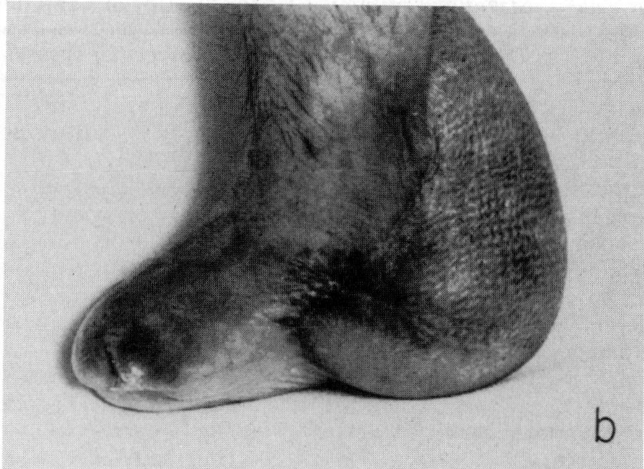

Figure 139–5. Extremities (hands *[A]* and foot *[B]*) of a 14-year-old boy who was observed by two physicians as his petechial rash progressed to "bruises" (purpura fulminans). These bruises were not recognized as the hallmarks of *N. meningitidis*–induced sepsis. In addition to the loss of extremities due to the necrotizing vasculitis of meningococcemia, the patient rapidly developed signs and symptoms characteristic of the acute meningitis syndrome.

with the first dose of antibiotic (0.6 mg · kg^{-1} · d^{-1} IV in four divided doses for the first 4 days of antibiotic treatment) is widely used to treat children age 2 months and older with bacterial meningitis. Deleterious effects of corticosteroids used as outlined have been rare. Routine corticosteroid use for adults is not advised.

Complications

Systemic complications may dominate the clinical course of acute bacterial meningitis. Forty per cent of patients with pneumococcal meningitis have concomitant sepsis. The sepsis is usually from an extra-CNS focus, such as pneumonia. Less commonly, sepsis represents seeding of the bloodstream from the infected meninges. Whether bacteremia precedes or follows meningeal infection, the sepsis demands immediate attention. General supportive measures are crucial. Other complications such as aspiration of gastric contents, seizures, and gastrointestinal bleeding must be monitored and prevented if possible.

When *Neisseria meningitidis* is causative, rhinorrhea or sore throat is often an antecedent, followed by fever, chills, and a petechial rash. Failure to recognize a febrile rash as meningococcemia may allow evolution to necrotizing vasculitis with loss of extremities (Fig. 139–5) or death. Progression to acute meningitis syndrome is not inevitable, but patients often have positive CSF cultures for *N. meningitidis* even when signs and symptoms of direct CNS involvement are lacking. Physiologic doses of steroids may be necessary when fulminant meningococcemia is complicated by hypotension due to adrenal insufficiency.[18]

As inflammatory exudate fills the ventricles and subarachnoid space, impairment of cranial and spinal nerve roots, cerebral infarction and edema, hydrocephalus, and subdural effusion may occur. As many as 15% of patients experience impaired ocular movement, and 11% develop hemiparesis or quadriparesis.[19] Fortunately, focal defects may resolve during recovery (Table 139–5).

Hydrocephalus can cause morbidity long after the infection has resolved. The availability of CT and MRI has improved management of this complication. Subdural effusions have been associated with *H. influenzae* meningitis in children; however, the importance of this complication and the need to aspirate such effusions are debatable. Cerebral infarction and edema have developed in the course of aggressive infection or delayed therapy.[19a] Anecdotal reports suggest that high-dose steroids may be lifesaving when intracranial pressure is markedly elevated.

Focal Central Nervous System Defects

Focal neurologic abnormalities or papilledema is unusual at presentation in pyogenic meningitis and suggests the presence of a focal lesion (see Figs. 139–3 and 139–4). Interpretation of CT, MRI, or electroencephalographic findings is central to treating such patients. Brain abscess, tumor, or herpetic encephalitis is best diagnosed with this information (Table 139–6). The absence of papilledema or focal neurologic defects in a patient with headache, fever, and progressive impairment of higher integrative functions suggests that bacterial meningitis is more likely and that lumbar puncture is needed. Uncal herniation is extremely unlikely in such a patient, and it is hazardous to delay a diagnostic lumbar puncture should pyogenic meningitis be present.

BRAIN ABSCESS

Pyogenic brain abscess is a localized suppurative infection of parenchymal CNS tissue and may involve any region from the cerebral cortex to the conus medullaris. Despite modern antibiotic therapy and refined surgical and radiographic techniques, mortality rates are approximately 15% to 25%. This poor prognosis is related to its relative infrequency and the technical difficulty of surgical intervention. Patients with altered sensoria on presentation clearly have a worse prognosis.[20] In most cases, CT or MRI provides sufficient information for optimal management. MRI is more

TABLE 139–5. Focal Neurologic Signs in Bacterial Meningitis

Early onset (defect is present at or shortly after presentation)
Often accompanied by focal or generalized seizures
Possibly related to meningeal vasculitis or cortical ischemia
Usually reversible
Late onset (defect develops late in course, often as patient is otherwise recovering)
Probably related to cortical vein thrombosis
May be reversible
Persisting (present on presentation and worsens during therapy)
Usually represents a major complication or mistaken diagnosis: brain abscess, herpes encephalitis, subdural empyema
Often requires a major change in therapy

TABLE 139–6. Differential Diagnosis of Central Nervous System Infection and Tumor

	Brain Abscess	*Bacterial Meningitis*	*Herpetic Encephalitis*	*Brain Tumor*
History				
Headache	Severe often focal	Severe generalized	Mild to severe	Absent to severe
Focal defect	Often	Occasional	Occasional	Usual
Progression	Days to weeks	Hours to days	Days	Days to months
Physical Examination				
Fever/degree	Usual/low grade	Always/high	Usual/variable	Rare
Early focal signs	Often	Occasional	Occasional	Usual
Pressure signs	Often	Rare	Occasional	Often
Distal infection	Often	Often	Unrelated	Unrelated
CT or MRI Scan				
Focal	Always*	No	Occasional	Always
Ring effect/onset	Often/late†	—	No	Often/early

*May be negative or nonspecific during first 48 hours of illness.
†Development of abscess wall will be delayed by steroid therapy.

sensitive for small or early lesions and better visualizes the cerebellum and brain stem.

Pathophysiology

A brain abscess begins as a localized area of parenchymal cellulitis (cerebritis), which evolves to necrosis and frank suppuration. The initial stage, characterized by vascular congestion, petechial hemorrhage, cerebral edema, and tissue softening, is demonstrable by MRI. As cerebritis progresses, CT findings become abnormal, revealing a capsule-like hyperemic zone surrounding the area of inflammation. In time, liquefaction results in frank abscess formation.

As the abscess matures, a dense capsule is formed. In relatively avascular areas of the brain, collagen formation is delayed. Once formed, however, the capsule resolves slowly. When necrosis is rapid and capsule formation delayed, as in the relatively avascular cerebral white matter, abscess rupture is more likely. In some cases, edema is the dominant process.

In the preantibiotic era, contiguous foci (middle ear, mastoids, and sinuses) caused most brain abscess. With the availability of antibiotics, however, such complications have become less common. An increasing proportion of cases is due to distant foci of infection or originate from unknown sites. With hematogenous seeding, abscesses tend to develop in the middle cerebral artery distribution. The etiologic pathogen relates to the route of infection (Table 139–7). The bacteria most often isolated from brain abscess are aerobic and anaerobic streptococci, although enteric gram-negative rods, staphylococci, pneumococci, and *Nocardia asteroides* may be present. Fungi such as *Aspergillus* and protozoa such as amebae can also be etiologic agents.[21–25]

Clinical Course

The variable signs and symptoms of brain abscess relate to variations in location, size, and rapidity of development. At one extreme, the course may span weeks, with few constitutional symptoms. In this setting, signs and symptoms of a space-occupying lesion predominate, and neoplasm is the primary diagnostic concern. In contrast, a previously asymptomatic brain abscess may rupture into the subarachnoid space, causing death within hours. The differential diagnosis in this setting includes an acute cerebral vascular event and pyogenic meningitis. However, brain abscess

TABLE 139–7. Brain Abscess

	Origin	*Organism**	*Incidence (% of Total)*	*Location*
Contiguous foci (70%)	Middle ear	ANA and A streptococci, *B. fragilis,* A GNR	35%	Temporal lobe
	Mastoids	A GNR, *B. fragilis,* ANA and A streptococci	15%	Cerebellum
	Sinuses	ANA streptococci, *Bacteroides,* staphylococci, *Hemophilus,* pneumococcus	15%	Frontal lobe
	Trauma	Staphylococci, ANA bacteria	5%	Site of trauma
Distal foci (30%)	Lungs	ANA streptococci, A GNR, *Nocardia*	10%	Occur at cortical junction along distribution of middle cerebral artery, involving frontal, pareital, and temporal lobes. Abscesses are often multiple.
	Right-to-Left shunts	Staphylococci, ANA and A streptococci	5%	
	Abdominal infections	A and ANA GNR	5%	
	Unknown sites	A and ANA streptococci	10%	

*Mixed infections are common.
Abbreviations: ANA = anaerobic; A = aerobic; GNR = gram-negative rods.

usually progresses subacutely for 7 to 14 days. Classic symptoms include excruciating headache, low-grade fever, and focal neurologic signs. Occasionally, a patient has no symptoms referable to the CNS, and the absence of fever does not preclude the diagnosis. Lumbar puncture may demonstrate increased cells and protein and normal or decreased glucose. However, organisms are identified in only 10% of cases. Because lumbar puncture may be life threatening in the presence of an expanding brain abscess, this procedure should be avoided when a focal lesion is likely.

Parameningeal foci cause brain abscess as the inflammatory process erodes through bone and meningeal tissues (see Table 139–7). Chronic otitis, sinusitis, or postsurgical and post-traumatic dural defects in a patient with progressive neurologic deterioration strongly suggest brain abscess.

Bacterial pathogens also invade neural tissues via hematogenous spread. The presence of chronic extrameningeal suppurative foci or illicit intravenous drug use predisposes to brain abscess. Pulmonary filtration helps protect the host from hematogenous seeding of the brain. However, when cyanotic heart disease or pulmonary arteriovenous fistulas are present, brain abscesses may occur.[26] About one fifth of patients have no recognized source of infection, and delayed diagnosis in these cases may increase mortality. Brain abscesses associated with endocarditis are rare but, when present, are often multiple and small. Rarely, bacterial meningitis causes intracerebral abscess.

The CNS complications of brain abscess relate to both the inflammation and the space-occupying lesion. Nonspecific complications include aspiration, gastrointestinal bleeding, and general inanition. The specific signs and symptoms of brain abscess relate to the space-occupying effect and may offer the most easily recognizable clues; however, even these findings may be absent or impossible to differentiate clinically from other causes of space-occupying lesions. When surrounding edema is excessive, aggressive therapy with corticosteroids is warranted. If a brain abscess ruptures into the subarachnoid space or into a cerebral ventricle, the patient will rapidly deteriorate.

Computed Tomography and Magnetic Resonance Imaging

CT and MRI techniques are particularly valuable in assessing brain abscesses. Changes in lesion size can be accurately monitored from week to week. Neurosurgical intervention can be guided by assessing proximity to vital neural structures. An expanding abscess may be aggressively drained, or conversely, a stable or shrinking abscess can be assiduously observed.

CT scanning has some limitations, particularly in the early cerebritis stage. In addition, the cerebellum, brain stem, and spinal cord may not be well visualized, and CT may not detect lesions of 1.5 cm or smaller. For such lesions, MRI scan enhanced with intravenous gadolinium is more sensitive. However, most symptomatic brain abscesses are detectable by CT, an exception being multiple small abscesses associated with endocarditis. Persons thus affected may have major functional impairment but only nonspecific changes on CT.

Although CT and MRI may assess the maturity of the abscess and associated capsule, misinterpretation can occur. Because the vascularity of the cerebral white matter is modest in comparison with gray matter, CT may erroneously suggest that capsule formation is lagging behind the inflammatory process in lesions involving the white matter. Steroid therapy may delay or even reverse CT findings by delaying true capsule formation.

Therapy

Combined antimicrobials and surgical drainage constitute the classic management of pyogenic brain abscesses. The antimicrobials must cross the blood-brain barrier and be administered for prolonged periods. Aspiration of the abscess is usually required to isolate the pathogen and to guide therapy. Positive cultures from blood or extra-CNS suppurative foci occasionally establish a presumptive etiologic diagnosis, allowing a preliminary therapeutic regimen to be instituted. Because neurologic status may change rapidly, frequent evaluation of patients is critical.

Brain abscess can resolve with antimicrobial therapy alone, and the use of CT has encouraged continuation of medical therapy without surgery in patients who are stable and in whom the cause has been determined by appropriate cultures.[27] However, neurosurgical intervention is indicated (1) in patients who deteriorate because of the space-occupying effect; (2) for aspiration and culture to define specific antimicrobial therapies; and (3) for abscesses that do not respond to medical therapy. Steroids should not be routinely used. However, in patients with edema and neurologic deterioration, high-dose steroids are indicated.

VIRAL INFECTIONS OF THE CENTRAL NERVOUS SYSTEM

All components of the CNS are vulnerable to viral infection. The resultant clinical syndrome may be meningitis, encephalitis, or myelitis. Acute viral meningitis is manifested by meningeal irritation, CSF pleocytosis, and an uncomplicated clinical course. Impairment of higher integrative functions dominates viral encephalitis. Personality changes may occur, with irritability and inability to concentrate. Patients may also develop fever, persisting headache, nausea, and vomiting. As a result of parenchymal involvement, CNS function may deteriorate over several days through confusion, lethargy, somnolence, and coma. Systemic symptoms become more prominent as CNS dysfunction worsens. Meningismus may develop at any point during viral encephalitis or may remain absent.

Pathophysiology

Viruses most commonly enter the CNS hematogenously. Virus may initially traverse mucous membranes (e.g., enteroviruses) or be inoculated into subcutaneous tissues (e.g., arthropod-borne viruses). After local replication within extraneural tissues, sustained viremia occurs. Alternatively, virus may gain access to the CNS by neuronal spread, as occurs when rabies virus spreads along peripheral nerves into the CNS. The olfactory tracts may provide a route of entry for herpes simplex virus.[28]

Individual viruses demonstrate affinities for different areas of the CNS. Enteroviruses and mumps viruses usually involve the ependyma and tissues of the subarachnoid space, producing meningeal irritation. In contrast, arthropod-borne and rabies viruses almost always involve the parenchyma and cause encephalitis. In older children and adults, herpes simplex virus type I characteristically causes temporal lobe encephalitis whereas herpes simplex virus type II more typically causes meningitis.[28] Such affinities are not absolute. For example, enteroviruses may on rare occasions cause encephalitis.

Acute Viral Meningitis

Many viruses cause meningitis. A pathogen usually cannot be isolated from adults with presumed viral meningitis, and the term *aseptic meningitis* describes this syndrome. Acute viral meningitis is common in neonates and young adults but is unusual after age 40.

Non-neonatal acute viral meningitis typically develops during the summer or fall in otherwise healthy young adults. For several days chills, myalgias, and malaise are followed by excruciating headache, photophobia, stiff neck, nausea, and vomiting. Lumbar puncture reveals clear fluid with normal glucose, mildly elevated protein, and lymphocytic pleocytosis. The illness resolves without sequelae. The meningeal symptoms last 7 to 10 days, with malaise persisting for as long as 6 weeks. Differentiation from bacterial or fungal infection is the primary goal of management (see Fig. 139–3). Therapy is entirely symptomatic.

Viral Encephalitis

A host of viral agents infect the parenchyma of the brain or spinal cord to produce encephalitis or myelitis, respectively. Both diseases impair neurologic function and may cause irreversible neuronal injury. Viral encephalitis is typically an acute febrile illness associated with headache, an altered level of consciousness disproportionate to systemic illness, behavioral or speech disturbances, and often neurologic signs such as seizures or hemiparesis. In contrast, viral myelitis spares higher integrative functions.

Noninfectious syndromes may mimic viral encephalitis and myelitis, and virtually any component of the CNS may be involved. Specific antiviral therapy is available for very few causes of encephalitis. When cerebral or spinal cord edema compromises CNS function, high-dose corticosteroids are indicated.

Herpes Encephalitis

Unlike most viral infections, herpes simplex encephalitis is amenable to antiviral therapy. This illness may occur at any age and tends to produce a rapidly devastating illness. Successful treatment requires prompt administration of intravenous acyclovir. The mortality of documented untreated infections may exceed 70%, although mild or asymptomatic cases may occur. The morbidity from surrounding cerebral edema may be considerable.

Herpes simplex encephalitis involves the temporal lobes in the vast majority of cases. This localization causes aphasia, anosmia, temporal lobe seizures, and focal neurologic defects. Such findings, often with a severe prodromal headache progressing to confusion, lethargy, or coma, suggest the diagnosis. Electroencephalography is superior to CT scan in detecting localization.[7] In some cases, MRI findings are abnormal when electroencephalography and CT are not diagnostic. Unfortunately, a wide range of signs and symptoms may occur. Preliminary studies suggest that a polymerase chain reaction performed on CSF is often diagnostic.[28a] Serology alone is not diagnostic, and CSF may be normal or nonspecifically abnormal. A rising titer of antibodies in the CSF may confirm the diagnosis but does not occur until 1 week or more into the illness. Empirical therapy with acyclovir is often used in critically ill patients with encephalitis and evidence of focal CNS involvement. Brain biopsy may be necessary if response to acyclovir is not prompt. A full 10-day course of antiviral therapy should be administered if herpes simplex encephalitis is suspected.[29]

Central Nervous System Infection and Patients with AIDS

CNS dysfunction is common in patients with acquired immunodeficiency syndrome (AIDS). Neurologic disease may be due to direct CNS involvement by many pathogens. CT or MRI and lumbar puncture are indicated for any patient with AIDS with significant headache or altered mental status, even when CNS symptoms do not dominate the picture. Because mass lesions are prevalent, lumbar puncture should generally be deferred until after CT or MRI. Common mass lesions in AIDS are toxoplasmosis, lymphoma, and progressive multifocal leukoencephalopathy. Enhancement after intravenous contrast favors toxoplasmosis or lymphoma and makes progressive multifocal leukoencephalopathy, at present untreatable, unlikely. The vast majority of patients with toxoplasmosis have detectable serum antibodies to *Toxoplasma gondii*, sometimes at low titer, and a negative test for serum antibody makes the diagnosis much less likely. Laboratories that assay *Toxoplasma* antibody by serial dilution should use an initial serum dilution of 1:2 or less. Toxoplasmosis usually responds dramatically to appropriate antimicrobials, although lifelong therapy is necessary to prevent relapse.

Cryptococcal meningitis is also common in AIDS. Almost all patients with AIDS with cryptococcal meningitis have detectable cryptococcal antigen in both serum and CSF, often at very high titer (e.g., >1:100,000). The optimal therapy for cryptococcal meningitis in AIDS is evolving but probably should include both amphotericin B and fluconazole.

PARADURAL ABSCESS

The epidural space is between the dura and the bony structures of the skull and vertebral column; the subdural space is between the subarachnoid membrane and the dura (see Fig. 139–2). Unlike the subarachnoid space, the paradural tissues are only potential spaces, with the arachnoid membrane and the dura resisting the spread of infection across their surfaces. Although subdural abscesses are more common within the cranium and epidural abscesses within the vertebral column, the causes, pathophysiology, and therapies are similar. These abscesses usually develop from a contiguous infection, surgery, or trauma.

In the skull, the epidural tissues are dense and epidural abscess is unusual. The subarachnoid membrane is less adherent to the dura, making the subdural space the more likely site of infection. The reverse is true in the vertebral column, where a thin layer of fat and blood vessels separate the dura from the vertebral bony structures. Here infection is more likely to involve the epidural space. Once established, infection may dissect within the epidural space for considerable distances.

Cranial subdural empyema may be clinically indistinguishable from a brain abscess. Subdural abscess is usually related to infection of the paranasal sinuses and less commonly to the ears or mastoids.[30] Trauma, surgical intervention, or hematogenous sources cause the remaining cases. Organisms common to sinusitis, including nonhemolytic streptococci, pneumococci, *Haemophilus*, anaerobes, and staphylococci, cause most infections. Gram-negative enteric bacilli may be associated with middle ear and mastoid infection.

An epidural abscess of the vertebral column classically progresses rapidly from spinal ache to paralysis.[31] Although such abscesses are most often caused by *Staphylococcus aureus*, unusual pathogens such as *Pseudomonas* have been frequently recognized in immunosuppressed patients and illicit drug users. Trauma or surgery of the vertebral column is a recognized cause of epidural abscess, and various organisms have been noted in this setting. Although most cases are community acquired, approximately one sixth occur postoperatively.

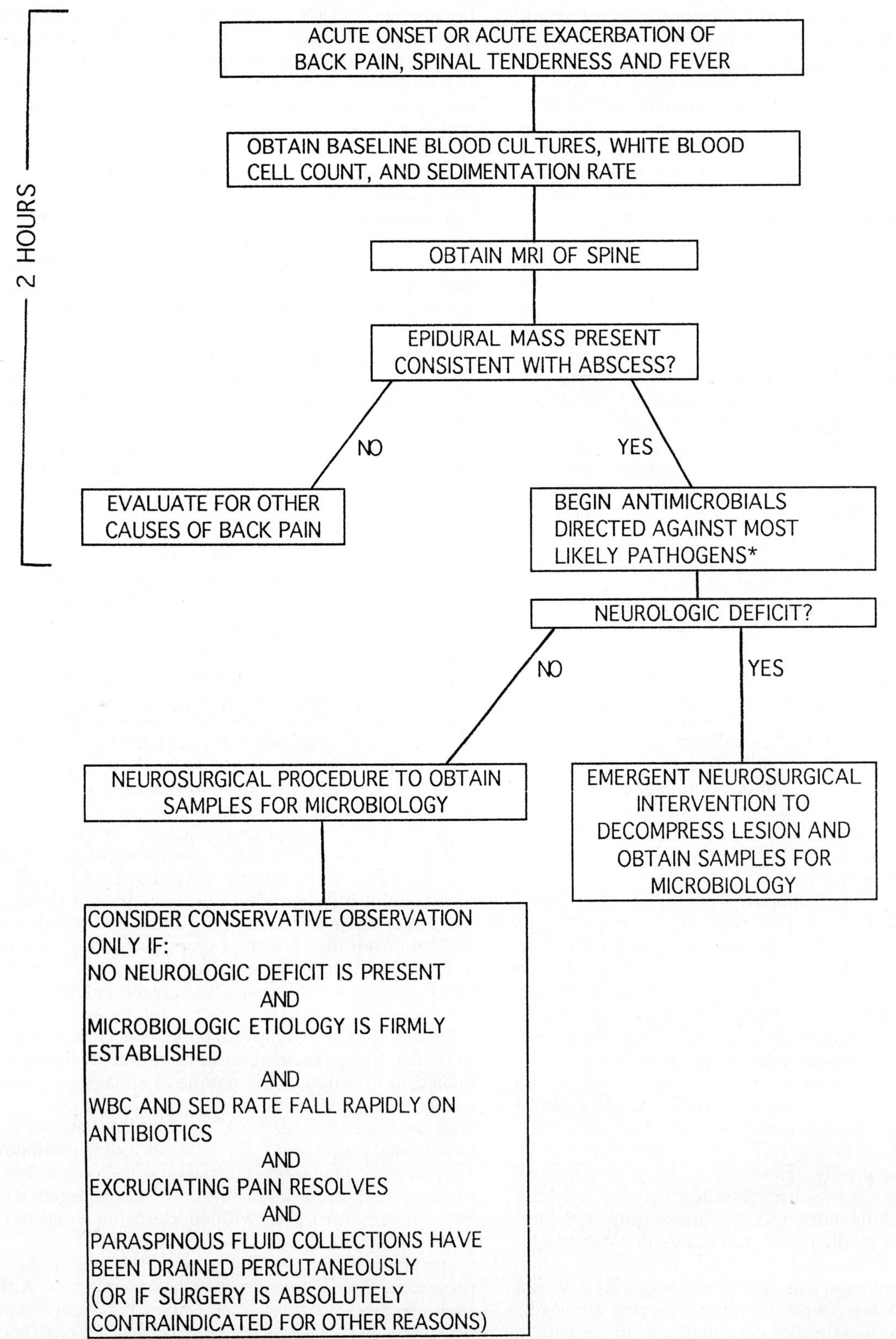

Figure 139–6. Algorithm for the management of patients with the spinal cord epidural abscess syndrome. If MRI cannot be performed, myelography (the lateral cervical approach may be required), high-contrast CT, or CT-myelography may be an acceptable alternative to localize an epidural abscess. (*If abscess drainage can be performed promptly, antimicrobial drugs may be withheld until specimens for microbiologic analysis are obtained; they can then be immediately administered in the operating room or radiology suite.)

Paradural abscesses tend to evolve rapidly, often producing irreversible damage to underlying neural structures. Antibiotics alone are rarely an option, and immediate neurosurgical drainage remains the mainstay of therapy. CT has greatly aided the management of subdural cranial abscess.

Spinal Epidural Abscess Syndrome

The spinal epidural abscess syndrome usually begins with localized severe spinal pain. Higher integrative functions generally remain intact; systemic manifestations are rarely severe enough to cause cortical dysfunction. Symptoms usually progress through four clinical phases: spinal ache, nerve root pain, radicular weakness, and paralysis. Back pain with fever, focal tenderness, and sensory or motor deficits strongly suggests this disease. The neck may be stiff, and a source of hematogenous seeding may be identified in three fourths of patients.

The rapidity of diagnosis depends on the severity of the signs and symptoms (Fig. 139–6). The diagnostic study of choice is MRI, which defines cord compression and the presence and extent of abscess, identifies drainable paraspinal fluid collections, and diagnoses concomitant vertebral osteomyelitis. Other procedures such as myelography and CT scanning may be used if MRI cannot be performed. Emergency neurosurgical intervention is generally considered mandatory for this infection, both to obtain tissue for microbiology and for decompression. Some patients have been successfully treated with antibiotics alone, without surgical intervention. Nonsurgical management might be considered if, on frequent examination, a patient does not develop weakness on antibiotic therapy, if severe pain does not persist, and if fever, peripheral white blood cell count, and sedimentation rate all decline on therapy.[32, 33] Unfortunately, some patients develop sudden neurologic impairment even weeks into conservative therapy, presumably secondary to vascular compromise of the cord. Neurologic defects require a more aggressive approach to management. Frequent neurologic examinations are mandatory for a patient with fever and recent severe back pain. The neurologic deficit may initially be limited to a loss of pain sensation in the perianal region (second sacral dermatome). Weakness indicates the need for immediate neurosurgical consultation and MRI. If myelography is performed, CSF should be obtained for examination.

Degenerative disease and metastatic tumor may mimic epidural abscess, especially if fever is present. A metastatic tumor of the spinal cord can rapidly produce severe neurologic deficits, and a history of malignancy may be suggestive. Metastatic tumors are often best treated with steroids and radiotherapy. If fever cannot be easily attributed to another site of infection or inflammation, MRI usually distinguishes among degenerative spinal disease, metastatic tumor, and epidural abscess. In some cases, exploratory surgery may be necessary for diagnosis. Other considerations include transverse myelitis or hematoma.

Spinal epidural abscess demands prompt antimicrobial therapy to minimize residual weakness or paralysis. Community-acquired abscesses are usually due to *S. aureus* and should be treated with nafcillin. If methicillin-resistant staphylococci are prevalent, vancomycin should be substituted. Recent urinary tract infection, decubitus ulcers, or vertebral surgery suggests the presence of gram-negative bacilli, and a third-generation cephalosporin, with or with-

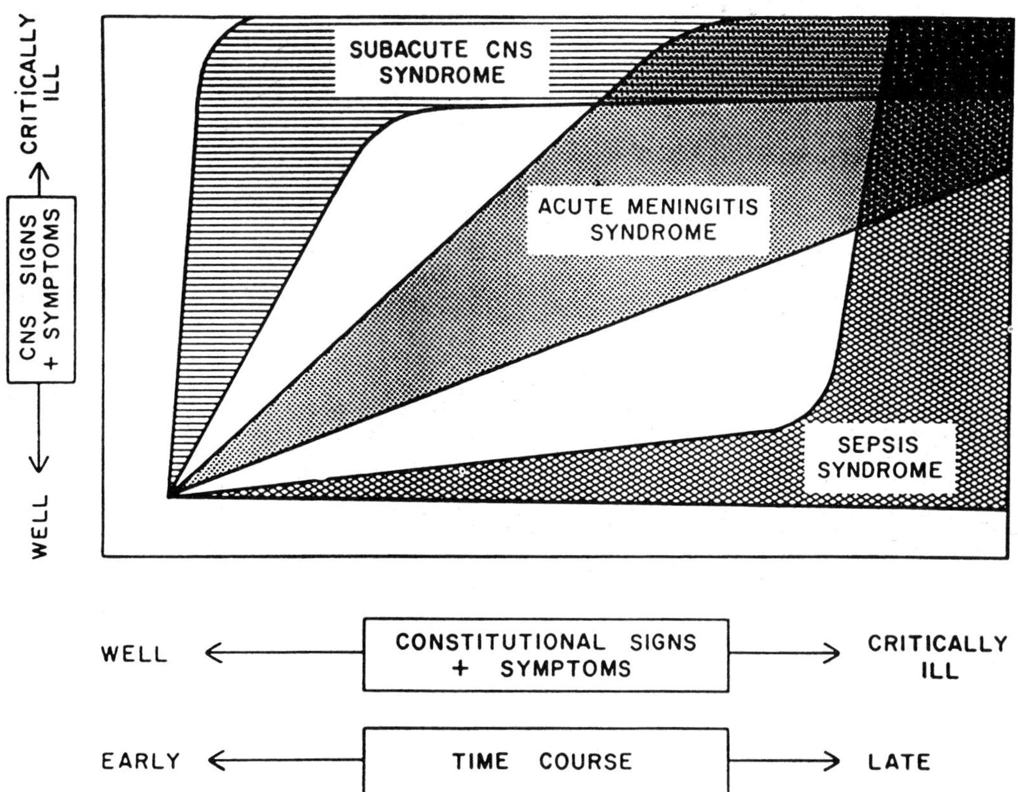

Figure 139–7. Graphic representation of the clinical presentations of the subacute CNS infections syndrome, the acute meningitis syndrome, and the sepsis syndrome. On the *vertical axis* is the spectrum of CNS signs and symptoms (e.g., loss of higher integrative functions or of focal sensory or motor deficits); on the *horizontal axis* is the spectrum of constitutional symptoms (e.g., fever and malaise). The *horizontal axis* also depicts the time-course of the different syndromes.

out an aminoglycoside, should be added. Treatment may be modified when culture results are available.

SEPSIS SYNDROME

In the sepsis syndrome, an acutely ill patient develops CNS dysfunction late in the course of illness. Gram-negative sepsis frequently produces this syndrome, and multiple organ failure may develop. Patients are not always observed early in the illness, and at presentation, signs and symptoms of CNS disease may dominate the illness (Fig. 139–7). In treating a patient, general supportive measures take precedence over CNS concerns. After a brief assessment, general life-support measures should correct hypotension, hypoxia, and anuria. As soon as easily accessible body fluid specimens are obtained for culture, broad-spectrum antimicrobials should be administered. At this point, a history should be carefully taken and physical examination performed and the patient treated as outlined for subacute CNS infection syndrome (see Fig. 139–4). Delays in directly assessing the CNS are justifiable only when the history has been adequate to document that a clear-cut systemic illness preceded the onset of CNS symptoms and signs. Otherwise, a more aggressive use of lumbar puncture and CT or MRI is warranted (see Figs. 139–3 or 139–4).

SUMMARY

Acute infection of the CNS may require drastic therapeutic maneuvers. Because the four major syndromes of CNS infection (i.e., acute meningitis syndrome, subacute CNS infection syndrome, spinal epidural abscess syndrome, and sepsis syndrome) differ in signs and symptoms as well as in approaches to definitive diagnosis and therapy, it is important to distinguish among them. Moreover, diverse infectious and noninfectious causes may produce similar syndromes in the CNS. For therapy to be effective, it must be instituted within minutes to hours of the initial evaluation. Thus, in the practice of critical care medicine involving CNS disease, therapy and diagnosis must be carefully coordinated to offer the earliest possible therapy for all likely disease processes while efficiently working to identify the specific disease process.

References

1. Mount LA: Congenital dermal sinuses. JAMA 1949; 139:1263.
2. Simberkoff MS, Moldover NH, Rahal JJ Jr: Absence of detectable bactericidal and opsonic activities in normal and infected human cerebrospinal fluids. J Lab Clin Med 1980; 95:362.
2a. Tunkel AR, Scheld WM: Pathogenesis and pathophysiology of bacterial meningitis. Clin Microbiol Rev 1993; 6:118.
3. Lepper MH, Dowling HF: Treatment of pneumococcal meningitis with penicillin compared with penicillin plus Aureomycin. Arch Intern Med 1951; 88:489.
4. Rahal JJ Jr, Simberkoff MS: Bactericidal and bacteriostatic action of chloramphenicol against meningeal pathogens. Antimicrob Agents Chemother 1976; 10:322.
4a. Baldwin LN, Henderson A, Thomas P, et al: Acute bacterial meningitis in young adults mistaken for substance abuse. Br Med J 1993; 306:775.
5. Durand ML, Calderwood SB, Weber DJ, et al: Acute bacterial meningitis: A review of 493 episodes. N Engl J Med 1993; 328:21.
6. Carpenter RR, Petersdorf RG: The clinical spectrum of bacterial meningitis. Am J Med 1962; 33:262.
7. Whitley RJ, Soong S, et al: Herpes simplex encephalitis. JAMA 1982; 247:317.
8. Whitley RJ, Alford CA, Hirsch MS, et al: Vidarabine versus acyclovir therapy in herpes simplex encephalitis. N Engl J Med 1986; 314:144.
9. Talan DA, Guterman JJ, Overturf GD, et al: Analysis of emergency department management of suspected bacterial meningitis. Ann Emerg Med 1989; 18:856–862.
10. Wenger JD, Hightower AW, Facklam RR, et al: Bacterial meningitis in the United States, 1986: Report of a multistate surveillance study. J Infect Dis 1990; 162:1316.
11. Friedland IR, Klugman KP: Failure of chloramphenicol therapy in penicillin-resistant pneumococcal meningitis. Lancet 1992; 339:405–408.
12. Congeni BL: Comparison of ceftriaxome and traditional therapy of bacterial meningitis. Antimicrob Agents Chemother 1984; 25:40.
13. Wright PF, Kaiser AB, Bowman CM, et al: The pharmacokinetics and efficacy of an aminoglycoside administered into the cerebral ventricles in neonates: Implications for further evaluation of this route of therapy in meningitis. J Infect Dis 1981; 143:141.
14. Lin T-Y, Chrane DF, Nelson JD, et al: Seven days of ceftriaxone therapy is as effective as ten days' treatment for bacterial meningitis. JAMA 1985; 253:3559–3563.
15. Lebel MH, Freij BJ, Syrogiannopoulos GA, et al: Dexamethasone therapy for bacterial meningitis—results of two double-blind, placebo-controlled trials. N Engl J Med 1988; 319:964–971.
16. Girgis NI, Farid Z, Mikhail IA, et al: Dexamethasone treatment for bacterial meningitis in children and adults. Pediatr Infect Dis J 1989; 8:848–851.
17. Odio CM, Faingezicht I, Paris M, et al: The beneficial effects of early dexamethasone administration in infants and children with bacterial meningitis. N Engl J Med 1991; 324:1525–1531.
18. Boswirth DC: Reversible adrenocortical insufficiency in fulminant meningococcemia. Arch Intern Med 1979; 139:823.
19. Dodge PR, Swartz MN: Bacterial meningitis—a review of selected aspects. N Engl J Med 1961; 272:954.
19a. Pfister HW, Feiden W, Einhaupl KM: Spectrum of complications during bacterial meningitis in adults. Results of a prospective clinical study. Arch Neurol 1993; 50:575.
20. Seydoux C, Francioli P: Bacterial brain abscesses: Factors influencing mortality and sequelae. Clin Infect Dis 1992; 15:394.
21. Garfield J: Management of supratentorial intracranial abscess: A review of 200 cases. Br Med J 1969; 2:7.
22. Brewer NS, MacCarty CS, Wellman WE: Brain abscess: A review of recent experience. Ann Intern Med 1975; 82:571.
23. Dreissen JJR, van Alphen HAM: Brain abscess and subdural empyema. J Neurol Neurosurg Psychiatry 1976; 39:481.
24. Jefferson AA, Keogh AJ: Intracranial abscesses: A review of treated patients over 20 years. Q J Med 1977; 1983:389.
25. Fischbein CA, Rosenthal A, Fischer EG, et al: Risk factors for brain abscess in patients with congenital heart disease. Am J Cardiol 1974; 34:97.
26. Press OW, Ramsey PG: Central nervous system infections associated with hereditary hemorrhagic telangiectasia. Am J Med 1984; 77:86–92.
27. Boom WH, Tuazon CU: Successful treatment of multiple brain abscesses with antibiotics alone. Rev Infect Dis 1985; 7:189–199.
28. Whitley RJ: Viral encephalitis. N Engl J Med 1990; 323:242.
28a. Anderson NE, Powell KF, Croxson MC: A polymerase chain reaction assay of cerebrospinal fluid in patients with suspected herpes simplex encephalitis. J Neurol Neurosurg Psychiatry 1993; 56:520.
29. Landry ML, Booss J, Hsiung GD: Duration of vidarabine therapy in biopsy-negative herpes simplex encephalitis. JAMA 1982; 247:332.
30. Kaufman DM, Miller MH, Steigbigel NH: Subdural empyema: Analysis of 17 recent cases and review of the literature. Medicine 1975; 54:485.
31. Baker AS, Ojemann RG, Swartz MN, et al: Spinal epidural abscess. N Engl J Med 1975; 293:463.
32. Wheeler D, Keiser P, Rigamonti D, et al: Medical management of spinal epidural abscesses—case report and review. Clin Infect Dis 1992; 15:22–27.
33. Baker AS, Ojemann RG, Baker RA: Editorial response to Wheeler et al—To decompress or not to decompress—spinal epidural abscess. Clin Infect Dis 1992; 15:28–29.

CHAPTER 140

Toxic Shock Syndrome

Charles J. Fisher, Jr., MD, FCCM • Leo A. Celi, MD

Toxic shock syndrome (TSS) is an acute febrile illness involving multiple organ systems and is associated with hypotension and rash. The syndrome typically occurs in young, previously healthy menstruating women using tampons and is characterized by the following clinical symptoms: fever (temperature 38.9°C or greater); syncope, hypotension, or shock; vomiting and watery diarrhea; diffuse inflammation of the mucous membranes; diffuse erythroderma or petechial skin rash; desquamation of the hands and feet during convalescence; and laboratory evidence of multiple organ dysfunction (Table 140–1).

Since the clinical entity and its association with *Staphylococcus aureus* were first described in 1978,[1] more than 3000 cases have been reported to the Centers for Disease Control in Atlanta. Although the majority of TSS cases are associated with menstruation, an increasing number are being reported in men and nonmenstruating women.[2] TSS has been linked with various types of staphylococcal infections, including empyema, surgical and postpartum infections, deep abcesses, head and neck infections, influenza-related respiratory tract infections, and staphylococcal colonization of mucous membranes.[3–6]

TABLE 140–1. Criteria for Diagnosis of Toxic Shock Syndrome: Confirmed Cases Meet All Six Criteria; Probable Cases Meet Five Criteria

1. Temperature ≥38.9° C (102° F)
2. Erythematous macular rash (occasionally petechial)
3. Desquamation of palms and soles during recovery phase*
4. Systolic blood pressure ≤90 mm Hg for adults or ≤ fifth percentile for age in children; or orthostatic syncope or orthostatic hypotension
5. Involvement of three or more organ systems
   - Gastrointestinal: vomiting and/or watery diarrhea at onset of illness
   - Mucous membrane: vaginal, oropharyngeal, or conjunctival hyperemia
   - Muscular: severe myalgia and/or creatine phosphokinase level more than twice the upper limit of normal
   - Renal: blood urea nitrogen or creatinine level at least twice the upper limit of normal, and/or urinary sediment with sterile pyuria (≥5 white blood cells per high-power field)
   - Hepatic: total bilirubin, serum glutamic-oxaloacetic transaminase, or serum glutamic-pyruvic transaminase at least twice the upper limit of normal
   - Hematologic: thrombocytopenia (platelet count ≤100,000/mm^3)
   - Central nervous system: disorientation or alterations in consciousness without focal findings and in the absence of hypotension and hyperpyrexia
   - Cardiopulmonary: hypoxemia, adult respiratory distress syndrome, or myocardial depression (cardiac index ≤3.3 $L/min \cdot m^2$)
   - Metabolic: serum calcium ≤7.0 mg/dL, serum phosphate ≤2.5 mg/dL, and total serum protein ≤5.0 mg/dL
6. Reasonable evidence for the absence of rickettsial disease, leptospirosis, meningococcemia, or rubeola

*Desquamation is obviously an unnecessary criterion in fatal cases.

ETIOLOGY AND PATHOPHYSIOLOGY

TSS is usually associated with the presence of or infection by *S. aureus* bacteria.[1, 3, 5, 7] *S. aureus* isolates from patients with the menstrual form of TSS elaborate low concentrations of hemolysin, lipase, and nuclease, thereby appearing relatively innocuous; however, they can produce large amounts of pyrogenic exotoxins.[8] Because most patients with TSS have a cutaneous infection that usually involves a mucous membrane and produces negative blood cultures, it has been postulated that the intravascular invasion of *S. aureus* is less important than the production, absorption, and action of its toxins.[9] More than 90% of *S. aureus* isolates from patients with TSS are phage-type 59/29 and elaborate large amounts of a unique exotoxin[10, 11] now called TSS toxin-1 (TSST-1). High-affinity receptors for TSST-1 on human epithelial cells and the toxin's rapid absorption via endocytosis support the possibility of its enhanced uptake from epithelial surfaces.[12] The frequent absence of a local inflammatory response in postoperative wounds associated with TSS further suggests that toxin rather than infection produces illnesses.[13, 14] Only 60% to 75% of *S. aureus* strains from nonmenstrual TSS elaborate TSST-1. In one study, enterotoxin B was the only toxin produced by 38% of isolates from patients with nonmenstrual TSS. In addition, three independent reports implicated enterotoxin C as a cause of nonmenstrual TSS.[15]

TSST-1 is a 22,000 to 25,000 molecular weight polypeptide protein that easily diffuses across intact mucous membranes and bears some resemblance to staphylococcal enterotoxins B and C.[16] TSST-1 and enterotoxins B and C are referred to as superantigens. Their biologic properties include induction of tumor necrosis factor, interleukin-1, and interferon-γ; induction of lymphocyte mitogenicity; enhancement of delayed-type hypersensitivity; blockade of reticuloendothelial cell clearance; enhancement of susceptibility to endotoxin shock; suppression of immunoglobulin production; and inhibition of neutrophil chemotaxis.[17] It is postulated that these superantigens either directly or indirectly cause myocardial dysfunction, peripheral vasodilation, and increased capillary permeability,[13] resulting in hypotension, oliguria, hypoxemia, and shock. Whether the multiorgan system dysfunction is a direct result of the toxin or secondary to prolonged organ ischemia is unclear.[15, 17]

The toxin-producing strain of *S. aureus* is found infrequently in patients without TSS,[8] and 80% of the normal adult population has high antibody titers to TSST-1.[10] By comparison, 95% of patients who develop TSS have low or no antibody titers to TSST-1. This observation implies that high titers are protective and suggests that it may be possible to serologically identify patients who are vulnerable to the development of TSS. Using animal models to confirm the causative role of TSST-1 in the pathogenesis of TSS has met with limited but promising success.[18] More work remains to be done in this field. It is possible that other bacteria act synergistically with *S. aureus* in the pathogenesis of TSS by producing endotoxin. *Escherichia coli* has frequently been co-isolated along with *S. aureus* from the vagina of women with menstrual TSS.[19]

EPIDEMIOLOGY

Eighty-four per cent of the reported cases of TSS are associated with menstruation.[2] In 1980, the peak incidence of menstrual TSS was 6 to 14 cases per 100,000 women; this rate has decreased by about two thirds. A history of tampon use continues to be present in 99% of menstruation-related cases.[2] Menstrual TSS occurs predominantly in white females (98%) under 25 years of age (65%), with an age range of 11 to 61 years and a mean age of 22 years. The case-fatality ratio for TSS has dropped from 10% in 1980 to between 2.6% and 3.5% currently.[2, 20] Epidemiologic studies have not linked *S. aureus* infection with any high-risk exogenous hygienic practice;[4] however, hygienic factors *not* associated with the development of TSS include the method of tampon insertion, the number of tampons used per day, and the length of time a tampon is kept in place. The use of hygienic products such as douches, feminine deodorants, and vaginal suppositories, the frequency of bathing with or without a tampon in place, and a patient's sexual history also do *not* have any specific association with the development of menstrual TSS.[4, 21]

An increased risk of developing menstrual TSS is noted with the use of highly absorbent tampons,[21] which alter the vaginal mucosa presumably by absorbing fluid from the vaginal epithelium. The intracellular bridges are thus disrupted in the vaginal mucosa, increasing its susceptibility to bacterial toxins. The polyester foam in these products effectively binds ionized magnesium and removes it from the vaginal environment. In vitro studies have demonstrated that the rate of TSST-1 production by TSS strains of *S. aureus* increases 12-fold in a low-magnesium medium.[22] Highly absorbent tampons have been removed from the market. Use of the contraceptive sponge has also been linked to TSS.[23]

The incidence of nonmenstrual TSS has remained relatively constant since 1980 and now represents one third of all cases,[2, 20] with one third of these occurring in males. The racial distribution of nonmenstrual TSS approximates that of the United States population; 87% of cases occur in whites. The mean age of patients with nonmenstrual TSS is significantly higher (27 y), and the case-fatality ratio is reportedly between 5%[2] and 16.7%.[20] Nonmenstrual TSS has been associated with nonsurgical cutaneous and subcutaneous infections (30%); abortion or childbirth (27%); postoperative infections (18%); nonmenstrual, nonpostpartum vaginal infections (5%); and various other sources of infection (20%).[2] Postoperative TSS usually becomes clinically evident 2 days after surgery. This delay may reflect a toxin-producing, subclinical incubation period. Postpartum TSS occurs either within 3 days of delivery or at least 14 days after delivery. Early-onset postpartum TSS is temporally similar to postoperative TSS, whereas late-onset postpartum TSS appears to be tampon related. *S. aureus* isolates from nonmenstrual cases are similar in all respects to *S. aureus* isolates from patients with menstrual TSS. The most common sites of infection in nonmenstrual TSS are the extremities, perianal region, and axillae.[7]

TSS cases have been reported in all 50 states of the United States and in many other countries, including Japan, Australia, New Zealand, Israel, Canada, South Africa, and most countries of Europe.

CLINICAL FEATURES

Initial symptoms typically consist of the rather sudden onset of fever, nausea, and vomiting, followed by watery diarrhea. This prodrome is usually associated with malaise and myalgias and may last 12 to 48 hours before development of acute illness (Fig. 140–1). The acute illness occurs precipitously and is associated with headache, fever, myalgias, orthostatic hypotension, hyperemic mucous membranes, and a diffuse erythematous macular rash (Fig. 140–2). The myalgias and muscle weakness are among the earliest, often the most painful, and in the case of weakness the most prolonged manifestations of TSS. The rash of TSS typically is blanching, nonpruritic, and macular, and is usually present at the time of presentation. It fades in about 3 days.[15] Patients often have diminished bowel sounds with a distended, diffusely tender abdomen suggesting peritoneal irritation. All patients develop a diffuse conjunctivitis with scleral injection and photophobia, which frequently progresses to subconjunctival hemorrhages or an exudative conjunctivitis. Additionally, most patients develop diffuse erythematous pharyngitis with a strawberry-colored tongue. During the convalescent period, desquamation of the palms and soles is noted (Fig. 140–3).

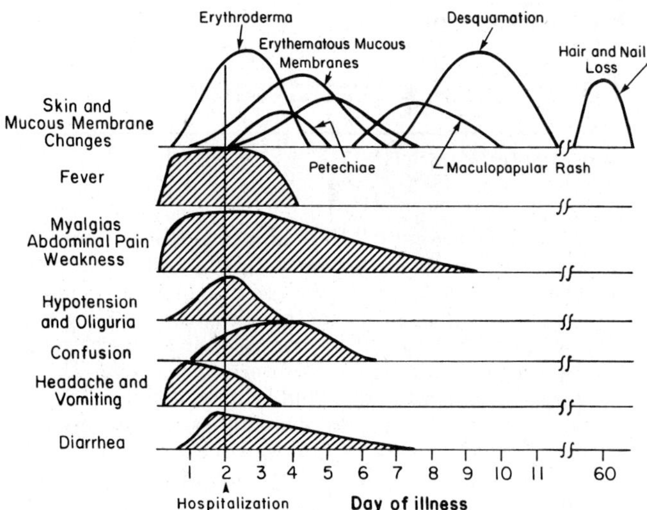

Figure 140–1. Composite line drawing of major clinical manifestations of TSS. (From Chesney PJ, Davis JP, Purdy WK, et al: Clinical manifestations of toxic shock syndrome. JAMA 1981; 246:741. Copyright 1981, American Medical Association.)

During the prodrome and at the beginning of acute illness, patients are exquisitely sensitive to deep touch, and the creatine phosphokinase level is often two to three times its normal value. During convalescence, muscle tenderness resolves and creatine phosphokinase level returns to normal. Creatine phosphokinase fractionation reveals no evidence of a myocardial source.

Most patients with TSS have renal dysfunction characterized by sterile pyuria, microscopic hematuria and proteinuria, and invariably oliguria. Oliguria is frequently accompanied by azotemia; blood urea nitrogen and creatine levels are greater than 40 mg/dL and 2.4 mg/dL, respectively.

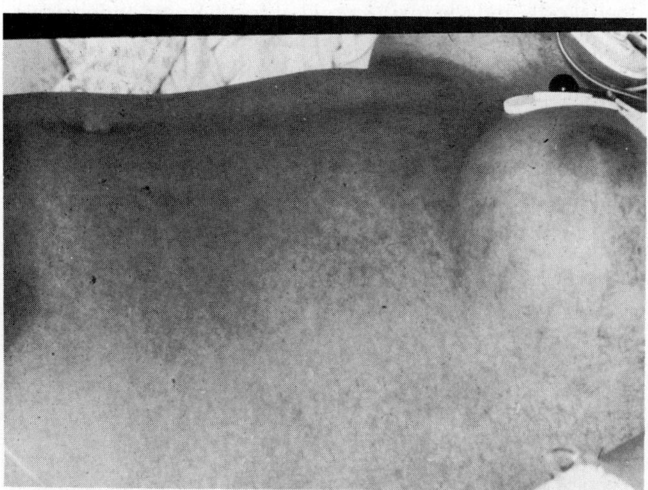

Figure 140–2. Typical erythematous macular, sunburn-like rash of TSS.

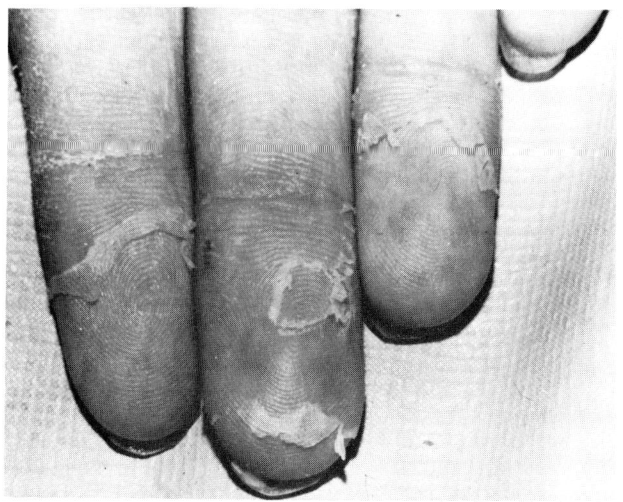

Figure 140–3. Characteristic desquamation of fingertips.

Potential mechanisms for the acute tubular necrosis observed in TSS include ischemic injury related to hypotension and the renal toxicity of tumor necrosis factor.[15]

Hepatobiliary abnormalities often elevate transaminases, bilirubin, and alkaline phosphatase levels. It is unclear whether these abnormalities are directly related to circulating bacterial toxins or hypotension. The elevated bilirubin cannot be explained by hemolysis, and the hepatobiliary tree is patent.

Platelet count frequently drops below 100,000/mm^3, and occasional profound thrombocytopenia may require platelet transfusion. The bone marrow of thrombocytopenic patients is hypercellular with respect to granulocytes but has normal numbers of megakaryocytes. This observation suggests either relative suppression of megakaryocyte precursors, with or without peripheral platelet consumption, or failure of platelet release from the bone marrow. Rarely noted is clinical or laboratory evidence of disseminated intravascular coagulation.

Most patients complain of severe headache, and many have a stiff neck and other clinical signs of meningeal irritation, including confusion, disorientation, hallucinations, and delirium. These symptoms may occur as late as 4 or 5 days after the onset of illness and may be due to mediator-induced cerebral edema. Cerebrospinal fluid from lumbar puncture is either normal or consistent with an aseptic meningitis. Generally, central nervous system findings resolve without sequelae. However, some patients report difficulty concentrating, persistent headache, and recent memory loss up to a year after acute illness.

Profound hypocalcemia may accompany hypoalbuminemia, but high serum levels of calcitonin have also been demonstrated.[24] Hypomagnesemia, by interfering with parathyroid hormone secretion and action, may also contribute to hypocalcemia.[15] Clinical tetany is rare. There is currently no explanation for the hypophosphatemia that is noted despite renal impairment.

Incipient circulatory abnormality may be manifested by extreme peripheral vasoconstriction with acrocyanosis, and all patients develop hypotension and tachycardia within 24 hours of symptom onset. In mild forms of TSS, the major complaint may be orthostatic syncope rather that hypotension. Although hypotension is generally responsive to vigorous fluid resuscitation, it sometimes is profound as a result of decreased vasomotor tone and nonhydrostatic leakage of protein-rich fluid from the microcirculation and may be accompanied by evidence of myocardial dysfunction, which peaks 24 to 48 hours after the onset of TSS. This coincides with a depressed cardiac index and echocardiographic evidence of left atrial and ventricular dilation and diffuse hypokinesis.[25, 26] Patients show no evidence of myocardial infarction or coronary vasculitis, although they frequently experience exertional fatigue during convalescence.

RECURRENT ILLNESS

Approximately one third of patients with TSS have a recurrent episode of TSS, and as many as six recurrences have been reported in a single patient.[20] In some patients, protective antibodies may not appear for a year or more. Recurrent disease is very rare in nonmenstrually associated cases. Most recurrent episodes occur within 3 months of the initial event, usually on the same relative menstrual day as the initial episode.[4] Antistaphylococcal antibiotics administered during the acute illness reduce the rate of recurrence, as does permanent discontinuation of tampon use.[4] These independent prophylactic measures are also synergistic. The criteria for the diagnosis of recurrence are less stringent than for the initial episode; recurrent TSS should be considered in any individual who was previously afflicted with TSS and who later develops suspicious symptoms (Table 140–2).

SEQUELAE

Commonly observed sequelae of TSS are late-onset rash, reversible patchy alopecia, telogen effluvium, prolonged weakness, fatigue and exercise intolerance, recurrent episodes of TSS, protracted myalgias, and carpal tunnel syndrome. Less commonly observed but problematic are the neuropsychologic sequelae of TSS, including persistent headache, confusion, memory loss, inability to compute, and loss of higher integrative functions.

PATHOLOGIC FINDINGS

Pathologic findings at postmortem examination are consistent with the hypothesis that the illness is caused by a staphylococcal toxin. Beneath its basal layer, the vaginal-cervical mucosa is separated by ulceration, severe vasodilation, inflammation, and thrombosis.[27] Bacterial invasion is minimum. The primary pulmonary findings are severe capillary congestion, intra-alveolar hemorrhage, atelectasis, and hyaline membrane formation. Periportal inflammation with microvesicular fatty changes and centrilobular congestion are observed in the liver, and pathologic findings in the kidneys are consistent with acute tubular necrosis. Histologic examination of the heart reveals interstitial edema, sparse peri-

TABLE 140–2. Criteria for Recurrence of Toxic Shock Syndrome

Major Criteria
- Temperature ≥38.9° C (102° F)
- Rash
- Mucous membrane hyperemia or myalgia
- Vomiting or diarrhea
- Systolic blood pressure ≥90 mm Hg for adults; orthostatic drop in diastolic blood pressure ≥15 mm Hg from lying to sitting; or orthostatic syncope

Definite Recurrence
- Desquamation and at least three of the major criteria

Probable Recurrence
- Desquamation and two of the major criteria
- Three of the major criteria associated with menstruation

vasculitis, and myofibrillar degeneration without evidence of myocarditis or infarction.

DIFFERENTIAL DIAGNOSIS

Although TSS can usually be easily recognized by the abrupt appearance of headache, gastrointestinal symptoms, and a desquamative rash associated with hypotension and multiorgan dysfunction, various infectious, toxic, or immunologic disorders can produce similar symptoms. These disorders include streptococcal or staphylococcal scarlet fever, leptospirosis, Rocky Mountain spotted fever, meningococcemia, hemolytic uremic syndrome, erythema multiforme, drug eruptions, septic shock, acute viral syndrome, gastroenteritis, rubeola, staphylococcal scalded skin syndrome, and Kawasaki's disease. Kawasaki's disease, also known as *mucocutaneous lymph node syndrome*, has many clinical similarities to TSS: fever unresponsive to antimicrobial drugs, conjunctivitis, pharyngitis, strawberry tongue, fissured lips, peripheral edema, cervical lymphadenopathy, and a desquamative erythematous rash on the extremities. The major differences between TSS and Kawasaki's disease are the hypotension associated with TSS and the lymphadenopathy and indurative nature of the rash on the extremities of patients with Kawasaki's disease.

The desquamation of the palms and soles seen in the convalescent phase of TSS frequently helps confirm the diagnosis and differentiate it from other entities. Serum assays for TSST-1 are purely investigational at this point, and no sensitive or specific diagnostic test currently exists for TSS.

TOXIC SHOCKLIKE SYNDROME

Increasing numbers of reports have described patients with invasive group A streptococcal infection who present with a clinical picture indistinguishable from that of TSS. This syndrome has been called either toxic shocklike syndrome or toxic streptococcal syndrome. In contrast to TSS, most cases of toxic shocklike syndrome are associated with severe streptococcal focal infection and frequently bacteremia. Desquamation is less frequently seen.[28]

The Centers for Disease Control criteria for this diagnosis are isolation of group A streptococci, hypotension, and two of the following clinical organ dysfunctions: renal insufficiency, coagulopathy, liver dysfunction, adult respiratory distress syndrome, soft-tissue necrosis, and a generalized erythematous rash.[29]

Of the isolates from patients with toxic shocklike syndrome, M types 1 and 3 were most common and 80% produced streptococcal pyrogen toxin A. This toxin displays significant amino acid similarity to and has the same biologic properties as TSST-1 and enterotoxins B and C, the so-called superantigens. Despite intensive therapy and early use of antibiotics, a mortality rate between 20% and 35% is currently reported.[28, 30]

TREATMENT

Fundamental in the management of hypotensive, critically ill patients with TSS is optimal intensive care that includes invasive hemodynamic monitoring, excellent bedside nursing, and early aggressive management of life-threatening manifestations, specifically those related to the serious hemodynamic compromise that develops in most patients. Generally, patients with TSS have an increased cardiac index and a low pulmonary capillary wedge pressure that respond to vigorous fluid resuscitation with crystalloid solution. The volume of fluid required varies with each patient but in severe cases may be greater than 20 L administered over 24 hours.[13, 31] Crystalloid solution is preferable to colloid solution during the stage of increased capillary permeability, and it has been suggested that patients with TSS resuscitated with colloid fluids are more likely to have abnormal findings on chest radiographs than patients receiving crystalloid.[31] Generally, oliguria and azotemia are easily reversible with vigorous volume resuscitation; however, renal failure occasionally persists, and a few patients may require hemodialysis.[32]

A few hypovolemic patients who do not respond to fluid therapy develop significant myocardial dysfunction 24 to 48 hours after the onset of illness. These patients require inotropic support with a vasoactive amine. A low normal cardiac index associated with signs of hypoperfusion and end-organ failure responds to treatment with dobutamine,[25] and low-dose dopamine may also be useful to maintain renal blood flow. High-dose dopamine should be used judiciously, particularly in the absence of adequate volume resuscitation. In the more severe cases, hypoxemia progresses to adult respiratory distress syndrome, necessitating mechanical ventilation with positive end-expiratory pressure. Antimicrobial therapy with a β-lactamase–resistant antistaphylococcal drug should be instituted after culture specimens are collected from sites such as the oropharynx, rectum, vagina, wounds, catheters, and other areas. Most agents ordinarily used for treating staphylococcal infections are effective if the organism is community acquired. Some hospital-acquired staphylococci associated with toxic shock may be resistant, however, and require treatment with vancomycin.

Occasionally, other specific therapy is required to correct hypocalcemia, acid-base imbalance, adult respiratory distress syndrome, acute renal failure, myocardial dysfunction, or disseminated intravascular coagulation with thrombocytopenia. Not all cases of TSS require intensive care; mild cases, particularly recurrences, require only supportive care, modest fluid replacement, and intravenous antibiotics. In menstrual TSS, early removal of the tampon is paramount. Some studies suggest that this should be followed by an irrigating douche to remove any unabsorbed toxin from the vaginal vault.[31]

The efficacy of high-dose intravenous corticosteroids has not been proved, although retrospective evidence suggests that they may reduce the duration and severity of disease if given early.[33]

Specific recommendations to enhance the elimination, breakdown, and reversal of the toxin await further investigation into the pathogenesis of TSS.

References

1. Todd J, Fishaut M, Kapral F, et al: Toxic shock syndrome associated with phage-group-1 staphylococci. Lancet 1978; ii:1116.
2. Chesney PJ, Bergdoll MS, Davis JP, et al: The disease spectrum, epidemiology and etiology of toxic shock syndrome. Annu Rev Microbiol 1984; 38:315.
3. Shands KN, Schmid GP, Dan BB, et al: Toxic shock syndrome in menstruating women: Its association with tampon use and *Staphylococcus aureus* and the clinical features in 52 cases. N Engl J Med 1980; 303:1436.
4. Davis JP, Osterholm MT, Helms CM, et al: Tri-state toxic shock syndrome study II. Clinical and laboratory findings. J Infect Dis 1982; 145:441.
5. Soravia C, Romand J, Herrmann M, et al: Group A beta-hemolytic *Streptococcus* septicemia: The toxic strep syndrome. Intensive Care Med 1993; 19:53.

6. Tolan R: Toxic shock syndrome complicating influenza A in a child: Case report and review. Clin Infect Dis 1993; 17:43.
7. Reingold AL, Hargrett NT, Dan BB, et al: Non-menstrual toxic shock syndrome: A review of 130 cases. Ann Intern Med 1982; 96:871.
8. Schlievert PM, Osterholm MT, Kelly JA, et al. Toxin and enzyme characterization of *Staphylococcus aureus* isolates from patients with and without toxic shock syndrome. Ann Intern Med 1982; 96:937.
9. Davis JP, Vergeront JM, Chesney PJ: Possible host-defense mechanisms in toxic shock syndrome. Ann Intern Med 1982; 96:986.
10. Bergdoll MS, Crass BA, Reiser RF, et al: An enterotoxin-like protein in *Staphylococcus aureus* strains from patients with toxic shock syndrome. Ann Intern Med 1982; 96:969.
11. Schlievert PM, Shands KN, Dan BB, et al: Identification and characterization of an exotoxin from *Staphylococcus aureus* associated with toxic shock syndrome. J Infect Dis 1981; 143:509.
12. Kushnaryov VM, MacDonald HS, Reiser R, et al: Staphylococcal toxic shock toxin specifically binds to cultured human epithelial cells and is rapidly internalized. Infect Immun 1984; 45:566.
13. Fisher CJ, Horowitz BZ, Nolan SM: The clinical spectrum of toxic shock syndrome. West J Med 1982; 135:175.
14. Bartlett PC, Reingold AL, Graham DR, et al: Toxic shock syndrome associated with surgical wound infections. JAMA 1982; 147:1448.
15. Freedman JD, Beer DJ: Expanding perspectives on the toxic shock syndrome. Adv Intern Med 1991; 36:363.
16. Reiser RF, Robbin RN, Khoe GP, et al: Purification and some physiochemical properties of toxic shock toxin. Biochem 1983; 22:3907.
17. Parsonnet J, Hickman RK, Eardly DD, et al: Induction of human interleukin-1 by toxic shock syndrome toxin-1. J Infect Dis 1985; 151:514.
18. Quimby F, Nguyen HT: Animal studies of toxic shock syndrome. CRC Crit Rev Microbiol 1985; 12:1.
19. Chow AW, Bartlett KH, Percival-Smith R, et al: Vaginal colonization with *Staphylococcus aureus* positive for toxic shock marker-protein and *Escherichia coli*. Rev Infect Dis 1989; 150:80.
20. Reingold AL: Toxic shock in the USA: Epidemiology. Postgrad Med J 1985; 61:23.
21. Osterholm MT, Davis JP, Gibson RW, et al: Toxic shock syndrome; relation to catamenial products, personal health and hygiene and sexual practices. Ann Intern Med 1982; 96:954.
22. Mills JT, Parsonnet J, Isai YC, et al: Control of production of toxic shock syndrome toxin by magnesium ion. J Infect Dis 1985; 151:1158.
23. Centers for Disease Control: Toxic-shock syndrome and the vaginal contraceptive sponge. MMWR 1984; 33:43.
24. Heimburger DC: Hyperthyrocalcitoninemia in toxic shock syndrome. South Med J 1981; 74:1265.
25. Fisher CJ, Horowitz BZ, Albertson TE: Cardiorespiratory failure in toxic shock syndrome: Effect of dobutamine. Crit Care Med 1985; 13:160.
26. Burns JR, Menapace FJ: Acute reversible cardiomyopathy complicating toxic shock syndrome. Arch Intern Med 1982; 142:1032.
27. Pars AL, Hergaldt AL, Blum D, et al: Pathologic findings in twelve cases of toxic shock syndrome. Ann Intern Med 1982; 96:852.
28. Hoge CW, Schwartz B, Talkington DF, et al: The changing epidemiology of invasive group A *Streptococcus* infections and the emergence of streptococcal toxic shock-like syndrome. JAMA 1993; 269:384.
29. CDC defines group A *Streptococcus* toxic shock syndrome. Am Fam Physician 1993; 47:1643.
30. Musser JM: Clinical relevance of *Streptococcus* pyrogenic exotoxins in streptococcal toxic shock-like syndrome and other severe invasive infections. Pediatr Ann 1992; 21:823.
31. Chesney PJ, Crass BA, Polyak MB, et al: Toxic shock syndrome: Management and long-term sequelae. Ann Intern Med 1982; 96:847.
32. Chesney RW, Chesney PJ, Davis JP, et al: Renal manifestations of staphylococcal toxic shock syndrome. Am J Med 1981; 71:583.
33. Todd JK, Ressman M, Caston SA, et al: Corticosteroid therapy for patients with toxic shock syndrome. JAMA 1984; 252:3399.

CHAPTER 141

Bacterial Pneumonia in Adult Respiratory Distress Syndrome

Jacqueline J. Coalson, PhD

MAGNITUDE OF THE PROBLEM

Adult respiratory distress syndrome (ARDS) is the clinical syndrome associated with the morphologic lesion termed *diffuse alveolar damage* (DAD). DAD evolves through exudative and proliferative/reparative stages in the human lung. The histopathology of these stages is uniform, despite wide differences in the clinical cause.[1] Pneumonia is the host's inflammatory response to the uncontrolled growth of microorganisms invading the lower respiratory tract and is histologically manifested by the presence of neutrophils and other effector cells in the peripheral bronchi and alveolar spaces. Until the early 1970s, it was generally believed that patients with ARDS died with hypoxemic respiratory failure with underlying proliferative fibrotic lung lesions as a consequence of the DAD process. In 1986, however, a pathologic review of 77 postmortem examinations in a study population with ARDS documented that more than 70% of the patients had evidence of bronchopneumonia at autopsy, and in 21%, it was the only lung finding. Only nine patients had severe pulmonary fibrosis (reparative DAD).[2] In this same ARDS study population, it was shown that multiple organ failure, death, and infection were highly interrelated, the most common cause of death being multiple organ failure rather than uncorrectable hypoxemia, of which only 2 of 141 patients died.[3, 4]

Lung infection not only is a common complication and a frequent cause of death in patients with acute lung injury but is a common initiating event of ARDS. Pneumonia and aspiration accounted for nearly 37% of the 741 patients with acute respiratory failure enrolled by the multiple centers in the extracorporeal membrane oxygenation (ECMO) trial.[5] These same two categories accounted for 66% of the 90 patients selected from this larger group of patients for randomization to ECMO or control treatment. In other studies, the percentage of patients with pneumonia has varied widely, probably dependent on how the patient populations were selected by the investigators.[6, 7]

Bacterial infection in nonpulmonary sites is significantly related to the problem of adult respiratory failure and nosocomial pneumonia. The pathogenesis of sepsis with its numerous cascading mediators is not only increasingly complex, but its definition also continues to undergo refinement. The terms *sepsis*, *sepsis syndrome*, and *septic shock* represent increasing degrees of illness severity; the increasing organ dysfunction associated with each occurs as a continuous rather than discrete entity. Initiators of sepsis include endotoxin, gram-positive or yeast cell products, enterotoxin, viral or fungal antigens, and toxic shock syndrome toxin-1. Whether or not sepsis can be initiated by noninfectious factors remains controversial, but most clinicians do accept that certain patients never experience bacteremia and others lack a source of documented infection even at autopsy. The lungs in septic patients can be the recipients of a metastatic blood-borne infection from another organ, the source of a clinically silent focus of pneumonia that "feeds" the septic process,[3] or the septic process via its widespread permeability defect can simply inactivate the lungs' local defenses and allow the lungs to acquire nosocomial pneumonia via aspi-

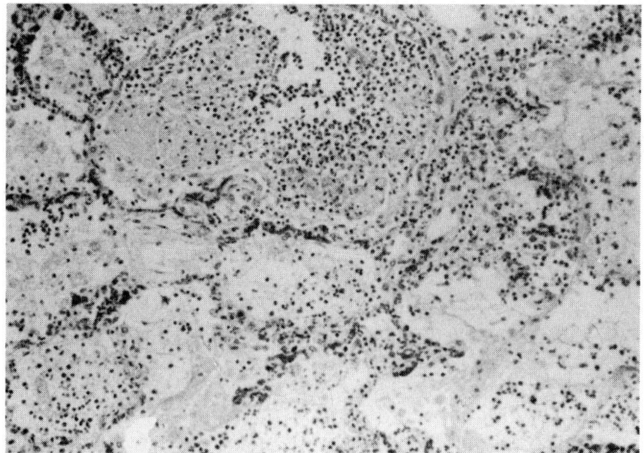

Figure 141–1. Lung specimen from a patient with documented sepsis who died 7 days after onset of ARDS. Alveolar walls are engorged with red blood cells. The alveolar spaces contain edema, fibrin strands, and numerous polymorphonuclear neutrophils (PMNs). (Hematoxylin and eosin, ×150.)

ration of oropharyngeal flora. All result in histologic evidence of pneumonia in the lungs of patients (Figs. 141–1 and 141–2).

Sepsis was thought to be the causative factor in approximately 15% of the patients with acute respiratory failure studied by the ECMO centers.[5] In surgical patients, especially after trauma, sepsis has been reported to account for as many as 90% of fatal cases of ARDS, clearly documenting that it is the most common cause of severe and ultimately fatal lung injury.[8] It is now clear that nosocomial pneumonia in patients with ARDS is frequently characterized by the sepsis syndrome and accompanied by multiple organ failure.[9, 10] The link between the systemic response induced by sepsis and multiple organ failure is no doubt complex, but tumor necrosis factor and interleukin-1 are important mediators along with activated neutrophils, complement, and various components of the coagulation system. Therefore, bacterial infection, either of the lung itself or sepsis originating at nonpulmonary sites, is the major contributor to the poor prognosis in patients with ARDS. Excellent reviews of the interrelationships between infection, sepsis, and multiple organ failure detail current knowledge.[11–13]

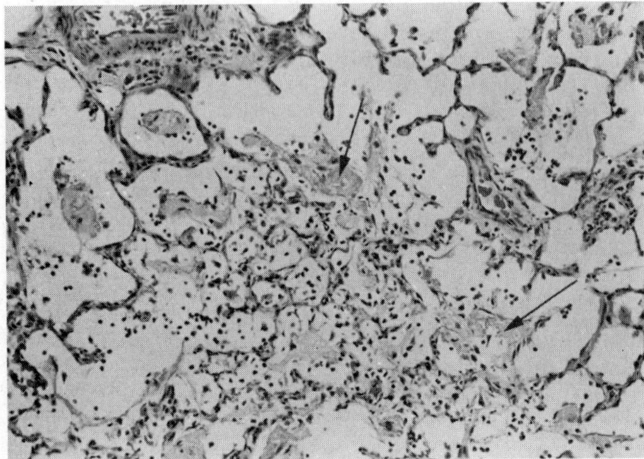

Figure 141–2. Baboon lung exposed to 80% oxygen for 11 days. Fibrin aggregates *(arrows)*, the result of exudative DAD, are intermixed with an "alveolitis" of alveolar macrophages and fewer PMNs. This is the most severe lesion manifested in this model. (Hematoxylin and eosin, ×150.)

The events that allow us to understand how pulmonary infection is manifested in a patient with ARDS mandate an understanding of the normal defense mechanisms in the lungs and how their disruption can result in patients' increased vulnerability to infection in the intensive care unit (ICU).

NORMAL DEFENSE MECHANISMS IN THE RESPIRATORY TRACT

The lungs can be challenged via the bloodstream and airway and, more rarely, by contiguous spread of infection. The filtration of potential injurants by the upper and lower respiratory tract is quite extraordinary (Table 141–1). The mucociliary apparatus, along with the important gag and cough reflexes, has a pivotal role in removing inhaled microbes. The lungs complement these defense mechanisms with several immunoglobulins, IgA at the airway level and IgG at the alveolar level, and other secretions including lysozyme, lactoferrin, surfactant, and fibronectin. The interrelated activities of these factors allow for entrapment and neutralization of microbes and their subsequent removal on the mucociliary blanket. Bronchus-associated lymphoid tissue and lymphocytes add needed immunologically competent cells. At the alveolar level, the alveolar macrophages function effectively in a normal host to remove those microbes smaller than 0.2 μm, which may bypass all of the airway physical and mechanical barriers in the airways. Alveolar macrophages, through various mediators (e.g., lymphokines, tumor necrosis factor, interleukin-1), also have an important role in recruiting inflammatory cells, a systemic response that enhances microbicidal activity. Bacterial adherence (binding of bacteria) to epithelial cells and interbacterial inhibition (receptor sites occupied by gram positives in normalcy) prevent colonization of the oropharynx and tracheobronchial tree with gram-negative organisms, an important but incompletely understood defense mechanism.

COLONIZATION OF THE RESPIRATORY TRACT

Nosocomial bacterial pneumonias develop in hospitalized patients and are due to a shift of flora that can be documented when patients become progressively sicker.[14] The endogenous microflora in the oropharynx of a healthy individual usually consists of nonpathogenic, gram-positive (*Streptococcus salivarius*, lactobacilli), and anaerobic bacteria.

TABLE 141–1. Defense Mechanisms of the Respiratory System

Normal oropharyngeal bacterial flora
Aerodynamic filtration
Airway reflexes
Cough
Gag
Bronchoconstriction
Mucociliary escalator
Oropharyngeal and airway secretions: saliva, mucus
Lactoferrin
Complement
Surfactant
Fibronectin
Alpha-antitrypsin
Lysozyme
Immunoglobulins A and G
Bronchus-associated lymphoid tissue lymphocytes
Alveolar macrophages

Colonization of the oropharynx in healthy individuals with gram-negative bacilli is very uncommon, occurring in only 1% to 6% of subjects. The same low incidence of gram-negative bacilli colonization is found among personnel caring for patients in ICUs. Colonization of the upper respiratory tract by gram-negative bacilli is mediated by alterations in the surface properties of the epithelial cells.[15, 16] Experimentally, it is known that after exposure to malnutrition, general surgery, or renal dysfunction, buccal cell adherence increases serially, probably as a result of an elaboration of proteases.[15, 17] The proteases remove the fibronectin on cell surfaces, then allowing adherence of gram-negative organisms.[17] The organisms most likely to spread during infections have specialized surfaces that enable them to adhere to cell surfaces (e.g., pili, fibrillae, lipotichoic acid, and so on). The risk factors responsible for oropharyngeal colonization with gram-negative bacilli include neutropenia, prior antibiotic therapy, alcoholism, azotemia, coma, diabetes, serious illness, hypotension, intubation, smoking, surgery, and neutralization of gastric acid.[15, 16]

In a prospective study of patients hospitalized in a medical ICU, Johanson and coworkers demonstrated that in those who developed nosocomial pneumonia, 85% had preceding gram-negative bacilli cultured from the oropharynx.[18] Critically ill patients also can exhibit colonization of the tracheobronchial tree. Tillotson and Finland examined 149 antibiotic-treated patients with primary pneumonia and found that 59% of these patients developed lower airway colonization with pathogenic bacteria (e.g., *Staphylococcus aureus, Klebsiella pneumoniae, Escherichia coli, Haemophilus influenzae, Pseudomonas aeruginosa,* and others).[19] In 48 patients treated with mechanical ventilation and endotracheal intubation, Schwartz and colleagues determined that by day 8 of illness, more than two thirds of the patients had gram-negative bacilli in their tracheal aspirates.[20] Niederman and associates examined patients with tracheostomies and showed that about half of the study group developed persistent colonization of the lower airways. In these colonized subjects, pneumonia occurred at a threefold greater frequency.[21] Although some of the non-Enterobacteriaceae *(Pseudomonas* and *Acinetobacter)* may be from an exogenous environmental source, the gram-negative bacilli that colonize the oropharynx and tracheobronchial tree of patients with ARDS are usually not acquired from an environmental source but are acquisitions from the gram-negative organisms that reside in a patient's gastrointestinal tract or are acquired from another patient's bacterial flora. These organisms are transmitted from patient to patient on the hands of personnel.[13]

TABLE 141–2. Pathogenetic Steps in Nosocomial Pneumonia Due to Gram-Negative Bacilli

Onset of Predisposing Factor(s)
Serious illness, surgery, antibiotics, etc., initiate proteases
Colonization (acquisition)
Adherence properties of the oropharyngeal and tracheobronchial airway epithelium are altered; gram-negative bacilli acquired.
Entry into Lungs
Aspiration of colonized upper-airway secretions or neutralized gastric secretions occurs.
Interaction with Defense Mechanisms
The host's inadequate local and systemic defenses allow bacterial multiplication.
Formation of Pneumonitic Inflammatory Exudate
Edema, inflammatory cell infiltrates, and bacterial products collect in airspaces.
Egress from Lungs
Spread can occur via the lymphatics and/or bloodstream.

PATHOGENESIS OF PNEUMONIA

The mechanisms by which secretions of the upper airway contaminate the lower respiratory tract via the airway depend on the route of delivery of microbe(s), and the status of the host's local and systemic defenses (Table 141–2). The manner by which bacteria are presented to the lungs is a primary determinant of whether or not infection will develop. Berendt showed in the squirrel monkey that the deposition of 10^7 *K. pneumoniae* in an aerosol failed to produce pneumonia, whereas 10^4 organisms, if delivered as a fluid bolus into the trachea, did produce pneumonia.[22] In humans, infection by inhalation of microbes probably occurs only in a few particular instances, such as in infection with *Legionella* organisms.

The probability of producing pneumonia using a bolus delivery is enhanced by an increase in either the number of bacteria instilled or the volume of the inoculum. If a bolus is delivered in a mucin suspension and is not removed, multiplication with persistence of bacteria occurs in the distal portion of lung and results in edema, inflammation, and accumulation of bacterial products. Experimentally, in normal animals, 10^7 and greater bacterial concentrations delivered as a bolus routinely induce pneumonia and can cause death of the animal.[23–25] However, patients with ARDS invariably have underlying lung lesions of DAD and may be injured by aspirated secretions containing smaller quantities of microbes.

Experimental settings that more closely mimic compromised patients in an ICU environment have been developed to assess how infection augments lung injury. Johanson and colleagues examined the effects of bacterial superinfection on injured hamster lungs pretreated with 100% oxygen. Inocula of both 10^3 and 10^6 organisms elicited pneumonias.[26] In an oleic acid–induced lung injury model in the baboon, animals that sustained a superimposed pneumonia and bacteremia had a precipitous clinical course when compared with baboons treated with oleic acid only.[27] Likewise, lung injury induced by 80% oxygen produces a mild DAD lesion in baboons during an 11-day period. However, if infection is induced by an intrabronchial inoculation of *P. aeruginosa* organisms on day 6, the animals sustain a severe lung injury, clearly documenting the detrimental effect of infection on a predamaged lung[28] (Fig. 141–3; see also Fig. 141–2).

Microaspiration of bacteria from a colonized oropharynx or tracheobronchial tree is the primary route of acquisition of microbes into the lung. Organisms that colonize the upper respiratory tract may be abundantly present in secretions. Concentrations of organisms in the oropharyngeal secretions may be as high as 10^8/mL,[13] so that aspiration of even small quantities of oropharyngeal secretions is sufficient to introduce a massive bacterial inoculum into the lungs. Aspiration of oropharyngeal secretions occurs in at least 45% of healthy individuals during sleep and in nearly all patients with impaired levels of consciousness.[29] Cuffed endotracheal tubes do not protect against aspiration of small volumes of secretions from the oropharynx because of the milking of small quantities around the endotracheal cuff during cycles of the respirator.[20] The endotracheal tube can also serve as a conduit of microbes from healthcare givers and equipment used in respiratory therapy. In fact, the risk of pneumonia is 6 to 21 times greater in intubated patients than in other hospitalized patients.[30] Finally, retrograde migration to the oropharynx from a stomach colonized with microbes can occur, after which aspiration into the lungs can result.[31–33] Acid-neutralizing therapy with antacids and

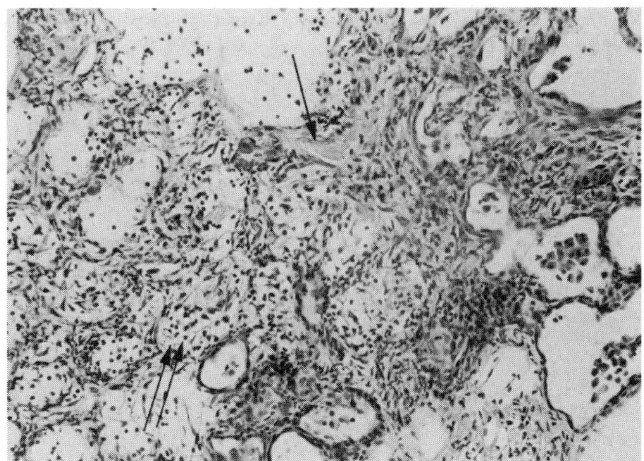

Figure 141–3. Baboon lung exposed to 80% oxygen for 6 days, followed by intrabronchial instillation of *Pseudomonas* organisms. A residual fibrin aggregate is identified *(arrow)*, but the alveoli are filled with organizing fibrous connective tissue *(double arrow)* that is infiltrated with both PMNs and mononuclear cells. (Hematoxylin and eosin, ×150.)

H_2 blockers allows gastric pH to rise, permitting gram-negative organisms in the stomach to increase exponentially.

Only certain patients with ARDS go on to develop pneumonia; it is assumed that their antibacterial defense mechanisms are impaired. The presence of endotracheal tubes that markedly reduce mucociliary transport and the presence of pulmonary edema and alveolar hypoxia that impair the bactericidal capacity of the lungs are among suggested mechanisms. Edema fluid can interfere with the bactericidal function of alveolar macrophages and the antibacterial function of surfactant by reducing its quantity and changing its functional characteristics.[34, 35] The interaction of bacilli with the alveolar macrophages and polymorphonuclear neutrophils (PMNs) within the alveolar space has been studied by a number of investigators.[13] Deposition of 10^9 organisms by aerosolization results in a rapid clearance and no infection with *S. aureus* and other gram-positive organisms.[36] Low-virulence organisms, such as those found in normal oropharyngeal flora, do not require PMNs or circulating antibody. However, inhalation of gram-negative bacilli is associated with a longer clearance time and a rapid recruitment of PMNs in distal airways.[37] Neutropenia is associated with a more impaired clearance of gram-negative bacilli than macrophage depletion.[38]

Nosocomial pneumonias in patients with ARDS are usually polymicrobial, because the organisms are selected from a larger group of colonizing pathogens in the tracheobronchial and oropharyngeal secretions.[4, 39] Why only certain organisms subsequently elicit pneumonia is not well understood. Enteric gram-negative bacilli are the predominant pathogens in patients with ARDS. Gram-negatives were found in 75% of the cases in Fagon and colleagues' study and in 56% of patients in Seidenfeld and associates' study, and in both, the most common gram-negative pathogen was *P. aeruginosa*.[4, 39] The specific risk factors identified with the causation of *P. aeruginosa*-induced pneumonia in patients with ARDS are leukopenia, corticosteroid therapy, intravascular monitoring devices, and respiratory therapy equipment.[15] Gram-positive isolates accounted for 52% and 32%, respectively, of the bacteria cultured from the patients in these two studies.

Calibration of the histologic findings of pneumonia with quantitative bacterial cultures of the lung has been experimentally carried out. In baboons and hamsters with either normal lungs or lungs damaged by oleic acid or oxygen, a correlation was found between the appearance of histologic pneumonia and greater than 10^4 colony-forming units (CFU) per gram of lung tissue.[26, 40] Lungs demonstrating fewer bacteria did not contain characteristic histologic foci of infection. In a patient study, bacterial infections of the lung that had been manifested clinically also contained at least 10^4 cfu/g of tissue.[41] The presence of more than 10^5 CFU/mL of exudate has been used by Bartlett to document the presence of lung pneumonia.[42]

CLINICAL ASPECTS OF PNEUMONIA

Among all the patients admitted to hospitals, infections of the respiratory tract represent one of the most common nosocomial infections, along with urinary tract and surgical wound infections.[43] The risk of respiratory tract infection, however, varies among different patient groups. Johanson and coworkers determined that the risk of nosocomial pneumonia in 213 patients admitted to medical ICUs was approximately 12%, including 24% of patients with acute respiratory failure.[18] More recently, Fagon and colleagues documented that the risk of infection increases with the duration of mechanical ventilation. In 567 patients treated with mechanical ventilation, the overall rate of infection was 9%, but the risk was 6.5% after 10 days, 19% after 20 days, and 28% after 30 days of ventilation.[39] Extensive data that define the risk or frequency of nosocomial pneumonia in specific patient populations such as ARDS are lacking, but several studies have come from various populations including medical/surgical, surgical, medical, or respiratory ICU populations. Only a few of these studies, however, have distinguished between pneumonia as a cause of ARDS and pneumonia that arises as a complication of ARDS. In 1975, Fulton and Jones observed that 45% of their patients had primary pneumonia and 50% had nosocomial pneumonias.[44] In Seidenfeld and associates' study, 21% of the patients had pneumonia that initiated ARDS and 53% had pneumonia as a complication during their hospital course.[4] Pneumonia was the cause in 33% and a complication in 34% of 583 patients with ARDS enrolled in the European collaborative study.[45]

The time criterion that has been used to separate community-acquired pneumonia from nosocomial pneumonia has been inadequately defined historically. Johanson and coworkers found that 50% of patients required at least 4 days of mechanical ventilation before colonization occurred.[18] Others have used 48 hours, 4 days, or no definite period.[46–48] Pneumonia developing within 4 days of ventilation has been designated as early onset and that after 4 days as late onset.[49] This definition has been reaffirmed by the European survey, in which 50% of pneumonias started before day 4. Langer and colleagues suggest that early-onset pneumonias most likely are secondary to aspiration whereas those after 4 days have a different pathogenesis.[49]

However, estimates of the frequency of lower respiratory tract infection in patients with ARDS are questionable because of inadequacy of current diagnostic techniques. The usual clinical criteria for diagnosis of nosocomial pneumonia include fever, leukocytosis, and purulent tracheobronchial secretions. However, each of these criteria is commonly encountered whether or not bacterial infection is present in patients with ARDS. This problem is further complicated by the fact that nearly all patients with acute respiratory failure have colonization of the respiratory tract with pathogenic organisms, usually gram-negative bacilli, so that the presence of these organisms in Gram's stains or cultures of respiratory tract secretions cannot be a reliable guide to the presence or absence of infection.

When Andrews and associates examined the accuracy of these criteria in an overall assessment in the diagnosis of nosocomial pneumonia among 30 patients who died with acute respiratory failure, the presence or the absence of bacterial pneumonia was misdiagnosed in 30% of the cases.[50] Pneumonias in the study were definitively diagnosed for purposes of comparison at autopsy by examining multiple sections of the lungs of patients who died with acute respiratory failure. Histologic pneumonias were diagnosed by the presence of an intense PMN inflammatory exudate that centers on terminal or respiratory bronchioles and extends into subjacent and surrounding alveoli. Of the 58% of patients with histologically diagnosed pneumonia, one third were judged clinically not to have pneumonia. Of the 42% without histologically proven pneumonia, one fifth were judged to have clinical evidence of pneumonia. Chastre and coworkers[51] also found that nosocomial pneumonias are underdiagnosed clinically when compared with histologic findings at autopsy.

Other investigators have since offered criteria to allow a definite diagnosis of pneumonia to be made clinically.[52] Salata and coworkers diagnose nosocomial pneumonia when a new or progressive pulmonary infiltrate develops with (1) positive pleural fluid or blood cultures for the same organism as in a tracheal aspirate, (2) radiographic cavitation, (3) histopathologic demonstration of pneumonia or necrosis, or (4) new fever, leukocytosis, and purulent tracheal aspirate.[53] Chastre and colleagues' criteria for pneumonia include (1) a positive pleural culture, (2) rapid cavitation of lung infiltrates, and (3) histopathologic demonstration of pneumonia.[51] Pham and associates diagnose nosocomial pneumonia if one of four criteria are present: (1) positive blood cultures unrelated to another source and obtained within 48 hours before or after bronchial sampling; (2) positive culture of empyema fluid; (3) computed tomography evidence of pulmonary abscess; or (4) pathologic evidence of pneumonia in postmortem study, within 3 days after sampling, that demonstrates abscess inflammation or areas of consolidation with intense PMN accumulations.[54] Meduri and colleagues' criteria include details that document the histologic presence of pnuemonia, clinical evidence, and growth of pathogen(s) in culture.[48] Most investigators advocate the usefulness of examining the cells from bronchoalveolar lavage (BAL) specimens microscopically for intracellular organisms. If more than 25% of the alveolar macrophages contain organisms, pneumonia is usually present.[48, 55]

The use of a protected specimen brush (PSB) and BAL to improve the diagnostic threshold has been attempted by several investigators. Using 10^3 CFU/mL as a breakpoint to define a positive PSB culture has proved useful in animal and human studies.[40, 48, 56] The PSB specimen, which samples as little as 0.001 mL of lung secretions, is diluted in 1 mL of holding medium for processing, and a growth of 10^3 CFU/mL represents 10^5 to 10^6 bacteria per milliliter. When properly used, the PSB specimen collects respiratory secretions with a minimum degree of contamination. The diagnostic thresholds of BAL range from 10^3 CFU/mL to 10^5 CFU/mL, so a colony count of 10^4 CFU/mL in a BAL specimen, considering a dilution factor of 10 to 100, represents 10^5 to 10^6 bacteria per milliliter.[46, 51] This technique is plagued by the problem of contamination with upper airway bacteria even in patients without pneumonia, and in 30% of patients, contaminants are found in high concentration.[46, 51] However, BAL recovers at least 5 to 10 times more organisms than are retrieved by PSB. Autopsy studies have shown that nosocomial pneumonia involves predominantly the posterior portions of the lower lobes but that the pneumonias are frequently disseminated into each lobe.[40, 57] Clinical studies supporting this observation have varied, however; several have reported sterility of different sample sites in lungs,[58, 59] whereas others have shown close correlation between culture samples when obtained from different lobes.[54, 60] The influence of antibiotic therapy on BAL and PSB samples is considerable, and efforts to obtain bronchoscopic specimens before starting antibiotic therapy are strongly recommended.

Meduri reviewed the diagnostic value of PSB and BAL in diagnosing pneumonia in ventilated patients.[61] Quantitative cultures of the PSB had an overall sensitivity and specificity between 70% and 90%. The combined clinical results of three studies that used quantitative cultures of BAL to diagnose pneumonias in ventilated patients show an overall sensitivity of 77% and a specificity of 69%, with a false-positive rate of 30% in patients without pneumonia. The protected BAL procedure has been used in 46 patients, 25 of whom were ventilated. Protected BAL quantitative cultures had a sensitivity and positive predictive value of 97% and a specificity and negative predictive value of 92%.[48] Gram's staining of cytocentrifuged BAL specimens is helpful in identifying the causative organism(s); intracellular organisms in 7% or more of the recovered alveolar cells identify 80% of patients as having pneumonia and only 4% of patients as not having pneumonia. With the use of these clinical modalities to diagnose pneumonia, several investigators in prospective studies have shown that quantitative cultures of either PSB or BAL specimens occur less frequently than is clinically suspected.[48, 56]

OUTCOME

The mortality rate of nosocomial pneumonia has been reported to be between 55% and 75% in mechanically ventilated patients.[10, 30, 32, 62] In ARDS study populations, the presence of infection of any source has been associated with a poor outcome and with multiple organ failure. Seidenfeld and colleagues demonstrated a survival rate of 67% in patients with no infection versus 21% when infection of any type was present. The mortality rate was 88% when pneumonia complicated ARDS in this study series.[4] In the ARDS patient population of Montgomery and coworkers, late deaths usually resulted from a hospital-acquired sepsis syndrome arising from the lungs and leading to multiple organ failure, whereas early deaths (before 72 hours) were most often due to a patient's underlying disease.[9]

Investigators have found that the mortality of nosocomial pneumonias of various causes differs. For example, Fagon and coworkers showed that the mortality of *Pseudomonas*, and *Acinetobacter* and *S. aureus* was greater than that of other types of gram-negative pneumonias.[39] Prior antibiotic therapy was more common in patients who developed *P. aeruginosa* and *Acinetobacter* species than other gram-negative pneumonias.[39] Celis and coworkers showed a higher mortality rate in a group of patients with gram-negative pneumonias due to high-risk causes than in patients with gram-negative pneumonias due to other causes.[30]

Treatment protocols for antibiotic coverage of patients with ARDS are beyond the scope of this chapter. In general, regimens that provide coverage for enteric gram-negative bacilli (i.e., *P. aeruginosa*, *Klebsiella* species, and *E. coli*) and against *S. aureus* should be selected for patients with ARDS and pneumonia, and vancomycin is administered if methicillin resistance is present. The European experience of selective digestive decontamination has successfully reduced the incidence of pneumonia, but the mortality rates due to multiple organ failure have not been altered. In baboon models of ARDS, Johanson and colleagues prevented pneumonia with the use of topical respiratory antibiotics.[40] The use of intravenous penicillin, along with topical polymyxin B, gentamicin, or both, reduced the severity of histologic pneumonia, and the bacterial loads (characterized by a bacterial index) were reduced. Concern remains, however, that the use of these approaches on a widespread basis might cause emergence of antibiotic-resistant strains in the ICU environment.

Niederman presents an excellent review on strategies for the prevention of pneumonia.[63] Future studies must address means to reduce bacterial adherence of gram-negative bacilli to airway cells. Development of antibodies against gram-negative bacteria would be helpful to use in patients who develop pneumonias. An important advance that would make a major impact on the emergence of the sepsis syndrome would be a means to enhance the integrity and intactness of the intestinal mucosa to prevent translocation of bacteria or bacterial products from the intestine. Anti-inflammatory agents are necessary to prevent the systemic infection from leading to multiple organ failure. Because of the complexity of the various clinical situations that can predispose patients to the development of nosocomial pneumonia, a multipronged approach undoubtedly must be developed for successful treatment of ARDS in the ICU setting.

References

1. Katzenstein AA, Askin FB: Surgical pathology of non-neoplastic lung disease. *In*: Major Problems in Pathology. 2nd ed. Bennington JL (Ed). Vol 13. Philadelphia, WB Saunders, 1990, pp 9–57.
2. Coalson JJ: Pathology of sepsis, septic shock and multiple organ failure. *In*: New Horizons: Perspectives on Sepsis and Septic Shock. Sibbald WJ, Sprung CL (Eds). Fullerton, CA, Society of Critical Care Medicine, 1986, pp 27–59.
3. Bell BC, Coalson JJ, Smith JD, et al: Multiple organ failure and infection in adult respiratory distress syndrome. Ann Intern Med 1983; 99:293.
4. Seidenfeld JJ, Pohl DF, Bell RD, et al: Incidence, site, and outcome of infections in patients with the adult respiratory distress syndrome. Am Rev Respir Dis 1986; 134:12.
5. Extracorporeal support for respiratory insufficiency: Collaborative study (December, 1979). National Heart, Lung, and Blood Institute, US Dept of Health, Education, and Welfare, Public Health Division, 1979.
6. Baumann WR, Jung RC, Koss M, et al: Incidence and mortality of adult respiratory distress syndrome: A prospective analysis from a large metropolitan hospital. Crit Care Med 1986; 14:1.
7. Fowler AA, Hamman RF, Good JT, et al: Adult respiratory distress syndrome: Risk with common predispositions. Ann Intern Med 1983; 98:593.
8. Walker L, Eiseman B: The changing pattern of post-traumatic respiratory distress syndrome. Ann Surg 1975; 181:693.
9. Montgomery AB, Stager MA, Carrico C, et al: Causes of mortality in patients with the adult respiratory distress syndrome. Am Rev Respir Dis 1985; 132:485.
10. Craven DE, Kunches LM, Kilinsky V, et al: Risk factors for pneumonia and fatality in patients receiving continuous mechanical ventilation. Am Rev Respir Dis 1986; 133:792.
11. Niederman MS, Fein AM: The interaction of infection and the adult respiratory distress syndrome. Crit Care Clin 1986; 2:471.
12. Niederman MS, Fein AM: Sepsis syndrome, the adult respiratory distress syndrome, and nosocomial pneumonia: A common clinical sequence. Clin Chest Med 1990; 11:633.
13. Johanson WG Jr: Bacterial infection in ARDS: Pathogenetic mechanisms and consequences. *In*: Textbook of Critical Care. 2nd ed. Shoemaker WC, Ayres S, Grenvik A (Eds). Philadelphia, WB Saunders, 1989, pp 845–853.
14. Johanson WG, Pierce AK, Sanford TP: Changing pharyngeal flora of hospitalized patients: Emergence of gram-negative bacilli. N Engl J Med 1969; 281:1137.
15. Higuchi JH, Johanson WG: The relationship between adherence of *Pseudomonas aeruginosa* to upper respiratory cells in vitro and susceptibility to colonization in vivo. J Lab Clin Med 1980; 95:698.
16. Palmer LB: Bacterial colonization: Pathogenesis and clinical significance. Clin Chest Med 1987; 8:455.
17. Woods DE, Straus DC, Johanson WG, et al: Role of salivary protease activity in adherence of gram-negative bacilli to mammalian buccal epithelial cells in vivo. J Clin Invest 1981; 68:1435.
18. Johanson WG Jr, Pierce AK, Sanford JP, et al: Nosocomial respiratory infections with gram-negative bacilli: The significance of colonization of the respiratory tract. Ann Intern Med 1972; 77:701.
19. Tillotson JR, Finland M: Bacterial colonization and clinical superinfection of the respiratory tract complicating antibiotic treatment of pneumonia. J Infect Dis 1969; 119:597.
20. Schwartz DB, Olson DE, Kauffman CA: Influence of aspiration on tracheal colonization following endotracheal intubation. Am Rev Respir Dis 1984; 129:A182.
21. Niederman MS, Ferranti RD, Ziegler A, et al: Respiratory infection complicating long-term tracheostomy: The implication of persistent gram-negative tracheobronchial colonization. Chest 1984; 85:39.
22. Berendt RF: Relationship of method of administration to respiratory virulence of *Klebsiella pneumoniae* for mice and squirrel monkeys. Infect Immun 1978; 20:581.
23. Ansfield MJ, Woods DE, Johanson WG Jr: Lung bacterial clearance in murine pneumococcal pneumonia. Infect Immun 1977; 17:195.
24. Toews GB, Gross GN, Pierce AK: The relationship or inoculum size to lung bacterial adherence and phagocytic cell response in mice. Am Rev Respir Dis 1979; 120:559.
25. Onofrio JM, Toews GB, Lipscomb MF, et al: Granulocyte-alveolar macrophage interaction in the pulmonary clearance of *Staphylococcus aureus*. Am Rev Respir Dis 1983; 127:335.
26. Johanson WG Jr, Higuchi JH, Woods DE, et al: Dissemination of *Pseudomonas aeruginosa* during lung infection: Role of oxygen-induced lung injury. Am Rev Respir Dis 1985; 132:358.
27. Campbell DG, Coalson JJ, Johanson WG Jr: The effect of bacterial superinfection on lung function after diffuse alveolar damage. Am Rev Respir Dis 1984; 129:974.
28. Coalson JJ, King RJ, Winter VT, et al: Oxygen and pneumonia-induced lung injury. I. Pathological and morphometric studies. J Appl Physiol 1989; 67:346.
29. Huxley EJ, Viroslav J, Gray WR, et al: Pharyneal aspiration in normal subjects and patients with depressed consciousness. Am J Med 1978; 64:564.
30. Celis R, Torres A, Gatell J, et al: Nosocomial pneumonia: A multivariable analysis of risk and prognosis. Chest 1988; 93:318.
31. Atherton ST, White DJ: Stomach as source of bacteria colonising respiratory tract during artificial ventilation. Lancet 1978; 2:968.
32. DuMoulin GC, Hedley-Whyte J, Paterson DG, et al: Aspiration of gastric bacteria in antacid-treated patients: A frequent cause of postoperative colonization of the airway. Lancet 1982; 1:242.
33. Pingleton SK, Hinthorn DR, Liu C: Enteral nutrition in patients receiving mechanical ventilation: Multiple sources of tracheal colonization include the stomach. Am J Med 1986; 80:827.
34. Juers J, Rogers RM, McCurdy JB: Enhancement of bactericidal capacity of alveolar macrophages by human "alveolar lining material." Clin Res 1975; 23:348.
35. LaForce FM: Effects of alveolar lining material on phagocytic and bacterial activity of lung macrophages against *Staphylococcus aureus*. J Lab Clin Med 1976; 88:691.
36. Huber GL, LaForce FM, Johanson WG Jr: Experimental models in pulmonary antimicrobial defenses. *In*: Respiratory Defense Mechanisms. Brain JD, Proctor DF, Reid L (Eds). New York, Marcel Dekker, 1977, pp 983–1022.
37. Pierce AK, Reynolds RC, Harris GD: Leukocytic response to inhaled bacteria. Am Rev Respir Dis 1977; 116:679.
38. Rehm SR, Gross GN, Pierce AK: Early bacterial clearance from murine lungs. Species-dependent phagocyte response. J Clin Invest 1980; 66:194.
39. Fagon JY, Chastre J, Domart Y, et al: Nosocomial pneumonia in patients receiving continuous mechanical ventilation: Prospec-

tive analysis of 52 episodes with use of a protected specimen brush and quantitative culture techniques. Am Rev Respir Dis 1989; 139:877.
40. Johanson WG Jr, Seidenfeld JJ, Gomez P, et al: Bacteriologic diagnosis of nosocomial pneumonia following prolonged mechanical ventilation. Am Rev Respir Dis 1988; 137:259.
41. Chastre J, Viau F, Brun P, et al. Prospective evaluation of the protected specimen brush for the diagnosis of pulmonary infections in ventilated patients. Am Rev Respir Dis 1984; 130:924.
42. Bartlett JG: Invasive diagnostic techniques in pulmonary infections. *In*: Respiratory Infections: Diagnosis and Management. 2nd ed. Pennington JE (Ed). New York, Raven Press, 1989, pp 52–68.
43. Centers for Disease Control: National nosocomial infections study report: Annual summary, 1984. MMWR 1986; 35:17S–29S.
44. Fulton RL, Jones CE: The cause of post-traumatic respiratory insufficiency in man. Surg Gynecol Obstet 1975; 140:179.
45. Carlet J, Hemmer M, Flandre P, et al: Infection and ARDS: A complex interaction: A prospective study of 583 patients. Am Rev Respir Dis 1989; 139:A270.
46. Torres A, De La Bellacasa JP, Xaubet A, et al: Diagnostic value of quantitative cultures of broncho-alveolar lavage and telescoping plugged catheters in mechanically ventilated patients with bacterial pneumonia. Am Rev Respir Dis 1989; 140:306.
47. Rodriguez De Castro F, Violan JS, Capuz BL, et al: Reliability of the bronchoscopic protected specimen brush in the diagnosis of pneumonia in mechanically ventilated patients. Crit Care Med 1991; 19:171.
48. Meduri GU, Beals D, Maijub G, et al: Protected bronchoalveolar lavage: A new bronchoscopic technique to retrieve uncontaminated distal airway secretions. Am Rev Respir Dis 1991; 143:855.
49. Langer M, Cigada M, Mandelli M, et al: Early onset pneumonia: A multicenter study in intensive care units. Intensive Care Med 1987; 13:342.
50. Andrews CP, Coalson JJ, Smith JD, et al: Diagnosis of nosocomial bacterial pneumonia in acute, diffuse lung injury. Chest 1981; 80:254.
51. Chastre J, Fagon JT, Soler P, et al: Diagnosis of nosocomial bacterial pneumonia in intubated patients undergoing ventilation: Comparison of the usefulness of bronchoalveolar lavage and the protected specimen brush. Am J Med 1988; 85:499.
52. Pingleton SK, Fagon JV, Leeper KV: Patient selection for clinical investigation of ventilator-associated pneumonia: Criteria for evaluating diagnostic techniques. Chest 1992; 102(Suppl 1):553S.
53. Salata RA, Lederman MM, Shales DM, et al: Diagnosis of nosocomial pneumonia in intubated, intensive care unit patients. Am Rev Respir Dis 1987; 135:426.
54. Pham LH, Brun-Buissson C, Legrand P, et al: Diagnosis of nosocomial pneumonia in mechanically ventilated patients: Comparison of a plugged telescoping catheter with the protected specimen brush. Am Rev Respir Dis 1991; 143:1055.
55. Chastre J, Fagon JY, Soler P, et al: Quantification of BAL cells containing intracellular bacteria rapidly identifies ventilated patients with nosocomial pneumonia. Chest 1989; 95:190S.
56. Fagon JY, Chastre J, Hance AJ, et al: Detection of nosocomial lung infection in ventilated patients: Use of a protected specimen brush and quantitative culture techniques in 147 patients. Am Rev Respir Dis 1988; 138:110.
57. Rouby JJ, Martin de Lassale E, Poete P, et al: Nosocomial bronchopneumonia in the critically ill: Histologic and bacteriologic aspects. Am Rev Respir Dis 1992; 146:1059.
58. Baughman RP, Thorpe JE, Staneck J, et al: Use of the protected specimen brush in patients with endotracheal or tracheostomy tubes. Chest 1987; 91:233.
59. Belenchia JM, Wunderink RG, Meduri GU, et al: Alternative causes of fever in ARDS patients suspected of having pneumonia. Am Rev Respir Dis 1991; 143:A683.
60. Pugin J, Auckenthaler R, Mili N, et al: Diagnosis of ventilator-associated pneumonia by bacteriologic analysis of bronchoscopic and nonbronchoscopic blind bronchoalveolar lavage fluid. Am Rev Respir Dis 1991; 143:1121.
61. Meduri GU: Ventilator-associated pneumonia in patients with respiratory failure. A diagnostic approach. Chest 1990; 97:1208.
62. Stevens RM, Teres D, Skillman JJ, et al: Pneumonia in an intensive care unit: A thirty-month experience. Arch Intern Med 1974; 134:106.
63. Niederman MS: Strategies for the prevention of pneumonia. Clin Chest Med 1987; 8:543.

CHAPTER 142A

Intra-Abdominal Sepsis

John M. Kellum, MD, FACS

HISTORICAL PERSPECTIVE

Postoperative or post-traumatic infection has supplanted hemorrhage as the leading cause of death in general surgical services. It has been estimated that the average cost of managing a postoperative infection in 1992 was $28,000, whereas that of an average intensive care unit stay for the treatment of infection complicated by organ system failure was $150,000.[1]

19th Century War Surgery

The history of surgical infection is really the history of war surgery. During the American Civil War, a gunshot wound to an extremity was tantamount to an amputation or to death from gas gangrene; a gunshot wound to the abdomen was almost uniformly fatal. Surgeons were not generally prepared to undertake celiotomy under such circumstances. Although Joseph Lister had described his antiseptic technique in the 1860s,[2] it was not widely accepted at military field hospitals of the day and, in fact, remained controversial well into the 1880s.[3]

20th Century War Surgery

In the 1880s, Billroth founded his famous surgical school in Vienna and demonstrated that gastrectomy was feasible using Lister's technique. However, at the time of World War I, the military war wound was still associated with an extremely high rate of fatal infection. On the Western Front alone, it was estimated that 50,000 German soldiers died from gas gangrene.[4]

Before World War I, Landsteiner had described the elements of the ABO blood type system.[5] However, during this war, surgeons had poor supplies of blood for transfusion and were ignorant of the volumes of blood needed to combat hemorrhagic shock. Alfred Blalock,[6] working at the Vanderbilt School of Medicine's surgical research laboratories in the 1930s, did pioneering work in the understanding of shock and blood replacement. Thus, by World War II, a much improved management of hemorrhagic problems prevailed; yet, the prevention and treatment of sepsis remained relatively primitive.

Although sulfa antibiotics and penicillin had been discovered before the beginning of World War II, their limited availability caused them to be of marginal benefit to the overall military medical effort. When penicillin became available in May of 1944, a reduction in case fatality rates for abdominal wounds and in the incidence of postoperative bacterial peritonitis was observed with its use as compared with the use of sulfonimides alone.[7] During the war, however, important policies were established with regard to the treatment of war wounds. Standardized methods of wide débridement of soft tissue wounds were developed and had a more profound effect on the reduction of cases of gas gangrene than did the availability of penicillin. In addition, after 1943 all colonic injuries were handled by colostomy[8]; this policy is credited with greatly reducing the death rate from intra-abdominal sepsis following this injury.

During the Korean and Vietnam wars, great improvements were made in expediting the evacuation of the wounded from the battlefield into appropriate field hospitals staffed by well-trained surgeons, nurses, and corpsmen.[9] The importance of massive intravenous therapy with crystalloid solutions early in the resuscitative effort to avoid acute renal failure was first appreciated during the Korean conflict.[1] Because antibiotics were widely used for the first time to prevent infection, a change in the character of wound pathogens became apparent. Instead of β-hemolytic streptococcus and *Clostridium perfringens,* surgeons encountered the scourge of the early 1950s: *Staphylococcus aureus.*

With the development of semisynthetic antibiotics with good staphylococcal coverage, the gram-negative aerobes like *Escherichia coli, Klebsiella pneumoniae,* and other Enterobacteriaceae emerged as important pathogens around the time of the Vietnam war, both in military and in civilian hospitals. The aerobic pathogens gradually changed with the progressive development of more powerful antibiotics. The havoc wreaked by *Pseudomonas aeruginosa* is a good example. On the other hand, the anaerobic pathogens remained the same with *Bacteroides fragilis,* whose virulence had originally been described by Meleney and coworkers[10] in the 1930s, still the important pathogen with regard to intra-abdominal sepsis.

Relationship Between Aerobic and Anaerobic Bacteria

Although many surgeons questioned the pathogenicity of anaerobic organisms, the experimental work of Weinstein and coworkers[11] demonstrated that the presence of *B. fragilis* was necessary to produce an experimental intra-abdominal abscess in rats, which developed on about the 7th day after mixed peritoneal contamination. On the other hand, gram-negative aerobes were more important in the early bacteremic, septic phase, which resulted in a 43% mortality within the first 3 days in this model. Thus, it appears that a synergistic relationship exists between aerobic and anaerobic bacterial species of the type usually encountered with mixed bacterial contamination from bowel injury or perforation. Gram-negative aerobes, such as *E. coli,* caused the early septic phase with the elaboration of endotoxin. Endotoxin is generally credited for the massive peripheral vasodilitation observed in septic shock with consequent subnormal peripheral vascular resistance and arterial hypotension. On the contrary, most obligate anaerobes, like *B. fragilis,* do not elaborate biologically active endotoxins, but are required for the establishment and maintenance of an intra-abdominal abscess.[11]

Antibiotic Prophylaxis of Colon Surgery

A major landmark in the successful prevention of intra-abdominal sepsis following elective surgery was the randomized, prospective, multicenter trial of an oral antibiotic combination, in addition to a mechanical bowel preparation, versus a mechanical bowel preparation *alone* before colon surgery.[12] Carried out at Veteran Administration Hospitals, this study demonstrated a highly significant improvement in the incidence of wound infections ($P<.001$), intra-abdominal abscesses ($P<.02$), and anastomotic leaks ($P<.05$) in the group receiving oral antibiotics. The antibiotics used were neomycin (aerobic microbe coverage) and erythromycin (anaerobic coverage) in three 1-g doses each.

Theory of Translocation of Bacteria Across the Bowel Wall

In 1985, Deitch and colleagues,[13] extending a theme of prior investigation going back over 100 years, reported that certain stressful clinical circumstances were accompanied by the overgrowth of luminal bacteria in the distal small intestine or colon and actual movement of bacteria or bacterial byproducts across the basement membrane with localization in the mesenteric lymph nodes and in the portal circulation in the rat. The circumstances included burns,[13] endotoxemia,[14] hemorrhagic shock,[15] intestinal ischemia,[16] obstructive jaundice,[17] malnutrition,[18] withdrawal of oral diet with substitution of total parenteral nutrition,[19] and a diet low in fiber.[20]

This model was proposed as a possible explanation for the persistence of septic signs and for the development of multiple organ failure in some severely ill patients who are recovering from severe trauma or peritonitis but have no other apparent source of infection. Earlier, Polk and Shields[21] had recommended routine laparotomy for abdominal surgery patients who manifested signs of organ dysfunction but no other apparent source of infection. However, Norton[22] reported that such laparotomies frequently yielded negative results and that once sequential, multiple organ system dysfunction was established, drainage of persistent abdominal collections rarely was associated with survival. Although the clinical relevance of bacterial translocation as a source of persistent sepsis and organ dysfunction is far from proven, the theory has opened up a renewed interest in the subject of what nutrients or humoral factors are important in the maintenance of gut integrity. Souba and associates,[23] drawing on the experimental work of Windmueller[24] and Wilmore and colleagues,[25] has presented clinical evidence that both glutamine (either enterally or parenterally administered) and enteral fiber are necessary to prevent the translocation of luminal bacteria in man. This idea had arisen from the laboratory finding that enterocytes in tissue culture appear to prefer glutamine, oxaloacetic acid, and other ketone bodies to glucose as a nutrient.[24]

DEMOGRAPHICS OF INTRA-ABDOMINAL SEPSIS

As reported by Saini and coworkers,[26] 61% of intra-abdominal abscesses in 100 consecutive patients treated at a Boston teaching hospital were from spontaneous intra-abdominal disease, whereas 10% were the result of trauma and 29% were complications of abdominal surgery. Of the 61 with spontaneous intra-abdominal causes, appendicitis occurred in 16 (26%); diverticulitis in 12 (20%); primary liver abscess in 7 (11%); perforated colon cancer in 6 (10%); Crohn's disease, perforated peptic ulcer, and pancreatitis in 3, each (5%); and miscellaneous causes in 11 (18%).

The mean age of patients with intra-abdominal infections was 56 years (range: 12–82 years).[26] Males exhibit a slight predominance of over females with respect to age (57% versus 43%, respectively).

In those patients who develop intra-abdominal sepsis as a complication of abdominal surgery, the overwhelming majority have surgery of the alimentary tract. In the series of Saini and coworkers,[26] for example, 73% of patients who developed intra-abdominal abscesses had gastrointestinal or biliary surgery; of this group, 73% had colonic operations. Given the normal flora of the gastrointestinal tract, which is demonstrated in Figure 142A–1, this preponderance of postoperative infections is not surprising. Whereas most infections in "clean" surgical procedures arise from exogenous bacterial contamination, most infections complicating "clean-contaminated" gastrointestinal operations result from endogenous contamination.

The distributions of abscesses are as shown in Figure 142A–2. The subphrenic collection remained the most common intra-abdominal abscess, followed by pelvic localization.[26]

RISK OF SEPSIS AND ANTIBIOTIC PROPHYLAXIS IN SURGERY PATIENTS

Both elective and emergency surgery can be stratified into four categories to predict the likelihood of postoperative infection. *Clean* surgical operations, those in which an incision passes through antiseptically prepared integument but does not cross mucous membranes, are associated with a wound infection rate of less than 2%.[27] Inguinal hernia repair is a common example. *Clean-contaminated* operations are those in which a mucous membrane is transected in such a manner that contamination is controlled. Most elective alimentary tract operations fall under this category, including cholecystectomy, pancreatectomy, and hepatectomy as well as intestinal procedures. Figure 142A–1 demonstrates the wide variation in the intestinal flora under normal, nondiseased conditions among the various regions of the gastrointestinal tract.[28] Because of the wide variation in potential inocula, the range of predicted infection rates is also wide (5–15%), depending on whether a surgeon is cutting across the pylorus (low level of inocula) or the colon (high level of inocula). *Contaminated* operations, the third category of infection risk, imply the transection of integument or mucous membrane in an uncontrolled fashion. Penetrating trauma of the abdomen may cause contamination, not only because it can cross a mucous membrane in an uncontrolled fashion but also because it can pass through unprepared integument and cause devascularization of soft tissue of the abdominal wall. The infection rates average around 20%. The fourth and final category, *dirty*, is associated with massive contamination or the crossing of prepared integument to deal with a grossly infected process such as a large diverticular abscess or osteomyelitis. If skin is closed in these cases, infection rates exceed 35%.

An appreciation of these principles allows the surgeon to prepare patients and to conduct operations in such a way as to lower the infection rates. The principles of prophylactic antibiotic use include:

1. The risk of infection of an operation should exceed the risk of side effects of the antibiotics used (generally about 5%) except in those instances, such as the placement of vascular prosthetic grafts, in which the implications of an infection are life-threatening.
2. Antibiotics must be given before the expected time of contamination so that antibiotic tissue levels in the wound and peritoneum are maximum at the time of contamination.
3. Antibiotic therapy should be tailored to cover the anticipated pathogens that will contaminate the wound or peritoneum.
4. If possible, antibiotics that are narrow in spectrum should be chosen to prevent the emergence of resistant strains that may lead to the development of nosocomial infections in the hospital environment. For example, a first-generation cephalosporin is usually preferable to a second-generation or third-generation cephalosporin in elective gallbladder surgery, since it can be expected to cover common bile pathogens and to provide coverage against both streptococci and staphylococci; this is superior to the coverage provided by the later-generation drugs. It is also significantly less expensive.
5. When performing operations requiring entrance into the distal half of the ileum or the colon, oral antibiotics effective against both aerobic and anaerobic organisms should be employed with a brief preoperative course to reduce the inoculum of contamination.

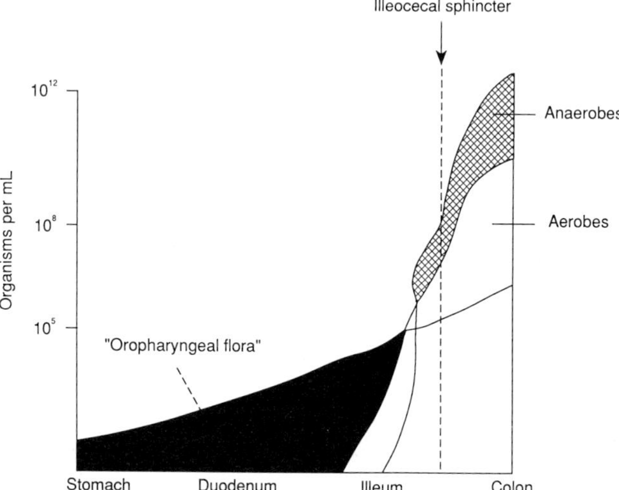

Figure 142A–1. The normal bacterial flora of the human alimentary tract. Although an exponential rise in the number of both aerobic and anaerobic microorganisms was observed in the distal one half on the ileum, the density of anaerobes exceeded that of aerobes by 10^3 organisms per milliliter of luminal fluid in the distal colon. (Modified with permission from a drawing by Sherwood A. Gorbach, M.D., Division of Infectious Diseases, Tufts New England Medical Center, Boston, MA.)

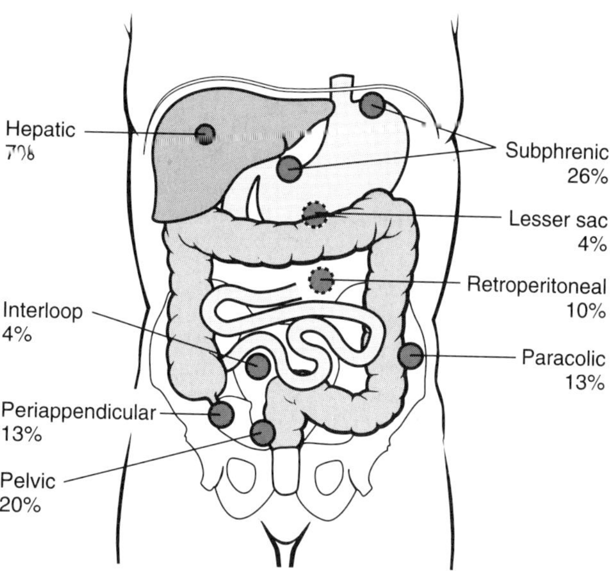

Figure 142A–2. The peritoneal location of 130 intra-abdominal abscesses in 100 consecutive patients treated at Tufts New England Medical Center Hospital (Boston, MA) is demonstrated. (From Saini S, Kellum JM, O'Leary MP, et al: Improved localization and survival in patients with intraabdominal abscesses. Am J Surg 1983; 145:138.)

BIOCHEMISTRY OF INTRA-ABDOMINAL SEPSIS

Endotoxin

Many of the gram-negative aerobic organisms, such as *E. coli,* liberate endotoxin, which is rapidly absorbed through the peritoneum into the circulation. Later, after the formation of an abscess, these same organisms can elaborate endotoxin, which is absorbed into the venous drainage of the abscess wall. In either case, the lipopolysaccharide component of endotoxin is thought to initiate the release of a cascade of mediators of the inflammatory process. It, in itself, appears to cause a profound collapse of vascular tone and systemic hypotension.

The most common form of endotoxin-induced hypotension is the hyperdynamic state, in which cardiac index is elevated and the patient's skin feels warm owing to a combination of fever and peripheral vosodilitation. Much less commonly, the cardiac index is depressed; this latter form is associated with a high early mortality rate.

Leukocyte and Platelet Mediators

Endotoxin exerts both local and systemic effects. When it invades the circulation, it activates macrophages, which in turn release tumor necrosis factor and interleukins.[1] It also activates platelets to release platelet-activating factor, which causes platelets to aggregate and causes localized vasoconstriction through the release of vasoactive substances such as serotonin.

Prostanoids

Through activation of leukocytes and platelets, inflammatory mediators such as prostacyclin and thromboxane are released.[1] These can give rise to pulmonary lesions that culminate in the development of adult respiratory distress syndrome. Sielaff and associates[29] demonstrated that in experimental septic shock in the pig, prior administration of ibuprofen—a prostaglandin synthetase inhibitor—largely blocks the characteristic pulmonary lesion seen in that model. The eicosanoids are also thought to be partly responsible for the microcirculatory damage of gastrointestinal mucosa seen in endotoxin-induced shock.[22] However, clinical evidence that ibuprofen improves sepsis outcome is still lacking.

Oxygen-Derived Free Radicals

Leukocytes contain vesicles that are rich in precursors of oxygen radicals. In clinical situations in which tissue ischemia is followed by reperfusion, (e.g., hemorrhagic or septic shock), xanthine oxidase catalyzes the conversion of hypoxanthine—itself a product of the effect of ischemia on tissue adenosine triphosphate—to oxidants and nonoxidative toxins. In addition, leukocytes adhere to vascular endothelial cells, resulting in neutrophil activation with elaboration of oxygen radicals and other toxins that cause a microcirculatory injury; this results in increased capillary permeability and interstitial edema. This theory is supported by the morphologic findings of adult respiratory distress syndrome, which is associated with interstitial edema and the presence of platelet, neutrophil, and fibrin debris in the pulmonary microcirculation.[1]

None of these mechanisms is mutually exclusive. Certainly, the elaboration of cytokines from activated macrophages and leukocytes is complementary to the microcirculatory theory of multiple organ failure. Furthermore, it is possible that bacterial translocation can initiate some of the macrophage activation and leukocyte adherence to endothelium that lead to organ dysfunction. The cellular and humoral mediators of multiple organ failure and bacterial translocation are given extensive treatment in other chapters in this textbook.

DIAGNOSIS OF INTRA-ABDOMINAL SEPSIS

Clinical

Patients with intra-abdominal abscesses from spontaneous abdominal disease frequently present with acute abdominal disorders. Examples are perforated appendicitis, acute diverticulitis, and perforated peptic ulcer. Classic clinical and laboratory findings of intra-abdominal abscess include fever (usually ≥102°F), leukocytosis, and localized abdominal tenderness. Postoperative abscesses are more difficult to diagnose because these signs are often present after abdominal surgery in patients without abscesses. In the series of Saini and coworkers,[26] clinical findings were the indication for operative drainage in 41% of patients with intra-abdominal abscesses.

Radiologic

Classic plain radiographic films of the abdomen may be helpful in the diagnosis. Such films may demonstrate abnormal collections of gas or fluid. Figure 142A–3 demonstrates an air-fluid level in a large left subphrenic abscess that was a complication of a perforated peptic ulcer.

Contrast gastrointestinal radiography may also diagnose and localize intra-abdominal abscesses. Figure 142A–4 dem-

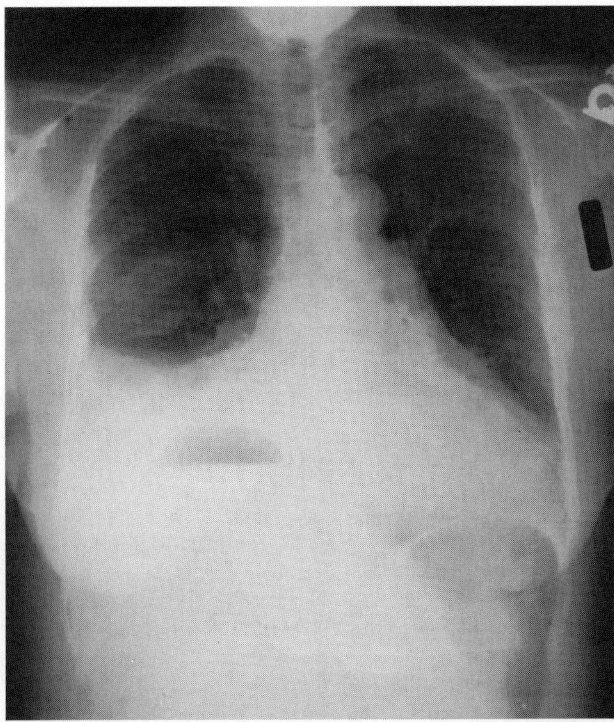

Figure 142A–3. This plain radiograph of the chest and upper abdomen demonstrates a right subdiaphragmatic abscess with an air-fluid level. This patient presented with right upper quadrant abdominal pain, right shoulder pain, and fever. At surgery, he was found to have a chronic, sealed-off, duodenal ulcer perforation as the cause of his abscess.

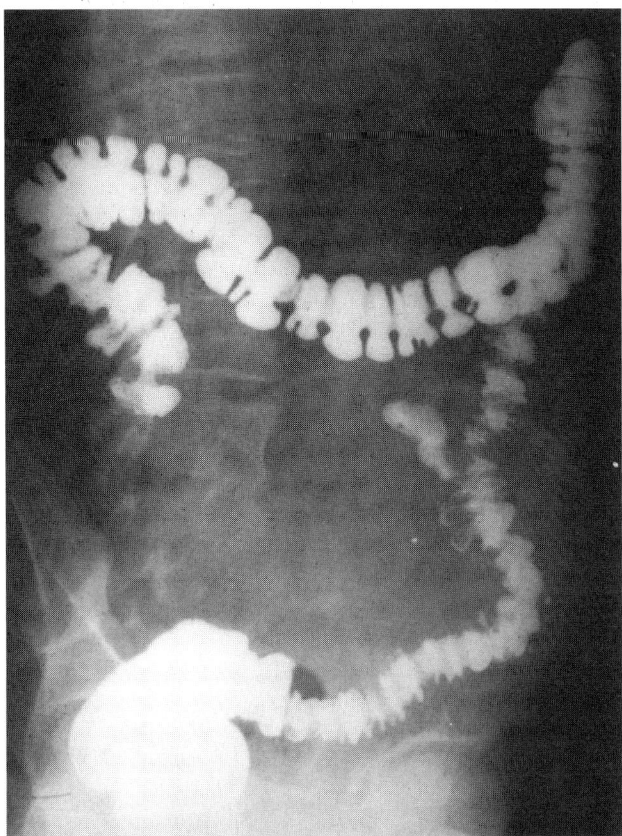

Figure 142A–4. A contrast radiograph of the colon (barium enema) demonstrates diverticulitis of the sigmoid colon with perforation into a pericolic abscess.

onstrates how a barium enema can localize a pericolic abscess in a patient with acute diverticulitis.

Modern imaging techniques, however, have revolutionized the diagnosis of intra-abdominal abscess. Saini and coworkers[26] reported that computed tomography was superior to both gallium scintigraphy and ultrasonography in accurate diagnosis (see Fig. 45–1*A*). The advantages of computed tomography include the ability to differentiate fluid and gas within an abscess from that inside the gastrointestinal lumen. They are superior to ultrasound techniques when the localization of an abscess was not previously suspected based on the clinical evidence, when dealing with a pelvic or interloop abscess, and, most importantly, when dealing with multiple intra-abdominal collections.[26] In patients with generalized peritoneal contamination, a fever occurring 5 or more days postoperatively and not explained by other causes (e.g., pulmonary atelectasis or pneumonia, urinary tract infection, wound infection, thrombophlebitis, intravenous catheter infection, or drug reaction) is an indication for computed tomography of the entire abdomen and pelvis. The reduced mortality for intra-abdominal abscess patients reported by Saini and coworkers[26] was attributed to early diagnosis, largely as a result of the availability of computed tomography, rather than to any improvement in the therapy for multiple organ failure. Recently, Goris and van Dalen[30] noted that the mortality for multiple organ failure has remained stubbornly constant at 60%.

THERAPY FOR INTRA-ABDOMINAL SEPSIS

Fluid/Pressor Therapy for Septic Shock

The reader is referred to Chapters 13 and 14 for a detailed treatment of this subject. In septic shock–related to intra-abdominal sepsis, the diagnosis is frequently established after the placement of a Swan-Ganz catheter for monitoring pulmonary capillary wedge pressure and cardiac output. The hypotension of septic shock, in contrast to that seen with hemorrhagic shock or cardiac failure, is usually associated with an elevated cardiac index and a markedly decreased systemic vascular resistance. Mixed venous oxygen content is usually high or normal, reflecting the presence of significant arteriovenous shunting and diminished cellular oxygen uptake associated with the septic state.

Antibiotics

In the early stages of intra-abdominal sepsis, the antibiotics used should be broad-spectrum and therapy aimed at covering potential aerobic gram-negative and anaerobic microorganisms. In a patient who has been in the hospital, and especially in the intensive care unit, for several days, the antibiotics should offer coverage for *P. aeruginosa*. If aminoglycosides are used, it is important to measure peak and trough levels after early dosing to avoid ototoxicity and nephrotoxicity. Prolonged dosing intervals can be calculated from readily available tables in the case of reduced renal function. (A detailed discussion of antibiotic therapy for surgical infection is included in Chapter 132.)

Drainage of Intra-Abdominal Abscesses

Although most abscesses require drainage, certain intra-abdominal abscesses can sometimes be cured with antibiotic therapy alone. For example, multiple small liver abscesses that occur secondary to cholangitis sometimes resolve with antibiotic therapy alone. The explanation for this is that liver abscesses, like some lung or brain abscesses, may communicate with the ductile system draining the organ and thus be partially drained. Small pericolic abscesses associated with acute diverticulitis often resolve with antibiotic therapy alone. Kellum and colleagues[31] reported that nearly 90% of patients with acute diverticulitis—all of whom are thought to have colonic microperforations and pericolic collections—are successfully treated with antibiotics alone and equally well if treated with either cefoxitin alone or a combination of gentamicin and clindamycin. Again, the communication of a pericolic abscess with a perforated diverticulum affords at least partial drainage. Since most intra-abdominal abscesses do not communicate with drainage conduits, they do not resolve without some form of drainage.

Percutaneous Catheter Drainage of Abscesses

Gerzof and coworkers[32] reported a highly successful series of patients treated with computed tomography–or ultrasound-guided placement of drainage catheters in intra-abdominal abscesses. In their report, the authors emphasized the importance of the following factors in the success of the technique:

1. That complete drainage of all abscesses or loculations is achieved.
2. That broad-spectrum antibiotic coverage is given prior to manipulation.
3. That follow-up imaging or contrast studies are carried out to document that the abscess completely resolves.
4. That a safe route for percutaneous catheter drainage of abdominal abscesses is available.
5. That surgical back-up is available.

In this series,[32] 61 (86%) of 71 abscesses in 67 patients were successfully drained. However, there were 11 complications (15%), and 6 deaths were attributable to sepsis (3 of these were related to inadequate drainage). Only one abscess recurred during the follow-up from 2 to 5 years.

This technique is particularly valuable in patients with unilocular, solitary abscesses and in those with organ failure or coagulopathy, in whom conventional surgical drainage carries a high risk of mortality. Contraindications to percutaneous catheter drainage of abdominal abscesses include a surgical abdomen in which intestinal perforation or gangrene is likely or in which the drainage route violates a hollow viscus or the pleural space.

Surgical Drainage and Drains

Saini and coworkers[26] reported that since the availability of computed tomography, the mortality rate for open surgical drainage has fallen from 30% to 12%. The complication rate was high (28% in this series of 100 consecutive patients), and complications included recurrent abscesses, enterocutaneous fistulas, and superinfection with resistant organisms. The authors noted that imaging tests made extraserous or regional surgical drainage more accurate, and thus they recommended this approach over transperitoneal drainage (through a vertical midline incision) because of a lower observed morbidity. Open drainage was preferable in patients with multiple abscesses, for computed tomography–localized interloop abscesses, and for most pelvic abscesses.

Whether to use any of various types of drains is largely a matter of the personal preference of the surgeon. Active suction drains have the advantage that negative pressure is used to continuously evacuate the contents of an abscess cavity and that less contamination occurs from the drain itself. Disadvantages include the tendency of suction drains to become plugged and the greater likelihood of some of the stiffer suction drains to erode into the intestines or blood vessels. Passive drains such as the redoubtable Penrose drain are less likely to become plugged, especially if they are placed through a large opening in the abdominal wall; they are also less likely to erode into vital structures. On the other hand, Penrose drains require more active management from the surgeon in that they must be moved frequently to avoid being walled off from the target collection. Another disadvantage is the potential for external contamination with their use.

Ancillary Therapies

Monoclonal antibodies against the lipopolysaccharide component of endotoxin have been developed and tested in man. Unfortunately, early promising data could not be substantiated in larger clinical trials; thus, these therapies have not been approved for widespread clinical use. Despite this setback, various biotechnology companies are developing these promising technologies. Antibodies to tumor necrosis factor, interleukins, and platelet-activating factor have been developed and clinical trials of their use in septic patients are beginning.

In addition, nonantibodies are being developed with monoclonal techniques to replace various deficient elements found in the patient with sepsis. For example, a monoclonally synthesized surfactant is being clinically tested in surgical patients with sepsis thought to be at high risk for adult respiratory distress syndrome.

Miscellaneous

One strategy that is still in the investigative phase involves the use of triiodothyronine to improve the inotropic action of the heart under the stress of septicemia. A second is the use of allopurinol to block the action of xanthine oxidase in catalyzing the production of oxygen radicals in the ischemia-reperfusion model of septic shock.

At the present time, it must be concluded that aggressive diagnosis and therapies, which are aimed at the prevention of sequential multiple organ system failure, should be the main goal of the surgeon treating peritonitis and intra-abdominal sepsis. Even if successful strategies are developed to combat the ravages of multiple organ failure, they will likely be extravagantly expensive not only in terms of financial costs, but, more importantly, in terms of patient morbidity.

References

1. Deitch EA: Multiple organ failure, pathophysiology and potential future therapy. Ann Surg 1992; 216:117–134.
2. Haagensen CD, Lloyd WEB: A Hundred Years of Medicine. New York, Sheridan House, 1943, pp 239–248.
3. Ravitch M: A Century of Surgery 1880–1980. Philadelphia, JB Lippincott, 1981.
4. Garrison FH: Notes on the History of Military Medicine. Washington, Association of Military Surgeons, 1922, pp 188–206.
5. Landsteiner K: Individual differences in human blood. Science 1931; 73:403.
6. Blalock A: Acute circulatory failure as exemplified by shock and hemorrhage. Surg Gynecol Obstet 1934; 58:551–561.
7. Drye JC: Penicillin and sulfonamide therapy (2410 casualties). *In:* Surgery in World War II: General Surgery. Vol 2. Coates JB, DeBakey ME (Eds). Washington D.C., Office of the Surgeon General, 1947, pp 197–201.
8. Hays SB: Policy on large bowel injuries. Circular Letter No. 178. Washington, D.C., Office of the Surgeon General, October 23, 1943.
9. Barrett O: U.S. medicine in Vietnam: The early years. *In:* Internal Medicine in Vietnam. Vol 2: General Medicine and Infectious Diseases. Ognibene AJ, Barrett O (Eds). Washington, D.C., Office of the Surgeon General, 1982, pp 21–38.
10. Meleney FL, Opps S, Harvey HD, et al: Peritonitis: II. Synergism of bacteria commonly found in peritoneal exudates. Arch Surg 1932; 25:709–721.
11. Weinstein WM, Onderdonk AH, Bartlett JG, et al: Experimental intra-abdominal abscesses in rats: Development of an experimental model. Infect Immun 1974; 10:1250–1255.
12. Clarke JS, Condon RE, Bentley DW, et al: Preoperative oral antibiotics reduce septic complications of colon operations: Results of a prospective, randomized double-blind clinical study. Am J Surg 1977; 186:251.
13. Deitch EA, Maejima K, Berg R: Effect of oral antibiotics and bacterial overgrowth on the translocation of the GI tract microflora in burned rats. J Trauma 1985; 25:385–392.
14. Deitch EA, Berg R, Specian R: Endotoxin promotes the translocation of bacteria from the gut. Arch Surg 122:185–190.
15. Baker JW, Deitch EA, Berg RD, et al: Hemorrhagic shock induces bacterial translocation from the gut. J Trauma 1988; 28:896–906.
16. Bennion RS, Wilson SE, Williams RA: Early portal anaerobic bacteremia in mesenteric ischemia. Arch Surg 1984; 119:151–155.
17. Deitch EA, Sittig K, Li M, et al: Obstructive jaundice promotes bacterial translocation from the gut. Am J Surg 1990; 159:79–84.
18. Deitch EA, Xu DZ, Qi L, et al: Protein malnutrition alone and in combination with endotoxin impairs systemic and gut-associated immunity. JPEN J Parenter Enteral Nutr 1992; 16:25–31.
19. Mainous M, Xu DZ, Lu Q, et al: Oral-TPN–induced bacterial translocation and impaired immune defenses are reversed by refeeding. Surgery 1991; 110:277–283.
20. Spaeth G, Berg RD, Specian RD, et al: Food without fiber promotes bacterial translocation from the gut. Surgery 1990; 108:240–246.
21. Polk HC, Shields CL: Remote organ failure: A valid sign of occult intra-abdominal infection. Surgery 1977; 81:310.
22. Norton LW: Does drainage of intra-abdominal pus reverse multiple organ failure? Am J Surg 1985; 149:347–350.
23. Souba WW, Scott TE, Wilmore DW: Intestinal consumption of intravenously administered fuels. JPEN J Parenter Enteral Nutr 1985; 9:18–22.
24. Windmueller HG: Glutamine utilization by the small intestine. Adv Enzymol 1982; 53:202–231.

25. Wilmore DW, Goodwin CW, Aulick LH, et al: Effect of injury and infection on visceral metabolism and circulation. Ann Surg 1980; 192:491.
26. Saini S, Kellum JM, O'Leary MP, et al: Improved localization and survival in patients with intraabdominal abscesses. Am J Surg 1983; 145:136–142.
27. Nichols RL: Classification of surgical wounds and nonoperative factors influencing surgical wound infection. *In:* Decision Making in Surgical Sepsis. Nichols RL, Hyslop NE, Bartlett JG (Eds). Philadelphia, BC Decker, 1991, pp 20–22.
28. Bartlett JG: The normal flora. *In:* Surgical Infections, Selective Antibiotic Therapy. Condon RE, Gorbach SL (Eds). Baltimore, Williams & Wilkins, 1981, pp 1–6.
29. Sielaff TD, Sugerman HJ, Tatum JL, et al: Successful treatment of adult respiratory distress syndrome by histamine and prostaglandin blockade in a porcine *Pseudomonas* model. Surgery 1987; 102:350–357.
30. Goris RJA, van Dalen R: Selective decontamination in the intensive care unit. *In:* Advances in Trauma and Critical Care. Vol 7. Maull KI (Ed). St. Louis, Mosby–Year Book, 1992, pp 61–78.
31. Kellum JM, Coppa GF, Way LR, et al: Randomized, prospective comparison of cefoxitin with gentamicin-clindamycin in the treatment of acute colonic diverticulitis. Clin Ther 1992; 14:376–384.
32. Gerzof SG, Robbins AH, Johnson WC, et al: Percutaneous catheter drainage of abdominal abscesses: A five-year experience. N Engl J Med 1981; 305:653–657.

CHAPTER 142B

Identification of Previously Undiagnosed Disease: Hantavirus Pulmonary Syndrome

Howard Levy, MD

Despite the advances that have been made in the diagnosis and treatment of infectious disease, a large number of organisms remain as candidates for novel infections. Emerging disorders include virulent forms of previously benign bacterial and viral infections, unusual presentations of disease in immunosuppressed patients, pathogen explanation of disease previously thought to be idiopathic, and novel disease caused by new human-pathogen contact. In the last two decades, we have have encountered Legionnaire's disease, acquired immunodeficiency syndrome (AIDS), and Lyme disease. During the same period, eosinophilia-myalgia syndrome was described and was related to a noninfectious cause—namely L-tryptophan ingestion.

Recognition of a new disease requires that it present in a cluster of patients so that astute physicians can observe its epidemic nature. In the absence of patient clustering, the disease presentation has to be sufficiently unusual to be discerned against the background clinical presentation of other similar diseases. Infectious pathogens and environmental stimuli are the leading candidates for the causation of any new disease.

In May 1993, an outbreak of acute illness associated with hantavirus infection was identified in the southwestern United States.[1,2] The disease was unusual both in its clustering and in its manifestation, which was sufficiently different from the usual presentation of adult respiratory distress syndrome and sepsis syndrome. The illness, *hantavirus pulmonary syndrome,* was characterized by a patient history of contact with rodents or rodent droppings followed a number of days later by fever, myalgias, and headache and then by cough and the rapid development of respiratory failure. Contact with the Centers for Disease Control and Prevention (CDC) was mandatory to establish disease causation and to initiate therapeutic and epidemiologic studies. Close collaboration of state, federal, and hospital personnel allowed rapid advances in gaining an understanding the disease, so that a mere 4 months after recognition of the first case, we had reached an understanding of the disease; equivalent levels of understanding had taken years to achieve with Legionnaire's disease and AIDS.

As of March 1, 1994, laboratory evidence of acute hantavirus infection had been confirmed in 64 patients in 16 states who had a similar clinical syndrome. Of these patients, 45% were women, 50% Native Americans, 40% non-Hispanic whites, 8% Hispanics, and 2% blacks. The median age of affected individuals was 31 years. Sixty per cent of the patients died. The pattern of serologic cross-reactivity to four different previously identified hantaviruses and the genetic sequences of virus amplified from patient tissues showed that these infections were due to a previously unknown hantavirus species. The majority of cases have occurred in the Four Corners Region where New Mexico, Arizona, Colorado and Utah meet, and this has led to a proposed designation of the virus as the *Four Corners virus.* The hantavirus involved has been isolated in cell culture, and it is considerably divergent from others in the group, indicating that it is not a recent mutation from the other hantaviruses but that previous infections had gone undiagnosed. In retrospect, the earliest identified infection occurred in 1975 in a patient from southern New Mexico; this patient survived the illness. This demonstrates that although the illness's presentation is unique, it took an epidemic to recognize the unusual presentation and mobilize resources to identify the causative agent.

The deer mouse *Peromyscus maniculatus* has been identified as the likely principal reservoir of this virus. Up to 30% of deer mice trapped in the outbreak area were found to be seropositive for this virus. Nucleotide sequence analyses of amplified deoxyribonucleic acid products from three-polymerase chain reaction (PCR)–positive humans and from six-PCR–positive *P. maniculatus* rodents trapped around the patients' dwellings are closely related and provide direct genetic evidence of the link between the hantavirus infection in the rodents and that in the human cases. The ability to use these extremely sensitive probes to search for microbial causes will almost certainly lead to the discovery of additional diseases in the future. Some patients were residents of areas outside of the recognized home range of *P. maniculatus,* but their viruses show significant genetic divergence from the prototypic strain. The identification of a high rate of seroprevalence in this species of rodent with an extremely wide range (sparing only portions of the Gulf states) suggests that human infections with hantavirus, although unrecognized prior to 1993, will remain an endemic problem in a large geographic area of the United States. It is likely that other animal rodent carriers that can explain disease occurrence outside of this range will be identified.

Before the 1993 outbreak of disease, there were four recognized members of the genus *Hantavirus* (family Bunyaviridae[3]): Hantaan, Puumala, Seoul, and Prospect Hill; each species has its own specific rodent reservoir. Isolation of the Hantaan virus, which causes hemorrhagic fever with renal syndrome, was reported in Korea in 1978.[4] The Seoul virus causes a milder form of the syndrome. The Hantaan, Puumala (cause of Nephropathia epidemica), and Seoul viruses are known human pathogens. The Prospect Hill virus, which was demonstrated in meadow voles, has not been associated with disease.

Cardiopulmonary dysfunction, ranging from mild hypoxemia with stable hemodynamics to rapid respiratory failure with shock, differentiates hantavirus pulmonary syndrome patients from patients with other hantavirus syndromes.[5] We have cared for 16 of the patients presenting with the disease and have observed a 36% death rate. Infection with this hantavirus can be either a short-term, mild process or a rapidly fatal disease, and intervention may result in recovery. On presentation, fever or chills were present in all 16 patients, and all but one patient had gastrointestinal complaints such as nausea or vomiting, abdominal pain, or diarrhea. Many patients were sent home with these symptoms only to return extremely ill later. Myalgias were seen in most, and headache in one half of patients. Many patients complained of cough on presentation, but dyspnea often was a late-developing symptom, occurring just prior to respiratory decompensation. The mean duration of symptoms before hospitalization was 4 days. Patients deteriorated rapidly, and the mean duration to death was an additional 3 days. All patients required oxygen on admission. Several had copious, amber-colored, nonpurulent pulmonary secretions that were always associated with diffuse pulmonary infiltrates observed on chest radiography. This fluid, suctioned directly from the trachea just after intubation, had a total protein ratio of edema fluid–to–serum of greater than 80%. Bronchoalveolar lavage fluid was remarkable for its absence of cellularity and for the inability to demonstrate the presence of viral protein in the fluid.

Many laboratory test results were abnormal at presentation. On the peripheral smear, a triad of thrombocytopenia, a left shift in the myeloid series, and the presence of large immunoblastoid lymphocytes are unique and characteristic for this disease and occurred in all patients on admission. Unusual constellations of symptoms or signs should be considered by clinicians as a possible indicator of novel disease. Hemoconcentration was notable, indicating generalized capillary leak, but hemoglobin concentration fell to anemic levels with adequate fluid resuscitation. Serum lactate levels became elevated at some point during the hospital course in a majority of patients. Those patients with peak lactate levels above 4 mmol/L died. All patients demonstrated mildly increased lactate dehydrogenase levels, and most had elevated aspartate aminotransferase concentrations. These levels rose twofold to fivefold greater than the upper limit of normal as the clinical picture worsened. Serum alanine aminotransferase was also elevated in most patients, although not as high as aspartate aminotransferase. Serum bilirubin and alkaline phosphatase typically were normal throughout the hospital course. Serum creatinine levels remained normal in all survivors, unlike in all other patients with previously described hantavirus infections, which have caused renal failure or insufficiency without pulmonary involvement.

Several parameters indicate the presence of severe gas exchange abnormalities. The ratio of arterial oxygen tension to fraction of inspired oxygen was low in all patients, and a majority of patients had nadir values less than 100. Fifty per cent of patients required mechanical ventilation, and high levels of positive end-expiratory pressure were required. The range of lowest measured total respiratory system compliance was from 11 to 27 mL/cm H_2O. Chest radiography in patients who had progression to respiratory failure initially showed bibasilar infiltrates, which rapidly spread to include all four quadrants of the lung. All patients developed pulmonary parenchymal infiltrates during the course of their illness. Large pleural effusions were noted in several patients, and this was recognized as being unusual for adult respiratory distress syndrome. Heart sizes were uniformly normal. The initial pulmonary artery wedge pressure in all patients was ≤8 mm Hg, and the ratio of tracheal to serum protein was greater than 80%[6]; this suggested that the edema was due to an increase in permeability of the pulmonary capillary bed and not to an increase in hydrostatic forces. Pulmonary edema, hyaline membranes, and a mononuclear infiltrate were noted at autopsy in those patients who died.

The occurrence of severe cardiopulmonary dysfunction appears to predict a poor prognosis. The hemodynamic profile of our patients who have progressed to shock differs from the typical profile of patients with septic shock[7] in that they demonstrated an early drop in cardiac index with raised systemic vascular resistance. Several authors have shown that characteristic hemodynamic measurements in both bacteremic and viremic shock include an increase in cardiac index and a low systemic vascular resistance.[8–10] These differences alerted us to the fact that we were dealing with a previously undiagnosed illness. Critically ill patients developed shock manifested by low mean arterial pressure. Initial pulmonary artery wedge pressure was low, and despite fluid resuscitation and inotropic support, the cardiac index was below cardiogenic shock values in patients who died, ranging between 3.2 and 2.6 L/m^2 per minute in survivors. The drop in cardiac index was associated with an elevation in the systemic vascular resistance index, a decrease in oxygen delivery, and a rise in serum lactate concentration. Clinical recovery was marked by an increase in the cardiac index to normal or supranormal levels and by a return of other measurements to normal values. Transthoracic echocardiograms showed moderate to severely depressed left ventricular systolic function in patients who died.

Although gas exchange abnormalities became quite severe in many patients, all patients could be adequately oxygenated throughout the course of their illness. Cardiogenic shock and pulseless electrical activity was the cause of death. The rapidity of death appeared to correlate with the rate of progression of hypoxemia and with pulmonary radiographic findings. Recovery in survivors was as rapid as the initial decline, and few patients who survived for 48 hours after hospital admission have died. Recovery has been complete with no significant residual deficits. No patients had multiple organ failure, renal failure, or hepatic failure; this emphasized the difference between this disease and other causes of systemic inflammatory response syndrome.

Management of patients with hantavirus pulmonary syndrome requires early diagnosis, as antiviral therapy requires sufficient time to be beneficial. Since the majority of cases occur in rural areas, early transfer to a regional intensive care unit is advisable, as we believe improving survival is related to the availability of more sophisticated care. Rapid diagnosis is available at the University of New Mexico, which has developed a test for antibodies in a three-antigen recombinant immunoblot assay for immunoglobulins M and G. Diagnostic serology and PCR testing are also available through the CDC in Atlanta.

When dealing with a disease of unknown and potentially infectious cause, the highest levels of precaution should be adopted. We maintained complete barrier nursing, and particle masks were required for all personnel entering the outside venting rooms until the cause of illness was clear. No case of person-to-person transmission has been documented, but we maintain universal precautions and respiratory isolation of all suspected cases because this disease, as for other hantaviral illnesses, is thought to be contracted by inhalation of infectious particles. Viral ribonucleic acid has not been detected in bronchial secretions, even by PCR analysis, but it is found in peripheral blood mononuclear cells.

In general, viruses belonging to the family Bunyaviridae have been sensitive in vitro to ribavirin (Virazole), but this drug is not licensed for use in the United States. Most of our patients have been treated under CDC protocol with intravenous ribavirin (Virazole). The fulminant course of hantavirus pulmonary syndrome by the time patients present to a medical center suggests that insufficient time is available for an antiviral agent to be effective. In addition, the low viral load implicates mechanisms such as immunologic and cytokine mediators as the predominant factor in disease, and not overwhelming viremia. If it becomes possible to identify patients very early in the disease course, then an antiviral agent such as ribivirin could have a role in aborting florid hantavirus pulmonary syndrome. The improving survival may be attributed to improved recognition of less severe cases or improved medical management.

When dealing with a new disease, patients must be presumptively treated for sepsis and given antibiotics that are used to treat a wide variety of the usual causes of infection. We include plague coverage in this broad spectrum, as the majority of patients presenting with similar findings will prove not to have hantavirus pulmonary syndrome although they did have rodent exposure. In the absence of any specific therapy, we have managed the patients as we do others with systemic inflammatory response syndrome. Close monitoring of oxygenation is extremely important so that timely intubation and mechanical ventilation can be provided when required. Because the status of patients with this viral infection can deteriorate very rapidly, we place a flow-directed pulmonary artery catheter as soon as it is clinically warranted. We maintain as low a wedge pressure as is compatible with satisfactory cardiac indices because of the extreme capillary leak. In place of continued fluid boluses, we use inotropic agents such as dopamine, dobutamine, and norepinephrine earlier in the resuscitation of these patients than in the usual patient with systemic inflammatory response syndrome. Transthoracic echocardiography allows early detection of severely decreased myocardial function. Cardiac arrhythmias, particularly any episodes of electromechanical dissociation, portend a poor outcome and are aggressively treated. Red blood cells are given to maintain oxygen delivery if hemoglobin concentration falls. Thrombocytopenia has not required support with platelet transfusion and increases as the clinical course improves. We monitor serum lactate levels closely and consider salvage therapy when these levels exceed 4 mmol/L, since this has uniformly correlated with poor outcome.

Salvage therapy should be considered in critically ill patients with this syndrome, as ribavirin therapy is often administered too late in the disease course to be beneficial. Bradykinin activation has been demonstrated in other hantavirus infections, and we have observed low levels of total and low-molecular-weight kininogen levels return to normal as the disease remitted. High-molecular-weight kininogen levels remained normal at all times. Bradykinin antagonist (Bradycor [Cortech, Denver, CO]) may be administered in a randomized, placebo-controlled protocol to critically ill patients with confirmed hantavirus pulmonary syndrome. We believe that extracorporeal membrane oxygenation therapy is another potential treatment modality, especially because it offers cardiovascular support. Because surviving patients with this illness recover rapidly, we anticipate that extracorporeal membrane oxygenation support would be short-term. One patient has been successfully treated with this modality.

This new disease presented an unusual challenge for our intensive care unit when six suspected cases occurred during the Memorial Day weekend, 1993, when it was difficult to mobilize resources. Intense media interest was focused on the outbreak and added stress to the difficulties of dealing with a disease of unknown cause, which was initially thought to be uniformly fatal. Press releases were provided to communicate advances in diagnosis and care and were extremely useful in helping to disseminate information about human-rodent contact as the cause of the disease and to assist in the prevention of potential new cases.

We believe that early intervention and careful support of abnormal physiology by standard intensive care medicine has improved survival in patients with hantavirus pulmonary syndrome, even in the absence of specific therapy. This disease has demonstrated that we can still expect outbreaks of novel infection as conventional diseases are controlled. New epidemics of viral disease are to be anticipated as viral evolution continues.[11] Careful attention to the principles of critical care medicine outlined in this book will most likely allow successful intervention against even the most formidable of diseases.

References

1. Centers for Disease Control and Prevention: Outbreak of acute illness—Southwestern United States, 1993. MMWR 1993; 42: 421–424.
2. Centers for Disease Control and Prevention: Update: Hantavirus Disease—United States, 1993. MMWR 1993; 42:612–614.
3. McKee KT Jr, LeDuc JW, Peters CJ: Hantaviruses. *In:* Textbook of Human Virology. 2nd ed. Belshe RB (Ed). St. Louis, Mosby-Year Book, 1991, pp 615–632.
4. Lee HW, Lee PW, Johnson KM: Isolation of the etiologic agent of Korean hemorrhagic fever. J Infect Dis 1978; 137:298–308.
5. McCormick JB: Diseases caused by hantaviruses. *In:* Hunter's Tropical Medicine. Strickland GT (Ed). Philadelphia, WB Saunders, 1991, pp 251–254.
6. Fein A, Grossman RF, Jones JG, et al: The value of edema fluid protein measurement in patients with pulmonary edema. Am J Med 1979; 67:32–38.
7. Parrillo JE: Pathogenetic mechanisms of septic shock. N Engl J Med 1993; 328:1471–1477.
8. Parker MM, Parrillo JE: Septic shock: Hemodynamics and pathogenesis. JAMA 1983; 250:3324–3327.
9. Okrent DG, Abraham E, Winston D: Cardiorespiratory patterns in viral septicemia. Am J Med 1987; 83:681–686.
10. Deutschman CS, Konstantinides FN, Tsai M, et al: Physiology and metabolism in isolated viral septicemia. Arch Surg 1987; 122:21–25.
11. Morse SS (Ed): Emerging Viruses. New York, Oxford University Press, 1993.

SECTION XI
HEMATOLOGY/ONCOLOGY

Stephen M. Ayres

CHAPTER 143

Diagnosis and Management of Bleeding Disorders

Nils U. Bang, MD

Approximately 80,000 patients in the United States die each year from uncontrollable generalized bleeding arising from congenital or acquired coagulation defects. Fifty per cent of all deaths in the United States can be attributed to thrombotic disorders, most frequently thrombi formed at sites of atheromatous lesions resulting in heart attacks and strokes, and to a sizable number of venous thromboembolisms. Considered together, generalized bleeding problems and thrombotic disorders transcend all subspecialties of medicine and surgery. Rapid establishment of an accurate diagnosis and institution of correct therapy represent one of the major challenges facing critical care physicians today.

The information gained from a careful history and physical examination almost never suffices to establish the correct diagnosis of an unknown bleeding disorder or a suspected case of venous thromboembolism. Diagnoses of coagulopathies are made in the laboratory. To make appropriate therapeutic decisions and to order the proper laboratory tests and interpret the results correctly, a critical care physician must have sufficient knowledge of the principal physiologic features of normal hemostasis and the pathophysiology of bleeding disorders and thrombotic events.

NORMAL HEMOSTASIS

In simplistic terms, the cessation of bleeding from a severed blood vessel occurs in two well-defined phases. At the site of vascular injury, blood platelets come in contact with subendothelial connective tissue, most notably microfibrils and collagen. Although platelets do not adhere to normal endothelial cells, they have a strong affinity for subendothelial connective tissue, particularly collagen, and they stick to the collagen exposed when a vessel is severed. Contact with collagen activates platelets, setting in motion a series of complex events—the generation of the prostaglandin thromboxane A_2 as well as activation of the cyclic adenosine monophosphate and inositol triphosphate–diacyl glycerol messenger systems. The net result is the secretion from the platelets of a number of substances normally stored in the so-called alpha granules and dense bodies readily visible in the platelet by electron microscopy. Released substances include adenine nucleotides, particularly adenosine diphosphate, catecholamines, serotonin, and thromboxane A_2, substances that all cause platelets to aggregate (i.e., cause more platelets to stick to the platelets already adhered to the collagen of the vessel wall). A platelet plug is eventually formed, constituting a temporary seal of the injured vessel. In order to make this seal permanent, fibrin must form in and around the platelet plug. The activated platelet undergoes dramatic membrane changes, making it possible to assemble clotting factors on the platelet surface that cooperatively generate large quantities of thrombin, the enzyme ultimately responsible for clotting fibrinogen. Thrombin also is a potent activator of platelets, thereby attracting more platelets to the aggregate and further consolidating the seal.

It is easy to comprehend that patients can bleed for three different reasons. If platelets are too scarce, insufficient platelets are available to form the initial hemostatic plug. If platelets are present in normal numbers but function abnormally, these platelets either adhere poorly to subendothelial connective tissue or activate sluggishly, thereby slowing down or abolishing the formation of an aggregate. Finally, if a patient's fibrin-forming mechanism is abnormal, the initial hemostatic plug forms normally; however, if little or no fibrin is available to reinforce the primary plug, platelets deaggregate, the plug washes away, and rebleeding is likely to occur.

PLATELET DISORDERS

Quantitative

The history and physical examination can offer clues about whether a patient suffers from a quantitative or qualitative platelet disorder or a disorder of fibrin formation. If a patient is admitted with a history or physical findings of spontaneous hemorrhages in the skin, petechiae and ecchymoses, mucous membrane bleeding including nosebleeds, or bleeding from the gastrointestinal tract, thrombocytopenia or a platelet function disorder should be considered. If, on the other hand, a patient appears with a history or physical findings of bleeding into the muscles, bones, or joints, a defect in the fibrin-forming mechanism may be primarily suspected. These rules are not without exception, however, and the precise diagnosis requires a laboratory examination. If a platelet count of less than 50,000 to 100,000 is diagnosed, the bone marrow examination should be conducted early to estimate bone marrow megakaryocytes to aid in the diagnosis of amegakaryocytic or megakaryocytic thrombocytopenia. The major reasons for decreased bone marrow megakaryocytes, listed in Table 143–1, include bone marrow infiltration by metastatic tumors, leukemic cells, and sometimes infectious granulomas; bone marrow dysplasia; bone marrow aplasia secondary to exposure to chemicals or drugs, particularly thiazide diuretics and ethanol; and ionizing radiation. Amegakaryocytic thrombocytopenia on rare occasions can be congenital or hereditary. Conditions producing thrombocytopenia at birth include constitutional aplastic anemia (Fanconi's syndrome), amegakaryocytic thrombocytopenia with congenital malformations (thrombocytopenia with absent radius syndrome), and sex-linked thrombocytopenia (Wiskott-Aldrich syndrome). Megaloblastic anemia secondary to folic acid or vitamin B_{12} deficiency produces ineffective megakaryocytopoiesis, which in severe cases can result in a sharply reduced number of

TABLE 143–1. Amegakaryocytic Thrombocytopenias

Bone marrow infiltration with:
- Tumor cells
- Leukemic cells
- Infectious granulomas (rare)

Bone marrow dysplasia
Myeloproliferative disorders (myelofibrosis)
Bone marrow aplasia
- Primary
- Secondary to chemicals, drugs (e.g., thiazide diuretics, ethanol), ionizing radiation

Hereditary disorders
- Fanconi's syndrome
- Thrombocytopenia with congenital malformations
- X-linked thrombocytopenia (Wiskott-Aldrich syndrome)

Ineffective megakaryocytopoiesis
- Vitamin B_{12} deficiency
- Folate deficiency
- Iron deficiency (rare)

megakaryocytes in the bone marrow. Likewise, severe iron deficiency anemia, which is frequently accompanied by thrombocytopenia, can occasionally result in ineffective megakaryocytopoiesis and decreased numbers of megakaryocytes in the bone marrow.

If a bone marrow examination demonstrates a normal or increased number of megakaryocytes, several differential diagnostic possibilities are considered (Table 143–2). Thrombocytopenia can occur because of altered distribution of platelets. Normally 20% of platelets reside in the spleen and 80% circulate in the blood. When the spleen is substantially enlarged for various reasons, the splenic pool increases (i.e., the number of platelets sequestered in the spleen increases). Depending on the degree of splenomegaly, the normal blood-to-spleen platelet distribution of 80%:20% can be reduced or in extreme cases reversed. Thus, if the physical examination has revealed substantial splenomegaly, this may already provide a clue to the pathophysiology of the thrombocytopenia at hand.

Thrombocytopenia frequently develops secondary to enhanced destruction of platelets in the periphery. With increased destruction of platelets, the normal bone marrow can boost platelet production up to 10-fold normal. However, when the rate of destruction in the periphery exceeds the capacity of the bone marrow to produce platelets, thrombocytopenia ensues. Thrombocytopenia often accompanies disseminated intravascular coagulation (DIC).

Thrombotic Thrombocytopenic Purpura

Thrombotic thrombocytopenic purpura (TTP) is a rare disorder in which platelets are consumed through deposition of thrombi in the microcirculation. The diagnosis is suspected if a patient is admitted with a constellation of renal impairment, central nervous system manifestations, fever, hemolytic anemia, and thrombocytopenia. The diagnosis can be confirmed in 70% to 80% of cases through gingival biopsy showing microvascular thrombi without evidence of vasculitis. Aggressive treatment combines plasma exchange, emergency splenectomy, and high-dose corticosteroids (1–3 g methylprednisolone per day). Some authorities recommend platelet function inhibitors.

TABLE 143–2. Megakaryocytic Thrombocytopenias

Altered distribution of platelets (splenomegaly)
Enhanced destruction of platelets in the circulation
- Disseminated intravascular coagulation
- Thrombotic thrombocytopenic purpura
- Hypersplenism
- Prosthetic heart valves
- Immune thrombocytopenias

Enhanced Peripheral Platelet Destruction

A large spleen may cause a reduction in platelet count because of a simple redistribution between peripheral and splenic pools. Patients with splenomegaly, such as encountered in portal hypertension, also show evidence of enhanced platelet destruction by the spleen, referred to as *hypersplenism*. Both platelets and red blood cells can be mechanically destroyed by artificial heart valves. Finally, platelets can be destroyed in the circulation through immune mechanisms (Table 143–3).

Idiopathic Autoimmune Thrombocytopenic Purpura

The diagnosis of idiopathic autoimmune thrombocytopenic purpura (ITP) is one of exclusion. About 90% of the cases of acute ITP occur in children and are characterized by abrupt onset of severe thrombocytopenia with a benign course resolving in more than 80% of cases within 6 weeks to 6 months. It is preceded by a viral illness in 60% to 80%, especially in children. Ten per cent of acute cases are in adults, and these patients also recover regardless of treatment. The use of treatment is controversial and may actually worsen the process. Plasmapheresis and splenectomy are sometimes required in refractory cases. Intravenous infusion of gamma globulin for 5 successive days has resulted in an elevation of platelets to normal within 5 to 10 days.

Reports have described dramatic responses to infusion of large intravenous doses of preimmune immunoglobulin G (IgG) in patients with ITP. Both intact and chemically modified monomeric IgG are now available. The recommended therapeutic dosage (400 mg/kg body weight for 5 days) has resulted in satisfactory elevation of platelet levels in about two thirds of patients. A summary of the literature concerning this therapy concluded that (1) unmodified IgG preparations are probably superior to modified preparations, (2) the treatment appears less effective in patients with disease of long duration, (3) the platelet count at the time of treatment is unrelated to the response, and (4) the duration of the response is longest in patients who achieve the highest initial elevation. It has also been shown that platelet-associated immunoglobulin levels approach normal. In acute ITP that occurs in children, treatment with IgG is often curative. However, of patients with chronic ITP, usually adults, who are treated with IgG, more than 90% experience recurrent thrombocytopenia within 1 to 4 weeks. The optimal treatment regimen is still a matter of debate and ranges from 165 $mg \cdot kg^{-1} \cdot d^{-1}$ for 5 days to 1 $g \cdot kg^{-1} \cdot d^{-1}$ for 2 days. It is also suggested that later intermittent booster injections of 1 g/kg for up to 6 months may lead to remissions. It is questioned whether this expensive form of therapy, although transiently effective, will be solidly established in the treatment of chronic ITP.

TABLE 143–3. Immune Thrombocytopenias

Secondary to:
- Multiple transfusions (isoantibodies)
- Drugs
- Post-transfusion (in PL1-negative individuals, alloantibodies)
- Lymphomas
- Chronic lymphocytic leukemia
- Collagen vascular disease
- Viral infections ("acute ITP")

Idiopathic thrombocytopenic purpura

Qualitative

A platelet functional disorder, congenital or acquired, is suspected in a patient with a positive bleeding history, petechiae, ecchymoses, mucous membrane bleeding, a tendency to bruise easily, perhaps a positive family history, and a normal platelet count. Three types of functional platelet syndromes are recognized: (1) Glanzmann's thrombasthenia and Bernard-Soulier syndrome, in which the absence of platelet membrane glycoprotein prevents the platelets from adhering to connective tissue to aggregate and to support clot retraction; (2) the storage pool defects previously known as thrombocytopathies, in which platelets in response to appropriate stimuli fail to release substances such as adenosine diphosphate necessary to propagate the aggregation reaction; and (3) von Willebrand's syndrome, which does not represent a primary platelet disorder but rather a defect of cofactor protein necessary for platelet adhesion to connective tissue. However, of far greater clinical significance are the drug-induced platelet functional disorders. Platelet dysfunction can also be caused by many classes of commonly used drugs, including the nonsteroidal anti-inflammatory agents (with aspirin heading the list), β-blockers, slow calcium channel blockers, local anesthetic-type antiarrhythmic drugs, and last but not least a number of frequently used β-lactam antibiotics.

DISORDERS OF THE COAGULATION SYSTEM

Normal Blood Coagulation

Figure 143–1 is a diagram of the coagulation system. According to international agreement, individual coagulation proteins are assigned Roman numerals and their activated

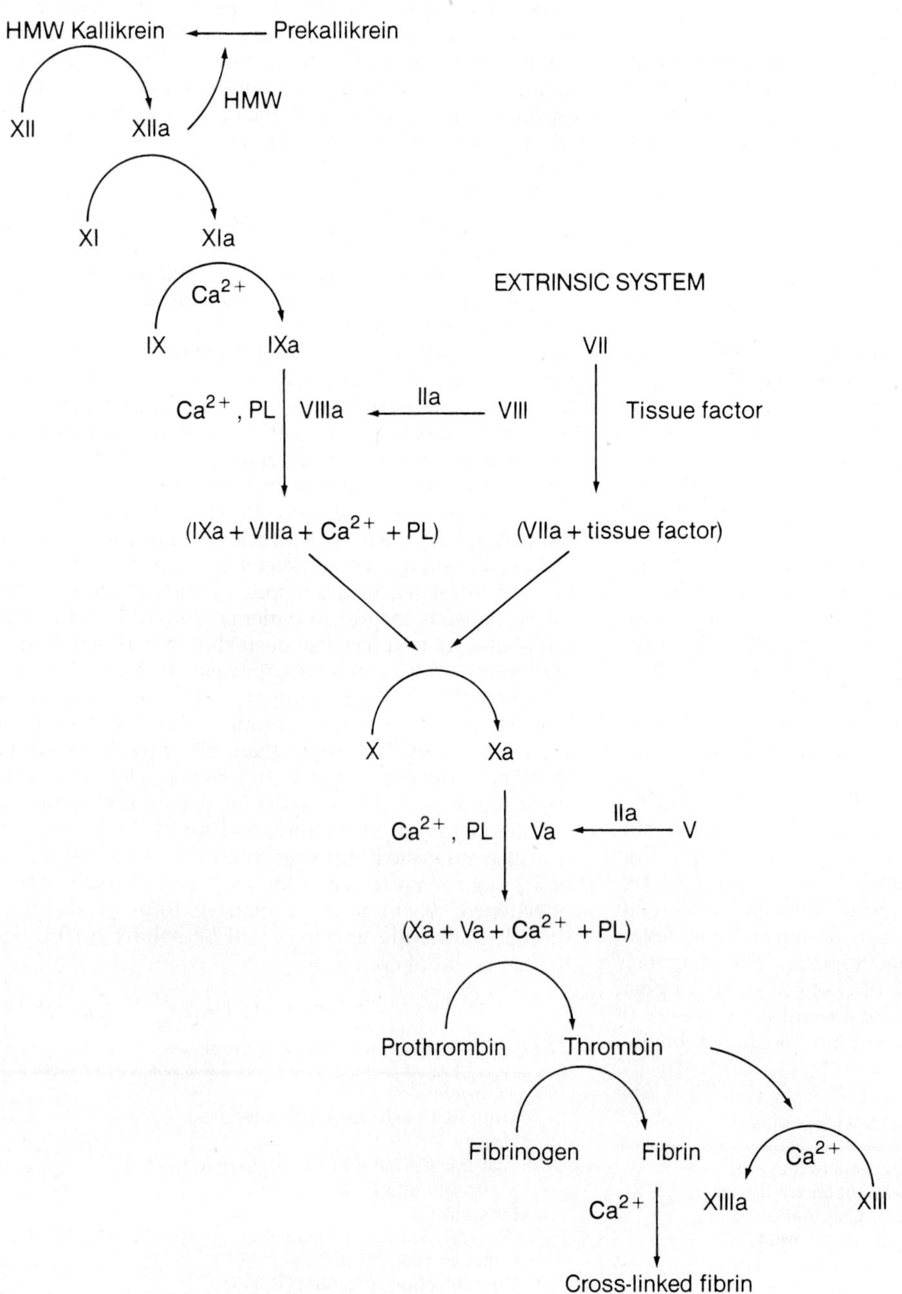

Figure 143–1. Diagram of the coagulation system (see text).

TABLE 143–4. Blood Coagulation Proteins

	Enzymes		
Final Substrate	*Transpeptidase*	*Serine Proteases*	***Cofactors***
Fibrinogen	Factor XIII	Factor XII	HMW kininogen
		Prekallikrein	
		Factor XI	
		Factor IX	Factor VII
		Factor X	Factor V
		Factor VII	Tissue factor
		Factor II	

Abbreviation: HMW = high-molecular-weight.

counterparts Roman numerals plus the letter a. Blood coagulation is best viewed as a chain reaction involving serine proteases and cofactors. The clotting factor serine proteases normally circulate as inactive proenzymes. When the first enzyme of this coagulation cascade is activated, the activated serine protease makes a clip and splits certain peptide bonds in the next proenzyme link in the chain, thereby activating it, and from this sequence of conversions of the inactive zymogen precursors to active serine proteases through limited proteolysis, the enzyme thrombin finally emerges. Thrombin makes four clips in the fibrinogen molecule, the soluble plasma protein precursor of fibrin converting fibrinogen into fibrin monomer. Fibrin monomer in turn spontaneously lines up with other fibrin molecules in a polymerization reaction, producing the insoluble network gel fibrin. Classically, two pathways of coagulation are recognized—an intrinsic and an extrinsic pathway. The intrinsic pathway is so named because it operates strictly with components contained in the blood. The extrinsic pathway is so named because it requires, in addition to blood components, tissue factor that comes in contact with blood clotting factors only under pathologic conditions, such as tissue trauma or acute and chronic inflammatory events, which make the tissue factor available on the surface of monocytes and endothelial cells. For certain steps in the chain reaction—that is, conversion of Factor IX into IXa by Factor XIa or VIIa, Factor X to Xa by Factor IXa or VIIa, and the conversion of prothrombin (Factor II) to thrombin (Factor IIa), calcium and a phospholipid bilayer membrane are required. Intrinsic as well as extrinsic blood coagulation does not occur without ionized calcium. Key steps in the coagulation reaction occur on cell surfaces. This interphase phenomenon can take place on platelets, monocytes, polymorphonuclear leukocytes, and even endothelial cells. The system operates very poorly in solution unless phospholipid liposomes, substituting for the cell bilayer membrane, are added. Table 143–4 depicts the biochemical classification of the proteins involved in blood coagulation. The final substrate in the reaction is fibrinogen, which is converted into fibrin by thrombin. The enzymes involved in coagulation are serine proteases such as trypsin, chymotrypsin, and plasmin, with one exception—namely, Factor XIII, or fibrin-stabilizing factor, which is a transpeptidase, an enzyme capable of forming new peptide bonds. This enzyme introduces new peptide bonds into fibrin, making the fibrin clot mechanically stronger as well as more resistant to degradation by proteolytic enzymes. The serine proteases of the system are Factor XII, or Hageman factor; prekallikrein; Factors XI, IX, X, and VII; and Factor II, or prothrombin. In addition, the system makes use of cofactors, proteins that in themselves possess no enzymatic activity but that boost the proteolytic activity of certain clotting factors. Thus, the protein high-M_r kininogen is important in helping activated Factor XII to activate Factor XI. Factor VIII is of crucial importance as a cofactor for activated Factor IX to activate Factor X. Factor V works in consort with Factor X to convert prothrombin into thrombin, and tissue factor is of major importance as a cofactor of Factor VII in the extrinsic pathway to activate Factor X. The two major cofactors, Factors V and VIII, possess little or no activity in themselves but become activated when exposed to minimum concentrations of thrombin or Factor Xa, which converts these cofactors to their active forms through limited proteolysis.

Figure 143–2 focuses on the earliest phases of the intrinsic pathway, the so-called contact system, to illustrate an important concept pertaining to plasma protease enzyme systems. The contact system of the blood coagulation system illustrates the general principle that plasma protein enzyme systems rarely if ever function in and of themselves but that they are interreacting systems sharing activators as well as inhibitors. To become activated, Hageman factor, or Factor XII, has to be adsorbed onto a negatively charged surface and to interact with two proteins, prekallikrein and high-M_r kininogen, long-known components of another system, the kallikrein-kinin system; the major function of this system is to produce bradykinin and other low-M_r kinins, which dilate small blood vessels, increase vascular permeability, and serve other functions in the acute or chronic inflammatory response to injury. By studying patients with genetic defi-

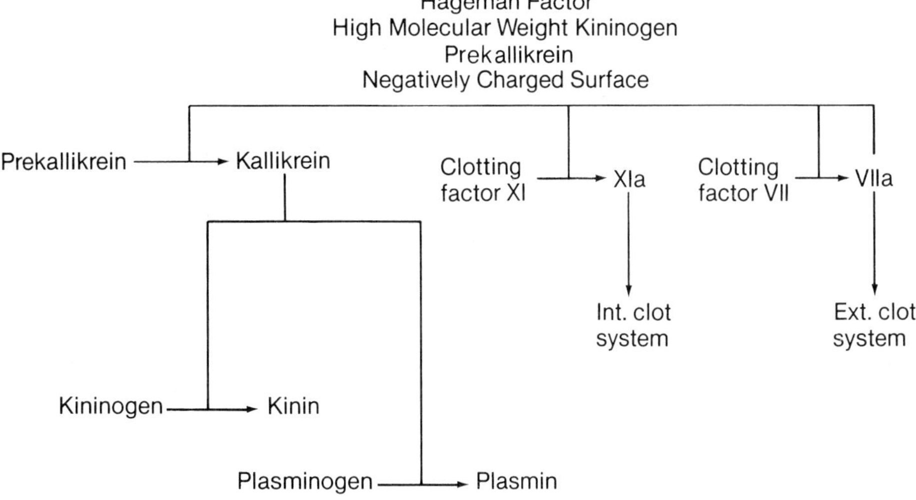

Figure 143–2. Reactions associated with "contact activation" of blood coagulation (see text). (Courtesy of J. H. Griffin, Ph.D.)

ciencies of either prekallikrein or high-molecular-weight kininogen, it became apparent that these proteins also serve as clotting factors, because patients with prekallikrein or high-molecular-weight kininogen deficiencies universally exhibit prolonged clotting times as measured in the test tube.

Once Hageman factor is activated, further activation of prekallikrein results, thereby producing the active serine protease, kallikrein. The production of kallikrein has two consequences: It releases bradykinin and vasoactive peptides from high-molecular-weight kininogen and it to some extent and through poorly defined mechanisms converts the fibrinolytic proenzyme plasminogen into fibrinolytically active plasmin. Hageman factor, once activated, converts the next zymogen in the clotting cascade, Factor XI, into activated Factor XI or XIa to produce activation of the intrinsic clotting system. As indicated in Figure 143–2, the activated Hageman factor, perhaps through activation of prekallikrein, is capable of activating the extrinsic clotting system such that the sharp division between intrinsic and extrinsic clotting mechanisms, which is very useful for practical laboratory purposes, probably is not tenable in human pathophysiology.

A perplexing dilemma in blood coagulation is that patients with identified Hageman factor, prekallikrein, or high-molecular-weight kininogen deficiency have no clinical bleeding problems although their blood exhibits markedly retarded coagulation in the test tube. Based on these discrepancies, the suggestion has been made and supported by persuasive experimental evidence that Factor XI adsorbed onto the platelet surface can undergo activation independently of activation of the contact system. However, neither the alternative activator nor the peptide bonds cleaved in this hypothetic activation step have been identified. It is also theoretically possible that the contact activation system, through activation of the fibrinolytic enzyme system, may activate the complement system, because work with purified proteins has shown that plasmin is capable of activating the C1S portion of the C1 complex of the classic pathway of complement activation independently of the C1Q component and immune complexes. A possible clinical corollary is that of Thai hemorrhagic fever (dengue), in which activation of the coagulation, fibrinolytic enzyme, and complement systems appears to occur in parallel.

The most important steps in the coagulation cascade are the IX-IXa, X-Xa, and prothrombin to thrombin conversions. Individual proteins and the diagnosis of their defects in hemophilia A and B and the more rarely encountered inherited clotting factor defects are discussed next.

In the practical diagnosis of an unknown defect of hemostasis, as previously mentioned, it generally holds that if a patient has petechiae, ecchymoses, and mucous membrane bleeding, with or without bleeding elsewhere, the physician should first consider a quantitative or qualitative platelet disorder. If, on the other hand, a patient is admitted with inappropriate bleeding into a muscle, bones, or joints, the physician should primarily suspect a defect in the fibrin-forming mechanism. If it is on a constitutional basis, it may be one of the hemophilias or other clotting disorders; if the history suggests otherwise, it may be one of the acquired coagulation disorders. It is essential to obtain a detailed history for a constitutional bleeding disorder. First, most inherited bleeding disorders, certainly hemophilia A and B, exist in all degrees of severity. The textbook picture largely refers to severe hemophilia with the frequent spontaneous hemorrhage into joints and tissues leading to crippling joint deformities. The clinical course of the mild to moderate cases of hemophilia is much less appreciated; diagnosis of these cases frequently is not made until serious or even life-threatening hemorrhage appears in conjunction with surgery or major injuries, to the surprise of the patient as well as the physician. In evaluating a bleeding history, it is therefore important to ask very specific questions about surgery and trauma. Hemophilia or other constitutional bleeding problems should be suspected if bleeding lasts for more than 24 hours after surgery. Recurrent bleeding after the first 24 hours greatly heightens the index of suspicion. Excessive postoperative bleeding limited to the first 24 hours as a rule is not due to hemophilia unless the patient had to be transfused during that time interval; unless that question is specifically asked, this information is not frequently volunteered. In obtaining a history for the neonatal period, it is important to realize that even severe hemophiliacs often endure the major trauma of delivery without bleeding complications. This protection of the newborn is not caused by transplacental transfer of maternal clotting factors, because the levels of clotting factors in severe hemophiliacs have been demonstrated to be zero in cord blood. This protection lasts for the first week or two of a child's life, and circumcision performed during the first few days of life of a hemophiliac may not cause excessive bleeding. The first symptom is a tendency to bruising occurring within the first 3 to 6 months of life. Toward the end of the first year, an affected child becomes more susceptible to injuries, and this is the time when serious bleeding abnormalities begin to occur in severely afflicted individuals.

A couple of points about the family history also need to be emphasized. The two major types of hemophilia, hemophilia A and B, are transmitted by the sex-linked recessive mode of inheritance. When a male carries the abnormal gene located in the X chromosome, he is affected by the disease. When a female carries the abnormal gene, she is a carrier. Therefore, all daughters of an affected man are carriers, as they inherit his abnormal X chromosome. None of his sons are affected, because they derive the single X chromosome from the mother. The offspring of a female carrier have a 50% chance of inheriting the abnormal X chromosome causing disease in the male and a carrier state in the female. Hemophilia A and B are the only two congenital bleeding disorders transmitted in this manner. Deficiencies in all other clotting factors as well as platelet function disorders are inherited by other mechanisms. Thus, all congenital bleeding disorders with the exception of hemophilia A and B affect males and females equally. However, it is very important to keep in mind that 25% to 30% of cases of hemophilia A and about 20% of cases of hemophilia B appear de novo—that is, with a negative family history. These de novo cases are almost always severe and must represent gene mutations in recent generations.

Thus, the diagnosis of a constitutional clotting factor deficiency can never be made by history or physical examination alone but requires a series of simple laboratory tests to be unequivocally established. Figure 143–3 is a simplified scheme that divides the clotting reactions into three different boxes. Clotting factors in box 1, Factors XII, XI, IX, and VIII (in addition to prekallikrein and high-molecular-weight kininogen), are the four factors strictly involved in the intrinsic mechanism. Box 2 contains only one clotting factor, namely Factor VII, the only factor needed in the extrinsic but not the intrinsic pathway. Box 3 contains four factors, X, V, II, and I—that is, factors required in the final activation steps that are common for both pathways, the extrinsic and the intrinsic. The box system is convenient because it tells you how to use two simple routine clotting tests, the prothrombin time test and the activated partial thromboplastin time (APTT) test, to help in the correct diagnosis of an

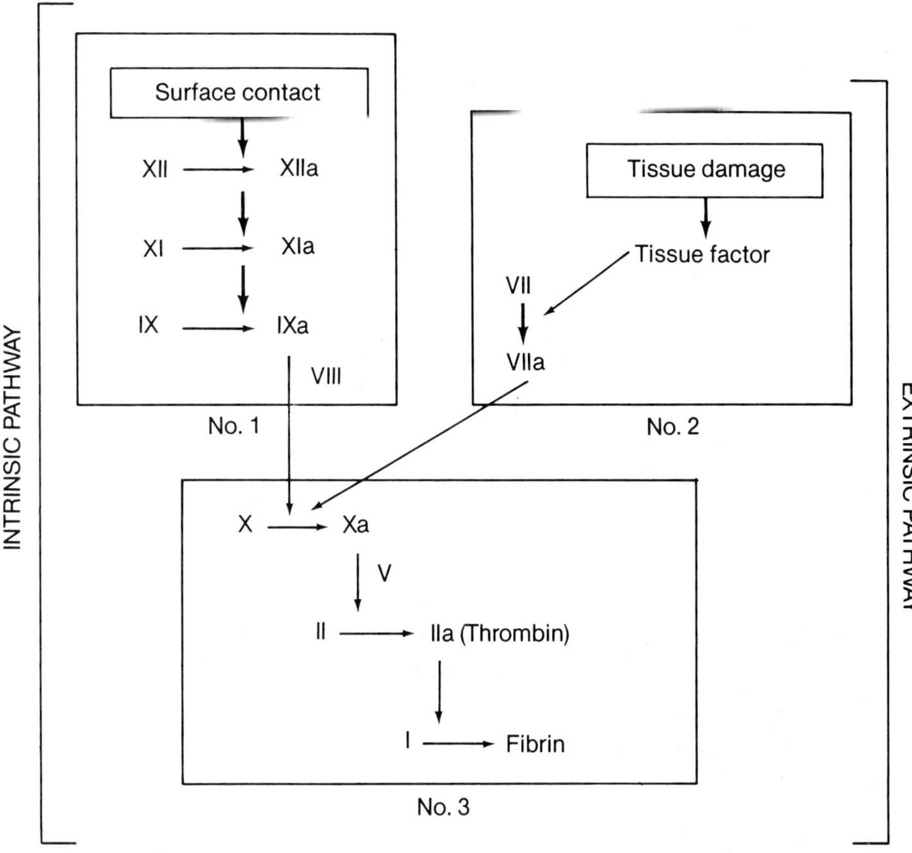

Figure 143–3. A simplified scheme of the clotting mechanism (see text).

CLOTTING FACTORS MEASURED IN THE PTT

Hageman (XII)
PTA (XI)
PTC (IX)
AHG (VIII)
Stuart (X)
Ac globulin (V)
Prothrombin (II)
Fibrinogen (I)

CLOTTING FACTORS MEASURED IN THE PRO-TIME

Proconvertin (VII)
Stuart factor (X)
Ac globulin (V)
Prothrombin (II)
Fibrinogen (I)

	POSSIBLE COAGULATION DEFECT
Patient 1. Pro-time normal, PTT prolonged	XII, XI, IX, VIII
Patient 2. Pro-time prolonged, PTT normal	VII
Patient 3. Pro-time prolonged, PTT prolonged	X, V, II, I

unknown constitutional bleeding disorder (Figs. 143–4 and 143–5). To determine the prothrombin time, mix the patient's plasma, a source of the tissue factor necessary to activate the extrinsic mechanism, and calcium ions. Prolongation of the prothrombin time denotes that the extrinsic pathway is no longer intact. The affected factor could be one of five—proconvertin, or Factor VII; Stuart factor, or Factor X; AC globulin, or Factor V; prothrombin, or Factor II; or fibrinogen, or Factor I. The prothrombin time does not measure factors that are strictly concerned with the intrinsic mechanism—Hageman factor, or Factor XII; PTA, or Factor XI; Christmas factor, or Factor IX; antihemophilic globulin, or Factor VIII. Note that Factors VIII and IX, which are deficient in the more common forms of hemophilia, are not picked up by the prothrombin time. Thus, the prothrombin time is perfectly normal in patients suffering from either hemophilia A or B. For the APTT test (Fig. 143–5), mix the patient's plasma and phospholipid liposomes mimicking cell membrane phospholipid bilayers and again calcium ions, without which intrinsic and extrinsic clotting is impossible. Negatively charged substances such as kaolin or celite or ellagic acid are also added to maximally activate Hageman factor, thereby ensuring maximum activation of the intrinsic coagulation mechanism. Prolongation of the partial thromboplastin time means a deficiency somewhere along the intrinsic pathway. One link in the chain is weak or missing. For instance, both Factor VIII and IX deficiency of hemophilia A and B result in prolongation of the APTT. The test becomes particularly valuable if combined with the prothrombin time.

The simplified coagulation scheme depicted in Figure 143–3 shows the three possible permutations that may be encountered in evaluating a patient with an unknown constitutional bleeding disorder. If for instance a patient shows a normal prothrombin time and a prolonged APTT, factor deficiency is precluded in boxes 2 and 3. The defect must be among Factors XII, XI, IX, and VIII, in box 1. All are strictly concerned with the intrinsic clotting mechanism. If a pro-

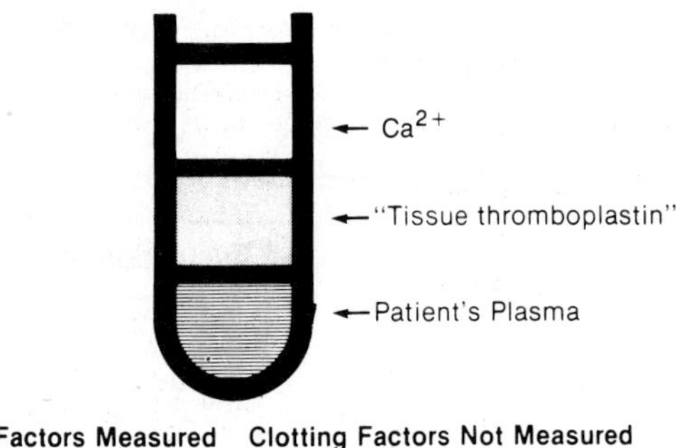

Clotting Factors Measured	Clotting Factors Not Measured
Proconvertin (VII)	Hageman (XII)
Stuart factor (X)	PTA (XI)
Ac globulin (V)	PTC (IX)
Prothrombin (II)	AHG (VIII)
Fibrinogen (I)	FSFV (XIII)
	Plate factors

Figure 143–4. Principles of the prothrombin time test.

longed prothrombin time and a normal APTT are found in another patient, abnormalities along the intrinsic pathway are precluded—that is, clotting factors contained in boxes 1 and 3. The only clotting factor abnormality producing this permutation is a deficiency in Factor VII. If both the prothrombin time and the APTT are prolonged, the defect must lie somewhere in that part of the activation sequence that is common to both pathways—that is, the clotting factors contained in box 3, clotting Factors X, V, II, and I. To localize the defect further, we make use of the so-called substituted APTT (Fig. 143–6). To treat a patient whose prothrombin time is normal and APTT grossly abnormal, a physician would suspect abnormal activities of one of four clotting factors strictly operative along the intrinsic pathway contained in box 1, Factors VIII, IX, XI, and XII. Illustrated in Figure 143–6 is the differential diagnosis between Factor VIII and Factor IX deficiency, hemophilia A and B. The patient's plasma, previously shown to produce a prolonged APTT, is admixed with plasmas known to be severely deficient in Factor VIII or Factor IX. In the modern laboratory, appropriate reagents from patients with known clotting factor deficiencies or plasma specimens from which a specific clotting factor has been removed through immunoabsorption are stored away in the freezer. High-quality reagents from these diagnostic tests are readily available through commercial sources. In this case, add to the unknown

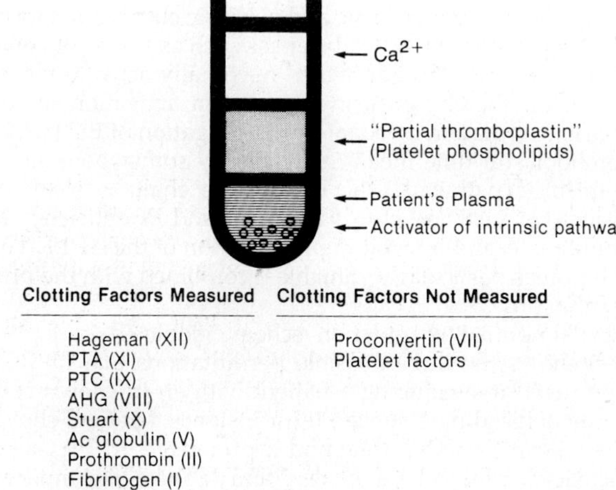

Figure 143–5. Principles of the activated partial thromboplastin time test.

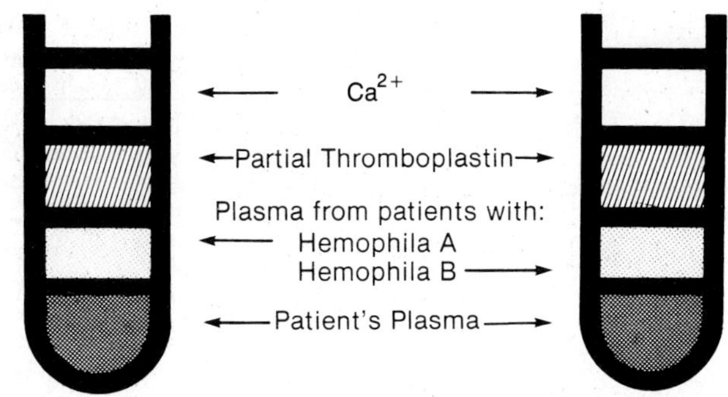

Figure 143–6. The differential diagnosis between hemophilia A and B (see text).

plasma, in turn, plasmas deficient in Factor VIII or Factor IX. If the prolonged APTT is corrected with hemophilia A plasma, the patient must suffer from hemophilia B. If, on the other hand, the prolonged APTT is corrected with hemophilia B but not hemophilia A plasma, the patient must suffer from hemophilia A. If no correction occurs with either hemophilia A or hemophilia B plasma, that patient may likely have deficiencies of either Factor XI or XII; this can be checked in the same fashion by performing APTTs on mixtures of aliquots of the patient's plasma and plasma grossly deficient in Factor XI or XII. If the patient's prothrombin time as well as APTT is abnormal, return to the clotting factors in box 3, the clotting factors common for both the extrinsic and intrinsic pathways. Using the same substitution strategy, the patient's plasma is tested in the APTT system mixed with plasma deficient in Factors V, X, and II. Congenital or acquired deficiency in fibrinogen is readily quantified in the test system where excess thrombin is added to the patient's plasma; fibrinogen can then be measured using a calibration curve and a standard plasma sample of predetermined fibrinogen content. In mild hemophilia, the APTT is occasionally at the upper limit of normal or marginally prolonged. In these cases, specific factor assays must be used. Clotting factor assays are variants of the APTT that essentially measure the degree to which a patient's plasma corrects the defect of a plasma known to contain zero or near zero levels of the clotting factor to be determined. Unfortunately, factor assays are not universally available in small hospital laboratories. Factor assays are not difficult to set up and standardize, and without the availability of factor assays, an emergency physician may occasionally face a serious dilemma in instituting correct therapy in a patient who has not been diagnosed as having mild hemophilia and who bleeds uncontrollably after trauma or during surgery.

LIVER DISEASE

The coagulation defects encountered in severe chronic liver disease are complex and multifactorial. The liver synthesizes all procoagulant proteins, with the possible exception of Factor VIII:c, and decreased synthesis of these proteins may in and of itself result in serious coagulation defects and bleeding problems. The synthesis of the vitamin K–dependent procoagulants is usually affected the earliest, followed by Factors V, XI, and XII. Cholestasis and malabsorption may further suppress the biosynthesis of vitamin K clotting factors; most clinicians would recommend a single test dose of 10 to 15 mg of vitamin K_1 to establish whether the clotting defect is in part correctable. Fibrinogen biosynthesis is maintained at normal levels until the very end, and a low level of fibrinogen in the absence of symptoms and signs of

DIC is of grave prognostic significance. Clotting Factor VIII levels always remain normal or elevated even in end-stage liver disease, and low levels of Factor VIII in liver disease strongly suggest the complication of DIC. A perplexing coagulation defect in liver disease is acquired dysfibrinogenemia, first demonstrated in patients with hepatoma but also demonstrated in a sizable number of patients with cirrhosis of the liver. The abnormal fibrinogen in liver disease is more heavily glycosylated than normal fibrinogen, with a sharp increase in total hexose, hexosamine, and sialic acid. This abnormal protein converts normally to fibrin monomer, but fibrin monomer polymerization is slow and inefficient. Because all clotting tests depend on the rate of appearance of a fibrin clot, an abnormal fibrinogen level can produce spuriously low values in clotting tests, such as the prothrombin time and the APTT. The diagnosis of dysfibrinogenemia is made in the special laboratory using the so-called thrombin clotting time and measuring fibrinogen through chronometric assays and immunoassays.

DISSEMINATED INTRAVASCULAR COAGULATION

Once considered a complication encountered occasionally in obstetric practice, DIC is currently a more commonly noted hematologic complication and occurs in association with disease states treated by the entire spectrum of medical and surgical practice. Today, with improved laboratory techniques, it is apparent that DIC exists in varying degrees ranging from life-threatening, acute, and severe to mild or more chronic. In acute DIC, fibrin deposition in the microcirculation and consumption of clotting factors and platelets occur more quickly than they can be synthesized by the liver and bone marrow. Consequently, the levels of circulating consumable clotting factors (fibrinogen and Factors V, VIII, XIII, and II) and circulating platelets sharply decrease. Compensatory fibrinolytic mechanisms are almost always operative; as a consequence, high levels of fibrinogen-fibrin split products are readily demonstrable in the serum of patients with acute DIC. In contrast, in chronic DIC, fibrin deposition and consumption of clotting factors are thought to proceed more slowly, to permit hepatic synthesis of clotting factors and even bone marrow production of platelets to keep pace. The body possesses an impressive capability for the compensatory production of platelets and clotting factors to maintain adequate hemostasis. Thus, the bone marrow can generate 10 times the usual number of platelets, and the liver can synthesize at least five times the amount of fibrinogen it produces under normal baseline conditions. The rate of synthesis may occasionally exceed the consumption rate, and the net result is the higher than normal levels of fibrinogen and Factors V, VIII, and XIII and platelet counts that may be normal or only mildly depressed. In chronic DIC states, compensatory fibrinolytic mechanisms are also active, producing high levels of fibrinogen-fibrin split products in the circulation. Unless suitable measurements for fibrinogen-fibrin split products are performed, the diagnosis of chronic DIC cannot be made in a significant number of cases. Table 143–5 summarizes the many clinical situations in which DIC can be encountered as a complication and underscores the magnitude of the problem.

TABLE 143–5. Disease States Associated with Disseminated Intravascular Coagulation

Category		*Clinical Situation*
Obstetric complications		Abruptio placentae
		Amniotic fluid embolism
		Dead fetus syndrome
		Eclampsia (preeclampsia?)
		Placenta previa
		Placenta accreta
		Abortion (hypertonic saline solution)
		Hydatid mole
		Extrauterine pregnancy
		Forceps delivery
		Normal delivery
Tissue trauma		Major surgery
		Major trauma and burns
		Fat embolism
		Rejection of transplants
		Heat stroke
Hemolytic processes		Transfusion of mismatched blood
		Drowning
		Acute hemolysis secondary infection
		Immune mechanisms
		Acid ingestion
Malignant neoplasms		Solid tumors
		Leukemias-lymphomas
Snakebites		Acute myocardial infarction (usually associated with cardiogenic shock)
Cardiovascular system		Circulatory collapse from any cause
		Severe progressive strokes
		Aortic aneurysms and Kasabach-Merritt syndrome (local intravascular coagulation)
Chronic liver disease		
Infections	Bacterial	Gram-negative meningococcal and pneumococcal septicemias
	Rickettsial	Rocky Mountain spotted fever
	Viral	Hemorrhagic smallpox, hemorrhagic fevers (Thai, Korean, and others)
	Mycotic	Acute histoplasmosis
	Parasitic	Malaria (particularly falciparum)
Miscellaneous		Acute and chronic renal disease (?)
		Collagen vascular disorders
		Thrombotic thrombocytopenic purpura (?)
		Hemolytic-uremic syndrome (?)
		Purpura fulminans
		Acute pancreatitis
		Allergic vasculitis
		Amyloidosis
		Polycythemia vera
		Thrombocythemia
		Ulcerative colitis

(From Bang NU: Disseminated intravascular coagulation. *In:* Laboratory Evaluation of Coagulation. Triplett DA [Ed]. Chicago, American Society of Clinical Pathologists Press, 1982.)

Pathogenesis

In many clinical situations, the basic mechanism in DIC is probably the availability of tissue factor in the circulation and the consequent activation of clotting via the extrinsic pathway. Whenever substantial and traumatic tissue damage or large areas of tissue necrosis occur, the possibility of complicating DIC must always be kept in mind. Tissue factor may not only enter blood vessels from surrounding damaged tissues but can also arise when cells in direct contact with circulating blood (i.e., monocytes and endothelial cells) are triggered to synthesize and express tissue factor on their cell membranes. This is most likely the mechanism responsible for the frequent occurrence of DIC in endotoxemia but may also be implicated in numerous other inflammatory states in which monokines such as interleukin-1 and tumor necrosis factor are synthesized and secreted. Other mechanisms implicated in DIC include the release of thromboplastin-like substances from red blood cells during acute hemolysis, particularly after transfusion of mismatched blood, and the secretion of certain proteases from leukemic or solid tumor cells capable of "bypassing" the normal coagulation mechanisms through direct activation of Factor X. Such proteases have been demonstrated particularly in acute promyelocytic leukemia, which carries an almost 100% risk for DIC and mucinous adenocarcinomas. In patients with solid tumors, DIC is usually chronic and the hemorrhagic tendency is usually mild, but major vessel thrombosis is a frequent complication.

Disseminated Intravascular Coagulation Versus Primary Fibrinolysis

It was previously reported that blood obtained from some patients clotted in the test tube but soon liquefied again. Subsequently, the connection was established between enhanced levels of fibrinolytic activity and bleeding under these conditions. In these clinical situations, the designation of pathologic or primary fibrinolytic states became popular. It has become increasingly obvious from critical reviews of previously published cases that the diagnosis of a primary fibrinolytic state is untenable in most cases; many investigators seriously question whether the bleeding resulting from primary fibrinolysis is a bona fide clinical entity. Most cases previously reported as primary fibrinolysis were later interpreted as being fibrinolysis secondary to DIC. At this time, most workers in the field tend to regard DIC as the primary event and fibrinolysis as the compensatory physiologic repair mechanism. Depending on the magnitude of the fibrinolytic response, whether it is feeble or whether it grossly overshoots, we may encounter a clinical picture in which either DIC or fibrinolysis predominates; however, an element of each process—clotting and lysis—is almost always present.

Disseminated Intravascular Coagulation in Liver Disease

Coagulation problems in acute and chronic parenchymal liver disease are numerous and difficult to sort out. Several mechanisms are responsible—for example, suppression of synthesis of procoagulant proteins, thrombocytopenia secondary to hypersplenism, acute ethanol intoxication, and folate deficiency, as well as the inability of the severely injured liver to clear activated clotting factors and fibrinolytic enzymes from the circulation. Although some have questioned the existence of DIC syndrome associated with severe, acute, and chronic liver disease, most clinicians today are convinced that DIC occurs with some frequency in liver disease, often representing a serious complication. Arguments in favor of the occurrence of the DIC syndrome in acute and chronic parenchymal liver disease are increased levels of fibrinogen-fibrin degradation products and shortened fibrinogen survival improved by heparin.

Diagnosis

In the acute forms of DIC, the diagnosis is strongly suspected from the findings of a combination of low-level fibrinogen, a prolonged prothrombin time, and an APTT reflecting low levels of consumable clotting Factors V, VIII, and II and thrombocytopenia. To substantiate the diagnosis, a test for fibrinogen-fibrin split products in serum by immunoassay (ThromboWellco test) is necessary.

In diagnosing the chronic forms of DIC, one cannot rely on low levels of fibrinogen, a prolonged prothrombin time and APTT, and a low platelet count. All of these variables may be normal or nearly normal, and the diagnosis can be made only through the demonstration of high levels of fibrinogen and fibrin split products in serum. Additional tests have been suggested to reflect the presence of soluble fibrin complexes in plasma, which are soluble intermediates between fibrinogen and fibrin. The addition of protamine sulfate or ethanol causes these soluble intermediates to form a gel. The protamine sulfate and ethanol gelation tests, when strongly positive, in most cases confirm the suspicion of DIC. However, a weakly positive result is not of great value because false positives and false negatives may occur.

High levels of fibrinogen-fibrin split products are not specific for DIC. In large aortic aneurysms, fibrin is being deposited and dissolved with rapid turnover, thereby producing high circulating levels of fibrinogen-fibrin split products. Similarly, in the giant hemangioma of the Kasabach-Merritt syndrome, fibrin turnover is rapid enough to elevate sharply the levels of fibrinogen-fibrin degradation products.

Fibrinogen-fibrin degradation products are elevated frequently in various acute and chronic glomerular disorders, most likely reflecting localized intravascular coagulation in renal glomeruli. Elevated fibrinogen-fibrin split products should not be considered evidence for DIC in the setting of acute or chronic renal disease. The one important exception to this rule is acute renal failure associated with shock from gram-negative septicemia or other causes in which renal glomeruli represent only one of many target organs for microcirculatory thrombosis. Of special importance is the recognition that DIC occurs as a complication of gram-negative septicemia of septic abortion because pregnant women are at a very high risk for the development of bilateral renal cortical necrosis in conjunction with DIC.

Clinical Features

In acute DIC, bleeding combined with multiple organ failure is usual. Frequent bleeding problems include severe gastrointestinal bleeding, hematuria, oozing from venipuncture sites, and large areas of ecchymoses. These bleeding problems are often accompanied by acute renal failure. Chronic DIC as observed in certain malignancies usually produces mild bleeding problems (with the exception of metastatic cancer of the prostate, which usually produces the more acute picture of DIC). Chronic DIC is often complicated by major vessel thrombosis, usually deep vein thrombosis or pulmonary embolism, which characteristically responds poorly to heparin or oral anticoagulant therapy and tends to be recurrent. In some instances, thrombosis of medium-sized arteries can occur, leading to gangrene of the lower extremities. Chronic DIC is occasionally accompanied by heavy fibrin deposition in renal glomeruli and the development of renal failure.

Treatment

The most controversial issue in DIC is therapy, and the controversies remain so deep that it is impossible to make specific recommendations at this time. Through the late 1950s, the recommended treatment was replacement with whole fresh blood, platelets, clotting factors such as fibrinogen, and fresh frozen plasma containing, in addition to fibrinogen, clotting Factors V and VIII. In the late 1950s, attention was focused mainly on the fibrinolytic component of DIC states; for that reason, the fibrinolytic enzyme system inhibitor ϵ-aminocaproic acid (EACA) (Amicar) was introduced as the specific treatment of choice for patients with hypofibrinogenemic hemorrhage. Although initial case reports were encouraging, subsequent experience has taught us differently. Between 1959 and 1968, the author personally treated 51 patients with DIC with Amicar, with an 80%

failure rate. Serious complications were occasionally encountered in the form of major vessel thrombosis, particularly thrombotic strokes; on two occasions, patients with cirrhosis of the liver and hypofibrinogenemic hemorrhage lapsed into hepatic coma during treatment with Amicar. It is likely that this complication occurs because EACA effectively competes with essential amino acids for transmembrane transport, thereby further reducing hepatocyte protein synthesis. Today there is almost universal agreement that EACA has little if any role in the treatment of DIC states.

In the early 1960s, treatment with heparin was instituted based on the reasoning that heparin would block the fundamental problem of enhanced clotting activity. Heparin given in doses ranging from 150 to 600 $U \cdot kg^{-1} \cdot d^{-1}$ and usually in combination with suitable replacement measures was the mainstay of treatment of DIC syndromes during the next 10 to 15 years. Widespread use of heparin was based almost entirely on anecdotal material, isolated case reports, and small uncontrolled clinical trials. A prospective controlled clinical trial has never been performed, and even retrospective analyses are lacking. Table 143–6 is a retrospective analysis of the outcome of heparin treatment in DIC from the author's laboratory, based on records from Indiana University Hospitals from 1966 to 1974. This series of cases has been broken into three categories: two categories of severe acute DIC and one group of patients with chronic DIC. Patients in all three groups received heparin in full dosages comparable to those given to patients with acute pulmonary embolism. One group of patients with acute DIC included those with meningococcal septicemia and the Waterhouse-Friderichsen syndrome, a specialized form of DIC producing bilateral adrenal cortical necrosis. This group comprised only three patients; however, in view of the grave prognosis in these cases, it was encouraging to note two survivors. Similar encouraging results have been reported by others. A larger group was composed of patients with acute severe DIC due to various causes. Most of these patients had cirrhosis of the liver or gram-negative septicemia. The series encompassed only six obstetric and surgical cases. For the whole group, the failure rate in heparin-treated patients was 90%. Twelve patients with chronic DIC were given treatment with heparin. Most had solid tumors, often presenting with deep vein thrombosis and mild bleeding diathesis with laboratory evidence of chronic DIC. This small group of patients fared somewhat better.

TABLE 143–6. Retrospective Analysis of Results of Heparin Treatment in Disseminated Intravascular Coagulation

Disseminated Intravascular Coagulation	*No. of Patients*	*After Heparin Therapy*	
		Improved	*Unchanged, Deteriorated, Died*
Acute			
Meningococcal septicemia, Waterhouse-Friderichsen syndrome	3	2	1
All other causes (mainly cirrhosis and/or gram-negative septicemia)	41	6	35
Chronic			
Major vessel thrombosis (mainly solid tumors)	12	7	5

(From Bang NU: Disseminated intravascular coagulation. *In:* Laboratory evaluation of Coagulation. Triplett DA [Ed]. Chicago, American Society of Clinical Pathologists Press, 1982.)

TABLE 143–7. Therapy for Disseminated Intravascular Coagulation

When Indicated	*Treatment*	*Degree of Certainty*
Always	Treat underlying disease when possible	Established
Almost never	ϵ-Aminocaproic acid (Amicar)	Established
Chronic DIC, with major vessel thrombosis	Heparin, full dose	Reasonable
Acute DIC	Substitution therapy and full-dose heparin	Most uncertain
	Antithrombin III preactivated with small doses of heparin in sufficient quantity to correct calculated antithrombin III deficiency	Speculative
	Platelet function inhibitors to prevent release of platelet factor 4	Speculative
	Cold-insoluble globulin to improve reticuloendothelial function	Speculative

(From Bang NU: Disseminated intravascular coagulation. *In:* Laboratory Evaluation of Coagulation. Triplett DA [Ed]. Chicago, American Society of Clinical Pathologists Press, 1982.)

Among the 12 patients, we saw definitive improvement in 7 after treatment with heparin. Based on these studies, we have at this point largely abandoned heparin as treatment in acute DIC at Indiana University Hospitals and currently use heparin only in patients with chronic DIC with concurrent major vessel thrombosis. Based on past failures and newer information, Table 143–7 summarizes the different modalities of treatment of DIC. The one most important principle in the treatment of DIC agreed on by everybody is to treat the underlying cause. If you can treat effectively an obstetric emergency or gram-negative septicemia, this is by far the most effective measure; in most instances, specific forms of treatment, such as heparin, need not be considered. One additional issue that has been resolved with reasonable certainty is that EACA, the fibrinolytic enzyme inhibitor, has little if any role in the treatment of DIC; in chronic DIC, limited experience demonstrates that heparin has some role. In acute DIC, with the possible exception of the special case of meningococcal septicemia, the author concluded from his figures that the therapeutic approach used earlier—full-dosage heparin combined with various replacement measures—is an unsatisfactory solution. The theoretic alternative of replacement of antithrombin III–heparin cofactor, which is often sharply reduced in DIC in combination with low-dose heparin, remains largely speculative. However, it is believed that the approach of treating DIC with purified antithrombin III and low-dose heparin should be tested in controlled clinical trials in an attempt to improve what has been a truly dismal record.

Suggested Reading

Hemostasis and Normal Platelet Function

Berndt MC, Caen JP: Platelet glycoproteins. Prog Haemost Thromb 1984; 7:111.

Colman RW: Platelet activation: Role of an ADP receptor. Semin Hematol 1986; 23:119.

Hardesty RM: Molecular mechanism of platelet adhesion. Adv Exp Med Biol 1985; 191:411.

Lawler J: The structural and functional properties of thrombospondin. Blood 1986; 67:1197.

Leung L, Nachman R: Molecular mechanisms of platelet aggregation. Annu Rev Med 1986; 37:179.
Marguerie GA, Ginsberg MH, Plow EF: Fibrinogen and platelet function. Adv Exp Med Biol 1985; 191:41.
Peerschke EI: The platelet fibrinogen receptor. Semin Hematol 1985; 22:241.
Shapiro SS: Characterization of factor VIII receptors. Adv Exp Med Biol 1985; 192:55.
Silverstein RL, Leung LL, Nachman RL: Thrombospondin: A versatile multifunctional glycoprotein. Arteriosclerosis 1986; 6:245.

Quantitative Platelet Disorders

Bussel JB, Pham LC: Intravenous treatment with gammaglobulin in adults with immune thrombocytopenic purpura: Review of the literature. Vox Sang 1987; 52:206.
Colvin BT: Thrombocytopenia. Clin Haematol 1985; 14:661.
Hamilton GC: Platelet count. Emerg Med Clin North Am 1986; 4:75.
Karpatkin S: Autoimmune thrombocytopenic purpura. Semin Hematol 1985; 22:260.
Kelton JG: Heparin-induced thrombocytopenia. Haemostasis 1986; 16:173.
Kulkarni GA, Pellegrini JR, Nathanson L: Thrombotic thrombocytopenic purpura. Am Fam Physician 1985; 31:141.
Machin SJ: Clinical annotation. Thrombotic thrombocytopenic purpura. Br J Haematol 1984; 56:191.
Martin JN Jr, Morrison JC, Files JC: Autoimmune thrombocytopenic purpura: Current concepts and recommended practices. Am J Obstet Gynecol 1984; 150:86.
Moore SB: Post-transfusion purpura: A brief review. Ir Med J 1985; 78:365.
Rote NS, Lau RJ: Immunologic thrombocytopenic purpura. Clin Obstet Gynecol 1985; 28:84.
Sheehan RG: Thrombopoiesis and thrombokinetics—an approach to the evaluation of thrombocytopenia. Am J Med Sci 1985; 289:168.
Shende A: Idopathic thrombocytopenic purpura in children. Pediatr Ann 1985; 14:609.
Sills RH: Thrombotic thrombocytopenic purpura. I. Pathophysiology and clinical manifestations. Am J Pediatr Hematol Oncol 1984; 6:425.

Qualitative Platelet Disorders and Platelet Function Tests

Bang NU, Kammer RB: Hematologic complications associated with beta-lactam antibiotics. Rev Infect Dis 1983; 5:S380.
Bussel JB, Hilgartner MW: The use and mechanism of action of intravenous immunoglobin in the treatment of immune haematologic disease. Br J Haematol 1984; 56:1.
Day HJ, Rao AK: Evaluation of platelet function. Semin Hematol 1986; 23:89.
Eisenstaedt R: Blood component therapy in the treatment of platelet disorders. Semin Hematol 1986; 23:1.
George JN, Nurden AT, Phillips DR: Molecular defects in interactions of platelets with the vessel wall. N Engl J Med 1984; 311:1084.
Lind SE: Prolonged bleeding time. Am J Med 1984; 77:305.
Rao AK, Holmsen H: Congenital disorders of platelet function. Semin Hematol 1986; 23:102.
White JG: Platelet granule disorders. CRC Crit Rev Oncol Hematol 1986; 4:337.

The Coagulation System and Coagulation Tests

Angelos MG, Hamilton GC: Coagulation studies: Prothrombin time, partial thromboplastin time, bleeding time. Emerg Med Clin North Am 1986; 4:95.
Bevers EM, Rosing J, Zwall RF: Development of procoagulant binding sites on the platelet surface. Adv Exp Med Biol 1985; 192:359.
Mann KG: Membrane-bound enzyme complexes in blood coagulation. Prog Hemost Thromb 1984; 7:1.
Mann KG: The biochemistry of coagulation. Clin Lab Med 1984; 4:207.
Walsh PN: Platelet-mediated coagulant protein interactions in hemostasis. Semin Hematol 1985; 22:178.

Acquired Coagulation Disorders

Bang NU: Disseminated intravascular coagulation. *In*: Laboratory Evaluation of Coagulation. Triplett DA (Ed). Chicago, American Society of Clinical Pathologists Press, 1982, p 143.
Bang NU, Tessler SS, Heidenreich RO, et al: Effects of moxalactam on blood coagulation and platelet function. Rev Infect Dis 1982; 4:S546.
Espinoza LR, Hartmann RC: Significance of the lupus anticoagulant. Am J Hematol 1986; 22:331.
Harris EN, Gharavi AE, Asherson RA, et al: Antiphospholipid antibodies: A review. Eur J Rheumatol Inflamm 1984; 7:5.
Kelly DA, Tuddenham EG: Haemostatic problems in liver disease. Gut 1986; 27:339.
Owen CA Jr, Bowie EJW: Chronic intravascular coagulation and fibrinolysis (ICF) syndromes (disseminated intravascular coagulation). Semin Thromb Hemost 1977; 3:4.
Rock WA Jr: Laboratory assessment of coagulation disorders in liver disease. Clin Lab Med 1984; 4:419.

CHAPTER 144

Diagnosis and Treatment of Venous Thromboembolism

Russel D. Hull, MBBS, MSc • Graham F. Pineo, MD
Gary E. Raskob, BSc, MSc

Venous thromboembolism (venous thrombosis, pulmonary embolism, or both) usually complicates the course of sick, hospitalized patients but may also affect ambulant and otherwise apparently healthy individuals.[1–3] Pulmonary embolism remains the commonest preventable cause of hospital death and is responsible for approximately 150,000 to 200,000 deaths per year in the United States. Most patients who die from pulmonary embolism succumb suddenly or within 2 hours of the acute event, before therapy can be initiated or can take effect.[4] Effective prophylaxis against venous thromboembolism is now available for most high-risk patients.[5–7] Prophylaxis is more effective in preventing death and morbidity from venous thromboembolism than is treatment of the established disease.

PATHOPHYSIOLOGY

Venous thrombi are composed predominantly of fibrin and red cells and have a variable platelet and leukocyte component. The formation, growth, and dissolution of venous thromboemboli represent a balance between various thrombogenic stimuli and several protective mechanisms. The factors that predispose to the development of venous thromboemboli are venous stasis, activation of blood coagulation, and vascular damage. The protective mechanisms that counteract these thrombogenic stimuli include (1) the inactivation of activated coagulation factors by circulating inhibitors (e.g., antithrombin III, α_2-macroglobulin, alpha$_1$ antitrypsin, and activated protein C); (2) clearance of activated coagulation factors and soluble fibrin polymer complexes by the reticuloendothelial system and by the liver; and (3) dissolution of fibrin by fibrinolytic enzymes derived from plasma and endothelial cells, and digestion of fibrin by leukocytes.

Various risk factors predispose to the development of venous thromboembolism (Table 144–1).

Pulmonary embolism originates from thrombi in the deep veins of the leg in 90% or more of patients.[8–12] Other, less common, sources of pulmonary embolism include the deep pelvic veins, the renal veins, the inferior vena cava, the right ventricle, and the axillary veins. Most clinically important pulmonary emboli arise from thrombi in the popliteal or

TABLE 144–1. Factors Predisposing to the Development of Venous Thromboembolism

Clinical Risk Factors
Surgical and nonsurgical trauma
Previous venous thromboembolism
Immobilization
Malignant disease
Heart disease
Leg paralysis
Age (>40 years)
Obesity
Estrogens
Parturition
Inherited or acquired abnormalities
Protein C deficiency
Protein S deficiency
Antithrombin-III deficiency
Dysfibrinogenemia
Heparin-induced thrombocytopenia

more proximal deep veins of the leg. Pulmonary embolism occurs in 50% of patients with objectively documented proximal vein thrombosis; many of these emboli are asymptomatic.[9] Usually, only part of the thrombus embolizes, and 50% to 70% of patients with angiographically documented pulmonary embolism have detectable deep venous thrombosis of the legs at the time of presentation. The clinical significance of pulmonary embolism depends on the size of the embolus and the cardiorespiratory reserve of the patient.[8]

CLINICAL FEATURES

The clinical features of venous thrombosis include leg pain, tenderness and swelling, a palpable cord, discoloration, venous distention, and prominence of the superficial veins, and cyanosis. The clinical diagnosis of venous thrombosis is highly nonspecific because none of the symptoms or signs is unique, and each may be caused by nonthrombotic disorders. Patients with relatively minor symptoms and signs may have extensive deep venous thrombi, whereas those with florid leg pain and swelling, suggesting extensive deep venous thrombosis, may have negative results on objective testing. Thus, objective testing is mandatory to confirm or exclude a diagnosis of venous thrombosis.[13]

The clinical presentation of pulmonary embolism depends on the size, location, and number of emboli, and on the patient's underlying cardiorespiratory reserve. The clinical manifestations of acute pulmonary embolism generally can be divided into several syndromes that overlap considerably: (1) transient dyspnea and tachypnea in the absence of other associated clinical manifestations; (2) pulmonary infarction or congestive atelectasis (also known as ischemic pneumonitis or incomplete infarction), which includes pleuritic chest pain, cough, hemoptysis, pleural effusion, and pulmonary infiltrates on chest x-ray study; (3) right ventricular failure associated with severe dyspnea and tachypnea; (4) cardiovascular collapse with hypotension, syncope, and coma (usually associated with massive pulmonary embolism); and (5) less common and highly nonspecific clinical features, including confusion and coma, pyrexia, wheezing, resistant cardiac failure, and unexplained arrhythmia.

It is now widely accepted that the clinical diagnosis of pulmonary embolism is highly nonspecific. Multiple studies indicate that in more than half of all patients with clinically suspected pulmonary embolism, the diagnosis is not confirmed by objective testing. Therefore, objective testing is mandatory to confirm or exclude the presence of pulmonary embolism.[14–16]

OBJECTIVE TESTS FOR THE DIAGNOSIS OF VENOUS THROMBOSIS

Various ancillary tests, such as chest x-ray study; arterial blood gas determination; electrocardiography; and laboratory tests, such as those for fibrinopeptide A, D-dimer, and serum lactate dehydrogenase, have a role in the diagnosis of venous thromboembolism, but they all lack sensitivity and specificity. The main role of these tests is to rule out other conditions that may mimic pulmonary embolism, such as acute myocardial infarction, pneumonia, or pneumothorax. Objective tests used in the diagnosis of venous thrombosis include impedance plethysmography (IPG), B-mode ultrasonography, duplex ultrasonography, and color-flow ultrasonography and ascending venography. Objective tests used in the diagnosis of pulmonary embolism include ventilation-perfusion lung scanning and pulmonary angiography.

Venography

Venography is the standard objective method for the diagnosis of venous thrombosis. Venography is a difficult technique to perform well and requires considerable experience to execute adequately and to interpret accurately. Certain venographic abnormalities have been used as criteria for the diagnosis of acute deep venous thrombosis.[13] The most reliable of these is the presence of an intraluminal filling defect that is constant in all x-ray films and is seen in numerous projections. Other venographic abnormalities, such as nonfilling of a segment of the deep venous system or nonfilling of the entire deep venous system above the knee, may be caused by technical artifacts, particularly if the dye is injected too far proximally into the dorsal foot vein. These artifacts may then be interpreted either as caused by thrombus because the vein is not filled or as normal because a filling defect is not seen. The common femoral, external iliac, and common iliac veins may not be adequately filled by ascending venography, which can lead to an incorrect diagnosis based on inadequate venography. In the case of nonfilling of an entire segment of the deep venous system, the diagnosis of acute or recurrent venous thrombosis must depend on the use of other tests, such as IPG or ultrasonography.[17]

Numerous problems are related to venography. Even in the best of circumstances, it may be impossible to cannulate a vein on the dorsum of the foot, making ascending venography impossible on one or both legs. If filling of the common femoral or iliac systems is inadequate, femoral venography may be necessary.

Venography is associated with many clinically troublesome side effects. Pain may occur in the foot while dye is being injected, or delayed pain may occur in the calf 1 or 2 days after injection. The procedure may be complicated by superficial phlebitis and even deep venous thrombosis in a small percentage of patients with normal results on venography (1–2%).[18] Other less common complications of venography include hypersensitivity to the radiopaque dye and local skin or tissue necrosis due to extravasation of dye at the injection site. Both nonionic and high ionic contrast media may cause or aggravate renal insufficiency in patients at high risk for these complications, such as those with established renal disease, hypertension, heart failure, diabetes, or multiple myeloma.[19, 20] The risks of venography must be carefully weighed in such circumstances and reviewed with the patient before venography is performed.

Impedance Plethysmography

IPG is sensitive and specific for proximal vein thrombosis in symptomatic patients, but it is insensitive to calf vein thrombosis.[21–23] In patients with clinically suspected venous thrombosis, positive IPG results can be used to make therapeutic decisions in the absence of clinical conditions known to produce false-positive results. A normal result excludes the diagnosis of proximal vein thrombosis but does not exclude calf vein thrombosis. This potential limitation can be overcome by serial IPG evaluations. The use of serial IPG is based on the concept now confirmed by clinical observation that calf vein thrombi are clinically important only when extension into the proximal veins occurs, at which point detection with IPG is possible. The effectiveness and safety of IPG have been evaluated by prospective clinical trials in patients with clinically suspected venous thrombosis. Based on the data provided by these studies, the following recommendations can be made: (1) a positive result on IPG is highly predictive of acute proximal vein thrombosis (positive predictive value >90%) and (2) withholding anticoagulant therapy is safe in symptomatic patients who have negative results by serial IPG for 10 to 14 days.[10, 21, 23]

Although IPG has a high sensitivity and specificity for the detection of symptomatic venous thrombosis, it lacks sensitivity for the detection of asymptomatic venous thrombosis in patients who have had surgery, such as total hip replacement, or in trauma patients. In such circumstances, the only reliable method for the detection of deep venous thrombosis is bilateral ascending venography.

IPG has certain limitations. False-positive results may occur in patients with disorders that interfere with arterial inflow or venous outflow. These disorders include severe congestive cardiac failure, constrictive pericarditis, severe arterial insufficiency, hypotension, and external compression of veins. Most of these disorders are readily recognized clinically. False-positive results may also occur if the test is performed incorrectly or if the patient is not relaxed. The test cannot be performed on some patients, such as those who are in plaster casts or who cannot be adequately positioned because of immobilization or pain.

Ultrasonography

Venous imaging using real-time, B-mode ultrasound with or without Doppler assessment is a promising technique for the evaluation of patients with clinically suspected deep venous thrombosis.[24–29] Prospective studies have shown that the single criterion of vein compressibility is highly sensitive and specific for the detection of proximal vein thrombosis (sensitivity and specificity, both >95%).[24–29] Other criteria, such as echogenicity or change in venous diameter during a Valsalva maneuver, are less useful for this purpose. The visualization of an echogenic band is highly sensitive but is nonspecific (specificity, 50%). The percentage of change in venous diameter during a Valsalva maneuver is both insensitive and nonspecific.

Real-time, B-mode venous ultrasonography is insensitive for the detection of isolated calf vein thrombosis, and, like IPG, serial testing using this method is required to detect proximal extension. B-mode venous ultrasound may fail to detect isolated iliac vein thrombi. This is a practical clinical limitation in patients in whom isolated vein thrombosis is common, such as pregnant patients with clinically suspected venous thrombosis. Color-flow imaging and other technologic advances have improved the ability of B-mode venous imaging to detect isolated iliac vein and calf vein thrombi.[29]

Doppler ultrasound and IPG are both highly sensitive and specific in the diagnosis of proximal vein thrombosis in symptomatic patients. However, Doppler ultrasonography is more sensitive to the detection of symptomatic calf vein thrombosis. Doppler ultrasonography is more reliable than IPG for detecting proximal vein thrombosis in patients with increased central venous pressure or arterial insufficiency. Doppler ultrasonography can be used in patients whose leg is in a plaster cast or external fixation, who are in traction, or who have had leg amputation.

Both IPG and Doppler ultrasonography have high sensitivity and specificity for the diagnosis of proximal vein thrombosis in symptomatic patients, but both lack sensitivity and specificity for the detection of asymptomatic venous thrombosis in patients who have undergone surgery.[30, 31] Ultrasonography is becoming more readily available, and, as the cost outlay for the equipment decreases, it will probably supplant IPG as the most popular noninvasive test for the detection of venous thrombosis.

OBJECTIVE TESTS FOR THE DIAGNOSIS OF PULMONARY EMBOLISM

Perfusion lung scanning is the key diagnostic test for patients with suspected pulmonary embolism. A normal perfusion scan result excludes clinically important pulmonary embolism.[32–34] An abnormal perfusion scan result, however, is nonspecific and may occur in conditions that produce either increased radiographic density (e.g., pneumonia, atelectasis, and pleural effusion) or regional reduction in ventilation (e.g., chronic obstructive lung disease, acute asthma, bronchial mucus plugs, and bronchitis, all of which are frequently associated with normal radiographic results).

Ventilation imaging was introduced to improve the specificity of an abnormal perfusion scan result by differentiating embolic occlusion of the pulmonary vasculature from perfusion defects occurring secondary to a primary disorder of ventilation.[35–37] This basic premise (that perfusion defects that ventilate normally [ventilation-perfusion mismatch] are due to pulmonary embolism, whereas matching ventilation-perfusion abnormalities are due to other conditions) has been shown to be incorrect by recent prospective clinical trials.[38, 39]

Ventilation lung scanning is helpful only if the perfusion defect is segmental or greater and is associated with ventilation mismatch; such patients have a high probability (≥86%) of pulmonary embolism confirmed by pulmonary angiography.[9, 35–38] Other abnormal findings on lung scans, such as matching ventilation-perfusion defects (either segmental or subsegmental), subsegmental defects with ventilation mismatch, or perfusion defects that correspond to an area of increased density on chest radiography (indeterminate perfusion scan results), are associated with a 20% to 40% frequency of pulmonary embolism.[9, 35] Further investigations, including pulmonary angiography and objective tests for venous thrombosis, are therefore required in patients who have indeterminate ventilation-perfusion scan findings.[9, 35, 39] Pulmonary angiography, or venography, or both, should be used when other approaches are unavailable or inconclusive. The morbidity associated with these tests is substantially less than that arising from unnecessary anticoagulant therapy and inappropriate hospitalization.

Pulmonary Angiography

Pulmonary angiography is the accepted diagnostic reference standard for pulmonary embolism.[40–42] The diagnosis is established if an intraluminal filling defect is constant on multiple films, or if abrupt termination (cut-off) of a vessel greater than 2 to 5 mm in diameter occurs and is constant on multiple films.[40, 41] Other abnormalities, such as oligemia, vessel pruning, and loss of filling of small vessels, are nonspecific and occur in many conditions, including pneumonia, atelectasis, bronchiectasis, emphysema, and pulmonary carcinoma.[40, 41]

In recent years, the diagnostic resolution of pulmonary angiography has markedly improved, and the risk to the patient decreased, by the use of selective catheterization and repeated injections of small volumes of dye. This technique is safe in the absence of severe chronic pulmonary hypertension or severe cardiac or respiratory decompensation.[43] Clinically significant complications, including tachyarrhythmias, endocardial or myocardial injury, cardiac perforation, cardiac arrest, and hypersensitivity reactions to contrast medium, occur in up to 3% to 4% of patients.[40, 43]

DIAGNOSIS AND TREATMENT OF PULMONARY EMBOLISM BASED ON OBJECTIVE TESTING FOR PROXIMAL DEEP VENOUS THROMBOSIS

At least 80% of patients with pulmonary embolism have thrombi originating in the lower leg veins.[8–12] Because of the diagnostic inaccuracy of noninvasive tests for pulmonary embolism, particularly in patients with indeterminate lung scan results, the concept of using objective tests for the detection of proximal venous thrombosis in the legs was developed in patients suspected of having pulmonary embolism.[14–16, 43] This combined strategy for the diagnosis and treatment of pulmonary embolus or venous thrombosis (e.g., venous thromboembolism) has been applied in prospective clinical trials.

Noninvasive tests, such as IPG or B-mode venous ultrasonography, have advantages because they are free of morbidity and are readily repeatable. Proximal vein thrombosis is revealed by IPG in 10% to 25% of patients with indeterminate results on ventilation-perfusion scans. This diagnostic ability has important implications for management: untreated or inadequately treated proximal vein thrombosis is associated with a high risk (20–50%) of recurrent venous thromboembolism.

A positive result on venography or noninvasive testing is an indication for therapy; however, the venographic result is negative in approximately 30% of patients with angiographically documented pulmonary embolism. Two possible explanations exist for this finding. First, pulmonary embolism may have originated from a source other than the deep veins of the legs. Alternatively, the emboli may have originated from the deep veins of the legs, but all or most of the thrombus embolized, leaving no residual thrombosis detectable at the time of presentation.

Patients with abnormal but indeterminate lung scan results and negative objective test results for venous thrombosis require pulmonary angiography to confirm or exclude pulmonary embolism. This diagnostic modality may, however, be impractical or unavailable. In patients who do not have severely limited cardiac or respiratory reserve, serial objective testing for proximal vein thrombosis is an alternative approach, based on the concept that clinically important recurrent pulmonary embolism is unlikely (<1%) in the absence of proximal vein thrombosis. This concept is supported by the findings of studies of the natural history of venous thrombosis and by clinical trials of noninvasive testing in patients with symptoms or signs suggesting deep venous thrombosis.[10, 21, 23] Furthermore, recent prospective studies indicate that the use of serial objective testing for proximal vein thrombosis is an effective and practical alternative to pulmonary angiography in patients with indeterminate lung scan results who have adequate cardiorespiratory reserve.[44–46]

Anticoagulant Therapy for Venous Thromboembolism

Anticoagulant drugs (heparin, warfarin, or both) are the mainstay of the management of venous thromboembolism. This chapter concentrates on the role of heparin and warfarin in the treatment of thromboembolism and does not discuss the role of thrombolysis, thrombectomy, or vena cava filters (see Chapter 64).

The objectives of treatment in patients with venous thromboembolism are (1) to prevent death from pulmonary embolism, (2) to prevent recurrent venous thromboembolism, and (3) to prevent postphlebitic syndrome.

Heparin

Heparin is a mixture of anionic glycosaminoglycans that have an average molecular weight of 10,000 to 17,000 D (range, 3,000 to 25,000 D). Heparin inhibits the coagulation pathway by numerous mechanisms, the most important of which is the inhibition of activated Factors XII, XI, IX, X, and II, that is, thrombin, with the greatest inhibition being on Factor X and thrombin.[47–49] The anticoagulant effect of heparin is also mediated by heparin cofactor II, which is independent of antithrombin III.[49] Heparin is well absorbed after subcutaneous injection, with peak levels appearing after injection and lasting up to 12 hours. The subcutaneous route of administration has been used in both prophylaxis and treatment, but continuous intravenous infusion is the preferred approach for treatment. Intermittent intravenous injection is associated with a greater risk of bleeding than other methods. The test most commonly used to monitor heparin therapy is the activated partial thromboplastin time (aPTT) test.

Monitoring of Heparin Therapy: Therapeutic Range

Clinical trials have established the need for initial heparin treatment in patients with proximal vein thrombosis.[50–52] Some investigators have shown than an adequate intensity of heparin treatment is required to prevent recurrent venous thromboembolism.[51, 52] This finding establishes both the need to monitor the anticoagulant response to heparin and the need to titrate the heparin dose in the individual patient, because the anticoagulant response to a standard dose of heparin varies widely between patients. (See later.)

It has become common clinical practice to adjust the heparin dose to maintain the result of the aPTT within a defined therapeutic range. Over the years, this therapeutic range has evolved based on clinical custom to the use of an upper and lower limit, which is an aPTT of 1.5 to 2.5 times the control value. The use of an aPTT ratio of 1.5 as the lower limit of the therapeutic range is supported by data from clinical trials. In contrast, until very recently, no firm evidence was reported from clinical trials to provide clear guidelines on the upper limit of the therapeutic range. The use of an upper limit and the clinical practice of reducing the heparin dose when the aPTT exceeds this limit have been based on clinical custom and the intuitive belief that this practice will minimize the risk of bleeding. Indeed, the dose of heparin given has been cited as one of the risk factors for bleeding during heparin therapy, but this observation was based on retrospective studies. Recently, data from rigorously designed clinical trials have become available that enable firm recommendations to be made about the appropriate therapeutic range for the aPTT. The findings indicate that failure to exceed the lower limit (aPTT ratio, 1.5) is associated with an unacceptably high risk of recurrent venous thromboembolism, but in contrast, no association exists between supratherapeutic aPTT responses and the risk of bleeding.

Lower Limit

Data from two randomized trials establish an aPTT ratio of 1.5 as the lower limit of the therapeutic range.[51, 52] The first trial evaluated the clinical outcomes in patients with proximal vein thrombosis who were treated either with continuous intravenous heparin or with intermittent subcutaneous heparin.[51] In both treatment groups, the heparin dose was adjusted to maintain the aPTT ratio above the predefined lower limit of 1 .5. The subcutaneous regimen resulted in an initial anticoagulant response below the lower limit in most (63%) patients and in a high frequency of recurrent venous thromboembolism (11 of 57 patients, or 19%). None of the patients above the therapeutic level developed a venous thromboembolism. In contrast, continuous intravenous heparin administration resulted in an adequate anticoagulant response in most (71%) patients and in a low frequency of recurrent thromboembolic events (3 of 58 patients, 5%); the recurrences in this group were also limited to patients with an initial subtherapeutic anticoagulant response. Thus, 13 of 53 patients (24.5%) with an aPTT response below the lower limit for 24 hours or longer had recurrent venous thromboembolism, compared with only 1 of 62 patients (1.6%) in whom an aPTT ratio of 1.5 or more was achieved ($P<.001$). These data represent a relative risk of 15:1 for recurrent venous thromboembolism for patients given inadequate initial heparin treatment (aPTT ratio <1.5).

These findings are strongly supported by a recent randomized trial that compared intravenously administered heparin with orally administered anticoagulants alone for the initial treatment of patients with proximal vein thrombosis.[52] The latter treatment group, by the nature of their treatment, have an inadequate aPTT for at least the first 48 hours because the onset of the anticoagulant effect of oral anticoagulants is delayed. Recurrent venous thromboembolism occurred in 11 of 55 patients (20%) treated with oral anticoagulants alone, compared with 3 of 50 patients (6%) who received initial intravenous heparin that was adjusted to maintain the aPTT above 1.5 times the control value ($P=.032$).

Upper Limit

New information about the upper limit of the therapeutic range for the aPTT has become available very recently.[53] Clinical outcomes were evaluated in patients with proximal vein thrombosis who were randomly assigned to receive initial treatment with either intravenous heparin alone or intravenous heparin with simultaneous warfarin sodium. Both regimens achieved adequate therapy in almost all patients, but the combined heparin and warfarin group received more intensive anticoagulation, and most of these patients exceeded the predefined upper limit (aPTT ratio, 2.5) for sustained periods of time. Thus, 69 of 99 patients (69%) in the group who received combined therapy had a supratherapeutic value (ratio ≥2.5) that persisted for 24 hours or more, compared with 24 of 100 patients (24%) who received heparin alone ($P<.001$). Despite this more intense therapy in the combined group, bleeding complications occurred with similar frequency in the two groups: 9 of 99 patients in the group given combined therapy (9.1%), compared with 12 of 100 patients (12.0%) in the group given heparin alone. Importantly, bleeding complications occurred in 8 of 93 patients (8.6%) who had supratherapeutic findings. Major bleeding occurred in 3 of 93 patients (3.2%) who had supratherapeutic aPTT findings (relative risk, 0.3; $P=.09$). Major bleeding occurred in 11% of patients considered to be high risk, but in only 1% of those considered to be low risk ($P=.007$). These findings demonstrate a lack of association between a supratherapeutic aPTT (ratio ≥2.5) and the risk of clinically important bleeding complications.

Need for Quality Assurance for Heparin Therapy

The current clinical practice of using an intuitive approach to heparin dose titration frequently results in inadequate therapy.[54, 55] For example, an audit of physician practice at three university-affiliated hospitals documented that 60% of patients failed to achieve an adequate aPTT (ratio, 1.5) during the first 24 hours of therapy, and 30% to 40% of patients continued to have subtherapeutic aPPTs over the next 3 to 4 days.[54] A startling finding was that in one third of patients in whom a subtherapeutic aPTT was found, no change in heparin dose occurred. These findings show that physician practices in the administration of intravenous heparin have been dominated by a desire to avoid supratherapeutic aPTTs because of the fear of bleeding complications, and much less concern existed over the risk of recurrent venous thromboembolism. This approach has been shown to result in the administration of inadequate therapy in most patients; the clinical trial data indicate that it is inappropriate, and indeed dangerous, because it places the patients at unacceptably high risk for recurrent venous thromboembolism.

We have recently completed a randomized clinical trial evaluating a prescriptive approach to intravenous heparin administration (Tables 144–2 and 144–3).[53] Patients were randomly assigned to initial heparin therapy alone or to heparin therapy with simultaneous warfarin sodium therapy. The objective of the prescriptive approach was to minimize the proportion of patients receiving subtherapeutic doses of heparin and to do so within 24 hours regardless of the concomitant use of oral anticoagulants. Only 2% and 1% of the patients had subtherapeutic aPPTs for more than 24 hours in the heparin and warfarin group and the heparin group, respectively. Recurrent venous thromboembolism (objectively documented) occurred infrequently in both groups (7%).

TABLE 144–2. Heparin Protocol

1. Administer initial intravenous heparin bolus: 5000 U.
2. Administer continuous intravenous heparin infusion: commence at 42 mL/h of 20,000 U (1680 U/h) in 500 mL of two-thirds dextrose and one-third saline (a 24-hour heparin dose of 40,320 U), except in the following patients, in whom heparin infusion is commenced at a rate of 31 mL/h (1240 U/h, a 24-hour dose of 29,760 U):
   - Patients who have undergone surgery within the previous 2 weeks.
   - Patients with a previous history of peptic ulcer disease or gastrointestinal or genitourinary bleeding.
   - Patients with recent stroke (i.e., thrombotic stroke within 2 weeks previously).
   - Patients with a platelet count < 150 × 10^9/L.
   - Patients with miscellaneous reasons for a high risk of bleeding (e.g., hepatic failure, renal failure, or vitamin K deficiency).
3. Adjust heparin dose by use of the aPTT. The aPTT test is performed in all patients as follows:
   - 4–6 hours after commencing heparin; the heparin dose is then adjusted according to the nomogram shown in Table 144–3.
   - 4–6 hours after the first dosage adjustment.
   - Then, as indicated by the nomogram for the first 24 hours of therapy.
   - Thereafter, is once daily, unless the patient is subtherapeutic,* in which case the aPTT test is repeated 4–6 hours after the heparin dose is increased.

aPTT = activated partial thromboplastin time.

*Subtherapeutic = aPTT <1.5 times the mean normal control value for the thromboplastin reagent being used.

TABLE 144–3. Intravenous Heparin Dose—Titration Nomogram for aPTT

	IV Infusion		
aPTT	*Rate Change (mL/h)*	*Dose Change (U/24 h)**	*Additional Action*
≤45	+6	+5760	Repeated aPTT test† in 4–6 h
46–54	+3	+2880	Repeated aPTT test in 4–6 h
55–85	0	0	None‡
86–110	−3	−2880	Stop heparin sodium treatment for 1 h; repeated aPTT test 4–6 h after heparin treatment is restarted
>110	−6	−5760	Stop heparin treatment for 1 h; repeated aPTT test 4–6 h after heparin treatment is restarted

(From Hull RD, Raskob GE, Rosenbloom D, et al: Optimal therapeutic level of heparin therapy in patients with venous thrombosis. Arch Intern Med 1992; 152:1589.)

*Heparin sodium concentration, 20,000 U in 500 mL = 40 U/mL.

†With the use of Actin-FS thromboplastin reagent (Dade, Mississauga, Ontario).

‡During the first 24 hours, repeated aPTT test in 4–6 hours. Thereafter, the aPTT is determined once daily, unless subtherapeutic.

aPTT = activated partial thromboplastin time; IV = intravenous.

Subcutaneous Heparin Compared with Continuous Intravenous Heparin

In the past, numerous randomized trials have compared the effectiveness and safety of heparin given by the subcutaneous and continuous intravenous routes.[56, 57] Investigators have concluded that subcutaneously administered heparin was as effective and as safe as intravenously administered heparin.[57] However, this meta-analysis has been criticized because of the selection of studies for review and because of the lack of data on aPTT values in patients receiving subcutaneous heparin.[58] In view of the well-established need to achieve a lower limit of the aPTT therapeutic range, heparin given by the subcutaneous route cannot be recommended in the initial treatment of proximal vein thrombosis.

Subcutaneous Adjusted-Dose Heparin for Long-Term Treatment

Adjusted-dose subcutaneous heparin is the long-term anticoagulant regimen of choice in pregnant patients, in certain patients at high risk of bleeding, and in patients who return to geographically remote areas in which long-term anticoagulant monitoring is unavailable or impractical (in whom the heparin dose is adjusted during the first few days of long-term therapy and then fixed).[59] The starting dose of long-term subcutaneous heparin is determined from the patient's initial intravenous heparin dose requirement. A starting subcutaneous dose equivalent to one third of the patient's 24-hour intravenous heparin dose is administered every 12 hours. The subcutaneous dose is adjusted during the first few days of long-term therapy to maintain the mid-interval aPTT (determined 6 hours after injection) at 1.5 times the control value. This level of anticoagulant response is usually achieved with a dose of 8000 to 12,000 U/12 h (mean dose, 10,000 U/12 h). In pregnant patients, larger doses may be required, and continued monitoring is desirable because of changes in heparin requirements throughout the course of pregnancy.

Adverse Effects

The side effects of heparin therapy include bleeding, thrombocytopenia, arterial thromboembolism, hypersensitivity, and osteoporosis. Bleeding, the commonest side effect of heparin, occurs in 5% to 10% of patients during initial continuous intravenous heparin therapy.[53] At particular risk are patients who have had recent surgery or trauma and those with an underlying hemostatic defect or predisposing clinical risk factor (e.g., unsuspected peptic ulcer or occult carcinoma). The risk of bleeding complications is greater in patients who receive intravenous heparin by intermittent injection than in those who receive continuous infusion.

The onset of thrombocytopenia, now a well-recognized complication of heparin therapy, usually occurs 7 to 10 days after heparin treatment is commenced but may occur earlier in patients previously exposed to heparin.[60] This complication has been seen with the low-molecular-weight (LMW) heparins as well. Although the exact incidence of this complication with these agents is as yet undetermined, it appears to be around 1% to 2%. Heparin-induced thrombocytopenia is commoner in patients receiving beef-lung heparin than in those receiving porcine-intestinal heparin. The thrombocytopenia may be moderate or severe, and the severe form is less common than the moderate form. The precise mechanism of heparin-induced thrombocytopenia is currently unknown but probably involves immune mechanisms, particularly in the severe forms of the disorder. It is currently unknown how frequently patients with moderate thrombocytopenia may progress to the severe form, which may include the added complication of arterial thrombosis. This complication may precede or coincide with the fall in platelet count. Heparin-induced thrombocytopenia with arterial thrombosis results in a high incidence of limb amputation and mortality. Therefore, heparin in all forms must be discontinued when heparin-induced thrombocytopenia is diagnosed. Alternate approaches to treatment include insertion of an inferior vena caval filter or the use of ancrod (Arvin),[61] a defibrinogenating extract of snake venom that produces effective anticoagulation while oral anticoagulants are being instituted. Another agent, a heparinoid consisting mainly of dermatan sulfate along with heparan and condroitin sulfate (ORG 10172-Organon, The Netherlands), does not cross-react with heparin during in vitro immunoassays and has been used effectively in a few patients with heparin-induced thrombocytopenia.[62, 63]

Osteoporosis occurs rarely in patients receiving long-term subcutaneous heparin therapy (more than 15,000 U of heparin per day for longer than 6 months).[64] The earliest clinical manifestation of heparin-associated osteoporosis is usually the onset of nonspecific low-back pain primarily involving the vertebrae or ribs; patients may also present with spontaneous fracture in these areas.

Hypersensitivity to heparin is uncommon and may take the form of a skin rash or, less commonly, anaphylaxis. Alopecia has been reported as a rare complication of heparin therapy. Serum transaminase levels may be moderately raised. Heparin-induced hypoaldosteronism is recognized but rare. Rarely, a bluish discoloration of the toes, associated with a burning sensation, has been reported.

Neutralization of Heparin Anticoagulant Effect

The anticoagulant effect of heparin can be immediately neutralized by intravenous injection of protamine sulfate. The appropriate neutralizing dose depends on the dose of heparin, its route of administration, and the time it is given. If protamine sulfate is used within minutes of an intravenous heparin injection, a full neutralizing dose (1 mg of protamine sulfate per 100 U of heparin) should be given. Because the plasma half-life of intravenously administered heparin is approximately 60 minutes, an injection of protamine sulfate in a bolus of more than 50 mg is seldom required. An occasional hypotensive response to protamine sulfate has been reported; therefore, it should be injected slowly over a 10- to 30-minute period. Treatment with protamine sulfate may need to be repeated because protamine is cleared from the blood more quickly than is heparin. After subcutaneous injection of heparin is administered, repeated small doses of protamine may be required because of prolonged heparin absorption from the subcutaneous depot.

Low-Molecular-Weight Heparin and Heparinoids

In recent years, LMW derivatives of commercial heparin have been prepared that have a mean molecular weight of 4000 to 5000 D, in contrast to unfractionated heparin, which has a mean molecular weight of 10,000 to 17,000 D. Pharmacokinetic studies and recent small clinical trials in selected patients with venous thrombosis indicate that the bioavailability of these LMW-heparin fractions after subcutaneous injection is very high.[65, 66] For example, investigators have reported that the bioavailability of LMW heparin after a subcutaneous injection of 120 IU/kg of Factor Xa to healthy volunteers was approximately 90% of an equivalent intravenous dose. The excellent bioavailability of LMW heparin, together with its half-life (anti–Factor Xa activity), which is longer than unfractionated heparin, suggests that it may be possible to develop an effective regimen for initial treatment with LMW heparin using once-daily subcutaneous injection.[67, 68] The anticoagulant response (Factor Xa units per milliliter) observed with a given dose of LMW heparin is highly correlated with body weight, so that LMW heparin is effective when given in standard doses (Factor Xa international units per kilogram) without laboratory monitoring.[67, 68]

Low-Molecular-Weight Heparin in the Treatment of Proximal Venous Thrombosis

The results of small trials comparing subcutaneously or intravenously administered LMW heparin with continuous intravenously administered heparin suggest that LMW heparin may have a role in treatment as well as in prophylaxis.[69] Four randomized clinical trials have compared LMW heparin given subcutaneously once or twice daily with continuous intravenously administered heparin.[70–73] In two of the European trials, Fraxiparine was given in a fixed dose subcutaneously twice a day and was compared with continuous intravenously administered heparin that was monitored by aPTT.[70, 71] Both studies used the Arnesen and Marder scales on repeat venography to assess efficacy, and in the collaborative European multicenter study, perfusion lung scans were performed on days 0 and 10. Both studies suggest that Fraxiparine was at least as effective as unfractionated heparin for the prevention of venographic extension of thrombosis.

A randomized trial compared the relative effectiveness and risk of bleeding of fixed-dose LMW heparin (Fraxiparine) with adjusted-dose intravenous unfractionated heparin in consecutive symptomatic patients with proximal vein thrombosis. The regimens were administered for 10 days, followed by oral warfarin sodium therapy for 3 months.[72] Patients in the LMW-heparin group received subcutaneous injections every 12 hours according to body weight (12,500 aXa Institute Choay units for patients <55 kg; 15,000 aXa Institute Choay units for patients between 55 and 80 kg; and 17,500 aXa Institute Choay units for patients >80 kg). Patients in the adjusted-dose intravenous heparin group received a continuous infusion to maintain the aPTT within 1.5 to 2.0 times the mean normal control value.[73] All patients had baseline perfusion lung scans and chest x-ray studies. Contrast venography was repeated on day 10, or earlier if new symptoms developed. The frequency of objectively diagnosed recurrent venous thromboembolism was comparable in the unfractionated heparin and the LMW-heparin groups: 12 (14%) versus 6 (7%) (95% confidence interval for the difference −3% to 15%; $P = .13$). Clinically evident bleeding occurred in 3.5% of patients receiving unfractionated heparin versus 1.1% of those receiving LMW heparin (>0.2). At 6-month follow-up, 12 deaths had occurred in the unfractionated heparin group, versus 6 in the Fraxiparine group; this difference was largely due to cancer deaths (8 of 18 in the unfractionated heparin group versus 1 of 15 in the LMW-heparin group).

In a multicenter, double-blind clinical trial, fixed-dose, subcutaneously administered LMW heparin (Logiparin, Novo-Nordisk, Sweden) (175 Factor Xa IU/kg) was compared with continuous intravenously administered heparin that was adjusted to maintain an aPTT of 1.5 times to 2.5 times the mean normal control value.[66] Oral warfarin sodium was started on day two. All patients had venographically proven proximal venous thrombosis and, at the time of entry, underwent ventilation perfusion lung scans, chest radiographs, and IPG. New episodes of venous thromboembolism were seen in six of 213 patients receiving LMW heparin (2.8%) and in 15 of 219 patients receiving intravenous unfractionated heparin (6.9%) ($P = .07$; 95% confidence interval for the difference 0.02% to 8.1%). Major bleeding associated with initial therapy occurred in one patient receiving LMW heparin (0.5%) and in 11 patients receiving intravenous unfractionated heparin (5.0%), a reduction in risk of 95% ($P = .006$). During long-term warfarin therapy, major hemorrhage was seen in five patients receiving LMW heparin (2.3%) and in none of those receiving intravenous heparin ($P = .028$). Ten patients who received LMW heparin (4.7%) died, compared with 21 patients who received intravenous unfractionated heparin (9.6%), a risk reduction of 51% ($P = .049$). The most striking difference was in abrupt deaths in patients with metastatic carcinoma, and most of these deaths occurred within the first 3 weeks. The long-term use of LMW heparin in place of warfarin sodium may have a greater impact on recurrent thromboembolic events, bleeding, and death, particularly in patients with metastatic carcinoma.

Taken together, the results of these studies provide strong evidence that LMW heparin given subcutaneously is as effective and as safe as unfractionated heparin in the treatment of proximal venous thrombosis.[72, 73] The decreased mortality rate, particularly in patients with metastatic carcinoma, was unexpected and requires confirmation in future prospective randomized trials.

Oral Anticoagulant Therapy

Two distinct chemical groups of oral anticoagulants exist: the 4-hydroxy coumarin derivatives (e.g., warfarin sodium) and the indane-1, 3-dione derivatives (e.g., phenindione). The coumarin derivatives are the oral anticoagulants of choice because they are associated with fewer nonhemorrhagic side effects than are the indanedione derivatives (see *Adverse Effects*).

Oral anticoagulants produce their anticoagulant effect by inhibiting the vitamin K–dependent γ-carboxylation of coagulation Factors II, VII, IX, and X.[74, 75] This effect results in the synthesis of immunologically detectable, but biologically inactive, forms of these coagulation proteins. Oral anticoagulants also inhibit the vitamin K–dependent γ-carboxylation of proteins C and S. Protein C circulates as a proenzyme that is activated on endothelial cells by the thrombin-thrombomodulin complex to form activated protein C. Activated protein C inhibits activated Factor VIII activity directly, and in the presence of protein S, it also inhibits activated Factor V. Therefore, vitamin K antagonists, such as warfarin sodium, create a biochemical paradox by producing an anticoagulant effect that results from the inhibition of procoagulants (Factors II, VII, IX, and X) and by producing a potentially thrombogenic effect by impairing the synthesis of naturally occurring inhibitors of coagulation (proteins C and S).

The anticoagulant effect of the vitamin K antagonists is delayed until the normal clotting factors are cleared from the circulation, and the peak effect does not occur until 36 to 72 hours after drug administration.[74, 75] With a 40-mg loading dose, Factor VII levels usually fall rapidly to less than 20% of normal, and sometimes to less than 10% of normal, for as long as 3 to 4 days. In some patients, suppression of Factor VII to this level is seen within 24 hours. Sick patients with impaired liver function or reduced vitamin K stores are particularly susceptible to large loading doses. Equilibrium levels of Factors II, IX, and X are not reached until about 1 week after the initiation of therapy. The equilibrium levels of these factors are not achieved quicker by use of a large loading dose (e.g., 40 mg). Therefore, the use of small initial daily doses (e.g., 10 mg) is the preferred approach for the initiation of warfarin treatment.

A 4- to 5-day overlap with intravenous heparin during the initiation of warfarin sodium therapy is important.[52] Experimental evidence indicates that the maximum antithrombotic effect of warfarin is delayed for as long as 5 days, even though the anticoagulant effect, reflected by an increase in the prothrombin time (due mainly to a reduction in Factor VII), may be evident within 2 to 3 days. Factor VII and protein C have similar short half-lives (approximately 4 to 5 hours). During the first 24 to 48 hours of warfarin sodium therapy, the levels of functional Factor VII and protein C fall, while the levels of functionally active Factors II, IX, and X remain relatively normal. Thus, during the first 24 to 48 hours of therapy, oral anticoagulants have the potential to be thrombogenic because the anticoagulant effect of minimally functional Factor VII is counteracted by the potentially thrombogenic effect of low levels of functional protein C with minimally decreased levels of functional Factors II, IX, and X. After 72 to 96 hours, the levels of functional Factors II, IX, and X fall, and the optimal anticoagulant activity of warfarin therapy is expressed. For these reasons, oral anticoagulant therapy must overlap with heparin therapy for 4 to 5 days even though the prothrombin time may be prolonged into the therapeutic range after 2 to 3 days.

Monitoring of Oral Anticoagulant Therapy

The laboratory test most commonly used to measure the effects of warfarin is the one-stage prothrombin time test, which is sensitive to reduced activity of Factors II, VII, and X but is insensitive to reduced activity of Factor IX. The optimal therapeutic range for oral anticoagulant therapy monitored by the prothrombin time test has been controversial because, until recently, it had not been adequately evaluated in clinical trials. Further confusion about the appropriate therapeutic range occurred because the different tissue thromboplastins used for measuring the prothrombin time vary considerably in sensitivity to the vitamin K–dependent clotting factors and in response to warfarin. Rabbit brain thromboplastin, which is widely used in North America, is less sensitive than is standardized human brain thromboplastin, which has been widely used in the United Kingdom and other parts of Europe. A prothrombin time ratio of 1.5 to 2.0 obtained with rabbit brain thromboplastin (i.e., the traditional therapeutic range in North America) is equivalent to a ratio of 4.0 to 6.0 obtained with human brain thromboplastin. Conversely, a two- to threefold increase in the prothrombin time obtained with standardized human brain thromboplastin is equivalent to a 1.25- to 1.5-fold increase in the prothrombin time obtained with rabbit brain thromboplastin, such as Simplastin or Dade-C.

To promote standardization of the prothrombin time for the monitoring of oral anticoagulant therapy, the World Health Organization has developed an international reference thromboplastin from human brain tissue and has recommended that the prothrombin time ratio be expressed as the international normalized ratio (INR).[76] The INR is the prothrombin time ratio obtained by testing of a given sample using the World Health Organization reference thromboplastin. For practical clinical purposes, the INR for a given plasma sample is equivalent to the prothrombin time ratio obtained using a standardized human brain thromboplastin known as the Manchester comparative reagent, which has been widely used in the United Kingdom. The currently recommended therapeutic range of 1.25 to 1.5 times the control value obtained with rabbit brain thromboplastin, such as Simplastin or Dade-C, corresponds to an INR of 2.0 to 3.0.[7]

In a survey of 53 hospital laboratories, only 21% reported prothrombin times as INR results, and 30% of hospitals could not provide data on the international sensitivity index of the thromboplastin being used. This study indicated that the current recommendations regarding the international sensitivity index and INR are being disregarded by most laboratories involved in the study and that anticoagulant monitoring would therefore be substandard.[77]

Warfarin Sodium

Warfarin sodium is administered in an initial dose of 10 mg/d for the first 2 days, and the daily dose is then adjusted according to the INR. Heparin therapy is discontinued on the fourth or fifth day after the initiation of warfarin therapy, provided that the INR is prolonged into the therapeutic range (INR, 2.0 to 3.0; prothrombin time, 1.25 to 1.5 times control value).

Once the anticoagulant effect and patient's warfarin dose requirements are stable, the INR is monitored weekly throughout the course of oral anticoagulant therapy. However, if factors that may produce an unpredictable response to warfarin are present (e.g., concomitant drug therapy), the INR should be monitored more frequently to minimize the risk of complications resulting from poor anticoagulant control.

Adverse Effects

The major side effect of oral anticoagulant therapy is bleeding.[78] Bleeding during well-controlled oral anticoagulant therapy is usually due to surgery or other forms of trauma, or to local lesions, such as peptic ulcer or carcinoma.[78] Spontaneous bleeding may occur if warfarin sodium is given in an excessive dose, resulting in marked prolongation of the INR; this bleeding may be severe and even life-threatening. The risk of bleeding can be substantially reduced by adjustment of the warfarin dose to achieve a less intense anticoagulant effect than has traditionally been used in North America (INR, 2.0 to 3.0; prothrombin time, 1.25 to 1.5 times control value obtained using a rabbit brain thromboplastin, such as Simplastin or Dade-C).[79]

Nonhemorrhagic side effects of oral anticoagulant differ according to whether coumarin derivatives (e.g., warfarin sodium) or indanediones are administered. Such side effects are uncommon with coumarin anticoagulants, and the coumarins are therefore the oral anticoagulants of choice.

Coumarin-induced skin necrosis is a rare but serious complication that requires immediate cessation of oral anticoagulant therapy.[80, 81] It usually occurs between 3 and 10 days after therapy has commenced, is commoner in women, and most often involves areas of abundant subcutaneous tissues, such as the abdomen, buttocks, thighs, and breast. The mechanism of coumarin-induced skin necrosis, which is associated with microvascular thrombosis, is uncertain but appears to be related, at least in some patients, to depression of protein C level. Patients with congenital deficiencies of protein C may be particularly prone to the development of coumarin skin necrosis.

Oral anticoagulants cross the placenta and may cause fetal malformations when used during pregnancy.[82–84] Two specific fetopathic syndromes are associated with oral anticoagulant administration during pregnancy. Treatment with oral anticoagulants during the sixth to twelfth weeks of gestation may induce the syndrome of warfarin embryopathy in the fetus. This syndrome consists of skeletal abnormalities ranging from stippled epiphyses to frank skeletal hypoplasia. Although most of the reported cases have occurred in infants of mothers receiving warfarin, this syndrome has also been reported to result from phenindanedione or acenocoumarin administration. Oral anticoagulant administration during the second or third trimester of pregnancy may result in central nervous system abnormalities in the fetus, including abnormalities of the ventricular system (Dandy-Walker malformation), dorsal midline dysplasia, and optic atrophy. Therefore, the use of oral anticoagulants is contraindicated at any time during pregnancy, and they should not be used in women planning a pregnancy. Adjusted-dose heparin can safely be given throughout pregnancy in patients with venous thromboembolism, and from that observation, indications have been extrapolated to include patients requiring anticoagulation to prevent systemic embolism from prosthetic heart valves.[83]

Factors that Interact with the Effects of Oral Anticoagulant Therapy

A large number of drugs interact with oral anticoagulants and may produce either a prolongation or a reduction in the anticoagulant effect (Table 144–4). Special care should be taken to adjust the dose of oral anticoagulants during the time that other drugs are being taken, to minimize the risk of inadequate anticoagulant control.

Increased sensitivity to oral anticoagulants occurs in patients with vitamin K deficiency or impaired liver function, and in those with thyrotoxicosis due to the more rapid metabolism of the vitamin K–dependent clotting factors.

TABLE 144–4. Drugs that Interact with Oral Anticoagulant Agents

Increase Anticoagulant Effect
Allopurinol
Anabolic steroids
Clofibrate
Co-trimoxazole (trimethoprim and sulphamethoxazole)
Dextrothyroxine
Neomycin
Nortriptyline
Phenyramidol
Quinidine
Salicylate
Sulphinpyrazone
Decrease Anticoagulant Effect
Barbiturates
Cholestyramine
Diuretics
Estrogens
Glutethimide
Griseofulvin
Phenytoin
Rifampicin

Antidote to Oral Anticoagulant Agents

The antidote to the vitamin K antagonists is vitamin K_1. If an excessive increase of the INR occurs, the treatment depends on the degree of the increase and whether or not the patient is bleeding. If the increase is mild and the patient is not bleeding, no specific treatment is necessary other than reduction in the warfarin dose. The INR can be expected to decrease during the next 24 hours with this approach. With more marked increase of the INR in patients who are not bleeding, treatment with small doses of vitamin K_1, given either orally or by subcutaneous injection (2.5 to 5.0 mg), could be considered. With very marked increase of the INR, particularly in a patient who is either actively bleeding or at risk for bleeding, the coagulation defect should be corrected.

Reported side effects of vitamin K include flushing, dizziness, tachycardia, hypotension, dyspnea, and sweating. Intravenous administration of vitamin K_1 should be performed with caution to avoid inducing an anaphylactoid reaction. The risk of anaphylactoid reaction can be reduced by slow administration of vitamin K_1, at a rate no faster than 1 mg/min IV. In most patients, intravenous administration of vitamin K_1 produces a demonstrable effect on the INR within 6 to 8 hours and corrects the increased INR within 12 to 24 hours. Because the half-life of vitamin K_1 is less than that of warfarin sodium, a repeat course of vitamin K_1 may be necessary. If bleeding is very severe and life threatening, vitamin K therapy can be supplemented with concentrates of Factors II, VII, IX, and X.

References

1. Dismuke SE, Wagner EH: Pulmonary embolism as a cause of death. The changing mortality in hospitalized patients. JAMA 1986; 255:2039.
2. Dalen JE, Alpert JS: Natural history of pulmonary embolism. Prog Cardiovasc Dis 1975; 17:259.
3. Anderson FA, Wheeler HB, Goldberg RJ, et al: A population-based perspective of the hospital incidence and case-fatality rates of deep vein thrombosis and pulmonary embolism. Arch Intern Med 1991; 151:933.
4. Donaldson GA, Williams C, Scanell J, et al: A reappraisal of the application of the Trendelenburg operation to massive fatal embolism. N Engl J Med 1963; 268:171.
5. Consensus Conference: Prevention of venous thrombosis and pulmonary embolism. JAMA 1986; 256:744.
6. International Multicentre Trial: Prevention of fatal postoperative pulmonary embolism by low doses of heparin. Lancet 1975; ii:45.
7. Hyers TN, Hull RD, Weg JG: Antithrombotic therapy for venous thromboembolic disease. Chest 1992; 102:391S.
8. Moser KM, LeMoine JR: Is embolic risk conditioned by location of deep venous thrombosis? Ann Intern Med 1981; 94:439.
9. Hull RD, Hirsh J, Carter CJ, et al: Pulmonary angiography, ventilation lung scanning, and venography for clinically suspected pulmonary embolism with abnormal perfusion lung scan. Ann Intern Med 1983; 98:891.
10. Huisman MV, Buller HR, ten Cate JW, et al: Serial impedance plethysmography for suspected deep-vein thrombosis in outpatients. The Amsterdam general practitioner study. N Engl J Med 1986; 314:823.
11. Nicolaides AN, Kakkar VV, Field ES, et al: The origin of deep vein thrombosis: A venographic study. Br J Radiol 1971; 44:653.
12. Hull RD, Hirsh J, Sackett DL, et al: Clinical validity of a nega-

tive venogram in patients with clinically suspected venous thrombosis. Circulation 1981; 64:622.

13. Rabinov K, Paulin S: Roentgen diagnosis of venous thrombosis in the leg. Arch Surg 1972; 104:134.
14. Bone RC: Ventilation/perfusion scan in pulmonary embolism. "The emperor is incompletely attired." J Am Med Assoc 1990; 263:2794.
15. Secker-Walker RH: On purple emperors, pulmonary embolism, and venous thrombosis. Ann Intern Med 1983; 98:1006.
16. Kelley MA, Carson JL, Palevsky HI, et al: Diagnosing pulmonary embolism: New facts and strategies. Ann Intern Med 1991; 114:300.
17. Hull RD, Secker-Walker RH, Hirsh J: Diagnosis of deep vein thrombosis. *In:* Thrombosis and Hemostasis: Basic Principles and Clinical Practice. 2nd Ed. Colman RW, Hirsh J, Marder VJ, et al (Eds). Philadelphia, JB Lippincott, 1987, p 1220.
18. Hull RD, Carter CJ, Jay RM, et al: The diagnosis of acute, recurrent, deep-vein thrombosis: A diagnostic challenge. Circulation 1983; 67:901.
19. Parfrey PS, Griffiths SM, Barrett BJ, et al: Contrast material-induced renal failure in patients with diabtes mellitus, renal insufficiency or both. N Engl J Med 1989; 320:143.
20. Schwab SJ, Hlarky MA, Pieper KS, et al: Contrast nephrotoxicity: A randomized controlled trial of a nonionic and an ionic radiographic contrast agent. N Engl J Med 1989; 320:149.
21. Hull RD, Hirsh J, Carter CJ, et al: A randomized trial of noninvasive diagnostic testing for clinically suspected deep-vein thrombosis: The diagnostic efficacy of impedance plethysmography. Ann Intern Med 1985; 102:21.
22. Hull RD, Taylor DW, Hirsh J, et al: Impedance plethysmography: The relationship between venous filling and sensitivity and specificity for proximal-vein thrombosis. Circulation 1978; 58:898.
23. Huisman MV, Buller HR, ten Cate JW, et al: Management of clinically suspected acute venous thrombosis in outpatients with serial impedance plethysmography in a community hospital setting. Arch Intern Med 1989; 149:511.
24. Cronan JJ, Dorfman GS, Scola FH, et al: Deep venous thrombosis: US assessment using vein compressibility. Radiology 1987; 162:191.
25. Lensing AWA, Prandoni P, Brandjes D, et al: Detection of deep-vein thrombosis by real-time B-mode ultrasonography. N Engl J Med 1989; 320:342.
26. Pedersen OM, Aslaksen A, Vik-Mo H, et al: Compression ultrasonography in hospitalized patients with suspected deep venous thrombosis. Arch Intern Med 1991; 151:2217.
27. Vaccaro JP, Cronan JJ, Dorfman GS: Outcome analysis of patients with normal compression US-examinations. Radiology 1990; 175:645.
28. Heijboer H, Brandjes D, Lensing AWA, et al: Efficacy of real-time B-mode ultrasonography versus impedance plethysmography in the diagnosis of deep vein thrombosis in symptomatic outpatients. Arch Intern Med 1992; 152:1901.
29. Rose SC, Zwiebel WJ, Nelson BD, et al: Symptomatic lower extremity deep venous thrombosis: Accuracy, limitations, and role of color duplex flow imaging in diagnosis. Radiology 1990; 175:639.
30. Ginsberg JS, Caco CC, Brill-Edwards P, et al: Venous thrombosis in patients who have undergone major hip or knee surgery: Detection with compression US and impedance plethysmography. Radiology 1991; 181:651.
31. Davidson B, Elliott GC, Lensing AWA: Low accuracy of color Doppler ultrasound to detect proximal leg vein thrombosis during screening of asymptomatic high-risk patients. Ann Intern Med 1992; 117:735.
32. Kipper MS, Moser KM, Kortman KE, et al: Long-term follow-up of patients with suspected pulmonary embolism and a normal lung scan. Chest 1985; 82:411.
33. Hull RD, Raskob GE, Coates G, et al: Clinical validity of a normal perfusion lung scan in patients with suspected pulmonary embolism. Chest 1990; 97:23.
34. PIOPED Investigators: Value of the ventilation/perfusion scan in acute pulmonary embolism: Results of the Prospective Investigation of Pulmonary Embolism Diagnosis (PIOPED). J Am Med Assoc 1990; 263:2753.
35. Alderson PO, Rujanavech N, Secker-Walker RH, et al: The role of ^{133}Xe ventilation studies in the scintigraphic detection of pulmonary embolism. Radiology 1976; 120:633.
36. McNeil BJ: Ventilation-perfusion studies and the diagnosis of pulmonary embolism: Concise communication. J Nucl Med 1980; 21:319.
37. Biello DR, Mattar AG, McKnight RC, et al: Ventilation-perfusion studies in suspected pulmonary embolism. Am J Radiol 1979; 133:1033.
38. Hull RD, Hirsh J, Carter CJ, et al: Diagnostic value of ventilation-perfusion lung scanning in patients with suspected pulmonary embolism. Chest 1985; 88:819.
39. Sasahara AA, Sharma GVRK, Parisi AF: New developments in the detection and prevention of venous thromboembolism. Am J Cardiol 1979; 43:1214.
40. Dalen JE, Brooks HL, Johnson LW, et al: Pulmonary angiography in acute pulmonary embolism. indications, techniques, and results in 367 patients. Am Heart J 1979; 81:175.
41. Bookstein JJ, Silver TM: The angiographic differential diagnosis of acute pulmonary embolism. Radiology 1974; 110:25.
42. Novelline RA, Oksana HB, Athanasoulis CA, et al: The clinical course of patients with suspected pulmonary embolism and a negative pulmonary arteriogram. Radiology 1978; 126:561.
43. Mills SR, Jackson DC, Older RA, et al: The incidence, etiologies, and avoidance of complications of pulmonary angiography in a large series. Radiology 1980; 136:295.
44. Stein PD, Hull RD, Saltzman HA, et al: Strategy for diagnosis of patients with suspected acute pulmonary embolism. Chest 1993;103:1553.
45. Hull RD, Raskob GE, Coates G, et al: A new non-invasive management strategy for patients with suspected pulmonary embolism. Arch Intern Med 1989; 149:2549.
46. Hull RD, Raskob GE, Ginsberg JS, et al: A definitive noninvasive strategy for the management of patients with suspected pulmonary embolism. Arch Intern Med 1993; 154:289.
47. Bjork I, Lindahl U: Mechanism of the anticoagulant action of heparin. Mol Cell Biochem 1982; 48:161.
48. Rosenberg RD: The heparin-antithrombin system: A natural anticoagulant mechanism. *In:* Thrombosis and Hemostasis: Basic Principles and Clinical Practice. 2nd ed. Colman RW, Hirsh J, Marder V, et al (Eds). Philadelphia, JB Lippincott, 1987, p 1373.
49. Hirsh J: Heparin. N Engl J Med 1991; 324:1565.
50. Salzman EW, Deykin D, Shapiro RM, et al: Management of heparin therapy: Controlled prospective trial. N Engl J Med 1975; 292:1046.
51. Hull RD, Raskob GE, Hirsh J, et al: Continuous intravenous heparin compared with intermittent subcutaneous heparin in the initial treatment of proximal-vein thrombosis. N Engl J Med 1986; 315:1109.
52. Brandjes DPM, Buller HR, Heijboer H, et al: Comparative trial of heparin and oral anticoagulants in the initial treatment of proximal deep vein thrombosis. N Engl J Med 1992; 327:1485.
53. Hull RD, Raskob GE, Rosenbloom D, et al: Optimal therapeutic level of heparin therapy in patients with venous thrombosis. Arch Intern Med 1992;152:1589.
54. Wheeler AP, Jaquiss RD, Newman JH: Physician practices in the treatment of pulmonary embolism and deep-venous thrombosis. Arch Intern Med 1988; 148:1321.
55. Cruickshank MK, Levine MN, Hirsh J, et al: A standard heparin nomogram for the management of heparin therapy. Arch Intern Med 1991; 151:333.
56. Pini M, Pattachini C, Quintavalla R, et al: Subcutaneous vs intravenous heparin in the treatment of deep venous thrombosis—A randomized clinical trial. Thromb Haemost 1990; 64:222.
57. Hommes DW, Bura A, Mazzolai L, et al: Subcutaneous heparin compared with continuous intravenous heparin administration in the initial treatment of deep vein thrombosis. Ann Intern Med 1992; 116:279.
58. Moser KM, Fedullo PF: Subcutaneous compared with intravenous heparin for deep vein thrombosis. Ann Intern Med 1992; 117:265.
59. Hull R, Delmore T, Carter C, et al: Adjusted subcutaneous heparin versus warfarin sodium in the long-term treatment of venous thrombosis. N Engl J Med 1982; 306:189.

60. Warkentin TE, Kelton JG: Heparin and platelets. Hematol Oncol Clin North Am 1990; 4:243.
61. Demers C, Ginsberg JS, Brill-Edwards P, et al: Rapid anticoagulation using ancrod for heparin-induced thrombocytopenia. Blood 1991; 78:2194.
62. Chong BH, Ismail F, Cade J, et al: Heparin-induced thrombocytopenia: Studies with a new low molecular weight heparinoid, Org 10172. Blood 1989; 73:1592.
63. Ortel TL, Gockerman JP, Califf RM, et al: Parenteral anticoagulation with the heparinoid Lomoparan (Org 10172) in patients with heparin induced thrombocytopenia and thrombosis. Thromb Haemost 1992; 67(3):292.
64. Howell R, Fidler J, Letsky E, et al: The risks of antenatal subcutaneous heparin prophylaxis: A controlled trial. Br J Obstet Gynaecol 1983; 90:1124.
65. Hirsh J, Levine MN: Low molecular weight heparin. Blood 1992; 79:1.
66. Verstraete M: Pharmacotherapeutic aspects of unfractionated and low molecular weight heparin. Drugs 1990; 40:498.
67. Bergqvist D, Hedner U, Sjorin E, et al: Anticoagulant effects of two types of low molecular weight heparin administered subcutaneously. Thromb Res 1983; 32:381.
68. Siegbahn A, Y-Hassan S, Boberg J, et al: Subcutaneous treatment of deep venous thrombosis with low molecular weight heparin. A dose finding study with LMWH-Novo. Thromb Res 1989; 55:767.
69. Albada J, Nieuwenhuis HK, Sixma JJ: Treatment of acute venous thromboembolism with low molecular weight heparin (Fragmin). Results of a double-blind randomized study. Circulation 1989; 80:935.
70. A Collaborative European Multicentre Study: A randomised trial of subcutaneous low molecular weight heparin (CY 216) compared with intravenous unfractionated heparin in the treatment of deep vein thrombosis. Thromb Haemost 1991; 65:251–256.
71. Lopaciuk S, Meissner AJ, Filipecki S, et al: Subcutaneous low-molecular-weight heparin versus subcutaneous unfractionated heparin in the treatment of deep vein thrombosis: A Polish multicenter trial. Thromb Haemost 1992; 68:14.
72. Prandoni P, Lensing AW, Buller HR, et al: Comparison of subcutaneous low-molecular-weight heparin with intravenous standard heparin in proximal deep-vein thrombosis. Lancet 1992; 339:441.
73. Hull RD, Raskob GE, Pineo GF, et al: Subcutaneous low-molecular weight heparin compared with continuous intravenous heparin in the treatment of proximal-vein thrombosis. N Engl J Med 1992; 326:975.
74. Vermeer C: Gamma-carboxyglutamate-containing proteins and the vitamin K-dependent carboxylase. Biochem J 1990; 266:625.
75. Furie B, Furie BC: Molecular basis of vitamin K-dependent gamma-carboxylation. Blood 1990; 75:1753.
76. Poller L, Tabener DA: Dosage and control of oral anticoagulants: An international study. Br J Haematol 1982; 51:479.
77. Bussey HI, Force RW, Bianco TM, et al: Reliance on prothrombin time ratios causes significant erors in anticoagulation therapy. Arch Intern Med 1992; 152:278.
78. Levine MN, Raskob GE, Hirsh J: Hemorrhagic complications of long term anticoagulant therapy. Chest 1989; 95(Suppl 2):26S.
79. Hull R, Hirsh J, Jay R, et al: Different intensities of oral anticoagulant therapy in the treatment of proximal-vein thrombosis. N Engl J Med 1982; 307:1676.
80. Grimaudo V, Gueissaz F, Hauert J, et al: Necrosis of skin induced by coumarin in a patient deficient in protein S. Br Med J 1989; 298:233.
81. Becker CG: Oral anticoagulant therapy and skin necrosis: Speculation on pathogenesis. Adv Exp Med Biol 1987; 214:217.
82. Hall JG, Pauli RM, Wilson KM: Maternal and fetal sequelae of anticoagulation during pregnancy. Am J Med 1980; 68:122.
83. Ginsberg JS, Hirsh J: Use of anticoagulants during pregnancy. Chest 1989; 95(Suppl 2):156S.
84. Iturbe-Alessio I, del Carmen Fonseca M, Mutchinik O, et al: Risks of anticoagulant therapy in pregnant women with artificial heart valves. N Engl J Med 1986; 315:1390.

CHAPTER 145

Bleeding Disorders of Childhood

David H. Ebb, MD • Gordon L. Bray, MD

Prompt restoration of adequate hemostasis in a bleeding child requires both an understanding of the basic elements of normal coagulation and a familiarity with the array of pathologic states that are common in children. This chapter provides a logical framework for the assessment and management of abnormal bleeding in children, with special emphasis on aspects of the hemostatic mechanism that are unique to children.

Although a carefully obtained history and physical examination may define an acquired cause of acute hemorrhage (e.g., infection, liver disease, or inadvertent ingestion of anticoagulant medications), no antecedent event may have occurred that suggests a bleeding tendency in the young patient with an inherited disorder of hemostasis. An otherwise healthy infant or child may never have encountered a hemostatic challenge sufficient to unmask an underlying bleeding disorder. Even the most exhaustive patient and family history may not identify a hemostatic disorder inherited in an autosomal recessive manner or one that is the result of a germline mutation in one or both parents. In addition, postnatal development of the hemostatic system over the first 3 to 4 years of life is associated with levels of coagulation factors that are different from adult standards. Failure to account for the physiologic differences in hemostasis between children and adults may lead to misdiagnosis and improper management of children who have excessive bleeding.

MAJOR COMPONENTS OF NORMAL HEMOSTASIS

The normal response to vascular injury includes reflex vasoconstriction, formation of a platelet plug that adheres to exposed subendothelial connective tissues (*primary hemostasis*), and consolidation of the platelet plug within a meshwork of polymerized fibrin (*coagulation mechanism*). Most causes of excessive bleeding can be classified according to whether either or both of these hemostatic components is abnormal. Defects in primary hemostasis result either from abnormal platelet function or from decreased platelet number. Abnormal coagulation reflects accelerated degradation of fibrin, resulting in inadequate clot stabilization, or it reflects decreased availability or function of one or more coagulation proteins. The distinction between primary hemostasis and coagulation is useful for a theoretic understanding of the hemostatic mechanism. In vivo, both occur simultaneously and are interdependent (Fig. 145–1).

INHERITED DISORDERS OF PRIMARY HEMOSTASIS

Thrombocytopenias

Normal platelet number is the same in infants, young children, and adults. Platelet production begins at the end of the first trimester, with normal adult levels (150,000–450,000/mm^3) established by 30 weeks' gestation.[1] Under normal circumstances, platelets are released into the plasma

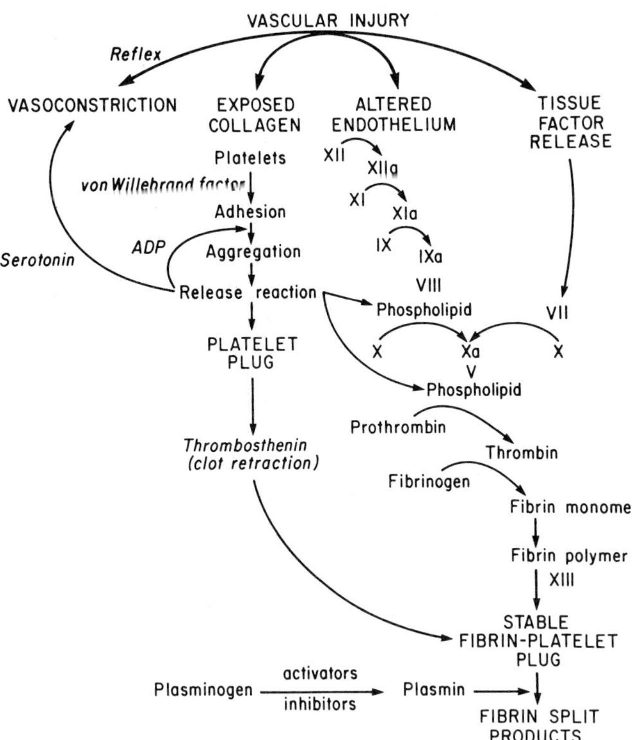

Figure 145–1. Diagrammatic representation of the hemostatic mechanism. (From Lusher JM: Diseases of coagulation: The fluid phase. *In:* Hematology of Infancy and Childhood. 3rd ed. Nathan DG, Oski FA [Eds]. Philadelphia, WB Saunders, 1987, p 1294.)

as anuclear cell fragments derived from polyploid megakaryocytes in the bone marrow. The circulating platelet has an average life span of 10 days.[2] Quantitative defects are caused by decreased production (e.g., bone marrow failure syndromes), increased consumption (e.g., hemorrhage, disseminated intravascular coagulation), peripheral destruction (e.g., immune-mediated processes), or splenic pooling.

Constitutional disorders of platelet production are relatively rare. Thrombocytopenia may present in early infancy as an isolated hematologic finding (e.g., amegakaryocytic thrombocytopenia) or as part of a syndrome marked by other phenotypic abnormalities (e.g., Wiskott-Aldrich syndrome or thrombocytopenia with absent radii syndrome). Aregenerative thrombocytopenia may also arise later in childhood as the initial hematologic manifestation of bone marrow failure. Syndromes causing such failure include Fanconi's aplastic anemia or dyskeratosis congenita.[3]

Wiskott-Aldrich syndrome is an X-linked disorder characterized by thrombocytopenia, eczema, progressive immunodeficiency involving both cellular and humoral immunity, and increased predisposition to lymphoid malignancies.[4] Platelets from patients with Wiskott-Aldrich syndrome are small, have decreased numbers of dense granules, and exhibit shortened survival. Hemorrhage and overwhelming infection are the commonest causes of early mortality in patients with Wiskott-Aldrich syndrome. Allogeneic bone marrow transplantation is curative of both the platelet and immunologic defects for patients who have a human leukocyte antigen–matched donor.[5] Splenectomy has been shown to result in a long-term increase in platelet number and size at the cost of an increased risk of bacterial sepsis.[6] Patients who fail to have a sustained response to splenectomy may respond to a combination of intravenous gamma G immunoglobulin (IgG) high-dose steroids, and vinca alkaloids, administered on an intermittent basis (Bray, 1987, unpublished data).

The thrombocytopenia with absent radii syndrome is characterized by forearm abnormalities, including absence or hypoplasia of the radii or ulnae, cardiac malformations in nearly one third of cases, transient leukemoid reactions, and thrombocytopenia that presents within the first 4 months of life.[7] Examination of bone marrow aspirates from affected infants reveals a marked decrease or absence of megakaryocytes, often in the presence of myeloid hyperplasia. Hemorrhagic complications tend to occur during the first year of life, with a bleeding-related mortality rate of 35%. Platelet transfusions are the only intervention available for managing bleeding in these children. To avoid allosensitization and refractoriness to platelet concentrates, platelet transfusions should be reserved for use in the acutely bleeding patient. Neither splenectomy nor pharmacologic intervention (steroids, intravenous IgG) are useful in this syndrome.[7] Interestingly, the platelet count begins to rise spontaneously after the first year of life, and thrombocytopenia partially or completely resolves. Affected children do not show an increased risk of bone marrow aplasia or malignancy.

Fanconi's aplastic anemia resembles thrombocytopenia with absent radii in its initial presentation, which includes thrombocytopenia and skeletal abnormalities involving the upper extremities. In contrast to patients with thrombocytopenia with absent radii, those with Fanconi's anemia typically present with thrombocytopenia at a mean age of 8 years and invariably progress to complete bone marrow failure over a period of months to years. In addition, patients have an increased predisposition to the development of malignancies (particularly myeloid leukemias) and often demonstrate radial anomalies that include the absence of thumbs.[3] In addition to hematologic and skeletal abnormalities, one third of Fanconi's anemia patients have renal anomalies. Cytogenetic studies reveal markedly increased spontaneous and mutagenic agent–induced chromosomal breaks, which is the single most reliable diagnostic finding. Because bone marrow transplantation is the treatment of choice, administration of blood products should be reserved for emergent situations in transplant candidates. Platelets should be administered only for acute bleeding.

Disorders of Platelet Function

Children with normal platelet counts who present with hemorrhage may have a qualitative defect in platelet function. Functional abnormalities may arise as a result of (1) defects in platelet membrane glycoproteins (e.g., glycoprotein Ib, glycoprotein IIb/IIIa) that mediate platelet-vessel wall and platelet-platelet interactions, (2) deficient or qualitatively abnormal plasma protein ligands (e.g., von Willebrand's factor [vWF], fibrinogen) required for effective platelet adhesion and aggregation, (3) platelet granule deficiencies, or (4) abnormalities in the generation of thromboxane A_2, the most potent physiologic agonist of platelet aggregation.

von Willebrand's Disease

vWF is a large, multimeric molecule that circulates in a noncovalent complex with Factor VIII. Binding of vWF to platelet membrane glycoprotein Ib is essential for effective platelet adhesion to exposed subendothelial collagen in damaged vessel walls.[8] Because vWF is the carrier protein for Factor VIII, decreased levels of vWF can result in correspondingly low levels of Factor VIII and in prolongation of the activated partial thromboplastin time (aPTT). vWF is synthesized in endothelial cells and megakaryocytes, where it is packaged in platelet alpha granules. Release of vWF from endothelial cell storage pools (e.g., Weibel-Palade bodies) can be induced by thrombin, epinephrine, and vasopressin analogues (e.g., desmopressin acetate [DDAVP]).[9]

von Willebrand's disease (vWD) is a group of disorders in which quantitative or qualitative abnormalities of vWF cause impaired adhesion of platelets to exposed subendothelial surfaces at sites of vascular injury. This defect in primary hemostasis underlies the bleeding diathesis observed in patients with vWD. Although patients with vWD have variable bleeding severity, affected patients typically present with easy bruisability, recurrent epistaxis, and other mucous membrane bleeding. Menorrhagia in postpubescent girls may lead to chronic blood loss and iron deficiency anemia. Excessive hemorrhage may follow surgery, dental procedures, or trauma, and even mild head injury carries a risk of intracranial hemorrhage. vWD is usually inherited in an autosomal dominant fashion, and males and females are affected in equal numbers. A small subset of patients with a severe form of the disease exhibit an autosomal recessive pattern of inheritance. Hemarthroses and muscle hematomas characteristic of the hemophilias (see later) are features of this severe (type III) variant of the disease.[8]

Diagnosis and Classification

Evaluation of the patient with suspected vWD should include a platelet count; a template bleeding time; assays of Factor VIII activity, vWF antigen, ristocetin cofactor activity,* and ristocetin-induced platelet aggregation; and analysis of vWF multimeric composition by sodium dodecyl sulfate (SDS) agarose gel electrophoresis (Table 145–1). Differentiating vWD subtypes is essential because the choice of therapy for bleeding depends on the specific subtype present.

Approximately 80% of vWD patients have type I disease, which is characterized by decreased amounts of structurally and functionally normal vWF.[10] Type I vWD the subtlest form of the disease, in which the bleeding time may be either normal or prolonged. Plasma levels of Factor VIII, vWF antigen, and ristocetin cofactor activity are decreased proportionately in type I vWD, and SDS agarose gels demonstrate normal vWF multimeric structure.[11] Patients with type II variants have decreased or absent levels of high-molecular-weight vWF multimers. Patients with subtype IIa vWD almost always exhibit prolonged bleeding times and have markedly diminished ristocetin cofactor activity, although their levels of Factor VIII activity and vWF antigen are usually normal. Patients with subtype IIb have mildly decreased ristocetin cofactor activity, and they demonstrate a distinctive *increase* in platelet aggregation when their platelet-rich plasma is incubated in the presence of low-dose ristocetin.[8, 11] Aggregation of autologous, platelet-rich plasma in response to low-dose ristocetin administration reflects the increased affinity of abnormal, type IIb vWF for platelet membranes and distinguishes type IIb vWD from types I and IIa. Type III vWD is the most severe form of the disease, affecting 1% to 3% of patients. Hemorrhagic complications are similar to those observed in patients with moderate hemophilia.[12] This variant is characterized by the complete absence of vWF antigen and ristocetin cofactor activity.

*Addition of the antibiotic ristocetin to plasma causes platelet aggregation by inducing the binding of platelet glycoprotein Ib to its ligand, vWF. When vWF is deficient or structurally abnormal, decreased aggregation of control platelets occurs in response to the addition of ristocetin to the patient's platelet-poor plasma. This observation forms the basis of the ristocetin cofactor activity assay. Decreased ristocetin cofactor activity is diagnostic of vWD.

Treatment and Prevention of Bleeding

Management of bleeding complications in patients with vWD requires prompt increase of vWF activity in plasma either by infusion of exogenous vWF or by stimulation of release of endogenous stores. Cryoprecipitate is the most commonly administered source of exogenous vWF. Because the levels of ristocetin cofactor activity in cryoprecipitate vary from bag to bag, dosing is somewhat empiric, and adjustments are based on clinical response.[13] As a general guideline, we suggest infusing one bag of cryoprecipitate for every 5 kg of body weight, up to a maximum of eight bags per dose. For severe or prolonged bleeding, cryoprecipitate should be given every 8 to 12 hours.

DDAVP is the treatment of choice for bleeding in most patients with type I, and in some patients with type IIa vWD.[14] DDAVP stimulates the release of vWF from Weibel-Palade bodies in endothelial cells. Because it is not a blood

TABLE 145–1. Results of Laboratory Studies in Patients with von Willebrand's Disease

Laboratory Test	*von Willebrand's Disease*			
	Type I	*Type IIa*	*Type IIb*	*Type III*
Bleeding time	Normal or prolonged	Usually prolonged	Usually prolonged	Always prolonged
Factor VIII:C	Normal or mildly decreased	Normal or mildly decreased	Usually normal	Always markedly decreased*
vWF antigen (Laurell assay)	Normal or mildly decreased	Normal or mildly decreased	Usually normal	Usually absent
Ristocetin-induced platelet aggregation	Usually normal	Usually decreased	Increased†	Markedly decreased to absent
Ristocetin cofactor activity	Normal or mildly to moderately decreased‡	Moderately to markedly decreased	Usually mildly to moderately decreased	Markedly decreased to absent
vWF multimeric analysis in SDS agarose gels	All MW multimers present and decreased proportionately	Absent of high and intermediate MW multimers; normal or increased low MW multimers	Absence of high mW multimers; normal or increased low and intermediate MW multimers	Lack of *all* MW multimers (high, intermediate, and low)

(From Bray GL: Inherited and acquired disorders of hemostasis. *In:* Textbook of Pediatric Critical Care. Holbrook PR [Ed]. Philadelphia, WB Saunders, 1993, pp 783–801.)

*Levels of factor VIII:C in most patients with type III vWD are comparable with those exhibited by patients with moderate-to-severe Factor VIII deficiency.

†A diagnostic feature of type IIb vWD is the ability of low concentrations of ristocetin (0.2–0.3 mg/mL) to cause aggregation in platelet-rich plasma.

‡Patients wtih type I vWD usually have proportionate decreases in plasma levels of VIII:C, vWF antigen, and ristocetin cofactor activity.

MW = molecular weight; vWD = von Willebrand's disease; vWF = von Willebrand's factor.

product, its use does not incur a risk of blood-borne viral infection. When administered intravenously (0.3 μg/kg over 15 to 30 minutes in 30 to 50 mL of normal saline) or subcutaneously, DDAVP stimulates a rapid, threefold to fivefold increase in Factor VIII, vWF antigen, and ristocetin cofactor activity. Repetitive use of DDAVP over short intervals leads to the development of tachyphylaxis due to depletion of endogenous vWF stores, thereby limiting its subsequent effectiveness. Frequent dosing can also lead to water retention and hyponatremia. For these reasons, DDAVP should be given no more frequently than once daily, and serum electrolyte levels should be carefully monitored. Patients with type III vWD do not respond to DDAVP, because they have no endogenous stores of vWF to mobilize. DDAVP is contraindicated in patients with type IIb because it stimulates the secretion of functionally abnormal vWF that promotes intravascular platelet aggregation and thrombocytopenia.[14]

Factor VIII concentrates that contain significant quantities of vWF represent a third therapeutic option. Several concentrates have been shown to contain hemostatic levels of structurally normal vWF.[15] Anecdotal evidence has been reported of its successful use in patients with types I and IIa vWD.

Defects in Platelet Membrane Glycoprotein Receptors

Bernard-Soulier Syndrome

Patients with Bernard-Soulier syndrome lack platelet membrane glycoprotein Ib, which mediates adhesion of platelets to subendothelium through the binding of vWF. Bernard-Soulier syndrome is characterized by moderate-to-severe mucocutaneous bleeding that presents early in life. Laboratory findings include mild-to-moderate thrombocytopenia, unusually large platelets noted on peripheral blood film, and prolonged bleeding time. In vitro assays of platelet aggregation reveal a normal response to adenosine diphosphate, epinephrine, and collagen, as well as a decreased response to thrombin. Platelets from individuals with Bernard-Soulier syndrome fail to aggregate in the presence of ristocetin.[16] Therapy for the bleeding patient with Bernard-Soulier syndrome is limited to platelet transfusions. However, because transfused platelets possess glycoprotein Ib, platelet concentrate use frequently results in the development of alloantibodies to glycoprotein Ib and subsequent refractoriness to platelet transfusions.[17]

Glanzmann's Thrombasthenia

Glanzmann's thrombasthenia is an autosomal recessive disorder characterized by prolonged bleeding time and early-onset mucocutaneous bleeding, despite a normal platelet count. Platelets from individuals with Glanzmann's thrombasthenia lack the membrane glycoprotein IIb/IIIa complex required for fibrinogen-mediated platelet-platelet interaction. Platelets in patients with this disorder adhere normally to injured vessel walls but are unable to extend the primary platelet plug by aggregating with each other. These platelets do not aggregate in vitro in the presence of physiologic agonists (adenosine diphosphate, epinephrine, thrombin, collagen) but do respond to the antibiotic ristocetin.[16] The same pattern of bleeding prolongation and impaired platelet aggregation is observed in patients with congenital afibrinogenemia, although this disorder is easily distinguished from Glanzmann's thrombasthenia by measurement of fibrinogen levels. Hemorrhagic complications in patients with Glanzmann's thrombasthenia are treated with platelet transfusions. The risk of antiglycoprotein IIb/IIIa alloantibody formation in these patients mandates a cautious approach to the use of platelet concentrates.[17] Menorrhagia in post-pubescent females often responds to treatment with oral contraceptives.

Platelet Granule Deficiencies

Absence or deficiency of platelet granules can produce a mild-to-moderate bleeding diathesis. Normal platelets contain three types of storage organelles: alpha granules, dense granules, and lysosomes. The constituents of alpha granules include platelet factor 4, β-thromboglobulin, platelet-derived growth factor, fibrinogen, Factor V, vWF, and high-molecular-weight kininogen. Dense granules are rich in adenosine diphosphate and adenosine triphosphate and, in addition, contain serotonin, phospholipase, and calcium.[18]

GRAY-PLATELET SYNDROME. Individuals with gray-platelet syndrome are severely deficient or completely lacking in alpha granules. Elevations of platelet factor 4 and β-thromboglobulin in plasma suggest that this syndrome is the result of a packaging defect rather than an intrinsic inability to synthesize alpha-granule constituents. The clinical features of gray-platelet syndrome include mild thrombocytopenia, prolonged bleeding time, and abnormal, thrombin-induced platelet aggregation and secretion.[18]

DENSE-GRANULE DEFICIENCY. Patients with dense-granule deficiency often have a history of easy bruising, epistaxis, gingival or gastrointestinal bleeding, menorrhagia, and excessive bleeding after surgical procedures. Platelets from some individuals with dense-granule defects have a concomitant deficiency of alpha granules. Characteristic laboratory findings include prolongation of bleeding time and failure to have a second wave of aggregation when platelets are stimulated by adenosine diphosphate or epinephrine.[7, 18] Treatment of hemorrhagic complications in these patients requires the infusion of platelet concentrates.

ACQUIRED DISORDERS OF PRIMARY HEMOSTASIS

Acquired disorders of primary hemostasis include both quantitative and functional platelet defects. Acquired thrombocytopenias are a consequence of impaired production, peripheral sequestration, or accelerated platelet destruction by immune or nonimmune mechanisms. Immune-mediated platelet destruction is caused by the binding of IgG—or less commonly by IgM and complement—resulting in the subsequent clearance of sensitized platelets by the reticuloendothelial system.

Neonatal Thrombocytopenia

Most often, thrombocytopenia in premature and full-term neonates is a consequence of accelerated platelet destruction due to infection or immune-mediated mechanisms. Severe thrombocytopenia can occur in infants who are infected by any of the TORCH viruses (toxoplasmosis, rubella, cytomegalovirus, or herpes simplex) or human immunodeficiency virus type 1 (HIV-1). Bacterial sepsis can trigger disseminated intravascular coagulation (DIC) and platelet consumption by acceleration of platelet adhesion to damaged blood vessels. Consumptive thrombocytopenia also occurs in the setting of birth asphyxia, preeclampsia, hyperbilirubinemia treated with phototherapy, meconium aspiration, neonatal respiratory distress syndrome, persistent pulmonary hypertension, necrotizing enterocolitis, or cyanotic congenital heart disease.[1] For all of the aforementioned conditions, acute bleeding is treated or prevented with platelet transfusions while the underlying disorder is being investigated and corrected. *Platelet concentrates must be irradiated to minimize the risk of graft-versus-host disease.*

Neonatal Immune Thrombocytopenia

Isolated thrombocytopenia in an otherwise healthy newborn should raise suspicion of an immune-mediated mechanism. Discrimination between alloimmune and isoimmune thrombocytopenia is essential for the selection of a suitable platelet donor for the neonate.

Alloimmune thrombocytopenia is the result of transplacental passage of maternal antiplatelet autoantibody. In such situations, the mother's platelet count is usually decreased but may be normal. The duration of thrombocytopenia in the infant is a function of the persistence of maternal antibody in the neonate's circulation. Because IgG has a half-life of 21 days, the infant's thrombocytopenia generally resolves within several days to weeks after parturition.[1]

Most infants born to mothers with immune thrombocytopenic purpura (ITP) are not severely thrombocytopenic and require no intervention other than close observation. In the event of life-threatening hemorrhage, platelet transfusions may promote hemostasis, although a sustained increment in platelet count may not occur because of the rapid clearance of sensitized donor platelets. For the severely thrombocytopenic newborn at risk for life-threatening hemorrhage, infusion of IgG (1 $g \cdot kg^{-1} \cdot d^{-1}$ for 2 to 3 days), either alone or in conjunction with corticosteroid administration (prednisolone, 2 mg/kg), may be the most effective therapy.[1]

Isoimmune thrombocytopenia occurs in infants whose mothers have normal platelet counts and no bleeding history. Hemorrhagic complications, such as gastrointestinal bleeding, hematuria, and hemoptysis frequently occur in conjunction with a platelet count of less than $20 \times 10^9/L$. The occurrence of intracranial hemorrhage in approximately 15% of severely thrombocytopenic newborns represents the greatest source of morbidity in affected infants.[1]

Isoimmune thrombocytopenia is the result of maternal exposure to paternally derived antigens on fetal platelets that are not present on maternal platelets. Maternal sensitization to foreign-platelet antigens results in the formation of antibodies directed against fetal platelets. Transplacental passage of antibodies results in fetal and neonatal thrombocytopenia. PL^{A1} is the most commonly implicated platelet antigen, causing 75% of cases of isoimmune thrombocytopenia. This antigen is found on the surface of platelets in 98% of the general population but is missing from the platelets of mothers with affected newborns. First-born infants are affected in nearly half the cases. Maternal sensitization can occur at any time during pregnancy, along with an attendant risk of antenatal intracranial hemorrhage. Infants born with platelet counts of less than $30 \times 10^9/L$ should be treated with platelet transfusions from a donor who is PL^{A1}-antigen negative. The best source of PL^{A1}-negative platelets is usually the patient's mother.[1] Isoimmune thrombocytopenia usually resolves within the first month of life.

Immune Thrombocytopenic Purpura

ITP is estimated to affect 20,000 children in the United States annually and has a peak incidence between 2 and 5 years of age. Patients commonly present with acute onset of petechiae and purpura, often 1 to 3 weeks after a nonspecific viral illness. Approximately 25% to 30% of affected children present with epistaxis, 5% of cases are complicated by gastrointestinal bleeding, and central nervous system (CNS) hemorrhage complicates 0.5% to 1.0% of cases.[20] Petechiae and purpura are the commonest findings on physical examination, and splenomegaly has been reported in 10% to 20% of patients. In contrast to adult-onset ITP, in which women are more commonly affected, no gender predilection exists in the pediatric form of the disease.

Laboratory Findings

Eighty per cent of patients with ITP present with platelet counts of less than $40 \times 10^9/L$.[7] Review of the peripheral blood film reveals decreased numbers of abnormally large platelets. Results of coagulation studies (prothrombin time, aPTT, fibrinogen, fibrin degradation products) are always normal. Examination of bone marrow aspirates typically reveals normal-to-increased numbers of megakaryocytes, consistent with increased platelet turnover. Although debate continues about the role of bone marrow aspiration in the diagnosis of acute ITP, nearly three fourths of pediatric hematologists continue to perform this study as part of their evaluation of ITP.[21] Bone marrow aspiration is strongly recommended in patients who present with splenomegaly, or before therapy with corticosteroids is initiated.

Natural History

More than 80% of children with ITP experience remission of their disease within several months of presentation. Chronic ITP is defined as a platelet count of less than $100 \times 10^9/L$ for longer than 6 months.[17] The pathogenesis of the acute and chronic forms of childhood ITP are different, with chronic ITP more closely resembling the adult form of the disease. Increased levels of platelet-associated IgG are found in approximately 90% of children with ITP; most of the immunoglobulin in patients with acute ITP is not platelet-specific autoantibody.[20] Recent studies suggest that high levels of platelet-associated IgG may reflect the rapid turnover of platelets and the mobilization of IgG from alpha granules to the platelet membrane. Hence, elevated platelet-associated IgG levels are primarily a consequence, and not a cause, of increased thrombolysis.[22] The temporal association of viral illness with the onset of acute ITP suggests that the latter may be triggered by antigen-antibody complexes adsorbed to the platelet membrane, prompting platelet clearance by reticuloendothial system macrophages.[17, 23]

The onset of chronic ITP may be more insidious than that of the acute form, often presenting without a history of a viral prodrome. Ten per cent to 20% of children with new-onset ITP ultimately develop chronic disease, with the greatest risk occurring in children older 10 years of age.[17] The pathogenesis of chronic ITP involves the formation of platelet-specific autoantibodies that bind to antigenic determinants on the platelet surface.[17]

Treatment

The debate among pediatric hematologists regarding the need for treatment of acute ITP in childhood reflects the generally benign nature of the disease and the high incidence of spontaneous recovery. This course is in contrast to that of adult ITP, in which 60% to 80% of patients ultimately require splenectomy.[20] The most commonly employed treatment options include oral prednisone or intravenous IgG administration. For the acutely bleeding child, IgG (1 $g \cdot kg^{-1} \cdot d^{-1}$ IV for 1 to 3 days) is the treatment of choice because of its rapid onset of action. Most children treated with intravenous IgG respond with an increase in platelet count within 1 week of initiation of therapy.

The mechanisms of action of intravenous IgG and corticosteroids remain incompletely understood. The effect of intravenous IgG may be mediated through the blockade of Fc receptors on macrophages, which prevents recognition and phagocytosis of opsonized platelets, or through idiotype-anti-idiotype interactions.[20] The mechanism of action of corticosteroids is even less well understood, although it appears to be multifactorial. Independent of their effect on platelet number, steroids may reduce bleeding risk in the thrombocytopenic patient by increasing microvascular stability.[2] Steroid-mediated increased platelet survival and subsequent resolution of thrombocytopenia have been attributed to suppression of antibody production by B lymphocytes and inhibition of phagocytosis of antibody-sensitized platelets.[7]

Platelet transfusions are indicated only in patients with life-threatening (e.g., CNS) hemorrhage. Donor platelets offer minimal benefit because of their rapid sensitization and subsequent clearance by the host reticuloendothelial system. In addition, donor platelets may stimulate alloantibody formation. If CNS bleeding requires neurosurgical evacuation, the patient should be prepared for emergency splenectomy and should be treated with intravenous IgG and bolus methylprednisolone administration.[17] Intraoperative infusion of platelet concentrates after interruption of the splenic blood supply maximizes the recovery and life span of donor platelets before craniotomy is performed. Because patients with ITP produce platelets at two to three times the rate of normal individuals, many patients exhibit a rapid increase in platelet count after ligation of the splenic pedicle.

Management guidelines for the thrombocytopenic child who does not have active bleeding are less clear. We recommend that children with platelet counts of less than 20 to 30 $\times$ 10^9/L be treated with prednisone at an initial dose of 2 $mg \cdot kg^{-1} \cdot d^{-1}$ for 1 to 3 weeks, followed by a gradual weaning of the dosage over 1 to 3 weeks. Because prolonged therapy with steroids can lead to fluid retention, osteoporosis, growth retardation, cushingoid features, and acne, children who either fail to improve or cannot sustain improvement when steroids are weaned should be treated with intermittent doses of intravenous IgG to maintain a platelet count of at least 30 to 40 $\times$ 10^9/L. Splenectomy may be considered for the child with chronic ITP (see later). Because of the high risk of postsplenectomy sepsis, splenectomy should be deferred, if possible, until affected children are 6 years of age. All patients should receive the polyvalent pneumococcal vaccine before splenectomy and penicillin prophylaxis after splenectomy.

Splenectomy leads to partial or complete remission of thrombocytopenia in approximately 75% of patients with chronic ITP.[17] Recurrence of thrombocytopenia after splenectomy is performed should prompt a search for an accessory spleen or spleens. Treatment options for splenectomy nonresponders include periodic infusions of IgG, alternate-day administration of steroids, or administration of vinca alkaloids (vincristine or vinblastine), cyclophosphamide, cyclosporine, IgG anti-D, or interferon α.[17]

HIV-Related Thrombocytopenia

Thrombocytopenia is a relatively common manifestation of HIV-1 infection. Although multiple etiologies exist for thrombocytopenia in patients with acquired immunodeficiency syndrome (e.g., infections, drugs), asymptomatic HIV-1–infected patients frequently develop a syndrome that is analogous to ITP. Although platelet-associated IgG levels are uniformly elevated in HIV-1–related ITP, the pathophysiology of platelet destruction is complex and multifaceted. Accelerated platelet destruction in homosexual men has been attributed to the adsorption of circulating immune complexes to platelet membranes, prompting their clearance by reticuloendothelial system macrophages. ITP in HIV-1–infected intravenous drug results from a combination of platelet-bound immune complexes and platelet-specific autoantibody formation. In HIV-1–infected people with hemophilia, ITP is predominantly a consequence of autoantibodies directed against platelet membrane glycoproteins.[23] Most patients exhibit normal-to-increased numbers of megakaryocytes on examination of bone marrow aspirates. Some thrombocytopenic patients exhibit decreased numbers of megakaryocytes in their bone marrow, or ineffective thrombopoiesis, or both, which may be a consequence of HIV-1 infection of megakaryocytes or deposition of immune complexes on their surfaces.[24]

Therapeutic options for patients with HIV-related thrombocytopenia are similar to those previously outlined for ITP. For bleeding patients, intravenous IgG administration is frequently effective, although increases in platelet count are transient, generally lasting 7–10 days. Corticosteroids are effective in a significant number of patients, although the effect is often not sustained. Steroid therapy may be complicated by the development of oropharyngeal candidiasis, reactivation of latent herpesvirus infection, and accelerated CD4+ lymphocyte depletion. Zidovudine may be the most effective medical therapy for patients with thrombocytopenia. The rapid rise in platelet count observed after the initiation of zidovudine has been attributed to its antiviral effect.[23] Splenectomy is reserved for patients who fail to respond to any of the aforementioned medical approaches.

Miscellaneous Causes of Acquired Thrombocytopenia

Infection

Thrombocytopenia is a common complication of systemic viral and bacterial infections, affecting 20% to 30% of patients with bacterial septicemia. Typically, the mechanism for development of thrombocytopenia is accelerated platelet clearance. Elevated levels of platelet-associated IgG and decreased platelet survival in both bacterial and viral (particularly Epstein-Barr virus) infections suggest an immune complex–mediated cause for the thrombocytopenia. Increased adhesion of platelets to exposed subendothelial surfaces of damaged blood vessels may contribute to thrombocytopenia in patients with bacterial sepsis.[7] Many patients with sepsis-associated thrombocytopenia do not experience concomitant consumptive coagulopathy.

Bone Marrow Infiltration

Thrombocytopenia secondary to decreased platelet production can result from the replacement of normal bone marrow by neoplastic or other infiltrative processes, such as the leukemias, neuroblastoma, and myeloproliferative, storage, and granulomatous disorders. Decreased production and increased consumption of platelets are associated with the virus-associated hemophagocytic syndrome, which is most frequently a consequence of acute cytomegalovirus or Epstein-Barr virus infection. Virus-associated hemophagocytic syndrome is characterized by histiocytic hyperplasia, sequestration of circulating platelets in the spleen and liver, and phagocytosis of hematopoietic precursors by medullary histiocytes.[25]

Pharmacologic Agents

Thrombocytopenia can be caused by decreased production or increased consumption of circulating platelets. The marrow-suppressive effects of chemotherapeutic agents used to treat cancer are well characterized and predictable. Thrombocytopenia secondary to myelosuppressive medications is treated with infusions of platelet concentrates in patients with active bleeding, or in those with platelet counts of less than 10 $\times$ 10^9/L. A higher threshold for platelet transfusion (20 $\times$ 10^9/L) is recommended for patients with brain tumors.[26]

Drug-mediated platelet consumption is usually idiosyncratic and typically results from an immune-mediated mechanism. Thrombocytopenia usually occurs days to weeks after the introduction of the offending drug. Re-exposure to the causative medication after resolution of the thrombocytopenia leads to a prompt decrease in platelet count. Specific mechanisms underlying the development of drug-induced thrombocytopenia include (1) binding of drug-antidrug antibody complexes to platelets; (2) binding of the drug directly to the platelet surface, prompting antibody attachment to the drug-platelet complex; (3) formation of platelet membrane neoantigens caused by binding of the drug to the platelet surface; or (4) formation of drug-induced platelet autoantibodies (e.g., those caused by methyldopa, quinidine, interferon).[7]

Although many drugs have been implicated in the development of drug-induced thrombocytopenia, this complication occurs most commonly in patients taking heparin. Quinidine, the penicillins, digoxin, valproic acid, and cimetidine have also been implicated in the development of idiosyncratic thrombocytopenia.[7, 27] Heparin is unique because of its ability to cause life-threatening arterial thrombosis with thrombocytopenia, and also because of the tendency for the thrombocytopenia to improve in some instances, despite continuation of heparin therapy. Heparin-induced thrombocytopenia occurs a mean of 10 days after its initiation, and it occurs more commonly in patients taking higher doses and in those treated with bovine preparations. If arterial thrombosis occurs, heparin should be immediately discontinued. A combination of low-molecular-weight heparin and antifibrinolytic therapy may be an effective alternative therapy in patients with arterial thrombosis until oral anticoagulants reach effective plasma levels.[27] In children with mild thrombocytopenia, heparin therapy may be continued, but careful attention should be paid to the patients' platelet count, and transition to oral anticoagulant therapy should occur as soon as possible.

Therapy for drug-induced thrombocytopenias consists of stopping the offending drug as soon as possible.[7]

Miscellaneous Causes of Platelet Dysfunction

Uremia

Hemorrhagic complications in uremic patients arise from impaired platelet–vessel wall interactions. Qualitative defects in plasma vWF and decreased levels of platelet vWF are believed to be the primary causes of uremic bleeding.[29] Additional factors contributing to the increased bleeding include platelet granule defects and impairment of platelet aggregation resulting from high concentrations of uremic retention products. Alterations in vessel wall endothelium lead to increased production of the platelet antagonist prostacyclin (PGI_2).[29] Patients characteristically exhibit petechiae, purpura, mucous membrane bleeding, prolonged bleeding times, and abnormal platelet aggregation.

Anemia has also been identified as a contributor to the hemostatic impairment occurring in uremic patients. Elevations in hematocrit value, achieved either through red blood cell transfusions or through the use of recombinant human erythropoietin, can lead to shortened bleeding time and decreased bleeding tendency. Increasing the hematocrit value to 30% may lead to displacement of circulating platelets toward the vessel wall, thereby facilitating their contact with the endothelium and improving hemostasis.[29]

Uremic bleeding diathesis is most effectively managed with a combination of dialysis and maintenance of an adequate hematocrit value.[29] In patients with persistent bleeding after dialysis or in those who are at high risk for hemorrhagic complications from elective surgery, bleeding risk can be further reduced with infusions of cryoprecipitate or DDAVP. Both measures increases plasma vWF levels, transiently decrease bleeding time, and probably reduce bleeding tendency.[14]

Extracorporeal Oxygenation

Children supported by cardiopulmonary bypass or extracorporeal membrane oxygenation are at risk for hemostatic derangements that can lead to excessive intraoperative and postoperative bleeding. Potential defects include impaired platelet function, mild (dilutional) thrombocytopenia, increased fibrinolysis, and inadequate neutralization of the anticoagulant heparin. Hypothermia can exacerbate thrombocytopenia as a result of splenic and hepatic platelet pooling, which is reversed when body temperature is normalized.[30]

Platelet dysfunction appears to be the primary cause of postoperative bleeding complications. As they pass through the oxygenator apparatus, platelets may undergo partial activation and may secrete their granular contents, causing partial depletion of alpha granules.[30] Platelet function is further impaired by plasma membrane–receptor defects that compromise the binding of plasma protein ligands, such as fibrinogen and vWF. The severity of platelet dysfunction appears to vary in proportion to the duration of bypass. Postoperative platelet transfusions are usually sufficient to control hemorrhage for all patients except those (approximately 3%) who require surgical re-exploration.[31] Controlled, randomized studies using preoperative infusions of the serine protease inhibitor aprotonin or intraoperative infusions of DDAVP in adults have demonstrated shortened bleeding times and decreased blood loss after cardiopulmonary bypass.[31, 32] Although these therapeutic adjuncts appear promising, their role in children remains to be established.

Pharmacologic Agents

Drug-induced platelet dysfunction rarely causes spontaneous hemorrhage unless it is superimposed on an underlying hemostatic disorder, such as thrombocytopenia or hemophilia. The most noteworthy drug effects on platelet function (e.g., those resulting from aspirin or nonsteroidal anti-inflammatory drug administration) are mediated through inhibition of platelet cyclooxygenase activity. Inactivation of cyclooxygenase inhibits the production of thromboxane A_2, a potent platelet agonist. The semisynthetic penicillins and cephalosporins can produce variable defects of in vitro platelet aggregation that are dose and duration dependent.[17] The clinical significance of these observations is unclear. Although inhibition of platelet function may be therapeutically desirable in specific contexts (e.g., prevention of recurrent myocardial infarction or stroke), unwanted platelet dysfunction is treated by withdrawal of the causative agent. Drugs that interfere with platelet function should be avoided, if possible, in patients with underlying congenital or acquired hemostatic deficits (Table 145–2).

INHERITED COAGULOPATHIES

Development of the Coagulation Mechanism

Clotting and fibrinolytic proteins are detectable in fetal plasma as early as 10 to 11 weeks of gestation, with the levels of most coagulation proteins rising in proportion to gestational age.[33] Although most coagulation plasma proteins approach adult levels by the time an individual is 6 months of age, as a group, they exhibit discordant developmental patterns.[34] For example, the mean levels of Factor VIII, vWF, and fibrinogen approximate the normal adult range by 30 weeks' gestation. In contrast, the levels of vitamin K–dependent coagulation proteins (Factors II, IX, and X and protein C) are significantly lower, ranging from 40%

TABLE 145–2. Commonly Used Drugs that Prolong Bleeding Time or Decrease In Vitro Platelet Aggregation

Antiplatelet Agents
Aspirin
Dipyridamole
Sulfinpyrazone
Ticlopidine
Antibiotics
Semisynthetic penicillins
Cephalosporins
Nonsteroidal Anti-inflammatory Agents
Ibuprofen
Naproxen
Indomethacin
Phenylbutazone
Miscellaneous
Heparin
Dextran sulfate
Glyceryl guaiacolate
Ethyl alcohol
Valproic acid
ω_3-J Polyunsaturated fatty acids
Phenothiazines

(From Bray GL: Inherited and acquired disorders of hemostasis. *In:* Textbook of Pediatric Clinical Care. Holbrook PR [Ed]. Philadelphia, WB Saunders, 1993, pp 783–801.)

to 66% of adult mean levels in full-term infants.[35] Significant differences exist also in neonatal, early childhood, and adult levels of the contact activation clotting factors (newborns have 30–50% of adult mean levels at term), the major coagulation protease inhibitors (protein C, protein S, antithrombin-TIII, and heparin cofactor II), and the activators and inhibitors of fibrinolysis.[35, 36] Some investigators have suggested that the lower risk for thrombosis in early childhood may be the result of the nearly twofold higher levels of the minor coagulation protease inhibitor, α_2-macroglobulin.[36] The relative infrequency of thrombosis in children may also result from lower levels of prothrombin, which alter the kinetics of clot formation in a protective manner.

Not surprisingly, in view of the physiologic differences in individual factor levels at different stages of development, results of coagulation screening tests must be interpreted in the context of age-specific norms. During the first 6 months of life, the acceptable upper limit of the aPTT is greater than that of the adult. This discrepancy is the result of the aforementioned age-dependent difference in concentration of the contact activation factors (Factor XII, Factor XI, high-molecular-weight kininogen, and prekallikrein). In contrast, upper-limit norms for prothrombin time are stable from shortly after birth through adulthood, reflecting the attainment of adult levels of Factor VII within the first week of life.[34] Recently established age-adjusted norms for factor levels and coagulation screening tests should improve diagnostic accuracy and enhance the appropriateness of interventions based on these assays. Table 145–3 lists the age-adjusted normal values for various components of the coagulation mechanism.

Hemophilias

Patients with hemophilia characteristically exhibit bleeding into joints and muscles after either minimal or no trauma. In all individuals with hemophilia, bleeding is the result of delayed thrombin generation, which in turn results in deficient clot formation.

Hemophilia A (Factor VIII deficiency) and hemophilia B (Factor IX deficiency) account for most inherited coagulopathies. Factor VIII deficiency is the cause of 80% to 85% of all cases of hemophilia, occurring in 1 in 5000 male births. Ten per cent to 15% of hemophilia results from Factor IX deficiency, occurring in 1 in 25,000 males. Nearly one third of newly diagnosed patients with hemophilia have no family history of coagulopathy, reflecting the common occurrence of spontaneous mutation in the genes for Factors VIII and IX.[37] Because the clinical manifestations of hemophilias A and B are indistinguishable, the correct diagnosis depends on the results of specific assays for Factors VIII and IX.

The frequency and severity of bleeding episodes in people with hemophilia is largely a function of the baseline coagulation factor level. Activity levels measure endogenous factor availability relative to a reference standard that is 100% of normal (100 IU/dL). Patients with factor levels greater than 5% of normal are mildly affected and bleed only in response to significant trauma or surgery. Severely affected patients with less than 1% of normal activity are prone to frequent, spontaneous episodes of bleeding.[37] Because mean Factor VIII levels in normal newborns are within the normal adult range, the diagnosis of Factor VIII deficiency—regardless of severity—is generally easy in early infancy.[34] In contrast, Factor IX levels consistent with mild deficiency overlap with those observed in normal newborns, potentially complicating the diagnosis of mild hemophilia B shortly after birth.[34]

Bleeding Manifestations

Many children with hemophilia, particularly those who are mildly or moderately affected, do not experience abnormal bleeding during the first year of life. The onset of abnormal bleeding often coincides with the attainment of motor development milestones, such as crawling or walking.[37] Some hemophilic infants initially present with significant bleeding after a forceps-assisted delivery or circumcision. The absence of abnormal bleeding after circumcision does not rule out the diagnosis of hemophilia, because only 30% of infants bleed excessively after this procedure.[12] As the child becomes increasingly mobile during the second year of life, the incidence of musculoskeletal bleeding generally increases. Typical presentations include excessive cutaneous bruising, bleeding from the nose and mouth, muscle hematomas in the extremities, and hemarthroses, most often involving the knees, elbows, and ankles.

Potentially life-threatening complications of hemophilia include CNS, retropharyngeal or retroperitoneal hemorrhage, and bleeding associated with episodes of multiple trauma, or surgery undertaken without adequate factor replacement. The incidence of CNS hemorrhage in patients with hemophilia has been reported to vary from 2.6% to 13.8%, with a case fatality rate ranging from 20% to 50%. Chronic neurologic deficits (seizure disorder, cognitive or motor deficits) occur in up to 50% of patients who survive CNS bleeding.[38] Intracranial bleeding in infants and children usually follows head trauma. In a large, retrospective study of infants with hemophilia, nearly 2% experienced CNS hemorrhage related to birth trauma either during or shortly after delivery, and an additional 1.9% exhibited intracranial hemorrhage within the first 4 weeks of life.[39] Because CNS bleeding is a relatively common problem in newborns, particularly in premature infants, the possibility of an inherited factor deficiency may be overlooked. Thus, Factor VIII and Factor IX levels should be assayed in any male infant with intracranial bleeding, regardless of whether a history of trauma or birth asphyxia is elicited.

Bleeding into the retropharyngeal space can lead to asphyxia due to extrinsic compression of the upper airway.

TABLE 145–3. Reference Values for Coagulation Tests in the Healthy Full-Term Infant During the First 6 Months of Life

*Coagulation Test**	*Day 1 (mean/range)*	*Day 5 (mean/range)*	*Day 30 (mean/range)*	*Day 90 (mean/range)*	*Day 180 (mean/range)*	*Adult (mean/range)*
PT (s)	13.0/10.1–15.9†	12.4/10.0–15.3†	11.8/10.0–14.3†	11.9/10.0–14.2†	12.3/10.7–13.9†	12.4/10.8–13.9
INR	1.00/0.53–1.62	0.89/0.53–1.48	0.79/0.53–1.26	0.81/0.53–1.26	0.88/0.61–1.17	0.89/0.64–1.17
aPTT (s)	42.9/31.3–54.5	42.6/25.4–59.8	40.4/32.0–55.2	37.1/29.0–50.1†	35.5/28.1–42.9†	33.5/26.6–40.3
TCT (s)	23.5/19.0–28.3†	23.1/18.0–29.2	24.3/19.4–29.2†	25.1/20.5–29.7†	25.5/19.8–31.2†	25.0/19.7–30.3
Fibrinogen (g/L)	2.83/1.67–3.99†	3.12/1.62–4.62†	2.70/1.62–3.78†	2.43/1.50–3.79†	2.51/1.50–3.87†	2.78/1.56–4.00
Procoagulation factors						
II (U/mL)	0.48/0.26–0.70	0.63/0.33–0.93	0.68/0.34–1.02	0.75/0.45–1.05	0.88/0.60–1.16	1.08/0.70–1.46
V (U/mL)	0.72/0.34–1.08	0.96/0.45–1.45	0.98/0.62–1.34	0.90/0.48–1.32	0.91/0.55–1.27	1.06/0.62–1.50
VII (U/mL)	0.66/0.28–1.04	0.89/0.35–1.43	0.90/0.42–1.38	0.91/0.39–1.43	0.87/0.47–1.27	1.05/0.67–1.43
VIII (U/mL)	1.00/0.50–1.78†	0.88/0.50–1.54†	0.91/0.50–1.57†	0.79/0.50–1.25†	0.73/0.50–1.09	0.99/0.50–1.49
IX (U/mL)	0.53/0.15–0.91	0.53/0.15–0.91	0.51/0.21–0.81	0.67/0.21–1.13	0.86/0.36–1.36	1.09/0.55–1.63
X (U/mL)	0.40/0.12–0.68	0.49/0.19–0.79	0.59/0.31–0.87	0.71/0.35–1.07	0.78/0.38–1.18	1.06/0.70–1.52
XI (U/mL)	0.38/0.10–0.66	0.55/0.23–0.87	0.53/0.27–0.79	0.69/0.41–0.97	0.86/0.49–1.34	0.97/0.67–1.27
XII (U/mL)	0.53/0.13–0.93	0.47/0.11–0.83	0.49/0.17–0.81	0.67/0.25–1.09	0.77/0.39–1.15	1.08/0.52–1.64
XIIIa (U/mL)	0.79/0.27–1.31	0.94/0.44/1.44†	0.93/0.39–1.47†	1.04/0.36–1.72†	1.04/0.46–1.62†	1.05/0.55–1.55
XIIIb (U/mL)	0.76/0.30–1.22	1.06/0.32–1.90	1.11/0.39–1.73†	1.16/0.48–1.84†	1.10/0.50–1.70†	0.97/0.57–1.37
vWF (U/mL)	1.53/0.50–2.87	1.40/0.50–2.54	1.28/0.50–2.46†	1.18/0.50–2.06	1.07/0.50–1.97	0.92/0.50–1.58
PK (U/mL)	0.37/0.18–0.69	0.48/0.20–0.76	0.57/0.23–0.91	0.73/0.41–1.05	0.86/0.56–1.16	1.12/0.62–1.62
HMWK (U/mL)	0.54/0.06–1.02	0.74/0.16–1.32	0.77/0.33–1.21	0.82/0.30–1.46†	0.82/0.36–1.28†	0.92/0.50–1.36

(Modified from Andrew M, Paes B, Milner R, et al: Development of the human coagulation system in the full-term infant. Blood 1987; 70:165–172.)

*All factors except fibrinogen are expressed as U/mL, where pooled plasma contains 1.0 U/mL. All reference values are expressed as mean and range, which encompass 95% of the population. Between 40 to 77 samples were assayed for each value for the newborn. Some measurements were skewed because of a disproportionate number of high values. The lower limit, which excludes the lower 2.5% of the population, has been given.

†Values that are indistinguishable from those of the adult.

aPTT = activated partial thromboplastin time; HMWK = high-molecular-weight kininogen; INR = international normalized ratio; PK = prekallikrein; PT = prothrombin time; TCT = thrombin-clotting time; vWF = von Willebrand's factor.

This complication may occur rapidly in infants because of their small upper-airway diameter. Older children may present with complaints of sore throat, dysphagia, or hoarse speech. Presenting manifestations in infants and toddlers may include nasal flaring, labored respirations, and inspiratory stridor suggestive of upper-airway obstruction. Diagnostic findings include abnormal widening of the retropharyngeal soft tissue shadow on lateral neck x-ray studies and increased lucency of the retropharyngeal soft tissues on computed tomographic scanning.[40]

Retroperitoneal hemorrhage occurring after blunt trauma to the abdomen or flank can lead to cardiovascular collapse due to extensive bleeding into the retroperitoneal space. Clinical manifestations include diffuse tenderness over the abdomen and back, accompanied by signs and symptoms of intravascular volume loss. Blood in the retroperitoneal cavity can be identified by either ultrasound or abdominal CT scan.[37, 41]

Limb-threatening bleeding complications of hemophilia include compartment syndromes caused by hematomas that compress neurovascular bundles. Bleeding into the iliopsoas muscle may be difficult to diagnose because of the localization of pain to the groin or lower abdomen, mimicking either hemarthrosis of the hip or acute appendicitis. Patients typically present with flexion and external rotation of the hip on the involved side. Compression of the femoral nerve can result in paresthesias along the anterior aspect of the thigh, quadriceps muscle paresis, and diminished patellar reflexes. Plain x-ray studies of the abdomen often reveal loss of the psoas muscle shadow. The presence of a hematoma can be confirmed with retroperitoneal ultrasound.[12, 37] Compartment syndrome can also arise in the forearm. Expanding intramuscular hematomas can compress the median and ulnar nerves, resulting in significant functional deficits in the hand.[37]

Treatment

Guidelines

Therapy for hemophilia-related bleeding depends on the severity of the factor deficiency; the location, severity and duration of the hemorrhagic event; the half-life of the coagulation product infused; and issues that may alter the pharmacokinetics of factor replacement, such as the presence of an inhibitor.

Products available for the treatment of bleeding in patients with hemophilia A include cryoprecipitate, lyophilized Factor VIII concentrates (either plasma derived or recombinant), and DDAVP. Cryoprecipitate is prepared by slow thawing of frozen plasma to 4°C after the plasma has been screened for evidence of HIV-1, hepatitis B, and hepatitis C virus infection. The cold insoluble (precipitated) fraction is rich in Factor VIII, vWF, and fibrinogen, making it useful for patients with hemophilia A, vWD, and primary or acquired hypofibrinogenemia. Each bag of cryoprecipitate contains 80 to 120 IU of Factor VIII.[42]

Factor VIII concentrates are available in either intermediate or high purity. Intermediate-purity products have relatively low specific activity (<15 IU/mg of protein) and often contain variable quantities of fibrinogen, fibronectin, and vWF. High-purity Factor VIII, either recombinant or plasma-derived, is prepared by monoclonal antibody–affinity chromatography and contains only Factor VIII and pasteurized human albumin, which is added as a stabilizer. Plasma from several thousand donors who are screened for HIV-1, hepatitis B and hepatitis C virus infection are required for each lot of Factor VIII concentrate manufactured. Factor VIII concentrates are either pasteurized or treated with a solvent-detergent suspension to inactivate lipid-enveloped viruses that may have eluded detection in the screening process. The combination of screening, purification, and viral inactivation measures has nearly eliminated the risk of viral transmission from the use of factor concentrates. Risk of infection by human blood–borne viruses is nonexistent when recombinant Factor VIII is employed.[42, 43] In light of these advances in purity and safety, replacement therapy for hemophilia A–related bleeding has moved away from the use of single donor cryoprecipitate and toward the use of virally inactivated, plasma-derived or recombinant Factor VIII preparations.[44]

The in vivo recovery, biologic half-life, and hemostatic

effectiveness of high-purity products are comparable to those of intermediate-purity preparations. Infusion of 1 U of Factor VIII per kilogram of body weight usually results in a 2% increment in plasma Factor VIII level 30 minutes after infusion, and the factor has a biologic half-life ranging from 12 to 15 hours.[37] Less than the expected recovery or half-life suggests the presence of an inhibitor to Factor VIII.

As noted earlier, DDAVP carries no risk of blood-borne viral infection, because it is not derived from human plasma. Infusion of DDAVP (0.3 μg/kg of body weight) generally increases Factor VIII levels to three to five times baseline levels. Patients with moderate-to-severe Factor VIII deficiency do not exhibit an adequate therapeutic response to DDAVP for most bleeding events.[14] Potential candidates for treatment (i.e., patients with baseline Factor VIII levels ≥10–15% of normal) should be infused with DDAVP to assess the extent of their response. Once the magnitude of response has been documented, the indication for DDAVP is determined by the severity of the bleeding episode and the desired plasma Factor VIII level. DDAVP is not recommended for the treatment of life-threatening hemorrhage.[14, 45]

Therapeutic options for patients with Factor IX deficiency include infusion of fresh frozen plasma (FFP) and Factor IX concentrates of intermediate or high purity. FFP provides 1 U of Factor IX activity per milliliter. In view of its low specific activity and the fluid limitations frequently imposed on critically ill children, FFP is often impractical as a means of Factor IX replacement therapy. In general, FFP use is limited to the treatment or prophylaxis of minor bleeding complications that require no more than a 10% to 15% increment in Factor IX activity over baseline levels.[42, 45]

Until recently, prothrombin complex concentrates (PCCs) were the only alternative to FFP for Factor IX replacement therapy. In addition to Factor IX, PCCs contain significant amounts of other vitamin K–dependent clotting proteins (Factor II, Factor X) and small quantities of activated clotting proteins. Factors II and X have in vivo half-lives that exceed that of Factor IX, leading to accumulation of these procoagulants when repeated doses of PCCs are used. Frequent infusions of PCCs carry a risk of thromboembolic complications and DIC that may be caused by the accumulation of activated clotting proteins and supraphysiologic levels of Factors II and X in plasma.[46] The risk of thrombosis is greatest in patients receiving large amounts of PCCs over a short period of time and in those with other risk factors for hypercoagulability, such as polycythemia, prolonged immobility, or advanced liver disease. The risk of thromboembolic complications may be decreased by the addition of heparin, given as 5 IU/mL of reconstituted factor concentrate, or 100 IU of heparin per 500 IU of Factor IX.[47, 48] In view of the risk for thrombosis with PCCs, their use should be avoided in newborns.

Two recently licensed high-purity Factor IX preparations provide highly specific activity for Factor IX and decreased concentrations of non–Factor IX proteins. These preparations are recommended for use in patients who require surgery, in those with chronic liver disease, or in those who sustain substantial crush injuries requiring prolonged factor replacement and immobilization.[46, 49]

The recovery and half-life of Factor IX differ from those of Factor VIII. Thirty minutes after infusion of 1 IU of Factor IX per kilogram, plasma levels rise by only 1%. The biologic half-life of Factor IX is 18 to 24 hours.[47, 50]

Major Bleeding Events and Preparation for Surgery

Patients with life- or limb-threatening hemorrhage require prompt correction of factor activity to 80% to 100% of normal, and maintenance of factors level in the range of 50% to 100% is usually indicated for several days to weeks thereafter. Patients with CNS bleeding should receive 2 weeks of uninterrupted factor replacement therapy. These individuals are at risk for rebleeding into the CNS for up to 6 months after the initial event.[45]

For patients with hemophilia A, 100% correction is achieved with a loading dose of 50 IU of Factor VIII per kilogram, followed by repeated infusions of 25 IU/kg every 12 to 15 hours. Alternately, a continuous infusion of Factor VIII at a dose of 2 to 3 $U \cdot kg^{-1} \cdot h^{-1}$ may be delivered after the initial loading dose.[45] Response to factor replacement should be carefully monitored both by clinical assessment and by regular assays of plasma Factor VIII levels. The management of major bleeding events in patients with hemophilia B is analogous to that of hemophilia A, requiring 80% to 100% correction of Factor IX activity. This goal is usually achieved with a loading dose of 80 to 100 IU/kg of Factor IX, followed by 40 to 50 U/kg every 18 to 24 hours.[12] When PCCs are used, patients should be closely monitored for evidence of DIC and thrombosis.

Preparation for surgical procedures follows similar guidelines for factor replacement as outlined for life-threatening hemorrhages. All surgical candidates should be screened preoperatively for the presence of inhibitors, to prevent potentially life-threatening bleeding due to suboptimal intraoperative factor recovery and half-life, as is discussed later. For major surgery, postoperative factor replacement should allow for maintenance of factor levels that are 50% of normal for 5 to 7 days, followed by levels of at least 30% for an additional week.[12]

Non–Life Threatening Hemorrhage and Minor Invasive Procedures

Less aggressive measures are required for the treatment of routine hemarthroses and hematomas, or for the preparation for minor surgical procedures, such as tooth extractions. For children undergoing dental extractions or presenting with gingival bleeding, adjunctive therapy with an antifibrinolytic agent (ε-aminocaproic acid or tranexamic acid) is often sufficient to maintain hemostasis after an initial infusion of factor concentrate. Antifibrinolytic therapy has not proved useful for the treatment of hemarthrosis. Use of these adjunctive measures is contraindicated in the setting of hematuria. Because of the increased risk of thrombosis, use of antifibrinolytic therapy in patients receiving PCCs should be deferred or avoided.[45] Specific dosing recommendations for both routine and major hemorrhagic events or surgical procedures are summarized in Table 145–4.

Complications

INHIBITORS. Approximately 22% to 33% of patients with hemophilia A and 2% to 3% of those with hemophilia B develop alloantibodies against Factors VIII and IX, respectively.[51, 52] Alloantibodies neutralize the functional activity of infused clotting proteins, resulting in the partial or complete failure of factor replacement therapy. Inhibitors occur principally in patients with moderate-to-severe factor deficiency (i.e., <5% factor activity), and most of these patients are initially identified in childhood or adolescence. Inhibitors are quantitated in a Bethesda assay, in which 1 U of inhibitory activity is the amount capable of neutralizing 50% of the factor activity present in a 1:1 mixture of patient and normal plasma that is incubated at 37°C for 2 hours.[53, 54]

Strategies for the treatment or prevention of bleeding in patients with inhibitors depend on the inhibitor titer at the time of the bleeding event, the presence or absence of an anamnestic response when the patient is challenged with the deficient clotting factor, and the type and severity of

TABLE 145–4. Treatment of Specific Hemorrhages in Hemophilia

Type of Bleed	*Hemophilia A*	*Hemophilia B*
Hemarthrosis*	20 U/kg FVIII concentrate†; 15 U/kg if treated early. Repeat dose the following day if bleed is severe.	30 U/kg FIX concentrate‡; 20 U/kg if treated early.
Muscle or significant subcutaneous hematoma	20 U/kg FVIII concentrate; may need treatment every other day until bleed is well controlled.	30 U/kg FIX concentrate; may need treatment every 2 or 3 days until bleeding is well controlled.‡
Mouth, deciduous tooth, or tooth extraction	20 U/kg FVIII concentrate; antifibrinolytic therapy; remove loose deciduous tooth.	30 U/kg concentrate; antifibrinolytic therapy§; remove loose deciduous tooth.
Epistaxis	Pressure for 15–20 min; pack with petroleum jelly gauze; antifibrinolytic therapy; 20 U/kg FVIII concentrate if aforementioned therapy fails.	Pressure for 15–20 min; pack with petroleum jelly gauze; antifibrinolytic therapy; 30 U/kg FIX concentrate if aforementioned therapy fails (4 h after antifibrinolytic dose).
Major surgery, life-threatening hemorrhage (e.g., CNS, GI, airway)	50 U/kg FVIII concentrate, then 25 U/kg q 12 h or continuous infusion to maintain FVIII >50 U/dL for 5–7 d, then >30 U/dL for 5–7 d.	80 U/kg FIX concentrate, then 20–40 U/kg every 12–24 h to maintain FIX >40 U/dL for 5–7 days, then >30 U/dL for 5–7 days.‡
Iliopsoas hemorrhage	50 U/kg FVIII concentrate, then 25 U/kg every 12 h until patient is asymptomatic, then 50 U/kg every other day for a total of 10–14 d.‖	80 U/kg FIX concentrate, then 20–40 U/kg every 12–24 h to maintain FIX >40 U/dL until patient is asymptomatic, then 30 U/kg every other day for a total of 10–14 days.‡‖
Hematuria	Bed rest; 1½ × maintenance fluids; if bleeding is not controlled in 1 or 2 days, 20 U/kg FVIII concentrate; if bleeding is not controlled, prednisone if patient is HIV negative.	Bed rest; 1½ × maintenance fluids; if bleeding is not controlled in 1 or 2 days, 30 U/kg FIX concentrate; if bleeding is not controlled, prednisone if patient is HIV negative.

(From Gill JC, Montgomery RR: Principles of therapy for hemostasis factor deficiencies. *In* Hematology of Infancy and Childhood. 4th ed. Nathan DG, Oski FA [Eds]. Philadelphia, WB Saunders, 1993, p. 1799.)

*For hip hemarthrosis, orthopedic evaluation for possible aspiration is advisable.

†For mild or moderate hemophilia, DDAVP, 0.3 μg/kg, should be used instead of FVIII concentrate if patient is known to respond with a hemostatic level of FVIII; if repeated doses are given, monitor FVIII levels for tachyphylaxis.

‡If repeated doses of FIX concentrate are given, add heparin, 100 U per 500 U of FIX; monitor antithrombin III and DIC parameters; when highly purified FIX concentrates are available, they are preferred.

§Do not give antifibrinolytic therapy until 4–6 hours after a dose of FIX concentrate.

‖Repeat radiologic assessment before discontinuation of therapy.

CNS = central nervous system; DDAVP = desmopressin acetate; DIC = disseminated intravascular coagulation; F = Factor; GI = gastrointestinal; HIV = human immunodeficiency virus.

hemorrhage. Patients who demonstrate a brisk anamnestic response after repeated exposure to infused factor are described as high responders. In contrast, those with inhibitors that are low in titer (<10 Bethesda units) and do not rise significantly after repeated exposure to the deficient factor are referred to as low responders. Low responders can spontaneously lose their antibody or can evolve into high responders, and high responders can revert to low-responder status.[45]

Life-threatening hemorrhage in low-responder patients can usually be managed by infusion of higher-than-normal doses of the deficient factor (e.g., bolus with 100 U/kg of Factor VIII, followed by continuous infusion of 10 to 20 $U \cdot kg^{-1} \cdot h^{-1}$) as a means of overwhelming the effects of the inhibitor. Factor levels should be monitored at 1 and 4 hours after the bolus infusion, and then at least once daily to determine the efficacy of the dosing schedule.[45] Patients who respond well to this regimen initially may become refractory, necessitating a switch to a different therapeutic approach.

Few universally accepted guidelines exist for the management of bleeding in high-responder patients. Although several potential treatment modalities exist for these patients, none predictably and consistently arrest (or prevent) bleeding.[49, 52] Management of bleeding complications in patients with high-responder inhibitors should always be carried out in consultation with a hematologist (preferably in a hemophilia treatment center) who is familiar with currently available treatment modalities (see references 55 to 59 for in-depth discussions of management strategies for high-responder inhibitors).

TRANSFUSION-TRANSMITTED INFECTIONS. Since the first reported cases of AIDS in people with hemophilia, infection by human blood–borne viruses (principally HIV-1 and hepatitis C virus) have emerged as the greatest cause of mortality in patients with hemophilia.[60, 61] Approximately 80% of patients with severe Factor VIII deficiency and 40% to 50% of patients with severe Factor IX deficiency have HIV-1 infection.[60] More than 80% of patients with severe hemophilia are seropositive for hepatitis C virus; most of these patients have chronic hepatitis C virus infection and thus are at significant risk for developing chronic active hepatitis, cirrhosis, and hepatocellular carcinoma over the course of years to decades.[58, 62, 63]

Other Inherited Coagulation Factor Deficiencies

Deficiencies of the contact activation factor XII, prekallikrein, or high-molecular-weight kininogen are rare conditions that cause a prolonged aPTT but do not predispose to abnormal bleeding. No specific measures are indicated in the critical care management of patients with a deficiency of one of these proteins. Deficiency of Factor XI is inherited in an autosomal fashion and occurs most frequently in individuals of Ashkenazi Jewish descent. Levels of Factor XI of less than 30% are associated with postoperative or posttraumatic bleeding complications. Because neither the degree of aPTT prolongation nor the baseline level of Factor XI correlate well with the risk of bleeding, Factor XI replacement is recommended for patients with levels of Factor XI that are less than 30% of normal who require surgery.[12]

Deficiencies of prothrombin, fibrinogen, or Factors V, VII,

X, and XIII are inherited in an autosomal fashion. All are associated with abnormal bleeding, with the severity and risk of hemorrhage reflecting the extent of deficiency. Deficiency of Factor V, Factor X, fibrinogen, or prothrombin is associated with prolongation of both the prothrombin time and the aPTT. Isolated prolongation of prothrombin time is characteristic of Factor VII deficiency. Abnormal bleeding occurs in patients with prothrombin levels of less than 30% and with Factor VII levels of less than 15% to 20%. Bleeding secondary to prothrombin deficiency usually responds to infusions of FFP or PCCs.[12] Likewise, Factor VII–deficient patients can be treated either with FFP or lyophilized concentrates that contain high levels of Factor VII.[12, 58] Clinically significant hypofibrinogenemia (<75mg/dL) may present in the neonatal period with gastrointestinal bleeding or extensive hematoma formation related to birth trauma, or the disorder may not become apparent until later in life, presenting with excessive postsurgical bleeding or wound dehiscence. Both FFP and cryoprecipitate can be used for fibrinogen replacement, although cryoprecipitate is a more concentrated source of this protein.[12] Severe deficiency of Factor XIII (<1% of normal) is associated with impaired clot stability. Clinical manifestations include prolonged oozing after separation of the umbilical stump, easy bruisability, mucous membrane bleeding, and poor wound healing. Patients with Factor XIII deficiency have normal prothrombin time, aPTT and thrombin time. Diagnosis depends on the demonstration of abnormally rapid clot lysis in the presence of 5 mol/L urea or 1% monochloracetic acid.[12]

ACQUIRED COAGULOPATHIES

Vitamin K Deficiency

Vitamin K is a cofactor that is required for the normal post-translational γ-carboxylation of prothrombin, Factor VII, Factor IX, Factor X, protein C, and protein S. In vitamin K–deficiency states, these coagulation proteins do not bind calcium normally, a prerequisite for their normal activation and function.[12] Factors contributing to vitamin K deficiency in the newborn include low placental transfer of vitamin K, low concentrations of vitamin K in breast milk, and lack of vitamin K_2 synthesis by intestinal flora at birth.[36] Symptomatic vitamin K deficiency generally presents within the first days to weeks of life in the form of hemorrhagic disease of the newborn. Early hemorrhagic disease of the newborn presents at or shortly after birth with the occurrence of cephalhematomas and intracranial, intrathoracic, or intra-abdominal hemorrhage. It is usually a consequence of maternal ingestion of vitamin K antagonists (e.g., warfarin, anticonvulsants, or antituberculous medications) before delivery.[44] Classic hemorrhagic disease of the newborn arises within the first week of life and often presents with cutaneous bruising, gastrointestinal bleeding, or excessive hemorrhage after circumcision in breastfed infants who do not receive vitamin K at birth.[44] The lower frequency of this disorder in formula-fed infants reflects the higher concentration of vitamin K in proprietary formulas compared with breast milk.[36] The routine administration of vitamin K at birth (0.5–1.0 mg IM) has significantly reduced the incidence of classic hemorrhagic disease of the newborn. Delayed hemorrhagic disease of the newborn may occur as late as 3 months of age, regardless of whether vitamin K is given at birth. It typically occurs in infants who are exclusively breastfed and develop a prolonged diarrheal illness or who are receiving broad-spectrum antimicrobial therapy. These infants commonly present with ecchymoses, mucous membrane bleeding, or excessive oozing after venipuncture.[36]

Hemorrhagic complications due to vitamin K deficiency can occur in older infants and in children as a result of fat malabsorption states (e.g., cystic fibrosis, celiac disease) or in children who are supported by total parenteral nutrition that lacks vitamin K supplementation.[44] Vitamin K deficiency may also present after the accidental or deliberate ingestion of warfarin-containing compounds (e.g., coumadin, rodenticides) and carries an attendant risk of bleeding that can last for days to months.[19, 47]

Patients with vitamin K deficiency should be treated with parenteral vitamin K_1 (e.g., Aquamephyton), given subcutaneously or by slow intravenous infusion at a dose of 1–5 mg. Resolution of bleeding symptoms is generally rapid (within 4 to 6 hours) and usually precedes improvement in the results of coagulation screening studies. Any infant or child with life-threatening hemorrhage due to vitamin K deficiency should also receive FFP to rapidly increase vitamin K–dependent clotting factor levels.[44]

Liver Disease

The coagulopathy that accompanies advanced liver disease reflects the liver's role in the production and regulation of most proteins required for normal coagulation. In addition to decreased biosynthesis of essential coagulation proteins, other contributors to impaired hemostasis in patients with advanced liver disease include (1) low-grade DIC due to diminished clearance of activated clotting factors, (2) thrombocytopenia due to hypersplenism, (3) increased fibrinolysis, and (4) platelet dysfunction secondary to increased concentrations of fibrin degradation products.[64]

Improved hemostasis in patients with liver failure can be achieved by infusions of FFP and cryoprecipitate. Correction of the prothrombin time and aPTT to 1.5 times their control values or less is usually sufficient to allow for minor diagnostic procedures, such as liver biopsy. Coagulation factor replacement with FFP and cryoprecipitate is only a temporizing measure in the treatment or prevention of excessive hemorrhage secondary to liver disease. Supplemental vitamin K administration is rarely successful unless a significant biliary obstructive component is present that leads to decreased absorption of dietary vitamin K.[47]

DISORDERS OF HEMOSTASIS INVOLVING PLATELETS AND CLOTTING FACTORS

Disseminated Intravascular Coagulation

DIC is the term given to describe the pathologic activation of the coagulation and fibrinolytic pathways that results in the systemic depletion of procoagulant, anticoagulant, and fibrinolytic proteins and carries an attendant risk of hemorrhage, thrombosis, or both. Common conditions that lead to DIC in children are summarized in Table 145–5.

Pathophysiology

DIC is triggered by two major mechanisms: vascular endothelial cell injury and parenchymal tissue damage leading to the exposure of tissue factor.[65] Injury to vascular endothelium results in the release of tissue plasminogen activator and the exposure of subendothelial adhesive proteins to circulating platelets and clotting factors. Plasma contact with negatively charged, subendothelial matrix leads to activation of Factor XII and initiation of the intrinsic coagulation pathway. Activated Factor XII (XIIa) mediates the activation of kallikrein from prekallikrein and hydrolyzes plasminogen to plasmin. Kallikrein catalyzes the cleavage of bradykinin from high-molecular-weight kininogen.

TABLE 145–5. Conditions That Commonly Trigger Acute Disseminated Intravascular Coagulation in Children

Neonatal Disorder
Intrauterine infections
Maternal toxemia
Abruptio placentae
Hyaline membrane disease, meconium aspiration
Necrotizing enterocolitis

Infections
Bacterial sepsis (either gram positive or gram negative)
Falciparum malaria
Rickettsial infections (e.g., Rocky Mountain spotted fever)
Disseminated fungal infections
Systemic viral infections (e.g, herpesvirus infections)

Other Illnesses
Hypovolemic shock
Acute (hypergranular) promyelocytic leukemia
Intravascular hemolytic transfusion reactions
Extensive burns or trauma
Intracranial injuries (e.g., gunshot wounds)
Hyperthermia or hypothermia
Proteolytic snake venoms (e.g., *Echis carinatus*)

Localized Consumptive Coagulopathy
Kasabach-Merritt syndrome (giant hemangioma, disseminated intravascular coagulation)
Hyperacute renal allograft rejection
Dead fetus syndrome

(From Bray GL: Inherited and acquired disorders of hemostasis. *In:* Textbook of Pediatric Critical Care. Holbrook PR [Ed]. Philadelphia, WB Saunders, 1993, pp 783–801.)

Bradykinin is a powerful vasodilator that plays an integral role in the development of the hypotension that is often associated with DIC.[65] Parenchymal tissue injury and necrosis result in the release of membrane-bound tissue factor that binds and activates Factor VII; Factor VIIa–tissue factor complex in turn activates Factors X and IX. Both mechanisms lead to the generation of circulating thrombin, which cleaves fibrinogen to soluble fibrin and activates platelet Factor V, Factor VIII, and Factor XIII. This combination of events results in hypofibrinogenemia, thrombocytopenia, depletion of plasma procoagulant levels, and activation of fibrinolysis. As a result, patients with DIC exhibit increased risk of hemorrhage, or formation of microthrombi, or both, resulting in ischemic tissue damage.[65]

Clinical Manifestations

Petechiae and purpura are the most consistent clinical manifestations of DIC, followed by mucosal bleeding from the nasopharynx, gastrointestinal, and genitourinary tracts. Hemorrhage into the CNS or pulmonary parenchyma may complicate cases of DIC that are especially severe and fulminant. Ischemia resulting from thrombus formation in distal extremities can lead to the gangrene and tissue sloughing that is characteristic of purpura fulminans. Ischemic thrombosis of the renal vasculature results in acute cortical necrosis and chronic renal failure. Bleeding complications of DIC are usually treated more successfully than are thrombotic complications, which frequently result in long-term functional disability, organ failure, or both.[66]

Diagnosis

Acute DIC is accompanied by varying degrees of thrombocytopenia, hypofibrinogenemia, and increased concentrations of fibrin degradation products in plasma. These conditions typically lead to prolongation of prothrombin time and aPTT.[66] Levels of prothrombin, Factor V, and Factor VIII are most frequently reduced in DIC. Levels of factor VIII are useful in discriminating between DIC and the coagulopathy associated with liver failure: Factor VIII levels are typically normal or elevated in most patients with liver failure.[12] Examination of the peripheral blood smear may reveal erythrocyte injury and fragmentation secondary to microangiopathic hemolysis.[66]

Treatment

The cornerstone of therapy for DIC is correction of its underlying cause. Life-threatening hemorrhagic complications can be averted with platelet transfusions in patients with severe thrombocytopenia (platelet count $<20{,}000/mm^3$). Infusions of FFP and cryoprecipitate are indicated for severe hypofibrinogenemia. Anticoagulation with heparin may be beneficial in patients with DIC in whom thrombosis predominates (e.g., those with purpura fulminans).[67] Anecdotal evidence suggests that heparin may ameliorate or prevent DIC in patients with acute promyelocytic leukemia, if therapy is initiated before the start of chemotherapy.[68] Intracranial hemorrhage should be regarded as an absolute contraindication to the use of heparin.

The recent licensure of antithrombin III concentrates has generated interest in their potential usefulness in the treatment of DIC. In a randomized trial comparing antithrombin III with heparin, antithrombin III significantly shortened the duration of DIC and improved survival in cases of advanced shock.[69] Although the role of antithrombin III concentrates in DIC have not been clearly defined, they appear to be most effective when endogenous antithrombin III levels are <70% of normal.[69]

DIAGNOSTIC APPROACH TO THE BLEEDING CHILD

In addition to the history and physical examination, several principles are useful in guiding the diagnostic evaluation in

TABLE 145–6. Clinical Features of the Two Main Groups of Hemostatic Disease

Clinical Findings	*Platelet or Vascular Defects*	*Plasma Coagulation Defects*
Common hemorrhagic symptoms	Epistaxis; petechiae; purpura; ecchymoses; gastrointestinal hemorrhage; menorrhagia	Deep tissue hemorrhages, especially hemarthroses and intramuscular bleeds
Bleeding from superficial cuts and abrasions	Often profuse and prolonged	Usually mild
Bleeding from deep cuts, lacerations, dental extractions	Onset immediate; often permanently arrested with local pressure; seldom rebleeds	Onset often delayed; not permanently controlled by local pressure; rebleeding likely to occur several hours after removal of local pressure
Spontaneous bleeding	Usually superficial; small and multiple loci of involvement	Usually a single locus; large and deep-seated hematomas or hemarthroses

(From Stuart M, Kelton J: The platelet: Quantitative and qualitative abnormalities. *In*: Hematology of Infancy and Childhood. 3rd ed. Nathan DG, Oski FA [Eds]. Philadelphia, WB Saunders, 1987, p. 1347.)

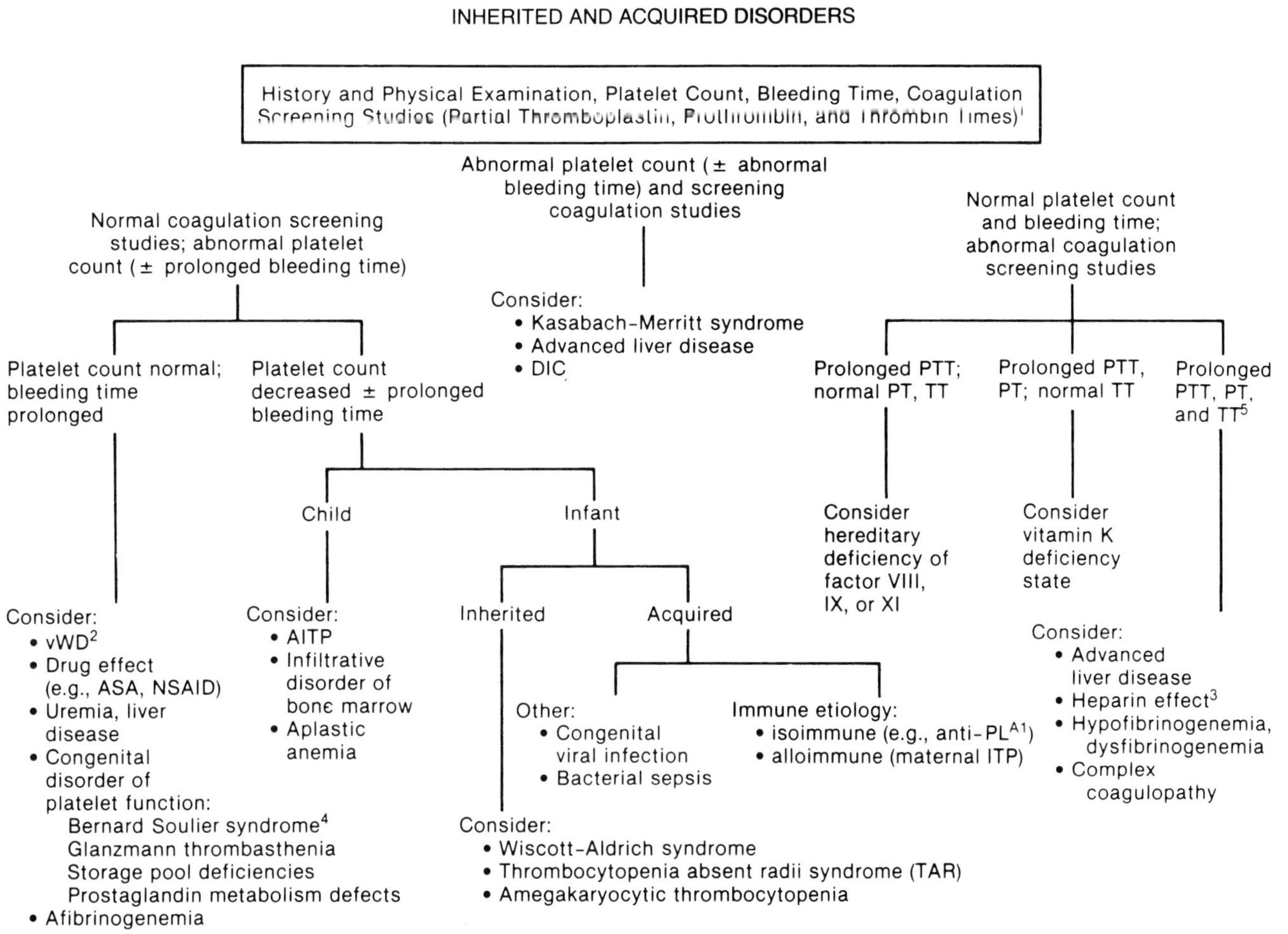

INHERITED AND ACQUIRED DISORDERS

History and Physical Examination, Platelet Count, Bleeding Time, Coagulation Screening Studies (Partial Thromboplastin, Prothrombin, and Thrombin Times)[1]

Normal coagulation screening studies; abnormal platelet count (± prolonged bleeding time)

- Platelet count normal; bleeding time prolonged
  - Consider:
    - vWD[2]
    - Drug effect (e.g., ASA, NSAID)
    - Uremia, liver disease
    - Congenital disorder of platelet function: Bernard Soulier syndrome[4], Glanzmann thrombasthenia, Storage pool deficiencies, Prostaglandin metabolism defects
    - Afibrinogenemia
- Platelet count decreased ± prolonged bleeding time
  - Child — Consider:
    - AITP
    - Infiltrative disorder of bone marrow
    - Aplastic anemia
  - Infant
    - Inherited — Consider:
      - Wiscott-Aldrich syndrome
      - Thrombocytopenia absent radii syndrome (TAR)
      - Amegakaryocytic thrombocytopenia
    - Acquired
      - Other:
        - Congenital viral infection
        - Bacterial sepsis
      - Immune etiology:
        - isoimmune (e.g., anti-PL[A1])
        - alloimmune (maternal ITP)

Abnormal platelet count (± abnormal bleeding time) and screening coagulation studies

- Consider:
  - Kasabach-Merritt syndrome
  - Advanced liver disease
  - DIC

Normal platelet count and bleeding time; abnormal coagulation screening studies

- Prolonged PTT; normal PT, TT — Consider hereditary deficiency of factor VIII, IX, or XI
- Prolonged PTT, PT; normal TT — Consider vitamin K deficiency state
- Prolonged PTT, PT, and TT[5] — Consider:
  - Advanced liver disease
  - Heparin effect[3]
  - Hypofibrinogenemia, dysfibrinogenemia
  - Complex coagulopathy

Figure 145–2. Algorithmic approach to the infant or child with a suspected bleeding disorder. (From Bray GL: Inherited and acquired disorders of hemostasis. *In:* Textbook of Pediatric Critical Care. Holbrook PR [Ed]. Philadelphia, WB Saunders, 1993, p 799.)

a child with abnormal bleeding. The presence of petechiae and purpura and/or mucosal bleeding suggests disorders of primary hemostasis (i.e., deficits in platelet number or function). Hemorrhages involving muscles and joints with swelling and impaired range of motion suggest the presence of coagulation factor deficiencies (Table 145–6).[70] Hemorrhagic complications that initially present in infancy or early childhood in an otherwise healthy child suggest an inherited rather than acquired cause.[70] Initial laboratory evaluation of a suspected bleeding disorder should include screening studies, such as a platelet count and determinations of prothrombin time, aPTT, and bleeding time. Examination of the peripheral blood smear may reveal the presence of platelet aggregates, a common finding in patients with spurious or anticoagulant-induced thrombocytopenia. Review of the peripheral smear may also reveal platelets that are abnormally large (e.g., ITP, Bernard-Soulier syndrome) or abnormally small (e.g., Wiskott-Aldrich syndrome). Despite its shortcomings, the bleeding time remains the best available test of platelet function in vivo. Results of bleeding time assessments should be interpreted cautiously because they may be influenced by medications that interfere with platelet function. A normal bleeding time does not preclude a defect in primary hemostasis in a child with a strong personal or family history of a bleeding disorder. Screening tests for the assessment of coagulation include prothrombin time, aPTT, and thrombin time. Heparin-contaminated samples drawn from indwelling catheters can significantly alter the results of these studies. For this reason, plasma for coagulation studies should be obtained by peripheral venipuncture whenever possible to ensure plasma sampling uncontaminated by heparin.

Figure 145–2 provides an algorithmic approach to evaluation of bleeding disorders in children.

References

1. Andrew M: Neonatal hematology. *In:* Hematology of Infancy and Childhood. 4th ed. Nathan DG, Oski FA (Eds). Philadelphia, WB Saunders, 1993, pp 115–153.
2. Hardin R: Physiology of coagulation: The platelet. *In:* Hematology of Infancy and Childhood. 3rd ed. Nathan DG, Oski FA (Eds). Philadelphia, WB Saunders, 1987, pp 1271–1292.
3. Alter BP, Young NS: The bone marrow failure syndromes. *In:* Hematology of Infancy and Childhood. 4th ed. Nathan DG, Oski FA (Eds). Philadelphia, WB Saunders, 1993, pp 216–316.
4. Perry GS IV, Spector BD, Schumann LM, et al: The Wiskott-Aldrich syndrome in the United States and Canada (1892–1979). J Pediatr 1980; 97:72.
5. Corash L, Shafer, Blaese RM: Platelet-associated immunoglobulin, platelet size, and the effect of splenectomy in the Wiskott-Aldrich syndrome. Blood 1985; 65:1439.
6. Lum LG, Tubergen DG, Corash L, et al: Splenectomy in the management of the thrombocytopenia of the Wiskott-Aldrich syndrome. N Engl J Med 1980; 302:892.
7. Stuart MJ, Kelton JG: The platelet: Quantitative and qualitative

abnormalities. *In:* Hematology of Infancy and Childhood. 3rd ed. Nathan DG, Oski FA (Eds). Philadelphia, WB Saunders, 1987, pp 1343–1478.
8. Miller JL: von Willebrand disease. Hematol Oncol Clin North Am 1990; 4(1):107.
9. Hardin RI and Wagner DD: Molecular and cellular biology of von Willebrand factor. *In:* Progress in Hemostasis and Thrombosis. Coller BS (Ed). Philadelphia, WB Saunders, 1989, pp 233–259.
10. Manno CS. Difficult pediatric diagnoses: Bruising and bleeding. Pediatr Clin North Am 1991; 38(3):637.
11. Montgomery RR, Coller BS: von Willebrand disease. *In:* Hemostasis and Thrombosis. Colman RW, Hirsh J, Marder VJ, et al (Eds). Philadelphia, JB Lippincott, 1994, pp 1134–1147.
12. Montgomery RR and Scott JP: Hemostasis: Diseases of the fluid phase. *In:* Hematology of Infancy and Childhood. 4th ed. Nathan DG, Oski FA (Eds). Philadelphia, WB Saunders, 1993, pp 1605–1650.
13. Coller BS: von Willebrand disease. *In:* Hemostasis and Thrombosis. 2nd ed. Colman RW, Hirsh J, Marder VJ, et al (Eds). Philadelphia, JB Lippincott, 1987, p 60–96.
14. Manucci PM: Desmopressin: A nontransfusional form of treatment for congenital and acquired bleeding disorders. Blood 1988; 72:1449.
15. Berntorp E and Nilsson IM: Use of a high purity factor VIII concentrate (Hemate P) in von Willebrand's disease. Vox Sang 1989; 56:212.
16. McEver RP: The clinical significance of platelet membrane glycoproteins. Hematol Oncol Clin North Am 1990; 4(1):87.
17. Beardsley DS: Platelet abnormalities in infancy and childhood. *In:* Hematology of Infancy and Childhood. 4th ed. Nathan DG, Oski FA (Eds). Philadelphia, WB Saunders, 1993, pp 1561–1604.
18. Rao AK: Congenital disorders of platelet function. Hematol Oncol Clin North Am 1990; 4(1):65.
19. Buchanan GR: Hemorrhagic diseases. *In:* Hematology of Infancy and Childhood. 3rd ed. Nathan DG, Oski FA (Eds). Philadelphia, WB Saunders, 1987, pp 104–127.
20. Bussel JB: Autoimmune thrombocytopenic purpura. Hematol Oncol Clin North Am 1990; 4(1):179.
21. Dubansky AS, Oski FA: Controversies in the management of acute idiopathic thrombocytopenic purpura: A survey of specialists. Pediatrics 1986; 77:49.
22. George JN: Platelet IgG: Its significance for the evaluation of thrombocytopenia and for understanding the origin of alpha-granule proteins. Blood 1990; 76:859.
23. Karpatkin S: HIV-1-related thrombocytopenia. Hematol Oncol Clin North Am 1990; 4(1):193.
24. Northfelt DW, Mitsuyasu RT: Hematologic complications of HIV infection. *In:* Pediatric AIDS: The Challenge of HIV Infection in Infants, Children and Adolescents. Pizzo PA, Wilfert CM (Eds). Baltimore, Williams & Wilkins, 1991, pp 337–345.
25. McClain K, Gehrz R, Grierson H, et al: Virus-associated histiocytic proliferations in children. Am J Pediatr Hematol Oncol 1988; 10(3):196.
26. Beutler E: Platelet transfusions: The 20,000/μL trigger. Blood 1993; 81(6):1411.
27. Warkentin TE, Kelton JG: Heparin and platelets. Hematol Oncol Clin North Am 1990; 4(1):243.
28. Gralnick HR, McKeown LP, Williams SB, et al: Plasma and platelet von Willebrand factor defects in uremia. Am J Med 1988; 85:806.
29. Carvalho AC: Acquired platelet dysfunction in patients with uremia. Hematol Oncol Clin North Am 1990; 4(1):129.
30. Haskes LA: Bleeding after cardiopulmonary bypass. N Engl J Med 1986; 314:1446.
31. Salzman EW, Weinstein MJ, Weintraub MD, et al: Treatment with desmopressin acetate to reduce blood loss after cardiac surgery. N Engl J Med 1986; 314:1402.
32. Bidstrup BP, Royston D, Sapsford TN, et al: Reduction in blood use after cardiopulmonary bypass with high dose aprotinin (Trasylol). J Thorac Cardiovasc Surg 1989; 97:364.
33. Andrew M, Castle V, Sagal S, et al: Clinical impact of neonatal thrombocytopenia. J Pediatr 1987; 110:457.
34. Andrew M, Paes B, Milner R, et al: Development of the human coagulation system in the full-term infant. Blood 1987; 70(1):165.
35. Andrew M, Paes B, Johnston M: Development of the hemostatic system in the neonate and young infant. Am J Pediatr Hematol Oncol 1990; 12:95.
36. Andrew M, Vegh P, Johnston M, et al: Maturation of the hemostatic system during childhood. Blood 1992; 80(8):1998.
37. Levine PH: The clinical manifestations of hemophilias A and B. *In:* Hemostasis and Thrombosis. 2nd ed. Colman RW, Hirsh J, Marder VJ, et al (Eds). Philadelphia, JB Lippincott, 1987, pp 97–111.
38. Bray GL, Luban NLC: Hemophilia presenting with intracranial hemorrhage. Am J Dis Child 1987; 141:1215.
39. Goldsmith JC, Kletzel M: Risk of birth-related intracranial hemorrhage in hemophilic newborns: Results of a North American survey (Abstract). Blood 1990; 76(suppl):1676a.
40. Bray GL, Nugent D: Hemorrhage involving the upper airway in hemophilia. Clin Pediatr 1986; 25:436.
41. Forbes CD, Madhok R: Genetic disorders of blood coagulation: Clinical presentation and management. *In:* Disorders of Hemostasis. 2nd ed. Ratnoff OD, Forbes CD (Eds). Philadelphia, WB Saunders, 1991, pp 141–202.
42. Lusher JM: Viral safety and inhibitor development associated with monoclonal antibody-purified F VIII C. Ann Hematol 1991; 63:138.
43. Bray GL: Recent developments in the biotechnology of plasma-derived and recombinant coagulation factor VIII. J Pediatr 1990; 117:503.
44. Bray GL: Normal and disordered coagulation in the neonate. Transfus Sci 1991; 12:231.
45. Gill JC, Montgomery RR: Principles of therapy for coagulation factor deficiencies. *In:* Hematology of Infancy and Childhood. 4th ed. Nathan DG, Oski FA (Eds). Philadelphia, WB Saunders, 1993, pp 1796–1818.
46. Kim HC, Matts L, Eisele J, et al: Monoclonal antibody-purified factor IX—Comparative thrombogenicity to prothrombin complex concentrate. Semin Hematol 1991; 28(3 suppl 6):15.
47. Lusher JM: Diseases of coagulation: The fluid phase. *In:* Hematology of Infancy and Childhood. 3rd ed. Nathan DG, Oski FA (Eds). Philadelphia, WB Saunders, 1987, pp 1293–1342.
48. Winter M: The practical management of hemophilia. Blood Rev 1992; 6:174.
49. Maunucci PM, Bauer KA, Gringeri A, et al: No activation of the common pathway of the coagulation cascade after a highly purified factor IX concentrate. Br J Haematol 1991; 79:766.
50. Rizza CR, Jones P: Management of patients with inherited blood coagulation defects. *In:* Haemostasis and Thrombosis. 2nd ed. Bloom AL, Thomas DP (Eds). Edinburgh, Churchill Livingstone, 1987, pp 465–493.
51. Ehrenforth S, Kreuz W, Scharrer I, et al: Incidence of development of factor VIII and factor IX inhibitors in haemophiliacs. Lancet 1992; 339:594.
52. Kasper CK: Treatment of factor VIII inhibitors. *In:* Progress in Hemostasis and Thrombosis. Coller BS (Ed). Philadelphia, WB Saunders, 1989, pp 57–86.
53. Kasper CK, Aledort LM, Counts RB, et al: A more uniform measurement of factor VIII inhibitors. Thromb Diath Haemorrh 1975; 34:869.
54. Kessler CM: An introduction to factor VIII inhibitors: Their detection and quantitation. Am J Med 1991; 91(suppl 5A):15.
55. Lozier JN, Santagostino E, Kasper C: Use of porcine factor VIII for surgical procedures in hemophilia A patients with inhibitors. Semin Hematol 1993; 30(2 suppl 1):10.
56. Sjamsoedin LJ, Heijnen L, Mauser-Bunschoten EP, et al: The effect of activated prothrombin-complex concentrate (FEIBA) on joint and muscle bleeding in patients with hemophilia A and antibodies to factor VIII. N Engl J Med 1981; 305:717.
57. Hedner U, Bjoern S, Bernvil SS, et al: Clinical experience with human plasma-derived factor VIIa in patients with hemophilia A and high titer inhibitors. Haemostasis 1989; 19:335.
58. Bloom AL: Progress in the management of hemophilia. Thromb Haemost 1991; 66(1):166.
59. Nilsson IM: The management of hemophilia in patients with inhibitors. Transfus Med Rev 1992; 6(4):285–293.
60. Pierce GF, Lusher JM, Brownstein AP, et al: The use of purified clotting factor concentrates in hemophilia. JAMA 1989; 261(23):3434.
61. Roberts HR: The treatment of hemophilia: Past tragedy and future promise. N Engl J Med 1989; 321(17):1188.

62. Cuthbert JA: Southwestern Internal Medicine Conference: Hepatitis C. Am J Med Sci 1990; 299(5):346.
63. Alter HJ, Purcell RH, Shih JW, et al: Detection of antibody to hepatitis C virus in prospectively followed transfusion recipients with acute and chronic non-A, non-B hepatitis. N Engl J Med 1989; 321(22):1494.
64. Mannucci PM, Forman SP: Hemostasis and liver disease. *In:* Hemostasis and Thrombosis. Colman RW, Hirsh J, Marder VJ, et al (Eds). Philadelphia, JB Lippincott, 1982, pp 595–601.
65. Marder VJ, Feinstein DI, Francis CW: Consumptive thrombohemorrhagic disorders. *In:* Hemostasis and Thrombosis. 3rd ed. Colman RW, Hirsh J, Marder VJ, et al (Eds). Philadelphia, JB Lippincott, 1994, pp 1023–1063.
66. Bick RL: Disseminated intravascular coagulation and related syndromes: A clinical review. Semin Thromb Hemost 1988; 14(4):299.
67. Feinstein DI: Treatment of disseminated intravascular coagulation. Semin Thromb Hemost 1988; 14(4):351.
68. Lisiewicz J: DIC in acute leukemia. Semin Thromb Hemost 1988; 14(4):343.
69. Vinazzer H: Therapeutic use of antithrombin III in shock and disseminated intravascular coagulation. Semin Thromb Hemost 1989; 15(3):347.
70. White GC II, Marder VJ, Colman RW, et al: Approach to the bleeding patient. *In:* Hemostasis and Thrombosis. 3rd ed. Colman RW, Hirsh J, Marder VJ, et al (Eds). Philadelphia, JB Lippincott, 1994, pp 1134–1147.

CHAPTER 146

Plasma and Blood Substitutes

Gail T. Tominaga, MD • Kenneth Waxman, MD, FACS

Plasma expansion is attained through intravenous infusion of blood or its components or blood and plasma substitutes. Crystalloids (electrolyte solutions containing sodium) have been shown to be effective but relatively inefficient plasma volume expanders. Once infused intravascularly, crystalloids distribute throughout the entire extracellular fluid space, of which only a relatively small portion is the plasma volume. Hence, large volumes of crystalloid fluids need to be infused to result in effective plasma volume expansion.

More effective plasma expansion can be attained with colloid fluids, which contain larger molecules that diffuse relatively slowly across the semi-permeable capillary membranes. The first colloid plasma substitutes were tested around the turn of the century, when a carbohydrate exudate from acacia trees was used as a volume expander. This was used clinically during World War I and proved to be highly antigenic.[1] Another colloid solution developed in the early 1900s is gelatin. Gelatins are used clinically in Europe but are unavailable in the United States. Problems with these solutions include rapid urinary excretion causing a short duration of plasma expansion, antigenicity, and anaphylaxis.[2]

One of the major disadvantages of colloid solutions is that they are unable to transport oxygen. Although not yet clinically available, two types of oxygen-carrying solutions have undergone investigation—perfluorochemical (PFC) emulsions and hemoglobin solutions. Attempts to develop a hemoglobin-based red blood cell (RBC) substitute have spanned many decades. Hemoglobin in solution has many characteristics of a potentially ideal plasma expander: (1) colloid osmotic effects, (2) oxygen-carrying and releasing capacity, (3) stability exceeding that of whole blood, (4) absence of type-specific RBC antigens, and (5) absence of viral contaminants of plasma. Blood, on the other hand, has several disadvantages: It (1) requires typing and crossmatching, (2) has a short half-life, (3) poses a risk of disease transmission, and (4) cannot be used as a perfusate for organ preservation because of its increased viscosity at low temperatures.

This chapter reviews two synthetic plasma substitutes currently available, dextran solutions and hydroxyethyl starch (HES), and two oxygen-carrying solutions, PFC emulsions and hemoglobin solutions.

DEXTRAN

Dextrans are polysaccharides produced by the conversion of sucrose into long glucose polymers by the bacterial enzyme dextransucrase. Clinically used dextrans are produced by the bacterium *Leuconostoc mesenteroides*. The molecules produced by the bacteria are very large, with molecular weights of several million. For intravenous infusion, partial acid hydrolysis produces dextran fractions within specific weight ranges. Two dextran solutions are most widely used, a 6% solution with an average molecular weight of 70,000 (dextran 70) and a 10% solution with an average molecular weight of 40,000 (dextran 40, or low-molecular-weight dextran). The dextrans can be efficiently produced in large quantities and stored for many years at room temperature either in powdered form or in solution.

Dextran is mainly secreted unchanged in the urine. The rate of renal excretion depends on the molecular size, with smaller dextran molecules being excreted rapidly and larger molecules excreted very slowly.[3] In patients with normal renal function, approximately 60% of infused dextran 40 is excreted into the urine within 6 hours and almost 70% within 24 hours.[4] Tubular absorption of dextran is negligible. Dextran molecules not excreted in the urine slowly diffuse into the interstitium, where uptake into the reticuloendothelial cells and slow metabolism to carbon dioxide occur.[5] Reticuloendothelial cell dysfunction as a result of this uptake has been postulated, but the clinical implication of this remains unproven.

Rapid renal excretion of dextran particles of molecular weight less than 50,000, along with tubular resorption of water, produces a highly viscous urine. Urine specific gravity may increase to extremely high levels (i.e., 1.088) in patients receiving dextran 40 infusions.[6] In patients with severe dehydration or impaired renal perfusion, the risk of acute renal failure is increased secondary to obstruction of the renal tubules by the highly viscous filtrate.[7] This can be avoided by concurrent administration of noncolloidal fluids.[8]

The plasma half-life of dextran solutions depends on their molecular size. Dextran 40 is excreted more rapidly than dextran 70, but dextran 40 solutions have a higher oncotic effect per gram infused and thus produce a more pronounced plasma volume expansion.

Dextrans are effective plasma expanders with efficacy equal or superior to albumin. A number of studies have shown this plasma volume expansion, with subsequent hemodynamic improvement.[9–13]

In addition to plasma volume expansion, dextran solutions have antithrombotic effects. These are probably mediated by inhibition of platelet and leukocyte aggregation as well as augmentation of blood flow in the microcirculation. Because a major pathophysiologic deficit after shock is decreased microcirculatory blood flow, administration of dextrans to patients in shock may offer a therapeutic advantage. This effect may be mediated by decreased blood viscosity by hemodilution or inhibition of RBC and platelet aggregation within the capillaries by low-molecular-weight dextran, which may reverse or prevent intravascular sludging.[14–16]

Anaphylactic reactions to dextran occur in 0.03% to 0.07% of patients and may be severe or even fatal.[17, 18] These reactions usually occur during infusion of the first 100 mL. Close monitoring during the initiation of dextran infusion is suggested. Isolated reports in the literature have described fetal deaths due to dextrans given maternally before or during delivery.[19, 20]

Dextran affects normal coagulation in a dose-related fashion. Low doses of dextran (<1.5 g/kg body weight) are not associated with clinical bleeding, but platelet adhesiveness and plasma levels of clotting factors are decreased. Larger doses of dextran have been associated with significant bleeding complications.[21] Such consideration limits its use in perioperative or bleeding patients to 1000 to 1500 mL in 24 hours. Precipitation of acute renal failure has been associated with significant bleeding complications, although this is controversial. Renal failure after dextran use is usually reported when renal perfusion is reduced or when preexisting renal damage is present. Hence, dextran administration is not recommended in patients with renal insufficiency.

Another potential problem reported with dextran infusion is subsequent difficulty in blood crossmatching. This effect may be due to the adherence of the dextrans to antigens on the RBC membrane. This problem can be avoided by obtaining a blood specimen for crossmatching before infusion.

Low-molecular-weight dextran has also been used effectively as a plasma substitute for priming in extracorporeal circulation.[22–23] In addition, dextrans have been studied and used as possible effective modalities in treating patients with myocardial ischemia, cerebral ischemia, and peripheral vascular disease and in maintaining vascular graft patency.

HYDROXYETHYL STARCH

Starch is the energy storage polysaccharide of plants and is analogous functionally and structurally to glycogen, the energy storage polysaccharide molecule of animals. Starch is composed of two types of glucose polymers: amylose, a linear molecule, and amylopectin, a highly branched molecule that structurally resembles glycogen. Amylopectin is well tolerated when infused intravascularly into animals but is rapidly hydrolyzed enzymatically, with a half-life of only 20 minutes. Modification of the starch molecule by hydroxyethylation, creating HES, has made it less susceptible to amylase hydrolysis and hence more stable within the plasma.[24]

There are several types of HES solutions, characterized by their average molecular weight and degree of substitution. The first developed solution, hetastarch, has a large mean molecular weight (69,000; range 10,000–100,000) with a wide range. This has implications when considering elimination of HES from the vascular space. Smaller molecules are excreted unchanged into the urine, whereas larger molecules slowly diffuse into the interstitium, where slow enzymatic degradation occurs. In normal subjects, HES is almost completely cleared from the plasma within 2 days (half-life is 17 h), yet only about 50% of the HES is eliminated from the body. The remaining HES is eliminated very slowly, and much of the initial dose persists in the reticuloendothelial cells for weeks after infusion.[24]

HES appears to be extremely well tolerated, with relatively infrequent and mild side effects. Allergic reactions to HES are uncommon; unlike dextran, HES is not antigenic. In one large series, the incidence of allergic reactions to HES was 0.085% in 16,405 infusions compared with 0.011% in 60,048 infusions for albumin infusion.[25] No fatal anaphylactic reactions to HES were reported in this study.

The only clinically important adverse effect of HES infusion appears to be some impairment of coagulation, which appears to be dose related. Low doses have no effect on coagulation, whereas moderate doses (20 mL/kg) may transiently decrease platelet counts, decrease fibrinogen levels, and prolong prothrombin time and partial thromboplastin time.[26] Platelet function, including adhesiveness, remains intact. Although these effects may be measured, there is no evidence of clinical bleeding problems with HES infusions of as much as 20 mL/kg.[27] There have been no controlled human studies of larger infusions with HES, but studies of animals have shown increased incisional bleeding, increased intraoperative blood loss, and spontaneous serosal bleeding when very large doses of HES are infused.[28]

A problem of unclear significance with HES infusion is occasional elevation of the serum amylase level. It is unclear if this hyperamylasemia is a result of subclinical pancreatitis, if HES acts as a physiologic stimulant to pancreatic amylase secretion, or if it results in amylase aggregation.[29] It is known that amylase-starch complexes form and can increase serum amylase to more than twice the normal values during a period of several days. Unlike dextrans, HES does not interfere with blood crossmatching, and it has no apparent adverse effect on renal function.[30]

The most commonly used HES is hetastarch, which is available as a 6% solution in physiologic salt solution and contains 60 g/L colloid and 154 mEq/L sodium and chloride. It has an osmolarity of 310 mOsm/L, pH of 5.5, and colloid oncotic pressure of 30 mm Hg.[31]

Pentastarch, a modification of the hetastarch formulation, has a lower average molecular weight, more homogeneous particle size, and less hydroxyethyl substitution. These changes allow for a more predictable, rapid excretion of pentastarch compared with hetastarch. Pentastarch theoretically poses less risk of reticuloendothelial impairment. In addition, larger volumes may have less effect on coagulation parameters.[32] Pentastarch is available as a 10% solution and has a colloid osmotic pressure of 40 mm Hg.

HES has been well studied for its efficacy as a plasma volume expander. Hetastarch (6% solution in saline) increases plasma volume from 71% to 230% of the volume infused.[31, 33–35] The colloid osmotic pressure is increased significantly after hetastarch infusion, thus explaining its ability to expand the plasma volume by more than the infused volume. The colloid osmotic pressure remains elevated for 2 to 5 days after HES infusion, corresponding to the plasma half-life of HES. In addition, pentastarch has a greater degree of volume expansion than either albumin or 6% hetastarch.[36]

In comparative studies of fluid therapy, infusing 6% HES solutions has increased central venous pressure, pulmonary capillary wedge pressure, cardiac output, and ventricular stroke work, with efficacy equivalent to that of 5% albumin infusion.[27, 37, 38] No bleeding problems were reported in these studies, including perioperative patients. HES, in particular pentastarch, has also been successfully used as a priming solution for cardiopulmonary bypass.[39]

HES has similarities and differences compared with dextran. Both dextran and HES effectively raise colloid osmotic pressure and plasma volume, although the plasma volume increase may be greater and somewhat more sustained after infusion of higher-molecular-weight dextrans. Dextrans are more useful agents in decreasing blood viscosity and increasing microcirculatory blood flow and thus have advantage as antithrombotic agents and as therapy for microcirculatory flow disturbances. HES, on the other hand, appears to be associated with fewer adverse effects, including a lower incidence of anaphylaxis, fewer bleeding problems, and no adverse renal effects.

PERFLUOROCHEMICAL EMULSIONS

Fluoridation of hydrocarbons generates a biologically inert liquid with high oxygen solubility. This solution differs from hemoglobin in that hemoglobin combines with oxygen whereas oxygen is dissolved in PFC emulsions. Oxygen is thereby supplied to tissues via simple diffusion after delivery by PFC emulsions. Its potential use as a blood substitute has been delayed because it requires suspension in an emulsion suitable for intravascular infusion.

In 1965, Clark and Gollan demonstrated that a mouse could survive when completely submerged in a PFC liquid equilibrated with oxygen at 1 atm.[40] In 1967, Sloviter and Kamimoto made a PFC emulsion with albumin and found that isolated, perfused brain preparations could be maintained with this emulsion as well as with blood.[41] In 1968, Geyer performed the first successful total exchange transfusions with rats, using a PFC emulsion made from perfluorotributylamine (FC47).[42] Significant problems occurred with these early emulsions, including prolonged tissue retention times (half-life of 895 days) and pulmonary and hepatic toxicity.

During the 1970s, an improved emulsion, Fluosol-DA 20% (Fluosol), was developed.[43] This emulsion is 20% PFC by weight and contains seven parts perfluorodecalin for short tissue dwell time and three parts perfluorotripropylamine for improved emulsion stability. Poloxamer 188 (Pluronic F-68) and egg yolk phospholipid are added as emulsifying agents, and HES is added to increase oncotic pressure. Fluosol must be stored frozen and infused within 24 hours of thawing.

PFC emulsions are eliminated unchanged through the airways. The particles of Fluosol-DA emulsion have a mean diameter of 0.1 μm. This small size allows elimination through the alveolar membrane. Some uptake of PFC emulsions occurs in the reticuloendothelial cells. The half-life of Fluosol is dose dependent. At a dose of 10 mL/kg, the circulatory half-life is approximately 8 hours; at a dose of 20 mL/kg, the plasma half-life is about 17 hours.[44, 45] Trace amounts of Fluosol are present in the liver and spleen for as long as 80 days after treatment. Accumulation of perfluorocarbons occurs on repeated administration. Therefore, administration more than once every 6 months is not recommended.

Because the oxygen dissolved in PFC emulsions is not bound as it is to hemoglobin, the amount of oxygen transported depends on the partial pressure of oxygen in the arterial blood ($Pa{O_2}$). Although PFCs have about 20 times the solubility for oxygen as plasma, significant volumes of oxygen are still dissolved only at high $Pa{O_2}$ values. Thus the clinical use of PFC emulsions requires good pulmonary function and high inspired oxygen concentrations. An advantage of this relatively low "affinity" of PFC for oxygen is that nearly all oxygen dissolved in PFC at arterial oxygen tensions is released to peripheral tissues at tissue oxygen tensions.

PFC emulsions improve peripheral blood flow by plasma volume expansion and possibly by improved microcirculatory flow. The small PFC emulsion particles (1/70th the size of RBCs) may flow through constricted areas of the microcirculation not accessible to RBCs. This characteristic may improve peripheral tissue oxygenation both by delivering oxygen dissolved in the PFC and by increasing plasma flow and delivery of the oxygen dissolved in plasma.

Fluosol was given to normal volunteers and tested in clinical trials in Japan in 1978.[46] It was first used in the United States in 1979, and limited trials have been performed, largely in anemic and bleeding patients who refused blood on religious grounds. Mitsuno and coworkers reported that Fluosol infusion did result in significant plasma volume expansion.[47] Tremper and Waxman and their colleagues reported small series of anemic patients who had some improvement in oxygen delivery and oxygen consumption after Fluosol administration.[48–49]

A number of adverse effects have possibly been related to administering PFC emulsion. These include transient leukopenia, elevated results of liver function tests, increased pulmonary arterial pressures, transient hypotension, and pulmonary failure.[49–51] It appears that an emulsifying agent in Fluosol, poloxamer 188, may be responsible for some of these adverse effects via activation of the complement system.[52]

The clinical usefulness of currently available PFC emulsion as a blood substitute has not been well established. A number of limitations of these solutions appear to be problematic. First, the volumes of PFC emulsion that have been infused have been limited, and with these volumes only a relatively small amount of oxygen can be dissolved. Therefore, its oxygen-transporting capability is limited. Second, the plasma half-life is relatively short. Third, the stability of the current emulsion limits the shelf life, even when stored frozen. Fourth, in order to dissolve significant volumes of oxygen in Fluosol, very high $Pa{O_2}$ must be achieved and adequate pulmonary function and high inspired oxygen concentrations are necessary. Finally, a number of possible adverse effects of Fluosol administration have been reported. Most of these limitations may be improved on when a better, biologically inert surfactant becomes available.[53]

There are potential therapeutic uses for PFC emulsions other than as blood substitutes. The most promising of these may be its use as a coronary artery angioplasty perfusate. Anderson and associates demonstrated significantly prolonged time to onset of angina, reduced duration of chest pain, and improved subjective evaluation of chest pain when Fluosol was infused through the central lumen of the angioplasty catheter in 29 patients with single-vessel disease and good cardiac function.[54] Cowley and colleagues evaluated the use of Fluosol in 38 high-risk cardiac patients (defined as those with unstable angina, a history of recent myocardial infarction, severe left ventricular dysfunction, multivessel disease, or high-risk lesions). Cardiac output declined less in Fluosol-treated patients than in controls. No adverse side effects attributable to Fluosol were noted.[55] Hence, intracoronary perfusion of Fluosol during angioplasty may ameliorate or prevent procedural ischemia in high-risk cardiac patients.

PFCs may also be used as radiation therapy enhancers,[56] as drug delivery solvents,[57] and as a radiologic contrast medium,[58] as well as for the acute treatment of myocardial or cerebral ischemia.[59]

Second-generation perfluorocarbon emulsions have been developed and are under investigation.[60, 60a] Potential continues to exist for these improved solutions as effective resuscitation fluids.

STROMA-FREE HEMOGLOBIN

Human Hemoglobin Solutions

The development of an ideal hemoglobin-derived blood substitute has eluded investigators for more than a century.

A persistent problem has been the inability to develop hemoglobin solutions that provide adequate oxygen and carbon dioxide exchange, while avoiding toxicity that precludes clinical safety and long-term survival.

Investigators in the 1940s and 1950s found hemoglobin solutions to be nephrotoxic and to cause alterations of blood coagulation and vasoconstriction.[61–64] In the late 1960s, Rabiner and associates reported that these toxic effects occurred because of contaminants derived from the RBC membrane.[65] The term *stroma-free hemoglobin* (SFH) was introduced by Rabiner and coworkers to describe the more highly purified hemoglobin solutions they had prepared. Although a misnomer, because some stroma is present, the name SFH has since become the standard nomenclature for stroma-removed hemoglobin solutions. Based on the results of these studies, a phase I clinical trial was performed in 1978 by administering 250 mL of stroma-free hemoglobin, containing 1.2% stroma, to eight healthy volunteers. It was found that the nearly complete removal of stromal contaminants reduced but did not completely prevent the development of toxic reactions.[66] It was also reported that hemoglobinuria, which was previously considered innocuous, was associated with decreases in urine volume and creatinine clearance. Investigators have traditionally focused on human hemoglobin solutions. The preparation of hemoglobin solutions generally consists of hemolysis of washed, outdated human RBCs, purification by crystallization and washing, and reconstitution for storage in solution or in dry form.[67] Although these preparations are relatively stable, gradual breakdown to methemoglobin occurs when they are stored at room temperature. Shelf life is greatly prolonged if SFH is stored frozen.

One of the major problems with the SFH preparations is increased affinity for oxygen compared with that of RBCs. The oxygen half-saturation (P_{50}) of SFH solutions varies from 12 to 16 mm Hg, compared with 26 to 27 mm Hg for fresh blood. This increased oxygen affinity, depicted by the left-shifted oxygen dissociation curve, is due to the loss of tetrameric hemoglobin, lack of 2,3-diphosphoglycerate (2,3-DPG), and a higher pH compared with the intracellular RBC pH. This increased affinity for oxygen by SFH solutions could lead to inadequate release of oxygen in the tissues, despite adequate circulating volumes of oxygen. Solutions to this problem have evolved. By reacting hemoglobin with pyridoxal-5′-phosphate, the P_{50} has been increased to 23 to 26 mm Hg.[68]

In addition, hemoglobin has been encapsulated with 2,3-DPG in liposomes, simulating RBCs. Liposome-encapsulated hemoglobin (LEH) has a normal hemoglobin dissociation curve and an increased half-life (16–24 h).[69] Inclusion of carbohydrate components such as gangliosides into the liposomal bilayer results in increased circulation times. As a result, these ganglioside-containing liposomes may exhibit reduced impact on the reticuloendothelial system. The LEH solutions have been shown to increase plasma half-life and can carry sufficient oxygen to sustain life,[69a] but safety has not yet been proved.

Another problem with SFH solutions is their relatively rapid clearance from the vascular space due to uptake by the reticuloendothelial system and to renal excretion. In experimental studies, SFH solutions have a plasma half-life of 2 to 4 hours.[67] Rapid loss of hemoglobin is also associated with a significant osmotic diuresis, resulting in intravascular volume depletion. To counter these effects, hemoglobin has been complexed to form larger-molecular-weight species.[70] Polymerization of hemoglobin has generally been carried out using random cross-linking agents, most commonly glutaraldehyde. This process has several disadvantages. A heterogeneous distribution of products is obtained, causing the protein to be modified at many different sites on the molecule. Most cross-linking agents are nonspecific and difficult to control and lead to increased oxygen affinity, highly variable material, increased antigenicity, and enhanced auto-oxidation.[71–73] In addition, polymers with a molecular weight greater than 500 behave like impurities and activate complement.[74, 75] To avoid this problem, selective polymerization is used. HbXL99α, a hemoglobin derivative produced by specific cross-linking between the α subunits, has been shown to have a markedly reduced rate of auto-oxidation.[76–77] Under physiologic conditions, the P_{50} of HbXL99α is 29 mm Hg, resulting in oxygen-transport characteristics similar to those of whole blood.[77] In addition, it was found that hemoglobin introduced into the circulating plasma was a factor in oxidative stress, and this could be controlled by concomitant administration of antioxidants or oxygen radical scavengers.[78]

Bovine Hemoglobin Solutions

The use of outdated banked blood or pedigree human donor blood as a hemoglobin source poses the problems of disease transmission risks and limited supply. Therefore, alternative sources of hemoglobin have been investigated. Bovine hemoglobin, in particular, has been extensively studied.

Bovine hemoglobin has several unique characteristics. First, bovine blood appears to avoid the risk of viral diseases associated with human blood and obviates supply constraints inherent with human hemoglobin preparations. Bovine hemoglobin has the additional physiologic advantage of not requiring 2,3-DPG to lower its oxygen affinity. Human hemoglobin must be modified by pyridoxylation to allow it to release oxygen in a stroma-free, 2,3-DPG–free environment, thus increasing the risk of contamination during preparation. In contrast, bovine hemoglobin does not require modification because it uses chloride ion to lower its oxygen affinity.[79] Fortunately, the chloride ion concentration of human plasma is adequate to decrease the oxygen affinity of bovine hemoglobin to a satisfactory level (P_{50} = 28 mm Hg) before polymerization.[80]

In 1983, Feola and colleagues reported that bovine hemoglobin, polymerized as well as unmodified, was an effective carrier of oxygen and capable of sustaining life in animals that had severe hemorrhage.[81] Subsequent studies showed that intravenous administration of bovine hemoglobin was safe if the hemoglobin was pure, selectively polymerized, and complemented with antioxidants or radical scavengers.[74, 75, 78, 82, 83] In addition, in 1988, Feola and associates demonstrated that bovine hemoglobin with these characteristics could be safely administered to humans. In 1992, a clinical trial was performed in Zaire.[84] Nine children with sickle cell anemia were transfused with a bovine hemoglobin solution (containing 10% hemoglobin) to 25% blood volume. No adverse reactions were reported. In addition, five patients with aplastic crisis had reticulocytosis in response to transfusion.

These initial studies make bovine hemoglobin solutions a potentially promising blood substitute.

Recombinant Hemoglobin Solutions

Use of recombinant DNA techniques to produce hemoglobin for use as a substitute offers several advantages: potentially unlimited supply, virus-free material, and the possibility of tailoring the properties of the hemoglobin. Nagai and coworkers were the first to produce human hemoglobin via recombinant methods.[85]

Human hemoglobin can currently be synthesized in *Escherichia coli*[86] and *Saccharomyces cerevisiae*[87] whose genomes have been modified to contain globin genes. However, these hemoglobins cannot be used as blood substitutes for several reasons. (1) Oxygen affinity is high, owing to the absence of 2,3-DPG, precluding sufficient oxygen unloading to the tissues; (2) they dissociate into α-β dimers[88] that are cleared rapidly by renal filtration or are rapidly oxidized to the nonfunctional methemoglobin form.

Soluble hemoglobin injected into the circulatory system cannot interact with 2,3-DPG in RBCs, making its oxygen affinity too high to support oxygen transport. Appropriate mutations in the globin genes resulting in the expression of a synthetic hemoglobin with low oxygen affinity, resembling that of normal blood, can be produced. The coexpression of β-globin chains and α-globin subunits linked by a peptide bond results in the direct synthesis of stabilized and fully functional hemoglobin tetramers.[89] Fusion of the two α-globin subunits increases the half-life of this hemoglobin molecule in vivo by preventing its dissociation into α-β dimers. Unlike hemoglobins that have been chemically cross-linked, genetically fused di-α-hemoglobin can be produced by simple microbial fermentation and purified without further modification.[90] Hence, this new recombinant hemoglobin is a strong potential candidate to develop for future use as a blood substitute.

CONCLUSION

Colloid fluid solutions are frequently used as plasma volume expanders in critically ill patients. Individual agents, including dextran and HES solutions, have unique advantages and disadvantages.

Concerns about the safety and availability of the national blood supply have rekindled interest in the development of blood substitutes. Clinical studies have dampened the initial enthusiasm for perfluorocarbon emulsions as blood substitutes. Primary concerns are the inadequate amount of oxygen that can be carried by PFCs, as well as their toxicity. Hemoglobin, in contrast, is capable of picking up enough oxygen from atmospheric air to be an efficient oxygen carrier under all environmental conditions. Several hemoglobin solutions have been formulated. The major issues delaying clinical application of hemoglobin solutions are those of safety, which remain to be tested.

References

1. Gruber VF: Blood replacement. Berlin, Springer, 1969, p. 21.
2. Saddler JM, Horsey PJ: The new generation gelatins. A review of their history, manufacture and properties. Anaesthesia 1987; 42:998–1004.
3. Arturson G, Wallenius G: The renal clearance of dextran of different molecular sizes in normal humans. Scand J Clin Lab Invest 1964; 16:81.
4. Arturson G, Granath K, Thoren L, et al: The renal excretion of low molecular weight dextran. Acta Chir Scand 1964; 127:543.
5. Atik M: The uses of dextran in surgery: A current evaluation. Surgery 1969; 65:548–562.
6. Langsjoen PH: Observations in the excretion of low molecular dextran. Angiology 1965; 16:148.
7. Matheson NA, Diomi P: Renal failure after the administration of dextran 40. Surg Gynecol Obstet 1970; 131:661–668.
8. Bergentz SE, Falkheden T, Olson S: Diuresis and urinary viscosity in dehydrated patients: Influence of dextran-40,000 with and without mannitol. Ann Surg 1965; 161:582.
9. Thoren L: Dextran as a plasma volume substitute. Prog Clin Biol Res 1978; 19:265–282.
10. Amundson B, Jennische E, Haljama EH: Skeletal muscle microcirculatory and cellular metabolic effects of whole blood, Ringer's acetate, and dextran to infusions in hemorrhagic shock. Circ Shock 1980; 7:111–120.
11. Gelin LE, Solvell L, Zeederfeldt B: The plasma volume expanding effect of low viscous dextran and macrodex. Acta Anaesthesiol Scand 1961, 122:309–323.
12. Shoemaker WC: Comparison of the relative effectiveness of whole blood transfusions and various types of fluid therapy in resuscitation. Crit Care Med 1976; 4:71–78.
13. Gelin LE, Davidson I: Plasma expanders and hemodilution in the treatment of hypovolemic shock. *In:* Pathophysiology of Shock, Anoxia, and Ischemia. Cowley RA, Trump BF (Eds). Baltimore, Williams & Wilkins, 1981, pp 454–463.
14. Dormandy JA: Influence of blood viscosity on blood flow and the effect of low molecular weight dextran. Br Med J 1971; 4:716–719.
15. Knisley MH, Bloch EH, Eliot TS, et al: Sludged blood. Science 1947; 106:431.
16. Bygdeman S, Eliasson R: Effect of dextran on platelet adhesiveness and aggregation. Scand J Clin Lab Invest 1967; 20:17–23.
17. Ring J, Messmer K: Incidence and severity of anaphylactoid reactions to colloid volume substitutes. Lancet 1977; 1:466–469.
18. Fordhoff A: Anaphylactoid reactions to dextran—a report of 133 cases. Acta Anaesthesiol Scand 1977; 21:161–167.
19. Barbier P, Jonville AP, Autret E, et al: Fetal risks with dextrans during delivery. Drug Safety 1992; 7:71–73.
20. Berg EM, Fasting S, Sellevold OF: Serious complications with dextran-70 despite hapten prophylaxis. Is it best avoided prior to delivery? Anesthesia 1991; 46:1033–1035.
21. Karlson KE, Garson AA, Shafton GW, et al: Increased blood loss associated with administration of certain plasma expanders: dextran 75, dextran 40, and hydroxyethyl starch. Surgery 1967; 62:670–678.
22. Long IM: Status of plasma expanders in open heart surgery. Dis Chest 1962; 41:578–581.
23. Woltjes J, deJong JC, tenDuis HJ, et al: The priming of extracorporeal circuits: The effect on canine blood elements. Transfusion 1979; 19:552–557.
24. Waxman K, Tremper KK, Mason GR: Blood and plasma substitutes: Plasma expansion and oxygen transport properties. West J Med 1985; 143:202–206.
25. Ring J, Messmer K: Incidence and severity of anaphylactoid reactions to colloid volume substitutes. Lancet 1977; 1:466–469.
26. Korttila K, Grohn P, Gordon A, et al: Effects of hydroxyethyl starch and dextran on plasma volume and blood hemostasis and coagulation. J Clin Pharmacol 1984; 24:273–282.
27. Puri VK, Paidipaty B, White L: Hydroxyethyl starch for resuscitation of patients with hypovolemia and shock. Crit Care Med 1981; 9:833–837.
28. Karlson KE, Garzon AA, Shafton GW, et al: Increased blood loss associated with administration of certain plasma expanders. Surgery 1967; 62:670–678.
29. Kohler H, Kirch W, Horstmann HJ: Formation of high molecular aggregates between serum amylase and colloidal plasma substitutes. Anaesthesist 1977; 26:623–627.
30. Thompson WL: Hydroxyethyl starch. Prog Clin Biol Res 1978; 19:283–292.
31. Haupt MT, Rackow EC: Colloid osmotic pressure and fluid resuscitation with hetastarch, albumin and saline solutions. Crit Care Med 1982; 10:159–162.
32. Strauss RG, Stansfield C, Henriksen RA, et al: Pentastarch may cause fewer effects on coagulation than hetastarch. Transfusion 1988; 28:257–260.
33. Killian JP: The effect of 6% HES, 4.5% dextran 60 and 5.5% oxgel on blood volume. Anaesthesist 1977; 24:193–197.
34. Lamke LO, Liljedahl SO: Plasma volume changes after infusion of various expanders. Resuscitation 1976; 5:93–102.
35. Metcalf W, Papadopoulos A, Tufaro R, et al: A clinical physiologic study of hydroxyethyl starch. Surg Gynecol Obstet 1970; 131:255–267.
36. Kohler H, Zschiedrich M, Clasen R, et al: The effects of 500 ml 10% hydroxyethyl starch 200/0.5 and 10% dextran 40 on blood volume, colloid osmotic pressure and renal function in human volunteers. Anaesthesist 1982; 31:61–67.
37. Lazrove S, Waxman K, Shippy C, et al: Hemodynamic, blood volume and oxygen transport responses to albumin and hydroxyethyl starch infusion in critically ill postoperative patients. Crit Care Med 1980; 8:302–306.

38. Moggio RA, Rha CC, Somberg ED, et al: Hemodynamic comparison of albumin hydroxyethyl starch in postoperative cardiac surgery patients. Crit Care Med 1983; 11:943–945.
39. London MJ, Franks M, Verrier ED, et al: The safety and efficacy of ten per cent pentastarch as a cardiopulmonary bypass priming solution. A randomized clinical trial. J Thorac Cardiovasc Surg 1992; 104:284–296.
40. Clark LC Jr, Gollan F: Survival of mammals breathing organic liquids equilibrated with oxygen at atmospheric pressure. Science 1966; 152:1755–1756.
41. Sloviter HA, Kamimoto T: Erythrocyte substitute for perfusion of brain. Nature 1967; 216:458–460.
42. Geyer RP: Whole animals perfusion with fluorocarbon dispersions. Fed Proc 1970; 29:1758–1763.
43. Yokoyama K, Yamanouchi K, Watanabe M, et al: Preparation of perfluorodecalin emulsion, an approach to the red cell substitute. Fed Proc 1975; 34:1478–1483.
44. Proceedings of the 4th International Symposium on Perfluorochemical Blood Substitutes, Kyoto, Japan, October 1978. Amsterdam, Elsevier, 1979.
45. Proceedings of the 5th International Symposium on Perfluorochemical Blood Substitutes, Mainz, Germany, 1981. Munich, Zuckerschwerdt Verlag, 1982.
46. Markowski H, Tenschev P, Frey R: Tolerance of an oxygen-carrying colloid plasma substitute in humans. Proceedings of the 4th International Symposium on Perfluorochemical Blood Substitutes, Kyoto, Japan, October 1978. Amsterdam, Excerpta Medica, 1979, pp 47–50.
47. Mitsuno T, Ohyanagi H, Naito R: Clinical studies of a perfluorochemical whole blood substitute (Fluosol-DA)—summary of 186 cases. Ann Surg 1982; 195:60–69.
48. Tremper KK, Friedman AE, Levine EM, et al: The preoperative treatment of severely anemic patients with a perfluorochemical oxygen-transport fluid, Fluosol DA. N Engl J Med 1982; 307:277–283.
49. Waxman K, Tremper KK, Cullen BF, et al: Perfluorocarbon infusion in bleeding patients refusing blood transfusions. Arch Surg 1984; 119:721–724.
50. Waxman K, Cheung CK, Mason GR: Hypotensive reaction after infusion of a perfluorochemical emulsion. Crit Care Med 1984; 119:721–724.
51. Police AM, Waxman K, Tominaga G: Pulmonary complications in three patients receiving Fluosol DA-20% following life-threatening blood loss. Crit Care Med 1985; 13:96–98.
52. Vercellotti GM, Hammerschmidt DE, Craddock PR, et al: Activation of plasma complement by perfluorocarbon artificial blood: Probable mechanism of adverse pulmonary reactions in treated patients and rationale for corticosteroid prophylaxis. Blood 1982; 59:1299–1304.
53. Clark LC Jr, Clark EW, Moore RE, et al: Room temperature-stable biocompatible fluorocarbon emulsions. Prog Clin Biol Res 1983; 122:169–180.
54. Anderson HV, Leimgruber PP, Roubin GS, et al: Distal coronary artery perfusion during percutaneous transluminal coronary angioplasty. Am Heart J 1985; 110:720–726.
55. Cowley MJ, Snow FR, DiSciascio G, et al: Perfluorochemical perfusion during coronary angioplasty in unstable and high-risk patients. Circulation 1990; 81(Suppl 3):IV27–34.
56. Morton JD, Porter E, Yabuki H, et al: Effects of a perfluorochemical emulsion on the response of BA1112 rat rhabdomyosarcomas to continuous low-dose-rate irradiation. Radiat Res 1990; 124:178–182.
57. Weber TR, Westfall SH, Webb LE, et al: The effects of perfluorochemicals on tumor growth and chemotherapy response. J Pediatr Surg 1987; 22:1187–1190.
58. Mattrey RF, Long DC: Potential role of PFOB in diagnostic imaging. Invest Radiol 1988; 23(Suppl 1):S298–301.
59. Rice HE, Virmani R, Hart CL, et al: Dose-dependent reduction of myocardial infarct size with the perfluorochemical fluosol-DA. Am Heart J 1990; 120:1039–1046.
60. Meinert H, Fackler R, Knoblich A, et al: On the perfluorocarbon emulsions of second generation. Biomater Artif Cells Immobilization Biotechnol 1992; 20:805–818.
60a. Goodin TH, Grossbard EB, Kaufman RJ, et al: A perfluorochemical emulsion for prehospital resuscitation of experimental hemorrhagic shock: A prospective, randomized, controlled study. Crit Care Med 1994; 22:680–689.
61. Amberson WR, Jennings JJ, Rhode CM: Clinical experience with hemoglobin saline solutions. J Appl Physiol 1949; 1:469–489.
62. Amberson WR: Blood substitutes. Biol Rev 1937; 12:46–74.
63. Brandt JL, Grank R, Lichtman HC: The effects of hemoglobin solutions on renal function in man. Blood 1951; 6:1152–1158.
64. Miller JH, McDonald RK: The effect of hemoglobin on renal function in the human. J Clin Invest 1951; 30:1033–1040.
65. Rabiner SF, Helbert JR, Lopas H, et al: Evaluation of stroma-free hemoglobin solution for use as a plasma expander. J Exp Med 1967; 126:1127–1142.
66. Savitsky JP, Doczi J, Black J, et al: A clinical safety trial of stroma-free hemoglobin. Clin Pharmacol Ther 1978; 23:73–80.
67. DeVenuto F, Friedman HI, Neville JR, et al: Appraisal of hemoglobin solution as a blood substitute. Surg Gynecol Obstet 1979; 149:417–436.
68. Yabuki A, Yamaji K, Ohki H, et al: Characterization of a pyridoxilated hemoglobin-polyoxyethylene conjugate as a physiologic oxygen carrier. Transfusion 1990; 30:516–520.
69. Rabinovici R, Rudolph AS, Ligler FS, et al: Liposome-encapsulated hemoglobin: An oxygen-carrying fluid. Circ Shock 1990; 32:1–17.
69a. Rabinovici R, Rudolph AS, Vernick K, et al: A new salutary resuscitative fluid: Liposome-encapsulated hemoglobin/hypertonic saline solution. J Trauma 1993; 35:121–127.
70. Sehgal LR, Gould SA, Rosen AL, et al: Polymerized pyridoxylated hemoglobin: A red cell substitute with normal oxygen capacity. Surgery 1984; 95:433–438.
71. Bunn FH, Esham WT, Bull RW: The renal handling of hemoglobin. J Exp Med 1969; 129:909–924.
72. Mok W, Chen DE, Mazur A: Cross linked hemoglobins as potential protein plasma extenders. Fed Proc 1975; 34:1458–1460.
73. Hedlund BE, Drayton CP, Alsop DS, et al: Polymerized hemoglobins. *In*: Transfusion Medicine: Recent Technological Advances. Murasaki K, Peetoom F (Eds). New York, Alan R Liss, 1986, pp 39–48.
74. Feola M, Simoni J, Canizaro PC, et al: The toxicity of polymerized hemoglobin solutions. Surg Gynecol Obstet 1988; 166:211–222.
75. Feola M, Simoni J, Dobke M, et al: Complement activation and the toxicity of stroma-free hemoglobin solutions in primates. Circ Shock 1988; 25:275–290.
76. Chatterjee R, Welty EV, Walder RY, et al: Isolation and characterization of a new hemoglobin derivative cross-linked between the alpha chains (lysine 99α-1 → lysine 99α-2). J Biol Chem 1986; 261:9929–9937.
77. Snyder SR, Welty EV, Walder RY, et al: HbXL99α: A hemoglobin derivate that is cross-linked between the alpha subunits is useful as a blood substitute. Proc Natl Acad Sci U S A 1987; 84:7280–7284.
78. Simoni J, Feola M, Canizaro PC: Generation of free oxygen radicals and the toxicity of hemoglobin solutions. Biomater Artif Cells Artif Organs 1990; 18:189–202.
79. Benesch RE, Benesch R, Renthal RD, et al: Affinity labelling of the polyphosphate binding site of hemoglobin. Biochemistry 1972; 11:3576–3582.
80. Fronticelli C, Bucci E, Orth C: Solvent regulation of oxygen affinity in hemoglobin. J Biol Chem 1984; 259:10841–10844.
81. Feola M, Gonzalez H, Canizaro PC, et al: Development of a bovine stroma-free hemoglobin solution as a blood substitute. Surg Obstet Gynecol 1983; 157:399–408.
82. Feola M, Simoni J, Canizaro PC: Quality control of hemoglobin solutions: I. The purity of hemoglobin before modification. Artif Organs 1991; 15:243–248.
83. Feola M, Simoni J, Canizaro PC: Immunological compatibility of hemoglobin solutions. Trasfus Sangue 1988; 33:121–128.
84. Feola M, Simoni J, Angelillo R, et al: Clinical trial of a hemoglobin based blood substitute in patients with sickle cell anemia. Surg Gynecol Obstet 1992; 174:379–386.
85. Nagai K, Thogersen HC: Generation of beta-globin by sequence-specific proteolysis of a hybrid protein produced in *Escherichia coli*. Nature 1984; 309:810–812.
86. Hoffman SJ, Looker DL, Roehrich JM, et al: Expression of fully functional tetrameric human hemoglobin in *Escherichia coli*. Proc Natl Acad Sci U S A 1990; 87:8521–8525.
87. Ogden JE, Coghlan D, Jones G, et al: Expression and assembly of functional human hemoglobin in *S. cerevisiae*. Biomater Artif Cells Immobization Biotechnol 1992; 20:473–475.

88. Ackers GK, Halvorson HR: The linkage between oxygenation and subsequent dissociation in human hemoglobin. Proc Natl Acad Sci U S A 1974; 71:4312–4316.
89. Looker D, Abbott-Brown D, Cozart P, et al: A human recombinant haemoglobin designed for use as a blood substitute. Nature 1992; 356:258–260.
90. Looker D, Mathews AJ, Neway JO, et al: Expression of recombinant human hemoglobin in *Escherichia coli*. Methods Enzymol 1994; 231:364–374.

CHAPTER 147

Intensive Care of the Cancer Patient

Graziano C. Carlon, MD

Despite advances in surgery, chemotherapy, and radiation therapy, the mortality rate for cancer in the United States has increased from 143 per 100,000 in 1930 to 171 per 100,000 in 1989.[1] This observation, however, is related to the sharp increase of a few very lethal malignancies, especially lung cancers. In the aggregate, 5-year survival after diagnosis of cancers has increased from 20% in 1930 to 40% in 1989. The large numbers of individuals affected guarantee that most physicians, including those practicing in critical care units, will be involved in the treatment of patients with malignancies. They may be required to manage life-threatening complications associated with the malignancy itself or presenting as side effects of treatment. The acute event may be the first manifestation of the disease; it may occur while the patient is being actively treated, with a reasonable expectation of success; or it may represent a terminal complication. These factors also influence management decisions. Finally, illnesses common to the general population may also affect cancer patients at any time, and a relationship to the underlying malignancy should not be automatically assumed.

This chapter describes complications of cancer and its treatment that may result in urgent consultation for admission to an intensive care unit (ICU). Both the major categories of malignancies and the most important therapeutic modalities are reviewed.

LIFE-THREATENING COMPLICATIONS OF CANCER

Hematologic Malignancies

Hematologic malignancies rarely present as acute events requiring intensive care. Usually, patients are admitted to the ICU for supportive treatment of complications that developed during therapy. Aggressive management of complications is justified by continuous improvement in the results of treatment. For instance, 5-year survival in childhood leukemia was 4% in 1970 and now exceeds 70%, thanks to advances in chemotherapy and bone marrow transplantation. The more benign forms of Hodgkin's disease have comparable cure rates, and the rate of permanent remission exceeds 50% for non-Hodgkin's lymphoma. These results have been largely achieved through very aggressive treatment modalities that carry their own risks of significant complications that may require intensive care.

Leukemias

Bleeding, sepsis, and neurologic dysfunction are occasional initial manifestations of acute leukemia that may require advanced life support. Replacement of blood volume; administration of coagulation factors, including platelets; and broad-spectrum antibiotics are the principal means of treatment. Resistance to infections is extremely limited, and antibiotics should be administered without delay at the first suspicion of bacterial contamination.[2] The therapeutic regimen should include an aminoglycoside, a penicillin active against gram-negative bacteria, and an agent that provides adequate coverage of staphylococcal species. Third- and fourth-generation cephalosporins are also commonly used, alone or in combination with aminoglycosides or quinolones.[3] Selection of specific agents should depend on patterns of sensitivity and antibiotic susceptibility in each hospital. Fungal infections can also be devastating in these patients. Antifungal therapy with intravenous amphotericin B is the only available treatment option, but mortality rate is very high when fungal dissemination to vital organs has occurred (Figs. 147–1 and 147–2).[4]

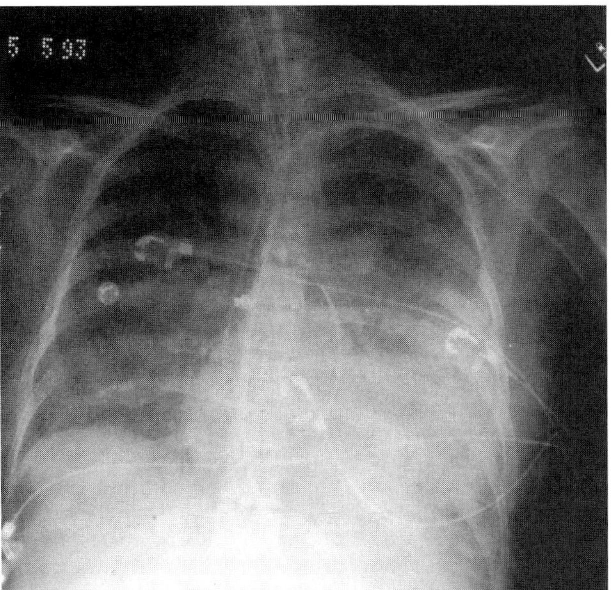

Figure 147–1. Chest radiograph of a patient with severe, disseminated fungal infection. The radiographic picture suggested the presence of pulmonary infiltrates.

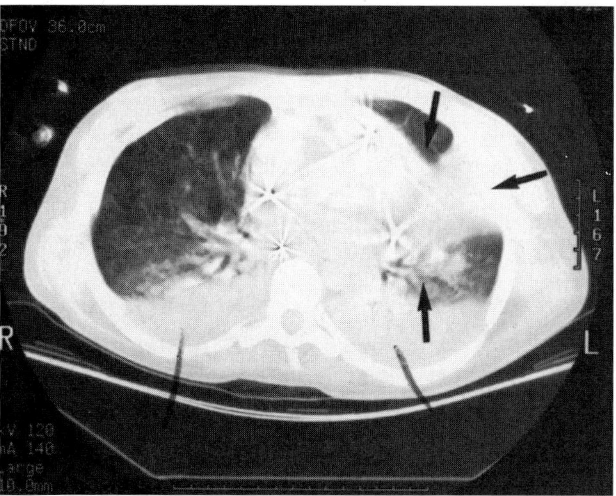

Figure 147–2. CT scan of the chest from the patient in Figure 147–1. The fungal mass is penetrating the pericardium and invading the myocardium.

Central venous, pulmonary artery, and systemic arterial access should be obtained only when clinically necessary, by use of the strictest aseptic precautions. Infection risks associated with indwelling catheters are well known. The lowest infection rates occur with implantable devices, especially those that are completely submerged under the skin, although they cannot be used for monitoring.[5] Once in place, catheters should not be manipulated; clinical studies have also indicated that routine substitution does not prevent infections, and this practice should no longer be used.[6]

Respiratory failure with hypoxemia and increased pulmonary venous admixture requiring mechanical ventilation and positive end-expiratory pressure is a particularly serious event in leukemic patients.[7] Occasionally, respiratory failure may be the first manifestation of the disease and may improve after chemotherapy (Fig. 147–3).[8] Radiographic evidence may be scanty because dense infiltrates cannot develop in the absence of white cells. The diagnosis is based on the absence of positive cultures, the identification of leukemic cells in bronchoalveolar lavage fluid, and the rapid improvement seen on chest x-ray study and in respiratory function after chemotherapy. More commonly, lung infiltrates are expressions of local or systemic sepsis, drug toxicity, hypersensitivity, or fluid overload. Acute respiratory distress requiring mechanical ventilation for more than 72 to 96 hours is associated with a mortality rate of 60% to 70% in these patients,[9] a figure that does not differ from those reported for the general population.[10]

Pulmonary parenchymal bleeding is a severe complication of the thrombocytopenia and other coagulation abnormalities frequently seen with systemic malignancies. Treatment includes replacement of clotting factors and early institution of mechanical ventilation.[11]

Acute promyelocytic leukemia is often associated with disseminated intravascular coagulation. Most authors recommend continuous intravenous infusion of low-dose heparin (7–10 $U \cdot kg^{-1} \cdot h^{-1}$) and cautious replacement of coagulation factors. The dangers of the disease and its therapy justify admitting patients to an ICU for close monitoring during the early phases of management. Because these patients are severely thrombocytopenic, sensitivity to heparin may be disproportionately increased, and frequent determination of partial thromboplastin time is required to regulate dosage. Often, intravascular coagulation subsides after the first course of chemotherapy.[12]

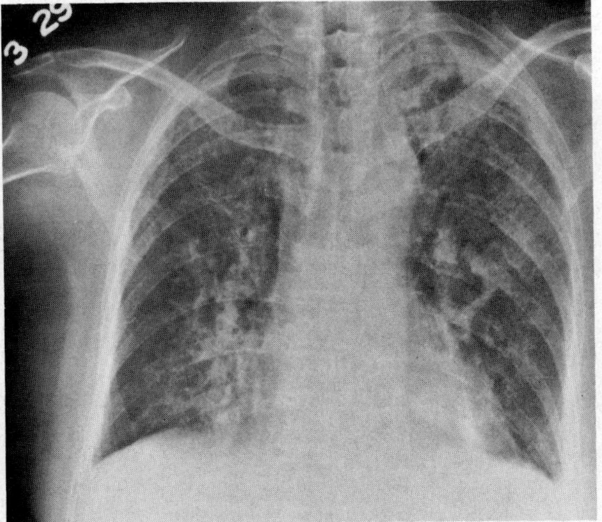

Figure 147–3. Chest radiograph of a patient with diffuse bilateral modular infiltrates. The radiograph cleared within a few days, subsequent to combination chemotherapy for the underlying acute myeloblastic leukemia.

Renal infiltrates, although common in patients with acute leukemia, rarely cause serious deterioration of renal function. Because many patients with systemic malignancies have reduced total body muscle mass, indices of renal function, such as serum creatinine, should be interpreted with caution. Nephrotoxic chemotherapy or antibiotics contribute to renal dysfunction, and dosages must be adjusted according to measured creatinine clearance and serum levels. A method that has proved effective is daily determination of creatinine clearance on the basis of 3-hour urine collections.[13]

Hyperviscosity syndromes, as seen in plasma cell myeloma, occasionally cause renal failure. Plasmapheresis rapidly reverses the associated symptomatology, but chemotherapy is needed to control the progression of the disease.

Lymphomas

Malignant lymphoma in the mediastinum can compress the superior vena cava, causing signs and symptoms of frightening gravity. Although usually slowly progressive, with ample time for the development of adequate collateral circulation, acute superior vena caval occlusion is a medical emergency that requires immediate intervention with radiation therapy, chemotherapy, or both.[14] Dramatic resolution may be seen in as little as 12 to 24 hours. Depending on the severity of the symptoms, performing a biopsy may not be possible before treatment begins. Whenever possible, however, specimens should be obtained first to confirm the histologic diagnosis and to guide subsequent treatment.

Infiltration of lung parenchyma by lymphoma is common and can be confused with chronic pulmonary infiltrates. Although it rarely causes respiratory failure severe enough to require mechanical ventilation, massive hemorrhage secondary to vascular invasion has been observed.

Expansion into and infiltration of other organs, such as the stomach, has also been described in patients with lymphomas. Massive bleeding is difficult to control both because surgical removal may be impossible and because effective therapy may result in rapid necrosis of the malignant infiltrate, precipitating hemorrhage or perforation.

Myelomas

The kidneys are often severely affected by multiple myeloma, particularly of the light-chain variety, and renal failure, once established, is usually not reversible.[15]

Hypercalcemia, a complication of myeloma and of tumors that metastasize to bones, may cause obtundation, coma, and in extreme cases, respiratory or cardiac arrest. Treatment includes intravenously administered balanced saline solutions to facilitate calcium elimination by increasing glomerular filtration, and intravenous furosemide (5–20 mg), which selectively inhibits calcium reabsorption.[16] Salmon calcitonin (80–150 U/kg given at 8- to 12-hour intervals) can rapidly lower serum calcium levels, but its usefulness is limited by early tachyphylaxis.[17] Corticosteroids (100–300 mg/d of hydrocortisone) are also useful in the treatment of hypercalcemia secondary to osteolytic processes. The antineoplastic antibiotic mithramycin effectively lowers calcium level through inhibition of osteoclast activity, but its action does not begin until 18 to 24 hours after administration, it has the potential of severe hypocalcemia, and it is often accompanied by a precipitous fall in platelet count.[18] More recently, biphosphonates have also been successfully used to lower serum calcium level.[19–21] Many myeloma patients are severely malnourished and have low serum albumin

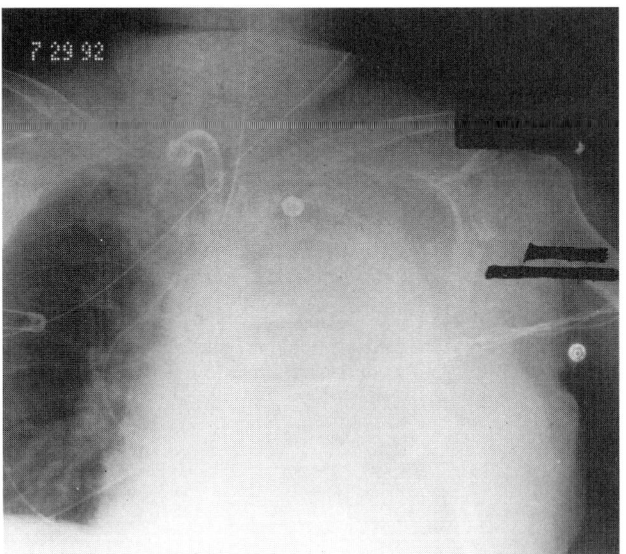

Figure 147–4. Chest radiograph of a patient with obstruction of the left mainstem bronchus secondary to adenocarcinoma of the lung. A brief period of support on mechanical ventilation allowed palliative laser vaporization of the obstruction and several months of survival for the patient.

levels; therefore, the ionized fraction of serum calcium represents a higher percentage of the total value. Estimation of ionized calcium concentration from the McLean-Hastings nomograms is far less accurate than direct determination with an ion-selective electrode.

Solid Tumors

Serious emergencies related to solid tumors or their treatment may arise at any time during the course of the disease. They commonly represent a terminal event, and decisions on the degree of support that should be given must include considerations of the likelihood of worthwhile palliation.

Central nervous system metastases are sometimes associated with coma and respiratory depression. Rapid resolution of symptoms is achieved with pharmacologic doses of steroids, preferably dexamethasone (24–100 mg/d given in four divided doses), followed by surgical excision, if appropriate, and whole-brain radiation therapy. The 2-year survival rate of patients with solitary brain metastasis from lung adenocarcinoma is as high as 40%.[22] Because at least temporary palliation can be obtained, ICU admission is justified in the absence of widespread disease.

Malignant invasion of the major bronchi or the trachea can usually be palliated by interstitial brachytherapy, external-beam radiation, or vaporization with the neodymium:yttrium-aluminum-garnet laser.[23] Intubation through the tumor or into the contralateral uninvolved bronchus may be required for support until the occlusion is at least partially relieved (Fig. 147–4).

Malignant mediastinal adenopathy can cause superior vena caval occlusion. Radiotherapy or chemotherapy is associated with considerable improvement in patients with lymphomas, but it is of short-term benefit in most solid tumors. Invasion of the heart chambers by metastatic lesions is rare but almost invariably fatal (Figs. 147–5 and 147–6).

Severe hepatic dysfunction rarely occurs with primary or metastatic disease, because 80% of the parenchyma can be replaced without appreciable change in laboratory values. Liver failure is invariably an irreversible terminal event.[24]

Renal failure from parenchymal invasion occurs rarely in solid tumor patients. Bilateral ureteral obstruction from malignant disease in the pelvis is commoner and leads to hydronephrosis and renal failure. Percutaneous or direct surgical relief of obstruction is often followed by massive postobstructive diuresis, which requires careful fluid and electrolyte replacement to avoid further renal damage.

CHEMOTHERAPY

During the past two decades, impressive advances have been made in the development of chemotherapeutic agents, increasing both the efficacy of the drugs and the spectrum of disease covered. Very few neoplasms are completely unresponsive to drug therapy. Chemotherapy alone may provide long-term or complete control of disease in acute child-

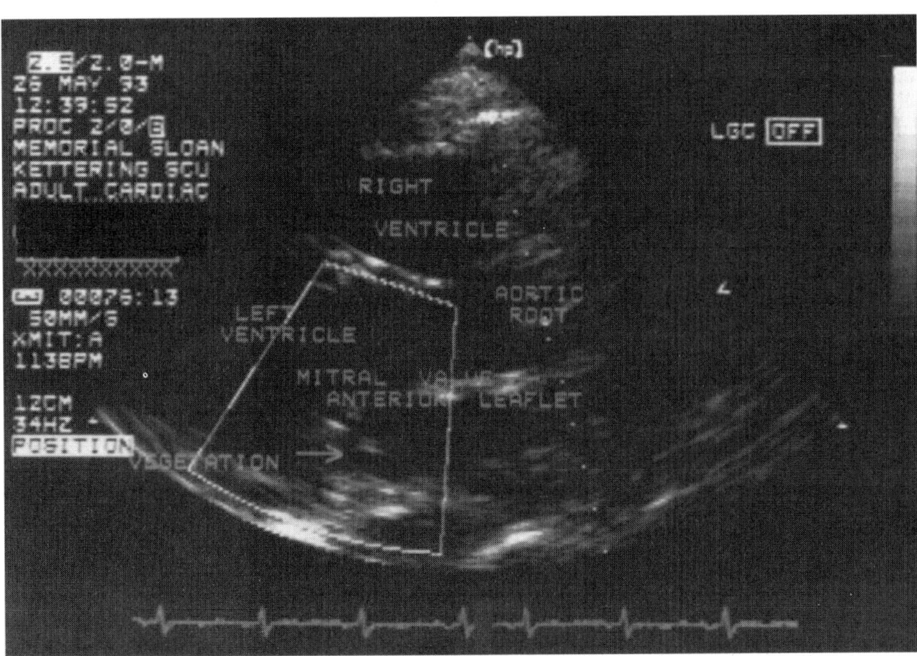

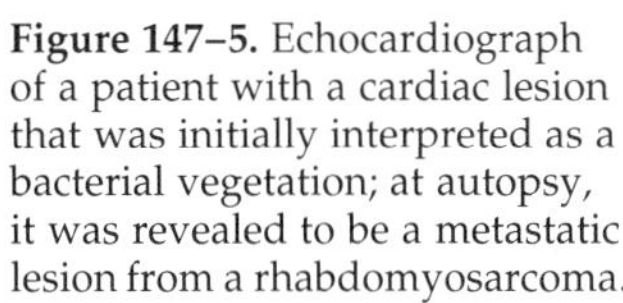
Figure 147–5. Echocardiograph of a patient with a cardiac lesion that was initially interpreted as a bacterial vegetation; at autopsy, it was revealed to be a metastatic lesion from a rhabdomyosarcoma.

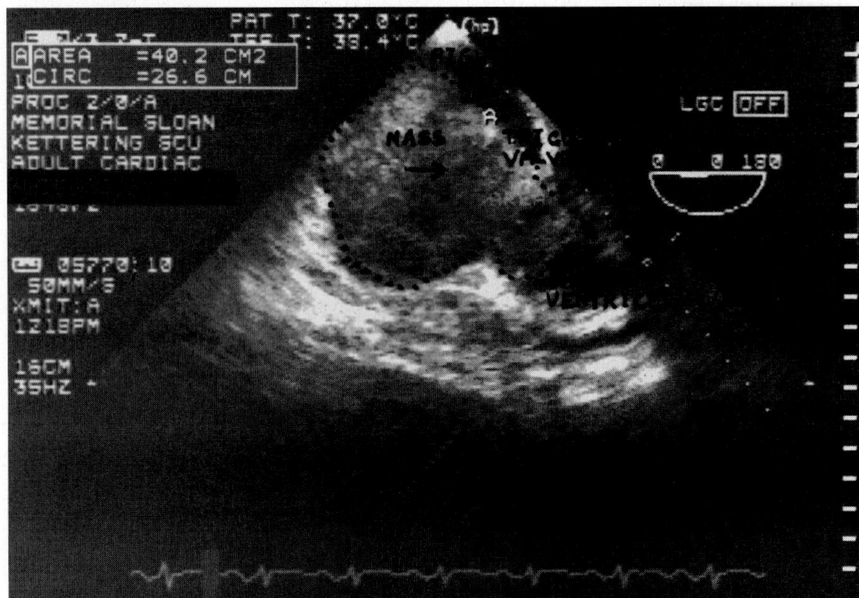

Figure 147–6. Rare, pedunculated metastatic lesion from a peripheral rhabdomyosarcoma, invading the right atrium and the posterior leaflet of the tricuspid valve. An attempt to remove the mass under bypass failed; the patient received a palliative anastomosis between the right innominate vein and the pulmonary artery to relieve blood flow obstruction.

hood leukemias, choriocarcinoma, Hodgkin's disease, and testicular carcinoma, and many other cancers have improved survival and disease-free intervals as a result of chemotherapy, used alone or in conjunction with surgery and radiotherapy.

Conceptually, chemotherapeutic agents should selectively destroy neoplastic cells by interfering with pathways of metabolism not shared by their normal counterparts. Unfortunately, such specificity is difficult to achieve, and healthy cells are also damaged during therapy. Drugs used in combination can have additive side effects that may be potentiated by other factors, such as malnutrition, prior radiation therapy, or surgery. Accordingly, critical care physicians should be familiar with the complications of commonly used chemotherapeutic agents.

Alkylating Agents

Alkylating agents form covalent bonds with preformed nucleic acids, and this interferes with their action. The prototype of this class of drug is *mechlorethamine* (nitrogen mustard), which is used primarily to treat disseminated Hodgkin's disease. Mechlorethamine causes nausea, vomiting, and bone marrow suppression.

Busulfan is used in the treatment of chronic myeloid leukemia. It is associated with an irreversible interstitial lung fibrosis that develops after months or even years of therapy. When busulfan is administered with nitrosoureas, however, its toxicity can be accelerated, and lung fibrosis may develop within a few weeks.[25]

Cyclophosphamide, one of the most versatile chemotherapeutic agents, is useful in the treatment of hematologic malignancies as well as solid tumors, neuroblastomas, and carcinomas of the breast, testis, lung, ovary, endometrium, and prostate. It can cause diffuse interstitial lung fibrosis after a few months to several years of therapy.[26] Respiratory failure associated with lung fibrosis is characterized by an inability to increase lung volume or to recruit collapsed alveoli despite increasing airway pressure. The high airway pressures caused by inelastic and fibrotic lung parenchyma frequently result in barotrauma. High-frequency jet ventilation has been useful in some patients, enabling the maintenance of satisfactory gas exchange, but the ultimate prognosis of these patients remains dismal.[27]

Cyclophosphamide is associated with myocardial toxicity when cumulative doses exceed 1800–2000 mg/m^2.[28] Active metabolites of cyclophosphamide are excreted in the urine, where they reach concentrations that are damaging to the bladder mucosa, causing severe hemorrhagic cystitis. Because cyclophosphamide increases water reabsorption by distal renal tubules and collecting ducts, hydration alone may not maintain a sufficient diuresis without the use of mannitol or other diuretics. Cyclophosphamide and other alkylating agents deplete plasma cholinesterase, probably by interfering with hepatic synthesis, thereby prolonging the duration of action of local anesthetics and depolarizing neuromuscular blocking drugs. Resolution of muscle paralysis after anesthesia may be prolonged unless this effect is considered.

Chlorambucil and *melphalan* are oral agents that cause myelosuppression and minimal nausea or vomiting. Melphalan is used to treat multiple myeloma and breast and ovarian carcinomas, and chlorambucil is used to treat the nodular forms of non-Hodgkin's lymphoma, chronic lymphatic leukemia, and ovarian carcinoma.[29]

Antimetabolites

Antimetabolites interfere with nucleic acid synthesis of new nucleic acids in actively dividing cells, such as those of the hematopoietic system. Most, if not all, antimetabolites cause severe myelosuppression and present the risk of life-threatening sepsis or hemorrhage.

Methotrexate competitively inhibits the action of folic acid, preventing nucleic acid formation and cellular replication. It is used to treat choriocarcinomas, acute lymphatic leukemia, sarcomas, and breast and lung carcinomas. Methotrexate is highly toxic to the liver, and serial liver biopsies have been recommended for early identification of liver damage during prolonged therapy. Renal failure has also been reported and is usually reversible. Mucositis and exfoliative dermatitis are common, and fluid loss or sepsis may follow loss of large areas of skin. Pulmonary toxicity, characterized by mild nondesquamative alveolitis and noncaseating granulomas, has been observed.[30] Intrathecal administration to control central nervous system involvement in childhood leukemia also has the potential for tissue damage. Folinic acid (citrovorum rescue factor) is given to minimize these toxic effects.

5-Fluorouracil, a pyrimidine antimetabolite, is the chemotherapeutic agent of choice for neoplasms of the gastrointestinal tract and is used in combination with other drugs in breast cancer. It is primarily complicated by myelosuppression. An analogue, 5-fluorodeoxyuridine, sometimes causes severe diarrhea that necessitates fluid and electrolyte support.

Vinca Alkaloids

Vincristine and *vinblastine*, alkaloids derived from plants of the periwinkle family, impair the synthesis of cellular microtubules. They are an effective treatment for Hodgkin's and non-Hodgkin's lymphomas, acute lymphoblastic leukemia, and some solid tumors, including Wilms' tumor and sarcomas. They are administered intravenously and are highly toxic to both the peripheral and the central nervous systems. Both the sensory and the motor neurons are affected, as are nonmyelinated sympathetic fibers. Orthostatic hypotension related to the loss of sympathetic tone is a common complication of vincristine administration. Prolonged ileus can develop after vincristine or vinblastine therapy and is usually a self-limiting complication that responds to conservative measures, although cecal dilatation may require emergency cecostomy or colonoscopic decompression to avoid perforation. At high doses, vinca alkaloids are powerful antidiuretics and can cause an inappropriate antidiuretic hormone syndrome, leading to severe hyponatremia. Severe skin necrosis develops with subcutaneous extravasation.[31]

Antineoplastic Antibiotics

Doxorubicin hydrochloride is an effective treatment for tumors of the ovary, breast, testicles, stomach, thyroid, and bladder. It is also effective against lymphomas, sarcomas, multiple myeloma, and acute myeloblastic leukemia. Toxicities of doxorubicin hydrochloride include myelosuppression, stomatitis, alopecia, and severe skin necrosis if extravasation occurs (Fig. 147–7). The most serious complication of this drug is the irreversible cardiomyopathy that often develops when doses exceed 550 mg/m^2.[32] With lower amounts, swelling of myofibril cytoplasm may cause temporary deterioration of cardiac function. Continued therapy causes further myocardial injury, leading to vacuolization, cellular necrosis, and eventually, fibrosis. Patients should be followed up with serial echocardiograms, electrocardiography-gated radionuclide scans, or endomyocardial biopsies. Information obtained from electrocardiographic tracings is usually nonspecific and identifies the presence of irreversible lesions only. Myelosuppression can be quite profound, consisting of absolute granulocyte counts below 250 mm^3 and platelet counts below 20,000 mm^3 for 14 to 21 days after doses of 90 to 120 mg/m^2 are administered; occasionally, pancytopenia may last as long as 5 weeks. Treatment of cardiac failure, once established, is difficult. Digitalis toxicity can develop rapidly because the number of cardiac receptors available to bind the drug is decreased by necrosis of myocardial cells. Other oral inotropes, such as amrinone, cause unacceptable side effects and are no longer used clinically.[33] Some benefits have been reported with the oral inotrope vasodilator flosequinan, but complications are also being observed with long-term administration of this agent.[34, 35] At this time, treatment of patients with heart failure secondary to anthracycline administration is best handled by afterload reduction; oral angiotensin-converting enzyme–II inhibitors can be helpful if blood pressure and renal function can be satisfactorily maintained.[36]

Actinomycin D is an effective treatment for Wilms' tumors, choriocarcinoma, neuroblastoma, and rhabdomyosarcoma; it is also effective in the combination chemotherapy of Ewing's sarcoma. Actinomycin D is defined as a "radiomimetic agent" because its modality of action is similar to that of ionizing radiation. When administered after radiation therapy, actinomycin D may reactivate or aggravate radiation-induced side effects, such as skin erythema, vascular necrosis, and radiation pneumonitis. A similar recall effect has also been described after therapy with other antineoplastic agents.[37] Severe nausea and vomiting, cardiac toxicity, and bone marrow suppression also occur.

Streptozotocin is used in the treatment of malignant pancreatic islet cell tumors, and it has a beneficial effect on hypoglycemia and, experimentally, in colonic adenocarcinoma. Its most serious toxicity is renal failure, which can be irreversible.[38]

Mithramycin is used to treat patients with metastatic testicular tumors other than seminoma. Toxic side effects include hemorrhage, hepatic toxicity, renal damage, hypocalcemia, stomatitis, and fever.

Mitomycin C has proved to be moderately effective against gastric and colon carcinomas. Major toxicities include nausea, diarrhea, and delayed bone marrow suppression.

Bleomycin is effective against solid tumors of the head and neck, lymphomas, and epidermoid tumors of the esophagus. It is exceptionally beneficial for the treatment of dys-

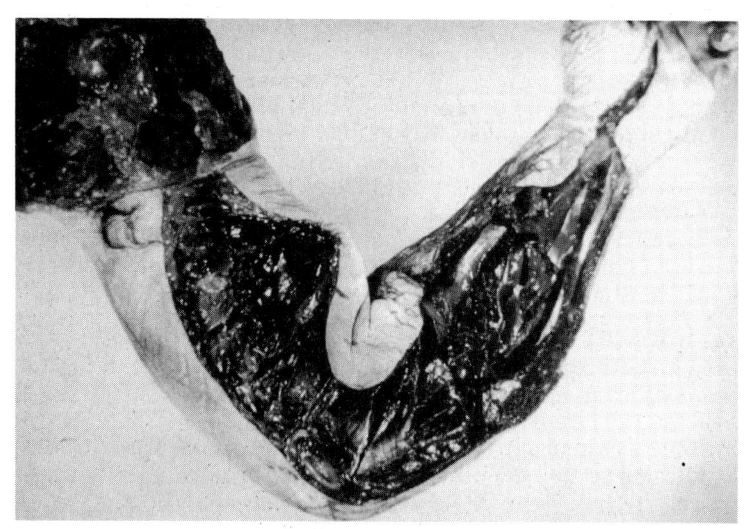

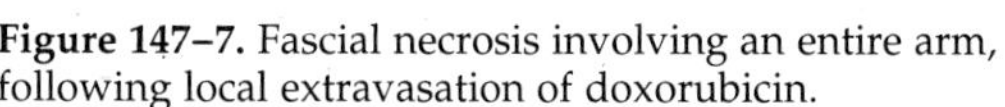

Figure 147–7. Fascial necrosis involving an entire arm, following local extravasation of doxorubicin.

germinomas when it is infused in high doses and in combination with other chemotherapeutic agents. The commonest complication of bleomycin therapy is acute interstitial pneumonitis, which is usually associated with cumulative doses greater than 350 mg/m^2;[39] however, severe respiratory failure has been reported after doses as low as 100 mg/m^2. The histopathology is characterized by alveolar and interstitial infiltrates, which are more prominent at the bases.[40] Diffusion abnormalities and restrictive lung disease persist 4 to 9 months after cessation of treatment. Although pulmonary function test results usually return to normal within 12 months of therapy, the lungs remain abnormally susceptible to nonspecific noxious agents, such as high levels of inspired oxygen and fluid overload.[41, 42] In patients with hypersensitivity to bleomycin, a single dose may cause severe exfoliative dermatitis, which occasionally results in sloughing of large areas of skin. In immunosuppressed patients, the consequences of this complication are obvious, and treatment follows all the dictates for management of massive second and third degree body burns.

Taxanes

Considerable enthusiasm has greeted the introduction of a new class of antineoplastic agent, the taxanes. These substances are the most promising representatives of antimicrotubular chemotherapy, an approach that directly interferes with mitosis during cell division.[43] Taxol, the first taxane used in humans, was initially applied to the treatment of ovarian cancer; more recently, it has been used for metastatic breast cancer, non–small cell lung cancer, and dysgerminomas. Phase I trials are being proposed for other neoplasms as well; indeed, taxanes may represent the major new drug category of the 1990s, as platinum compounds were in the 1980s and anthracyclines in the 1970s.

A limitation to Taxol use is that the substance can be obtained only from the bark of the partially endangered California Yew tree.[44] In the past year, however, significant success has been obtained from deriving taxotere, an analog of Taxol with nearly identical antitumoral activity, from the renewable needles of the American and European Yew trees.[45] It seems reasonable to anticipate that the number of patients receiving taxanes will rapidly increase in the near future. Taxane administration has not been associated with specific organ injury, even though patients have complained of many problems, such as neurologic deficits or typhlitis.[46] The main complication associated with taxanes has been severe bone marrow suppression, which is usually the dose-limiting complication. As taxanes become more widely used, additional complications may appear; at this time, however, taxanes are often given to patients with advanced disease, who are more susceptible to nonspecific adverse effects. Some complications may also be related to the solvent medium, ricinic acid; early phase I trials were occasionally suspended until treatment for hypersensitivity to ricinic acid was added.[47]

Tamoxifen

Tamoxifen has been used for many years in the treatment of metastatic breast cancer. Renewed interest has now developed because of a large, prospective study that is attempting to determine its efficacy in the prophylaxis of breast cancer in high-risk individuals. Even though no life-threatening complications have been reported after tamoxifen administration, its proposed administration to healthy individuals requires especially close monitoring for unexpected complications.[48]

Miscellaneous Agents

The *nitrosoureas* carmustine, lomustine (CCNU), and methyl-CCNU probably act as alkylating agents. They are among the few substances that have activity against brain tumors because they are lipid soluble and can cross the blood-brain barrier. CCNU is effective in the treatment of lymphomas; carmustine, in lymphomas, multiple myeloma, and oat-cell carcinoma. Methyl-CCNU is being investigated as a treatment for gastrointestinal carcinomas. Nitrosoureas induce severe myelotoxicity, which is the dose-limiting factor. Myelosuppression is prolonged (4–5 weeks) and is potentiated by repeated doses. Hepatotoxicity and pulmonary hypersensitivity have been reported.

Another agent, cis-*diamminedichloroplatinum* (*cis*-platinum) is an effective treatment for testicular, ovarian, bladder, and head and neck cancers, and for soft tissue sarcomas and lymphomas.[49] Synergy between *cis*-platinum and other agents, particularly adriamycin, has been experimentally shown. This drug is very nephrotoxic and invariably causes some deterioration of renal function. Failure to maintain high urinary flow (> 2 $mL \cdot kg^{-1} \cdot h^{-1}$) for 24 to 48 hours after administration of *cis*-platinum results in a high incidence of acute tubular necrosis that is often irreversible. Isolated reports have been published of cardiac failure and seizures following *cis*-platinum administration.[50] New platinum compounds, such as carboplatinum, have been associated with fewer renal and neurologic side effects.

Procarbazine, an oral agent, is used to treat lymphomas, brain tumors, melanoma, and oat-cell carcinoma. Toxicities include nausea, vomiting, bone marrow suppression, and skin rash.

L-*Asparaginase* is useful only in the treatment of acute lymphoblastic leukemia. It can cause severe but reversible depression of albumin synthesis,[51] central nervous system abnormalities, anorexia, nausea, vomiting, and pancreatitis. Anaphylactic reactions, sometimes extremely severe, occur in 5% to 20% of patients.

Dimethyltriazeno-imidazole carboxamide is used intravenously in the treatment of malignant melanoma, but antineoplastic activity has also been observed in lymphomas, sarcomas, and oat-cell carcinoma. Its side-effects include nausea, vomiting, delayed myelosuppression, and a flulike syndrome.

Human lymphocytic interferon, which has been synthesized by human cells for protection from viral infections, has become the subject of intensive clinical studies in the past few years. Previously available only in minute quantities, interferon can now be obtained from the microorganism *Escherichia coli* by recombinant DNA techniques.[52] Interest in interferon is based on the theory that some malignancies may be induced by virally mediated changes in cellular nucleic acids. Patients treated with interferon may require ICU admission because of complications of their underlying disease. Serious side effects of interferon administration include hypotension, weakness, bone marrow suppression, and hyperthermia.[53] Supportive therapy and discontinuation of treatment are often required to reverse the symptoms.

Cytokines

Because cancer represents uncontrolled cellular development, some research has focused on the utilization of substances that interfere with cellular growth and multiplication. Furthermore, destruction of cancerous and other abnormal cells is a task usually accomplished by T lymphocytes. Therapeutic opportunities may exist through the improvement of the ability of lymphocytes to attack cancer cells.

Tumor necrosis factor is probably generated by activated macrophages[54] and can now be produced in large quantities by recombinant DNA methodology. In human applications, tumor necrosis factor has caused serious febrile reactions[55] and severe metabolic acidosis, at times lethal. Despite these adverse effects, tumor necrosis factor has shown some antineoplastic activity in various solid tumors, thus opening a new avenue in antineoplastic research therapy. Patients receiving tumor necrosis factor may require ICU admission for treatment of consequent hypotension and renal failure.

Adoptive Immunotherapy

Interleukin and lymphokine-activated killer cells are used alone or, more often, in combination in the treatment of aggressive malignancies, including hepatomas and melanomas. Severe complications ranging from renal failure to cardiovascular collapse and respiratory failure have been reported with the use of these substances and may precipitate admission to the ICU.[56-58] Recent research has demonstrated the involvement of cytokines in the pathogenesis of septic shock; these findings may explain the similarity of symptoms observed after exogenous administration of these drugs for antitumoral purposes with the classical manifestation of septic shock.[59] This modality of cancer treatment is promising because it is based on the enhancement of natural defenses against cancer; however, caution is needed until all potential side effects have been identified.

Clinical Drug Trials

The commonest chemotherapeutic agents, their indications, and the major complications associated with their administration have been described. New agents are continuously being developed, and their introduction into clinical use follows a precise methodology that is designed to acquire extensive clinical information while minimizing potential complications. Three phases can be identified in the development process.

Phase I Drugs

Experimental chemotherapeutic agents that have proved effective in animal models are introduced through a phase I trial. A drug is administered at predetermined doses to patients who have not responded to all other forms of therapy, regardless of the underlying disease. The dangers of taking these agents are substantial: organ damage in human beings may be more severe than in experimental animals, systems and organs not affected in animals may be injured in humans, and unpredictable reactions may develop at any time. In most institutions, patients who receive phase I drugs are not considered candidates for admission to the ICU. A delicate ethical problem develops when a patient whose disease had been considered irreversible exhibits a positive response to a phase I drug and subsequently develops life-threatening complications as a consequence of the therapy administered. Refusing advanced life support may result in iatrogenic death while the underlying disease is improving. The balance between allocation of scarce ICU resources, patient rights, and potential benefits originating from better understanding of the therapy should be assessed on an individual basis. Inflexible restrictive rules should be avoided.

Phase II Drugs

Phase II drugs are agents that have proved effective in phase I studies. During phase II trials, drugs are tested in specific types of malignancy, and their efficacy is quantitatively determined.

A major risk for patients receiving a phase II drug is toxicity occurring as doses are carefully escalated. Unexpected complications during phase II trials can occur, as evidenced by events that followed trials of two agents that have since been withdrawn because of unacceptable side effects. Succinilated acinetobacter glutaminase asparaginase, a metabolic inhibitor similar to L-asparaginase, had demonstrated antineoplastic activity in acute leukemia. In humans, however, treatment with high doses resulted in severe metabolic acidosis secondary to lactate accumulation. Coma, possibly due to inhibition of glutamic acid synthesis or generation of false neurotransmitters, also developed. Although both conditions were reversible with appropriate therapy (respiratory support, hydration, and bicarbonate administration), the benefits did not justify the risks of side effects, and the use of the drug was abandoned. 2,3-Deoxycoformycin was also introduced for the treatment of acute leukemias. Unexpected toxic effects included severe renal and respiratory failure that required hemodialysis and mechanical ventilation. The pulmonary complications suggested hypersensitivity pneumonitis and resolved within 48 hours with high-dose steroid therapy.[60] None of the complications observed with high doses of these two agents had been anticipated from the results of animal experiments and phase I trials.

Treatment of patients receiving phase II drugs presents the same ethical problems as treatment with phase I drugs. Allocation of an ICU bed must be evaluated in each individual case.

Phase III Drugs

Substances that have successfully completed a phase II trial are compared with standard therapy for efficacy. Unexpected complications are uncommon at this stage, and patients enrolled in phase III trials should be considered for admission to ICUs.

Combination Chemotherapy

Whereas single-agent chemotherapy was the common treatment modality during the early phases of drug management of neoplasms, current protocols are based on the use of multiple agents in combination, each with a different mechanism of action and toxicity. Neoplasms in which combination chemotherapy has proved successful include Hodgkin's disease, diffuse non-Hodgkin's lymphomas, acute leukemias, and disseminated testicular and breast tumors.

When such protocols are designed, the following criteria apply:

1. Each drug should have some antitumoral activity when used alone.
2. Each drug should have a different mechanism of action.
3. Toxic effects should not be additive, so that each drug may be used at full dose.

Despite these precautions, however, the possibility remains that more serious complications will develop when multiple drugs are administered simultaneously. Patients receiving aggressive combination therapy are therefore likelier to require admission to an ICU than those receiving single agents. In some centers, oncology wards include intermediate care units, where intensive nursing care can be provided.

Adjuvant Chemotherapy

Solid tumors that have been successfully resected are the subject of prospective trials to determine whether chemotherapy agents, used alone or in combination, are effective in preventing local or systemic recurrence. This concept is known as *adjuvant therapy*, and results to date are not as encouraging as it had been hoped. Toxicity is related to the dosage schedule and the agents used.

RADIATION THERAPY

Radiation therapy alone can be curative for stage I Hodgkin's disease or early breast cancer. More commonly, it is used in association with surgery, or chemotherapy, or both, to achieve local and/or regional control. Radiation therapy is also useful for the symptomatic relief of metastatic bone diseases, multiple brain metastases, and spinal cord compression.

Factors such as bulk, site, growth rate, and vascularity determine the responsiveness of a tumor to ionizing radiation. The sensitivity of adjacent tissues to high-energy particles is often the limiting factor in treatment. In recent years, the availability of computerized techniques to define the field of radiation and of more accurate methods to deliver the ionizing particles has increased the effective dose that can be safely administered and has greatly reduced the incidence of complications.

The diseases in which radiation therapy can offer definitive cure, prolongation of life, or worthwhile palliation are many, but potentially dangerous side effects must always be considered because all tissues, particularly those with higher cell turnover, are subject to injury.

Radiation damage is characterized histologically by diffuse microvascular thrombosis with necrosis of surrounding tissues, thereby explaining such diverse complications of radiation therapy as myocardial infarction, renal failure, skin necrosis, and injury to major vessels, such as the thoracic and abdominal aorta.[61]

Critical care physicians should be familiar with the extraordinary range of morbid changes associated with radiation therapy because complications may develop into life-threatening circumstances that require ICU admission.

Radiation pneumonitis is probably the commonest adverse effect of ionizing radiation that may require ICU support. Developing 3 to 6 months after treatment, it may lead to acute respiratory failure or to permanent functional limitation from interstitial fibrosis.

Injuries to other organs may also occur, precipitating frustrating problems of management that fortunately are rarely life threatening. The gastrointestinal tract is highly susceptible to radiation injury. Severe malabsorption and diarrhea, with marked derangement of fluid and electrolyte balance, may follow a course of radiation therapy. Although the process is usually self-limiting and reversible, it may progress for weeks and months after termination of therapy. In a few extreme cases, patients otherwise cured become permanently unable to tolerate enteral feedings and must be supplemented by total parenteral nutrition. The most catastrophic complications pertain to obstruction, bleeding, enteric fistulas, or perforation, which often require emergency surgery.

Some antineoplastic agents (cyclophosphamide, methotrexate, doxorubicin, actinomycin D, bleomycin, carmustine) may cause a recall phenomenon when given to a patient who has been exposed to radiation; injury, sometimes severe, develops in organs irradiated months and even years earlier.[62, 63] Damage during the initial course of therapy was often not apparent at the time of treatment.

The central and peripheral nervous systems are not immune from radiation damage. These tissues have a rich capillary network and are extremely susceptible to oxygen deprivation. Brain necrosis, transverse necrotizing myelitis, paraplegia, and tetraplegia have been associated with radiation therapy.

Steroid administration can limit most adverse side effects of radiation therapy. Although radiation pneumonitis can be entirely eliminated by simultaneously administered steroid treatment,[64] a recall phenomenon almost invariably occurs once steroids are withdrawn. The pneumonic process is then as severe or more severe than if steroids had never been given. Resumption of steroids is the only option and often must be continued for life. At present, a consensus advises against the prophylactic use of steroids.[65]

HYPERTHERMIA

There is experimental, and to a lesser degree, clinical, evidence that elevated body temperature is more damaging to cancerous than normal tissues. This susceptibility has been identified for the cells of many solid tumors and systemic malignancies. Therapeutic exploitation of this selective sensitivity has been the subject of recent laboratory investigations and some cautiously enthusiastic clinical trials. After the insertion of an arteriovenous shunt, blood is circulated through an extracorporeal heat exchanger, and body temperature is raised to 41.5 to 42°C for 2 to 4 hours. Life-threatening complications may develop quite rapidly at these temperatures, and close observation is mandatory. Admission to an ICU or another comparable location may be advisable prior to treatment.

The response of major organ systems to controlled hyperthermia has been carefully investigated. Pulmonary artery catheterization and thermodilution cardiac output measurements have indicated that cardiac compromise is uncommon, even in patients with a history of heart disease.[66] Minor arrhythmias have been reported and are attributed to the significant electrolyte imbalance that may occur with hyperthermia. Hypokalemia can be severe, sustained by the hyperventilation and respiratory alkalosis that is induced by elevated temperature and increased potassium loss through the urine. Hemolysis has not been detected, but coagulation abnormalities, including increased prothrombin time, partial thromboplastin time, and decreased platelet count, are commonly reported. Measurement of fibrin-degradation products indicates a modest but continuous process of disseminated intravascular coagulation. Patients with extensive metastatic liver disease are reported to have a very high incidence of serious complications from hyperthermia. Acute myelopathy and irreversible demyelinization have developed, resulting in limb paralysis.[67]

Cellular phagocytosis is decreased when temperature exceeds 41.5°C, and patients become more susceptible to bacterial infections.

For most patients, in experienced hands and with very close monitoring, hyperthermia is a safe, although experimental, form of therapy. However, despite several years of applications, indications for hyperthermia have not been expanded, and the role of this form of therapy may remain limited.[68, 69]

INDICATIONS FOR SURGICAL CONSULTATION

In critically ill cancer patients, the surgeon most frequently intervenes to resolve acute complications of the disease or its treatment.

Epistaxis is common in severely thrombocytopenic patients and is usually associated with dehydrated mucous membranes or nasogastric intubation. Most bleeding originates in the anterior nasal septum and can be managed by hemostatic packs, cauterization, and platelet transfusions for severe thrombocytopenia. Occasionally, Foley catheter tamponade or postnasal packs with an antibiotic ointment–impregnated gauze tampon, anchored anteriorly by silk sutures tied over a dental roll, are required to treat more serious hemorrhage. Impaired drainage leads to sinusitis or middle ear infection, further aggravated by leukopenia and colonization by opportunistic organisms.

Airway obstruction is a relatively common cause of emergency admission. This complication can be associated with a previously undiagnosed cancer of the oropharynx, the base of the tongue, or the larynx; bilateral vocal cord paralysis; or extrinsic pressure on the trachea from mediastinal lymphoma. Traumatic endotracheal intubation may induce bleeding or edema, further compromising an airway that is partially occluded by tumor. A carefully performed tracheotomy or cricothyroidotomy with the patient under local anesthesia is preferred.[70]

Although most surgeons still favor to perform a tracheotomy in the operating room, adequate instrumentation and lighting should be available for this purpose in an ICU. Transportation of critically ill patients can be dangerous and time consuming and should be avoided whenever possible.

The ideal timing of elective tracheostomy is controversial; in some cancer patients, this intervention may be advisable when ventilatory support will exceed 5 to 7 days. Elective tracheostomy lessens the amount of sedation needed, provides greater comfort, and decreases the risk of blood, originating from the lower airway or trachea, coagulating in the endotracheal tube of thrombocytopenic patients (Fig. 147–8). Meticulous surgical technique using electrocautery and suture ligation of all potential bleeders permits tracheotomy, even in patients with severe coagulation abnormalities.[71]

Hemoptysis, or sudden bleeding, from an endotracheal tube, is an alarming and often terminal event in severely thrombocytopenic patients who have hematologic malignancies or disseminated intravascular coagulation. Occasionally, it may be related to necrosis of an endobronchial tumor, and resection or cauterization by neodymium:yttrium-aluminum-garnet laser is useful to control bleeding or to ease severe dyspnea. Esophageal cancers may cause acute respiratory embarrassment by erosion and fistulization into the trachea or left mainstem bronchus. Esophageal exclusion is required to prevent further aspiration of oral and gastric secretions.

Airway compression by germ cell tumors, malignant thymomas, or lymphoma of the mediastinum may cause acute dyspnea. Associated superior vena caval obstruction is not a contraindication to a biopsy of palpable supraclavicular disease or to an anterior mediastinotomy to obtain tissue for histologic and cell marker analysis before therapy is instituted. If general anesthesia is necessary, the endotracheal tube should not be removed until the patient is fully awake and able to sit up, because muscle relaxation and tracheal compression may cause acute asphyxia. Occasionally, the tube must remain in place for 48 to 72 hours, until chemotherapy or radiotherapy partially opens the airway; this situation most commonly results from malignant lymphoma, and response to therapy is often rapid and dramatic.

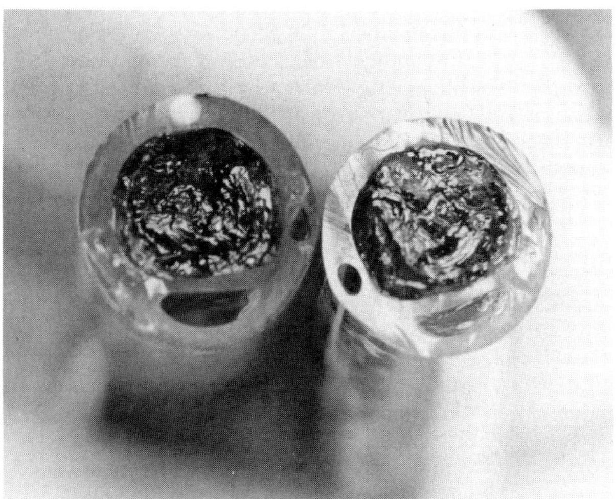

Figure 147–8. Section of an endotracheal tube completely obstructed by a large clot in a patient with less than 20,000 platelet/mm^3.

Hemorrhage from major vessels of the head and neck is an occasional but dramatic sequela to radiation therapy, surgery, and orocutaneous fistula formation.[72] Attempts to control bleeding locally are rarely successful, because the site is usually at the base of an infected necrotic tumor, and bleeding is from branches of the external carotid artery. Bilateral ligation is necessary to preclude collateral circulation. Carotid artery rupture from tumor erosion or skin flap necrosis is particularly catastrophic. It is usually heralded by minor oozing and never occurs in the presence of intact skin or mucosa. Direct finger pressure over the bleeding site while avoiding complete occlusion and any attempt to directly suture the vessel is mandatory. Time should be taken to restore blood volume and to transport the patient to the operating room. Ligation in patients with hypovolemia and hypotension is likely to result in hemiplegia. The correct procedure is to ligate the carotid artery above and below the site of the rupture, excising the fistulized segment.

Drug extravasation with cellulitis, ulceration, and necrosis of skin is now rarely seen, because of improved methods of vascular access for chemotherapy. Toxic drugs infiltrating the tissues around a venipuncture site can result in full-thickness loss of skin and subcutaneous tissue and in damage to adjacent nerves, muscle, and tendons. This situation has been most commonly reported with doxorubicin (Adriamycin) therapy but has occurred with actinomycin D, mithramycin, mitomycin C, vinca alkaloids, and streptozocin. Prompt recognition, early excision of the necrotic area under fluorescein control, and coverage with skin grafts or local flap rotation minimize injury and hasten rehabilitation.

Postoperative wound infections are a potential source of serious sepsis and often have an insidious presentation. Leukopenia and corticosteroid therapy minimize traditional signs at the site of incision, thereby delaying recognition. Often, the first sign is a foul smelling, watery stain on the dressing, with edema of the incisional margins but little or no cellulitis. Opening the skin incision down to the fascia may release large volumes of purulent, necrotic material or enteric drainage.

Necrotizing soft tissue infections, particularly of the perineum, genitals, and perianal region, can arise as a result of seemingly minor rectal fissures, perirectal abscesses, urethral infections, decubitus ulcers, or surgical procedures. Leukemic patients are particularly susceptible to this catastrophic complication and may present with fulminant gangrene of the perineum and scrotum. These necrotizing infections are caused by a mixed spectrum of aerobic and anaerobic bacteria,[73] and broad-spectrum intravenous antibiotics must be promptly instituted while all tissues of questionable viability are aggressively debrided. If the infection is of rectal or perianal origin, a defunctionalized proximal colostomy is often required.

Appropriate intervention for these infections may be delayed because the initial presentation is deceptively benign. Early recognition is essential if fulminant progression, both local and systemic, is to be avoided. When invasive sepsis develops during the neutropenic nadir of chemotherapy, toxemia and multiple-organ system failure usually defy all supportive efforts, and survival is rare.

Malignant pleural effusions that accumulate rapidly require catheter or tube drainage at a controlled rate to avoid re-expansion pulmonary edema; ultrasonographic guidance is useful if the effusion is loculated.

Acute pneumothorax has occurred after necrosis of metastatic lung lesions that were sensitive to chemotherapy. This condition can lead to subcutaneous emphysema and pneumomediastinum that requires insertion of a chest tube.

Esophageal perforation is a rare complication of instrumentation or vomiting after chemotherapy. The treatment of choice consists of immediate left thoracotomy, closure of the perforation, buttressing with a pleural flap, copious irrigation, and adequate drainage of the pleural cavity. Operative intervention is favored over conservative drainage, which should be restricted to minimally symptomatic patients with locally contained perforation and no signs of sepsis. Initially, the size of the perforation and the extent of the pleural and mediastinal contamination may not be apparent, even with contrast studies or esophagoscopy.

Pericardiocentesis is indicated to obtain fluid for diagnostic study or to relieve *acute cardiac tamponade.* Occasionally, surgery is necessary to treat recurrent or loculated effusions or complications of the procedure, such as laceration of the myocardium, coronary arteries, or veins. Subxyphoid pericardiotomy is preferred when a definitive procedure is required to drain loculated fluid and to obtain tissue for biopsy.

ABDOMINAL COMPLICATIONS

The abdomen remains now, as it was at the time of Hippocrates, the testing ground of surgeons' judgment and skill. The aphorism of the great master, aptly quoted by Welch, notes, "The art is long, life is short, decision difficult and delay perilous."[74] When referring to the acute abdomen, those words apply now as then and acquire an even greater significance in immunocompromised patients.

Evaluation of an acute abdominal process in a cancer patient requires a thorough review of the stage of malignancy and all therapy received to date. Radiation, prior surgery, and recent chemotherapy influence the differential diagnosis, the timing of exploration, the surgical procedure, and the perioperative support measures.

Signs and symptoms may result from gastrointestinal toxicity of chemotherapeutic agents,[75] or they may be masked by them. Pseudo-obstructive adynamic ileus, typhlitis,[76] necrotizing enteropathy, or "ileocecal syndrome"[77] are common examples of acute abdominal processes. Corticosteroids are implicated in acute peritonitis due to perforation of a gastric or duodenal ulcer and often mask signs of spontaneous enteric or colonic perforation from other causes. Fecal contamination can exist without localizing signs when patients are undergoing steroid therapy. Marrow ablation, immunosuppression, coagulopathies, and infection with bacterial, viral, fungal, or parasitic organisms add to the diagnostic and therapeutic confusion. "The simplest operative concepts of diversion, drainage and decompression may be the only procedures to be performed; complicated resectional or anastomotic operations may be doomed to failure by the underlying nature of the disease or the patient's status."[78]

Physical examination repeated at frequent intervals is required to detect subtle changes. The obtunded patient is unable to express pain, and localizing signs are often muted or absent. Slight leukocytosis with a leftward shift may be all the defense a depressed marrow can muster. Local responses to an inflammatory stimulus are inadequate to contain the insult, and septicemia rapidly supervenes. Positive blood cultures, acute chemical diabetes, progressive renal impairment, hypovolemia, and tactic acidosis are common laboratory findings at the time of surgical intervention; these conditions result from delayed recognition and consultation.

Diagnostic procedures include plain, sitting, or lateral films of the abdomen, ultrasonography, gallium-67 citrate imaging, and technetium-99m studies of the hepatobiliary system. Indium-labeled white blood cells and platelets have been used for scintigraphic localization of septic foci. Ultrasonography and computed tomography with contrast media facilitate diagnosis and help guide percutaneous drainage of abdominal abscesses, obviating surgical exploration in many critically ill patients. In addition to angiography and interventional radiology, the surgeon has the option of peritoneal lavage or peritoneoscopy as aids in diagnosis. The latter procedure can be performed safely, using small-bore endoscopes with improved optics after administration of platelets if necessary. This minimally invasive procedure has been helpful in recognizing painful hepatomegaly from congestion or metastasis, mesenteric ischemia, acute cholecystitis, intra-abdominal bleeding, and purulent peritonitis.

Common causes of right upper-quadrant pain include metastases, leukemic infiltrates or abscesses in the liver, acute hepatitis, and suppurative cholangitis due to primary or metastatic malignant obstruction of the extrahepatic biliary tree.[79] Early recognition and prompt percutaneous, transhepatic, or surgical drainage of the common bile duct is mandatory. Fulminant sepsis, encephalopathy, and disseminated intravascular coagulation may develop in just a few hours, leading to multiple organ failure and death.

Acalculous cholecystitis and empyema of the gallbladder may develop insidiously and, if unrecognized, may lead to septic decompensation.[80] Ultrasonography is the most reliable means of confirming this diagnosis. Surgical or percutaneous computed tomographically guided drainage must not be delayed, to avoid perforation. This diagnosis is particularly difficult in obtunded patients.

Hemorrhagic enteritis in leukemic patients may be associated with herpes, cytomegalovirus, fungal infestation, uremia, coagulation defects, or antimetabolite toxicity. Other parasitic infections that cause diarrhea in patients undergoing steroid therapy include strongyloidiasis and giardiasis. Leukemic infiltrates of the mucosa or submucosa are prone to ulceration or perforation during a course of chemotherapy. Agranulocytic necrosis may occur after transmural bacterial invasion of the bowel wall. The various manifestations of necrotizing enteropathy, particularly ileocecal syndrome, are common reasons for surgical consultation. These lesions cause bleeding, perforation, or obstruction and act as portals of entry for gram-negative bacteria. Surgery should not be denied on the basis of pancytopenia alone unless the patient has not responded to all reasonable antileukemic therapy. Conservative management carries a mortality of almost 100%, whereas salvage is possible with physiologic and pharmacologic support given in concert with aggressive operative intervention.

Cecal perforation from leukemic infiltrates in the ileocecal wall requires right hemicolectomy and primary anastomosis or diversion. Colonic pseudo-obstruction seen in association with multiple organ failure, electrolyte imbalance, or renal failure may lead to perforation unless colonoscopy or cecostomy is performed when the dilation exceeds 10 to 12 cm on a plain x-ray film of the abdomen. The possibility that Ogilvie's syndrome is actually a paraneoplastic neuropathy of the gastrointestinal tract is discussed by Schuffler and coworkers.[81]

Gastrointestinal tract obstruction occurring as a complication of prior surgery, radiation therapy, or recurrent disease usually develops during an ICU admission for other reasons. Differentiating mechanical obstruction from paralytic ileus can be quite difficult in these patients, many of whom have serious metabolic derangements and may have received opiates, vinca alkaloids, or both. The physician must be aware of gastric atony and aspiration, a frequent reason for ICU referral.

Penetrating, obstructing, and perforating carcinomas of the colon and rectum require an aggressive surgical approach. In patients surviving "curative" resections, penetrating and obstructing lesions were associated with a 5-year survival rate that was the same as that for the curative resection group as a whole (40%), whereas those with perforating lesions had roughly half this life expectancy. The operative mortalities in these groups were considerably higher, justifying intensive postoperative care.[82]

Acute mesenteric ischemia, a catastrophic consequence of embolism, arterial or venous thrombosis, or low-flow states, occurs most commonly in the elderly. This condition is of concern in the critically ill cancer patient who is admitted to the ICU with complications associated with obtundation, hypercoagulability, sepsis, and hypoperfusion. Increasing awareness of nonocclusive mesenteric ischemia secondary to inadequate perfusion has been due to the work of Boley and colleagues,[83] who have done much to elucidate the mechanism of acute mesenteric vascular occlusion. These researchers have raised the survival rate in patients with this diagnosis to over 50% because of an aggressive diagnostic and therapeutic protocol and have shown increased bowel salvage and improved quality of life among survivors.

Massive hepatic bleeding may occur without warning as a result of rupture of primary malignant tumors, metastases, adenomas, or hemangiomas. Effective chemotherapy leads to tumor necrosis, hemorrhage, distention of the liver capsule, and spontaneous intra-abdominal bleeding. Emergency exploration and lobectomy is the preferable treatment, but hepatic artery ligation and packing may be the only treatment possible in the thrombocytopenic patient or in the patient in whom metastases are multiple and bilateral.

Hematuria is most commonly associated with thrombocytopenia, other coagulopathies, radiation cystitis, and cyclophosphamide-induced hemorrhagic cystitis. The last condition is a potentially life-threatening complication related to the interaction of cyclophosphamide metabolites and bladder epithelium. Serious hemorrhage can usually be avoided by maintenance of a high urine output with frequent voiding. Diuresis is continued for 24 hours after the conclusion of chemotherapy administration, with parenteral infusions of 3000 mL/m^2 per day and furosemide, 5 to 10 mg every 8 to 12 hours. An electrolyte solution, such as D5 .045NS plus 40 mEq of potassium hydrochloride and 1 g of magnesium sulfate per liter, usually maintains electrolyte balance. *N*-acetyl cysteine (5% in saline) has been used for bladder irrigation to minimize the effect of toxic metabolites. Cystoscopic electrocoagulation or instillation of 4% formaldehyde solution may be required, and, on rare occasions, urinary diversion alone or with cystectomy has been necessary.

EVALUATING SEVERITY OF DISEASE

The decision to withhold or terminate therapy is one of the most difficult confronted by a physician. By training and tradition, those who practice medicine strive to defeat disease, not yield to it, and this concept is strongly rooted not only in the medical profession, but also in the expectations of patients. In ancient Egypt, physicians to the royal household were symbolically executed whenever a pharaoh died. Their names were changed, and a papyrus bearing their old names was ceremonially burned. The clear implication was that a physician who failed to prevent death, regardless of the circumstances, committed a crime serious enough to be punished by death. This symbolism has been replaced in recent years by the threat of legal prosecution whenever a perception of failure of the medical art is entertained by a patient.

Until recently, when major organ systems failed, death was unavoidable, regardless of the feelings and expectations of patients and physicians. Today, the very advances of medicine that permit prolongation of life are forcing doctors and health authorities to develop criteria that limit indiscriminate use of extraordinary life-support techniques. The development of just, humane, and universally accepted criteria for the allocation of finite resources first requires objective criteria to measure both acuity of illness and likelihood of survival.

In the past 20 years, many attempts have been made to develop such objective techniques. The Therapeutic Intervention Scoring System was the first method that attempted to quantify disease based on the amount of care provided to patients, both inside and outside the ICU.[84, 85] Since then, many other instruments have been proposed that have been based on nursing interventions, physiologic variables, and previous medical history. Each method has generated varying degrees of interest[86–88]; currently, the Society of Critical Care Medicine is attempting to sponsor a large, multicenter, outcome-evaluation study; commercial groups are also involved in these projects, and federal officials have suggested that objective measures of outcome may ultimately receive official sanction and may be used to allocate scarce resources. Despite these considerations, however, the proliferation of measurement techniques and the minimal clinical impact they have had 20 years after the introduction of the Therapeutic Intervention Scoring System, emphasize the difficulties involved in transferring into practice theoretical considerations of limitations of care.

All scoring and measuring systems reach the same general conclusion and generate the same self-evident graphics; sick patients use many resources and have a poor outcome (Fig. 147–9). All methods, however, reach conclusions regarding outcome only after ICU admission and are probabilistic in nature.[89] In a society in which the well-being of the individual is usually placed above that of the State, and therefore of the aggregate of all individuals, limitation of care can take place only on a voluntary basis. Although considerable savings could be realized by denying ICU admission or continued care to patients with less than a 15% to 20% chance of survival, the likelihood that such a cutoff point would be voluntarily accepted by a significant number of individuals is nonexistent. Reducing the cutoff point to much lower probabilities of survival, such as 1% to 2%, may result in greater acceptance but would also negate all economic and organizational benefits.[90] Ultimately, only a change in society's perception of the right of individuals to demand treatment may permit the establishment of enforceable guidelines to limit or deny care. For the time being, predictive methods remain an interesting but strictly academic field of investigation.[91] Physicians cannot rely on these methods to determine the type and the extent of care that critically ill patients, including those with underlying malignancies, should receive. Decisions must continue to be based on experience and conscience.[92]

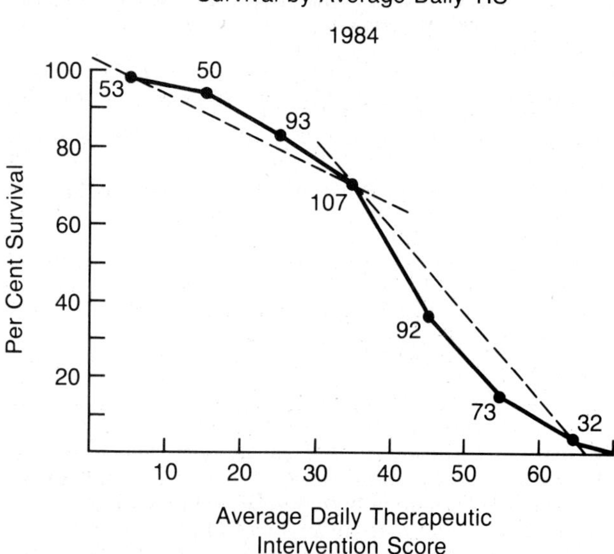

Figure 147–9. Survival rates of patients, based on average daily therapeutic intervention scores (ADTIS).

References

1. American Cancer Society: Cancer Facts and Figures—1993. Atlanta, American Cancer Society, 1993.
2. Dekker AW, Rozenberg-Arska M, Sxma JJ, et al: Prevention of infection by trimethoprim-sulfamethoxazole plus amphotericin B in patients with acute non-lymphoblastic leukemia. Ann Intern Med 1981; 95:555.
3. Barza M: Imipenem: First of a new class of beta lactam antibiotics. Ann Intern Med 1985; 103:552–560.
4. Tollemar J, Ringden O, Andersson S, et al: Prophylactic use of liposomal, amphotericin B (AmBisome) against fungal infections: A randomized trial in bone marrow transplant recipients. Transplant Proc 1993; 25:1495–1497.
5. LaQuaglia MP, Lucas A, Thaler HT, et al: A prospective analysis of vascular access device-related infections in children. J Pediatr Surg 1992; 27:840–842.
6. Groeger JS, Lucas AB, Coit D, et al: A prospective randomized evaluation of the effect of silver impregnated subcutaneous cuffs for preventing tunneled chronic venous access catheter infections in cancer patients. Ann Surg 1993; 218:206–210.
7. Bodey GP: Pulmonary infiltrates in acute leukemias. Chest 1979; 75:298.
8. Prakash UB, Divertie MB, Banks PM: Aggressive therapy in acute respiratory failure from pulmonary infiltrates. Chest 1979; 73:345.
9. Carlon GC, Howland WS, Ray C, et al: High frequency jet ventilation: A prospective randomized evaluation. Chest 1983; 84:551.
10. Cunningham AJ: Acute respiratory distress syndrome—Two decades later. Yale J Biol Med 1991; 64:387–402.
11. Snow RM, Miller WC, Rice DL, et al: Respiratory failure in cancer patients. JAMA 1979; 241:2039.
12. Rosenthal RL: Acute promyelocytic leukemia associated with hypofibrinogenemia. Blood 1963; 21:495.
13. Carlon GC, Scheiner E, Colaco FM, et al: Nephrotoxic antibiotics in patients with renal failure. Guidelines for debilitated patients. Crit Care Med 1979; 7:1.
14. Perez CA, Present CA, Van Amburg AL III, et al: Management of superior vena cava syndrome. Semin Oncol 1978; 5:123.
15. Martinez-Maldonado M, Yium DM, Suki WM, et al: Renal complications of multiple myeloma: Pathophysiology and some aspects of clinical management. J Chronic Dis 1971; 24:221.
16. Suki WM, Yium JJ, Von Minden M, et al: Acute treatment of hypercalcemia with furosemide. N Engl J Med 1970; 282:839.
17. Vaughn CB, Vaitkevicius VK: The effects of calcitonin in hypercalcemia in patients with malignancy. Cancer 1974; 34:1268.
18. Godfrey TE: Mithramycin for hypercalcemia of malignant disease. Calif Med 1971; 115:1.
19. Burckhardt P, Thiebaud D, Perey L, et al: Treatment of tumor-induced osteolysis by APD. Recent Results. Cancer Res 1989; 116:54–66.
20. Theiault RL: Management of hypercalcemia in breast cancer. Oncology 1990; 4:43–46.
21. Clemens MR, Fessele K, Heim ME: Multiple myeloma: Effect of daily dichloromethylene biphosphate on skeletal complications. Ann Hemat 1993; 66:141–146.
22. Posner JB: Neurologic complications of systemic cancer. Med Clin North Am 1971; 55:265.
23. Joyner LR, Maran PG, Sarama R, et al: Neodymium-YAG laser treatment of intrabronchial lesions. Chest 1985; 87:418–427.
24. Fortner JC, McLean B, Kim DK, et al: The seventies evolution in liver surgery for cancer. Cancer 1981; 47:2162.
25. Hankins DG, Sander S, MacDonald FM, et al: Pulmonary toxicity recurring after a six week course of busulfan therapy and after subsequent therapy with uracil mustard. Chest 1978; 73:415.
26. Friedman MA, Carter JB: Serious toxicities associated with chemotherapy. Semin Oncol 1978; 5:193.
27. Carlon GC, Kahn RC, Howland WS, et al: Clinical experience with high frequency jet ventilation. Crit Care Med 1981; 9:1.
28. Pierri MK: Heart disease and cancer. *In*: Critical Care of the Cancer Patient. Howland WS, Carlon GC (Eds). Chicago, Year Book Medical Publishers, 1985, pp 61–85.
29. Chabner BA, Myers CE, Olivero VT: Clinical pharmacology of anticancer drugs. Semin Oncol 1978; 4:165.
30. Rosenow EC III: The spectrum of drug-induced pulmonary disease. Ann Intern Med 1972; 77:977.
31. Gottlieb RJ, Cottner J: Vincristine induced bladder atony. Cancer 1971; 28:674.
32. Bristow MR, Mason JW, Billingham ME, et al: Doxorubicin cardiomyopathy evaluation by phonocardiography, endomyocardial biopsy and cardiac catheterization. Ann Intern Med 1978; 88:168.
33. Leier CV: Current status of non-digitalis positive inotropic drugs. Am J Cardiol 1992; 69:120G–128G.
34. Barnett DB: Flosequinan. Lancet 1993; 341:733–736.
35. Noble J, Farrer M, McComb JM: Flosequinan and arrhythmogenesis. Lancet 1993; 341:1100.
36. Swedberg K: Reduction in mortality by pharmacological therapy in congestive heart failure. Circulation 1993; 87:IV126–129.
37. Einhorn L, Krause M, Horseback N, et al: Enhanced pulmonary toxicity with bleomycin and radiotherapy in oat cell lung cancer. Cancer 1976; 37:2414.
38. Moertel CG, Reitmier RJ, Schutt AJ, et al: Phase II study of streptozotocin (NSC-85998) in the treatment of advanced gastrointestinal cancer. Chemotherapy Rep 1971; 55:303.
39. Luna MA, Bedrossian CWM, Lichtiger B, et al: Interstitial pneumonitis associated with bleomycin therapy. Am J Clin Pathol 1972; 58:501.
40. Bernet JM, Reich JD: Bleomycin. Ann Intern Med 1979; 90:945.
41. Goldiner PL, Carlon GC, Cvitkovic E, et al: Factors influencing morbidity and mortality in patients treated with bleomycin. Br Med J 1978; 1:1664.
42. Gilson AJ, Sahn SA: Reactivation of bleomycin lung toxicity following oxygen administration. Chest 1985; 88:304–306.
43. Rowinsky EK, Onetto N, Canetta RM, et al: Taxol: The first of the taxanes, an important new class of antitumor agents. Semin Oncol 1992; 19:646–662.
44. Runowicz CD, Wiernik PH, Einzig AI, et al: Taxol in ovarian cancer. Cancer 1993; 71:1591–1596.
45. Bissett D, Setanoians A, Cassidy J, et al: Phase 1 and pharmacokinetic study of taxotere (RP 56976) administered as a 24-hour infusion. Cancer Res 1993; 53:523–527.
46. Pestalozzi BC, Sotos GA, Choyke PL, et al: Typhlitis resulting from treatment with taxol and doxorubicin in patients with metastatic breast cancer. Cancer 1993; 71:1797–1800.
47. Chang AY, Kim K, Glick J, et al: Phase II study of Taxol, merbarone and piroxantrone in stage IV non–small-cell lung cancer: The Eastern Cooperative Oncology Group. J Natl Cancer Inst 1993; 85:388–394.
48. Rubens RD: Metastatic breast cancer and its complications. Curr Opin Oncol 1992; 4:1050–1054.

49. Einhorn LH, William SD: The role of *cis*-platinum in solid tumor therapy. N Engl J Med 1979; 330:284.
50. Rosenzweig M, Von Hoff DD, Slavik M, et al: *Cis*-diamminedichloroplatinum. Ann Intern Med 1977; 86:803.
51. Haskell CM, Canellos GI, Loventhal BD, et al: L-asparaginase toxicity. Cancer Res 1968; 24:74.
52. Sherwin SA, Mayer D, Ochs JJ, et al: Recombinant leukocyte A interferon in advanced breast cancer. Ann Intern Med 1983; 98:598.
53. Scott G, Secher DS, Flowers D, et al: Toxicity of interferon. Br Med J 1981; 282:1345.
54. Zacharchuck CM, Drysdale BE, Mayer MM, et al: Macrophage-mediated cytotoxicity: Role of a soluble macrophage cytotoxic factor similar to lymphotoxin and tumor necrosis factor. Proc Natl Acad Sci USA 1983; 80:6341–6345.
55. Khan A: Preclinical and Phase I clinical trials with lymphotoxin. *In*: Human Lymphokines. New York, Academic Press, 1982, pp 621–630.
56. Redman BG, Flaherty L, Martino S, et al: Effect of calcium replacement on the hemodynamic changes associated with high dose interleukin-2 therapy. Am J Clin Oncol 1992; 15:340–343.
57. Feinfeld DA, D'Agati V, Dutcher JP, et al: Interstitial nephritis in a patient receiving adoptive immunotherapy with recombinant interleukin-2 and lymphokine-activated killer cells. Am J Nephrol 1991; 11:489–492.
58. Farrell MM: The challenge of adult respiratory distress syndrome during interleukin-2 immunotherapy. Oncol Nurs Forum 1992; 19:475–480.
59. Giroir BP: Mediation of septic shock: New approaches for interrupting the endogenous inflammatory cascade. Crit Care Med 1993; 21:780–789.
60. Kahn RC, Carlon GC, Miller D, et al: Acute respiratory failure due to 2,3′-deoxycoformycin. Intensive Care Med 1982; 8:101.
61. Moreynolds RA, Gold GL, Roberts WC: Coronary heart disease after mediastinal irradiation for Hodgkin's disease. Am J Med 1976; 60:39.
62. Schreml W, Bargon G, Anger B, et al: Progrediente Lungfibrose unter Kombinationstherapie mit BCNU. Blut 1978; 36:353.
63. Lamoureux KB: Increased clinically symptomatic pulmonary radiation reactions with adjuvant chemotherapy. Cancer Chemother Res 1974; 58:705.
64. Casciari RJ, Berman JJ, Glauser FL: Acute febrile illness associated with bilateral pulmonary infiltrates after irradiation in a patient with Hodgkin's disease. South Med J 1977; 70:345.
65. Wara WM, Phillips TL, Margolis LW, et al: Radiation pneumonitis: A new approach to the derivation of time-dose factors. Cancer 1973; 32:547.
66. Bull JM, Lees D, Schuette W, et al: Whole body hyperthermia: A phase I trial of a potential adjuvant to chemotherapy. Ann Intern Med 1979; 90:317.
67. Douglas MA, Parks LC, Bebin J: Sudden myelopathy secondary to therapeutic total-body hyperthermia after spinal cord irradiation. Med Intell 1977; 304:583.
68. Yoshikawa T, Kokura S, Tainaka K, et al: The role of active oxygen species and lipid peroxidation in the antitumor effect of hyperthermia. Cancer Res 1993; 53:2326–2329.
69. Ben-Yosef R, Kapp DS: Persistent and/or late complications of combined radiation therapy and hyperthermia. Int J Hyperthermia 1992; 8:733–745.
70. Greisz H, Quarnstrom O, Willen R: Elective cricothyroidotomy: A clinical and histopathological study. Crit Care Med 1982; 10:387–389.
71. Turnbull AD, Carlon G: Airway management in the thrombocytopenic cancer patient with acute respiratory failure. Crit Care Med 1979; 7:76–77.
72. Strong EW: Head and neck emergencies. Curr Probl Cancer 1979; 4:36–41.
73. Dellinger EP: Severe necrotizing soft tissue infections: Multiple disease entities requiring a common approach. JAMA 1981; 246:1717–1721.
74. Welch CE: Foreword. *In*: Acute Disorders of the Abdomen. Sreenivas VI (Ed). New York, Springer-Verlag, 1980, pp vii–viii.
75. Mitchell EP, Schein PS: Gastrointestinal toxicity of chemotherapeutic agents. Semin Oncol 1982; 9:52–64.
76. Varki SP, Armitage JO, Feagler JR: Typhlitis in acute leukemia. Cancer 1979; 32:695–697.
77. Sherman NJ, Woolley MM: The ileocecal syndrome in acute childhood leukemia. Arch Surg 1973; 107:39–42.
78. Wilson RE: Surgical emergencies. *In*: Cancer: Principles and Practice of Oncology. DeVita VT, Hellman S, Rosenberg SA (Eds). Philadelphia, JB Lippincott, 1982, pp 1604–1616.
79. Weissglas IS, Brown RA: Acute suppurative cholangitis secondary to malignant obstruction. Can J Surg 1981; 24:468–470.
80. Smith JP, Bodai BI: Empyema of the gallbladder: Potential consequence of medical intensive care. Crit Care Med 1982; 10:451–452.
81. Schuffler MD, Baird HW, Fleming CR: Intestinal pseudo-obstruction as the presenting manifestation of small-cell carcinoma of the lung: A paraneoplastic neuropathy of the gastrointestinal tract. Ann Intern Med 1983; 98:129–134.
82. Kelley WE Jr, Brown PW, Lawrence W Jr: Penetrating obstructing and perforating carcinomas of the colon and rectum. Arch Surg 1981; 116:381–384.
83. Boley SJ, Brandt LJ, Veith FJ: Ischemic disorders of the intestines. Curr Probl Surg 1978; 15:1–85.
84. Cullen W, Civetta JM, Briggs BA, et al: Therapeutic intervention scoring system: A method for quantitative comparison of patient care. Crit Care Med 1974; 2:57.
85. Silverman DG, Goldiner PL, Kaye BA, et al: The therapeutic intervention scoring system: An application to acutely ill cancer patients. Crit Care Med 1975; 3:222–225.
86. Rockwood K, Noseworthy TW, Gibney RTN, et al: One-year outcome of elderly and young patients admitted to intensive care units. Crit Care Med 1993; 21:687–691.
87. Lemeshow S, Teres D, Avrunin JS, et al: Refining intensive care unit outcome prediction by using changing probabilities of mortality. Crit Care Med 1988; 16:470–477.
88. Chalfin DB, Carlon GC: Age and utilization of ICU resources of critically ill cancer patients. Crit Care Med 1990; 18:694–698.
89. Zaren B, Bergstrom R: Survival of intensive care patients: II. Prognostic factors from the patient's medical history. Acta Anaesthesiol Scand 1988; 32:101–107.
90. Jecker NS: Futility and rationing. Am J Med 1992; 92:189–196.
91. Swenson MD: Scarcity in the intensive care unit: Principles of justice for rationing ICU beds. Am J Med 1992; 92:551–555.
92. Yarbro JW: Changing cancer care in the 1990s and the cost. Cancer 1991; 67:1718–1727.

SECTION XII
TRAUMA

William C. Shoemaker • Kenneth Waxman

CHAPTER 148
Epidemiology of Trauma

Dennis L. Kelleher, PhD • Arthur L. Trask, MD, FACS

Traumatic injury in America is to a large extent preventable. As in the investigation of acute diseases, the epidemiologic study of traumatic injury leads to an increased understanding of the trauma process, to the identification of potential predictors of its clinical course and outcome, and to the formulation of effective preventive strategies. However, traditional epidemiologic methods have been applied to trauma only within the last 40 years.[1]

Traumatic injury is a probabilistic function of a specific population at risk, in a specific risk environment, with a specific level of risk protection. The causative agent of trauma is energy, principally kinetic, that leads to a forcible disruption of normal anatomy or physiology. Traumatic injury can be analyzed on a population as well as on an individual basis. From an epidemiologic perspective, the essential element in the assessment of trauma is the systematic collection of data. The primary data elements are injury severity, injury frequency, and the social significance of the injury. Also important are who is being injured, how persons are being injured, and where the injury is taking place and under what circumstances. Such data are indispensable for comparing local injury rates with state, regional, and national norms and for evaluating potential interventions.

This chapter discusses the epidemiology of trauma, emphasizing the sources of data available for the study of traumatic injury. Also discussed are methods that are available to describe more fully the medical health hazard of trauma. An understanding of the epidemiology of trauma increases the potential for optimal care of the trauma patient as well as the number of opportunities for secondary and primary prevention.

OVERVIEW OF TRAUMA EPIDEMIOLOGY

Epidemiologic assessment of traumatic injury provides the critical care specialist with the most reliable estimates of patient numbers, injury type, severity of injury, clinical outcome, and potential for complications. It also provides reliable estimates of national, regional, and local trends in the type and severity of traumatic injury, which can prove invaluable for long-term planning of a critical care facility. In addition, injury trends are essential for identifying the crucial resources for a critical care unit, such as personnel, equipment, and training requirements. With the computer support available at most hospitals today, reliable projections of critical care requirements based on local trauma statistics are readily available and can be used to define local hospital priorities for optimal critical care.

TRAUMA MORTALITY

With a traumatic injury, the severity of injury and the availability of an effective trauma care system define the initial clinical course.[3a] In 1983, Trunkey described the trimodal distribution of trauma death as a function of time after injury.[2, 3] The model, based on a retrospective analysis of trauma deaths in San Francisco over a 2-year period, identified three distinct peaks in mortality.

The first peak, occurring within the first hour, describes fatal injuries for which provision of immediate medical care is minimally effective. These injuries include lacerations to the brain or major blood vessels. Patients in this early phase usually do not reach the hospital alive. Over 50% of all trauma deaths occur in the first phase.

The second peak in mortality, from 1 to 4 hours, includes patients for whom immediate definitive medical treatment may save their lives. Deaths during this period are the result of significant head injury, severe hemorrhage, or other multiple injuries. The prevention of deaths in this second phase is the primary goal of an effective regional trauma care system. The development of the American College of Surgeons Committee on Trauma's "Resources for Optimal Care of the Injured Patient"[4] and its Advanced Trauma Life Support curriculum are directed specifically at improving both prehospital and initial hospital treatment for the trauma patients at risk in this category.

The third peak in trauma mortality occurs over the period of 1 to 5 weeks. Sepsis and multiple organ failure predominate as causes of death for patients in this group. Early and optimal critical care for the patients at risk in this third phase reduces the number of patients who die from these causes.

INJURY CLASSIFICATION

Trauma can range from an uncomplicated single injury to extremely complex multiple injuries. An understanding of trauma requires consideration of three essential elements of injury classification: mechanism of injury, severity of injury, and projected clinical outcome.

Mechanism of Injury

Two classes of traumatic injury have been defined: blunt and penetrating. *Blunt trauma* is a distributed dissipation of kinetic energy either by concussion or by deceleration. Blunt trauma can lead to direct contusing injury, shearing, vascular disruption, and indirect lacerations secondary to skeletal fractures. *Penetrating trauma* is a more focal dissipation of a projectile's kinetic energy that leads to direct-impact lacerations and fractures.

A narrower classification scheme for trauma is analysis of the mechanism of injury. Mechanism of injury describes the physical forces and the environment in which trauma occurs. For example, motor vehicle collision describes one mechanism of injury. However, the mechanism of injury can be further described by specifics of the injury event such as vehicle speed and whether the vehicle's occupant was wearing a seat belt. Such microanalysis of mechanism of injury is codified by the E-Code descriptors of the International Classification of Diseases (ICD)–9 convention. Mechanism of injury analysis is extremely important in identifying potential injury prevention programs.

Severity of Injury

Efforts to develop better prognostic indicators for trauma require better clinical descriptive measures for traumatic injury. Wisner has recently reviewed the history of the development of injury scoring.[5] Initial scoring for triage purposes emphasized an inventory of the wounds sustained. It was thought that such an inventory would adequately describe the clinical state of the trauma patient. The *Injury Severity Score* (ISS) is a scaled measure of the anatomic injury sustained. As with burn calculations, the ISS is calculated on a body part basis. An international convention sponsored by the Association for Advancement of Automotive Medicine developed a scoring procedure for traumatic injury. The type and severity of injury to an organ or tissue is assigned an *Abbreviated Injury Score* (AIS). The maximal AIS for each body part is squared, and the highest three body part scores are summed to yield the ISS.[6]

Prediction of Outcome

As a measure of anatomic injury, ISS has proved to be less predictive of clinical course and outcome than two more recent measures: the *Trauma Score* (TS) and the *Revised Trauma Score* (RTS).[5] Both the TS and RTS rely on physiologic measures of injury rather than on anatomic disruption. The RTS has been shown to be a more reliable predictor of outcome and is based on three physiologic measures: the *Glasgow Coma Scale* score (a measure of neurologic status), respiratory rate, and systolic blood pressure.

A third measure has been developed to relate anatomic injury (ISS) and physiologic status (RTS). The *TRISS* plot (RTS on the y-axis, ISS on the x-axis) allows a hospital to directly relate its clinical outcomes with population-based outcome statistics. A probability of survival line, calculated from data of the *Major Trauma Outcome Study* (MTOS), overlays the TRISS plot and identifies outlying patients; this provides a valuable quality assurance measure for trauma personnel.

In addition to the above measures, a knowledge of injury "clustering" can aid the trauma physician in evaluating more fully the clinical course of an injured patient. Certain types of injuries co-occur with a high frequency. Knowledge of injury clusters can significantly reduce missed injuries. An example of an injury clustering phenomenon is blunt trauma to the chest suffered during a car crash. The basic forces of impact are dissipated simultaneously on the two body regions, leading frequently to associated lower extremity fractures.

Populations at Risk

The clinical cycle of trauma begins with the description of a population at risk. Large-scale studies of accident incidence rates, morbidity, and mortality have defined demographic, socioeconomic, behavioral, legal, and product-related factors that influence the incidence and severity of traumatic injury.[5a] Figure 148–1 describes the demographic relationship between child age and sex and bicycle/motor vehicle–related fatalities. Age and sex were found to be major determinants of the frequency of fatal bicycle-related injuries. Figure 148–2 relates the incidence of homicide-related mortality in young American males. Teenage black males are 10-fold more likely to die of homicide than are white males. Figure 148–3 demonstrates the impact of personal behavior on trauma rates. In 1991, 20% of all fatal or severe injury car crashes in America involved alcohol as a contributing factor. The rate of alcohol involvement was threefold greater for fatal crashes than for property damage alone. Emphasis on prevention of drunk driving and raising of the legal drinking age have markedly reduced the rate of alcohol-related car crashes over the last 10 years. Figure 148–4 dramatically portrays the potential impact of laws specifically enacted to reduce trauma rates by increasing protection from injury.[5b, 5c] Between 1966 and 1969, 40 states passed some form of motorcycle helmet law. Motorcycle fatalities decreased in number coincidently with passage of those laws. However, 27 states repealed or weakened those laws in the late 1970s. Motorcycle fatalities rose dramatically following repeal.

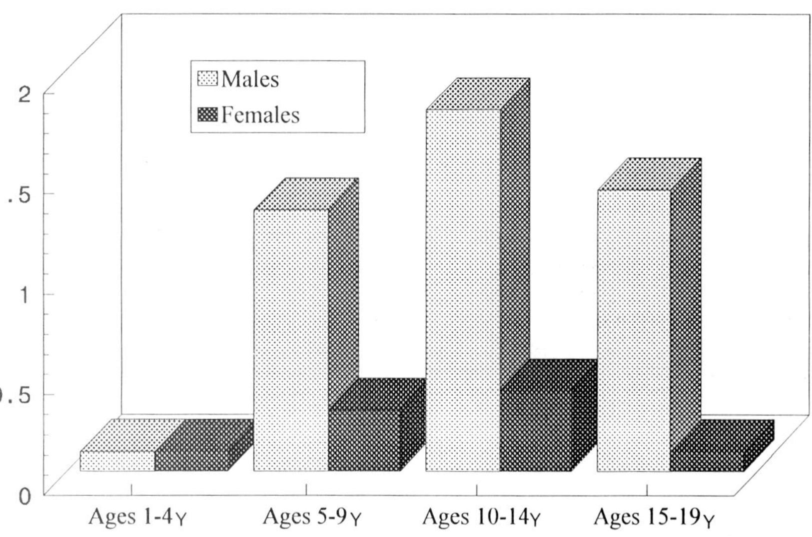

Figure 148–1. This graph describes the age and sex dependence of mortality for bicycle and motor vehicle collisions. The mortality rate of young males is fourfold greater than that of young females (per 100,000 children). (Redrawn from Children's Safety Network. [1991]: A Data Book of Child and Adolescent Injury. Washington, DC, National Center for Education in Maternal and Child Health, 1991.)

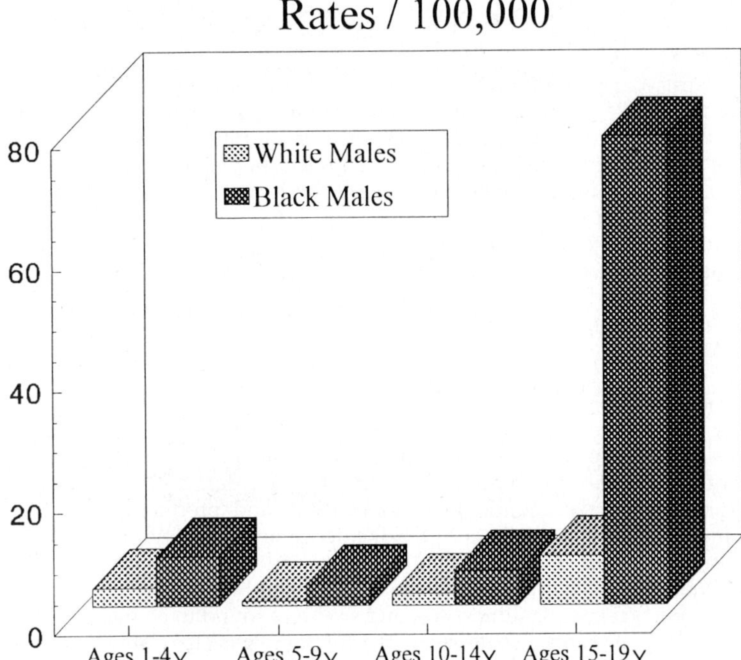

Figure 148–2. This graph compares the homicide mortality rates for young white males with those of young black males. Teenage black males have a homicide mortality that is 10-fold greater than that of teenage white males. (Redrawn from Children's Safety Network. [1991]: A Data Book of Child and Adolescent Injury. Washington, DC, National Center for Education in Maternal and Child Health, 1991.)

These examples illustrate the wide utility of trauma epidemiology in describing the injury environment and in suggesting preventive strategies.

National Statistics on Trauma Injuries

National statistics on the incidence, severity, and outcome of major trauma in the United States were difficult to abstract until recently. Responsibility for collecting injury statistics varies by federal agency. Statistics on motor vehicle accidents are the responsibility of the Department of Transportation; occupational injuries of the Department of Labor; and home and recreation injuries of the National Safety Council. Each of these agencies publishes annual reports on the incidence, prevention, and economic cost of traumatic injury.

An excellent example of a national data base is the national statistical survey of motor vehicle crashes maintained by the Department of Transportation. National statistics on the incidence of injuries due to motor vehicle crashes are available from the National Highway Traffic Safety Administration (NHTSA). NHTSA annually publishes the Fatal Accident Reporting System (FARS) report. The FARS report documents motor vehicle crash statistics on a state-by-state basis. The principal emphasis of this report is fatalities. Included are national estimates for drivers, passengers, pedes-

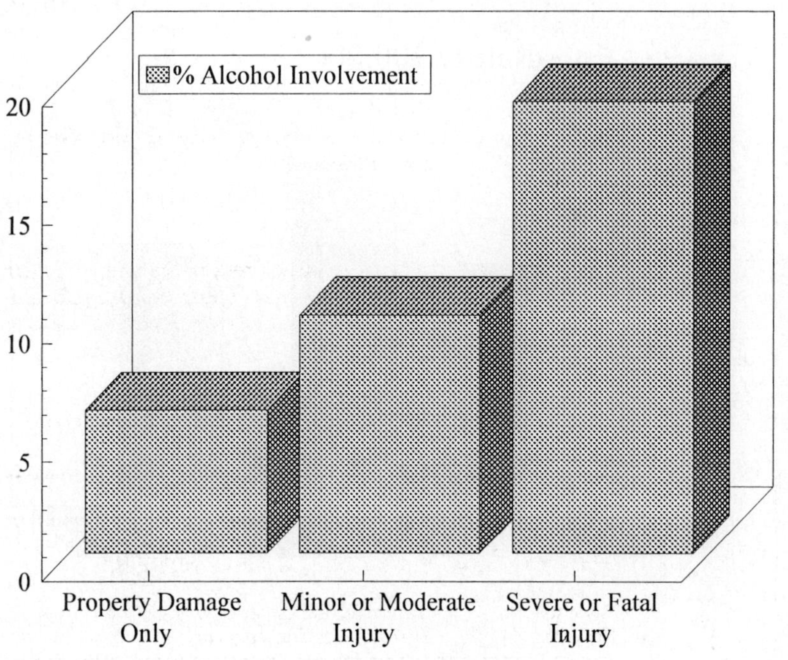

Figure 148–3. Per cent of motor vehicle crashes in 1991 in which alcohol was identified as a contributing factor. (Redrawn from General Estimates System, 1991. Washington, DC, National Highway Traffic Safety Administration, US Department of Transportation publication DOT HS 807954, 1993.)

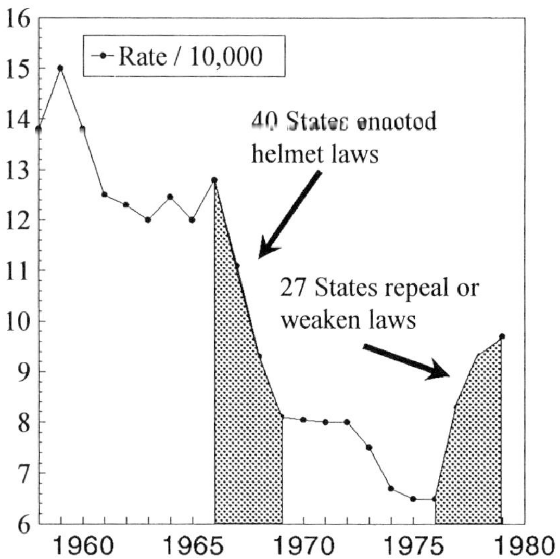

Figure 148–4. Impact of motorcycle helmet laws on motorcycle fatalities. (Redrawn from The Effectiveness of Motorcycle Helmets in Preventing Fatalities [Report and Research Note]. Washington, DC, National Highway Traffic Safety Administration, US Department of Transportation publication DOT HS 807416, 1989.)

trians, and motorcyclists with respect to injury and fatality. Other data reported include seat belt use, consumption of alcohol, type of vehicle, and certain demographic information.

NHTSA has recently extended the FARS data base by establishing the *National Accident Sampling System* (NASS), a statistically based survey of reported accidents. The NASS collects detailed information on the injuries and medical outcomes of motor vehicle crashes through its *Crashworthiness Data System.* The Crashworthiness Data System is considered essential for assessing the effectiveness of automobile design and safety regulations, such as seat belt laws. It can also provide valuable national estimates of motor vehicle injury incidence, severity, and outcome.

An important component missing from each of these reporting systems is data on the clinical course and outcome of traumatic injury. The American College of Surgeons Committee on Trauma, in collaboration with hospitals in the United States and Canada, coordinated the *Major Trauma Outcome Study* (MTOS).[7] The MTOS collected trauma registry data from more than 120 designated trauma centers and hospitals on injury mechanism, injury diagnosis, injury severity, duration of hospital stay, and clinical outcome. The MTOS data base includes over 120,000 trauma patient records and serves as the principal population data base for developing predictive models of clinical outcome following trauma. In 1990, Champion and coworkers published the first large-scale analyses of the MTOS data.[7] These analyses form the basis for establishing the national norms of trauma care outcome. The outcome statistics from MTOS are an essential component of any trauma care quality-improvement program.

With discontinuance of the large-scale data collection of MTOS, nationwide trauma statistics now are available only from disparate sources. Current federal legislation mandates a comprehensive interagency program of trauma research. The legislation further mandates that a National Trauma Registry be established to provide a continuous national statistical survey of trauma.

It is important to keep in mind that national injury data bases, such as NASS and MTOS, are principally of value in creating national norms. *The most clinically relevant data for injury incidence, severity, and outcome are those collected at the local hospital level.*

Hospital-Based Trauma Registries

Hospitals that maintain a trauma registry have access to the most clinically valuable data on the epidemiology of trauma. The ability to define the local hospital experience in terms of trauma incidence and outcome is essential for proper allocation of resources, training, and quality of care improvement. Trauma registries began as isolated initiatives by interested emergency physicians and trauma surgeons using existing data base applications. With the development of trauma registry computer programs for personal computers in the 1980s, it became possible for all hospitals to collect empirical data on the local trauma experience. Most of the programs that are available also include a variety of additional features that allow the hospital to compare its local experience (incidence, outcome, complication rate) with the national results of the MTOS (Table 148–1).

National Trauma Statistics for Selected Injuries

Other chapters in this textbook provide more detailed information on the optimal assessment and management of trauma injuries. However, an overview of the magnitude of trauma's impact on healthcare and society is essential.

Motor Vehicle Collisions

Motor vehicle collisions represent the single most common major injury–producing mechanism. In 1991, 6.11 million motor vehicle crashes occurred in the United States. Of these, more than 2 million led to moderate, severe, or fatal injuries. Although the trend over the preceding 3 years does indicate a decrease in accident occurrence, the absolute magnitude of injury and death due to motor vehicle mishaps is staggering.

In 1991, 3.13 million persons were injured in motor vehicles crashes. Fifteen per cent, or 470,000, of the injuries sustained were severe or fatal. Of the 3.13 million persons involved, 2.96 million were occupants of a motor vehicle. Another 170,000 pedestrians, pedicyclists, and other persons were injured. In 1991, one person was either killed or injured by a motor vehicle crash in the United States every 10 seconds. The estimated cost to society of motor vehicle deaths through lost productivity annually exceeds that for any other single cause of death.[8]

Burns

Burns account for approximately 2 million injuries per year in the United States. Of those who sustain injury, approximately 70,000 require some form of emergency treatment or

TABLE 148–1. Selected Hospital Trauma Registries: Personal Computer–Based Programs

Register	*Source*
TRACS	American College of Surgeons (Chicago, IL)
Hospital Trauma Register	Richard Cales, MD (Alameda, CA)
Trauma One	Lancet Technology (Cambridge, MA)
Collector	Tri-Analytics, Inc. (Bel Air, MD)

hospitalization. Almost 6000 persons per year die of burn injuries. An important consideration is that 21,000 of those burn victims requiring hospitalization were children and youths younger than the age of 20 years.[9] Children younger than the age of 5 years have a 2.5-fold greater risk of dying from a burn injury than the population as a whole.

Falls

The National Safety Council estimates that 12 million persons are injured in falls each year.[10] Principal injuries that are associated with falls from height include upper and lower extremity fractures (including heal and foot fractures), skull fractures, intracerebral hemorrhage, vertebral fractures (particularly lumbar), and lacerations.

Handguns and Violence

The increasing availability and use of handguns in America has dramatically altered the probability that one will become a victim of penetrating trauma. Coincident with the increased availability and use of handguns is the sharp increase in urban violence associated with narcotics trafficking. Penetrating trauma by gunshot or stabbing now represents approximately 40% of the trauma cases in some urban trauma centers.[3]

SUMMARY

The application of traditional epidemiologic methods to traumatic injury can significantly improve our understanding of the mechanism of injury, the clinical presentation of injury, the initial and long-term clinical course of injury, and the probability of survival following injury. Comprehensive epidemiologic data also provide the basis for quality improvement in trauma critical care. A detailed analysis of a local hospital's trauma patient experience, when compared with the national norms of the MTOS, currently provides the best available quality of care standard for trauma critical care.

References

1. Gordon JE: The epidemiology of accidents. Am J Public Health 1949; 39:504–515.
2. Trunkey DD: Trauma. Sci Am 1983; 249:28.
3. Trunkey DD, Blaisdell FW: Epidemiology of trauma. *In*: Scientific American Medicine, Care of the Surgical Patient. Wilmore DW, Brennan MF, Harken AH, et al (Eds). New York, Scientific American, 1993.
3a. Shackford SR, Mackersie RC, Holbrook TL, et al: The epidemiology of traumatic death: A population based analysis. Arch Surg 1993; 128:571.
4. American College of Surgeons Committee on Trauma: Resources for Optimal Care of the Injured Patient. Chicago, American College of Surgeons, 1990.
5. Wisner DH: History and current status of trauma scoring systems. Arch Surg 1992; 127:111.
5a. Stylianos S, Eichelberger MR: Pediatric trauma: Prevention strategies. Pediatr Clin North Am 1993; 40:1359.
5b. US Department of Transportation: National Highway Traffic Safety Administration, General Estimate System, 1991. US Department of Transportation, Washington, DC, 1992.
5c. Cameron MH, Vulcan AP, Finch CF, et al: Mandatory bicycle helmet use following a decade of helmet promotion in Victoria, Australia: An evaluation. Accident Anal Prev 1994; 26:325.
6. Association for Advancement of Automotive Medicine: The Abbreviated Injury Scale, 1990, Revision. Des Plaines, IL, Association for Advancement of Automotive Medicine. 1990.
7. Champion HR, Copes WS, Sacco WJ, et al: The major trauma outcome study: Establishing national norms for trauma care. J Trauma 1990; 30:1356–1365.
8. US Department of Transportation: National Highway Traffic Safety Administration, General Estimate System, 1991. US Department of Transportation, Washington, DC, 1993.
9. Children's Safety Network: A Data Book of Child and Adolescent Injury. Washington, DC, National Center for Education in Maternal and Child Health, 1991.
10. National Safety Council: Accident Fact Book, 1986 Edition. Chicago, National Safety Council, 1986.

CHAPTER 149

Initial Assessment of the Multiple Trauma Patient

Edmund J. Rutherford, MD • Loren D. Nelson, MD

The role of the intensive care unit (ICU) in the management of the critically injured patient includes continuation of the resuscitation and evaluation initiated in the emergency department and operating room. It is essential that ongoing resuscitation be continuously evaluated and that adjustments be made as needed.

Trauma is a multisystem disease that results in a loss of normal homeostatic mechanisms and that places the patient in a situation of increased and abnormal physiologic demands. At the same time, access to normal metabolic substrates is removed. Pain, blood loss, fluid shifts, and sepsis all compound the physiologic abnormalities of injury.

Goal-directed physiologic monitoring is necessary to provide early warning of the potential problems of occult injuries, infection, sepsis, multiple organ failure, and other life-threatening complications. Monitoring of an injured patient should include a goal-directed survey of all organ systems and an in-depth review of the systems most likely to suffer from direct trauma or secondary injury related to hypoxia, hypoperfusion, or sepsis.

CLOSED HEAD INJURIES

Head injuries are a major contributor to the morbidity and mortality of trauma patients. Patients with a Glasgow Coma Scale score less than or equal to 8 have a mortality of 30.8%, whereas those with a score greater than 8 have a mortality rate of 0.9%.[1] Patients with a score less than or equal to 8 should be considered for intracranial pressure (ICP) monitoring.[1a] ICP monitoring measures the pressure within the skull exerted by the brain, blood, and cerebrospinal fluid. An increase in ICP may reduce cerebral perfusion pressure (CPP) to the point at which cerebral blood flow is reduced and cerebral oxygen delivery is inadequate. CPP can be calculated as the difference between mean arterial pressure (MAP) and ICP (CPP = MAP − ICP). An inadequate CPP may be treated by raising mean arterial pressure or decreasing ICP. ICP may be measured by several means. Subarachnoid bolts and intraventricular catheters connected to fluid-filled pressure transducers have been in use for years.

Fiberoptic technology has been applied to ICP monitoring (Camino, San Diego, CA). Advantages include the absence of a fluid column, which minimizes artifact and may reduce risk of infection. Comparison of the various sites for ICP monitor use is shown in Table 149–1. Normal ICP is 10 to 15 mm Hg, and concern should arise when the ICP is greater than 20 mm Hg. This must be evaluated in the

TABLE 149–1. Comparison of Sites for Intracranial Pressure Monitoring

	Advantages	*Disadvantages*
Epidural	Ease of insertion No dural penetration Low risk of infection	Unable to drain CSF Questionable accuracy
Subarachnoid bolt	Useful if ventricles are small No penetration of brain Decreased risk of infection	Unable to drain CSF Requires intact skull
Intraventricular catheter	Reliable measurement Access to CSF	Difficulty locating ventricle Risk of infection Risk of intracerebral bleeding or edema
Intraparenchymal monitor	Ease of insertion Low risk of infection Useful if ventricles are small May provide most accurate ICP	Unable to drain CSF Risk of bleeding

(Adapted from Hollingsworth P, Vos H, Daily EK: Use of fiber-optic pressure transducer for intracranial pressure measurements: A preliminary report.
Abbreviations: CSF = cerebrospinal fluid; ICP = intracranial pressure.

context of the CPP, which should be maintained at greater than 50 mm Hg and possibly as high as 70 to 80 mm Hg.[2]

As with all monitors, placement of a foreign body into a sterile environment is associated with a risk of infection. Historically, the infectious risk of ICP monitors is about 10% and varies with several factors, including the type of monitor and duration of use.[3] The infectious risk presented by both gram-positive and gram-negative organisms increases after 3 to 5 days of monitor use. Since there is variation among possible infectious organisms and a lack of demonstrable benefit from prophylactic antibiotics,[3] the use of antibiotics should be individualized.

Patients with head injuries are at increased risk for other infectious complications. This may be a result of their altered level of consciousness and of their need for long-term ventilator support. Pulmonary infection is the most common cause of sepsis and requires early recognition and treatment.[4] These patients are also at a low but increased risk for post-traumatic seizures, which can be improved with phenytoin therapy during the first week.[5] Although these patients are still at an increased risk for post-traumatic seizures after the first week, no statistical decrease in incidence in patients treated with phenytoin at 1 or 2 years has been observed, and a negative cognitive effect with impaired neurobehavior performance occurs in the severely injured patient.[6]

Another medication dilemma is the choice of sedation and pain control in the obtunded and often combative patient. Although the importance of the ability to follow the neurologic examination cannot be overemphasized, withholding analgesics for these patients, who often have other significant injuries, can worsen their agitation and increase oxygen demand. Adequate pain control and sedation can be accomplished with the use of narcotics whose effects can be pharmacologically reversed. If the neurologic examination has deteriorated, repeat brain computed tomography (CT) should be considered.

The initial management of a patient with suspected significant head injury and altered consciousness is tracheal intubation, hyperventilation to an arterial carbon dioxide tension of 25 to 30 mm Hg, and judicious isotonic fluid administration (normal saline at 0.75 to 1 $mL \cdot k^{-1} \cdot h^{-1}$). If the patient has an abnormal brain CT scan showing focal or generalized injury as well as a Glasgow Coma Scale score of less than or equal to 8 without intoxicants, placement of an ICP monitor should be considered. If ICP is greater than 20, continued hyperventilation, fluid resuscitation with isotonic or hypertonic solutions, and elevation of the head of the bed should be maintained. Mannitol (0.25–1 g/kg)[7] is given rapidly (over 10–15 minutes) and repeated every 4 to 6 hours (0.25–0.5 g/kg) while serum sodium concentrations (goal: 150–155 mEq/L) and serum osmolality (goal: 310–320 mOsm/kg) are followed every 6 hours. Steroids are of no benefit and are even potentially harmful in head injury.[8] Cerebral vasodilators (nitroprusside, nitroglycerin, and others) are avoided. If the treatment is needed for a significant period of time or must be maximized in a potentially unstable patient, pulmonary artery catheterization is used to optimize systemic oxygen transport. If ICP is still not controlled, barbiturate-induced coma may be considered to make the patient areflexic with an isoelectric electroencephalogram.[9] This approach may require the use of inotropes to maintain systemic oxygen transport.

SPINAL CORD INJURIES

All trauma patients should be considered to have a spinal injury until proven otherwise. This is particularly problematic for those patients who are unresponsive and unable to be assessed clinically. Lateral cervical spine radiography, even when demonstrating all seven vertebrae, has a sensitivity of only 0.85[10] of detecting significant injury (Fig. 149–1). An anterior-posterior view and an open-mouth odontoid view must be used to rule out more than 99% of cervical bone injuries. Patients who have a cervical spine injury or are obtunded should be evaluated for concomitant thoracic lumbar spine injuries. If a spine injury is identified on physical examination or plain films, further diagnostic studies (CT, magnetic resonance imaging) are often indicated.

Patients in whom a spine injury is suspected, confirmed, or cannot be ruled out should be transported with the greatest of caution. The cervical spine should be immobilized, and the patient should be moved in a manner that prevents flexion, extension, or rotation of the potentially injured areas. Airway manipulations should be performed with in-line stabilization of the cervical spine. The care of patients with a spinal cord injury begins with rapid diagnosis and initiation of methylprednisolone therapy within 8 hours of injury.[11] An initial bolus of 30 mg/kg followed by 5.4 $mg \cdot kg^{-1} \cdot h^{-1}$ for 23 hours results in a statistically significant improvement in motor function, sensation to pinprick, and touch at 6 months.

Patients with a neurologic deficit have unique hemodynamic problems. Because of the unopposed parasympathetic outflow, these patients are vasodilated with a low systemic vascular resistance, low blood pressure, and, at

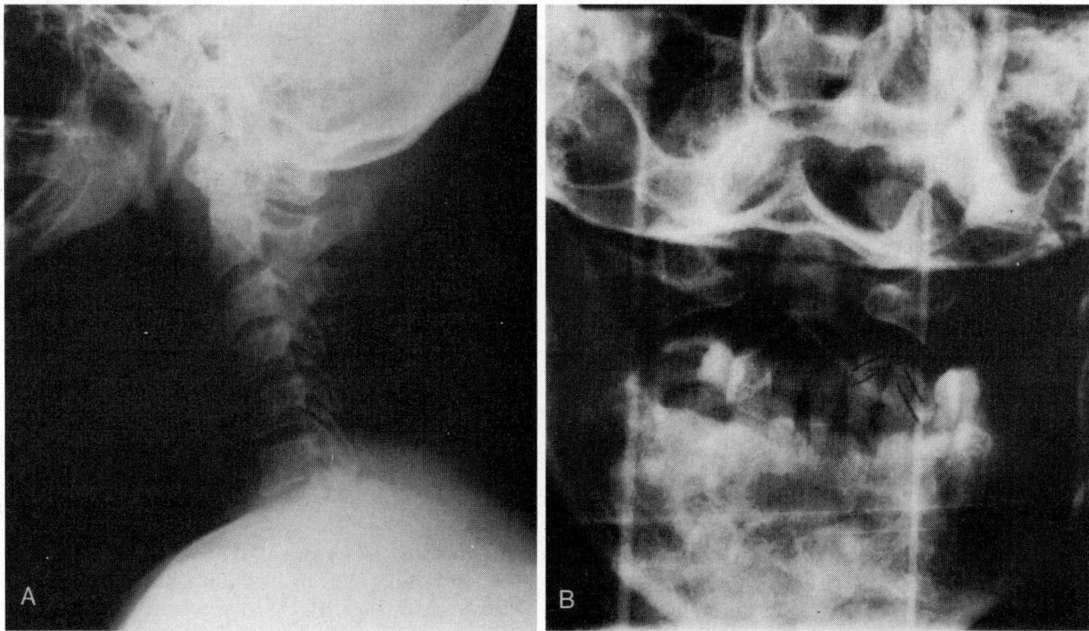

Figure 149–1. *A*, Lateral radiograph of a normal cervical spine (to C-6). *B*, This C-2 fracture noted only on the open-mouth odontoid view.

times, bradycardia. In high cervical spine injuries, cardiac sympathetic nerve functions are lost, and bradycardia and low cardiac output may occur. Cardiac output may be elevated in low spinal cord injuries. The low systemic vascular resistance places patients at risk for uncontrolled heat loss; thus, attention to temperature is critical, particularly in patients with other injuries. If perfusion is inadequate, sympathomimetics with both alpha and beta effects, such as dopamine, are usually effective. Pure alpha antagonists have a role in low spinal cord injuries when the heart rate and contractility are not problematic.

Because of the loss of intercostal function, tidal volume and negative inspiratory force are decreased. This, coupled with difficulty in mobilizing secretions and loss of abdominal expiratory muscle function, makes the patient prone to atelectasis and pulmonary infection. Prophylactic intubation can be avoided with early and aggressive pulmonary toilet. Oscillating beds such as the Roto-Rest (Kinetic Concepts, San Antonio, TX) improve pulmonary toilet and pulmonary shunt fraction.[12] When intubation is necessary, minimal support should be used to maximize spontaneous ventilatory activity and preserve ventilatory muscle strength.

CHEST TRAUMA

Twenty-five per cent of trauma deaths are caused by chest injuries.[13] Because of the potential substantial impact of intervention, the chest radiograph is of critical importance in the trauma patient. In addition to identifying the presence of a hemopneumothorax, important findings must be sought and ruled out on the trauma chest radiograph (Figs. 149–2 and 149–3).

Rib fractures are the most common thoracic injury, and the presence of multiple rib fractures increases the likelihood of other injuries and complications as well as the need for possible operative intervention and critical care manage-

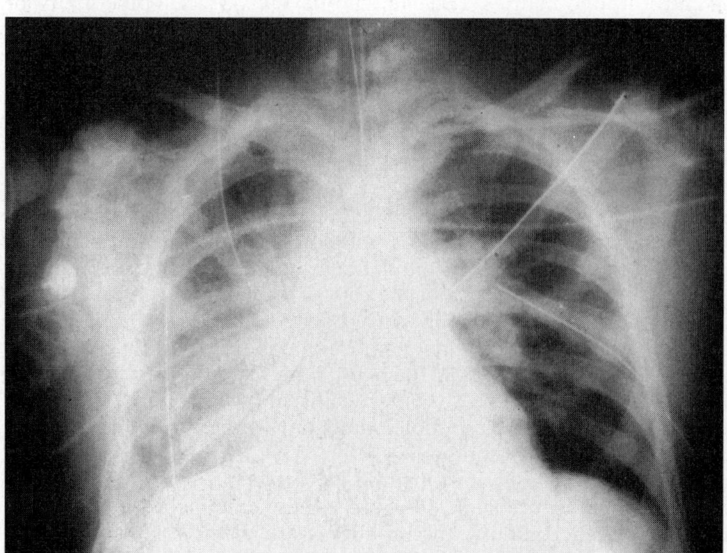

Figure 149–2. Radiograph of multiple rib fractures and pulmonary contusion.

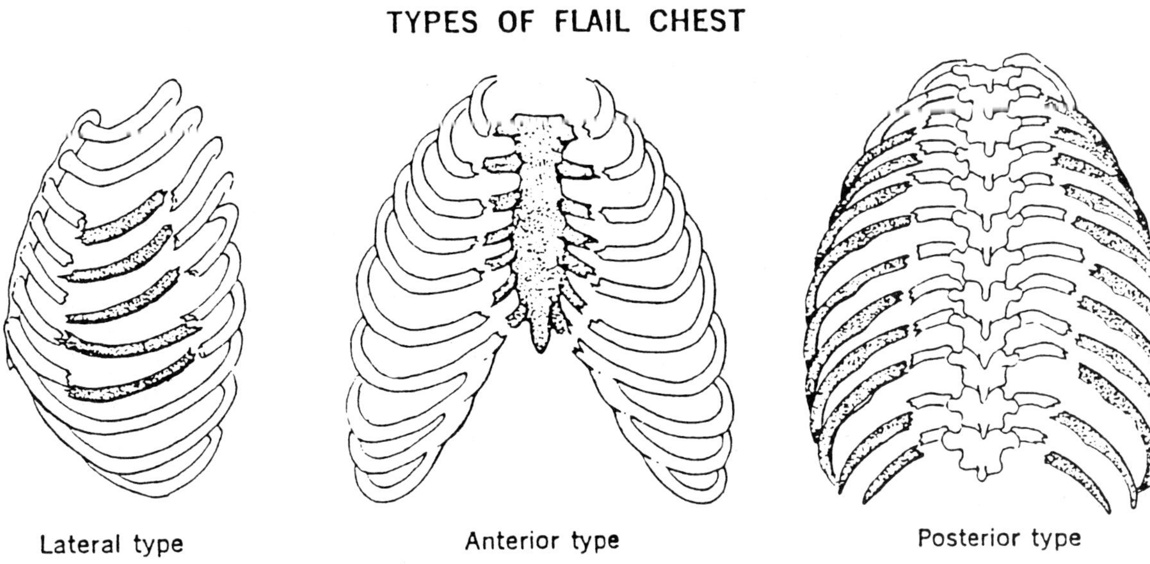

TYPES OF FLAIL CHEST

Lateral type | Anterior type | Posterior type

Figure 149–3. Types of flail chest. (From Naclerio EA: Chest Injuries: Physiologic Principles and Emergency Management. Orlando, Grune & Stratton, 1971, p 217.)

ment.[14] The most common clinical consequence of rib fractures or penetrating chest trauma that requires intervention is a pneumothorax or a hemothorax, or both. The majority of pneumothoraces and hemothoraces only require placement of a large-bore (e.g., 38-French) chest tube connected to an underwater seal/collection system (Fig. 149–4). A large-bore chest tube is preferred because of the propensity for smaller tubes to become obstructed by clot. Rarely, operative intervention may be required for large air leaks, which may signal major tracheobronchial injuries, or for persistent air leaks. A hemothorax that initially drains more than 1500 mL of blood or continues to drain more than 200 mL per hour may necessitate thoracotomy.[13] The most common ICU problems in patients with chest trauma include pain control, management of pulmonary contusion, and flail chest.

Pain control has a major impact on patients with chest injuries and allows improved pulmonary toilet. A patient-controlled analgesia device may provide adequate pain control with minimal invasiveness and personnel resources. Epidural narcotics are effective in the treatment of the pain of rib fractures and other thoracic trauma. Epidural analgesics have a longer duration of action and have been known to improve forced expiratory volume in 1 second, arterial oxygen tension, and alveolar-arterial oxygen tension difference compared with intravenous or intramuscular analgesics.[15, 16] Side effects include pruritus, urinary retention, hypotension, and respiratory system depression.

Pulmonary contusion (see Fig. 149–2) is a major factor in the morbidity and mortality of patients with chest trauma.[17] Although the number of fractures does not correlate with the severity of pulmonary injury,[18] rib, scapular, and sternal fractures are important markers of the magnitude of injury, and their presence should increase the suspicion of underlying injury. Likewise, the extent of pulmonary contusion on the initial chest radiograph does not correlate with the

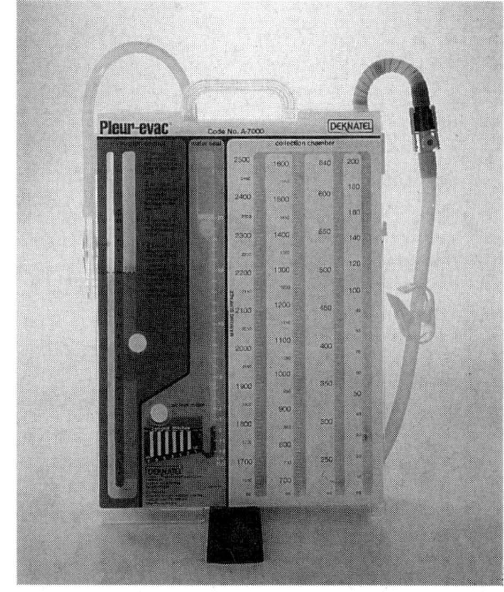

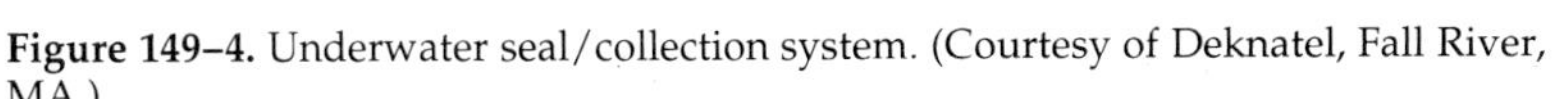
Figure 149–4. Underwater seal/collection system. (Courtesy of Deknatel, Fall River, MA.)

need for intubation or with mortality.[19] Patients with pulmonary contusion should be intubated, and ventilatory support instituted on the basis of their clinical status. Arterial blood gas analysis and pulse oximetry may be helpful. Nonventilating oxygenation support and continuous positive airway pressure by facemask may be useful in selected patients. Risk factors that have been shown to increase the likelihood for the need of tracheal intubation are an initial respiratory rate greater than 25 breaths per minute, a pulse rate greater than 100 beats per minute, a systolic blood pressure less than 100 mm Hg, and the presence of other injuries.[18] Ventilatory support includes increasing levels of positive end-expiratory pressure until oxygen saturation is satisfactory. Fluid resuscitation should be tempered, but not at the expense of delaying the restoration of adequate perfusion.

Like pulmonary contusion, flail chest has been associated with an increased mortality.[17] Defined as "paradoxical ventilatory movement," a flail chest generally requires at least two segmental fractures in each of three adjacent ribs (see Fig. 149–3). The treatment of flail chest has evolved over the last 35 years from towel clip traction to nonselective internal pneumatic stabilization to selective ventilator therapy.[20] The emphasis of the management of patients with flail chest is on the underlying pulmonary injury, pulmonary toilet, and pain control. The instability of the chest wall does not preclude adequate spontaneous ventilation. The paradoxical movement may even increase with adequate pain control. For those patients requiring ventilatory support, intermittent mandatory ventilation and positive end-expiratory pressure have been shown to improve functional residual capacity and oxygenation and to decrease the mean duration of mechanical ventilatory support.[21, 22] Operative stabilization of the chest wall is rarely necessary.

The spectrum of cardiac injuries ranges from concussion (injury without demonstrable pathologic changes) and contusion to rupture of the papillary muscles or of any of the cardiac chambers or septae.[23] Myocardial injury is believed to be common, often with minimal morbidity.[24] The diagnosis and significance of myocardial contusion is controversial. Multiple tests have been advocated, including electrocardiography, creatine phosphokinase isoenzyme assays, echocardiography, and radionuclide studies. Electrocardiography is neither sensitive nor specific,[25] and the correlation of creatine phosphokinase isoenzymes with cardiac contusion is poor.[26] The clinical usefulness of routine echocardiography and radionuclide studies has also been questioned.[27] Even when results are positive, the diagnosis of myocardial contusion has little impact on morbidity.[28] Since the major concern in myocardial contusion is dysrhythmias, most occurring within 12 hours of injury,[29] it is reasonable to monitor patients at risk for 24 hours with additional testing modalities (usually echocardiography) when clinically indicated. Myocardial contusion leading to left ventricular failure is uncommon but is associated with a high mortality. Pulmonary artery catheterization may be necessary for the titration of inotropes and vasodilators when ventricular dysfunction is suspected.

ABDOMINAL TRAUMA

Abdominal trauma is the most frequent cause of treatable, early, life-threatening hemorrhage in the injured patient. Patients may have unreliable findings on abdominal examination due to intoxicants, head injury, or paraplegia. Diagnostic peritoneal lavage and CT of the abdomen can be complementary, but typically only one diagnostic test is utilized. The relative merits of each test is beyond the scope of this chapter, but a prerequisite for CT is hemodynamic stability. Pain medication must be withheld in these patients to prevent obscuration of findings on physical examination either until a decision has been made for operative exploration or until the abdomen has been adequately evaluated and the need for serial abdominal examinations satisfied. The most common injury requiring abdominal intervention in blunt trauma is that of the spleen. Since the report of overwhelming postsplenectomy sepsis by King and Shumacker,[30, 31] efforts have been directed toward splenic salvage by nonoperative management, splenorrhaphy, and partial splenectomy.

The spectrum of liver injuries and their subsequent management vary greatly (Fig. 149–5). For limited blunt injuries, nonoperative management has been demonstrated to be safe with proper patient selection and close follow-up.[32] Patients must be hemodynamically stable, have adequate venous access, and should be monitored in the ICU with serial hematocrit determination. The management of severe injuries is more complex and ranges from tractotomy (with ligation of vessels and bile ducts), to resection, packing of the abdomen with laparotomy packs, temporary closure of the abdomen, and planned re-exploration when hypothermia and coagulopathy have been corrected.[33a, 33b, 33c] Hypothermia and coagulopathy represent the most common complications.

Hypothermia is a major contributor to coagulopathy and mortality.[34] Correction of hypothermia can be difficult. Useful techniques include warming of the external environment, use of heat shields and warming blankets, closing body cavities and covering exposed body areas to decrease further heat loss, addition of a humidifier to the ventilator circuit, and warming of all intravenous fluids.[34a] Rarely, irrigating body cavities with warm fluid via chest tubes or peritoneal lavage, or cardiopulmonary bypass is necessary.[35] Other complications of major hepatic trauma include hyperpyrexia, prolonged biliary leak, late hemorrhage, and hypoglycemia.[36]

Renal contusion is one of the most common urinary tract injuries after blunt trauma. The majority of renal contusions resolve without intervention or sequelae. The most common manifestation is hematuria, but significant injuries can occur in the absence of hematuria.[37] Patients with blood at the urethral meatus, scrotal hematoma, or a high-riding prostate gland should undergo retrograde urethrography before insertion of a Foley catheter to evaluate the possibility of urethral disruption. The upper urinary tract is evaluated

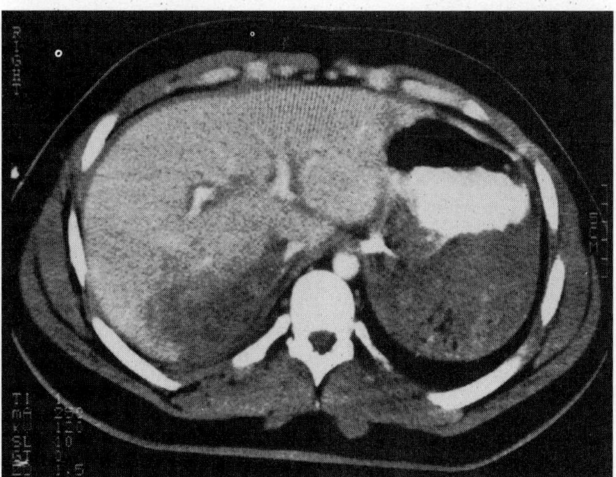

Figure 149–5. A CT scan demonstrating liver injury.

with either intravenous pyelography or CT with an intravenous contrast medium. CT assesses parenchymal injuries and provides information about other retroperitoneal structures.[38]

The magnitude of renal injury correlates with the occurrence of complications, renal failure, and death.[39] The most common causes of renal failure are hypoperfusion and nephrotoxic drugs.[40] Another cause to be kept in mind when evaluating trauma patients is rhabdomyolysis from crush injuries and ischemia. A positive result for blood on urine dipstick testing without red blood cells microscopically demonstrates myoglobinuria until proven otherwise. The most common causes of death are sepsis and multiple organ failure. Renal failure may also be associated with decreased filtration caused by increased intra-abdominal pressure.[41] Intra-abdominal pressure can be measured by instilling fluid into the bladder to create a fluid column (up to 300 mL), clamping the urinary catheter, and transducing the pressure. An intra-abdominal pressure greater than 30 mm Hg may cause sufficient renal parenchymal and venous compression to induce renal and other organ dysfunction. The increased pressure may be due to edema, ongoing bleeding, ascites, or placement of laparotomy packs and may necessitate opening of the abdomen.[41a] Adequate volume resuscitation and maintenance of renal oxygen delivery remain the key to preventing post-traumatic renal failure.

In blunt trauma, small bowel and colon injuries are less frequent than are solid viscus injuries, but they are becoming more common with increased use of seatbelts. The evaluation of these injuries can be difficult because CT is neither sensitive nor specific.[42] Diagnostic peritoneal lavage may also be negative. Delay of diagnosis increases morbidity. Finally, intervention requires a high index of suspicion, particularly in patients with a seatbelt contusion. Findings of increased abdominal pain, abdominal tenderness, and fever, especially in the first 24 hours after injury, should raise suspicion.

Pancreatic injuries can be difficult to diagnose and contribute significantly to morbidity and mortality. Since the pancreas is a retroperitoneal organ, diagnostic peritoneal lavage may not show any evidence of pancreatic injury. Amylase and lipase determinations are also of limited usefulness.[43] Successful treatment requires a high index of suspicion, identification of ductal injuries, and appropriate resection and drainage. Complications include intra-abdominal abscesses, fistulas, pseudocysts, and pancreatic insufficiency.

Duodenal injuries also can be difficult to diagnose. The nondiagnostic peritoneal lavage and delayed diagnosis can result in increased morbidity and mortality.[44] A CT scan with enteral contrast may demonstrate extravasation as well as extraluminal gas. Postoperative complications are similar to pancreatic injuries, most commonly fistulas and intra-abdominal abscesses. Parenteral nutrition is an important adjunct in the treatment of pancreatic and duodenal injuries.

ORTHOPEDIC AND EXTREMITY INJURIES

Pelvic fractures are common and may be a source of potential morbidity as well as mortality (Fig. 149–6). The mortality rate associated with open pelvic fractures is as high as 50%. For this reason, an anterior-posterior view of the pelvis is included in the routine radiographs of the blunt trauma patient. Bleeding from pelvic fractures can be massive. Because of the difficulty of controlling the source of bleeding, opening the retroperitoneal hematoma from a pelvic fracture should be avoided. Placement of an external fixator stabilizes the bone fragments and decreases blood loss.

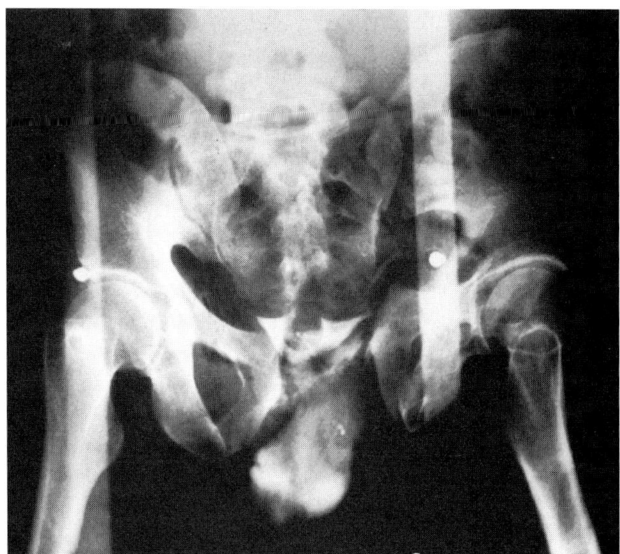

Figure 149–6. Open-book pelvic fracture with extravasation of dye from the genitourinary tract.

When external fixation is not indicated, the pneumatic antishock garment or military antishock trousers may be inflated to 30 to 40 mm Hg to help stabilize the pelvis and to induce venous tamponade. Although most bleeding is of venous origin, an arteriogram with embolization of bleeding points may be helpful in patients with persistent bleeding (usually a loss of greater than 6 units).[45] Patients with open pelvic fractures should be considered for diverting colostomy.

Many trauma patients have associated extremity fractures, and although they may not be immediately life threatening, they can have a major impact on outcome. Studies comparing early versus delayed stabilization demonstrate a decrease in the occurrence of adult respiratory distress syndrome, fat embolism, pneumonia, the number of days in the ICU and hospital, and the cost for patients having early stabilization (within 24 hours of injury).[46, 47] If early operative stabilization cannot be accomplished, skeletal traction should be instituted and maintained. Complications predisposed by the immobilization, such as pressure ulcers and deep venous thrombosis, should be monitored.

Extremity fractures and dislocations also predispose to vascular injuries. Perfusion of an extremity and signs of compartment syndromes must be monitored. An arteriogram is the gold standard for evaluation, but Doppler ultrasound examination may be a good screening modality. Neurologic deficits are the most common long-term sequelae.[48] If a compartment syndrome is suspected, the compartment pressure should be measured; if the pressure is elevated, fasciotomies should be performed. Compartment pressures can easily be performed at the bedside with a handheld or bedside monitor (Fig. 149–7). Normal compartment pressures range from 0 to 8 mm Hg. Decompression should be considered for pressures greater than 30 mm Hg.[49] Prolonged compartment syndromes may result in permanent muscle or nerve injury, rhabdomyolysis, or loss of the extremity.

OTHER CRITICAL CARE ISSUES

Trauma patients are at an increased risk for many of the same problems that affect other ICU patients. Immobiliza-

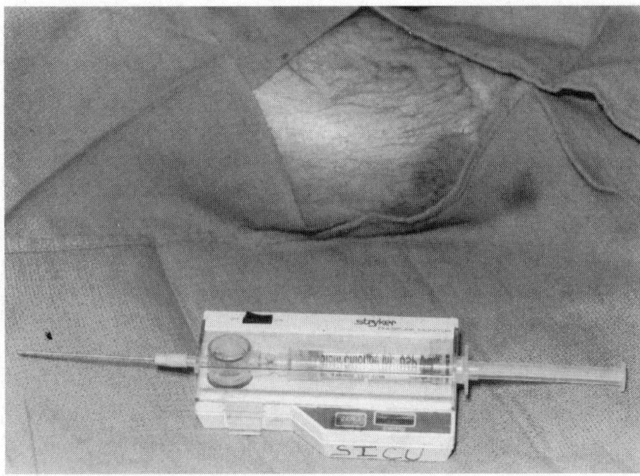

Figure 149–7. Stryker monitor for measuring compartment pressures.

tion predisposes these patients to deep venous thrombosis and pressure ulcers. Prophylactic measures for deep venous thrombosis that involve the use of anticoagulants may be contraindicated by the presence of other injuries, such as intracranial bleeding. In patients with lower extremity injuries, pneumatic compression stockings (Fig. 149–8) may be placed on the upper extremities to achieve some systemic fibrinolysis. Prophylactic vena cava filtration may be considered.

Pressure ulcers can occur early, even in young patients, particularly when such patients are kept on backboards because spinal injury has yet to be excluded. A patient should be taken off the backboard soon after arrival in the ICU, and precautions that include in-line stabilization and log-rolling should be instituted until spinal injury can be excluded.

Trauma patients are also at risk for the same infectious complications as other critically ill patients. This is in part due to the availability of a multitude of invasive devices and in part to the nonelective and sometimes less-than-sterile circumstances in which they were placed. All central lines placed in the emergency department should be considered contaminated and replaced or removed within the first 24 hours. Other causes of infectious processes to be considered include pneumonia, urinary tract infection, sinusitis (particularly with the use of nasoendotracheal tubes), intra-abdominal abscesses, and acalculous cholecystitis.

Multiple organ failure may be the ultimate expression of infectious complications. The development of multiple organ failure is associated with a high rate of mortality and should prompt a search for occult infection.[50] Because the gastrointestinal tract appears to be the reservoir for the pathogens of multiple organ failure, strategies to prevent breakdown of mucosal barriers and translocation, such as early enteral nutrition[51] and selective gut decontamination, may be helpful.

SUMMARY

Because of the magnitude of trauma and the size of the population affected, early assessment of the injured patient and prompt intervention has a great potential impact in economic terms and in respect to morbidity. To avoid the missing of injuries and to enhance a positive outcome, assessment should be systematic and goal directed. The most common injuries and potential complications should be kept in mind, and priorities should be established based on the most life-threatening injuries. Because trauma management is a multidisciplinary field, communication among all providers of care—the trauma team, the ICU service, subspecialists, nurses, ancillary services, and family members—is crucial. Care of the injured patient can be challenging, rewarding, and satisfying.

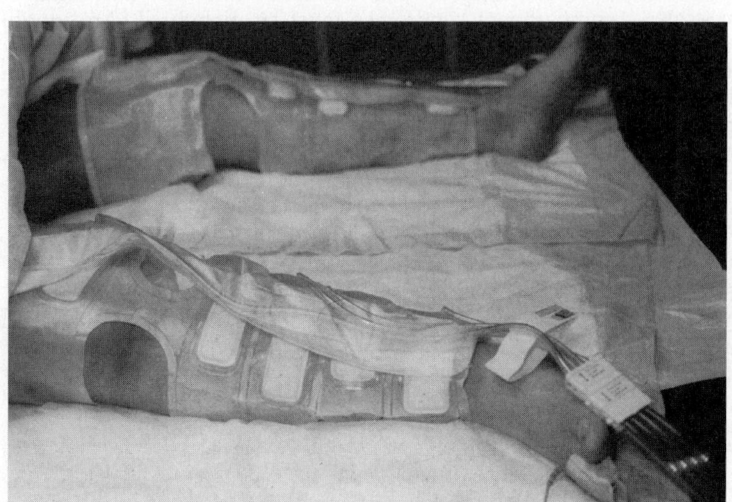

Figure 149–8. Pneumatic compression stockings.

References

1. Baxt WG, Moody P: The differential survival of trauma patients. J Trauma 1987; 27:602.

1a. Eddy VA, Vitsky JL, Rutherford EJ, et al: Aggressive use of ICP monitoring is safe and alters patient care. Am Surg 1994 (in press).

2. Rosner MJ, Daughton S: Cerebral perfusion pressure management in head injury. J Trauma 1990; 30:933.

3. Aucoin PJ, Kotilainen HR, Gantz NM, et al: Intracranial pressure monitors: Epidemiologic study of risk factors and infections. Am J Med 1986; 80:369.

4. Helling TS, Ebans LL, Fowler DL, et al: Infectious complications in patients with severe head injury. J Trauma 1988; 28:1575.

5. Temkim NR, Dikman SS, Wilensky AJ, et al: A randomized, double-blind study of phenytoin for the prevention of post-traumatic seizures. N Engl J Med 1990; 323:497.

6. Dikman SS, Temkin NR, Miller B, et al: Neurobehavioral effects of phenytoin prophylaxis of post-traumatic seizures. JAMA 1991; 265:1271.

7. Muizelear JP, Wei EP, Kontos HA, et al: Mannitol causes compensatory cerebral vasoconstriction and vasodilation on response to blood viscosity changes. J Neurosurg 1983; 59:822.

8. Dearden NM, Gibson JS, McDowell DG, et al: Effect of high-dose dexamethasone on outcome from severe head injury. J Neurosurg 1986; 64:81.

9. Rogers MC, Kirsch JR: Current concepts in brain resuscitation. JAMA 1989; 261:3143.

10. Ross SE, Schwab CW, David ET, et al: Clearing the cervical spine: Initial radiologic evaluation. J Trauma 1987; 27:1055.

11. Bracken MB, Shepard MJ, Collins WF, et al: A randomized, controlled trial of methylprednisolone or naloxone in the treatment of acute spinal cord injury. N Engl J Med 1990; 322:1405.

12. Nelson LD, Anderson HB: Physiologic effects of steep positioning in the surgical intensive care unit. Arch Surg 1989; 124:352.

13. Committee on Trauma of the American College of Surgeons: Advanced Trauma Life Support Course. Chicago, American College of Surgeons, 1989.

14. Lee RB, Morris JA Jr, Parker RS: Presence of three or more rib fractures as an indicator of need for interhospital transfer. J Trauma 1989; 29:795.

15. Bromage PR, Camporesi E, Chestnut D: Epidural narcotics for postoperative analgesia. Anesth Analg 1980; 59:473.

16. Rybro L, Schurizek BA, Petersen TK, et al: Postoperative analgesia and lung function: A comparison of intramuscular with epidural morphine. Acta Anaesthesiol Scand 1982; 26:514.

17. Clark GC, Schecter WP, Trunkey DD: Variables affecting outcome in blunt chest trauma: Flail chest vs. pulmonary contusion. J Trauma 1988; 28:298.

18. Barone JE, Pizzi WS, Nealon TF Jr, et al: Indications for intubation in blunt chest trauma. J Trauma 1986; 26:334.

19. Johnson JA, Cogbill TH, Winga ER: Determinants of outcome after pulmonary contusion. J Trauma 1986; 26:695.

20. Trinkle JK, Richardson JD, Franz JL, et al: Management of flail chest without mechanical ventilation. Ann Thorac Surg 1975; 19:355.

21. Sladen A, Aldredge CF, Albarran R: PEEP vs. ZEEP in the treatment of flail chest injuries. Crit Care Med 1973; 4:187.

22. Cullen P, Modell JH, Kirby RR, et al: Treatment of flail chest: Use of intermittent mandatory ventilation and positive end-expiratory pressure. Arch Surg 1975; 110:1099.

23. Bright EF, Beck CS: Nonpenetrating wounds of the heart: A clinical and experimental study. Am Heart J 1935; 10:293.

24. Parmley LF, Manion WC, Mattingly TW: Nonpenetrating traumatic injury of the heart. Circulation 1958; 18:371.

25. Harley OP, Mena I, Narahara KA, et al: Traumatic myocardial dysfunction. J Thorac Cardiovasc Surg 1984; 87:386.

26. Fabian TC, Cicala RS, Croce MA, et al: A prospective evaluation of myocardial contusion: Relationship between CPK and cardiac dysfunction. J Trauma 1990; 30:920.

27. Hossack KF, Moreno CA, Vanway CW, et al: Frequency of cardiac contusion in nonpenetrating chest injury. Am J Cardiol 1988; 61:391.

28. Ross P Jr, Degutis L, Baker CC: Cardiac contusion: The effect on operative management of the patient with trauma injuries. Arch Surg 1989; 124:506.

29. Baxter BT, Moore EE, Moore FA, et al: A plea for sensible management of myocardial contusion. Am J Surg 1989; 158:557.

30. King H, Shumacker HB Jr: Splenic studies: I. susceptibility to infection after splenectomy performed in infancy. Ann Surg 1952; 136:239.

31. Scher KS, Wroczynski FAS, Jones CW: Protection from post-splenectomy sepsis: Effect of prophylactic penicillin and pneumococcal vaccine on clearance of type 3 *Pneumococcus*. Surgery 1983; 93:792.

32. Meyer AA, Crass RA, Lin RC Jr, et al: Selective nonoperative management of blunt liver injury using computed tomography. Arch Surg 1985; 120:550.

33. Feliciano DV, Mattox KL, Burch JM, et al: Packing for control of hepatic hemorrhage. J Trauma 1986; 26:738.

33a. Morris JA Jr, Eddy VA, Rutherford EJ: The staged celiotomy: Damage control. Trauma Q 1993; 10:60.

33b. Morris JA Jr, Eddy VA, Blinman TA, et al: The staged celiotomy for trauma: Issues in unpacking and reconstruction. Ann Surg 1993; 217:576.

33c. Talbert S, Scalea TM, Rutherford EJ, et al: The staged celiotomy: Unpacking. Trauma Q 1993; 10:88.

34. Jurkovich GJ, Greiser WB, Luterman A, et al: Hypothermia in trauma victims: An ominous predictor of survival. J Trauma 1987; 27:1019.

34a. Eddy V, Morris JA Jr: Secondary resuscitation: An organ systems approach. Trauma Q 1993; 10:71.

35. Jurkovich GJ: Hypothermia in the trauma patient. Adv Trauma 1989; 4:111.

36. Cogbill TH, Moore EE, Jurkovich GJ, et al: Severe hepatic trauma: A multi-center experience with 1335 liver injuries. J Trauma 1988; 28:1433.

37. Clark DE, Georgitis JW, Ray FS: Renal artery injuries caused by blunt trauma. Surgery 1981; 90:87.

38. Vieira J, Smith CS, Cass AS, et al: Diagnosis of renal injury with computed tomography. Minn Med 1986; 69:207.

39. Carroll PR, Klostermen PW, McAninch JW: Surgical management of renal trauma: Analysis of risk factors, technique, and outcome. J Trauma 1988; 28:1071.

40. Morris JA Jr, Mucha P Jr, Ross SE, et al: Acute posttraumatic renal failure: A multicenter perspective. J Trauma 1991; 31:1584.

41. Richards WO, Scovill W, Shin B, et al: Acute renal failure associated with increased intra-abdominal pressure. Ann Surg 1983; 197:183.

41a. Eddy VA, Key SP, Morris JA Jr: Abdominal compartment syndrome: Etiology, detection, and management. J Tenn Med Assoc 1994; 87:55.

42. Sherck JP, Oakes DD: Small bowel injuries missed by computed tomography. J Trauma 1988; 28:1096.

43. Buechter KJ, Arnold M, Steele B, et al: The use of serum amylase and lipase in evaluating and managing blunt abdominal trauma. Am Surg 1990; 56:204.

44. Levinson MA, Petersen SR, Sheldon GF, et al: Duodenal trauma: Experience of a trauma center. J Trauma 1984; 24:475.

45. Panetta T, Sclafani SJA, Goldstein AS, et al: Percutaneous transcatheter embolization for massive bleeding from pelvic fractures. J Trauma 1985; 25:1021.

46. Johnson KD, Cadambi A, Seibert GB: Incidence of adult respiratory distress syndrome in patients with multiple musculoskeletal injuries: Effect of early operative stabilization of fractures. J Trauma 1985; 25:375.

47. Behrman SW, Fabian TC, Kudsk KA, et al: Improved outcome with femur fractures: Early versus delayed fixation. J Trauma 1990; 30:792.

48. Feliciano DV, Herskowitz K, O'Gorman RB, et al: Management of vascular injuries in the lower extremities. J Trauma 1988; 28:319.

49. Mubarak SJ, Owen CA, Hargens AR, et al: Acute compartment syndromes: Diagnosis and treatment with the aid of the Wick catheter. J Bone Joint Surg 1978; 60A:1091.

50. Fry DE, Pearlstein L, Fulton RL, et al: Multiple system organ failure: The role of uncontrolled infection. Arch Surg 1980; 115:136.

51. Baker CC, Degutis LC: Trauma and multiple organ failure: The clinical challenge. Trauma Management. *In*: Kreis DJ Jr, Gomez GA (Eds). Boston, Little, Brown and Co, 1989, pp 473–489.

CHAPTER 150

Preoperative Assessment of Critically Ill Patients

H. David Reines, MD, FACS, FCCM

A complete physiologic assessment of a critically ill patient before surgical intervention is frequently not possible. However, optimizing the cardiorespiratory system with therapeutic interventions and correcting metabolic deficiencies can significantly influence surgical outcome. Unlike preoperative evaluation of the elective surgical patient, the physician may not have the luxury of time to fully explore the causes of problems. Critically ill patients are by definition high risk; however, not all high-risk patients are critically ill. The patient who has been designated as a New York Heart Association Class 3 may be at home until his or her surgery, whereas a 23-year-old male gunshot victim who has sepsis with adult respiratory distress syndrome developed his pathology over a relatively short period of time and may already be in the intensive care unit (ICU)[1] (Table 150–1).

Critically ill patients requiring surgery fall into several broad categories, according to where they are in the system and what their underlying pathology is. Severely injured patients in the emergency room represent an entirely different spectrum of preoperative problems than does the preoperative, elective aortic aneurysm repair patient in the ICU or the postoperative cardiac bypass patient who develops acalculous cholecystitis.

Assessment of any patient begins with recording a complete history and performing a physical examination. Appropriate hemodynamic monitoring, appropriate laboratory investigation, therapeutic interventions to optimize or correct reparable defects, and safe transportation to and from the operating room are performed as time and the patient's condition permit.

The American Society of Anesthesiologists risk assessment criteria have withstood the test of time as an easy, if somewhat inexact, classification system[2] (Table 150–2). The majority of critically ill patients are either Class IV or V, and they frequently qualify as emergency patients as well. Another system for classifying patients has been proposed by the American College of Surgeons:[3]

CLASS I. Surgery is immediately required if a patient is to survive. Such surgery includes repair of an exsanguinating hemorrhage from trauma or of a ruptured aortic aneurysm. In such cases, the prime concern is to preserve life; optimization of cardiovascular and laboratory parameters may not be possible. Preoperative monitoring takes a secondary position to resuscitation when the source of bleeding must be controlled.

CLASS II. Surgery is urgent and clearly indicated—for example, for peritonitis secondary to perforated viscus, for an intraperitoneal abscess with systemic sepsis, or for hypotension secondary to small bowel obstruction or ischemic bowel associated with low-flow states. In these cases, optimizing a patient preoperatively may protect him or her during the surgical procedure and decrease the incidence of postoperative complications, especially multiple organ failure. The delay need not be prolonged. However, optimizing oxygen delivery by increasing intravascular volume or diuresis or by beginning inotropic support may decrease morbidity and mortality markedly.[4]

CLASS III. This class includes patients who are critically ill before a relatively elective procedure, such as those with poor myocardial function who have an ischemic ulcer on the leg. In these circumstances, elective admission to the ICU to correct reparable defects and to optimize cardiovascular function can decrease postoperative morbidity significantly.[5]

TABLE 150–1. The Old New York Heart Association Classification of Heart Failure Determined by Amount of Symptoms (Dyspnea and Fatigue)

Class 1	No symptoms
Class 2	Symptoms with ordinary activity
Class 3	Symptoms with less than ordinary activity
Class 4	Symptoms at rest

(From New York Heart Association, Criteria Committee: Nomenclature and Criteria for Diagnosis of Disease of the Heart and Great Vessels. 7th ed. Boston, Little, Brown and Co, 1973.)

Prior to 1973, the New York Heart Association recommended "Functional Capacity" be displayed in the complete cardiovascular disease diagnosis. Functional Capacity was determined for patients with angina pectoris or heart failure, according to the amount of effort required to produce chest discomfort or dyspnea and/or fatigue. This classification was abandoned in 1973. Because there is still a need for such a classification, the Canadian Cardiovascular Society classification of angina pectoris and the old New York Heart Association classification of heart failure are recommended. In either case, the designation should be displayed in the "Physiology" category of the complete cardiovascular diagnosis rather than listed separately under the abandoned Functional Capacity category. The new "Cardiac Status and Prognosis" category, which replaced the old "Functional Capacity," is determined by using all available data rather than symptoms alone. (From Hurst JN, Schlant RC, Rackley CE, et al: The Heart: Arteries and Veins. 7th ed. New York, McGraw-Hill, 1989, p 120.)

TABLE 150–2. American Society of Anesthesiologists Physical Status Scale

Class I	A normal healthy individual
Class II	A patient with mild systemic disease
Class III	A patient with severe systemic disease that is not incapacitating
Class IV	A patient with incapacitating systemic disease that is a constant threat to life
Class V	A moribund patient who is not expected to survive 24 h with or without operation
E	Added for emergency procedures

(Modified from American Society of Anesthesiologists: New classification of physical status. Anesthesiology 1963; 24:111.)

CARDIOVASCULAR SYSTEM

The purpose of the cardiovascular system is to deliver nutrients, especially oxygen, to the tissues. As defined by Goldman and coworkers in 1977, classic cardiac risk factors for elective surgery are congestive heart failure, recent myocardial infarction, and major arrhythmias.[6] Severe angina, hemodynamically significant valvular disease, and severe hypertension also represent cardiac risk factors. Critically ill patients undergoing surgical intervention may manifest cardiac insufficiency in more subtle ways than can be determined based on data from the history and physical examination alone. The evaluation of this patient population based on clinical criteria correctly estimates left ventricular filling pressures (pulmonary capillary wedge pressure) in only 50% of patients.[7] Furthermore, Shoemaker and Berlauk and their associates have demonstrated that optimization of oxygen delivery and cardiac index preoperatively can markedly improve outcome.[4, 5, 8]

Cardiac Risk Factors

The most widely accepted risk for a major postoperative cardiac event is recent myocardial infarction (MI). The definition of "recent" and the results of surgery in these patients have changed significantly since the mid-1970s. A large series conducted in 1972[9] showed a 20% incidence in MI if surgery was performed within 3 months of an MI; this resulted in a 69% mortality among these patients. The incidence dropped to 11% at 6 months and to 6% at more than 6 months.[10] Wells and Kaplan[11] reported no recurrent infarction in 48 patients with a recent MI when they were treated aggressively based on invasive hemodynamic monitoring. Rao and colleagues also confirmed that careful preoperative monitoring and correction of the existing cardiac problems could significantly lower postoperative cardiovascular morbidity and mortality.[12]

Coronary disease can be established based on electrocardiographic data and a history of angina or MI; however, if coronary disease is demonstrated, then a more thorough examination must be undertaken. Echocardiography is a useful screening test; however, exercise testing with thallium perfusion imaging can identify occult ischemia that cannot be detected with the use of less sophisticated techniques.[13] A positive stress test result should be followed by coronary arteriography if time allows. Preoperative coronary angioplasty or coronary artery surgery has been shown to be protective in the perioperative period. A study by Crawford and colleagues demonstrated a marked decrease in postoperative mortality and morbidity in patients with significant coronary artery disease amenable to preoperative correction who required noncardiac procedures.[14]

More recently, the Coronary Artery Surgery Study registry was reviewed to identify variables that affect operative mortality and cardiovascular morbidity for noncardiac procedures following coronary artery bypass surgery.[15] Noncardiac procedures were performed on 1600 patients following coronary arteriography. Three groups of patients were identified: Group 1 patients had no coronary artery disease (n = 399); group 2 patients were to undergo coronary artery bypass (n = 743); and group 3 patients had coronary disease but were not to undergo bypass (n = 458). Compared with patients in group 1, groups 2 and 3 were older, more symptomatic (with angina pectoris), had higher left ventricular end-diastolic pressures, and a higher incidence of previous MI. Total operative mortality was 1.3%. A statistically higher mortality was noted in group 3 patients (2.4%, P = .0009) than in those who had undergone coronary artery bypass. The mortality rates for groups 1 and 2 were statistically similar (0.5% and 0.9%, respectively). The incidence of nonfatal cardiovascular complications was 10.3%, although group 3 patients experienced an increased incidence of chest pain. No other differences were discernible among the three groups. Factors that were associated with increased mortality were history of prior MI, a high left ventricular score, preoperative use of nitrates, congestive heart failure, male sex, diabetes, age, dyspnea on exertion, and left ventricular hypertrophy based on electrocardiography. The authors concluded that coronary artery bypass should be undertaken before noncardiac surgery is undertaken in these patients.

Bishop and coworkers prospectively studied 253 high-risk surgical patients using previously defined criteria such as severe cardiorespiratory illness, extensive oncologic procedures, massive acute blood loss, sepsis, hemodynamic instability secondary to intra-abdominal catastrophe, respiratory failure requiring mechanical ventilation, acute renal failure, severe aortic disease, and hepatic failure.[16] Of this group, 64 patients (25%) died. From their data, the authors designed a randomized prospective study of high-risk patients. The patients were allocated to a control group in which "normal" hemodynamic and oxygen transport values were maintained or to a protocol group in which "supranormal" values were maintained (cardiac index [CI] > 4.5 L/min · m^2, oxygen delivery [$\dot{D}O_2$] > 600 mL/min · m^2, [$\dot{V}O_2$] > 170 mL/min · m^2). The patients were studied perioperatively, and oxygen deficit preoperatively and postoperatively was calculated. Although CI was raised only to 4.2 ± 1.2 L/min · m^2, $\dot{D}O_2$ was increased to 666 ± 131 mL/min · m^2 when fluids and inotropes were given. Mortality and organ failure were significantly reduced in the protocol group.

TABLE 150–3. Incidence of Multiple Organ Failure*

	Number of Patients with MOF (%)	
	Baseline $\dot{V}O_2$ <150 mL/min · m^2	*Baseline $\dot{V}O_2$ >150 mL/min · m^2*
12-h $\dot{V}O_2$ <150 mL/min · m^2	9/11 (82%)	3/4 (75%)
12-h $\dot{V}O_2$ >150 mL/min · m^2	3/10 (30%)	1/14 (7%)

(From Moore FA, Haenel JB, Moore EE, et al: Incommensurate oxygen consumption in response to maximal oxygen availability predicts postinjury multiple organ failure. J Trauma 1992; 33:58–65.)

*The incidence of multiple organ failure (MOF) was stratified by the patients' baseline $\dot{V}O_2$ (<150 versus >150) and 12-h $\dot{V}O_2$ (<150 versus >150).

A similar study performed by Moore and associates prospectively examined 39 severely injured patients at high risk for multiple organ failure.[17] Their high-risk factors included massive transfusion in the first 24 hours, multiple fractures, and combined flail chest–pulmonary contusion with early hypoxemia. A resuscitation protocol to maximize oxygen transport was initiated using as goals a $\dot{D}O_2$ greater than 600 mL/min · m^2 and a $\dot{V}O_2$ greater than 150 mL/min · m^2. To achieve these goals, arterial saturations of greater than 90% to 92%, a pulmonary capillary wedge pressure of 15 to 18 mm H_2O, and a hematocrit of 35% were maintained. If $\dot{D}O_2$ was not attained, low-dose inotropic support was initiated. Patients were grouped by baseline $\dot{V}O_2$ (Table 150–3). Only 7% of those who had $\dot{V}O_2$ greater than 150 mL/min · m^2 at baseline and maintained that value died, whereas 82% of patients with a low $\dot{V}O_2$ at baseline that was not corrected developed multiple organ failure. Multiple organ failure risk factors also included persistently elevated lactate levels.

A randomized prospective study of a homogeneous population of high-risk patients has demonstrated the efficacy of utilizing invasive monitoring to optimize cardiac dynamics and significantly decrease morbidity and mortality. Berlauk and colleagues studied a group of peripheral vascular disease patients before bypass surgery. The patients were randomized to one of three groups: no pulmonary artery pressure monitoring, pulmonary artery pressure monitoring preinduction, and pulmonary artery pressure monitoring 12 hours preoperatively with optimization to prevalues. Management of the last group was performed with the use of fluids and inotropes to achieve a pulmonary capillary wedge pressure of 8–15 mm Hg, CI greater than 2.8 L/min · m^2, and a systemic vascular resistance of 1100 dyne · s/cm^5 · m^2. Significant decrease in cardiac events and mortality occurred after patients were optimized preoperatively. If a patient's cardiac status could not be improved, then the surgical procedure was aborted[5] (Fig. 150–1).

The conclusion drawn from these studies was that routine hemodynamic measurements are insufficient to adequately assess cardiovascular status in critically ill patients. Opti-

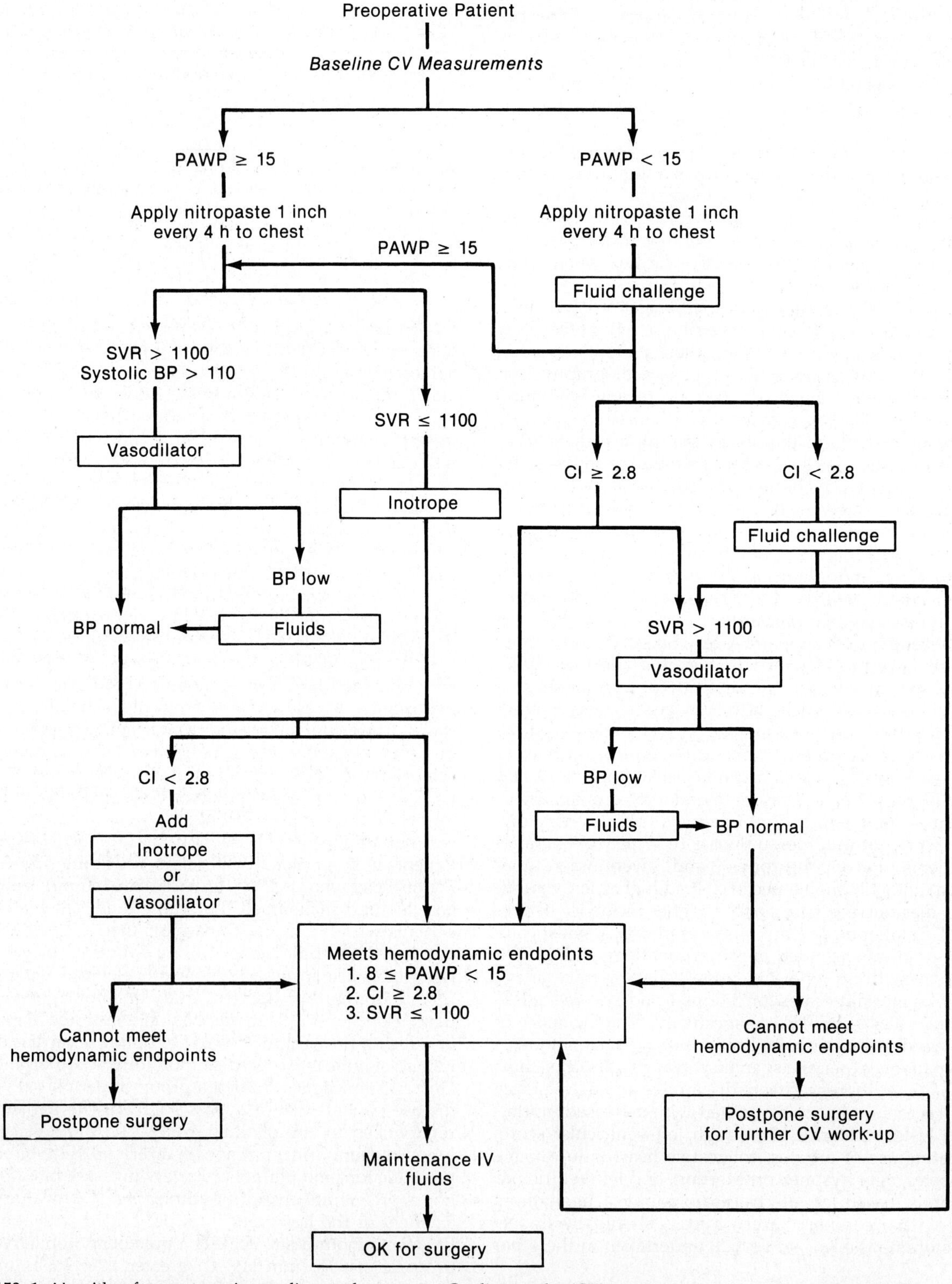

Figure 150–1. Algorithm for preoperative cardiovascular tune-up. Cardiovascular (CV) measurements were repeated after each intervention. Inotropes: dobutamine or dopamine. Vasodilators: nitroglycerin or nitroprusside. *Abbreviations*: BP = blood pressure; PAWP = pulmonary artery wedge pressure; SVR = systemic vascular resistance; CI = cardiac index. Measurement units are millimeters of mercury (mm Hg) for pressure, dyne · s/cm^{-5} · m^2 for resistance, and L/min per square meter for CI.

mizing oxygen delivery and utilization can decrease mortality and the occurrence of multiple organ failure. The inability to optimize these parameters is a poor prognostic sign that may preclude operative intervention. The judicious use of fluids and inotropes in these critically ill patients can improve surgical outcomes.

PULMONARY EVALUATIONS

The evaluation of pulmonary risk should encompass both chronic risk factors as well as those acutely related to the underlying disease process.

Chronic preexisting pulmonary pathology can be classified based on differentiation between restrictive and obstructive lung disease. Factors such as asthma and other bronchoreactive diseases can be controlled preoperatively. Patients with abnormalities that cannot be improved, such as those with decreased total lung volume associated with pulmonary fibrosis, need to have a baseline determined to establish reasonable postoperative goals.

The standard risk factors should be elucidated. These include tobacco use, dyspnea on exertion, asthma, chronic obstructive pulmonary disease, environmental exposure to pollutants, neuromuscular disease, and morbid obesity with hypoventilation. Routine physical examination that reveals increased anteroposterior diameter, expiratory wheezes, hyper-resonance, and other stigmata of chronic obstructive pulmonary disease need to be identified. The most important tests are a chest radiography and pulmonary function screening tests. A forced vital capacity less than 50% predicted, a forced expiratory volume in 1 second of 0.8 to 1 L (or < 60% predicted), or an abnormal ratio of forced vital capacity to forced expiratory volume in 1 second are predictors of increased morbidity and mortality.[18] Although Miller and colleagues have developed risk criteria based on pulmonary functions for patients undergoing lung resection,[19] Cain and coworkers studied 106 patients undergoing open heart surgery and found no correlation between preoperative pulmonary function test results and the incidence of pulmonary complications.[20]

Many of the studies quoted in the literature were performed before the availability of modern ventilation–anesthesia techniques, especially epidural and patient-controlled pain management in the modern ICU.[21, 22] For patients undergoing lung resections, determinations of total lung capacity and maximal breathing capacities as well as of split lung functions with and without bronchodilator use are important.[23] Arterial blood gas analysis is helpful to determine baseline values.[21, 22]

The second category of patients are those with acute pulmonary problems, such as pulmonary contusion, thoracic wall trauma, acute bronchial obstruction that results in atelectasis and pneumonia as well as those requiring preoperative mechanical ventilation. Optimizing these patients' status is frequently not possible. The liberal use of intraoperative and perioperative therapeutic bronchoscopy, optimizing positive end-expiratory pressure, adequate pain relief, and vigorous pulmonary toilet helps to minimize the occurrence of major complications.

PREOPERATIVE NUTRITIONAL STATUS

The majority of trauma patients admitted to the emergency department are nutritionally replete; however, a large percentage of critically ill patients requiring emergent surgery do have nutritional deficits. Patients with a history of recent weight loss, patients who are unable to eat (e.g., those with esophageal cancer), and hypermetabolic patients who require hyperalimentation are frequently malnourished. Measurement of transferrin, prealbumin and serum albumin levels and determination of total lymphocyte counts are all helpful in assessing the status of a patient, whereas weight and anthropometric measurements are frequently unable to be performed because of edema and third-space losses.[24, 25] One randomized prospective study of Veterans Administration patients did not demonstrate an effect on the elective surgical complication rate when preoperative hyperalimentation was utilized.[26] In this study, 395 malnourished men were randomized to either receive preoperative total parenteral nutrition or nothing. The rates of major complications were similar in both groups (25.5% versus 24.6%, respectively) as were the 90-day mortality rates. Infectious complications were higher in the total parenteral nutrition group (14.4% versus 6.4%, respectively; $P = .01$). Severely malnourished patients, however, had fewer noninfectious complications than did nourished patients (5% versus 43, respectively; $P = .03$) and no concomitant increase in infectious complications. The authors concluded that hyperalimentation should be reserved for severely malnourished patients as defined by a nutrition risk index score of less than 83.5. Scores were obtained by the formula: $1.519 \times$ serum albumin in grams per liter $+ 0.417 \times$ current/usual weight $\times 100$. Serum albumin and prealbumin abnormalities were also important.

Despite findings of this study, alimenting critically ill patients in the ICU by the enteral or the parenteral route intuitively has an impact on wound healing, infection complications, and nitrogen balance. Eliminating the problems of central vein hyperalimentation through the utilization of early enteral feeding has been shown to decrease the rate of infectious complications in stressed patients.[27]

RENAL AND ELECTROLYTE STATUS

Patients with renal insufficiency have metabolic and fluid derangements, poor blood platelet function, and a propensity for infectious complications.

Electrolyte status must be normalized preoperatively. Hypokalemia with arrhythmias or a level of potassium less than 3.0 mEq/L should be treated with administration of potassium chloride solution at a rate of 20 to 40 mEq/h with arrhythmia monitoring. Similarly, severe hypokalemia with rhythm disturbances, hyperkalemia with rhythm disturbances, or a potassium level greater than 5.5 mEq/L indicates the need for urgent therapy with bicarbonate, insulin glucose, and calcium with concomitant administration of binding agents such as sodium polystyrene sulfonate (Kayexelate) orally or by enema. Hyponatremia with a sodium level less than 120 mEq/L should be treated with fluid restriction and diuretics, if time allows. If the patient is symptomatic or requires emergent surgery, a 3% sodium chloride solution can be carefully administered to correct the problem. Acid-base abnormalities that are amenable to therapy should be corrected, as should magnesium and calcium depletion.

Patients in acute or chronic renal failure should undergo dialysis within the 24-hour period preoperatively.[28] Volume status is critical because these patients may be volume-overloaded before dialysis and severely depleted after dialysis. Cardiovascular monitoring is essential to the determination of volume status. Correction of anemia with blood and blood products should be undertaken preoperatively and intraoperatively to increase oxygen-carrying capacity while causing the least detrimental effects on cardiac function and work.

NEUROLOGIC STATUS

Alterations in neurologic function are common in patients with critical illness. A full mental status evaluation and neurologic examination should be undertaken before surgery. The ability of the patient to sign an operative consent form must be determined. If a focal process or evidence of increased cerebral pressure is discovered, then appropriate computed tomography or magnetic resonance imaging should be utilized to localize the problem and to guide therapy. Lumbar puncture should be performed for meningitis once cerebral edema has been ruled out.

The role of carotid artery disease in postoperative morbidity is controversial.[29] Carotid bruits or symptoms of carotid disease are found in 15% of patients older than 55 years of age.[30] Data from the literature imply that asymptomatic patients with narrowing of the carotid arteries of greater than 50% are at significant risk for neurologic events; preoperative carotid artery surgery may be indicated in this population.[31]

OBESITY

Morbidly obese patients, especially those with hypoventilation syndrome or pulmonary hypertension, are at high risk owing to problems unique to their obese state. Prem and coworkers reported a mortality rate of up to 20% among morbidly obese patients undergoing hysterectomy for malignancy.[32] Fowkes and associates demonstrated a mortality rate of 2.1% in morbidly obese patients undergoing elective surgical procedures,[33] whereas Sugerman and colleagues reported a 0.5% mortality rate for gastric bypass procedures.[34] Invasive cardiovascular monitoring should be performed on any morbidly obese patient with sleep apnea, hyperventilation, or hypoventilation syndrome, and on those with pulmonary hypertension and hypoxia. Frequently, this population is fluid overloaded, and vigorous diuresis may be necessary preoperatively.[34] Cardiac output and CI are frequently elevated preoperatively; however, surgery appears to reduce ventricular performance in obese patients more than in nonobese patients.[35] Therefore, preoperative cardiovascular and pulmonary monitoring should be undertaken in the subset of obese patients who demonstrate cardiopulmonary difficulties.

AGE

Overall perioperative mortality for elective surgical procedures is 0.5% if no concomitant medical conditions are present. An age of over 70 years raises this rate to 1.25% to 2.5%.[36] This increase, however, may be due primarily to an increase in the incidence of concurrent disease in the elderly.

SUMMARY

The critically ill patient is at obvious high risk for complications during and following any surgical procedure. The degree of preparation for surgery depends in great part on the urgency of the procedure. The status of a patient who is to undergo an elective tracheostomy and percutaneous gastrostomy can be optimized more easily than that of a hypotensive gunshot victim or that of a patient with a ruptured aneurysm. A full laboratory profile should include a complete blood count, determination of electrolytes and acid-base status, measurement of magnesium, calcium, and glucose levels, and a clotting profile that includes a bleeding time.[37] Routine chest radiography and other appropriate views should be performed. Optimization of cardiovascular system status, especially of $\dot{D}O_2$ and volume status, appear to be helpful in preventing postoperative mortality and multiple system organ failure. Diligent care is necessary if critically ill patients are to be guided through the perturbations of their illness. Optimizing the parameters that are amenable to therapy preoperatively yields best results; therefore, attempts to achieve optimization should be made before the patient is brought to the operating room.

References

1. New York Heart Association, Criteria Committee: Nomenclature and Criteria for Diagnosis of Disease of the Heart and Great Vessels. 7th ed. Boston, Little, Brown and Co, 1973.
2. American Society Anesthesiologists: New classification of physical status. Anesthesiology 1963; 24:111.
3. Wolfe BM, Suda S, Moore PG: Preparation of the ICU patient for operation. *In*: Care of the Surgical Patient. Vol 1. New York, Scientific American, 1993, pp 1–13.
4. Shoemaker WC, Appel PL, Kram HB, et al: Prospective trial of supranormal values of survivors as therapeutic goals in high-risk surgical patients. Chest 1988; 94:1176–1186.
5. Berlauk JF, Abrams JH, Gilmour IJ, et al: Preoperative optimization of cardiovascular hemodynamics improves outcome in peripheral vascular surgery: A prospective, randomized clinical trial. Ann Surg 1991; 214:298–299.
6. Goldman L, Caldera DL, Nussbaum SR, et al: Multifactorial index of cardiac risk in noncardiac surgical procedures. N Engl J Med 1977; 297:845–850.
7. Raper R, Sibbald WJ: Misled by the wedge? The Swan-Ganz catheter and left ventricular preload. Chest 1986; 89:427–434.
8. Shoemaker WC, Appel PL, Kram HB: Role of oxygen debt in the development of organ failure sepsis, and death in high-risk surgical patients. Chest 1992; 102:208–215.
9. Tarhan S, Moffitt EA, Taylor WF, et al: Myocardial infarction after general anesthesia. JAMA 1972; 220:1451–1454.
10. Steen PA, Tinker JA, Tarhan S: Myocardial reinfarction after anesthesia and surgery. JAMA 1978; 239:2566–2570.
11. Wells PH, Kaplan JA: Optimal management of patients with ischemic heart disease for noncardiac surgery by complementary anesthesiologist and cardiologist interaction. Am Heart J 1981; 102:1029–1037.
12. Rao TL, Jacobs KH, El-Etr AA: Reinfarction following anesthesia in patients with myocardial infarction. Anesthesiology 1983; 59:499–505.
13. Baron JF, Mundler O, Bertrand M, et al: Dipyridamole-thallium scintigraphy and gated radionuclide angiography to assess cardiac risk before abdominal aortic surgery. N Engl J Med 1994; 330:663–669.
14. Crawford ES, Morris GC Jr, Howell JF, et al: Operative risk in patients with previous coronary artery bypass. Ann Thorac Surg 1978; 26:215–221.
15. Foster ED, Davis KB, Carpenter JA, et al: Risk of noncardiac operation in patients with defined coronary disease: The Coronary Artery Surgery Study (CASS) registry experience. Ann Thorac Surg 1986; 41:42–50.
16. Bishop MH, Shoemaker WC, Appel PL, et al: Relationship between supranormal circulatory values, time delays, and outcome in severely traumatized patients. Crit Care Med 1993; 21:56–63.
17. Moore FA, Haenel JB, Moore EE, et al: Incommensurate oxygen consumption in response to maximal oxygen availability predicts postinjury multiple organ failure. J Trauma 1992; 33:58–65.
18. Gass GD, Olsen GN: Preoperative pulmonary function testing to predict postoperative morbidity and mortality. Chest 1986; 89:127–135.
19. Miller JI, Grossman GD, Hatcher CR: Pulmonary function test criteria for operability and pulmonary resection. Surg Gynecol Obstet 1981; 153:893–895.
20. Cain HD, Stevens PM, Adinaya R: Preoperative pulmonary function and complications after cardiovascular surgery. Chest 1979; 76:130–135.
21. Stein M, Kootu GM, Simon M, et al: Pulmonary evaluation of surgical patients. JAMA 1962; 181:765–770.

22. Gracey DR, Divertie B, Didier E: Preoperative pulmonary preparation of patients with chronic obstructive pulmonary disease: A prospective study. Chest 1979; 76:123–129.
23. Miller WF, Wu N, Johnson RL Jr: Convenient method of evaluating pulmonary ventilatory function with single breath. Anesthesiology 1956; 17:480–493.
24. Blackburn GL, Bistrian BR, Maini BS, et al: Nutritional and metabolic assessment of the hospitalized patient. JPEN J Parenter Enteral Nutr 1977; 1:11–22.
25. Baker JP, Detsky AS, Wesson DE, et al: Nutritional assessment: A comparison of clinical judgment and objective measurements. N Engl J Med 1982; 306:969–972.
26. The Veterans Affairs Total Parenteral Nutrition Cooperative Study Group: Perioperative total parenteral nutrition in surgical patients. N Engl J Med 1991; 325:525–532.
27. Moore FA, Moore EE, Jones TN, et al: TEN versus TPN following major abdominal trauma: Reduced septic mortality. J Trauma 1989; 29:916–922.
28. Bonner J: Medical complications of the long-term dialysis patient: Perioperative treatment in hemodialysis patients. *In*: Oxford Textbook of Clinical Nephrology. Vol 2. Cameron S, Davison AM, Grunefeld JP, et al (Eds). New York, Oxford University Press, 1992; pp 1451–1452.
29. Wolf PA, Kannel WB, Sorlie P, et al: Asymptomatic carotid bruit and risk of stroke: The Framingham Study. JAMA 1981; 245:1442–1445.
30. Ropper AH, Wechsler LR, Wilson LS: Carotid bruit and risk of stroke in elective surgery. N Engl J Med 1982; 307:1388–1390.
31. Hobson RW II, Weiss DG, Fields WS, et al: Efficacy of carotid endarterectomy for asymptomatic carotid stenosis: The Veterans Affairs Cooperative Study Group. N Engl J Med 1992; 328:221–227.
32. Prem KA, Menshala MN, McKelvey J: Operative treatment of adenocarcinoma of the endometrium in obese women. Am J Obstet Gynecol 1965; 92:16–22.
33. Fowkes FG, Lunn JN, Farrow SC, et al: Epidemiology in anaesthesia: III. Mortality risk in patients with coexisting physical disease. Br J Anaesth 1982; 54:819–825.
34. Sugerman HJ, Baron PL, Fairman RP, et al: Hemodynamic dysfunction in obesity: Hypoventilation syndrome and the effects of treatment with surgically induced weight loss. Ann Surg 1988; 207:604–613.
35. Amad KH, Brennan JC, Alexander JK: The cardiac pathology of chronic exogenous obesity. Circulation 1965; 32:740–745.
36. Cohen MM, Duncan PG, Tate RB: Does anesthesia contribute to operative mortality? JAMA 1988; 260:2859–2863.
37. Velanovich V: Preoperative laboratory screening based on age, gender, and concomitant medical diseases. Surgery 1994; 115:56–61.

CHAPTER 151

Physiologic Response To Injury

Kenneth Waxman, MD, FACS

The purpose of this chapter is to examine the physiologic changes that occur following trauma and operations. Such consideration is important for this text because the critical illness that may follow trauma or operation can best be understood only if the usual physiologic responses to surgical and accidental trauma are appreciated. Furthermore, it is increasingly clear that the critical illness that may follow complicated trauma or operation is to a large extent mediated by exaggeration and imbalance of those physiologic compensations that normally occur. Thus, consideration of the physiologic changes that normally occur improves not only our understanding of recovery from uncomplicated trauma or operation but also our ability to provide effective treatment when complications occur.

Cuthbertson defined two phases of the metabolic response to trauma, an *ebb phase* and a *flow phase*.[1] Moore subsequently divided the flow phase into *catabolic* and *anabolic* stages.[2] The ebb phase occurs during the first several hours after injury and is characterized by hypovolemia, low blood flow, and the initial compensatory physiologic reactions to trauma and shock. Once resuscitation is complete and perfusion re-established, the flow phase begins. It is characterized by a hyperdynamic stress response, fluid retention and edema, catabolism, and hypermetabolism. This catabolic stage may last for days to weeks, depending on the severity of injury. Once volume deficits have been eliminated, wounds have closed, and infection has been controlled, the anabolic stage begins. This is characterized by a return to normal hemodynamics, diuresis, the reaccumulation of protein, the reaccumulation of body fat, and the restoration of body function. The anabolic stage generally is longer than the catabolic stage and may be weeks in duration.

The initial stress responses to trauma are deeply rooted in our biologic nature. These responses are first initiated by the perception of trauma, which may be either conscious or unconscious (as during anesthesia). The experiencing of injury and pain or even the anticipation of a dangerous situation initiates protective and recovery responses, both psychologic and physiologic. The responses include protective behaviors such as immobilization, withdrawal, and antagonism. In addition, a physiologic cascade is initiated; this includes neurologic, neurohormonal, cardiovascular, immunologic, and metabolic responses to trauma; these responses are examined in this chapter.

Two general points may be made about the stress response. First, the degree of the psychologic and physiologic responses are proportionate to the extent of shock and injury; they tend to be minimal for minor injury or operation and extensive for major accidental or surgical trauma. Signals that are initiated in injured or ischemic tissues communicate the extent of injury systemically. These signals are beginning to be understood and appear to be key in determining the extent of the stress response. Second, these stress responses may be necessary for recovery and are thus of survival value. However, when trauma is severe, the resultant physiologic responses are extensive and sustained. These same responses may then become injurious and contribute to a progression to critical illness and death.

STIMULI THAT INITIATE THE PHYSIOLOGIC RESPONSES TO TRAUMA

The stress response is initiated not only by injury but also by acute blood loss, shock, hypoxia, acidosis, and hypothermia. Furthermore, it can be initiated by psychologic stressors.[3–6] Fear alone initiates many aspects of the stress response, including sympathetic and neurohormonal responses, altered microcirculatory blood flow, and altered coagulation and immune function. It appears that psychologic stressors such as fear activate centrally mediated responses to trauma just as physical stressors do.

Another important stimulus that activates the stress response is pain.[7] Afferent nerve signals from injured tissues converge on the hypothalamus and stimulate the hypothalamic-pituitary axis, resulting in cortisol secretion. Pain is also a potent initiator of the sympathoadrenal axis, so that sympathetic tone and adrenal secretion of catechols are immediately activated by painful stimuli. The fact that pain is not experienced during anesthesia may be an important reason why extensive trauma of major operations is often so well tolerated, whereas a similar amount of tissue injury incurred during accidental trauma may cause a much more severe physiologic response.[8, 9] The importance of neural afferents from the site of tissue injury is confirmed in paraplegic humans, in whom the usual perioperative rise in cortisol level is not seen if the operation is carried out below the level of spinal cord damage.[3]

Another initiator of the stress response is hemorrhage and intravascular hypovolemia.[10, 11] Hemorrhage results in the stimulation of volume and pressure receptors, which activate the central nervous system. The response tends to be proportionate to the amount of shock; both the degree and duration of blood volume deficit are, thus, important determinants of the degree of physiologic response to injury. Furthermore, as hemorrhage and hypovolemia decrease cardiac output, tissue ischemia may result. Tissue ischemia is also an important activator of physiologic responses to injury, not only because it may potentiate activation of the centrally mediated stress responses, but also because tissue ischemia initiates potent local responses, such as elucidation of mediators and activation of cells.

Other initiators of the stress response are hypoxemia, acidosis, and hypercarbia. Chemoreceptors located in the aorta and carotid body are activated by changes in PO_2, PCO_2, or pH.[12] In addition, decreased blood flow causes tissue hypoxia and acidosis, which results in activation of the same receptors; these chemoreceptors thus indirectly sense low blood flow. Therefore, low blood flow results in activation of both chemoreceptors and baroreceptors, which then contribute to the initiation of central stress responses.

Hypothermia, which frequently occurs following trauma or during surgery, is sensed directly by the preoptic area of the hypothalamus and triggers the hypothalamic-pituitary axis.[13, 14] Thus, hypothermia may augment the stress response.

Another very important initiator of the physiologic responses to trauma is the wound itself. Tissue injury results in the production of afferent nerve signals that stimulate the sympathoadrenal axis as well as the hypothalamic-pituitary axis.[3] Of additional importance, however, are local processes that occur within the wound or ischemic tissues. These processes are critical in initiating both local and systemic responses that affect metabolism, coagulation, inflammation, and immunity. The extent of these responses is determined by the size of the wound or by the extent of ischemic injury.

These responses to injury and ischemia act in coordination as signals that communicate systemically in a quantitative manner. Hence, the physiologic reaction is proportionate to the magnitude of injury.[15]

MEDIATORS OF THE RESPONSES TO TRAUMA

Sympathoadrenal Axis

Activation of the sympathetic nervous system occurs when afferent nerve signals reach the brain following the presentation of a number of stimuli such as fear, pain, wounding, hemorrhage, and hypovolemia.[16–19] The adrenal medulla is stimulated whenever the sympathetic nervous system is stimulated because release of both epinephrine and norepinephrine is triggered by splanchnic sympathetic nerves that synapse directly with adrenal medullary cells. Catecholamines exert a multitude of effects, including an increase in blood pressure and heart rate, enhancement of cardiac contractility, an increase in minute ventilation, and vasoconstriction throughout the arterial and venous circulation. Catecholamines also affect pancreatic hormone release and affect glucose, amino acid, and fat metabolism.

Although these neurogenic and circulating catecholamine effects are of immediate survival value following major injury, prolonged and excessive stimulation of the sympathoadrenal axis may lead to adverse physiologic effects. Prolonged elevation of sympathetic tone and increase in catecholamine secretion may contribute to severe and uneven arteriolar vasoconstriction. In turn, this may reduce microcirculatory blood flow, impairing delivery of oxygen and metabolic substrate to the tissues. Furthermore, whereas an immediate effect of an increase in sympathetic tone is the redistribution of intravascular volume from the venous capacitance vessels, which increases central blood volume, the vasoconstricting effects on postcapillary venules may subsequently result in an increase in intraluminal capillary pressure. This contributes to loss of intravascular volume, intravascular hypovolemia, and edema formation. In addition, a prolonged increase in sympathoadrenal tone contributes to the catabolic metabolic state characteristic of severe trauma.

Hypothalamic-Pituitary-Adrenal Axis

Adrenal secretion of cortisol is central to the stress response.[2, 3, 7, 19–22] This secretion is mediated by the hypothalamic-pituitary-adrenal axis. This reflex arc is activated by stimuli, including fear, pain, hypotension, hypovolemia, and tissue injury. Neural afferent signals converge on the hypothalamus and provoke release of corticotropin-releasing factor, which stimulates adrenocorticotropic hormone (ACTH) secretion from the anterior lobe of the pituitary gland. Other substances also may modulate the release of corticotropin-releasing factor or have a direct effect themselves; these substances include vasopressin, angiotensin II, norepinephrine, and inhaled anesthetics. Endotoxemia also has an effect. ACTH is derived from a larger precursor called *proopiomelanocortin*. Besides ACTH, cleavage products of proopiomelanocortin include β-endorphin, β-lipotropin, and α-melanocyte–stimulating hormone. ACTH and β-endorphin are released simultaneously and in equimolar amounts from the same anterior pituitary cells. The target organ for ACTH is the adrenal cortex, in which it stimulates synthesis and release of cortisol. The degree of hypercortisolism parallels the degree of injury and classically has been used as a marker for the degree of stress response. The effects of glucocorticoid release into the circulation include sodium retention, insulin resistance, gluconeogenesis, lipolysis, and protein catabolism. Cortisol causes demargination of leukocytes and also inhibits the activity of phospholipase A, thereby down-regulating prostaglandin synthesis. Furthermore, elevation of cortisol levels enhances the catabolic effects of tumor necrosis factor (TNF) and interleukin-6 (IL-6). Like catecholamines, cortisol is important for recovery from acute injury. However, severe trauma with an extended injury response results in prolonged cortisol secretion, which has many detrimental effects and may contribute to a progression from the adaptive stress response toward critical illness.

Antidiuretic Hormone

Loss of blood volume is sensed by atrial receptors, whereas decreased pressure is sensed by baroreceptors in the carotid, aortic, and pulmonary arteries; the signals are communicated to the hypothalamus. Nerve fibers from the hypothalamus directly synapse with cells in the posterior lobe of the pituitary gland, triggering release of antidiuretic hormone.

Antidiuretic hormone is a potent vasoconstrictor and thus has pressor effect. Antidiuretic hormone also acts on renal collecting ducts to promote reabsorption of water, which causes water retention.[23, 24]

Renin-Angiotensin

Following trauma, when blood flow through the kidneys is decreased, the juxtaglomerular cells secrete renin. Renin enzymatically cleaves a precursor protein to form angiotensin I, which is further cleaved to form angiotensin II. Angiotensin II is an extremely potent vasoconstrictor and has significant pressor effect. It also directly acts on the kidney to induce a decrease in salt and water excretion. Angiotensin II also stimulates the secretion of aldosterone, which further causes decreased excretion of both salt and water.[23, 25, 26]

Endogenous Opioids

Endogenous opioids are released from the pituitary gland as part of the initial stress response in an amount equimolar to that of ACTH. In addition, endorphins are released into the circulation from the adrenal glands in response to sympathetic stimulation.[27–29] The most evident role of endogenous opioids is to decrease pain. Endogenous opioids have other actions as well. For example, opioids modulate catecholamine release from the adrenal medulla, and they may exert inhibitory feedback on pituitary activation and decrease ACTH release. Furthermore, β-endorphin directly increases the secretion of insulin. Thus, the opioids may be important as counter-regulatory inhibitors of the stress response in addition to minimizing sensation of pain. Furthermore, the endogenous opioids may modulate normal neutrophil and lymphocyte function (including T cell function) and activate neutrophils, thus acting as modulators of the immune system and linking central nervous system responses to immune responses.[30] Negative effects of endogenous opioids on circulation and immune function have been postulated, and endorphins have also been implicated as mediators that may worsen brain injury.[31]

Locally Produced Mediators

In addition to mediators that are activated centrally, important mediator substances arise from sites of tissue injury and cause both local and systemic effects.

An important initiating event for the production of local mediators is endothelial disruption at sites of injury and ischemia.[32] Subendothelial collagen and basement membrane exposed by such endothelial disruption activate circulating Hageman factor (Factor XII). Hageman factor initiates coagulation via the intrinsic pathway. Activation of the protein clotting system also activates the kinin and plasmin systems.[33] In addition, activated Hageman factor triggers activation of the complement cascade, which initiates inflammation.[34, 35] Another important set of processes activated by injury, ischemia, and endothelial disruption is arachidonic acid metabolism; this metabolism results in substances such as prostaglandins and leukotrienes, which are potent mediators of vascular tone, and cause inflammation, cellular activation, and coagulation.[36, 37]

Another byproduct of arachidonic release from the cell membrane is platelet activating factor, which is a potent stimulator of platelet and neutrophil activation.[38, 39] Hence, platelet activating factor contributes to microvascular thrombosis at the site of injury (and perhaps systemically). Activation of neutrophils by platelet activating factor further contributes to tissue injury and inflammation.

Activation of coagulation and inflammation at sites of injury is an essential component of healing and recovery. However, these local processes may also amplify into systemic responses after major trauma, such that increased coagulation and inflammation manifest in tissues and organs distant from the sites of injury.[40] Cellular elements are fundamental to this amplification process as well. In particular, activation of monocytes and macrophages, with the resultant activation of cytokine cascades, helps to mediate many of the systemic, immunologic, and metabolic effects after trauma.[41, 42] Of particular importance may be TNF, IL-1, IL-6, and IL-8, which may be important mediators of the inflammatory and metabolic processes that occur after trauma. In addition, the activation of neutrophils by local mediators at the sites of injury as well as by cytokines may have an important contribution to both local and distant capillary occlusion and inflammation.[43–45]

Another important mediator after shock and trauma may be reperfusion injury.[46] Tissues that have been ischemic because of shock or tissue injury release toxic oxygen radicals on reperfusion, which may initiate both local and systemic tissue injury. The extent of this effect is directly proportionate to the degree of shock and tissue injury. Hence, reperfusion injury may be another important mediator of the systemic manifestations of shock and injury.

The gut may play a central role in the elaboration of mediators.[46] As the gut mucosa is highly sensitive to low blood flow following shock and trauma, it is subject to early injury. Gut ischemia may lead to the direct elaboration of inflammatory and reperfusion products. Furthermore, the gut mucosal barrier function may be quickly lost; as a result, bacteria and endotoxin may enter the portal circulation. This may lead to activation of cytokine cascades within the macrophages of the mesentery and liver.

THE PHYSIOLOGIC RESPONSES

Psychologic Response

Following major trauma, patients exhibit characteristic behaviors.[47, 48] These include immobilization, when patients are fearful of moving or interacting; withdrawal, when patients may cease being aware of their environment and become incommunicative; and antagonism, when patients may resist interaction and display hostility to those around them. During this time, patients experience anxiety, which tends to persist for the duration of the catabolic phase of their recovery.

Altered Vital Signs

Following trauma or major operation, vital signs are not normal; patients are typically febrile, hypertensive, tachycardiac, and tachypneic.

Fever is common in the hours and days following resuscitation from moderate to severe trauma or major operations. It may be caused by tissue inflammation and cytokine release.[49] Early fever is a normal and expected part of the physiologic response and does not indicate that infection is present. However, fever may persist for many days, and infection must be suspected as part of the differential diagnosis at this time. However, fever due to a noninfectious inflammatory response or to stimulation of the central nervous system in patients with head injury may persist without infectious cause.

Following fluid resuscitation after trauma, blood pressure may be low, normal, or high. Blood pressure correlates poorly with either blood volume or flow.[50] Tachycardia is caused by sympathetic stimulation and high levels of circulating catecholamines.[51] Following severe trauma, tachycardia typically persists even after hypovolemia has been corrected and pain controlled. This stress tachycardia may persist for days or weeks, and the return of heart rate toward the normal range often correlates with the onset of the anabolic phase of the flow period. In severe trauma or shock, however, tachycardia may not occur, and heart rate may be normal or decreased; this may seriously impair the compensatory hyperdynamic physiologic response that is necessary for recovery.

Increased minute ventilation, which is reflected by both the presence of tachypnea and an increase in tidal volume, is also an expected response following major operation or injury.[52] It is driven by increased catecholamine levels and sympathetic tone as well as by increased oxygen consumption and carbon dioxide production following trauma. In patients with very severe injury or limited pulmonary reserve, increased ventilatory demands may lead to the need for ventilatory support.

Urine output is often diminished early after trauma or operation because of hypovolemia, a decrease in renal blood flow, and a hormonal milieu that leads to sodium and water reabsorption. However, opposing factors tend to increase urine output, particularly the osmotic diuretic effects of the hyperglycemia that occurs following major trauma. In addition, resuscitation with large volumes of crystalloid solutions as well as commonly used osmotically active agents such as radiologic contrast media and mannitol increase urine output. Interpretation of urine output may be further complicated by the possibility of the early and occult onset of oliguric or nonoliguric renal failure. Thus, urine output may be decreased, normal, or increased following trauma, and may not accurately reflect the intravascular volume.[53]

Edema

The initial responses to trauma contribute to the preservation of body fluids. Vasoconstriction mediated by both the sympathetic nervous system and circulating hormones helps to reduce blood loss. Catecholamines, cortisol, aldosterone, and angiotensin II promote sodium retention, whereas antidiuretic hormone as well as aldosterone and angiotensin II promote water retention. Thus, after mild to moderate trauma, blood volume, interstitial volume, and intracellular volumes are preserved. However, with severe and prolonged trauma and stress, marked disturbances of the distribution of body water occur; there is flux of salt and water from the intravascular into the interstitial space. This results in intravascular hypovolemia, even though an excess of total body salt and water as well as edema are present. An important cause of edema formation in the site of injury is inflammation with loss of capillary integrity. Inflammation within the wound, however, is only part of the phenomenon, because edema soon becomes generalized and is present within tissues distant from the injury.[54] This systemic edema formation does not necessarily involve capillary endothelial damage and protein leakage but may also be due to altered capillary physiology, leading to salt and water loss. The presence of circulating and local vasoactive mediators and an increase in sympathetic tone for prolonged periods cause postcapillary venular vasoconstriction and a resultant increase in intraluminal capillary pressure. Hypoproteinemia also decreases intravascular oncotic pressure. These factors, in addition to inflammation, increase the egress of salt and water from the capillaries. The magnitude of edema formation tends to be proportionate to the severity of injury and is progressive as long as the stress state persists. In order to maintain intravascular volume during this period, large volumes of intravenous fluids must be given, and maintenance of positive fluid balance is required. In fact, the more the edema progresses, the greater the amounts of fluid that are required to maintain intravascular volume because the volume of distribution of salt and water into the interstitium increases. It is difficult to clinically assess the intravascular volume in such patients; intravascular hypovolemia is frequently inadequately corrected in this setting.

Increased Cardiac Output

The initial stress response tends to maintain blood pressure by vasoconstriction, even if circulating blood volume is significantly decreased. Heart rate and cardiac contractility are increased, and this tends to maintain cardiac output. However, the combination of blood loss and fluid shifts from the intravascular into the interstitial spaces often results in decreased preload, such that cardiac output is decreased in the hours following trauma. This may be exacerbated during anesthesia, as nearly all anesthetic agents are cardiac depressants. As bleeding is controlled and resuscitation restores intravascular volume, cardiac output reaches supernormal levels and a hyperdynamic circulatory state is reached.[55, 56] This state is characterized by rapid heart rate, increased blood pressure, and increased cardiac output. The intensity of this hyperdynamic state and its duration are generally proportionate to the severity of shock and trauma or to the magnitude of operation. The return of the circulation to normal is an important indicator that recovery is progressing and that the stress response to trauma is waning.

Impaired Oxygen Transport

Microcirculatory blood flow may be markedly altered early following trauma. Vasoconstriction, mediated by sympathetic nerves, circulating catecholamines, vasopressin, angiotensin II, and local vasoconstrictors (such as kinins, histamines, and prostanoids) may be pronounced. Nitrogen oxide is a potent vasodilator produced by endothelium; it is possible that decreased nitrogen oxide production may also decrease microcirculatory flow after trauma.[57] Within constricted capillary beds, the tendency for endothelial adherence of circulating cells is increased, particularly that of polymorphonuclear leukocytes and platelets; this tendency may be augmented by activation and an increase in the adhesiveness of these cells by such mediators as platelet activating factor, TNF, IL-1, and complement as well as by the stress hormones and neurotransmitters.[58] The combination of microcirculatory vasoconstriction and leukocyte and platelet adhesion to the endothelium of constricted capillaries leads to a decrease in tissue perfusion in certain areas. This disturbance may be further exacerbated by the activated clotting system after trauma, particularly in areas of microcirculatory stasis; intravascular thrombosis within small vessels results. Another factor that may contribute to impaired oxygen transport to the cells is edema formation. An increased distance for oxygen diffusion between capillaries and cells may have an adverse effect on the delivery of both oxygen and nutritional substrate, particularly if such an increase is combined with altered microcirculatory blood flow.

Hypermetabolism

Following trauma, energy demands increase to supernormal levels.[1, 2, 50, 56, 59] Metabolism, as measured by oxygen consumption, increases to supernormal levels. The degree of hypermetabolism is generally related to severity of injury. Following major elective operation, patients may increase metabolic rates by 10% to 25%; in contrast, following major injury, patients may more than double basal metabolic rates. This hypermetabolic state is closely related to the hyperdynamic circulatory state; that is, those patients with very high metabolic requirements require greatly increased oxygen delivery and, thus, a hyperdynamic circulation with supernormal cardiac outputs. As oxygen consumption increases, so too does carbon dioxide production. Therefore, an increase in minute ventilation is needed; this is achieved through increases in both tidal volume and respiratory rate mediated by sympathetic nerves and circulating catecholamines.

Inflammatory substances, such as cytokines, are important mediators of the post-traumatic hypermetabolic state. TNF, IL-1, and IL-6 have been studied best. Wilmore[2] has shown, in volunteers, that the creation of sterile inflammation by injection of an inflammatory agent leads to many of the components of the hypermetabolic stress response. However, the complete manifestation of the stress response to injury was seen only when the hormones cortisol, glucagon, and epinephrine were infused in the presence of inflammation. Hence, the hypermetabolic response appears to be mediated by a combination of central stress responses and tissue inflammation.

The importance of inflammatory mediators in the post-traumatic hypermetabolic state is further suggested by a striking clinical similarity between trauma and sepsis. Fever, chills, shivering, and altered sensorium are frequent and expected responses to trauma just as they are to sepsis; they may be due to many of the same mediators. As a result, making a clinical diagnosis of infection following trauma may be exceedingly difficult.

Altered Protein Metabolism

Following severe trauma, marked alterations of protein metabolism occur.[59, 60] Total-body protein catabolism is increased, particularly within skeletal muscles. Total-body protein synthesis is also increased, particularly hepatic synthesis of acute-phase proteins. The mediators of altered protein metabolism include the stress hormones, the sympathetic nervous system, and cytokines, particularly TNF, IL-1, and IL-6. In addition, growth hormone may have an important role. Growth hormone exerts potent anabolic effects to increase the incorporation of amino acid into protein. The biologic activity of growth hormone is mediated by peptides called *somatomedins*, which are produced in the liver. A decrease in the production of somatomedin and somatomedin inhibitors as well as of complement and prostanoids may all interfere with growth hormone activity after trauma.

The amino acids necessary to fuel hepatic protein synthesis are derived from peripheral protein breakdown, particularly that of skeletal muscle. The increase in protein synthesis occurs to a lesser degree than does catabolism. Hence, a net loss of protein mass and a loss of nitrogen in the urine occur; the latter loss can be measured as negative nitrogen balance. Following severe injury, protein breakdown results in a significant loss of muscle mass and may progress to the loss of visceral protein mass as well. The wound appears to be spared to some extent; wound inflammation and some degree of healing tend to progress despite the existence of a catabolic state. Nonetheless, if it is severe, post-trauma catabolism can seriously impair wound healing. With aggressive nutritional support, protein synthesis may be sufficiently enhanced to achieve nitrogen equilibrium; however, a high rate of protein breakdown persists for the duration of the stress response, regardless of nutritional support.

The nature of both protein breakdown and of protein synthesis following injury is complex. For example, following muscle protein breakdown, amino acids are not simply released into the circulation. Rather, the branched-chain amino acids valine, leucine, and isoleucine are converted within the muscle into glutamate and keto acids. Glutamate may be metabolized within muscle to glutamine or alanine, whereas keto acids may be utilized by muscle for energy. The result is that the concentration of amino acids released into the circulation may be altered, with a relative increase of alanine and glutamine and a relative decrease of branched-chain amino acids. Glutamine is tissue trophic, particularly for the gut mucosa, and is rapidly cleared, such that in severe stress states glutamine levels may be decreased (despite increased production). Increased glutamine uptake is stimulated by both TNF and IL-1.

The nature of protein synthesis is also altered following injury. Despite increased amino acid uptake by the liver, the synthesis of albumin is depressed. A large portion of the amino acids are utilized for energy production by gluconeogenesis, with a resultant increase in urea production. Nonetheless, an overall increase in hepatic protein synthesis, with a shift toward synthesis of acute-phase proteins (e.g., proteins of inflammation, fibrinogen, and haptoglobin). This alteration in hepatic protein synthesis is importantly influenced by the stress hormones as well as by inflammatory cytokines.[62]

Altered Glucose Metabolism

The stress hormones cortisol, glucagon, and epinephrine increase the breakdown of glycogen to glucose; this response rapidly depletes glycogen stores following injury.[2, 59, 63, 64] Glucose is also produced by gluconeogenesis from alanine and other amino acids released by skeletal muscle breakdown. Hence, skeletal muscle breakdown in the stress state also contributes to increased glucose production. As the wound consumes much of the available glucose, and as anaerobic metabolism predominates in injured tissue, much of the glucose is converted to lactate; lactate is recycled in the liver in the Cori cycle, fueling additional glucose production. The energy to resynthesize glucose comes primarily from fat oxidation in the liver; hence, fat stores are also depleted by processes to produce glucose. The net effect of increased glucose production is to increase extracellular glucose concentrations. The increase in glucose provides energy for wounds and the inflammatory process; macrophages and leukocytes also utilize the increase in glucose following injury.

Insulin levels are initially low following injury, but subsequently increase to normal or supernormal levels. Nonetheless, following severe injury, hyperglycemia persists. This insulin resistance may be primarily due to the persistent elevation of glucagon, cortisol, and epinephrine levels. Insulin has as two of its major functions inhibition of the rate of hepatic glucose production and stimulation of glucose uptake in peripheral tissues. Therefore, the insulin resistance of the stress state may be central to persistent hyperglycemia as well as to muscle, fat, and glycogen breakdown.

Altered Fat Metabolism

In health, lipids constitute more than 80% of stored fuel reserves. Most tissues can readily use fatty acids as substrates for energy metabolism, preserving glucose substrate for the brain, red blood cells, and cells of inflammation and wound healing. Following injury, fat is oxidized at an accelerated rate; this effect is mediated by sympathetic stimulation, increase in epinephrine, glucagon, and cortisol levels, and insulin resistance.[64] A high intracellular concentration of fatty acids as well as elevated glucagon levels inhibit fatty acid synthesis. Hence, fatty acids are released into the circulation and become available as energy substrate. However, there are limitations to fat mobilization following stress. For example, increased lactate stimulates re-esterification within the adiposities, resulting in the futile (and energy-requiring) cycling of fat. Further, hyperglycemia may inhibit lipolysis and also may stimulate re-esterification.[65] In summary, although the stress response generally results in mobilization of fat into free fatty acids, there are important limitations to this effect.

Altered Coagulation and Inflammation

Important changes of coagulation occur following injury, including activation of both clotting and fibrinolytic systems. However, early after major injury, impairment of clotting often occurs: after blood loss and fluid replacement with banked blood or crystalloid fluids, circulating protein clotting factors and platelets are diluted. In addition, hypothermia, which frequently occurs following injury and operation, markedly impairs clotting. These factors tend to impair clotting early after injury. However, the clotting system is simultaneously activated.[66, 67] This activation is triggered by the release of tissue thromboplastin by injured tissue; this activates the extrinsic coagulation system. Subendothelial collagen and basement membrane exposed by trauma activate Hageman factor (Factor XII) to initiate coagulation (the intrinsic pathway). Activation of the protein clotting system also activates the kinin and plasmin systems. Activated Factor XII cleaves kininogen into bradykinin, a substance that disrupts endothelium; this contributes to edema, inflammation, and clotting. Activated factor XII also leads to conversion of plasminogen into plasmin.

Trauma, through its activation of Factor XII and kinin, also triggers complement activation. Kinin also activates complement. Adrenergic discharge, the stress hormones, stimulation of arachidonic acid metabolism, and activation of the clotting and complement cascades initiate and amplify coagulation and inflammation at the site of tissue damage. These processes are amplified further by platelets, monocytes, macrophages, and neutrophils.

Leukocytosis

Trauma is usually followed by leukocytosis, especially granulocytosis. Lymphocyte counts may be decreased, whereas monocyte counts may be increased. This pattern mimics that of sepsis, but it often occurs without infection. In addition to the increase in circulating neutrophil concentrations, an increase in the numbers of neutrophils within the capillary beds also appears to occur early after trauma. This effect may be initiated by the early vasoconstriction after injury and shock. In severe trauma, this effect may predominate, and leukopenia may be seen. Most of the neutrophils initially trapped in the microcirculation are probably subsequently released; this contributes to leukocytosis. However, a variable number of neutrophils may remain in the capillaries, particularly if resuscitation is delayed; these neutrophils may then be primed by tissue mediators and contribute to tissue ischemia and inflammation.

Altered Immunity

Following trauma, the immune response is markedly altered. The extent of immune disturbance is proportionate to the magnitude of injury or operation. The abnormalities seen after trauma or operation include a decrease in antibody response, a decrease in neutrophil chemotaxis, a decrease in delayed-type hypersensitivity, an increase in neutrophil adherence, an increase in serum immunosuppressive factors, a decrease in fibronectin levels, and a reduction in serum opsonic activity.[68, 69] The alterations of immunity are mediated by many factors, including the central neurohormonal stress response, activation of suppressor monocytes, and substances released by the inflammatory response, such as prostaglandins and cytokines.

THE ANABOLIC PHASE OF THE FLOW CYCLE

The second phase of the flow cycle of injury represents the anabolic and recovery phase of the injury response. During this period, each physiologic alteration that occurred during the catabolic phase may be reversed.

The onset of the recovery phase is heralded by a sense of well-being. Catecholamine and cortisol levels return to normal, as do temperature, heart rate, and blood pressure. Respiratory demands decrease; patients who required mechanical ventilatory support can usually be weaned from ventilators. Patients have increased urine output and negative fluid balances, and edema resolves. Metabolic demands decrease. Gut function improves, and appetite returns. Visceral and muscle protein is re-synthesized, allowing recovery of organ function and physical rehabilitation.

This reversal process does not occur quickly. The anabolic phase of recovery generally takes longer than the acute injury and catabolic phases, and thus may last many days or weeks. During this period, patients require psychologic support, nutritional support, and physical rehabilitation for complete recovery to occur. Often, the psychologic effects of trauma are the slowest to recover: a post-traumatic stress syndrome may result.[47, 70]

SUMMARY

Trauma, either accidental or surgical, results in alteration of nearly all physiologic systems. The stress response to trauma is triggered by the psychologic and physical perception of pain, injury, and shock. The response is mediated by the central nervous system, circulating hormones, substances produced in response to local inflammation acting both locally and systemically, and activated circulating cells. The magnitude of this response and its duration are proportionate to the degree of injury. Anesthesia diminishes the perception of injury and may thus diminish the magnitude of the stress response to injury.

During successful recovery, all physiologic disturbances may be reversed. However, following severe trauma, the stress response may require intensive interventional support and may thus be perceived as critical illness. As physiologic reserve is already stressed by trauma, complications superimposed upon this process are of major significance and often lead to severe illness or death. Only with an understanding of the usual physiologic responses to injury can these complications be recognized, understood in context, and optimally managed.

References

1. Cuthbertson DP: Post-shock metabolic responses. Lancet 1942; i:433.

2. Wilmore DW: Homeostasis: Bodily changes in trauma and surgery. *In*: Textbook of Surgery. 13th ed. Sabiston DC Jr (Ed). Philadelphia, WB Saunders, 1986, pp 23–37.
3. Hume DM, Egdahl RH: The importance of the brain in the endocrine response to injury. Ann Surg 1959; 150:697–712.
4. Rose RM: Endocrine responses to stressful psychologic events. Psychiatr Clin North Am 1980; 3:251–277.
5. Vielacres EC, Hollifield M, Katon WJ, et al: Sympathetic nervous system activity in panic disorder. Psychol Res 1987; 21:213–221.
6. Salmon P, Pear S, Smith CC, et al: The relationship of preoperative distress to endocrine and subjective responses to surgery: Support for Janis' theory. J Behav Mod 1988; 11:599–613.
7. Gann DS, Lilly MP: The neuroendocrine response to multiple trauma. World J Surg 1983; 7:101–118.
8. Kehlet H, Brandt MR, Rem J: Role of neurogenic stimuli in mediating the endocrine-metabolic response to surgery. JPEN J Parenter Enteral Nutr 1980; 4:152.
9. Zaloga GP: Catecholamines in anesthetic and surgical stress. Int Anesthesiol Clin 1988; 26:187–198.
10. DeMaria EJ, Lilly MP, Gann DS: Potential hormonal responses in a model of traumatic injury. J Surg Res 1987; 43:45–51.
11. Rea RF, Hamdan M, Clary MP, et al: Comparison of muscle sympathetic responses to hemorrhage and lower body negative pressure in humans. J Appl Physiol 1991; 70:1401–1405.
12. Cunningham DJ: Studies on arterial chemoreceptors in man. J Physiol 1987; 385:1–26.
13. Stotman GJ, Jed EH, Burchard KW: Adverse effects of hypothermia in post-operative patients. Am J Surg 1985; 149:495–501.
14. Reed HL, Chernow B, Lake CR, et al: Alterations in sympathetic nervous system activity with intraoperative hypothermia during coronary artery bypass surgery. Chest 1989; 95:616–622.
15. Bitterman H, Kinarty A, Lazarovich H, et al: Acute release of cytokines is proportional to tissue injury induced by surgical trauma and shock in rats. J Clin Immunol 1991; 11:184–192.
16. Jäättelä A, Ahlo A, Avihainen V, et al: Plasma catecholamines in severely injured patients: A prospective study on 45 patients with multiple injuries. Br J Surg 1975; 177:62.
17. Hutter JB, Pflug AE, Porte D: Mechanisms of plasma catecholamines increases during surgical stress in man. J Clin Endocrinol Metab 1977; 45:936.
18. Maddens M, Sowers J: Catecholamines in critical care. Crit Care Clin 1987; 3:871–872.
19. Breslow MJ, Ligier B: Hyperadrenergic states. Crit Care Med 1991; 19:1566–1579.
20. Darmaun D, Matthews PE, Bier DM: Physiologic hypercortisolemia increases proteolysis, glutamine and alanine production. Am J Physiol 1988; 255:E366–E373.
21. Harris MJ, Baker RT, McRoberts JW, et al: The adrenal response to trauma, operation, and cosyntropin stimulation. Surg Gynecol Obstet 1990; 170:513–516.
22. DePadova F, Pozzi C, Tonere MJ, et al: Selective and early increase of IL-1 inhibitors, IL-6 and cortisol after elective surgery. Clin Exp Immunol 1991; 85:137–142.
23. Hilton JG, Marullo DS: Trauma-induced increases in plasma vasopressin and angiotensin II. Life Sci 1987; 41:2195–3000.
24. Judd BA, Haycock GB, Dalton RN, et al: Anti-diuretic hormone following surgery in children. Acta Paediatr Scand 1990; 79:491–496.
25. Udelsman R, Norton JA, Jelenich SE, et al: Responses of the hypothalamic-pituitary-adrenal and renin-angiotensin axes and the sympathetic system during controlled surgical and anesthetic stress. J Clin Endocrinol Metab 1987; 64:986–994.
26. Starc TJ, Staluip SA: Time course changes of plasma renin activity and catecholamines during hemorrhage in conscious sheep. Circ Shock 1987; 21:129–140.
27. Risch SC, Kalin NH, Janowsky DS, et al: Co-release of ACTH and beta-endorphin immuno-reactivity in human subjects in response to central cholinergic stimulation. Science 1983; 222:77.
28. Schadt JC: Sympathetic and hemodynamic adjustments to hemorrhage: A possible role for endogenous opioid peptides. Resuscitation 1989; 18:219–228.
29. Lloyd DA, Teich S, Rowe NI: Serum endorphin levels in injured children. Surg Gynecol Obstet 1991; 172:449–452.
30. Deitch EA, Xu D, Bridges RM: Opioids modulate human neutrophil and lymphocyte function: Thermal injury alters plasma beta-endorphin levels. Surgery 1988; 104:41–48.
31. McIntosch TK, Hayes RL, Dewittl DS, et al: Endogenous opioids may mediate secondary damage after experimental brain injury. Am J Physiol 1987; 253:E565–E574.
32. McEver RP: Role of the endothelium on the inflammatory response. *In*: Critical Care: State of the Art. Vol 12. Fullerton, CA, Society of Critical Care Medicine, 1991, pp 121–138.
33. Ellis EF, Holt SA, Wei EP, Kontas HA: Kinins induce abnormal vascular reactivity. Am J Physiol 1988; 255:397–400.
34. Fosse E, Mollnes TE, Aasen AO, et al: Complement activation following multiple injuries. Acta Chir Scand 1987; 153:325–330.
35. Zimmerman T, Laszik Z, Nagy S, et al: The role of the complement system in the pathogenesis of multiple organ failure in shock. Prog Clin Biol Res 1989; 308:291–297.
36. Kuehl FA, Egan RW: Prostaglandins, arachidonic acid, and inflammation. Science 1980; 210:978–984.
37. Vane JR, Botting RM: Prostaglandins, prostacyclin, thromboxane and leukotrienes: The arachidonic acid cascade. *In*: Critical Care: State of the Art. Vol 12. Fullerton, CA, Society of Critical Care Medicine, 1989, pp 1–23.
38. Feuerstein G, Siren AL: Platelet-activation factor and shock. Prog Biochem Pharm 1988; 22:181–190.
39. Feuerstein G, Jue TL, Lysko PG: Platelet-activating factor: A putative mediator in central nervous system injury. Stroke 1990; 21:90–94.
40. Nuytinck HK, Offermass XJ, Kubat K, et al: Whole-body inflammation in trauma patients: An autopsy study. Arch Surg 1988; 123:1519–1524.
41. Michie HR, Wilmore DW: Sepsis, signals, and surgical sequelae (a hypothesis). Arch Surg 1990; 125:531–536.
42. Eslcay RL, Grino M, Chen HT: Interleukins, signal transduction, and the immune system–mediated stress response. Adv Exper Med Biol 1990; 274:331–343.
43. Christou NV, Tellado JM: In-vitro polymorphonuclear neutrophil function in surgical patients does not correlate with energy but with "activity" processes such as sepsis or trauma. 1989; Surgery 106:718–722.
44. Tanaka H, Ogura H, Yokata J, et al: Acceleration of superoxide production from leukocytes in trauma patients. Ann Surg 1991; 214:187–192.
45. Leff JA, Repine JE: Blood cells and ischemia-reperfusion injury. Blood Cells 1990; 16:183–191.
46. Wilmore DW, Smith RJ, O'Dwyer ST, et al: The gut: A central organ after surgical stress. Surgery 1988; 104:917–923.
47. Weisalth L: The stressors and the post-traumatic stress syndrome after an industrial disaster. Acta Psychiatr Scand 1989; 355:25–37.
48. Achterberg J, Kenner C, Casey P: Behavioral strategies for the reduction of pain and anxiety associated with orthopedic trauma. Biofeedback Self Regul 1989; 14:101–114.
49. Briese E, Cabana CM: Stress hyperthermia: Physiological arguments that it is a fever. Physiol and Behav 1991; 49:1153–1157.
50. Shoemaker WC: Pathophysiology, monitoring, outcome prediction, and therapy of shock states. Crit Care Clin 1987; 3:307–357.
51. Bahnsor RR, Anduole GL, Clayman RJ, et al: Catecholamine excess: Probable cause of post-operative tachycardia following retroperitoneal lymph node dissection for testicular carcinoma. J Surg Oncol 1989; 42:132–135.
52. Tulla H, Takala J, Alhaoa E, et al: Respiratory changes after open-heart surgery. Intensive Care Med 1991; 17:365–369.
53. Sladen RN: Effect of anesthesia and surgery on renal function. Crit Care Clin 1987; 3:373–393.
54. Demling RH, Lalonde C, Liu YP, et al: The lung inflammatory response to thermal injury: Relationship between physiologic and histologic changes. Surgery 1989; 106:52–59.
55. Clowes GHA, Del Guerco LR, Barwinsky J: The cardiac output in response to surgical trauma. Arch Surg 1960; 81:212–222.
56. Waxman K: Hemodynamic and metabolic changes during and following operation. Crit Care Clin 1987; 3:241–250.
57. Ochoa JB, Udekwa AO, Billiar TR, et al: Nitrogen oxide levels in patients after trauma and during sepsis. Am Surg 1991; 214:621–626.

58. Davis JM, Albert JD, Tracy KJ, et al: Increased neutrophil mobilization and decreased chemotaxis during cortisol and epinephrine infusions. J Trauma 1991; 31:725–731.
59. Cerra FB: Hypermetabolism–organ failure syndrome: A metabolic response to injury. Crit Care Clin 1989; 5:289–302.
60. Ressey PQ, Jian ZM, Johnson DJ, et al: Post-traumatic skeletal muscle proteolysis: The role of the hormonal environment. World J Surg 1989; 13:465–470.
61. Hall K, Tally M: The somatomedin-insulin–like growth factors. J Intern Med 1989; 225:47–54.
62. Bankey PE, Mazuski JE, Ortiz M, et al: Hepatic acute phase protein synthesis is indirectly regulated by tumor necrosis factor. J Trauma 1990; 30:1181–1187.
63. Wolfe RR, Klein S, Herndon DN, et al: Substrate cycling in thermogenesis and amplification of net substrate flux in human volunteers and burned patients. J Trauma 1990; 30:56–59.
64. Long CL, Nelson KM, Atkin JM, et al: A physiologic basis for the provision of fuel mixtures in normal and stressed patients. J Trauma 1990; 30:1077–1085.
65. Jeevanandam M, Young DH, Schuler WR: Nutritional impact on the energy cost of fat fuel mobilization in poly-trauma patients. J Trauma 1990; 30:147–154.
66. Greenberg CS, Sane DC: Coagulation problems in critical care medicine. *In*: Critical Care Medicine: State of the Art. Vol 11. Fullerton, CA, Society of Critical Care Medicine, 1990, pp 187–215.
67. Meakins JL: Host defense mechanisms in surgical patients: Effect of surgery and trauma. Acta Chir Scand 1989; 550:43–51.
68. Christou NV: Immune system dysfunction in multiple organ failure. *In*: Critical Care Medicine: State of the Art. Vol 9. Fullerton, CA, Society of Critical Care Medicine, 1988, pp 143–160.
69. Grunert BK, Smith CJ, Swine CA, et al: Early psychological aspects of severe hand injury. J Hand Surg 1988; 13:177–180.

CHAPTER 152

Anesthesia in the High-Risk Patient

Steven J. Barker, PhD, MD

A proverb among anesthesiologists states: "There may be minor operations, but there are no minor anesthetics." Even though all generalizations are false (including this one), anesthesia in trauma and other critically ill patients obviously engenders serious risks. These patients may have injuries that are life threatening and yet are not diagnosed when anesthesia is administered. They are not "optimized" for surgery in the sense of chronically ill patients undergoing elective procedures, in whom we have the luxury of obtaining consults from specialists and multiple laboratory studies for the purpose of adjusting medical therapy. Their intravascular volume status is often unknown, but they are usually hypovolemic. The medical histories are incomplete or nonexistent. Despite all of these factors, the anesthesiologist must administer anesthetic agents and other toxic drugs in doses that are, one hopes, sublethal.

In this chapter, some of the primary anesthetic considerations in critically ill patients, with emphasis on the acute trauma victim, are reviewed. This subject could occupy several volumes, and this discussion is not presented in great depth or detail. However, the viewpoint of the anesthesiologist in evaluating and treating these patients is presented in the hope that this knowledge will benefit all members of the critical care team.

PREOPERATIVE EVALUATION

History and Physical Examination

The preanesthetic evaluation of the trauma victim can begin before the patient reaches the emergency room. The nature and time of the injury, vital signs in the field, and paramedic therapy are important data that are often available by radio. In the ideal trauma center, an anesthesiologist is a member of the resuscitation team in the emergency room.[1] During the early resuscitation and evaluation, some history can usually be obtained from the patient or family as well as from paramedics or police.

Much of the information the anesthesiologist needs is the same as that being sought by the surgeon: the nature and extent of all injuries, vital signs and level of consciousness since the accident, and adequacy of the airway, ventilation, and circulation. In addition, the anesthesiologist must try to acquire other data that will affect anesthetic management. These include (1) all medications being taken and for what reason, (2) the status of any chronic medical problems, (3) surgical and anesthetic history, (4) use of alcohol, tobacco, or recreational drugs, and (5) relevant family history such as malignant hyperthermia. Even though "when did you eat last?" will always be asked, the anesthesiologist must treat every trauma patient and most other critically ill patients as having a full stomach.

Although complete data in all of these categories are rarely available, the astute clinician can collect much of it by being observant. In most trauma centers, a severity score of some sort is known before the patient's arrival. Table 152–1 shows the two most common systems in current use: the Glasgow Coma Scale (GCS) and the Trauma Score (TS).[2] The GCS is a neurologic status scale that is incorporated into the TS along with other scales for circulation and respiration. The neurologic assessment is particularly impor-

TABLE 152–1. Patient Severity Scales: Glasgow Coma Scale and Trauma Score

Glasgow Coma Scale		*Trauma Score*	
Eye Opening		*Systolic Blood Pressure (mm Hg)*	
Spontaneous	4	≥90	4
To voice	3	70–89	3
To pain	2	50–69	2
None	1	0–49	1
		No pulse	0
Verbal Responses		*Capillary Refill*	
Oriented	5	Normal	2
Confused	4	Delayed	1
Inappropriate words	3	None	0
Incomprehensible words	2		
None	1		
Motor Response		*Respiratory Rate (per minute)*	
Obeys command	6	10–24	4
Localizes pain	5	24–35	3
Withdraws (pain)	4	≥36	2
Flexion (pain)	3	1–9	1
Extension (pain)	2	None	0
None	1		
		Respiratory Expansion	
		Normal	1
		Retractive	0
		Glasgow Coma Scale	
		14–15	5
		11–13	4
		8–10	3
		5–7	2
		3–4	1
Totals	3–15		1–16

(Glasgow Coma Scale adapted with permission from Morris JA, Auerbach PS, Marshall GA, et al: The trauma score as a triage tool in the prehospital setting. JAMA 1986; 256:1319. Copyright 1986, American Medical Association.)

T	Trauma
I	Infection
P	Poison
P	Psychiatric
S	Shock
on	
A	Alcohol
E	Epilepsy
I	Insulin
O	Opiates
U	Urea/Metabolic

Figure 152–1. The differential diagnosis of altered mental status in the emergency room based on the mnemonic device "TIPPS on AEIOU."

tant to the anesthesiologist because it will often determine the urgency of obtaining a secured airway. A useful mnemonic for possible causes of altered level of consciousness, TIPPS on AEIOU, is shown in Figure 152–1.

The physical examination of the acute trauma victim is heavily influenced by urgency and available time. The seriously injured patient may require surgical intervention as quickly as he or she can be taken to the operating room, but even this situation permits a degree of preanesthetic examination. The assessment may begin with the ABCs: *A*irway, *B*reathing, and *C*irculation. Ask the patient to take a deep breath. The response to this simple command gives some indication of neurologic status (GCS) as well as the adequacy of both the airway and respirations. If no breath occurs, positive-pressure ventilation by mask should begin immediately, and preparations should be made for endotracheal intubation. While observing the response to the "breathe" command, one should palpate a radial pulse for rate, fullness, and intensity and auscultate a blood pressure as soon as possible. One must not wait for a measurement via an automated sphygmomanometer, which can cycle for several minutes before it is determined that there is no blood pressure.

If the patient exhibits adequate respirations and pulse, he or she is stable enough to continue the physical examination while being observed for stridor, retractions, or evidence of circulatory or neurologic changes. At this time, the patient should be receiving supplemental oxygen by mask and should be monitored by continuous pulse oximetry and electrocardiogram (ECG). The examination should proceed with an assessment of the intravascular volume status. Shock, whether hypovolemic or other, is a general state of inadequate tissue perfusion, which should be evident by clinical manifestations.[3] These include pallor, peripheral cyanosis, tachycardia and tachypnea, diaphoresis, oliguria, and disorientation. In the infant or small child, systolic blood pressure may be an indicator of volume status. Normal values of blood pressure and heart rate versus age are listed in Table 152–2. The adult autonomic system can usually maintain supine blood pressure near normal values until the acute volume deficit is 30% or more, making blood pressure a poor volume indicator in adult patients. Orthostatic testing is a more sensitive diagnostic of volume status but should be performed with caution in the trauma patient.[4] Tachycardia is an indicator of moderate volume deficits in adults, although this will also be influenced by pain and other factors.

Patients with neck injuries may suffer from spinal shock, during which hypotension may not be accompanied by tachycardia. Spinal shock is caused by a disruption of sympathetic outflow and manifests as low vascular resistance with increased intravascular capacity. Thus, the patient is functionally hypovolemic even if no blood has been lost. Initial hemoglobin or hematocrit values are of little help in determining acute blood loss; a patient in hypovolemic shock from acute hemorrhage may have a normal hemoglobin. Early bladder catheterization is very helpful in monitoring volume status and also provides indications of renal injuries.

Although hypotension in trauma patients usually signifies hypovolemia, the possibility of pericardial tamponade in chest trauma cannot be ignored. If this diagnosis is missed, the patient will surely die. Look for clinical signs of tamponade: hypotension with a quiet heart, jugular venous distention that increases with inspiration (Kussmaul's sign), dull sternal percussion, paradoxical pulse, electrical alternans, and diastolic equalization of filling pressures. Be wary also of other causes of hypotension in the acute trauma patient: tension pneumothorax (especially with rib fractures), pulmonary embolism (fractures, crush injuries), aortic tear or dissection, hypoxemia, acidosis, and even myocardial infarction. (Ask yourself, for example, "Why did the patient fall down the stairs?") Obviously, for any of these findings, prompt treatment must begin while the examination proceeds.

As preoperative preparation continues, the patient's neurologic status must be continually monitored for any deterioration in GCS, pupil reactivity, or motor and sensory function. The blunt trauma patient should be considered to have an unstable cervical spine until it is ruled out by both neurologic examination and a lateral radiograph in which C-7 is well visualized,[5] as shown in Figure 152–2. While awaiting radiographs in the spontaneously breathing patient, look for flaccidity, loss of rectal tone, diaphragmatic breathing, or hypotension with bradycardia (spinal shock). Radiographs alone cannot rule out cervical spine injury in a

TABLE 152–2. Normal Values of Blood Pressure and Heart Rate Versus Age

Age (year)	*Blood Pressure (mm Hg)* Systolic	*Blood Pressure (mm Hg)* Diastolic	*Heart Rate (beats per minute)*	
Newborn			120	
1	70	45	120	
2	80	60	110	
4	85	60	100	
6	90	60	100	
8	95	62	90	
10	100	65	90	
			Male	Female
12	108	67	85	90
14	112	70	80	85
16	118	75	75	80
18	120	80	70	75

(Adapted with permission from Stewart DJ: Manual of Pediatric Anesthesia. New York, Churchill Livingstone, 1979, pp 11–12.)

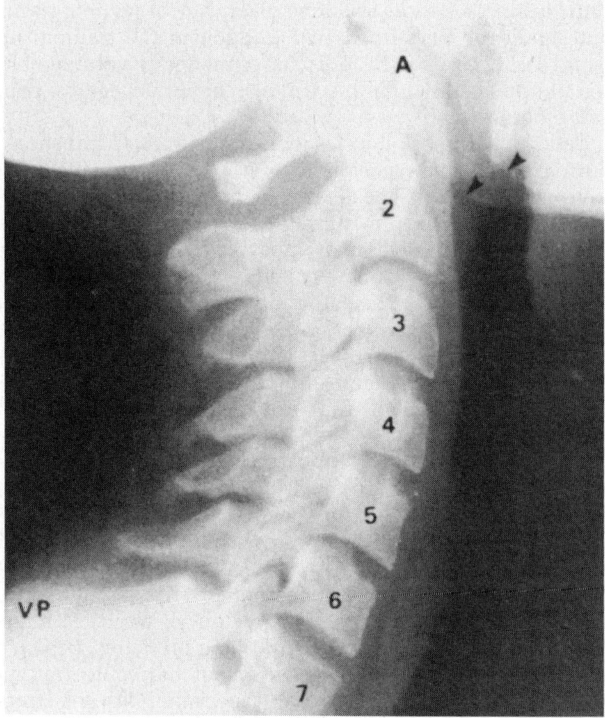

Figure 152–2. A normal lateral radiograph of the neck. Note the relationships of the numbered vertebral bodies, the anterior arch of C-1 (A), and the length of the spinous process of the vertebra prominens (VP), or C-7. (From Anderson JE: Grant's Atlas of Anatomy. Baltimore, Williams & Wilkins, 1978, p 5-4.)

comatose patient.[6] The physical examination should also be guided by the mechanism of injury or disease. Blunt trauma requires careful monitoring of pulmonary status (pulmonary contusion, pneumothorax) as well as circulation (myocardial contusion, aortic injury). Penetrating trauma demands early attention to potential injuries along the wound track, particularly those that may involve the heart or major vessels, viscera (especially liver or spleen), and airway.

In the nontrauma critical care patient who requires a surgical procedure, the anesthetic evaluation must also begin with the ABCs and neurologic status and then focus on the disease processes that make the patient critically ill. In the patient with gastrointestinal hemorrhage, one must perform an ongoing evaluation of intravascular volume, hemoglobin, and coagulation function. The intracerebral hemorrhage patient requires close attention to ventilation, with early institution of mechanical hyperventilation and other intracranial pressure (ICP) reduction maneuvers. The septic surgical patient demands continuous monitoring of both circulation and oxygenation, often including pulmonary artery catheterization to measure cardiac output and systemic vascular resistance.

Laboratory Studies

As with the history and physical examination, the required preanesthetic laboratory studies will be influenced by the time available to await the results. Whereas a patient with a bleeding aortic aneurysm must undergo surgery without delay, a patient with a closed femur fracture can await any indicated laboratory tests. When time permits, all trauma patients should have lateral cervical spine and anteroposterior chest radiographs, blood hemoglobin, and ECG. Other routine tests for major trauma include serum electrolyte determination, arterial blood gas analysis, coagulation profile (or at least platelet count), and urinalysis. Emergency surgery should not be delayed while awaiting the results of this second group.

For any case of blunt trauma and all but the most minor penetrating trauma, a blood specimen should be sent to the blood bank on admission. Criteria for obtaining a "type and screen," as opposed to a full type and crossmatch, will vary among institutions and with severity of injury. For example, at the University of California Irvine Medical Center, a type and screen takes about 20 minutes and type and crossmatch requires 30 to 40 minutes. Type-specific blood will cause a serious transfusion reaction in about 1 in 10,000 units; after a partial crossmatch the incidence is even lower.[7] Longer waiting times may be expected for platelet concentrates (30–60 minutes) and fresh frozen plasma (45 minutes).

PREPARATION

The success of an emergency anesthetic in the critically ill patient depends on careful preparation of both the patient and the operating suite. The operating room, which is often overlooked, should first be made warm. Virtually all trauma patients are hypothermic before surgery, and many become more so intraoperatively. Hypothermia causes peripheral vasoconstriction, dysrhythmias, coagulopathy, and shivering, leading to increased metabolic rate (see later discussion). Once established, hypothermia is difficult to reverse in the operating room. For major trauma, we recommend warming the operating room to about 30°C (86°F) before the patient enters the room. Because all intravenous fluids (especially blood) must be warmed to 37°C, appropriate high-volume fluid warmers must be set up in advance. A warming blanket should be placed on the operating table, and the ventilator circuit should include a functioning heater-humidifier.

In addition to a carefully checked anesthesia machine and ventilator, the required monitors (see later discussion) must be set up and calibrated before the patient enters the room. The anesthesia supply cart must include an appropriate assortment of laryngoscopes and endotracheal tubes as well as ventilating masks and airways. Drugs drawn into syringes should include rapid induction agents (thiopental, ketamine, etomidate), muscle relaxants, and pressors (epinephrine, phenylephrine). Airway equipment and emergency drugs should be located on top of the supply cart in an organized fashion, as shown in Figure 152–3. Antidysrhythmics, narcotics, and sedative-hypnotics should be in the cart. Large-bore (14- and 16-gauge) intravenous cannulas and 8-French or larger introducer sets for central access must also be at hand. Equipment for rapid institution of transtracheal jet ventilation (TTV) should be present, including a source of oxygen at approximately 50 psi with a push-button valve. Finally, a suction source with a large, rigid tip must be at the head of the operating table.

Preoperative preparation of the critically ill patient will usually concentrate on ensuring adequate oxygenation and perfusion. In the trauma patient, ensuring perfusion usually implies volume resuscitation. In head-injury patients, prevention of increased ICP also assumes a high priority. If there is any question regarding either oxygenation or ICP, the trachea should be intubated and mechanical ventilation instituted before the patient comes to the operating room. Criteria for early intubation and controlled ventilation are listed in Table 152–3. The obtunded or comatose patient should be hyperventilated to partial pressure of arterial carbon dioxide ($Pa{CO_2}$) values of 24 to 28 mm Hg, and pharmacologic therapy for ICP control (mannitol or furosemide)

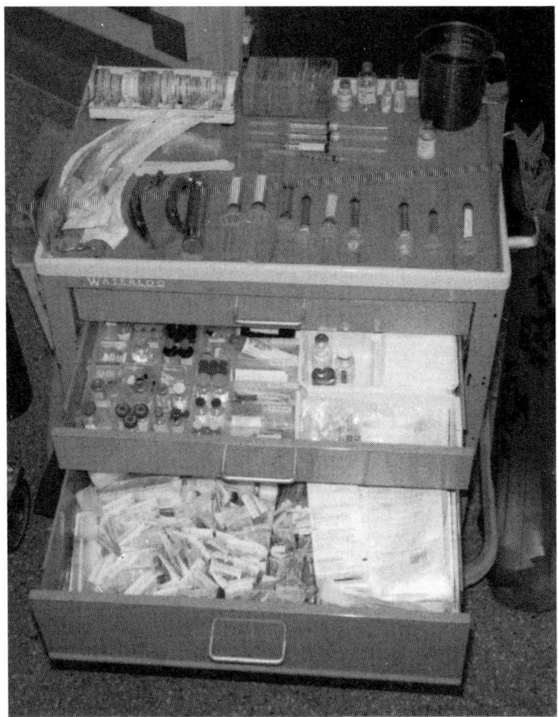

Figure 152–3. A well-prepared anesthesia supply cart. Airway equipment and drugs in syringes are organized clearly on the top of the cart.

should be instituted if volume status permits. Cervical spine precautions (including a collar) should be continued on all trauma patients unless the spine has been "cleared" by both radiography and neurologic examination (see prior discussion).

Adequate intravenous access should be established before the patient comes to the operating room. In the adult trauma patient, this implies a minimum of two 14- or 16-gauge peripheral cannulas placed in noninjured extremities. For patients with undiagnosed thoracic or abdominal injuries, one or more central cannulas of the "introducer" type are recommended. These can be inserted via the internal jugular, subclavian, or femoral route; obviously, they should not be inserted into or distal to injured vessels. Thus, the femoral approach should generally be avoided in suspected abdominal injuries. A 7-French introducer is a good volume catheter unless a pulmonary artery catheter is passed through it. An intra-arterial cannula should be inserted as early as possible for any craniotomy or thoracotomy and should be considered for any exploratory laparotomy.

Sedative or analgesic premedication should be used with extreme caution, particularly in the trauma setting. No sedative/analgesic drugs should be given to a nonintubated patient whose neurologic, respiratory, or hemodynamic status may be unstable. This criterion will eliminate most trauma patients, except those with isolated, painful, peripheral injuries, such as lacerations or fractures. If time permits, the trauma patient should receive preoperative antacid therapy, but only clear antacids (e.g., sodium citrate) should be used. Cimetidine and metoclopramide may be helpful only if they can be given 30 to 60 minutes before induction.[8] Metoclopramide is contraindicated in the acute abdomen. Emptying the stomach by means of a nasogastric tube is a reasonable precaution in many patients.

TABLE 152–3. Criteria for Early Endotracheal Intubation and Mechanical Ventilation of Trauma and Critically Ill Patients

1. Cardiac arrest
2. Clinical signs of shock
3. Hypoxia
4. Hypercarbia
5. Signs of developing airway obstruction
6. Head injury with decreased mental status
7. Burn injury with singed nasal hairs or soot in airway
8. Combativeness
9. Chest trauma with dyspnea

MONITORING

Required monitors for critically ill patients during anesthesia can be divided into two categories: noninvasive and invasive. Noninvasive monitors are virtually risk free, and a basic array of these should be used on every patient. These include ECG, sphygmomanometer, pulse oximeter, capnograph, core temperature probe, and stethoscope. The ECG should provide at least two continuous waveforms for monitoring of rate and rhythm and for diagnosis of ischemia. The combination of leads II and V_5 is probably the most sensitive for ischemia detection, and monitors with continuous ST-segment analysis may be helpful.[9] Although ST analysis may be the most reliable of the routine monitors for ischemia detection, it does not give the earliest possible warning of diminished coronary perfusion. As shown in Figure 152–4, the onset of ST changes may occur 10 minutes after the beginning of wall-motion abnormalities following partial coronary occlusion.

Automated sphygmomanometers are in such widespread use today that newly trained anesthesiologists may have little experience interpreting Korotkoff's sounds. However, the automated instruments often require unacceptably long measurement times in unstable patients, and they are least reliable during hypovolemic shock. The manual sphygmomanometer is still the best alternative to an arterial cannula in these patients, and its use as a back-up to the automated device is encouraged.

Pulse oximetry must be used continuously on the critically ill patient throughout the perioperative period, and capnography must be used during every general anesthetic. Both are considered minimum standards of intraoperative care by the American Society of Anesthesiologists.[10] Continuous temperature monitoring is also a minimum standard, and in the critically ill patient one must ensure that core temperature (esophageal or rectal) rather than skin temperature is being monitored.

Transcutaneous oxygen ($Ptco_2$) is a noninvasive monitor of the oxygen tension on heated skin. $Ptco_2$ is sensitive to skin perfusion as well as to arterial oxygen tension (Pao_2), and it will, therefore, change with volume status in the hypovolemic patient. The restoration of $Ptco_2$ to its "normal" value of roughly 80% of Pao_2 is one indication of adequate volume resuscitation.[11]

Although technically an invasive device, the urinary catheter should be considered a required monitor for all but the most superficially injured trauma patients. The catheter should be connected to a collection system that permits urine volume to be periodically measured to within 2 to 5 mL rather than to a simple uncalibrated urine bag. Urine volume measured every 15 to 30 minutes provides an important indication of both volume status and renal function. In addition, the appearance of hematuria or hemoglobinuria can warn of renal injury or transfusion reaction.

The most common invasive monitor in critically ill pa-

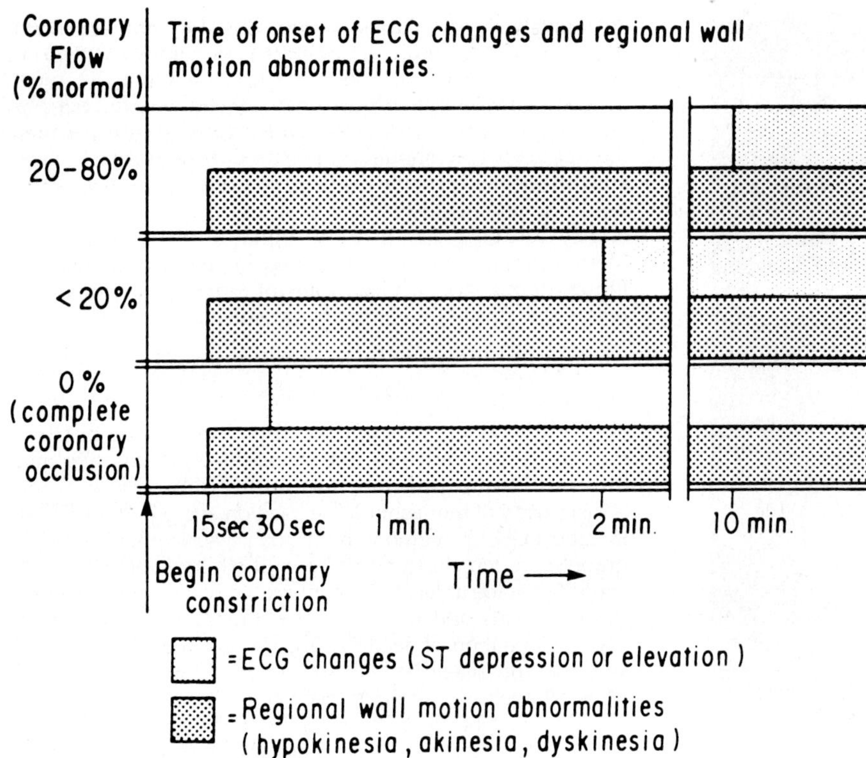

Figure 152–4. The temporal relationship between varying degrees of sudden coronary constriction and the onset of both ST-segment changes and regional wall motion abnormalities. ST-segment changes may occur 10 minutes or longer after a sudden decrease in coronary perfusion, whereas wall motion changes are almost immediate. (From Clements FM, DeBruijn NP: Electrocardiography: Monitoring for ischemia. *In:* Clinical Monitoring. Lake CL (Ed). Philadelphia, WB Saunders, 1990, p 41.)

tients is the arterial cannula, which should be inserted preoperatively (time permitting) in any patient with hemodynamic instability or questionable oxygenation/ventilation status. A rare exception to this policy may be the patient with bleeding aortic aneurysm who must be anesthetized quickly and without preoperative painful stimulation. The distal radial artery is the most common site used, but in the absence of distal pulses the brachial or axillary artery is acceptable with a low incidence of complications. The femoral artery is less convenient and carries a greater risk of

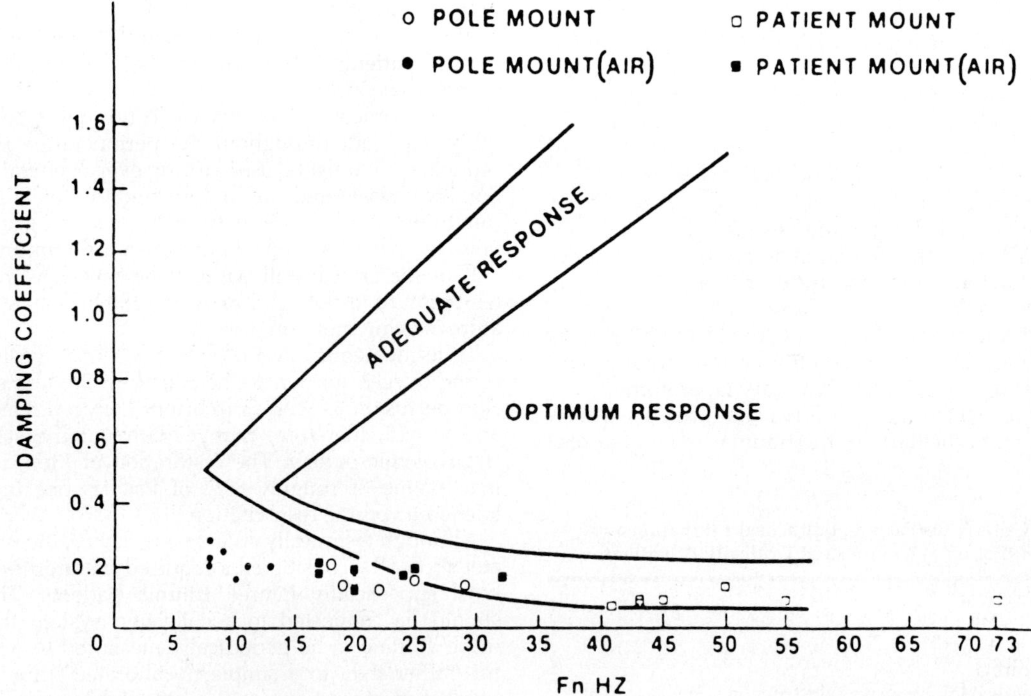

Figure 152–5. The relationship between damping coefficient and resonant frequency required to maintain an adequate response in a transducer and fluid-filled tubing pressure monitoring system. Data points represent seven disposable transducer-tubing systems with two different tubing lengths, with and without the presence of air bubbles in the system. (From Hunziker P: Accuracy and dynamic response of disposable pressure transducer–tubing systems. Can J Anaesth 1987; 34:409.)

infection, but it is an acceptable site if the upper extremity cannot be cannulated. All transducers and fluid-filled tubing pressure monitoring systems are subject to artifacts that distort the waveform and may cause errors in pressure measurement. The user should be aware of the resonant frequency and damping coefficient of the measurement system and the effects these values will have on the pressure waveform. Figure 152–5 illustrates the desired relationship between resonant frequency and damping coefficient for adequate system response and shows data points from several common disposable transducer-tubing systems.

Central venous pressure monitoring should be considered in patients who are hemodynamically unstable or who may have significant hemorrhage. In serious abdominal or pelvic trauma, the femoral veins should be avoided, as noted previously. In blunt chest trauma, particularly with rib fractures, the risk of pneumothorax must be considered when using the internal jugular or subclavian approach. Central venous cannulas should be of the introducer type, which allow the passage of a pulmonary artery catheter through a sheath. Pulmonary artery catheterization may be indicated in cases of massive transfusion (e.g., liver injuries), impaired left ventricular function (myocardial contusion or infarction), pulmonary edema, or radical changes in vascular resistance (sepsis). Table 152–4 lists some common indications for perioperative pulmonary artery catheterization. Pulmonary artery oximetry, which provides continuous monitoring of mixed venous oxygen saturation, can also be helpful in critically ill patients. Continuous ICP monitoring should be considered in the patient with a closed head injury and altered mental status. The risks of invasive monitoring must always be weighed against the potential benefits in critically ill patients.[12, 13]

AIRWAY MANAGEMENT

Management of the airway of the critically ill patient is one of the greatest challenges facing the anesthesiologist. Trauma patients and all others with possible intestinal ileus must be considered to have full stomachs and, hence, are at high risk for pulmonary aspiration. Because they are often hypovolemic, they may not tolerate a "rapid-sequence induction" in which intravenous anesthetics and muscle relaxants are given as a bolus to secure the airway quickly. Furthermore, these patients may have airway or central nervous system injuries that impair their ability to breathe adequately. Their injuries or their anatomy may also make them difficult to intubate by direct laryngoscopy.[14] Cervical spine trauma can put them at risk for spinal cord injury during intubation. The anesthesiologist must often act quickly and with incomplete patient data to secure a deteriorating airway. Despite the risk of aspiration or spinal cord injury, the avoidance of hypoxemia takes the highest priority at all times.

TABLE 152–4. Indications for Perioperative Pulmonary Artery Catheterization and Monitoring

Major procedures involving large fluid shifts and/or blood loss in patients with coronary artery disease
Patients with recent myocardial infarctions or unstable angina
Patients with poor left ventricular function (congestive heart failure)
Patients in hypovolemic, cardiogenic, or septic shock, or with multiple organ failure
Massive trauma cases
Patients with right heart failure, COPD, pulmonary hypertension, or pulmonary embolism
Patients requiring high levels of positive end-expiratory pressure
Hemodynamically unstable patients requiring inotropes or intra-aortic balloon counterpulsation
Patients undergoing surgery of the aorta requiring cross-clamping
Patients undergoing hepatic transplantation
Patients with massive ascites undergoing portocaval shunts

(From Saidman LJ, Smith NT: Monitoring in Anesthesia. Boston, Butterworth-Heinemann, 1993.)

Abbreviation: COPD = chronic obstructive pulmonary disease.

The initial assessment of the critically ill patient described previously concentrates on mental status, the ability and desire to breathe, and circulation. Early in this assessment, the following question must be answered: "Do I need a secured airway now, or can it wait until the induction of anesthesia in the operating room?" Indications for obtaining a secured airway early include poor ventilation or oxygenation, decreased or changing mental status, signs of developing airway obstruction (stridor, snoring, and so on), possible airway burns (soot in nares, singed nasal hairs), shock, or combativeness requiring sedation. Early recognition of developing obstruction requires constant attention. The patient who is apneic or obstructed requires immediate airway intervention, whereas the comatose, stable, breathing patient can afford a more deliberate approach.

If an immediate secured airway is required (apnea or obstruction), then orotracheal intubation under direct laryngoscopy is the method of first choice.[1] Manual cervical spine stabilization should be maintained by a properly trained assistant,[15, 16] and cricoid pressure (Sellick's maneuver) should be applied during both intubation and mask ventilation, as illustrated in Figure 152–6. Although it is preferable to avoid positive-pressure mask ventilation in full-stomach patients because it increases the risk of aspiration, avoidance of hypoxia holds top priority. Proper cricoid pressure (see Fig. 152–6) helps prevent both air insufflation into the stomach and regurgitation of stomach contents into the pharynx. Anesthetic drugs and muscle relaxants should be used only as needed and are subject to the considerations discussed later.

If orotracheal intubation is not possible and an immediate airway is needed, then either TTV or emergency cricothyroidotomy should be accomplished without delay. Using a 14-gauge intravenous cannula inserted through the cricoid membrane and a source of oxygen at 30 to 50 psi, TTV can maintain both adequate oxygenation and ventilation in most patients.[17] It is an excellent way to "buy time" for establishing a more permanent, secured airway by endotracheal intubation or formal tracheostomy. A cricothyroidotomy can also be performed quickly in the apneic patient, but a surgical tracheostomy requires too much time in this situation.[18]

In the less emergent scenario of the breathing patient who needs a secured airway, several options can be considered. Blind nasal intubation can be performed on the awake, cooperative patient, but it is rarely the method of choice in acute trauma. Stimulation of the gag reflex can cause vomiting and aspiration, and epistaxis can obscure visualization during subsequent intubation attempts.[19] Because studies have shown that direct orotracheal intubation can be accomplished safely in the uncleared cervical spine using manual stabilization, there is little incentive for attempting the nasal route in these patients.[1, 15] Other options include fiberoptic-assisted, retrograde, and blind oral intubation using an intubating stylet. The technique selected depends on the degree of urgency, the patient's anatomy, and the nature of the injuries.[14] Fiberoptic-assisted intubation is usually not a good choice when the pharynx is filled with blood from facial injuries.

The question of how and when to "clear" the cervical

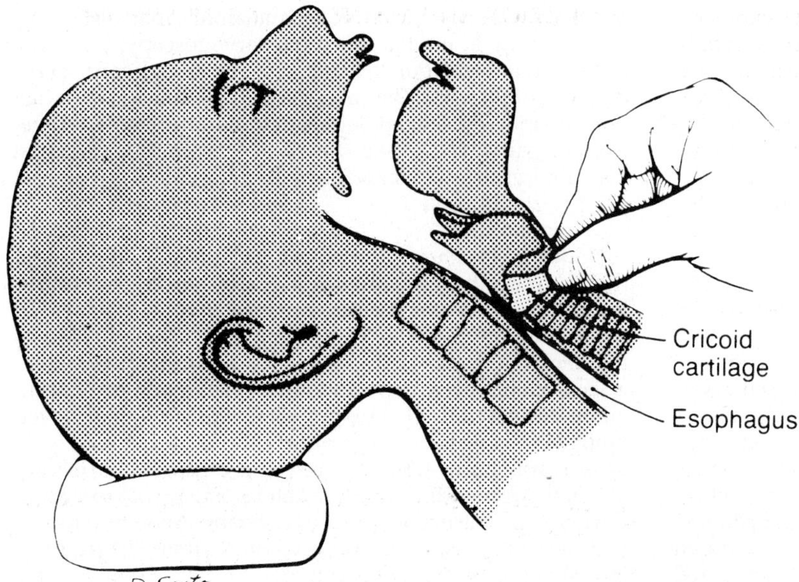

Figure 152–6. The Sellick maneuver is the application of pressure by the thumb and index finger to the cricoid cartilage. Properly executed, this maneuver occludes the esophagus and can prevent aspiration of gastric contents.

spine is important in blunt trauma patients, particularly victims of motor vehicle accidents. If the patient is apneic or in shock or has rapidly changing mental status or massive facial injuries that will soon jeopardize the airway, intubation should be performed without delay using manual stabilization, as described previously. If the patient is awake and cooperative, a neurologic examination and a lateral cervical spine radiograph are indicated. If the examination is normal and the radiograph shows no injury with adequate visualization of the seventh cervical vertebra (C-7), then the cervical spine can be considered normal for purposes of airway management.[20] If C-7 is not visualized, the radiograph can be repeated once if time permits. In the comatose or obtunded patient, the cervical spine cannot be considered cleared by single-view radiography in the absence of a neurologic examination. One retrospective study concluded that 17% of spinal cord injuries occur without radiologic evidence of bone injury.[7] Our policy is to treat the cervical spine as unstable during intubation unless both the radiograph and neurologic examinations are normal.

The American Society of Anesthesiologists formed a Difficult Airway Task Force in 1990, which produced the airway algorithm shown in Figure 152–7.[21] Most of this protocol is applicable to trauma and other critically ill patients, but the option to "awaken" after failed intubation may not exist. Awake intubation options should be considered in difficult airways, but these require some degree of patient cooperation. Whatever intubating technique is selected,

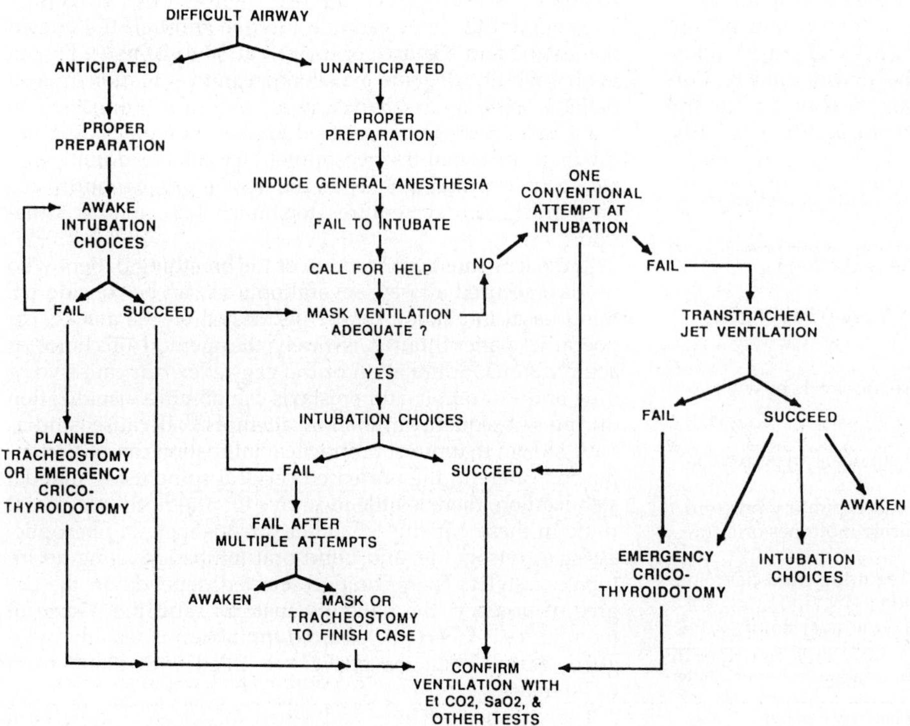

Figure 152–7. The Difficult Airway Algorithm of the American Society of Anesthesiologists. (From Benumof JL: Management of the difficult airway: The ASA algorithm. *In:* Review Course Lectures. International Anesthesia Research Society, 1993. Baltimore, Williams & Wilkins, 1993, pp 83–91.)

some general principles should be applied. Full-stomach patients must be intubated either while awake or by rapid-sequence induction, described later. The use of antacids and histamine$_2$ blockers has been discussed. Time permitting, the patient should breathe 100% oxygen by mask for at least 2 minutes before intubation or induction of anesthesia. After intubation, positive-pressure ventilation with 100% oxygen should be maintained until it is certain that fraction of inspired oxygen (FIO_2) can be safely reduced.

Anesthetics or muscle relaxants, if needed to secure the airway, must be used with caution in critically ill patients. Drugs may be required to facilitate intubation in the alert or uncooperative patient, or they may be indicated to prevent dangerous increases in ICP in the head-injury patient. If a hypnotic agent such as thiopental must be used in a trauma patient, the method of choice is rapid-sequence induction, in which the hypnotic and succinylcholine are given as a rapid intravenous bolus while cricoid pressure is maintained until the airway is secured.[22] Rapid sequence minimizes the risk of pulmonary aspiration, but it entails hemodynamic changes that may not be tolerated by the hypovolemic patient. A patient who is 20% to 30% intravascular volume depleted may have a normal supine blood pressure, yet 4 to 5 mg/kg of IV thiopental given to this patient may lead to cardiac arrest. Alternatives in the moderately hypovolemic patient include lower dose thiopental (1–2 mg/kg), etomidate, and ketamine. Etomidate, 0.2 to 0.3 mg/kg IV, decreases blood pressure less than an equipotent dose of thiopental, but, like thiopental, it is a myocardial depressant and has the additional property of adrenocortical suppression.[23] Ketamine, 1 to 2 mg/kg IV, tends to maintain blood pressure by means of its sympathomimetic property, which also lends it a bronchodilating effect. However, its direct myocardial depression will be manifest in the hypovolemic patient who is already at maximum sympathetic outflow.[24] Furthermore, ketamine is contraindicated in the head-injury patient because of its potential to increase ICP. The patient with clinical signs of shock should receive none of these hypnotic drugs. Intubation should be accomplished in this case with muscle relaxant, either alone or combined with a small dose of narcotic (e.g., fentanyl, 1–3 μg/kg). Table 152–5 shows some intravenous agents commonly used for securing the airway, along with their indications and contraindications.

All drugs to facilitate intubation should be given intravenously if possible, preferably via a central vein. If venous access is not available and intubation must be accomplished immediately, ketamine and succinylcholine can be given intramuscularly. This is an undesirable alternative because absorption will be slowed in the patient who is in shock, and several minutes may elapse before acceptable intubating conditions are obtained. During this period, the airway is unprotected, and the risk of pulmonary aspiration is greatly increased.

INDUCTION AND MAINTENANCE OF ANESTHESIA

All agents that produce the state of general anesthesia are, simply put, poisons. Every anesthetic agent available today will cause death if used in overdose, and the lethal dose varies with the patient and disease. This issue is paramount in the critically ill patient because the "therapeutic window" of many drugs becomes small or vanishes. The task, then, is to select which poisons will be best tolerated in the patient and procedure at hand, to keep the doses within their therapeutic range, and to counteract negative side effects as they develop. This requires a thorough knowledge of the patient's injuries, diseases, allergies, and all medications or drugs being taken. As noted previously, much of this medical history may be unavailable in the trauma patient, and the anesthesiologist is forced to make educated guesses on the patient's status.

The normovolemic (<10% volume deficit), normotensive, otherwise healthy trauma patient who requires general anesthesia will tolerate a standard rapid-sequence induction with thiopental, 4 to 5 mg/kg, and succinylcholine, 1 mg/kg (see Table 152–5). Although succinylcholine remains the muscle relaxant that achieves good intubating conditions most rapidly, its side effects and contraindications must be well understood by the user. It can cause both tachydysrhythmias and bradydysrhythmias, including asystole and ventricular tachycardia or fibrillation. Its potassium-releasing property contraindicates succinylcholine in patients with (1) severe burns or crush injuries that are more than 24 hours old, (2) highly elevated serum potassium, (3) denervating diseases (major stroke, multiple sclerosis, and so on), (4) serious intra-abdominal infection, and (5) myotonic dystrophy.

Cricoid pressure should be maintained throughout the induction until proper placement of the endotracheal tube has been verified both by capnography and auscultation of bilateral breath sounds.[22] Volatile agents, nitrous oxide, and narcotics can all be used for maintenance of anesthesia. However, even in straightforward cases, the anesthesiologist must be prepared to change techniques rapidly as the patient's status changes. Trauma patients often exhibit a "golden period" of 1 or 2 hours, followed by rapid decompensation. Many factors can change patient status intraoperatively, including continued hemorrhage, pericardial tamponade, myocardial contusion or infarction, aortic injury, pulmonary contusion, pneumothorax, pulmonary embolism, and subdural or subarachnoid hemorrhage, to name a few. There is no place for complacency in giving anesthesia to the critically ill patient.

The patient who has lost 15% to 25% of blood volume, even if normotensive, should have anesthesia induced in a more conservative fashion (see Table 152–5). Ketamine or etomidate can be used as described previously, in doses that are reduced as volume deficit increases.[24] Although keta-

TABLE 152–5. Intravenous Agents Used to Provide Sedation/Anesthesia for Securing the Airway in Critically Ill Patients

Agent	*Dose*	*Indications*	*Contraindications*
Thiopental	2–5 mg/kg	Intubation in awake, normovolemic patient	>10% volume depletion, shock, CHF, porphyria
Etomidate	0.2–0.3 mg/kg	Intubation in mildly hypovolemic patient	>15–20% volume depletion, adrenal suppression
Ketamine	1–2 mg/kg	Intubation in mild to moderate hypovolemia, asthma, bronchospasm	>20–25% volume depletion, increased intracranial pressure
Fentanyl	1–3 μg/kg	Intubation in serious hypovolemia with signs of shock	Hypertensive response not blocked; hypotension may worsen in shock

Abbreviation: CHF = congestive heart failure.

mine is absolutely contraindicated in head-injury patients, succinylcholine is not, and it should be used in every rapid-sequence induction. These moderately hypovolemic patients will often not tolerate volatile anesthetic agents, and maintenance will involve either a nitrous-narcotic technique or narcotic alone until intravascular volume is restored.

The severely hypovolemic patient who has lost 30% or more of blood volume will exhibit clinical signs of shock. If this patient must come to surgery before the volume deficit can be corrected, then he or she should be intubated either with no drugs or with muscle relaxant alone. Once the airway is secured, small doses of intravenous narcotic (e.g., fentanyl) should be carefully titrated as circulating volume is restored. Benzodiazepines (diazepam or midazolam) may be used for their amnestic effects, but these can also worsen hypotension and must be given with caution. The goal in these patients is to correct hypovolemia as soon as possible and gradually add more anesthetic drugs as tolerated.

Regional anesthesia is an option that is too often overlooked in critically ill and trauma patients. A regional block may be an excellent choice for peripheral surgical procedures in these patients, providing three guidelines are strictly followed. First, the patient must not be hypovolemic or have significant ongoing hemorrhage when a central regional (subarachnoid or epidural block) is performed.[25] Second, the patient must not have a coagulopathy. Third, the patient should be alert and cooperative and have a normal neurologic examination, must not be intoxicated or under the influence of drugs, and must be able to breathe normally and protect the airway in the position required for surgery. Continuous catheter techniques are advantageous because they allow the anesthetic dose to be titrated slowly and provide an excellent vehicle for postoperative pain therapy. Regional anesthesia permits continuous monitoring of neurologic status and may provide improved blood flow to injured extremities.[26]

FLUID MANAGEMENT

Fluid therapy is an essential component of anesthetic care in all critically ill patients, particularly trauma victims. The intravascular volume of these patients is often far from normal, and it can change rapidly during the perioperative period. Anesthetic agents themselves change the "functional" volume status by increasing intravascular capacity. Volume status must be monitored continuously throughout the perioperative period, as described previously. In addition to the volume monitors already discussed, increased alveolar dead space or "wasted ventilation" is an indicator of hypovolemia. Arterial blood gas analysis will reveal a developing metabolic acidosis when significant hypovolemia persists for more than a few minutes.

The first requirement of fluid therapy is adequate vascular access. If intravenous access cannot be obtained initially because of hypovolemia, fluids can be given through an intraosseous needle inserted into the bone marrow of the tibia.[27] Central venous access should then be established as soon as possible. If a military antishock trousers suit is in use, it should not be deflated until fluid resuscitation is in progress and basic monitors are functioning. Deflation should be accomplished slowly and cautiously—first the abdominal binder and then one leg at a time—while vital signs are continuously monitored.

All resuscitation fluids should be warmed to 37°C. Most trauma patients are hypothermic when they reach the hospital, and resuscitation can worsen this condition if intravenous fluids are not warmed. Pressurization devices should be available for large-bore intravenous catheters to provide rapid infusion. A satisfactory fluid-warming and infusion system should be capable of giving a unit of blood (450 mL) in fewer than 2 minutes. One of the pressurization and fluid-warming systems that meets these requirements is shown in Figure 152–8.

In choosing the initial resuscitation fluid, the following priorities must be considered. In the trauma patient, the restoration of circulating volume is always the first priority. It is unlikely for a previously healthy trauma patient to die acutely of anemia, but many die of hypovolemic shock. Recent experience with Jehovah's Witness patients has reinforced this principle. At the University of California Irvine Medical Center, patients with hematocrit values as low as 6% (hemoglobin = 2 g/dL) have survived. After volume status has been stabilized, the second priority is the restoration of blood oxygen-carrying capacity. Because oxygen-carrying blood substitutes are not yet commercially available, this requires the transfusion of red blood cells (RBCs) when oxygen-carrying capacity is inadequate. The third priority in fluid therapy is the normalization of coagulation status, which may require the transfusion of platelets, fresh frozen plasma, or other blood components.

During the initial resuscitation, the goal is to achieve adequate circulating volume. How much is enough? In answering this, the clinician must consider that (1) acute blood loss is usually underestimated, (2) tissue losses during surgical exposure amount to 4 to 8 $mL \cdot kg^{-1} \cdot h^{-1}$, (3) crystalloid replacement must be two to three times the volume of

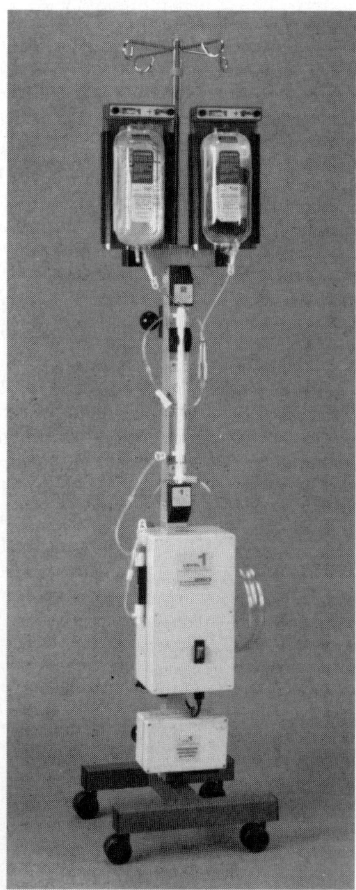

Figure 152–8. The Level I Fluid Management System (Level I Technologies, Inc., Marshfield, MA). Given adequate intravenous access, this system can infuse one unit (450 mL) of blood in less than 1 minute while maintaining a delivery temperature of 37°C. Other similar systems are commercially available.

blood loss, and (4) most anesthetics increase intravascular capacity. These factors tend to result in inadequate volume replacement, which can cause continued vital organ hypoperfusion, acute renal failure, worsening acidosis, and cardiovascular collapse.[28] On the other hand, giving too much fluid can produce volume overload and mild pulmonary edema in the recovery room. In most trauma patients, it is safer to give too much fluid rather than too little; that is, furosemide (Lasix) in the recovery room is preferable to cardiopulmonary resuscitation in the operating room. In other critical patients with known ventricular dysfunction, fluid overload can have more serious consequences.

The first intravenous fluid given to trauma victims is usually crystalloid. The composition of the commonly used crystalloid solutions is shown in Table 152–6. Crystalloids can provide rapid volume replacement with balanced electrolyte solutions; they are not allergenic, immunogenic, or toxic; they quickly restore urine output, keep blood viscosity low, and present less danger of overload because they can be rapidly diuresed. On the other hand, crystalloids do not carry oxygen; they redistribute to the entire extracellular fluid volume within an hour and thereby contribute more to peripheral and pulmonary edema, can produce dilutional coagulopathies, and require larger infusion volumes than colloids (two to three times blood loss). Some studies advocated hypertonic saline as a resuscitation solution, but this technique has its own complications and is not widely accepted at present.[29]

Colloids include all blood products, high-molecular-weight dextran, albumin, and hetastarch solutions such as Hespan. Only colloids can carry oxygen or replace lost coagulation factors; they may remain intravascular longer and thus create less edema, may increase cardiac output more than crystalloids,[30] and can replace that which is lost: whole blood. On the negative side, colloids can cause allergic or immune reactions; some carry risk of infection (hepatitis, human immunodeficiency virus); they can cause electrolyte imbalances; and some have toxic effects (citrate toxicity, nephrotoxicity, crossmatch problems, coagulopathy). Transfusion reactions from incompatible blood products are life-threatening complications that can occur at the worst possible time in the critical patient. The controversy between crystalloid and colloid will continue, and there are no patient outcome studies that prove either side of the argument.[31–34]

Although volume loss can be corrected with either crystalloid or colloid, defects in oxygen-carrying capacity or coagulation can be corrected only by colloids. Although fully crossmatched whole blood is the ideal replacement product for acute hemorrhage, this is often not available. If partially crossmatched or O-negative blood must be used in an emergency, it may be safer to use packed erythrocytes (PRBCs) to minimize the transfusion of plasma antibodies. When using PRBCs to improve oxygen-carrying capacity, one should not rely on an arbitrary hemoglobin threshold below which transfusion is begun. The acceptable hemoglobin value will depend on the nature of the patient's injuries or disease, general health, and the rate at which blood is being lost or is expected to be lost. In a healthy, young patient with a traumatic amputation and no further bleeding, a hemoglobin value of 8 might be acceptable. The same patient with a rigid, swollen abdomen should be receiving transfusion at the time of incision.

The most common coagulopathy in trauma patients is dilutional thrombocytopenia, resulting from replacement of lost blood with anything other than whole blood.[35] The decision to transfuse platelets should be based on a measured thrombocytopenia in the presence of abnormal bleeding rather than an arbitrary criterion such as number of PRBC units given. The platelet count should normally be kept above 70,000 in the operating room. The level in most previously healthy patients will remain above this value until they have received more than one full blood volume of colloid. Platelets sequestered in the spleen and reticuloendothelial system are released during stress, thus ameliorating the decrease in platelet count caused by blood loss. Figure 152–9 shows the percentage of decrease in measured platelet count plotted as a function of the number of blood volumes transfused.[36] These data from both adult and pediatric patients show that the actual platelet decrease is less than would be expected on the basis of simple dilution of the blood volume.

Deficiencies of fibrinogen or other coagulation factors usually appear later than thrombocytopenia, and replacement therapy should be guided by measured laboratory values such as prothrombin and partial thromboplastin time (PTT). In particular, fresh frozen plasma should be transfused when abnormal coagulation values are measured, not according to the number of PRBC units given and never as a volume expander. During rapid, uncontrolled hemorrhage, the anesthesiologist and surgeon must anticipate specific blood component needs, allowing for the time required by the blood bank to produce the required component.

PERIOPERATIVE COMPLICATIONS

The list of possible anesthetic-related perioperative complications is almost endless. Described briefly here are only three adverse events, selected because they often occur in trauma and other critically ill patients.

TABLE 152–6. Commonly Used Intravenous Crystalloid Solutions and Their Ingredients

Ingredient	*Normal Saline*	*Ringer's Lactate*	*Normosol R (pH 7.4)*	*5% Dextrose in Water*	*5% Dextrose in ½ NS*	*10% Dextrose in Water*
Na (mEq/L)	154	130	140	—	77	—
K	—	4	5	—	—	—
Cl	154	109	98	—	77	—
Ca	—	3	—	—	—	—
Mg	—	—	3	—	—	—
Lactate	—	28	—	—	—	—
pH	5.7	6.7	7.4	5.0	4.9	4.9
mOsm/L	308	273	295	253	407	505
Dextrose (g/L)	—	—	—	50	50	100
Calories/L	—	9	18	170	170	340

Abbreviations: Na = sodium; K = potassium; Cl = chloride; Ca = calcium; Mg = magnesium; NS = normal saline.

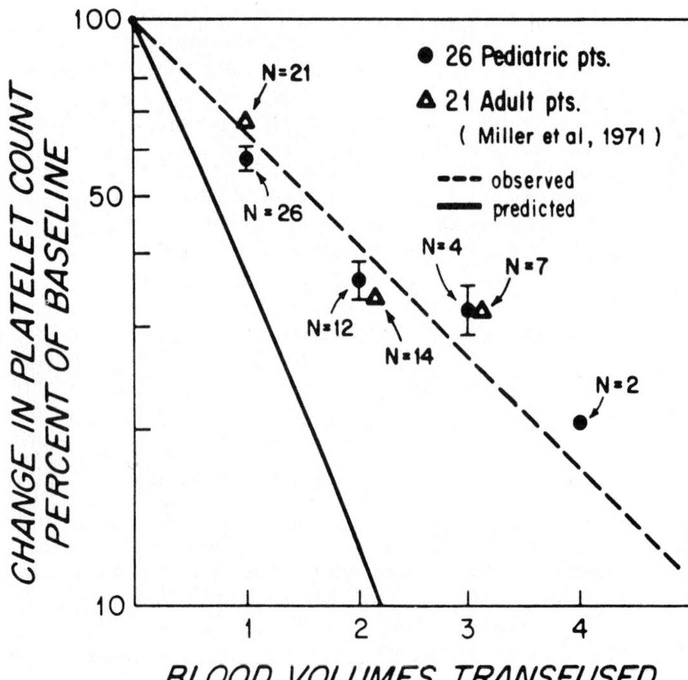

Figure 152–9. Percentage decrease in platelet count plotted as a function of the number of blood volumes of non–platelet-containing solution transfused. Data points with best-fit *(dashed line)* represent two studies of 26 pediatric and 21 adult patients. The *solid line* is expected change based on the simple dilution of blood volume. The difference results from the release of platelets from the spleen and reticuloendothelial system. (From Cote CJ, Lui LM, Szyfelbein SK, et al: Changes in serial platelet counts following massive blood transfusion in pediatric patients. Anesthesiology 1985; 62:197–201.)

Disseminated Intravascular Coagulation

In addition to the more common dilutional coagulopathies discussed previously, trauma and other critically ill patients are at risk for disseminated intravascular coagulation (DIC) or "consumption coagulopathy." The hallmark of this process is generalized activation of the coagulation cascade, causing rapid consumption of platelets, fibrinogen, and Factors V and VIII.[35, 37] This results in diffuse, uncontrollable bleeding from the entire surgical field, possibly accompanied by diffuse intravascular thrombosis and organ ischemia. Intravascular fibrin formation activates the fibrinolytic system, causing an elevation in fibrin–split products (FSP), which in turn produces platelet dysfunction. The diagnosis of DIC is confirmed by clinical evidence of bleeding accompanied by a decreased platelet count, decreased fibrinogen level (usually less than 150 mg/dL), and positive fibrin–split products. Activated PTT (aPTT) is generally abnormal because of consumption of Factors V and VIII. DIC may occur without the presence of elevated FSP because these are rapidly removed from circulation by the liver.[37]

DIC is apparently triggered by a phospholipid not normally present in the circulation: platelet Factor III, or tissue thromboplastin. Patients at risk include those with vascular endothelial damage resulting from burns, trauma, extensive surgery, or shock. Also at risk are patients with obstetric complications (abruption, amniotic fluid embolism, fetal demise), or sepsis. Possible causes of DIC are listed according to category in Table 152–7. As long as phospholipid triggers circulate, the DIC process will continue. Therapy is, therefore, aimed first at the underlying cause, which is easier said than done. In fetal demise, this is accomplished by removal of the dead fetus and placenta. In serious trauma or burns, the damaged vascular endothelium often cannot be removed. Step two in therapy is replacement of consumed blood constituents, primarily platelets, fibrinogen, and Factors V and VIII. This requires transfusion of platelet concentrates, fresh frozen plasma, and occasionally cryoprecipitate.[38] The goal of replacement therapy is to maintain a platelet count of at least 100,000, a normal aPTT, and a fibrinogen level of at least 200 mg/dL. The third possible step in therapy, the use of heparin, is reserved for disorders of the coagulation cascade and is generally not appropriate in surgical patients.

Hypothermia

Hypothermia is almost unavoidable in trauma patients because most are hypothermic before they reach the operating room, and anesthesia further compromises their thermoregulatory mechanisms. General anesthesia lowers the threshold temperature at which hypothermic corrective responses begin, thus converting to some extent to poikilotherms. Anesthesia also reduces cutaneous vasoconstriction, which normally helps to conserve heat, and muscle relaxants block the shivering response.

Hypothermia has many physiologic effects, some of which may be beneficial in the critically ill.[39] Metabolism

TABLE 152–7. Possible Causes of Disseminated Intravascular Coagulation*

Disorders of Vascular Integrity
Burns
Vasculitis
Dissecting aortic aneurysm
Circulating Immune Complexes
Sepsis
Toxemia of pregnancy
Immune complex disease processes
Release of Tissue Phospholipids into Circulation
Massive crush injuries
Necrotic malignant tissue
Massive hemolysis
Obstetric complications
Amniotic fluid embolism
Fetal demise
Abruptio placentae

*All causes involve a loss of localization of the hemostatic process.

decreases by 8% per degree Celsius, and reaches one half of normal values at 28°C. Oxygen demand is reduced correspondingly so that low organ perfusion may be better tolerated. Blood flow is also shifted away from the extremities and muscles, with a larger fraction perfusing the heart and brain. Decreased cardiac output accompanied by sinus bradycardia may have a beneficial effect on the myocardial oxygen supply-demand balance.

These potential benefits of hypothermia are generally outweighed by its deleterious effects in critically ill patients undergoing surgery. In addition to sinus bradycardia, the ECG may show atrial fibrillation, prolonged PR and QT intervals, and widened QRS. Below 28°C, more serious dysrhythmias ensue, including nodal rhythm, frequent premature ventricular contractions, atrioventricular block, and refractory ventricular fibrillation.[40] Increased sympathetic tone can cause heart rate and blood pressure to increase under light levels of anesthesia. Myocardial contractility increases as temperature falls, reaching its maximum at 28°C.[41] Hypoxic pulmonary vasoconstriction is attenuated by hypothermia and at 30°C is less than one half of normal response.[42] Plasma volume is decreased because of an apparent transcapillary fluid shift, thus worsening preexisting hypovolemia. Blood viscosity is increased by both the direct effect of temperature and hemoconcentration as a result of decreased plasma volume. Of special concern in trauma patients, hypothermia causes platelet dysfunction and thrombocytopenia, with the latter resulting from platelet sequestration in the liver.[43] Both are usually reversible by rewarming. Effects of hypothermia on other coagulation factors are unclear, but severe hypothermia is a possible cause of DIC (see prior discussion).

Given the dangers of accidental hypothermia, particularly in trauma patients, one must make every attempt to prevent or correct it. The operating room should be kept warm, respired gases should be both warmed and humidified, all intravenous replacement fluids and irrigation should be warmed to 37°C, and a warming blanket should be placed between the patient and the operating table. Air-filled patient warmers, such as the Bair Hugger, may also be helpful as long as they do not obstruct the surgical field.

Pulmonary Aspiration

Pulmonary aspiration of gastric contents is responsible for up to 20% of all anesthetic-related deaths. The overall mortality from aspiration in several studies is about 5%,[44] but mortality as high as 70% has been reported. Trauma patients are at particularly high risk for aspiration for several reasons. They are frequently obtunded or comatose and have impaired protective airway reflexes. They must always be considered to have full stomachs because gastric emptying virtually ceases at the time of the injury. They may also have anatomic risk factors such as increased intragastric pressure, diaphragmatic rupture, airway injury, and so on. Aspiration can take place at any time during or after traumatic injury, but the risk is greatest when the airway is unprotected and the patient is obtunded. For this reason, a protected airway (i.e., a cuffed endotracheal tube) should be established as soon as possible in the obtunded trauma patient.

The pathophysiology of aspiration depends on the nature and volume of the aspirate.[45] Nonacid liquids (pH >2.5) such as blood or saliva will cause few histologic abnormalities, but they can still produce laryngospasm, bronchospasm, and loss of surfactant. Acid liquid aspiration produces extensive atelectasis, alveolocapillary breakdown with intra-alveolar hemorrhage, and interstitial edema. Significant hypoxemia and pulmonary hypertension can occur early, with minimal change in pH or partial pressure of carbon dioxide. If the aspirate is nonacid with particulates, early hypoxemia can be more severe and is often accompanied by an increase in Pa_{CO_2} and a decrease in pH. An inflammatory response ensues in the bronchioles and alveolar ducts, and granulomas may form around aspirated particles. Acid particulate is the most damaging aspirate, causing severe hemorrhagic pulmonary edema and alveolar septal necrosis. Severe hypoxemia and hypercarbia are combined with systemic hypotension and pulmonary hypertension. Mortality is high and can occur early, particularly in critically ill patients.[46]

Clinical signs of aspiration include vomitus in the oropharynx, wheezing, cyanosis, coughing, hypoxemia, pulmonary edema, and hypotension. Chest x-ray films may show nothing at all or may show changes only after several hours.[44] Diffuse bilateral infiltrates can indicate significant aspiration, and their resolution seems to parallel the clinical course. Any of these signs may appear late or not at all, but the most suggestive one is sudden hypoxemia with no other explanation.

Given the serious consequences of aspiration, its prevention is a key component of anesthetic management. Although the accepted nothing by mouth (NPO) guidelines for elective operations may be changing,[47] there is no doubt that trauma or other critically ill patients expecting emergency surgery must be kept NPO. Prophylactic antacids to increase gastric pH are appropriate, but particulate antacids should never be used. As shown in Figure 152–10, the hypoxemia resulting from particulate antacid aspiration is almost as severe as that caused by acid aspirate.[48] In contrast, nonparticulate antacids are relatively benign when aspirated. In the alert, cooperative patient, we recommend sodium citrate (0.30 mol, 30 mL) or Alka-Seltzer (two tablets in 30 mL) given 15 to 30 minutes before surgery.

The period of greatest risk for aspiration is that between inducing general anesthesia and securing the airway with a cuffed endotracheal tube. This time should be minimized in all trauma patients by using rapid-sequence induction, as described previously. Properly applied cricoid pressure during induction can prevent vomiting even when esophageal pressure reaches 100 cm H_2O, and it should never be released until the endotracheal cuff is inflated and proper positioning has been confirmed by breath sounds.[22] If vomiting occurs before intubation despite cricoid pressure, the head should be turned to the side and the oropharynx cleared by suction before laryngoscopy. After the airway has been secured, a nasogastric tube should be used to empty the stomach as much as possible before extubation. The trauma patient should not be extubated until he or she is awake enough to follow commands.

If the patient aspirates despite these precautions, therapy should depend on the severity and course of the lesion. Very mild aspiration may require nothing more than supplemental oxygen and monitoring of arterial blood gases. If the patient fails to maintain a Pa_{O_2} value greater than 70 mm Hg despite an F_{IO_2} of 0.5, more aggressive treatment should be considered. The mainstay of therapy in such cases is continuous positive airway pressure (CPAP), which should be titrated to minimize intrapulmonary shunt. Although CPAP can be provided by facemask, this technique requires patient cooperation and does not protect from further aspiration. Patients with severely impaired compliance may also require mechanical ventilation to maintain acceptable blood gas values. Response to therapy can be determined by monitoring intrapulmonary shunt, compliance, work of breathing, and alveolar dead space. F_{IO_2} should be reduced to values less than 0.4 before reducing CPAP.

Bronchoscopy is not indicated unless significant solid ma-

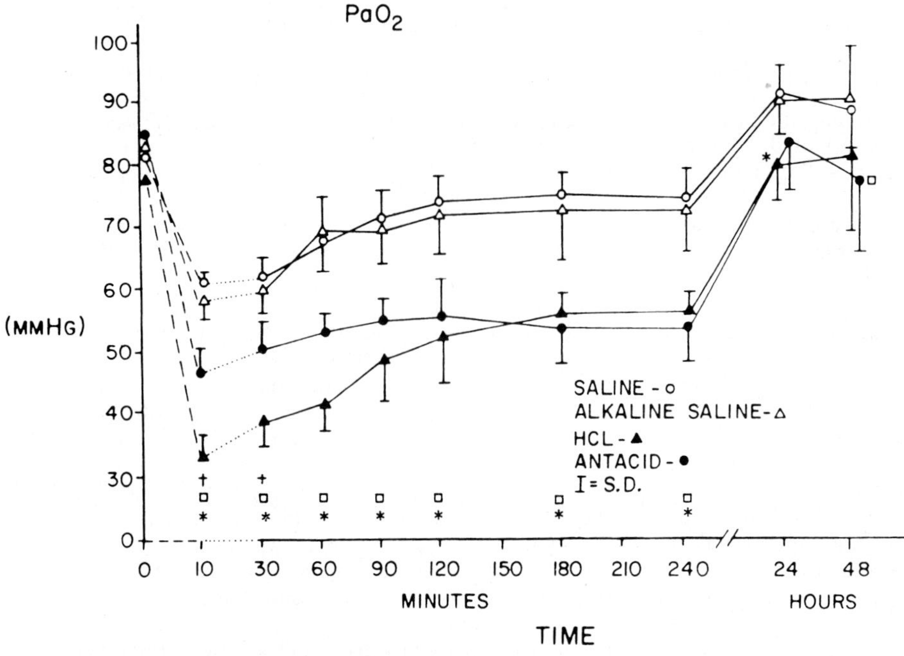

Figure 152–10. Pa_{O_2} values plotted versus time in animals that aspirated saline, alkaline saline (pH = 8.3), hydrochloric acid, and particulate antacid. The Pa_{O_2} decrease resulting from antacid aspiration is almost as severe as that from acid aspiration. Note that the two curves are significantly different only at 10 and 30 minutes following aspiration. (From Gibbs CP, Schwartz DJ, Wynne JW, et al: Antacid pulmonary aspiration in the dog. Anesthesiology 1979; 51:380.)

terial has been aspirated. Prophylactic antibiotics are also not indicated for most aspirations and may be harmful by altering the normal respiratory flora.[49] Antibiotics should be reserved for secondary bacterial pneumonia from known pathogens or suspected feculent aspiration. Although steroid therapy has been used in the past, there is no evidence that it improves outcome, and it is not recommended for routine treatment of aspiration.

Only three of the anesthetic-related complications that commonly occur in the critically ill are discussed. Some of the other complications, such as transfusion reaction, acute renal failure, sepsis, and pulmonary embolism, are discussed elsewhere in this text. Malignant hyperthermia is another very serious anesthetic complication, discussion of which is beyond the scope of this chapter. Several excellent reviews of this familial disease are available.[50–52]

CONCLUSIONS

Critically ill patients, including trauma victims, often have no unused reserves in cardiac or pulmonary function. The additional stress created by general or even regional anesthesia may be more than these patients can tolerate. To minimize the high anesthetic risk in the critically ill, clinicians must know as much as possible about their disease process, the functioning of major organ systems, and the nature of the expected surgical stress. The anesthetic plan must account for these factors by avoiding drugs or techniques that would worsen the patient's preexisting problems. Appropriate monitoring of cardiopulmonary function should be established before anesthetic induction. Possible anesthetic or surgical complications must be anticipated, and therapeutic options (e.g., blood products) must be made available before the start of the procedure.

In this chapter, the anesthetic considerations for taking a critically ill patient to the operating room have been surveyed only briefly. There are several good references providing more detail on anesthetic problems in patients with specific diseases or compromised organ systems[53] or in patients undergoing specific surgical procedures.[54, 55] An intelligent, well-trained, and alert anesthesiologist can effectively minimize anesthetic risk in the critically ill.

References

1. Scannell G, Waxman K, Tominaga G, et al: Orotracheal intubation in trauma patients with cervical fractures. Arch Surg 1993; 128:903–906.
2. Morris JA, Auerbach PS, Marshall GA, et al: The trauma score as a triage tool in the prehospital setting. JAMA 1986; 256:1319.
3. Moss GS, Saletta JD: Traumatic shock in man. N Engl J Med 1974; 290:724.
4. Knopp R, Claypool R, Leonardi D: Use of the tilt test in measuring acute blood loss. Ann Emerg Med 1980; 9:72.
5. Crosby ET: The adult cervical spine: Implications for airway management. Can J Anaesth 1990; 37:77.
6. Streitwieser DR, Knopp R, Wales LR, et al: Accuracy of standard radiographic views in detecting cervical spine fractures. Ann Emerg Med 1983; 12:538–542.
7. Polesky HS, Walker RH (Eds): Safety and Transfusion Practices. Northfield, IL, College of American Pathologists, 1982.
8. Solanki DR, Suresh M, Ethridge HC: The effects of intravenous cimetidine and metoclopramide on gastric volume and pH. Anesth Analg 1984; 63:599.
9. Kaplan JA, King SB III: The precordial electrocardiographic lead (V_5) in patients who have coronary artery disease. Anesthesiology 1976; 45:570–574.
10. American Society of Anesthesia, House of Delegates: Standards for Basic Intraoperative Monitoring: ASA Directory. Philadelphia, JB Lippincott, 1988.
11. Tremper KK, Barker SJ: Transcutaneous oxygen measurement: Experimental studies and adult applications. Anesthesiol clin 1987; 25:67–96.
12. Saidman LJ, Smith NT: Monitoring in Anesthesia. 3rd ed. Boston, Butterworth, 1993.
13. Lake CL: Clinical Monitoring. Philadelphia, WB Saunders, 1990.
14. Benumof JL: Management of the difficult adult airway. Anesthesiology 1991; 75:1087.

15. Holley J, Jorden R: Airway management in patients with unstable cervical spine fractures. Ann Emerg Med 1989; 18:1237–1239.
16. Jorden R: Airway management. Emerg Med Clin North Am 1988; 6:671–686.
17. Benumof JL, Scheller MS: The importance of transtracheal jet ventilation in the management of the difficult airway. Anesthesiology 1989; 71:769–778.
18. DeLaurier GA, Hawkins ML, Treat RC, et al: Acute airway management: Role of cricothyroidotomy. Ann Surg 1990; 56:12–15.
19. Danzi DF, Thomas DM: Nasotracheal intubation in the emergency department. Crit Care Med 1980; 8:677–679.
20. American College of Surgeons: Advanced Trauma Life Support Manual. Chicago, American College of Surgeons, 1993.
21. Benumof JL: Management of the difficult airway: The ASA algorithm: Review Course Lectures, International Anesthesia Research Society, 1993. Baltimore, Williams & Wilkins, 1993.
22. Sellick BA: Cricoid pressure to control the regurgitation of stomach contents during induction of anesthesia. Lancet 1961; 2:404.
23. Fragen RJ, Shanks CA, Molteni A, et al: Effects of etomidate on hormonal responses to surgical stress. Anesthesiology 1984; 61:652.
24. White PF, Way WL, Trevor AJ: Ketamine: Its pharmacology and therapeutic uses. Anesthesiology 1982; 56:119.
25. Kennedy WF, Bonica JJ, Akamatsu TJ, et al: Cardiovascular and respiratory effects of subarachnoid block in the presence of acute blood loss. Anesthesiology 1968; 29:29.
26. Modig J, Borg T, Karlstrom G, et al: Thromboembolism after total hip replacement: Role of epidural and general anesthesia. Anesth Analg 1983; 62:174–180.
27. Harte FA, Chalmers PC, Walsh RF, et al: Intraosseous fluid administration: A parenteral alternative in pediatric resuscitation. Anesth Analg 1987; 66:687–689.
28. Shoemaker WC, Appel PL, Kram HB: Tissue oxygen debt as a determinant of lethal and nonlethal postoperative organ failure. Crit Care Med 1988; 16:1117.
29. Layon J, Duncan D, Gallager TJ, et al: Hypertonic saline as a resuscitation solution in hemorrhagic shock. Anesth Analg 1987; 66:154.
30. Shires GT III, Peitzman AB, Albert SA, et al: Response of extravascular lung water to intraoperative fluids. Ann Surg 1983; 197:515.
31. Virgilio RW, Rice CL: Crystalloid versus colloid resuscitation: Is one better? A randomized clinical study. Surgery 1979; 85:129.
32. Giesecke AH, Jenkins MT: Fluid therapy. Clin Anesth 1976; 11:57.
33. Velanovich V: Crystalloid versus colloid fluid resuscitation: A meta-analysis of mortality. Surgery 1989; 105:65.
34. Hankeln K, Radel C, Beez M, et al: Comparison of hydroxyethyl starch and lactated Ringer's solution on hemodynamics and oxygen transport of critically ill patients in prospective crossover studies. Crit Care Med 1989; 17:133.
35. Miller RD, Robbins TO, Tong MJ, et al: Coagulation defects associated with massive blood transfusion. Ann Surg 1971; 174:794.
36. Cote CJ, Liu LM, Szyfelbein SK, et al: Changes in serial platelet counts following massive blood transfusion in pediatric patients. Anesthesiology 1985; 62:197–201.
37. Murray DJ, Olson J, Strauss R, et al: Coagulation changes during packed red blood cell replacement of major blood loss. Anesthesiology 1988; 69:839.
38. Fischbach DP, Fogdall RP: Coagulation: The Essentials. Baltimore, Williams & Wilkins, 1981.
39. Wong KC: Physiology and pharmacology of hypothermia. West J Med 1983; 138:227.
40. Rittenhouse EA, Mohri H, Dillard D, et al: Deep hypothermia in cardiovascular surgery: Current review. Ann Thorac Surg 1974; 17:63.
41. Covino BG, Beavers WR: Changes in cardiac contractility during immersion hypothermia. Am J Physiol 1958; 195:433.
42. Benumof JL, Wahrenbrock EA: Dependency of hypoxic pulmonary vasoconstriction on temperature. J Appl Physiol 1977; 42:56.
43. Hessel EA II, Schmer G, Dillard DH: Platelet kinetics during deep hypothermia. J Surg Res 1980; 28:23.
44. Olsson GL, Hallen B, Hambraeus-Jonzon K: Aspiration during anaesthesia: A computer-aided study of 185,358 anaesthetics. Acta Anesth Scand 1986; 30:84.
45. Awe WC, Fletcher WS, Jacob SW: The pathophysiology of aspiration pneumonitis. Surgery 1966; 60:232.
46. Schwartz DJ, Wynne JW, Gibbs CP, et al: The pulmonary consequences of aspiration of gastric contents at pH values greater than 2.5. Am Rev Respir Dis 1980; 121:119.
47. Cote CJ: NPO after midnight for children: A reappraisal. Anesthesiology 1990; 72:589–592.
48. Gibbs CP, Schwartz DJ, Wynne JW, et al: Antacid pulmonary aspiration in the dog. Anesthesiology 1979; 51:380.
49. Wynne JW, Modell JH: Respiratory aspiration of stomach contents. Ann Intern Med 1977; 87:466.
50. Gronert GA: Malignant hyperthermia. Anesthesiology 1980; 53:395.
51. Britt BA (Ed): Malignant Hyperthermia. Boston, Martinus Nijhoff, 1987.
52. Gronert GA, Rosenberg H: Management of patients in whom trismus occurs following succinylcholine. Anesthesiology 1988; 68:653.
53. Stoelting RK, Dierdorf SF, McCammon RL: Anesthesia and Co-Existing Disease. New York, Churchill Livingstone, 1988.
54. Miller RD (Ed): Anesthesia. 3rd ed. New York, Churchill Livingstone, 1990.
55. Barash PG, Cullen BF, Stoelting RK: Clinical anesthesia. 2nd ed. Philadelphia, JB Lippincott, 1992.

CHAPTER 153

Intraoperative and Postoperative Transfusion Therapy

A. Gerson Greenburg, MD, PhD

A continuous and adequate supply of oxygen to tissues is a prerequisite for human survival. In a very real sense, humans are obligate aerobic organisms. Independent of etiologic mechanisms, all forms of the "shock syndrome" are characterized by inadequate oxygen delivery to tissues often associated with impaired oxygen utilization. How inadequate oxygen delivery to tissues is affected depends very much on which element of this complex system is altered.[1–4] What is particularly important for patient management in the intra- and postoperative periods is an appreciation of the components of the oxygen delivery system and an understanding of how they can be manipulated to accomplish a specific therapeutic objective.

In this chapter the concepts that make up the oxygen delivery system are briefly reviewed to put into context the possible therapeutic interventions for the time frames in question. Next, the products and techniques currently available for augmenting oxygen delivery are discussed, with some background data on risk and disease transmission associated with blood transfusion. Then a rationale is offered for when to apply the various options intraoperatively and postoperatively in the context of a risk-benefit analysis for the situation. An afterword provides a glimpse into the future, the era of red blood cell (RBC) substitutes, and offers a brief overview of this evolving and dynamic field; someday it could be the first-line response in the intensive care unit (ICU) or operating room (OR) to the need for increasing oxygen delivery.

Ultimately, the clinical decision to offer RBC transfusion in any specific situation depends on the answer to two specific questions: Does this patient need a transfusion? Should I transfuse this patient? The answer to the first question depends very much on analysis of the data that establish the presence or absence of adequate oxygen delivery. In a very real sense, it is a scientific approach to making the decision, certainly appropriate in today's high-technology ORs and ICUs. The decision to administer the transfusion—assuming it is indicated—is a judgment issue highly based on an assessment of risk. That risk is to the patient if a transfusion is given and includes all of the issues of transfusion reaction, incompatibility, transmission of infectious disease, and other, perhaps unknown items. The decision to not administer a transfusion is also a "judgment call." In this instance, whether the anemic state or inadequate oxygen delivery impairs the recovery process or affects the patient's overall outcome becomes the issue. It is accepted that the state of inadequate global oxygen delivery can be defined; it is less well accepted that the limits of that determination are known such that an absolute transfusion trigger can be identified.

Every clinician should weigh these issues when deciding to transfuse. The philosophic aspects of this argument are relative to patient care because there may be an effect on outcome, either positive or adverse, if these issues are not considered.

OXYGEN DELIVERY SYSTEM

The transfer of oxygen from the alveolus in the lung to the intracellular mitochondria is quite complex. There are many membrane systems with active and passive transport mechanisms involved. Transfer of oxygen across the pulmonary alveolocapillary membrane is a subject unto itself and is detailed elsewhere in this volume (see Chapters 35 and 87). Diseases that limit the diffusion of oxygen produce systemic hypoxia manifested as arterial oxygen desaturation. There is a relationship between saturation and oxygen content shown in the following equation, where Cao_2 is arterial oxygen content, Sao_2 is arterial oxygen saturation, Pao_2 is partial pressure of oxygen in arterial blood, and Hb is hemoglobin concentration in grams per deciliter:

$$Cao_2 = Hb \times 1.34 \times Sao_2 + Pao_2 \times 0.0031$$

It is clear that the major determinants of Cao_2 are Hb and Sao_2. Except in rare hemoglobinopathies, inadequate saturation usually reflects pulmonary gas exchange problems. Moreover, if blood is 100% saturated, there is an upper limit to oxygen content, assuming hyperbaric conditions are not present. The oxygen-carrying capacity reflects the maximum amount of oxygen that can be carried given full saturation; it has no specific clinical application at this time. The easiest method for increasing the oxygen content of arterial blood is the addition of hemoglobin.[5]

The delivery of oxygen ($\dot{D}o_2$) is most dependent on hemodynamics because it is defined as the product of flow, cardiac output, and arterial oxygen content. It describes overall $\dot{D}o_2$ and does not account for redistribution or specific tissue microcirculatory adjustments. Its measurement can serve as a good guide for overall patient management as long as the errors in the measurements are appreciated.[6] Although technically feasible, measuring tissue-specific $\dot{D}o_2$ has not attained clinical application.

Oxygen consumption ($\dot{V}o_2$) on a global or total body basis is assumed to be the product of cardiac output and the arteriovenous oxygen content difference. Like $\dot{D}o_2$, it is subject to measurement error in each of the variables and is sensitive to regional flow distribution and metabolic activity. Any situation that increases metabolic activity such as agitation, fever, major burns, or significant tissue injury will increase $\dot{V}o_2$. Measuring tissue-specific oxygen utilization is not in wide clinical use.

The oxygen extraction ratio (OER) is defined as the ratio of global oxygen consumption and global oxygen delivery. It reflects the efficiency of tissue oxygen use but clearly represents other variables including flow, oxygen-carrying capacity, and oxygen content. Normally between 0.25 and 0.30, the OER, when increased, most likely reflects poor flow with increased extraction, whereas values below 0.25 generally indicate high flow and poor extraction, or tissue inability to consume and use oxygen.

Another factor influencing $\dot{D}o_2$ is the position of the oxyhemoglobin dissociation curve, which is primarily regulated by intraerythrocytic 2, 3-diphosphoglyceric acid and plasma pH. The shape of the curve determines the P_{50} (the oxygen tension at which the hemoglobin is 50% saturated) and has an effect on oxygen availability. In this context, oxygen availability refers to the oxygen being present but bound so tightly to the Hb that it is not accessible for use; the result is a functional decrease in oxygen delivery. The normal P_{50} is 27.5 ± 1.0 mm Hg, and variations of 3.0 mm Hg in either direction are not actually of clinical significance.[7–9]

When $\dot{V}o_2$ is plotted against $\dot{D}o_2$, there appears to be a critical level of $\dot{D}o_2$ below which tissue is deprived of oxygen. To this point, working backward from adequate $\dot{D}o_2$, $\dot{V}o_2$ appears relatively stable. However, further diminution of $\dot{D}o_2$ significantly decreases $\dot{V}o_2$ in a near-linear fashion; $\dot{V}o_2$ is said to be flow dependent.[10] The point at which $\dot{V}o_2$ changes from flow dependent to flow independent is called the *critical oxygen delivery point* and has implications for transfusion therapy as well as overall critical care. At this point of $\dot{D}o_2$, lactic acid accumulation is noted, reflecting a switch from aerobic to anaerobic metabolism in the tissues. Below this critical $\dot{D}o_2$, the OER begins to increase exponentially, reflecting a decrease in $\dot{D}o_2$. If these variables are used to monitor patients, adequate $\dot{D}o_2$, however achieved, is defined as any value above the critical oxygen delivery point. Maintaining $\dot{D}o_2$, therefore, should obviate the problems of inadequate oxygen delivery.

RESPONSES TO DECREASED OXYGEN DELIVERY

When the state of decreased $\dot{D}o_2$ is present, physiologic compensation occurs at many levels. Intracellularly, less energy is produced from glucose consumption—2 mol of adenosine triphosphate instead of 36 mol in the aerobic conditions—with the resulting intracellular acidosis producing cellular dysfunction initially, which can, in fact, progress to tissue and organ failure (see Chapter 35). The effect of this cellular and eventual tissue and organism acidosis is clear; unreversed, it could lead to cell death. The effects of acidosis on intracellular communication systems—mediators, initiators, effectors—is not well defined but is assumed to be undesirable and detrimental. Siegel and colleagues reported on the interaction of these variables with specific respect to outcome.[11]

It is important to note that lactic acidosis can be detected at the point of critical $\dot{D}o_2$, where the OER increases and the $\dot{D}o_2$ decreases. The convergence of two or three variables on one specific $\dot{D}o_2$ value is particularly interesting because the critical $\dot{D}o_2$ point could then be considered a possible transfusion trigger. Obviously, this approach and analysis apply mostly to the ICU and OR because the necessary measurements are readily obtained there.

It is easier to appreciate the global compensatory mechanisms for a decreased $\dot{D}O_2$. Because $\dot{D}O_2$ is the product of cardiac output and CaO_2, the latter a function of Hb concentration, any acute decrease in Hb or intravascular volume increases cardiac output as compensation. This relationship is generally linear over the clinically relevant range, assuming that intercurrent disease, age, and pharmacologic agents do not prevent the homeostatic mechanisms from being activated. Interventions that increase cardiac output—preload, contractility, afterload—may be used to improve $\dot{D}O_2$ without reverting to RBC transfusion provided the patient has sufficient cardiovascular reserve.

The idea of improving $\dot{D}O_2$ by first increasing cardiac output is based on the $\dot{D}O_2$ physiology previously explored. The limitation is clearly the ability of the heart to meet the increased demands. Cardiac physiology is complex and not the subject of this chapter (see Chapter 46). However, certain aspects of cardiac physiology are relevant to deciding when to transfuse a patient because if the heart has limited reserves and cannot provide adequate $\dot{D}O_2$, it may be more appropriate to transfuse RBCs early.[12]

It is generally accepted that adequate coronary flow is required for proper cardiac muscle function. It is further assumed that aging naturally limits cardiac reserve, the ability to respond to acute stress or increased flow demands. Figure 153–1 expresses some of the key cardiac physiology involved, especially coronary flow because it is influenced by decreases in blood volume and coronary artery disease. The main point of this diagram is the graphic demonstration of a significant decrease in coronary artery blood flow associated with hypovolemia in the presence of coronary artery disease. Abstracted from basic science concepts relative to coronary blood flow, it is relevant to the clinical situation; a heart with limited coronary flow is not able to provide the necessary increases in cardiac output to afford an adequate global $\dot{D}O_2$.

TRANSFUSION TRIGGER

Even a cursory appreciation of the previous discussion would lead one to conclude that an absolute value for a transfusion trigger does not exist. The transfusion trigger is a dynamic variable, governed by many factors including cardiovascular status, vascular volume, and Hb concentration. A patient with adequate global $\dot{D}O_2$, flow-independent oxygen consumption, a normal oxygen extraction ratio, and no lactic acidosis has no obvious indication for an RBC transfusion.[13, 16] Applying the principles of $\dot{D}O_2$ physiology

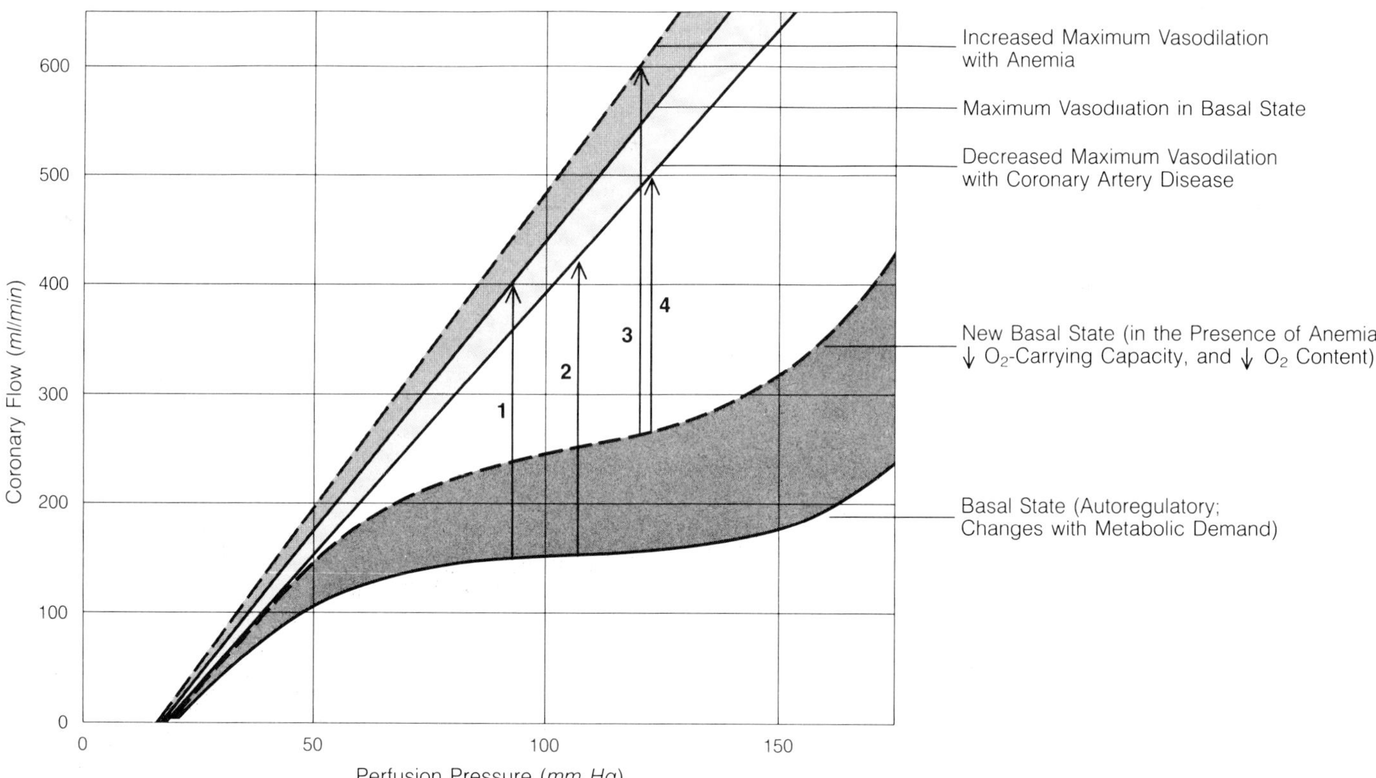

Figure 153–1. The coronary reserve concept[14, 15] describes pressure-flow relations and the influence of coronary artery disease or anemia, or both, on the coronary circulation. The basal autoregulatory state is essentially a flow-dependent–flow-independent situation for this particular vascular bed. When anemia is superimposed, thereby decreasing oxygen-carrying capacity and oxygen content, the basal curve shifts upward to meet the new baseline state, which resets the autoregulator. A minor increase in flow is possible with maximum vasodilation because of the anemia (shown in *dark gray*), but basal flow needs exceed the increase provided by this vasodilation. Similarly, if the coronary circuit is unable to dilate because of intrinsic disease or physiology, maximum dilation is not possible, and the flow response is limited (shown in *light gray*). Normal reserve is shown as line 1; it is the potential dilation available to meet flow requirements of any change in metabolic demand above basal levels. Reserve in the presence of coronary disease is shown in line 2; at similar pressure, a decrease in flow is noted. Normal reserve in the presence of anemia is indicated by line 3, and reserve in the presence of both coronary disease and anemia is shown as line 4. Note the significant decreases in reserve associated with disease or anemia, or both, and their influence on coronary flow. (From Greenburg AG: Indications for transfusion. *In:* Care of the Surgical Patient. Section I, Subsection 6. Wilmore DW (Ed). New York, Scientific American, Inc.)

to deciding the indications for transfusion is a proper scientific approach; new transfusion options on the horizon (e.g., Hb solutions) will be given based on these concepts. The future holds the promise of transfusing grams of Hb, not units of blood or RBCs, as is the current practice. Beyond the scope of the current chapter, the idea of RBC substitutes—various forms of Hb solutions or perfluorocarbons—for use intra- and postoperatively is noted for completeness.[17]

It should be noted that Schneider and colleagues, over a decade ago, integrated many of these ideas and established a transfusion nomogram interrelating the key variables.[7] Somewhat cumbersome to use, the idea of matching the indication for transfusion to patient needs was presented. It was one other way of exploring the elements of this important problem.

PRODUCTS AND TECHNIQUES FOR EFFECTING INCREASED OXYGEN DELIVERY

Clearly, any intervention that increases cardiac output will, by definition, increase $\dot{D}O_2$. Thus, agents used to increase preload, contractility, or afterload may be used to augment $\dot{D}O_2$, up to a point. Chapters 12 and 13 noted the limits of this approach in terms of age and coronary disease–related cardiac physiology specifically, and such discussion is not repeated here.

Increasing preload using intravascular volume loading or expansion—crystalloid or colloid—has a long and honorable history. It is still applicable in the intra- and perioperative periods. Variations of the approach include hypertonic saline and hypertonic/hyperoncotic solutions currently being evaluated in acute resuscitation but not yet widely used intra- or postoperatively.[18–20]

Transfusion of RBCs is the standard, widely used, clinically accepted method of increasing $\dot{D}O_2$ and may, for now, be the best and most appropriate treatment in specific situations. Correction of any underlying deficit in the $\dot{D}O_2$ system of specific disease states also would improve $\dot{D}O_2$; the goal would be normalization of $\dot{V}O_2$ reflected by a normal OER. In the operating room and ICU, the first step for increasing $\dot{D}O_2$ is optimization of the hemodynamic variables associated with $\dot{D}O_2$.

RISKS OF TRANSFUSION OF RED BLOOD CELLS

All treatment decisions are associated with some degree of risk including the decision to not treat if that is believed to be appropriate. Because of great concern about the transmission of infectious disease by RBC transfusion, especially human immunodeficiency virus (HIV), newer concepts of transfusion triggers and indications for transfusion are evolving. It is a difficult argument to refute. However, the publicity surrounding the risks of HIV and acquired immunodeficiency syndrome with blood transfusion has forced attention on appropriate transfusion alternatives and methods to decrease or eliminate the risks. Withholding a transfusion until it is absolutely indicated is reasonable if the point of necessity could be easily identified; unfortunately, this point is not readily apparent outside the areas of sophisticated monitoring. Thus, the conservative stance is frequently assumed; some patients who need transfusions are denied them, whereas others who may not require them are transfused, perhaps inappropriately.

The risks of transfusion per unit of blood or blood component transfused is shown in Table 153–1, after Valeri.[21–23] These are population estimates based on literature reviews[24, 25] and estimates of donor pool population positivity for infectious disease markers.[21, 23, 26–29] Of note, the most commonly transmitted viral agent associated with blood transfusion is cytomegalovirus (CMV); its true prevalence is difficult to estimate.[30] Fortunately, this virus is harbored in white blood cells, and modern transfusion techniques—component therapy—minimize exposure to these cells, thereby limiting risk. Although CMV is rarely of clinical significance, a patient with immune system compromise is more likely to show signs of CMV infection if it is present. Recall that many ICU patients are postoperative or post-trauma or have prolonged illnesses and are, in fact, immunosuppressed, increasing their risk for CMV infection if exposed. The range of infectious diseases transmitted by RBC transfusion is great.[22, 23, 31]

TABLE 153–1. Estimated Risk per Unit Blood or Blood Component Transfused*

Variable	*Risk*
Immediate	
Allergic	
Fever, chills, urticaria	1:100
Immunologic	
Hemolytic, nonfatal	1:6000
Hemolytic, fatal	1:100,000
Delayed	
Infectious	
Hepatitis C virus	1:3,300
HTLV-1, HTLV-2	1:50,000
Hepatitis B virus	1:200,000
HIV-1	1:225,000

*Data compiled from Valeri[21] and Gillon and Greenburg.[22, 23]

Abbreviations: HTLV = human T-cell lymphotrophic virus; HIV = human immunodeficiency virus.

There are other complications of transfusion therapy not easily classified as immune or infectious disease related. They are associated with the logistics of transfusion, the techniques, and the equipment used. Many of these issues are exaggerated with autotransfusion.[32]

The dilutional coagulopathy and disseminated intravascular coagulation may be technique specific as are reinfusion of anticoagulant and air embolism. Certainly, the issue of dilutional coagulopathy associated with massive transfusion therapy is well known; in some ways, that is a separate topic with its own unique problems.[33, 34] The coagulopathy of massive transfusion is dilutional but needs to be treated only if symptomatic; the appropriate therapy is transfusion of platelets for the bleeding indication and not prophylactically. The coagulopathy of autotransfusion is also dilutional, but platelet activation plays a role.

Other aspects of complications of transfusion therapy often overlooked are related to hypothermia, especially exaggerated with rapid transfusion of cold bank RBCs. Warming the blood, if possible, is desirable. Of note, hypothermia is particularly related to bleeding. The coagulation system appears to be truly thermodynamically regulated; when temperatures are below the optimal 37°C, the coagulation system begins to fail. It is best to maintain patients at normothermic levels to obviate this problem. The coagulopathy induced by hypothermia is believed to be primarily related to platelet dysfunction.[35–37]

It must also be noted that transfused bank blood has a significant concentration of potassium (20–50 mEq/L) as a result of RBC lysis during storage. If infused rapidly, cardiac dysrhythmia is possible, aggravated, of course, in the presence of hypothermia, both affecting cardiac excitability. An excess of citrate—the primary anticoagulant of stored blood—can bind serum calcium, decreasing it and inducing cardiac dysfunction. This is not a problem if the RBC infusion rate is less than 100 mL/min; when the infusion rate exceeds this level, supplemental calcium in the form of gluconate may be required. The rate- and volume-related transfusion problems are well documented and should always be considered. In general, these are not issues for elective surgical procedures because rarely are the volumes large. An area of recent concern is an apparent immune suppressive effect of transfusion therapy. Initially perceived as a benefit in renal transplantation,[38] where history of transfusion correlated to increased graft survival, it was later seen to be a liability with respect to survival in patients with malignant disease.[22, 23, 39] Using colon cancer as a model, transfusion appeared to induce an immune suppression that was adversely related to survival in terms of recurrence and longevity.[40–42] If transfusions are immunosuppressive, then the host is placed at increased risk, and infectious complications as well as the tumor-related factors could affect outcome. It is important to appreciate the mechanisms of this immune suppression so future therapy can be aimed at minimizing or eliminating the impact. Clearly, RBC substitute solutions will be required to meet this standard when tested clinically.

The induced immune suppression is related to the volume of allogeneic blood infused; the greater the quantity infused, the more pronounced and prolonged the effect.[43] An issue in the era of autologous donation and autotransfusion is whether the technique or process plays a role. One study failed to demonstrate an outcome difference between techniques (autologous versus allogeneic) but did show a survival advantage if no transfusion was required.[42] The act of transfusion may be more critical than the form used to deliver the product in terms of immune system alterations.[21] The mechanisms proposed to explain this effect implicate both cellular and plasma components of blood. Changes in suppressor T cells (e.g., number and function), cytokine production, monocyte function, and natural killer cell function are postulated.[44, 45]

It is generally assumed there is an increased risk of infection after allogeneic transfusion.[39] It is difficult to sort the effects of trauma from the effects of transfusion on the host defense system. At this time, the problem is assumed to be multidimensional, with many factors at play. If, indeed, the act of transfusion is immunosuppressive, independent of the technique used, its use should be minimized. Then, when making the transfusion decision, this factor must be weighed against the hemodynamic consequences of not transfusing with altered $\dot{D}O_2$ and an impact on host defenses. Clearly, the decision process is complex and requires analysis of many variables at once before ordering a transfusion. A series of tradeoffs—risks and benefits—must be considered each time a transfusion is considered.

RED BLOOD CELL TRANSFUSION OPTIONS

The options for RBC transfusion late in the 20th century are many. Not all are applicable to every situation, and many require significant preplanning to use them effectively. The RBC options for use in emergency situations are more limited than those available for elective surgical procedures. Autologous blood is perceived to be safest, at least with respect to transmission of infectious disease, but there is always a risk of clerical error and a major transfusion reaction. Homologous RBCs will most probably be used in urgent and emergency situations; they come in a variety of forms with various levels of treatment to minimize complications. The list of variations for autologous RBC products continues to expand as newer, more efficient technologic solutions are put into general use. Various forms of autotransfusion are now available for use: preoperative autologous blood donation with or without erythropoietin augmentation, intra- and postoperative cell salvage, and intraoperative hemodilution. Some are clearly not applicable to emergency situations or the ICU, whereas others have much broader general application. Table 153–2 lists the various forms of homologous RBCs that can be infused. The differences in terms of oxygen-carrying capacity are relatively small. The real differences are in the quantity of non-RBC material infused (e.g., protein, dead cells, debris), which could lead to undesirable side effects.

TABLE 153–2. Homologous Red Blood Cells (RBCs)

Whole blood
Packed RBCs
Leukocyte-free RBCs
Adenine stored RBCs
Washed packed RBCs
Frozen packed RBCs
Rejuvenated frozen packed RBCs

There are few, if any, indications for the use of whole blood. Component therapy is not only appropriate because of its specificity—treating a specific deficiency—but it is desirable because it conserves resources, maximizing the usefulness of a single unit of blood for many patients. Blood undergoes many tests before it can be released for use. These are shown in Table 153–3. To accomplish all of these tests requires time, and the unique properties of "fresh whole blood" may be lost when 24 hours are required to ensure the safety of the product.

All solutions of packed RBCs (PRBCs) deliver about 200 mL of RBCs; thus, they all increase oxygen-carrying capacity equally. Factors that influence oxygen availability changes in P_{50} are related to length of storage and type of storage solution/preservatives and anticoagulant used. A discussion of this issue is beyond the scope of this chapter. Generally, the blood bank dispenses the older units first. Special preservatives (e.g., adenine) are used to maintain "normal" RBC metabolic activity in storage; this approach is generally effective, and old blood (e.g., 35 days stored) is useful and has a good circulating half-life when infused. Washing RBCs and depleting them of white blood cells are techniques used to decrease the incidence of allergic transfusion reactions and future immunologic complications. The removal of debris and old RBCs does accomplish this.

Freezing RBCs is an alternative to liquid storage. Useful cells within their liquid storage life or outdated cells subjected to rejuvenation can be stored in the frozen state. This is most appropriate for O-negative universal donor and autologous predeposit situations but may be applied to rare

TABLE 153–3. Tests on Donor Units

Syphilis
Viral hepatitis
Hepatitis B surface antigen and antibody to hepatitis B core antigen
Antibody to hepatitis C; ALT surrogate marker of liver infection
Retroviruses
Antibody to HIV-1 (anti-HIV-1) and HIV-2 (anti-HIV-2)
Antibody to HTLV-I/II

Abbreviations: ALT = alanine aminotransferase; HIV = human immunodeficiency virus; HTLV = human T-cell lymphotrophic virus.

TABLE 153–4. Autologous Transfusion Options

Preoperative autodonation with or without erythropoietin augmentation
Intraoperative hemodilution
Cell salvage: intraoperative, postoperative

blood types as well. The freezing and thawing process adds to the complexity of the transfusion therapy. The cryoprotectant must be removed by sequential washings, which actually provides a cleaner solution of RBCs and removes the excess debris in the process. Once defrosted and washed, the shelf life of frozen cells is limited. The work of Valeri is seminal in this area.[46]

Table 153–4 lists the various forms of autotransfusion. As noted, the rationale for the use of autologous blood is clear; it is safe relative to transmission of infectious disease. Whether it is safe relative to placing the immune system/host defense mechanism at risk is less well accepted.[39–41, 43–45] Transfusion of old, dysfunctional RBCs appears to be a major part of the immunocompromise problem whether the cells are homologous or autologous. Patients scheduled for elective surgery in which a significant blood loss is anticipated and in whom there is concern that the cardiovascular reserve is insufficient should be considered candidates for autologous predeposit autodonation. Blood loss for a given procedure by a surgeon is usually predictable; this datum is the basis for defining a maximum surgical blood ordering schedule (MBOS).[47] The MBOS matches resources to needs, improving blood banking efficiency. It also affords a means of providing a "type and screen" specimen to the laboratory/blood bank if blood is needed unexpectedly for a case that usually does not require it.

Autologous predeposit blood is removed over a period of days to weeks before a planned operative procedure such that the first unit will be outdated after the planned surgical date.[48, 49] Donor criteria appear to be somewhat arbitrary; hematocrit of 33% or Hb of 11 g/dL makes a patient eligible. The ability to withstand an acute blood loss of 200 to 450 mL and tolerate a vasovagal reaction are also important criteria.[50] Provided the iron substrate is available and nutrition is adequate, a unit of RBCs can be withdrawn every 7 days. Elderly patients with and without cardiac disease apparently tolerate this procedure. It is not yet clear whether adding erythropoietin to the regimen is effective.[49] If autologous predeposit is combined with intraoperative hemodilution and cell salvage when appropriate, enough autologous RBCs for most major elective cases can be accumulated.

An understanding of the normal erythropoietic response will provide a basis for considering the use of recombinant erythropoietin in the postoperative period. Surgery and trauma in general suppress erythropoiesis.[51] Normal erythropoiesis will not be operative in a hypotensive, immunosuppressed patient subject to acute hemorrhagic anemia, all most likely superimposed on a chronic disease state, which is a not uncommon intensive care scenario. The role of recombinant erythropoietin in critical care is not clear. Effectiveness and safety must be shown in return for a potentially high cost.[52, 53]

The concept of intraoperative hemodilution pioneered by Messmer is finally gaining wider application.[54] An acute normovolemic anemia is induced by removing RBCs and replenishing the intravascular space with crystalloid (preferred), colloid, or a combination of the two to maintain the intravascular volume. Seated in the scientific principles of $\dot{D}O_2$ physiology, hemodilution appears to be well tolerated by all patient populations. Used alone, it can provide three to four units of RBCs—in the form of whole blood—although usually only one to three units are taken. As noted, when combined with predeposit autotransfusion, a significant volume of autologous blood is available for any given patient. Usually the blood is withdrawn in the operating room and kept there, at room temperature, for a maximum of 4 hours; if reinfusion is to occur later, the blood must be labeled and properly stored. It does not require the usual testing for donor units.[55]

Clearly, the level of hemodilution is finite; at some point $\dot{D}O_2$ is compromised and anaerobic metabolism begins. Moreover, the technique relies heavily on cardiovascular status: specifically, the ability of the heart to increase cardiac output in response to new demands. Similarly, adequate renal function is required to permit off loading of the diluent. The interactions of these variables and their optimization are very much related to identification of an appropriate transfusion trigger.[56] Before universal application, more effort is required to explore this technique, its range of application, and, more critically, its limits. Case reports are helpful in focusing on this problem, and a critical editorial perspective is helpful in defining the limits.[57, 58]

Intraoperative RBC salvage should be considered for all elective surgeries in which blood loss of two units or more is expected and for all emergency cases in which infection and contamination with bowel contents or malignant cells are not present. It is a safe, cost-effective method that decreases demands on the blood bank. It is particularly effective in vascular and cardiac procedures, total joint replacement, liver transplantation, spine surgery, and certain gynecologic operations.[59, 60]

Modern autotransfusion devices are of two major types, with real differences in cost as well as quality of infused, salvaged RBCs. Systems that collect and wash RBCs are preferred even if there is an additional cost because the final product is more desirable. The use of a filter is mandatory, and the benefit of washing cells in eliminating coagulopathies has been reported.[61–63]

Perioperative salvage—drainage from chest tubes or mediastinal tubes—is a good method of conserving the blood supply while minimizing some of the risks of transfusion. The salvaged RBCs can be infused directly or after washing.[64]

Autotransfusion and the use of autologous blood are useful techniques for blood conservation and patient safety. In the early 1990s, a panel of experts was assembled and their views were published.[32] In this document, most of the key issues surrounding this technique and the various options were discussed.

TRANSFUSION IN EMERGENCY AND URGENT RESUSCITATION SITUATIONS

Acute massive hemorrhage either intraoperatively or postoperatively is generally treated with major volume resuscitation including crystalloids, colloids, and then some form of RBC transfusion. The choice of which RBCs to use with special reference to type and the need for crossmatching has been of interest for many years. Generally, when 30% or more of the circulating blood volume is lost, there is the requirement to add RBCs to the resuscitation effort.

Type-Specific Red Blood Cells

Type-specific, uncrossmatched PRBCs are the preferred and logical choice in this situation. Typing of blood is relatively rapid (5–7 minutes), and available units can be on the way for use shortly thereafter. Several studies demonstrated the safety of this approach, its effectiveness, and the low incidence of transfusion reaction.[65, 66] Type-specific uncrossmatched blood can cause a transfusion reaction in previously transfused patients and multiparous women. Both groups are at risk because they may harbor undetected antibodies; the risks are perceived to be small. It is important to note that delays in administration of type-specific RBCs are due to the time it takes to transport specimens and RBCs, not the time it takes to type the specimen.

Type O, Rh-Negative Red Blood Cells

Lacking the major ABO cellular antigens, type O RBCs can theoretically be administered without fear of a major ABO incompatibility reaction. With the advent of blood component therapy, the plasma component of a unit of PRBCs is very small, and the risk of minor transfusion reactions (donor serum against recipient cells) is diminished. Type O, Rh-negative blood is the universal donor, usually given as PRBCs. After receiving large quantities of universal RBCs, patients with type A, B, or AB blood may have transfusion reactions when subsequently administered RBCs typed and crossmatched to their initial, preuniversal donor transfusion specimen. It is possible that subsequent crossmatching would be complicated because of the admixture of RBCs in the patient. These reactions, potentially real, are fortunately quite rare. The use of type-specific RBCs would obviate any of these problems.

Type O, Rh-Positive Red Blood Cells

In men and in women beyond the childbearing age, in whom antibody formation is less of a problem, type O, Rh-positive blood is another universal donor. This concept is advocated because it would increase the donor pool and augment the national blood supply. Only about 8% of the U.S. population has type O, Rh-negative blood, a rather limited pool. Patients who are Rh negative do not have preexisting antibodies to the Rh antigen and thus will not have an immediate transfusion reaction if given Rh-positive RBCs. Rh-negative multiparous women and previously transfused Rh-negative patients are at increased risk, however. About 70% of Rh-negative individuals who receive Rh-positive RBCs will acquire anti-D antibodies. Indeed, few patients are in this situation. One interesting study found a 1% incidence of preformed, clinically significant antibodies in 449 trauma patients; none of these were anti-Rh.[67]

Type O, Rh-positive blood should be considered the third option after type-specific uncrossmatched and type O, Rh-negative blood for emergency RBC replacement.[68]

APPLICATIONS OF THE OPTIONS FOR RED BLOOD CELL TRANSFUSION

Many transfusion options are available for use in both the OR and ICU. As part of optimizing the oxygen delivery system, transfusion with RBCs is still a major and appropriate technique. In deciding which options to use, a number of variables must be considered: elective or emergency procedure, estimated blood loss, patient's overall state of health with particular reference to cardiovascular and pulmonary systems, and the possibility of an underlying anemia. The latter is of concern because it will eliminate the use of certain predeposit autologous options for elective surgery.

At the initial scheduling of a surgical procedure, an assessment of the likelihood of perioperative transfusion is made. On the basis of data accumulated through MBOS,[47, 69] it is very likely the transfusion requirement can be closely approximated. The widest range of transfusion options are available for the patient who has no anemia at the time. Because autologous blood is safe with respect to transmission of infectious disease, its use is desirable. Of note, blood drawn for autologous transfusion is fully tested even though in most instances it generally will never be turned into the general donor pool; the unit is allowed to reach expiration and is then discarded. Clearly, patients who are ineligible to donate for the general pool can provide acceptable units for self-use assuming all other criteria for autologous predeposit are met. Moreover, blood collected as autologous predeposit is usually labeled differently to minimize inadvertent and potentially lethal introduction into the general pool. A major cause of lethal transfusion reaction continues to be clerical error resulting in the patient receiving the wrong unit of RBCs. Anything that minimizes this risk is a positive quality control measure and should be encouraged.

The addition of recombinant human erythropoietin (r-HuEPO) to the regimen of autologous predeposit has been noted previously. Still a costly therapy, it may have a use in this arena. It can be argued that the MBOS and proper planning for the operative aspects of a procedure can cover the needs in a nonanemic patient with adequate iron stores. The anemic patient population may be more appropriate for this adjunctive therapy. In addition, the perioperative uses of r-HuEPO for vascular, orthopedic, oncologic, and cardiac surgery are just being explored.

Acute normovolemic hemodilution is an excellent technique for elective surgical procedures and some urgent cases in which there has not been a significant hypovolemic period or major blood loss. An option applicable in the OR only, it is clearly an effective technique that minimizes risks to the patient and places minimal demands on the blood bank. The risk of transmission of infectious disease is minimized, and other forms of transfusion reactions should be eliminated. A wider use of the technique has been encouraged, and gradually there has been acceptance and wider application. When acute normovolemic hemodilution is used in combination with predeposit autologous and RBC salvage, it is possible to acquire six to eight units of a patient's blood for use in a single perioperative period, an idea worthy of consideration because so few common procedures actually use more blood than this.

Intraoperative RBC salvage is a major advance in hemotherapy, and developing technology will no doubt further refine and improve the technique in the years to come. Washing the RBCs effectively eliminates some of the complications, especially the coagulopathy. In the systems used to recycle mediastinal or chest tube drainage, the risk of infusing an excessive amount of anticoagulant exists and must always be considered a potential risk. The rate of loss and reinfusion plays a role in determining the incidence of this significant complication.

Most autologous transfusion options cannot be applied in the emergency surgical situation. Intraoperative RBC salvage is helpful provided there is no contamination with bowel contents. Cell salvage in emergency surgery for repair of aortic aneurysms is desirable. The general risks of the cell salvage techniques are the potential to induce a coagulopathy, overdilution, infusion of excessive anticoagulant, and the potential to infuse cell fragments, proteins, protein fragments, and other "debris," which could have toxic consequences on many key host systems, including the host defense mechanism generally.

ALLOGENEIC TRANSFUSION OPTIONS

Traditional transfusion for nearly a century has been allogeneic—homologous—RBCs evolving from whole blood to mostly, if not exclusively, PRBCs. The risk of transfusion with this family of agents has been explored previously.

Although clinicians are primarily concerned with transmission of infectious disease, many other toxic side effects and complications can arise from allogeneic RBC transfusion. Although the risks are reasonably low for a population as a whole, when a complication or adverse event does occur, it has real impact.

Because patients are aware of this directed donor option, surgeons and intensive care physicians need to be alert to its use. By selecting donors, a given patient believes the risk of transmission of infectious disease is minimized. Patients and their families need to be made aware of the potential for blood group incompatibility and that not all patient-selected donors will necessarily have compatible blood. Blood collected through directed donation is fully processed and tested before release; this process has no short cuts. Full crossmatching is expected. There are complexities of directed donations that limit its application. The potential for immunization is real for the recipient, and women of child-bearing age and bone marrow transplant recipients could be at increased risk if given blood from a family member. To minimize this possibility, some centers irradiate the blood before infusion. Like autologous blood, directed donations are not usually crossed over into the general blood pool once their need has expired. Because these two classes do not fit the group of "voluntary donor," it is safer to not enter these units into the general blood banking pool.[24, 25]

RBCs typed and crossmatched to a recipient are the first line of allogeneic units generally available. Given sufficient time to accomplish the task, this blood is usually "safe" from the potential of a major transfusion reaction. It is also safe to the extent it is tested for the potential of infectious disease transmission. Unfortunately, there is always the risk of clerical error with resulting mortality.[70, 71] The concept of immune suppression associated with RBC transfusion therapy being a positive or a negative factor needs to be noted again. Analytically, one should question the basis for this problem. Two options appear: the act of transfusion or the transfused product. If the problem arises from the act of transfusion, then one would expect to see immune depression even in patients receiving autologous blood. Lending support to the argument is the linkage of the immune suppression to an impaired reticuloendothelial system most likely associated with the clearance of old, crenated RBCs.

Using allogeneic RBCs is the option of choice in emergency situations, and when an urgent elective surgical procedure is scheduled, the time available for planned preoperative autologous donation is limited. Intraoperatively, in an emergency, this may be the only option, possibly supplemented with intraoperative salvage provided the patient meets the accepted criteria.

RBC transfusion has an inherent finite risk. Ideally, that risk should be minimized by the use of alternatives directed at improving $\dot{D}O_2$ and autologous RBCs whenever possible. The latter is more appropriate for planned elective surgery and should be encouraged. There are still many patients who find themselves in the OR on an urgent or even emergency basis when time to prepare autologous units is not available.

Some postoperative patients who have had the luxury of time to achieve autologous predeposit and to whom all of the units were not returned may be in an ICU when they develop significant bleeding and hypovolemia requiring an RBC transfusion; for them, the stored, unused autologous units are ideal. Whenever possible, the use of intraoperative hemodilution is now encouraged; for urgent and emergency cases, this technique has very limited application. For now, it has no place as a perioperative transfusion option in the ICU.

The decision to transfuse is complex and requires the decision maker to weigh many options, using an often incomplete data base. If the cardiovascular system can accommodate a decreased oxygen-carrying capacity—acute anemia—without untoward effects, then optimization of hemodynamics is the necessary first step if the bleeding is controlled. In the ICU and OR, where there is sophisticated monitoring equipment, a more accurate assessment of a transfusion trigger threshold may be attained. This is usually accomplished in the context of reaching a therapeutic goal relative to $\dot{D}O_2$ rather than optimization of intravascular volume and restoration of blood volume, both difficult to measure accurately.

In the absence of measurable variables and defined parameters, the decision to transfuse usually results in an assessment of the risk of not transfusing against the well-defined transfusion risks previously noted. This interesting topic has been explored recently and the issues presented in an interesting way. Many practitioners do not appreciate all of the risks and potential tradeoffs of the $\dot{D}O_2$ system and the role transfusion therapy plays in this important decision.[28, 31, 39, 72]

A LOOK AT THE FUTURE

In a society driven by technology, it is reasonable to assume that a substitute for RBCs will at some time be available. Ongoing concern about the safety of the blood supply, an emerging world community, and transfusion logistics will all converge to bring this family of products to the marketplace. It is not the intent of this chapter to review this area in detail; rather, an overview is presented so the reader will be familiar with the concepts as these products begin to enter clinical trials and application. A relatively complete review has been published.[15]

The concept behind oxygen-carrying RBC substitutes is to augment oxygen-carrying capacity. Thus, these solutions need to carry and off load oxygen in an effective and efficient manner without inducing toxicity or physiologic consequences perceived as detrimental. The general categories of RBC substitute solutions are shown in Table 153–5.

Independent of the source of the material—synthetic or biologic—there are potential problems related to the production, storage, administration, and biologic response for each group of agents. Some problems will be unique to a specific concept, but most are universal when it relates to the response to transfusion.[73] Factors to be considered as potential toxins include purity of the starting materials and final product, sterilization, storage modalities, and stability as well as the purification/clean-up techniques applied during manufacture. When an unexpected finding is seen clinically—hypertension, bradycardia, coagulopathy, altered renal function—after low-dose infusion of experimental agents, the toxicity could be related to other aspects: the modified molecule, the molecular modifier and its metabo-

TABLE 153–5. General Categories/Classes of Red Blood Cell Substitute Solution

Metalloporphyrins
Liposome-embedded heme
Encapsulated hemoglobin
Modified red blood cells
Perfluorocarbon emulsions
Chemically modified hemoglobin tetramers
Conjugated hemoglobins
Polymerized hemoglobin

lites, iron overload, or contaminants such as solution residuals or "fellow travelers." More recently, there is concern that the solution has an inherent pharmacologic effect, especially hemoglobin-based products, partially related to the binding of nitric oxide or other small molecules with significant vasoactivity. At this writing, these are being evaluated.[74]

Metalloporphyrins and embedded heme liposomes are interesting avenues for exploration and could yield good results over time. The liposome is being extensively explored, and some reports are encouraging but not conclusive.[75] In this case, the addition of hypertonic saline confounds rather than simplifies the analysis of the solution's effectiveness. The idea of modifying all RBCs to be universal donors is intriguing because it could eliminate a form of risk; unfortunately, the product is not yet sufficiently stable for widespread application.

The two areas of greatest effort continue to be fluorocarbons and hemoglobin-based solutions.[76-79]

A number of hemoglobin-based solutions are in various phases of clinical testing. The most recent products appear to be clean and relatively free of the toxicity seen with earlier, less pure materials. Whether they will achieve full clinical application is, of course, to be determined in the future. At this time, there are at least 11 modifiers or families of modifiers and four or five cross-linkers for hemoglobin being explored. The size of the molecule, degree of polymerization (the preferred form), and purity are all significantly improved over previous materials.[15] As this field evolves and the products improve, the current materials or updated versions of them will be able to play a major role in augmenting or replacing $\dot{D}O_2$ system components in the perioperative period.

References

1. Renzi RM, Kaye W, Greenburg AG: Oxygen utilization in the critically ill patient in surgical intensive care. *In:* Barie PS, Shires GT (Eds). VI. Boston, Little, Brown and Co, 1993, pp 211–226.
2. Cheng EY: Disease processes affecting oxygen transport and consumption. Probl Crit Care 1972; 6:366–374.
3. Greenburg AG: Pathophysiology of shock. *In:* The Physiologic Basis of Modern Critical Care. Miller TA (Ed). St. Louis, CV Mosby, 1988, pp 154–172.
4. Holcroft JW, Robinson MK: Shock. *In:* Care of the Surgical Patient. Wilmore DW, Brennan MF, Harken AH, et al (Eds). New York, Scientific American, 1988–1992, pp 1–37.
5. Gutierrez G: Cellular oxygen requirements. Probl Crit Care 1992; 6:347–365.
6. Bartlett RH, Decker RE: Oxygen kinetics: Pitfalls in clinical research. J Crit Care 1990; 5:77.
7. Schneider AJ, Stockman III JA, Oski FA: Transfusion nomogram: An application of physiology to clinical decisions regarding the use of blood. Crit Care Med 1981; 9:949.
8. Harken AH, Woods M: The influence of oxyhemoglobin affinity on tissue oxygen consumption. Ann Surg 1976; 183:130.
9. Greenburg AG, Pricolo VE: Life threatening acid based disorders. *In:* Care of the Surgical Patient. Wilmore DW (Ed). New York, Scientific American, 1989.
10. Shibutani K, Komatsu T, Kubal K, et al: Critical level of oxygen delivery in anesthetized man. Crit Care Med 1983; 11:640.
11. Dunham CM, Siegel JH, Weireter L, et al: Oxygen debt and metabolic acidemia as quantitative predictors of mortality and the severity of the ischemic insult in hemorrhagic shock. Crit Care Med 1991; 19:231–243.
12. Wei JY: Age and the cardiovascular system. N Engl J Med 1992; 327:1735–1739.
13. Greenburg AG: Indications for transfusion. *In:* Care of the Surgical Patient. Wilmore DW (Ed). New York, Scientific American, 1991.
14. Hoffman JIE: Maximal coronary flow and the concept of coronary vascular reserve. Circulation 1984; 70:153.
15. Biro GP: Blood substitutes and the heart: A critical view. *In:* International Symposium on Artificial Blood Substitutes. DeStasio G (Ed). Osperaliero, "Divenere," USL BA/11, Bari Carbonara, Italy, 1987, p 233.
16. Babineau TJ, Dzik WH, Borlase BC, et al: Reevaluation of current transfusion practices in patients in surgical intensive care units. Am J Surg 1992; 164:22–25.
17. Greenburg AG: Alternatives to conventional uses of blood products. *In:* Critical Care Medicine: State of the Art. Vol. 13. Carlson EW, Reines HD (Eds). Anaheim, CA, Society of Critical Care Medicine, 1992, pp 325–351.
18. Krausz MM, Ravid A, Feigen E, et al: The effect of heat load and dehydration on hypertonic saline solution treatment of uncontrolled hemorrhage shock. Surg Gynecol Obstet 1993; 177:583–592.
19. Holcroft JW, Vassor MJ, Turner JE, et al: 3% NaCl and 7.5% NaCl/dextran 70 in the resuscitation of severely injured patients. Ann Surg 1987; 206:279–288.
20. Maningas P, Mattox K, Pepe P, et al: Hypertonic saline dextran solutions for the pre-hospital management of hypovolemia. Am J Surg 1989; 157:528–534.
21. Valeri CR: Transfusion medicine and surgical practice. ACS Bull 1993; 78:19–24.
22. Gillon J, Greenburg AG: Transfusions: Infectious complications. Infect Med 1992; 9:19.
23. Gillon J, Greenburg AG: Transfusions: Immunologic, volume-related and storage-related complications. Infect Med 1993; 10:41–44.
24. Goldfinger D: Directed blood donations: Pro. Transfusion 1989; 29:70–74.
25. Page PL: Directed blood donations: Con. Transfusion 1989; 29:65–69.
26. Seidl S, Kuhul P: Transmission of diseases by blood transfusion. World J Surg 1987; 11:30–35.
27. Donahue JG, Munoz A, Ness MP, et al: The declining risk of post-transfusion hepatitis C virus infection. N Engl J Med 1992; 327:369–373.
28. Carson JL, Russell LB, Tarragin MI, et al: The risks of blood transfusion: The relative influence of acquired immunodeficiency syndrome and non-A, non-B hepatitis. Am J Med 1992; 92:45–52.
29. Heymann SJ, Brewer TF, Fineberg HV, et al: How safe is safe enough? New infections in the U.S. blood supply. Ann Intern Med 1992; 117:612–614.
30. Wilhelm JA, Matter L, Schopfer K: The risk of transmitting cytomegalovirus to patients receiving blood transfusions. J Infect Dis 1986; 154:169–171.
31. Goodnough LT, Shuck JM: Risks, options, and informed consent for blood transfusion in elective surgery. Am J Surg 1990; 159:602–609.
32. The use of autologous blood: Special communication. JAMA 1990; 263:414.
33. Counts RB, Haisch C, Simon TL, et al: Hemostasis in massively transfused trauma patients. Ann Surg 1979; 190:91–99.
34. Harrigan C, Lucas CE, Ledgerwood AM, et al: Serial changes in primary hemostasis after massive transfusion. Surgery 1985; 98:836–843.
35. Valeri CR, Cassidy G, Khuri SF, et al: Hypothermia: Induced reversible platelet dysfunction. Ann Surg 1987; 205:175–181.
36. Valeri CR, MacGregor H, Pompei F, et al: Acquired abnormalities of platelet function. N Engl J Med 1991; 324:1670.
37. Reed RL, Johnston TD, Hudson JD, et al: The disparity between hypothermic coagulopathy and clotting studies. J Trauma 1992; 33:465–470.
38. Opelz G, Sengar DPS, Mickey MR, et al: Effect of blood transfusion on subsequent kidney transplants. Transplant Proc 1973; 3:253–259.
39. Collins JA: Current status of blood therapy in surgery. Adv Surg 1989; 22:75.
40. Burrows L, Tarter P: Effect of blood transfusion on colonic malignancy recurrence rate. Lancet 1982; 2:662.
41. Francis DMA: Relationship between blood transfusion and tumour behavior. Br J Surg 1991; 78:1420–1428.
42. Busch ORC, Hop WCJ, Hoynck-Ven Papendrecht MAW, et al: Blood transfusion and prognosis in colorectal cancer. N Engl J Med 1993; 328:1372–1376.

43. Kerman RH, Agostino G, Van Buren CT, et al: Effect of blood transfusions on graft survival and immune responsiveness. Trans Proc 1983; 15:1022–1025.
44. Smith DM Jr: Immunosuppressive effects of blood transfusion. Clin Lab Med 1992; 12:723–741.
45. Waymack JP, Gugliuzza K, Dong Y-L, et al: Effect of blood transfusion on immune function: IX. Effect on lymphocyte metabolism. J Surg Res 1993; 55:269–272.
46. Valeri CR: Frozen red blood cells. *In:* Principles of Transfusion Medicine. Rossi EC, Simon TL, Moss GS (Eds). Baltimore, Williams & Wilkins, 1991.
47. Stehling LC: Pre-operative blood ordering. Int Anesthesiol Clin 1982; 20:45.
48. Toy PTC, Strauss RG, Stemling LC, et al: Pre-deposited autologous blood for elective surgery. N Engl J Med 1987; 316:517.
49. Goodnough LT, Rudnick S, Price TH, et al: Increased pre-operative collection of autologous blood with recombinant human erythropoietin therapy. N Engl J Med 1989; 321:1163.
50. Ruetz PP, Johnson SA, Callahan R, et al: Fainting: A review of its mechanisms and a study of blood donors. Medicine 1967; 46:363.
51. Howard RJ, Simmons RL: Acquired immunological deficiencies after trauma and surgical procedures. Surg Gynecol Obstet 1974; 138:771.
52. Rosen AL, Gould SA, Sehgal LR, et al: Erythropoietic response to acute anemia. Crit Care Med 1990; 18:298.
53. Levine EA, Rosen AL, Sehgal LR, et al: Treatment of acute post-operative anemia with recombinant human erythropoietin. J Trauma 1989; 29:1134.
54. Messmer K: Hemodilution. Surg Clin North Am 1975; 55:659.
55. Messmer K: Pre-operative hemodilution. *In:* Principles of Transfusion Medicine. Rossi EC, Simon TL, Moss GS (Eds). Baltimore, Williams & Wilkins, 1991.
56. Rudowski R, Greenburg AG, Kaye W, et al: Unpublished data, 1992.
57. van Woerkeus ECSM, Trouwborst A, van Lanschol JJB: Profound hemodilution: What is the critical level of hemodilution at which oxygen delivery-dependent oxygen consumption starts in an anesthetized human? Anesth Analg 1992; 75:818–821.
58. Leone BJ, Spahn DR: Anemia, hemodilution and oxygen delivery. Anesth Analg 1992; 75:651–653.
59. Kruskall M: Intra-operative autotransfusion. *In:* Principles of Transfusion Medicine. Rossi ER, Simon TL, Moss GS (Eds). Baltimore, Williams & Wilkins, 1991.
60. Giordano GF, Giordano DM, Wallace BH, et al: An analysis of 9,918 consecutive peri-operative autotransfusions. Surg Gynecol Obstet 1993; 176:103.
61. Griffith LD, Billman GF, Daily PO, et al: Apparent coagulopathy caused by infusion of mediastinal blood and its prevention by washing of the infusate. Ann Thorac Surg 1989; 47:400.
62. Horst HM, Dlugos S, Fath JJ, et al: Coagulopathy and intra-operative blood salvage (IBS). J Trauma 1992; 32:646.
63. Bull BS, Bull MH: Enhancing the safety of intra-operative RBC salvage. J Trauma 1989; 29:320.
64. Lapore V, Radegran K: Autotransfusion of mediastinal blood in cardiac surgery. Scand J Thorac Cardiovasc Surg 1989; 23:47.
65. Blumberg N, Bove JR: Uncross matched blood for emergency transfusion. JAMA 1978; 240:2057.
66. Gervin AS, Fisher RP: Resuscitation of human patients with type-specific uncross matched blood. J Trauma 1984; 24:327.
67. Schmidt PJ, Leparc GF, Samia CT: Use of RH-positive blood in emergency situations. Surg Gynecol Obstet 1988; 167:229–233.
68. Schwab CW, Shayne JP, Turner J: Immediate resuscitation with type-O unmatched blood: A two-year prospective exercise. J Trauma 1986; 26:897–902.
69. American Society of Anesthesiologists: Questions and Answers About Transfusion Practices. 2nd ed. Park Ridge, IL, American Society of Anesthesiologists, 1992.
70. Honig CL, Bove JR: Transfusion: Associated fatalities: Review of the bureau of biologic reports, 1976–1978. Transfusion 1980; 20:653–661.
71. Myhre BA: Fatalities from blood transfusion. JAMA 1980; 244:1333–1335.
72. Silberstein LE, Kruskall MS, Stehling LC: Strategies for the review of transfusion practices. JAMA 1989; 262: 1993–1997.
73. Greenburg AG, Kim HW: Evaluating new red cell substitutes: Critical analysis of toxicity models. Biomater Artif Cells Immobil Biotech 1992; 20:575–580.
74. Hedlund B: Free hemoglobin solutions may aggravate oxygen radical mediated reperfusion industry (Abstract). Biomater Artif Cells Immobil Biotech 1991; 19:394.
75. Rabinovicci RU, Rudolph AS, Vernick J, et al: A new salutary resuscitative fluid: Liposome encapsulated hemoglobin/hypertonic saline solution. J Trauma 1993; 35:121–127.
76. Geyer RP: Perfluorocarbons as oxygen transport vehicles. Biomater Artif Cells Artif Organs 1988; 16:31.
77. Reiss KG, Aurlen C, Greiner J, et al: Design synthesis and evaluation of fluorocarbons. Biomater Artif Cells Artif Organs 1988; 16:421.
78. Chang TMS: Blood substitutes based on modified hemoglobin prepared by encapsulation or cross linking: An overview. Biomater Artif Cells Immobil Biotech 1992; 20:159–182.
79. Riess JG: Overview of progress in fluorocarbon approach to in vivo oxygen delivery. Biomater Artif Cells Immobil Biotech 1992; 20:183–204.

CHAPTER 154

Intraoperative Hemostasis

Harry B. Kram, MD, FCCM

The failure to achieve intraoperative hemostasis can rapidly produce life-threatening consequences. Even if circulating blood volume deficits are replaced before hypovolemia produces shock, the loss of coagulation factors may have already set the stage for future bleeding and further complications. Thus, the cardinal rule is to control exsanguinating hemorrhage and restore circulatory intravascular volume as rapidly as possible.

Surgical bleeding, even when not excessive, is still a hazard because it obstructs the surgeon's view of the operative field and thus increases the risk of inadvertent damage to the surrounding structures. The importance of adequate hemostasis was recognized even by the earliest surgeons; Celsus (circa 30 A.D.) first reported hemostasis by suture ligation, and Galen of Pergamum (circa 150 A.D.) used cautery to control bleeding. Early in the 14th century, Henri de Mondeville recommended attaining hemostatically dry wounds and using sharp, clean knives and needles to perform surgery. During the 15th century, Bertapaglia of Padua advocated isolated suture ligation instead of en masse ligation of tissue and was the first to describe suture ligation of a single blood vessel.[1] Ambroise Paré, in 1552, popularized the suture ligation principle rather than indiscriminate cauterization for hemostasis. In 1840, Porta demonstrated the superiority of catgut suture material, and Joseph Lister, in 1867, developed the antiseptic gut ligature.[1]

In 1911, Harvey Cushing[2] used silver clips, well-solidified blood clots, and bits of raw muscle to effect hemostasis during cerebral surgery; at Cushing's suggestion, Grey[3] experimented with fibrin obtained from sheep's blood. Samuel Harvey found sheep fibrin ideal from the standpoint of hemostasis and absorption, but its application was deemed difficult; consequently, he converted the fibrin of beef blood obtained from a local slaughterhouse into a paperlike hemostatic material that had greater ease in handling and preservation.[4] William Halsted, in 1913, advocated the superiority of a fine silk suture over catgut and recommended incorporating minimal tissue in the suture when transfixing tissues and blood vessels to control hemorrhage.[5]

TECHNIQUES

Techniques to achieve intraoperative hemostasis may be classified as follows: (1) manual compression, (2) mechanical tamponade, (3) sutures, clips, and ligatures, (4) clamps and shunts, (5) thermal and laser energy, (6) hemostatic agents, and (7) tissue adhesives. Management of intraoperative bleeding secondary to nonmechanical causes such as inherited clotting abnormalities, coagulopathies, and fibrinolysis is beyond the scope of this chapter.

Manual Compression

The simplest method for rapidly controlling hemorrhage from an isolated bleeding point is digital compression. Direct digital pressure over a bleeding laceration in a large blood vessel is often the most expedient, least traumatic, and easiest technique to obtain hemostasis while definitive suture repair is performed. Cardiac stab wounds, for example, may be managed with several properly placed sutures while an assistant applies digital pressure to the spurting ventricle. Clamping of the ventricular wall is contraindicated because of the potential for injuring critical coronary vessels and is often ineffective because the ventricular wall is easily torn by the injudicious use of traumatic clamps. Use of atraumatic vascular clamps has greatly reduced the potential for causing intimal damage to blood vessels during clamping, but no clamp is totally atraumatic; the finger, on the other hand, may be the penultimate atraumatic hemostat. Manual compression techniques rely on reduction in blood flow to the bleeding area, which allows clotting to proceed. Although this may also be accomplished through the use of tourniquets, direct pressure is recommended to avoid the extensive tissue damage associated with prolonged tourniquet application.

The Pringle maneuver of compressing the hepatic artery and portal vein in the hepatoduodenal ligament between the index finger in Morrison's canal and the anteriorly placed thumb is a time-proven example of manual compression to achieve intraoperative hemostasis from the transected cystic or hepatic artery during open-gallbladder surgery. An atraumatic vascular clamp may also be used to perform the Pringle maneuver to help control liver bleeding with trauma or resection; after temporary inflow occlusion, it may be easier to control specific intrahepatic bleeding sources. Occlusion of total hepatic inflow for longer than 15 to 20 minutes under normothermic conditions has been condemned by some,[6] but others safely performed normothermic occlusion for extended periods during elective hepatic resections.[7] Local hypothermia[8] and high-dose steroids[9] have also been used to extend inflow occlusion time safely. If it is necessary to occlude blood flow to the liver for an extended period of time, the vascular occlusion can be briefly and intermittently interrupted.

Mechanical Tamponade

Mechanical tamponade, in its simple form, consists of applying pads and packs to a bleeding site with sufficient pressure so as to slow or halt hemorrhage and to enable blood clots to form. Most cases of intra-abdominal organ bleeding can be initially controlled by temporary packing to allow time to correct hypovolemia, acidosis, hypothermia, and cardiac arrhythmias. In some severe injuries, mechanical tamponade with or without manual compression may decrease bleeding sufficiently to allow repair or ligation of bleeding sources.

The use of compression packing can also be used for extended periods of time postoperatively, if necessary. Several studies confirmed the value of prolonged packing of severe liver injuries with re-exploration and removal of the packs at 1 to 7 days.[10–12] Specific indications for liver packing are extensive bilobar injuries and refractory coagulopathy.[12] This technique of hemostasis was less than satisfactory when used during World War II, usually because of intra-abdominal infectious complications. However, in present civilian practice, it may be lifesaving and is not associated with excessive rates of infection, but early removal of the packs is important in minimizing the risk of intra-abdominal infection.[10, 11] Packing allows time to correct hemodynamic abnormalities, coagulation deficits, and hypothermia as well as to evaluate other associated injuries.

The viable pedicle omental pack has been used to tamponade hepatic,[13] splenic,[14, 15] and other intra-abdominal injuries. A pedicle flap of greater omentum is fashioned and sutured into place for mild to moderate bleeding tamponade.

Mechanical tamponade has also been applied externally in patients experiencing exsanguination from pelvic fractures as an alternative to surgical exploration. The use of military antishock trousers (MAST) in these circumstances is a simple, effective method.[16, 17] Although it is not uncommon to leave the MAST suit inflated for up to 48 hours or longer with pressures of 25 to 50 mm Hg,[16] potential problems include pressure necrosis,[18] compartment syndromes,[19] and severe hypotension from rapid deflation of the MAST suit.[16]

Mechanical tamponade by the abdominal wall often occurs naturally with massive hemoperitoneum in the trauma patient with a tense, distended abdomen. This "autotamponade" may slow intra-abdominal hemorrhage but may also compromise cardiorespiratory function by impairing venous return to the heart and diaphragmatic excursions. Surgical incision of the abdominal wall relieves abdominal autotamponade but may be associated with immediate exacerbation of intra-abdominal bleeding, hypotensive shock, and cardiac arrest. This may occur so rapidly as to suggest air embolus. Supraceliac abdominal aortic cross-clamping through the gastrohepatic ligament or preliminary left thoracotomy with intrathoracic aortic cross-clamping may be useful for massive exsanguinating hemorrhage.[20]

Sutures, Clips, and Ligatures

Nonabsorbable sutures are resistant to enzymatic digestion or hydrolysis, whereas absorbable sutures are not. In general, absorbable sutures are obtained from natural collagen or are synthetic copolymers of lactide and glycolide or a homopolymer of glycolide.[1] Nonabsorbable sutures may be made of silk, cotton, or synthetic materials; the most widely used is silk. However, silk may be absorbed over long periods of time. The ultimate absorption of suture material is determined by its size and composition, by the condition of the tissues being sutured, and by the general health and status of the patient.[21]

Generally, multifilament sutures are easier to handle and tie than are monofilament sutures; surgical steel and polypropylene are monofilaments requiring careful placement of the knots to prevent kinking and subsequent fracture of the suture. Monofilament or absorbable sutures are usually recommended for use in potentially infected wounds. Polypropylene, nylon, and absorbable polyglycolic acid suture materials have the lowest incidence of infection in bacteria-contaminated tissue studied in the rat model.[1] The degradation products of nylon and polyglycolic acid appear to have antibacterial properties, whereas the physiologic inertness of polypropylene probably accounts for its ability to maintain a low incidence of infection. A polyglycolic acid mesh is also available for use in the treatment of bleeding splenic injuries.[15, 22]

The use of metallic clips as ligatures of bleeding blood vessels was first popularized by Harvey Cushing,[2] who used silver U-shaped wires to control bleeding from meningeal vessels. Various types and sizes of stainless steel clips may be applied by a specially designed clip holder. The advantages of clipping bleeding vessels compared with using ligatures are increased speed and the ability to ligate bleeders in locations that are otherwise inaccessible or difficult to reach. The metallic clips may also act as permanent radiographic markers of the surgical site when postoperative radiation therapy is required.

Recently, staples have been used to achieve rapid control of hemorrhage and to provide hemostasis in otherwise inaccessible areas. A mechanical stapling device, such as the ligating and dividing stapler, places two clips of stainless steel on either side of a dividing blade and simultaneously ligates and divides tissues between its jaws. These staplers contain multiple clips, allowing for rapid, repetitive use. Staplers may not be suitable to control bleeding from large blood vessels and internal organs.

The individual ligature is a permanent method for establishing complete hemostasis of a single bleeding vessel. A simple ligature is all that is necessary for most small arteries and veins, but large arteries may require a transfixing suture to ensure adequate control.

Ligation of the hepatic artery is occasionally required to stem bleeding after hepatic trauma when conventional methods are unsuccessful.[23–25] Survival after hepatic artery ligation is dependent on increased extraction of oxygen by tissues of the portal circulation, the existence or development of collateral blood flow, and the presence of anomalous vessels.[26, 27] Only when local control of hemostasis is impossible should the common hepatic artery or its branch to the affected lobe be ligated. In patients in whom the common hepatic or right hepatic artery is ligated, cholecystectomy should be performed.[10, 28]

The ligation of a major artery or vein may be performed to control hemorrhage secondary to vascular trauma. Although harmless in some areas, major vascular ligation may result in devastating consequences in other body areas and should be performed only when more conservative efforts at establishing hemostasis fail. Sequelae of major arterial ligations include organ ischemia, necrosis, and local infection. Complications after major venous ligation include local venous hypertension, edema, and loss of function (Tables 154–1 to 154–4).[29]

Clamps and Shunts

The temporary clamping of blood vessels to effect hemostasis is basically a form of mechanical tamponade. Although various atraumatic clamps have been designed for this, none are absolutely atraumatic. Moreover, varying degrees of intimal damage can occur when major blood vessels are temporarily clamped. Only the minimum amount of pressure required to occlude flow should be applied.

Surgical clamps are available in various sizes and configurations for use on different size vessels and locations. In some instances, a folded gauze sponge held tightly within the steel clamps of a ring hemostat may be used to compress major blood vessels, such as the vena cava and iliac veins. A simple tourniquet useful in obtaining hepatic hemostasis may be constructed using a large DeBakey aortic clamp and a 1.88-cm (¾-inch) Penrose drain. The Lin compression clamp[30, 31] and the Storm-Longmire clamp[32, 33] are examples of instruments designed to decrease blood loss during major hepatic resections; they are but a few of the many specialized clamps designed to control bleeding.

Major hepatic bleeding that continues despite the Pringle maneuver implicates injured hepatic veins with blood loss from the inferior vena cava. A variety of shunts, with and without balloons, for insertion into the vena cava both above and below the diaphragm have been proposed[34]; they function by stopping the hepatic venous bleeding yet allowing inferior vena caval blood to return to the heart (Fig. 154–1). They are usually inserted in conjunction with clamping of the porta hepatis (Pringle maneuver). Shunts inserted downward from above the diaphragm are secured by placing a pursestring suture around a right atrial appendage incision. Shunts inserted upward from below the diaphragm consist either of a Foley catheter or a straight piece of plastic tubing placed upward through an incision in the inferior vena cava. An alternative method for achieving vascular isolation of bleeding hepatic venous injuries involves the placement of four vascular clamps: one across the porta hepatis, one across the aorta above the celiac axis, one across the supradiaphragmatic inferior vena cava via a pericardiotomy, and one across the suprarenal inferior vena cava.[35] Yellin and colleagues[35] demonstrated that in dogs this is simpler, faster, and associated with less blood loss than inferior vena caval shunts. The disadvantage of this technique is depressed cardiac output secondary to obstructed inferior vena caval venous return that may result in cardiac arrest.

Temporary intravascular shunts are also valuable in sur-

TABLE 154–1. Percentage of Brain Ischemia After Ligation of Various Arteries

Artery	%
Internal carotid	40
Common carotid	20
Vertebral	8
Innominate	5

(Data from Ehrichs E: Major vascular ligations. *In*: Prognosis of Surgical Disease. Eiseman B [Ed]. Philadelphia, WB Saunders, 1980.)

TABLE 154–2. Percentage of Liver Ischemia After Ligation of Various Arteries

Artery	%
Right hepatic	10
Left hepatic	36
Common hepatic	10
Proper hepatic	12
Celiac	0

(Data from Ehrichs E: Major vascular ligations. *In*: Prognosis of Surgical Disease. Eiseman B [Ed]. Philadelphia, WB Saunders, 1980.)

TABLE 154–3. Percentage of Intestinal Ischemia After Ligation of Various Arteries

Artery	%
Superior mesenteric	100
Inferior mesenteric	2

(Data from Ehrichs E: Major vascular ligations. *In*: Prognosis of Surgical Disease. Eiseman B [Ed]. Philadelphia, WB Saunders, 1980.)

TABLE 154–4. Percentage of Distal Necrosis Requiring Amputation after Ligation of Various Arteries

Artery	%
Axillary	43
Subclavian	30
Brachial (above profunda)	55
Brachial (below profunda)	25
Radial	5
Ulnar	2
Radial and ulnar	40
Common iliac	53
External iliac	45
Common femoral	80
Deep femoral	0
Superficial femoral	55
Popliteal	70
Posterior tibial	14
Anterior tibial	8
Anterior and posterior tibial	70

(Data from Ehrichs E: Major vascular ligations. *In*: Prognosis of Surgical Disease. Eiseman B [Ed]. Philadelphia, WB Saunders, 1980.)

gery involving the potential for central nervous system ischemia (e.g., carotid endarterectomy). The Javid shunt,[36] a straight tube that is secured in place with a specially designed clamp or silk suture, and the Pruitt-Inahara shunt,[37] a T shunt with balloons, are examples of plastic tubes that may be used to maintain carotid arterial blood flow while minimizing blood loss during carotid arterial surgery. Their use during carotid endarterectomy maintains carotid arterial perfusion to the brain with minimal blood loss.

Thermal and Laser Energy

Although Galen favored cautery as the ideal technique of effecting hemostasis of bleeding tissues almost 2000 years ago, it was not until 1928 that Cushing used an electrocautery unit designed by W. T. Bovie to establish cerebral hemostasis. The development of nonflammable anesthetics increased the popularity of the Bovie cautery unit in the 1960s and led to its widespread acceptance in today's operating room setting.[38] The Bovie converts electrical energy into thermal energy. By concentrating a large amount of current into a small area, a high-current density generates a high resistance and intense heat. As the current spreads out through the tissues, resistance and heat production decrease. The current leaves the body through a grounding electrode, usually in the form of a plate; the plate should be placed over a large muscle mass close to the operative field, avoiding bony prominences and irregular contours, and should be large enough to prevent a concentration of current that would cause burning of the adjacent skin.

The degree of coagulation or cutting is determined by the waveform of the current. Coagulation is best achieved using damped, interrupted sinusoidal waves, whereas cutting is achieved most efficiently by an undamped, continuous sinusoidal waveform. A waveform of interrupted, undamped sinusoidal waves produces a mixture of coagulation and cutting. When using the Bovie electrocautery unit, more tissue damage is seen in dense avascular tissue than in vascular tissue because blood flow effectively conducts heat away from the coagulation site. When vessels are seen during Bovie cutting, they may be grasped with forceps and coagulated through the forceps before their division. Electrocautery processes are more efficient if the tip of the instrument is smooth and clean, because differences in surface area affect current density. The major advantages of electrocautery are its speed and efficiency; the disadvantages are tissue necrosis, delays in the wound healing process, and decreased wound strength.

Cooling of tissues has been used to produce hemostasis, as exemplified by the use of ice-water lavage to control bleeding from esophageal or gastric mucosa nonoperatively. Direct cooling increases blood viscosity and produces vasoconstriction, both of which decrease blood flow to the affected vessels. Systemic temperatures less than 35°C, however, should be avoided because they may predispose to ventricular arrhythmias. Cryogenic surgery uses localized extreme cooling to about −200°C and has been applied effectively in patients undergoing neurosurgery. At extremely low temperatures, the tissues undergo cryogenic necrosis as lipoproteins denature, resulting in hemostasis.

The laser, in contrast to electrocautery, converts light energy, rather than electrical energy, into thermal energy, which in turn vaporizes tissue water. The hemostatic qualities of the laser relate to the coagulum formed on the cut surface of the exposed tissue and to protein denaturation. Fidler and associates[39] used the carbon dioxide laser for hemostasis in experimental exsanguinating liver injuries; there was equally good healing and less extensive damage to liver tissue than with Bovie or suture methods. Similarly, White and colleagues[40] used a neodymium:yttrium-aluminum-garnet laser to weld incisions in arteries and veins

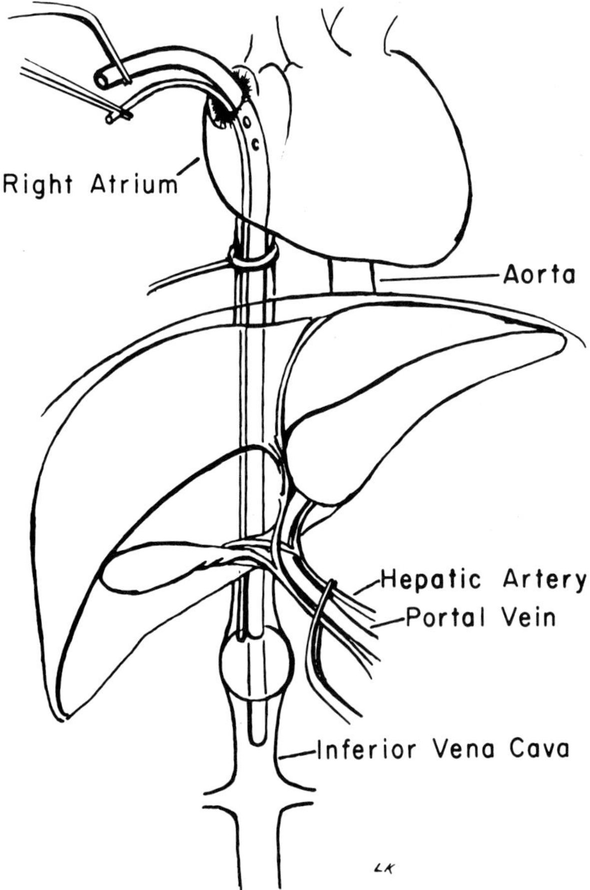

Figure 154–1. Use of an endotracheal tube as an atriocaval shunt for the intraoperative management of retrohepatic inferior vena cava injuries. Note that holes have been cut into the intra-atrial portion of the endotracheal tube for blood return to the heart. Clamping of the hepatic artery and portal vein within the hepaticoduodenal ligament (Pringle maneuver) to decrease hepatic inflow is shown.

under controlled experimental conditions and found more rapid healing compared with sutured blood vessels.

Hemostatic Agents

Most solid hemostatic agents work by providing a scaffold or network of interstices that entrap platelets and blood components that provide for organization of a clot. Mason and Read[41] demonstrated that platelets are probably more important than the soluble clotting factors in the hemostatic reaction. Liquid hemostatic agents, such as epinephrine and thrombin, act by vasoconstriction and stimulation of the clotting cascade, respectively; they are usually used for controlling mucosal or parenchymal oozing. The most widely used solid hemostatic agents available in the United States today include gelatin foam sponge, oxidized cellulose, and microfibrillar collagen. These hemostatic agents are aided by manual compression or mechanical tamponade during and after application.

Gelatin foam, made from denatured animal gelatin, is available as a sponge that is usually soaked in thrombin immediately before use. The sponge has no significant hemostatic action in and of itself; its effects are mainly related to direct contact between blood and sponge by the pressure exerted on the wound surface. It is believed to be less effective as a hemostatic agent compared with oxidized cellulose and microfibrillar collagen in cases of moderate to severe hemorrhage.[42] Oxidized regenerated cellulose and microfibrillar collagen work by aggregating platelets in thrombi contained with their interstices and are thus effective in the presence of heparin. Oxidized regenerated cellulose is available as a sheet, whereas microfibrillar collagen is available as a powder or nonwoven web form. Although relatively inert, both substances stimulate a chronic inflammatory response and require phagocytosis to be removed from the body.

Hemostatic agents left in contaminated wounds potentiate infection and should be used in the smallest quantities possible. Hinman and Babcock[43] showed that a bacterial inoculum insufficient to produce infection in the absence of foreign bodies may produce overwhelming infection in the presence of foreign bodies. Oxidized cellulose was found to be superior to gelatin sponge and microfibrillar collagen in resisting infection.[44–46]

Tissue Adhesives

Tissue adhesives are synthetic or natural chemicals used to glue bleeding sites. Methyl-2-cyanoacrylate (Eastman 910) is a synthetic tissue adhesive developed in the 1960s as a hemostatic agent[47]; unfortunately, significant histotoxicity has limited its use.[48] Although various modifications of the latter compound led to less tissue inflammatory reaction,[49] cyanoacrylates are still regarded as unacceptable for general human use in the United States.

Studies performed over the past decade have indicated that the use of highly concentrated human fibrinogen in conjunction with thrombin, Factor XIII, and calcium chloride results in the formation of a natural fibrin glue that lacks significant tissue reactivity or toxicity.[50–57] Historic studies by Ingraham and colleagues[55] found that the extent of tissue reaction to a single silk suture was considerably greater than that caused by large amounts of fibrin; they also found considerably greater tissue reaction to bone wax or raw muscle than to fibrin. Although not yet available for commercial use in the United States, this adhesive has been found to be extremely effective in establishing parenchymal organ hemostasis.[52, 56, 58–60] Controlled experimental studies comparing fibrin glue with oxidized regenerated cellulose for sealing synthetic graft-arterial anastomoses has shown fibrin glue to be significantly superior to oxidized cellulose in establishing complete hemostasis and preventing recurrent bleeding postoperatively.[57] Methods for preparing autologous fibrin glue have also been devised,[61, 62] but their tensile strength is inferior to that of nonautologous, highly concentrated fibrinogen mixtures. Combined fibrin glue–collagen patches have also been used for hemostasis.[63]

In summary, the failure to achieve intraoperative hemostasis may be life threatening. The control of hemorrhage, by whatever method, is of paramount importance and should be performed as expediently as possible along with the restoration of circulating intravascular volume.

References

1. Shackelford RT, Zuidema GD: Surgery of the Alimentary Tract. 2nd ed. Philadelphia, WB Saunders, 1981, pp 535–600.
2. Cushing H: The control of bleeding in operations for brain tumors. Ann Surg 1911; 54:1.
3. Grey EG: Fibrin as a hemostatic in cerebral surgery. Surg Gynecol Obstet 1915; 21:452.
4. Harvey SC: Fibrin paper as a hemostatic agent. Ann Surg 1918; 68:66.
5. Halsted WS: The employment of fine silk in preference to catgut and the advantages of transfixing tissues and vessels in controlling hemorrhage. JAMA 1913; 60:1119.
6. Reffuci FL: The effects of temporary occlusion of the afferent hepatic circulation in dogs. Surgery 1953; 33:342.
7. Huguet C, Nordlinger B, Bloch P, et al: Tolerance of the human liver to prolonged normothermic ischemia. Arch Surg 1978; 113:1448.
8. Bernhard WF, McMurrey JD, Curtis GW: Feasibility of partial hepatic resection under hypothermia. N Engl J Med 1955; 253:159.
9. Santiago Delphín EA, Figueroa I, López R, et al: Protective effect of steroids on liver ischemia. Ann Surg 1975; 41:683.
10. Walt AJ: The mythology of hepatic trauma—or Babel revisited. Am J Surg 1978; 135:12.
11. Svoboda JA, Peter T, Dang CV, et al: Severe liver trauma in the face of coagulopathy: A case for temporary packing and early reexploration. Am J Surg 1982; 144:717.
12. Moore EE: Critical decisions in the management of hepatic trauma. Am J Surg 1984; 148:712.
13. Stone HH, Lamb JM: Use of the pedicled omentum as an autogenous pack for control of hemorrhage in major injuries of the liver. Surg Gynecol Obstet 1975; 141:92.
14. Sherman R: Rationale for and methods of splenic preservation following trauma. Surg Clin North Am 1981; 61:127.
15. Cooper MJ, Williamson RCN: Splenectomy: Indications, hazards, and alternatives. Br J Surg 1984; 71:173.
16. Mucha P: Pelvic fractures. Probl Gen Surg 1984; 1:154.
17. McLaughlin AP, McCullough DL, Kerr WS, et al: The use of external counterpressure (G-suit) in the management of traumatic retroperitoneal hemorrhage. J Urol 1977; 107:940.
18. Godbout B, Burchard KW, Slotman GJ, et al: Crush syndrome with death following pneumatic antishock garment application. J Trauma 1984; 24:1052.
19. Williams TM, Knopf R, Ellyson JH: Compartment syndrome after anti-shock trouser use without lower extremity trauma. J Trauma 1982; 22:595.
20. Ledgerwood AM, Kazmers M, Lucas CE: The role of thoracic aortic occlusion for massive hemoperitoneum. J Trauma 1976; 16:610.
21. Postlethwait RW, Schauble JF, Dillon ML, et al: Wound healing: II. An evaluation of surgical suture material. Surg Gynecol Obstet 1959; 108:555.
22. Delany HM, Porreca F, Mitsudo S, et al: Splenic capping: An experimental study of a new technique for splenorrhaphy using woven polyglycolic acid mesh. Ann Surg 1982; 196:187.
23. Graham RR, Cannell D: Accidental ligation of the hepatic artery. Br J Surg 1933; 20:566.
24. Madding GF, Kennedy PA: Hepatic artery ligation. Surg Clin North Am 1972; 52:719.

25. Mays ET: Lobar dearterialization for exsanguinating wounds of the liver. J Trauma 1972; 12:397.
26. Tygstrup N, Winkler K, Melengaard K, et al: Determination of the hepatic arterial blood flow and oxygen supply in man by clamping the hepatic artery during surgery. J Clin Invest 1962; 41:447.
27. Bengmark S, Rosengren K: Angiographic study of the collateral circulation to the liver after ligation of the hepatic artery in man. Am J Surg 1970; 119:620.
28. Aaron S, Fulton RL, Mays ET: Selective ligation of the hepatic artery for trauma of the liver. Surg Gynecol Obstet 1975; 141:187.
29. Ehrichs E: Major vascular ligation. *In:* Prognosis of Surgical Disease. Eiseman B (Ed). Philadelphia, WB Saunders, 1980, pp 102–105.
30. Lin TY: Results in 107 hepatic lobectomies with a preliminary report on the use of a clamp to reduce blood loss. Ann Surg 1973; 177:413.
31. Ryan WH, Hummel BW, McClelland RN: Reduction in the morbidity and mortality of major hepatic resection. Am J Surg 1982; 144:740.
32. Storm FK, Longmire WP: A simplified clamp for hepatic resection. Surg Gynecol Obstet 1971; 133:103.
33. Longmire WP, Trout HH, Greenfield J, et al: Elective hepatic surgery. Ann Surg 1974; 179:712.
34. Anderson CB, Ballinger WF: Abdominal injuries. *In:* The Management of Trauma. 4th ed. Zuidema GD, Rutherford RB, Ballinger WF (Eds). Philadelphia, WB Saunders, 1985, pp 449–504.
35. Yellin AE, Chaffee CB, Donovan AJ: Vascular isolation in treatment of juxtahepatic venous injuries. Arch Surg 1971; 102:566.
36. Rob CG: Reconstruction of the internal carotid artery: An update. Surg Rounds 1981; 4:40.
37. Pruitt JC: 1009 consecutive carotid endarterectomies using local anesthesia, EEG, and selective shunting with Pruitt-Inahara carotid shunt. Contemp Surg 1983; 23:49.
38. Glover JL: The Bovie: A new look at an enduring technology. Am Coll Surg Bull 1986; 71:4.
39. Fidler JP, Hoefer RW, Polanyi TG, et al: Laser surgery in exsanguinating liver injury. Ann Surg 1975; 181:74.
40. White RA, Abergel R, Lyons R, et al: Comparison of laser welded and sutured venotomies and arteriotomies. Biomater Trans 1986; 9:140.
41. Mason RG, Read MS: Some effects of a microcrystalline collagen preparation on blood. Haemostasis 1974; 3:31.
42. Abbott WM, Austen WG: The effectiveness and mechanism of collagen-induced topical hemostasis. Surgery 1975; 78:723.
43. Hinman F, Babcock KO: Local reaction to oxidized cellulose and gelatin hemostatic agents in experimentally contaminated renal wounds. Surgery 1949; 26:633.
44. Dineen P: Antibacterial activity of oxidized regenerated cellulose. Surg Gynecol Obstet 1976; 142:481.
45. Scher KS, Coil JA: Effects of oxidized cellulose and microfibrillar collagen on infection. Surgery 1982; 91:301.
46. Dineen P: The effect of oxidized regenerated cellulose on experimental intravascular infection. Surgery 1977; 82:575.
47. Nathan HS, Nachlas MM, Solomon RD, et al: Non-suture closure of arterial incisions using a rapidly polymerizing adhesive. Ann Surg 1960; 152:648.
48. Raekallio J, Seligman AM: Acute reaction to arterial adhesive in healing skin wounds. J Surg Res 1964; 4:124.
49. Lehman RA, Hayes GJ: The toxicity of alkyl-2-cyanoacrylate tissue adhesives: Brain and blood vessels. Surgery 1967; 61:915.
50. Staindl O: The healing of wounds and scar formation under the influence of a tissue adhesion system with fibrinogen, thrombin, and coagulation Factor XIII. Arch Otorhinolaryngol 1979; 222:241.
51. Redl H, Schlag G, Dinges DP, et al: Background and methods of "fibrin sealing." *In:* Biomaterials. Winter GD, Fibbons DF, Plenk HC (Eds). New York, John Wiley & Sons, 1982, pp 669–676.
52. Kram HB, Shoemaker WC, Hino ST, et al: Splenic salvage using biologic glue. Arch Surg 1984; 119:1309.
53. Kram HB, Shoemaker WC, Hino ST, et al: Tracheal repair with fibrin glue. J Thorac Cardiovasc Surg 1985; 90:771.
54. Kram HB, Garces MA, Klein ST, et al: Common bile duct anastomosis using fibrin glue. Arch Surg 1985; 120:1250.
55. Ingraham FD, Bailey OT, Nulsen FE: Studies on fibrin foam as a hemostatic agent in neurosurgery, with special reference to its comparison with muscle. J Neurosurg 1944; 1:171.
56. Kram HB, Reuben BI, Fleming AW, et al: Use of fibrin glue in hepatic trauma. J Trauma 1988; 28:1195–1201.
57. Kram HB, Nugent P, Reuben BI, et al: Fibrin glue sealing of polytetrafluoroethylene vascular graft anastomoses: Comparison with oxidized cellulose. J Vasc Surg 1988; 8:563–568.
58. Kram HB, Nathan RC, Mackabee JR, et al: Clinical use of nonautologous fibrin glue. Am Surg 1988; 9:510–513.
59. Kram HB, del Junco T, Clark SR, et al: Techniques of splenic preservation using fibrin glue. J Trauma 1990; 30:97–101.
60. Kram HB, Shoemaker WC, Clark SR, et al: Spraying of aerosolized fibrin glue in the treatment of nonsuturable hemorrhage. Am Surg 1991; 57:381–384.
61. Gestring GR, Lerner R: Autologous fibrinogen for tissue-adhesion, hemostasis and embolization. Vasc Surg 1983; 17:294.
62. Dresdale A, Rose EA, Jeevanandam V, et al: Preparation of fibrin glue from single-donor fresh-frozen plasma. Surgery 1985; 97:750.
63. Scheele J, Gentsch HH, Matteson E: Splenic repair by fibrin tissue adhesive and collagen fleece. Surgery 1984; 95:6.

CHAPTER 155

Thoracic Injuries

Robert F. Wilson, MD, FACS, FCCM

Chest injuries are directly responsible for more than 25% of the trauma deaths that occur annually, and they contribute significantly to at least another 25% of these fatalities.[1, 2] Patients with chest trauma who have shock or respiratory distress when first seen in the hospital have a particularly high mortality rate. In one series, 11% required endotracheal intubation soon after arrival in the emergency department (ED) and 58% of these patients died.[3] If shock was present with the ventilatory difficulty, the mortality rate was 73%.

MASSIVE SUBCUTANEOUS EMPHYSEMA

Subcutaneous emphysema is usually caused by injuries to lung parenchyma. Air can also reach the chest wall by dissecting back along an injured bronchus into the hilum and mediastinum and then into the extrapleural spaces. Rarely, subcutaneous emphysema may be caused by injury to the esophagus or pharynx. In addition, if a patient with subcutaneous emphysema is to be placed on a ventilator, it is prudent to assume that there is an underlying pneumothorax, and a chest tube should be inserted on the sides in which this is present.

INJURY TO THE CHEST WALL

Probing of chest wounds to determine their depth or direction is inadvisable because it may damage underlying structures and cause a pneumothorax or recurrent bleeding. Small open-chest wounds can act as one-way valves, allowing air to enter during inspiration and thereby causing an increasing pneumothorax. If the chest wound is two-thirds the cross-sectional area of the upper airway, air will preferentially enter the chest through the wound rather than through the tracheobronchial tree. Open, sucking wounds of the chest should be covered immediately by a sterile, airtight dressing, and a chest tube should be inserted simultaneously at a separate site to relieve the associated pneumothorax.

RIB FRACTURES

Simple Fractures

Fractures should be assumed to be present in any patient who has pain and localized tenderness over the ribs after chest trauma. Up to 40% of rib fractures (particularly the anterior and lateral portions of the first four ribs) may not visualize for 7 to 14 days after injury.[4]

The principal diagnostic goal with clinically suspected rib fractures is the detection of significant complications, especially hemopneumothorax, pulmonary contusion, and major vascular injury. A single upright posteroanterior (PA) chest x-ray film has the greatest yield in detecting fractures and associated injuries or complications. If the PA view does not show a suspected pneumothorax, the patient should have inspiratory and expiratory PA or apical-lordotic views. Delayed pneumothorax or hemothorax may occasionally develop more than 6 to 12 hours after the initial injury.

Severe chest wall pain can often be relieved by blocking the intercostal nerves of the ribs involved plus two ribs above and two below with a long-acting local anesthetic such as 0.5% bupivacaine hydrochloride (Marcaine) mixed with an equal quantity of 2% lidocaine with epinephrine. Any residual tender spots are also injected with the local anesthetic. Epidural analgesia, however, is usually more effective.[5]

First- and Second-Rib Fractures

It takes great force to fracture the first or second ribs. In one series, 40% of patients with fractures of the first and second ribs had myocardial contusion, bronchial tears, or major vascular injury.[6] Although a first- or second-rib fracture in itself is not an indication for a thoracic aortogram, fractures of the first rib are associated with higher mortality rates (15–30%) than are fractures of the other ribs because of the frequent severe associated injuries.[7]

Multiple and Lower Rib Fractures

Patients with three or more rib fractures have increased mortality and morbidity rates and should generally be seen in a trauma center.[8] If a patient with fractures of ribs 9, 10, or 11 is hypotensive, intra-abdominal bleeding must be suspected. In one series of 783 patients with fractured ribs, 71% of the patients admitted in shock had a ruptured intra-abdominal viscus.[7]

FLAIL CHEST

Pathophysiology

Segmental rib fractures (i.e., fractures of the same rib in two or more locations) of three or more adjacent ribs anteriorly or laterally often result in the phenomenon known as flail chest. Pendelluft (a ventilatory phenomenon described by Brauer in 1909 referring to movement of air back and forth between the injured and uninjured lungs) was considered to be an important cause of the hypoxemia seen with flail chest, but it is clinically significant only in rare circumstances when the upper airway is partially obstructed. Although the flail segment increases the work of breathing, the main cause of the hypoxemia in flail chest patients is the underlying lung contusion.[9]

Treatment

Nonventilatory Therapy

Patients with mild to moderate flail chest and little or no underlying pulmonary contusion can often be managed without ventilator assistance; however, it must be remembered that the lung changes and the flail will tend to get worse during the next 24 to 48 hours,[10] especially if excess fluid is given or the patient does not cough and take deep breaths adequately.

Ventilatory Support

Death in patients with flail chest is primarily due to associated injuries,[11] but delayed or inadequate ventilatory support can greatly increase mortality rates.[12] Our indications for early ventilatory assistance with flail chest include shock, three or more associated injuries, severe head injury, previous severe pulmonary disease, fracture of eight or more ribs, or age greater than 65 years.[12] Patients with only one of these problems and early ventilatory assistance had a mortality rate of only 7%; however, if ventilatory assistance was delayed until there was clinical evidence of respiratory failure, the mortality rate was 69%.[12] Operative stabilization of the chest wall is rarely needed but should be considered if a thoracotomy is performed for another reason or when mechanical ventilation is very difficult or undesirable.[13]

STERNAL FRACTURES

Sternal fractures may be associated with flail chest or other severe injuries, including myocardial contusions, in up to 50% to 60% of patients.[14] In such patients with severe trauma, electrocardiograms (ECG), monitoring of creatine kinase–MB (CK-MB) levels, and evaluation of abnormal myocardial motion are warranted. However, studies suggest that sternal fractures are only occasionally associated with severe underlying injuries.[14a, 14b]

TRAUMATIC ASPHYXIA

Sudden severe crushing of the chest, especially by heavy weights, may result in the "masque ecchymotique" described by Ollivier, a French pathologist in 1837. This entity includes subconjunctival hemorrhage plus petechiae, edema, and cyanosis of the head, neck, and upper extremities.[15] Although these patients may look moribund initially, the neurologic impairment is usually only temporary, and long-term morbidity is due primarily to associated injuries.[16]

INJURIES TO THE LUNGS

Pulmonary Contusions

The main pathologic change in pulmonary contusion is capillary damage, resulting in increased interstitial and intra-alveolar fluid, which causes a progressive decrease in lung compliance and increasing physiologic shunting and hypoxemia for at least 24 to 48 hours. Areas of opacification on chest x-ray film taken within 6 hours of blunt chest trauma are usually considered to be pulmonary contusions; however, at thoracotomy the extent of the lung injury is usually much larger than suspected radiologically. As a general rule, the chest x-ray film changes lag at least 24 hours behind the blood gas changes.

Treatment of pulmonary contusions is similar to that for flail chest and primarily involves maintenance of adequate ventilation. Chest physiotherapy, intercostal nerve or epidural blocks, and nasotracheal suction are used as needed.

Ventilatory assistance is occasionally required, especially if there are severe other injuries, particularly to the brain. Survival is primarily determined by the associated injuries and the patient's age.[17] Patients who have a unilateral lung injury and who respond poorly to conventional mechanical ventilation may benefit from synchronous independent lung ventilation provided through a double-lumen endobronchial catheter.[18]

Systemic Air Embolism

In patients with penetrating chest wounds, particularly those causing hemoptysis, positive-pressure ventilation must be used with care. High ventilatory pressures may force air from an injured bronchus into an adjacent open pulmonary vein, producing systemic air emboli. This probably accounts for many of the arrhythmias and sudden deaths that occur after intubation of patients with penetrating chest wounds.

If systemic air embolism occurs, the patient should be turned onto the left side (unless there is bleeding in the right lung) and the head should be lowered. If the patient does not respond promptly to nonoperative therapy, a thoracotomy should be performed to clamp the injured area of lung and then aspirate air from the heart and aorta.[19] Open-heart massage with clamping of the ascending aorta or cardiopulmonary bypass may be required to push air out of the coronary arteries.

Intrabronchial Bleeding

Intrabronchial bleeding is poorly tolerated and can rapidly cause death by flooding alveoli. This causes severe hypoxemia but relatively little change in partial pressure of arterial carbon dioxide or airway resistance.[20] Noninvolved lung must be kept as free of blood as possible, and nasotracheal suction and bronchoscopy should be used as often as necessary. A thoracotomy, if done, should be performed with the patient lying flat to prevent the noninjured lung from being flooded.

If the bleeding is severe, a double-lumen endotracheal (Carlens) tube can be used to confine the bleeding to one lung. In some instances, the bleeding can be controlled only by occluding the involved bronchus with a Fogarty arterial balloon catheter or by packing it with gauze until the bleeding site can be controlled surgically.

Hemothorax

Cause

The high concentration of thromboplastin and the low arterial pressures combine to reduce bleeding from torn lung parenchyma. Consequently, if there is continued significant intrathoracic bleeding after penetrating trauma, it is usually from severe lung injuries or damaged major vessels.

Diagnosis

Fluid collections greater than 300 mL can usually be seen on good upright chest x-ray films. If the patient is supine, up to 500 to 1000 mL of blood may not be apparent radiologically.

Treatment

Closed Thoracostomy (Chest Tube) Drainage

Blood in the pleural cavity should generally be removed as completely and rapidly as possible. Not only may a hemothorax restrict ventilation and venous return, but the clots also release fibrinolytic and fibrinogenolytic substances that act as anticoagulants and contribute to continued intrathoracic bleeding. A small, stable hemothorax does not always have to be removed, but it should be carefully observed. A large (32- to 40-French) chest tube is ideal for draining a hemothorax. If the hemothorax persists and there is minimal chest tube drainage, the chest tube either is occluded by clots or is not inserted into the proper area and should be replaced. Decubitus chest films showing a fluid shift indicate that some blood is unclotted and may be at least partially removed by another chest tube.

Although there continues to be controversy about the need for antibiotics in patients requiring a chest tube for a traumatic hemothorax or pneumothorax, data from the six available double-blind prospective studies showed a clear reduction in the incidence of pneumonia and empyema (18% [41/234] versus 3% [7/238]) when antibiotics were given while the chest tube is in place.[21–26a] These findings were confirmed in a meta-analysis.[27] Studies by Cant and colleagues[28] suggested that antibiotics given for 24 hours are adequate, and, according to Demetriades and associates,[29] only one dose of antibiotic needs to be given.

Autotransfusion

In patients with massive bleeding into a body cavity, autotransfusion can reduce the need for bank blood and decrease the risks associated with its use. Intrathoracic bleeding is generally ideal for autotransfusion because there is usually no contamination of the blood by bile or intestinal contents.

Thoracotomy

Only 5% to 15% of patients with penetrating chest wounds require a thoracotomy because of continuing intrathoracic hemorrhage causing (1) unstable vital signs, (2) chest tube drainage greater than 1500 to 2000 mL, (3) chest tube drainage exceeding 300 mL/h for more than 3 hours, or (4) the chest to remain more than half full of blood on x-ray film.[30, 31]

Occasionally, when the chest tube is initially inserted, blood will emerge at an alarmingly rapid rate. If the patient's condition improves as the blood is removed and resuscitation fluids are given, continuing chest tube drainage and monitoring the patient are in order. However, if the patient's vital signs deteriorate as the blood is removed, the chest tube should be clamped and the patient taken directly to surgery. If the patient has a cardiac arrest in the ED or is too unstable to move to the operating room (OR) safely, an ED thoracotomy should be performed.[32, 33]

Decortication

There has been increasing enthusiasm for early removal of large, persisting hemothoraces to prevent later empyema or fibrothorax.[30] However, most hemothoraces will almost completely resorb spontaneously within 3 to 4 weeks. A retained hemothorax should be evacuated if it (1) occupies more than a third of one hemithorax, (2) causes atelectasis of a lobe or two or more segments, or (3) is associated with spiking fever exceeding 101°F. In selected cases, this may be done early with a thoracoscope.[30a] Delay beyond 4 weeks may result in a very tenacious peel and significant bleeding because adjacent capillaries have begun to grow into the fibrous tissue.

Pneumothorax

Pathophysiology

Collections of air or blood within the pleural cavity reduce vital capacity and increase intrathoracic pressure, thereby decreasing minute ventilation and venous return to the heart. If there is any obstruction to the upper airway or if the patient has torn blebs or chronic obstructive lung disease, additional air may be forced into the pleural cavity during expiration, causing a tension pneumothorax with intrapleural pressures exceeding atmospheric pressure. A pneumothorax is not apt to cause severe symptoms unless it (1) is a tension pneumothorax, (2) occupies more than 40% of one hemithorax, or (3) occurs in a patient with shock or preexisting cardiopulmonary disease.

Diagnosis

If a pneumothorax is suspected, apical-lordotic films may allow better visualization of the apex. Occasionally, a small pneumothorax is not apparent on chest x-ray films but is seen on a computed tomographic (CT) scan of the chest or abdomen. This is referred to as an *occult pneumothorax.*[34]

If a tension pneumothorax is suspected because the patient is in severe respiratory distress with decreased breath sounds, hyperresonance on one side of the chest, and displacement of the mediastinum (trachea) to the other side, insertion of a large needle into the involved side may help confirm the diagnosis and provide temporary relief until a chest tube can be inserted.

Treatment

Observation

A pneumothorax that is "occult" or small (less than 1.0 cm wide and confined to the upper third of the chest) and is unchanged on two chest x-ray films taken 4 to 6 hours apart in an asymptomatic individual can be treated by observation alone; however, if the patient cannot be observed closely or is put on a ventilator, a chest tube or pleural catheter should be inserted.

Chest Tube Drainage

If only a pneumothorax is present, a small to moderate-sized (24- to 28-French) chest tube may be inserted anteriorly in the second intercostal space in the midclavicular line; however, a high midaxillary tube is generally safer and preferable. Occasionally, a small catheter with a stopcock and syringe may be used to aspirate a pneumothorax.[35]

The intrathoracic position of the chest tube and the amount of air or fluid remaining in the pleural cavity should be checked with an upright portable chest film as soon as possible after the tube is inserted. If the patient must go to the radiology department for the x-ray film, the chest tube should not be clamped because a continuing air leak could collapse the lung and cause a tension pneumothorax. While the tube is unclamped, the water-seal drainage bottle should be kept 1 to 2 feet lower than the patient's chest.

Serial chest films and careful recording of the volume of blood loss and the size of the air leak are important guides to the functioning of the chest tubes. If a chest tube becomes blocked and a significant pneumothorax or hemithorax is still present, the tube should be replaced.

The chest tube can usually be removed if there has been no air leak and less than 100 mL of fluid drainage for the previous 24 hours. However, if the patient is on a ventilator and the peak inspiratory pressures exceed 40 to 50 cm H_2O, most physicians would prefer to keep the chest tubes in to act as a safety valve in case a new pneumothorax suddenly develops.

Complications

Continued Air Leak

In general, a patient can tolerate a small or moderate-sized pneumothorax without complications if there is no continuing air leak. An air leak will usually stop within 24 to 48 hours if the lung is completely expanded and the visceral and parietal pleura are in contact. However, if a combination of pneumothorax and continued air leak is not corrected within 24 to 48 hours, the incidence of empyema and bronchopleural fistula is greatly increased. Recently, autologous fibrin gel has been administered via a chest tube to control traumatic bronchopleural fistulas successfully.[36]

Continued Pneumothorax

The most frequent reasons for failure to evacuate a pneumothorax rapidly and completely are (1) improper position of the chest tubes, (2) an inadequate number of chest tubes, or (3) inadequate suction. An air leak and pneumothorax persisting in spite of two well-placed chest tubes attached to 20- to 30-cm H_2O suction are generally due to (1) occlusion of bronchi with secretions or a foreign body, (2) a tear of one of the larger bronchi, or (3) a large tear of the lung parenchyma. Under such circumstances, emergency bronchoscopy should be performed to clear the bronchi and identify any damage to the tracheobronchial tree.

Post-Traumatic Pulmonary Pseudocyst

Occasionally after trauma, an airspace without a bronchial or pleural connection develops within the injured lung parenchyma. This may cause cough, chest pain, leukocytosis, and low-grade fever. Most of these resolve spontaneously over a few weeks or months. If they enlarge or become infected, resection or drainage may be required.[37]

Pneumomediastinum

Pneumomediastinum can be an important finding in patients with chest trauma. Subcutaneous emphysema in the neck should make one look closely for this problem. The diagnosis of pneumomediastinum should also be suspected from the presence of a crunching sound (Hamman's sign) over the heart during systole. This finding is present in about 50% of patients with pneumomediastinum and is accentuated when the patient is in the left lateral decubitus position. Bruit de moulin, a loud precordial murmur caused by turbulence of air and fluid in the pericardial cavity, may also be heard.

There is usually little or no disability from a pneumomediastinum, except perhaps in the newborn; rarely, a tension pneumopericardium may develop in older individuals.[38] Even with few symptoms, one must look closely for an injury to the airways or the digestive tract.

TRACHEOBRONCHIAL INJURIES

Lower Trachea and Major Bronchi

Most blunt injuries to bronchi are due to rapid deceleration and shearing of mobile bronchi from relatively fixed proximal structures.[39] However, forced expiration against a closed glottis or compression against the vertebral column may also play a role, particularly in tracheal lacerations.

Injuries to the trachea or major bronchi should be suspected if there is massive subcutaneous or mediastinal emphysema or if there is a persistent pneumothorax with a continuing large air leak.[39] On bronchoscopy, the usual injury is a transverse tear in a mainstem bronchus or at the origin of an upper lobe bronchus. The characteristic injury in the trachea is a vertical tear in the membranous portion near its attachment to the tracheal cartilages.

If the lung expands and the air leak stops, partial lacerations of the bronchi involving more than a third of the circumference may be missed initially but will often result in repeated pulmonary infections or severe bronchial stenosis. Low tracheal and major bronchial lacerations require thoracotomy and direct repair as soon as feasible. The tracheobronchial repair should be assessed by tomograms, bronchoscopy, or bronchogram in 3 months or sooner if any obstructive symptoms develop.

ENDOTRACHEAL FLAME BURNS

Many patients requiring prolonged ventilatory support have a tracheostomy performed, usually sometime between days 5 and 14. Because many of these patients require a fraction of inspired oxygen greater than 0.30 during the procedure, the endotracheal tube may become ignited if electrocautery is used to control tracheal bleeding.[40] The resulting tracheobronchial burn is usually fatal.

CARDIAC TRAUMA

Penetrating Injury

Pathophysiology

Most patients who reach the hospital alive after penetrating cardiac trauma have relatively small cardiac injuries, and a pericardial tamponade is often present to help stop the bleeding from the heart.[41] However, the tamponade can also cause shock because of reduced diastolic filling of the heart, and its effects on survival are not clear-cut.[42] There is also an occasional case in which pericardial tamponade after a penetrating injury may be delayed for weeks or months.[43]

Diagnosis

Clinical Features

All patients in shock with a penetrating chest wound between the midclavicular line on the right and midaxillary line on the left should be considered to have a cardiac injury until proven otherwise. Beck's triad (distended neck veins, decreased blood pressure (BP), and depressed heart tones) can be very deceptive, and many false-positive and false-negative results occur.[41] With hypovolemia, the neck veins will usually not be distended until or unless the blood volume is at least partially restored. Furthermore, chest injuries can cause the patient to breathe abnormally or strain, thereby raising the central venous pressure and distending the neck veins in the absence of tamponade. Muffled heart sounds are the least reliable sign in Beck's triad. Paradoxical pulse, characterized by a drop in systolic BP of more than 10 to 15 mm Hg during normal inspiration, should also suggest tamponade.

Chest X-Ray Films

A chest x-ray film should be obtained for every trauma victim before going to the OR; however, x-ray films are of little help in diagnosing cardiac injury except in the unusual case with intrapericardial air. Because the average acute tamponade has only 150 to 200 mL of blood and clots, significant enlargement of the cardiac shadow is unusual.[41]

Echocardiography

Echocardiography can be helpful in diagnosing the presence of pericardial blood. However, this test is often not immediately available, and there are occasional false-negative results.[41a, 41b]

Subxiphoid Pericardial Window

Another alternative for diagnosing tamponade and a cardiac injury is exploration via a subxiphoid pericardial window. If blood is found, the incision can be extended up as a midsternotomy to repair the cardiac damage. If a patient has a stab wound over the precordium and the patient has been hemodynamically stable, a subxiphoid pericardial window will reveal an injury in up to 18% of patients.[44, 45]

Treatment

Fluid

The quickest way to correct hypotension caused by pericardial tamponade is to increase preload by rapid infusion of intravenous fluids; however, if the increased preload and intracardiac pressures restart bleeding from the cardiac wound before thoracotomy, the patient's condition can rapidly deteriorate.[46]

Pericardiocentesis

If it is not possible to perform a thoracotomy almost immediately, a pericardiocentesis should be performed. Pericardiocentesis is primarily a diagnostic procedure, but removal of as little as 5 to 10 mL of blood from the pericardium may increase stroke volume by 25% or more, with a dramatic improvement in cardiac output and BP.

Almost all pericardiocenteses are done via the paraxiphoid approach with an 18-gauge, 10-cm spinal needle. Generally, a large portion of the blood in the pericardial cavity is clotted; consequently, one can usually remove only 3 to 5 mL of blood at a time without manipulating the needle. If 20 mL of blood can be drawn out easily and rapidly, it usually indicates that the blood is being aspirated from the right ventricle.

If an immediate thoracotomy is not planned, a plastic catheter can be used for the pericardiocentesis and left in place for continuing drainage of the intrapericardial blood until the cardiac wound is repaired. At least 25% of patients with acute tamponade will have a negative pericardiocentesis; therefore, if there is a strong suspicion of tamponade in a stable patient but the pericardiocentesis is negative, a thoracotomy should be performed promptly.

THORACOTOMY

Prompt thoracotomy to relieve pericardial tamponade and repair the wound in the heart, preferably in the OR, is the treatment of choice for cardiac wounds causing bleeding and tamponade.[47] In many instances, however, the patient has had a cardiac arrest or is in such severe shock that it seems unlikely that the patient will tolerate transfer to the OR.

An ED thoracotomy for penetrating cardiac injuries is generally recommended for patients who are (1) clinically dead on arrival to the ED but who had some signs of life in transit (32% survival) or (2) deteriorating and with no obtainable BP (33% survival).[48] ED thoracotomies for patients with no signs of life at the scene or within 5 minutes of arrival in the hospital are futile. Cardiac arrest from blunt trauma or brain or abdominal injuries is also almost uniformly fatal.[48, 49]

Coronary Artery Injuries

Ligation of the cut ends of lacerated coronary arteries is the treatment of choice for small vessels. Injured proximal coronary arteries may also be ligated if there is no evidence of cardiovascular dysfunction. However, such patients must be observed closely. If arrhythmias, myocardial infarction, or impaired hemodynamic function develops, an aortocoronary bypass with coronary artery bypass grafting should be performed.

Injuries to Great Arteries in the Chest

Injuries to the great arteries in the chest are uncommon in patients who reach the hospital alive. Diagnosis can be difficult, and a high index of suspicion and arteriography are often required in stable patients to make this diagnosis. If the injury involves a vessel supplying blood to the head and complete clamping of the artery is required for its repair, the stump (distal vessel) pressure should be measured. If the stump pressure is less than 50 mm Hg or cannot be measured, it is prudent to insert a temporary external or internal shunt to ensure adequate blood flow to the brain.[50] With some injuries, it may be prudent to bypass the area of the injury with a graft before entering the hematoma. Carotid injuries should probably be repaired unless the vessel is already occluded distally.

BLUNT CARDIAC TRAUMA

Myocardial Contusion

Cardiac trauma is the most frequent unsuspected visceral injury responsible for death in fatally injured accident victims.[51] In carefully monitored patients admitted to the hospital with severe blunt chest trauma, the incidence of myocardial contusion causing a dangerous arrhythmia or impaired cardiac function is probably about 10% to 20%.[52, 53]

Diagnosis

Clinical Features

A tachycardia that is out of proportion to the degree of trauma or blood loss may be the first tip to the diagnosis. Other helpful physical signs may include a friction rub or abnormality in the heart sounds. Occasionally, an irregular rhythm caused by premature atrial or ventricular contractions or atrial fibrillation may occur.

Electrocardiogram

ST-T wave abnormalities caused by myocardial contusion are present on admission or develop within 12 hours in many but not all patients with myocardial contusion. Significant arrhythmias developing after 24 hours is very uncommon. Continuous Holter monitoring for 3 to 5 days has revealed "significant arrhythmias" (SARRs), usually short runs of ventricular tachycardia, in up to 78% of patients with such monitoring; however, the effect, if any, of SARRs on outcome was not clear.[54]

Enzymes

Serum glutamic oxaloacetic transamine, lactate dehydrogenase, and creatine phosphokinase (CPK) levels are often elevated in patients with severe blunt chest trauma because of injuries to the liver, lung, bone, brain, and skeletal muscle. In most centers, an MB fraction greater than 5% is considered evidence of myocardial injury; however, it is increasingly suggested that this not be routinely used for diagnosis.[54]

Other Studies

X-ray film or clinical evidence of a fractured sternum should make one look closely for myocardial contusion. Radionuclide angiography (RNA)[52] or two-dimensional echocardiography[55] may pick up dyskinesia or akinesia of the ventricles that may not be apparent otherwise. In one study,[52] almost two thirds of the patients with ventricular wall-motion abnormalities on RNA had normal ECG and CK-MB studies.

Insertion of a pulmonary artery catheter and determinations of ventricular function curves with fluid loading may reveal subclinical myocardial dysfunction as reflected by a relatively flat cardiac function curve.[56]

Treatment

If a myocardial contusion is suspected, most patients are admitted for early detection and treatment of complications, especially arrhythmias and congestive heart failure. However, if the myocardial contusion is an isolated injury, complications are uncommon and intensive care unit (ICU) monitoring is generally not needed. Indeed, it has been suggested that the term *myocardial contusion* be abandoned and the term *blunt cardiac injury* be substituted.[57] Furthermore, it has been suggested that asymptomatic patients with "blunt cardiac injury with minor ECG or enzyme abnormality" not be admitted to an ICU for extensive monitoring.[57] Nevertheless, if abnormal heart wall motion is noted on a two-dimensional echocardiogram or RNA, the patient is at increased risk for the development of shock and arrhythmias during general anesthesia for up to a month after the injury.[58] In such patients hypotension that is not responding to fluid loading and inotropes should be treated with intra-aortic balloon pumping.

Pericardial Injury and Effusions

Pericardial injury should be suspected if there is ECG or other evidence of myocardial damage. However, a normal ECG does not rule out traumatic pericarditis with an effusion. In some instances, only echocardiography or autopsy may provide the diagnosis. Tamponade resulting from effusion may occur within minutes or as late as weeks or months after the injury.[59] Retained pericardial blood can also cause later constrictive pericarditis. If nonclotting blood is found on pericardiocentesis, a thoracotomy is generally in order, preferably with cardiopulmonary bypass available.

Cardiac Rupture

Shock not responding promptly to fluid replacement or transfusions after blunt chest trauma may represent pericardial tamponade from a ruptured cardiac chamber.[60] In patients reaching the hospital alive, the injury is usually a tear in the superior or inferior vena cava at its junction with the atrium. Other sites include the junction of the atrial appendage with the right atrium or the anterior surface of the right ventricle. Prompt control of the bleeding site with a fingertip, large vascular clamp, or Foley catheter before definitive suture closure may be lifesaving.

Septal Defects

Septal defects after blunt chest trauma are rare but should be looked for carefully if there is evidence of myocardial damage. The muscular interventricular septum near the apex is particularly susceptible to perforation after blunt trauma. The triad of chest trauma, systolic murmur, and an infarct pattern on ECG should suggest an interventricular septal defect.

Although small, traumatic ventricular septal defects (VSDs) may close spontaneously,[61] surgical repair, preferably 6 to 8 weeks after the trauma, is the treatment of choice. The presence of poorly controlled congestive heart failure requires earlier operation.

Valve Injuries

Rupture of the aortic valve is the most common valvular lesion in patients who survive nonpenetrating cardiac injury. Blunt trauma rarely may also lacerate a papillary muscle or the chordae tendineae of the mitral valve. The prognosis for traumatic rupture of a mitral papillary muscle or mitral valve leaflet is grave, and death usually occurs within a few hours or days after injury.[62] The tricuspid valve is rarely involved in blunt trauma. Tricuspid insufficiency does not usually cause a significant hemodynamic problem unless the patient has pulmonary hypertension, but early repair is recommended.[63]

Follow-Up

It is important that patients with proven or suspected cardiac injury be closely observed throughout their hospitalization and have follow-up for undiagnosed injuries or complications, particularly for post-traumatic pericarditis, VSD, valvular defects, and ventricular aneurysms.

TRAUMATIC RUPTURE OF THE AORTA

Natural History

Of an estimated 8000 patients who have a traumatic rupture of the aorta (TRA) annually, 80% to 90% die within a few minutes of their injury.[51] Of the patients who survive at least 1 hour and are not treated for their TRA, 30% die within 6 hours, 40% within 24 hours, 72% within 8 days, 83% within 3 weeks, and 90% within 10 weeks.

Location

In automobile accident patients who reach the hospital alive, at least 90% of aortic injuries occur just distal to the left subclavian artery.[51] The next most common site of thoracic great vessel injury in such patients is the innominate artery at its origin or the left subclavian artery at the first rib. Tears in the lower descending aorta are very rare, but they tend to occur adjacent to severely comminuted fractures of vertebral bodies.

Diagnosis

Clinical Features

About one third of the patients with TRA have little or no external evidence of chest trauma. In the other two thirds, multiple severe extrathoracic injuries often distract the physician. Consequently, if aortic transection is to be diagnosed early, it must be suspected in any patient who has been in a high-speed motor vehicle accident.[30]

Clinical findings that suggest the diagnosis of TRA include (1) a systolic murmur over the precordium or the back; (2) voice change because of pressure on the left recurrent laryngeal nerve; (3) hypertension in the upper extremities; and (4) weak pulses in the lower extremities.

The most frequent radiologic finding with TRA is widening of the superior mediastinum adjacent to the aortic knob. A false appearance of mediastinal widening can easily be obtained, however, if the chest x-ray films are taken anteroposterior instead of PA, less than 100 cm from the x-ray film machine, with the patient lying flat, and with poor inspiration. The optimal chest x-ray film is an upright PA film taken at 6 feet at full inspiration with the patient leaning forward 10° to 12°.

The most accurate chest x-ray film signs of TRA include deviation of the esophagus to the right and a blurred or obscured aortic knob. In one study of 86 patients with blunt trauma,[64] there were no instances of TRA if the aortic contour was normal, and there was no deviation of the trachea or nasogastric tube.

Other x-ray film signs include apical cap, downward displacement of the left mainstem bronchus, obliteration of the usual clear space between the aortic knob and the left pulmonary artery, and displacement of the right paraspinous interface.[64] Although fractures of the first or second ribs have been thought to be associated with an increased incidence of traumatic aortic rupture, this assumption is increasingly questioned.[30]

Unfortunately, widened mediastinum and other radiologic changes may not be apparent on the chest x-ray film for several hours in up to a third of patients.[65] Consequently, serial chest films should be taken in any patient with severe chest or upper abdominal trauma at 6- to 8-hour intervals during the first day and then daily for the next 3 days.

Aortography

If an aortic rupture is suspected because of the mechanism of injury or clinical or chest x-ray film changes, an aortogram should be performed. While waiting for the aortogram, it is important to not let the patient with a suspected TRA become hypertensive or gag or strain excessively. Because of an increasing tendency to obtain aortograms with even mild suspicion of TRA, more than 95% of the aortograms now performed to rule out blunt injury to the aorta or its major branches are negative.

Although the aortogram is the gold standard for diagnosis of thoracic great artery injury, it will occasionally provide false-positive (primarily because of a ductus bump) or false-negative results. During the aortogram, in addition to getting a good view of the aortic isthmus with a left anterior oblique view, the entire aorta and its branches should be visualized to rule out the less common locations of traumatic ruptures or multiple injuries that might otherwise be missed. If the patient is in shock or has a very large or a rapidly expanding mediastinal hematoma, the patient should be taken directly to the OR without aortography.

In a report by Waugh and Sacharias,[66] it was noted that local complications with conventional angiography may occur in up to 23.2% of patients and systemic complications may occur in up to 9.4%. Although the rates of amputation (0.1%) or death (0.3%) resulting from transfemoral studies are relatively low,[67] if they occur in an individual with a negative study, the indications for the aortogram are apt to be questioned. Death has also occurred in at least two instances when the angiographic catheter was manipulated through the aorta at the level of a tear.[68] If angiography is performed in a hospital where relatively few cases are seen each year, the incidence of complications is increased up to 32-fold.[67]

Computed Tomographic Scans

Over the past few years, there has been some enthusiasm for using contrast-enhanced CT scans as a screening test. A CT scan showing no adjacent hematoma or other evidence of vascular injury is unusual in patients with thoracic great vessel injuries. In fact, this author is not aware of such a case in the literature, except for two reported by Miller and colleagues[69] and two by Durham and associates.[70] Miller's cases are somewhat questionable because one involved misreading by a resident at night and in the other no intravenous contrast was used. Durham's cases may have been missed on suboptimal films. Nevertheless, CT scans can be used for screening or diagnosis, preferably with spiral CT angiography or electron-beam CT angiography.[71]

Transesophageal Ultrasonography

Transesophageal ultrasonography if available, can be performed on a cooperative patient without excessive gagging or vomiting and can be a great help in the early diagnosis of intrathoracic problems after severe chest trauma. Investigators have found that it can easily visualize hematomas around the great vessels and may even detect some aortic injuries directly.[72,73]

Treatment

Nonoperative Management or Delayed Surgery

Many patients with TRA have multiple injuries and are at extremely high risk for emergency repair. By carefully controlling blood pressure, using α- or β-blockers as needed, several surgeons have been able to either delay surgery until the conditions were optimal[74, 75] or avoid surgery completely because the aortic injuries were nonthreatening in appearance.[76]

"Clamp and Sew"

In a few centers with extensive experience with thoracic aortic surgery, the aortic repair may be preferentially performed by a rapid "clamp and sew" technique without an external shunt or cardiopulmonary bypass.[30] Under these circumstances, an intravenous infusion of an α- and β-blocker may be used to keep the systolic BP in the upper portion of the body less than 150 to 180 mm Hg to diminish the chances of intracerebral hemorrhage or left-sided heart failure while the aorta is clamped. The operation must be rapid and precise because clamping of the descending aorta for more than 30 minutes without perfusion of the distal aorta greatly increases the risk of damage to the spinal cord and abdominal viscera. Paraplegia after cross-clamping of the thoracic aorta is probably due to prolonged ischemia to the distal spinal cord, but other factors also play a role. The clamp and sew technique without any bypass or shunt can also cause significant hemodynamic and metabolic changes.[77]

Cardiopulmonary Bypass

Repair of traumatic rupture of the thoracic aorta is often performed under partial bypass because it allows increased time for a meticulous, unhurried repair and reduces the risk of ischemic damage to the spinal cord and abdominal viscera. If the patient's condition is stable, transfer to a hospital where cardiopulmonary bypass is available is wise just in case problems develop during the repair. The usual circuit, from the femoral vein to the femoral artery, requires an oxygenator and heparin, which increases the risk of dangerous bleeding into injuries of the brain, eyes, or retroperitoneum.

Recent use of a special vortex (Biomedicus) bypass pump with catheters in the left atrium and femoral artery may be particularly helpful and safe because no oxygenator and no heparin are required. In the four published series using this technique, there have been only two (7%) deaths and no paraplegia.[78–81]

External Shunts

An alternative to cardiopulmonary bypass is a shunt to divert blood around the involved aorta.[82] The proximal end of the tubing (filled with heparinized saline) can be inserted into the ascending aorta, the aortic arch, or the apex of the heart. The distal end can be inserted into the mid or lower descending thoracic aorta or the femoral artery. If special heparin-coated polyvinyl tubing is used, the patient may not have to be exposed to the risk of systemic heparinization. Using this technique in patients with acute TRA, Verdant and colleagues[82] achieved a survival rate of greater than 95% and no paraplegia.

ESOPHAGEAL INJURIES

Isolated Injuries

Lacerations of the esophagus occur most frequently during endoscopic biopsy or dilatation of a narrowed or obstructed esophagus.[83] The esophagus can also be injured by swallowed foreign bodies. Injury to the esophagus by external trauma is seen only rarely in patients who reach the hospital alive.

If esophageal injury is suspected, an esophagogram should be performed. Many physicians prefer a water-soluble radiopaque material, such as Gastrografin, because it causes less reaction than barium if it leaks into surrounding tissues. However, with such contrast material there is at least a 25% incidence of false-negative results,[84] which are less likely with barium. In addition, if the water-soluble radiopaque material is aspirated into the lungs, it can cause a more severe pneumonitis than barium.

Flexible esophagoscopy is being performed increasingly for diagnosis, but it may miss more than 20% of injuries, even if combined with an esophagogram. Winter and Weigelt[85] believed that rigid esophagoscopy is more accurate than examination with a flexible scope. Bronchoscopy should also be performed to rule out associated tracheobronchial injuries.

If treatment is delayed beyond 24 hours, primary closure of a torn esophagus is usually not advisable because local edema, tissue necrosis, and infection make secure suturing and primary healing unlikely. If mediastinitis develops, it may be rapidly fatal unless the site is drained early and adequately. Whether or not a repair is attempted, continuous complete drainage of the stomach (preferably with a gastrostomy tube) and the adjacent mediastinum (with chest tubes) is important and may be necessary for up to several weeks.

In spite of all the technical and nutritional advances in recent years, the mortality rate of esophageal injuries is about 5% to 25% for those treated definitively within 12 hours and 25% to 66% or higher for those treated after 24 hours.[86, 87] As a consequence, there is increased interest in resecting the injured esophagus except in early, uncomplicated cases.[88]

Caustic Ingestions

Pathophysiology

Ingestion of caustic material, such as lye, can cause severe inflammation and occasional full-thickness necrosis of the esophagus. Even if there is minimal injury to the lips, mouth, or pharynx, alkali may cause severe damage to the esophagus, causing necrosis and perforation or severe strictures. Efforts to neutralize the alkali or remove it by stimulating vomiting or with a nasogastric tube can cause even worse injury.

Swallowed acid tends to coagulate protein, which limits its further penetration into tissues. Consequently, it tends to cause its most severe injuries in the dependent portions of the stomach.

Diagnosis

Many patients with caustic ingestion have severe pain and respiratory distress when first seen, and they may require vigorous resuscitation before any diagnostic studies are performed. Severe injury is found in about 50% of patients who have dysphagia, vomiting, or drooling. If none of these three clinical findings are present, the chances of a significant esophageal injury are very small.[89] Nevertheless, to determine conclusively whether there is severe injury and a high risk of stricture, esophagoscopy down to the first area of severe damage is advocated.

Treatment

Until very recently, patients with severe caustic injury to the esophagus were routinely treated with glucocorticoids, antacids, and antibiotics to reduce the amount of stricture formation. However, in the only prospective clinical trial published, no statistically significant advantage to steroids was found.[90] Because the risks of steroid use may outweigh the potential benefits, some investigators have recommended that steroids not be used for caustic tissue injury.[91] Interestingly, a review of the literature described in detail esophageal injury in which steroids were given for 2 weeks or not at all and showed a reduced incidence of strictures in second-degree and third-degree burns (24% [54/228] vs 52% [13/25] $P < 01$).[92]

THORACIC DUCT INJURIES

Chylothorax is usually the result of thoracic surgery or penetrating trauma. Because the major portion of the thoracic duct in the chest is slightly to the right of the midline, injuries to the thoracic duct usually cause a right chylothorax. Thoracic duct leakage in the chest may result in the loss of 1500 to 2500 mL/d of a clear (if the patient is under nothing by mouth orders) or milky-white odorless fluid containing lymphocytes (not polymorphonuclear leukocytes) and fat globules (demonstrated by Sudan III) or chylomicrons (demonstrated by lipoprotein electrophoresis) with minimal cholesterol.[93]

Adequate drainage of the pleural cavity with a chest tube for several days usually results in spontaneous closure of the fistula. If the fistula persists and is large, intravenous hyperalimentation with nasogastric suction may help by reducing the amount of chyle draining and by preventing the protein malnutrition that can rapidly develop in these patients. If the patient is allowed to eat, a strict, no-fat diet or a diet in which fat is given only as a medium-chain triglyceride is preferred.[94] If the drainage is greater than 1500 mL/d and leads to metabolic and nutritional problems or persists for more than 14 days, surgery is generally indicated.

References

1. LoCicero J, Mattox KL: Epidemiology of chest trauma. Surg Clin North Am 1989; 59:15.
2. Santavirta S, Arajarvi E: Ruptures of the heart in seatbelt wearers. J Trauma 1992; 32:275.
3. Wilson RF, Gibson DEB, Antonenko D: Shock and acute respiratory failure after chest trauma. J Trauma 1977; 17:697.
4. Freed HA, Chields NN: Most frequently overlooked radiographically apparent fractures in a teaching hospital emergency department. Ann Emerg Med 1984; 13:900.
5. Luchette FA, Radfshar MR, Kaiser R, et al: Prospective evaluation of epidural versus intrapleural catheters for analgesia in chest wall trauma. J Trauma 1993; 35:165.
6. Wilson JM, Thomas AN, Goodman PC, et al: Severe chest trauma: Morbidity implications of first and second rib fracture in 120 patients. Arch Surg 1978; 113:846.
7. Bassett JS, Gibson RD, Wilson RF: Blunt injuries to the chest. J Trauma 1968; 8:418.
8. Lee RB, Bass SM, Morris JA, et al: Three or more rib fractures as an indicator for transfer to a Level I trauma center: A population-based study. J Trauma 1990; 30:689.
9. Trinkle JK, Richardson JD, Franz JL, et al: Management of flail chest without mechanical ventilation. Ann Thorac Surg 1975; 19:355.
10. Landercasper J, Cogbill TH, Strutt PJ: Delayed diagnosis of flail chest. Crit Care Med 1990; 18:611.
11. Freedland M, Wilson RF, Bender JS, et al: The management of flail chest injury: Factors affecting outcome. J Trauma 1990; 12:1460.
12. Sankaran S, Wilson RF: Factors affecting prognosis in patients with flail chest. J Thorac Cardiovasc Surg 1970; 60:402.
13. Landreneau RJ, Hinson JM Jr, Hazelrigg SR, et al: Strut fixation of an extensive flail chest. Ann Thorac Surg 1991; 51:473.
14. Wojcik JB, Morgan AS: Sternal fractures: Their natural history. Ann Emerg Med 1988; 17:912.

14a. Brookes JG, Dunn RJ, Rogers IR: Sternal fractures: A retrospective analysis of 272 cases. J Trauma 1993; 35:46.

14b. Hills MW, Delparado AM, Dean SA: Sternal fractures: Associated injuries and management. J Trauma 1993; 35:55.

15. Rosato RM, Shapiro MJ, Keegan MJ, et al: Cardiac injury complicating traumatic asphyxia. J Trauma 1991; 31:1387.
16. Jongewaard WR, Cogbill TH, Landercasper J: Neurologic consequences of traumatic asphyxia. J Trauma 1992; 32:28.
17. Stellin G: Survival in trauma victims with pulmonary contusion. Am Surg 1981; 57:780.
18. Adoumie R, Shennib H, Brown R, et al: Differential lung ventilation: Applications beyond the operating room. J Thorac Cardiovasc Surg 1993; 105:229.
19. Yee ES, Verrier ED, Thomas AN: Management of air embolism in blunt and penetrating chest trauma. J Thorac Cardiovasc Surg 1983; 85:661.
20. Wilson RF, Soullier GW, Wiencek RG: Hemoptysis in trauma. J Trauma 1987; 27:1123.
21. Grover FL, Richardson JD, Fewel JG, et al: Prophylactic antibiotics in the treatment of penetrating chest wounds. J Thorac Cardiovasc Surg 1977; 74:528.
22. Stone HH, Panagiotis NS, Hooper CA: Cefamandole for prophylaxis against infection in closed tube thoracostomy. J Trauma 1981; 21:975.
23. Mandal AK, Montano J, Thadepalli H: Prophylactic antibiotics and no antibiotics compared in penetrating chest trauma. J Trauma 1985; 25:639.
24. LeBlanc KA, Tucker WY: Prophylactic antibiotics and closed tube thoracostomy. Surg Gynecol Obstet 1985; 160:259.
25. LoCurto JJ Jr, Tischler CD, Swan KG, et al: Tube thoracostomy and trauma: Antibiotics or not? J Trauma 1986; 26:1067.
26. Brunner RG, Vinsant GO, Alexander RH, et al: The role of antibiotic therapy in the prevention of empyema in patients with an isolated chest injury (ISS 9–10): A prospective study. J Trauma 1990; 30:1148.

26a. Wilson RF, Janning SW: Antibiotic Therapy for Surgery-Related Infections. 2nd ed. Springfield, NJ, Scientific Therapeutics Information, 1994, pp 29–31.

27. Fallon WF, Wears RL: Prophylactic antibiotics for the prevention of infectious complications including empyema following tube thoracostomy for trauma: Results of meta-analysis. J Trauma 1992; 33:110.
28. Cant PJ, Smyth S, Smart DO: Antibiotic prophylaxis is indicated for chest stab wounds requiring closed tube thoracostomy. Br J Surg 1993; 80:464.
29. Demetriades D, Breckon V, Breckon C, et al: Antibiotic prophylaxis in penetrating injuries of the chest. Ann R Coll Surg Engl 1991; 73:348.
30. Mattox KL: Approaches to trauma involving the major vessels of the thorax. Surg Clin North Am 1989; 69:77.

30a. O'Brien J, Cohen M, Solit R, et al: Thoracoscopic drainage and decortication as definitive treatment for empyema thoracis following penetrating chest injury. J Trauma 1994; 36:536.

31. Mansour MA, Moore EE, Moore FA, et al: Exigent postinjury thoracotomy: Analysis of blunt versus penetrating trauma. Surg Gynecol Obstet 1992; 175:97.
32. Esposito TJ, Jurkovich GJ, Rice C, et al: Reappraisal of emergency room thoracotomy in a changing environment. J Trauma 1991; 31:881.
33. Ivatury RR, Kazigo J, Rohman M, et al: "Directed" emergency room thoracotomy: A prognostic prerequisite for survival. J Trauma 1991; 31:1076.
34. Collins JC, Levine G, Waxman K: Occult traumatic pneumothorax: Immediate tube thoracostomy versus expectant management. Am Surg 1992; 58:743.
35. Obeid FN, Shapiro MJ, Richardson HH, et al: Catheter aspiration for simple pneumothorax (CASP) in the outpatient management of simple traumatic pneumothorax. J Trauma 1985; 25:882.
36. Nicholas JM, Dulchavsky SA: Successful use of autologous fibrin gel in traumatic bronchopleural fistula: Case report. J Trauma 1992; 32:87.
37. Carroll K, Cheeseman SH, Fink MP, et al: Secondary infection of post-traumatic pulmonary cavity lesions in adolescents and young adults: Role of computed tomography and operative debridement and drainage. J Trauma 1989; 29:109.
38. Hudgens S, McGraw J, Craun M: Two cases of tension pneu-

mopericardium following blunt chest injury. J Trauma 1991; 31:1408.
39. Taskinen SO, Salo JA, Halttunen PEA, et al: Tracheobronchial rupture due to blunt chest trauma: A follow-up study. Ann Thorac Surg 1989; 48:846.
40. Lew EO, Mittleman RE, Murray D: Endotracheal tube ignition by electrocautery during tracheostomy: Case report with autopsy findings. J Forensic Sci 1991; 36:1586.
41. Wilson RF, Bassett JS: Penetrating wounds of the pericardium or its contents. JAMA 1966; 195:513.
41a. Bolton JWR, Bynoe RP, Lazar HL, et al: Two-dimensional echocardiography in the evaluation of penetrating intrapericardial injuries. Ann Thorac Surg 1993; 56:506.
41b. Aaland MO, Bryan EC III, Sherman R: Two-dimensional echocardiogram in hemodynamically stable victims of penetrating precordial trauma. Ann Surg 1994; 60:412.
42. Buckman RF, Badellino MM, Mauro LH, et al: Penetrating cardiac wounds: Prospective study of factors influencing initial resuscitation. J Trauma 1993; 34:717.
43. Aaland MO, Sherman RT: Delayed pericardial tamponade in penetrating chest trauma: Case report. J Trauma 1991; 31:1563.
44. Duncan AO, Scalea TM, Sclafani SJ, et al: Evaluation of occult cardiac injuries using subxiphoid pericardial window. J Trauma 1989; 29:955.
45. Mayor-Davies JA, Britz RS: Subxiphoid pericardial windows: Helpful in selected cases. J Trauma 1990; 30:1399.
46. Gyhra A, Pierart J, Torres P, et al: Experimental cardiac tamponade with a myocardial wound: The effect of rapid intravenous infusion of saline. J Trauma 1992; 33:25.
47. Washington B, Wilson RF, Steiger Z: Emergency thoracotomies for penetrating trauma. Curr Surg 1984; 41:14.
48. Rohman M, Ivatury RR, Steichen FM, et al: Emergency room thoracotomy for penetrating cardiac injuries. J Trauma 1983; 23:570.
49. Lorenz HP, Steinmetz B, Lieberman J, et al: Emergency thoracotomy: Survival correlates with physiologic status. J Trauma 1992; 32:780.
50. Marvasti MA, Parker FB Jr, Bredenbery CE: Injuries to arterial branches of the aortic arch. Thorac Cardiovasc Surg 1984; 32:293.
51. Parmley LF, Manion WC, Mattingly TW: Non-penetrating traumatic injury to the heart. Circulation 1958; 18:371.
52. Sutherland GR, Driedger AA, Holliday RL, et al: Frequency of myocardial injury after blunt chest trauma as evaluated by radionuclide angiography. Am J Cardiol 1983; 52:1099.
53. McLean RF, Devitt JH, Dubbin J, et al: Incidence of abnormal RNA studies and dysrhythmias in patients with blunt chest trauma. J Trauma 1991; 31:968.
54. Paone RF, Peacock JB, Smith DLT: Diagnosis of myocardial contusion. South Med J 1993; 86:867.
55. King RM, Mucha P Jr, Seward JB, et al: Cardiac contusion: A new diagnostic approach utilizing two-dimension echocardiography. J Trauma 1983; 23:610.
56. Torres-Mirabal P, Gruenberg JC, Talbert JF, et al: Ventricular function of myocardial contusion: A preliminary study. AJR 1972; 115:281.
57. Mattox KL, Flint LM, Carrico CJ: Blunt cardiac injury (formerly termed "myocardial contusion") (Editorial). J Trauma 1992; 33:649.
58. Frazee RC, Mucha P, Farnell MB, et al: Objective evaluation of blunt cardiac trauma. J Trauma 1986; 26:510.
59. Solomon D: Delayed cardiac tamponade after blunt chest trauma: Case report. J Trauma 1991; 31:1322.
60. Calhoon JH, Hoffman TH, Trinkle JK, et al: Management of blunt rupture of the heart. J Trauma 1986; 26:495.
61. Krajcer Z, Cooley DA, Leachman RD: Ventricular septal defect following blunt trauma: Spontaneous closure of residual defect after surgical repair. Cathet Cardiovasc Diagn 1977; 3:409.
62. Al Kasab A, Westaby S, Al Zaibag MA, et al: Traumatic papillary muscle dysfunction: Attempted mitral-valve repair and eventual prosthetic replacement. Eur Heart J 1988; 9:1030.
63. Dontigny L, Baillot R, Panneton J, et al: Surgical repair of traumatic tricuspid insufficiency: Report of three cases. J Trauma 1992; 33:266.
64. Peters DR, Gamsu G: Displacement of the right paraspinous interface: A radiographic sign of acute traumatic rupture of the thoracic aorta. Radiology 1980; 134:599.
65. Wilson RF, Arbulu A, Basset J, et al: Acute mediastinal widening following blunt chest trauma: Critical decisions. Arch Surg 1972; 104:551.
66. Waugh JR, Sacharias N: Arteriographic complications in the DSA eras. Radiology 1992; 182:243.
67. Hessel SJ, Adams DF, Abrams HL: Complications of angiography. Radiology 1981; 138:273.
68. LaBerge JM, Jeffrey RB: Aortic lacerations: Fatal complications of thoracic aortography. Radiology 1987; 165:367.
69. Miller FB, Richardson JD, Thomas HA, et al: Role of CT in diagnosis of major arterial injury after blunt thoracic trauma. Surgery 1989; 106:596.
70. Durham RM, Zuckerman D, Wolverson M, et al: Computed tomography as a screening exam in patients with suspected blunt aortic injury. J Trauma 1993; 35:161.
71. Raptopoulos V: Chest CT for aortic injury: Maybe not for everyone. AJR Am J Roentgenol 1994; 162:1053.
72. Shapiro MJ, Yanofsky SD, Trapp J, et al: Cardiovascular evaluation in blunt thoracic trauma using transesophageal echocardiography (TEE). J Trauma 1991; 31:835.
73. Kearney PA, Smith W, Johnson SB, et al: Use of transesophageal echocardiography in the evaluation of traumatic aortic injury. J Trauma 1993; 34:696.
74. Stiles QR, Cohimia GS, Smith JH, et al: Management of injuries of the thoracic and abdominal aorta. Am J Surg 1985; 150:132.
75. Hilgenberg AD, Logan DL, Akins CW, et al: Blunt injuries of the thoracic aorta. Ann Thorac Surg 1992; 53:233.
76. Fisher RG, Oria RA, Mattos KL, et al: Conservative management of aortic lacerations due to blunt trauma. J Trauma 1990; 30:1562.
77. Van Normal GA, Pavlin EG, Eddy AC, et al: Hemodynamic and metabolic effects of aortic unclamping following emergency surgery for traumatic thoracic aortic tears in shunted and unshunted patients. J Trauma 1991; 31:1007.
78. Oliver HF, Mahler TD, Liebler GA, et al: Use of the Bio-Medicus centrifugal pump in traumatic tears of the thoracic aorta. Ann Thorac Surg 1984; 38:586.
79. Hess PJ, Howe HR, Robicsek F, et al: Traumatic tears of the thoracic aorta: Improved results using the Bio-Medicus pump. Ann Thorac Surg 1989; 48:6.
80. Walls JT, Curtis JJ, Boley T: Sarns centrifugal pump for repair of thoracic aortic injury: Case reports. J Trauma 1989; 29:1283.
81. McCroskey BL, Moore EE, Moore FA, et al: A unified approach to the torn thoracic aorta. Am J Surg 1991; 162:473.
82. Verdant A, Page A, Cossett R, et al: Surgery of the descending thoracic aorta: Spinal cord protection with the Gott shunt. Ann Thorac Surg 1988; 46:147.
83. Jones WG, Ginsberg RJ: Esophageal perforation: A continuing challenge. Ann Thorac Surg 1992; 53:534.
84. Glatterer MS Jr, Toon RS, Ellestad C, et al: Management of blunt and penetrating external esophageal trauma. J Trauma 1985; 25:601.
85. Winter RP, Weigelt JA: Cervical esophageal trauma, incidence and cause of esophageal fistulas. Arch Surg 1990; 125:849.
86. Wilson RF, Steiger Z: Oesophageal Injuries. *In:* Trauma Surgery. 4th ed. Champion HR, Robbs JV, Trunkey DD (Eds). London, Butterworths, 1989, pp 327–340.
87. Richardson JD, Martin LF, Borzotta AP, et al: Unifying concepts in treatment of esophageal leaks. Am J Surg 1985; 149:157.
88. Tilanus HW, Bossuyt P, Schattenkerk ME, et al: Treatment of oesophageal perforation: A multivariate analysis. Br J Surg 1991; 78:582.
89. Crain EF, Gershel JC, Mezey AP: Caustic ingestions: Symptoms as predictors of esophageal injury. Am J Dis Child 1984; 138:863.
90. Hawkins DB, Demeter MJ, Barnett TE: Caustic ingestion: Controversies in management: A review of 214 cases. Laryngoscope 1980; 90:98.
91. Ferguson MK, Migliore M, Staszak VM, et al: Early evaluation and therapy for caustic esophageal injury. Am J Surg 1989; 157:116.
92. Howell JM, Dalsey WC, Hartsell FW, et al: Steroids for the treatment of corrosive esophageal injury: A statistical analysis of past studies. Am J Emerg Med 1992; 10:421.
93. Robinson CLN: The management of chylothorax. Ann Thorac Surg 1986; 39:90.
94. Ramzy AI, Rodriguez A, Cowley RA: Pitfalls in the management of traumatic chylothorax. J Trauma 1982; 22:513.

CHAPTER 156

Abdominal and Pelvic Trauma

Marc J. Shapiro, MD · Rodney M. Durham, MD
John E. Mazuski, MD, PhD

From this chapter, the clinician will have a better understanding of the significance of injuries to the abdomen and pelvis. The abdominal and pelvic cavities are considered together because of the direct communication of intra-abdominal contents. Ten per cent of deaths from penetrating and blunt trauma are directly due to injuries in this region. Gunshot wounds to the abdomen lead to intraperitoneal penetration in 90% of cases, and stab wounds lead to intraperitoneal penetration in 30% to 40%. Overall mortality rates from intra-abdominal gunshot wounds are approximately 5% and for stab wounds 2%. Blunt trauma leads to abdominal operative intervention 10% of the time in the civilian population. The mortality rate in blunt trauma is usually not solely related to the intra-abdominal injury but rather to an associated injury such as severe head or chest injury. Before further discussion can begin, the anatomy must be defined.[1]

ANATOMY

Because of the attachments of the diaphragm and its changing position during ventilation, the boundaries of the intraperitoneal cavity are not constant. For this reason, penetrating injuries that occur below the fourth intercostal interspace anteriorly, the fifth interspace in the midaxillary line, and the sixth interspace posteriorly or below the tip of the scapula have the possibility of entering the abdomen. The lower extent of the pelvis is the perineal area, which anteriorly extends to the inguinal ligament attachments at the anterosuperior iliac spine. The lateral border of the abdomen lies roughly at the level of the anterior axillary line.

There are four intraperitoneal areas: (1) the intrathoracic portion of the peritoneal cavity is protected by the rib cage and includes the liver, gallbladder, stomach, transverse colon, and spleen, (2) the intra-abdominal cavity contains the bulk of the abdominal hollow viscera including small bowel, ascending and descending colon, and omentum, (3) the pelvis, which is protected by the pelvic girdle, contains the rectum, bladder, iliac vessels, and internal female genitalia, and (4) the retroperitoneum contains the aorta, inferior vena cava, pancreas, kidneys, ureters, parts of the duodenum, and large bowel.

MECHANISM OF INJURY

Motor vehicle accidents account for approximately 50% of blunt abdominal injuries; other contributing causes include falls, assaults, contact sports, and crush injuries. The severity of injury is related to the offending agent and the amount of energy produced and dissipated. Kinetic energy is defined as $MV^2/2G$, where M is the mass of the projectile, V is the velocity of the projectile, and G is the gravitational force exerted. High-velocity weapons with a muzzle velocity of more than 2000 feet/s create devastating injury. A rapid deceleration injury can cause a shearing effect, leading to avulsion of solid viscera with hemoperitoneum. Lap belt restraints may cause sudden elevation in intra-abdominal pressure, leading to hollow viscus rupture or mesenteric tears. In blunt trauma, the incidence of specific organ injury is as follows: spleen, 25% to 35%; liver, 15% to 25%; kidneys, 10% to 15%; and retroperitoneal hematoma, 10% to 15%. In penetrating abdominal trauma, the incidence of specific organ injury is as follows: small bowel, 30% to 35%; mesentery and omentum, 15% to 20%; liver, 15% to 20%; colon, 10%; and diaphragm, 10%.[1]

Regardless of the mechanism of injury, an adequate history is crucial to provide insight as to what might be injured. For instance, in a deceleration automobile crash, a driver wearing a lap belt may experience a sudden increase in intra-abdominal pressure, leading to small bowel perforation, or may be compressed against the steering wheel, sustaining a fractured sternum and cardiac contusion.[2] In penetrating injuries, the identification of entry and exit sites can give the clinician a crude idea of what may be injured; however, bullets do not travel in straight lines and there is more than meets the eye in connecting point A and point B and treating only those areas that lay between.

The clinician should also be knowledgeable in child abuse; children may repeatedly present to the emergency room under the guise of having sustained some form of nonabusive trauma. Major blunt abdominal trauma resulting from child abuse can be lethal, with reported mortality rates up to 50%. Suspicion should peak when continued injury lacks explanation, stories appear to be changing, unexplained or inappropriate blame is assigned to another individual, a discrepancy exists between history and physical examination, the injury pattern delays child development, or there is an obvious delay in seeking healthcare.[3]

INITIAL APPROACH

The initial approach to all victims of injury is the same, with airway, breathing, circulation, and resuscitation being performed concurrently. Laboratory evaluation should be ordered as soon as intravenous catheterization is begun, with blood being withdrawn for the blood chemistries listed in Table 156–1. A history should be obtained, including medical and surgical history, present medications, history of drug and alcohol abuse, and allergies. Unfortunately, the physical examination may be misleading in that 23% to 36% of patients with intraperitoneal injuries will lack significant findings.[4] Inspection for lacerations, ecchymosis, or abrasions may provide subtle clues of internal abdominal injuries. Auscultation of the abdominal cavity has been found to be unreliable because the presence or absence of bowel sounds lacks correlation with specific abdominal findings and, in fact, should be used only as point of reference for subsequent examinations. Tympany by percussion may denote presence of pathologic intra-abdominal air, although this may be hard to distinguish from physiologic intraluminal air. Dullness to percussion may be due to intra-abdomi-

TABLE 156–1. Blood Chemistries for Major Trauma

Type and crossmatch six units packed cells
Complete blood cell count
Electrolytes
Blood sugar
Blood urea nitrogen
Creatinine
Amylase (for blunt and penetrating abdominal)
Prothrombin time
Partial thromboplastin time
Urinalysis
(Alcohol)
(Drug screen)
Other

TABLE 156–2. Ancillary Evaluation Aids

Local exploration	Intravenous pyelogram
Plain radiographs	Liver/spleen scan
Computed tomographic scanning	Laparoscopy
Diagnostic peritoneal lavage	Laparotomy
Ultrasonography	

nal hemorrhage or may be a normal physiologic finding in an individual who has recently consumed a large meal.

The physical examination is a continuous process and should be repeated periodically as the work-up is being completed. Interpretation of the abdominal examination in a paralyzed or intoxicated patient or in a patient euphoric from illicit drug use will also be unreliable. The physical findings most associated with internal injuries in blunt trauma include abdominal tenderness and guarding in as many as 75% of patients. Peritoneal signs of rebound, rigidity, and tenderness only occur in approximately 28% of patients with an acute abdomen. Thus, other diagnostic tests need to be performed, although, in the case of an unstable patient or one with obvious penetration of the intra-abdominal cavity from a gunshot wound, further work-up should be minimized because the patient needs to go to the operating room (OR) in an expeditious fashion. During the physical examination, a nasogastric (NG) tube should be placed if there is no obvious maxillofacial injury, bleeding diathesis, or other contraindications; otherwise, an orogastric tube is necessary. A rectal examination should also be included in the physical to evaluate whether the prostate is free floating or high riding or if there is evidence of rectal bleeding. When the rectal examination is normal and there is no blood at the urethral meatus or evidence of a scrotal hematoma, a Foley catheter may be placed and urinalysis obtained. Additional ancillary laboratory tests such as those listed in Table 156–2 can prove helpful in identifying other areas of injury.

DIAGNOSTIC MODALITIES

History, physical, and laboratory examinations continue, with additional testing being performed as outlined in Table 156–2. Significant findings on physical examination may be absent or misleading in up to 45% of patients with intraperitoneal injury.[5, 6] In patients who have sustained blunt abdominal trauma, urgent celiotomy is indicated in those with abdominal distention, hypotension, overt peritonitis, or obvious signs of visceral injury. The approaches to evaluating penetrating and blunt trauma are different and are presented as such.

Before 1965, abdominal paracentesis was performed to evaluate for the presence of hemoperitoneum. However, because of a low sensitivity in accuracy and a high rate of false-negative results, other means of evaluation were scrutinized. In 1965, diagnostic peritoneal lavage (DPL) was introduced as a means of evaluating victims with abdominal trauma. Commonly used criteria include a red blood cell (RBC) count of more than 100,000 cells/mm^3, a white blood cell count of greater than 500 cells/mm^3, an elevated amylase level, and the presence of bile or other intra-abdominal debris.[6] When DPL amylase and alkaline phosphatase levels are elevated in the presence of a history consistent with possible small-bowel injury, laparotomy should strongly be considered.[7]

Before placing the DPL catheter, bladder and gastric decompression should be accomplished. If lavage fluid drains from the Foley catheter, the gastric tube, or a chest tube, the patient needs to undergo prompt laparotomy. DPL has an accuracy rate of greater than 98%, has a rate of false-positive and false-negative results of less than 4%, and, when done using the open technique, has a complication rate of less than 5%. Quicker DPLs use the percutaneous or Seldinger techniques. However, there is a learning curve when these techniques are used, reflected by an initial increased complication rate. DPL is useful in the hemodynamically unstable patient whose condition precludes transport. In the uncooperative patient who cannot be sedated, who has intravenous contrast allergy, or whose computed tomographic (CT) scan is equivocal, DPL is a good diagnostic tool.

Early in the 1980s, CT scanning began to have a prominent role in trauma. The CT scan is relatively noninvasive, identifying specific organ injury and function, and allows for the evaluation of the retroperitoneum. It can be used in a sequential fashion comparing progression or resolution of injury. Generally, intravenous and oral contrast is administered to a hemodynamically stable patient in the radiology suite. In the patient with a positive DPL, the nontherapeutic laparotomy rate may decrease from 25% to 6% with CT scanning by defining specific organ injury and quantitating intra-abdominal blood. In addition, the CT scan may identify false-positive DPL results caused by retroperitoneal or nonsurgical pelvic sources of hemorrhage. Limitations of CT scan include inability to evaluate bowel perforation, which may occur in up to 4% of major blunt abdominal trauma. Disadvantages of CT scan include the necessity for specialized personnel and equipment, 20 to 30 minutes to perform the abdominal and pelvic CT, movement of the patient out of the resuscitation bay, limitation to patient access, and an increase in cost over DPL. CT scan interpretation is user dependent.[8]

Six areas in the abdomen and pelvis identified by CT scan help quantitate hemoperitoneum, which is difficult to do with DPL. Blood tends to pool in the following six dependent areas: (1) Morison's pouch (superior to the right kidney, inferior to the liver); (2) left subphrenic space; (3) right subphrenic space; (4) right pericolic gutter; (5) left pericolic gutter; and (6) the pelvic cul-de-sac. In general, a small collection of blood correlates with approximately 100 to 200 cc in any of these spaces. A moderate collection of blood in two spaces plus the pelvis corresponds with 250 to 500 cc, and collections of more than 500 cc may accumulate in the pelvis.

DPL and CT scanning can be complementary in evaluating blunt abdominal trauma.[9] DPL and CT are associated with unnecessary laparotomy rates of 15.5% and 0.8%, respectively and inappropriate observation rates of 1.7% and 6.9%, respectively. DPL is not as specific as CT scan, although both have a sensitivity of 99%. CT accuracy is 98%, whereas DPL accuracy is 92%.[10] DPL can also be done in a serial manner within the intensive care unit (ICU). Because CT scans are not portable, DPL is attractive for patients who are undergoing extensive monitoring procedures in the ICU. When equivocal, the catheter can be left in place and the patient relavaged. Abdominal CT and DPL should not be used in patients who are undergoing celiotomy and may be misleading in obese patients and those with subcutaneous emphysema.

Enthusiasm exists in the pediatric population for the use of CT scan over DPL in a hemodynamically stable and non–life-threatened injured child. The likelihood of abdominal injury is heightened when three or more of the following clinical indications exist: gross hematuria, lap belt injury, bicycle injury, abdominal tenderness, or trauma score of 12 or less.[11, 12]

Ultrasonography is used in Europe and Japan for the evaluation of blunt abdominal trauma. Accuracy is upward of 100%, sensitivity is 84%, and specificity is 98%.[13] Approximately 70 cc of intraperitoneal blood is necessary for visualization on ultrasonographic scan, with a 20% to 25% incidence of failure to detect spleen or liver injury.[4] Advantages of ultrasonography include its portability, rapidity, relative low cost, and repeat ability. Limitations include use in patients who are uncooperative and in those with rib fractures or hollow viscus injury and operator dependency.[14]

Abdominal and pelvic angiography for abdominal and pelvic trauma aids in identifying and controlling arterial bleeding from pelvic fractures and, on rare occasion, intra-abdominal visceral bleeding. Disadvantages of angiography include the necessity of performing the study in the radiology suite, nephrotoxic intravenous dye load, and contrast allergies to the dye. Special personnel and equipment are required, the test is expensive, and it does not evaluate for hollow viscus injury.

The usefulness of laparoscopy for trauma is not established. Theoretically, this procedure could be performed in the emergency department or ICU with local or inhalational anesthesia if the patient is cooperative. Presently, laparoscopy is used diagnostically to determine whether intra-abdominal penetration has occurred. However, limitations include inability to visualize the entire small bowel and the spleen and poor visualization in the presence of ongoing hemorrhage. Although the reported complication rate is low, we have produced a tension pneumothorax in one patient with a diaphragmatic injury and tension pneumopericardium in another patient with a penetrating pericardial injury. This procedure will most likely have limited usefulness and will serve to complement CT scan, DPL, and ultrasonography.[15, 16, 16a, 16b]

For penetrating trauma, a more direct approach is generally used. Mandatory exploratory laparotomy for all abdominal stab wounds is no longer universally practiced. Frequently, treatment involves local exploration in the emergency department with the potential for discharge if the peritoneal cavity is not violated. Penetration into the abdominal cavity from a stab wound can be evaluated by different means. A patient may undergo prompt laparotomy, or a DPL may be performed to evaluate the patient further, although there is debate in terms of the number of RBCs needed (1000–100,000/cm^3) to lead one to laparotomy. CT scanning misses small-bowel injuries, the most common organ injured in stab wounds. Ultrasonography and laparoscopy have limitations in visualization of small-bowel injuries as well. Some investigators believe that peritoneal penetration, air under the diaphragm, evisceration of omentum or bowel, blood found on abdominal paracentesis, and shock on admission are not absolute indications for surgery, although these theories are not universally accepted. Rather, careful initial and repeated clinical examination should be used.[17]

Posterior stab wounds are more difficult to explore locally. CT scanning is 89% sensitive, 98% specific, and 97% accurate in evaluating stab wounds to the back.[18] Depending on clinical findings, many of these patients are admitted and observed without further work-up unless their clinical condition changes or abnormalities, such as hematuria, are found.

For the most part, gunshot wounds to the abdomen are explored. Although there are a few who will observe and perform DPL or abdominal CT to evaluate these patients further, exploration is the standard.[19]

Liver-spleen scanning has lost favor in evaluating blunt trauma patients with the advent of CT scanning. Patients with hepatic or splenic injury who are not operated on can be monitored by CT scan or ultrasonography. Intravenous pyelogram (IVP) has been replaced by CT scanning with intravenous contrast. Trauma patients are prone to aerophagia with unprepared bowel, making IVP resolution limited. Urethra and bladder injuries are discussed subsequently.

ANTIBIOTICS

Major trauma increases neutrophil adherence, decreases chemotaxis, impairs phagocytosis, and decreases bactericidal activity. Injury leads to fibronectin deficiency, decreased levels of complement and immunoglobulins, and a decrease in cell-mediated immunity. All this promotes infection. Surgical wounds are defined as clean (no injuries, operation occurring less than 6 hours since injury), clean contaminated, or contaminated (colon injury, operation occurring more than 6 hours since injury), with infection rates of 3.2%, 8.1%, and 24.6%, respectively. Weigelt found penetrating wounds to have an overall infection rate of 10.9%; gunshot wounds, 15.3%; stab wounds, 10.9%; shotgun wounds, 11.7%; and blunt abdominal trauma, 7.1%. The wound infection rate without prophylactic antibiotics is 21% versus 11% with prophylactic antibiotics. Delayed primary closure infection rates were 21.7% and secondary closure rates were 24% in comparison to 5.2% with primary closure in the clean-contaminated group.[20]

Subcutaneous wound infections are treated by opening the wound, irrigating, debriding, and packing. Surrounding cellulitis, subfascial infection, or the use of prosthetic material dictates the need for antibiotics. *Staphylococcus aureus* is the most common offending organism.

Fever occurs in approximately one half of patients sustaining significant intra-abdominal injury. Evaluation includes physical examination, which may be nonrevealing, and radiographs such as CT or ultrasonography. Intra-abdominal abscess formation tends to manifest at approximately 7 to 10 days postoperatively. Percutaneous or surgical drainage of infected material should be performed; antibiotics should not be relied on solely.

Antibiotic use in trauma differs from that in elective surgery. The incidence of postinjury infection is 24% in major penetrating injuries, and many deaths from penetrating abdominal trauma are related to infection. Studies in the early 1970s demonstrated that preoperative antibiotics for penetrating trauma decreased infection rates from 30% to 7%. Although the type of antibiotic is frequently less critical than adequate serum blood levels before surgery, single antibiotics such as the cephalosporins have been shown to have equivalent or better results in preventing intra-abdominal abscesses and wound infection than antibiotic combinations such as clindamycin, gentamicin, or tobramycin.[21, 21a] In a prospective study of 515 patients, Fabian and coworkers found that only 24 hours of therapy were necessary for all cases of penetrating abdominal trauma.[22] Higher doses of prophylactic antibiotics may be necessary in the severely injured patient because intravascular volume and volume of distribution are increased as a result of aggressive resuscitation.[23] When Feliciano compared 31 groups in 14 publications undergoing various antibiotic trials during abdominal traumatic surgical procedures, the abscess rate was 4.4% and wound infection rate was 5.1%.[21] Risk factors for the development of infection include perioperative shock, massive blood transfusion, high severity of injury, left-sided colon injury with colostomy, more than one intra-abdominal organ injury, old age, presence of immunosuppression, and a catabolic nutritional state. Abdominal trauma with associated open fractures increases the risk of infection, especially if the fracture is severe with soft-tissue damage. Such patients will benefit from broad-spectrum parenteral antibiotic therapy, although the duration of administration is still debatable.[21b]

STOMACH

Injuries to the stomach are more common with penetrating injuries than blunt injuries (7–20% vs. 0.4–1.7%). The stomach is unique in that the flora and bacteria within the stomach are pH dependent, with bacterial counts being less than 10^3 organisms/mL. When the pH is less than 4, organisms found include streptococci, lactobacilli, micrococci, staphylococci, and oral bacteroides. At higher pH levels, neutralized either by food or the use of neutralizing agents such as histamine$_2$ (H_2) blockers and antacids, predominant organisms include *Streptococcus viridans, Bacteroides melaninogenicus* and *B. asaccharolyticus,* staphylococci, and *Neisseria.*[24]

The most likely mechanism of gastric injury from blunt trauma is from sudden and acute increase in intraluminal pressure secondary to a direct blow to the full stomach (an empty stomach lies relatively protected within the inferior margins of the rib cage). Perforation usually occurs along the anterior greater curvature of the stomach. Fifty per cent to 80% of patients with blunt gastric rupture will present with signs of peritoneal irritation or shock. Free abdominal air is found in less than two thirds of patients, although aerophagia may lead to intragastric air. Blood in the NG tube is ominous but not pathognomonic for gastric injury because blood may be seen after placement of the NG tube.[24] Complications related to penetrating gastric injuries have been associated with age, gunshot wounds, and the use of two or more units of blood.[25] Because of the low bacterial load within the stomach, gastric injuries early on generally do not lead to sepsis, which is different from missed colon injuries, as discussed subsequently.

DUODENUM

Because of its partial retroperitoneal location, duodenal injuries are frequently difficult to recognize. A high index of suspicion is required when evaluating patients after significant blunt or penetrating upper abdominal injury because a delay in diagnosis significantly increases mortality. Penetrating wounds account for a majority of injuries to the duodenum. Blunt trauma leads to duodenal rupture by crushing, bursting, or shearing effects. Early mortality in duodenal injury is secondary to hypovolemic hemorrhagic shock, whereas late mortality is related to other associated injuries or sepsis. Approximately 50% of individuals with duodenal injury will have hyperamylasemia. However, amylase, although sensitive, is not specific, being positive in patients who have maxillofacial glandular injuries. If the injury is retroperitoneal, a negative peritoneal lavage may not exclude a duodenal laceration.

Plain radiographs rarely show intraperitoneal, retroperitoneal, or intrabiliary air. Obliteration of the right psoas margin, right scoliosis, and retroperitoneal air around the kidney suggest duodenal injury. Pneumoperitoneum can be exaggerated by injecting air through the NG tube before obtaining a plain upright and left lateral decubitus abdominal radiograph. A water-soluble upper gastrointestinal (GI) study, with the patient specifically placed in the right lateral decubitus position, may show the injury. CT scan may not reveal the injury, even with contrast.[26]

Treatment of duodenal injury is surgical. Morbidity is associated with a large defect (>75% of the circumference), injury to the first or second portion of the duodenum, a delay in operation of more than 24 hours after injury, and adjacent common bile duct injury.[27]

Postoperative care includes volume resuscitation and GI decompression with suction until bowel function returns. Duodenal fistulization may occur in up to 14% of patients.[26] Once the fistula is identified, gastric decompression is used to decrease duodenal stimulation. An H_2 blocker may decrease gastric output, and somatostatin may decrease pancreatic secretion. Surrounding skin is protected from maceration because of activated enzymes. Nutritional support is provided either enterally distal to the fistula or parenterally. If 4 to 6 weeks of medical management are not successful, operative intervention is strongly considered. During the period of fistulization, blood gases should be monitored, as should electrolytes because electrolyte and acid-base abnormalities are frequent, especially with high-output fistulas.

SMALL BOWEL

The small bowel is approximately 22 feet long with the jejunum in the upper two fifths and the ileum in the lower three fifths. Of the wounds that penetrate the peritoneal cavity, the small bowel is the most commonly injured intra-abdominal organ, sustaining injury in 80% of abdominal gunshot wounds and in 30% of stab wounds. In severe blunt abdominal trauma, the small bowel is the third most common organ injured, after the spleen and liver, sustaining injury in 5% to 15% of cases, primarily from crushing injuries related to seat belt usage, shearing from sudden deceleration injuries, or bursting because of a potential closed loop. Blunt abdominal trauma in children may lead to an intramural hematoma of the small bowel (especially duodenum), which is compressed between the abdominal wall and the vertebrae. Under these circumstances, the diagnosis can be made from an upper GI series demonstrating obstruction or delayed passage and deformity. In the absence of other serious injuries, treatment is conservative.[28]

As with the stomach, the physical examination may be nonrevealing in identifying small-bowel injury. In addition, the neutral pH and low bacterial count of the succus entericus provoke only a minimal inflammatory response initially. Blood serology and plain radiographs are generally not helpful, and many times, free air will not be seen. CT scanning misses intestinal injury because findings are very subtle or nonspecific.[29] The presence of GI contents with DPL makes this test useful.

When perforation of the small bowel is recognized, operation is mandatory. Perioperative antibiotics are administered, NG decompression is undertaken, and, once hemodynamic instability is corrected, the patient is taken to the operating room. The amount of NG drainage should be monitored and replaced with balanced electrolyte solution. Resectional therapy or primary repair may be undertaken. Surgical complications include bleeding, wound infection, repair breakdown, anastomotic failure, fistulization, abscess, or obstruction. Postoperatively, a patient may exhibit signs and symptoms of leakage with fever, tachycardia, leukocytosis, peritonitis, or external fistulization. The presence of multiple organ failure or persistent fever after abdominal surgery with temperature spikes and tachycardia should lead one to consider performing a CT scan to look for an abdominal abscess. Once infection is identified, antibiotics should be continued. Abscesses can be drained by percutaneous, radiographically guided drainage or through operation. When a wound infection occurs, the incision is opened and debridement may be necessary. In general, a superficial wound infection should be treated locally without antibiotics.

COLON

The large intestine is approximately 6 feet long and is injured in less than 5% of all blunt abdominal trauma victims and about in 15% of victims with penetrating trauma.[30] Recognition of colon injury is hampered by the fact that physical findings may be delayed, CT scanning may miss injuries, and DPL may not pick up retroperitoneal colon injury. Therapy has changed through the years, moving away from colostomy, because the morbidity and mortality from colostomy and colostomy closure appear to be higher than those for primary repair.[31, 32] A majority of injuries are repaired primarily, even up to 12 hours after injury. Perioperative antibiotics are administered and NG decompression is continued until evidence of peristalsis appears. Risks factors for infection from colon injury include two to four units of blood transfused, elderly, two or more associated injuries, injury to the spleen, shock, and significant contamination. In the presence of gross contamination, wound infection frequently occurs; thus, the wound should be left open or delayed primary closure considered.[31]

The presence of fever and leukocytosis after postoperative day 5 may be related to a leak resulting from the colon repair. Symptomology consistent with peritonitis dictates the need for relaparotomy. Rectal examination may disclose fluctuance from a pelvic abscess, or CT scan may confirm an intra-abdominal abscess. If rectal contrast is to be used, it should be water soluble and administered gently. The presence of a retained foreign body (e.g., bullet) that has gone through the colon increases the likelihood of an associated abscess, necessitating operation to remove the foreign body and drain the abscess.[33] Antibiotic coverage initially for a colon-related abscess should include anaerobic coverage for bacteroides. In the presence of a wound infection or massive contamination, the skin incision should be opened. Sutures may have to be removed to allow for granulation of an infected wound, dealing with the secondary ventral hernia once the patient has recovered.

LIVER

As a large structure, the liver is vulnerable because of its location in the upper abdomen. Hepatic injury occurs in 15% to 20% of blunt abdominal trauma, 40% of abdominal stab wounds, and 30% of abdominal gunshot wounds. Compression of the liver between the ribs and spine and shearing at fixed points secondary to rapid deceleration are seen with blunt trauma. Mechanism of injury is important because penetrating abdominal trauma is treated more often surgically than blunt abdominal trauma.[34]

Pediatric patients have been treated successfully for many years without operative intervention, particularly with the improvement and accessibility of CT scanning. A similar approach has been applied for blunt adult injury.[35] In the hemodynamically stable patient, CT scanning provides quantitative and qualitative information not only about the liver but about other intra-abdominal organs as well, and comparison can be made with subsequent scans. In the hemodynamically stable patient with a closed head injury, spinal cord injury, or equivocal abdominal examination secondary to illicit drug use and in the presence of hematuria or pelvic fractures, CT scanning can provide additional information.[34] The unstable patient, however, should undergo DPL in the emergency department or the ICU when there is concern of intra-abdominal hemorrhage. DPL, although specific for blood, is not sensitive in defining the source of bleeding. Radionuclide scanning and arteriography for the most part have been replaced by CT scanning, although embolization of hepatic bleeding may, on rare occasion, still be required. The role of laparoscopy in the emergency department or ICU still needs to be defined. Variables such as operator experience and the ability to visualize the anatomy in the presence of hemoperitoneum limit its use.

When there is concern about intra-abdominal penetration from a stab wound, local exploration in the emergency department and possibly DPL may be performed to decrease the number of nontherapeutic laparotomies. Gunshot wounds to the upper abdomen require operative exploration. Obtaining plain radiographs should not delay the procedure, although they may be helpful in locating a foreign object such as a bullet.

Table 156–3 outlines the grading scale for hepatic injuries. A hemodynamically stable patient with grade I to III injury may be treated nonoperatively with initial bed rest and gastric decompression in the presence of an ileus. Prophylactic antibiotics are not given. Repeat CT scans, or ultrasonography, or both, are performed weekly during hospitalization or more frequently if there is evidence of blood loss, such as a fall in the hematocrit level. Although there is no hard and fast rule for when laparotomy is performed after conservatively monitoring a hepatic injury, many will agree that continuing need for transfusion (more than two to four units of blood within 24 hours), a deterioration in vital signs in a patient with an isolated liver injury, an increase in abdominal tenderness with signs of peritonitis, or a worsening CT scan dictates laparotomy. Grade IV, V, and VI injuries usually require prompt laparotomy.[34, 34a]

Postoperative complications are minimized by continuing resuscitation, including blood if necessary, maintaining normothermia, and ensuring hemostasis. Patients with major hepatic injuries requiring perihepatic packing are at risk for oliguric renal failure and intra-abdominal sepsis. Continued resuscitation in the ICU may be necessary, with the patient's condition being optimized with the use of pulmonary artery and arterial catheters.[34b]

A common early complication of major hepatic injury is consumption coagulopathy. By correcting hypothermia, metabolic acidosis, and coagulopathy, the chance of successful control of bleeding with relaparotomy is improved. Angiography, although not routinely performed, should be considered in the case of continued hemorrhage. Intra-ab-

TABLE 156–3. Hepatic Injury Grading

Grade		*Description*
I	Hematoma:	Subcapsular nonexpanding: <10% surface area
	Laceration:	Minor parenchymal or nonbleeding capsule: <1 cm deep
	Treatment:	Usually observation
II	Hematoma:	Subcapsular nonexpanding: 10–50% surface area
	Laceration:	Nonexpanding: <3 cm deep, <10 cm long
	Treatment:	Observation, hepatorrhaphy
III	Hematoma:	Subcapsular: >50%, expanding; >2 cm intraparenchymal
	Laceration:	>3 cm deep
	Treatment:	Observation, hepatorrhaphy, debridement/resection
IV	Hematoma:	Ruptured central hematoma
	Laceration:	25–75% lobar destruction
	Treatment:	Debridement/resection
V	Laceration:	75% lobar destruction
	Vascular:	Juxtahepatic venous injuries
	Treatment:	Debridement/resection
VI	Vascular:	Hepatic avulsion
	Treatment:	Hepatic transplant

(Adapted with permission from Moore EE: Organ injury scaling: Spleen, liver, and kidney. J Trauma 1989; 29:1664–1666.)

dominal distention resulting from hemoperitoneum and an engorged liver elevates the diaphragm and increases intra-abdominal pressure, contributing to respiratory failure and pneumonia. Increased abdominal pressure can also have an adverse effect on effective renal blood flow, leading to renal failure.

The rate of intra-abdominal infection is dependent on the magnitude of injury and the success of repair, and it varies between 1.9% and 17%. Drainage is frequently performed in severe injury using a closed-suction system. Factors associated with intra-abdominal abscess formation from hepatic injury, in addition to the severity of injury and the type of drainage, include transfusion of more than six units of blood and the presence of three or more organ injuries.[36] Although postoperative fever is not uncommon in patients sustaining major hepatic injury, continued, ongoing evaluation is necessary if pyrexia persists after the third postoperative day. CT scanning has been helpful in identifying abnormal fluid collections, which can be drained percutaneously under radiographic guidance. In some instances, reexploration may be necessary. Persistent pyrexia may be due to reabsorbed, devitalized hepatic parenchyma in patients who had debridement, placement of deep parenchymal sutures, or selective vascular ligation of liver structures. In most instances, these high temperatures will resolve within 5 days of initial operation.

Hemobilia—blood within the biliary system—may manifest itself with jaundice or GI bleeding days to weeks after injury. Arterial embolization angiographically has been used successfully for hemobilia and is the initial procedure of choice.[37] Blood coming directly from hepatic drains immediately after surgery is due to either coagulopathy or surgical bleeding, or both. Bleeding that occurs several days to weeks after injury may be secondary to erosion of a drain into the liver or vascular bleeding.

Biliary fistulas occur in up to 10% of patients with major hepatic injury. Most will close within weeks if there is no distal biliary obstruction. A persistent fistula should be evaluated with a fistulogram or endoscopic retrograde cholangiopancreatography (ERCP). When a major intrahepatic duct or common bile duct is involved, operative intervention with resection or reconstruction is necessary. Patients with a persistent cough productive of bile may have a bronchobiliary fistula between the right diaphragm and dome of the liver, necessitating operation to control the fistula.

With major hepatic injury, gluconeogenesis is impaired and hypoglycemia may be seen in 4% of patients. Thus, serum blood sugar levels should be monitored and hypertonic glucose administered when hypoglycemia exists. The occurrence of encephalopathy resulting from hepatic failure days after injury must be distinguished from administered ICU medications. When the liver is the cause, the exogenous nitrogen load from nutritional support should be decreased.

The patient who continues to have a complex postoperative course needs to have the liver included in the evaluation because necrosis or occlusion of venous outflow may occur after major hepatic injury. Angiography or radionuclide scanning may further define the problem. The overall mortality rate of 10% to 15% in hepatic injuries is due to shock- or transfusion-related coagulopathy perioperatively. Further evaluation necessitates continued clinical acumen and serial CT scanning. Early nutritional support and continued aggressive resuscitation, as well as awareness of the potential for postoperative sepsis, are crucial for managing patients with hepatic injury.

SPLEEN

The spleen is a very vascular structure, becoming morphologically mature during the first year of life and reaching its maximal weight at puberty. It contains 25% of the total lymphoid mass of the body, and the total splenic circulation is 150 to 250 mL/min, consuming 5% of the cardiac index. Preservation of the spleen, when possible, is the primary therapeutic goal. As an important immunologic organ, the spleen is a major site for immunoglobulin (Ig) M and opsonin production, which helps clear antigen and bacteria. The spleen serves as a biologic filter, removing bacteria and abnormal and aged RBCs. With splenectomy, there is a decrease in IgM levels, and the greatest reduction in bacterial clearance occurs with encapsulated gram-positive bacteria.[38, 39]

Diagnosing splenic injury by physical examination alone is 65% accurate. Patient complaints include left upper quadrant tenderness or referred left shoulder pain, known as Kehr's sign. The presence of left lower rib fractures in blunt trauma should raise the possibility of splenic injury. Hematocrit decreases may be delayed, even with massive splenic injury. Although 20% of patients with fractures of the left 8th to 10th ribs may have a splenic injury, abdominal plain films are nonspecific. Stable patients may undergo contrast-enhanced CT scans with a high degree of accuracy; however, these scans do require time for preparation and expertise for interpretation. Ultrasonography is a rapid, noninvasive test, although its resolution is poorer than that of CT; its images are limited by dressings, tubes, wounds, and ileus. Patient positioning and manipulation of the left upper quadrant also render ultrasonography difficult. Radionuclide liver/spleen scans have less resolution than CT scans, and anatomic variance may falsely suggest injury. Angiography is invasive, time consuming, and expensive and requires expertise and movement of the trauma patient to a specialized area; this has limited utilization in evaluating isolated splenic injury. In the unstable patient, DPL remains the standard for diagnosing intra-abdominal injuries. However, its low specificity does not localize the site of injury and may lead to nontherapeutic laparotomy. Thus, CT scan presently is the best modality for evaluating splenic injury in the stable patient. A useful classification system of splenic injuries is listed in Table 156–4.

Conservative management is the preferred approach for splenic injury; the best candidates are those younger than 55 years with a grade I to III injury, no other major concomitant injuries, and no abnormal mental status changes precluding continued abdominal assessment. However, if the patient becomes unstable after volume replacement, has

TABLE 156–4. Grading Splenic Injury

Grade		*Description*
I	Hematoma:	Subcapsular nonexpanding: <10% surface area
	Laceration:	Minor parenchymal or capsule, nonbleeding: <1 cm deep
	Treatment:	Usually observation
II	Hematoma:	Subcapsular nonexpanding: 10–50% surface area
	Laceration:	Capsular: bleeding
	Treatment:	Observation, splenorrhaphy
III	Hematoma:	Subcapsular: >50%, expanding; >2 cm intraparenchymal
	Laceration:	>3 cm deep
	Treatment:	Observation, splenorrhaphy, splenectomy
IV	Hematoma:	Intraparenchymal bleeding
	Laceration:	>25% devascularization
	Treatment:	Partial or total splenectomy
V	Shattered or devascularized spleen	
	Treatment:	Splenectomy

(Adapted with permission from Moore EE: Organ injury scaling: Spleen, liver, and kidney. J Trauma 1989; 29:1664–1666.)

other obvious associated abdominal injuries, cannot be evaluated, or has an equivocal abdominal examination, laparotomy with possible splenic salvage should be considered. Nonoperative therapy is successful in 90% of children, being attributed to a thicker splenic capsule, hemostatic properties of the splenic capsule, and the presence of myoepithelial cells, which may have constrictive properties in the capsule.[38] Serial CT scans are performed in children in the first week, with close monitoring of vital signs and hematocrit. Transfusions rarely are given for hematocrits greater than 25%. Nonoperative management is abandoned when blood requirements exceed 20 mL/kg or approximately 30% of blood volume. Fewer adults are successfully observed, and our policy generally is that, if more than two units of blood are transfused within 24 hours for an isolated splenic injury, the patient undergoes laparotomy. Because of the complementary nature of DPL and CT in blunt trauma, the incidence of delayed splenic rupture is less than 1%. In a selective literature review, 70% of pediatric patients were eligible for nonoperative management; of these, 89% were successfully managed in this fashion. Of the adults managed nonoperatively, 69% were treated successfully.[38]

When operative intervention is indicated, the surgeon will try to salvage the spleen by partial splenectomy or splenorrhaphy. In the unstable patient, the patient with continued blood loss, or in the grade V spleen (see Table 156–4), splenectomy is usually performed. Postoperative complications include blood transfusion reactions, ileus, atelectasis, pneumonia, and left pleural effusion. Drains are not used for isolated splenic injuries. Reactive thrombocytosis occurs 2 to 10 days after splenectomy, resolving in 2 to 12 weeks. When platelet counts exceed 1.5 million, the use of an antiplatelet agent should be considered.

Overwhelming postsplenectomy infection (OPSI) has occurred in children who have undergone splenectomy. The incidence of lethal OPSI in nontrauma pediatric patients is 0.86%, and the mortality rate for trauma-related, splenectomized children is 0.56%. The risk of lethal OPSI in a 4-year-old child is two and one-half times that of an older child. OPSI has a rapid onset, with a 12- to 18-hour prodrome of sore throat, fever, and malaise rapidly progressing to headache, vomiting, worsening fever, and, within hours, convulsion, coma, and death. The risk of OPSI in adults after splenectomy for isolated splenic injury is low but increases with degree of injury and in the presence of certain associated injuries such as pancreatic, colon, central nervous system, and extremity fractures.[40, 41] The predominant organism is pneumococcus, although meningococcus or influenza bacillus may be the offending agent. Because splenectomized patients are at increased risk for the development of late major septic complications, a vaccine against several pneumococcal capsular antigens (Pneumovax) should be administered to patients generally during their first outpatient visit. In the unreliable population not prone to return for follow-up care, the vaccine should be administered before discharge. Animal studies have shown that daily penicillin prophylaxis is as effective as penicillin given at the first sign of infection. Penicillin is used prophylactically when invasive procedures or dental work are performed.[39, 40]

When observed, patients remain at bed rest for approximately 3 days if the injuries are less than grade III, and they are usually able to be discharged within a week. The length of convalescence at home is still a matter of debate, although repeat CT scan or ultrasonography can be performed at 1 month to monitor resolution of the splenic injury.

PANCREAS

Approximately 90% of patients with pancreatic injuries will have at least one other associated injury, averaging three and one half associated intra-abdominal injuries per patient. Two thirds of pancreatic injuries are penetrating and one third are blunt, with findings ranging from simple contusion to complete disruption of the gland. In blunt trauma, approximately 60% of the injuries to the pancreas are due to the impact of the steering wheel on the upper epigastric region incurred during an automobile accident; however, only 8% of blunt abdominal injuries with hyperamylasemia have a pancreatic injury and 40% with pancreatic injury have a normal initial serum amylase. Serum isoamylase has likewise not been helpful in distinguishing pancreatic from salivary gland injury.[42] Serum lipase levels also have no role. Because of the retroperitoneal location of the pancreas, clinical evaluation and DPL may not be helpful. Abdominal CT scans have a sensitivity and specificity in excess of 80%, although CT is user dependent. ERCP may delineate pancreatic ductal injuries but also is operator dependent. Thus, a high index of suspicion must always exist when there is concern about pancreatic injury.

Alpha (glucagon), beta (insulin), and delta (gastrin) islet cells are responsible for the endocrine state of the gland. Excision of greater than 90% of pancreatic substance is required before deficiency is seen, because there is hypertrophy and increased physiologic activity of the remaining islet cells after resection. Removal of more than 90% of the pancreas after trauma will most likely produce diabetes, however.

Pancreatic injuries are identified primarily at the time of laparotomy for hemorrhage and other associated injuries. When a pancreatic injury is recognized, intervention should be undertaken because mortality rates may be as high as 10% to 25% and morbidity rates 30% to 40%.[42] Contusions and simple lacerations are treated with closed-suction drainage, which is continued until the patient is eating and drainage is negligible. Distal transection of the gland is treated with distal pancreatectomy, and proximal transection or parenchymal injury with probable duct injury is treated with distal resection or pancreatic-enteric reconstruction. Combined pancreatic and duodenal injury carries even higher morbidity and mortality than either injury alone, necessitating procedures such as active sump drainage of the pancreas with pyloric-duodenal exclusion, pancreaticoduodenectomy (Whipple procedure), or duct ligation.

Enteral feedings distal to an anastomosis should begin shortly after surgery if the rest of the GI tract is intact. Somatostatin may be given to decrease pancreatic exocrine secretions. Complications occur postoperatively in up to one third of patients and include minor fistulas with an output of less than 200 mL/d, which usually spontaneously resolve. High-output fistulas (>500 mL/d) may require surgical intervention. Electrolytes and acid-base status should be continuously monitored when fistulas are present. In addition, a low-fat, high-pH elemental feeding will lead to less pancreatic stimulation. If there is an increase in fistula output with enteral feedings, parenteral nutrition should be used.

Pancreatic abscesses occur in less than 5% of injuries, although intra-abdominal abscess and wound infection with pancreatic injury occur in up to 35% of patients. Surgical debridement may be performed in the ICU, although, on occasion, treatment might require only percutaneous closed drainage. Secondary hemorrhage requiring blood transfusion may occur in up to 10% of pancreatic injuries, particularly in the presence of devitalized necrotic pancreatic tissue. In such instances, blood replacement therapy is initiated and reoperation considered.

Post-traumatic pseudocysts occur in less than 5% of patients, usually weeks after injury. Many pseudocysts can be treated with percutaneous drainage, although those communicating with the main pancreatic duct usually require operative intervention. Children are prone to the development of traumatic pancreatitis and pseudocysts. They are treated conservatively, with some pseudocysts drained externally.[43] Postoperative pancreatitis is seen in up to 13% of patients yet rarely progresses to hemorrhagic pancreatitis, which has a high mortality rate.

Necrotizing pancreatitis is a life-threatening problem treated with surgical debridement and drainage. The abdominal cavity is usually left open, and continued ICU bedside lavage is performed. Antibiotics are given in the presence of infection and modified according to pancreatic tissue cultures. When pancreatic infection occurs or persists weeks after injury, fungal colonization may occur. Nutrition should be maintained and the skin protected from activated pancreatic enzymes to prevent maceration. Many of these wounds are allowed to granulate, leaving the patient with a hernia that can be dealt with on an elective basis.

GENITOURINARY TRACT

The kidneys and ureters are retroperitoneal, and the bladder is primarily extraperitoneal, making evaluation by clinical examination unreliable. Most injuries to the genitourinary tract are discovered fortuitously or during the work-up of traumatic hematuria. In the absence of symptoms or shock, the use of a urinary dipstick serves as a reliable screen for the presence or absence of hematuria.[44] The number of RBCs on urinalysis correlating with significant renal injury is debatable, being up to 50 RBCs per high-power field.[45, 46] However, there may not be any RBCs seen with total ureteral transection. In blunt trauma, blood at the urethral meatus (also applies to females), scrotal hematoma, or a high-floating prostate on rectal examination suggests urethral injury, and a urethrograph should be performed before placement of a Foley catheter. In a male, an 18-gauge catheter is placed in the meatus and 30 mL of contrast is given, obtaining oblique views. Once a Foley catheter is placed, a cystogram with 300 mL of contrast (obtain prevoid and postvoid films, lateral and anteroposterior) should be performed to determine whether a bladder injury exists. Extraperitoneal bladder perforation is treated conservatively with bladder decompression through suprapubic cystostomy or Foley catheter.

CT scanning with contrast has replaced IVP in screening for renal and ureteral injuries; it can disclose a lack of perfusion to the kidney from vascular injury. When identified, such an injury needs to be operatively repaired within 6 hours. Contained parenchymal injuries to the kidney may be seen on CT scan and observed. Intraperitoneal renal injury, caliceal renal injury, ureteral transection, and intraperitoneal bladder perforation are repaired urgently by laparotomy, with which other associated intra-abdominal injuries can also be managed. When used, IVP using 1.5 to 2 mL/kg of water-soluble intravenous contrast should be given as a bolus injection and a scout film and subsequent films at 1, 3, 10, and 20 minutes obtained either in the emergency room, OR, or ICU.

If nephrectomy is required, mild elevation of creatinine will be seen for 48 hours. Compensation from the remaining functioning kidney will eventually normalize the creatinine. Maintaining effective renal blood flow is crucial with any renal injury. Low-dose dopamine (2–4 $\mu g \cdot kg^{-1} \cdot min^{-1}$) may produce renal vasodilation and improve renal blood flow. Nephrotoxic drugs should be used judiciously. Depending on other injuries, when a conservative approach is taken, volume resuscitation continues.

PELVIC FRACTURES

A mortality rate of up to 50% from massive pelvic fractures has been reported, with a complication rate of 74%.[47] Frequently, other associated injuries are responsible for the poor outcome. In severely injured patients with pelvic hemorrhage, early intervention is crucial. Pneumatic antishock garments have been used for periods up to 72 hours, although the complication of compartment syndrome exists.[48] An external fixator can be applied quickly at any time, although not all pelvic fractures respond to external fixation. Percutaneous transcatheter arterial embolization has been used when four or more units of blood transfusion within 24 hours or six or more units of blood transfusion within 48 hours are required in an unstable pelvic fracture patient with a negative or borderline DPL or for a large pelvic retroperitoneal hematoma discovered at the time of celiotomy.[49] The incidence of vascular injuries with high-energy pelvic fractures is significant as is injury to the lumbosacral nerve plexus, bladder, urethra, lower GI tract, and reproductive organs.[49a] Sepsis after a delay in recognition of injuries from pelvic fracture spicules penetrating the GI tract has been reported.[50]

Continued hemorrhage refractive to fixatures and embolization and penetrating pelvic injuries require laparotomy. Frequently, oozing from the pelvic venous plexus is refractive to pressure, hemostatic agents, packing, and even bilateral internal iliac artery ligation. On rare occasion, packs are left in the abdomen for 48 hours. Internal pelvic fixation can also be used depending on the clinical state of the patient.

The majority of patients with pelvic fractures are treated conservatively with bed rest or unilateral nonweightbearing for about 6 weeks. Numerous studies demonstrated that the frequency of deep venous thrombosis (DVT) in patients with hip fractures and total hip and knee arthroplasty may be as high as 40% to 60%, with mortality from acute pulmonary embolization ranging from 0.5% to 2%.[51] Similarly, pelvic fractures are likely to be associated with an appreciable frequency of DVT partly because many of these patients require prolonged immobilization; thus, prophylaxis should be initiated early. DVT prophylaxis includes pneumatic compression stockings, use of heparin (or low-molecular-weight heparin), aspirin, or other anticoagulants. Early mobilization is ideal if possible. Continued resuscitation and repeat CT scanning or repeat angiography may be needed if extraperitoneal bleeding persists. Rarely, hemicorporectomy has been required to control bleeding.

PREGNANT PATIENT

Approximately 6% of all pregnancies are complicated by trauma. The priorities for management of the pregnant patient are no different than those of the nonpregnant patient; the mother should be stabilized before the stabilization of the fetus. The physiologic changes during pregnancy can influence outcome. Blood volume steadily increases by the 28th week to 40% to 50% above normal. The so-called physiologic anemia of pregnancy is due to the smaller increase in RBC mass in relation to plasma volume. Thus, significant blood loss may not be recognized in the pregnant patient because of delay in hypotension.[52]

By the end of the first trimester, cardiac output increases by 30%, heart rate increases by 15 to 20 beats per minute, and blood pressure may drop by 10 to 15 mm Hg. Positioning of the pregnant patient is crucial because after 20 weeks of gestation the uterus may occlude the inferior vena cava (IVC), thus decreasing pelvic and cardiac output by 25% in a supine patient. By manually displacing the uterus to the left and positioning the patient in a left lateral position, pressure is taken off the IVC.

As a result of displacement of the diaphragm superiorly in pregnancy, functional residual capacity is decreased 25%, although tidal volume is increased by 40%.[52] Minute volume ventilation rises approximately 50% with a decrease in partial pressure of arterial carbon dioxide to approximately 32 mm Hg. Serum bicarbonate decreases and arterial pH rises, leading to a chronic state of compensated respiratory alkalosis and a decrease in buffering capacity. This diminution of buffering may aggravate the acidosis of shock.

As a result of decreased gastric motility and decreased gastroesophageal sphincter tone, vomiting and delayed gastric emptying occur in the pregnant patient. Thus, gastric decompression with suction should be performed early. The gravid uterus may compress the urinary tract with an increase in bladder capacity and delayed bladder emptying, promoting urinary stasis and sepsis.

A complete blood count, screening for blood type and antibodies, and the Kleihauer-Betke stain are required in most patients. If the mother is Rh negative, Rh immunoglobulin should be administered. A leukocytosis of 20,000 cells/mm^3 with normal differential count occurs by term. An increase in coagulation Factors VII, VIII, and IX and plasma fibrinogen, coupled with a decrease in plasminogen activator, promotes clotting. Thus, antiembolism devices such as pneumatic compression stockings and subcutaneous heparin should be initiated early. Abruptio placentae may release thromboplastic substances and initiate fulminant intravascular coagulation.[52]

Radiographic evaluation in the pregnant patient raises different concerns. Approximately 30% of the dose absorbed by the mother is transmitted to the fetus. Radiation exposure to the mother of .05 Gy or less is still considered safe, with teratogenic risks being greatest during organogenesis, the second to eighth week after conception. Abdominal and perineal shields are used when possible as is ultrasonography.[52]

During pregnancy, the weight of the pituitary gland may increase by 30% to 50%. Shock may cause necrosis of the anterior pituitary, resulting in pituitary insufficiency. Eclampsia, a complication of pregnancy with seizures and hypertension, may mimic head injury. In the presence of hyperreflexia, eclampsia must be considered.

Continuous fetal monitoring should be used in the ICU. Hemodynamic monitoring may be necessary in an attempt to optimize fluids for the pregnant patient. Vaginal bleeding may be indicative of placental separation secondary to direct injury or vaginal/uterine injury secondary to pelvic fractures. Associated factors in predicting fetal demise include direct uteroplacental fetal injury, maternal shock, pelvic fracture, maternal severe head injury, and hypoxia.[53] Continued, thorough evaluation of mother and fetus is mandatory.

POSTOPERATIVE COMPLICATIONS AND REOPERATION IN ABDOMINAL AND PELVIC TRAUMA

Complications may be minimized by taking patients with obvious intra-abdominal injuries directly to the OR and continuing resuscitation in concert with laparotomy. Additional diagnostic studies, if possible, should be delayed until the patient returns to the ICU, unless the outcome of surgery will be altered on the basis of the study. The most common complication occurs usually within 24 hours of injury.[54] When persistent hypotension, tachycardia, abdominal distention, or bloody drainage from abdominal drain sites exists in a noncoagulopathic normothermic patient, reoperation should urgently be performed. When hemorrhage is occurring, platelet counts should be maintained above 35,000 to 50,000, and coagulation parameters should be monitored closely. Fresh frozen plasma should be infused for a prolonged prothrombin time and partial thromboplastin time. In those patients in whom packing is required, continued aggressive resuscitation with blood and component therapy is necessary, with repeat laparotomy scheduled in 24 to 48 hours.

On occasion, the abdominal or pelvic injury may be missed with early signs of hypovolemic hemorrhagic shock. A hollow viscous injury may be missed and not be evident until 5 days after laparotomy. The presence of bile from drains or other unusual drainage warrants prompt re-evaluation radiographically or surgically. Early development of the adult respiratory distress syndrome may also suggest a missed intra-abdominal injury or ongoing intra-abdominal catastrophe. The presence of devitalized tissue or GI injury may lead to bacterial contamination of the abdominal cavity despite perioperative broad-spectrum antibiotics with reoperation necessary to debride, repair, and drain. A wound infection, or less frequently necrotizing fasciitis, may occur with a closed abdominal incision. Wound infections can be treated easily by opening up the wound, whereas necrotizing fasciitis requires wide operative debridement as well as antibiotics.

As discussed, abdominal abscess formation may have many causes. Peritonitis mandates prompt surgical intervention, whereas fluid collections may be treated radiographically with percutaneous drainage. Intakes and outputs, such as from fistulas or drains, in addition to NG and Foley catheter drainage, need to be tabulated to guide fluid therapy. Drainage should be controlled and electrolytes monitored closely with nutritional support maintained. An adynamic ileus persisting for 7 days after laparotomy should raise the concern of a postoperative bowel obstruction. This can be confirmed using water-soluble contrast material given orally or through the NG tube.

The onset of right upper quadrant pain, tenderness, and fever or an increase in bilirubin in the ICU may suggest acute acalculous cholecystitis, which is prevalent in older men, especially those who have sustained major trauma.[55] If suspected, ultrasonography should be performed. If there is evidence of gallbladder wall thickening of 4 mm or greater, pericholecystic fluid, subserosal edema in the absence of ascites, intramural gas or sloughing of the mucosal membrane, acute acalculous cholecystitis should be considered. The presence of biliary sludge is a soft sign.[55] A hepatoiminodiacetic acid scan in ICU patients generally shows nonvisualization of the gallbladder because the GI tract is not being used for nutrition.

The intensivist should always be aware that a deterioration in a patient's state may be due to an intra-abdominal catastrophe that was not recognized on admission. Clinical examination, laboratory tests, interpretation of hemodynamic values, and ancillary tests all need to be coordinated at the bedside and a plan carried out if the patient is to undergo these examinations safely outside of the ICU or requires a trip to the OR.

References

1. Moore EE, Mattox KL, Feliciano DV: Trauma. 2nd ed. Norwalk, CT, Appleton & Lange, 1991.
2. McAnena OJ, Moore EE, Marx JA: Initial evaluation of the pa-

tient with blunt abdominal trauma. Surg Clin North Am 1990; 70:495.
3. Cooper A, Floyd T, Barlow B, et al: Major blunt abdominal trauma due to child abuse. J Trauma 1988; 28:1483.
4. Feliciano DV: Diagnostic modalities in abdominal trauma: Peritoneal lavage, ultrasonography, computed tomography scanning, and arteriography. Surg Clin North Am 1991; 71:241.
5. McConnell DB, Trunkey DD: Nonoperative management of abdominal trauma. Surg Clin North Am 1990; 70:677.
6. Thal ER, Meyer DM: The evaluation of blunt abdominal trauma: Computed tomography scan, lavage, or sonography? Adv Surg 1991; 24:201.
7. McAnena OJ, Marx JA, Moore EE: Peritoneal lavage enzyme determinations following blunt and penetrating abdominal trauma. J Trauma 1991; 31:1161.
8. Mirvis SE, Shanmuganathan K: Abdominal computed tomography in blunt trauma. Semin Roentgenol 1992; 27:150.
9. Sorkey AJ, Farnell MB, Williams HJ, et al: The complementary roles of diagnostic peritoneal lavage and computed tomography in the evaluation of blunt abdominal trauma. Surgery 1989; 106:794.
10. Meredith JW, Ditesheim JA, Stonehouse S, et al: Computed tomography and diagnostic peritoneal lavage: Complementary roles in blunt trauma. Am Surg 1992; 58:44.
11. Taylor GA, Eichelberger MR, O'Donnell R, et al: Indications for computed tomography in children with blunt abdominal trauma. Ann Surg 1991; 213:212.
12. Taylor GA, Eichelberger MR: Clinical variables associated with high risk of associated abdominal injury (Letter to the editor). Ann Surg 1992; 216:99.
13. Wening JV: Evaluation of ultrasound, lavage, and computed tomography in blunt abdominal trauma. Surg Endosc 1989; 3:152.
14. Hoffmann R, Nerlich M, Muggia-Sullam M, et al: Blunt abdominal trauma in cases of multiple trauma evaluated by ultrasonography: A prospective analysis of 291 patients. J Trauma 1992; 32:452.
15. Livingston DH, Tortella BJ, Blackwood J, et al: The role of laparoscopy in abdominal trauma. J Trauma 1992; 33:471.
16. Sosa JL, Sims D, Martin L, et al: Laparoscopic evaluation of tangential abdominal gunshot wounds. Arch Surg 1992; 127:109.
16a. Ivatury RR, Simon RJ, Weksler B, et al: Laparoscopy in the evaluation of the intrathoracic abdomen after penetrating injury. J Trauma 1992; 33:101.
16b. Brandt CP, Priebe PP, Jacobs DG: Potential of laparoscopy to reduce non-therapeutic trauma laparotomies. Am Surg 1994; 60:416.
17. Demetriades D, Rabinowitz B: Indications for operation in abdominal stab wounds: A prospective study of 651 patients. Ann Surg 1987; 205:129.
18. Meyer DM, Thal ER, Weigelt JA, et al: The role of abdominal CT in the evaluation of stab wounds to the back. J Trauma 1989; 29:1226.
19. Lowe RJ, Saletta JD, Read DR, et al: Should laparotomy be mandatory or selective in gunshot wounds of the abdomen? J Trauma 1977; 17:903.
20. Weigelt JA: Risk of wound infections in trauma patients. Am J Surg 1985; 150:782.
21. Feliciano DV, Spjut-Patrinely V: Pre-, intra-, and postoperative antibiotics. Surg Clin North Am 1990; 70:689.
21a. DiPiro JT, Fortson NS: Combination antibiotic therapy in the management of intra-abdominal infection. Am J Surg 1993; 165:825.
21b. Nichols RL, Smith JW, Robertson GD, et al: Prospective alterations in therapy for penetrating abdominal trauma. Arch Surg 1993; 128:55.
22. Fabian TC, Croce MA, Payne LW, et al: Duration of antibiotic therapy for penetrating abdominal trauma: A prospective trial. Surgery 1992; 112:788.
23. Reed RL, Ericsson CD, Wu A, et al: The pharmacokinetics of prophylactic antibiotics in trauma. J Trauma 1992; 32:21.
24. Durham R: Management of gastric injuries. Surg Clin North Am 1990; 70:517.
25. Durham RM, Olson S, Weigelt JA: Penetrating injuries to the stomach. Surg Gynecol Obstet 1991; 172:298.
26. Weigelt JA: Duodenal injuries. Surg Clin North Am 1990; 70:529.
27. Snyder WH, Weigelt JA, Watkins WL, et al: The surgical management of duodenal trauma. Arch Surg 1980; 115:422.
28. Stevens SL, Maull KI: Small bowel injuries. Surg Clin North Am 1990; 70:541.
29. Sherck JP, Oakes DD: Intestinal injuries missed by computed tomography. J Trauma 1990; 30:1.
30. Ross SE, Cobean RA, Hoyt DB, et al: Blunt colonic injury: A multicenter review. J Trauma 1992; 33:379.
31. Huber PJ, Thal ER: Management of colon injuries. Surg Clin North Am 1990; 70:561.
32. Burch JM, Brock JC, Gevirtzman L, et al: The injured colon. Ann Surg 1986; 203:701.
33. Poret HA, Fabian TC, Croce MA, et al: Analysis of septic morbidity following gunshot wounds to the colon: The missile is an adjuvant for abscess. J Trauma 1991; 31:1088.
34. Feliciano DV, Pachter HL: Hepatic trauma revisited. Curr Probl Surg 1989; 26:459.
34a. Meredith JW, Young JS, Bowling J, et al: Nonoperative management of blunt hepatic trauma: The exception or the rule. J Trauma 1994; 36:529.
34b. Abou-Khalil B, Scalea TM, Trooskin SZ, et al: Hemodynamic responses to shock in young trauma patients: Need for invasive monitoring. Crit Care Med 1994; 22:633.
35. Delius RE, Frankel W, Coran AG: A comparison between operative and nonoperative management of blunt injuries to the liver and spleen in adult and pediatric patients. Surgery 1989; 106:788.
36. Noyes LD, Doyle DJ, McSwain NE Jr: Septic complications associated with the use of peritoneal drains in liver trauma. J Trauma 1988; 28:337.
37. Czerniak A, Thompson JN, Hemingway AP, et al: Hemobilia. Arch Surg 1988; 123:718.
38. Shackford SR, Molin M: Management of splenic injuries. Surg Clin North Am 1990; 70:595.
39. Lucas CE: Splenic trauma. Ann Surg 1991; 213:98.
40. Malangoni MA, Dillon LD, Klamer TW, et al: Factors influencing the risk of early and late serious infection in adults after splenectomy for trauma. Surgery 1984; 96:775.
41. O'Neal BJ, McDonald JC: The risk of sepsis in the asplenic adult. Ann Surg 1981; 194:775.
42. Jurkovich GJ, Carrico CJ: Pancreatic trauma. Surg Clin North Am 1990; 70:575.
43. Warner RL, Othersen HB, Smith CD: Traumatic pancreatitis and pseudocyst in children: Current management. J Trauma 1989; 29:597.
44. Kennedy TJ, McConnell JD, Thal ER: Urine dipstick vs. microscopic urinalysis in the evaluation of abdominal trauma. J Trauma 1988; 28:615.
45. Klein S, Johs S, Fujitani R, et al: Hematuria following blunt abdominal trauma. Arch Surg 1988; 123:1173.
46. Stalker HP, Kaufman RA, Stedje K: The significance of hematuria in children after blunt abdominal trauma. AJR 1990; 154:569.
47. Trafton PG: Pelvic ring injuries. Surg Clin North Am 1990; 70:655.
48. McSwain NE Jr: Pneumatic anti-shock garment: State of the art 1988. Ann Emerg Med 1988; 17:506.
49. Panetta T, Sclafani SJA, Goldstein AS, et al: Percutaneous transcatheter embolization for massive bleeding from pelvic fractures. J Trauma 1985; 25:1021.
49a. Gruen GS, Leit ME, Gruen RJ, et al: The acute management of hemodynamically unstable multiple trauma patients with pelvic ring fractures. J Trauma 1994; 36:706.
50. Shapiro MJ, Wolverson MK: Perforation of the retroperitoneal sigmoid colon secondary to fracture-dislocation of the left sacroiliac joint. J Trauma 1989; 29:694.
51. White RH, Goulet JA, Bray TJ, et al: Deep-vein thrombosis after fracture of the pelvis: Assessment with serial duplex-ultrasound screening. J Bone Joint Surg 1990; 72A:495.
52. Pearlman MD, Tintinalli JE, Lorenz RP: Blunt trauma during pregnancy. N Engl J Med 1990; 323:1609.
53. Kissinger DP, Rozycki GS, Morris JA Jr, et al: Trauma in pregnancy: Predicting pregnancy outcome. Arch Surg 1991; 126:1079.
54. Ledgerwood AM, Lucas CE: Postoperative complications of abdominal trauma. Surg Clin North Am 1990; 70:715.
55. Shapiro MJ, Luchtefeld WB, Kurzweil S, et al: Acute acalculous cholecystitis in the critically ill. Am Surg 1994; 60:335.

CHAPTER 157

Management of Head Trauma

Ross Bullock, MD, PhD • John D. Ward, MD, FCCM

Modern management of brain-injured patients requires intensive care, usually for many days. Appropriate management requires an understanding of the pathophysiologic mechanisms that damage the brain and the mechanisms by which delayed secondary brain damage may occur, as well as an awareness of the interaction between systemic injuries and the injured brain. Management in an intensive care unit (ICU) is required for two groups of head-injured patients: (1) those with severe primary brain injuries sufficient to produce coma or to require intracranial surgery, for whom ICU management is directed at the brain injury primarily, and (2) patients who have sustained multisystem trauma with a coexisting moderate head injury, who are also at significant risk of delayed secondary brain damage and require ICU management to optimize recovery.[1]

The aims of ICU management for patients with brain trauma are twofold: (1) to detect and treat those complications of the primary injury that may cause delayed brain damage and (2) to provide the optimal conditions for natural recovery of brain function.

At present, no specific pharmacologic therapy has been conclusively shown to improve outcome after traumatic brain injury, but it is likely that several such agents may emerge in the near future based on ongoing clinical trials.[2,3] The impact of such specific forms of therapy cannot, however, be fully realized unless optimal management of cerebral and systemic hemodynamic and metabolic parameters is achieved by ICU therapy during the crucial first hours and days after injury.

CAUSES OF BRAIN DAMAGE DUE TO CEREBRAL TRAUMA

Primary Brain Injury

Shear forces due to postimpact acceleration-deceleration events are particularly harmful to the brain in comparison with other organs because of its soft consistency, mobility within the closed skull, and lack of fibrous tissue restraint.[4] Primary impact damage causes *focal cerebral contusions*, present in as many as 80% of injuries and usually maximum over the orbital and temporal surfaces of the anterior part of the brain.[5,6] Tensile damage to axons in both gray and white matter causes both reversible and nonreversible ultrastructural changes in the axolemma and axoplasm, which may lead to *diffuse axonal injury*.[7,8] When this process is widespread, it carries a particularly poor prognosis associated with severe disability, death, or persistent vegetative state.[7]

Reversible post-traumatic axonal dysfunction is poorly understood, but it may be the mechanism by which most neurologic recovery occurs after head trauma.[8]

Intracranial Hematoma

Intracranial hematomas occur in about 30% to 40% of severely head-injured patients and may be extracranial (subdural, epidural) or intracerebral.[4] The majority of intracranial hematomas probably develop within the first hour after impact. However, better resuscitation and earlier computed tomographic (CT) scanning have demonstrated that a significant number of patients, particularly those with early post-traumatic hypotension and coagulation disorders, may develop hematoma hours and even occasionally days after the injury.[4]

SECONDARY INTRACRANIAL DAMAGE

Hypoxic-Ischemic Brain Damage

Hypoxic-ischemic brain damage is widespread in 80% to 90% of patients who die after head injury.[5,9] In most patients, it is predominantly focal, occurring in relation to contusions and hematomas, but it may also be caused by metabolic changes (discussed later), by raising intracranial pressure (ICP), and most significantly by extracranial events such as hypoxemia and hypotension.[1] *The primary focus of ICU management for brain-injured patients is prevention of delayed development of hypoxic-ischemic brain damage.*

BIOCHEMICAL EVENTS LEADING TO DELAYED DAMAGE AFTER BRAIN TRAUMA

Ionic Flux

Evidence from animal models suggests that massive ion flux occurs across neuronal and astrocytic membranes in the first minutes after impact[10] (Fig. 157–1). Efflux of potassium and influx of sodium into neurons occur, and the subsequent astrocytic and neuronal metabolic response that is required to normalize these ionic changes seems to be predominantly a result of anaerobic glycolysis.[11] This leads to marked cerebral acidosis because of generation of lactate and hydrogen ions. These ionic events may generate astrocytic swelling and an increase in brain stiffness, together with whole-brain swelling and increase in ICP in some circumstances.

Calcium Flux

Calcium flux into neurons may occur after brain trauma owing to release of excitatory amino acids (glutamate and aspartate), and this may cause early or late damage to intracellular systems.[12]

Delayed damage to neurons, astrocytes, and endothelial cells of the microvasculature may result from free radical generation. Laboratory evidence suggests that this may be facilitated by the presence of free iron in the tissues, by reperfusion of previously ischemic tissue, by changes in second-messenger systems such as phospholipase C, and by ischemic damage to free radical–quenching enzymes.[12,13]

OTHER HEMODYNAMIC AND METABOLIC FACTORS CAUSING DELAYED DAMAGE

Cerebral Blood Flow

The authors performed early tomographic cerebral blood flow (CBF) measurements in severely head-injured patients within the first few hours of injury, and 30% of these patients demonstrated sufficiently low CBF levels to cause failure of aerobic neuronal and astrocytic metabolism.[14,15] This then leads to cessation of ionic and neurotransmitter homeostasis and consequent cell swelling. The cause of this early reduction in CBF is not known.[14]

Cerebral Autoregulation

Cerebrovascular autoregulatory mechanisms in normal individuals maintain CBF constant despite wide fluctuations

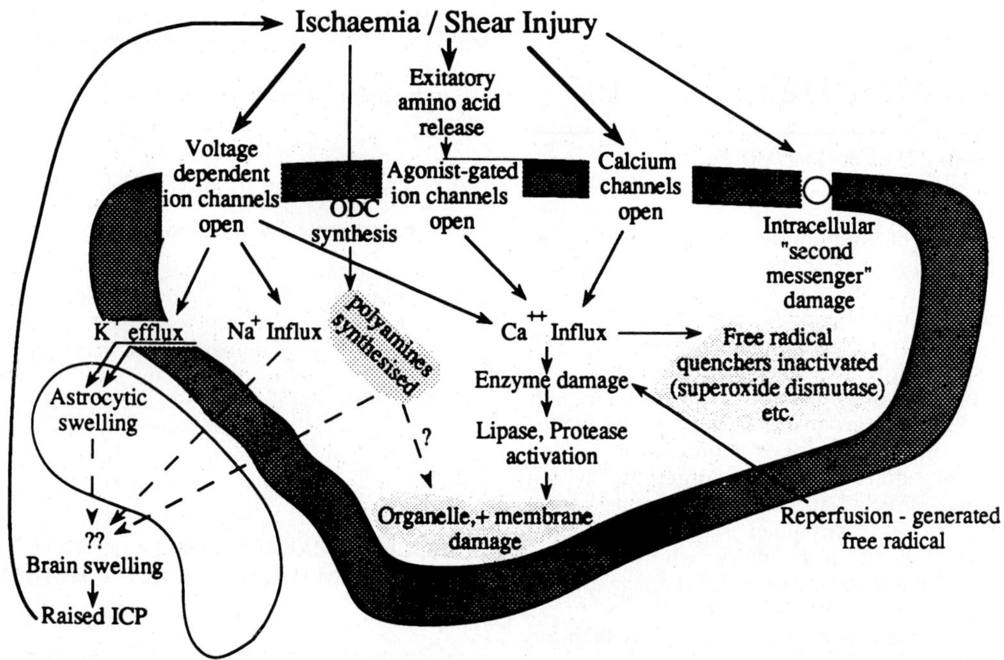

Figure 157–1. Schematic outline of biochemical events which may be responsible for neuronal and astrocytic changes after head trauma. (Reprinted from Bullock R: Opportunities for neuroprotective drugs in clinical management of head injury. J Emerg Med 1993; 11:23–30, with kind permission from Elsevier Science Ltd., The Boulevard, Langford Lane, Kidlington OX5 1GB, UK.)

in mean arterial blood pressure, ranging from 50 to 150 mm Hg. This autoregulatory capacity is lost for a period, which may be as long as several days in severely injured patients (Fig. 157–2). Head-injured patients are thus predisposed to ischemic brain damage at levels of mean arterial pressure that would be considered satisfactory in a normal individual.[1, 16, 17]

RAISED INTRACRANIAL PRESSURE AND BRAIN SWELLING

High ICP may jeopardize perfusion of the whole brain, and clear evidence from several studies shows that prolonged periods of reduced cerebral perfusion pressure, even at levels of 50 to 60 mm Hg, have an adverse effect on prognosis.[18, 19]

SYSTEMIC HYPOXEMIA

Systemic hypoxemia is a common consequence of pneumothorax, aspiration pneumonia, and adult respiratory distress syndrome in patients with head and multiple injuries, and early hypoxemic episodes can significantly jeopardize outcome in head-injured patients.[1, 20]

HYPERGLYCEMIA

Laboratory studies and studies of patients with stroke have now shown that hyperglycemia (a normal stress response to multiple trauma) increases neuronal damage after global brain ischemia. No evidence yet shows that therapeutic normalization of blood glucose is beneficial.[19]

HYPERTHERMIA

Laboratory studies have shown that increases in brain temperature may exacerbate neuronal death owing to a sublethal ischemic insult in models of both focal and global ischemia.[21] Some evidence suggests that brain temperature may rise 1° to 2°C higher than body core temperature after severe head injury. Moderate hypothermia therefore is an important modality in the treatment of head-injured patients. A trial of moderate hypothermia in severe head trauma is currently in progress, and preliminary data suggest that moderate hypothermia (32°C) is beneficial for outcome.[22]

ABNORMALITIES OF THE BLOOD-BRAIN BARRIER

Clinical studies have now shown that the blood-brain barrier becomes permeable to small molecules in the region of focal cerebral contusions after head injury.[23] Because this process appears to be maximum several days after the injury, the theoretic risk exists that circulating drugs and metabolites may easily gain access to the brain, particularly around contusions, during the period that patients with head trauma receive ICU therapy.

INITIAL EVALUATION AND STABILIZATION

Significant brain injuries are followed by periods of apnea, the duration of which increases with the severity of the injury.[17] Because of this factor, combined with one or more of the mechanisms referred to earlier, as many as 30% of patients with severe head injuries and multiple trauma are hypoxic or ischemic by the time they reach the emergency room.[1, 14] The first priority for prehospital and emergency room treatment of patients with head injury and multiple trauma, therefore, is to establish and maintain adequate cerebral oxygenation and perfusion. Severely head-injured patients who do not obey commands or speak should therefore be intubated after a brief neurologic and systemic assessment. Intubation should be performed in a rigid cervical collar to prevent cervical cord damage due to an occult cervical spine injury. Respiration should be maintained by artificial ventilation, and intravenous access should be obtained as soon as possible by the most appropriate means—usually a large-bore peripheral line and a central venous line. Blood pressure should be maintained by rapid infusion of both crystalloid and colloid plasma volume expanders to achieve adequate central venous pressure (8–10 cm H_2O). Pressor agents, such as dopamine or dobutamine, should be used without hesitation even during this early phase, once plasma volume has been restored and active internal bleeding has been diagnosed (by peritoneal lavage and chest radiograph) and treated. Continuous pulse oximetry and early blood gas analysis should be performed as soon as possible in the emergency room or before, in order to diagnose and treat early hypoxemia. Chest and cervical spine radiographs are thus mandatory for all head-injured patients who are unable to speak or obey commands.

COMPUTED TOMOGRAPHIC SCANNING

CT scanning, although clearly the most important diagnostic modality for head-injured patients, should be delayed until adequate blood pressure (mean arterial blood pressure > 80 mm Hg) and cerebral oxygenation have been achieved. When a CT scanner is situated in the emergency room, however, it may be possible for these activities to be carried out concomitantly. Modern CT facilities require only a few minutes to scan the whole brain, and the cervical spine may be studied at the same time when findings on the plain radiograph are suspicious or inconclusive. In addition to its use for diagnosing intracranial hematoma, the CT scan can also provide useful information about the presence or absence of raised ICP. Effacement of the basal cisterns is almost always present when ICP is greater than 20 mm Hg.[24] The prognosis is most favorable when hematomas are diagnosed by CT scan and removed *before* they can cause neurologic deterioration due to raised ICP or local mass effect.[4] With the increased use of CT scanning in less severely head-injured patients, smaller mass lesions such as cerebral contusions or "smear" subdural hematomas are being found more frequently. Treatment of these patients may sometimes be difficult. In some circumstances, ICP monitoring, together with subsequent CT scanning at intervals, may assist the neurosurgeon in determining which of these patients requires surgical evacuation of their mass lesion.[4]

SURGERY

When surgical evacuation of an intracranial mass lesion is required, skilled and rapid teamwork are mandatory to allow safe anesthesia with adequate monitoring, consistent with evacuation of the hematoma *as rapidly as possible.* When patients develop signs of transtentorial herniation (fixed, dilated pupil together with increasing blood pressure and decreasing pulse rate), the situation is particularly dangerous. Hematoma evacuation must be performed as rapidly as possible, but hypotension during the procedure must also be prevented, particularly at the moment when the dura is opened. This is best achieved by administration of 20% mannitol (1 g or 5 mL/kg body weight), given as rapidly as possible, as soon as an intracranial hematoma is diagnosed on CT. Preanesthetic monitoring should include an arterial catheter, a large-bore central venous line, at least one peripheral line, and an indwelling bladder catheter. In cases that are herniating, these may be established on the operating table while the neurosurgeon makes a temporal bur hole under local anesthesia to initiate clot removal. Halothane and any hypotensive anesthetic agents should be avoided. Bleeding at the time of hematoma evacuation must be anticipated, and sufficient transfusion should be given to maintain a normal circulating blood volume.

Immediate abdominal or thoracic surgery is occasionally necessary to achieve hemodynamic stability before the CT scan can be obtained. Under these circumstances, if pupil dilatation develops, an intraoperative ventricular tap may be performed to facilitate ICP measurement. A ventriculogram, using 2 to 5 mL of air, may be performed using an anteroposterior plain skull radiograph to detect midline shift and mass effect. Exploratory bur holes can thus be performed during the same surgery, if needed.

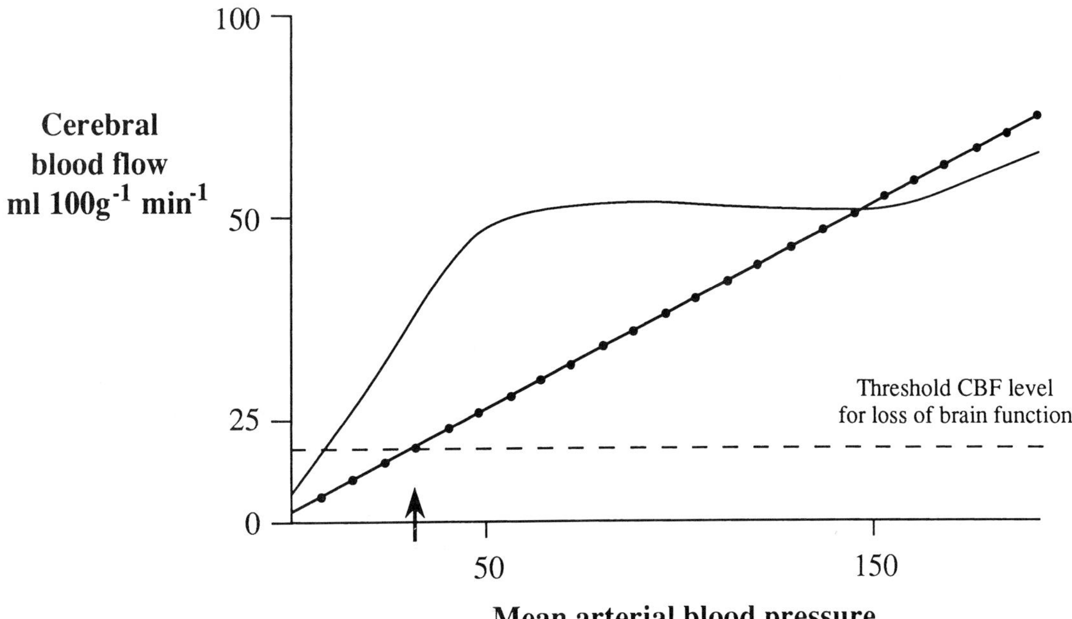

Figure 157–2. Autoregulatory curve for global cerebral blood flow versus mean arterial pressure. *Key:* solid line = normal curve; dotted line = "pressure passive" nonautoregulatory curve seen in severe head injury patients. Note that ischemic brain damage may develop at mean arterial blood pressure levels of from 40 to 50 mm Hg (when intracranial pressure is normal) or higher (when intracranial pressure is high).

HEAD INJURY MANAGEMENT IN THE INTENSIVE CARE UNIT

Monitoring

Monitoring is aimed at early detection of cerebral hemodynamic, systemic, or metabolic changes that may induce secondary brain damage. No single monitoring technique has been found to be satisfactory, and increasing numbers of monitoring techniques are becoming available for brain-injured patients. The ideal monitoring modality should be accurate, robust, and noninvasive. It should detect harmful events *before* they occur and should be continuously applicable and inexpensive.

With the increasing use of artificial ventilation, pharmacologic paralysis, and sedative drugs in head-injured patients, the role of neurologic evaluation by an ICU nurse using such instruments as the Glasgow Coma Scale has diminished. Nevertheless, careful hourly evaluation of pupils, motor responses, and hemodynamic parameters (discussed later) still constitutes the mainstay of ICU management, and continuous one-to-one patient-to-nurse care is the hallmark of the optimal ICU environment.

SYSTEMIC MONITORING

As outlined elsewhere in this volume, continuous monitoring of blood pressure (systolic, diastolic, and mean) and arterial oxygen saturation, either by pulse oximetry or indwelling oxygen-sensing electrodes, is mandatory for optimal hemodynamic management. In addition, head-injured patients benefit from continuous measurement of end-tidal carbon dioxide (CO_2) and core temperature.

INTRACRANIAL PRESSURE MONITORING

Although the origin of raised ICP within the milieu of brain damage mechanisms after brain trauma is still debated, rational management of the injured brain depends on a knowledge of continuous cerebral perfusion pressure, which in turn can only be obtained by monitoring ICP and mean arterial blood pressure together. Indications for ICP monitoring are listed in Table 157–1.

TABLE 157–1. Indications for Intracranial Monitoring After Cranial Trauma*

Coma (Glasgow Coma Scale score 9 or less), evidence of raised pressure on CT scan (basal cistern effacement, midline shift) or any CT abnormality
Postcraniotomy (for mass lesion)
Intracranial mass lesion with space-occupying effect on CT scan (even in conscious patients)
Coma and multiple trauma or thoracic injury requiring ventilation for several days (even when CT scan is normal)

*Mean arterial pressure should also be measured and cerebral perfusion pressure displayed.

ICP may be monitored using an intraventricular catheter, which allows therapeutic cerebrospinal fluid drainage when pressure is high. Fiberoptic ICP sensors are now available for either intraparenchymal or intraventricular use, and these systems are easy to insert at the bedside using a twist-drill technique.[25] Extradural and subdural sensors are generally regarded as highly inaccurate, particularly when ICP is high.[26]

CONTINUOUS JUGULAR VEIN OXYGEN SATURATION MONITORING

Laser-assisted spectrophotometric techniques allow continuous measurement of venous oxygen saturation, using fine-bore catheters. These catheters may be placed within the jugular bulb, thus allowing continous monitoring of cerebral arteriovenous oxygen differences (PaO_2–PAO_2) by comparison with arterial oxygen saturation.[27] Continuous jugular oxygen saturation (SIO_2) techniques are particularly of value in detecting brain ischemia due to poor brain perfusion (widening of the PaO_2–JvO_2 to levels >8.5 mL/100 mL). Their main value may be in guiding hyperventilation therapy in patients in whom high ICP is suspected to be due to cerebral hyperemia. This technique is also useful for confirming the diagnosis of cerebral hyperemia (PaO_2–JvO_2 <4 mL/100 mL) and assessing its response to hyperventilation and drug therapy (Fig. 157–3).

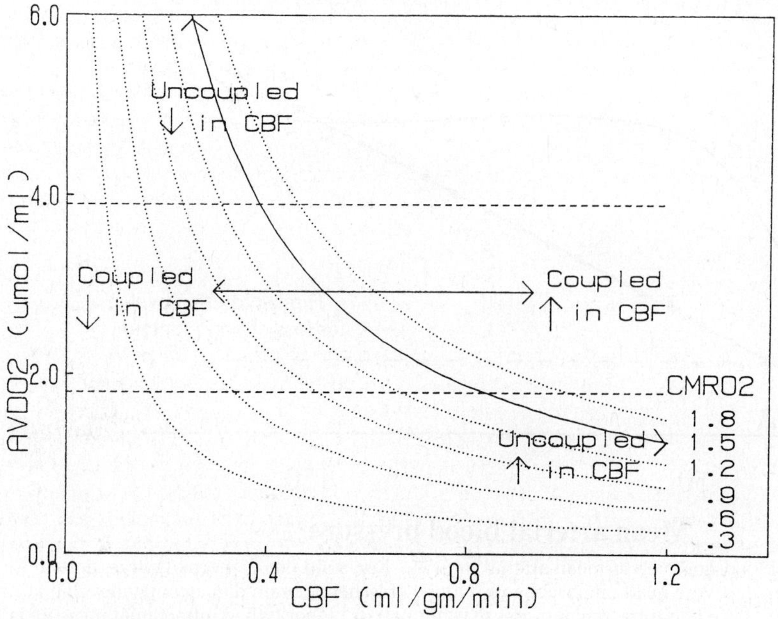

Figure 157–3. Diagram to show the relationship between cerebral arteriovenous oxygen differences ($AVDO_2$) and cerebral blood flow. (After Robertson CS, Narayan RK, Goksalau L, et al: Cerebral arteriovenous oxygen difference as an estimate of cerebral blood flow in comatose patients. J Neurosurg 1989; 70:222.)

ELECTROENCEPHALOGRAPHIC MONITORING

Technology is now available for continuous monitoring of multichannel "paperless" electroencephalographic (EEG) techniques that may display as spectoral frequencies of different rhythm patterns or as simple bar graphs of activity. These methods are expensive, and their benefits have not been validated.[28] Simpler equipment (cerebral function monitors) is available to depict the amplitude of crude EEG activity in each hemisphere. Because of the difficulty in interpreting EEG patterns after head injury and the complexity of pharmacologic interventions in head-injured patients, EEG has not made a major impact on management.

CEREBRAL BLOOD FLOW MONITORING

CBF monitoring may be continuously performed using the laser Doppler technique, after craniotomy. Cerebral blood flow may also be measured intermittently using xenon 133 inhalation techniques, or it may be assessed using completely noninvasive transcranial Doppler methods. Transcranial Doppler techniques may also yield information about intracranial compliance and ICP, which cause typical changes in the waveform pattern (Fig. 157–4).[29]

EVOKED POTENTIAL MONITORING

Somatosensory and motor evoked potentials have been measured frequently in head-injured patients both continuously and intermittently. Changes in the evoked potential patterns correlate well with outcome, and these techniques are useful in predicting patients in whom recovery is unlikely. They have not, however, become widely used in guiding *therapy*.[30]

PULMONARY ARTERY WEDGE PRESSURE MEASUREMENT

Increasing emphasis is being placed on the need to maintain cerebral perfusion pressure at levels of 70 mm Hg or greater in severely head-injured patients.[18] Inotropic support is thus more often needed to maintain cardiac output and blood pressure at the required levels. Under these circumstances, pulmonary artery wedge pressure measurements are particularly useful for titrating volume preload to left and right heart output. Pulmonary artery wedge pressure measurement is also useful in those patients who develop severe respiratory complication, such as adult respiratory distress syndrome (see Chapter 92).

OTHER LABORATORY PARAMETERS

Frequent arterial blood gas analysis is mandatory to guide respiratory therapy, and measurements of serum osmolarity may be required every 12 hours or even every 6 hours in patients who are receiving mannitol therapy for raised ICP, in order to detect hyperosmolarity. Blood glucose, urea, and electrolyte values also require evaluation every 6 to 12 hours, and hyperglycemia (blood glucose levels exceeding 150 mg/100 mL) should be cautiously treated by low-dose insulin, as needed, to maintain normoglycemia.

FLUID AND ELECTROLYTE THERAPY

Adequate circulating volumes should be maintained using central venous pressure monitoring (optimal central venous pressure 6–12 cm H_2O in paralyzed ventilated patients), 4.5% saline/5% dextrose, or normal saline or lactated Ringer's are suitable solutions. A minimum fluid volume of 3 L/d should be maintained, but some patients may require considerably larger volumes (up to 5–6 L/d or more) in order to maintain adequate cerebral perfusion pressures. Colloid solutions, such as fresh frozen plasma, Plasmanate, or albumin, all are suitable for this purpose.

NUTRITION

Head injury alone increases nitrogen loss and body mass catabolism. This is further exacerbated when multiple injuries are present. The process may be mediated by excessive catecholamine output from the posterior hypothalamus, as part of the stress response. Support for early nutrition to try to offset these losses in head-injured patients therefore has some basis.[31] This can usually be achieved (when abdominal surgery has not been performed) by the use of continuous drip feeding using fine-bore nasogastric and nasojejunal tubes. With careful titration of the feed volume and strength, it is often possible to establish feeding the day after injury. This may need to be delayed in patients who have multiple injuries and have undergone laparotomy. Factors that often delay establishment of gastric feeding include large doses of muscle relaxant and opiate drugs, which should therefore be used in the lowest necessary doses. Early placement of a feeding gastrostomy or jejunostomy should be considered whenever a head-injured patient undergoes laparotomy or when tracheostomy is needed. A percutaneous endoscopic gastrojejunostomy is often the optimal technique, and it reduces risks of undetected aspiration pneumonitis.

It is seldom necessary to resort to parenteral nutrition in patients with severe head trauma. It has not been possible to demonstrate an improvement in outcome with the elective use of early parenteral nutrition in head-injured patients.[19]

RESPIRATORY THERAPY

The aims of respiratory therapy in head-injured patients are (1) to maintain optimal oxygenation of the injured brain and avoid episodes of desaturation and (2) to control the alveolar partial pressure of CO_2 (P_{ACO_2}) and thus influence CBF and ICP. In patients who retain the cerebrovascular CO_2 response, a reduction in ICP of 1.3 mm Hg may be achieved for each 1 mm Hg P_{ACO_2} reduction. When the cerebrovascular responses are compromised, however, as is frequently the case after head trauma, this is less predictable.[16]

Hyperventilation is an effective method for short-term control of ICP, particularly when it is due to cerebral vascular engorgement (hyperemia). Cerebral hyperemia complicates about 45% of cases of severe head injury and is particularly common in children and those with acute subdural hematoma and global brain swelling on the CT scan (see Fig. 157–4).[20]

In a controlled clinical trial at the Medical College of Virginia, the effects of *prophylactic* hyperventilation were tested against ventilation to normocapnia (arterial partial pressure of CO_2 [Pa_{CO_2}] 35–40 mm Hg). Hyperventilation failed to improve outcome; indeed, outcome was slightly worse for those patients in the hyperventilation group.[32, 33] When hyperventilation (Pa_{CO_2} >32 mm Hg) is required in order to control rising ICP, then monitoring of the Pa_{O_2}–Jv_{O_2} should be performed, preferably using the continuous jugular bulb technique. Reduction in S_{IO_2} to levels less than 55% to 60% may indicate that hyperventilation is harmful, by inducing cerebral vasoconstriction and ischemia. Whenever artificial ventilation is used, chest physiotherapy and frequent radiographic surveillance of the chest are manda-

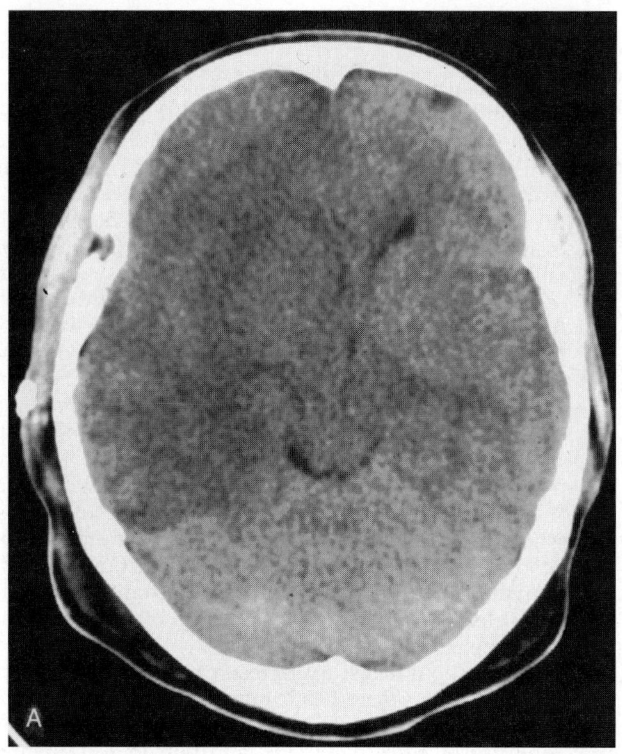

Figure 157–4. CT scan appearances demonstrating hemispheric brain swelling after removal of acute subdural hematoma *(A)*, and corresponding CBF patterns, indicating transient cerebral hyperemia *(B)*. *Abbreviations:* CBF (probe) = CBF measured by cortical Doppler flow probe; MCA velocity = transcranial Doppler changes in middle cerebral artery; CBF (Xe-CT) = blood flow measured by xenon-enhanced CT method.

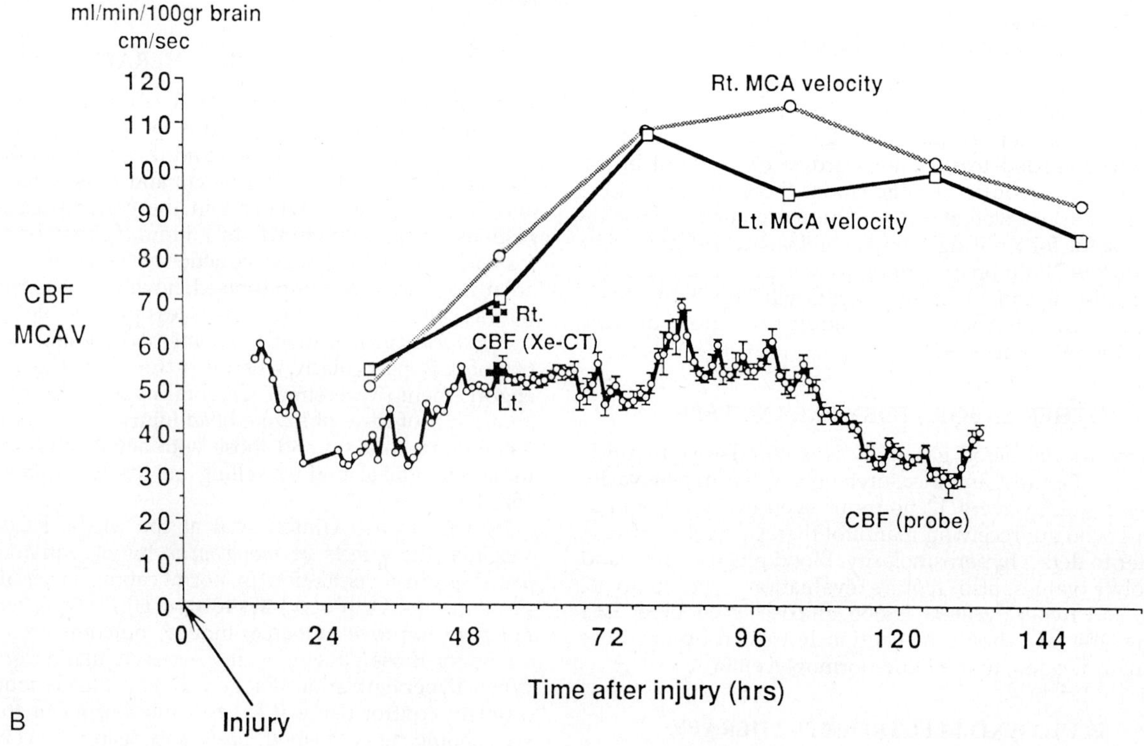

tory to prevent atelectasis and hypostatic pneumonia. Postural therapy using such adjuncts as the Rotorest bed are advantageous in preventing atelectasis and decubitus skin ulceration while improving nursing efficiency because turning patients is not necessary. These measures do not increase ICP. Cerebral venous drainage and ICP control may be optimal with 20 degrees of head elevation.

MANAGEMENT OF HIGH INTRACRANIAL PRESSURE

When ICP exceeds 20 mm Hg for more than a few minutes at a time (as occurs during suctioning, physiotherapy, weaning from the respirator, and so on), then action must be taken. Once hypercapnia and excessive end-tidal airway pressures have been excluded (usually due to "fighting the ventilator"), then the first stage of management for raised ICP is to exclude a new mass lesion or enlargement of a preexisting cerebral contusion. A CT scan must therefore be performed without delay. When a significant mass lesion is present, then the optimal form of management is usually surgical excision, when this is feasible. The decision may be difficult, however, and a trial of medical management may be preferred, particularly when the mass lesion is located in the dominant hemisphere.[4] Table 157–2 outlines the ICP management algorithm in use at the Medical College of Virginia. Mannitol may be administered in repeated bolus doses until the serum osmolarity approaches 320 mOsm/L. When ventricular drainage is possible, then this measure should be used intermittently, with alternating periods of drainage and pressure monitoring. If these measures fail, then moderate hypothermia should be induced, cooling the patient with a cooling blanket, ice packs, and neuromuscular paralysis until the core temperature is around 32°C. Hyperventilation can then be used if needed, as described earlier.

BARBITURATE THERAPY

Although barbiturates are still used in many ICUs (including the authors') as a last resort to manage high ICP, it has been shown in randomized controlled studies that *prophylactic* administration of barbiturates was ineffective in improving outcome after severe head injury.[34–36] Pentobarbital is usually administered in an initial dose of 5 to 10 mg/kg, usually given as a bolus dose of 50 mg initially, until the EEG shows burst suppression. Further intermittent intravenous doses can then be administered to maintain blood levels between 3.0 and 4.5 mg/dL. Because of slow clearance of barbiturates from the system after administration is withdrawn, other agents such as etomidate and propofol have been tried as measures to control ICP by reducing brain metabolism.[37] Although both of these agents are significantly shorter acting than barbiturates, they may also cause hypotension and require concomitant administration of inotropes.

Several well-conducted, controlled trials have shown that conventional steroids have no place in the management of ICP due to head injury.[38]

It is widely held that uncontrollable ICP (which develops

TABLE 157–2. Management Algorithm for Raised Intracranial Pressure at the Medical College of Virginia

Treatment Objective: To minimize time that ICP is >20 mm Hg while maintaining CPP >70 mm Hg

Level 1: Sedation/paralysis
Maintained until ICP is <20 mm Hg for a 12-h period with no additional therapy
- Morphine, q 1 h, 4 mg/dose; or IV drip with 250 mg in 250 mL at 4 mg/h
- Vecuronium, q 1 h, 6–10 mg/dose; or continuous infusion to maintain paralysis
- Pa_{CO_2} maintained at 35 ±

Level 2: Drain cerebrospinal fluid if ICP is >20 mm Hg for 5 min
- Continue management of ICP with drainage as long as it is effective
- If drainage is poor, ensure catheter position is optimal in ventricle

Level 3: Mannitol
If ICP is >20 mm Hg for 5 min and cannot be controlled with drainage, give mannitol, 50–100 g IV push; continue with mannitol therapy as needed until osmolarity reaches 320

Level 4: If ICP is >25 mm Hg for 5 min and cannot be managed with mannitol or if cerebral perfusion pressure is <50 mm Hg
- Begin *controlled hypothermia* to maintain core temperature at 92°F (also requires daily surveillance of blood cultures). Then:

A. Hypertensive therapy
Patients without parenchymal contusions:
Induce hypertension with phenylephrine and other pressor agents as needed to maintain systemic blood pressure ≥180 mm Hg
Patients with parenchymal contusions:
Induce hypertension to systemic blood pressure of 150–170 mm Hg

B. Aggressive hyperventilation (Pa_{O_2}–P_{AO_2} < 8)
If ICP exceeds 25 mm Hg for 5 min and cannot be managed with hyperventilation to P_{CO_2} 30 mm Hg, aggressively hyperventilate to reduce ICP, guided by S_{IO_2} (Keep S_{IO_2} >55%)

Level 5: Hypnotics
If ICP stays >25 mm Hg for 5 min with osmolarity >320

A. Etomidate
- Repeat CT scan
- Give etomidate, 40 mg IV push
  Start at 40 mg/h and titrate etomidate dose to burst suppression on EEG
- Monitor renal function

B. Phenobarbital
If ICP stays >30 mm Hg for >5 min with osmolarity >320 and there was no response to etomidate
- Pentobarbital, 5–10 mg/kg IV over 60 min, then titrate to burst suppression on EEG, and blood levels of 3–4.5 mg/dL are reached

in about 15–20% of patients admitted to an ICU with severe head injury) is an indicator that the underlying brain damage sustained at the time of injury was overwhelming. In frequent cases, however, ICP rises uncontrollably even in patients who had *spoken* at some time after their injury, suggesting that delayed and therefore *treatable* mechanisms are responsible for these increases in ICP. Research techniques are making it possible to determine the relative contribution of cerebrovascular engorgement and neuronal and astrocytic swelling to raised ICP after severe head injury. It may thus be possible in the future to target ICP therapy to whichever of these mechanisms is shown to be operative.

MANAGEMENT OF RESPIRATORY COMPLICATIONS

Management of aspiration pneumonitis, hypostatic pneumonia, and adult respiratory distress syndrome is addressed in other chapters. Prophylactic antibiotic therapy directed at preventing chest infection should not be given to all head-injured patients. Pulmonary surveillance by frequent blood and sputum cultures, chest radiography, and arterial blood gas analysis should instead be performed. Only if evidence of a pneumonic process is found should antibiotics be given.

NEUROPROTECTIVE DRUGS

Laboratory studies have yielded a number of potent neuroprotective compounds that are capable of reducing ischemic brain damage due to focal and global cerebral ischemic events.[2, 3] These compounds have also shown the ability to improve functional outcome and mortality rates in rodents subjected to traumatic brain injury. Large-scale phase III efficacy studies are now under way with free radical–scavenging compounds, glutamate antagonists, and calcium channel blockers. If efficacy is demonstrated in any of these studies, then the treatment of head-injured patients may be profoundly altered. Emergency squads and rapid-response teams may be equipped with these agents to permit administration as soon as possible after injury.

In an important large trial investigating acute spinal cord injury, administration of methylprednisolone, 30 mg/kg within the first 6 hours of injury, was shown to improve outcome significantly.[39]

OUTCOME EVALUATION AND QUALITY CONTROL

The outcome after both severe and moderate head injuries was compared in a major survey of trauma centers across the United States.[40] The outcomes were found to vary from 43% below expected to 52% above expectation, across the 41 centers studied, when the severity of the injuries was stratified. However, when the difference between observed and expected outcome was compared by center, it was found that 70% of the variation in outcome was seen in moderate rather than severe head injuries and that outcome varied enormously from center to center. It is thus clear that the quality of treatment that head-injured patients receive in the first hours and days after their injury exerts a profound effect on outcome.

It is imperative that the ever-increasing range of neuromonitoring and therapeutic modalities that are becoming available for head-injured patients be evaluated by the controlled clinical trial format in order to conclusively demonstrate benefit within an increasingly cost-conscious healthcare environment. Such trials are facilitated by multicenter head injury care networks, such as the Traumatic Coma Data Bank group, and the American Brain Injury Trials Consortium, in which head injury care is broadly standardized.

Physicians who provide acute care for head-injured patients are now presented with the challenge of translating the enormous laboratory advances in understanding of brain metabolism, pathophysiology, and neuroprotection into optimal forms of diagnosis, monitoring, and therapy for head-injured patients.

References

1. Miller JD, Sweet R, Narayan R, et al: Early insults to the injured brain. JAMA 1978; 25:240–439.
2. Bullock R: Opportunities for neuroprotective drugs in clinical management of head injury. J Emerg Med 1993; 11:23–30.
3. Bullock R, Fujisawa H: The role of glutamate antagonists for the treatment of CNS injury. J Neurotrauma 1992; 9:S443–S462.
4. Bullock R, Teasdale GM: Surgical management of traumatic intracranial hematomas. *In:* Handbook of Clinical Neurology. Vol 13(57). Head Injury. Braakman R (Ed). Amsterdam, Elsevier, 1990, pp 259–297.
5. Adams H, Graham DI: The pathology of blunt head injuries. *In:* Scientific Foundations of Neurology. Critchley M, O'Leary JL, Jennett B (Eds). Philadelphia, FA Davis, 1972, pp 478–491.
6. Gennarelli TA, Thibault LE: Biomechanics of acute subdural hematoma. J Trauma 1982; 22:680–686.
7. Adams J, Graham D, Murray L, et al: Diffuse axonal injury due to nonmissile head injury in humans: An analysis of 45 cases. Ann Neurol 1982; 12:557–563.
8. Povlishock J: The morphopathologic responses to experimental head injuries of varying severity. *In:* Central Nervous System Trauma Status Report. Becker D, Povlishock J (Eds). Richmond, Byrd Press, 1985, pp 55–79.
9. Graham DI, Adams JH, Doyle D: Ischemic brain damage in fatal nonmissile head injuries. J Neurol Sci 1978; 39:213–234.
10. Katayama Y, Becker DP, Tamura T, et al: Massive increases in intracellular potassium and the indiscriminate release of glutamate following concussive brain injury. J Neurosurg 1990; 73:889–900.
11. Andersen BJ, Marmarou A: Post-traumatic selective stimulation of glycolysis. Brain Res 1992; 585:184–189.
12. Siesjo BK: Pathophysiology and treatment of focal cerebral ischemia. Part 1: Pathophysiology. J Neurosurg 1992; 77:169–185.
13. Delahunty TM: Mild traumatic brain injury enhances muscarinic receptor linked inositol phosphate production in rat hippocampus. Brain Res 1992; 594:307–310.
14. Bouma GJ, Muizelaar JP, Stringer WA: Ultra early evaluation of regional cerebral blood flow in severely head injured patients using stable xenon-enhanced computerized tomography. J Neurosurg 1992; 77:360–368.
15. Muizelaar JP, Becker DP, Lutz HA, et al: Cerebral ischemia after severe head injury: Its role in determining clinical status and the possible treatment. *In:* Advances in Neurotraumatology. Villani R, Papo I, Griovanelli M, et al (Eds). Amsterdam, Excerpta Medica, 1982, pp 92–98.
16. Enevoldsen EM, Jensen FT: Autoregulation and CO_2 responses of cerebral blood flow in patients with acute head injury. J Neurosurg 1978; 48:689–703.
17. Gennarelli TA, Segama H, Wald U, et al: Physiological response to angular acceleration of the head. *In:* Head Injury—Basic and Clinical Aspects. Grossman RG, Gildenberg PL (Eds). New York, Raven Press, 1982, pp 129–139.
18. Contant CF, Robertson CS, Gopinath SP, et al: Determination of clinically important thresholds in continuously monitored patients with head injury. J Neurotrauma 1993; 10(Suppl 1):S57.
19. Luerssen TG, Marshall LF: The medical management of head injury. *In:* Handbook of Clinical Neurology. Vol 13(57). Head Injury. Braakman R (Ed). Amsterdam, Elsevier, 1990, pp 207–247.
20. Muizelaar JP, Marmarou A, DeSalles AF, et al: Cerebral blood flow and metabolism in severely head injured children. Part 1: Relationship with GCS, outcome, ICP and PVI. J Neurosurg 1989; 71:63–71.
21. Ginzberg M, Sternau L, Globus M, et al: Therapeutic modulation of brain temperature: Relevance to ischemic brain injury. Cerebrovasc Brain Metab Rev 1992; 4:189–225.
22. Marion DW, Obrist WD, Cavlier P, et al: The use of moderate

therapeutic hypothermia for patients with severe head injuries: A preliminary report. J Neurosurg 1993; 79:354–362.
23. Bullock R, Statham P, Patterson J, et al: Vasogenic edema after focal human head injury—a SPECT mapping study. *In:* Brain Oedema. Reulen HJ, Baethmann A, Marmarou A (Eds). Springer-Verlag, Berlin, 1990, pp 286–289.
24. Toutant SM, Klauber MR, Marshall LF, et al: Absent or compressed basal cisterns on first CT scan: Ominous predictors of outcome in severe head injury. J Neurosurg 1984; 61:691–694.
25. Ostrup RC, Luerssen TG, Marshall LF: Continuous monitoring of intracranial pressure with a miniaturized fiberoptic device. J Neurosurg 1987; 67:206–211.
26. Mendelow AD, Rowan JO, Murray L: A clinical comparison of subdural screw pressure measurements with ventricular pressure. J Neurosurg 1983; 58:45–49.
27. Robertson CS, Narayan RK, Goksalau L, et al: Cerebral arteriovenous oxygen difference as an estimate of cerebral blood flow in comatose patients. J Neurosurg 1989; 70:222–230.
28. Moulton RJ, Marmarou A, Ronen J, et al: Spectral analysis of the EEG in craniocerebral trauma. Can J Neurol Sci 1988; 15:82–86.
29. Hassler W, Steinmetz H, Gawlaowski J: Transcranial Doppler ultrasonography in raised intracranial pressure and in intracranial circulatory arrest. J Neurosurg 1988; 68:745–751.
30. Greenberg RP, Becker DP, Miller JD, et al: Evaluation of brain function in severe human head trauma with multimodality evoked potentials. Part 2: Localization of brain dysfunction and correlation with post-traumatic neurological condition. J Neurosurg 1977; 47:150–162.
31. Young B, Ott L, Norton J, et al: Metabolic and nutritional sequelae in the non-steroid treated head injury patient. Neurosurgery 1985; 17:784.
32. Muizelaar JP, Marmarou A, Ward JD, et al: Adverse effects of prolonged hyperventilation in patients with severe head injury: A randomized clinical trial. J Neurosurg 1991; 75:731–739.
33. Ward JD, Choi S, Marmarou A, et al: Effect of prophylactic hyperventilation on outcome in patients with severe head injury. *In:* Intracranial Pressure VII. Hoff JT, Betz AL (Eds). Berlin, Springer-Verlag, 1989, pp 631–633.
34. Marshall LF, Smith RW, Shapiro HM: The outcome with aggressive treatment in severe head injuries. Part II. Acute and chronic barbiturate administration in the management of head injury. J Neurosurg 1979; 50:26.
35. Shapiro HM, Wyle SR, Loeser J: Barbiturates—augmented hypothermia for persistent hypertension. J Neurosurg 1974; 40:90.
36. Ward JD, Becker DP, Miller JD, et al: Failure of prophylactic barbiturate coma in the treatment of severe head injury. J Neurosurg 1985; 62:383.
37. Batjer Hunt H: Cerebral protective effects of etomidate: Experimental and clinical aspects. Cerebrovasc Brain Metab Rev 1993; 5:17–31.
38. Todd NV, Teasdale GM: Steroids in human head injury: Clinical studies. *In:* Steroids in Diseases of the Central Nervous System. Capildeo R (Ed). New York, John Wiley & Sons, 1989, pp 151–161.
39. Bracken MB, Shepard MJ, Collins WF, et al: A randomized controlled trial of methylprednisolone or naloxone in the treatment of acute spinal cord injury: Results of the second National Acute Spinal Cord Injury Study. N Engl J Med 1990; 322:1405–1411.
40. Klauber MR, Marshall LF, Luerssen JG, et al: Determinants of head injury mortality: Importance of the low risk patient. Neurosurgery 1984; 24:31–36.

CHAPTER 158

Acute Spinal Cord Trauma

Rosemary Hickey, MD • Tod B. Sloan, MD, PhD
Maurice S. Albin, MD, MSc (Anesth)

EPIDEMIOLOGY

The incidence of spinal cord injury (SCI) appears to range from 12.4 to 53.4 per million population in the United States. Injuries sustained in vehicular accidents account for about one half of these. Annually, acute SCI accounts for at least 12,000 cases of paraplegia and quadriplegia in the United States. About 4000 of these patients die before reaching a hospital, and 1000 die during hospitalization. Approximately 4000 cases of traumatic quadriplegia are added to the national pool each year, and it is estimated that in 1988, about 177,000 persons suffering from traumatic SCI resided in the United States.[1] Contributing to the problem of SCIs due to motor vehicle accidents is the fact that at least 50% of the deaths are alcohol related, and ethanol has been shown to exacerbate intracranial and SCI lesions.[2, 3]

Epidemiologic data from many countries seem to indicate that the etiologic factors causing SCI are (in order of decreasing incidence) vehicular accidents, falls while on or off the job, and sports injuries (particularly diving injuries). There appears to be a much higher incidence of SCI in males, with most patients ranging in age from 15 to 35 years. Not surprisingly, younger and middle-aged persons suffer from occupational injuries whereas older persons are more likely to suffer SCI after falls at home. SCI occurs relatively infrequently in the pediatric population, accounting for approximately 5% to 10% of all spinal injuries. This low incidence can be explained by certain anatomic and biomechanical factors of the pediatric spine, including its increased mobility secondary to ligamentous laxity. A different injury profile is also noted in pediatric patients, with young children sustaining a greater proportion of both SCI without radiologic abnormality and upper cervical cord injury. Elderly patients with preexisting cervical degenerative disease may be susceptible to SCI with even minor trauma, and in some instances the injury may escape detection.

ANATOMIC AND VASCULAR CONSIDERATIONS

Spinal Cord Circulation

Anatomically, the substance of the spinal cord is supplied by branches from a number of major vessels, including the vertebral and posterocerebellar arteries. Regional perfusion is provided by branches from the thoracic and abdominal aorta as well as from the deep cervical, intercostal, lumbar, and lateral sacral arteries. Lateral spinal arteries, originating from all of these parent vessels, eventually terminate in the anterior and posterior radicular arteries. The anterior radicular artery entering at each side of the cord with each anterior root (only six to eight of these vessels are of significant caliber) joins with the anterior spinal artery, which descends on the ventral surface of the cord after its formation from branches of both vertebral arteries. Within the cranium, small branches of the vertebral or posterior-inferior cerebellar arteries continue caudally over the dorsal surface of the cord, usually as two small vessels known as the posterior spinal arteries. Only five to eight of the posterior radicular arteries are of sufficient size to provide meaningful perfusion to the cord. The largest radicular arteries, both anterior and posterior branches, usually enter the cord circulation in the upper lumbar region. Although the venous drainage of the spinal cord may be variable, its anatomic pattern is similar to that of the arteries.

Autoregulation of Spinal Cord Blood Flow

Studies investigating the effect of varying perfusion pressure on spinal cord blood flow (SCBF) have demonstrated that SCBF is maintained over a wide blood pressure range by autoregulation. Hickey and colleagues found that autoregulation of the spinal cord closely paralleled that of the brain and occurred between spinal cord perfusion pressures of 60 and 120 mm Hg.[4] Below the lower and above the upper limits, SCBF became directly dependent on perfusion pressure. After SCI, autoregulation is altered or completely lost. Guha and associates reported the effects of experimental SCI on autoregulation. They found that after mild SCI, SCBF was lower than that in control animals and the lower limit of autoregulation was increased. Severe SCI resulted in a marked decrease in SCBF and a loss of autoregulation.[5]

These autoregulatory responses may be particularly important in view of the tenuous blood supply to certain areas of the cord. Wide spacing of the radicular arteries supplying the spinal cord leaves large "watershed" areas along the course of the anterior spinal artery, and these areas are vulnerable to ischemia. In these watershed areas, the arterial inflow is precarious and interruption of blood flow can have serious ischemic consequences. The tenuous blood supply to the cord, its interruption after injury, and alterations in autoregulation all point out the potential adverse consequences of allowing sustained arterial hypotension in patients with acute SCI.

PATHOPHYSIOLOGY OF INJURY

Acute spinal cord neuronal damage is probably the consequence of two types of injury. First is the direct mechanical injury from the traumatic impact. Secondary injury results from the vascular and chemical processes set in motion by the initial impact. Although various methods and medications have successfully reduced the degree of secondary injury in experimental animals, attempts to resuscitate the human spinal cord after injury have been disappointing.

The changes in the spinal cord of humans after injury appear to be similar to those changes in experimental injury.[6] In animal studies, the physiologic changes are the same, regardless of the mechanism of injury (impact or compression).[6] Various studies have shown that the most consistent early change is in SCBF.[7] By 10 minutes, hypoperfusion has been identified in the posterocentral part of the cord. Although hyperemia is occasionally observed after trauma, blood flow is always decreased when moderate to severe injury occurs. By 2 hours after injury, perfusion of the intrinsic arteries of the cord is markedly decreased.

The first visual change after injury is petechial hemorrhage in the gray matter, which occurs within minutes. The hemorrhage appears to circumscribe a single blood vessel. For more severe impacts, the degree of hemorrhage extends circumferentially in proportion to the magnitude of impact. As early as 1 hour after trauma, central chromatolysis, microvacuolation, and ischemic injury occur in the anterior horn cells. The changes in the gray matter of the cord are similar to changes in the cerebral cortex after ischemic injury and are consistent with microvascular injury. The post-traumatic change in the white matter is mainly edema around the vascular structures. The edema is primarily of the vasogenic type (e.g., fluid of low protein content leaking from the blood vessels). The edema spreads and reaches the pial surface by 6 hours. Vasogenic edema is predominant for the first 24 hours but can contribute to cord swelling for 9 days. In addition, by 30 minutes, the axoplasm of the neurons shows changes consistent with axoplasmic stasis and axonal membrane failure.

After 8 to 24 hours, an inflammatory response begins, with infiltration of polymorphonuclear neutrophils in the area of hemorrhage. The inflammatory response appears to parallel the degree of hemorrhage and continues for 72 hours after trauma.

Indirect experimental evidence lends support to the hypothesis that hyperoxia is a factor in the pathogenesis of neuronal injury in the spinal cord. When SCI was induced by ischemia and reperfusion was conducted without excessive oxygenation, metabolic and functional recovery improved.[8, 9]

Various other studies suggest that a cascade of destructive events ensues, resulting in spinal cord damage. The mechanisms of injury appear to be similar to those in the brain. These include a central role for calcium, excitotoxic neurotransmitters, prostanoids, and free radicals. Interestingly, the major target organ of these reactive radicals appears to be the microvasculature. Studies using antioxidants in experimental SCI suggest that oxygen radical injury may be a major contributor to postinjury hypoperfusion.[10–12] Other mechanisms in addition to oxygen radicals probably contribute to hypoperfusion after injury. That calcium flux is one of these mechanisms is implied by the observation that calcium channel blockers and cyclooxygenase inhibitors reduce the decrease in spinal white matter blood flow after concussion.

CLINICAL PATTERNS OF SPINAL CORD INJURY

Depending on the degree of severity and type of injury, the resultant SCI may produce several syndromes relating to neurologic damage. Aside from bony injury without neurologic injury (intact), classification of neurologic injury patterns is based on the degree and distribution of neurologic dysfunction. In complete SCI, total paralysis and loss of sensation result from complete interruption of the ascending and descending pathways below the level of the lesion. Functional levels of complete lesions have been classified by Stauffer and Bell.[13] High cervical lesions with damage to the brain stem to C-1 are termed *pentaplegia.* These patients have paralysis of the lower cranial nerves and accessory muscles, as well as sensory and motor loss in the arms and legs. Respiratory quadriplegics have functional levels at C-2 to C-3, leaving face and neck sensation intact and retaining control of the sternocleidomastoid, trapezius, and accessory muscles. These patients require ventilatory support, because diaphragmatic control is lost. Quadriplegia involves motor and sensory loss in legs (injury to C-4 to C-8), and paraplegia involves loss in the legs only (injury to T-1 to S-1). Perineal paraplegia involves loss of sacral roots S-2 to S-5, causing bowel, bladder, and sexual dysfunction.

In an incomplete injury, some of the sensory or motor fibers below the lesion are preserved. Incomplete injuries can be delineated according to the anatomic damage sustained and include the following symptom complexes.[14] The anterior cord syndrome is characterized by paralysis with hypesthesia and hypalgesia below the level of injury but preservation of position sense, vibration sense, and light touch. Anterior compression of the spinal cord affects the lateral corticospinal tract and spinothalamic tract but preserves the posterior columns. Central cord syndrome occurs when cellular destruction in the center of the cord is more extensive than in the periphery, giving a disproportionate degree of motor paralysis in the upper extremities as compared with the lower. This is accompanied by various degrees of sensory loss. Central destruction of the spinal cord due to hemorrhage or necrosis is noted, with sparing of the peripheral leg area in the lateral corticospinal tract.

Brown-Séquard syndrome is a lesion of the lateral half of the spinal cord and is manifested by ipsilateral paresis and contralateral loss of pain and temperature sensation. The cauda equina syndrome involves peripheral nerves instead of the spinal cord directly. When complete, it includes paralysis of the lower extremities, sensory loss, and bowel and bladder dysfunction. When incomplete, symptoms may include sciatica, numbness, and patchy sensation or bowel and bladder dysfunction with saddle anesthesia. Because peripheral nerves possess the ability to regenerate when compared with the spinal cord, the prognosis for recovery from this syndrome appears to be better.

One specialized form of incomplete lesion is sacral sparing. In affected persons, the lesion appears to be complete except for the presence of function in the sacral area, such as rectal tone, perianal sensation, or deep touch. Identification of this condition, as well as differentiation of other incomplete lesions, is important in that the prognosis is often more favorable than for complete lesions if aggressive early care is provided.[15]

PHYSIOLOGIC DISTURBANCES

Multiple system dysfunction may occur after SCI (Table 158–1). Dysfunction of the pulmonary and cardiovascular system is especially important. Fluid and electrolyte imbalance, loss of temperature control, and associated injuries also complicate SCI.

Pulmonary System

Pulmonary complications are a major cause of morbidity and mortality after acute SCI. An epidemiologic study of 5131 patients sustaining SCIs between 1973 and 1980 determined that pneumonia was the overall leading cause of death after SCI.[16]

With SCI, dysfunction of any or all of the muscles of respiration may occur, depending on the level of injury. Damage to cord segments C-3 to C-5 involves the phrenic nerve nuclei, and when the lesion is above C-4, voluntary diaphragmatic respiration mediated by the phrenic nerve is not possible.[13] Patients with low-level cervical quadriplegia with intact phrenic nerve nuclei also have respiratory impairment. They lack the proper intercostal muscle activity necessary to stabilize the rib cage, and diaphragmatic contraction may result in a paradoxic inward motion of the upper thorax during inspiration. Abdominal muscle dysfunction also occurs, leading to the inability to achieve normal residual volumes during expiration.[17] Hemorrhage and edema may extend the level of neurologic dysfunction above the initial level of injury, leading to delayed deterioration in respiratory function.

A reduction in vital capacity occurs between 1 and 5 days after cervical SCI and gradually improves over time. Other alterations in pulmonary mechanics in quadriplegic patients include a reduction in total lung capacity, expiratory reserve volume, and forced expiratory flow rates with an increase in residual volume and the work of breathing. As a result of these alterations, patients are subject to retention of secretions, atelectasis, increased ventilation-perfusion mismatch, and poor ability to sigh and cough. Retention of secretions may require nasotracheal suctioning or fiberoptic bronchoscopy. An abdominal push maneuver in which a patient's expiratory effort is assisted by posterior and cephalad abdominal pressure has been shown to improve peak expiratory flow rates during attempts to cough. In contrast to noninjured patients, a change in body position from the upright to supine position may improve ventilatory function in quadriplegic patients. This results from an improvement in vital capacity due to a reduction in residual volume (residual volume is abnormally elevated in quadriplegic patients) from the effect of gravity on the abdominal contents.

In addition to the altered ventilatory function intrinsic to patients with SCI, other insults may also compromise ventilation. Associated chest trauma at the time of injury may result in a pneumothorax, hemothorax, or pulmonary contusion. Gastric atony secondary to spinal shock may cause a large gastric air bubble that limits diaphragmatic excursion and increases the risk of aspiration. Aspiration is a particular risk in patients who have depressed consciousness due to associated head injury. Pulmonary embolism secondary to deep venous thrombosis may occur as a consequence of bed rest, immobilization, and muscle paralysis.

The incidence of pulmonary edema is increased in patients with acute SCI. In animal studies of cervical cord transection, an increase in extravascular lung water has been demonstrated, suggesting alterations in pulmonary permeability after SCI.[18] Pulmonary edema attributed to autonomic dysfunction at the time of injury (neurogenic pulmonary edema) has also been noted in humans. Although the exact mechanisms leading to pulmonary edema are not fully understood, patients with cervical SCI are particularly vulnerable to this complication and require meticulous management of volume status.

Pulmonary therapy emphasizing the prevention, recognition, and treatment of secretion retention is valuable in quadriplegic patients. This includes frequent repositioning, deep-breathing exercises, incentive spirometry, chest percussion, assisted coughing, and serial pulmonary function testing.[19] When secretion retention is noted, intermittent positive-pressure breathing, bronchodilators, and in some instances fiberoptic bronchoscopy may be used to clear secretions.[19]

TABLE 158–1. Physiologic Disturbances Associated with Acute Spinal Cord Injury

- Pulmonary
  - Respiratory muscle dysfunction (↓ vital capacity, ↓ total lung capacity, ↓ expiratory reserve volume, ↑ residual volume, ↑ work of breathing)
  - Chest trauma
  - Aspiration
  - Pulmonary edema
  - Pulmonary embolism
- Cardiovascular
  - Loss of sympathetics to heart (T-1 to T-4)
  - Loss of vascular tone
  - Myocardial injury
  - Blood loss with trauma
- Fluid and electrolyte
  - Respiratory acidosis
  - Hypercalcemia
  - Altered response to succinylcholine chloride
- Loss of temperature control
  - Poikilothermia
- Associated injuries

Cardiovascular System

SCI is characterized by autonomic dysfunction that interferes with maintenance of cardiovascular stability. Experimental studies of animals have shown that an initial increase in mean arterial pressure follows injury and may be accompanied by cardiac ectopic beats and blocked by α-adrenergic blocking agents. This initial hypertensive response documented in animals has not been detected in humans, probably because of the time delay from injury to examination. After the initial period of hypertension, hemodynamic changes consistent with sympathetic denervation occur. Loss of sympathetic innervation to the heart at T-1 through T-4 cord levels leaves the parasympathetic cardiac innervation via the vagus unopposed, resulting in bradycardia. Elimination of sympathetic arterial tone results in hypotension. Cellular damage to the myocardium may also contribute to cardiovascular instability.

Bradycardia associated with SCI is most frequent in patients with a complete injury at the cervical level. It generally resolves by 3 to 5 weeks after injury and does not require permanent pacemaker therapy. Bradycardia is a frequent occurrence with suctioning or changes in body position. Vagal stimulation that cannot be compensated for by an integrated sympathetic response may be the mechanism underlying bradycardia associated with these events. Hypoxemia also has a role during tracheal suctioning. Treatment of bradycardiac episodes is with vagolytic therapy (atropine, propantheline bromide) and, if associated with tracheal suctioning, increased ventilation and oxygenation. In patients with symptomatic bradycardia not responding to medical measures, cardiac pacing may be necessary.

Hypotension associated with SCI may present a difficult management problem. The use of a pulmonary artery catheter is helpful in guiding management of hypotension and volume replacement in these patients. Fluid volume is optimized with volume infusion, and if hypotension persists, vasoconstrictors are then added.[20]

Fluid and Electrolytes

Electrolyte balance may be affected by pH alterations such as respiratory acidosis due to alveolar hypoventilation. Metabolic alkalosis due to loss of gastric hydrochloride from nasogastric suction may occur, as may hypochloremia due to vomiting or gastric suction. Alterations in calcium balance may also be encountered. Immobility leads to increased mobilization of calcium from bone, hypercalciuria, and in some instances hypercalcemia. Hypercalciuria leads to the formation of renal calculi and renal parenchymal damage.

Temperature Control

Body temperature may approach that of the environment (poikilothermia) owing to loss of the ability to sweat in hot environments or vasoconstriction in cooler environments. These patients are prone to excessive heat loss during surgical procedures and easily become hypothermic.

Associated Injuries

Approximately half of all patients with traumatic SCI also sustain other injuries. The possibility of concomitant head injury and SCI should always be considered, necessitating immobilization of the head and neck until SCI can be precluded in head trauma victims. Chest trauma may also occur, resulting in fractured ribs, pulmonary contusions, hemothorax, or pneumothorax. The diagnosis of intra-abdominal injuries, which occur in approximately 5% of patients sustaining blunt cervical SCI, may be particularly difficult. The loss of abdominal muscle tone and sensation as well as the hypotension that may be associated with acute cervical SCI masks the typical signs of blood loss due to abdominal injury. Musculoskeletal injuries including long-bone fractures (with the possibility of fat emboli) as well as pelvic fractures and hip fracture-dislocation may also occur.

Spinal Shock

The syndrome of spinal shock is characterized by the absence of all cutaneous and tendon reflexes below the level of the lesion. Patients exhibit flaccid paralysis and evidence of interruption of sympathetic pathways including bradycardia, hypotension, and decreased systemic vascular resistance. Sympathetic interruption associated with spinal shock also leads to gastric atony, dilation, and ileus, which require nasogastric suctioning, and bladder atony, which requires indwelling or intermittent catheterization. The duration of areflexia is variable but is usually 3 to 6 weeks in adults. Reappearance of the anal and bulbocavernosus reflexes heralds the return of spinal reflex activity, which generally occurs in a distal-to-cephalad direction.

ASSESSMENT OF PATIENTS WITH SPINAL CORD INJURY

As with any patient, a thorough evaluation is important for patients with SCI. Four basic considerations about the spinal injury are (1) spinal stability, (2) time since the neural injury, (3) spinal level of injury, and (4) degree of neural injury.

Problems of Spinal Instability

The degree of spinal instability is important in that neurologic injury may be aggravated by improper management. Of particular concern are patients who are unstable as a result of malfusion (when corrective surgery was not performed or stabilization procedures were ineffective), because their instability may be overlooked. In some acute cases, muscle spasm may partially splint the bony instability, protecting the patient until anesthesia or muscle relaxants eliminate that effect. Identifying an unstable spine is critical in planning patient care in traction devices.

Problems Relating to the Time After Injury

During the acute phase, associated injuries and the presence of a full stomach warrant attention in addition to the spinal injury. After 24 hours, the possibility of excessive potassium release following the administration of succinylcholine must be considered. Here, with major muscle denervation, the number of postsynaptic receptors becomes increased, as if to amplify any small neuromuscular signal that may be present. When depolarized by succinylcholine, pores on the neuromuscular junction open like a sieve, allowing massive exodus of stored intracellular potassium. Lethal levels of serum potassium have been reported (as high as 14 mEq/L) after neurologic injury, as soon as 3 days after injury, and as late as 6 months after injury. Because experimental studies suggest that the change may happen shortly after injury, it would appear prudent to avoid succinylcholine between 1 day and 1 year after SCI when denervation of muscle has occurred.

As the time after injury progresses into the phase of chronic spinal injury, uncontrolled spinal reflexes may pose problems. Two hyperreflexic syndromes are identifiable. First, muscle spasms may occur as a result of hyperactive spinal reflexes controlling muscle tone. Without the tempering influence of cortical, brain stem, and cerebellar influences, uncontrolled spasms of muscle activity may result. This "mass reflex" may make treatment of unanesthetized patients difficult.

The second syndrome of hyperreflexia is due to autonomic vascular reflexes. Usually beginning 2 to 3 weeks after injury, afferent impulses to the spinal cord may elicit unchecked sympathetic efferent activity.[21] The afferent stimulation is typically due to distention or manipulation of hollow organs (notably the bowel or bladder), although it can be elicited by other sensory stimulation (such as skin sensation). Spinal reflex activity elicits autonomic efferent activity, which causes vasoconstriction in the affected region of the body. The result is an influx of blood into the circulation proportionate to the volume of contracted vasculature. This results in hypertension if more blood volume is introduced into the circulation than can be accommodated by vasodilatation in the unaffected vasculature. For complete neurologic injuries below the seventh thoracic vertebra, the arms and abdominal viscera are able to dilate and compensate such that vasoconstriction below T-8 is not accompanied by hypertension. At higher spinal levels, however, hypertension is observed in 65% to 85% of patients, despite upper-extremity vasodilation. For neurologic levels below T-4, baroreceptor-mediated bradycardia usually accompanies the hypertension. However, at higher levels, tachycardia can result if the sympathetic innervation of the heart is included in the autonomic efferent activity. The typical symptoms of this "autonomic hypertension" are headache and nasal stuffiness (from vasodilatation), as well as vague feelings of discomfort. More serious sequelae, such as cerebral hemorrhage, convulsions, and coma, may also occur.

Autonomic hypertension may become a problem during stimulating procedures. For patients in whom this is known to be a problem, specific sensory nerves (such as the pudendal) can be blocked or interruption of the efferent output may be more effective. Intravenous agents such as ganglionic blockers (e.g., trimethaphan), direct-acting vasodilating agents (e.g., sodium nitroprusside), or β- and α-β–blockers (e.g., esmolol or labetalol) can be titrated to correct the blood pressure until the inciting problem is corrected. The hypertensive episode can often be stopped by eliminating a bowel or bladder distention that may be the inciting stimulus.

Patients with chronic SCI have many of the problems that pertain to other chronically debilitated patients. For example, most of these patients develop gastric erosions that may be aggravated by steroids. As with any chronically immobilized patient, hypercalcemia can occur in cervical SCI. The changes in calcium metabolism can lead to osteoporosis, hypercalciuria, and renal calculi, but hypercalcemia is somewhat rare. Hypercalcemia is most common in male adolescents with high cervical lesions 1 to 12 weeks after injury and may contribute to reduced renal function. This may be manifested as early as 10 days after injury. Cardiac conduction defects may occur with calcium levels exceeding 12 mg/dL, and levels as high as 16 mg/dL have been reported.

Problems Relating to the Level of Injury

The issue of neurologic dysfunction can be considered by examining the problems of a complete spinal injury, because the injury level varies with the anatomic level (Table 158–2). Clearly, patients who are intact have few problems related to neural dysfunction. Patients with incomplete lesions have intermediate types and severity of the problems described as follows for complete spinal cord lesions.

Patients with a cauda equina lesion are often overlooked, because gross neurologic function appears normal. However, the loss of bowel and bladder function can have serious consequences. Acutely, urinary tract infection can cause systemic derangements such as fever. Chronically, recurrent infections may cause pyelonephritis and renal insufficiency. These as well as other chronic infections can cause amyloidosis, leading to organ dysfunction secondary to amyloid deposition. Renal deposition can lead to renal insufficiency, and adrenal insufficiency has been noted. Regardless of the cause, these renal consequences contribute significantly to the long-term morbidity and mortality of patients with SCI. Bowel problems tend to be more significant if a bowel regimen is not optimal. Improper management can result in fluid and electrolyte disturbances.

TABLE 158–2. Problems Associated with Severe Spinal Cord Injury at Different Levels*

- High cervical
  - Ventilation
- Low cervical
  - Intubation
  - Limited cardiovascular reserves
- High thoracic
  - Reduced alveolar ventilation
  - Loss of cardiac sympathetics (T-1 to T-4)
  - Autonomic hypertension (T-7; chronic phase)
- Low thoracic
  - Loss of abdominal muscles
  - Reduced expiratory reserves
  - Bowel and gastric distention (acute phase)
- Lumbar
  - Hypercalciuria
  - Poor vascular reserves
  - Decubitus ulcers (chronic phase)
  - Loss of temperature regulation
  - Mass reflex (chronic phase)
  - Deep venous thrombosis, pulmonary embolism
  - Hyperkalemia associated with succinylcholine (1 d–1 y)
- Sacral
  - Loss of bowel function
    - Alteration in fluid and electrolyte function
  - Loss of bladder function
    - Infection, renal failure
    - Amyloidosis

*A lesion at any level shares the problems of all lower-level injuries.

In addition to these complications, patients with injury of the lumbar cord face further concerns because of the loss of neural control of the legs. Denervation of muscle is associated with hyperkalemia after succinylcholine. Loss of sympathetic tone in the legs causes passive heat loss and gain through the skin surface, as well as a reduction in the ability of the vascular system to compensate for alterations in vascular volume. Chronically, the problem of reflex muscle spasms may make management difficult. The loss of muscle tone leads to flexion contractures and fixed deformities that may make nursing difficult. Finally, decubitus ulcers over the buttocks lead to chronic infections and associated systemic sequelae.

Injury in the thoracic column is attended by a loss of pulmonary reserve for coughing and clearing of secretions. The loss of abdominal and intercostal musculature can contribute to an increased risk of pulmonary morbidity, as detailed earlier. Immediately after injury, bowel and gastric distention can contribute to reduced pulmonary reserves. When the level of injury ascends above T-7, autonomic reflexes in the chronic cases can lead to hypertensive episodes. In the high thoracic region (T-1 to T-4), the loss of sympathetic tone of the heart may cause bradycardia owing to the relative imbalance of sympathetic and vagal influences.

Some acutely injured patients may experience severe bradycardia and even asystole when maneuvers such as airway manipulation increase vagal tone. As noted earlier (see *Cardiovascular System*), treatment is with vagolytic therapy and, when associated with tracheal suctioning, increased ventilation and oxygen. Injuries to the cervical region may cause ventilatory difficulty requiring ventilatory support and intubation while also making airway management difficult. Acutely injured patients may have neck instability, placing the spinal cord at risk for injury with neck manipulation associated with intubation. This risk may attend instabilities as low as T-4 and as high as the odontoid. Only one third of all cervical fractures are associated with posterior ligamentous injury, in which the spine is more unstable when flexed than when extended (i.e., less likely to sustain SCI during extension). Devices applied for stabilization, such as a halo brace, may make conventional direct laryngoscopy impossible. Once the spine is stabilized, these patients may have limited neck motion due to bony fusion. This may make intubation difficult, depending on a patient's anatomy.

In the midcervical region, the loss of arm musculature causes further loss of tone in the vascular beds, leading to increased heat exchange with the environment and lack of cardiovascular reserves. In these patients, pulmonary artery catheters may be necessary in the acute phase to manage fluids, because excessive volume infusion may result in congestive heart failure whereas insufficient fluids may not allow adequate cardiac performance. Hypotension and cardiac arrest have been reported with position change. Once the fluid volume is stabilized, patients without cardiac disease do not usually require invasive monitoring until other circumstances (such as surgery) alter their vascular dynamics. Lesions in the high cervical region can cause marked impairment of ventilation because innervation of the diaphragm via the phrenic nerve (C-3 to C-5) is impaired by injury or edema from lower levels. Acutely, these patients may need ventilatory support and tracheostomy, and chronic supportive therapy may be required.

Assessment of Neurologic Injury

In addition to a careful neurologic examination, objective assessment of neurologic function by sensory or motor evoked potentials can be a valuable adjunct in patient assessment. In comatose or obtunded patients, detailed clinical assessment may not be possible, making objective testing the only available option. In awake patients, these methods allow an objective assessment. The objective value of the tests allows removal of examiner or patient bias (e.g., a patient may deny loss of sensation or feel sensation that is mechanically referred from lower testing areas to more cephalad regions). In addition, these techniques may be more sensitive to residual function than a patient's ability to perceive. These techniques are thus invaluable to identify incomplete lesions (i.e., areas of function in a patient who is otherwise neurologically complete) or to document the daily progression of neurologic changes.

The sensory tract can be assessed using somatosensory evoked potentials (SSEPs) or dermatomal evoked potentials.[22] SSEPs are measured after repetitive electric stimulation of a peripheral nerve. The resulting nervous signal is recorded as it traverses the nervous system through the peripheral nerve, spinal cord, and brain stem and finally passes into the sensory cortex. The SSEP signal travels the spinal cord primarily via the posterior columns, which mediate proprioception and vibration. The choice of peripheral nerve for stimulation depends on several factors. The use of a mixed motor-sensory nerve may offer considerable advantage over a pure sensory nerve, because stimulation can be verified by visible motor movement. It is important to recognize that the nerve chosen enters via discrete roots. Median (C-6 to C-7) or ulnar (C-8) nerves are used when possible because they have greater amplitude than do lower-extremity responses. Likewise, the common peroneal nerve (L-4 to L-5) has greater amplitude than does the posterior tibial nerve (L-4 to S-2). However, posterior tibial nerve stimulation can be verified by recording in the popliteal fossa, just as median and ulnar stimulation can be verified by recording over the brachial plexus (Erb's point) when motor activity is not possible (i.e., with pharmacologic neuromuscular paralysis).

One notable variation of the SSEP is the dermatomal evoked potential, in which stimulation is conducted of dermatomal regions. Recording between and including C-4 to S-5 has been noted. This can allow assessment of individual nerve roots of multiroot peripheral nerves where the SSEP may be normal despite severe injury to a portion of the roots. It can also be used to assess regions of the spinal column that are not assessed by major nerves (especially the sacral regions).

Motor Tract Monitoring

SSEP and dermatomal evoked potential monitoring assess the tracts of the sensory paths in the posterior columns (tracts serving proprioception and vibration). Because this represents a highly select neural tract, damage to other regions of the spinal cord could occur without changes. The motor tracts of the anterior spinal cord are topographically removed from the sensory tracts, and the vascular supply is by a separate vascular system.

The third technique, motor evoked potentials, is currently in an evolutionary stage. Similar to the end-to-end technique of the SSEP, the motor cortex can be excited by a stimulation current placed by bilateral scalp electrodes or a palate-cortex pair. Alternatively, the cortex can be stimulated via an electromagnetic discharge over the motor cortex. Electric potentials traveling in the motor tracts can be recorded at the spinal cord, peripheral nerve, or muscle and used as an index of motor pathway viability. The potential hazards of the stimulation current, however, are not fully known.

DRUG THERAPY

To date, treatment strategies for SCI have largely focused on reducing the degree of secondary injury or attempting to promote regeneration of the damaged neurons. Various studies demonstrate that the neural tracts of the injured cord are largely intact after injury.[23] Animal experiments support the concept that motor function can recover to normal levels with as little as 4% to 6% of the cortical neurons having connection to the cord. If axonal survival exceeds 6%, full motor function is possible.[24] This observation suggests that even a marginal improvement in neuronal survival may markedly improve function. Because the gray matter may be more sensitive to injury than white matter (because the metabolic rate is higher than in the surrounding white matter) and it is therefore more dependent on a higher SCBF, strategies to improve SCI outcome may revolve around improving gray matter viability.

Unfortunately, a major disparity exists between experimental SCI and clinical human injury with respect to treatment success.[25] The most commonly offered explanation for this disparity is that the methods used for resuscitation require application before or very shortly after the injury (i.e., before the cascade of destructive events is initiated). Because inevitable delays are generally associated with emergency medical care, irreversible events have begun. If this is the explanation, then these methods of resuscitation should be effective for SCI that occurs during surgery, when application is possible before or very shortly after the injury.

The concept of early intervention is also supported by microscopic studies of the spinal cord after injury. Despite functional paralysis, during a brief period after injury, even the electron microscope can detect only minimum changes. This period is followed by vasogenic edema that spreads concentrically from the central gray matter. Hemorrhages develop, notably in the central gray matter. They appear to be associated with a breakdown in the vascular wall integrity and may be promoted by system hypertension. It is possible that reductions in SCBF that occur 30 to 60 minutes after injury contribute to the disintegration of the neurons with time and that elimination of such flow restrictions could lessen the injury.

At present, methylprednisolone is considered routine in spinal injury after a multicenter, randomized, placebo-controlled trial in acute spinal cord injury (National Acute Spinal Cord Injury Study, or NASCIS II). One hundred sixty-two patients received methylprednisolone, 30 mg/kg, followed by a continuous infusion of 5.4 $mg \cdot kg^{-1} \cdot h^{-1}$ for the next 23 hours. Improvement in motor neurologic scores was noted at 6 weeks, 6 months, and 1 year in patients with complete as well as incomplete lesions,[26] provided the drug was started within 8 hours of injury. It should be noted, however, that motor and sensory evaluations in this study were made on the basis of neurologic examination and not on functional ability.

The neuroprotective effects of steroids have been reviewed by Hall[27] and are not dependent on steroid receptors. The mechanism probably is inhibition of lipid peroxidation. Compounds with the steroid nucleus but without glucocorticoid effects have now been synthesized (21-aminosteroids). One compound, tirilazad (U-74006F), appears to be particularly promising in experimental cerebral ischemia[28] and SCI and is currently in phase II clinical trials. Also under investigation are gangliosides, complex acidic glycosphingolipids found in high concentration in central nervous system cell membranes.[29] In experimental neurologic injury, gangliosides (GM_1) have been found to promote healing and regeneration and may offer future benefit for patients with SCI.

INTUBATION

Various methods are available for securing the airway when intubation is necessary.[30] If time allows, awake intubation allows continuous assessment of neurologic function and may avoid some medications associated with potassium release (succinylcholine) or ventilatory depression. This generally can be accomplished using fiberoptic or blind techniques. In general, barring a skull base fracture, the nasal route is favored, particularly if prolonged ventilation is anticipated or anatomic considerations (such as lower facial fractures) suggest an oral technique will be difficult. To accomplish the nasal intubation, prior use of an anticholinergic for drying is useful. Judicious use of intravenous sedation (e.g., midazolam) and analgesia (e.g., fentanyl) is often helpful. However, elderly individuals or severely injured patients may tolerate only minimal doses. The procedure may be performed without intravenous sedation if a patient is instructed about the procedure and excellent topical anesthesia is applied. For the nasal route, 4% to 5% cocaine or 0.2% phenylephrine hydrochloride in 4% lidocaine applied to the nasal mucosa shrinks the turbinates and topically anesthetizes the nasal passage.

Additional anesthesia (lidocaine jelly or ointment or local anesthesia spray) applied to the posterior tongue may be helpful but is not essential. Anesthesia of the vocal cords and larynx is also provided to prevent a patient from coughing up or swallowing the fiberoptic. This may be done with the transtracheal injection of 2 to 4 mL of 4% lidocaine applied percutaneously via the cricothyroid membrane. The transtracheal injection may be accomplished using a 20-gauge catheter with the needle removed after insertion, because the needle tip might injure the vocal cords owing to their proximity. To anesthetize the larynx above the vocal cords, some authorities prefer the use of a superior laryngeal nerve block. This is done by injecting 2 mL of 2% lidocaine into the thyrohyoid membrane bilaterally, superiorly off the lateral wing of the thyroid cartilage. These techniques allow the blind nasal or fiberoptic-guided nasal technique to be accomplished more easily.

If a patient is at risk for aspiration, the transtracheal technique may not be optimal, because laryngeal anesthesia allows the airway to be unprotected for several minutes. An approach that lessens the risk of aspiration is to anesthetize only the nasal mucosa initially; then, when the fiberoptic tip is just above the vocal cords, 2 to 4 mL of 4% lidocaine is sprayed through the working channel of the fiberoptic scope. After 60 to 90 seconds, adequate anesthesia allows passage of the scope, thus minimizing the unprotected period. This latter technique is also quite useful in patients with anterior neck abnormalities that contraindicate a transtracheal approach.

In some patients, particularly those in acute need of airway protection or ventilation, an awake oral approach may be the preferred technique. In patients with midface trauma or with basilar skull fractures (often suggested by Battle's sign, "raccoon eyes," associated head trauma, and pneumocephalus on computed tomography), the nasal route is generally contraindicated. The oral route may also be preferred when intubation is likely to be brief, because nasal trauma and associated bleeding can be avoided. Local anesthesia for awake oral intubation requires local anesthesia of the tongue and posterior pharynx. This can be accomplished using aerosolized local anesthesia, local anesthetic ointments placed on the tongue, or viscous lidocaine jelly. Additional anesthesia of the larynx as described earlier is also useful. A specialized oral airway is available for fiberoptically guided oral intubation. It assists in guiding the endotracheal tube around the base of the tongue and prevents a patient from biting down on the fiberoptic scope.

For patients with unstable cervical lesions (perhaps as low as T-4), direct laryngoscopy is generally not the method of choice because extension may cause further SCI. In an emergency situation, however, intubation may need to be accomplished without adequate time to prepare the patient. Here, the need to provide ventilation and oxygenation may preclude a controlled awake intubation. In these cases, surgical access to the airway via a cricothyrotomy or tracheostomy after jet ventilation may be needed if facial trauma or neck instability precludes oral intubation. In the most extreme cases, direct laryngoscopy may be the only method by which the airway can be accessed rapidly enough. In these cases, traction devices to realign the cervical spine (e.g., Gardner-Wells tongs or halo traction) may not have been placed, and an assistant should provide axial traction and attempt to minimize head extension during the laryngoscopy. In this case, the assistant should apply axial traction of 5 to 10 lb at the mastoid area, pulling while keeping the head and neck aligned.[31] For unstable lower cervical spinal injuries, traction may be applied at the midpoint of a line connecting the lateral edge of the eye and the external auditory meatus.[32] For unstable C1–C2 lesions, stabilization of the head to minimize motion and extension may be preferable, as traction may produce excessive distraction.

Various studies have evaluated direct laryngoscopy with oral intubation in cervical injury patients in acute need of airway placement.[30–32] Interestingly, when midline axial traction is applied, the production of neurologic injury is not common. One explanation for the apparent safety is that most extension in the cervical spine during intubation appears to be above C-4 but the majority of cervical spine injuries are below C-3 (>78%). In addition, many injured patients have ligamentous disruption posteriorly with preserved ligaments anteriorly (as many as one third of patients), such that extension is less of a potential hazard. Thus, although the preferred method of intubation is an awake procedure so that neurologic function can be documented, direct laryngoscopy with in-line traction appears to be a safe alternative in an acute situation. In a retrospective study of 150 patients with traumatic cervical spine injuries undergoing operative stabilization, Suderman and colleagues noted no differences in neurologic outcome whether intubation was performed while a patient was awake or under general anesthesia or when comparing oral intubation with all other techniques.[33]

RESPIRATORY CARE

If immediate intubation is not necessary, aggressive chest physiotherapy is required to maintain pulmonary function. This can take the form of incentive spirometry, aerosol therapy to a preset limit by pressure-driven nebulizer, percussion and vibration, chest physiotherapy to treat any areas of infiltrate or atelectasis, limited postural drainage, frequent changes of position, warm mist humidification of oxygen-enriched air delivered through wide-bore tubing, and avoidance of anticholinergics.

Retention of secretions may require blind nasal tracheal suctioning with a soft suction catheter; if a major lung segment appears to be collapsed as a result of a mucus plug, fiberoptic bronchoscopy may be indicated. During such maneuvers, care must be taken to avoid severe bradyarrhythmias due to abnormal tracheal reflexes. Increased ventilation and oxygenation before suctioning may be preventive, because these responses may be due to unrecognized borderline hypoxemia exacerbated by a tracheal suctioning procedure. Assistance with coughing can be provided with an abdominal push maneuver. Use of an abdominal corset when a patient is upright enables the diaphragm to assume its normal resting position and improves its function.

Gastric stasis and intestinal atony accompany spinal shock in many cases. This can lead to abdominal distention, increasing the risk of aspiration. Passage of a nasogastric tube and control of the gastric pH are desirable. However, the combination of antacids, hydrogen ion loss in gastric aspirate, the metabolic effect of diuretic therapy, and maintenance of ionic balance in total parenteral nutrition by addition of acetate can lead to significant metabolic alkalosis. Once the base excess is greater than 9 or 10, respiratory compensation for the metabolic alkalosis is a risk. This may result in hypoventilation, further loss of lung volume, and increased ventilation-perfusion mismatch. If this complication develops, the cause of the alkalosis must be recognized and eliminated.

VENTILATORY SUPPORT

If respiratory function continues to deteriorate despite all the foregoing therapeutic interventions, intubation and ventilation should not be delayed too long. Physicians may tend to withhold ventilator support if a patient has been breathing adequately for 24 to 48 hours because of the fear that the patient will remain ventilator dependent. However, although respiratory function may gradually deteriorate initially, the authors' experience has shown that some time later the patient will return to the same respiratory parameters as exhibited immediately after injury. To delay excessively the provision of ventilator support leads to patients' anxiety, dyspnea, exhaustion, and unnecessary retention of secretions. The result may be loss of lung volume and further deterioration in static pulmonary compliance, and these changes may allow a significant pulmonary infection to become established.

Once the decision is made to ventilate a patient, the authors use ventilator settings that provide close to full respiratory support, requiring only relatively modest respiratory work from a patient. It is desirable to use a ventilator that imposes minimum respiratory work when a patient takes a spontaneous breath; the Siemens 900C (Siemens, Stockholm, Sweden) has proved very suitable. The authors use the ventilator in synchronized intermittent mandatory ventilation mode and do not add the pressure support component unless lung volumes are very low or compliance is excessively compromised by pulmonary interstitial edema or infiltrates. A low level of positive end-expiratory pressure (+5 cm H_2O) is added as soon as cardiovascular stability is attained.

WEANING FROM VENTILATION

Weaning parameters of forced vital capacity, negative inspiratory force, and oxygenation index are checked daily. As pulmonary function and mechanics improve, weaning from mechanical ventilation can proceed. Satisfaction of weaning parameters often occurs between the 10th and 21st days after injury. Weaning criteria, as noted by Mackenzie and Ducker,[34] are listed in Table 158–3. A gradual weaning technique with progressive reduction in the synchronized intermittent mandatory ventilation rate is generally used, although once weaning parameters are met, a rapid-interval weaning technique may also be very effective.

Because of possible laryngeal incompetence, enteral feedings are suspended in the periextubation period (e.g., from 4 h before until 12 h after extubation). Patients are encouraged to take sips of water at an early stage and proceed to a normal diet as tolerated. Tracheostomy is seldom indicated, and patients may be cared for while intubated for as long as 3 weeks without problems.

If weaning proves unsuccessful, patients may be main-

TABLE 158–3. Weaning Criteria

Parameter	*Acceptable Value*
Maximum inspiratory force	> − 20 cm H_2O
Maximum expiratory force	> + 20 cm H_2O
Vital capacity	> 1000 mL
Expiratory flow	> 10 L/s (level dependent)
PaO_2/FIO_2	> 250
V_{DS}/V_T	< .55
Lung thorax compliance	> 30 mL/cm H_2O

(From Mackenzie CF, Ducker TB: Cervical spinal cord injury. *In:* Clinical Controversies in Neuroanestheisa and Neurosurgery. Matjesko J, Katz J [Eds]. New York, Grune & Stratton, 1986, pp 77–134.)

tained on small portable ventilators, thus permitting discharge from the hospital. A permanent tracheostomy is required for these patients. An alternative approach for patients with high quadriplegia is electric stimulation of the phrenic nerve.[35] Before this approach is considered, the viability of the phrenic nerve is determined by percutaneous stimulation of the nerve carried out under fluoroscopic observation of diaphragm movements.[35]

CONCLUSION

Throughout all of the phases after spinal injury, these patients can present numerous challenges. With attentive care, many of the potentially life-threatening complications of SCI can be acutely managed, to assist patients through an often long and difficult hospitalization. Major advances in patient care, such as those available in specialized spinal care trauma centers, have improved the outlook for acute management and rehabilitation of these patients. Perhaps the best hope for long-term improvement in outcome rests in prevention. When proper care is provided, many of these patients live very productive lives.

References

1. Harvey C, Rothschild BB, Asmann AJ, et al: New estimates of traumatic SCI prevalence: A survey-based approach. Paraplegia 1990; 28:537.
2. Flamm ES, Demopoulos HB, Seligman ML, et al: Ethanol potentiation of central nervous system trauma. J Neurosurg 1977; 46:328.
3. Albin MS, Bunegin L: An experimental study of craniocerebral trauma during ethanol intoxication. Crit Care Med 1986; 14:841.
4. Hickey R, Albin M, Bunegin L, et al: Autoregulation of spinal cord and cerebral blood flow: Is the spinal cord a microcosm of the brain? Stroke 1987; 17:1183.
5. Guha A, Tator C, Rochon J: Spinal cord blood flow and systemic blood pressure after experimental spinal cord injury in rats. Stroke 1989; 20:372.
6. Means ED, Anderson DK: Pathophysiology of acute spinal cord injury. *In:* Handbook of the Spinal Cord. Davidoff FA (Ed). New York, Marcel Dekker, 1987, pp 19–61.
7. Sandler AN, Tator CH: Effect of acute spinal cord compression injury on regional spinal cord blood flow in primates. J Neurosurg 1976; 45:660.
8. Marsala M, Danielisova V, Chavko M, et al: Improvement of energy state and basic modifications of neuropathological damage in rabbits as a result of graded postischemic spinal cord reoxygenation. Exp Neurol 1989; 105:93.
9. Danielisova V, Marsala M, Chavko M, et al: Postischemic hypoxia improves metabolic and functional recovery of the spinal cord. Neurology 1990; 40:1125.
10. Young W: Blood flow, metabolic and neurophysiological mechanisms in spinal cord injury. *In:* Central Nervous System Trauma Status Report. Povlishock JT, Becker DB (Eds). Bethesda, NIH, 1983, pp 463–474.
11. Hall EG, Wolf DL: A pharmacological analysis of the pathophysiological mechanisms of posttraumatic spinal cord ischemia. J Neurosurg 1986; 64:951.
12. Hall ED, Wolf DL: Post-traumatic spinal cord ischemia: Relationship to injury severity and physiological parameters. CNS Trauma 1987; 4:15.
13. Stauffer ES, Bell GD: Traumatic respiratory quadriplegia and pentaplegia. Orthop Clin North Am 1978; 9:1081.
14. Maroon JC, Abla AA: Classification of acute spinal cord injury, neurological evaluation and neurosurgical considerations. Crit Care Clin 1987; 3:655.
15. Schrader S, Sloan TB, Toleikis JR: Detection of sacral sparing in acute spinal cord injury. Spine 1987; 12:533.
16. DeVivo MJ, Kartus PL, Stover SL, et al: Cause of death for patients with spinal cord injuries. Arch Intern Med 1989; 149:1761.
17. Luce JM, Culver BH: Respiratory muscle function in health and disease. Chest 1982; 81:82.
18. Albin MS, Bunegin L, Wolf S: Brain and lungs at risk after cervical spinal cord transection: Intracranial pressure, brain water, blood-brain barrier permeability, cerebral blood flow and extravascular lung water changes. Surg Neurol 1985; 24:191.
19. McMichan JC, Michel L, Westbrook PR: Pulmonary dysfunction following traumatic quadriplegia. Recognition, prevention and treatment. JAMA 1980; 243:528.
20. Mackenzie CF, Shin B, Krishnaprasad D, et al: Assessment of cardiac and respiratory function during surgery on patients with acute quadriplegia. J Neurosurg 1985; 62:843.
21. Schonwald G, Fish K, Perkash I: Cardiovascular complications during anesthesia in chronic spinal cord injured patients. Anesthesiology 1985; 55:550.
22. Sloan TB, Toleikis JR, Koht A: Evaluation of spinal cord function by means of evoked potentials. *In:* Surgery of Spine Trauma. Meyer PR (Ed). New York, Churchill Livingstone, 1989, pp 121–136.
23. Kakulas A: The applied neurobiology of human spinal cord injury: A review. Paraplegia 1988; 26:371.
24. Young W: Recovery mechanisms in spinal cord injury: Implications for regenerative therapy. *In:* Neural Regeneration and Transplantation, Frontier of Clinical Neuroscience. Vol 6. Seil FJ (Ed). New York, Alan R Liss, 1989, pp 157–169.
25. Fernandez E, Pallini R, Marchese E, et al: Experimental studies on spinal cord injuries in the last fifteen years. Neurol Res 1991; 13:138.
26. Bracken MB, Shepard MJ, Collins WF, et al: A randomized, controlled trial of methylprednisolone or naloxone in the treatment of acute spinal-cord injury. N Engl J Med 1990; 322:1405.
27. Hall ED: The neuroprotective pharmacology of methylprednisolone. J Neurosurg 1992; 76:13.
28. Perkins WJ, Milde LN, Milde JH, et al: Pretreatment with U74006F improves neurologic outcome following complete cerebral ischemia in dogs. Stroke 1991; 22:902.
29. Rodden FA, Weigandt H, Bauer BL: Gangliosides; the relevance of current research to neurosurgery. J Neurosurg 1991; 74:606.
30. Wood PR: Managing the airway in cervical spine injury—a review of the advanced trauma life support protocol. Anaesthesia 1992; 47:792.
31. Albin MS, Bunegin L, Gilbert J, et al: Anesthesia for spinal cord injury. Probl Anesth 1990; 4:138.
32. Magnaes B: Clinical recording of pressure on the spinal cord and cauda equina. J Neurosurg 1982; 57:64.
33. Suderman VS, Crosby ET, Lui A: Elective oral tracheal intubation in cervical spine-injured adults. Can J Anaesth 1991; 38:785.
34. Mackenzie CF, Ducker TB: Cervical spinal cord injury. *In:* Clinical Controversies in Neuroanesthesia and Neurosurgery. Matjesko J, Katz J (Eds). New York, Grune & Stratton, 1986, pp 77–134.
35. Sharkey PC, Halter JA, Nakajima K: Electrophrenic respiration in patients with high quadriplegia. Neurosurgery 1989; 24:529.

CHAPTER 159

Pediatric Trauma (Basic Principles)

Arthur Cooper, MD

Trauma causes more deaths among children aged 1 to 14 years than all other illnesses combined, annually claiming the lives of nearly 10,000 children nationwide. The magnitude of the problem is staggering: 80% of those with fatal injuries die before hospital admission[1] (hence the recent focus on injury prevention and prehospital care), yet trauma is still responsible for some 10% of all pediatric hospitalizations[2] and about 15% of all pediatric intensive care unit (ICU) admissions.[3] For those who do survive to hospital

TABLE 159–1. Pediatric Trauma Score

	Coded Value		
Patient Characteristics	*+2*	*+1*	*−1*
Weight (kg)	>20	10–20	<20
Airway	Normal	Maintained	Unmaintained
Systolic blood pressure (mm Hg)	>90	50–90	<50
Central nervous system	Awake	Obtunded	Coma
Open wound	None	Minor	Major
Skeletal trauma	None	Closed	Open, multiple

(From Tepas JJ, Mollitt DL, Talbert JL, et al: The pediatric trauma score as a predictor of injury severity in the injured child. J Pediatr Surg 1987; 22:14–18.)

admission, critical care may be vital to ultimate outcome. In fact, major trauma is one of the few conditions for which tertiary pediatric intensive care has been proved beneficial.[4]

Critical care specialists who encounter children infrequently require a working knowledge of important differences between pediatric and adult trauma care. The goal of this chapter is to provide that information and to describe how these differences affect the critical management of children with multiple injuries. Fundamental to this knowledge are the concepts that (1) although the similarities far outnumber the differences, understanding these differences is vital to proper management and (2) critical management should begin in the field, must continue in the emergency department, radiologic suite, operating room, and ICU, and is the responsibility not of a single individual or specialty but of a multidisciplinary team of providers—each of whose members is expert in a certain phase of pediatric trauma care and can rightly lay claim to the title of "pediatric traumatologist" in that discipline. The team leader should be a surgeon with experience in and commitment to the care both of trauma victims and of children. However, because nonoperative treatment is so frequently employed in the management of major pediatric trauma, critical care specialists can expect to have an active role—and at times the leading role—in facilitating optimal recovery of injured children and their families.

IMPORTANT DIFFERENCES

The mortality rate in childhood injuries serious enough to warrant trauma center care is about 3%.[5] Head injury is responsible for 75% of the deaths[5, 6]; truncal injury is associated with a fatal outcome in no more than 15% of all cases of major pediatric trauma but is seldom the immediate cause of death (except in penetrating trauma).[7] Although the overall mortality rate due to trauma is lower among children than it is among adults, children require hospitalization for traumatic injury at a rate that approaches that of adults.[1] Mortality is lowest in hospitals that make pediatric trauma care a priority[4, 8–10]; children at risk of death or disability, as judged by the Pediatric[11] (Table 159–1) or Revised[12] Trauma Score or other proven indicators of serious injury[13] (anatomic, physiologic, and mechanism of injury criteria) should be transported to such facilities where available[14] (Table 159–2).

Mechanisms and Patterns of Injury

Compared with adults, injured children are subject to a different spectrum of injury, which, when coupled with the immature anatomic features and physiologic responses of a child, produces distinct patterns of injury that are unique to childhood (Table 159–3).[5] Blunt injury cases exceed cases of penetrating injury by a ratio of 7:1; penetrating injury is more often fatal. Deaths typically are caused by motor vehicle–related injuries and gunshot wounds. Most blunt trauma in childhood is sustained unintentionally, but 7% is due to physical assault and 3% to physical abuse; physical abuse should be suspected whenever a delay in obtaining treatment is unexplained or when the history is vague or otherwise incompatible with the observed physical findings.

Motor vehicle trauma, the principal blunt injury category, may result in injuries to pedestrians and occupants; in the former, fracture of the midshaft of the femur often is associated with closed head and torso injuries (the Waddell triad), whereas in the latter, closed head and cervical spine injuries (in unrestrained children) and lap belt injuries (in improperly restrained children) are predominant.[15, 16] Falls from extreme heights also result in head, long-bone, and torso injuries, their severity directly related to the magni-

TABLE 159–2. Possible Indications for Transfer to a Pediatric Trauma Center

History of Injury
Patient thrown from a moving vehicle
Falls from >15 ft
Extrication time >20 min
Passenger cabin of vehicle invaded >12 in
Death of another passenger
Accident in a hostile environment (e.g., heat, cold water)

Anatomic Injuries
Combined system injury
Penetrating injury of the groin or neck
Three or more long-bone fractures
Fractures of the axial skeleton
Amputation (other than digits)
Persistent hypotension
Severe head trauma
Maxillofacial or upper airway injury
Central nervous system injury with prolonged loss of consciousness, posturing, or paralysis
Spinal cord injury with neurologic deficit
Unstable chest injury
Blunt or penetrating trauma to the chest or abdomen
Burns, flame or inhalation

System Considerations
Necessary service or specialist not available
No beds available
Need for pediatric ICU care
Multiple casualties
Family request
Paramedic judgment
Severity scores: Trauma score 12 or less; or revised trauma score 11 or less; or pediatric trauma score 8 or less

(From Harris BH, Barlow BA, Ballantine TV, et al: American Pediatric Surgical Association: Principles of pediatric trauma care. J Pediatr Surg 1992; 27:423–426.)

TABLE 159–3. Causes of Injury in Major Pediatric Trauma

By Circumstance	Frequency (%)	Mortality (%)
Accident	89	3
Assault	7	5
Child abuse	3	12
Self injury	1	26
Other	1	8
By Type	***Frequency (%)***	***Mortality (%)***
Blunt	86	3
Penetrating	12	5
Crush	1	6
Other	1	18
By Mechanisms	***Frequency (%)***	***Mortality (%)***
Fall	27	4
Motor vehicle occupant	18	5
Motor vehicle pedestrian	15	5
Bicycle	9	2
Sport	5	<1
Gunshot wound	5	10
Stabbing	5	1
Struck	4	2
Beating	3	7
Motorcycle	1	4
Animal bite	1	<1
All-terrain vehicle/ recreational vehicle	1	2
Other	5	7

(From DiScala C, Brooke MM, Barlow B, et al: National Pediatric Trauma Registry Biannual Report. Boston, Tufts University Rehabilitation and Childhood Trauma Research and Training Center, 1993.)

tude of vertical displacement.[17, 18] Bicycle-related trauma may include closed head injury after an unprotected fall from a moving bicycle or upper abdominal visceral injury associated with a fall against the handlebars.[19, 20] Abuse-related injuries, when severe enough to warrant trauma care, typically involve the head, skeleton, and soft tissues; injuries to intrathoracic and intra-abdominal organs, which are less common, are confined chiefly to the chest wall and upper abdominal viscera and present with characteristic patterns that are both diagnostic and prognostic of mortality.[21]

Anatomic and Physiologic Considerations

Many factors render a child vulnerable to these types of injuries. A child's head is proportionately larger than an adult's (thus ensuring that whenever a child is struck by or thrown from a moving car or falls from a height or a moving bicycle, he or she will land head first), and the bones of the head are softer (allowing forces of impact to be transmitted directly to the brain). The cervical spine is more flexible (accounting for a lower incidence of vertebral injury but, paradoxically, a similar incidence of spinal cord injury), and the axial skeleton is weaker (accounting for a higher incidence of long-bone fractures). Together, these factors—especially a child's more cephalad center of gravity—explain the relatively greater importance of the central neuraxis in the epidemiology, pathology, and physiology of major pediatric trauma (Table 159–4).[6] Indeed, given the poorer protection afforded to the internal organs by the truncal wall, intrathoracic and intra-abdominal injuries are surprisingly infrequent in childhood.[7]

Children are also subject to a distinctive pattern of traumatic brain injury, the leading cause of mortality and morbidity in pediatric trauma.[6] Diffuse brain injuries, particularly (1) cerebral swelling associated with the loss of cerebral pressure autoregulation, which may result from both severe impact and cerebral anoxia (and is associated with cerebral arteriolar vasomotor paralysis, increased cerebral blood volume, and increased intracranial pressure), and (2) axonal (white matter) shearing associated with marked deceleration injuries (such as violent shaking), are far more common in childhood than in later years. In contrast, although focal areas of cerebral (gray matter) contusion or laceration may occur (in a coup-contrecoup pattern) adjacent to bony prominences after concussive injuries (typically in the frontal and temporal lobes), major intracranial hemorrhage (epidural, subdural, and intracerebral hematomas) is uncommon and often is of insufficient volume to warrant surgical evacuation. Still, it must be noted that subdural hematomas in infants, in the absence of a history suggestive of traumatic injury, may be indicative of child abuse (particularly when associated with retinal hemorrhages) and commonly result from tearing of the bridging meningeal veins that may be associated with the whiplash shaken impact syndrome.[22]

Cervical spine injury is an uncommon event in pediatric trauma, occurring at a rate of 1.8 per 100,000 population,[23] in contrast to closed head injury, which occurs at a rate of 185 per 100,000 population.[24] When cervical spine injury does occur, it is more frequent at levels (C-2, C-1, and the occipitoatlantal junction) above those whose nerve roots give rise to diaphragmatic innervation (C-4), predisposing

TABLE 159–4. Frequency and Mortality of Injuries in Major Pediatric Trauma

By Body Region	Frequency (%)	Mortality (%)
Multiple	43	5
Extremities	20	0
Head and neck	18	5
External	12	0
Abdomen	3	1
Face	2	0
Thorax	1	3
By Anatomic Diagnosis	***Frequency (%)***	***Mortality (%)***
Head injury	29	*
Fracture	23	*
Open wound	16	*
Superficial wound	11	*
Contusion	8	*
Thoracic/abdominal injury	8	*
Spine injury	2	*
Other	5	*

(From DiScala C, Brooke MM, Barlow B, et al: National Pediatric Trauma Registry Biannual Report. Boston, Tufts University Rehabilitation and Childhood Trauma Research and Training Center, 1993.)

*Cannot be accurately determined, because there are 77,480 diagnoses among the 32,574 patients enrolled in NPTR-2 as of October 1993.

children to respiratory arrest as well as paralysis. The increased momentum produced by the proportionately larger head of a child, the greater elasticity of the spinal ligaments, and the more horizontal apposition of the cervical vertebrae appear largely responsible for this somewhat different spectrum of injuries: "locking" of the lower cervical vertebrae is quite rare, whereas subluxation (with or without dislocation) and odontoid fractures are more common. Subluxation without dislocation (spinal cord injury without radiographic abnormality) may be caused by either lateral shearing or axial stretching and accounts for as many as 20% of pediatric spinal cord injuries,[25, 26] as well as a large number of prehospital deaths that were previously attributed to head trauma itself.[27]

Chest injuries also pose special problems in childhood, because the plasticity of the cartilaginous ribs allows impacting forces to be transmitted directly to underlying intrathoracic structures. It is not uncommon for children to sustain pulmonary or myocardial contusions without rib fractures or external signs of trauma such as ecchymoses or petechiae. However, although less likely to sustain rib fractures, a child is at greater risk of ventilatory and circulatory compromise both from tension pneumohemothorax (the most common immediately life-threatening chest injury) and from large posterior flail segments, owing to the greater mobility of the mediastinum in childhood. Moreover, a child's ability to compensate for such respiratory derangements is limited by (1) larger oxygen consumption but smaller functional reserve capacity (which make a child more susceptible to hypoxia), (2) lesser pulmonary compliance yet greater chest wall compliance (which dictate a chiefly tachypneic response to hypoxia), and (3) horizontally aligned ribs and rudimentary intercostal musculature (which make a small child a diaphragmatic breather).

Abdominal injuries also are different in childhood. The overall smaller size of the abdomen predisposes a child to multiple rather than single injuries as energy is dissipated from a blunt force. The flexible ribs cover only the uppermost portion of the abdomen, and the thinner abdominal wall provides little protection to the proportionately larger solid organs of the upper abdomen. These facts account for the higher incidence of upper abdominal injuries observed in children, including those to the pancreas (traumatic pancreatitis and pancreatic pseudocyst)[7]; however, the capsules of the other solid upper abdominal viscera (liver, spleen, and kidneys) are thicker and more elastic, leading to a lower incidence of shattering injuries and a higher rate of spontaneous cessation of bleeding, hence a greater reliance on nonoperative management.[28–30] Finally, acute gastric dilatation due to air swallowing is also more common in childhood,[31] predisposing a child to significant ventilatory and circulatory compromise by (1) limiting diaphragmatic motion, (2) increasing risk of aspiration, and (3) causing vagally mediated dampening of the normal tachycardiac response to hypovolemia.

Bone injuries, too, vary from the typical adult pattern. Because cortical bone in childhood is highly porous and easily disrupted and the periosteum is more elastic and vascular, the incidence of incomplete fractures (torus and greenstick fractures) and complete but nondisplaced fractures is higher. Other factors that make skeletal trauma in childhood unique include (1) a rapid rate of healing and freedom from non-union; (2) a tendency to remodel in the plane of the fracture, although not in the rotational plane; (3) a high incidence of ischemic vascular injuries, particularly about the elbow, which, even if they do not immediately threaten the limb, may cause disfiguring contracture; (4) a low incidence of associated ligamentous injuries; and (5) long-term growth disturbances associated both with fractures involving the physeal growth plate (undergrowth) and with fractures involving the diaphyses of long bones (overgrowth).[32] The most frequent long-bone injuries sustained by victims of major trauma are fractures of the femur and tibia associated with pedestrian motor vehicle trauma and the Waddell triad of injuries, underscoring the need for also carefully searching for head and torso injuries in any child who sustains a femur fracture on being struck by a moving vehicle. *Isolated* femur fractures in children are rarely if ever associated with significant blood loss: The average decline in hematocrit is only 3% and the maximum reduction about 6%, neither of which is sufficient to cause shock; thus, if signs of shock are present, a diligent search must be made for another source of bleeding, which is usually found in the abdomen.[33]

The most important difference between children and adults with respect to major trauma, however, relates to the airway. The pediatric airway is narrower at all levels and is more easily obstructed not only by mucus, blood, and particulate matter but also (owing to the larger tongue and smaller jaw) by a child's own soft tissues—especially when head trauma causes unconsciousness, leading to a loss of tone in the muscles of the head and neck. In this way, a relatively mild primary brain injury is converted to a far more damaging secondary brain injury, as the hypoxia produced by soft-tissue obstruction of the upper airway (as the tongue and epiglottis fall across the laryngeal inlet) contributes to the loss of cerebral pressure autoregulation, leading to the vicious downward spiral of diffuse cerebral swelling, increased intracranial pressure, and uncal herniation. In short, major pediatric trauma is perhaps more a disorder of airway and breathing than of the circulation: Indeed, although shock often occurs in addition to respiratory insufficiency (to the marked detriment of the patient), only 8% of child trauma victims with significant mortality risk, as indicated by a Pediatric Trauma Score of 8 or less, are hypotensive.[34] Thus, critical care specialists must take into account the relative infrequency of hemodynamic versus neuroventilatory impairment (whether primary or secondary) in a child, adopting strategies that (1) promote aggressive resuscitation of the central nervous system and (2) prevent overzealous restoration of the circulating blood volume.

Among children who do present with significant hypovolemia, however, another key difference from adults is a child's ability to compensate for the physiologic derangements induced by hemorrhagic shock. The remarkable ability of a child to maintain afterload in the hypovolemic state by means of peripheral vasoconstriction (thereby maintaining perfusion of the core organs) leads to what has been called the "deceptive" presentation of shock in a pediatric patient: The child remains normotensive and appears well perfused until some 25% to 30% of circulating blood volume has been lost. This unique capacity to vigorously preserve hemodynamic stability comes at a high price, however, because anaerobic metabolism and lactic acidosis accompany diversion of blood flow from peripheral tissues, increasing work of breathing and decreasing myocardial contractility, ultimately limiting a child's ability to sustain this compensatory response for a prolonged period. This fact underscores an important caveat in pediatric trauma management: Because the severity of pediatric shock can easily be underestimated in the early stages, the diagnosis and treatment must be based on abnormalities in the physical signs of tissue perfusion, ahead of blood pressure. Hypotension (defined in children older than 1 year of age as systolic blood pressure $<$ [70 + twice the child's age in years]) is a late sign of shock in a child and implies that the compensatory mechanisms have already failed and that death of the child is imminent.

INITIAL MANAGEMENT

The approach to resuscitation of child trauma victims is similar to that for adults. Initial attention is directed to maintenance of the airway, breathing, and circulation, including control of bleeding and treatment of shock, and management of immediately life-threatening chest injuries. Initial assessment and management should be guided by consensus protocols.[35–37] However, it is also important that a qualified surgeon experienced in the management of childhood trauma be involved as early as possible in the course of the resuscitation, for two reasons: (1) The need for surgical management of pediatric trauma is great, despite the limited role of operative management in intracranial and intra-abdominal injuries[38]; and (2) the major iatrogenic causes of mortality in pediatric trauma, in addition to mismanagement of initial resuscitation, have been the failure to recognize internal bleeding (intracranial and intra-abdominal) in a timely manner (delaying needed operation)[39] and the failure to recognize that internal bleeding is not present (promoting dangerous overhydration).

Primary Survey and Resuscitation

High-concentration oxygen must be given to every trauma victim via a nonrebreathing mask (if the patient is alert and breathing spontaneously) or by means of assisted ventilation. Care should be taken to stabilize the cervical spine in the neutral position to prevent potential (re)injury to the cervical spinal cord[40]; this may require placing a thin layer of padding beneath the torso and extremities of a young child, whose prominent occiput may force the neck into slight flexion when positioned supine on a flat surface. Intubation and hyperventilation are required if the modified Glasgow[41] or Adelaide[42] Pediatric Coma Scale (developed and validated for use in infants and young children whose verbal abilities are limited) score is 8 or less (Tables 159–5 and 159–6). The oropharyngeal route is preferred for emergency intubation in pediatric patients. Needle or surgical cricothyrotomy is rarely required, because cervical spine injuries are uncommon and usually stable.

External hemorrhage is controlled next (by direct pressure), and life-threatening chest injuries (particularly tension pneumothorax) are treated or precluded (by the same methods used in adults). Venous access is then obtained using large-bore plastic cannulas at peripheral sites (or a bone marrow aspiration needle in the anterior tibial bone marrow of a young child in whom venous access cannot readily be obtained). Blood samples are sent for type and crossmatch, and hemodynamic status is carefully assessed. If simple hypovolemia (compensated shock) is present, lactated Ringer's solution (20 mL/kg) is infused as rapidly as possible and should be repeated if a child does not promptly stabilize; if frank hypotension (decompensated shock) is present or if a child responds poorly or transiently to crystalloid (40 mL/kg), packed red blood cells (10 mL/kg) should be given immediately (and repeated as necessary) and the child prepared for emergency operation. Neither military antishock trousers[43] nor resuscitative thoracotomy[44] appears advantageous in initial resuscitation, and neither is currently advocated for this purpose (although military antishock trousers may be useful for temporary control of retroperitineal hemorrhage in severe comminuted pelvic fractures,[45] and resuscitative thoractomy may be lifesaving in penetrating thoracic injuries and blunt aortic rupture).

TABLE 159–5. Adelaide Pediatric Coma Scale

Patient Characteristics	*Coded Value*
Eye opening	
Spontaneous	4
To speech	3
To pain	2
None	1
Best verbal response	
Oriented	5
Words	4
Vocal sounds	3
Cries	2
None	1
Best motor response	
Obeys commands	5
Localizes pain	4
Flexion to pain	3
Extension to pain	2
None	1
Total*	3–14
*Normal aggregate score	
0–6 months	9
6–12 months	11
1–2 years	12
2–5 years	13
>5 years	14

(Adapted from Simpson DA, Cockington RA, Hanieh A, et al: Head injuries in infants and young children: The value of the Paediatric Coma Scale. Childs Nerv Syst 1991; 7:185. Copyright Springer-Verlag, 1991.)

The primary survey and resuscitation phases of the trauma response are conducted concurrently. Once the airway has been secured, external bleeding has been controlled, immediately life-threatening chest injuries have been treated or precluded, and vascular access has been obtained, a nasogastric tube (or an orogastric tube, if severe facial trauma is present or a basilar skull fracture is suspected[46]) is inserted to relieve gastric dilatation. A Foley catheter is also inserted at this time, unless the child has been fully stabilized or catheter placement is contraindicated by the presence of blood at the meatus, discoloration of the scrotum, or displaced fractures of the pubic sym-

TABLE 159–6. Modified Glasgow Coma Scale

Patient Characteristics	*Coded Value*
Best motor response	
Obeys	6
Localizes	5
Withdraws	4
Abnormal flexion	3
Extensor response	2
Nil	1
Verbal response	
Oriented	5
Confused conversation	4
Inappropriate words	3
Incomprehensible sounds	2
Nil	1
Eye opening	
Spontaneous	4
To speech	3
To pain	2
Nil	1
Total	3–15

(From Bruce DA, Raphaely RC, Goldberg AI, et al: Pathophysiology, treatment and outcome following severe head injury in children. Childs Brain 1979; 5:174–191.)

physis. Ongoing administration of fluid or blood is guided by hemodynamic response to initial therapy: In children with evidence of active hemorrhage, sufficient blood should be given to maintain a hematocrit of 30% in preparation for emergency operation; in children who rapidly stabilize, fluid should be titrated to maintain a urine output of 1 $mL \cdot kg^{-1} \cdot h^{-1}$ (2 $mL \cdot kg^{-1} \cdot h^{-1}$ in infants or if myoglobinuria is present), and transfusion withheld unless the hematocrit drifts below 20%.

Adequate circulating blood volume has been achieved when blood pressure has returned to normal (defined in children older than 1 year of age as systolic blood pressure = [90 + twice the child's age in years]) and no signs of inadequate peripheral perfusion are present. If a child fails to improve despite seemingly adequate initial volume resuscitation and there are no signs to suggest intra-abdominal or pelvic bleeding, other forms of shock must be considered, particularly obstructive shock due to missed tension pneumothorax. Such conditions must be treated if found. Still, most children in decompensated (hypotensive) shock are victims of unrecognized hemorrhage, which can be reversed only if promptly recognized and appropriately treated by means of rapid transfusion and immediate surgical intervention.

Secondary Survey and Evaluation

Once primary assessment has been completed and resuscitation is well under way, secondary assessment should be undertaken. To be sure no injuries escape detection, this must include both complete exposure of the patient and logrolling, especially with penetrating trauma; however, special care must be taken with a child, whose ratio of body surface area to mass is larger than in an adult, to avoid the development of hypothermia. A careful head-to-toe examination, as for an adult, is the cornerstone of this phase of the trauma response and addresses all organ systems; it includes appropriate laboratory and radiologic examinations. Features unique to child trauma victims are emphasized next.

PHYSICAL ASSESSMENT. Immediate loss of consciousness is usual in diffuse axonal shearing; progressive but rapid deterioration is suggestive of diffuse cerebral swelling. Cervical spine tenderness, swelling, spasm, and torticollis are suggestive of vertebral injury, but their absence does not preclude associated spinal cord trauma; the doll's-eyes maneuver therefore should be avoided in examining a comatose child, even if a lateral cervical spine radiograph appears normal (because of the possibility of spinal cord injury without radiographic abnormality). Cold-water calorics may be used instead. Both upper abdominal distention due to unrelieved gastric dilatation and intercostal nerve injuries associated with lower rib fractures can mimic peritonitis. Most important, the absence of external signs does not rule out the presence of internal truncal injury.

LABORATORY EVALUATION. Serial hematocrit measurements provide an accurate estimate of the extent of ongoing blood loss, so long as hemodynamic stability is maintained. Serum transaminase[47] and amylase determinations may yield important clues with respect to contusions of the liver and spleen (which is contiguous with the tail of the pancreas). Urine that is grossly bloody or that contains more than 20 red blood cells per high-power field on microscopic examination suggests injury to the kidneys.[48] Hematuria is also a signal marker of injury severity, because significant injury to the fairly well-protected kidneys is associated with injury to other intra-abdominal organs in as many as 80% of cases.

RADIOLOGIC EXAMINATION. A lateral cervical spine radiograph cannot rule out spinal cord injury (thus is not a prerequisite to emergency intubation, which should proceed as indicated, taking appropriate spinal precautions), nor can it definitively preclude bony abnormality (particularly odontoid fracture, the most common cause of vertebral injury in childhood). Hence, it is not required as part of the initial evaluation of a comatose child. Likewise, skull radiographs are a poor marker of brain injury and need not be obtained as part of the initial evaluation of a comatose child unless a depressed skull fracture is suspected. Thus, computed tomographic (CT) scans of the head are usually the first imaging studies performed on a child who has sustained significant head injury (modified Glasgow or Adelaide Pediatric Coma Scale score ≤13, unconsciousness >5 min) or has signs of increased intracranial pressure (severe headache, drowsiness, vomiting) and should be repeated some 24 to 36 hours after admission for a child who remains comatose, to determine if a previously documented injury has progressed or a previously undocumented injury has appeared. CT scans of the cervical spine may be obtained concomitantly with scans of the head if vertebral injury is strongly suspected but also can miss odontoid fracture. Magnetic resonance imaging is reserved for late confirmation of diffuse cerebral white matter shearing and spinal cord injuries suspected on the basis of clinical examination, as well as for acute spinal cord injuries that have not been demonstrated using other radiologic techniques. Double-contrast CT scans of the abdomen (Table 159–7), including the lower chest, are obtained when signs suggest intra-abdominal bleeding, when shock in the field has responded to volume resuscitation, or when the mechanism of injury suggests that significant intra-abdominal injury may be present. However, no child should be taken to the radiography department if he or she is not hemodynamically stable or is not continuously monitored and attended by a physician capable of definitive management of the pediatric airway, particularly if sedatives or neuromuscular blocking agents are required to complete the examinations.

DIAGNOSTIC PERITONEAL LAVAGE. Most children with splenic and hepatic lacerations heal spontaneously without the need for laparotomy. Thus, diagnostic peritoneal lavage is rarely helpful in pediatric blunt abdominal trauma, because the need for laparotomy is determined not by the presence or absence of intraperitoneal blood but by the ongoing transfusion requirement. Its use is therefore reserved for patients who are unconscious or about to undergo general anesthesia for operative treatment of intracranial or musculoskeletal injuries. It also has no place in the management of hemodynamically unstable patients who require laparotomy, adding little to what is already known and

TABLE 159–7. Doses of Contrast Agents for Computed Tomography of Abdomen

Intravenous Contrast	*Oral Contrast*
Meglumine diatrizoate (Hypaque), 60%	Diatrizoate sodium (Hypaque), 1.5%
A rapid IV bolus:	PO or via NG tube:
0–9 y, 2 mL/kg	0–2 y, 60 mL
>9 y, 50 mL (followed by 50–100 mL IV infusion)	3–5 y, 120 mL
	6–9 y, 180 mL
	>9 y, 300–400 mL

(Adapted by permission from Kane NM, Cronan JJ, Dorfman GS, et al: Pediatric abdominal trauma: Evaluation by computed tomography. Pediatrics 1988; 82:11–15.)

serving only to delay definitive operation.[49] It is occasionally useful for diagnosis of hollow visceral injury.[50]

ACUTE MANAGEMENT

The overall morbidity and mortality of major pediatric trauma are closely linked with the functional outcome of the brain injury that typically occurs after significant blunt impact. Fortunately, the results of treatment of severe closed head trauma are decidedly better in children than in adults.[24, 51, 52] This advantage is ablated if associated injuries are severe enough to cause hypotension, but most children with severe closed head trauma do not have such injuries. Thus, optimal resuscitation of the injured brain is the primary goal of all phases of initial pediatric trauma management—in the field, in transport, in the emergency department, in the operating room, and especially in the ICU—and takes precedence over all but exsanguinating hemorrhage.

With the exception of the soft-tissue upper-airway obstruction that accompanies head injury severe enough to produce coma (discussed earlier), most instances of respiratory insufficiency are due to injuries of the upper airway or chest. Similarly, most instances of decompensated (hypotensive) shock observed in children, in the absence of tension pneumothorax (which causes both respiratory insufficiency and shock), are due to intra-abdominal bleeding, major pelvic fractures, or spinal cord trauma. Most children with major blunt trauma can initially be managed by nonoperative means. However, "nonoperative" does not mean "nonsurgical," because, as in appendicitis, mature surgical judgment is needed to determine whether or when operation may be required and, if so, what type of operation should be performed.[53] Definitive treatment of commonly encountered pediatric injuries is summarized next.

Head

Acute collections of epidural or subdural blood of sufficient size to cause mass effect require immediate surgical evacuation. Closed linear skull fractures are managed expectantly; open fractures and depressed fractures that invade the cranial vault by a distance equal to the thickness of the adjacent calavarium require intravenous antibiotics and operative treatment. Basilar skull fractures should be suspected on the basis of clinical signs (raccoon eyes, the Battle sign, hemotympanum, cerebrospinal fluid rhinorrhea or otorrhea), because radiographic studies are rarely diagnostic. Antibiotics should not be given to patients with cerebrospinal fluid leaks, however, unless fever develops, and operative control of cerebrospinal fluid leaks is required only for children whose drainage does not cease spontaneously within 2 to 3 weeks. Concussions, which in young children may be heralded by impact seizures rather than loss of consciousness, require no specific treatment unless the level of consciousness is persistently altered. Impact seizures also require no specific treatment unless they persist, but they do not usually occur in the absence of significant anatomic injury and therefore serve as a marker of serious intracranial pathology (see Chapter 172).

Spinal Cord

The cervical region is most frequently affected, with 50% of affected patients dying before reaching the hospital or during hospitalization. Of the remainder, most remain disabled with little hope of recovery, despite recent preliminary evidence that high-dose methylprednisolone (30 $mg \cdot kg^{-1} \cdot 15\ min^{-1}$ loading dose followed by 5.4 $mg \cdot kg^{-1} \cdot h^{-1}$ constant infusion) given immediately on recognition of injury may hold some promise in mitigating the effects of the primary injury.[54] The primary injury is responsible for most of the morbidity, but secondary injury may occur if the head and neck are not properly stabilized in the neutral position (discussed earlier), for which both a semi-rigid extrication collar and a commercially available head immobilizer are required. In addition to high-dose methylprednisolone, acute care of spinal cord injury focuses on treatment of neurogenic shock, which typically is present in both spinal shock (reversible) and frank spinal cord disruption (irreversible). Associated fractures to vertebral structures anterior to the spinal cord, which usually are stable, are treated by continuous immobilization until full healing occurs. Fractures to vertebral pedicles and facet joints are usually unstable and are treated by mild skeletal traction using Gardner-Wells tongs, followed by surgical fusion of damaged vertebrae. Both anterior and posterior fractures may escape detection until a full cervical spine series (anteroposterior, lateral, and odontoid views) is obtained and hence cannot be presumed absent until definitively precluded by appropriate radiologic studies (properly supervised flexion-extension views, fluoroscopy, radionuclide scan, or magnetic resonance imaging), particularly if clinical signs of vertebral injury are present (discussed earlier).

Chest

Most chest injuries can be managed expectantly or by means of tube thoracostomy; in the latter case, care should be taken to create a tunnel of adequate length, because a child's thin chest wall provides an ineffective seal around the catheter. However, despite the lower incidence of rib fractures and higher incidence of pulmonary contusions that are also associated with the thinner chest wall in children than in adults, truly life-threatening pulmonary contusions are encountered infrequently in childhood. Adult respiratory distress syndrome, or post-traumatic pulmonary insufficiency, may be encountered when pulmonary contusion is complicated by gastric aspiration or initial resuscitation is complicated by overhydration; the role of corticosteroids in the management of this syndrome is of no proven benefit and may worsen the outcome of patients with gastric aspiration, but extracorporeal membrane oxygenation may hold some promise in the treatment of this condition.[55] Finally, a higher incidence of traumatic asphyxia is also observed in children than in adults. Although no treatment is required other than supportive care, traumatic asphyxia reflects the extreme severity of blunt forces applied to the chest and mandates an especially thorough search for intrathoracic injury.

Abdomen

Acute management of intra-abdominal and genitourinary injuries in children is chiefly nonoperative; injuries requiring operation, however, are treated as in adults. Bleeding from hepatic and splenic injuries is mostly self-limited, laparotomy being reserved for instances when a patient presents in decompensated (hypotensive) shock or the transfusion requirement exceeds 40 mL/kg of body weight (half the circulating blood volume) within 24 hours of injury. Laparotomy for management of renal, pancreatic, gastrointestinal, and genitourinary injuries is performed as indicated (Table 159–8). Pancreatic pseudocyst occurs with greater frequency in children than in adults and is heralded by the development of a tender epigastric mass 3 to 5 days after upper abdominal trauma; patients who develop pan-

TABLE 159–8. Indications for Early Operation in Pediatric Abdominal Trauma

Blunt
Hemodynamic instability despite adequate volume resuscitation
Transfusion requirement >50% of estimated blood volume
Physical signs of peritonitis
Endoscopic evidence of rectal tear
Radiologic evidence of intraperitoneal or retroperitoneal gas
Radiologic evidence of gastrointestinal perforation
Radiologic evidence of intraperitoneal bladder rupture
Radiologic evidence of renovascular pedicle injury
Radiologic evidence of pancreatic transection
Bile, bacteria, stool, or >500 WBCs/mm^3 on peritoneal lavage

Penetrating
All gunshot wounds
All stab wounds associated with evisceration; blood in stomach, urine, or rectum; physical signs of shock or peritonitis; radiologic evidence of intraperitoneal or retroperitoneal gas
All suspected thoracoabdominal injuries (unless precluded by laparoscopy or thoracoscopy)
Bile, bacteria, stool, or >500 WBCs/mm^3 on peritoneal lavage

Abbreviation: WBCs = white blood cells.

creatic pseudocysts require 6 to 8 weeks of complete bowel rest and total parenteral nutrition in preparation for a surgical drainage procedure.

Skeleton

Long-bone fractures are rarely life threatening, and the general care of a patient takes precedence; however, early stabilization serves both to decrease a patient's discomfort and to limit the amount of blood loss. Closed treatment predominates for fractures of the clavicle, upper extremity, tibia, and femur (in infants and toddlers); fractures of the femur increasingly involve the use of external fixation (in school-age children) and intramedullary rods (in adolescents). Operative treatment is required for open fractures (for debridement and irrigation), displaced supracondylar fractures (because of their association with ischemic vascular injury), and major or displaced physeal fractures (which must be reduced anatomically). Fortunately, owing to the ability of most long-bone fractures in children to remodel, reductions need not be perfectly anatomic. Remodeling is limited in torus and greenstick fractures, because the hyperemia typical of complete fractures is unlikely to occur.

Penetrating Injuries

Penetrating injuries in children are being encountered in ever greater numbers. Management by experienced surgeons is required, and all such children should be referred to a trauma center with pediatric capabilities if available. All penetrating wounds must be treated as infected; once swelling has subsided, accessible missile fragments—particularly those in contact with cerebrospinal or joint fluid—should be removed to prevent the subsequent development of lead posioning.[56] Early involvement of social services, psychiatric support, and responsible law enforcement and child welfare agencies is mandatory; the initial history is rarely accurate when injuries are nonaccidental.

INTENSIVE CARE

Critical management of specific injuries depends on the type, extent, and severity of these injuries. In unstable patients, surgical intervention usually precedes ICU admission, whereas in stable patients, definitive therapy is directed by the appropriate specialist(s) after ICU admission. Children who have head, chest, abdominal, or skeletal injuries and who present in coma, respiratory insufficiency, or shock or who require ongoing resuscitation should be admitted to the ICU for further treatment, whether or not operation is first performed. Such children should receive no oral intake (because of the temporary paralytic ileus that often accompanies blunt abdominal trauma and in case general anesthesia should later be required) and, assuming both normal hydration and hemodynamic stability, should receive intravenous fluids at the maintenance rate (Table 159–9), except in cases of brain or solid abdominal visceral injury (discussed later). Intravenous lines inserted in the field and in the emergency department should be replaced to prevent the development of septic complications.

An important goal of critical care management, once physiologic stability is achieved, is avoidance of further deterioration, and monitoring must be designed to warn the critical care team of impending deterioration. For children with potential respiratory insufficiency, this should include frequent determination of vital signs, continuous measurement of arterial oxygen saturation, and measurement of arterial blood gases (as needed). For children with potential circulatory embarrassment, it should include frequent examination for signs of tissue hypoperfusion; ongoing measurement of systolic, diastolic, and mean blood pressure; and, if necessary, determination of central venous or pulmonary artery pressure. Similarly, urinary output and the volume of external losses of blood or fluid (particularly intrathoracic hemorrhage) should be recorded hourly, and abdominal girth (at the level of the umbilicus) should be recorded hourly if there is any question about intra-abdominal hemorrhage. Critical care management of specific injuries is discussed next.

Head

The functional status of the central neuraxis is the primary determinant of outcome after pediatric trauma. Thus, acute care of head injury should constitute the main focus of ICU management. The general principles of ICU management of traumatic brain injury in children and adults are the same; however, because diffuse brain injuries are more common in children than in adults, the emphasis in treatment is nonoperative. Surgically remediable causes of increased intracranial pressure must be aggressively treated if found, just as in adults; otherwise, treatment is directed at mitigating the effects of the increased intracranial pressure so commonly associated with traumatic brain injury in children while ensuring that ventilation, oxygenation, and perfusion are maintained. Other medically remediable complications of severe head trauma, such as the syndrome of inappropriate antidiuretic hormone secretion and severe hypoglycemia, must also be aggressively treated if found, again as in adults. The details of management of increased intracranial pressure are discussed in Chapter 172.

TABLE 159–9. Maintenance Fluid Requirements in Children

Body Weight	*Daily Fluid Requirement*
0–10 kg	100 mL/kg
10–20 kg	1000 mL (first 10 kg) + 50 mL/kg (10–20 kg)
>20 kg	1500 mL (first 20 kg) + 20 mL/kg (>20 kg)

(From Holliday MA, Segar WE: Maintenance need for water in parenteral fluid therapy. Pediatrics 1957; 19:823–832.)

Spinal Cord

ICU management of patients with spinal cord injuries is chiefly supportive. Patients with associated vertebral injury are treated as indicated (discussed earlier); those with definite or suspected spinal cord injury should continue to receive high-dose methylprednisolone, together with prophylactic antacid therapy (discussed later), until neurologic function has stabilized. Patients with documented spinal cord injuries, complete or partial, should be cared for on alternating-pressure or air-fluidizing mattresses to prevent the development of decubitus ulcers. Those with neurogenic bladders require an indwelling Foley catheter, followed by clean intermittent catheterization once stable, to prevent the development of urinary stasis and subsequent infection of the upper tracts. Finally, patients with quadriplegia or paraplegia at the midthoracic level or above are subject to pulmonary infections secondary to paralysis of the intercostal muscles. Such conditions also contraindicate the use of depolarizing neuromuscular blocking agents such as succinylcholine, owing to denervation hyperkalemia, which first appears 3 days after injury and may persist for as long as 1 year.

Chest

Definitive management of the respiratory insufficiency that accompanies severe chest injury is expectant. The least amount of artificial respiratory support necessary to maintain the arterial partial pressure of oxygen at 70 to 80 mm Hg is used to minimize the effects of oxygen toxicity and retard the development of resorption atelectasis. Continuous positive airway pressure or positive end-expiratory pressure should be used for maintenance of arterial oxygen tension and functional residual capacity whenever the fraction of inspired oxygen exceeds 40%, but adverse effects of positive end-expiratory pressure on the circulation must be avoided. If fresh bronchial or pulmonary suture lines or pneumothoraces are present, special efforts should be made to keep the peak inspiratory pressure below 20 to 25 cm H_2O when positive-pressure ventilation must be used. Naturally, spontaneous ventilation is preferred, and extubation should be accomplished as soon as it is feasible. Pulmonary contusions can be expected to resolve spontaneously within 7 to 10 days. Adult respiratory distress syndrome is best avoided and the effects of neurogenic pulmonary edema (when present) mitigated through the judicious use of crystalloid fluid and appropriate diuresis as indicated. Indications for early thoracotomy include ongoing hemorrhage (in excess of 2 to 4 $mL \cdot kg^{-1} \cdot h^{-1}$ from the chest tube) and massive air leak; indications for late thoracotomy include trapped lung and persistent air leak.

Abdomen

Nonoperative treatment of hemodynamically stable children with lacerations of the solid viscera of the upper abdomen requires a minimum of 7 to 10 days of strict bed rest, the first 1 to 3 days of which should be spent in the ICU. If respiratory care is required, incentive spirometry is preferred, because clots that are organizing may be disturbed by vigorous chest physiotherapy. During this interval, excessive palpation of the abdomen should be avoided. Antipneumococcal vaccine should be given if the spleen is disrupted (as well as penicillin prophylaxis if splenectomy is performed to prevent overwhelming postsplenectomy infection). The stomach should be kept decompressed to prevent reactivation of splenic bleeding due to stretching of the short gastric vessels that can accompany gastric dilatation. Serial hematocrit values should be measured regularly until stable, and elevated serum enzyme levels and urinalysis that is positive for blood or myoglobin should be rechecked at intervals until normal. A repeat CT scan should be obtained before hospital discharge, to document the progress of healing in injuries that are severe. Dilutional coagulopathies should be anticipated when the tranfusion requirement exceeds 80 mL/kg (the equivalent of one entire circulating blood volume); they may be prevented through early and effective control of intra-abdominal bleeding (discussed earlier). Administration of platelet concentrates, fresh frozen plasma, and intravenous calcium supplements should be guided by the results of the platelet count, the partial thromboplastin time, and the ionized calcium level.

Skeleton

Initial ICU care of skeletal injuries consists of careful immobilization and, in extremity fractures, serial observation for signs of neurovascular compromise. Fracture-associated arterial insufficiency is recognized by the presence of a pulse deficit, but detection of compartment syndromes may require measurement of tissue pulp pressure. Fasciotomy is indicated when this pressure exceeds 40 cm H_2O. Traumatic fat embolism secondary to long-bone fracture and rhabdomyolysis as a sequela of severe crush injury, though rare, can be associated with major pediatric trauma; supportive treatment of both conditions is indicated. Ongoing ICU care of skeletal injuries should focus on prevention of friction burns and bed sores and early provision of rehabilitative services.

Somatic Support

Long-term ICU treatment of children with major injuries also involves nutritional support, of nitrogen perhaps more than energy, and, in patients who are not eating, antacid therapy using both topical and systemic agents to avoid gastric stress ulcer bleeding. Children with hematomas of the liver, spleen, or pelvis may develop low-grade fever as these are resorbed; however, high spiking temperatures should occasion a search for a fever source, such as infected hematomas or effusions or pelvic osteomyelitis. Children with large retroperitoneal hematomas due to pelvic fractures may develop hypertension on rare occasions, presumably as a result of pressure on the renal vessels. The condition may require temporary use of antihypertensive agents but invariably resolves without the need for surgical decompression. Children with chest tubes or long-term indwelling Foley catheters are at risk for systemic infection and should receive prophylactic or suppressive antibiotics as long as the tube is required. Multiple organ system failure is a rare complication of major pediatric trauma, and use of enteral feedings to preserve the integrity of the gut mucosal barrier may be preventive.

Psychic Support

Efforts must also be made to attend to the emotional needs of injured children and their families. In addition to loss of control over their child's destiny, parents of seriously injured children may also feel enormous guilt, whether or not these feelings are warranted. Critical care providers should therefore attempt to create as normal an environment as possible for children and allow parents to participate meaningfully in ICU care. In so doing, critical interventions are facilitated because children perceive that parents and providers are working together to ensure an optimal recovery.

Interhospital Transport

Pediatric victims of multisystem trauma should undergo direct primary transport from the injury scene to a trauma center with pediatric critical care capabilities. If this proves impossible, secondary transport from the initial receiving hospital to the pediatric trauma center may be necessary. Transport providers must, at a minimum, be capable of critical pediatric assessment and monitoring and must be highly skilled in the techniques of pediatric endotracheal intubation and vascular access, as well as fluid and drug administration in critically ill and injured children.[57, 58] Whenever possible, therefore, interhospital transport of such patients should be conducted by specialized pediatric transport teams staffed by physicians and nurses with special training in pediatric critical care treatment and transport.[59, 60]

References

1. Cooper A, Barlow B, Davidson L, et al: Epidemiology of pediatric trauma: Importance of population-based statistics. J Pediatr Surg 1992; 27:149–154.
2. Graves EJ: Detailed Diagnoses and Procedures, National Hospital Discharge Survey, 1989. Vital Health Stat [13] 1991; 108:1–236.
3. Klem SA, Pollack MM, Glass NL, et al: Resource use, efficiency, and outcome prediction in pediatric intensive care of trauma patients. J Trauma 1990; 30:32–36.
4. Pollack MM, Alexander SR, Clarke N, et al: Improved outcomes from tertiary center pediatric intensive care: A statewide comparison of tertiary and nontertiary facilities. Crit Care Med 1991; 19:150–159.
5. DiScala C, Brooke MM, Barlow B, et al: National Pediatric Trauma Registry Biannual Report. Boston, Tufts University Rehabilitation and Childhood Trauma Research and Training Center, 1993.
6. Tepas JJ, DiScala C, Ramenofsky ML, et al: Mortality and head injury: The pediatric perspective. J Pediatr Surg 1990; 25:92–96.
7. Cooper A, Barlow B, DiScala C, et al: Mortality and truncal injury: The pediatric perspective. J Pediatr Surg 1994; 29:33–38.
8. Nakayama DK, Copes WS, Sacco W: Differences in trauma care among pediatric and nonpediatric trauma centers. J Pediatr Surg 1992; 27:427–431.
9. Hall JR, Reyes HM, Meller JL, et al: Traumatic death in urban children, revisited. Am J Dis Child 1993; 147:102–107.
10. Cooper A, Barlow B, DiScala C, et al: Efficacy of pediatric trauma care: Results of a population-based study. J Pediatr Surg 1993; 28:299–305.
11. Tepas JJ, Ramenofsky ML, Mollitt DL, et al: The pediatric trauma score as a predictor of injury severity: An objective assessment. J Trauma 1988; 28:425–429.
12. Kaufmann CR, Maier RV, Rivara FP, et al: Evaluation of the pediatric trauma score. JAMA 1990; 263:69–72.
13. American College of Surgeons Committee on Trauma: Resources for Optimal Care of the Injured Patient: 1993. Chicago, American College of Surgeons, 1993, pp 19–23.
14. Harris BH, Barlow BA, Ballantine TV, et al: American Pediatric Surgical Association: Principles of pediatric trauma care. J Pediatr Surg 1992; 27:423–426.
15. Christoffel KK, Tanz R: Motor vehicle injury in childhood. Pediatr Rev 1983; 4:247–254.
16. Newman KD, Bowman LM, Eichelberger MR: The lap belt complex: Intestinal and lumbar spine injury in children. J Trauma 1990; 30:1133–1140.
17. Barlow B, Niemirska M, Gandhi R: Ten years of experience with falls from a height in children. J Pediatr Surg 1983; 18:509–511.
18. Roshkow JE, Haller JO, Hotson GC, et al: Imaging evaluation of children after falls from a height: Review of 45 cases. Radiology 1990; 175:359–363.
19. Selbst SM, Alexander D, Ruddy R: Bicycle-related injuries. Am J Dis Child 1987; 141:140–144.
20. Sparnon AL, Ford WDA: Bicycle handlebar injuries in children. J Pediatr Surg 1986; 21:118–119.
21. Cooper A, Floyd T, Barlow B, et al: Major blunt abdominal trauma due to child abuse. J Trauma 1988; 28:1483–1486.
22. Duhaime AC, Gennarelli TA, Thibault LE, et al: The shaken baby syndrome: A clinical, pathological and biomechanical study. J Neurosurg 1987; 66:409–415.
23. Kewalramani LS, Kraus JF, Sterling HM: Acute spinal-cord lesions in a pediatric population: Epidemiological and clinical features. Paraplegia 1980; 18:206–219.
24. Kraus JF, Fife D, Cox P: Incidence, severity and external causes of pediatric brain injury. Am J Dis Child 1986; 140:687–693.
25. Sneed RC, Stover SL: Undiagnosed spinal cord injuries in brain-injured children. Am J Dis Child 1988; 142:965–967.
26. Dachling P, Pollack IF: Spinal cord injury without radiographic abnormality in children—the SCIWORA syndrome. J Trauma 1989; 29:654–664.
27. Bohn D, Armstrong A, Becker L, et al: Cervical spine injuries in children. J Trauma 1990; 30:463–469.
28. Oldham KT, Guice KS, Ryckman F, et al: Blunt liver injury in childhood: Evolution of therapy and current perspective. Surgery 1986; 100:542–549.
29. Pearl RH, Wesson DE, Spence LJ, et al: Splenic injury: A 5-year update with improved results and changing criteria for conservative management. J Pediatr Surg 1989; 24:121–125.
30. Cosentino CM, Luck SR, Barthel MJ, et al: Transfusion requirements in conservative nonoperative management of blunt splenic and hepatic injuries during childhood. J Pediatr Surg 1990; 25:950–954.
31. Cogbill TH, Bintz M, Johnson JA, et al: Acute gastric dilatation after trauma. J Trauma 1987; 27:1113–1117.
32. Rockwood CA, Wilkins KE, King RE (Eds): Fractures in Children. 3rd ed. Philadelphia, JB Lippincott, 1984.
33. Barlow B, Niemirska M, Gandhi R, et al: Response to injury in children with closed femur fractures. J Trauma 1987; 27:429–430.
34. Cooper A, Barlow B, DiScala C: Mortality and physiologic instability: The pediatric perspective. J Trauma (in press).
35. American College of Surgeons Committee on Trauma: Advanced Trauma Life Support Student Manual. 6th ed. Chicago, American College of Surgeons, 1992.
36. American Academy of Pediatrics and American College of Emergency Physicians Joint Task Force on Advanced Pediatric Life Support: Advanced Pediatric Life Support. 2nd ed. Elk Grove Village IL, and Dallas, American Academy of Pediatrics and American College of Emergency Physicians, 1993.
37. American Heart Association and American Academy of Pediatrics Working Group on Pediatric Resuscitation: Textbook of Pediatric Advanced Life Support. 2nd ed. Dallas, American Heart Association, 1994.
38. Kaufmann CR, Rivara FP, Maier RV: Pediatric trauma: Need for surgical management. J Trauma 1989; 29:1120–1126.
39. Dykes EH, Spence LJ, Young JG, et al: Preventable pediatric trauma deaths in a metropolitan region. J Pediatr Surg 1989; 24:107–111.
40. Herzenberg JE, Hensinger RN, Dedrick DK, et al: Emergency transport and positioning of young children who have an injury of the cervical spine. J Bone Joint Surg 1989; 71-A:15–22.
41. Bruce DA, Raphaely RC, Goldberg AI: Pathophysiology, treatment, and outcome following severe head injury in children. Childs Brain 1979; 5:174–191.
42. Simpson DA, Cockington RA, Hanieh A, et al: Head injuries in infants and young children: The value of the Paediatric Coma Scale. Childs Nerv Syst 1991; 7:183–190.
43. Cooper A, Barlow B, DiScala C, et al: Efficacy of MAST use in children who present in hypotensive shock (abstract). J Trauma 1992; 33:151.
44. Beaver BL, Colombani PM, Buck JR, et al: Efficacy of emergency room thoracotomy in pediatric trauma. J Pediatr Surg 1987; 22:19–23.
45. Garcia V, Eichelberger M, Ziegler M, et al: Use of military antishock trouser in a child. J Pediatr Surg 1981; 16:544–546.
46. Fletcher SA, Henderson LT, Miner ME, et al: The successful removal of intracranial nasogastric tubes. J Trauma 1987; 27:948–952.
47. Oldham KT, Guice KS, Kaufman RA, et al: Blunt hepatic injury and elevated hepatic enzymes: A clinical correlation in children. J Pediatr Surg 1984; 19:457–461.

48. Lieu TA, Fleisher GR, Mahboubi S, et al: Hematuria and clinical findings as indications for intravenous pyelography in pediatric blunt renal trauma. Pediatrics 1988; 82:216–222.
49. Powell RW, Green JB, Ochsner MG, et al: Peritoneal lavage in pediatric patients sustaining blunt abdominal trauma: A reappraisal. J Trauma 1987; 27:6–10.
50. Cobb LM, Vinocur CD, Wagner CW, et al: Intestinal perforation due to blunt trauma in children in an era of increased nonoperative treatment. J Trauma 1986; 26:461–463.
51. Kraus JF, Fife D, Conroy C: Pediatric brain injuries: The nature, clinical course, and early outcomes in a defined United States' population. Pediatrics 1987; 80:501–507.
52. Luerssen TG, Klauber MR, Marshall LF: Outcome from head injury related to the patient's age: A longitudinal prospective study of adult and pediatric head injury. J Neurosurg 1988; 68:409–416.
53. Haller JA: Emergency medical services for children: What is the pediatric surgeon's role? Pediatrics 1987; 79:576–581.
54. Bracken MB, Shepard MJ, Collins WF, et al: A randomized, controlled trial of methylprednisolone or naloxone in the treatment of acute spinal cord injury. N Engl J Med 1990; 322:1405–1411.
55. Weber TR, Tracy TF, Connors R, et al: Prolonged extracorporeal support for nonneonatal respiratory failure. J Pediatr Surg 1992; 27:1100–1105.
56. Selbst SM, Henretig F, Fee MA, et al: Lead poisoning in a child with a gunshot wound. Pediatrics 1986; 77:413–416.
57. Smith DF, Hackel A: Selection criteria for pediatric critical care transport teams. Crit Care Med 1983; 11:10–12.
58. MacNab AJ: Optimal escort for interhospital transport of pediatric emergencies. J Trauma 1991; 31:205–209.
59. American Academy of Pediatrics, Committee on Hospital Care: Guidelines for air and ground transportation of pediatric patients. Pediatrics 1986; 78:943–950.
60. Day S, McCloskey K, Orr R, et al: Pediatric interhospital critical care transport: Consensus of a national leadership conference. Pediatrics 1991; 88:696–704.

CHAPTER 160

Critical Care of Wounds and Wounded Patients

Thomas K. Hunt, MD • David D. Zabel, MD

For centuries, clinicians believed wound healing to be an immutable process that could, at best, be maintained at "normal" by attention to nutrition. Modern knowledge, however, reveals that healing is an amazingly complex collection of normal coping processes that is easily and commonly impaired and falls short of its full potential unless actively supported. The once heretical dream that clinicians might actually enhance wound healing over traditional expectations is now a fact. Nevertheless, unnecessary infections in wounds and failure to heal continue to occur because medical thought has not accommodated to the new knowledge.

The aims of this chapter are to outline the modern view of healing mechanisms and to point out how practitioners of intensive care medicine can protect and even enhance healing and resistance to bacterial infection.

THE NATURE OF REPAIR

Healing follows an intense disruption of the normal extracellular environment in which local blood perfusion is interrupted and, as a consequence, coagulation and inflammation are recruited. Eventually, healing forms a new circulation (angiogenesis) and with it a new extracellular matrix made mainly of collagen and proteoglycans. The end of normal wound healing coincides with restoration of a normal extracellular environment, but in some cases, repair may continue to the point of excessive scar. One must recognize at the onset that repair and resistance to infection in the wound site are complex, made up of redundant mechanisms and remarkably dependent first on circulatory factors and then on nutrition (Fig. 160–1).

Coagulation/Hemostasis

The first stimulus to wound healing is probably activation of tissue complement, which attracts polymorphonuclear leukocytes to defend against infection. The next stimulus emerges from the coagulation process. Hageman factor is activated. Thrombin (itself a mitogen and angiogenic stimulus) causes platelets to release platelet-derived growth factor, platelet factor 4 transforming growth factor-β (TGF-β), and insulin-like growth factor-1 (IGF-1), all of which stimulate fibroblast replication.[1] Polymerization of fibrinogen to fibrin is followed by fibrinolysis and release of peptides (particularly fibrinopeptide E) that are chemotactic mainly to monocytes. Fibrin itself activates monocytes to release cytokines. Macrophages also produce some of the growth factors found in platelets.[1–3] Plasmin, which digests the fibrin, also digests basement membranes of vessels, an event that is essential to angiogenesis.[4] Next follows a complex set of proteolytic events in which preexisting matrix is digested.

Coagulation, however useful, also exerts a price. When bleeding of cut vessels is ended by hemostasis, the local microvasculature is not only compromised by injury but is also clotted back to the nearest undamaged pathway for blood, thus further diminishing the vascular supply at the edge of the injury. Bruising or crushing trauma extensively injures the vascular supply and produces large volumes of ischemic tissue.

Inflammation

The initial cellular reaction is composed of polymorphonuclear leukocytes. A few days later, macrophages predominate. The polymorphonuclear cells contribute mainly to resistance to infection and matrix digestion. Their absence seriously impairs only resistance to infection. On the other hand, all forms of repair are severely impeded by the absence of monocytes, more specifically, tissue macrophages.[2, 3]

Macrophages, with some help from lymphocytes, release a number of so-called growth factors or cytokines* when stimulated by injured tissue, fibrin, foreign bodies, and especially the low oxygen and high lactate concentrations found in wounds. These substances, in turn, stimulate growth and migration of fibroblasts and endothelial cells.[4–6] The exact details are unknown, but TGF-β, interleukin-1, interleukin-6, interleukin-8, tumor necrosis factor-α (TNF-α), IGF-1,[7] and monocyte/macrophage-derived growth factor[8] have been traced to macrophages. With the addition of these substances and probably others like them, the local environment begins to encourage cell growth as well as to attract inflammatory cells, new fibroblasts, and endothelial cells into the conditioned area. Many of the growth factors are also *chemattractants*. Some of them, TNF and interleukin-1, for example, also serve as messengers to the liver and

*For present purposes, *growth factor* and *cytokine* are synonymous.

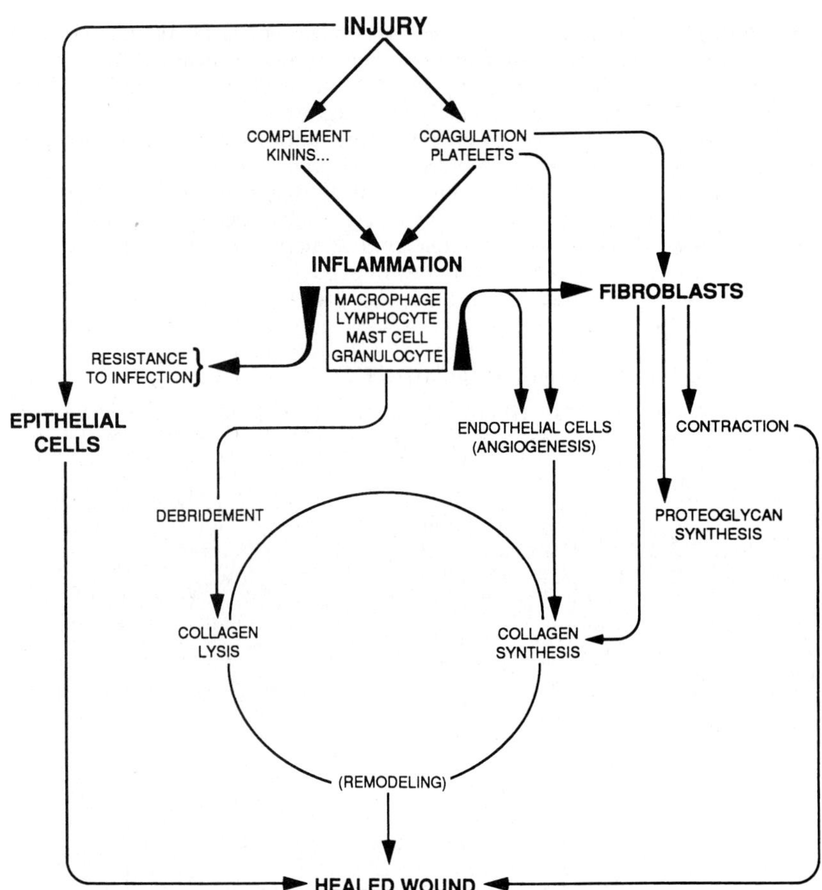

Figure 160–1. Schematic representation of wound healing. The mainstream of repair is an obligate sequence involving injury; coagulation/complement; inflammation; increased cell replication of fibroblasts, epithelium, and vascular endothelium; synthesis of extracellular protein and proteoglycans; the balance of collagen lysis and collagen synthesis; remodeling; and quiescence. (From Zabel DD, Hunt TK: Skin, peritoneum, and colonic healing processes. Perspect Colon Rectal Surg 1993; 6:191–224.)

other distant tissues to produce the so-called acute-phase response.

In what appears to be one of the key processes that define wound healing, granulocytes and macrophages are activated or "primed" on entering the wound space. Among other consequences of this event is the rapid conversion of molecular (dissolved) oxygen to superoxide, which is extremely important to resistance to infection. The net reaction (simplified) is as follows:

$$\text{Glucose} + O_2 \rightarrow O_2^- + \text{lactate} + H^+$$

The critical enzyme in this set of reactions is an NADPH-linked oxygenase. This is a central event in healing and accomplishes three important steps: (1) It contributes superoxide, which is essential to intraleukocytic killing of bacteria. (2) It consumes oxygen, and the resulting hypoxia later limits new matrix formation and leads to vulnerability to infection. (3) It produces lactate and stimulates collagen synthesis and angiogenesis (discussed later).

Macrophages and granulocytes also release proteolysins, including several collagenases. Ordinarily, this serves useful functions such as debridement of denatured tissue, remodeling of the new scar tissue so that it can acquire strength without undue mass, and assistance of angiogenesis. On the other hand, it will become clear later that the synthetic responses require hemodynamic and respiratory support whereas proteolysis has no such requirement. If the synthetic processes are delayed, these lytic enzymes can literally erode the new and surrounding normal tissues.

Fibroplasia

After a few days, under the intense stimulation of the wound environment, fibroblasts migrate in and multiply. They become the dominant cells at the wound edge, where they synthesize and deposit the collagen and proteoglycans, which eventually connect the edges of the wound and give it strength. Fibroblasts originate locally.[9]

Fibroblast replication rates are proportional to oxygen availability. The partial pressure of oxygen (Po_2) optimum is about 50 mm Hg. It will become apparent later that the Po_2 of the tissue at the edge of the wound space, where fibroblasts replicate and later function, is controlled by the rate of local perfusion and arterial Po_2 (Pao_2).

Neovascularization

Reparative cells cannot effectively replicate, resist infection, or deposit a new connective matrix without angiogenesis to replace the damaged vascular supply. New vessels in the form of blind-ended capillaries emerge from normal tissue moving toward the wound space, leaving behind a maturing circulation. All new vessels start as endothelial cell buds from venules that follow the lead of macrophages and fibroblasts.[10, 11] The original tight network of capillaries coalesces, and some vessels become as large as 3 to 5 mm in diameter in the final scar.[6, 12]

Neovascularization also follows the steep oxygen gradient that characterizes wounds. The major angiogenic stimulus in wounds is derived from macrophages, which produce one or more chemattractants, angiogenic polypeptide(s) when placed in a hyperlactated or hypoxic environment.[13, 14] Under experimental conditions, angiogenesis stops when the oxygen gradient is reversed.[15]

The Wound Module

By the end of the third or fourth day, full-thickness wounds have a characteristic cellular architecture.[16] A layer of macrophages surrounds the wound space. Beneath this is a layer of immature fibroblasts. Under these is a layer of replicating fibroblasts, which characteristically lie just on the injury side of the most distal functioning vessel and accompany the proliferating endothelial buds. Behind the budding vessels are mature fibroblasts and the earliest visible traces of scar collagen (Fig. 160–2).

This wound module advances into the wound space, drawn inward by products of activated macrophages, and supports its new vessels with new collagenous matrix. The vascular unit is best seen clinically in so-called cutting cones of healing fractures, in which osteoclasts (bone macrophages) literally cut through old bone, drawing endothelial cells behind them in order to meet vessels from the other side of the fracture.

Dead spaces, from which products of injury have long since disappeared, heal until filled. This happens for several reasons: First, immature vessels leak fibrin, which activates macrophages to produce growth and chemoattractant factors. Second, the growth of vessels follows the oxygen and lactate gradients (mentioned earlier). These elicit TNF-α, TGF-β, and interleukin-1 from macrophages, which in turn make more lactate in response to epidermal growth factor, IGF-1, and possibly others.[14, 17, 18] Healing continues until the new vessels unite with others, establish mature circulatory loops, stop leaking fibrin, and decrease the lactate gradient. As circulations unite, the oxygen and lactate gradients are obliterated. If foreign bodies, antigen-antibody complexes, infection, or other processes continue to elicit inflammation, the gradients do not disappear and healing continues—perhaps to excessive scarring.

Collagen Synthesis

The mechanical mainstay of repair in humans is regeneration of connective tissue. The strength of this connective tissue is based on collagen polymers, or fibers which in turn are composed of long, thin monomers in the form of triple helices measuring approximately 289 by 1.4 nm. Fibroblasts release the monomers into the extracellular space, where they polymerize and eventually literally glue the sides of the wound together.[9]

Assembly of the collagen monomer begins with synthesis of three alpha chains, which are long sequences of trimers with the basic structure of glycine-X-R, in which X is often proline, hydroxyproline, lysine, or hydroxylysine. The gene, however, does not code for hydroxylysine or hydroxyproline. Instead, some of its prolines and lysines are hydroxylated as each growing alpha chain comes off the polyribosome and is inserted into the endoplasmic reticulum.[19] These clinically significant reactions are catalyzed by prolyl and lysyl hydroxylase and require molecular oxygen, ferrous iron, ascorbic acid, and oxoglutarate. If a minimum number of prolines are not hydroxylated, the alpha chains cannot form the thermostable triple helix that characterizes the collagen monomer and therefore cannot be exported from the cell. If the triple helix fails to form, the alpha chains are instead degraded intracellularly. Without hydroxylysines, a later step in which the monomers cross-bind and provide strength to the final fiber cannot occur. The amount of oxygen that is available for these hydroxylations controls the rate at which collagen is deposited into the extracellular space and the rate at which wounds can support new vessels and gain strength.[20]

The major stimulus for collagen formation is closely related to the low oxidation-reduction potential in the healing area. This low potential is due largely to the high concentration of lactate that is contributed by leukocytes during *aerobic* glycolysis.[21] Lactate dihydroascorbate is the reduced form of ascorbate. It stimulates the formation of collagen-synthesizing enzymes and collagen synthesis in aerobic fibroblast cultures.[21] The mechanism is complex and depends

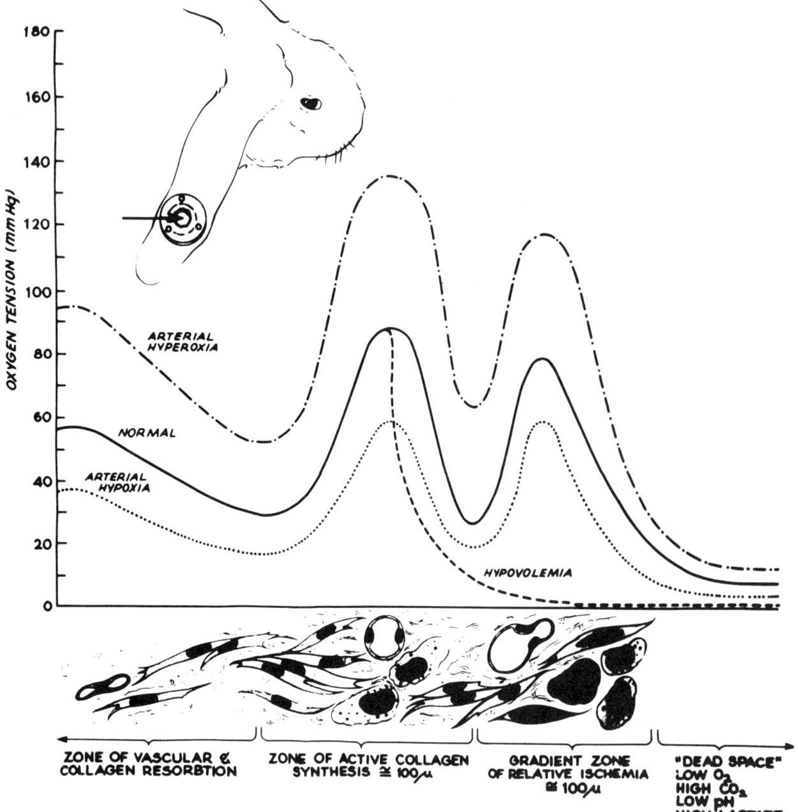

Figure 160–2. A schematic view of the cross-section of tissue growing into a rabbit's ear chamber. To make these chambers, a hole is made in the rabbit's ear, and the hole is sandwiched between glass and Teflon membranes. The diagram shows a cross-section of the tissue growing into the hole. Oxygen tension was measured with a microoxygen electrode. Note the peaks of oxygen tension over the functioning vessels and the important long gradient into the dead space. The cells abutting the dead space are macrophages. Just behind them are immature fibroblasts. Multiplying fibroblasts are always found at a PO_2 of 30 to 40 mm Hg. Behind the capillaries are more mature fibroblasts and fibrillar collagen. Ahead of the advancing capillary arcade is an antigenically but not morphologically identifiable collagen gel. Note that in hypovolemia, the most distal capillary usually closes down. As hypovolemia increases, the remainder of the capillaries closes down in sequence.

on the rate at which nicotinamide can be removed from the oxidized form of nicotinamide-adenine dinucleotide (NAD+) (*not* the reduced form [NADH]) to form adenosine diphosphoribose (ADPR). Various forms of ADPR normally suppress collagen gene expression and post-translational prolyl hydroxylation. However, when lactate accumulates, the NAD+ pool shrinks, the inhibitory ADPR is removed, collagen messenger ribonucleic acid production rises, and synthesis ensues.[21] Thereafter, the critical hydroxylations (similarly controlled by ADPR) that control export and depend on oxygen occur (Fig. 160–3).

Herein lies a critical point for clinical care that at first appears paradoxical. The mechanism for collagen synthesis and deposition relies on a low NAD+ (i.e., a low oxyredox potential). However, collagen deposition is critically dependent on Po_2. The paradox is resolved by the fact that the low NAD+ is a direct consequence of the lactate released (aerobically) by leukocytes. When Pao_2 is elevated, little effect on either Po_2 or lactate is noted in the wound space. A larger effect on Po_2 is observed in the zone of collagen synthesis. For this reason, elevating Pao_2 raises collagen deposition without materially changing the oxyredox state.

The Michaelis constant (K_m) for oxygen of prolyl hydroxylase is about Po_2 of 25, and the Vmax occurs at about Po_2 of 200.[20] The clinical consequence of this is that full collagen synthetic capacity is not reached under ordinary circumstances—even in normal individuals breathing air at 1 atm pressure. Experimental data in human surgical patients are consistent. Collagen deposition is a function of Po_2 throughout the clinical range and higher (Fig. 160–4). As will be seen later, resistance to infection is similarly related to Po_2.[16, 22–25] This suggests that the practice of tolerating low Pao_2 in fear of oxygen toxicity carries a potential penalty of infection and poor healing.

Other requirements for collagen synthesis are amino acids for its structure, glucose to meet the energy needs of protein synthesis, iron, and ascorbate (to transfer oxygen for proline and lysine hydroxylation). Sulfated amino acids and lysine are also requirements, as is vitamin A. Other vitamins are probably also needed, if only for energy metabolism.[26] For unknown reasons, arginine in high doses markedly stimulates collagen deposition.[27]

Growth factors, particularly IGF-1 and TGF-β, also stimulate collagen synthesis and deposition.[28, 29] Mechanisms are unknown, except that some evidence unites this observation with the ADPR system—namely, that IGF-1 inhibits ADPR synthetase.*

Collagen Lysis

Collagen turns over rapidly in wounds and areas of inflammation. The lytic mechanisms are not entirely understood but almost certainly consist of three basic components. One mechanism begins with collagenases that are normally released by inflammatory cells and fibroblasts during catabolic situations such as starvation, stress, and inflammation.

*Unpublished observation of Z. Hussain, PhD and E.M. Spencer, MD.

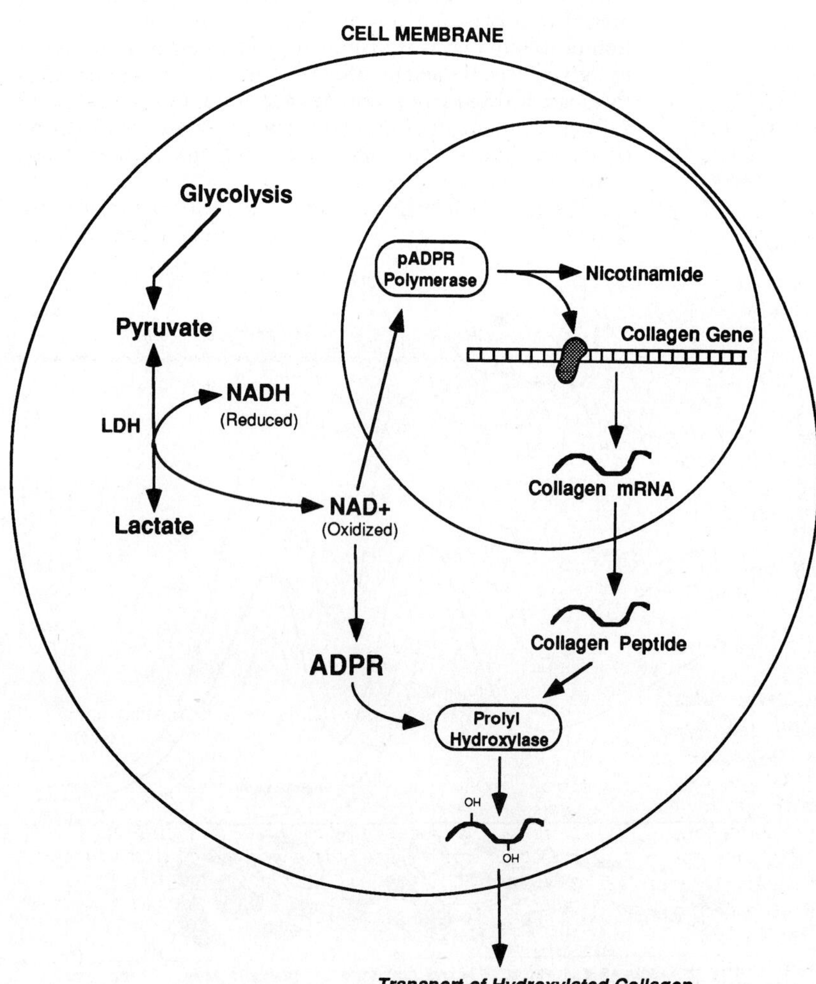

Figure 160–3. Schematic diagram of the metabolic control of collagen synthesis. The hypoxic and hyperlactated wound environment reduces NAD+ via lactic dehydrogenase (LDH). Thus, the synthesis of nuclear pADPR and cytoplasmic ADPR, which can be made *only* from NAD+, is significantly reduced. This, in turn, initiates the repression of collagen gene expression and the inhibition of cytoplasmic prolyl hydroxylase. As a result, both collagen transcription and prolyl hydroxylase are activated; this leads to the enhanced production of hydroxylated collagen peptide, provided that vitamin C and oxygen are present as substrate for prolyl hydroxylase. Some evidence implicates a negative action of certain growth factors on the "denicotinamidization" reactions; this negative action enhances collagen synthesis pADPR production. (From Zabel DD, Hunt TK: Skin, peritoneum, and colonic healing processes. Perspect Colon Rectal Surg 1993; 6:191–224.)

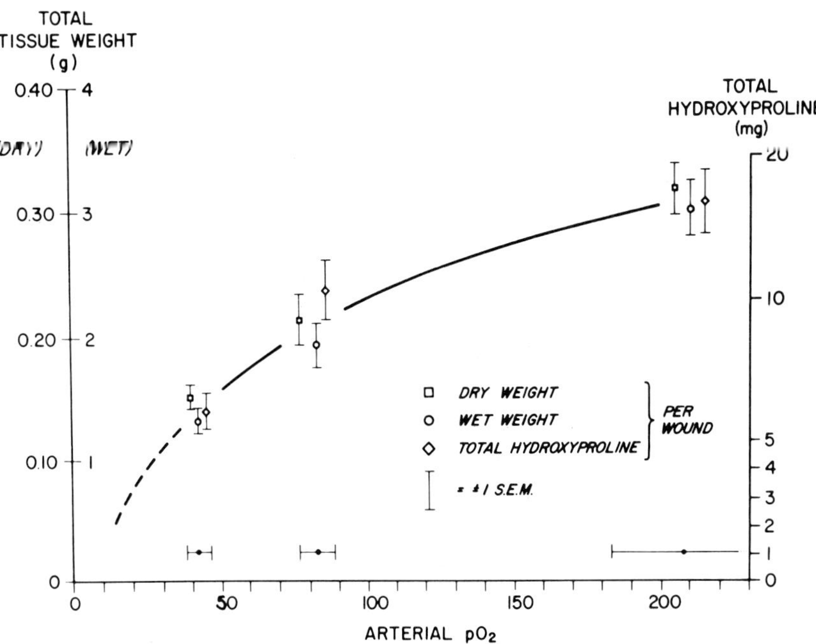

Figure 160–4. Total dry weight, wet weight, and hydroxyproline (collagen) content of tissue taken from wound cylinders and placed subcutaneously in rabbits that were allowed to breathe either 12% oxygen, air, or 40% oxygen. The increase in tissue weight of between 80 and 210 mm Hg is due to the increase in the partial pressure of oxygen rather than to the small increase of hemoglobin-bound oxygen in that range. (From Hunt TK, Pai MP: Effect of varying ambient oxygen tensions on wound metabolism and collagen synthesis. Surg Gynecol Obstet 1972; 135:561. By permission of Surgery, Gynecology & Obstetrics.)

A group of lysosomal enzymes also cleaves collagen during inflammation. These enzymes are normally found mainly in the phagosomes of leukocytes, but they can and do leak into the extracellular space. The plasmin/plasminogen system also has a role.

Wound edge fusion depends on net collagen synthesis and deposition. If lysis predominates, healing may stop or even regress. The balance between collagen synthesis and lysis is delicate enough to be influenced in either direction, particularly by circulatory status and nutrition (Table 160–1). Collagen synthesis consumes energy and nutrients and depends heavily on vascular resources. Collagen lysis, on the other hand, uses little if any vital resources and is activated in ischemia.

Epithelization

The epithelia that eventually cover the surfaces of wounds are led largely by growth factors released by their own stem cells. For instance, squamous epithelization is led by keratinocytes, which release growth factors much as macrophages do. As epithelium advances over healing wounds, the underlying connective tissue contracts and mitotic and synthetic activity in the deeper tissue begins to recede.[19] This effect is conspicuously absent in excessive scarring. Epithelization is easily hindered, especially in zinc and vitamin A deficiencies and during anti-inflammatory steroid therapy.[30] Epithelization is also oxygen dependent, for reasons that are unknown.[31]

Wound surfaces exposed to ambient conditions usually dry out and form eschars. Because eschar cannot support overlying cells, epithelium must proceed underneath by enzymatically cleaving the boundary between eschar and live tissue. This is a slow process. On the other hand, epithelia migrate quickly over moist, viable surfaces. For this reason, new dressing techniques have been designed to retain the moisture and the extracellular milieu that foster repair. They are truly improvements over the old wet-to-dry gauze dressings. Open wounds should not be allowed to desiccate. Simple, water-impermeable plastic films (Tegaderm, for instance) on donor site wounds enhance epithelization by more than 20%.[32]

WOUND INFECTION AND IMMUNITY

Many years of surgical experience have demonstrated that the incidence of wound infection is inversely proportional to the vascularity of the wounded tissue. Wounds of the tongue, although frequent, rarely become infected. Infection of face or neck wounds is also as rare and less frequent than infection in the extremities. Muscle is rarely infected, and then only when ischemic. Subcutaneous tissues of the trunk and limbs, which have the least blood supply, are most commonly the site of infection.

Resistance to infection is one of the most important contributions of healing. The first break in the host defense

TABLE 160–1. Factors Affecting Collagen Metabolism

Factors that decrease collagen synthesis
Preoperative
Starvation (protein depletion)
Steroids
Infection
Associated injuries
Hypoxia
Radiation injury
Uremia
Diabetes
Advanced age
Operative
Tissue injury
Poor blood supply
Poor apposition of surrounding tissues (pelvic anastomosis)
Postoperative
Starvation
Hypovolemia
Hypoxia
Drugs, e.g., actinomycin, 5-fluorouracil, methotrexate
Factors that increase collagen lysis (all are active before and after operation)
Starvation
Severe trauma
Inflammation
Infection
Steroids

occurs when cutaneous (or mucosal) immune mechanisms are broached. Clearly, rapid repair is the ultimate defense mechanism. Early closure of large, open wounds such as burns is an important strategy and goal.

In one way or another, most of the known immune functions contribute to host defenses. However, one of the distinctive properties of healing is its dependence on nonspecific immunity. This becomes apparent because one aspect of nonspecific immunity, oxidative bacterial killing, is put at great disadvantage in wounds and therefore becomes a conspicuous vulnerability.

As noted, leukocytes are immediately attracted into wounds, where complement factors assist them in seeking out bacteria. Contact is made, and phagocytosis occurs. Leukocyte granules fuse with the developing phagosome and release into it so-called nonoxidative killing substances such as defensins, cationic protein, myeloperoxidase, lactoferrin, and others, which are toxic to bacteria. All this occurs with apparently equal efficiency in anaerobic and aerobic environments. The nonoxidative system is remarkably efficient, and organisms that are sensitive to it are rarely causes of wound infections. Some organisms—staphylococci, for instance—are less susceptible than others.

Phagocytosis also activates the so-called oxidative killing system. This begins with a burst of oxygen consumption, which may rise more than 50 times above the baseline level. This is due to assembly ("activation") of the components of the NADPH-linked oxygenase of leukocytes.[33] As noted earlier, the reactants are glucose and molecular oxygen. The products—superoxide, lactate, and hydrogen ion—are secreted into phagocytic vacuoles. Note that this constitutes *aerobic* glycolysis. Superoxide kills some bacteria. Superoxide that is not immediately fixed onto bacterial membranes is dismutated to hydrogen peroxide. Peroxide, halide, and myeloperoxidase (from the granule fusion) form hypohalites such as hypochlorite, which are also toxic to bacteria. Excess peroxide is then reconverted to molecular oxygen and presumably recycled. Clearly, this is a fast-moving set of reactions that maintains a pool of bactericidal oxygen radicals (Fig. 160–5).

The size of the radical pool is determined by the rate at which oxygen is converted to superoxide by the NADPH-linked oxygenase. The K_m with respect to oxygen is about 50 mm Hg. In plain terms, this means that the rate of superoxide production for bactericidal purposes occurs at only half maximum speed at 50 mm Hg and is maximum only when intracellular PO_2 is about 500 mm Hg. Therefore, bacterial killing capacity is limited by PO_2 in the range from 0 to about 500 mm Hg. In clinical terms, this means that no one breathing air at only 1 atm can kill bacteria at maximum rate. Certainly, in the oxygen-starved environment of wounds, bacterial killing is seriously impaired. This appears to be the Achilles heel of wounds.

We know that the lack of superoxide production presents a serious clinical problem because children who inherit a deficiency of the NADPH-linked oxygenase (chronic granulomatous disease) die of infections early in life unless constantly protected by antibiotics.[34] Even with antibiotics, they are plagued with infections by organisms that are commonly those found to infect wounds (i.e., *Staphylococcus aureus*, group A *Streptococcus*, *Escherichia coli*, *Pseudomonas aeruginosa*, and some *Proteus* species). In short, a lack of the substrate, oxygen, is equivalent to a lack of the NADPH-linked oxidase, the local equivalent of chronic granulomatous disease (Figs. 160–6 and 160–7).

Killing capacity is also limited somewhat by pH. If extracellular pH is low, the pH of the phagosome is similarly low, and the backpressure of mass action limits superoxide production. The pH optimum is rather broad, and pH is probably not as important to bacterial killing as oxygen until severe acidosis is reached.[35]

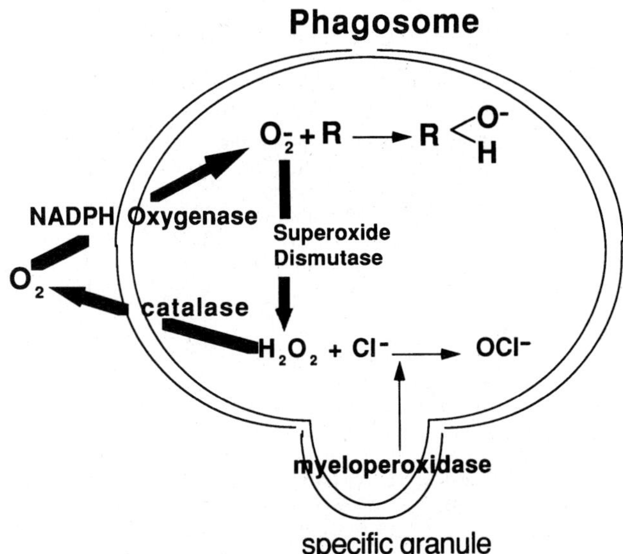

Figure 160–5. A schematic diagram of a phagocytic vacuole of a polymorphonuclear leukocyte. Dissolved oxygen is converted to superoxide by the NADPH -linked oxygenase. Superoxide may then be converted to a family of radicals or to hydrogen peroxide (H_2O_2) by superoxide dismutase. The latter can then be enzymatically converted to hypochlorite; alternatively, it can be catalyzed to be transported extracellularly as dissolved oxygen, which can start the cycle over again. (From Zabel DD, Hunt TK: Skin, peritoneum, and colonic healing processes. Perspect Colon Rectal Surg 1993; 6:191–224.)

Hypoxia also potentiates infection in other ways. Data are emerging to show that hypoxia is a stimulus for TNF and

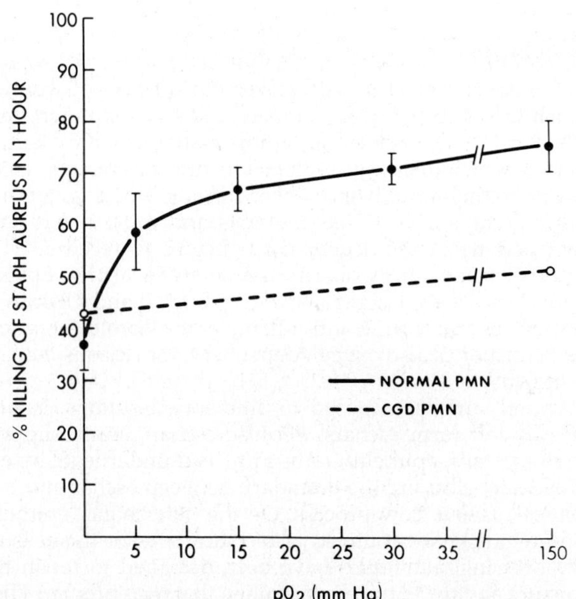

Figure 160–6. The bactericidal capacity of normal leukocytes and of those from patients with chronic granulomatous disease. Cell function decreases as PO_2 falls, especially below 30 mm Hg. Normal cells essentially "acquire" chronic granulomatous disease as oxygen disappears from the environment.

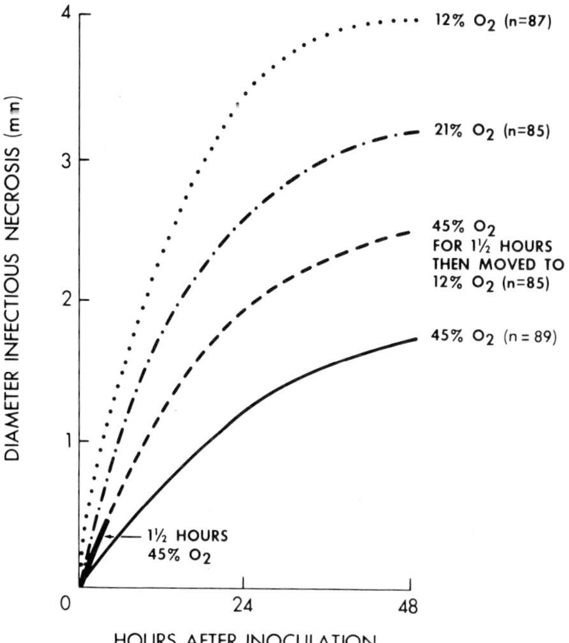

Figure 160–7. *Escherichia coli* was injected into the dermis of guinea pigs allowed to breathe 12% oxygen, air, or 45% oxygen. Only about 3% of the test injections in hypoxic animals showed no detectable necrosis, 20% showed no necrosis in air, and 50% showed no necrosis in 45% oxygen. These differences are highly significant. Breathing 45% oxygen for only 1.5 hours immediately after injection reduced the size and frequency of lesions.

interleukin-1 secretion by leukocytes in culture. Cytokines are clearly made in wounds, and almost certainly they perform a useful normal function in stimulating acute-phase protein synthesis in the liver after injury. However, cytokines also have well-known deleterious functions when excessively stimulated. Extensive hypoxic tissue after multiple injuries theoretically could lead to excessive levels of cytokines. This might be the first of the two "hits" that are usually necessary to produce the full syndrome of sepsis and multiple organ failure. It could be the only one necessary in elderly or already ill patients. The only two known and useful therapeutic responses when this circumstance arises are to (1) reperfuse and reoxygenate or (2) debride the ischemic tissue.[36] They are not mutually exclusive.

Large open wounds as are encountered in burns depress immune functions in several other ways. Leukocyte turnover becomes massive and prolonged, and nutritional demands increase. Contamination is prolonged and increased in number and type of organisms, and the specific immune system is brought more into play. Injury-related defects of this system are disclosed by the fact that extensively burned patients become infected by organisms that do not flourish in simple wounds and are not killed by either oxidative or nonoxidative functions of granulocytes. In burned or severely traumatized patients, saprophytic and fungal infections became more troublesome.

A last defect in wound immunity relates to the great distances that bloodborne antibacterial substances such as antibiotics and antibodies must diffuse in order to reach the source of bacteria in the wound space. Entry of antibiotics into wounds, for instance, is delayed by about 90 minutes over entry into normal subcutaneous tissue. Patients who are to undergo operation and who need antibiotics should have them before operation, and well before operation (6–8 h) if an infected wound is to be encountered.

PHYSIOLOGY OF REPARATIVE TISSUE

The circulatory physiology of tissues changes with injury. Tissues with variable blood flow and high peak oxygen demands have a high capillary density. For good reason, therefore, diffusion does not normally limit transport of oxygen, hydrogen ion, carbon dioxide (CO_2), or even lactate. In the heart, for example, the greatest distance oxygen or CO_2 might have to diffuse to reach its destination is less than 8 μm, less than the diameter of a red blood cell. The mean intercapillary distance in the subcutaneous tissue of the abdomen or legs, on the other hand, may be 50 μm or more.

When tissue is divided by a sharp scalpel (the most favorable injury), an ischemic zone of about twice the intercapillary distance is created by the injury and hemostasis. In the heart, this presents little problem, and healing is exceptionally efficient and free of infection. However, in the connective tissues of the trunk and extremities, diffusion distances become 80 to 120 μm, and diffusion then limits nutrition. Capillary Po_2, which is the driving force to diffusion, rather than the total quantity of hemoglobin-bound oxygen, then becomes the major limiting determinant of oxygen delivery. Removal of CO_2, lactate, and H^+ is seriously impeded.

The importance of Po_2 and the relative lack of importance of hemoglobin and total oxygen delivery to wounds are emphasized further by two other facts: First, as noted earlier, the rates of three enzymes that are vital to wounds, prolyl and lysyl hydroxylases and the NADPH-linked oxygenase of leukocytes, are dependent on Po_2 throughout the range from 0 to more than 200 mm Hg. Second, wounds use relatively little oxygen and use it at a constant rate. This means that Po_2 is highly manipulable but only by variations in Pao_2 and perfusion and *not* by blood hemoglobin. There are many proofs of this. The simplest tells most of the story. Mean Po_2 in small wounds in well-perfused patients is easily influenced by changes in Pao_2 but is insensitive to changes in hemoglobin over a wide range.[37] When Pao_2 rises above about 300 mm Hg, mean Po_2 in the center of well-perfused wounds (which is about 10 mm Hg above the Po_2 of venous blood draining from the wound) often rises over 100 mm Hg, indicating that no hemoglobin-bound oxygen is used at that Pao_2. At normal perfusion rate, the extraction ratio in subcutaneous wounds of the trunk is about ½ to 1 vol%.

Clearly, it is clinically profitable to maintain a high Po_2 in wounded tissue. A high Pao_2 is important, but it is not sufficient to achieve this. Perfusion must also be adequate (Fig. 160–8).[37] In mathematic terms, if oxygen extraction remains constant (as it does in wounds), tissue Po_2 approaches Pao_2 as flow approaches infinity.[38] The way to maintain a high local Po_2 is, therefore, to maintain a high flow of blood at a high Po_2 and keep the extraction ratio as low as possible. For wound-healing purposes, this means that pulmonary function and cardiac output are important. It also means—and this has been overlooked by most clinicians—that local vasoconstriction mediated by the sympathetic nervous system, smoking, and drugs, which lead to α-adrenergic overactivity and vasoconstriction, are obstacles to maintaining the high tissue Po_2 that is necessary for prompt repair and to prevent infection.

The mean Po_2 in a small test wound in an unoperated volunteer's arm is about 65 mm Hg.[38] In response to breathing approximately 70% oxygen, it rises to about 100 mm Hg. In contrast, the mean Po_2 in the same site in most patients immediately after a major operation is about 45 mm Hg and during oxygen breathing usually rises only about 15 mm Hg. The response to oxygen breathing postoperatively is particularly indicative of the state of peripheral

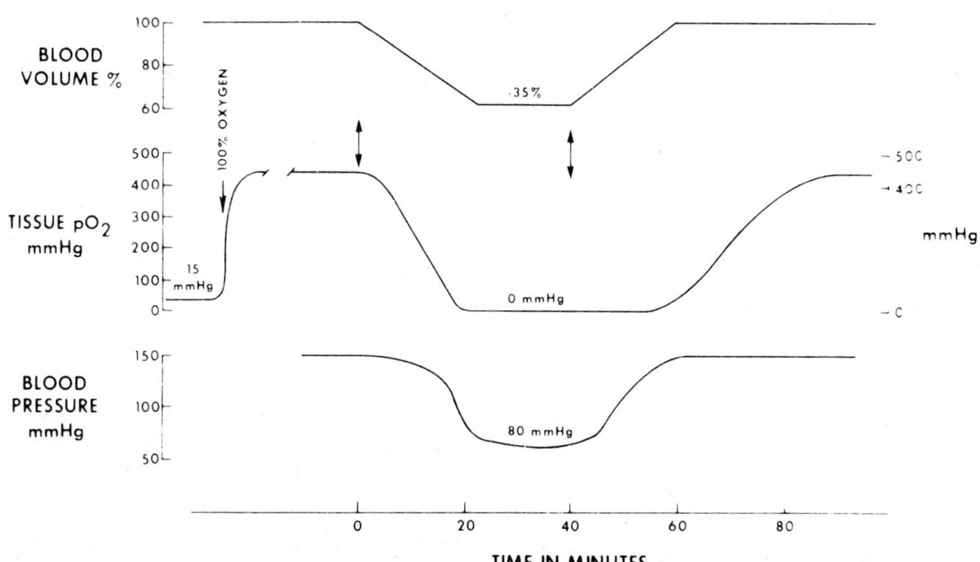

Figure 160–8. In this experiment, a calibratable macroelectrode was placed under the flank skin of a dog, and wound Po_2 was measured as the wound healed. The wound was several weeks old at the time this experiment was begun, and this accounted for the rather high basal Po_2 and the rather large response to oxygen breathing. Less mature wounds are less responsive to oxygen. At the first *double-headed arrow,* blood was removed in stepwise fashion. At the second *double-headed arrow,* volume loss was replaced by infusion of dextran. At the end of the experiment, the wound-tissue Po_2 was the same as it was before the blood loss, despite the fact that the hematocrit had fallen from 40% to approximately 25%.

perfusion and is depressed by vasoconstriction due to sympathetic nervous activity. The major mediators of sympathetic activity—contracted blood volume, pain, cold, and fear—all are conspicuously present in the postoperative and critical care environment (Fig. 160–9).[39] Wound Po_2 falls quickly in response to cold and rises on rewarming. The response to pain relief is less obvious because it is difficult to measure pain and to assess the side effects of narcotic administration.

Baseline Po_2 falls about 30% in volunteers after smoking

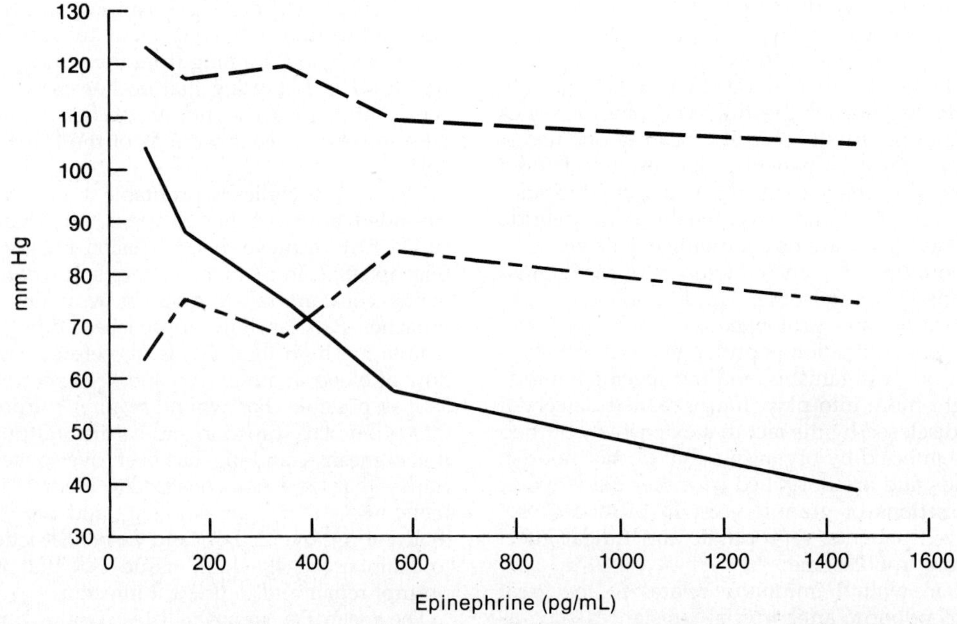

Figure 160–9. Oxygen supply to wounds and nonwounded tissue depends on the concentration of inspired oxygen, cardiac and pulmonary function, oxygen-carrying capacity of the blood, vascular tone, and diffusion of oxygen from capillaries into tissue. In this experiment, subcutaneous oxygen tension *(solid line),* pulse *(irregularly dashed line),* and Pao_2 *(regularly dashed line)* were continuously monitored in human volunteers during administration of varying concentrations of infused epinephrine. Subcutaneous oxygen tension fell as the plasma concentration of epinephrine increased. Pulse and Pao_2 did not markedly change. Postoperative patients who are cold, anxious, and in pain experience a similar stimulation of sympathetic nerves and also have lower subcutaneous wound oxygen tensions. The y axis refers to mm Hg Po_2 and pulse rate. (From Jensen JA, Jonsson K, Goodson WH, et al: Epinephrine lowers subcutaneous wound oxygen tension. Curr Surg 1985; 42:472.)

one cigarette and remains low for most of an hour.[40] Systemic administration of α-adrenergic agents, depending on dose, reduces mean wound Po_2 in volunteers to as low as 10 or 15 mm Hg even while the subjects breathe oxygen. Patients taking diuretics often are tissue hypoxic. The authors have observed wound/tissue Po_2 to rise in response to discontinuation of β-adrenergic blocking agents and administration of α-blockers. Many questions about the effects of vasoactive drugs on tissue oxygen remain to be answered.

By measurement with microprobes, wound pH and Po_2 are heterogeneous. Histograms of tissue Po_2 obtained by microelectrodes show a wide distribution with many zones measured at zero Po_2. Near functioning vessels, Po_2 may be quite high. As perfusion falls, the number of anoxic zones increases, and it seems reasonable to assume that resistance to infection diminishes in proportion to the number and size of these severely hypoxic zones (see Fig. 160–2). A failure of the mean to rise in response to a rise in Pao_2 implies the presence of anoxic zones.

Tissue partial pressure of CO_2 (Pco_2) has been measured less extensively than Po_2. In general, it changes as a reciprocal of Po_2, and in dead space wounds the mean is approximately 70 to 80 mm Hg. Lactate in wound fluid is not greatly influenced by changes in Po_2, implying that aerobic glycolysis by leukocytes is the most important source of lactate. Large wounds such as burns release large amounts of lactate into venous blood and recirculate it to the liver.[41] This incurs a significant circulatory and metabolic burden and accounts for some of the hypermetabolism of injury. Activation of the reticuloendothelial system (i.e., increased oxygen consumption by macrophages and endothelial cells, activated by injury) probably accounts for a greater fraction of hypermetabolism.

The nature of a wound affects its oxygen economy. The more severe the wound, the lower the oxygen supply in relation to demand. In needle wounds, Pco_2 is usually about 50 mm Hg, whereas in dead space wounds in the same patients it is between 30 and 40 mm Hg (Fig. 160–10).[42] Po_2 decreases in all wounds during the first few days as inflammation develops and fibroblasts accumulate.

INTENSIVE CARE OF WOUNDED PATIENTS

Many drugs and techniques help preserve or even accelerate wound healing, but time after time, perfusion of the injured area with well-oxygenated blood has been found to be primarily important. In practice, this translates into maintaining a high cardiac output, usually by keeping blood volume at an optimal level, avoiding pain, and preventing cold and fear, all designed to avert peripheral vasoconstriction and boost peripheral flow.

Maintaining a cardiac output suitable for repair is perhaps the most challenging task. When healing and resistance to tissue infections are major goals, care may deviate somewhat from that given to patients who have acute cardiac or pulmonary disease as sole problems. When wounds and cardiopulmonary problems are present, central pressure monitoring may be useful in achieving the best possible peripheral perfusion and oxygenation consistent with cardiopulmonary reserve. However, central pressures themselves bear little or no relation to peripheral perfusion. It is important to remember that the periphery, which is where infectable wounds are, accounts physiologically for a minority of blood flow even in the absence of muscular activity, and the sympathetic nervous system governs peripheral flow.* The contribution of peripheral venous blood to mixed venous Po_2, for instance, is small, and considerable vasoconstriction must occur before mixed venous Po_2 reflects it.[43]

The sympathetic nervous system is usually the major obstacle to flow. Catecholamine levels and, by association, sympathetic tone, both ordinarily low during anesthesia, rise dramatically as pain and cold are experienced. Cold leads to peripheral vasoconstriction and hence tissue hypoxia. Warmth does the opposite, and in fact, this is one of the principles behind transcutaneous oximetry. Cold vasoconstriction causes a transient, deceptive increase in urine output. Aggressive warming with forced-air warming blankets returns tissue Po_2 toward normal. Because of the increased urine volume during hypothermia, however, warming may be difficult and may replace cold vasoconstriction with hypovolemic vasoconstriction. Therefore, increased fluid replacement may also become necessary both to facilitate warming and to maintain peripheral perfusion. Pain is also a problem. Fortunately, new techniques of pain relief, epidural analgesia, for instance, show real promise of avoiding autonomic vasoconstriction and tissue hypoxia due to pain-induced vasoconstriction.

*Do not confuse *peripheral resistance* (which is total resistance) with this expression *peripheral flow*, which refers to blood flow in skin, bones, muscle, and fascia.

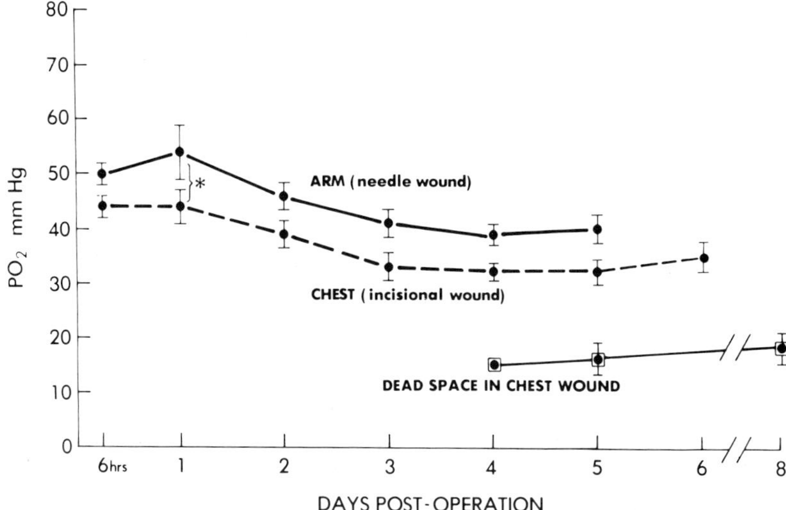

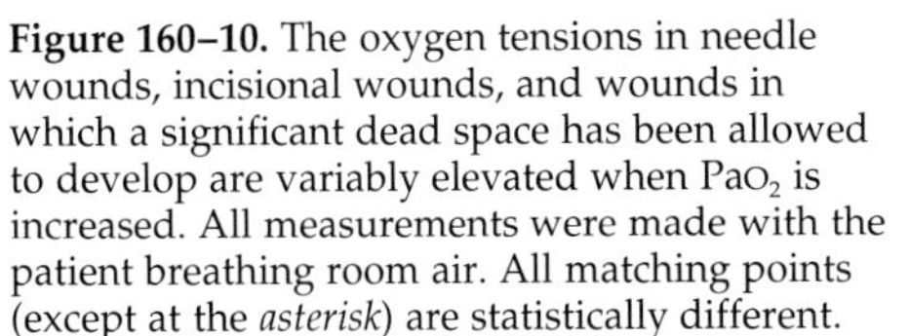

Figure 160–10. The oxygen tensions in needle wounds, incisional wounds, and wounds in which a significant dead space has been allowed to develop are variably elevated when Pao_2 is increased. All measurements were made with the patient breathing room air. All matching points (except at the *asterisk*) are statistically different.

The nature of the sympathetic nervous system is such that any one of these stimuli—hypovolemia, pain, cold, and fear—can lead to vasoconstriction *by itself*. To ensure peripheral flow, therefore, one must control all, and all at the same time. In clinical studies, this goal is currently reached in about half of patients in postoperative recovery rooms.[44, 45] Clearly, this record can be improved.

After acute trauma, third-space losses and hormonal changes, including cytokine release, lead to large fluid requirements. When patients after major surgery or injury are resuscitated to the usual criteria—that is, normal pulse, blood pressure, and urine output—their peripheral (wound) Po_2 values frequently remain low and are uninfluenced by changes in fraction of inspired oxygen.[46] By definition, these values are equated to poor peripheral perfusion in the presence of normal vital signs.

For some time, fluid infusion rates in postoperative patients have been keyed to peripheral tissue Po_2. This measure has often shown the need to give more fluid than otherwise seems necessary.[47] On occasion, some edema and pleural effusion appear to be the price of adequate peripheral tissue oxygenation. Fears of pulmonary edema are thus raised, and if cardiac reserve is severely limited, those fears may be realized. If this is the case, it may be necessary to use other technology such as pulmonary artery catheterization, positive-pressure breathing, and cardiotonic drugs to achieve the most advantageous combination of functions. On the other hand, when tissue oxygenation normalizes, fluid replacement can safely be reduced even when urine output is low, and fluid overload can thus be prevented. One should keep in mind that in following a policy of fluid restriction, today's caution to avoid cardiac failure or pulmonary edema may become tomorrow's defeat when infection or wound breakdown occurs.

One of the important lessons learned from measuring peripheral tissue Po_2 is that urine output does not reflect peripheral perfusion. In a series of trials, various clinical indexes of peripheral perfusion were compared with subcutaneous oximetry, which is an unwarmed quantitative measure of wound/peripheral Po_2. Such indexes as capillary return over the glabella or the patellas, eye globe turgor, and postural changes were moderately useful indexes of perfusion as estimated by various clinicians in that they correlated with subcutaneous Po_2 and its response to oxygen breathing.[47] However, a clinician's perception of peripheral perfusion was associated randomly with respect to tissue Po_2 because physicians held urine output in high esteem and were misled by it. Neither high nor low urine volumes correlated well with peripheral tissue Po_2.

In short, present orthodox intensive care methods are not keyed to peripheral wound perfusion and Po_2. Therefore, they do not necessarily ensure adequate peripheral perfusion and Po_2 to ensure healing or resistance to infection. When healing and tissue infections are problematic, one should consider measuring peripheral tissue Po_2. Clinical methods are becoming available.[37]

ANEMIC PATIENTS

Wound healing in anemic patients is rarely improved by transfusion of blood or blood cells unless anemia is very severe (hematocrit $<15\%$) or unless cardiac output cannot compensate normally. This has been shown in many clinical and laboratory studies. Correcting circulating blood volume deficits is more important than correcting anemia,[48] as illustrated by satisfactory wound healing following saline-replaced blood loss in Jehovah's Witnesses. Wound Po_2 and responses to breathing oxygen can be normal in patients with severe anemia,[49] and wound Po_2 has not been affected by increasing the packed cell volume in the range from 17 to 25 vol% in these patients.

When anemia is associated with a blood flow problem, as in patients with sickle cell anemia, the precipitous decrease in tissue Po_2 during removal of blood for transfusion can be avoided by saline infusion before and during replacement of blood. Considerations of wound healing should not be used as an indication for transfusion unless hematocrit falls below about 20% or cardiac or brain function is threatened by critical stenoses in major feeding vessels.

ANTIBIOTIC THERAPY

To be effective, preventive antibiotics must be given before operation or very soon after injury. Antibiotics given later appear to have little value.[50] Normal tissues are saturated by antibiotics in minutes; however, peak antibiotic concentrations are not reached in wound tissue until 1.5 hours after intravenous bolus doses and 4 to 6 hours after starting a constant infusion.[50] During the first 3 hours after injury, leukocytes are swept up into fibrin clots. This activity is thought to impair spread of infection, but on the other hand, it promotes abscess formation. Unfortunately, it also inhibits diffusion of antibiotics to where the bacteria are. Thus, the efficacy of antibiotics given late after wounding is further impaired.

NUTRITION

Nutrition affects both healing and immunity to infection. Unfortunately, the relationships are vague. Sound surgical judgment depends on nutritional assessment. When possible, most surgeons postpone major elective operations until patients are nutritionally ready, although what "ready" means is far from clear. Readiness does not require weight gain. It appears mainly to mean that pools of rapidly turning over substances are restored. A few days' repletion even of chronic losses seems to restore wound healing.[51] The corollary is that acute *starvation*, even for a few days, is surgically important.

Calorie and protein needs are also governed by the extent of injury and infection. Patients recovering from uncomplicated cardiac surgery need little protein and only minimum calories, whereas patients who have had simple colostomies for peritonitis resulting from diverticulitis may need supplements for both. Convincing arguments have been made for preoperative nutritional supplementation to enhance immunity when a patient has suffered severe infection or severe injury or has lost significant weight in a short time.[52]

Vitamins A and D, riboflavin, niacin, pyridoxal, and ascorbic acid all are essential for wound healing, as are zinc, copper, manganese, and iron (Table 160–2). Methionine or cysteine and lysine are essential, and many of the deleterious effects of protein depletion can be corrected by giving adequate amounts of these amino acids.[26] Glutamine and arginine seem particularly important. Arginine in large doses enhances collagen deposition even in normal volunteers.[27] Some commercial dietary supplements are constituted accordingly.

Immediately postoperatively, nutrition is rarely so important that it cannot be limited to dextrose, water, salt, vitamins, and minerals in favor of more pressing critical care needs. Total parenteral nutrition is often helpful, but if it interferes with support of vital organs, it can usually be omitted for a few days. Early resumption of *enteral* feeding is highly desirable.[52]

Vitamin A, often useful in counteracting the tendency of

TABLE 160–2. Roles of Vitamins and Minerals in Wound Healing

Vitamin/Mineral	*Role in Wound Healing*
C	Hydroxylation of proline and lysine Collagen lysis/deposition Reduction of oxygen to superoxide Capillary membrane stability
B_1	Cofactor for lysyl oxidase
B_5	Cell replication
B_6	Osteoblastic/osteoclastic activity
A	Epithelial growth Synthesis of glycoproteins Cellular immunity Collagen synthesis
D	Bone repair
E	Membrane stabilization Antioxidant properties
K	Coagulation
Mg	Enzyme cofactor
Zn	Cofactor for ribonucleic acid and deoxyribonucleic acid polymerase Immune function
Fe	Hydroxylation of lysine and proline

anti-inflammatory steroids to suppress repair, can be given intravenously at up to 10,000 to 15,000 units daily (or orally 25,000 units) for about a week.[53] About 1 g of ascorbic acid a day is usually sufficient. Zinc levels fall in response to anti-inflammatory steroids, and 50 to 100 mg can be given intravenously each day for a week or so. Zinc is also likely to be low in patients with gastrointestinal fistulas and chronic diarrhea and in patients who have had a number of operations in quick succession.

TIMING AND PRIORITIES

Many disagreements between critical care specialists and surgeons hinge on the issue of priorities and timing. It is tempting to follow a "safe" course with respect to cardiopulmonary function. However, temporizing measures that keep patients volume contracted may only postpone disaster, because poor perfusion and hypoxia due to hypovolemia are not necessarily preferable to mild or moderate heart failure. In difficult surgical cases, wound healing is often the key to a patient's survival, and a well-healed wound that is free of infection reflects not only correct surgical technique but also excellent and immediate postoperative wound care. In short, the responsibility is no longer in the hands of the surgeon alone.

References

1. Knighton DR, Hunt TK, Thakral KK, et al: Role of platelets and fibrin in the healing sequence. Ann Surg 1982; 196:379.
2. Leibovich SJ, Ross R: The role of macrophages in wound repair. Am J Pathol 1975; 78:71.
3. Stein JM, Levenson SM: Effect of the inflammatory reaction on subsequent wound healing. Surg Forum 1966; 17:484.
4. Hunt TK, Knighton DR, Thakral KK, et al: Studies on inflammation and wound healing. Angiogenesis and collagen synthesis stimulated in vivo by resident and activated wound macrophages. Surgery 1984; 96:48.
5. Rifkin DB, Moscatelli D, Gross J, et al. Proteases, angiogenesis and invasion. *In:* Cancer Invasion and Metastases; Biologic and Therapeutic Aspects. Nicolson SL, Milas L (Eds). New York, Raven Press, 1984.
6. Knighton D, Oredsson S, Banda M, et al: Regulation of repair. Hypoxic control of macrophage-mediated angiogenesis. *In:* Soft and Hard Tissue Repair: Biological and Clinical Aspects. Hunt TK, Heppenstall RB, Pines E, et al (Eds). New York, Praeger Scientific Publications, 1984, pp 41–49.
7. Karey P, Sirbasku DA: Human platelet derived mitogens. II. Localization of insulin-like growth factor I to the alpha-granule and release in response to thrombin. Blood 1989; 74:1093–1111.
8. Dvonch V, Murphey RJ, Matsuoka J, et al: Changes in growth factor levels in human wound fluid. Surgery 1992; 112:18–23.
9. Hunt TK, van Winkle W Jr: Normal repair. *In:* Fundamentals of Wound Management in Surgery. Hunt TK, Dunphy JE (Eds). New York, Appleton-Century-Crofts, 1979, pp 2–67.
10. Schoefl G: Electron microscopic observations on the regeneration of blood vessels after injury. Ann N Y Acad Sci 1964; 116:789–802.
11. Ausprunk DH, Folkman J: Migration and proliferation of endothelial cells in preformed and newly formed blood vessels during tumor angiogenesis. Microvasc Res 1977; 14:53–65.
12. Polverini PH, Cotran RS, Gimbrone MA, et al: Activated macrophages induce vascular proliferation. Nature 1977; 269–804.
13. Knighton DR, Hunt TK, Scheuenstuhl H, et al: Oxygen tension regulates the expression of angiogenesis factor by macrophages. Science 1983; 221:1283.
14. Jensen JA, Hunt TK, Scheuenstuhl H, et al: Effect of lactate, pyruvate, and pH on secretion of angiogenesis and mitogenesis factors by macrophages. Lab Invest 1986; 54:574.
15. Knighton DR, Silver IA, Hunt TK: Regulation of wound-healing angiogenesis—effect of oxygen gradients and inspired oxygen concentration. Surgery 1981; 90:262.
16. Silver IA: The physiology of wound healing. *In:* Wound Healing and Wound Infection: Theory and Surgical Practice. Hunt TK (Ed). New York, Appleton-Century-Crofts, 1980, pp 11–31.
17. Schultz G, Grant M: Neovascular growth factors. Eye 1991; 5:170–180.
18. Polverini P, Cotran R, Gimbrone M: Activated macrophages induce vascular proliferation. Nature 1977; 269:804–806.
19. Hunt TK: The physiology of wound healing. Ann Emerg Med 1988; 17:1265–1273.
20. Hutton J, Tappel A, Udenfriend S: Cofactor and substrate requirements of collagen proline hydroxylase. Arch Biochem 1967; 118:231–234.
21. Hussain M, Ghani P, Hunt TK: Inhibition of prolyl hydroxylase by poly(ADP-ribose) and phosphoribosyl-AMP. Possible role of ADP-ribosylation in intracellular prolyl hydroxylase regulation. J Biol Chem 1989; 264:7450–7455.
22. Niinikoski J: Oxygen and wound healing. Clin Plast Surg 1977; 4:361.
23. Hunt TK, Pai MP: Effect of varying ambient oxygen tensions on wound metabolism and collagen synthesis. Surg Gynecol Obstet 1972; 135:561–567.
24. Renvall S, Niinikoski J: Intraperitoneal oxygen and carbon dioxide tensions in experimental adhesion disease and peritonitis. Am J Surg 1975; 130:286.
25. Hunt TK, Niinikoski J, Zederfeldt BH, et al: Oxygen in wound healing enhancement: Cellular effects of oxygen. *In:* Hyperbaric Oxygen Therapy. Davis JC, Hunt TK (Eds). Bethesda, Undersea Medical Society, 1977, pp 11–22.
26. Levenson SM, Seifter E, van Winkle W Jr: Nutrition. *In:* Fundamentals of Wound Management. Hunt TK, Dunphy JF (Eds). New York, Appleton-Century-Crofts, 1979, pp 286–363.
27. Barbul A, Lazarou S, Efron D, et al: Arginine enhances wound healing and lymphocyte immune responses in humans. Surgery 1990; 108:331–336.
28. Ignotz R, Endo T, Massague J: Regulation of fibronectin and type I collagen mRNA levels by transforming growth factor beta. J Biol Chem 1987; 262:6443–6446.
29. Goldstein R, Poliks C, Pilch P, et al: Stimulation of collagen formation by insulin and insulin-like growth factor 1 in cultures of human fibroblasts. Endocrinology 1989; 124:964–970.
30. Hunt TK: Disorders of repair and their management. *In:* Fundamentals of Wound Management in Surgery. Hunt TK, Dunphy JE (Eds). New York, Appleton-Century-Crofts, 1979, pp 68–168.
31. Medawar PS: The behavior of mammalian skin epithelium under strictly anaerobic conditions. Q J Microsc Sci 1947; 88:27.
32. Eaglstein WH: Experiences with biosynthetic dressings. J Am Acad Dermatol 1985; 12:434–440.
33. Babior B: The respiratory burst oxidase. Adv Enzymol Relat Areas Mol Biol 1992; 65:49–95.

34. Knighton DR, Halliday B, Hunt TK: Oxygen as an antibiotic: A comparison of the effect of inspired oxygen concentration and antibiotic administration on in vivo bacterial clearance. Arch Surg 1986; 121:191.
35. Lehrer R, Ganz T, Selsted M, et al: Neutrophils and host defense (Clinical conference). Ann Intern Med 1988; 109:127–142.
36. Border J, Bone L: Multiple trauma: Major extremity wounds and their immediate management and its consequences. Adv Surg 1988; 21:263–291.
37. Jonsson K, Jensen J, Goodson W, et al: Tissue oxygenation, anemia, and perfusion in relation to wound healing in surgical patients. Ann Surg 1991; 214:605–613.
38. Jonsson K, Jensen JA, Goodson WH, et al: Assessment of perfusion in postoperative patients using tissue oxygen measurements. Br J Surg 1987; 74:263–267.
39. Jensen JA, Jonsson K, Goodson WH, et al: Epinephrine lowers subcutaneous wound oxygen tension. Curr Surg 1985; 42:472–474.
40. Jensen JA, Goodson WH, Hopf HW, et al: Cigarette smoking decreases tissue oxygen. Arch Surg 1991; 126:1131–1134.
41. Wilmore D: Pathophysiology of the hypermetabolic response to burn injury. J Trauma 1990; 30(Suppl 12):S4–6.
42. Goodson WH, Andrews WS, Thakral KK, et al: Wound oxygen tension of large vs. small wounds in man. Surg Forum 1979; 30:93.
43. Sheldon CA, Cerra FB, Bohnoff N, et al: Peripheral postcapillary venous pressure: A new, more sensitive monitor of effective blood volume during hemorrhagic shock and resuscitation. Surgery 1983; 111:399–406.
44. Gottrup F, Gellett S, Kirkegaard L, et al: Effect of hemorrhage and resuscitation on subcutaneous, conjunctival, and transcutaneous oxygen tension in relation to hemodynamic variables. Crit Care Med 1988; 17:904–907.
45. Gosain A, Rabkin J, Reymond J, et al: Tissue oxygen tension and other indicators of blood loss or organ perfusion during graded hemorrhage. Surgery 1991; 109:523–532.
46. Fiddian-Green R, Haglund U, Gutierrez G, et al: Goals for the resuscitation of shock. Crit Care Med 1993; 21(Suppl 2):S25–31.
47. Jensen JA, Riggs K, Vasconez LO, et al: Clinical assessment of postoperative peripheral perfusion. Surg Forum 1987; 38:66–67.
48. Heughan C, Grislis G, Hunt TK: The effect of anemia on wound healing. Ann Surg 1974; 179:163.
49. Jensen JA, Goodson WH III, Vasconez L, et al: Wound healing in anemia: A case report. West J Med 1986; 144:465.
50. Ehrlich HP, Lick V, Hunt TK: Kinetics of cephaloridine in experimental wounds. Am J Med Sci 1973; 265:33.
51. Windsor J, Knight G, Hill G: Wound healing response in surgical patients: Recent food intake is more important than nutritional status. Br J Surg 1988; 75:135–137.
52. Meakins JL: Host defense mechanisms, wound healing and infection. *In:* Fundamentals of Wound Management. Hunt TK, Dunphy JE (Eds). New York, Appleton-Century-Crofts, 1979, pp 242–285.
53. Hunt TK, Ehrlich HP, Garcia JA, et al: Effect of vitamin A on reversing the inhibitor effect of cortisone on healing of open wounds in animals and man. Ann Surg 1969; 170:633.

CHAPTER 161

Acute Pain in the Intensive Care Unit

Carl Anthony Hess, MD

The management of pain from acute tissue injury has been a medical dilemma throughout history. Initial treatments were widely spiritual, and historical pain remedies reflected the current interpretation of pain pathways at the time (Fig. 161–1). Modern thinking has developed a progressive scientific approach to understanding nociceptive pathways, and pain is now accepted as a true physiologic phenomenon. The process of pain transmission is multifaceted, and research continues to provide further understanding of its mechanisms. With knowledge and appreciation of the neurophysiologic basis for pain, it would seem obvious that interest in its adequate treatment would follow closely. Unfortunately, traditional bias and misconceptions have retarded the devotion of full attention to the adequate treatment of acute pain. Only recently have discovery and appreciation of the benefits of acute pain management been realized. In addition to the obvious emotional and psychologic benefit to the patients in pain, there is evidence of physiologic improvement, decreased morbidity, and favorable outcome with the superior control of acute pain. With this realization comes scrutiny of traditionally inadequate pain treatment regimens and motivation toward the development of better systemic and regional techniques and drug delivery technology. This chapter reviews the adequate treatment of pain in the acute setting, emphasizing the favorable impact of adequate pain control and discussing treatment options that maximize patient benefit.

The definitions of pain are many and varied. The International Association for the Study of Pain defines pain as an "unpleasant sensory and emotional experience associated with actual or potential tissue damage." This definition reflects the physiologic purpose of pain—that is, survival. Pain transmission is triggered by tissue injury or the threat of tissue damage, and protective mechanisms are elicited to prevent or minimize the injury. Such mechanisms are beneficial to some extent. However, a point is reached, especially in postoperative or post-traumatic acute pain, at which these mechanisms, which are designed to protect, cause ultimate detriment to the patient. Given that pain is an emotional as well as sensory experience, it seems that other affective mechanisms combine with neurophysiologic transmission to act at the expense of outcome.

PAIN PATHWAYS AND MECHANISMS

Painful impulses are known to stimulate peripheral pain receptors, known as *nociceptors*, that transmit impulses via specialized peripheral afferent pain fibers to the spinal cord and into the brain. Subsequently, mechanisms are activated to prevent injury (behavior) and to minimize perceived pain (endogenous analgesia) (Fig. 161–2). A key element, missing in early descriptions of pain, is the role of spinal cord modulation in pain transmission, which is now considered a major focus of specialized acute pain intervention. Modulation of pain impulses is known to occur through several dorsal horn mechanisms. These include local activation or inhibition of nociceptive impulses, release of neurotransmitters that promote pain or provide analgesia, and transmission to ascending excitatory and to descending inhibitory tracts.

Chemical modulation of pain transmission occurs via several neurotransmitter-receptor systems that have been shown to affect spinal processing of nociceptive input. Excitatory neurotransmitters (e.g., substance P) are active in the spinal cord and enhance pain transmission. The inhibitory elements are the opioids, the α_2-adrenergic fibers, γ-aminobutyric acid, and the serotoninergic and adenosinergic receptors. Endogenous neurotransmitters, like exogenously administered analgesics, work on dorsal horn neurons to inhibit excitatory transmitter release and to consequently decrease pain transmission and perception.

Pathways originating in the periphery and projecting through dorsal root ganglia to dorsal horn neurons and higher centers are illustrated in Figure 161–3. Note the site of action for various pain treatment techniques. These pain treatment modalities are discussed in detail later in this chapter.

PHYSIOLOGIC CONSEQUENCES OF ANESTHESIA AND SURGERY

The importance of acute pain management is illustrated by the physical derangements brought on by acute tissue injury and their potential for improvement—most notably, pulmonary, cardiac, neuroendocrine, and vascular aberrations that can lead to increased morbidity and poor outcome. Figure 161–4 illustrates these pathophysiologic changes and their consequences.

TRADITIONAL PAIN TREATMENT REGIMENS: INADEQUACY OF ACUTE PAIN TREATMENT

Despite rapid progress in the development of new and more effective acute pain treatment techniques, a large number of patients continue to receive traditional limited therapies consisting of pro re nata (prn) intramuscular or intravenous opioid analgesia. In 1973, Marks and Sachar demonstrated that 73% of medical inpatients were in moderate to severe distress despite their receiving an analgesic regimen of prn intramuscular meperidine.[1] Underdosing of analgesia for acute pain was emphasized, with only 1 patient out of 37 receiving doses greater than 75 mg. No adjustment of dosage for weight, increased pain frequency, or previous response was made, and physician concern over addiction and respiratory depression contributed to inadequate pain relief. In a follow-up study in 1980, Cohen demonstrated a 75% rate of moderate to severe distress in surgical patients despite prn intramuscular narcotic regimens.[2] Nursing choices reflected similar irrational concerns (e.g., no adjustment for weight or previous response), and the philosophy was that complete pain relief was not the goal.

The ineffectiveness of prn intramuscular opioids should be intuitive. Patients need to express the need for pain relief before steps leading to analgesic administration are initiated. This results in an excessive time delay from the time of pain onset to the time of analgesia. Nursing response, patient evaluation, and preparation and administration of analgesic medications may take as long as 1 hour. Following administration, drug uptake and subsequent blood levels fluctuate dramatically and are unpredictable when the intramuscular route is used. Rapid changes in drug blood levels result in systemic analgesic levels in the subanalgesic range as well as in the excessive range, leading to adverse side effects. Clearance rapidly brings drug blood levels down through the analgesic range to subtherapeutic levels, the patient experiences recurrent pain, and the cycle begins again.

The incorrect choice of medications represents a dramatic example of misconceptions that result in inadequate pain control. Specifically, paralyzing agents have been used for analgesia and sedation in critically ill patients who are ventilator dependent. Besides subjecting patients to the suffering of untreated pain, this practice produces additional emotional trauma in awake, paralyzed patients who are also in pain. In their article entitled "Paralyzed With Pain," Loper and coworkers reported the prevalent misuse of paralyzing agents in an intensive care unit (ICU) setting.[3] Their survey revealed that 5% to 10% of physicians and nurses advocated the use of pancuronium for analgesia and that a much higher percentage (50–70%) advocated its use for anxiolysis. Additional individuals reported that although they did not advocate its use for analgesia, they were unaware that pancuronium contained no analgesic properties. Coincidently, 80% of physicians in the survey advocated the use of diazepam for analgesia. These results exposed a commonly held misconception that muscular paralysis represents a calm and painless state and that sedation is a good method of pain control. This is certainly not the case; neuromuscular blocking agents and benzodiazepines have no analgesic effect, and patients in the survey reported the terrifying experience of being paralyzed and not knowing why. In addition, paralyzing agents have no anxiolytic properties and should be administered with a medication properly designed for anxiety control, such as benzodiazepine, to prevent the recall of distressing experiences in the ICU—most notably, awake paralysis.

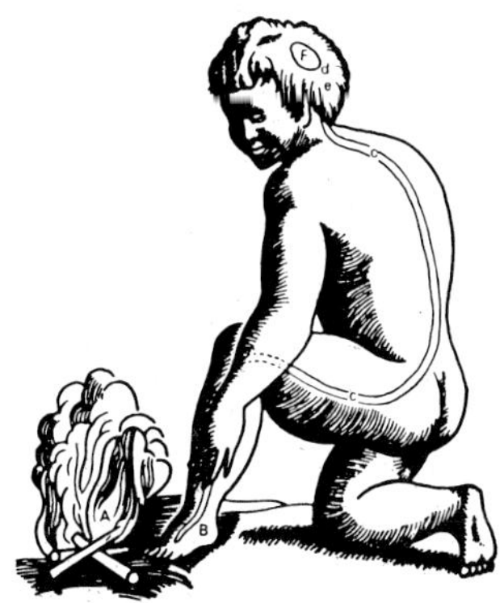

Figure 161–1. Descartes pain concept as illustrated by his model of a boy with his foot in a fire. His was the first theory to include the peripheral afferent nerves, spinal cord, and brain as the primary elements in pain transmission. (Reprinted with permission from Melzak R, Wall PD: Pain mechanisms: A new theory. Science 1965; 15:971. Copyright 1965, American Association for the Advancement of Science. Adapted from Descartes, R: "L'Homme" [Paris, 1644], as translated by M. Foster in *Lectures on the History of Physiology During the 16th, 17th, and 18th Centuries* [Cambridge, England, Cambridge University Press, 1901.])

PAIN MANAGEMENT FOR ACUTE TISSUE INJURY

Systemic Opiates

Despite traditional inadequacies and the development of nonopioid pain treatment modalities, systemic opioid anal-

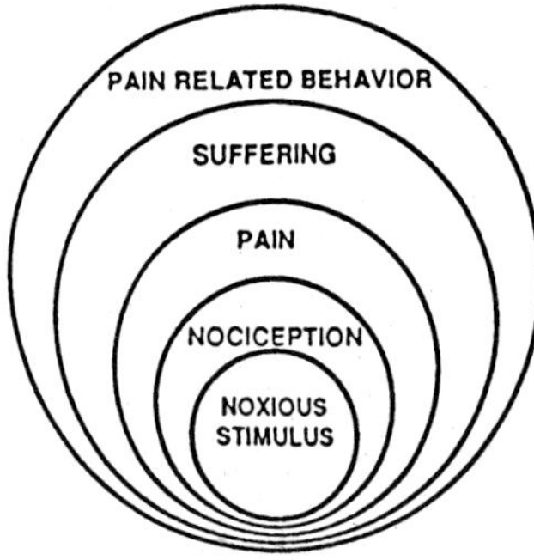

Figure 161–2. A multidimensional model of pain assessment. Evaluation and measurement are often difficult because pain is a highly subjective, multidimensional experience that combines sensory and affective components. Noxious stimuli result in pain perception, with afferent neural transmission characterizing space, time, and intensity of the stimulus. Emotional components are elicited in response to this painful experience and result in the patient's suffering. This is exhibited as pain-related behavior. Many factors affect both the sensory and emotional aspects of pain and thus affect pain behavior. Of all the components in the multidimensional model, pain-related behavior alone has potential for assessment and measurement. (From Loeser JD: Concepts of pain. *In*: Chronic Low Back Pain. Stanton-Hicks M, Boas R (eds). New York, Raven Press, 1982, p 124. Reprinted with permission.)

TABLE 161–1. Systemic Opioid Analgesics for Acute Pain Management

	Equianalgesic Doses (mg)*	*Half-Life (h)*	*Peak Effect (h)*	*Duration (h)*
Pure Agonists				
Morphine	10 IM	2–3	0.45–1	3–6
	20–60 PO		1.5–2	4–7
Meperidine	75 IM	2–3	0.5–1	3–4
	300 PO	—	1–2	3–6
Hydromorphone	1.5 IM	2–3	0.5–1	3–4
	7.5 PO	—	1–2	3–4
Levorphanol	2 IM	12–15	0.5–1	3–6
Methadone	10 IM	15–190	0.5–1.5	4–6
	20 PO			
Codeine	130 IM	2–3	1.5–2	3–6
	200 PO			
Partial Agonists				
Buprenorphine	0.4	2–5	0.5–1	4–6
Mixed Agonist-Antagonists				
Pentazocine	60 IM	2–3	0.5–1	3–6
	180 PO	—	1–2	3–6
Nalbuphine	10 IM	4–6	0.5–1	3–6
Butorphanol	2 IM	2–3	0.5–1	3–4

*Dose that provides analgesia equivalent to 10 mg of intramuscular morphine. Analgesic requirements and tolerance are widely variable according to patient's condition and severity of injury. Medication should be administered in low doses initially and titrated carefully to analgesic effect and to cardiovascular and respiratory status.

Abbreviations: IM = intramuscular; PO = per os.

gesia appropriately continues to be the mainstay of postoperative pain control. If given in regimens that consistently maintain blood levels in the analgesic range, systemic opiates can be a safe and beneficial method of relieving postsurgical pain. Continuous opioid infusions or patient-controlled analgesia (PCA) regimens seem to provide superior analgesia as well as the physical and emotional benefits inherent with adequate pain relief.

Opioid analgesics act on multiple opiate receptors in the central nervous system, spinal cord, and peripheral nervous system. Varying interactions with these receptors result in different pharmacologic profiles among the systemic opiates. The opiate receptors most often involved in supraspinal and spinal analgesia as well as in narcotic side effects are the mu and kappa receptors. Drugs acting at opiate receptors are divided into *agonists, agonists-antagonists,* and *partial agonists* (Table 161–1). Pure antagonists are used for narcotic reversal (e.g., naloxone). Examples of opioid agonists are the common systemic narcotics morphine, hydromorphone, meperidine and methadone as well as the newer synthetic opiates fentanyl and sufentanil. Partial agonists include codeine and buprenorphine, and agonists-antagonists include pentazocine, nalbuphine, butorphanol, and the newer drug dezocine. Analgesia is most profound with the pure opioid agonists and seems to reach a plateau with partial agonists and agonists-antagonists. However, opiate side effects appear to parallel the amount of agonist activity and are diminished with accompanying antagonism. Table 161–1 shows commonly used narcotic analgesics with dosage equivalence and duration of action.

SIDE EFFECTS OF OPIATES. The side effects of systemic opiates are the limiting factor in their use in critically ill patients, multiple trauma victims, and patients undergoing extensive operations. Most notable are respiratory depression and hypotension. Maximal respiratory depression occurs within the first 10 minutes after intravenous administration of morphine but may be delayed for 30 minutes following an intramuscular injection. An accompanying increase in arterial carbon dioxide tension and a decrease in lung volumes follow administration of an analgesic dose. In addition, morphine depresses the cough reflex, inhibiting the clearance of secretions and possibly contributing to postoperative atelectasis. Hypotension occurs with the maintenance of therapeutic analgesic levels of morphine, likely from histamine-induced arteriolar and venous dilatation. Drugs associated with less histamine release, such as fentanyl, seem to provide analgesia with more hemodynamic stability in these patients.

Other side effects of the use of systemic narcotics include nausea and vomiting, pruritus, urinary retention, and gastrointestinal dysfunction.

Systemic opiate therapy may be used in an effective manner postoperatively. In patients who are critically ill, hemodynamically unstable, or unable to operate a PCA device for various reasons or in whom other techniques are unfeasible or contraindicated, the intermittent administration of systemic opiates is an effective method of postoperative pain control. Knowledge of the spectrum of postoperative pain management regimens is required to tailor treatment to each individual patient and to provide the most effective analgesic with a maximum of safety and a minimum of side effects. However, it must be recognized that some patients, despite their receiving the best possible traditional narcotic regimen, continue to experience significant postoperative pain and are therefore subject to the detriments of inadequate pain relief or to dangerous side effects from excessive doses. Extensive surgery of the upper abdomen or thorax may render a patient uncomfortable and unable to ambulate or give good respiratory effort. In such a patient, more specialized techniques such as PCA, central neural blockade with local anesthetics or spinal opiates, peripheral nerve blocks, or intrapleural catheters may need to be considered.

PATIENT-CONTROLLED ANALGESIA

PCA with parenteral medications consists of a set dosage of a drug given at a set interval by patient demand, with or without an accompanying continuous infusion. PCA has been available for almost 10 years.[4] PCA technology has since developed rapidly, and its popularity has increased

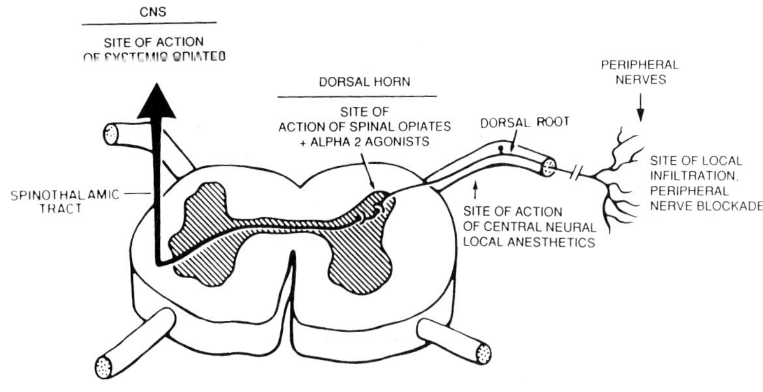

Figure 161–3. Anatomy of pain transmission and sites of analgesic action. The pain of acute tissue injury may be attenuated at many levels and by many actions. This includes blockade of peripheral nerve afferent transmission, blunting of sympathetic ganglia, dorsal root blockade by epidural or intrathecal local anesthetics, and receptor-mediated dorsal horn mechanisms (via opiates and alpha$_2$ agonists). These mechanisms result in diminished pain transmission contralaterally to ascending spinothalamic tract neurons and, consequently, in fewer impulses traveling to higher centers in the brain. Finally, central nervous system (CNS) analgesic levels of systemic medications afford pain relief from central receptor mechanisms. (Adapted from Badner NH: Epidural agents for postoperative anaglesia. Anesthesiol Clin North Am 1992; 10:322.)

dramatically. Traditional agents such as morphine and meperidine are the most common medications used in PCA devices. Therefore, the increasing use of PCA reflects recognition of the inefficiency of conventional parenteral regimens and the appreciation that more consistent, effective drug blood levels are delivered by the PCA route of administration.[5]

Intramuscular injections lead to inconsistent plasma concentrations of medication. Onset and time to peak plasma concentration can vary up to sevenfold with repeated injections and with varying patient populations. With continuous intravenous infusions or patient-controlled dosing of opioids, a more consistent opioid plasma concentration is achieved.[6] When a patient's plasma concentration of a drug falls below the minimal analgesic concentration, the patient begins to feel pain, administers an on demand dose, and rapidly restores the plasma level of the analgesic to within the analgesic range (Fig. 161–5).

In addition to consistent blood levels of drug, the psychologic benefit received by patients who feel some control over their pain treatment regimen cannot be underestimated. Pharmacokinetic and pharmacodynamic factors appear to be less important in a patient's decision for demand dosing than psychologic considerations. If a patient is an acceptable candidate for PCA, analgesia is superior and a lower overall drug dosage is needed.[5]

General Guidelines for Use

PCA devices have several variables of administration. The PCA or demand dose is of fixed size and is intermittently administered by the patient at a preset lockout interval. The PCA dose is the small quantity of analgesic given immediately upon the patient's self-evaluation and conclusion that he or she needs pain medication. The lockout interval is the time period allowable between PCA doses within which the device does not administer any analgesic. In addition, many PCA devices are equipped with 1-hour and 4-hour total dosage limits designed for added safety.

Many different opioids can be used in PCA regimens. Nonopioid medications are also being investigated for patient-controlled use. Although largely empirical, guidelines for PCA administration of commonly used opioid narcotics are listed in Table 161–2.

Side Effects and Complications

Problems encountered with the use of PCA are related to side effects of the medications themselves and to mechanical or operator error. The incidence of opiate side effects does not appear to be any different than with other methods of narcotic administration.

CENTRAL NEURAL BLOCKADE

Postoperative pain control with central neural local anesthetics has been in use since the 1940s. Unfortunately, the administration of local anesthetics in the intrathecal or epidural space is associated with dramatic cardiovascular side effects that accompany the superior analgesia that the drugs provide. Clinical use of intraspinal morphine as a pain management modality began in the late 1970s. This has subsequently led to the popularity of intraspinal opiate use postoperatively because of the superior analgesia provided segmentally with greater cardiovascular stability. Although less severe than those of local anesthetics, the side effects of spinal opiates are varied, the most disconcerting of which is the occurrence of late respiratory depression. Because of this potentially fatal side effect, the use of other drugs and drug combinations has been proposed. These include opiate analgesics that are more lipid-soluble, agonist-antagonist narcotics, combinations of narcotics and local anesthetics, and non-narcotic analgesics such as the alpha$_2$-agonist clonidine. Each analgesic or analgesic combination has its merits, but no one drug or drug combination has been used without complication. The following sections summarize the advantages and disadvantages of the intraspinal medications commonly used for postoperative pain control.

Central Neural Blockade with Local Anesthetics

Before the advent of indwelling catheters for intrathecal and epidural use, local anesthesia was provided in single-shot injections that lasted from 3 to 4 hours in the best of circumstances. This complete neural blockade was effective for intraoperative use and proved superior in providing analgesia upon emergence.[7] However, before catheters were

TABLE 161–2. Guidelines for Patient-Controlled Analgesia with Various Opioid Analgesics*

Drug (Concentration)	*Demand Dose*	*Lockout Interval (min)*
Morphine (1 mg/mL)	0.5–3.0 mg	5–12
Meperidine (10 mg/mL)	5–30 mg	5–12
Fentanyl (10 μg/mL)	10–20 μg	5–10
Hydromorphone (0.2 mg/mL)	0.05–0.25 mg	5–10
Methadone (1 mg/mL)	0.5–2.5 mg	8–20
Nalbuphine (1 mg/mL)	1–5 mg	5–10

(Adapted from Ferrante FM: Patient-controlled analgesia. Anesthesiol Clin North Am 1992; 10:292.)

*Analgesic requirements vary widely among patients. Age, severe underlying disease, and individual response may make dosage adjustment necessary.

used, the benefit could not be extended into the postoperative period, when pain control is most important.

The sites of intrathecal and epidural local anesthetic administration are in the area of the dorsal root (see Fig. 161–1). Small postganglionic sympathetic fibers are blocked first, followed by sensory fibers, and finally by motor nerve fibers. Intensity of blockade is dependent on the volume and concentration of the local anesthetic given. Despite providing excellent analgesia, this neural blockade often becomes problematic postoperatively because of its profound cardiovascular effects. Hypotension caused by central neural local anesthetics is of particular concern in critically ill patients or in those undergoing major surgeries with ongoing blood loss and fluid shifts.

Epidural local anesthesia for postoperative pain has been reported for abdominal, thoracic, and orthopedic surgeries.[7] In addition, the use of local anesthetics in thoracic epidural catheters has been shown to decrease the need for mechanical ventilation following multiple rib fractures.[8] Infusions of 0.5% bupivicaine or 1.5% lidocaine not only provide superior analgesia for multiple types of surgery, but also show beneficial effects on pulmonary and endocrine function. Use of epidural analgesia has been associated with shorter time to ambulation, decreased hospital stay, and lower incidence of pulmonary complications in selected patients.[9] Similarly, patients undergoing lower abdominal surgery were shown to have decreased values for the indices of the stress response whereas those undergoing upper abdominal operations did not consistently show this benefit.[10]

In light of the superior analgesia and potential physiologic benefits, local anesthetic analgesia via the epidural or intrathecal route seems ideal. However, the side effects of cardiovascular instability and motor weakness prohibit its use in many patients. The same studies that showed beneficial effects also revealed high incidences of hypotension in patients receiving intermittent bolus or continuous infusion of local anesthetics. In addition, a large percentage of patients develop motor blockade that precluded ambulation even when more a dilute local anesthetic concentration was used. Because cardiovascular stability and early ambulation are emphasized as the mainstays of postoperative analgesic benefit, the use of moderate to high concentrations of local anesthetic given by bolus or infusion is not consistently practiced, especially in the ICU setting.

SPINAL OPIATE ANALGESIA

The term "spinal opiate analgesia" refers to either intrathecal or epidural administration of a narcotic analgesic. Since the advent of its clinical use, rapid progress has been made in management techniques that use spinal opiate analgesia, and this modality has consistently proved itself to provide superior analgesic efficacy and a reduction in the perioperative morbidity associated with poor pain control. The undesirable side effects of hypotension and motor weakness associated with local anesthetics are avoided with spinal opiate therapy, but awareness of the side effects of these spinal medications is still important.

No single opiate medication has proved itself to be vastly superior to others with regard to analgesic efficacy, improvement of perioperative morbidity, and incidence of side effects. Commonly used opiate analgesics include morphine, meperidine, fentanyl, and sufentanil, and management differences are related to physicochemical properties of the drug selected (e.g., its lipid solubility), catheter placement, and dosing guidelines (Table 161–3). Nonopiate analgesics or opiate agonists-antagonists have also been used with varying degrees of success, as have opioid and local anesthetic combinations.

Morphine

Morphine was the first opiate described for spinal opiate therapy and has become the standard to which all other spinal analgesics are compared. Site of action of morphine, as with other spinal opiates, appears to be on opiate receptors in the dorsal horn of the spinal cord.[11] Epidural morphine administration has demonstrated analgesia superior to that of conventionally administered parenteral narcotics.[12] In addition, profound analgesia extends into the postoperative period.

Morphine is the least lipid soluble of all the commonly used spinal opiates, having an octanol/water partition coefficient of 1.42. Its onset of action is therefore delayed for 45 to 60 minutes while it penetrates through the dura into the substantia gelatinosa of the dorsal horn. This drug is advantageous not only because of its extended duration of action but also because it can be administered in the low lumbar region for high abdominal or thoracic procedures. Larger doses are needed for lumbar administration (4–8 mg for thoracotomy versus 2–5 mg for lower abdominal procedures). A continuous infusion may also be used (0.1 mg/mL at a rate of 3–10 mL/h). However, given the long duration of action afforded by morphine's lipid insolubility and pharmacokinetic profile, epidural infusions of the drug may be less practical than administration of the more lipid-soluble agents.

Side effects and complications of intraspinal morphine are

TABLE 161–3. Spinal Opiates for the Treatment of Acute Pain

Drug	*Single Dose* (mg)*	*Infusion Rate† (mg/h)*	*Onset (min)*	*Duration of Single Dose‡ (h)*
Epidural				
Morphine	1–6	0.1–1.0	30	6–24
Meperidine	20–100	5–20	5	2–6
Hydromorphone	1–2	0.1–0.2	15	10–16
Fentanyl	0.025–0.10	0.025–0.10	5	2–4
Sufentanil	0.01–0.06	0.01–0.05	5	2–4
Intrathecal				
Morphine	0.1–0.5		15	8–24
Meperidine	10–30			10–24
Fentanyl	0.005–0.025		5	3–6
Sufentanil	0.004–0.0075		5	2–6

(Adapted from Ready LB: Intraspinal opioid analgesia in the perioperative period. Anesthesiol Clin North Am 1992; 10:150.)
*Low doses may be effective when administered to the elderly or when injected in the cervical or thoracic region.
†If combining with a local anesthetic, consider 0.0625% bupivacaine. Be wary of cardiovascular effects.
‡Duration of analgesia varies widely; higher doses produce longer duration. (Individual doses may vary, adjustment should be made according to patient physical status and pain management requirements.)
Lipid solubility: Morphine < Hydromorphine << Meperidine << Fentanyl < Sufentanil.

the same as those of other commonly used spinal opiates and include nausea and vomiting, pruritus, urinary retention, and early and late respiratory depression. Because of its persistence in the cerebrospinal fluid, the incidence and severity of side effects appear to be greater than those of more lipid-soluble opiates. Late respiratory depression has been the most dramatic side effect of intraspinally administered morphine, with early case reports of patient morbidity and mortality. Much attention has been directed to the issue of clinical safety regarding the use of intraspinal morphine. Three large studies reviewing 15,000 patients found an incidence of late respiratory depression of less than 1%.[13–15] Numerous articles published after these studies reported similarly low rates; others have advocated its safe use despite this complication if adequate vigilance protocols are followed.[16] Late respiratory depression appears to be the result of cephalad migration of morphine in the cerebrospinal fluid, which is less likely with the more lipid-soluble opiates. Respiratory depression can occur up to 24 hours following the administration of morphine (see Table 161–4 for predisposing factors).

Other complications occur commonly postsurgically and should not be solely attributed to intraspinal administration of morphine. Nausea and vomiting have been reported to occur in 30% to 40% of patients receiving epidural morphine. Urinary retention, which occurs in 5% to 40% of patients, is due to bladder detrusor muscle dysfunction and may be less of an issue in the intensive care setting because critically ill patients or those undergoing large procedures commonly have indwelling urinary catheters. Pruritus is variable, occurring in 10% to 90% of cases, and, although it is not histamine mediated, it responds to intravenous administration of diphenhydramide (Benadryl). If refractory, intravenous infusions of small doses of naloxone may be administered to counteract side effects independent of analgesic effect.

TABLE 161–4. Factors Predisposing to the Development of Respiratory Depression Following Intraspinal Opioid Administration*

Hydrophilic drug (e.g., morphine)
Large/repeat doses
Use of parenteral opioids or other central nervous system depressants
Elderly or debilitated patients
Coexisting respiratory disease
Thoracic epidural analgesia
High sensitivity to opioids (i.e., no previous exposure to opioids)
Intrathecal administration
Raised intrathoracic pressure (e.g., with controlled ventilation, coughing, vomiting)

(Adapted from Cousins MJ, Mather LE: Intrathecal and epidural administration of opioids. Anesthesiology 1984; 61:276–310.)

*Factors present should indicate the use of high vigilance protocols (i.e., ICU admission, monitored bed, and respiratory monitoring).

Meperidine

Meperidine displays the physicochemical advantages of greater lipid solubility and an octanol/water partition coefficient many times that of morphine. This affords meperidine a quicker onset of action (15–30 minutes), lesser degree of cephalad spread (potentially fewer side effects), and a shorter duration of action (4–6 hours), which lends practicality to continuous infusion. In addition, meperidine has the distinct advantage of possessing local anesthetic properties and is the only opiate to have been used as a sole anesthetic when given intrathecally.[17] Unfortunately, this local anesthetic effect is not clinically evident when meperidine is given epidurally, and its analgesic and side effect profiles are not significantly different from those of the more lipid-soluble opiate analgesics. Nonetheless, meperidine represents a practical option in intrathecal or epidural administration, offering all the advantages of the other spinal opiates. It can be used in bolus form or as a continuous infusion and shows potential for combination with dilute local anesthetic solutions.

Fentanyl

Fentanyl is a synthetic opioid agonist that contains the same chemical nucleus as morphine but which is manufactured synthetically rather than by chemical modification. Fentanyl is approximately 100-fold more potent than morphine and is 500-fold more lipid-soluble. These physicochemical properties afford fentanyl a rapid onset of analgesia and a short duration of action. With higher lipid solubility, cephalad migration is minimal because of diffusion into the lipid layers of the dura before significant spread can occur. For this reason, larger doses need to be administered via a lumbar epidural catheter to provide analgesia for upper abdominal and thoracic surgery (100–200 μg), whereas lower doses are adequate for lower operations. Because of its short duration of action, fentanyl is an ideal drug to be used in a continuous infusion through an epidural catheter. Using a concentration between 4 μg/mL and 10 μg/mL, an infusion of 0.5 to 1.0 $\mu g \cdot kg^{-1} \cdot h^{-1}$ is administered for postoperative pain. Epidural infusion is less likely to result in rapid or significant accumulation of systemic fentanyl levels if lumbar epidural catheters are used for low abdominal and peripheral surgeries, or if thoracic epidural catheters are used for upper abdominal and thoracic procedures.

Problems encountered with epidural fentanyl infusions occur when lumbar epidural catheters are used for extensive abdominal procedures or thoracotomies, and these problems are related to the high lipid solubility of the drug. Using a low epidural catheter, larger doses (1–1.5 $\mu g \cdot kg^{-1} \cdot h^{-1}$) are required for analgesia. This results in rapidly distributed systemic fentanyl concentrations similar to those required for intravenous fentanyl analgesia. It has been suggested that this analgesic regimen may be nothing more than a modified form of intravenous therapy.[18] Consistent reports of this effect indicate that epidural fentanyl infusions require insertion of the epidural catheter in close proximity to the surgical dermatomes affected.

Sufentanil

Sufentanil is a newer-generation synthetic opiate that is reported to be five- to sevenfold as potent as fentanyl when given systemically. Sufentanil has twice the lipid solubility of fentanyl and initially showed great promise as a successor to epidural fentanyl. Sufentanil provides excellent analgesia, a short onset of action (<15 minutes), and a duration of action that is longer than that of fentanyl (4–6 hours). Epidural dosing guidelines have revealed that sufentanil potency in the epidural space is only twice that of fentanyl. This is attributable to a higher degree of nonspecific uptake by lipophilic tissues.[19]

Given its high lipid solubility and short duration of action, sufentanil has been used in intermittent bolus, continuous epidural infusions, and even in PCA devices. Boluses of 30 to 50 μg for upper abdominal or thoracic surgery and 15 to 30 μg for peripheral surgeries are required for analgesia. Epidural infusion rates to 0.15 to 0.30 $\mu g \cdot kg^{-1} \cdot h^{-1}$ are sufficient when a dilute 1-μg/mL solution is used. Given the high degree of lipid solubility and systemic absorption from continuous epidural infusions, the issue of plasma concentrations of sufentanil with continuous infusions has been raised. Although sufentanil has not been as extensively investigated as fentanyl, significant systemic levels have been reported and may represent a lack of true advantage of sufentanil over fentanyl in continuous infusions.[20]

Opioid–Local Anesthetic Combinations

Problems arising from spinal opiate side effects and systemic absorption have led to the use of narcotic–local anesthetic combinations. This practice aims to minimize the dose of spinally administered opiates and, in turn, the problems associated with their use. In addition, some evidence shows that the addition of dilute local anesthetic solutions improves analgesia. Several investigations[19] have indicated that analgesia obtained from epidural infusions of fentanyl or sufentanil was enhanced when used with dilute solutions of bupivacaine. Similarly, epidural infusions of hydromorphone with more dilute bupivacaine solutions were superior to use of hydromorphone alone for cesarean section pain. There have been conflicting reports, however, that epidural morphine combined with bupivacaine has no advantage over epidural morphine alone in terms of analgesia, total narcotic requirement, or side effects following thoracotomy or upper abdominal surgery or cesarean section. Similar results have been found with fentanyl-bupivacaine combinations.

Addition of local anesthetics to spinal opiate infusions or boluses may enhance analgesia without clinical signs of local anesthetic blockade. However, benefit may also stem from coincident sympathetic or sensory blockade achieved with a local anesthetic solution. The benefit in superior analgesia and decreased spinal opiate requirement may come at the expense of the potentially deleterious local anesthetic side effects of hypotension, motor weakness, and inability to ambulate. The importance of the analgesic regimen therefore needs to be factored into the total plan of patient care and tailored individually to each patient's needs following acute tissue injury.

INFLUENCE ON OUTCOME

Outcome is a primary consideration in pain treatment. Patient outcome is expressed in terms of overall well-being as well as of morbidity and mortality. The goals of acute pain management should be (1) to optimize the emotional and psychologic well-being of the patient and of his or her family (patient satisfaction), (2) to provide superior pain relief with a minimum of side effects from the medication or technique, (3) to restore or maintain preoperative physiologic function, and (4) to minimize postoperative complications and thereby shorten the duration of the ICU or hospital stay. The challenge of acute pain management is to accomplish these goals in an efficient, safe, and cost-effective manner. Although no firm conclusion can be offered at present, it is indicated that adequate acute pain management by PCA, the use of spinal opiates, or peripheral or central neural blockade shows benefit over previously used regimens in postoperative recovery as well as in providing superior analgesia and optimal patient satisfaction.

PCA has demonstrated outcome advantages in terms of decreased confusion, restoration of pulmonary function, fewer pulmonary complications, shorter time to ambulation, and shortened hospital stay.[21–23]

Since the advent of spinal opiate analgesia, the beneficial effects of spinal opiate therapy on the physiologic derangements of acute tissue injury have been consistently demonstrated. In addition to providing favorable outcome regarding pulmonary complications,[24–26] the cardiovascular system,[27–29] neuroendocrine stress response,[10] and vascular complications,[27, 30, 31] superior analgesia with spinal opiates has demonstrated the ability to decrease the time needed for mechanical ventilation, the duration of intensive care, and the duration of hospital stay and to lower the total cost of hospitalization.

The economic impact of the benefits provided by adequately treated acute pain is only indicated by the results of outcome studies. It is evident that epidural analgesia in critically ill patients has the potential to diminish morbidity and thereby to minimize the necessity for medical intervention and support. In addition to statistically significant diminution in hospital and ICU stays as well as in ventilator time, cost analyses are being presented in the literature more frequently. Adoption of more effective pain management techniques and the development of acute pain services are emerging as cost-effective alternatives to traditional parenteral narcotic techniques and represent a compassionate endeavor to optimize patient comfort.

REGIONAL BLOCKADE

Side effects such as sedation, respiratory depression, nausea, gastrointestinal dysfunction, potential cardiovascular depression, and difficulty in monitoring mental status in head injury patients often make the use of systemic narcotics a poor option in the treatment of acute pain. Preexisting conditions (e.g., critical illness, central nervous system disease, anatomic considerations, coagulopathy) may render the use of spinal opiates impractical. As a result, many critically ill patients do not receive any pain treatment or are undertreated. If the use of systemic opioids is to be avoided, regional anesthetic techniques can provide excellent analgesia and help maintain patients alert and cooperative. Local anesthetics can be administered for local infiltration, intravenous regional anesthesia, peripheral nerve blocks, and central neural blockade. Regional techniques exist for virtually every indication and location of pain (Table 161–5).

Local Infiltration

Local infiltration is perhaps the simplest method for providing extended wound analgesia. Local anesthetic can be administered by subcutaneous infiltration for analgesia of minor injuries, along the surgical edges of postoperative wounds, infused continuously through implanted catheters inserted at surgical sites, and even injected into a fracture hematoma for reduction. Fears have been expressed that injections of local anesthetics into a wound may interfere with the normal healing process. However, no evidence supports that wound healing is delayed or that infection is introduced by this technique. Bupivacaine 0.25% is the preferred local anesthetic. Epinephrine-containing local anesthetics should be avoided because of the possibility of decreased blood flow and theoretic risks of delayed wound healing.

Intravenous Regional Blockade

Although seldom used for analgesia in the postoperative or post-traumatic patient, the intravenous regional technique is extremely useful for manipulation of limb fractures or for simple surgical procedures. The advantages of the technique are that it is simple, has a rapid onset and controllable duration of action, provides some muscle relaxation, and is safe when given by experienced personnel. The procedure involves placement of a double tourniquet on the proximal extremity and the intravenous administration of large volumes of dilute local anesthetic distally (40 or 50 mL of a 0.5% lidocaine solution for an upper extremity or a lower extremity, respectively). Systemic levels of local anesthetic can result from tourniquet leakage or from its inadvertent release. Bupivacaine is not recommended for this reason.

Peripheral Nerve Blockade

Peripheral nerve blockade for pain in trauma or postoperative patients is often not considered, either because of the inexperience of available personnel in performing the blockade or because of surgical time constraints. The techniques of peripheral nerve blockade produce effective, long-lasting analgesia with a minimum of side effects. Appropriate blocks exist for almost all areas of the body. With the use of a long-acting local anesthetic such as bupivacaine, analgesia may last up to 24 hours. Catheter techniques have been described for several peripheral blocks, including those of the intercostal space, interpleural space, femoral nerve, and brachial plexus.

Intercostal Blockade

Intercostal blockade is simple and effective and has been extensively used to provide pain relief for patients with fractured ribs, blunt trauma, and upper abdominal and thoracic surgery. Because of significant pain, these patients often have poor respiratory effort and an ineffective cough and risk respiratory failure, which necessitates intubation and mechanical ventilation. Systemic opioid analgesia is often problematic in these patients because of its respiratory depressant and cough suppressant actions. Consistent evidence indicates that intercostal nerve block reduces the requirements of opioids and improves pulmonary function after injury.[32]

Intercostal blockade has advantages over interpleural and thoracic epidural blockades in that it is technically easier to perform and is not associated with the side effects of epidural blockade such as hypotension, motor weakness, and urinary retention. Disadvantages of intercostal blocks include the fact that multiple levels are frequently involved, and thus multiple injection sites are needed. Furthermore, unless a continuous infusion catheter is inserted, intercostal blocks must be repeated frequently (although analgesia up to 24 hours has been obtained with bupivacaine). An inherent risk of pneumothorax, a potentially fatal complication in patients with severe respiratory compromise, also exists. Because of rapid absorption into intercostal vessels, significant systemic levels of local anesthetics may result with large or repeated doses, and this can result in profound cardiovascular or central nervous system effects.

Continuous intercostal analgesia provided via indwelling catheter has been used successfully to treat pain following upper abdominal surgery, thoracic surgery, and chest trauma, especially that caused by fractured ribs.[33] The obvious advantage is provision of prolonged analgesia without the need for multiple blocks and their associated risks. Local anesthetic provided through an indwelling catheter in a single intercostal space spreads cephalad and caudad to provide analgesia at several levels for multiple areas of injury.

Interpleural Blockade

Administration of local anesthetics via a percutaneous catheter placed between the visceral and parietal pleura provides good unilateral thoracic dermatomal analgesia. Interpleural analgesia has been used successfully in managing various types of pain in the thorax and upper abdomen, including pain after cholecystectomy and thoracotomy that is caused by multiple rib fractures.[34] The mechanism of action of interpleural analgesia is still uncertain. Possibilities include diffusion of local anesthetic through the parietal pleura, with subsequent spread superficially to block the intercostal nerves and posteromedially to block nerve roots and sympathetic ganglia in the paravertebral space. Direct local anesthetic action may also occur on pleural nerve endings.

Contraindications to this block include a recent thoracic infection with pleuritis and fibrosis of the pleura. Inflammation and increased vascularity can increase absorption and the systemic toxicity of the local anesthetics. Although the presence of thoracostomy tubes does not preclude use

TABLE 161–5. Regional Blocks for Management of Acute Pain

Region	*Block*
Head/neck	Occipital nerve Cervical epidural Superficial cervical plexus Local infiltration
Shoulder	Interscalene plexus Local infiltration
Chest	Intercostal Thoracic epidural Interpleural
Arm	Brachial plexus IV regional Peripheral nerve (radial, median, ulnar) Local infiltration
Abdomen	Upper: Intercostal Interpleural catheter Wound infiltration Thoracic epidural Lower: Wound infiltration Thoracic/lumbar epidural
Groin (hernia)	Ilioinguinal Iliohypogastric Local infiltration Lumbar epidural
Flank (nephrectomy)	Thoracic/lumbar epidural Intercostal Paravertebral somatic
Hand	Brachial plexus Elbow/wrist (radial, median, ulnar nerves) IV regional
Fingers	Digital Wrist
Anogenital	Caudal Epidural Penile
Anterior thigh (skin graft)	Lateral femoral cutaneous
Thigh/knee	Femoral/sciatic/obturator nerve Lumbar epidural Local infiltration
Leg	Femoral/sciatic nerve Lumbar epidural Knee (saphenous, common peroneal nerves) IV regional Local infiltration
Feet	Lumbar epidural Ankle Local
Toes	Digital Ankle

Abbreviation: IV = intravenous.

of this technique (chest tubes can actually be used to deliver the local anesthetic), it works best in situations in which no such drains are required. The degree of sensory anesthesia obtained with interpleural block is inconsistent. Frequently, pinprick sensation is well maintained, despite adequate analgesia. The greatest utility of this technique appears to be in circumstances that contraindicate the use of other regional anesthesia techniques, such as when severe vertebral injuries are present and accompanied by multiple rib fractures.

Femoral/Sciatic Blockade

Femoral nerve blockade has been used to provide analgesia and muscle relaxation for femoral fractures and after total knee arthroplasty.[35] The extent of analgesia depends on the fracture site. Excellent pain relief can be obtained for midshaft fractures, good relief for lower-third fractures, and partial relief for upper-third fractures. The method can be extended to give continuous analgesia for several days with insertion of a catheter into the femoral sheath and administration of dilute local anesthetics (e.g., 0.125–0.25% bupivacaine solution). By increasing the volume of injectate and encouraging cephalad spread, the femoral nerve block can include the lateral femoral cutaneous and obturator nerves, thus providing more complete analgesia for the upper thigh.

Except for injuries to the foot, blockade of the sciatic nerve alone is of little value in providing analgesia. Combined sciatic and femoral blocks, however, provide excellent anesthesia below the knee for significant lower extremity trauma, multiple fracture sites, and dislocations around the ankle.

Brachial Plexus Blockade

Brachial plexus blockade can be performed via the axillary, infraclavicular, interscalene, and supraclavicular routes.[36] The choice of technique depends on the site of the injury and on the patient's ability to move the arm. In general, higher lesions (e.g., upper-arm injury, dislocated shoulder) require analgesia extending into the C-5 dermatome, and this is best achieved with an interscalene approach. The axillary approach is also very popular and has been used successfully in both adults and children. As with other techniques, continuous infusion of local anesthetic can be used to prolong neural blockade. This is particularly useful following reimplantation procedures or other vascular injuries that result in diminished blood flow and vasospasm. The prolonged chemical sympathectomy provided by brachial plexus blockade permits improved blood flow to the area of injury. Incomplete analgesia in the hand with these techniques can be remedied by supplemental blockade of the individual nerves (i.e., radial, median, or ulnar) at the elbow or wrist.

Other Peripheral Nerve Blocks

Multiple nerve blocks have applications in acute pain management of postoperative, post-traumatic, or critically ill patients.[37] Ilioinguinal-iliohypogastric nerve blocks are useful after femoral groin area manipulation or hernia repair. A wrist block is easy to perform by blocking the median, radial, and ulnar nerves at the wrist. Indications for this block include lacerations or fractures of the digits and pending incision for removal of abscess of the digits. An ankle block is likewise easy to perform; it requires blockade of five nerves at the ankle: the tibial, sural, saphenous, superficial, and deep peroneal nerve. Indications for this block include the relief of pain in the sole or the dorsum of the foot. Psoas compartment lumbar plexus blockade is another alternative for lower extremity analgesia and is often used in conjunction with sciatic nerve blockade for complete anesthesia of the leg.

SPECIAL CASES

Patients with Multiple Trauma

Patients with varying degree of trauma and postoperative patients suffer similarly from the pain of acute tissue injury. The management of pain in the case of uncontrolled tissue injury can be difficult and complex, and adverse outcomes can result from overtreatment or undertreatment of this pain. Obviously, in the acute phase of trauma, immediate attention must be given to the stabilization of a patient's respiratory and cardiovascular status. Treatment of pain is appropriately deferred until the patient is stabilized and the extent of his or her injury is fully investigated and diagnosed. Acute pain from trauma results in profound and sustained catecholamine release that may support the blood pressure and cardiac output in a patient who has sustained large blood losses. Once respiratory and volume status has been restored, the slow titration of intravenously administered opioids for pain management is appropriate. This is performed under careful critical observation for respiratory effects, myocardial depression, and hypotension.

Acute injury causes immobility of the injured area. This inhibits movement of an injured extremity, spine, or ribs secondary to pain. Many of these injuries are sufficiently so painful that systemic narcotics must be used in doses large enough to render them potentially dangerous owing to the side effects that they can produce. In this scenario, any number of regional analgesic techniques may be employed to prevent or reduce the use of systemic narcotics for pain relief. Local infiltration, peripheral nerve blockade, or central neural blockade with a local anesthetic or opiates may be employed safely alone or in combination with systemic analgesics.

Burn Patients

Patients presenting with burn injuries offer a challenge to the physicians and medical staff involved in their care. The pain from burn injuries is grossly undertreated. The primary method of pain management in these patients should be the intravenous administration of opioids. As in acute trauma, this should be started only after a secured airway has been ensured and stable hemodynamics have been established. In general, full thickness burns are not painful, but partial thickness burns are extremely painful. Patients with severe burn trauma have two types of pain. First, constant pain from the burn injury occurs at rest and with the performance of daily activities. This pain should be managed around-the-clock with opioid regimens. Second, procedures necessary for burn treatment are associated with severe pain. These include débridement, dressing changes, hydrotherapy, and physical therapy. This pain should be managed with the tailoring of a drug regimen that is specific to both the patient and to the procedure. Pain management during these procedures may include the use of opioids alone or in combination with anxiolytics or dissociative anesthesia with ketamine. Many clinicians use fentanyl as the opioid of choice during procedures, with initial doses in the range of 1 to 6 μg/kg with the addition of midazolam, 0.08 mg/kg, in divided doses. Although ketamine can be given intravenously or intramuscularly, it is best to avoid intramuscular drug regimens in burn patients. Intravenous doses

TABLE 161–6. Pharmacokinetics of Selected Analgesic and Sedative Agents

Agent	*Volume of Distribution (L/kg)*	*Plasma Protein Binding (%)*	*Hepatic Clearance* ($mL \cdot kg^{-1} \cdot min^{-1}$)	*Renal Excretion Free Drug (%)*	*Elimination Half-Life (min)*	*Active/Toxic Metabolites*	*Drug Activity*	
							Hepatic failure	*Renal failure*
Morphine	3.2	30	14.7	10	114	Yes	+	+ +
Meperidine	3.8	60	15.1	5	180–250	Yes	+ +	+ + +
Fentanyl	4.1	84	11.6	8	200	No	+	+
Sufentanil	4.5	92.5	12.7	1–2	148–164	Yes	+ +	+ + +
Methadone	6	90	2.8	5	35 h	No	+ + +	+
Lidocaine	1.3	70	0.95 L/min	NA	96	Yes	+ +	+ + +
Bupivacaine	2.0	95	0.47 L/min	NA	210	No	+ +	+ +
Ketorolac	0.2	99	4.0	58	300–310	No	+	+ +
Diazepam	1.5	98	0.3	5	21–37	Yes	+ +	+ +
Midazolam	1.5	98	6–8	5	60–200 h	No	+ +	No change

(Data from Sinatra RS: Pain management in patients suffering from major organ failure. *In:* Acute Pain: Mechanisms and Management. Sinatra RS, Hord AH, Ginsberg B, et al [Eds]. St. Louis, Mosby-Year Book, 1992; Stoelting RK: Opioid agonists and antagonists. *In*: Pharmacology and Physiology in Anesthetic Practice. Stoelting RK [Ed]). Philadelphia, JB Lippincott, 1987; *and* Micaela M, Buckley T, Brogden RN: Ketorolac: A review of its pharmacodynamic and pharmacokinetic properties, and therapeutic potential. Drugs 1990; 39:86–109.)

Key: + = mild; + + = moderate; + + + = major potentiation of activity; NA = not available.

for ketamine can be titrated using 0.5 to 1.0 mg/kg. Ketamine should be used in combination with anxiolytics to abate the increased incidence of hallucinations and excitement. Although many nonpharmacologic therapeutic modalities have been tried, including hypnosis, relaxation training, biofeedback, distraction techniques, and transcutaneous electrical nerve stimulation therapy, excruciating pain associated with burn injuries appears to require more aggressive intervention.

Patients with Major Organ Failure

Many patients suffering from major organ failure receive suboptimal pain management because of fear on the part of caregivers that treatment may worsen an already critical condition.[38] With major organ dysfunction, significant changes can occur in the pharmacokinetic profile of analgesic medication. Volume of distribution, clearance, and excretion are affected by organ failure, and these effects are exaggerated by drug administration. Table 161–6 summarizes the pharmacokinetics of different drugs and the pharmacodynamic changes associated with hepatic and renal failure. Acute pain management for significant, specific organ dysfunction is discussed in the following sections.

Central Nervous System

Central nervous system trauma or disease represents a challenge to the providers of acute pain control particularly for patients who have disruption of the blood-brain barrier and increased intracranial pressure. Controversy exists as to whether these patients should receive opioid agents. The concern over opioid-induced increase in arterial carbon dioxide tension and subsequent elevation of intracranial pressure has led many clinicians to avoid the use of these agents. Use of meperidine should be avoided, since active metabolites may induce seizure activity. Central neural blockade (epidural or intrathecal) carries the risk of dural puncture, which causes brain stem herniation. Some physicians have employed transcutaneous electrical stimulation and ketorolac as adjuvant therapy for pain relief.

Pulmonary Failure

Patients with severe pulmonary conditions (e.g., chronic obstructive pulmonary disease, restrictive lung disease, and pulmonary hypertension) who sustain multiple trauma or who undergo thoracic or abdominal procedures are excellent candidates for continuous epidural opiate infusions. This technique may better preserve pulmonary function postoperatively compared with intravenous opioid administration. Administration of ketorolac and transcutaneous electrical nerve stimulation application to supplement opioid use have had good results. Other modalities include placement of interpleural catheters, intercostal nerve blockade, or continuous intercostal infusions with extreme caution directed toward the risk of pneumothorax.

Cardiac Failure

Patients with severe ischemic heart disease recovering from noncardiac surgery can avoid ischemic events if proper pain management is provided. Epidurally and intrathecally administered opioids suppress the catecholamine response to pain more effectively than intravenously administered opioids. Patients who receive intravenous therapy should be given intravenous opioids carefully titrated to analgesia and side effects. Individuals with severely depressed cardiac function who receive intravenous morphine are susceptible to hypotension. Meperidine should be used with caution in these patients because its vagolytic action may induce tachycardia, hypertension, and subsequent ischemia.

Liver Failure

In patients with liver disease, it is difficult to quantitate the extent of dysfunction in metabolism and biotransformation until the late stages of liver failure. Thus, the physician must always be concerned with analgesic overdosage in these patients. The capability of the liver to synthesize may be compromised to the point that a coagulopathy develops, and this renders regional analgesia impractical. However, if no contraindications to catheter placement exist, spinal opiate therapy is acceptable and provides excellent benefits for patients with hepatic failure. Intrathecal administration of morphine (0.25–0.5 mg) provides superior analgesia and a duration similar to that of intravenous doses 100-fold greater and infused through a PCA device. With epidural analgesia, when a local anesthetic is added to an opioid agent, care must be taken that the patient does not reach toxic serum concentrations of local anesthetic. If coagulopathy exists or if the surgical site does not permit the use of regional analgesia, intravenous fentanyl administered continuously or by a PCA device can be a safe alternative (see Table 161–6).

TABLE 161–7. Guidelines for Postoperative Analgesia with Opioids in Children

Route	*Drug*	*Dose**
Continuous IV	Morphine	0.05–0.06 mg · kg^{-1} · h^{-1}
	Meperidine	0.5–0.6 mg · kg^{-1} · h^{-1}
	Fentanyl	2–4 μg · kg^{-1} · h^{-1}
Intermittent IV†	Morphine	0.08–0.1 mg/kg every 2 h
	Meperidine	0.8–1 mg/kg/every 2 h
PO	Codeine	0.5–1 mg/kg every 4 h
	Morphine	0.3 mg/kg every 4 h
IM‡	Morphine	0.1–0.15 mg/kg every 3–4 h
	Meperidine	1–1.5 mg/kg every 3–4 h

(Adapted from Berde CB: Pediatric postoperative pain management. Pediatr Clin North Am 1989; 36:924.)

*For nonintubated patients in the first 3 months of life, or for other patients with an increased tendency for respiratory depression, starting doses should be diminished by at least a factor of 3 to 4 from doses recommended here, and facilities for intensive observation and respiratory support should be available.

†Intravenous boluses should be administered slowly (e.g., over 15 to 20 minutes).

‡Individual response varies. Doses should be carefully titrated and adjusted according to patients' physical status and analgesic requirements.

Renal Failure

Epidural or intrathecal administration of morphine in renal failure patients offers several advantages over systemic narcotics, including superior analgesia, low dosage requirements, minimum accumulation, and absence of renal toxicity. Intravenous opioid administration must be conducted with great care. Intravenous use of meperidine and sufentanil carries the potential for accumulation of active metabolites that are renally excreted. PCA with fentanyl represents an excellent option in renal failure patients because the analgesia is adequate and the renally excreted metabolites have minimal activity. The renal activity of ketorolac, although likely insignificant in the acute setting, should discourage its use in patients with renal failure (see Table 161–6).

PEDIATRIC PATIENTS

Traditional bias against treating pain in the postoperative period is exaggerated in the pediatric population because of additional misconceptions that children do not experience pain in the same manner as do adults. In 1968, Swaffard and Allen reported that only 2 of 60 children in their surgical ward required pain medications.[39] They stated that "pediatric patients seldom need medication for relief of pain. They tolerate discomfort well." In 1977, Eland and Anderson were the first to challenge these practices and to document the extent of this bias.[40] Their study revealed that many children were not only undertreated but also that some were not treated at all, despite their having severe injuries (e.g., traumatic amputation of the foot) or having undergone major surgeries (e.g., heminephrectomy). Consistent disparity exists between the number of pain medication doses given to adults and that given to pediatric patients undergoing similar procedures. The undertreatment of pain in pediatric patients exists not only in the postoperative arena; inadequate relief is given to children suffering from burn wounds, infants undergoing circumcision, and children requiring diagnostic procedures such as bone marrow aspiration. Possible explanations for inadequate pain control in pediatric patients include incorrect assumptions, traditional attitudes, the complexity of pain assessment, and the lack of research and training in this area.[41]

Pain Management in Children

Assessment of pediatric pain can be very difficult. Crying may persist because of postoperative pain or because of fear, anxiety, or loneliness. Accurate interpretation of pain behavior remains the biggest challenge in properly treating pain in pediatric patients. Once the extent of pain has been established, various modalities for treatment exist. Nonpharmacologic treatment includes appropriate teaching and guidance offered in the preoperative period. Other tools include imagery, hypnosis, and distraction techniques that are helpful in treating the postoperative pain of children in various age groups. Transcutaneous electrical nerve stimulation therapy has been used alone or in combination with analgesic therapy to alleviate the pain of tissue injury.

Despite these nonpharmacologic interventions, systemic analgesic therapy is the mainstay of pediatric pain control. Management of mild to moderate forms of postoperative pain includes use of the first line of drugs, the nonopiate analgesics that include acetaminophen and nonsteroidal anti-inflammatory agents. Acetaminophen has a high therapeutic ratio and very few contraindications. Doses range from 10 to 15 mg/kg perorally or 15 to 20 mg/kg rectally every 4 hours. Several of the nonsteroidal agents provide excellent pain relief. Although these medications cause platelet dysfunction, gastritis, and renal pathology, side effects are rare with short-term postoperative use. If pain persists, opioid analgesia may be required. Narcotic analgesics provide excellent relief if given in sufficient amounts at effective intervals. Table 161–7 lists the various starting doses of opioids for pediatric use. These agents may be administered by various routes, including the oral, rectal, intranasal, transdermal, intravenous, intramuscular, epidural, and intrathecal routes. Intramuscular injections are particularly distressing to pediatric patients to the point that they may deny having pain to avoid receiving an injection. PCA is now considered an excellent alternative to intermittent intramuscular or intravenous injection in pediatric patients. The literature suggests that if properly selected, children benefit from all the advantages of the regimen in terms of the maintenance of consistent drug levels, superior analgesia, and improved emotional status. Some centers routinely use PCA devices on patients as young as 6 years of age.[42]

Regional analgesia has increased the possibilities for pain treatment in children. Pain management for painful pediatric procedures such as lumbar puncture, suturing lacerations, bone marrow aspirations, circumcisions, and biopsies and for pain associated with trauma and surgery are indications for the use of the regional analgesic techniques. Optimum management and outcome depend on the minimization of emotional as well as physical trauma. Psychologic and behavioral strategies combined with pharmacologic treatment modalities can be utilized successfully to accomplish a procedure without significant pain or suffering.

Pediatric patients need not suffer from the pain of acute tissue injury despite the traditional inadequacy of pain management in the pediatric population. Most pain management techniques for adults are appropriate for children. As in the adult population, physiologic disturbance and poor outcome may result from inadequately treated pain in children, and the importance of adequate treatment cannot be overemphasized.

CONCLUSIONS

In summary, inadequate acute pain relief from tissue injury can have detrimental physiologic effects that are additive to the original insult (see Fig. 161–4). This includes delayed recovery from surgery or trauma, increased morbidity, and

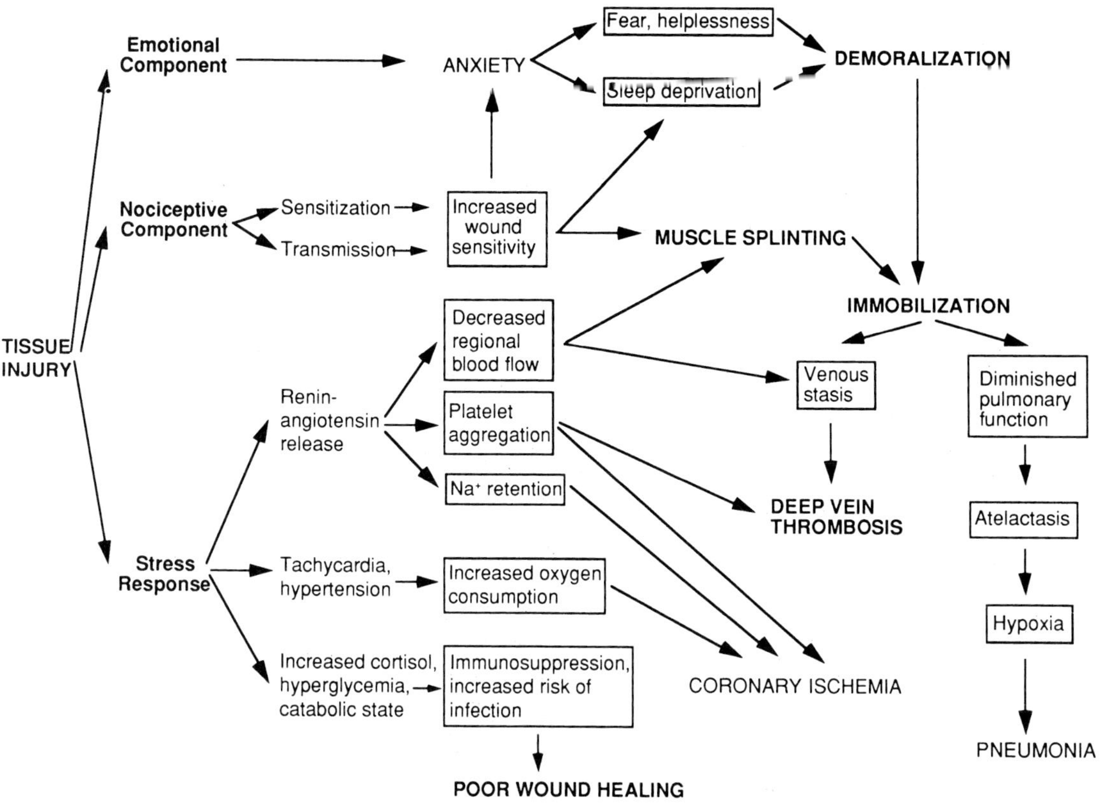

Figure 161–4. Overview of the physiologic consequences of acute tissue injury, including multisystem responses, key target organs, and contributors to morbidity, mortality, and poor outcome. (Adapted from Sinatra RS: Pathophysiology of acute pain. *In*: Acute Pain Mechanisms and Management. Sinatra RS, Hord AH, Ginsberg B, et al (Eds). St. Louis, Mosby-Year Book, 1992, pp 44–57.)

poor pulmonary function postoperatively. Splinting secondary to pain, inability to clear secretions, and reactivity of the bronchial tree lead to atelectasis and pulmonary complications. Accelerated catecholamine release increases systemic vascular resistance, increases cardiac stroke work, and worsens myocardial oxygen supply-demand ratios. Hypercoagulation leads to significant thromboembolic phenomena and vascular compromise. The stress response leads to excessive protein wasting and poor wound healing. Patient anguish and suffering may lead to agitation, increasing the possibility of inadvertent extubation, disconnection of arterial and intravenous lines, and difficulty in the provision of effective nursing care. It is necessary to realize that the true importance of adequate acute pain management lies in outcome as well as in patient satisfaction; thus, we must use all pain treatment techniques, drugs, and drug delivery technology that are at our disposal to adequately treat the pain of tissue injury.

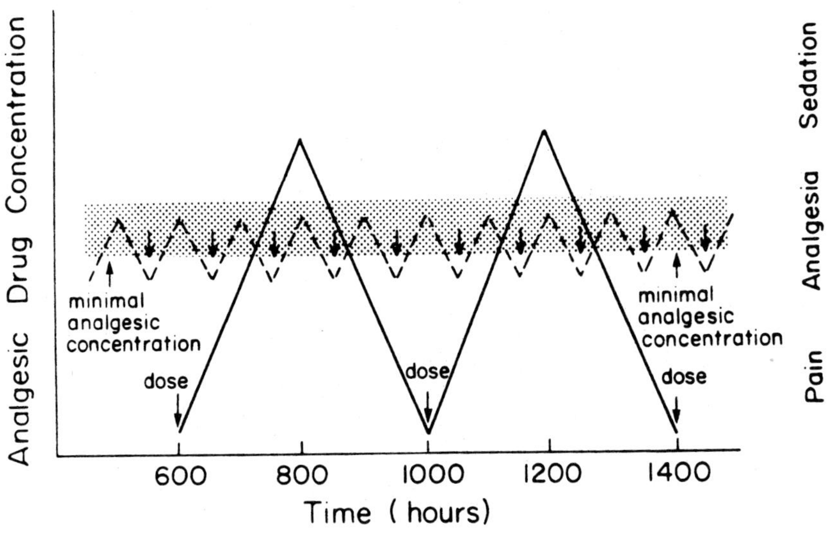

Figure 161–5. The archetypal model of PCA. The comparative relation between analgesic drug concentrations, dosing intervals, and analgesic response between PCA and periodic intramuscular narcotic administration illustrates the theoretic benefit derived from PCA and the inefficiency of traditional regimens. PCA drug concentration is represented by the *dashed line*, and intramuscular opioid concentration is represented by the *solid line*. The frequent, small, and on-demand dosing of PCA affords maintenance of drug concentrations more consistently within analgesic levels. In contrast, intramuscular administration shows high variability, with the majority of concentrations in the subanalgesic or superanalgesic range; this results in unrelieved pain or side effects. (From Ferrante FM, Orav EJ, Rocco AG, et al: A statistical model for pain in patient-controlled analgesia and conventional intramuscular opioid regimens. Anesth Analg 1988; 67:457–461.)

References

1. Marks RM, Sachar EJ: Undertreatment of medical inpatients with narcotic analgesics. Ann Intern Med 1973; 78:173.
2. Cohen FL: Postsurgical pain relief: Patients' status and nurses' medication choices. Pain 1980; 9:265.
3. Loper KA, Butler S, Nessley M, et al: Clinical note: Paralyzed with pain: The need for education. Pain 1989; 37:315.
4. White PF: Patient-controlled analgesia: A new approach to management of postoperative pain. Semin Anesth 1985; 4:255.
5. Bollish SJ, Collins CL, Kirking DM, et al: Efficacy of patient-controlled versus conventional analgesia for postoperative pain. Clin Pharm 1985; 4:48.
6. Ferrante FM, Orav EJ, Rocco AG: A statistical model for pain in patient-controlled analgesia and conventional intramuscular opioid regimens. Anesth Analg 1988; 67:457.
7. Gregg R: Spinal analgesia: Management of postoperative pain. Anesthesiol Clin North Am 1989; 7:79.
8. Dittman M, Steenblock U, Kranzlin M, et al: Epidural analgesia or mechanical ventilation for multiple rib fractures. Intensive Care Med 1982; 8:89.
9. Buckley FP, Robinson NB, Simonowitz DA, et al: Anaesthesia in the morbidity obese. Anaesthesia 1983; 38:840.
10. Kehlet H: The stress response to anesthesia and surgery: Release mechanisms and modifying factors. Clin Anaesthesiol 1984; 2:315.
11. Yaksh TL: Spinal opiate analgesia: Characteristics and principles of action. Pain 1981; 11:293.
12. Logas WG, El-Baz N, El-Ganzouri A, et al: Continuous thoracic epidural analgesia for post-operative pain relief following thoracotomy: A randomized prospective study. Anesthesiology 1987; 67:787.
13. Rawal N, Arner S, Gustafsson LL, et al: Present state of extradural and intrathecal opioid analgesia in Sweden. Br J Anaesth 1987; 59:791.
14. Ready LB, Loper KA, Nessley M, et al: Postoperative epidural morphine is safe on surgical wards. Anesthesiology 1991; 75:452.
15. Stenseth R, Sellevold O, Breivik H: Epidural morphine for postoperative pain: Experience with 1085 patients. Acta Anaesthesiol Scand 1985; 29:148.
16. Cross DA, Hunt JB: Feasibility of epidural morphine postoperative analgesia in a small community hospital. Anesth Analg 1991; 72:765.
17. Paech MJ: Epidural pethidine or fentanyl during caesarean section: A double-blind comparison. Anaesth Intensive Care 1989; 17:157.
18. Loper KA, Ready LB, Downey M, et al: Epidural and intravenous fentanyl infusions are clinically equivalent after knee surgery. Anesth Analg 1990; 70:72.
19. Badner NH: Epidural agents for postoperative analgesia. Anesthesiol Clin North Am 1992; 10:321.
20. Cohen SE, Tan S, White PF: Sufentanil analgesia following cesarean section: Epidural versus intravenous administration. Anaesthesiology 1988; 68:129.
21. Egbert AM, Leland HP, Short LM, et al: Randomized trial of postoperative patient-controlled analgesia vs. intramuscular narcotics on frail elderly men. Arch Intern Med 1990; 150:1897.
22. Wayslak TJ, Abbott FV, English MJM, et al: Reduction of postoperative morbidity following patient-controlled morphine. Can J Anaesth 1990; 37:726.
23. Scalley RD, Berquist K, Cochran RS: Patient-controlled analgesia in orthopedic procedures. Orthop Rev 1988; 17:1106.
24. Bromage PR, Camporesi E, Chestnut D: Epidural narcotics for postoperative analgesia. Anesth Analg 1980; 59:473.
25. Cuschieri RJ, Morran CG, Howie DC, et al: Postoperative pain and pulmonary complications: Comparison of three analgesic regimens. Br J Surg 1985; 72:495.
26. Rawal N, Sjostrand UM, Christoffersson E, et al: Comparison of intramuscular and epidural morphine for postoperative analgesia in the grossly obese: Influence on postoperative ambulation and pulmonary function. Anesth Analg 1984; 63:583.
27. Yeager MD, Glass DD, Neff RK, et al: Epidural anesthesia and analgesia in high-risk surgical patients. Anesthesiology 1987; 66:729.
28. Vanstrum GS, Bjornson KM, Ilko R: Postoperative effects of intrathecal morphine in coronary artery bypass surgery. Anesth Analg 1988; 76:261.
29. El-Baz N, Goldin M: Continuous epidural infusion of morphine for pain relief after cardiac operations. J Thorac Cardiovasc Surg 1987; 93:878.
30. Modig J, Borg T, Bagge L, et al: Role of epidural and of general anesthesia in fibrinolysis and coagulation after total hip replacement. Br J Anaesth 1983; 55:625.
31. Simpson IJ, Radford SG, Forster SJ, et al: The fibrinolytic effects of anesthesia. Anesthesiology 1982; 37:3.
32. Faust RJ, Nauss LA: Post-thoracotomy intercostal block: Comparison of its effect on pulmonary function with those of intramuscular meperidine. Anesth Analg 1976; 55:542.
33. Murphy DF: Intercostal nerve blockade for fractured ribs and post-operative analgesia: Description of a new technique. Reg Anesth 1983; 8:151.
34. Covino BG: Interpleural regional analgesia. Anesth Analg 1988; 67:427.
35. Hord AJ, Roberson JR, Thompson WF, et al: Evaluation of continuous femoral nerve analgesia after primary total knee arthroplasty. Anesth Analg 1990; 70:S164.
36. Bridenbaugh LD: The upper extremity: Somatic blockade. *In*: Neural Blockade in Clinical Anesthesia and Management of Pain. 2nd ed. Cousins MJ (Ed). Philadelphia, JB Lippincott, 1988, pp 387–415.
37. Pither C, Hartrick C: Post-operative pain. *In*: Handbook in Regional Anesthesiology. Raj PP (Ed). Chicago, Churchill Livingstone, 1985.
38. Sinatra RS: Pain management in patients suffering from major organ failure. *In*: Acute Pain: Mechanisms and Management. Sinatra RS (Ed). St. Louis, Mosby-Year Book, 1992, pp 399–421.
39. Swafford L, Allen D: Pain relief in the pediatric patient. Med Clin North Am 1968; 52:131.
40. Eland JM, Anderson JE: The experience of pain in children. *In*: Pain: A Source Book for Nurses and Other Health Professionals. Jacox A (Ed). Boston, Little, Brown and Co, 1977.
41. Schecter NL: The undertreatment of pain in children: An overview. Pediatr Clin North Am 1989; 36:781–794.
42. Berde CB: Pediatric postoperative pain management. Pediatr Clin North Am 1989; 36:921–940.

CHAPTER 162

Management of the Burn Patient

Robert H. Demling, MD

Burn injuries remain a leading cause of mortality and severe long-term dysfunction, especially in children and young adults. The incidence of severe burns remains highest among those aged 18 to 30 years, with men predominating over women by a ratio of 8 to 1.[1–3]

Many advances have been made in burn management, and these advances have resulted in a marked decrease in mortality, especially in patients of young age. Burns that involve 70% to 80% of the body's surface used to be 100% fatal. Now, the mortality rate is reported to be less than 50% by many burn centers. The major advances have been in two areas. The first is in the rapid and safe removal of burn tissue before the onset of infection and wound closure, using available autologous skin and liberal use of temporary skin substitutes; this is followed by optimization of the rate of wound healing with the use of scientific principles. The second advance has been in the areas of critical care management, which allows the patient to avoid major organ failure, especially pulmonary failure, during the wound healing period. Preventive medicine is the key to success. It is now well established that treatment of organ failure in the presence of remaining burn tissue is extremely difficult in view of the fact that the organ failure, especially respiratory failure, is perpetuated by the inflammation and infection in a wound. In addition, a persistent immunodeficient state and increased skin and lung colonization by infectious organisms leads to a high risk of continued nosocomial infection. Multisystem organ failure in the burn patient has a mortality of nearly 100% compared with 50% to 70% in the non–burn trauma patient. Elderly burn patients are particularly vulnerable to organ failure and mortality, with the major problem being the limitation of cardiopulmonary reserve required to cope with the burn-induced stress response.[1–4]

The importance of critical care management is emphasized by the fact that the leading cause of death in burn patients is no longer burn wound sepsis but respiratory failure. Pulmonary problems, of course, are particularly common after smoke inhalation, which markedly increases the mortality rate.

Because of the importance of preventing complications in order to optimize survival and take advantage of the new developments in wound management, a clear understanding of burn-induced disease is essential. Post-burn problems occurring over the time course of injury are remarkably predictable, and this predictability can be used to avoid major problems before they evolve.

The simplest and most accurate way to clarify the post-burn pathophysiology is to divide the post-burn period into three very well-defined periods:

1. The resuscitation period (0–36 hours)
2. The postresuscitation period (2–5 days)
3. The inflammation-infection period (from 6 days to wound closure)

Treatment among these phases changes dramatically, as does a patient's physiology; this chapter discusses the changes that occur in each of these phases.

THE RESUSCITATION PERIOD

Three key components of management are important in the resuscitation period:

1. Airway and pulmonary support
2. Cardiovascular support
3. Wound management

Airway and Pulmonary Problems

Airway and lung dysfunction are of particular concern immediately after burn. Although clinical evidence of such dysfunction is often delayed in onset, early preventive measures need to be initiated to avoid potentially life-threatening problems. Lung and airway problems are most evident in patients who have suffered a smoke inhalation injury, but airway problems can also readily develop in the absence of smoke exposure, especially if the patient has sustained full-thickness burns to face and neck.[4–7]

Smoke inhalation injury complex can be divided into phases that are based not on the time of the injury but rather on the timing of manifestation of the injury (Table 162–1).

A hypoxic insult, carbon monoxide, and cyanide toxicity are evident immediately after injury. The major difficulty in making the diagnosis is the misinterpretation of symptoms that usually fit a host of other disease processes—in particular, central nervous system–related impairments, such as those caused by alcohol and drug abuse or by head injury. Maintaining a high index of suspicion is mandatory. Clues to the diagnosis of carbon monoxide toxicity include a *measured* oxygen saturation of hemoglobin that is lower than predicted by the oxygen tension and the presence of an unexplained increase in anion gap metabolic acidosis. Verification is accomplished by assessing carboxyhemoglobin level (normal level: <5%). The value often underestimates the initial magnitude of the carbon monoxide toxicity, as invariably initial emergency care responders begin to displace the carbon monoxide with oxygen at the scene of injury. Continued oxygen administration (90–100%) is required. Cyanide poisoning is more difficult to diagnose because blood cyanide levels are often not readily available. Restoration and maintenance of perfusion allow the cyanide to be metabolized. Treatment with sodium nitrate, followed by sodium thiosulfate therapy, can be initiated if high cyanide levels are evident or suspected.[14]

Upper airway injury from heat and chemicals in smoke can be detected simply by direct laryngoscopy (injury is indicated by a reddened mucosa). However, the degree of injury and risk of subsequent edema cannot be accurately predicted by initial findings. In the absence of a burn—in particular, a facial burn—the injury can often be treated without intubation. A body burn injury, however, markedly increases the upper airways edema process, especially when large amounts of fluids are infused.

The additional presence of a deep facial burn will lead to massive facial edema over the next 12 to 18 hours, making it extremely difficult to intubate the patient later, if necessary. Therefore, early *elective* intubation is indicated when deep facial burns and any evidence of an airway injury exist. Intubation is often indicated when only deep facial burns are present (Table 162–2). This would certainly be the case if a large body burn is also present, necessitating early excision and grafting beginning in the next several days. Intubation required for the operation would be extremely difficult and hazardous. Since the first 5 days are the optimum time for surgery, waiting for facial edema to resolve so that a "safe" intubation can be performed would result in later morbidity from unresected burn.[8]

The pulmonary response to a chemical burn to the lower airway is initially bronchorrhea, bronchoconstriction, small airways closure, and marked ventilation-perfusion mismatch.[4–6, 9] Atelectasis is also very common. Endotracheal intubation is often indicated for pulmonary toilet, airway protection, and for positive-pressure ventilatory support.[8, 10] Pulmonary dysfunction can also occur with deep burns to the chest wall, which produce a restrictive defect and necessitate chest wall escharotomy (Fig. 162–1). It is often difficult to distinguish the pulmonary effects of a stiff chest wall from those caused by increased airways resistance.

Cardiovascular Support

The massive fluid losses from a skin burn are the result of three processes. The first is the alteration in vascular permeability, which results from heat and vasoactive mediators in

TABLE 162–1. Phases of Smoke Inhalation Injury

Process	*Onset of Symptoms*
Hypoxia injury from low amount of inspired oxygen in the fire	Immediate
Carbon monoxide and cyanide toxicity	Immediate
Upper airway impairment from heat and chemicals	Delayed for 6–18 hrs
Lower airway injury from chemicals in smoke	Delayed for hrs to days

TABLE 162–2. Initial Assessment of Airway (to Intubate or Not to Intubate)

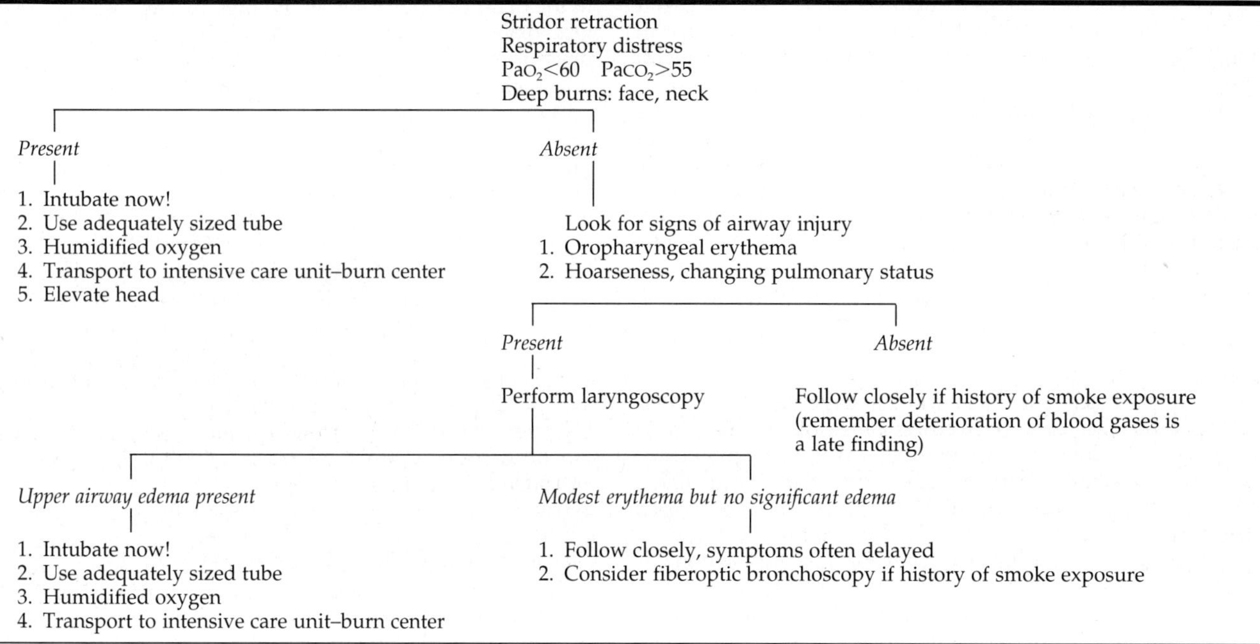

Stridor retraction
Respiratory distress
$Pa_{O_2}<60$ $Pa_{CO_2}>55$
Deep burns: face, neck

Present

1. Intubate now!
2. Use adequately sized tube
3. Humidified oxygen
4. Transport to intensive care unit–burn center
5. Elevate head

Absent

Look for signs of airway injury
1. Oropharyngeal erythema
2. Hoarseness, changing pulmonary status

Present

Perform laryngoscopy

Absent

Follow closely if history of smoke exposure (remember deterioration of blood gases is a late finding)

Upper airway edema present

1. Intubate now!
2. Use adequately sized tube
3. Humidified oxygen
4. Transport to intensive care unit–burn center

Modest erythema but no significant edema

1. Follow closely, symptoms often delayed
2. Consider fiberoptic bronchoscopy if history of smoke exposure

(Modified from Demling RH, Lalonde C: Airway and pulmonary abnormalities. *In:* Burn Trauma. Blaisdell FW, Trunkey DD [Eds]. New York, Thieme, 1989, p 10.)

burn tissue, that leads to a loss of plasma. The second is a marked increase in negative interstitial forces, either increased osmotic pressure or a negative interstitial pressure, both of which markedly accentuate the initial fluid shifts. The third source of volume loss is a fluid shift into non–burn interstitium as a result of burn-induced hypoproteinemia. A component of decreased cardiac contractility is also seen in patients with large burns.[11–13]

Several abnormalities may contribute to a decrease in cardiac output. Positive-pressure breathing and loss of water and plasma lead to a decreased preload. Release of catecholamines and other systemic vasoconstrictors may increase systemic vascular resistance and afterload. Alterations in contractility are unusual and occur mostly with large-area third-degree burns.

The purpose of formulas used to guide fluid resuscitation is at least to assist in the estimation of needs. However, after the initial decision has been made as to the type of fluids to be given and the rate at which they are to be administered, subsequent replacement is dictated by an ongoing assessment of perfusion, not by a mathematic equation. Isotonic crystalloid solution is the initial fluid of choice. The first 24-hour fluid need is often estimated based on the following formula: 4 mL of fluid × % of body surface burned × patient's body weight in kilograms. One half of the result is given in the first 8 hours. Since the fluid losses are ongoing, the rate of tissue edema is dependent on the rate of fluid infusion. Thus, excessive edema can be easily produced. The parameters of adequacy of perfusion become the key elements. In a young patient, a pulse rate of 120 beats per minute or less, a systolic blood pressure of 100 mm Hg (or a mean blood pressure of approximately 85 mm Hg), a urine output of 0.5 $mL \cdot kg^{-1} \cdot h^{-1}$, a correction of a base deficit, and a mixed or central venous oxygen saturation of hemoglobin exceeding 60% are together very reliable parameters. The risks of infection and thrombotic complications usually preclude the routine use of pulmonary artery catheters. The exception would be the elderly patient, in whom preexisting cardiac or pulmonary dysfunction make clinical assessment unreliable. Lactated Ringer's solution is the initial fluid to be given. Protein- or non–protein-containing colloid solutions can be infused immediately if perfusion with crystalloid solution alone is inadequate.[11] The fluids should be infused at a constant rate rather than as a bolus, since the latter simply increases the rate of plasma loss into the burn tissue because the burn tissue capillaries leak for days.

Figure 162–1. Preferred sites of escharotomy. (From Demling RH, LaLonde C: Airway and pulmonary abnormalities. *In:* Burn Trauma. Blaisdell FW, Trunkey DD [Eds]. New York, Thieme, 1989, p 19.)

TABLE 162–3. Specific Resuscitation Guidelines

Patient <40 years old and <50% total body surface burned; no smoke inhalation	*Patient <40 years old and >60% total body surface burned with or without smoke inhalation*	*Patient not responding to fluid alone*
1. Can give isotonic crystalloid solution for 24 h as primary fluid 2. Begin replacing protein deficit at 12–18 h (1–2 $mL \cdot kg^{-1} \cdot h^{-1}$)	1. Use isotonic crystalloid solutions as primary fluid 2. Add colloid solution from beginning (2 $mL \cdot kg^{-1} \cdot h^{-1}$) 3. Consider hypertonic saline early 4. May need to add renal dose dopamine	1. Look for pulmonary problem, increased airway pressure 2. Consider inotrope beta agonist first choice 3. Consider use of blood as volume expander
Patient with burn and severe smoke inhalation	*Patient >40 or <5 years old with large burn*	*Patient in shock*
1. Will usually need combination of crystalloid and colloid solutions to maintain hemodynamic stability, especially with increasing need for positive pressure 2. Consider low-dose dopamine if urine output poor despite large volume infusion	1. Isotonic crystalloid solution primary fluid 2. Add colloid from beginning (nonprotein or protein) to maintain stability 3. Consider careful use of hypertonic saline 4. May need to add inotropic support	1. Give colloid solution (5% albumin dextran) along with crystalloid solution until shock corrected 2. Then use crystalloid solution as primary fluid

(Modified from Demling RH, LaLonde C: Restoration and maintenance of hemodynamic stability. *In:* Burn Trauma. Blaisdell FW, Trunkey DD (Eds). New York, Thieme, 1989, p 41.)

Red blood cell mass may also be decreased as a result of the damage of red blood cells by heat; acute hemolysis as well as external losses from escharotomies and possible other trauma consequently occur. Hematocrit is often a false indicator of blood volume, since severe plasma volume loss and some red blood cell loss leads to a normal hematocrit, even though a severe decrease in blood volume could be present. Red blood cell transfusion is often very useful in restoring hemodynamic stability in patients who do not respond to crystalloid and colloid solutions alone.

A coagulopathy is also often present; it is manifest as a hypercoagulable state in those with modest burns and as a hypocoagulable state in patients with a massive burn owing to a consumptive coagulopathy.[14]

Renal and splanchnic blood flow are more selectively decreased, and levels of antidiuretic hormones, such as aldosterone, are increased.[15] Low-dose dopamine therapy can be very useful to help restore renal and splanchnic blood flow and to prevent an excessive infusion of fluids to increase a marginal urine output when all other aspects of perfusion appear adequate (Table 162–3).

Wound Management

Assessing the size and depth of the wound is the next priority (Fig. 162–2). Decisions as to the subsequent operative management are best made in the early resuscitation period, since the ideal time for excision is before the onset of wound inflammation.

The specific management of the wound, the choice of topical antibiotics, and related topics are not covered in this chapter. However, it is important to point out that heat loss is a major problem in burn patients and that a warm environment is mandatory for patients with large burn lest they experience severe hypothermia.[16] Since glucose stores are depleted very early in such patients, no energy reserves are available to increase body heat and to counteract the low body temperature.

THE POSTRESUSCITATION PERIOD

In general, this period—from 2 to 5 days after burn injury—is the ideal time to initiate aggressive wound excision and closure. For this to occur, the patient must be hemodynamically stable, which means that an optimum initial resuscitation is required. Hypovolemia or uncontrolled respiratory dysfunction, especially the absence of a good airway, markedly increases operative risks. It is also important to recognize that this "grace period" is short-lived and that once wound colonization, inflammation, and profound hypermetabolism develop, operative risks again escalate, especially in the presence of any lung or cardiac problems. To optimize cardiopulmonary function, an understanding of the physiologic changes that occur during this period is necessary.

Airway and Pulmonary Support

In the presence of smoke inhalation, this period is one of continuing problems, with small-airway plugging from secretions and alveolar atelectasis resulting in an increased shunt fraction.[4–6] Airway edema and increased airways reactivity are still present and often necessitate partial mechanical ventilatory support and positive end-expiratory pressure.[8–10] Nosocomial pneumonia is usually not a high-risk factor at this time, but it does become a major problem toward the end of the first week, as oropharyngeal colonization by pathogenic organisms develops.

Major fluid balance problems again develop during this period. Fluid shifting back into the circulation from tissue edema can lead to hypervolemia, which can, of course, aggravate the pulmonary problem. However, as fragile as the lung may be at this point, the marked increase in carbon dioxide production and in the risk of infection (which will occur in the subsequent weeks) worsens. Therefore, moderate lung dysfunction is not a contraindication to operative intervention.[8]

It is extremely important that the operative procedures be kept short, (i.e., <2 hours) and that optimal pulmonary support be provided, including positive end-expiratory pressure. Initiation of systemic antibiotic therapy early when signs of bacterial tracheobronchitis are observed is also critical because local lung defenses have been substantially diminished as a result of mucosal injury to the airway. The use of prophylactic antibiotics in the absence of any evidence of airways infection is contraindicated.

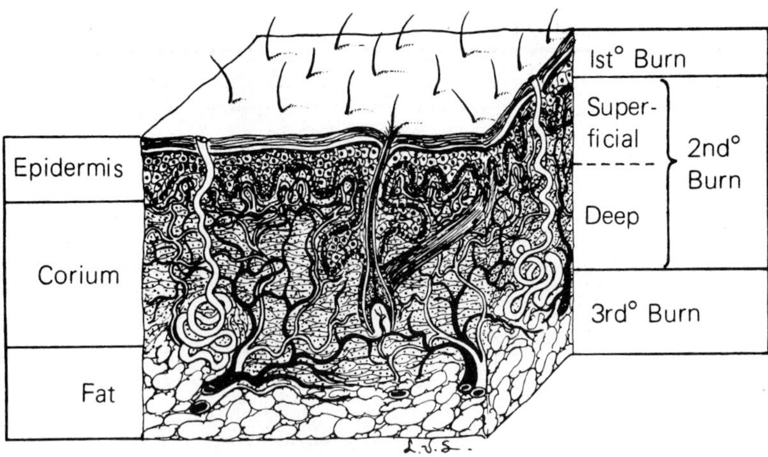

Figure 162–2. Diagram of a cross-section of skin demonstrating epidermis and corium (dermis) and burn depth. (From Demling RH, LaLonde C: Management of the burn wound. *In:* Burn Trauma. Blaisdell FW, Trunkey DD [Eds]. New York, Thieme, 1989, p 43.)

Cardiovascular Support

This period is characterized by major fluid shifts in both directions, as well as by a progressive decrease in red blood cell mass in large body burns (Fig. 162–3). Losses of plasma into burn tissue in deep burns and from the wound surface in superficial burns continue. The higher the capillary pressure, the greater the plasma losses. In addition, a marked and continued evaporative water loss from the wound surface occurs. Losses per hour can be estimated from the following formula:

Loss in millimeters per hour = (25 + % of body surface burned) × body surface area in square meters

Fluid gains include those of resorbing edema. Much of the edema fluid is sequestered in poorly perfused tissues, so that resorption is slow at first, particularly for patients with third-degree burns. Resorption is much more rapid in those with second-degree burns, especially as wound blood flow increases.

Hypotonic salt solution with added potassium, calories, and protein should be used to replace evaporative and urinary losses. The hematocrit should be maintained above 30% by infusing packed red blood cells, whereas surgical losses should be replaced with red blood cells and plasma. Administration of additional crystalloid solution for these losses is contraindicated. Electrolyte replacement should be guided by plasma levels; however, in general, sodium intake should be limited and potassium intake increased. Plasma albumin should be maintained greater than 2.5 g/dL and amino acids and lipids added to maintain nutritional status.

Red blood cell injury caused by heat and oxidants, as evidenced by membrane lipid peroxidation,[17] results in a rapid clearance of injured cells by the reticuloendothelial system. In addition, red blood cell production is markedly impaired and is comparable with that seen with any severe chronic disease.[14] One hypothesis is that the bone marrow stem cells are being diverted into formation of inflammatory cells, markedly diminishing the precursor cells available for hematopoiesis. A decreasing hematocrit in the absence of a focus of blood loss is therefore typical of a major burn. A hemoglobin level of 10 to 11 g/dL is typical by days 3 to 4 after injury. This decrease in red blood cell mass from the burn itself makes an assessment of the blood loss from another site (e.g., a fracture or a ruptured spleen) very difficult. Therefore, a complete trauma work-up must be considered early if warranted by the circumstances of injury.

Monitoring volume by the same perfusion parameters as during resuscitation can be very misleading. When wound inflammation begins to evolve after day 3, heart rate increases, reflecting a hyperdynamic state and not necessarily a hypovolemic state. In addition, as the solute byproducts of injured cells are cleared by the kidney, an osmotic diuresis can develop. Urine output may appear excellent, but unless its specific gravity is checked, a misinterpretation of the value may occur. A high specific gravity, as is commonly present, and a high urine output may indicate the need for giving more fluid rather than less so as to keep up with the osmotic diuresis.

The fluids used during this time should also contain nutrients and be hypotonic in terms of salt content to restore nutrients and to replace water loss. Protein colloid solutions and red blood cells are needed to replace ongoing losses.

CHANGING PATTERN OF FLUID GAINS VERSUS LOSSES DURING POSTRESUSCITATION PERIOD

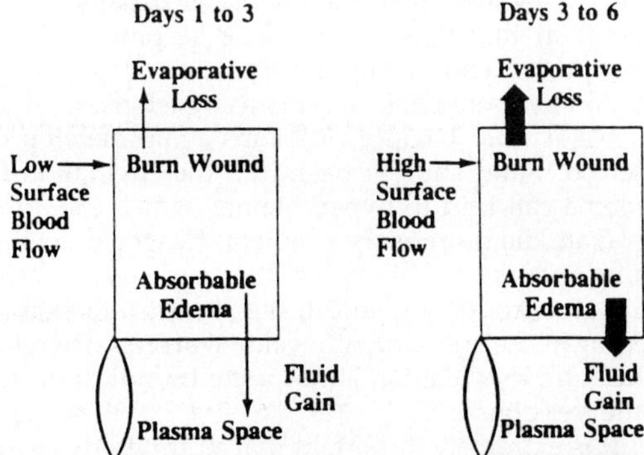

Figure 162–3. Schematic drawing of fluid shifts over time following burn. On days 1 to 3, the shift is mostly out of the plasma space into burn, with some evaporative losses; in contrast, on days 3 to 6, fluid is reabsorbed but with additional evaporative losses. (From Demling RH, LaLonde C: Maintaining hemodynamic stability. *In:* Burn Trauma. Blaisdell FW, Trunkey DD [Eds]. New York, Thieme, 1989, p 87.)

Wound Management

In addition to the use of topical antibiotics twice daily, excision of burn tissue and skin closure are performed during this period. A consumptive coagulopathy is often present on days 2 and 3, and coagulation factors and platelets are often needed, at least with the first excision. Operation duration must be kept short (i.e., <2 hours), and the operating room environment must be kept as warm as the intensive care or burn unit environment. Blood loss can be substantial, but losses for the same area excised in the first 3 to 4 days are less than one half of those seen with excisions after 1 week, when wound hypervascularity develops. Since the wounds are invariably colonized by organisms, usually *Staphylococcus aureus,* perioperative antibiotic coverage is indicated.[18] Other microorganisms are also commonly isolated. The enterococci are found in 55% of patients, *Escherichia coli* in 40%, *Pseudomonas aeruginosa* in 25%, *Candida albicans* in 40%, and β-hemolytic streptococci in 5%. A first-generation cephalosporin is usually adequate. All wounds should be considered to be contaminated.

THE INFLAMMATION–INFECTION PERIOD

The hypermetabolic response to injury begins at about 4 to 5 days after injury and peaks at about 7 to 10 days.[19–21] The process does not require infection, but, of course, infection is a major complication in burn patients. Unfortunately, it is extremely difficult to distinguish burn inflammation–induced hypermetabolism from an infection-induced process.

This period is by far the most difficult period for management, taxing the decision-making skills of even the most experienced burn treatment expert.

Airway and Pulmonary Support

The smoke-injured lung remains prone to pneumonia for weeks after injury until the mucociliary border is restored.[21] Nosocomial pneumonia is, therefore, a major problem during this period. Bacteria may reach the patient by hand transfer from other people, burn wounds, respiratory therapy equipment, and the change in normal flora associated with antimicrobial therapy. Changes in host defenses further increase the incidence of pneumonia in burn patients. Impaired cough, the presence of an endotracheal tube, alterations in consciousness, smoke inhalation, pulmonary congestion with increases in interstitial and alveolar water, and decreased systemic immune function may all enhance the likelihood of pneumonia development. In addition, the marked increase in metabolic rate results in a concomitant increase in carbon dioxide production, which increases the work of breathing. The addition of increased carbon dioxide production to a lung already injured can result in rapid deterioration, especially as fatigue develops. The need for vigorous pulmonary toilet combined with an increase in minute ventilation often requires partial ventilatory assistance, at least until the lung inflammation resolves. Recognition of these increased demands is particularly important in the operating room and during patient transport severe hypercarbia is to be avoided. Sepsis- or inflammation-induced adult respiratory distress syndrome is also a prominent problem during this period.

Respiratory failure may be prevented by the use of intermittent mandatory ventilation or continuous positive airway pressure. An adequate blood volume prevents alveolar collapse and minimizes decrements in dead space. Carbon dioxide production should be reduced by limiting excess carbohydrate intake, controlling temperature, and avoiding the provocation of unnecessary anxiety and pain in the patient.

Cardiovascular Support

Maintaining adequate fluid replacement for evaporative water loss and for blood and plasma loss from débridements is required. The hyperthermic response to inflammation with or without infection further accentuates the evaporative losses from the wound.

Cardiac output is often more than double normal in order to supply the necessary increased oxygen demands. In addition, blood flow to burn tissue is increased two- to threefold greater than normal. Elderly patients with limited cardiac reserve often develop myocardial dysfunction as work load exceeds functional ability. The need for inotropic support is much more common during this period than during the initial resuscitation (Table 162–4).

Metabolic Support

Maintenance of adequate nutrition is critical during this period because the severe hypermetabolism and catabolism initiated by inflammation result in a severe loss of muscle mass and impaired wound healing if not aggressively managed. The ideal route, of course, is the gastrointestinal tract. Some parenteral nutrition may also be required, but this can usually be given in the form of a peripheral vein solution in view of the increased water requirements of the burn patient[19–21] (Table 162–5).

Infection Control

Nosocomial infection is particularly prevalent during this period in view of the combination of host immunosuppres-

TABLE 162–4. Hemodynamic Support

Restore and maintain adequate oxygen delivery	*Maintain fluid and electrolyte balance*	*Avoid excess stress*
1. Replace red blood cell losses to maintain hematocrit at more than 30	1. Replace increased water losses (evaporative and urinary)	1. Avoid excess temperature (>102°f) for sustained periods
2. Maintain serum albumin 2.5 g/dL or higher	2. Replace electrolyte losses (especially increased gastrointestinal, diarrhea, nitrogen losses)	2. Avoid excess heat loss
3. Maintain cardiac index approximately 1.5–2.0 times normal	3. Replace extracellular fluid losses, which shift into cells with nutrition (especially K^+, PO_4^-)	3. Avoid excess pain, anxiety
4. If lactic acidosis is present, increase oxygen delivery		4. Ensure adequate rest
5. Keep arterial oxygen saturation greater than 90%		

(Modified from Demling RH, Lalonde C: Hemodynamic and metabolic support. *In:* Burn Trauma. Blaisdell FW, Trunkey DD [Eds]. New York, Thieme, 1989, p 176.)

TABLE 162–5. Metabolic Support

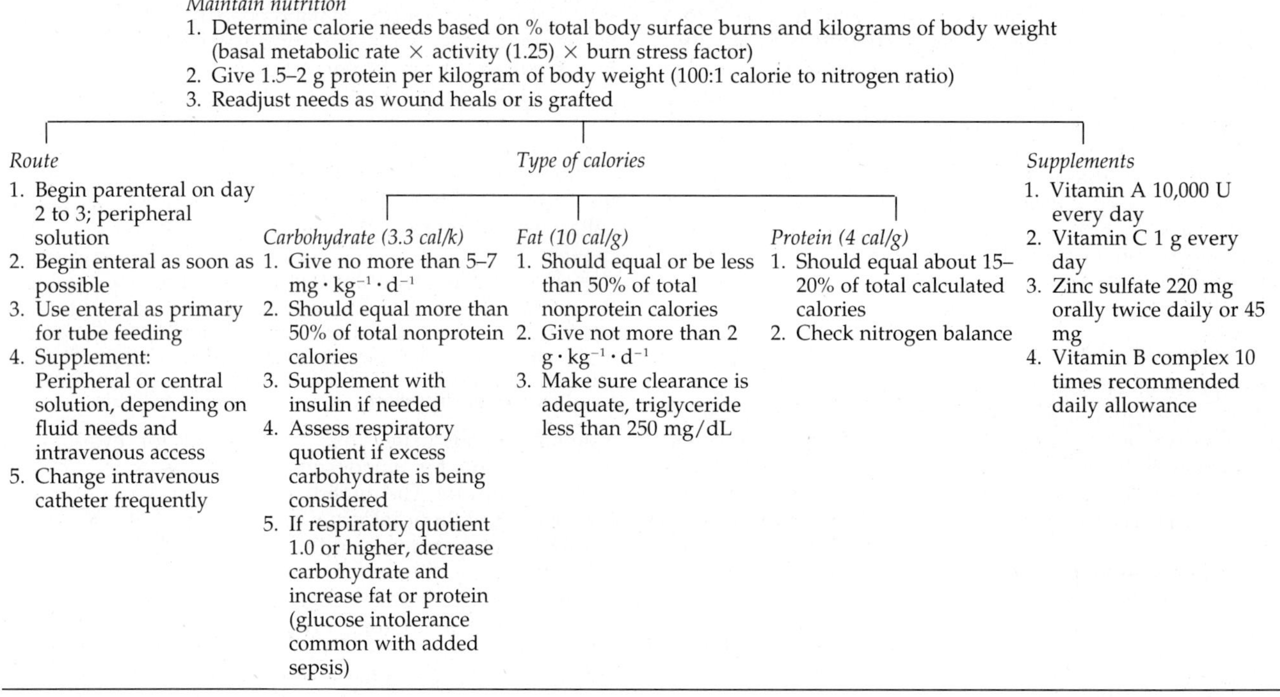

Maintain nutrition

1. Determine calorie needs based on % total body surface burns and kilograms of body weight (basal metabolic rate × activity (1.25) × burn stress factor)
2. Give 1.5–2 g protein per kilogram of body weight (100:1 calorie to nitrogen ratio)
3. Readjust needs as wound heals or is grafted

Route	*Type of calories*			*Supplements*
	Carbohydrate (3.3 cal/k)	*Fat (10 cal/g)*	*Protein (4 cal/g)*	
1. Begin parenteral on day 2 to 3; peripheral solution	1. Give no more than 5–7 $mg \cdot kg^{-1} \cdot d^{-1}$	1. Should equal or be less than 50% of total nonprotein calories	1. Should equal about 15–20% of total calculated calories	1. Vitamin A 10,000 U every day
2. Begin enteral as soon as possible	2. Should equal more than 50% of total nonprotein calories	2. Give not more than 2 $g \cdot kg^{-1} \cdot d^{-1}$	2. Check nitrogen balance	2. Vitamin C 1 g every day
3. Use enteral as primary for tube feeding	3. Supplement with insulin if needed	3. Make sure clearance is adequate, triglyceride less than 250 mg/dL		3. Zinc sulfate 220 mg orally twice daily or 45 mg
4. Supplement: Peripheral or central solution, depending on fluid needs and intravenous access	4. Assess respiratory quotient if excess carbohydrate is being considered			4. Vitamin B complex 10 times recommended daily allowance
5. Change intravenous catheter frequently	5. If respiratory quotient 1.0 or higher, decrease carbohydrate and increase fat or protein (glucose intolerance common with added sepsis)			

(Modified from Demling RH, Lalonde C: Hemodynamic and metabolic support. *In:* Burn Trauma. Blaisdell FW, Trunkey DD [Eds]. New York, Thieme, 1989, p 177.)

sion and bacterial colonization. The burn wound is best managed by the use of topical antibiotics during this phase. Systemic antibiotics for the burn wound are only indicated if there is evidence of an invasive burn infection as diagnosed by burn wound biopsy or for perioperative management.

Vascular catheter sepsis is a major problem that can only be controlled by frequent catheter replacement (i.e., every 4 days) and by removal of monitoring lines (e.g., arterial lines) as soon as possible. Nosocomial pneumonia is a particularly common problem in the burn and inhalation injury patient. Since the entire tracheobronchial tree is usually injured, multiple areas of the lung may develop a pneumonia if early treatment is not initiated. An increase in the quantity and purulence of sputum with an increase in white blood cell count and bacteria on Gram's staining of a deep sputum sample is usually sufficient evidence to support initiation of antibiotic therapy.

Wound Management

In order to assess a wound for infection, the definition of infection must be well understood. Burn wounds are never sterile, even in the presence of topical agents or systemic antibiotics.[22] The presence of bacteria only on the wound surface or in the nonviable tissue itself is termed *colonization.* Colonization may be by a single type of organism or by organisms of multiple types. Although endotoxin may be released locally and some is absorbed, the bacteria themselves are not invading underlying viable tissue. "Infection" of the wound, or *local wound sepsis,* is the term used to indicate beginning invasion of the underlying viable tissue. With progression, the viable tissue and its blood vessels are invaded, and "septicemia" develops. Endotoxemia can also produce a picture of sepsis, and endotoxin absorption can occur without the need for bacterial invasion of blood vessels. The risk of infection's overcoming local defenses is high when the blood flow in the subeschar space is marginal, as occurs before neovascularization and granulation tissue formation. After several weeks, when the highly vascularized granulation tissue develops at the interface, local resistance to invasive infection increases. Inflammation of the wound will be present as a result of the response to the nonviable and injured tissue.

The most common organism involved in wound infection, particularly in the first week, is *S. aureus.*[23, 24] Beta-hemolytic streptococcal infection can also be seen early, but the organism is recovered in fewer than 5% of burn patients. Infection with gram-negative organisms is more evident after the first week. *P. aeruginosa* is present on the wounds of approximately 20% to 30% of burn patients. *E. coli, Proteus* species, or *Klebsiella* species are also noted in about 25% of burn wounds. Enterococci and *C. albicans* are microorganisms that are now seen with increasing frequency. Each is now observed in the wounds of about 50% of burn patients.[18]

The clinical diagnosis of a wound infection can be quite difficult to make. Fever, leukocytosis, tachycardia, and intermittent temperature spikes are characteristically seen in the burn patient with or without infection. A sudden accentuation of these abnormalities can be taken as an indication of the presence of infection someplace. Common characteristics of invasive burn infection (burn wound sepsis) relative to the most common organisms involved are presented.[23]

A conversion of the burn wound in the first several days is usually not bacterial in origin and may actually not be deepening at all but rather a simple buildup of surface exudate. After this time, however, conversion is usually due to an increase in bacterial content, particularly of *S. aureus,* during the first week. Wound purulence is a reliable indicator of infection only if the purulence is in the subeschar space. What looks like purulence on the surface when the dressing is initially removed is often simply surface exudate

TABLE 162–6. Summary of Daily Burn Care

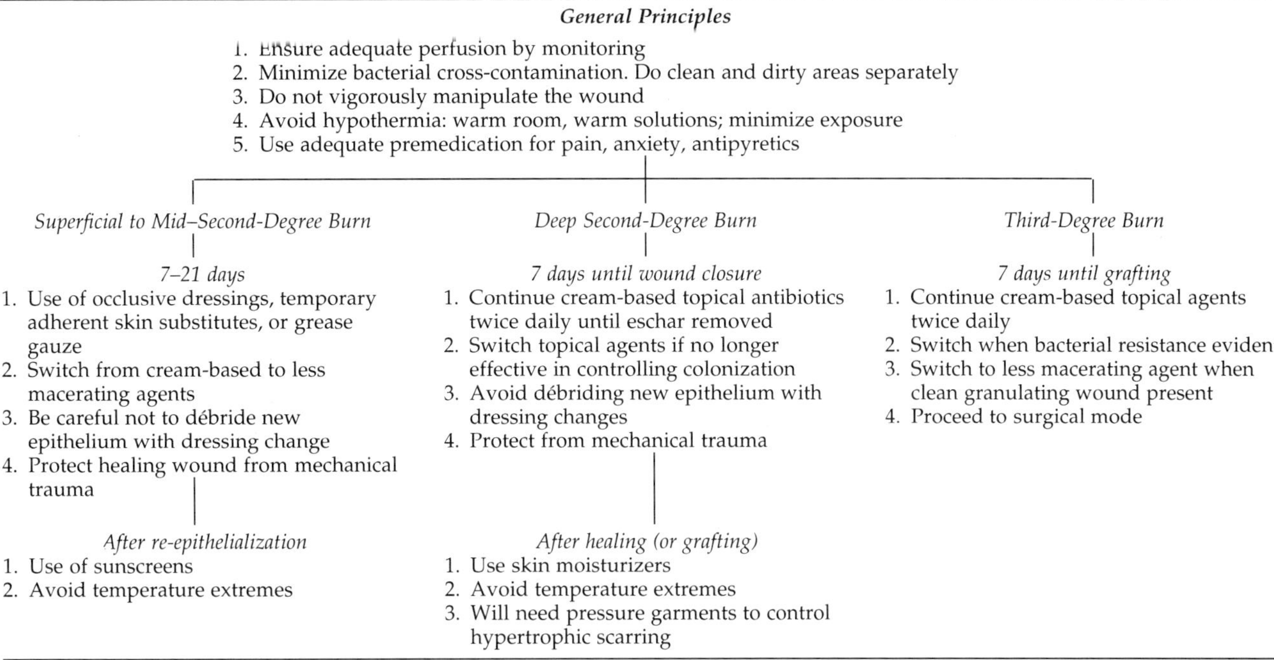

General Principles

1. Ensure adequate perfusion by monitoring
2. Minimize bacterial cross-contamination. Do clean and dirty areas separately
3. Do not vigorously manipulate the wound
4. Avoid hypothermia: warm room, warm solutions; minimize exposure
5. Use adequate premedication for pain, anxiety, antipyretics

Superficial to Mid–Second-Degree Burn	*Deep Second-Degree Burn*	*Third-Degree Burn*
7–21 days	*7 days until wound closure*	*7 days until grafting*
1. Use of occlusive dressings, temporary adherent skin substitutes, or grease gauze 2. Switch from cream-based to less macerating agents 3. Be careful not to débride new epithelium with dressing change 4. Protect healing wound from mechanical trauma	1. Continue cream-based topical antibiotics twice daily until eschar removed 2. Switch topical agents if no longer effective in controlling colonization 3. Avoid débriding new epithelium with dressing changes 4. Protect from mechanical trauma	1. Continue cream-based topical agents twice daily 2. Switch when bacterial resistance evident 3. Switch to less macerating agent when clean granulating wound present 4. Proceed to surgical mode
After re-epithelialization	*After healing (or grafting)*	
1. Use of sunscreens 2. Avoid temperature extremes	1. Use skin moisturizers 2. Avoid temperature extremes 3. Will need pressure garments to control hypertrophic scarring	

(Modified from Demling RH, Lalonde C: Management of the Burn Wound. *In:* Burn Trauma. Blaisdell FW, Trunkey DD [Eds]. New York, Thieme, 1989, p 191.)

mixed with residue of the topical antibiotic. Exudate is especially prominent with the use of silver sulfadiazine. The results of wound inspection are more valid after the previously applied topical agent and surface exudate have been wiped off.

Surface cultures of the wound invariably demonstrate growth of some bacteria. It is impossible to distinguish a surface bacterial colonization from that of a wound infection based on the results of surface cultures. However, identification of the type of bacteria that has colonized on the surface is useful for assessment of the effectiveness of the topical agents being used. Cultures are taken after the wound exudate has been removed. The wound is colonized and subsequently infected most commonly by *S. aureus* within the first week, with gram-negative organisms being more prevalent beginning in the second week.

The most reliable method of diagnosing a burn wound infection is bacterial analysis of a burn wound biopsy. A small, full-thickness portion of eschar is removed using a punch biopsy instrument or scalpel. The biopsy must include some underlying viable subcutaneous tissue. Two techniques can then be applied. The quantitative bacterial count of the biopsy material is one method. It has been established that 10^5 organisms per gram of tissue is the bacterial load that is preinvasive. The same quantitation is considered to indicate infection in the urinary tract (i.e., >100,000 organisms per milliliter). Fewer than 10^5 organisms is indicative of colonization, whereas 10^5 or more indicates infection with a high potential for progression to wound sepsis.

Gentle daily débridement is the appropriate management during this period for burn tissue not yet excised. A granulation tissue bed then develops; the tissue bed is more resistant to infection and is used as the appropriate bed for a skin graft. Aggressive surgical débridement of infected tissue, although sometimes necessary, frequently leads to postoperative bacteremia and hemodynamic instability, which must be anticipated (Table 162–6).

REHABILITATION

Exercise routines, including active and passive range-of-motion exercise of all burned and nonburned areas, is necessary shortly after a patient's admission if permanent loss of function in burned joints is to be avoided. This activity must be considered a high priority in daily management because many losses in function cannot be regained once scar tissue has been deposited across joint surfaces and once muscles have been allowed to atrophy. Maintenance of muscle mass and mobility is critical to the optimization of outcome.

SUMMARY

The burn-injured patient is at high risk for major infection and organ failure complications as a result of the burn and of the host response to injury. Marked improvements in critical care management and outcome are based almost entirely on early aggressive efforts toward prevention rather than on the treatment of complications owing to an improvement of our knowledge of the disease process. The objective is for the burn care team to control the local and systemic burn response, and not for the burn injury process to control the care being provided. A working knowledge of the burn injury and its evolution over time is essential if optimal results are to be obtained.

References

1. Demling RH: Burn management. *In:* Pre and Post-Operative Care. Wilmore D (Ed). New York, Scientific American, 1991.
2. Demling RH: Medical progress: Burns. N Engl J Med 1985; 313:1389.
3. Demling RH: Improved survival after massive burns. J Trauma 1983; 23:179.
4. Cahalane M, Demling RH: Early respiratory abnormalities from smoke inhalation. JAMA 1984; 251:771.
5. Moylan J, Alexander G: Diagnosis and treatment of inhalation injury. World J Surg 1978; 2:185.

6. Head J: Inhalation injury in burns. Am J Surg 1990; 139:508.
7. Thompson P, Herndon D, Traber D, et al: Effect on mortality of inhalation injury. J Trauma 1986; 28:163.
8. Demling RH: Effect of early burn excision and grafting on pulmonary function. J Trauma 1984; 24:830.
9. Venus B, Matsuda T, Copiozo J: Prophylactic intubation and continuous positive airway pressure in the management of inhalation injury in burn victims. Crit Care Med 1981; 9:519.
10. Robinson W, Hudson L, Robertson H: Ventilation and perfusion alterations after smoke inhalation injury. Surgery 1982; 90:305.
11. Demling RH: Fluid resuscitation after major burns. JAMA 1983; 250:1438.
12. Arturson G: Microvascular permeability to macromolecules in thermal injury. Acta Physiol Scand 1979; 463:111.
13. Harms B, Bodai B, Demling RH: Microvascular fluid and protein flux in pulmonary and systemic circulations after thermal injury. Microvasc Res 1982; 23:77.
14. Peterson V, Robinson W: Hematologic changes in burn patients. *In:* The Art and Science of Burn Care. Boswick J (Ed). Rockville, MD, Aspen Publications, 1987.
15. Deitch E: Intestinal permeability is increased in burn patients shortly after injury. Surgery 1990; 107:411.
16. Wilmore D, Mason A, Johnson D: Effect of ambient temperatures on heat production and heat loss in burn patients. J Appl Physiol 1975; 38:593.
17. Sasaki J, Cottam G, Baxter C: Lipid peroxidation following thermal injury. J Burn Care Rehabil 1983; 4:251.
18. Yurt R, Mason A, Pruitt B: Increased susceptibility to infection related to extent of burn injury. Arch Surg 1984; 119:183.
19. Alexander J: The role of infection in the burn patient. *In:* The Art and Science of Burn Care. Boswick J (Ed). Rockville, MD, Aspen Publications, 1987, pp 103–112.
20. Jahoor F, Herndon D, Wolfe R: Role of insulin and glucagon in the response of glucose and alanine kinetics in burn injured patients. J Clin Invest 1986; 78:807.
21. Saffle J, Medina E, Raymond J: Use of indirect calorimetry in the nutritional management of burned patients. J Trauma 1985; 25:32.
22. Pruitt B, Erickson D, Morris A: Progressive pulmonary insufficiency and other pulmonary complications of thermal injury. J Trauma 1975; 15:369.
23. Boxx W, Brand D, Acampara D: Effectiveness of prophylactic antibiotics in the treatment of burns. J Trauma 1985; 25:224.
24. Demling RH, LaLonde C: Infection and sepsis. *In:* Burn Trauma. Demling RH, LaLonde C (Eds). New York, Thieme Publishers, 1989, pp 193–207.

CHAPTER 163

Smoke Inhalation Injury

Robert H. Demling, MD

The inhalation of smoke is a common cause of morbidity and mortality, especially in view of the large number of fires that occur each year and the risk of smoke exposure that they present. It is now well established that the leading cause of death in fires is the inhalation of smoke, and not burn injury—a fact confirmed by fires in multistory buildings in which the fire itself may be confined to a small area but the smoke from the fire rapidly fills the entire structure.

Smoke injury is also the cause of more than half of the deaths among burn patients. Respiratory failure is now the leading cause of death in burn patients, with the smoke inhalation insult being the predominant factor in the subsequent lung damage.[1–3] Since patients with smoke exposure are commonly transported directly or transferred to large urban hospitals, especially those with a trauma center or burn center, a working knowledge of the disease process among the members of emergency rooms as well as critical care, trauma, and burn units is necessary if optimal care is to be ensured.

The disease process itself is quite complex and is best understood if the lung dysfunction is described in terms of time postinjury because the disease process and its treatment vary tremendously from initial presentation to resolution or progression over ensuing weeks or months, especially in the presence of a burn. Therefore, the smoke inhalation injury with and without burn injury is discussed in regard to both its general pathophysiology, presentation, and treatment and its specific management during the following three postinsult phases:

1. Early resuscitation phase (0 to 36 hours)
2. Postresuscitation phase (2 to 5 days)
3. Inflammation-infection phase (usually 5 days to lung healing and burn wound closure)

GENERAL PATHOPHYSIOLOGY

The smoke inhalation complex consists of a direct lung injury component and a systemic component, even with smoke inhalation alone. Both components are worsened by the presence of a body burn.[4–6]

Lung Component

The injury to the lung itself is dependent on the components of the smoke inhaled, the degree of smoke exposure, and the lung's response to the insult.[7–9]

Components of Smoke

The injury caused by *heat* is usually confined to the area above the vocal cords except for in the very rare instance of long-term exposure or exposure to steam. The *gas phase* contains a host of toxins, including carbon monoxide, cyanide gas, acids, and aldehydes. Oxidants are also clearly present in the gas phase. These agents produce both a systemic response and local airways injury. The vapors in large part are mucous membrane irritants that cause intense bronchorrhea, bronchoconstriction, and airways edema. The process often peaks hours after injury, although patients with preexisting airways reactivity disease can develop very early, intense bronchoconstriction. The *particulate phase injury* exposure to lung is dependent on particle size and a patient's breathing pattern.[10–12] The particle deposition depends on particle size. Particles range from 0.1 to 15 μm in diameter, depending on the heat of the smoke and on what was burning. Particles 3 to 5 μm in diameter appear to predominate based on the findings of many smoke inhalation studies. In general, particles greater than 5 μm are cleared by the nasopharynx if the patient is able to breathe nasally. With mouth breathing, most of the larger particles deposit in the larynx, trachea, and large airways. Particles smaller than 5 μm deposit in both large and small airways and in the alveoli. The degree of deposition in the distal regions of the lung is promoted by deep breathing, as would occur in an attenuated hypoxic patient or in a patient who actively attempted to escape insult. In contrast to the short duration of injury in the gas phase, particles can adhere to the mucosa and perpetuate the local tissue injury. In turn, particle clearance is impeded by the impairment of mucociliary action, which also perpetuates the injury.

Of major importance is the fact that kinds of smoke from different environments vary dramatically in their toxicity. Examples of extremely toxic smoke include that produced from the burning of automobile interiors, upholstery, and

TABLE 163–1. Common Toxic Elements in Housefire Smoke

Gas	*Source*	*Effect*
Carbon monoxide	Any organic matter	Tissue hypoxia
Carbon dioxide	Any organic matter	Narcosis
Nitrogen dioxide	Wallpaper, wood	Bronchial irritation Dizziness Pulmonary edema
Hydrogen chloride (phosgene)	Plastics (polyvinylchloride)	Severe mucosal irritation
Hydrogen cyanide	Wool, silk, nylons (polyurethane)	Headache Respiratory failure Coma
Benzene	Petroleum plastics	Mucosal irritation Coma
Aldehydes	Wood, cotton, paper	Severe mucosal damage Extensive lung damage
Ammonia	Nylon	Mucosal irritation

(From Demling RH, Lalonde C: Airway and pulmonary abnormalities. *In*: Burn Trauma. Blaisdell FW, Trunkey DD [Eds]. New York, Thieme, 1989, p 11.)

chemicals (e.g., in chemical factory fires), of which hydrocarbons are a major component (Table 163–1).

Degree of Smoke Exposure

The degree of smoke exposure is dependent on the mass of smoke inhaled, the depth of breathing, and the time of exposure.[13] Unfortunately, the only marker we have at present to roughly define this exposure is the time spent in the smoke environment, neurologic status, and carbon monoxide toxicity. In fact, a high carboxyhemoglobin level (i.e., >40%) produces an obtunded state and provides evidence that exposure time is quite long.[14] This assumes other factors that cause obtundation, namely, head injury, drugs, and alcoholism, are not present. As far as the basic mechanism of injury, a clear proportional increase in the degree of initial lung injury occurs with increases in smoke exposure.

Lung Response (General Pathophysiology)

The degree of initial and late injury is in large part related to the status of the lung before injury. A lung with any element of reactive airways disease or chronic changes (e.g, those caused by smoking) likely reacts to smoke exposure more intensely than does a healthy lung. In addition, the inflammatory response caused by the injury produces much of the subsequent damage. The inflammatory response is very individualized, depending on available mediator precursors and available defenses such as the presence of antioxidants and antiproteases[15] (Table 163–2).

The mechanism of the airways and parenchymal injury is very complex. The agents toxic to cells that are present on the particles lead to a number of pathologic events. First, direct mucosal injury; loss of ciliary activity; and subsequent impairment of particle, mucous and, later, bacterial clearance occur. Second, very early bronchial blood flow as well as increased bronchial vessel permeability markedly increases; this leads to submucosal edema and vascular engorgement that narrow airways lumina.[16] Third, tissue destruction resulting from these factors as well as a secondary inflammatory response ensue. The result is a slough of mucosa in both large and small airways and a marked increase in mucus production (Fig. 163–1).

TABLE 163–2. Secondary Mediators Involved

1. *Oxidants* from inflammatory cells or produced by reaction of smoke toxins with mucosa.
2. *Arachidonic acid metabolites*, both prostanoids and leukotrienes, producing both bronchoconstriction and altered permeability.
3. *Protease* release from inflammation in the presence of decreased antiprotease activity.
4. *Cytokines* (TNF-IL-1) released from injured mast cells.
5. *Increased neuropeptide production*: substance P, bradykinin, calcitonin-related gene peptide, leading to bronchoconstriction, bronchorrhea, altered airways vessel permeability.
6. Decreased *neutral endopeptidase* production as a result of mucosal damage.

A vast array of mediators are likely involved (see Chapters 17, 18, 19, and 22). Oxidants and oxidant-activated eicosanoid and leukotriene production are known to be present.[9, 15] The release of neutrophil proteases may be involved in the mucosal slough itself. Clearly, agents described generally as the neuropeptides are also involved.[17] The many neuropeptides produced below the mucosa are potent bronchoconstrictors and can increase blood flow and alter permeability. The major attenuation of these agents occurs with the mucosal production of other neutralizing neuropeptides that are severely damaged and may lead to an unchecked progression of the mucosal injury (see Table 163–2).

The role of injury to the alveolocapillary membrane remains unclear. In most animal models, neutrophil sequestration is evident in the alveolocapillary membrane; alveolar flooding is also present, although the alveolar flooding is usually found only with massive and usually early fatal injuries.[18, 19] Most studies have demonstrated that flooding around the more injured small airways and retrograde filling of alveoli from airways edema are more likely. This concept is best corroborated by the fact that alveolar edema in man is not commonly seen in the initial 24 to 36 hours of resuscitation when massive amounts of fluid are infused, especially in the presence of a burn. It is more likely that a second insult occurring 2 to 3 days after injury causes the activation of lung inflammation with later alveolocapillary leak. Certainly, clearance of excess parenchymal fluid is impaired owing to injury of lymphatics in the interstitium caused by the airways injury. Therefore, the lung is more susceptible to fluid accumulation.

Alveolar injury that leads to atelectasis certainly is involved with exposures to smoke.[20] Oxidants and other toxins are known to deactivate surfactant, resulting in alveolar instability and, in turn, collapse and increased shunt.

Systemic Component (with or Without Burn)

The smoke injury produces both early and late systemic changes (Table 163–3).

Early Changes

The initial smoke insult produces a general impairment in systemic blood flow due to a decrease in cardiac index and

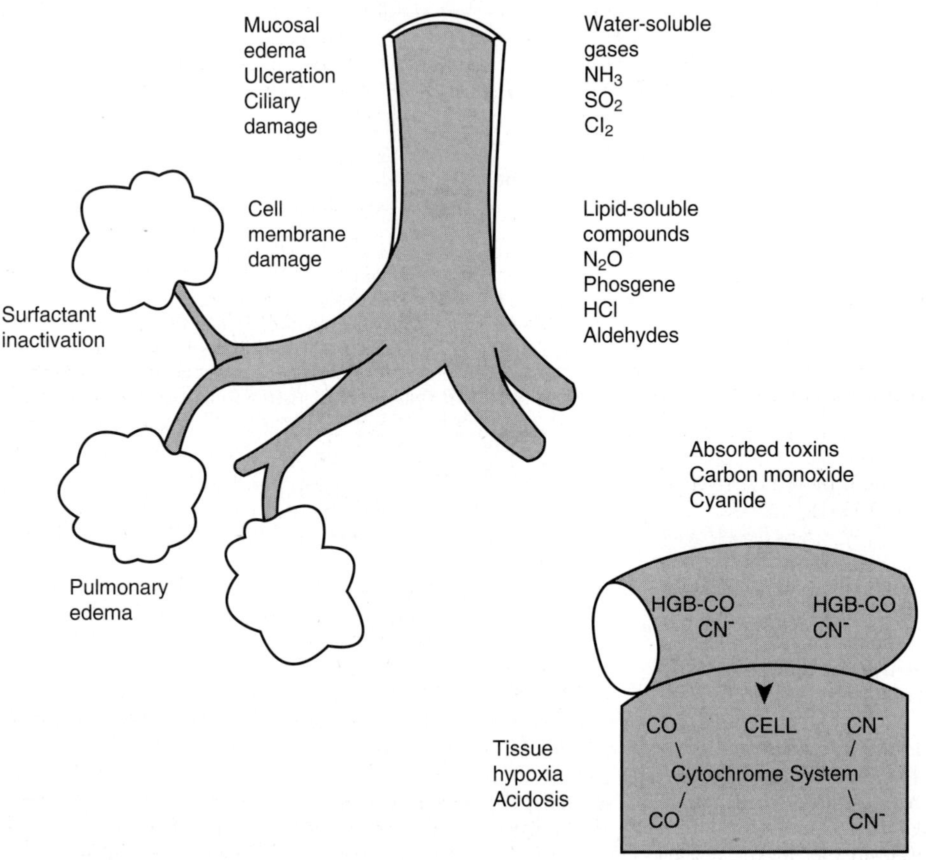

Figure 163–1. Diagram demonstrating the mechanism of smoke inhalation injury. Water-soluble gases primarily affect the upper airways mucosa, whereas lipid-soluble compounds involve areas deeper in the lung (they are transported on carbon particles). These agents can lead to surfactant inactivation and, with extreme exposures, to alveolar edema. (From Demling RH, Lalonde C: Airway and pulmonary abnormalities. *In:* Burn Trauma. Blaisdell FW, Trunkey DD [Eds]. New York, Thieme, 1989, p 4.)

in filling pressures. The decrease in cardiac index is multifactorial and includes an initial anoxic episode, carbon monoxide and cyanide toxicity, and a decrease in blood volume due in part to an increased loss of fluid and protein into lung and systemic tissue.[6, 21]

Treatment during the resuscitation period involves the infusion of isotonic crystalloid or colloid solutions, or both, at a rate needed to restore and maintain adequate perfusion based on standard markers. Fluid requirements may well approach those needed in the presence of a moderate burn.[22] The addition of a burn markedly increases fluid and protein losses in excess of those predicted for burn alone.[21] Smoke inhalation is now recognized to increase the rate of burn edema formation significantly. Decreasing fluid intake in an attempt to keep the lung "dry" is known only to increase cardiopulmonary instability and morbidity.[4]

TABLE 163–3. Systemic Response to Smoke Inhalation

Early Changes
- Decreased oxygenation from carboxyhemoglobin, cyanide
- Decreased perfusion from blood volume losses secondary to altered microvessels
- Accentuation of burn edema and burn fluid requirements
- Increased oxygen consumption

Late Changes
- Development of a systemic inflammatory resposne compatible with the "sepsis syndrome"
- Hyperdynamic hypermetabolic state, maldistribution of blood flow, increased risk of other organ dysfunciton
- Increased risks of systemic infection, both in burn wound and in lung

Late Effects

After 2 to 3 days, the lung—and, in particular, the airways—becomes a massive focus of inflammation that presents all of the signs and symptoms seen with a large inflammatory focus: namely, a hyperdynamic state, an increase in oxygen demands, and maldistribution of blood flow. The presence of a nosocomial pneumonia certainly amplifies this response. The addition of a body burn markedly increases the risk of both lung infection and burn infection owing to both an increase in immunosuppression and an increase in the risk of cross-contamination.[23] This problem is of particular concern in the presence of a face and neck burn. Treatment is similar to that for any inflammation-induced disease and includes optimization of systemic perfusion and maintenance of nutrition and immune defenses. In the case of burn, this means early burn excision.[24]

EARLY RESUSCITATION PHASE

The appropriate diagnosis and treatment of this phase basically dictate the subsequent course of the disease.[3, 25–27]

Diagnosis

The diagnosis is, first and foremost, an index of suspicion because history may be unavailable or unreliable. Of course, any patient with a history of significant exposure to smoke is considered to have a smoke inhalation injury until it can be proved otherwise. A long exposure time is not required

TABLE 163–4. Symptoms of Carbon Monoxide Intoxication

Carboxyhemoglobin Level (%)	*Symptoms*
0–5	Normal value
15–20	Headache, confusion
20–40	Disorientation, fatigue, nausea, visual changes
40–60	Hallucination, combativeness, coma, shock state
≥60	Mortality > 50%

(From Demling RH, Lalonde C: Airway and pulmonary abnormalities. *In*: Burn Trauma. Blaisdell FW, Trunkey DD [Eds]. New York, Thieme, 1989, pp 6, 7.)

if the smoke is particularly toxic, as is that from the burning mattresses or upholstery from which gases such as cyanide are released in large quantities. A particularly important symptom is a lack of consciousness at the scene of injury because an unconscious or disoriented state can readily be caused by smoke and because the victim is likely to consume more smoke once he or she is unconscious or confused. Initial physical findings of carbonaceous sputum, facial burn, singed nasal hairs, or respiratory symptoms such as coughing or wheezing are diagnostic signs; however, lung dysfunction is often delayed in onset and may not be present. Initial blood gas measurements are often normal, with the exception that a decrease in measured arterial oxygen saturation and metabolic acidosis due to carbon monoxide are present. The initial chest radiograph is also usually relatively normal, since the initial injury is primarily to the airways, not to the parenchyma, and often requires several days before radiographic changes of atelectasis, increased water, and focal infiltrates become evident.[28]

Pathophysiology and Treatment

The initial injury process has four components.

Hypoxia from Low Fraction of Inspired Oxygen

The inspired air in a fire has a decreased oxygen tension (PO_2) in view of oxygen utilization during combustion. The fraction of inspired oxygen (FIO_2) frequently reaches 0.1, leading to an alveolar PO_2 (PaO_2) of 50 to 60 mm Hg and, in turn, to an arterial oxygen utilization tension (PaO_2) of less than 40 mm Hg. The hypoxic insult can lead to severe organ dysfunction (in particular, brain dysfunction) as a result of both ischemia and subsequent reperfusion injury. A brief neurologic study using the Glasgow Coma Scale is a part of the initial evaluation. Treatment involves the immediate administration of high-flow oxygen. A persistent neurologic dysfunction after reversal of carbon monoxide toxicity and hypovolemia may well reflect the initial hypoxic insult.

Carbon Monoxide and Cyanide Toxicity

Carbon monoxide toxicity is one of the leading causes of death in fires (Tables 163–4 and 163–5). While oxygen is used during combustion, carbon monoxide is released, that is, it is a basic byproduct of combustion. Carbon monoxide is rapidly transported across the alveolar membrane and preferentially binds with the hemoglobin molecule in place of oxygen. In addition, carbon monoxide shifts the hemoglobin-oxygen curve to the left, thereby impairing oxygen unloading at the tissue level. The result is a major impairment in oxygen delivery, since 98% of oxygen is carried to the tissues on hemoglobin. With prolonged exposure, carbon monoxide can also saturate cells, binding to cytochrome oxidase and thereby further impairing mitochondrial function and adenosine triphosphate production. Production of hydrocyanide, the gaseous form of cyanide, is a well-recognized cause of morbidity and mortality, especially with the burning of synthetic substances such as polyurethane.[29] Although cyanide can be absorbed through the gastrointestinal tract or skin, it is most dangerous when aerosolized and inhaled because of its rapid absorption across the large surface area of the lung. The hydrocyanide then binds to the cytochrome system, thereby inhibiting cell metabolism and adenosine triphosphate production. All cells, in particular those of the liver, have a detoxication process for hydrocyanide in which the enzyme rhodanese converts hydrocyanide to thiocyanate. The thiocyanate is then excreted in the urine. This protective system can be overcome by the presence of a large amount of cyanide, especially if the patient is also hypovolemic, since hypovolemia impairs cyanide metabolism and clearance.

SYMPTOMS. Symptoms of carbon monoxide toxicity are usually not present until carboxyhemoglobin level exceeds 15%—that is, 15% of the hemoglobin is bound to carbon monoxide rather than to oxygen.[14] One symptom is a decrease in tissue oxygenation, with initial manifestations being neurologic owing to the impairment of cerebral oxy-

TABLE 163–5. Treatment of Carbon Monoxide and Cyanide Toxicity

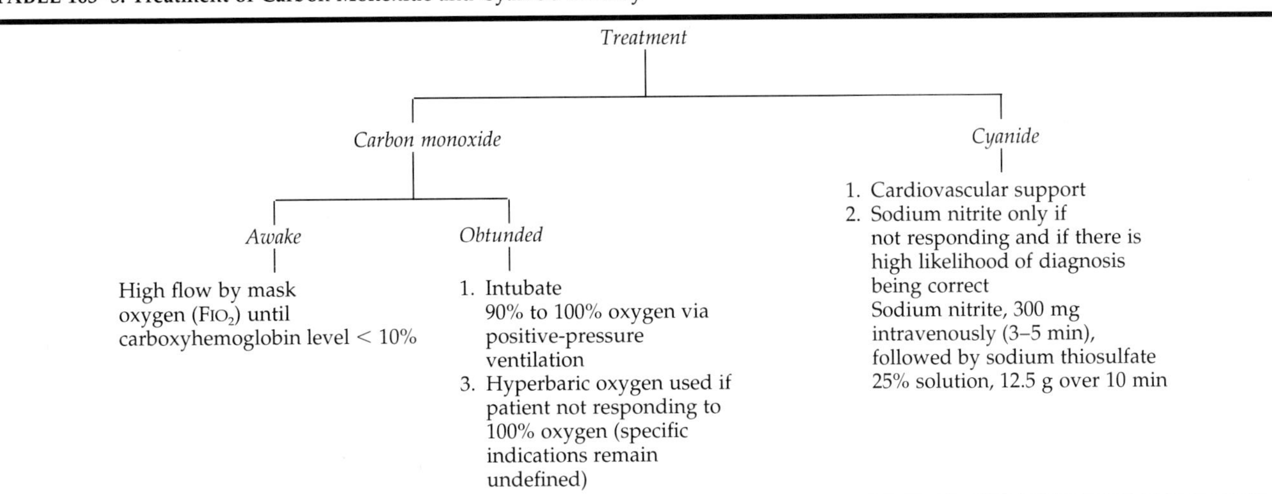

(From Demling RH, Lalonde C: Airway and pulmonary abnormalities. *In*: Burn Trauma. Blaisdell FW, Trunkey DD [Eds]. New York, Thieme, 1989, pp 6, 7.)

genation. Major myocardial dysfunction can also develop from the initial myocardial ischemia, especially in patients with preexisting coronary artery disease. In addition, the neurologic dysfunction caused by carbon monoxide exposure can lead to progressive and permanent cerebral dysfunction. Frequently, a patient awakens transiently after severe inhalation injury only to have progressive neurologic deterioration 24 to 48 hours later. This process is believed to be caused by prolonged brain hypoxia from both the presence of carbon monoxide and the low environmental oxygen tension. Cyanide toxicity presents in a very similar fashion to that of carbon monoxide, with profound metabolic acidosis and obtundation occurring in severe cases. Diagnosis, however, is more difficult because cyanide levels are not always readily available or very reliable.[29]

DIAGNOSIS. Carbon monoxide toxicity is measured based on carboxyhemoglobin level. The persistence of a metabolic acidosis in a patient with adequate volume resuscitation and cardiac output suggests persistent carbon monoxide (or cyanide) impairment of oxygen utilization and delivery. However, hypovolemia and other cell poisons cannot be excluded. Arterial oxygen tension remains relatively normal because the chemical alteration of hemoglobin or of the cytochrome system by carbon monoxide does not affect the amount of oxygen dissolved in arterial plasma. The measured oxygen saturation of hemoglobin is markedly decreased relative to the PO_2. Oxygen saturation is less than that expected based on the measured PaO_2.

Therefore, if a discrepancy exists between the measured PaO_2 and the measured oxygen saturation, carbon monoxide toxicity is present until it can be proved otherwise. A high carboxyhemoglobin level is also indicative of a significant smoke exposure, and therefore a chemical burn to the airways is likely to be present. A low carboxyhemoglobin level does not always indicate a minimal smoke exposure because the administration of oxygen at the scene of the fire can displace some of the carbon monoxide before the patient arrives at the emergency room. Blood cyanide levels can be measured to make the diagnosis of cyanide toxicity. Normal cyanide levels in smokers are less than 0.1 mg/L. A lethal level is considered to be about 1 mg/L.[29]

TREATMENT. Treatment of carbon monoxide toxicity consists of the early displacement of carbon monoxide from hemoglobin by administration of 90% to 100% oxygen. The half-life of carboxyhemoglobin in the patient breathing 20% oxygen is about 120 to 200 minutes, whereas its half-life when he or she breathes 90% to 100% high-flow oxygen is 30 minutes; that is, the concentration of carboxyhemoglobin is reduced by approximately 50% every 30 minutes if an oxygen concentration of 90% to 100% is used. Oxygen administration is required for all patients with major burns until carbon monoxide toxicity can be ruled out or until carboxyhemoglobin levels return to normal.

Administration of hyperbaric oxygen (2–3 atmospheres) produces an even more rapid displacement of carbon monoxide and is most useful in patients who have had prolonged exposure (i.e., when carbon monoxide is also present in the mitochondria, since carbon monoxide is more difficult to displace from the cytochrome system). The drawback of hyperbaric oxygen use is the inability to adequately treat the whole patient when he or she is isolated in a hyperbaric chamber. Hyperbaric oxygen is best used in patients who have severe neurologic compromise and high carboxyhemoglobin level—that is, greater than 50%—but no major burns or severe pulmonary injury and who do not respond to high-flow oxygen with clearance of symptoms. However, the vast majority of cases can be successfully managed by simply using 90% to 100% oxygen.

Endotracheal intubation and the use of 90% to 100% oxygen with mechanical ventilatory assistance are indicated for those patients with impaired neurologic function and a high carboxyhemoglobin level. This patient group not only needs more aggressive attempts toward displacement of carboxyhemoglobin using positive pressure at a high FIO_2 but is also at a high risk for aspiration, as are any neurologically impaired patients.

In general, for patients with cyanide poisoning, cardiopulmonary support is usually sufficient treatment, since the liver clears the cyanide from circulation via the enzyme rhodanese. Sodium nitrate is used in severe cases (300 mg intravenously over 5–10 minutes), especially in those in which the diagnosis is made based on blood levels. Methemoglobin is produced by the nitrite, which, in turn, binds the cyanide. However, methemoglobin does not transport oxygen, and a tissue hypoxia can develop; this is similar to the original cyanide effect. Ordinarily, thiosulfate, which binds the cyanide to form thiocyanate, is also given. One must be reasonably sure of the diagnosis of cyanide toxicity before giving sodium nitrite.

Upper Airways Obstruction from Tissue Edema (Internal and External)

Direct injury caused by the inhalation of air heated to a temperature of 150°C or higher ordinarily manifests as burns to the face, oropharynx, and upper airway (above the vocal cords). Even superheated air is rapidly cooled before it reaches the lower respiratory tract because of the tremendous heat exchanging efficiency of the oropharynx and nasopharynx.[3]

Heat produces an immediate injury to the airway mucosa, resulting in edema, erythema, and ulceration. Although these mucosal changes may be anatomically present shortly after the burn, physiologic alterations do not occur until the edema is sufficient to produce clinical evidence of impaired upper airway patency. This may not occur for 12 to 18 hours. The presence of a body burn magnifies the injury to airways in direct proportion to the size and depth of the skin burn. The massive fluid requirements necessary to treat the skin burn are in part responsible, as are mediators released from the burned skin.

Another compounding injury is any face or neck burn that produces marked anatomic distortion and, in the case of a deep neck burn, external compression on the larynx. A particularly dangerous injury is the third-degree facial burn in which minimal external edema is present. The absence of external edema is caused by the inelasticity of third-degree burns, which does not allow expansion. Intraoral edema in this case is usually massive but unrecognized unless sought. A more superficial burn causes massive external edema but may produce much less mucosal edema and airway compromise. The effects of deep facial burns on airway maintenance are:

1. Airway obstruction because of intraoral and laryngeal edema
2. Anatomic distortion because of face and neck edema, which increases the difficulty of endotracheal intubation
3. Oral edema, which decreases clearance of intraoral secretions
4. Impaired protection of the airway caused by aspiration

The local edema process usually resolves within 4 to 5 days.

SYMPTOMS. Symptoms of obstruction—namely, stridor, dyspnea, increased work of breathing, and eventually cyanosis—do not develop until a critical narrowing of the airway is present.[3, 25–27] Upper airway noise indicative of an increase in turbulent airflow often precedes obstruction. It is difficult to distinguish noise caused by a narrowed airway from that caused by an increase in oral and nasal secretions resulting from smoke irritation. The airway edema and the external burn edema process have a parallel time course, so that by the time symptoms of airway edema develop, external and internal anatomic distortion will have become extensive.

DIAGNOSIS. A history must be obtained regarding the nature of the burn. This information may not always be available from the emergency medical service transport team if a patient has been transferred from another emergency room rather than from the scene of injury and if he or she cannot provide the information. Inspection of the oropharynx in the search for soot or evidence of a heat injury should be performed on every burn victim. A number of techniques have been used to assess further the degree of injury and to determine the need for endotracheal intubation. Fiberoptic bronchoscopy or laryngoscopy can determine whether physical evidence of pharyngeal or laryngeal mucosal injury is present (namely, erythema and edema). Laryngoscopy is the more rapid and less complicated diagnostic tool. Unfortunately, unless serial studies are performed, neither of these tests can accurately predict the severity of subsequent airway compromise, since the edema is progressive during the first 18 to 24 hours after injury.[25]

TREATMENT. Maintenance of an adequate airway is essential for successful early management. Four standard criteria ("the four Ps") must be satisfied if endotracheal intubation is to be made possible:

1. Maintenance of airway *p*atency
2. *P*rotection against aspiration
3. *P*ulmonary toilet to decrease mucous plugging and the risk of infection
4. *P*ositive-pressure ventilation

The upper airways injury can meet at least the first two criteria and frequently the third if the patient fatigues and cannot clear secretions (see Table 163–5).

Intubation of the trachea is not without its own complications because the cough mechanism is impaired, especially in patients with good respiratory mechanics. In addition, intubation increases the risk of nosocomial infection. A decision must be made in the initial assessment as to whether the airway can be managed safely without an endotracheal tube. When in doubt, it is safer to intubate.[3, 30]

Chemical Burn to Upper and Lower Airways

This aspect of inhalation injury is often an extension of the upper airways injury just described but is generally much more serious than that produced by heat alone. Alveolar edema is not a major component of the early disease state and is therefore less responsible for the early impairment of gas exchange than are atelectasis and airway closure. Several clinical studies have verified that lung water content is significantly increased only after massive inhalation injury in which damage has extended to the very small airways. The increase in airways fluid caused by mucosal irritation looks and acts physiologically like any increase in alveolar water content. Alveolar flooding in this severe case may well be due to retrograde flow of bronchorrhea. A body burn markedly potentiates the inhalation-induced lung dysfunction caused by chemical injury. The mortality rate for patients with severe inhalation injury alone is 5% to 8%. The mortality rate of the combination of a major burn and smoke inhalation far exceeds that of either injury alone.[3, 4, 22–24]

SYMPTOMS. Symptoms may be absent at the time of admission, with the true magnitude of the degree of injury only becoming evident after 24 to 48 hours. Early symptoms usually consist of bronchospasm manifested as wheezing and bronchorrhea. An intense initial bronchorrhea caused by the irritation of the airway mucosa in combination with the increase in oral and nasal secretions can give the appearance of fulminant pulmonary edema. The presence of soot in the lung secretions is certainly evidence of smoke exposure but is not a necessary finding. Early bronchospasm and bronchiolar edema initiated by the irritant gases cause a marked decrease in lung compliance and an increase in the work of breathing. Impairment of the clearance of secretions accentuates the problem. The resultant ventilation-perfusion mismatch creates impaired gas exchange and an increase in the alveolar-arterial oxygen gradient and in minute ventilation.[31]

DIAGNOSIS. Diagnostic indications are a history of closed space exposure, physical findings (soot, presence of symptoms), an increase in carboxyhemoglobin level, direct visualization of injury (with laryngoscopy), fiberoptic bronchoscopy, and indirect visualization (with ventilation-perfusion xenon scanning). Physical findings on admission that suggest smoke exposure include facial burn, the presence of soot in the sputum, dyspnea, coughing, wheezing, and bronchorrhea. If present, these findings are helpful in establishing diagnosis. However, many patients demonstrate a minimum of symptoms early after injury, and only when airways edema develops do symptoms become evident. An elevated carboxyhemoglobin level indicates an exposure to the elements in smoke. Visualization of the upper and lower airways by fiberoptic bronchoscopy can provide information on the anatomic extent of injury, but initial observations have not been found to prognosticate accurately the magnitude of injury to allow anticipation of the subsequent course.

TREATMENT. Initial treatment of a chemical burn consists of aggressive upper airway maintenance and pulmonary support, which includes maintenance of small airway patency and the removal of soot and mucopurulent secretions. Careful and well-monitored fluid resuscitation is necessary if accentuation of the process is to be avoided. Undervolume resuscitation aggravates the pulmonary dysfunction as much as does over-resuscitation.[4, 22] The addition of positive end-expiratory pressure is frequently necessary to maintain small airway patency and an adequate functional residual capacity by assisting in holding the edematous airway open until edema resolves. Early endotracheal intubation and positive end-expiratory pressure have been reported to decrease the incidence of lung-related deaths after severe burns and smoke inhalation.[30] Positive-pressure support should be initiated before severe respiratory compromise occurs, since prevention of airway closure is much more readily accomplished than is the reopening of collapsed airways. A large enough tube (i.e., one with at least a 7-mm internal diameter) should be used in adults because very thick secretions develop as a result of the lung injury. If the tube initially introduced is too small, it will be very dangerous to change once massive facial and airway edema develops. Although the nasotracheal route may be more comfortable to the patient, the tube size may need to be compromised, which may lead to problems for secretion clearance later. The continued use of additional humidified oxygen to maintain adequate oxygen delivery as well as to assist in the clearance of secretions is indicated. Elevation of the patient's head and chest 20° to 30° is also helpful (see Table 162–2).

Bronchospasm can be treated with bronchodilators, either administered parenterally or in an aerosol. Intravenous aminophylline, although a good bronchodilator, is frequently limited in its usefulness because of the tachycardia observed in the early postburn period. Beginning about 18 to 24 hours after a burn injury, an increase in airway resistance is often due to bronchiolar edema and airway plugging rather than to bronchospasm. The impaired gas exchange often responds to further increases in positive end-expiratory pressure and to bronchodilators. Use of prophylactic antibiotics is not indicated.

The injured airways mucosa frequently becomes colonized by bacteria, especially if an endotracheal tube is present. Prophylactic antibiotics use will only lead to overgrowth of more resistant organisms. It is now well demonstrated that the early use of high-dose corticosteroids in the presence of a body burn increases rather than decreases the morbidity and mortality of smoke inhalation.[32]

Impaired Chest Wall Compliance

A reduction in chest wall compliance may accompany reductions in pulmonary compliance. Respiratory excursion can be markedly impaired by a burn to the chest wall. The process is most evident with a circumferential third-degree burn. The loss of elasticity in the chest wall due to the burn tissue markedly increases the work of breathing required to maintain functional residual capacity and an adequate tidal volume. As more subeschar edema develops and compresses the chest wall, the end-expiratory intrathoracic volume begins to decrease. Edema from a second-degree burn is also sufficient to alter lung mechanics. The loose areolar tissue in the axilla and lateral chest wall sequester large amounts of edema fluid, leading to development of a very heavy and tense chest wall. Full-thickness burns produce a more severe limitation because tissue expansion is markedly impaired and intrathoracic volume becomes compressed. The result is a significant increase in work of breathing and hypoventilation. Maximum respiratory effort is frequently required just to maintain adequate gas exchange. Any process that compromises the necessary increase in inspiratory force and muscle activity, such as hypoxia, hypovolemia, pain, or sedation, increases the work of breathing, increases the development of atelectasis, and produces hypoventilation. Ventilation-perfusion abnormalities may be increased if a patient is mechanically ventilated because the positive pressure delivered to the airway cannot adequately be distributed to noncompliant regions of the lung.

DIAGNOSIS. Symptoms may not be clearly evident until edema formation peaks at about 10 to 12 hours. The first clinical evidence of the chest wall restrictive defect is often labored breathing followed by a rapid respiratory deterioration, particularly in the patient who is not receiving ventilator support. With the combination of chest burn and inhalation injury, it is very difficult to distinguish the degree of impairment in total lung compliance caused by the increase in airway edema and bronchospasm compared with that due to impairment of the chest wall.

TREATMENT. The three main treatment principles are:

1. Recognition of the problem
2. Control of the tissue edema process (elevation of upper body if hemodynamically stable)
3. Surgical decompression of chest wall constriction

Common Pitfalls in Initial Pulmonary Support

1. The use of initial arterial oxygen tension to reflect the adequacy of oxygenation
2. The use of a small nasotracheal tube in the presence of smoke inhalation injury
3. Endotracheal intubation without addition of some positive end-expiratory pressure
4. Fluid restriction in a patient with a burn and an inhalation injury

POSTRESUSCITATION PHASE

This period is often "the calm before the storm." Early symptoms are resolving, but the peak tracheobronchial mucosal slough and bronchopneumonia have not yet appeared.

Continued Upper Airway Obstruction

PATHOPHYSIOLOGY. Upper airway and facial edema caused by the heat-induced tissue and mucosal damage begins to resolve between days 2 and 4 in patients with superficial injuries. However, in those with full-thickness burns, edema, both external and that in the oropharynx and larynx, resolve more slowly. Occasionally, excision of deep neck eschar is necessary to allow expansion of the underlying soft tissue, which in turn restores venous drainage and allows edema formation.

Increasing Tracheobronchitis

PATHOPHYSIOLOGY. With a severe injury, the damaged mucosa becomes necrotic at 3 to 4 days after injury and begins to slough. The increase in viscous secretions can lead to distal airway obstruction, atelectasis, and a high risk for the rapid development of bronchopneumonia. As airways inflammation increases over the next several days, a diffuse interstitial edema can develop.[28] Even modest volume overload potentiates the edema process during this period. The

TABLE 163–6. Pathophysiology of Chemical Tracheobronchitis (2 to 6 Days)

Large and small airways, edema, spasm	*Increased secretions*
1. Decreased dynamic compliance 2. Increased work 3. Decreased functional residual capacity 4. Atelectasis and increased shunt (hypoxemia) 5. Parenchymal involvement 6. Increased risk of edema with any hypervolemia	1. Increased work 2. Airways plugging by secretions 3. Increasing shunt (hypoxemia) 4. Increased risk of infection tracheobronchial colonization, pneumonia, sepsis)
Increased minute ventilation	*Evidence of sepsis syndrome*
1. Increasing dead space 2. Increasing carbon dioxide production	1. Lung inflammation 2. Lung infection

(From Demling RH, Lalonde C: Pulmonary abnormalities. *In*: Burn Trauma. Blaisdell FW, Trunkey DD [Eds]. New York, Thieme, 1989, p 74.)

magnitude of the pulmonary infection is in large part dependent on the status of host defenses and the aggressiveness of pulmonary support. If infection can be controlled and secretions cleared, the acute process will resolve over the next 7 to 10 days. However, the risk of infection persists for several weeks, extending well into the inflammation period[2, 3, 23] (Table 163–6).

SYMPTOMS. In the first several days after injury, remaining soot continues to be present in the airways secretions. Diffuse rhonchi are usually present once inflammation has developed. Evidence of tracheobronchitis followed by that of bronchopneumonia is common in a substantial number of patients. The characteristics of the symptom complex are as follows:

Change of sputum from loose to mucopurulent
Evidence of necrotic tissue in sputum
Increase in the work of breathing
Alteration of gas exchange
Visualization of infiltrates on radiography (late finding)

Do not underestimate the magnitude of injury based on initial presentation, since lung function may be deceptively good on day 2 and only deteriorate rapidly on days 3 and 4. Chest radiographic findings invariably underestimate the magnitude of the chemical inhalation–induced airways injury.

TREATMENT. The clearance of soot, mucopurulent exudate, and sloughing mucosa is essential to avoid progression of the lung injury. An endotracheal tube may be necessary if clearance of secretions is inadequate. If the injury is severe, especially if a large burn is present, early tracheostomy through nonburned skin on a previously excised and grafted neck burn significantly improves secretion clearance and helps to more safely secure the airway. Ventilator assistance may also be necessary if the patient is fatigued and if gas exchange worsens. The continuous rotation bed is ideal for the patient with an inhalation injury and a large body burn in whom side movement is difficult because of the pain and stiffness that result from tissue edema. The constant postural drainage assists in the removal of airway plugs (Table 163–7).

Infection surveillance is crucial during this early period if a bacterial bronchitis is to be detected before the development of a pneumonia. Sputum smears and monitoring of the character of the sputum are useful early guides. Systemic antibiotics are not given prophylactically, but they are administered when a bacterial process becomes evident.

Common Pitfalls

Extubating Too Soon

Resolution of facial edema does not always correspond with resolution of airways edema. In addition, many pulmonary problems necessitate creation of an artificial airway in the burn patient. Look at the whole picture!

Underestimating the Lower Airways Injury

Once the initial airways edema is resolving, a quiet period (the "calm before the storm") often occurs; the period precedes bacterial tracheobronchitis and the resultant bronchopneumonia. An appreciation of impending problems results in more aggressive preventive measures.

Failure to Provide Adequate Postanesthetic Support

The major burn patient, especially one with a chest burn, must put forth a large work effort to maintain adequate ventilation. The work loading increases as hypermetabolism and increased carbon dioxide production result. A general anesthetic impairs diaphragmatic motion, decreases functional reserve capacity, and decreases maximum inspiratory

TABLE 163–7. Assess for Lower Airway Injury (to Ventilate or Not to Ventilate with Positive Pressure)

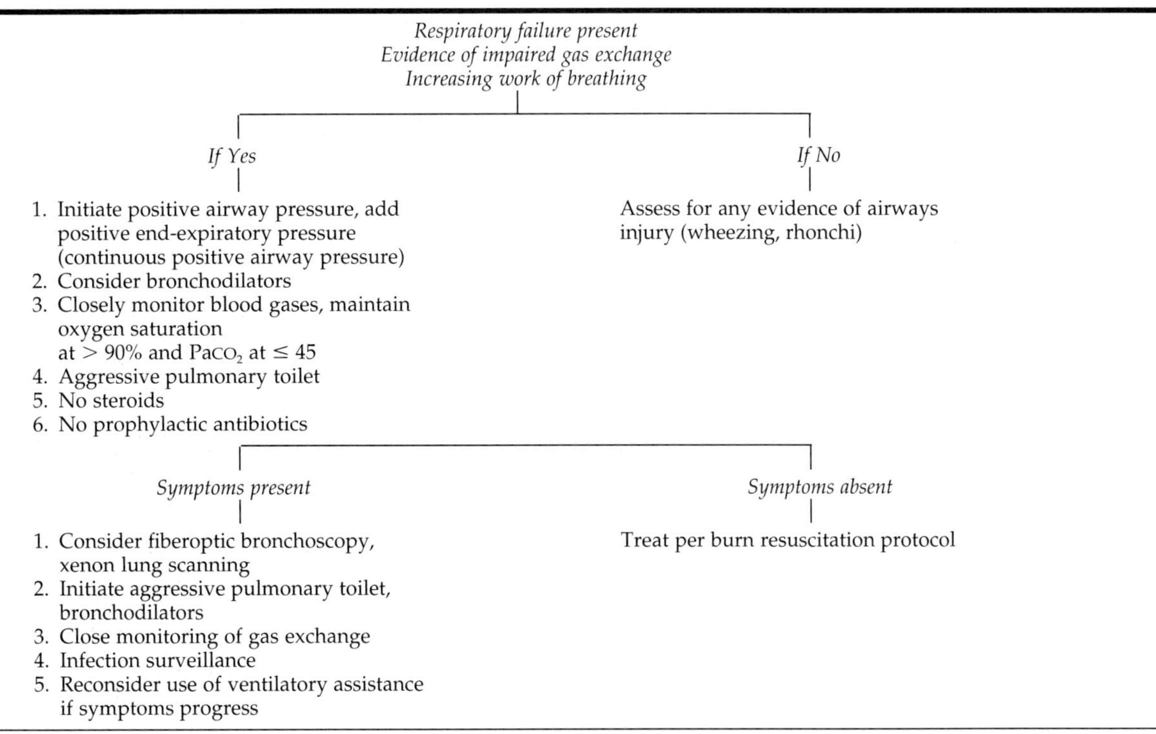

Respiratory failure present
Evidence of impaired gas exchange
Increasing work of breathing

If Yes

1. Initiate positive airway pressure, add positive end-expiratory pressure (continuous positive airway pressure)
2. Consider bronchodilators
3. Closely monitor blood gases, maintain oxygen saturation at > 90% and Pa_{CO_2} at ≤ 45
4. Aggressive pulmonary toilet
5. No steroids
6. No prophylactic antibiotics

If No

Assess for any evidence of airways injury (wheezing, rhonchi)

Symptoms present

1. Consider fiberoptic bronchoscopy, xenon lung scanning
2. Initiate aggressive pulmonary toilet, bronchodilators
3. Close monitoring of gas exchange
4. Infection surveillance
5. Reconsider use of ventilatory assistance if symptoms progress

Symptoms absent

Treat per burn resuscitation protocol

(Modified from Demling RH, Lalonde C: Airway and pulmonary abnormalities. *In*: Burn Trauma. Blaisdell FW, Trunkey DD [Eds]. New York, Thieme, 1989, p 16.)

force; all of these factors can result in significant postoperative pulmonary dysfunction.[24] The use of muscle relaxants should be kept to a minimum. Ideal management is to maintain support (e.g., provide continuous positive airway pressure) until full restoration of preoperative mechanics and of gas exchange has occurred.

Underestimating the Effect of Chest Wall Stiffness on Lung Function

Underestimation of the increased work of breathing is created by a rigid chest wall, even when the presence of normal lung parenchyma leads to fatigue, airway collapse, and secondary infection. This process is particularly likely to occur in the early postanesthesia period.[33]

INFLAMMATION-INFECTION PHASE

Pulmonary problems remain a major cause of morbidity and mortality during this phase. Pulmonary failure and pulmonary sepsis exceed burn wound sepsis as a cause of mortality.

Three major processes occur during this period: (1) nosocomial pneumonia, (2) hypermetabolism-induced respiratory fatigue (power failure), and (3) adult respiratory distress syndrome (low-pressure pulmonary edema). These three processes are closely interrelated. The burn patient is very susceptible to infection, particularly after a smoke-inhalation injury. The hypermetabolic state produces a marked increase in oxygen needs and in carbon dioxide production. The increase in work demands on the lung as a gas-exchanging organ can exceed the adequacy of lung function. Adult respiratory distress syndrome is a severe complication of the sepsis process, which is very difficult to reverse in the burn patient.[34]

Nosocomial Pneumonia

Pathophysiology

Burn patients with a combination of inhalation injury and a major body burn are at the greatest risk for pneumonia, with a rate of incidence that exceeds 50%. The high incidence results from the presence of virulent organisms in the intensive care unit environment and from the immunosuppressed state of the burn patient.[23] Since eradication of an established pneumonia in the smoke inhalation and burn patient is very difficult, prevention is of primary importance. Preventive measures focus on two areas: improvement of systemic defenses and improvement of local lung defenses.

Improvement of Systemic Host Defenses

Maintenance of adequate oxygen delivery to the burn wound tissue and to other tissue at risk for infection is necessary. It is achieved by optimizing blood volume, hemoglobin level, and cardiac output. Nutritional status must be maintained both by providing adequate calories and protein and by using the correct mix of nutrients. In addition, underlying chronic diseases that are also immunosuppressive, such as diabetes, must be controlled as much as possible.

Improvement of Local Lung Defenses

Maintaining an adequate cough mechanism is of utmost importance in the patient at risk for pneumonia, particularly in the absence of positive-pressure support, since a greater risk for hypoventilation and atelectasis exists. Analgesics and sedation must be used carefully. It is necessary to provide adequate pain relief, especially if splinting due to a chest wall burn is present.

If continued intubation is expected to be necessary for many weeks, conversion to a tracheostomy within the first several days greatly assists in the clearance of secretions. The tracheostomy should not be placed through burned tissue. If the neck is burned, early excision and grafting of the neck area is indicated; the subsequent tracheostomy can be performed through the skin graft in 24 to 48 hours[33] (Table 163–8).

Hypermetabolism-Induced Respiratory Fatigue (Power Failure)

PATHOPHYSIOLOGY. The increase in oxygen consumption and carbon dioxide production during this period requires an increase in gas exchange relative to that seen in the previous periods.[35] A 50% to 100% increase in carbon dioxide production is seen in patients with burns covering in excess of 50% of the total body surface. In addition, the severe catabolism, initiated by the inflammatory response, can lead not only to extremity weakness but also to weakness of the chest wall muscle. Chronic pain and anxiety lead to sleep deprivation and fatigue. Common causes of impaired oxygenation during this period are heart failure that leads to lung edema and hypoventilation-induced atelectasis as fatigue develops. The major problem during this period is usually not hypoxemia but rather hypercapnia

TABLE 163–8. Treatment of Tracheobronchitis

Increased airways resistance (edema)	*Increased secretions: Bacterial colonization*
1. Positive-pressure assistance to increase functional residual capacity 2. Consider bronchodilators 3. Avoid congestive heart failure, volume overload	1. Aggressive pulmonary toilet, and consider early tracheostomy in severe cases, especially with large burns (postural changes extremely important) 2. Infection surveillance, daily sputum smear 3. Assess for antibiotic use; do not wait for radiographic findings of infiltrate before initiating empiric therapy, if sputum indicative of infection
Do not produce hypovolemia in an attempt to correct airways edema	

(From Demling RH, Lalonde C: Pulmonary abnormalities. *In*: Burn Trauma. Blaisdell FW, Trunkey DD [Eds]. New York, Thieme, 1989, p 77.)

TABLE 163–9. Mechanism of Power Failure

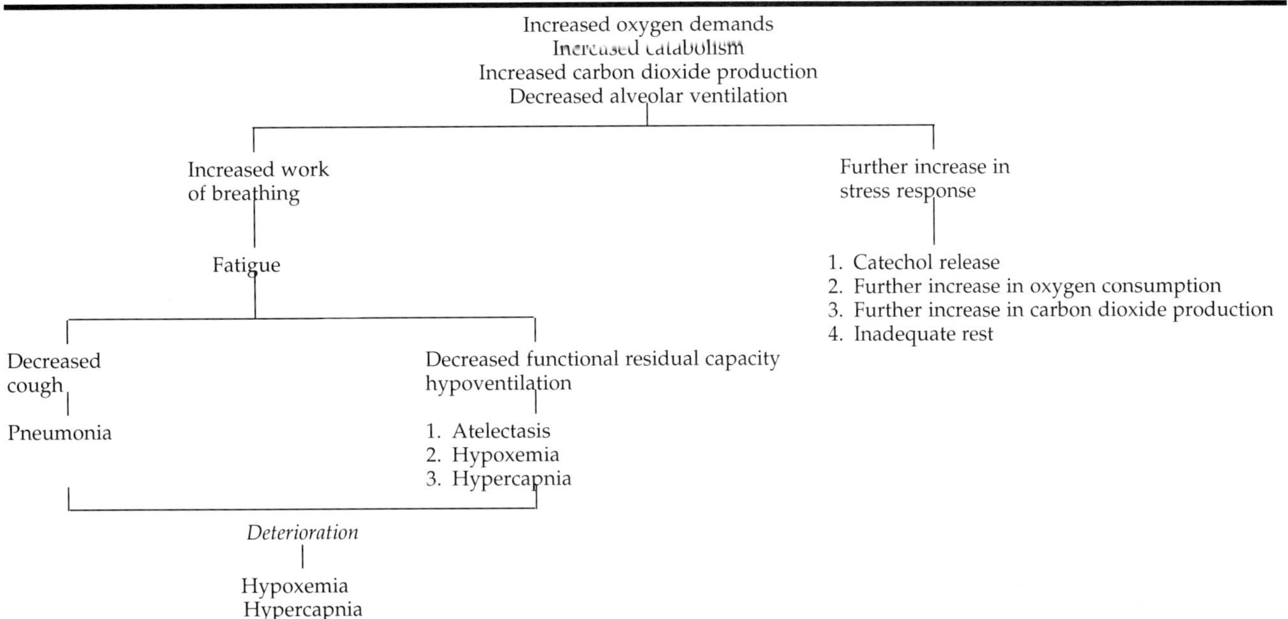

(From Demling RH, Lalonde C: Pulmonary abnormalities. *In*: Burn Trauma. Blaisdell FW, Trunkey DD [Eds]. New York, Thieme, 1989, p 158.)

because carbon dioxide removal is directly dependent on alveolar minute ventilation. A doubling of carbon dioxide production means a doubling of alveolar ventilation to maintain a normal Pa_{CO_2}. Increased ventilation means increased work of breathing, especially if a decrease in compliance or an increase in dead space is also present. Increased tidal volumes require an increased inspiratory force, and the added work must be sustained 24 hours a day. If fatigue develops, impaired clearance of secretions will also occur, and this can lead to nosocomial pneumonia as well as to hypercapnia.

The "power failure" syndrome commonly occurs is in the perioperative period. Underestimation of increased ventilatory needs can lead to the development of hypercapnia during the anesthesia period. An increase in Pa_{CO_2} produces an intense catechol release, anxiety, and a further increase in oxygen demands and carbon dioxide production. However, an additional increase in carbon dioxide level will also be produced if an excess amount of carbohydrate is infused (Table 163–9).

TREATMENT. Controlling lung edema and infection while maintaining nutrition and adequate rest as well as chest wall exercise are key components. Fatigue and early evidence of respiratory compromise can be treated with assisted ventilatory support.

Partial ventilatory support via a tracheostomy may be useful, especially if the anticipated problem is expected to last several weeks, as is the case with a large body burn.[36] In addition, added ventilatory support should be provided in the early postoperative period until a patient can resume sufficient spontaneous ventilation.

Adult Respiratory Distress Syndrome (Low Pressure Pulmonary Edema)

In general, this form of adult respiratory distress syndrome is a combination of both airways and alveolar involvement and is highly lethal.

Common Pitfalls

1. Underestimation of the risks for pneumonia
2. Underestimation of increased ventilatory requirements in the perioperative period
3. Underestimation of the workload of breathing during the hypermetabolic state
4. Underutilization of the tracheostomy

References

1. Cope O: Management of the Coconut Grove burns at the Massachusetts General Hospital. Ann Surg 1943; 117:801–809.
2. Clark W, Reid W, Gelmour W, et al: Mortality probability in victims of fire trauma: Revised equation to include inhalation injury. Br Med J 1986; 292:1303–1308.
3. Cahalane M, Demling R: Early respiratory abnormalities from smoke inhalation. JAMA 1984; 251:771–776.
4. Zawacki B, Jung R, Joyce J, et al: Smoke, burns, and the natural history of inhalation injury in fire victims. Ann Surg 1977; 185:100–110.
5. Schuelen J, Munster A: The parkland formula in patients with burns and inhalation injury. J Trauma 1982; 22:869–884.
6. Lalonde C, Knox J, Youn YK, et al: Burn edema is accentuated by a moderate smoke inhalation injury in sheep. Surgery 1992; 112:908–917.
7. Crapo R: Smoke inhalation injuries. JAMA 1981; 246:1694–1698.
8. Loke J: The toxic environment and its medical implications with special emphasis on smoke inhalation. *In:* Pathophysiology and Treatment of Inhalation Injuries. Loke J (Ed.) New York, Marcel Dekker, 1988, pp 453–489.
9. Youn YK, Lalonde C, Demling RH: Oxidants and pathophysiology of burn and smoke inhalation injury. Free Rad Biol Med 1992; 12:409–415.
10. Brain J, Valberg P: Deposition of aerosol in the respiratory tract. Am Rev Respir Dis 1979; 120:1325–1371.
11. Dennis W: The Effect of Breathing Rate on the Deposition of Particles in the Human Respiratory Tract. *In:* Inhaled Particles III. Walton W (Ed.) Surrey, England, Urwin Brothers, 1971, pp 91–102.
12. Heyder J, Gebhart J, Rudolf G, et al: Deposition of particles in

the human respiratory tract in the size range of 0.0005–15 μm. J Aerosol Sci 1986; 17:811–825.
13. Morrow P: Deposition and retention models for internal dosimetry of the human respiratory tract. Health Phys 1966; 12:173–207.
14. Watanabe K, Makino K: The role of carbon monoxide poisoning in the production of inhalation burns. Ann Plast Surg 1985; 14:284–294.
15. Church D, Pryor W: Free radical chemistry of cigarette smoke and its toxicological implications. Environ Health Perspect 1985; 64:111–126.
16. Stothert J, Ashley K, Kramer G, et al: Intrapulmonary distribution of bronchial blood flow after moderate smoke inhalation. J Appl Physiol 1990; 69:1734–1739.
17. Barnes P, Baraniuk J, Belvisi M: Neuropeptides in the respiratory tract. Am Rev Respir Dis 1991; 144:1187–1198.
18. Tranbaugh R, Elings V, Christensen J, et al: Effect of inhalation injury on lung water accumulation. J Trauma 1983; 23:597–603.
19. Herndon D, Barrow R, Traber D, et al: Extravascular lung water changes following smoke inhalation and massive burn injury. Surgery 1987; 102:341–348.
20. Nieman G, Clark W, Wax S, et al: The effect of smoke inhalation on pulmonary surfactant. Ann Surg 1980; 191:171–181.
21. Navar P, Saffle J, Warden G: Effect of inhalation injury on fluid resuscitation requirements after thermal injury. Am J Surg 1985; 150:716–721.
22. Herndon D, Traber D, Traber L: The effect of resuscitation on inhalation injury. Surgery 1986; 100:248–254.
23. Shirani K, Pruitt B, Mason A: The influence of inhalation injury and pneumonia on burn mortality. Ann Surg 1986; 205:82–86.
24. Demling RH: Effect of early burn excision and grafting on pulmonary function. J Trauma 1984; 24:830–837.
25. Schneider W, Berger A, Machnder P: Diagnostic and therapeutic possibilities for fiberoptic bronchoscopy in inhalation injury. Burns 1988; 14:53–57.
26. Moylan J: Inhalation injury. J Trauma 1981; 21:720–728.
27. Haponik E, Summer W: Respiratory complications in the burned patient: Diagnosis and management of inhalation injury. J Crit Care 1987; 2:121–128.
28. Coblentz C, Chiles C, Putnam C: Radiologic evaluation. *In:* Respiratory Injury: Smoke Inhalation and Burns. Haponik E, Munster A (Eds). New York, McGraw-Hill, 1990, pp 179–195.
29. Vogel S, Sultan T: Cyanide poisoning. Clin Toxicol 1981; 18:367–372.
30. Venus B, Matsuda T, Copioza J, et al: Prophylactic intubation and continuous positive airway pressure in the management of inhalation injury in burn victims. Crit Care Med 1981; 9:519–524.
31. Robinson N, Hudson L, Robertson H: Ventilation and perfusion alterations after smoke inhalation injury. Surgery 1981; 90:352–360.
32. Robinson N, Hudson L, Rum M: Steroid therapy following isolated smoke inhalation injury. J Trauma 1982; 22:876–880.
33. Demling RH, Crawford G, Lind L, et al: Restrictive pulmonary dysfunction caused by the grafted chest and abdominal burn. Crit Care Med 1988; 16:743–747.
34. Marshall W, Dimick A: The natural history of major burns with multiple subsystem failure. J Trauma 1983; 23:102–105.
35. Molnar J, Wolfe R, Burke J: Burns: Metabolism and nutritional therapy in thermal injury. *In:* Nutritional Support of Medical Practice. Schneider H (Ed). Philadelphia, JB Lippincott, 1983, pp 266–281.
36. Hunt J, Purdue G, Gunning T: Is tracheostomy warranted in the burn patient? Indications and complications. J Burn Care Rehabil 1986; 7:492–497.

CHAPTER 164

Hypothermia and Cold-Related Injuries

Eric H. Hubli, MD • Robert H. Demling, MD

HYPOTHERMIA

Hypothermia is defined as a decrease in core body temperature below 35°C (95°F).[1–3] The causes of hypothermia may be categorized as either accidental or iatrogenic. *Iatrogenic hypothermia* is caused by the deliberate use of cold to depress core body temperature in a controlled fashion over a designated period of time as an adjunct to medical care (e.g., as during cardiopulmonary bypass).[2, 4] The term *accidental hypothermia* implies the existence of normal thermoregulatory control and can be defined as an undesired decrease in core body temperature due to exposure to an ambient temperature that is less than core body temperature. The heat loss responsible for hypothermia occurs in three ways: radiation, conduction, and convection. *Radiation* implies thermal loss in the form of infrared radiation. *Conduction* loss occurs as a result of direct body contact with a colder surface. *Convection* loss occurs whenever the rate of temperature decrease is dependent on the flow of environmental air or fluid across a surface, which decreases surface temperature.

Many factors other than exposure contribute to or predispose a patient to the development of hypothermia (Table 164–1). These include metabolic disease, central nervous

TABLE 164–1. Factors That Predispose to Hypothermia

Metabolic	*Age*
Hypothyroidism	Neonate
Hypopituitarism	Elderly
Myxedema	*Miscellaneous*
Renal failure/uremia	Erythroderma
Hypoglycemia	Sepsis
Hypothalamic disorders	Trauma
Diabetes mellitus	Burns
Alcohol abuse	Water exposure
Malnutrition	Previous cold exposure
CNS/Mental Status	
CNS injury (spinal cord or brain injury)	
Psychiatric disease	
Wernicke's encephalopathy	
Alzheimer's disease	
Alcohol abuse	
Drug overdose	
Medications	
General anesthesia	
Benzodiazepines	
Paralytics	
Antidepressants	
Barbiturates	
Narcotics	
Reserpine	
Anticholinergics	
Salicylates/antiprostaglandins	
Phenothiazines	
Diuretics	
Alpha-, beta-blockers	
Calcium channel blockers	
Organophosphates	

Abbreviation: CNS = central nervous system.

system disorders, medications, recreational drugs, mental and psychiatric illness, associated trauma or surgery, infection, age, and alcohol abuse. Special attention should be devoted to the last two of these factors because of their increasing importance with respect to hypothermia. Alcohol abuse remains the primary culprit in non–war-related hypothermia. Alcohol increases susceptibility to hypothermia by depressing the sensorium and decreasing shivering as well as by causing vasodilatation, which further increases heat loss. The body's protective mechanisms against the cold are therefore bypassed.

Age is also a prominent factor in hypothermia.[5] Neonates have been known to be susceptible owing to their high ratio of body surface area to body size. Insight into the physiologic changes that occur in the aged has revealed many factors that increase their risk of hypothermia. As age increases, the ability to generate heat from metabolic activity decreases. Inability to mount an appropriate physiologic response to cold is also caused by a decrease in cardiac output, the presence of peripheral vascular disease, and the effects of vasoactive and cardiac medications. Finally, heat loss may be increased owing to a blunting of adaptive responses associated with alterations in sensorium and an increase in radiant heat loss due to a reduction in the amount of subcutaneous fat.

Pathophysiology

Humans are homeotherms that can independently maintain a core body temperature of between 97 and 99°F (36.1 and 37.2°C) in the face of ambient variants, which range from 60 to 130°F. Outside of these limits, temperature extremes are adjusted by means of compensatory mechanisms that depend on behavior modification. The homeostatic core body temperature of 98.6°F (37°C) is maintained by the anterior preoptic region of the hypothalamus, which receives afferent spinothalamic input and mediates efferent sympathetic response.

In the face of a mild-to-moderate decrease in core body temperature to 90 to 94°F (32–35°C), the hypothalamus initiates a sympathetic and catecholamine response that leads to an increase in cardiac output, basal metabolic rate, oxygen consumption, and intermittent peripheral vasoconstriction. Isometric muscle contractions in the form of shivering generate up to a fivefold increase in peripheral heat production. As core body temperature continues to decrease below the hypothermic range of 90 to 94°F (32–35°C), a generalized downward metabolic spiral begins. Basal metabolic rate falls as do blood pressure and cardiac output because of a decrease in cardiac contractility that occurs secondary to a cold-induced reduction in inotropic and chronotropic response. Central blood volumes increase owing to peripheral vasoconstriction, and this, coupled with cold-induced renal dysfunction, leads to a "cold diuresis." Hematocrit and creatinine and blood urea nitrogen levels all increase. Respiratory rate slows, and mental status becomes sluggish. Purposeful activity decreases because of central nervous system changes and an inhibition of peripheral sensory and motor nerve function. The rate of cooling increases as baseline compensatory mechanisms fail.

As core body temperature enters the range of 80.6 to 89.6°F (27–32°C), physiological abnormalities progress. Shivering stops below 89.6°F (32°C). Myocardial electrophysiology usually reveals bradycardia associated with decreased sinoatrial node response. The pathognomonic J (or Osborne) wave also becomes evident. Myocardial excitability increases, and atrial fibrillation is common. A continued rise in blood viscosity occurs because of a pathologic diuresis and cooling, which increase viscosity by 2% for each 1°C decrease in temperature. The oxygen dissociation curve shifts to the left, and oxygen delivery is further decreased. However, cellular needs may be adequately met as oxygen solubility in plasma increases and as cell oxygen demand decreases owing to a lower basal metabolic rate. Especially relevant is the fact that cerebral oxygen demand decreases 6% for each 1°C fall in temperature; this protects the brain from damage due to the low-flow state.

Coagulation abnormalities are also present.[6] Initial changes include qualitative and quantitative platelet changes. Platelets are transiently sequestered in the liver and spleen.

Blood acid-base and electrolyte anomalies indigenous to hypothermia have been recently characterized.[7] Impairment of the Na^+-K^+ adenosine triphosphate pump leads to hyponatremia and hyperkalemia.[8] Blood pH can fall in response to an increase in lactate production.

When severe hypothermia (<80°F [<26.7°C]) develops just before a coma state occurs, peripheral vasoconstriction diminishes and surface rewarming takes place. Patients experience a subjective rewarming phenomenon, and some display a pattern of "paradoxical undressing."[9] After this, further cooling occurs rapidly. Patients may become apneic, have a low or unmeasurable blood pressure, and develop profound bradycardia or asystole. In this setting, ventricular excitability is great, and care must be taken to prevent ventricular fibrillation. A patient may appear lifeless; however, no patient should be pronounced dead until rewarming to 35°C has been completed.

Diagnosis

Hypothermia is primarily a diagnosis of suspicion and should be strongly considered in a patient with a history of prolonged cold exposure or body immersion, bradycardia, and slow respiration. Confirmation of diagnosis is made on the basis of the use of a low-reading thermometer and the exclusion of other metabolic derangements. Recent use of the low-reading thermometer has greatly increased our understanding of hypothermia. Before the early 1980s, these thermometers were not widely used.

Therapy

Prevention

Prevention is always the best therapy. In either the outdoor or hospital setting, limiting exposure to cool temperatures, maximizing body coverage, careful temperature monitoring, and the intake of warm fluids (intravenously or perorally) minimize the risk of hypothermia.

Before Hospital Admission

In the preadmission setting, therapy is directed toward prevention of further heat loss, with removal of wet clothing and wrapping of the patient in a dry blanket. When available, warmed intravenous fluid and warmed humidified oxygen should be administered. High oxygen tension and limited patient movement decrease the likelihood that ventricular fibrillation will occur during transport. If patients display bradycardia and slow respiratory function, care should be limited to observation. Asystolic patients should receive a modified cardiopulmonary resuscitation. Compressions should be longer and slower and have increased relaxation intervals to compensate for the decreased blood flow associated with increased blood viscosity.

Initial Resuscitation

Initial evaluation and care based on the fundamentals of trauma resuscitation are always warranted. If a patient is breathing spontaneously, warm humidified oxygen (100% at 42°C) should be administered. If the patient is apneic, careful intubation should be performed. Pretreatment with 100% oxygen by facemask and 500 mg (or 5–10 mg/kg) of bretylium tosylate decreases the likelihood of ventricular fibrillation. Mechanical ventilation should be instituted, and the hypothermic state should be monitored on the basis of blood gas values, with parameters set to maintain blood gas status appropriately for the patient's size and weight. Arterial blood gas readings should be corrected for physiologic shifts that are observed with hypothermia. For each 1°C decrease in temperature from 37°C, pH increases by 0.015, carbon dioxide tension decreases by 5%, and arterial oxygen tension decreases by 7%. As such, the alkalotic state noted in hypothermia should be expected and promoted to maintain the intracellular neutrality needed to ensure proper enzymatic and cellular function.

Venous access should be obtained, and electrocardiographic monitoring should be performed as the patient is being exposed and subsequently wrapped in blankets. Central venous catheters are helpful in monitoring central venous pressures and as a means of administering warm fluid directly to the heart. During insertion, care must be taken not to pass the guide wire or the catheter into the ventricle; otherwise, fibrillation may occur. The use of Swan-Ganz catheters is contraindicated.

Warmed intravenous fluids (42°C) consisting of normal saline, with or without dextrose, are recommended. Potassium-containing fluids such as lactated Ringer's solution are not recommended because hypothermic patients may be hyperkalemic because of dysfunction of the Na^+-K^+ adenosine triphosphate pump. Thiamine and folate should be administered prophylactically owing to the high correlation of alcohol abuse and hypothermia. Patient movement should be kept to a minimum because of cardiac irritability.

Laboratory examination of baseline blood values should be performed, and electrocardiograms should be obtained. Many hematologic and physiologic parameters have been evaluated for their prognostic ability with respect to patient survival. To date, potassium, lactate, amylase, and blood sugar levels, initial temperature, respiratory rate, heart rate, and initial blood pressure have not proved prognostic. As such, resuscitation must be attempted in all hypothermic patients until core body temperature increases to 35°C.

Rewarming

Two rewarming techniques can be used for hypothermic patients: passive rewarming and active rewarming.[2, 10] *Passive rewarming* relies on endogenous heat generation and ambient temperature to raise core body temperature slowly at a rate of approximately 0.5 to 2.0°C per hour. This form of rewarming is indicated in the mildly hypothermic, hemodynamically stable patient. Broader application of this technique to moderate and severely hypothermic patients who were hemodynamically stable has met with good results.

The term *active rewarming* implies the use of heat sources to raise core body temperature. These sources may be administered by internal or external means. External heat sources such as heat shields, warming blankets, and immersion baths can be perilous to a patient for a number of reasons. First, rapid rewarming of the shell can cause peripheral vasodilatation with associated shunting of cold, hyperkalemic, lactate-rich blood to the core. This can precipitate rewarming shock, cardiac arrhythmias, or asystole. Also, when a warm bath is used, cardiac compressions are at best difficult to perform, and defibrillation is impossible. Owing to these factors, internal means of rewarming are preferred.

Many forms of internal rewarming have been utilized. Choice of method is best addressed at each institution, taking into account a patient's condition and the therapeutic modalities available.

The Stable Patient

The most basic form of internal rewarming consists of administering heated, moist oxygen (42°C) and warm intravenous fluids as well as body coverage with a dry blanket. With this method, body temperature should rise by 1 to 2°C per hour. If a more rapid temperature rise is desired or if moderate to severe hypothermia is present, more rapid rewarming can be achieved with the use of nasogastric and rectal lavage with warmed fluids (temperature rises 5–10°C per hour). Bretylium tosylate may be administered prophylactically.

The Unstable Patient

In unstable or asystolic patients, more aggressive rewarming may be warranted. Peritoneal lavage with fluids warmed to 45°C raises temperature by 15 to 20°C per hour. Initially, a lavage catheter is placed, and 1 L of warm saline is administered. Unilateral closed pleural lavage with an anterior midclavicular chest tube and an inferior axillary chest tube accomplishes a similar warming trend with the added advantage of rapid cardiac rewarming.

Direct cardiac rewarming via median sternotomy and mediastinal irrigation has also proved effective. This method offers the added advantage of direct access to the heart and great vessels in the event that cardiopulmonary bypass is needed.

Extracorporeal bypass using femoral access is an excellent technique for rapid rewarming because it allows for a controlled temperature rise and provides an external pump in the event of cardiac dysfunction.[2–4] These systems have even been tied into dialysis circuits as a means of maintaining homeostasis. The major disadvantage of this rewarming technique is the inherent need for heparinization, which limits its use to patients without concomitant severe traumatic injuries. New rewarming techniques that involve the use of heparinless extracorporeal bypass and a Bio-Medicus pump, continuous arteriovenous rewarming by direct patient pressure, and extracorporeal diathermy (ultrasound) offer new approaches to patient care.

COLD URTICARIA

Cold urticaria describes a syndrome in which exposure to cold leads to urticaria and angioedema.[11] In certain subsets of patients, anaphylaxis may occur, causing hypotension, tachycardia, shock, and even death. Although limited cold exposure can act as a trigger, most anaphylactic responses are associated with aquatic activity. Cold urticaria syndromes may be classified as familial or acquired. Diagnosis is confirmed by history and a positive result on the cold stimulation test (exposure to a cold source leads to a formation of a wheal and flare response). Stimulus response times are analyzed to determine the severity of disease. Management consists of prevention, that is, decreasing exposure to cold and eliminating aquatic activities. Cold tolerance induction and medications such as antihistamines, cyproheptadine, doxepin, ketotifen, epinephrine, corticosteroids, and doxantrazole have all proved effective.

LOCAL COLD INJURIES: FROSTBITE

Frostbite is the most severe of the local cold injuries, and it involves freezing of the affected tissues.[12–14] Freezing uniformly begins when tissue temperature reaches −2°C; how-

TABLE 164–2. Risk Factors Associated with Frostbite Injury

Blood Flow–Related	*Age*
Peripheral vascular disease	Elderly
Cardiac disease	Very young
CNS/Mental Status	*Race*
Dementia/history of psychiatric illness	Black > White
CNS injury (spinal cord or brain)	
	Miscellaneous
Medications	Ethanol
Same as for hypothermia (see Table 164–1)	Previous cold exposure
	Tobacco use
Vasoconstrictors	Malnutrition

ever, the effects of cold exposure may be increased in the presence of wind or moisture, which can increase convection and conductive loss (water dissipates heat 32 times faster than does air). An example of this is that a temperature of −6.7°C (44°F) in the presence of a 40-mile/h wind has the same tissue effects as an air temperature of −40°C in the presence of a 2-mile/h wind.

There are two classifications of frostbite injury. The first is clinically based and categorizes injury as *superficial* (if only the skin and subcutaneous tissue are frozen) or *deep* (if underlying tissue is frozen). The second classification grades frostbite injury by degree. *First-degree injury* consists of hyperemia and edema. *Second-degree injury* is characterized by hyperemia, edema, and clear blister formation. *Third-degree injury* displays hyperemia, edema, and hemorrhagic blister formation, whereas *fourth-degree injury* presents with complete tissue necrosis and gangrene.[15]

Risk factors for frostbite are similar to those for hypothermia; however, the effect of wind chill can drastically increase the severity of injury (Table 164–2).

Pathophysiology

As tissue temperature decreases in the face of cold exposure, the body responds with a cyclic pattern of peripheral vasoconstriction followed by vasodilatation. This 7- to 10-minute sequence, known as the *hunting reflex,* helps to minimize heat loss while adequate shell perfusion is maintained. As core temperature decreases further, this reflex is bypassed because the body preferentially maintains core temperature. As such, peripheral vessels remain constricted, shell/extremity temperature begins to decrease, and at −2°C a plateau is reached. Ice crystals begin to form in the interstitial space. This creates an osmotic gradient and a fluid shift from the cell into the interstitium that leads to cellular dehydration. Chondrocytes show direct freeze injury. On a microscopic level, vascular integrity is lost as microvascular endothelial cells separate from the internal elastic lamina. Intercellular junctions increase in size owing to cellular constriction associated with freezing and dehydration. Arterioles are the first to show damage, but venule damage soon follows. These changes increase vascular permeability and lead to subendothelial collagen exposure.[15] Once ice crystal formation has reached its peak (a process limited by fluid availability), tissue temperature drops and begins to equilibrate with ambient temperature.

Rapid freezing, such as that associated with contact with an extremely cold metal or liquid, causes a different pathophysiologic response. This response is characterized by ice crystal formation within the intracellular space. This, in turn, leads to direct cellular injury and tissue death.

Thawing/Rewarming

Tissue damage and loss cannot be explained solely based on the changes caused during the initial freeze. Only chondrocytes show direct freeze injury. Some other factors must be involved; indeed, in the rewarming phase, a series of mediators serve to amplify the effects of earlier cellular changes.

As tissue is rewarmed, reperfusion commences. Ice crystals begin to dissolve, and cellular swelling occurs as a result of intracellular fluid shifts. Endothelial damage spreads into the entire microvascular tree. Capillary leaks lead to interstitial edema and red blood cell extravasation. Red blood cell sludging, vasoconstriction, and platelet aggregation further compromise blood flow. Platelet activation and degranulation occur in response to endothelial damage. Histamine, serotonin, bradykinin, and white blood cell chemoattractants are released. Arachidonic acid pathways are activated, and vasoconstrictive substrates such as thromboxane A_2 and prostaglandin $F_{2\alpha}$ are formed. This combination of events increases cellular and tissue death by increasing tissue hypoxia. The effects of oxygen free radicals on this series of events are as yet undetermined; however, the release of oxidants has been documented.

Therapy

Before Hospital Admission

The extent of preadmission care is dictated by the availability of secondary aid. Generally, rewarming is contraindicated in a setting in which a potential for refreezing exists because refreezing dramatically increases tissue damage. Patients may utilize the affected body part; however, care should be taken to minimize trauma to the desensitized area.

Hospital Care

After overall patient status has been assessed and total body rewarming has commenced, the frostbitten area should be rapidly rewarmed by placing the affected part in a warm water bath (42°C) for approximately 30 minutes. Care should be taken to document appropriate water temperature. Never rewarm with a direct heat source because thermal injury may occur.

Rewarming can be extremely painful, and narcotics may be needed to relieve a patient's pain. Tetanus prophylaxis should be administered according to protocol. After rewarming, wounds should be assessed for possible débridement. Clear blisters may be removed. Hemorrhagic blisters represent deeper tissue involvement and should be left intact. The affected area should be elevated, if possible, in order to decrease tissue edema. Use of systemic antibiotics is controversial but in general should be limited to patients with documented or suspected infections.

Follow-up care consists of active physiotherapy and twice-daily hydrotherapy with judicious wound débridement. Surgical management should be of an expectant nature. Escharotomy is warranted if vascular compromise occurs. Early débridement or amputation may be necessary if the affected tissue is causing uncontrollable sepsis or disseminated intravascular coagulation. Otherwise, surgical intervention consists of débridement and reconstruction approximately 30 to 60 days after injury. This allows for adequate tissue demarcation and minimizes tissue loss.

Concomitant fractures or dislocations can be addressed at the time of arrival. Dislocations should be reduced, and closed fractures set with posterior splints. Open fractures warrant intraoperative management.

Adjuvant Therapy

Many forms of adjuvant therapy have been explored. Aloe vera, a thromboxane synthetase inhibitor, and ibuprofen, a cyclooxygenase inhibitor, appear to be effective in reducing the inflammatory response by blocking the formation of thromboxane A_2 and prostaglandin $F_{2\alpha}$. Arterial dilators such as reserpine, tolazoline, and nifedipine have been used but have not been proved to be effective. Antiplatelet and thrombolytic agents such as dextran, heparin, urokinase, and streptokinase have also shown little clinical efficacy. Studies on animal models using the calmodulin antagonists trifluoroperazine hydrochloride and thioridazine have shown good results. Also, free radical scavengers such as dimethyl sulfoxide and superoxide dismutase may have potential. Further trials for both products are needed.

Finally, attempts at chemical and surgical sympathectomy and, more recently, electrostimulation of the spinal cord have yielded mixed results. Although sympathectomy may offer benefits in decreasing sequelae of frostbite, its usefulness with regard to tissue salvage has yet to be demonstrated.

Complications and Side Effects

Sequelae of frostbite vary in degree of severity; a physician must watch for hypersensitivity to cold, hyperhidrosis, Raynaud's disease, peripheral neuropathy, atrophy of nails, hair, or muscle, and possible bone deformity.

IMMERSION FOOT AND TRENCH FOOT

Immersion foot and trench foot represent a multifactorial process in which conductive heat loss due to moisture combines with poor vascular flow secondary to immobility and constriction to produce a cold injury in an extremity exposed to temperatures of 50°F (10°C) or less. Symptoms include numbness, tingling, pain, and itching. Initially, the skin is swollen and red. This gradually gives way to a gray-blue discoloration. After a few days, a hyperemic state sets in. Two to 6 weeks later, these symptoms gradually subside, and the patient is left with a cold-sensitive extremity. Superficial gangrene may be noted.

Management is similar to that for a second-degree burn. Limb elevation and careful wound management are essential. Physical therapy is used to maintain range of motion.

OPHTHALMIC COLD INJURIES

Corneal injury due to freezing associated with high wind chill situations and to exposure to reflected ultraviolet radiation at high altitude can cause keratitis combined with opacification and corneal pitting. Prevention with appropriate eyewear is the treatment of choice. However, in the presence of such injury, aggressive ophthalmologic intervention with cycloplegia, mydriasis, and antibiotics is essential for a good result.[3]

References

1. Britt D, Dascombe W, Rodriguez A: New horizons in management of hypothermia and frostbite injury. Surg Clin of North Am 1991; 71:345–370.
2. DelRossi A, Cernaianu A, Vertrees R, et al: Heparinless extracorporeal bypass for treatment of hypothermia. J Trauma 1991; 30:79–82.
3. Edlich R, Chang D, Birk K, et al: Cold injuries. Compr Ther 1989; 15:13–21.
4. Gentilello L, Cortes V, Moujaes S, et al: Continuous arteriovenous rewarming: Experimental results and thermodynamic model simulation of treatment for hypothermia. J Trauma 1990; 30:1436–1449.
5. Wongsurawat N, David B, Morley J: Thermoregulatory failure in the elderly. J Am Geriatr Soc 1990; 38:900–906.
6. Patt A, McCroskey B, Moore E: Hypothermia-induced coagulopathies in trauma. Vasc Trauma 1988; 68:775–785.
7. Swain J: Hypothermia and blood pH. Arch Intern Med 1988; 148:1643–1645.
8. Schaller M, Fischer A, Perret C: Hyperkalemia. JAMA 1990; 264:1842–1845.
9. Sivaloganathan S: Paradoxical undressing and hypothermia. Med Sci Law 1986; 26:225–228.
10. Hall K, Syverud S: Closed thoracic cavity lavage in the treatment of severe hypothermia in human beings. Ann Emerg Med 1990; 19:204–206.
11. Wanderer A: Cold urticaria syndromes: Historical background, diagnostic classification, clinical and laboratory characteristics, pathogenesis, and management. J Allergy Clin Immunol 1990; 85:965–977.
12. Arregui R, Morandeira JR, Martinez G, et al: Epidural neurostimulation in the treatment of frostbite. PACE Pacing Clin Electrophysiol 1989; 12:713–717.
13. Beitner, R, Chen-Zion M, Sofer-Bassukevitz Y, et al: Treatment of frostbite with the calmoduling antagonists thioridazine and trifluoperazine. Gen Pharmacol 1989; 20:641–646.
14. Vogel J, Dellon L: Frostbite injuries of the hand. Clin Plast Surg 1989; 16:565–576.
15. Marzella L, Jesudass R, Manson P, et al: Morphologic characterization of acute injury to vascular endothelium of skin after frostbite. Plast Reconstr Surg 1989; 83:67–75.

Suggested Readings

Manning B, Stollerman G: Hypothermia in the elderly. Hosp Pract 1993; 26:53–70.

Mileski W, Raymond J, Winn R, et al: Inhibition of leukocyte adherence and aggregation for treatment of severe cold injury in rabbits. Am Physiol Soc 1993; 74:1432–1435.

Weinberg A: Hypothermia. Ann Emerg Med 1993; 22:370–377.

CHAPTER 165

The Hyperthermic Syndromes

Stephen M. Ayres, MD • Richard L. Keenan, MD

Fever in the critically ill patient is almost always considered to be a manifestation of infection and a possible harbinger of either sepsis or septic shock. Although most fever encountered in the intensive care unit is a response to microbial invasion, some fevers are due to either exposure to high temperatures or abnormalities in the thermoregulatory apparatus. Since the mid-1940s, at least six major summer heat waves in the United States have produced large numbers of heat-related deaths and seriously taxed the resources of physicians who were unprepared for the human ravages of high ambient temperatures. High body temperatures may be observed in certain clinical entities such as meningitis, falciparum malaria, cerebrovascular accidents near the hypothalamus, and multiple organ system failure. A body temperature of greater than 106°F (41.1°C) during a period of high ambient temperatures combined with an early elevation of liver enzyme levels suggests the possibility of heat stroke. Since cooling is also indicated in other patients with high temperatures, the cooling should be instituted immediately while the diagnosis is being clarified.

Human body temperature is maintained within close limits by a balance between heat production and heat dissipation. Heat is normally generated by muscular activity and metabolic reactions. It is dissipated by a mixture of radiation, convection, conduction, and evaporation.[1] Significant heat injury can occur in athletes, military personnel working in hot environments, and those whose occupations require vigorous activity. Experienced physicians in St. Louis have long observed that roofers were in particular exposed to heat stress and that heat injury among them could be considered an early warning sign that others in the population might soon be at risk. Heat injury can also occur in resting and unacclimated individuals who are elderly or who have abnormalities in their temperature-regulating system because of intercurrent disease. Two specific heat injury syndromes are malignant hyperthermia during general anesthesia and the neuroleptic malignant syndrome. The former is due to a genetic defect, and the latter to an unusual reaction to psychotropic drugs such as the phenothiazines.

TEMPERATURE REGULATION

Radiation and convection account for about 75% of heat losses at room temperature if an individual is undressed. The wearing of clothing significantly decreases such losses. Heat loss by these mechanisms decreases as ambient temperature reaches body temperature; ambient temperatures above body temperature actually increase the heat of the body. The unique evaporative loss by sweating accounts for only 25% of heat loss at room temperature but becomes the dominant mechanism at high ambient temperatures. High humidity reduces evaporative losses, explaining why the heat syndromes are particularly common in hot, humid environments.[1]

When ambient temperatures rise, activation of hypothalamic centers leads to cutaneous vasodilation with shunting of blood away from the liver and splanchnic area in an apparent effort to contain visceral heat production to a limited region. Vasodilation enhances sweat gland activity and permits the loss of up to 1.5 L of sweat per hour in the unacclimated person. Such vasodilation increases cardiac output and stresses the heart; cardiovascular disease may limit the necessary increase in cardiac output and reduces the ability of an individual to tolerate acute heat stress. Acclimation occurs after about 1 week of prolonged heat exposure and is associated with a substantial increase in sweat volume and with a reduction in sweat sodium content of 6% to 7%. Plasma volume also increases, underscoring the need for persons to increase fluid intake when in hot environments. Heart disease limits the body's adaptive response to prolonged heat exposure and increased humidity and explains the vulnerability of the sick and the elderly to heat injury.

The importance of intact hypothalamic integrating centers is demonstrated by the neuroleptic malignant syndrome, which is associated with the use of phenothiazines and certain other dopamine inhibitors by certain sensitive individuals. Caroff and coworkers[2] have suggested that neuroleptic malignant syndrome "may be part of a group of syndromes which, by a combination of central and peripheral mechanisms culminate in a final common pathway of skeletal muscle hypermetabolism and hyperthermia." The syndrome can usually be differentiated from the environmental heat syndromes by the associated rigidity characteristic of phenothiazine use.

THE CONSEQUENCES OF EXPOSURE IN HOT ENVIRONMENTS

The three classic heat-related syndromes are heat cramps, heat exhaustion, and heat stroke. Heat exhaustion is found in young people during heavy exercise and appears to be related to the excessive loss of sodium chloride in the sweat. Salt losses can be considerable because the sweat content of salt in unacclimated individuals is 30 to 50 mEq/L compared with 5 mEq/L in acclimated people.

The syndromes of heat exhaustion and heat stroke are closely related; heat stroke is diagnosed when rectal temperature exceeds 106°F (41.1°C) and when evidence of vascular insufficiency (i.e., the "stroke" symptoms) is present. The cutoff point of 106°F is obviously arbitrary, but it is an important sign that immediate attempts at cooling are necessary because the uncoupling of oxidative phosphorylation and the failure of enzyme systems occur when the core body temperature reaches 107°C. At that temperature, cell membranes become more permeable, sodium leaks into the cells, and adenosine triphosphate stores are depleted.[3]

Heat exhaustion follows vigorous exercise in young individuals and the failure of an appropriate cardiovascular response in the elderly. Diuretics (fluid loss), anticholinergics (inhibition of sweating), phenothiazines, cyclic antidepressants, monoamine oxidase inhibitors, lithium, antihistamines, sympathomimetics, hallucinogens, ethanol, salicylates, and glutethimide have all been recognized as agents that predispose to heat injury. Fluid depletion and hemoconcentration is observed in both the young and the old, although elderly patients with cardiovascular disease may have volume status that is close to normal. Individuals present with a temperature of 100 to 103°F, profuse sweating, postural hypotension, fatigue, and thirst. A relatively normal mental status distinguishes them from individuals with heat stroke. Fluid replacement with normal saline and rest in a cool place is usually sufficient to reverse the symptoms. Rest and a cool environment may be sufficient in the elderly; oral fluids should be tried before resorting to the careful use of intravenous fluids.[4]

Acute neurologic abnormalities are the hallmark of heat stroke, and any individual with mental status or neurologic changes and a high body temperature should be considered to have the syndrome.[4] Other manifestations include lethargy, fatigue, dizziness, nausea, and vomiting. Body temperatures are greater than 103°F (39.4°C) and may be greater than 107°F (41.6°C). Tissue damage begins with temperatures above that level. A hot but dry skin is caused by sweat gland damage and is considered a classic sign, but many patients present with hot and moist skin. In addition to mental status and neurologic changes, patients have evidence of multiple organ system dysfunction.

Liver damage is extremely common, and early elevation of the levels of liver enzymes such as serum glutamic-oxaloacetic transaminase and serum glutamate pyruvate transaminase is a useful sign of heat stroke.[5] Pulmonary edema, disseminated intravascular coagulation, cardiovascular abnormalities, and acute renal failure are common after initial cooling and stabilization. Fluid management becomes critical because cooling results in a redistribution of blood volume from the periphery to the central organs.

Pulmonary edema due to cardiovascular dysfunction, the adult acute respiratory distress syndrome, and a variety of pneumonias can all occur. The combination of disseminated intravascular coagulation and respiratory failure suggests the diagnosis of adult acute respiratory distress syndrome and the possible development of multiple organ system failure.[6] Tek and Olshaker[4] emphasized the importance of disseminated intravascular coagulation with respect to both diagnosis and outcome. The usual indicators for disseminated intravascular coagulation should be monitored closely. The authors suggest that heparin therapy, although controversial, may be useful.

Acute renal failure has been found in up to 35% of patients with heat stroke and may be caused by a "combination of direct thermal injury, hypotension, shock from cardiovascular collapse, and rhabdomyolysis."[7] Rhabdomyolysis should be treated with alkalinization and mannitol, furosemide, and fluid therapy.[7]

Major electrolyte abnormalities are observed on hospital admission, and electrolyte shifts during treatment are common. Hypophosphatemia, hypocalcemia, hypoglycemia, and infections are common. Calcium replacement is probably not indicated unless levels are extremely low because infused calcium may be distributed to injured muscle. Infections such as pneumonia may complicate the syndrome and could lead to a confusion in diagnosis.

The high mortality observed with delayed treatment can be reduced if a patient is rapidly cooled.[8] Immersion in a tub filled with ice water is the most efficient way to produce rapid cooling, although cold packs or frequent sponging may also be used. Emergency rooms in areas where high ambient temperatures are common should have both extra-long rectal thermometers for the measurement of high temperatures and stainless steel tubs for quick cooling. Patients must be rubbed to maintain vasodilation.

The peripheral vasoconstriction associated with immersion in ice water may have an adverse effects in individuals with cardiovascular dysfunction and has led some clinicians to consider alternative cooling methods.[9] Evaporation of 1 g of water consumes seven times as much heat as does the melting of 1 g of ice and does not produce peripheral vasoconstriction. The Makkah Body Cooling Unit[10] is a refinement of the evaporative cooling method that was developed to treat heat syndromes in the large number of pilgrims who travel to Mecca. Rapid cooling rates were observed, and the method is probably the best available at the present time; however, it may be impractical for the intermittently encountered heat stress disasters treated in hospitals throughout the United States and in other countries.

THE STEAMY ST. LOUIS SUMMER OF 1980

Experience with prolonged elevation of ambient temperatures has shown how deadly this situation can be. On July 1, 1980, the day that the Department of Medicine at St. Louis University took over the medical service at the St. Louis City Hospital, an incredible heat wave struck both St. Louis and Kansas City, Missouri. The ambient temperature in St. Louis was above 100°F (38.9°C) for 16 days and frequently was as high as 102 to 104°F. The humidity was high. In Kansas City, the ambient temperature was above 108°F (42.2°C) on 10 days.

Complicating the medical situation was the fact that the St. Louis City Hospital was not air conditioned. The city had lived through disastrous heat spells in the past, but for some reason the city government officials had refused to install what had become standard hospital equipment in other hospitals throughout the country. The inability of the aged sick, particularly those given diuretics, antihypertensive agents, and tranquilizers, to withstand heat stress was soon to set the stage for a disaster of tragic proportion. Bodies piled up in the morgue, but patients who were fortunate enough to reach the emergency room alive survived because of vigorous cooling with crushed ice and careful attention to fluid losses. In all, 81 patients seen at St. Louis City Hospital had body temperatures greater than 105°F and were diagnosed as having heat stroke. The low death rate of 7% was probably an American record.

The newly appointed chief of the medical service at St. Louis City Hospital, Dr. Joseph Marr, and his associate, Dr. Peter Geiss, described their method of treatment.[11] Patients with high temperatures were covered with ice, and their rectal temperatures were monitored. Intravenous fluids were administered as needed, and patients were removed from the ice baths when their rectal temperature had decreased to 100 to 101°F. Neither ice water enemas nor renal dialysis were necessary, and shivering was prevented by removing the ice before the patients reached a normal temperature. Shivering reduces heat loss and can be eliminated by the administration of chlorpromazine; however, Marr observed that removal of a patient from the cooling tub at the prescribed temperature also prevented shivering. Most patients were not volume-depleted, and excessive fluid replacement was not needed. Specific problems such as respiratory failure were treated in the usual manner.

The medical staff at St. Louis City Hospital faced an unusual situation because the hospital was not air conditioned. Their experience illustrates the importance of the ambient temperature. It was soon noted that a large majority of the patients who had been successfully cooled in the emergency room developed heat-related complaints and high body temperatures after they were admitted to the non–air-conditioned wards. The staff responded by maintaining fluid balance with continuous intravenous infusions and by packing patients in ice water–soaked sheets as had been done in the emergency room.

The heat continued. It was intolerable in the morning, became murderous by afternoon, and persisted in the seemingly airless wards throughout the night. Patients forgot elemental modesty and sat or lay prostrate in their beds, frequently wearing nothing at all. While the city government seemed unable to cope with the situation, the military moved in with several massive self-contained military cooling units. The cooling machines, which were normally used to cool military aircraft in desert conditions, were set up outside St. Louis City Hospital. Their large hoses were run from street level to at least three separate patient areas of the hospital. For once, the large multipatient ward construction was advantageous. Cooling of a series of private rooms could not have been accomplished as easily.

Nurses and physicians reported an almost miraculous improvement in patients' spirits and statuses. Fevers dropped, fluid requirements were lessened, and serious conditions improved. The cooling units were designed for combat situations and produced considerable noise, but cold noise was preferred to hot sleep, and the patients gradually improved.

Epidemiologic study later described the magnitude of the disaster.[12] There were 308 excess deaths in St. Louis and 236 in Kansas City during July 1980. Death rates were 56.8% and 65.2% in July 1980 compared with death rates in July 1978 in St. Louis and Kansas City, respectively. Heat stroke rates were 10- to 12-fold greater in individuals over 65 years of age compared with younger people; the death rate was sixfold greater in people of low socioeconomic status who had little access to air-conditioned environments compared with more affluent individuals.

Hyperthermia from elevated ambient temperature can complicate the lives of ill patients living in many cities of the United States each summer. Only an understanding of the hazards and manifestations of environmental hyperthermia can help physicians distinguish between the fever of infection and heat exhaustion or heat stroke.

MALIGNANT HYPERTHERMIA

During the first half of the 20th century, patients occasionally died while undergoing surgery as a result of extreme fevers (body temperatures exceeding 42°C). In an era without air conditioning in hospitals, the source of fever was assumed to be environmental. However, a case report in

1960 suggested that at least some fevers were due to a previously unrecognized syndrome involving muscle hypermetabolism triggered by anesthetic agents. The disorder appeared to be familial.[13] Numerous similar case reports followed. Shortly thereafter, a similar, genetically determined syndrome in pigs well known to meat packers as stress hyperthermia was described.[14] Malignant hyperthermia (MH) is now recognized as a disease of muscle metabolism, in which intracellular calcium levels are increased as a result of exposure to certain triggering agents.[15] This, in turn, results in increased adenosine triphosphatase activity with depletion of adenosine triphosphate, actin-myosin coupling, which causes intense muscle contraction, breakdown of glucose with a sharp increase in oxygen consumption, production of carbon dioxide, and production of heat. Once begun, progression is rapid. If the patient is left untreated, severe acidosis and hyperthermia can occur in minutes. Ventricular fibrillation is typically the terminal event.

The gene responsible for MH is located on chromosome 19 in humans.[16] It is believed to occur in about 1 in 50,000 persons. Known triggering agents include the depolarizing muscle relaxant succinylcholine and all of the volatile inhalation anesthetics, including ether, halothane, enflurane, and isoflurane. In general, the intravenous anesthetic agents, including the nondepolarizing relaxants such as pancuronium and vecuronium, are not triggers. In susceptible pigs, stress alone is a sufficient trigger. However, stress and other environmental agents, including chemicals, have not been documented as triggers of MH in humans. Thus, the disease seems to be limited to patients undergoing general anesthesia. Prevention is an important aspect of management. Susceptible patients may be identified through the recording of a careful preanesthetic history that includes questioning about any family history of adverse anesthetic events. Known triggering agents should be avoided in susceptible patients once they are identified. Patients with Duchenne type muscular dystrophy and possibly other rare myopathies also are susceptible.[17] During anesthesia, unexplained tachycardia and elevated end-expiratory carbon dioxide levels should be considered warning signs, and continuous temperature monitoring should be performed.

Diagnosis of MH is currently best made by the observation of an actual episode. Muscle rigidity (especially that of the masseter), high fever following the administration of triggering agents, hypercarbia despite adequate ventilation, myoglobinemia, myoglobinuria, and marked elevation of creatine kinase values are all typical. Unfortunately, no convenient laboratory test specific for MH is yet available. A muscle contracture test that requires sampling of fresh muscle is available in a few centers and is reasonably specific. A definitive deoxyribonucleic acid–based test is currently in development.[18]

Treatment of an MH episode includes the use of dantrolene, a hydantoin derivative that inhibits the release of calcium from sarcoplasmic reticulum. Intravenous administration of dantrolene in sufficient dosage (2.5–10 mg/kg) immediately aborts the syndrome. Dantrolene may also be given prophylactically (2.5 mg/kg) preoperatively; the avoidance of triggering agents is also recommended. Nonspecific therapy may include surface cooling as well as lavage of open body cavities with cold saline.

References

1. O'Donnell TF Jr, Clowes GH: The circulatory abnormalities of heat stroke. N Engl J Med 1972; 287:734–737.
2. Caroff SN, Mann SC, Lazarus A, et al: Neuroleptic malignant syndrome: Diagnostic issues. Psych Ann 1991; 21:130–147.
3. Yarbrough BE, Hubbard RW: Heat related illness. *In:* Management of Wilderness and Environmental Emergencies. Auerbach PS, Geehr EC (Eds). St. Louis, CV Mosby, 1989, pp 119–143.
4. Tek D, Olshaker JS: Heat illness. Emerg Med Clin North Am 1991; 10:299–308.
5. Rubel CR: Hepatic injury associated with heatstroke. Ann Clin Lab Sci 1984; 14:130–136.
6. El Kassimi FA, Al-Mashadani SA, Akhtar J: Adult respiratory distress syndrome and disseminated intravascular coagulation complicating heat stroke. Chest 1986; 90:571–574.
7. Curley G, Irwin RS: Disorders of temperature control: Part I. Hyperthermia. Intensive Care Med 1986; 1:5–14.
8. O'Donnell TF: Acute heatstroke: Epidemiologic, biochemical, renal and coagulation studies. JAMA 1975; 234:824–828.
9. Magazanik A, Epstein Y, Udassin R, et al: Tap water: An efficient method for cooling heatstroke victims—a model in dogs. Aviat Space Environ Med 1980; 51:864–866.
10. Weiner, J, Khogali M: A physiologic body cooling unit for treatment of heat stroke. Lancet 1980; ii:507–509.
11. Geiss P, Marr JJ: Management of heat injury syndromes. *In:* Critical Care State of the Art. Anaheim, CA, Society of Critical Care Medicine, 1982.
12. Jones TS, Liang AP, Kilbourne EM, et al: Morbidity and mortality associated with the July 1980 heat wave in St Louis and Kansas City, Mo. JAMA 1982; 247:3328–3331.
13. Denborough MA, Lovell RH: Anaesthesia deaths in a family. Lancet 1960; ii:45.
14. Berman MC, Harrison HH, Bull AB, et al: Changes underlying halothane-induced malignant hyperpyrexia in Landrace pigs. Nature 1970; 224:653–655.
15. MacLennan DH, Phillips MS: Malignant hyperthermia. Science 1992; 256:789–794.
16. Ball SP, Johnson KJ: The genetics of malignant hyperthermia. J Med Genet 1993; 30:89–93.
17. Wedel DJ: Malignant hyperthermia and neuromuscular disease. Neuromuscul Disord 1992; 2:157–164.
18. Levitt RC: Prospects for the diagnosis of malignant hyperthermia susceptibility using molecular genetic approaches. Anesthesiology 1992; 76:1039–1048.

SECTION XIII
CENTRAL NERVOUS SYSTEM

Ake Grenvik • William C. Shoemaker

CHAPTER 166
Critical Care Neurology

Lawrence R. Wechsler, MD • Allan H. Ropper, MD

Since the early 1980s, neurologic critical care has undergone enormous development. Dedicated neurologic neurosurgical intensive care units (ICUs) have become commonplace. Our understanding of the pathophysiology of brain injury and advances in monitoring techniques have resulted in improved treatment and, it is hoped, improved survival. Neurologic intensive care medicine has become a discipline of its own.

A common problem encountered in neurologic-neurosurgical ICUs is raised intracranial pressure (ICP). Monitoring of ICP and treatment of intracranial hypertension requires knowledge of intracranial dynamics and of the effects of variations in physiologic parameters. Coma, respiratory failure, hemorrhagic or ischemic stroke, and general medical problems that complicate neurologic illnesses also frequently lead to admission to a neurologic-neurosurgical ICU. Metabolic encephalopathies are probably more commonly encountered in medical or surgical ICUs but fall under the purview of neurologic critical care. In most cases, optimal care requires a team approach that includes intensivists, medical and surgical subspecialists, specially trained nurses, and ancillary personnel.

Whether dedicated neurologic ICUs improve outcome has not been established, but the benefit of specially trained staff attending to life-threatening neurologic problems in a controlled setting should be apparent. Alterations in brain function are often the most difficult problems for family members to understand, and the neurologic ICU staff can provide valuable support in such situations. The standards of practice developed in neurologic ICUs are equally applicable to neurologically ill patients in general medical or surgical units when a dedicated neurologic ICU is not available.

PHYSIOLOGY OF RAISED INTRACRANIAL PRESSURE

The intracranial compartment consists of brain (80%), cerebrospinal fluid (10%), and blood (10%). Addition of a space-occupying lesion initially results in a compensatory reduction in one of these components. When compensatory mechanisms are exhausted, ICP begins to rise. Shift of cerebrospinal fluid from the intracranial compartment through the foramen magnum to the spinal subarachnoid space counteracts the early effects of an intracranial mass. Tissue shifts, such as that caused by uncal herniation, block this pathway, leading to rapid elevations of ICP. Changes in cerebral blood volume also occur with raised ICP. Most of the blood volume resides in the venous circulation,[1] with venous blood volume falling in response to raised ICP. The brain itself has very little capacity to compensate for these changes. Intracellular dehydration can occur, but this event adds little available intracranial volume. *Compliance* represents the change in ICP for any given increment in intracranial volume (Fig. 166–1). When brain compliance is low, small changes in intracranial volume result in large changes in ICP because of the lack of ability of the brain to compensate.

As ICP rises, cerebral perfusion pressure (CPP) falls, eventually resulting in cerebral ischemia. CPP is defined as mean arterial pressure minus ICP. CPP normally ranges from 70 to 100 mm Hg. When CPP falls below 30 to 40 mm Hg, ischemia occurs, ultimately leading to neuronal death. ICP alone has no direct deleterious effects on brain function. Injury results from cerebral ischemia and from tissue shifts that result from pressure vectors. ICP is less than 10 mm Hg in normal individuals, and levels of 50 to 60 mm Hg are usually associated with cerebral ischemia. Transient elevations in ICP occur periodically (plateau waves) and can lead to ischemic damage and sudden herniation, even when baseline ICP is relatively normal. When brain compliance is low, marked increases in ICP can occur during these episodes. Lundberg type A plateau waves are usually the most damaging because of the high levels of ICP attained and the prolonged duration. They occur more frequently at night or in the early morning, when monitoring may not be as frequent.[2] The cause of plateau waves is unclear, but most evidence points to a vascular mechanism.[3]

Tissue shifts occur in patients with intracranial mass lesions as a result of pressure gradients and movement of brain tissue across dural boundaries. Brain herniation may occur across the midline under the falx (subfalcian herniation), through the tentorial opening (uncal herniation), and into the foramen magnum (tonsillar herniation). Brain stem signs are observed in association with herniation of brain tissue that occurs as a result of compression of neural structures and as a result of vascular compression with secon-

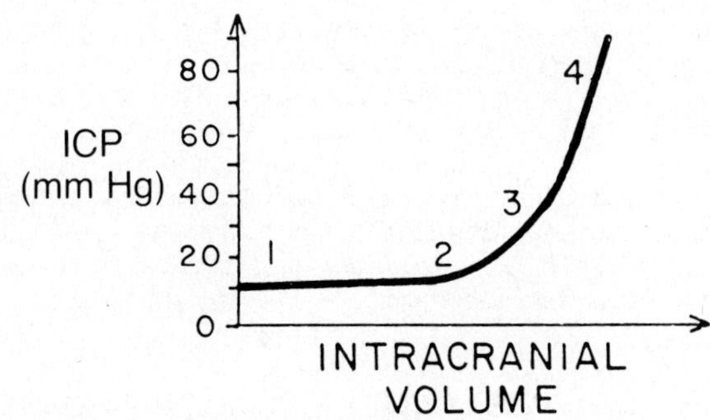

Figure 166–1. Relationship between intracranial volume and ICP. The change in ICP for any given increase in intracranial volume depends on the existing compensatory mechanisms. (From Shapiro HM: Intracranial hypertension: Therapeutic and anesthetic considerations. Anesthesiology 1975; 43:447.)

dary ischemia. These signs are discussed in detail elsewhere.[4] Although downward shifts of tissue are associated with neurologic signs, the orderly rostral-to-caudal progression of brain stem abnormalities described by Plum and Posner[4] is rarely seen in practice. Some evidence suggests that horizontal shifts are more important predictors of level of consciousness than is downward herniation.[5] In patients with acute brain lesions, displacement of the pineal body seen on computed tomography correlates with a diminished level of consciousness.[5] If obtundation is out of proportion to the pineal shift, other causes for stupor or coma should be sought.

Considerable reserve exists in blood flow to the brain. Changes in brain function do not typically occur until cerebral blood flow (CBF) falls from normal levels of approximately 50 to 18 $mL \cdot 100\ g^{-1} \cdot min^{-1}$.[6] As CBF falls below this threshold, electrical activity within neurons ceases, and available energy is used to maintain membrane pump functions. When CBF drops further, basic cellular integrity can no longer be supported, membrane pump function fails, and ionic gradients begin to break down, causing intracellular edema and cell death.[7] In animal models of acute focal cerebral ischemia, infarction depends not only on the absolute level of CBF but also on the duration of ischemia.[8]

Under normal conditions, cerebral metabolism is closely coupled to CBF.[9] Factors that stimulate cerebral activity, such as pain, excessive external stimulation, and seizures, increase metabolic demands and therefore increase CBF. Cerebral blood volume also increases, resulting in raised ICP when compliance is low.

Changes in $Paco_2$ have a dramatic effect on CBF. Decreases in $Paco_2$ quickly decrease CBF, although this effect is transitory. Carbon dioxide crosses the blood-brain barrier rapidly, but the hydrogen ion cannot pass this barrier, resulting in an increase in CSF pH that normalizes over several hours. CBF initially falls and then returns to normal over the same time course.[10] Increases in $Paco_2$ cause an increase in CBF that also returns to normal over several hours. Although extreme hyperventilation causes marked reductions in CBF, ischemia does not usually occur in the normal brain.[11, 12] Whether the same holds true for injured brain, however, is unknown.

The partial pressure of oxygen affects CBF only in its extremes. A Pao_2 of less than 50 mm Hg may stimulate CBF by increasing production of lactate. A very high Pao_2 decreases CBF, although the magnitude of this reduction is small. CBF decreases by 6% for every degree of reduction in temperature,[13] whereas fever increases CBF in a linear fashion up to 42°C.[14] At higher temperatures, direct toxic injury to brain occurs. The effects of hypotension and hypertension on CBF are mitigated by autoregulation within a range of blood pressures. In normotensive individuals, changes in mean arterial pressure between 60 and 130 mm Hg are accompanied by compensatory changes in vascular tone, thereby maintaining cerebral blood flow. This range may be shifted to a higher level in patients with hypertension. Beyond these limits, CBF follows blood pressure passively, increasing or decreasing significantly in response to blood pressure changes. Abnormal brain regions may lose autoregulation and CBF varies directly in proportion to mean arterial pressure changes under these conditions.

GENERAL CARE OF THE NEUROLOGIC PATIENT

Meticulous attention to the details of daily care helps avoid the complications of prolonged ICU stay. Stuporous or comatose patients require special attention to the care of their skin, eyes, and bladder. Methylcellulose artificial tears prevent corneal desiccation and ulceration, and intermittent bladder catheterization performed under sterile conditions minimizes the risk of urinary tract infection. Frequent turning of the patient is necessary to prevent skin breakdown. Patients with neuropathies such as the Guillain-Barré syndrome must be positioned in such a way to avert pressure on nerves that can lead to compression neuropathies.

Intubation may be necessary in patients with impaired consciousness to protect the airway from aspiration and to provide adequate gas exchange with assisted ventilation. Neurologic diseases involving the brain stem impair pharyngeal function and predispose to aspiration. Airway protection may also be necessary in the first few days after a large hemispheric stroke. Early intubation and mechanical ventilation should be considered in patients in whom long apneic periods accompany irregular respirations, and in those with frequent vomiting. The timing of tracheostomy for clearance of secretions and airway protection varies, depending on the prognosis for neurologic recovery. Many patients who have had a stroke recover function within 7 to 10 days, thus avoiding the need for tracheostomy.

Fever in patients who have had a brain insult nearly always results from infection. Pneumonia and urinary tract infections are the commonest causes of fever in patients with depressed consciousness.[15, 16] The supine position, a decreased cough, a diminished gag reflex, and shallow breathing pattern may predispose to the development of atelectasis. Routine chest physiotherapy should help prevent atelectasis and subsequent fever.

Dehydration often accompanies osmotic therapy used for the reduction of ICP. Electrolytes and osmolarity must be regularly monitored to prevent complications related to hyperosmolarity.[17, 18] In addition, large volumes of hypotonic fluids may aggravate cerebral edema. Therefore, normal saline is recommended for intravenous infusions. Deep venous thrombosis and sepsis complicate neurologic illnesses, generally after the first week, contributing to late mortality.

THERAPY FOR RAISED INTRACRANIAL PRESSURE

In patients who have had brain injury, control of ICP is critical to avoid secondary brain damage from tissue shifts and to prevent ischemia. CPP is the major determinant of CBF. Clinical signs cannot be relied on to detect reduced CPP that may result in ischemia. Focal signs, such as pupillary dilation or posturing, may occur in patients with normal ICP; however, raised ICP may be present in the absence of neurologic changes.[19] In addition, middle fossa lesions typically compress the brain stem at lower ICP levels than those affected by supratentorial masses. The typical Cushing's response of hypertension, bradycardia, and respiratory abnormalities usually occurs quite late in patients with raised ICP.[20]

Blood pressure may fluctuate without concomitant changes in ICP, thereby increasing or reducing CPP. When autoregulation is impaired, ICP changes passively with blood pressure, and no change in CPP occurs. Increases in blood pressure may worsen edema without significantly benefiting CPP. Thus, direct measurement of ICP is necessary for the determination of CPP and for the evaluation of the effects of therapeutic maneuvers. In addition, errors in therapy, such as in the administration of medications or intravenous fluids that raise ICP, can be avoided by ICP monitoring.

In patients with head injury, raised ICP is associated with poor outcome, and brain death is a common consequence.[21–23] ICP elevation may simply reflect the extent of underlying brain damage, and some studies have revealed no improvement in outcome after treatment of ICP.[24] However, control of ICP occasionally leads to improvement. Debate continues over the question of whether use of ICP monitoring to guide therapy is more effective than empiric ICP treatment. Theoretically, management based on ICP monitoring should reduce unnecessary treatment that could be harmful and thus avoid transient reductions in CPP. This benefit, however, has yet to be demonstrated in clinical trials.

Patients with intracerebral hemorrhage[25] and ischemic stroke[26] also have poor outcome when ICP is raised. The benefits of ICP monitoring and treatment are unproved, but it at least provides a guide for medical therapy and may help the clinician decide on the timing of surgical intervention.[27–29] However, ICP monitoring should be reserved for stuporous or comatose patients, particularly those with evidence of tissue shifts on computed tomography and a reasonable likelihood of functional recovery.[30] In all cases in which ICP monitoring is employed, physician and nursing personnel should be experienced in the interpretation and management of ICP monitoring devices and should be knowledgeable about therapeutic options.

Hyperventilation Therapy

The mainstays of conventional medical therapy for raised ICP include hyperventilation and osmotic agents. Hyperventilation rapidly reduces ICP by vasoconstriction and reduction of cerebral blood volume. An almost immediate reduction in ICP occurs, followed by further decrements that reach a maximum after approximately 30 minutes. As discussed previously, however, the duration of ICP reduction is typically brief. In some patients, hyperventilation is ineffective, which usually signifies severe brain injury, with little remaining normal brain to respond to the effects of hyperventilation.[31] Initial reduction of $Paco_2$ to 25 to 30 mm Hg is preferable and should produce a decrease in ICP. Further rapid reductions in $Paco_2$ can be obtained with additional hyperventilation when sudden pressure spikes or subsequent rises in ICP occur. Once Pao_2 has been reduced, hyperventilation should be continued, despite loss of effectiveness. Allowing $Paco_2$ to rise when ICP has returned to the previous baseline level may result in a dangerous rise in ICP. However, induced hyperventilation may paradoxically lead to increased ICP if positive intrathoracic pressure is transmitted to the intracranial compartment, such as occurs in a patient with low brain compliance.[32] This effect may exceed the decrease in ICP that results from hypocapnia. Raising the head may be helpful in this situation, although the effect of head position on ICP and CPP in individual cases is variable.[33, 34]

The CSF alkalosis induced by hyperventilation is gradually compensated for and is probably complete within 24 hours. Recent clinical data suggest that the addition of weak bases and buffers such as tromethamine sustains the effects of alkalosis on cerebral vessel caliber and assists in buffering lactate, an effect that is associated with poor outcome after head injury. In one recent study of head-injured patients, short-term outcome was improved by the addition of tromethamine to hyperventilation, although long-term outcome did not differ at 12 months.[35] If sustained hyperventilation is required, adding a buffer lends a theoretic advantage, although this treatment has not become current practice, probably because the benefit is marginal.

Osmotic Therapy

Osmotic agents have multiple effects on the brain and cerebral circulation that might contribute to ICP control. Water is drawn out of the brain across the blood-brain barrier as a result of the osmotic gradient, but other factors, such as viscosity changes or decreased CSF production, may also play at least a minor role in ICP reductions. Volume depletion should be avoided when osmotic agents are used because hypotension and reduced cardiac output compromise CBF. Fluid restriction contributes to volume depletion, but limiting free water is necessary. Mannitol is the most commonly used osmotic agent. Small doses of mannitol reduce ICP as effectively as large doses, although the duration of action is longer with large doses.[36] ICP reduction occurs 10 to 20 minutes after administration and reaches a maximum approximately 60 minutes after infusion.[37] Intracranial compliance improves after mannitol administration,[38] with this change occurring more quickly than the ICP reduction. Rebound increases in ICP have been reported after mannitol withdrawal but were seen rarely in large series of patients treated for raised ICP.[37, 39] Osmolarity should be monitored frequently during mannitol therapy, and the dose should be tailored to cause a specific level of osmolality. An initial increase to 290 to 300 mOsm/kg is usually adequate to reduce ICP.[40] If ICP continues to rise, additional increases in osmolality as high as 320 mOsm/kg may provide additional benefit. Although further reduction of ICP may be achieved with osmolarity beyond this level, complications, such as volume depletion, hypotension, electrolyte disturbances, and hyperglycemia, often outweigh the benefits. Mannitol produces an initial increase in CBF, possibly as a result of viscosity effects, that is usually not clinically significant.[41, 42] Diuretics such as furosemide do not have this initial effect on CBF and therefore may help obtain acute ICP reductions.[43, 44] However, the ability of diuretics to maintain ICP reduction is uncertain. Other osmotic agents, such as glycerol, hypertonic saline, and urea, can be used to increase osmolality but are less effective than mannitol and cause more toxicity. At present, mannitol is the preferred osmotic agent for the treatment of raised ICP.

Corticosteroid Therapy

Corticosteroids reduce cerebral edema surrounding tumors but are less reliably effective for edema in other conditions. High doses of steroids improved survival after head trauma in one study,[45] but these results have not been confirmed by other studies. Any effect on ICP is delayed for at least several hours, although an improvement in compliance may occur more quickly.[46] Corticosteroids have not been beneficial in patients with acute ischemic stroke.[47, 48] In a small, randomized study of patients with intracerebral hemorrhage, no improvement in outcome occurred after 3 weeks in those treated with steroids,[49] and a higher frequency of medical complications occurred in the steroid treatment group. Although the studies on corticosteroid use are small and methodologically flawed, current evidence argues against the routine use of steroids for acute ischemic or hemorrhagic stroke.

Blood Pressure Control

Blood pressure control in patients with intracranial hypertension remains an important but poorly investigated area. In normal brain regions, autoregulation prevents changes in cerebral blood volume and minimizes ICP variations that occur with blood pressure fluctuations. However, in damaged areas of brain, elevations in blood pressure may increase hydrostatic pressure and may contribute to edema formation. Hypotension may reduce ICP but not improve CPP because of the concomitant drop in mean arterial pressure (Fig. 166–2). The work of Rosner and Becker[50] suggests

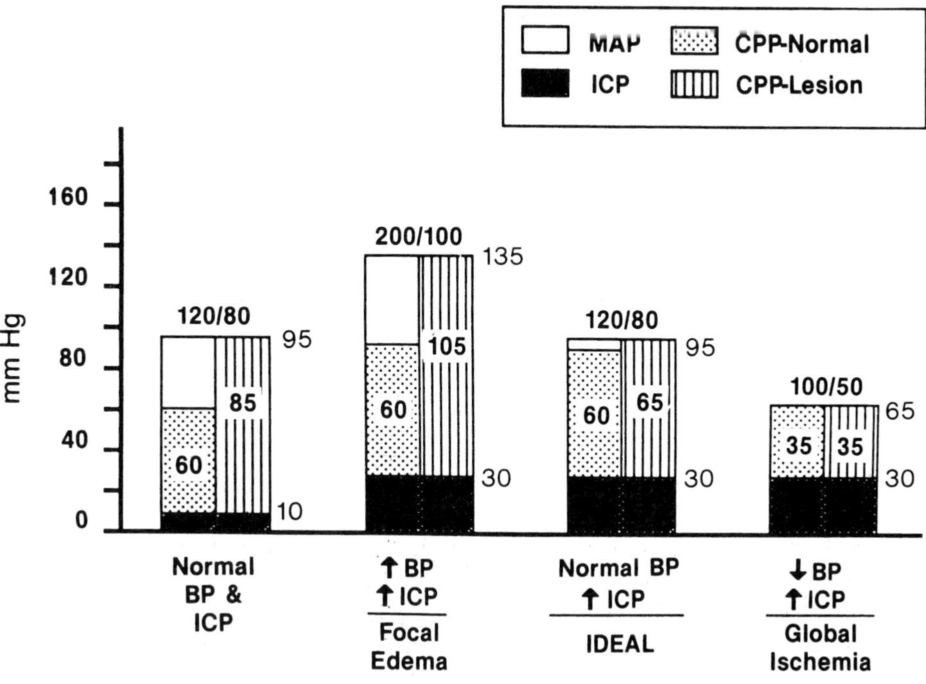

Figure 166–2. Effects of blood pressure (BP) changes on CPP in patients with elevated ICP. The left side of each *vertical bar* represents normal areas of brain, whereas the right side represents damaged areas with loss of autoregulation. The *first bar* indicates normal levels of CPP. The *second bar* illustrates the effects of elevated BP. CPP is preserved by autoregulation in normal areas but rises greatly in damaged areas, thus contributing to edema formation. The *third bar* shows effects of normalization of BP with raised ICP. CPP levels in damaged areas return to normal levels, thus maintaining adequate perfusion but minimizing edema. The *fourth bar* illustrates the effects of hypotension with compromise of CPP in normal and damaged brain. (From Ropper AH, Rockoff MA: Physiology and clinical aspects of raised intracranial pressure. *In:* Neurological and Neurosurgical Intensive Care. Ropper AH [Ed]. New York, Raven Press, 1993, p 37.)

that mild hypotension may be deleterious because it can trigger cerebral vasodilation and plateau waves. Moreover, a hypertensive spike can abort the plateau wave and lower ICP. This concept has theoretic support, but the use of pressors to lower ICP has not yet found its way into standard practice. Ideally, CPP should be maintained in the range of 60 to 70 mm/Hg to minimize deleterious effects on cerebral edema while maximizing perfusion. Monitoring of ICP allows this parameter to be optimized, rather than requiring adjustment of treatment based on peripheral measures of blood pressure without knowledge of the actual CPP.

Miscellaneous Therapies

Other interventions can help maximize ICP control in patients whose conditions are unstable. Fever increases metabolic rate and therefore CBF, contributing to ICP elevations. Temperature should therefore be lowered to the normal range with antipyretics and cooling blankets when needed. The optimal head position for the treatment of patients with raised ICP is controversial. Raising the head 30° from horizontal usually lowers ICP, but this effect may be offset by reduced CPP and by hypoperfusion. Some studies indicate that plateau waves occur more frequently when the head is elevated.[33, 34] When ICP monitoring is performed, direct measurements of ICP and CPP dictate the optimal head position. Agitation and seizures increase cerebral metabolism and CBF and should be aggressively treated. Ventricular catheters can be used to remove CSF, but compression of the ventricles by mass effect can limit the usefulness of this technique.

CEREBRAL MONITORING

Monitoring cerebral function has assumed an increasingly important role in the care of critically ill patients with neurologic illnesses. Change in neurologic status is the primary guide to therapy, but in comatose patients or in those receiving paralytic agents, electrophysiologic monitoring provides an alternative means of detecting changes in neurologic function. Electrophysiologic monitoring may be more sensitive than is clinical examination in detecting abnormalities, and, in fact, abnormalities may precede clinical changes. Treatments that suppress neurologic activity, such as high-dose barbiturate administration, do not alter evoked potentials,[51, 52] allowing monitoring to continue in this setting. Electrophysiologic tests may also provide prognostic information that contributes to important decisions regarding continuation of care.

Electroencephalography

Electroencephalography (EEG) is easily accomplished in an ICU but requires constant attention by nursing and technical personnel to maintain optimal signals, as well as a trained observer to avoid misinterpretation of artifacts. The raw EEG tracing is prone to misinterpretation because usually only one or two channels can be continuously monitored, and considerable expertise is needed to detect subtle changes. Computerized analysis of EEG recordings generates more manageable information in the form of compressed spectral array.[53] Specific aspects of the EEG, such as spectral edge (frequency below which lies 90% of EEG power), content of specific frequencies, or frequency ratios, can be plotted against time for trend analysis. These techniques allow EEG patterns to be followed for variability.

Experience with EEG monitoring during carotid surgery suggests that this technique may be useful for detecting early ischemia. Significant changes[54] in the EEG occur when blood flow falls below 18 $mL \cdot 100g^{-1} \cdot min^{-1}$ and becomes isoelectric when blood flow is in the 12 to 15 $mL \cdot 100\ g^{-1} \cdot min^{-1}$ range.[55] The spectral edges and amplitudes of specific frequencies have correlated with reduced perfusion in some studies,[56, 57] but large-scale, well-designed trials have not been conducted. Most monitoring has been performed in the patients undergoing carotid artery or cardiac surgery, and it is not clear that EEG can be applied to continuous monitoring of critically ill patients in the ICU. EEG and compressed spectral array are prone to artifacts in the ICU, which makes routine interpretations difficult except by the most highly trained personnel.

Specific EEG or compressed spectral array patterns may provide prognostic information. In patients with head injury, invariant low frequency and amplitude records are associated with a poor prognosis,[58, 59] whereas a greater percentage of those with cycling patterns improve. In some studies, interhemispheric amplitude asymmetries[58] and changes in frequency power helped predict outcome.[60, 61] Alpha coma, a pattern of alpha activity resembling normal alpha but extending over a broader range (typically 8–13 Hz) occurs most commonly after anoxic-ischemic injury and carries an extremely poor prognosis.[62, 63] Pontine infarcts and fast activity induced by medications occasionally cause a similar pattern, but the prognosis for these states is quite different. "Spindle coma," the presence of spindle activity despite unresponsiveness, is often associated with a good outcome.[64]

Although compressed spectral array and EEG trend monitors are currently available, their impact on treatment remains unclear. EEG data have been used successfully by some investigators to predict cerebral ischemia[65] and response to therapy,[66] but more experience is needed. In addition, other techniques, such as xenon blood flow or transcranial Doppler studies, may be better suited to this application. Nonetheless, EEG remains a useful technique to detect nonconvulsive status or to follow electrical status and the effects of treatment in paralyzed patients.[67]

Evoked Potentials

Brain stem auditory evoked potentials (BAEPs) and somatosensory evoked potentials (SSEPs) are the most commonly monitored evoked potentials. BAEPs are technically easier to record and obtain a consistent tracing than are SSEPs. They are also more resistant to anesthesia and barbiturates than are SSEPs.[68, 69] BAEPs consist of five identifiable waves generated from specific brain stem structures along the auditory pathways. Wave I represents potentials generated by the eighth nerve. Other waves originate from the cochlear nucleus, the superior olive, the lateral lemniscus, and the inferior colliculus.[70] Lesions above the midbrain do not result in BAEP abnormalities unless tissue shifts occur with disturbance of lower brain stem function. Brain stem lesions are also rarely found with normal BAEPs if the auditory pathways are spared. These anatomic limitations must be considered in patients with brain injury and normal BAEPs. The complete absence of BAEPs cannot be used as evidence of brain stem pathology. If wave I is not present, the integrity of the brain stem cannot be determined, however, the presence of wave I without waves II through V implies significant pathology of the brain stem auditory pathways. Unilateral abnormalities suggest localization of lesions to one side.

SSEPs are obtained by electrical stimulation of the median, ulnar, peroneal, or tibial nerves. Upper extremity nerves are most commonly used for this monitoring. Waves are generated from the brachial plexus, the upper cervical cord, the dorsal column nuclei, the ventroposterior thalamus, and the sensory cortex.[70] Cortically generated potentials are most important for monitoring applications, including head injury, global anoxia, and ischemia. These waves reflect the integrity of the primary sensory cortex and by extrapolation, the entire hemisphere. Like BAEPs, potentials from the dorsal column nuclei must be present for conclusions to be made based on the absence of cortical waves. SSEPs are also relatively resistant to high-dose barbiturate administration,[71] allowing monitoring of neurologic function during barbiturate coma.

Evoked potentials may also provide prognostic information. The absence of waves II through V on BAEPs has been associated with poor outcome in patients with head injury,[72, 73] but when wave I is absent or BAEPs are normal, prognosis cannot be determined. SSEP abnormalities correlate strongly with outcome. Bilateral absence of cortical waves almost invariably implies a poor prognosis when potentials from dorsal column nuclei are maintained.[74, 75] Combining results of BAEPs and SSEPs may improve the overall accuracy of either test alone.[76–78]

Both BAEPs and SSEPs have been used as confirmatory tests to support the diagnosis of brain death. This support

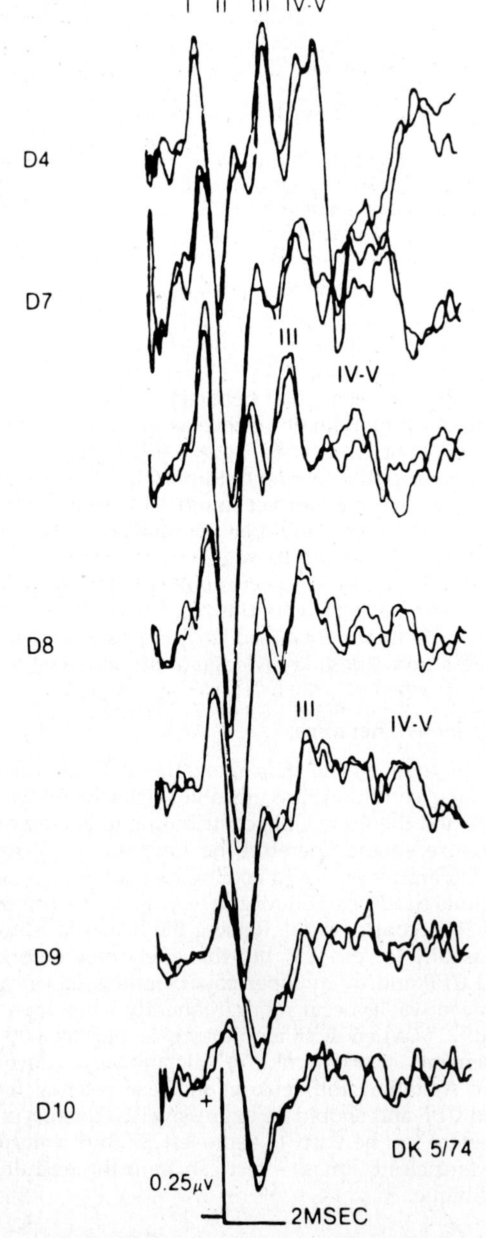

Figure 166–3. Brain stem auditory evoked potentials from a patient with severe anoxia on day 4 (D4). Waves I through V are initially identifiable; however, on subsequent recordings, the later waves gradually disappear, a finding associated with clinical deterioration. On day 9 (D9), the patient met the clinical criteria for brain death, and only wave I was evident. (From Starr A: Auditory brainstem responses in brain death. Brain 1976; 99:543–554, by permission of Oxford University Press.)

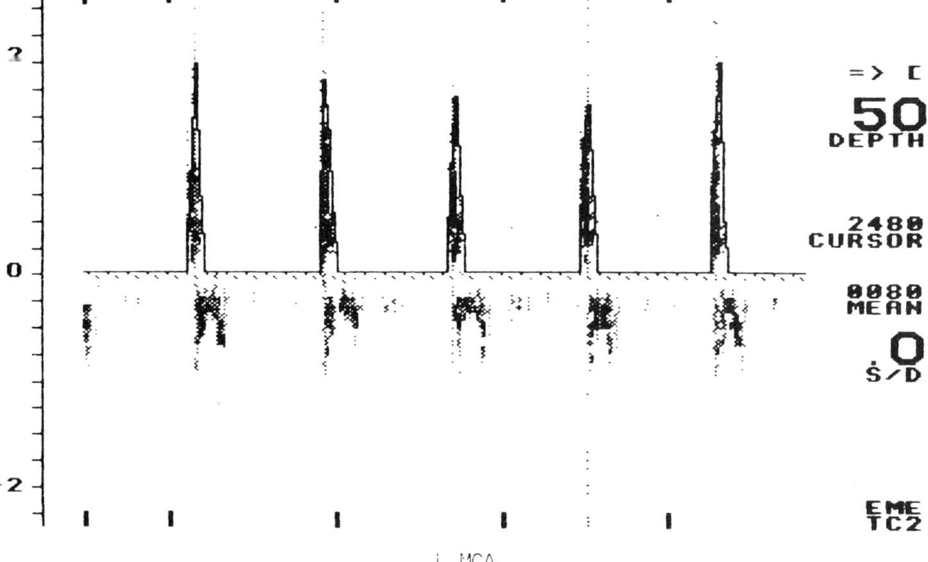

Figure 166–4. TCD recording from the middle cerebral artery in brain death. There is a brief systolic spike, with reversed flow during diastole.

is particularly useful when barbiturate levels are high because cortical waves on SSEPs and waves II through V on BAEPs are typically preserved when coma results from barbiturate intake. Absence of these waves with preservation of wave I on BAEP and dorsal column nuclei potentials on SSEP confirms severe cortical and brain stem damage (Fig. 166–3).[74] SSEPs are usually more useful because wave I on BAEPs is absent more often in brain death than are dorsal column nuclei potentials on SSEPs.[74]

In patients with raised ICP, loss of BAEP wave V suggests midbrain compression due to tissue shifts.[79, 80] BAEP abnormalities may also predict midbrain hemorrhage in patients with severe head injury and signs of midbrain pathology.[81] In some patients with brain stem strokes, abnormal BAEPs correlated with an unstable clinical course.[82] SSEPs are lost in patients with severe hemispheric ischemia[83, 84] and may be useful to monitor cerebral function during carotid endarterectomy or in the ICU for longer-term use. The relative advantages of evoked potentials, EEG and transcranial Doppler ultrasound for these purposes have not been established.

Transcranial Doppler Ultrasound

Evaluation of the intracranial arterial circulation by transcranial Doppler (TCD) ultrasound has provided new approaches to the monitoring of critically ill patients with neurologic disease. This technique uses a 2-MHz ultrasound probe affixed to the temporal area above the zygomatic arch. TCD ultrasound is well suited to ICU applications because it is noninvasive and because unlimited studies can be performed at the patient's bedside without known risk to the patient. From the temporal window, the middle cerebral artery (MCA), the anterior cerebral artery, and the posterior cerebral artery can be insonated. The basilar and vertebral arteries are examined via the occipital window, and the intracranial internal carotid artery and the ophthalmic arteries are approached through the orbital window. During monitoring, the probe is usually focused on one middle cerebral artery, and velocity is monitored continuously. Simultaneous bilateral middle cerebral artery monitoring is also now available. Trend-monitoring software allows rapid read-out of velocity changes. Other physiologic parameters,

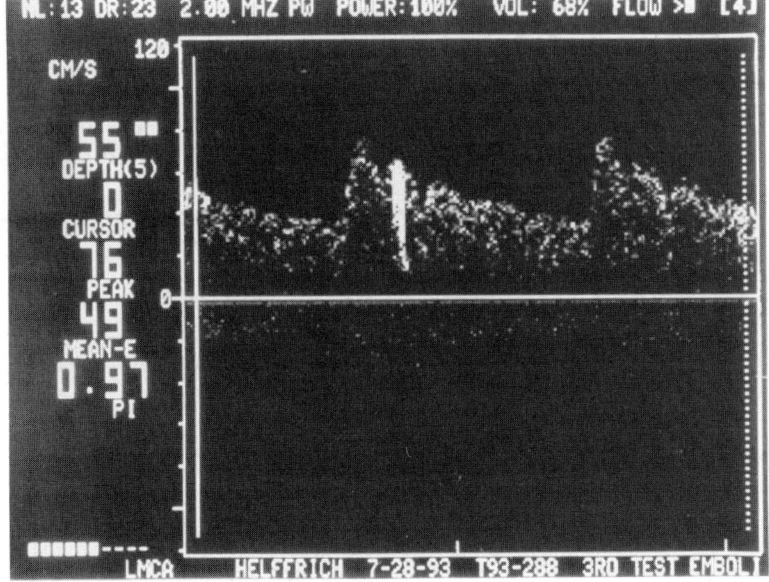

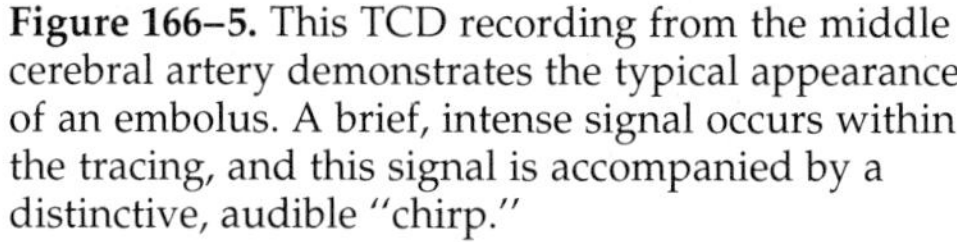
Figure 166–5. This TCD recording from the middle cerebral artery demonstrates the typical appearance of an embolus. A brief, intense signal occurs within the tracing, and this signal is accompanied by a distinctive, audible "chirp."

such as blood pressure or ICP, can be monitored simultaneously and correlated directly with velocity changes.

Characteristic changes occur in the velocity curve when ICP is elevated. Mean flow velocity decreases and pulsatility index ([peak velocity − end-diastolic velocity]/mean velocity) increases with rising ICP.[85, 86] When ICP reaches levels approaching the mean arterial pressure, TCD ultrasound demonstrates brief systolic spikes or a reverberating pattern with reversed flow during diastole (Fig. 166–4).[87, 88] TCD ultrasound has been used as an ancillary test to support the diagnosis of brain death when clinical criteria alone are insufficient. The to-and-fro TCD ultrasound flow patterns are highly associated with brain death,[88] although rare examples of minimally preserved brain stem function have been reported.[89] Identical findings should be recorded from multiple intracranial arteries (both middle cerebral arteries or at least one middle cerebral artery and the basilar artery) because similar patterns can be seen with occlusion of a single artery.[90]

Changes in velocity curves over time may reflect ICP changes, but TCD ultrasound cannot be used to determine absolute ICP. In patients with subarachnoid hemorrhage, the resistive index, another measure of pulsatility, reflects ICP increases even with coexistent vasospasm, when velocity increases simultaneously.[91] When the resistive index is below 0.5 (normal levels), mean velocity changes can be used to monitor the severity of vasospasm without any effect of ICP on the velocity curve. Changes in TCD tracings reflecting ICP variations may also occasionally help guide therapy in patients with large strokes who are poor candidates or at high risk of undesirable side effects with direct ICP monitoring. Changes in Pa_{CO_2}, hematocrit value, and

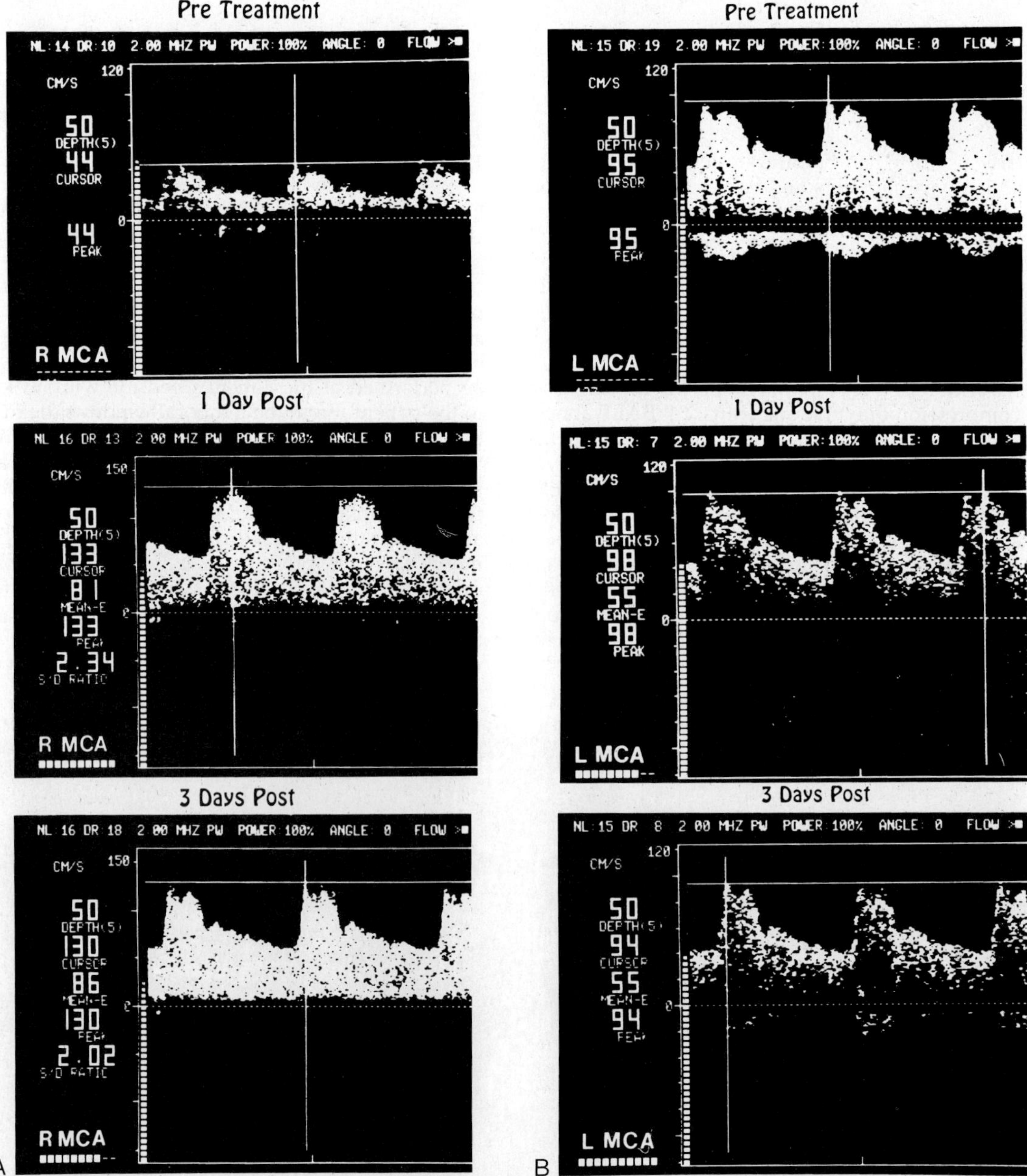

Figure 166–6. *A*, TCD recordings from the right middle cerebral artery before and after recanalization with intravenous tissue plasminogen activator (tPA). Initial waveforms demonstrate reduced peak velocity with increased pulsatility due to an increase in peripheral vascular resistance. After thrombolysis, middle cerebral artery waveforms normalize and transiently show increased velocity, most likely due to hyperemia. *B*, Recordings from the normal left middle cerebral artery in the same patient for comparison.

cardiac output alter TCD velocities, and these parameters should be recorded during TCD ultrasound monitoring so that velocity changes are properly interpreted.

TCD ultrasound monitoring has also been applied to patients with cerebrovascular disease. Intraoperative monitoring of middle cerebral artery velocity during carotid endarterectomy may identify patients at risk for stroke during carotid artery clamping.[92] In the immediate postoperative period, a sudden fall in middle cerebral artery velocity suggests reocclusion, possibly necessitating exploration of the endarterectomy site. Marked increases in velocity occasionally occur in the first few days after surgery, indicating hyperemia that is sometimes associated with intracerebral hemorrhage.[93] Recognition of hyperperfusion and careful blood pressure control help prevent this serious complication.

Emboli passing through the intracranial circulation produce a brief, high-intensity signal within the Doppler spectrum (Fig. 166–5).[94] Detection of emboli in the intracranial circulation ipsilateral to a recent carotid endarterectomy raises the suspicion of residual thrombus at the operative site. Emboli are found by TCD ultrasound monitoring more commonly in patients who have had a stroke, particularly in those with atrial fibrillation,[95, 96] and may predict risk for additional ischemic events.

Intra-arterial or intravenous administration of thrombolytic agents has recently been studied for the treatment of acute ischemic stroke.[97–99] TCD ultrasound monitoring provides an excellent method for the identification of occluded intracerebral arteries and allows the progress of thrombolysis to be monitored without the need for repeat arteriography (Fig. 166–6).[100] Recanalization can be documented by return of antegrade flow, and therapy can then be tailored to the time course of reperfusion. As acute stroke therapy improves, TCD ultrasound monitoring will likely play an increasingly important role.

References

1. Shenkin HA, Bouzarth WF: Clinical methods of reducing intracranial pressure. Role of the cerebral circulation. N Engl J Med 1970; 282:1465–1471.
2. Lundberg N, Cronqvist S, Kjallquist A: Clinical investigations on interactions between intracranial pressure and intracranial hemodynamics. Prog Brain Res 1958; 30:69–75.
3. Rosner MJ, Becker DP: Origin and evolution of plateau waves. J Neurosurg 1984; 60:312–324.
4. Plum F, Posner JB: The Diagnosis of Stupor and Coma. Philadelphia, FA Davis, 1980.
5. Ropper AH: Lateral displacement of the brain and level of consciousness in patients with an acute hemispheral mass. N Engl J Med 1986; 314:953–958.
6. Astrup J, Siesjo BK, Symon L: Thresholds in cerebral ischemia—The ischemic penumbra. Stroke 1981; 12:723.
7. Astrup J, Symon L, Branston NM, et al: Cortical evoked potentials and extracellular K^+ and H^+ at critical levels of brain ischemia. Stroke 1977; 8:51.
8. Jones TH, Morawetz RB, Crowell RM, et al: Thresholds of focal cerebral ischemia in awake monkeys. J Neurosurg 1981; 54:773.
9. Raichle M: Sensori-motor area increase of oxygen uptake and blood flow in the human brain during contralateral hand exercise. *In:* Brain Work: The Coupling of Function, Metabolism and Blood Flow in the Brain. Ingvar DH, Lassen NA (Eds). New York, Academic Press, 1975, pp 372–376.
10. Agnoli A: Adaptation of CBF during induced chronic normoxic respiratory acidosis. Scand J Clin Lab Invest 1968; 8(Suppl 102):D.
11. Harp JR, Wolman H: Cerebral metabolic effects of hyperventilation and deliberate hypotension. Br J Anaesth 1973; 45:256–261.
12. Campkin TV, Baker RG, Pabora M, et al: Acid-base changes in arterial blood and cerebrospinal fluid during craniotomy and hyperventilation. Br J Anaesth 1974; 46:263–271.
13. Albert FN, Fazekas JF: Cerebral haemodynamics and metabolism during induced hypothermia. Anesth Analg 1956; 35:381–388.
14. Clasen RA, Pandolfi S, Liang I, et al: Experimental study of relation of fever to cerebral edema. J Neurosurg 1974; 41:516–558.
15. Hindfelt B: The prognostic significance of subfebrility and fever in ischemic cerebral infarction. Acta Neurol Scand 1976; 53:72.
16. Przelomski MM, Roth RM, Gleckman RA, et al: Fever in the wake of a stroke. Neurology 1986; 36:427.
17. Feig PU, McCardy DK: The hypertonic state. N Engl J Med 1977; 297:1444.
18. Maccario M: Neurologic dysfunction associated with nonketotic hyperglycemia. Arch Neurol 1968; 19:525.
19. Bruce DA, Berman WA, Schut L: Cerebrospinal fluid pressure monitoring in children: Physiology, pathology and clinical usefulness. Adv Pediatr 1977; 24:233–290.
20. McDowall DG: Monitoring the brain. Anesthesiology 1976; 45:117–134.
21. Marshall LF, Smith RW, Shapiro HM: The outcome of aggressive treatment in severe head injuries: Part I. The significance of intracranial pressure monitoring. J Neurosurg 1979; 50:20–25.
22. Marshall LF, Smith RW, Shapiro HM: The outcome of aggressive treatment in severe head injuries: Part II. Acute and chronic barbiturate administration in the management of head injury. J Neurosurg 1979; 50:26–30.
23. Miller JD, Becker DP, Ward JD: Significance of intracranial hypertension in severe head injury. J Neurosurg 1977; 47:503–516.
24. Stuart GG, Merry GS, Smith JA, et al: Severe head injury managed without intracranial pressure monitoring. J Neurosurg 1983; 59:601–605.
25. Ropper AH, King RB: Intracranial pressure in comatose patients with intracerebral hemorrhage. Arch Neurol 1984; 41:725–728.
26. Ropper AH, Shafran B: Brain edema after stroke: Clinical syndrome and intracranial pressure. Arch Neurol 1984; 41:26–29.
27. Kaneko M, Koba T, Yokoyama T: Early surgical treatment for hypertensive intracerebral hemorrhage. J Neurosurg 1977; 46:579–583.
28. Kaneko M, Tanaka K, Shimada T, et al: Long-term evaluation of ultra-early operation for hypertensive intracerebral hemorrhage in 100 cases. J Neurosurg 1983; 58:838–842.
29. Rengachary S, Batnitzky S, Morantz RA, et al: Hemicraniectomy for acute massive cerebral infarction. Neurosurgery 1981; 8:321–328.
30. Ropper AH: Neurological intensive care. *In:* Handbook of Clinical Neurology. Vascular Diseases. Part II. Vinken PJ, Bruyn GW, Klawans HL (Eds). Amsterdam, The Netherlands, Elsevier, 1989, pp 203–232.
31. Schalen W, Messeter K, Nordstrom CH: Cerebral vasoreactivity and the prediction of outcome in severe traumatic brain lesions. Acta Anaesthesiol Scand 1991; 35:113–122.
32. Apuzzp MLJ, Weiss MH, Petersons V, et al: effect of positive end expiratory pressure ventilation on intracranial pressure in man. J Neurosurg 1977; 46:227–232.
33. Durward QJ, Amacher AL, Del Maestro RF, et al: Cerebral and cardiovascular responses to changes in head elevation in patients with intracranial hypertension. J Neurosurg 1983; 59:938–944.
34. Rosner MJ, Coley IB: Cerebral perfusion pressure, intracranial pressure and head elevation. J Neurosurg 1986; 65:636–641.
35. Muizelaar JP, Marmarou A, Ward JD, et al: Adverse effects of prolonged hyperventilation in patients with severe head injury: A randomized clinical trial. J Neurosurg 1991; 75:731–739.
36. Marshall LF, Smith RW, Rauscher LA, et al: Mannitol dose requirements in brain-injured patients. J Neurosurg 1978; 48:169–172.
37. James HE, Langfitt TW, Kumar V, et al: Treatment of intracranial hypertension: Analysis of 105 consecutive continuous recordings of intracranial pressure. Acta Neurochir (Wien) 1977; 36:189–200.
38. Miller JD, Leech P: Effects of mannitol and steroid therapy on intracranial volume-pressure relationships in patients. J Neurosurg 1975; 42:274–281.

39. Goluboff B, Shankin A, Haft H: The effects of mannitol and urea on cerebral hemodynamics and cerebrospinal fluid pressure. Neurology 1964; 14:891–898.
40. Marshall LF, Smith RW, Rauscher LA, et al: Mannitol dose requirements in brain-injured patients. J Neurosurg 1978; 48:162–172.
41. Bruce DA, Langfitt TW, Miller JD, et al: Regional cerebral blood flow, intracranial pressure, and brain metabolism in comatose patients. J Neurosurg 1973; 38:131–144.
42. Jafar JJ, Johns LM, Mullan SF: The effect of mannitol on cerebral blood flow. J Neurosurg 1986; 64:754–759.
43. Cottrell JE, Robustelli A, Post K, et al: Furosemide- and mannitol-induced changes in intracranial pressure and serum osmolality and electrolytes. Anesthesia 1977; 47:28–30.
44. Wilkinson HA, Wepsic JG, Austin G: Diuretic synergy in the treatment of acute experimental cerebral edema. J Neurosurg 1977; 34:203–208.
45. Faupel G, Reulen HJ, Muller D, et al: Double-blind study on the effects of steroids on severe closed head injury. *In:* Dynamics of Brain Edema. Pappius HM, Feidel W (Eds). Berlin, Springer-Verlag, 1976, pp 337–343.
46. Miller JD, Leech P: Effects of mannitol and steroid therapy on intracranial volume-pressure relationships in patients. J Neurosurg 1975; 42:274–281.
47. Bauer RB, Tellez H: Dexamethasone as treatment in cerebrovascular disease: Part 2. A controlled study in acute cerebral infarction. Stroke 1973; 4:547–555.
48. Norris JW, Hachinski VC: Megadose steroid therapy in ischemic stroke. Stroke 1985; 16:150.
49. Poungvarin N, Bhoopat W, Viriyavejakul A, et al: Effects of dexamethasone in primary supratentorial hemorrhage. N Engl J Med 1987; 316:1229–1233.
50. Rosner MJ, Becker DP: Origin and evolution of plateau waves. J Neurosurg 1984; 60:312–324.
51. Drummond JC, Todd MM, Sangu M: The effect of high dose sodium thiopental on brain stem auditory and median nerve somatosensory evoked responses in humans. Anesthesiology 1985; 63:249–254.
52. Newlon PG, Greenberg RP, Enas GG, et al: Effects of therapeutic pentobarbital coma on multimodality EPs recorded from severely head-injured patients. Neurosurgery 1983; 12:613–619.
53. Bickford RG: Newer methods of recording and analyzing EEG. *In:* Current Practice of Clinical Electroencephalography. Klass DW, Daly DD (Eds). New York, Raven Press, 1979, pp 451–480.
54. Sharbrough FW, Sundt TM Jr: The value of simultaneous EEG and blood flow monitoring during carotid endarterectomy. Electroencephalogr Clin Neurophysiol 1979; 37:423.
55. Sundt TM Jr, Sharbrough FW, Anderson RE, et al: Cerebral blood flow measurements and electroencephalograms during carotid endarterectomy. J Neurosurg 1974; 41:310–320.
56. Prior PF: Polygraphic monitoring in prevention of ischaemic brain damage during surgery and intensive care. Electroencephalogr Clin Neurophysiol Suppl 1987; 39:221–226.
57. Pronk RAF: Data processing for monitoring brain function during anesthesia and surgery. Electroencephalog Clin Neurophysiol Suppl 1987; 39:215–220.
58. Bricolo A, Turrazzi S, Faccioli F, et al: Clinical application of compressed spectral array in long-term EEG monitoring of comatose patients. Electroencephalogr Clin Neurophysiol 1978; 45:211–225.
59. Bricolo A, Turrazzi S, Faccioli F: Combined clinical and EEG examinations for assessment of severity of acute head injuries. Acta Neurochir Suppl (Wien) 1979; 28:35–39.
60. Steudel WI, Kruger J: Using the frequency analysis of the EEG for prognosis in severe brain injuries. Adv Neurosurg 1978; 5:36–43.
61. Steudel WI, Kruger J: Using the spectral analysis of the EEG for prognosis of severe brain injuries in the first post-traumatic week. Acta Neurochir Suppl (Wien) 1979; 28:40–42.
62. Moller M: Alpha-pattern coma and survival after cardiac arrest. Electroencephalogr Clin Neurophysiol 1978; 44:518–522.
63. Sorensen K, Thomassen A, Wernberg M: Prognostic significance of alpha frequency EEG rhythm in coma after cardiac arrest. J Neurol Neurosurg Psychiatry 1978; 41:840–842.
64. Bergamasco B, Bergamini L, Doriguzzi T, et al: EEG sleep patterns as a prognostic criterion in posttraumatic coma. Electroencephalogr Clin Neurophysiol 1968; 24:374–377.
65. Suzuki A, Yoshioka K, Yasui N: Clinical application of EEG topography in cerebral ischemia: Detection of functional reversibility and hemodynamics. Brain Topogr 1990; 3:167–174.
66. Jordan K: Correlative xenon-enhanced CT cerebral blood flow (XeCTCBF) and EEG to functionally stratify acute cerebral infarction. Neurology 1991; 41(Suppl 1):336.
67. Borel C, Hanley D: Neurologic intensive care unit monitoring. Crit Care Clin 1985; 1:223–239.
68. Sutton LN, Frewen T, March R, et al: The effects of deep barbiturate coma on multimodality evoked potentials recorded from severely head-injured patients. J Neurosurg 1982; 57:178–185.
69. Newlon PD, Greenberg RP, Enas GG, et al: Effects of therapeutic pentobarbital coma on multimodality EPs recorded from severely head-injured patients. Neurosurgery 1983; 12:613–619.
70. Chiappa KH, Hock DB: Electrophysiologic monitoring. *In:* Neurological and Neurosurgical Intensive Care. Ropper AH (Ed). New York, Raven Press, 1993, pp 147–183.
71. Drummond JC, Todd MM, Sangu M: The effect of high dose sodium thiopental on brain stem auditory and median nerve somatosensory evoked responses in humans. Anesthesiology 1985; 63:249–254.
72. Seales DM, Rossiter VS, Weinstein ME: Brainstem auditory evoked responses in patients comatose as a result of blunt head injury. J Trauma 1979; 19:347–353.
73. Karnaze DS, Marshall LF, Mccarthy CS, et al: Localizing and prognostic value of auditory evoked responses in coma after closed head injury. Neurology 1982; 32:299–302.
74. Goldie WD, Chiappa KH, Young RR, et al: Brainstem auditory and short-latency somatosensory evoked responses in brain death. Neurology 1981; 31:248–256.
75. Hume AL, Cant BR, Shaw NA: Central somatosensory conduction time in comatose patients. Ann Neurol 1979; 5:379–384.
76. Frank LM, Furgiuele TL, Etheridge JE Jr: Prediction of chronic vegetative state in children using evoked potentials. Neurology 1985; 35:931–934.
77. Lindsay KW, Carlin J, Kennedy I, et al: Evoked potentials in severe head injury—Analysis and relation to outcome. J Neurol Neurosurg Psychiatry 1981; 44:796–802.
78. Narayan RK, Greenberg RP, Miller JD, et al: Improved confidence of outcome prediction in severe head injury. A comparative analysis of the clinical examination, multimodality evoked potentials, CT scanning, and intracranial pressure. J Neurosurg 1981; 54:751–762.
79. Nagao S, Roccaforte P, Moody RA: Acute intracranial hypertension and auditory brain-stem responses. J Neurosurg 1979; 51:846–851.
80. Ropper AH, Shafran B: Brain edema after stroke: Clinical syndrome and intracranial pressure. Arch Neurol 1984; 41:26–29.
81. Ropper AH, Miller DC: Acute traumatic midbrain hemorrhage. Ann Neurol 1985; 18:80–86.
82. Stern BJ, Krumholz A, Weiss H, et al: Evaluation of brainstem stroke using brainstem auditory evoked responses. Stroke 1982; 13:705–711.
83. Branstom NM, Symon L, Crockard HA, et al: Relationship between the cortical evoked potential and local cortical blood flow following acute middle cerebral artery occlusion in the baboon. Exp Neurol 1974; 45:195–208.
84. Ropper AH: Evoked potentials in cerebral ischemia. Stroke 1986; 17:3–5.
85. Klingelhofer J, Conrad B, Benecke R, et al: Intracranial flow patterns at increasing intracranial pressure. Klin Wochenschr 1987; 65:542–545.
86. Klingelhofer J, Conrad B, Benecke R, et al: Evaluation of intracranial pressure from transcranial Doppler studies in cerebral disease. J Neurol 1988; 235:159–162.
87. Ropper AH, Kehne SM, Wechsler L: Transcranial Doppler in brain death. Neurology 1987; 37:1733–1735.
88. Petty GW, Mohr JP, Pedley TA, et al: The role of transcranial Doppler in confirming brain death: Sensitivity, specificity, and suggestions for performance and interpretation. Neurology 1990; 40:300–303.

89. Pillay PK, Willberger J: Transcranial Doppler evaluation of brain death. Neurosurgery 1989; 25:481–482.
90. Williams MA, Razumovsky AY, Diringer M, et al: Transcranial Doppler ultrasonography in the intensive care unit. *In:* Transcranial Doppler Ultrasonography. Babikian VL, Wechsler LR, (Eds). St. Louis, Mosby, 1993, pp 175–189.
91. Klingelhofer J, Sander D, Holzgraefe M, et al: Cerebral vasospasm evaluated by transcranial Doppler ultrasonography at different intracranial pressures. J Neurosurg 1991; 75:752–758.
92. Halsey JH Jr: Risks and benefits of shunting in carotid endarterectomy. Stroke 1992; 23:1583–1587.
93. Powers AD, Smith RR, Graeber MC: Transcranial Doppler monitoring of cerebral blood flow velocities during surgical occlusion of the carotid artery. Neurosurgery 1989; 25:383–389.
94. Spencer MP, Thomas GI, Nicholls SC, et al: Detection of middle cerebral artery emboli during carotid endarterectomy using transcranial Doppler ultrasonography. Stroke 1990; 21:415–423.
95. Tegeler CH, Hitchings LP, Leighton VJ, et al: Carotid ultrasound emboli monitoring in stroke: Initial clinical experience. J Neuroimaging 1991; 1:61.
96. Tegeler CH, Leighton VJ, Barber CC, et al: Nonoperative clinical use of carotid artery Doppler emboli detection. J Neuroimaging 1991; 1:162.
97. del Zoppo GJ, Poeck K, Pessin MS, et al: Recombinant tissue plasminogen activator in acute thrombotic and embolic stroke. Ann Neurol 1992; 32:78–86.
98. Haley EC Jr, Brott TG, Sheppard GL, et al: Pilot randomized trial of tissue plasminogen activator in acute ischemic stroke. Stroke 1993; 24:1000–1004.
99. Jungreis CA, Wechsler LR, Horton JA: Intracranial thrombolysis via a catheter embedded in the clot. Stroke 1989; 20:1578–1580.
100. Karnik R, Stelzer P, Slany J: Transcranial Doppler sonography monitoring of local intra-arterial thrombolysis in acute occlusion of the middle cerebral artery. Stroke 1992; 23:284–287.

CHAPTER 167

The Critical Care of the Neurosurgical Patient

Thomas C. Witt, MD • Thomas G. Luerssen, MD, FACS, FAAP
Lawrence F. Marshall, MD

The response of the central nervous system to injury is relatively stereotyped, in spite of the wide variety of insults it can suffer. However, in contrast to most other organ systems, the brain is also quite susceptible to secondary insults. Thus, whereas the effects of spontaneous intracranial hemorrhages, neoplasms, infections, and other disorders are quite well characterized and understood, the brain and spinal cord are potentially quite vulnerable to ischemia, hypoxia, and hypocarbia. In addition, operative procedures on these tissues also produce unique effects that can be anticipated but not quite avoided. Thus, the interaction of the primary reaction to injury, the consequences of secondary insult to the nervous system, and the milieu in which treatment occurs determines how a patient will ultimately fare. The foundation of the basic management of the critically ill neurosurgical patient is a systematic ongoing plan to mitigate the effects of the primary insult and to prevent further brain dysfunction or injury. Because these patients may experience a relatively large number of secondary or tertiary events, a high level of vigilance is required. In addition, because of the brain's unique susceptibility to ischemia and hypoxia, much of our effort in the critical care environment is devoted to these potential complications.

The brain and spinal cord require a high level of perfusion with adequate fuel to function normally. Systemic hypovolemia, hypotension, hypoxia, hypoglycemia, and hyperglycemia, even of a relatively brief duration, may have catastrophic results. An adequate physiochemical environment must be sustained because of the complex interaction between the extracellular and intracellular milieu. Because of the injured brain's unique susceptibility to such events as sedation and abnormalities of electrolyte concentration, these processes must be avoided. Furthermore, the time window is relatively small for the successful treatment of most systemic complications, such as infection. Each Celsius degree of fever results in a dramatic increase in the metabolic rate of the tissue, and this increase may be deleterious in the patient who already is at the borderline between adequate and inadequate substrate delivery. Infection is also a potentially unique problem, not only because of the intensive care unit environment but also because patients with traumatic injuries, who make up the commonest group found in the neurosurgical or critical care unit, have immunosuppression as a result of their injury. Most late deaths in neurosurgical patients who have critical illnesses are due to sepsis, resulting either from pneumonia or from a systemic infection.[1]

Other issues that are unique to the neurosurgical patient are the development of deep venous thrombosis, with the risk of pulmonary embolus and the relatively high risk posed by anticoagulation. Thus, the patient who has undergone recent craniotomy is at risk for rehemorrhage, although this risk has probably been somewhat exaggerated.[2, 3] Most patients can receive prophylactic anticoagulation after 24 to 48 hours. Although each practitioner of a specialty deems his or her patients unique, the brain, because of its high metabolic rate and complex function, is indeed uniquely susceptible to insults in a time course that is much more rapid and potentially catastrophic than for most other organ systems. The focus of this chapter, therefore, is to describe the pathophysiology of the brain and its relationship to injury and the mechanisms by which these secondary insults to the brain and spinal cord, particularly ischemia and swelling, can be avoided.

Under normal conditions, cerebral blood flow in humans is approximately 50 mL/100 g of brain tissue per minute.[4] Furthermore, the vasculature of the brain possesses the ability to autoregulate cerebral blood flow at a fairly constant rate and over a wide range of systemic mean arterial pressures.[5] Although the exact mechanisms governing autoregulation are not completely understood, the main factors appear to be an intrinsic vascular smooth muscle response to stretch and relaxation, the local concentration of various tissue metabolites, and the direct neural control of vascular tone.[6] Two very potent regulators of cerebral blood flow are arterial P_{CO_2} and P_{O_2}. Elevation of the arterial P_{CO_2} by 15 mm Hg can result in a mean cerebral blood flow increase of 75%.[7] Conversely, the common therapeutic manipulation of decreasing P_{CO_2} by a similar amount is associated with a cerebral blood flow decrease of as much as 33%.[8] Although cerebrovascular tone is clearly sensitive to a wide range of P_{CO_2} levels, its sensitivity to arterial oxygen tension is restricted to the more extreme levels of hypoxia and hyperoxia. Thus, a reduction in P_{O_2} to 50 mm Hg results in about a doubling of cerebral blood flow, whereas inhalation of 100% oxygen produces only a mild vasoconstriction and a 15% decrease in cerebral blood flow.[7]

The cerebrovascular tone also determines, to some extent, the total cerebral blood volume. Because the intracranial contents are enclosed in a rigid container, the cerebral blood volume, the volume of cerebrospinal fluid (CSF), and the volume of brain must exist in equilibrium. At a certain point, the addition of any further abnormal volume, which occurs with certain pathologic processes such as hemorrhage or tumor, results in increases of intracranial pressure (ICP), unless a compensatory reduction occurs in one of the normal components. This compensation of intracranial volume can be measured and expressed as a mathematical relationship termed *intracranial compliance.* If the brain's compliance is low, then the compensatory decrease in intracranial volume is insufficient, and ICP rises. As compensatory reserves are exhausted and ICP increases, cerebral ischemia results.

ICP and mean arterial blood pressure are indirect indicators of the degree of cerebral blood flow, and their relationship can give an estimation of cerebral perfusion pressure. *Cerebral perfusion pressure* has been defined as the difference between mean arterial blood pressure and ICP. In adults, cerebral perfusion pressure should be maintained at a level greater than 65 mm Hg, if possible.

The relationship between ICP, blood pressure, and cerebral perfusion is complicated and is still undergoing active clinical and basic research. Clearly, elevated ICP can result in a diminished cerebral perfusion pressure and progressive brain dysfunction due to ischemia. However, neurologic catastrophes can occur at normal ICPs in patients with temporal lobe or posterior fossa lesions. Furthermore, focusing entirely on cerebral perfusion pressure may be too simplistic. In the analysis of the Traumatic Coma Data Bank, investigators found that the proportions of time a patient experienced ICPs greater than 20 mm Hg and the proportions of time that blood pressures were less than 80 mm Hg were correlated with poor outcome. However, a diminished cerebral perfusion pressure by itself was not necessarily correlated with poor outcome.[9] In contrast, aggressive control of ICP and cerebral perfusion pressure has been shown to be associated with improved patient outcome.[9–15] Once ICP is greater than 20 mm Hg, many patients exhibit a significantly decreased ability to tolerate additional increases in intracranial volume.[16] Patients with sustained ICPs of greater than 40 mm Hg virtually always show some clinical neurologic deterioration.[10]

PREVENTION OF ISCHEMIA DUE TO INTRACRANIAL HYPERTENSION

One of the simplest methods for reducing ICP is the promotion of normal cerebral venous drainage. Decreasing the cerebral venous pressure can be accomplished by raising the head of the patient's bed by 15° to 30°.[17] Furthermore, careful attention to head position by maintaining it in the neutral position enhances cerebral venous drainage. If the head is turned to one side, if a cervical spine immobilization device is poorly fitted, or if the tape securing an endotracheal tube is too tight, the patient's jugular venous drainage may be impaired.[18]

Some studies have found an inconsistent response of ICP to head elevation. Occasionally, head elevation results in an elevation of ICP. Some investigators have suggested that head elevation may induce a shift of brain tissue toward the foramen magnum and thereby impede the outflow of CSF.[19] Rosner and Coley[20] have postulated that in the patient with intracranial hypertension, head elevation will usually result in a greater decrease in mean arterial pressure at head level than in ICP and will thus produce a net decrease in cerebral perfusion pressure. In contrast, Feldman and coworkers[21] have clearly demonstrated that in the normovolemic patient, head elevation usually results in a reduction in ICP.[21] We believe that occasionally, the demonstration by Rosner and colleagues is true: cerebral perfusion pressure can be maximized and the frequency of delta ICP waves minimized if the head of the patient's bed is kept flat. Thus, because a variability exists in the response of ICP to head elevation, the optimal degree of head elevation should be individualized for each neurosurgical patient.[19, 22]

BRAIN EDEMA

Reactive edema can occur in many circumstances. Cerebral edema becomes clinically significant when it results in a focal mass effect or when it produces a global elevation in ICP and therefore impairs the cerebral perfusion. Vasogenic edema is commonly seen surrounding tumors, abscesses, intraparenchymal hemorrhages, and contusions. Interestingly, cytotoxic edema occurs not only in ischemic and hypoxic injuries but also in head injury. Recent studies using magnetic resonance imaging have shown that very little evidence of barrier disturbance is present early after acute head injury. Vasogenic edema in head injury appears to occur after the first 2 to 3 days rather than, as was previously thought, much earlier.

Vasogenic edema from tumors and abscesses can be extremely responsive to the administration of systemic corticosteroids. It has been known for many years that the administration of dexamethasone significantly improves postoperative outcomes in patients undergoing resections of cerebral neoplasm associated with surrounding edema.[23, 24] Similar responses are seen in patients with cerebral abscesses.[25] In contrast, the administration of corticosteroids for brain injury or intracranial hemorrhages does not appear to significantly affect either the process or the ultimate outcome.[26–28]

Osmotic diuresis can also effectively lower ICP in most pathologic processes. The most widely used osmotic diuretic, mannitol, administered in doses of 0.25 to 1 g/kg, effectively lowers ICP. Mannitol is thought to create a relative osmotic load in the intravascular space and to extract both extracellular and intracellular water from the brain.[29] However, growing evidence indicates that mannitol may also induce vasoconstriction by altering blood viscosity and local oxygen delivery.[30] Close attention must be paid to serum osmolality and electrolytes when mannitol is used, particularly when it is administered frequently or in large doses. Hypernatremia, hyperosmolality, and hypokalemia can be associated with prolonged administration of mannitol, and the drug should not be administered if the serum sodium level exceeds 150 mEq/dL or if the serum osmolality exceeds 320 mOsm/kg. Also, the diuresis resulting from mannitol administration may exacerbate hypovolemia and hypotension.

The loop diuretic furosemide has been used alone[31] and in combination with mannitol[32, 33] to achieve similar reductions in ICP, especially in patients undergoing craniotomy. Some studies have indicated that the combination of these two drugs results in a larger and more sustained decrease in ICP than the use of either drug alone.[34, 35]

Patients whose conditions are rapidly deteriorating from elevated ICP and who do not respond to the immediate therapies outlined earlier should undergo endotracheal intubation and mechanical ventilation. As a patient's level of consciousness falls, the patient becomes unable to prevent airway obstruction or aspiration. Endotracheal intubation should be performed in a controlled fashion to prevent a reflex elevation of systemic arterial blood pressure and venous pressure. Surges in blood pressure that are commonly seen during intubation can be blocked by rapid administration of a hypnotic medication, such as thiopental at 3 to 5 mg/kg, followed by a nondepolarizing neuromuscular paralytic agent. Although succinylcholine, a depolarizing neuromuscular blockade agent, can be used in the acutely deteriorating patient, its use should be avoided in those with chronic motor deficits because of the increased risk of significant hyperkalemia, which occurs as potassium is released from chronically denervated muscles. During ventilation, cerebral venous return is enhanced by the use of relatively large tidal volumes (i.e., approximately 15 mL/kg) and a relatively low ventilatory rate (i.e., approximately 12 breaths per minute). Positive end-expiratory pressure can be used at low levels in patients with good intracranial compliance.[22] Respiratory therapy maneuvers, such as postural drainage and percussion, should be used as long as the procedures do not produce prolonged or dangerous increases in ICP. Pulmonary toilet should be meticulous, and the reflex sympathetic responses associated with endotracheal suctioning may be effectively blocked by the intermittent administration of intravenous lidocaine at 1.5 mg/kg for a minute or two before the patient is suctioned.[36, 37]

Hyperventilation is an effective means of reducing ICP, but the effects of mechanical hyperventilation appear to decrease over time. Considerable controversy exists regarding the relative risk for cerebral ischemia under circumstances in which regional cerebral blood flow is already compromised by hyperventilation. Muizelaar and associates[38] have argued, on the basis of the results of a small clinical trial, that hyperventilation produces transient adverse effects on the outcome of severe head injury. However, Cruz,[39] in a study of continuous monitoring of systemic and cerebral oxygenation in patients with acute brain injury, showed that hyperventilation often improves cerebral oxygen metabolism, particularly in patients with post-traumatic cerebral "luxury perfusion." In fact, in such patients, the outcome is significantly improved when hyperventilation is employed. Cruz has coined the term *optimal hyperventilation* and perhaps, as in the area of head position, most patients will benefit, although occasionally patients may be made worse by hyperventilation. The recent development of monitors of cerebral oxygen consumption may help to identify patients who are at risk for ischemia.[39]

Drainage of ventricular CSF and, in rare instances, drainage of lumbar subarachnoid CSF can effectively lower ICP. Clearly, any pathologic process associated with ventricular enlargement is best treated by CSF drainage. The placement of ventricular catheters can occur at the patient's bedside, in the intensive care unit, or in the operating room. The management of continuous or intermittent drainage has been described elsewhere.[22, 40] Ventricular catheters carry two major disadvantages: the risk of hemorrhage and the risk of infection. The risk of intraparenchymal hemorrhage during catheter placement is felt to be approximately 1%.[41, 42] The risk of CSF infection from a ventriculostomy has been reported to be between 2% and 7% in most centers. The risk of infection appears to increase with prolonged placement. However, the administration of prophylactic antibiotics or the empirical placement of new ventricular catheters has not clearly altered that rate of infection.[43–45]

Intracranial hypertension, particularly that resulting from brain swelling that is refractory to all other therapies, often responds to the administration of high doses of barbiturates. Dearden and Miller[46] showed that in head-injured patients in whom the pattern of injury is one of diffuse rather than of focal brain damage, barbiturates are more effective than mannitol in reducing ICP. The same statement is true for propofol, indicating that hypnotics are likely to be more effective in this pattern of brain injury, which is often associated with cerebral hyperemia and luxury perfusion.

Barbiturates cause depression of neuronal activity and significant slowing of brain waves on the electroencephalogram. The concomitant decrease in the brain's utilization of oxygen results in a significant decrease in cerebral blood flow and volume.[47, 48] The administration of barbiturates may also limit the formation of edema and may provide some protection for neurons at risk of ischemia. However, the administration of systemic high-dose barbiturates is associated with significant morbidity. Hemodynamic instability is common, especially in patients who are hypovolemic. At extremely high doses of barbiturates, myocardial contractility may be impaired. Therefore, all patients who are to receive high-dose barbiturate therapy would benefit from the placement of a central venous pressure monitor or a Swan-Ganz monitor. Meticulous attention to the maintenance of appropriate intravascular volume, especially before the administration of loading doses of barbiturates, is essential.

Barbiturates also may increase the patient's risk for infection. In vitro studies have demonstrated that barbiturates decrease lymphocyte responsiveness, phagocytosis, and peripheral proliferation.[49, 50]

Barbiturates may increase the risk for pneumonia by impairing tracheobronchial reflexes. Additional side effects of barbiturates include hypothermia and decreased gastric motility.[51, 52]

Barbiturate therapy is initiated with loading doses of 3 to 10 mg/kg of body weight of pentobarbital. The loading dose should be given relatively slowly, in increments of 50 to 100 mg, to blunt the hypotensive response. Concomitant use of fluid and volume support, as well as vasopressors, may be necessary to maintain a satisfactory arterial pressure. Maintenance doses of barbiturates (1–4 $mg \cdot kg^{-1} \cdot h^{-1}$) can be used for extended periods, as long as the patient is hemodynamically stable. Increased hepatic enzyme activity may require escalation of doses to maintain the therapeutic effect.[53, 54] The goal of barbiturate therapy is to effectively reduce ICP without producing hypotension or impairing cerebral perfusion. Marshall and Bowers[52] have indicated that serum pentobarbital levels of greater than 5 mg/dL have no further benefit and are associated with significant complications. Electroencephalographic monitoring may be helpful to follow the therapeutic effects of barbiturates. Some investigators report the titration of barbiturates to electroencephalographic activity either to the point of burst suppression or when electrocerebral silence occurs, and this level is associated with the maximum effect of barbiturates.[47, 53, 55]

Barbiturates must be tapered slowly when they are discontinued; lethal rebound intracranial hypertension can occur if barbiturate therapy is stopped suddenly. The withdrawal of barbiturates over 3 to 5 days has generally been found to be safe.[52] Once barbiturates have been withdrawn, the neurologic effects may take a further 24 to 72 hours to clear.[53]

PREVENTION OF ISCHEMIA DUE TO CEREBRAL VASOSPASM

Cerebral vasospasm is an arteriopathy that results in marked narrowing of the cerebral arteries or arterioles and can produce profound cerebral ischemia. Although vasospasm can occur in many situations, including head injury,[52, 56] and after craniotomies for tumors and unruptured aneurysms,[58] it is most often life threatening after aneurysmal subarachnoid hemorrhage. The cause of cerebral vasospasm is not understood, although intense effort has been directed at attempting to determine the pathophysiologic mechanisms that underlie this process. Several vasoactive substances released from the breakdown of blood products in the subarachnoid space are suspected to contribute to the development of this arteriopathy.[56–59] Furthermore, several studies have shown a correlation between the amount and distribution of subarachnoid blood and the incidence and location of the vasospasm.[60–66] Cerebral vasospasm can occur immediately after hemorrhage but is generally seen as a delayed response to intracranial hemorrhage. Most often, this response occurs 4 to 10 days after the initial hemorrhage. Patients at risk for cerebral vasospasm can be monitored with noninvasive transcranial Doppler ultrasound. As the Doppler ultrasound demonstrates an increased flow velocity through the cerebral arteries that suggests vasospasm, specific therapies can be introduced.

Normal blood flow velocity obtained with transcranial Doppler ultrasound is in the range of 30 to 80 cm/s in the middle cerebral artery distribution, the vessel most easily insonated.[67] As mentioned, the flow velocity may increase before the clinical signs of cerebral ischemia appear.[65] In patients with aneurysmal subarachnoid hemorrhage, a ratio of flow velocities of 3:1 (comparing the middle cerebral artery with the internal carotid artery) is evidence of cerebral vasospasm. Alternatively, some investigators believe that flow velocities of greater than 120 cm/s often correlate with angiographically visible vasospasm and that a mean velocity of greater than 200 cm/s is usually associated with a greater than 50% reduction in cerebrovascular diameter.[68]

The availability of Doppler methodology has permitted a much more rational and systematic approach to patients with cerebral vasospasm. In addition to avoiding hypovolemia and hypotension in such patients (which is an interesting irony because 20 years ago patients with aneurysmal subarachnoid hemorrhage were often treated with dehydration and induced hypotension), a series of strategies have been developed to try to enhance cerebral perfusion. These strategies augment cerebral blood volume and cerebral blood pressure and alter the rheologic aspects of the circulation by hemodilution. In patients with an unclipped cerebral aneurysm, aggressive volume expansion and hypertension may increase the risk of aneurysmal hemorrhage. However, if the patient's aneurysm is clipped, hypervolemic therapy can be instituted at the first sign of vasospasm, either when detected by transcranial Doppler ultrasound or cerebral angiogram, or at the initial sign of neurologic deterioration. Hypervolemia can be induced by the administration of crystalloid, colloid, or whole blood until the central venous pressure is 8 to 12 mm Hg, or the pulmonary artery wedge pressure is 14 to 20 mm Hg, or both.[69–71] The goal is to achieve the maximum cardiac filling pressures that will optimize cardiac output without producing pulmonary edema. The use of a central venous catheter or a Swan-Ganz catheter is mandatory. In some patients, a hypervolemic state may be difficult to maintain because of diuresis. Kassell and coworkers[70] advocate the use of subcutaneous doses of aqueous vasopressin to prevent this diuresis.

Cerebral blood flow may be further enhanced by the institution of controlled hypertension. Vasopressors, such as aramine,[72] dopamine,[70, 73, 74] and phenylephrine,[71, 74] as well as inotropic agents, such as dobutamine and digoxin,[70] have been used to maintain systolic blood pressures between 150 and 200 mm Hg.[69, 73, 74] Cardiac output may be further enhanced by the administration of atropine, which blocks the reflex vagal depression of heart rate.[70] The induction of hypervolemic hypertension should be maintained at least until the end of the high-risk period of vasospasm, which may be up to 14 days after the hemorrhage. At that time, the treatments can be slowly weaned while hypotension and hypovolemia are still avoided.

The use of hemodilution to improve cerebral blood flow in vasospasm remains controversial.[69] Hemodilution as a means of treating cerebral vasospasm is based on the principle that blood viscosity increases as the hematocrit value rises.[75] Although the optimal hematocrit value in patients with cerebral vasospasm and ischemia has yet to be conclusively determined, some authors advocate maintaining it in the range of 33% to 40%.[69, 70]

Recently, vasospasm has been effectively treated by the administration of calcium channel blockers, specifically nimodipine. Several large clinical series of patients with subarachnoid hemorrhage have shown that the administration of nimodipine reduces the incidence of ischemic deficits and results in improved functional outcome.[76–81] In these studies, nimodipine was administered intravenously at a rate of 2 mg/h for 12 to 14 days and then orally at 45 to 60 mg every 4 hours for 7 days.[78, 80, 81] In other studies, it was administrated as an oral medication at 60 to 90 mg every 4 hours for a total of 21 days.[76, 77] Although the exact mechanism of action of nimodipine is unclear, it has been suggested that this drug blocks the influx of calcium to vascular smooth muscle cells and inhibits their contraction. This effect is relatively selective for the cerebral vasculature,[82] although the drug has been shown to cause systemic hypotension. Although some studies have failed to demonstrate a difference in the degree of angiographically visible vasospasm in patients treated with nimodipine compared with those not treated with this agent, studies using transcranial Doppler ultrasound have shown decreased flow velocities in the treatment group.[76–78, 80] Some investigators have postulated that nimodipine may act on smaller-caliber arteries beyond the resolution of cerebral angiography.[77] Furthermore, because the influx of calcium ions been suggested to play a role in ischemic cellular death,[83] nimodipine may have a separate neuronal protective effect in patients with vasospasm.[77]

In certain situations, hypertension must be assiduously avoided. Patients with ruptured but unclipped cerebral aneurysms should not have a systolic blood pressure greater than 160 mm Hg.[69, 70] In areas of traumatically injured brain where autoregulation is impaired, the blood-brain barrier may be further disrupted in areas of hypertension; therefore, cerebral edema may be aggravated.[84] Furthermore, patients who have undergone craniotomies for resection of various masses are at risk for intraparenchymal hemorrhages when blood pressure is uncontrolled. The exact limits of blood pressure should be individualized, depending on the pathologic process and the patient's premorbid average systemic blood pressure. The lower limit of mean arterial pressure for adequate cerebral perfusion is higher in chronically hypertensive patients than in normotensive patients.[85] This fact is particularly important in the treatment of patients with hypertensive intracranial hemorrhages. These hemorrhages commonly occur in central regions of the brain in which blood pressures are greater than 200 mm Hg. Although these patients require expeditious reduction of their blood pressure to prevent additional hemorrhage, the systolic blood pressure should not be reduced below 130 to 140 mm Hg.

Strict blood pressure control is extremely critical in patients who have undergone resection of large arteriovenous malformations. These patients are at risk for intraparenchymal hemorrhage due to rupture of tenuously cauterized blood vessels. They are also at risk for a phenomenon that has been termed *normal–perfusion-pressure breakthrough bleeding*. This entity, first described by Spetzler and associates,[86] can cause devastating complications after successful resection of arteriovenous malformations. The chronic diversion of blood supply in the region of the high-flow arteriovenous malformation renders the adjacent brain relatively ischemic. The vessels in the area of relative ischemia are, therefore, chronically dilated. When the arteriovenous malformation is resected, these chronically dilated vessels are faced with a marked increase in cerebral blood flow and intravascular pressures. Because these vessels cannot autoregulate in response to this increased blood flow, vascular congestion with severe brain swelling can result. If the vessel walls are extremely weak, frank hemorrhage can occur. Eventually, these blood vessels regain the ability to regulate cerebral blood flow, although the recovery may take as long as 2 weeks.[87]

Normal–perfusion-pressure breakthrough can be prevented by a staged resection of the arteriovenous malformation. However, meticulous control of the blood pressure is also necessary.[87–91] Controlled hypotension has been achieved by use of nitroprusside, nitroglycerin, hydralazine, nifedipine, β-blockers, and labetalol.[92] Vasodilatory drugs also cause intracerebral vasodilation and accordingly can increase ICP. However, this theoretical side effect is uncommonly encountered. β-Blockers and labetalol apparently do not cause significant cerebral vasodilation and may be the initial drugs of choice for the control of elevations of blood pressure in neurosurgical patients.

PREVENTION OF SECONDARY SPINAL CORD INJURY

Only a few specific treatments are available for the prevention of secondary injury to the spinal cord. When a fracture results in instability of the spine, efforts must be made to immobilize the spine and to restore normal alignment. In the patient with an acute spinal cord injury, a large, multicenter, randomized, double-blinded clinical trial has shown that administration of high doses of methylprednisolone (30 mg/kg of body weight given as a bolus, followed by 5.4 mg/kg of body weight per hour over a period of 24 hours) results in significant recovery of motor function as long as the drug is given within 8 hours of the injury.[93] Methylprednisolone is believed to exert its effect by inhibiting lipid peroxidation induced by free radical formation at the injury site.[94] Patients with injury to the cauda equina or to an isolated nerve root and patients with gunshot wounds to the spine were excluded from this study.

In patients with nontraumatic compressive lesions of the spinal cord (e.g., tumors, epidural abscesses, and disk herniations), administration of high-dose dexamethasone (20 mg every 6 hours) can help to temporarily reduce the deficits related to vasogenic edema.

CONCLUSION

In summary, patients with central nervous system injuries of any type are uniquely vulnerable to secondary insults, particularly ischemia and hypoxia. Thus, a systematic and rational approach clearly understood by all medical personnel involved in the care of these patients is essential to maximize recovery and to minimize complications. Without such meticulous planning, the improved results from our remarkably improved understanding of the neurochemical mechanisms underlying brain injury will not be translatable into further improved outcomes.

References

1. Helling TS, Evans LL, Fowler DL, et al: Infectious complications in patients with severe head injury. J Trauma 1988; 28:1575.
2. Frim DM, Barker FG, Puletti CE, et al: Postoperative low-dose heparin decreases thromboembolic complications in neurosurgical patients. Neurosurgery 1992; 30:830.
3. Persson AV, Davis RJ, Vallavicencio JL: Deep venous thrombosis and pulmonary embolism. Surg Clin North Am 1991; 71:1195
4. Kety SS, Schmidt CF: The nitrous oxide method for the quantitative determination of cerebral blood flow in man: Theory, procedure and normal values. J Clin Invest 1948; 27:476.
5. Lassen NA: Cerebral blood flow and oxygen consumption in man. Physiol Rev 1959; 39:183.
6. Chehrazi BB, Youmans JR: Cerebral blood flow in clinical neurosurgery. *In*: Neurological Surgery. 3rd ed. Youmans JR (Ed). Philadelphia, WB Saunders, 1990, pp 696–740.
7. Kety SS, Schmidt CF: The effects of altered arterial tensions of carbon dioxide and oxygen on cerebral blood flow and cerebral oxygen consumption of normal young men. J Clin Invest 1948; 27:484.
8. Kety SS, Schmidt CF: The effects of active and passive hyperventilation on cerebral blood flow, cerebral oxygen consumption, cardiac output, and blood pressure of normal young men. J Clin Invest 1946; 25:107.
9. Marmarou A, Anderson RL, Ward JD, et al: Impact of ICP instability and hypotension on outcome in patients with severe head trauma. J Neurosurg 1991; 75:S59.
10. Miller JD, Becker DP, Ward JD, et al: Significance of intracranial hypertension in severe head injury. J Neurosurg 1977; 47:503.
11. Becker DP, Miller JD, Ward JD, et al: The outcome from severe head injury with early diagnosis and intensive management. J Neurosurg 1977; 47:491.
12. Marshall LF, Smith RW, Shapiro HM: The outcome with aggressive treatment in severe head injuries. J Neurosurg 1979; 50:20.
13. Miller JD, Butterworth JF, Gudeman SK: Further experience in the management of severe head injury. J Neurosurg 1981; 54:289.
14. Saul TG, Ducker TB: Effect of intracranial pressure monitoring and aggressive treatment on mortality in severe head injury. J Neurosurg 1982; 56:498.
15. Bruce DA, Schut L, Bruno LA, et al: Outcome following severe head injuries in children. J Neurosurg 1978; 48:679.
16. Marmarou A, Tabaddor K: Intracranial pressure: Physiology and pathophysiology. *In*: Head Injury. 2nd ed. Cooper PR (Ed). Baltimore, Williams & Wilkins, 1987, pp 159–176.
17. Durward QJ, Amacher AL, Del Maestro RF, et al: Cerebral and cardiovascular responses to changes in head elevation in patients with intracranial hypertension. J Neurosurg 1983; 59:938.
18. Shapiro HM: Intracranial hypertension: Therapeutic and anesthetic considerations. Anesthesiology 1975; 43:445.
19. Ropper AH, O'Rourke D, Kennedy SK: Head position, intracranial pressure, and compliance. Neurology 1982; 32:1288.
20. Rosner MJ, Coley IB: Cerebral perfusion pressure, intracranial pressure, and head elevation. J Neurosurg 1985; 65:636.
21. Feldman Z, Kanter MJ, Robertson CS, et al: Effect of head elevation on intracranial pressure, cerebral perfusion pressure, and cerebral blood flow in head injured patients. J Neurosurg 1992; 76:207.
22. Becker DP, Gade GF, Young HF, et al: Diagnosis and treatment of head injury in adults. *In*: Neurological Surgery. 3rd ed. Youmans JR (Ed). Philadelphia, WB Saunders, 1990, pp 2017–2148.
23. French LA, Galicich JH: The use of steroids for control of cerebral edema. Clin Neurosurg 1962; 10:212.
24. Renaudin J, Fewer D, Wilson CB, et al: Dose dependency of Decadron in patients with partially excised brain tumors. J Neurosurg 1973; 39:302.
25. Osenbach RK, Loftus CM: Diagnosis and management of brain abscess. Neurosurg Clin North Am 1992; 3:403.
26. Gudeman SK, Miller JD, Becker DP: Failure of high-dose steroid therapy to influence intracranial pressure in patients with severe head injury. J Neurosurg 1979; 51:301.
27. Cooper PR, Moody S, Clark WK, et al: Dexamethasone and

severe head injury: A prospective double-blind study. J Neurosurg 1979; 51:307.
28. Dearden NM, Gibson JS, McDowall DG, et al: Effect of high-dose dexamethasone on outcome from severe head injury. J Neurosurg 1986; 64:81.
29. Nath F, Galbraith S: The effect of mannitol on cerebral white matter content. J Neurosurg 1986; 65:41.
30. Muizelaar JP, Lutz HA, Becker DP: Effect of mannitol on ICP and CBF and correlation with pressure autoregulation in severely head-injured patients. J Neurosurg 1984; 61:700.
31. Samson D, Beyer CW: Furosemide in the intraoperative reduction of intracranial pressure in the patient with subarachnoid hemorrhage. Neurosurgery 1982; 10:167.
32. Cottrell JE, Robustelli A, Post K, et al: Furosemide and mannitol-induced changes in intracranial pressure and serum osmolality and electrolytes. Anesthesiology 1977; 47:28.
33. Schettini A, Stahurski B, Young HF: Osmotic and osmotic-loop diuresis in brain surgery: Effects on plasma and CSF electrolytes and ion excretion. J Neurosurg 1982; 56:679.
34. Wilkinson HA, Rosenfeld S: Furosemide and mannitol in the treatment of acute experimental intracranial hypertension. Neurosurgery 1983; 12:405.
35. Pollay M, Fullenwider C, Roberts PA, et al: Effect of mannitol and furosemide on blood-brain osmotic gradient and intracranial pressure. J Neurosurg 1983; 59:945.
36. Donegan MF, Bedford RF: Intravenously administered lidocaine prevents intracranial hypertension during endotracheal suctioning. Anesthesiology 1980; 52:516.
37. Yano M, Nishiyama H, Yokota H, et al: Effect of lidocaine on ICP response to endotracheal suctioning. Anesthesiology 1986; 64:651.
38. Muizelaar JP, Maramarou A, Ward JD: Adverse effects of prolonged hyperventilation in patients with severe head injury: A randomized clinical trial. J Neurosurg 1991; 75:731–739.
39. Cruz J: Combined continuous monitoring of systemic and cerebral oxygenation in acute brain injury: Preliminary observations. Crit Care Med 1993; 21:1225–1232.
40. Chesnut RM, Marshall LF: Treatment of abnormal intracranial pressure. Neurosurg Clin North Am 1991; 2:267.
41. Narayan RK, Kishore PRS, Becker DP, et al: Intracranial pressure: To monitor or not to monitor? A review of our experience with severe head injury. J Neurosurg 1982; 56:650.
42. North B, Reilly P: Comparison among three methods of intracranial pressure recording. Neurosurgery 1986; 18:730.
43. Mayhall CG, Archer NH, Lamb VA, et al: Ventriculostomy-related infections: A prospective epidemiologic study. N Engl J Med 1984; 310:553.
44. Aucoin PJ, Kotilainen HR, Gantz NM, et al: Intracranial pressure monitors. Epidemiologic study of risk factors and infections. Am J Med 1986; 80:369.
45. Kanter RK, Weiner LB: Ventriculostomy-related infections. N Engl J Med 1984; 311:987.
46. Dearden NM, Miller JD: Paired comparison of hypnotic and osmotic therapy in the reduction of raised intracranial pressure (ICP) after severe head injury. *In*: Intracranial Pressure VII. Hoff JT (Ed). New York, Springer-Verlag, 1989, pp 474–481.
47. Kassell NF, Hitchon PW, Gerk MK, et al: Alterations in cerebral blood flow, oxygen metabolism, and electrical activity produced by high dose sodium thiopental. Neurosurgery 1980; 7:598.
48. Pierce EC, Lambertsen CJ, Deutsch S, et al: Cerebral circulation and metabolism during thiopental anesthesia and hyperventilation in man. J Clin Invest 1962; 41:1664.
49. Neuwelt EA, Kikuchi K, Hill SA, et al: Barbiturate inhibition of lymphocyte function. Differing effects of various barbiturates used to induce coma. J Neurosurg 1982; 56:254.
50. Moudgil GC: Effect of premedicants, intravenous anesthetic agents and local anesthetics on phagocytosis in vitro. Can J Anaesth 1981; 28:597.
51. Shapiro HM, Wyte SR, Loeser J: Barbiturate-augmented hypothermia for reduction of persistent intracranial hypertension. J Neurosurg 1974; 40:90.
52. Marshall LF, Bowers SA: Medical management of head injury. Clin Neurosurg 1981; 29:312.
53. Kassell NF, Peerless SJ, Drake CG, et al: Treatment of ischemic deficits from cerebral vasospasm with high dose barbiturate therapy. Neurosurgery 1980; 7:593.
54. Sawada Y, Sugimoto H, Kobayashi H, et al: Acute tolerance to high-dose barbiturate treatment in patients with severe head injuries. Anesthesiology 1982; 56:53.
55. Newlon PG, Greenberg RP, Enas GG, et al: Effects of therapeutic pentobarbital coma on multimodality evoked potentials recorded from severely head-injured patients. Neurosurgery 1983; 12:613.
56. Grolimund P, Weber M, Seiler RW, et al: Time course of cerebral vasospasm after severe head injury. Lancet 1988; i:1173.
57. Suwanwela C, Suwanwela N: Intracranial arterial narrowing and spasm in acute head injury. J Neurosurg 1972; 36:314.
58. Wilkins RH: Cerebral vasospasm in conditions other than subarachnoid hemorrhage. Neurosurg Clin North Am 1990; 1:329.
59. Weir B: The history of cerebral vasospasm. Neurosurg Clin North Am 1990; 1:265.
60. Heros RC, Zervas NT, Varsos V: Cerebral vasospasm after subarachnoid hemorrhage: An update. Ann Neurol 1983; 14:599.
61. Fisher CM, Kistler JP, Davis JM: Relation of cerebral vasospasm to subarachnoid hemorrhage visualized by computerized tomographic scanning. Neurosurgery 1980; 6:1.
62. Hijdra A, van Gijn J, Nagelkerke NJD, et al: Prediction of delayed cerebral ischemia, rebleeding, and outcome after aneurysmal subarachnoid hemorrhage. Stroke 1988; 19:1250.
63. Mizukami M, Takemae T, Tazawa T, et al: Value of computed tomography in the prediction of cerebral vasospasm after aneurysm rupture. Neurosurgery 1980; 7:583.
64. Adams HP, Kassell NF, Torner JC, et al: Predicting cerebral ischemia after aneurysmal subarachnoid hemorrhage: Influences of clinical condition, CT results, and antifibrinolytic therapy. Neurology 1987; 37:1586.
65. Harders AG, Gilsbach JM: Time course of blood velocity changes related to vasospasm in the circle of Willis measured by transcranial Doppler ultrasound. J Neurosurg 1987; 66:718.
66. Seiler RW, Grolimund P, Aaslid R, et al: Cerebral vasospasm evaluated by transcranial ultrasound correlated with clinical grade and CT-visualized subarachnoid hemorrhage. J Neurosurg 1986; 64:594.
67. Aaslid R, Huber P, Nornes H: Evaluation of cerebrovascular spasm with transcranial Doppler ultrasound. J Neurosurg 1984; 60:37.
68. Newell DW, Winn HR: Transcranial Doppler in cerebral vasospasm. Neurosurg Clin North Am 1990; 1:319.
69. Awad IA, Carter LP, Spetzler RF, et al: Clinical vasospasm after subarachnoid hemorrhage: Response to hypervolemic hemodilution and arterial hypertension. Stroke 1987; 18:365.
70. Kassell NF, Peerless SJ, Durward QJ, et al: Treatment of ischemic deficits from vasospasm with intravascular volume expansion and induced arterial hypertension. Neurosurgery 1982; 11:337.
71. Solomon RA, Fink ME, Lennihan L: Early aneurysm surgery and prophylactic hypervolemic hypertensive therapy for the treatment of aneurysmal subarachnoid hemorrhage. Neurosurgery 1988; 23:699.
72. Rosenstein J, Suzuki M, Symon L, et al: Clinical use of a portable bedside cerebral blood flow machine in the management of aneurysmal subarachnoid hemorrhage. Neurosurgery 1984; 15:519.
73. Levy ML, Giannotta SL: Induced hypertension and hypervolemia for treatment of cerebral vasospasm. Neurosurg Clin North Am 1990; 1:357.
74. Giannotta SL, McGillicuddy JE, Kindt GW: Diagnosis and treatment of postoperative cerebral vasospasm. Surg Neurol 1977; 8:286.
75. Thomas DJ, Marshall J, Russell RW, et al: Effect of hematocrit on cerebral blood flow in man. Lancet 1977; ii:941.
76. Philippon J, Grob R, Dagreou F, et al: Prevention of vasospasm in subarachnoid hemorrhage. A controlled study with nimodipine. Acta Neurochir (Wien) 1986; 82:110.
77. Petruk KC, West M, Mohr G, et al: Nimodipine treatment in poor-grade aneurysm patients. Results of a multicenter double-blind placebo-controlled trial. J Neurosurg 1988; 68:505.
78. Ljunggren B, Brandt L, Saveland H, et al: Outcome in 60 consecutive patients treated with early aneurysm operation and intravenous nimodipine. J Neurosurg 1984; 61:864.
79. Allen GS, Ahn HS, Preziosi TJ, et al: Cerebral arterial spasm—A controlled trial of nimodipine in patients with subarachnoid hemorrhage. N Engl J Med 1983; 308:619.

80. Seiler RW, Grolimund P, Zurbruegg HR: Evaluation of the calcium-antagonist nimodipine for the prevention of vasospasm after aneurysmal subarachnoid hemorrhage. A prospective transcranial Doppler ultrasound study. Acta Neurochir (Wien) 1987; 85:7.
81. Auer LM: Acute operation and preventive nimodipine improve outcome in patients with ruptured cerebral aneurysms. Neurosurgery 1984; 15:57.
82. Allen GS, Gross CJ, Henderson LM, et al: Cerebral arterial spasm: Part 4. In vitro effects of temperature, serotonin analogues, large nonphysiological concentrations of serotonin, and extracellular calcium and magnesium on serotonin-induced contractions of the canine basilar artery. J Neurosurg 1976; 44:585.
83. Siesjo BK: Cerebral circulation and metabolism. J Neurosurg 1984; 60:883.
84. Marsh ML, Marshall LF, Shapiro HM: Neurosurgical intensive care. Anesthesiology 1977; 47:149.
85. Lassen NA: Control of cerebral circulation in health and disease. Circ Res 1974; 34:749.
86. Spetzler RF, Wilson CB, Weinstein P, et al: Normal perfusion pressure breakthrough theory. Clin Neurosurg 1977; 25:651.
87. Hassler W, Gilsbach J: Intra- and perioperative aspects of the hemodynamics of supratentorial AV-malformations. Acta Neurochir (Wien) 1984; 73:35.
88. U HS: Microsurgical excision of paraventricular arteriovenous malformations. Neurosurgery 1985; 16:293.
89. Ojemann RG, Heros RC, Crowell RM: Arteriovenous malformations of the brain. *In*: Surgical Management of Cerebrovascular Disease. 2nd ed. Baltimore, Williams & Wilkins, 1988, pp 347–413.
90. Sugita K, Takayasu M: Arteriovenous malformations—General considerations. *In*: Brain Surgery: Complication Avoidance and Management. Apuzzo MLJ (Ed). New York, Churchill Livingstone, 1993, pp 1113–1117.
91. Stein BM, Kader A: Intracranial arteriovenous malformations. Clin Neurosurg 1991; 39:76.
92. Ropper AH, Rockoff MA: Treatment of intracranial hypertension. *In*: Neurological and Neurosurgical Intensive Care. Ropper AH, Kennedy SF (Eds). Rockville, MD, Aspen Publishers, 1988, pp 23–41.
93. Bracken MB, Shepard MJ, Collins WF, et al: Methylprednisolone or naloxone treatment after acute spinal cord injury: 1-year follow-up data. Results of the Second National Acute Spinal Cord Injury Study. J Neurosurg 1992; 76:23.
94. Hall ED: The neuroprotective pharmacology of methylprednisolone. J Neurosurg 1992; 76:13.

CHAPTER 168

Cerebral Vascular Emergencies

Sidney Starkman, MD • Bruce Dobkin, MD

Although only a modest proportion of the half million individuals who suffer an acute stroke in the United States each year require admission to a critical care unit, the near-future availability of pharmacologic interventions that enhance cerebral perfusion and protect ischemic neurons may increase the need for early critical care to use and monitor the effects of these agents. Patients with subarachnoid hemorrhage (SAH), large intracerebral hemorrhage (ICH), increased intracranial pressure (ICP), or progressive hemispheric or brain stem ischemic stroke are usually admitted to critical care units. Coma, respiratory compromise, and threatening medical, especially cardiac, disease also require special monitoring. In about 3% of non-neurologic intensive care patients, stroke complicates their course.[1]

CLASSIFICATION OF STROKE

Options for the management of stroke[2] increasingly depend upon the cause. Strokes are commonly categorized as being ischemic resulting from large arterial atherothrombosis (35%), small penetrating vessel disease (20%), and cardioembolism (25%); as being hemorrhagic (15%); or as having other causes (5%).

Ischemic Strokes

Ischemic strokes are caused by a reduction in blood supply to brain parenchyma. This category includes strokes due to acute thrombosis, to hypoperfusion distal to a stenosed or occluded artery, to embolism (cardiogenic, paradoxical, and artery-to-artery), and occasionally to profound systemic hypotension that produces infarction in the vulnerable "watershed" regions between cerebral artery territories. About 30% of ischemic strokes are preceded by a transient ischemic attack (TIA), in which symptoms usually resolve within 20 minutes but can last hours.

Ischemic strokes caused by cardiogenic emboli are commonly encountered by critical care specialists.[3] The emboli originate from mural thrombi associated with atrial fibrillation, acute myocardial infarction (primarily anterior), ventricular aneurysm, and dilated cardiomyopathy. Cardiac surgery, cardiac catheterization, prosthetic cardiac valves, and valvular heart disease are other causes. Infectious and nonbacterial thrombotic endocarditis are rarer causes. Direct or indirect trauma to carotid or vertebral arteries can cause the vessel to dissect and cause thromboemboli or occlusion. After serious trauma, fat emboli (from long bone fractures) and air emboli can produce cerebral infarction.

Hemorrhagic Strokes

Hemorrhagic strokes include SAH and ICH. SAH often results from the rupture of a saccular (berry) aneurysm. Spontaneous ICH is characteristically produced by the rupture of small, hypertension-damaged arteries in the brain parenchyma. In the elderly, amyloid angiopathy can cause lobar hemorrhages. An arteriovenous malformation can bleed superficially into the subarachnoid space or intracerebrally, as can an aneurysm. ICH is a complication in about 2% of patients receiving warfarin anticoagulation. About 1% of patients given thrombolytic treatment for acute myocardial infarction have cerebral bleeding. ICH is associated with the use of certain drugs, such as cocaine, amphetamine, and phencyclidine. Brain tumors can hemorrhage. In sickle cell disease, hemorrhagic and ischemic strokes occur. Cerebral venous sinus thrombosis is an uncommon stroke syndrome consisting of headache, focal deficits, and seizures; it is primarily seen in elderly debilitated patients and in pregnant or postpartum women.

CLINICAL FEATURES

The abrupt onset of focal cerebral dysfunction should be treated as a medical emergency so that brain injury can be minimized and complications reduced. Common symptoms include hemiparesis, aphasia, incoordination, paralysis or sensory loss of one or more limbs, hemianopsia, monocular visual loss, diplopia, dysarthria, and ataxia. The appearance of any of these signs with nausea, clumsiness, vertigo, unilateral hearing loss, vomiting, or photophobia mandates consideration of stroke. A marked change in the level or state of consciousness, for example, stupor, coma, confusion, delirium, or seizure, may develop. Headache is more commonly associated with hemorrhagic than ischemic stroke and can be a prominent symptom in arterial dissection. Sudden onset of a severe headache with or without change in mental status must prompt consideration of an SAH. Acute ataxia, vomiting, and vertigo, particularly when accompanied by acute headache, may indicate a stroke in the cerebellum.

A precise diagnosis determines the appropriate initial therapy and helps select interventions that could prevent future strokes. The history, the risk factors, the temporal features of the disorder, and the results of patient's physical and neurologic examination determine the direction of the evaluation. One aim is to distinguish between ischemia, hemorrhage, and masqueraders of stroke. Another is to localize the lesion as a cortical, subcortical, or brain stem stroke. Temporal features can help distinguish between embolic and thrombotic stroke, but not reliably. For example, in cardioembolic stroke, which most often involves the middle cerebral artery stem or its branches, the onset is sudden in most cases; in a small number of cases, the onset is progressive over 12 to 24 hours. Symptoms and signs of a large-artery thrombotic stroke may fluctuate or worsen in a step wise fashion in 20% of patients. The presence of TIAs in the same distribution as the stroke, especially repetitive, stereotyped TIAs, points to occlusive disease.[4] Thrombotic occlusion of small, penetrating arteries to the deep brain matter, including the internal capsule, basal ganglia, thalamus, and pons causes lesions commonly smaller than 1 cm (lacunae). Lacunar stroke can progress and is preceded by TIAs in nearly 25% of cases. In SAH, the onset of symptoms is rather abrupt. With ICH, focal symptoms usually peak within minutes, although bleeding can continue in 30% of patients in the first few hours.[5]

Differential Diagnosis of Stroke

The differential diagnosis of stroke includes metabolic and toxic diseases. For example, hypoglycemia can produce a focal neurologic deficit. An unwitnessed seizure may be followed by a transient postictal motor deficit. A subdural hematoma resulting from head trauma can masquerade as a stroke; however, a patient may also suffer a fall and a subsequent head injury because of a stroke. Other neuromedical problems that can be mistaken for stroke include migraine complicated by hemiparesis, basilar migraine with associated neurologic signs, brain tumor, exacerbation of underlying dementia, metabolic encephalopathy, carpal tunnel syndrome associated with hand numbness, and brachial plexopathy with arm weakness. Even relatively mild secondary factors, such as infection or electrolyte abnormalities, may allow previous stroke deficits to re-emerge. Of interest, nearly 10% of cancer patients suffer from cerebrovascular disease; the clinical presentation of an encephalopathy is as common as that of an acute focal deficit in this population.[6]

Initial Assessment

Initial laboratory tests usually include complete blood count; platelet count; determinations of prothrombin time, partial thromboplastin time, and erythrocyte sedimentation rate; syphilis serology; renal and liver function tests; chest radiography; and electrocardiography. Sodium and glucose levels, blood urea nitrogen level, osmolality, and sometimes, arterial blood gases are monitored. Antiphospholipid antibodies and additional coagulation studies may be indicated. The neurologic examination should be repeated frequently to assess improvement or deterioration in neurologic status.

DIAGNOSTIC TESTING

Noncontrast computed tomography (CT) is the usual initial diagnostic test in the acute stroke patient. CT usually detects an ICH, as well as other intracranial mass lesions, such as subdural hematoma, tumor, and abscess. The hyperdense artery sign on CT may localize an acute thrombus.[7] Infarction may first be detected on CT 6 to 12 hours after stroke onset. When symptoms progress in the ischemic stroke patient, repeat CT scans may reveal the development of hemorrhagic infarction or mass effect secondary to cerebral edema. In ICH, follow-up late CT may reveal an underlying tumor or an arteriovenous malformation. In the hemorrhagic stroke patient whose condition deteriorates, CT may demonstrate cerebral edema, rebleeding, or hydrocephalus.

Magnetic resonance imaging detects ischemic stroke earlier than does CT, but 6 to 12 hours may be needed to assess the extent of the ischemic injury. In the detection of lacunar stroke and cerebellar and brain stem infarction, magnetic resonance imaging is superior to CT. Magnetic resonance imaging may not detect acute bleeding as readily as does CT, but it may reveal an underlying tumor or an arteriovenous malformation.

The most available noninvasive studies for atherothrombotic diseases are the carotid duplex scan and the transcranial Doppler ultrasound. The carotid duplex scan, depending on technical competence, provides reliable imaging of the carotid bifurcation by combining ultrasound imaging with Doppler flow.[8] The transcranial Doppler ultrasound detects, with about 80% sensitivity, severe stenoses and occlusions of the intracranial carotid, middle cerebral, and vertebrobasilar arteries. Vasospasm after SAH can be monitored by transcranial Doppler ultrasound.[9, 10]

The use of echocardiography should be limited to patients with a suspected cardiac source of emboli. Transthoracic two-dimensional echocardiography can detect a valvular or mural source of emboli. It may detect a patent foramen ovale or an atrial septal defect. Transesophageal echocardiography is superior to transthoracic two-dimensional echocardiography to image the left atrium and left atrial appendage for thrombi, to detect a septal defect, and to assess the aorta as sources of emboli.[11]

Lumbar puncture is usually not indicated in the stroke patient. However, it is valuable for the diagnosis of suspected SAH when the CT result is negative. Also, it is performed when the diagnosis of bacterial meningitis or septic embolism is being considered.

Magnetic resonance angiography may be especially useful in the detection of carotid bifurcation, vertebrobasilar and middle cerebral artery occlusive disease, and aneurysms. In patients with TIAs and mild stroke, angiography is particularly valuable[12] to distinguish between atherothrombotic and cardioembolic stroke. If performed within 24 hours of onset, it may detect an embolus before its lysis and migration. Angiography is indicated in younger patients and in those in whom an unusual cause is suspected, such as cervicocephalic dissection, fibromuscular dysplasia, and vasculitis. When extracranial carotid surgery is being planned, angiography is usually indicated to optimally assess the bifurcation and to detect tandem arterial lesions. In SAH, angiography defines the feeders to an arteriovenous malformation, visualizes the aneurysm that bled, locates other aneurysms, and detects vasospasm. In venous sinus thrombosis, angiography is diagnostic, although CT, magnetic resonance imaging, and magnetic resonance angiography may also detect this disorder.

GENERAL MANAGEMENT

Critical care management of stroke patients includes close observation of unstable patients, monitoring of hemodynamic and pulmonary parameters, and treatment for brain swelling and increased ICP.[13] The mortality and morbidity of patients with acute stroke may be reduced when careful attention is paid to aeration, hydration, and nutrition, and when measures are taken to prevent infection, decubitus ulcers, and venous thrombosis. Blood pressure, intravascular volume, temperature, oxygenation, and glucose level must be monitored.

Airway Management and Oxygenation

Strokes that depress level of consciousness and affect lower bulbar function can limit the patient's ability to maintain and protect the airway. The risk of hypoxia, hypoventilation with hypercapnia, and aspiration also increases. Prophylactic intubation may be needed in these patients. Hypoxia may cause additional cellular injury, especially in cerebral tissue that is hypoperfused. Common causes of hypoxia include aspiration pneumonia, pulmonary embolism, congestive heart failure, and obstructive breathing patterns.

Intracranial Pressure

Fever, overhydration, hypoxia, hypercapnia, agitation, increased central venous pressure, increased mean airway pressure, and impairment of venous outflow by compression of neck veins or awkward neck position can affect ICP. The head should be elevated to 30°.[2] If ICP is being monitored, optimal position should be determined by varying the head position. Stool softeners may prevent straining, which can also affect ICP. Despite their antivasogenic cerebral edema and free radical scavenging properties, glucocorticoids have not demonstrated a beneficial effect in the treatment of acute stroke. Glycerol and dextran have had equivocal efficacy.

Patients with elevated ICP and declining level of consciousness or other signs of herniation should be intubated and hyperventilated to a Pco_2 of 25 to 30 mm Hg. Coughing, gagging, or agitation during intubation or suctioning can cause rises in blood pressure and ICP; these rises can be blunted by pretreatment with intravenous lidocaine. Mannitol osmotic therapy also reduces ICP.

Blood Pressure

Management of blood pressure is one of the most important considerations in the critical care of stroke patients.[13a] In a healthy brain, cerebral blood flow is autoregulated to protect the tissue from fluctuations in blood pressure and to provide adequate cerebral perfusion. With chronic hypertension, autoregulation is maintained, but at higher blood pressure levels. In the injured brain region, the blood vessels may lose their ability to autoregulate in response to alterations in blood pressure, carbon dioxide tension, or hypoxia. Consequently, cerebral perfusion depends on mean arterial blood pressure and ICP. Lowering the systemic blood pressure can produce clinical deterioration. In the case of ischemic stroke, hypertension should not be treated acutely unless the mean arterial blood pressure (diastolic + ⅓ [systolic − diastolic] = pulse pressure) is greater than 140 mm Hg or the systolic pressure exceeds 200 mm Hg. The initially elevated blood pressure usually falls spontaneously within 12 to 72 hours.[14, 15] Often, relief of pain, agitation, hypoxia, and vomiting are sufficient to induce normal levels of blood pressure. In the case of SAH, rebleeding and mortality rates are higher if the blood pressure is elevated soon after the ictus. Blood pressure should be aggressively controlled preoperatively. Antihypertensive agents should be used if bed rest, sedation, and measures to avoid straining and coughing are not sufficient.

The management of hypertension in patients with ICH is similar to that of patients with ischemic infarction. Areas of the brain adjacent to an intracerebral hematoma may become ischemic, partly from mass effect. Acute therapy for hypertension could lead to additional decreases in perfusion.[16] Persistent, severe hypertension might cause additional bleeding into the hematoma. Careful treatment of severe hypertension should be pursued if the patient is in danger of myocardial, aortic, or renal damage associated with the hypertension.

Only parenteral drugs should be used acutely. Common agents include nitroprusside, administered by constant infusion, and β-blockers, such as labetalol, administered parenterally. The latter drug has a half-life of 6 hours. The disadvantage of nitroprusside is that it is a cerebral vasodilator and can cause an increase in ICP, particularly in patients who already have cerebral swelling or a mass effect from a hematoma. Nitroprusside, however, is readily titratable and has a rapid onset and offset.

Intravascular Volume

Optimization of cardiac output and treatment of hypovolemia should be important priorities in the maintenance of cerebral perfusion pressure. Dehydration and hemoconcentration should be avoided. Administration of fluids may reduce blood viscosity and improve cerebral perfusion. Care must be taken to avoid hyponatremia and free-water overload, which can exacerbate cerebral edema after a large infarction or an ICH; therefore, normal saline should be administered. Studies of hypervolemic and normovolemic hemodilution have not shown a clear benefit, although no study has achieved the goal of a hematocrit value of about 33% to 35% within 12 hours of the stroke.[17] Volume expansion and even venesection should be considered when the hematocrit value is greater than 50%, especially in progressing ischemic stroke.

Temperature

Hyperthermia increases cerebral blood flow and volume, resulting in elevated ICP. Treatment should be aggressive and immediate. Of course, fever is most often an indicator of infectious disease and is usually not a manifestation of cerebral or hypothalamic injury.

Blood Glucose Level

Both hyperglycemia and hypoglycemia may be harmful. Hyperglycemia in the acute phase of stroke is associated with poor outcome.[18] Glucose levels above 200 mg/dL should be treated with insulin, although the benefit of strict glucose management in acute stroke is controversial.

TREATMENT OF ISCHEMIC STROKE

At present, no therapies can ameliorate the damage caused by an ischemic injury.[19, 20, 20a] Investigational strategies are directed toward thrombolysis and neuronal protection.

Antithrombotic Therapy

Antithrombotic therapy with anticoagulants, such as heparin and warfarin, is frequently employed, but its benefit in acute and progressing stroke is uncertain.[21] Heparin is also used for recent TIA and for early prevention of recurrent cardioembolism.[22, 23] In addition, heparin is sometimes used after acute thrombosis of a large vessel to prevent the extension of thrombus intracranially. It is administered intravenously without a bolus in instances in which a greater than one third hemispheric infarction is present. Generally, nothing is gained from anticoagulation, and some risk of clinically significant hemorrhage into an infarct exists when the results of the examination or imaging studies point to a two thirds or greater area of hemispheric infarction, especially in the elderly or the hypertensive patient. In arterial dissection with significant vessel narrowing, heparin may be useful in preventing thrombosis and embolism. In cerebral venous thrombosis, heparin seems to have some benefit, even in patients with some intracranial hemorrhage related to the venous occlusions, but the results of clinical trials are pending.[24]

Patients with small cardioembolic strokes whose CT scan at about 48 hours after the event does not show hemorrhagic transformation can be given anticoagulants. Asymptomatic spontaneous hemorrhagic transformation commonly appears in the infarcted region within the first few days. After a large cardioembolic stroke, anticoagulation is most safely withheld for 5 to 7 days after cerebral infarction. If a CT scan shows no significant area of hemorrhage into the infarct, the drug can be started; but, remarkably, clinical deterioration is unusual in patients who are receiving heparin and have a patchy hemorrhagic stroke.[25] An International Stroke Trial comparing aspirin, heparin, and their combination as treatment for acute ischemic stroke is under way. Also, low-molecular-weight heparinoids, which appear less likely to cause bleeding complications, are under clinical investigation.[26]

Antithrombotic therapy with the antiplatelet medications aspirin and ticlopidine is widely used in patients not receiving anticoagulant drugs. Although studies have not proved their efficacy in acute stroke, both agents help prevent recurrent stroke and stroke after atherothrombotic TIA.

Studies of fibrinolytic therapy with ancrod, recombinant tissue plasminogen activator, streptokinase, and urokinase for acute arterial occlusions suggest potential, but still uncertain, benefits of these products.

Neuronal Protection

A major focus of current stroke research is the use of "neuroprotective agents" to reduce neuronal injury after the onset of ischemia.[27] Neuroprotective therapy is partly based on the notion that calcium flux and calcium-activated enzymes contribute to neuronal insult after ischemia by triggering a cascade of events that lead to cell death. In a healthy neuron, free calcium is usually excluded from the cytosol. Intracellular levels increase after ischemia because of calcium flux into the cell and liberation of intracellular stores. In addition, calcium-activated proteases and phospholipases produce free radicals, which destroy the cell membrane. One trigger for calcium influx into neurons is the excitatory neurotransmitter glutamate, whose release is induced by ischemia.[27a] Glutamate receptor antagonists reduce ischemic neuronal injury in animal models; however, the mechanism may actually be improved regional cerebral blood flow rather than neuroprotection.[28, 29] Several drugs whose actions are aimed at correcting these abnormalities are currently under clinical evaluation. Calcium channel blockers may benefit patients treated within 6 hours of the onset of ischemic stroke. Studies in humans have not revealed a clear benefit when the drug was started 12 to 24 hours after onset.[30] Nimodipine has been shown to be of benefit in patients after SAH, although the mechanism for this effect is uncertain. Other investigational drugs, including free radical scavengers, such as the 21-aminosteroids, are being tested.[30a]

TREATMENT OF INTRACEREBRAL HEMORRHAGE

Surgery for ICH remains controversial. When a hematoma causes progressive deterioration secondary to mass effect, evacuation should be considered. Cerebellar hemorrhages often present as a surgical emergency. They can cause brain stem compression, can halt respiration, and can result in death. Also, acute hydrocephalus may occur if the cerebellum impinges on the fourth ventricle. Surgical evacuation of large cerebellar hemorrhages should be performed before consciousness is greatly decreased.[31] Patients with small cerebellar hemorrhage and no hydrocephalus can be treated by close observation. Those with more superficial lobar hematomas or accessible subcortical intracranial hemorrhages can improve after surgical intervention. An alert patient with ICH whose level of consciousness declines may warrant emergent surgical evacuation. Patients with large, deep hematomas affecting the basal ganglia and brain stem do not usually benefit from surgery.[32] Intraventricular hemorrhage is not itself an ominous sign but may result in hydrocephalus. Ventriculostomy should be considered early in patients with acute hydrocephalus and in some patients with intracerebral hematomas whose conditions are deteriorating. Prognosis is usually poor for elderly patients who have large hematomas and a decreased level of consciousness. With the advent of stereotactic surgery and the use of thrombolytics for clot dissolution, the role of surgery in ICH could increase.

TREATMENT OF SUBARACHNOID HEMORRHAGE

After the rupture of an intracranial aneurysm, aneurysmal rebleeding, vasospasm, and hydrocephalus commonly occur, with associated morbidity and mortality.[33, 34] The risk of aneurysmal rebleeding, which has an associated mortality of about 30%, is highest within the first 48 hours. Rebleeding is prevented by microsurgical clipping of the aneurysm. When the aneurysm is surgically inaccessible, such as an intracavernous aneurysm, an interventional neuroradiologist can ablate the aneurysm with balloon occlusion or coil thrombosis. The timing of the aneurysm clipping is controversial, but earlier aneurysm surgery can result in improved outcome.[35, 36] Patients with mild deficits (Hunt and Hess grades I–III[37]) are generally operated on within the first 24 to 48 hours.[38] Stuporous and comatose patients at Hunt and Hess grades IV and V can significantly improve after clot evacuation and treatment of hydrocephalus. Presurgical therapy usually involves careful control of blood pressure and administration of mild sedatives, anticonvulsants, and stool softeners.

The incidence and extent of delayed-onset cerebral vasospasm following SAH correlates with the amount of bleeding visualized by CT. The vasospasm, angiographically seen in 75% of SAH patients, can result in ischemic injury. It is treated prophylactically with calcium channel blockers, such as nimodipine.[39] When SAH is identified, noncomatose patients should be given nimodipine orally or via nasogastric tube, and the therapy should continue for 21 days. Nimopidine improves outcome in SAH without a decrease in the incidence and the severity of arteriographically detected vasospasm.[40] Avoid hypotension usually associated with volume contraction. After the aneurysm is clipped, intracisternal injection of tissue plasminogen activator may enhance the clearing of blood from the subarachnoid space and thus prevent vasospasm.[41–43] Once the aneurysm is successfully clipped, the combination of hypervolemic and hypertensive therapy can reduce morbidity in the patient who develops symptomatic vasospasm after surgery. Volume expansion is accomplished via administration of saline solution with colloid. A Swan-Ganz catheter may be needed for hemodynamic monitoring of optimal cardiac output. Controlled increase of arterial blood pressure by 10% to 15% using the vasopressors dopamine or dobutamine may, over hours, reverse the neurologic deficit from vasospasm. Percutaneous transluminal balloon angioplasty can be beneficial in selected patients who have persistent arterial narrowing.

Hydrocephalus occurring after SAH can be acute, subacute, and delayed. Acute obstructive hydrocephalus may develop after intraventricular hemorrhage or when blood is deposited in the basal cisterns. Continual coma or abrupt onset of stupor may indicate the presence of hydrocephalus; it should be diagnosed by CT or MRI and should be treated immediately by ventriculostomy. Continuous cerebrospinal fluid drainage can be accomplished with repeated lumbar punctures or a ventriculoperitoneal shunt. Subacute hydrocephalus may develop in the first few days to a week after SAH and is characterized by the gradual, although sometimes acute, onset of stupor. Delayed hydrocephalus occurs 10 days to months after hemorrhage and is characterized by gait apraxia, urinary incontinence, and cognitive dysfunction. Therapy via ventriculoperitoneal drainage can reverse most impairments.

Hyponatremia commonly occurs after SAH, as does volume contraction. Regulation of antidiuretic hormone is disturbed, and plasma atrial natriuretic factor level is elevated. Administration of fluids in excess of maintenance levels prevents the development of volume depletion, but not hyponatremia.[44] The hyponatremia is treated with hypertonic saline and a diuretic.

The surgical treatment of arteriovenous malformations is complicated by their size and their location. Combined preoperative endovascular embolization and various surgical and radiosurgical techniques are used.[45]

COMPLICATIONS

Most stroke patients, with the exception of hemorrhagic patients, die from complications related to the stroke rather than from the stroke itself.[46–48] Death in the first 2 weeks after infarction is usually due to cerebral edema and transtentorial herniation or cardiac and pulmonary complications. Complications of acute stroke can be divided into two categories: neurologic and nonneurologic.

Neurologic

Cerebral Edema and Transtentorial Herniation

Transtentorial herniation is the leading cause of death within the first week of hemorrhagic and ischemic strokes. Edema, which is mostly intracellular, complicates 20% of large hemispheric infarctions and produces brain stem compression. The cerebral edema usually becomes clinically important 2 to 5 days after the onset of the stroke.[13] The earliest signs of transtentorial herniation are a change in the patient's level of consciousness and ipsilateral pupil dilatation. A large cerebellar infarction that swells can rapidly lead to lethargy and brain stem signs.[49] Efforts to lower the ICP and to decrease the swelling should be made immediately. Surgical removal of an edematous cerebellum may be life saving, and the residual deficit is usually negligible.[50]

Seizures

Approximately 5% to 7% of stroke patients have a seizure within 24 hours of the stroke. These early, often focal, seizures are not associated with a higher mortality rate or a worse functional outcome, although the risk of developing late epilepsy may be elevated. Neurologic worsening is common following a seizure that occurs after a stroke. This situation calls for anticonvulsant therapy in the long term after a first or repeated seizure beyond the first few days.

Nonneurologic

Cardiac Arrhythmias and Myocardial Infarction

Atrial fibrillation occurs in approximately 18% of patients who have a cerebral infarction or hemorrhage. Four per cent of patients have more serious arrhythmias. Patients thought to have cardiac arrhythmias should undergo electrocardiographic monitoring. Acute myocardial infarction occurs concomitantly with stroke onset in up to 3% of patients.[51] Of interest, fewer than 2% of patients with acute myocardial infarction develop ischemic strokes, and 85% of such strokes occur within the first month.[52]

Pneumonia

Because pneumonia is the leading cause of death in the weeks that follow cerebral infarction or hemorrhage, its prevention is particularly important. Although it may be clinically inapparent, aspiration is likelier to occur in patients with bilateral strokes, but it occurs initially after unilateral strokes in almost 50% of patients. Patients at risk for developing pneumonia should sit upright at 30°. Therapies include pulmonary toilet, encouragement of coughing, and postural drainage. Oral feeding should be avoided until the patient can swallow without coughing and can cough on command. In patients with obvious impairment of oropharyngeal control, tube feedings are needed until aspiration can no longer be detected by examination or by barium swallow and until oral intake provides greater than 800 cal/d. A Dobbhoff tube can be used in patients who remain too lethargic to safely swallow and in patients who are alert but have dysphagia. Because predicting the duration of the dysphagia is difficult, placement of a percutaneous gastrojejunostomy can be postponed, particularly if inpatient rehabilitation is planned.

Deep Venous Thrombosis

Weakness and immobility substantially increase the risk of deep venous thrombosis (DVT), especially in the paretic leg; the incidence of subclinical DVT is as high as 75% up to 2 weeks after a stroke. Diagnosis can be difficult because some patients are asymptomatic and unable to complain as a result of impaired speech or altered consciousness. Mortality can be higher in acute stroke patients who develop DVT than in those patients who do not.[53] Early mobilization is important in preventing DVT. The National Institutes of Health consensus conference on the prevention of venous thrombosis and pulmonary embolism recommends prophylaxis with low-dose heparin, 5000 U every 12 hours SC, in nonambulatory stroke patients who have no contraindications.[53] Low-molecular-weight heparinoids are being studied in the prevention of DVT. Patients with a hemorrhagic stroke or other contraindications benefit from external pneumatic compression and elastic stockings.

Pulmonary Embolism

Pulmonary embolism is the fourth commonest cause of death in patients who have had a stroke. It usually occurs when the DVT involves the vessels proximal to the popliteal vein. Once a diagnosis of pulmonary embolism is made, definitive anticoagulant treatment should be initiated; in situations in which anticoagulation is risky or contraindicated, insertion of a filter or inferior vena caval ligation may be needed.

Urinary Disorders

Urinary incontinence is a common problem after stroke, occurring initially in 60% of patients. However, 6 months after a stroke, only 15% remain incontinent, a level similar to that seen in the general elderly population. Urinary incontinence seen in the first week after a stroke may have prognostic significance, causing a higher morbidity and mortality. Urinary tract infections are common.

SECONDARY PREVENTION AFTER TRANSIENT ISCHEMIC ATTACK AND ISCHEMIC STROKE

Approximately 11% of patients with atherothrombotic stroke have a recurrent stroke within the first year. A recurrent stroke is associated with a longer hospital stay and higher mortality.[54] Prevention of recurrent stroke involves directing attention to the risk factors for stroke.[55–58] Nearly one third of untreated TIAs result in ischemic stroke; of these, 20% do so within a month, and 50% do so in the year after the first episode.

Suggested pharmacologic interventions include administration of aspirin[59] or ticlopidine.[60, 61] Investigators debate whether the daily aspirin dose should be low (30 to 80 mg) or high (325 to 1300 mg).[62] Patients with atrial fibrillation are usually treated with warfarin.

Carotid endarterectomy is beneficial after TIA or nondisabling stroke in patients with a bifurcation stenosis of 70% or more.[63, 64]

REHABILITATION

Twenty per cent to 30% of stroke survivors are likely to require inpatient rehabilitation. Motivated patients who require moderate-to-maximum assistance in mobility and self-care are excellent candidates for a short-term rehabilitation program. The goal of such rehabilitation is to reach a level of function sufficiently independent to avoid nursing home placement. The social worker, therapists, and family should be involved early in discharge planning.[65]

CONCLUSION

Stroke therapy may be entering a golden age in which new pharmacologic agents, advanced imaging and perfusion technology, and multicenter national and international clinical trials could lead to treatments that reduce morbidity.[66, 67] Public education is needed to encourage risk factor reduction and to increase awareness of the signs and symptoms of stroke. Some emerging therapies may have to be applied within 90 minutes of a stroke and others within 6 hours.[68–70] Neurologists, neurosurgeons, neuroradiologists, emergency physicians, and critical care specialists, along with rehabilitation professionals and family members, need to work together to lessen impairments and to improve the quality of life of stroke patients.

ACKNOWLEDGMENT

The authors wish to express their gratitude to Danica Barron, whose research efforts and assistance in the preparation of this chapter proved invaluable.

References

1. Bleck TP, Smith MC, Pierre-Louis SJC, et al: Neurologic complications of critical medical illnesses. Crit Care Med 1993; 21:98.
2. Grotta JC: Medical progress: Current medical and surgical therapy for cerebrovascular disease. N Engl J Med 1987; 317:1505.
3. Levine SR: Acute cerebral ischemia in a critical care unit. Arch Intern Med 1989; 149:90.
4. Dobkin B: Orthostatic hypotension as a risk factor for symptomatic cerebrovascular disease. Neurology 1989; 38:30.
5. Broderick JP, Brott TG, Tomsick T, et al: Ultra-early evaluation of intracranial hemorrhage. J Neurosurg 1990; 72:195.
6. Rogers LR: Cerebrovascular complications in cancer patients. Neurol Clin 1991; 9:889.
7. Leys D, Pruvo JP, Godefroy O, et al: Prevalence and significance of hyperdense middle cerebral artery in acute stroke. Stroke 1992; 23:317.
8. Sutton-Tyrell K, Wolfson SK Jr, Thompson T, et al: Measurement of variability in duplex scanning. Stroke 1992; 23:215.
9. Caplan LR, Brass LM, DeWitt LD, et al: Transcranial Doppler ultrasound: Present status. Neurology 1990; 40:696.
10. Petty GW, Wiebers DO, Meissner I: Transcranial Doppler ultrasonography: Clinical applications in cerebrovascular disease. Mayo Clin Proc 1990; 65:1350.
11. De Rook FA, Comess KA, Albers GW, et al: Transesophageal echocardiography in the evaluation of stroke. Ann Intern Med 1992; 117:11.
12. Caplan L, Wolpert S: Arteriography in occlusive strokes. AJNR Am J Neuroradiol 1991; 120:593.
13. Wechsler LR, Ropper AH: Management of stroke in the intensive care unit. Semin Neurol 1986; 6:324.
13a. Lisk DR, Grotta JC, Lamki LM, et al: Should hypertension be treated after acute stroke? A randomized controlled trial using single photon emission computed tomography. Arch Neurol 1993; 50:855.
14. Broderick J, Brott T, Barsan W, et al: Blood pressure during the first hours of acute focal cerebral ischemia. Neurology 1990; 40(Suppl 1):145.
15. Brott T, Reed RL: Intensive care for acute stroke in a community hospital setting: The first 24 hours. Stroke 1989; 20:694.
16. Powers WJ: Acute hypertension after stroke. The scientific basis for treatment decisions. Neurology 1993; 43:461.
17. The Hemodilution in Stroke Study Group: Hypervolemic hemodilution treatment of acute stroke. Results of a randomized multicenter trial using pentastarch. Stroke 1989; 20:317.
18. Pulsinelli WA, Levy DE, Sigsbee B, et al: Increased damage after ischemic stroke in patients with hyperglycemia with or without established diabetes mellitus. Am J Med 1983; 74:540.
19. Barsan WG, Brott TG, Olinger CP, et al: Early treatment for acute ischemic stroke. Ann Intern Med 1989; 222:449.
20. Biller J: Medical management of acute cerebral ischemia. Neurol Clin 1992; 10:63.
20a. Adams HP, Brott TG, Crowell RM, et al: Guidelines for the management of patients with acute ischemic stroke: A statement for healthcare professionals from a special writing group of the Stroke Council, American Heart Association. Stroke 1994; 25:1901.
21. Haley EC Jr, Kassell NF, Torner JC: Failure of heparin to prevent progression in progressing ischemic stroke. Stroke 1988; 19:10.
22. Rothrock JF, Hart RG: Antithrombotic therapy in cerebrovascular disease. Ann Intern Med 1991; 115:885.
23. Sherman DG, Dyken ML, Fisher M: Antithrombotic therapy for cerebrovascular disorders. Chest 1992; 102:529S.
24. Pessin MS, Estol CJ, Lafranchise F, et al: Safety of anticoagulation after hemorrhagic infarction. Neurology 1993; 43:1298.
25. Einhaupl KM, Villringer A, Meister W, et al: Heparin treatment in sinus venous thrombosis. Lancet 1991; 338:597.
26. Massey EW, Biller J, Davis JN, et al: Large-dose infusions of heparinoid ORG 10172 in ischemic stroke. Stroke 1990; 21:1289.
27. Zivin, JA, Choi DW: Stroke therapy. Sci Am 1991; 265:56.
27a. Stuart LA, Rosenberg PA: Excitatory amino acids as a final common pathway for neurologic disorders. N Engl J Med 1994; 330:613.
28. Buchan A: Advances in cerebral ischemia: Experimental approaches. Neurol Clin 1992; 10:49.
29. Smith SE, Meldrum B: Cerebroprotective effect of a non-*N*-methyl-D-aspartate antagonist, GYKI 52:466, after focal ischemia in rat. Stroke 1992; 23:861.
30. The American Nimodipine Study Group: Clinical trial of nimodipine in acute ischemic stroke. Stroke 1992; 23:3.
30a. The STIPAS Investigators: Safety study of tirilazad mesylate in

patients with acute ischemic stroke (STIPAS). Stroke 1994; 25:418.
31. Auer LM, Auer T, Sayama I: Indications for surgical treatment of cerebellar hemorrhage and infarction. Acta Neurochir (Wien) 1986; 79:74.
32. Batjer HH, Reisch JS, Allen BC, et al: Failure of surgery to improve outcome in hypertensive putaminal hemorrhage: A prospective randomized trial. Arch Neurol 1990; 47:1013.
33. Kirsch JR, Diringer MN, Borel CO, et al: Cerebral aneurysms: Mechanisms of injury and critical care interventions. Crit Care Clin 1989; 5:755.
34. Whiting DM, Barnett GH, Little JR: Management of subarachnoid hemorrhage in the critical care unit. Cleve Clin J Med 1989; 56:775.
35. Haley EC Jr, Kassell NF, Torner JC, et al: The international cooperative study on the timing of aneurysm surgery: The North American experience. Stroke 1992; 23:205.
36. Kassell NF, Torner JC, Haley EC Jr, et al: The international cooperative study on the timing of aneurysm surgery: Part I. Overall management results. J Neurosurg 1990; 73:18.
37. Hunt RC, Hess RN: Surgical risk as related to time of intervention in the repair of intracranial aneurysms. J Neurosurg 1968; 28:1920.
38. Solomon RA, Onesti ST, Klebanoff L: Relationship between the timing of aneurysm surgery and the development of delayed cerebral ischaemia. J Neurosurg 1991; 75:56.
39. Phillippon J, Grob R, Dagreau F, et al: Prevention of vasospasm in subarachnoid hemorrhage: A controlled study with nimodipine. Acta Neurochir (Wien) 1986; 82:110.
40. Pickard JD, Murray GD, Illingworth R, et al: Effect of oral nimodipine on cerebral infarction and outcome after subarachnoid haemorrhage. British Aneurysm Nimodipine Trial. Br Med J 1989; 298:636.
41. Finlay JM, Weir BKA, Kassell NF, et al: Intracisternal recombinant tissue plasminogen activator after aneurysmal subarachnoid haemorrhage. J Neurosurg 1991; 75:181.
42. Ohman J, Servo A, Heiskanen O: Effect of intrathecal fibrinolytic therapy on clot lysis and vasospasm in patients with aneurysmal subarachnoid haemorrhage. J Neurosurg 1991; 75:197.
43. Zambramski JM, Spetzler RF, Lee KS, et al: Phase I trial of tissue plasminogen activator for the prevention of vasospasm in patients with aneurysmal subarachnoid haemorrhage. J Neurosurg 1991; 75:189.
44. Diringer MN, Wu KC, Verbalis JG, et al: Hypervolemic therapy prevents volume contraction but not hyponatremia following subarachnoid hemorrhage. Ann Neurol 1992; 31:543.
45. Vinuela F, Dion JE, Duckwiler G: Combined endovascular embolization and surgery in the management of cerebral arteriovenous malformations: Experience with 101 cases. J Neurosurg 1991; 75:856.
46. Brown M, Glassenberg M: Mortality factors in patients with acute stroke. JAMA 1973; 224:1493.
47. Chambers BR, Norris JW, Shurvell BL, et al: Prognosis of acute stroke. Neurology 1987; 37:221.
48. Silver FL, Norris JW, Lewis AJ, et al: Early mortality following stroke: A prospective review. Stroke 1984; 15:492.
49. MacDonell RAL, Kalnins RM, Donnan GA: Cerebellar infarction natural history, prognosis and pathology. Stroke 1987; 18:849.
50. Heros RC: Surgical treatment of cerebellar infarction. Stroke 1992; 23:937.
51. Behar S, Tanne D, Abinader E: Cerebrovascular accident complicating acute myocardial infarction: Incidence, clinical significance and short- and long-term mortality rates. The SPRINT Study Group. Am J Med 1991; 91:45.
52. Landi G, Dangelo A, Boccardi E, et al: Venous thromboembolism in acute stroke: Prognostic importance of hypercoagulability. Arch Neurol 1992; 49:279.
53. Consensus conference on prevention of venous thrombosis and pulmonary embolism. JAMA 1986; 256:744.
54. American Hospital Association Statistics Table 12A. Chicago, American Hospital Association, 1992, p 214.
55. Shinton R, Beevers G: Meta-analysis of relation between cigarette smoking and stroke. Br Med J 1989; 298:789.
56. Stroke Prevention in Atrial Fibrillation Investigators: Stroke Prevention in Atrial Fibrillation Study: Final results. Circulation 1991; 84:527.
56a. Stroke Prevention in Atrial Fibrillation Investigators: Warfarin versus aspirin for prevention of thromboembolism in atrial fibrillation: Stroke Prevention in Atrial Fibrillation II Study. Lancet 1994; 343:687.
57. Systolic Hypertension in the Elderly Program Cooperative Research Group: Prevention of stroke by antihypertensive drug treatment in older persons with isolated systolic hypertension: Final results of the Systolic Hypertension in the Elderly Program. JAMA 1991; 265:3255.
58. Wolf PA, Belanger AJ, D'Agostino RB: Management of risk factors. Neurol Clin 1992; 10:177.
59. Warlow C: Secondary prevention of stroke. Lancet 1992; 339:724.
60. Gent M, Blakely JA, Easton JD, et al: The Canadian American Ticlopidine Study (CATS) in thromboembolic stroke. Lancet 1989; i:1215.
61. Hass WK, Easton JD, Adams HP Jr, et al: A randomized trial comparing ticlopidine hydrochloride with aspirin for the prevention of stroke in high-risk patients. N Engl J Med 1989; 321:501.
62. Van Gijn J: Aspirin-dose and indications in modern stroke prevention. Neurol Clin 1992; 10:193.
63. North American Symptomatic Carotid Endarterectomy Trial Collaborators: Beneficial effect of carotid endarterectomy in symptomatic patients with high-grade carotid stenosis. N Engl J Med 1991; 325:445.
64. European Carotid Surgery Trialists' Collaborative Group: MRC European Surgery Trial: Interim results for symptomatic patients with severe (70–99%) or with mild (0–29%) carotid stenosis. Lancet 1991; 337:1235.
65. Dobkin BH: The rehabilitation of elderly stroke patients. Clin Geriatr Med 1991; 7:507.
66. Fisher M, Bogousslavsky J: Evolving toward effective therapy for acute ischemic stroke. JAMA 1993; 270:360.
67. Hallenbeck JM, Frerichs KU: Stroke therapy. Arch Neurol 1993; 50:768.
68. National Stroke Association Consensus Statement: Emergency evaluation and treatment. Stroke: The first six hours. J Stroke Cerebrovasc Dis 1993; 3:133.
69. Scheinberg P: The biologic basis for the treatment of acute stroke. Neurology 1991; 41:1867.
70. Camarata PJ, Heros RC, Latchaw RE: "Brain attack": The rationale for treating stroke as a medical emergency. Neurosurgery 1994; 34:144.

CHAPTER 169A

Seizures in the Critically Ill

Thomas P. Bleck, MD, FCCM

Seizures complicate the course of about 3% of adult intensive care unit (ICU) patients admitted for non-neurologic conditions. The medical and economic impact of these seizures confers importance on them out of proportion to their incidence. A seizure is often the first indication of a central nervous system (CNS) complication; thus, its rapid diagnosis is mandatory. In addition, since epilepsy affects 2% of the population, patients with preexisting seizures occasionally enter the ICU for treatment of other problems. Since the initial treatment of these patients is the province of the intensivist, he or she must be familiar with seizure management as it affects the critically ill patient. Patients developing status epilepticus (SE) often require the care of a critical care specialist in addition to that of a neurologist.

Seizures have been recognized at least since Hippocratic times, but their relatively high rate of occurrence in critically ill patients has only recently been recognized. Seizures complicating critical care treatments (e.g., lidocaine use) are also a recent phenomenon. Early attempts at treatment included the use of bromide[1] and morphine[2] as well as ice applications. Barbiturates were first employed in 1912, and phenytoin in 1937.[3] Paraldehyde was popular in the next two decades.[4] More recently, emphasis has shifted toward the benzodiazepines, which were pioneered in the 1960s.[5]

EPIDEMIOLOGY

Limited data are available on the epidemiology of seizures in the ICU. A 10-year retrospective study of all ICU patients with seizures at the Mayo Clinic revealed that 7 patients had seizures per 1000 ICU admissions.[6] Our 2-year prospective study of medical ICU patients identified 35 with seizures per 1000 admissions.[7] These two studies are not exactly comparable, as the patient populations and methods of detection differed in each. Seizures are probably even more frequent in pediatric ICUs.

Certain ICU patients are at higher risk for seizures, but the degree to which they are has not been quantitated. Theophylline frequently produces seizures or SE if it has been inadvisedly rapidly loaded or if high concentrations of the drug occur; however, occasionally these complications arise at "therapeutic" levels. Renal failure or an altered blood-brain barrier increases the likelihood of seizures for patients receiving imipenem-cilastatin, but other patients receiving this antibiotic (or γ-aminobutyric acid [GABA] antagonists like penicillin) are also at risk. Transplant recipients, especially those receiving cyclosporin, are also at increased risk, as are those who rapidly become hypo-osmolar for any reason. Nonketotic hyperglycemia patients have an unusual predisposition toward partial seizures and partial SE.

Incidence estimates for generalized convulsive SE (GCSE) in the United States vary from 50,000 cases per year[8] to 250,000 cases per year.[9, 9a] Some portion of the difference can be accounted for by different definitions; however, the latter estimate represents the only population-based data available and may be more accurate. Mortality estimates similarly vary from 1% to 2% in the former study to 22% in the latter. This disagreement follows from a conceptual discordance: the smaller number describes mortality that the authors directly attribute to SE, whereas the larger figure estimates the overall mortality rate, even though death was frequently caused by the underlying disease rather than by SE itself. For example, the study of DeLorenzo and coworkers[9] included SE due to anoxia in its SE mortality estimate. In many of the reports surveyed in the earlier review,[8] such patients would not have been included.

Many risk factors emerged from the Richmond study.[9, 9a] SE lasting longer than 1 hour carried a mortality rate of 32% compared with 2.7% for SE with a duration of less than 1 hour. SE caused by anoxia resulted in 70% mortality in adults but less than 10% mortality in children. The commonest cause of SE in adults was stroke, followed by withdrawal from antiepileptic drug therapy, cryptogenic SE, and SE related to alcohol withdrawal, anoxia, and metabolic disorders. Systemic infection was the commonest cause of SE in childhood, followed by congenital anomalies, anoxia, metabolic problems, anticonvulsant withdrawal, CNS infections, and trauma.

The data in Table 169A–1, based on 20 years of experience at the San Francisco General Hospital,[10–12] are of interest because almost all patients with SE in the city of San Francisco who begin to have seizures outside of a hospital are transported there. About 10% of epilepsy patients present with SE,[13] and nearly 20% of seizure patients experience an episode of SE within 5 years of their first seizure.[9]

CLASSIFICATION

The most frequently used classification scheme is that of the International League Against Epilepsy[14] (Table 169A–2). This scheme allows classification based on clinical criteria without inferring cause. *Simple partial seizures* start focally in the cerebral cortex, without invading other structures. The patient is aware throughout the episode and appears otherwise unchanged. Bilateral limbic dysfunction produces a *complex partial seizure;* awareness and ability to interact are diminished (but may not be completely abolished). *Automatisms* (movements that a patient makes without awareness) may occur. *Secondary generalization* results from invasion by epileptic electrical activity of the other hemisphere or subcortical structures.

Primary generalized seizures arise from the cerebral cortex and diencephalon at the same time; no focal phenomena are visible, and consciousness is lost at the onset. *Absence seizures* are frequently confined to childhood; they consist of the abrupt onset of a blank stare that usually lasts 5 to 15 seconds, after which the patient abruptly returns to normal. *Atypical absence seizures* occur in children with the Lennox-Gastaut syndrome. *Myoclonic seizures* start with brief synchronous jerks, without alteration of consciousness initially, followed by a generalized convulsion. They frequently occur in the genetic epilepsies; in the ICU, they commonly follow anoxia or metabolic disturbances.[15] *Tonic-clonic seizures* start with tonic extension, evolve to bilaterally syn-

TABLE 169A–1. Etiologies of Status Epilepticus at the San Francisco General Hospital

	1970–1980 (%)		*1980–1989 (%)*	
Cause	*Prior Seizures*	*No Prior Seizures*	*Prior Seizures*	*No Prior Seizures*
Ethanol-related	11	4	25	12
Anticonvulsant noncompliance	27	0	41	0
Drug toxicity	0	10	5	10
Refractory epilepsy	NA	NA	8	0
CNS infection*	0	4	2	10
Trauma	1	2	2	6
Tumor	0	4	2	7
Metabolic*	3	5	2	4
Stroke*	4	11	2	5
Anoxia*	0	4	0	6
Other	11	5	3	5

(Data from Lowenstein DH, Alldredge BK: Status epilepticus in an urban public hospital in the 1980s. Neurology 1993; 42:483–488.)
*Conditions most likely to result in ICU admission.
Abbreviation: NA = not applicable.

TABLE 169A–2. International Classification of Epileptic Seizures

- Partial seizures (seizures beginning locally)
  - Simple partial seizures (consciousness not impaired)
    - with motor symptoms
    - with somatosensory or special sensory symptoms
    - with autonomic symptoms
    - with psychic symptoms
  - Complex partial seizures (with impairment of consciousness)
    - beginning as simple partial seizures and progressing to impairment of consciousness
      - without automatisms
      - with automatisms
    - with impairment of consciousness at onset
      - with no other features
      - with features of simple partial seizures
      - with automatisms
  - Partial seizures (simple or complex), secondarily generalized
- Primary generalized seizures (bilaterally symmetric, without localized onset)
  - Absence seizures
    - true absence ("petit mal")
    - atypical absence
  - Myoclonic seizures
  - Clonic seizures
  - Tonic seizures
  - Tonic-clonic seizures ("grand mal")
  - Atonic seizures
- Unclassified seizures

(Adapted from Bleck TP: Status epilepticus. *In*: Textbook of Clinical Neuropharmacology. 2nd ed. Klawans HL, Goetz CG, Tanner CM [Eds]. New York, Raven Press, 1992, pp 65–73.)

chronous clonus, and conclude with a postictal phase. Clinical judgment is required to apply this classification system in the ICU. Patients in whom consciousness has already been altered by drugs, hypotension, sepsis, or intracranial pathology may be difficult to classify concerning the nature of their partial seizures.

SE is classified by a similar system that has been altered to match observable clinical phenomena (Table 169A–3).[16] *GCSE* is the commonest type of SE encountered in the ICU and poses the greatest risk to a patient. It may either be primarily generalized, as in the drug-intoxicated patient, or be secondarily generalized, as in the brain abscess patient who develops GCSE. *Nonconvulsive SE* (NCSE) in the ICU frequently follows partially treated GCSE. Some use the term for all cases of SE that involve altered consciousness without convulsive movements; this blurs the distinctions among absence SE, partially treated GCSE, and complex partial SE (CPSE), which have different causes and treatments. Epilepsia partialis continua (a special form of partial SE in which repetitive movements affect a small area of the body) sometimes lasts for months or years.

PATHOGENESIS AND PATHOPHYSIOLOGY

The reported "causes" of SE can be divided into predispositions and precipitants. Predispositions are static conditions that increase the likelihood of SE's occurring in the presence of a precipitant. Precipitants are events that can produce SE in most, if not all, people, but tend to affect those with predispositions at lesser degrees of severity (e.g., those with barbiturate withdrawal). The causes and effects of SE at the cellular, brain, and systemic levels are interrelated, but their individual analysis is useful for understanding them and their therapeutic implications. Longer SE durations produce more profound alterations with an increasing likelihood of permanence and of becoming refractory to treatment. The processes involved in a single seizure and the transition to SE have been reviewed.[17]

The ionic events of a seizure follow the opening of ion channels coupled to excitatory amino acid receptors. From the standpoint of the intensivist, three channels are particularly important because their activation may raise intracellular free calcium to toxic concentrations: alpha-amino-3-hydroxy-5-methyl-4-isoxazole propionic acid (AMPA), *N*-methyl-D-aspartate (NMDA), and metabotropic channels. These excitatory amino acid systems are crucial for learning and memory. Many drugs that block these systems are available but are too toxic for chronic use. The deleterious consequences of SE and the brief period for which they would be needed suggest that such agents may have a role in SE. Counter-regulatory ionic events are also triggered by the epileptiform discharge, such as the activation of inhibitory interneurons, which suppress excited neurons via $GABA_A$ synapses.

The cellular effects of excessive excitatory amino acid channel activity include (1) the generation of toxic concentrations of intracellular free calcium; (2) activation of autolytic enzyme systems; (3) production of oxygen free radicals; (4) generation of nitric oxide, which both enhances subsequent excitation and serves as a toxin; (5) phosphorylation of enzyme and receptor systems, which makes subsequent seizures more likely; and (6) an increase in intracellular osmolality, which produces neuronal swelling. If adenosine triphosphate production fails, membrane ion exchange ceases, and neurons swell further. These events produce the neuronal damage associated with SE.

Many other biophysical and biochemical alterations occur during and after SE. The intense neuronal activity activates immediate-early genes and produces heat shock proteins, providing indications of the deleterious effects of SE and insight into the mechanisms of neuronal protection.[18] Wasterlain and associates have summarized mechanisms by which SE damages the nervous system.[19] Absence SE is an exception among these conditions; it consists of rhythmically increased inhibition and does not produce clinical or pathologic abnormalities.

The mechanisms that terminate seizure activity are poorly understood. The leading candidates are inhibitory mechanisms, primarily GABAergic neuronal systems. Clinical observation supports the contention that human SE frequently

TABLE 169A–3. Clinical Classification of Status Epilepticus

- Generalized seizures
  - GCSE
    - Primary generalized SE
      - Tonic-clonic SE
      - Myoclonic SE
      - Clonic-tonic-clonic SE
    - Secondarily generalized SE
      - Partial seizure with secondary generalization
      - Tonic SE
  - NCSE
    - Absence SE ("petit mal" status)
    - Atypical absence SE (e.g., in the Lennox syndrome)
    - Atonic SE
    - NCSE as a sequela of partially treated GCSE
- Partial SE
  - Simple partial SE
    - Typical
    - Epilepsia partialis continua
  - CPSE
- Neonatal SE

(Adapted from Lothman EW: The biochemical basis and pathophysiology of status epilepticus. Neurology 1990; 40[Suppl 2]:13–23.)

follows withdrawal from the use of GABA agonists (e.g., benzodiazepines).

The electrical phenomena of SE at the whole brain level, as seen in the scalp electroencephalogram, reflect the seizure type that initiates SE (e.g., absence SE begins with a 3-Hz wave-and-spike pattern). During SE, this rhythm slows, but the wave-and-spike characteristic remains. GCSE goes through a sequence of electrographic changes (Table 169A–4).[20] The initial discharge becomes less well formed, implying that neuronal firing loses synchrony. The sustained depolarizations that characterize SE alter the extracellular milieu, most importantly by raising extracellular potassium levels. The excess potassium ejected during SE exceeds the buffering ability of astrocytes. Raising extracellular potassium level potentiates the production of more seizures.

The increased cellular activity of SE elevates demand for oxygen and glucose, and blood flow initially increases. After about 20 minutes, however, energy supplies become exhausted. This causes local catabolism to support ion pumps (in an attempt to restore the internal milieu); this is a major cause of epileptic brain damage. The brain contains systems to terminate seizure activity; GABAergic interneurons and inhibitory thalamic neurons are both important in this respect.

SE produces neuropathology even in patients who are paralyzed, ventilated, and maintained at normal temperature and blood pressure. The hippocampus, a crucial area for memory, contains the most susceptible neurons, but other regions are also vulnerable. In addition to damaging the CNS, GCSE produces life-threatening systemic effects.[21] Systemic and pulmonary arterial pressures rise dramatically at seizure onset. Epinephrine and cortisol prompt further elevations and also produce hyperglycemia. Muscular work raises blood lactate levels. Breathing is impaired by both airway obstruction and abnormal diaphragmatic contractions. Carbon dioxide excretion falls while its production increases markedly. Muscular work accelerates heat production; concomitantly, skin blood flow falls. This combination can raise core temperature dangerously.

The combined respiratory and metabolic acidoses frequently lower the arterial blood pH to 6.9 or lower.[21a] The acidosis may produce hyperkalemia; in addition to its deleterious effects on cardiac electrophysiology, the elevated extracellular potassium level helps propagate seizure activity. Coupled with hypoxemia and the elevation of circulating catecholamine concentrations, these conditions rarely can produce cardiac arrest. This sequence probably accounts for some cases of epileptic sudden death; neurogenic pulmonary edema is the likely cause of many others. The severity of the acidosis may prompt consideration of bicarbonate administration. When this is attempted, however, the likelihood of the occurrence of pulmonary edema is inordinately high. Rapid termination of seizure activity is the most appropriate treatment; the restitution of ventilation and the metabolism of lactate quickly restore a normal pH.

After about 20 minutes, motor activity begins to diminish, and ventilation usually improves. Body temperature may continue to increase, however. Hyperglycemia diminishes; after 1 hour, gluconeogenesis can fail, producing hypoglycemia. GCSE patients often aspirate oral or gastric contents, producing pneumonia. Rhabdomyolysis is common and may lead to renal failure. Compression fractures, joint dislocations, and tendon avulsions are other sequelae.

CLINICAL MANIFESTATIONS

Three problems complicate seizure recognition: (1) the occurrence of complex partial seizures in the setting of impaired awareness, (2) the occurrence of seizures in patients receiving pharmacologically induced paralysis, and (3) misinterpretation of other abnormal movements as seizures. ICU patients often have depressed consciousness in the absence of seizures owing to their disease, its complications (such as septic encephalopathy[22]), or drug use. A further decline in alertness may reflect a seizure; an electroencephalogram is required to confirm that one has occurred.

Patients receiving neuromuscular junction blocking agents do not manifest the usual signs of seizures. Since most such patients receive sedation with GABA agonists, the likelihood of seizures is small. One nondepolarizing agent, atracurium, has a metabolite that is potentially epileptogenic in some animals. No human electroencephalographic studies have been performed to determine whether patients are susceptible. Autonomic signs of seizures (hypertension, tachycardia, pupillary dilation) may also be the effects of pain or the response to inadequate sedation. Hence, patients who have a potential for seizures (e.g., those with intracranial pathology) and who manifest these signs should undergo electroencephalography. The actual incidence of this problem is unknown.

Abnormal movements can occur in patients with metabolic disturbances or anoxia. Some can be distinguished from seizures by observation, but if doubt about their nature persists, electroencephalography should be performed. Psychiatric disturbances in the ICU occasionally resemble complex partial seizures. Prolonged electroencephalographic monitoring may be required if the problem is intermittent.

Manifestations of Status Epilepticus

The manifestations of SE depend on the type and, for partial SE, the cortical area of abnormality. Table 169A–3 presents the types of SE encountered and focuses on those seen most frequently in the ICU.

Primary GCSE begins as tonic extension of the trunk and

TABLE 169A–4. Electroencephalographic and Clinical Correlations in Generalized Convulsive Status Epilepticus

Stage	*Typical Clinical Manifestations**	*Electroencephalographic Features*
1	Tonic-clonic convulsions; hypertension and hyperglycemia common	Discrete seizures with interictal slowing
2	Low- or medium-amplitude clonic activity, with rare convulsions	Waxing and waning of ictal discharges
3	Slight but frequent clonic activity, often confined to the eyes, face, or hands	Continuous ictal discharges
4	Rare episodes of slight clonic activity; hypotension and hypoglycemia become manifest	Continuous ictal discharges punctuated by flat periods
5	Coma without other manifestations of seizure activity	Periodic epileptiform discharges on a flat background

(Data from Treiman DM: Generalized convulsive status epilepticus in the adult. Epilepsia 1993; 34[Suppl 1]:S2–S11.)

*The clinical manifestations may vary considerably, depending on the underlying neuropathophysiologic process (and its anatomy), systemic diseases, and medications. In particular, stages of the electrographic progression may be sufficiently brief to be overlooked. Partially treating SE may dissociate the clinical and electrographic features.

extremities without preceding focal activity. No aura is reported, and consciousness is immediately lost. After several seconds of tonic extension, the extremities start to vibrate; clonic (rhythmic) extension of the extremities quickly follows. This phase wanes in intensity over a few minutes. The patient may then repeat the cycle of tonus followed by clonic movements, or continue to have intermittent bursts of clonic activity without recovery. Less common forms of GCSE are *myoclonic SE* (bursts of myoclonic jerks that increase in intensity and lead to a convulsion) and *clonic-tonic-clonic SE* (clonic activity precedes the first tonic contraction). Myoclonic SE is usually seen in patients with anoxic encephalopathy or metabolic disturbances.

Secondarily generalized SE begins with a partial seizure and progresses to convulsive activity. The initial focal clinical activity may be overlooked. This seizure type implies the presence of a structural lesion, so care must be taken to elicit evidence of lateralized movements.

Of the several forms of generalized NCSE, the one of greatest importance to intensivists is NCSE as a sequel of inadequately treated GCSE.[22a] When a patient with GCSE is treated with anticonvulsants (often in inadequate doses), visible convulsive activity may stop, but the electrochemical seizure continues. Patients begin to awaken within 15 to 20 minutes after the successful termination of SE; many regain consciousness much faster. Patients who do not start to awaken after 20 minutes should be assumed to have entered NCSE. Careful observation may disclose slight clonic activity. NCSE is an extremely dangerous problem because the destructive effects of SE continue even without obvious motor activity. NCSE demands emergent treatment with electroencephalographic monitoring to prevent further cerebral damage, since no clinical criteria are available to indicate whether therapy is effective.

Partial SE in ICU patients often follows a stroke or occurs with the rapid expansion of brain masses. Clonic motor activity is most easily recognized, but the seizure takes on the characteristics of adjacent functional tissue. Therefore, somatosensory or special sensory manifestations occur, and the ICU patient may be unable to report such symptoms. *Aphasic SE* occurs when a seizure begins in a language area, and it may resemble a stroke. Epilepsia partialis continua involves repetitive movements that are confined to a small region of the body. It may be seen with nonketotic hyperglycemia or with focal brain disease; anticonvulsant treatment is seldom useful. Complex partial SE presents with diminished awareness. The diagnosis often comes as a surprise when an electroencephalogram is obtained.

DIAGNOSTIC APPROACH

When an ICU patient has a seizure, one has a natural tendency to try to stop the event. This leads to both diagnostic obscuration and iatrogenic complication. Beyond protecting the patient from harm, very little can be done sufficiently rapidly to influence the course of the seizure. Padded tongue blades or similar items should not be placed in the mouth; they are more likely to obstruct the airway than to preserve it. The seizures of most patients stop before any medication can reach the brain in an effective concentration.

Observation is the most important activity to perform when a patient has a single seizure. This is the time to collect evidence of a partial onset in order to implicate structural brain disease. The postictal examination is similarly valuable; language, motor, sensory, or reflex abnormalities after an apparently generalized seizure are evidence of focal pathology.

Seizures in ICU patients have several potential causes that must be investigated. Drugs are a major cause of ICU seizures, especially in the setting of diminished renal or hepatic function or when the blood brain barrier is breached. Drug withdrawal is also a frequent offender. Although ethanol withdrawal is common, discontinuing any hypnosedative agent may prompt convulsions 1 to 3 days later. One report suggests that narcotic withdrawal may produce seizures in the critically ill.[6]

The physical examination should emphasize the areas listed earlier for the postictal examination. Evidence of cardiovascular disease or systemic infection should be sought, and the skin and fundi closely examined. Illicit drug screening should be performed on patients with unexplained seizures. Cocaine is becoming a major cause of seizures.[23] Electrolytes and serum osmolality should also be measured. However, hypocalcemia rarely causes seizures beyond the neonatal period; its identification on analysis must signal the end of the diagnostic work-up. Hypomagnesemia has an equally unwarranted reputation as the cause of seizures in malnourished alcoholic patients.

The need for imaging studies for these patients has been an area of uncertainty. A prospective study of neurologic complications in medical ICU patients determined that 38 of 61 patients (62%) had a vascular, infectious, or neoplastic explanation for their seizures. Hence, computed tomography or magnetic resonance imaging should be performed on most ICU patients with new seizures. Hypoglycemia and nonketotic hyperglycemia can produce seizures, and patients with these conditions might be treated for metabolic disturbances and observed if they do not present other evidence of focal disease. With current technology, there are almost no patients who cannot undergo computed tomography scanning. Although magnetic resonance imaging is preferable in most situations, the presence of the magnetic field precludes the use of infusion pumps and other metallic devices. Whether to administer contrast media for computed tomography depends on the clinical setting and on the appearance of the unenhanced CT scan.

Electroencephalography is a vital diagnostic tool for evaluating the seizure patient.[23a] Partial seizures usually have electroencephalographic abnormalities that begin in the area of the cortex that produces the seizures. Primary generalized seizures appear to start over the entire cortex simultaneously. Postictal slowing or depressed amplitude provide clues as to the focal cause of the seizures, and epileptiform activity helps to classify the type of seizure and to guide treatment. In patients who do not begin to awaken soon after seizures have apparently been controlled, emergent electroencephalography is necessary to exclude NCSE (Fig. 169A–1).

Considering the causes of seizures in the ICU setting, patients who need cerebrospinal fluid analysis usually require computed tomography first. When CNS infection is suspected, empiric antibiotic treatment should be started while these studies are being performed.

In contrast to the patient with a single or a few seizures, the SE patient requires concomitant diagnostic and therapeutic efforts. Although 20 minutes of continuous or recurrent seizure activity usually define SE, one should not stand by waiting for this period to pass before starting treatment. Since most seizures stop within 2 to 3 minutes, it is reasonable to start treatment after 5 minutes of continuous seizure activity or after the second or third seizure occurs without recovery between the spells.

GCSE can rarely be confused with decerebrate posturing, but observation usually makes the distinction straightforward. Tetanus patients are awake during their spasms and flex rather than extend their arms as seizure patients do.[18]

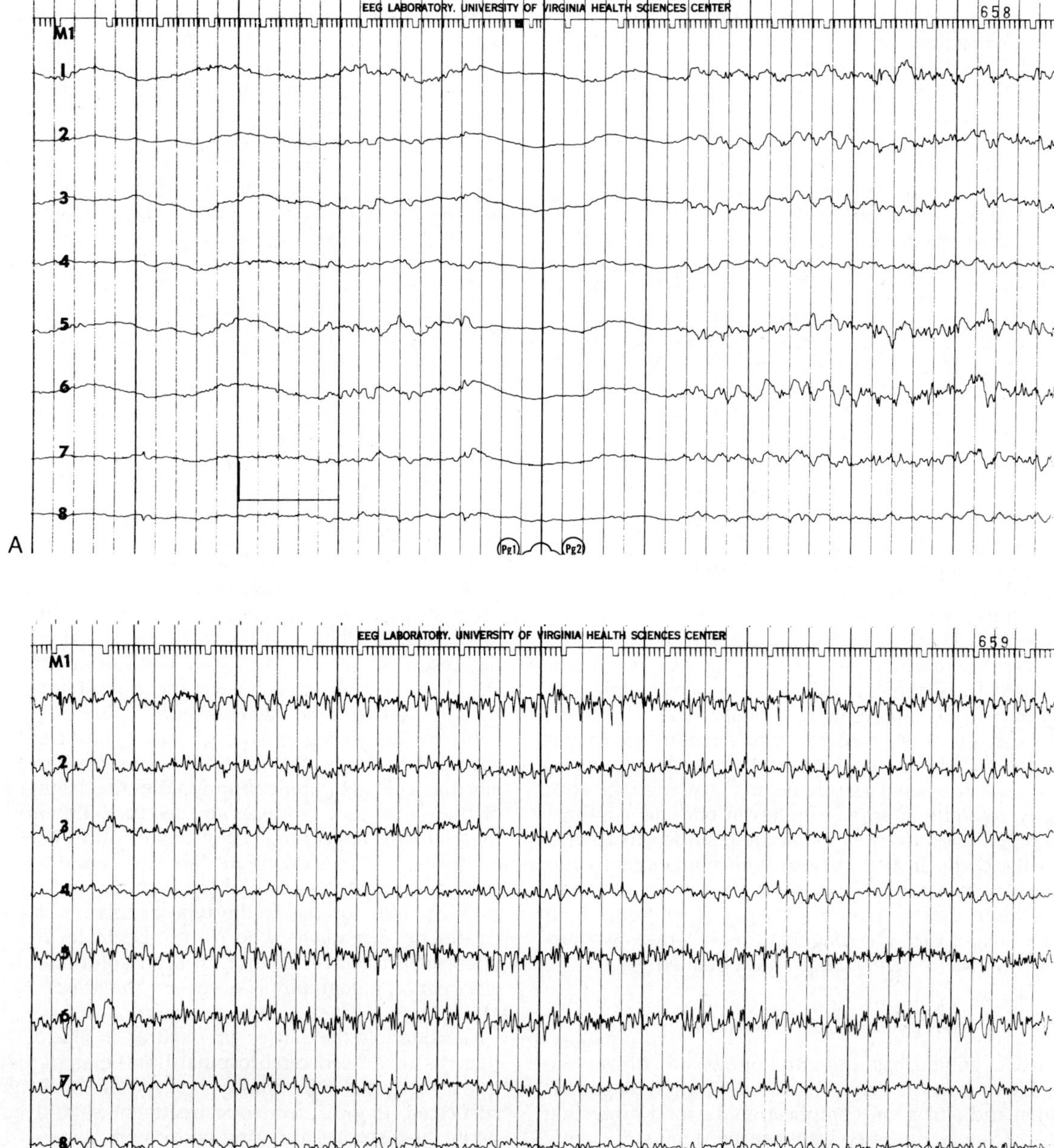

Figure 169A–1. EEG recording during SE. *A,* The onset of the seizure. *B–D,* Evolution of a seizure. (Montage: longitudinal bipolar; channels 1–4, left temporal, and channels 5–8, left parasagittal; calibration: vertical, 50 μV; horizontal, 1 s.)

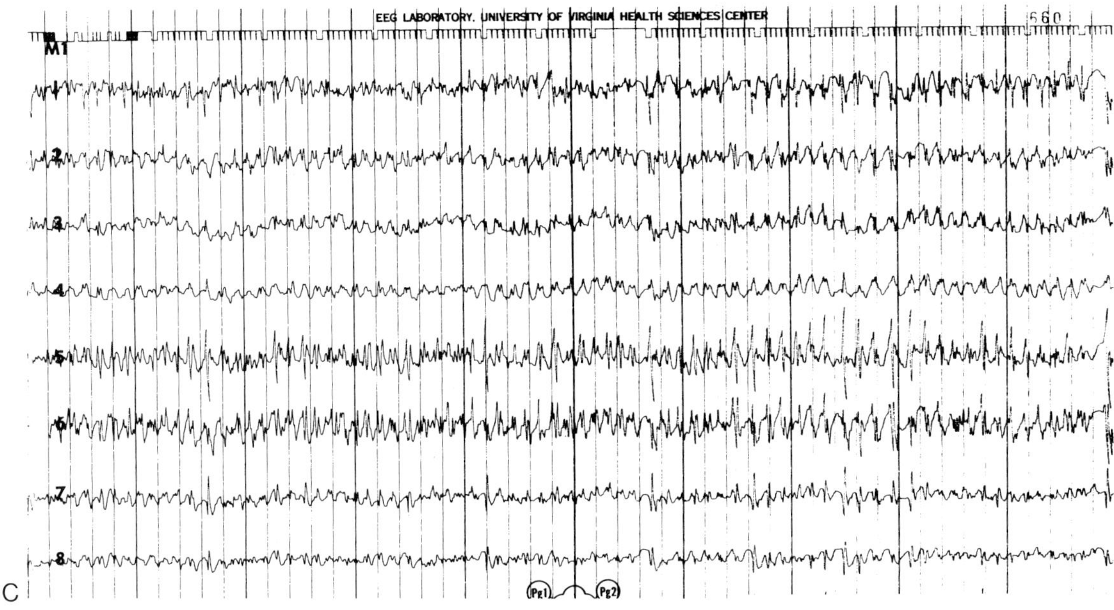

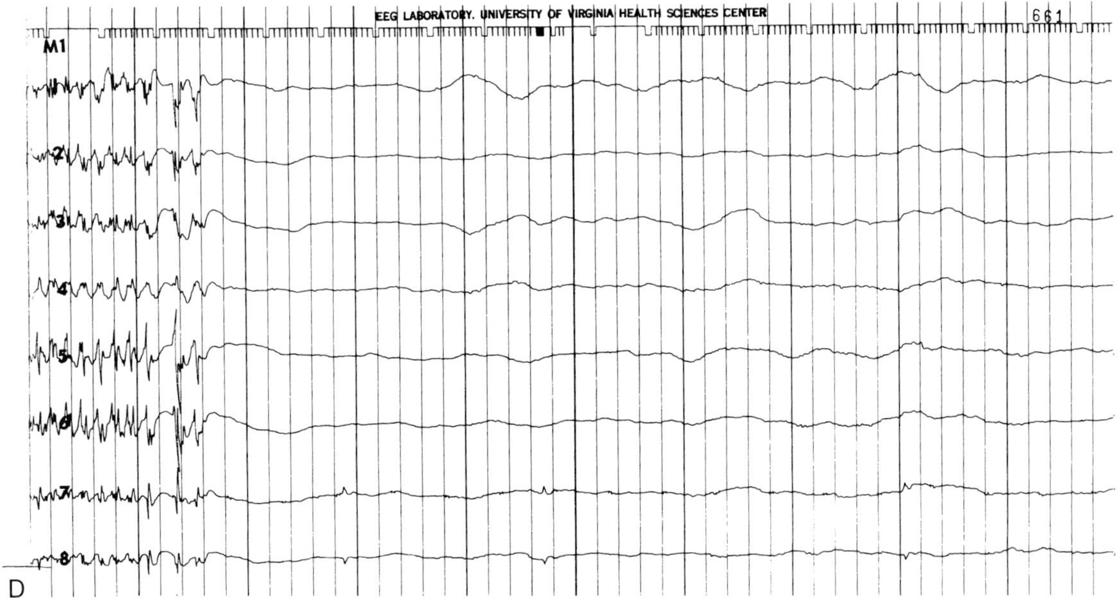

Figure 169A–1 *Continued*

Treatment for SE should not be delayed to obtain an electroencephalogram. A variety of findings may be present on the EEG, depending on the type of SE and its duration (see Table 169A–4). CPSE patients are often without such organized discharges of GCSE; instead, they have waxing and waning rhythmic activity in one or several brain regions. A diagnostic trial of intravenous benzodiazepine therapy is often necessary to diagnose CPSE. Patients developing refractory SE or having seizures during neuromuscular junction blockade require continuous electroencephalographic monitoring.

MANAGEMENT APPROACH

Making the decision to administer anticonvulsants to an ICU patient who experiences one or a few seizures requires consideration of a provisional cause, estimation of the likelihood of recurrence, and recognition of the utility and limitations of anticonvulsants. For example, the occurrence of seizures during ethanol withdrawal does not indicate the need for chronic treatment, and giving phenytoin does not prevent further withdrawal convulsions. The patient may need prophylaxis against delirium tremens, but the few seizures themselves seldom require treatment. Patients with convulsions during barbiturate or benzodiazepine withdrawal, in contrast, should usually receive short-term treatment with lorazepam to prevent SE. Seizures due to drugs or metabolic disorders should also be treated briefly but not chronically. Figure 169A–2 shows a management algorithm for SE.

The ICU patient with CNS disease who has even one seizure should usually be given chronic anticonvulsant therapy, and this approach should be reviewed before he or she is discharged. Initiating this treatment after the first *unprovoked* seizure helps prevent subsequent epilepsy.[24] Starting therapy after the first seizure in a critically ill patient at risk for seizure recurrence may be even more important, especially if his or her condition would be seriously complicated by a convulsion. In the ICU setting, phenytoin is frequently selected owing to its ease of administration and its lack of sedative effects. Hypotension and arrhythmias, which may complicate rapid administration, can usually be prevented by slowing the infusion to less than 25 mg/min. Because of the rare but possible occurrence of third-degree atrioventricular block, an external cardiac pacemaker should be available when patients with conduction abnormalities receive intravenous phenytoin. A phenytoin precursor presently in phase III clinical trials (fosphenytoin) will probably supplant phenytoin because it is safer and easier to administer. The serum phenytoin concentration should be kept within the "therapeutic" range of 10 to 20 μg/mL (corresponding to an unbound or "free" concentration of 1–2 μg/mL) unless further seizures occur; the level may then be increased until signs of toxicity are observed. Failure to prevent seizures at a total concentration of 25 μg/mL is usually an indication to add phenobarbital to the regimen.

Phenytoin is approximately 90% protein bound in normal hosts. Patients with renal dysfunction have lower total phenytoin levels at a given dose because the drug is displaced from binding sites, but the unbound level of the drug is not affected. Thus, renal failure patients, and perhaps others who are receiving highly protein-bound drugs (which compete for binding), may benefit from determination of free phenytoin level. Only the free fraction is metabolized, so the dose is not altered with changes in renal function. The clearance half-time with normal liver function varies from about 12 to 20 hours (intravenous form) to over 24 hours (extended-release capsules), so that a new steady-state serum concentration occurs within 3 to 6 days. Phenytoin need not be given more frequently than every 12 hours. Hepatic dysfunction mandates decrease of the maintenance dose.[24a] Hypersensitivity is the major adverse effect of concern to the intensivist. This may manifest itself solely as fever but commonly includes rash and eosinophilia. Adverse reactions to phenytoin and other anticonvulsants have been reviewed elsewhere.[25]

Phenobarbital remains a useful anticonvulsant for those intolerant to phenytoin or who have persistent seizures after

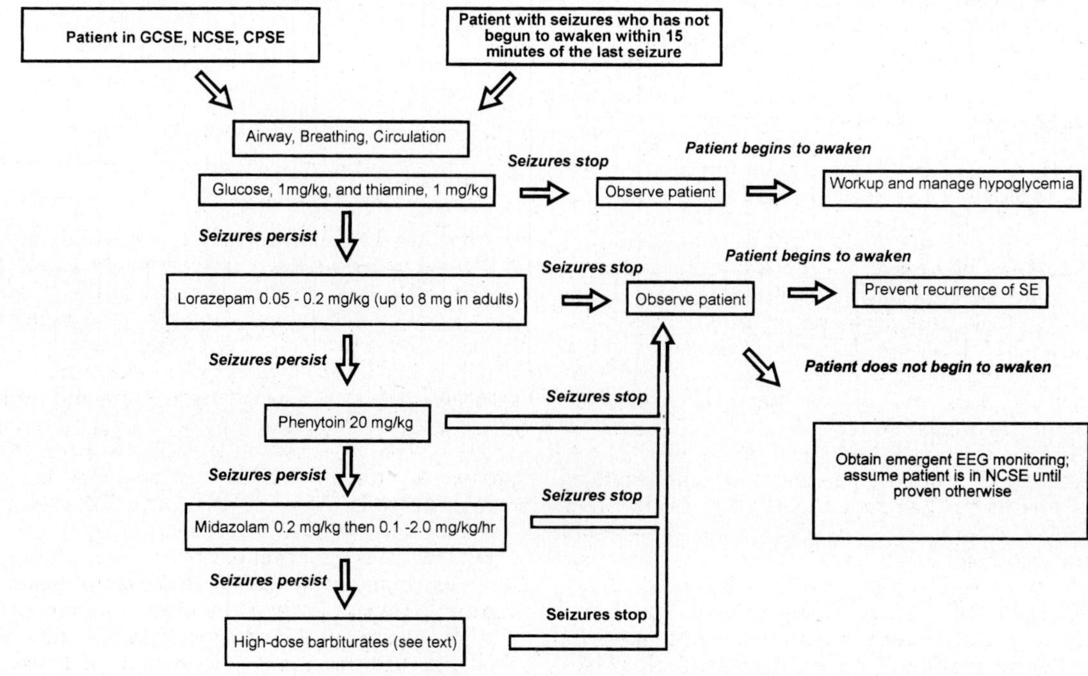

Figure 169A–2. Management algorithm for SE.

TABLE 169A–5. Suggested Protocol for Treating Status Epilepticus

I. Establish an airway, provide oxygen, and ensure ventilation. If neuromuscular junction blockade is required for intubation, use a short-acting agent (e.g., succinylcholine or vecuronium).

II. Determine blood pressure. If the patient is hypotensive, begin volume replacement or the use of vasoactive agents (or both) as indicated. GCSE patients who present with hypotension usually require admission to a critical care unit. (Hypertension should not be treated until SE is controlled, since terminating SE usually substantially corrects it, and many of the agents used to terminate SE can produce hypotension.)

III. Unless the patient is known to be normo- or hyperglycemic, administer dextrose (1 mg/kg) and thiamine (1 mg/kg).

IV. Terminate SE. The following sequence is recommended (see text for details); be cognizant of the potential of these drugs to eliminate the visible convulsive movements of GCSE when leaving the patient in nonconvulsive SE. Patients who do not begin to respond to external stimuli 15 minutes after the apparent termination of GCSE should be considered at risk for nonconvulsive SE and should undergo emergent electroencephalographic monitoring.

   A. Give lorazepam, 0.05–0.2 mg/kg at a rate of 0.04 mg/kg per minute. This drug should be diluted in an equal volume of the solution being used for intravenous infusion, as it is quite viscous. Most adult patients who respond do so by a total administered dose of 8 mg. The latency of effect is debated, but lack of response after 5 minutes should indicate failure.

   B. If SE persists after lorazepam administration, begin phenytoin, 20 mg/kg at a rate of 0.3 mg/kg per minute. If the patient tolerates this infusion rate, it may be increased to a maximum of 50 mg/min. Hypotension and arrhythmias are the major concern. Many investigators believe that an additional 5 mg/kg dose of phenytoin should be administered before the next line of therapy is attempted.

   C. If SE persists, administer midazolam, 0.2 mg/kg as a bolus, followed by an infusion of 0.1–2.0 mg/kg per hour to achieve seizure control (as determined by electroencephalographic monitoring). Intubate the patient at this stage if this has not already been accomplished. A patient reaching this stage should be treated in a critical care unit.

   D. Should the patient not be controlled with midazolam, administer pentobarbital, 12 mg/kg at a rate of 0.2–0.4 mg/kg per minute as tolerated, followed by an infusion of 0.25–2.0 mg/kg per hour as determined by electroencephalographic monitoring (with an initial goal of burst-suppression; in some cases, an isoelectric electroencephalogram may be required to eliminate all seizures). Most patients require systemic and pulmonary artery catheterization, with fluid and vasoactive drug therapy as indicated to maintain blood pressure. Other complications of this treatment are discussed in the text.

V. Prevent recurrence of SE. The choice of drugs depends greatly on the cause of SE and/or the patient's medical and social situation. In general, patients not previously receiving anticonvulsants whose SE is easily controlled often respond well to chronic treatment with phenytoin or carbamazepine. In contrast, others (e.g., patients with acute encephalitis) require two or three anticonvulsants at "toxic" levels (e.g., phenobarbital at greater than 100 μg/mL) to be weaned from midazolam or pentobarbital and may still have occasional seizures.

VI. Treat complications.

   A. Rhabdomyolysis should be treated with vigorous saline diuresis to prevent acute renal failure; urinary alkalization may be a useful adjunct. If definitive treatment of GCSE takes longer than expected because of hypotension or arrhythmias, neuromuscular junction blockade under electroencephalographic monitoring might be considered.

   B. Hyperthermia usually remits rapidly after termination of SE. External cooling usually suffices if the core temperature remains elevated. In rare instances, cool peritoneal lavage or extracorporeal blood cooling may be required. High-dose pentobarbital generally produces poikilothermy.

   C. The treatment of cerebral edema occurring secondary to SE has not been well studied. When substantial edema is present, one should suspect that SE and cerebral edema are both manifestations of the same underlying condition. Hyperventilation and mannitol may be valuable if edema is life threatening. Edema due to SE is vasogenic in origin; thus, steroids may be useful as well.

---

adequate phenytoin administration. The target for phenobarbital in the ICU should be a serum concentration of 20 to 40 μg/mL. Hepatic and renal dysfunction alter phenobarbital metabolism. Since its usual clearance half-time is about 96 hours, maintenance doses of this agent should be provided once a day. A steady-state level takes about 3 weeks to become established. Sedation is the major adverse effect; allergy to the drug occurs rarely.

Carbamazepine therapy is seldom started in the ICU because its insolubility precludes parenteral formulation. Oral loading in conscious patients may produce coma that lasts several days. This drug causes hyponatremia in patients who receive it chronically.

GCSE obviously constitutes a medical emergency; however, NCSE and CPSE are also emergencies but are more difficult to recognize. In each circumstance, one must act quickly to prevent additional cerebral damage. Table 169A–5 presents a sample management scheme.[26] Patients with simple partial SE or epilepsia partialis continua are at less risk for the development of widespread cerebral damage and are also less likely to respond to the aggressive approach outlined in Table 169A–5. In these patients, correcting underlying problems, such as nonketotic hyperosmolar hyperglycemia, is crucial. Errors in terminating SE include (1) inadequate dosing of effective drugs and (2) continued use of drugs that are ineffective in the patient being treated. The first point most frequently applies to phenytoin use; the proverbial "gram of Dilantin (trademark for phenytoin manufactured by Parke-Davis, Morris Plains, NJ)" is inadequate for those weighing more than 50 kg.

Lorazepam is our agent of first choice for terminating SE. A current study comparing four choices of treatment (lorazepam; diazepam followed by phenytoin; phenytoin alone; and phenobarbital) should provide information on the best choice of first-line agent. Advantages of lorazepam over diazepam are its duration of action against SE (4–14 hours as opposed to 20 minutes) and its higher initial response rate. One group reported that children receiving diazepam for SE more often required intubation and mechanical ventilation than did comparable children receiving lorazepam.[27] Europeans often use midazolam or clonazepam initially. Midazolam is very useful for refractory SE.[28] Respiratory depression is the major adverse effect of this class of drugs, especially when they are given together with barbiturates or paraldehyde.

Phenytoin is a very effective anti-SE agent but cannot be delivered rapidly enough to be considered a first-line agent. It has a long duration of action when an adequate dose is given (a 20-mg/kg dose produces a serum level >20 μg/mL for 24 hours). Adding 5 mg/kg if 20 mg/kg fails to stop SE may be useful.[29] If the patient is no longer in SE during phenytoin administration, a slower rate should be employed.

Some advocate the use of phenobarbital as a first-line drug,[30] but it has typically been used as a third-line agent, after administration of a benzodiazepine and phenytoin.[31] Although this approach has been widely accepted by the neurologic community, we rarely use phenobarbital for two reasons. First, only a small percentage of patients who have failed treatment with two anticonvulsants respond to a third conventional agent[12]; second, at least an additional 20 minutes are required to obtain control in the few patients who do respond. Phenobarbital remains an important drug in the management of simple partial SE and for patients who are being weaned from high-dose midazolam or anesthetic barbiturates.

Pentobarbital and thiopental are usually reserved for refractory SE. Although these drugs are effective in sufficiently large doses, their side effects can limit their use[32] and may be fatal.[33] However, they are important when other modalities have failed (Table 169A–5).

Although intravenous paraldehyde has been abandoned, this agent is still useful. The current formulation is licensed only for enteral use. It can be given every 3 hours either through a Teflon-coated nasogastric tube or rectally via a rubber catheter. The enteral form can be filtered for intramuscular injection; it should be given deeply into the lateral gluteal muscles, with special care taken to avoid the sciatic nerves. This route of administration should be confined to a few doses, when rectal or oral treatment is not feasible.

Isoflurane, an inhaled anesthetic, controls refractory SE; however, it is difficult to deliver such a gas outside the operating suite or the recovery area.[34] It has no known advantage over intravenous anticonvulsants and can raise intracranial pressure.

Propofol has been reported effective in the treatment of refractory SE but has not been directly compared with other compounds.[35] It may offer a lower risk of ventilatory depression and promote more rapid awakening compared with other drugs when it is discontinued.

PROGNOSIS

Wijdicks and Sharbrough have reported that 34% of patients experiencing a seizure died during that hospitalization.[6] Our prospective study of neurologic complications in medical ICU patients showed that having even one seizure while in the ICU for a non-neurologic reason doubled in-hospital mortality.[10] This effect on prognosis primarily reflected the cause of the seizure.[35a]

Three major factors determine outcome in patients with SE: the type of SE, its cause, and its duration. GCSE has the worst prognosis for neurologic recovery; myoclonic SE following an anoxic episode carries a very poor prognosis for survival. CPSE can produce limbic system damage, usually manifested as a memory disturbance. Most studies of outcome concentrate on GCSE mortality. Hauser, summarizing data available in 1990, suggested that mortality rates vary from 1% to 53%.[8] Those studies attempting to distinguish mortality due to SE from that caused by underlying disease attribute rates of 1% to 7% to SE and rates of 2% to 25% to its cause. Population-based studies in Richmond showed that the mortality rate associated with SE lasting longer than 1 hour increased 10-fold over that for SE lasting less than 1 hour.[9, 9a] Causes associated with increased mortality included anoxia, intracranial hemorrhages, tumors, infections, and trauma.

Limited data are available concerning the functional abilities of GCSE survivors, and no data reliably permit a distinction between the effects of SE and those of its causes. One review concluded that intellectual ability declined as a consequence of SE.[36] Survivors of SE frequently seem to have memory and behavioral disorders out of proportion to the structural damage produced by the cause of their seizures. A wealth of experimental data support this observation, emphasizing strongly the rapid and effective control of SE. Case reports of severe memory deficits following prolonged CPSE have also been published.[35] Whether treatment of SE reduces the risk of subsequent epilepsy remains uncertain. Experimental studies indicate that SE lowers the threshold for subsequent seizures.[37]

References

1. Wilks S: Bromide and iodide of potassium in epilepsy. Med Times and Gaz (Lond) 1861; 2:635–636.
2. Gowers WR: Epilepsy and Other Chronic Convulsive Diseases: Their Causes, Symptoms, and Treatment. London, J and A Churchill, 1881.
3. Bleck TP, Klawans HL: Mechanisms of epilepsy and anticonvulsant action. *In:* Textbook of Clinical Neuropharmacology. Klawans HL, Goetz CG, Tanner CM (Eds). New York, Raven Press, 1992, pp 23–30.
4. Weschler IS: Intravenous injection of paraldehyde for control of convulsions. JAMA 1940; 114:2198.
5. Gastaut H, Naquet R, Poiré R, et al: Treatment of status epilepticus with diazepam (Valium). Epilepsia 1965; 6:167–182.
6. Wijdicks EFM, Sharbrough FW: New-onset seizures in critically ill patients. Neurology 1993; 43:1042–1044.
7. Bleck TP, Smith MC, Pierre-Louis JC, et al: Neurologic complications of critical medical illnesses. Crit Care Med 1993; 21:98–103.
8. Hauser WA: Status epilepticus: Epidemiologic considerations. Neurology 1990; 40(Suppl 2):9–13.
9. DeLorenzo RJ, Towne AR, Pellock JM, et al: Status epilepticus in children, adults, and the elderly. Epilepsia 1992; 33(Suppl 4):S15–S25.

9a. Towne AR, Pellock JM, Ko D, et al: Determinants of mortality in status epilepticus. Epilepsia 1994; 35:27–34.

10. Aminoff MJ, Simon RP: Status epilepticus: Causes, clinical features and consequences in 98 patients. Am J Med 1980; 69:657–666.
11. Lowenstein DH, Alldredge BK: Status epilepticus in an urban public hospital in the 1980s. Neurology 1993; 42:483–488.
12. Bleck TP: Status epilepticus. University Reports on Epilepsy 1992; 1:1–7.
13. Ettinger AB, Shinnar S: New-onset seizures in an elderly hospitalized population. Neurology 1993; 43:489–492.
14. Commission on Classification and Terminology of the International League Against Epilepsy: Proposal for revised clinical and electroencephalographic classification of epileptic seizures. Epilepsia 1981; 22:489–501.
15. Bleck TP: Metabolic encephalopathy. *In:* Emergent and Urgent Neurology. Weiner WJ (Ed). Philadelphia, JB Lippincott, 1991, pp 27–57.
16. Bleck TP: Status epilepticus. *In:* Textbook of Clinical Neuropharmacology. 2nd ed. Klawans HL, Goetz CG, Tanner CM (Eds). New York, Raven Press, 1992, pp 65–73.

17. Lothman EW: The biochemical basis and pathophysiology of status epilepticus. Neurology 1990; 40(Suppl 2):13–23.
18. Lowenstein DH, Simon RP, Sharp FR: The pattern of 72-kDa heat shock protein–like immunoreactivity in the rat brain following fluothyl-induced status epilepticus. Brain Res 1990; 531:173–182.
19. Wasterlain CG, Fujikawa DG, Penix L, et al: Pathophysiological mechanisms of brain damage from status epilepticus. Epilepsia 1993; 34(Suppl 1):S37–S53.
20. Treiman DM: Generalized convulsive status epilepticus in the adult. Epilepsia 1993; 34(Suppl 1):S2–S11.
21. Walton NY: Systemic effects of generalized convulsive status epilepticus. Epilepsia 1993; 34(Suppl 1):S54–S58.
21a. Brivet F, Bernardin M, Cherin P, et al: Hyperchloremic acidosis during grand mal seizure lactic acidosis. Intensive Care Med 1994; 20:27–31.
22. Bolton CF, Young GB, Zochodne DW: The neurologic complications of sepsis. Ann Neurol 1993; 33:94–100.
22a. Granner MA, Lee SI: Nonconvulsive status epilepticus: EEG analysis in a large series. Epilepsia 1994; 35:42–47.
23. Rowbotham MC, Lowenstein DH: Neurologic complications of cocaine use. Annu Rev Med 1990; 41:417–422.
23a. Jordan KG: Continuous EEG and evoked potential monitoring in the neuroscience intensive care unit. J Clin Neurophysiol 1993; 10:445–475.
24. First Seizure Trial Group: Randomized clinical trial of the efficacy of antiepileptic drugs in reducing the risk of relapse after a first unprovoked tonic-clonic seizure. Neurology 1993; 43:478–483.
24a. Lindow J, Wijdicks EF: Phenytoin toxicity associated with hypoalbuminemia in critically ill patients. Chest 1994; 105:602–604.
25. Smith MC, Bleck TP: Toxicity of anticonvulsants. *In:* Textbook of Clinical Neuropharmacology. 2nd ed. Klawans HL, Goetz CG, Tanner CM (Eds). New York, Raven Press, 1992, pp 45–64.
26. Bleck TP, Lothman EW: Status epilepticus. *In:* Principles and Practice of Neurocritical Care. Hanley DF, Hacke W, Teasdale G (Eds). Baltimore, Williams & Wilkins, 1994.
27. Chuilli DA, Ternfrup TE, Kanter RK: The influence of diazepam or lorazepam on the frequency of endotracheal intubation in childhood status epilepticus. J Emerg Med 1991; 9:13–17.
28. Kumar A, Bleck TP: Intravenous midazolam for the treatment of refractory status epilepticus. Crit Care Med 1992; 20:483–488.
29. Osorio I, Reed RC: Treatment of refractory generalized tonic-clonic status epilepticus with pentobarbital anesthesia after high-dose phenytoin. Epilepsia 1989; 30:464–471.
30. Shaner DM, McCurdy SA, Herring MO, et al: Treatment of status epilepticus: A prospective comparison of diazepam and phenytoin versus phenobarbital and optional phenytoin. Neurology 1988; 38:202–206.
31. Working Group on Status Epilepticus: Treatment of generalized convulsive status epilepticus. JAMA 1993; 270:854–859.
32. Yaffe K, Lowenstein DH: Prognostic factors of pentobarbital therapy for refractory generalized status epilepticus. Neurology 1993; 43:895–900.
33. Bleck TP: High-dose pentobarbital treatment of refractory status epilepticus: A meta-analysis of published studies. Epilepsia 1992; 33:5.
34. Bleck TP: Therapy for status epilepticus. Clin Neuropharmacol 1983; 6:255–268.
35. Treiman DM, Delgado-Escueta AV: Complex partial status epilepticus. Adv Neurol 1983; 34:69–81.
35a. Shorvon S: The outcome of tonic-clonic status epilepticus. Curr Opin Neurol 1994; 7:93–95.
36. Dodrill CB, Wilensky AJ: Intellectual impairment as an outcome of status epilepticus. Neurology 1990; 40(Suppl 2):23–27.
37. Lothman EW, Bertram EH: Epileptogenic effects of status epilepticus. Epilepsia 1993; 34(Suppl 1):S59–S70.

CHAPTER 169B

Status Epilepticus in Children

Joseph M. Scheller, MD

Status epilepticus (SE) in neonates (younger than 1 month of age) is a separate topic and is not addressed in this chapter. In this chapter, those patients between the ages of 1 month and 18 years are considered.

SE has been studied at several institutions in the 1980s, and these institutions' reports[1–3] form the backbone of our current understanding of the condition. No randomized, controlled trials of anticonvulsant treatments for SE in children have been conducted; thus, recommendations are based on clinical experience and adult data. As for adults, diazepam (0.3 mg/kg), lorazepam (0.1 mg/kg), phenytoin (20 mg/kg), or phenobarbital (15 mg/kg) can be used intravenously for initial treatment. If the first drug is not effective, a second is tried. If seizures are still not controlled, then barbiturate coma is induced.

IMPORTANT POINTS REGARDING STATUS EPILEPTICUS IN CHILDREN

Intravenous access in children is often difficult to achieve. Table 169B–1 lists medications that can be tried when an intravenous line cannot be started.

Three to 5% of all children, most often between the ages of 6 months to 5 years, experience febrile seizures—that is, seizures precipitated by a febrile illness that has not directly affected the central nervous system. Five per cent of these seizures are long enough to be classified as status epilepticus.[4, 5] Thus, a fairly large percentage (estimated at 25%) of cases of SE in children are related to routine infections such as otitis, gastroenteritis, sinusitis, pharyngitis, and pneumonia, and a much smaller percentage to more serious infections such as meningitis and encephalitis.

Fifty to 75% of children with SE have no previous history of any seizures, whereas another 10% to 20% of children have had a previous episode of SE. A rapidly taken medical history should determine whether a history of seizures or previous neurologic abnormality exists. Tables 169B–2 through 169B–5 list the most common causes of SE once this information is known. A few clinical points need to be remembered when these tables are used.

Table 169B–2 lists the most likely cause for SE when a child is previously normal with no history of seizures. The category of central nervous system infection includes disorders that may not cause dramatic abnormalities of the cerebrospinal fluid, such as herpes encephalitis and Lyme disease. Toxic conditions commonly seen in pediatrics are the result of accidental ingestions of prescribed or illegal drugs found in the home. A common metabolic abnormality is hyper- or hyponatremia due to inappropriate treatment of mild diarrhea. Nonaccidental trauma (child abuse) must be suspected in any infant in whom the symptom severity does not fit the history given by the child's caretaker. Infants who have been severely shaken may suffer brain hemorrhages that can cause SE.[6] These children may not have skin or bone evidence of trauma, but retinal hemorrhages are often noted on funduscopic examination.[7]

Table 169B–3 lists common causes of SE in those children who have been previously diagnosed as being neurologically abnormal. Most of these children have already had

TABLE 169B–1. Drugs That Are Effective for Childhood Status Epilepticus When an Intravenous Line Cannot Be Placed

Diazepam (IV solution)	0.5 mg/kg PR
Lorazepam	0.5 mg/kg PR
Paraldehyde	0.3 mL/kg PR (mixed 1:1 with oil)
Valproate	20 mg/kg PR (mixed 1:1 with water)
Carbamazepine	5 mg/kg NG

Abbreviations: IV = intravenous; PR = per rectum; NG = nasogastric.

TABLE 169B–2. Causes of Status Epilepticus in Children with No History of Seizures and Normal Neurologic Development

Fever with no central nervous system infection (febrile seizure)
Central nervous system infection
Toxic/metabolic
Head trauma (accidental and nonacccidental)
Familial epileptic syndrome
Idiopathic

TABLE 169B–3. Status Epilepticus in Children with No Seizure History and Abnormal Neurologic Development

V-P shunt obstruction
Ex-premature infant with a history of intracranial bleeding
Previous central nervous system infection
Previous traumatic brain injury
Chromosomal abnormality/syndrome
Congenital brain maldevelopment or infection
Cerebral palsy

TABLE 169B–4. Status Epilepticus in Children with a History of Seizures and Normal Neurologic Development

Nontherapeutic blood levels of anticonvulsant
Superimposed acute illness

TABLE 169B–5. Status Epilepticus in Children with a History of Seizures and Abnormal Neurologic Development

Nontherapeutic blood levels of anticonvulsant
Superimposed acute illness
Intractable epilepsy
Progressive degenerating neurologic condition
Idiopathic

neuroimaging tests, and repeat studies should be ordered on their admission to the intensive care unit only if a superimposed illness is suspected, such as cerebritis or a blocked or infected V-P shunt.

Tables 169B–4 and 169B–5 list the most likely causes for SE when the child has had seizures in the past. If a subtherapeutic level of anticonvulsant is discovered, an initial reaction might be to accuse the caregiver of missing one or more doses of the drug. Although this does happen, more commonly the child has developed gastroenteritis, and the resultant vomiting or diarrhea has led to poor drug absorption. For reasons that are not clear, a superimposed childhood illness may trigger seizures even when anticonvulsant levels are therapeutic.

PROGNOSIS

The mortality rate for childhood SE is between 3% and 7%.[1–3] One third of children who developed SE as part of an acute central nervous system insult or progressive neurologic problem will have new neurologic deficits as a result of the SE. New neurologic deficits and later intellectual problems are rare (incidence: 2–5%) in others with SE.

Children who had an episode of febrile SE have about a 10% to 21% chance of developing epilepsy (recurrent unprovoked afebrile seizures).[5, 8] Children whose first unprovoked seizure was SE have a 30% chance of developing epilepsy within the next 2 years.[1]

References

1. Maytal J, Shinnar S, Moshe SL, et al: Low morbidity and mortality of status epilepticus in children. Pediatrics 1989; 83:323–331.
2. Phillips SA, Shanahan RJ: Etiology and mortality of status epilepticus in children. Arch Neurol 1989; 46:74–76.
3. Dunn DW: Status epilepticus in children. J Child Neurol 1988; 3:167–173.
4. Hauser WA: Status epilepticus: Epidemiologic considerations. Neurology 1990; 40(Suppl 2):9–13.
5. Verity CM, Ross EM, Golding J: Outcome of childhood status epilepticus and lengthy febrile convulsions: Findings of national cohort study. Br Med J 1993; 307:225–228.
6. Duhaime AC, Gennarelli TA, Thibault LE: The shaken baby syndrome: A clinical, pathological, and biomedical study. J Neurosurg 1987; 66:409–417.
7. Lambert SR, Johnson TE, Hoyt CS: Optic nerve and retinal hemorrhages associated with the shaken baby syndrome. Arch Ophthalmol 1986; 104:1509–1515.
8. Verity CM, Golding J: Risk of epilepsy after febrile convulsions: a national cohort study. Br Med J 1991; 303:1373–1376.

CHAPTER 170

Postoperative Confusion

Jill D. Kaplan, MD, • *Allan H. Ropper, MD*

Postoperative confusion is a common and potentially life-threatening condition that is often misdiagnosed, is mistaken for a worsening dementia, or is mistakenly called "intensive care unit psychosis." The acute confusional state (ACS) may represent the initial or the only sign of a serious underlying illness, such as acute myocardial infarction, pulmonary embolism, pneumonia, or sepsis. The list of conditions associated with postoperative confusion is extensive because virtually any illness complicating the postoperative course may cause confusion, especially in the elderly, in whom confusion is a more common presenting sign of illness than is fever, pain, or tachycardia.[1] The relatively stereotypic mental status changes of ACS reflect a nonspecific response to pathogenic insults.[2, 3] Postoperative confusion is infrequently caused by a primary neurologic event; a combination of toxic or metabolic abnormalities is usually responsible, such as drug effects or withdrawal, electrolyte imbalance, hypoxia, acid-base disorders, hepatic and renal failure, hyperglycemia and hypoglycemia, and cardiac or pulmonary insufficiency.[3–5] It is usually obvious to the nursing staff when a patient is confused postoperatively, although findings may initially be subtle. Evaluating the patient efficiently is critical because most mental status alterations are reversible, and the underlying conditions, if uncorrected, may be associated with significant morbidity. The agitated patient may remove sutures, intravenous lines, or nasogastric tubes, further impairing electrolyte balance and nutrition. A fall may cause a fracture or a subdural hematoma. Pulmonary emboli and deep venous thrombosis can result from prolonged immobilization as the patient lapses into stupor or is sedated for agitation. Patients with postoperative confusion have lengthened hospital stays, greater need for long-term care after discharge, and more medical complications, such as urinary tract infections, feeding problems, and decubitus ulcers.[6]

This chapter defines the terminology of postoperative confusion, reviews the factors associated with the condition, and describes how to clinically evaluate the confused postoperative patient. Laboratory studies, differential diagnosis, and pathophysiology are then discussed, followed by prognosis and treatment.

DEFINITION

Postoperative confusion is a confusing topic, largely because of the ambiguity of the nearly 30 different terms used to describe the syndrome. Encephalopathy, organic mental syndrome, acute brain failure, beclouded state, delirium, and ACS have all been used to describe mental status changes. Even the most accepted terms—ACS and delirium—are not universally employed, with psychiatrists favoring the former and neurologists and gerontologists, the latter.

In this chapter, *confusion* is used as a general term to denote a state characterized principally by a disturbance of attention. Disorientation, increased distractibility, inability to register immediate events and to recall them later, or inability to maintain a coherent stream of thought are the most salient features. Rapid fluctuations may occur from one hour to the next, and symptoms may worsen nocturnally, which is termed *sundowning*. Although diminished alertness and reduced activity are common, irritability and restlessness may also occur. In advanced stages, confusion is accompanied by decreased alertness or drowsiness, then evolves into stupor, and finally, coma. *Stupor* is a state of unresponsiveness from which a patient can be aroused only by vigorous and repeated stimuli. In *coma*, the patient appears asleep and is incapable of sensing or responding to inner needs or external stimuli.

Overactivity of psychomotor and autonomic nervous system functions defines *delirium*, which we refer to as a special type of confusional state in which perceptual disturbances are prominent. Vivid hallucinations and delusions, insomnia, and a heightened alertness may occur in this state. As in the archetypal alcohol withdrawal patient, tremulousness and jerky movements are usually present, along with dilated pupils, flushed facies, tachycardia, and diaphoresis.

INCIDENCE AND ASSOCIATED FACTORS

The incidence and risk factors for postoperative confusion are not well defined, despite a growing literature on the subject. Different studies have arrived at opposite conclusions concerning the basic facts and predisposing features. These discrepancies are accounted for by differences in diagnostic criteria, patient selection, types of surgery, and study design. Mental status changes have reportedly followed coronary artery bypass in 3%[7] to 79%[8] of patients; they have followed orthopedic surgery in 28%[9] to 61%[6]; and lung transplantation, in 73% of patients.[10] Most reports have found no greater likelihood of a patient's developing cognitive impairment after intracardiac surgery than after coronary bypass procedures,[11–14] but others have disagreed.[15]

Studies of cardiac procedures, the surgery most frequently assessed for postoperative neurologic complications, have produced the most conflicting results. Retrospective studies almost certainly give falsely low prevalences of below 3%[7, 16, 17] for postoperative confusion, whereas prospective studies cite incidences between 11% and 34%.[11–15, 18] Most studies have used a battery of neuropsychologic tests to measure cognitive impairment[8, 11, 12, 16, 19] but have not specifically addressed the diagnosis of confusion or delirium. Although 79% of coronary bypass patients were found to have postoperative cognitive deterioration by neuropsychologic testing in one large study, over half of the patients denied difficulty and were clinically asymptomatic.[8]

The roles of various factors associated with the development of confusion after cardiac surgery have been debated. Older patients are at greater risk than others for the development of cognitive impairment according to some studies,[11, 12, 15] but results contradicting this finding have been reported by others.[13, 16, 19] One study of 312 coronary bypass patients found that a history of transient ischemic attacks, stroke, diabetes mellitus, or peripheral vascular disease correlated with the development of moderate-to-severe neuropsychologic impairment[19]; however, these preoperative factors have not been associated with postoperative confusion in another large study.[13] Similarly, prior myocardial infarction[14] or poor cardiac function[12] have been found to predispose to cognitive impairment or, in other studies, to have no association.[13, 19] The preadmission use of propranolol and chlordiazepoxide has also been correlated with impaired postoperative mental function.[12]

The significance of intraoperative technical factors during cardiac surgery has been controversial. Cardiopulmonary bypass time in excess of 2 hours,[11, 13, 14, 19] prolonged aortic cross-clamp time,[10, 12] mean arterial pressure below 40 to 50 mm Hg,[11, 13, 14, 16, 19] and minimum hematocrit level[13, 19] have not been related to postoperative mental status changes in most studies, but others have reported a correlation with perfusion time greater than 2 hours,[12, 16] operation lasting over 7 hours,[12] minimum hemaglobin level,[19] or unexpected intraoperative events, such as massive bleeding.[16]

Conflicting evidence has also been reported about postoperative factors associated with confusion after cardiac surgery. Hypotension[19] and the use of pressors postoperatively[13] have been associated with cognitive impairment in some reports, but the use of an intra-aortic balloon pump (a marker for hypotensive and severely ill patients) has not been a factor,[7, 19] except in one study.[13] Mental status changes have variably been associated with postoperative electrolyte abnormalities,[12] but not with infections.[19]

Drugs with anticholinergic effects are often associated with confusion.[6, 9, 18, 20–23] In a study of postcardiotomy delirium, most of the 34% of patients who developed delirium had high serum levels of anticholinergic drugs, whereas those who remained cognitively normal had low levels. As anticholinergic drug levels increased, progressive impairment of cognitive function occurred on the "Mini-Mental State" examination.[18] Anticholinergic eye drops may contribute to the up to 16% incidence of delirium after cataract surgery.[24]

Psychoactive medicines, which are associated with risk of falls and hip fractures,[25, 26] have been associated with confusion after orthopedic surgery also.[6, 9, 23] Some authors have correlated a history of depression[6, 23]; prior stroke, dementia or old age[6]; severe perioperative hypotension[6]; and early postoperative hypoxemia[23] with the development of confusion after orthopedic surgery.

The ACS that followed cardiac transplantation was most often due to systemic infection in a study in which 54% of patients developed neurologic complications.[27] Alternatively, high cyclosporine levels and cardiopulmonary bypass were predictive of confusion after lung transplantation in a small retrospective study in which most patients developed delirium.[10]

To summarize, despite a massive amount of literature on the topic, little consistent data regarding postoperative confusion exist. Incidence and associated factors depend on the diagnostic criteria used to define the mental status abnormalities, but also on the patient population, the type of surgery, and the study design. Prospective investigations may help to clarify risk factors and prevalence in the future.

CLINICAL APPROACH

Accurate mental status and neurologic examination must begin *before* the patient is confused. An accurate history taken from the patient and the family is essential, including questions about prior strokes or mental decline and whether or not the patient balances his or her checkbook, shops alone, or drives a car. Are there any lateralizing findings, such as hemiparesis, that suggest a prior stroke? This information is valuable later, when the physician tries to decipher which physical findings are new. The clinical approach for the evaluation of the postoperatively confused patient is outlined in Table 170–1.

TABLE 170–1. Examination of the Confused Patient

History (from family and patient)
- Baseline mental status (balances checkbook, shops independently, or drives)
- Previous medical illnesses (diabetes mellitus, heart disease, or liver disease)
- Previous stroke
- Previous psychiatric history
- Substance abuse (alcohol, sedative-hypnotics)

General Physical Examination
- Vital signs (respiratory pattern, e.g., Cheyne-Stokes)
- Evidence of acute or chronic systemic illness
- Nuchal rigidity
- Evidence of head trauma

Neurologic Examination
- *Mental Status Examination*
  - Level of consciousness (e.g., is hyperalert, alert, lethargic, stuporous, comatose)
  - Attention (can give months or days in reverse order)
  - Language (comprehends yes/no questions and conveys meaning without errors)
  - Memory (remembers details from hospitalization or a short story)
  - Visuospatial (can draw a clock, shows spatial neglect)
- *Cranial Nerves*
  - Pupillary reaction and size
  - Extraocular movements (gaze preference)
  - Facial symmetry
- *Motor System*
  - Pronator "drift"
  - Fine finger movements
  - Gait (walks on heels and toes)
  - Spontaneous (e.g., tremor, myoclonus, asterixis)

General Examination

The physician should begin the examination by observing the patient casually for asymmetries of movement, gaze preference, or neglect of visual space. If no "focal" or lateralizing motor or sensory signs are present, a stroke or a primary neurologic process is less likely to be present, with a few exceptions, such as meningitis, or small, widespread brain emboli from endocarditis.

Vital signs can provide an important clue to diagnosis. Fever should not be attributed to atelectasis without a thorough search for an occult infection; a brain lesion disturbing the hypothalamus, or "central fever," is an extremely rare cause of pyrexia. Alcohol or barbiturate intoxication, extracellular fluid depletion, and myxedema may cause hypothermia. Decreased respiratory rate may point to barbiturate or morphine toxicity, or rarely to hypothyroidism, whereas tachypnea suggests pneumonia, pulmonary edema, or diabetic or uremic acidosis. Although hyperventilation can result from brain stem lesions, most commonly it is a compensation for primary pulmonary dysfunction. *Cheyne-Stokes breathing*, a regular crescendo-decrescendo cycle between which an apneic period may occur, occurs commonly in patients with deep bilateral cerebral lesions or a massive supratentorial lesion, but it is also common in those with metabolic disturbances or congestive heart failure. Hypotension commonly occurs in patients in states of depressed alertness, particularly in those with sepsis, internal hemorrhage, diabetes, myocardial infarction, or alcohol or barbiturate intoxication. Hypertensive encephalopathy is an uncommon cause of postoperative confusion. When increased blood pressure is combined with bradycardia, known as the Cushing effect, increased intracranial pressure is likely. The stigmata of chronic alcoholism, such as spider telangiectasias, palmar erythema, hepatosplenomegaly, and caput medusae, may be evident. The physician may misdiagnose the acutely delirious postoperative patient who is not known to be an alcoholic.

Mental Status Examination

The mental status examination can be directed by initial observations and can be abbreviated if language or attention deficits are obvious. Assessment should be systematic and should include level of consciousness, attention, language, memory, and visuospatial skills.

Level of Consciousness and Affect

The physician should begin by noting the state of consciousness and attention because abnormalities in these areas limit the interpretation of cognitive tests that follow. Attention should be tested formally, as outlined later, rather than by casual observation. Speech and writing may appear incoherent or comprehension impaired in the inattentive patient, leading to the mistaken diagnosis of aphasia, amnesia, or inability to calculate. The states of normal alertness, lethargy, stupor, and coma represent a continuum. Affect should also be considered; a lack of concern about a deficit may be a sign of right parietal lobe stroke, frontal lobe disease, or underlying depression.

Attention

Attention is easily tested by asking the patient to recite the months of the year in reverse order, or days of the week, if months prove to be too difficult. Questions about number span are also useful. The normal person should be able to repeat a sequence of six digits forward and four digits backward, after hearing them recited at the rate of 1 per second.[28] Serial subtraction of 7 from 100 is a less consistent measure of attention.

Language

Formal language testing is not necessary if the patient can understand the examiner and can convey meaning through fluent speech without malformed or inappropriate words, known as *paraphasias*. If the patient is aphasic, testing of spontaneous speech output, comprehension, repetition, naming, reading, and writing should be performed. Comprehension is best tested with questions requiring yes or no responses, such as "Do monkeys fly?" or "Does April come before March?" Naming difficulty is not helpful for localization, because it may occur with metabolic derangements as well as with aphasia.

Memory

Memory can be examined informally through questions about current events or the hospitalization. If this information is accurate, no further probing is needed. When the patient is given three words or a short story to recall, the patient should be asked to repeat the information until he or she can do so without prompting. Memory, the retention of learned information, cannot be tested unless the information is first registered. The patient with *Korsakoff's psychosis*, the mental manifestation of Wernicke's disease, has a striking inability to memorize new facts but is otherwise alert, attentive, and able to recall distant events. *Wernicke's disease*, seen mostly in alcoholics, is characterized by nystagmus, gaze palsies, gait ataxia, and mental confusion. Although Wernicke's disease and Korsakoff's psychosis are associated with thiamine deficiency, they may also appear in patients with lesions of the diencephalon or temporal lobes. A korsakoffian type of impairment of retentive memory may also be a feature of anoxic encephalopathy and Alzheimer's disease.

Visuospatial Ability

Visuospatial skills, which are a right parietal lobe function, can be tested by asking the patient to copy a solid cube or to put numbers inside a large circle (of at least a 5-inch diameter, to detect a spatial neglect) that represents a clock.[28]

Neurologic Examination

Neurologic examination can be directed to three key areas: eyes, face, and motor function. Asymmetries in these areas may point to a focal brain lesion. The pupils and their reaction to light, ocular movements, visual fields, optic discs, and symmetry of facial movements should be assessed. Normal pupils indicate that the midbrain is intact, which is usually the case in patients with drug intoxication and metabolic disorders. Exceptions include opiate (e.g., heroin and morphine) intoxication, which causes pinpoint pupils that barely react to light, and atropine excess, which causes widely dilated and fixed pupils. Visual fields can be assessed by noting if the patient blinks to threat from either side.

Integrity of the motor system can be determined by having the patient outstretch the arms, palms upward, and then observing for pronation (drift). Slowness of fine finger movements, such as tapping on the thumb with the index finger, indicates corticospinal tract difficulty. If the patient can walk on heels and toes, important leg weakness is unlikely.

Tremor, myoclonus, or asterixis are important clues to a toxic or metabolic state, and each occurs individually in 15% to 25% of patients who are encephalopathic from sepsis.[29] *Tremor* refers to a regular, rhythmic oscillation of a part of the body around a fixed point, usually in one plane. The tremor of metabolic encephalopathy is coarse and less regular, occurring at a rate of 8 to 10 per second, and is usually absent at rest.[30] Sudden, nonrhythmic, asymmetric twitching of parts or groups of muscles is seen with *myoclonus*, particularly in the postanoxic and uremic states or with the use of haloperidol. Widespread lightning-like contractions, or *myoclonus multiplex*, can be triggered by sensory stimuli, such as loud noises, or by an abrupt touch to the body, and usually signifies a severe metabolic disturbance. Arrhythmic lapses of sustained posture, or *asterixis*, is elicited by asking the patient to hold the arms outstretched with the hands dorsiflexed at the wrists. Asterixis occurs not only with hepatic encephalopathy but also with hypercapnia, uremia, and other metabolic and toxic encephalopathies, particularly after phenytoin administration.

Laboratory Analysis and Radiologic Imaging

Three neurologic studies are useful, in different circumstances, in the evaluation of the confused patient: (1) cranial computed tomography or magnetic resonance imaging, (2) lumbar puncture, and (3) electroencephalography (EEG). Computed tomography provides important information if asymmetries are present on examination or if a focal process is suspected, such as a subdural hematoma following a fall. Computed tomography must always be performed before the lumbar puncture in such cases, or if increased intracranial pressure is suspected.

Lumbar puncture may be life saving in the case of bacterial meningitis, which may occur in the absence of a stiff neck. It should be performed in patients with both confusion and unexplained fever, or in patients in whom meningitis is highly suspected, such as in those who have undergone neurosurgery. Lumbar puncture may also be critical if a subarachnoid hemorrhage is suspected because computed tomography may not detect up to 15% of intracranial bleeds. The physician must carefully record the opening pressure before sending the fluid for protein, glucose, cell count analysis in the first and fourth tubes, and for microscopic analyses.

EEG is one of the most useful diagnostic tests for postoperative confusion. Not all conditions that cause confusion have the same effect on the EEG, even though slowing of the background rhythm is common in patients with alterations of consciousness. Barbiturate intoxication and effects of other sedatives may induce increased frequency and amplitude on the EEG, whereas delirium tremens and Wernicke-Korsakoff disease cause surprisingly little or no change on the EEG. Bilaterally synchronous, large, sharp "triphasic waves" are characteristic of hepatic encephalopathy but may also appear in patients with renal or pulmonary failure. Sharp waves, or "spikes" (fast waves of high amplitude), may be detected if seizures are thought to be present. A normal EEG result in a patient whose responses are slow and who is inattentive supports the diagnosis of depression, whereas mild but diffuse slow-wave abnormalities occur with profound dementia.

Other laboratory tests should include determinations of electrolyte, glucose, and calcium levels; white blood cell count; hematocrit value, and both urine and serum toxin screenings. Additional laboratory tests may be useful, including determinations of arterial blood gases and ammonia and phosphate levels, liver and thyroid function tests, coagulation screenings, blood and urine cultures, urinalysis, electrocardiography and chest x-ray studies.

DIFFERENTIAL DIAGNOSIS

The list of conditions associated with postoperative confusion is extensive, as previously emphasized. A full list of differential diagnoses appears in Table 175–1.

Focal findings on neurologic examination are useful for determining the cause of the confusion. Nonfocal findings suggest that the primary source of the ACS lies outside the central nervous system. In such cases, tremor, asterixis, or myoclonus suggest a toxic or metabolic etiology, especially hypoxia. Postoperative hypoxia, infection, hyperglycemia, metabolic acidosis or alkalosis, renal or hepatic failure, hyponatremia, and drug intoxication or withdrawal are conditions without lateralizing signs that are commonly associated with ACS. Thiamine deficiency, which is responsible for the symptoms of the Wernicke-Korsakoff syndrome, may produce confusion in the undernourished patient, especially after the administration of glucose.

Infections usually do not cause focal neurologic findings and must be aggressively pursued, even in the absence of fever; meningeal signs may not be present in the stuporous patient. The commonest diagnostic error made by physicians in a retrospective cardiac transplantation study was to mistakenly ascribe unrecognized central nervous system infection to metabolic disturbances or to "intensive care unit psychosis".[27] Neurologic disorders occurred in over 50% of transplant recipients, and infection was the commonest cause. The term *septic encephalopathy* has been introduced by Young and colleagues[31] to denote the mental status changes that accompany systemic infection in the absence of other organ failure or overt involvement of the brain or meninges. Clinical or EEG evidence of diffuse cerebral dysfunction has been found in over 70% of patients with positive blood cultures.[31] Often, a polyneuropathy becomes evident as the confusional state abates, and patients may have unexplained difficulty in weaning from mechanical ventilation.[31]

Medications are among the most commonly cited causes of postoperative confusion. Drug toxicity is especially common in the elderly patient with a compensated dementia, impaired renal or hepatic function, or a known increased sensitivity to medications. Anticholinergic drugs, such as atropine, antihistamines, and antiparkinsonian agents, are frequently implicated,[6, 18, 20–22] as discussed later. Cimetidine may produce confusional states[32, 33] but also inhibits the cytochrome P-450 enzyme system and thus increases the toxicity of drugs metabolized by the liver, such as bendzodizepines, barbiturates, lidocaine, and narcotic analgesics.[34] Mental status abnormalities have occurred in 5% of patients given 40 mg/d of prednisone and in up to 20% of patients given 80 mg/d.[34] Drugs commonly associated with postoperative confusion are listed in Table 170–2.

TABLE 170–2. Drugs Commonly Used Postoperatively That Have Been Associated with Confusion

Anticholinergic agents	Methyldopa
Anticonvulsants	Metoclopramide
Antihistamines	Metronidazole
Benzodiazepines	Narcotic agents
Captopril	Nitroprusside sodium
Cephalosporins	Nonsteroidal anti-inflammatory agents
Cimetidine	Penicillin
Ciprofloxacin	Procainamide
Clonidine	Propranolol
Corticosteroids	Quinidine sulfate
Digitalis	Ranitidine
Imipenem-cilastin	Theophylline
Ketoconazole	Trimethoprim-sulfamethoxazole
Lidocaine	

Patients with neurologic causes of postoperative confusion usually have focal signs, except patients with meningitis; encephalitis; small, widespread emboli from endocarditis; and a few small stroke syndromes, as discussed later. A toxic or metabolic derangement, especially hypoglycemia or hyperglycemia, may also cause focal signs, either sui generis or reappearing from a prior stroke. Focal findings may also result from a subdural hematoma caused by patient's unwitnessed fall, or they may be seen after a "spontaneous" hematoma occurs in a patient who is taking an anticoagulant or has a blood dyscrasia.

Two particular strokes, right middle cerebral artery and left posterior cerebral artery infarction, may present with confusion and few other findings and are often difficult to detect in the inattentive patient.[35–38] Visual field loss, hemisensory deficit, inability to read (but ability to write), and anomia most severe for colors are seen after bilateral or dominant-hemisphere posterior cerebral artery strokes.[35] Signs of right middle cerebral artery strokes include visual field loss, neglect of visual stimuli on the left side of space, and less often, slight drift of the outstretched left arm or mild left face and hand weakness.[36, 37]

MECHANISMS/PATHOPHYSIOLOGY

Such a wide diversity of conditions are associated with postoperative confusion that a common pathophysiology is unlikely. Attention can be disturbed by many different mechanisms, not all of which are fully understood. Cerebral metabolism is reduced in all metabolic disorders that produce decreased consciousness.[4] A subsequent reduced synthesis of neurotransmitters and especially of acetylcholine may result,[39] thereby playing a central role in causing an ACS. Interference with cholinergic transmission also occurs as a result of exposure to toxins and drugs that produce confusional states, such as antihistamines, antidepressants, neuroleptics, and antiparkinsonian drugs. Raised serum levels of anticholinergic drugs were found in most of the 34% of patients who developed postcardiotomy delirium in one study, whereas those who remained cognitively normal had low levels.[19] Drugs such as alcohol, barbiturates, phenytoin, and phenothiazines exert direct effects on neuronal membranes in the cerebrum and diencephalon,[4] where impairment of the reticular activation system may reduce arousal.

The mental status changes associated with infection may be due to bacterial products or to cytokines,[29, 40] messengers released from macrophages and lymphoctes during sepsis. Cytokines may directly affect brain function, increase procoagulant activity, cause capillary leakage with tissue edema, and alter the blood-brain barrier.[29]

Focal brain lesions of the inferior posterior parietal, temporal, or inferior frontostriatal regions of the right middle cerebral artery,[36–38] or of the posterior hippocampus, parahippocampal, and occipitotemporal gyri of the left posterior cerebral artery territory[35] also cause ACS. Strokes in these areas usually result from emboli, most often of a cardiac source.[37] The attention deficit resulting from these strokes may be caused by the disconnection of limbic structures from cortical input.[35–37]

TREATMENT

Therapy is generally aimed at reversible medical disorders, but symptomatic treatment may also be needed to protect the agitated patient from injury. Fluid and electrolyte balance, blood volume, perfusion pressure, oxygenation, and infection all require close attention postoperatively. "Polypharmacy" should be avoided, and all nonessential drugs, especially those with psychoactive properties, should be withdrawn. Sedative-hypnotic drugs should not be used unless alcohol or benzodiazepine withdrawal is being treated.

Agitation is best controlled by nonpharmacologic means, whenever possible. The physician should encourage the presence of a family member, explain all procedures in detail, arrange nursing procedures to maximize uninterrupted sleep, keep the room dimly lit, and replace eyeglasses and hearing aids to avoid loss of sensory cues.

Haloperidol is the drug of choice for rapid control of agitation when nonpharmacologic measures fail, with a few exceptions. Because it has minimum effect on respiration and blood pressure, unlike the benzodiazepines, it is the ideal treatment for severely ill patients with cardiovascular or respiratory compromise. Although not yet approved by the Food and Drug Administration, its intravenous use is usually advised and can be arranged through the hospital's human studies committee. Intramuscular injection may also be effective but is less favorable because drug absorption may be slower and erratic by this route, especially in cases of hypotension, and may also interfere with the interpretation of muscle enzyme studies. The initial intravenous dose of haloperidol varies with the degree of delirium: 0.5 to 2 mg for mild agitation, 2 to 5 mg for moderate agitation, and 10 to 20 mg, given slowly, for severe agitation.[34] Heparin infusions should be stopped because heparin sodium forms a precipitate when it is combined with haloperidol lactate; intravenous lines or heparin locks should be flushed with 0.9% saline before and after haloperidol infusion. Because the onset of action takes 10 to 30 minutes, repeat doses should be given at intervals of no less than 20 to 30 minutes. The dose may be repeated, if the desired effect is not achieved 30 minutes after the initial dose. If the agitated delirium is still uncontrolled 30 minutes after the second dose, the initial dose should be doubled and can be given every 30 minutes until the patient is calm. Alternatively, if the patient is severly agitated, each successive dose may be doubled and given every 30 minutes until the patient is calm.[34]

Haloperidol administered intravenously rarely causes extrapyramidal symptoms, such as occur after oral administration.[34] Dystonic reactions are the commonest extrapyramidal symptoms, usually involving face and neck, and they respond to anticholinergic therapy (e.g., diphenydramine or benztropine).

Neuroleptics are not the best treatment for anticholinergic delirium, hepatic encephalopathy, or alcohol or benzodiazepine withdrawal. They are also contraindicated in coma. Anticholinergic drugs should be discontinued and supportive care provided for patients with anticholinergic delirium; parenteral physostigmine may be useful in life-threatening cases but can cause side effects, such as cardiac arrhythmias and respiratory depression. In hepatic encephalopathy, a short-acting benzodiazepine that requires little liver degradation (e.g., oxazepam) is recommended. Benzodiazepines are the drugs of choice in the treatment of alcohol or benzodiazepine withdrawal.

PROGNOSIS

Several factors are often simultaneously responsible for postoperative confusion, but because these reverse with time, the patient is usually left without residual damage. Shortcomings not previously noted by the family, however, may suddenly become apparent. In the elderly, usually a considerable delay (days to months) occurs between the resolution of the underlying metabolic derangement or drug effect and the recovery of mental function. Furthermore, the elderly[3] and those who have anoxic brain damage may not regain a normal mental state or return to the original level of functioning.

References

1. Lipowski ZJ: Delirium in the elderly patient. N Engl J Med 1989; 320:578.
2. Chedru C, Geschwind N: Disorders of higher cortical functions in acute confusional states. Cortex 1972; 8:395.
3. Mesulam MM: Disordered mental states in the postoperative period. Urol Clin North Am 1976; 3:199.
4. Adams RD, Victor M: Principles of Neurology. New York, McGraw-Hill, 1989.
5. Heilman KM, Valenstein E, Watson RT: Behavioral aspects of neurological disease: Attentional, intentional, and emotional disorders. *In*: Clinical Neurology. Joynt RJ (Ed). Philadelphia, JB Lippincott, 1990, pp 1–35.
6. Gustafson Y, Berggren D, Brannstrom B, et al: Acute confusional states in elderly patients treated for femoral neck fracture. J Am Geriatr Soc 1988; 36:525.
7. Coffey CE, Massey EW, Roberts KB, et al: Natural history of cerebral complications of coronary artery bypass graft surgery. Neurology 1983; 33:1416.
8. Shaw PJ, Bates D, Cartlidge NEF, et al: Early intellectual dysfunction following coronary bypass surgery. Q J Med 1986; 58:59.
9. Rogers MP, Liang MH, Daltroy LH, et al: Delirium after elective orthopedic surgery: Risk factors and natural history. Int J Psychiatry Med 1989; 19:109.
10. Craven JL: Postoperative organic mental syndromes in lung transplant recipients. J Heart Lung Transplant 1990; 9:129.
11. Townes BD, Bashein G, Hornbein TF, et al: Neurobehavioral outcomes in cardiac operations. J Thorac Cardiovasc Surg 1989; 98:774.
12. Savagneau JA, Stanton BA, Jenkins CD, et al: Neuropsychological dysfunction following elective cardiac operation. J Thorac Cardiovasc Surg 1982; 84:585.
13. Breuer AC, Furlan AJ, Hanson MR, et al: Central nervous system complications of coronary artery bypass graft surgery: Prospective analysis of 41 patients. Stroke 1983; 14:682.
14. Kornfeld DS, Heller SS, Frank KA, et al: Delirium after coronary artery bypass surgery. J Thorac Cardiovasc Surg 1978; 76:93.
15. Slogoff S, Girgis KZ, Keats AS: Etiologic factors in neuropsychiatric complications associated with cardiopulmonary bypass. Anesth Analg 1982; 61:903.
16. Sotaniemi KA, Juolasmaa A, Hokkanen ET: Neuropsychological outcome after open-heart surgery. Arch Neurol 1981; 38:2.
17. Coupal P, Morin P, Paiement B: Delirium after surgery with extra-corporeal circulation. Can J Anaesth 1981; 28:350.
18. Tune LE, Damlouji N, Holland A, et al: Association of postoperative delirium with raised serum levels of anticholinergic drugs. Lancet 1981; ii:651.
19. Shaw PJ, Bates D, Cartlidge NEF, et al: An analysis of factors predisposing to neurological injury in patients undergoing coronary bypass operations. Q J Med 1989; 72:633.
20. Golinger RC, Peet T, Tune LE: Association of elevated plasma anticholinergic activity with delirium in surgical patients. Am J Psychiatry 1987; 144:1218.
21. Greenblatt DJ, Shader RI: Anticholinergics. N Engl J Med 1973; 288:1215.
22. Francis J, Martin D, Kapoor WN: A prospective study of delirium in hospitalized elderly. JAMA 1990; 263:1097.
23. Berggren D, Gustafson Y, Eriksson B, et al: Postoperative confusion after anesthesia in elderly patients with femoral neck fractures. Anesth Analg 1987; 66:497.
24. Chung F, Lavelle PA, McDonald S, et al: Cognitive impairment after neuroleptanalgesia in cataract surgery. Anesth Analg 1989; 68:614.
25. Ray WA, Griffin MR, Schaffner W, et al: Psychotropic drug use and the risk of hip fracture. N Engl J Med 1987; 316:363.
26. Tinetti ME, Speechley M, Ginter SF: Risk factors for falls among elderly persons living in the community. N Engl J Med 1988; 319:1701.

27. Hotson JR, Pedley TA: The neurological complications of cardiac transplantation. Brain 1976; 99:673.
28. Mesulam MM: Principles of Behavioral Neurology. Philadelphia, FA Davis, 1988.
29. Young CB, Bolton CF: The neurology of sepsis. Neurol Chron 1992; 2:1.
30. Plum F, Posner JB: The Diagnosis of Stupor and Coma. Philadelphia, FA Davis, 1982.
31. Young GB, Bolton CF, Austin TW, et al: The encephalopathy associated with septic illness. Clin Invest Med 1990; 13:297.
32. Adler LE, Sudju L, Wilets G: Cimetidine toxicity manifested as paranoia and hallucinations. Am J Psychiatry 1980; 137:1112.
33. Schentag JJ, Cerra FB, Calleri G: Pharmacokinetic and clinical studies in patients with cimetidine-induced mental confusion. Lancet 1979; i:177.
34. Fish DN: Treatment of delirium in the critically ill patient. Clin Pharm 1991; 10:456.
35. Devinsky O, Bear D, Volpe BT: Confusional states following posterior cerebral artery infarction. Arch Neurol 1988; 45:160.
36. Mesulam MM, Waxman SG, Geschwind N, et al: Acute confusional states with right middle cerebral artery infarctions. J Neurol Neurosurg Psychiatry 1976; 39:84.
37. Caplan LR, Kelly M, Kase CS, et al: Infarcts of the inferior division of the right middle cerebral artery: Mirror image of Wernicke's aphasia. Neurology 1986; 36:1015.
38. Mori E, Yamadori A: Acute confusional state and acute agitated delirium. Arch Neurol 1987; 44:1139.
39. Engel GL, Romano J: Delirium, a syndrome of cerebral insufficiency. J Chronic Dis 1959; 9:260.
40. Dinarello CA: Interleukin-1 and the pathogenesis of the acute-phase response. N Engl J Med 1984; 311:1413.

CHAPTER 171

Evaluation of the Comatose Patient

Jonathan D. Root, MD • Fred Plum, MD

Altered states of consciousness generate some of the commonest emergency room visits and intensive care admissions. Rapid assessment of the underlying mechanisms, that is, the pathophysiology of the change in sensorium, is essential to the initiation of effective life-saving measures. Consciousness may be defined as the "state of awareness of the self and the environment"[1] and requires two intact physiologic components: wakefulness and cognitive function. Most disorders regarded as acute disturbances of consciousness are, in fact, impairments of arousal that create circumstances under which the brain's capacity for consciousness cannot be tested. Chronic unconsciousness following severe cerebral injury, by contrast, can occur during full wakefulness in the condition called the *vegetative state.* Coma represents the most profound acute perturbation of arousal and consists of a state of uninterruptable, sleeplike unresponsiveness. Stupor may be considered a slightly less ominous sign because vigorous external noxious stimulation leads to brief arousal. Alterations in arousal level may be brief, lasting several seconds or minutes, or sustained, lasting several hours or longer; this chapter discusses states that produce prolonged periods of unarousability requiring intensive evaluation and care.

ANATOMY, PATHOLOGY, PATHOPHYSIOLOGY

The arousal state is governed by a combination of cortical and brain stem function. Arousal mechanisms arise from the rostral one third of the pontine tegmentum and hypothalamus and project activating signals forward to the thalamus and cortex.[2] The system contains adrenergic, cholinergic, serotonergic, and other ascending fiber systems, no one of which has been isolated as the singular arousal neurotransmitter.[3] Thalamic relay nuclei include the medial, intralaminar, and reticular nuclei, which in turn send diffuse projections to the cerebral cortex.[4] Furthermore, the cortex feeds back on the thalamic nuclei to contribute an important self-cycling loop to arousal mechanisms.[5] Acute, severe damage either to the ascending brain stem–thalamic activating system or to the corticothalamocortical loop is capable of producing an unarousable state. Consciousness depends on continuous interaction between the mechanisms that provide arousal and awareness. The cerebrum provides for cognition and self-excitation, and the brain stem and thalamus provide the activating mechanism.[5] Reciprocal interaction of these structures allows for maintenance of consciousness. Therefore, a depressed level of consciousness can result from dysfunction of brain stem activating mechanisms, or impaired cerebral hemispheres, or both. Reduction of arousal and attention results in sustained impairment of consciousness and in changes in an individual's normal sleep-wake cycle.

Structural Lesions Causing Coma

The causes of coma may be divided into structural and nonstructural disorders. Structural disease of the intracranial contents sufficient to produce coma may be located in either the supratentorial or the infratentorial compartments. Mass lesions sufficient to produce coma do so by disruption of brain stem–hypothalamic activating mechanisms through a shift or compression of deep-lying intracranial contents; this event may occur either by halting of axoplasmic flow or by production of sustained depolarization because of ischemia or hemorrhage. Factors contributing to the degree and rate of loss of arousal include the location and size of the lesion and any associated inflammatory or reactive tissue surrounding the lesion. Cerebral mass lesions displace normal intracranial contents, altering the normal physiology of the brain's cerebrospinal fluid production and resorption as well as its vascular supply. These changes, in turn, can engender an increased bulk of the tissue, a reduction in intracranial compliance, and an additional shift or herniation of intracerebral structures. Increased intracranial pressure commonly reflects these abnormalities, although it is not, of itself, necessarily dangerous. In many patients with acutely received or developing intracranial mass lesions, cerebrovascular autoregulation deteriorates, potentially resulting in recurrent, abrupt increases in intracranial pressure (pressure waves), which further compromise cerebral blood flow in critically injured areas.

Two herniation syndromes are recognized that delineate the mechanism by which supratentorial lesions produce coma. In both, the acuteness of injury dictates whether actual anatomic changes precede (in slowly developing lesions) or parallel the patient's descent into stupor or coma. *Downward transtentorial herniation* can be centrally or unilaterally predominant. Central herniation most often accompanies deep or midline supratentorial masses, large hemispheric infarctions, or extra-axial mass lesions and results in compression of brain stem activating systems in the thalamus and midbrain. Plum and Posner have outlined the successive pathologic and clinical stages.[1] Pathologically, bilateral, symmetric displacement of the supratentorial contents occurs through the incisura or tentorial notch (which separates the anterior-middle cranial fossa from the posterior fossa) into the subtentorial region. Arousal is impaired early, pupils become small (to 3 mm) and reactive, and bilateral corticospinal tract dysfunction develops. Periodic (Cheyne-Stokes) breathing, grasp reflexes, roving eye movements, or depressed escape of oculocephalic reflexes often accompany the process. Decorticate (flexor) or decerebrate posturing is common. Without appropriate therapy to interrupt these events at the deep diencephalic stage, central herniation usually progresses to compress the midbrain, leading to deep coma and to pupils' becoming midposition (3–5 mm) and unreactive to light, signifying both sympathetic and parasympathetic denervation. Spontaneous eye movements cease and become increasingly difficult to elicit by either oculovestibular or oculocephalic maneuvers. Spontaneous decerebrate posturing may occur as midbrain destruction progresses. Once this stage is reached, recovery becomes unlikely. As the wave of downward compression-ischemia advances, it destroys pontine and medullary function, resulting in bizarre breathing patterns and absent reflex eye movements. Eventually, autonomic cardiovascular and respiratory functions cease as medullary centers fail.

Uncal herniation most often accompanies laterally placed hemispheric lesions, which produce side-to-side brain displacement as well as transtentorial herniation. Signs and symptoms are characterized by focal hemispheric dysfunction (aphasia, hemiparesis, seizures), leading to unilateral (usually ipsilateral) compression paralysis of the third cranial nerve. Signs of uncal herniation include pupillary enlargement and diminished reaction to light as the uncus of the temporal lobe first protrudes into the tentorial notch.[1, 6] Shortly after the pupil dilates, more severe oculomotor paresis develops, and the eye turns outward and downward. The ipsilateral posterior cerebral artery may become compressed, causing ipsilateral occipital lobe ischemia. Unchecked, the temporal lobe compresses the midbrain, resulting in loss of consciousness and bilateral or contralateral decerebrate posturing. Ipsilateral to the intracranial lesion, a hemiparesis may develop if the opposite cerebral peduncle becomes compressed against the contralateral tentorial edge. Brain stem signs then become symmetric, and herniation proceeds in the same pattern as occurs with central herniation, with progressive rostrocaudal brain stem dysfunction.

Both of these herniation syndromes eventually disrupt central brain stem and posterior diencephalic activating systems. Results of magnetic resonance imaging (MRI) or postmortem studies in such patients confirm the presence of brain stem buckling, midbrain compression, and brain stem infarction and hemorrhage.[7] Direct mass effect or a differential pressure gradient between compartments (and not the absolute level of intracranial pressure) leads to displacement of intracranial contents, with potentially fatal consequences. Blockage of cerebrospinal fluid outflow may lead to obstructive hydrocephalus, increased intracranial pressure, and herniation of supratentorial contents into the subtentorial compartment.

Subtentorial lesions produce coma by direct destruction of tegmental pontomesencephalic activating systems, by compression of these structures, or by squeezing of the medulla downward sufficiently to push the brain stem and cerebellar tonsils into the foramen magnum, thereby causing cardiorespiratory collapse. Acute intrinsic lesions of the brain stem, usually consisting of hemorrhage or ischemia, often cause the abrupt onset of coma and are invariably associated with abnormal neuro-ophthalmologic function. Pupils may be pinpoint as a result of disruption of pontine sympathetic pathways, or they may be dilated as a result of destruction of the third cranial nerve nuclei or its intra-axial exiting fibers. Dysconjugate eye movements and nystagmus occur frequently, and vertical eye movements are relatively preserved. Ocular bobbing signifies pontine damage.

Affected patients develop signs of abnormal corticospinal tract function and may be quadriplegic; flaccidity in the upper extremities and flexor responses in the lower extremities often accompany midbrain-pontine damage.[1] Pathologically, basilar artery thrombosis or emboli to the basilar artery leads to asymmetric infarction of the brain stem, with involvement of the ascending reticular activating system and the neighboring densely packed neuropil, as well as the ascending and descending motor and sensory tracts. Infarction of the midline thalamic nuclei secondary to thrombosis of the apex of the basilar artery may produce coma without other obvious brain stem signs. Hemorrhages into the basis pontis spare consciousness but produce neuro-ophthalmic signs and motor dysfunction. Extension of the hemorrhage into the rostral pontine tegmentum usually results in stupor or coma. Basilar migraine, described by Bickerstaff,[8, 9] may produce an alteration of consciousness secondary to dysregulation of brain stem activating centers. Other intrinsic brain stem lesions (e.g., those caused by tumor, abscess, granuloma, demyelination) tend to progress slowly and usually spare arousal mechanisms; they may, however, reduce attention and other cognitive mechanisms, leading to a state of akinetic mutism. Rapidly developing, extensive central pontine myelinolysis may cause acute coma by extension into the pontine tegmentum.

Extra-axial posterior fossa lesions may produce coma by compression of brain stem activating mechanisms or by upward herniation. Signs of compression of the pons may be difficult to distinguish from intrinsic lesions, but they are often accompanied by headache, vomiting, and hypertension due to a Cushing response. Upward transtentorial herniation by the mesencephalon is initially characterized by coma, reactive miotic pupils, asymmetric or absent caloric responses, and decerebrate posturing; caudal-rostral brain stem dysfunction then occurs, with midbrain failure and accompanying midposition, fixed pupils.[10] Causes of brain stem compression include cerebellar hemorrhages, infarctions and infections, rapidly expanding cerebellar or fourth ventricular tumors, or rarely, subtentorial epidural or subdural hematomas. Lateral ventricular drainage aimed at relieving obstructive hydrocephalus associated with posterior fossa masses sometimes precipitates acute upward transtentorial herniation (as was discussed by Reich and coworkers[7]).[11]

Downward herniation of the cerebellar tonsils through the foramen magnum may cause acute medullary dysfunction and abrupt respiratory and circulatory collapse. Less severe impaction of the tonsils in the foramen magnum can lead to obstructive hydrocephalus and consequent bihemispheric dysfunction with alteration in level of consciousness. Accompanying signs include headache, vertical nystagmus, nausea, vomiting, lower cranial nerve signs, ataxia, and irregular breathing. Lumbar puncture in this setting carries a considerable risk of catastrophic consequences.[7] Diagnostic MRI followed by surgical decompression of the posterior fossa and possibly ventricular drainage are recommended.

Nonstructural Disorders Causing Coma

Nonstructural disorders, including metabolic or toxic disturbances, produce coma by diffusely depressing the function of brain stem and cerebral arousal mechanisms. Metabolic coma can be of abrupt onset, such as that occurring with toxic drug ingestion, surgical level anesthesia, or cardiac arrest, or it may progress slowly after a period of confusion and inattention. The main symptoms of metabolic encephalopathy are disturbances in arousability and cognitive function. Other symptoms include abnormalities in the normal sleep-wake cycle, autonomic disturbances, and abnormal respiratory variations, depending on the cause of the encephalopathy. The commonest distinguishing clinical feature of metabolic or toxic encephalopathy is the preservation of pupillary reflexes, except in incidents involving overdoses of anticholinergic agents or near-fatal anoxia; lack of pupillary reactivity requires a search for an underlying structural lesion. The remainder of the neurologic examination shows evidence of bilateral cerebral cognitive and arousal dysfunction, with varying degrees of brain stem dysregulation. Deeply comatose patients who have no imaged or clinical evidence of brain stem or hemispheric function and no known cause for their coma must be assumed to have suffered accidental or intentional self-poisoning. Metabolic disturbances particularly affect patients with serious systemic illnesses, those who have undergone complicated surgery, and, especially, those of advanced age. Special attention should be given to a historical evaluation of the patient's previous medical and psychiatric illnesses and the use of potentially intoxicating drugs.

The clinical characteristics of metabolic encephalopathy reflect evidence of multilevel central nervous system dysfunction. At the outset, many patients demonstrate abnormalities in cognition that are at least as severe as their disturbance of arousal. Misperception, disorientation, multimodality hallucinations, poor concentration and memory, and occasionally, hypervigilance may progress to profound stupor or coma; the individual's level of consciousness often fluctuates between examinations. Motor signs, when they exist, are most often symmetric and bilateral; patients often suffer from tremor, asterixis, and multifocal myoclonus. Spontaneous motor activity ranges from bradykinesia, in cases of sedative overdose and endogenous metabolic disturbances, to hyperactivity, in states of drug withdrawal or overdose of stimulating agents, such as cocaine and phencyclidine. Sensory abnormalities rarely occur. Seizures occur particularly in states of drug withdrawal associated with cortical disease. Focal seizures may occur without underlying substrate abnormalities in patients with hypoglycemia, hypocalcemia or hypercalcemia, hepatic encephalopathy, uremia, or toxic ingestion. Autonomic dysregulation and hypothermia occur in patients who have sedative drug overdoses, hypoglycemia, and myxedema. Hyperthermia occurs in withdrawal states, particularly delirium tremens, anticholinergic overdose, infection, neuroleptic malignant syndrome, or malignant hyperthermia. The legion causes of metabolic or toxic encephalopathy are detailed in Table 171–1.

Coma is not a permanent state; all patients who survive beyond the stage of acute, systemic complications reawaken and either proceed to recovery (with none or varying degrees of disability) or plateau at a vegetative level. The vegetative state may be defined as chronic wakefulness without awareness and may be a consequence of various pathologic insults, including stroke, trauma, poisoning, infections, hypoxia-ischemia, hypoglycemia, or degenerative disease.[12] Pathologically, extensive damage to the cortical mantle, thalamus, and cerebellum is seen, usually with limited or no direct brain stem destruction.[13] Metabolic studies performed with positron-emission tomography confirm the profound depression of glucose utilization by the cerebral cortex in vegetative patients, with values approaching those found during deep, barbiturate-induced anesthesia.[14] Clinically, vegetative patients appear to be awake and to have cyclical sleep patterns; however, such individuals do not show evidence of cognitive function or learned behavioral responses to external stimulation. Vegetative patients may feature spontaneous eye opening and eye movements and stereotypic facial and limb movements; however, they are unable to demonstrate speech or comprehension, and they lack purposeful activity. Vegetative patients generate normal body temperatures, are doubly incontinent, and usually have normally functioning cardiovascular, respiratory, and digestive systems. Nutritional support via enteral feedings can prolong survival for an indefinite period. Crucial in determining the existence of the vegetative state is the exclusion of the presence of the locked-in syndrome; in this latter condition, the patient is awake and aware but is unable to communicate because of total muscular paralysis. The patient may have some ability to move the eyelids, thereby permitting a coded form of communication. Positron-emission tomographic studies demonstrate mild diminishment in central glucose utilization as compared with that in control subjects.[14] Pathologically, this condition may be produced by lesions of descending motor pathways in the ventral pontine or inframedullary bulbar regions; it rarely occurs with severe, inflammatory acute demyelinating or axonal polyneuropathies.

The term persistent vegetative state defines the condition as lasting for at least 1 month after traumatic or nontraumatic brain injury. Accurate diagnosis of the persistent vegetative state requires extended observation of the patient to assess behavioral responses to external stimulation and to demonstrate cognitive unawareness. Misdiagnosis in 18 of 49 patients in persistent vegetative states referred to a rehabilitation center was documented by Childs and colleagues.[15] Although inaccurate diagnosis may have resulted from an unclear definition of persistent vegetative state that was applied by the referring physicians, misdiagnosis occurred significantly more often in patients who suffered a traumatic brain insult and whose injury occurred at least 3 months before transfer for rehabilitation. Accurate reclassification of patients was accomplished in 14 of 18 patients by the third day of observation.[15] Prognostic considerations of patients in a persistent vegetative state are considered later.

NEURODIAGNOSTIC EVALUATION

Careful but rapid assessment is essential in comatose patients. The neurodiagnostic evaluation begins with a sharply focused history and physical examination. Immediate attention is directed at maintenance of adequate respiratory and cardiovascular function and securing of appropriate blood studies, as is discussed later. Then, further investigation may be necessary to document the location of the lesion and to provide guidance for therapeutic intervention. Such studies provide anatomic assessment, functional assessment, or both, of the central nervous system. Two types of imaging techniques provide helpful information for defining the anatomic localization of lesions that produce coma: computed tomography (CT) and MRI. MRI is technically more difficult but allows relatively rapid assessment of intracranial contents and is particularly helpful in defining abnormalities in the posterior fossa, which may be obscured by bone artifact inherent in CT scanning. MRI provides visualization of anatomic lesions, such as those resulting from acute stroke, encephalitis, central pontine myelinolysis, and traumatic shear injury, with greater resolution and at an earlier time than CT scanning. The injection of the paramagnetic substance gadolinium helps delineate areas of blood-brain barrier breakdown and may augment the sensitivity of the scanning technique. Sagittal MRI views are particularly useful in the documentation of the degree of supratentorial or infratentorial herniations and may enable intervention before clinical deterioration (Fig. 171–1).[7] Newer MRI techniques allow for functional imaging of the central nervous system by measurement of cerebral blood flow to a particu-

TABLE 171–1. Metabolic or Toxic Causes of Stupor or Coma

I. Endogenous disorders
  A. Deprivation of substrate
    1. Hypoxia with normal cerebral blood flow
      a) Diminished oxygen tension secondary to pulmonary disease
      b) Diminished oxygen content
        (1) Anemia
        (2) Carbon dioxide poisoning
        (3) Altitude sickness
        (4) Anesthetic accidents
        (5) Cyanide poisoning
    2. Ischemia
      a) Diminished cerebral blood flow to diffuse brain regions
      b) Shock secondary to hemorrhagic hypovolemia, sepsis, cardiac arrest, pulmonary embolism, or diminished peripheral vascular resistance
      c) Increase in cerebrovascular resistance
        (1) Hyperventilation
        (2) Hyperviscosity syndrome
        (3) Vasospasm secondary to subarachnoid hemorrhage
        (4) Vessel occlusion
          i) Disseminated intravascular coagulation
          ii) Vasculitis
          iii) Multiple emboli secondary to subacute bacterial endocarditis, aortic disease, fat emboli
          iv) Cardiopulmonary bypass
          v) Platelet disorder
          vi) Thrombotic thrombocytopenic purpura
        (5) Failure of autoregulation
        (6) Hypertensive encephalopathy
    3. Hypoglycemia
    4. Cofactor deficiency
      a) Thiamine
      b) Vitamin B_{12}
      c) Pyridoxine
  B. Organ dysfunction with secondary brain dysregulation
    1. Liver
      a) Hepatic encephalopathy
      b) Reye's syndrome
      c) Urea cycle disorders
    2. Kidney
    3. Lung
    4. Endocrine
      a) Parahypopituitarism
      b) Hyperthyroidism or hypothyroidism
      c) Hyperparathyroidism or hypoparathyroidism
      d) Hyperadrenalism or hypoadrenalism
      e) Diabetes
        (1) Ketoacidosis
    5. Other
      a) Porphyria
      b) Sepsis
      c) Paraneoplastic encephalopathy secondary to cancer

II. Abnormalities of osmolality or acid-base status
III. Abnormalities of temperature regulation
  A. Hypothermia
  B. Hyperthermia
    1. Neuroleptic malignant syndrome
    2. Heat stroke
IV. Infections or inflammation of the central nervous system
  A. Encephalitis
  B. Leptomeningitis
  C. Parainfectious encephalomyelitis
V. Seizures and postictal states
VI. Concussion
VII. Exogenous poisons
  A. Alcohol or sedative drugs
  B. Acid poisons
    1. Ethylene glycol
    2. Methyl alcohol
    3. Paraldehyde
  C. Psychotropic drugs
    1. Opiates
    2. Cocaine
    3. Amphetamines
    4. Lithium
    5. Tricyclic antidepressants and anticholinergic agents
    6. Phenothiazines
    7. Mescaline
    8. Monoamine oxidase inhibitors
  D. Other
    1. Anticonvulsants
    2. Salicylates
    3. Cimetidine
    4. Steroids
    5. Cardiac glycosides
    6. Ciguatera toxin
VIII. Intensive care unit psychosis

lar region; future application of this technique may allow rapid determination of diminished cerebral blood flow, such as occurs in stroke or vasospasm, and will probably be useful in assessing the effect of therapeutic interventions.

CT remains the most readily accessible neuroradiographic technique for rapid assessment of intracranial contents. The technique is indispensable in the management of acute head injury. CT can delineate calvarial fractures and intracranial hematomas (epidural, subdural, intraparenchymal, intraventricular, subarachnoid), which may require acute neurosurgical intervention. The technique should be employed before cerebrospinal fluid is removed for examination in nearly all incidences of coma caused by suspected meningitis, encephalitis, or posterior fossa lesion. CT scanning without contrast enhancement should be used to assess patients suspected of having an intracranial hemorrhage, ischemic stroke of at least 12 hours' duration, or hydrocephalus. The addition of iodinated contrast material highlights areas of blood-brain barrier breakdown, particularly those caused by tumors, meningitis, abscesses, and acute or subacute stroke. CT scanning may, however, underestimate the degree of intracranial compartmental herniation, which is better assessed by MRI.[7]

Fever in an acutely comatose patient suggests infection, either meningitis or encephalitis. After precautions are taken to rule out intracranial mass lesions, a lumbar puncture may then be performed with the patient in the decubitis position, and the cerebrospinal fluid may be sent for appro-

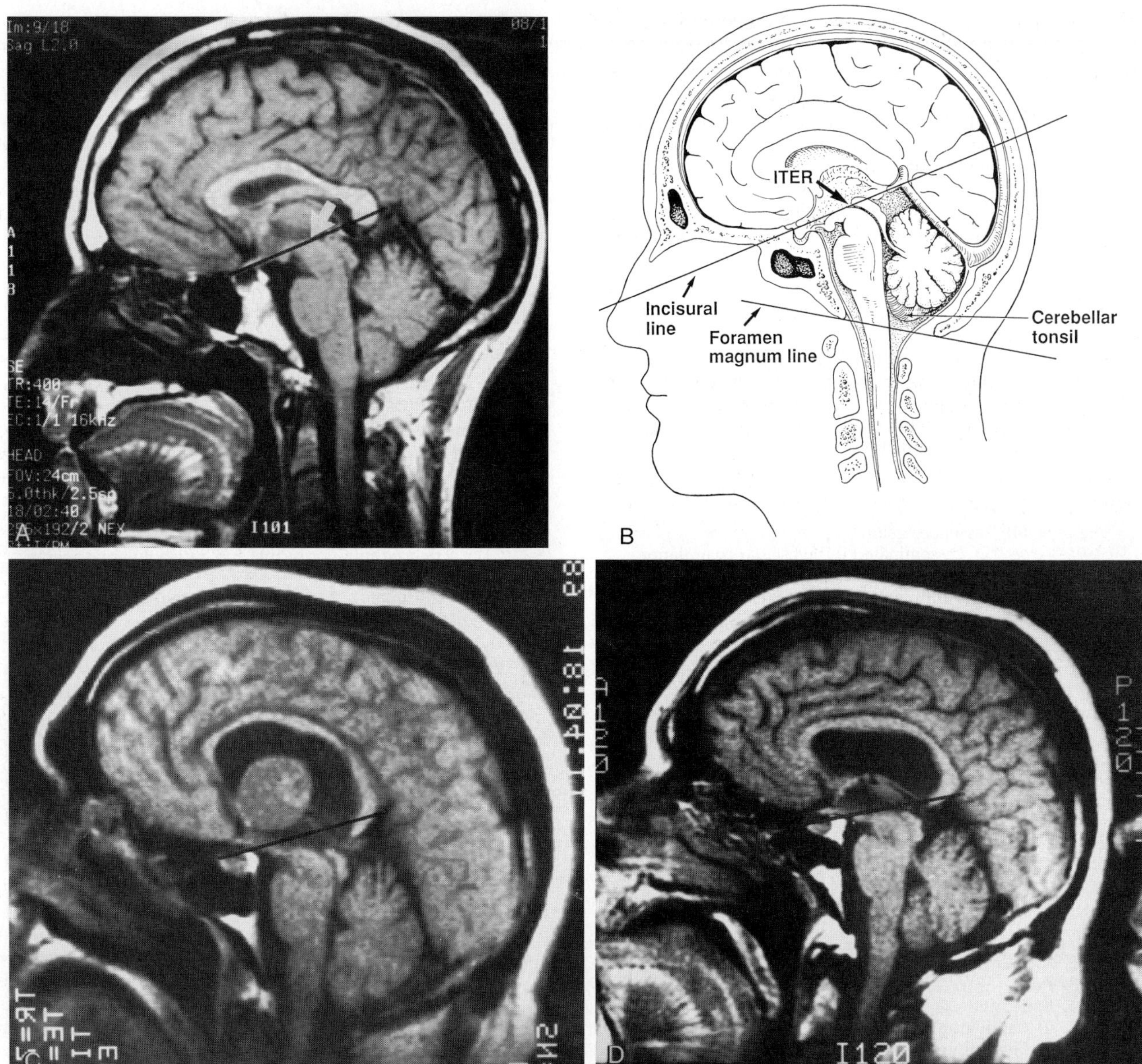

Figure 171–1. Midsagittal MRI views of a normal adult brain and of a brain with reversible downward transtentorial herniation. MRI view of a normal adult male brain *(A)* with accompanying diagram *(B)*. The opening of the tentorium of the cerebellum or anterior cerebellar notch lies along a line (incisural line) defined anteriorly by the anterior tubercle of the sella turcica and posteriorly by the junction of the Galen's vein, the inferior sagittal sinus, and the confluence of the straight sinus. The proximal opening of the aqueduct of Sylvius, the iter *(arrow)*, lies within 2 mm of the incisural line.[7] The foramen magnum line is defined between the inferior tip of the clivus anteriorly and the bony base of the posterior lip of the foramen magnum. *C*, A 47-year-old male who experienced 1 week of headache, nausea, vomiting, and gait ataxia presented with abrupt onset coma, palsy of cranial nerve III, hyperreflexia, and extensor plantar responses bilaterally. MRI revealed a third ventricular mass, obstructive hydrocephalus, and displacement of the iter inferiorly by 6.5 mm. The cerebellar tonsils were not displaced. *D*, Subsequent MRI view in the patient in *B* 2 weeks after surgical removal of a colloid cyst. The iter is 1.2 mm below the incisural line. The patient had full neurologic recovery. (*A*, *C*, and *D* reprinted with permission from Reich JB, Sierra J, Camp W, et al: Magnetic resonance imaging measurements and clinical changes accompanying transtentorial and foramen magnum brain herniation. Ann Neurol 1993; 33:159–170.)

priate studies. Rarely, hyperthermia may complicate direct central nervous system injuries, particularly subarachnoid, intraventricular, and intraparenchymal hemorrhages. Severe hyperthermia alone may also cause coma, as occurs in malignant hyperthermia secondary to anesthesia and the neuroleptic malignant syndrome.

Electroencephalography (EEG) possesses only selective value over brain imaging in identifying causes of coma. Patients with metabolic or toxic encephalopathies may have bilateral, symmetric slow or fast activity on the EEG, depending on the cause of the encephalopathy. Overdosage with sedative hypnotics may produce rapid beta activity (>13 Hz). In hepatic encephalopathy, a characteristic slowing into the theta (4–7 Hz) or delta (1–3 Hz) range occurs that is accompanied by paroxysmal or triphasic waves. Focally destructive lesions, such as those caused by stroke, tumor, abscess, and herpes encephalitis, show focal slow activity and, sometimes, periodic lateralized epileptiform discharges. A continuous EEG alpha pattern in a patient in an unresponsive coma implies a poor prognosis.[16] Such tracings occur most often in patients with either postanoxic encephalopathy or acute pontine tegmental damage. The EEG is indispensable in the evaluation of nonconvulsive generalized status epilepticus and multiple complex partial seizures, both of which produce alterations in cognitive function and level of arousal. An EEG may also aid in locating the initiating epileptogenic site of a lesion in a patient with postictal confusion. Occasionally, an EEG may be necessary to differentiate psychogenic unresponsiveness from true coma; a normally reactive EEG in an unresponsive patient excludes organic brain disease.

Continuous EEG monitoring in the intensive care unit setting has revealed evidence of a high incidence of unsuspected electrographic seizures in critically ill neurologic patients.[17, 18] Treatment of the seizures as well as the underlying condition may enhance both the rapidity of recovery and the prognosis. Continuous EEG monitoring should be employed in patients treated for status epilepticus because the clinical examination is insufficiently sensitive to ascertain the presence and frequency of subclinical electrographic seizures. Only through this technique can the continuation of potentially dangerous seizure activity and the need for appropriate intervention be recognized.

Assessment and manipulation of intracranial pressure may be necessary during intensive management of brain-injured patients. Options include measurement of subdural, subarachnoid, intraventricular, or intraparenchymal pressures. Drainage of cerebrospinal fluid may relieve high intracranial pressures in patients with diminished cerebral compliance and, therefore, compromised central perfusion. We favor placement of a ventriculostomy because it allows accurate measurements of intraventricular intracranial pressure and it provides a mechanism for cerebrospinal fluid drainage. Patients with moderate-to-severe head trauma, acute hydrocephalus, Reye's syndrome, and occasionally, encephalitis often are best treated with a ventriculostomy into the lateral ventricle. Monitoring of intracranial pressure allows therapeutic intervention before clinical deterioration occurs in patients with diminished intracranial compliance; whether the routine practice of this procedure alters prognosis is not certain. Measurement of intracranial pressure, however, allows calculation of cerebral perfusion pressure, a critical determinant of cerebral blood flow and therefore oxygen and substrate delivery. The rate of complications with this technique is low. Our experience suggests that the risk of ventricular infection increases with time. We recommend removing or changing catheters every 5 to 7 days. The organism that most commonly causes catheter-related ventriculitis has been *Staphylococcus epidermidis*.

MANAGEMENT

Management of the comatose patient may be divided into two categories: emergent and serial.[19, 20] As noted, emergent therapy must be applied even as diagnostic evaluation is being carried out to prevent irreparable central nervous system injury; adequate cardiorespiratory function must be preserved so that tissue hypoxia does not develop. For deeply comatose patients, we recommend early endotracheal intubation to ensure adequate ventilatory support and airway protection. Extreme care must be taken to prevent neck movement in patients whose coma is secondary to head trauma. Arterial blood oxygen saturation greater than 90% and normocarbia (unless clear evidence of cerebral herniation is ascertained) must be maintained through alteration of ventilator settings; positive end-expiratory pressure should be avoided when increased intracranial pressure may be present. Circulation should be maintained by appropriate fluid management, using lactated Ringer's solution except when normal saline is used for the management of cerebral herniation. Mean arterial pressures are kept at 80 to 90 mm Hg with fluids and pressors, and urine output should be at least 0.5 $mL \cdot kg^{-1} \cdot h^{-1}$. A nasogastric tube is placed to facilitate gastric lavage, to prevent regurgitation, and to allow for eventual enteral feeding. Within a few minutes of the patient's arrival at the hospital, blood should be obtained for biochemical analysis, including studies of glucose level, blood gases, electrolyte level, renal and hepatic function, calcium level, and complete blood count. Thiamine, 100 mg IM, and 50% glucose solution, 50 mL IV, are given immediately thereafter. Blood and urine should be obtained shortly after admission to be analyzed for toxic substances. Naloxone is given empirically to reverse a potential narcotic overdose. If a drug overdose is suspected, then flumazenil, a benzodiazepine antagonist, should be given intravenously. Patients who respond to any of these treatments must be watched carefully for recurrent lethargy or coma because several of the various antidotes do not sustain arousal in instances of moderate-to-severe poisoning.[21, 22]

Further therapy depends on the clinical situation and the continued evaluation of the patient. Electrocardiography should be performed to ascertain evidence of a possible myocardial infarction or arrhythmia that may have caused a cardiac arrest and hypoxic-ischemic brain injury; deeply inverted T waves throughout the precordium may occur in subarachnoid hemorrhage and may indicate that a primary central nervous system event is the cause of coma. Body temperature should be obtained; hypothermia may accompany Wernicke's disease, drug overdose (particularly sedative-hypnotics), near-drowning, hypoglycemia, hypothyroidism, or profound sepsis. Hyperthermia most often indicates an infection and demands an investigation for meningitis, encephalitis, or a cerebral abscess. Hyperthermia also may be caused by subarachnoid, intraparenchymal, or intraventricular hemorrhage; drug overdose with agents with anticholinergic properties; and heat exposure. After appropriate cultures are obtained, patients thought to have active infection should receive antimicrobial agents to minimize further damage to the central nervous system. Correction to normothermia should be undertaken gradually in the hypothermic patient to prevent cardiac dysrhythmias and is essential in patients with hyperthermia greater than 40° Celsius, which itself may exacerbate a central nervous system injury by increasing metabolic demands. Focal and generalized seizures should be controlled with a combination of benzodiazepines and other longer-acting anticonvulsants (phenytoin, barbiturates); generalized status epilepticus may itself cause coma and may produce irreversible brain damage unless it is aggressively managed.[23] In instances of a particular drug intoxication, specific antidotes should be applied (Table 171–2).

Once emergency resuscitation procedures are completed, and if the clinical examination suggests a nonmetabolic cause for the coma, an emergent CT scan should be obtained. Transtentorial herniation usually can be identified on horizontal-plane CT: any disfiguration of the normal shape of the ambient cisterns, which usually become narrowed or occluded as supratentorial structures descend into the tentorial incisura, is evidence of this disorder. Should a mass be found and signs of herniation be clinically apparent, therapy designed to lower intracranial pressure should be rapidly employed and its effects on clinical signs evaluated. Therapy should include temporarily inducing hyperventilation to a P_{CO_2} of 25 to 30 mm Hg, raising the head of

TABLE 171–2. Neurologic Manifestations of Common Drug Poisoning

Drug	*Signs and Symptoms*	*Diagnostic Test*	*Treatment*
Sedative Hypnotics Benzodiazepines Barbiturates Chloral hydrate Meprobamate Ethchlorvynol (Placidyl)	Confusion; lethargy; ataxia; nystagmus; hypothermia; dysarthria; respiratory depression; coma. Pupillary reactions preserved except in instances of deep barbiturate coma. Possible withdrawal seizures.	Blood	Supportive care; gastric lavage; flumazenil for benzodiazepine overdose; hemoperfusion for extreme barbiturate intoxication.
Glutethimide	As above, except pupils may be fixed at different degrees of dilatation, anticholinergic signs, hyperthermia.	Blood	As above.
Methaqualone	Agitation; hypertonic; hyper-reflexia; ataxia; hallucinations; convulsions.	Blood	As above.
Ethanol	Confusion; agitation; delirium; ataxia; nystagmus; dysarthria; coma.	Blood, breath	Supportive care; lavage if within 1 hour of ingestion; thiamine; glucose. Treat withdrawal with benzodiazepines.
Opioids	Lethargy; small reactive pupils; hypothermia; hypotension; urinary retention; shallow, irregular respirations; convulsions.	Urine Response to naloxone	Naloxone, 0.4 mg IV or IM; continuous naloxone infusion, if necessary. Supportive care with intubation as necessary. Lavage if overdose is by ingestion.
Stimulants Amphetamine Methylphenidate Cocaine	Hypervigilance; paranoia; violent behavior; tremulousness; dilated pupils; hyperthermia; tachycardia or arrhythmias; focal neurologic signs secondary to CNS stroke or hemorrhage; seizures	Blood, urine	Supportive care; sedation with benzodiazepines. Treat hypertensive crisis with sodium nitroprusside or labetalol. Watch for rhabdomyolysis.
Psychedelics (LSD, mescaline, PCP)	Delirium; delusions; marked agitation; hallucinations; hyperactivity; dilated pupils; hyper-reflexia; nystagmus.	Blood Measure PCP levels in gastric juice	Gastric lavage; charcoal. Benzodiazepines and haloperidol for sedation.
Antidepressants Tricyclic antidepressants	Anticholinergic effects: dry mouth; agitation; restlessness; ataxia; tachycardia or arrhythmias; hyperthermia; hysteria; convulsions; mydriasis.	Blood, urine	Cardiac monitoring; gastric lavage; charcoal; mild systemic alkalinization. Physostigmine for refractory arrhythmias. Anticonvulsants for seizures.
Monoamine oxidase inhibitors	Drowsiness; ataxia; seizures; hypertensive crisis. Hypotension with severe overdose.		Symptomatic care; gastric lavage; avoid narcotics.
Neuroleptics	Dystonia; drowsiness; coma; convulsions; hypotension; miosis; tremor; hypothermia; neuroleptic malignant syndrome.	Urine	Gastric lavage. Treat extrapyramidal signs with diphenhydramine or benztropine mesylate. Treat neuroleptic malignant syndrome with dantrolene or bromocriptine.
Lithium	Lethargy; tremulousness; weakness; polyuria; polydipsia; ataxia; seizures; coma.	Blood	Hemodialysis for delirium, seizures, or coma.
Methanol, Ethylene glycol	Drunkenness; hyperventilation; stupor; convulsions; coma. Blindness with methanol use.	Blood	Symptomatic care; gastric lavage; ethanol infusion; hemodialysis. For methanol intoxication, 4-methylpyrazole under investigation.
Antihistamines	Anticholinergic effects: dry mucosa; flushed skin; hyperthermia; dilated pupils; delirium; hallucinations; seizures; coma.		Supportive care; gastric lavage; control of seizures with benzodiazepines; physostigmine for life-threatening anticholinergic effects.
Organophosphates	Cholinergic crisis: cramps; excessive secretions; diarrhea; bronchoconstriction. Later, tremulousness; fasciculations; weakness; convulsions; hypertension; tachycardia; confusion; anxiety; coma.	RBC cholinesterase level	Symptomatic care; decontamination; atropine; pralidoxime

TABLE 171–2. Neurologic Manifestations of Common Drug Poisoning *Continued*

Drug	*Signs and Symptoms*	*Diagnostic Test*	*Treatment*
Carbon monoxide	Confusion; agitation; headache; convulsions; coma, respiratory failure; cardiovascular collapse.	History Carboxyhemoglobin level	Remove patient from area; 100% oxygen until carboxyhemoglobin levels fall to <5%. Hyperbaric oxygen if central nervous system affected. Treat cerebral edema with hyperventilation, diuretics, and cerebrospinal fluid drainage, if necessary.
Salicylate	Tinnitus; hyperpnea; confusion; convulsions; coma; hyperthermia.	Blood	Supportive care; gastric lavage; charcoal; systemic alkalinization; hemodialysis for coma or seizures.
Cyanide	Agitation; confusion; headache; vertigo; hypertension; hypotension; seizures; paralysis; apnea; coma.	Blood	Amyl nitrate; sodium nitrate; sodium thiosulfate; 100% oxygen; hyperbaric oxygen for refractory signs. Vitamin B_{12} injection.
Anticonvulsants Phenytoin Carbamazepine Phenobarbital (see Barbiturates) Valproic acid Primidone Ethosuximide Felbamate Clonazepam (see Benzodiazepines)	Drowsiness; ataxia; nystagmus; tremulousness; coma. Dysrhythmias with carbamazepine or phenytoin overdose.	Blood Ammonia level in patients taking valproic acid.	Supportive care; gastric lavage; charcoal. Watch for withdrawal seizures.

(Adapted from Plum F: Disturbances of consciousness and arousal. *In*: Cecil Textbook of Medicine. 19th ed. Wyngaarden JB, Smith LH Jr, Bennett JC [Eds]. Philadelphia, WB Saunders, 1992, pp 2048–2059; Mofenson HC, Caraccio R, Greenshen J: Acute poisonings. *In*: Conn's Current Therapy 1993. Rakel RE [Ed]. Philadelphia, WB Saunders, 1993, pp 1148–1192; Olson KR: Toxicology screens and asymptomatic poisoning. *In*: Current Practice of Emergency Medicine. Callahan ML [Ed]. Philadelphia, BC Decker, 1991, pp 1138–1142, *and* Linden CH: Antidotes in poisoning. *In*: Current Practice of Emergency Medicine. Callahan ML [Ed]. Philadelphia, BC Decker, 1991, pp 1146–1162.

the bed to 30°, administering diuretics (mannitol, 1 g/kg IV), surgical decompression of extracerebral hematomas, and administration of steroids (dexamethasone, 20–40 mg/d) in instances of tumors with vasogenic edema. Drainage of cerebrospinal fluid may be undertaken via a ventriculostomy in patients who are unresponsive to other techniques to lower intracranial pressure or in those with acute hydrocephalus who have an expected favorable prognosis. Maintenance of cerebral blood flow (and thus substrate delivery) through adequate cerebral perfusion pressure and cardiac output is most critical to the prevention of secondary brain injury. Accordingly, once transient signs of herniation have been corrected, ventilation should be *slowly* reduced to bring Pa_{CO_2} levels back to 32 to 35 mm Hg. To continue at lower levels eliminates the chance of using hyperventilation to meet recurring episodes of raised intracranial pressure or herniation.

Serial management of coma should be directed at treating the disease or diseases causing the comatose state and at preventing complications. Effective care demands meticulous attention to the maintenance of tissue perfusion and oxygenation, the documentation and anticipation of acute neurologic events (particularly diminished cerebral perfusion, herniation, or seizures), aggressive, rapid treatment of initial or subsequent infections, and prevention of agitation. Most intensive care units attempt to prevent venous thrombosis by using either full-length leg pneumatic compression boots or subcutaneous heparin. Nutritional needs can be met by initiating enteral or parenteral feedings within 24 to 36 hours after admission. Eye protection using lubricants and taping the lids shut can prevent corneal injury.

PROGNOSIS

Evaluation of the comatose patient necessitates an estimate of prognosis. Appropriate prognostication is essential for providing early, informed discussion with loved ones and for rationing intensive services in hopeless instances. Prognosis in nontraumatic coma depends on the cause of the coma, the clinical signs at presentation and subsequent neurologic examinations, and the length of time the patient is comatose.[27–29] The overall prognosis of nontraumatic coma is poor: only 16% of 500 patients studied by Levy and associates[27] regained independent life during the first year after presentation. The remainder of this cohort either died without recovery from coma (61%), remained in a persistent vegetative state (12%), or became permanently dependent on others for daily living (11%). The longer a coma persists, the lower the chance for recovery; patients surviving in coma for a week without conflicting variables (sedation) rarely recover: only 1 of 38 patients made a good recovery at one year. Total mortality at 1 year was 88%. Remember, however, that the longer one waits to issue a reliable prognosis to the family, the more difficult it becomes to deal with a cognitively hopeless future simply by reducing intensive care measures. The early establishment of a highly probable outcome ideally should be made within the first 24 hours after hospital admission. Prognosis depends on the etiology of nontraumatic coma. Patients in coma secondary to cerebrovascular disease or subarachnoid hemorrhage had only a 9% chance of achieving independent function, followed by patients suffering a cardiopulmonary arrest (12%). One third of patients with metabolic dysfunction, particularly hepatic encephalopathy, did well, regaining independent activity. The severity of signs of brain stem dysfunction on admission inversely correlates with the chance of good recovery in nontraumatic coma.[27, 28] Absent pupillary responses at any time after onset and absent caloric reflexes 1 day after onset indicated a poor prognosis (<2% recovery). No patient with absent pupillary light reflexes, corneal reflexes, caloric or oculocephalic responses, or lack of a motor response to noxious stimulation at 3 days after onset ever regained independent function. Patients who did recover were those who within 1 to 3 days spoke any words, opened their eyes to noise, or had spontaneous eye movements.

Except in the case of carbon monoxide poisoning, patients in coma caused by exogenous agents that depress brain activity carry an overall good prognosis, unless medical complications compound the poisoning. Despite absent brain stem reflexes and electrocerebral silence on EEG, patients with deep, sedative drug intoxication may expect to make a complete recovery, barring additional medical insults. Therefore, in the emergent situation, all undiagnosed patients should be supported vigorously until the precise cause of the coma can be fully elucidated.

Prognosis in traumatic coma is slightly better than in nontraumatic coma. Jennett and colleagues[30] reported that approximately 40% of 1000 patients with coma lasting more than 6 hours recovered to moderate disability or made a good recovery at 6 months. A worse prognosis was associated with increasing age, especially over 60 years, the presence of an intracranial hematoma, or autonomic dysregulation. Recovery correlated inversely with Glasgow coma score; particularly poor prognostic signs within the first 24 hours of coma were nonreactive pupils and absent eye movements: 90% of such patients either died or recovered only to a vegetative state. Intracranial hypertension (intracranial pressure > 20 mm Hg) occurring after head injury is associated with increased mortality independent of other factors that are considered predictive of neurologic outcome.[31]

The development of the vegetative state carries an ominous prognosis; once it appears, few recover completely. Patients whose vegetative state is caused by head trauma or subarachnoid hemorrhage have a more favorable prognosis than those whose vegetative state is caused by asphyxia. A multi-society task force found that among trauma patients, 52% of adults in a persistent vegetative state recovered some degree of consciousness within 6 months. Few recovered after that time, but younger trauma victims did better than older ones. Similarly, Groswasser and Sazbon[33] indicated that among 134 men and women whose vegetative state (induced by trauma) persisted 1 month, 54% regained consciousness.[33] Of these, about half managed to care for their daily needs, but only eight became independently employed. Statistics for recovery from nontraumatic coma are even worse. Of 100 such patients studied by Sazbon and coworkers,[34] only two children and one adult ever became independent in daily living tasks. Forty-six percent died within the first postonset year, and 68% died within 6 years. The results in both the traumatic and nontraumatic cases provide important information to help physicians and families to reach ethical decisions about caring for overwhelmingly brain-damaged patients.

References

1. Plum F, Posner JB: The Diagnosis of Stupor and Coma. 3rd ed. Philadelphia, FA Davis, 1980.
2. Plum F: Coma and related global disturbances of the human conscious state. *In*: Cerebral Cortex. Vol 9. Peters A (Ed). New York, Plenum Publishing, 1990, pp 359–425.
3. Denoyer M, Sallanon M, Birda L, et al: Neurotoxic lesion of the mesencephalic reticular formation and/or the posterior hypothalamus does not alter waking in the cat. Brain Res 1991; 539:287–303.
4. Steriade M, McCarly RW: Brain Stem Control of Wakefulness and Sleep. New York, Plenum Publishing, 1990.
5. McCormick DA, Von Krosigk M: Corticothalamic activation modulates thalamic firing through glutamate "metabotropic" receptors. Proc Natl Acad Sci USA 1992; 89:2774–2778.
6. Ropper AH, Cole D, Locris DN: Clinicopathologic correlation in a case of pupillary dilation from cerebral hemorrhage. Arch Neurol 1991, 48:1166–1169.
7. Reich JB, Sierra J, Camp W, et al: Magnetic resonance imaging measurements and clinical changes accompanying transtentorial and foramen magnum brain herniation. Arch Neurol 1993; 33:159–170.
8. Bickerstaff ER: Basilar artery migraine. Lancet 1961; i:15–17.
9. Bickerstaff ER: Impairment of consciousness in migraine. Lancet 1961; ii:1057–1059.
10. Cuneo RA, Caronna JJ, Pitts L, et al: Upward transtentorial herniation: Seven cases and a literature review. Arch Neurol 1979; 36:618–623.
11. Kase CS, Wolf PA: Cerebellar infarction: Upward transtentorial herniation after ventriculostomy. Stroke 1993; 24:1096–1098.
12. Council on Scientific Affairs and Council on Ethical and Judicial Affairs: Persistent vegetative state and the decision to withdraw or withhold life support. JAMA 1990; 263:426–430.
13. Dougherty JH Jr, Rawlinson DG, Levy DE, et al: Hypoxic-ischemic brain injury and the vegetative state: Clinical and neuropathologic correlation. Neurology 1981; 31:991–997.
14. Levy DE, Sidtis JJ, Rottenberg DA, et al: Differences in cerebral blood flow and glucose utilization in vegetative versus locked-in patients. Ann Neurol 1987; 22:673–682.
15. Childs NL, Mercer WN, Childs HW: Accuracy of diagnosis of persistent vegetative state. Neurology 1993; 43:1465–1467.
16. Westmoreland B, Klass DW, Sharbrough FW, et al: Alpha-coma: Electroencephalopathic, clinical, pathologic, and etiologic correlations. Arch Neurol 1975; 32:713–718.
17. Jordan KG: Nonconvulsive seizures (NCS) and nonconvulsive status epilepticus (NCSE) detected by continuous EEG monitoring in the Neuro ICU (NICU-CEEG). Neurology 1992; 42(Suppl 3):194.
18. Lowenstein DH, Aminoff MJ: Clinical and EEG features of status epilepticus in comatose patients. Neurology 1992; 42:100–104.
19. Plum F: Disturbances of consciousness and arousal. *In*: Cecil Textbook of Medicine. 19th ed. Wyngaarden JB, Smith LH Jr, Bennett JC (Eds). Philadelphia, WB Saunders, 1992, pp 2048–2059.
20. Caronna JJ: The comatose patient: Diagnosis, treatment, and prognosis. *In*: Handbook of Critical Care Neurology and Neurosurgery. Henning RJ, Jackson DL (Eds). New York, Praeger Publishers, 1985, pp 113–126.
21. Hojer J, Baehrendtz S, Mattel G, et al: Diagnostic utility of flumazenil in coma with suspected poisoning: A double blind, randomised controlled study. Br Med J 1990; 301:1308–1311.
22. Winkler E, Shlomo A, Kriger D, et al: Use of flumazenil in the diagnosis and treatment of patients with coma of unknown etiology. Crit Care Med 1993; 21:538–542.
23. Working Group on Status Epilepticus: Treatment of convulsive status epilepticus. JAMA 1993; 270:854–859.
24. Mofenson HC, Caraccio R, Greenshen J: Acute poisonings. *In*: Conn's Current Therapy 1993. Rakel RE (Ed). Philadelphia, WB Saunders, 1993, pp 1148–1192.
25. Olson KR: Toxicology screens and asymptomatic poisoning. *In*: Current Practice of Emergency Medicine. Philadelphia, Callaham ML (Ed). BC Decker, 1991, pp 1138–1142.
26. Linden CH: Antidotes in poisoning. *In*: Current Practice of Emergency Medicine, Callaham ML (Ed). Philadelphia, BC Decker, 1991, pp 1146–1162.
27. Levy DE, Bates D, Caronna JJ, et al: Prognosis in nontraumatic coma. Ann Intern Med 1981; 94:293–301.
28. Levy DE, Caronna JJ, Singer BH, et al: Predicting outcome from hypoxic-ischemic coma. JAMA 1985; 253:1420–1426.
29. Levy DE: Disorders of consciousness. *In*: Prognosis of Neurological Disorders. Evans RW, Baskin DS, Yatsu FM (Eds). New York, Oxford University Press, 1992, pp 353–358.

30. Jennett B, Teasdale G, Braakman R, et al: Prognosis of patients with severe head injury. Neurosurgery 1979; 4:283–301.
31. Chesnut RM, Marshall LF: Management of head injury: Treatment of abnormal intracranial pressure. Neurosurg Clin North Am 1991; 2:267–284.
32. The Multi-Society Task Force on PVS (Ashwal S. and Cranford R., co-chairmen): Medical aspects of the persistent vegetative state. New Engl J Med 1994; 330:1499–1508, and 1572–1579.
33. Groswasser Z, Sazbon L: Outcome in 134 patients with prolonged post-traumatic unawareness. J Neurosurg 1990; 72:81–84.
34. Sazbon L, Zagreba F, Ronen J, et al: Course and outcome of patients in a vegetative state of nontraumatic etiology. J Neurol Neurosurg Psychiatry 1993; 56:407–409.

CHAPTER 172

Pediatric Neurosurgical Emergencies

D.A. Bruce, MB, ChB • Dale Swift, MD • Charles Teo, MD
William J. Morris, MD

Most neurosurgical catastrophes, sudden disasters, are a result of elevated intracranial pressure (ICP). Thus, a brief outline of the normal physiologic mechanisms that maintain the balance between pressure and volume inside the dural sac is necessary to understand what occurs under pathologic circumstances.

The intradural space consists of the intraspinal space plus the intracranial space. The volume of this space in an adult is approximately 1700 mL, of which approximately 10% is spinal fluid, 10% blood volume, and 80% brain and spinal cord tissue. In a neonate, this volume is about 400 mL. Because the spinal dural sac is not always fully distended, some increase in volume of the intradural space can be achieved at the expense of compression of the spinal epidural veins, thus permitting some distention of the spinal dural sac. In an infant with an open fontanelle and open sutures, some small increase in volume of the intradural space can be achieved by separation of the sutures and distention of the fontanelle. This increase in space is not very significant if the rise in intracranial volume is rapid. Once the dural sac is fully distended, any further increase in volume of one component of the intracranial space must be offset by a decrease in volume of one of the other components. The contents of the intracranial space are brain, blood, and spinal fluid. When using a formula to represent the intracranial volume-pressure relationships, a term is often included to represent the presence of any other intracranial mass (e.g., tumor or hematoma):

$$V_{csf} + V_{blood} + V_{brain} + V_{other} = V_{constant} = V_{eq} + V_e \quad \text{[Equation 1]}$$

This relationship is graphically represented in Figure 172–1. Thus, with a pathologic increase in one component, the others are decreased to maintain a constant pressure. The most effective compensation is displacement of cerebrospinal fluid (CSF) from the cranial space to the spinal space and reabsorption of CSF across the arachnoid villi. As the ICP rises, some decrease in CSF production may occur, further aiding compensation. The second major volume compensation is that of the intracranial pial blood volume. As volume rises in one of the other components, the pial blood volume is displaced into the venous sinuses, thereby serv-

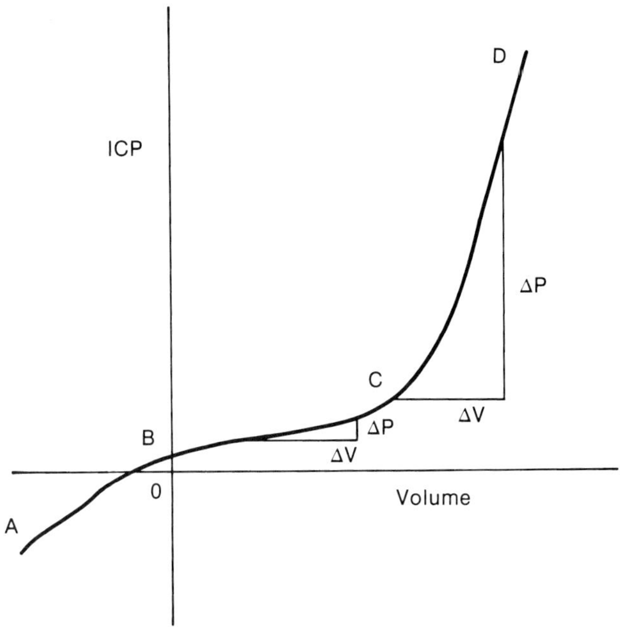

Figure 172–1. An idealized pressure-volume curve. The area on the left below 0, AB, represents the period when the spinal sac is not fully distended; BC—the period of volume compensation; and CD—the period of exhausted compensation.

ing to maintain the ICP. Finally, the brain itself can be compressed to compensate for increases in volume. This is most easily demonstrated in the setting of acute hydrocephalus, when the brain is compressed by the CSF resulting in ventricular enlargement; or in acute epidural hematoma, when the brain is compressed and distorted by the mass of the hematoma. The compressibility of the brain depends on several factors that affect the elasticity of the brain. These include the water content, the degree of myelination, and the vascular turgor from systemic arterial pressure. As a result of these compensatory mechanisms, a certain increase in one component of the intracranial space can occur with little change in the ICP. The volume increase that can be tolerated depends on the rate of increase and the components that are increasing. Once this volume is exceeded, any further increase in volume is tolerated less well, and some increase in pressure occurs because less and less volume compensation can occur. This is best demonstrated in Figure 172–1, which illustrates a biexponential curve showing a segment of little change in pressure despite an increase in volume, followed by a progressively steeper increase in pressure for each equal change in volume. This later segment is the area of limited or absent volume compensation and is increasingly dependent on the elastic properties of the intracranial contents to prevent major increases in ICP.

The intradural space is divided into a series of compartments by the foramen magnum and the folds of the dura, the falx, and the tentorium. The frontal fossa is separated from the middle fossa by the lesser wing of the sphenoid bone. The right half of the supratentorial space is separated from the left by the falx cerebri, and the supratentorial space is separated from the infratentorial space by the tentorium. Finally, the intracranial space becomes the intraspinal canal at the foramen magnum. The compartments are important because rises in pressure in one compartment can result in distortion and displacement of brain into another compartment, with consequent tissue and vascular compression that can result in brain dysfunction and brain damage. Frontal mass lesion can cause herniation across the lesser wing of the sphenoid, with resultant compression of the intracranial carotid artery and subsequent ischemia (transalar herniation). Expanding lesions on one side of the supratentorial space can cause herniation from one side to the other under the falx cerebri, with compression of the anterior cerebral arteries and resultant ischemia (subfalcine herniation). The most frequent cerebral herniation occurs at the tentorial hiatus, with distortion and displacement of the mesial temporal lobe or lobes, forcing the parahippocampal gyrus through the tentorial notch, and compression of the brain stem–perforating vessels, the posterior cerebral arteries, and the perforating vessels to the thalamus (transtentorial herniation). A mass in the posterior fossa can occasionally cause herniation of the cerebellar vermis upward through the tentorial notch and compression of the brain stem and posterior cerebral and thalamic perforating vessels (upward herniation). This is most frequently precipitated by drainage of the lateral ventricles in the presence of a posterior fossa mass. Finally, herniation can occur at the foramen magnum, with displacement of the cerebellar tonsils through the foramen magnum and compression of the medulla and the vertebral and posterior inferior cerebellar arteries (foramen magnum or tonsillar herniation). It is clinically difficult to diagnose transalar herniation or subfalcine herniation, which usually occur in the presence of loss of consciousness. Transtentorial herniation is recognized by a progression of symptoms that usually begin with increasingly severe headache followed by somnolence and eventually loss of consciousness. The signs are of pupillary dilatation, usually of the ipsilateral pupil (80%) due to compression of cranial nerve III, hemiparesis of the opposite side due to compression, and ischemia of the cerebral peduncle. If the lesion is untreated, dilatation of the opposite pupil occurs, with bilateral compression of cranial nerve III, bilateral hemiparesis, decerebrate posturing, bradycardia, hypertension, and ultimately apnea and death as a result of progressive compression of the brain stem pons and medulla. In children, the initial hemiparesis occurs on the side ipsilateral to the herniation 50% of the time, presumably because of the anatomy of the tentorial notch. This can cause clinical confusion that is easily resolved with a neuroimaging study. Foramen magnum herniation may be identified by complaints of headache and neck pain. The pain may initially be relieved by extension of the neck. As herniation progresses, the medulla oblongata is compressed with resulting hypertension, bradycardia, bradypnea, and finally apnea. The onset of apnea may be preceded only by severe headache or neck pain with no clinical signs.

As well as causing distortion and focal vascular compression, elevated ICP can affect general cerebral blood flow (CBF). The cerebral blood vessels exhibit autoregulation to changes in perfusion pressure. Perfusion pressure (CPP) is

$$CPP = MAP - MICP$$

where MAP is mean arterial pressure and MICP is mean intracranial pressure. The cerebral vessels respond to decrease in perfusion pressure by vasodilating, decreasing resistance to flow and thus maintaining the same CBF despite either a decline in arterial pressure or an increase in ICP. The exact limits of autoregulation are not known through the period of infancy and childhood but probably range between 35 and 40 mm Hg at the lower end and greater than 100 mm Hg at the upper end. Below the limits of autoregulation, the CBF falls as the CPP is lowered. Cerebral metabolism is preserved to a CBF of about 50% of normal, after which some degree of cerebral ischemia begins. As blood flow falls below 25% of normal, irreversible damage begins. Thus, autoregulation is a further brain-protective mechanism against increased ICP. Trauma in children often leaves autoregulation intact, whereas ischemia seems more likely to abolish autoregulation, making the CBF more sensitive to small changes in the CPP. Unfortunately, the status of autoregulation is not known in the clinical setting, and thus therapy is directed at maintaining normal or nearly normal ICP and MAP in the hope that this will preserve CBF. If the ICP is high enough or the MAP low enough, the CPP will be inadequate to maintain cerebral perfusion and cerebral ischemia will result. The grossest manifestation of this deficit is the cessation of CBF and death of the brain and thus the child.[2]

The common denominator for many neurosurgical catastrophes is intracranial hypertension, with resultant cerebral herniation and focal ischemia or globally elevated ICP and diffuse cerebral ischemia. A cycle of problems occurs as the ICP becomes increased. As noted earlier, during the early period of compensation, the addition of volume to the cranium may be tolerated. Over time, however, as compensation becomes exhausted, the addition of a similar volume may result in a pressure wave that may rise to the level of the arterial pressure and result in cessation of CBF. As cerebral herniation progresses and the subarachnoid spaces are occluded, the transmission of pressure with the craniospinal axis is impeded, once again setting the stage for a much larger increase in pressure for any given increase in volume. The frequent waves of ICP may further abolish pressure autoregulation and make the brain more prone to ischemia at the same CPP. A progressive loss of compensatory ability often follows an intracranial catastrophe, and an increase in pressure that was tolerated in the first few hours after the insult may not be tolerated 24 hours later because of the gradual exhaustion of the compensatory mechanisms.

In a clinical setting it is rare that the balance between one intracranial component and the others is preserved because alterations in volume in all three components often occur in the same direction at the same time. After head injury, subarachnoid hemorrhage blocks the CSF pathways, interfering with pressure transmission, and increases CSF outflow resistance by clogging the arachnoid villi. CSF volume thus can increase. Intracranial hematomas or contusions result in increased brain volume, and the cerebral blood volume is increased as a result of hyperemia—that is, all three components are affected at the same time, resulting in a very limited compensatory ability and therefore early and common increases in ICP. A similar series of events, disturbance of the balance of equilibrium in several of the components of the intracranial space at the same time, occurs with many of the lesions that result in the need for urgent neurosurgical treatment. The course of compensatory loss of the volume-pressure homeostasis is typically that of intermittent waves of ICP rather than stable high pressure. Thus, signs and symptoms can wax and wane, leading a physician to a false sense of security about the urgency for therapy.

Before any surgical intervention, resuscitation of a child with a neurosurgical catastrophe addresses the usual concerns of airway patency, bleeding, and circulation. Specific therapy to lower the ICP (e.g., mannitol or glycerol) depends on the evidence of elevated ICP and the history of rapid deterioration of level of consciousness with signs of cerebral herniation. The history is often the deciding factor, because absolute signs of intracranial hypertension are few and may not be present, depending on the rate of increase in ICP. Papilledema is a sure sign of intracranial hypertension but is often absent because of the rapidity of the onset of symptoms or because the anatomy of the subarachnoid space in the optic nerve is such that papilledema does not occur. After trauma, acute loss of consciousness is rarely the result of increased ICP, and there is no indication for routinely giving an osmotic diuretic to children in coma after head trauma. When intracranial hypertension is suspected in a comatose child, endotracheal intubation is performed after bag and mask hyperventilation with 100% oxygen, followed by a nondepolarizing, short-acting muscle relaxant and sodium pentothal or a similar anesthetic. The head is maintained in the midline, and if the blood pressure is adequate, the head is elevated 20% to 30%. If continued elevation of the ICP is an immediate concern, an ICP monitor can easily be placed after early resuscitation.

TRAUMA

Traumatic lesions that require surgical therapy in children are rare, occurring in 20% to 30% of children with a Glasgow Coma Scale score of 8 or less. Traumatic unconsciousness is a neurologic emergency but usually is not the result of elevated ICP and does not require surgical intervention but rather rapid resuscitation. Lesions that may require immediate surgery are the intracranial hematomas, compound depressed skull fractures, and penetrating trauma.

Birth Trauma

All forms of intracranial hematomas are encountered in the neonatal period, but all are rare. Epidural hematomas occur in the supratentorial and infratentorial spaces and, if producing cerebral compression, require evacuation. Before any surgery is performed on a neonate, clotting studies must be performed and abnormalities corrected if necessary. Subdural hematomas are a major problem to handle surgically, and if they are not large, efforts to control the ICP medically should usually be attempted before resorting to surgery. Most intracerebral hematomas in neonates are hemorrhagic infarctions or venous hemorrhages, and surgery is rarely indicated. The brain is 90% water, and hemostasis can be very difficult; the pia mater and cerebral vessels can be peeled off the brain by the sucker, resulting in increased damage. Once again, surgery is a last-resort measure in most cases.

Non–Birth-Related Trauma

Compound Depressed Skull Fracture

Compound depressed skull fractures are open wounds of the brain and require urgent surgical debridement as soon as a patient is stabilized. These fractures are the most common reason for surgery after trauma in children. The aim of the surgery is to debride the brain of contamination including bone fragments, remove any associated hematomas, repair the dura to prevent cerebral herniation, and reconstruct the skull either with the fragments present or with split cranial bone. It is usually possible to replace the fragments and avoid the need for a second reconstructive operation. Other forms of penetrating skull trauma require surgical exploration (e.g., dog bites, dart injuries). Gunshot wounds of the head and brain are increasingly common in children and usually require surgery to debride the bone fragments from the brain, remove intracranial hematomas, and repair the dura and cranium. The indications depend on whether or not a child is likely to survive the injury, because little is to be gained by operating on a child who is clearly going to die after surgery.

Epidural Hematoma

Epidural hematomas are either venous as a result of bleeding from the diploic space of the skull after fracture or arterial from rupture of branches of the middle meningeal or posterior meningeal arteries. They are found in 6% to 8% of children who undergo computed tomography (CT) scanning after head injury. The children are almost equally divided into three groups, one third never being unconscious, one third being unconscious from the time of injury, and one third demonstrating a lucid period followed by unconsciousness. Early CT scan to identify the lesion is important because the recovery is closely correlated with the level of consciousness at the time of surgical evacuation and the presence of other cerebral injury. In children younger than 8 years, the location of the typical epidural hematoma is rather higher in the parietal and temporal parietal area than the typical anterior temporal location in adults, and thus blindly placing bur holes is rarely advisable. A CT scan should be obtained whenever possible to pinpoint the exact location of the lesion and to identify other intracranial lesions. If a child with a skull fracture is showing signs of rapidly progressing herniation and if time does not permit a CT scan and surgery must be done emergently, the center of the craniotomy should be over the center of the fracture. Most epidural hematomas require surgical removal by craniotomy, but small lesions (especially frontal ones) in the presence of normal consciousness can often be treated conservatively.

Subdural Hematomas

Subdural hematomas are usually the result of tearing of the bridging cortical veins due to acceleration-deceleration injury or tearing of the cerebral cortex and cortical arteries. The incidence varies from 5% to 30% in children hospitalized for head injury. The highest frequency is in children younger than 1 year, and the cause is usually child abuse. In infants and toddlers, the lesions are usually small and bilateral and do not require surgery. In a child who has an open fontanelle and is in extremis, the fontanelle can be tapped and bloody fluid removed, acutely lowering the ICP. The major problem is usually the underlying brain swelling, and treatment with ICP monitoring and medical management of the ICP is the mainstay of therapy. The finding of a subdural hematoma and retinal hemorrhages is pathognomonic of child abuse, except when a high-speed accident has occurred and has been witnessed (e.g., automobile accident). In an older child, subdural hematomas are a result of severe acceleration-deceleration injuries and are due to tears of the cerebral cortex and arterial rupture. They are usually associated with severe brain swelling and elevated ICP, and the clinical picture is usually of a comatose child. Many of these lesions do not require surgery, because the problem is to control the brain swelling and ICP. In general, if the brain distortion is considerably more than the width of the subdural hematoma and the subdural hematoma is less than 1 cm, surgery is not performed; however, the indications for surgery vary with the condition of the individual child and the neurosurgeon's individual criteria for surgery in this setting. Even if surgery is performed, postoperative brain swelling can be expected, and ICP monitoring and medical control of the ICP are likely to be necessary in an intensive care unit.

Intracerebral Hematomas and Contusions

Most intracerebral hematomas occur with severe head trauma and often in association with diffuse axonal injury. They are encountered in 3% to 5% of postinjury CT scans in children who usually have a Glasgow Coma Scale score of less than 8. Many are in the deep white mater or basal ganglia, and it is rare that surgical evacuation is necessary or advisable. These children are at risk for elevated ICP and may require intense medical treatment to control brain swelling and edema.[2] Large, more superficial hematomas are occasionally identified, and they may require surgical evacuation to control herniation and severely elevated ICP. Surgery if necessary should focus on resection of the hematoma, preserving as much brain tissue as possible. Acute cerebral contusions are relatively rarely reported after head injury in children and in general do not need surgical resection, primarily because of the need to remove brain that often can recover. In follow-up studies of children with moderate or severe head injuries, a high incidence of contusions has been identified (50%), the majority in the frontal area, followed by the anterior temporal tip.[3] Although some of these lesions were visible on the original CT scan, the majority were not. The latter are also clearly not surgical lesions and require no specific early intervention.

Post-traumatic subarachnoid hemorrhage, brain swelling, brain edema, arterial spasm, and focal strokes do not require surgery.[4] The delayed traumatic lesions that can require acute surgery are delayed intracranial hemorrhage, after 7 to 10 days; ruptured traumatic aneurysm, with a peak incidence around 10 to 14 days; and post-traumatic hydrocephalus, which can occur anytime up to 1 year after the trauma but most commonly requires a shunt in the first 3 months.

VASCULAR LESIONS

Early high-output cardiac failure in neonates can occur with vascular shunting lesions in the cranium. The most frequent is the vein of Galen aneurysm, which is a malformation of the vessels that supply the choroid plexus of the third ventricle. It usually is not a true arteriovenous malformation (AVM) but is a direct shunting of branches of any or all of the following vessels into the vein of Galen: anterior cerebral, posterior lateral and medial choroidal, thalamic and hypothalamic perforators, posterior cerebral, anterior choroidal, and least likely the middle cerebral. The term *aneurysm* is misleading: The aneurysm is of the internal cerebral veins or the vein of Galen and the straight sinus and is not arterial. This lesion rarely bleeds in the first few months of life, and the problem is to control the heart failure. This can often be accomplished by medical means. If it cannot, then selective embolization of particular arterial feeders with coils or balloons may help cut down the flow and permit control of the cardiac failure. Another option is embolization of the venous aneurysm via a transvenous route or directly through the torcula. Rarely is open operation to control the feeders successful in the first few days of life. If the heart failure can be controlled for 6 weeks or more and the failure should recur, direct surgery to occlude the direct shunting arteries can be successfully accomplished at this age. The options for venous or arterial embolization remain open and are possibly less dangerous options, although the risks of hemorrhage, pulmonary embolization by the coils, and heart attack remain concerns with any mode of therapy.

Other arteriovenous shunts that occur in neonates usually affect the dura mater, with or without cerebral involvement. Early treatment focuses on control of the heart failure with embolization if necessary. Early open surgery is rarely advisable because of the high risk of excessive blood loss.

Arteriovenous Malformations

Arteriovenous malformations are congenital anomalies of the vascular system and can occur anywhere in the cerebrum, brain stem, cerebellum, and spinal cord. Lesions in the spinal cord are rare in children. AVMs result in neurosurgical emergencies as a result of rupture of usually venous components of the AVM and ensuing acute hemorrhage of blood at arterial pressure into the cerebral substance or the ventricular system. They are four times more likely to be the cause of intracranial hemorrhage in children than are aneurysms.[5] The result is a sudden increase in ICP manifested clinically by the sudden onset of severe headache or sudden loss of consciousness. The signs and symptoms depend on the location of the hemorrhage and can include hemiparesis, aphasia, hemisensory loss, hemianopia if the hemorrhage occurs into the supratentorial brain, or focal brain stem symptoms if the hemorrhage is in the posterior fossa. The only manifestation may be the acute onset of coma. The mortality from the first bleed has been reported to be as high as 24% in children.[5] Standard resuscitation is followed by a CT scan to confirm the diagnosis of intraventricular or intraparenchymal hemorrhage. Treatment varies depending on the clinical state of the patient. With signs of progressive herniation and impending death, acute evacuation of the hematoma may be necessary. Although obtaining an angiogram to identify the anatomy of the AVM is ideal, this is not always possible because of the rate of neurologic deterioration, which cannot be reversed despite hyperventilation and osmotic diuretics. The aim of surgery is evacuation of the clot to provide relief of the ICP and reverse any herniation. If an obvious AVM is encountered and is small, it may be possible to remove it also; more often, the safer course is to stop after evacuation of the clot. Arteriography can be performed and then a second operation to resect the lesion.

Acute rebleeding from an AVM is rare, and urgent surgery therefore is not necessary to prevent a rebleed. If the blood is predominantly in the ventricle, an intraventricular catheter is required to monitor the ICP and provide for CSF drainage. Acutely, as little CSF as possible is drained to prevent the catheter's becoming clogged by blood clot. The ICP is controlled by a combination of therapy. When a patient is stable and has recovered consciousness, arteriography and definitive therapy can be undertaken. When the clot is parenchymal and the ICP and herniation can be controlled by medical means, it is advisable to postpone surgery until the clot has liquefied and the brain swelling and edema have subsided. This hiatus makes the surgery much safer and allows adequate investigation and planning of therapy. Therapy is either surgery, surgery preceded by embolization, or, for smaller deep lesions, focused radiation therapy. In a small percentage of cases, no obvious site of hemorrhage is identified. A repeat arteriogram some months later is required to be certain that a small lesion was not present but compressed by the acute hemorrhage. The rebleed rate for AVMs is 2% per year. In children in whom no lesion is identified, the rebleed rate is close to zero.[6]

Aneurysm

As noted earlier, intracranial hemorrhage in children is less frequently a result of rupture of an aneurysm than of an AVM.[7] Aneurysms may be congenital or mycotic and may be found on the feeding arteries of an AVM. Aneurysms occur in the subarachnoid space, and thus subarachnoid hemorrhage rather than intraparenchymal hemorrhage is the usual result of rupture. The signs and symptoms are typically sudden onset of unendurable headache followed by stiff neck and photophobia and in about 50% of cases by coma. Diagnosis is made on the history, which in a child triggers the performance of a CT scan to rule out a parenchymal clot such as would occur with an AVM. The CT findings may appear normal or may show subarachnoid hemorrhage. The definitive diagnosis is made by lumbar puncture.

Because aneurysms tend to rebleed in 24 to 48 hours,[8–10] the next step in diagnosis is cerebral arteriography. Magnetic resonance imaging (MRI) angiography is not adequate to visualize a small aneurysm. Although the most common location is at the bifurcation of the carotid, many aneurysms occur distally in children, and they are often giant. Mycotic aneurysms in particular occur on the distal branches of the cerebral vessels, and the rare post-traumatic aneurysm can occur on any vessel but is most frequently on the anterior cerebral artery. The grading system[11] for aneurysms in adults is quite adequate for children, and aneurysms grade III or higher are usually treated by acute surgery to clip or trap the aneurysm before rebleeding, because with each rebleed the mortality rate rises. After rebleeding, the next major complication is cerebral ischemia as a result of cerebrovascular spasm.[12] This is treated by volume expansion, calcium blockers, and induced arterial hypertension.[12, 13] Because of the need for elevating the blood pressure to treat spasm, it is currently believed that early clipping of the aneurysm makes this therapy to reverse or prevent ischemia safer. The use of free radical scavengers has been reported to markedly improve outcome in patients with subarachnoid hemorrhage.

Rarely, acute hemorrhage from the nose, mouth, or ear can occur as a result of a traumatic aneurysm of the internal carotid artery. It requires emergency arteriography and either embolization or surgical ligation, depending on the location of the lesion.

Cavernous Angiomas and Venous Angiomas

Although both cavernous and venous angiomas can present with the acute onset of a new neurologic deficit and headache, it is rare that they require emergency surgery. Venous angiomas are most likely when the hematoma is in the posterior fossa, where brain stem compression can be sufficiently severe to require treatment by clot removal. In venous angiomas, the large draining vein should not be occluded because it is often the only venous drainage from a large area of the cerebellum.

The diagnosis is usually established on a noncontrast CT scan, which shows acute hemorrhage, and a contrast scan, which in the case of a cavernoma may demonstrate enhancement and in the case of a venous angioma shows the large vein and often its tributaries. Both these lesions are well demonstrated on an MRI scan, which shows evidence of old hemorrhage and the surrounding edema. Cerebral arteriography usually shows no lesion in the case of the cavernous malformation and the caput of draining veins and the single large vein of the venous angioma. Acute hydrocephalus can occur as a result of posterior fossa hematoma and may require treatment with a ventriculostomy. The ventricle should be drained slowly, and the supratentorial pressure should be kept above 15 mm Hg to prevent upward herniation of the cerebellar vermis. This is true whenever a ventricular drain is required for relief of acute hydrocephalus secondary to a posterior fossa mass. Anticonvulsants are necessary if a patient presents with seizures, and corticosteroids are helpful to treat the cerebral edema that is often present. It is rare that severe intracranial hypertension is present. In most cases, definitive resection of the cavernous angioma is the treatment of choice once the hematoma and brain edema have subsided. The best treatment for venous angiomas often is to leave them alone unless repeated bleeding occurs, in which case a small AVM is often present and may be resected.

CONGENITAL LESIONS

Most congenital anomalies of the central nervous system are not true neurosurgical emergencies but are often considered by the family to be catastrophes and therefore require acute pediatric neurosurgical consultation.

Craniofacial Anomalies

The severe anomalies of the craniofacial skeleton that engender an often horrific reaction are those that involve amniotic band syndromes, facial clefts, cloverleaf skull appearance, or congenital absence of the nose or eyes. Children with severe Crouzon's, Apert's, or Pfeiffer's syndromes also appear dramatically abnormal, and a correct initial diagnosis often is not made. Despite their appearance, few of these children require emergency neurosurgery. The acute problem is most often the airway, because choanal atresia or marked hypoplasia of the midface may interfere with ventilation. Endotracheal intubation can be very difficult, and a tracheostomy may occasionally be required to save a child's life. The globes of the eyes occasionally are completely dislocated out of the orbit, with closure of the lids posterior to the globe. This results in exposure and ischemia and requires treatment, first with lubricant and plastic wrap to keep the conjunctiva moist. Rarely is tarsorraphy adequate because of the degree of exorbitism, and early surgery with supraorbital rim advancement and tarsorraphy is occasionally the only way to obtain some coverage for the eyes.

Newborns with the cloverleaf skull anomaly usually have hydrocephalus and generalized suture closure, and many of these children require a surgical craniectomy or a shunt in the first week of life. In general, craniofacial surgery for children with severe anomalies is delayed until after 4 months of age unless they show evidence of intracranial hypertension. It is almost impossible to correct any aspect of the facial anomaly before 4 months, even in the upper orbital area.

Encephalocoeles

Encephalocoeles occur at a rate of 1:10,000 live births in North America, and about 70% occur in the posterior region of the cranium and are either supratentorial or infratentorial. Although often presenting with a dramatic external appearance, most encephalocoeles are not surgical emergencies; however, those that are not completely skin covered and are leaking CSF or displaying visible brain tissue require urgent closure in 24 hours if the general condition of the neonate is otherwise stable. The exposed lesion is covered with sterile saline-soaked sponges, and broad-spectrum antibiotics are begun. CT or MRI scan or both are required to define the anatomy of the encephalocoele and the intracranial brain. Prognosis is best correlated with the size and anatomic appearance of the residual intracranial brain rather than the size of the encephalocoele. The more normal the size of the head and the appearance of the brain, the more favorable the prognosis. The herniated cerebral tissue is not normal, and no effort is made to replace it within the cranial cavity; the abnormal tissue is removed, sparing the intracranial vasculature, and the dura closed. Hydrocephalus is common but usually does not need therapy in the first few days. With severe hydrocephalus, it is preferable to insert a shunt and decompress the brain before performing a definitive operation on the encephalocoele. Anterior encephalocoeles in the nose or mouth, often in association with a cleft palate, can produce acute airway obstruction and feeding problems that require tracheostomy for emergency management of the airway. In such cases, it is advisable to postpone definitive surgery for as long as several months if possible to make the surgery safer.

Aplasia Cutis Congenita

Aplasia cutis congenita is an area of the skull where bone and skin fail to form, leaving exposed and occasionally slightly herniating dura, most commonly in the midline, associated with a suture or venous sinus. This is not an encephalocoele and, because the dura is intact, often can be treated conservatively until a child is older, at which time surgery to rotate skin over the lesion is usually necessary. Smaller lesions can be treated by immediate surgical closure of the skin.

Teratomas and Choristomas

Teratomas and choristomas are rare lesions, but they can present at birth as an emergency because of airway obstruction or feeding problems. The most common location is in the tongue or fauces. These lesions are usually small at birth and grow rapidly in the first few days of life, yet they are rarely malignant. Tracheostomy and a feeding tube are often required during the early life-threatening phase. Those that come to neurosurgical attention usually involve the intracranial space and exit from the cranium through the cranial nerve foramina, most frequently the trigeminal or superior or inferior orbital fissures, and present in the mouth and neck. These lesions can usually be completely removed in a single operation in the first few months of life, with cure of the lesions. It is unclear whether these should be categorized as congenital or neoplastic lesions, and in some cases true tumors are found. These children should be treated only by craniofacial teams with the support systems to perform such surgery and, if necessary, to carry out reconstruction in infants.[14]

Myelomeningocele

Failure of closure of the skin, muscle, bone, and spinal cord constitutes a myelomeningocele. These can occur at any level of the spinal canal but are most frequent in the lumbar area. These lesions frequently have disruption of the thin covering of arachnoid over the placode and are leaking CSF. There is no real emergency about closing these lesions, but in most pediatric neurosurgical centers they are closed within 24 to 48 hours after birth, assuming that the neonate is otherwise stable.[15] If closure is to be delayed more than a few hours, the lesions are covered with sterile saline-soaked sponges, and broad-spectrum antibiotics are begun.

Hydrocephalus

It is unusual for a newborn with hydrocephalus to present a neurosurgical emergency. Because hydrocephalus is present prenatally, the brain accommodates and the sutures may be split and the cranium significantly enlarged. Thus, there is usually time to make an accurate diagnosis of the cause of the hydrocephalus and to shunt the lesion electively. With signs such as apnea or bradycardia that are believed to be the result of increased ICP, the ventricle can easily be tapped through the fontanelle and the pressure relieved until an elective shunt can be placed.

Acute hydrocephalus due to congenital and acquired causes can present later in life, in a child with closed sutures. In this case, rapid diagnosis and therapy may be required to prevent either death or serious brain damage because the cranium cannot expand, and by the time a child presents for medical care, the compensatory mechanisms are usually exhausted and waves of ICP elevation occur, posing the risk of sudden death. This is true also of children who have a CSF shunt in place and in whom a shunt malfunction has occurred. The difficulty with diagnosis in this group of patients is the lack of definitive signs that confirm the diagnosis. The diagnosis of shunt malfunction or acute intracranial hypertension due to hydrocephalus is essentially based on the history and often confirmed only by a neuroimaging study, CT or MRI scan, that shows ventricular dilatation. In a small group of children with shunts, the ventricles do not enlarge or enlarge only minimally in the presence of a shunt dysfunction, *slit ventricle syndrome.*[16, 17] In these children, it is important to compare their current scan with a previous scan if possible and, if not, to act again on the history and assume a shunt malfunction.

Because autoregulation of CBF is typically intact in a child presenting with acute hydrocephalus, the ICP waves that occur are often unassociated with any signs. The symptoms are of severe, episodic headache that may be associated with vomiting or visual obscurations. The major pain may be behind the eyes or in the back of the neck as a result of tonsillar herniation. The headache may be relieved by vomiting, because this triggers hyperventilation and thus a decrease in ICP that can abort the pressure wave. If a child is not having a wave of pressure at the time of the examination, he or she may appear perfectly normal, and even with a wave of high pressure there may be nothing to identify other than the pain of the headache, which is of course subjective to the patient. The examination may reveal papilledema, but as mentioned earlier, the absence of papilledema does not rule out intracranial hypertension of a life-threatening degree. Decreased level of consciousness either accompanying the headache or continuously may occur, as may a stiff neck due to tonsillar herniation, cranial nerve VI palsy due to diffuse ICP, or more rarely a cranial nerve III palsy. Visual acuity may be decreased as a result of chronic papilledema, or optic atrophy may be present. Vital signs changes such as bradycardia and hypertension may occur but are often late manifestations that occur only at the time of brain stem decompensation and cannot be relied on as clinical indicators of increased ICP. The only way to confirm or refute the diagnosis is to obtain a CT scan and to look for evidence of ventricular enlargement. When elevated ICP is suspected, it is always preferable to avoid sedation of the child if possible or, if sedation is needed, to give the least amount possible and to realize that sedation may lead to decreased ventilation, increased arterial partial pressure of carbon dioxide, and precipitation of further pressure waves. A plan to treat these should be in place before sedation. When hydrocephalus is present, some urgent therapy is required to abort the waves of increased ICP. Therapy ranges from acute administration of corticosteroids in those patients with a tumor to ventriculostomy or an emergency shunt procedure. In patients without a tumor or preexisting shunt and in whom an acute or chronic CNS infectious process is not suspected, the ideal treatment is insertion of a shunt as an emergency procedure. This is the final as well as the initial therapy and avoids the risk of an infection from a temporary ventriculostomy. The critical factor is to appreciate the urgency of the situation and not procrastinate.

In children with a preexisting shunt, a radiographic shunt survey to evaluate the intactness and position of the shunt system is necessary in addition to the scan. If there is question about a shunt block, the shunt system can be tapped and the site of block identified as proximal or distal to the shunt reservoir. In children with the slit ventricle syndrome, when very little fluid is present in the ventricle and the ability to remove fluid is therefore limited, it is often better to test the proximal catheter by back-injecting contrast medium into the ventricle to establish the patency of the proximal shunt catheter. The distal end of the shunt can be checked by measuring the runoff pressure with a manometer. When the shunt is blocked proximal to the valve system such that CSF cannot be withdrawn, it is safer to revise the shunt immediately rather than to wait until the next day. If the shunt is blocked distal to the valve, adequate ventricular decompression can be attained by tapping the reservoir and removing CSF. In this setting, the shunt revision may be postponed until the next convenient opening in the operating schedule, and Diamox and dexamethasone may be used to slow CSF production during the waiting period. Any severe headaches need to be treated by further fluid withdrawal from the shunt and not treated with narcotics; if headaches persevere, shunt revision is urgently required.

NEOPLASIA

In only a few cases are brain tumors neurosurgical catastrophes, but these must be rapidly identified and treated. Even in the authors' hospital, the occasional child dies in the intensive care unit or on the ward as a result of a pressure wave associated with a brain tumor. These children are usually admitted with a history of headache, nausea, and vomiting, and they suffer herniation while awaiting workup for a suspected gastrointestinal lesion. This unfortunate scenario develops despite the availability of CT and MRI scans. Others are admitted and a lesion identified on scan, but the symptoms of increased ICP are ignored because of the absence of objective signs, only to result in clinical herniation and occasionally death. The problem is exactly as described in children with hydrocephalus, in whom autoregulation of CBF is intact and very high pressures can be tolerated without apparent signs. Many of the tumors that present this way are posterior fossa tumors producing hydrocephalus. In 5% to 10% of cases of tumor, hemorrhage occurs into the tumor, producing acute deterioration that is no different from that related to other types of intracranial hemorrhage.[18] Tumors in the supratentorial compartment are usually easier to diagnose because of accompanying local signs (e.g., hemiparesis, visual field cut). Rarely is an emergency operation necessary, but in the presence of progressive herniation, repeated pressure waves, or unconsciousness, rapid surgical debulking may be required. As noted previously, ventricular drainage in the presence of a large posterior fossa tumor can result in upward herniation; thus, resection of the tumor may be required at the time of insertion of the ventricular drain. In patients with less acute symptoms, corticosteroids usually bring about rapid clinical improvement, permitting surgery to be performed electively.

A final presentation of tumor that requires emergency surgery is the rapid progression of visual loss. This may be due to local compression of the optic nerves, chiasm, or tracts by tumor and can occur as a result of hemorrhage into such tumors as optic gliomas or pituitary tumors or can simply result from a tumor mass, as in craniopharyngioma or meningioma. Such rapid visual loss that is the result of local compression is an indication for emergency surgical decompression of the optic apparatus. The other setting in which rapid visual loss can occur results from papilledema. In this setting, ventricular drainage or shunting plus steroids is usually chosen over emergency tumor resection in an effort to lower the ICP gradually and prevent the acute blindness that can occasionally occur after posterior fossa decompression. Rarely in children do tumors erode into adjacent structures, but epistaxis or bleeding from the ear occasionally is the first manifestation of a large skull base tumor. Although these rarely require acute neurosurgical intervention, if bleeding is severe or hard to control, CT or MRI scan may be necessary to make the diagnosis and acute embolization or vessel ligation may be necessary to attain hemostasis.

INFECTION

The most frequent setting in which an infectious process requires emergency neurosurgery is that of a brain abscess.[19, 20] The presentation is either with focal neurologic deficit or the signs of intracranial hypertension. The aim of therapy is dual: to obtain a specimen for culture and to evacuate any intracranial mass. CT scan usually identifies the lesion, and the therapy is increasingly often stereotaxic drainage with or without leaving a catheter in situ for further drainage if necessary. It is rare that an attempt at abscess removal is performed as the primary procedure, unless the abscess is very large and superficially located in the brain. Even then, because of the surrounding edema, it is generally preferable simply to drain the lesion, treat with antibiotics, and monitor on scan. Indeed, in many cases, craniotomy is never necessary and the abscess can be treated simply by antibiotics with or without repeated needle drainage.

Subdural Empyema and Epidural Empyema

Epidural empyema usually occurs with either severe air sinus infections or osteomyelitis of the skull.[21] The mass effect is usually small, and acute drainage is only rarely necessary. In the frontal area, drainage of the frontal sinus often results in drainage of the epidural abscess also.

Subdural empyema is a much more catastrophic situation, with underlying pial and often cerebral inflammation, septic thrombophlebitis, and brain edema. In the past, this was always treated by urgent craniotomy and aspiration of the pus.[21, 22] Currently, with earlier diagnosis as a result of CT scan, bur hole aspiration for culture and immediate relief of mass effect is often all that is required, followed by antibiotics and corticosteroids. In children, the subdural empyema commonly recurs at different locations and may require repeated surgery, which may be extensive craniotomy if resolution is not achieved by medical management. Small lesions may require no surgery.

Meningitis

It is rare that meningitis is an acute neurosurgical emergency, but acute hydrocephalus can occur with bacterial meningitis, requiring ventricular drainage. This is most often the case in tuberculous meningitis but does occur with the more common infections.

Viral Encephalitis

Despite antiviral agents, brain biopsy is occasionally necessary in focal encephalitis to aid in diagnosis and choice of therapy. Biopsy is more often performed only in more chronic encephalitis associated with other immune disturbances, such as in organ transplant recipients or a child with acquired immunodeficiency syndrome.

Shunt Infection

Most shunt infections do not require emergency shunt removal but shunt tap and appropriate antibiotics. In children with an acute abdomen as a result of the shunt infection, emergency exteriorization of the abdominal end of the shunt may be required. When the infecting organism is *Staphylococcus,* the shunt usually requires elective removal and replacement. With other organisms, the shunt can often be saved.

SPINE CATASTROPHES

Most acute surgical problems of the spinal canal and cord are a result of trauma or neoplasia. The majority of spinal injuries do not require emergency neurosurgical intervention other than external stabilization with a halo device or skull tongs.[23] Children with deteriorating neurological findings and evidence of spinal cord compression on CT or MRI are the ones most likely to require surgical decompression and stabilization. Penetrating injuries of the spine usually require surgical exploration, although this is often not the case for bullet wounds.

Spinal cord compression by tumor is usually slowly progressive, but worsening can occur suddenly. A child who is complaining of difficulty standing or walking or who has back pain plus incontinence must be taken seriously, and a careful examination and appropriate neuroimaging performed, usually MRI scan. It is rare for such complaints to be hysterical, yet children are still sent out of emergency departments only to return with a complete spinal cord lesion. The importance of early identification of spinal cord compression is that the greater the amount of neurologic deficit present preoperatively, the less the chance for neurologic recovery. The lesions that most often produce spinal cord compression and that present acutely are neuroblastoma, lymphoma, bone tumors (e.g., aneurysmal bone cysts), and least often intrinsic spinal cord tumors. While awaiting surgery, corticosteroids are begun. Vascular lesions of the spinal cord are uncommon in children, but rare aneurysms, cavernous angiomas, and AVMs do occur and can present either as acute subarachnoid hemorrhage or acute spinal cord lesion. The possibility of a spinal cord lesion must be kept in mind if no intracranial site for hemorrhage is found. These spinal vascular lesions can usually be operated on electively, but with an acute intraspinal hematoma, emergency surgery may be indicated after appropriate neuroradiologic studies have defined the pathology.

POSTOPERATIVE

The postoperative catastrophes that are encountered depend on the location and type of surgery performed but fall into several categories: hemorrhage, edema, cerebrovascular spasm or occlusion, new neurologic deficits, seizures, and metabolic problems.

The results of postoperative hemorrhage are similar to acute intracranial hemorrhage (described earlier). After posterior fossa surgery, the largest danger is acute hydrocephalus, which can be manifested only as a headache until a fatal pressure wave occurs. As with other causes of hydrocephalus, the medical personnel caring for children who have undergone posterior fossa surgery must be aware of the lack of signs associated with hydrocephalus and must be ready to repeat the CT scan to identify ventricular enlargement. Treatment is usually with ventricular drainage. Local signs of posterior fossa compression—swallowing difficulty, diplopia, cranial nerve palsies, occasional mutism, or deteriorating consciousness—may require direct evacuation of a posterior fossa clot. Intraventricular hemorrhage, like posterior fossa hemorrhage, can produce only headache and pressure waves or may result in the sudden onset of coma. Treatment is usually symptomatic, consisting of ventricular drainage and control of the ICP until the clot resolves. Intracerebral or epidural hemorrhage requires surgical evacuation if large enough to produce symptoms and signs. Arterial spasm is usually associated with aneurysm or AVM surgery, and its treatment has been discussed. Brain edema usually develops over several days, and rarely is the treatment surgical. Steroids, ventilation, sedative drugs, and osmotic agents all may be required in severe cases. Seizures are uncommon in the postoperative period, but when they occur should be vigorously treated. It is always necessary to check blood glucose, calcium, and electrolyte levels, because if one of these is the cause, anticonvulsants may not be necessary. If no metabolic derangements are found, the drug of choice is phenytoin.

Most acute metabolic problems are related to disturbances of pituitary axis function. Diabetes insipidus is the most frequent and occurs when the pituitary stalk is manipulated or divided, as in resection of craniopharyngioma. By combing careful fluid management and, if necessary intravenous 1-deamino-(8-D-arginine)-vasopressin, effective control of serum sodium and osmolality can usually be achieved.

BRAIN DEATH

The diagnosis and confirmation of death as a result of irreversible brain damage are no more difficult in children than in adults.[24] Minimum anecdotal evidence suggests that in premature infants and neonates and possibly in the first 1 month of life, the signs of brain death (absent neurologic findings, lack of ventilation, flat electroencephalogram, absent CBF) can occur yet survival and recovery of the infant still be possible.[25] After that period, however, the absence of all neurologic function other than spinal reflexes for greater than 6 hours, ICP equal to the arterial pressure for longer than 1 hour, the absence of CBF, and a flat electroencephalogram all are as meaningful in a child as in an adult. Other than the ICP equal to the arterial pressure and the absence of CBF, the other determinants of death are dependent on a known history or diagnosis of the event precipitating the death and the absolute absence of any medication or drugs that could influence the results of the examination. There is no reason to prolong the life-support process in a dead child, and the reasons for failing to act by declaring death and removing the cardiovascular support from a dead child are almost always based on the inability of the medical attendants to accept the state of affairs. The situation is no more reversible in a child than in an adult, and a disservice is done to the family by not permitting them to start the grieving process despite the fact that death has occurred. Finally, despite the apparent difficulty some physicians still have in approaching families for organ donation, studies have shown that this ability to help a living child in a situation of despair is often the one event that can help the family feel that something good has come from the tragedy.

References

1. Avezaat CJJ, Van Eijhdhoven JHM: Cerebrospinal fluid pulse pressure and craniospinal dynamics. A theoretical and experimental study. The Hague, A Gonabloed en zoon, 1984.
2. Bruce DA: Pathophysiology of intracranial pressure. *In*: Diseases of the Nervous System. Vol 2. Asbury AK, McKhann GM, McDonald WI (Eds). Philadelphia, WB Saunders, 1986, pp 1044–1062.
3. Mendelsohn D, Levin HS, Bruce D, et al: Late MRI after head injury in children: Relationship to clinical features and outcome. Childs Nerv Syst 1992; 8:445–452.
4. Bruce DA: Head Injuries in the pediatric population. Curr Probl Pediatr 1990; 20:67–107.
5. Humphreys RP: Special article: Hemorrhagic stroke in childhood. Riv Neurosci Pediatr 1986; 2:1.
6. Ondra SL, Troupp H, George ED, et al: The natural history of symptomatic arteriovenous malformations of the brain: A 24 year follow up assessment. J Neurosurg 1990; 73:387–391.

7. Meyer FB, Sundt TM, Fode NC, et al: Cerebral aneurysms in childhood and adolesence. J Neurosurg 1989; 70:420–425.
8. Hijdra A, vanGijn J, Nagelkerke NJ, et al. Prediction of delayed cerebral ischemia, rebleeding and outcome after aneurysmal subarchnoid hemorrhage. Stroke 1988; 19:1250–1256.
9. Kassell NF, Torner JC, Haley C Jr, et al: The international cooperative study of the timing of aneurysm surgery. Part I: Overall management results. J Neurosurg 1990; 73:18–36.
10. Kassell NF, Torner JC, Jane JA, et al: The international cooperative study of the timing of aneurysm surgery. Part 2: Surgical results. J Neurosurg 1990; 73:37–47.
11. Drake CG: Report of world federation of neurological surgeons committee on a universal subarachnoid grading scale. J Neurosurg 1988; 68:985–990.
12. Kassell NF, Peerless SJ, Durward QJ, et al: Treatment of ischemic deficits from vasospasm with intravascular volume expansion and induced arterial hypertension. Neurosurgery 1982; 11:337–343.
13. Petruk KC, West M, Mohr G, et al: Nimodipine treatment in poor grade aneurysm patients; results of a multicenter double-blind placebo controlled trial. J Neurosurg 1988; 68:505–517.
14. Fearon JA, Munro IR, Bruce DA, et al: Massive teratomas involving the cranial base: Treatment and outcome—a two-center report. Plast Reconstr Surg 1992; 91:223–228.
15. Charney E, Weller S, Sutton JN, et al: Management of the newborn with myelomeningocele: Time for a decision making process. Pediatrics 1985; 75:58–64.
16. Coker SB: Cyclic vomiting and the slit ventricle syndrome. Pediatr Neurol 1987; 3:297–299.
17. Serlo W, Heikkinen E, Saukkonen AL, et al: Classification and management of the slit ventricle syndrome. Childs Nerv Syst 1985; 1:194–199.
18. Laurent JP, Bruce DA, Schut L: Hemorrhagic brain tumors in pediatric patients. Childs Brain 1981; 8:263–266.
19. Hirsch JF, Roux FX, Sainte-Rose C, et al: Brain abscess in childhood. A study of 34 cases treated by puncture and antibiotics. Childs Brain 1983; 10:251–255.
20. Neilsen H: Cerebral abscess in children. Neuropediatrics 1983; 14:76–81.
21. Smith HP, Hendrick EB: Subdural empyema and epidural abscess in children. J Neurosurg 1983; 58:392–395.
22. Hockley AD, Williams B: Surgical management of subdural empyema. Childs Brain 1983; 10:294–297.
23. Dickman CA, Rekate HL, Sonntag VKH, et al: Pediatric spinal trauma: Vertebral column and spinal cord injuries in children. Pediatr Neurosci 1989; 15:237–256.
24. Determination of brain death. Ad hoc committee on brain death. J Pediatr 1987; 100:15–19.
25. Volpe JJ: Brain death determination in the newborn. Pediatrics 1987; 80:292–297.

CHAPTER 173

Controversies in Brain Death Certification

David J. Powner, MD • *Joseph M. Darby, MD*
Ake Grenvik, MD, PhD

Although brain death was first described clinically nearly 40 years ago,[1, 2] its definition, diagnosis, and certification remain controversial. Partly because of incomplete information and nonuniform practice,[3, 4] controversy and at times conflict encompass

1. Defining death as a physical and/or philosophical event[5]
2. Selecting reliable testing methods to confidently identify when death has occurred
3. Deciding who may make the clinical diagnosis and certification of death

Uncertainty and indecision concurrently arise owing to difficulty in defining life. If life is either the presence of cellular processes or the accumulation of cellular activity into measurable neuronal function or cognitive perception or a spiritual essence, then its absence, death, must be evaluated in very different ways. Similarly, if the purpose of diagnosing death is to obtain organs for transplantation, different standards, procedures, and even personnel may be applied than are used, for example, during the terminal withdrawal of life support. This chapter reviews many of these controversies, not intending to resolve disputes but to provide physicians with the information needed to participate comfortably in brain death confirmation and certification or to decline to participate.

CARDIORESPIRATORY CRITERIA FOR DEATH

Traditional criteria for defining death require cessation of cardiac and respiratory function. This definition has been historically supported by observable disintegration of the body after loss of those bodily functions identified as the properties of life. Discoloration, rigidity, and decomposition of the body are objective endpoints that are generally accepted as criteria for the absence of life. These measures were used historically before the pivotal role of cardiorespiratory function was acknowledged and accurate measures of those functions were available. Fear of pronouncing death when a patient was actually alive led to prolonged periods of observation before burial. That same concern remains today because death has been redefined and its criteria are not as easily measured as are cardiac and respiratory parameters.

BRAIN CRITERIA FOR DEATH—OVERVIEW

Decapitation represents an extreme example of an instance in which a person is considered deceased despite the brief continuation of cardiopulmonary function.[1] Otherwise, society accepted only cardiorespiratory criteria until the technologic capacity to sustain cardiopulmonary function after severe brain injury forced physicians and society to address the separation of cardiorespiratory and neurologic survival. Reasons for addressing this separation included justification for making further clinical decisions such as discontinuation of cardiopulmonary support and the improved survival of recipients after transplantation of organs from donors with a heartbeat. Excellent reviews of the evolution of that confrontation[1, 6] summarize the process leading to the Uniform Determination of Death Act, which is the basis for most state statutes in the United States:

"An individual who has sustained either (1) irreversible cessation of circulatory and respiratory functions, or (2) irreversible cessation of all functions of the entire brain, including the brainstem, is dead."

Through practice, public opinion, policy, legal precedence, and statute, the equivalency of a patient's death and the death of some or all components of the brain has been accepted in most countries of the world. This acceptance, in part, reflects:

- The inability of central nervous system neurons to undergo cell division to replace other neurons lost to injury or disease
- The lack of an extracorporeal method to substitute for lost brain function as exists for renal function with hemodialysis or cardiac function with circulatory assist devices
- The inability to transplant this vital organ

TABLE 173–1. Group/Institutional Policies Advocating Whole-Brain Criteria for Death and Requiring Cerebral Testing*

American Neurological Association
Harvard Medical School
Medical College of Virginia
National Institutes of Health—Collaborative Study on Cerebral Survival
Rutgers Medical School
University of Bonn Klinik
University of Pennsylvania
Swedish groups
Japanese Ministry of Health and Welfare[8]

*See Powner[7] for primary citations except as added in this table.

Whole-Brain Criteria

The equivalence of life to the function of the entire brain forms the foundation of these criteria for death. Thus, a person may be declared deceased only when all functions of the entire brain are determined to be irrevocably absent. Implied therein is the permanency of an irrevocable state, testing of all parts of the brain, and the assumption that all testing is valid to avoid an unacceptable false determination of death.

A large number of diagnostic methods have been proposed to attempt valid testing, absent neuronal function, and irreversibility. Table 173–1 lists some of the numerous authoritative groups that have published whole-brain criteria. Each set of criteria requires that certain agents or conditions known to depress brain function reversibly (Table 173–2) be absent before testing is started. All criteria stipulate that a careful neurologic examination using standard methods demonstrate no response to verbal stimulation, no seizures, no decerebrate or decorticate posturing, no reaction to painful stimuli administered over cranial nerve afferent tracts, no cranial nerve reflexes, and no respiratory effort when hypercarbia or hypoxemia is present. Table 173–3 lists specific criteria and methodologic considerations for testing; these apply not only to whole-brain standards but also to brain stem criteria discussed later.

Some criteria mandate repeated examinations at a specified interval or require a known cause of brain failure to imply irreversibility. In addition to a neurologic examination, single or repetitive confirmatory tests may be required to further document absent neuronal function or lack of intracranial blood flow. Whole-brain criteria require specific evidence of death of the cerebrum. This is often documented either by electroencephalography (EEG) or through evaluation of cerebral blood flow. Table 173–4 lists those tests of the cerebrum or other parts of the brain that may be advocated in conjunction with the neurologic examination to document absent functions of the entire brain. Tests dependent on neuronal function are valid only when those confounding factors listed in Table 173–2 are absent. Tests of anatomic blood flow are used when some confounding factor (e.g., drugs) is or may be present. The clinical and technical limits of each confirmatory test must be understood. Examples include the following:

1. Xenon and technetium radionuclide blood flow studies primarily assess only cerebral flow and poorly visualize the

TABLE 173–2. Confounding Agents/Conditions That Must Be Absent Before Brain Death Testing*

- Shock/hypotension
- Hypothermia <32°C
- Drugs known to alter neurologic and/or neuromuscular function or electroencephalographic testing:
  - Anesthetics
  - Paralytics
  - Methaqualone
  - Barbiturates
  - Diazepam
  - High-dose bretylium[9]
  - Mecloqualone
  - Amitriptyline[10]
  - Meprobamate
  - Trichloroethylene
  - Alcohols
- Brain stem encephalitis[11]
- Guillain-Barré syndrome[12]
- Encephalopathies associated with hepatic failure, uremia, and hyperosmolar coma
- Severe hypophosphatemia

*See Powner[7] for primary citations except as added in this table.

TABLE 173–3. Examination Criteria and Methods*

1. Absent spontaneous movement, decorticate or decerebrate posturing; lack of seizures, shivering, response to verbal stimuli, response to noxious stimuli administered through a cranial nerve pathway. Spinal reflexes may persist.
2. Absent pupillary reflex to direct and consensual light; pupils need not be equal or dilated. The pupillary reflex may be selectively altered by eye trauma, cataracts, high-dose dopamine, glutethimide, scopolamine, atropine, or monoamine oxidase inhibitors.
3. Absent corneal, oculocephalic, cough, and gag reflexes. The corneal reflex may be altered as a result of any type of facial weakness.
4. Absent oculovestibular reflex when tested with 20 to 50 mL of ice water irrigated into an external auditory canal clear of cerumen after elevating the patient's head 30°. Labyrinthine injury or disease, anticholinergics, anticonvulsants, tricyclic antidepressants, and some sedatives may alter responses.
5. Failure of the heart rate to increase by more than 5 beats per minute after 1–2 mg IV of atropine has been used to further assess the vagal nerve and nuclei.
6. Absent respiratory efforts in the presence of hypercarbia (partial pressure of carbon dioxide >50–60 mm Hg) or, in rare circumstances, carefully monitored hypoxemia. Many protocols for apnea testing[13] have been advocated to prevent hypoxemia during testing.

*See Powner[7] for original citations except as added in this table. Neurologic examination can be performed only when those factors listed in Table 173–2 are absent.

TABLE 173–4. Confirmatory Tests in Whole-Brain Criteria*

- Evaluate neuronal function:
  - Electroencephalogram or cerebral function monitor
  - Evoked potentials[13a]
  - Biochemical tests of cerebrospinal fluid or jugular venous blood
- Evaluate intracranial blood flow:
  - Contrast angiography, magnetic resonance[14] or computed tomography imaging
  - Radionuclide perfusion studies using technetium cranial radionuclide angiography and technetium-HMPAO scintigraphy[15]
  - Xenon-enhanced computed tomography[16]
  - Digital subtraction angiography/venography
  - Ophthalmic artery blood flow
  - Transcranial Doppler study[17]
- Miscellaneous:
  - Intracranial pressure higher than systolic blood pressure[18]
  - Sustained cerebral perfusion pressure <5 mm Hg[18]

*See Powner[7] for primary citations except as added in this table.

posterior fossa and vertebral artery circulation. Variant flow patterns in both tests may limit interpretation when present.

2. EEG testing must be done at maximum gain in accord with standards established by the American Electroencephalographic Society.[1] Technical issues and inter-rater variability may affect reliability.[19]

3. Brain stem auditory evoked potentials evaluate only the brain stem and should be performed after apnea testing.[20, 21]

4. Extracranial Doppler testing of blood flow should be attempted only when the systolic blood pressure is greater than 100 mm Hg.[21]

5. The intracranial pressure may be lower than systolic blood pressure.[22]

Intertest precision in patients with absent brain function on clinical examination was evaluated by comparing the EEG, brain stem auditory evoked potentials, and findings on extracranial Doppler ultrasonography and digital subtraction angiography.[21] Although agreement was reached in most of the 50 cases studied, variation between the tests persisted in some patients because of either technical limitations or actual disparities in results. The investigators concluded that the only reliable assessment of brain death using whole-brain criteria depends on four-vessel angiography.[21]

If all testing criteria are met, other standards may address the specific process of certification. In some cases, brain death may be certified by one or more physicians who have prescribed expertise in this area and who have or do not have a primary or consultative relationship with the patient. Various concerns about a potential conflict of interest for a certifying physician during organ donation may further limit a physician's participation.

Despite such elaborate standards and procedures, considerable evidence shows that in some patients, residual neuronal function continues even though a patient has fulfilled whole-brain criteria. Such evidence includes:

1. Maintenance of body temperature (i.e., not all patients become poikilothermic[23])

2. Spontaneous depolarizations detected by deeply placed electrodes despite an isoelectric cortical EEG[1]

3. Continuing or inducible pituitary and/or hypothalamic hormone production after four-vessel angiography has shown no flow[24, 25]

4. Resumption of blood flow after relief of obstructing lesions[1] and postmortem examination in patients whose brain death was confirmed by the absence of flow during angiography

Therefore, those who demand the most precise documentation that all cellular function of the entire brain is absent before confirming brain death acknowledge that no set of criteria is sufficiently detailed for that purpose. Most commonly, the potential that residual cellular and tissue function may exist is recognized but not specifically sought.

Cerebral Criteria

Loss of cerebral or "neocortical" function while brain stem function persists has not traditionally been accepted as equivalent to death although vigorously advocated by some.[26, 26a] This proposition states that the critical element of life is the organized cognition originating from the cerebrum, which provides "personhood" as the unique feature of human life.[26, 26a] Cognition implies awareness to identify oneself and often is measured as the ability to follow complex commands requiring the intellectual integration of afferent stimuli and efferent actions. Permanent loss of personhood would, therefore, identify a loss of the essential element of the human quality and permit the declaration of death for the purposes of withdrawal of supportive therapies and, potentially, for organ donation. Testing of cerebral function requires absence of cognitive responses but not necessarily coma. Eye opening and a state of apparent alertness may be accepted as long as integrated awareness is absent. Some objective assessment of cerebral anatomy such as computed tomography or magnetic resonance imaging scans or blood flow may be used. Although current blood flow measurements and computed tomography or magnetic resonance imaging may diagnose extreme cases of anatomic ischemia and tissue reabsorption, intermediate levels of injury remain difficult to quantify and accurately prognosticate by these tests. Proton emission tomography scans that demonstrate extremely low cerebral oxygen uptake in cortical layers are a new technique used to evaluate neocortical cellular function.

A major concern of opponents of the use of cerebral criteria is that the permanence of cerebral dysfunction cannot be predicted in most clinical circumstances.[27] Prolonged states of absent cognition followed by awakening among patients who have metabolic encephalopathy and who have been thought to be in a vegetative state support that position. Opponents of the use of only cerebral criteria to define brain death also raise the so-called slippery slope argument in which noncognitive patients may be declared dead using progressively less stringent criteria in response to increasing external pressures to do so (e.g., from fiscal or transplantation sources).

A category of noncognitive patients, anencephalic infants, deserves special mention. Some propose that because these patients lack cortical tissue entirely, they have never experienced cognition and thus could not regain it, nor could they ever acquire any integrated responses. Therefore, the proposition is forwarded that these individuals have never been nor could they ever be "alive,"[28] even though they may appear alert and apparently may respond to comforting measures. This position has been legally supported for the purposes of renal transplantation in Germany.[29]

Although anencephalic infants often experience cardiorespiratory failure soon after birth, attempts to provide that support until complete brain stem failure occurs and the infant fulfills the whole-brain criteria for death have not led to successful organ removal for transplantation.[30] Therefore, advocates of transplantation of organs from anencephalic infants have proposed changes in statutes that define death or permit procurement of anatomic gifts. Such changes would expressly allow use of anencephalic neonates as donors before whole-brain or brain stem criteria for death are fulfilled. Physiologic and anatomic variations within the diagnosis of anencephaly, the declining incidence of this abnormality, limitations in the ability to transplant these small organs, and a large number of ethical concerns about the personhood status of anencephalic infants have limited any resolution of this controversy.[31]

Brain Stem Criteria

Criteria documenting absent brain stem function have been accepted as equivalent to a patient's death within the United Kingdom since the mid-1970s and are directly or indirectly accepted by the groups/institutions shown in Table 173–5. These groups do not or no longer *require* cerebral testing beyond that provided by the standard neurological examination. Interruption of the reticular activating fibers within the brain stem presumes a noncognitive state. Absent spontaneous breathing leads to asystole if mechanical ventilation

TABLE 173–5. Groups/Institutional Policies Accepting Brain Stem Testing or Not Requiring Separate Tests of the Cerebrum*

Medical Colleges of the United Kingdom
United States Navy
National Board of Health—Finland
Prince Henry Hospital, Sydney, Australia
University of Minnesota
University of Pittsburgh
Royal College of Surgeons (Dublin)
President's Commission for the Study of Problems in Medicine and Biomedical and Behavioral Research

*See Powner[7] for primary citations.

is not provided. Criteria established by the Conference of Medical Royal Colleges[32] are nearly identical to those for evaluation of the brain stem within the whole-brain criteria (see Table 173–3) but do not require examination of the cerebrum beyond clinical confirmation of absent cognition. They emphasize the same exclusions (see Table 173–2) to ensure validity of testing and demand that patients be noncognitive as a result of a known cause that would be sufficient to assume an irreversible condition. These, as all criteria, assume that all reasonable therapeutic interventions have been attempted to treat the underlying brain injury. Requirements for retesting and decisions about who may be responsible for certification of death may be added at the local level.

Documented cases of continued low-amplitude EEG activity[1, 33] and cerebral blood flow[6] exist in patients who have fulfilled these criteria. It is not considered, however, that such findings bestow cognition.

BRAIN DEATH IN CHILDREN

The criteria described earlier generally are restricted to adults and children older than 5 to 7 years. Specific criteria considered useful in infants and young children have been published by the Task Force for the Determination of Brain Death in Children[34, 34a] and are presented in Table 173–6. Most practicing pediatric intensivists responding to a survey strongly rely on clinical examination, EEG, and radionuclide testing and repeat a single clinical examination within 12 to 24 hours.[35] Evaluation of preterm and full-term newborns[36] demonstrates the variability of EEG and radionuclide findings as compared with the physical examination in that age group and emphasizes that phenobarbital may dramatically alter neuronal function. Xenon–computed tomography guidelines have also been proposed for children older than 1 month as follows: (1) Flow less than 5 mL/min per 100 g of brain tissue is consistent with no flow as recorded by radionuclide studies; (2) flow less than 10 mL/min per 100 g of brain tissue is consistent with clinical brain death; (3) flow greater than 10 to 15 mL/min per 100 g of brain tissue is associated with potential for survival.[37]

TABLE 173–6. Guidelines Useful for Brain Death Evaluation in Children

Prerequisite to evaluation:
- History of cause of coma eliminates reversible conditions (similar to Table 173–2)

Physical examination criteria:
- Coma (loss of consciousness, vocalization, and volitional activity)
- Apnea using standardized testing
- Absent brain stem function:
  - Midposition or fully dilated pupils unresponsive to light
  - Absent spontaneous eye movements, oculocephalic and oculovestibular reflexes
  - Absent movement of bulbar musculature
  - Absent corneal, gag, cough, sucking, and rooting reflexes
  - Flaccid tone and absent spontaneous or induced movements except for those caused by spinal cord reflexes
  - Findings on examination should be consistent with brain death during entire observation and testing period as below

Age-specific observation period and retesting:
- 7 d of age to 2 mo—two examinations and EEGs separated by 48 h
- 2 mo to 1 y of age—two examinations and EEGs separated by at least 24 h or initial examination plus isoelectric EEG followed by cerebral radionuclide study confirming no cerebral blood flow
- Older than 1 y of age—two examinations at least 12 h apart, with EEG and cerebral radionuclide studies optional

(From Guidelines for determination of brain death in children. Arch Neurol 1987; 44:587.)

SUMMARY

The equivalence of a person's death with absent function of a portion or the entirety of that person's brain has largely been accepted as an alternative to traditional cardiorespiratory criteria. Controversy continues about which part(s) of the brain must be without function, the methods of assessment, the political or bureaucratic processes of death certification, and the importance of continuing residual neuronal activity at a cellular or functional level despite completion of the most detailed whole-brain criteria.

As medical and social standards evolve and produce changes in fiscal, ethical, and transplantation priorities, it seems apparent that these controversies will intensify rather than abate. The essence of such discussion returns, in part, to the elemental issue of the personal and societal value placed on life, its definition and preservation. As each social group determines and re-examines those definitions and priorities, further variations within the concomitant description of death will likely emerge. Life and death and their consequences therefore continue to be based on societal as well as physiologic criteria. Spiritual or theologic absolutes likewise form a part of the societal matrix but appear to be a progressively smaller voice in the discussions.

The individual critical care practitioner is, therefore, often called on not only to influence the larger debate but also to develop and implement many local policies that reflect global and regional perspectives. It is hoped that this chapter will assist in identifying issues relevant to those perspectives and the important task of understanding brain death.

References

1. Pallis C: Brainstem death: The evolution of a concept. Semin Thorac Cardiovasc Surg 1990; 2:135.
2. Grenvik A: Brain death and organ transplantation, a 40-year review. Opuscula Medica (Stockh) 1992; 37:33.
3. Black PM, Zervas NT: Declaration of brain death in neurosurgical and neurologic practice. Neurosurgery 1984; 15:170.
4. Youngner SJ, Landefeld S, Coulton CJ, et al: Brain death and organ retrieval: A cross-sectional survey of knowledge and concepts among health professionals. JAMA 1989; 261:2205.
5. Catherwood JF: Rosencrantz and Guildenstern are "dead"? J Med Ethics 1992; 18:34.
6. Darby J, Yonas H, Brenner RP: Brainstem death with persistent EEG activity: Evaluation by xenon-enhanced computed tomography. Crit Care Med 1987; 15:519.
7. Powner DJ: The diagnosis of brain death in the adult patient. J Intensive Care Med 1987; 2:181.
8. Takeuchi K, Takeshita H, Takakura K, et al: Evolution of criteria for determination of brain death in Japan. Acta Neurochir (Wien) 1987; 87:93.

9. Thompson AE, Sussmane JB: Bretylium intoxication resembling clinical brain death. Crit Care Med 1989; 17:194.
10. Yang KL, Dantzker DR: Reversible brain death: A manifestation of amitriptyline overdose. Chest 1991; 99:1037.
11. Chandler JM, Brilli RJ: Brainstem encephalitis imitating brain death. Crit Care Med 1991; 19:977.
12. Hassan T, Mumford C: Guillain-Barré syndrome mistaken for brain stem death. Postgrad Med J 1991; 67:280.
13. Benzel EC, Mashburn JP, Conrad S, et al: Apnea testing for the determination of brain death: A modified protocol. J Neurosurg 1992; 76:1029.
13a. Macho C: Multimodality evoked potentials and electroretinography in a test battery for an early diagnosis of brain death. J Neurosurg Sci 1993; 37:125.
14. Aichner F, Felber S, Birbamer G, et al: Magnetic resonance: A noninvasive approach to metabolism, circulation, and morphology in human brain death. Ann Neurol 1992; 32:507.
15. de la Riva A, Gonzalez FM, Llamas-Elvira JM, et al: Diagnosis of brain death: Superiority of perfusion studies with 99 Tc^{m}-HMPAO over conventional radionuclide cerebral angiography. Br J Radiol 1992; 65:289.
16. Pistoia F, Johnson DW, Darby JM, et al: The role of xenon CT measurements of cerebral blood flow in the clinical determination of brain death. AJNR 1991; 12:97.
17. Feri M, Ralli L, Felici M, et al: Transcranial Doppler and brain death diagnosis. Crit Care Med 1994; 22:1120.
18. Dominguez-Roldan JM, Murillo-Cabezas F, Munoz-Sanchez A, et al: Is intracranial hypertension useful in the diagnosis of brain death? Transplant Proc 1992; 24:31.
19. Buchner H, Schuchardt V: Reliability of electroencephalogram in the diagnosis of brain death. Eur Neurol 1990; 30:138.
20. Firsching R, Frowein RA, Wilhelms S, et al: Brain death: Practicability of evoked potentials. Neurosurg Rev 1992; 15:249.
21. Nau R, Prange HW, Klingel Lofer J, et al: Results of four technical investigations in fifty clinically brain dead patients. Intensive Care Med 1992; 18:82.
22. Richard KE, Nanassis K, Frowein RA: Intracranial pressure: A reliable criterion of brain death? Neurosurg Rev 1989; 12(Suppl 1):287.
23. Jastremski M, Powner DJ, Snyder JV, et al: Problems in brain death determination. Forensic Sci 1978; 11:201.
24. Sugimoto T, Sakano T, Kinoshita Y, et al: Morphological and functional alterations of the hypothalamic-pituitary system in brain death with long term bodily living. Acta Neurochir (Wien) 1992; 115:31.
25. Arita K, Uozumi T, Oki S, et al: The function of the hypothalamo-pituitary axis in brain dead patients. Acta Neurochir (Wien) 1993; 123:64.
26. Cranford RE, Smith DR: Consciousness: The most critical moral (constitutional) standard for human personhood. Am J Law Med 1987; 13:233.
26a. Lizza JP: Persons and death: What's metaphysically wrong with our current statutory definition of death? J Med Philos 1993; 18:351.
27. Young B, Blume W, Lynch A: Brain death and the persistent vegetative state: Similarities and contrasts. Can J Neurol Sci 1989; 16:388.
28. Diaz JH: The anencephalic organ donor: A challenge to existing moral and statutory laws. Crit Care Med 1993; 21:1781.
29. Holzgreve W, Beller FK, Buchholz B, et al: Kidney transplantation from anencephalic donors. N Engl J Med 1987; 316:1069.
30. Peabody JL, Emergy JR, Ashwal S: Experience with anencephalic infants as prospective organ donors. N Engl J Med 1989; 321:344.
31. Shewmon DA, Capron AM, Peacock WJ, et al: The use of anencephalic infants as organ sources. JAMA 1989; 261:1773.
32. Diagnosis of brain death: Statement issued by the honorary secretary of the Conference of Medical Royal Colleges and their Faculties in the United Kingdom on 11 October 1976. Br Med J 1976; 2:1187.
33. Ogata J, Imakita M, Yutani C, et al: Primary brainstem death: A clinico-pathological study. J Neurol Neurosurg Psychiatry 1988; 51:646.
34. Guidelines for determination of brain death in children. Arch Neurol 1987; 44:587.
34a. Farrell MM, Levin DL: Brain death in the pediatric patient. Historical, sociological, medical, religious, cultural, legal, and ethical considerations. Crit Care Med 1993; 21:1951.
35. Lynch J, Eldadah MK: Brain-death criteria currently used by pediatric intensivists. Clin Pediatr 1992; 31:457.
36. Ashwal S, Schneider S: Brain death in the newborn. Pediatrics 1989; 84:429.
37. Ashwal S, Schneider S, Thompson J: Xenon computed tomography measuring cerebral blood flow in the determination of brain death in children. Ann Neurol 1989; 25:539.

CHAPTER 174

Neuromuscular Disorders in Critical Care

Thomas P. Bleck, MD, FCCM

Disturbed neuromuscular function may be the cause of a patient's presentation to an intensive care unit (e.g., botulism), may be the consequence of another critical illness (e.g., critical illness polyneuropathy), or may result from various therapeutic measures used by the intensivist (e.g., neuromuscular junction blockade). This chapter addresses the first two of these classes of illness; it focuses primarily on respiratory failure as a consequence of neuromuscular disease but also addresses autonomic dysfunction occurring in this setting. To facilitate understanding of the concepts involved, it commences with a brief review of the aspects of neuromuscular transmission that become deranged in the disorders discussed in this chapter.

NEUROMUSCULAR ASPECTS OF RESPIRATION

Nervous system activity destined to produce motor output is conducted to the lower motor neuron, also known as the alpha motor neuron. The cell bodies of these neurons are located in the brain stem (for the cranial musculature) and the spinal cord (for the rest of the body). These neurons receive various excitatory and inhibitory inputs. Axons of these neurons travel through the subarachnoid space, penetrate the dura mater, and travel (usually in concert with other types of nerves) to the muscles they innervate. These axons are myelinated, and myelinization accelerates neuromuscular transmission. The axon terminates on a number of muscle fibers; this group is called the *motor unit.* The axon communicates with the muscle via a specialized area termed the *neuromuscular junction.* On the presynaptic side of the neuromuscular junction, the neurotransmitter *acetylcholine* is synthesized, packaged in vesicles, and stored for release. Depolarization of the axon opens presynaptic calcium channels, which activate the molecular machinery responsible for drawing the vesicles to the presynaptic membrane, with which they fuse and release their contents into the synaptic cleft. The acetylcholine then activates its postsynaptic receptor, producing an influx of sodium, which depolarizes the muscle. This depolarization releases calcium ions from the sarcoplasmic reticulum, causing contraction of the muscle. After activating the acetylcholine receptor complex, the acetylcholine molecule is degraded by *cholinesterase*; the choline released by this reaction is then recycled by the presynaptic neuron.

Three muscle groups may be defined based on their importance for respiration: the upper airway muscles (muscles of the palate and the pharynx and the genioglossus muscle);

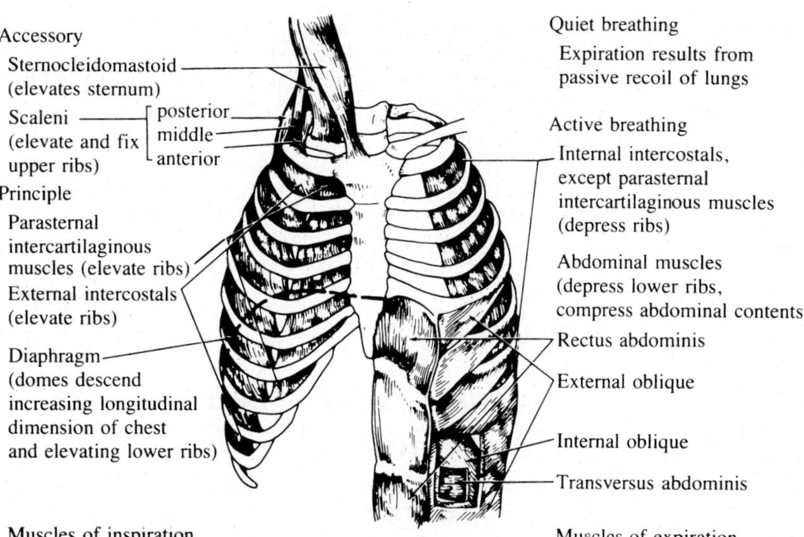

Figure 174–1. Major respiratory muscles. Inspiratory muscles are indicated on the left, and expiratory muscles are indicated on the right. (From Garrity ER: Respiratory failure due to disorders of the chest wall and respiratory muscles. *In*: Respiratory Intensive Care. MacDonnell KF, Fahey PJ, Segal MS [Eds]. Boston, Little, Brown and Co, 1987, p 313. Published by Little, Brown and Company.)

the inspiratory muscles (sternomastoid, diaphragm, scalenes, and parasternal intercostals); and the expiratory muscles (internal intercostal muscles, except for the parasternals, and abdominal muscles) (Fig. 174–1).[1] The upper-airway muscles receive their innervation from the lower cranial nerves. Sternomastoid innervation arrives predominantly from cranial nerve XI, with a small contribution from C-2. The phrenic nerve originates from cell bodies located between C-3 and C-5, with a maximum contribution from C-4, and innervates the diaphragm. Innervation to the scalenes arises from C-4 to C-8, whereas that of the parasternal intercostals is from T-1 to T-7. The intercostal muscles receive innervation from T-1 to T-12, and the abdominal musculature from T-7 to L-1. Reference to this innervation scheme is important in understanding the effects of spinal cord and nerve root injuries on respiration and for the differential diagnosis of disorders producing apparently diffuse weakness.

RECOGNITION OF NEUROMUSCULAR RESPIRATORY FAILURE

Patients experiencing respiratory dysfunction due to neuromuscular disease typically present with a combination of upper-airway dysfunction and diminished tidal volume (VT). Difficulty with swallowing liquids, including respiratory secretions, is the most typical presentation of pharyngeal weakness, although some patients have an equal or greater degree of difficulty with solid food. A hoarse or nasal voice may also signal problems with the upper airway. These conditions are noted in patients who are at risk for aspiration and presage difficulty with attempts at negative-pressure ventilation (cuirass[2] or iron lung), because the weakened muscles may not be able to keep the airway open as the pressure falls. Paradoxical abdominal movement (inward movement of the abdomen during inspiration) is an important sign of diaphragmatic weakness.[3]

Loss of VT occurs most dramatically with diaphragmatic weakness but also follows insults that affect the ability of the paraspinal intercostals to keep the chest wall expanded against negative intrapleural pressure. This is most apparent in patients with lower cervical spinal cord injuries; they frequently develop atelectasis despite preserved phrenic nerve function (this problem usually diminishes over weeks as the muscles develop spasticity).

Patients with progressive generalized weakness (e.g., with the Guillain-Barré syndrome [GBS]) commonly begin to lose VT before developing upper-airway weakness. In order to maintain minute ventilation and therefore carbon dioxide excretion, a patient's respiratory rate increases; this rate is thus one of the most important clinical parameters to monitor. As the vital capacity (VC) falls from the norm of about 65 mL/kg to about 30 mL/kg, the patient's cough weakens and clearing secretions becomes difficult. A further decrease of VC to 20 to 25 mL/kg results in an impaired ability to sigh, with progressive atelectasis; hypoxemia may be present because of ventilation-perfusion mismatching and because an increasing percentage of VT is used to ventilate dead space. Before the VC reaches 15 mL/kg, a patient should be in an intensive care unit because respiratory failure is imminent, and endotracheal intubation should be considered. The precise point at which mechanical ventilation is necessary varies with the patient, the underlying condition, and especially the likelihood of a rapid response to treatment. Regardless of the VC, indications for intubation include evidence of fatigue, hypoxemia despite supplemental oxygen administration, and difficulty with secretions. Although a rising arterial partial pressure of carbon dioxide (Pa_{CO_2}) usually suggests the need for intubation and mechanical ventilation, occasional patients (e.g., those with myasthenia gravis [MG]) can be managed under very close observation in an intensive care unit without such assistance or with less invasive techniques (e.g., bilevel positive airway pressure [biPAP]).

In addition to the VC, trended measurements of the maximum inspiratory pressure (PImax, more typically recorded as negative inspiratory force [NIF]) are useful indicators of ventilatory capacity. Inability to maintain a PImax greater than 20 to 25 cm H_2O usually indicates a need for mechanical ventilatory assistance. Although the maximum expiratory pressure (PEmax) is a more sensitive indicator of weakness,[4] it has not proved to be as useful as an indicator of the need for mechanical ventilation. A more detailed discussion of these variables and their use may be found in Chapters 73 and 76.[5]

Because a patient with neuromuscular respiratory failure has intact ventilatory drive,[6] the fall in VT is initially matched by an increase in respiratory rate, keeping the Pa_{CO_2} normal or low until the VC becomes dangerously small. Many patients initially maintain their Pa_{CO_2} in the range of 35 mm Hg because of either a subjective sense of dyspnea at low VT, or hypoxia from atelectasis and increasing dead space. When the $Pa{CO_2}$ begins to rise in this circumstance, abrupt respiratory failure may be imminent.

The modest degree of hypoxia in most of these patients worsens when the $Pa{CO_2}$ begins to rise, displacing more oxygen from the alveolar gas; however, aspiration, pneumonia, and pulmonary embolism are also frequent causes of hypoxemia in these patients. To determine the relative contributions of these conditions to a patient's hypoxemia, one can use a simplified version of the alveolar air equation (for derivation, see Chapters 73 and 76):

$$P_{AO_2} = P_{IO_2} - (Pa_{CO_2}/R)$$

where P_{IO_2} is the partial pressure of inspired oxygen (in room air, 150 mm Hg) and R is the respiratory quotient (on most diets, about 0.8). This allows one to estimate the alveolar-arterial oxygen difference ($P_{AO_2} - Pa_{O_2}$). Under ideal circumstances in young people, this value is about 10 mm Hg in room air but rises to about 100 mm Hg at a fraction of inspired oxygen of 1.0. The alveolar air equation allows one to factor out the contribution of hypercarbia to the decrease in arterial partial pressure of oxygen (Pa_{O_2}); it should be used to determine whether there is a cause of significant hypoxemia in addition to the displacement of oxygen by carbon dioxide.

Patients with weakness of the orbicularis oris may have artifactually low VC and NIF measurements because they cannot form a tight seal around the devices' mouthpieces. The need for nursing and respiratory therapy personnel who are experienced in the care of these patients is thus underscored, especially the need for physicians to observe these patients directly rather than relying solely on reported measurements. The physical findings associated with neuromuscular respiratory failure are reviewed in detail in Chapters 73 and 76.[7] Among the most important findings are rapid, shallow breathing[7a]; the recruitment of accessory muscles; and paradoxical movement of the abdomen during the respiratory cycle. Fluoroscopy of the diaphragm is occasionally valuable for the diagnosis of diaphragmatic dysfunction.[8]

Autonomic dysfunction frequently accompanies some of the neuromuscular disorders requiring critical care. GBS (discussed later) represents one of the best examples. Autonomic problems may arise synchronously with weakness or may follow the onset of the motor disorder by a week or more.

DIFFERENTIAL DIAGNOSIS OF NEUROMUSCULAR DISORDERS

A wide spectrum of neuromuscular diseases may result in ventilatory failure; Table 174–1 presents an anatomically oriented list of diagnostic possibilities. Only the most common disorders can be discussed in this chapter. Consult a recent review of this subject[9, 10] or the references listed in Table 174–1 for more details. Some of the diseases listed (e.g., the Lambert-Eaton syndrome) rarely cause respiratory

TABLE 174–1. Neuromuscular Causes of Acute Respiratory Failure

Location	*Disorder*	*Associated Autonomic Dysfunction?*
Spinal cord	Tetanus[13]	Frequently
Anterior horn cell	Amyotrophic lateral sclerosis[14]	No
	Poliomyelitis	No
	Rabies	Frequently
Peripheral nerve	Guillain-Barré syndrome	Frequently
	Critical illness polyneuropathy and related conditions[15]	Sometimes
	Diphtheria	No (associated with myocardiopathy)
	Porphyria	Occasionally
	Ciguatera	Sometimes
	Saxitoxin poisoning	No
	Tetrodotoxin (pufferfish) poisoning	No
	Paraneoplastic neuropathy[16]	No
	Thallium poisoning	No
	Buckthorn polyneuropathy	No
Neuromuscular junction	Myasthenia gravis	No
	Botulism[17]	Frequently
	Lambert-Eaton myasthenic syndrome[18]	No
	Hypermagnesemia[19]	No
	Organophosphate poisoning	No
	Tick paralysis	No
	Snakebite	No
Muscle	Polymyositis	No
	Dermatomyositis	No
	Critical illness myopathy[20]	No
	Myopathy associated with pharmacologic neuromuscular junction blockade	No
	Eosinophilia-myalgia syndrome[22]	No
	Muscular dystrophies[23]	No (but cardiac rhythm disturbances common)
	Carnitine palmitoyl transferase deficiency	No
	Nemaline myopathy[24]	No
	Acid maltase deficiency[25]	No
	Mitochondrial myopathy[26]	No
	Acute hypokalemic paralysis	No
	Stonefish myotoxin poisoning	No
	Barium poisoning	No
	Rhabdomyolysis	No

failure on their own but may be contributing causes in the presence of other conditions,[11] such as neuromuscular junction blockade intended only for the duration of a surgical procedure.[12]

Guillain-Barré Syndrome

GBS (also called *acute inflammatory polyneuropathy* or *polyradiculoneuritis*) is a predominantly motor peripheral neuropathy of acute onset, presumably due to antibodies directed against peripheral nerve components. Approximately 1.7 cases occur per 100,000 population per year.[27] Most patients suffer a demyelinating neuropathy, but in about 5% of cases the condition is a primary axonopathy.[27a] Numerous antecedents have been implicated[28]; the more frequent are listed in Table 174–2.

The initial findings of patients with GBS are weakness, usually most marked in the legs, associated with sensory complaints but without objective signs of sensory dysfunction.[27b] Deep tendon reflexes may be absent on presentation, but this finding may take several days to develop. The cerebrospinal fluid typically reveals an elevated protein content; this may not be present until the second week of illness. The major reason to examine the cerebrospinal fluid is to preclude other diagnoses; on occasion, a pleocytosis is present, suggesting the possibility of acute human immunodeficiency virus infection. Findings on electromyographic studies, which may be normal initially, typically show multifocal conduction blocks, slowed conduction velocity, and impaired or absent responses on tests of proximal (e.g., nerve root) function.

Differential diagnostic considerations for patients with suspected GBS are primarily those listed in the peripheral nerve section of Table 174–1.

Treatment for patients with GBS includes (1) management of ventilatory failure; (2) management of autonomic dysfunction; (3) meticulous nursing care; (4) psychologic support; (5) physical and occupational therapy; (6) prevention of deep venous thrombosis; (7) nutritional support; (8) early planning for rehabilitation; and (9) treatment of the immunologic lesion that produced the condition. Patients who are developing respiratory failure with GBS should generally be intubated when the VC falls to about 15 mL/kg or when difficulty with secretions begins, because the response to treatment is slow. If a patient has been immobile for several days before intubation and neuromuscular junction blockade is needed, a nondepolarizing agent should be used to avoid transient hyperkalemia. Oral intubation is again being viewed as preferable to the nasal route, because the endotracheal tube is frequently required for a week or longer, raising the risk of sinusitis.

Many patients are too weak to trigger the ventilator; in such cases, the assist/control mode is initiated. Weaning patients with GBS from mechanical ventilation must wait for adequate improvement in strength. The author usually shifts to pressure support ventilation for weaning, although evidence of its superiority over intermittent mandatory ventilation or synchronized intermittent mandatory ventilation modes is at present only anecdotal. Although the majority of patients require mechanical ventilation for less than 4 weeks, as many as 20% need 2 or more months of support before they can breathe without assistance. Improvement in VC to greater than 15 mL/kg and in NIF to greater than 25 cm H_2O suggests that a patient has improved adequately to begin weaning. A formula using a combination of ventilatory and gas exchange variables may allow more accurate determination of a patient's ability to be weaned.[29]

Autonomic dysfunction is most typically manifested as a hypersympathetic state and is often heralded by unexplained sinus tachycardia. The blood pressure may fluctuate wildly. Rare patients experience bradycardiac episodes, which may require temporary pacing. Autonomic surges during tracheal suctioning or due to a distended viscus may be very dramatic and should be minimized. Autonomic failure and pulmonary embolism are now the major causes of mortality in GBS.

Nursing care for patients with GBS is similar to that for other paralyzed ventilated patients, but special care must be taken to remember that these patients are completely lucid. In addition to explaining the procedures carefully, arranging for distractions during the daytime (e.g., television, movies, conversation, visitors) and adequate sleep at night are very important. For the most severely affected patients, sedation should be considered. In concert with physical and occupational therapists, passive exercise should be performed frequently throughout the day.

Deep venous thrombosis is a significant danger for patients with GBS. Episodic arterial desaturation is a common event, presumably due to transient mucus plugging, which means that submassive pulmonary emboli may be overlooked. Adjusted-dose heparin (to slightly prolong the partial thromboplastin time) and sequential compression devices should be used; therapeutic anticoagulation may be considered. The risk of fatal pulmonary embolism extends through the initial period of improvement until patients are ambulatory.

Nutritional support should commence as soon as a patient is admitted, with appropriate concern for the risk of aspiration.[30] Most mechanically ventilated patients with GBS can be fed via soft, small-caliber feeding tubes; autonomic dysfunction affecting the gut occasionally requires total parenteral nutrition.

The only specific treatment for GBS is an attempt to remove the autoantibody that is presumed to underlie the

TABLE 174–2. Major Antecedent Causes of Guillain-Barré Syndrome

Frequent	*Infrequent*	*Questionable*
Upper respiratory tract infections	Mycoplasma infection	Hepatitis B vaccine
Diarrheal illness due to *Campylobacter jejuni*	*Leptospira icterohaemorrhagiae* infection	Influenza vaccine
Cytomegalovirus infection	Surgery	Hyperthermia
Epstein-Barr virus infection	Salmonellosis	Epidural anesthesia
Hepatitis A infection	Rabies vaccine	
Hepatitis B infection	Tetanus toxoid	
Hepatitis C infection	Bacille Calmette-Guérin immunization	
Human immunodeficiency virus infection	Sarcoidosis	
Borrelia burgdorferi infection	Systemic lupus erythematosus	
	Lymphoma	
	Trauma	

peripheral nerve lesion.[31] Plasma exchange is the accepted treatment, usually consisting of five treatments over 10 days.[32] The optimal schedule for exchanges was the subject of a recently completed French trial, the result of which should be available shortly. Albumin is the preferred replacement solution.[33] Interest in high-dose intravenous immunoglobulin as an equivalent or superior treatment for GBS[34] has been tempered by reports of disease progression[35] and severe relapses.[36] At present, a multinational trial comparing these treatment strategies is in progress. Until these results are available, plasma exchange remains the treatment of choice.[37] Prednisone or immunosuppressive agents are not useful.[38] Combinations of treatments are being studied.[38a] When a specific cause (e.g., Lyme disease) is found, its appropriate treatment may speed recovery.

Myasthenia Gravis

MG is a consequence of an autoimmune attack on the neuromuscular junction, producing weakness by impairing neuromuscular transmission. The reported prevalence is as high as 5 cases per 100,000 population, but only a small fraction of these patients develop respiratory failure. MG has a predilection to affect young women and older men. The thymus is typically involved in the immunopathogenesis, with thymomas present in about 10% of patients and thymic hyperplasia in the majority of the remainder. Intensivists may encounter myasthenic patients in crisis (either myasthenic or cholinergic), with resultant respiratory failure; as a consequence of aspiration; with a complication of immunosuppressive treatment; or for postoperative care after a thymectomy.

MG typically involves weakness of ocular muscles, producing ptosis and diplopia, and it frequently produces dysphagia. This diagnosis should be considered in patients who have acute respiratory failure with these cranial nerve findings. In this setting, botulism (which is also a disorder of neuromuscular transmission) is an important differential diagnostic concern.[17] However, the bulk of patients with MG and respiratory failure already have received the diagnosis.[39] In addition to myasthenic crisis (worsening of the disease), intensivists must consider cholinergic crisis (overtreatment with anticholinesterase) as a cause of declining ventilatory function. This distinction is often made by blinded administration of a short-acting anticholinesterase (e.g., edrophonium, 10 mg) and a placebo, with pre- and post-test measures of strength (e.g., VC or NIF) and neuromuscular transmission (by electromyography). The test should be conducted with the assistance of an experienced neurologist, because many variables affect its interpretation. It should be carried out only in a setting where airway and ventilatory support are at hand, because patients in cholinergic crisis may become apneic during the test. A positive test result (e.g., strength improves) suggests that a higher dose of an anticholinesterase (e.g., pyridostigmine) may be useful. If a patient becomes weaker, the dose should be reduced. Some experienced neurointensivists doubt that oral anticholinesterase agents in usual doses produce cholinergic crises,[39] suggesting that this test may be of little value.

Patients who are developing ventilatory failure with MG but are not experiencing upper-airway problems may at times be managed with "permissive hypercapnea" under close observation in an intensive care unit. The criteria for intubation and mechanical ventilation are similar to those discussed earlier for GBS. If the upper airway is competent and the patient is not experiencing difficulty handling secretions, intermittent nasal biPAP may be a useful temporizing measure. However, the majority of patients who develop hypercapnea in myasthenic crisis require intubation, as do those who are becoming fatigued. If corticosteroid treatment is to be instituted, the likelihood of transient worsening should be anticipated and the patient closely observed for the first several days for signs of ventilatory failure.

TABLE 174–3. Drugs That May Increase Weakness in Myasthenia Gravis

Definite	*Likely*	*Rare or Questionable*
Neomycin	Gentamicin	Ciprofloxacin
Streptomycin	Amikacin	Atenolol
Kanamycin	Tobramycin	
Lincomycin	Lidocaine	
Quinidine	Phenytoin	
	Propranolol	
	Phenothiazines	
	Lithium	

Once a patient is committed to mechanical ventilation, many experts withdraw anticholinesterase treatment for several days. Corticosteroids or other immunosuppresants are continued. Enteral feeding and pulmonary embolism prophylaxis are started, and the patient is allowed to rest for 2 to 4 days. The details of ventilatory support and the weaning strategy are similar to those for the GBS. If a patient is not weaned within 1 week, the anticholinesterase agent is typically reintroduced at a lower dose. The role of plasma exchange in managing acute exacerbations of MG remains controversial, but this technique appears useful as a short-term measure. Corticosteroids (e.g., prednisone, $1 \text{ mg} \cdot \text{kg}^{-1} \cdot \text{d}^{-1}$) are begun in patients who have not been receiving them. The details of treating these challenging patients have been reviewed.[39]

A large number of drugs are reported to worsen or unmask MG[40]; the more important ones are listed in Table 174–3. The disease also affects the response to pharmacologic neuromuscular junction blockade; patients are exceptionally sensitive to nondepolarizing agents but resistant to depolarizing agents.[41]

The value of thymectomy in the long-term management of MG is clear; however, a patient in acute respiratory failure is generally considered a poor operative risk, and the procedure is delayed until a patient's condition has improved.[41a] Post-thymectomy pain control and ventilatory function can be improved by postoperative epidural morphine administration.[42]

Critical Illness Polyneuropathy and Myopathy

During the past decade, several investigators have reported a predominantly axonal neuropathy that delays ventilatory weaning in patients who are otherwise recovering from a critical illness, most frequently one involving sepsis.[43] Witt and coworkers prospectively studied 43 consecutive patients with sepsis and multiple organ failure, of whom 70% showed electrophysiologic evidence of a sensorimotor axonal neuropathy.[44] Fifteen of the patients experienced difficulty weaning from mechanical ventilation as a consequence of their neuropathy. More recent studies have uncovered a wide variety of neurologic problems that delay weaning but for which the eventual prognosis is relatively positive.[45] A separate myopathy of critical illness has also been recognized.[20]

References

1. Garrity ER. Respiratory failure due to disorders of the chest wall and respiratory muscles. *In*: Respiratory Intensive Care. MacDonnell KF, Fahey PJ, Segal MS (Eds). Boston, Little, Brown & Co, 1987, pp 312–320.

2. Jackson M, Kinnear W, King M, et al: The effect of five years of nocturnal cuirass-assisted ventilation in chest wall disease. Eur Respir J 1993; 6:630–635.
3. Mier-Jedrzejowicz AK, Brophy C, Moxham J, et al: Assessment of diaphragm weakness. Am Rev Respir Dis 1988; 137:977–883.
4. Black LF, Hyatt RE: Maximal static respiratory pressures in generalized neuromuscular disease. Am Rev Respir Dis 1971; 103:641–650.
5. Alex CG, Tobin MJ. Assessment of pulmonary function in critically ill patients. *In*: Textbook of Critical Care. 3rd ed. Ayres SM, Grenvik A, Holbrook PR, et al (Eds). Philadelphia, WB Saunders (in press).
6. Borel CO, Teitelbaum JS, Hanley DF: Ventilatory failure and carbon dioxide response in ventilatory failure due to myasthenia gravis and Guillain-Barré syndrome. Crit Care Med 1993; 21:1717–1726.
7. Rochester DF, Truwit JD: Respiratory muscle failure in critical illness. *In*: Textbook of Critical Care. 3rd ed. Ayres SM, Grenvik A, Holbrook PR, et al (Eds). Philadelphia, WB Saunders (in press).
7a. Yang KL, Tobin MJ: A prospective study of indexes predicting the outcome of trials of weaning from mechanical ventilation. N Engl J Med 1991; 324:1445–1450.
8. Loh L, Goldman M, Newsom-Davis J: The assessment of diaphragm function. Medicine 1977; 56:165–169.
9. Bennett DA, Bleck TP: Diagnosis and treatment of neuromuscular causes of respiratory failure. Clin Neuropharmacol 1988; 11:303–347.
10. Kelly BJ, Luce JM: The diagnosis and management of neuromuscular diseases causing respiratory failure. Chest 1991; 99:1485–1494.
11. Bleck TP, Smith MC, Pierre-Louis JC, et al: Neurologic complications of critical medical illnesses. Crit Care Med 1993; 21:98–103.
12. Breucking E, Mortier W: Anesthesia in neuromuscular diseases. Acta Anaesthesiol Belg 1990; 127–132.
13. Bleck TP: Tetanus. *In*: Infections of the Central Nervous System. Scheld WM, Whitley RJ, Durack DT (Eds). New York, Raven Press, 1991, pp 603–624.
14. Kuisma MJ, Saarinen KV, Teirmaa HT: Undiagnosed amyotrophic lateral sclerosis and respiratory failure. Acta Anaesthesiol Scand 1993; 37:628–630.
15. Gorson KC, Ropper AH: Acute respiratory failure neuropathy: A variant of critical illness polyneuropathy. Crit Care Med 1993; 21:267–271.
16. Dalmau J, Graus F, Rosenblum MK, et al: Anti-Hu-associated paraneoplastic encephalomyelitis/sensory neuropathy. A clinical study of 71 patients. Medicine 1992; 71:5–72.
17. Bleck TP: *Clostridium botulinum*. *In*: Principles and Practice of Infectious Diseases. Mandell GM, Bennett JE, Dolin R (Eds). New York, Churchill Livingstone (in press).
18. Peolsi G, Perili V, Sollazzi L, et al: Lambert-Eaton myasthenic syndrome: A clinical contribution. Acta Anaesthesiol Belg 1991; 42:41–44.
19. Gambling DR, Birmingham CL, Jenkins LC: Magnesium and the anaesthetist. Can J Anesth 1988; 35:644–654.
20. Zochodne DW, Ramsay DA, Saly V, et al: Acute necrotizing myopathy of intensive care: Electrophysiological studies. Muscle Nerve 1994; 17:285–292.
21. Waclawik AJ, Sufit RL, Beinlich BR, et al: Acute myopathy with selective degeneration of myosin filaments following status asthmaticus treated with methylprednisolone and vecuronium. Neuromuscular Disorders 1992; 2:19–26.
22. Swygert LA, Back EE, Auerbach SB, et al: Eosinophilia-myalgia syndrome: Mortality data from the US national surveillance system. J Rheumatol 1993; 20:1711–1717.
23. Curran FJ, Colbert AP: Ventilator management in Duchenne muscular dystrophy and postpoliomyelitis syndrome: Twelve years' experience. Arch Phys Med Rehabil 1989; 70:180–185.
24. Sasaki M, Yoneyama H, Nonaka I: Respiratory involvement in nemaline myopathy. Pediatr Neurol 1990; 6:425–427.
25. Barohn RJ, McVey AL, DiMauro S: Adult acid maltase deficiency. Muscle Nerve 1993; 16:672–676.
26. Kim GW, Kim SM, Sunwoo IN, et al: Two cases of mitochondrial myopathy with predominantly respiratory dysfunction. Yonsei Med J 1991; 32:184–189.
27. Ropper AH: Critical care of Guillain-Barré syndrome. *In*: Neurological and Neurosurgical Intensive Care. Ropper AH (Eds). New York, Raven Press, 1993, pp 363–382.
27a. Gupta SK, Taly AB, Suresh TG, et al: Acute idiopathic axonal neuropathy (AIAN): A clinical and electrophysiological observation. Acta Neurol Scand 1994; 89:220–224.
27b. Hughes RA: The spectrum of acquired demyelinating polyradiculoneuropathy. Acta Neurol Belg 1994; 94:128–132.
28. Ropper AH, Wijdicks EFM, Truax BT: Guillain-Barré Syndrome. Philadelphia, FA Davis, 1991.
29. Jabour ER, Rabil DM, Truwit JD, et al: Evaluation of a new weaning index based on ventilatory endurance and the efficiency of gas exchange. Am Rev Respir Dis 1991; 144:531–537.
30. Roubenoff RA, Borel CO, Hanley DF: Hypermetabolism and hypercatabolism in Guillain-Barré syndrome. JPEN J Parenter Enteral Nutr 1992; 16:464–472.
31. Bleck TP: Treatment strategies for the Guillain-Barré syndrome. Crit Care Med 1993; 21:641–643.
32. Guillain-Barré Study Group: Plasmapheresis and acute Guillain-Barré syndrome. Neurology 1985; 35:1096–1104.
33. French Cooperative Group on Plasma Exchange in Guillain-Barré Syndrome. Role of replacement fluids. Ann Neurol 1987; 22:753–761.
34. van der Meché FGA, Schmitz PIM, Dutch Guillain-Barré Study Group: A randomized trial comparing intravenous immune globulin and plasma exchange in Guillain-Barré syndrome. N Engl J Med 1992; 326:1123–1129.
35. Castro LHM, Ropper AH: Human immune globulin infusion in Guillain-Barré syndrome: Worsening during and after treatment. Neurology 1993; 43:1034–1036.
36. Irani DN, Cornblath DR, Chaudry V, et al: Relapse in Guillain-Barré syndrome after treatment with human immune globulin. Neurology 1993; 43:873–875.
37. Bleck TP: IVIg for GBS: Potential problems in the alphabet soup. Neurology 1993; 43:857–858.
38. Buchman AS: Inflammatory demyelinating polyneuropathies. *In*: Textbook of Clinical Neuropharmacology and Therapeutics. Klawans HL, Goetz CG, Tanner CM (Eds). New York, Raven Press, 1992, pp 497–504.
38a. The Dutch Guillain-Barré Study Group: Treatment of Guillain-Barré syndrome with high-dose immune globulins combined with methylprednisolone: A pilot study. Ann Neurol 1994; 35:749–752.
39. Fink ME: Treatment of the critically ill patient with myasthenia gravis. *In*: Neurological and Neurosurgical Intensive Care. Ropper AH (Ed). New York, Raven Press, 1993, pp 351–362.
40. Wright RB: Myasthenia. *In*: Textbook of Clinical Neuropharmacology and Therapeutics. Klawans HL, Goetz CG, Tanner CM (Eds). New York, Raven Press, 1992, pp 505–516.
41. Cullen DJ, Bigatello LM, DeMonaco HJ: Anesthetic pharmacology and critical care. *In*: The Pharmacologic Approach to the Critically Ill Patient. Chernow B (Ed). Baltimore, Williams & Wilkins, 1994, pp 291–308.
41a. Turani E, Szathmary I, Molnar J, et al: Myasthenia gravis: Prognostic significance of clinical data in the prediction of post-thymectomy respiratory crises. Acta Chir Hung 1992–1993; 33:353–360.
42. Kirsch JR, Diringer MN, Borel CO, et al: Preoperative lumbar epidural morphine improves postoperative analgesia and ventilatory function after transsternal thymectomy in patients with myasthenia gravis. Crit Care Med 1991; 19:1474–1479.
43. Bleck TP: Neurologic complications of critical illness. *In*: Neurological and Neurosurgical Intensive Care. Ropper AH (Ed). New York, Raven Press, 1993, pp 193–201.
44. Witt NJ, Zochodne DW, Bolton CF, et al: Peripheral nerve function in sepsis and multiple organ failure. Chest 1991; 99:145–152.
45. Kelly BJ, Matthay MA: Prevalence and severity of neurologic dysfunction in critically ill patients. Influence on need for continued mechanical ventilation. Chest 1993; 104:1818–1824.

CHAPTER 175

Psychiatric Problems of the Critically Ill Patient

Ned H. Cassem, MD

Life-threatening illness in itself is difficult enough to manage, but the difficulty of management and the jeopardy of patients can be dramatically increased when critically ill patients develop abnormal mental states.[1] Agitation in particular, threatening indwelling lines, catheters, pacing wires, and other therapeutic or monitoring technologies, is usually the hallmark warning sign for a clinician. Derangements of emotion, cognition, and behavior are common in critical care settings and require prompt attention.

DIFFERENTIAL DIAGNOSIS

No treatment can proceed without a careful diagnostic evaluation. In critical care settings as in emergency wards, a clinician can routinely call to mind seven conditions just to make sure a patient is not suffering from one of them. These are states in which intervention needs to be especially prompt, because prolonged failure to make the diagnosis may result in permanent central nervous system (CNS) damage: (1) Wernicke's disease, (2) hypoxia, (3) hypoglycemia, (4) hypertensive encephalopathy, (5) intracerebral hemorrhage, (6) meningitis/encephalitis, and (7) poisoning, whether exogenous or iatrogenic. Other, less urgent but still acute conditions requiring intervention include subdural hematoma, septicemia, subacute bacterial endocarditis, hepatic or renal failure, thyrotoxicoma/myxedema, delirium tremens, anticholinergic psychosis, and complex partial seizures, particularly complex partial status epilepticus. Once a consultant has eliminated these basic illnesses as possible causes of a patient's disturbed brain function, time can be allowed for a more systematic approach to the differential diagnosis. An excellent comprehensive differential diagnosis list compiled by Ludwig (Table 175–1)[2] has been slightly expanded. A quick review of this list is warranted even when the consultant is relatively sure of a diagnosis.

TABLE 175–1. Differential Diagnosis of Brain Dysfunction in Critical Care Patients (Ludwig's Differential Diagnosis of the Confusion-Delirium-Dementia-Coma Complex)

General Cause	*Specific Causes*
Vascular	Hypertensive encephalopathy; cerebral arteriosclerosis; intracranial hemorrhage or thromboses; circulatory collapse (shock); systemic lupus erythematosus; polyarteritis nodosa; thrombotic thrombocytopenic purpura
Infectious	Encephalitis; meningitis; general paresis; human immunodeficiency virus
Neoplastic	Space-occupying lesions such as gliomas, meningiomas, abscesses
Degenerative	Senile and presenile dementias such as Alzheimer's or Pick's dementia, Huntington's chorea, Wilson's disease
Intoxication	Chronic intoxication or withdrawal effect of sedative-hypnotic drugs such as bromides, opiates, tranquilizers, anticholinergics, dissociative anesthetics, anticonvulsants
Congenital	Epilepsy; postictal states; aneurysm
Traumatic	Subdural and epidural hematomas; contusion; laceration; postoperative trauma; heat stroke
Intraventricular	Normal-pressure hydrocephalus
Vitamin deficiency	Deficiencies of thiamine (Wernicke-Korsakoff), niacin (pellagra), vitamin B_{12} (pernicious anemia)
Endocrine-metabolic	Diabetic coma and shock; uremia; myxedema; hyperthyroidism, parathyroid dysfunction; hypoglycemia; hepatic failure; porphyria; severe electrolyte or acid-base disturbances; remote side effect of carcinoma; Cushing's syndrome; Wilson's disease
Metals	Heavy metals (lead, manganese, mercury); carbon monoxide; toxins
Anoxia	Hypoxia and anoxia secondary to pulmonary or cardiac failure, anesthesia, anemia
Depression, other	Depressive pseudodementia; hysteria; catatonia

(From Ludwig AM: Principles of Clinical Psychiatry. New York, Free Press, 1980, p 234.)

Psychiatric symptoms in the realm of thought, emotion, or behavior have many possible causes, particularly in a critical care setting. These causes can be grouped into four categories. First, the abnormality may arise from the CNS effect of a patient's medical illness or its treatment (e.g., the abnormalities produced by hypoxia). Second, the abnormality may be an effect of the medical illness on a patient's mind (the subjective CNS), as in a patient who thinks he or she is "washed up" after a myocardial infarction. Third, the disturbance may arise from the mind primarily, as in a conversion or factitious symptom. A patient may exaggerate about pain in order to get more narcotics. Finally, the abnormality may be a result of interactions between the sick patient and his or her environment or family—for example, a patient who has no complaints until his or her family arrives, at which time he or she promptly assumes the countenance of acute distress and complains continuously. For these reasons, a psychiatric consultant must become acquainted with the disease of the individual patient and, like a renal or infectious disease consultant, begin by reviewing the chart completely. This includes the old chart, no matter how extensive. Some patients have had prior psychiatric consultations and have presented similar difficulties. Other patients have had no psychiatric consultations but have caused considerable trouble for their caregivers on prior admissions, much of which may be extensively documented. The comprehensive consultation should then include the following: (1) a summary of a patient's illness and the reason for psychiatric consultation; (2) the family psychiatric history, especially any major affective disorder, panic or agoraphobia, or alcoholism; (3) a patient's past psychiatric history, especially prior episodes of depression, anxiety, mania, phobia, and alcohol or drug abuse; (4) relevant psychosocial factors; (5) current medications and laboratory values; (6) past medical history; (7) examination results and impression, with or without formulation and differential diagnosis; and (8) treatment plan. The treatment plan should include further diagnostic recommendations, such as thyroid function tests; the recommended psychopharmacologic treatments, such as administration of an antidepressant; behavioral/psychosocial treatment recommendations, such as limit setting or family intervention;

psychotherapeutic treatment, such as clarification and support; goals and projected plans; and guarantee of regular follow-up for as long as indicated.

Because some psychiatric disorders tend to have a hereditary pattern, such as major affective disorder and panic disorder, the family history can be of diagnostic help. If a patient's immediate relatives have suffered from depression, anxiety, or mania, the patient is more vulnerable to affective disorder. Examination of current and past medications is mandatory, because pharmacologic agents can produce abnormal psychiatric symptoms either from their presence in the patient in therapeutic quantities, in overdose quantities, or in withdrawal. Moreover, these considerations must be routinely considered, especially in patients whose drugs have been stopped because of surgery or hospitalization or whose drug orders have not been transmitted during transfer. Alcohol as well as barbiturates, narcotics, benzodiazepines, meprobamate, tricyclic antidepressants, neuroleptics, and other psychotropic medications are regularly associated with withdrawal symptoms if abruptly terminated. Steroids, anticonvulsants, methylphenidate, β-blockers, and clonidine are also associated with withdrawal symptoms.[3]

Intensive care unit (ICU) psychosis is a popular diagnosis often conferred on patients exhibiting abnormal behavior in a critical care setting. Acute "functional" psychosis in a critical care setting is rare. The term is invoked to imply that the environmental features of critical care settings are themselves capable of inducing psychosis. The rationale given for this is either sensory deprivation or monotony. In point of fact, the use of this diagnosis usually means that the cause of a delirium is simply unknown. There would be more justification for ascribing acute panic to psychotic thoughts if, for example, it were established that a patient's father died at the same age of the same disease in the same hospital during the same month. When used as a convenient diagnostic catch-all term, however, *ICU psychosis* has more risks than benefits because it tends to discourage thoughts of differential diagnosis and the search for a specific treatment.

DRUGS ASSOCIATED WITH CLINICAL DELIRIUM

Of all causes of altered mental status, drugs are probably the most common. Some, such as lidocaine, are quite predictable in their ability to cause an encephalopathic state, and the relationship is clearly dose related. Others, such as antibiotics, are much rarer causes of delirium and usually affect only someone whose brain is already vulnerable, as in a patient with a low seizure threshold.[4] Table 175–2 lists some drugs in clinical use that have been associated with delirium.

The number of drugs that can be involved either in direct toxic actions or in toxic effects because of drug interactions are numerous, potentially bewildering, and constantly changing. Certain sources provide regular reviews of published summaries and updates.[5] Critical care physicians in the local facility are commonly aware of these hazards.

The usual treatment is to discontinue or reduce the drug. This is sometimes not possible. For example, in a patient who has life-threatening ventricular irritability and for whom lidocaine seems essential at a high rate of infusion, there may be no way that one can immediately reduce the dose even though the etiologic connection with agitation is clear. Treatment of nonspecific delirium, specifically use of intravenous haloperidol, can proceed while the lidocaine is maintained. However, the CNS derangement will not cease until the drug is reduced to a nontoxic level or withdrawn. Once a florid delirium with lidocaine begins, reduction of the dose to a prior level that was not toxic may not eliminate the delirium.

Elderly patients are more susceptible to the toxic actions of many of these drugs, and some of those listed in Table 175–2 have been reported to cause delirium only in elderly patients (e.g., nonsteroidal anti-inflammatory drugs and eye drop and nose drop preparations).[6]

An anticholinergic psychosis can be reversed by intravenous physostigmine in doses of 0.5 to 2 mg administered parenterally. Caution is essential for patients in critical care settings, however, because their autonomic nervous systems are generally less stable than those of patients who have developed an anticholinergic psychosis because of a voluntary overdose. Moreover, if a reasonably large systemic amount of anticholinergic drug is clearing the system slowly (as in a patient who has renal failure and excessive scopolamine levels), the therapeutic effect of physostigmine, although sometimes quite dramatic, is usually short lived. The cholinergic reaction to intravenously administered physostigmine can cause profound bradycardia and hypotension, thereby multiplying the complications instead of reducing them. It should also be noted, on the other hand, that a continuous intravenous infusion of physostigmine has been successfully used to manage a case of anticholinergic poisoning.[7] Because of the diagnostic value of physostigmine, one may wish to use it even though its effects will not be permanently therapeutic. If one were to use an intravenous injection of 1 mg of physostigmine, protection against excessive cholinergic reaction could be provided by preceding this injection with an intravenous injection of 0.2 mg of glycopyrrolate. This anticholinergic agent does not cross the blood-brain barrier and should protect a patient from the peripheral cholinergic actions of physostigmine.

Figure 175–1 presents a decision tree or quasi algorithm according to which the diagnosis and treatment of specific abnormalities can be conceptualized and can proceed.

Generally speaking, the diagnostic and therapeutic considerations contained in this summary algorithm have been considered by the physicians in the critical care unit before the arrival of a psychiatric consultant. It is the obligation of the consultant to reconsider all organic possibilities that may have caused a patient's psychiatric symptoms. The psychiatric symptoms are sometimes so bizarre or so offensive that the prior diagnostic efforts were distracted. Idealistically, one hopes that agitation in a critically ill patient can be traced to one of the specific causes outlined in this differential diagnosis. Most of the time, many known factors that could impair CNS function are identified, but their exact contributions are not clear, some of their elements are beyond correction, and efforts to correct other abnormalities have not resulted in any clearly therapeutic response. At this point, the treatment of choice is the treatment for nonspecific delirium.

MANAGEMENT OF SPECIFIC PROBLEMS

Reactions to myocardial infarction can serve as a model for the type and pattern of emotional reactions to an acute critical illness (Fig. 175–2).[8] A patient who has had a myocardial infarction typically exhibits fear and anxiety during and after admission. As symptoms stabilize or subside, some patients may decide that the symptoms were not so severe or were even a false alarm. A few of these patients may even insist on signing out of the hospital. After diagnostic tests confirm the presence of myocardial infarction, feelings of despondency begin. These are normal, correctly classified as "uncomplicated bereavement," but some patients later develop major depression. As the hospitalization

TABLE 175–2. Drugs in Clinical Use That Have Been Associated with Delirium

- β-Adrenergic blockers
  - Albuterol
  - Atenolol
  - Betaxolol
  - Propranolol
  - Timolol
- γ-Aminobutyric acid (GABA) agonists
  - Baclofen
  - Benzodiazepines
- Antiarrhythmics
  - Amiodarone
  - Disopyramide
  - Flecainide
  - Lidocaine
  - Mexiletine
  - Procainamide
  - Quinidine
  - Tocainide
- Antibacterials, antifungals, anthelmintics
  - Aminoglycosides
  - Amodiaquine
  - Amphotericin B
  - Cephalosporins
  - Chloramphenicol
  - Chloroquine
  - Colistin
  - Dapsone
  - Ethambutol
  - Gentamicin
  - Isoniazid
  - Ketoconazole
  - Mefloquine
  - Metronidazole
  - Nalidixic acid
  - Norfloxacin
  - Podophyllin resin (topical)
  - Quinacrine
  - Rifampin
  - Sulfonamides
  - Tetracyclines
  - Thiabendazole
  - Ticarcillin
  - Tobramycin
  - Trimethoprim-sulfamethoxazole
  - Vancomycin
  - Zidovudine
- Anticholinergics
  - Atropine
  - Belladonna alkaloids
  - Benztropine
  - Diphenhydramine
  - Eye and nose drops
  - Scopolamine
  - Thioridazine
  - Trihexyphenidyl
- Anticonvulsants
  - Phenytoin
- Antihistamines
- Antihypertensives
  - Captopril
  - Clonidine
  - Methyldopa
  - Polythiazide
  - Prazosin
  - Reserpine
- Anti-inflammatory drugs, nonsteroidal
  - Flurbiprofen
  - Ibuprofen
  - Indomethacin
  - Naproxen
  - Sulindac
- Antiparkinsonian agents
  - Amantadine
  - Bromocriptine
  - Levodopa
  - Pergolide
- Antiviral agents
  - Acyclovir
  - Interferon
- Baclofen
- Barbiturates
- Caffeine
- Calcium channel blockers
  - Diltiazem
  - Nifedipine
  - Verapamil
- Clomiphene
- Contrast media
  - Iopamidol
  - Metrizamide
- Cyclobenzaprine
- Diethyltoluamide
- Digitalis preparations
- Disulfiram
- Dronabinol
- Ergotamine
- Histamine H_2 antagonists
  - Cimetidine
  - Famotidine
  - Ranitidine
- Immunosuppressives
  - Aminoglutethamide
  - L-Asparaginase
  - 5-Azacytidine
  - Chlorambucil
  - Ciprofloxacin
  - Cyclosporine
  - Cytarabine (high-dose)
  - Dacarbazine
  - Ethionamide
  - 5-Fluorouracil
  - Interferon-α
  - Methenamine
  - Methotrexate (high-dose)
  - Procarbazine
  - Tamoxifen
  - Vinblastine
  - Vincristine
- Ketamine
- Lithium
- Monoamine oxidase inhibitors
  - Isoniazid
  - Phenelzine
  - Procarbazine
- Narcotic analgesics
  - Buprenorphine
  - Meperidine (normeperidine)
- Pentazocine
- Retinoids
  - Etretinate
  - Isoretinoin
- Steroids
  - Adrenocorticotropic hormone (ACTH)
  - Anabolic steroids
- Sympathomimetics
  - Aminophylline
  - Amphetamines
  - Cocaine
  - Ephedrine
  - Phenylephrine
  - Phenylpropanolamine
  - Theophylline
- Tricyclic antidepressants
  - Amitriptyline
  - Clomipramine
  - Desipramine
  - Imipramine
  - Maprotiline
  - Nortriptyline
  - Protriptyline
  - Trimipramine

(Adapted from Cassem NH, Hackett TP: The setting of intensive care. *In*: Massachusetts General Hospital Handbook of General Psychiatry. Cassem NH [Ed]. St. Louis, Mosby-Year Book; 1991, pp 373–399.)

progresses, personality problems such as passive-aggressive behavior may complicate interactions between the patient and hospital personnel and, as with problems with fear, denial, or depression, lead to psychiatric consultation.

This conceptualization can be of practical assistance in caring for patients in a critical care unit. For example, if a patient seems impossible to deal with on the day of admission to an ICU, the reason is very likely underlying fright. Nothing else destroys personality or behavior quite like panic. Staff members often comment 3 or 4 days later that this patient seems like a completely different (improved) person. On the other hand, when patients become impossible to deal with only after 4 or 5 days in the unit and no new and frightening event has occurred, their behavior probably reflects a lifelong style of coping with stress. In contrast to patients who are frightened when admitted, those who demonstrate personality problems later (such as dependent patients who constantly have the call light on) are not likely to become favorites of the staff, no matter how long they stay in the unit. By nature they have typically handled threats to their self-esteem with hostility or machismo intimidation, and they can be expected to continue to do so in a critical care setting. The delay in emergence of these character-related interpersonal problems (a "civil in-

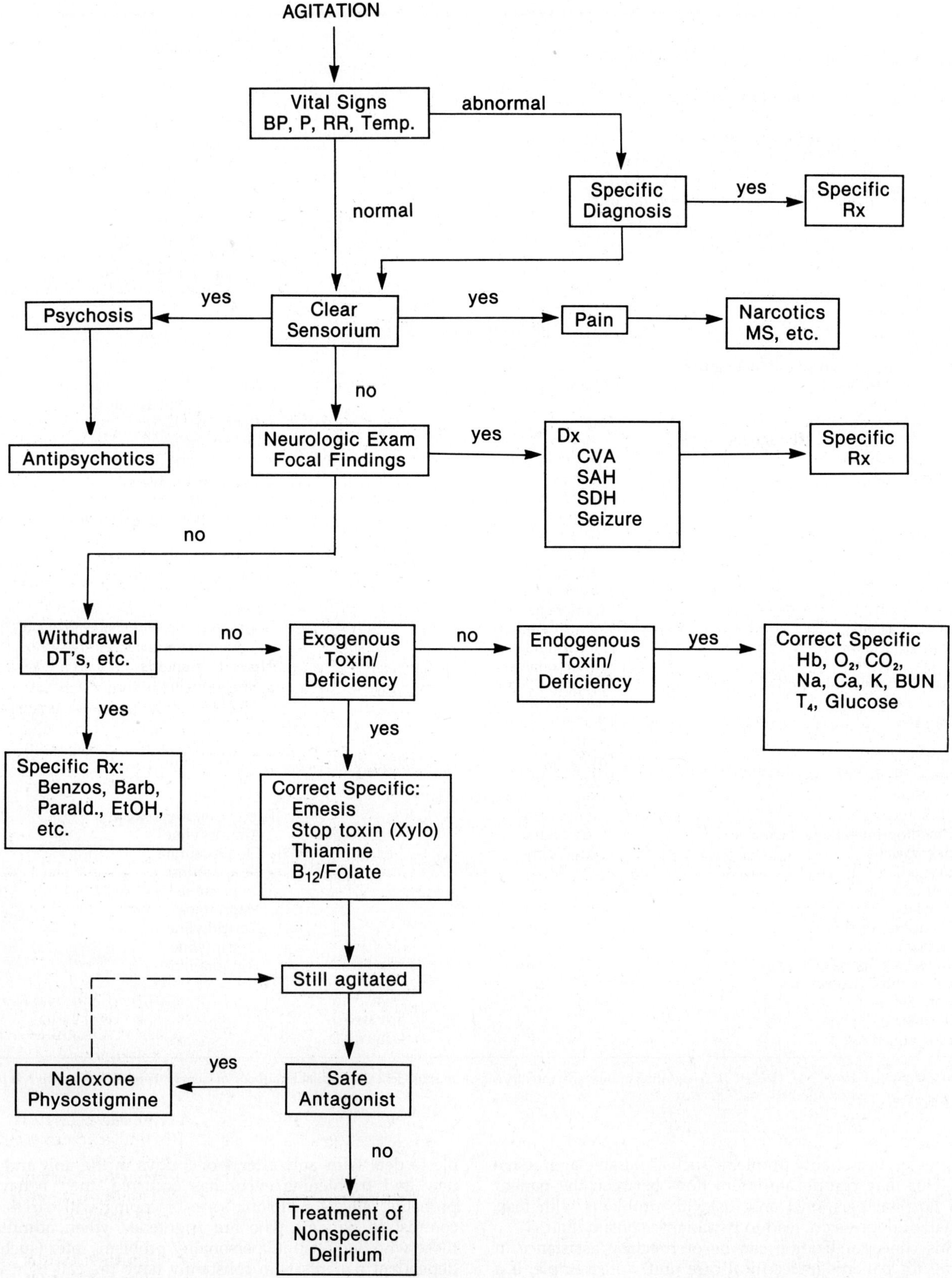

Figure 175–1. Decision tree for the diagnosis and treatment of specific abnormalities. *Abbreviations*: BP = blood pressure; P = pulse; RR = respiratory rate; MS = morphine sulfate; CVA = cerebrovascular accident; SAH = subarachnoid hemorrhage; SDH = subdural hematoma; DT's = delirium tremens; Hb = hemoglobin; BUN = blood urea nitrogen; EtOH = ethanol. (Reprinted from Cassem NH: Psychiatric and ethical issues in the critical care unit. *In:* Current Therapy in Critical Care Medicine. Parrillo JE (Ed). Toronto, BC Decker, 1987, p 334, by courtesy of Marcel Dekker, Inc.)

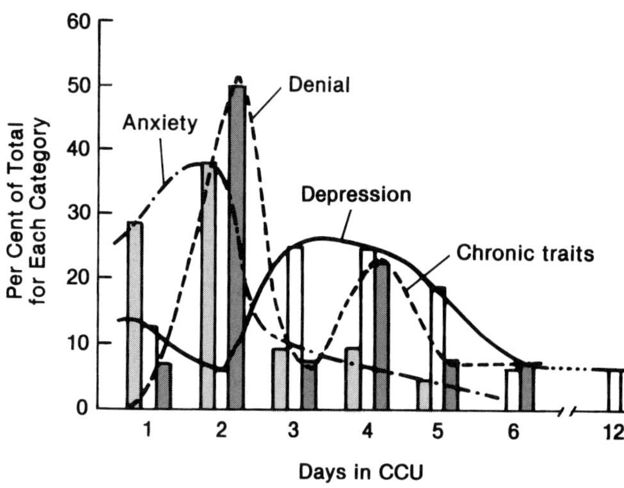

Figure 175–2. Hypothetical sequence of emotional and behavioral reactions of a coronary care unit (CCU) patient derived from the timing of consultation requests for emotional difficulties in 149 coronary patients admitted over a 15-month period. Most problems during the first 2 days stemmed from fear and anxiety. Denial (primarily manifested by the desire to sign out) followed shortly thereafter and promoted the request for psychiatric consultation. Despondency, sometimes persistent, was not far behind, peaking on days 3, 4, and 5. A final group of management requests was related mostly to dependency issues and tended to emerge on or after day 4. (From Cassem NH, Hackett TP: Psychiatric consultation in a coronary unit. Ann Intern Med 1971; 75:13.)

terval") is intriguing but not explained. It is possible that these patients suspend regressive or manipulative interpersonal dealings while their life hangs in balance, because the threat of death is more important and immediate than the fear of something else, such as dependency.

Fear and Anxiety

Admission to an ICU setting is invariably associated with life-threatening disease. Even after the fear of death has ceased to haunt their consciousness, patients may fear that they will be maimed by the illness or by its treatments. This fear may assume many guises: verbosity, outbursts of anger, paranoia, and silent withdrawal all are behaviors typically produced by fear.

Treatments of fear include medication and the dialogue of quiet reassurance. Unless panic has begun to encroach on rationality, the drugs of choice are the benzodiazepines (Table 175–3). If a patient's condition is one in which autonomic lability may be a hazard (e.g., myocardial infarction), routine prescription of one of these agents is warranted whether the patient looks anxious or not. Even when autonomic lability is not a hazard, the anxiety that accompanies severe acute medical illness is the most common indication for benzodiazepines.

How swiftly the drug acts, its rate of onset, is determined by its lipid solubility. Of the benzodiazepines available, diazepam probably produces a high blood level most rapidly and is of particular value for patients who need to feel tranquilization quickly. About 8% of patients given tranquilizers complain of feeling sedated. Although these patients may be experiencing a cumulative excessive dose, they are more likely reacting to the drug's rapid absorption and would better tolerate the slow, steady accumulation of a less lipid-soluble benzodiazepine such as oxazepam.

Clorazepate and prazepam are two long-acting benzodi-

TABLE 175–3. Benzodiazepines: Duration of Action, Metabolic Half-Life, and Active Metabolites

	Half-Life (h)	*Onset of Action*	*Metabolized to*
Short-acting			
Oxazepam (Serax)	5–15	Slow	—
Lorazepam (Ativan)	10–20	Intermediate	—
Temazepam (Restoril)	9–12	Slow	—
Alprazolam (Xanax)	12–15	Intermediate	α-Hydroxyalprazolam
Triazolam (Halcion)	2–3	Intermediate	α-Hydroxytriazolam
Estazolam (ProSom)	10–24	Intermediate	4-Hydroxyestazolam 1-Oxo-estazolam
Midazolam (Versed)	1.5–2.5	Rapid	1-Hydroxymethyl m.
Moderately long			
Diazepam (Valium)	26–53	Rapid	*N*-desmethyldiazepam
Chlordiazepoxide (Librium)	8–28	Intermediate	Desmethylchlordiazepoxide Demoxepam *N*-desmethyldiazepam
Halazepam (Paxipam)	14	Intermediate	*N*-desmethyldiazepam
Clonazepam (Klonopin)	20–80	Slow	(five metabolites)
Long			
Clorazepate (Tranxene)	30–200	Rapid	*N*-desmethyldiazepam
Prazepam (Centrax)	30–200	Slow	*N*-desmethyldiazepam
Very long			
Flurazepam (Dalmane)	40–150	Rapid Rapid Rapid	*N*-desalkylflurazepam Hydroxyethylflurazepam Flurazepam aldehyde
Quazepam (Doral)	40–150	Rapid	2-Oxo *N*-desalkylflurazepam

azepines that are not active in their original form. They both have the same metabolite, *N*-desmethyldiazepam, which is the only metabolite that produces psychotropic effects. Clorazepate, however, produces high blood levels within the first hour, whereas prazepam enters the system slowly. By 4 hours, the concentration of desmethyldiazepam is essentially the same for both these agents.[9] The choice of such an agent is made according to whether a patient wants to feel an effect quickly or wants the effect to be imperceptible.

When using longer-acting agents such as diazepam, whose half-life varies between 20 and 60 hours, a physician can assume that saturation has been attained after 2 or 3 days and can administer only a bedtime or twice-daily dose thereafter. However, if a patient's anxiety responds more favorably to repeated dosing, three or four divided doses a day may remain clinically preferable. Parenteral forms of chlordiazepoxide and diazepam are available, but intramuscular absorption of these two agents is erratic, less completely absorbed than in oral form, and should be avoided. Oral or cautious intravenous administration is recommended.

Most benzodiazepines can, on rare occasions and in sufficient dose, produce paradoxical rage or hostility. This should not discourage their use, even in hostile patients. Agitated elderly patients, however, can become more confused when given benzodiazepines. Because the half-lives of these agents tend to become longer with age, shorter-acting agents are recommended for elderly patients: oxazepam, lorazepam, and temazepam. Lorazepam and midazolam are the only short-acting drugs currently available for parenteral use and for that reason have special value in critical care units. Both are more expensive than diazepam, and fiscal constraints often require that their use be minimized. Diazepam's effectiveness is the gold standard of this drug class; it just stays in the system longer. Midazolam should never be used outside a monitored setting.

A general rule is to prescribe the simplest and shortest-acting effective drug (e.g., 15 mg of oxazepam given three or four times per day). With the physician's permission, the nurse can withhold this if it seems excessive or report if the patient seems undermedicated. One of the most sensitive measures of a dose's adequacy is the perception of the critical care nurse. A nurse who cares for a patient for an entire 8-hour shift is generally able to see whether the patient appears to be growing more anxious or has begun to sleep all the time and is becoming harder to arouse and engage.

Slow accumulation of metabolites is a problem worth worrying about. Because the metabolism of these agents and their metabolites requires oxidative enzyme processes, those patients with hepatic impairment are at greatest risk to accumulate excessive and toxic doses. Hence, another major advantage of the three short-acting benzodiazepines—oxazepam, lorazepam, and temazepam—is that for inactivation they require only glucuronide conjugation by the liver. Even in patients with advanced cirrhosis, this metabolic step is quite simply achieved, and the half-lives of these agents in patients with liver failure remain essentially the same as in patients with normal hepatic function. When a cirrhotic alcoholic patient with delirium tremens requires intravenous treatment, lorazepam is the benzodiazepine of choice.

When abuse potential is a concern, evidence suggests that the greatest potential of risk occurs with diazepam, lorazepam, and alprazolam and the least risk appears to be associated with oxazepam.[10] Halazepam, clorazepate, and clonazepam may have lower abuse potential. In acutely ill patients, however, the abuse potential of these agents is far outweighed by their benefits.

If a patient's fear is sufficiently intense to impair reason or if a patient appears to be in a state of panic or (transient) psychosis, a *neuroleptic* agent (discussed later) is the drug of choice. Panicky individuals are barely in control, and the benzodiazepines can sometimes further compromise an already diminished ability to cope.

Clarification, explanation, and *reassurance* can also have very soothing effects on anxious patients, particularly when fear stems from threatening or erroneous conceptions of disease. Questions such as "Have you ever known anyone with these symptoms?" or "What is your idea of a heart attack?" can be used to uncover misconceptions. When a family member has died of the same condition, his or her age at death may figure heavily in patients' fear; patients often expect that fate will take them at the same age.

After false ideas have been corrected, it is important to mention positive aspects of the treatment plan. For example, patients with cardiac disease might be assured that myocardial healing is complete in 5 to 6 weeks and that normal activities will be resumed along with an exercise program. Even when the prognosis is grave, as in lung cancer, a calm statement of the treatments planned to counteract and contain the malignancy is important to anxious patients. The more ominous the prognosis, the more important it is to encourage patients to specify the fear so that specific and *valid* reassurance (e.g., that medication can control pain) can be given. False reassurance is not recommended because it robs physicians of credibility and, therefore, of the ability to reassure patients later in the illness. Equanimity has perhaps the most soothing effect on patients. Anxious patients have a way of making people who take care of them anxious, and a vicious circle may develop. A calm person can break that deleterious interaction.

Denial and the Threat to Sign Out

Denial allows acutely ill patients to avoid panic by minimizing or precluding the threatening implications of their disease.[11] If panic sets in, patients may get the urge to flee; threatening to sign out therefore especially reflects fear and anxiety. Although the threat to sign out can mean that an individual does not take the illness seriously, it should be assumed to be a manifestation of panic unless proved otherwise.

Because such persons are desperate and often irrational, antagonism flares when efforts are made to detain them. Patients should not be threatened or given the idea that they are being cornered. Sitting on a chair so that one is physically lower than patients, speaking in a gentle and quiet voice, and emphasizing the positive aspects of proposed treatment are likely to be most effective. A gentle approach is essential. For example, a physician might begin by saying, "I am not here to force you to do anything; what I ask is that you let me know your point of view and then let me know that you understand mine."

Seriously ill patients need to hear the truth in direct but quiet, calm terms. They must understand that their illness is manageable if they stay in the hospital: "Your heart is damaged and needs to be carefully monitored to avoid further damage and risk, but it's much like the process of cement setting. At first it's fragile when freshly poured, but if given the chance to firm up it can hold up a building. The same can be true of your heart muscle if you give it a chance to repair itself." As patients calm down, they may respond to questions about the source of their fear.

Before talking to patients who threaten to sign out, a physician should ask that the family be mobilized immediately. Their appearance and pleading with patients, even when hysterical, may induce them to stay. Even if patients become calm, they should be medicated promptly, most often with an antipsychotic such as haloperidol.

Most of these patients (at least the ones who would be able to leave the hospital under their own power) are not mentally incompetent, and requesting a formal psychiatric evaluation may be inappropriate. Having patients sign out against medical advice is also usually unnecessary if the conversation and circumstances are carefully documented in the chart and furthermore is of no value as a punitive measure. Even if patients leave, they should be told that they are welcome to the appropriate treatment whenever they change their mind and choose to return. The emphasis is always on *what is best for the patient*—both in one's conversation with the patient and in making practical judgments about how to handle signing out. This can help undercut the accusation some of these patients make that the physician is only interested in a power struggle.

Delirium

Acute delirium is one of the most common psychiatric problems of critical care. Twenty years ago, it was routine to administer atropine to patients newly admitted to a coronary care unit when they developed bradycardia. Some of these patients, particularly older ones with some preexisting organic brain disease, developed an acute delirium. For such patients, parenteral propantheline bromide (Pro-Banthine), a quaternary ammonium compound that does not cross the blood-brain barrier and is equally effective in treating bradycardia, was substituted. This can still be done, but problems are seldom so simple. The drugs that may be causing the delirium, such as lidocaine or prednisone, often cannot be changed without possible detriment to a patient. Alternatively, pain may be the cause of agitation in a delirious patient. Morphine sulfate can relieve pain but may be contraindicated by an associated decrease in blood pressure or respiratory rate.

Psychosocial measures are not effective in treating a bona fide delirium of uncertain or unknown cause. In these cases, treatment options include administration of various drugs up to and including neuromuscular blocking agents with or without or the use of physical restraints. However, restraints are likely to be in place already, particularly if critical lines have been jeopardized by agitation. Moreover, paralytic drugs such as pancuronium bromide require use of mechanical ventilation, which increases the risk of respiratory compromise in postoperative patients. Delirium is therefore usually treated with an antipsychotic such as haloperidol, often in combination with a benzodiazepine.

Drug Treatment of Delirium

Because agitated critically ill patients may harm themselves by pulling out pacemaker wires, pumps, sutures, the endotracheal tube, or other therapeutic lifelines, the decrease of agitation is the treatment goal against which any drug's effects are titrated. Benzodiazepines are often effective in mild agitation and in practice are tried first, as 2.5 mg of intravenous diazepam. Especially in higher doses, these agents can cause or exacerbate confusion in older patients. This occurs much less often with antipsychotics, unless the chosen drug has high anticholinergic properties, such as thioridazine.

Haloperidol is probably the antipsychotic most commonly used to treat agitated delirium in a critical care setting. Its effects on blood pressure, pulmonary artery pressure, heart rate, and respiration are milder than those of the benzodiazepines, making it an excellent agent for severely ill patients with impaired cardiorespiratory status.[1, 12, 13]

Although haloperidol can be administered orally or parenterally, acute delirium with extreme agitation requires parenteral medication. Intravenous administration is preferable to intramuscular administration because drug absorption may be poor in distal muscles if a patient's delirium is associated with circulatory compromise or borderline shock. The deltoid is probably preferable to the gluteal muscle for intramuscular injection, but neither is as reliable as the intravenous route. Second, agitated patients are commonly paranoid, and repeated painful intramuscular injections may increase their sense of being attacked by enemy forces. Third, intramuscular injections can complicate interpretations of muscle enzyme studies if enzyme fractionation is not available. Fourth, and most important, haloperidol is less likely to produce extrapyramidal side effects when given intravenously than intramuscularly or orally,[14] at least for patients without a prior serious psychiatric disorder.

In contrast to the immediately observable sedation produced by intravenous diazepam, intravenous haloperidol has a mean distribution time of 11 minutes in normal volunteers[15]; this may be even longer in critically ill patients. The mean half-life of intravenous haloperidol's subsequent, slower phase, is 14 hours. This is still a more rapid metabolic rate than the overall mean half-lives of 21 and 24 hours for intramuscular and oral doses, respectively. The oral dose has about half the potency of the parenteral dose; therefore, 10 mg of haloperidol by mouth corresponds to 5 mg intravenously or intramuscularly.

Haloperidol has not been approved by the Food and Drug Administration for intravenous administration. Any drug can be used for a patient and is justified as "innovative therapy." For critical care units wishing to use intravenous haloperidol, one approach would be to present this desire to the hospital's independent review board or human studies committee with request to use the drug with careful monitoring of results based on the fact that it is the drug of choice for the patient's welfare, is the safest drug, and is justifiable as innovative therapy. After a period of monitoring, the committee can choose to make the use of the drug routine in that particular hospital.

In Europe, intravenous haloperidol has been used to treat delirium tremens and acute psychosis and to premedicate patients scheduled for electroconvulsive therapy. Its use has been associated with few side effects on blood pressure, heart rate, respiratory rate, or urine output, as well as with very few extrapyramidal side effects. The reason for the latter is not known. Studies of the use of intravenous haloperidol in psychiatric patients have not shown that these side effects were fewer. The reason for their more rare appearance after intravenous administration in medically ill patients may be that many medically ill patients have other circulating medications that are protective, especially the benzodiazepines, or that patients with psychiatric disorders, especially schizophrenia, are more susceptible to the side effects.[14]

Before administration of intravenous haloperidol, the intravenous line should be flushed with 2 mL of normal saline. Phenytoin precipitates haloperidol, and mixing the two in the same line must be avoided. Haloperidol may occasionally precipitate with heparin, and because all lines in critical care units are usually heparinized, the 2-mL flush is advised. The initial bolus dose of haloperidol varies from 0.5 to 20 mg but is usually 2 mg for mild agitation, 5 mg for moderate, and 10 mg for severe. The only time when a consultant would use a higher initial dose is when a patient has already been unsuccessfully treated with reasonable doses of haloperidol. To account for haloperidol's lag time, doses are usually staggered by at least a 30-minute interval.

If a 5-mg dose does not calm an agitated patient after 30 minutes, 10 mg should be administered. Partial control of agitation is usually not adequate and only prolongs the delirium or guarantees excessive doses of haloperidol after the delirium is under control.

After calm is achieved, agitation should be the sign for a repeat dose. Ideally, the total dose of haloperidol on the second day should be a fraction of that on day 1. After complete lucidity has been achieved, patients need to be protected from delirium only at night, by small doses of haloperidol (1–3 mg), which can be given orally. As in the treatment of delirium tremens, consultants are advised to stop the agitation quickly and completely at the outset rather than barely keep up with it over several days. The maximum total dose of intravenous haloperidol to be used as an upper limit has not been established, although intravenous administration of single-bolus doses of 150 mg has been used in the author's institution and up to 985 mg total has been used in a 24-hour period.[16] The highest doses have been required for delirious patients on the intra-aortic balloon pump.[17] A continuous infusion of haloperidol has also been used to treat severe, refractory delirium.[18]

Hypotensive episodes after administration of intravenous haloperidol are rare and almost invariably are caused by hypovolemia. This ordinarily is easily checked in patients who are in an ICU and who have indwelling pulmonary artery catheters, but because agitation is likely to return, volume replacement is necessary before administering further doses. Veins suffer no local caustic effects. Intravenous haloperidol is generally safe for epileptic patients and victims of head trauma, unless psychotropic drugs are contraindicated by the need for careful neurologic monitoring. Although intravenous haloperidol may be administered without mishap to patients receiving epinephrine drips, after very large doses of haloperidol a pressor other than epinephrine, such as norepinephrine, should be used to avoid unopposed β-adrenergic activity.

Intravenous haloperidol does not block a dopamine-mediated increase in renal blood flow. It also appears to be the safest agent for patients with chronic obstructive pulmonary disease.

Several centers have found intravenous haloperidol use to be associated with the development of torsades de pointes ventricular tachycardia.[19–21] The reason is not clear, although particular caution is urged in the presence of low levels of potassium and magnesium, prolonged QT interval, hepatic compromise, or specific cardiac abnormality (mitral valve prolapse, dilated ventricle). Progressive QT widening after haloperidol administration may presage the danger. Although the incidence remains small, 4 of 1100 cases in one unit,[20] all reports are very recent. Terfenadine and astemizole, popular newer antihistamines, have caused torsades de pointes, usually when taken in overdose or concurrently with drugs that slowed their metabolism. History of their recent use should be sought.

An alternative agent to haloperidol is intravenous droperidol, an agent already approved by the Food and Drug Administration for intravenous administration. This agent, however, is a much more potent α_1-adrenergic antagonist and is more likely to lead to difficulties with hypotension, particularly when it is combined with other agents. One such instance arose at the author's institution when droperidol was used as an intravenous antiemetic for cancer patients simultaneously receiving oral tetrahydrocannabinol. In one study, both droperidol and haloperidol were administered in equal doses to agitated emergency department patients; intramuscular droperidol achieved more rapid control than intramuscular haloperidol, and no difference was noted when the drugs were used by the intravenous route.[22]

Critically ill patients with human immunodeficiency virus infection may be more susceptible to the extrapyramidal side effects of haloperidol, including neuroleptic malignant syndrome,[23–25] leading an experienced group to recommend molindone. The latter is associated with fewer such effects, is available only in oral preparation, and can be prescribed as 25 mg once or twice a day or, in a more acute situation, 25 mg every hour until calm.

Intravenous diazepam is routinely used to treat agitated states, particularly delirium tremens, as are intravenous chlordiazepoxide and lorazepam. Any of these intravenous benzodiazepines may be a useful adjunct in the treatment of acute nonspecific delirium. A common, effective regimen for treating agitation combines haloperidol with intravenous lorazepam, either simultaneously, 1 to 2 mg lorazepam with 10 mg haloperidol, or alternately.[26]

Intravenous alcohol is also extremely effective in the treatment of alcohol withdrawal states. Its disadvantage is that it is toxic in itself to both the liver and brain, although its use can be quite safe if these organs do not already show extensive damage (and sometimes is quite safe even when they do). A 5% solution of alcohol mixed with 5% dextrose in water run at 1 mL/min has a calming effect amazingly quickly. Other parenteral neuroleptic drugs for the treatment of agitation are thiothixene, trifluoperazine, fluphenazine, and chlorpromazine. Chlorpromazine is extremely effective, but its very potent α-blocking properties can be exceedingly dangerous for critically ill patients. When administered intravenously or intramuscularly, it can abruptly decrease total peripheral resistance and cause a precipitous decline in cardiac output. Nevertheless, intravenous use in small doses (e.g., 10 mg) can be both safe and effective.

Despondency

In any serious illness, the mind itself sustains an injury, as though the illness (e.g., myocardial infarction) produced an ego infarction. This psychic damage, called despondency, is distinct from depression, which is a major affective disorder. Even when recovery of the diseased organ is complete, recovery of self-esteem appears to take somewhat longer, and despondency tends to become a serious problem in critically ill patients the longer they stay in a unit. In patients with myocardial infarction, the myocardial scar is fully formed in 5 to 6 weeks but the recovery of psychologic well-being often requires 2 to 3 months.

Despondency is a mixture of dread, bitterness, and despair that causes patients to see themselves as broken, scarred, and ruined. Work and relationships seem jeopardized. Disappointment with what has and has not been accomplished haunts the individual, who may now feel old and a failure. The disease may not have killed these patients, but they feel it has crippled their career and personal aspirations. Concerns of this kind become apparent rather early in acute illness and may prompt consultation requests by the second or third day of hospitalization.

Feeling better is the best antidote for illness-induced acute despondencies. In the interim, patients should be encouraged but never forced to express any concerns about the damage done by the illness. Some patients are upset merely to find such depressive concerns in their consciousness and even worry that this signals a "nervous breakdown." It is essential to let them know that such concerns are normal emotional counterparts to physical illness that will fluctuate in their intensity and probably disappear gradually as health returns. Patients are also reassured to hear about any rehabilitation plans while still in the acute phase of recovery.

Major Depression

Of the various types of depression, critical care is concerned only with those conditions that require specific treatment (i.e., major depression, depression with mania or manic symptoms, and depression with psychotic symptoms). The diagnostic criteria for a depressive episode are as follows: (1) sleep disturbance, including any type of insomnia or hypersomnia (early morning awakening is especially significant); (2) loss of interest in usually stimulating activities such as job, hobbies, or social activities; (3) guilt feelings or feelings of self-reproach or worthlessness; (4) decreased energy and feelings of tiredness or exhaustion; (5) impaired concentration, decreased ability to think, slow or mixed-up thinking, and indecisiveness; (6) disturbed appetite accompanied by weight loss or gain; (7) psychomotor agitation or retardation; and (8) recurrent thoughts of death or suicide, including the wish to be dead. Patients ordinarily must possess at least four of these eight symptoms for 2 weeks to qualify for the diagnosis of major depression. Even if a patient has not been in the ICU this long, he or she may have been depressed before admission.

The presence of a distinguishable loss or life event is not necessary for a diagnosis of major depression. Patients may actually deny being depressed, ascribing symptoms of fatigue, poor appetite, and sleep disturbance to the primary disease. If neither patients' illnesses nor their medications are entirely responsible for depressive symptoms, somatic treatment is indicated.

If patients are lethargic, hard to mobilize, and listless and seems to show no investment in their care-taking regimen, an excellent and safe choice for treatment would be a psychostimulant: either 2.5 to 20 mg of dextroamphetamine sulfate or 2.5 to 20 mg of methylphenidate.[26, 27] These drugs can be extremely helpful in mobilizing a person who appears to have recovered physiologically from a long illness but who lacks motivation. They are helpful both therapeutically and diagnostically. If, for example, one is not sure whether an element of major depression exists, one excellent way to probe for this is with a test dose of a psychostimulant. For example, a patient could be given 5 mg of dexedrine once in the morning. Switching to a tricyclic or conventional antidepressant is not necessary immediately. Some patients improve with psychostimulant therapy alone, become mobilized, and achieve recovery. Other patients require addition of a traditional antidepressant, particularly if they are having a great deal of difficulty sleeping at night. For such patients, a tricyclic antidepressant such as doxepin may be tried. A starting dose of 25 mg is used the first night, increasing nightly by 25 mg until an adequate sleep dose is achieved. Other sedative antidepressants that can be helpful are nortriptyline, 10 or 25 mg, and trazodone, 50 mg, at bedtime.

In addition to their slow onset of therapeutic effect, the tricyclic antidepressants have three major drawbacks.[28] First, they cause orthostatic hypotension. Free of this side effect are the serotonin-specific reuptake inhibitors, fluoxetine (Prozac), paroxetine (Paxil), and sertraline (Zoloft); bupropion (Wellbutrin); and safest of the traditional tricyclics, nortriptyline. The most common offenders in this category are imipramine, chlormipramine, amitriptyline, and desipramine. Second, all antidepressants except monoamine oxidase inhibitors, trazodone, the serotonin-specific reuptake inhibitors, and bupropion have anticholinergic effects. Most potent are amitriptyline and protriptyline (in fact, in vitro, 9 mg of amitriptyline is equal in potency to 1 mg of atropine). Finally, tricyclic antidepressants can prolong cardiac conduction, particularly in the His-Purkinje system. The electrocardiogram usually shows slightly prolonged PR, QRS, and QT segments and a slightly flattened T wave.[29] Those patients of particular concern, of course, are those with an acutely unstable conduction system of any kind. Prolongation of the corrected QT interval, an effect of tricyclic antidepressants, can contribute to the development of arrhythmias (discussed earlier). Those agents that appear to lack association with cardiac arrhythmias or dysfunction include the serotonin-specific reuptake inhibitors, bupropion, the monoamine oxidase inhibitors, and the psychostimulants.

For critically ill patients who appear to be depressed, a trial of a psychostimulant is a reasonable beginning. If the response is partial or ineffective, then agents that can be used are nortriptyline, starting at 25 mg and increasing every week by 25 mg to 50 or 75 mg nightly, aiming for a therapeutic plasma level between 50 and 150 ng/mL. The serotonin-specific reuptake inhibitors can be given once a day at any time: fluoxetine 20 mg, paroxetine 20 mg, or sertraline 50 mg. Fluoxetine and paroxetine require metabolic oxidation by the cytochrome P_{450} enzyme system and can thereby cause decreased metabolism and higher levels of other drugs, such as the benzodiazepines. Sertraline appears to do this to a significantly lesser extent. Bupropion can be started at a dose of 50 or 75 mg, and, given two or three times a day, increased to a total dose between 200 and 400 mg daily.

Anxiety That Inhibits Weaning from a Ventilator

The multimodal treatment of anxiety related to weaning from a ventilator often begins with a benzodiazepine such as lorazepam administered before weaning periods or a neuroleptic such as haloperidol if the patient appears to be near panic. Droperidol has also been helpful for breaking status asthmaticus, with distinct improvements in pulmonary function.[30] Again, if haloperidol or droperidol is used, the intravenous route is recommended.

Persons who suffer acute and chronic respiratory failure and therefore require prolonged mechanical ventilation may become so anxious when the weaning process begins that psychiatric assistance is requested. Even though a patient is physically ready for weaning, anxiety can transiently increase metabolic demands and cardiac work until further weaning is contraindicated.

Most behavioral exercises for relaxation encourage the subject to take slow, deep, easy breaths. This is one of the quickest and surest ways of inducing relaxation for most people, but it is exactly what patients with respiratory problems cannot do and precisely what makes them so anxious. Multimodal treatment of this difficulty often begins with a benzodiazepine administered before weaning periods or an antipsychotic such as haloperidol if a patient appears to be near panic. Patients themselves can indicate whether a drug is effective and which drug is most helpful. In some cases, it may be possible to use a mixture of nitrous oxide if the respiratory physician or anesthesiologist is present to administer it. Hypnosis or relaxation techniques have often been helpful in distracting patients from the weaning process. In this case, the instruction to breathe easily is better omitted from the hypnotic suggestion; patients should be encouraged to concentrate either on a tranquil scene such as a beach or on a single concept (mantra).[31] Finally, patients may be helped by the explanation that the weaning process itself can be expected to produce anxiety. Despondency as well as anxiety can become a problem with impeding weaning; therefore, the remarks in the foregoing section on despondency may apply here as well.

The psychologic state of patients who require paralysis by neuromuscular blocking agents can be monitored by heart rate, blood pressure, changes in sweating, or patients' tears. Habitually addressing patients whenever approaching the bedside is orienting and reassuring. Analgesics should be supplied if there is any risk of pain, and some antianxiety agent should be administered regularly, usually a benzodiazepine. Sublingual lorazepam, oxazepam by nasogastric tube, and a bolus of intravenous diazepam every 6 hours all are ways of addressing this problem.

The Difficult Patient: Refusal to Obey the Rules

Rule violators harass physicians and nurses by their refusal to comply with treatment regimens. These are the patients who drink water while under strict limitation of intake, get out of bed when confined to strict bed rest, or smoke against orders. Paradoxically, such individuals are often dependent persons who react by hyperindependent behavior when placed in a dependent position. Finding such an individual doing pushups at the bedside or chinups on the overhanging bar, the physician is usually barraged with criticism about the overprotective attitude of the nurses. Physicians should try to restore a sense of control in these individuals whenever possible while avoiding fights over limits—for example, "Look, no one here really has any intention or ability to play policeman. We can only explain the nature of your illness and how to make it better; after that, we depend on you to let us know how we can get the job done." On some issues, the staff can bend, but if compromise is medically contraindicated, it is usually helpful to let patients know that no one can make them do anything they do not want to do, and when they do not comply, it is they and not their caregivers who suffer. For example, "Your Pronestyl and gentamicin should be taken on schedule for your own safety, but your Valium and Colace can be postponed or refused." Any such statement is meant to reassure patients that they are respected and that the treatment regimen is not intended to be an act of oppression. Gentle humor, exaggerated in the direction of acknowledging what the patient can do, can at times defuse some of the anger and soften conflict when used naturally—for example, "If you feel you must stand up to void, OK; let us know. But you're forbidden to do a handstand from your intravenous pole until we can sell tickets so spectators can watch."

Hostile Patients

Anger and aggression are usually aroused by threat or damage to self-esteem. Hostility or outrage is thus a common emotion in critically ill patients, especially those who have been in an ICU for more than 2 weeks.

When presented as a frontal assault ("You never told me I'd be confined to my back [or lose my hair or be nauseated] most of the time."), anger is at least a direct, albeit heated, response to disease. Pent-up anger tends to discharge itself indirectly on more tangible targets, such as a noisy roommate, the night staff, or the hospital food. In either case, the physician should quietly listen to the grievance, gently ask for the details ("You may be right that my explanation [or warnings] were incomplete. What do you recall?"), and offer sincere regret for whatever has damaged the self-esteem ("Nausea may well be the worst discomfort there is"; "I wish there were some way hair loss could be avoided"). A common mistake is attempting to reassure or mitigate the anger too quickly ("It is only temporary; it will grow [or come back]"), because this misses the point. Another tactical error is saying, "I understand"; this often makes patients more angry, because they believe that no one understands their unique affliction. By contrast, the gentle hearing-out process often quiets the wrath. A physician may even be able to say something like, "You know, even if these treatments had no unpleasant effects, it's bad enough to have this disease in the first place." Patients may then take that opportunity to vent some anger on the primary culprit, the disease itself. At least both physician and patient are in full agreement on that point.

Subtle hostility and devious aggression are much harder to deal with, primarily because they are disguised. Physicians often find themselves increasingly annoyed with patients. Angry patients provoke this annoyance in numerous ways: by demeaning implications (repeating after every proposed intervention, "Are you saying you can't do anything for me, then?"), by obsequiousness (every fifth word is "Doctor"), by ignoring what is being said (looking out the window as soon as the physician starts to speak), or by being passive-aggressive (the patient is compliant and agreeable to the physicians and nurses but tells friends and family that overworked staff members don't answer the call bell for an hour or that the well-meaning nurse didn't mean to infiltrate his intravenous line but just slipped).

The style of expressing anger is molded by a patient's personality. If a patient can admit the hostility and describe it, the process described earlier for open anger can proceed: hearing out details, sympathy for the wounded ego, and reminder that the disease is the culprit. Uncontrolled anger inappropriately vented on a spouse, nurses, or others is usually embarrassing, and patients may be thankful to those who help them control their feelings and thereby preserve their self-respect. If patients do not admit hostility, physicians can help them acknowledge it directly ("I sense you're more angry than you've let on"), followed by the evidence ("Your comments regularly make your family mad at all of us"; "Every time I start to say something, you appear to tune out"). Even if this attempt is not successful, at least a physician has let patients know they are responsible for their own behavior. This is especially effective when physicians have been able to keep their own hostility under control.

Some patients are not just temporarily angry; they may be habitual help rejectors. Others have personality disorders, such as borderline personalities, that are so severe that no physician should attempt to handle them without the help of a psychiatrist. These individuals are extremely manipulative help rejectors who are expert at engaging others in conflict-ridden relationships and often provoke staff conflicts. These patients work extremely hard to interfere with the help being given them.[32]

In summary, the golden rule of treating hostile patients is not to accept blame for the disease and in a kindly but firm way to remind patients and their families that all treatment is for their benefit, even when a cure cannot be guaranteed. For example, "Because you deserve the best treatment available for your condition, we'll do our best to see that you receive it (even when you try to interfere)."

RITES OF PASSAGE: TRANSFER OUT OF A CRITICAL CARE SETTING

Patients with heart disease experience a dramatic rise in catecholamine excretion on the day of transfer out of the coronary care unit.[33] Transfer from an ICU to a general ward is generally both bad and good news for patients—bad, because it means reduced coverage and observation; good, because it means that their condition has improved. Ideally, the discharge date should be made definite at least 24 hours in advance. Explicit warnings about less frequent checks and fewer nurses should be accompanied by the assurance that intensive care is no longer necessary. In essence, increased independence should be represented as a reward rather than a hazard.

SUMMARY

Psychiatric contributions to the recovery of critically ill patients begin with relief of behavioral, cognitive, or affective disturbances caused by medical problems. Thus, CNS disorders may be alleviated by restoring physiologic equilibria, such as glucose levels or oxygen tensions, or by adding a specific psychopharmacologic agent, such as haloperidol for delirium. The mind is then helped to recover by specific diagnosis and treatment of any psychiatric disorder; supportive psychotherapy; behavioral therapy, such as hypnosis and relaxation; veterinary or limbic therapy (the "laying-on of hands" or "talking a person down"); and preparation for the transition from the critical care unit to the next phase of hospitalization. The ICU environment is optimized for recovery by addition of windows, clocks, or calendars; changing lighting schedules to approximate day and night; noise reduction; addition of music, photos, or ear phones; and the tailoring of visiting schedules to meet patients' needs. Finally, patients' family and social network is assessed and, when possible, integrated into the treatment and support of patients.

The psychiatric consultation particularly emphasizes a history of psychiatric disorders in patients or their families, as well as historical determinants such as an anniversary reaction, the meaning of the illness to patients, recent stresses, the nature of patients' social support network, their premorbid personality, issues of secondary gain and the profit derived from the symptoms of being sick, and the possibility of other causes such as conversion, malingering, or factitial illness. The therapeutic approach is multimodal and closely integrated with the rest of patients' critical care.

References

1. Cassem NH, Hackett TP: The setting of intensive care. *In*: Massachusetts General Hospital Handbook of General Hospital Psychiatry. 3rd ed. Cassem NH (Ed). St Louis, Mosby-Year Book, 1991, pp 373–399.
2. Ludwig AM: Principles of Clinical Psychiatry. New York, Free Press, 1980, p 234.
3. Adler LE, Bell J, Kirch D, et al: Psychosis associated with clonidine withdrawal. Am J Psychiatry 1982; 139:110.
4. Snavely SR, Hodges GR: The neurotoxicity of antibacterial agents. Ann Intern Med 1984; 101:92–104.
5. Drugs that Cause Psychiatric Symptoms. Med Lett 1993; 35:65–70.
6. Tolefson GD, Garvey MJ: Indomethacin and prostaglandins: Their behavioral relationships in an acute toxic psychosis. J Clin Psychopharmacol 1982; 2:62–64.
7. Stern TA: Continuous infusion of physostigmine in anticholinergic delirium: Case report. J Clin Psychiatry 1983; 44:463–464.
8. Cassem NH, Hackett TP: Psychiatric consultation in a coronary unit. Ann Intern Med 1971; 75:9.
9. Greenblatt DJ: Pharmacokinetic comparisons. Psychosomatics 1980; 21(Suppl):9.
10. Griffiths RR, Wolf B: Relative abuse liability of different benzodiazepines in drug abusers. J Clin Psychopharmacol 1990; 10:237–243.
11. Hackett TP, Cassem NH, Wishnie HA: The coronary care unit: An appraisal of its psychological hazards. N Engl J Med 1968; 279:1365.
12. Sos J, Cassem NH: The intravenous use of haloperidol for acute delirium in intensive care settings. *In*: Psychic and Neurological Dysfunctions After Open Heart Surgery. Speidel H, Rodewald G (Eds). Stuttgart, George Thieme Verlag, 1980, pp 196–199.
13. Cassem NH, Lake CR, Boyer WF: Psychopharmacology in the ICU. *In*: The Pharmacologic Approach to the Critically Ill Patient. Chernow B (Ed). Baltimore, Williams & Wilkins, 1994.
14. Menza MA, Murray GB, Holmes VF, et al: Decreased extrapyramidal symptoms with intravenous haloperidol. J Clin Psychiatry 1987; 48:278–280.
15. Forsman A, Ohman R: Pharmacokinetic studies on haloperidol in man. Curr Ther Res 1976; 10:319.
16. Tesar GE, Murray GB, Cassem NH: Use of high-dose intravenous haloperidol in the treatment of agitated cardiac patients. J Clin Psychopharmacol 1985; 5:344–347.
17. Sanders KM, Stern TA, O'Gara PT, et al: Delirium after intraaortic balloon pump therapy. Psychosomatics 1992; 33:35–41.
18. Fernandez F, Holmes VF, Adams F, et al: Treatment of severe, refractory agitation with a haloperidol drip. J Clin Psychiatry 1988; 49:239–241.
19. Metzger E, Friedman R: Prolongation of the corrected QT and torsades de pointes cardiac arrhythmia associated with intravenous haloperidol in the medically ill. J Clin Psychopharmacol 1993; 13:128–132.
20. Wilt JL, Minnema AM, Johnson RF, et al: Torsade de pointes associated with the use of intravenous haloperidol. Ann Intern Med 1993; 119:391–394.
21. Hunt N, Stern TA: The association between intravenous haloperidol and torsades de pointes: Three cases and a review of the literature. Psychosomatics (in press).
22. Thomas H Jr, Schwartz E, Petrilli R: Droperidol versus haloperidol for chemical restraint of agitated and combative patients. Ann Emerg Med 1992; 21:407–413.
23. Fernandez F, Levy JK, Mansell PWA: Management of delirium in terminally ill AIDS patients. Int J Psychiatry Med 1989; 19:165–172.
24. Breitbart W, Marotta RF, Call P: AIDS and neuroleptic malignant syndrome. Lancet 1988; 2:1488–1489.
25. Fernandez F, Levy JK: The use of molindone in the treatment of psychotic and delirious patients infected with the human immunodeficiency virus. Case Reports. Gen Hosp Psychiatry 1993; 15:31–35.
26. Adams F, Fernandez F, Andersson BS: Emergency pharmacotherapy of delirium in the critically ill cancer patient: Intravenous combination drug approach. Psychosomatics 1986; 27(Suppl 1):33–37.
27. Masand P, Pickett P, Murray GB: Psychostimulants for secondary depression in medical illness. Psychosomatics 1991; 32:203–208.
28. Cassem NH: Depression. *In*: Massachusetts General Hospital Handbook of General Hospital Psychiatry. 3rd ed. Cassem NH (Ed). St Louis, Mosby-Year Book, 1991, pp 237–268.
29. Giardina EGV, Bigger JT, Glassman AH, et al: The electrocardiographic and anti-arrhythmic effects of imipramine hydrochloride at therapeutic plasma concentrations. Circulation 1979; 60:1045.
30. Prezant DJ, Aldrich TK: Intravenous droperidol for treatment of status asthmaticus. Crit Care Med 1988; 16:96–97.
31. Benson HA. The Relaxation Response. New York, Morrow & Co, 1975.
32. Groves JE: Management of the borderline patient on a medical or surgical ward: The psychiatric consultant's role. Int J Psychiatry Med 1975; 6:337.
33. Klein RF: Transfer from a coronary care unit: Some adverse responses. Arch Intern Med 1968; 122:104.

SECTION XIV
TRANSPLANTATION

Ake Grenvik

CHAPTER 176

History and Organization of Organ Transplantation

Brian A. Broznick, CPTC • Susan A. Stuart, RN, BSN, CPTC
Ake Grenvik, MD, PhD

During the past decade, transplantation has evolved from an experimental process to an accepted lifesaving therapy. The ability to replace a diseased organ with a healthy one from a living or cadaveric donor has in some respects become routine. In the United States alone, on the average, someone receives a solid-organ transplant every 32 minutes.[1] It must be noted, however, that even though more patients are afforded a second chance at life today than 10 years ago, more patients also die awaiting their chance at transplantation. Every 3 to 4 hours of each day, another patient dies before being provided this lifesaving gift.[1] Additionally, hundreds of thousands of individuals each year receive a cornea transplant, bone graft, skin graft, or other type of human tissue that provides severely disabled individuals with the ability to lead a productive and active life. However, the need for cadaveric organs and tissues continues to exceed the numbers donated.

Success rates in organ transplantation have reached heights of greater than 80% 1-year survival.[2] However, the successes have not come without obstacles along the way. Before 1980, advances in transplantation were painfully slow. During the latter part of the 1960s and well into the 1970s, a 1-year renal allograft survival rate of 65% was achieved but also carried a recipient mortality rate as high as 20%.[2a]

New discoveries in the field of immunology and development of better immunosuppressive therapy led to greater success rates in transplantation and a decline in patient mortality. Since both graft and patient survival have greatly increased, physicians have become more willing to recommend transplantation to their patients. Unfortunately, waiting lists for transplantation have more than doubled during the past 5 years.[3] Two factors that inhibit the growth of this field of medicine are (1) not ensuring that every family is given the opportunity to donate organs or tissues when appropriate and (2) families refusing to donate organs and tissues when the opportunity arises.

In July 1994, over 35,000 individuals were awaiting some type of solid-organ transplant. Because of the number of patients waiting and the lack of available organs, a formalized distribution system and organization of transplant centers and affiliated organizations had to be developed. Such arrangements need to take into account the limitations of preservation and transplant center resources, but most importantly, they have to keep patients' needs in mind. To achieve public trust and support of transplantation, a fair and equitable distribution system of available organs had to be organized.

This chapter recounts the development of the system that exists in the United States today, along with achievements that have been gained.

THE EARLY YEARS

Clinical trials in transplantation began approximately four decades ago. Achievements were made rapidly. In 1945, for example, Landsteiner, Hufnagel, and Hume performed what some consider a transplant by connecting a cadaveric kidney to a brachial artery and cephalic vein of a woman who was experiencing acute renal failure. Forty-eight hours later, the graft was removed. No significant amounts of urine were produced, but fortunately the patient's own kidneys resumed function within a few hours of the procedure.[4] In 1954, Murray and associates performed the first successful kidney transplant between two identical twins.[5] The technique used by this team was adapted for similar procedures in allotransplantation of other organs. Murray was awarded the Nobel Prize in Medicine in 1990 for his pioneering transplantation research, together with Thomas, who initiated and refined the technique for bone marrow transplantation.[6] Through the 1960s, organ retrieval, surgical technique, and immunosuppression witnessed further important developments. The most common problems confronting transplantation were rejection and infection. In the late 1960s, Starzl and associates began clinical trials using antilymphocyte serum to counteract rejection.[7] During this same time period, different transfusion techniques on prospective kidney recipients and removal of the patient's spleen were carried out. Although these procedures did provide some benefits, partially through donor-specific transfusions, the risk of sensitizing a patient against a transplanted graft was also identified.

THE ROLE OF HISTOCOMPATIBILITY

Compatibility in transplantation surgery became increasingly obvious during the 1960s. It was observed that a recipient's and donor's tissue types were critical to the outcome of a transplanted graft. The human leukocyte antigen (HLA) system was discovered by a large number of renowned researchers, and the designation "HLA" was agreed on at a World Health Organization meeting in New York in 1968.[8] It soon became apparent that a large recipient pool would be necessary to obtain the best HLA match between donated organs and the waiting patients. However, during this time, relatively few patients were waiting for kidney transplantation. Because renal transplantation was still considered experimental, only a few centers funded by United States National Institutes of Health grants were performing transplant procedures.

FORMATION OF A TRANSPLANTATION SYSTEM

In the late 1960s, a regional transplant system began to take form. Successful sharing of kidneys based on HLA matching was accomplished, but few transplant centers participated. The Medical College of Virginia, the University of Virginia,

Duke University, and Johns Hopkins University were initially involved. In 1968, what was probably the first long-distance transport of a donor organ took place when a kidney was sent from Richmond, Virginia, to Atlanta, Georgia, where it was successfully transplanted. Transportation for this mission was carried out by the Virginia Air National Guard based in Richmond. During this period, preservation of kidneys consisted of simple cold-storage techniques, which permitted only brief organ preservation, making time a critical factor between procurement and transplantation.

In 1969, the Medical College of Virginia applied for and was awarded a contract from the Kidney Disease Control Agency (KDC) of the Public Health Service, with Dr. David Hume designated as the principal investigator. Other participating centers included Duke University, Georgetown University, University of North Carolina, University of Maryland, University of Virginia, Johns Hopkins University, Emory University, and Danville Memorial Hospital. This particular contract specified a feasibility study to be conducted regarding the recovery of kidneys in a remote location, preservation of these organs, and identification of HLA specificity of the donor and the best-matched recipient for the organs. At the same time, techniques for expanding the preservation time of kidneys were also being developed, using pulsatile perfusion.

A considerable number of projects were initiated simultaneously in the early phase of the KDC contract. Policies were developed for kidney sharing, studies were begun to determine the best means of kidney preservation, and thought was given to designing a computerized system for recipient matching with donated organs. The General Electric time-sharing system was ultimately selected to work with the originating centers to develop this matching system. Each original member was equipped with a terminal to connect it with the GE system, which became operational in late 1969 under the name The Southeastern Regional Organ Procurement Program (SEROPP).* At the time the system became operational, fewer than 100 patients were awaiting transplantation. As with any new system, flaws were identified, but the new system did represent the first on-line computer matching technique, operating over a fairly large geographic area. Formal criteria were developed for transplantation of donated kidneys based on the best available match. Several patients were on occasion identified with equal matches, and tie-breaking criteria were developed using patient waiting times. Thus, the patient who waited the longest was offered first opportunity for transplantation. It became apparent that funding and reimbursement were to become extremely important for the success of this system. Transplant centers began to discuss finances with insurance companies and the federal government. Acquisition charges for recovery, preservation, and transportation of kidneys were developed at this time.

Because SEROPP demonstrated success, it grew in importance. By showing better success rates in transplantation and development of more refined techniques for organ preservation, the number of programs performing transplants continued to grow, and the majority of these programs joined SEROPP. Some of the financial restraints were lifted in 1972, when amendments to Medicare legislation allowed for payment of cost incurred for dialysis treatment as well as kidney procurement, transportation, and transplantation.

ORGAN-SHARING SYSTEMS DEVELOP

In 1975, charter members of SEROPP decided to incorporate into a new organization known as the Southeastern Organ Procurement Foundation (SEOPF). The computer programs that were developed and remaining funds from the original KDC contract were transferred to SEOPF. During this time, other organ-sharing systems were making their appearance in the United States and in Europe. Euro-Transplant, as well as programs in the United Kingdom, Germany, France, and Scandinavian countries, were being developed. It soon became evident to all involved that transplantation and organ sharing could not be contained within one geographic boundary but had to be expanded to include entire nations or possibly even continents. The need for this type of expansion was recognized in the United States by SEOPF, whose board of directors authorized the organization and incorporation of the United Network for Organ Sharing (UNOS).

THE GROWTH YEARS

Clinical successes in other types of organ transplants were also achieved. However, two major obstacles continued to plague the transplant community—graft rejection and organ shortage. During this time, many new developments took place. Improved surgical techniques and organ preservation and development of new immunosuppressant drugs caused a tremendous growth in this field during the latter part of the 1970s and the early 1980s. In 1976, Borel outlined the immunosuppressive properties of cyclosporine, which offered new hope for transplant recipients.[9] Specifically, this drug possessed selectivity for T lymphocytes and proved far more effective than agents previously used. The initial trials with cyclosporine were conducted by Calne and colleagues.[10] Their findings, however, suggested that cyclosporine was highly toxic. Further investigative studies conducted by Starzl and coworkers indicated that cyclosporine could be safely used and could be an effective immunosuppressive drug for combating organ rejection.[11] Indeed, the development and use of cyclosporine made transplantation a useful and lifesaving form of therapy in the early 1980s. Success rates for heart and liver transplantation achieved during this time had only been previously accomplished with renal transplantation. With this increased success rate in transplantation, more and more suitable recipients were identified. A mechanism was needed to ensure equitable sharing of all organs. It was not uncommon during the early part of the 1980s to encounter individuals bidding for lifesaving organs on television or radio or in the printed media. Livers needed for children awaiting transplantation were commonly announced in the media during this time. In addition, during this time, instances of inequitable organ distribution were being described. Although a well-organized and responsibly fair system was in place, the public demanded greater accountability and equitability in organ distribution and transplantation.

FEDERAL GOVERNMENT RESPONSE

In 1984, in response to public pressure, the United States Congress passed Public Law 98-507. This law commonly became known as the National Transplant Act.[12] The law called for the formation of a task force on organ procurement and transplantation, which was charged with the comprehensive examination of all aspects of human organ donation, procurement, and transplantation. The task force's role was to assess current public and private efforts to secure organs for transplantation and identify factors that diminished the number of organs available. In addition, the task force was to evaluate the problems in coordinating the procurement of transplantation organs and tissues. This act further established procedures for certifying organ procurement organizations (OPOs). The task force would report to

*Armata T: History of the Southeastern Organ Procurement Foundation "SEOPF" (Personal communications). December 1992.

and work under the Secretary of Health and Human Services. Requirement for OPOs were expanded to include specific criteria regarding board composition, defined geographic areas for organ procurement, equitable allocation of organs recovered, and fiscal responsibilities. Additionally, the law called for the establishment of a nationwide organ procurement and transplant network (OPTN) to which all transplant centers, organ procurement organizations, and histocompatibility laboratories would have to belong. For the first time, all entities involved in transplantation would come together under one central organization. In addition, a scientific registry was established to provide accurate data on transplantation numbers, graft survival, and equity in organ sharing.

The task force published its written report in April 1986.[13] Most of the recommendations were implemented within a 2-year period. Certification of OPOs were initiated, and a 1-year contract was offered for the development and implementation of the OPTN. This contract, along with the scientific registry contract, was awarded to UNOS, based in Richmond, Virginia. By the end of the first fiscal year, UNOS had implemented a nationwide organ distribution system, and the network became fully operational in October 1987.

UNITED NETWORK FOR ORGAN SHARING

UNOS now represents a formalized system for organ distribution. Besides maintaining a 24-hour, 365-day service to facilitate the placement of available organs with waiting recipients, UNOS developed membership criteria, organ recovery standards, and qualifications for transplant surgeons and physicians. Histocompatibility needs and OPO requirements were also established. A board of directors was elected, comprising not only healthcare professionals involved in the transplant arena but also the lay public, delegates from voluntary health organizations, and perhaps most importantly, patient representatives.

Independent registries for kidney, liver, heart, lung, pancreas, and bone marrow transplantation were incorporated into UNOS. Information on all organ donors and recipients became available under one unified system. This system, for the first time, allowed for the collection of comprehensive statistics that provide quality assurance and further advancement and refinement of transplantation technology.

One of the most difficult tasks that faced UNOS as a new contractor for the OPTN was establishing a fair and equitable system for distributing available organs. During the start-up time of UNOS, Starzl and associates in Pittsburgh instituted a system for equitable organ allocation.[14] This system provided "points" or "credits" to transplantation candidates based on waiting time accrued, quality of antigen match, logistic considerations, and urgency. Because this system proved fairly effective in Pittsburgh, it was adopted by UNOS. Subsequent changes in the system have been made, but it remains fairly intact today. Under this system, each organ is matched somewhat differently. Kidneys, for example, are matched by ABO compatibility, tissue antigen matching, a negative serum–white blood cell crossmatch between donor and recipient, and waiting time. The patient with the best match, especially in relation to the donor's HLA, receives the kidney. Livers are distributed in a different manner. Because there is no effective, permanent mechanical support for patients with end-stage liver disease, histocompatibility is usually not tested before transplantation. The patients are selected based on compatibility of blood type and organ size. Waiting time and urgency of need are also factors that have important roles in the selection of recipients for liver transplantation. Four different categories exist for prioritizing these patients. The most urgent category is status four. Patients in this category are those who are hospitalized, in critical condition, and whose life expectancy is less than 72 hours. All of these patients must be receiving intensive care. The next most critical category is status three, which is reserved for patients who are hospitalized but not in an intensive care unit. These patients cannot care for themselves at home and must wait in the hospital for an available organ. After status three are status two patients—those patients who are home bound but do not have the ability to work and may need some specialized care. The final category is status one, which is reserved for patients who have been identified as having end-stage liver disease but are still fairly self-sufficient.

For patients awaiting heart transplantation, only two categories are recognized. Status one is reserved for patients in the most critical condition. These are patients who are hospitalized and need some type of supportive measure, either a mechanical support device or inotropic drug support. Status two includes all patients awaiting transplantation outside the hospital. Hearts, like livers, are matched by ABO compatibility and size. Waiting time also has an important role in heart transplantation.

For those awaiting lung transplantation, no categorization currently exists. These patients are matched solely on ABO and size compatibility. The only other factor that is taken into consideration is the length of waiting time. This is also true of patients awaiting combined heart-lung transplants.

Pancreases are distributed in a somewhat different manner from other nonrenal organs but in a manner similar to that of kidneys. Because most individuals believe that histocompatibility is important, pancreas recipients have similar criteria to meet as do those awaiting renal transplantation. In many cases, patients receive a combined kidney-pancreas transplant.

With the exception of a perfectly matched kidney, distribution of organs is carried out locally first, then regionally, and finally nationally. Organs recovered within an OPO service area are first offered to patients waiting for transplantation at centers to which the OPO has an affiliation. If for some reason the organs cannot be allocated locally, they are offered to patients within the region in which the OPO resides. Currently, 11 regions have been designated throughout the United States. If regional allocation is not feasible, organs are entered into the national pool.

ORGAN DONATION ISSUES

Although progress has been made in ensuring equitable distribution of donated organs, increasing survival rates for patients receiving a transplant, providing better immunosuppressive drugs, and improving preservation of organs, one major problem remains in ensuring everyone an opportunity for transplant—the shortage of suitable organs for transplantation.

UNOS was recently requested, as part of the OPTN contract, to develop methods for increasing organ donation. The first step taken by UNOS was to study factors that led to increased accomplishments by some OPOs. Although all areas of operation of OPOs were reviewed, very few conclusions could be drawn to distinguish why some OPOs perform better than others.[15] It was apparent, however, that a close relationship between organ procurement coordinators and donor hospitals did have a positive effect on increasing donation within these hospitals. The number of years of experience of the executive director of the OPO and the type of background of this individual also seemed related to increased donation. After this study, the committee within

UNOS that carried out this survey recommended that OPOs develop a way to identify their specific donor pool. Additionally, potential donor availability studies should be undertaken by every OPO, with subsequent strategies to maximize donation developed based on obtained data. The committee also believed that it was important to examine the operations of those OPOs with the highest procurement rates and disseminate its findings to all other OPOs.

UNOS has also invited most organizations involved in transplantation to develop a national campaign for increasing organ donation. This coalition has been accepted by the National Advertising Council and is receiving nearly $30 million of free advertising between 1994 and 1996. It is hoped that this will stimulate an increase in organ donation.

In January 1994, nearly 36,000 patients were waiting for some type of solid-organ transplant: 26,681 patients were awaiting a kidney transplant, 3492 a liver, 2935 a heart, 212 a pancreas transplant, 1008 combined kidney-pancreas, 205 combined heart-lung transplants, and 1467 a single or double lung transplant. At least one of these patients is dying every 4 hours. In 1993, there were 4895 organ donors, resulting in 15,461 organ donations. However, this represents an increase in donation of only 8% over 1992. Therefore, the gap between the number of patients receiving transplants and the number of patients awaiting transplantation continues to increase.[16] Intensified work needs to be carried out to gain public acceptance of donation if all patients awaiting transplantation are to be afforded an opportunity for continued life.

Organ donation, as mentioned before, is not keeping pace with the rapidly increasing need. Difficult decisions continue to arise regarding organ allocation. One issue that needs to be further addressed in the near future is recipient selection criteria. Scientific evidence does suggest that healthier patients at the time of transplantation benefit more than do critically ill patients. Although the tendency has been to treat critically ill patients first because of the shortage of available organs, this policy may need to be revised in the very near future.

A well-designed and well-executed approach needs to be planned in regard to both professional and public education. Thousands of organs are wasted needlessly every year, simply because of lack of understanding and no request for the organs being made at the time of death. Healthcare professionals, including physicians such as neurologists, intensivists, traumatologists, anesthesiologists, and surgeons, must shoulder the responsibility for donor identification. They do not, however, need to assume responsibility for approaching families. Organ procurement coordinators are specifically trained and readily available to do this. Additionally, new avenues of donation must be explored. By increasing the donor pool, more patients in need of transplantation can receive treatment.

WHAT THE FUTURE MIGHT HOLD

Under the current criteria, approximately 12,000 potential organ donors exist in the United States in any given year,[17] but only about 4500 donations take place annually. One of the most important factors inhibiting an increase in this number is simply the fact that many families are never asked. The second largest problem is that nearly 50% of individuals approached say no.

A possible way to provide more organs for transplantation is to look at other nontraditional types of donations. The criteria used in regard to organ donation have been greatly expanded in the past few years. Organs are increasingly being recovered from patients in their late 60s and 70s. Most of these organs are kidneys but in some cases also livers. Additionally, patients with a history of diabetes or hypertension are no longer ruled out for donation. Although these disease processes may affect some organ systems, they do not affect all. Many organs can be recovered from these patients and transplanted successfully.

The use of living organ donors may be expanded in the future. Although living donation was for many years limited to kidneys, the tail of the pancreas of living donors has been used and lobes of livers or lungs have also been recovered and transplanted (e.g., from parents to their children). Even a heart can be procured from a living donor. This occurs when a patient receives a combined heart-lung transplant. If the heart of the recipient of a heart-lung block is healthy, it may be transplanted into a second recipient, so-called domino transplantation.

Although difficult medicolegal problems surround donation of organs from anencephalic infants, this particular type of patient can also be used for possible donation. Many parents of anencephalic babies wish to see a donation carried out to provide some meaning to the birth of such a grossly deformed child. In some countries, such as Germany, anencephalic infants are not considered to be alive and procurement of organs is permitted while the heart is still beating and the organs perfused. Successful kidney transplantation from such cases has been reported.[18]

Another potential for increasing the donor pool is to return to organ recovery from non-heartbeating donors, which was commonly used in the 1960s. This is frequently done in those Asian countries where brain death is not yet recognized as death of the individual. Some Western countries (e.g., Holland) have continued to use non-heartbeating donors primarily for kidneys. In the United States, this donor category includes those patients who suffered lethal brain injuries but who are not certified brain dead and are under evaluation for brain death when cardiac arrest occurs. If consent has been obtained, the patient is transported to the operating room for immediate organ recovery. However, death must be certified on the basis of cessation of cardiopulmonary function before removal of donated organs.

Another category comprises terminally ill patients whose family has made a conscious decision to have life-support treatment withdrawn and in addition wish to donate organs. After cessation of cardiopulmonary function, the patients are declared dead and organ recovery can take place.

Non-heartbeating donors may also be patients who are admitted to the hospital in full cardiac arrest and cardiopulmonary resuscitation is either unsuccessful, contraindicated, or unwanted by the patient or his or her surrogate. If agreement has been reached in advance or if the patient's surrogate agrees to organ donation at the time, an aortic cannula can be inserted via the femoral artery for infusion of cold preservation solution. Similarly, an inferior vena cava cannula is inserted for drainage. The patient can then be taken to the operating room for urgent organ recovery.

In some occasional situations, patients who have undergone cardiac surgery cannot be weaned successfully from cardiopulmonary bypass. In many of these cases, cardiopulmonary bypass has been stopped and the patients have been certified dead, based on cardiopulmonary criteria. If consent for donation is obtained, these patients may also provide lifesaving organs for transplantation.

The foregoing are examples of possible indications for increasing the donor pool. These and other potential donor categories will no doubt continue to be discussed as the need for organs continues to outstrip the number of organs available for transplantation.

SUMMARY

During the past 40 years, transplantation has become a highly beneficial form of therapy, but this achievement has come at great cost. Only by ensuring equitable access to organs can this fascinating and rapidly changing medical field continue its successful growth. Trust and support are of utmost importance if this lifesaving therapy is to be offered to the many thousands of patients in need. Although the future is bright for most transplant recipients, it is not for those who die waiting for a second chance at life. As we gain more knowledge and experience in transplantation, new avenues must be explored to meet the needs of these patients. Xenografting and cell transplantation are two new areas that are being explored. The controversies about these types of procedures are numerous, but promising experiments continue to be carried out. Efforts by both involved healthcare professionals and the lay public need to increase significantly if transplantation is to advance further.

References

1. UNOS Update, Special Edition, Vol 8, Issue 12, December 1992.
2. Vaughn W, Daily O, Ellison M, et al: UNOS 1991 Annual Scientific Registry Report.

2a. Ellison M, Daily O, Breen T: UNOS 1993 Annual Scientific Registry Report.

3. UNOS Update, Special Edition, Vol 8, Issue 12, December 1992.
4. Hume DM, Merrill JP, Miller BF, et al: Experiences with renal homotransplantation in the human: Report of nine cases. J Clin Invest 1955; 34:327.
5. Murray JE, Merrill JB, Harrison JH: Renal homotransplantation in identical twins. Surg Forum 1955; 6:432.
6. Thomas ED, Ashley CA, Lochte HL, et al: Intravenous infusion of bone marrow in patients receiving radiation and chemotherapy. N Engl J Med 1957; 257:491.
7. Starzl TE, Marchioro TL, Porter KA, et al: The use of heterologous anti-lymphoid agents in canine renal and liver homotransplantation in a human renal transplantation. Surg Gynecol Obstet 1967; 124:301.
8. Terasaki PL (Ed): History of HLA: 10 Recollections. Los Angeles, UCLA Tissue Typing Laboratory, 1990.
9. Borel J: Comparative study of in vitro and in vivo drug effects on cell-mediated cytotoxicity. Immunology 1976; 31:631.
10. Calne RY, White D, Rolles K: Prolonged survival of pig orthotopic heart grafts treated with cyclosporine A. Lancet 1978; 1:1183.
11. Starzl TE, Weil R III, Iwatsuki S, et al: The use of cyclosporine A and prednisone in cadaver transplantation. Surg Gynecol Obstet 1980; 151:17.
12. "National Transplant Act," Public Law 98-507, US Congress, 1984.
13. Jonasson O: Organ Transplantation Issues and Recommendations. Report of the Task Force in Organ Transplantation, April, 1986, US Department of Health and Human Services, Public Health Service, Human Resources and Service Administration.
14. Starzl TE, Shapiro R, Tepperman C: The point system for organ distribution. Transplant Proc 1989; 21:3432–3436.
15. Alexander JW, Broznick B, Ferguson R: Organ Procurement Organization Function: UNOS newsletter, September, 1992, Vol 8, Issue 9:2–25.
16. Association of Organ Procurement Organizations (AOPO) Voluntary Fax 1993 Survey Report, January 1994.
17. Nathan HM, Jarrell BE, Broznick BA, et al: Estimated potential organ donor pool in Pennsylvania. Nephrology News and Issues 1990; 4:22.
18. Holzgreve W, Beller FK, Uchholz B, et al: Kidney transplantation from anencephalic donor. N Engl J Med 1987; 316:1068.

CHAPTER 177

Organ Donor Categories and Management

Christina I. Klufas, MD • David J. Powner, MD
Joseph M. Darby, MD • Keith L. Stein, MD, FCCP, FCCM
Ake Grenvik, MD, PhD

Refined surgical techniques, improved immunosuppression, and advancements in critical care therapy have permitted organ transplantation to become the definitive treatment for some end-stage organ diseases, genetic defects, and malignancies. However, transplantation is often limited by a lack of acceptable donor organs, and, in contrast to remarkable recipient survival rates, patients frequently die while awaiting organs. For example, at the end of 1992, more than 22,000 potential recipients were waiting in the United States for a renal transplant. However, during the entire year of 1992, only 10,108 such transplants were performed. Of these, 7698 were cadaveric organs, and the remainder were kidneys from living related donors. Throughout 1992, only 4521 cadaver donors were available, for a potential maximum of 9042 kidneys, which would be just a little greater than 40% of the demand.[1] By the middle of 1994, more than 35,000 potential recipients were awaiting organ transplantation.[1a] These data highlight the need to increase donor organ supply and maximize the efficiency of organ procurement.[2]

Efforts to increase donor organ availability have been primarily focused on educating the general public and healthcare professionals about organ donation needs. Numerous surveys show that most private citizens have positive views about organ donation,[3, 4] and yet the actual number of donors remains low. Legislative attempts at improving organ procurement have likewise not been successful. The Uniform Anatomical Gift Act and required request law enacted in several states initially stimulated increases in organ donation, but these gains were not maintained.[5] The doctrine of presumed consent has been proposed as another method to increase donor availability. Under this doctrine, all patients would be assumed to grant permission for donation unless specific written directives to the contrary have been provided. This approach is based on survey data indicating that most patients are more inclined to donate their own organs than to agree to donate organs from a family member. Similarly, the use of presumed consent is proposed for organ procurement from patients sustaining irreversible cardiac arrest, anencephalics, and fetuses.[6, 7] However, medical, legal, and ethical concerns currently limit the free use of presumed consent and similar methods of increasing organ supply in the United States.

During the initial decade of organ transplantation, which began with renal transplantation in 1954, organ sources were limited to living, related donors or cadaveric, nonheartbeating donors.[8] After the acceptance of death based on brain death criteria, organ retrieval from cadaveric, heartbeating, brain-dead donors has become the major source of organs for transplantation.[9]

The goal of organ donor management is to secure organs that will function optimally in the recipient. Despite normal biochemical, hematologic, and serologic assessment before transplantation, early failure of the implanted organ occurs in some recipients. This failure is not due to infection, surgical errors, transport, immunologic hyperacute rejection, or

TABLE 177–1. Organ Donor Categories

Heartbeating Donors
Brain dead
Living, related
Living, unrelated
Anencephalic
Non-Heartbeating Donors
Animal Donors

recognized physiologic imbalances. Although the causes of primary organ failure are not entirely known, in situ ischemic injury to donor organs after brain injury or during the development of brain death likely contributes. For example, Darracott-Cankovic and associates[10] used quantitative birefringence microscopy to show that, despite similar age, sex, incidence of cardiac arrest, and level of inotropic support, 43% of procured hearts have impaired function before removal from brain-dead donors. Death from cardiac failure and the requirement for inotropic support after implantation are significantly higher in recipients of these hearts when compared with recipients of hearts showing normal birefringence. Increased emphasis on careful donor management may, therefore, decrease the incidence of primary organ failure in the recipient.

In this chapter, we define two broad categories of organ donors (Table 177–1) and discuss treatment goals and methods for those donors commonly admitted to the intensive care unit.[11, 12] The intensivist is often in a position to identify the potential donor, participate in treatment of the initial disease or injury, and ensure sound physiologic management during development of and after established brain death. Through these important steps of donor identification and proper treatment, critical care physicians can have a vital role in increasing organ supply, improving the quality of donated organs, and extending the survival of the recipient.

GENERAL CONSIDERATIONS

All dying patients may be evaluated as potential donors except those with an extracranial malignancy, untreated septicemia, viral hepatitis, active tuberculosis, and positive human immunodeficiency virus serology. Age criteria, once limited, are now less emphasized because organs from older patients have proven acceptable, particularly for older recipients.[13] Organs from donors older than 55 years may be assessed by organ-specific biomedical studies and by inspection at the time of procurement. Donors with chronic diseases (e.g., diabetes or hypertension) should not be automatically excluded unless harmful end-organ effects are present.

The purpose of donor screening is to secure organs that will function optimally in the recipient and perhaps avoid complications of immunologic rejection and primary organ failure. Criteria to determine suitability of individual organs are discussed in subsequent chapters.

Heartbeating Donors

Anencephalic Donors

Anencephalic infants are born without a cerebrum but often with sufficient brain stem activity to sustain cardiac and respiratory function. By current definition in the United States, they are not brain dead. However, because they have neither the capacity for cognition or ability to experience human senses nor the possibility to ever acquire those characteristics of "personhood," philosophic questions have been raised as to whether they are truly "alive."[14] (See Chapter 173.)

Because death by cessation of cardiorespiratory function is inevitable in anencephalic infants, it has been proposed that they be considered organ donors. Management as donors has been approached in three ways: full life support until brain death has occurred using traditional criteria; minimal support until severe hemodynamic or respiratory instability has produced brain stem death, after which cardiopulmonary support is instituted and brain death diagnosed; or removal of organs while on full support and before brain stem functioning has ceased.[15] Each option has limitations. When full support is initiated soon after birth, deterioration of the brain stem may not occur for a prolonged period of time during which infection or other complications may intervene and limit organ function.[16] If cardiopulmonary function is not supported, hypotension may produce organ ischemia before brain stem death occurs, making the organs unsuitable for transplantation. Although successful renal transplantation from anencephalic donors has been reported when cardiopulmonary support has been provided and the kidneys have been removed while brain stem function continues,[17] this method is controversial because continued function of the brain stem excludes certification of death by most criteria.

None of these options is currently practiced in the United States. Opposition to the use of anencephalic infants as donors is based on reluctance to consider these patients to be dead and on the low numbers of potential donations from this organ donor category. Because the diagnosis of anencephaly in utero can be made by ultrasound examination, abortions are more common and the number of infants born alive with anencephaly is low and declining.[15] The option of prolonging gestation when anencephaly is recognized in utero solely for the subsequent procurement of usable organs has been uniformly decried.

Living, Related Donors

The first successful kidney transplant from a living, related donor was accomplished in 1954 by Murray and colleagues.[18] Living, related donors remained the preferred source of organs in kidney transplantation because of the minimal risks for the donor and better results with such donors compared with cadaveric donors.[19] However, as cadaveric organ transplantation from heartbeating, brain-dead donors improved, a trend developed in the United States away from living donors and toward brain-dead donors. Of 10,108 kidneys transplanted in 1992, 24% were from living donors compared with 31.3% in 1982.[1, 2] Living, related donors, therefore, have been used less except in pediatric cases when transplantation is preferred before dialysis[20] and in countries where cadaveric donor supply is limited or an organ-sharing system is not yet established. However, because of the current organ shortage, living donors are again increasingly being used because of their past success. Organ transplantation from living donors has now expanded beyond renal transplantation to include one lung or a single lobe[21] and parts of the pancreas or liver. Even the heart may be transplanted from living patients as in the "domino" procedure during which a heart-lung recipient donates a native healthy heart for transplantation into another heart recipient.[22]

With living donors, specifically related donors, the recipient's waiting period for an organ is minimized. The potential donor is easily identified, and only suitability testing is needed. Thereafter, the transplant can be scheduled at the appropriate time in the progression of the recipient's disease rather than being determined by the availability of an organ and the waiting list status of the recipient. Other technical advantages include minimizing procurement and preservation injury to the transplanted organs and providing sufficient time to complete ABO and human leukocyte antigen matching.

The well-being of the donor must also be considered during this type of transplantation because there may be short- and long-term risks, although these are low. Donor mortality after unilateral nephrectomy is less than 0.1%,[23] and long-term studies have noted the development of proteinuria or hypertension in a small number of kidney donors. It is important to note that donors of one paired organ are fully evaluated for normal functioning of both organs before procurement. Living donors have also contributed segments of the pancreas, liver, lung, and small intestine. These procedures technically are more complex than donor nephrectomy and may be associated with greater risk for the donor. At the University of Chicago, left lateral segmentectomies in 45 living, related donors of liver grafts resulted in no donor deaths.[24] However, potential morbidity after liver resection includes hemorrhage, leakage of bile, incidental splenectomy, infection, and complications from anesthesia.[25] These risks to the donor may be deemed acceptable when contrasted with the benefits to the recipient.[26]

Living, Unrelated Donors

Improved immunosuppressive therapy allows another possibility for transplantation (i.e., living, unrelated organ donation). Although bone marrow transplantation and blood transfusion from donors unrelated to their recipients are common, the idea of solid organ donation from unrelated, living donors has not met with wide social acceptance. There are two types of living, unrelated donor relationships: the genetically separate yet emotionally related (e.g., husband and wife) and the unrelated, unconnected donor. One important difference between living donors and cadaveric donors is that the donation from a living donor is usually made for a specific patient rather than into an organ pool to be anonymously matched to the recipient by an organ procurement agency. Therefore, organ suitability/matching must be ensured early. It has been proposed that if a living donor is immunologically incompatible with the related recipient and the willingness to donate exists, an organ donation will be made and matched to an unknown recipient.[27] The donor's willingness to donate if the intended recipient is immunologically incompatible usually changes, however, so that donations into an anonymous pool are rare.

Recipient and organ survival after donation from living, unrelated donors is similar to that from mismatched, living, related and brain-dead donors.[28–30] One study, however, suggests that the organs from an unrelated donor have better survival than those from brain-dead, heartbeating cadavers.[30]

Public concern about the commercial sale of donor organs has been focused particularly on living, unrelated donors.[31] Payment for organs has been condemned and is unlawful in many countries, including the United States. This danger, however, should not discourage appropriate development of other options within this category.

Brain-Dead Donors

Head injury is the cause of death in approximately 77% of brain-dead organ donors,[32] with motor vehicle fatalities yielding the greatest proportion of viable organs.[12] Intracranial hemorrhage, brain tumor, and anoxic injury cause brain death in most other donors. The critical care physician most commonly participates in organ donation through the care of such patients with catastrophic brain injury and who, despite maximum treatment, progress to brain death. Treatment priorities initially directed toward maintenance or recovery of physiologic homeostasis for the patient continue after brain death, but the emphasis changes from brain-oriented treatment to maintaining optimal organ function. Thus, treatment goals form a continuum of patient and family support throughout the entire treatment time and yet expand to include the recipient's needs after brain death of the donor occurs. Hemodynamic instability, fluid or electrolyte imbalance, and other consequences of brain death may jeopardize donor organ homeostasis and, therefore, require the timely diagnosis of brain death and removal of organs.[33] The diagnosis and certification of brain death are discussed elsewhere in this text (see Chapter 174).

As reviewed earlier in this chapter, experimental and histological data suggest that injury to organs may occur in the donor. Donor organs may be affected by various pathophysiologic changes, particularly those of a hypercatecholamine state during the evolution of brain death.[32, 34, 35] In cases of severe brain injury, the possibility and even likelihood of brain death can and should be recognized early. As in any disease process in which alternative outcomes are possible and acknowledged, accepting the possibility that the patient may become an organ donor before certifying brain death is not unethical or improper. Therapy directed toward organ support even before brain death while attempting to maximize treatment of the primary injury or disease so as to restore normal brain function is, likewise, not unethical. So long as any therapy does not diminish the primary goal of restoring brain function, it may be considered as part of the primary patient care plan. Therefore, it is appropriate to prevent or treat regional or systematic catecholamine surges and other hormonal or metabolic changes occurring after severe brain injury. In so doing, the physician may prevent or minimize the hemodynamic or physiologic instability that may influence recovery of the patient and likewise injure organs that may be subsequently donated and transplanted.

Hemodynamic Changes

Cardiovascular instability is commonly present in patients with severe brain injury,[36] especially immediately before and after brain death. This instability has been attributed to an increase in circulating and regional myocardial catecholamines, loss of arterial neurohumoral regulation, and intravascular volume derangements. Described and demonstrated in the baboon model,[37] acute intracranial hypertension appears to cause a progressive increase in activity of the sympathetic nervous system, cardiac tachyarrhythmias, and systemic hypertension. Bradyarrhythmias may be seen after the intracranial pressure increases further during brain herniation. Ischemic injury to the heart is postulated to occur as a result of coronary arteriolar vasoconstriction caused by the intense regional sympathetic nervous system discharge.

Histologic myocardial contraction bands are suggested to be evidence of this ischemia and occur in experimental models of brain death precipitated by acute herniation.[37] Contraction bands may be seen in other conditions associated with high catecholamine levels but are not diagnostic and have even been suggested to be artifacts produced during tissue preparation.[38] High catecholamine levels have also been associated with neurogenic pulmonary edema.[39] Secondary injury to the heart, vasodilation caused by a form of "cerebrospinal disconnection" (similar to "spinal shock"), endorphin release,[40] or other hormonal abnormalities[41] may produce hypotension after brain death. A sequence of marked hypertension followed by severe hypotension is uniformly reproducible in animals and occurs in approximately 50% of patients during the evolution of brain death.

In baboons, the hemodynamic changes, histologic contraction bands, and pulmonary edema noted previously are reduced after the baboons are treated with calcium channel or β-receptor blockade before induction of brain death.[42] These agents have not been used in patients for this purpose, and there is no evidence in animals that this therapy would improve the function of the heart or other organs after transplantation.

The goal of conventional treatment in the organ donor is to maintain an optimal tissue oxygen delivery. Invasive hemodynamic monitoring (i.e., systemic arterial and central venous or pulmonary artery pressures) is usually essential for adequate fluid resuscitation and titration of therapy. Radial arterial catheters are preferred in multiple organ procurement because the femoral site may be eliminated from monitoring during some organ procurement procedures. Pulmonary artery catheters, although not routinely required, may be placed for assessment of right ventricular function and pulmonary artery pressures before lung or heart procurement or if the status of the intravascular volume is unclear. Infection, a risk with any invasive catheter, and the possibility of direct endocardial injury with a pulmonary artery catheter should be carefully considered. Care must be taken to avoid treating one organ at the expense of another because a careful balance of treatment is needed when multiple organs are to be obtained. For example, volume loading to maintain high intravascular volume and urine output to preserve renal function may induce ventricular distention or pulmonary congestion and harm the heart and lungs.

Hypotension should first be treated by volume expansion. The choice of crystalloid, colloid, or blood products depends on coexisting electrolyte abnormalities, disorders of free water conservation, or anemia. Vasoactive drugs should be chosen carefully and used judiciously to avoid vasoconstriction and possible ischemic damage to donor organs. Low-dose dopamine at less than 5 $\mu g \cdot kg^{-1} \cdot min^{-1}$ causes vasodilation of renal, mesenteric, and coronary arterial beds and has been used to decrease the effect of vasoconstriction of other simultaneously used vasoactive agents in organ donors.[43] Dopamine at less than 10 $\mu g \cdot kg^{-1} \cdot min^{-1}$ has also been shown not to affect allograft function adversely after transplantation.[44, 45] Use of norepinephrine is discouraged because of vasoconstriction of regional vascular beds. Low-dose epinephrine and vasopressin have been used to maintain blood pressure and decrease urinary loss from diabetes insipidus in brain-dead patients with normal liver and renal function.[46]

Reperfusion injury after correction of hypoperfusion in the donor may influence organ function. The use of free radical scavengers, such as superoxide dismutase, allopurinol, and mannitol,[47] has been suggested. Administration of these agents and the extent of reperfusion injury in the donated organ are still being investigated.

Cardiac Arrest

Although cardiovascular and pulmonary support is continued, cardiac arrest may occur after brain death. Its incidence varies, as does the time interval between brain death and cardiac arrest (from 24–72 hours to as long as months[43, 48]). Cardiac arrest is usually preceded by ventricular fibrillation or bradycardia, leading to asystole. Cardiac arrest itself does not exclude organ donation, but failure to promptly re-establish oxygen delivery leads to ischemic damage, rendering donor organs useless. Epinephrine, isoproterenol, or transcutaneous or transvenous pacing are chosen as chronotropic agents because atropine is ineffective after loss of the function of the vagal nuclei. If cardiac function cannot be quickly re-established, open cardiac massage, cardiopulmonary bypass (CPB),[49] or emergent organ removal should be considered.

Respiratory Care

Maintaining optimal pulmonary function is important not only when the lungs are obtained for transplantation but also to maintain adequate gas exchange in support of other vital organs being considered. Standard therapy and goals are appropriate for these patients, including prevention of mucous accumulation and atelectasis, positioning of the endotracheal tube so as to avoid injury to the area of subsequent tracheal anastomoses in a potential lung donor, close monitoring of fluid balance to avoid pulmonary congestion, and maintenance of minute ventilation to normalize arterial pH. Because the brain-dead donor is often hypothermic, a slightly alkalemic pH may help maintain better organ function.[32]

Arterial oxygen saturation should be kept above 95% through administration of supplemental oxygen and positive end-expiratory pressure (PEEP). The changing pulmonary and cardiovascular status of the donor will determine the titration of either therapy and may impose a maximum beyond which further increases in oxygen or PEEP become detrimental rather than beneficial. For example, administration of excessive PEEP to improve oxygenation may reduce cardiac output and oxygen delivery to all organs, whereas high levels of inspired oxygen and PEEP may both injure the lung directly.

Fluid Therapy

Volume replacement is essential to replace increased urinary losses resulting from osmotic or diuretic therapy, physiologic diuresis of previously administered fluids, or diabetes insipidus. Diabetes insipidus does not develop in all brain-dead donors[36] but when present may result in significant hypotonic polyuria that, without treatment, leads to hyperosmolality, electrolyte abnormalities, hypovolemia, and hemodynamic instability. The patient's free water deficit should be corrected with hypotonic solutions. Dextrose-containing fluids should be avoided so as to prevent significant hyperglycemia, which may promote further osmotic diuresis. Concomitant electrolyte disturbances such as hypokalemia should be corrected. Exogenous vasopressin may be required to replace circulating antidiuretic hormone after brain death. Intravenous desmopressin acetate (DDAVP) is recommended in divided doses of 2 to 4 μg daily. Alternatively, a continuous intravenous infusion of aqueous pitressin may be used and titrated to its lowest effective dose. Urine output should be maintained at 100 to 250 mL/h (1–2 $mL \cdot kg^{-1} \cdot h^{-1}$) and excessive volume losses replaced hourly.

Temperature Control

Brain-dead patients may lose temperature regulation after loss of hypothalamic function and become hypothermic. Adverse effects of hypothermia include ventricular arrhythmias, coagulopathy, cold-induced polyuria, and regional vasoconstriction. Passive exogenous rewarming through use of aluminum foil blankets, heating inspired gas, or warmed intravenous fluids may be required. Overly aggressive rewarming should be avoided because it may increase oxygen consumption.[32] The best approach to temperature management is to prevent hypothermia by preventing heat loss.

Endocrine Changes

Hormonal changes before, during the evolution of, and after brain death may greatly influence the patient's physiologic homeostasis. The hypercatecholamine state, as previously discussed, has significant hemodynamic consequences. Altered thyroid hormone levels noted after severe injury of any type and after brain death may be significant, although data suggest that there is not an actual reduction in thyroid hormone beyond that characteristic of the euthyroid sick syndrome.[37, 41] The benefits of thyroid hormone administration have not yet been conclusively shown. Disruption of the hypothalamic-pituitary axis after brain death also seems logical. However, variable levels of cortisol and pituitary hormones have been reported, suggesting that the axis may remain intact or that residual stores of hormone are still available after brain death.[32]

Management of the brain-dead organ donor involves understanding intricate physiologic interactions between all organ systems. These derangements and the consequences of the instituted interventions will affect the organs being considered for procurement and may subsequently alter organ function after transplantation.

Non-Heartbeating Donors

Multiple organ procurement from brain-dead donors has become increasingly successful, but the demand for organs has not been met by this category alone. Although organ procurement from non-heartbeating donors has the disadvantage of possible hypotension preceding cardiac arrest and, therefore, potentially longer warm ischemia times after cessation of effective circulatory function, such donors are accepted in Europe and Japan.[50–52] Categories of non-heartbeating donors include patients who have sustained a cardiac arrest and those in whom cardiac arrest is immanent or may be expected soon after withdrawal of treatment.

Because of the concerns about injury to donor organs during prolonged warm ischemia time, one urgent goal is to induce mild to moderate hypothermia before cardiac arrest followed by rapid cooling with preservation fluids immediately after cardiac arrest. Hypoperfusion during hypothermia is better tolerated by organ donors because of a reduction in tissue metabolism and energy consumption induced by the hypothermia.[53] Cooling by noninvasive methods is less effective than the use of cooled intravascular fluids.[54, 55] Therefore, permission for placement of vascular catheters for in situ cooling and organ preservation as well as for the donation must be obtained urgently from the appropriate family member or surrogate.

Ideally, if donation can be anticipated, catheter insertion should be performed before cardiac arrest. If a cardiac arrest has occurred unexpectedly, valuable time may be lost in searching for family members or surrogates to give consent. This situation also requires a decision by the family under extreme stress, which itself may cause the family to decline permission for donation. Therefore, in some areas (i.e., the Regional Organ Bank of Illinois), placement of catheters with infusion of cooling solution has been advocated based on presumed consent.[56] After cooling has been initiated, more time is available for discussion and consideration of organ procurement by the family.

Initiating in situ cooling of abdominal organs in deceased patients with identified organ donor cards has also been suggested; warm ischemia is converted to less injurious cold ischemia while relatives are found for final consent to procure organs suitable for transplantation.

Twenty-two patients had been placed on CPB at the University of Pittsburgh Medical Center during unsuccessful attempts to resuscitate them from cardiac arrest.[9, 49] Four patients survived, and three recovered full neurologic function. In others, brain death developed; these patients were evaluated for organ donation or remained in coma, dependent on CPB. CPB was later withdrawn from these patients after consideration for organ donation as non-heartbeating donors.[57] Patients who regain brain function but remain dependent on CPB should be evaluated for heart transplantation as potential recipients.

At the University of Pittsburgh Medical Center, a protocol has also been established for terminally ill patients to become organ donors.[58] The approved policy honors the patient's or family's decision to forgo life-sustaining treatment and to donate organs after death. Patients in whom cardiac arrest is considered imminent after withdrawal of cardiopulmonary support are considered for donation. Within this protocol, discussion with the patient or family and planning may take place over a suitable time period to permit fully informed consent. The policy stipulates that discussion of organ donation not be initiated until after the decision for withdrawal of life support is made. Thereafter, organ donation is requested, and if the patient is accepted as a suitable donor, he or she is moved to the operating room where cardiopulmonary support is withdrawn. After 2 minutes of ventricular fibrillation, asystole, or electromechanical dissociation, the patient is pronounced dead and organ procurement is initiated. It is important to appreciate that this short period of cardiac arrest is sufficient for certification of death only in cases in which cardiopulmonary resuscitation is unwanted or contraindicated.

Maintaining patient comfort as treatment is withdrawn is an important part of the policy as is support for family or friends because they are not present with the patient at the time of death. Physician and nurse staffing in the operating room is provided from the intensive care unit to avoid any perceived conflict of interest. Operating room personnel, including the procuring transplant surgeons, are not present during withdrawal of life support.

A group similar to terminally ill patients who request withdrawal of life support are those patients with lethal brain injury and hemodynamic instability but who are not brain dead. These patients may undergo similar withdrawal of life support in the operating room with organ procurement after cardiac arrest. Alternatively, patients with lethal brain injury and cardiovascular instability may be placed on CPB, especially when hemodynamic instability prohibits timely completion of brain death determination. After CPB is initiated, brain death may be certified and organs then procured from a brain-dead donor as opposed to a non-heartbeating donor. If brain death criteria are not met but death is nonetheless deemed inevitable, CPB can be withdrawn and organ procurement approached as in other non-heartbeating donors.

Finally, patients who do not wish to receive cardiopulmonary resuscitation and have never been placed on life support may request to become organ donors after death. The circumstances surrounding the death of such patients will determine whether organ procurement is feasible. If cardiac arrest occurs in a situation in which CPB can be quickly initiated or catheters rapidly placed for in situ cooling, organs from these patients may be removed and successfully transplanted.

Animal Donors

Xenografting was initially attempted 25 years ago when primate kidneys were transplanted into humans.[59, 60] Advancements in immunosuppression have made further attempts at xenotransplantation more realistic although not yet successful.

Technical difficulties and philosophic concerns surrounding use of higher primates for organ transplantation in humans distinguish this category of donor organs from the others. Continued investigation of this potential donor category will answer further questions about control of rejection[61] and may increase the organ pool available for recipients.

SUMMARY

Although patients are surviving longer with end-stage organ disease as a result of bridging devices such as dialysis machines and ventricular assist devices, transplantation continues to offer a superior long-term solution to many forms of end-stage single organ failure. To facilitate such efforts, more potential donors must be identified including brain-dead, non-heartbeating, living related, and living unrelated donors. Alternative organ donor options, such as animal donors, must be investigated further. It is hoped that, in the near future, all patients awaiting a second chance to live through some form of organ transplantation can be offered this opportunity.

To ensure procurement of the best functioning organs with minimal risk of failure after transplantation, skillful management of identified donors is required so that in situ injury does not complicate procurement, preservation, transplantation, or subsequent organ function. Critical care physicians play an important role in organ transplantation through their timely identification of potential donors and by providing those patients with optimal care throughout their hospitalization.

References

1. UNOS Update. 1993; 9:41. (Available from P.O. Box 13770, Richmond, VA 23225.)
1a. UNOS Update. 1994; 10:37.
2. Evans RW, Orians CE, Ascher NL: The potential supply of organ donors: An assessment of the efficiency of organ procurement efforts in the United States. JAMA 1992; 267:239.
3. Manninen DL, Evans RW: Public attitudes and behavior regarding organ donation. JAMA 1985; 253:311.
4. American Council on Transplantation: The US Public's Attitudes Toward Organ Transplants/Organ Donation. Princeton, NJ, The Gallup Organization, Inc, 1985.
5. Virnig BA, Caplan AL: Required request: What difference has it made? Transplant Proc 1992; 24:2155.
6. Cohen C: The case for presumed consent to transplant human organs after death. Transplant Proc 1992; 24:2168.
7. Peabody J, Emery JR, Ashwal S: Experience with anencephalic infants as prospective organ donors. N Engl J Med 1989; 321:344.
8. Murray JE: Forty years of transplantation: Merely a prologue. Transplant Proc 1992; 24:1647.
9. Grenvik A: Brain death and organ transplantation: A 40 year review. Opuscula Medica 1992; 37:33.
10. Darracott-Cankovic S, Stovin P, Wheeldon D, et al: Effect of donor heart damage on survival after transplantation. Eur J Cardiothorac Surg 1989; 3:525.
11. Gore SM, Cable DJ, Holland AJ: Organ donation from intensive care units in England and Wales: Two year confidential audit of deaths in intensive care unit. Br Med J 1992; 304:349–355.
12. Waller JA, Haisch CE, Skelly JM: Potential availability of transplantable organs according to factors associated with type of injury event. Accid Anal Prev 1992; 24:193–200.
13. Alexander JW: High risk donors: Diabetics, the elderly, and others. Transplant Proc 1992; 24:2221.
14. Cefalo RC, Ingelhardt MT: The use of fetal and anencephalic tissue for transplantation. J Med Philos 1989; 14:25.
15. Medical Task Force on Anencephaly: The infant with anencephaly. N Engl J Med 1990; 332:669.
16. Peabody JL, Emery KR, Ashwal S: Experience with anencephalic infants as prospective organ donors. N Engl J Med 1989; 321:344.
17. Holzgreve W, Beller FK, Buchholz B, et al: Kidney transplantation from anencephalic donors. N Engl J Med 1987; 316:1068.
18. Merrill J, Murray J, Harrison J, et al: Successful homotransplantation of the human kidney between identical twins. JAMA 1956; 160:277.
19. Spital A, Spital M, Spital R: The living kidney donor: Alive and well. Arch Intern Med 1986; 146:1993.
20. Shmueli D, Bar-Nathan N, Nakadre R: Eleven years of renal transplantation in children (Israel). Transplant Proc 1992; 24:1841.
21. Goldsmith MF: Mother to child: First living donor lung transplant. JAMA 1990; 264:2724.
22. Smith JA, Williams JJ, Rabinov M, et al: Combined heart-lung transplantation including the "domino" donor procedure in the single lung transplant era. Transplant Proc 1992; 24:2264.
23. Ogden DA: Consequences of renal donation in man. Am J Kidney Dis 1983; 2:501.
24. Siegher M: Liver transplantation using living donors. Transplant Proc 1992; 24:2223.
25. Busuttil R: Living related liver donation: Con. Transplant Proc 1991; 23:43.
26. Ethics of organ transplantation from living donors. Transplant Proc 1992; 24:2236.
27. Rapaport F, Cortesini R: The past, present and future of organ transplantation with special needs in kidney procurement and donation. Transplant Proc 1985; 17:3.
28. Berlocca P, Alfain D, Bruzzone P, et al: Is unrelated living donor a valid organ source in renal transplantation under CyA therapy? Transplant Proc 1991; 23:912.
29. Sesso R, Klag M, Ancao M, et al: Kidney transplantation from living unrelated donors. Ann Intern Med 1992; 117:983–989.
30. Francis DMA, Walker RG, Miller RJ, et al: Living related and living unrelated kidney transplantation using low-dose triple immunosuppression. Transplant Proc 1992; 24:1887.
31. Council of the Transplantation Society: Commercialization in transplantation: The problems and some guidelines for practice. (Editorial). Transplantation 1986; 41:1.
32. Darby JM, Stein K, Grenvik A, et al: Approach to management of the heartbeating brain dead organ donor. JAMA 1989; 261:2222.
33. Powner DJ: The diagnosis of brain death in the adult patient. J Intensive Care Med 1987; 2:181.
34. Mackersie RC: Organ procurement and brain death in trauma patients. J Intensive Care Med 1989; 4:137.
35. Payen D, Quintin L, Plaisance P, et al: Head injury: Clonidine decreases plasma catecholamines. Crit Care Med 1990; 18:392.
36. Jastremski M, Powner DJ, Snyder JV, et al: Problems in brain death determination. Forensic Sci 1978; 11:201.
37. Novitzky D, Wicomb WN, Cooper DKC, et al: Electrocardiographic hemodynamic and endocrine changes occurring during experimental brain death in the Chacma baboon. J Heart Transplant 1984; 4:63.
38. Kinoshita Y, Okamoto K, Yahata K, et al: Clinical and pathological changes of the heart in brain death maintained with vasopressin and epinephrine. Pathol Res Pract 1990; 186:173.
39. Malik AB: Mechanisms of neurogenic pulmonary edema. Circ Res 1985; 57:1.
40. Toledo-Pereyra LH, Castellano J, Finkelstein I: Improved donor kidney function and hemodynamics following naloxone administration. Transplant Proc 1988; 20:733.
41. Powner D, Hendrich A, Lagler R, et al: Hormonal changes in brain dead patients. Crit Care Med 1990; 18:702.
42. Novitzky D, Cooper DKC, Rose AG, et al: Prevention of myocardial injury by pretreatment with verapamil hydrochloride prior to experimental brain death. Am J Emerg Med 1987; 5:11.
43. Soifer BE, Gelb A: The multiple organ donor: Identification and management. Ann Intern Med 1989; 110:814.
44. Trento A, Hardesty RL, Griffith BP: Early function of cardiac homografts: Relationship to hemodynamics in the donor and length of ischemic period. Circulation 1986; 74:77.

45. Whelchel JD, Diethelm AG, Phillips MG, et al: Effect of high dose dopamine in cadaver donor management on delayed graft function and graft survival following renal transplantation. Transplant Proc 1986; 18:523.
46. Iwai A, Sakano T, Uenishi M, et al: Effects of vasopressin and catecholamines on the maintenance of circulatory stability in brain dead patients. Transplantation 1989; 48:613.
47. Hernandez LA, Ceragen N: Role of antioxidents in organ preservation and transplantation. Crit Care Med 1988; 16:543.
48. Powner DJ, Jastremski M, Lagler R: Continuing care of multiorgan donor patients. J Intensive Care Med 1989; 4:75.
49. Tisherman SA, Grenvik A, Safar P: Cardiopulmonary-cerebral resuscitation: Advanced and prolonged life support with emergency cardiopulmonary bypass. Acta Anaesthesiol Scand 1990; 34(Suppl 94):63.
50. Koostra G, Wijnen R, van Hooff JP, et al: Twenty percent more kidneys through a non-heart beating program. Transplant Proc 1991; 23:910.
51. Koostra G, Wynen R, VanHoof JP: The non-heart beating kidney donor: Of any help in developing countries. Transplant Proc 1992; 24:2040.
52. Kozaki M, Matsuno N, Tamaki T, et al: Procurement of kidney grafts from non-heart beating donors. Transplant Proc 1991; 23:2575.
53. Hochacka PW: Defense strategies against hypoxia and hypothermia. Science 1986; 231:234.
54. Maessen JG, VanDer Vusse GJ, Koostra G: New approach to preservation of non-heart beating donor kidneys: Total body cooling. Transplant Proc 1987; 19:4159.
55. Hoshino T, Koyama M, Onoto R, et al: Transplantation of livers from non-heart beating donors is possible by core cooling technique. Transplant Proc 1989; 21:3519.
56. UNOS Update. 1992; 8:15. (Available from P.O. Box 13770, Richmond, VA 23225.)
57. DeVita M, Snyder JV: Development of the University of Pittsburgh Medical Center policy for the care of terminally ill patients who may become organ donors after death following removal of life support. Kennedy Institute Ethics J 1993; 3:131.
58. Youngner SJ, Arnold RM: Ethical, psychosocial, and public policy implications of procuring organs from non-heartbeating cadaver donors. JAMA 1993; 269:2769.
59. Najarian JS: Overview of in vivo xenotransplantation studies: Prospects for the future. Transplant Proc 1992; 24:733.
60. Reemtsma K: Xenografts. Transplant Proc 1992; 24:2225.
61. Bach FH: Xenotransplantation: A view to the future. Transplant Proc 1993; 25:25.

CHAPTER 178

Multiple Organ Procurement

Ignazio Roberto Marino, MD • Howard R. Doyle, MD
Yoogoo Kang, MD • Robert L. Kormos, MD
Thomas E. Starzl, MD, PhD

Solid organ transplantation (heart, lung, liver, kidney, pancreas, and intestine) has become a successful and widely accepted treatment for a variety of conditions. However, the shortage of cadaveric organs is hindering the larger use of this therapeutic option. In spite of the progressive evolution of public and professional understanding and acceptance of organ donation during the past 30 years, only a little more than 25% of all potential brain-dead organ donors will actually come to donation.[1–3] As of July 31, 1993, there were 31,868 transplant candidates on the United Network for Organ Sharing (UNOS) waiting list,[4] representing an increase of 330% from December 1986 (9632). At the same time, the supply of organ donors underwent a marginal increase between 1986 and 1991 (from approximately 4000 to 4500) and has been stable in the past 2 years, with 4534 in 1992[5–7] (Fig. 178–1). It is also estimated that every day seven potential organ recipients in the United States will die before a suitable organ is found.[8] Consequently, although the need has increased dramatically, we observe with mounting concern the persistent wastage of available organs and the death of potential recipients. These are both mainly related to unwillingness to donate or a lack of awareness regarding donation as well as delays or failure by the medical staff to consider organ donation.[3] In addition, there are other forces at work that have significantly decreased organ availability for the sicker patients, such as a policy implemented by UNOS in 1991 that substantially changed previous allocation criteria.[9] As a result of this, there is now an even more limited number of organs available for the most severely ill patients, and some advocate their outright exclusion from transplant candidacy in favor of the elective cases.[10, 10a]

Many routes have been explored in an attempt to remedy this situation, including the development of artificial organs,[11] utilization of living donors even for extrarenal organs,[12, 13] xenotransplantation,[14–17] and non-heartbeating donors.[18] However, a more immediate impact on organ shortage could be effected by improving our current mechanisms for organ recovery and the management of potential donors.

ORGAN RECOVERY

Standardized criteria for the determination of brain death were defined by the Ad Hoc Committee of the Harvard Medical School[19] and have been the subject of a more recent report.[20] The concept of brain death and the management of the brain-dead donor are discussed in detail in Chapter 177.

Once a potential organ donor is identified, the multiple organ procurement process should be triggered. This starts by contacting the local Organ Procurement Organization (OPO) as soon as the irreversibility of brain injury has been established. In 1992, there were 68 OPOs and 266 transplant centers in the United States. These represent the largest organ procurement and transplant network in the world. Most intensive care units (ICUs) have the telephone number of the local agency available. However, the telephone number and location of the area's OPO can be obtained from the UNOS, which has a 24-hour telephone hotline (800-243-6667). These OPOs, originally set up to organize the recovery of kidneys, coordinate the complex logistics of multiple organ recovery and their distribution within a predetermined geographic area. They are also responsible for the payment of all charges incurred during the process of organ donation, ensuring that donor families are not billed for any of them. Once contacted, the local OPO will send a procurement coordinator to the referring hospital. These coordinators perform a number of administrative and technical functions, covering every aspect of the donation process. On receiving a referral, they will perform an evaluation and discuss organ donation with the potential donor's family, making sure the relatives have a complete and satisfactory explanation of the diagnosis of brain death and a clear understanding of the organ procurement process. Families should be informed separately but as soon as possible after the irreversibility of the lethal brain damage has been established and be given a clear explanation of the prognosis. This will give them time to accept the patient's death and allow them to deal with their grief. It is extremely important to respect this phase because it has been demonstrated that consent for donation increases from 18% to 60% if the family is allowed to deal with the concept of brain death first and

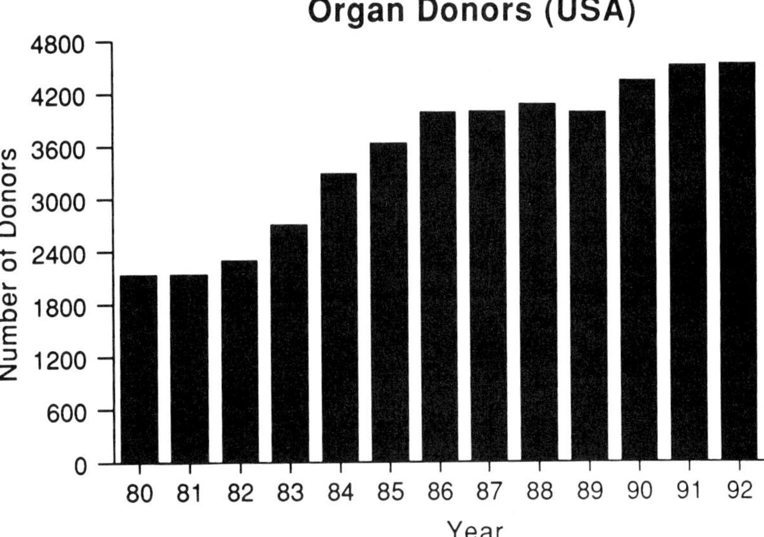

Figure 178–1. Organ donor supply in the United States from 1980 through 1992. (Modified from Evans RW: Organ procurement expenditures and the role of financial incentives. JAMA 1993; 269:3113–3118. Copyright 1993, American Medical Association.)

the issue of organ donation is brought up later.[3] Religious beliefs about human life, the dead body, and life after death are extremely important considerations for those involved in organ donation and transplantation. No major religion specifically prohibits organ donation, although in some situations there may be restrictions. Table 178–1 summarizes some of the major religious and cultural beliefs associated with organ donation and transplantation.[21] Families may feel the need to discuss the matter with a church representative before making a decision.

If the family decides to donate, a consent for donation form is supplied by the hospital or by the procurement coordinator and is completed and signed by the next of kin. In addition, the coordinator sees to it that all medicolegal requirements are met, from adequate documentation of brain death in the chart to securing permission from the coroner when necessary. Medical staff privileges for the recovery teams are also arranged. Hospitals differ in their policies for granting such privileges. Some hospitals do not consider the organ procurement as a surgical procedure because a determination of brain death has been made. In this circumstance, temporary privileges are not required for outside surgeons.

At the same time, the procurement coordinator assumes control of three main activities: (1) donor evaluation, (2) coordination of donor and recipient matching, (3) donor operation and organ preservation and shipment to the recipients' hospitals. The role of the coordinator in each of these is critical because the most important issue in organ procurement, once the decision to proceed has been made, is to have someone who "directs traffic," maintaining clear lines of communication between the members of the different teams involved. A lack of communication at this point can disrupt donor care and compromise organ stability.

TABLE 178–1. Major Religious and Cultural Beliefs Associated with Organ Donation and Transplantation

Group	*Donation*	*Transplantation*
Amish	Reluctant if transplant outcome uncertain	Acceptable for the well-being of the candidate
Baha'i	Acceptable	Acceptable
Baptist	Individual decision	Acceptable
Buddhist	Individual decision	Buddha's teachings on the middle path (i.e., the avoidance of extremes) could be applicable to this
Christian Science	Individual decision	Individual decision
Episcopal	Encouraged	Encouraged
Evangelical Covenant	Encouraged	Encouraged
Greek Orthodox	Acceptable (although not for research)	Acceptable for the well-being of the candidate
Gypsies	Against	Against
Hinduism	Individual decision	Individual decision
Islam	Acceptable (organs of Moslem donors must be transplanted immediately and not stored in organ banks)	Acceptable
Jehovah's Witnesses	Individual decision (not encouraged)	May be considered acceptable (organs should be completely drained of blood before transplantation)
Judaism	Encouraged	Encouraged
Latter-day Saints	Individual decision	Individual decision
Protestant denominations	Individual decision	Acceptable
Religious Society of Friends (Quakers)	Individual decision	Individual decision
Roman Catholicism	Encouraged	Acceptable
Unitarian Universalist	Acceptable	Acceptable
United Methodist	Encouraged	Acceptable

Donor Information — Donor ID# — UNOS ID#

Name ______ Admitting Date: ______ Referral Date: ______

Age: ______ Sex: ______ Race: ______ Recovery Date: ______ Clamp Time: ______ AM/PM

Date of Birth: ______ Hospital: ______

Next of Kin: ______ City/State: ______

Relationship: ______ Referred By: ______

Address: ______ Phone #: ______

Program: ______

Program 24 hr #: ______

Next of Kin Phone: ______ Attending: ______

Consulting: ______

Medical Records No.: ______

Pronouncement Date: ______ Time: ______

Consent For: ______

Cause of Death: ______

Past Medical History: (Complete history please)

Heart Disease: (Y/N) ______

Liver Disease: (Y/N) ______

Renal Disease: (Y/N) ______

Diabetes: (Y/N) ______

Neurological: (Y/N) ______

Cancer: (Y/N) ______

Lung Disease: (Y/N) ______

Arthritis or Joint Disease: (Y/N) ______

Recent Flu-like Symptoms: (Y/N) ______

Unexplained Weight Loss: (Y/N) ______

Toxic Exposure: (Y/N) ______

Drug Use: Prescribed or Other: (Y/N) ______

Alcohol Abuse: (Y/N) ______

Smoker: (Y/N) ______

Blood Transfusion History: (x 2 yrs.) (Y/N) ______

Previous Surgery: (Y/N) ______

Immunization or Vaccinated: (x 6 mo.) (Y/N) ______

Travel outside U.S.A. since 1977: (Y/N) ______

Homosexual or Bisexual: (Y/N) ______

Received pit-hGh: (Y/N) ______

Recent Infections: (Y/N) (if yes give treatment) ______

G.I. Disorders: (Y/N) ______

Hematologic Disorders: (Y/N) ______

Under Physician's Care: (Y/N) ______

Physician, Phone #, Address: ______

Donor Information — Donor ID#

ABO: ______ HLA: ______ DR: ______ LE Type: ______ WT: ______ HT: ______

Chest Cir: ______ Girth: ______ RC/BRR: ______ LC/BLR: ______

Hospital History (include E.R., V/S, Arrests, O.R. Procedures, Injuries, Infection, ect.)

EKG, Echo & Cardiac Consult:

Chemistries

Date				
BUN				
Creat.				
T. Bil.				
D. Bil.				
SGOT				
SGPT				
LDH				
GGT				
Amylase				
CPK				
Glucose				
Hgb/Hct.				
PT				
PTT				
Plat.				
WBC				

Urinalysis

Date			
Color			
Appear.			
pH			
Sp. Grav.			
Glucose			
Protein			
Blood			
RBC			
WBC			
Epith.			
Casts			
Bact.			

ABG'S & Lytes

Date			
pH			
PO2			
PCO2			
O2 Sat.			
FIO2			
PEEP			
VT			
Rate			
Na +			
K +			
Cl -			
Ca ++			

Blood Pressure (Note B/P< 90.Time)	Urine Output (Note Anuria/Oliguria)	Med. During ADM
		Blood & Blood Products

Serology

Date	Time	Test	Pre	Post Result	Local/Import	Reported By	Reported To
		RPR/VDRL					
		HBs Ag					
		HAA					
		HIV					
		HTLV-I					
		CMV					
		HCV					

Cultures (Blood, Urine, Sputum) Date, Results

Figure 178–2. Donor data sheet used by the Western Pennsylvania Organ Procurement Organization, CORE (Center for Organ Recovery and Education). (Courtesy of Brian Broznick.)

Therefore, the needs and protocols of the individual teams should be discussed in detail before any donor surgery is begun. In addition, if possible, the logistic arrangements between teams should be expedited so that no time constraints are placed on the host team. On the other hand, the host team must be tolerant because different organs often have to be flown to distant parts of the country, and some recipient surgery may be quite complex and time consuming. To facilitate matters, the host team should make available basic information on the donor to expedite the evaluation by the visiting teams (Fig. 178–2).

DONOR EVALUATION AND MANAGEMENT

There are very few absolute contraindications to organ donation, and they can be grouped into three broad categories: (1) severe trauma, (2) malignancy outside of the central nervous system (CNS), and (3) active infections. The first category, trauma, refers only to injury to the organ itself and will not preclude donation of those organs that are not affected. Malignancy other than primary CNS tumors will also disqualify the prospective donor. An important group of exclusionary criteria is the presence of active infections. Systemic sepsis, active tuberculosis, viral encephalitis, and Guillain-Barré syndrome are contraindications to organ donation as are active hepatitis and the presence of the hepatitis B surface antigen. Past infection with hepatitis B virus, as evidenced by the presence of antibodies, does not preclude donation. Whether organs should be used if the donor has hepatitis C antibodies has been the subject of controversy in the last few years. There is evidence in the literature of hepatitis C virus (HCV) transmission after transplantation.[22] However, the donor shortage is so serious at this time that HCV-positive donors need to be considered at least for lifesaving organs such as the liver, heart, and lungs.[23] Policies concerning other organs such as the kidney and pancreas are currently being debated.[22, 24]

The human immunodeficiency virus (HIV) has had a great impact on the field of transplantation, and donors who test positive for HIV antibody are rejected. Prospective donors should also have a venereal disease research laboratory (VDRL) test and should have cytomegalovirus (CMV) titers determined as soon as possible. The significance of a positive VDRL is difficult to ascertain, but it is our practice to treat recipients of VDRL-positive donors with a course of benzathine penicillin. The CMV status of the donor has prognostic significance regarding the incidence, and severity, of subsequent CMV infections. Recipients of organs harvested from seronegative donors have a reduced chance of acquiring a CMV infection, regardless of their own serologic status.[25–27] Epstein-Barr and herpes varicella zoster virus (VZV) are not part of the usual viral screening. The only situation in which these viruses become relevant is when the donor has active disease related to them (infectious mononucleosis or systemic VZV infection). If this is the case, organ donation should not be considered.

Donors with infections under control or those affecting organs not specifically considered for donation (i.e., an abdominal organ donor suffering from pneumonia) may still be suitable. Children who die as a result of bacterial meningitis related to *Haemophilus influenzae* or *Neisseria meningitidis* can still be considered for donation if the organism and its sensitivity are known beforehand.

Prolonged organ ischemia related to severe hypotension or cardiac arrest might represent a contraindication to donation. However, it is the policy of the Pittsburgh Transplantation Institute to critically evaluate all donors, including those with cardiac arrest and prolonged cardiopulmonary resuscitation (CPR). In fact, many of these donors have been found acceptable by post-CPR physiologic and biochemical criteria, and their organs have been successfully transplanted.[18, 28, 29]

TABLE 178–2. Age Guidelines for Organ and Tissue Donation Used at the Pittsburgh Transplantation Institute

Organ/Tissue	*Age*
Heart	≤60 y*
Heart-lungs	≤60 y*
Lungs	≤60 y*
Kidney	1 mo–75 y*
Liver	≤75 y*
Pancreas	≤65 y*
Intestine†	
Bone	15–65 y
Bone marrow	≤75 y
Cornea	1–65 y
Skin	15–65 y
Heart valves	≤55 y

*Donors beyond these age limits could be accepted on the basis of the individual organ function.

†No age limits have been set for intestinal donors. Intestines should be available from most organ donors and are always evaluated on an individual basis.

Other patients who may not be acceptable as donors are those with a long-standing history of diabetes mellitus, hypertension, and cardiac or peripheral vascular disease. Again, however, the donor and organ viability should be assessed on a case by case basis, and a patient who is not acceptable as a heart or lung donor might still be an excellent abdominal organ donor. Sometimes the suitability of individual organs can be assessed only after direct examination by the donor surgeon at the time of procurement.

The donor age deserves special mention. The chronologic age is less important than the physiologic age when assessing for specific organ donation. For some organs, age may not be an important limiting factor.[30, 30a] The liver is, in a certain way, protected from aging, and we have successfully used livers from donors as old as 75 years. Popper, in 1985, dedicated an extensive review to the aging of the liver.[31] According to his study, the liver's great functional reserve, its regenerative capacity, and its large blood supply are the key factors in delaying its aging compared with other organs. Table 178–2 shows the age guidelines for individual organs used in our institution. In general, it is rare to find a suitable heart or lung allograft from donors older than 60 years because of the increased incidence of coronary artery disease and chronic pulmonary disease.

In summary, given the enormous need for organs and the very few criteria that absolutely disqualify a potential donor, the local OPO should be contacted in virtually every case. Figure 178–2 shows the data collection form used by the Center for Organ Recovery and Education, the western Pennsylvania, southern New York, and West Virginia organ procurement agency). These data should be promptly faxed to those involved in the evaluation process.

Individual Organ Assessment: Abdominal Organs

The criteria used to determine the suitability of kidneys are very flexible. As shown in Table 178–2, a kidney donor can be between 1 month and 75 years of age. Serum creatinine and blood urea nitrogen (BUN) are used as markers of donor renal function and should be normal. Obviously, donors with chronic renal disease are not considered for kidney donation. However, patients with transient creatinine and BUN elevations related to dehydration or hypotension, or both, are not excluded from kidney donation if the BUN and creatinine fall after appropriate volume correction.

Attempts at predicting liver allograft function after transplantation based on donor information have met with little success. The diverse literature[23, 32–43a] devoted to the topic is testimony to our lack of a clear understanding, one that can translate into well-informed decision making during donor evaluation. As a rule, the donor should have normal or near-normal serum aspartate aminotransferase (AST), serum alanine aminotransferase (ALT), bilirubin, and prothrombin time, but we have successfully used livers from donors with AST and ALT that were 10 times greater than the upper limit of normal. The important parameter is not an isolated AST or ALT value, but the trend established since the ICU admission.[44] The bilirubin can be elevated as a result of massive blood transfusions used during the resuscitation of a shock patient. A history of hepatitis or alcoholism is certainly a warning sign but does not preclude the use of the liver. In general, in the case of a marginal liver donor, the intraoperative assessment by the donor surgeon is the best single piece of information.

There is only one absolute exclusion criterion in the evaluation of a pancreas donor: a history of diabetes mellitus. Amylase elevations have been seen in as many as 39% of pancreas donors, without any evidence of pancreatitis, and thus isolated hyperamylasemia does not contraindicate the use of the pancreas.[45] The serum glucose may be falsely elevated in donors receiving steroid therapy or as a result of decreased circulating insulin.[46]

Intestinal transplantaton is emerging as a valuable modality for the treatment of patients with intestinal failure. Early in 1993, UNOS formed a subcommittee responsible for systematizing the listing of recipients, helping identify suitable donors, and establishing guidelines for the equitable allocation of intestinal grafts at both local and national levels. Because of the time constraints, it is impossible to perform a functional assessment of the donor bowel. Relatively young age, hemodynamic stability, and donor-recipient size match are the critical parameters used in evaluating an intestinal donor.[47] At our institution, preference was initially given to infant and juvenile donors with stable hemodynamics. However, the age range has been gradually expanded provided the donor is stable and receiving minimal vasopressor support ($\leq$10 $\mu g \cdot kg^{-1} \cdot min^{-1}$ of dopamine). Size matching is always given special consideration. A majority of intestinal transplant recipients have undergone extensive intestinal resections, leading to a significant reduction in the size of the abdominal cavity. Therefore, donors are chosen that are 15% to 40% smaller in body weight than the selected recipients.[47]

Individual Organ Assessment: Thoracic Organs

Besides a negative history of cardiac disease and a normal chest x-ray film, the donor should have a normal heart physical examination and 12-lead electrocardiogram. However, a number of electrocardiographic changes might be detected in brain-dead patients, which do not preclude thoracic organ donation.[48, 49] A brain-dead patient who is able to maintain a systolic blood pressure greater than 90 mm Hg with a dopamine requirement less than 10 $\mu g \cdot kg^{-1} \cdot min^{-1}$ is considered a suitable candidate for heart donation.[50, 51] Cardiac isoenzymes are recommended in case of chest trauma, to rule out myocardial contusion, and when the potential donor has suffered a cardiac arrest or prolonged hypotension. Clearly, in male donors older than 35 years, the incidence of coronary artery disease increases, especially in the face of risk factors such as hypercholesterolemia, family history of heart disease, and a history of smoking. Coronary angiography may be helpful in the evaluation of high-risk and older donors, but it is not routinely required, and most hospitals will find the logistics of performing it prohibitive. Therefore, a decision will have to be made based on a cardiologic consultation, evaluating the history, electrocardiogram, and echocardiogram. As is the case for the liver, and because of the severe shortage, it is prudent even in high-risk donors to have the heart examined on the operating table after sternotomy. Visualizing and palpating the coronary arteries will give a significant amount of information with respect to the incidence of coronary artery disease. If plaques are felt along the left main coronary artery or left anterior descending artery, the heart, in most cases, will not be suitable for transplantation. In extreme cases of a very sick recipient, however, the transplant team may make a decision to take this heart, and isolated cases of coronary artery bypass being performed at the time of transplantation have been reported. Indeed, reports exist that, in cases of isolated mild coronary artery disease, the donor allograft functions well with no increase in early mortality.

Transesophageal echocardiography has been demonstrated to be an important adjuvant in the evaluation of a potential cardiac donor. Severe cardiac hypertrophy, valvular defects, and global myocardial dysfunction or segmental wall abnormalities have been diagnosed in what appeared to be otherwise reasonable cardiac donors. At this time, limited information is available about the use of such hearts, and in most cases it is prudent to avoid the use of a heart with demonstrated wall-motion abnormalities.[52] In general, minor changes in the electrocardiogram or echocardiogram, localized infection,[53] transitory hypotension, brief cardiac arrest, and thoracic trauma do not contraindicate heart donation. The importance of donor-recipient weight mismatch greater than 20% is critical only in the face of high pulmonary vascular resistance. In carefully selected donors, survival after transplantation with a donor between 40 and 55 years of age is no different than that observed in the case of younger donors.[54] As the limits for donor selection are extended, it becomes more evident that it is safe to extend donor age up to 55 to 60 years and ischemic time further than 4 to 5 hours.[55–57]

The presence or absence of cardiac or cardiopulmonary arrest in itself is not a contraindication to the use of a heart for transplantation. Especially in the pediatric population, it has been found that even in donors who have undergone extended CPR (up to 125 min) as long as cardiac function at the time of cardiectomy is normal, there does not appear to be an increased risk for performance of the heart or survival of the recipient after transplantation.

All of the selection criteria mentioned in the case of a heart donor also apply to heart-lung or isolated single or double lung donors. In addition, a donor is not acceptable for lung or heart-lung donation when there is a history of heavy smoking, chronic lung disease, or pulmonary aspiration. The height, weight, and chest circumference of the heart-lung donor should closely match those of the recipient. A number of physiologic parameters can be used when assessing a lung donor, including the partial pressure of arterial oxygen/fraction of inspired oxygen (PaO_2/FIO_2) ratio ($\geq$250 mm Hg) and peak airway pressure (<30 cm H_2O with 15 mL/kg of tidal volume and 5 cm H_2O of positive end-expiratory pressure [PEEP]).[58–60] Aspiration pneumonia is frequent in the brain-dead patient, and thus the character of the sputum is a critical piece of information. The role of bronchoscopy is still being debated; it is considered mandatory by some authors,[61] whereas others believe it is indicated only when there is a question of foreign body aspiration or to obtain sputum for Gram's stain and culture.[46] Bronchoscopy will provide, however, important culture information to guide appropriate antibiotic therapy after transplantation. In cases in which frank purulence is noted on bronchoscopy, the lungs will not be suitable. However, it is conceivable that one lung may be salvaged for transplantation from a set in which one appears to be more infected than the other.

COORDINATION OF DONOR AND RECIPIENT MATCHING

Once the coordinator finishes the donor evaluation, there are still many hours of intense work before completing the process. After obtaining the appropriate consent, therapeutic efforts should be geared to protect the donated organs until the actual retrieval can be carried out. Their integrity should be maintained by optimal organ perfusion, avoidance of further damage, and subsequent removal and preservation with minimal ischemic injury. Care of the donor during organ procurement, therefore, requires a continuation of the intensive care that was provided before brain death was declared followed by a precise surgical procurement procedure. Whereas in the 1970s and early 1980s donor management mainly, if not exclusively, addressed kidney function, the patient now must always be approached as a multiple organ donor, and this can present a real challenge to the physician managing the case. The physician should keep the patient hemodynamically stable, with optimal organ perfusion and oxygenation. This is not easy because of the loss of many body reflexes and the dramatic changes in the hormonal milieu.[62] Several studies have shown a significant reduction of cortisol,[63] insulin,[63] and thyroid hormones.[48, 63–67] Also, 50% to 70% of brain-dead patients suffer from diabetes insipidus.[68, 69] A number of protocols that call for the use of hormones such as triiodothyronine, cortisol, or insulin during donor management[46, 49, 64, 66, 67, 70] have given conflicting results. The details of donor management are provided in Chapter 177 and are not repeated here. We stress only a few points we believe to be important. Adequate perfusion should always be maintained while keeping the use of vasoactive drugs to a minimum. This may require the administration of several liters of fluid to obtain adequate filling pressures. Replacement therapy with fresh frozen plasma, platelets, and cryoprecipitate may be used if a serious bleeding diathesis is present. However, even if fibrinolysis is suspected, ε-aminocaproic acid should be avoided because it can induce microvascular thrombosis in the donor organs.

During this phase, the procurement coordinator asks local transplant programs about their needs for organs. Under the current system, local programs have first priority, and only when organs are not used locally are inquiries made at the regional and national levels. An exception to this rule is when a prospective kidney recipient, who resides in another region, is found to have a so-called "six antigen match." These kidneys have to be sent away, with the receiving transplant center "paying back" at a later date. Organ allocation is a very complicated and controversial subject, and what system should be used is presently being debated.[10] As of this writing, amendments to the National Organ Transplant Act are being discussed in the Congress, and it is not clear what changes will be implemented. A point system for renal transplantation was developed in Pittsburgh in 1985 that gave credit points to renal transplant candidates. Credits were acquired for time waiting, quality of antigen match, degree of immunologic sensitization, medical urgency, and logistic considerations of getting the donor organ and the recipient together within the time limitations of safe organ preservation. The system went into effect in western Pennsylvania on January 1, 1986.[9] Although initially adopted by UNOS on November 1, 1987, the point system never went into effect at the national level because of difficulties encountered in reconciling it to myriad local interests. A similar point system was developed for liver transplantation, having been in place at Pittsburgh since January 1987. Our experience with organ allocation based on point systems, in which organs go to those who have been waiting longer or who are sicker, has been most favorable.[10, 10a] Graft and patient survivals have not suffered by giving organs to sicker or older patients. At the same time, our observations provide some assurance that the concepts of equitable access and efficient use of a scarce societal resource are not mutually exclusive.

Human leukocyte antigen (HLA) matching is not a critical issue for extrarenal organs. However, we routinely perform HLA typing on all extrarenal organs, a practice that is at variance with what most other institutions do in this country. Although it is expensive, we consider it important because it allows us to determine the presence of microchimerism in the recipient, information that may be extremely useful in the future when deciding how to manage the immunosuppression.[71]

When the recipients for all the abdominal and thoracic organs are identified, an operating room (OR) time in the donor hospital is arranged. The procurement coordinator contacts the recipient institutions to arrange for the simultaneous arrival of all the harvesting teams. Kidneys have been procured by local teams for many years and shipped if not used locally. Today, a similar practice is being adopted in the United States for other organs, particularly livers.[72]

The intestinal donor should receive intravenous ampicillin and cefotaxime at the appropriate doses when first evaluated and every 6 hours after that. The last dose is given in the OR at the time of harvesting. Also, polyethylene glycol-electrolyte solution (GoLYTELY) is administered through the nasogastric tube to flush the intestine. The total amount ranges from 250 to 2000 mL, depending on the recipient's body size (250 mL in the infant and 2000 mL in the adult) and the administration rate is 10 to 30 mL/min. After the intestinal flushing, an antibiotic mixture that includes polymyxin E (100 mg), tobramycin (80 mg), and amphotericin B (500 mg) is given through the nasogastric tube every 4 hours until procurement. In pediatric donors, the doses are halved, whereas infants receive only one fourth of the dose. Newborns receive no intestinal preparation. If preharvest flushing cannot be performed, this is done after procurement, using cold Ringer's lactate. Also, polymyxin B or kanamycin can be substituted for polymyxin E if the latter is not available at the donor hospital.

MULTIPLE ORGAN DONOR OPERATION

Anesthesia

The donor operation can be time consuming, and the role of the anesthesiologist is very important, especially if we compare the multiple organ procurement that is now usually performed with those carried out in the past, when the kidneys were often the only organs removed. A complete review of the anesthetic aspects of organ donation was recently published,[73] and we restrict ourselves to its salient points.

The goal of medical management during organ procurement is to avoid ischemic organ damage by optimizing organ perfusion. Therefore, care of the donor is a continuation of the intensive care that was provided before brain death (see Chapter 177). The most important issue is the clear communication between the members of the procurement team because the surgical procedure and procurement protocol may differ depending on the procurement team and the specific organ. For the preoperative evaluation of the donor, the anesthesiologist should review the medical and surgical histories, including the cause of brain death, condition and supportive measures of vital organs, drug allergies, and medications. Cardiopulmonary function is assessed by means of the hemodynamic profile, requirement of inotropic support, efficiency of gas exchange, degree of ventilatory support, chest radiograph, electrocardiogram, arterial blood gas tensions, and acid-base state. Renal function is evaluated by urine output, BUN, and serum levels of creatinine and electrolytes. Hepatic function is evaluated by AST, ALT, and bilirubin, and pancreatic function is evaluated by blood glucose level and serum amylase. Hemoglobin concentration and the blood type of the donor are identified to prepare blood products. In addition, the validity of brain death certification, consent from family members, and permission from the coroner are verified. The transition from the ICU to the OR is a crucial period, and the donor is continuously monitored, ventilated, and treated.

Intraoperative care of the donor is essentially similar to that of other critically ill patients undergoing major surgery, although management of pathophysiologic changes unique to the donor should be clearly understood. In general, equipment and medications routinely available for general anesthesia are satisfactory for the management of donors. However, a volume ventilator may be needed for donors requiring high levels of PEEP or airway pressure. The OR should be kept warm, and a warming blanket and blood warmer are necessary to prevent hypothermia. A large volume of crystalloids and colloid solutions (e.g., 5% albumin, plasma protein fraction, or hetastarch) and five units of packed red blood cells should be prepared. The electrocardiogram is monitored, preferably using lead V_5, to detect arrhythmias or myocardial ischemia, particularly in heart donors. Blood pressure is monitored by an indwelling catheter in the radial artery or brachial artery. The femoral artery cannulation is avoided because the aorta will be cross-clamped. Central venous pressure (CVP) monitoring is essential,[74] and a pulmonary arterial catheter is useful in unstable donors. Two-dimensional transesophageal echocardiography may be used to assess preload and cardiac contractility in unstable heart donors. Urine output and body temperature are monitored, and all or some of the following laboratory tests may be needed: hemoglobin and hematocrit, arterial blood gas tensions and acid-base state, serum electrolytes, ionized calcium, lactate, and blood glucose level.

General anesthetics are required to blunt sympathetic response that occurs during surgery.[75] This so-called mass reflex is caused by neurogenic vasoconstriction and stimulation of the adrenal medulla by the spinal reflex arc and manifests as tachycardia hypertension, perspiration, and involuntary movements. These movements, also known as "Lazarus sign" (includes arm and hand movements toward the body) can be very disturbing to those involved in the organ recovery, and muscle relaxants should be administered ahead of time.

Isoflurane is the agent of choice because the degree of myocardial depression is less than with other inhalation agents. Halothane is avoided in liver donors because hepatotoxicity may be a concern in the presence of potential hepatic ischemia. Enflurane is avoided in kidney donors because it increases the blood level of inorganic fluoride. Short-acting narcotics such as fentanyl (5–10 μg/kg) may be used in hemodynamically unstable donors. In addition, muscle relaxants (pancuronium bromide, 0.05–0.1 mg/kg, or vecuronium bromide, 0.05–0.1 mg/kg) are required to provide satisfactory abdominal muscle relaxation and to abolish involuntary movements. Other pharmacologic interventions include systemic heparinization (300–500 U/kg) before cannulation of the aorta, mannitol (0.25–0.5 g/kg), and furosemide (40 mg) to induce diuresis before division of the renal pedicle and prevent ischemia-induced acute tubular necrosis.[76–78] Alpha-adrenergic receptor blockers, such as phenoxybenzamine hydrochloride, may be used to promote renal vasodilation and prevent vasospasm.[79] However, these blockers are not recommended in multiple organ procurement because their effects on other organs are unknown. Prophylactic administration of antibiotics such as broad-spectrum cephalosporins is recommended by some centers,[80, 81] although its efficacy is controversial.[44, 82]

Specific goals of ventilatory care are to maintain a PaO_2 between 70 and 100 mm Hg, an oxygen saturation of arterial hemoglobin greater than 95%, and a partial pressure of arterial carbon dioxide within the range of 35 to 45 mm Hg to avoid pulmonary complications. In hypothermic donors, a mild respiratory alkalosis (pH 7.4–7.5) may be preferred to improve tissue perfusion.[83, 84] This goal frequently is achieved by ventilating with a tidal volume of 10 to 15 mL/kg, a respiratory rate of fewer than 20 breaths per minute, FIO_2 of 30% to 40%, and a low level of PEEP (<5 cm H_2O). However, when pulmonary complications interfere with gas exchange, the tidal volume is increased up to 20 mL/kg, the respiratory rate is increased up to 20 breaths per minute, and the PEEP is increased up to 10 cm H_2O. In general, an increase in FIO_2 is preferred to an excessive tidal volume and high PEEP to maintain venous return and splanchnic blood flow.

The goal of circulatory care is to preserve perfusion of all organs that are to be procured by maintaining systolic blood pressure between 100 and 120 mm Hg, with a CVP less than 10 cm H_2O and minimal vasopressor support.[48, 85, 86] Hypotension (systolic blood pressure <80 mm Hg or mean arterial pressure <40 mm Hg) is associated with an increased incidence of acute tubular necrosis and nonfunction of the donor kidneys[87, 88] as well as poor function of the liver.[89] However, maintaining a satisfactory blood pressure is difficult to achieve at times because of altered circulatory physiology in the brain-dead donors. Preload frequently is decreased because of blood loss, vasomotor paralysis, diuretic therapy, or diabetes insipidus. Tachycardia, bradycardia, and arrhythmias caused by massive sympathetic discharge are not unusual, and myocardial contractility frequently is impaired by myocytolysis, coronary spasm, and reduction of myocardial energy storage.[90] Afterload may be increased by excessive sympathetic tone or decreased by vasomotor paralysis.

Intravascular volume is adjusted with the guidance of the CVP (<10 cm H_2O). Fluid deficit is corrected with the infusion of a balanced electrolyte solution (e.g., lactated Ringer's) or a colloid solution (5% albumin or hetastarch).[91] Urine output and insensible losses are replaced by a hypotonic solution with glucose (e.g., 5% dextrose in 0.45% sodium chloride [NaCl], 1 $mL \cdot kg^{-1} \cdot h^{-1}$). Adjustment of intravascular volume may decrease the need for vasopressors in many cases,[92] but acute volume expansion may increase myocardial oxygen consumption, congestive heart failure, arrhythmias, and the need for inotropic support because the compliance of the heart is decreased in most donors.[88] Excessive urine output (>200–250 mL/h) is replaced by a hypotonic electrolyte solution with supplementation of potassium chloride (KCl, 20 mmol/L). When hypotension persists even after adequate volume replacement, vasopressors may be required. Dopamine hydrochloride (2–5 $\mu g \cdot kg^{-1} \cdot min^{-1}$ and up to 10 $\mu g \cdot kg^{-1} \cdot min^{-1}$) is the first choice to improve cardiac contractility. Other inotropes include dobutamine hydrochloride (2–10 $\mu g \cdot kg^{-1} \cdot min^{-1}$) and isoproterenol hydrochloride (0.1–1 $\mu g \cdot kg^{-1} \cdot min^{-1}$), but these drugs may dilate peripheral vascular beds, decreasing blood pressure. Alpha vasopressors (phenylephrine hydrochloride, norepinephrine bitartrate, or metaraminol bitartrate) are avoided because they may decrease splanchnic and coronary blood flow.[93, 94] In addition, the oxygen-carrying capacity to the peripheral tissues is improved by transfusion of packed red blood cells (1–3 U) to maintain the hematocrit between 25% and 30%.[95]

Severe cases of tachycardia and hypertension caused by the mass reflex may be controlled by the administration of general anesthetics, a beta antagonist, such as labetalol hydrochloride or esmolol hydrochloride, or a calcium channel blocker, such as verapamil hydrochloride.[63] Occasionally, an α-blocker such as hydralazine or sodium nitroprusside may be given to reduce afterload. Supraventricular or ventricular arrhythmias are treated with conventional antiarrhythmic drugs. Circulatory arrest, which occurs in 10% of potential donors and in 66% of referred donors,[96] is treated according to conventional circulatory resuscitative measures, but if bradycardia is a concern, a direct-acting agent such as isoproterenol or epinephrine is used because donors are unresponsive to centrally acting chronotropic drugs, such as atropine.

Progressive hypothermia, which is seen in up to 86% of donors because of the loss of hypothalamic function,[48] results in sinus bradycardia, atrioventricular dissociation, and ventricular arrhythmias. At a temperature lower than 28°C, prolonged PR and QT intervals and wide QRS complexes are replaced by T-wave inversion, ST-segment depression, and rise of ventricular fibrillation. Other effects of hypothermia are a leftward shift in the hemoglobin-oxygen dissociation curve, an increase in blood viscosity, decrease in splanchnic blood flow and glomerular filtration, hyperglycemia, and metabolic and respiratory acidosis. Body temperature is kept within the normal range (>35°C) by increasing the room temperature, infusing all fluids through a blood warmer, and using a warming blanket and a heated humidifier in the inspiratory limb of the ventilation circuit.

Adequate diuresis (>0.5 $mL \cdot kg^{-1} \cdot h^{-1}$, preferably 1 to 1.5 $mL \cdot kg^{-1} \cdot h^{-1}$) is important because urine output is an indirect indication of preload and is a prognostic indicator for renal graft and hepatic function.[97] The administration of fluid or dopamine may be effective in maintaining adequate renal perfusion and diuresis. However, a high dose of dopamine (>10 $\mu g \cdot kg^{-1} \cdot min^{-1}$) may lead to acute tubular necrosis and nonfunction of the renal graft.[87] For persistent oliguria, furosemide (1–2 mg/kg) and mannitol (0.5 g/kg) may be administered. Diabetes insipidus, caused by a nonfunctioning pituitary gland, results in polyuria, hypovolemia, and electrolyte imbalance. Excessive urine output is replaced with a hypotonic solution (0.45% NaCl with KCl, 20 mmol/L), and supplemental antidiuretic hormone is administered to maintain urine output in the range of 100 to 250 mL/h. The synthetic analog of vasopressin, desmopressin acetate (DDAVP), is preferred (0.5–1 U/h) because of its long duration of action and a low pressor/antidiuretic effect ratio.[98] However, the pressor activity in excessive doses of desmopressin acetate may increase the risk of acute tubular necrosis[99] and reduce hepatic blood flow.[100] Desmopressin acetate increases the sensitivity to catecholamines,[100] and catecholamine doses should be reduced when desmopressin acetate is given to the donor. Hyperglycemia is a complication of diabetes insipidus and is treated by an infusion of insulin (5–10 U).

Metabolic acidosis caused by inadequate tissue perfusion may be compounded by respiratory acidosis. Because of potential myocardial depression, metabolic acidosis is corrected by administration of sodium bicarbonate. When hypernatremia is a concern, tromethamine, or tris(hydroxymethyl) aminomethane (THAM) may be used (0.3 mol THAM [mL] = body weight [kg] × base deficit [mmol/L]) instead of sodium bicarbonate. Electrolyte imbalances (hypernatremia, hypokalemia, hypocalcemia, hypophosphatemia, and hypomagnesemia) caused by fluid shifts and diabetes insipidus may result in arrhythmias and myocardial dysfunction. Hypernatremia and hypokalemia are treated by administration of a hyponatremic solution (0.45% NaCl) and KCl (20 mmol/L). Ionized hypocalcemia caused by large blood transfusions is corrected by the administration of calcium chloride or calcium gluconate to preserve cardiac contractility. Hypomagnesemia is treated with magnesium sulfate (50 mg/kg) also to preserve myocardial contractility.[101] Glucose metabolism is relatively well maintained, although hyperglycemia may occur as the result of a decreased level of insulin and as a complication of diabetes insipidus. Serum levels of triiodothyronine, insulin, and cortisol are low in animal models, and the administration of triiodothyronine improves hemodynamic stability by maintaining myocardial stores of energy and glycogen. However, the beneficial role of triiodothyronine is unclear in clinical settings.[49, 65]

Coagulopathy may occur in organ donors. Dilutional coagulopathy is caused by the shift of intravascular volume, consumption coagulopathy may result from the release of tissue thromboplastin from injured tissues and the ischemic organs, and fibrinolysis results from intravascular coagulation or the release of tissue plasminogen activator from the ischemic tissues. Disseminated intravascular coagulation has been reported in 80% of donors with head injury,[102] but its clinical significance is unknown. Coagulation abnormalities are treated conservatively.

Once cardioplegia is induced, no further supportive care is necessary. After cross-clamping of the aorta (the time is recorded by the procurement coordinator [Fig. 178–3]), mechanical ventilation and monitoring are discontinued, and all cannulas are removed. The organs are swiftly removed in the following sequence: heart, lungs, liver, pancreas, intestine, and kidneys. No supportive care is needed for procurement of corneas or bones because these tissues tolerate a prolonged ischemia without significant injury.

Donor Operation

Before starting a multiple organ procurement, it is mandatory that the different surgical teams discuss the techniques and sequence they want to adopt. A detailed discussion of the surgical procedure is critical because, after aortic cross-clamping, time is of the essence. Everything should proceed as smoothly and expeditiously as possible to minimize organ damage. The basic principle of any donor operation is the core cooling of the organs to be removed. Cooling of a solid organ at the time of donor circulatory arrest was described for experimental liver transplantation 35 years ago.[103] It was then promptly applied to kidney preservation in clinical transplantation,[104] and it still represents the single most important aspect of any organ preservation technique.

Recovery Data — Donor ID#

Surgeons Renal: ______ Assisting: ______

Hepatic: ______ ______

Cardiac: ______ ______

Heart/Lung: ______ ______

Pancreas: ______ ______

Coordinators/Technicians (Tissue): ______ ______

______ ______

In O.R. ______ AM/PM Incision ______ AM/PM Depart O.R. (0) ______ AM/PM Depart O.R. (T) ______ AM/PM

Condition During Surgery (include: Blood Pressure, Urine Output, Complications, Comments)

______

______

______

Operating Room Drugs (include dosage and time)

Methyprednisolone: ______ Mannitol: ______ Furosemide: ______

Heparin: ______ Vasodilator: ______ Blood Products ______

Antibiotics: ______ Others: ______

Nephrectomy Data

En Bloc: Y/N In Situ: Y/N

Flush Sol'n: ______ Vol: ______

Final Flush (Sol'n Vol): ______

Storage Sol'n: ______

	R	L
Art Clamp:	______	______
Flush Start	______	______
Flush End:	______	______
Warm Ischemia Time	______	______
Clamps Off:	______	______
Cold Ischemia Time	______	______

Hepatectomy Data

Precool Start ______

Sol'n/Vol: ______

Portal Flush Start: ______

Sol'n/Vol: ______

Aortic Flush Start: ______

Sol'n/Vol: ______

Final Flush (Sol'n/Vol) ______

Clamps Off: ______

Cold Ischemia Time ______

Anatomy: ______

______

Cardiectomy Data

Infusion Start: ______

Sol'n/Vol. ______

Clamps Off: ______

Cold Ischemia Time ______

Heart Lung Data

Infusion Start (R) ______

Sol'nVol: ______

Infusion Start (L) ______

Sol'n/Vol: ______

Clamps Off: ______

Cold Ischemia Time ______

Single or Double Lung Data

Infusion Start: ______

Sol'n/Vol. ______

Clamps Off: ______

Cold Ischemia Time ______

Pancreas Data

Infusion Start: ______

Sol'n/Vol. ______

Final Flush; (Sol'n/Vol) ______

Clamps Off: ______

Cold Ischemia Time ______

Anatomy ______

Renal Anatomy

R ______ L ______

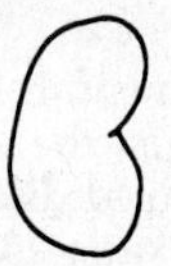

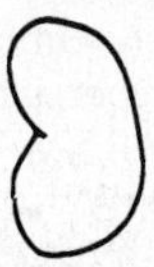

Biopsy Results: ______

Organs and Tissues Recovered (Check appropriate box and circle "T" for Transplant, "R" for Research)

☐ **R-KI** T/R ☐ **L-KI** T/R ☐ **LI** T/R ☐ **LU** T/R ☐ **PA** T/R ☐ **HR** T/R ☐ **HV** T/R ☐ **MV** T/R ☐ **Bones** T/R

☐ **BM** T/R ☐ **Veins** T/R ☐ **Skin** T/R ☐ **Cornea** T/R ☐ **INT** T/R ☐ **Other** T/R

Figure 178–3. Intraoperative data collection sheet used by the Western Pennsylvania Organ Procurement Organization, CORE. (Courtesy of Brian Broznick.)

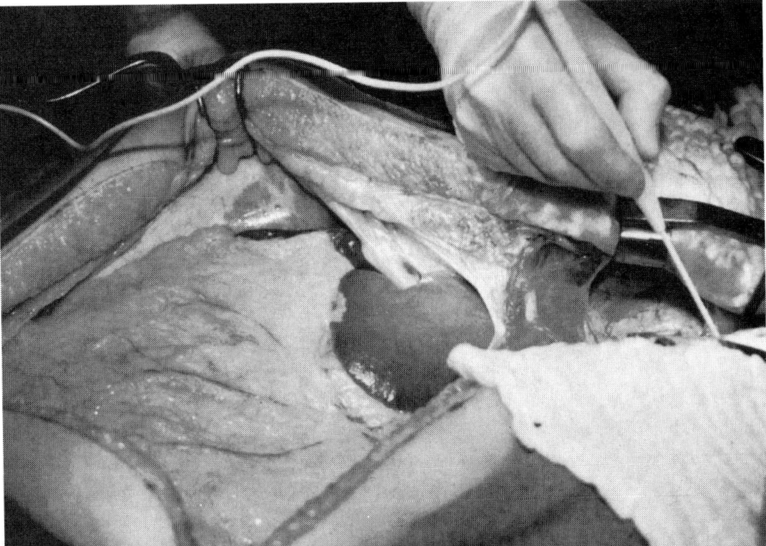

Figure 178–4. Intraoperative photograph showing the total midline incision used for multiple organ procurement. (See Color Plate Section of this textbook.) (Courtesy of Andrei Stieber, MD.)

The first solution used was chilled Ringer's lactate, replaced in the late 1960s by the so-called Collins' solution, characterized by an electrolyte composition close to the intracellular one.[105] This solution was successfully used for about 20 years until the introduction of the University of Wisconsin solution,[106, 107] which extended the duration of organ viability. The easiest way to achieve almost immediate internal core cooling of the donor organs is by in situ infusion of the preservation solution, chilled to 4°C, at the time of the circulatory arrest. The remaining technical aspects of organ retrieval are secondary to this critical maneuver.

The surgical procedure for multiple cadaveric organ pro-

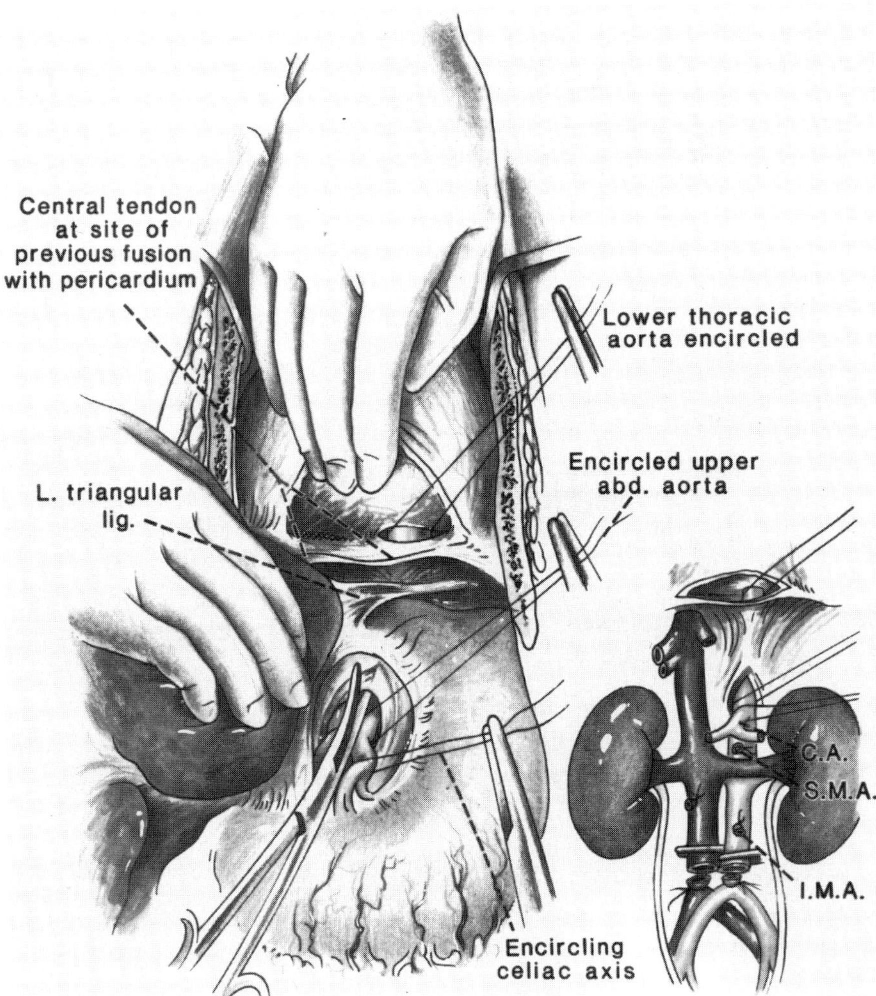

Figure 178–5. The aorta is dissected and encircled just above (or, alternatively, just below) the diaphragm. *Abbreviations*: L. triangular lig. = left triangular ligament; Encircled upper abd. aorta = encircled upper abdominal aorta; C.A. = celiac axis; S.M.A. = superior mesenteric artery; I.M.A. = inferior mesenteric artery. (See Color Plate Section of this textbook.)

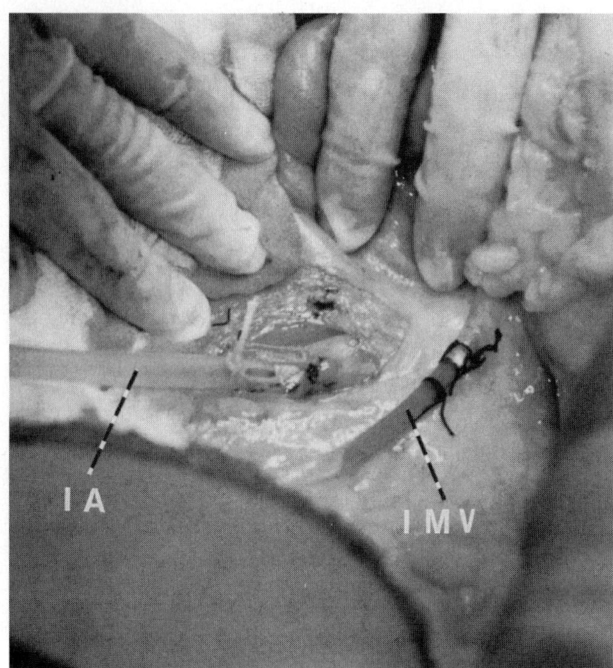

Figure 178–6. Intraoperative photograph showing the donor inferior mesenteric vein (IMV) and the infrarenal aorta (IA) dissected and cannulated for the cold perfusion. (See Color Plate Section of this textbook.) (Courtesy of Andrei Stieber, MD.)

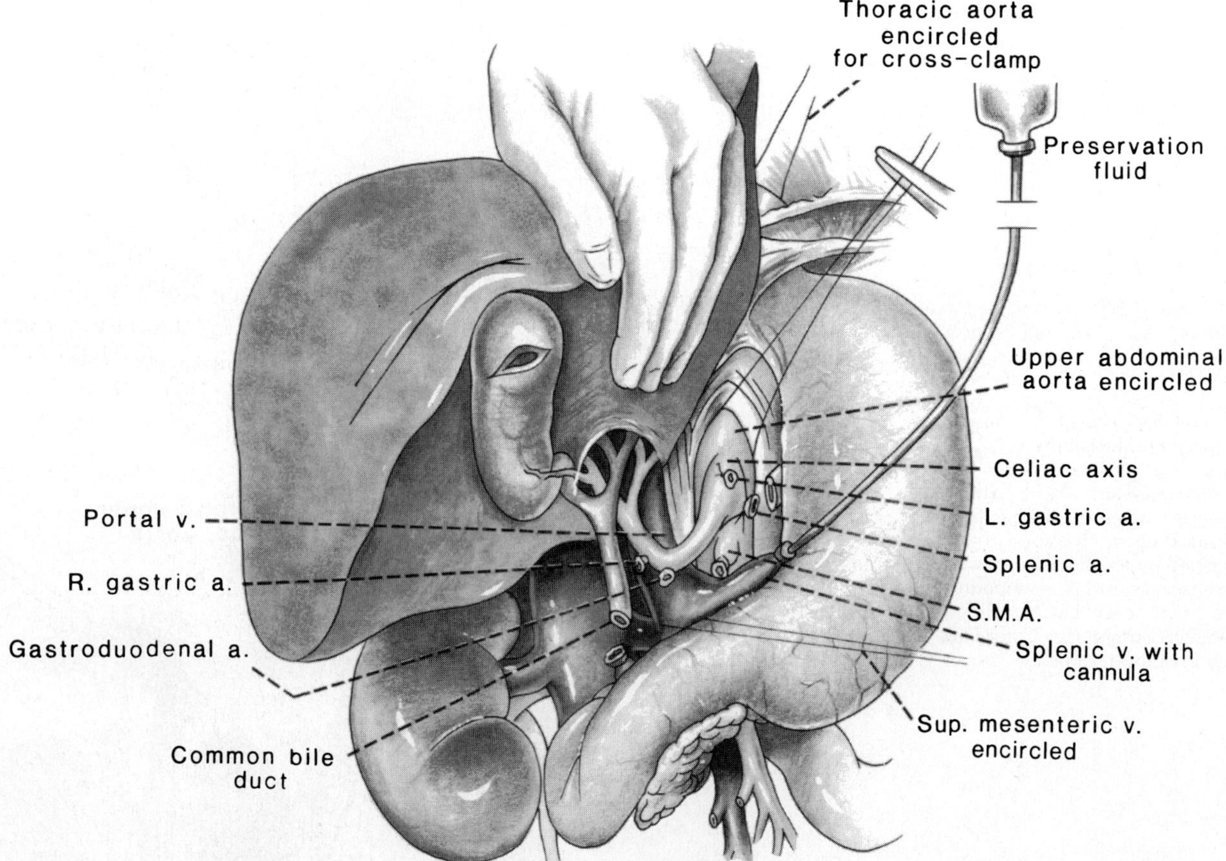

Figure 178–7. Liver hilar dissection, transection of the common bile duct, and incision of the gallbladder fundus to prevent autolysis of the mucosa of the biliary tract. In this drawing, the splenic vein is cannulated; however, the inferior mesenteric vein can be cannulated alternatively, as shown in Figure 178–6. *Abbreviations*: Portal v. = portal vein; R. gastric a. = right gastric artery; Gastroduodenal a. = gastroduodenal artery; L. gastric a. = left gastric artery; Splenic a. = splenic artery; S.M.A. = superior mesenteric artery; Splenic v. with cannula = splenic vein with cannula; Sup. mesenteric v. encircled = superior mesenteric vein encircled. (See Color Plate Section of this textbook.)

curement has undergone a progressive evolution. In 1984, when procurement of extrarenal organs was becoming more common, a technique was published by the Pittsburgh group[108] that required a meticulous in vivo dissection of the donor organs and extensive manipulation of the abdominal viscera. A subsequent refinement of this technique was introduced in 1986.[109] This improved technique is the method in use today, and it is basically characterized by a "no-touch en bloc removal" of the core cooled solid organs. The technical details of this operation lie outside the scope of this chapter, and we only describe the major points.

A complete midline incision is performed from the suprasternal notch to the pubis (Fig. 178–4). As soon as the thoracic and abdominal organs are visualized, the procurement coordinator collects the first information on the appearance of the donor organs and relays it to the local OPO so that they can be made available to the recipient teams. The aorta is then exposed and encircled either immediately above or below the diaphragm (Fig. 178–5). The inferior mesenteric vein is encircled and cannulated for infusion of the cold portal perfusate. The aorta is then dissected for 2 cm at the level of the origin of the inferior mesenteric artery, which is tied and divided. The aorta is encircled at this level and prepared for cannulation. Figure 178–6 shows the donor inferior mesenteric vein and the infrarenal aorta cannulated for the cold perfusate. The common bile duct is tied distally and transected close to the upper margin of the duodenum, and the gallbladder is incised and washed free of bile to prevent autolysis of the mucosa of the biliary tract. The arterial anatomy of the liver should be carefully examined for possible anomalies. Prior knowledge of any anomaly will be extremely helpful in preventing mistakes during organ removal. At this point the basic initial dissection is completed (Fig. 178–7), and the thoracic team prepares the chest organs for removal. The pleural spaces are opened widely after initial mediastinal dissection. Very little initial dissection is done around the inferior and superior vena cava and aorta other than to place sutures for the expected cannulation of the aorta for cardioplegia or the main pulmonary artery if the lungs are being harvested as well. The lungs are quickly examined through the pleural spaces, and very little dissection is required thereafter. It should be noted that the donor's heart so far has continued beating spontaneously and maintained circulation of all organs.

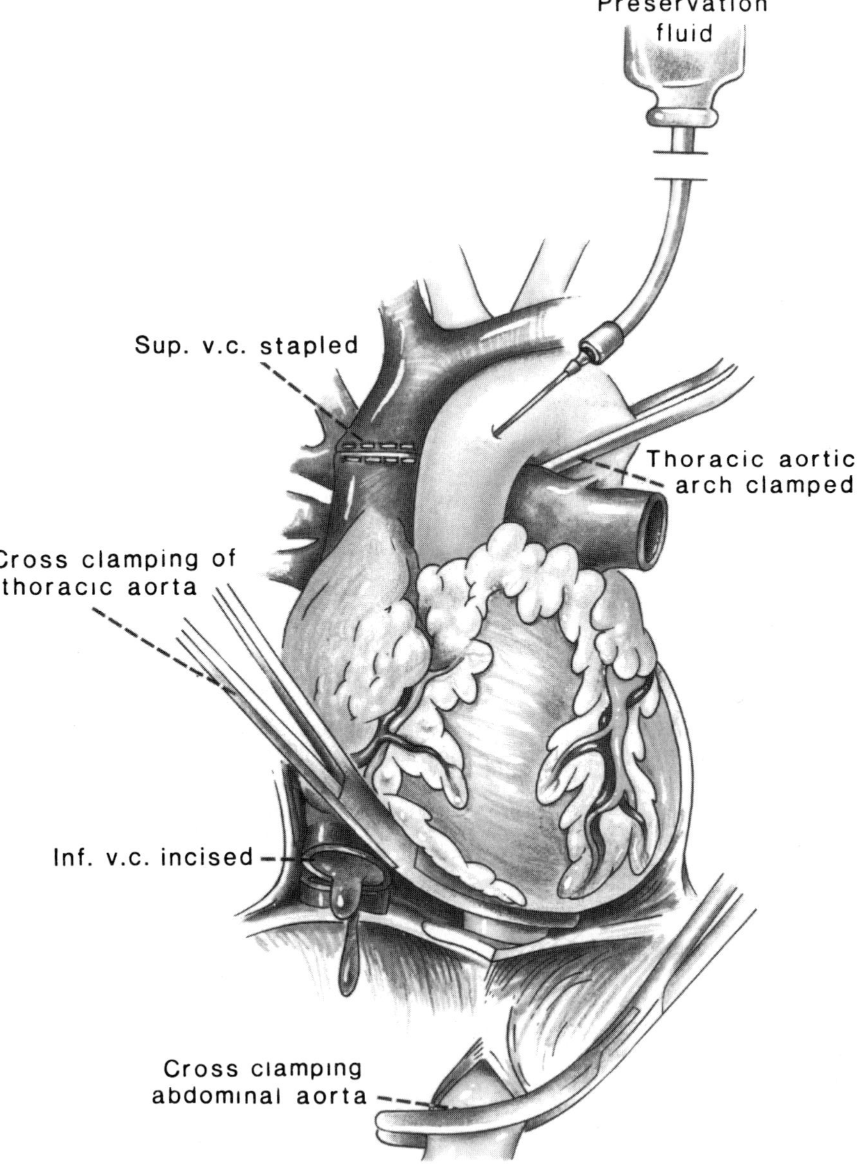

Figure 178–8. Occlusion of the superior vena cava inflow and simultaneous clamping of the aorta proximal to the innominate artery. The aorta is also simultaneously clamped just above or below the diaphragm. Cardioplegic solution infused through the ascending aorta is allowed to run only in the heart. *Abbreviations*: Sup. v.c. stapled = superior vena cava stapled; Inf. v.c. incised = inferior vena cava incised. (See Color Plate Section of this textbook.)

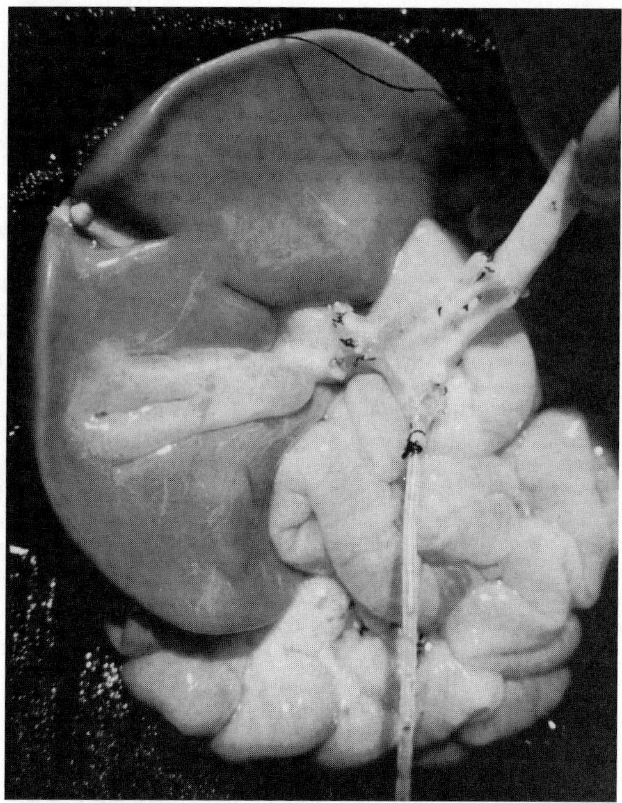

Figure 178–9. En bloc harvesting of liver and small bowel from a pediatric donor. (See Color Plate Section of this textbook.)

As soon as the thoracic team completes their dissection, 300 to 500 U/kg of heparin are given intravenously, and the aorta is cannulated after ligating it distal to the inferior mesenteric artery (see Fig. 178–6). The thoracic team then occludes the superior vena cava, and the aorta is simultaneously clamped proximal to the innominate artery and just above or below the diaphragm (Fig. 178–8). The cold infusion is started, the inferior vena cava is vented, and the heart is separately perfused with cold cardioplegic solution. The heart is removed first. If the lungs are being harvested simultaneously, cold flush is started through the pulmonary artery, venting the solution through the left atrial appendage. Once cardioplegic solution has been administered, the aorta is transected, and the rest of the lung perfusion solution is allowed to drain through the open aorta. Mediastinal dissecton is then carried out, removing the lungs and heart en bloc if the block is to be used for a heart-lung transplant. The more common situation is one in which the heart is harvested by one group and lungs are to be used for separate transplants. In this situation, once the cardioplegia and lung perfusion have been completed, the heart is carefully dissected by the two teams, ensuring that enough pulmonary artery and left atrial cuff remain on both the heart and the lungs, making them both available for transplantation. Once the heart has been removed, the lung team can then proceed with extraction of the lungs.

During this phase, the abdominal organs are untouched while they are exsanguinated and the cold perfusion is continued. After removal of the thoracic organs, the abdominal team proceeds with the final dissection and removal of the liver, pancreas, intestine, and kidneys. The technical steps have been outlined elsewhere by us[47, 108–111] and others.[112–114] After the organ recovery, long segments of the iliac arteries and veins, inferior vena cava, and aorta[115] (and carotid arteries in children) should always be removed and stored under hypothermic conditions. This ensures the ability to deal with all possible vascular problems that might be encountered during the recipient operations.[115–119a]

With the development of the intestinal and multivisceral transplant program at the University of Pittsburgh (see Chapter 185), a technique was developed for the removal of essentially the entire abdominal visceral bloc (Fig. 178–9).[47, 119b] Anatomic considerations are fundamental during intestinal and multivisceral procurement because recipients require different types of intestinal transplantation (isolated small bowel, liver and small bowel, true multivisceral, and so on) based on different disease and needs.[119b] These procurement techniques do not interfere with those of other organs. In our first 35 intestinal donor operations, there were 62 kidneys, 35 livers, 18 hearts, and 3 lungs procured simultaneously.[47]

At the end of the operation, the procurement coordinator completes the form shown in Figure 178–3. These data are of critical importance for the recipient operations and subsequent follow-up of the transplanted patients, which are the endpoints of a successful multiple organ procurement.

ACKNOWLEDGMENT

This research was aided by research grants from the Veterans Administration and National Institutes of Health project grant no. DK 29961.

References

1. Data from United Network for Organ Sharing Research Department. UNOS Update 1992; 8:20–27.
2. Evans RW, Orians CE, Ascher NL: The potential supply of organ donors. JAMA 1992; 267:239–246.
3. Garrison RN, Bentley FR, Raque GH, et al: There is an answer to the shortage of organ donors. Surg Gynecol Obstet 1991; 173:391–396.
4. UNOS Update 1993; 9:23.
5. Evans RW: Organ procurement expenditures and the role of financial incentives. JAMA 1993; 269:3113–3118.
6. Orians CE, Evans RW, Ascher NL: Estimates of organ-specific donor availability for the United States. Transplant Proc 1993; 25:1541–1542.
7. Campbell JR, Layne JA: The donor dilemma: The lifelink foundation approach. UNOS Update 1993; 9:16.
8. Donation and Transplantation: Medical School Curriculum. Richmond, VA, UNOS, 1992.
9. Starzl TE, Shapiro R, Teperman L: The point system for organ distribution. Transplant Proc 1989; 21(Suppl 3):3432–3436.
10. Eghtesad B, Bronsther O, Starzl TE, et al: Disease gravity and urgency of need as guidelines for liver allocation. Hepatology 1994; 20:56S–62S.
10a. Marino IR, Doyle HR, Rakela J, et al: Orthotopic liver transplantation: Indications and results. *In*: Diseases of the Biliary Tract and Pancreas. Hess W, Cirenei, A, Rohner A, et al (Eds). Padua, Italy, Piccin Publisher, 1994 (in press).
11. Galletti PM: Bioartificial organs. J Artif Org 1992; 16:55–60.
12. Caplan A: Must I be my brother's keeper? Ethical issues in the use of living donors as sources of liver and other solid organs. Transplant Proc 1993; 25:1997–2000.
13. Kirchner SA: Living related lung transplantation: A new observation in single lung transplantation. AORN J 1991; 54:712–714.
14. Cooper DKC, Kemp E, Reemtsma K, et al (Eds): Xenotransplantation: The Transplantation of Organs and Tissues Between Species. Berlin, Springer-Verlag, 1991.
15. Starzl TE, Fung J, Tzakis A, et al: Baboon to human liver transplantation. Lancet 1993; 341:65–71.
16. Starzl TE, Tzakis A, Fung JJ, et al: Human liver xenotransplantation. Xeno. A Review of Xenotransplantation and Related Topics 1993; 1:4–7.

17. Marino IR, Tzakis AG, Fung JJ, et al: Liver xenotransplantation. *In*: Surgical Technology International. Braverman MH, Tawes RL (Eds). San Francisco, Surgical Technology International, Thomas F. Laszlo Publisher, 1993, pp 139–144.
18. Anaise D, Rapaport FT. Use of non-heart-beating cadaver donors in clinical organ transplantation logistics, ethics and legal consideration. Transplant Proc 1993; 25:2153–2155.
19. Ad Hoc Committee of the Harvard Medical School: A definition of irreversible coma. Report of the Ad Hoc Committee of the Harvard Medical School to examine the definition of brain death. JAMA 1968; 205:337–340.
20. Guidelines for the determination of death: Report of the medical consultants on the diagnosis of death to the President's Commission for the Study of Ethical Problems in Medicine and Biomedical and Behavioral Research. JAMA 1981; 246:2184–2186.
21. Childress J: Attitudes of major western religious traditions towards uses of the human body and its parts. *In*: Justice and the Holy: Essays in Honor of Walter Harrelson. Knight DA, Paris PJ (Eds). Atlanta, Scholar Press, 1989.
22. Pereira BJG, Levey AS, Kirkman RL: Hepatitis C-positive individuals are not suitable for organ donation. Transplant Immunol Lett 1993; 9:3–17.
23. Pruim J, Klompmaker IDSJ, Haagsma EB, et al: Selection criteria for liver donation: A review. Transplant Int 1993; 6:226–235.
24. Roth D: Hepatitis C-positive individuals are suitable for organ donation. Transplant Immunol Lett 1993; 9:2–6.
25. Fox AS, Tolpin MD, Baker AL, et al: Seropositivity in liver transplant recipients as a predictor of cytomegalovirus disease. J Infect Dis 1988; 157:383–385.
26. Haagsma EB, Klompmaker IJ, Grond J: Herpes virus infection after orthotopic liver transplantation. Transplant Proc 1987; 19:4054–4056.
27. Rakela J, Wiesner RH, Taswell HF, et al: Incidence of cytomegalovirus infection and its relationship to donor-recipient serologic status in liver transplantation. Transplant Proc 1987; 19:2399–2402.
28. Yanaga K, Kakizoe S, Ikeda T, et al: Procurement of liver allografts from non-heart beating donors. Transplant Proc 1990; 22:275–278.
29. Yanaga K, Tzakis AG, Starzl TE: Personal experience with procurement of 131 liver allografts. Transplant Int 1989; 2:137–142.
30. Teperman L, Podesta L, Mieles L, et al: The successful use of older donors for liver transplantation. JAMA 1989; 262:2837.
30a. Marino IR, Doyle HR, Doria C, et al: Outcome of liver transplantation using donors 60 to 79 years of age. Transplant Proc 1995 (in press).
31. Popper H: Aging and the liver. *In*: Progress in Liver Diseases. Vol 8. Popper H, Levy GL (Eds). New York, Grune & Stratton, 1985, pp 659–683.
32. Kakizoe S, Yanaga K, Starzl TE, et al: Frozen section of liver biopsy for the evaluation of liver allografts. Transplant Proc 1990; 22:416–417.
33. Kakizoe S, Yanaga K, Starzl TE, et al: Evaluation of protocol before transplantation and after reperfusion biopsies from human orthotopic liver allografts: Considerations of preservation and early immunological injury. Hepatology 1990; 11:932–941.
34. Adam R, Azourlay D, Astarciuglu I, et al: Reliability of the MEGX test in the selection of liver grafts. Transplant Proc 1991; 23:2470–2471.
35. Bowers JL, Teramoto K, Clouse ME: 31P NMR assessment of orthotopic liver transplant viability: The effect of warm ischemia (Abstract). Presented at the 10th Annual Meeting of the Society of Magnetic Resonance in Medicine, San Francisco, 1991.
36. Kanetsuna Y, Fujita S, Tojimbara T, et al: Usefulness of 31P-MRS as a method of evaluating the viability of preserved and transplanted rat liver. Transplant Int 1992; 5(Suppl 1):S379–S381.
37. Oellerich M, Burdelski M, Ringe B, et al: Lignocaine metabolite formation as a measure of pre-transplant liver function. Lancet 1989; 1:640–642.
38. Ozaki N, Gubernatis G, Ringe B, et al: Arterial blood ketone body ratio as an indicator for viability of donor livers. Transplant Proc 1991; 23:2487–2489.
39. Reding R, Feyaerts A, Wallemacq P, et al: Liver graft assessment in organ donors by the lidocaine monoethyglycinexylidide test is unreliable. Br J Surg 1992; 79(Suppl 1):S142.
40. Schroeder TJ, Gremse DA, Mansour ME, et al: Lidocaine metabolism as an index of liver function in hepatic transplant donors and recipients. Transplant Proc 1989; 21:2299–2301.
41. Yamaoka Y, Taki Y, Gubernatis G, et al: Evaluation of the liver graft before procurement: Significance of arterial ketone body ratio in brain-dead patients. Transplant Int 1990; 3:78–81.
42. Burdelski M, Oellerich M, Raude E, et al: A novel approach to assessment of liver function in donors. Transplant Proc 1988; 20(Suppl 1):591–593.
43. Makowka L, Gordon RD, Todo S, et al: Analysis of donor criteria for the prediction of outcome in clinical liver transplantation. Transplant Proc 1987; 19:2378–2382.
43a. Marino IR, Doyle HR, Aldrighetti L, et al: Effect of donor age and sex on the outcome of liver transplantation. Lancet (in press).
44. Stock PG, Najarian JS, Ascher NL: Liver transplantation. *In*: Critical Care State of the Art. Gallagher TJ, Shoemaker WC (Eds). Fullerton, CA, Society of Critical Care Medicine, 1988, pp 21–24.
45. Hesse UJ, Najarian JS, Sutherland DER: Amylase activity and pancreas transplants. Lancet 1985; 2:726–728.
46. Darby JM, Stein K, Grenvik A, et al: Approach to management of the heart beating brain dead organ donor. JAMA 1989; 261:2222–2228.
47. Furukawa H, Casavilla A, Kadry Z, et al: Basic considerations for the procurement of intestinal grafts. Proceedings of the Third International Symposium on Small Bowel Transplantation, Paris, November 3–6, 1993.
48. Griepp RB, Stinson EB, Clark DA, et al: The cardiac donor. Surg Gynecol Obstet 1971; 133:792–798.
49. Novitzky D, Cooper DKC, Reichart B: Hemodynamic and metabolic responses to hormonal therapy in brain dead potential organ donors. Transplantation 1987; 43:852–854.
50. Copeland JG, Emery RW, Levinson MM, et al: Selection of patients for cardiac transplantation. Circulation 1987; 75:2–9.
51. Renlund DG, Bristow MR, Lee HR, et al: Medical aspects of cardiac transplantation. J Cardiothorac Anesth 1988; 2:500–512.
52. Stoddard MF, Logaker RA: The role of transesophageal echocardiography in cardiac donor screening. Am Heart J 1993; 125:1676–1681.
53. Lammermeier DE, Sweeney MS, Haupt HE, et al: Use of potentially infected donor hearts for cardiac transplantation. Ann Thorac Surg 1990; 50:222–225.
54. Luciani GB, Livi U, Faggian G, et al: Clinical results of heart transplantation in recipients over 55. J Heart Lung Transplant 1992; 11:1177–1183.
55. Pflugfelder PW, Singh NR, McKenzie FN, et al: Extending cardiac allograft ischemic time and donor age: Effect on survival and long-term cardiac function. J Cardiovasc Surg (Torino) 1991; 32:46–49.
56. Menkis AH, Novick RJ, Kostuk WJ, et al: Successful use of the "unacceptable" heart donor. J Heart Lung Transplant 1991; 10:28–32.
57. Sweeney MS, Lammermeier DE, Frazier OH, et al: Extension of donor criteria in cardiac transplantation: Surgical risk versus supply-side economics. Ann Thorac Surg 1990; 50:7–10.
58. Harjula A, Starnes VA, Oyer PE, et al: Proper donor selection for heart-lung transplantation. J Thorac Cardiovasc Surg 1987; 94:874–880.
59. Tarazi RY, Bonser RS, Jamieson SW: Heart-lung transplantation. *In*: Critical Care State of the Art. Gallagher TJ (Ed). Fullerton, CA, Society of Critical Care Medicine, 1988, pp 55–72.
60. Todd RJ: Pulmonary transplantation. *In*: Critical Care State of the Art. Gallagher TJ (Ed). Fullerton, CA, Society of Critical Care Medicine, 1988, pp 41–53.
61. Detterbeck FC, Mill MR, Williams W, et al: Organ donation and the management of the multiple organ donor. Contemp Surg 1993; 42:281–285.
62. Soifer BE, Gelb AW: The multiple organ donor: Identification and management. Ann Intern Med 1989; 110:814–823.

63. Novitzky D, Wicomb WN, Cooper DKC, et al: Electrocardiographic, hemodynamic, and endocrine changes occurring during experimental brain death in the Chacma baboon. J Heart Transplant 1984; 4:63–69.
64. Pennefather SH, Bullock RE: Triiodothyronine treatment in brain-dead multiorgan donors: A controlled study. Transplantation 1993; 55:1443.
65. Macoviak JA, McDougall IR, Bayer MF, et al: Significance of thyroid dysfunction in human cardiac allograft procurement. Transplantation 1987; 43:824–826.
66. Gifford RRM, Weaver AS, Burg JE, et al: Thyroid hormone levels in heart and kidney cadaver donors. J Heart Transplant 1986; 5:249–253.
67. Wahlers T, Fieguth HG, Jurmann M, et al: Does hormone depletion of organ donors impair myocardial function after cardiac transplantation? Transplant Proc 1988; 20(Suppl 1):792–794.
68. Nygaard CE, Townsend RN, Diamond DL: Organ donor management and organ outcome: A six-year review from a level I trauma center. J Trauma 1990; 30:728–732.
69. Bodenham A, Park GR: Care of the multiple organ donor. Intensive Care Med 1989; 15:340–348.
70. Novitzky D, Cooper DKC, Morrell D, et al: Change from aerobic to anaerobic metabolism after brain death, and reversal following triiodothyronine therapy. Transplantation 1988; 45:32–36.
71. Starzl TE, Demetris AJ, Trucco M, et al: Cell migration and chimerism after whole organ transplantation: The basis of graft acceptance. Hepatology 1993; 17:1127–1152.
72. Miller CM, Teodorescu V, Harrington M, et al: Regional procurement and export of hepatic allografts for transplantation. Mt Sinai J Med 1990; 57:93–96.
73. Kang YG, Kormos RL, Casavilla A: Organ procurement from donors with brain death. *In*: Trauma Anesthesia and Critical Care. Grande C (Ed). Philadelphia, WB Saunders, 1993, pp 1013–1024.
74. Luksza AR: Brain-dead kidney donor: Selection, care, and administration. Br Med J 1979; 1:1316–1319.
75. Wetzel RC, Setzer N, Stiff JL, et al: Hemodynamic responses in brain dead organ donor patients. Anesth Analg 1985; 64:125–128.
76. Dahlager JL, Bilde T: The integrity of tubular cell function after preservation in Collin's solution: Canine kidneys. Transplantation 1976; 21:365–369.
77. Rijksen JFWB: Preservation of Canine Kidneys: The Effect of Various Preservation Fluids on Renal Morphology and Function. 1972. Master's thesis, University of Leiden, The Netherlands.
78. Schloerb PR, Postel J, Mortiz ED, et al: Hypothermic storage of the canine kidneys for 48 hours in a low chloride solution. Surg Gynecol Obstet 1975; 141:545–548.
79. Miller CH, Alexander JW, Smith EJ, et al: Salutary effect of phentolamine (Regitine) on renal vasoconstriction in donor kidneys: Experimental and clinical studies. Transplantation 1974; 17:201–210.
80. Abramowicz M: The choice of antimicrobial drugs. Med Lett 1982; 24:21–23.
81. Abramowicz M: Choice of cephalosporins. Med Lett 1983; 25:57–60.
82. Schuler S, Parnt R, Warnecke H, et al: Extended donor criteria for heart transplantation. J Heart Transplant 1988; 7:326–330.
83. Kroncke GM, Nichols RD, Mendenhall JT, et al: Ectothermic philosophy of acid-base balance to prevent fibrillation during hypothermia. Arch Surg 1986; 121:303–304.
84. Swain JA: Hypothermia and blood pH: A review. Arch Intern Med 1988; 148:1643–1646.
85. Flanigan WJ, Ardon LF, Brewer TE, et al: Etiology and diagnosis of early post-transplantation oliguria. Am J Surg 1976; 132:808–815.
86. Toledo-Pereyra LH, Simmons RL, Olson LC, et al: Cadaver kidney transplantation effect of hypotension and donor pretreatment with methylprednisolone and phenoxybenzamine. Minn Med 1979; 62:159–161.
87. Whelchel JD, Diethelm AG, Phillips MG, et al: The effect of high-dose dopamine in cadaver donor management on delayed graft function and graft survival following renal transplantation. Transplant Proc 1986; 18:523–527.
88. Wicomb WN, Cooper DKC, Lanza RP, et al: The effects of brain death and 24 hours storage by hypothermic perfusion on donor heart function in the pig. J Thorac Cardiovasc Surg 1986; 91:896–909.
89. Busuttil RW, Goldstein LI, Danovitch GM, et al: Liver transplantation today. Ann Intern Med 1986; 104:377–389.
90. Novitzky D, Rose AG, Cooper DKC: Injury of myocardial conduction tissue and coronary artery smooth muscle following brain death in the baboon. Transplantation 1988; 45:964–966.
91. Davidson I, Berglin E, Brynger H: Perioperative fluid regimen, blood and plasma volumes, and colloid changes in living-related donors. Transplant Proc 1984; 16:18–19.
92. Kormos RL, Donato W, Hardesty RL, et al: The influence of donor organ stability and ischemia time on subsequent cardiac recipient survival. Transplant Proc 1988; 20:980–983.
93. Slapak M: The immediate care of potential donors for cadaveric organ transplantation. Anaesthesia 1978; 33:700–709.
94. Levinson MM, Copeland JG: The organ donor: Physiology, maintenance, and procurement considerations. Contemp Anesth Pract 1987; 10:31–45.
95. Hardesty RL, Griffith BP: Multiple cadaveric organ procurement for transplantation with emphasis on the heart. Surg Clin North Am 1986; 66:451–457.
96. Emery RW, Cork RC, Levinson MM, et al: The cardiac donor: A six-year experience. Ann Thorac Surg 1986; 41:356–362.
97. Lucas BA, Vaughn WK, Spees EK, et al: Identification of donor factors predisposing to high discard rates of cadaver kidneys and increased graft loss within one year post transplantation. Transplantation 1987; 43:253–258.
98. Richardson DW, Robinson AG: Desmopressin. Ann Intern Med 1985; 103:228–239.
99. Schneider A, Toledo-Pereyra LH, Seichner WD, et al: Effect of dopamine and pitressin on kidneys procured and harvested for transplantation. Transplantation 1983; 36:110–111.
100. Cowley AW, Monos E, Guyton AS: Interaction of vasopressin and the baroreceptor reflex system in the regulation of arterial blood pressure in the dog. Circ Res 1974; 34:505–514.
101. Davis S, Olichwier KK, Chakko SC: Reversible depression of myocardial performance in hypophosphatemia. Am J Med Sci 1988; 295:183–187.
102. Kaufman HH, Hui KS, Mattson JC, et al: Clinicopathologic correlations of disseminated intravascular coagulation in patients with severe head injury. Neurosurgery 1984; 15:34–42.
103. Starzl TE, Kaupp HA Jr, Brock DR, et al: Reconstructive problems in canine liver homotransplantation with special reference to the postoperative role of hepatic venous flow. Surg Gynecol Obstet 1960; 111:733–743.
104. Starzl TE: Experience in Renal Transplantation. Philadelphia, WB Saunders, 1964.
105. Collins GM, Bravo-Shugarman M, Terasaki PI: Kidney preservation for transportation. Lancet 1969; 2:1219–1222.
106. Belzer FO, Southard JH: Principles of solid organ preservation by cold storage. Transplantation 1988; 45:673–676.
107. Todo S, Tzakis A, Starzl TE: Preservation of livers with UW or Euro Collin's solution (Letter to the editor). Transplantation 1988; 46:925–926.
108. Starzl TE, Hakala TR, Shaw BW Jr, et al: A flexible procedure for multiple cadaveric organ procurement. Surg Gynecol Obstet 1984; 158:223–230.
109. Starzl TE, Miller C, Broznick B, et al: An improved technique for multiple organ harvesting. Surg Gynecol Obstet 1987; 165:343–348.
110. Starzl TE, Miller CM, Rapaport FT: Organ procurement. *In*: Care of the Surgical Patient. Wilmore DW, Brennan MF, Harken AH, et al (Eds). New York, Scientific American, 1990, pp 1–14.
111. Yanaga K, Podesta L, Broznick B, et al: Multiple organ recovery for transplantation. *In*: Atlas of Organ Transplantation. Starzl TE, Shapiro R, Simmons RL (Eds). New York, Gower Medical Publishing, 1992, pp 3.2–3.49.
112. Schwartz ME, Podesta L, Morris M, et al: Donor management, techniques and procurement. *In*: The Handbook of Transplantation Management. Makowka L (Ed). Austin, TX, R.G. Landes Company, 1991, pp 44–71.
113. Marsh CL, Perkins JD, Sutherland DE, et al: Combined hepatic and pancreaticoduodenal procurement for transplantation. Surg Gynecol Obstet 1989; 168:254–258.

114. Esquivel CO, Nakazato PZ, Concepcion W: Liver transplantation: Modern techniques in donor and recipient operations. *In*: Surgical Technology International. Braverman MH (Ed). San Francisco, Surgical Technology International, Thomas F Laszlo Publisher, 1992, pp 315–321.
115. Starzl TE, Halgrimson CG, Koep LJ, et al: Vascular homografts from cadaveric organ donors. Surg Gynecol Obstet 1979; 149:76–77.
116. Todo S, Makowka L, Tzakis AG, et al: Hepatic artery in liver transplantation. Transplant Proc 1987; 19:2406–2411.
117. Tzakis A, Mazzaferro V, Pan C, et al: Renal artery reconstruction for harvesting injuries in kidney transplantation: With particular reference to the use of vascular allografts. Transplant Int 1988; 1:80–85.
118. Tzakis A, Todo S, Starzl TE: The anterior route for arterial graft conduits in liver transplantation (Letter to the editor). Transplant Int 1989; 2:121.
119. Stieber AC, Zetti G, Todo S, et al: The spectrum of portal vein thrombosis. Ann Surg 1991; 213:199–206.
119a. Marino IR, Doyle HR, Starzl TE: Surgical technique of orthotopic liver transplantation. *In*: Diseases of the Biliary Tract and Pancreas. Hess W, Cirenei A, Rohner A, et al (Eds). Padula, Italy, Piccin Publisher, 1994 (in press).
119b. Scotti-Foglieni C, Marino IR, Starzl TE, et al: Human intestinal-multivisceral transplantation. *In*: Liver Transplantation. D'Amico DF, Bassi N, Tedeschi U, et al (Eds). Milan, Masson, 1994, pp 235–254.

CHAPTER 179

Principles of Immunosuppression

Alan J. Rosenbloom, MD • John J. Fung, MD, PhD

BASIC PRINCIPLES OF IMMUNOSUPPRESSION

A reasonable definition of optimal immunosuppression in transplantation is that level of treatment that achieves graft acceptance with the least possible suppression of systemic immunity. Once this level has been achieved, there is no advantage to more immunosuppression. In fact, there is considerable potential for harm. This harm comes from the increasing probability of infection (see Chapter 134 on infections in immunosuppressed patients) and malignancy, in addition to other side effects, which are inherent risks with all the immunosuppressants currently available. Achieving this optimal level of immunosuppression is difficult. There are presently no diagnostic tests that can accurately quantify the actual degree of suppression of immunity. Hence, the titration of immunosuppression retains an element of trial and error. In practice, over- or underimmunosuppression almost invariably becomes apparent only in retrospect.

The timing, dosing, and selection of immunosuppressive agents differ widely. Most immunosuppressive regimens combine drugs, often with different modes of action and toxicities, allowing lower doses of each drug. Currently, transplantation immunosuppression is dominated by four classes of drugs: corticosteroids, cytokine suppressive agents, cytotoxic agents, and antilymphocyte antibodies.

The use of cyclosporin A (CyA) with steroids forms the backbone of most immunosuppressive regimens. An antiproliferative agent or an antilymphocyte antibody, or both, may be added. When acute cellular rejection occurs, it is common to treat with brief, high doses of steroids or antilymphocyte antibodies or both.

The early postoperative period in general calls for the greatest degree of immunosuppression. Many patients, over the long run, can maintain graft acceptance with less drug as time goes on. It has been shown that a few patients can be completely withdrawn from therapy without rejection; unfortunately, there currently is no way to identify which patients are good candidates for this maneuver.

BASIC SCIENCE REVIEW

Lymphocytes are preprogrammed to recognize foreign antigen during their development in the thymus. Antigen specificity is determined by an antigen-binding unit on the T cell surface: the T cell receptor (TCR). The specificity of the binding site of the TCR results from its amino acid composition. The gene sequence coding for the TCR rearranges during development, such that each T cell ends up with a different TCR binding specificity. Because the gene rearrangements are completely random, a huge library of binding sites capable of recognizing both "self" and "foreign" molecules is generated. Thymocytes with TCRs that bind to "self" molecules are subsequently destroyed by a poorly understood mechanism.

Lymphocytes recirculate at a rate of 1% to 2% per hour, migrating through all tissues of the body. Recirculation routes are not random. Specialized cell-surface "homing" molecules on T lymphocytes mediate attachment to specific endothelial molecules in targeted tissues. Once inside tissue, antigen-presenting cells (APCs) such as macrophages make intimate contact with the lymphocytes and present foreign antigen that has been processed intracellularly by the APC. The APC phagocytoses foreign protein and enzymatically cleaves it to the size of small peptides 8 to 12 amino acids in length. These peptides are loaded onto a class of specialized carrier molecules, known as the major histocompatibility complex (MHC) molecules. The MHC molecule carries the peptide fragment to the cell surface, where it is displayed to T cells.

On the T cell surface is the TCR. The TCR associates with an "accessory" molecule, either CD4 or CD8. The TCR interacts with the peptide fragment and the CD4 or CD8 interacts with the MHC molecule on the APC. This interaction produces the signal that initiates the proliferation of T cell clones recognizing the particular antigen fragments of foreign protein. It is the requirement for antigen presentation by APCs bearing an MHC molecule specific to the host that is the basis for MHC-restricted antigen recognition.

Antigen-directed proliferation of T cell clones is absolutely required for an effective immune response. It is the key to the production of large numbers of T cells specific for foreign antigen. It is driven by a positive feedback loop between T cells and a soluble hormone. Cells recognizing antigen make the potent growth factor (interleukin [IL]-2) and, simultaneously, become responsive to IL-2 by making IL-2 receptor. This dual synthesis allows the cells to stimulate their own "autocrine" clonal expansion.

During an ongoing immune response, proliferating T cells recruit many other cell types and immune mechanisms into action. T cells produce IL-1 through 6, IL-9, and IL-10 as well as interferons, tumor necrosis factor (TNF)-α and TNF-β, granulocyte colony-stimulating factor (G-CSF), and granulocyte-monocyte colony-stimulating factor (GM-CSF).[1] These substances have at least three important functions. First, cytokines can attract and activate other leukocytes. For example, CD4 helper T cell cytokines attract macrophages and CD8-bearing cytotoxic lymphocytes into rejecting allografts.[2] They also trigger macrophage activation and CD8 lymphocyte cell maturation. The resulting multicellular tissue infiltration has traditionally been referred to as delayed-type hypersensitivity (DTH). CD4 helper T cell cytokines are also responsible for the activation of B cells and thus, indirectly, for the majority of antibody production. Second, cytokines up-regulate both MHC molecules on tissues and adhesion molecules on endothelium. This aids in the entry and accumulation of leukocytes in the tissue and an accelerated recognition of "foreign" molecules. Third, cytokines activate distant organ responses, such as the hepatic acute-phase response, bone marrow phagocyte synthesis, and the hypothalamic-pituitary axis, producing the systemic signs of inflammation.

Once the antigen is consumed or removed, the process down-regulates. A number of sensitized memory T cells remain and contribute to a stronger secondary response on rechallenge with the same antigen.

In the case of transplanted solid organs, donor T lymphocytes enter the graft rapidly. Conversely, recipient APC cells also exit the graft immediately after reperfusion. Thus, recipient lymphocytes potentially become sensitized to donor (foreign) antigens both inside and outside of the transplanted organ.

Recently, evidence has suggested the existence of at least two subpopulations of CD4-bearing T cells in humans. Helper T subset one (Th1) cells preferentially drive cell-mediated immunity. Helper T subset two (Th2) cells stimulate B cell antigen production. The two subsets produce a different, but overlapping, set of cytokines. Some of the Th1 cytokines down-regulate the production of Th2 cytokines and vice versa. Hence, the two distinct responses represented by these subsets are somewhat mutually exclusive. The predominance of one subset or the other is believed to influence the character of the immune response to a particular challenge. The mechanisms that determine the choice between Th1 and Th2 are under investigation.

As molecular knowledge has advanced, a greater understanding of how many immunosuppressants work has evolved. More importantly, new strategies are guided by this knowledge, resulting in new drugs. Virtually every known step of the immune process can be targeted, and many new drugs are now in various stages of development.

SPECIFIC AGENTS

Corticosteroids

Corticosteroids are extensively used in brief but high doses for the reversal of acute rejection episodes. They are also almost invariably a part of multidrug maintenance regimens.[3]

Prednisone has a somewhat variable oral bioavailability of about 80%. The serum half-life of both prednisone and methylprednisolone is 3 hours. However, suppression of cytokine production, likely to be a key effect, persists for 24 hours or more. There is no fixed dosing regimen. Rather, doses are titrated by effect and local custom. A preoperative dose of 250 to 1000 mg may be given followed by 20 to 200 mg/d during the first week. Acute rejection may be treated with one to three high doses, 250 mg to 1 g IV methylprednisolone, or by a tapering regimen starting at 200 mg/d and reducing to baseline maintenance doses over 3 to 6 days. There is evidence to suggest that lower doses than those traditionally used can be equally effective. By combination regimens, steroids can often be reduced to 10 or 20 mg/d or less, including therapy every other day.

Corticosteroids have broad effects on many cell types. They interfere with the production of IL-1 and IL-2, blocking the early steps of T cell activation. Multiple other immune effects occur, including (1) antagonism of inflammatory mechanisms by stabilization of leukocyte lysosomal membranes, decreased capillary permeability, and inhibition of histamine release and the kinin, and complement systems; (2) drastic reduction of lymphocyte traffic and circulating immunoglobulin levels and reduction in numbers of neutrophils and eosinophils; and (3) inhibition of leukocyte adhesion to endothelium.

Prednisone and prednisolone have much less mineralocorticoid effect than the naturally occurring glucocorticoids. However, sodium retention, edema, hypertension, potassium loss, and hypokalemic alkalosis can be seen with prolonged use of these drugs. Suppression of the pituitary-adrenal axis can be seen with all steroids but is variable between patients. Acute adrenal insufficiency can develop unexpectedly if the patient is stressed, even up to 12 months after stopping steroids.

Unfortunately, the ill effects of corticosteroids are numerous and cause considerable morbidity. An increased incidence of serious infections is well documented. Impaired fibroblast growth and collagen synthesis contribute to poor wound healing. Hence, surgical wounds and anastomoses are at increased risk, and gastrointestinal (GI) ulcerations tend to heal slowly, with an increased risk of perforation and rebleeding. Spontaneous GI ulceration occurs in approximately 2% of patients on steroids. As a result of suppression of signs of inflammation, the diagnosis of intra-abdominal infection and peritonitis can be significantly delayed, with disastrous consequences. Decompensation of glucose tolerance is often dramatic. Generalized protein catabolism and bone demineralization can produce a debilitated state. Atherosclerosis may be accelerated. The risk of cataract and increased intraocular pressure (glaucoma) is increased. Central nervous system (CNS) effects such as euphoria and mood swings are well known. Soft-tissue and dermatologic changes such as fat redistribution, skin atrophy, and striae produce the characteristic cushingoid appearance.

Cytotoxic Drugs

Agents commonly used for immunosuppression in transplantation include antimetabolites,[4] such as azathioprine (AZA), and alkylating agents, such as cyclophosphamide (CPM). AZA, a thio analog of the purine adenine, inhibits purine metabolism. Purines are required for deoxyribonucleic acid (DNA) and ribonucleic acid (RNA) synthesis. Also, AZA can be incorporated into DNA in place of natural purines. The altered molecule does not function properly, allowing strand breaks in the chromosomes. Thus, not surprisingly, AZA is most toxic to proliferating cells that are making new DNA. In contrast, CPM nonspecifically damages cellular macromolecules by alkylating them, particularly DNA. Thus, CPM is toxic to both resting and dividing cells. The precise mechanism of immunosuppression mediated by cytotoxic drugs is unknown. However, the antiproliferative effects on lymphocytes are believed to inhibit the generation of antigen-specific T cell clones.

Azathioprine

AZA[3,5,6] can be used in maintenance of immunosuppressive regimens. It has no usefulness in the treatment of acute rejection episodes.

The oral bioavailability of AZA is about 40%. The metabolism of AZA is complex. The parent drug is inactive but is rapidly converted to several metabolites. Thio-inosinic acid is an inhibitor of purine synthesis. The 6-thioguanine nucleotides (TGN) are known to incorporate into DNA. TGN has a very long tissue half-life, perhaps on the order of 13 days. On this basis, once-daily dosage is logical. The final inactive end metabolite is 6-thiouric acid, which is excreted by the kidneys. With congenital deficiency of the enzyme thiopurine methyltransferase (1 in 300 patients), or renal failure, accumulation of TGN causes increased toxicity. The drug is usually given orally. The starting dose is between 3 and 5 mg/kg as a single daily oral dose. It can be given intravenously at half the dose for brief periods. Typical maintenance oral dosage after transplantation is 2 to 3 mg/kg daily. Tapering to 1 to 2 $mg \cdot kg^{-1} \cdot d^{-1}$ is often possible as time goes on. In combination regimens, AZA can be reduced to as low as 0.25 to 0.5 $mg \cdot kg^{-1} \cdot d^{-1}$.

Dose-limiting myelosuppression usually occurs 1 to 2 weeks into therapy. Pancytopenia and thrombocytopenia with megaloblastic anemia is the pattern usually seen. White blood cell counts below 3000 cells/mm^3 mandate discontinuation or reduction of the drug. As with other antiproliferative drugs, nausea, vomiting, and hair loss may occur. Hepatic injury can occur in two patterns: a reversible hepatitis and a rare but serious hepatic veno-occlusive disease, which can cause irreparable damage. AZA therapy has also been associated with an increased risk of pancreatitis believed to be due to a hypersensitivity reaction. The role of AZA, however, has been questioned in both of these.[7, 8] Hypersensitivity to AZA has been reported to cause a variety of manifestations. Diagnosis of these disorders has been largely on clinical grounds.

Allopurinol inhibits xanthene oxidase, one of the enzymes involved in degradation of AZA metabolites, and can increase its toxicity.

Cyclophosphamide

CPM has been used in place of AZA, particularly when there is suspected AZA-associated hepatitis. CPM is also the most widely used preparatory treatment for bone marrow transplantation. It is useful at high doses both to incapacitate the recipient's immune system, preventing rejection of the grafted marrow, and in neoplastic diseases requiring marrow transplantation as effective chemotherapy.

Oral CPM is well absorbed (87–96%); peak concentrations are reached in 1 hour.[9] CPM is activated by metabolism in the liver. Several metabolites are formed. The ultimately active metabolite phosphoramide mustard is eliminated by spontaneous hydrolysis with an intracellular half-life of 40 to 50 minutes. Blood half-life is about 5 to 7 hours. Neither impaired renal function nor liver failure requires dosage adjustment. CPM is removed by hemodialysis. CPM used in transplant regimens is administered at low doses (3–5 $mg \cdot kg^{-1} \cdot d^{-1}$), which is significantly less than doses used for chemotherapy (60 $mg \cdot kg^{-1} \cdot d^{-1}$).

As with all antiproliferative agents, patients can experience nausea, vomiting, and hair loss. Hemorrhagic cystitis is a well-known side effect of CPM, but the reported incidence is very variable (0.5–40%). It can be limited by giving thiosulfate or, apparently equally well, with aggressive hydration.

Side effects are considerably more common and serious with the high-dose therapy used for bone marrow transplantation. Virtually all patients experience nausea, vomiting, and hair loss. As many as 15% of patients experience clinically significant cardiac dysfunction. Infertility has also been associated with these doses.

CPM levels or effects can be increased by use of allopurinol and cimetidine but not ranitidine. CPM potentiates the effects of succinylcholine.

Cytokine Suppressive Agents

When a T lymphocyte is activated by antigen, a coordinated program of multiple gene activations is set in motion; this program eventuates in the proliferation of the activated cell. CyA blocks the transcription of 10 genes of at least 60 that are activated. Some of these are IL-2, IL-3, and IL-4, granulocyte-macrophage colony-stimulating factor, and interferon γ. The inhibition of the production of IL-2, which acts as a potent T cell growth factor, is a key effect and has been extensively studied. The drug is known to block the activation of the IL-2 gene, ultimately preventing the synthesis of IL-2. At this level, both CyA and FK-506 act similarly; further, they both interfere with the binding of specific transcription factors to the promoter (control region) of the IL-2 gene, preventing RNA synthesis.[10] The intracellular pathways leading to action on the gene are complex and incompletely understood.

The occurrence of CyA-like substances appears to be remarkably universal and evolutionarily conserved. Specific receptors for CyA are present in most cells. They have even been observed in a wide range of cell types in plants. As these drugs are studied in greater detail, it becomes clear that they have multiple effects on many processes in lymphocytes and other cells as well.

Cyclosporine

Before the introduction of CyA, immunosuppression protocols relied heavily on steroids and cytotoxic drugs. These regimens had the disadvantage of producing broad suppression of the immune and inflammatory cascades. CyA introduced a new era of immunosuppression, with potent, relatively specific, noncytotoxic suppression of T cell activation.

The drug is insoluble in water and thus must be dissolved in an organic solvent. Oral bioavailability is about 30%, with much variability (range = 10–60%). Small intestinal absorption decreases with bowel dysfunction or reduced bile flow.[11] The volume of distribution of CyA is large and variable. Hepatic metabolism is the only significant elimination mechanism. Drug alteration is via the cytochrome P450 IIIA enzymes. The mean terminal half-life with normal liver function is 19 hours. At least 17 metabolites are identifiable, and at least a few are immunosuppressive although of considerably less potency than the parent compound. Half-life increases with hepatic failure and is changed significantly by coadministration of a large number of other drugs that can cause unexpected increased or decreased serum levels, by induction, or by competitive inhibition of P450.[12] Many other drugs are also additive to CyA renal toxicity (Table 179–1). For all these reasons, it is essential that levels be monitored regularly and dosage adjusted accordingly.

Monitoring CyA levels is not without problems. Measuring CyA in blood or plasma with radioimmunoassay (RIA) or high-pressure liquid chromatography (HPLC) gives different results. No method is clearly superior; thus, there is no universally accepted blood level. Target levels may vary widely from center to center. Roughly, desired levels, by mode of testing,[13] are (1) RIA in serum or plasma, 150 to 250 ng/mL at the time of transplantation, tapered to 50 to 100 ng/mL at 3 to 6 months and (2) HPLC in whole blood, 100 to 300 ng/mL initially, tapered to 80 to 200 ng/mL.

CyA administration is typically begun 12 to 24 hours before heart or kidney transplantation and just after graft reperfusion in liver allograft recipients. A typical dose is 4 to 5 $mg \cdot kg^{-1} \cdot d^{-1}$ IV. This amount can be given in two divided doses each over 2 to 6 hours. Alternatively, some centers prefer to use slow, continuous infusion over 24 hours. The changeover to oral dosing usually requires a dose three times higher (i.e., about 12–15 mg/kg). After 1 to 2 weeks, the dosage can be slowly tapered as a result of equilibration within body fat stores. Many patients are tapered to as low as 3 mg/kg by 6 months after transplant. Liver transplant patients with a T tube, which diverts some

TABLE 179–1. Drug Interactions with Cyclosporine

Increase Cyclosporine Levels		*Decrease Cyclosporine Levels*	*Enhance Cyclosporine Nephrotoxicity*
Ketoconazole	Fluconazole	Phenytoin	Aminoglycosides
Norfloxacin	Metoclopramide	Phenobarbital	Amphotericin B
Erythromycin	Verapamil	Carbamazepine	Trimethoprim
Diltiazem	Nicardipine	Valproic acid	Melphalan
Methylprednisolone	Prednisolone	Nafcillin	Acyclovir
Methyltestosterone	Levonorgestrel	Rifampin	Ganciclovir
Warfarin	Ethanol		Doxorubicin
Imipenem/cilastatin			Digoxin
			Furosemide
			Metolazone
			Indomethacin

(From Chan GL, Gruber SA, Skjei KL, et al: Principles of immunosuppression. Crit Care Clin 1990; 6:841–892.)

of the bile flow, require higher oral doses because of decreased absorption.

Several adverse effects are seen early with the administration of CyA. Significant acute nephrotoxicity, probably resulting from vasoconstrictive effects on the afferent arterioles of the kidney,[14] is a major problem. The mechanism of this effect is under debate.[15] This nephrotoxicity is transient and reversible with a decrease of dosage or discontinuation of drug.[16] The incidence of nephrotoxicity varies from approximately 25% to 32%, 37%, and 38% in kidney, heart, and liver transplant patients, respectively.[17] Hypertension occurs frequently, within weeks of commencing therapy. The incidence varies widely in different patient populations, between 10% and 80%.[18] It is hypothesized that this is due to a vasoconstrictive effect of CyA both in the renal and systemic circulations[19] perhaps caused by antagonism of endothelium-derived relaxation factors or increased synthesis of endothelin, a vasoconstrictor. Physiologically, the hypertension is responsive to sodium restriction; therapies incorporating diuretics or calcium channel blockers have been advocated.[18] Minor neurotoxicity (tremor) is common (10–55%) and may improve over time without a change in therapy.

More severe symptoms such as seizures and encephalopathy have also been associated with CyA, but it is frequently not clear if the association is causal.[20] Several reports detail a rare syndrome of confusion and cortical blindness in both liver and bone marrow transplant patients.[15] Hypomagnesemia and hypocholesterolemia are believed to be risk factors for CyA neurotoxicity.[15] CyA is diabetogenic, although analysis of this effect is confounded by the frequent concomitant use of steroids with CyA.[15] Other metabolic effects include hypochloremic alkalosis and changes in serum potassium, magnesium, prolactin, and testosterone.[21] Hepatotoxicity, manifested by an increased cholestatic tendency, may be quite common,[15] but a reduction in dosage often improves this effect, and it does not appear to be a major problem. Connective tissue side effects of CyA are common and can be distressing to the patient. These include hirsutism, seen over 2 to 4 weeks in 20% to 45%, gingival hyperplasia in 4% to 16%, and coarsening of facial features.[22]

Chronic administration of CyA has been associated with a nonreversible nephrotoxicity. The incidence is estimated at 15% to 40%.[23] The pathologic lesion resembles nephrosclerosis.[14, 24]

FK-506

The largest experience with FK as a maintenance drug is at the University of Pittsburgh Medical Center. About 1600 patients were on FK as of March 1992.[25] In terms of the suppression of alloimmunity, FK appears to have at least the same as, and possibly more immunosuppressive efficacy than CyA. On a weight-to-weight basis, FK is more potent than CyA by a factor of 10 to 15 times. Experiences in patients after liver,[26] kidney,[27] and heart[28] transplantation have been reported.

The role of FK as a maintenance immunosuppression is not yet determined. The major question is that of superiority over CyA. Clearly, both drugs are highly effective immunosuppressants; the ultimate deciding factor may be the side effects and toxicity associated with the two agents. Precise quantitation of FK toxicity and analysis of its comparability to CyA are confounded by multiple factors. Early studies with FK used doses that were too high. The complex and variable pharmacokinetics of FK, as with CyA, makes estimation of appropriate dosing difficult and blood level measurement very important. Multiple technical difficulties in obtaining and interpreting FK levels further complicated early use of the drug. These are gradually being resolved. As the drug enters wider usage, and as laboratory monitoring methodology improves, a clearer picture will inevitably emerge.

In the treatment of acute resistant or chronic rejection, experience with FK rescue has been variable. Patients selected have been resistant to CyA, steroids, and usually antilymphocyte antibodies and AZA. Response rates of 70% to 85% have been reported for resistant acute cellular rejection.[29, 30] Resistant chronic rejection responded less well.[30] In one study,[31] the response of chronic rejection depended on the degree of injury present when starting rescue therapy. The finding on biopsy of "early" chronic rejection predicted a high degree of success with FK. More advanced changes predicted less success.

Absorption of an oral dose of FK is variable (5–67%). GI absorption of FK is less dependent on bile flow than is that of CyA; therefore, there is no need to decrease the dose when the T tube is clamped after liver transplantation.[32] The drug is metabolized by the liver, and elimination is markedly slowed with liver dysfunction. In one study of liver transplant patients,[32] the half-life ranged from 3.5 to 40.5 hours. The volume of distribution also varied widely from 5.6 to 65 L/kg body weight. FK inhibits the hepatic cytochrome P450 reductase, which metabolizes it, potentially decreasing its own metabolism[33] and causing an increase in blood levels. The clinical importance of this phenomenon is unknown. Inhibitors of P450 may increase FK blood levels by inhibiting cytochrome P450 activity. Conversely, inducers of P450 may decrease FK levels.[32] Because FK can cause significant toxicity, the frequent determination of levels is crucial, particularly in patients with hepatic dysfunction.

FK is initially started intravenously with a slow, continuous infusion over 24 hours.[34] The initial dose is 0.05 mg·kg^{-1}·d^{-1} for liver transplants, 0.10 mg·kg^{-1}·d^{-1} for kidney transplants, and 0.15 mg·kg^{-1}·d^{-1} for small-bowel transplants. When the patient can take oral FK, the intravenous drug is discontinued, and the oral dose is started at 0.15 mg·kg^{-1}·d^{-1} in two divided doses.[35] Subsequent dosing is modified to maintain FK levels between 1 and 2 ng/mL by plasma monitoring. FK has nephrotoxicity potential, and the degree of its expression is dependent on other factors such as use of other nephrotoxic drugs, pretransplant renal function, and factors associated with the development of acute tubular necrosis (ATN) such as hypotension. The mechanism is not yet clear. Increased endothelin synthesis may play a role.[36] Early studies suggest that this effect reverses with lowering the dose or changing to the oral route, or both.[37] The incidence of long-term renal injury, as seen with CyA, is unknown.

Hypertension appears less common than with CyA, with approximately 50% of the incidence in comparison.[35]

Neurotoxicity appears comparable to CyA; both minor and major toxicities are seen.[38] Minor toxicity, such as tremor, insomnia, and dysethesias, is common and, as with CyA, is seen in about 20% to 30% of patients. Major toxicity such as encephalopathy, which can progress to coma, seizures, psychosis, and other neurologic deficit, is less common, being estimated at 3% to 5%, depending on the organ type being transplanted. After liver transplantation, patients are particularly prone to major neurotoxicity (approximately 8%), whereas major neurotoxicity is rarely seen with heart, lung, or kidney transplants.

GI side effects including diarrhea, anorexia, bloating, and flatulence are similar to those seen with CyA. FK is also similarly diabetogenic (10–20%). Both drugs inhibit insulin release in a rat model. Hyperkalemia, sometimes severe enough to prompt the use of fludrocortisone acetate (Florinef), has been noted with FK.[30] Studies in rats reveal some hepatotoxicity, but the clinical significance is not known.

One of the major advantages of FK appears to be the ability to use less steroid; thus, regimens with FK may produce less diabetes and hypertension overall.

There are, as with CyA, many ways to measure FK levels. The first method described used enzyme-linked immunosorbent assay with solid-phase extraction in plasma.[25] Turnaround time for FK levels is between 24 and 48 hours. The drug is trapped at high concentration inside red blood cells in a temperature-dependent fashion. Thus, whole blood levels can be 8 to 10 times higher than plasma levels with much variability (3.6–39).[32] Somewhat higher, more consistent plasma levels can be obtained by equilibration of the sample at 37°C before analysis. HPLC and mass spectroscopy are being investigated, as is the use of whole blood. One study of whole blood versus plasma[39] showed that whole blood levels were more stable and more reliably elevated with nephrotoxicity than were plasma levels.

Rapamycin

The use of rapamycin (RPM)[10,40,41] has yet to be determined. The drug is clearly an extraordinarily potent immunosuppressant. It inhibits DTH and both B and T cell responses to alloantigen. In animal models, RPM prolongs the survival of MHC-incompatible grafts and can halt ongoing rejection. The mechanism of action differs significantly from either FK or CyA in that RPM does not block transcription of cytokine messenger RNA but rather inhibits the translation of these in RNAs. There is evidence that the drug may be synergistic with CyA and perhaps additive with FK, although under some conditions RPM and FK are mutually antagonistic.[42]

RPM has a poor bioavailability after oral administration. Very low plasma levels (currently below detection) are therapeutic. The issues of drug delivery, stability, and monitoring remain problematic and require resolution before RPM can be introduced for human use.

Antilymphocyte Antibodies

Antilymphocyte antibodies,[17,43] such as antilymphocyte globulin (ALG), were first produced by immunizing animals against purified lymphocyte preparations, producing multispecificity polyclonal antibodies. Antibodies cross-reacting with other cellular molecules in blood were removed by extensive absorption to blood components. Because of variability between immunized animals, substantial amounts of ALG are pooled to produce a more homogeneous preparation. Many of the limitations of antithymocyte globulin (ATG) preparations were related to their variability in potency; leukopenia, thrombocytopenia, and anemia seen with those products were due to contaminating antibodies. Hybridoma technology later allowed the development of single-specificity monoclonal antibodies (e.g., OKT3 directed against one particular epitome of a single cell-surface molecule). These drugs are much more uniform, standardized, and potent.

The place of immunoglobulin therapy in immunosuppressive regimens is in a state of flux. These agents were originally shown effective in the reversal of acute rejection. For this use, OKT3 has been shown to be more effective than high doses of steroids. More recently, these drugs have been introduced into some maintenance regimens and have been used in other situations.

The strategy of using antilymphocyte antibodies immediately after transplantation has been referred to as "prophylactic" or "induction" therapy. This practice is based on the concept that early incapacitation of the immune system may theoretically reduce the propensity for subsequent rejection. This strategy has been described in heart,[44] liver,[45] and kidney[46] transplantation. Claimed benefits are a delay in the time to onset of acute rejection, fewer episodes of rejection, and no significant increase in infectious complications in these studies. The related concept of "sequential" therapy was introduced in response to the significant renal toxicity of CyA seen in liver, heart, and kidney transplantation. The practice is to use antibody therapy in the first 1 to 2 weeks after transplantation in lieu of CyA. It is during this period that renal injury is most likely to occur from a variety of insults. Cyclosporine is begun later. Proponents cite a reduced incidence of early renal dysfunction.[47,48] The impact of this strategy on long-term renal function is much less clear.

This early intensification of immunosuppression is not universally accepted. Some voice concern over the well-known associations of antilymphocyte antibody therapy and immunosuppression in general with infection and malignancy.[49,50] Others describe no benefit, greater expense,[51] or the successful use of regimens avoiding induction altogether.[52] Compromise strategies involve using prophylaxis only in high-risk patients[53] and use of one dose of OKT3, followed by early evaluation of renal function; antibody is discontinued unless ATN is imminent.[54]

Immunoglobulin therapy is given either intravenously or intramuscularly. Equine ATG is given in the dosage range of 10 to 15 mg/kg in a single daily dose. Therapy of acute rejection is usually continued for 14 days. With OKT3, the dose of 5 mg/d for 10 to 14 days is typical. Prophylactic OKT3 regimens use the same dose usually for 7 to 10 days of therapy. Polyclonal preparations cause a high incidence of febrile reactions with the first few doses. Antihistamines, antipyretics, and sometimes steroids are given in preparation. Because the antibodies react with other blood cells, leukopenia (about 14%) and thrombocytopenia (about 30%) are seen. Anaphylaxis occurs in fewer than 1%. Nonetheless, a skin test prior to use is recommended. Skin rash is a fairly frequent occurrence (10–30%).

OKT3 is by far the most extensively studied of the monoclonal antibodies. On the first one or two doses, there is a large intravascular release of cytokines by lymphocytes. This "first dose effect" frequently causes fever, chills, tachycardia, gastrointestinal disturbances, bronchospasm, and elevation or depression of blood pressure. These effects can be blocked to a large extent by pretreatment with a 1 g IV bolus of solumedrol 15 to 60 minutes prior to OKT3 infusion.[55] Individuals vary in the amount of endogenous antibody they form directed against the mouse antibody. Intermediate and high responders form a significant titer of blocking antibodies. This antibody production can be decreased by continuing other immunosuppressive therapy during monoclonal antibody administration. Retreatment can often succeed if higher doses of antibody are used for subsequent administration. The very highest antibody responders, probably about 5% to 20% of patients, form high-titer antibodies and fail even increased dose therapy. Some[43] advocate following CD3+ cell counts with flow cytometry in patients on OKT3. If CD3+ cells reach 10%, it is recommended that OKT3 be either increased in dosage (to as much as 15 mg/d) or discontinued. Others suggest monitoring anti-OKT3 antibody titers.[56]

Antibodies to surface molecules on lymphocytes interfere with lymphocyte function in the immune response by several possible mechanisms. Lymphocytes are known to be both removed from the circulation rapidly after treatment with antilymphocyte antibodies and phenotypically and functionally altered. Treatment with OKT3 (anti-CD3 specific for CD3, which is a protein closely associated with the T cell receptor complex) has been shown to modulate the CD3/TCR, causing cocapping and internalization of the complex. After the initial disappearance of cells bearing the target molecule, those lymphocytes reappearing do not display the molecule on the surface despite the fact that they are capable of producing it, unless OKT3 therapy is halted for at least 48 hours. Obviously, lymphocytes without the antigen receptor cannot react to antigen.

The potent suppression of T lymphocyte populations is known to be associated with an increased incidence of viral infection and lymphoproliferative disorders. It is not clear whether antibody therapy is any worse than other immunosuppression in producing these. Some evidence suggests that problems arise because antibodies are used for too long a time[47] or too late in the course of resistant rejection when the immunosuppression burden is already high.[57]

Other Agents

Mycophenolic Acid and RS-61443

Interference with purine metabolism is known to cause immunosuppression. The antibiotic mycophenolic acid (MPA)[58] inhibits inosine monophosphate dehydrogenase, which is involved in the de novo synthesis of guanosine monophosphate. MPA may also interfere with the expression of adhesion molecules on leukocytes. A modified form of MPA designated RS-61443 (RS6) was synthesized in an attempt to provide more stability and better bioavailability. The drug has been tested in animal models and in human trials. It was shown to have effect in 6 of 9 patients with steroid and antilymphocyte antibody resistant rejection.[59] It was also effective as part of a quadruple induction (ALG, steroid, CyA, and RS6) with triple maintenance (steroid, CyA, and RS6) in renal transplant recipients. In a very small trial using RS6 and prednisone in four liver transplantation patients who could not tolerate CyA, the drug was successful in controlling rejection in a two-drug regimen with prednisone.[60]

The use of RS6 remains to be determined. It would be logical to use the drug in a fashion similar to AZA. The antiproliferative effect may be more specific than AZA with less toxicity. The drug effect appears to be at least additive with CyA. The ability to block humoral responses effectively may make the drug useful in antibody-mediated processes. The following adverse effects were encountered in these studies: gastritis in 1 of 48, ileus in 3 of 48, nausea and vomiting in 2 of 48. This was in contrast to previous dog studies wherein major GI toxicity was noted. No significant nephrotoxicity, hepatotoxicity, or bone marrow suppression was noted in this small study.

Mizoribine

Mizoribine (MZB),[61] also known as Bredinin, is an adenosine analog. Like RS6 and MPA, MZB is an inhibitor of the enzyme inosine monophosphate dehydrogenase.

MZB has been used[62, 63] as a maintenance agent in combination with CyA and steroids primarily in renal transplant patients. The drug appears to have advantages over AZA, in particular less myelotoxicity and hepatotoxicity.[64]

The drug is administered once daily at an oral dose of 50 to 300 mg/d. With a normal GI tract, peak blood levels are achieved 2 to 3 hours after an oral dose. Absorption of MZB is delayed in the presence of GI disease. The major elimination pathway of MZB is renal. There is little hepatic metabolism, and 85% of a dose is excreted unchanged in the urine. Clearance of the drug is thus markedly affected by renal failure. In 26 renal transplant patients with an average creatinine clearance of 50 mL/min (range = 22–93 mL/min), the half-life was 4 hours (range = 1.6–8.2 hours).

Brequinar

Brequinar (BQR)[65, 66] is an antimetabolite with broad antineoplastic activity that has been tested in humans with cancer. It is an inhibitor of dihydrorotate dehydrogenase, a mitochondrial enzyme in the de novo synthesis pathway of pyrimidines. Dose-limiting toxicities were due to thrombocytopenia and a severe desquamative dermatitis. The antiproliferative effects of the drug appear to be mediated by the depletion of pyrimidine precursors needed for DNA and RNA synthesis. BQR is a potent immunosuppressant in a rat model[67] and appears to act synergistically, at least in vitro, with CyA and RPM.[68]

15-Deoxyspergualin

Deoxyspergualin (DSG)[69–72] was discovered by a drug development program investigating antitumor agents in Japan. The drug was shown to be very active against lymphoid tumors only and later was shown to be immunosuppressive. The molecular basis for the action of DSG is unknown but appears to be different than that of all previously known immunosuppressant drugs.

DSG has performed well in animal models of xenograft transplantation and did better than FK or CyA. In a human trial[72] with one haplotype-matched renal transplant, the incidence of accelerated rejection was significantly decreased when DSG was combined with CyA.

The drug must be given intravenously. In renal transplant patients, the half-life varied between 39 and 55 hours, which was about twice that seen in prior studies in cancer patients.

In a human trial in which DSG was used for reversal of rejection, doses ranging from 80 to 220 mg/m^2 per day were used. The optimal dose appeared to be 180 mg/m^2 per day. In a small comparative study, the drug appeared similar in efficacy to OKT3 for the reversal of steroid-resistant rejection.[73] In other studies in which DSG was used in combination with AZA, CyA, and steroids for maintenance of immunosuppression, doses of 3 to 5 mg$\cdot$kg$^{-1}\cdot$d^{-1} were used.

Toxicity is decreased by slow infusion over 4 to 5 hours. The toxic effects seen in transplanted patients have been CNS (facial dysesthesias), GI (anorexia, nausea), reversible bone marrow suppression (lymphocytes and thrombocytes), and reversible hypotension. The bone marrow suppression appears to be the most significant side effect.

References

1. Male D, Champion B, Cooke A, et al: Advanced Immunology. 2nd ed. London, Gower, 1991.
2. Hall BM: Cells mediating allograft rejection. Transplantation 1991; 51:1141–1151.
3. Chan GL, Gruber SA, Skjei KL, et al: Principles of immunosuppression. Crit Care Clin 1990; 6:841–892.
4. Goust JM, Stevenson HC, Galbraith RM, et al: Immunosuppression and immunomodulation. Immunol Series 1990; 50:481–498.
5. Chan GL, Erdmann GR, Gruber SA, et al: Azathioprine metabolism: Pharmacokinetics of 6-mercaptopurine, 6-thiouric acid and 6-thioguanine nucleotides in renal transplant patients. J Clin Pharmacol 1990; 30:358–363.
6. Boitard C, Bach JF: Long-term complications of conventional immunosuppressive treatment. Adv Nephrol 1989; 18:335–354.
7. Lia-no F, Moreno A, Matesanz R, et al: Veno-occlusive hepatic disease of the liver in renal transplantation: Is azathioprine the cause? (see comments). Nephron 1989; 51:509–516.
8. Frick TW, Fryd DS, Goodale RL, et al: Lack of association between azathioprine and acute pancreatitis in renal. Lancet 1991; 337:251–252.
9. Moore MJ: Clinical pharmacokinetics of cyclophosphamide. Clin Pharmacokinet 1991; 20:194–208.
10. Henderson DJ, Naya I, Bundick RV, et al: Comparison of the effects of FK-506, cyclosporin A and rapamycin on IL-2 production. Immunology 1991; 73:316–321.
11. Freeman DJ: Pharmacology and pharmacokinetics of cyclosporine. Clin Biochem 1991; 24:9–14.
12. Watkins PB: The role of cytochromes P-450 in cyclosporine metabolism. J Am Acad Dermatol 1990; 23:1301–1309.
13. Keown PA: Optimizing cyclosporine therapy: Dose, levels, and monitoring. Transplant Proc 1988; 20:382–389.
14. Remuzzi G, Bertani T: Renal vascular and thrombotic effects of cyclosporine. Am J Kidney Dis 1989; 13:261–272.
15. Rush DN: Cyclosporine toxicity to organs other than the kidney. Clin Biochem 1991; 24:101–105.
16. Keown PA, Stiller CR, Wallace AC: Effect of cyclosporine on the kidney. J Pediatr 1987; 111:1029–1033.
17. American Hospital Formulary Service: AHFS Drug Information 91. 33rd ed. Bethesda, MD, American Society of Hospital Pharmacists, 1991.
18. Luke RG: Mechanism of cyclosporine-induced hypertension. Am J Hypertens 1991; 4:468–471.
19. Mason J: The pathophysiology of Sandimmune (cyclosporine) in man and animals. Pediatr Nephrol 1990; 4:554–574.
20. Mason J: The pathophysiology of Sandimmune (cyclosporine) in man and animals. Pediatr Nephrol 1990; 4:686–704.
21. Scott JP, Higenbottam TW: Adverse reactions and interactions of cyclosporin. Med Toxicol Adverse Drug Exp 1988; 3:107–127.
22. Reznick VM, Lyons Jones K, Durham BL, et al: Changes in facial appearance during cyclosporine treatment. Lancet 1987; 1:1405–1407.
23. Lorber MI: Cyclosporine: Lessons learned—Future strategies. Clin Transplant 1991; 5:505–516.
24. Kopp JB, Klotman PE: Cellular and molecular mechanisms of cyclosporin nephrotoxicity. J Am Soc Nephrol 1990; 1:162–179.
25. Warty VS, Venkataramanan R, Zendehrouh P, et al: Practical aspects of FK506 analysis (Pittsburgh experience). Transplant Proc 1992; 23:2730–2731.
26. Fung J, Abu-Elmagd K, Jain A, et al: A randomized trial of primary liver transplantation under immunosuppression with FK-506 vs cyclosporine. Transplant Proc 1992; 23:2977–2983.
27. Shapiro R, Jordan M, Scantlebury V, et al: FK506 in clinical kidney transplantation. Transplant Proc 1992; 23:3065–3067.
28. Armitage JM, Kormos RL, Fung J, et al: The clinical trial of FK506 as primary and rescue immunosuppression in adult cardiac transplantation. Transplant Proc 1992; 23:3054–3057.
29. Jensen CWB, Scantlebury V, Fung J, et al: FK506 conversion of renal allografts failing cyclosporine immunosuppression. Transplant Proc 1992; 23:3078–3081.
30. Lewis WD, Jenkins RL, Burke PA, et al: FK506 rescue therapy in liver transplant patients with drug resistant rejection. Transplant Proc 1992; 23:2989–2991.
31. Shaw BW, Markin R, Stratta R, et al: FK506 rescue treatment of acute and chronic rejection in liver allograft recipients. Transplant Proc 1992; 23:2994–2995.
32. Venkataramanan R, Jain A, Warty VS, et al: Pharmacokinetics of FK506 in transplant patients. Transplant Proc 1992; 23:2736–2740.
33. Vincent SH, Wang RW, Karanam BV, et al: Effects of the immunosuppressant FK-506 and its analog FK-520 on hepatic and renal cytochrome P450 mixed-function oxidase. Biochem Pharmacol 1991; 41:1325–1330.
34. Abu-Elmagd K, Fung J, Draviam R, et al: Four hour versus 24 hour intravenous infusion of FK506 in liver transplantation. Transplant Proc 1992; 23:2767–2770.
35. Fung JJ, Abu-Elmagd K, Todo S, et al: FK506 in clinical organ transplantation. Clin Transplant 1991; 5:517–522.
36. Moutabarrik A, Ishibashi M, Kameoka H, et al: FK506 mechanism of nephrotoxicity: Stimulatory effect on endothelin secretion by cultured kidney cells. Transplant Proc 1992; 23:3133–3136.
37. McCauley J, Takaya S, Fung J, et al: The question of FK 506 nephrotoxicity after liver transplantation. Transplant Proc 1991; 23:1444–1447.
38. Eidelman BH, Abu-Elmagd K, Wilson J, et al: Neurologic complications of FK-506. Transplant Proc 1991; 23:3175–3178.
39. Japanese FK506 Study Group: Japanese study of FK506 on kidney transplantation: The benefit of monitoring the whole blood FK506 concentration. Transplant Proc 1992; 23:3085–3088.
40. Morris RE: Rapamycins: Antifungal, antitumor, antiproliferative and immunosuppressive macrolides. Transplant Rev 1992; 6:39–87.
41. Morris RE, Meiser BM, Wu J, et al: Use of rapamycin for the suppression of alloimmune reactions in vivo: Schedule dependence, tolerance induction, synergy with cyclosporine and FK 506, and effect on host-versus-graft and graft-versus-host reactions. Transplant Proc 1991; 23:521–524.
42. Dumont FJ, Melino MR, Staruch MJ, et al: The immunosuppressive macrolides FK-506 and rapamycin act as reciprocal antagonists in murine T cells. J Immunol 1990; 144:1418–1424.
43. Kreis H, Legendre C, Chatenoud L: OKT3 in organ transplantation. Transplant Rev 1991; 5:181–199.
44. Prieto M, Lake KD, Pritzker MR, et al: OKT3 induction and steroid-free maintenance immunosuppression for treatment of high-risk heart transplant recipients. J Heart Lung Transplant 1991; 10:901–911.
45. Millis JM, McDiarmid SV, Hiatt JR, et al: Randomized prospective trial of OKT3 for early prophylaxis of rejection after liver transplantation. Transplantation 1989; 47:82–88.
46. Goldman M, Abramowicz D, De Pauw L, et al: Beneficial effects of prophylactic OKT3 in cadaver kidney transplantation: Comparison with cyclosporin A in a single-center prospective randomized study. Transplant Proc 1991; 23:1046–1047.
47. Stratta RJ, D'Alessandro AM, Armbrust MJ, et al: Sequential antilymphocyte globulin/cyclosporine immunosuppression in cadaveric renal transplantation: Effect of duration of ALG therapy. Transplantation 1989; 47:96–102.
48. Benvenisty AI, Cohen D, Stegall MD, et al: Improved results using OKT3 as induction immunosuppression in renal allograft recipients with delayed graft function. Transplantation 1990; 49:321–327.

49. Cockfield SM, Preiksaitis J, Harvey E, et al: Is sequential use of ALG and OKT3 in renal transplants associated with an increased incidence of fulminant posttransplant lymphoproliferative disorder? Transplant Proc 1991; 23:1106–1107.
50. Taylor RM: Monoclonal and polyclonal antibodies: Clinical aspects. Immunol Lett 1991; 29:113–116.
51. Barr ML, Sanchez JA, Seche LA, et al: Anti-CD3 monoclonal antibody induction therapy: Immunological equivalency with triple-drug therapy in heart transplantation. Circulation 1990; 82:IV291–IV294.
52. Menkis AH, McKenzie FN, Thomson D, et al: Benefits of avoidance of induction immunosuppression in heart transplantation. J Heart Transplant 1989; 8:311–314.
53. Macris MP, Van Buren CT, Sweeney MS, et al: Selective use of OKT3 in heart transplantation with the use of risk factor analysis. J Heart Transplant 1989; 8:296–302.
54. Thistlethwaite JR Jr, Heffron TG, Stuart JK, et al: Selective OKT3 induction therapy in adult cadaveric-donor renal transplant recipients. Am J Kidney Dis 1989; 14:28–34.
55. Chatenoud L, Gerran C, Legendre C, et al: In vivo cell activation following OKT3 administration. Transplantation 1990; 49:697–702.
56. Schroeder TJ, Hariharan S, First MR: Antibody response to OKT3 and methods for monitoring. Transplant Proc 1993; 25:77–80.
57. D'Alessandro AM, Pirsch JD, Stratta RJ, et al: OKT3 salvage therapy in a quadruple immunosuppressive protocol in cadaveric renal transplantation. Transplantation 1989; 47:297–300.
58. Sollinger HW, Eugui EM, Allison AC: RS-61443: Mechanism of action, experimental and early clinical results. Clin Transplant 1991; 5:523–526.
59. Sollinger HW, Deierhoi MH, Belzer FO, et al: RS-61433: A phase I clinical trial and pilot rescue study. Transplantation 1992; 53:428–432.
60. Freise CE, Hebert M, Osorio RW, et al: Maintenance immunosuppression with prednisone and RS-61443 alone following liver transplantation. Transplant Proc 1993; 25:1758–1759.
61. Turka LA, Dayton J, Sinclair G, et al: Guanine ribonucleotide depletion inhibits T cell activation: Mechanism of action of the immunosuppressive drug mizoribine. J Clin Invest 1991; 87:940–948.
62. Amemiya H, Suzuki S, Watanabe H, et al: Synergistically enhanced immunosuppressive effect by combined use of cyclosporine and mizoribine. Transplant Proc 1989; 21:956–958.
63. Kokado Y, Ishibashi M, Jiang H, et al: A new triple-drug induction therapy with low dose cyclosporine, mizoribine and prednisolone in renal transplantation. Transplant Proc 1989; 21:1575–1578.
64. Mita K, Akiyama N, Nagao T, et al: Advantages of mizoribine over azathioprine in combination therapy with cyclosporine for renal transplantation. Transplant Proc 1990; 22:1679–1681.
65. Anderson LW, Strong JM, Cysyk RL: Cellular pharmacology of DUP-785: A new anticancer agent. Cancer Communications 1989; 1:381–387.
66. Arteaga CL, Brown TD, Kuhn JG, et al: Phase I clinical and pharmacokinetic trial of brequinar sodium (DuP 785; NSC 368390). Cancer Res 1989; 49:4648–4653.
67. Cramer DV, Chapman FA, Jaffee BD, et al: The effect of a new immunosuppressive drug, brequinar sodium, on heart, liver and kidney allograft rejection in the rat. Transplantation 1992; 53:303–308.
68. Kahan BD, Tejpal N, Gibbons-Stubbers S, et al: The synergistic interactions in vitro and in vivo of brequinar sodium with cyclosporine or rapamycin alone and in triple combination. Transplantation 1993; 55:894–900.
69. Takahashi K, Ota K, Tanabe K, et al: Effect of a novel immunosuppressive agent, deoxyspergualin, on rejection in kidney transplant recipients. Transplant Proc 1990; 22:1606–1612.
70. Ochiai T, Nakajima K, Sakamoto K, et al: Comparative studies on the immunosuppressive activity of FK506, 15-deoxyspergualin, and cyclosporine. Transplant Proc 1989; 21:829–832.
71. Okazaki H, Sato T, Jimbo M, et al: Prophylactic use of deoxyspergualin in living related renal transplantation. Transplant Proc 1991; 23:1094–1095.
72. Koyama I, Amemiya H, Taguchi Y, et al: Prophylactic use of deoxyspergualin in a quadruple immunosuppressive protocol in renal transplantation. Transplant Proc 1991; 23:1096–1098.
73. Okubo M, Tamura K, Kamata K, et al: 15-Deoxyspergualin "rescue therapy" for methylprednisolone-resistant rejection of renal transplants as compared with anti-T cell monoclonal antibody (OKT3). Transplantation 1993; 55:505–508.

CHAPTER 180

Critical Care of Kidney Transplant Recipients

Lakshmipathi Chelluri, MD • Ronald Shapiro, MD
Jerry McCauley, MD

The kidney continues to be the most commonly transplanted solid organ; nearly 10,000 transplants are performed annually in the United States. The combination of better immunosuppression and infection prophylaxis has led to current results of 1-year patient survival in the 90% to 100% range and 1-year graft survival of 75% to 90% for recipients of cadaveric organs. For patients receiving a kidney from a living donor, even better results can be obtained.[1, 2] Kidney transplantation is a less expensive therapy than dialysis for patients with end-stage renal disease and is associated with both an improved quality of life and economic rehabilitation.[3, 4]

The surgical techniques and principles of perioperative management for kidney transplant recipients have been standardized, and most patients do not, in fact, need monitoring in the intensive care unit (ICU). Patients with specific medical problems or those experiencing complications during the preoperative or postoperative period may require management in an ICU. This chapter describes the care of straightforward patients undergoing kidney transplantation and those complications requiring management in an ICU.

PREOPERATIVE EVALUATION

Evaluation of patients for kidney transplantation is usually done on an outpatient basis.[5] Potential candidates meet with the transplant surgeon, nephrologist, social worker, and coordinator. A history and complete physical examination are recorded, and certain laboratory tests are performed. Important elements of the history include questions about previous transplants, complications after transplantation, blood transfusions, urologic problems, and dialysis status. Patients need not be on dialysis to undergo transplantation because progression to end-stage renal disease may lead to evaluation and transplantation before dialysis becomes necessary. Additional medical problems, such as diabetes mellitus, cardiac or pulmonary disease, liver, pancreatic, or other gastrointestinal problems, neurologic or musculoskeletal disorders, infections, and malignancies, are all specifically addressed. Active infections or malignancies are absolute contraindications to transplantation. All diabetics undergo noninvasive evaluation for coronary artery disease beginning with a stress or adenosine thallium test. Cardiac catheterization is also performed, if necessary. Patients with significant coronary artery disease may even require coronary artery bypass grafting before transplantation.[6–9] A psychosocial evaluation by the social worker is of enormous importance, particularly with regard to issues of compliance and recreational drug use.

Routine laboratory studies, in addition to the usual chemistry and hematology panels, include serologic evaluation for cytomegalovirus (CMV), hepatitis A, B, and C, and human immunodeficiency virus. Human leukocyte antigen typing is performed, and panel-reactive antibody levels are assessed to measure the degree of presensitization. Routine radiologic studies, in addition to a chest x-ray film, include ultrasonography of the gallbladder and native kidneys. A voiding cystourethrogram is performed only if indicated. Other tests, such as noninvasive peripheral arterial Doppler examination, pulmonary function tests, and upper and lower digestive tract endoscopy, are performed when necessary.

There is no absolute lower or upper age limit for renal transplantation. Recipients have ranged in age from 8 months to 78 years. When the evaluation is completed, patients are presented before the evaluation committee, and a decision is made to include the patient on the waiting list, reject the patient, or order further tests.

Once a patient is on the waiting list, the dialysis unit sends blood on a monthly basis for cross-matching. Kidneys are allocated according to a computerized point system that takes into account quality of antigen matching, waiting time, and the panel-reactive antibody level. Patients of a suitable blood type are crossmatched when a kidney becomes available, and the patient who is highest on the list with a negative crossmatch receives the organ. The system is formally unbiased with regard to gender, age, race, and socioeconomic status.

PERIOPERATIVE MANAGEMENT

When a kidney becomes available, the selected recipient is admitted to the hospital and immediately evaluated by the surgeon, nephrologist, and anesthesiologist. In addition to an interval history and physical examination, routine tests such as serum electrolytes, blood urea nitrogen, creatinine, an electrocardiogram, and a chest radiograph are obtained. Hyperkalemia and pulmonary edema on physical examination or chest radiograph, or both, are indications for preoperative dialysis. Although mild hyperkalemia (potassium ion <5.5 mEq/L) may be treated with an ion exchange (Kayexalate) enema, dialysis is generally preferred because an ion exchange may not be effective rapidly enough and can impose an additional sodium load and might precipitate or worsen pulmonary edema. Anticoagulation during dialysis is limited to prevent bleeding complications during and after surgery.

In the absence of significant cardiopulmonary dysfunction, central venous (CVP) and noninvasive arterial pressure monitoring are used. Diabetic patients with autonomic neuropathy may have a higher risk of experiencing cardiovascular instability and may require additional hemodynamic monitoring.[10] Patients are maintained in a euvolemic state during surgery with guidance from CVP monitoring. The diseased kidneys are not usually removed unless they are infected or if there is a specific indication for nephrectomy.[11]

Kidneys are generally transplanted with a heterotopic position in the iliac fossa. The external iliac artery and vein are exposed retroperitoneally. The renal vein and artery are then anastomosed, usually end to side to the iliac vessels. Intravenous furosemide (1 mg/kg) and mannitol (1 g/kg) are given while the vascular anastomoses are being performed. Systolic arterial pressure is maintained between 120 and 140 mm Hg to ensure adequate perfusion of the transplanted kidney. After revascularization of the allograft, the transplanted ureter is implanted into the recipient's bladder. Antibiotic prophylaxis with a first-generation cephalosporin, both systemic and topical, is routine.

In the immediate postoperative period, urine output is used to guide fluid replacement. Kidneys function variably after transplantation; some kidneys have an immediate diuresis with urine volumes exceeding 1000 mL/h, and some make no urine at all. For patients with urine output greater than 300 mL/h, 80% of the urine volume is replaced with normal saline, or 5% or 1% glucose with half normal saline (some surgeons prefer to add some bicarbonate to the intravenous fluid). For patients with a urine output less than 300 mL/h, all volume is replaced with the same solution. Additional fluid is generally not indicated. Specifically, in patients with negligible urine output, accounting for insensible losses by giving 40 mL/h is discouraged because it can be associated with fluid overload and the development of pulmonary edema. In diabetic patients, insulin therapy is guided by frequent blood sugar monitoring. Occasionally, an insulin drip is necessary.

General postoperative care is not particularly different from that of nontransplant patients. An oral diet is resumed after return of gastrointestinal function. Intravenous fluids can be discontinued once a patient is tolerating oral fluids well. Wound care differs only in that skin staples are left for 3 weeks instead of 1 week to account for slower healing with steroid medication.

Transplant patients require a large number of medications in the initial post-transplant period. Immunosuppressive agents, such as cyclosporine, azathioprine, and prednisone, are given to prevent rejection. Antilymphocyte preparations, such as OKT3 or antithymocyte globulin (ATG), are used for induction in some centers, whereas elsewhere they are used only for rejection. Conventional cyclosporine-based therapy has been associated with 1-year patient survival between 90% and 100% and 1-year graft survival of 75% to 90%. The variability is a function of patient selection, skill in adjusting immunosuppression, and quality of follow-up. Cyclosporine is associated with a number of side effects; the most important of these is nephrotoxicity, although hypertension, metabolic problems, and cosmetic derangements are also seen.[12] New immunosuppressive agents are being evaluated in clinical trials worldwide. These include FK-506, an agent somewhat similar in its mechanism of action to cyclosporine, and RS-61443, a mycophenolic acid derivative, which is being evaluated as a substitute for azathioprine.[13, 14] Several other agents are at an earlier stage of development.

In addition to antirejection medication, patients routinely receive drugs to prevent opportunistic infections, such as nystatin (Mycostatin) (*Candida*), acyclovir (herpes simplex and cytomegalovirus), and trimethoprim-sulfamethoxazole (*Pneumocystis carinii*). Other agents are taken to prevent peptic ulcer disease (histamine$_2$ [h$_2$] receptor blockers, antacids, sucralfate), maintain electrolyte levels (calcium, phosphorus, magnesium supplements), or treat metabolic derangements (allopurinol). Over time, many of these medications can be tapered or eliminated.

INDICATIONS FOR ADMISSION TO THE INTENSIVE CARE UNIT

Most patients undergoing renal transplantation do not need postoperative intensive care. The indications for admission to an ICU can be classified into those occurring during the operative and early postoperative periods and those occurring in the late postoperative period (i.e., longer than 3 months after transplantation).

Indications for Perioperative Intensive Care

Cardiac

Patients with significant cardiac dysfunction (i.e., a left ventricular ejection fraction less than 30%) or significant coronary artery disease may need perioperative hemodynamic monitoring. This is usually accomplished with a Swan-Ganz catheter inserted via a jugular vein and a radial arterial catheter. Although the femoral artery and vein can be cannulated for such monitoring, care should be taken not to cannulate the femoral vessels on the same side as the transplant. Maintaining adequate cardiac filling pressures and using inotropic agents can improve cardiac function and facilitate management of these patients during the perioperative period. Patients with hemodynamic instability during the operation need postoperative monitoring and assessment in the ICU for myocardial injury. Iatrogenic pulmonary edema secondary to fluid overload during the transplantation is a complication that should be avoided. Occasionally, emergency dialysis may be required to remove excess fluid and improve pulmonary gas exchange.

Hypertension

Hypertension requiring parenteral therapy is occasionally necessary and can be the result of sudden inadvertent withdrawal of antihypertensive medications or excessive fluid administration. Often, reinstitution of the pretransplant antihypertensive medications and the occasional use of sublingual nifedipine (10 mg) are sufficient. Occasionally, intravenous nitroprusside is needed. In such cases, it is necessary to monitor thiocyanate levels, particularly when the allograft is functioning poorly. Labetolol and esmolol are useful in controlling blood pressure but can be problematic because β-blockers can cause hyperkalemia.[15]

Pulmonary

Most of the patients undergoing renal transplantation are extubated postoperatively and do not need mechanical ventilatory support or intensive respiratory care. Patients with significant pulmonary dysfunction preoperatively on the other hand may need prolonged mechanical ventilation or respiratory therapy with bronchodilators.

Renal Failure

Allograft dysfunction is not an uncommon problem. Oliguria in the early postoperative period may be due to prolonged ischemia or problems with the donor before organ recovery; hypovolemia, vascular thrombosis, and hyperacute rejection. In addition, external obstruction secondary to hematoma or obstruction of the ureter or Foley catheter can also be causes of low or no urine output postoperatively. Renal flow scans and ultrasonography are useful in assessing blood flow of the renal vessels and kidney function. Allograft function usually improves over time (7–21 days) if the cause of oliguria is acute tubular necrosis. Fluid restriction and close monitoring of electrolytes are needed in patients with oliguria or anuria. Pulmonary edema and hyperkalemia are the important complications that obviously require immediate therapy. Hemodynamically stable patients can undergo hemodialysis to remove fluid; in hemodynamically unstable patients, bicarbonate-buffered dialysate solutions, which are associated with less hemodynamic instability than acetate-buffered solution, could be used.[16–19] Patients who have been on peritoneal dialysis preoperatively can be put on low-volume, frequent-exchange peritoneal dialysis if peritoneal integrity has been maintained during the transplantation procedure. Hypoxemia is one of the complications of dialysis. Therefore, patients with significant pulmonary dysfunction may need an increase in supplemental oxygen during hemodialysis.[20] In critically ill patients who may not be able to tolerate dialysis, continuous renal replacement therapy techniques such as continuous arteriovenous or venovenous hemofiltration with or without dialysis and slow continuous ultrafiltration with or without dialysis are useful. These methods of renal replacement therapy are particularly useful in patients who receive large volumes of fluid because of parenteral nutrition and antibiotic therapy.[21, 22] At our medical center, continuous renal replacement therapy is performed with a double-lumen venous catheter and a roller pump to achieve the desired flow through the system.

Hyperkalemia

Hyperkalemia during the postoperative period may be caused by tissue trauma during surgery, excessive bleeding, and transfusions and occasionally by the use of β-blockers for treatment of hypertension. Beta-blockade prevents entry of potassium into the cell and may promote hyperkalemia.[15] Although ion exchange resins can be used to decrease serum potassium levels, they have high sodium content and may worsen pulmonary edema. Dialysis is the treatment of choice in patients with hyperkalemia, particularly when hyperkalemia is associated with fluid overload.

Rejection

One of the common causes of graft dysfunction is rejection, which can occur in up to 50% or more of patients. Current immunosuppressive therapy at the University of Pittsburgh Medical Center includes FK-506 and steroids as primary therapy. A trial is in progress to assess the utility of adding azathioprine. FK-506 is a new immunosuppressive agent and has been shown to be comparable to cyclosporine in its ability to prevent rejection. FK-506 is more potent and probably somewhat more efficacious than cyclosporine. It allows the eventual elimination of steroids in 30% to 40% of patients. It is comparable to cyclosporine in terms of nephrotoxicity, neurotoxicity, and diabetogenicity. The incidence of hypertension may be less, and hypercholesterolemia occurs less frequently than in patients on cyclosporine. Both cyclosporine and FK-506 have significant dose-related toxicity and significant drug interactions.[23–26] Blood or plasma levels of these drugs should be monitored closely to avoid such problems.

Rejection is categorized into hyperacute, accelerated, acute, or chronic. Hyperacute rejection is rare and should never occur with the availability of pretransplant cross-matching techniques; it is mediated by preformed antibodies. These antibodies bind to the donor organ endothelium and initiate a cascade of events that lead to graft thrombosis within minutes of transplantation. When it occurs, immediate allograft nephrectomy is required. Accelerated rejection is similar to hyperacute rejection but occurs within the first few days (rather than minutes) after transplantation. The outcome is usually, but not always, the same as with hyperacute rejection. Acute rejection generally occurs from 1 week to several months after transplantation (although it can also occur later) and can manifest itself as a rise in creatinine with or without decreasing urine volume. Definitive diagnosis is made by kidney biopsy. Acute rejection is managed by steroids or antilymphocyte preparations, such as OKT3 or ATG. Patients receiving OKT3 need to be monitored closely because OKT3 can cause fever, an increase in cardiac output, and a decrease in systemic vascular resistance (mediated by cytokine release, especially tumor necrosis factor), hypotension, pulmonary edema, and, rarely, anaphylactic shock.[27–32] Chronic rejection occurs late after transplantation; it is poorly understood and difficult to treat and leads to eventual loss of the allograft.

Technical Complications

Technical complications are unusual but need to be recognized early and may require operative intervention. Postoperative bleeding may be secondary to inadequate hemostasis or a bleeding diathesis secondary to uremia. Desmopressin acetate, or DDAVP (0.3 μg/kg), conjugated estrogens intravenously (0.6 mg·kg^{-1}·d^{-1} for 5 days), hemodialysis, and cryoprecipitate have been shown to improve platelet function and decrease perioperative bleeding. In the uncomplicated transplantation, they are rarely needed.[33–36]

Vascular complications include arterial or venous thrombosis, stenosis, and disruption. Arteriostenosis may occur late after surgery and can be treated with angioplasty. The other vascular complications usually result in loss of the allograft. Ureteral complications include urinary leak secondary to technical error or ureteral ischemia, resulting in necrosis, or ureterostenosis with obstruction. These complications usually require reoperation. A lymphocele may occur because of the disruption of lymphatics and can manifest itself as ipsilateral leg edema with a fluid collection around the kidney on ultrasonographic examination. Lymphocele is usually treated by the creation of a peritoneal window to drain the lymph into the peritoneal cavity.

Indications for Late Postoperative Intensive Care

Late complications requiring intensive care are usually related to immunosuppression and its complications, most importantly the development of opportunistic infections.[37, 38]

Infectious Complications

Infection is the most common complication of immunosuppression and the leading cause of death. Patients are at particularly high risk for various infections during the first few months after transplantation because of the heavier immunosuppression during this period. Peterson reported that about one third of transplant patients acquired an infection within 4 years after transplantation; half of the infections were viral, and one third were bacterial.[39] An important principle in renal transplantation patients with severe infectious complications is that the kidney is expendable; immunosuppression is routinely discontinued if there is any question of life-threatening infection.

Bacterial Infections

Although opportunistic infections are common in immunosuppressed patients, bacterial infections are also relatively common. Early and aggressive antibiotic therapy is crucial; at the same time, care must be taken not to overuse antibiotics because of the development of resistance or antibiotic-associated diarrhea (pseudomembranous colitis). Wound infections are rare, and deep infections should never occur with appropriate antibiotic prophylaxis. Urinary tract infections are not uncommon and must be treated aggressively to prevent ascending infections; bladder catheterization should be avoided if possible.

Mycobacterial infections are unusual but can be life-threatening. Patients with a positive purified protein derivative test should receive prophylaxis with isoniazid and vitamin B_6 for 1 year after transplantation. Any transplant patient admitted with a new pneumonia should be placed in respiratory isolation until three sputum samples are negative for acid-fast bacilli by smear and staining. Bronchoalveolar lavage (BAL) may be necessary to make a diagnosis. Treatment of active tuberculosis includes three- or four-drug therapy (isoniazid, ethambutol, pyrazinamide, and rifampin) and cessation of immunosuppression. *Legionella* pneumonia can be nosocomial or community acquired.[40] Traditional treatment with high-dose erythromycin has more recently been replaced by the quinolones, ciprofloxacin or ofloxacin. Immunosuppression is also usually decreased. Prophylactic trimethoprim-sulfamethoxazole therapy for *P. carinii* (see later discussion) may be useful for preventing *Legionella* infections.

Viral Infections

Viral infections are the most common infections after transplantation. Four main types of viruses are recognized[41–45]; the herpes viruses (Epstein-Barr virus, CMV, herpes zoster varicella, and herpes simplex), adenovirus, papovavirus, and viral hepatitis. CMV is the most common viral infection. To prevent CMV infection, all transplant patients receive high-dose oral acyclovir (800 mg orally four times a day) postoperatively, if the renal function is normal, for the first 6 months; seronegative recipients with seropositive donor kidneys receive anti-CMV hyperimmunoglobulin (CytoGam).[46, 47] In patients who acquire CMV despite these prophylactic measures, intravenous ganciclovir, 5 mg/kg twice daily, with adjustment for renal dysfunction, is given. The clinical spectrum of CMV ranges from asymptomatic infection to serious systemic disease. Death used to be seen in the preganciclovir era but should be rare today.

CMV can occur as a primary infection in a seronegative recipient of a kidney from seropositive donor or can occur as a reactivation infection. Early diagnosis is made by BAL or upper gastrointestinal biopsy. Presence of CMV early antigen in the BAL fluid or in the gastric biopsy with compatible clinical symptoms and signs is an indication for treatment with ganciclovir.[48, 49] A number of studies have shown that ganciclovir is effective in treating CMV infections. The prognosis of CMV pneumonia is grave if oxygenation is poor and mechanical ventilatory support is required. In patients with severe systemic CMV disease, immunosuppression should be stopped, even if it results in the loss of the allograft.[50–52]

Herpes simplex infections usually present as mucocutaneous infections; low-dose acyclovir (200 mg orally twice daily) is effective prophylaxis. Active infections respond to intravenous acyclovir. Herpes zoster varicella infections (shingles) usually present as a vesicular rash along a single dermatome. Intravenous acyclovir (10 mg/kg every 8 hours with adjustment for renal dysfunction) is the treatment of choice. Epstein-Barr virus can be associated with post-transplant lymphoproliferative disorder, which can result in serious systemic complications, multiple organ failure, or death. Immunosuppressive therapy is withdrawn and high-dose intravenous acyclovir (500 mg/m^2 every 8 hours) or possibly ganciclovir is administered.

Protozoal Infections

P. carinii is the most common protozoal pathogen causing pneumonia in immunosuppressed patients. Prophylactic therapy with trimethoprim-sulfamethoxazole (80/400 mg) given once or twice a day or inhalational pentamidine (300 mg once a month) essentially eliminates the disease. Established pneumonia is treated with cessation of immunosuppression and intravenous trimethoprim/sulfamethoxazole (20 mg·kg^{-1}·d^{-1} with adjustment for renal dysfunction) or pentamidine (4 mg·kg^{-1}·d^{-1}). Patients with renal dysfunction and oliguria require close monitoring in view of the high obligatory fluid requirements associated with administration of these drugs. Patients with severe pulmonary infection require mechanical ventilatory support and have a poor prognosis.[53, 54]

Fungal Infections

In immunosuppressed patients, saprophytic fungi can cause infections.[55–59] *Candida* is the most common fungal pathogen. Oral candidiasis is prevented by low-dose oral nystatin (5 mL four times a day). *Candida* esophagitis can respond to high-dose oral nystatin (20 mL four times a day), although a short course of amphotericin B (0.25 $mg \cdot kg^{-1} \cdot d^{-1}$ for 3 to 5 days) is often also necessary. Rarely, *Candida* infection can present as a mycotic pseudoaneurysm of the arterial suture line of the allograft. This can result in massive hemorrhage. Usual treatment for this consists of allograft nephrectomy and ligation of the iliac artery; arterial bypass may also be necessary. Systemic fungal infections resulting in pneumonia or brain abscesses are found in debilitated patients who have received a great deal of immunosuppression and multiple broad-spectrum antibiotics. *Mucor, Aspergillus,* or *Cryptococcus* may be the cause of other important fungal infections and can cause severe pulmonary and cerebral complications. Systemic fungal infections are usually treated with full-dose amphotericin B. Other fungal agents such as flucytosine and fluconazole may be useful adjunctive agents. Patients with brain abscesses may require more aggressive treatment with drainage and placement of an Ommaya reservoir for direct delivery of the drugs into the cerebrospinal fluid or actual resection of the lesion; the mortality is extremely high.

Gastrointestinal Complications

The range of gastrointestinal problems after transplantation is enormous and is considered by specific organ.[60–63]

Esophagus

The most common esophageal problem, *Candida* esophagitis, was previously discussed. Esophageal reflux, usually a preexisting problem, can be exacerbated by steroids and is treated with the same agents used for peptic ulcer disease.

Stomach and Duodenum

The stomach is often the site of post-transplant complications. The necessity for high-dose steroids makes peptic ulcer disease more likely. Routine prophylaxis with H_2 blockers, sucralfate, and antacids will minimize the incidence of ulcer formation. Omeprazole is effective when breakthrough occurs. Patients can present with bleeding or, less commonly, perforation, but these should be uncommon with adequate prophylaxis.[64] CMV, discussed previously, can affect both the stomach and duodenum; diagnosis and treatment are described previously. Diabetics are prone to gastroparesis; metaclopramide is often effective in managing this problem. In some patients, erythromycin, 250 mg three times daily, has been found to be useful.[65]

Small Intestine and Colon

The large intestine is more often the source of complications than the small intestine.[66–70] Exacerbations of preexisting disease, such as diverticulitis or even occult carcinoma, can occur and are handled according to standard surgical principles. Immunosuppression may have to be decreased or eliminated temporarily. An important early colonic problem is pseudo-obstruction or Ogilvie's syndrome. It tends to occur in patients with nonfunctioning kidneys and can lead to perforation, most commonly of the cecum. This is a devastating complication that can result in sepsis or even death. Avoidance is the goal; when it does occur, early, aggressive colonoscopy with placement of a decompression tube can be of enormous help in preventing perforation. Perforation is treated according to the usual surgical principles. Invasive CMV disease in the colon can present as bleeding, particularly from a cecal ulcer. Post-transplant lymphoproliferative disease can present as single or multiple masses in the colon or small intestine, or both, with or without bleeding. Both are treated as described previously.

Liver

Viral hepatitis secondary to hepatitis B or C is an important cause of morbidity or mortality after renal transplantation. Patients with quiescent preexisting disease can have exacerbation related to immunosuppression. New-onset disease can also occur. Progression to end-stage liver disease and the need for liver transplantation, although not common, can certainly occur. Treatment with interferon-alpha has been tried with rather disappointing results. Although generally a less serious problem, gallbladder disease can be a source of significant morbidity. Gallstones noted in the pretransplant evaluation are best treated with cholecystectomy before transplantation. Post-transplant complications of preexisting cholelithiasis can include acute inflammation, pancreatitis, and even perforation. New formation of gallstones after transplantation is not uncommon, particularly under cyclosporine immunosuppression. The availability of laparoscopic cholecystectomy is an attractive option in the immunosuppressed transplant patient. An important point should be made in patients taking cyclosporine who require common bile duct exploration. An open T tube will significantly decrease cyclosporine levels, and appropriate dosage adjustment is required.

Pancreatitis

Pancreatitis after transplantation can be related to multiple causes. The most important offender is steroids, although azathioprine, pentamidine, and trimethoprim-sulfamethoxazole can also cause pancreatitis in addition to hypercalcemia or biliary disease.[71–73] Post-transplant pancreatitis can be a serious problem and can lead to severe morbidity or even mortality. Withdrawal of the offending agent and supportive care, with attention to fluid and electrolyte balance and adequate nutrition, will usually lead to resolution. Immunosuppression may need to be reduced or temporarily stopped as well. Somatostatin may be useful in the treatment of severe pancreatitis.[74, 75]

Neurologic Complications

Neurologic complications are usually related to drug toxicity or infections.[76–79] Metabolic encephalopathy, hypertensive encephalopathy, cerebrovascular events, and new-onset seizures have all been reported. Infections can be caused by *Listeria, Cryptococcus, Nocardia, Aspergillus,* and *Mucor. Toxoplasma,* Coccidia, CMV, and herpes infections are also reported. Cerebral hemorrhage can occur secondary to septic emboli or intracerebral aneurysms. Early detection and aggressive management are needed to improve survival. Seizures after transplantation may be related to inadvertent withdrawal of antiseizure medications or to drug toxicity or metabolic problems. Traditional antiseizure medications, such as phenobarbital or diphenylhydantoin, can, by virtue of accelerating the cytochrome P_{450} pathway in the liver, lead to a marked decrease in cyclosporine levels, thus necessitating increased dose requirements guided by the close monitoring of serum levels.

SUMMARY

The majority of the patients undergoing renal transplantation have relatively unremarkable postoperative courses and can often be discharged from the hospital within 1 to 2 weeks. This chapter has summarized both routine management and management of complications resulting in admission to the ICU. Close collaboration among the transplant surgeon, nephrologist, and intensivist is needed to provide optimal care and improve outcome.

References

1. Living Unrelated Kidney Donation Advocated. UNOS Update 1992; 8:6.

2. Takemoto S, Terasaki PI, Cecka JM, et al: Survival of nationally shared, HLA-matched kidney transplants from cadaveric donors. N Engl J Med 1992; 327:834.
3. Eggers P: Comparison of treatment costs between dialysis and transplantation. Semin Nephrol 1992; 12:284.
4. Simmons RG, Anderson CR, Abress LK: Quality of life and rehabilitation differences among four end-stage renal disease therapy groups. Scand J Urol Nephrol 1990; 131:7.
5. Hunt J: Pretransplant evaluation and outcome. Semin Nephrol 1992; 12:227.
6. Braun WE, Phillips D, Vidt DG, et al: Coronary arteriography and coronary artery disease in 99 diabetic and nondiabetic patients on chronic hemodialysis or renal transplantation programs. Transplant Proc 1981; 13:128.
7. Najarian JS, Sutherland DE, Simmons RL, et al: Kidney transplantation for the uremic diabetic patient. Surg Gynecol Obstet 1977; 144:682.
8. Philipson JD, Carpenter BJ, Itzkoff J, et al: Evaluation of cardiovascular risk for renal transplantation in diabetic patients. Am J Med 1986; 81:630.
9. Weinrauch LA, D'elia JA, Monaco AP, et al: Preoperative evaluation for diabetic renal transplantation: Impact of clinical, laboratory, and echocardiographic parameters on patient and allograft survival. Am J Med 1992; 93:19.
10. Burgos LG, Ebert TJ, Asiddao C, et al: Increased intraoperative cardiovascular morbidity in diabetics with autonomic neuropathy. Anesthesiology 1989; 70:591.
11. Darby CR, Cranston D, Raine AE, et al: Bilateral nephrectomy before transplantation: Indications, surgical approach, morbidity and mortality. Br J Surg 1991; 78:305.
12. Kahan BD: Cyclosporine. N Engl J Med 1989; 321:1725.
13. Starzl TE, Fung JJ, Jordan M, et al: Kidney transplantation under FK 506. JAMA 1990; 264:63.
14. Shapiro R, Jordan M, Scantlebury V, et al: FK 506 in clinical kidney transplantation. Transplant Proc 1991; 23:3065.
15. Bia MJ, Lu D, Tyler K, et al: Beta adrenergic control of extrarenal potassium disposal: A beta-2 mediated phenomenon. Nephron 1986; 43:117.
16. Hampl H, Paeprer H, Unger V, et al: Hemodynamic changes during hemodialysis, sequential ultrafiltration, and hemofiltration. Kidney Int 1980; 18:S83.
17. Campese VM: Cardiovascular instability during hemodialysis. Kidney Int 1988; 33:S186.
18. Hakim RM, Pontzer MA, Tilton D, et al: Effects of acetate and bicarbonate dialysate in stable chronic dialysis patients. Kidney Int 1985; 28:535.
19. La Greca G, Feriani M, Bragantini L, et al: Effects of acetate and bicarbonate dialysate on vascular stability: A prospective multicenter study. Int J Artif Organs 1987; 10:157.
20. Broe M, DeBacker W: Pathophysiology of hemodialysis-associated hypoxemia. Adv Nephrol 1989; 18:297.
21. Lauer A, Alvis R, Avram M: Hemodynamic consequences of continuous arteriovenous hemofiltration. Am J Kidney Dis 1988; 12:110.
22. Stevens PE, Davies SP, Brown EA, et al: Continuous arteriovenous hemodialysis in critically ill patients. Lancet 1988; ii:150.
23. Pirsch JD, Kalayoglu M, D'Alessandro AM, et al: Pulmonary infiltrates and eosinophilia in an FK 506 liver transplant recipient. Transplant Proc 1991; 23:3195.
24. Fung JJ, Alesiani M, Abu-Elmagd K, et al: Adverse effects associated with the use of FK 506. Transplant Proc 1991; 23:3105.
25. Ichihashi T, Naoe T, Yoshida H, et al: Hemolytic uremic syndrome during FK 506 therapy. Lancet 1992; 340:60.
26. Baciewicz AM, Baciewicz FA: Cyclosporine pharmacokinetic drug interactions. Am J Surg 1989; 157:264.
27. Ortho Multicenter Transplant Study Group: A randomized clinical trial of OKT3 monoclonal antibody for acute rejection of cadaveric renal transplants. N Engl J Med 1985; 313:337.
28. Norman DJ, Barry JM, Bennett WM, et al: The use of OKT3 in cadaveric renal transplantation for rejection that is unresponsive to conventional anti-rejection therapy. Am J Kidney Dis 1988; 11:90.
29. Deierhoi MH, Barber HW, Curtis JJ, et al: A comparison of OKT3 antibody and corticosteroids in the treatment of acute renal allograft rejection. Am J Kidney Dis 1988; 11:86.
30. Thistlethwaite JR, Stuart JK, Mayes JT, et al: Monitoring and complications of monoclonal therapy: complications and monitoring of OKT3 therapy. Am J Kidney Dis 1988; 11:112.
31. Stein KL, Ladowski J, Kormos R, et al: The cardiopulmonary response to OKT3 in orthotopic cardiac transplant recipients. Chest 1989; 95:817.
32. Abramowicz D, Crusiaux A, Goldman M: Anaphylactic shock after retreatment with OKT3 monoclonal antibody. N Engl J Med 1992; 327:736.
33. Mannucci PM, Remuzzi G, Pusineri F, et al: Deamino-8-D-arginine vasopressin shortens the bleeding time in uremia. N Engl J Med 1983; 308:8.
34. Remuzzi G: Bleeding disorders in uremia: Pathophysiology and treatment. Adv Nephrol 1989; 18:171.
35. Shemin D, Elnour M, Amarantes B, et al: Oral estrogens decrease bleeding time and improve clinical bleeding in patients with renal failure. Am J Med 1990; 89:436.
36. Greger B, Bockhorn H, Reeb A, et al: Treatment of perioperative bleeding after kidney transplantation by conjugated estrogen. Transplant Proc 1987; 19:3704.
37. Boitard C, Bach JF: Long-term complications of conventional immunosuppressive treatment. Adv Nephrol 1989; 18:335.
38. Gottesdiener KM: Transplanted infections: Donor-to-host transmission with the allograft. Ann Intern Med 1989; 110:1001.
39. Peterson PK, Ferguson R, Fryd DS, et al: Infectious diseases in hospitalized renal transplant recipients: A prospective study of a complex and evolving problem. Medicine 1982; 61:360.
40. Wilczek H, Kallings I, Nystrom B, et al: Nosocomial legionnaires' disease following renal transplantation. Transplantation 1987; 43:847.
41. Englund JA, Sullivan CJ, Jordan C, et al: Respiratory syncytial virus infection in immunocompromised adults. Ann Intern Med 1988; 109:203.
42. Sherry MK, Klainer AS, Wolff M, et al: Herpetic tracheobronchitis. Ann Intern Med 1988; 109:229.
43. Jenkins D, Wicks A: Herpes simplex esophagitis in a renal transplant patient: The need for antiviral therapy. Am J Gastroenterol 1988; 83:331.
44. Kharsa G, Degott C, Degos F, et al: Fulminant hepatitis in renal transplant recipients. Transplantation 1987; 44:221.
45. Quarto M, Germinario C, Fontana A, et al: HIV transmission through kidney transplantation from a living related donor. N Engl J Med 1989; 320:1754.
46. Balfour HH, Chace BA, Stapleton JT, et al: A randomized, placebo-controlled trial of oral acyclovir for the prevention of cytomegalovirus disease in recipients of renal allografts. N Engl J Med 1989; 320:1381.
47. Farrugia E, Schwab TR: Management and prevention of cytomegalovirus infection after renal transplantation. Mayo Clin Proc 1992; 67:879.
48. Crawford SW, Bowden RA, Hackman RC, et al: Rapid detection of cytomegalovirus pulmonary infection by bronchoalveolar lavage and centrifugation culture. Ann Intern Med 1988; 108:180.
49. Pisani RJ, Wright AJ: Clinical utility of bronchoalveolar lavage in immunocompromised hosts. Mayo Clin Proc 1992; 67:221.
50. Crumpacker C, Marlowe S, Zhang JL, et al: Treatment of cytomegalovirus pneumonia. Rev Infect Dis 1988; 10:S538.
51. Boston Renal Transplant CMV Study Group: Gancyclovir for treatment of renal transplant-associated primary cytomegalovirus pneumonia. J Infect Dis 1988; 157:187.
52. Paya CV, Hermans PE, Smith TF, et al: Efficacy of gancyclovir in liver and kidney transplant recipients with severe cytomegalovirus infection. Transplantation 1988; 46:229.
53. Masur H: Prevention and treatment of pneumocystis pneumonia. N Engl J Med 1992; 327:1853.
54. Fox BC, Sollinger HW, Belzer FO, et al: A prospective, randomized, double-blind study of trimethoprim-sulfamethoxazole for prophylaxis of infection in renal transplantation: Clinical efficacy, absorption of trimethoprim-sulfamethoxazole, effects on the microflora, and the cost-benefit of prophylaxis. Am J Med 1990; 89:255.
55. Chugh KS, Sakhuja V, Jain S, et al: Fungal infections in renal allograft recipients. Transplant Proc 1992; 24:1940.
56. Terrell CL, Hermans PE: Antifungal agents used for deep-seated mycotic infections. Mayo Clin Proc 1987; 62:1116.
57. Wong-Beringer A, Jacobs RA, Guglielmo BJ: Treatment of funguria. JAMA 1992; 267:2780.

58. Perfect JR, Durack DT, Gallis HA: Cryptococcemia. Medicine 1983; 62:98.
59. Morduchowicz G, Shmueli D, Shapira Z, et al: Rhinocerebral mucormycosis in renal transplant recipients: Report of three cases and review of the literature. Rev Infect Dis 1986; 8:441.
60. Tavli S, Kekec Y, Tokyay R, et al: Severe surgical complications after kidney transplantation. Transplant Proc 1992; 24:1859.
61. Santiago-Deplin EA, Morales-Otero LA, Gonzalez ZA: Gastrointestinal complications and appendicitis after kidney transplantation. Transplant Proc 1989; 21:3745.
62. Castaneda MA, Garvin PJ: General surgical procedures in renal allograft recipients. Am J Surg 1986; 152:717.
63. Komorowski RA, Cohen EB, Kauffman HM, et al: Gastrointestinal complications in renal transplant recipients. Am J Clin Pathol 1986; 86:161.
64. Sarosdy MF, Saylor R, Dittman W, et al: Upper gastrointestinal bleeding following renal transplantation. Urology 1985; 26:347.
65. Janssens J, Peeters TL, Vantrappen G, et al: Improvement of gastric emptying in diabetic gastroparesis by erythromycin. N Engl J Med 1990; 322:1028.
66. Lao A, Bach D: Colonic complications in renal transplant recipients. Dis Colon Rectum 1988; 31:130.
67. Stylianos S, Forde KA, Benvenisty AI, et al: Lower gastrointestinal hemorrhage in renal transplant recipients. Arch Surg 1988; 123:739.
68. Murphy BJ, Weinfeld A: Innocuous pneumatosis intestinalis of the right colon in renal transplant recipients: Report of three cases. Dis Colon Rectum 1987; 30:816.
69. Lillemoe KD, Romolo JL, Hamilton SR, et al: Intestinal necrosis due to sodium polystyrene (Kayexalate) in sorbitol enemas: Clinical and experimental support for the hypothesis. Surgery 1987; 101:267.
70. Wooton FT, Rhodes DF, Lee WM, et al: Colonic necrosis with Kayexalate-sorbitol enemas after renal transplantation. Ann Intern Med 1989; 111:947.
71. Fernandez JA, Rosenberg JC: Post-transplantation pancreatitis. Surg Gynecol Obstet 1976; 143:795.
72. Hart CC: Aerosolized pentamidine and pancreatitis. Ann Intern Med 1989; 111:691.
73. Antonow DR: Acute pancreatitis associated with trimethoprim-sulfamethoxazole. Ann Intern Med 1986; 104:363.
74. D'Amico D, Favia G, Biasiato R, et al: The use of somatostatin in acute pancreatitis: Results of a multicenter trial. Hepatogastroenterology 1990; 37:92.
75. Gjorup I, Roikjaer O, Andersen B, et al: A double-blinded multicenter trial of somatostatin in the treatment of acute pancreatitis. Surg Gynecol Obstet 1992; 175:397.
76. Bruno A, Adams HP: Neurologic problems in renal transplant recipients. Neurol Clin 1988; 6:305.
77. Gottrand F, Largilliere C, Farriaux J: Cyclosporine neurotoxicity. N Engl J Med 1991; 324:1744.
78. Eck P, Silver SM, Clark EC: Acute renal failure and coma after a high dose of oral acyclovir. N Engl J Med 1991; 325:1178.
79. Eidelman BH, Abu-Elmagd K, Wilson J, et al: Neurologic complications of FK 506. Transplant Proc 1991; 23:3175.

CHAPTER 181

Intensive Care of Liver Transplant Recipients

David J. Kramer, MD • Robert Selby, MD
John J. Fung, MD, PhD

Liver transplantation (OLTX) has become a recognized therapeutic option for patients with end-stage liver disease (ESLD). It affords the opportunity for a disabled person to return to a full and active life. Although expensive, OLTX may well be more cost effective than the routine medical care of terminally ill liver failure patients.[1,2] The first OLTX in humans was performed by Starzl in 1963.[3] However, significant progress could not occur until the advent of more potent immunosuppressives. Still, the success of OLTX and its acceptance as routine were not acknowledged until 1981 with the introduction of cyclosporin A(CyA).[4] Technical improvements in surgical approach and organ preservation, combined with increasingly sophisticated anesthetic and intensive care management, have provided early survival rates of nearly 90%.

CANDIDATE SELECTION

Optimal candidates are those for whom the risk of surgery is far outweighed by the potential for improvements in their quality of life. Furthermore, the risk of recurrence of the primary disease should be low.[5,6] Not surprisingly, those who are at the highest risk for surgery also achieve the greatest gains when they survive. Unfortunately, such patients have a higher mortality and require significantly greater resources, particularly intensive care and rehabilitation. Achieving an appropriate balance is largely a factor of institutional bias and donor organ availability. Indeed, programs in the nascent stages should not be expected to assume the care of high-risk patients until they have demonstrated mastery of basic cases. This should not mean that the more difficult patients are not cared for but rather that they should be referred to centers with more experience. Organ allocation plays a pivotal role. When donors are available or a change in technique suddenly makes available previously discarded organs, the threshold for working with high-risk patients can be lowered. However, when organs are scarce or not distributed according to need, patients who are at high risk often wait until transplantation is no longer feasible.

At the University of Pittsburgh, there are few absolute contraindications to OLTX. However, factors have been identified that significantly increase the risk and should be recognized as relative contraindications (Table 181–1). From the surgical perspective, prior right upper quadrant abdominal surgery, particularly biliary reconstruction, results in a more technically difficult procedure. Patients who are sicker (U.S. United Network Organ Sharing status 4),[7] particularly those with fulminant hepatic failure, fare worse. In that regard, those with higher Acute Physiology and Chronic Health Evaluation II scores, those in the intensive care unit (ICU), and particularly those requiring mechanical ventilation or hemodialysis, or both, fare worst. Not surprisingly,

TABLE 181–1. Contraindications to Liver Transplantation

Absolute	*Relative*
Extrahepatic malignancy	Cholangiocarcinoma
Infection for which the liver is not the source	HIV infection (in the absence of AIDS)
Hepatitis B with active replication	Hepatitis B without evidence of active replication
Brain death (in patients with FHF)	Elevated intracranial pressure associated with hemodynamic instability in FHF
	Portal venous thrombosis
	Extrahepatic organ system failure not related to the ESLD
	Pulmonary hypertension
	Hepatopulmonary syndrome

Abbreviations: HIV = human immunodeficiency virus; AIDS = acquired immunodeficiency syndrome; FHF = fulminant hepatic failure; ESLD = end-stage liver disease.

medical therapy in such circumstances is even less successful.

Patients with cirrhosis and underlying hepatocellular carcinomas are candidates for OLTX if the disease is limited to the liver and the lesions are small, there is no evidence for major intrahepatic venous invasion, the disease is unilobar, and nodal disease is absent. Extensive radiologic staging of these patients to stratify them into tumor stages is imperative so that the risk of postoperative recurrence can be estimated. Patients with biliary tract malignancy, such as cholangiocarcinoma, have a very high rate of recurrence.[8, 9] Whether more extensive resection, including the liver, a portion of small bowel, and pancreas, will be more successful in controlling recurrence of these tumors is doubtful.[10, 11]

Patients with chronic hepatitis B virus (HBV) have a near-universal recurrence of the disease in the graft.[12] The time course may be highly varied, and some have argued that the enormity of the problem from a worldwide perspective, the speed with which viral inhibitors are being developed, and the varied post-transplant courses mandate an attempt at OLTX.[13, 14] Adjuvant therapy with hepatitis B immune globulin[15] has been reported of benefit, particularly when guided by titers. However, the benefit accrued is small, and other inhibitors such as thymosin are under active investigation.[16] For reasons that are unclear, patients transplanted with HBV fare worse at each postoperative stage than those with other causes of ESLD. Some have speculated that this is a systemic disease accounting for both the high rate of reinfection and the decreased survival. At present, patients with evidence of active viral replication including serum HBV deoxyribonucleic acid and/or who are hepatitis E antigen positive are not currently considered for OLTX at our center (University of Pittsburgh Medical Center).

Although a disastrous course might be expected for patients who are infected with the human immunodeficiency virus (HIV) at the time of OLTX, given the need for additional immunosuppression, this has not been the case. Indeed, the survival is lower than for HIV-negative patients receiving OLTX but only slightly.[8, 17] Concern is greatest for the operating surgeons, anesthesiologists, and intensivists who routinely perform invasive procedures on such patients as well as for ICU nurses and other personnel caring for these patients. At our center, only those with advanced disease—acquired immunodeficiency syndrome (AIDS)–related complex or established AIDS—are denied OLTX.

Patients with thrombosed portal veins present a formidable surgical challenge. These patients need to have superior mesenteric artery (SMA) arteriography with venous phase studies to demonstrate patency of the superior mesenteric vein. SMA occlusion precludes liver transplantation.

Fulminant hepatic failure (FHF)—liver failure with encephalopathy in a patient without previously known liver disease developing within an 8-week period[18]—is increasingly being managed with OLTX. With this surgical option, the survival has improved from 20% to 75%.[19, 20] Such patients are often critically ill at the time of transplantation. They require intensive hemodynamic and neurologic monitoring preoperatively. In particular, intracranial pressure monitoring[21–25] and cerebral blood flow determination are routinely used at our institution. Some patients may improve with supportive care (e.g., patients with acetaminophen intoxication, *Amanita* poisoning, or hepatitis A) but most will deteriorate. Progressive encephalopathy with sustained intracranial hypertension resulting in inadequate cerebral perfusion precludes successful OLTX because brain death will result. Such patients are also prone to the development of pancreatitis, which, when severe, makes OLTX unacceptably risky. Cardiovascular instability,[26] atrial and ventricular arrhythmias,[27] and respiratory insufficiency are common complications of FHF and make the operative risk significantly higher. Patients who require high-dose vasopressor support (e.g., more than 1 $\mu g \cdot kg^{-1} \cdot min^{-1}$ of epinephrine) and those with severe adult respiratory distress syndrome (ARDS) (e.g., requiring more than 10 cm positive end-expiratory pressure [PEEP] or fraction of inspired oxygen [F_{IO_2}] >70%) have an unacceptable operative risk. Pancreatitis, which is common in patients with FHF, should resolve before proceeding with OLTX.

Patients with ESLD severe enough to make them eligible for OLTX often deteriorate precipitously and require admission to the ICU. Common precipitants include infection, (particularly pneumonia and spontaneous bacterial peritonitis) and gastrointestinal bleeding (from esophageal and gastric varices, portal hypertensive gastropathy, gastric and duodenal ulceration, and so on). Although these events herald the impending demise of the patient and intensify the search for an organ, they also further compromise the potential recipient and may lead to multisystem organ failure (MSOF) and subsequently death.

The decision regarding when a patient is "too sick" to undergo OLTX is complex. Patients with unresolved extrahepatic infection and those with high vasopressor requirements should not undergo transplantation. Although they might survive the operation, the graft is likely to fail quickly, resulting in the patient's death. Short of this disastrous scenario, we have successfully managed patients requiring dialytic support for renal failure, mechanical ventilation, severe encephalopathy (grade IV), profound coagulopathies, and MSOF with OLTX. Usually, with good graft function, MSOF will resolve.

DONOR SELECTION AND OPERATION

Assessing potential graft function in a donor is still very inexact. Potential donors who have malignancy or are infected with HIV or hepatitis B are eliminated. Other considerations include age greater than 65 years (although some have clearly functioned acceptably) and direct hepatic trauma. Evidence of chronic liver disease in the donor should be sought but often may not be evident until gross inspection or after procurement. Donor livers with biopsy-proven microvesicular steatosis are not routinely accepted. Liver function tests are not sufficiently discriminatory to use to decline a graft. Other measures such as lidocaine clearance[28, 29] are not routinely available within a short enough time frame.

Brain death results in marked changes in homeostasis for the donor. Hemodynamic instability is common and may result in part from massive fluid loss caused by diabetes insipidus. Correction with desmopressin and adequate hemodynamic monitoring and intervention are essential to preserving vital organ function. Anesthetic techniques to blunt the response to surgical stimulation are essential.

A skilled surgical dissection with rapid identification of the hepatic vessels,[30] including the hepatic arterial anomalies present in 20% of the population, cannulation and perfusion with (University of Wisconsin) solution, and rapid cooling are essential for graft preservation. Although a cold ischemia time of less than 16 hours is preferable, up to 24 hours will still enable adequate graft function.[31]

RECIPIENT OPERATION

The recipient operation has become a highly refined surgical procedure. Improvements in anesthetic and surgical practice have made evident the importance of the other factors described previously—candidate selection and donor organ quality—in the eventual outcome for the recipient. The surgical procedure may be divided into three stages: hepatectomy, anhepatic, and postreperfusion. Each involves special consideration by the anesthesiologist and surgeon.

Monitoring for such cases includes pulse oximetry, electrocardiography, arterial pressure (often from two vessels), and pulmonary arterial pressures. Maintenance of large-bore central venous catheters (e.g., two 8.5-French introducers) and the ability to infuse whole blood at up to 2 L/min as with the rapid infusion system are essential to maintain hemodynamic stability during the occasional massive blood loss. More extensive monitoring is indicated in select cases. Right ventricular function may be compromised by the presence of pulmonary hypertension, which may develop acutely during reperfusion.[32–35] Titration of intravenous fluid and vasopressors may be more effectively guided by the right ventricular ejection fraction and end-diastolic volume. These values may be obtained by use of the REF1 oximetric pulmonary artery catheter (Baxter-Edwards). Additional cardiovascular assessment is provided by the frequent use of transesophageal echocardiography. This provides a dynamic on-line picture to the anesthesiologist to assess the adequacy of resuscitation. In patients with FHF, who are prone to experience intracranial hypertension, intracranial pressure monitoring is essential. Although cerebral blood flow measurements are difficult to obtain in the operating room, the arterial-jugular venous oxygen content difference may be used as a surrogate. Cerebral blood flow may also be assessed by use of transcranial Doppler ultrasound to measure the velocity of flow in the middle cerebral artery. Continuous electroencephalography (EEG) and compressed spectral array are currently under investigation as monitoring techniques in this setting.

Anesthesia is often induced with etomidate and maintained with a balanced technique of inhalational agents (isoflurane), muscle relaxation (vecuronium), and judicious use of narcotics (fentanyl) and benzodiazepines (midazolam).[36]

Monitoring of the coagulation capacity of the recipient is complicated by the presence of profound derangements and the need for rapid correction. Depleted coagulation factors and thrombocytopenia are common. Furthermore, excessive fibrinolysis, which may be evident early in the procedure but not of clinical import, may assume a major role after significant blood loss and particularly on reperfusion. Standard measures of coagulation prove to be very sensitive, too much so to address the question of what to transfuse to abate the medical bleeding and often too slow. Kang and colleagues introduced the thromboelastograph for routine use during OLTX. It provides the anesthesiologist with a rapid assessment of the coagulation status, the presence or absence of fibrinolysis, and the effects of intervention with protamine or ε-aminocaproic acid, an inhibitor of fibrinolysis.[37–39]

The surgical procedure involves meticulous dissection, which is often hampered by severe portal hypertension with substantial bleeding from venous collaterals. Insufficient control results in significant blood loss. Identification of the hilar structures may be complicated by adhesions from prior biliary tract surgery. Recipient vessel patency and the adequacy of blood flow must be assessed before placing the graft into the surgical field. An arterial graft for the hepatic artery may be chosen when the recipient anatomy is anomalous or of diminished caliber or when the presence of atherosclerosis makes stenosis of the celiac trunk or native hepatic artery likely. Other indications include a marked size discrepancy and inadequate donor length. Portal venous thrombosis may be managed with a "jump" graft placed on the superior mesenteric vein if the portal vein cannot be "declotted."[40] The donor and recipient caval veins are usually anastomosed end to end above and below the liver.

However, an alternative technique, "piggyback,"[41–43] may be preferred in settings of marked hemodynamic instability—using only portal bypass—or when there is a marked size discrepancy between donor and recipient. The technique requires isolating the hepatic veins of the recipient without interrupting flow in the inferior vena cava (IVC). Venovenous bypass is routinely used in our center (Fig.

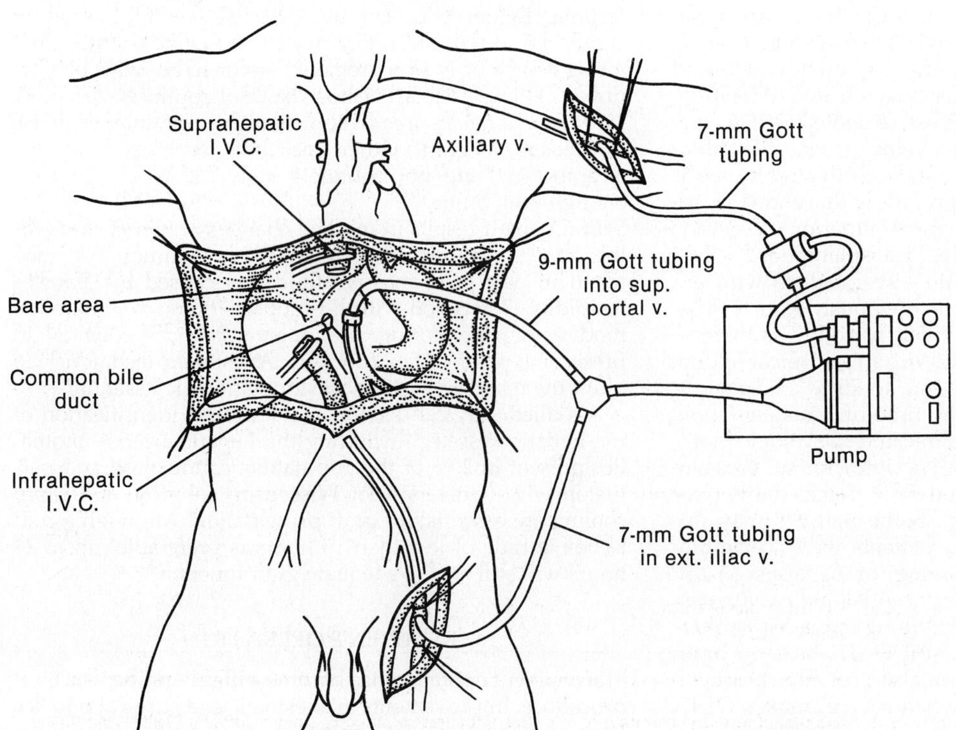

Figure 181–1. Venovenous bypass. *Abbreviations:* I.V.C. = inferior vena cava; ext. iliac v. = external iliac vein. (From Starzl TE, Griffith BP, Shaw BW Jr, et al: Veno-venous bypass without systemic anticoagulation for transplantation of the human liver. Surg Gynecol Obstet 1985; 160:270, by permission of Surgery, Gynecology, & Obstetrics.)

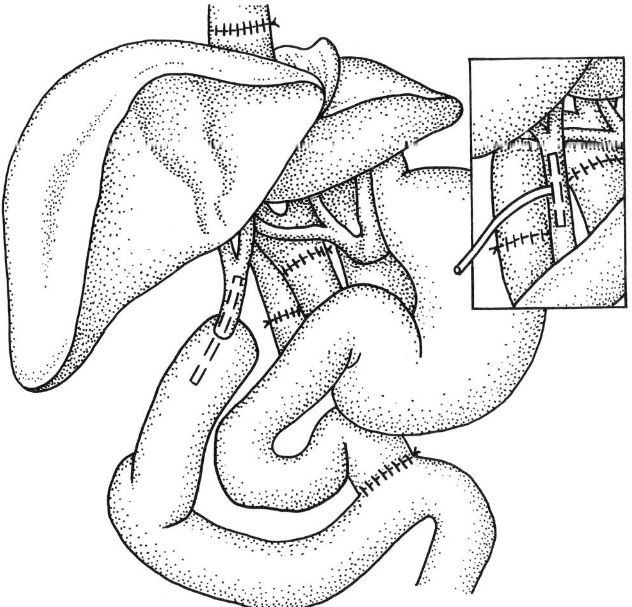

Figure 181–2. Choledochojejunostomy and choledochocholedochostomy. (Reprinted with permission from Starzl TE, Demetrius AJ, Van Thiel D: Liver transplantation. N Engl J Med 1989; 321:1014, 1092.)

181–1) to minimize hemodynamic instability, portal hypertension, and venous congestion of the intestines, which occur routinely in its absence.[44] The biliary anastomosis is fashioned after the vascular anastomoses are completed and the graft reperfused. Two options currently used are a choledochocholedochostomy or creating a midjejunal Roux-en-Y limb with a choledochojejunostomy (Fig. 181–2). The former is faster and aesthetically (anatomically) more pleasing. Unfortunately, there is a significant restenosis rate. Care must also be taken not to create such an anastomosis when the bile duct is involved in the primary disease process, as with primary sclerosing cholangitis.

In approximately 10% of patients, reperfusion will be accompanied by near-complete cardiovascular collapse.[45] Although the exact mechanism is undefined, marked shifts occur in electrolytes (hyperkalemia and hypocalcemia) and temperature perhaps in reaction to the preservative solution. A hypocontractile left ventricle complicates the loss of vasomotor tone. Volume resuscitation and inotropes (epinephrine) with replenishment of calcium guided by ionized calcium analysis are usually sufficient to recover. Fortunately, this event is usually short lived. However, significant insult to the graft, heart, kidneys, and brain may occur and require postoperative attention.

POSTOPERATIVE MANAGEMENT

As might be surmised from the preceding discussion, the postoperative management of the OLTX recipient is largely governed by the patient's preoperative condition, the adequacy of the donor organ, and operative success of the recipient surgical and anesthetic teams. Indeed, the function of the graft is the dominant factor in the recovery of the patient.

Liver Allograft Function

Early graft function is usually assessed by measurement of total bilirubin, transaminases, canalicular enzymes, and clotting factors. The schematic presented by the University of Toronto is useful for assessing graft function by these parameters (Table 181–2).[46] Parameters such as the arterial ketone body ratio (AKBR)[47] and oxygen consumption[48] correlate with graft survival. However, even in a recent retrospective review of our patients, Doyle and colleagues were unable to define a unique predictor with adequate sensitivity and specificity to use for an individual OLTX recipient.[49] Other techniques, such as neural network modeling, are under active investigation.[50]

Typically, an elevated bilirubin level in the first few days reflects preoperative values and the consequence of the harvest itself. In the absence of severe harvest injury, it typically falls to normal during the first week. Transaminases aspartate aminotransferase and alanine aminotransferase often show an injury pattern with elevations during the first 3 days, which return to normal slowly thereafter. Canalicular enzymes (gamma-glutamyl transpeptidase and alkaline phosphatase) typically rise to four or five times normal and return to normal over the course of the next few weeks. Marked injury that occurs during the procurement and is believed to reflect an ischemic insult results in a more extreme and more prolonged abnormality. Thus, the transaminase will peak higher, the bilirubin will remain abnormal, sometimes for weeks, and the canalicular enzymes will be elevated for a prolonged period. Unless irreversibly damaged, synthetic function seems to normalize after the third day and the AKBR returns toward 1.0. Although the values may normalize, occasionally graft dysfunction may be evidenced only by the patient's failure to thrive. In particular, MSOF may develop or fail to resolve. Retransplantation may be the only option.

Knowledge of the details of procurement and implantation should color the interpretation of liver function abnormalities in the early postoperative period. Technical problems should always be sought before an immunologic mechanism is incriminated. Even with the widespread use of percutaneous liver biopsy, histologic impressions will prove incorrect when a vascular or biliary duct problem is present. Furthermore, a misdiagnosed technical problem that is treated inadvertently as rejection results in the inten-

TABLE 181–2. Classification of Graft Function After OLTX

Variable	*Grade I*	*Grade II*	*Grade III*	*Grade IV*
SGOT SGPT	<1000	>1000 initially <1000 at 48 h	>2500 for ≥ 48 h	>2500 rising
PT	Normal	Mild prolongation	Very abnormal	Severe coagulopathy
Bile	>40 mL/d	>40 mL/d	<40 mL/d minimal	None

Abbreviations: OLTX = liver transplantation; SGOT = serum glutamic-oxaloacetic transaminase; SGPT = serum glutamate pyruvate transaminase; PT = prothrombin time.

(Data from Greig PD, Woolf GM, Sinclair SB, et al: Treatment of primary liver graft nonfunction with prostaglandin E_1. Transplantation 1989; 48:447–453.)

sification of a patient's immunosuppressive regimen and places him or her at grave risk for infectious complications. One caveat is that, although some processes produce a typical enzyme pattern, these patterns are not sufficiently sensitive and specific to avoid a diagnostic work-up.

The diagnostic work-up for a patient in the perioperative period with liver function abnormalities should include a Doppler ultrasound examination to determine vessel patency. Concern about the adequacy of flow should prompt an angiogram. Other abnormalities are often present but not specific. Early occlusion of the hepatic artery may be approached surgically with nearly 50% graft salvage rate.[51] It presents with a precipitous deterioration in a patient's hemodynamic status, abrupt development of respiratory failure (ARDS), and severe coagulopathy, all associated with markedly elevated transaminase. Bacteremia is common. Hepatic artery thrombosis, which occurs later in the patient's postoperative course, is often less dramatic in its presentation.[52] Indeed, some patients are asymptomatic. Others show destruction of the biliary duct system with multiple intrahepatic strictures, bilomas, and often intrahepatic abscesses. Recurrent bacteremia, in the absence of another source, may be the only suggestive indication of hepatic artery thrombosis.

The presentation of portal venous thrombosis is usually much less dramatic. In the early postoperative period, the most frequent manifestation is persistent ascites. Enteric congestion and bleeding as a consequence of portal hypertension may also occur. Later, a thrombosed portal vein should be considered if the patient presents with variceal hemorrhage. Although IVC occlusion related to thrombosis in the retrohepatic vena cava does occur, it is uncommon. More common are anastomotic strictures. Stenosis at the lower anastomosis of the IVC is manifest solely by lower extremity edema and renal dysfunction. Stenosis at the upper anastomosis may present as a syndrome similar to Budd-Chiari, with marked passive congestion of the liver, ascites, lower extremity edema, and renal failure. The diagnosis may be suggested by ultrasound examination, but more commonly the clinical picture prompts a catheterization and measurement under fluoroscopy of the IVC pressures above and below the anastomoses. When strictures are diagnosed, the approach is commonly surgical, but balloon dilatation has been accomplished in some cases.

Competency of the biliary tract should be confirmed by cholangiography, which is simple when a T tube drains the choledochostomy but must be performed percutaneously in patients with choledochojejunostomy, in which T tubes are not used, or when elevated canalicular enzymes and persistent jaundice are unexplained. Disruption of the biliary anastomosis is rare but typically occurs near the end of the first week and may indicate thrombosis of the hepatic artery, which interrupts the blood supply to the donor part of the choledochus. It may be heralded by developing sepsis syndrome and disproportionate rise in the bilirubin.

Graft rejection may occur at any point after OLTX. Hyperacute rejection is noticeably rare, if it occurs at all with OLTX. Nevertheless, a humoral component of rejection may be evidenced by antibody deposition in the arterial endothelium and by persistence or recrudescence of a positive crossmatch.[53] More commonly, acute cellular rejection (ACR) develops. This is often evident after the first week but has occurred within the first few days and several years after OLTX. Thus, its usual description as "acute" is a misnomer. Although a periductal lymphocytic infiltrate associated with the development of a cellular infiltrate around the central veins is the histologic criterion for the diagnosis of ACR,[54] such changes may be evident to a lesser degree even in the absence of clinical abnormalities. In a graft with stable function, rejection is typically associated with a rise in bilirubin associated with elevations in the transaminases and canalicular enzymes. Other clinical findings include signs of the sepsis syndrome, diarrhea, sudden increasing ascites, and laboratory findings of thrombocytopenia, hemolysis, and eosinophilia. Chronic rejection, also a misnomer because it may occur at any point, is the development of arteriopathy and vanishing bile ducts. Its presentation is insidious, and signs of terminal liver disease may develop slowly.

The approach to rejection is divided into two phases: prophylaxis and treatment.[54a] Prophylaxis is achieved by the combination of corticosteroids and CyA or FK-506. Azathioprine, used before the advent of newer immunosuppressives, is reserved for patients with recurrent rejection episodes or for those unable to tolerate necessary doses of the newer agents. Newer immunosuppressive agents and techniques are under development. The current regimen at the University of Pittsburgh is outlined in Table 181–3. The regimen for prophylaxis is initiated during surgery with 1 g of IV methylprednisolone. Crossmatch-negative recipients are treated with 20 mg daily in addition to FK-506 or CyA. OKT3 is reserved for the treatment of ACR resistant to steroids.[55] The approach for crossmatch-positive patients includes an additional methylprednisolone taper over 6 days. When mild, ACR is treated with a bolus of methylprednisolone and increased FK-506 administration. If this is not adequate, we elect to use the steroid taper. OKT3 is used when rejection resistant to these measures is evident. It is used for a short course, and the FK-506 dosage is increased. Usually, chronic rejection is not amenable to intensification of therapy. One exception appears to be the improvement in graft function, which occasionally attends the switch from CyA to FK-506.[56]

TABLE 181–3. Immunosuppression for OLTX Recipients: University of Pittsburgh

Agent	*Dose*	*Timing*
Methylprednisolone	1 g	Intraoperative
	20 mg	Daily
Crossmatch (+)	200 mg; taper to 20 mg	First 6 days
FK-506*	0.075 mg/kg IV	Continuous infusion over 24 h until oral intake
	0.15 mg/kg PO	Twice daily
Cyclosporine A*	6 mg/kg IV	Continuous infusion over 24 h until oral intake
	10 mg/kg PO	Twice daily
Azathioprine†	2 mg/kg PO or IV	Daily
OKT3	5–10 mg/mL	Daily for 3–5 days for treatment of ACR

*Either FK-506 or cyclosporine A is selected.
†Used in addition to cyclosporine A or FK-506.
Abbreviations: OLTX = liver transplantation; IV = intravenous; PO = oral; ACR = acute cellular rejection.

The major side effects of CyA and FK-506 are similar in that both cause significant nephrotoxicity and neurotoxicity. The insults to the kidneys incurred by the transplant procedure and the immunosuppressive regimen are evident in more than 90% of patients.[57] Ten percent require some dialytic intervention, and a few will require long-term hemodialysis. Neurotoxicity is more evident in the elderly and is compounded by electrolyte disturbances, particularly hyponatremia and hypomagnesemia.[58] Impairments range from a mild expressive aphasia to tremors to confusion, coma, and seizures. Other side effects of CyA such as hypertension and hirsutism are less common with FK-506. Because FK-506 is a more potent agent, many patients are able to have corticosteroids tapered, if not completely discontinued.[68, 68b]

Abnormal liver function may attend systemic illness. For example, marked hyperbilirubinemia may occur with septic episodes, even in the nontransplanted host. Infections may or may not directly involve the liver. However, jaundice may occur with the development of pneumonia or may herald the presence of an abscess. Other systemic processes, such as disseminated fungal infections (*Candida* or *Aspergillus*) and herpes virus infections such as herpes simplex or herpes zoster, may result in profound derangement of liver function. A systemic process that may also affect the liver is lymphoma. A unique post-transplant lymphoproliferative disease (PTLD) has been described in these patients and may involve the liver.

HEMODYNAMIC CHANGES

The characteristic hemodynamic changes of ESLD resolve slowly after OLTX. The exact timing is unresolved, and the controversy likely reflects the preoperative state of some of the patients. Thus, these problems may resolve more slowly in patients with profoundly deranged liver function and incipient if not established MSOF than in recipients who are less sick at the time of transplantation. A vasodilated hyperdynamic state is typical[59–63] and rarely normalizes completely in the immediate postoperative period. Patients who are unable to mount a hyperdynamic response fare worse, such as those who have sustained an ischemic cardiac injury or those with a restrictive cardiomyopathy, as may be seen in amyloidosis or in hemochromatosis. This observation has also been made in other postsurgical, critically ill patients. However, the magnitude of the hemodynamic changes in the patient with ESLD in the post-OLTX phase is much greater.

Marked elevation in right-sided cardiac pressures compromises allograft function. Hepatic congestion results in hyperbilirubinemia. Portal pressure is elevated simultaneously, perhaps resulting in bacterial translocation and endotoxemia with further graft dysfunction. A depressed cardiac output causes decreased hepatic arterial and portal flow and allograft ischemia. Careful management of intravascular volume, with ventricular filling pressures optimized by cardiac output or stroke work index, is combined with judicious use of inotropes.

The selection of inotropic and vasopressor agents is governed by the degree of arterial vasodilation and cardiac dysfunction. Although we favor dopamine and dobutamine, alone or in combination, it is clear that more potent agents such as norepinephrine and epinephrine may be required. In the setting of pulmonary hypertension with predominantly right-sided heart failure, more intensive monitoring of ventricular size and function with transesophageal echocardiography, including measurement of the right ventricular ejection fraction, is essential to guide titration of intravascular volume and vasoactive medication.

Marked arterial vasodilation, which requires treatment with vasopressors, particularly when it occurs in the face of improving graft function, should prompt an evaluation for a focus of inflammation:infection, pancreatitis, and graft rejection.

In the differential diagnosis of the low cardiac output syndrome associated with high filling pressures, cardiac tamponade should be excluded at an early stage. There are surgical and medical factors that increase the potential for tamponade. These include the superior aspect of the Mercedes incision, which may violate the pericardial parietal reflection, right atrial engraftment of the inferior vena cava anastomosis, and the medical complications of depressed coagulation, thrombocytopenia, and renal failure. It is crucial for the intensivist considering this diagnosis in such a setting to appreciate that tamponade physiology may present with a deceptively normal cardiac output, calculated systemic vascular resistance, and arterial venous oxygen content difference. This paradox reflects the hyperdynamic, vasodilated state present before the onset of tamponade.

Hypertension may occur in the postoperative period. It commonly reflects inadequate analgesia or sedation,[12] impaired gas exchange, and hypoglycemia, although hypotension is more common. However, hypertension may persist once these factors are addressed and attention should then be focused on cyclosporine[64, 65] and FK-506. Given the vasoconstrictive properties of both medications, one likely mechanism is activation of the renin-angiotensin pathway. This complication occurs more commonly with cyclosporine than with FK-506—30% versus 10%—and is more resistant to antihypertensive therapy.[66–68a] Antihypertensive therapy is initiated for systolic blood pressure greater than 160 mm Hg or diastolic blood pressure greater than 95 mm Hg and consists of calcium channel blockade with nifedipine or combined β- and α-blockade with labetalol. Long-term management rests on a combination of angiotensin-converting enzyme (ACE) inhibition, β-blockade, and calcium channel blockade. Hypertension resistant to the first-line agents is usually managed with stronger vasodilators such as nitroprusside perhaps in combination with β-blockade.

PULMONARY CONSIDERATIONS

Pulmonary complications of ESLD are common and relate to the combination of physiologic and immunologic derangements, which are practically always present.[69] Thus, atelectasis, pleural effusions, reduced functional residual capacity, and limited vital capacity related to ascites are often present preoperatively. The operative procedure in the upper abdomen, placement of a "normal" sized graft in the site of a shrunken, cirrhotic liver, and postoperative ileus may further decrease vital capacity. Inadequate pain control results in splinting and atelectasis and increases the risk of pneumonia. However, long-term pulmonary sequelae are rare, and most patients have improved pulmonary function tests when studied more than 1 year after OLTX.

The prompt evaluation of pulmonary infiltrates in these patients is mandatory. Although a primary pneumonic process should be considered, many pulmonary infiltrates do not reflect infection. Pulmonary edema—hydrostatic and nonhydrostatic—is common. Nonhydrostatic pulmonary edema, ARDS, when associated with decreased lung compliance and increased FIO_2, may result from a primary pulmonary infection but more commonly is associated with intra-abdominal inflammation such as peritonitis and pancreatitis. Graft failure, whether caused by rejection or primary nonfunction or a vascular catastrophe, as occurs with hepatic artery thrombosis, may also produce ARDS. When liver failure per se is identified as the cause, ARDS will resolve after transplantation. ARDS may also develop during treatment of rejection with OKT3.[70]

We routinely use bronchoscopic techniques to aid the clinical assessment of pulmonary infiltrates and to establish the diagnosis of pneumonia. Despite the severe derangements of coagulation present in these patients, bronchoalveolar lavage (BAL) has been performed without significant hemorrhage in any patient. Quantitative cultures are performed, and bacterial isolates in excess of 100,000 colony-forming units (CFU)/mL are considered positive. We have found that the BAL, although sensitive, lacks specificity because the bronchoscope may be contaminated by passage through the upper airway or endotracheal tube. We frequently use a protected brush specimen (PBS) in patients with less severe coagulopathy. Quantitative cultures are obtained, and isolates in excess of 1000 CFU/mL are considered positive. Complications have been rare. In more than 100 patients, PBS has resulted in minor bleeding (controlled at the time of bronchoscopy) in four patients and major hemorrhage in one patient in whom the profound coagulopathy, thrombocytopenia, and uremia would normally present a contraindication to PBS, although these procedures can be completed within 15 minutes and transient worsening of gas exchange may occur. In only one third of cases suspected of pneumonia did we obtain bronchoscopic confirmation. Although antibiotic administration confounds the results in some patients; in most cases, negative results force an evaluation for other sites of infection or inflammation.

Liver-lung interactions have been described by Matuschak and associates.[71] Two specific pulmonary complications—the hepatopulmonary syndrome and pulmonary hypertension—may also develop in patients with liver disease, specifically portosystemic shunting resulting from portal hypertension.

Cyanosis has been recognized in patients with cirrhosis.[72] Several explanations have been tendered. Anatomic right-to-left shunts have been described: intrapulmonary[73, 74] and between the portal venous system and pulmonary veins via esophageal veins.[75] An increase in closing volume, resulting in air trapping, has been observed. A leftward shift of the oxyhemoglobin saturation curve has been observed.[76] However, the realization that many patients have a diffusion defect and that hypoxic pulmonary vasoconstriction is impaired, combined with anatomic studies showing dilated intrapulmonary capillaries[77] and multiple inert gas studies showing significant ventilation-perfusion mismatch, has led to the following understanding. Patients with the hepatopulmonary syndrome have dilated capillaries, which cause a diffusion impairment. Furthermore, an increased dispersion in the ventilation-perfusion relation results in a mismatch such that many poorly ventilated units are excessively perfused.[78] This does not constitute a true right-to-left shunt, which explains the observation that hyperoxia will result from prolonged exposure to high FIO_2. The most useful preoperative test is contrast echocardiography, a "bubble" study. Early appearance of contrast in the left atrium is diagnostic.[79] Such patients may be successfully transplanted with resolution of the shunt, although they may have a prolonged postoperative ICU stay. High FIO_2 may be required to maintain adequate arterial saturation. Oxygen consumption must be minimized. Once graft function is restored, gas exchange improves, although more than a year may be required for complete resolution.

Pulmonary hypertension occurs more commonly in patients with cirrhosis than in controls. No precipitant has been identified. The histopathologic abnormalities in the lungs are typical of primary pulmonary hypertension, which is a clinical diagnosis of exclusion. Once the diagnoses of left ventricular failure, intracardiac shunting with increased cardiac output, autoimmune disease, and pulmonary embolism have been eliminated, liver-related pulmonary hypertension should be considered. The picture may become clouded when the process evolves to right ventricular failure with secondary hepatic congestion. Measures to manipulate pulmonary artery pressures have been complicated by systemic hypotension and frustrated when the pulmonary artery pressures are unchanged, a consequence of decreased vascular resistance and elevated cardiac output. Systemic hypotension may result in right ventricular ischemia and worsened right ventricular function. Trials of prostacyclin therapy are being conducted in patients with pulmonary hypertension without liver disease, but the potential benefit to liver patients remains to be defined. Although patients with mild pulmonary hypertension (see Table 181–4 for definitions) undergo OLTX without significant complications, the picture is bleak for those with moderate to severe pulmonary hypertension. One patient with moderate pulmonary hypertension has survived 1 year. Repeat right-sided heart catheterization demonstrated resolution of pulmonary hypertension. However, most OLTX patients have died. Such patients tolerate massive fluid shifts poorly. Right ventricular overload and failure develop abruptly, particularly upon reperfusion of the graft. This rapidly compromises the graft, resulting in massive liver and bowel congestion. Low cardiac output results in graft ischemia. These patients succumb quickly in the face of acute MSOF. Such patients are not currently considered candidates for liver transplantation (Fig. 181–3). However, means to support the right ventricle more aggressively such as a right ventricular assist device, extracorporeal membrane oxygenation, or pharmacologic measures such as inhaled nitric oxide are being considered.

Mechanical ventilatory support is often required for these patients preoperatively. Intubation may be required because the patient cannot protect the airway because of encephalopathy or massive upper gastrointestinal hemorrhage. Respiratory failure may be precipitated by volume overload and pulmonary edema, infection with high ventilatory requirements, or profound muscle weakness. These same factors govern the decision about extubation. One must balance the risk of pulmonary infection associated with an endotracheal tube and impaired clearance of secretions with the risks of aspiration and infection resulting from poor cough effort after extubation. The patient should have a clear mental state and improving liver function values before extubation. The median duration of intubation after transplantation is between 2 and 3 days. Prolonged mechanical ventilation invariably reflects an infectious complication or marginal graft function. Ventilator dependence may result from multiple insults and resolves as the primary process is treated and as the benefits of physical therapy and nutritional support are realized. In the management of hypoxemia, the benefit accrued from increased mean airway

TABLE 181–4. Pulmonary Hypertension and Liver Disease

Category	*Mean PA Pressure (mm Hg)*	*Systolic PA Pressure (mm Hg)*
Mild	25–34	35–44
Moderate	35–44	45–59
Severe	45–75	60–100
Very severe	>75	>100

Abbreviation: PA = pulmonary artery.

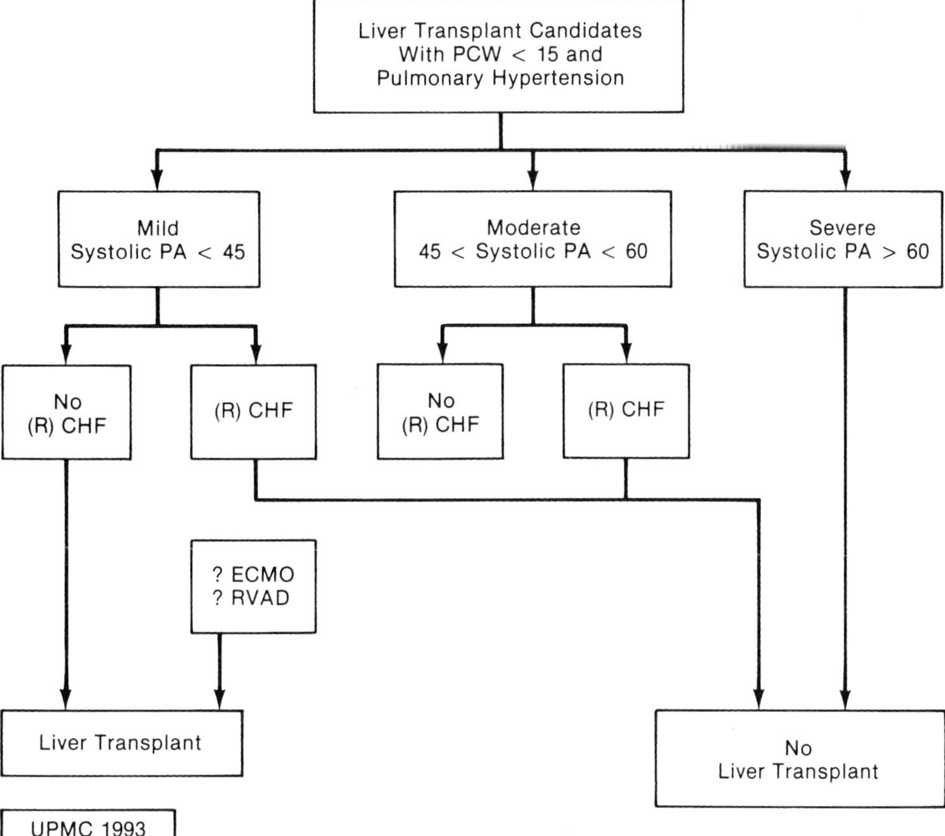

Figure 181–3. Management algorithm for patients with ESLD and pulmonary hypertension. *Abbreviations:* PCW = pulmonary capillary wedge pressure; PA = pulmonary artery; CHF = congestive heart failure; ECMO = extra corporeal membrane oxygenation; RVAD = right ventricular assist device.

pressure obtained with PEEP or decreased expiratory time must be weighed against its variable effect on right atrial pressure, which, in addition to the effect on venous return, is reflected in the hepatic venous and portal venous pressures. In the setting of hypoxemia, in which airway pressure is efficiently reflected in venous pressure, as in patients with intrapulmonary shunt, we favor increasing the FIO_2 rather than raising the airway pressure.

RENAL CONSIDERATIONS

Renal dysfunction in patients with liver disease is frequently unrecognized. Liver dysfunction and malnutrition make elevations in blood urea nitrogen and creatinine unimpressive despite significant derangements in glomerular filtration. In the post-transplant period, several factors conspire to impair renal function, including preoperative renal failure such as the hepatorenal syndrome, episodic hypotension resulting in tubular damage, medication such as cyclosporine, FK-506, and vasopressors, which cause renal arterial vasoconstriction, and medications such as amphotericin, which causes tubular damage.[80] Furthermore, liver allograft dysfunction may lead to a functional impairment of the kidneys analogous to the hepatorenal syndrome. Dialytic support is required in approximately 10% of patients and is usually temporary. We prefer to use continuous ultrafiltration with or without dialysis to manage fluid balance in hemodynamically unstable patients with renal failure. Once discharged from the ICU, such patients are managed with conventional hemodialysis. Protective measures such as perioperative dopamine, calcium channel blockade, and prostaglandin E_1 have not been efficacious in our setting when applied indiscriminantly.

GASTROINTESTINAL CONSIDERATIONS

Enteral nutrition may be started early in the postoperative period in the patient with a choledochocholedochostomy, whereas it is usually deferred for 72 hours in patients with a choledochojejunostomy, because the latter also have a jejunojejunostomy (see Fig. 181–2). When parenteral nutrition is required, we use crystalline amino acids and supply one third of the nonprotein calories as fat. This minimizes glucose intolerance, which is common in the early post-OLTX period.

Upper gastrointestinal bleeding in the OLTX recipient is uncommon, but prompt investigation is mandatory when it occurs. Gastritis and stress ulceration are common causes. Recurrence of esophageal and gastric varices often reflects diminished portal vein blood flow or thrombosis. Bleeding distal to the ligament of Treitz may be from the site of the jejunojejunostomy. Surgical control may be problematic, and we elect to optimize the coagulation status and hemodynamics before re-exploration.

Bleeding from the gastrointestinal tract weeks or months after surgery should prompt a work-up for infectious causes such as cytomegalovirus (CMV) or *Clostridium difficile* enterocolitis. However, in addition to the considerations outlined previously, bleeding may be a manifestation of neoplastic gastrointestinal involvement with lymphoma (PTLD). Patients may acquire fistulas from a hepatic arterial graft or splenic artery aneurysms. Angiography may confirm the diagnosis in more stable patients but should not delay exploration because rapid operative intervention is mandatory.

Pancreatitis is a feared complication of OLTX. Although nearly 20% of patients will demonstrate biochemical abnormalities such as elevated amylase or lipase levels, only 5% will have clinically significant pancreatitis.[81] Conservative measures are usually effective in mild cases. Management of severe pancreatitis is as controversial in this setting as in the patient without OLTX. The role of somatostatin and operative débridement with continuous lavage remains to be defined.

NEUROLOGIC CONSIDERATIONS

Patients with minimal pretransplant hepatic encephalopathy who have an uncomplicated operation and receive a good graft usually have rapid normalization of neurologic function after the effects of general anesthesia have resolved. Changes in mental status in such patients require aggressive evaluation. Most commonly, the side effects of immunosuppressives such as CyA and FK-506 may be identified and resolve with adjustment of medication. Focal deficits make embolic or hemorrhagic complications a concern. Intracranial infection is rare in the early postoperative period but must be ruled out in the patient who presents with headache and confusion.

Patients with early graft dysfunction also often have changes in mentation. Graft swelling may result in some portal congestion and portosystemic shunting. Frequently, this is difficult to demonstrate. Routine measures that result in lower ammonia levels are ineffective. Flumazenil may produce a more awake but still encephalopathic patient. The exact mechanism remains to be elucidated. Medication side effects assume a much greater role in such patients. Clearance of commonly used immunosuppressives, analgesics, and sedatives-hypnotics is impaired. The amnestic effects of some agents may compound the problem. We favor short-acting narcotics such as fentanyl for analgesia and short-acting benzodiazepines such as midazolam for sedation. Severe agitation often does not respond to such measures until the patient is unconscious. Haloperidol or droperidol is preferred in such settings. Careful cardiac monitoring is required during parenteral use because ventricular arrhythmias may develop, albeit rarely. An alternative approach to sedation, low-dose propofol, is rapidly gaining favor in other patient populations.[82] However, data in patients with liver failure are limited. Furthermore, propofol appears to increase hepatic oxygen consumption. In a severely injured graft, such an effect may prove injurious. Further study is warranted.

A small but significant incidence of seizures has been recognized in this population. Medications play a major role in the differential diagnosis because several lower the seizure threshold, including CyA, FK-506, OKT3, and haloperidol.[83, 84] Electrolyte abnormalities such as hyponatremia and hypomagnesemia are common and further lower the seizure threshold. Hypoglycemia must also be considered and rapidly treated. Although we elect to correct such abnormalities in the early postoperative period, it is unclear whether efforts at oral replenishment of magnesium are effective later in the course. Sometimes such electrolyte abnormalities are the only causative factor identified.

Nonconvulsive or akinetic seizures, although rare, are much more common in this ICU population than in others. It is essential that seizures, in fact status epilepticus, be considered among the differential diagnoses of the comatose patient. We enjoy strong electroencephalographic support and frequently monitor such patients for prolonged periods to define the process and to determine the effects of therapy.

Patients with FHF require special neurologic consideration. Such patients have some elements of gamma-aminobutyric acid–mediated portosystemic encephalopathy[85] of chronic liver disease but importantly also have intracranial hypertension and cerebral edema.[86] We elect to routinely monitor patients in grade III and grade IV coma with an epidural intracranial pressure monitor and measure cerebral blood flow with the inhalation xenon techniques during computed tomographic (CT) scanning and cerebral oxygen consumption after placing a jugular bulb catheter for oxygen content determination.[87] Continuous EEG monitoring is added once pentobarbital has been required to control intracranial hypertension. Patients are considered viable candidates for OLTX as long as EEG activity is preserved and adequate cerebral perfusion pressure can be maintained with sustained cerebral blood flow. Intraoperative monitoring includes these measures, combined with the transcranial Doppler examinations,[88] which facilitate moment-to-moment titration of anesthetics and vasopressors. Although the initial period of graft reperfusion is the most hazardous, cerebral hyperemia and intracranial hypertension may persist for several days postoperatively. These abnormalities usually resolve with good graft function. Such intensive neurologic monitoring and careful exclusion of candidates who are at high risk for herniation have resulted in only one postoperative brain death and no apparent neurologic sequelae even in patients transplanted in grade IV coma.

INFECTIOUS COMPLICATIONS

Rejection of the allograft is treated aggressively when it develops. Such measures are complicated by the parallel development of infections. Heavily immunosuppressed patients die not of rejection but of infection. Within that framework, it should be appreciated that the patient with liver failure who undergoes liver transplantation is at tremendous risk for infection. In the early postoperative period, bacterial and fungal infections are common. The most frequently involved areas are the operative site and the lungs. Perioperative antimicrobial prophylaxis is currently provided as 48 hours of ampicillin and cefotaxime. Prophylactic regimens vary among centers. The most common microorganisms isolated in our infected patients are *Pseudomonas, Acinetobacter, Klebsiella, Enterobacter, Staphylococcus, Enterococcus,* and *Candida.* Unfortunately, antimicrobial resistance is common, and isolates in patients who die of an infectious process are occasionally resistant to all known antimicrobials.[89] Fungal colonization is also common. Patients with prolonged, difficult surgical procedures who are heavily transfused seem to be at higher risk for fungal infection as are patients who undergo retransplantation.[90, 91] We currently use low-dose amphotericin (10–20 mg/d) for 14 days, although its efficacy is unproved and fungal infections remain a significant problem.

Later after transplantation, infections reflect the specific effects of immunosuppressive agents on T cell function. Although bacterial and fungal infections occur, a greater emphasis on viral and opportunistic pathogens becomes necessary. Pneumonia caused by *Pneumocystis carinii* was common before the advent of routine prophylaxis with trimethoprim-sulfamethoxazole. Its occurrence now is restricted to those for whom prophylactic measures have been stopped.

CMV infections are common in the transplant population.[92, 93] However, the clinical severity of infection—whether it is asymptomatic, presents with a viral syndrome, involves only one organ such as the lungs, gastrointestinal tract, or liver, or involves multiple organs—is highly variable. Those patients who are seronegative before OLTX and who receive an organ from a seropositive donor are at highest risk for CMV infection. Whether patients who are seropositive before OLTX experience reactivation of latent virus or are infected by another CMV strain is a matter of some debate. In addition to the morbidity and mortality attributed directly to CMV, it should be appreciated that patients with CMV disease also have a higher frequency of bacterial and fungal infections. It is not clear whether it is CMV per se or the antecedent heavy immunosuppression, particularly with OKT3—associated with a higher incidence of CMV—that is the cause.

Prophylactic measures to prevent symptomatic CMV disease are under investigation. One regimen recently studied at our institution involved 2 weeks of ganciclovir followed by high-dose acyclovir versus high-dose acyclovir alone.[94] At 24 weeks CMV infection was evident in 60% and disease in 40% of those treated with acyclovir alone, but in the ganciclovir group infection decreased to 28% and disease decreased to 12%. Surprisingly, these benefits were not realized in the highest risk group:donor positive, recipient negative. Additional measures such as CMV immunoglobulin administration are under investigation.[95]

ENDOCRINE CONSIDERATIONS

Hyperglycemia is common in the early postoperative period and reflects the combination of stress and administration of corticosteroids. Patients are routinely managed with continuous infusions of insulin, with the dose adjusted according to a sliding scale. Conversion to six doses daily and then to twice daily therapy with regular and NPH insulin is achieved after discharge from the ICU in those patients who manifest glucose intolerance. Although lower doses of steroids are rejoined with CyA and FK-506, both of these drugs also impair glucose tolerance. The recognition that increased atherosclerosis occurs in transplant recipients makes a tightly controlled blood glucose level desirable. Unfortunately, hypoglycemia may be precipitated by liver allograft failure because gluconeogenesis is impaired. The sudden development of marked hyperglycemia or symptomatic hypoglycemia, which is not iatrogenic, should prompt an evaluation for infection.

Adrenal insufficiency is well recognized in patients receiving steroids. An additional factor to consider in these patients is that the right adrenal gland is often sacrificed during the transplant procedure. Adrenal gland infection may be caused by CMV. Adrenal hemorrhage has been observed in patients with profound coagulopathy and in those with gram-negative sepsis. A depressed cortisol response to the corticotropin analog, cosyntropin, has been a useful diagnostic adjunct for the clinical decision whether to maintain corticosteroid supplementation.

Thyroid dysfunction, particularly hypothyroidism, is common in patients with primary biliary cirrhosis and in autoimmune hepatitis. Sometimes this diagnosis is not considered preoperatively and becomes apparent in the postoperative period as changes in mental status, depressed cardiac output, and arrhythmias, which prompt evaluation.

As with other critical illness, the euthyroid sick syndrome is commonly identified in OLTX patients when a low thyroxine and normal thyroid-stimulating hormone are noted. When newly diagnosed and treated, an addisonian crisis can be averted with adequate corticosteroid replacement.

CONCLUSION

Patients with terminal liver disease can undergo successful transplantation. With adequate organ availability, even critically ill patients with ESLD have dramatic improvement. Intensive care of such patients is demanding but highly rewarding. Developments in the future will focus on better candidate selection and alternative means of immunosuppression. Determining how sick someone needs to be before a lifesaving transplant should be withheld requires understanding the chance of such a patient's survival, graded for quality of life. This must be compared with transplanting a less sick patient who must assume the current risk of the procedure versus the greater but delayed risk of waiting. The intensivist must be an active participant in this review such that the enormous expense of intensive care is focused on those patients who can successfully undergo OLTX.

References

1. Gordon RD, Starzl TE: Changing perspectives on liver transplantation in 1988. *In:* Clinical Transplants. Terasaki PI (Ed). Los Angeles, UCLA Tissue Typing Laboratory, 1988.
2. National Institutes of Health Consensus Conference on Liver Transplantation. Bethesda, MD, 1983.
3. Starzl TE, Porter KA, Brettschneider L, et al: Clinical and pathologic observations after orthotopic transplantation of the human liver. Surg Gynecol Obstet 1969; 128:327.
4. Iwatsuki S, Starzl TE, Todo S, et al: Experience in 1000 liver transplants under cyclosporin-steroid therapy: A survival report. Transplant Proc 1988; 20(Suppl 1):498.
5. Van Thiel DH, Gavaler JS: Recurrent disease in patients with liver transplantation: When does it occur and how can we be sure? Hepatology 1987; 7:181.
6. Polson RJ, Portmann B, Neuberger J, et al: Evidence for disease recurrence after liver transplantation for primary biliary cirrhosis: Clinical and histologic follow up studies. Gastroenterology 1989; 97:715.
7. UNOS Update. 1989; 5:1.
8. Starzl TE, Demetrius AJ, Van Thiel D: Liver transplantation (parts I and II). N Engl J Med 1989; 321:1014–1092.
9. Koneru B, Cassavila A, Bowman J, et al: Liver transplantation for malignant tumors. Gastroenterol Clin North Am 1988; 17:177.
10. Starzl TE, Todo S, Tsakis A, et al: Abdominal organ cluster transplantation for the treatment of upper abdominal malignancies. Ann Surg 1989; 210:374.
11. Starzl TE, Towe M, Todo S, et al: Transplantation of multiple abdominal viscera. JAMA 1989; 261:1449.
12. Dindzans VJ, Schade RR, Van Thiel DH: Medical problems before and after transplantation. Gastroenterol Clin North Am 1988; 17:19.
13. Todo S, Demetrius AJ, Van Thiel D, et al: Orthotopic liver transplantation for patients with hepatitis B virus (HBV) related disease. Hepatology 1991; 13:619–626.
14. Lauchart W, Muller R, Pichlmayer R: Long-term immunoprophylaxis of hepatitis B virus reinfection in recipients of human liver allografts. Transplant Proc 1987; 19:4051.
15. Lauchart W, Muller R, Pichlmayer R: Long-term immunoprophylaxis of hepatitis B virus reinfection in recipients of human liver allografts. Transplant Proc 1987; 19:4051.
16. Mutchnick MG, Appelman HD, Chung HT, et al: Thymosin treatment of chronic hepatitis B: A placebo controlled pilot trial. Hepatology 1991; 14:409–415.
17. Dummer SJ, Erb S, Breinig M, et al: Infection with human immunodeficiency virus in the Pittsburgh transplant population. Transplantation 1990; 47:134.
18. Trey C, Davidson CS: The management of fulminant hepatic failure. *In:* Progress in Liver Disease. Popper H, Shaffner F (Eds). New York, Grune & Stratton, 1970.
19. Bismuth H, Samuel D, Guenheim J, et al: Emergency liver transplantation for fulminant hepatitis. Ann Intern Med 1987; 107:337.
20. Kramer DJ, Aggarwald S, Martin M, et al: Fulminant hepatic failure: Management options. Transplant Proc 1991; 23:1895–1898.
21. O'Grady JG, Gimson AES, O'Brien CJ, et al: Controlled trials of charcoal hemoperfusion and prognostic factors in fulminant hepatic failure. Gastroenterology 1988; 94:1186.

22. O'Grady JG, Alexander GJM, Hayllar KM, et al: Early indicators of prognosis in fulminant hepatic failure. Gastroenterology 1989; 97:439.
23. Potter D, Peachey T, Eason J, et al: Intracranial pressure monitoring during orthotopic liver transplantation for acute liver failure. Transplant Proc 1989; 21:3528.
24. Canalese J, Gimson AES, Davis C, et al: Controlled trial of dexamethasone and mannitol for the cerebral oedema of fulminant hepatic failure. Gut 1982; 23:625.
25. Forbes A, Alexander GJ, O'Grady JG, et al: Thiopental infusion in the treatment of intracranial hypertension complicating fulminant hepatic failure. Hepatology 1989; 10:306.
26. Abelmann WH, Kowalski HJ, McNeely WF: Cardiovascular studies during acute infectious hepatitis. Gastroenterology 1954; 27:61.
27. Weston MJ, Talbot IC, Howorth PJN, et al: Frequency of arrhythmias and other cardiac abnormalities in FHF. Br Heart J 1976; 38:1179–1188.
28. Oellerich M, Raude E, Burdelski M, et al: Monoethylglycine xylidede formation kinetics: A novel approach to assessment of liver function. J Clin Chem Clin Biochem 1987; 25:845–853.
29. Burdelski M, Oellerich M, Lamesch P, et al: Evaluation of quantitative liver function tests in liver donors. Transplant Proc 1987; 19:3838–3839.
30. Starzl TE, Hakala TR, Shaw B, et al: A flexible procedure for multiple cadaveric organ procurement. Surg Gynecol Obstet 1984; 158:223.
31. Todo S, Nery J, Yanaga K, et al: Extended preservation of human liver grafts with UW solution. JAMA 1989; 261:711.
32. Dewolf A: Does ventricular dysfunction occur during liver transplantation? Transplant Proc 1991; 23:1922–1923.
33. Kang Y, Freeman J, Aggarwal S, et al: Hemodynamic instability during liver transplantation. Transplant Proc 1989; 21:3489–3492.
34. Dewolf A, Gasior T, Kang Y: Pulmonary hypertension in a patient undergoing liver transplantation. Transplant Proc 1991; 23:2000–2001.
35. Dewolf A, Begliomin B, Gasior T, et al: Right ventricular function during liver transplantation. Anesth Analg 1993; 76:562–568.
36. Stoelting RK, Blitt CD, Cohen PJ, et al: Hepatic dysfunction after isoflurane anesthesia. Anesth Analg 1987; 66:147.
37. Kang YG, Martin DJ, Marquez J, et al: Intraoperative changes in blood coagulation and thromboelastographic monitoring in liver transplantation. Anesth Analg 1985; 64:888.
38. Marquez JM, Martin D: Anesthesia for liver transplantation. *In:* Hepatic Transplantation: Anesthetic and Perioperative Management. Winter PM, Kang YG (Eds). New York, Praeger, 1986.
39. Rettke SR, Chantigian RC, Janossy TA, et al: Anesthesia approach to hepatic transplantation. Mayo Clin Proc 1989; 64:224.
40. Tzakis A, Todo S, Stieber A, et al: Venous jump grafts for liver transplantation in patients with portal vein thrombosis. Transplantation 1989; 48:530–531.
41. Figueras J, Sabate A, Fabregat J, et al: Hemodynamics during the anhepatic phase in orthotopic liver transplantation with vena cava presentation: A comparative study. Transplant Proc 1983; 25:2588–2589.
42. Kang Y: Hemodynamic changes during intra-abdominal organ transplantation. Transplant Proc 1993; 25:2583–2587.
43. Stieber AC, Marsh JW Jr, Starzl TE: Preservation of the retrohepatic vena cava during recipient hepatectomy for orthotopic transplantation of the liver. Surg Gynecol Obstet 1989; 168:542–544.
44. Denmark W, Shaw BW, Starzl TE, et al: Veno-venous bypass without systemic anticoagulation in canine and human liver transplantation. Surg Forum 1983; 34:380.
45. Aggarwal S, Kang Y, Freeman J, et al: Post reperfusion syndrome: Cardiovascular collapse following hepatic reperfusion during liver transplantation. Transplant Proc 1987; 19:54–55.
46. Greig P, Woolf GM, Sinclair SB, et al: Treatment of primary liver graft nonfunction with prostaglandin E_1. Transplantation 1989; 48:447–453.
47. Asonuma K, Takaya S, Selby R, et al: The clinical significance of the arterial ketone body ratio as an early indicator of graft viability in human liver transplantation. Transplantation 1991; 51:164–171.
48. Takaya S, Nonami T, Selby R, et al: The relationship of systemic hemodynamics and oxygen consumption to early allograft failure after liver transplantation. Transplant Int 1993; 6:73–76.
49. Doyle HR, Marino IR, Jabbour N, et al: Early death or retransplantation in adults to following orthotopic liver transplantation: Can outcome be predicted? Transplantation (in press).
50. Doyle HR, Dvorchik I, Mitchell S, et al: Predicting outcome after liver transplantation: A connectionist approach. Ann Surg 1994; 219:408–415.
51. Yanaga K, Lebeau G, Marsh JW, et al: Hepatic artery reconstruction for hepatic artery thrombosis after orthotopic liver transplantation. Arch Surg 1990; 125:628–631.
52. Yanaga K, Makowka L, Starzl TE: Is hepatic artery thrombosis after liver transplantation really a surgical complication? Transplant Proc 1989; 21:511.
53. Mañez R, Kobayashi M, Takaya S, et al: Humoral rejection associated with antidonor lymphocytotoxic antibodies following liver transplantation. Transplant Proc 1993; 25:888–890.
54. Starzl TE, Demetris AJ: Liver transplantation: A 31-Year Perspective. Chicago, Year Book Medical Publishers, 1990.
54a. Rosenbloom AJ, Kramer DJ, Stern KL, et al: Immunosupressive therapy of transplant patients. *In:* The Pharmacologic Approach to the Critically Ill Patient. 3rd ed. Chernow B (Ed). Baltimore, Williams & Wilkins, 1994.
55. Starzl TE, Iwatsuki S, Shaw B, et al: Orthotopic liver transplantation in 1984. Transplant Proc 1985; 17:250.
56. Demetrius AJ, Fung JJ, Todo S, et al: Conversion of liver allograft recipients from cyclosporin to FK 506 immunosuppressive therapy: A clinicopathologic study of 96 patients. Transplantation 1992; 53:1056–1062.
57. McCauley J, Van Thiel D, Starzl TE, et al: Acute and chronic renal failure after liver transplantation. Nephron 1990; 55:121.
58. Thompson CB, Sullivan KM, June CH, et al: Association between cyclosporin neurotoxicity and hypomagnesaemia. Lancet 1984; 2:1116.
59. Bayley TJ, Segel N, Bishop JM: The circulatory changes in patients with cirrhosis of the liver at rest and during exercise. Clin Sci 1964; 26:227.
60. Kowalski HJ, Abelmann WH: The cardiac output at rest in Laennec's cirrhosis. J Clin Invest 1953; 32:1025.
61. Murray JF, Dawson AM, Sherlock S: Circulatory changes in chronic liver disease. Am J Med 1958; 24:358.
62. Claypool JG, Delp M, Lin TK: Hemodynamic studies in patients with Laennec's cirrhosis. Am J Med Sci 1957; 234:48.
63. Martin D: Hemodynamic monitoring during liver transplantation. *In:* Hepatic Transplantation: Anesthetic and Perioperative Management. Winter PM, Kang YG (Eds). New York, Praeger, 1986.
64. Curtis JJ, Luke RG, Jones P, et al: Hypertension in cyclosporin treated renal transplant recipients is sodium dependent. Am J Med 1988; 85:134.
65. Bennett WM, Porter GA: Cyclosporin-associated hypertension (Editorial). Am J Med 1988; 85:131.
66. Fung J, Todo S, Abu-Elmagd K, et al: Randomized trial in primary liver transplantation under immunosuppression in FK 506 or cyclosporin. Transplantation Proc 1993; 25:1130.
67. McCauley J, Fung JJ, Brown H, et al: Renal function after conversion from cyclosporin to FK 506 in liver transplant patients. Transplant Proc 1991; 23:3148–3149.
68. Todo S, Fung JJ, Tzakis A, et al: One hundred ten consecutive primary orthotopic liver transplants under FK 506 in adults. Transplant Proc 1991; 23:1397–1402.
68a. European FK506 Multicentre Liver Study Group: Randomized trial of FK506 and cyclosporin in prevention of liver allograft rejection. Lancet 1994; 344:423–428.
69. Krowka MJ, Cortese DA: Pulmonary aspects of chronic liver disease and liver transplantation. Mayo Clin Proc 1985; 60:407–418.
70. Fagon JY, Chastre J: Hospital acquired pneumonia. *In:* Pathophysiologic Foundations of Critical Care. Pinsky MR, Dhamaut JF (Eds). Baltimore, Williams & Wilkins, 1993.
71. Matuschak GM, Rinaldo JE, Pinsky MR, et al: Effect of end-stage liver failure on the incidence and resolution of the adult respiratory distress syndrome. J Crit Care 1987; 2:162.
72. Krowka MJ, Cortese DA: Pulmonary aspects of liver disease and liver transplantation. Clin Chest Med 1987; 10:593–616.

73. Hales MR: Multiple small arteriovenous fistulas of the lungs. Am J Pathol 1956; 32:927–943.
74. Robin ED, Laman D, Horn BR, et al: Platypnea related to orthodeoxin caused by true vascular lung shunts. N Engl J Med 1976; 294:941–943.
75. Calabresi P, Abelmann WH: Portocaval and portopulmonary anastomosis in Laennec's cirrhosis in heart failure. J Clin Invest 1957; 36:1257–1265.
76. Caldwell PRB, Fritts HW, Courmans A: Oxyhemoglobin dissociation curve in liver disease. J Appl Physiol 1965; 20:316–320.
77. Davis HH, Schwartz DJ, Letrak SS, et al: Alveolar capillary oxygen disequilibrium in hepatic cirrhosis. Chest 1978; 73:507–511.
78. Rodriguez-Roisin R, Roca J, August AGN, et al: Gas exchange and pulmonary vascular reactivity in patients with liver cirrhosis. Am Rev Respir Dis 1987; 135:1085.
79. Dansky HM, Schwinger ME, Cohen MV: Using contrast enhanced echocardiography to identify abnormal pulmonary arteriovenous connections in patients with hypoxemia. Chest 1992; 102:1690–1692.
80. McCauley J, Van Thiel D, Starzl TE, et al: Acute and chronic renal failure after liver transplantation. Nephron 1990; 55:121.
81. Alexander JA, Demetrius AJ, Gavaler JS, et al: Pancreatitis following liver transplantation. Transplantation 1988; 45:1062.
82. Carmichael FJ, Crawford MW, Khayyam N, et al: Effect of propofol infusion on splanchnic hemodynamics and liver oxygen consumption in the rat: A dose response study. Anesthesiology 1993; 79:1051–1060.
83. de Groen PC, Aksamit AJ, Rakela J, et al: Central nervous system toxicity after liver transplantation. N Engl J Med 1987; 318:861.
84. Adams DH, Gunson B, Honigsberger L, et al: Neurologic complications following liver transplantation. Lancet 1987; *i*:949–951.
85. Jones EA, Basile AS, Mullen KD, et al: Flumazonil: Potential implications for hepatic encephalopathy. Pharmacotherapy 1990; 45:331–343.
86. Ware AJ, D'Agostiono AN, Combes B: Cerebral edema: A major complication of massive hepatic necrosis. Gastroenterology 1971; 61:877.
87. Aggarwal S, Kramer D, Yonas H, et al: Cerebral hemodynamic and metabolic changes in fulminant hepatic failure. Hepatology 1994; 19:80–87.
88. Aggarwal S, Witt JP, Kang Y, et al: Transcranial Doppler waveform analysis: A new approach to predict ICP in patients with fulminant hepatic failure. Hepatology 1993; 18:735.
89. Linden P, Pasculle AW, Kusne S, et al: Therapy and clinical outcome of vancomycin resistant enterococcus faecium (VREF) in a liver transplant recipient population. Proceedings of the 32nd Interscience Conference on Antimicrobial Agents and Chemotherapy, Los Angeles, October 1992.
90. Kusne S, Dummer JS, Singh N, et al: Infection after liver transplantation: An analysis of 101 consecutive cases. Medicine 1988; 67:132.
91. Kusne S, Dummer JS, Singh N, et al: Fungal infections in liver transplantation recipients. Transplantation 1985; 40:347.
92. Balfour HH, Chace BA, Stapleton JT, et al: A randomized, placebo-controlled trial of oral acyclovir for the prevention of cytomegalovirus disease in recipients of renal allografts. N Engl J Med 1989; 320:1381.
93. Pomeroy C, Englund JA: Cytomegalovirus: Epidemiology and infection control. Am J Infect Control 1987; 15:107.
94. Martin M, Mañez R, Linden P, et al: A prospective randomized trial comparing sequential ganciclovir-high dose acyclovir to high dose acyclovir for prevention of cytomegalovirus disease in adult liver transplant recipients. Transplantation (in press).
95. Syndman DR, Werner BG, Heinze-Lacey B, et al: Use of cytomegalovirus immunoglobulin to prevent cytomegalovirus disease in renal transplant recipients. N Engl J Med 1987; 317:1049.

CHAPTER 182

Intensive Care of the Cardiac Transplant Recipient

Keith L. Stein, MD, FCCP, FCCM • John M. Armitage, MD
G. Daniel Martich, MD, FCCP • Robert L. Hardesty, MD
Robert L. Kormos, MD • Bartley P. Griffith, MD

HISTORICAL PRELUDE

A persistent cause of death in the United States, cardiovascular illnesses claim more than 800,000 victims per year. Particularly in the last decade, the ongoing search for the treatment of individuals afflicted with end-stage cardiac disease has resulted in transplantation evolving into a lifesaving procedure with low intra- and postoperative mortality and high-quality, long-term survival. One-year actuarial survival now exceeds 80% (Fig. 182–1). Despite a critical lack of available organs, the popularity and growing success of transplantation (since the pioneering technical achievements of prominent surgeons including Christian Barnard[1] and Denton Cooley[2]) are attributable to the concurrent advancement in organ preservation and surgical implantation skills along with enhanced immunomodulation.

Coincident with the enhanced efficacy of human heart transplantation has been the rapid proliferation of medical centers active in this area. The number of such sites in the United States has burgeoned from only 5 in 1981 to 70 in 1986 and to more than 150 in 1994. With this growth has come an expanding interest in, and need for familiarity with, the procedures and characteristics of perioperative support unique to these critically ill patients.

PATIENT SELECTION AND DEMOGRAPHICS

Current indications for cardiac transplantation include end-stage cardiomyopathy, either idiopathic or ischemic, resulting in New York Heart Association class IV symptoms and a left ventricular ejection fraction of less than 20% (Table 182–1). Whereas in the early 1980s the predominant predisposition was idiopathic disease, ischemic disease is currently the most significant factor and an older patient population the primary recipient group. Other less common indications include valvular heart disease, isolated cardiac

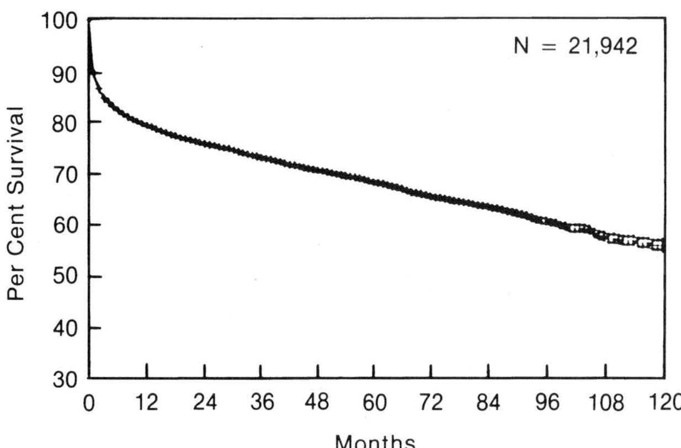

Figure 182–1. Actuarial survival curve of all orthotopic heart transplants performed between 1967 and 1992. (From Kaye MP: Actuarial survival: Hearts 1967–1992. Heart Lung Transplant 1993; 12:543.)

TABLE 182–1. Recipient Selection Criteria

New York Heart Association class IV symptoms
End-stage cardiomyopathy: ischemic, idiopathic, valvular, other
Left ventricular ejection fraction ≤20%
Preservation of other vital visceral functions
Contraindications: active infection, severe pulmonary hypertension, psychological or social instability

amyloidosis,[3] congenital anomalies, and sarcoidosis. Recently, we have been evaluating as possible transplant recipients patients with unreconstructible coronary vascular disease who suffer angina at rest.

Selection criteria continue to evolve as our understanding grows of the risk factors that adversely affect survival. Generally, prospective recipients must have significant preservation of their other vital visceral organ function. In the past, age, obesity, elevated pulmonary vascular resistance (PVR), insulin-dependent diabetes mellitus, presence of active infection, previous cardiac surgery, recent pulmonary embolism (PE), and systemic disease have all been applied as restrictive criteria. However, the advent of new immunosuppressives such as cyclosporine A (CyA) and FK-506, improved surgical technique, and enhanced understanding of perioperative support have eliminated most of these barriers. For example, the recipient age limit continues to expand; in selected cases, recipients are now older than 65 years. Even the presence of preexisting neoplastic diseases is no longer an absolute contraindication to heart transplantation.[4]

Of the aforementioned concerns, the most important one that remains is elevated PVR. When PVR is greater than 5 Wood units or the transpulmonary gradient (TPG) is greater than 15 mm Hg (and unresponsive to prostaglandin E_1 infusion),[5] acute right ventricular (RV) failure may occur soon after implantation of the normal donor heart (which has never been previously exposed to elevated RV afterload).[5a] Compensatory maneuvers to ameliorate this problem include the use of oversized donor hearts or occasionally heterotopic heart transplantation. Potential candidates with a persistent TPG of greater than 15 mm Hg are unlikely to be accepted as recipients.

Impairment of other vital organ function may also preclude successful transplantation. Thus, low creatinine clearance or pulmonary function tests showing a severe limitation of forced expiratory volume in 1 second (FEV_1) or FEV–forced vital capacity (FVC) ratio requires careful consideration. Diabetics requiring more than 50 units of insulin per day for control or evidencing sequelae such as significant vasculopathy are probably also poor recipient candidates.

POSTOPERATIVE CARE

Electrocardiography and Monitoring

The anastomosis of the new heart to native circulation normally requires a residual remnant of both native atria to be left intact (Fig. 182–2). This may occasionally complicate interpretation of the postoperative electrocardiogram (ECG) by the apparent presence of two autonomous atrial depolarizations: the nontransmitted P waves of the native atria and the sinoatrial node activity of the donor heart. However, the most common early postoperative rhythm is sinus tachycardia, facilitating discrimination between the two P wave sites.[6] Maneuvers that enhance patient vagal tone will only affect the still innervated native atrial remnants but cannot alter the ventricular rate of the denervated donor's heart.

Initially, and particularly in the absence of pharmacologic intervention, the intrinsic rate of the denervated heart may be quite slow. As a direct consequence of hypothermic cardioplegic preservation in concert with possible ischemia and preservation injury, ventricular contractility and stroke volume are frequently impaired, and cardiac output is limited. Both myocardial and systemic oxygen delivery become heart rate dependent.[7] Thorough invasive monitoring is always applied, including left ventricular preload (as crudely assessed by pulmonary arterial occlusion pressure), myocardial performance (cardiac index), and effective peripheral oxygen delivery (hourly urine output, serum pH and lactate, mixed venous oxygen tension). To focus on RV function specifically (end-systolic and diastolic volumes), the ejection fraction Swan-Ganz catheter (REF-1, Baxter-Edwards) is sometimes used.[8] Trans-esophageal echocardiography is also useful to evaluate ventricular distension and regional myocardial performance. Intra- and postoperative use of intra-arterial cannulation and pulse oximetry is routine.

Initial Cardiovascular Support

Support of the recently transplanted heart begins intraoperatively during separation from cardiopulmonary bypass (CPB). The donor heart is rewarmed from the profoundly hypothermic state (used for preservation) at the completion of the four surgical anastomoses (left and right atria, pulmonary artery, aorta). In this sluggish state, the heart requires inotropic support (Table 182–2). Therapy is focused on chronotropy to elevate the heart rate to greater than 90

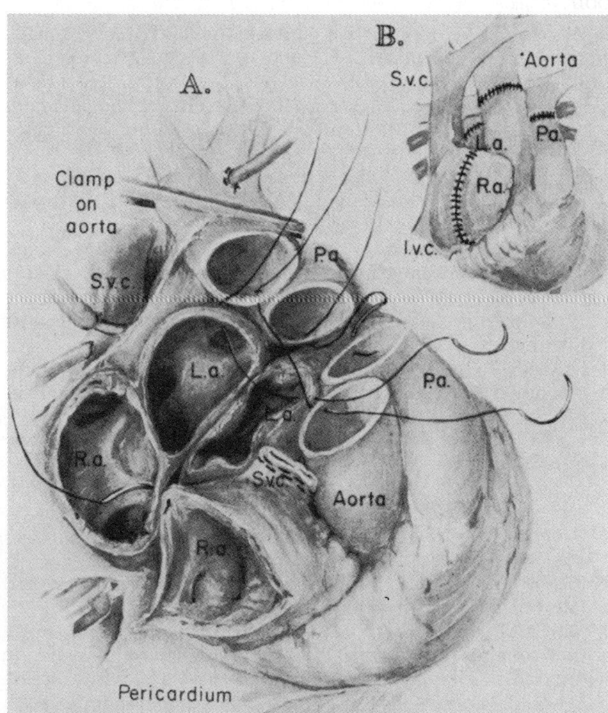

Figure 182–2. Technique for orthotopic cardiac transplantation. *A*, Implantation requires biatrial anastomoses beginning with the left atrium. End-to-end anastomosis between donor and native aortas is performed next. The aortic crossclamp is then removed; this restores blood flow to the graft. The pulmonary artery anastomosis can be completed during the period of rewarming and reperfusion of the graft. *B*, Completed anastomoses. *Abbreviations:* S.V.C. = superior vena cava; R.a. = right atrium; L.a. = left atrium; P.a. = pulmonary artery; I.v.c. = inferior vena cava.

TABLE 182–2. General Guidelines for Postoperative Support: Cardiovascular

Chronotropy/inotropy: dobutamine
Pulmonary hypertension: prostaglandin E_1
Volume repletion
Arrhythmias: procainamide, lidocaine

beats per minute and inotropy to maintain the cardiac index at more than 2.5 L/min · m². An element of transient RV dysfunction is common, particularly when exacerbated by the presence of mild chronic pulmonary hypertension. Left ventricular contractility may also be impaired in some patients.[9] This constellation of problems responds particularly well to the combined $beta_1$–$beta_2$ agonists isoproterenol and dobutamine. Our preference is for dobutamine, which, although less potent, is less of a peripheral vasodilator and thus less of a hypotensive agent. With continuous infusion of the synthetic exogenous catecholamine dobutamine at 5 to 10 $\mu g \cdot kg^{-1} \cdot min^{-1}$, the heart rate predictably rises.[10] The simultaneous reduction in PVR, in conjunction with improved contractility, results in improved ejection fraction and a consequent decrease in ventricular (end-systolic and end-diastolic) volumes and wall tension. Additional inotropic therapy with agents including epinephrine, dopamine, amrinone, and levarterenol is infrequently necessary.

Two specific entities in particular may induce severe ventricular decompensation in this early postoperative period. Hyperacute rejection, which is both rare and difficult to diagnose, had occurred in 19 of our first 450 patients. This lethal complication either may present in the operating room immediately after reperfusion of the graft or may follow a more insidious course marked by a progressive rise in central venous pressure with concomitant decline in cardiac index seemingly unresponsive to pharmacotherapy. In our series, only one of these patients survived after heroic support with the Jarvik-7 total artificial heart, plasmapheresis, and subsequent retransplantation.[11–13] This complication is exceedingly rare today.

The second major concern in this period is that of recalcitrant pulmonary hypertension. The newly transplanted heart unaccustomed to this stress of significant RV afterload may suffer acute RV failure. The administration of intravenous prostaglandin E_1 has been beneficial[13a] as described for patients with this problem related to mitral valve disease and coronary artery bypass grafting.[14, 15] In addition, the use of moderately "oversized" donor hearts in patients with elevated pretransplant PVR has also been effective in limiting the risk of early postoperative right-sided heart failure and death. Fortunately, secondary pulmonary hypertension usually resolves rapidly after transplant, and persistent instability is rare.[16]

Heterotopic heart transplantation refers to the technique of connecting the donor heart to the recipient heart in parallel. The native heart remains in its anatomic location, and the donor heart is placed in the right chest with the four anastomoses connecting left atrium to left atrium and right atrium to right atrium, both side to side, and the aorta to aorta and pulmonary artery to pulmonary artery, with these great vessel anastomoses end to side, as illustrated in Figure 182–3. Because of the long distance, it is also necessary to use a graft for the pulmonary artery anastomosis. This transplantation technique was originally used with the hope that native cardiac function would improve in patients with idiopathic cardiomyopathy. However, the results with heterotopic heart transplantation are far inferior to orthotopic transplantation with the native heart replaced by the donor heart. Therefore, heterotopic heart transplantation is rarely used today and only occasionally in recipients who would otherwise be excluded because of prohibitively high PVR (greater than 8 Wood units).

The critical care medicine practitioner will appreciate the uniqueness of the clinical problems of a heterotopic heart transplant recipient in the intensive care unit (ICU). With two hearts in the chest, usually beating at different rates and frequently also different rhythms, two distinct ECGs will be displayed (Fig. 182–4). These are best recognized by placing electrodes laterally to the left for the native heart and to the right for the donor heart. Similarly, chest x-ray examination will reveal two cardiac silhouettes, with the donor heart appearing as a "tumor" in the right chest (Fig. 182–5). Postoperative morbidity is influenced by compression of the right lower lung lobe by the donor heart with increased risk of atelectasis and subsequent pneumonia. Chronic anticoagulation is also indicated because of the tendency for thrombus formation in the diseased native heart with a high risk of major systemic embolization.

Occasionally, aggressive support with intra-aortic balloon counterpulsation[17] or ventricular assist devices[18, 19, 19a] may be deemed appropriate. However, enthusiasm for these highly invasive maneuvers must be tempered by their significant hazards including infection in the immunosuppressed recipient and their limited likelihood of success.

Stroke volume development by the transplanted heart is exquisitely dependent on the maintenance of adequate intravascular volume (preload), as approximated by measurement of central venous and pulmonary artery occlusion pressure. More specific assessment of RV end-diastolic volume as a reflection of preload through the use of the rapid response REF-1 catheter mentioned previously is sometimes used.

Despite the inherent risks associated with the transfusion of blood products (including transmission of viral hepatitis C and cytomegalovirus), optimal cellular oxygen delivery probably necessitates a hemoglobin concentration of approximately 10 g/dL. As in other postsurgical groups, the search for the optimal and safe red blood cell volume continues, and transfusion thresholds must be individualized.

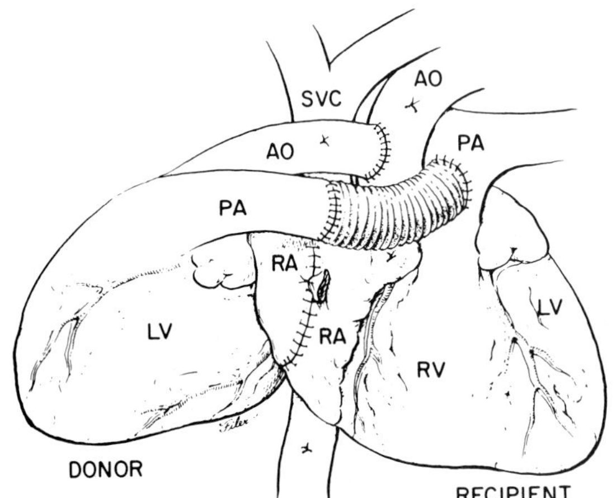

Figure 182–3. Completed anastomoses of a heterotopic cardiac transplantation. The native heart is connected to the donor heart with side-to-side anastomoses between the right atria and between the left atria. The aorta and pulmonary arteries are anastomosed using an end-to-side technique which usually requires a graft for the pulmonary artery anastomosis. *Abbreviations:* AO = aorta; LV = left ventricle; RV = right ventricle.

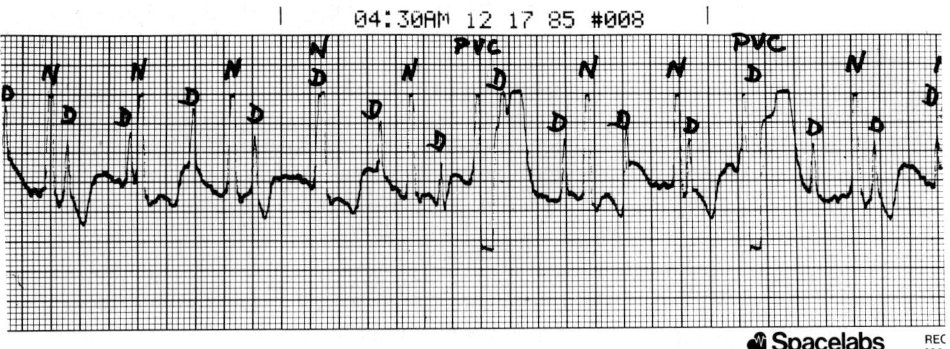

Figure 182–4. Electrocardiogram rhythm strip from a patient who received a heterotopic heart transplant. The donor heart's rate (D) is 138 beats per minute, whereas the native heart's rate (N) is 96 beats per minute with occasional premature ventricular contractions.

Surgical Complications Associated with Heart Transplantation

Although additional corrective surgery is rarely required after cardiac transplantation, four circumstances may necessitate surgical intervention: (1) technical complications related to cardiac implantation; (2) complications of endomyocardial biopsy; (3) sternal dehiscence or infectious mediastinitis; and (4) general and vascular surgical complications after cardiac transplantation. The latter two are included in the later discussion of asepsis, fever, and sepsis.

Atrial septal defects may occur if the atria, which must hold two suture lines during implantation, are placed under undue tension. In addition, reopening of a probe patent foramen ovale may occur with RV strain and elevated right atrial pressure. Although rarely of major clinical significance, a patent foramen ovale is carefully sought and repaired intraoperatively when found to avoid right-to-left shunting with arterial hypoxemia.

When the heart is empty, as during reimplantation, precise orientation between new and native vascular structures may be difficult. Pulmonary artery torsion and obstruction may result from rotational misalignment. This extremely rare entity is most often recognized immediately after separation from CPB, although delayed diagnosis has been reported.[20] Repair of such misalignment requires reinstitution of CPB.

The pericardium may be huge in recipients who have dilated cardiomyopathies. The potential space left between this sac and the small transplanted heart sets the stage for a bloody postoperative pericardial effusion and delayed tamponade. This complication has been virtually eliminated by operative excision of a portion of the pericardium, thus creating pericardial drainage.

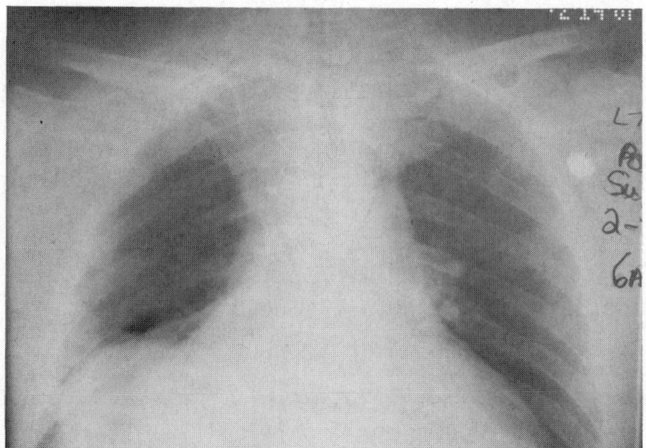

Figure 182–5. Postoperative chest radiograph of heterotopic heart transplant patient. "Tumor-like" opacity on the right side of the chest is the heterotopic heart; the native heart remains in its natural position.

Although surprisingly rare, perforation of the wall of the right ventricle can occur during endomyocardial biopsy (for rejection surveillance). The right ventricle is most susceptible to perforation early postoperatively, when it is dilated, and before maturation of mediastinal and pericardial adhesions. Thus, the first postoperative biopsy is considered the most risky and is routinely performed in the operating room, with provisions made for urgent therapy of tamponade if it occurs. Coronary artery RV fistulas may also rarely result from transmural biopsies,[21] as can fistulas to cardiac veins.[22] They are generally small and do not require therapy. More "routine" complications such as pneumothorax and hemothorax have also occurred in the setting of myocardial biopsy.

Antiarrhythmic Therapy

The transplanted donor heart is deprived of all normal autonomic innervation of both sympathetic and parasympathetic origin. This denervated state appears to be a permanent condition in most individuals,[23] although anecdotal reports such as the occurrence of angina after transplantation may indicate rare exceptions to this permanence.[24] As a result of the denervated state, the most frequent rhythm exhibited in the early postoperative period is sinus bradycardia or low-grade atrioventricular (AV) nodal block. The heart rate must, therefore, be supported with positive chronotropic agents during the early postoperative period, generally for 2 to 5 days.

Recent experience suggests that fewer than 10% of these patients experience persistent bradyarrhythmias requiring implantation of a permanent pacemaker before hospital discharge.[25] In addition, any of the commonly noted postcardiac surgical arrhythmias may be exhibited and in fact may be more common in the denervated heart.

In applying antiarrhythmic therapy, it must be appreciated that any medications or interventions (such as vagal maneuvers) that act via the autonomic nervous system will not elicit the normally anticipated response.

Pharmacologic Agents

Atropine

Through its direct action on the vagal nuclei of the brain stem, atropine normally is a cardioaccelerator. However, in the denervated transplanted heart, atropine is devoid of any cardiac effects. To increase heart rate, it is instead necessary to directly stimulate β receptors by administration of intravenous beta agonists such as isoproterenol or dobutamine.

Digoxin

Digoxin exhibits both positive inotropic and antiarrhythmic properties. Because of its long half-life and low therapeutic dose–toxic dose ratio, it is infrequently used in the ICU solely for its inotropic effects. It is frequently administered to control the rate of ventricular response to atrial fibrillation in other cardiac surgical patients. The effect of digoxin to diminish AV nodal conduction and hence reduce the ventricular rate is primarily due to an augmentation of vagal tone, which is absent in the transplanted heart. Digoxin is, therefore, not very useful in the acute control of atrial fibrillation in the heart transplant recipient. It does continue to play a role in the long-term rate control of atrial fibrillation as a result of the gradual (nonvagally mediated) depression of AV nodal transmission that occurs after chronic oral digoxin administration.[26]

Lidocaine

Lidocaine's effects on the cardiac rhythm are virtually independent of the autonomic nervous system.[27] Consequently, it is useful for the control of ventricular ectopy in the heart transplant patient. However, because lidocaine clearance is dependent on hepatic metabolic degradation, toxicity may occur more commonly in transplant recipients who are poorly perfused.[28] This toxicity initially may be manifest as subtle disturbance in central nervous system function. Beginning as confusion or sedation, this disturbance, if unrecognized, may progress to seizures or respiratory arrest as circulating lidocaine levels rise. The threat of toxicity is limited when serum levels remain below 5 μg/mL.

Phenytoin

Phenytoin's action as an antiarrhythmic drug for suppressing ventricular irritability closely parallels that of lidocaine, rendering it similarly useful in transplant recipients.[29] Despite the apparently complex interaction of phenytoin with the autonomic nervous system, it retains its effect through predominantly direct action on the heart. As with lidocaine, hepatic degradation may be impaired by hepatic insufficiency or hypoperfusion, resulting in elevated circulating levels. It is also important to note that phenytoin increases the rate of metabolism of cyclosporine, necessitating close attention to the circulating levels of this immunosuppressive agent.

Quinidine

The properties of quinidine are partially dependent on the autonomic nervous system. For example, the typical acceleration in heart rate is the result of an atropine-like vagal inhibition, thus absent in this patient population. Quinidine's suppression of automaticity in the Purkinje system is a direct effect, as is the increase in action potential duration and refractory period.[30] Thus, suppression of reentrant arrhythmias, such as supraventricular tachycardias or atrial flutter, can still be effectively achieved in heart transplantation patients.

Procainamide

As with quinidine, procainamide exhibits direct electrophysiologic suppression of the myocardial activation system. It is an extremely useful drug for the acute control of both atrial and ventricular tachyarrhythmias. Careful attention must be paid to serum levels, including the active metabolite *N*-acetyl procainamide[31] (particularly in patients with renal insufficiency) because the negative inotropic effect of this drug on the transplanted heart is especially evident.

Bretylium

Originally released as an antihypertensive agent, bretylium has profound autonomic effects, although its direct effect on the transplanted heart is less predictable. Immediately after administration, hypertension may result from the release of circulating catecholamines. The rise in blood pressure may be exaggerated by the lack of normal cardiac compensatory mechanisms. The clinically useful antiarrhythmic properties of bretylium are poorly understood and may depend significantly on an intact autonomic system. Consequently, this drug is rarely used in the cardiac transplant population and is reserved for circumstances in which more consistently effective therapies for ventricular tachycardia or fibrillation have proven ineffective. Eliminated unchanged in the urine, bretylium may thus have prolonged action in patients with renal insufficiency.

Verapamil

Verapamil's calcium-entry blocking properties are most effective when the calcium channels are in either the open or inactivated position. Therefore, it is most therapeutic when the channel activity is highest: at the sinoatrial and AV nodes of the heart.[32] Verapamil is an excellent medication for the treatment of supraventricular tachyarrhythmias.[33, 34] It is equally effective in its direct action on the denervated transplanted heart. However, extreme caution is advisable when using verapamil in the early post-transplant period because of its profound negative inotropic activity, particularly in patients with left ventricular dysfunction.[35] Severe myocardial depression has also been reported with concomitant administration of quinidine, disopyramide, or β-blockers. Verapamil infusion, rather than intermittent bolus administration, may be advantageous because control of supraventricular tachycardia in critically ill patients may be achieved with minimal side effects even in the face of significant heart disease.[36] As a result of hepatic clearance, verapamil effects may be accentuated by impaired hepatic function or perfusion.

Esmolol

Although β-blockers are rarely indicated in this period of myocardial dysfunction, rare patients may exhibit severe supraventricular tachyarrhythmias that significantly impair ventricular filling (particularly with poor diastolic compliance). Under these unique circumstances, acute rate control with the β_1 selective receptor blocker esmolol may be indicated. Esmolol may be used for rapid rate control because intravenous titration is facilitated by its very short half-life of about 9 minutes. Generally, however, β-blocker therapy is best avoided in the early postoperative period.

Pulmonary Support and Dysfunction

With separation from CPB and immediately after several 15- to 20-mL/kg body weight sighs, mechanical ventilation is instituted at a minute ventilation of 100 mL/kg divided into breaths of 12 mL/kg tidal volume (Table 182–3). An initial fractional inspired oxygen concentration (FIO_2) of 0.9 and positive end-expiratory pressure (PEEP) of 5 cm H_2O are routinely applied. Attempts are made to rapidly diminish the FIO_2 to 0.5 as dictated by digital pulse oximetry and intermittent arterial blood gas analyses.

TABLE 182–3. General Guidelines for Postoperative Support: Pulmonary

Minute ventilation of 100 mL/kg
Positive end-expiratory pressure of 5 cm H_2O
Minimize fraction of inspired oxygen
Rewarm to avoid shivering
Wean to extubate 3–18 hours
Respiratory failure: cardiogenic; noncardiogenic pulmonary edema; sepsis; diaphragmatic paresis

Recovery from post-CPB hypothermia involves a marked increase in metabolic rate. This often necessitates an increase in delivered minute ventilation to avoid respiratory acidosis. Shivering is associated with massive increases in oxygen consumption,[37] a problem best avoided through the judicious administration of sedation and temporary pharmacologic neuromuscular blockade. Heated humidifiers in the ventilator circuit help to restore normothermia quickly.

In the absence of other complications, weaning from ventilatory support toward planned extubation follows a routine course. Standard extubation criteria include the presence of a neurologic state adequate to protect and clear the airway, cardiovascular stability with sufficient cellular oxygen delivery, a spontaneous minute ventilation of less than 30% above normal without tachypnea, normocarbia, and adequate arterial oxygen saturation on a PEEP of 5 cm H_2O and FIO_2 of 0.5 or lower.[38] Most patients can be extubated within 12 to 18 hours of surgery.

Unilateral diaphragmatic paresis may present as early postoperative impairment of mechanical sufficiency, evidenced by limited inspiratory force and FVC of less than 15 mL/kg body weight. Although more frequent on the left side and usually attributed to hypothermic injury to the phrenic nerve as it lies outside the posterior pericardium, this lesion may affect the right diaphragm or, rarely, both diaphragms. As a paresis, the compromise is usually transient with significant resolution within the first 7 to 10 days postoperatively. Even when the diaphragm remains unilaterally paretic, sufficient ventilatory reserve allows extubation in most patients. Occasionally, prolonged mechanical ventilation and consideration of diaphragmatic plication may be necessary.

Persistent pulmonary dysfunction with hypoxemia and depressed static pulmonary compliance are particularly significant in these immunosuppressed patients. Under these circumstances, abnormal chest radiographs revealing parenchymal infiltrates of uncertain cause require prompt evaluation. Concern over the balance between the potential lethality of delaying treatment of a pneumonia and the possible toxicities of antibiotics necessitates heroic attempts at early accurate diagnosis including fiberoptic bronchoscopy with bronchoalveolar lavage or transbronchial biopsy or both. Rarely, open lung biopsy is indicated.

Atelectasis with characteristic radiographic changes suggestive of focal loss of lung volume is particularly common after the prolonged periods of nonventilation experienced during CPB. Left lower lobe atelectasis occurs frequently and may be the first suggestion of phrenic nerve injury (described previously). Significant hypoxemia may result from increased intrapulmonary shunt, which may be exacerbated when compromise of the normal hypoxic pulmonary vasoconstriction mechanism for matching ventilation and perfusion occurs during administration of circulating vasodilators or vasodilatory inotropes.[39] Therapy is directed at the reopening of collapsed lung units through application of PEEP and chest physiotherapy and manipulation of airway pressure. Recalcitrant areas of atelectasis may respond to therapeutic bronchoscopy with evacuation of tenacious secretions.[40]

Radiographic infiltrates that are unresponsive to the aforementioned therapy, particularly if the patient exhibits fever and leukocytosis, suggest that pulmonary infection is likely.[41] Identification of the specific pathogens is often difficult.[42] Sputum cultures, whether from expectorated samples or from endotracheal tube suctioning, are generally unreliable. A better correlation between the cultured organisms and true pathogens has been reported with the transbronchoscopic protected brush technique and bronchoalveolar lavage for quantitative culture results.[43] Current treatment while awaiting culture results is empiric and is guided by epidemiologic data and a high clinical index of suspicion. Because gram-negative bacilli are the most likely pathogens in the first month after transplantation, broad-spectrum antipseudomonal antibiotics are frequently used, with the response to treatment as a marker of the appropriateness of specific therapy. Despite their relative rarity, close attention to possible opportunistic (e.g., *Pneumocystis*), fungal (e.g., *Aspergillus*), viral (e.g., cytomegalovirus, herpes), and other (*Staphylococcus, Legionella*) infections is always appropriate.[44, 45]

Acute cardiac dysfunction may present as cardiogenic pulmonary edema with delayed-onset pulmonary decompensation. The possibility of rejection and consequent need for further immunomodulation is then assessed by urgent endomyocardial biopsy.[46] PE must be considered in those patients who have undergone prolonged postoperative bed rest in the absence of specific attention to prevention of deep venous thrombophlebitis (DVT)[47] (although the incidence of DVT and PE is considered rare after full heparinization during CPB).

One must consider that septicemia from distant sites including the urinary tract or biliary tree may also precipitate acute respiratory failure.[48] The diagnosis of noncardiogenic pulmonary edema (also known as adult respiratory distress syndrome, or ARDS) is strongly suggested by the sudden appearance of characteristic bilateral pulmonary infiltrates on chest x-ray film in association with hypoxemia and low static pulmonary compliance in the absence of an elevated pulmonary artery occlusion pressure.[49] The onset of ARDS may necessitate provision of continuous positive airway pressure via facemask or reinstitution of endotracheal intubation for full ventilatory support. Concomitant administration of antimicrobial therapy aimed at the suspected specific pathogens is essential.

Metabolic Considerations and Renal Protection

The chronic administration of diuretics, often a mainstay of the treatment of congestive heart failure, is frequently associated with hypomagnesemia[50] (Table 182–4). Intraoperative administration of osmotic diuretics such as mannitol may further deplete this ion. As a cause of hypokalemia, or concomitant with it, this magnesium depletion can be associated with tachyarrhythmias and may exacerbate myocardial dysfunction.[51] As with hypokalemia, prolongation of the PR and QT intervals, widened QRS complex, ST-segment depression, and T-wave inversion are seen on ECG. Intravenous administration of magnesium sulfate promptly reverses these changes and improves hemodynamic stability. Intravenous magnesium repletion should not be too vigorous or rapid, however, because vasodilation and hypotension may result.

Other consequences of magnesium deficiency include coronary arterial spasm,[52] laryngeal spasm with stridor, ane-

TABLE 182–4. General Guidelines for Postoperative Support: Metabolic, Renal, and Coagulation

Replete magnesium, phosphate, potassium, chloride
Early respiratory alkalosis, later hypochloremic metabolic alkalosis
Low dose dopamine infusion
Reverse heparin with protamine, replete coagulation factors as needed
Consider desmopressin acetate (DDAVP), positive end-expiratory pressure, and surgical re-exploration

mia, and central nervous system or renal dysfunction.[53, 54] Prevention is achieved through early repletion and continued daily administration of magnesium supplements titrated to the clinical course and serum magnesium levels.

Hypophosphatemia frequently occurs in the postoperative course and is at least partially attributable to the acute increase in extracellular fluid volume experienced during CPB. Also contributing to the decline in serum phosphate are the administration of exogenous catecholamines and inappropriate urinary losses during spontaneous diuresis after moderate hypothermia. Both hypokalemia and hypomagnesemia also contribute to hypophosphatemia. Of the many clinical consequences, the most relevant include compromised myocardial performance,[55] platelet and leukocyte dysfunction, central nervous system impairment, and prolonged respiratory insufficiency.[56] In addition, depletion of 2,3-diphosphoglycerate will significantly decrease the P_{50} of hemoglobin saturation, compromising cellular oxygen availability. Adenosine triphosphate depletion may also occur. The potentially lethal complications of profound hypophosphatemia are readily avoided by judicious repletion of phosphate[57] through delivery of potassium or sodium phosphate solutions into the central circulation.

After heart transplantation, metabolic derangements usually occur in two phases. In the first 8 to 12 hours postoperatively, respiratory alkalosis may be apparent, particularly in the hypothermic phase of recovery. In 48 to 72 hours, this is followed by a metabolic alkalosis that is typically associated with low serum chloride and hypokalemia. After confirmation of a low urine chloride excretion (less than 10 mEq/L), repletion of potassium and chloride will usually result in correction. A simultaneous bicarbonate diuresis initiated by intravenous acetazolamide may accelerate correction, particularly in patients whose compensatory hypoventilation is impairing adequate gas exchange.[58, 59]

Preservation of renal function is a high priority. Recovery from the moderate hypothermia of CPB is frequently marked by a notable diuresis. This limits the value of monitoring urine output as an index of perfusion adequacy in the first 6 to 12 hours of postoperative intensive care. With the multiplicity of anticipated insults to renal function, including hypoperfusion, possible administration of aminoglycosides, and immunosuppressive therapy with cyclosporine or FK-506, early administration of small doses of dopamine ($1–2\ \mu g \cdot kg^{-1} \cdot min^{-1}$) may be beneficial through renal and splanchnic vasodilation or maintained diuresis (without significant tachycardia), or both.[60–62] Renal failure, particularly if oliguric in nature, contributes significantly to morbidity and mortality, with overall hospital mortality greater than 50% in those with a coexistent acute cardiac illness.[63]

Bleeding and Coagulopathies

As in all cardiac surgical patients, excessive postoperative bleeding may result in life-threatening consequences including tamponade. Although extensive bleeding requiring reoperation is relatively rare (and probably carries an incidence similar to coronary artery bypass surgery of less than 4%[64]), moderate chest tube drainage (>200 mL of blood per hour) in the early postoperative period is common and multifactorial. Such bleeding requires prompt evaluation and treatment (Table 182–4).

Heparin, through its actions including activation of antithrombin III,[65] effectively inhibits clot formation during CPB. Reversal of its action by neutralization with protamine sulfate administered intravenously begins in the operating room and may continue in the ICU. Protamine therapy is rarely complicated by severe adverse reactions such as profound hypotension with vasodilation and heart failure, noncardiogenic pulmonary edema, pulmonary vasoconstriction, and bronchospasm.[66, 67] Some of these responses result from the elaboration of complement fraction C5a and the prostanoid thromboxane.[68, 69] Whatever the mechanism, caution in using protamine (particularly in those patients previously exposed to protamine in neutral protamine Hagedorn insulin preparations and in vasectomized men) is appropriate. Titration of protamine is accomplished by measurement of the activated clotting time (ACT) with generation of an individualized dose-response curve[70] or by a protamine titration assay.[71] The goal is to normalize the ACT at approximately 100 to 120 seconds. Despite this therapy, release of lipid-bound heparin postoperatively may lead to reanticoagulation and bleeding, requiring reassessment of clot formation in the ICU.[72]

The multifactorial nature of postcardiac surgical bleeding is illustrated by the variety of coagulopathies that may occur including dilution or consumption of clotting factors, thrombocytopenia and thrombocytopathy, and even fibrinolysis. Hemorrhage may also result from disruption of any one of the four vascular anastomoses between the host and donor (i.e., the aortic, pulmonary arterial, left and right atrial suture lines) as well as at the ascending aortic cannulation site. Rapid correction of intrinsic clotting abnormalities by assessment of, and routine therapy for, abnormal prothrombin, partial thromboplastin time, and platelet count is essential. Desmopressin acetate (DDAVP; 1-deamino-8-D arginine vasopressin), a synthetic vasopressin analog, has been shown to reduce blood loss significantly in some patients undergoing complex (nontransplant) cardiac operations.[73] However, this has not been uniformly substantiated in subsequent studies, and routine administration is unlikely to be of value. Functioning perhaps through increases in plasma levels of von Willebrand factor and improved platelet adhesiveness, desmopressin acetate in a dose of 0.3 μg/kg body weight IV may still be a useful adjunct in the bleeding patient.

Persistent bleeding has been found by some to diminish (while correcting the existing coagulopathy) through the judicious application of low levels (10–20 cm H_2O) of PEEP.[74, 75] Other investigators failed to demonstrate such a beneficial effect, particularly when PEEP is applied prophylactically.[76, 77] One must be particularly aware of the potentially deleterious effects of PEEP on RV afterload, compliance, and function when considering this therapy for control of bleeding after heart transplantation.

Should bleeding persist at a brisk rate (>200 mL/h with a chest or mediastinal tube hematocrit of greater than one-half the circulating hematocrit), surgical re-exploration is necessary. In situations of imminent cardiac tamponade or arrest, emergency thoracotomy in the surgical ICU is required. At least in nontransplant cardiac surgical populations, this procedure is lifesaving and probably complicated by a wound infection rate of only 5%.[78] Transesophageal echocardiography is an important method for discriminating between regional tamponade and severe myocardial dysfunction.[78a]

Immunosuppressive Therapy

A detailed discussion of immunosuppressive therapy is outside the scope of this chapter but is well summarized elsewhere.[79] Certain aspects peculiar to cardiac transplant recipients require further comment (Table 182–5).

Current immunosuppression therapy begins with azathioprine administration (4 mg/kg IV) just before the ini-

TABLE 182–5. General Guidelines for Postoperative Support: Immunosuppression

Azathioprine
Steroids
Cyclosporine A or FK-506
Rejection: bolus steroids; sometimes rabbit antithymocyte globulin or OKT3

tiation of surgery. Methylprednisolone (7 mg/kg IV) is delivered at the time of aortic cross-clamp removal. Postoperative therapy follows with methylprednisolone, 5 mg/kg in three divided doses over the first 24 hours, and then a dose of 0.15 mg/kg of prednisone per day orally. In some patients, azathioprine may be continued at 2.5 $mg \cdot kg^{-1} \cdot d^{-1}$ via nasogastric tube or orally, titrated chronically to maintain the white blood cell count greater than 5000/mL.[91]

CyA, perhaps through selective activation of T suppressor cells and inhibition of cytotoxic T cell proliferation, has contributed significantly to the long-term survival of orthotopic heart transplant recipients. It has potentiated an increase in the 1-year survival from 60%[80] to 80% to 85%.[81] On the basis of experience suggesting a decrease in renal dysfunction after earlier therapy, this agent is now begun 12 hours postoperatively when the patient is physiologically stable. Dosing is targeted at whole blood levels of 600 to 800 ng/dL by radioimmunoassay technique. The inherent risks of nephro-, neuro-, and hepatotoxicity are well described.[82–85] Nephrotoxicity has been further reduced by the continuation of azathioprine postoperatively, which has allowed a decrease in the maintenance dosage of both steroids and CyA.[86] A rather unique response to CyA in the orthotopic heart transplant recipient is the almost universal occurrence of systemic hypertension related to its use.[87] This hypertension is easily controlled with antihypertensive agents including diuretics and hydralazine and typically appears approximately 50 days postoperatively. The mechanism seems to be related to altered vascular compliance or fluid balance (perhaps associated with subclinical renal impairment) and appears independent of the renin-angiotensin axis. Further, no adverse effects on organ perfusion have occurred as long as diastolic blood pressure is maintained at or near normal levels.

At least in an animal model, CyA can increase pentobarbital hypnosis and fentanyl analgesia by an unknown mechanism.[88] Thus, it is prudent to monitor the patient's response to analgesic and sedative medications carefully, particularly after extubation.

In some institutions, early postoperative immunosuppression involves the use of either rabbit antithymocyte globulin (RATG) or the murine-derived monoclonal antibody OKT3. Begun within 72 hours of operation, daily intramuscular dosing of 100 mg of RATG into the thigh is associated with few noticeable systemic side effects other than chills, fever, and thrombocytopenia.[89] Complaints are usually limited to local inflammation responsive to symptomatic therapy and early mobilization. Serum sickness, hemolysis, and anaphylaxis are rare consequences of this therapy. The monoclonal antibody OKT3[90, 91] has more profound systemic effects. During its initial use in renal transplant recipients, there were reports of frequent flulike syndromes and occasionally dyspnea and possible cardiovascular compromise attributed to ventricular strain.[92] We have seen a remarkably high incidence of hypoxemia (more than two thirds of the patients) after intravenous administration. Fever, tachycardia, and transient alterations in cardiac output and peripheral perfusion also may appear at different times within the first 10 hours after OKT3 administration. Hemodynamic compromise sometimes requires reinstitution or an increase in inotropic or vasopressor support. This response, which is unique to the first (and rarely second) dose of OKT3,[93] has limited its use to rescue antirejection therapy.

FK-506, a potent immunosuppressive macrolide,[94] is currently being evaluated at the University of Pittsburgh Medical Center[95, 95a] as a primary immunosuppressive agent in conjunction with low-dose steroids. Early results suggest more effective rejection prophylaxis and perhaps less nephrotoxicity than cyclosporine-based regimens. Typically started as an intravenous drip of 0.075 mg/kg over the first 24 to 72 hours, target serum levels of 0.8 to 1.0 ng/mL are achieved. Oral maintenance doses are subsequently instituted.

Monitoring for rejection revolves around the appropriate use of endomyocardial biopsies along with right-sided heart catheterization periodically in the postoperative period.[46] These procedures are performed by the cardiac surgeons every week in the immediate postoperative period. Additional biopsies are specifically done when the suspicion of a rejection episode is high such as in the presence of unexplained fever, tachycardia, arrhythmias, or altered perfusion state. Echocardiography may also provide insight into rejection pathophysiology,[95b] as suggested by shortening of the duration of isovolemic relaxation.[96, 97] Once incipient rejection has been confirmed, therapy with bolus steroids or a course of RATG, or both, is initiated.[98, 99] After the first 6 to 9 months, the incidence of rejection markedly decreases.

Asepsis, Fever, and Infection

The immunosuppressed state of the transplant recipient requires compulsive attention to the avoidance of infection and, failing that, its prompt diagnosis and eradication (Table 182–6). Perioperative antibiotic prophylaxis, often with a first- or second-generation cephalosporin, does not diminish the need for meticulous sterile technique when introducing invasive devices. This is particularly true when traversing the normal skin barrier for central venous access or invading body cavities as with a urinary drainage catheter. These devices remain a threat as pathways for infection as long as they are in place. Thus, prompt removal is appropriate as soon as deemed medically safe. Mechanical circulatory assist devices, when used for pretransplant stabilization, strongly predispose the patient to the development of nonviral infections.[100]

The onset of fever, particularly in the presence of leukocytosis with immature white blood cells, requires instant evaluation. Attribution of these symptoms and signs to atelectasis in the presence of steroid therapy is safe only after careful elimination of other more sinister possibilities. Except for the aggressiveness required in the work-up and the inclusion of many opportunistic pathogens (such as *Pneumocystis*, herpes, fungi, *Legionella*, and viruses such as cytomegalovirus[101]) in the differential, the evaluation follows normal logical pathways and must include radiography and carefully acquired cultures.[102]

General surgical complications are particularly common

TABLE 182–6. General Guidelines for Postoperative Support: Sepsis

Aggressive diagnostic evaluation: cultures, early bronchoscopy, abdominal ultrasound, computed tomographic or magnetic resonance imaging scan, sinus films
Suspect common (bacterial) and opportunistic pathogens (e.g., cytomegalovirus, *Pneumocystis carinii* pneumonia, *Listeria*, *Legionella*, fungi)

in this transplant population, occurring in 28% of the patients undergoing transplantation at the University of Pittsburgh between 1980 and 1985.[103] These problems included sigmoid perforation, small-bowel perforation, acute calculous cholecystitis, pancreatitis, and cecal ulceration. The notable mortality associated with these lesions (10 of 40 such patients) illustrates the need for early aggressive diagnosis (using ultrasonography and abdominal computed tomographic scan or magnetic resonance imaging) and operative intervention as appropriate.[104, 105]

Mediastinitis is a particularly serious complication of heart transplantation, with an incidence as high as 7.5% in one early study. The incidence is currently less than 3% overall, 5% when an intra-aortic balloon pump is used for preoperative support, and as high as 43% after support with the total artificial heart.[106] Several unique aspects of this problem include (1) its frequently late occurrence (4 to 6 weeks postoperatively) after augmentation of the immunosuppressive regimen in response to acute rejection; (2) its relatively asymptomatic presentation with little temperature or white blood cell elevation, or an unstable sternum; (3) its treatment with mediastinal 5% povidone-iodine solution irrigation; and (4) its follow-up by serial chest CT scans.[107] Although the typical pathogen is *Staphylococcus*, gram-negative bacteria and *Mycoplasma hominis* have also been reported. Infection remains a prevalent life-threatening complication of heart transplantation and must be pursued relentlessly.

OUTCOME AND THE FUTURE

Actuarial survival rates after cardiac transplantation continue to rise and are now greater than 85% at 1 year. The more experienced transplant centers achieve the highest success. Quality of life estimates are in progress but suggest generally high patient satisfaction in many important areas including return to productive life. Immunosuppressive therapy continues to evolve with FK-506, rapamycin, and immunomodulation (e.g., anti-tumor necrosis factor[108]) in the future.

Although cardiac transplantation is a lifesaving procedure, it is not a panacea. Chronic rejection and the early development of accelerated endothelial coronary vascular disease, perhaps secondary to rejection, cytomegalovirus, and endothelialitis,[109, 110] seriously impair the function of many donor hearts within 5 years of implantation,[111] necessitating angioplasty, bypass surgery, or consideration of retransplantation.[112] Infectious complications also contribute to nonsurvival. As the application of sophisticated transplantation techniques increases in scope, so must the understanding of, and familiarity with, the nuances of perioperative critical care support. Most discouragingly, the list of potential recipients lengthens and mortality on waiting lists increases and the availability of donor organs has failed to increase significantly.[113, 113a] Interest in xenotransplantation[114, 115] and evolution of mechanical cardiac circulatory assist devices thus remain essential.

References

1. Barnard CN: A human cardiac transplant: An interim report of a successful operation performed at Groote Schur Hospital, Capetown. S Afr Med J 1967; 41:1271.
2. Cooley DA, Bloodwell RD, Hallman GL, et al: Organ transplantation for advanced cardiopulmonary disease. Ann Thorac Surg 1969; 8:30.
3. Hosenpud JD, Uretsky BF, Griffith BP, et al: Successful intermediate-term outcome for patients with cardiac amyloidosis undergoing heart transplantation: Results of a multicenter survey. J Heart Transplant 1990; 9:346.
4. Edwards BS, Hunt SA, Fowler MB, et al: Cardiac transplantation in patients with preexisting neoplastic diseases. Am J Cardiol 1990; 65:501.
5. Murali S, Reddy PS, Armitage JA: The effect of prostaglandins E_1 on the transpulmonary gradient of heart transplant candidates. Circulation 1988; 78:250.
5a. Murali S, Kormos RL, Uretsky BF, et al: Preoperative pulmonary hemodynamics and early mortality after orthotopic cardiac transplantation: The Pittsburgh experience. Am Heart J 1993; 126:896.
6. Goodman DJ, Rossen RM, Rider AK, et al: The effect of cycle length on cardiac refractory periods in the denervated human heart. Am Heart J 1976; 91:332.
7. Stinson EB, Caves PK, Griepp RB, et al: Hemodynamic observations in the period after human heart transplantation. J Thorac Cardiovasc Surg 1975; 69:264.
8. Gasior TA, Armitage J, Stein K, et al: Right ventricular performance in the transplanted heart. Anesthesiology 1989; 71:A85.
9. von Scheidt W, Neudert J, Erdmann E, et al: Contractility of the transplanted, denervated human heart. Am Heart J 1991; 121:1480.
10. Ingels NB Jr, Ricci DR, Daughters GT II, et al: Effects of heart rate augmentation on left ventricular volumes and cardiac output of the transplanted human heart. Circulation 1977; 56(Suppl II):32.
11. Jacquet L, Stein K, Kormos R, et al: Hyperacute rejection following heart transplantation: Clinical hemodynamic evolution. Chest 1989; 96:233S.
12. Griffith BP, Hardesty RL, Kormos RL, et al: Temporary use of the Jarvik-7 total artificial heart before transplantation. N Engl J Med 1987; 316:130.
13. Farrar DJ, Hill D, Gray LA, et al: Heterotopic prosthetic ventricles as a bridge to cardiac transplantation. N Engl J Med 1988; 318:333.
13a. Vincent JL, Carlier E, Pinsky MR, et al: Prostaglandins E_1 infusion for right ventricular failure after cardiac transplantation. J Thorac Cardiovasc Surg 1992; 103:33.
14. D'Ambria MN, LaRaia PJ, Philbin DM, et al: Prostaglandins E_1: A new therapy for refractory right heart failure and pulmonary hypertension after mitral valve replacement. J Thorac Cardiovasc Surg 1985; 89:567.
15. Dewirst WE: Prostaglandins E_1 for refractory right heart failure after coronary artery grafting. J Cardiothorac Anesth 1988; 2:56.
16. Bhatia SJS, Kirshenbaum JM, Shermin RJ, et al: Time course of resolution of pulmonary hypertension and right ventricular remodeling after orthotopic cardiac transplantation. Circulation 1987; 76:819.
17. Sanfelippo PM, Baker NH, Ewy HG, et al: Experience with intraaortic balloon counterpulsation. Ann Thorac Surg 1986; 41:36.
18. Zumbro GL, Kitchens WR, Shearer G, et al: Mechanical assistance for cardiogenic shock following cardiac surgery, mycardial infarction, and cardiac transplantation. Ann Thorac Surg 1987; 44:11.
19. Hetzer R, Hennig E, Schiessler A, et al: Mechanical circulatory support and heart transplantation. J Heart Lung Transplant 1992; 11:S175.
19a. Pennington DG, McBride LR, Peigh PS, et al: Eight years' experience with bridging to cardiac transplantation. J Thorac Cardiovasc Surg 1994; 107:472.
20. DeMarchena E, Futterman L, Wozniak P, et al: Pulmonary artery torsion: A potentially lethal complication after orthotopic cardiac transplantation. Heart Transplantation 1989; 8:499.
21. Sandu JS, Uretsky BF, Zerbe TR, et al: Coronary artery fistula in the heart transplant patient: A potential complication of endomyocardial biopsy. Circulation 1989; 79:350.
22. Yeoh JK, Anderson ST, Federman J, et al: Coronary artery to middle cardiac vein fistula following endomyocardial biopsy in a heart transplant patient. Cathet Cardiovasc Diagn 1991; 24:108.
23. Mason JW, Stinson EB, Harrison DC: Autonomic nervous system and arrhythmias: Studies in the transplanted denervated human heart. Cardiology 1976; 61:75.

24. Stark RP, McGinn AL, Wilson RF: Chest pain in cardiac-transplant recipients: Evidence of sensory reinnervation after cardiac transplantation. N Engl J Med 1991; 324:1791.
25. Scott CD, Omar I, McComb JM, et al: Long-term pacing in heart transplant recipients is usually unnecessary. PACE 1991; 14:1792.
26. Ricci DR, Orlick AE, Reitz BA, et al: Depressant effect of digoxin on atrioventricular conduction in man. Circulation 1978; 57:898.
27. Goodman A, Gilman L: The Pharmacologic Basis of Therapeutics. 7th ed. New York, Macmillan, 1985, p 723.
28. Thomson PD, Melmon KL, Richardson JA, et al: Lidocaine pharmacokinetics in advanced heart failure, liver disease and renal failure in humans. Ann Intern Med 1973; 78:499.
29. Winkle RA, Glantz SA, Harrison DC: Pharmacologic therapy of ventricular arrhythmias. Am J Cardiol 1975; 36:629.
30. Mason JW, Winkle RA, Rider AK, et al: The electrophysiologic effects of quinidine in the transplanted human heart. J Clin Invest 1977; 59:481.
31. Galeazzi RL, Benet LZ, Sheiner LB: Relationship between the pharmacokinetics and pharmacodynamics of procainamide. Clin Pharmacol Ther 1976; 20:278.
32. Linden J, Brooker G: The influence of resting membrane potential on the effect of verapamil on atria. J Mol Cell Cardiol 1980; 12:325.
33. Singh BN, Collett JT, Chew CYC: New perspectives in the pharmacologic therapy of cardiac arrhythmias. Prog Cardiovasc Dis 1980; 22:243.
34. Antman EM, Stone PH, Muller JE, et al: Calcium channel blocking agents in the treatment of cardiovascular disorders: Part I. Basic and clinical electrophysiologic studies. Ann Intern Med 1980; 93:857.
35. Edward JD, Kishen R: Significance and management of intractable supraventricular arrhythmias in critically ill patients. Crit Care Med 1986; 14:280.
36. Barabarash RA, Bauman JL, Lukazewski AA, et al: Verapamil infusions in the treatment of atrial tachyarrhythmias. Crit Care Med 1986; 14:886.
37. Guffin A, Girard D, Kaplan JA: Shivering following cardiac surgery: Hemodynamic changes and reversal. J Cardiothorac Anesth 1987; 1:24.
38. Hall JB, Wood LDH: Liberation of the patient from mechanical ventilation. JAMA 1987; 257:1621.
39. Mulroy M, Fairley HB: Effect of dopamine on intrapulmonary shunt fraction and oxygen transport in acute pulmonary failure. Am Rev Respir Dis 1977; 115:S143.
40. Lindholm C-E, Ollman B, Snyder JV, et al: Flexible fiberoptic bronchoscopy in critical care medicine: Diagnosis, therapy and complications. Crit Care Med 1974; 2:250.
41. Schulman L, Smith C, Drusin R, et al: Respiratory complications of cardiac transplantation. Ann J Med Sci 1988; 296:1.
42. Singer C, Armstrong D, Rosen PP, et al: Diffuse pulmonary infiltrate in immunosuppressed patients: A prospective study of 80 cases. Am J Med 1979; 66:110.
43. Stover DE, Zaman MB, Haidu SI, et al: Bronchoalveolar lavage in the diagnosis of diffuse pulmonary infiltrates in the immunosuppressed host. Ann Intern Med 1985; 101:1.
44. Collaborative DHPG Treatment Study Group: Treatment of serious cytomegalovirus infections with 9-(1,3-dihydroxy-2-propoxymethyl) quinine in patients with AIDS and other immunodeficiencies. N Engl J Med 1986; 314:801.
45. Dummer JS: Infectious complications of transplantation: Historical background and immunosuppression. Cardiovasc Clin North Am 1990; 20:163.
46. Billingham ME: Diagnosis of cardiac rejection by endomyocardial biopsy. J Heart Transplant 1980; 1:25.
47. Mohr DN, Ryn JH, Litin SC, et al: Recent advances in the management of venous thromboembolism. Mayo Clin Proc 1988; 63:281.
48. Fein AM, Lippman M, Holtzman H, et al: The risk factors, incidence and prognosis of ARDS in septicemia. Chest 1983; 83:40.
49. Fowler AA, Hamman RF, Good TF, et al: Adult respiratory distress syndrome: Risk with common predisposition. Ann Intern Med 1983; 98:593.
50. Reinhart RA, Desbeins NA: Hypomagnesemia in patients entering the ICU. Crit Care Med 1985; 13:506.
51. Burch GE, Giles TD: The importance of magnesium deficiency in cardiovascular disease. Am Heart J 1977; 94:649.
52. Turlapty PDMV, Altura BM: Magnesium deficiency produces spasms of coronary arteries: Relationship to etiology of sudden death ischemic heart disease. Science 1980; 208:198.
53. Schneeberger EE, Morrison AB: The nephropathy of experimental magnesium deficiency. Lab Invest 1965; 14:674.
54. Chernow B, Smith J, Rainey TG, et al: Hypomagnesemia: Implications for the critical care specialist. Crit Care Med 1982; 10:193.
55. Davis SV, Olichwier HK, Chakko SC: Reversible depression of myocardial performance in hypophosphatemia. Am J Med Sci 1988; 295:183.
56. Newman JH, Neff TA, Ziporin P: Acute respiratory failure associated with hypophosphatemia. N Engl J Med 1977; 296:1101.
57. Goldstein J, Vincent J-L, Leclerc J-L, et al: Hypophosphatemia after cardiothoracic surgery. Intensive Care Med 1985; 11:114.
58. Hodgkin JE, Soeprono FF, Chan DM: Incidence of metabolic alkalemia in hospitalized patients. Crit Care Med 1980; 12:725.
59. Berthelson P: Cardiovascular performance and oxyhemoglobin dissociation after acetazolamide in metabolic alkalosis. Intensive Care Med 1982; 8:269.
60. Goldberg LI: Cardiovascular and renal actions of dopamine: Potential clinical implications. Pharmacol Rev 1972; 24:1.
61. Beregovich J, Bianchi C, Rubler S, et al: Dose-related hemodynamic and renal effects of dopamine in congestive heart failure. Am Heart J 1974; 87:550.
62. Hilberman M, Maseda J, Stinson EB, et al: The diuretic properties of dopamine in patients after open-heart operations. Anesthesiology 1984; 61:489.
63. Rasmussen HH, Pitt EA, Ibils LS, et al: Prediction of outcome in acute renal failure by discriminant analysis of clinical variables. Arch Intern Med 1985; 145:2015.
64. Cosgrove DM, Loop FD, Lytle BW, et al: Determinants of blood utilization during myocardial revascularization. Ann Thorac Surg 1985; 40:380.
65. Rosenberg RD: Actions and interactions of anti-thrombin and heparin. N Engl J Med 1975; 292:146.
66. Olinger GN, Becker RM, Bonchek LJ: Noncardiogenic pulmonary edema and peripheral vascular collapse following cardiopulmonary bypass: Rare protamine reaction! Ann Thorac Surg 1980; 29:20.
67. Shapira N, Schaff HV, Piebler JM, et al: Cardiovascular effects of protamine sulfate in man. J Thorac Cardiovasc Surg 1982; 84:505.
68. Cavarocchi NC, Schaff HV, Orszulak TA, et al: Evidence for complement activitation by protamine-heparin interaction after cardiopulmonary bypass. Surgery 1985; 98:525.
69. Morel DR, Zapol WM, Thomas SJ, et al: C5a and thromboxane generation associated with pulmonary vaso- and bronchoconstriction during protamine reversal of heparin. Anesthesiology 1987; 66:597.
70. Bull BS, Huse W, Brauer F, et al: Heparin therapy during extracorporeal circulation: II. The use of dose-response curve to individualize heparin and protamine dosage. J Thorac Cardiovasc Surg 1975; 69:685.
71. LaDuca F, Mills D, Thompson S, et al: Neutralization of heparin using a protamine titration assay and the activated clotting time test. J Extra Corp Technol 1984; 19:358.
72. Kaul TK, Crow MJ: Heparin administration during extracorporeal circulation: Heparin rebound and postoperative bleeding. J Thorac Cardiovasc Surg 1979; 78:95.
73. Salzman EW, Weinstein MJ, Weintraup RM, et al: Treatment with desmopressin acetate to reduce blood loss after cardiac surgery. N Engl J Med 1986; 314:1402.
74. Ilabac PA, Ochsner JL, Mills NL: Positive end-expiratory pressure in the management of the patient with a postoperative bleeding heart. Ann Thorac Surg 1980; 30:281.
75. Hoffman WS, Tumasello DN, MacVaugh H: Control of postcardiotomy bleeding with PEEP. Ann Thorac Surg 1982; 34:71.
76. Zurick AM, Urzua J, Ghaths M, et al: Failure of positive end-expiratory pressure to decrease postoperative bleeding after cardiac surgery. Ann Thorac Surg 1982; 34:608.
77. Murphy DA, Finlayson DC, Craver JE, et al: Effect of positive end-expiratory pressure on excessive mediastinal bleeding

after cardiac operations. J Thorac Cardiovasc Surg 1983; 86:865.
78. McKowen RL, Magovern GJ, Liebler GA, et al: Infectious complications and cost-effectiveness of open resuscitation in the surgical intensive care unit after cardiac surgery. Ann Thorac Surg 1985; 40:386
78a. Ziady GM, Bjerke RJ, Armitage JM, et al: Diastolic mitral regurgitation and severe tricuspid regurgitation as a cause of low cardiac output and hypotension early after heart transplantation. J Am Soc Echo 1994; 7(suppl):S59.
79. Council on Scientific Affairs: Introduction to the management of immunosuppression. JAMA 1987; 257:1781.
80. Gaudiani VA, Stinson EB, Alderman E, et al: Long-term survival and function after cardiac transplantation. Ann Surg 1981; 194:381.
81. Goldstein JP, Wechsler AS: Heart transplantation. J Heart Transplant 1985; 20:46.
82. Myers BD, Ross J, Newton L, et al: Cyclosporine-associated chronic nephropathy. N Engl J Med 1984; 311:699.
83. Hardesty RI, Griffith BP, Debski RF, et al: Experience with cyclosporine in cardiac transplantation. Transplant Proc 1983; 15:2553.
84. Klintmalm GBG, Iwatzuki S, Starzl TE: Cyclosporine A hepatotoxicity in 66 renal allograft recipients. Transplantation 1981; 32:488.
85. Schade RR, Guglielmi A, Van Thiel DH, et al: Cholestasis in heart transplant recipients treated with cyclosporine. Transplant Proc 1983; 15:2757.
86. Griffith BP, Hardesty RL, Lee A, et al: Management of cyclosporine toxicity by reduced dosage and azathioprine. J Heart Transplant 1985; 4:410.
87. Thompson ME, Shapiro AP, Johnsen AM, et al: New onset of hypertension following cardiac transplantation: A preliminary report and analysis. Transplant Proc 1983; 215:2573.
88. Cirella VN, Panuck CB, Lee YJ, et al: Effects of cyclosporine on anesthetic action. Anesth Analg 1987; 66:703.
89. Cosimi AB: The clinical usefulness of antilymphocyte antibodies. Transplant Proc 1983; 15:583.
90. Gilbert EM, Eiswirth CC, Renlund DG, et al: Use of orthoclone OKT3 monoclonal antibody in cardiac transplantation: Early experience with rejection prophylaxis and treatment of refractory rejection. Transplant Proc 1987; 19:45.
91. Delmonico FL, Cosimi AB: Monoclonal antibody treatment of human allograft recipients. Surg Gynecol Obstet 1988; 166:89.
92. Ortho Multicenter Transplant Study Group: A randomized clinical trial of OKT3 monoclonal antibody for acute rejection of cadaveric renal transplants. N Engl J Med 1985; 313:337.
93. Stein KL, Ladowski J, Kormos R, et al: The cardiopulmonary response to OKT3 in orthotopic cardiac transplant recipients. Chest 1989; 95:817.
94. Todo S, Murase N, Podesta U, et al: Effect of FK 506 in experimental organ transplantation. Transplant Proc 1988; 20:215.
95. Armitage JA, Kormos RL, Griffith BP, et al: A clinical trial of FK 506 as primary and rescue immunosuppression in cardiac transplantation. Transplant Proc 1991; 23:1149.
95a. Armitage JM, Kormos RL, Morita S, et al: Clinical trial of FK506 immunosuppression in adult cardiac transplantation. Ann Thorac Surg 1992; 54:205.
95b. Fan C, Mather P, Panidis JP, et al: Effect of transplant heart rejection and its treatment on systolic and diastolic left ventricular function as assessed by two-dimensional and Doppler echocardiography. J Am Soc Echo 1994; 7(supplement):S59.
96. Dawkins KD, Oldershaw PJ, Billingham ME, et al: Changes in diastolic function as a non-invasive marker of cardiac allograft rejection. J Heart Transplant 1984; 3:286.
97. St. Goar FG, Gibbons R, Schnittger I, et al: Left ventricular diastolic function: Doppler echocardiographic changes soon after cardiac transplantation. Circulation 1990; 82:872.
98. McGregor CGA, Jamieson SW, Oyer PE, et al: Heart transplantation at Stanford University. J Heart Transplant 1984; 4:31.
99. Griffith BP, Hardesty RL, Bahnson HT: Powerful but limited immunosuppression for cardiac transplantation with cyclosporine and low-dose steroid. J Thorac Cardiovasc Surg 1984; 87:35.
100. Hsu J, Griffith B, Dowling R, et al: Infections in mortally ill cardiac transplant recipients. J Thorac Cardiovasc Surg 1989; 98:506.
101. Rice PS, Kudesia G, Price C, et al: Diagnosis of cytomegalovirus infection in heart transplant recipients. J Clin Pathol 1992; 45:636.
102. Mammana RB, Petersen EA, Fuller JK, et al: Pulmonary infections in cardiac transplant patients: Modes of diagnosis, complication and effectiveness of therapy. Ann Thorac Surg 1983; 36:700.
103. Steed DL, Brown B, Reilly JJ, et al: General surgical complications in heart and heart-lung transplantation. Surgery 1985; 98:739.
104. Leitman IM, Paull DE, Barie PS, et al: Intra-abdominal complications of cardiopulmonary bypass operations. Surg Gynecol Obstet 1987; 165:251.
105. Colon R, Frazier OH, Kahan BD, et al: Complications in cardiac transplant patients requiring general surgery. Surgery 1988; 103:32.
106. Trento A, Dummer GS, Hardesty RL, et al: Mediastinitis following heart transplantation. Incidence, treatment and results. J Heart Transplant 1984; 3:336.
107. Griffith BP, Kormos RL, Hardesty RL, et al: The artificial heart: Infection related morbidity and its effect on transplantation. Ann Thorac Surg 1988; 45:409.
108. Bolling SF, Kunkel SL, Lin H: Prolongation of cardiac allograft survival in rats by anti-TNF and cyclosporine combination therapy. Transplantation 1992; 53:283.
109. Normann SJ, Salomon DR, Leelachaikul P, et al: Acute vascular rejection of the coronary arteries in human heart transplantation: Pathology and correlations with immunosuppression and cytomegalovirus infection. J Heart Lung Transplant 1991; 10:674.
110. Hruban RH, Beschorner WE, Baumgartner WA, et al: Accelerated arteriosclerosis in heart transplant recipients is associated with a T-lymphocyte-mediated endothelialitis. Am J Pathol 1990; 137:871.
111. Uretsky BF, Murali S, Redd PS, et al: Development of coronary artery disease in cardiac transplant patients receiving immunosuppressive therapy with cyclosporine prednisone. Circulation 1987; 76:827.
112. Neish AS, Loh E, Schoen FJ: Myocardial changes in cardiac transplant-associated coronary arteriosclerosis: Potential for timely diagnosis. J Am Coll Cardiol 1992; 19:586.
113. Darby JM, Stein KL, Grenvik A, et al: Approach to the management of the heart-beating "brain dead" organ donor. JAMA 1989; 261:2222.
113a. Livi U, Bortolotti U, Luciani GB, et al: Donor shortage in heart transplantation: Is extension of donor age limits justified? J Thorac Cardiovasc Surg 1994; 107:1346.
114. Hammer C, Schultz A, Pratschke J, et al: Bridging to transplant: Allogeneic heart transplantation after xenografting. J Heart Lung Transplant 1992; 11:S182.
115. Kawanchi M, Gundry SR, Alonso de Begona J, et al: Prolonged survival of orthotopically transplanted heart xenograft in infant baboons. J Thorac Cardiovasc Surg 1993; 106:779.

CHAPTER 183

Lung Transplantation: Thirty Years of Progress

Morris I. Bierman, MD • Keith L. Stein, MD, FCCP, FCCM
James Dauber, MD • Robert L. Hardesty, MD
Bartley P. Griffith, MD

Thirty years ago, the transplantation of a single lung from a donor with pulmonary edema into a recipient with squamous cell carcinoma of the lung was first described.[1] Since then, progress in lung transplantation has been slow relative to that in the transplantation of other organs. Nevertheless, major advances in preservation, surgical technique, and immunosuppression have now made lung transplantation a viable option for patients with end-stage pulmonary disease. The ability to perform single, double, or heart-lung transplantation allows the procedure to be tailored to the needs of the recipient. As with other organs, the scarcity of donors limits the number of available transplants and requires the maximum utilization of all donor lungs that become available.

PREOPERATIVE EVALUATION

Recipient Selection

The criteria for recipient selection are similar among the large transplant centers.[2–4] These criteria can be organized into three areas that are crucial in determining the suitability of an individual for lung transplantation. They are assessment of the patient's general medical condition, his or her specific pulmonary disorder, and psychosocial factors.

General Medical Condition

The patient's general medical condition is assessed by determining any factors that may affect the transplantation procedure or its long-term success. Patients with severe systemic illnesses such as malignant diseases, poorly controlled diabetes mellitus, or hypertension are generally not considered for transplantation. Those with severe systemic manifestations of their respiratory condition (e.g., sarcoidosis, vasculitis) are also poor candidates for transplantation.

Although not as important as a physiologic assessment, age is an important consideration in determining a patient's suitability for lung transplantation. In general, patients considered for single lung transplantation are younger than 60 years of age, and those considered for double lung or heart-lung transplantation are younger than 50 years.[2, 3]

A cardiovascular assessment is a crucial part of the evaluation. A general evaluation of right and left ventricular function is performed with nuclear imaging techniques. A left ventricular ejection fraction less than 35% suggests the need for heart-lung transplantation. Right ventricular dysfunction is a common occurrence in patients with end-stage pulmonary vascular or parenchymal disease and may be reversible with transplantation.[5] The lower limit of right ventricular function that would preclude transplantation as well as other factors that determine the reversibility of right ventricular function remain to be defined.[6] Patients with pulmonary vascular diseases undergo right-sided heart catheterization to assess accurately the degree of pulmonary hypertension. Left-sided heart catheterization with coronary angiography is performed in all patients who are considered to be at risk for coronary artery disease. Cardiac catheterization is also crucial to determine the exact nature of cardiac defects in patients with congenital heart disease who are being considered for heart-lung or isolated lung transplantation.

An assessment of baseline renal and hepatic function is also performed because the surgical procedure and immunosuppressive agents may have important effects on the kidney and liver. Renal function is assessed by measuring the levels of blood urea nitrogen and creatinine as well as creatinine clearance. Hepatic function is assessed by measuring the levels of serum bilirubin, transaminases, and alkaline phosphatase.

Potential recipients also undergo serologic screening for herpes simplex virus, cytomegalovirus, Epstein-Barr virus, and toxoplasmosis. Such screening is crucial for the administration of specific prophylactic agents following transplantation.

Pulmonary Assessment

A wide variety of diseases may be considered as indications for lung transplantation. Pulmonary parenchymal diseases such as cystic fibrosis, emphysematous lung disease, and idiopathic pulmonary fibrosis are the most common indications for most lung transplantation procedures (Fig. 183–1).[7] In the past, patients with primary pulmonary hypertension and Eisenmenger's syndrome generally received a heart-lung transplant. However, as heart-lung en bloc transplants have become more difficult to acquire, increasing numbers of these patients are now receiving single or double lung allografts for these conditions. Simple cardiac defects, such as an atrial septal defect, a patent ductus arteriosus, or a ventricular septal defect, may be corrected at the time of lung transplantation.

The optimal timing of transplantation during the course of the patient's illness can be difficult to determine. The patient should not be so desperately ill that surviving the procedure is unlikely, yet all possible medical and surgical therapies for the patient's illness should have been tried before he or she is considered for transplantation. This "transplant window"[2] is best estimated based on knowledge of the natural history of the primary disease, close following of the progress of the patient's individual course, the performance of serial evaluations as appropriate (e.g., pulmonary function tests, exercise testing), and monitoring of the patient's functional status. Once cachexia, inactivity, and multisystem dysfunction occur, the probability of success greatly decreases. Patients usually have a life expectancy of from 1 to 2 years at the time they are considered for transplantation, which coincides with the range of the waiting period for an organ in most centers.

Several therapies for pulmonary disease may have an impact on the transplantation procedure. Patients who have had a previous thoracotomy (e.g., biopsy, pulmonary resection, or pleurectomy) may have extensive mediastinal and pleural adhesions. These adhesions may slow the removal of the native lungs if they involve crucial structures (e.g., phrenic nerves), and they can be the source of troublesome hemorrhage. Prior thoracic procedures are thus a contraindication to heart-lung transplantation, which requires cardiopulmonary bypass with its attendant anticoagulation. In single and double lung transplantation, they are only relative contraindications because cardiopulmonary bypass can usually be avoided.

Corticosteroids are anti-inflammatory agents that are used to treat various pulmonary diseases. However, some centers maintain that these drugs may interfere with the healing of airway anastomoses[8, 9] and that they should be withdrawn from patients before lung transplantation.[2, 3] This is a controversial issue because the early use of corticosteroids may be beneficial by reducing early episodes of rejection. Because withdrawal of these agents is impossible in many patients, other centers merely require that their dosage be minimized (e.g., limited to less than 20 mg/d of prednisone). Patients with severe toxicity from chronic steroid therapy are generally not considered for transplantation.

The chronic or recurrent administration of antibiotics also plays an important role in the treatment of several pulmonary diseases—most notably, cystic fibrosis. Such patients are often colonized with highly resistant organisms. Preoperative determination of the sensitivity patterns of these organisms is crucial if rational antibiotic prophylaxis is to be provided during the postoperative period.

Psychosocial Assessment

The transplantation process can be a source of considerable stress to a patient who already must contend with the hardships and limitations of end-stage lung disease. Psychiatric disorders are common in lung transplant candidates and can range from mood disorders to substance abuse.[10] Different factors have a role during the various stages of the

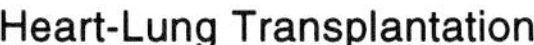

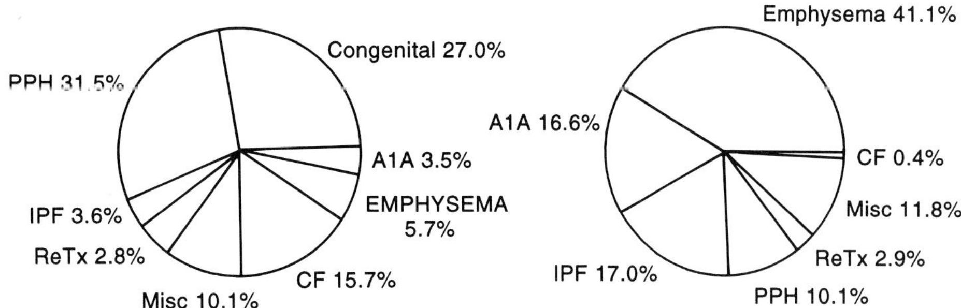

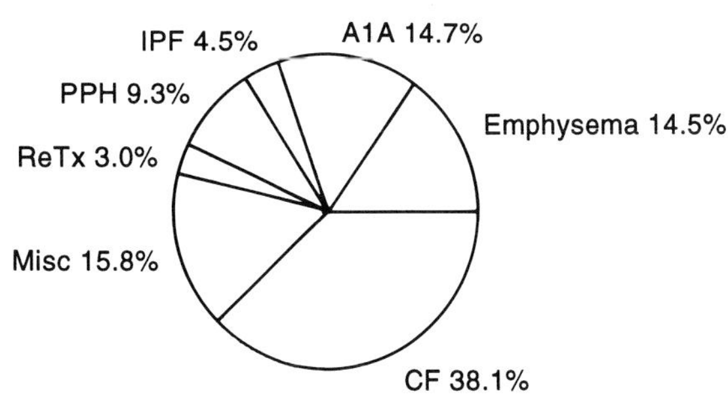

Figure 183–1. Indications for lung transplantation in adults. *Abbreviations*: PPH = primary pulmonary hypertension; IPF = ideopathic pulmonary fibrosis; ReTx = retransplantation; CF = cystic fibrosis; A1A = alpha$_1$-antitrypsin deficiency. (From Hosenpud JD, Novick RJ, Breen TJ, et al: The registry of the International Society for Heart and Lung Transplantation: Eleventh official report—1994. J Heart Lung Transplant 1994; 13:561.)

process (e.g., evaluation for transplantation, perioperative care, long-term care, and rehabilitation). A stable personality and strong family support are necessary to cope with the added stress at any stage. Extensive interviews with the potential recipient (occasionally requiring formal psychiatric evaluation) are necessary to assess the ability of the patient and his or her family to cope with these challenges.

Donor Selection

As with many other types of organ transplants, the availability of suitable donors is a major factor limiting the widespread application of the procedure. It has been estimated that lungs acceptable for transplantation are found in only 15% of potential donors.[11]

Ideally, potential donors must have no history of smoking or chronic lung disease. In addition they must be without systemic illness, such as sepsis or malignancy, that could potentially affect the recipient. They must be without serologic evidence of hepatitis, syphilis, and human immunodeficiency virus. The lungs themselves must have no evidence of injury or infection, as demonstrated by a clear chest radiograph; good gas exchange, as determined by blood gas analysis; and normal pulmonary mechanics. Bronchoscopy is generally performed to ensure that the airways are free of purulent secretions, inflammation, aspirated material, or other pathology.[11a]

Once the donor organs have been found to be acceptable, a recipient is matched on the basis of immunologic compatibility (ABO blood type) and size. Size is assessed based on the donor's height, weight, and thoracic dimensions as determined by chest radiographic examination. In heart-lung and double lung transplantation, it is particularly important to avoid the use of lungs that are too large because compressive atelectasis and marked hemodynamic instability can result. In single lung transplantation, an oversized lung may be transplanted on the recipient's left side, where the hemidiaphragm can descend somewhat to accommodate it.[12] Once the donor transplant is found to be compatible, airway cultures are obtained to guide the use of perioperative antibiotics. Serologic studies for cytomegalovirus, Epstein-Barr virus, herpes simplex virus, and toxoplasmosis are performed. Because of the scarcity of organs, these studies are not used prospectively to match recipients but rather to guide the postoperative use of prophylactic measures such as ganciclovir administration.

OPERATIVE ISSUES

Lung Preservation

Although rapid advances in surgical technique and immunosuppression have increased the clinical success of lung and heart-lung transplantation, many issues surrounding lung preservation remain poorly understood. The earliest procedures required that the donor be brought to the transplant center so that the lungs could be removed and immediately placed into the recipient without the need for preservation.[13] Distant procurement of organs was necessary to expand the donor pool and simplify the procedure; hence, various techniques for lung preservation have been used. Direct comparison of these techniques has been difficult because of the lack of consensus concerning an appropriate experimental model, transplantation technique, and measures of the adequacy of preservation. Nevertheless, a few common principles have emerged.[13a]

Hypothermic Preservation

Normothermic preservation of an autoperfused heart-lung en bloc transplant has been successfully used in the past as a means of distant organ procurement.[14] Because this method was technically complex, hypothermic techniques were developed that allow ischemic times of 4 to 6 hours.[15]

Hypothermia is crucial to slow cellular metabolism and to depress the activity of intracellular enzymes that lead to cell death during ischemic preservation.[15] Two methods have been used to achieve pulmonary hypothermia. Core cooling of the donor can be accomplished by placing the donor on cardiopulmonary bypass.[16, 17] This technique is complex because it may require that a portable cardiopulmonary bypass unit be brought to the donor hospital. Furthermore, once hypothermic cardiac arrest occurs, pulmonary perfusion ceases and bronchial arterial perfusion becomes uncertain. Therefore, uniform pulmonary cooling may be impossible to achieve with cardiopulmonary bypass alone. For these reasons this technique has not been widely applied.

The most common technique for achieving hypothermia involves flushing the donor lung with a cold preservative solution through the pulmonary artery after the lung has been removed. Generally, a vasodilator such as prostacyclin or prostaglandin E_1 is also used to ensure uniform perfusion of the organ with the hypothermic solution. The preservative flush may include modified Euro-Collins, blood-based, low potassium–dextran, or University of Wisconsin solutions.[18]

For transport to the recipient, the lungs are placed in cold saline or ice. The ideal temperature has not been established, nor has it been determined whether the lungs should be inflated or remain deflated during transport.[18] Furthermore, the role of supplemental oxygen for inflating donor lungs for transport has not been established.

Adjunctive Measures

Several other measures have also been considered to reduce the injury to the lung during preservation and reperfusion. The inflammatory cascades that lead to such injury have been poorly defined. Nevertheless, a variety of anti-inflammatory agents have been used during various stages of procurement and reimplantation of the lungs.[18] For example, not only are prostaglandin E_1 and prostacyclin used in many centers for their vasodilatory properties as outlined earlier, but these agents also have anti-inflammatory effects that may be beneficial.[19, 20] Similarly, corticosteroids have been shown to be of some benefit in animal models.[21]

Cytotoxic oxygen free radicals are widely believed to play an important role in ischemia-reperfusion injury to the lung.[20] Various measures have been contemplated as means of preventing free radical injury. For example, because leukocytes may be a source of the free radicals, leukocyte depletion using filters during procurement and reimplantation has been proposed.[22] The application of such techniques is likely to be limited, as they require that cardiopulmonary bypass be used in both the donor and the patient. A much more practical approach would be to administer agents that act as scavengers of free radicals, such as allopurinol,[23] superoxide dismutase,[24] catalase,[25] and dimethylthiourea.[26] In addition, because iron plays a role in the generation of free radicals, chelating agents such as deferoxamine[27] may be useful. Each of these agents has been shown to be of benefit in animal models, but they have not been widely applied to transplantation in humans.

Transplantation Options

Initially, lung transplantation was performed only as a heart-lung combination. Although effective, it was impractical for patients with isolated lung disease, and as heart transplantation became increasingly widespread, the availability of heart-lung en bloc transplants was reduced. Single and double lung transplantations eliminated the need for extraneous heart transplantation and expanded the use of available donor lungs. Lobar transplantation from both cadavers and living, related donors has been performed on small numbers of pediatric patients.[28] The availability of each of these choices allows the operation to be tailored to the needs of the individual patient.

Heart-lung transplantation is currently performed for patients with complex congenital heart disease. Also, it is performed for those patients with pulmonary parenchymal or vascular disease that is combined with coronary artery disease or poor left ventricular function (e.g., left ventricular ejection fraction ≤35%). Double lung transplantation must be utilized for septic pulmonary disease (e.g., cystic fibrosis, bronchiectasis) because the allograft would be at risk for infectious complications if a single lung transplant was performed. Other indications for double lung transplantation include primary pulmonary hypertension and secondary pulmonary hypertension due to simple cardiac defects, which may be corrected at the time of transplantation. In addition, double lung transplantation may be indicated for bullous emphysema.

Single lung transplantation has been performed in patients with various parenchymal and vascular pulmonary diseases. It was once believed to be contraindicated in cases of emphysematous lung disease because of concerns about severe hyperinflation of the remaining native lung and ventilation-perfusion mismatch.[29] However, subsequent experience showed that such concerns were overemphasized and that the procedure could be performed in patients with emphysema due to chronic obstructive pulmonary disease or $alpha_1$-antitrypsin deficiency. Although such patients may not achieve as large an improvement in lung volume as those receiving double lung transplants, they do experience a significant improvement in gas exchange and exercise tolerance.[30, 31] Given the scarcity of donor organs, single lung transplantation for emphysema is a reasonable option.

Single lung transplantation has recently been performed for patients with pulmonary hypertensive disorders. Following transplantation, most of the blood flow is directed toward the allograft, whereas ventilation is directed to both lungs. Nevertheless, these patients have experienced decreases in their pulmonary artery pressures, improvements in gas exchange, and recovery of right ventricular function.[32] Of concern, however, is the increased operative risk and the lack of reserve afforded by the native lung should infection or rejection occur in the allograft.[33] In such circumstances, ventilation-perfusion mismatch can result in severe hypoxemia.

For single lung transplantation, few guidelines exist for determining which of the native lungs to replace. One approach is to perform preoperative ventilation-perfusion scanning. If ventilation and perfusion are significantly decreased on one side, that side's lung is generally chosen to be replaced. In emphysematous patients, it may be preferable to select the right lung for transplantation. The high compliance of the native lung, coupled with expiratory airflow limitation, can cause hyperinflation and compression of the newly transplanted lung. Compression is less likely to occur if the native lung remains in the left side of the chest because of the ability of the left hemidiaphragm to descend in order to accommodate the hyperinflated lung.

Technical Considerations

Cardiopulmonary Bypass

Cardiopulmonary bypass, although associated with risks and complications, is a necessary part of heart-lung or single lung transplantation performed for pulmonary hypertension. When double lung transplantation was initially described, en bloc implantation of both lungs simultaneously

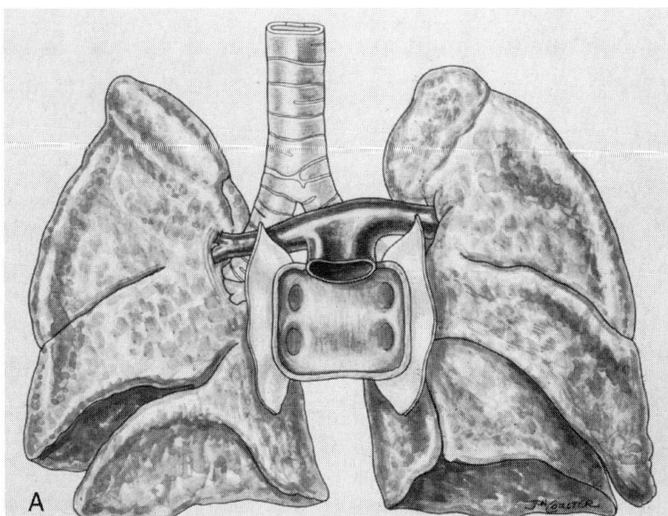

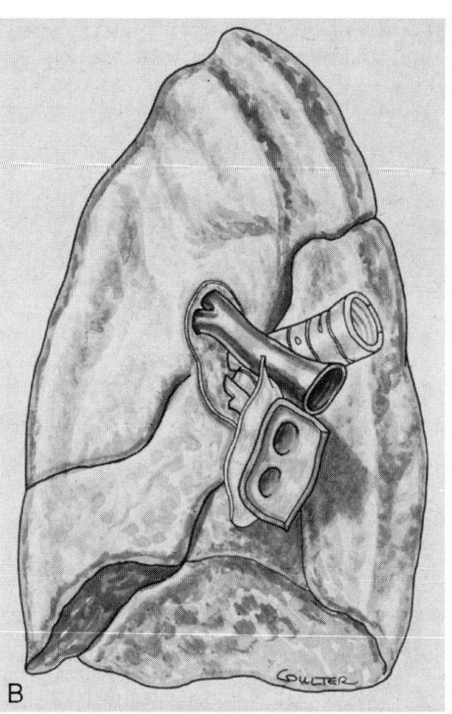

Figure 183–2. *A,* In the donor, the lungs are removed with the airway divided at the trachea, the pulmonary artery severed proximal to its bifurcation, and the pulmonary veins harvested as a cuff of the left atrium. *B,* Division of the mainstem bronchi, pulmonary artery, and atrial cuff yields the right and left lungs for implantation. The right lung is shown here.

also necessitated the use of bypass.[34] This procedure was later refined, and each lung is now implanted individually[35, 36] (Fig. 183–2). If a preoperative perfusion scan indicates a marked discrepancy between the right and left lung of the recipient, then the lung with the least perfusion is replaced first. As each lung is isolated, its pulmonary artery is clamped, and the effects on the recipient's hemodynamic status and ability to maintain acceptable gas exchange are closely monitored. If tolerated, cardiopulmonary bypass can be successfully avoided. A similar approach is taken with single lung transplantation[37, 38] such that cardiopulmonary bypass is reserved for those recipients who are unable to tolerate single lung ventilation using the contralateral native lung.

Incision

Heart-lung transplantation is performed through a standard median sternotomy. A lateral thoracotomy through the fifth or sixth intercostal space is used for single lung transplantation. For double lung transplantation, a bilateral thoracotomy or "clamshell" incision is used (Fig. 183–3); this requires division and ligature of both internal mammary arteries.

Airway Anastomoses

The integrity of the airway anastomoses has been a major concern in pulmonary transplantation. Complications such as dehiscence and stricture have necessitated several changes in surgical technique. The blood supply to the large airways comes from the bronchial circulation, which originates from the aorta and upper intercostal arteries.[39] During removal of the lungs, this supply is interrupted so that the airways become dependent on deoxygenated pulmonary arterial blood after transplantation. Consequently, ischemia is believed to play a major role in the development of airway complications.

Several measures can enhance the integrity and vascularity of the airway anastomoses. Dissection about the airways is minimized during removal of the native lungs to preserve the bronchial circulation as much as possible. Reconnection of the donor bronchial circulation to the recipient aorta has been performed but is technically complex and increases the duration of the procedure.[40] Although the tracheal anastomosis performed with heart-lung transplantation has proved to be relatively free of complications, the same anastomosis performed for double lung transplantation has been less successful.[41] The reasons for this discrepancy are unclear, although it may relate to the loss of coronary-carinal collateral vessels that supply the lower trachea. Nevertheless, for double lung transplantation, bilateral bronchial anastomoses are preferred.[35, 36, 42, 43] Generally, the airways are joined by telescoping the mainstem bronchus of the donor airway into that of the recipient[44] to reinforce the juncture (Fig. 183–4). Prior to the development of the telescoping technique, many centers chose to wrap the anastomoses in either omentum or a pedicle of intercostal muscle or internal mammary artery.[45] This was to provide additional reinforcement, contain any potential dehiscence, and improve revascularization.

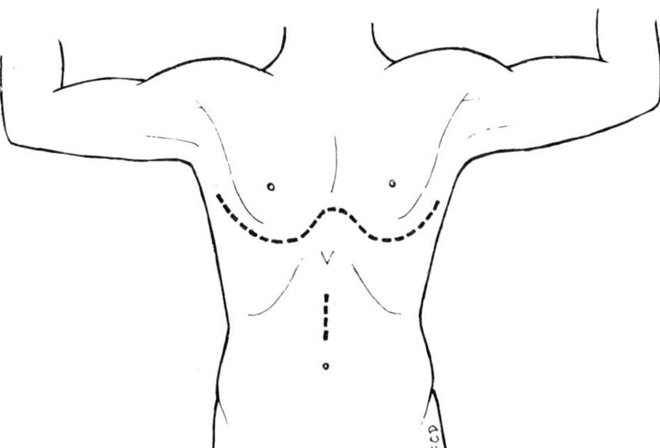

Figure 183–3. The "clam shell" incision used for double lung transplantation. The midline abdominal incision is made, should the surgeon wish to use an omentopexy. (From Egan TM, Detterbeck FC: Technique and results of double lung transplantation. Chest Surg Clin North Am 1993; 3:89–111.)

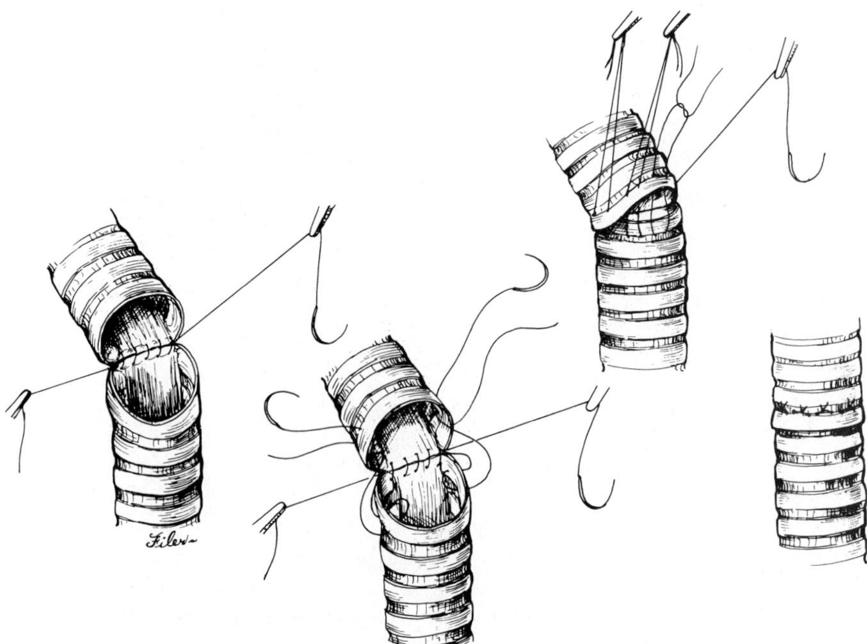

Figure 183–4. The anastomosis of the airway begins with a continuous approximation of the membranous portions and is completed with the placement of interrupted horizontal mattress sutures from the larger airway in such a way that the smaller is telescoped. (From Griffith BP, Magee MJ: Single lung transplantation. Chest Surg Clin North Am 1993; 3:75–88.)

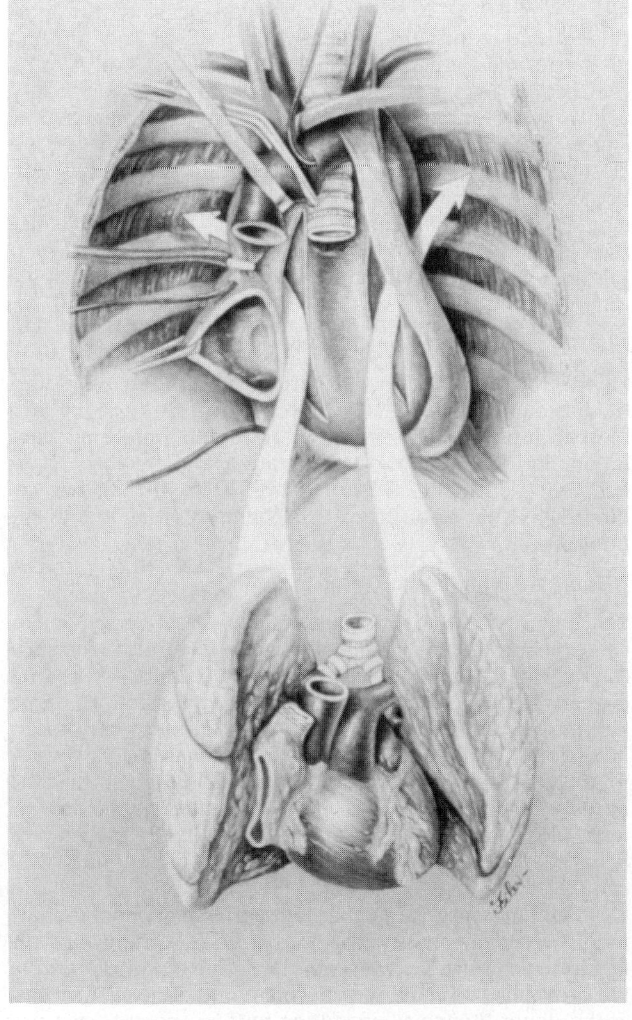

Figure 183–5. With heart-lung transplantation, the donor organs are inserted with anastomoses of the trachea, aorta, and right atrial cuff.

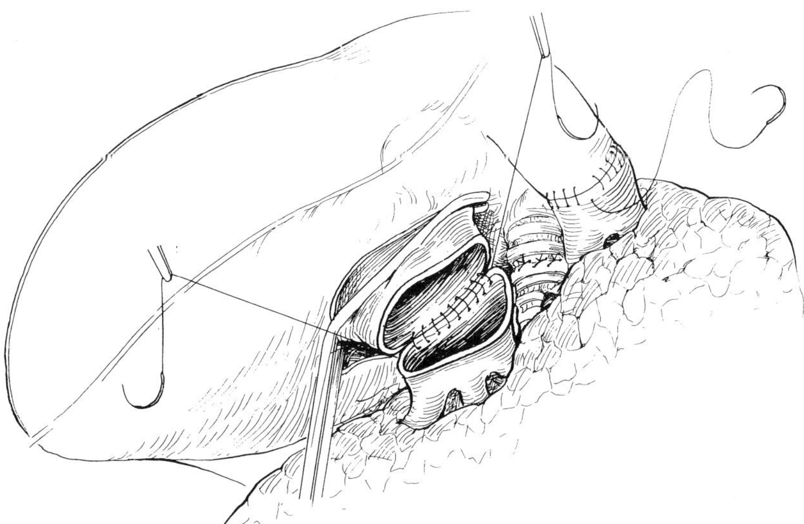

Figure 183–6. Completion of a left lung transplantation. The atrial cuff of the donor is being sewn to that of the recipient. The bronchial and pulmonary arterial anastomoses are completed. (From Griffith BP, Magee MJ: Single lung transplantation. Chest Surg Clin North Am 1993; 3:75–88.)

Vascular Anastomoses

In heart-lung transplantation, the aorta and a cuff of right atrium containing the vena cavae comprise the vascular anastomoses (Fig. 183–5). In single lung and sequential double lung procedures, the pulmonary artery of the side to be transplanted is joined to the pulmonary artery segment of the donor. Pulmonary veins are procured with a cuff of donor left atrium that is joined to the left atrium of the recipient (Fig. 183–6). The characteristics of the anastomoses can be assessed postoperatively with transesophageal echocardiography, radionuclide perfusion scanning, or pulmonary angiography.

MANAGEMENT IN THE INTENSIVE CARE UNIT

Respiratory Management

The basic principles of airway and ventilatory management in the lung transplant recipient are no different than those for other critically ill patients. Adequate oxygenation is ensured with administration of supplemental oxygen and positive end-expiratory pressure. Control of the partial pressure of carbon dioxide in arterial blood ($Paco_2$) and pH is achieved by providing an adequate minute ventilation at the lowest airway pressures possible. The $Paco_2$ is adjusted to maintain the pH. Patients who were hypercapnic preoperatively usually remain so temporarily after transplantation. The $Paco_2$ gradually normalizes over several weeks as the medullary respiratory centers re-equilibrate. Extubation generally occurs within 48 hours, when conventional criteria are met and the patient is able to protect the airway.

Varying degrees of respiratory insufficiency may develop in the early postoperative period. Numerous factors can cause respiratory failure at this time, and these are outlined in Table 183–1. The development of infiltrates on the chest radiograph in the early postoperative period combined with poor gas exchange and abnormal respiratory mechanics was referred to as the "re-implantation" response in early publications.[46] As Table 183–1 demonstrates, several factors can potentially cause such infiltrates.

Preservation-Reperfusion Injury

Injuries caused by preservation or reperfusion result in infiltrates in the transplanted lung or lungs in the immediate postoperative period. They may be accompanied by various degrees of gas exchange impairment and abnormal compliance. Depending on the severity of the injury, recovery may occur within just a few hours or may be prolonged for weeks.

Pulmonary Edema

The transplanted lung is particularly susceptible to the development of pulmonary edema in the postoperative period for several reasons. First, the increase in intravascular and total body volume required to maintain hemodynamic stability during the procedure results in hydrostatic forces that favor the formation of pulmonary edema. Any cardiac dysfunction that is present can exacerbate this problem. Additional postoperative fluid requirements, such as transfusions for hemorrhage or blood products to correct coagulopathy, also contribute to volume overload. Second, increases in capillary permeability related to preservation-reperfusion injury or the use of cardiopulmonary bypass[47] also increase lung water volumes. Third, pulmonary edema is common in single lung transplantation patients, in whom the transplanted lung must immediately accept all of the cardiac output (e.g., pulmonary hypertension).[32] Fourth, disordered fluid clearance related to the disruption of the pulmonary lymphatic circulation may play a role in the development of pulmonary edema.

For these reasons, fluid administration is minimized in the postoperative period. When necessary, vasoactive agents are added to maintain blood pressure. Diuretics are administered as soon as the patient is hemodynamically stable.

The possibility of pulmonary venous obstruction must also be considered when pulmonary edema develops in the transplanted lung.[48] This may occur as a result of kinking of the pulmonary veins or of thrombosis of a narrow venous anastomosis. When pulmonary venous obstruction is diagnosed, surgical correction is necessary. The diagnosis can be

TABLE 183–1. Causes of Respiratory Insufficiency After Lung Transplantation

Causes
Preservation injury
Reperfusion injury
Pulmonary edema
Pulmonary venous obstruction
Ventilation-perfusion mismatch
Hyperinflation
Pneumonia
Rejection
Phrenic nerve dysfunction

made at the bedside by measuring pulmonary venous flow from the transplanted lung using Doppler transesophageal echocardiography. Alternatively, the delayed transit of contrast medium may be detected with pulmonary angiography.[49]

Ventilation-Perfusion Mismatch

In patients receiving a single lung transplant, ventilation-perfusion mismatch can lead to significantly abnormal gas exchange. This may occur whenever the allograft receives most of the pulmonary perfusion. For example, in patients with primary or secondary pulmonary hypertension, perfusion scans generally show that most of the blood flow tends toward the transplanted lung in the immediate postoperative period. Because differences in respiratory compliance between the two lungs are usually small, ventilation is usually equally split. This results in suboptimal gas exchange, although usually not to such an extreme that the patient is impaired.

Ventilation-perfusion mismatch can become a serious problem should infiltrates develop in the transplanted lung for any reason (e.g., preservation injury, rejection, pneumonia). In such cases, ventilation tends toward the native lung, whereas most of the pulmonary blood flow continues to the transplanted lung. Severe hypoxemia and hypercapnia can result. Differential lung ventilation with the selective application of positive end-expiratory pressure and other techniques may be necessary to achieve adequate oxygenation and ventilation.

Hyperinflation

When single lung transplantation is performed for an emphysematous state, the patient is left with markedly different respiratory mechanics in each hemithorax. The transplanted lung has either normal mechanics or varying degrees of restrictive physiology if injuries such as pulmonary edema or rejection occur. In contrast, the native, emphysematous lung has obstructive physiology that necessitates a long expiratory time for full emptying because of expiratory airflow limitation and high compliance. Furthermore, increased compliance results in the direction of a disproportionate amount of the tidal volume to this lung. The situation is exacerbated if the compliance of the allograft deteriorates, causing even more of the tidal volume to be directed toward the native lung. This abnormal distribution of the tidal volume, coupled with the need for a prolonged expiratory time, can create serious hyperinflation.

The major consequence of this hyperinflation is progressive compression of the allograft. If this condition remains unrecognized, the mediastinum can be shifted to such an extent that hemodynamic collapse results. This problem is best managed by performing differential lung ventilation using a double-lumen tracheobronchial tube, with the tidal volumes, flow rates, and inspiratory-expiratory ratios customized to each lung. The administration of bronchodilators to the native lung must be continued. Finally, because positive-pressure ventilation exacerbates these problems, extubation should occur as soon as the patient is clinically able to support himself or herself with spontaneous breathing.

Pneumonia

The lung transplant recipient is susceptible to pneumonia for several reasons. First, immunosuppression, a necessary part of transplantation, is used to prevent episodes of rejection. Second, the clearance of secretions from the transplanted lung may be poor because of impaired ciliary motility related to the denervation of the transplanted lung and to the physical barrier posed by the airway anastomoses. Third, with disruption of the lymphatic circulation, the normal migration of immune effector cells is altered. Fourth, colonization or infection of the donor lung can infect the recipient. Fifth, the recipient's native airways (e.g., the proximal trachea and sinuses) may be a source of infection to the newly transplanted lung.

Pneumonia is quite common in the early postoperative period. It must be suspected whenever the patient develops a localized infiltrate, especially if it is accompanied by fever and leukocytosis. The diagnosis is made rapidly by using bronchoscopy with bronchoalveolar lavage or protected brush catheters to obtain samples for Gram's staining and for quantitative cultures of the airways.

Rejection

Episodes of acute rejection during the first 30 days after lung transplantation are common; according to a recent series,[50] the average number of episodes per patient is 1.2. Rejection most commonly occurs from 2 to 4 weeks following transplantation, although in some patients it may be seen within days of the procedure. Acute rejection of the lung is indicated by the abrupt appearance of infiltrates accompanied by worsening gas exchange and pulmonary mechanics. Fever and leukocytosis may also occur, raising concern about infection. Bronchoscopy is essential not only to establish the diagnosis but also to exclude infection.[51] A transbronchial biopsy is required because the findings of bronchoalveolar lavage are not unique to rejection.

Phrenic Nerve Injury

Patients with inflammatory lung disease or recurrent respiratory infections may develop dense pleural adhesions. During removal of the recipient's native lungs, these adhesions may obscure vital structures, such as the phrenic nerve, causing them to be inadvertently cut or severed. The phrenic nerve can also be damaged if excessive traction is placed on it during manipulation of the lungs. Absence of phrenic nerve function results in serious diaphragmatic insufficiency that may slow weaning from mechanical ventilation.

Hemodynamic Management

The principles of hemodynamic management for transplant recipients are similar to those for other critically ill patients. The goals are to ensure adequate organ perfusion as evidenced by an adequate blood pressure; cardiac index; mixed venous oxygen saturation; and end-organ function. The only exception is that volume administration is kept to the minimum necessary to achieve these goals. Vasoactive agents are added when appropriate to maintain the mean arterial pressure. Inotropic agents are needed to support the heart in cases of heart-lung transplantation and may be needed to support the right side of the heart in other forms of lung transplantation, especially when the patient has preexisting right ventricular dysfunction. Vasodilators such as prostaglandin E_1 are occasionally necessary to control pulmonary artery pressure.

Supraventricular arrhythmias such as atrial fibrillation may occur following pulmonary transplantation. These are managed with conventional means.

Hemorrhage

Postoperative bleeding was a major contributor to morbidity and mortality in the early transplantation experience.[52] Brisk bleeding created hemodynamic problems and greatly increased fluid requirements, which contributed to postoperative graft dysfunction. Furthermore, if the hemorrhage was not well drained, the transplanted lung was compressed by the intrathoracic hematoma.

Patients at risk for bleeding include those with extensive

pleural adhesions, those with Eisenmenger's syndrome and extensive mediastinal vessels, and those who receive heparinization that is necessary for cardiopulmonary bypass. The ability to avoid bypass has been a major factor in reducing the incidence of hemorrhage after lung transplantation.

Renal Management

Renal function is optimized through support of the circulation, as described previously. Because of the need to minimize lung water, patients receive diuretics as soon as they are hemodynamically stable. Nephrotoxic medications such as cyclosporine or FK-506 are not given until an adequate urine output has been demonstrated.

Gastrointestinal Considerations

All transplant patients receive prophylaxis against upper gastrointestinal stress ulceration. Enteral feedings are begun as soon as normal bowel function is evident. Of major concern, however, is the management of patients with cystic fibrosis who must be maintained on the same bowel regimen they were receiving at home. Pancreatic enzyme supplements should be restarted as soon as the patient begins enteral feeding.

Infectious Disease Considerations

Infectious complications are important causes of both early and late complications. Prophylactic antibiotics and other agents play an important role in preventing such problems. These measures are summarized in Table 183–2.

Bacterial pneumonia is the most common infectious complication in the early postoperative period. Bacterial colonization in the donor may influence the development of infections in the recipient.[53] Because many donors are at risk for aspiration as well as nosocomial pneumonia, prophylactic antibiotics are aimed at organisms that cause these infections (e.g., clindamycin with a third-generation cephalosporin). The administration of antibiotics is continued until results of cultures from the donor trachea are obtained. If bacterial growth in the donor is demonstrated, the antibiotic regimen in the recipient is modified as necessary and continued for 7 days.

TABLE 183–2. Postoperative Prophylaxis Following Lung Transplantation

Organism	*Prophylaxis*
Bacteria (pneumonia)	
Routine	Ceftazidime/clindamycin
Cystic fibrosis	Antibiotics directed against organisms isolated in preoperative or intraoperative cultures
Bronchiectasis	Antibiotics directed against organisms isolated in preoperative or intraoperative cultures
Candida species	
+ Donor culture	Fluconazole or amphotericin B
Cytomegalovirus serology	
D^+ R^-	Ganciclovir for 3 mo
D^- R^+	Ganciclovir for 6 wk
D^+ R^+	Ganciclovir for 6 wk
Pneumocystis carinii	Trimethoprim/sulfamethoxazole
Herpes simplex virus serology	
D^+ R^-	Acyclovir or ganciclovir if cytomegalovirus prophylaxis also required
D^- R^+	
D^+ R^+	
Toxoplasmosis	
Heart-lung recipient D^+ R^-	Clindamycin/pyrimethamine/folinic acid or sulfadiazine/pyrimethamine/folinic acid

Abbreviations: D = donor; R = recipient.

In patients with cystic fibrosis, the antibiotics are chosen to cover organisms with which the patient has had prior infections, either according to cultures obtained during the pretransplantation evaluation or as guided by recipient tracheal cultures obtained at the time of transplantation. Resistant pseudomonal organisms, such as *Pseudomonas cepacia,* are difficult to manage.[54] In patients with these organisms, antibiotic therapy is often continued until the patient has been extubated and is doing well. Special attention must be devoted to the treatment of sinus infections, as they may serve as a reservoir for recurrent pulmonary infection.

Cultures indicating a heavy growth of *Candida* in the donor have been linked to invasive candidiasis in the recipient.[53] Prophylactic, low-dose amphotericin B (0.3 $mg \cdot kg^{-1} \cdot d^{-1}$) or fluconazole is appropriate in these patients for 4 to 6 weeks.

At the time of transplantation, serologic studies are performed on the donor to assess the recipient's risk for cytomegalovirus infections. Patients who are seronegative and receive organs from seropositive donors require prophylaxis against primary infection. Ganciclovir therapy is started on the second postoperative day and continued for 2 to 3 months.[55, 56] Patients who are already seropositive at the time of transplantation are at risk for reactivation[57] and also require antiviral prophylaxis. Ganciclovir is started within 1 week after transplantation and is continued for 6 weeks.

Patients who are seronegative for cytomegalovirus are also at risk of acquiring primary cytomegalovirus infections from blood products. The use of seronegative blood products in these patients may reduce the incidence of cytomegalovirus infections.[58]

Immunosuppression

Immunosuppression for the lung transplant recipient consists of corticosteroids, azathioprine, and either cyclosporin or FK-506. Cytolytic agents such as OKT3, Minnesota antilymphocyte globulin, and rabbit antithymocyte globulin are used in some centers[29] but may increase the risk of cytomegalovirus disease[59] without increasing overall survival.[51] The intensity of the immunosuppression fluctuates, depending on the presence of active rejection or serious infection. Azathioprine administration is started in the immediate postoperative period. Cyclosporine or FK-506 is started intravenously as soon as the patient demonstrates adequate urine output; it is then given orally when the patient can take liquids. The serum levels of both of these medications must be monitored closely, as they may vary widely with the state of the patient's intestinal absorption and of his or her hepatic and renal function. Furthermore, the concomitant administration of other drugs can affect serum levels by interfering with or potentiating hepatic metabolism.

Some studies indicate that corticosteroids may interfere with the healing of the airway anastomoses.[7, 8] For this reason, some transplant centers require that patients who are taking corticosteroids preoperatively be weaned from them before transplantation. These centers withhold corticosteroids for 1 or 2 weeks after transplantation to allow the airway to heal. Other centers are not as strict and use varying amounts of corticosteroids in the perioperative period.

Acute episodes of rejection are treated with large doses of methylprednisolone (e.g., 1 g/d) over 3 days. Patients usually respond rapidly, with improvements in radiographically observed infiltrates, gas exchange, and pulmonary mechanics. Improvement can be seen in as little as 24 hours. In the past, corticosteroid treatment was often used empirically when rejection was suspected and when an infectious cause for the patient's deterioration was believed to be unlikely.

Since the safety and efficacy of transbronchial biopsy in establishing the diagnosis of rejection have been confirmed,[51, 60] empiric treatment should generally be avoided.

LATE COMPLICATIONS

Infection

Infection is a constant risk in the immunosuppressed transplant recipient. Increased vigilance for infectious complications is especially important after periods of augmented immunosuppression for the treatment of acute or chronic rejection. Although bacterial infections are of the greatest concern in the early postoperative period, after 30 days other infections must be considered.

Cytomegalovirus

Infections with cytomegalovirus are quite common in lung transplant recipients. Those with cytomegalovirus infection can exhibit various manifestations, ranging from asymptomatic viral shedding to virulent pulmonary infection. The disease may be localized to the allograft or widely disseminated. Seronegative patients receiving seropositive organs are at the highest risk for cytomegalovirus-related morbidity and mortality.[56] Secondary infections in seropositive recipients are common but are generally less serious.[58] Ganciclovir prophylaxis has been successful in reducing the incidence of cytomegalovirus disease in high-risk patients.[55]

Pneumocystis Carinii

Pulmonary infection with *Pneumocystis carinii* has become unusual since the advent of prophylaxis,[61] generally the oral administration of trimethoprim-sulfamethoxazole three times per week. The diagnosis should be suspected whenever the patient has diffuse infiltrates in the transplanted lung or lungs. Fiberoptic bronchoscopy with bronchoalveolar lavage is necessary, and usually sufficient, to establish the diagnosis.

Fungus

A variety of fungal infections may plague transplant recipients. Patients whose culture of the donor airway reveals *Candida* species are at risk for developing systemic candidiasis,[53] as are patients who have prolonged stays in the intensive care unit that involve treatment with potent antibiotics. Primary *Candida* infection of the transplanted lung is rare, although a mycotic aneurysm of a vascular anastomosis has been described.[62]

Aspergillus species have also been a source of late fungal infection in lung transplant recipients. In patients receiving a single lung transplant, it is important to exclude colonization with this organism as part of the preoperative evaluation. As in any immunocompromised patient, it can be difficult to distinguish between colonization and true infection. When isolated, the significance of the organism must not be underestimated, especially for pathogenic species such as *A. fumagatus, A. flavus,* and *A. niger.* Aggressive therapy with amphotericin B or itraconazole may be indicated.

Toxoplasmosis

In heart-lung transplantation, the transmission of toxoplasmosis by the allograft must be considered when a seronegative patient receives seropositive organs. Prophylaxis is administered with either clindamycin or a combination of sulfadiazine and pyrimethamine with folinic acid to reduce marrow suppression.

Chronic Rejection

Acute cellular rejection generally presents as the abrupt onset of infiltrates, worsening gas exchange, abnormal pulmonary mechanics, and, occasionally, systemic symptoms such as fever. In contrast, the syndrome of chronic rejection has a much more insidious presentation: an increase in dyspnea and cough accompanied by a decline in pulmonary function. The chest radiograph generally shows no infiltrates, and no systemic manifestations exist. Pathologically chronic rejection is characterized by obliterative bronchiolitis, which can usually be diagnosed by transbronchial biopsy (occasionally, an open lung biopsy is necessary). This syndrome has complicated all forms of lung transplantation (single lung, double lung, and heart-lung), having a prevalence of 20% to 40% in long-term survivors.[63] It is a major source of late morbidity and mortality.

An immunologic contribution to obliterative bronchiolitis has been suggested by studies of lymphocytes recovered during bronchoalveolar lavage. Increased donor-specific alloreactivity is strongly associated with acute rejection and to a lesser degree with chronic rejection.[64, 65] Episodes of acute rejection, cytomegalovirus pneumonitis, and severe ischemic airway injury place patients at risk for the subsequent development of obliterative bronchiolitis.[64, 66] The progression of obliterative bronchiolitis may be slowed with the application of augmented immunosuppression.[67–69]

Patients are monitored with serial pulmonary function tests that are often performed with hand-held spirometers in the patient's home. A decline in flow rates and vital capacity can indicate either rejection or new infection.[50, 70] Any unexplained dyspnea must be investigated, especially if accompanied by a decrease in the forced expiratory volume in 1 second. Transbronchial biopsy is then performed to establish the diagnosis. Newly diagnosed chronic rejection is usually treated with pulses of corticosteroids. Persistent cases require the use of antilymphocyte globulins or monoclonal antibodies. These have included rabbit antithymocyte globulin, Minnesota antilymphocyte globulin, or OKT3. Unfortunately, relapse is common.[63] Refractory cases have been treated with total lymphoid irradiation at the University of Pittsburgh, but the efficacy of this approach remains to be established. In cases that proceed to serious respiratory debility, retransplantation must be considered.

A relationship may exist between the development of obliterative bronchiolitis and infections with cytomegalovirus, *P. carinii,* and Epstein-Barr virus.[71] In one series of patients, cytomegalovirus infection was common in those who developed obliterative bronchiolits. Furthermore, evidence of increased lymphocytic activity against donor cells was noted in most of the patients who developed cytomegalovirus infection.[72] It has been speculated that the immunologic response against these pathogens may heighten host sensitivity to the allograft. Prophylaxis against infections of this type may therefore be crucial in preventing chronic rejection.

Airway Complications

Late stricture of the airway anastomoses may occur in a minority of patients.[72a] It is believed to arise from inadequate revascularization of the airway with resultant ischemia. Varying degrees of ischemic injury can be noted on bronchoscopic examination performed in the early postoperative period. Generally, these resolve without specific therapy, although some progress to stricture and potentially critical airway obstruction.[73] Once a diagnosis has been made, treatment consists of either stenting the airway to maintain patency or the laser removal of granulation tissue.[74, 75]

Post-Transplantation Lymphoproliferative Disorder

The post-transplantation lymphoproliferative disorder represents a neoplastic response of recipient lymphocytes to the immunomodulation required in transplant recipients.

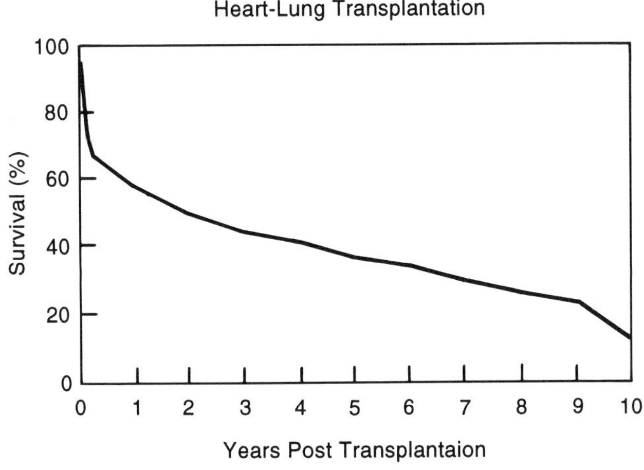

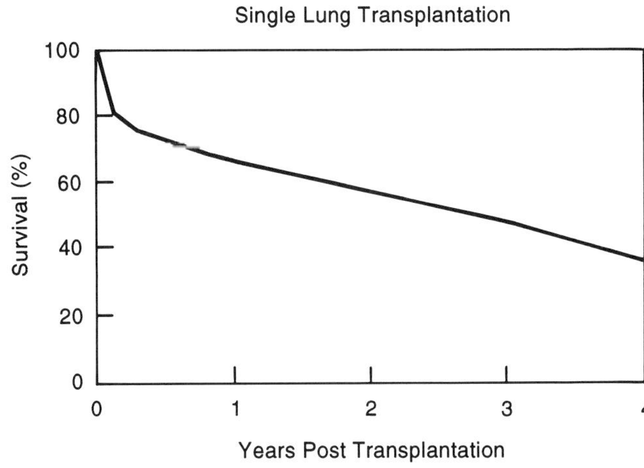

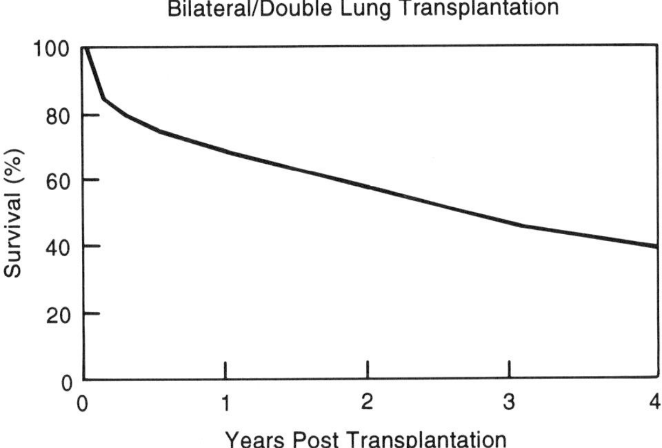

Figure 183–7. Adult lung transplantation: actuarial survival. (From Hosenpud JD, Novick RJ, Breen TJ, et al: The registry of the International Society for Heart and Lung Transplantation: Eleventh official report—1994. J Heart Lung Transplant 1994; 13:561.)

Infection with Epstein-Barr virus may be associated with the development of this complication.[76] It may appear as a systemic illness or localized to the transplanted lung. Treatment requires a reduction in the level of immunosuppression, although this increases the risk of acute or virulent chronic rejection. In localized cases, retransplantation is an option, although the long-term success of such procedures has not been determined.

OUTCOME

The International Society for Heart and Lung Transplantation has maintained a registry that contains data on patients who have received heart, lung, and heart-lung transplants since 1983. Information on 1567 heart-lung, 1943 single lung, and 943 double lung transplantations has been collected as of December 1993.[7]

The actuarial survival curves for single, double, and heart-lung transplant recipients are shown in Figure 183–7. It is of interest that the bilateral single lung technique for replacing both lungs confers a statistically significant survival advantage compared with the en bloc replacement of both lungs.[7]

Overall, infection remains the most common cause of mortality[80] both in the early and late postoperative periods.[77] Bacterial infections are most common in the early postoperative period, with viral and fungal infections being the most important causes of late infectious deaths.[77] Another important cause of mortality is early nonspecific graft dysfunction,[80] which emphasizes the need for improved techniques of graft preservation. Acute rejection is an unusual cause of early mortality. However, chronic rejection manifested by obliterative bronchiolitis has been a significant cause of late deaths.[77] Obliterative bronchiolitis represents a major obstacle to long-term success following lung transplantation.

References

1. Hardy JD, Webb WR, Dalton ML, et al: Lung homotransplantation in man. JAMA 1963; 186:99–108.
2. Marshall SE, Kramer MR, Lewiston NJ, et al: Selection and evaluation of recipients for heart-lung transplantation. Chest 1990; 98:1488–1494.
3. Egan TM, Trulock EP, Boychuk J, et al: Analysis of referrals for lung transplantation: The Washington University Lung Transplantation Group. Chest 1991; 99:867.
4. Morrison DL, Maurer JR, Grossman RF: Preoperative assessment for lung transplantation. Clin Chest Med 1990; 11:207–215.
5. Carere R, Patterson GA, Liu P, et al: Right and left ventricular performance after single and double lung transplantation. J Thorac Cardiovasc Surg 1991; 102:115–122.
6. Jain D, Zaret BL: Assessment of right ventricular function: Role of nuclear imaging techniques. Cardiology Clinics 1992; 10:23–39.
7. Hosenpud JD, Novick RJ, Breen TJ, et al: The registry of the

International Society for Heart and Lung Transplantation: Eleventh official report—1994. J Heart Lung Transplant 1994; 13:561–570.
8. Goldberg M, Lima O, Morgan E, et al: A comparison between cyclosporine A and methylprednisolone plus azathioprine on bronchial healing following canine lung autotransplantation. J Thorac Cardiovasc Surg 1983; 85:821–826.
9. Lima O, Cooper JD, Peters WJ, et al: Effects of methylprednisolone and azathioprine on bronchial healing following lung autotransplantation. J Thorac Cardiovasc Surg 1981; 82:211–215.
10. Craven JL, Bright J, Dear CL: Psychiatric, psychosocial and rehabilitative aspects of lung transplantation. Clin Chest Med 1990; 11:247–257.
11. Harjula A, Baldwin JC, Starnes V, et al: Proper donor selection for heart-lung transplantation: The Stanford experience. J Thorac Cardiovasc Surg 1987; 94:874–880.
11a. Riou B, Guesde R, Jacquens Y, et al: Fiberoptic bronchoscopy in brain-dead organ donors. Am J Respir Crit Care Med 1994; 150:558–560.
12. Miyoshi S, Schaefers HJ, Trulock EP, et al: Donor selection for single and double lung transplantation: Chest size matching and other factors influencing posttransplantation vital capacity. Chest 1990; 98:308–313.
13. Pearson FG: Lung transplantation: Samuel Jason Mixter lecture. Arch Surg 1989; 124:535.
13a. Kirk AJ, Colquhoun IW, Dark JH: Lung preservation: A review of current practice and future directions. Ann Thorac Surg 1993; 56:990–1000.
14. Hardesty RL, Griffith BP: Autoperfusion of the heart and lungs for preservation during distant procurement. J Thorac Cardiovasc Surg 1987; 93:11–18.
15. Cooper JD, Vreim CE: NHLBI workshop summary: Biology of lung preservation for transplantation. Am Rev Respir Dis 1992; 146:803–807.
16. Baumgartner WA, Williams GM, Fraser CD, et al: Cardiopulmonary bypass with profound hypothermia: An optimal preservation method for multiorgan procurement. Transplantation 1989; 48:882–886.
17. Yacoub MH, Khaghani A, Banner N, et al: Distant organ procurement for heat and lung transplantation. Transplant Proc 1989; 21:2548–2550.
18. Novick RJ, Menkis AH, McKenzie FN: New trends in lung preservation: A collective review. J Heart Lung Transplant 1992; 11:377–392.
19. Harjula AL, Baldwin JC, Stinson ET, et al: Clinical heart-lung preservation with prostaglandin E-1. Transplant Proc 1987; 19:4101–4102.
20. Griffith BP, Zenati M: The pulmonary donor. Clin Chest Med 1990; 11:217–226.
21. Hooper TL, Jones MT, Thomson DS, et al: Modulation of ischemic lung injury by corticosteroids. Transplantation 1990; 50:530–532.
22. Pillai R, Bando K, Schueler S, et al: Leukocyte depletion results in excellent heart-lung function after 12 hours of storage. Ann Thorac Surg 1990; 50:211–214.
23. Bonser RS, Fragomeni LS, Harris K, et al: Acute physiologic changes after extended pulmonary preservation. J Heart Transplant 1990; 9:220–229.
24. Bando K, Tago M, Teraoka H, et al: Extended cardiopulmonary preservation for heart-lung transplantation: A comparative study of superoxide dismutase. J Heart Transplant 1989; 8:59–66.
25. Paull DE, Keagy BA, Kron EJ, et al: Reperfusion injury in the lung preserved for twenty-four hours. Ann Thorac Surg 1989; 47:187–192.
26. Detterbeck FC, Keagy BA, Paull DE, et al: Oxygen free radical scavengers decrease reperfusion injury in lung transplantation. Ann Thorac Surg 1990; 50:204–210.
27. Conte JV, Katz NM, Foegh ML, et al: Iron chelation therapy and lung transplantation: Effects of deferoxamine on lung preservation in canine single lung transplantation. J Thorac Cardiovasc Surg 1991; 101:1024–1029.
28. Starnes VA, Lewiston JN, Luikart H, et al: Current trends in lung transplantation: Lobar transplantation and expanded use of single lungs. J Thorac Cardiovasc Surg 1992; 104:1060–1066.
29. Stevens PM, Johnson PC, Bell RL, et al: Regional ventilation and perfusion after lung transplantation in patients with emphysema. N Engl J Med 1970; 282:245–249.
30. Low DE, Trulock EP, Kaiser LR, et al: Morbidity, mortality and early results of single versus bilateral lung transplantation for emphysema. J Thorac Cardiovasc Surg 1992; 103:1119–1126.
31. Patterson GA, Maurer JR, Williams TJ: Comparison of outcomes of double and single lung transplantation for obstructive lung disease: The Toronto Lung Transplant Group. J Thorac Cardiovasc Surg 1991; 101:623–632.
32. Pasque MK, Kaiser LR, Dressler C, et al: Single lung transplantation for pulmonary hypertension: Technical aspects and immediate hemodynamic results. J Thorac Cardiovasc Surg 1992; 103:475–481.
33. Levine SM, Jenkinson SG, Bryan CL, et al: Ventilation-perfusion inequalities during graft rejection in patients undergoing single lung transplantation for primary pulmonary hypertension. Chest 1992; 101:401–405.
34. Patterson GA, Cooper JD, Goldman B, et al: Technique of successful clinical double-lung transplantation. Ann Thorac Surg 1988; 45:626–633.
35. Pasque MK, Cooper JD, Kaiser LR, et al: Improved technique for bilateral lung transplantation: Rationale and initial clinical experience. Ann Thorac Surg 1990; 49:785–791.
36. Bisson A, Bonnette P: A new technique for double lung transplantation: "Bilateral single lung" transplantation. J Thorac Cardiovasc Surg 1992; 103:40–46.
37. Raffin L, Michel-Cherqui M, Sperandio M, et al: Anesthesia for bilateral lung transplantation without cardiopulmonary bypass: Initial experience and review of intraoperative problems. J Cardiothorac Vasc Anesth 1992; 6:409–417.
38. Hirt SW, Haverich A, Wahlers T, et al: Predictive criteria for the need of extracorporeal circulation in single-lung transplantation. Ann Thorac Surg 1992; 54:676–680.
39. Schreinemakers HH, Weder W, Miyoshi S, et al: Direct revascularization of bronchial arteries for lung transplantation: An anatomical study. Ann Thorac Surg 1990; 49:44–54.
40. Couraud L, Baudet E, Martigne C, et al: Bronchial revascularization in double-lung transplantation: A series of eight patients: Bordeaux Lung and Heart-Lung Transplant Group. Ann Thorac Surg 1992; 53:88–94.
41. Patterson GA, Todd TR, Cooper JD, et al: Airway complications after double lung transplantation: Toronto Lung Transplant Group. J Thorac Cardiovasc Surg 1990; 99:14–21.
42. Metras D, Noirclerc M, Baillant A, et al: Double lung transplant: The role of bilateral bronchial suture. Transplant Proc 1990; 22:1477–1478.
43. Kaiser LR, Pasque MK, Trulock EP: Bilateral sequential lung transplantation: The procedure of choice for double-lung replacement. Ann Thorac Surg 1991; 52:438–446.
44. Calhoon JH, Grover FL, Gibbons WJ, et al: Single lung transplantation: Alternative indications and technique. J Thorac Cardiovasc Surg 1991; 101:816–825.
45. Turrentine MW, Kesler KA, Wright CD, et al: Effect of omental, intercostal, and internal mammary artery pedicle wraps on bronchial healing. Ann Thorac Surg 1990; 49:574–579.
46. Reitz BA, Wallwork JL, Hunt SA, et al: Heart-lung transplantation: Successful therapy for patients with pulmonary vascular disease. N Engl J Med 306:557.
47. Royston D, Minty BD, Higenbottam T, et al: The effect of surgery with cardiopulmonary bypass on alveolar-capillary barrier function in human beings. Ann Thorac Surg 1985; 40:139–143.
48. Haydock DA, Trulock EP, Kaiser LR: Management of dysfunction in the transplanted lung: Experience with seven clinical cases: Washington University Lung Transplant Group. Ann Thorac Surg 1992; 53:635–641.
49. Malden ES, Kaiser LR, Gutierrez FR: Pulmonary vein obstruction following single lung transplantation. Chest 1992; 102:645–647.
50. Griffith BP, Hardesty RL, Armitage JM, et al: Acute rejection of lung allografts with various immunosuppressive protocols. Ann Thorac Surg 1992; 54:846–851.
51. Scott JP, Fradet G, Smyth RL, et al: Prospective study of transbronchial biopsies in the management of heart-lung and single lung transplant patients. J Heart Lung Transplant 1991; 10:626–637.
52. Griffith BP, Hardesty RL, Trento A, et al: Heart-lung transplan-

tation: Lessons learned and future hopes. Ann Thorac Surg 1987; 43:6–16.
53. Zenati M, Dowling RD, Dummer JS, et al: Influence of the donor lung on development of early infections in lung transplant recipients. J Heart Transplant 1990; 9:502–509.
54. Ramirez JC, Patterson GA, Winton TL, et al: Bilateral lung transplantation for cystic fibrosis: The Toronto Lung Transplant Group. J Thorac Cardiovasc Surg 1992; 103:287–294.
55. Duncan SR, Paradis IL, Dauber JH, et al: Ganciclovir prophylaxis for cytomegalovirus infection in pulmonary allograft recipients. Am Rev Respir Dis 1992; 146:1213–1215.
56. Ettinger NA, Bailey TC, Trulock EP, et al: Cytomegalovirus infection and pneumonitis: Impact after isolated lung transplantation. Am Rev Respir Dis 1993; 147:1017–1023.
57. Smyth RL, Sinclair J, Scott JP, et al: Infection and reactivation with cytomegalovirus strains in lung transplant recipients. Transplantation 1991; 52:480–482.
58. Duncan AJ, Dummer JS, Paradis IL, et al: Cytomegalovirus infection and survival in lung transplant recipients. J Heart Lung Transplant 1991; 10:638–646.
59. Calhoon JH, Nichols L, Davis R, et al: Single lung transplantation: Factors in postoperative cytomegalovirus infection. J Thorac Cardiovasc Surg 1992; 103:21–26.
60. Higenbottam T, Stewart S, Penketh A, et al: Transbronchial lung biopsy for the diagnosis of rejection in heart-lung transplant patients. Transplantation 1988; 46:532–539.
61. Kramer MR, Stoehr C, Lewiston NJ, et al: Trimethoprim-sulfamethoxazole prophylaxis for pneumocystis carinii infections in heart-lung and lung transplantation: How effective and for how long? Transplantation 1992; 53:586–589.
62. Dowling RD, Baladi N, Zenati M, et al: Disruption of the aortic anastomosis following heart-lung transplantation. Ann Thorac Surg 1990; 49:118.
63. Trulock EP: Management of lung transplant rejection. Chest 1993; 103:1566–1576.
64. Zeevi A, Rabinowich H, Yousem SA, et al: Presence of donor-specific alloreactivity in histologically normal lung allografts is predictive of subsequent bronchiolitis obliterans. Transplant Proc 1991; 23:1128–1129.
65. Rabinowich H, Zeevi A, Paradis IL, et al: Proliferative responses of bronchoalveolar lavage lymphocytes from heart-lung transplant patients. Transplantation 1990; 49:115–121.
66. Clelland C, Higenbottam T, Otulana B, et al: Histologic prognostic indicators for lung allografts of heart-lung transplants. J Heart Transplant 1990; 9:177–186.
67. Glanville AR, Baldwin JC, Burke CN, et al: Obliterative bronchiolitis after heart-lung transplantation: Apparent arrest by augmented immunosuppression. Ann Intern Med 1987; 107:300–304.
68. Allen MD, Burke CM, McGregor CG, et al: Steroid-responsive bronchiolitis after human heart-lung transplantation. J Thorac Cardiovasc Surg 1986; 92:449–451.
69. Griffith BP, Paradis IL, Zeevi A, et al: Immunologically mediated disease of the airways after pulmonary transplantation. Ann Surg 1988; 208:371–378.
70. Otulana BA, Higenbottam T, Scott J, et al: Lung function associated with histologically diagnosed acute lung rejection and pulmonary infection in heart-lung transplant recipients. Am Rev Respir Dis 1990; 142:329–332.
71. Dauber JH, Paradis IL, Dummer JS: Infectious complications in pulmonary allograft recipients. Clin Chest Med 1990; 11:291–308.
72. Keenan RJ, Lega ME, Dummer S, et al: Cytomegalovirus serologic status and postoperative infection correlated with risk of developing chronic rejection after pulmonary transplantation. Transplantation 1991; 51:433–438.
72a. Griffith BP, Magee MJ, Gonzalez IF, et al: Anastomotic pitfalls in lung transplantation. J Thorac Cardiovasc Surg 1994; 107:743–754.
73. Schafers HJ, Haydock DA, Cooper JD: The prevalence and management of bronchial anastomotic complications in lung transplantation. J Thorac Cardiovasc Surg 1991; 101:1044–1052.
74. Colt HG, Janssen JP, Dumon JF, et al: Endoscopic management of bronchial stenosis after double lung transplantation. Chest 1992; 102:10–16.
75. Cooper JD, Pearson FG, Patterson GA, et al: Use of silicone stents in the management of airway problems. Ann Thorac Surg 1989; 47:371–378.
76. Penn I: Immunosuppression: A contributing factor in lymphoma formation. Clin Transplant 1992; 6:214–219.
77. de Hoyos AL, Patterson GA, Maurer JR, et al: Pulmonary transplantation: Early and late results: The Toronto Lung Transplant Group. J Thorac Cardiovasc Surg 1992; 103:295–306.
78. Griffith BP, Magee MJ: Single lung transplantation. Chest Surg Clin 1993; 3:75–88.
79. Trento A, Griffith BP, Hardesty RL: Heart-lung transplantation. *In*: Textbook of Critical Care. 2nd ed. Shoemaker WC, Ayres S, Grenvik A, et al (Eds). Philadelphia, WB Saunders, 1989, pp 1343–1348.
80. Kaye MP: The registry of the International Society for Heart and Lung Transplantation: Tenth official report—1993. J Heart Lung Transplant 1993; 12:541–548.

CHAPTER 184

Pancreas and Islet Cell Transplantation

Derek C. Angus, MB, ChB, MPH • David J. Kramer, MD
Camillo Ricordi, MD • Andreas G. Tzakis, MD

With advances in both surgical technique and immunosuppression, pancreatic solid organ transplantation (PTX) and islet cell transplantation (ITX) are becoming increasingly viable clinical options in the management of pancreatic endocrine insufficiency. Certain fundamental questions remain unanswered, however, such as the long-term effects of both the transplants and the consequent immunosuppression on the late sequelae of diabetes mellitus. Because there is probably enough support to justify increased utilization of these procedures across the country, the critical care physician will be ever more likely to encounter patients with pancreatic transplants in the intensive care unit (ICU). Therefore, we summarize broadly the questions that remain unanswered in PTX and ITX that may have relevance for the intensivist. There is currently insufficient experience to recommend strongly a particular approach to the ICU management of these patients, but we also highlight some of the difficulties and hazards encountered and the approaches taken in the care of these patients.

BACKGROUND

Diabetes is the most common endocrine disease in the world, with an incidence of up to 16/100,000 in childhood, a prevalence of 260/100,000 by the age of 20 years, and a cumulative risk of 1050/100,000 for type 1 diabetes and 10,030/100,000 for type 2 diabetes by the age of 70 years.[1, 2] Despite extensive study of insulin administration, glucose control, and careful surveillance for complications, the outcome for diabetes remains somewhat gloomy. It is the fourth leading cause of disease-related death in Western countries with a resultant morbidity that is both severely debilitating for the patient and a significant strain on national health resources.[3] It is the underlying cause of renal failure in up to 40% of all new patients requiring dialysis and is the leading cause of blindness in adults in Western countries.[4]

Type 1 diabetes mellitus is characterized by the progressive destruction of the beta cells within the islets of Langerhans, leading to insufficient insulin secretion and worsening glucose control. This destruction is autoimmune mediated and is associated with both human leukocyte antigen (HLA) inheritance and environmental factors, but the exact stimulus to autoimmunity remains unclear.[5] Exogenous insulin therapy is the mainstay of management. Although reasonable glucose control can be achieved, there is a significant burden placed on patient lifestyle, and, more importantly, the long-term sequelae of diabetes are not avoided. Consequently, researchers have long been interested in the possibility of replacing the pancreas or islets with the goals of avoiding exogenous insulin therapy and reducing or avoiding the devastating consequences of renal impairment, small-vessel disease, advanced atheroma, and neuropathy.

The first recorded attempt to replace pancreatic tissue was in 1893 when Watson Williams, a surgeon in Bristol, England, transplanted two pieces of freshly harvested sheep pancreas into the breast and abdominal wall of a 15-year-old boy unfortunately without success.[6] Several decades later, in 1966, surgeons at the University of Minnesota performed pancreatic transplantation in two patients, achieving normoglycemia in one up to 6 months postoperatively.[7] However, more than 10 years passed before pancreatic transplantation became more than an occasional research procedure, largely because of improvements in surgical technique and advances in immunosuppression, including the advent of cyclosporin A.[8–10] Since then, the annual rate, as recorded by the International Pancreas Transplant Registry, has steadily climbed with more than 600 procedures in 1990. The U.S. United Network Organ Sharing Registry reported that current 1-year patient and graft survival rates are 91% and 72%, respectively, and 80% and 57%, respectively, at 3 years.[9] It is significant that these figures are comparable with other organ transplant success rates.

The modern approach to islet transplantation was pioneered by Moskalewski as well as by Lacy and Kostianovisky, who developed the procedures for isolation of the islets from the exocrine tissue.[11, 12] In 1967 Lacy published the technique for pancreatic distention and infusion of a collagenase suspension, which remains the basis of islet separation today. However, until 1984, there were no reports of successful implantation of islets as determined by an increase in basal C peptide release still observable at 1 month after transplant.[13] Twenty-six adult cases were reported between 1985 and 1989 in which only 30% demonstrated basal C peptide production at 1 week and less than 20% at 1 month. None of these cases have shown long-term C peptide production.[14] In August 1990, Tzakis and colleagues published the first series of successful islet transplants in humans.[15] The series included only nine patients, and there are only a handful of centers around the world that are likely to emulate these results in the next few years. However, the potential benefit of islet transplantation is enormous, and this first success is likely to be followed by a significant increase in research and development in this field. In 1990, in addition to the Pittsburgh study, four other groups (Edmonton, Milan, Paris, and St. Louis) all reported cases of islet transplants with long-term insulin independence.[14, 16–18]

INDICATIONS

PTX is most commonly performed in combination with a kidney transplant for patients with diabetes mellitus and end-stage renal failure.[8, 9, 19] Isolated PTX is usually performed in patients who already have kidney transplants and are thus already receiving immunosuppression. However, both PTX and ITX have been performed on patients either as single procedures or as part of multivisceral procedures (not including renal transplantation). The usual indications for these latter groups are upper abdominal malignancy or prior extensive resection after trauma or Crohn's disease.[15] Finally, several groups have also reported their results with segmental or partial pancreatic and islet autotransplantation in patients with chronic pancreatitis.[20–23] With the exception of PTX combined with or after kidney transplantation, PTX and ITX are still generally considered experimental procedures.[8, 19]

SURGICAL TECHNIQUE

Pancreatic Solid Organ Transplantation

Both whole and partial PTXs have been performed, but, for reasons of surgical convenience, the most common approach is to transplant the entire organ. The graft is placed in the peritoneal space to allow absorption of the significant exocrine "sweat" that can occur in the early postoperative phase.[24] Initially, when placed in the retroperitoneal space, tryptic secretions caused severe abscess and fistula formation. Although drainage into the duodenum seems desirable, the risk of anastomotic leak in patients on high-dose steroids plus the desire to monitor graft function through assessment of the exocrine secretion rate has led most centers to drain exocrine secretions via a cuff of donor duodenum into the recipient bladder. The donor superior mesenteric artery and celiac axis are connected to the iliac artery, and the donor portal vein is anastomosed to the iliac veins, resulting in systemic drainage of the pancreatic endocrine secretions (Fig. 184–1).

Islet Cell Transplantation

ITX is a significantly less invasive procedure capable of being performed in the radiology suite. The main problems associated with ITX technique are isolation, purification, and choice of implantation site.

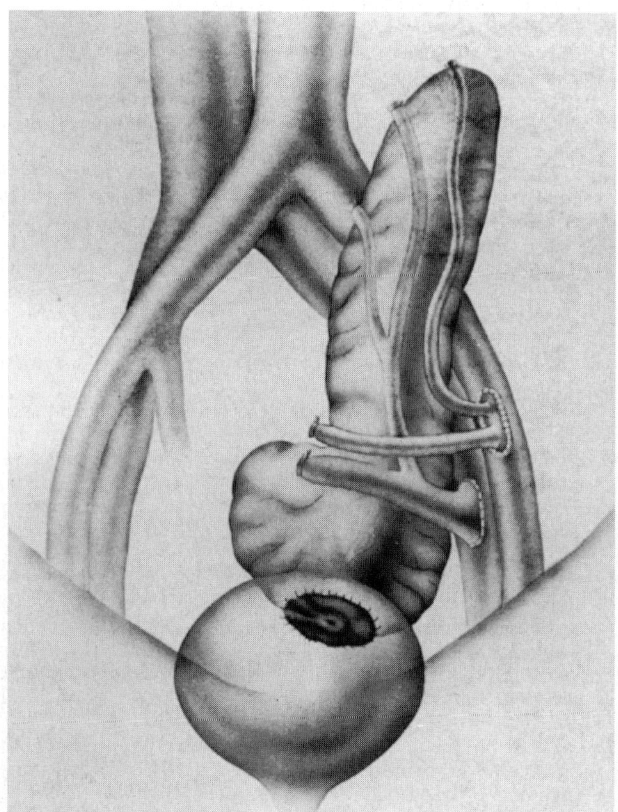

Figure 184–1. Whole pancreatic transplantation with pancreaticocystostomy (without use of a donor duodenal cuff). (From Sollinger HW, Folkert OB: Pancreas transplantation with urinary tract drainage. *In:* Pancreatic Transplantation. CG Groth (Ed). Philadelphia, WB Saunders, 1988, p 137.)

Islet Isolation

To harvest islets successfully, the entire pancreas gland must be procured from the donor and then dissolved into particles small enough to survive in a culture medium in which oxygen and other metabolic substrates can be exchanged with waste products across cell membranes by diffusion.[25] Furthermore, during the cleaving process, trauma to the islets must be minimized.[26] Initially, two techniques were used: digestion by the enzyme collagenase (in which the pancreatic skeleton is dissolved allowing release of the islets) or mechanical dissociation (in which the tissue is subjected to prolonged oscillation). The use of collagenase allows excellent cleavage between exocrine and endocrine tissues in the pancreas.[12] However, the main disadvantage is that prolonged contact with the enzyme may produce toxic effects to the islets, resulting in a decreased yield. Mechanical dissociation is obviously free of any chemical toxicity; however, this technique subjects the islets to potentially harmful shear and compression forces.

Today, an automated method combining both collagenase and mechanical oscillation is used (Fig. 184–2).[26] When this method, which was used successfully in rodent models, was applied to large mammalian and human pancreata, the technique produced rather contaminated mixtures with a relatively low yield of islets. A significant breakthrough was the introduction of ductal perfusion of collagenase.[27] The pancreas is distended with a collagenase mixture, and the exocrine skeleton of the pancreas can be rapidly dissolved, leaving relatively untraumatized islets. The entire preparation is washed continually with Hank's solution containing 2% fetal calf serum to ensure clearing of the collagenase. The islets are then separated using Ficoll density-gradient centrifugation. This technique is now widely adopted throughout centers engaged in ITX.[28]

Islet Yield and Measurement

Experiments in dogs show that overt diabetes is seen when less than 10% of the pancreas is left.[29] In humans, subtotal pancreatectomies leaving 5% of the pancreas usually result in diabetes.[30] Thus, it is assumed that at least 10% of the normal islet mass must be replaced if one is to expect return to normal glucose tolerance.[25] However, individual islets vary greatly in diameter, and, even if a volume of islets is estimated correctly, this is not necessarily a guarantee of viability. There have been several methods proposed to determine islet yields. Currently, there remains no uniform acceptance of an in vitro method to determine viability because techniques such as the insulin-amylase ratio continue to have significant difficulties.[25] However, there is now a consensus with regard to the measurement of islets.[28] Individual islets vary greatly in diameter from less than 50 mm to 500 mm (representing a 1000-fold increase in volume), and because the yields necessary for transplantation in large mammals and humans are too large to allow a complete count, a multisampling technique has been developed.[31] In each sample, examined by microscopy, islets are classed into different groups depending on their diameter. The volume in each class of diameter range is then added, and the total yield is expressed as the number of 150-mm islet equivalents. To ensure an accurate count by this technique, it is important that multiple samples are included, drawn from a solution in which the islets are suspended evenly. This technique does not accurately reflect purity (although this can be gauged at microscopy) nor does it assess viability. The only meaningful way to determine viability is post-transplant evaluation of islet function.

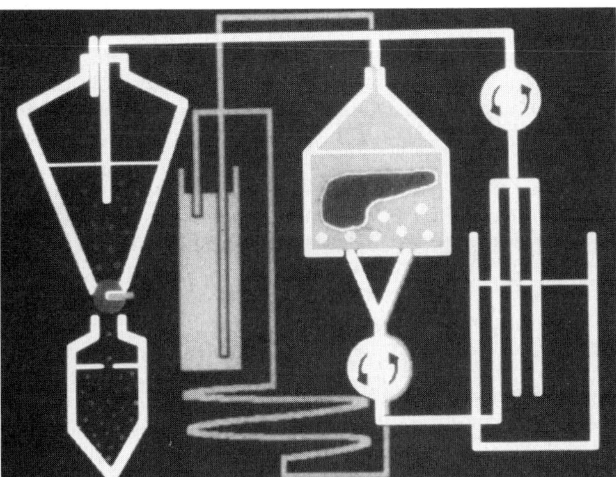

Figure 184–2. Schematic diagram of modern automated islet isolation.

Islet Transplantation Site

In earlier studies in rodents, dogs, and nonhuman primates, islets have been implanted in many different sites including the skin, thymus, spleen, portal circulation, and kidney subcapsule.[32–36] Alternative sites of implantation may be considered with regard to later access, immunologic privilege, anatomic mimicry, vascularity, and convenience.

Although results remain inconclusive, certain patterns are emerging. Subcutaneous sites are largely a poor choice because of the relatively low vascularization with the resultant failure of, or reduction in, implantation.[32] In contrast, more vascular sites, such as the liver, spleen, and kidney subcapsule, have been associated with greater success.[33–35]

With regard to whether the islets are drained by either portal or systemic circulation, results are conflicting. However, it appears that the islets are more metabolically effective when drained by the portal venous system.[37, 38] Initial studies in humans of intraportal infusions were associated with extreme morbidity, including hypotension and death.[39] However, these side effects were attributed to impurity of the islet preparation, and intraportal infusion is currently the preferred route of administration with minimal complications reported (Fig. 184–3).[15–18]

Future alternatives include the use of immunoprivileged sites such as the testis or central nervous system and organelles (neovascular structures formed after implantation of collagen coated fibers and growth factors in serous spaces such as the peritoneum).[40–42] Immunoprivileged sites may allow for reduced exogenous immunosuppression, and organelles may provide highly vascular sites with relatively easy access, thus allowing improved monitoring for rejection and function.

Combined Kidney-Pancreas Transplantation

Figure 184–4 highlights the surgical procedure for combined kidney-pancreas transplantation. The pancreas is embedded in the right iliac fossa and anastomosed as described previously for a solitary PTX. The kidney is placed in the opposite fossa through a separate oblique lower abdominal incision.

Multivisceral Transplantation

Obviously, the exact site and anastomoses in multivisceral transplantation are dependent on which organs are re-

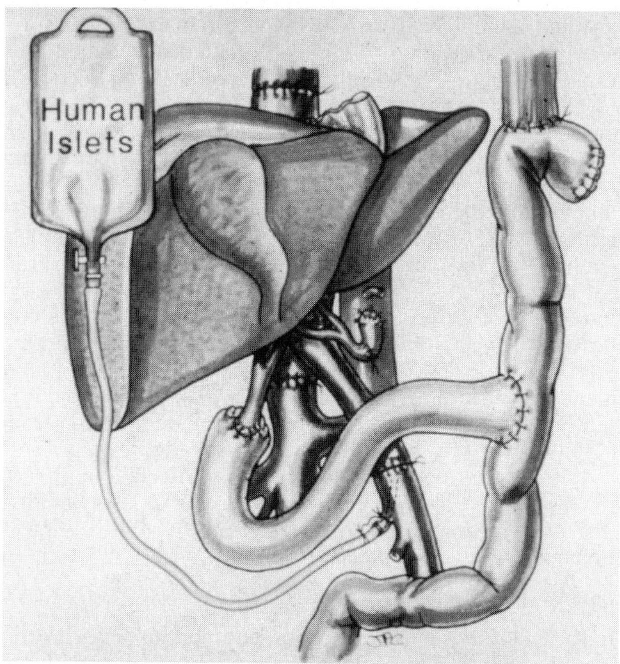

Figure 184–3. Liver and pancreatic islet transplantation after upper abdominal exenteration.

moved and which are replaced. The procedures performed in Pittsburgh have included resection and transplantation of the liver, pancreas, spleen, some or all of the stomach, duodenum, jejunum, ileum, and, in some, partial colon. Usually, the donor graft comprises the liver, duodenum, pancreas or islets, small bowel, and sometimes a section of right colon. A gastrojejunostomy is performed with the donor duodenum left as a blind loop into which the donor biliary tree and pancreatic duct are drained. A Silastic catheter is placed

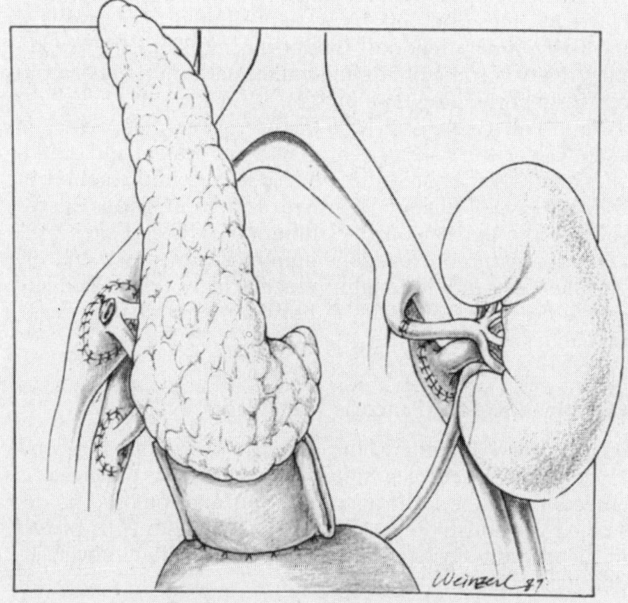

Figure 184–4. Combined pancreatic and renal transplantation with pancreaticoduodenocystostomy. (From Corry RJ: Pancreatico-duodenal transplantation with urinary tract drainage. *In*: Pancreatic Transplantation. CG Groth (Ed). Philadelphia, WB Saunders, 1988, p 150.)

into the duodenum to facilitate drainage. A distal ileostomy is then fashioned to be followed by reconnection to the recipient colon at a later date, or there is a primary anastomosis at the distal end of the bowel graft to the recipient colon with a side ileostomy to allow partial drainage. This procedure allows pancreatic venous drainage to enter the donor portal system as opposed to the systemic drainage in isolated pancreas or combined pancreas-kidney transplantation. The potential benefits of portal drainage are outlined later. Figure 184–3 shows an example of one surgical procedure used in multivisceral transplantation and resection.

METABOLIC CONTROL

PTX and ITX are not lifesaving procedures. Their primary indication is the reversal from a diabetic state to a normal state of glucose metabolism on the assumption that this will result in a reduction of the long-term complications of diabetes.[25] Therefore, the ultimate determination of the success of pancreatic transplantation is based on the presence of long-term glucose control and avoidance of diabetic complications.

There is considerable evidence that PTX improves sugar control. Fasting and postcibal blood glucose levels and hemoglobin A_{1c} levels have been shown to fall largely within normal ranges and remain so for a period of years.[43–53] However, systemic insulin levels are two to three times higher than normal because of concomitant steroid administration and, more importantly, the systemic venous drainage of the donor pancreas.[44, 52, 54] PTX also appears to improve counterregulation of glucose partially, including a reduction in the incidence of hypoglycemic attacks compared with patients receiving exogenous insulin administration alone. This has been attributed predominantly to an improvement in pancreatic glucagon control as opposed to enhanced catecholamine release.[8, 45, 53, 55, 56] The elevated systemic insulin levels have raised concern regarding possible adverse effects on serum lipid metabolism. However, preliminary evidence suggests that, if anything, PTX appears to confer a beneficial effect on lipid metabolism with a reduction in low-density lipoproteins and an increase in high-density lipoproteins.[57]

There is less evidence regarding the ability of ITX to achieve good metabolic control. Several studies attempting long-term follow-up of animals that have received islet transplantation show a late return to hyperglycemia.[58] It has been postulated that this is more likely to occur when glucose control in the initial postoperative period is suboptimal, thereby stressing the islets during implantation, a period of proposed graft vulnerability. Unfortunately, these studies are hampered by an inability to determine whether a sufficient volume of islets has been successfully implanted and whether those islets have remained free from rejection and, therefore, able to function optimally throughout follow-up.

In most early reports of human ITX recipients, the recipient pancreas remained in place, thus confusing the ability to determine to what extent serum insulin and C peptide levels were due to the donor islets. Tzakis and coworkers published their results with a series of patients who underwent upper abdominal exenteration.[15] Thus, these patients were rendered undisputedly diabetic before receiving multivisceral transplants including intraportal ITX. Basal and intravenous glucagon–stimulated C peptide responses were measured intraoperatively after exenteration and liver transplantation but before islet infusion. As expected, there was no C peptide response in any of the patients. Patients received between 105,000 and 562,000 150-mm islet equivalents each and were immunosuppressed with FK-506 and prednisone. All patients demonstrated C peptide response both immediately after the procedure and up to 6 months later.

Better prognostication of the ability of ITX to achieve good metabolic control will depend on our capability to define more accurately the total islet yield, the percentage of that yield that implants successfully, and, thereafter, the percentage that remains functional despite episodes of rejection or other stresses to the islets.

REJECTION

The cornerstone of diagnostic techniques in the identification of solid organ rejection is graft biopsy. However, for a variety of reasons including accessibility, risk of bleeding, and risk of ductal leakage, biopsy is not a practical technique in PTX.[59] Likewise, monitoring of endocrine function is of limited value because decreased blood sugar control usually occurs late in the course of rejection. Commonly, therefore, urinary amylase is measured, taking advantage of the surgical drainage of the graft into the bladder. The interpretation of urinary amylase results, however, is confounded by the patient's fluid status (and consequent urine production) and nutritional status. Some centers, therefore, propose direct cannulation of the pancreatic duct to aspirate and assess pure exocrine secretion. This technique, however, is not yet adopted widely, is cumbersome, and is not without risk.

Islet cells behave in a manner similar to that of skin allografts with regard to their disposition to immunogenicity.[34] Therefore, if transplanted across a major HLA group, rapid rejection will ensue unless immunosuppressives are administered. Furthermore, evidence suggests that islet cell function is critically sensitive to rejection with little reserve capacity.[25] Treatment with immunosuppressive agents such as cyclosporine has had mixed results in rodent experiments.[60, 61] However, more recent studies with parenteral cyclosporine and close blood level monitoring offer greater promise. Unfortunately, cyclosporine and other immunosuppressives including steroids compromise islet function.[62] Therefore, alternative approaches have been used.

One method is to enclose islets in biocompatible membranes. Experiments of membranes made of polyvinyl polymer and hydrogel have demonstrated encouraging results.[63, 64] These membranes have pores large enough to allow diffusion of insulin and other metabolites but too small to allow entry of cells or antibodies. One problem, however, is the development of a fibrin sheath around the membrane, resulting in subsequent dysfunction. If this technique could become successful, then the islets need not be allografts but indeed could be xenografts. This would then solve the problem of limited supply because widespread use of islet allografts for diabetes will certainly be severely limited by the lack of donors.[25]

Other approaches involve desensitization procedures, such as transplanting a renal allograft first into the recipient but maintaining the islets in vitro for several weeks during which time it is hoped that the recipient would acquire a degree of tolerance.[65] Alternatively, rejection may be avoided through multiple small-volume donors. Preliminary evidence suggests that a certain volume of islets is required (>50 islets) before rejection is encountered. Although this is clearly insufficient to reverse hyperglycemia, multiple harvesting of 50-islet aliquots from different donors might potentially circumvent rejection.[66] Finally, it has been postulated that, because the beta cells themselves are relatively nonimmunogenic, if a solution could be produced that was 100% pure, rejection may not be encountered.[67]

Clearly, significant work is required in this area and, until then, avoidance of rejection in humans will be attempted with the use of immunosuppressives. Regrettably, the diagnosis of rejection will remain difficult because we currently do not use any techniques of implantation in humans that allow subsequent islet analysis. Thus, the diagnosis of rejection after PTX and ITX can usually be supported only by the concurrent diagnosis of rejection in organs that can be biopsied: the kidney and liver. Although this is the only practical method in use today, a 10% to 20% incidence of rejection in isolated PTX has been posited.[68] Clearly, therefore, there is a need for more definitive methods for the diagnosis of rejection in PTX and ITX.

RECURRENCE OF DIABETES

Although results in PTX and ITX over recent years have been encouraging, there is as yet insufficient follow-up time to determine whether patients with type 1 diabetes mellitus will develop an alloimmune response against the implanted islets (either in the whole organ or when transplanted separately), mimicking the destruction of the native islets. In studies using the BB rat (which is thought to represent a model for type 1 diabetes mellitus), there is evidence both for and against major histocompatibility restriction of the autoimmune process seen in diabetes.[69, 70] If diabetes proves to be restricted to the host's HLA status, transplantation across major histocompatibility barriers may result in protection of the grafted islets from the autoimmune process. However, this interesting concept remains unanswered.

EFFECT ON CHRONIC DIABETIC COMPLICATIONS

The influence of PTX and ITX on long-term complications of diabetes mellitus remains unclear. Ramsay and colleagues conducted a 5-year follow-up of 22 patients who received successful PTX and 16 who received unsuccessful grafts.[46] Retinopathy was halted by years 4 and 5 in the group with successful PTX. However, the differences between the groups were not statistically significant. Similar findings have been reported by others.[47, 48] PTX does appear to confer protection against the development of diabetic nephropathy for a simultaneously transplanted kidney.[49] PTX years after a kidney transplant, when compared with kidney transplant alone, also appeared to be beneficial, with decreased mesangial and glomerular deposition.[8] There is also some preliminary evidence that PTX may halt or even reverse somatic and autonomic neuropathy.[50, 51, 71] Unfortunately, there is little evidence in humans regarding the long-term effects of ITX. Results in animal experiments have not clarified this dilemma. Using a rat model in which diabetes is induced experimentally with rapid renal changes, islet transplantation has been shown to prevent or reverse some but not all of the pathologic renal changes.[72, 73] Clearly, for both PTX and ITX, definitive information regarding the effects on the long-term sequelae of diabetes mellitus is required.

INTENSIVE CARE UNIT MANAGEMENT

The principles of postoperative management include routine ICU care, strict glucose control, careful monitoring for rejection, and nutrition.

Routine Intensive Care Unit Care

Much of the postoperative management of patients receiving ITX or PTX, either singly or in combination with other solid organs, consists of the provision of standard ICU care. This includes careful attention to nosocomial infection, multiple system organ function, and provision of supportive therapy as indicated (e.g., blood and blood products for bleeding complications) while the patient is weaned from the ventilator and rehabilitated.

Glucose Control

Although there is currently little experience in long-term follow-up of human ITX recipients, evidence in rodents suggests that the survival of the islets may be dependent on the avoidance of hyperglycemia in the initial phases. Therefore, it is important to strive for careful glucose control in the postoperative period.[25] This can be somewhat problematic. Patients who have received a concomitant liver transplant often have compromised liver function initially, and a potential complication is profound hypoglycemia. Such patients are also receiving immunosuppressive agents. Cyclosporine, FK-506, and prednisone all exert a diabetogenic effect, potentially stressing the transplanted islets.[62, 74] Our policy for blood glucose control in orthotopic liver transplant recipients is to maintain the glucose at levels greater than 200 mg/L, preferring hyperglycemia to hypoglycemia because the latter might not be diagnosed easily in the comatose or sedated patient. To achieve a suitable compromise in those receiving an ITX, we measure blood sugar very frequently, either hourly or every 2 hours for the first few days postoperatively. Furthermore, nearly all patients are controlled with a continuous intravenous insulin infusion. It is not clear whether PTX recipients require such close scrutiny of blood sugar levels.

Immunosuppression

The usual immunosuppressive regimen for PTX recipients is a combination of cyclosporine, prednisone, and azathioprine. Successful ITX has also been reported in humans using this regimen.[16–18] However, the largest series of ITX patients reported to date were managed with FK-506 as the primary agent. Whether treated with FK-506 or cyclosporin A, patients usually also receive a 5-day tapered course of steroids. Episodes of rejection are treated with either increased doses of FK-506 or steroids. Refractory rejection is usually managed with the murine T cell antibody OKT3. Rejection is most commonly suspected by evidence of impaired function or biochemical abnormalities of the solid organ (increased liver function test values, increased blood urea nitrogen or creatinine, electrolyte imbalance, or anuria). The diagnosis is confirmed by organ biopsy. PTX rejection may also be suspected by decreased urinary amylase secretion, but this diagnosis can be difficult to make, as discussed previously. There is currently no way to assess islet cell rejection directly when the cells are infused via the portal system unless an islet is coincidentally seen on liver biopsy. Islet cell rejection is, therefore, presumed to be possible when there is evidence of rejection elsewhere. Future possibilities for rejection monitoring include the use of organelles for transplantation at accessible sites, allowing multiple biopsies.[14] Meanwhile, the only way of determining islet rejection, as opposed to liver or kidney rejection, is to measure serum C peptide levels or to document insulin secretion failure. Unfortunately, these methods lack sufficient sensitivity because, by the time they become abnormal, islet function may be lost.[25] The alternative approach of managing patients with higher levels of immunosuppression in case of rejection is not currently favored because the marked increase in risk from life-threatening infection probably outweighs the potential benefit.

Nutrition

The management of nutritional repletion following PTX and ITX varies among institutions. In Pittsburgh, all patients are treated with total parenteral nutrition (TPN), which is commenced early in the postoperative period. Insulin is mixed in the TPN solution and additional supplements are given intravenously as required. When patients are able, they are allowed tube feedings or a normal diet as tolerated. Those patients who have undergone abdominal exenteration have understandable digestive difficulties, and transfer to a normal diet is difficult. Almost all have lost significant body weight in the first 3 months after transplant despite vigorous attempts to maintain adequate nutrition.[75]

CONCLUSIONS

PTX has clearly moved into the clinical arena as a viable treatment option for patients with diabetes and end-stage kidney or liver disease. Survival rates for both patient and graft are equivalent to those for other transplanted solid organs and, although not all questions are answered regarding its influence on the long-term sequelae of diabetes, patient quality of life is clearly improved. Expansion of PTX to other patient populations remains controversial, especially because of concerns related to long-term immunosuppression. This has led to increased efforts in the field of ITX, where immunosuppression may not be required. There have been exciting results in the last 3 years, and the next decade may well see the first large-scale studies in ITX. The challenge for these studies will be to improve methods for the isolation and measurement of islets, the subsequent monitoring of islet function, and the presence or absence of rejection or recurrent disease. Meanwhile, work must continue in PTX to determine a more feasible method to diagnose rejection. For the critical care physician, a knowledge of the surgical techniques and methods by which postoperative graft function can be monitored will, when combined with sound critical care, allow optimal management of these seemingly complex patients.

References

1. Laporte RE, Fishbein HA, Drash AL, et al: The Pittsburgh insulin-dependent diabetes mellitus (IDDM) registry: The incidence of insulin-dependent diabetes mellitus in Allegheny County, Pennsylvania (1965–1976). Diabetes 1981; 30:270.
2. Krolewski AS, Warram JH, Rand LI, et al: Epidemiologic approach to the etiology of type I diabetes mellitus and its complications. N Engl J Med 1987; 317:1390.
3. Harris MI, Hanaman RS (Eds): Diabetes in America. National Institutes of Health publication no. 85-1468. Bethesda, MD, National Institutes of Health, 1985.
4. Goetz FC, Elick B, Fryd D, et al: Renal transplantation in diabetes. Clin Endocrinol Metab 1986; 15:807.
5. Eisenbarth GS: Type I diabetes mellitus. N Engl J Med 1986; 314:1360.
6. Williams PW: Notes on diabetes treated with and by grafts of sheep's pancreas. Br Med J, December 8, 1894, p 1303.
7. Kelly WD, Lillehei RC, Merke FK, et al: Allotransplantation of the pancreas and duodenum along with the kidney in diabetic nephropathy. Surgery 1967; 61:827.
8. Robertson RP: Pancreatic and islet transplantation for diabetes: Cures or curiosities? N Engl J Med 1992; 327:1861.
9. Sutherland DER, Gruessner A, Moudry-Munns K: Report on results of pancreas transplantation in the United States October 1987 to October 1991 from the United Network for Organ Sharing Registry. *In:* Clinical Transplants 1991. Terasaki PI (Ed). Los Angeles, UCLA Tissue Typing Laboratory, 1991.
10. Sutherland DER, Dunn DL, Goetz FC, et al: A 10-year experience with 290 pancreas transplants at a single institution. Ann Surg 1989; 210:274.

11. Moskalewski S: Isolation and culture of the islets of Langerhans of the guinea pig. Gen Comp Endocr 1965; 5:342.
12. Lacy PE, Kostianovisky M: A method for the isolation of intact islets of Langerhans from the rat pancreas. Diabetes 1967; 16:35.
13. Hering BJ, Bretzel RG, Federlin K: Current status of clinical islet transplantation. Horm Metab Res 1988; 20:537.
14. Ricordi C, Starzl TE: Cellular transplants. Transplant Proc 1991; 23:73.
15. Tzakis AG, Ricordi C, Alejandro R, et al: Pancreatic islet transplantation after upper abdominal exenteration and liver replacement. Lancet 1990; 336:402.
16. Warnock GL, Kneteman MN, Ryan E, et al: Normoglycaemia after transplantation of freshly isolated and cryopreserved pancreatic islets in type 1 (insulin-dependent) diabetes mellitus. Diabetologia 1991; 34:55.
17. Altman JJ, Cugneno PH, Tesier C, et al: Epiploic flap: A new site for islet implantation in man. Horm Metab Res 1991; 25:136.
18. Scharp DW, Lacy PE, Santiago JV, et al: Insulin independence after islet transplantation into type I diabetic patient. Diabetes 1990; 39:515.
19. London NJ, Bell PR: Pancreas and islet transplantation. Br J Surg 1992; 79:6.
20. Dafoe DC, Naji A, Perloff LJ, et al: Pancreatic and islet autotransplantation. Hepatogastroenterol 1990; 37:307.
21. Hogle HH, Reemtsma K: Pancreatic autotransplantation following resection. Surgery 1987; 83:359.
22. Rossi RL, Heiss FW, Watkins E Jr, et al: Segmental pancreatic autotransplantation with pancreatic ductal occlusion after near-total or total pancreatic resection for chronic pancreatitis. Ann Surg 1986; 203:626.
23. McDonald JC, Rohr MS, Tucker WY: Recent experience with autotransplantation of the kidney, jejunum and pancreas. Ann Surg 1983; 197:678.
24. Margreiter R, Ofner D, Reinl E, et al: Pancreas transplantation: A critical appraisal. Transplant Proc 1992; 24:2383.
25. Gray DWR, Morris PJ: Developments in isolated pancreatic islet transplantation. Transplantation 1987; 43:321.
26. Ricordi C, Lacy PE, Finke EH, et al: Automated method for isolation of human pancreatic islets. Diabetes 1988; 37:413.
27. Horaguchi A, Merrell RC: Preparation of viable islet cells from dogs by a new method. Diabetes 1981; 30:455.
28. Ricordi C, Gray DWR, Hering BJ, et al: Islet isolation assessment in man and large animals. Acta Diabetol Lat 1990; 27:185.
29. Sun AM, Coddling JA, Haist RE: A study of glucose tolerance and insulin response in partially depancreatectomized dogs. Diabetes 1974; 23:424.
30. Child CG, Frey CHJ, Fry WJ: A reappraisal of removal of ninety-five percent of the distal portion of the pancreas. Surg Gynecol Obstet 1969; 129:49.
31. Marchetti P, Finke EH, Gerasimiu-Vazeou A: Automated large-scale isolation, in vitro function and xenotransplantation of porcine islets of Langerhans. Transplantation 1991; 52:209–213.
32. Gray BN, Watkins E: Isolated islet transplantation in experimental diabetes. Aust J Exp Biol Med Sci 1976; 54:57.
33. Kemp CB, Knight MJ, Scharp DW, et al: Effect of transplantation site on the results of pancreatic islets isografts in diabetic rats. Diabetologia 1973; 9:486.
34. Finch DR, Wise PH, Morris PJ: Successful intra-splenic transplantation of sygeneic and allogeneic isolated pancreatic islets. Diabetologia 1977; 13:195.
35. Reece-Smith H, DuToit DF, McShane P, et al: Prolonged survival of pancreatic islet allografts transplanted beneath the renal capsule. Transplantation 1981; 31:305.
36. Posselt AM, Barker CF, Tomaszewski JE, et al: Induction of donor-specific unresponsiveness by intrathymic islet transplantation. Science 1990; 249:1293.
37. Matas AJ, Payne WD, Grotting JC, et al: Portal venous systemic transplantation of dispersed neonatal pancreas. Transplantation 1977; 24:333.
38. Squifflet JP, Sutherland DE, Florack G, et al: Physiologic comparison of segmental pancreas and islet transplants in rats. Transplant Proc 1985; 17:378.
39. Mehigan DG, Bell WR, Zuidema CG, et al: Disseminated intravascular coagulation and portal hypertension following pancreatic islet autotransplantation. Ann Surg 1980; 191:287.
40. Tze WJ, Tai J: Intrathecal allotransplantation of pancreatic endocrine cells in diabetic rats. Transplantation 1986; 41:531.
41. Bobzein B, Yasunami Y, Majercik M, et al: Intratesticular transplants of islet xenografts (rat to mouse). Diabetes 1983; 32:213.
42. Thompson JA, Haudenschild CC, Anderson KD, et al: Heparin-binding growth factor 1 induces the formation of organoid neovascular structures in vivo. Proc Natl Acad Sci USA 1989; 86:7928.
43. Possa G, Traeger J, Dubernard JM, et al: Endocrine responses of type 1 (insulin-dependent) diabetic patients following successful pancreas transplantation. Diabetologia 1983; 24:244.
44. Diem P, Abid M, Redmon JB, et al: Systemic venous drainage of pancreas allografts as independent cause of hyperinsulinemia in type 1 diabetic recipients. Diabetes 1990; 39:534.
45. Katz H, Homan M, Velosa J, et al: Effects of pancreas transplantation on postprandial glucose metabolism. N Engl J Med 1991; 325:1278.
46. Ramsay RC, Goetz FC, Sutherland DER, et al: Progression of diabetic retinopathy after pancreas transplantation for insulin-dependent diabetes mellitus. N Engl J Med 1988; 318:208.
47. Petersen MR, Vine AK, University of Michigan Pancreas Transplant Evaluation Committee: Progression of diabetic retinopathy after pancreas transplantation. Ophthalmology 1990; 97:496.
48. Schneider A, Meyer-Schwickerath E, Nusser J, et al: Diabetic retinopathy and pancreas transplantation: A 3-year follow-up. Diabetologia 1991; 34(Suppl 1):S95.
49. Bohman S-O, Tyden G, Wilczek H, et al: Prevention of kidney graft diabetic nephropathy by pancreas transplantation in man. Diabetes 1985; 34:306.
50. Kennedy WR, Navarro X, Goetz FC, et al: Effects of pancreatic transplantation on diabetic neuropathy. N Engl J Med 1990; 322:1031.
51. Gaber A, Cardoso S, Pearson S, et al: Improvement in autonomic function following combined pancreas-kidney transplantation. Transplant Proc 1991; 23:1660.
52. Osei K, Henry ML, O'Dorisio TM, et al: Physiological and pharmacological stimulation of pancreatic islet hormone secretion in type I diabetic pancreas allograft recipients. Diabetes 1990; 30:1235.
53. Diem P, Redmon JB, Abid M, et al: Glucagon, catecholamine and pancreatic polypeptide secretion in type I diabetic recipients of pancreas allografts. J Clin Invest 1990; 86:2008.
54. Luzi L, Secchi A, Facchini F, et al: Reduction of insulin resistance by combined kidney-pancreas transplantation in type I (insulin-dependent) diabetic patients. Diabetologia 1990; 33:549.
55. Gerich JE, Langlois M, Noacco C, et al: Lack of glucagon response to hypoglycemia in diabetes: Evidence for an intrinsic pancreatic alpha cell defect. Science 1973; 182:171.
56. Benson JW Jr, Johnson DG, Palmer JP, et al: Glucagon and catecholamine secretion during hypoglycemia in normal and diabetic man. J Clin Endocrinol Metab 1977; 44:459.
57. La Rocca E, Secchi A, Parlavecchia M, et al: Lipid metabolism after successful kidney and pancreatic transplantation. Transplant Proc 1991; 23:1672.
58. Ziegler MM, Reckard CR, Barker CF: Long term metabolic and immunological considerations in transplantation of pancreatic islets. J Surg Res 1974; 16:575.
59. Tydén G: Pancreatic graft rejection. *In:* Pancreatic Transplantation. Groth CG (Ed): Philadelphia, WB Saunders, 1988, p 249.
60. Morris PJ, Finch DR, Garvey JF, et al: Suppression of rejection of allogeneic islet tissue in the rat. Diabetes 1986; 29(Suppl):107.
61. Dibelius A, Konigsberger H, Walter P, et al: Prolonged reversal of diabetes in the rat by transplantation of allogeneic islets from a single donor and cyclosporine treatment. Transplantation 1986; 41:426.
62. Hahn JH, Laube F, Lucke S, et al: Toxic effects of cyclosporine on the endocrine pancreas of Wistar rats. Transplantation 1986; 41:44.
63. Altman JJ, Houlbert D, Callard P, et al: Long-term plasma glucose normalization in experimental diabetic rats with macroencapsulated implants of benign human insulinomas. Diabetes 1986; 35:625.
64. Taunton-Rigby A: Transplantation of encapsulated islets. Transplant Proc 1986; 18:1861.
65. Gray DW, Reece-Smith H, Fairbrother B, et al: Isolated pancreatic islet allografts in rats rendered immunologically unresponsive to renal allografts: The effect of the site of transplantation. Transplantation 1984; 37:434.
66. Ohzato H, Porter J, Monaco AP, et al: Fifty islets maintain

euglycemia and survive longer than 200 islets in allogeneic and xenogeneic diabetic hosts. Transplant Proc 1993; 25:953–954.
67. Gotoh M, Maki T, Satomi S, et al: Immunological characteristics of purified islet grafts. Transplantation 1986; 42:387.
68. Klima G, Königsrainer A, Schmid T, et al: Is the pancreas rejected independently of the kidney after combined pancreatic-renal transplantation? Transplant Proc 1988; 20:665.
69. Prowse SJ, Bellgrau D, Lafferty KJ: Islet allografts are destroyed by disease recurrence in the spontaneously diabetic BB rat. Diabetes 1986; 35:110.
70. Markmann JF, Posselt AM, Bassiri H, et al: Major-histocompatibility-complex restricted and nonrestricted autoimmune effector mechanisms in BB rats. Transplantation 1991; 52:662–667.
71. Navarro X, Kennedy WR, Loewenson RB, et al: Influence of pancreas transplantation on cardiorespiratory reflexes, nerve conduction, and mortality in diabetes mellitus. Diabetes 1990; 39:802.
72. Weber CJ, Silva FG, Hardy MA, et al: Effect of islet transplantation on renal function and morphology of short- and long-term diabetic rats. Transplant Proc 1979; 11:549.
73. Gotzche O, Gunderson HJ, Osterby R: Irreversibility of glomerular basement membrane accumulation despite reversibility of renal hypertrophy with islet transplantation in early diabetes. Diabetes 1981; 30:481.
74. Fung JJ, Alessini M, Abu-Elmagd K, et al: Adverse effects associated with the use of FK 506. Transplant Proc 1991; 23:3105.
75. Tzakis AG: Personal communication, 1991.

CHAPTER 185

Intestinal and Multiple Organ Transplantation

Jorge Reyes, MD • Robert Selby, MD • Kareem Abu-Elmagd, MD
Andreas G. Tzakis, MD • Satoru Todo, MD
Adrian Casavilla, MD • Thomas E. Starzl, MD, PhD

The concept and practice of intestinal transplantation were born together with those for kidney and liver transplantation. After the introduction of cyclosporin A, transplantation of these other organs enjoyed rapid clinical applicability. Success with intestinal transplantation, however, remained blurred because of a high incidence of graft loss due to rejection, infection, and technical complications.[1]

The first experimental attempts at intestinal transplantation were reported by Lillehei and coworkers in 1959 as an isolated organ graft in dogs.[2] One year later, Starzl and Kaupp included the small bowel as part of a multivisceral graft in dogs (liver, stomach, pancreaticoduodenal complex, small and large intestine).[3] The first human application of a modified form of this operation was the transplantation of a "cluster" of organs in 1989.[4] This allograft consisted of liver and pancreaticoduodenal complex after upper abdominal exenteration for malignancy (Fig. 185–1). Viability of varying lengths of intestine with these clusters was proven, as was evidence of regeneration after severe rejection-induced injury. The inclusion of the liver in this type of graft was believed to protect the other organs transplanted from the same donor against rejection.[3, 5, 6]

In 1987, a 3-year-old girl received a multivisceral abdominal graft that contained the stomach, duodenum, pancreas, small bowel, colon, and liver. She had an extended survival of 6 months with intestinal graft function.[7] An even longer survival of 1 year was obtained in a recipient of a liver and small bowel graft treated by Grant and associates.[8] Until

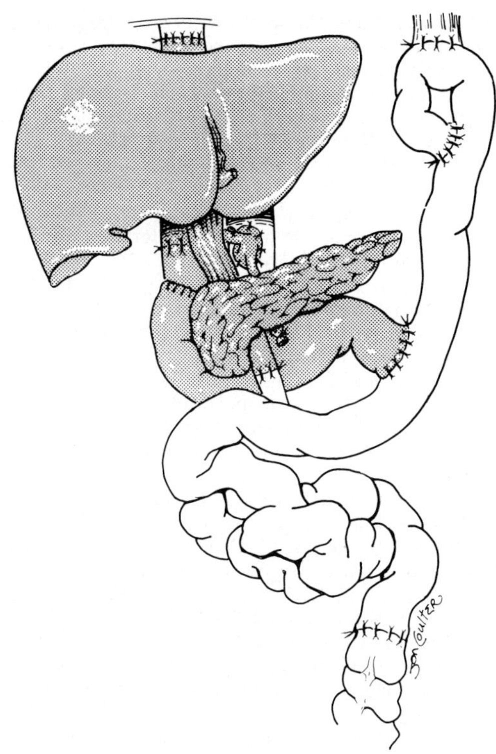

Figure 185–1. Cluster allograft (*shaded portion*), including the liver, pancreas, and duodenal segment of small intestine. (From Starzl TE, Todo S, Tzakis A, et al: Abdominal organ cluster transplantation for the treatment of upper abdominal malignancies. Ann Surg 1989; 210:374–386.)

1990, there had been only two survivors of isolated cadaveric intestinal grafting.[9, 10]

INDICATIONS

Loss of intestinal function may be acute (e.g., necrotizing enterocolitis, volvulus, mesenteric thrombosis) or chronic (e.g., Crohn's disease, radiation enteritis). Candidate classification can be approached with an arbitrary division of surgical and nonsurgical cause. Patients with surgical causes generally suffer from loss of bowel length after resections for atresias, infarctions (e.g., volvulus, vascular catastrophes, necrotizing enterocolitis), or strictures and fistulas as with Crohn's disease. With nonsurgical causes of intestinal failure, the anatomic length and gross morphology may be normal. These causes include motility disorders (e.g., intestinal pseudo-obstruction, Hirschsprung's disease), absorptive insufficiencies (e.g., microvillus inclusion disease), polyposis syndromes, and incarcerating desmoid tumors.

Total parenteral nutrition has become the standard of care for patients who are unable to maintain a normal nutritional state by use of the gastrointestinal tract alone (intestinal failure).[11] Transplantation of the intestine either alone or accompanied by other intra-abdominal organs (liver, stomach, pancreas) may be beneficial in these patients, since the stability and duration of total parenteral nutrition therapy varies, depending on complicating factors such as infection, metabolic disorders, difficulty with vascular access, and liver dysfunction.[11]

The decision regarding allograft composition focuses on the integrity of the remaining gut and other abdominal organs, both functionally and anatomically. Guidelines used

TABLE 185–1. Partial and Complete Intestinal Allografts

Organ Transplanted	*Indication*
Multivisceral (stomach, duodenum, pancreas, liver, small bowel, colon)	Pseudo-obstruction/aganglionosis syndrome with hepatic failure; diffuse splanchnic venous thrombosis and hepatic failure
Liver and small intestine	Hepatic failure after prolonged hyperalimentation for short gut syndrome
Liver, duodenum, and pancreas (organ cluster transplantation)	After upper abdominal exenteration for malignancy
Small intestine	Congenital or acquired absence or dysfunction

in substantiating the need for concomitant liver replacement in these intestinal transplantation candidates are biochemical dysfunction (hyperbilirubinemia, transaminase abnormalities, hypoalbuminemia, and coagulopathy), pathologic processes (fibrosis or cirrhosis on liver biopsy), and the clinical presence of portal hypertension as manifested by hepatosplenomegaly, ascites, or esophageal varices. Patients deficient in protein S, protein C, and antithrombin III (liver-derived) should receive a combined liver–small intestine allograft. Recipients lacking these substances develop diffuse thromboses within the splanchnic system and undergo transplantation for mesenteric venous hypertension rather than for intestinal insufficiency.[12] Patients with motility disorders that involve the entire gastrointestinal tract are candidates for replacement of this entire system (Table 185–1).

Table 185–2 lists the causes for intestinal failure in patients who underwent transplantation at the University of Pittsburgh. Inability to continue total parenteral nutrition because of the development of hepatic cirrhosis and venous access limitations were the most frequent indications for transplantation.

ABDOMINAL VISCERAL PROCUREMENT

The safe procurement of multiple visceral organs, either en bloc or as separate components, hinges on a few fundamental precepts. Conceptually, the focus is to isolate and cool the organs, thus preserving their vascular and parenchymal anatomy. Multivisceral en bloc retrieval including the stomach, duodenum, pancreas, liver, and small intestine is the parent operation, and the assembled components have been likened by Starzl and colleagues to a large clump of individual grapes from the whole.[13] An appreciation of the fundamental strategy of multivisceral organ retrieval leads to an understanding of the lesser variant operations—that is, liver, small intestine, combined liver–small intestine, and organ cluster (liver, duodenum, and pancreas) transplantation. A more complete discussion of the specifics of organ procurement is presented in Chapter 178

TABLE 185–2. Indications for Composite and Isolated Intestinal Transplantation in 33 Patients at the University of Pittsburgh from May 1990 to January 1993

Pediatric Patients (48%)		*Adult Patients (52%)*	
Necrotizing enterocolitis	29%	Crohn's disease	31%
Gastroschisis	21%	Thrombolytic disorder	25%
Volvulus	17%	Trauma	16%
Pseudo-obstruction	13%	Pseudo-obstruction	9%
Hirschsprung's disease	7%	Radiation enteritis	6%
Intestinal atresia	7%	Desmoid tumor	5%
Microvillus inclusion disease	3%	Familial polyposis	4%
Malrotation	3%	Volvulus	4%

RECIPIENT OPERATIONS

Most patients who need intestinal or multiorgan replacements have had multiple forays into the abdominal cavity for intestinal resections, lengthening procedures, and treatment of complications. This results in volume contraction of the abdominal cavity and severe adhesions. For this reason, the organs of the donor need to be smaller than those of the recipient to allow proper abdominal closure.

Previous operations may complicate the removal of the recipient's organs, especially if cirrhosis, portal hypertension, or inferior vena caval thromboses are present, all of which may be sequelae of the original disease or of prior operations. The recipient's operation consists of removal of the failed organs with exposure of the vascular anatomy and, finally, allograft implantation. Following is a brief description of the salient features of the recipient operations.

Multivisceral Transplantation

After essentially abdominal exenteration and exposure of the retroperitoneal aorta and inferior vena cava have been performed, the multivisceral graft (Fig. 185–2) is connected by its vascular attachments: first the suprahepatic attachment, then infrahepatic vena caval connections, and finally the arterioaortic anastomosis. The recipient's portal vein and its outflow and inflow organs (gastrointestinal tract, pancreas, and liver) are removed with the enterectomy. The donor portal vein retains its continuity via the liver in the procurement of the allograft; thus, no portal vein anastomosis is required in this procedure.

Restoration of intestinal continuity requires an esophagogastric anastomosis and a coloenteric anastomosis with the distal ileum allograft. Initially, the patient also receives an ileostomy (see Fig. 185–2). Takedown of the ileostomy can be performed after several months, when oral nutrition is consistently adequate, a stable immunosuppressant regimen has been achieved, and the need for frequent endoscopic surveillance has lessened.

Liver–Small Bowel

Liver and small intestine are removed in these patients, but the remainder of the foregut (stomach, duodenum, pancreas) is retained. When possible, the liver is removed with the retrohepatic vena cava preserved in situ.[14] After the enterectomy, the composite allograft is implanted by anastomosing the suprahepatic vena cava of the donor (including the hepatic veins) end-to-side to the recipient's vena cava. The donor infrahepatic vena cava can then be ligated. The double arterial stem of the celiac and superior mesenteric arteries (using the Carrel button technique) are connected to the infrarenal aorta with subsequent graft reperfusion. Since the axial stem of the portal vein between the donor organs has remained intact, all that is required for the completion of portal flow is attachment of the portal vein of the remnant foregut in the recipient to the intact portal stem of the donor (Fig. 185–3). This may not be possible, however, because of size discrepancy or difficult anatomic relationships between donor and recipient portal veins. In this case, a permanent portocaval shunt is per-

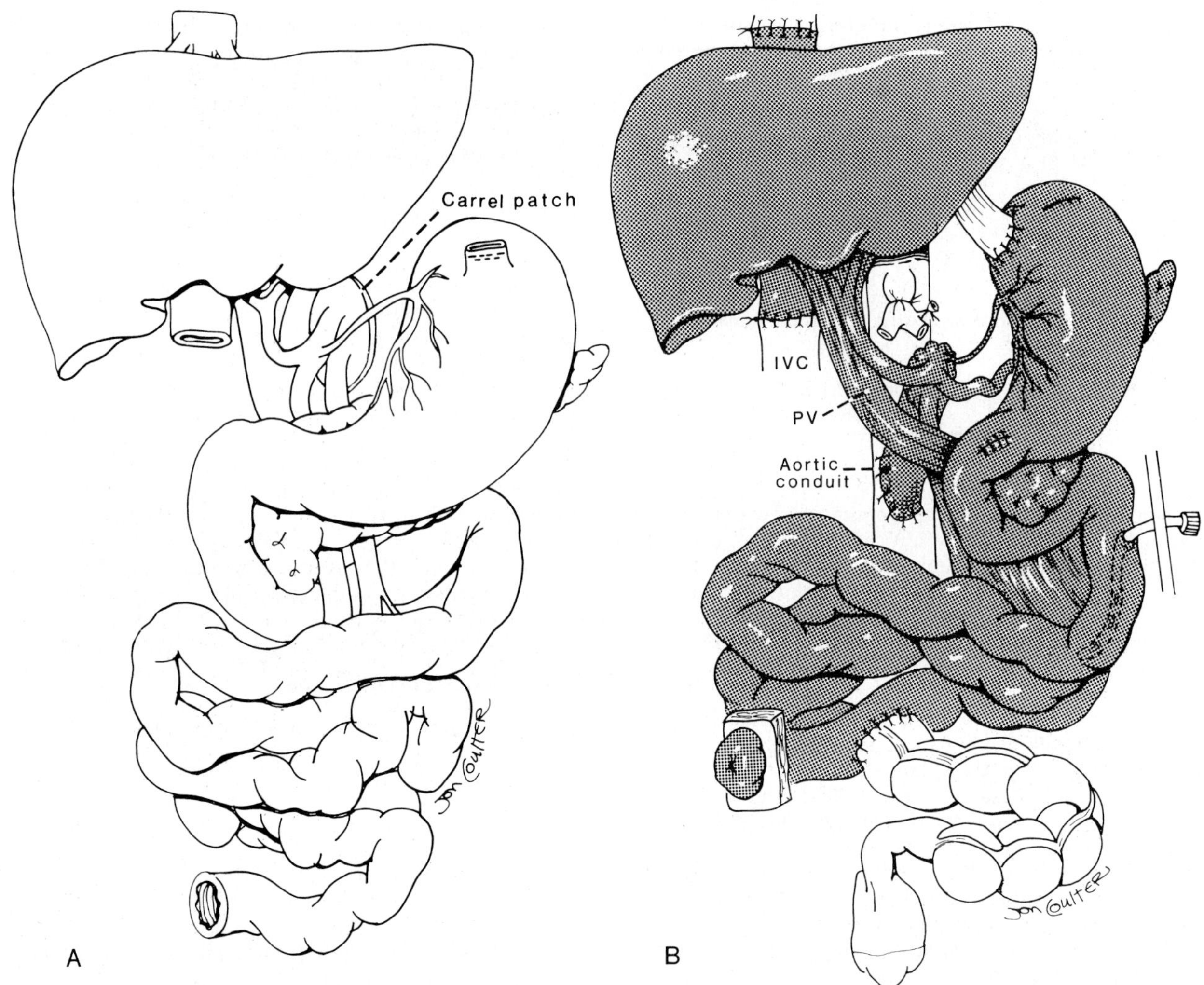

Figure 185–2. Diagrams of multivisceral donor organs before (*A*) and after (*B*) implantation show the suprahepatic and infrahepatic vena caval and arterioaortic anastomoses. *Abbreviations*: IVC = inferior vena cava; PV = portal vein. (From Starzl TE, Todo S, Tzakis A, et al: The many faces of multivisceral transplantation. Surg Gynecol Obstet 1991; 172:335–344. By permission of Surgery, Gynecology & Obstetrics.)

formed. The intestinal anastomoses are then completed with a proximal jejunojejunostomy, ileocolostomy, and Roux-en-Y biliary anastomoses (see Fig. 185–3). A temporary distal ileostomy is also provided.

Isolated Small Bowel

After wide exposure, the recipient's small intestine is removed from the ligament of Treitz to the colon. The superior mesenteric artery of the donor bowel is sewn to the infrarenal aorta, and the donor superior mesenteric vein to the recipient portal vein or, alternatively, the donor superior mesenteric vein is anastomosed to the recipient's inferior vena cava (Fig. 185–4). Reperfusion of the graft is effected after the vascular anastomoses. Intestinal continuity is completed with proximal and distal anastomoses, and access to the ileum for endoscopic examination is provided by a temporary chimney ileostomy.[15]

Cold ischemia refers to the time between procurement and implantation of the allograft; for best results, whenever a segment of the intestine is included, this period should be less than 10 hours to avoid preservation injury. Warm ischemic time for the allograft (sewing-in time) is about 30 minutes and is also a determinant of preservation injury to the intestine.

IMMUNOSUPPRESSION

Immunosuppression is similar in recipients of small bowel, liver–small bowel, cluster, and multivisceral transplants. One gram of intravenous hydrocortisone (for children) or methylprednisolone (for adults) is given immediately after graft reperfusion. Administration of FK-506 (0.15–0.2 mg · kg^{-1} · d^{-1}) is then begun by continuous intravenous infusion, with steady-state plasma levels between 2 and 3 ng/mL as targets. A steroid taper of methylprednisolone is started at a dose of 100 mg (for children) or 200 mg (for adults) and reduced over a period of 5 days to 10 mg (for children) or 20 mg (for adults) per day. In some cases, azathioprine may be added to mitigate the nephrotoxicity and neurotoxicity of the FK-506. As gastrointestinal motility resumes, oral FK-506 given twice daily may be used to supplement the intravenous regimen, which is gradually tapered.

Induction therapy as well as chronic maintenance therapy involves the use of two and often three drugs. However, if organ tolerance with minimal rejection episodes is demonstrated, gradual reduction and even cessation of steroid therapy may be possible.

Prostaglandin E_1 (Prostin) is administered, 0.003 to 0.009 mg · kg^{-1} · min^{-1}, for the first 5 postoperative days. This is

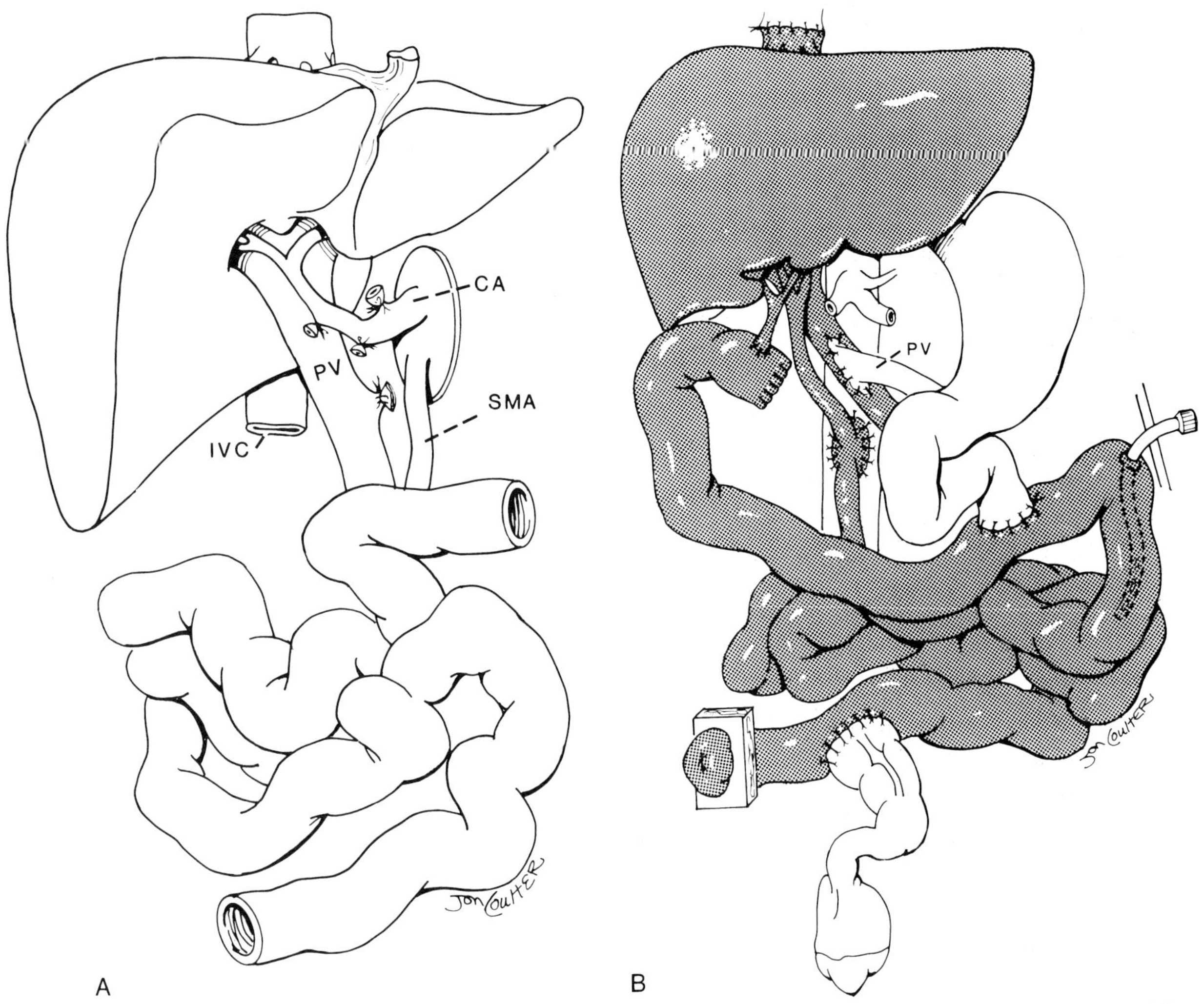

Figure 185–3. Combined liver–small intestinal allograft. *A,* After removal from donor; note the intact portal venous axial stem and the common origin from the aortic patch of the celiac and superior mesenteric arteries (CA and SMA, respectively). *B,* After transplantation, a single upper caval and arterioaortic anastomosis is done before reperfusion. Recipient PV to donor PV shunt allows venous outflow of retained pancreas and stomach from recipient. (From Starzl TE, Todo S, Tzakis A, et al: The many faces of multivisceral transplantation. Surg Gynecol Obstet 1991; 172:335–344. By permission of Surgery, Gynecology & Obstetrics.)

given both for its beneficial effects on renal perfusion as well as for its prevention of microvascular thromboses, the damage-mediating event in acute cellular rejection and procurement injury.[16]

POSTOPERATIVE CARE

Recipients of multivisceral, liver–small bowel, or cluster grafts commonly suffer from severe liver failure. Therefore, the care with respect to lungs, infection surveillance, and liver graft function is similar to that for routine liver transplant recipients. Recipients of isolated small bowel transplants who have stable liver function have a lesser preoperative medical acuity.

Ventilatory Management

Extubation can often be accomplished within 48 hours of transplantation. Unusual circumstances such as graft malfunction, sepsis, inability to close the abdominal wall, or severe preoperative hepatic failure may prevent early extubation. Since the operation is quite long (8–18 hours) and the patients are often in a weakened nutritional state preoperatively, a careful assessment of weaning parameters is required. The negative inspiratory force, forced vital capacity, and spontaneous minute ventilation are most important. It is wise to observe the patients for several hours while they remain intubated on continuous positive airway pressure to make certain that they can tolerate the withdrawal of mechanical support and extubation. Incisional pain, ascites, and pleural effusions may compromise ventilation and the ability to cough. Muscle wasting and malnutrition, partial or complete paralysis of the right hemidiaphragm,[17] and occasional discrepancies in donor/recipient size that produce an increased intra-abdominal volume with compression of the thoracic cavity may be factors responsible for respiratory impairment. These patients often require low doses of intravenous narcotics, repeated thoracentesis and paracentesis, and supplemental extensive respiratory therapy if they are to avoid the need for reintubation. Many patients have required tracheostomies because of the need for prolonged ventilatory support.

Renal Function

Early following transplantation, there is significant interstitial accumulation of fluid into the graft, lung, and peripheral tissues; this accumulation peaks at 48 to 72 hours. Extensive

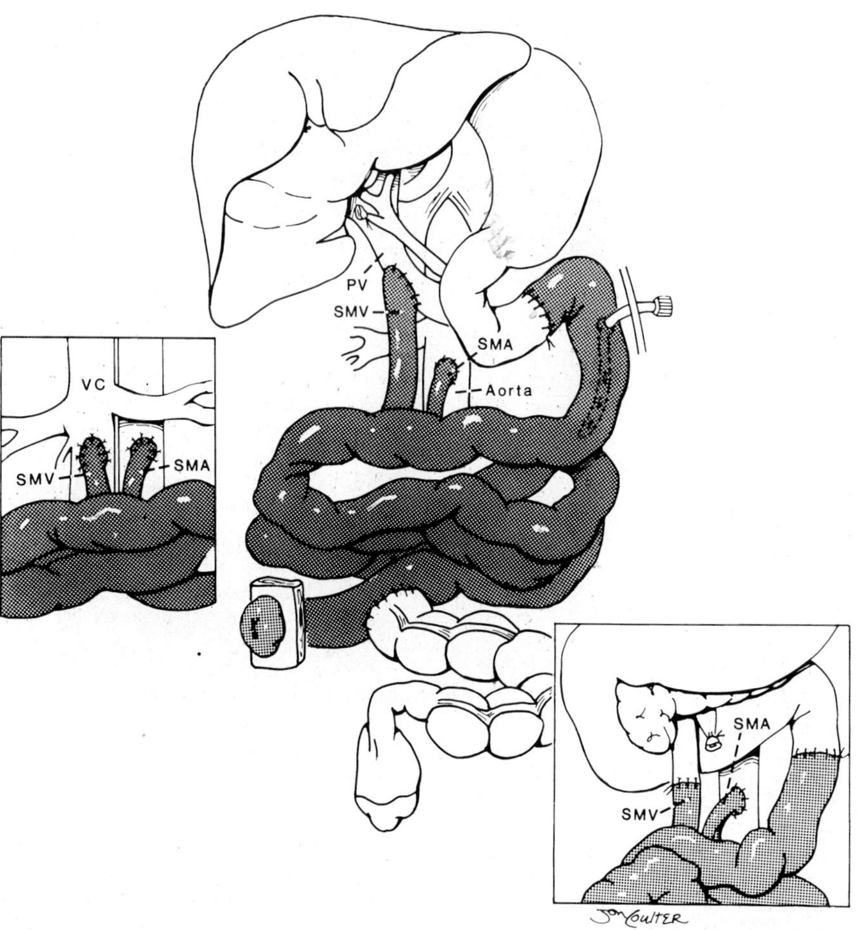

Figure 185–4. Illustration of an isolated small bowel graft showing mesenteric venous and arterial connections. The distal ileal chimney allows easy access to bowel mucosa. (From Todo S, Tzakis A, Abu-Elmagd K, et al: Intestinal transplantation in composite visceral grafts or alone. Ann Surg 1992; 216:223–234.)

volume shifts into the transplanted bowel (related to preservation injury) and heavy ascites production (related to mesenteric lymphatic leakage) lead to intravascular volume depletion, which can exacerbate the nephrotoxicity of FK-506 and certain antibiotics. Continuous central venous pressure measurement, often for weeks following transplantation, provides important information for maximizing graft perfusion and preserving the integrity of the kidneys.

Infection Control

Recipients of isolated or composite small bowel grafts receive prophylactic, broad-spectrum intravenous antibiotics. Any history of recent nosocomial infections before transplantation should be addressed with the administration of appropriate specific antibiotics. Colonizing organisms growing from enterocutaneous fistulous tracts should be treated perioperatively.

All recipients are given a "cocktail" of oral nonabsorbable antibiotics every 6 hours for 1 month; the mix includes amphotericin B, gentamicin, and polymixin E and is intended to achieve selective bowel decontamination.[18] Surveillance stool cultures are performed every 3 days. If any organisms grow in quantitative cultures to colonies of greater than 10^8 organisms and if the patient demonstrates signs of systemic sepsis, or if there is ongoing acute cellular rejection of the allograft, then specifically directed intravenous antibiotics are added to the regimen to treat the presumed translocating organisms. This most commonly occurs during episodes of acute rejection, when the mucosal barrier of the allograft has been immunologically damaged.

Routine prophylaxis to prevent cytomegalovirus infection includes a 2-week course of intravenous ganciclovir while lifetime oral trimethoprim-sulfamethoxazole is used as prophylaxis for pneumocystis pneumonia.

Nutritional Support

Standard total parental nutrition formulas are tapered gradually as oral or enteral feedings (via gastric or jejunal tube) are advanced. Tube feedings are initiated with an isotonic dipeptide formula containing medium-chain triglycerides and glutamine. This is later converted to a lactose- and gluten-free diet that contains dietary fibers to promote normalization of intestinal motility and function. Most patients do not voluntarily eat adequate amounts early after the operation; therefore, enteral supplementation is required when the intestinal tract becomes functional. This resistance to resumption of oral feedings has been particularly impressive in pediatric recipients.[19]

Assessment of Graft Status

A judgment of the anatomic and functional integrity of the graft begins in the operating room. The normal appearance of the mesentery and intestine is pink and nonedematous with the intestine occasionally demonstrating contractions. Alterations from this appearance can be observed in the operating room and in the ileal stoma postoperatively.

Surveillance for intestinal graft rejection focuses on clinical evaluation and gross morphologic examination of the stoma and the distal ileum with enteroscopy. Endoscopic evaluations are performed routinely twice a week through the allograft ileostomy, whereas upper endoscopy is performed as indicated. Grossly, the bowel reacts to insult in nonspecific ways with edema, cyanosis, congestion, and increased stomal output; these alterations should signal a broad differential to include preservation injury, systemic sepsis, rejection, and enteritis.

The stomal output is assessed for volume, consistency, and the presence of reducing substances, which can be seen in the event of rejection, bacterial overgrowth, or malabsorption. Typical stomal output of a clear, watery effluent within the first week of implantation is 1 to 2 L/d for adults and 40 to 60 mL/kg per day for children. If these volumes are exceeded and no significant pathology is present, paregoric, loperamide, pectin, somatostatin, or oral antibiotics may be utilized singly or in combination to control the diarrhea. The presence of blood in the stool is always an ominous sign and must be assumed to indicate rejection until it is proved otherwise.

Serum tests are important to give indications of possible anatomic injury to the liver (bilirubin, aspartate aminotransferase, and alanine aminotransferase), but no such tests exist for the intestinal grafts. Serum markers for nutritional adequacy and anabolic status (transferrin, albumin, retinoic acid) are of limited value, whereas specific tests of the absorptive ability of the graft are good measures of overall function. Assessment of small bowel function relies on absorption studies of D-xylose and FK-506 and on the quantitation of fat in the stool. Most patients develop satisfactory absorption curves for D-xylose within the first postoperative month, with absorption improving over time. Abnormal results obtained after 1 month should always prompt an aggressive search for underlying pathology, especially rejection. The maintenance of satisfactory FK-506 plasma trough levels of 2 to 3 ng/mL on oral therapy alone is a good indicator of adequate absorption. In our patients, this has occurred at a mean of 28 days after transplantation and tends to be delayed longer in recipients of multivisceral grafts.[19] The excretion of fat in the stool has been abnormal in almost all patients. However, clinical steatorrhea has not been a problem.

Radiologic evaluations by standard barium gastrointestinal examination are valuable in assessing mucosal pattern and motility and are performed routinely after the first postoperative week. A normal mucosal pattern is expected. Intestinal transit time is around 2 hours. Intestinal graft rejection, when mild, can be suspected when evidence of mucosal edema exists. Severe rejection, with exfoliation of the mucosa, ablates the normal mucosal pattern and can be seen as segments of "tubulized" intestine and strictures (Fig. 185–5).

COMPLICATIONS

Before a description of the variety of potential complications, it is important to have a general perspective on the care of these patients. Comprehensive management of intestinal recipients requires a multidisciplinary approach by surgeons, anesthesiologists, nurses, critical care physicians, pathologists, and a host of internal medicine subspecialists. Easy access to diagnostic and therapeutic modalities, including mechanical ventilation, hemodialysis, bronchoscopy, gastrointestinal endoscopy, thromboelastography, percutaneous cholangiography, ultrasonography, invasive and noninvasive contrast radiography, and sophisticated hemodynamic monitoring systems, is paramount.

More important than the above, however, is a vigilance about patient care and attention to detail, on the part of both physicians and nurses. Problems in these patients can originate from a multiplicity of sources. Several assumptions can be made in these patients based on our experience:

1. Preoperative deterioration of physical performance status predisposes to various organ system failure that persists in the postoperative period even though allograft function may be acceptable.
2. Transplant patients are labor intensive and require aggressive respiratory therapy, nutritional and antibiotic sup-

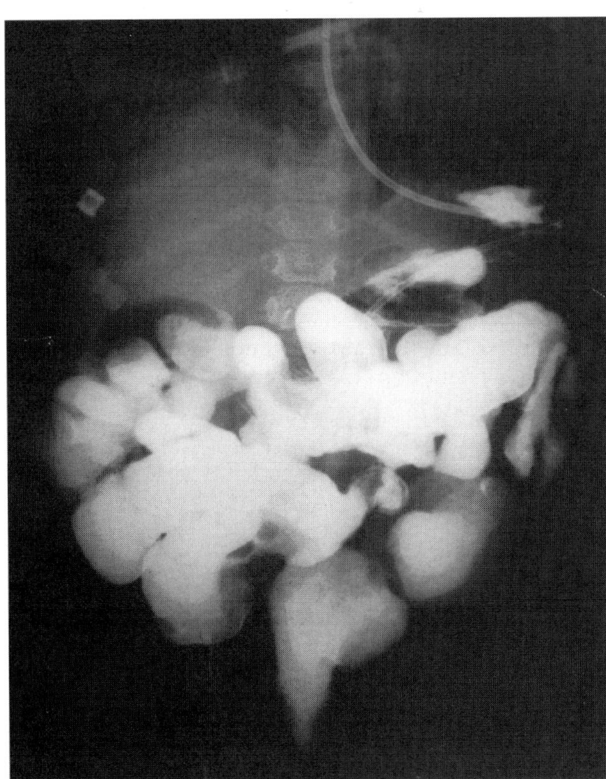

Figure 185–5. Severely damaged allograft intestine in a recipient of a liver–small bowel after multiple episodes of rejection. Diffuse tubulized gut, strictures, and significant distention of the native duodenum are seen.

port, fluid management, and nursing care, often for prolonged periods in the intensive care unit.

3. Immunotherapy doses in patients with multivisceral transplants tend to be higher than in patients with single organ transplants.

4. The majority of patients develop episodes of infection and rejection after transplantation, often concomitantly. Any subjective complaints or objective abnormalities should be vigorously pursued until a cause is found or until they resolve.

Graft Rejection

Intestinal allograft rejection can present as an array of symptoms that include fever, abdominal pain, distention, nausea, vomiting, and a sudden increase in stomal output. The stoma may become edematous, erythematous, and friable. Gastrointestinal bleeding can occur in cases of severe uncontrollable rejection in which ulcerations and sloughing of the intestinal mucosa occur. Septic shock or acute respiratory distress syndrome may develop. Bacterial or fungal translocation can occur during intestinal allograft rejection due to disruption of the intestinal mucosal barrier. Gut decontamination must be instituted during these episodes.[20]

Endoscopically, the transplanted intestinal mucosa loses its velvety appearance. It may become hyperemic or dusky, as well as hypoperistaltic. Erythema may be focal or diffuse. The mucosa becomes friable, and diffuse ulcerations appear (Fig. 185–6).

Histologically, there is a variable presence of lamina propria edema and villous blunting. However, the mononuclear cell infiltrates and cryptitis with apoptosis and regeneration are necessary for establishing the diagnosis of rejection. Neutrophils, eosinophils, and macrophages may be seen traversing the muscularis mucosa.[21] The degree of epithelial and crypt cell damage varies. Complete mucosal sloughing and crypt destruction are seen in grafts with severe rejection. The mucosal surface is partially replaced by inflammatory pseudomembranes and granulation tissue (Fig. 185–7). This may precipitate continuous blood loss as well as intermittent septic episodes from the damaged intestine.

Chronic rejection has been observed in patients with persistent intractable rejection episodes. Clinically progressive weight loss, chronic diarrhea, intermittent fever, and gastrointestinal bleeding dominate the presentation. Histologically, villous blunting, focal ulcerations, epithelial metaplasia and scant cellular infiltrate are present on endoscopic mucosal biopsies. Full-thickness intestinal biopsies show obliterative thickening of intestinal arterioles.

The incidence of acute intestinal allograft rejection during the first 90 days after transplantation is reported to be 80% in isolated small bowel recipients and 77% in liver–small bowel recipients. The incidence of acute liver allograft rejection in liver–small bowel recipients is 55%.[21]

Graft rejection is treated initially with bolus steroid therapy (intravenous hydrocortisone or methylprednisolone) in cases of mild rejection, with a steroid taper in cases of moderate to severe rejection. The FK-506 trough levels in plasma should reach 2 to 3 ng/mL by either the oral or intravenous routes. OKT3 is used when rejection has progressed with a steroid taper; however, it should be entertained as the initial therapeutic agent in cases of severe mucosal injury and crypt damage.

Postoperative Hemorrhage

Coagulopathy is more often an intraoperative problem that relates to liver dysfunction, qualitative and quantitative platelet defects, and fibrinolysis.[22] Intraoperative bleeding is furthered by vascularized adhesions from previous surgery and portal hypertension. Temporary graft reperfusion coagulopathy mediated by plasminogen activators from the graft may occur.[23] Efforts are taken to normalize these global aspects of coagulation by the end of the operative procedure so that in the absence of liver dysfunction, the coagulopathy is usually minor in the postoperative period. Postoperative intra-abdominal bleeding is most often a technical problem, arising from vascular anastomoses or extensive, raw peritoneal surfaces. Certainly, coagulation should be normalized if postoperative bleeding occurs; if bleeding is proved, the origin should be presumed surgical and managed as such by early exploration.

Biliary Complications

Continuity of the biliary axis is preserved in multivisceral and cluster grafts, whereas liver–small bowel and isolated small bowel grafts require Roux-en-Y choledochojejunostomy. Correspondingly, these grafts can develop biliary system–related surgical complications (i.e., leaks and obstructions).

Biliary leaks usually occur within the first 2 weeks after small bowel transplantation and may herald their presence with bilious drainage from the abdominal wound or drains or merely with unexplained sepsis. The response to external bilious drainage should be immediate exploration with surgical revision of the biliary dehiscence. In the case of unexplained sepsis in any intestinal transplant recipient, all surgical anastomoses should be radiographically inspected (with percutaneous cholangiography), and if leakage is suspected, they should be openly revised. There is no place for percutaneous diversion of biliary or intestinal leakage in these patients, since both wound healing and antimicrobial immunity are impaired by multimodal immunotherapy.

Biliary obstruction generally follows an anastomotic stricture and is a delayed complication, but any clinical picture

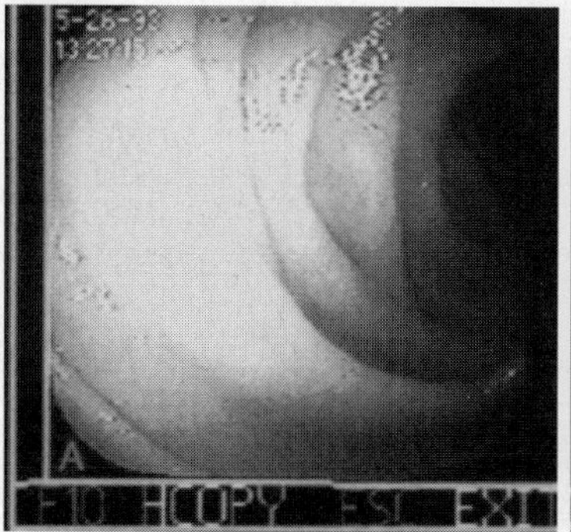

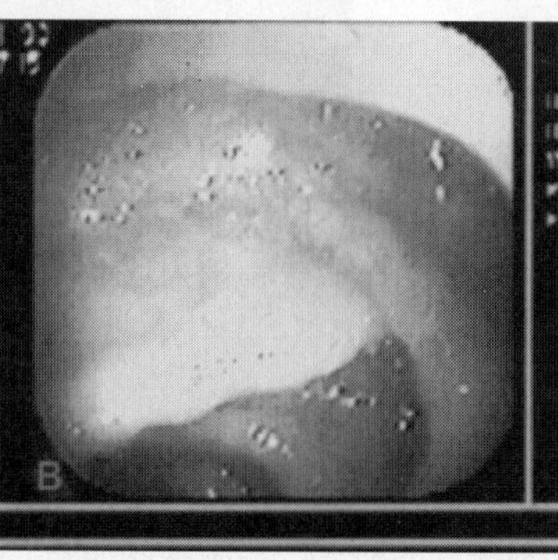

Figure 185–6. *A,* Normal endoscopic appearance of transplanted small intestine. *B,* Moderate acute cellular rejection of an intestinal allograft demonstrating diffuse edema and focal erythema. (See Color Plate Section of this textbook.)

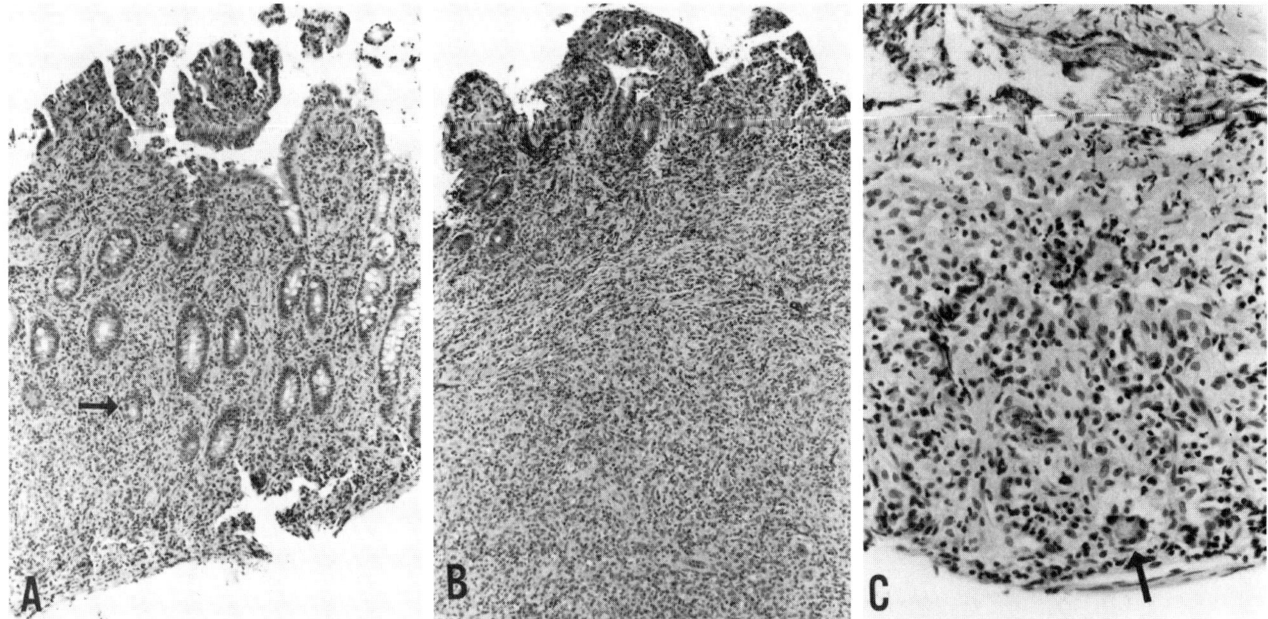

Figure 185–7. Acute cellular rejection. *A*, Endoscopic biopsy obtained 14 days after transplantation showed widening of the lamina propria with increased mononuclear cells, which were often cuffed around small vessels and infiltrating the crypt epithelium (*arrow*; hematoxylin and eosin, 140×). *B*, The reaction was more intense in biopsies that contained lymphoid nodules and where blastogenesis, focal ulcerations, congestion, and neutrophil plugging of capillaries were also seen (moderate acute cellular rejection; hematoxylin and eosin, 140×). *C*, Uncontrolled acute rejection eventually resulted in widespread mucosal destruction; the mucosa was replaced by granulation tissue. Note the overlying inflammatory pseudomembrane (*arrow*; hematoxylin and eosin, 350×).

that resembles cholangitis or biliary obstruction should be followed with cholangiography to prove patency, regardless of the timing after transplantation.

Vascular Complications

Major arterial thrombosis is a disastrous complication that leads to massive necrosis of the organs correspondingly supplied. Elevation of hepatic enzymes and pallor of the intestinal stoma are accompanied by clinical deterioration, fulminant sepsis, and hepatic coma. Isolated small bowel grafts can be removed with the expectation of patient recovery, but in patients with composite grafts, the event is usually fatal. Patency of the arteries can be rapidly confirmed with Doppler ultrasound examination.

Since the superior mesenteric vein–portal vein axis is preserved in the composite grafts, venous outflow thrombosis is less likely to occur in patients with them. Isolated small bowel grafts have an anastomosis of these veins that can potentially occlude. Ascites, stomal congestion, and, ultimately, mesenteric infarction would be the ultimate result.

Neither of these problems produces subtle clinical signs, and diagnosis should be prompt and obvious. In our series, thrombosis of the hepatic artery has occurred in a pediatric recipient of a liver–small bowel graft, with consequent hepatic gangrene. This patient required retransplantation of the liver component of the graft, even though a full liver–small bowel graft was desirable.

Incomplete obstruction of major inflow or outflow vessels may be suspected on biopsy or based on clinical and laboratory evidence of organ dysfunction. Contrast vascular studies are confirmatory, and the correction is surgical or, in some cases, with balloon dilatation.

Gastrointestinal Complications

Gastrointestinal bleeding after intestinal transplantation is an ominous sign that requires prompt attention. Rejection is the most probable cause and should be immediately diagnosed or ruled out on the basis of enteroscopic biopsy results. The diagnosis of rejection relies not only on histologic evidence but also on the endoscopic appearance (see Figs. 185–6 and 185–7). However, in the absence of any pathology on endoscopy and with other supporting clinical evidence of rejection, the patient should still be treated for acute rejection.

Leakage of either the proximal or distal gastrointestinal anastomosis can occur in any recipient, but it is more common in pediatric patients than in adults. Any fresh surgical margin, including native duodenal and colonic stumps and gastrostomy sites, are vulnerable to poor wound healing and subsequent leakage. Presentation is often dramatic (florid sepsis), and confirmation is with radiologic contrast imaging. Surgical revision, evacuation of peritoneal soilage, and often re-exploration are required to eliminate the contamination effectively. Again, sepsis without an obvious source should prompt the performance of contrast studies to document the integrity of all gastrointestinal anastomoses; if the findings are inconclusive, diagnostic laparotomy is indicated.

Native gastric atony and pylorospasm that produce early satiety or vomiting are common and self-limiting. Hypermotility of the allograft intestine occurs early after transplantation; in the absence of rejection or bacterial overgrowth, it can be controlled with agents such as paregoric, loperamide, or pectin. Sudden changes in intestinal motility, particularly when accompanied by abdominal distention and vomiting in the case of decreased motility, should initiate a search for rejection.

Infections

The frequency of infectious complications is high and is responsible for significant morbidity and mortality after intestinal transplantation. This reflects the relatively higher level of immunosuppression required to maintain the graft

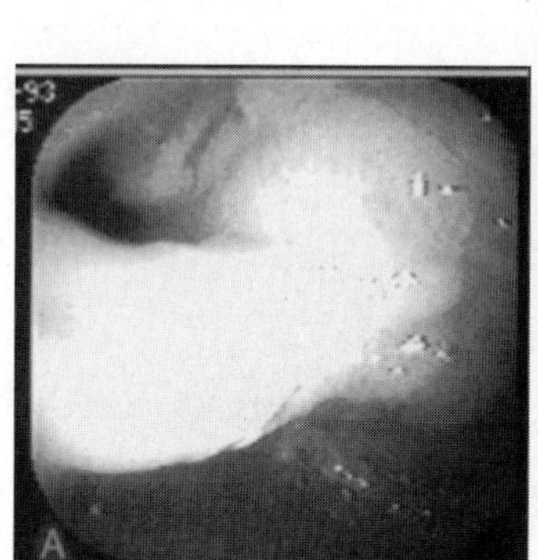

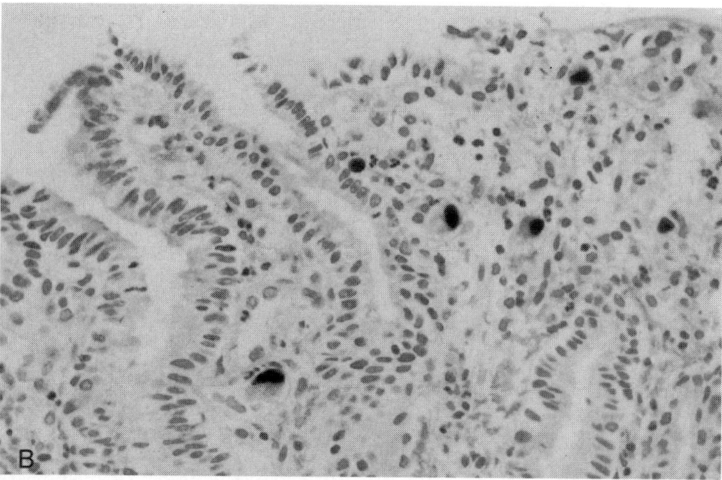

Figure 185–8. *A,* Endoscopic appearance of cytomegaloviral enteritis is characterized by hyperemic erosions. *B,* The diagnosis was confirmed histologically by the presence of characteristic inclusions, by staining for viral antigens, or both. Note the focal neutrophilic inflammation (immunoperoxidase for cytomegalovirus antigens, 350×). (See Color Plate Section of this textbook.)

in these intestinal recipients.[18] Other predisposing factors include the severity of the preoperative liver failure (in multivisceral and liver–small bowel recipients) as well as the presence of intra-abdominal, pulmonary, or intravenous line–induced sepsis before transplantation. Also, technically more difficult transplantation procedures with increased operative time, transfusion requirements, and likelihood of re-exploration reflect the advanced disease of these patients. Recipients of small bowel grafts have the lowest incidence of complications because of the more elective nature of their candidacy.

Infectious pathogens include bacteria, fungi, and viruses. Infections that present clinically relate (in order of frequency) to intravenous lines, the abdominal wound, deep abdominal abscesses, peritonitis, and pneumonia. Bacterial translocation in grafts damaged by rejection illustrates the need for concomitant antirejection and antimicrobial therapy and is a frequent source of infection.

Of the bacterial pathogens, staphylococci and enterococci are common, whereas gram-negative rods usually accompany polymicrobial infections. Not uncommonly, separate sources of infection occur simultaneously, or mixed infections from the same source are present. This leads to multiple antibiotic regimens and sets the stage for the development of resistant organisms. Particularly problematic has been the nascent strain of panresistant enterococci. Persistence of a physiologic hyperdynamic state in a patient being treated for proven infection should raise the suspicion of retained phlegmonous material in the abdomen or the possibility of rejection.

Fungal infections become problematic after heavy treatment for rejection, massive antibiotic usage, intestinal leaks, and multiple surgical explorations. The authors routinely employ low-dose amphotericin B prophylaxis in patients with these complications. Established fungal infections require long-term, full-dose antibiotic therapy and reduction or cessation of immunotherapy. All persistently septic recipients are potential candidates for moderation of immunosuppressant dosages if no coexistent cellular rejection is present.

Clinical cytomegalovirus infection is commonly seen in adult intestinal graft recipients and often involves the allograft intestine (65% of the time). A cytomegalovirus-positive donor graft transplanted into a cytomegalovirus-negative recipient is a significant risk factor, but intense baseline immunosuppression with high FK-506 levels and cumulative doses of pulse steroids is a constant feature. Clinical presentation has generally been enteritis of variable severity with focal ulcerations and bleeding (Fig. 185–8). Neither prophylactic courses of ganciclovir therapy nor passive administration of immunoglobulin has been effective in preventing cytomegalovirus infection. Avoidance of cytomegalovirus-positive grafts in cytomegalovirus-negative recipients and the reduction of immunosuppression are our present strategy for controlling cytomegalovirus infections in intestinal graft recipients.

Less commonly, respiratory syncytial virus, adenovirus, and parainfluenza virus have occurred in the pediatric population. All viral infections are opportunistic and have as a "common denominator" the need for aggressive treatment of rejection episodes in complicated patients with high Acute Physiologic and Chronic Health Evaluation scores.

Post-transplantation lymphoproliferative disease associated with the Epstein-Barr virus has occurred in three children (6% of all patients and 11% of pediatric patients) and resulted in one fatality. These patients presented with multifocal disease and were treated with intravenous acyclovir or ganciclovir as well as with cessation of immunosuppression. Rejection of the intestinal allograft may occur during the recovery phase and should be treated with steroids and reinstitution of FK-506 immunosuppression.[24]

Under the best of circumstances, the outlay of financial and time expenditures in composite and isolated small bowel transplant recipients is impressive. For best possible results, candidates who are nutritionally optimal and free of active infection should be selected. Donor organs should be discarded if they are less than perfect. Even with technically perfect operations, the managing physicians should expect a panoply of postoperative difficulties and be prepared to support these patients in all ways for an indefinite period of time. Managing the balance between excessive and inadequate immunosuppression in the face of potentially virulent infections, the pursuit of rejection and sources of infection, and maintenance of comprehensive critical care support are the most challenging tasks.

References

1. Grant D: Intestinal transplantation: Current status. Transplant Proc 1989; 21:2869–2871.

2. Lillehei RC, Goott B, Miller FA: The physiologic response of the small bowel of the dog to ischemia including prolonged in vitro preservation of the bowel with successful replacement and survival. Ann Surg 1959; 150:543.
3. Starzl TE, Kaupp HA Jr: Mass homotransplantation of abdominal organs in dogs. Surg Forum 1960; 11:28–30.
4. Starzl TE, Todo S, Tzakis A, et al: Abdominal organ cluster transplantation for the treatment of upper abdominal malignancies. Ann Surg 1989; 210:374–386.
5. Calne RY, Sells RA, Pena JR, et al: Introduction of immunologic tolerance by porcine liver allograft. Nature 1969; 223:472–474.
6. Kamada N, Davies HS, Wight D, et al: Liver transplantation in the rat: Biochemical and histological evidence of complete tolerance induction in nonrejector strains. Transplantation 1983; 35:304–311.
7. Starzl TE, Rowe M, Todo S, et al: Transplantation of multiple abdominal viscera. JAMA 1989; 261:1449–1457.
8. Grant D, Wall W, Mimeault R, et al: Successful small-bowel/liver transplantation. Lancet 1990; 335:181–184.
9. Goulet OK, Revillon Y, Jan D, et al: Small-bowel transplantation in children. Transplant Proc 1990; 22:2499.
10. Deltz E, Schroeder P, Gebhard H, et al: Successful clinical small bowel transplantation: Report of a case. Clin Transplant 1989; 3:89.
11. Oasis, Home Nutrition Support Patient Registry Annual Report—1989 Data. Albany, NY, The Oley Foundation, 1991.
12. Casella JF, Lewis JH, Bontempo FA, et al: Successful treatment for homozygous protein C deficiency by hepatic transplantation. Lancet 1988; i:435–438.
13. Starzl TE, Todo S, Tzakis A, et al: The many faces of multivisceral transplantation. Surg Gynecol Obstet 1991; 172:335–344.
14. Tzakis A, Todo S, Starzl TE: Piggyback orthotopic liver transplantation with preservation of the inferior vena cava. Ann Surg 1989; 210:649–652.
15. Todo S, Tzakis A, Abu-Elmagd K, et al: Intestinal transplantation in composite visceral grafts or alone. Ann Surg 1992; 216:223–234.
16. Takaya S, Iwaki Y, Starzl TE: Liver transplantation in positive cytotoxic crossmatch cases using FK506, high dose steroids, and prostaglandin E_1. Transplantation 1991; 54:927–933.
17. Karavias D, Jabbour N, Felekouras E, et al: Right diaphragmatic paralysis following orthotopic liver transplantation. Submitted.
18. Reyes J, Abu-Elmagd K, Tzakis A, et al: Infectious complications after human small bowel transplantation. Transplant Proc 1992; 24:1249–1250.
18a. Green M, Reyes J, Nour B, et al: Early infectious complications of liver-intestinal transplantation in children: Preliminary analysis. Transplant Proc 1994; 26:1420–1421.
19. Reyes J, Tzakis AG, Todo S, et al: Nutritional management of intestinal transplant recipients. Transplant Proc 1993; 25:1200–1201.
20. Abu-Elmagd K, Tzakis A, Todo S, et al: Monitoring and treatment of intestinal allograft rejection in humans. Transplant Proc 1993; 25:1202–1203.
21. Nakamura K, Abu-Elmagd K, Todo S, et al: Pathology of human small intestinal transplantation: Alone or in combination with the liver. Submitted.
22. Kang YG, Martin DJ, Marquez JM, et al: Intraoperative changes in blood coagulation and thromboelastographic monitoring in liver transplantation. Anesth Analg 1985; 64:888.
23. Stahl RL, Duncan A, Hooks MA, et al: A hypercoagulable state follows orthotopic liver transplantation. Hepatology 1990; 12:553.
24. Reyes J, Tzakis A, Bonet H, et al: Lymphoproliferative disease after intestinal transplantation under FK506 immunosuppression. Transplant Proc 1994; 26:1426–1427.

CHAPTER 186

Bone Marrow Transplantation

Edward D. Ball, MD • Elana J. Bloom, MD
Albert D. Donnenberg, PhD • Steven M. Pincus, MD, PhD
Witold B. Rybka, MD • Margarida deMagalhaes-Silverman, MD

Bone marrow transplantation (BMT) is increasingly used in the treatment of certain malignant as well as nonmalignant disorders (Table 186–1). The basic strategy is to give very high doses of drugs or radiation or both to ablate malignant cells or the host's lymphohematopoietic system, followed by infusion of normal stem cells. The source of these cells can be a human leukocyte antigen (HLA)-identical sibling or a partially or fully HLA-identical related or matched unrelated donor (MUD). These are called allogeneic BMT. A twin donor is sometimes used (syngeneic transplant). In autologous BMT, the recipient's bone marrow (BM) or blood-derived stem cells are used. The choice between an autologous or allogeneic BMT depends on many issues, including the disease state, the availability of a suitable donor, and the risk-benefit analysis for each patient. The age of BMT recipients has been increasing. Allogeneic BMT is now performed in patients up to 55 years of age. Autologous BMT can probably be performed up to age 70. This chapter reviews the major indications and problems associated with BMT and attempts to address the main issues in treatment of patients undergoing BMT.

INDICATIONS

The indications for BMT are steadily increasing. BMT was first applied to the leukemias and immune deficiency disorders (including aplastic anemia), but the indications have expanded to include lymphoma, solid tumors, and genetic diseases. As BMT becomes safer, the indications and the numbers of patients treated will most likely continue to increase. Some of the current indications for BMT are shown in Table 186–1.

ACUTE LEUKEMIA. Complete remission (CR) rates of 70% to 80% are achieved in the majority of patients with acute myelogenous leukemia (AML). Cure of AML can only be obtained with additional therapy. Direct comparisons of the different modalities of treatment for patients with AML in first CR have been difficult to assess. It is yet unclear whether BMT (autologous or allogeneic from HLA-identical sibling) would result in long-term leukemia-free survival superior to that with chemotherapy in patients with AML in first CR when various prognostic variables are taken into account.[1] Studies addressing this issue are under way.

TABLE 186–1. Disorders Treated with Bone Marrow Transplantation

Malignant Disorders
Acute leukemia
Chronic myelogenous leukemia
Myelodysplastic syndrome
Lymphomas
Solid tumors
Nonmalignant Disorders
Aplastic anemia
Immunologic disorders
Hemoglobinopathies
Metabolic disorders

Patients who suffer a relapse can often achieve a second CR with further induction chemotherapy but are rarely cured. Patients undergoing transplantation in second or subsequent CR or early relapse have a 30% to 50% disease-free survival (DFS) after allogeneic or autologous BMT.[2]

For adults with acute lymphoblastic leukemia (ALL), CR rates of 75% to 95% can be obtained using intensive regimens. The use of allogeneic BMT in first CR in adults with ALL is also controversial.[3] An analysis in the International Bone Marrow Transplant Registry showed a 5-year leukemia-free survival probability of 38% with chemotherapy alone and of 44% with allogeneic BMT. Some groups, however, recommend allogeneic BMT for adults who have certain high-risk factors and ALL in first CR. As with AML, patients with ALL who suffer relapse or those who have resistant disease have a poor prognosis. About 30% of these patients may be salvaged by allogeneic BMT. Autologous BMT for ALL yields fewer long-term periods of DFS.[3] The National Marrow Donor Program reported on the use of MUD transplants in acute leukemia (AML and ALL). The probability of DFS at 1.5 years was 45% in 58 patients in first and second CR and 19% in 98 patients with more advanced disease.

LYMPHOMAS. Most data on BMT in lymphoma are from autologous BMT; relatively few HLA-identical transplants are reported.[4, 5] Patients who have aggressive non-Hodgkin's lymphoma and are not cured with their initial chemotherapy regimen have a poor outcome. During the past few years, high-dose chemotherapy with autologous or allogeneic BMT has been increasingly used. Patients whose tumor fails to respond initially with chemotherapy have an extremely poor prognosis even when high-dose chemotherapy is used.[4] Patients who achieve an initial complete response and then suffer relapse are those in whom the results of high-dose chemotherapy are most encouraging. The real question for these patients suffering relapse is whether BMT is better than conventional therapy. Prospective trials are under way to answer this question.

In advanced Hodgkin's disease, high-dose chemotherapy with BM rescue has been used.[5a] Results from retrospective studies have shown efficacy of this strategy in disease refractory to front-line therapy, in early relapse, and even in second or subsequent CR.

CHRONIC MYELOGENOUS LEUKEMIA. BMT using marrow from related donors or MUD is the only known curative therapy for chronic myelogenous leukemia (CML).[6] Using an HLA-identical sibling, 50% to 65% of patients in the chronic phase can be cured. When patients undergo transplantation in accelerated phase, only 15% to 30% are expected to be cured, and if BMT is performed in patients in blast crisis, approximately 10% of the patients are expected to have long-term DFS. Best results with allogeneic BMT in CML are obtained in persons who are younger than 20 years and who receive a transplant in chronic phase within the first year of diagnosis. For patients who do not have an HLA-identical sibling, BMT with an HLA-identical MUD is an option.[7] The data on 102 consecutive patients who had CML and who received an allogeneic BMT from a MUD have been published. A 29% DFS at 2½ years was observed. Interest has been expressed in the possibility that patients with CML may be cured by high-dose chemotherapy followed by autologous rescue with BM or blood-derived stem cells.[7a] Data from numerous sources suggest that benign Philadelphia chromosome–negative hematopoietic stem cells exist with their malignant counterparts in a vast majority of patients with CML.

APLASTIC ANEMIA. Among nonmalignant disorders, the largest number of allogeneic BMT have been carried out for the treatment of severe aplastic anemia. With supportive treatment alone, only 20% to 30% of patients with severe aplastic anemia will be alive 2 years after diagnosis.[8] If an allogeneic BMT from an HLA-identical donor is performed soon after the diagnosis in a nontransfused patient, the long-term survival exceeds 80%. Transfused patients have a probability of survival of about 60% to 70%. BMT from HLA-identical MUD has also been performed in patients with severe aplastic anemia. A report from five centers on 40 unrelated BMT for severe aplastic anemia reported a 28% survival rate.

MYELODYSPLASTIC SYNDROME. Patients with myelodysplastic syndrome represent a treatment challenge. No specific effective therapy currently exists for this syndrome. Allogeneic BMT has been used in patients who have myelodysplastic syndrome and are younger than 50 years and have a histocompatible donor.[9] DFS at 3 years is estimated at 45%. Autologous BMT has been tested in a few patients whose MDS has transformed into acute leukemia, but early results are not encouraging.

GERM CELL TUMORS. Approximately 30% of patients with germ cell tumors suffer a relapse or are unresponsive to first-line chemotherapy. For patients who fail to experience a complete response to initial induction therapy or who fail standard-dose salvage chemotherapy, dose-intensive therapy with autologous BMT is an option. A review of the published literature shows that this approach results in a durable, complete response (3–42 mo) in about 10% to 20% of heavily pretreated patients and represents a curative option in patients who otherwise would die of their disease.

BREAST CANCER. Metastatic breast cancer is essentially incurable. The overall median survival of afflicted women is about 2 years. High-dose chemotherapy followed by autologous BMT or peripheral stem cell rescue has been used in patients with metastatic hormone-unresponsive breast cancer. When such a strategy is used in heavily pretreated patients with refractory metastatic disease, the results are dismal and the responses obtained are not durable. The most recent generation of clinical studies with high-dose chemotherapy has included a standard-dose induction regimen implemented to the point of maximum response, followed by the administration of high-dose chemotherapy as consolidation.[10, 11] The complete response rate achieved with this strategy is about 50%, and 20% to 30% of women are in continuous complete response with a follow-up interval of 18 to 40 months from the time of BMT. Based on the high complete response rates and durable remissions in patients with metastatic disease, trials of primary or adjuvant intensive therapy and autologous BMT were initiated in patients with locally advanced breast cancer (inflammatory or stage III or stage II disease with more than 10 positive nodes). These women have 85% probability of relapse within 10 years. Randomized trials assessing the efficacy of dose-intensive therapy and autologous BMT in stage II (with 10 or more positive nodes), III, and IV breast cancer are under way.

OTHER SOLID TUMORS. Intensive therapy with autologous BMT has been tried for patients with other solid tumors. Trials of dose-intensive therapy for sarcomas, gliomas, and malignant melanomas have not shown any significant benefit. However, early results of high-dose chemotherapy with BMT or peripheral stem cell rescue in patients with ovarian cancer or neuroblastoma are encouraging.

MANIPULATION OF THE GRAFT

Tumor Cell Purging

Because autologous BMT may contain occult tumor cells that could contribute to relapse, various methods to deplete tumor cells from autografts have been developed. Purging of BM is commonly used in autologous BMT for leukemia, lymphoma, neuroblastoma, and breast cancer. The most commonly used methods use chemical agents or monoclonal antibodies (mAb).

Cyclophosphamide congeners, including mafosfamid and 4-hydroperoxycyclophosphamide (4-HC), have been extensively used for BM purging in the leukemias,[12] lymphoma, and breast cancer.[13] These compounds are cytotoxic to both lymphoid and myeloid leukemia cells, including normal colony-forming cells (hematopoietic progenitors). Long-term BM cultures indicate that earlier progenitor cells are spared, and clinical BMT has shown that BM repopulation after myeloablative therapy does occur. Purging with 4-HC has been applied to autologous BMT in AML, ALL, breast cancer, and lymphoma.

A large number of murine mAb reactive with antigens present on hematopoietic and solid tumors are available for purging of malignant cells from BM.[14] Complement-mediated (C′) lysis has been the most frequently used method of achieving tumor cell lysis with mAb. Repeated treatment with mAb and C′ is capable of removing four to six logs of tumor cells.[15] It is important that the mAb not react with and destroy large numbers of normal BM hematopoietic progenitor cells.

Monoclonal antibody purging has been used for the treatment of AML, ALL, lymphoma, breast cancer, and neuroblastoma. Patients who have AML and undergo transplantation with autologous BM purged with two mAb (PM-81 and AML-2-23) in second and third CR experienced a 3-year DFS of 50%.[16] Similarly, patients with malignant lymphoma undergoing autologous BMT with B1 and B4 mAb and C′ purged BM had a 50% probability of remaining disease free 37.8 months after BMT. Purging was monitored by polymerase chain reaction, focusing on the bcl2 transcript.[17] If the polymerase chain reaction was not rendered negative after purging, the relapse rate was much higher.

An alternative method of purging involves the use of magnetic microspheres, or magnetic colloids. The method consists of reacting the target cells with mAb followed by incubation with antimouse immunoglobulin-coated immunomagnetic beads. Alternatively, the mAb may be conjugated or absorbed onto the immunomagnetic beads directly. The magnetized cellular particles are then passed over a magnet, which removes the magnetized particles and allows the unbound cells to pass through into a collection system. This method has also been applied to the removal of lymphoma cells, small-cell carcinoma of the lung cells, neuroblastoma cells, and breast carcinoma cells.[13, 18]

Another alternative to BM purging is to enrich for hematopoietic stem cells. This may be accomplished using mAb to the CD34 antigen, which is expressed on hematopoietic progenitor cells and probably the true stem cell.[19] Immunoabsorption column-based approaches using the CD34 mAb 12.8 to enrich for hematopoietic progenitors for autologous BMT have been developed. Enriched CD34-positive cells have been successfully used to reconstitute BM after myeloablative chemotherapy in patients with metastatic breast cancer and neuroblastoma.[20]

The evaluation of BM purging is problematic because relapse can occur from failure to eradicate cells both in vivo and in vitro. Evaluation of purging in lymphoma is aided by the common existence of the translocation t(14;18) with rearrangement of the bcl-2 proto-oncogene. Relapse was more common in cases of malignant lymphoma in which residual disease was still present, as shown by polymerase chain reaction amplification of the t(14;18) breakpoint after BM purging with mAb and C′.[17] Genetically tagged BM cells from patients with AML were present in leukemia cells at relapse, suggesting that occult leukemia cells in the BM are capable of contributing to relapse.[21]

T Cell Depletion

Elimination of mature T lymphocytes from the BM allografts by various methods has markedly reduced the incidence and severity of acute and chronic graft-versus-host disease (GVHD). The incidence of acute GVHD has been reduced to 10% to 11% in recipients of T cell–depleted HLA-matched BM grafts. Significant reductions have also been noted in partially matched familial and MUD transplant recipients. To date, elimination of this life-threatening complication through allograft T cell depletion has not lived up to its potential for improving the overall success of allogeneic BMT. Increased incidence of graft failure and increased leukemic relapse in some diseases, most notably CML, have offset the advantages of GVHD ablation to the extent that in the aggregate, DFS in T cell–depleted and T cell–replete allogeneic BMT is similar. This observation suggests that T cell depletion, as currently practiced, may not be equally indicated in all instances of allogeneic BMT. Factors such as the source of the graft (partially matched familial or MUD) or a patient's age can affect GVHD incidence, severity, or consequent morbidity and mortality. Thus, T cell depletion may be of significant benefit for particular diseases or risk groups.

Various methods have been proposed for T cell depletion. Among the most widely used are mAb-based negative selection techniques, separation based on lectin-mediated agglutination, and physical separation by size and density. Remarkably, similar success in elimination of acute GVHD has been reported for all of these processes, providing that they achieved a T cell reduction on the order of 2 logs. Interpretation of reported differences in the incidence of T cell depletion–related complications are hampered by differences in patient selection and the small sample size of diagnosis-specific groups in individual studies.

Monoclonal Antibody-Based Methods

Monoclonal antibodies represent an important tool for graft processing. Monoclonal antibodies directed against determinants expressed on T cells, T cell subsets, as well as non–T lymphocytes have been used alone and in combination in clinical trials. These include OKT3 (anti-CD3), Campath-1 (CDw52), anti-CD2, -CD3, -CD4, -CD5, -CD6, and -CD8 plus Tp44, CT2 (anti-CD2), anti-CD6 plus -CD8,[22] anti-CD2, -CD5 plus -CD7, anti-CD5 alone, and anti-CD8 alone.[23] Several different mAb-based technologies are available for T cell depletion. These include incubation with complement, antiglobulin-conjugated magnetic beads, conjugation to immunotoxins, and conjugation to solid-phase substrates. Most of these methods, when optimally applied, yield a depletion of two to three orders of magnitude[24] and thus are sufficient to prevent GVHD in the majority of HLA-matched BMT.

Soybean Agglutinin and E-Rosette Depletion

Agglutination using a lectin derived from soybeans (SBA) formed the basis for the first clinically successful implementation of BMT with lymphocyte-depleted BM. Preclinical experiments using human BM revealed that the majority of clonogenic myeloid cells are SBA negative and that SBA could be used to agglutinate and deplete a wide variety of lineage-committed cells including lymphocytes. Addition of a second round of depletion using treated sheep red blood cells, which bind to T cells via the T cell–specific surface determinant CD2, permitted up to 3 logs of T cell depletion.

The SBA positive fraction is irradiated and infused with the SBA negative/E-rosette–negative fraction (about 5 × 10^7 cells/kg).

Elutriation

Counterflow centrifugal elutriation (CCE) separates cells on the basis of size and density. It takes advantage of the observation that the majority of myeloid clonogenic cells can be isolated in a "large-cell" fraction that is depleted of lymphocytes. The method is rapid and reproducible and does not destroy the lymphocyte-rich fractions. Protocols initiated at the Johns Hopkins Oncology Center and the Pittsburgh Cancer Institute have standardized the degree of lymphocyte depletion by adding back a specified number of lymphocytes determined on the basis of a recipient's ideal body weight. The rationale is to recover some of the beneficial effects of graft lymphocytes (promotion of engraftment, antileukemic effect) while preventing GVHD. At a dose of 0.5 × 10^6 lymphocytes per kilogram,[25] no patients receiving BM from a matched sibling died of or developed organ GVHD (≥stage II) or chronic GVHD. The incidence of grade 1 GVHD was 15%. Stable engraftment occurred in 95%. Overall actuarial 2-year survival for 60 high-risk patients receiving CCE-engineered BM was 50%. Combining data from two published trials of CCE-lymphocyte depletion,[25] DFS was dependent on the original diagnosis: 60% (at 24 mo) in acute leukemias but only 21% in CML.[26]

GRAFT-VERSUS-HOST DISEASE

GVHD is a complication of transplantation unique to allogeneic BMT. It occurs if the following requirements are met: (1) immunologically competent donor T lymphocytes are present in the graft, (2) they recognize host alloantigens as incompatible, and (3) the host lacks immunocompetence to mount an effective immunologic reaction (i.e., rejection) against these attacking cells.[27] This may occur despite a donor being an HLA-identical sibling and having nonreactive in vitro testing by mixed lymphocytic culture. However, GVHD increases in frequency and severity with the use of a MUD, presumably because of histocompatibility differences undetected by current HLA testing. GVHD in syngeneic (identical twin) and autologous BMT may also occur. It is thought to be due to autoreactivity (i.e., failure to develop mechanisms of self-tolerance).

Effector Cells and Target Antigens

Unmanipulated BM allografts typically contain 2 to 5 billion mature T cells. Animal data and clinical experience indicate that the effector cells that mediate acute GVHD make up a potent but small subpopulation of these mature T cells. In animal models of major histocompatibility complex (MHC) mismatched allogeneic BMT, CD8+ T cells are responsible for GVHD directed against MHC class I differences, and CD4+ T cells account for MHC class II–specific disease. In humans, the great majority of allogeneic BMT performed to date have relied on the availability of fully MHC-matched sibling donors. Despite this, more than half of the recipients of grafts obtained from these matched sibling donors develop clinically significant GVHD. The target antigens of such responses are presumed to be minor histocompatibility determinants. Although animal models provide support for the GVHD directed against minor histocompatibility antigens, the absence or presence of GVHD cannot be predicted solely on the basis of such genetic disparities. In patients receiving second allogeneic BMT from the same matched sibling donor, GVHD outcomes in the first and second transplants were often discordant.[27]

Incidence and Risk

Despite modern serologic and molecular HLA typing techniques to confirm compatibility of donor and recipient, GVHD continues to be a major cause of morbidity and mortality associated with BMT. Clinically significant GVHD incidence is 45% (25–70%) in patients receiving HLA-identical sibling BM and occurs in virtually all recipients of incompatible or MUD BM. Risk factors for development of GVHD include HLA disparity, female-to-male (donor-recipient) transplant, older age, and prophylaxis regimens or T cell depletion used for prevention of GVHD. In addition, the type of leukemia, viral infections, cytomegalovirus (CMV) status, HLA type, donor alloimmunity (pregnancy or transfusion), splenectomy, and T cell dose have been reported to affect the risk of GVHD.[28]

The spectrum of GVHD encompasses two forms: acute GVHD and chronic GVHD. They are distinctive with respect to rate of progression, time of onset, and response to treatment. However, because acute GVHD may be the greatest risk factor for developing chronic GVHD, prevention of both forms is logical.

Prophylaxis of GVHD consists of immunosuppressives such as corticosteroids, methotrexate, and cyclosporin. Methotrexate and cyclosporin are equally effective in preventing GVHD, and a combination of both drugs is better than either drug alone, resulting in improved survival. The addition of corticosteroids to methotrexate, cyclosporin, or antithymocyte globulin is more effective than any single-drug therapy. Administration of intravenous immunoglobulin and pentoxifylline and elimination of T lymphocytes from the donor BM before transplantation (T cell depletion) have been associated with a reduction in the incidence of GVHD. Total elimination of GVHD in patients with leukemia may cause loss of graft-versus-leukemia effect, resulting in increased relapse rates and adverse effects on long-term survival. Experimental prophylactic agents include thalidomide, zolimomab artiox (Xomazyme-CD5), tacrolimus (FK-506), and mAb against lymphocyte cytokine receptors on T lymphocytes (e.g., anti-interleukin-2-receptor antibody). Current research efforts are also directed toward elimination of GVHD without compromising the graft-versus-leukemia effect.

Acute Graft-Versus-Host Disease

Acute GVHD, which generally occurs within the first 100 days after allogeneic transplant, may affect the skin, gastrointestinal (GI) tract, and liver. The first manifestation is often an erythematous maculopapular rash involving face, neck, palms, and soles, associated with pain or tingling of the extremities. This may be accompanied by fever and flu-like symptoms. The rash may be localized or may involve the entire body with formation of bullae and desquamation. Insensible fluid loss and superinfection are critical care issues in the face of epidermolysis of GVHD. The characteristic progression of rash (distal to proximal), pruritus, and onset coinciding with early engraftment help a clinician differentiate acute GVHD from drug eruptions, chemotherapy effect, and infectious skin diseases. However, biopsy is mandatory to confirm the diagnosis.

Immunopathology of Acute Graft-Versus-Host Disease

Cutaneous acute GVHD is recognized histologically by epidermal necrosis and dyskeratosis, as well as perivascular

TABLE 186–2. Clinical Staging of Acute Graft-Versus-Host Disease

Grade	*Skin*	*Liver*	*Gut*
I	<25% body surface area	Bilirubin 2–3 mg/dL	Diarrhea 500–1000 mL/d
II	25–50% body surface area	Bilirubin 3–6 mg/dL	Diarrhea 1000–1500 mL/d
III	Generalized	Bilirubin 6–15 mg/dL	Diarrhea >1500 mL/d
IV	Desquamation	Bilirubin >15 mg/dL	Ileus

mononuclear cell infiltration of the dermis and lower epidermis. Although immunohistochemical studies have identified the preponderance of these mononuclear cells as T lymphocytes,[29] natural killer (NK) cells have also been observed. Attempts to characterize the T cell–target cell interactions underlying GVHD have led to identification of intercellular adhesion molecules and HLA-DR expression on keratinocytes, as well as the detection of T cells bearing a determinant associated with skin localization. The hypothesis that epidermal destruction is mediated directly by cytotoxic T cells is supported by the observation that a high proportion of CD8+ T cells detected in cutaneous GVHD lesions are serine protease positive (i.e, putative cytotoxic effector cells). Despite this evidence, a controlled prospective study failed to reveal differences in the distribution of lymphocytes in skin biopsy samples from recipients of BM autografts and recipients of allografts (with and without acute GVHD).

Intestinal GVHD presents as secretory, often bloody diarrhea with cramping abdominal pain, nausea, and vomiting. Despite stopping oral intake, high stool volumes (several liters per day) persist. (This diarrhea may overlap temporally with that caused by chemotherapy-induced damage to mucosa.) Stool studies reveal no pathogens and few, if any, leukocytes. Superimposed viral or fungal infection is not rare and must also be ruled out. Radiologic studies (generally not required for diagnosis) reveal a thickened bowel wall, loss of haustral markings, and rapid transit time. Computed tomography scans show thickened bowel. Histologic confirmation of GVHD is necessary and may be done by sigmoidoscopy. However, the upper GI tract may be involved also (with or without symptoms of anorexia, dyspepsia, or food intolerance); therefore, upper and lower endoscopic biopsies are recommended.[30, 31]

Liver involvement may occur simultaneously or follow the onset of rash by several days, with elevated bilirubin and alkaline phosphatase levels and subsequent elevation of transaminases. Differential diagnosis includes veno-occlusive disease (VOD) of the liver, gallstones, and cholestasis caused by total parenteral support or drugs (including cyclosporin). If coagulation and platelet support is adequate, histologic confirmation by liver biopsy should be made in equivocal cases such as those without diagnostic skin or gut histology.

Clinical staging of each organ site (Table 186–2) and grading (Table 186–3) of overall GVHD status uses relatively gross measurements yet has significant prognostic value, with grades III to IV associated with significant mortality.

TABLE 186–3. Clinical Grade of Graft-Versus-Host Disease

Grade	
I	Skin + to + +, no gut or liver involvement
II	Skin + to + + +, gut + or liver + (or both)
III	Skin + + to + + +, gut + + to + + + or liver + + to + + + (or both)
IV	Any organ + + + +

Treatment of Graft-Versus-Host Disease

Although literature and trials of GVHD prophylaxis abound, fewer studies have been conducted for treatment of GVHD and results are less than satisfactory. Once established, GVHD is difficult to cure. Corticosteroids (methylprednisolone, 2–5 mg · kg^{-1} · d^{-1} IV in divided doses) and intravenous cyclosporin together are first-line treatments with overall response rates less than 50% for grades III to IV GVHD.[32] Complete response rates of 20% are found using conventional prophylaxis therapy for acute GVHD in MUD transplant recipients.[33] Infections, fluid retention, and hyperglycemia while on high-dose steroids may further compromise these patients. For patients who fail initial treatment of GVHD, second-line therapies may include FK-506 (tacrolimus), Xomazyme-H65 (anti-CD5 mAb, conjugated to the cytotoxic enzyme ricin A), antithymocyte globulin, antitumor necrosis factor-α mAb (BC7), anti-T cell mAb (OKT3), and interleukin-2 receptor mAb.[34] Results have varied, but in general, skin and gut GVHD may be responsive to second-line therapy; however, only skin GVHD shows appreciable CR (up to 40–50%). Sandostatin (Sandoz Pharmaceutical Corporation), a synthetic somatostatin analog useful in some secretory diarrheal diseases, has been beneficial as an adjunct therapy for acute GVHD of the intestine.[35] Critical care management of these patients includes total parenteral nutrition support (to avoid a catabolic state) and slow reintroduction of low-fat, lactose-free diets. A formal "GVHD diet" has been proposed for this purpose.

The effect of acute GVHD on immune reconstitution has been difficult to assess. It typically occurs at a time when T cell responses are markedly reduced, and it is treated by prompt initiation of immunosuppressive therapy. These agents exert variable effects on the adoptive transfer of donor immunity. Experimental immunization of BM donors and recipients was undertaken to determine the effects of two immunoprophylactic regimens, independent of GVHD. These studies indicated that the combination of cyclosporin and methylprednisolone did not prevent transfer of donor responses to recall antigens but virtually eliminated transfer of primary immunity to novel antigens. In contrast, cyclophosphamide plus methylprednisolone spared responses to a novel antigen (sheep erythrocytes) but blunted the transfer of tetanus toxoid–specific memory cells. It is not clear whether GVHD-induced immunopathology results in increased susceptibility to infection or the presence of viral infections in the early post-BMT period predisposes to acute GVHD. With these caveats in mind, the pace of T cell and B cell reconstitution is retarded in patients with GVHD. This may be explained in part by alloimmune alteration of lymph node architecture.[36] Chronic GVHD is clearly immnosuppressive and is often accompanied by systemic effects on the immune system such as dysregulation of immunoglobulin synthesis, lymphopenia, and functional asplenism. Because patients with significant chronic GVHD are at greatest risk of significant bacterial infections, immunization with pneumococcal, meningococcal, and *Haemophilus influenzae* type B vaccines is desirable. Although no information on the efficacy of immunization in this group is available, it would predictably be considerably lower than that in the absence of chronic GVHD. Successful immunization with tetanus and diphtheria toxoids has been reported in a proportion of patients with chronic GVHD.[37]

Autologous Graft-Versus-Host Disease

Anecdotal reports of GVHD-like skin rashes in autologous BMT have since been confirmed by the observation that a syndrome indistinguishable from cutaneous GVHD can be reproducibly elicited by administration of cyclosporin in the post-BMT period. Ongoing clinical trials are designed to determine whether this GVHD-like syndrome is associated with an antileukemic effect, as it appears to be in allogeneic BMT.

Chronic Graft-Versus-Host Disease

Chronic GVHD (Table 186–4), a late complication of allogeneic BMT, occurs in 60% of patients surviving more than 100 days after BMT. This syndrome resembles an autoimmune disorder involving lacrimal and salivary glands, with dry eyes and mouth (Sjögren-like syndrome), and skin fibrosis, with damage to adnexal structures (sweat glands, hair follicles, subcutaneous nerves) and hyper- or hypopigmentation of the skin. The GI tract may be involved with lichenoid oral mucosal changes, esophageal constriction with web formation, malabsorption, weight loss, and liver function abnormalities of cholestasis. Muscles and joints may be involved with myositis, polyserositis, and joint contractures. These manifestations may be chronically debilitating, but pulmonary involvement with bronchiolitis obliterans is most life threatening.[38] The BM graft and immune system are often affected by GVHD. Thrombocytopenia is correlated with poor outcome of chronic GVHD,[39] and immunoglobulin replacement may be helpful in preventing recurrent infections.

Treatment of chronic GVHD has relied largely on steroids. A regimen of alternating-day steroids and cyclosporin has been proposed for refractory disease. However, more potent or additional immunosuppression is often needed for this chronic, debilitating disorder. FK-506 (tacrolimus) has been used successfully at the University of Pittsburgh in patients with severe chronic GVHD including severe liver GVHD and bronchiolitis obliterans.[40] Other agents and modalities include thalidomide, ursodeoxycholic acid, photopheresis, and psoralin ultraviolet A.[41, 42]

New Approaches

Prediction of Graft-Versus-Host Disease

The ability to predict the outcome of GVHD would offer obvious advantages in donor selection and in choice of prophylactic strategy. The use of an assay involving cocultivation of primed donor lymphocytes with a patient's skin[43] has permitted prospective identification of patients with a sixfold higher relative risk of acute GVHD of stage II or greater. A positive or inconclusive result in this skin explant assay has been used as an inclusion criterion for a clinical trial of T cell depletion.[25] Another approach has been to assess the ability of BM donors to mount mixed lymphocyte reactions against histocompatibility antigens expressed on "third-party" transformed B cell lines. This entirely nonspecific evaluation of donor alloreactivity identified patients with a 4.5-fold relative risk of developing GVHD of grades II to IV.

Once the BMT has been performed, careful monitoring of the clinical parameters used to stage acute GVHD can provide information about the likelihood of disease progression.[44] Peak values for extent of rash, bilirubin, and daily stool output were usually reached earlier than 40 days after BMT. In 69 patients with biopsy-proven acute GVHD, the magnitude of these peak values was predictive of disease progression.

Graft Engineering

In graft engineering, BM grafts with defined hematopoietic and immunologic characteristics are formulated. Current examples of graft engineering include efforts to control the T cell dose, to augment the stem cell content of T cell–depleted allografts, or to eliminate specific T cell subsets. Among the latter are exclusion of CD5+ T cells (and consequent inclusion of CD5− mature T cells and NK cells), exclusion of CD8+ T cells (and inclusion of CD4+ T cells and CD8− NK cells),[23] and exclusion of CD4+ T cells (and inclusion of NK cells and CD8+ T cells). As the diversity of approaches demonstrates, these attempts are only first approximations of the ultimate goal, which is to formulate a preparation that reliably and rapidly engrafts, has enhanced antitumor and antimicrobial activity, and is tolerant of the host. Although benefit may be derived from further manipulating BM ablative or postgrafting immunosuppressive regimens, it is likely that the next significant increment in clinical benefit will require integration of physical and immunologic separation technologies. These may be combined with in vitro expansion of immune effectors and in vivo cytokine administration to provide the desired therapeutic effects.

TABLE 186–4. Chronic Graft-Versus-Host Disease

Limited
Localized skin involvement
Hepatic dysfunction
Extensive
Generalized skin involvement
Local skin and/or hepatic dysfunction plus:
- Liver with histology of cirrhosis or chronic aggressive hepatitis
- Eye involvement
- Oral mucosa or salivary gland
- Other target organ involvement

INFECTIOUS COMPLICATIONS OF BONE MARROW TRANSPLANTATION

Despite advances in the management of infectious complications of BMT, infections remain the most frequent cause of morbidity and mortality after BMT.[45] The infections most commonly developing after BMT occur during specific periods that are related to the immunocompetence of the patient and are termed the *early, middle,* and *late* periods of infectious risk (Table 186–5).

The *early period* after BMT is marked by severe neutropenia, lymphopenia, mucositis, and gastroenteritis due to the toxicity of the chemotherapy and radiation therapy. Further immunosuppression due to the prophylactic measures used to prevent acute GVHD also increase the infectious risk in allogeneic BMT. Common pathogens during the first month after BMT are *Staphylococcus, Streptococcus,* herpes simplex virus (HSV), and *Candida.* After mucositis and neutropenia have resolved, the risk of bacterial infection decreases. However, humoral and cellular immunodeficiencies persist for long periods after BMT and are especially severe in patients being treated for acute or chronic GVHD. The *middle period,* from engraftment until 100 days after BMT, is

TABLE 186–5. Peak Incidence of Infections After Bone Marrow Transplantation

Early (<30 d)	*Middle (30–100 d)*	*Late (>100 d)*
Staphylococcus	*Aspergillus*	Pneumococcus
Streptococcus	*Pneumocystis carinii*	*Haemophilus influenzae*
Gram-negative enterics	*Toxoplasma gondii*	Varicella-zoster
Candida albicans	Cytomegalovirus	
Herpes simplex	Adenovirus	
	JK virus	

characterized by infections due to CMV, *Pneumocystis carinii,* and *Aspergillus* species. During the *late period* after BMT, herpes zoster and encapsulated bacterial infections are prominent. In the absence of chronic GVHD, cellular and humoral immunity return to normal over a 1- to 2-year period.

Major reductions in infectious complications after BMT have been achieved by using the strategies of prophylactic and empirical antibiotic therapy.[45] Reverse isolation and strict hand washing are other approaches that are generally accepted as standard practice to decrease nosocomial transmission of infection. The use of chlorhexidine and nystatin mouthwashes also reduces the infectious risk posed by mucositis due to the suppression of oral flora.

Bacterial Infections

Gram-positive bacteria remain a common cause of morbidity in BMT and an occasional cause of mortality. The use of multilumen central venous catheters has resulted in an increased incidence of staphylococcal bacteremia. Furthermore, with the widespread use of prophylactic antibiotics for gram-negative bacteria, there has been a relative increase in the frequency of bacteremia due to gram-positive isolates. The use of vancomycin prophylactically has been very effective in reducing documented gram-positive infections.[46] Streptococcal bacteremia also occurs frequently in neutropenic patients who are not receiving prophylactic gram-positive coverage.[47] Sepsis and death due to *Streptococcus mitis* have been reported in neutropenic patients after BMT. Risk factors are severe mucositis, young age, and lack of prophylaxis for gram-positive organisms. Therefore, initiation of gram-positive coverage at first neutropenic fever is highly recommended if prophylaxis is not used. Sinopulmonary pneumococcal infections frequently occur in the late period after BMT owing to the impairment in opsonization and functional asplenia. Prophylaxis with trimethoprim-sulfamethoxazole several days a week prevents this complication.

Neutropenic patients are especially prone to infections due to gram-negative bacteria. The mucositis and gastroenteritis present during neutropenia allow easy access of enteric organisms into the bloodstream. Historically, the first neutropenic fever was caused by *Escherichia coli, Klebsiella, Pseudomonas,* or other facultative anaerobes. Neutropenic patients with BMT must immediately be given broad-spectrum gram-negative antibiotic coverage at the sign of first fever. Traditionally, a semi-synthetic penicillin or an antipseudomonal cephalosporin has been combined with an aminoglycoside. The nephrotoxicity of the aminoglycoside can be avoided by the use of either imipenem-cilastatin or double β-lactam regimens. Both approaches have been demonstrated to be equally effective as aminoglycoside-containing regimens for empirical initial therapy in febrile neutropenic patients.[48, 49]

Because of the frequency and severity of gram-negative infections in neutropenic hosts, much effort has been devoted to developing effective prophylaxis. The agents with the greatest success in achieving gram-negative prophylaxis are the fluoroquinolones. The effectiveness of oral ciprofloxacin prophylaxis after BMT compared with placebo was demonstrated in a small randomized trial.[50] In a large randomized trial that contained significant numbers of neutropenic BMT recipients with hematologic malignancies, ciprofloxacin was found to be superior to norfloxacin in decreasing the incidence of documented gram-negative bacteremia. The ciprofloxacin arm also had a lower incidence of neutropenic fevers. The prophylactic antibiotic can be discontinued at the time of first neutropenic fever when broad-spectrum gram-negative coverage is initiated, or, if a patient remains afebrile, when neutropenia resolves.

Fungal Infections

BMT recipients are at high risk for mucositis or invasive fungal infections due to neutropenia. They are often receiving therapy with corticosteroids and have an indwelling central venous catheter. The most frequent pathogens are *Candida* species, especially *Candida albicans,* and *Aspergillus* species. Less commonly encountered are fusaridiosis and mucormycosis.

Antifungal therapy continues to rely on amphotericin B; however, the response of documented aspergillosis to amphotericin in a neutropenic host is rather poor. Survival and response rates are improved when amphotericin is begun empirically in patients with febrile neutropenia not responding to broad-spectrum antibacterial antibiotics.[51] Because of the toxicity of standard amphotericin, efforts to find alternatives have been ongoing. A liposomal formulation of amphotericin B has significantly less toxicity yet appears to retain activity. Effectiveness of liposomal amphotericin for treatment of documented fungal infections in BMT recipients has not yet been established. The use of liposomal amphotericin B prophylactically in BMT recipients was studied in a randomized, placebo-controlled trial.[52] The investigators concluded that prophylactic liposomal amphotericin B was well tolerated, reduced fungal colonization, and reduced the incidence of systemic fungal infections.

Fluconazole has been efficacious as antifungal prophylaxis for *Candida* when started at the beginning of neutropenia.[53] The overall frequency of *Candida* colonization and infection was markedly reduced compared with retrospective controls. Interestingly, an increased incidence of *Candida krusei* infections resistant to fluconazole has been reported.[53, 54] An alternative to fluconazole may be itraconazole, which has activity against *Aspergillus* in vitro, but it is not yet known whether it will be as effective as amphotericin clinically.

Viral Infections

The herpesviruses are the most frequent cause of viral infection in BMT recipients. Members of the herpesvirus family include CMV, HSV, varicella-zoster virus (VZV), human herpesvirus 6, and Epstein-Barr virus. These infections are usually caused by reactivation of dormant virus. Other viruses that may occur after BMT include the BK and JC viruses, adenovirus, and respiratory syncytial virus. Post-BMT viral hepatitis is much less frequent than previously, owing to the screening of blood products for hepatitis C.

The most common infectious cause of death after allogeneic BMT is CMV infection. The most life-threatening presentation is CMV pneumonia, which has been fatal in as many as 85% of affected patients. CMV can also cause gastroenteritis, BM suppression, hepatitis, and less commonly retinitis or encephalitis. CMV infection may be manifested only by fever and viremia. Most CMV infections occur during the middle period of infectious risk. More than half of CMV-seropositive patients develop CMV infection if no prophylaxis is used. Other risk factors for CMV infection include severe GVHD and the use of total-body irradiation in the preparative regimen. The risk of CMV infection in seronegative patients can be eliminated by the use of a seronegative BM donor and seronegative blood products for transfusion.[55] Another major warning sign of CMV pneumonia is the development of CMV viremia in surveillance blood cultures.[56]

The definitive diagnosis of CMV pneumonia can be difficult to obtain, because it usually requires lung biopsy. The presence of viral inclusion bodies in cytology specimens obtained by bronchoalveolar lavage (BAL) or the culture of CMV from BAL fluid is sufficient for a presumptive diagnosis of CMV pneumonia in patients with interstitial pneumonitis.

Treatment of CMV pneumonia has been more satisfying since the demonstration that the combination of ganciclovir and intravenous immune globulin can reduce the mortality of this infection.[57] Those patients in whom therapy is initiated early are most likely to benefit. Research efforts have attempted to identify those patients who have early CMV infections and to target them for treatment. One approach was to perform BAL on all asymptomatic patients on day 35 after BMT. Asymptomatic CMV infection of the lungs was identified as a major risk factor for CMV pneumonia.[58] Those patients who were randomized to prophylactic ganciclovir did not develop CMV pneumonia. Another study used CMV excretion at any site as a basis for randomization to placebo or ganciclovir. The researchers concluded that early treatment with ganciclovir reduced CMV disease and improved survival.

Two trials of ganciclovir prophylaxis for all patients seropositive for CMV were reported. Patients were randomly assigned to receive ganciclovir or placebo at the time of engraftment. In one study, ganciclovir was also given for 1 week before BMT.[59] Both studies demonstrated a decrease in the incidence and severity of CMV infection in the patients receiving ganciclovir.[59, 60] Both studies also identified neutropenia as the major toxicity associated with ganciclovir therapy. Despite the reduction in significant CMV disease, survival was not improved by the use of ganciclovir prophylactically. Therefore, the best approach to treating BMT recipients seropositive for CMV has yet to be determined. The use of hematopoietic growth factors in combination with ganciclovir may abrogate the neutropenia caused by this drug. An alternative to ganciclovir may be foscarnet. Foscarnet lacks BM toxicity and has been demonstrated to be effective for CMV retinitis in patients with acquired immunodeficiency syndrome. Foscarnet is currently undergoing clinical trials in BMT recipients.

HSV infection had previously been a frequent complication in BMT recipients for several weeks after BMT. With the common use of prophylactic acyclovir, HSV infections are usually not encountered until prophylaxis has ended. Both oral and genital HSV infections occur. Reinstitution of acyclovir is generally effective therapy. In a case report, an acyclovir-resistant HSV infection in a BMT recipient was successfully treated with foscarnet. Human herpesvirus 6 infection has only recently been identified as a possible pathogen in pediatric and adult patients.[61] Isolation of the virus is associated with fever, skin rash, and BM suppression.

Approximately one third of BMT recipients who are seropositive for VZV will develop shingles, generally during the late period after BMT. The frequency of VZV infection appears to be similar for allogeneic and autologous BMT recipients.[62] Disseminated disease and involvement of multiple dermatomes are frequent presentations in BMT recipients compared with the general population. Acyclovir is effective therapy and should be given intravenously in complicated cases. If oral acyclovir is used, the patient must be monitored closely for any progression of lesions.

BK virus and JC virus are occasional causes of cystitis after BMT during the middle period of infectious risk. BK viruria is much more common and is associated with hemorrhagic cystitis.[63] Adenovirus is associated with interstitial pneumonia with the same time-course as CMV. No effective therapy for adenovirus pneumonia has been found, and this infection is usually fatal. Respiratory syncytial virus can cause an upper respiratory tract infection and pneumonia and caused an outbreak in a BMT center. Ribavirin has generally been used to treat this infection, although it is not clear whether the drug is effective in this setting.

Protozoal Infections

P. carinii is a frequent pathogen in immunocompromised hosts and can cause lethal pneumonia in BMT recipients. *P. carinii* pneumonia (PCP) usually ocurs during the middle period after BMT.[64] Patients at highest risk are those who have not received prophylaxis for PCP or in whom prophylaxis was discontinued. Patients present with a cough, fever, dyspnea, and an interstitial process on chest radiograph. In order to confirm the diagnosis, it is necessary to obtain BAL fluid or a lung biopsy sample. Trimethoprim-sulfamethoxazole remains the treatment of choice for PCP. The use of adjunctive corticosteroids has improved survival in patients with acquired immunodeficiency syndrome using PCP and should be considered in BMT recipients with moderate or severe pneumonia. Survival remains poor, with only one third of patients surviving PCP.[64] Survival is improved in patients in whom therapy is initiated promptly, in those who develop PCP more than 6 months after BMT, and in those in whom PCP is the only pathogen identified.

Toxoplasmosis is an occasional cause of death after BMT, with 31 cases reported in the literature.[65] A high index of suspicion should occur when patients present with central nervous system (CNS) symptoms such as hemiplegia, meningitis, or confusion. Unfortunately, some present with nonspecific signs such as fever alone, and the diagnosis is not made until autopsy. Almost all cases occur in patients who are seropositive for *Toxoplasma gondii* before BMT or for whom serologic status was not determined. Because most donors were seronegative in the reported cases, reactivation of latent infection appears to be the principal cause of disease. Most infections develop during the second and third month after BMT. Diagnosis is confirmed by parasitemia, brain biopsy, or autopsy in most cases. Isolation of *T. gondii* from cerebrospinal fluid or BAL fluid has also been reported. Therapy with pyrimethamine-sulfadiazine can be successful, but responders are at risk for relapse.

NONINFECTIOUS COMPLICATIONS OF BONE MARROW TRANSPLANTATION

A significant proportion of complications of BMT arise from the toxicity of the chemotherapy and irradiation used in BMT induction regimens. In fact, it is the intent of most such regimens to approach but not to exceed lethal dose, limiting toxicity for organ systems other than the BM. In addition, the toxicity of supportive treatments compounds the complexity of the situation. The success of BMT, then, depends on successfully maintaining patients through such critical complications. Intensive care facilities are used aggressively to achieve these ends.

Specific end-organ toxicities may be the primary source of dysfunction or may complicate dysfunction due to other toxicities. Each major toxicity must be judged individually in terms of reversibility when developing a therapeutic plan. The combination of all toxicities and their inter-relationships define the practical issues of the success of acute supportive therapy.

Neurologic Complications

Neurologic complications occur frequently after BMT, affecting as many as 70% of both adults and children.[66] The majority experience reversible metabolic encephalopathy. Autopsy studies have established the importance of cerebrovascular lesions, including hematoma, hemorrhagic necrosis, and infarction. Nonbacterial thrombotic endocarditis is the most frequent cause of embolization.

Acute CNS toxicity can be encountered with the initial cytoreductive regimen. Mechlorethamine is particularly toxic, acutely causing confusion, disorientation, headache, hallucinations, lethargy, tremor, paraplegia, seizure, and vertigo. Later manifestations include personality change, confusion, seizure, diplopia, and dementia. Radiologic studies reveal ventricular enlargement and cerebral atrophy, and electroencephalograms show diffuse slowing. Carmustine can also be associated with direct CNS toxicity. Busulfan induces seizures, and two thirds of patients show epileptiform activity on electroencephalography despite prophylaxis. Irradiation can produce a reversible syndrome of somnolence associated with lethargy, irritability, headache, low-grade fever, GI disturbance, and depression. Lhermitte's sign has been observed after irradiation and BMT. A particularly devastating complication of irradiation and intrathecal methotrexate is multifocal leukoencephalopathy, an extensive irreversible demyelination of the cerebral white matter associated with cerebral atrophy.[67] Late cognitive dysfunction has been reported in both children and adults.[68]

Cyclosporin is associated with several CNS toxicities. Seizures occur in association with the hypomagnesemia produced by cyclosporin. Reversible abnormalities include mental confusion, a motor spinal cord syndrome, a cerebellar-like syndrome,[69] and optic disk edema. Concurrent use of cyclosporin and corticosteroids is associated with a syndrome of hypertension, severe visual disturbances including blindness, seizures, and occipital lobe density, as well as changes on brain computed tomography or nuclear magnetic resonance imaging.[70] A frequent association is noted with the presence of microangiopathic hemolytic anemia. These abnormalities usually clear after cessation of cyclosporin; however, cyclosporin has been reinitiated subsequently at reduced dose without recurrence of these abnormalities.

Acute demyelinating polyneuropathy can occur de novo or can be exacerbated after BMT.[71] In addition, autonomic neuropathy has also been observed.

Mucosal and Gastrointestinal Complications

Oral and GI mucositis is a frequent, severe complication of intensive cytotoxic therapy.[72] Nausea and diarrhea accompany administration of both high-dose chemotherapy and irradiation but diminish rapidly after the delivery of the agent is completed. Extensive mucosal ulceration develops during the 10 to 14 days after treatment, however, leading to recurrence of both symptoms. Pain in the oropharynx can be debilitating, requiring massive narcotic analgesia. In both adolescents and adults, patient-controlled analgesia results in improved palliation of pain and decreased analgesic requirements.[73] Topical antibiotic treatment leads to suppression of bacterial and fungal mouth flora but does not alter the course of mucositis.[74] The airway can be compromised by secretions and local edema. In severe cases, tracheal intubation can be very difficult. Involvement of the GI tract leads to diarrhea, abdominal pain, and intestinal bleeding.[75] Ulceration of the GI tract produces cholera-like fluid losses. The severe intestinal ulceration is frequently associated with sepsis, and necrotizing enterocolitis accompanies the most severe cases. The severe thrombocytopenia present throughout this phase complicates GI bleeding. Despite its severity, this complication is usually self-limited, resolving promptly with reconstitution of adequate neutrophil and platelet levels.

Pulmonary Complications

Although infections are the predominant cause of severe pulmonary toxicity after BMT, similar dysfunction has been attributed directly to chemotherapy and irradiation.[76] Drug-induced interstitial pneumonia can occur with cyclophosphamide, carmustine, and busulfan. Idiopathic interstitial pneumonia, complicating the use of total-body irradiation, is dependent on total dose. Lung shielding to attenuate the total dose to the lung has been effective in decreasing this complication.[77] High irradiation dose rates may increase the incidence of idiopathic interstitial pneumonia, although the overall incidence of interstitial pneumonia is not affected. Prior radiotherapy to the chest associated with the use of total-body irradiation increases the risk of interstitial pneumonia. Treatment for this complication is generally ineffective. Patients requiring ventilatory support show reversibility only if rapid extubation, within 4 days, is possible. Progressive interstitial pneumonia is uniformly fatal. Pulmonary function testing before BMT can identify patients at increased risk,[78] and post-BMT monitoring of diffusing capacity[79] or increased lung density on computed tomography may provide early diagnosis of affected patients.

Diffuse alveolar hemorrhage produces a syndrome of progressive dyspnea, hypoxia, cough, and diffuse consolidation on chest radiograph. It is differentiated from interstitial pneumonia by a very early onset in the post-BMT course and by the finding of hemorrhage on BAL. This complication is generally fatal, although reversal has occurred with high-dose corticosteroids.[80]

Cardiac Complications

The major cardiac complications are also related to the dose-limiting toxicity of cytotoxic therapy. Cyclophosphamide at 200 mg/kg is dose limiting for the heart, causing myocardial edema, fibrosis, and cellular hypertrophy,[81] as well as fibrinous pericarditis. Patients with more rapid in vivo activation of cyclophosphamide are more prone to this disorder.[82] A similar complication is seen with ifosfamide at doses of 10 to 18 g/m^2.[83] Severely affected individuals develop intractable congestive failure, usually in the first 2 weeks after BMT. In others, the changes are subclinical, consisting of an increase in left ventricular mass and impaired systolic and diastolic left ventricular function. These changes return to normal 1 year after BMT. Most patients will have had extensive use of anthracyclines before BMT. The myocardial fibrosis can lead to a baseline deficit that is subsequently exacerbated by fluid overload or compromised pulmonary function. Congestive failure can be a component of interstitial pneumonia or hepatic VOD. In this setting, strict attention must be given to the risk of fluid overload.

Nonbacterial thrombotic endocarditis following BMT occurs at a higher frequency in autopsy series than in clinical reports, being found in approximately 8% of patients.

Hepatic Complications

Hepatic VOD is a severe liver injury characterized by progressive fibrous obliteration of the lumina of small intrahepatic venules associated with centrilobular hepatocyte degeneration and sinusoidal fibrosis, resulting in portal hypertension and liver failure. An injury to the endothelium is followed by activation of coagulation. Risk factors include preexisting liver disease and elevated serum levels of glutamate-oxalate transaminase before BMT, as well as the use of methotrexate,[84] bulsulfan,[85] carmustine, and mitomycin C. The diagnosis when made on clinical grounds is accurate in approximately 20% of patients.[85] The exact definition of the clinical criteria for VOD is important, because slight alterations in definition can lead to observed differences of 8% to 32% in the same group of patients.[86] Patients with high early mortality are defined by the occurrence of hyperbilirubinemia greater than 34 mmol/L before day 21 after BMT, together with *two* of the following: hepatomegaly, weight gain greater than 5% of baseline, or ascites.[86] The diagnosis is confirmed by biopsy, but this is often precluded by the unstable condition of the patient, including the presence of increased platelet consumption attributed to this disorder.[87] Endovenous biopsy offers an alternative. Sonograms of the liver and portal circulation showing abnormalities of flow may help in establishing the diagnosis. Prophylactic therapy has been attempted with heparin, prostaglandin E_1, and ursodiol, a hydrophilic bile salt, with initially promising results, although a larger trial of heparin has not confirmed benefit. Thrombolytic therapy with recombinant human tissue plasminogen activator can reverse established severe VOD.

Nodular regenerative hyperplasia, which can be confused with VOD, is a more common disorder after BMT. Although severe VOD is associated with high mortality, this disorder usually has a benign course.

Renal Complications

Acute renal failure frequently occurs after allogeneic BMT.[88] Simple doubling of the serum creatinine level occurs in 53% of patients, and as many as 24% require dialysis. The potential for drug interactions is great. Cyclosporin nephrotoxicity is noted more frequently after BMT than after heart transplantation,[89] possibly indicating an interaction with the cytoreductive regimens used in BMT. The use of amphotericin B in addition to cyclosporin markedly increases the risk of renal failure. In autologous BMT, acute renal failure can occur with infusion of large amounts of hemolysate in the cryopreserved BM.[90] Late renal failure has been attributed to radiation nephritis. The onset of renal insufficiency, anemia, and hypertension occurs at a median of 9 months after BMT. Pentoxifylline, a xanthine derivative capable of downregulating tumor necrosis factor-α production, may modify renal injury due to these causes.[91]

Hemorrhagic cystitis is a frequent complication of high-dose cyclophosphamide, affecting not only the bladder but the renal pelvis and ureters as well.[92] The use of either sodium-2-mercaptoethane sulfonate or forced saline diuresis during cyclophosphamide administration decreases the incidence and severity of this complication.[93, 94] Bladder irrigation by an indwelling catheter has been ineffective.

Hematologic Complications

Hemolytic-uremic syndrome, characterized by intravascular hemolysis, thrombocytopenia, and renal failure, can arise in association with both cyclosporin and FK-506. In addition, this syndrome has been noted after autologous BMT.[95] The outcome in severe cases is usually fatal. Treatment with vincristine and plasma exchange has generally provided transient benefit.

Allogeneic platelet sensitization requires strategies for platelet matching to allow adequate support. In an acute-care setting, this can frequently be a difficult problem because the usual adequate hemostatic levels of 50,000 or 100,000 platelets per microliter are difficult to achieve and maintain. This complicates respiratory management, causing pulmonary and CNS hemorrhage. Coagulopathy complicating thrombocytopenia can be attributed to vitamin K deficiency secondary to the use of broad-spectrum antibiotics or liver failure.

Endocrine and Metabolic Complications

Endocrine dysfunction following BMT has been studied primarily in children. Compensated hypothyroidism occurs in approximately 25% of children at a median time of 1 year after BMT. Growth hormone deficiency can be the cause of growth retardation. Sterility occurs with radiation regimens in postpubertal individuals, and delay of secondary sexual characteristics is observed in children receiving a transplant before puberty. The extensive use of corticosteroids in the immediate post-BMT period and the multiplicity of organ systems showing abnormal signs make acute adrenal insufficiency hard to assess. Acutely ill patients should be assessed for adequacy of corticosteroid replacement.

The immediate post-BMT period is also associated with severe metabolic stress secondary to anorexia, mucositis, enteritis, and infection. Prophylactic total parenteral nutrition has been useful to manage this complication. A combination of partial parenteral nutrition and enteral nutrition has also been used successfully.[96] The total energy requirements for such support are uncertain. Although the normal practice is to exceed basal energy expenditure, replacement at basal levels is sufficient to maintain body weight and serum albumin, with a lesser derangement of sodium and potassium balance. Increasing nitrogen dose without increasing calories can improve maintenance of body weight. Glutamine supplementation of parenteral nutrition can attenuate the fluid retention and expansion of the extracellular fluid compartment commonly encountered with standard parenteral formulations. In addition, nitrogen balance is improved and the incidence of infection decreased with glutamine supplementation.[97]

Intensive Care Considerations

BMT units are generally organized as acute-care settings dedicated to the management of the complications of high-dose chemoradiotherapy as well as the consequences of prolonged myelosuppression. The onset of severe renal, cardiac, or pulmonary failure usually necessitates an escalation of intervention, often leading to intubation and mechanical ventilation. The decision for the extent and duration of intensive care support must be judged on the basis of the reversibility of each process affecting a patient. Seemingly severe complications involving BM failure before expected engraftment, such as acute renal failure and acute sepsis, can in fact be reversed with adequate supportive care. Invasive monitoring by intra-arterial catheterization and pulmonary artery catheterization can be maintained in the setting of neutropenia and thrombocytopenia, provided strict sterile precautions are observed and adequate hemostasis is achieved. If possible, coagulopathy should be reversed and a platelet level of 50,000/μl should be maintained. However, because these levels cannot always be achieved, care should be taken to optimize these parameters as much as possible and to achieve effective local hemostatic control. Reverse isolation and full neutropenic precautions are often compromised in an acute-care setting. An attempt should be made to maintain them while patients remain neutropenic. However, once neutropenia is resolved, continued isolation techniques should focus on preventing nosocomial infections in an immunocompromised host, such as *P. carinii* and CMV infections, rather than continued precautions aimed at neutropenia alone. Segregation of BMT recipients from other infected patients in an intensive care unit is important.

The occurrence of multiple irreversible organ failure should be considered differently, because acute support has little success in this setting. Failure of more than three organ systems, septic shock, and mechanical ventilation are associated with a high mortality.[98] In patients with respiratory failure, prolonged ventilatory support for more than 4 to 7 days is generally associated with a fatal outcome.[98, 99]

CONCLUSION

BMT is increasingly used successfully to treat various malignant as well as nonmalignant diseases. The toxicity of BMT has been reduced by the use of antibiotics, better transfusion support, more informed use of cytoreductive agents, prophylaxis of GVHD, the use of cytokines and peripheral blood stem cells, and selection of patients for BMT earlier in the course of their diseases. Limitations of BMT continue to be the difficulty in controlling GVHD and relapse of malignant diseases. Current research on the use of cytokines, immunomodulatory agents such as interleukin-2 and mAb, and new preparative regimens offer the hope of continued improvement in outcomes. Moreover, BMT is likely to become a means of correcting certain genetic diseases by gene transfer approaches.[100]

References

1. Begg C, Pilot L, McGlave P: Bone marrow transplantation versus chemotherapy in acute non-lymphocytic leukemia: A meta-analytical review. Eur J Cancer Clin Oncol 1989; 25:1519.
2. Selvaggi KJ, Wilson J, Mills LE, et al: Improved outcome for high-risk acute myeloid leukemia patients using autologous bone marrow transplantation and monoclonal antibody purged bone marrow. Blood 1994; 83:1698–1705.
3. Ramsay N, Kersey J: Indications for marrow transplantation in acute lymphoblastic leukemia. Blood 1990; 75:815.
4. Gulati S, Shank B, Black P, et al: Autologous bone marrow transplantation for patients with poor prognosis lymphoma. J Clin Oncol 1988; 6:1303.
5. Sheperd JD, Barnett MJ, Connors JM, et al: Allogeneic bone marrow transplantation for poor prognosis non-Hodgkin's lymphoma. Br Med J 1993; 12:591–596.
6. Thomas ED, Clift R: Indications for marrow transplantation in chronic myelogenous leukemia. Blood 1989; 73:861.
7. McGlave P, Bartsh G, Anasetti C, et al: Unrelated donor marrow transplantation therapy for chronic myelogenous leukemia: Initial experience of the National Marrow Donor Program. Blood 1993; 81:453–550.

7a. Bierman PJ, Vose JM, Armitage JD: Autologous transplantation for Hodgkin's disease: Coming of age? Blood 1994; 83:1161–1164.

8. Katsanis E, Ramsay N: Treatment of acquired severe aplastic anemia. Am J Pediatr Hematol Oncol 1989; 11:360.
9. Appelbaum F, Barrall J, Storb R, et al: Bone marrow transplantation for patients with myelodysplasia: Pretreatment variables and outcome. Ann Intern Med 1990; 112:590.
10. Antman K, Ayash L, Elias A, et al: A phase II study of high-dose cyclophosphamide, thiotepa, and carboplatin with autologous marrow support in women with measurable advanced breast cancer responding to standard-dose therapy. J Clin Oncol 1992; 10:102.
11. Peters WP, Ross M, Vredenburgh JJ, et al: High-dose chemotherapy and autologous bone marrow support as consolidation after standard-dose adjuvent therapy for high-risk primary breast cancer. J Clin Oncol 1993; 1:1132–1143.

11a. Carella AM, Podesta M, Frasoni F, et al: Collection of "normal" blood repopulating cells during early hematopoietic recovery after intensive conventional chemotherapy in chronic myelogenous leukemia. Bone Marrow Transplant 1993; 12:167–171.

12. Yeager A, Kaizer H, Santos G, et al: Autologous bone marrow transplantation in patients with acute nonlymphocytic leukemia using ex-vivo marrow treatment with 4-hydroperoxycyclophosphamide. N Engl J Med 1986; 315:141.
13. Shpall E, Bast RJ, Joines W, et al: Immunomagnetic purging of breast cancer from bone marrow for autologous transplantation. Bone Marrow Transplant 1991; 7:145.
14. Ball E: Immunophenotyping of acute myeloid leukemia cells. Clin Lab Med 1990; 10:721.
15. Howell A, Fogg-Leach M, Davis B, et al: Continuous infusion of complement by an automated cell processor enhances cytotoxicity of monoclonal antibody sensitized leukemia cells. Bone Marrow Transplant 1989; 4:317.
16. Ball ED, Rybka WB: Autologous bone marrow transplantation for adult acute leukemia. Hematol Oncol Clin North Am 1993; 7:201.
17. Gribben J, Freedman A, Neuberg D, et al: Immunologic purging of marrow assessed by PCR before autologous bone marrow transplantation for B-cell lymphoma. N Engl J Med 1991; 325:1525.
18. Vredenburgh J, Simpson W, Memoli V, et al: Reactivity of anti-CD15 monoclonal antibody PM-81 with breast cancer and elimination of breast cancer cells from human bone marrow by PM-81 and immunomagnetic beads. Cancer Res 1991; 51:2451.
19. Civin C, Strauss L, Brovall C, et al: Antigenic analysis of hematopoiesis. III. A hematopoietic progenitor cell surface antigen defined by a monoclonal antibody raised against KG-1a cells. J Immunol 1984; 133:157.
20. Berenson RJ, Bensinger WI, Hill RS, et al: Engraftment after infusion of CD34+ marrow cells in patients with breast cancer or neuroblastoma. Blood 1991; 77:1717.
21. Brenner MK, Rill DR, Moen RC, et al: Gene-marking to trace origin of relapse after autologous bone-marrow transplantation. Lancet 1993; 341:85.
22. Patterson J, Prentice HG, Brenner MK, et al: Graft rejection following HLA matched T-lymphocyte depleted bone marrow transplantation. Br J Haematol 1986; 63:221.
23. Champlin R, Ho W, Gajewski J, et al: Selective depletion of CD8+ T lymphocytes for prevention of graft-versus-host disease after allogeneic bone marrow transplantation. Blood 1990; 76:418.
24. Poynton C: T cell depletion in bone marrow transplantation. Bone Marrow Transplant 1988; 3:265.
25. Wagner JE, Santos GW, Noga SJ, et al: Bone marrow graft engineering by counterflow centrifugal elutriation: Results of a phase I–II clinical trial. Blood 1990; 75:1370.
26. Noga SJ, Wagner JE, Santos GW, et al: Allograft lymphocyte-dose modification with counterflow centrifugal elutriation (CCE): Effects on chronic GVHD and survival in a case/control study. Blood 1991; 78:227.
27. Gale RP, Horowitz MM, Butturini A, et al: What determines who develops graft-versus-host disease: The graft or the host (or both)? Bone Marrow Transplant 1992; 10:99.

28. Weisdorf D, Hakke R, Blazar B, et al: Risk factors for acute graft-versus-host disease in histocompatible donor bone marrow transplantation. Transplantation 1991; 51:1197.
29. Sloane JP, Thomas JA, Imrie SF, et al: Morphological and immunohistological changes in the skin in allogeneic bone marrow recipients. J Clin Pathol 1984; 37:919.
30. Roy J, Snover D, Weisdorf S, et al: Simultaneous upper and lower endoscopic biopsy in the diagnosis of intestinal graft-versus-host disease. Transplantation 1991; 51:642.
31. Weisdorf DJ, Snover DC, Haake R, et al: Acute upper gastrointestinal graft-versus-host disease: Clinical significance and response to immunosuppressive therapy. Blood 1990; 76:624.
32. Martin PJ, Schoch G, Fisher L, et al: A retrospective analysis of therapy for acute graft-versus-host disease: Initial treatment. Blood 1990; 76:1464.
33. Roy J, McGlave PB, Filipovich AH, et al: Acute graft-versus-host disease following unrelated bone marrow transplantation: Failure of conventional therapy. Bone Marrow Transplant 1992; 10:77.
34. Hiraoka A, Masaoka T, Asano S, et al: Phase II study of FK506 for allogeneic bone marrow transplantation. Bone Marrow Transplant 1992; 10:707.
35. Ely P, Dunitz J, Rogosheske J, et al: Use of a somatostatin analogue, octreotide acetate, in the management of acute gastrointestinal graft-versus-host disease. Am J Med 1991; 90:707.
36. Sale GE, Anderson P, Browne M, et al: Abnormal CD4:CD8 ratios and delayed germinal center reconstitution in lymph nodes of human graft recipients with graft-versus-host disease (GVHD): An immunohistological study. Exp Hematol 1992; 20:1017.
37. Ljungman P, Wilkund-Hammarsten M, Duraj V, et al: Response to tetanus toxoid immunization after allogeneic bone marrow transplantation. J Infect Dis 1990; 162:496.
38. Holland HK, Wingard JR, Beschorner WE, et al: Bronchiolitis obliterans in bone marrow transplantation and its relationship to chronic graft-v-host disease and low serum IgG. Blood 1988; 72:621.
39. Sullivan KM, Witherspoon RP, Storb R, et al: Prednisone and azathioprine compared with prednisone and placebo for treatment of chronic graft-v-host disease: Prognostic influence of prolonged thrombocytopenia after allogeneic marrow transplantation. Blood 1988; 72:546.
40. Tzakis AG, Abu-Elmagd A, Fung JJ, et al: FK 506 rescue in chronic graft-versus-host disease after bone marrow transplantation. Transplant Proc 1991; 23:3225.
41. Vogelsang G, Farmer ER, Hess AD, et al: Thalidomide for the treatment of chronic graft-versus-host disease. N Engl J Med 1992; 326:1055.
42. Bloom EJ, Telang GH, Jegasothy BV: Extracorporeal chemophotopheresis (ECPP) in treatment of chronic graft-versus-host disease (C-GVHD) after allogeneic bone marrow transplantation. Proc Am Soc Clin Oncol 1991; 10:229.
43. Vogelsang GB, Hess AD, Berkman AW, et al: An in vitro predictive test for graft-versus-host disease in patients with genotypic HLA-identical bone marrow transplants. N Engl J Med 1985; 313:645.
44. Darmstadt GL, Donnenberg AD, Vogelsang GB, et al: Clinical, laboratory, and histopathologic indicators of the development of progressive acute graft-versus-host disease. J Invest Dermatol 1992; 99:397.
45. Karp J, Merz W, Dick J, et al: Strategies to prevent or control infections after bone marrow transplants. Bone Marrow Transplant 1991; 8:1.
46. Attal M, Schlaifer D, Rubie H, et al: Prevention of gram-positive infections after bone marrow transplantation by systemic vancomycin: A prospective, randomized trial. J Clin Oncol 1991; 9:865.
47. Valteau D, Hartmann O, Brugieres L, et al: Streptococcal septicaemia following autologous bone marrow transplantation in children treated with high-dose chemotherapy. Bone Marrow Transplant 1991; 7:415.
48. Rolston KV, Berkey P, Bodey GP, et al: A comparison of imipenem to ceftazidime with or without amikacin as empiric therapy in febrile neutropenic patients. Arch Intern Med 1992; 152:283.
49. Winston D, Ho W, Bruckner D, et al: Beta-lactam antibiotic therapy in febrile granulocytopenic patients: A randomized trial comparing cefoperazone plus piperacillin, ceftazidime plus piperacillin, and imipenem alone. Ann Intern Med 1991; 115:849.
50. Lew MA, Kehoe K, Ritz J, et al: Prophylaxis of bacterial infections with ciprofloxacin in patients undergoing bone marrow transplantation. Transplantation 1991; 51:630.
51. Karp JE, Merz WG, Charache P: Response to empiric amphotericin B during antileukemic therapy-induced granulocytopenia. Rev Infect Dis 1991; 13:592.
52. Tollemar J, Ringden O, Andersson S, et al: Prophylactic use of liposomal amphotericin B (AmBisome) against fungal infections: A randomized trial in bone marrow transplant recipients. Transplant Proc 1993; 25:1495.
53. Goodman JL, Winston DJ, Greenfield RA, et al: A controlled trial of fluconazole to prevent fungal infections in patients undergoing bone marrow transplantation. N Engl J Med 1992; 326:845.
54. Wingard J, Merz W, Rinaldi M, et al: Increase in *Candida krusei* infection among patients with bone marrow transplantation and neutropenia treated prophylactically with fluconazole. N Engl J Med 1991; 325:1274.
55. Bowden RA, Slichter SJ, Sayers MH, et al: Use of leukocyte-depleted platelets and cytomegalovirus-seronegative red blood cells for prevention of primary cytomegalovirus infection after marrow transplant. Blood 1991; 78:246.
56. Ljungman P, Aschan J, Azinge JN, et al: Cytomegalovirus viraemia and specific T-helper cell responses as predictors of disease after allogeneic marrow transplantation. Br J Haematol 1993; 83:118.
57. Emanuel D, Cunningham I, Jules-Elysee K, et al: Cytomegalovirus pneumonia after bone marrow transplantation successfully treated with the combination of ganciclovir and high-dose intravenous immune globulin. Ann Intern Med 1988; 109:777.
58. Schmidt GM, Horak DA, Niland JC, et al: A randomized, controlled trial of prophylactic ganciclovir for cytomegalovirus pulmonary infection in recipients of allogeneic bone marrow transplants. N Engl J Med 1991; 324:1005.
59. Winston DJ, Ho WG, Bartoni K, et al: Ganciclovir prophylaxis of cytomegalovirus infection and disease in allogeneic bone marrow transplant recipients. Ann Intern Med 1993; 118:179.
60. Goodrich JM, Bowden RA, Fisher L, et al: Ganciclovir prophylaxis to prevent cytomegalovirus disease after allogeneic marrow transplant. Ann Intern Med 1993; 118:173.
61. Drobyski WR, Dunne WM, Burd EM, et al: Human herpesvirus-6 (HHV-6) infection in allogeneic bone marrow transplant recipients: Evidence of a marrow-suppressive role for HHV-6 in vivo. J Infect Dis 1993; 167:735.
62. Schuchter LM, Wingard JR, Piantadosi S, et al: Herpes zoster infection after autologous bone marrow transplantation. Blood 1989; 74:1424.
63. Arthur RR, Shah KV, Charache P, et al: BK and JC virus infections in bone marrow transplants. J Infect Dis 1988; 158: 563.
64. Tuan IZ, Dennison D, Weisdorf DJ: *Pneumocystis carinii* pneumonitis following bone marrow transplantation. Bone Marrow Transplant 1992; 10:267.
65. Derouin F, Devergie A, Auber P, et al: Toxoplasmosis in bone marrow-transplant recipients: Report of seven cases and review. Clin Infect Dis 1992; 15:267.
66. Patchell RA, White CL III, Clark AW, et al: Neurologic complications of bone marrow transplantation. Neurology 1985; 35:300.
67. Thompson CB, Sanders JE, Flournoy N, et al: The risks of central nervous system relapse and leukoencephalopathy in patients receiving marrow transplants for acute leukemia. Blood 1986; 67:195.
68. Andrykowski MA, Altmaier EM, Barnett RL, et al: Cognitive dysfunction in adult survivors of allogeneic marrow transplantation: Relationship to dose to total body radiation. Bone Marrow Transplant 1990; 6:269.
69. Atkinson K, Biggs J, Darveniza P, et al: Cyclosporin-associated central nervous system toxicity after allogeneic bone marrow transplantation. Transplantation 1984; 38:34.
70. Reece DE, Frei-Lahr DA, Shepherd JD, et al: Neurologic com-

plications in allogeneic bone marrow transplant patients receiving cyclosporin. Bone Marrow Transplant 1991; 8:393.
71. Eliashiv S, Brenner T, Abramsky O, et al: Acute inflammatory demyelination polyneuropathy following bone marrow transplantation. Bone Marrow Transplant 1991; 8:315.
72. Carl W, Higby DJ: Oral manifestations bone marrow transplantation. Am J Clin Oncol 1985; 8:81.
73. Hill HF, Mackie AM, Coda BA, et al: Patient-controlled analgesic administration. A comparison of steady-state morphine infusions with bolus doses. Cancer 1991; 67:873.
74. Epstein JB, Vickars L, Spinelli J, et al: Efficacy of chlorhexidine and nystatin rinses in prevention of oral complications in leukemia and bone marrow transplantation. Oral Surg Oral Med Oral Pathol 1992; 73:682.
75. Wolford JL, McDonald GB: A problem-oriented approach to intestinal and liver disease after marrow transplantation. J Clin Gastroenterol 1988; 10:419.
76. Masaoka T, Ramsay NK, Rimm AA, et al: Risk factors for interstitial pneumonia following bone marrow transplantation for severe aplastic anemia. Br J Haematol 1989; 71:535.
77. Labar B, Bogdanic V, Nemet D, et al: Total body irradiation with or without lung shielding for allogeneic bone marrow transplantation. Bone Marrow Transplant 1992; 9:343.
78. Ghalie R, Szidon JP, Thompson L, et al: Evaluation of pulmonary complications after bone marrow transplantation: The role of pretransplant pulmonary function tests. Bone Marrow Transplant 1992; 10:359.
79. Milburn HJ, Prentice HG, duBois RM: Can lung function measurements be used to predict which patients will be at risk of developing interstitial pneumonitis after bone marrow transplantation? Thorax 1992; 47:421.
80. Chao NJ, Duncan SR, Long GD, et al: Corticosteroid therapy for diffuse alveolar hemorrhage in autologous bone marrow transplant recipients. Ann Intern Med 1991; 114:145.
81. Kupari M, Volin L, Suokas A, et al: Cardiac involvement in bone marrow transplantation: Electrocardiographic changes, arrhythmias, heart failure and autopsy findings. Bone Marrow Transplant 1990; 5:91.
82. Ayash LJ, Wright JE, Tretyakov O, et al: Cyclophosphamide pharmacokinetics: Correlation with cardiac toxicity and tumor response. J Clin Oncol 1992; 10:995.
83. Quezado ZM, Wilson WH, Cunnion RE, et al: High-dose ifosfamide is associated with severe, reversible cardiac dysfunction. Ann Intern Med 1993; 118:31.
84. Essell JH, Thompson JM, Harman GS, et al: Marked increase in veno-occlusive disease of the liver associated with methotrexate use for graft-versus-host disease prophylaxis in tients receiving busulfan/cyclophosphamide. Blood 1992; 79: 2784.
85. Meresse V, Hartmann O, Vassal G, et al: Risk factors for hepatic veno-occlusive disease after a high-dose busulfan-containing regimens followed by autologous bone marrow transplantation: A study in 136 children. Bone Marrow Transplant 1992; 10:135.
86. Blostein MD, Paltiel OB, Thibault A, et al: A comparison of clinical criteria for the diagnosis of veno-occlusive disease of the liver after bone marrow transplantation. Bone Marrow Transplant 1992; 10:439.
87. Rio B, Andreu G, Nicod A, et al: Thrombocytopenia in veno-occlusive disease after bone marrow transplantation. Blood 1986; 67:1773.
88. Zager RA, O'Quigley J, Zager BK, et al: Acute renal failure following bone marrow transplantation: A retrospective study of 272 patients. Am J Kidney Dis 1989; 13:210.
89. Nizze H, Mihatsch MJ, Zollinger HU, et al: Cyclosporine-associated nephropathy in patients with heart and bone marrow transplants. Clin Nephrol 1988; 30:248.
90. Smith DM, Weisenburger DD, Bierman P, et al: Acute renal failure associated with autologous bone marrow transplantation. Bone Marrow Transplantation 1987; 2:195.
91. Bianco JA, Appelbaum FR, Nemunaitis J, et al: Phase I-II trial of pentoxifylline for the prevention of transplant-related toxicities following bone marrow transplantation. Blood 1991; 78:1205.
92. Efros M, Ahmed T, Choudhury M: Cyclophosphamide-induced hemorrhagic pyelitis and ureteritis associated with cystitis in marrow transplantation. J Urol 1990; 144:1231.
93. Hows JM, Mehta A, Ward L, et al: Comparison of mesna with forced diuresis to prevent cyclophosphamide induced haemorrhagic cystitis in marrow transplantation: A prospective randomised study. Br J Cancer 1984; 50:753.
94. Shepherd JD, Pringle LE, Barnett MJ, et al: Mesna versus hyperhydration for the prevention of cyclophosphamide-induced hemorrhagic cystitis in bone marrow transplantation. J Clin Oncol 1991; 9:2016.
95. Rabinowe SN, Soiffer RJ, Tarbell NJ, et al: Hemolytic-uremic syndrome following bone marrow transplantation in adults for hematologic malignancies. Blood 1991; 77:1837.
96. Mulder PO, Bouman JG, Gietema JA, et al: Hyperalimentation in autologous bone marrow transplantation for solid tumors. Comparison of total parenteral versus partial parenteral plus enteral nutrition. Cancer 1989; 64:2045.
97. Ziegler TR, Young LS, Benfell K, et al: Clinical and metabolic efficacy of glutamine-supplemented parenteral nutrition after bone marrow transplantation. A randomized, double-blind, controlled study. Ann Intern Med 1992; 116:821.
98. Torrecilla C, Cortes JL, Chamorro C, et al: Prognostic assessment of the acute complications of bone marrow transplantation requiring intensive therapy. Intensive Care Med 1988; 14:393.
99. Afessa B, Tefferi A, Hoagland HC, et al: Outcome of recipients of bone marrow transplants who require intensive-care unit support. Mayo Clin Proceed 1992; 67:117.
100. Mulligan RC: The basic science of gene therapy. Science 1993; 260:926.

CHAPTER 187

General Surgical Complications in Transplant Patients

Kenneth K. W. Lee, MD • *David L. Steed, MD*

Transplantation is now an accepted treatment for end-stage heart, lung, liver, and kidney disease. As immunosuppressive therapy continues to improve, transplantation of other organs such as the small intestine and pancreas is likely to increase as well. Prevention and treatment of organ rejection and infectious complications continue to be the major concerns after organ transplantation. General surgical complications also frequently arise, however, and are a cause of significant morbidity and mortality among organ transplant recipients. In renal, heart, and heart-lung transplantation, in which the gastrointestinal (GI) tract is not disturbed by the transplant procedure itself, general surgical complications have been reported in 9.5% to 45% of graft recipients, requiring operation in 46% to 71% and resulting in a mortality rate of 8% to 17%.[1–7]

For a general surgeon, a transplant recipient poses two challenges: management of common problems in the setting of post-transplant immunosuppression and identification and treatment of the specific problems, both common and uncommon, to which a transplant recipient is particularly susceptible. The general surgical problems arising in transplant recipients encompass the full range occurring in a general patient population. Early diagnosis and aggressive treatment with operative intervention as necessary, combined with careful titration of immunosuppressive therapy to minimize rejection while avoiding oversuppression, can achieve a successful outcome. Two series, for example, have shown no differences in survival between heart or heart-lung transplant recipients suffering GI complications compared with the entire transplant population.[1, 2] Elective operation is well tolerated, and emergency operation, when necessary, may be lifesaving.

The presentation of an acute surgical illness in a transplant recipient may be subtle and masked by the patient's continuing immunosuppressive therapy. Unexplained fever, leukocytosis, or sepsis or the development of new abdominal complaints, particularly after heart, heart-lung, or kidney transplantation, should alert a physician to the possibility of a surgical illness and prompt a thorough evaluation. A detailed history should be obtained, and a complete physical examination including ear, throat, rectal, and pelvic examinations performed. Common problems such as perirectal abscesses[5] and phlebitis at catheter sites must be considered, because in immunosuppressed transplant recipients they may become sources of serious infections. Routine laboratory tests and radiographic and endoscopic studies should be pursued until a definitive diagnosis is obtained and the need for surgical intervention determined. When a diagnosis cannot be established, diagnostic laparoscopy or peritoneal lavage should be strongly considered.

The constellation of general surgical problems to which a transplant recipient is particularly susceptible arises from two factors: technical features of the transplant operation itself and long-term immunosuppressive therapy. Thus, patients undergoing heart or heart-lung transplantation are at risk for complications resulting from cardiopulmonary bypass, such as acute pancreatitis[8] or GI bleeding, whereas liver transplant recipients may develop complications relating to venovenous bypass. All transplant recipients are at risk for complications of chronic immunosuppression such as opportunistic infections and post-transplant lymphoproliferative disorders.

ESOPHAGUS

Esophagitis may occur among transplant recipients and produce symptoms of dysphagia and epigastric discomfort and may be complicated by bleeding. Rarely, however, does it require surgical intervention. In a series of 153 heart and 6 heart-lung transplant recipients, esophagitis was suspected and biopsy proven in 19 (12.4%).[4] As among nontransplant patients, peptic ulcerations may develop in transplant recipients and can be similarly managed using antacids, histamine receptor antagonists, and proton pump antagonists. Commonly, however, esophageal ulcerations in transplant recipients are due to a viral or fungal cause.[4, 6, 9] Although such ulcerations have also been recognized in otherwise normal individuals, immunosuppressive and antibiotic therapy predispose transplant recipients to these lesions and to similar lesions elsewhere in the GI tract.[10] In a second series of 340 heart transplant recipients, 6 of 20 patients undergoing upper endoscopy were found to have esophagitis; in 3 of these 6 patients, a viral cause was identified.[9] Similarly, among 13 renal transplant recipients found to have esophagitis, the cause was herpesvirus in 5, *Candida* in 2, and cytomegalovirus (CMV) in 1.[6]

Viral ulcerations of the esophagus typically appear as discrete, well-rounded, punched-out ulcerations with raised edges.[9] The diagnosis can in most instances be established by the typical light microscopic appearance of ballooning degeneration, eosinophilic nuclear inclusions, and multinucleated giant cells seen on biopsy specimens. Acyclovir and 9-(1,3-dihydroxy-2-proproxymethyl) guanine (DHPG) are usually effective treatment despite continuing immunosuppressive therapy.[9a]

Candida esophagitis is typically symptomatic, most commonly causing dysphagia, which may be accompanied by retrosternal pain, nausea, vomiting, or GI bleeding. Diagnosis is best established by upper endoscopy, because it reveals typical candidal lesions consisting of white plaques overlying friable erythematous mucosa and permits biopsy of the lesions to determine if tissue infiltration by yeast hyphae is present.[11] Treatment of *Candida* esophagitis should be promptly initiated to relieve its symptoms, to prevent dissemination in the setting of chronic immunosuppression, and to prevent local complications such as stricture formation[12] or perforation.[13] Topical (oral) therapy may be effective and may also be useful prophylaxis in transplant recipients.[9] Systemic therapy consisting of ketoconazole or amphotericin B is indicated when topical therapy fails, for extensive or disseminated infection, and for chronic esophagitis.

STOMACH AND DUODENUM

The stomach and duodenum may be affected by the same processes as the esophagus but more commonly require surgical intervention for treatment of major hemorrhage or perforation. As in the esophagus, gastroduodenal ulceration may be due to an infectious or peptic cause. A high incidence (6–24%) of peptic ulcer disease has frequently been described in renal transplant recipients[14–17] and has also been reported among heart and heart-lung transplant recipients.[1, 3, 9] The pathogenesis of peptic ulceration after transplantation is unclear and may be multifactorial. Higher basal and maximal acid output[14] and serum gastrin levels[18] have been reported in renal transplant recipients; depletion of gastric mucosal histamine such as occurs in patients with duodenal ulcers has been demonstrated in renal transplant recipients.[16] An association between transplant rejection or dysfunction and peptic ulcer disease has also been noted.[17] Exogenous steroids given as immunosuppression additionally heighten the risk of peptic ulceration. Of interest, Knechtle and colleagues[17] observed a reduction in peptic ulcer disease among renal transplant recipients after cyclosporin was added to the immunosuppressive regimen.

CMV and less frequently herpesvirus may also cause gastric or duodenal ulceration and may contribute to the high incidence of gastric and duodenal ulceration frequently reported. In renal transplant recipients, Cohen and associates[19] found evidence of active CMV infection in several ulcers that were believed to be of acid-pepsin origin. Other investigators have noted a high incidence of CMV inclusions in gastric and duodenal mucosa of renal transplant recipients despite the absence of symptoms or endoscopic abnormalities.[20] Gastric and duodenal ulceration has also been associated with invasive *Candida* infections.[4] The manifestations of gastroduodenal ulcerations of infectious cause are identical to those of acid-pepsin origin: epigastric pain, bleeding, and perforation.

Because of the high incidence of peptic ulcer disease, prophylaxis consisting of histamine receptor antagonists is routine in most transplant centers. Prophylactic antiulcer surgery in transplant candidates or recipients has also been proposed for patients with a prior history of peptic ulcer disease or hyperchlorhydria. Owens and coworkers[21] reviewed data on 1853 renal allograft recipients from 12 centers and found that the incidence of post-transplant peptic ulcer disease was significantly reduced in patients operated on for their peptic ulcer disease before transplantation in comparison with patients not undergoing operation. Linder and colleagues[22] similarly observed that pretransplant operation for peptic ulcer disease reduced the incidence of post-transplant peptic ulcer disease. In contrast, Haffner and associates failed to find benefit when proximal gastric vagotomy was performed prophylactically in renal transplant recipients with hyperchlorhydria.[23] Although these data suggest a possible role for prophylactic ulcer surgery in transplant candidates with a history of peptic ulcer disease, they are derived from the pre–H_2 receptor antagonist era and therefore may no longer be pertinent.

Epigastric pain or discomfort or upper GI bleeding should prompt an evaluation that includes esophagogastroduodenoscopy. Intensified treatment should be instituted if gastritis, duodenitis, or frank ulcers are found. Biopsy specimens should be obtained from ulcers and appropriate antiviral or antifungal therapy added if an infectious cause is demonstrated. Biopsy material should also be obtained to preclude the presence of a lymphoproliferative disorder[3] or other neoplasm involving the stomach. Bleeding or perforation requires aggressive evaluation and treatment as in nontransplant patients.

In addition to ulcerative abnormalities, other disorders may affect the stomach and duodenum in transplant recipients. Poor gastric emptying may occur after thoracic organ transplantation and presumably results from injury to the vagus nerves; persistent symptoms may require a surgical drainage procedure.[2, 7]

BILIARY TRACT

Several reports have found a high incidence of cholelithiasis among organ transplant recipients and particularly among heart transplant recipients. Spes and colleagues[24] found that among 27 heart transplant recipients shown to be free of gallstones before transplantation, gallstones developed in 9 after transplantation, and of these, 7 developed gallstones within 1 year of transplantation. In a review of 159 patients undergoing heart transplantation, Steck and coworkers[25] found a lower incidence of de novo cholelithiasis but an overall incidence of 29.6% among the 141 patients in whom the status of the biliary tract was known. Girardet and associates[26] similarly observed a low incidence of de novo cholelithiasis (3.3%) but a high overall incidence (39.3%).

Cyclosporin itself may significantly contribute to the development of gallstones after transplantation. Experimentally, cyclosporin causes decreased bile flow and bile acid secretion.[27, 28, 28a] Cholestasis has also been demonstrated in heart transplant recipients treated with cyclosporin.[29] Lorber and coworkers[30] have found a significant increase in the development of gallstones in renal transplant recipients whose immunosuppressive regimen included cyclosporin in comparison with those whose regimen did not include cyclosporin.

Several other factors may also contribute to the high incidence of cholelithiasis among transplant recipients. Gallbladder stasis may result during times of serious illness such as immediately after transplantation or during episodes of graft rejection, particularly if parenteral nutrition is used or enteral nutrition is limited; gallbladder stasis has been shown to promote the development of gallstones.[31, 32] Coronary artery disease, a common basis for heart transplantation, may also be a risk factor for cholelithiasis.[33] A higher incidence of cholelithiasis has been observed among diabetic heart transplant recipients[24]; interestingly, glucose administration may potentiate cyclosporin-induced cholestasis.

Symptomatic cholelithiasis in transplant candidates should be treated by cholecystectomy if the patient's condition permits. Most nonthoracic organ transplant candidates can tolerate cholecystectomy without difficulty; laparoscopic surgical techniques combined with endoscopic methods may hasten recovery and lessen postoperative discomfort. In contrast, cholecystectomy in thoracic organ transplant candidates may often be a procedure with high morbidity and is best deferred until after transplantation when the patient's cardiac and pulmonary function is improved. Nonoperative alternatives should be considered in such high-risk patients. Endoscopic papillotomy effectively reduces the risk of recurrent gallstone pancreatitis, a potentially lethal complication in an immunosuppressed transplant recipient, although the risk of subsequent cholecystitis may be heightened, warranting cholecystectomy after transplantation. Percutaneous cholecystostomy may be effective treatment for acute cholecystitis.

When treatment of gallstones cannot be delayed until after transplantation, careful anesthetic management may reduce postoperative morbidity and mortality in heart or lung transplant candidates.[26, 34] Epidural anesthesia may be useful for conduct of the operation, particularly if a laparoscopic surgical technique is used, and for postoperative analgesia. When general anesthesia is used, high-dose narcotic anesthesia is appropriate because of its minimum effect on cardiac filling pressures, contractility, and afterload. Invasive monitoring with pulmonary and systemic arterial catheters should be routinely used; transesophageal echocardiography permits accurate intraoperative assessment of myocardial contractility and wall motion. In selected patients, preoperative placement and perioperative use of an intra-aortic balloon pump may be beneficial.

Treatment of asymptomatic cholelithiasis in transplant recipients remains controversial. In their series of 141 patients, Steck and colleagues[25] found that among 16 patients with asymptomatic gallstones identified on ultrasonography performed before heart transplantation, only 1 patient required a cholecystectomy 28 months after transplantation. The remaining 15 patients had not developed significant symptoms during a mean follow-up of 21 months. In total, seven patients underwent cholecystectomy for cholecystitis,[3] recurrent biliary colic,[2] or recurrent gallstone pancreatitis[2] after heart transplantation. No deaths occurred among these patients. One patient developed postoperative pneumonia, one developed recurrent abdominal pain and elevated liver function values, and a third developed severe pancreatitis complicated by pseudocyst formation and was hospitalized for 75 days after cholecystectomy. Based on these results, Steck and coworkers concluded that cholecystectomy can be safely performed for symptomatic cholelithiasis after heart transplantation but that screening ultrasonography and prophylactic cholecystectomy are not indicated in heart transplant recipients with asymptomatic cholelithiasis.

In contrast, Sekela and coworkers[35] reviewed a series of 24 consecutive patients who underwent biliary tract surgery after cardiac transplantation. Seventeen patients underwent elective cholecystectomy and operative cholangiography for symptomatic or asymptomatic cholelithiasis and experienced no deaths or complications; common bile duct exploration was required in one of these patients. In contrast, three of seven patients requiring urgent operation died of complications of biliary tract disease. In addition to cholecystectomy and cholangiography, three patients required common bile duct exploration and two required pancreatic debridement. Significantly, all three deaths occurred in patients who had no prior biliary tract symptoms. Based on these results, Sekela and coworkers also concluded that elective cholecystectomy is safe in cardiac transplant recipients but recommended that all patients be screened for cholelithiasis and that elective cholecystectomy be performed in all patients found to have cholelithiasis. They recommend that cholecystectomy be performed once recovery from the transplantation procedure is complete if rejection is well controlled or before the end of this post-transplantation period if symptoms are evident. Girardet and associates[26] also advocate treatment of asymptomatic gallstones in heart transplant recipients. In a series of 31 patients undergoing heart transplantation, 4 patients with previously asymptomatic cholelithiasis developed biliary complications requiring emergency or urgent surgery, and 2 of the 4 patients died. In contrast, five other patients with asymptomatic cholelithiasis who underwent elective biliary surgery all had uncomplicated postoperative courses.

Together, these studies demonstrate that elective biliary surgery can be safely performed in transplant recipients. Given the potential for serious morbidity or mortality when biliary tract disease becomes symptomatic in transplant recipients, an aggressive approach to diagnosis of asymptomatic cholelithiasis appears warranted. If detected, elective cholecystectomy should be undertaken, with the timing of operation determined by the patient's condition. Pretransplant operation, if a patient's condition permits, is preferable because it avoids potential complications resulting from ongoing immunosuppressive therapy as well as risk to the transplanted organ should perioperative complications arise and require reductions in the transplant recipient's baseline immunosuppressive therapy. Use of laparoscopic surgical techniques combined as necessary with endoscopic techniques minimizes the potential for wound-related complications and facilitates rapid recovery from elective cholecystectomy.

PANCREAS

Acute pancreatitis is an infrequent but serious complication of organ transplantation. In a collective review of 1321 patients undergoing renal transplantation through 1968, 23 (1.7%) cases of acute pancreatitis resulting in 12 (52%) deaths were found.[36] More recent reports have noted a similar incidence and mortality of acute pancreatitis after renal transplantation despite advances in immunosuppressive therapy and postoperative care.[37–39, 39a] Acute pancreatitis has also been recognized as an early complication in most series of heart or heart-lung transplantation. Pancreatitis occurred in 8 of 178 heart transplant recipients reported by Merrell and colleagues.[5] Steed and associates found pancreatitis in 2 of 143 undergoing heart or heart-lung transplants. Three additional patients were found at autopsy to have severe pancreatitis that had not been recognized before death.[7] Watson and coworkers similarly reported pancreatitis in 8 of 429 heart and heart-lung transplant recipients with the mean time of onset 12 days after transplantation; at autopsy, 4 additional patients were found to have severe pancreatitis.[1] Finally, in a review of 176 patients who died after cardiac or cardiopulmonary transplantation, 15 cases of pancreatitis were identified; interestingly, in 11 of the 15 cases the diagnosis was clinically inapparent.[40]

Acute pancreatitis after organ transplantation may arise from various causes. Gallstones and alcohol, the most common causes of acute pancreatitis in the general population, may similarly cause pancreatitis among transplant recipients. A number of other factors, however, relate to the transplant operation itself, the underlying health of the transplant recipient, or post-transplant therapy or complications that particularly predispose transplant recipients or candidates to the development of acute pancreatitis. Among heart or lung transplant recipients, acute pancreatitis in the early postoperative period may result from cardiopulmonary bypass.[8] Orthotopic renal transplantation in which a left nephrectomy is performed and the graft is revascularized using the splenic vessels of the recipient may also risk direct surgical trauma to the pancreas and the subsequent development of pancreatitis.[39]

Transplant recipients may also be predisposed to the development of acute pancreatitis by virtue of coexisting medical conditions. Postmortem studies have emphasized the frequency of anatomic abnormalities in the pancreas of patients with end-stage renal disease (ESRD).[41, 42] More recently, Rutsky and coworkers reported the incidence of acute pancreatitis in patients with ESRD without renal transplantation to be higher than previously recognized.[43] In a study of 1001 patients with ESRD, the 10-year incidence of pancreatitis was 2.3% and the overall mortality 20.8%; in contrast, the overall prevalence of acute pancreatitis in the United States based on autopsy data is approximately 0.5%. The basis for this increased incidence of pancreatitis in patients with ESRD without transplantation is uncertain. Hypertriglyceridemia and hyperlipidemia have been associated with the development of acute pancreatitis[44, 45]; they are frequently present in patients undergoing maintenance dialysis and in patients with coronary artery disease and may contribute to the incidence of acute pancreatitis in renal or cardiac transplant recipients. Hyperparathyroidism and hypercalcemia are also frequently observed in ESRD and may persist after renal transplantation and contribute to a higher risk of acute pancreatitis.[46, 47] In a series of 224 renal transplant recipients, acute pancreatitis occurred in 4 of 37 hypercalcemic patients but in only 4 of 187 normocalcemic patients.[48]

Immunosuppressive therapy given after transplantation may also predispose transplant recipients to the development of acute pancreatitis. Corticosteroids have frequently been implicated in the development of acute pancreatitis.[49–51] A causal relationship between acute pancreatitis and azathioprine (Imuran) has been widely reported[52–55]; a relationship between azathioprine and acute pancreatitis in transplant recipients was first noted by Hume.[56] The association between acute pancreatitis and azathioprine therapy in transplant recipients has been questioned, however, and a causal role for cyclosporin suggested. In experimental studies, cyclosporin worsens the histologic abnormalities observed with caerulein-induced acute pancreatitis.[57] Two retrospective studies[57, 58] have shown a lower incidence of post-transplant acute pancreatitis in renal transplant recipients treated with azathioprine (0.5% and 0.96%) in comparison with patients treated with cyclosporin (3.8% and 7.7%). In a prospective randomized comparison of patients treated with azathioprine or cyclosporin after renal transplantation, no significant differences were observed in the incidence of acute pancreatitis or hyperamylasemia.[59]

Finally, infection by viruses[60] such as the mumps virus or coxsackievirus may cause acute pancreatitis. In transplant recipients, CMV infection of the pancreas may arise as a complication of immunosuppressive therapy and result in acute pancreatitis.[61]

Early diagnosis and treatment of acute pancreatitis and prompt recognition of the development of complications of acute pancreatitis are essential in transplant recipients. Serum amylase levels may be elevated owing to persistent renal insufficiency; amylase-creatinine clearance ratios and serum lipase levels may be more useful for the diagnosis of acute pancreatitis. Imaging studies of the pancreas are very important: dynamic computed tomography (CT) performed by rapid bolus infusion of intravenous contrast as the pancreas is imaged reveals pancreatic edema and peripancreatic inflammatory changes consistent with acute pancreatitis. More importantly, dynamic CT scanning permits differentiation between acute interstitial edematous pancreatitis and acute necrotizing pancreatitis, because with the latter the intravenous contrast fails to enhance areas of pancreatic necrosis. In the absence of pancreatic necrosis, the incidence of pancreatic infection, the need for surgical intervention, and the overall morbidity and mortality of acute pancreatitis are very low, whereas the presence of pancreatic necrosis significantly increases the risk of each of these developments. Beger,[62] for example, has reported his experience with 897 patients: among 679 patients with interstitial edematous pancreatitis, 3 (0.4%) required operation, with an overall mortality of 0.8%; among 157 patients with necrotizing pancreatitis, 132 (84%) required operation, with an overall mortality of approximately 10%. In other series, the mortality from necrotizing pancreatitis has ranged from 10% to 59%. Imaging by dynamic CT scanning or ultrasonography is also useful for identification and monitoring of acute pancreatitis-associated fluid collections and pancreatic pseudocysts.

Acute pancreatitis in a transplant recipient should be treated as in a nontransplant patient, by withdrawal of oral intake and administration of intravenous fluid. Causes of acute pancreatitis should be sought and should include ultrasonographic examination of the gallbladder. If possible, medications that might contribute to the development of pancreatitis should be discontinued or reduced in dose; however, because these medications are likely to constitute a patient's immunosuppressive therapy, significant alterations in treatment may not be possible. In the absence of pancreatic necrosis or development of complications such as a persistent symptomatic or complicated acute peripancreatic fluid collection, further treatment is usually unnecessary. With resolution of symptoms and biochemical abnormalities, oral intake can gradually be reinstituted. Failure of signs and symptoms to resolve or redevelopment of signs and symptoms as oral intake is reinstituted warrants further investigation with dynamic CT scanning and possibly endoscopic retrograde cholangiopancreatography.

Management of necrotizing pancreatitis is controversial. Infected pancreatic necrosis requires surgical intervention. Several investigators, however, have proposed that noninfected pancreatic necrosis can be successfully managed nonoperatively.[62, 63] These investigators recommend percutaneous radiologically guided aspiration of areas of necrosis when infection is suspected and operation when infection is confirmed or if a patient's clinical condition fails to respond to nonoperative therapy. Other investigators have maintained that pancreatic necrosis requires operation irrespective of the presence or absence of infection.[64] Optimal treatment of transplant recipients with necrotizing pancreatitis has not been defined. However, given the increased susceptibility to infection resulting from chronic immunosuppressive therapy and the significant morbidity and mortality associated with pancreatic infections, early surgical intervention consisting of pancreatic necrosectomy should be strongly considered.

Similarly, treatment of complications of acute pancreatitis such as pseudocysts has not been defined. Reports suggest that in nontransplant patients, the incidence of bleeding, rupture, or infection of pseudocysts is lower than previously thought and that expectant nonoperative management may be appropriate for pseudocysts that are nonenlarging and asymptomatic.[65, 66] In the absence of comparable data in transplant recipients, definitive treatment of persistent pseudocysts should be considered to avoid the heightened morbidity associated with a pseudocyst complication.

SMALL INTESTINE, COLON, AND RECTUM

The incidence of major colorectal complications after renal transplantation is approximately 2% to 3%.[67, 68] A wide range of surgical problems involving the small or large intestine may arise. These include common conditions such as appendicitis or diverticulitis, as well as conditions to which transplant recipients are particularly susceptible, such as CMV-induced cecal ulcerations and post-transplant lymphoproliferative disorders. Accordingly, treatment of intestinal problems after transplantation comprises management of common problems in the setting of chronic immunosuppressive therapy and management of specific problems arising as a consequence of the patient's transplant.

Chronic immunosuppression in transplant recipients predisposes them to development of unusual infections that may be life threatening.[68a] Opportunistic infections of the intestine by *Aspergillus*,[69] *Histoplasma*,[70] and *Mycobacterium*[71] have been reported, presenting as GI bleeding or perforation. Neutropenic enterocolitis in which mucosal ulceration of the bowel wall occurs in association with invasion by clostridial organisms has also been described after transplantation.[71] CMV infection may cause ulceration of the colon, especially in the cecum, and present as lower GI bleeding or perforation.[72] Mortality from bleeding cecal ulcers may be high: in a series of nine renal transplant recipients with bleeding cecal ulcers due to CMV, only one patient survived.[72] As with other causes of lower GI bleeding in transplant recipients, aggressive diagnosis using colonoscopy and angiography should be undertaken. Treatment with DHPG should be instituted and immunosuppressive therapy reduced if possible; early operation should be performed for continued bleeding.

Fulminant *Clostridium difficile* colitis may also occur in transplant recipients and present as overwhelming sepsis; colonoscopy and fecal studies are typically diagnostic. CT scans characteristically demonstrate diffuse colonic wall thickening and may reveal ascites. Of interest, either diarrhea or obstipation may be present. Initial treatment consists of enteral vancomycin and parenteral metronidazole; total abdominal colectomy with end-ileostomy should be performed if a patient develops hemodynamic instability or respiratory insufficiency or fails to respond promptly to medical therapy.[73, 73a, 73b]

Lower GI bleeding in transplant recipients is uncommon but carries a high mortality. In a review of 16 series concerned with GI complications in more than 4000 renal transplant recipients, Stylianos and colleagues[67] identified 38 patients with lower GI bleeding. In 16 patients, bleeding resulted from opportunistic infection of the colon by fungi or CMV. In 15 patients, bleeding resulted from pseudomembranous, ischemic, or uremic colitis, and in 7 patients bleeding resulted from ulcers of undetermined cause. Only 12 patients (38%) were treated operatively, and the overall mortality was 72%, leading the authors to recommend early diagnosis, withdrawal of immunosuppression, and early operative intervention for significant continued bleeding. Accurate diagnosis of the cause of bleeding is important because it determines appropriate adjunctive therapy such as DHPG or amphotericin.

Colonic perforation may also occur after transplantation; several series of renal transplant recipients have reported an approximate incidence of 1% to 2%. Earlier series reported mortality rates of 50% to 70%, but lower rates have been reported.[74–76] Several risk factors for perforation have been suggested. Diverticular disease is the most common cause of colonic perforation in renal transplant recipients. Prophylactic colonic resection in transplant recipients with diverticular disease has been suggested,[74] but there is little evidence to support this recommendation. It is also uncertain whether more stringent indications for surgery should be applied to transplant recipients who experience an uncomplicated episode of acute diverticulitis. Colonic infection, as noted earlier, may result in acute perforation. Colonic pseudo-obstruction,[77] constipation exacerbated by ingestion of aluminum-containing antacids, fecal impaction, colonic ischemia, and uremia itself may also be contributing factors.[75]

Early diagnosis followed by prompt resuscitation and surgical treatment is required for successful treatment of colonic perforations after transplantation. Resection with exteriorization as an ileostomy or colostomy should be performed. Broad antibiotic coverage should be given, and where appropriate, antiviral or antifungal therapy should be initiated. Immunosuppressive therapy should be reduced until the risk of perioperative infection has been minimized. To prevent colonic perforation, aggressive use of colonoscopic decompression of the colon when pseudo-obstruction is present, avoidance of constipation, and judicious use of immunosuppressive therapy may be beneficial.

After transplantation, a family of tumors that are most commonly of B cell origin may arise. These tumors are referred to as post-transplant lymphoproliferative disorders (PTLDs), and although such tumors may arise throughout the body, including the transplanted organ, they are of particular importance in the small and large intestine, because in these locations such tumors may result in obstruction, perforation, or bleeding and necessitate surgical intervention. PTLDs are believed to arise as a consequence of chronic immunosuppression; additionally, infection by the Epstein-Barr virus is believed to be an important cofactor in the development of these tumors.

The overall incidence of PTLDs is uncertain. Nalesnik and colleagues[78] have reported frequencies of 1.0%, 1.8%, 2.2%, and 4.6% for kidney, heart, liver, and heart-lung transplant recipients, respectively. However, Malatack and associates[79] have monitored 132 pediatric liver transplant recipients for the development of PTLD and calculated an onset rate of 2.8% per year with a cumulative risk of almost 20% by 7 years. The relative importance of specific immunosuppressive agents in the development of PTLD has not been fully defined: azathioprine, cyclosporin, FK-506, and OKT3 all have been linked to the development of PTLD.[80]

Three patterns of clinical presentation have been broadly described for PTLD[80]: (1) fulminant, rapidly progressive polyclonal disease, which often leads to death of the patient; (2) single or metastatic clonal tumors, which progress despite immune modulation; and (3) single or multiple clonal or nonclonal tumors, which often respond to immune modulation. The most common subset of PTLD—and for a general surgeon the most important—consists of single or multiple tumors with a predilection for extranodal sites, particularly the GI tract, brain, and transplanted organ. GI tract involvement may manifest itself as perforation, bleeding, or obstruction occurring as the initial presentation or after treatment.

Reduction of immunosuppressive therapy is the primary mode of treatment for both clonal and nonclonal PTLD. Acyclovir,[81] ganciclovir,[82] and interferon-α[83] have also been used for treatment of PTLD. Surgical intervention is indicated for perforation, uncontrolled bleeding, or unremitting obstruction and entails limited resection of the affected bowel segment. Other areas of disease generally should not be resected but rather treated postoperatively by modulation of the immunosuppressive regimen and antiviral therapy; however, prophylactic resection may sometimes be warranted in order to avoid perforation during subsequent treatment.

VASCULAR COMPLICATIONS

As patients live longer after heart transplantation, an accelerated form of coronary atherosclerosis has been recognized. Accelerated peripheral vascular disease has also been reported. In a large series of patients who had undergone cardiac transplantation, peripheral vascular disease appeared in 10% within 3 years of the heart transplantation.[84] This included 6% with occlusive disease and 4% with abdominal aortic aneurysm. One patient had a vertebral artery dissection.

Patients undergoing heart transplantation commonly have the risk factors associated with atherosclerosis. Forty-one per cent of patients undergoing heart transplantation have sustained hypertension, 23% have hyperlipidemia, 14% have diabetes mellitus, and 36% are older than 50 years.[84] A history before transplantation of ischemic cardiomyopathy is also predictive of the development of peripheral vascular disease. The development of peripheral vascular disease after transplantation does not appear to correlate with a pretransplant history of hyperlipidemia or hypertension, and thus, those at risk for peripheral vascular disease after heart transplantation likely cannot be recognized before transplantation simply by identifying risk factors.

Hypertension after transplantation is not uncommon, because immunosuppressive medications, specifically prednisone and cyclosporin, may initiate or aggravate hypertension.[85, 86] Hyperlipidemia is also associated with immunosuppressive agents. In addition, a reduced creatinine clearance, perhaps related to immunosuppression, may aggravate hyperlipidemia.[87] Agents that reduce lipid levels, such as lovastatin, gemfibrozil, clofibrate, and nicotinic acid, have been reported to cause myopathy with subsequent rhabdomyolysis and renal failure in heart transplant recipients.[88] Therefore, these agents must be used with extreme caution in this setting.

A higher incidence of infrarenal abdominal aortic aneurysm has been reported in patients undergoing heart transplantation for ischemic heart disease.[89] After transplantation, the average expansion rate was greater than that for nontransplant patients, suggesting that patients with abdominal aortic aneurysms require close follow-up after heart transplantation. Finally, patients undergoing heart transplantation may also have vascular complications related to the use of an intra-aortic balloon pump or artificial heart device; in these settings, peripheral ischemia may result from emboli or arterial damage occurring at the time of insertion of the device.

SUMMARY

In summary, transplant recipients are particularly susceptible to many common as well as uncommon general and vascular surgical problems. Early diagnosis and aggressive treatment, combined with careful titration of immunosuppressive therapy to minimize graft rejection while avoiding oversuppression, can usually achieve a successful outcome of these problems.

References

1. Watson CJE, Jamieson NV, Johnston PS, et al: Early abdominal complications following heart and heart-lung transplantation. Br J Surg 1991; 78:699–704.
2. Augustine SM, Yeo CJ, Buchman TG, et al: Gastrointestinal complications in heart and in heart-lung transplant patients. J Heart Lung Transplant 1991; 10:547–556.
3. Welch RW, Yokoyama Y, Cooper DKC, et al: The gastrointestinal management of patients undergoing heart transplantation. Okla State Med Assoc 1991; 84:557–562.
4. Villar HV, Neal DD, Levinson M, et al: Gastrointestinal complications after human transplantation and mechanical heart replacement. Am J Surg 1989; 157:168–174.
5. Merrell SW, Ames SA, Nelson EW, et al: Major abdominal complications following cardiac transplantation. Arch Surg 1989; 124:889–894.
6. Komorowski RA, Cohen EB, Kauffman HM, et al: Gastrointestinal complications in renal transplant recipients. Am J Clin Pathol 1986; 86:161–167.
7. Steed DL, Brown B, Reilly JJ, et al: General surgical complications in heart and heart-lung transplantation. Surgery 1985; 98:739–745.

8. Rose DM, Ranson JHC, Cunningham JN, et al: Patterns of severe pancreatic injury following cardiopulmonary bypass. Ann Surg 1984; 199:168–172.
9. Johnson R, Peitzman AB, Webster MW, et al: Upper gastrointestinal endoscopy after cardiac transplantation. Surgery 1988; 103:300–304.
9a. Stratta RJ: Clinical patterns and treatment of cytomegalovirus infection after solid-organ transplantation. Trans Proc 1993; 25(Suppl 4):15–21.
10. Rubin RH, Cosimi AB, Tolkoff-Rubin NE, et al: Infectious disease syndromes attributable to cytomegalovirus and their significance among renal transplant recipients. Transplantation 1977; 24:458–464.
11. Bolivar R, Bodey GP: Candidiasis of the gastrointestinal tract. *In:* Candidiasis. Bodey GP, Fainstein V (Eds). New York, Raven Press, 1985, pp 181–201.
12. Orringer MB, Sloan H: Monilial esophagitis: An increasingly frequent cause of esophageal stenosis? Ann Thorac Surg 1978; 26:364–374.
13. Jones JM, Glass NR, Belzer FC: Fatal *Candida* esophagitis in two diabetic patients after renal transplantation. Arch Surg 1982; 117:499–501.
14. Chisholm GD, Mee AD, Williams G, et al: Peptic ulceration, gastric secretion, and renal transplantation. Br Med J 1977; 1:1630–1633.
15. Sarodsky MF, Cruz AB, Saylor R, et al: Upper gastrointestinal bleeding following renal transplantation. Urology 1985; 26:347–350.
16. Timoney AG, Man WK, Spencer J, et al: Histamine and duodenal ulceration in renal transplant recipients. Gut 1989; 30:65–71.
17. Knechtle SJ, Kempf K, Bollinger RR: Peptic ulcer disease following renal transplantation. Transplant Proc 1987; 19:2233–2236.
18. El Ghonaimy E, Barsoun R, Soliman M, et al: Serum gastrin in chronic renal failure: Morphological and physiological considerations. Nephron 1985; 39:86–94.
19. Cohen EB, Komorowski RA, Kauffman HM, et al: Unexpectedly high incidence of cytomegalovirus infection in apparent peptic ulcers in renal transplant recipients. Surgery 1985; 97:606–612.
20. Franzin G, Muolo A, Griminelli T: Cytomegalovirus inclusions in the gastroduodenal mucosa of patients after renal transplantation. Gut 1981; 22:698–701.
21. Owens ML, Passara E, Wilson SE, et al: Treatment of peptic ulcer disease in the renal transplant patient. Ann Surg 1977; 186:17–21.
22. Linder MM, Kosters W, Rethel R: Prophylactic gastric operations in uremic patients prior to renal transplantation. World J Surg 1979; 3:501–504.
23. Haffner JFW, Jakobsen A, Flatmark AL: Upper gastrointestinal bleeding in renal transplant recipients: The role of prophylactic gastric surgery. World J Surg 1983; 7:738–742.
24. Spes CH, Angermann CE, Beyer RW, et al: Increased incidence of cholelithiasis in heart transplant recipients receiving cyclosporin therapy. J Heart Transplant 1990; 9:404–407.
25. Steck TB, Costanzo-Nordin MR, Keshavarzian A: Prevalence and management of cholelithiasis in heart transplant patients. J Heart Lung Transplant 1991; 10:1029–1032.
26. Girardet RE, Rosenbloom P, DeWeese BM, et al: Significance of asymptomatic biliary tract disease in heart transplant recipients. J Heart Transplant 1989; 8:391–398.
27. Stone BG, Udani M, Sanghvi A, et al: Cyclosporin A–induced cholestasis: The mechanism in a rat model. Gastroenterology 1987; 93:344–351.
28. LeThai B, Dumont M, Michel A, et al: Cholestatic effect of cyclosporin in the rat. Transplantation 1988; 46:510–512.
28a. Azer SA, Stacey NH: Cyclosporine-induced interference with uptake of bile acids by human hepatocytes. Trans Proc 1993; 25:2892–2893.
29. Schade RR, Guglielmi A, Van Thiel DH, et al: Cholestasis in heart transplantation recipients treated with cyclosporin. Transplant Proc 1983; 15:2757–2760.
30. Lorber MI, Van Buren SM, Flechner SM, et al: Hepatobiliary complications of cyclosporin therapy following renal transplantation. Transplant Proc 1987; 19:1808–1810.
31. Roslyn JJ, Pitt HA, Mann LL, et al: Gallbladder disease in patients on long-term parenteral nutrition. Gastroenterology 1983; 84:148–154.
32. Bernhoft RA, Pelligrini CA, Brodercik WC, et al: Pigment sludge and stone formation in the acutely ligated dog gallbladder. Gastroenterology 1983; 85:1166–1171.
33. Bortnichak EA, Freeman DH, Ostfeld AM, et al: The association between cholesterol cholelithiasis and coronary heart disease in Framingham, Massachusetts. Am J Epidemiol 1985; 121:19–28.
34. Boline GB, Gifford RRM, Yang HC, et al: Cholecystectomy in the potential heart transplant patient. J Heart Lung Transplant 1991; 10:269–274.
35. Sekela ME, Hutchins DA, Young JB, et al: Biliary surgery after cardiac transplantation. Arch Surg 1991; 126:571–573.
36. Johnson WC, Nasbeth DC: Pancreatitis in renal transplantation. Ann Surg 1970; 171:309–314.
37. Frick TW, Fryd DS, Sutherland DER, et al: Hypercalcemia associated with pancreatitis and hyperamylasemia in renal transplant recipients. Am J Surg 1987; 154:487–489.
38. Salem RR, Williams G, Blumgart LH: Acute pancreatitis following renal transplantation. Dig Surg 1985; 2:126–130.
39. Fernandez-Cruz L, Targarona EM, Cugat E, et al: Acute pancreatitis after renal transplantation. Br J Surg 1989; 76:1132–1135.
39a. Fang J-T, Huang C-C, Lai M-K, et al: Acute pancreatitis after renal transplantation. Trans Proc 1994; 26:1993–1994.
40. Aziz S, Bergdahl L, Baldwin JC, et al: Pancreatitis after cardiac and cardiopulmonary transplantation. Surgery 1985; 97:653–660.
41. Baggenstoss AH: The pancreas in uremia: A histopathologic study. Am J Pathol 1948; 24:1003–1011.
42. Avram MM, Iancu M: Pancreatic disease in uremia and parathyroid hormone excess. Nephron 1982; 32:60–62.
43. Rutsky EA, Robards M, Van Duke JA, et al: Acute pancreatitis in patients with end-stage renal disease without transplantation. Arch Intern Med 1986; 146:1741–1745.
44. Saharia P, Margolis S, Zuidema GD, et al: Acute pancreatitis with hyperlipemia: Studies with an isolated perfused canine pancreas. Surgery 1977; 82:60–67.
45. Brunzell J, Schrott H: Interaction of familial and secondary causes of hypertriglyceridemia: Role in pancreatitis. Clin Res 1973; 21:723.
46. Mixter CG, Keynes WM, Cope O: Further experience with pancreatitis as a diagnostic clue to hyperparathyroidism. N Engl J Med 1962; 266:265–272.
47. Reeve TS, Delbridge LW: Pancreatitis following parathyroid surgery. Ann Surg 1982; 195:158–162.
48. Frick TW, Fryd DS, Sutherland DER, et al: Hypercalcemia associated with pancreatitis and hyperamylasemia in renal transplant recipients. Am J Surg 1987; 154:487–489.
49. Bencosme SA, Lazarus SS: Pancreas of cortisone-treated rabbits: Pathogenic study. AMA Arch Pathol 1956; 62:285–295.
50. Nelp WB: Acute pancreatitis associated with steroid therapy. Arch Intern Med 1961; 108:102–110.
51. Carone FA, Liebow AA: Acute pancreatic lesions in patients treated with ACTH and adrenal corticoids. N Engl J Med 1957; 257:690–697.
52. Kawanishi H, Rudolph E, Bull FE: Azathioprine-induced acute pancreatitis. N Engl J Med 1972; 289:357.
53. Paloyan D, Levin B, Simonowitz D. Azathioprine-associated acute pancreatitis. Am J Dig Dis 1977; 22:839–840.
54. Scarpelli DG: Toxicology of the pancreas. Toxicol Appl Pharmacol 1989; 101:534–554.
55. Banarjee AK, Patel KJ, Grainger SL: Drug induced acute pancreatitis—a critical review. Med Toxicol Adverse Drug Exp 1989; 4:186–198.
56. Hume DM: Progress in clinical renal homotransplantation. Adv Surg 1966; 2:419–498.
57. Kenmochi T, Asano T, Shimada H, et al: Clinical and experimental studies of acute pancreatitis after renal transplantation. Transplant Proc 1992; 24:1578–1580.
58. Yoshimura N, Nakai I, Ohmori Y, et al: Effect of cyclosporin on the endocrine and exocrine pancreas in kidney transplant recipients. Am J Kidney Dis 1988; 12:11–17.
59. Frick TW, Fryd DS, Goodale RL, et al: Lack of association between azathioprine and acute pancreatitis in renal transplantation patients. Lancet 1991; 337:251–252.
60. Durr G: Acute pancreatitis. *In:* The Exocrine Pancreas. Howat H, Sarles H (Eds). Philadelphia, WB Saunders, 1979, p 352.
61. Margreiter R, Schmid T, Dunser M, et al: Cytomegalovirus

(CMV)-pancreatitis: A rare complication after pancreas transplantation. Transplant Proc 1991; 23:1619–1622.
62. Beger HG: Surgery in acute pancreatitis. Hepatogastroenterology 1991; 38:92–96.
63. Bradley EL III, Allen K: A prospective longitudinal study of observation versus surgical intervention in the management of necrotizing pancreatitis. Am J Surg 1991; 161:19–25.
64. Rattner DW, Legermate DA, Lee MJ, et al: Early surgical debridement of symptomatic pancreatic necrosis is beneficial irrespective of infection. Am J Surg 1992; 163:105–110.
65. Vitas GJ, Sarr MG: Selected management of pancreatic pseudocysts: Operative versus expectant management. Surgery 1992; 111:123–130.
66. Yeo CJ, Bastidas JA, Lynch-Nyhan A, et al: The natural history of pancreatic pseudocysts documented by computed tomography. Surg Gynecol Obstet 1990; 170:411–417.
67. Stylianos S, Forde KA, Benvenisty AI, et al: Lower gastrointestinal hemorrhage in renal transplant recipients. Arch Surg 1988; 123:739–744.
68. Flanigan RC, Reckard CR, Lucas BA: Colonic complications of renal transplantation. J Urol 1988; 139:503–506.
68a. Van Laethem JL, Bourgeois N, Gelin M, et al: Digestive tract infections in kidney and liver transplantation in a single institution. Transplant 1993; 55:433–435.
69. Kinder RB, Jourdan MH: Disseminated aspergillosis and bleeding colonic ulcers in renal transplant patient. J R Soc Med 1985; 78:338–339.
70. Brett MT, Kwan JTC, Bending MR: Caecal perforation in a renal transplant patient with disseminated histoplasmosis. J Clin Pathol 1988; 41:992–995.
71. Frankel AH, Barker F, Williams G, et al: Neutropenic enterocolitis in a renal transplant patient. Transplantation 1991; 52:913–914.
72. Sutherland DER, Chan FY, Foucar E, et al: The bleeding cecal ulcer in transplant patients. Surgery 1979; 86:386–398.
73. Medich DS, Lee KKW, Simmons RL, et al: Laparotomy for fulminant pseudomembranous colitis. Arch Surg 1992; 127:847–853.
73a. Kelly CB, Pothoulakis C, LaMont JT: *Clostridium difficile* colitis. N Engl J Med 1994; 330:257–262.
73b. Lipsett PA, Samantaray DK, Tam ML, et al: Pseudomembranous colitis: A surgical disease? Surgery 1994; 116:491–496.
74. Carson SD, Krom RAF, Uchida K, et al: Colon perforation after kidney transplantation. Ann Surg 1978; 188:109–113.
75. Church JM, Braun WE, Novick AC, et al: Perforation of the colon in renal homograft recipients. Ann Surg 1986; 203:69–76.
76. Nghiem DD, Corry RJ: Colorectal perforation in renal transplant recipients. Am Surg 1983; 49:554–557.
77. Stratta RJ, Starling JR, D'Alessandro AM, et al: Acute colonic ileus (pseudo-obstruction) in renal transplant recipients. Surgery 1988; 104:616–623.
78. Nalesnik MA, Jaffe R, Starzl TE, et al: The pathology of posttransplant lymphoproliferative disorders occurring in the setting of cyclosporin A–prednisone immunosuppression. Am J Pathol 1988; 133:173.
79. Malatack JJ, Gartner JC, Urbach AH, et al: Orthotopic liver transplantation, Epstein-Barr virus, cyclosporin, and lymphoproliferative disease: A growing concern. J Pediatr 1991; 118:667.
80. Nalesnik MA: Lymphoproliferative disease in organ transplant recipients. Springer Semin Immunopathol 1991; 13:199–216.
81. Hanto DW, Frizzera G, Gajl-Peczalska KJ, et al: Epstein-Barr virus, immunodeficiency, and B cell proliferation. Transplantation 1985; 39:461.
82. Pirsch JD, Stratta RJ, Sollinger HW, et al: Treatment of severe Epstein-Barr virus-induced lymphoproliferative syndrome with ganciclovir: Two cases after solid organ transplantation. Am J Med 1989; 86:241.
83. Sharpir RS, Chauvenet A, McGuire W, et al: Treatment of B-cell lymphoproliferative disorders with interferon-alpha and intravenous gamma globulin. N Engl J Med 1988; 318:1334.
84. Bull DA, Hunter GC, Copeland JG, et al: Peripheral vascular disease in heart transplant recipients. J Vasc Surg 1992; 16:546.
85. Ozdogan E, Banner N, Fitzgerald MB, et al: Factors influencing the development of hypertension after transplantation. J Heart Transplant 1990; 9:548.
86. Luke RG: Mechanism of cyclosporin-induced hypertension. Am J Hypertens 1991; 4:468.
87. Higgins RM, Ratcliffe PJ. Hypercholesterolemia and vascular disease after transplantation. Transplant Rev 1991; 5:131.
88. East C, Alivizatos PA, Grundy SM, et al: Rhabdomyolysis in patients receiving lovastatin after cardiac transplantation. N Engl J Med 1988; 318:47.
89. Piotrowski JJ, McIntyre KE, Hunter GC, et al: Abdominal aortic aneurysm in the patient undergoing cardiac transplantation. J Vasc Surg 1991; 14:460.

CHAPTER 188

Future of Transplantation (Including Xenografting)

John J. Fung, MD, PhD • *Ronald Shapiro, MD*
Ake Grenvik, MD, PhD • *Forrest Dodson, MD*
Thomas E. Starzl, MD, PhD

In Chapter 176, a detailed history of organ transplantation is provided. However, in order to appreciate and understand the forces that will drive advances in transplantation into the next century, this chapter focuses on a few of the past developments in transplantation that have helped to shape current transplant practices (Fig. 188–1). The beginning of solid-organ transplantation can be traced back to the technical achievement of Alexis Carrel. In 1902, he described the techniques of vascular anastomosis, thus ushering in accounts of autologous and homologous transplantation.[1] Although a number of animal-to-human kidney transplants were reported in the ensuing three decades, a human donor organ was not used until 1933, by the Russian surgeon Voronoy.[2] This and other attempts at using human kidneys for transplantation failed owing to acute tubular necrosis and rejection. The first successful human transplant occurred on December 23, 1954, and was performed by the Boston team of Moore, Murray, Merrill and Harrison. The use of an identical twin kidney from one brother to another was the immunologic advantage that distinguished the early successes in kidney transplantation from those that otherwise were doomed to fail.[3]

Gibson and Medawar ascribed an immunologic basis to the rejection of tissues between genetically nonidentical individuals.[4] In 1960, Calne used azathioprine, developed several years earlier by Burroughs-Wellcome, in attempts to gain success in unrelated kidney transplantation using immunosuppressive agents.[5] Starzl and Marchioro then modified the immunosuppressive regimen by adding corticosteroids for rejection and began routinely to achieve success.[6] This success led to increasing attempts at human kidney transplantation, aggravating the shortage of organs to use for transplantation. A number of attempts at animal-to-human transplantation were performed. The longest survivor was a 23-year-old woman who lived for 9 months after receiving kidneys from a chimpanzee.[7]

In 1968, the Ad Hoc Committee of the Harvard School of Medicine proposed the concept of "irreversible coma."[8] Further clarification of the pathophysiology of irreversible brain stem injury and subsequent somatic death followed, as did objective criteria to document irreversible brain injury. The brain death concept has eventually been accepted throughout the United States (see Chapter 173). The details of brain death evaluation and certification vary from state to state

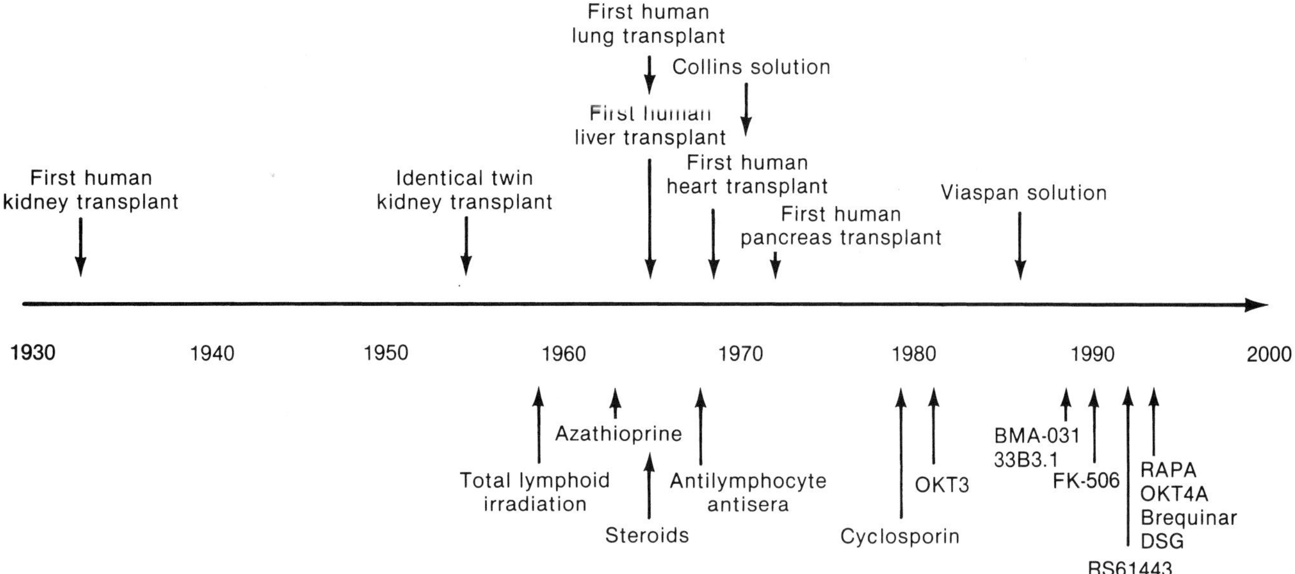

Figure 188–1. Abbreviated chronologic summary of significant milestones in transplantation.

but require a clinical picture of coma not due to medication (e.g., alcohol) or physical reasons (e.g., hypothermia) and lack of cranial nerve reflexes. Confirmatory tests are used to document the absence of blood flow to the brain and the lack of cerebral and brain stem electric activity. The use of brain-dead donors, with optimal hemodynamic parameters, offers the possibility of improved quality organs with minimum warm ischemia damage. This has also allowed procurement of extrarenal organs in a systematic manner.[9] Another improvement in the area of donor management was the development of preservation solutions, first Collin's solution[10] and currently Viaspan, developed by Belzer and coworkers at the University of Wisconsin[11] (see Chapter 178).

The next advancement in the field of transplantation came with the discovery of the immunosuppressive qualities of cyclosporin, described by Borel and colleagues.[12] Clinical trials were conducted in England by Calne and colleagues[13] and shortly thereafter in the United States by Starzl and colleagues.[14] The combination of cyclosporin and steroids was soon introduced into clinical transplantation, and the impact on liver, heart, and kidney transplantation was felt almost overnight. With the introduction of cyclosporin into clinical transplantation, survival rates for patients and grafts improved dramatically (see Chapter 179). Nevertheless, allograft rejection and the consequences of treatment of rejection continue to be the most common causes of retransplantation and death. Clinical rejection occurs in as many as 80% of solid-organ allograft recipients, who are maintained on cyclosporin and steroid therapy. In addition, a number of toxicities, including nephrotoxicity, may limit the optimal use of cyclosporin. Chronic renal damage and functional impairment have been shown to occur in transplant recipients, and hypertension, requiring antihypertensive therapy, occurs in the majority of these patients. Alterations in clinical immunosuppression to prevent or reverse these and other side effects have included: (1) reduction of cyclosporin dose or (2) addition of azathioprine, antilymphocyte antibodies, or other agents, with concomitant reductions in the cyclosporin dose. These methodologies have their inherent dangers, increasing susceptibility to both rejection and infection.

Organ transplantation is currently accepted as a therapeutic modality for treatment of various end-stage organ diseases. Kidney transplantation has been paid by Medicare and the End-Stage Renal Disease Program for almost 15 years. Liver, heart, and heart-lung transplantation have been paid by a majority of third-party insurances for more than 10 years. Medicare has also recognized the benefits of these procedures and has developed entitlement programs covering these procedures. Pancreas, lung, and intestinal transplantation have not yet been universally subscribed to by third-party payers, but as experience is accumulated and the efficacy of these procedures is proved, it is likely that these procedures will likewise be covered by Medicare. As experience in organ transplantation grows and the experimental procedures also become accepted, the pressure exerted on a limited donor pool continues to increase. Donors who have not previously been used are being considered, and more attention is focused on artificial support systems and the area of xenotransplantation.

The purpose of this concluding chapter to this section of the book is to put into perspective some of the areas of research and development that may affect the future of transplantation. Reference to other chapters in this book provides a more detailed description of developments in those areas, which are worth mentioning in the context of future developments in the field of organ transplantation. It is not possible in this chapter to mention all of the various fields that may affect the future of transplantation, and failure to discuss an area of interest does not in any way suggest that such an area is not of importance.

UPDATE ON THE SUCCESS OF SOLID-ORGAN TRANSPLANTATION

In 1984, the National Transplant Act was passed by the Congress of the United States. This act called for formation of an organ procurement network and a scientific registry (see Chapter 176). In 1987, the United Network of Organ Sharing was awarded a contract from Health Resources and Services Administration to maintain a scientific registry for organ transplantation. One of the purposes of the registry is to collect and analyze data regarding the success of organ transplantation and the factors that are important in determining success. This registry represents one of the first attempts to examine the role of donor and recipient characteristics, as well as center-specific parameters, that affect organ transplantation. The factors that have been analyzed have included age and race of the recipient, risk factors in the recipient population, and the medical urgency of the recipient population. These were then applied to national and center-specific outcomes. In 1992, the first Report of Center-Specific Graft and Patient Survival Rates was published.[15] A second report is expected in late 1994, using additional risk factors that have been added since the first report. The following data have been abstracted from published United Network of Organ Sharing statistics for the United States experiences, including the period from October 1, 1987, and December 31, 1991. In all organ transplant types, the registry has recorded an improvement in patient and graft survival during the period of time that has been analyzed. This is in part related to improvement in medical management, increased experience at the individual transplant centers, and changing recipient characteristics.

Kidney

The overall 1-year patient survival rate for cadaveric kidney transplants was 93%, which was slightly lower at 90% by 2 years after transplantation. The 1- and 2-year graft survival rates were 79% and 73%, respectively. Patients whose kidney allograft fails can be placed back on dialysis support, accounting for the significant differences between patient and graft survival. Factors that adversely affect the success of cadaveric kidney transplants appear to be (1) repeat transplant (approximately 6% worse 2-year graft survival than first-time kidney transplants); (2) blacks as recipients (approximately 7–9% worse 2-year graft survival as compared with white recipients); (3) poor histocompatibility (HLA) matching (12% worse 2-year graft survival in the worst match as compared with the best match); and (4) very young (<5 y of age) or very old (>65 y of age) recipients. The corresponding biologic explanations for these risk factors include (1) increased likelihood of sensitization of the recipient in repeated transplantation; (2) worse matching characteristics of the black versus white populations; (3) role of histocompatibility, as determined by HLA matching, in the intensity of the rejection process; and (4) concurrent medical problems in the elderly or increased technical complications in the very young.

Living donors have been used for kidney transplantation since the earliest attempts at kidney transplantation. The overall graft and patient survival rates for recipients of living donor kidneys are better than for recipients of cadaveric kidney transplants. The 1- and 2-year patient survival rates for living donor recipients were 93% and 90%, respectively. The corresponding 1- and 2-year graft survival rates were 91% and 87%. Many of the risk factors that adversely influenced graft survival in cadaveric kidney recipients also apply in living donor recipients. The biologic explanation for the improvement in the graft and patient survival in the living donor group as compared with the cadaveric organ recipients is principally related to closer HLA matching and better quality kidney allografts, with improved early graft function. The onset of early acute tubular necrosis after kidney transplantation, either from preservation or immunologic causes, has a deleterious effect on graft survival.

Liver

The 1- and 2-year patient survival rates after liver transplantation are 74% and 69%, respectively. The corresponding graft survival rates are 67% and 62%. Unlike failure of kidney transplantation, failure of a liver graft results in a patient's death unless these patients undergo retransplantation. The risk factors associated with poorer outcomes include (1) older (>65 y of age) recipient age (2-y patient survival 7% less than the mean survival); (2) repeat transplants (2-y survival for recipient of previous transplants was 24% less than for those receiving only one transplant); (3) Asian race (2-y survival 17% less than for the mean survival); and (4) degree of medical illness at the time of liver transplantation (2-y survival of the most critically ill was 28% less than for those with little stigmata of liver disease). For graft survival, the risk factors were similar, although the very young (<5 y of age) recipients had the lowest graft survival (2-y graft survival 3% less than the mean graft survival). The corresponding biologic explanations for these risk factors include (1) concurrent medical conditions in the elderly; (2) increased severity of illness in those receiving more than one liver transplant; (3) higher incidence of hepatitis B and C, as well as the presence of primary liver tumors, in the Asian recipients, as compared with other races; and (4) higher risk in more ill patients related to other organ system involvement, such as respiratory or renal failure. In the pediatric population, a higher rate of technical complications is ascribed to the higher graft loss in this group. For several risk factors, the penalty in patient and graft survival appears to occur in the immediate post-transplant period, without a disproportionate loss after the first 3 months.

Heart

The 1- and 2-year patient survival rates after heart transplantation were 82% and 77%, respectively. The corresponding graft survival rates were 81% and 76%. The similarity between patient and graft survival in heart transplantation is due to the limited retransplantations performed. Unlike kidney or liver transplantation, the principal risk factor that adversely affects both patients and graft survival appears to be very young age (<5 y). Both the patient and graft survival rates were 13% less in this age group as compared with the mean survival. Severity of medical illness at the time of heart transplantation also predicted patient and graft survival, with patients having the most critical need for heart transplantation having a 23% worse 2-year outcome than those receiving transplantation with minimum impact of their heart disease. Finally, women have approximately 3% to 4% worse patient and graft survival than do men. The corresponding biologic explanations for these risk factors include (1) difficulty in obtaining heart grafts of appropriate size for the young and for women and (2) the presence of concurrent medical illnesses in those who are critically in need of heart transplantation, as well as the use of biomechanical devices to maintain these patients until transplantation.

Pancreas

Pancreas transplantation has been used in three scenarios: (1) pancreas alone, as treatment of type I juvenile-onset diabetes mellitus, without overt renal failure, (2) pancreas combined with simultaneous kidney transplantation (SPK), for diabetic patients with renal failure, and (3) pancreas after successful kidney transplantation (PAK). Overall, the 1- and 2-year graft function rates for all pancreas transplants are 73% and 65%, respectively. In the national experience, patients undergoing SPK have fared the best, with 1- and 2-year graft survival rates of 78% and 71%, compared with 50% and 40% for pancreas alone and 47% and 37% for PAK.

The biologic explanation for these differences lies in the difficulties in assessing pancreas rejection. In pancreas transplantation, elevation of the serum glucose is often a late sign of rejection, because only 10% of the islet mass may be present before overt diabetes mellitus reappears. Thus, reversal of rejection may not recover sufficient islet function to ensure long-term graft function. In SPK, the kidney has been used as a "window" to assess pancreas rejection. It has been assumed that treatment of kidney rejection will also treat rejection of the pancreas, which is occurring at the same time. In PAK, monitoring of pancreas rejection has been less successful, especially when the HLA of the original kidney donor and the HLA for the pancreas donor are significantly different.

The 1- and 2-year patient survival rates for pancreas transplantation are 89% and 84%, respectively. For SPK, the corresponding survival rates are 90% and 85%, which are approximately 5% to 7% worse than for patients who receive kidney grafts alone. The increased morbidity and mortality of adding a pancreas transplant at the time of kidney transplantation are related to technical factors in pancreas grafting, such as a higher rate of infections after pancreas transplantation.

Heart-Lung

The number of heart-lung transplants has actually fallen in the past 4 years, in part because of a shift of some of these candidates toward lung transplantation. The patient survival is almost identical to that for the graft survival, because retransplantation is rare. The 1- and 2-year survival rates are 55% and 48%, respectively. Because experience with this procedure is limited, detailed analysis of the risk factors is meaningless.

Lung

The patient survival rate after lung transplantation is also similar to the graft survival, owing to the limited experience with retransplantation. The 1- and 2-year patient survival rates are 67% and 58%, respectively. The corresponding graft survival rates are 66% and 53%. Males tend to have a poorer patient and graft survival (approximately 11–12% less than 2-y survival, as compared with women). The biologic explanation for this is not clear but may be related to differences in the indications for lung transplantation between males and females.

Controversies

One of the principal controversies about the meaning of these data is the effect on national policies regarding organ allocation and possible restriction of transplant services to select groups of recipients.[16, 17] Some have argued that the transplant community should restrict transplants to those who have the greatest likelihood of long-term survival, whereas others have viewed transplantation as a means to provide lifesaving therapy to those who have the most to gain (i.e., the most critically ill).

IMMUNOLOGIC ADVANCES

Several new developments in the area of immunology and immunosuppression promise to affect organ transplantation in the near future. Although Chapter 179 has been devoted to the discussion of immunosuppressive agents, attention is given here to two new agents that may be released for general use within the next 24 months.

Chimerism

Billingham and colleagues first associated tolerance to skin grafting with hematopoietic mixing or chimerism in freemartin cattle and subsequently verified this finding by injecting viable allogeneic spleen cells into fetuses of the recipient strain.[18, 19] Ildstad and Sachs demonstrated the ability to duplicate mixed allogeneic lymphodendritic chimerism and subsequent tolerance by allogeneic bone marrow transplantation.[20] The concept of natural microchimerism, which develops after solid-organ transplantation, was first suggested by clinical observations of acquisition of delayed-type hypersensitivity in recipients after successful kidney transplantation.[21] This hypothesis was documented years later, after technologic advances allowed for detection of small numbers of donor cells (outside of the grafted organ), using immunostaining or polymerase chain reactions, in which donor deoxyribonucleic acid is amplified.[22] This pattern of migration of donor-derived cells after transplantation was subsequently found in experimental animal models[23] and in other human organ transplant models, such as liver and small-bowel transplantation.

The functionality of these cells was suggested in a study by Starzl and coworkers, in which an unexpected benefit of transplantation of the liver for type IV glycogen storage disease resulted in reversal of the deposition of the insoluble defective polysaccharide.[22] In this study, donor-derived cells were detected in the heart and other tissues in two patients receiving liver transplants for glycogen storage disease type IV. Similar findings were noted in a transplant recipient with a deficiency of the lysosomal enzyme B glucocerebrosidase, which causes type 1 Gaucher's disease.

A more systematic survey of long-term survivors after liver transplantation was performed using immunostaining and polymerase chain reaction.[24] In a group of 22 surviving liver transplant recipients who received transplants more than 10 years before being studied, all demonstrated systemic tissue microchimerism. The immunologic privilege of the liver, its ability to induce systemic hyporesponsiveness and to protect other organs from rejection, may lie in the relative abundance of migratory cells in the liver as compared with other organs, such as the kidney and heart. If this hypothesis is correct, then strategies can be developed to identify the cell type and the optimal source of these cells and to enhance the migration of these cells, in an attempt to accentuate the immunomodulating effect of these cells on the recipient immune response.

The effect of the migratory donor cells on the recipient immune response is not clear. It is likely that a number of factors determine the ultimate effect of these cells on allograft survival. If insufficient immunosuppression is given in the early phases after transplantation, then these cells may be immunogenic and may accentuate the rejection process. If the recipient is made immunoincompetent shortly before transplantation, either by cytoablation or by an imbalance in the number of immunocompetent donor cells given, then a graft-versus-host disease process may occur, in turn further suppressing the immunocompetence of the recipient.[25] If an appropriate balance of immunosuppression is given, along with a sufficient number of migratory cells or their precursor stem cells, then a phase in which the donor cells can migrate and take residence in the recipient follows a phase in which peripheral anergy or coexistence may occur.

A number of observations have suggested that a source of these cells are of bone marrow or hematogenous in origin. Donor-specific blood transfusions (DST) have been shown to enhance long-term graft survival in living donor kidney transplants since the 1970s. Cochrum and colleagues reported that DST enhanced 1-year graft survival from 57%

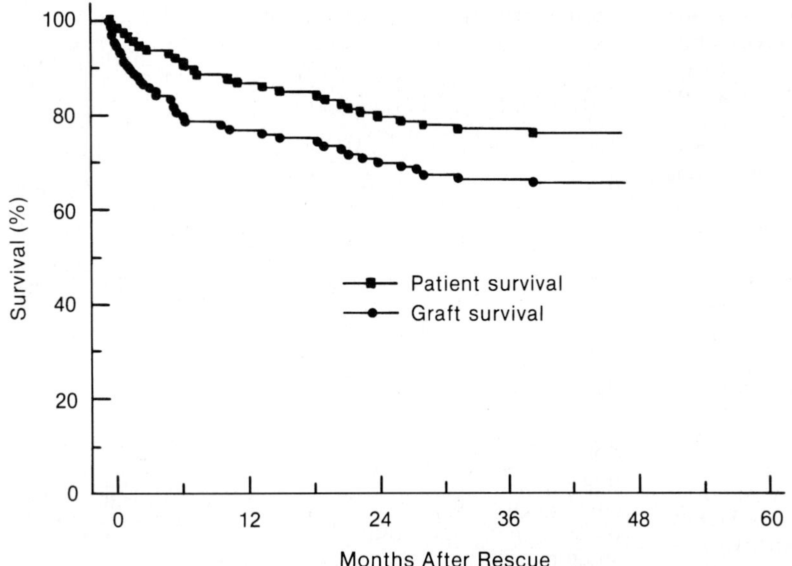

Figure 188–2. Kaplan-Meier estimates of patient and liver allograft survival in patients on cyclosporin who were converted to FK-506 therapy for biopsy-documented chronic rejection.

to 95%.[26] Even in the cyclosporin era, Salvatierra and coworkers reported a 1-year graft survival of 93% in DST-treated patients, as compared with 82% in non-DST patients.[27] In addition, the work of the University of Wisconsin group also shows a benefit of DST infusion in reducing rejection and the need for steroids.[28] Protocols have been developed to infuse donor bone marrow at the time of solid-organ transplantation. The authors are currently using cadaveric bone marrow infusion, along with solid-organ transplantation, in attempts to enhance the chimerism observed after solid-organ transplantation alone.

FK-506 (Prograf)

FK-506 (Fujisawa Pharmaceutical, Osaka, Japan) is a new immunosuppressive agent that is a macrolide antibiotic produced by the fungus *Streptomyces tsukubaensis.* The molecular structure of FK-506 is unrelated to cyclosporin, and the two drugs have different cytosolic binding sites.[29, 30] Although both drugs inhibit T lymphocyte activation, there is a practical difference in the use of these agents. The ability of FK-506 to be used to reverse ongoing, established rejection is not a characteristic of cyclosporin. The first use of FK-506 was for the indication of uncontrolled liver allograft rejection that was therefore considered treatment failure of conventional immunosuppression. The results of this experience revealed a marked ability to reverse ongoing rejection, even in cases in which chronic changes were observed.[31–36] Between 50% and 70% of patients treated by conversion to FK-506 had both clinical and histopathologic responses. In a long-term follow-up of 113 patients with chronic rejection, 75% of patients were still alive 3 years after FK-506 conversion, and 65% of liver allografts were still functioning (Fig. 188–2).[36] Liver and kidney functions before FK-506 conversion and at 1, 2, and 3 years after FK-506 conversion are shown in Table 188–1.

The United States Multicenter FK-506 Liver Study Group analyzed the prognostic factors for successful conversion from cyclosporin to FK-506–based immunosuppressive therapy for refractory rejection.[37] At 1 month after conversion, 54% of patients were noted to have complete or partial response or to be clinically improved. By 6 months after conversion, this benefit was noted in 67% of patients, and at 1 year in 86%. In this series in which the most refractory rejections were converted from cyclosporin to FK-506, the 1-year actuarial graft and patient survival rates after conversion were 50% and 72%, respectively.

Three randomized trials have been performed, comparing FK-506 with cyclosporin in primary liver transplantation. Although each trial had unique features regarding the im-

TABLE 188–1. Liver and Renal Functions*

	Before Conversion				
	All Patients	*Excluding Failure*	*1 Year*	*2 Years*	*3 Years*
Liver Function					
Bilirubin (mg/dL)	4.4	3.8	0.8	0.8	0.9
Serum glutamic-pyruvic transaminase (IU)	268	232	83	93	62
Serum glutamic-oxaloacetic transaminase (IU)	186	160	63	67	56
Alkaline phosphatase (IU)	250	243	241	212	224
γ-Glutamyl transpeptidase (IU)	445	448	409	342	207
Renal Function					
Blood urea nitrogen (mg/dL)	31.5		32.2	31.1	30.1
Creatinine (mg/dL)	1.6		2.5	1.7	1.8

*All values listed are the mean.

munosuppressive regimens, the characteristics of the patient groups and treatment of rejection, one of the primary endpoints was the failure of the defined treatment to prevent and control rejection. In the University of Pittsburgh series, low-risk candidates were randomized to FK-506 with steroids as compared with cyclosporin with steroids.[38] One hundred fifty-four patients were enrolled between February 17, 1990, and December 30, 1991. The 1-year patient and graft survival rates, as analyzed by intent to treat, were 92% and 88%, respectively, for FK-506, compared with 85% and 79%, respectively, for cyclosporin. The follow-up at 2 years revealed that the modest increase in patient and graft survival in the FK-506 limb was retained and that the good results in the cyclosporin limb were due, in part, to the ability of FK-506 to treat rejection in the cyclosporin group (Fig. 188–3). The freedom from rejection was statistically greater in the FK-506–treated group than in the cyclosporin-treated group. In addition, the freedom from steroid use and the lower incidence of hypertension were prominent features of patients treated with FK-506. The results in this single-center study have been compared with two other ongoing randomized liver transplant trials in both the United States and Europe (preliminary data presented at the International Liver Transplantation Society, Toronto, Canada, October 1993). In each series, more than 500 patients were entered into the combined limbs. Using a regimented FK-506 treatment arm, the early preliminary results support the findings at the University of Pittsburgh. The European study demonstrated an enhanced patient and graft survival in the FK-506 limb as compared with the cyclosporin limb. Although the patient survival was similar in both groups in the American study, a slight benefit in graft survival was noted in the FK-506 limb. Both studies found less rejection in the FK-506 limb, and the overall dosing of steroids was less in the FK-506 limb.

The application of FK-506 rescue therapy to kidney transplantation was an extension of the experience gained in liver transplantation. The main difference between the two organ systems is the predominance of arteriopathy and sclerosis of epithelial structures in the kidney allografts undergoing

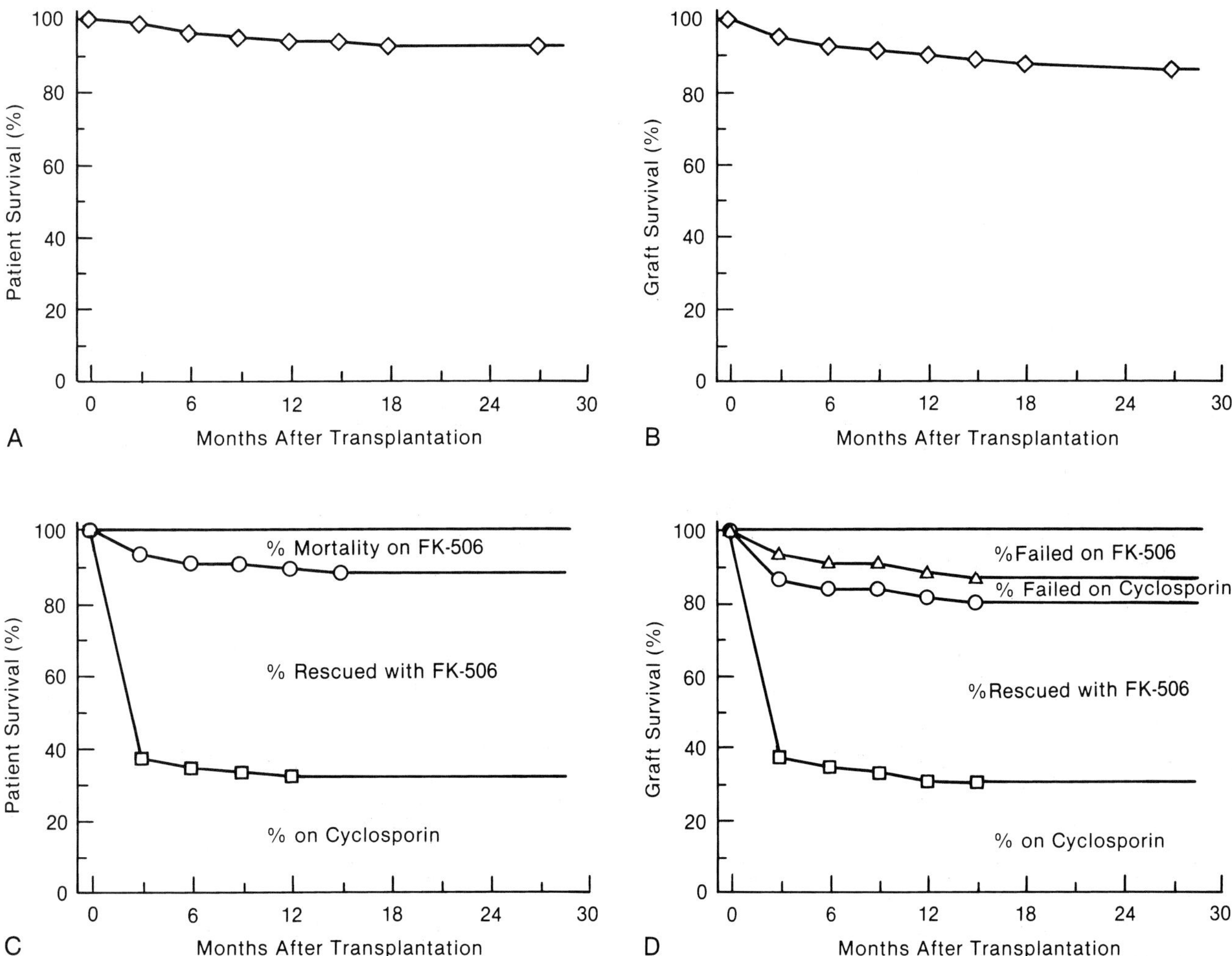

Figure 188–3. *A*, Kaplan-Meier estimate of patient survival in 79 patients randomized to FK-506 therapy and steroid therapy following liver transplantation (from February 1990 to December 1991). *B*, Corresponding graft survival in the FK-506 randomized liver transplant recipients. *C*, Kaplan-Meier estimate of patient survival in 75 patients randomized to cyclosporin therapy and steroid therapy following liver transplantation (from February 1990 to December 1991). "% Mortality on FK-506" represents the loss of patients originally treated with cyclosporin but required FK-506 conversion, and who ultimately died. "% Rescued with FK-506" represents patients initially randomized to receive cyclosporin but who were converted to FK-506 therapy following transplantation. "% on Cyclosporin" represents the group of patients who remain on cyclosporin therapy. *D*, Corresponding graft survival in patients initially randomized to cyclosporin therapy. "% Failed on Cyclosporin" represents those grafts lost in patients who were still on cyclosporin therapy at the time of retransplantation.

chronic rejection. This was found to limit the ability of FK-506 to rescue grafts with this pathologic finding. In a series of 35 patients, those with ongoing acute cellular rejection had a successful conversion rate of 71% whereas those with stigmata of chronic rejection were not able to be rescued.[39] Those with living related kidney transplants had a higher rate of rescue (73%) than those with cadaveric grafts (50%), probably related to an earlier referral for FK-506 rescue therapy.

A randomized trial using FK-506 in a double-drug regimen (FK-506 and steroids) versus a triple-drug regimen (FK-506, steroids, and azathioprine) was performed in kidney transplantation at the University of Pittsburgh.[40] Two hundred four patients were enrolled, and there were no specific exclusion criteria based on immunologic or transplant history. Thirty per cent of the patients were undergoing retransplantation, with 17% of the recipients being sensitized (per cent reactive antibody [PRA] >40%). The 1-year actuarial patient and graft survival rates for the two-drug versus three-drug regimen were 95% and 90% versus 91% and 82%, respectively. No differences were noted in the kidney function with the mean serum creatinine level of 1.8 ± 0.8 mg/dL. The rejection rate in the three-drug regimen was less than that for the two-drug regimen (37% vs. 51%), although this was not statistically significant ($P = 0.07$). Crossover from one group to another was not uncommon. Twenty-five per cent of the two-drug group were given azathioprine, principally because of rejection, and 45% of the three-drug group required discontinuation of azathioprine because of leukopenia or hepatic dysfunction.

Armitage and coworkers at the University of Pittsburgh reported their experience with FK-506–based immunosuppression after heart transplantation.[41, 42] In eight patients, FK-506 was used as rescue therapy for patients suffering from persistent, refractory cardiac rejection on cyclosporin, azathioprine, and steroids. All of these eight patients had received and failed one or more courses of antilymphocyte therapy while receiving cyclosporin therapy. In keeping with the previous experiences with rescue therapy, all of these patients had demonstrated improvement in the histopathology after FK-506 conversion.

Seventy-two primary adult patients were given FK-506 as primary immunosuppression after heart transplantation.[42] The 1-year patient and graft survival rate was 92%. The freedom from rejection at 90 days was 41% and at 180 days was 34%. Renal dysfunction was frequently noted, and the mean serum creatinine level at 6 months after transplantation was 2.2 mg/dL. The incidence of diastolic hypertension was 54% but was considered mild, because treatment consisted of a single agent in all cases. The incidence of new-onset diabetes was 20% in this group of patients.

FK-506 is not without its limitations. Toxicity profiles for FK-506 are similar to that of cyclosporin, perhaps because of similar mechanisms of action. A detailed analysis and review of the adverse effects of FK-506 are beyond the scope of this discourse. Readers are referred to detailed reports of FK-506 adverse effects.[43, 44] Both FK-506 and cyclosporin administration have been associated with side effects, many of which are similar and some of which are peculiar to a given organ transplant.

RS61443 (Mycophenolate Mofetil)

RS61443 (Syntex Research, Palo Alto, CA) is an analog of mycophenolic acid with enhanced oral bioavailability.[45] Like mycophenolic acid, RS61443 inhibits inosine monophosphate dehydrogenase and guanosine monophosphate synthetase, both key enzymes that regulate the purine nucleotide salvage pathway.[46] It has in vitro inhibitory effects on both B and T lymphocytes.[47]

Mycophenolic acid was initially used as an agent for the treatment of refractory psoriasis.[48] This drug was relatively well tolerated, the principal side effects being leukopenia, mucositis, and gastrointestinal upset. Patients reportedly had a higher incidence of upper respiratory tract infections, and long-term patients had a higher incidence of skin cancers. RS61443 has been studied in clinical trials for treatment of refractory rheumatoid arthritis, in transplant trials as primary therapy along with cyclosporin and steroids, in kidney transplantation, as well as in rescue therapy in patients with refractory organ rejection.[49] Preliminary results suggest that this drug is relatively well tolerated in doses up to 3.5 to 4.0 g/d. Results of several randomized studies of RS61443 in primary organ transplantation are not available. Several rescue studies have suggested that RS61443 is capable of stabilizing or reversing ongoing rejection in as many as 80% of cases when added to cyclosporin-based immunosuppression.

APPLICATIONS TO NEW ORGAN TRANSPLANTATION

One way to assess the impact of a new immunosuppressive agent in transplantation is the ability to successfully transplant organs that were not considered feasible with standard immunosuppression. This was certainly the situation when cyclosporin was introduced to liver transplantation. Chapters 183 through 185 deal with the topics of lung, pancreas, and intestinal transplantation, and a brief reference to the impact of FK-506 in these organ transplants is provided here.

Intestinal Transplantation

Success with intestinal transplantation under cyclosporin immunosuppression has been sporadic.[50–52] A growing experience of small-bowel transplantation, either alone or combined with other abdominal organs, has been accumulated under FK-506 at the University of Pittsburgh.[53–55] Small-bowel allografts have been transplanted alone ($n = 9$), together with liver ($n = 16$), or as part of a multivisceral cluster ($n = 3$). In these 28 patients, 82% were alive at a median follow-up of 9 months. Graft survival was 76% at the same period. Graft function was satisfactory, with 84% of survivors being totally enterally sufficient and the other 16% relying on supplemental parenteral nutrition. Rejection was not uncommon, with 90% of the patients having at least one rejection episode of the intestinal allograft. Rejection has been treated by additional steroids and addition of azathioprine; however, antilymphocyte preparations have been used occasionally.

Lung Transplantation

Lung transplantation is a rapidly developing procedure that has been limited because of technical, preservation, and immunologic reasons. A prospective randomized trial of primary adult pulmonary transplantation was conducted at the University of Pittsburgh.[56] Azathioprine was combined with either FK-506 or cyclosporin, resorting to using steroids only if the recipient encountered more than one episode of rejection. Twenty-eight patients were randomized to FK-506, and 29 patients were randomized to cyclosporin. The 6-month graft survival was statistically better in the FK-506 group than in the cyclosporin group (86% vs. 69%, respectively, $P < 0.05$). Twenty-one per cent of the patients receiving FK-

506 were rejection free at 6 months, as compared with only 3% of the cyclosporin recipients.

Islet Cell Transplantation

Treatment of type I diabetes mellitus with islet cell transplantation is the goal of pancreas transplantation. The morbidity and mortality associated with transplantation of the exocrine component of whole-pancreas transplantation are well known. Ricordi and coworkers have developed an automated system of enzymatic and mechnical separation that has improved previous methods for islet cell isolation.[57] Application of this technique has proved to be applicable to clinical situations by infusion of purified islets into liver allografts, during combined liver-islet transplantation, and has shown long-term islet function in selected cases of surgically induced diabetes mellitus. The early experience with islet transplantation for treatment of juvenile onset type I diabetes mellitus has been less successful, although C-peptide secretion was almost uniformly observed.[58] At the University of Minnesota, three cases of exogenous insulin freedom have been noted in patients undergoing combined kidney-islet cell transplantation.* The technical and immunologic factors are still being investigated.

ADVANCES AND INNOVATIONS IN SUPPORT SYSTEMS—EXPANSION OF THE DONOR POOL

Extracorporeal Liver Assist Device

Acute liver insufficiency can present as either fulminant hepatic failure (FHF) or primary nonfunction of liver allografts (PNF) after liver transplantation. The clinical presentation is acute liver failure complicated by hepatic encephalopathy in a previously healthy person (FHF) or after liver transplantation (PNF). Survival from either FHF or PNF is poor, particularly in patients suffering advanced encephalopathy with development of hepatorenal syndrome, systemic lactic acidosis, and severe coagulopathy. The morbidity and mortality of FHF and PNF cannot be underestimated. FHF has a mortality rate of 60% to 95%, with higher mortality from viral and toxic exposure FHF, lower in patients with acetaminophen overdose. PNF occurs in 10% of patients after liver transplantation, and contributing factors include donor instability and length of preservation times, although many PNF cases have no predisposing factors. Mortality associated with PNF is approximately 40% to 50%, even after retransplantation.

The epidemiology of FHF in the United States was reviewed at the Fulminant Hepatic Failure Workshop as part of the National Digestive Diseases Advisory Board, held February 1993. The overall incidence of FHF is approximately 2000 cases per year. The incidence of PNF is approximately 200 to 300 cases per year. Management of both PNF and FHF is challenging and aimed at prevention and treatment of complications including infections, brain edema, hemodynamic instability, pulmonary and renal failure, acid-base disturbances, and coagulopathy. Orthotopic liver transplantation has increasingly been used for selected patients with FHF, whereas orthotopic retransplantation is the only procedure of choice in patients with PNF.

The concept of using mechanical devices to maintain patients with PNF or FHF until transplantation is an attractive one. Nevertheless, dialysis and charcoal hemoperfusion are not of proven benefit, because the multiple biochemical functions are not being replaced, and their use has not resulted in decreased mortality in patients with FHF.[59, 60]

*Sutherland D: Personal communication, 1993.

Three proposed systems have used a hybrid device containing metabolically active liver cells.

Laboratory models have attempted to use primary hepatocyte cultures, isolated from either animal or human livers; however, the inability to grow such cells in vitro has limited the practicality of this source of cells. Rozga and coworkers have used a liver support system consisting of plasma separation and perfusion through a charcoal filter and hollow-fiber cartridge using porcine hepatocytes attached to collagen-coated dextran microcarrier beads, which are then placed into the extracapillary space of a hollow-fiber cartridge. Plasma is passed through the intracapillary space, and the porcine hepatocytes are separated from the plasma by the cartridge membrane. In a case report of a patient with FHF, total hepatectomy with extracorporeal liver support was able to support the patient until orthotopic liver transplantation could successfully be completed.[61] In this case, intracranial pressures and serum ammonia were thought to be controlled with the use of the porcine hepatocyte–extracorporeal liver assist device (ELAD) system.

The system described by Shatford and coworkers at the University of Minnesota is similar in theory to the porcine hepatocyte–ELAD but uses rat hepatocytes in a collagen gel placed in the lumen of hollow-fiber cartridges.[62] Blood is passed through the extracapillary space, but the hepatocytes are protected from immune damage by the cartridge membrane.[63] This system has not yet been used in human trials.

The third ELAD system is based on the use of a subclone of HepG2 (Hep G2/C3), which is a human hepatoblastoma cell line and expresses nearly normal levels of several central metabolic pathways and has the morphology and polarity characteristic of human hepatocytes.[64] Hep G2/C3 can be grown in hollow-fiber cartridges, with the intention of developing an extracorporeal liver assist device (C3-ELAD). Six human patients have been treated with C3-ELAD.[65, 66] Two were on a compassionate basis, and four under a Food and Drug Administration–approved protocol. All of the patients had advanced encephalopathy at the onset of therapy, and all were in an intensive care unit. The devices were used between 24 hours and 6 days. Improved clinical status, such as mental status, was noted in three of the six patients. One patient recovered completely from FHF, apparently as a result of C3-ELAD. Two other patients improved but died of non–liver-related causes, one from sepsis 3 days after discontinuation of C3-ELAD therapy and the other of brain death after a period of hypotension not thought to be related to C3-ELAD therapy. The remaining three patients died, one during an unrelated diagnostic procedure, one as a result of technical inability to continue C3-ELAD therapy, and one as a result of advanced metabolic derangements related to liver failure.

Non–Heartbeating Donors

Before the acceptance of brain death, donors were required to have cessation of heart function in order to procure organs for transplantation. In some countries where brain death legislation has not been passed, such as Japan, non–heartbeating donors (NHBD) represent a principal source of organs for transplantation. Two distinct populations of NHBD have been identified, one after uncontrolled cardiopulmonary arrest and the other under conditions of removal from life support, without having fulfilled criteria for brain death. The first situation would require immediate procurement or infusion of preservation solution into the pronounced individual in a setting where family consent may not be available. Such a pilot study has been initiated by the Regional Organ Bank of Illinois, based on in situ perfusion of the abdominal aorta with a double-balloon catheter.[67]

The second situation is that of using patients who do not fulfill brain death criteria but in whom an express wish has been made by either the patient or family to remove life support and to have the patient become an organ donor after declaration of death. Such a protocol has been developed by the University of Pittsburgh Medical Center and the Center for Organ Recovery and Education, which is the organ procurement organization associated with the geographic area of Pittsburgh. This protocol was developed in response to a perception that some families wished to have the right to terminate life support and to donate organs, if so desired. A 2-year process of internal and external review, development of guidelines, and passage by two ethics committees resulted in a protocol that has been in effect since 1992. The protocol emphasizes that "Patients or their surrogates can decide to forgo life-sustaining treatment and the Guidelines authorize comfort measure for patients wishing to forgo such treatment. Furthermore, all patients have the right to elect organ donation in the event of their death. . . . The purpose of this document is to provide an auditable, ethically justifiable policy that respects the rights of the donor while maximizing the possibility for successful organ donation." The details of this protocol are worth discussing, because they may form a foundation for further developments in this field. The interest in using NHBD is highlighted by the increasing development of protocols among organ procurement organizations around the country.

A number of principles of the approved NHBD protocol have been implemented to ensure that patients, healthcare providers, and potential recipients are safeguarded. The most important principles are summarized below:

1. "Decisions concerning the treatment and management of the patients . . . must be made separately from and prior to the decision of organ donation. . . . Patients shall be considered for organ donation . . . only when the patient or surrogate initiates discussion of organ donation."
2. "It is the health care professional's primary responsibility to optimize the patient's care. . . . It is an important objective of this policy that the interest in procuring organs does not interfere with optimal patient management."
3. "Appropriate candidates for organ donation shall be limited to those patients on life-sustaining treatment in whom withdrawal of that therapy is likely to result in death within a short period of time."
4. "Health care professionals shall not be required to participate in the procedures described below. . . ."

Other important points that should be emphasized follow: (1) The process of initiating discussion must come from the patient or surrogate, in order to minimize any perception of conflict of interest. (2) The situation must be reviewed by an ethics representative. (3) The protocol requires full informed consent with the patient or surrogate. (4) If removal of life support does leads to an "unacceptable prolonged warm ischemia time," as determined by the organ procurement organization or procuring surgeon, then donation may be canceled. (5) Pronouncement of death must be by an intensivist without any clinical or research interest with the transplant program. (6) Transplant physicians will not be involved in the management of these patients before declaration of death. Nevertheless, the NHBD has already generated a number of controversial ethical discussions.[68]

A report by Yokoyama and coworkers, in Japan, revealed that the 1-year graft survival of 110 kidney allografts taken from NHBD were similar to those reported in brain-dead heartbeating donors.[69] At the University of Pittsburgh, similar results have been obtained for both kidney and liver allografts taken from NHBD.[69a] It is too early to extrapolate the potential impact on the donor pool using NHBD.

Xenotransplantation

In order to understand the trends in the development of xenotransplantation, it is important to realize that potential donors for cross-species transplantation into humans can be separated into two groups. We can consider that donors are either discordant or concordant. A discordant combination is characterized by the presence of a preformed antibody in the recipient, usually at high titers, that reacts and causes hyperacute rejection of the donor organ. On the other hand, concordant combinations are generally characterized by low or nonexistent antibodies, so that the resultant rejection process resembles that of an allograft.[70] As an example, transplants from primates into humans are usually concordant whereas cross-species transplants from a pig into a human would be discordant.

From animals studies, the concordant combinations usually reject their organs in a different time frame than discordant combinations. Livers and hearts from an untreated discordant combination are rejected by antibodies within minutes to hours after revascularization. These organs would be rejected days to weeks after transplantation in an untreated concordant combination. We also realize that liver grafts are less susceptible to antibody-mediated injury than are kidney or heart grafts. This difference has been used in more recent attempts at clinical xenotransplantation, with the expectation that liver xenografts may be more likely to succeed than other types of xenografts.

Using this train of thought, liver xenografts may be envisioned in three different clinical settings. The first would be to use liver xenografts as a temporary support, either until the liver recovers from injury or as a bridge to transplantation. These organs could be perfused outside of the recipient, in an ex vivo manner. This was reported in a number of early experiences in the 1960s and again more recently by the Johns Hopkins University and Duke University groups. Second, heterotopic liver xenotransplantation might be envisioned as a bridging method until an appropriate human liver is found. Finally, permanent orthotopic replacement of a diseased liver with a liver xenograft can be considered as a definitive procedure and one that may potentially expand the donor pool.

Several general therapeutic considerations may be taken into account in xenotransplantation. The first deals directly with the selection of an appropriate donor species. If an initial high titer of cytotoxic antibodies is noted in the recipient, then these antibodies must be depleted. This can be done either specifically, by immunoabsorption, or nonspecifically, by removing plasma immunoglobulins. Once a suitable environment is created, in which the likelihood of hyperacute rejection is reduced, then one must sustain a low titer of cytotoxic xenoantibody levels in the early posttransplant period, usually by pharmacologic methods. The second consideration is to minimize the inflammatory cascades that amplify the immune system. Specifically, complement activation leads to a number of inflammatory mediators, which are difficult to control. Agents that can interfere with this cascade and the subsequent inflammatory mediators must be developed. Finally, sustained suppression of cell-mediated rejection is important, in order to minimize the long-term damage to the xenograft that may occur via lymphocyte-derived cytokines.

Other considerations regarding the success of xenotransplants depend on the compatibility of proteins between the donor and recipient species, as well as potential infectious disease drawbacks. These are areas of immense interest in those studying xenotransplantation. Although three liver xenotransplantations have failed, the longest remaining viable for 72 days, important facts about the pathology, immunology, compatibility, and physiology were obtained and will aid in future attempts.[71, 72]

CONCLUSIONS

The field of transplantation has grown tremendously in the past 40 years since the first successful human transplant. A better understanding of the immune mechanisms that cause graft damage, as well as new immunosuppressive agents, has helped put transplantation in a therapeutic realm. Unfortunately, with the success of transplantation, the scarcity of donor organs remains one of the principal limitations for broader applications. In this area, efforts have been made to expand the donor pool, either by using donors who fall outside of the criteria once applied to living donors or to xenotransplantation. Each of the next advances in the expansion of the donor pool is likely to generate controversy and will require careful scientific approaches to ensure the safety of the recipients. Other developments in the area of bioartificial or totally artificial support devices are of significant interest, because successful development will solve the organ shortage problem.

References

1. Carrel A: La technique operatoire des anastomse vasculares et la transplantation des visceres. Lyon Medicine 1902; 98:859.
2. Voronoy VV: Blocking the reticuloendothelial system in man in some forms of mercuric chloride intoxication and transplantation of the cadaver kidney as a method of treatment for the anuria resulting from the intoxication. Transplant Sci 1991; 1:71.
3. Merrill JP, Murray JE, Harrison JH, et al: Successful homotransplantation of the human kidney between identical twins. JAMA 1956; 160:277.
4. Gibson T, Medawar PB: Fate of skin homografts in man. J Anat 1942; 77:299.
5. Calne RY, Murray JE: Inhibition of the rejection of renal homografts in dogs by Burroughs Wellcome 57-222. Surg Forum 1961; 12:118.
6. Starzl TE, Marchioro TL, Waddell WR: The reversal of rejection in human renal homografts with subsequent development of homograft tolerance. Surg Gynecol Obstet 1963; 117:385.
7. Reemtsma K, McCracken BH, Schlegel JU, et al: Renal heterotransplantation in man. Ann Surg 1964; 160:384.
8. Report of the Ad Hoc Committee of the Harvard Medical School: A definition of irreversible coma. JAMA 1968; 205:537.
9. Starzl TE, Miller C, Broznick B, et al: An improved technique for multiple organ harvesting. Surg Gynecol Obstet 1987; 165:343.
10. Collins GM, Bravo-Shugarman M, Terasaki PI: Kidney preservation for transportation. Lancet 1969; 2:1219.
11. Belzer FO, Southard JH: Principles of solid organ preservation by cold storage. Transplantation 1988; 45:673.
12. Borel JF, Feurer C, Gubler HU, et al: Biological effects of cyclosporin A: A new antilymphocytic agent. Agents Actions 1976; 6:468.
13. Calne RY, Rolles K, White DJG, et al: Cyclosporin A initially as the only immunosuppressant in 34 recipients of cadaveric organs: 32 kidneys, 2 pancreas, and 2 livers. Lancet 1979; 2:1022.
14. Starzl TE, Weil R, Iwatsuki S, et al: The use of cyclosporin A and prednisone in cadaveric kidney transplantation. Surg Gynecol Obstet 1980; 151:17.
15. U.S. Department of Health and Human Services: 1991 Report of Center-Specific Graft and Patient Survival Rates. Washington, DC, U.S. Department of Health and Human Services, 1991.
16. Gaston RS, Ayres I, Dooley LG, et al: Racial equity in renal transplantation: The disparate impact of HLA-based allocation. JAMA 1993; 270:1352–1356.
17. Bronsther O, Fung JJ, Tzalis A, et al: Prioritization and organ distribution for liver transplantation. JAMA 1994; 271:140–143.
18. Billingham R, Lampkin G, Medawar P, et al: Tolerance of homografts, twin diagnosis, and the freemartin condition in cattle. Heredity 1956; 6:201
19. Billingham RE, Brent L, Medawar PB: "Actively acquired tolerance" of foreign cells. Nature 1953; 172:603.
20. Ildstad ST, Sachs DH: Reconstitution with syngeneic plus allogeneic or xenogeneic bone marrow leads to specific acceptance of allografts or xenografts. Nature 1984; 307:168.
21. Wilson WEC, Kirkpatrick CH: Immunologic aspects of renal homotransplantation. *In:* Experience in Renal Transplantation. Starzl TE (Ed). Philadelphia, WB Saunders, 1964, p 239.
22. Starzl TE, Demetris AJ, Trucco M, et al: Chimerism after liver transplantation for Type IV glycogen storage disease and Type I Gaucher's disease. N Engl J Med 1992; 328:745.
23. Murase N, Demetris AJ, Woo J, et al: Lymphocyte traffic and graft-versus-host disease after fully allogeneic small bowel transplantation. Transplant Proc 1991; 23:3246.
24. Starzl TE, Demetris AJ, Trucco M, et al: Systemic chimerism in human female recipients of male livers. Lancet 1992; 340:876.
25. Starzl TE, Demetris AJ, Trucco M, et al: Cell migration and chimerism after whole organ transplantation: The basis of graft acceptance. Hepatology 1993; 17:1127.
26. Cochrum KC, Salvatierra O, Belzer FO: Correlations between MLC stimulation and graft survival in living related and cadaver transplants. Ann Surg 1974; 180:617.
27. Salvatierra O, Metzer J, Vincenti F: Donor-specific blood transfusions versus cyclosporine—the DST story. Transplant Proc 1987; 19:160.
28. Reed A, Pirsch JD, Armbrust MJ, et al: A comparison of donor-specific and random transfusions in living-related renal transplantation and their effect on steroid withdrawal. Transplant Proc 1991; 23:1321.
29. Siekierka JJ, Hung SHY, Poe M, et al: A cytosolic binding protein for the immunosuppressant FK506 has peptidyl-prolyl isomerase activity but is distinct from cyclophillin. Nature 1989; 341:755–757.
30. Harding MW, Galat A, Uehling DE, et al: A receptor for the immunosuppressant FK506 is cis-trans peptidyl-prolyl isomerase. Nature 1989; 341:758–760.
31. Fung JJ, Todo S, Jain A, et al: Conversion from cyclosporin to FK506 in liver allograft recipients with cyclosporine related complications. Transplant Proc 1990; 22:6–12.
32. Fung JJ, Todo S, Tzakis A, et al: Conversion of liver allograft recipients from cyclosporine to FK506 based immunosuppression: Benefits and pitfalls. Transplant Proc 1991; 23:14–21.
33. Winkler M, Ringe B, Gerstenkorn C, et al: Use of FK506 for treatment of chronic rejection after liver transplantation. Transplant Proc 1991; 23:2984.
34. D'Alessandro AM, Kalayoglu M, Pirsch JD, et al: FK506 rescue therapy for resistant rejection episodes in liver transplant recipients. Transplant Proc 1991; 23:2987.
35. Holland R, Sorrell M, Langnas A, et al: Chronic rejection in liver transplant recipients: Does conversion to FK506 confer a survival benefit? Hepatology 1993; 18:74A.
36. Fung JJ, Jain A, Hamad I, et al: Long term effects of FK506 following conversion from cyclosporine to FK506 for chronic rejection in liver transplant recipients. Hepatology 1993; 18:74A.
37. McDiarmid SV, Klintmalm G, Busuttil RW: FK506 rescue therapy in liver transplantation: Outcome and complications. Transplant Proc 1991; 23:2996.
38. Fung J, Todo S, Abu-Elmagd K, et al: A randomized trial in primary liver transplantation under immunosuppression with FK506 or cyclosporine. Transplant Proc 1993; 25:1130.
39. Jordan ML, Shapiro R, Jensen CWB, et al: FK506 conversion of renal allografts failing cyclosporine immunosuppression. Transplant Proc 1991; 23:3078–3081.
40. Shapiro R, Jordan J, Scantlebury V, et al: Randomized trial of FK506/prednisone vs. FK506/azathioprine/prednisone after renal transplantation: Preliminary report. Transplant Proc 1991; 25:669.
41. Armitage JM, Kormos RL, Fung J, et al: The clinical trial of FK506 as primary immunosuppression in adult cardiac transplantation. Transplant Proc 1991; 23:3054–3057.

42. Armitage JM, Kormos RL, Morita S, et al: Clinical trial of FK506 immunosuppression in adult cardiac transplantation. Ann Thorac Surg 1992; 54:205–211.
43. Cillo U, Alessiani M, Fung JJ, et al: Major adverse effects of FK506 used as an immunosuppressive agent after liver transplantation. Transplant Proc 1993; 25:628–634.
44. Fung JJ, Alessiani M, Abu-Elmagd K, et al: Adverse effects associated with the use of FK506. Transplant Proc 1991; 23:3105–3108.
45. Lee WA, Gu L, Miksztal AR, et al: Bioavailability improvement of mycophenolic acid through amino ester derivation. Pharmacol Res 1990; 7:161.
46. Franklin TJ, Cool JM: The inhibition of nucleic acid synthesis by mycophenolic acid. Biochem J 1969; 113:515.
47. Allison AC, Almquist SJ, Muller CD, et al: In vitro immunosuppressive effects of mycophenolic acid and an ester prodrug, RS-61443. Transplant Proc 1991; 23(Suppl):10.
48. Mariani R, Fleischmajer R, Schragger AH, et al: Mycophenolic acid in the treatment of psoriasis. Arch Dermatol 1977; 113:930.
49. Sollinger HW, Deierholi MH, Belzer FO, et al: RS-61443—a phase I clinical trial and pilot rescue study. Transplantation 1992; 53:428.
50. Deltz E, Schroeder P, Gebhardt H, et al: Successful clinical small bowel transplantation: Report of a case. Clin Transplant 1989; 3:89–91.
51. Grant D, Wall W, Mimeault R, et al: Successful small bowel/liver transplantation. Lancet 1990; 335:181.
52. Schroeder P, Goulet O, Lear PA: Small bowel transplantation: European experience (Letter). Lancet 1990; 336:110.
53. Todo S, Tzakis AG, Abu-Elmagd K, et al: Cadaveric small bowel and small bowel-liver transplantation in humans. Transplantation 1992; 53:369–376.
54. Todo S, Tzakis AG, Abu-Elmagd K, et al: Intestinal transplantation in composite visceral grafts or alone. Ann Surg 1992; 216:223–234.
55. Abu-Elmagd K, Fung JJ, Reyes J, et al: Management of intestinal transplantation in humans. Transplant Proc 1992; 24:1243–1244.
56. Griffith BP, Bando K, Hardesty RL, et al: Prospective randomized trial of FK506 versus cyclosporine after human pulmonary transplantation. Transplantation 1994; 57:848–851.
57. Ricordi C, Lacy PE, Finke EH, et al: An automated method for the isolation of human pancreatic islets. Diabetes 1988; 37:413.
58. Ricordi C, Carroll PB, Tzalid AG, et al: Outcome of human islet isolation and allotransplantation in 23 consecutive cases. Diabetes Nutr Metab (in press).
59. Hughes RH, Williams R: Clinical experience with charcoal hemoperfusion and resin hemoperfusion. Semin Liver Dis 1986; 6:164–173.
60. O'Grady JG, Gimson AES, O'Brien CJ, et al: Controlled trials of charcoal hemoperfusion and prognostic factors in fulminant hepatic failure. Gastroenterology 1989; 94:1186–1192.
61. Rozga J, Podesta L, LePage E, et al: Control of cerebral edema by total hepatectomy and extracorporeal liver support in fulminant hepatic failure. Lancet 1993; 342:898.
62. Shatford RA, Nyberg SL, Meier SJ, et al: Hepatocyte function in a hollow fiber bioreactor: A potential bioartificial liver. J Surg Res 1992; 53:549.
63. Nyberg SL, Platt JL, Shirabe K, et al: Immunoprotection of xenocytes in a hollow fiber bioartificial liver. ASAIO J 1992; 38:M463.
64. Thrift RN, Forte TM, Cahoon BE, et al: Characterization of lipoproteins produced by the human liver cell line, HepG2, under defined conditions. J Lipid Res 1986; 27:236–250.
65. Sussman NL, Chong MG, Koussayer T, et al: Reversal of fulminant hepatic failure using an extracorporeal liver assist device. Hepatology 1992; 16:60–65.
66. Sussman NL, Gislason GT, Conlin CA, et al: Use of the Hepatix Extracorporeal liver assist device in the treatment of fulminant hepatic failure. Hepatology 1993; 18:65A.
67. Anaise D, Smith R, Ishimaru M, et al: An approach to organ salvage from non-heartbeating donors under existing legal and ethical requirements for transplantation. Transplant Proc 1990; 22:290.
68. Youngner SJ, Arnold RM: Ethical, psychosocial, and public policy implications of procuring organs from non-heart-beating cadaver donors. JAMA 1993; 269:2769.
69. Yokoyama I, Uchida K, Tominaga Y, et al: Ten-year experience in the use of double balloon catheter for kidney procurement from non-heart beating donors in cadaveric kidney transplant. Clin Transplant 1993; 7:258.
69a. Casavilla A, Ramirez C, Shapiro R, et al: Experience with liver and kidney allografts from non–heart beating donors (in press).
70. Calne RY: Organ transplantation between widely disparate species. Transplant Proc 1970; 2:550.
71. Starzl TE, Fung J, Tzakis A, et al: Baboon-to-human liver transplantation. Lancet 1993; 341:65.
72. Nalesnik MA, Fung JJ, Starzl TE, et al: Pathology studies in two baboon to human liver xenograft cases. Abstract presented at the Second International Congress on Xenotransplantation, Cambridge, England, September 1993.
73. Makowaka L, Wu GD, Hoffman A, et al: Immunohistopathologic lesions associated with the rejection of a pig-to-human xenograft. Abstract presented at the Second International Congress on Xenotransplantation, Cambridge, England, September 1993.

SECTION XV

ISSUES IN PATIENT CARE

Joann I. Lamb

CHAPTER 189

Aspects of Critical Care Nursing Practice: Looking Back to Face the Challenge of the Future

Carole Birdsall, EdD, RN, CCRN

Critical care practice has evolved into a strong specialty within the healthcare arena during the past 25 years. The Society for Critical Care Medicine (SCCM) and the American Association of Critical-Care Nurses (AACN) combined have one of the largest memberships of any other specialty in healthcare. In its infancy, critical care practice was an unknown science attracting practitioners who were fascinated and intrigued by the uncharted waters of intensive care. With the advent of the thermodilution pulmonary artery catheter, the intra-aortic balloon pump, and advanced pharmacologic and surgical interventions, resuscitating and sustaining life for critically ill patients became reality. Now, widespread transplantation of multiple organs, continued technologic advances in pharmacology, space age diagnostic and therapeutic interventions, and interfaced computer applications at the bedside have created a highly technical environment. This environment is fraught with risk to patients and caregivers alike. Because of the nature of the environment and the mandates of managing the technology, humanistic care is often problematic. Concern for this issue led to a consensus conference on humane care in 1990 sponsored jointly by the SCCM and AACN.[1] This conference identified the need for addressing humane care in the critical care work environment. The challenge to critical care practitioners is to be proactive rather than reactive to the changes that will be necessary in the future to meet these mandates. Rather than moving into the next century with ambiguous goals, it is time to look back and use what is known about selected aspects of critical care nursing practice to face the challenge of the future.

LOOKING BACK

In 1969, Abdellah stated, "the goals of the ICU team are, first, the preservation of life; second, the restoration of the patient to his maximal functional capacity; and third, a decrease in the overall morbidity."[2] Despite a span of 25 years, these goals are still applicable. Although these goals seem simplistic, the complexity of critical care practice has changed markedly in the past decade, making outcomes less predictable. Many factors influenced this complexity and led to change in critical care practice. For commentary, several aspects of the past can be broadly grouped into changes affecting healthcare delivery, factors influencing productivity and motivation, and issues around communication.

Changes Affecting Healthcare Delivery

The past decade witnessed enormous change in healthcare policy. Legislative and judicial decisions about patient care issues abound. Questions about resource allocation in an era of cost containment are part of a daily dilemma for practitioners. Although the cost of healthcare services continues to rise, reflecting about 12% of the gross national product, growing numbers of Americans are without health insurance and without access to healthcare.[3] Uncertainty, healthcare reform, and ongoing change are influencing practice.

The healthcare environment itself is currently in crisis. The prospective reimbursement system based on diagnosis-related groups (DRGs) has negatively affected the fiscal status of most institutions. Disallowed inpatient services have resulted in a burgeoning growth in outpatient and home care with a corresponding compression of acuity within the institution. Many large inner-city hospitals serving the poor have reported an increased burden of bad debt and are struggling with inadequate income to meet demands for services. The professional salary within the urban institution often is less competitive than private and for-profit institutions in the same area, and recruiting qualified staff is more problematic. In addition, the cost of delivering care is greater in large metropolitan areas owing to the higher cost of living and the larger salaries. On the other side of the coin, DRG compression has forced many rural and smaller community hospitals to close, thus placing a greater burden on the existing services.

Because of DRG compression and disallowed services, the patient mix in hospitals has become more acute. The patient mix in any given institution helps influence the way care is practiced. When the acuity is high, the requirement for nursing care hours per patient increases. However, because of rising costs and demand for nursing services, qualified staff to fill this demand may be unavailable or money to pay for the services may be inadequate. The end result is practice shortcuts or lack of quality care.

The population requiring critical care is also changing. Patients are older and younger than ever before and require increasingly complex care of multisystem problems in an environment fraught with stiff legislation, rationed resources, and uncertainty. The aging population is significant in that older patients have more comorbidity leading to a greater number of complications.[3, 4] Further, a patient from a lower socioeconomic status without health insurance coverage has limited access to healthcare, and when hospitalization is needed, this individual may require more care because of preexisting unaddressed problems.

The proliferation of technology used in modern healthcare is well documented.[3, 5] Hospitals often market themselves as providing the newest or latest equipment to a public who often equates the technology with quality care. The highly technical critical care environment has become an expectation of the institution, the public, and the caregivers. As the amount of equipment has increased, the technology needed to support a patient in crisis has become greater. For each added item, the risk for iatrogenic injury has increased. The immediate past became an era of litigation associated with iatrogenic injury resulting in increased insurance costs. Issues of rationing resources have now come to the forefront and may negatively affect the future research and development of new technology.

The latest nursing shortage has resulted in a needed increase in nursing salaries. However, in combination with bad debt and limited income, many institutions have been forced to downsize the mix of professional to nonprofessional nursing staff to meet these salary demands. When downsizing is necessary, ancillary and support personnel are often cut back, resulting in diminished services to the existing nursing units. The nursing staff picks up and fills in for the failure of services, thus increasing the amount of non-nursing tasks required and the workload of the nursing staff and leading to professional dissatisfaction.

Practice changes result from an expanding body of knowledge evolving from advances in recombinant medications, technologic instrumentation, and ongoing research. These changes require ongoing staff development to maintain the appropriate level of knowledge and skills for staff. At the same time, cost containment has forced many staff education departments to downsize. Thus, as education needs increase, fewer individuals are available to meet them. These changes in combination with increased legislation and regulation mandate that institutions explore new ways of teaching adult learners and evaluate the outcomes of this endeavor with research.

Career Options

Staff nurses who practice in critical care have varied backgrounds with respect to education, experience, and commitment to the specialty. In urban areas, this is further compounded by cultural diversity. Practitioners see their careers developing in different ways. Critical care practice hones exceptional clinical skills. In most settings, the skills acquired as a critical care practitioner lend themselves to superior performance in other clinical areas in nursing. Thus, experienced critical care nurses are a welcome addition to other fields. As graduate nurses move from novice to expert[6] in nursing, career opportunities at the bedside are limited owing to a salary ceiling and staff nurse titles. Therefore, career-minded individuals often seek promotion up and away from patients. The type of clinical experience obtained in critical care nursing is excellent, and critical care practice may be used as a stepping stone to a rich and varied nursing career, often in other areas.

Job satisfaction and career advancement are goals sought by practitioners in different ways.[7–8] For recruitment and retention purposes, hospitals offer tuition benefits for furthering education.[7–9] Many critical care nurses take advantage of this opportunity and return to school to earn a baccalaureate, masters, or doctoral degree. As an individual acquires advanced education, a desire for a change, for an independent autonomous practice, or to earn more money can lead a practitioner to seek employment in nursing administration or other nonhospital fields. Thus, many critical care practitioners choose to leave bedside practice to achieve upward career mobility. Continual recruitment of new staff into critical care practice is thus needed to fill the places of those who have moved upward.

On the other hand, many critical care nurses are at an age when family and child rearing are of paramount importance. Thus, hoping and planning for better things for their children, these married female practitioners have different goals. They remain at the bedside with a firm commitment to make a difference in practice. Most juggle a career, child rearing, homemaking, and marriage with little or no household help and limited access to child-care services. Although many are unable to go back to school for a formal advanced education, they invest in critical care certification and ongoing continuing education as a means to stay current and enhance their knowledge. The role of certification in critical care practice has demonstrated how valued these expert practitioners are with respect to patient outcomes.[10] Thus, when an experienced critical care practitioner leaves a unit, the loss is not just a nurse but an expert who the field can ill afford to lose.

Factors Influencing Productivity and Motivation

The 12-Hour Shift

One of the factors influencing productivity and motivation in critical care nursing is the issue of continuity of care and the 12-hour shift. One advantage of this shift is convenience for a nurse in that, on average, a nurse need only come to work three times in any given week while maintaining full-time employment. Given the current move for enhanced concern for patients, perhaps the 12-hour shift needs to be readdressed. Research showed that when nurse-patient contact is limited, patients scored nurses lower on empathy and nonverbal communication than the nurses self-reported.[11] Contact was determined by the number of times a nurse cared for a particular patient. The 12-hour shift interferes with continuity of care by preventing the bonding that occurs when a nurse and patient or family build a nurse-person relationship. Rising acuity and shortened length of stay in combination with a 12-hour shift make continuity of care problematic for all patients. It can be argued that patients in a critical care unit have a shorter length of stay than medical-surgical patients and that continuity of care thus is not an issue. More research is needed, however, because it is well known that a 12-hour shift can be counterproductive to quality care owing to fatigue at the end of the period. These points raise questions about the efficacy of continuing with a practice that has limited benefit to patient care. Whether the 12-hour shift will endure is not clear. Further research addressing lack of continuity, nurses' fatigue, and negative patient outcomes is needed.

Care Delivery

Questions about nursing care delivery systems are being researched. Organized nursing continues to attempt to bring about change in the delivery of care and in institutional operations. Further understanding about the impact of manipulating the environments in which nurses practice is needed. Although the emphasis on patient-centered care[10, 12] in the current milieu implies flexibility, institutions and departments of nursing are relatively inflexible. Decisions about standards of care and modes of nursing care delivery directly affect patients and their families. The decisions also influence medical practice and the organization itself. Dissatisfaction with the critical care environment identified by patients and their families cannot be ignored while addressing nursing practice; neither can mandates from administration or concerns expressed by the medical community. All of these groups are involved in care delivery. Thus, any change made by nursing in the workplace directly affects many other people. In the same way, changes made by ancillary departments or physicians influence the way nursing care is delivered.

The one individual responsible for interpreting all of this change to staff is the head nurse or nurse manager for the individual critical care unit. A head nurse who anticipates, communicates, collaborates, and plans for change becomes a facilitator who ensures that critical care nursing practice is constantly evolving while simultaneously ensuring that it is well grounded in scientific theory based on relevant research.

Effective critical care nursing leaders with good management skills recognize the need to foster an environment of humanistic care[1, 13, 14] while simultaneously recognizing the interdependence of the relationships between physician, patient and family, ancillary departments, and nursing staff. The question arises, How can a critical care nursing leader maintain this multiple focus and still achieve the outcomes mandated by public policy, institutional needs, and regulatory agencies? The answer is vested in a commitment on the part of leaders to use a combination of theory, skill, and expectations based on the single-minded philosophy that quality nursing care is the only product provided by the critical care unit.[15–17]

Maslow's Theory

Maslow's hierarchy of needs[18] can be used as a framework to assess the status of patients, families, and staff in the critical care environment. Maslow stated that to achieve the highest level of personal growth, all needs below the level of self-actualization must be met. Thus, for each individual in the unit, physiologic needs, security and safety, love and belonging, and self-esteem require fulfillment before self-actualization can occur. Each of these needs as they relate to the critical care environment is important. Physiologic needs require no definition, but nursing staff who are tired, hungry, or thirsty cannot function at their optimal level. This is equally true for family, visitors, and physicians. All nursing staff are assigned meal breaks, and adherence to these times is an expectation. Unfortunately, family, significant others, and other healthcare workers are not assigned breaks. Therefore, fluids and access to juice, coffee, or tea for all people is a necessity. Relationships between people suffer when one or more of an individual's basic physiologic needs are not met. Thus, consideration for the needs of all persons in the unit, access to food and fluid, and the ability of the institution to help meet physiologic needs are incorporated in a humane work environment.

An environment that is safe and secure is needed before staff can focus on providing quality critical care. Herzberg's[18] two-factor achievement theory can be triangulated with Maslow's theory to provide concrete examples for application in critical care. Herzberg[18] defined hygiene factors and stated that these arise and prevent self-motivation. Poor working conditions represent an example of a factor that prevents staff from self-motivating and doing a good job. When the unit is not physically safe or when staff believe they are not safe, these hygiene factors emerge. Frequent needle sticks, low back injuries, or staff complaints about low wages are red flags that suggest that safety and security needs of the staff are not being fully addressed.

A sense of love and belonging is also important. Individuals in a critical care unit must feel as if they are part of a team and belong to the unit in order to perform at their best. Collaborative practice efforts help fulfill these needs. Incorporating all staff into the overall unit goals, formal and informal mechanisms of communication, and celebrations of festive or recognition events foster a sense of love and belonging that provides an impetus for continued quality improvement. Self-esteem and belief in oneself continue to promote positive outcomes in achievement. All individuals, regardless of their role within the critical care unit, must be treated with respect to ensure that each person's contribution to the work of the unit is valued. When an individual's self-esteem is threatened, the individual may believe that he or she is not welcomed or wanted. Thus, the individual may not feel safe or secure in the working environment and may not work productively. When individuals believe that the work they do is valued, they feel pride and are self-motivated. Finally, with full development of an individual's abilities and ambitions in a humanistic caring environment comes self-actualization. In this type of environment, all people thrive and optimal outcomes for both staff and patients are a reality.[15, 16, 18]

Communication Issues

Changing trends illustrate that we are a nation of diverse cultures. This cultural diversity creates problems in communication and understanding, often resulting in poor tolerance of another's beliefs, inadvertent errors, or lack of respect for and trust in others. When individuals feel as if they have been misunderstood or slighted, it is not important whether they are patients, family members, or staff members. While an individual feels this way, all subsequent communication is problematic. Barriers to effective communication usually result from lack of clarity in verbal interchange and real or perceived nonverbal communication differences.[11] In a critical care environment, all individuals feel stress. The degree of stress affects effective communication. Some people have poor communication skills, whereas others are very sensitive and astute when it comes to interpreting messages received. The differences in skills can lead to misinterpretation or anger. For example, when confronted by a concerned or angry physician or family member, a nurse can easily react in a way that leads to a negative interchange. This occurs more frequently when staff nurses have not had their own personal physiologic needs met and when they feel insecure or poorly supported by others.

All healthcare providers who have not had physiologic needs met or who are overtired from a long or very stressful day are at risk for causing communication barriers. Nonverbal communication such as sighing when asked a question, using facial grimaces when completing a task, or making a face when walking away from another individual evokes negative responses in an observer. These behaviors are unacceptable comportment. Consistent, direct, and timely communication as well as positive attitudes and behaviors contribute to effective patient-focused care.

Fostering the right attitude among staff is another subtle responsibility of the unit leaders. All individuals who are not members of the team must be treated as guests in the critical care unit to provide a framework for a successful beginning. Expressions of trust and respect are paramount requirements for all members of the team. When individuals show trust and respect, team cohesiveness and positive communication result. The tenet or belief is that effective quality patient-focused care outcomes occur in a professional environment supported by appropriate resources.[14, 16, 19] The way nursing leaders and physicians interact with the care providers contributes to outcomes. The classic work completed by Knaus and colleagues[20] clearly demonstrated that mortality improved when physicians and nurses effectively communicated with each other. Unless attention is given to staff and patients alike, outcomes may not be optimal in the critical care unit.[13, 14]

PRACTICE MANDATES AND RESEARCH ENDEAVORS

If practice as it is applied to critically ill patients is to evolve, it must be supported by personnel, resources, and an expanded body of knowledge based on research. Research endeavors directed at the delivery of care as well as patient outcomes is justified.[21] Several practice mandates must be addressed simultaneously with healthcare reform. The Joint Commission for the Accreditation of Healthcare Organizations (JCAHO) has recommended that hospitals consider use of a career ladder as a mechanism to foster quality care.[17] A career ladder based on acquisition of knowledge with salary commensurate with experience is needed to keep critical care practitioners at the bedside. In addition, implementation and ongoing evaluation of standards of care are needed. Current JCAHO regulations mandate written standards be available to staff.[17] As practice evolves, critical care nursing standards can lead the way toward a better understanding of how these standards affect the outcomes of patient care when implemented appropriately.

Alspach's[22] work on competency-based critical care orientation and education contributed significantly to cost-effective change. Alas, not all hospitals use this approach. In fact, in some hospitals, instructors traditionally give repetitive lectures month after month with no thought about the waste of personnel when orienting an experienced critical care practitioner and make no attempt to evaluate critical thinking in staff. Both competency and competency-based education are shared responsibilities of the clinical instructor and masters-prepared clinical nurse specialist. The interface of these roles as well as the outcome of the competency-based education needs further delineation. Issues about ways to ensure clinical competency, evaluate staff performance, and measure productivity are unresolved.[16, 23] Further, nursing academe and service continue on a dichotomous course. The resolution of this problem will contribute to the survival of nursing as a strong profession within the healthcare field in the next century.

Redundant written documentation including flow sheets in an era of automation and computerization abounds. The interface of critical care documentation to the hospital information system is evolving, but further research into the best way of storing and evaluating the abundance of information gleaned from continuous monitoring of many parameters is still in its infancy. Improved methods of documentation that are research based are needed to illustrate how professional nursing positively affects outcomes. Research projects directed at evaluating the modalities of nursing care with methods for documentation and teaching may provide improved practice for the next generation of critical care nurses.

Nursing research focused on the outcomes of the care provided is necessary to ensure that practice is based on scientific inquiry and that this practice justifies the cost of the care provided. Thus, changes in the workplace that address these issues need further exploration. Those factors leading to positive outcomes for patients must be documented and evaluated. Active staff participation in clinically relevant quality assessment and improvement committees provides a mechanism to initiate this work. Patient outcomes related to independent nursing practice including ambulation, feeding, hygiene, and rest and sleep patterns of critically ill patients are not fully understood. The impact of these issues on patients' outcome requires investigation.

THE FUTURE

The way that care is delivered continues to evolve.[4, 12, 13] As cost containment compresses the healthcare delivery system even more, financial reasons will necessitate that varied levels of technical and professional personnel work together in a critical care unit.[3, 23] Nurses committed to practice will be expert clinicians who have superior communication skills and who demonstrate their competence by certification. Goals for some include advanced education and active participation in multidisciplinary clinical research.

Nursing leaders responsive to the internal drive and upward mobility desires of critical care nurses are necessary.[8, 23] Leaders who address ways to enhance growth from novice to expert and research that shows others how this is achieved are important.[6] Defining new ways to help staff self-motivate and teaching effective communication skills to all team members in critical care can result in positive outcomes. Recognition of the value of experienced critical care nurses, institutional and medical support for increased decision making at the bedside, and a reasonable salary package for a career in critical care are needed.[10] These factors help ensure that practitioners will desire and can afford to stay at the bedside, contributing to the care of critically ill patients. Other innovative changes are needed to reform the healthcare system. The organizational climate is changing. Nursing practice is relinquishing old habits. There is growing awareness that empowering the nurse at the bedside does improve outcomes.[19] Humane leadership and management enhance both staff and patient-family satisfaction.[8, 13] Hence, growth and change with a shift in focus are emerging. A humane environment offering holistic care for patients and families and an exciting, safe, but challenging workplace for caregivers are inevitable.

References

1. Harvey MA, Ninos NP, Adler DC, et al: Results of the Consensus Conference on Fostering More Humane Critical Care-Creating a Healing Environment. Critical Care—State of the Art. Anaheim, CA, Society of Critical Care Medicine, pp 197–228.
2. Meltzer LE, Abdellah FG, Kitchell JR: Concepts and Practices of Intensive Care for Nurse Specialists. 2nd ed. Bowie, MD, Charles Press Publishers, 1969.
3. Ellstrom KE, Macar-Hinson M: The critical care patient: Characteristics and external environmental influences. *In:* Managing the Environment in Critical Care Nursing. Spicer JG, Robinson, MA (Eds). Baltimore, MD, Williams & Wilkins, 1990, pp 162–172.

3a. Dunn DL, Chen M: Uncompensated hospital care payment and access for the uninsured: Evidence from New Jersey. Health Serv Res 1994; 29:113.

4. Rudy E, Grenvik A: Future of critical care. Am J Crit Care 1992; 1:33.
5. Groeger JS, Strosberg MA, Halpern NA, et al: Descriptive analysis of critical care units in the United States. Crit Care Med 1992; 2:846.
6. Benner P, Tanner C, Chesla C: From beginner to expert: Gaining a differentiated clinical world in critical care nursing. Adv Nurs Sci 1992; 14:13.

6a. English I: Intuition as a function of the expert nurse: A critique of Benner's novice to expert model. J Adv Nurs 1993; 18:387.

7. Bruce JA: Reward strategies for the retention of professional nurses. Ann Arbor, MI, Doctoral Dissertation, University of Michigan, number PUZ9100508, 1990.
8. Stechmiller JK, Yarandi HN: Job satisfaction among critical care nurses. Am J Crit Care 1992; 3:37.

8a. Boumans NPG, Landeweerd JA: Working in an intensive or non–intensive care unit: Does it make any difference? Heart Lung 1994; 24:71.

9. Blegen MA: Nurses's job satisfaction: A meta-analysis of related variables. Nurs Res 1993; 42:36.
10. Mitchell PH, Armstrong S: American Association of Critical-Care Nurses Demonstration Project: Profile of excellence in critical care nursing. Heart Lung 1989; 18:219.
11. Birdsall C: Self-reported and patient-reported nonverbal communication and empathy levels of nurses. Ann Arbor, MI, Doctoral Dissertation, University of Michigan, number 9136355, 1991.
12. Daly B, Phelps C, Rudy E: A nurse managed special care unit. J Nurs Adm 1991; 21:31.

12a. Challenges in critical care nursing: Helping patient and families cope. Crit Care Nurs Suppl, August, 1993, p 4.
13. Rushton CH: Humanism in critical care: A blueprint for change. Pediatr Nurs 1991; 17:399.
14. Sorrells-Jones J: Caring for the caregivers: A wellness and renewal project. Nurs Admin Q 1993; 17:61.
15. Birdsall C: Performance, time and energy. *In:* Management Issues in Critical Care. Birdsall C (Ed). St Louis, Mosby-Year Book, 1991, pp 55–68.
16. McNeese-Smith D: The impact of leadership upon productivity. Nurs Econ 1992; 10:393.
17. Joint Commission Manual for Accreditation of Healthcare Organizations. The 1993 Joint Commission Accreditation Manual for Hospitals. Oakbrook Terrace, IL, 1993.
18. Ahmadian A: Motivation: In search of a better way. J Hum Behav Learn 1987; 4:17.
19. Chandler G: The source and process of empowerment. Nurs Admin Q 1992; 16:65.
20. Knaus WM, Draper EA, Wagner DP, et al: An evaluation of outcomes from intensive care in major medical centers. Ann Intern Med 1986; 104:410–418.
21. The future of outcomes research. Bus Hlth 1992; 10:29.
22. Alspach JG (Ed). Education Standards for Critical Care Nursing. St Louis, CV Mosby, 1986.
23. Kelly LY: The Nursing Experience: Trends, Challenges, and Transitions. 2nd ed. New York, McGraw-Hill, 1992.
23a. Ritchie J, Hagel C: Managing change: Introducing ancillary caregivers to the ICU. Nurs Manage 1993; 24:64a.

CHAPTER 190

The Impact of Healthcare and Technology Trends on Critical Care Practice

Ginger Schafer Wlody, RN, EdD, FCCM

The next 20 years will be a critical time in healthcare and in the specialty practice of caring for the critically ill. Global shifts in power, immigration, the changing economic and political climates, and soaring healthcare costs will continue to affect delivery of critical care.

This chapter discusses current and future trends that affect the practice of critical care and puts forth multidisciplinary strategies for critical care nurses to assist in maximizing resources. These strategies are designed to address the changing healthcare environment by assuming a proactive stance. Global trends and United States trends are addressed first, followed by healthcare costs and factors affecting those costs. Subsequently, technology and its benefits and liabilities are addressed. Guidelines for technology assessment are presented, and finally, the role of the nurse manager in creating a safe, healing environment is discussed. Four major strategies for maximizing resources in the current and future critical care environment are presented.

GLOBAL TRENDS

In discussions of healthcare and the future, it is important to note global trends that affect healthcare and subsequently critical care practice. Worldwide societal and economic changes are occurring at an accelerating rate.

A mosaic society is emerging, in which minorities are the majority, jobs are information based rather than industrial, high-technology skills are required, the population is aging, women outnumber men, and illiteracy is growing. The globe continues to shrink as communication technology advances. Whatever affects one country soon affects another. The impact of the European Common Market will change the way business is conducted across the European borders. Economic and communication changes subsequently affect healthcare changes. The economic rise of the Asian Pacific rim countries is startling, and Naisbett and Aburdene[1] refer to the Pacific rim as a powerful global presence. Scientific advances in one country are quickly adapted in other countries across the globe. Diseases, too, spread rapidly. The travels of the human immunodeficiency virus were traced from Africa to all nations of the world. We all are struck with problems related to acquired immunodeficiency syndrome, which has had an awesome impact on the world population. It is projected that in the year 2001, the total number of cases of acquired immunodeficiency syndrome worldwide will be 6 million.[2] In the future, medical and nursing advances in healthcare and the accompanying technology will continue to have global implications rather than affects on regional and local practice only.

HEALTHCARE TRENDS IN THE UNITED STATES

Although global changes affect the practice of critical care, this chapter focuses on critical care in the United States. Current healthcare trends in the United States can be divided into six areas: trends related to the financial climate, changes in healthcare services, technologic advances, changes in healthcare management, an emerging concept of an "ethical environment," and a mushrooming legal environment. Triage, resource allocation, and rationing will occur in various forms.

Technologic and scientific advances in healthcare have propelled complex financial issues to the forefront of concern. As we have increased our ability to diagnose and treat illness and to sustain life indefinitely, we have encountered increasing financial and ethical dilemmas. The current state of technology reveals that advances have occurred in every aspect of medical treatment and healthcare. As we have become more proficient in prolonging life, replacing body parts, and treating specific illnesses, we have learned that each new technology engenders a multitude of conflicts, dilemmas, and legal and financial questions. Consideration of ethical issues will have an increasingly important role in healthcare. Another important trend that will affect the delivery of critical care services more directly in the future is the growing aging population. "Estimates of the number of older Americans who will need specialized care by the year 2000 and the number of physicians who will be trained to provide that care foretell a serious disparity."[3] It is estimated that the number of people over 85 years old, now 2.1 million, will double by the end of the century. The healthcare needs of this aging population differ substantially from those of younger patients.[4]

OVERALL HEALTHCARE TRENDS

Overall healthcare trends include downsizing of American hospitals, increased patient acuity, increased complexity of home care, increased use of ambulatory services, and delivery of services to more underprivileged people. For example, ambulatory surgery centers that began in the early 1970s have increased in number dramatically since that time. Procedures such as cholecystectomy are frequently performed on an outpatient basis. Reimbursement policies have changed the way healthcare is delivered, because reimbursement for ambulatory procedures has increased but for hospital procedures has decreased.[5] The number of hospital beds devoted to care of the critically ill has increased tremendously, a trend that probably will continue as more healthcare services are delivered to the chronically ill at home. The increased numbers of human immunodeficiency virus–infected patients will cause changes in hospital services for these patients and may or may not include increased critical care services. Use of improved techniques and continued progress related to organ transplantation have been notable during the past decade, and transplant recipients will continue to require critical care services. Noninvasive technologic devices will increase, thereby decreasing costs and risks related to invasive procedures. McIntyre and colleagues have described a nonivasive method of predicting pulmonary capillary wedge pressure.[6]

Other advances in technology, such as increased use of genetic engineering to create new drugs and solve other healthcare problems, will continue. These trends in healthcare then require changes in educational needs and delivery systems for patient care. A paradigm shift in the methods of patient care management and payment systems is seen as necessary by most analysts in the healthcare field today. Technology advances will also result in escalating computerization of systems and trends toward use of bedside computers for all data gathering and analysis.

Current Healthcare Trends

Naisbett and Aburdene[1] said, "We're poised on the threshold of a great era of biotechnology." Major directions in biotechnology today will affect critical care nursing and include

- Genetic manipulation of crops and farm animals
- Identification and manipulation of inherited characteristics
- Genetic engineering to conquer diseases for which there are now no cures.

According to the Commerce Department, a decade of cost containment has done little to slow spiraling healthcare costs, and in 1990, United States health spending reached 661.3 billion dollars.[7] Problems related to widespread lack of insurance, an aging population, and immigration waves of low-income minorities make restructuring of the United States healthcare system inevitable. In 1989, private and public payers spent $230.1 billion on hospital services, an increase of 9.1% over 1988, and in 1989, spending on physician care rose 13% and totaled 119.4 billion dollars.[7]

Advanced medical equipment and technology are viewed as a strategic tool used to attract both physicians and patients to a hospital or healthcare institution. Healthcare institutions demonstrate their belief in the importance of technology by their rising technologic investment. Healthcare providers spent 8.25 billion dollars on capital equipment in 1988, compared with 8.21 billion dollars in 1987.[8] In fact, as mentioned, the most widely blamed culprit for the increases in healthcare costs is technology.[9] In the United States, 60% to 70% of medical professionals currently practice in specialties and 30% to 40% are in general practice. These ratios will change drastically, with a shift to general practice and physicians employed by others.[10]

Critical Care Trends

Critical care services will be expanded to care for patients at home. Patients will be discharged while connected to ventilators and receiving vasoactive drugs and using other high-technology patient care equipment. Fewer invasive procedures will be performed on critically ill patients, but more assist devices such as pulmonary or cardiac assist devices will be used. Increased telemetry and intermediate care (step-down units) to cope with the increasing number of high-acuity patients will be available. Critical care physicians may increasingly choose to work for hospitals or large practice groups.

FINANCIAL CLIMATE AND TRENDS

Since 1968, hospital care expenditures have rapidly increased as a result of inflation in prices of medical goods and services and a high intensity of medical care provided to a larger population. In 1988, healthcare expenditures were almost 12% of the gross national product,[11] and in 1991 this figure was as high as 14%.[12] Many view technology as the main cause of these increases.

Healthcare costs continue to escalate, and no apparent end is in sight. These costs accounted for 14% of the gross national product in 1993 and will soar upward toward 20% or greater if drastic actions and are not soon taken. Healthcare costs in other countries are lower than in the United States[12] (Fig. 190–1). The state of Oregon is the first of the states to attempt to restructure healthcare completely at the state level. At a meeting in Sacramento in 1991, John Kitzhaber, president of the Oregon state senate, told the California Health Forum that the United States health system is "fundamentally flawed and failing." He noted that "thirty-five million Americans are without health insurance in a system that spends 1.5 billion daily."[12]

Problems that affect financial trends in our current healthcare system include lack of universal access to care, cost shifting (disguised as cost containment), increasing use of technology with limited assessment of new technology, and lack of motivation in congress to change the system. The state of Oregon has implemented a state healthcare system that will provide a basic level of benefits to all citizens based on effectiveness of care rather than ability to pay. The Oregon plan, the first of its kind in the country, based its public policy on several assumptions (Table 190–1).

The Health Care Services Commission in Oregon established the priority list for services, which were then ap-

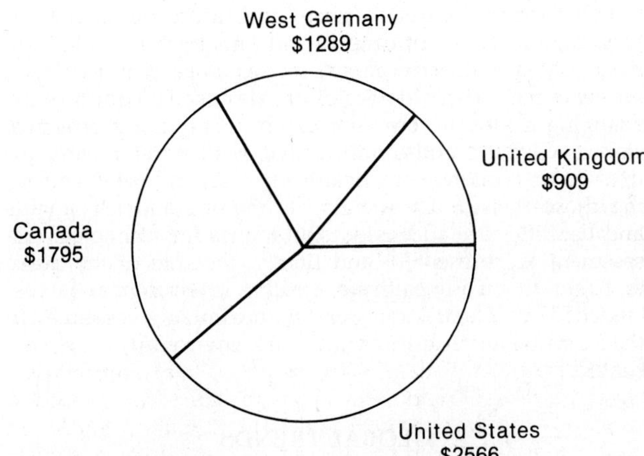

Figure 190–1. United States per capita healthcare spending compared with that of other countries (in US dollars [1990]). (Data from "Don't expect healthcare reform any time soon." USA Today, April 6, 1993, p 11A.) Copyright Ginger Schafer Wlody, RN, EdD, FCCM.

TABLE 190–1. Assumptions in the Oregon Healthcare Proposal

- Healthcare allocations are made as part of the overall budgetary allocation process
- Clear accountability
- Universal access for all citizens
- Society must finance a certain level of care for those who cannot afford it themselves
- There is a clearly defined process to determine the basic level of care
- Healthcare must be publicly debated
- Creation of incentives to use effective medical procedures
- Funding is explicit and economically sustainable

Data from Editor: Treatment for the American health care system: Universal access? Calif Hosp 1991; 18:25.

proved by the governor. Kitzhaber stated, "hospitals don't drive the costs of health care up, physicians do, by sending patients there."[12]

Changes in Healthcare Costs and Services

Current reimbursement policies are creating changes in the way healthcare is delivered. Reimbursement for outpatient ambulatory services has increased, whereas inpatient hospital reimbursement has lessened. This mechanism of reimbursement has forced hospitals to convert many procedures from inpatient to outpatient classifications.[5] Hospital beds in America will be closed or eliminated.[10] Problems related to recruitment and retention of professional nurses have also changed the way care is delivered to patients. Shortages of qualified personnel have led to new initiatives and programs such as managed care or case management. The American Association of Critical Care Nurses projects that 400,000 nurses will be required to meet the demands in the 21st century.[13] Non-nursing activities will be increasingly delegated to nonlicensed personnel such as patient technicians. Critical care education will increase the emphasis on management and training for both physician and nurse managers.

CHANGING SOCIETAL BELIEFS ABOUT HEALTHCARE

Although technologic advances have occurred with great rapidity during the past 25 years, societal and cultural belief systems have not kept pace. During this time span, societal changes have occurred in attitudes toward access to care, beliefs about the infallibility of physicians, attitudes toward death and dying, informed consent, and the handicapped. Universal access to care was a major issue in the early 1960s, when the concepts of Medicare and the Great Society deemed that everyone was entitled to equal access to care. President Lyndon Johnson took advantage of the Democratic gains in the 1964 congressional elections to push through landmark healthcare legislation. Medicare was established to provide care for the aged and disabled, and Medicaid was created to guarantee some medical care for the indigent.[14] In the late 1960s, the phrase *healthcare industry* began to be heard, and national health expenditures reached 46.3 billion dollars in 1966 and then 75 billion dollars in 1970.[14] President Jimmy Carter made an effort to impose price controls on hospitals in 1979, but the bill was narrowly defeated in Congress. Attention shifted in the Reagan administration to the idea of economic incentives for efficiency.

Today our society has returned to the concept of limited access to care, with patients having personal responsibility to provide for their own care. The phrase "equal access to care" has been replaced by "equitable access" to care.[15] On October 1, 1983, the Medicare program began phasing in a new plan to pay hospitals on the basis of diagnosis-related groups of illnesses. In this model, Medicare pays hospitals a set fee for each diagnostic category, with the incentive of retaining any monies if care is provided more efficiently or for less cost. The idea was to slow the growth of expenditures of hospital care, which form the bulk of Medicare costs.[16] A study by Russell and Manning found that prospective payment reduced Medicare's hospital costs substantially.[16] However, technology acquisitions have not yet been limited, so these technologies continue to be purchased and billed as direct patient care costs. Thus, the competitive environment between healthcare institutions was born.

The foregoing are macroallocation issues, which deal with patients in the aggregate. Microallocation issues affect individual patients and their healthcare providers. Scarce or decreased resources have the effect of forcing those in the healthcare field to make difficult choices in a strained economy.

The Ethical Environment

Three major struggles are seen as primary between the individual, the caregivers, and society. The three broad major ethical issues that will continue to plague us in critical care into the 21st century are those related to the struggle between autonomy of the individual and beneficence, between autonomy of the individual and utilitarianism, and individual rights in general. A disparity in level of healthcare services currently exists. As resources become more scarce, with increased government control of physicians and healthcare, individual choices will surely become more limited.

We are currently in an era of strong patient rights, and patients are frequently able to choose the level and type of care they want. In the future, our choices will be more limited in order to gain a more universal level of healthcare services. Problems will affect critical care nurses, patients, physicians and healthcare organizations. These struggles relate to the increasing number of patients requiring care (increased aging population, increased numbers of patients with acquired immunodeficiency syndrome) and to scarce resources.

Patient autonomy needs to be preserved as much as possible, and yet a physician's ability to practice must be sustained as much as is required. Informed consent has been greatly expanded. The Patient Self-Determination act of 1990 requires that patients receive information on advance directives, and it should result in patients' wishes being followed when they are unable to make decisions. Surrogates will be more readily identified, thus shortening delays in decisions altering care and withdrawal of care.

The struggle will continue between patients and families on one hand and the healthcare team on the other. An ever-changing balance will emerge in which patient autonomy is preserved. Other ethical struggles that will affect those of us in critical care include issues related to physician-assisted suicide and euthanasia. Supporters of these measures have become increasingly vocal, and an assisted suicide referendum was only narrowly defeated in California in the 1992 election.

The third major ethical struggle relates to maximizing resources. As the costs of healthcare delivery and services have increased, the ability to ensure that healthcare needs of all citizens are met has decreased. Scarce resources will necessitate use of decision-making strategies that although localized need to be coordinated, perhaps on regional or national levels. Decisions made at the local level are best and support the public demand to maintain local control.

TECHNOLOGIC ADVANCES IN CRITICAL CARE

According to Downs,[17] "Advances in technology have detrimental effects on critical care, particularly by encouraging a de-emphasis on the importance of clinical observation." He observes that students frequently fail to recognize signs of respiratory distress in tachypneic patients when their chest radiograph appears normal and their arterial blood gas oxygenation appears adequate.

Definitions

Technology is the popular word used to describe the apparatus and the procedures that are based on modern science, in contrast to the supposedly simpler and more humane healing arts. Diagnostic technology, in contrast to therapeutic technology, involves the use of expensive "scientific" machines, radioisotopes, electronics, and the like to make diagnoses. Therapeutic technology is viewed (in the popular context) as referring to complex surgical procedures such as organ transplantation and insertion of devices such as pacemakers or to specialized procedures such as dialysis therapy.[9] Medical technology assessment means (at a minimum) a systematic evaluation of safety and efficacy but may also include evaluations of economic, social, and ethical factors.[18]

Technologic Problems

The current healthcare environment is such that technologic and scientific advances have propelled complex issues to the forefront of concern. Technologic advances have leaped beyond society's ability to cope with the financial and ethical dilemmas they have induced. Technology is not inherently evil,[1] but the way in which we use it is key.

Anderson and Steinberg[19] describe the technologic arsenal already in place in hospitals and relate it to the eagerness with which physicians have incorporated new procedures into their practice and the frequency with which new technologic procedures have become part of patient-physician encounters. Technologic advances, although they are awesome and provide help for many patients, also require tremendous investments in highly skilled personnel and costly equipment to support them. Ramifications of the technologic imperative rampant in healthcare today will be discussed, as will problems related to developing, introducing, assessing, and using new technologies. Additionally, current and proposed models of technology assessment will be explored.

A growing trend in critical care is expansion of the field of organ transplantation. The field is so specialized that Cedars Sinai Medical Center in Los Angeles, for example, has a newsletter for its transplantation services. Organ transplantation has rapidly moved from an experimental therapy to the standard of care for some end-stage kidney, heart, lung, and liver diseases. As the benefits of transplantation have become increasingly apparent and the medical barriers have fallen, the demand for transplantation has grown rapidly, far outstripping the supply of organs.[20] As transplantation options expand, the need for critical care nurses in the field of transplantation increases. Critical care nurses are involved in preparing patients and their families for the transplant as well as for the postoperative care and the psychologic and social adjustments required. The number of organ transplants has been phenomenal during the past decade and will continue to grow exponentially in future decades as awareness increases.

An increasing number of types of organs are donated, and the shortage of organs in the United States today is chronic. More than 22,000 men, women, and children are waiting for organ transplantations. Of those, 5000 will die before an organ becomes available.[21] Randall[22] estimates that as many as 30% of the more than 3000 patients now awaiting heart or liver transplantation will die before an organ donor can be found. Although 15,000 people die annually under circumstances that would allow them to become organ donors, fewer than 4000 donations occurred.

THE TECHNOLOGIC IMPERATIVE

Ronald Bayer, associate for policy studies at the Hastings Institute, noted that, "As technology becomes available there is an ineluctable dynamic that makes it intolerable to have the technology and not use it."[15] He goes on to say that once one subset of the population has access to a technology, society finds it intolerable to see people dying in need of it. This was demonstrated by the case of a young child whose insurance would not pay for an experimental procedure to treat her fatal condition. The family sued the insurance company and appeared on television to garner support for their cause. Within hospitals, there is also a similar compulsion to use high-technology interventions. Administrators blame a pervasive American infatuation with technology and continue to purchase new items as soon as they become available.

Koenig[23] discusses the technologic imperative, stating that many believe that the mere existence of a dramatic new medical device provides a mandate for its continued use. She studied the social processes that contribute to the operation of a technologic imperative in medical practice and found a social "routinization" of a technical medical procedure and the creation of social rituals related to the technology. These social rituals support the continued use of a technology and its acceptance as "normal." Koenig found that the "new" standard of care became a moral as well as a technical obligation. Siegal[24] reviewed the development of coronary care units as a paradigm for the uncritical acceptance of technology in medical services. Studies comparing coronary care units with other settings for treatment of acute myocardial infarction in which intensive care is not shown to offer a consistent benefit over more conservative treatment are described. The author relates the proliferation of coronary care units to corporate involvement in medical research as corporations involved with monitoring devices strongly supported the development of coronary care units.

Problems Related to Inadequate Technology Assessment

This immediate and enthusiastic acceptance of new technology, or technologic imperative, creates a host of problems related to inadequate assessment, increased cost, lack of expertise, technology diffusion, and inadequate planning. Profits from use of new technologies are very high, and many large hospitals rush to be the first to have the latest in the technologic arsenal. Inadequate assessment of the device or technique sometimes results. The Los Angeles Times,[25] in a front page story, described the 1984 purchase by Humana of six lithotripters at 1.6 million dollars each soon after their approval by the federal government. Lithotripters are machines that pulverize kidney stones by shock waves. The technique is successful, but only a limited number of patients have kidney stones. Lithotripter owners soon began looking for additional uses for their machines and focused on the one million Americans yearly who have gallbladder attacks caused by gallstones. Studies from clinical trials now show that lithotripters worked for only 10% to 25% of patients with gallstones, thus necessitating surgery in the majority of patients. The treatments also caused disturbing side effects, such as hematuria and hypertension. This example points up the fact that expensive new technology is used with few guidelines and little agreement on usage. A model for technology assessment in critical care should include such factors as technologic capability, range of possible uses, therapeutic impact, diagnostic and therapeutic accuracy, impact on the healthcare providers, and patient outcome.

New technologies usually do not decrease costs at all; rather, physicians add the new technology to their armamentarium and use several methods of diagnosis instead of one. For example, a computed tomography scanner or magnetic resonance imager may be much more accurate that conventional radiography at detecting blood clots in the brain, but physicians more often than not use all three. The costs then quickly get out of hand, about $500 for the computed tomography scan, $900 for the magnetic resonance image, and $60 for a conventional radiograph.[25]

A third concern related to the rate of introduction of new technology is the need for standards for training for those who use it. Researchers believe that a new technology frequently becomes available and is introduced to the medical community so rapidly that those who acquire a new device, administer a new drug, or perform a new procedure are not sufficiently knowledgeable to use it effectively.

The diffusion of a new technology into practice is a fourth problem that has been described.[26] Because technology assessment involves not only examining technologies before they are released but also their diffusion into practice once they have been released, follow-up studies must be performed. Anderson and Lomas[26] analyzed the use of coronary artery bypass grafting in the province of Ontario, Canada. They found that the annual number of procedures increased 52% during a 7-year period between 1979 and 1985. Interestingly, large increases in rates of coronary artery bypass grafting in the over-65 population accounted for more than half of this increase in procedures, yet increased rates of surgery in this population were unlikely to be caused by increased prevalence of coronary artery disease. The researchers thought that the increase was related to a change in clinical attitude toward the use of coronary artery bypass grafts.

A fifth problem related to rapid use of new technology in healthcare focuses on inadequate planning. Because the reimbursement system fosters the use of technology related to patient procedures rather than new technology to cut the cost of caring for patients in the hospital, capital purchases focus on technologic devices for which the patients can be directly charged. For example, hospital information systems are lagging far behind available technology.[27] Bedside data information systems would provide safer, more efficient care by nursing and other personnel, but a hospital leader when interviewed stated, "I see nobody really willing to go into investment to put in bedside computers, which would certainly cut down on the problem of charting and improve the quality of care."[27] These data information systems would also act to help alleviate the nursing shortage that most hospitals have felt in recent years. Costly, rapidly emerging technologies that are seen as essential preclude planning for and purchasing everyday equipment. Thus, available funds go toward the new technologies.

Current and Proposed Approaches to Technology Assessment

Technology assessment is frustrating to hospital executives, who know that they must examine new technologies for their clinical use, their cost effectiveness, and their fit within hospital marketing strategies.[28] Formal technology assessment procedures are used in the largest medical centers, but small rural institutions simply do not have adequate resources for technology assessment. Hospitals frequently rely on their physicians for information related to emerging technologies, but this practice too is becoming problematic as the fast pace of change occurs. Some multihospital or large hospital systems have directors of technology assessment. Others use committees of physicians and administrators supplemented by a staff of researchers,[29] and in very small hospitals, a chief executive officer makes decisions related to technology acquisition.

A number of approaches to technology assessment have been recommended. Patricia Harris, Secretary of Department of Health and Human Services in 1980, announced that new health technologies should be subjected to cost-benefit analyses before financing their wide distribution.[29] Dorsey recommends some expectation of minimum benefit in terms of longevity, improved functional capacity, or socially useful productivity to justify the application of a very expensive technology.[30] Disler[31] suggests development of a system of distribution of technology that would focus on the benefit that a particular technology would confer on a given group, on the basis of certain health standards. Re[32] believes that it does not appear possible to wait for all technologies to be thoroughly tested by means of studies of cost and efficacy before they are introduced into clinical use. He states that somehow a "golden mean" must be found—a new approach that would reduce excessive use while "fostering innovation and providing for a pluralistic evaluation of technology . . . seeking care that has been demonstrated to be effective on the basis of cost-efficacy analysis."

Groups that are involved in technology assessment or that have information to guide others include the U.S. Office of Technology Assessment, the Advanced Treatment and Bionics Institute (a private organization), the American Hospital Association's Division of Clinical Services and Technology, the Institute of Medicine's Council on Health Care Technology, and the Johns Hopkins Program for Medical Technology and Practice Assessment. These programs are costly, particularly for smaller institutions, because of the added expertise and paperwork required.

Guyatt[33] has proposed guidelines for assessment of technology (Table 190–2). These criteria would help to establish whether a diagnostic technology was ready for dissemination. These six criteria can be considered to form a hierarchy of progressively more rigorous evaluation. Models such as that presented by Guyatt[33] should be developed and used to prevent unnecessary escalation of healthcare costs.

The Future

As costs escalate, issues related to technologic therapy will be addressed at an increasing rate. According to Perry,[27] hospitals that have large Medicare/Medicaid populations will not be able to afford to buy technology. Transplantation costs will continue to escalate as the demand for replacement of defective body parts increases. In 1985, more than a million people received artificial body parts.[34] That number currently is greatly increased and will continue to escalate. Questions such as the following may be raised:

TABLE 190–2. Guidelines for Technology Assessment

Criterion	*Definition*
Technologic capability	The ability of the technology to perform to specifications in a laboratory setting has been demonstrated.
Range of possible uses	The technology promises to provide important diagnostic information in a number of clinical situations.
Diagnostic accuracy	The technology provides information that allows the health worker to make a more accurate assessment about the presence and severity of disease.
Impact of the healthcare provider	The technology results in healthcare workers being more confident of their diagnoses and thereby decreases anxiety and increases comfort for the healthcare provider.
Therapeutic impact	The therapeutic decisions made by the healthcare providers are altered as a result of application of the technology.
Patient outcome	Application of the technology results in benefits to the patient.

(Data from Guyatt G: Guidelines for the general and economic evaluation of health care technologies. Soc Sci Med 1986; 22:393–428.)

1. How much healthcare technology do Americans want?
2. How much healthcare technology are we willing to pay for?
3. Will our pervasive American infatuation with high technology come at the expense of the elderly, the disabled, and the mentally ill who need less "glamorous" care?
4. Can we accept cost containment in healthcare?
5. Can we and will we establish an equitable process of rationing?
6. Will use of increasingly complex technology continue to drive our healthcare system and overshadow healthcare efficacy or patients' needs?
7. Will mechanisms of technology assessment that are "fair" be developed in our capitalistic, profit-oriented society?
8. Will healthcare institutions use mechanisms/models of technology assessment?

Society will continue to struggle with these issues. Consumers will identify their priorities and communicate these to government and healthcare leaders, physicians, nurses, and insurers.

MANAGEMENT ENVIRONMENT FOR THE FUTURE

Management in critical care is affected by hospital/medical center and university governing bodies (for those in affiliated teaching centers). Management trends include greater involvement of the workers, quality improvement and effectiveness, and increasing attention to selection of effective, well-prepared managers. Leadership is committed to increased effectiveness and a focus on meeting customers' needs. These concepts were promoted by Deming in the United States and then became popular in Japan during the 1980s. Today the concepts of total quality improvement and total quality management are being espoused by healthcare leaders and those who set the standards in hospitals, the Joint Commission Association for Health Care Organizations. Other management trends include use of concepts related to total quality management or total quality improvement, a movement from quality assurance to quality assessment and improvement, use of interdisciplinary healthcare teams for solving problems that prevent effective delivery of patient care, and a focus on recruitment and retention of professional critical care nurses. Rosabeth Moss Kanter, formerly editor of the *Harvard Business Review*,[35] recommends a newer model of managing businesses in the future. She recommends fewer levels of hierarchy to achieve more contact between top and bottom, more focus on teamwork across areas, more interest in external alliances, more sharing of resources with other organizations, and more stimulation of creativity.

In order to create the intensive care unit of the future, creation of a clinical practice environment that promotes excellence in patient care and that intertwines components of the healing environment, professional practice environment, financial environment, and interactive/communication environments is necessary.

Clinical practice is the essence of patient care. To manage it, factors that create a patient-centered environment must be present. Critical care managers today are in the throes of a highly technical and competitive healthcare market, and they need to be both effective and efficient. It is important to assist critical care managers to create an environment that, although highly technical, is nevertheless compassionate and humanistic. Nurse managers must have the concepts, tools, and strategies to create a clinical practice environment in which excellence in patient care is not only highly valued but implemented. A patient-centered, "customer-oriented" healing environment created by nurse managers empowers staff to deliver excellence in patient care, an excellence that is based on recognized standards, shared processes, and measurable outcomes.

Knowledge, methods, and systems to assist the critical care manager need to be in place so that he or she is able to meet the challenges of managing nursing care for a group of critically ill individuals. It is helpful to use the nursing role framework of CARE components—clinical, administrative, research, and educational roles of nursing. The components of a healing environment, from the practical new methodologies related to total quality improvement to the philosophy of total quality management, are important to consider. By implementing management strategies, resource use will be maximized and patient care will be enhanced.

SUMMARY

In summary, major changes in healthcare must occur now. As healthcare costs continue to soar, more than 30% of people in the United States remain uninsured. Global trends have been addressed, and multidisciplinary strategies for critical care nurses at the hospital or unit level have been put forth. As we move toward the 21st century, nurses have unique opportunities to create an environment where patients' needs can be met. In the current healthcare environment where managers are challenged daily by economic, administrative, and ethical issues, it is essential to create and sustain excellence in management of critically ill patients. A patient-centered, customer-oriented, healing environment created by nurse managers empowers staff to deliver excellence in patient care—excellence that is based on recognized standards, shared processes, and measurable outcomes.

Strategies for maximizing resources at the hospital and the unit level include nurse-physician collaboration, creation of a healing environment, development of a professional practice environment, survival of the economic environment, and creation of an interactive environment. Specific activities to support these strategies have been discussed. Future healthcare changes aimed at cost containment include streamlined healthcare services, regionalization of care, decreases in the overall number of hospital beds, increase in the number of critical care and intermediate care units (step-down units), and increased appropriate use of technology at the bedside.

References

1. Naisbett J, Aburdene P: Megatrends 2000: Ten Directions for the 1990's. New York, William Morrow & Co, 1990.
2. Chulay M: Critical care nursing in the 21st century. Cleveland Clinic Symposium. Cleveland, OH, April 5, 1993.
3. Rowe JW, Grossman E, Bond E: Academic geriatrics for the year 2000: An IOM report. N Engl J Med 1992; 316:1425–1428.
4. Schneider EL, Williams TF: Geriatrics and gerontology: Imperatives in education and training. Ann Intern Med 1986; 104:432–435.
5. Ferguson A: Critical care nurses magnified in crystal ball of health care. National Employment Review, 1991, pp 36, 46.
6. McIntyre K, Vita J, Lambrew C, et al: A noninvasive method of predicting pulmonary-capillary wedge pressure. N Engl J Med 1992; 327:1715–1720.
7. Rehm A: Legislative update (Organizational letter). Newport Beach, CA, American Association of Critical Care, Nurses. 1990.
8. Wagner S: Promoting high tech equipment. Modern Health Care, November 17, 1989, pp 39–50.
9. McGregor M: Technology and the allocation of resources. N Engl J Med 1989; 320:118–120.
10. "Don't expect health care reform any time soon." USA Today, April 6, 1993, p 11A.
11. Reagan M: Health care rationing: What does it mean? N Engl J Med 1988; 319:149–151.
12. Health costs keep skyrocketing. USA Today, April 6, 1993, p 11A.
13. American Association of Critical Care Nurses: Summary analysis of critical care nurse supply and requirements. Newport Beach, CA, AACN, 1988.
14. Millenson M: Health care in America. Modern Health Care, September 9, 1988, pp 58–74.
15. Richards G: Technology, costs and rationing issues. Hospitals, June 1, 1984, pp 80–86.
16. Russell L, Manning CL: The effects of prospective payment on medicine expenditures. N Engl J Med 1989; 320:439–444.
17. Downs J: Crisis and challenge (Editorial). Crit Care Med 1984; 12:843.
18. Rose M, Liebenluft RF: Antitrust implications of medical technology assessment. N Engl J Med 1989; 314:1490–1493.
19. Anderson G, Steinberg E: To buy or not to buy? Technology acquisition under prospective payment. N Engl J Med 1984; 311:182–185.
20. Margreiter R: What can be done about the insufficient supply of grafts? Transplant Proc 1987; 19:79–87.
21. Evans SA: Organ donors needed. The Tallahassee Opinion, May 7, 1991, p 4.
22. Randall T: Too few human organs for transplantation, too many in need . . . and the gap widens. JAMA 1991; 265:1223–1227.
23. Koenig B: The technological imperative in medical practice: The social creation of a routine treatment. *In:* Biomedicine Examined. Locke M, Gordon D (Eds). Boston, Kluwer, 1988.
24. Siegal DM: The high cost of medical technology: Getting at the heart of the matter. Med Care 1987; 25:979–987.
25. Chen R: Technology costs. Los Angeles Times. Feb. 28, 1990, p 1.
26. Anderson G, Lomas J: Monitoring the diffusion of a technology: Coronary artery bypass surgery in Ontario. Am J Public Health 1988; 78:251–254
27. Perry L: Challenges of '89. Modern Health Care, January 6, 1989, pp 28–36.
28. Souhrada L: System executives overcome barriers in technology assessment. Hospitals, August 5, 1989.
29. Evans RW: Health care technology and the inevitability of resource allocation and rationing decisions. JAMA 1983; 249:2047–2052.
30. Dorsey DB: The other health care revolution. Arch Pathol Med 1986; 110:264–268.
31. Disler DG: Rationing scarce resources. N Engl J Med 1989; 320:1629–1630.
32. Re R: Technology and the allocation of resources (Letter to the editor). N Engl J Med 1989; 32:1629.
33. Guyatt G: Guidelines for the general and economic evaluation of health care technologies. Soc Sci Med 1986; 22:393–408.
34. Editor: Glamour Magazine. 1985, p 456.
35. Flower J: How to be a business athlete; a conversation with Rosabeth Moss Kanter. Healthcare Forum J, January-February 1990, pp 39–42.

CHAPTER 191

Building Bedside Collaborative Practice

Maurene A. Harvey, RN, MPH, CCRN, FCCM • Dane J. Nichols, MD
Richard W. Carlson, MD, PhD

In the last half of the twentieth century, the industrialized world has rapidly evolved under the pressure of social forces and scientific advances. We now operate in an increasingly sophisticated environment in which specialization and communication have a dominant influence on human activity. As the division of labor increases within our society, so does the need for mechanisms to integrate complex behavior into a functional whole.

Historically, health care delivery systems have been slow to adapt to this changing environment. The inertia displayed by these systems seems rooted in the broad trusteeship for health care that is assumed by the medical profession.[1] Physicians have traditionally directed all aspects of care through a vertical hierarchy in which communication and planning are unidirectional. In this arrangement, allied health professionals have a restricted scope of activities and are dependent on the physician's direction for providing various aspects of care (Fig. 191–1).

However, changing practice environments have led to a greater reliance on the knowledge, expertise, and services provided by other practitioners, especially the professional nurse. In fact, patients are often admitted to hospitals because they require nursing care. In addition, as nurses and other caregivers involved in critical care (such as respiratory therapists) have developed distinct identities through parallel research and professional activities, their contributions have affected patient management to an ever-greater extent. This movement has necessitated the development of integrated health care practices. Moreover, as society assumes a larger role in shaping health care policy, providers find themselves under increasing economic and regulatory pres-

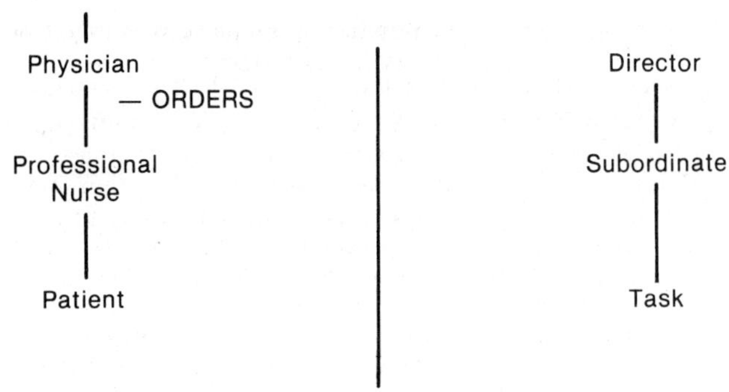

Figure 191–1. Traditional, hierarchal medical model.

sure to provide comprehensive, efficient, and effective care. This is particularly true in the highly complex and technical environment of the modern special care unit.

Both nurses and physicians have come to realize that communication and a collegial relationship are essential for effective practice. However, interactions among those involved in patient care are often less than optimal, as pointed out by Prescott and coworkers.[2] Factors cited by her as contributing to poor working relationships included changing economic and social status, shared practice domains, and unfamiliarity with other professions.

The historical divisions between professional groups have attracted attention on a national level and have led to programs designed to foster bedside collaboration. As described by Weiss and Davis, "Collaboration represents the optimum of maintaining assertiveness while cooperating. Balancing these elements allows the knowledge and skills of both professions to synergistically influence the care being provided."[3] Such collaboration led to horizontal organizational models in which participants (clinicians) are viewed as partners or colleagues in the provision of care (Fig. 191–2).

In this chapter, we explore the growth of collaborative practice models in response to various influences, the associated outcomes, and the means to implement these models in day-to-day practice, with special reference to the intensive care unit (ICU).

HISTORICAL PERSPECTIVES

In the late 1960s and early 1970s, the social dimension of the nurse-physician relationship was explored in numerous studies.[1, 4–6] Physicians clearly had a dominant position in the hospital environment, and both nurses' and physicians' behavior preserved this order. In response to the developing interest in collaboration, the American Medical Association and the American Nursing Association formed the National Joint Practice Commission (NJPC) in 1972 to identify factors that promote close working relationships.[7] Many practice models evolved from the NJPC; however, five essential elements were recognized as prerequisites to effective collaboration (Table 191–1). In 1977, under the guidance of the NJPC, a demonstration project was developed in which clinical elements incorporating these ideas were simultaneously introduced into certain hospital settings. Several years after the practice environment was restructured, participants were surveyed regarding their preference for practice models. Although objective measures of performance were not obtained, general support existed for collaborative practice, and satisfaction with patient outcome was high in those involved in the project.[8]

TABLE 191–1. Five Essential Prerequisites to Effective Collaboration

1. Communication
2. Competence
3. Accountability
4. Trust
5. Administrative support

(Adapted from Devereux P: Essential elements of nurse-physician collaboration. J Nurs Adm 1981; 11:19–23.)

Following the NJPC's lead, the Society of Critical Care Medicine and the American Association of Critical Care Nurses (AACN) established a task force in 1982 to identify factors necessary to foster collaboration in the intensive care environment. The task force, or the Interorganization Liaison Group (ILG), has met at intervals since that time and has prepared several position papers, which have subsequently been adopted by each parent organization. The first result of their activities was a joint practice statement released in 1982 (Table 191–2). The statement stressed the importance of physician and nurse autonomy in their respective fields, as well as the accountability of all health care professionals. The statement also affirmed that nurse and physician directors of a unit should have equal authority in the organization of critical care units.[9] These societies continue to explore various practice models as part of their ongoing commitment to problem solving and collaboration. Accordingly, the ILG has developed position statements on other topics of mutual concern that have been subsequently affirmed by both the Society of Critical Care Medicine and the AACN.[10, 11]

Endorsement of a multidisciplinary approach to critical care also came from a consensus conference held at the National Institutes of Health in 1983.[12] Collegial practice was supported at all levels, and the conference attendees recommended that the organizational structure within the ICU facilitate collaborative activity. In addition, the Joint Commission on Accreditation of Hospital Organization recognized the value of integrated practice by mandating a multidisciplinary approach to the management of critical care units.[13]

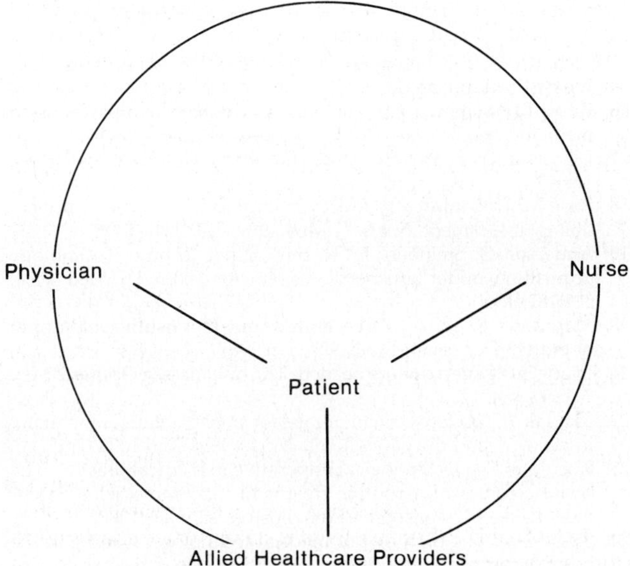

Figure 191–2. Collaborative or horizontal medical model.

TABLE 191–2. Jointly Approved SCCM/AACN Position Statement—1982

Principles:

1. Responsibility and accountability for effective functioning of critical care unit must be vested in physician and nurse directors who are on an equal decision-making level.
2. These directors must be appropriately prepared and educated. In addition to competence in patient management, they need knowledge and experience in the following areas: management principles, resource management, and skills in interpersonal relationships (including conflict resolution).
3. The organizational structure of a critical care unit must ensure that physicians are autonomous when dealing with issues that affect medical practice.
4. The organizational structure of a critical care unit must ensure that physicians are autonomous when dealing with issues that affect nursing practice.
5. Some aspects of patient care require interdependence between physicians and nurses. These aspects must be identified and addressed jointly.
6. Every critically ill person requires medical and nursing care. The services of additional disciplines may also be required in specific situations. To provide a holistic approach, the care delivered by other health team members must be coordinated by the physician and nurse directors.
7. Unit support services must be organized to enable the directors to optimally carry out their primary responsibilities in the practice of their respective disciplines (i.e., patient care).
8. The directors are accountable for the evaluation of the quality and efficiency of care and the financial provision of that care. They must develop a unit-specific system for the evaluation of care on a timely basis.
9. The directors are responsible for creating and maintaining an environment in which individuals have opportunities to realize their potentials.
10. Close collaboration between the directors is essential for successful management. This collaboration can be enhanced by daily rounds, weekly meetings, and other means that will ensure continuous, open communication.

COLLABORATIVE PRACTICE AND OUTCOME

Although support for joint practice activity is high in demonstration models, objective assessment of improved patient outcome has been infrequently reported. In a landmark study completed in 1986, Knaus and colleagues[14] evaluated the outcome of over 5000 patients cared for in various intensive care environments. Using the APACHE II (Acute Physiology and Chronic Health Evaluation) scoring system to stratify risks, the investigators found significant differences in institutional outcomes that were not predicted on the basis of severity of illness. An analysis of variables suggested that this unexplained outcome was not dependent on technologic capability but was influenced by administrative structure. Those units with the highest degree of staff involvement and physician-nurse interaction demonstrated the most favorable mortality ratio, suggesting that the process of care influenced patient outcome.

A second project performed under the auspices of the AACN attempted to measure and relate various aspects of unit structure, process, and outcome. The demonstration unit was established in a small, nonprofit, community-based hospital and emphasized decentralized administration, expertise through critical care certification, participation in decision making, and broad guidelines for nursing autonomy.[15] Standardized mortality ratios were derived from the APACHE II scoring systems. The results revealed a strikingly favorable difference from the anticipated mortality for the demonstration unit, supporting the belief that organizational characteristics can significantly affect outcome. Moreover, when patient and nursing opinions were gauged by various measurement tools, a high degree of satisfaction was demonstrated in both groups. This finding translated into lower-than-expected turnover in nursing staff and a decreased use of nurse-controlled consumable supplies.[15]

Many studies that have reviewed factors affecting nursing retention have demonstrated that collaborative practice ranks high on the list of qualities that nurses deem important.[16, 17] When one considers that the estimated cost for recruitment and training of a nurse in a specialty care area may be as high as $20,000, the economic effect of nursing retention on an institution can be significant.[18] Additional work further supports the notion that increased collaboration may be associated with positive outcomes in the intensive care environment.[19, 20] For example, Baggs[19] demonstrated that transfer decisions that were jointly agreed on were associated with decreased readmission rates in the ICU and in lower in-hospital mortality.

Finally, it seems reasonable to conclude that patients and families will be more likely to be satisfied and to trust caregivers in an atmosphere of cooperative enterprise. Achieving these goals remains an active area of investigation for nursing and administrative researchers.

Current Status

Despite empirical and objective support for collaborative practice, the pace to implement collaborative models on a larger scale has been slow. Enduring patterns of physician dominance and nurse deference, together with a heightened sense of competition between professional groups, have retarded progress in this area.[2]

Many reports have commented on the causes of these interprofessional conflicts and the social forces that abet them.[1, 2, 5, 6] Clearly, therefore, these relationships are not static but change in response to social and scientific advances. In particular, the past 30 years have been very turbulent for the nursing profession. The nurse's role and the perception of that role by society have changed. In addition, during this interval, the professional and educational evolution of the professional nurse has been dramatic. Nevertheless, these changes added new dimensions to the practice of nursing and have brought about a heightened awareness of the profession's contribution to health care. These events have come at a time when greater demands are placed on the professional nurse as a result of emerging technologies, higher patient acuity, and rising societal expectations. Despite these influences, nurses continue to perceive their primary task in a positive light.[21–23]

In the critical care environment, the nursing profession has responded to these challenges principally through educational initiatives and team building, thereby leading to a greater sense of autonomy and clarity of purpose. Formalization of the nursing process has been developed in the AACN's "Standards for Nursing Care of the Critically Ill."[24] Under these guidelines, the profession has increasing responsibility for the coordination of care and the evaluation of the patient's response to the disease process and for associated interventions.

The character of nursing practice is evolving through the use of nurse practitioners, primary care nurses, and clinical nurse specialists. Accordingly, conflict related to the nurse-physician relationship will inevitably occur. Physicians, unlike their nursing counterparts, who are enjoying a professional ascendancy, have witnessed the erosion of their historical prerogatives on many fronts. The patient-consumer is demanding a greater say in health care decisions. The legal profession and the insurance industry are increasingly reviewing patient management and outcomes. Cumbersome government regulations and changing reimbursement patterns are also affecting the manner in which physicians deliver care. Additional sources of conflict come from administrators who regulate these areas, both within and outside the hospital setting. Thus, the pre-eminent rule of the doctor is often eroded. Some physicians may therefore be threatened by collaborative practice.

Problems may also develop related to the manner in which nurses and physicians organize their time. Nurses plan their activities around the total needs of one or two patients. Constant attendance at the patient's bedside allows the nurse to assess a patient's needs and responses. Conversely, physicians have divided interests that limit their contact with patients. Thus, they rely on nursing personnel to summarize data and provide ongoing assessment of patient status.

Competitive interactions have unfortunately become a natural outgrowth of these changing professional relationships. In a large descriptive study, Prescott and associates[2] found that conflict resolution in these situations is often dominated by aggressive, inflexible postures, with settlement occurring through imposed authority. Collaboration and accommodation emerged as alternative strategies that represented varying degrees of assertiveness and cooperation. Of the two, accommodation occurred more frequently than collaboration in the nurse-physician relationship, particularly in situations in which patient welfare was not an issue. Unfortunately, these authors found few examples of collaboration in problem solving. In fact, collaboration occurred in only 14% of instances as perceived by physicians, whereas nurses described 7% of their interactions as collaborative. Compromise and avoidance complete the repertoire of alternative responses to conflict resolution. However, these options are perceived as least desirable and are resorted to infrequently. It is important, however, to realize that disagreement and competition are not always undesirable; in fact, these situations are often associated with positive outcomes. Nevertheless, flexible postures, with an emphasis on problem solving, are more beneficial to all participants. In the ideal collaborative practice model, all groups receive recognition, and key concerns are not compromised.

Within the past few years, physicians have become increasingly forced to adapt to multidisciplinary efforts. Currently, many physicians work in groups, and they frequently interact not only with other physicians but also with other health care providers. This trend appears to be gaining momentum. Physicians may therefore be more likely to accept a collaborative, mutually respectful relationship with the professional critical care nurse than they were a few years ago.

Components of Collaborative Practice

The body of knowledge concerning collaboration can be traced to the fields of group and institutional psychology and to industrial management. Communication, competence, and accountability were identified as factors that led to team building in interdisciplinary settings.[7] Trust and administrative support are cofactors that help to secure a stable working relationship. These five factors are necessary for creating effective collaboration in business, industry, and health care settings.

The development of collaboration using these essential factors has a defined natural history, beginning with the movement away from practice in isolation toward practice in concert with other health care providers. Increasing contact favors open communication, which is essential for staff development. Increasing contact can automatically lead to increased collaboration and communication, whether consciously pursued or not. However, communication is much more likely to be optimal when it reflects a deliberate effort to identify and clarify goals and mutually overlapping roles. Through interchange of ideas and expertise, practitioners become familiar with the nature and the scope of the other's practice. In this way, each practitioner is better able to assess individual competence. Once clinical expertise is demonstrated, trust can be established, and negotiation of new roles for both parties within the critical care environment can take place. In this regard, areas of nursing activities that are dependent, independent, and interdependent, as outlined in the AACN standards of care, must be clearly established (Table 191–3). Dependent nursing interventions are defined as those primarily directed by physicians through orders and medical care plans. Independent intervention by nurses are those that are unique to nursing, such as nursing assessment and diagnosis, teaching, counseling, and manipulation of the patient's environment. Interdependent activities reflect areas of shared interest and therefore include quality assurance and mutual responsibility for unit operation, organization, and administration. By analyzing the ICU environment, one can find increasing evidence of interdependent activities between nurses and physicians.

If dependent, independent, and interdependent areas of activity are considered, a clearer understanding of professional obligations and responsibilities emerges. A greater emphasis on shared structure and interactions may have not only professional and ethical implications but also legal ones, as suggested by Helm and Mazur.[25] All participants must be willing to accept legal and moral responsibility for their own actions, as well as, to some extent, the actions of the whole team caring for the patient.

Implementing Collaborative Practice

Organizational Structure

Collaborative practices do not arise spontaneously but grow out of commitment to a cooperative enterprise and dedication to comprehensive care. These themes need to be anchored in an organizational and managerial structure that facilitates team building.

The organizational factors identified by the NJPC that contribute to collaboration include primary nursing and clear definitions of the unit's environment. That is, each unit must identify the patient population it best serves and must attempt to minimize care for other patients who do not match the facilities and expertise of the unit.

TABLE 191–3. Classification of Nursing Functions in Relation to Physician Activities

Dependent
Is directed by physicians by means of orders and medical care plan
Independent
Performs unique nursing assessment and diagnosis
Develops care plans and outcomes
Supervises and delegates nursing functions
Interdependent
Has areas of shared responsibility, e.g., quality assurance, unit administration and operation, and technology acquisition

(Adapted from Kuhn R [Ed]. Outcome Standards for Nursing Care of the Critically Ill. Newport Beach, CA, American Association of Critical Care Nurses, 1990, pp 163–164.)

The mix of professional and technical personnel in the unit may also affect the organization and the effectiveness of the unit. A difference of opinion exists over whether or not units should use nursing support personnel, as well as how to achieve acceptable delegation of nursing tasks while ensuring responsibility and quality of care.[16, 17] The NJCP concluded that the registered nurse is ideally situated to implement and evaluate all aspects of care and to serve as the pivotal knowledge broker for other health care providers. Others, including the ILG and ultimately the AACN, have defined support personnel in the ICU and have developed a framework for their use.[10, 11]

Defining the nature of the population to be served is also a key consideration in the implementation of primary nursing in a critical care setting. If patient needs are accurately characterized, nursing requirements can be assessed, mechanisms can be developed to adjust to changing patient acuity, and teams with the appropriate mix of skills can be created. Controlled access through clearly articulated admission and discharge policies aids in the definition of unit goals and in the preservation of unit integrity.

Managerial factors can be divided into two broad categories: programming and feedback mechanisms. The first involves standardization of work and skills (i.e., the development of procedures and protocols), thereby allowing the organization to respond to routine situations in a predictable manner. Through the development of stereotyped responses, a high level of staff coordination and cooperation can be achieved, as witnessed in modern cardiovascular ICUs.

Feedback mechanisms become important when novel situations are encountered. In the intensive care environment, a high degree of patient instability and uncertainty about outcome may exist. In these instances, programmed responses cannot be relied on to cover all contingencies. Therefore, the organizational structure must allow for discretionary activity, means for self-adjustment, and development. Standardization of knowledge and skills is an important first step in this process. Corrective, positive feedback through supervision and group coordination can optimize patient outcome.[14]

Implementation

Incorporating these ideas into the day-to-day activities of specialty care areas continues to be a challenge. Both the nursing and the medical staff must be prepared for this period of transition. In the process of developing these frameworks, the team members in each unit should discuss issues, shared values, and potential areas of conflict. Each service should develop a mission statement to define the practice model, create standards of care, outline admission and discharge criteria, and develop protocols for caring for patients with difficult problems, such as severe or recurring pain or terminal illness. Other steps endorsed by the NJPC include integration of the patient record, encouragement of nurses' decision making, development of joint practice committees, and creation of joint care review panels.[7] Because separate nurse and physician progress notes are eliminated, team members are encouraged to read the evaluations of others. This plan also provides a formal means of communication between the nurse and the physician. Unnecessary duplication of information can also be avoided. The next step is independent clinical decision making, which allows the nursing staff to take full advantage of their clinical skills. In this regard, areas in which independent assessment and judgment may be employed must be clearly delineated. Nursing practice policies should be specifically tailored to the needs and requirements of a particular area and must be jointly crafted by nurse and physician administrators in keeping with legislated practice boundaries.[26]

A strong, ongoing commitment from the administration and the nursing and medicine departments is essential for the continued development of this practice model. Such commitment may take the form of seminars and workshops that define areas of competence, update skills, or stress concepts of professional practice. Support can also be demonstrated through the creation of joint-practice committees charged with the continuous monitoring of nurse-physician relationships and the evolvement of strategies that support joint practice. These committees should have a balanced rotating membership to decrease the opportunity for any one group to dominate the team's agenda.[27] By ongoing self-examination, these groups develop a certain structure, definition, and direction that deflects attention from the individual members and sharpens the focus of the process of health care delivery. This model can also be buttressed through joint record review, in which nurses and physicians together scrutinize the care provided to patients. This form of collaboration also provides an opportunity for the development of informal and formal clinical case conferences, which in turn reinforce practice guidelines, develop group competence, and promote clinical problem solving. The geographic assignment of others routinely involved in patient care, such as dietitians, pharmacists, and respiratory therapists, also contributes to the team identity.

The use of a consultant in team development provides yet another alternative. With no vested interest, the consultant can take a neutral view of team functions, working relationships, and patterns of communication and can identify strengths and weaknesses of the group.[28] Activities or individuals that have a negative influence on group development can be identified, and remedial action can be taken. Attention has recently focused on strategies that individuals can use to develop team orientation. Recognizing social and job-related stressors and evolving strategies to mollify their effects is one step that can avoid the consequences of unrelated events' spilling over into the workplace and exaggerating interpersonal conflicts. Learning to feel tension as it develops and taking measures to reduce stress may prevent such overreactions and the negative work-related interactions or perceptions that ensue.

Minimizing the inevitable effects of individual conflicts and personal biases is particularly difficult in intensive care, where the ego strength of nurses and physicians attracted to the specialty is typically quite high. They are often accustomed to independent decision making and have a high sense of accountability. In these situations, sensitivity to each other's perspective can be fostered by role-playing activities incorporated into unit retreats, orientation of new nurses and physicians, grand rounds presentations, and basic critical care education. Mechanisms should also be established to diffuse any unresolved conflicts without exacerbating them. Third parties on ad hoc committees are useful in this regard as long as they are professionally balanced and otherwise neutral. The focus should not be to select a winner or a loser, but to provide the best available alternative. When guided by the motto, "there are no problems in life, only unselected alternatives," no issue appears insurmountable.

COLLABORATIVE PRACTICE IN ACTION

In response to the perceived need for greater interdisciplinary cooperation in the management of the hopelessly ill, practitioners at Detroit Receiving Hospital developed the Comprehensive Supportive Care Team in 1985.[20, 29, 30] The team consists of a clinical nurse specialist and a limited number of rotating physicians who, in collaboration, provide broad support for the hopelessly ill patient and family. Specific plans are jointly developed that satisfy both nursing and medical goals. The team evaluates and revises the therapeutic plan in response to the patient's changing needs. Nursing, pastoral care, and social services staff are encouraged to participate in the decision-making process to ensure that the comfort and the psychologic and spiritual aspects of care are being satisfied. Close contact with the family is maintained through a designated team spokesman. The patient remains on the service until death, discharge, or significant change in status occurs that necessitates re-evaluation. Since its inception, the Comprehensive Supportive Care Team has provided consistent care to more than one thousand patients. Despite the nature of the population being served, acceptance and satisfaction among team and family members remains high. Moreover, by identifying the special needs of this group, costly care has been curtailed, resulting in better resource allocation within the institution.[20, 29]

CONCLUSIONS

The ICU is a dynamic environment that requires a coordinated effort to optimize patient outcome. Through conscientiously applied principles of collaboration, the integration of medicine, nursing, and allied health practices can be achieved while the interests of each are preserved.

Concrete steps that can be taken toward this practice model have been detailed by the NCPC, the ILG, and other interdisciplinary organizations. The effectiveness of these policies and techniques have been demonstrated in numerous settings and can be expected to be a common feature of future hospital environments as providers explore ways to control costs, provide comprehensive care, promote professionalism, and insure patient and family satisfaction.

References

1. McGraw RW: Interdisciplinary teamwork for medical care and health services: Components in organization. Ann Intern Med 1968; 69(4):821–835.
2. Prescott P, Bowen S: Nurse/physician relationships. Ann Intern Med 1985; 103:127–133.
3. Weiss S, Davis P: Validity and reliability of the collaborative practice scales. Nurs Res 1985; 34:299–305.
4. Stein L: The Doctor/nurse game. Arch Gen Psychiatry 1967; 16:699–703.
5. Pellegrino ED: What's wrong with the nurse-physician relationship in today's hospitals? A physician's view. Hospitals 1966; 40:70–80.
6. Bates B: Doctor and nurse: Changing roles and relations. N Engl J Med 1970; 283:129–134.
7. Devereux P: Essential elements of nurse-physician collaboration. J Nurs Adm 1981; 11:19–23.
8. Devereux P: Does joint practice work? J Nurs Adm 1981; 11:39–43.
9. Interorganization Liason Group: Focus on Critical Care 1983; 10:43–44.
10. Wlody G: Focus on Critical Care 1984; 11:43–45.
11. American Association of Critical Care Nurses: Focus on Critical Care 1989; 16:327–328.
12. Critical Care Medicine: Consensus conference. JAMA 1983; 250(6):798–804.
13. Joint Commission on Accreditation of Hospitals: Accreditation Manual of Hospitals. Chicago, The Joint Commission on Accreditation of Hospitals, 1982, p 182.
14. Knaus W, Draper E, Wagner D, et al: An evaluation of outcome from intensive care in major medical centers. Ann Intern Med 1986; 104:410–418.
15. Mitchell P, Armstrong S, Simpson T, et al: American Association of Critical Care Nurses Demonstration Project: Profile of excellence in critical care nursing. Heart Lung 1989; 18(3):219–237.
16. Baggs J, Ryan S: ICU Nurse-physician collaboration and nursing satisfaction. Nurs Econ 1990; 8(6):386–392.
17. Everly GS, Fulcione R: Perceived dimensions of job satisfaction for staff registered nurses. Nurs Res 1976; 25:346–348.
18. Evans SA, Carlson R: Nurse/physician collaboration: Solving the nursing shortage crisis. Am J Crit Care 1992; 1:25–32.
19. Baggs JG: The association between interdisciplinary collaboration and patient outcomes in a medical intensive care unit. Heart Lung 1992; 21:18–24.
20. Carlson RW, Devich L, Frank R: Development of a comprehensive supportive care team for the hopelessly ill on a university hospital service. JAMA 1988; 259:378–383.
21. Mohl PC, Denny NR, Mote TA, et al: Hospital unit stressors that affect nurses: Primary task vs. social factors. Psychosomatics 1992; 23:366–374.
22. Cronin-Stubbs D, Rooks C: The stress, social support and burnout of critical care nurses: The results of research. Heart Lung 1985; 14:31–39.
23. Martino JH, MacIntosh NJ: Effects of patient characteristics and technology on job satisfaction and stress of intensive care and intensive care nurses. Heart Lung 1985; 14:300–301.
24. Kuhn R (Ed): Outcome Standards for Nursing Care of the Critically Ill. Newport Beach, CA, American Association of Critical Care Nurses, 1990, pp 163–164.
25. Helms A, Mazur D: Physician collaboration dilemma. Dimens Crit Care Nurs 1992; 11(4):213–216.
26. Carlson RW, Haupt MT: Organization of critical care services. Acute Care 1989; 13:2–43.
27. Burchell RC, Thomas D, Smith H: Some considerations for implementing collaborative practice. Am J Med 1983; 74:9–13.
28. Chamberlain J: The use of a consultant in team development. J Contin Educ Nurs 1976; 7(5):25–29.
29. Field BE, Devich L, Carlson RW: Impact of a comprehensive supportive care team on management of hopelessly ill patients with multiple organ failure. Chest 1989; 96:353–356.
30. Campbell ML, Carlson RW: Terminal weaning from mechanical ventilation: Ethical and practical considerations for management. J Crit Care 1992; 1(3):52–56.

CHAPTER 192

Preventing Complications in the Intensive Care Unit

Elizabeth A. Henneman, RN, MS, CCRN • Paul E. Bellamy, MD

The critically ill patient provides the health care team with many challenges, among the greatest of which is the prevention of complications. An increased awareness of the cost of complications associated with intensive care management has led to a heightened interest in the scientific examination of interventions aimed at ameliorating these complications.

Preventing all complications in an intensive care unit (ICU) is, of course, impossible. Minimizing complications, however, demands that ICU personnel adopt an aggressive approach in managing what are sometimes considered the mundane aspects of patient care, such as skin care or line maintenance. Successful complication prevention requires a multidisciplinary commitment to the development and monitoring of standards of care with a preventive focus. Standards of care should reflect current research findings and should be appropriate for the population of the unit. These standards should incorporate nationally or internationally set standards when available or applicable, such as *International Standards for Safety in the Intensive Care Unit*[1] and the Society of Critical Care Medicine's *Guidelines for Standards of Care for Patients with Acute Respiratory Failure on Mechanical Ventilatory Support*.[2] In addition to being theoretically sound, these standards must also be feasible for the fast-paced, chaotic ICU environment. The effectiveness of the standards in achieving goals must also be continually evaluated through a unit-based program (e.g., continuous quality improvement).

Prevention of complications in the ICU must be initiated as early as possible in the patient's admission process, or before admission (e.g., in patients undergoing elective surgery), when feasible. Standardized admission order forms are useful to ensure that certain procedures are routinely carried out, especially in settings in which a significant learning curve exists, such as in teaching hospitals.

The variety and number of potential complications in critically ill patients is tremendous. This chapter reviews those that occur most commonly, are pertinent to most critically ill patients, and are predictable and therefore preventable in most cases. These complications include skin and mucosal breakdown, musculoskeletal injury, pulmonary complications, nosocomial infections, and ICU psychosis. No attempt has been made to cover the almost limitless list of complications that may arise in critically ill patients secondary to their illness or treatment. For example, complications associated with disease processes (e.g., arrhythmias), procedures (e.g., pneumothorax), treatments (e.g., fluid overload), and surgeries (e.g., bleeding) are not covered. Stress ulcers and pulmonary embolism, two of the commonest complications seen in ICU patients, are not covered in this section because they are addressed in other chapters in this text.

SKIN AND MUCOSAL BREAKDOWN

Alterations in the integrity of the skin and mucous membranes are among the best-recognized complications of critically ill patients. They are visible and constant reminders of the consequence of clinicians' actions or inactions. The patient in the ICU is at risk for skin and mucosal problems because of the underlying illness and ICU treatment modalities. Table 192–1 lists risk factors commonly seen in critically ill patients that may lead to the development of skin and mucosal injury.

TABLE 192–1. Risk Factors for the Development of Skin and Mucosal Injury in Critically Ill Patients

Risk factor
Immobility
Decreased oxygen delivery or consumption
Impaired nutritional status
Extremes of age (<1 y, >60 y)
Obesity
Edema
Diabetes mellitus
Immunosuppression
Infection
Decreased level of consciousness
Impaired sensation
Hyperthermia or hypothermia
Pre-existing illness (e.g., disseminated intravascular coagulopathy)
Incontinence
Use of invasive therapies
Nasogastric tubes
Endotracheal or tracheostomy tubes
Rectal tubes
Use of vasopressor medications

Pressure Ulcer

Pressure ulcers are lesions caused by unrelieved pressure that results in damage to underlying tissue. The "cost" of a pressure ulcer is high, both to the patient and to the institution. The incidence of pressure ulcers in the critical care setting has been reported to be as high as 40%.[3] Prevention of pressure ulcers requires multidisciplinary standards of care that recognize the potential for all critically ill patients to develop this complication. A comprehensive care plan demands early assessment, intervention, and evaluation of skin integrity. Unfortunately, because of the critical nature of the patient's condition at admission to the ICU, skin issues generally receive low priority. The patient who survives a critical disease yet dies from sepsis secondary to a pressure ulcer is a sad reminder of the irony of this situation.

Assessment of the patient's risk for pressure ulcer development should be performed as early as possible in the patient's hospital stay. Elective surgery patients should be evaluated preoperatively, and preventive interventions should be begun before their operation. For example, heart surgery patients, who are at risk for sacral pressure ulcers, should have special dressings or padding placed over that area preoperatively in preparation for lying flat on their back for prolonged periods. Tools to determine a patient's risk for developing pressure ulcers have been devised; however, the predictive ability of these tools in critically ill patients has not been well established. Modification and testing of these tools remains a high research priority. In the interim, staff should identify patients who are at risk for the development of pressure ulcers (Table 192–1) and should have guidelines available to assist them in choosing the most appropriate preventive therapy.

Interventions to prevent skin breakdown must also be initiated early in the patient's ICU course. Unit standards should address preventive measures appropriate for various patient populations. The most effective standards are those that delineate specific (e.g., mattress overlay) rather than vague (e.g., skin care precautions) interventions.

Because pressure ulcers are caused by immobility, interventions to decrease this complication are typically aimed at maximizing mobility. Unfortunately, many critically ill patients must remain relatively immobile. As a result, much effort has been directed at determining ways of decreasing or relieving pressure in these immobile patients.

Debate continues over the most effective method of pressure reduction and relief, and various mattress overlays, replacement mattresses, and specialty beds are now marketed for this purpose. Table 192–2 lists these products, their indications, and their advantages and disadvantages.

The cost-benefit ratio for the use of these products prophylactically has yet to be determined. However, the high risk of ulcers in the critically ill patient has led some experts to suggest the use of universal pressure ulcer precautions, that is, special pressure reduction beds for all critically ill patients. The significant cost associated with the use of special beds demands that an assessment of the individual patient's needs be ongoing to determine appropriate strategies for pressure reduction. For example, the use of a mattress overlay at a one-time nominal charge seems a reasonable preventive approach for all critically ill patients. However, the decision to use a very expensive, low-air-loss bed requires serious consideration of the cost-benefit ratio. As the patient's condition changes, the appropriateness of all pres-

TABLE 192–2. Pressure Reduction and Relief Devices

Device	*Indications*	*Advantages*	*Disadvantages*	*Comments*
Mattress Overlay	Patients with low-to-moderate risk who are expected to be on bed rest > 24 h. May be used as a prophylactic strategy on all ICU beds.			
Foam (3–4 inches thick and of appropriate density)*		Comfortable. One-time charge or low cost. No daily maintenance. Less user error than with plastic overlays. Less friction and shear than with standard hospital bed.	Potentially flammable. Difficult to reposition patient. Difficult to fit sheets wtih thick mattresses. Added height makes getting patient out of bed difficult. Require incontinence devices to prevent permanent soiling.	
Plastic		One-time charge or low cost. Potentially more effective than foam with heavy patients. Easy to clean.	Ensuring proper inflation level is cumbersome and subjective. Increased perspiration. Patient discomfort. Leaks if punctured.	
Water overlay		One-time charge or low cost. Conforms to body contours.	Cumbersome set-up process. Set-up time required. Leaks if punctured. May reduce effectiveness of CPR.	
Alternating-Pressure Mattress		Provides alternating pressure. Easy to clean. User friendly.	Increased perspiration from plastic. Motor requires an electric source.	
Replacement Mattress		No maintenance by nursing staff.	Initial cost.	Used in place of hospital mattress. Designed for multiple patient use.
Low–Air-Loss Bed	Patients who are immobile and cannot be turned at regular intervals or who are at high risk in other areas.	Surface fabrics are low-friction materials. Built-in scales available on most models.	High daily cost. Reduce patient mobility (patient "sinks" in bed). Difficult to transfer in and out of bed. Difficult to transfer patient in bed (heavy). Difficult to perform CPR.	Consists of multiple rows of air-filled cushions that can be programmed for each patient to provide maximum pressure relief. Tissue interface pressures are maintained below the recommended 25 mm Hg.
Air-Fluidized Bed	Immobility associated with wounds (e.g., stage IV pressure ulcers, burns, or grafts).	Pressure relief.	Potential dehydration from high air flow. Spontaneous patient movement restricted. Difficult to secure Fowler position (uses foam wedges, which slip). Difficult patient transfer in and out of bed. Bed extremely heavy. Cleaning process cumbersome (beads blown into air).	A fluidlike environment is created by passing air under silicone-coated beads, which are covered by a semipermeable sheet.
Pulsating Bed		Pressure relief plus potential for improved venous return.	See above for air loss.	
Kinetic Therapy				
Oscillating bed: low–air-loss	Severe hemodynamic instability or pulmonary conditions that would benefit from frequent turning schedule.	May be effective in management of pulmonary process.	High Cost. Conscious patients may not tolerate constant motion or turning.	Air cushions are alternately inflated and deflated to allow for gentle patient turning, or the bed frame rotates.

*Two-inch foam eggcrate mattresses do not reduce pressure and are intended for patient comfort only.
CPR = cardiopulmonary resuscitation; ICU = intensive care unit.

sure-reduction strategies must be examined and interventions made accordingly.

Clinical practice guidelines have been published that provide both the clinicians and the patients with useful information on the prevention of pressure ulcers in adults.[9] These guidelines may be useful when unit-based standards are developed for pressure ulcer prevention.

Device-Related Injury

The use of invasive therapies in critical care is plagued by numerous potential complications involving skin and mucosal injury. Indwelling devices, such as endotracheal, tracheostomy, nasogastric, and rectal tubes, present special problems in critically ill patients.

Endotracheal Tubes

The introduction of low-pressure cuffs on endotracheal tubes has allowed these tubes to be left in place for longer periods of time with less concern for tracheal damage. However, this practice increases the patient's risk for the development of pressure sores on the mouth or nares. This problem is compounded when monitoring devices (e.g., end-tidal carbon dioxide monitors) are clamped onto the endotracheal tube, causing additional traction and pressure. Furthermore, skin breakdown may occur on the face from the adhesive tape used to secure the tube, and lip necrosis may occur when the lip is caught between the tube and the tape.

Management of this problem requires unit standards that call for frequent tube repositioning, support to decrease traction on the endotracheal tube, and facial skin protection. Our standard is to reposition oral endotracheal tubes from side to side every 24 to 48 hours. Rolled up towels are used to prop up ventilator tubing to prevent traction on the mouth or nose from the ventilator circuitry and heavy attachments. To protect the skin, we apply Duoderm (Conva Tec, Princeton, NJ) under the tape on the face of any patient who may require long-term intubation or who has friable skin (Fig. 192–1). An alternative method would be to use Velcro endotracheal tube holders; however, we have not had success with this method in mobile or agitated patients.

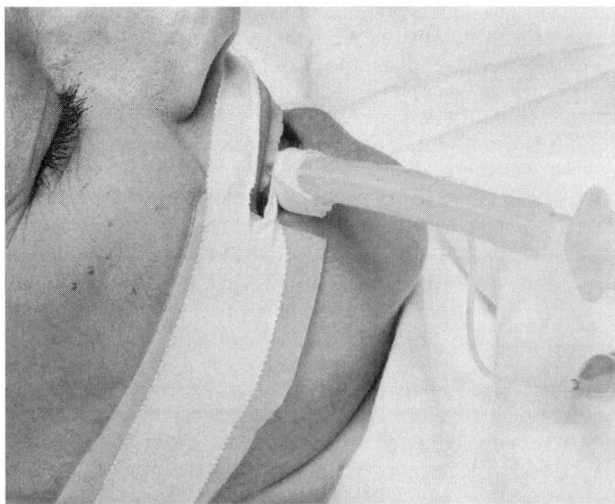

Figure 192–1. Use of a protective barrier under adhesive tape decreases the incidence of skin breakdown in high-risk patients (e.g., those undergoing long-term intubation, or those with friable skin).

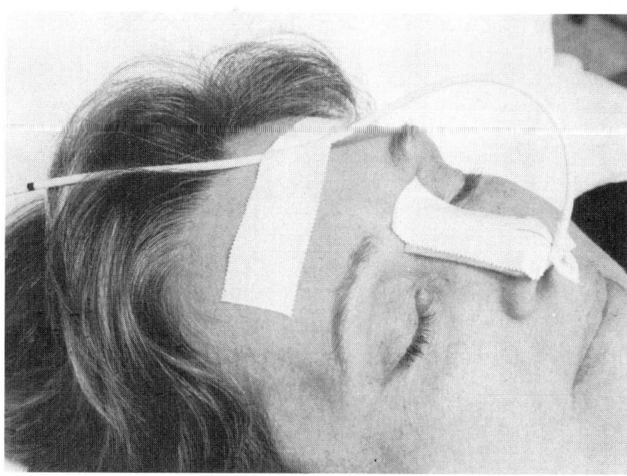

Figure 192–2. Incorrect positioning of a nasogastric tube. Note that upward flexion of the tube places pressure on patient's nares.

Tracheostomy Tubes

The problem of traction caused by the weight of ventilator tubing and other devices also occurs with tracheostomy tubes. Because patients with these tubes are often more mobile than those with ventilator tubes, extra care must be taken during transfers and repositioning to ensure that the tubes are positioned properly.

Tracheostomy tubes pose the additional problem of skin breakdown, which can occur secondary to secretions that ooze from the tracheostomy incision and from twill ties applied too tightly. The combination of the two (wet, tight tracheostomy ties) can seriously macerate the skin. Products are now available that use wide, soft material with Velcro fasteners, which we have found to be quite effective in securing tracheostomy tubes.

Feeding Tubes

Most skin breakdown problems resulting from feeding tubes can be avoided with proper positioning and taping. In an effort to adequately secure tubes, tubes are often flexed upward, out of the patient's face. This maneuver can result in an upward traction on the patient's nares and eventual skin breakdown at the nostril (Figs. 192–2 and 192–3). Although usually not life threatening, this complication causes an avoidable disfiguration and is an unfortunate re-

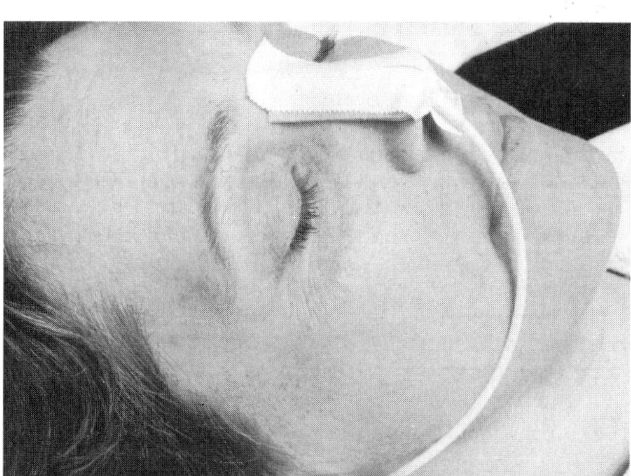

Figure 192–3. Correct nasogastric tube positioning. Note also the use of a protective barrier under the adhesive tape.

minder of the patient's stay in the ICU. Protective skin barriers, such as those previously recommended for endotracheal tubes, are useful in decreasing the skin breakdown associated with these tubes.

Rectal Tubes

Rectal tubes are used in critically ill patients with unrelenting diarrhea. Although the goal of these tubes is to increase patient comfort and decrease skin breakdown, other consequences to their use must be considered. The high pressure of the cuff used to prevent dislodgment of the tube can cause breakdown of the rectal mucosa and damage to the sphincter. Appropriate use of these tubes demands that a strict schedule of balloon deflation be adhered to (e.g., every 4 hours for a half hour). Alternatives to rectal tubes, such as rectal bags, should be attempted whenever possible.

Wound Drainage or Fistulas

Exudates from draining wounds or enterocutaneous fistulas can be extremely irritating to surrounding skin. Gastrointestinal contents (e.g., bile) pose serious threats to skin integrity. Prevention of skin breakdown requires that the surrounding skin be meticulously cleared of exudate. This goal is accomplished via frequent dressing changes and the use of protective skin barriers, such as transparent or hydroocclusive dressings. Gravity drainage bags are often useful for channeling large amounts of drainage away from the skin.

MUSCULOSKELETAL COMPLICATIONS

Contractures and footdrop are two of the commonest musculoskeletal complications seen in critically ill patients. These problems can be even more severe in the elderly and in those with neuromuscular disorders. Most of these problems result from the muscular weakness that develops after prolonged periods of immobility.

The use of neuromuscular junction–blocking agents is now considered an important adjunct in the treatment of patients with severe respiratory failure or increased intracranial pressure. These drugs have been associated with muscular weakness and prolonged paralysis.[5] As a result, even greater attention should be paid in these patients to aggressive preventive management of muscular atrophy.

Prevention of musculoskeletal complications requires frequent repositioning of the limbs and passive range-of-motion exercises. Maintaining proper body alignment and performing passive range-of-motion exercises is typically the responsibility of the critical care nurse, who integrates these interventions into other aspects of the patient's care (e.g., bathing). However, involvement of the physical therapist can be vital to ensuring a comprehensive care plan for the patient. In addition to evaluating the appropriateness and effectiveness of the range-of-motion exercises, the physical therapist can also evaluate the patient's progress and can make recommendations that address the patient's ongoing needs.

Family members who have expressed an interest in participating in the patient's care should be given instructions on performing simple range-of-motion exercises. Posting exercise instructions (i.e., "how-to" diagrams) and schedules can help motivate staff, patients, and families to adhere to these regimens.

PULMONARY COMPLICATIONS

The critically ill patient is at high risk for the development of pulmonary complications secondary to their disease process, surgery, or debilitation, or from the use of equipment that supports the patient through his or her illness (e.g., ventilators, endotracheal tubes). Guidelines have been developed by the Society of Critical Care Medicine that delineate standards of care for patients with acute respiratory failure.[2] Implementation of these guidelines may help decrease the number of pulmonary complications by standardizing the management of this high-risk patient population. The following section reviews some common complications seen in the ICU: atelectasis, nosocomial pneumonia, and unplanned extubation.

Atelectasis

The patient who is immobile or unable to breathe deeply may develop atelectasis, a complication that is commonly seen in the postoperative period, especially after abdominal or thoracic surgery. The mainstay of prophylaxis for atelectasis is to encourage the patient to breathe deeply on a regular basis. Although this recommendation seems straightforward, this goal is hampered in the very ill patient, whose consciousness may be altered, whose mobility is limited, and who is in pain.

In the awake patient, deep breathing is usually sufficient for preventing atelectasis. Maintaining a sustained maximal inspiration has been found to be the optimal means of preventing pulmonary complications in the postoperative period.[6, 7] Devices such as incentive spirometers may help motivate the patient but are of little value unless they are accompanied by specific instructions, monitoring, and support from the nurse or respiratory therapist.

The patient with a decreased level of consciousness requires alternative forms of therapy to prevent atelectasis, including frequent repositioning, intermittent positive-pressure breathing, and chest physiotherapy. Turning the patient from side to side either manually or via kinetic therapy helps to prevent atelectasis in the dependent lung. The routine use of intermittent positive-pressure ventilation in the awake, cooperative postoperative patient is inappropriate; incentive spirometry is as effective and is less costly. However, intermittent positive-pressure ventilation is indicated when the patient is unable to spontaneously perform deep-breathing maneuvers.

The routine use of chest physiotherapy (postural drainage, vibration, percussion) for the prevention of atelectasis has not been supported by research. However, atelectasis secondary to mucus plugs has been shown to be reversed with the use of chest physiotherapy.[8] The routine use of chest physiotherapy in all postoperative or ICU patients should be replaced by thoughtful consideration of each patient's needs. In many instances, deep breathing and increased mobility adequately prevent atelectasis.

Pain is often a major obstacle to patient compliance with deep-breathing maneuvers. Effective pain management and the use of pillows to splint incisions may help ensure patient cooperation. The use of patient-controlled anesthesia devices allows the patient to maintain control over pain relief during planned deep-breathing maneuvers.

Nosocomial Pneumonia

The ICU is the hospital setting in which most nosocomial pneumonias develop. The occurrence of a nosocomial infection has been demonstrated to increase the risk of death in the critically ill patient.[8a] Risk factors related to both the ICU patient and the environment are noted in Table 192–3. Traditional strategies for preventing pneumonia were aimed at optimizing the patient's potential to fight infection and at managing the environment to prevent the introduction of organisms and cross-contamination. Despite these efforts,

TABLE 192–3. Risk Factors for Nosocomial Infections in Critically Ill Patients

Immobility
Impaired nutritional status
Extremes of age (<1 y, >60 y)
Diabetes mellitus
Immunosuppression
Decreased level of consciousness
Decreased cardiac output
Use of invasive therapies
Nasogastric tubes
Endotracheal or tracheostomy tubes
Rectal tubes
Vascular access devices
Use of mechanical ventilation
Proximity of patients

the incidence of nosocomial infection remains high, especially in patients receiving mechanical ventilation.[9, 10] New research suggests that colonization of the patient's gastrointestinal tract plays a major role in the development of pneumonia, and efforts have been directed at developing methods to decrease this phenomenon.

Patients who are intubated and receiving mechanical ventilation are especially vulnerable to the development of pneumonia because they lack normal protective mechanisms, such as a cough reflex and functional cilia. Endotracheal and nasogastric tubes also inhibit normal mechanisms, such as chewing and swallowing, that prevent colonization of the oral cavity. Patients with depressed levels of consciousness resulting from sedation or neurologic injury are at risk for aspiration of these colonized organisms.

Because patients in the ICU are also at risk for the development of gastric stress ulcers and bleeding, they often receive prophylactic histamine$_2$ blockers or antacids. Antacids have been demonstrated to increase the risk of pneumonia in patients receiving mechanical ventilation, presumably by increasing the pH to a level (>4) that is inadequate for the inhibition of bacterial growth.[9]

Other researchers have suggested that aspiration of contaminated nasopharyngeal secretions may not be the major causative factor in the pathogenesis of nosocomial pneumonia. Recent findings indicate that ischemic mucosal injury and the associated translocation of enteric bacteria may play a more critical role.[11] Clearly, more research is needed regarding the pathogenic mechanisms active in the development of nosocomial pneumonia before optimal strategies can be created for reducing the frequency of this complication.

Interventions aimed at maximizing patient defenses have included meticulous mouth care and methods of preventing the stasis of secretions, which offer a reservoir for the growth of organisms. Routine interventions include turning, coughing, deep breathing, chest physiotherapy, and more recently, the use of kinetic beds. Although these techniques may be theoretically sound, their effectiveness in the prevention of pneumonia is not consistently supported in the literature.

The most recent technologic advance in the prevention of pneumonia has been the development of kinetic, or "self-rotating," beds. The enthusiasm for the use of these beds is based on the notion that if frequent turning is good for the patient, then constant turning is better. Several of these beds allow repositioning of patients who otherwise could not be turned (e.g., those with unstable spinal injuries). A variety of these beds exist. Some beds alternately inflate or deflate cushions in the mattress to gently reposition the patient, whereas in others, the entire bed frame moves. The newest models incorporate pressure-relief features as well as kinetic therapy. Few data exist to support the efficacy of these beds in improving such outcomes as decreased incidence of pressure ulcers, length of hospital stay, or decreased rate of mortality.[12]

Managing the environment to prevent nosocomial infection requires that appropriate standards exist regarding infection control. The Centers for Disease Control (CDC) offers guidelines for the development of these standards.[13] Significant progress can be made in the prevention of pneumonia if strict adherence to regimens designed to prevent cross-contamination are in place. Of these, proper handwashing is the most important procedure for the prevention of nosocomial infection.

Recent attention in the area of prevention of nosocomial pneumonia has been directed at eradicating organisms in the gastrointestinal tract, a technique called selective decontamination of the digestive tract. This intervention is based on the theory that respiratory infections appear to be related to colonization of the upper gastrointestinal tract and to subsequent spillover of gastrointestinal contents into the respiratory tract. Research supports the effectiveness of selective decontamination of the digestive tract in decreasing colonization and infection rates in various patient populations.[14, 15] However, data supporting the relationship between selective decontamination of the gastrointestinal tract and patient outcome remain controversial.[15a, 15b] Nonetheless, interest in the use of selective decontamination of the digestive tract is high and is worthy of further investigation to determine which patient groups would benefit from this intervention.

Aspiration pneumonia is a significant concern in ICU patients. Routine procedures, such as checking placement of nasogastric tubes before feedings and properly positioning the patient, can be effective in decreasing the incidence of aspiration pneumonia.

Although it is routinely used to ensure correct nasogastric tube placement or to measure nasogastric aspirate, aspiration of gastric contents is not always a reliable method for these determinations. Using this technique in patients with small-bore feeding tubes is fraught with problems because the tubing collapses down onto itself when aspiration is attempted. A chest radiograph should always be obtained to verify placement of small-bore tubes prior to the initiation of tube feedings.

Clinicians often erroneously assume that an inflated cuff on the endotracheal tube prevents aspiration of gastric contents into the lungs. As a result, patients may be placed inappropriately in the supine position, which increases their risk for aspiration. Research suggests that placing the patient at a 45° angle can be effective in reducing aspiration of gastric contents.[16]

Unplanned Extubation

Regardless of how well an endotracheal tube is secured, partial or complete unplanned extubation commonly occurs. Partial extubations typically occur in patients who are agitated and restless, who mouth the tube, slowly moving it up and out of the correct position. Partial extubation may also occur in a patient who has a strong cough or during repositioning of the tube. Unplanned extubations, in which the entire tube comes out, generally occur in agitated or confused patients.

The basic requisite for the prevention of either type of extubation is avoidance of situations that lead to anxiety and confusion. Every attempt must be made to inform the patient about the purpose of the endotracheal tube, if possible before the tube is inserted. Procedures (e.g., suctioning) should be explained to patients before they are performed so that the patients know what to expect. Judicious use of sedatives in addition to explanations is frequently warranted. However, indiscriminate application of restraints (either physical or chemical) for all intubated patients should be discouraged.

The position of the endotracheal tube at the lips should be noted and documented intermittently to ensure that partial extubations do not occur. Patients with a strong cough may benefit from more frequent suctioning or from the addition of intratracheal lidocaine (Xylocaine) if secretions are not the cause of the cough. All endotracheal tube repositioning should be performed with two staff members present, one to secure the tube and the other to apply the tape.

NOSOCOMIAL INFECTION

Decreasing the incidence of hospital-acquired infection is one of the greatest challenges facing ICU clinicians. Prevention of hospital-acquired infection requires strict adherence to basic principles of infection control and demands that meticulous attention be paid to procedures and other therapies that place the patient at risk. This section addresses the importance of general infection control measures in the control of nosocomial infection and provides recommendations for the management of indwelling catheters and intravascular lines.

The CDC has developed guidelines that are useful for setting policy standards in ICUs. These include guidelines for the prevention and control of nosocomial infections[13]; guidelines for the prevention of intravascular infections[17]; guidelines for the prevention of catheter-associated urinary tract infections[18]; and guidelines for the prevention of surgical wound infections.[19]

The CDC ranks its recommendations numerically from category 1 to category 3, depending on how well the recommendation is supported by research. Category 1 measures, for example, are strongly supported by studies deemed well designed or viewed effective by a majority of expert reviewers. These recommendations should be supplemented with techniques supported by the most current research findings if they are to be incorporated into unit-based standards.

An important infection control issue is the transmission of organisms between patients in the ICU. Many hospitals have drafted sophisticated policies aimed at reducing the spread of infection (e.g., isolation precautions; use of masks, gowns, gloves; and special airflow requirements). Despite these policies, cross-contamination of patients remains a significant issue in many ICUs. Surprisingly, the most basic infection control measures are frequently ignored or are erratically practiced by hospital personnel. The best example of this laxity is handwashing. The CDC guidelines for the prevention and control of nosocomial infection contain numerous category 1 recommendations regarding the washing of hands before and after patient contact.[13] Nonetheless, compliance with straightforward handwashing protocols is traditionally poor in the ICU. Failure to comply with such protocols can be devastating when staff care for infected and immunocompromised patients simultaneously. Improving staff compliance with handwashing protocols requires an understanding of the importance of such measures, the availability of adequate handwashing resources (e.g., sinks, nonirritating soaps), and appropriate role modeling by senior staff (e.g., attending physicians, unit managers).

Indwelling catheters (e.g., urinary) and intravenous lines have become integral components of the treatment of critically ill patients. Unfortunately, they are not without risks, the most common of which is the potential for introducing infection. Essential to the prevention of complications in the ICU patient is the judicious use of these catheters and intravenous lines; thoughtful consideration of the risk-benefit ratio associated with their use should be made in each patient situation.

TABLE 192–4. Summary of Category 1 Centers for Disease Control Recommendations for the Management of Urinary Catheters

1. Educate personnel in correct technique for catheter insertion and care.
2. Catheterize only when necessary.
3. Emphasize handwashing.
4. Insert catheter using sterile technique and equipment.
5. Secure catheter properly.
6. Maintain closed, sterile drainage.
7. Obtain urine samples aseptically.
8. Maintain unobstructed urine flow.

Indwelling Urinary Catheters

Careful monitoring of fluid intake and output in critically ill patients frequently necessitates the use of indwelling urinary catheters. Prevention of infections associated with their use requires that standards be set for their insertion, maintenance, and removal. The CDC guidelines for the prevention of catheter-associated urinary tract infections include numerous category 1 recommendations for the appropriate management of indwelling catheters, including the use of aseptic technique for catheter insertion and the maintenance of closed drainage systems (Table 192–4).[18]

Intravenous and Intra-arterial Catheters

A significant amount of research has been conducted on the reduction of infections associated with the use of intravenous and intra-arterial catheters. Potential risk factors and techniques for preventing infection have been identified. Recent interest has focused on the development of new types of catheters that will decrease the incidence of colonization of the catheter itself.

Critically ill patients are at high risk for the development of catheter-related infections. Because many of the patient risk factors cannot be altered, most investigators have attempted to determine methods of catheter management that decrease infection rates. Catheter management involves many factors: choice of catheter site, catheter placement technique (i.e., skill of the individual placing the catheter), type of placement (percutaneous versus cutdown), and catheter material. Catheter management also includes maintenance issues such as length of catheter placement, dressing changes, and line and site care.

Emphasis on the prevention of intravascular line infection is currently being placed on measures that reduce colonization of the insertion site and the catheter. Examples of methods that decrease site colonization include the use of strict protocols for mask, gown, and gloves during insertion; the use of effective cutaneous antiseptics; and the application of an iodophor topically on the insertion site. The latest approach to reducing catheter colonization has been the development of an antiseptic-coated catheter.[20]

The routine removal and replacement of catheters (e.g., every 3 to 5 days) in patients who show no evidence of catheter-related infection has been disputed. New evidence suggests that catheters can be left in place for prolonged periods of time, exchanged over a guide wire if a new catheter is needed, and removed completely only when signs of catheter-related sepsis exist.[21, 22] Table 192–5 is an example

TABLE 192–5. Standards of Care for the Placement and Maintenance of Arterial Catheters in the Intensive Care Unit

Preferred Sites	*Duration at Site*	*GWX Criteria (always culture catheter segment)*	*Removal Criteria*	*Insertion Standards*	*Site Care Standards*	*Hub/Injection Port/Tubing*
Radial, femoral, axillary, pedal (avoid in elderly or in patients with vascular disease and diabetes)	Indefinite	Evidence for site infection, e.g., inflammation Damped waveform Inability to withdraw blood to confirm catheter-related sepsis Note: no GWX for axillary site	Ischemia of distal extremity Unsafe location (brachial) Evidence for microembolization When evidence of catheter sepsis is present: post-GWX C&S ≥15 colonies with positive blood cultures Grossly infected site When catheter-related sepsis is likely to be present (e.g., in patients with fever, hypotension without other explanation)	Cap, mask, and gloves Sterile field	Scrub exit site with 3 alcohol and 3 povidone-iodine swabs. Apply povidone-iodine ointment to site. Dress with gauze (change daily) or transparent dressing (change on Monday, Wednesday, Friday).	Scrub with alcohol or povidone-iodine for 30 seconds before entering port for blood drawing Change tubing every 72 hours Change intravenous fluid every 24 hours

(Courtesy of the UCLA Medical Center, Los Angeles, CA.)
Abbreviations: GWX = guide wire exchange; C&S = culture and sensitivity; VAMP = venous arterial blood management protection.

of a unit-based standard for invasive vascular catheter management.

INTENSIVE CARE UNIT PSYCHOSIS

The psychologic complications of ICU care are perhaps the least understood and yet potentially the most devastating of all complications. *ICU psychosis* is the term traditionally used to describe the delirium that occurs between the third and seventh day in the ICU.[23] This delirium has been described as a fluctuating state of consciousness characterized by such features as fatigue, confusion, distraction, anxiety, and hallucinations. Some investigators have suggested that the development of ICU psychosis is related to three factors: the patient, the pharmacologic agents used, and the ICU environment. The fact that ICU psychosis typically resolves within 2 days after ICU discharge suggests that modification of the ICU environment and routines may significantly affect the patient's psychologic outcome.[23]

TABLE 192–6. Factors Contributing to Intensive Care Unit Psychosis and Preventive Interventions

Problem: Unfamiliar environment or personnel
Solution:
1. Orient patient and family to ICU as soon as possible after admission (preoperatively for elective surgery patients).
2. Use patient-family information booklets or videos as needed (e.g., American Association of Critical-Care Nurses booklet, *It's Critical That You Know**).
3. Minimize the number of personnel that come into contact with the patient.
4. Adopt models of care that maximize consistency of staff and promote continuity of care (e.g., primary nursing).

Problem: Lack of patient or family control over environment
Solution:
1. Provide patient and family with ongoing information regarding diagnosis, treatment plan, and prognosis. Use simple, straightforward communication style. Avoid medical jargon.
2. Allow patient and family decision making regarding care plan and daily activities (e.g., number and amount of visitors, bathing times, aggressiveness of care).

Problem: Isolation
Solution:
1. Institute unrestricted visiting practices: modify based on patient and family needs
2. Encourage family participation in routine activities (e.g., mouth care, foot massage).
3. Encourage family to bring in "comfort" items from home (e.g., pillow, drawings, photographs).
4. Ensure that patient has a means of communicating needs to staff (e.g., call bell, communication board).
5. If patient requires isolation precautions, provide patient and family with explanation as to need and purpose of such measures. Avoid unnecessary isolation procedures.

Problem: Noise
Solution:
1. Limit staff conversation at the bedside to patient and family discussions and necessary patient care discussion.
2. Adjust audible bedside alarms to appropriate level. Set alarm limits to reasonable levels.

Problem: Altered sleep patterns
Solution:
1. Cluster activities and interventions to allow for periods of uninterrupted sleep.
2. Obtain vital signs and perform interventions only as necessary.
3. Maximize the use of natural lighting. Dim lights at night.
4. Plan activities to allow sleep at night (e.g., wean during day if fatigue is an issue).
5. Administer sleep medications as needed.

*American Association of Critical-Care Nurses: It's Critical That You Know: A Resource for Families of Critically Ill Patients. Newport Beach, CA, American Association of Critical Care Nurses, 1987.

ICU = intensive care unit.

TABLE 192–7. Problems Encountered with Pain Management in Critically Ill Patients and Solutions

Problem: Inability to assess pain in noncommunicative patient
Solution:
1. Be alert to routine circumstances, procedures, and interventions that may cause pain (e.g., immobility, turning, weighing, blood drawing, suctioning).
2. Assess for signs and symptoms of acute pain (e.g., increased heart rate, blood pressure, and respiratory rate; cool clammy skin; crying, moaning, grimacing). Be aware that over time, adaptation occurs, and these signs may no longer be present.

Problem: Pain medication withheld because of concerns of hypotension and/or respiratory depression
Solution:
1. Be aware that severe pain may contribute to hypotension.
2. Monitor blood pressure frequently during narcotic administration (especially in patients with cardiac disease, hypovolemia, and pre-existing hypotension).
3. Slowly administer small, incremental dosages of narcotics intravenously.
4. Monitor respiratory rate frequently during narcotic administration. Use apnea monitors as needed.

Table 192–6 lists some of the common etiologies of ICU psychosis and suggests methods of preventing or minimizing this complication. In general, the patient and the family must be included in the patient's day-to-day care, and most importantly, they must be given clear, consistent information about the patient's progress and treatment plan. This communication often requires that the ICU staff repeat the same information (e.g., time and place when orienting the patient) several times a day or shift. Even more effort is required when patients are intubated and cannot communicate easily. In some instances, a pencil and paper are all that is needed for the patient to write down questions and concerns. In other instances, the patient may not be able to write, and more creative approaches for facilitating communication must be used, such as eye blinks or communication boards.

The patient should be given as much control as possible over his or her environment and schedule. All too frequently, the patient's schedule (e.g., preparing laboratory blood work, bathing, eating, weaning) is based on the convenience of the staff rather than on the needs of the patient.

Pain and discomfort are complications that may exacerbate ICU psychosis. Unfortunately, pain is frequently viewed as an inevitable consequence of being critically ill. A common sentiment expressed in critical care units is the notion that "a little pain is a small price to pay for wellness." Inadequately managed pain, however, not only contributes to delirium but also has a negative effect on the patient's physiologic state.

Effective management of pain in the critically ill patient presents challenges, but not insurmountable ones. Communication difficulties and unstable cardiopulmonary function are but two of the many obstacles that impede optimal pain management in the critically ill. Table 192–7 suggests strategies for providing appropriate pain management in the ICU. Patients who are unable to communicate their pain because of such factors as sedation, neurologic injury, or the use of a paralytic agent, are at a disadvantage in the ICU because they cannot express their complaints nor can they give feedback on the effectiveness of the pain medications they have been given. Research suggests that many patients with diagnoses not typically associated with pain (e.g., congestive heart failure, chronic obstructive pulmonary disease, cirrhosis) described having moderate-to-severe pain that was often inadequately treated.[24]

Although many tools for rating pain have been developed, they are typically too cumbersome to use or are not applicable to many ICU patients. Clinicians in the ICU must rely on indirect physiologic indices of pain, such as increased heart rate or blood pressure. Unfortunately, many other situations can lead to alterations in these variables besides pain, and they are valid indices only during the very acute period.

CONCLUSIONS

Preventing complications in the ICU requires the concerted efforts of a highly skilled, multidisciplinary group. Unit-based standards of care and a preventive approach are important for ensuring that early assessment and intervention are carried out for all patients. Ongoing evaluation of these standards, through quality-improvement monitoring, is necessary to ensure that the desired patient outcomes are achieved.

References

1. The International Task Force on Safety in the Intensive Care Unit: International standards for safety in the intensive care unit. Crit Care Med 1993; 21:453–456.
2. Task Force on Guidelines, Society of Critical Care Medicine: Guidelines for Standards of Care for Patients with Acute Respiratory Failure on Mechanical Ventilatory Support. Anaheim, CA, Society of Critical Care Medicine, 1990.
3. Bergstrom N, Demuth PJ, Braden BJ: A clinical trial of the Braden scale for predicting pressure sore risk. Nurs Clin North Am 1987; 22:417–428.
4. Pressure Ulcers in Adults: Prediction and Prevention. Clinical Practice Guideline No. 3. Rockville, MD, US Dept. of Health and Human Services: Agency for Health Care Policy and Research, 1992, publication No. 92-0047.
5. Gooch JL, Suchyta MR, Balbierz JM, et al: Prolonged paralysis after treatment with neuromuscular junction blocking agents. Crit Care Med 1991; 19:1125–1131.
6. Breslin E: Prevention and treatment of pulmonary complications in patients after surgery of the upper abdomen. Heart Lung 1981; 10:511–519.
7. Risser N: Preoperative and postoperative care to prevent pulmonary complication. Heart Lung 1980; 9:57–67.
8. Sutton P, Pavia D, Bateman J, et al: Chest physiotherapy: A review. Eur J Respir Dis 1982; 62:188–210.
8a. Bueno-Cavanillas A, Delgado-Rodriguez M, Lopez-Luque A, et al: Influence of nosocomical infection on mortality rate in an intensive care unit. Crit Care Med 1994; 22:55–60.
9. Du Moulin GC, Paterson DG, Hedley-Whyte J, et al: Aspiration of gastric bacteria in antacid-treated patients: A frequent cause of postoperative colonization of the airway. Lancet 1982; i:242–245.
10. Jimenez P, Torres A, Rodriguez-Roisin R, et al: Incidence and etiology of pneumonia acquired during mechanical ventilation. Crit Care Med 1989; 17:882–885.
11. Fiddian-Green RG, Baker S: Nosocomial pneumonia in the critically ill: Product of aspiration or translocation. Crit Care Med 1992; 19:763–769.
12. Choi SC, Nelson LD: Kinetic therapy in critically ill patients: Combined results based on meta-analysis. J Crit Care 1992; 7:57–62.
13. Gardner JS, Favero MS: CDC guidelines for the prevention and control of nosocomial infections. Guidelines for handwashing and hospital environmental control. Am J Infect Control 1986; 14:110–129.
14. Rodriguez-Roldan JM, Altuna-Cuesta A, Lopez A, et al: Prevention of nosocomial lung infection in ventilated patients: Use of an antimicrobial pharyngeal nonabsorbable paste. Crit Care Med 1990; 18:1239–1242.
15. Hartenauer U, Thulig B, Diemer W, et al: Effect of selective flora suppression on colonization, infection, and mortality in critically ill patients: 'A one year, prospective consecutive study. Crit Care Med 1991; 19:463–473.
15a. Hammond JM, Potgieter PD, Saunders GL: Selective decontamination of the digestive tract in multiple trauma patients—Is there a role? Results of a prospective, double-blind, randomized trial. Crit Care Med 1994; 22:33–39.
15b. Tetteroo GWM, Wagenvoort JHI, Mulder PGH, et al: Decreased mortality rate and length of hospital stay in surgical intensive care unit patients with successful selective decontamination of the gut. Crit Care Med 1994; 21:1692–1698.
16. Torres A, Serra-Batlles J, Ros E, et al: Pulmonary aspiration of gastric contents in patients receiving mechanical ventilation: The effect of body position. Am Coll Physicians 1992; 116:540–543.
17. Centers for Disease Control: Guidelines for Prevention of Intravascular Infections. Atlanta, GA, Centers for Disease Control, 1981.
18. Centers for Disease Control: Guidelines for Prevention of Catheter Associated Urinary Tract Infections. Atlanta, GA, Centers for Disease Control, 1981.
19. Garner J: CDC guidelines for the prevention and control of nosocomial infections. Guidelines for prevention of surgical wound infections. Am J Infect Control 1986; 14:71–80.
20. Maki DG, Wheeler SJ, Stolz SM, et al: Clinical Trial of a Novel Antiseptic-Coated Central Venous Catheter. Presented at Thirty-first Interscience Conference on Antimicrobial Agents and Chemotherapy. Chicago, October 1991.
21. Mermel LA, McCormick RD, Springman SR, et al: The pathogenesis and epidemiology of catheter related infection with pulmonary artery Swan-Ganz catheters: A prospective study utilizing molecular subtyping. Am J Med 1991; 91(Suppl 3B): 189–205.
22. Eyer S, Brummitt C, Crossly K, et al: Catheter related sepsis: Prospective, randomized study of three methods of long term catheter maintenance. Crit Care Med 1990; 18:10.
23. Ballard KS: Identification of environmental stressors for patients in a surgical intensive care unit. Issues Mental Health Nurs 1981; 3:89–108.
24. Desbiens NA, Wu AW, Bergner M, et al. and the SUPPORT Investigators: The six month pain experience of critically and seriously ill hospitalized adult patients. Clin Res 1992; 40:555A.
25. American Association of Critical Care Nurses: It's Critical That You Know: A Resource for Families of Critically Ill Patients. Newport Beach, CA, American Association of Critical Care Nurses, 1987.

CHAPTER 193

Stress Management of Staff, Family, and Patients

Sandra Lookinland, PhD, RN

Stressors inherent in an intensive care setting and the coping strategies used to deal with the distress have been extensively studied. The original work on this topic conducted in the 1970s focused on the environmental stressors encountered by intensive care unit (ICU) nurses that were shown to affect their physical and psychologic health and to be costly in terms of staff turnover.[1, 2] Later work questioned whether stress was totally context dependent or whether it was also possibly related to nurses' personal and social characteristics.

Research conducted in the late 1970s and 1980s centered around the needs of families of the critically ill. Molter's[3] initial descriptive study published in 1979 was replicated by Leske in 1986.[4] In a follow-up study, the psychometric properties of the Critical Care Family Needs Inventory were established.[5] As the use of ICUs increased over time, investigators began to study the stressors experienced and the coping strategies used by critically ill neonates, children, and adults.[6–8]

The body of literature addressing management of ICU stressors by patients, families, and staff continues to grow. The theoretic framework used and the implications of these findings for nursing practice are presented and areas for future research are identified in this chapter.

STRESS AND COPING FRAMEWORK

Stress

An individual experiences a person-environment transaction as stressful if the event is cognitively appraised as threatening to his or her well-being and as straining and surpassing coping resources.[9] Stressful events exist on a continuum ranging from major life events, such as a critical illness, to daily hassles. Daily hassles refer to ordinarily stressful person-environment transactions that occur in day-to-day living. Individuals perceive an event as stressful only if they determine it to have an impact on them. Therefore, one person's stressor may not affect another person who has the same person-environment transaction.

In initial assessment of the stressor, certain conditioning variables, including prior exposure to the stressor, self-esteem, nutritional status, and genetic predisposition, can affect the individual's cognitive appraisal of the event. If the conditioning variables are positive, they can serve as situational support. In addition, if prior effective coping behaviors are used and the threat of loss is not too overwhelming, the individual will handle the challenge adaptively. In summary, whether or not a single event becomes a stressor depends on the nature of the stressor itself (harm, threat, or challenge), on whether the event is perceived as stressful, and on the availability of situational supports and effective coping mechanisms.[10]

Coping

Coping strategies are thoughts and acts that the individual uses to handle the demands of stressful person-environment transactions; they are considered to be the mediator between the stressful event and its outcome. Two categories of coping strategies have been identified: problem focused and emotion focused. If the coping strategy chosen to handle the stressful situation is problem focused, the person will direct thoughts and actions toward altering the upsetting person-environment transaction. Emotion-focused coping strategies, however, are used to regulate the accompanying distressful emotions. If maladaptive coping methods are used, the outcomes can heighten the initial stressor. Most individuals tend to use both problem-focused and emotion-focused strategies during stressful life events.[11]

Problem-focused coping includes the confrontive (interpersonal) and cognitive (intrapersonal) forms. Emotion-focused strategies include distancing, escape-avoidance, self-control, positive appraisal, and acceptance of responsibility. When individuals seek social support (emotional, informational, or tangible aid from another person), they are using a combination of problem- and emotion-focused strategies.[12]

The types of strategies chosen depend on the person's primary and secondary appraisal of the event. Primary and secondary appraisals overlap somewhat because appraisal is ongoing and mediates the entire coping process. Reappraisal can occur as a result of a change in the primary appraisal or in the stressor itself. During primary appraisal, the personal significance of the event is determined (i.e., is the event harmful, beneficial, or relevant?). Later, during secondary appraisal, options or coping methods that might change the person-environment relationship are evaluated.[13]

An individual's choice during primary appraisal of coping options depends on the degree of threat to self-esteem. If individuals determine that their self-worth is at stake, they use confrontive coping, escape-avoidance, self-control, and acceptance of responsibility. In stressful encounters that are perceived to be highly changeable (secondary appraisal), people tend to choose more problem solving and positive reappraisal strategies and fewer escape-avoidance ones. People faced with physical health threats choose seeking social support as their primary coping behavior, followed in frequency by wishful thinking, avoidance, and self-blame.[14]

Developmental Perspective

Daily hassles encountered both at home and at work by young adults are strongly associated with negative health outcomes and subjective perceptions of well-being. In fact, daily hassles affect health outcomes more severely than do major life events in the young.[15]

Although young adults experience more major life events and daily hassles than do the aged, the hassles of the elderly are likelier to be centered around health and home maintenance issues. Young adults are likelier to appraise their health and family stressors as changeable than are the elderly. In a comparative study of young adults and retired elderly people, young adults were found to use more active, interpersonal, problem-focused forms of coping (confrontive coping, problem solving, and seeking of more social support) than were their elderly counterparts.[16] The retired group were likelier to use passive, intrapersonal, emotion-focused coping (distancing, acceptance of responsibility, and positive reappraisal). Only when dealing with health events were the elderly subjects more confrontive than the young adults. Older people are generally less likely to react with hostility or to rely on escapist fantasy when dealing with stress than are younger adults.

In contrast, other empirical studies have supported the contextual interpretation of age-related coping. The contextual interpretation suggests that differences in coping styles are a result of the changes people must cope with as they age rather than age itself.[17] Age is not the sole determinant of an individual's ability to cope or of his or her choice of coping style. Rather, it is more a function of the different types of stressors, such as events representing loss, that occur as one ages.

Although the elderly may experience fewer major life events than younger family members, the outside stressors they face are likelier to be related to loss. Daily hassles were found to occur less frequently in 65- to 75-year-old individuals than in other age groups, but they were more strongly related to distress than were major life events.[18] Even though daily hassles are thought to cause more stress in all age groups, the overall determinant of outcome is how the individual is able to cope with the distress. Ability to cope and psychologic well-being are strongly related.[19]

NEONATES

Many potential environmental, physiologic, and procedural neonatal stressors have been identified in the neonatal ICU. These factors include bright light, high levels of noise, and sensory deprivation.[6, 20, 21]

Some studies have focused on the stressors associated with treatment interventions. Routine nursing procedures, such as heel sticks and ventilator weaning, have been shown to cause physiologic stress in the neonate.[22] Neurobehavioral assessment performed at discharge can be accompanied by elevated cortisol levels and decreased growth hormone levels.[23, 24]

Stress-reducing techniques used by neonatal nurses in the ICU have been investigated. Intermittent, gentle tactile contact by the caregiver resulted in greater weight gains and activity levels, fewer ventilator days, fewer startle responses, and shorter hospitalizations.[25, 26] Non-nutritive sucking has been found to calm neonates during painful procedures, and the use of nonoscillating waterbeds decreases energy expenditure in preterm infants.[27, 28]

In a longitudinal study conducted 6 months after their children's discharge, mothers of critically ill infants were asked to recall the hospitalization. Mothers' remembrances were more painful if the infant was more severely ill, if the mother perceived problems dealing with neonatal ICU staff, and if mothers experienced less attachment with their infants.[29] In contrast, mothers who reported pleasant memories reported having found a purpose for the hospitalization and having felt more in control over the situation than those whose experiences were perceived as negative.

CHILDREN

A critically ill child perceives hospitalization as a stressful event, involving both physiologic and psychologic stressors.[30] An early study of physiologic stressors reported that steroid levels in children who were undergoing cardiotomy rose just before surgery and suture removal.[31] Behavioral indicators of psychologic stress in hospitalized children vary from appearing passive and withdrawn (showing fear, bewilderment) to kicking, screaming, and biting (showing anxiety, distress).[32]

In the preoperative period, both preschoolers and school-aged children tend to use orienting behavior as their main coping strategy.[33] During this period, the children seek information to accurately assess the situation.

Postoperatively, school-aged children use inactive behavior and attempts to control as means of coping. Children may withdraw both from parents and from nurses if the environment is perceived as stressful, or they may engage in overactive motor activity, such as throwing temper tantrums, resisting, and lashing out.[34] Children aged 7 to 14 years who were recovering from open-heart surgery expressed feelings about treatments and procedures, people, events, furnishings, and general impressions of the unit as a means of coping with hospitalization and surgery.[35] It is not known if children perceive these phenomena as threatening, however.

Nurses can support the coping mechanisms of critically ill children by using stress immunization and relaxation techniques.[36, 37] However, the most effective influence on the child's cognitive appraisal and on the child's ability to cope adaptively may be the presence of supportive parents.[7, 38] Absence of the nuclear family from the ICU has been shown to be detrimental to the child's adaptive coping.[39] Parents are able to provide emotional, tangible (physical care), and informational support.[40] Parents who ineffectively cope themselves, however, can offer little help to their child.[41]

NURSING CARE OF FAMILIES WITH CRITICALLY ILL INFANTS OR CHILDREN

Admission of an infant or a child into an ICU not only is a threat to the patient but also represents a crisis to the family unit as a whole. Some researchers have suggested that the nurse is caring for two entities during the hospitalization—the child and the parents.[42] The usual parental role as primary caregiver is usurped during the child's hospitalization, leading to high levels of anxiety.

Several authors have explicated strategies for caring for distressed parents of critically ill infants. Most suggest that nursing interventions be centered around supporting parents as they resolve three major issues—coping with loss, overcoming barriers to bonding, and obtaining adequate information about the infant's current and future needs.

During a child's critical illness, families must deal not only with the possibility of losing a loved one but also with such daily hassles as arranging child care for other children, obtaining transportation to the hospital, and dealing with financial concerns.[43] Parental stressors in the ICU have been identified as errors in communication, witnessed child care procedures, the child's appearance and reactions, contextual stimuli, absence of social support by friends, feelings of siblings, and role disruption.[44–48]

Parents have also identified loss of parenting role, uncertainty over outcome, and receipt of inconsistent information as stressors in a pediatric ICU.[49] If the critical illness occurred unexpectedly, parents experienced more stress and were less able to cope with the necessary therapeutic interventions.[46] Some researchers have found that parents who had knowledge of similar illness situations or had been exposed to ICUs in the past experienced less stress, whereas others reported that prior ICU experience did little to alleviate stress.[50, 51]

In a replication study of parental needs of critically ill children, Kirschbaum[52] found that parents reported needs for information and for assurance of good care similar to those reported by families of critically ill adults. In addition, parents' being recognized in their child's recovery and helping with the child's physical care were seen as very important.[52]

In a recent study, parents of critically ill children in the pediatric ICU again identified their strong need for informational support. Parents reported that the strongest need was for frequent, honest information about their child's condition. Expected outcomes must be explained in understandable terms. Anxieties were lessened if parents received comprehensive information, were with the sick child (unrestricted visiting hours), and were reassured that the child was receiving the highest level of care possible.[53]

In a study of critically ill neonates in Scotland, the perception of the role of grandparents by parents, nurses, and physicians was investigated. The presence of grandparents was hypothesized to lend social support and to buffer parental stress.[54] Both nurses and doctors believed that the grandparents' primary role was to provide emotional support and practical help for the parents. Parents agreed that grandparents were to provide social support but were to become active only at the parents' request. Only one third of the parent respondents felt that an appropriate grandparental role was to keep the home running smoothly, in contrast to the perceptions of most of the nurses and doctors. Parents disliked grandparents' attempts to advise or inform them. Overall role expectations were highest for the maternal grandmother.

Parents resent restricted visiting: they prefer having open visiting privileges and being allowed to be involved with care of their child (mutual participation model).[45, 55] Receiving accurate and truthful information was foremost with parents, as mentioned earlier, followed by being with the child, being given a place to rest near the pediatric ICU, being assured of appropriate interventions, and having active participation in the child's care.[56]

Coping strategies used by parents are independent of the category of the stressor. Individual family values, beliefs, expectations, and motivations all affect parents' appraisal of the threat and their choice of coping behaviors. Emotion-focused strategies tended to be used more often than did problem-focused strategies. The two most commonly identified means of coping were seeking social support and positively reappraising the event.[49] Another helpful coping strategy was being near the child as much as possible.[51] Parents who demonstrated cohesion and adaptability exhibited positive family chararacteristics and adjusted better to the child's intensive care hospitalization.[57]

A new philosophy of care, called *family-centered care,* has been proposed that combines humaneness with the high technology of pediatric and neonatal ICUs.[58] The role of the family is integrated into the health care needs of infants and children. To provide guidelines for the implementation of this philosophy, the Association for the Care of Children's Health has identified eight core elements[59]:

1. Recognition that the family is the constant in the child's life, whereas health care delivery personnel may vary.
2. Promotion of collaboration between parents and professionals.
3. Sharing of consistent information with parents on an ongoing basis and in a supportive manner.
4. Implementation of policies and programs that provide emotional and financial support for families.
5. Recognition of family strengths and respect for individual methods of coping.
6. Incorporation of developmental and emotional needs of the patient and family into the health care delivery system.
7. Encouragement of parent-to-parent support.
8. Provision of a health care delivery system that is flexible, accessible, and responsive to family needs.

The strategies proposed to attain each of these individual goals is beyond the scope of this review. The reader is referred to the article by Rushton[60] for a practice-oriented discussion of family-centered care in the intensive care unit.

CRITICALLY ILL ADULTS

Common indices of injury severity used as predictors of survival in trauma patients have not been useful for estimating long-term psychosocial adjustment and functional disability.[8] Rather, the patient's subjective appraisal of the injury was a better predictor of long-term outcome than were demographic variables or medical indices of injury severity. A significant amount of stress was found in the sample after the injury (mean = 15 months). Stress was related to the family environment and to the employment and financial consequences suffered as a result of the injury. Because of the nature of the research design used, causality could not be determined; that is, a supportive family environment might predict a more positive outcome, but a poorer outcome could conversely predict a disrupted family environment. Each event is likely to occur simultaneously when a family member experiences massive trauma. Of all demographic and socioeconomic variables evaluated, educational level was the only variable found to be positively related to better long-term functioning.

Patients recovering from coronary artery bypass grafting were found to use fewer coping strategies 6 weeks after the bypass than they were 1 week after the bypass.[61] The coping behaviors used most frequently included seeking social support, being problem focused, blaming self, and engaging in wishful thinking and avoidance.

Based on these findings, nurses can assist patients in dealing with their subjective interpretation of the traumatic event because modes of coping arise from the individual's cognitive appraisal of the stressor.[62] Different patients may view similar events quite differently, resulting in different consequences for long-term adjustment.[63] Early intervention should emphasize realistic perception of the event. This approach maximizes patients' ability to realistically evaluate their circumstances and to formulate realistic future expectations. Nurses can support adaptive problem-focused or emotion-focused coping strategies used by patients to handle the internal conflict caused by the traumatic event.

NURSING CARE OF FAMILIES OF CRITICALLY ILL ADULTS

Interest in the effect that critical illness has on the family began when it was realized that many family needs were not being met in critical care units. By necessity, nurses' energies were directed toward the patient, leaving little time to help families cope with the threatening event. Most families also expect nurses' attention to be focused on the needs of their loved one.[64] (At times, families are even seen to cause stress among nurses.[65]) If family stress is unrelieved, noncompliance with the treatment regimen can occur, causing a negative effect on recovery.[66]

Since Molter's seminal study[3] of family needs, interest in the area of family stressors and needs has been revived. Using a phenomenologic approach, Titler and colleagues[67] questioned the impact that ICU admission had on the family and the patient. Incongruencies were found between reports of the family and those of the patient and between the perceptions of the family and those of the nurses. The themes that emerged included (1) lack of communication, (2) protection of children from harmful information, (3) perceived overwhelming threat, (4) disruption of normalcy at home, (5) change in family relationships, and (6) role conflict and overload. Surprisingly, lack of communication had not been identified as a family need in previous studies.[4, 68]

Validating the psychometric properties of the Critical Care Family Needs Inventory, Leske[5] reported five dimensions of family needs: support, comfort, information, proximity, and assurance. To confirm and extend the results of previous studies using the Critical Care Family Needs Inventory, Price and coworkers[69] conducted a study in an inner city setting. This study was unique because of its large sample size and its use of ethnically diverse subjects. Their findings were consistent with previous investigations, with one exception. The urban poor did not rank "to feel there was hope" highly, which could possibly be attributed to the acuteness of their family member's illness.

Spouses of patients undergoing coronary artery bypass grafting reported that insensitivity and impersonalization by hospital staff, disrupted family life, lack of support within the family, and financial concerns contributed to stress.[70] Families identified nonsupportive behaviors by the nurse as being stressful. Successful nurses' interventions were found to be based on Lazarus' stress and coping theory and the identified needs of the patient's family.[71]

To determine whether nurses accurately perceive the needs of the family in the ICU, studies of nurses' perceptions were undertaken. O'Malley and associates[72] found that nurses believed that they had time to meet family needs, and that most nurses felt that family needs were important, but that cognitive needs superseded personal, physical, and psychologic needs.[72] Other studies reported that nurses do not accurately perceive the needs of the family. Family members also expressed discomfort in making their needs known to the caregiver. Incongruence existed between nurses' and families' perceptions, but most identified that family needs were met in the ICU.[73, 74]

CLINICAL IMPLICATIONS OF FAMILY STRESS

Based on interviews with nurses, investigators found that nurses understand little of the impact that critical illness has on family members.[75] Because of this lack of understanding, any intervention that might be undertaken would be misguided. Critical care nurses' responsibilities should include assessment of families' needs, identification of families at risk for ineffective coping, and identification of strategies to support the psychologic needs of the family.

The first step in family assessment is to determine past functioning of the family unit based on their interactions. According to family theory, a dysfunctional family system must be differentiated from temporarily ineffective coping in a functional family system. Kleeman[64] suggested areas to be assessed when determining functional status. These areas include levels of chronic anxiety within the family, how family members emotionally relate to one another, communication skills of family members, and multigenerational patterns. A dysfunctional family may demonstrate high levels of dependence, low levels of individual self-esteem, ineffective coping styles, and extremely rigid family relationships.[64]

The next step involves assessment of the family's perception of the threatening event and their emotional responses to the critical illness. Better patient outcomes occur in families with more cohesion and expressiveness and less conflict. Other family characteristics found to be helpful include independence, intellectual-cultural orientation, active-recreational orientation, and organization.[8] If nurses assume they understand how the family feels, interventions may fail. Patients in families that are judged to be functioning at a suboptimal level on several of the dimensions should be considered to be at risk for poor long-term recovery.

The final step is mobilization of past adaptive family coping mechanisms. Even well-functioning families may require help with the long-term adjustment to the stress caused by a severe injury. Early referral to counseling services may assist them in functioning more adaptively during the crisis and postcrisis periods.

Reasons for failure of nurses to meet family needs include lack of understanding of these needs, lack of knowledge concerning correct intervention, feelings of inadequacy concerning communication skills, and discomfort when faced with issues of bereavement and grief. In this era of consumer advocacy, the family must be included when a plan of care is instituted. Families have expressed a desire to be involved in the care of the patient, and, indeed, meeting this family need would actually save the nurse time.[73]

Possibly, many of the stressors ICU nurses encounter when dealing with patients and families could be reduced if their nursing care were grounded in a stress-and-coping paradigm. If theory-based care plans addressed family needs, nurses could choose appropriate interventions that were research based, would meet patient and family concerns, and at the same time would lessen environmental stressors for the nurse.

ICU NURSES' STRESSORS

Because of the visual and psychologic stressors facing nurses working in a burn unit, Tringali suggested that a psychiatric nurse be available to provide the necessary support.[76] In a small, exploratory pilot study, the highest stresses encountered by burn unit nurses had an emotional component[77] and included dealing with patients perceived as not being invested in their recovery and handling daily emotional issues related to pain, children, and death. In a study comparing burn and nonburn nurses, nonburn nurses were found to be more stressed and anxious, but both groups were equally satisfied with their jobs.[78] Psychosocial variables contributed more than 50% of the variance in job stress, whereas work setting (burn versus nonburn unit) contributed less than 6%. Work in a burn unit appears to contribute less to job stress than do such factors as nonwork stress and available emotional support.

In a German study, most ICU nurses handled work-setting stressors individually rather than as a group and used active, external actions as coping strategies.[79] Situations in which nurses coped actively were experienced as satisfactory. In patient scenarios that were perceived as personally stressful, nurses used passive coping strategies. Use of passive coping behaviors was related to nurse discontentment.

Physical environment, professional and interpersonal environment, and patient care stressors were evaluated in a multiunit study of general, neurologic, and cardiac ICU nurses.[80] Little variability was found between units. The most severe stressors reported by nurses, regardless of work area, were in patient care. Respondents reported the following stressors as most severe and occurring most frequently: too many interruptions, lack of respect or consideration from physicians, and need for rapid decision making with physicians not arriving soon enough in a crisis. No relationship was found between outside life stressors experienced by the nurses and the frequency or severity of work-setting stressors. These findings are consistent with those reported in community-based studies. Daily work hassles that occur most frequently (too many interruptions and slow laboratory results) contributed more to overall stress than did the more severe major work events (work overload and dealing with dying patients).

At work, an individual's perception of social support combined with coping ability can affect how stressful events are experienced. In 16 hospitals in the Netherlands, social support and coping were found to have a direct effect on the work situation and nurses' reactions to it. A main effect was seen with the coping measures of active problem solving and palliative behavior, whereas comforting cognitions were found to moderate or buffer nurses' reactions to the work situation. Nurses who used palliative behavior and comforting cognitions in times of stress reported more health complaints. On the other hand, those who received more social support in the work setting experienced higher job satisfaction and significance and reported fewer health complaints.[81]

Clinical Implications

Although much controversy exists in the literature over the factors responsible for burnout, agreement does exist that promoting autonomy and participation in decision making buffers work-related stress in the ICU. Innovative techniques to enhance recruitment and retention have focused on these buffers. Factors that have been shown to improve self-actualization include the institution of decentralized decision making, primary nursing, and clinical ladder advancement[82]; encouragement of collaborative practice by managers[83]; and provision of incentives for school attendance.[84]

NEEDS FOR FUTURE NURSING RESEARCH

Although needs of patients and families have been consistently identified in the literature, the suggestions derived from this research continue to be largely ignored in practice. Examples would be the family's desire for open visiting hours or for involvement in the patient's care. Open visiting hours are not in place universally, nor are families routinely asked to participate in their loved one's care. Studies that explore the reasons why these simple interventions are not widely used are needed.

Few studies have examined the stressors experienced and effective coping strategies used by ethnically diverse patients and their families. Only one study was found that included subjects other than white, middle-class individuals in the sample.[69] There remains a paucity of research on these individuals' needs, in spite of the growing ethnic diversity in the United States.

Studies have inferred that stressors and coping styles are gender neutral. Because most spousal studies have dealt with women, future studies must address the needs of male spouses as well. As the female population begins to grow older than at any time in history, ICU nurses will be faced with new challenges dealing with family members of the aged.[84a]

Little of the nursing literature addresses age-related changes associated with critical illness. Considering the changing age demographics predicted for the 21st century, the number of elderly patients cared for in the ICU will increase dramatically. The time has come to study more than the physiologic and psychologic responses of the elderly to chronic illnesses. Applied studies should be conducted using a total life-span approach.

Some of the lack of consistency in existing studies may be attributed to lack of refinement of underlying concepts. Interventional studies may have begun too early, and further qualitative studies are needed. Until the late 1980s, most study designs were quantitative. The recent qualitative studies have discovered new themes that might help account for some of the variance reported in previous studies. In this time of retrenchment and dwindling resources in health care, we must continue to provide quality patient care that is research based and is responsive to patient and family needs in a cost-effective manner.[85]

References

1. Hay D, Oken D: The psychological stresses of intensive care unit nursing. Psychosom Med 1972; 34:109.
2. Gentry W, Foster S, Froehling S: Psychologic response to situational stress in intensive and non-intensive nursing. Heart Lung 1972; 1:793.
3. Molter N: Needs of the relatives of critically ill patients: A descriptive study. Heart Lung 1979; 8:332.
4. Leske J: The needs of relatives of critically ill patients: A follow-up. Heart Lung 1986; 13:231.
5. Leske J: Internal psychometric properties of critical care family needs inventory. Heart Lung 1991; 20:236.
6. Glass P, Avery G, Subramanian K, et al: Effect of bright light in the hospital nursery on the incidence of retinopathy of prematurity. N Engl J Med 1985; 313:401.
7. Broome M: Working with the family of a critically ill child. Heart Lung 1985; 14:368.
8. Landsman I, Baum C, Arnkoff D: The psychosocial consequences of traumatic injury. J Behav Med 1990; 13:561.
9. Lazarus RS, Folkman S: Stress, Appraisal and Coping. 1st ed. New York, Springer, 1984, pp 55–81.
10. Lazarus RS: Cognitive and coping process in emotion. *In:* Stress and Coping: An Anthology. 1st ed. Monat A, Lazarus RS (Eds). New York, Columbia University Press, 1977, pp 144–158.
11. Folkman S, Lazarus RS: If it changes it must be process: Studies of emotions and coping during three stages of a college examination. J Pers Soc Psychol 1985; 50:571.
12. Stone AA, Neale JM: New measure of daily coping: Development and preliminary results. J Pers Soc Psychol 1984; 46:892.
13. Folkman S, Lazarus RS: An analysis of coping in a middle-aged community sample. J Health Soc Behav 1980; 21:219.
14. Folkman S, Lazarus RS, Dunkel-Schetter C, et al: Appraisal, coping, health status and psychological symptoms. The dynamics of a stressful encounter: Cognitive appraisal, coping and encounter outcomes. J Pers Soc Psychol 1986; 50:992.
15. DeLongis A, Coyne JC, Dakof G, et al: Relationship of daily hassles, uplifts and major life events to health status. Health Psychol 1982; 1:119.
16. Folkman S, Lazarus RS, Pimley S, et al: Age differences in stress and coping processes. Psychol Aging 1987; 2:171.
17. McCrae RR: Age differences in the use of coping mechanisms. J Gerontol 1982; 37:454.
18. Holahan CK, Holahan CJ, Belk S: Adjustment in aging: The roles of life stress, hassles and self-efficacy. Health Psychol 1984; 3:315.
19. Folkman S, Lazarus RS, Gruen R, et al: Appraisal, coping, health status, and psychological symptoms. J Pers Soc Psychol 1986; 50:571.
20. Gottfried A, Wallace-Lande P, Sherman-Brown S, et al: Physical and social environment of newborn infants in special care units. Science 1981; 214:673.
21. Rothchild B: Incubator isolation as a possible continuing factor to the high incidence of emotional disturbance among premature born persons. J Genet Psychol 1966; 110:287.
22. Long J, Alistair G, Phillip A, et al: Excessive handling as a cause of hypoxemia. Pediatrics 1980; 65:203.
23. Gunnar M, Isensee J, Fust S: Adrenocortical activity and the Brazelton Neonatal Assessment Scale: Moderating effects of the newborn's biobehavioral status. Child Dev 1987; 58:1448.
24. Schanberg S, Field T: Sensory deprivation stress and supplemental stimulation in the rat pup and the preterm human neonate. Child Dev 1987; 58:1431.
25. Field T, Schanberg S, Scafidi F, et al: Tactile/kinesthetic stimulation effects on preterm neonates. Pediatrics 1986; 77:654.
26. Jay S: The effects of gentle human touch on mechanically ventilated very short gestation infants. Matern Child Nurs J 1982; 11:199.
27. Field T, Goldson E: Pacifying effects of nonnutritive sucking on term and preterm neonates during heel sticks. Pediatrics 1984; 74:1012.
28. Deiriggi P: Effects of waterbed flotation on indicators of energy expenditure in preterm infants. Nurs Res 1990; 39:140.
29. Affleck G, Tennen H, Rowe J, et al: Mothers' remembrances of newborn intensive care: A predictive study. J Pediatr Psych 1990; 15:67.
30. Kidder C: Reestablishing health: Factors influencing the child's recovery in pediatric intensive care. J Pediatr Nurs 1989; 4:96.
31. Barnes M, Kenny R, Call T, et al: Measurement in management of anxiety in children for open heart surgery. Pediatrics 1972; 49:250.
32. Carty R: Observed behaviors of preschoolers in intensive care. Pediatr Nurs 1980; 6:21.
33. Savedra M, Tesler M: Coping strategies of hospitalized school-age children. West Nurs Res 1981; 3:371.
34. Carty R: Children's reaction to the ICU. *In:* The ICU Environment: Directions for Nursing. 1st ed. Noble M (Ed). Reston, VA, Reston Publishing, 1982, pp 99–125.
35. Barnes C: Levels of consciousness indicated by responses of children to phenomena in the intensive care unit. Matern Child Nurs J 1975; 4:215.
36. LaMontagne L, Pawlak R: Stress and coping of parents of children in a pediatric intensive care unit. Heart Lung 1990; 19:416.
37. Poster E: Stress immunization: Technique to help children cope with hospitalization. Matern Child Nurs J 1983; 12:119.
38. Rennick J: Reestablishing the parental role in a pediatric intensive care unit. J Pediatr Nurs 1986; 1:40.
39. May J: A psychiatric study of a pediatric intensive therapy unit. Clin Pediatr (Phila) 1972; 11:76.

40. Schaefer C, Coyne JC, Lazarus RS: The health-related functions of social support. J Behav Med 1982; 4:381.
41. Etzler C: Parent's reactions to pediatric critical care settings: A review of the literature. Issues Compr Pediatr Nurs 1984; 7:319.
42. Oehler J, Davidson M: Job stress and burnout in acute and nonacute pediatric nurses. Am J Crit Care 1992; 1:81.
43. Hodovanic B, Reardon D, Reese W, et al: Family crisis intervention program in the medical intensive care unit. Heart Lung 1984; 13:243.
44. Carter M, Miles M, Buford T, et al: Parental environmental stress in pediatric intensive care units. Dimens Crit Care Nurs 1985; 4:180.
45. Johnson P, Nelson G, Brunnquell D: Parent and nurse perceptions of parent stressors in the pediatric intensive care unit. Child Health Care 1988; 17:98.
46. Curley M: Effects of nursing mutual participation model of care on parental stress in the pediatric intensive care unit. Heart Lung 1988; 17:682.
47. Miles M, Carter M: Assessing parental stress in intensive care units. MCN Am J Matern Child Nurs 1983; 8:354.
48. Carnevale F: A description of stressors and coping strategies among parents of critically ill children—A preliminary study. Intensive Care Nurs 1990; 6:4.
49. Miles M, Carter M, Spicher C, et al: Maternal and paternal stress reactions when a child is hospitalized in a pediatric intensive care unit. Iss Compr Pediatr Nurs 1984; 7:333.
50. Tse A, Perez-Woods R, Opie N: Children's admissions to the intensive care unit: Parents' attitudes and expectations of outcome. Child Health Care 1987; 16:68.
51. Miles M, Carter M: Coping strategies used by parents during their child's hospitalization in an intensive care unit. Child Health Care 1985; 14:14.
52. Kirschbaum M: Needs of parents of critically ill children. Dimens Crit Care Nurs 1990; 9:344.
53. Farrell MF, Frost C: The most important needs of parents of critically ill children: Parent's perception. Intensive Crit Care Nurs 1992; 8:130.
54. McHaffie HE: Social support in the neonatal intensive care unit. J Adv Nurs 1992; 17:179.
55. Proctor D: Relationship between visiting policy in a pediatric intensive care unit and parental anxiety. Child Health Care 1987; 16:13.
56. Kasper J, Nyamathi A: Parents of children in the pediatric intensive care unit: What are their needs? Heart Lung 1988; 17:574.
57. Pilichi L: Family adaptation during a pediatric intensive care hospitalization. J Pediatr Nurs 1989; 4:268.
58. Koop C: Children with Special Health Care Needs—Campaign 87. Washington, DC, U.S. Dept. of Health and Human Services, 1987, pp 8–10.
59. Shelton T, Jeppson E, Johnson B: Family-Centered Care for Children with Special Health Care Needs. Washington, DC, Association for Care of Children's Health, 1987, pp 34–49.
60. Rushton C: Strategies for family-centered care in the critical care setting. Pediatr Nurs 1990; 16:195.
61. Redeker NS: A description of the nature and dynamics of coping following coronary artery bypass surgery. Scholar Inquiry Nurs Pract 1992; 6:63.
62. Lazarus RS, Folkman S: Coping and adaptation. *In:* The Handbook of Behavioral Medicine. 1st ed. Gentry WD (Ed). New York, Guilford, 1984, pp 282–325.
63. Bulman R, Wortman C: Attributions of blame and coping in the "real world": Severe accident victims react to their lot. J Pers Soc Psychol 1977; 35:351.
64. Kleeman K: Families in crisis due to multiple trauma. Crit Care Nurs Clin North Am 1989; 1:23.
65. Garner D, Stewart N: Staff involvement with families of patients in critical-care units. Heart Lung 1978; 7:105.
66. McIvor D, Thompson F: Self-perceived needs of family members with a relative in the ICU. Intensive Care Nurse 1988; 4:139.
67. Titler M, Cohen M, Craft M: Impact of adult critical care hospitalizations: Perceptions of patients, spouses, children and nurses. Heart Lung 1991; 20:174.
68. Norris L, Grove S: Investigation of selected psychosocial needs of family members of critically ill adult patients. Heart Lung 1986; 15:194.
69. Price D, Forrester A, Murphy P, et al: Critical care family needs in an urban teaching medical center. Heart Lung 1991; 20:183.
70. Artinian N: Stress experience of spouses of patients having coronary artery bypass during hospitalization and 6 weeks after discharge. Heart Lung 1991; 20:52.
71. O'Keefe B, Gilliss C: Family care in the coronary care unit: An analysis of clinical nurse specialist intervention. Heart Lung 1988; 17:191.
72. O'Malley P, Favaloro R, Anderson B, et al: Critical care nurse perceptions of family needs. Heart Lung 1991; 20:189.
73. Dockter B, Black D, Hovell M: Families and intensive care nurses comparison of perceptions. Patient Educ Counsel 1988; 12:29.
74. Lynn-McHale D, Bellinger A: Need satisfaction levels of family members of critical care patients and accuracy of nurse's perceptions. Heart Lung 1988; 17:447.
75. Caine R: Families in crisis: Making the critical difference. Focus Crit Care 1989; 16:184.
76. Tringali R: The role of the psychiatric nurse consultant on a burn unit. Issues Ment Health Nurs 1982; 4:17.
77. Lewis KF, Poppe S, Twomey J, et al: Survey of perceived stressors and coping strategies among burn unit nurses. Burns 1990; 16:109.
78. Rikli PA: Psychosocial determinants of chronic stress in nursing. Ann Arbor, 1987, Dissertation.
79. Becker-Carus C, Gunthner G: Stress and situation specific coping behavior in intensive care unit nursing staff. Work Stress 1989; 3:353.
80. Spoth R, Konewko P: Intensive care staff stressors and life event changes across multiple setting and work units. Heart Lung 1987; 16:278.
81. Boumans NPG, Landeweerd JA: The role of social support and coping behavior in nursing work: Main or buffering effect. Work Stress 1992; 6:191.
82. Doering L: Recruitment and retention: Successful strategies in critical care. Heart Lung 1990; 19:220.
83. Baggs J, Ryan S: ICU nurse-physician collaboration and nursing satisfaction. Nurs Econ 1990; 8:386.
84. Blix A, Lookinland S: Fit between motivational style and job demands as a correlate in the development of burnout in registered nurses. Unpublished manuscript.
84a. Lookinland S, Anson K: Perpetuation of ages and attitudes in current and future health care personnel: Implications for elder care. J Adv Nurs 1994 (in press).
85. Gipe BT: Clinical cost awareness: Unshrouding the mystery of healthcare expenses. Cost & Quality 1994; 1:4.

CHAPTER 194

Families in Critical Care: Environment, Needs, and Barriers to Care*

Claudia Bartz, PhD, RN

While the efforts of critical care providers focus on the patient, the family struggles to cope with the experience of having a loved one be seriously ill. Whether the patient is an emergent or nonemergent admission, the family needs information and support as well as help with making decisions related to the critical care experience. The purposes of this chapter are to (1) provide guidance for critical care providers to work with families in helpful and positive

*The opinions or assertions in this chapter are the private views of the author and are not to be construed as official or as reflecting the views of the Department of the Army or the Department of Defense.

ways and (2) challenge critical care providers to overcome the barriers to integrating the family into the patient's critical care experience. *Family* is defined as the social unit closely connected to the patient through love, or legal ties, or both.

CRITICAL CARE PROVIDERS

Physicians and nurses are essential to families, who feel vulnerable as they encounter critical care. Families need the timely and honest information that physicians and nurses can provide. Constant sensitivity to families, who face overwhelming physical patient care requirements, can help to sustain the humanistic and compassionate side of critical care providers' work. Physicians address the technology of critical care, identifying and treating medical problems from cellular to systemic levels. Physicians can explain to families the medical plan of care, the patient's response to that plan, and the risks and benefits of treatment modalities for continued care. Nurses orchestrate the timing of critical care, nurturing patients and assisting them in mobilizing their own strengths toward recovery. Nurses can aid families by explaining the hospital's layout and the unit's appearance, and by providing information, comfort, and support throughout the patient's critical care experience.

Other health care professionals, including social workers, psychiatrists, and psychologists, can make important contributions to the care of families. Social workers can guide the family through the maze of clinical and administrative rules and policies. If the family has a religious affiliation, a chaplain or lay worker from that denomination may be a valuable source of support and may also be a safe conduit between the family and the physicians and nurses. Hospital administrative staff can support the family members directly, as they face the financial implications of critical care, and indirectly, through the provision of adequate gathering areas near the critical care units.

Comfort with death should be explored with the family before the event, if possible. A recent survey[1] found that 95% of survey respondents (n=600) stated that "do not resuscitate" orders were discussed with the patient or family. In addition to making the family aware of the imminence of death, care providers need to ascertain how the family is coping with this supreme stressor. When death occurs in critical care, the family needs support both from their own social support network and from the direct care providers and psychologic-social-spiritual team of providers interacting with the family. Care providers' knowledge of how to access the family's social support network can also be helpful as the patient's condition deteriorates.

FAMILY CONTACT WITH CRITICAL CARE

The family's level of knowledge and comfort when faced with critical care is based on their prior experience, on media exposure, and on their normal coping mechanisms. Care providers should try to sustain hope and hope-inspiring strategies, such as spiritual beliefs and practices, among families. The family usually want to be near the patient, a need that creates tension between family and care providers throughout the critical care experience. The family wonders whether or not they will return to normal and even what is normal anymore.

As far as families are concerned, critical care admissions can be divided into emergent and nonemergent admissions. Emergent admissions can result from trauma, overdose or self-inflicted injury, or unpredicted complications of medical therapy. In any case, the family experiences crisis resulting from the fast-paced events that led to the critical care admission, and they may demonstrate such responses as denial, rationalization, guilt, anger, helplessness, or physical illness. Nonemergent admissions can result from pathophysiology related to chronic disease or to the requirement for preoperative and postoperative care. In these cases, the family may experience conflicting emotions regarding continued support of the patient and the financial and social drain on themselves.

Care providers support families by recognizing the tremendous changes the family is experiencing relative to themselves as well as to the patient. Parents of neonates in the neonatal intensive care unit said the most stressful aspect of that environment was the alteration in their parental role.[2] Families experience disrupted role relationships during critical illness.[3]

The family unit may already be strained before its contact with critical care. Financial strains may be magnified because of the cost of hospitalization and also because of lost income and extra living expenses, such as lodging requirements, during the family member's illness. Work responsibilities continue for family members who are employed, decreasing the time available for coping with the stress of critical illness or injury. If the patient was the main financial support, the family may be twice devastated: once from the critical illness or injury and once from the concern for meeting the regular and added financial commitments.

Social strains may increase when the family wonders whether the patient shouldn't have avoided the accident or have done more to prevent the crisis, for example, by changing cardiac risk behaviors. Families with conflicted role relationships before the critical illness event may have worsening interactions as they struggle with decisions and feelings of anger and powerlessness. Critical care providers may find themselves in the middle of these conflicted role relationships. Power plays and battles over control diminish a family's ability to communicate effectively with care providers about the patient's or the family's needs.

The lack of control and information, and the need to wait (for care, for decisions, for interventions), generate myriad emotions. Families may be frightened, hostile, confused, depressed, or apathetic. The family may minimize the seriousness of the event, avoiding important issues or becoming over-involved with other things. Their internal relationships may change, both between adults and between adults and children, as the critical illness goes on.

FAMILY NEEDS

Seminal work on critical care family needs was begun by Molter[4] and continues today. The internal psychometric properties of Molter's Critical Care Family Needs Inventory include Cronbach's alpha of 0.92.[5] Factor analysis has validated five categories in the Critical Care Family Needs Inventory labeled support, comfort, information, proximity, and assurance.[5] Hickey[6] reviewed the research literature on family needs, comparing rank-ordered needs across the eight primary studies that were replicable. Hickey found that the most important thing that critical care families can be given is information, and the most important emotion that can be instilled in families is hope.

Information About Environment

Families need information about the hospital and critical care environments. Critical care providers should periodically take the time to recall their first exposure to the critical care unit and to the family waiting area. A crucial question at the start, for example, may be how to get from the parking lot to the unit waiting area. Families may experience fear, surprise, or revulsion at the sights, sounds, and smells surrounding the patient. Questions abound. Where should I stand or sit? What are the machines and lights? What is all the noise, and which sounds are important? Why does the patient look like that? Who should I talk with?

Care providers and administrators should critically assess the family waiting area for adequacy of size, comfort, food availability, privacy availability, and toileting facilities. Are telephones readily available? Is there an area in addition to the main waiting room where families can be given bad news in private or be left to grieve in private? The stress of visiting the patient in a strange and sometimes chaotic area is amplified when families have to wait in uncomfortable surroundings.

Information About Visiting

Families need proximity to the patient.[5, 7] A recent study[8] found that open visiting hours significantly improved family satisfaction and that the addition of a preprinted information booklet enhanced these families' knowledge about the critical care event. Every critical care unit has a visiting policy for frequency and numbers of people allowed per visit. Even when clearly communicated at the onset of the critical care admission, the visiting policy often becomes unclear and frustrating. Staff interpret the policy in different ways, causing uncertainty and perhaps anger among the family. Families may start to struggle over who should visit.

Care providers should look at their reactions to visiting family members. Some providers may find it easier to keep the family at a distance, even though the family's need for information and comfort is often best met by having the family at the patient's bedside. Longer, more frequent visiting times should increase, rather than threaten, care providers' competence through increased motivation to be knowledgeable enough to answer tough questions about the medical and nursing care regimens. Because of their constant presence, nurses especially can be seen as caretakers and teachers rather than as technicians in the critical care environment.

Information for Making Decisions

Families need information to help them make decisions regarding the patient and themselves. The family is expected to make decisions constantly during the family member's critical illness. The family's ability to make decisions depends on how they normally approach decisions and on how well they are coping with the family member's critical illness or injury. Coping can be problem focused (including confrontation, problem solving, and social support) or emotion focused (including reappraisal, self-control, escape-avoidance, responsibility, and distancing).[9] Care providers must be attuned to families' responses to stress and must identify those families at risk for ineffective coping.[10]

All care providers, including administrators and chaplains, need to listen and respond to families' feelings and emotions supportively and nondefensively. The physician-nurse team is generally responsible for coordinating the participation of other direct and indirect care providers. Families' expressions of hope indicate increasing mastery over feelings of vulnerability or uncertainty regarding the family member's critical care.

Families are expected to make personal, financial, medical, ethical, and legal decisions when a family member is critically ill or injured.[11] Personal decisions include issues related to working and activities of daily living (transportation, lodging, and meals). To further complicate coping strategies, family plans change. The question of what to tell the children may cause intense anxiety among families. Financial decisions include those directly related to the cost of the family member's care and those arising from the necessities of living—employment, loans, mortgages, car payments, taxes, bank and investment accounts. The spouse who made all the decisions may now be noncontributory, requiring the previously passive spouse to learn to manage the family's finances.

The consent needed for medical treatment decisions requires a balance of technologic capability with quality of life as well as a consideration of what the patient would want. The family's informed consent for procedures, consultations, treatment trials, transportation, or discharge may be constrained by physical, cognitive, psychologic, or social factors. For example, the family may have strong views against continuing procedures that do not seem to help the patient, while the direct care providers continue to intervene, hoping for success and improvement in the patient's condition.

Basic American values, such as personal dignity, modesty, and comfort are often at odds with available technology, leaving the family to decide what would be best for the patient. The family is asked to make the difficult judgment of what quality of life would be satisfactory to the patient. The patient's present and future quality of life should be a fundamental element in discussions that require treatment decisions from family members and care providers. Sixty-seven per cent of respondents to a Society of Critical Care Medicine survey[1] stated that quality of life as viewed by the patient was the most important factor in making decisions to withhold or withdraw therapy.

Families say repeatedly that they want frequent and detailed communication from the physician. They want to know the patient's condition, plan of care, diagnostic and treatment options, and evidence of improvement or deterioration. They are more comfortable and less worried if they know that the patient is receiving the best possible care. They want to be called at home, at any time of the day or night, whenever anything about the patient changes.

Ethical and legal decisions made during the stress of a family member's critical care are the most difficult ones for the family. The care provider–family interaction during these times should be one of exquisite communication, understanding, and support. However, ethical issues, such as discontinuation of life support systems and readiness for organ or tissue donation, are often mired in families' ineffective coping patterns and are clouded by care providers' beliefs, values, and prior experiences with these issues. Parental nonconcurrence with the care providers' views about the most appropriate care for a child, for example, demonstrates the extreme difficulty of resolving some ethical issues.[12]

The recent attention to advance directives,[13] or living wills and durable powers of attorney, may alleviate some of the ethical decision making expected of families of critically ill patients. A values history[14] has been proposed as a tool physicians can use to elicit an explicit identification of values and an articulation of advance directives based on the patient's values. Decisions regarding treatment are to be based on the patient's right to act based on his or her own values. For a noncompetent patient, autonomy is preserved if the surrogate acts on the basis of known beliefs and values of the patient.

Living wills, which by 1991 were authorized for use by

statutes in 41 states and the District of Columbia, go into effect when the patient has no reasonable hope of recovery and is unable to participate in decisions for care. The language of living wills is generally vague, however, and provides guidance rather than a checklist of what or what not to do should the holder of the living will require critical care.

The durable power of attorney, based on statutes in all states and the District of Columbia, provides for a surrogate decision maker in the event of the holder's requiring critical care. The surrogate has as much guidance as the person (patient) has decided on before the critical illness or injury, ranging from broad to specific directions, perhaps even including chance remarks made by the person prior to becoming a patient.

A theory of medical ethics that emphasizes autonomy[15, 16] can help critical care providers to work through "do not resuscitate" decisions with families. Veatch[15] describes three contracts that frame ethical issues. The first contract stipulates general principles for human interaction between individuals in a society, exemplified by open, honest, and supportive communication among family members. The second contract is between the society's professionals and the society's members and has implied equality and mutuality based on designated roles. Care providers and families would be expected to have productive interactions that are focused on helping the patient and the family during the patient's critical care. The third contract is between health professionals and patients. Critically ill or injured patients have a right to the most complete information that they can comprehend during each phase of their care.

BARRIERS TO FAMILY CARE

In spite of the extensive research on family needs, barriers to family care remain. Three barriers addressed here are the mystique of technology, the challenge of communication, and competing beliefs and values.

As the identification and resolution of ethical issues becomes a more integral part of the plan of care, providers are recognizing that families are often the patient's only voice when hard questions concerning, for example, allocation of resources or quality of life, arise. As more patients are moved out of intensive care units and discharged from hospitals with substantial care needs remaining, families again are essential to sustaining and continuing the patients' progress toward recovery.

Yet, families are frustrated.[17] Families are kept out of units (e.g., "the patient had a restless night; the family hung around the door of the unit all night"), are kept uninformed (e.g., "the doctor will have to tell you," "the specialist will have to tell you," "more tests will need to be performed before we know for sure"), and are generally condescended to (e.g., "this is very complicated, we don't want you to worry"). Family needs have been sufficiently identified through research; now, the needs lists should be used to study critical care practice and to change it as indicated.[18] Craft and Willadsen[19] have begun such work by assessing the content validity of interventions used by nurses in their work with families.

Mystique of Technology

Family involvement in the care of the ill or injured has decreased as technologic diagnosis and treatment capability has increased. Reasons given for excluding families from critical care units might include such items as: (1) "we are too busy to worry about the family," (2) "they wouldn't understand what we were doing," (3) "they would think we were mean and uncaring and were inflicting unnecessary pain," (4) "they expect television-style critical care with its control, perfection, and happy outcomes," and (5) "they would be in the way, an interference with our routines." Some care providers have come to believe that the family's presence at the patient's bedside connotes scrutiny and evaluation of the care providers' technical capabilities. Care providers must not forget that the patient, and not spectacular technology, is the family's primary focus.

In a multidisciplinary effort, care providers need to evaluate whether they are using technology as a barrier to family visiting and family care. What rules for visiting are influenced by real technologic concerns? The evaluation might include determining how often reasons such as the five listed earlier are used in the unit. What explanations to families are inadequate because they are based on the assumption that families cannot comprehend sophisticated diagnostic and treatment technology?

Care providers can further assess whether and how patients are treated differently in the family's presence. Are procedures explained to the patient only when the family is present? If differences are found, for example, in the use of touch and in the consideration of the patient's modesty throughout technologic interventions, the assessment should explore why differences occur and whether these differences are appropriate. Another area to explore for differences would be whether and why the tone and content of staff interactions changes when the family is present.

Challenge of Communication

Research on family needs indicates that the need for information may be the most important need identified. Communication between sender and receiver is an immensely complex phenomenon in normal circumstances (e.g., two friends talking) and becomes even more complex in situations involving critical illness or injury. The care provider's communications integrate feelings (I am in charge, I am in control), rules (never get involved, never show emotions), and emotions (another patient dying on my watch). When the family member responds, the care provider filters and interprets the responses, places them on a positive/acceptable to negative/unacceptable continuum, and responds therapeutically or nontherapeutically, depending on his or her capability. Therapeutic responses could include the identification of feelings; restatement; clarification; and expressing of concern, support, and empathy.[20] Nontherapeutic responses could include arguing, defensiveness, and brusque reality orientation.[20]

When family members' communications are interpreted to suit the care provider's perception of the situation, barriers to meeting family needs may be magnified. For example, when a care provider has a communication barrier with the family, the family's questions may be interpreted as interference or criticism of the course of events and the plan for care. Families' uncooperativeness or nonadherence may be interpreted as sabotage of the care provider's efforts. In addition, families' confusion or lack of understanding may be attributed to an intellectual deficit. When the care provider is comfortable enough to receive families' communications and reflect perceptions back to the family to check accuracy when necessary, these situations may need to be considered in a more positive, productive light. For example, questions may demonstrate intense interest, nonadherence may demonstrate social or financial inability, and confusion may demonstrate that the care provider's verbal and nonverbal communications are not clear and consistent.

Critical care allows sub-barriers to be thrown up by care providers who have not developed their communication and interpersonal skills to the point that they are comfortable talking with families. These sub-barriers could include the use of acronyms or technical terms so that, predictably, "the family never understands me." Gaming is another sub-barrier, in which the provider says "it's not my patient," or "haven't we talked about that already," or "where was the family when I wanted to talk with them?" Time control is another effective sub-barrier. The care provider has commitments so pressing that the family never knows when they may be talked with at all, much less when they will receive consistent and timely information.

As with the barrier of technology, the barrier of communication can be lessened if care providers look at and listen to their patterns of interaction. Schedules or other patient care requirements should be assessed to determine whether they legitimately excuse the care provider from talking with families. Care providers can audiotape their interactions with families and can evaluate whether what they said and how they said it are congruent with their recollections of the interaction.

Competing Beliefs and Values

Critical care providers bring their beliefs and values into a unit or unit complex, where a set of values evolves as staff have varying degrees of impact due to positional power, personal power, and the credibility of longevity. Every critical care provider has experienced situations that involve questions about resource allocation, treatment failure, quality of life, and organ donation. The family, on the other hand, has little if any experience with these kinds of questions. Because the care providers have thought about and have weighed their opinions on these topics, they may assume (especially if time is short) that they know what is best for the patient and, by extension, the family. Providers judge each patient's needs and chances in the context of all the previous similar patients they have treated. Families usually want what is best for their loved one, but they do not have the benefit of an experiential context within which to frame the decision.

The increased emphasis on patient autonomy (e.g., the 1991 Patient Self-Determination Act[13]) comes in the midst of this clash between experienced, opinionated care providers and inexperienced but intimately concerned families. Now patients may want freedom from suffering, comfort, and palliation. Families, on the other hand, may want the patient's survival and continued life support. Care providers want to prevent failure at all costs while espousing commitment to the patient's quality of life and sensible use of available resources.

Organ donation is one example of a situation in which competing beliefs and values pose a barrier to the meeting of families' needs for information and support. Individual care providers have their own views on organ donation. Physicians and nurses may influence their peers for or against organ donations so that the philosophy of a unit evolves toward a predictable degree of support for donation. An institution committed to supporting transplantation programs will likely exert a strong pro-donor influence. When a critically ill or injured person meets the criteria for death, family members will be subject to queries about organ donation. When unit staff are confident of their position, open and honest discussion can occur with the family. The family can then be allowed to respond as they feel with no fear of reprisal.

If the family suggests or insists on organ donation, they risk meeting responses ranging from provider disinterest to provider zealotry. If congruency occurs and the family is totally supported in the decision to approve donation, the family can have some control over their relative's critical care. If the family makes the offer to a unit staff member who is not interested in organ donation, the family's hope that something good can come from the awfulness of critical illness or injury is lost. Regardless of the family's decision, they risk encountering a barrier (conflict with that unit's view) that care providers may use to excuse their inadequate attentions to the family until the critical illness is ended.

SUMMARY

Families need information and support from all care providers and administrators involved with critical care. The intimidating environment and the overwhelming requirements for decision making are a challenge to even the strongest families when faced with a family member's critical care. Care providers need to assess themselves and their practice for the presence of barriers to providing considerate and helpful care to their patients' families.

References

1. Sprung CL, Armstrong C, Bailey MA, et al: Attitudes of critical care medicine professionals concerning forgoing life-sustaining treatments. Crit Care Med 1992; 20:320.
2. Miles MS, Funk SG, Kasper MA: The stress response of mothers and fathers of preterm infants. Res Nurs Health 1992; 15:261.
3. Titler MG, Cohen MZ, Craft MJ: Impact of adult critical care hospitalization: Perceptions of patients, spouses, children and nurses. Heart Lung 1991; 20:174.
4. Molter NC: Needs of relatives of critically ill patients: A descriptive study. Heart Lung 1979; 8:332.
5. Leske JS: Internal psychometric properties of the Critical Care Family Needs Inventory. Heart Lung 1991; 20:236.
6. Hickey M: What are the needs of families of critically ill patients? A review of the literature since 1976. Heart Lung 1990; 19:401.
7. Marsden C: Family-centered critical care: An option or obligation? Am J Crit Care 1992; 1:115.
8. Henneman EA, McKenzie JB, Dewa CS: An evaluation of interventions for meeting the information needs of families of critically ill patients. Am J Crit Care 1992; 1:85.
9. LaMontagne LL, Pawlak R: Stress and coping of parents of children in a pediatric unit. Heart Lung 1990; 19:416.
10. Schlump-Urquhart SR: Families experiencing a traumatic accident: Implications and nursing management. Clin Issues Crit Care Nurs 1990; 1:522.
11. Mirr MP: Factors affecting decisions made by family members of patients with severe head injury. Heart Lung 1991; 20:228.
12. Nelson LJ, Nelson RM: Ethics and the provision of futile, harmful, or burdensome treatment to children. Crit Care Med 1992; 20:427.
13. Marsden C: Making patient self determination a reality in critical care. Am J Crit Care 1992; 1:122.
14. Doukas DJ, McCullough LB: The values history—The evaluation of the patient's values and advance directives. J Fam Pract 1991; 32:145.
15. Veatch RM: A Theory of Medical Ethics. New York, Basic Books, 1983.
16. Ott BB, Nieswiadomy RM: Support of patient autonomy in the do not resuscitate decision. Heart Lung 1991; 20:66.
17. Alspach G: Visions of healthcare: A view from the other side. Crit Care Nurs 1992; 12:13.
18. Dracup K, Bryan-Brown CW: An open door policy in ICU. Am J Crit Care 1992; 1:16.
19. Craft MJ, Willadsen JA: Interventions related to family. Nurs Clin North Am 1992; 27:517.
20. Johnson L: Communication: The key to crisis prevention in pediatric death. Crit Care Nurs 1992; 12:23.

SECTION XVI
ORGANIZATION AND MANAGEMENT OF CRITICAL CARE

Joann I. Lamb • Stephen M. Ayres

CHAPTER 195
The Utilization and Allocation of Critical Care Resources

I. Alan Fein, MD • Sandra L. Fein, MA, RN

The specialty of critical care medicine is coming of age in a time when all healthcare in the United States is undergoing dramatic change. The confluence of multiple forces, including an aging population, a battered economy, technologic advances, and a general awareness that the per capita cost of healthcare in America far exceeds that of other nations, has acutely forced a reassessment of healthcare delivery. Indeed, the military-industrial complex of the 1950s and 1960s has now been replaced by the medical-industrial complex as arguably the single predominant industry in this country. Whereas the restructuring of this industry has been ongoing for some years now, resulting in a free-market melange of private practice, health maintenance organizations (HMOs), preferred provider organizations (PPOs), independent practice associations (IPAs), and managed care associations, the demand for change will only accelerate in the immediate future. By its very nature an expensive, technology-driven specialty, critical care will be at the center of the vortex of evolution.

The demand for reform of healthcare is driven by two powerful forces: the first, and perhaps most potent, is the rapidly escalating cost of healthcare delivery, clashing with an economy in flux; the second is an aging yet educated population whose expectations of the miracles of modern science border on the unrealistic. Healthcare costs in the United States approached one trillion dollars in 1993, more than 14% of the gross domestic product, and they are increasing at a rate several times that of inflation. This has caused the public and legislators to take serious notice, and many echo the sentiments of a former Governor of Colorado Richard Lamm, who said, "Medical care is a fiscal black hole into which a nation can pour endless wealth. We should not transfer more national assets to health care."[1]

Serious federal attempts to reform healthcare and control costs began in the early 1970s. One of the major efforts was the passage of the Health Planning and Resource Development Act by Congress in 1974. This gave states and local agencies the authority to review hospital capital expenditures through "certificates of need." The goal was ostensibly to reduce costs by eliminating duplication of services and by generally making institutions "think twice" before they undertake major capital purchases or engage in new construction. It has been estimated that this process has slowed the rate of increase of expenditures by 2% to 3% at best and has significantly increased bureaucracy.[2] Despite all efforts, including the introduction of the Medicare Prospective Payment System in 1983, healthcare expenditures continued to rise at a rate estimated at three- to fivefold that of inflation. By 1990, the United States was spending $2566 per capita on healthcare—more than twice the average of the Organization for Economic Cooperation and Development, our European counterparts. The United States outspent Canada by 45%, France by 67%, Germany by 73%, Japan by 119%, and the United Kingdom by some 164%.[3] What makes these figures remarkable is that despite these extraordinary expenditures, the United States ranked 9th in hospitalizations per capita of 11 Western industrialized nations examined, 9th in life expectancy at birth for women (11th out of 11 for men), 11th of 11 for both infant mortality and the incidence of low infant birth weight. Indeed, Sweden's infant mortality rate was 58% that of the United States.[4] In an attempt to explain these apparent discrepancies and to bring the problem in focus, one healthcare analyst at a national public policy forum suggested that,

> *The areas where the United States has excelled are principally those areas fueled by our inflated spending in health care: medical technology, high-tech therapies, and for-profit medical provider systems. Unfortunately, with an estimated 36 million people uninsured, and an equal number reportedly under-insured, the population as a whole has not received the benefits of this success. In fact, the focus by our leading health care institutions and the media on the success of unusual, high-tech, and expensive therapies serves to underscore the inequities in our current system, where many have limited access to these technologies.*[5]

Intense examination of the American healthcare system is already underway, and those segments consuming disproportionately large amounts of the healthcare funds are being examined most closely. As critical care accounts for over 20% of acute care hospital charges and for about 1% of the nation's gross domestic product,[6] it is inevitable that it will come under the most careful scrutiny of any segment of the medical industry. A number of studies have already shown that most healthcare expenditures are incurred during the last few months of life, suggesting that allocation of resources is less than appropriate.[7] Surprisingly, for a field that represents such a disproportionately large amount of this nation's resources, very little is known about the efficacy, appropriateness, allocation, or even the utilization of these expenditures. Indeed, in a national point-in-time survey of intensive care units (ICUs), the response rate was only 38.7%.[8] It might be speculated that this survey was biased in that the more functional and organized units would be more likely to respond than those without well-organized leadership. Indeed, the entire issue of the relationships among organization, efficacy, and performance has yet to be clarified.

As the intensity of the healthcare crisis has increased, discussion of "rationing" healthcare services has become widespread and now permeates the literature. Although the rationing of healthcare services remains a politically dangerous concept, de facto rationing by practitioners and policy makers is generally conceded to be common.[9] National public policy seminars have addressed the issue, and one state, Oregon, is engaging in what has been described as "social experimentation" with the rationing of Medicaid expenditures.[10]

In the 1980s, Oregon, like many other states, found that the Medicaid budget was far from adequate and that some 450,000 Oregonians were left without healthcare coverage. During the 1987 legislative session, Oregon lawmakers decided that the state could no longer afford to spend its Medicaid dollars on high-cost, low-success treatment modalities, such as bone marrow transplantation, if it were to provide more poor Oregonians with healthcare coverage. Several months later, a young boy receiving Medicaid benefits died when he was denied a bone marrow transplantation procedure. This event elicited a widespread debate that became the focus of tremendous media attention. A variety of committees were established to study the healthcare issue, including numerous public forums, and by 1989, the Oregon Health Plan was passed by the legislature. The approved plan languished in bureaucracy as federal action was awaited. In 1993, Oregon obtained a federal waiver that allowed it to proceed with the reallocation of Medicaid funds and that would do the following:

- extend Medicaid eligibility to all persons with incomes below the federal poverty level;
- define a basic minimum healthcare package based on a rank-ordered listing of 709 paired medical conditions and treatments (treatments were ranked according to estimates of clinical effectiveness, social importance, and quality-of-life);
- provide a liability shield for medical providers that protects them from both criminal and civil prosecution as well as from professional disciplinary action when they do not provide those services that the legislature has chosen not to fund.

The Oregon Health Plan has great implications for how critical care is provided, regardless of its ultimate success or failure. It has already significantly raised public consciousness of the problems that arise from an increasing demand for a supply of resources that is no longer unlimited. The term "rationing" has now become part of the public policy lexicon and has become the subject of much media attention. It is now common to discuss openly and rationally sensitive issues that were commonly avoided just a few years ago. As the debate expands and both the general public and the medical and nursing communities become better informed, it becomes possible to develop meaningful policies and solutions to these difficult problems.

When the issue of rationing medical care for the critically ill was discussed at public policy development seminars held at the Brookings Institution in 1986 and in 1991, two recurrent themes became apparent:

- Can improved ICU management, quality care, efficiency, and cost containment make unnecessary a national policy that restricts costly but beneficial life-sustaining care, or will critical care units be the motivating force in the evolution of a system similar to that in Great Britain, where beneficial services are limited by overall centralized government budgeting?
- Should physicians be the ultimate gatekeepers for society in distributing medical services, or should they remain merely the agents for the patients' own medical goals, as called for in Hippocratic tradition? Who else should participate in decisions to limit beneficial services, if at all?[11]

Critical care is an expensive resource that must be managed effectively if we are to avoid compromising the quality of care delivered. Although there is general agreement about this, there is little agreement and less information about what constitutes quality care and, even more so, cost-effective care. Consequently, rationing not only exists but is growing. Medical ethicists have taken up the issue of rationing and the allocation of resources; the proliferation of papers on the subject attests to this. However, it is the attending physician, nurse, and patient who are caught between the hammer of reality and the anvil of policy, and this is even more true for the nurse and physician directors of critical care units. Their primary responsibility in managing the units is to ensure the appropriateness of care, the quality of care, and, ultimately, the allocation of care and of valued scarce resources.

APPROPRIATENESS OF CARE

It has been suggested,[10, 11] and it is probably safe to assume, that if all healthcare rendered were appropriate, rationing would not need to be discussed. "Appropriateness" is a difficult term to define and even more difficult to measure. A group from the RAND Corporation attempted a large-scale survey and meta-analysis of the literature to assess the "appropriateness" in healthcare delivery.[12] They were confronted with a lack of information and low-quality information in the literature, but their findings nonetheless are interesting. "Appropriate care" can generally be defined as care whose benefits exceed its cost or negative consequences. The definition and measurement of benefit and cost remain elusive yet important goals. Benefits usually include increased longevity, improved quality of life, decreased pain and anxiety, and improved functional capacity. Costs should be separated into monetary and nonmonetary categories. Nonmonetary costs, or risks, generally include morbidity, mortality, decreased quality of life, pain, and anxiety. The RAND group suggested that three approaches can be used to assess appropriateness, the first two being explicit approaches: the *benefit-risk approach,* which excludes monetary cost; the *benefit-cost approach,* which incorporates the cost both to the patient and society; and the *implicit approach,* which relies on the physician who provides service to judge its appropriateness. This last approach is even more subjective than the first two, and has the additional hazard of potentially being influenced by monetary benefits to the rating physician. The RAND group found ". . . at least double-digit levels of inappropriate care [in every study] . . . In particular, perhaps as much as one fifth to one quarter of acute care services were felt to be used for equivocal or inappropriate reasons."[12] Although most of the studies examined were not of the ICU setting, there is little to suggest that the findings there would be different.

A key paper by Robin published in 1983[13] critically examined the workings of ICUs and specifically excluded any discussion of cost effectiveness. He questioned whether critical care resources were in fact properly utilized. He suggested that five subpopulations of patients are found in ICUs:

1. Terminally or hopelessly ill patients for whom intensive care simply prolongs the process of dying;
2. Seriously ill patients who will benefit significantly from improvements in the quantity and quality of life by the interventions provided them in the ICU;
3. Patients who will recover whether care is provided in the critical care unit or elsewhere;
4. Patients whose lives are shortened or who are made less well specifically because of ICU-related iatrogenic complications;
5. Patients whose lives are shortened or who are made

less well because of iatrogenic misadventures not necessarily attributed to their ICU admission.

Robin's concern was that despite the extraordinary expenditures and resources allocated to the care of the critically ill, very little information concerns outcomes and appropriateness of care. There was and continues to be a spectacular paucity of information regarding the utilization of our resources. As Robin concluded,

The purpose of patient management is to optimize the possibility of happy and productive lives for patients. Much of ICU management, like much of modern medicine, may function tangentially to this main purpose. Physicians do harm as well as good. It is important to recognize this, not for the purpose of mea culpa, *but so that the harm can be detected and minimized. The actual balance between good and harm has not been established in ICUs. Many patients admitted are irreversibly ill and some would benefit maximally by not being admitted to an ICU. Some patients are clearly salvaged by ICU admission; others are clearly harmed. The relative distribution of these patients is important to establish in guiding our approach to ICUs generally.*[13]

Since Robin's comments were published in 1983, awareness of the need to examine healthcare delivery practices for the critically ill has increased, and numerous studies and commentaries, especially in the area of medical ethics, have been made. Indeed, a veritable proliferation of papers focuses largely on those groups of patients who Robin identified as either not benefiting or actually suffering as a result of admission to the ICU. The withdrawal and withholding of care have received attention, as has the concept of futile care. Identifying patients for whom further care or admission to the ICU would be futile is important to ensure the appropriate utilization of a scarce resource. The difficulty arises in defining "futile care" and in identifying those patients with a high degree of certainty. Schneiderman and colleagues commented that "futile care" is not necessarily a hopeless effort but rather interventions whose expectation of success "is either predictably or empirically so unlikely that its exact probability is often incalculable."[14] How mortality prediction models such as the *Acute Physiology and Chronic Health Evaluation* (APACHE) and *the Mortality Probability Model* (MPM) tools figure into the decision-making process remains to be seen, but they have already contributed significantly to the discussion.[15] The applicability of statistical tools that may be 95% or 99% reliable to real world decisions raises thorny moral, ethical, and social issues. Considering the economic forces that drive medicine today, the dilemmas become especially difficult for those forced to make decisions at the bedside. In an editorial published in 1992, Schuster said:

Ethical principles, for all their illumination, don't always shine with the same intensity—nor should they. We must learn to distinguish 'everything that can be done' from 'everything that should be done.' Making the distinction is not easy—and that's OK. It doesn't bother me at all that these decisions are tough, gut-wrenching, anxiety-provoking. But that is part of our responsibility—and it's about time that we began to accept it.[16]

UTILIZATION OF CRITICAL CARE UNITS

Although it is estimated that more than 4000 critical care units exist in the United States[8] and that these units consume about 1% of the national gross domestic product, it is remarkable that so little hard information is available regarding the utilization of these expensive resources. It is more than likely that, apart from the types of inappropriate care discussed above, some populations of patients admitted to critical care units could be cared for in less costly environments. This information is slowly coming to light, and it is clear that a need exists for a national database of information about how the critically ill are cared for in the United States.

Henning and colleagues reviewed 706 medical-surgical ICU patients and found that 40% of medical and 30% of surgical ICU admissions never received any intervention and were admitted strictly for monitoring purposes. They characterized patients using the *Acute Physiology Score* and found that patients with low scores received significantly fewer interventions.[17] They also found that as many as 45% of all ICU patients were admitted because they were believed to be at risk for medical or postoperative complication, yet fewer than one third of them actually required therapeutic interventions. They concluded that the organization and design of critical care units should include provisions for these "low-intervention patients," possibly in the form of intermediate or step-down monitoring units.

Oye and Bellamy[18] also found skewed distributions of resource consumption. They observed that some 41% of patients admitted to ICUs received no acute interventions but found that these patients consumed less than 10% of resources as measured using the Therapeutic Intervention Scoring System. They found that reducing the number of patients admitted for monitoring purposes would have relatively little impact on overall hospital charges and, consequently, costs. However, the top 8% of admitted patients accounted for some 50% of all resource consumption, and their mortality rate was 70.6%. They concluded that the key to improved utilization was a ". . . better understanding of the prognosis by physicians, patients, and their families . . . [to] reduce the amount of futile care. One approach to this is to regularly reassess the prognosis after patients are admitted to the unit. An additional approach is to discuss diagnosis, prognosis, and likelihood of benefit from treatment with hospitalized patients at risk for transfer to the ICU." However, surveys have shown that the majority of patients who wanted to communicate with their physician about life support had not done so.[19]

It would seem that careful examination and documentation of current practices in critical care on a large scale is urgently needed to assess the type of care delivered and the patient populations receiving it. Indeed, as Chernow titled an editorial, "The practice of critical care: Describing who we are, evaluating what we do, and computing the cost,"[20] the need for information is acute. Only when this need has been satisfied can guidelines for the appropriateness of care be developed.

QUALITY OF CARE

Measuring and assessing the quality of care delivered is an essential component of the management of critical care units. It appears that for adult medical-surgical patients, two objective measures are emerging that can be used for quality care assessment. The MPM II[21] provides information regarding the likelihood of survival at the time of admission to the ICU based on 15 objective variables. The APACHE III assesses severity of illness and probability of both survival and ICU length of stay based on 17 physiologic variables, age, and up to 7 comorbid conditions occurring during the first day of ICU stay.[22] The *Pediatric Risk of Mortality* (PRISM) has been used to compare and assess pediatric ICUs. These tools and the process of outcomes prediction are discussed in detail elsewhere in this book (see Chapter 198).

Although these tools have been tested in hundreds of hospitals worldwide, they are not widely in practice. In fact, there is no consensus as to how these tools should be used. Can they be used to determine admission to or discharge from units?[22a, 22b] Can they be used to determine when to discontinue life support? Can they be used in selecting likely candidates for triage? or Are they simply devices for retrospective analysis of the aggregate quality of care delivered to select patient populations? The discussion continues, but few unambiguous answers are available at this time.[22c] Although these tools are measures of expected mortality, it is less than clear that this is the only or best index of quality. To date, a universally accepted definition of a "high-performance" critical care unit has not been established. Cost and resource utilization are at least two other important reflections of performance, but they are not easily measured, if they can be measured at all. It would seem imperative that a range of performance measures be developed and agreed upon and that the process of unit management be evaluated as well. Some methodologies have already been proposed to meet these needs.[22d]

Zimmerman and colleagues[23] studied in detail the organizational structures of nine ICUs as part of a larger study of 42 units located throughout the United States. Using the APACHE III scoring system, they attempted to relate organizational structure with efficiency and risk-adjusted survival. They were able to characterize superior organizational practices that seemed to be more prevalent in better-performing ICUs, defining "high performance" as the attainment of superior risk-adjusted mortality ranks; that is, in high-performance units, the actual survival rates of patients exceeded the predicted survival rates. They found that "superior organizational practices among these ICUs were related to a patient-centered culture, strong medical and nursing leadership, effective communication and coordination, and open, collaborative approaches to solving problems and managing conflict."[23] These units typically had strong shared visions; empowered nursing staffs; ongoing educational programs, a strong sense of collegiality among nurses, physicians, and administrative staff; supportive, visible leadership; and a generally defined concept of collaborative practice. In lower-performance units, less collaboration was present, management was "top-down" and remote, and staff were more concerned about hospital rules, procedural issues, job security, hours, and pay than about patients and their well-being. However, this study was not able to relate efficacy with efficiency or efficacy and efficiency with organizational characteristics. This could be a result of the small number of units studied or of the inadequacy of the measures of performance and organization. If the extensive case studies performed in the non–healthcare business world are at all valid, strong cause-and-effect relationships exist among organization, management, and performance. Critical care units are extraordinarily complex environments with multiple constituencies and stakeholders. It will be difficult but not impossible to identify measurable parameters of performance, efficiency, cost, appropriateness, culture, and organization as well as perceived elements such as patient, family and staff satisfaction, leadership, communication, coordination, and collaboration; management of critical care units in the era of healthcare reform will depend on these measures' being well defined, accepted, validated, and reliable in the near future.

ALLOCATION OF CARE

Even in the best of circumstances, when resources are used appropriately and effectively, the demand may and inevitably will occasionally exceed the supply. The responsibility to triage—that is, to ensure adequate care and the appropriate allocation of scarce resources—falls directly on the shoulders of the unit directors. The Joint Commission on Accreditation of Healthcare Organizations mandates the appointment of unit directors and that there be written, functional policies that govern action when the patient population's demands exceed operational capacity.[24] This was mandated in response to the growing realization that the allocation of resources is typically performed in an ad hoc manner, and not necessarily with initial consideration of the best interests of the patient or the population as a whole. A revealing study by Marshall and colleagues of the admission practices of a surgical ICU during times of overcrowding concluded that "surgical attending physicians rarely used other open in-house ICU beds when surgical ICU beds were unavailable. Political power, medical provincialism, and income maximization overrode medical suitability in the provision of critical care services."[25] It is highly unlikely that this study represented an isolated, anomalous situation.

The need to allocate resources in a reasonable manner has legal implications. Thus far, the courts have had little to say on the issue, but this is likely to change. A few cases have already come to light, and more are to be expected. A prime example is the case of a young trauma victim who was admitted to an ICU in Florida several years ago. The unit was overcrowded, and during the night she was accidentally disconnected from her ventilator and suffered irreversible brain damage. A lawsuit was brought before a court, and during the trial that followed, it became apparent that inadequate staffing was largely the result of an alleged failure to triage. After the woman's admission, a nearly brain-dead patient was kept in the unit rather than being transferred to a regular ward, and two new patients were admitted rather than being diverted to another institution. The court ruled that the hospital was obligated to triage in order to continue to provide an appropriate level of care to patients already admitted.[26] Commenting on the court's decision, Englehardt and Rie said,

> *Depending on what probability of what benefits is afforded a patient already in a bed, the time of discharge can be advanced hour by hour in order to make a bed available to a newcomer who may be in slightly greater need or have a slightly greater likelihood of benefiting by admission.*[27]

The very concept of allocating scarce resources and determining "medical suitability" (i.e., who lives and who dies) invokes many medical, legal, and ethical issues that have been explored extensively in the literature. Teres reviewed many of these issues from a practical perspective and offered the following suggestions:

1. *An ICU medical director, designee, or supervisory nurse should be empowered as the gatekeeping office.*
2. *The basis for regulating admission, discharge, or triage from the special care unit should be medical suitability (from the utilitarian or egalitarian view) [conditions of limited medical suitability include:*
   high-probability estimate of hospital mortality
   persistent vegetative state
   full DNR (patient has failed aggressive medical therapy)
   patient is clinically unsalvageable (no marginal benefit)
   rapidly fatal underlying condition
   Alzheimer's disease]
   During high-level triage when all ICU patients are receiving active therapy, these decisions should override the individual primary physician-patient relationship.
3. *The guidelines should follow the "congestive heart failure" treatment analogy:*
   a. *preload reduction: hold high risk patients in the post-anesthesia care unit of Emergency Department, postpone surgery, hold transfers in outlying ICUs;*
   b. *improve cardiac performance: increase efficiency and decrease workload per patient by performing fewer invasive procedures and transporting fewer patients for abdominal CAT scans;*
   c. *afterload reduction: keep unstable patients in the post-anesthesia care unit, send sicker patients to intermediate care units, send "stable" ventilator-dependent patients to general medical-surgical units, and transfer or resolve issues regarding 'hopeless' patients.*[28]

The great difficulty for ICU directors is that triage and rationing place them in a position in which a serious potential for conflict of interest exists, especially if the director is personally caring for patients in the critical care unit. As one observer commented, "Physicians cannot serve two masters . . . [they] are required to do everything they believe may benefit each patient without regard to costs or other social considerations . . . It is society, not the individual practitioner that must make the decision to limit the availability of medical care."[29] In an extensive discussion of utilization strategies for ICUs, Kalb and Miller suggested that although this concept is firmly entrenched and ". . . precludes physicians from rationing in their role as care givers, it does not preclude hospital-based rationing policies, nor does it preclude physician involvement in setting hospital policy."[30] Taking this one step further, it becomes obvious that hospitals must not only have clear and unambiguous policies regarding the allocation of resources but that the role of the critical care unit directors must also be clearly defined to maximize effectiveness and minimize the possibility of conflicts of interest.

MANAGING UNITS

The issues confronting critical care units are both legion and complex and will have serious consequences in the future if they are not vigorously confronted. As the problems of ensuring appropriate care, quality care, and the allocation of resources are examined, it is apparent not only that these issues have economic, medical, legal, and ethical implications but also that they are closely interrelated. None of these issues can be considered in isolation. Rather, they are systematic problem areas that are closely interconnected and interdependent. To deal with these issues in a timely manner, the critical care unit must be viewed as a single system, an organization with multiple constituents and stakeholders embedded within the larger framework of the hospital and its stakeholders, which in turn constitute the regional and national healthcare economies.

Critical care providers have long dealt solely with the disease processes of individual patients. Patients must now be regarded as part of a larger whole, and a systems approach to care provision must be entertained. The challenge to every hospital and to every director of a critical care unit is to effect change so that decision-making policies regarding the appropriateness, quality, and allocation of care can be instituted. The patient, the critical care unit, society, and the allocation of care are all inextricably interrelated. As Zimmerman and colleagues concluded, critical care ". . . will continue to be costly and the ethical issues surrounding the use of ICU resources will continue to grow. ICUs will need to become organizationally and managerially competent in order to deal with these challenges."[23]

Implementing a management structure that can deal effectively with these issues is simple in theory but difficult in practice. A primary function of the management structure is to align and develop the internal capabilities and policies of the critical care unit with the pressures and forces generated by the multiple external environments within which the unit is embedded. Every critical care unit has a particular culture that resists change, as do the practices of medicine and nursing themselves. Implementing concepts such as Total Quality Management or patient-focused care, or even acceptance of the idea of employing a full-time intensivist/director of critical care, requires a significant change in thinking—that is, a change in the organizational culture of not only the ICU but also of the medical staff, the nurses, the ancillary staff, and the hospital administrators. The forces of change, driven by the healthcare economic crisis, mandate that critical care units can no longer be managed in the laissez faire mode of the past. The future requires that a comprehensive, multidisciplinary, systematic approach be taken to the management of all health care, but especially to those areas that demand the most resources. Critical care specialists must provide the leadership to ensure the optimal utilization and allocation of these vital resources.

References

1. Lamm R: "The crisis in health care." New York Times, February 19, 1987.
2. Dranove D, Cone K: Do state rate setting regulations really lower hospital expenses? J Health Econ 1985; 4:159–165.
3. Scheiber G, Pouillier J-P: International health spending: Issues and trends. Health Affairs 1991; 10:109.
4. Center for Health Policy Research, American Medical Association: International Health Systems: A Chartbook Perspective. Chicago, American Medical Association, 1991, pp 12–25.
5. Taylor R: Rationing healthcare in other countries. Unpublished paper presented at the Employee Benefit Research Institute (EBRI) Education and Research Fund Policy Forum: Rationing Health Care—Making Choices and Allocating Resources in the Health Care Delivery System: Implications for Access, Quality, and Costs. Washington, DC, December 1, 1992.
6. Intensive care units (ICUs): Clinical outcomes, costs, and decision-making. Health Technology Case Study 28. Washington, DC, Congress of the United States, Office of Technology Assessment, 1984.
7. Gaumer GL, Stavins J: Medicare use in the last 90 days of life. Health Serv Res 1992; 26:725–742.
8. Groeger JS, Guntupalli KK, Strosberg M, et al: Descriptive analysis of critical care units in the United States: Patient characteristics and intensive care unit utilization. Crit Care Med 1993; 21:279–291.
9. Strauss MJ, LoGerfo JP, Yeltlatzie JA, et al: Rationing of intensive care unit services: An everyday occurrence. JAMA 1986; 225:1143–1146.
10. Strosberg MA, Weiner JM, Baker R, et al: Rationing America's Medical Care: The Oregon Plan and Beyond. Washington, DC, The Brookings Institution Press, 1992.
11. Strosberg MA, Fein IA, Carroll JD (Eds): Rationing of Medical Care for the Critically Ill. Washington, DC, The Brookings Institution Press, 1989.
12. Brook RH, Kamberg CJ, Mayer-Oakes A, et al: Appropriateness of acute medical care for the elderly: An analysis of the literature. *In:* Health Care Quality Management for the 21st Century. Couch JB (Ed). Tampa, American College of Physician Executives, 1991.
13. Robin ED: A critical look at critical care. Crit Care Med 1983; 11:144–148.
14. Schneiderman LJ, Jecker NS, Jonsen AR: Medical futility: Its meaning and ethical implications. Ann Intern Med 1990; 112:949–954.
15. Knaus WA, Wagner DP, Lynn J: Short-term mortality predictions for critically ill hospitalized adults: Science and ethics. Science 1991; 253:1–6.
16. Schuster DP: Everything that should be done—Not everything that can be done. Am Rev Respir Dis 1992; 145:508–509.
17. Henning RJ, McClish D, Daly B, et al: Clinical characteristics and resource utilization of ICU patients: Implications for organization of intensive care. Crit Care Med 1987; 15:264–267.
18. Oye RK, Bellamy PE: Patterns of resource consumption in medical intensive care. Chest 1991; 99:685–689.
19. Frankl D, Oye RK, Bellamy PE: Attitudes of hospitalized patients toward life support: A survey of 200 medical inpatients. Am J Med 1989; 86:845–848.
20. Chernow B: The practice of critical care: Describing who we are, evaluating what we do, and computing the cost. Crit Care Med 1993; 21:1413–1415.
21. Lemeshow S, Teres D, Klar J, et al: Mortality probability models (MPM II) based on an international cohort of intensive care patients. JAMA 1993; 270:2478–2486.

22. Knaus WA, Wagner DP, Zimmerman JE, et al: Variations in mortality and length of stay in intensive care units. Ann Intern Med 1993; 118:753–761.
22a. Zimmerman JE, Wagner DP, Draper EA, et al: Improving intensive care unit discharge decisions: Supplementing physician judgement with predictions of next day risk for life support. Crit Care Med 1994; 22:1373–1384.
22b. Bone RC, McElwee NE, Eubanks DH, et al: Analysis of indications for early discharge from the intensive care unit. Clinical Efficacy Assessment Project: American College of Physicians. Chest 1993; 104:1812–1817.
22c. Cullen DJ, Chernow B: Predicting outcome in critically ill patients. Crit Care Med 1994; 22:1345–1348.
22d. Rapoport J, Teres D, Lemeshow S, et al: A method for assessing the clinical performance and cost-effectiveness of intensive care units: A multicenter inception cohort study. Crit Care Med 1994; 22:1385–1391.
23. Zimmerman JE, Shortell SM, Rousseau DM, et al: Improving intensive care: Observations based on organizational case studies in nine units: A prospective, multicenter study. Crit Care Med 1993; 21:1443–1451.
24. Joint Commission on Healthcare Organizations: Accreditation Manual for Hospitals: Special Care Units. Chicago, Joint Commission on Healthcare Organizations, 1992.
25. Marshall MF, Schwenzer KJ, Orsina M, et al: Influence of political power, medical provincialism, and economic incentives on the rationing of surgical intensive care beds. Crit Care Med 1992; 20:387–394.
26. *Von Stettina v Florida Medical Center,* 2 Fla Supp 2d 55 (Fla 17th Cir 1982) a 436 So Rptr 3rd 1022 (1983).
27. Englehardt HT, Rie MA: Intensive care units, scarce resources, and conflicting principles of justice. JAMA 1986; 255:1159–1164.
28. Teres D: Civilian triage in the intensive care unit: The ritual of the last bed. Crit Care Med 1993; 21:598–606.
29. Levinsky NG: The doctor's master. N Engl J Med 1984; 311:1573–1575.
30. Kalb ME, Miller DH: Utilization strategies for intensive care units. JAMA 1989; 261:2389–2395.

CHAPTER 196

Computers in the Intensive Care Unit: A Match Meant to Be!

Reed M. Gardner, PhD • Dean F. Sittig, PhD
Terry P. Clemmer, MD

The care of critically ill patients places exceptional demands on physicians and nurses. As a result of their medical problems, patients in intensive care units (ICUs) are monitored with elaborate bedside monitors and are subjected to a wide variety of laboratory tests. Therapy is complex, timing of treatment is critical, and careful documentation of the care given is essential. A large volume of data must be stored, processed, and used for clinical decision making. The tremendous growth in the volume of medical information, the demand for cost-effective care, and the need to document and justify why clinical decisions are made have placed a large burden on the medical care team. Patients, payers, the public, and healthcare policy makers are increasingly demanding accountability, insisting that complete and accurate records be kept by physicians, nurses, and therapists who care for the critically ill.[1–6]

Since the late 1960s, rapid development in computer technology has occurred, with remarkable reductions in computer cost (from $500,000 to less than $5000) and size (from room-sized units to laptop models) as well as an almost 1000-fold improvement in computing speed and a reduction in power consumption.[7, 8] Approximately every 1.5 years, the performance-to-price ratio for computers doubles. The latest (Pentium) silicon microprocessor chip announced by Intel (Portland, OR) executes 100 million instructions per second and contains 3 million transistors, all within the area of a postage stamp. In just over 12 years since the original IBM personal computer was introduced, computing speed has increased 20-fold, the number of components for computers 150-fold, and the computing capability 500-fold. With the increasing capability and decreasing cost of computing, the possibility of using computers to help solve the problem of data collection, storage, and decision-making support needs of the ICU is very attractive. It seems apparent that, as the complexity of critical care increases and the cost of computer hardware decreases, every ICU will soon use not just one but several interconnected microcomputers.

ICUs have become an integral part of most hospitals. Their concentration on the treatment of the critically ill has made the acquisition and proper use of data extremely important. In the modern ICU, computerized monitoring devices and recording systems are common. This chapter outlines how computers can be used for record keeping and decision making.

COMPUTERIZED RECORD KEEPING

Barnett[9] recently reviewed the application of computers to ambulatory practice and quoted Florence Nightingale's 1873 book entitled *Notes on a Hospital:*

> *In attempt to arrive at the truth, I have applied everywhere for information, but in scarcely any instance have I been able to obtain hospital records fit for any purpose of comparison. If they could be obtained, they would enable us to decide many other questions besides the one alluded to. They would show the subscribers how their money was being spent, what good was really being done with it, or whether the money was not doing mischief rather than good.*

It is surprising that Florence Nightingale's comments are still applicable over 120 years later. The same holds true for today's ambulatory and ICU patients' records.

The medical record remains the principal instrument for ensuring the continuity of patient care. The Institute of Medicine of the National Academy of Sciences declared that a computer-based patient record was an essential technology for healthcare in the United States.[10, 11] Information in the record should be easily retrievable and reviewable in a temporal relationship with the associated data. There is a real need to integrate and organize patients' records to optimize medical data review and decision making.[12–15] As the central focus of the care process, the traditional handwritten medical record has several limitations:

1. It might be physically unavailable because it can only be used by one person at one location at any given time.
2. It is often poorly organized, with information available only in the order that it was recorded. Also, this information is often illegible. Thus, information retrieval may be impossible, slow, or susceptible to error.[6]
3. Retrieval of data from the record for research is time consuming and cumbersome because it must be done manually.[16]
4. The everincreasing number of bedside computerized instruments present data in electronic form, and this data must be read by a human and written onto the record.

In complicated cases, the conventional record is less helpful than a structured flow chart. Whiting-O'Keefe and associates have shown that structured records are easier to review, decrease review time, and improve information flow.[13] Criticisms of manual records are especially germane to the critical care medical records because of the large amount of data collected and the pressure to make prompt treatment decisions in the ICU. The importance of having a unified medical record has been demonstrated by a study conducted at LDS Hospital (Salt Lake City, UT).[17] In this study, detailed records were kept of the data used by physicians to make treatment decisions during teaching "rounds" in a shock-trauma ICU (Fig. 196–1). It was a surprise to find that laboratory data (42%) were the most frequently used data (clinical laboratory: 33%; blood gas values: 9%), since physiologic bedside monitors have become synonymous with the modern ICU. Drug and fluid balance data were next (22%), followed by clinicians' observations (21%); the bedside physiologic monitor accounted for only 13% of the data used in making therapeutic decisions during teaching rounds. These findings also provide evidence that data from several sources, not just from the traditional physiologic bedside monitoring devices, must be communicated and integrated into a unified medical record to permit effective decision making and treatment in the ICU.

INTEGRATED INTENSIVE CARE UNIT COMPUTER RECORDS

Computer charting in the ICU must support multiple types of data collection to be effective. As can be seen in Figure 196–1, a large portion of the data needed to make decisions is from "physical" tasks, such as administration of a medication or auscultation of breath or heart sounds. At present, most data of this type must be entered manually. Thus, for computer charting systems to be successful, computers must be able to collect a wide variety of data from bedside monitors as well as from nurses and physicians at the bedside. Unfortunately, in the past, most attempts at computerized charting have dealt only with a limited set of data, such as that acquired from electronic bedside monitors.

Figure 196–2 illustrates the complexity of ICU charting. The patient record (chart) must document the actions taken by the medical staff to fulfill both medical and legal requirements (#1 and #2). In addition, much of the data that are logged on the chart are used for management (#3) and billing (#4) purposes. Many computer systems have ignored these requirements and unwittingly force the clinical staff to double-chart. Efficient management in hospitals is a must, especially with the public's current awareness of healthcare issues in the United States.[18–22] Hospitals now have strong incentives to know the cost of procedures and to control these costs. As a result, knowing a patient's acuity (i.e., how sick he or she is) is a necessity, not a luxury; this knowledge makes it possible to project nursing staff needs and to account for the care of patients based on acuity rather than on a fixed room charge.

Communication of information (#5) to and from other departments within a hospital is mandatory. Convenient and timely access to clinical and administrative information from a physician's home or office via modem and a personal computer link is essential. A computerized record allows this type of communication. Since the computerized ICU record is stored in the system, it is also readily available for concurrent or retrospective research purposes (#6). Continuity of care is particularly important for critically ill patients, who are generally cared for by a team of physicians, nurses, and therapists who frequently communicate data to one another. For example, a laboratory technician calls a ward clerk, who reports data to a nurse, who in turn passes the information on to a physician, who then makes a decision based on the data. Each step in this "human" transmission process is subject to delay and error.

For computers to be most useful in the ICU, an integrated patient data management system must exist.[23] Even though excellent progress has been made in the field of computerization in the ICU, many challenges have yet to be faced. These challenges and opportunities are discussed in the sections that follow.

Development of Better Data Entry Techniques

Computerization of patient monitoring and of all available patient data requires further development of data entry methods. At present, a ballpoint pen and a blank piece of paper provide a fast, easy, familiar, and convenient method for physicians, nurses, and others to chart patient information. Unfortunately, the conventional handwritten chart has many deficiencies, as noted earlier. However, the ease and flexibility of charting with the usual manual method are still the standard against which ICU computer charting is compared. Therefore, data entry methods that are efficient and effective for data recording and review must be developed. It is highly likely that such methods will include some of the newer screen and graphic functions that have become

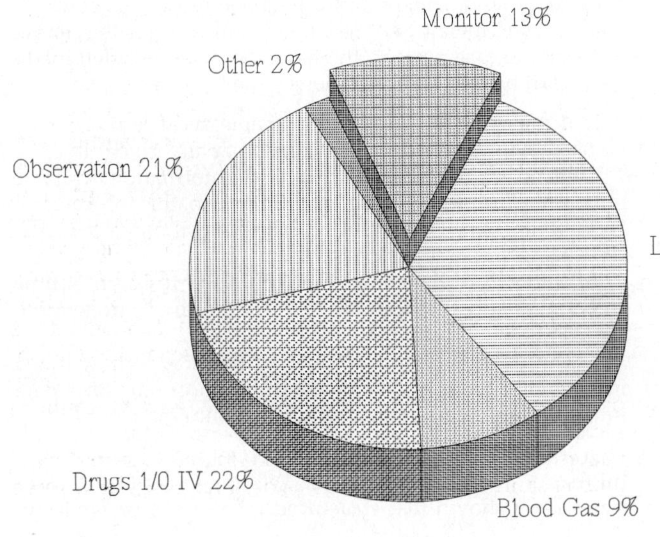

Figure 196–1. A pie chart showing data used for clinical decision-making by physicians during teaching rounds in a shock-trauma ICU. (From Bradshaw KE, Gardner RM, Clemmer TP, et al: Physician decision-making: Evaluation of data used in a computerized ICU. Int J Clin Monit Comput 1984; 1:81. Reprinted by permission of Kluwer Academic Publishers.)

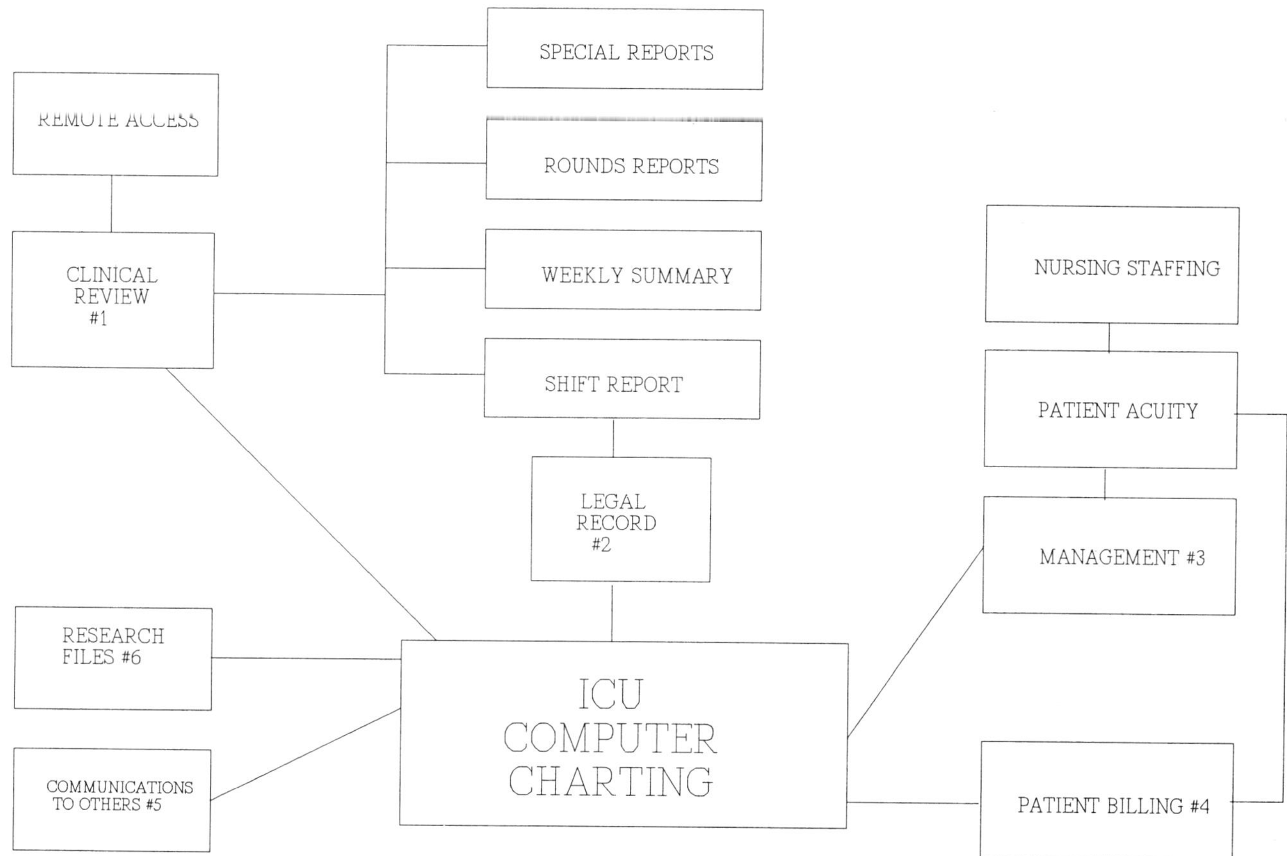

Figure 196–2. A block diagram showing the six major areas where computerized ICU charting interacts with nurses and physicians to make patient care more functional and efficient. See the text for an explanation of each function.

available with personal computers.[7] These devices include the mouse and floating cursor, light pens, and touch-sensitive monitor screens. Although each of these aids may help in entering data, the largest payoff is likely to be gained from a "smart" system. With a smart system, the terminal or work station at the bedside knows a great deal about a patient: his or her condition; what drugs have been prescribed with their dose, route of administration, and schedule; and the personal preferences of the physician caring for the patient. Thus, by being "smart," the computer system is able to present quickly personalized data entry and review menus, helping a nurse or physician to customize the care process. Also, innovative methods, such as "charting by exception," must be explored as healthcare providers become more aware of what the essential frequency of need and content of the chart should be.

Physicians, nurses, and therapists collect a large amount of data by making frequent observations, performing tests, and checking continuous monitoring equipment. Physicians generally prescribe complicated therapy for ICU patients. As a result, enormous amounts of clinical data accumulate. Physicians can miss important events and trends if accumulated data are not presented in a compact, well-organized format. In addition, the problems of managing these patients have been made even more challenging by economic pressures to reduce the cost of care.[18–22]

Figure 196–3 shows how nurses in a thoracic ICU (post–open heart surgery patients) spend their working day. As one would expect, nurses spend the majority of their time providing direct patient care (48%). Another 19% of their time (over 2 hours and 15 minutes per 12-hour shift) is spent documenting (charting).[24] The next most frequent activity (7%) is the communication of patient status information to other members of the healthcare team. Through the use of a good hospital computer system, the quality, accuracy, and ease of data communication within the ICU can be improved.[25, 26] An opportunity to reduce the data-handling time of the nursing staff also exists.

Standardization of Data Transfer Among Computers

Communication is one of the most important tasks of the healthcare professional. Data underlie the making of every medical decision. Except for personal observations made by and acted upon by physicians, nurses, and therapists at the bedside, all patient data must be communicated. Often, the data are communicated through several people and by several media before they get to the appropriate medical decision maker. Each step in the process, especially if it involves a handwritten record, can also result in delays and errors. Computers can solve these problems and are being used in more and more healthcare facilities to enhance communication. As can be noted in Figures 196–1 and 196–2, much of the data used to manage the treatment of patients comes from locations other than the bedside, such as the clinical laboratory. If ICU data are to be integrated with data from other computer systems, such as laboratory data, communications standards become crucial. Standards are now being developed that will make the task of "sharing" data among multiple computers in a hospital easier and more

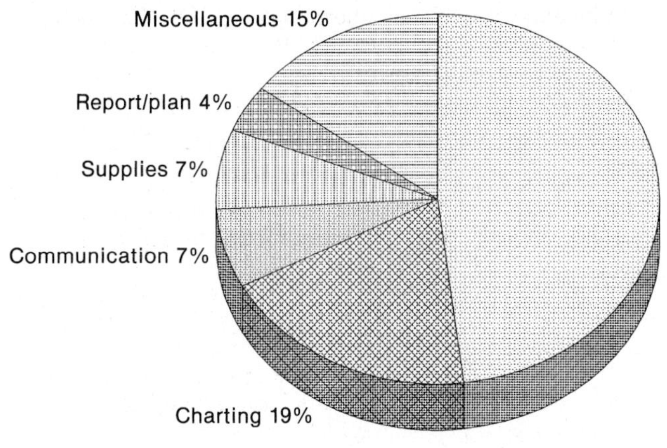

Figure 196–3. A pie chart indicating how nurses spend their time in a thoracic surgery ICU.

efficient.[27–34] Also, methods for better protecting patients' privacy in regard to computerized records are becoming highly advanced.[15, 33]

Medical Information Bus

By 1993, virtually every bedside patient monitor or support device (e.g., intravenous infusion pumps, ventilators, pulse oximeters, and physiological monitors) contained at least one and sometimes several microcomputers. However, since each device was usually made by a different manufacturer, it typically had its own display and was designed to work by itself, or "stand alone." As a result, common practice required that a nurse or therapist read data from the computer display of one of these devices (e.g., a pulse oximeter) and then manually enter the data into a computer terminal to get the data into the ICU's data base computer. An integrated "medical information bus (MIB)" that permits electronic acquisition of data from many different devices would be welcomed by all healthcare providers. Such a system would permit "real-time" data acquisition with little effort and almost no data entry errors. Currently, a committee of the Institute of Electrical and Electronic Engineers (IEEE) is working on the development of a standard for the MIB (IEEE Standard P1073).[27–30] The MIB communications system permits connection of each individual bedside device into a network, allowing almost instantaneous communication with each device. The communication technology being developed will allow the connection of a variety of bedside devices to a main computer and will automatically record their data.

The potential for more accurate and timely data acquisition as well as for labor reduction is enticing. However, the following problems still exist[27–30]:

1. The IEEE has not yet completed its standardization of the MIB standard. However, several of the initial standards have been written and approved.
2. Complex electrical device interfacing problems exist because there is no standard.
3. Complex "people" issues related to data acquisition exist; these include data ownership (e.g., should a nurse or a respiratory therapist enter a patient's fraction of inspired oxygen?), timely recording of data (what is "timely recording"? within 1 minute, 5 minutes, or 1 hour after the data is known?), and the selection and entry of representative data (should one select the high, low, or some other value for the recording interval selected?).

In our work and in that of Gravenstein and his colleagues, many of these issues are now being addressed.[30, 31] Based on several years of experimentation and experience, we have recently made recommendations about these issues.[31]

Better Data and Patient Quality Control Methods

In recent years, the work of Demming[34a] and others has been used to help improve the quality of many of the consumer products we purchase, such as automobiles and television sets. For medicine, Berwick tells us, "Real improvement in quality depends, according to the Theory of Continuous Quality Improvement, on understanding and revising the production process on the basis of data about processes themselves. Every process produces information on the basis of which the process can be improved."[35]

A computerized record remains the principal instrument for ensuring the continuity of care. Several authors have demonstrated that computerized methods can improve the quality of ICU patient care by alerting, reminding, and directing.[36–41] For example, Tate and associates have shown that computerized laboratory alerting leads to a significant increase in the proportion of patients in life-threatening situations who receive appropriate care and reduces the duration of the life-threatening alert condition as well as the length of stay in the hospital.[39] Elliott has shown that the computerized quality assurance monitors of respiratory therapy technologists improve staff member performance when measured against the department's stated policies and procedures.[40] Using computerized methods, Classen and associates found that adverse drug events in a general hospital were actually 80 times more prevalent than was originally thought based on the manual reporting of such events.[41]

DECISION MAKING AND ACCESS TO A MEDICAL KNOWLEDGE BASE

Guidelines for patient care have become widely discussed and applied.[42–46] In 1991, the Society of Critical Care Medicine embraced the concept of using guidelines for care.[46] Guidelines serve to ensure universal delivery of specific and well-accepted standards of care. Guidelines also ensure a minimum level of competence on the part of care providers and that the equipment and surroundings provided within an ICU are adequate. Although the use of computers has not yet been incorporated into formal guidelines, on the basis of the continuous quality improvement topics discussed earlier in this chapter, it is clear that computers can be used as devices to assist in the following of guidelines and improvement of patient care in the ICU.

The mark of a good physician is the ability to make sound clinical judgments. Medical decision making has traditionally been considered an artful and intuitive process rather than a scientific process. In recent years, however, computerized medical decision making has gained greater acceptance.[47–55] Indeed, the discussion of artificial intelligence is commonplace in medicine today. Use of the computer to assist in the complex task of medical decision making in the ICU has just begun.[47]

Computer-assisted decision support has been used in the ICUs at LDS Hospital in Salt Lake City for several years.[48–55] Figure 196–4 is a block diagram of the Health Evaluation through Logical Processing (HELP) computer system used at LDS Hospital. For an ICU patient, the HELP system collects and integrates data from a wide variety of sources. The data are automatically processed by the HELP decision-making system to determine whether the new information by itself or in combination with other data in the patient record, such as laboratory results or a previously generated decision, leads to a new medical decision. These computer-generated medical decisions are based on criteria (knowledge base) stored on the hard drive.

The HELP decision-making system has been used in the following areas: (1) interpretation (e.g., blood gas and hemodynamic parameter interpretation); (2) diagnosis; (3) alerting (i.e., the notification of life-threatening events); and (4) suggestion of treatment.

Development of Methods to "Standardize" Care

The development of algorithms for the care of the critically ill is a new and developing field. Use of the computer to provide clinical treatment instructions to physicians and other caregivers is appealing. Making treatment recommendations using computer methods is currently the most feasible. The art of medicine must be combined with the sciences of medicine to develop the best set of treatment strategies so that the best medical care can be made available to all. Chapter 101 presents further detail of the use of computerized algorithms for patient care.

DEVELOPMENT OF INTENSIVE CARE UNIT PATIENT DATA MANAGEMENT SYSTEMS

Until 1993, the development of computerized patient data management systems has taken place primarily in universi-

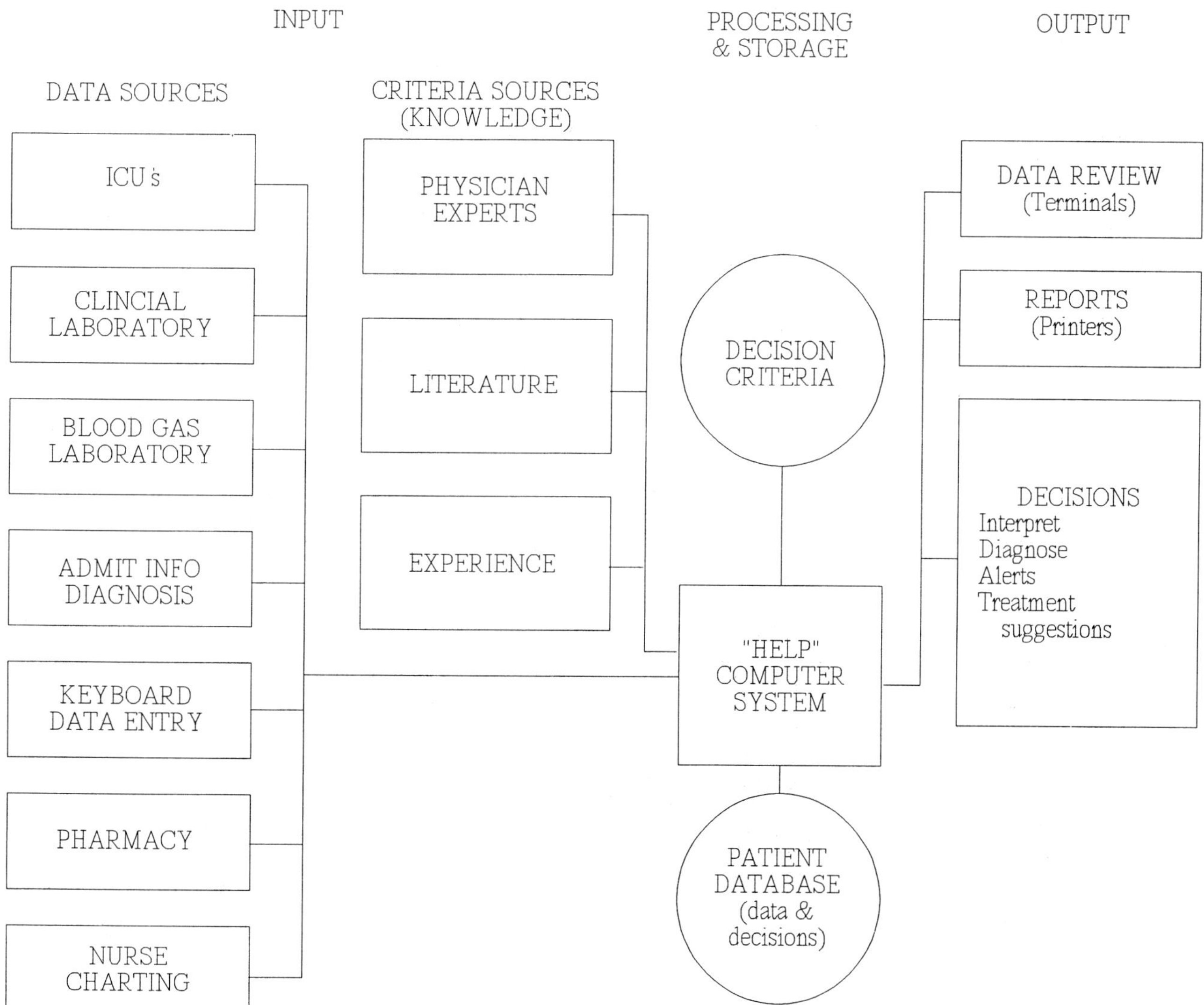

Figure 196–4. Patient data flows into the HELP decision-making computer system from a variety of data sources. The decision-making criteria (knowledge base) are then automatically applied to the data, giving an output of computer-aided decisions. A variety of outputs are generated, including information for review on computer terminals, printed reports, and possible medical decisions.

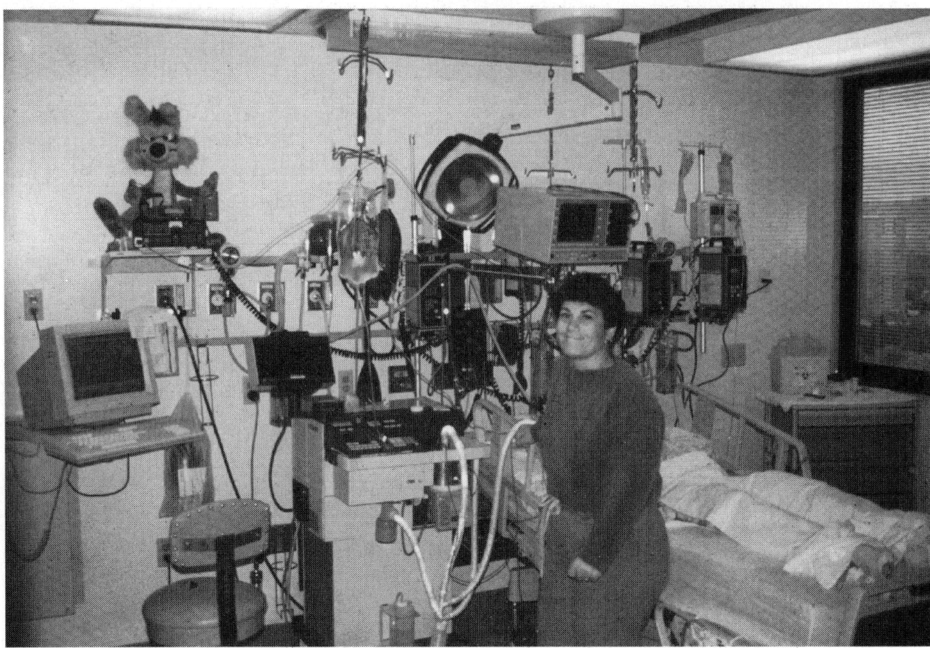

Figure 196–5. A photograph of a patient's room showing a computer terminal at each bedside. Also note the box in the center above the bed; this box is the Medical Information Bus bedside interface. Intravenous pumps, pulse oximeters, and ventilators are connected to the computer system through the Medical Information Bus. (See Color Plate Section of this textbook.)

ties and medical schools and their affiliated hospitals. As a result of the interest and excitement of having computer-assisted care in the ICU, several commercial vendors became interested in the marketing of such systems. A number of commercially available computerized ICU systems that have decision-support capabilities are beginning to become available.

EXAMPLES OF COMPUTERIZED DISPLAYS AND REPORTS

Figure 196–5 shows the scene in our ICU; each ICU room has a patient bed, a bedside terminal, and MIB connections. To satisfy the needs of physicians, nurses, therapists, and others caring for a patient, both bedside terminal screen reviews (displays) and printed reports are generated. To meet the clinical management needs required by critically ill patients and to generate an adequate legal record, most computerized patient data management systems generate printed reports for inclusion in the conventional paper medical record. In the future, a true "electronic" and "paperless" record may replace paper records entirely. However, for the moment, the limitations of display size and the convenience of paper outweigh the technologic advantages of a "paperless" data review.

A few examples of display screen formats and printed

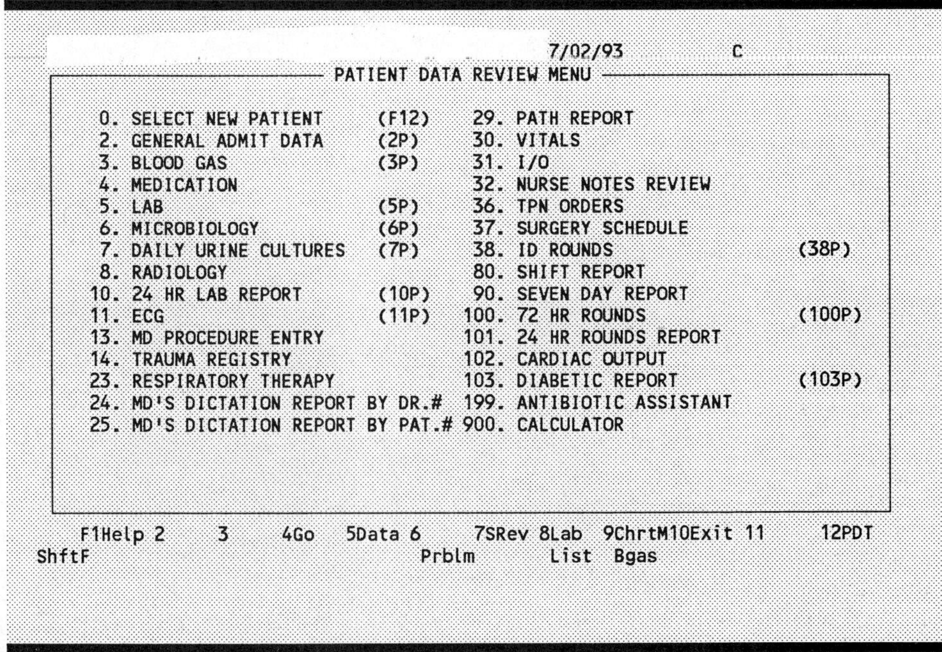

```
                                            7/02/93          C
                       PATIENT DATA REVIEW MENU

    0. SELECT NEW PATIENT      (F12)    29. PATH REPORT
    2. GENERAL ADMIT DATA      (2P)     30. VITALS
    3. BLOOD GAS               (3P)     31. I/O
    4. MEDICATION                       32. NURSE NOTES REVIEW
    5. LAB                     (5P)     36. TPN ORDERS
    6. MICROBIOLOGY            (6P)     37. SURGERY SCHEDULE
    7. DAILY URINE CULTURES    (7P)     38. ID ROUNDS               (38P)
    8. RADIOLOGY                        80. SHIFT REPORT
   10. 24 HR LAB REPORT        (10P)    90. SEVEN DAY REPORT
   11. ECG                     (11P)   100. 72 HR ROUNDS            (100P)
   13. MD PROCEDURE ENTRY              101. 24 HR ROUNDS REPORT
   14. TRAUMA REGISTRY                 102. CARDIAC OUTPUT
   23. RESPIRATORY THERAPY             103. DIABETIC REPORT         (103P)
   24. MD'S DICTATION REPORT BY DR.#   199. ANTIBIOTIC ASSISTANT
   25. MD'S DICTATION REPORT BY PAT.#  900. CALCULATOR

  F1Help 2      3     4Go    5Data 6      7SRev 8Lab  9ChrtM10Exit 11     12PDT
ShftF                               Prblm       List  Bgas
```

Figure 196–6. Terminal MENU.

```
                                                I 07/02/93           C   ADMT DIAGNOSIS: MULTIPLE INJURIES     REPORT DATE: 07/05/93
DR.                           SEX: M   AGE:  25   HEIGHT: 175   WEIGHT:  95.00   APACHE II:    0   MOF:    0  BSA:  2.10
                                                      ICU 24 HOURS ROUNDS REPORT
 CARDIOVASCULAR:  0
   LAST/MAX/MIN   SP:128/161/106   DP: 89/111/ 69   MP:105/135/ 82   HR: 90/150/ 90 | CPK                 CPK-MB
   TIME                CO    CI    HR   SV   SI    VP  MSP  MP  SVR LWI  PW  PA  PVR   RWI  | LACT    2.7 (03:45)
   JUL 05 06:00   7.00  3.33  106  67  32 16.0M 111 101 13  44  16  44  3.0  12.6

 RENAL, FLUIDS, LYTES:  0
   IN   2554 CRYST   2174  COLLOID         BLOOD       NG/PO    380   NA   147 (03:45) K    3.6  (03:45)  CL    112 (03:45)
   OUT  3692 URINE   2225  NGOUT      225  DRAINS   20                CO2 23.0 (03:45) BUN   17  (03:45)  CRE    .9 (03:45)
   NET -1138 WT     95.00  WT-CHG          LOSS   1222 STOOL          OSM              CRCL        UNA      S.G.  1.020

 RESPIRATORY:  0
                pH    PCO2    HCO3    BE    HB   CO/MT   PO2   SO2   O2CT   %O2   AVO2  VO2   C.O. A-a  QS/QT  PK/ PL/PP  MR/SR
   05 05:05 A  7.42   34.4    22.1   -1.1  11.5   2/ 1    81    94   15.3    40                     117          0/  0/ 5  15/ 0
          SAMPLE # 13, TEMP 37.5, BREATHING STATUS : ASSIST/CONTROL

            VENT  MODE  VR   Vt   O2%   PF  IP    MAP  PK   PL  PP  m-Vt  c-Vt  s-Vt  MR  SR  TR  m-VE  s-VE  t-VE  Cth   Pc
   05 12:25  B-II  A/C  15  750   40    50             36   30   5   830   715        15          10.7              28.6
   05 05:34  B-II  A/C  15  750   40    50             38   32   5   920   798        15          12.0              29.6
   -- NO SPONTANEOUS PARAMETERS WITHIN THE LAST 24 HOURS --

  F5-Print   F6-Notes   SF6-X Ray   F7-Vitals   SF7-Resp   F8-Lab   SF8-Urine   F9-Micro   SF9-B Gas   F11-Hemo   F12-New Patient
```

Figure 196–7. Twenty-four–hour ROUNDS (top).

reports are presented to illustrate the convenience and the advantages of computerized data review and reporting. The patient reviewed was a 25-year-old man who sustained an accidental injury and who was admitted to our Shock Trauma Unit.

Most computer systems are "menu"-driven; this means that the clinical user chooses a selection from a menu similar to that shown in Figure 196–6. For example, choosing option 101, the "24 HR ROUNDS REPORT," would yield the display shown in Figure 196–7. This terminal display shows data organized by physiologic system. Note that the blood pressures, cardiac output, and enzyme values related to cardiac function are shown. Data in this rounds report come from a wide variety of locations, including the admitting office, the medical records department, the bedside monitor, the nursing charting input, the chemistry laboratory, the blood gas laboratory, and the respiratory therapy department. The second screen of the record is shown in Figure 196–8 and presents data from the neurologic and psychologic assessment (note the Glasgow Scale Score of 14) as well as other data. Figure 196–9 shows the results of microbiologic analysis and the fact that there was a "positive micro result" along with the medication data. Typically, the 24-hour rounds report is printed; however, display terminal review is most convenient for physicians who access the computer system from their homes or offices.

If a physician wanted to review more detailed hemodynamic data while reviewing the 24-hour rounds report from the terminal, he or she could push the F11 key on the extended keyboard and within a few seconds would see the display shown in Figure 196–10. Note the computerized interpretation of the hemodynamic results as well as the listing of cardioactive medications (dopamine in this case) relevant to the results.

Pressing the F8 key would yield the laboratory results. An example screen is shown in Figure 196–11. Note that high and low values are marked with an H or an L, respectively. On the actual screen, these values are highlighted in

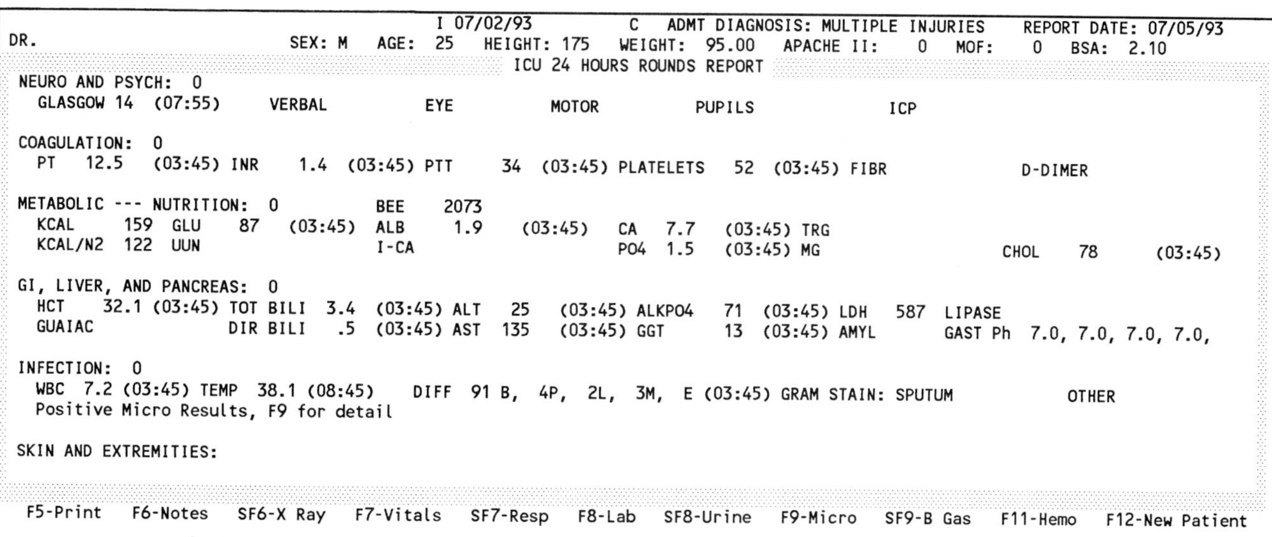

```
                                                I 07/02/93           C   ADMT DIAGNOSIS: MULTIPLE INJURIES     REPORT DATE: 07/05/93
DR.                           SEX: M   AGE:  25   HEIGHT: 175   WEIGHT:  95.00   APACHE II:    0   MOF:    0  BSA:  2.10
                                                      ICU 24 HOURS ROUNDS REPORT
 NEURO AND PSYCH:  0
   GLASGOW 14  (07:55)     VERBAL          EYE          MOTOR          PUPILS             ICP

 COAGULATION:  0
   PT   12.5   (03:45) INR    1.4  (03:45) PTT    34  (03:45) PLATELETS   52  (03:45) FIBR             D-DIMER

 METABOLIC --- NUTRITION:  0           BEE    2073
   KCAL     159  GLU    87   (03:45)  ALB     1.9    (03:45)   CA   7.7   (03:45) TRG
   KCAL/N2  122  UUN                  I-CA                     PO4  1.5   (03:45) MG                CHOL    78      (03:45)

 GI, LIVER, AND PANCREAS:  0
   HCT   32.1 (03:45) TOT BILI  3.4  (03:45) ALT   25   (03:45) ALKPO4   71  (03:45) LDH   587  LIPASE
   GUAIAC             DIR BILI   .5  (03:45) AST  135   (03:45) GGT      13  (03:45) AMYL       GAST Ph  7.0, 7.0, 7.0, 7.0,

 INFECTION:  0
   WBC  7.2 (03:45) TEMP  38.1 (08:45)   DIFF  91 B,  4P,  2L,  3M,  E (03:45) GRAM STAIN: SPUTUM        OTHER
   Positive Micro Results, F9 for detail

 SKIN AND EXTREMITIES:

  F5-Print   F6-Notes   SF6-X Ray   F7-Vitals   SF7-Resp   F8-Lab   SF8-Urine   F9-Micro   SF9-B Gas   F11-Hemo   F12-New Patient
```

Figure 196–8. Twenty-four–hour ROUNDS (middle).

```
                                     I 07/02/93          C    ADMT DIAGNOSIS: MULTIPLE INJURIES     REPORT DATE: 07/05/93
DR.                      SEX: M   AGE:  25   HEIGHT: 175   WEIGHT:  95.00   APACHE II:    0   MOF:    0   BSA:  2.10
                                          ICU 24 HOURS ROUNDS REPORT

INFECTION:  0
  WBC  7.2 (03:45) TEMP  38.1 (08:45)    DIFF  91 B,  4P,  2L,  3M,  E (03:45) GRAM STAIN: SPUTUM              OTHER
  Positive Micro Results, F9 for detail

SKIN AND EXTREMITIES:

MEDICATIONS:
  MORPHINE, INJ                 30.00    DOPAMINE, INJ                    .00    TAP WATER, LIQUID          60.00
  MIDAZOLAM (VERSED), INJ       15.00    RANITIDINE HCL (ZANTAC),     150.00    JEVITY, LIQUID            150.00
  METRONIDAZOLE (FLAGYL),     2000.00    POTASSIUM CHLORIDE, INJ       43.46    TAP WATER, LIQUID         150.00
  CEFTAZIDIME (FORTAZ), IN    3000.00    POTASSIUM PHOSPHATE, INJ       9.00
  VANCOMYCIN (VANCOCIN), I    2000.00    MAGNESIUM SULFATE 50%, I       1.00

TUBES:
  VEN ________  ART ________  SG ________  NG ________  FOLEY ________  ET ________  TRACH ________  DRAIN________
  CHEST ____________  RECTAL ______  JEJUNAL ________  DIALYSIS ________  OTHER ______________________________

                                  --- End of Report ---

  F5-Print  F6-Notes  SF6-X Ray  F7-Vitals  SF7-Resp  F8-Lab  SF8-Urine  F9-Micro  SF9-B Gas  F11-Hemo  F12-New Patient
```

Figure 196–9. Twenty-four–hour ROUNDS (bottom).

color to make them clearly visible. All laboratory results are available, but only the chemistry data are shown here.

Figure 196–12 shows a transcribed radiography report for the patient. Typically, after the film is read and observations are dictated, on-screen review is available within 1 hour. Figure 196–13 shows an example of nursing notes for the patient. Figure 196–14 shows a typical respiratory therapy display screen. All of the reports noted can also be printed.

A shift report is generated for each 12-hour period. Figure 196–15 is a shift report for the same patient. Note that vital signs (all automatically acquired with the MIB) are shown graphically, and fluid intake and output results are shown for the most current 12 hours and are summarized for an entire 24-hour period. In this case, the patient has a 5856 net balance gain. Since the patient was not weighed, a comparison of weight gain or loss cannot be made with fluid status. Below the vital sign graphics are measurement data. Some of the data are acquired automatically, and some are entered manually. Laboratory data are transmitted from the laboratory computer system to the ICU-HELP system. At the bottom of the screen, the medications that have been given are shown, with the amounts and times indicated graphically. The infusions are noted next. For example, infusion of dopamine, 4.40 $\mu g \cdot kg^{-1} \cdot min^{-1}$, was begun at 2200 hrs. The infusion data comes from intravenous infusion pumps with MIB interfaces. Next, blood gas data with computerized interpretations are presented. Note also that if arterial and venous blood gas values are available for the same time

Text continued on page 1769

```
                                             I 25Y M  07/02/93
HT 175 CM  WT 95.00 KG   BSA 2.10  SQM        DR CHRISTENSEN, B

TIME              CO    CI   HR  SV  SI  MP  MSP PA   RA  PW  PVR SVR  RWI  LWI
NORMAL HI        7.3  3.50   89 101  48 105  123 19    5  12  1.0  18  11.0  85
NORMAL LOW       2.9  2.80   49  47  38  70   80  9    1   4  0.5  12   8.0  48
------------------------ Review/Print Cardiac Output ------------------------
JUL 05 06:00     7.0  3.33 104  67  32  98  111 31   10  10  3.0  13  12.6  44
           LV PARAMETERS ARE WITHIN NORMAL LIMITS

JUL 04 04:00     7.4  3.41 111  67  31  86   98 37   12  12  3.4  10  13.0  36
           MILD LV DYSFUNCTION

JUL 03 04:00     7.6  4.00 116  66  34  64   77 33   12  16  2.2   7  12.7  29
            JUL 03 03:52  DOPAMINE (INTROPIN) 10.70 MCG/KG/MIN
            MODERATE LV DYSFUNCTION

JUL 02 22:10     5.1  2.68 114  45  24  66   77 31   14  16  2.9  10   6.7  19
            JUL 02 22:00  DOPAMINE (INTROPIN)  4.40 MCG/KG/MIN
            MODERATE LV DYSFUNCTION

>

                                  F9 - SCROLL
```

Figure 196–10. Hemodynamics.

C

CHEM 7

DATE	TIME		NA MMOL/L	K MMOL/L	CL MMOL/L	CO2 MMOL/L	BUN MG/DL	GLU MG/DL	CREAT MG/DL
05JUL	03:45	SE	**147H**	3.6	112	23	17	87	.9
04JUL	04:05	SE	146	3.6	**113H**	22	**22H**	71	1.0
03JUL	23:00	SE	144	3.8	**115H**	**19L**	**21H**	80	1.1
03JUL	03:55	SE	145	3.6	112	20	**22H**	101	1.2

CHEM 13

DATE	TIME		URAC MG/DL	TPRT GM/DL	ALB GM/DL	CA MG/DL	PHOS MG/L	CHOL MG/DL	TBIL MG/DL	DBIL MG/DL	ALKP IU/L	GGT U/L	LDH U/L	AST U/L	ALT U/L
05JUL	03:45	SE	4.6	**4.3L**	**1.9L**	**7.7L**	**1.5L**	78	**3.4H**	**.5H**	71	13	**587H**	**135H**	25
04JUL	04:05	SE	4.2	**4.3L**	**2.1L**	**7.6L**	**1.9L**	65	**7.4H**	**1.1H**	53	15	**632H**	**149H**	21
03JUL	03:55	SE	4.4	**4.0L**	**2.1L**	**7.0L**	2.6	71	**4.1H**	**.9H**	35	17	**534H**	**103H**	19
02JUL	09:50	SE	5.6	**3.8L**	**2.1L**	**7.2L**	**4.6H**	49	**3.3H**	.3	22L	15	**796H**	**139H**	26

LACTIC ACID, PLASMA (VENOUS)

DATE	TIME		LA-PLS MMOL/L
05JUL	03:45	PL	**2.7H**
04JUL	04:05	PL	**3.7H**

Figure 196–11. Laboratory data.

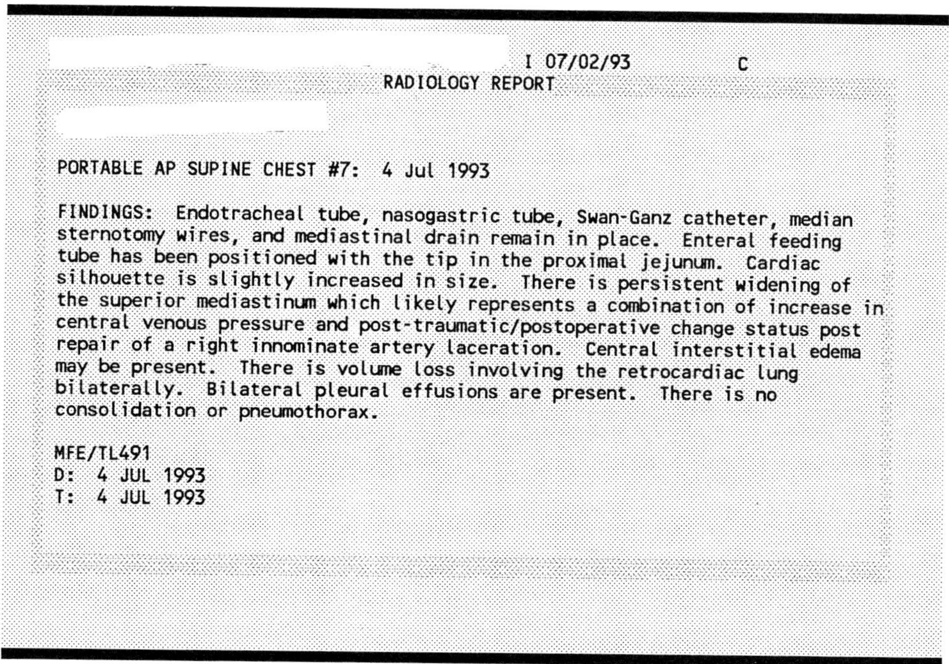

I 07/02/93 C

RADIOLOGY REPORT

PORTABLE AP SUPINE CHEST #7: 4 Jul 1993

FINDINGS: Endotracheal tube, nasogastric tube, Swan-Ganz catheter, median sternotomy wires, and mediastinal drain remain in place. Enteral feeding tube has been positioned with the tip in the proximal jejunum. Cardiac silhouette is slightly increased in size. There is persistent widening of the superior mediastinum which likely represents a combination of increase in central venous pressure and post-traumatic/postoperative change status post repair of a right innominate artery laceration. Central interstitial edema may be present. There is volume loss involving the retrocardiac lung bilaterally. Bilateral pleural effusions are present. There is no consolidation or pneumothorax.

MFE/TL491
D: 4 JUL 1993
T: 4 JUL 1993

Figure 196–12. Radiology report.

FLOOR COMMENTS

NAME· NO. ROOM:
DR. SEX: M AGE: 25 HEIGHT: 175 cm WEIGHT: 95.00 kg BSA:2.10 SQM
ADMIT DIAGNOSIS: MULTIPLE INJURIES ADMIT DATE: JUL 02 05:23

DATE/TIME	ACTION	
05 JUL 12:07	EMOTIONAL SUPPORT	: Emotional support - patient, Emotional support - family, Vented feelings, Discussed hospitalization, Discussed treatment, Discussed disease process, Tim spent 5 min. (es)
05 JUL 12:01	GU OUPUT	: Foley cath out 185 ml, Amber, Clear Mean BP 103
	OXIMETRY	: STO2 (finger): 95
05 JUL 11:16	INVASIVE LINES & TUBES	: Cordis, Right, Jugular, Dressing changed, Time spent 5 min. (D), Betadine, None, Clean, Dry
05 JUL 11:13	INVASIVE LINES & TUBES	: Opticath swan, Right, Jugular, Removed
05 JUL 10:59	TUBE/DRAIN MANAGEMENT	: Small ga. feed tube, Comment: FULL STRENGTH JEVITY
05 JUL 10:00	IRRIGATION	: Small ga. feeding tube, Tube feed infuse rate: 30 cc/hr
05 JUL 09:59	GU OUPUT	: Foley cath out 160 ml, Amber, Clear Mean BP 104
	OXIMETRY	: SVO2: 65, STO2 (finger): 92

Press <Enter> for more data, <Esc> to quit, F6 = Search time, F7 = Print, F12 = New patient

Figure 196–13. Nurse comments.

C

RESPIRATORY CARE CHARTING

07/05/93

VENTILATOR MONITORING

	VENT	MODE	VR	Vt	O2	PF	IP	TEMP	IE RATIO	PK	PL	MAP	PP	m-Vt	c-Vt	s-Vt	MR	SR	TR	m-VE	s-VE	t-VE	Cth	aOX	vOX	Pc	CF
05 12:25	B-II	A/C	15	750	40	50		35.0	1: 2.8	36	30		5	830	716		15			10.7			28.6	95			3.7
05 09:57	B-II	A/C	15	750	40	50		35.0	1: 2.8	36	28		5	710	596		15			8.9			25.9	93			3.7
05 07:25	B-II	A/C	15	750	40	50		35.0	1: 2.6	35	32		5	910	799		15			12.0			29.6	95		20	3.7
05 05:34	B-II	A/C	15	750	40	50		35.0	1: 2.8	38	32		5	920	798		15			12.0			29.6	94	66		3.7
05 03:41	B-II	A/C	15	750	40	50		35.0	1: 2.7	40	33		5	880	751		15			11.3			26.8	91	62		3.7
05 01:42	B-II	A/C	15	750	40	50		35.0	1: 2.9	37	30		5	780	620		15			9.3			24.8	95	63		5.0

07/05/93	DUR/ENTRY	OBSERVATIONS
05 12:25	10/12:26	- INTERFACE: ORALTRACH TUBE; ALARMS CHECKED; TEMP SETTING: 35.0; POSITION: SEMI-FOWLER; PATIENT CONDITION: CALM THERAPIST: LARRY RRT
05 09:57	10/09:58	- INTERFACE: ORALTRACH TUBE; ALARMS CHECKED; TEMP SETTING: 35.0; POSITION: SEMI-FOWLER; PATIENT CONDITION: CALM THERAPIST: LARRY RRT
05 07:25	10/07:27	- INTERFACE: ORALTRACH TUBE; ALARMS CHECKED; TEMP SETTING: 35.0; POSITION: SEMI-FOWLER; PATIENT CONDITION: CALM THERAPIST: LARRY RRT
05 05:34	5/05:36	- INTERFACE: ORALTRACH TUBE; ALARMS CHECKED; TEMP SETTING: 35.0; POSITION: SEMI-FOWLER; PATIENT CONDITION: SEMI CONSCIOUS, CALM; THERAPIST: TED RRT

------------ Press <Enter> for more...

Press <Enter> to continue, <Esc> to quit, <Page Up>, <Page Down>, arrow keys, <F5> to change search time, <F6> to print

Figure 196–14. Respiratory therapy data.

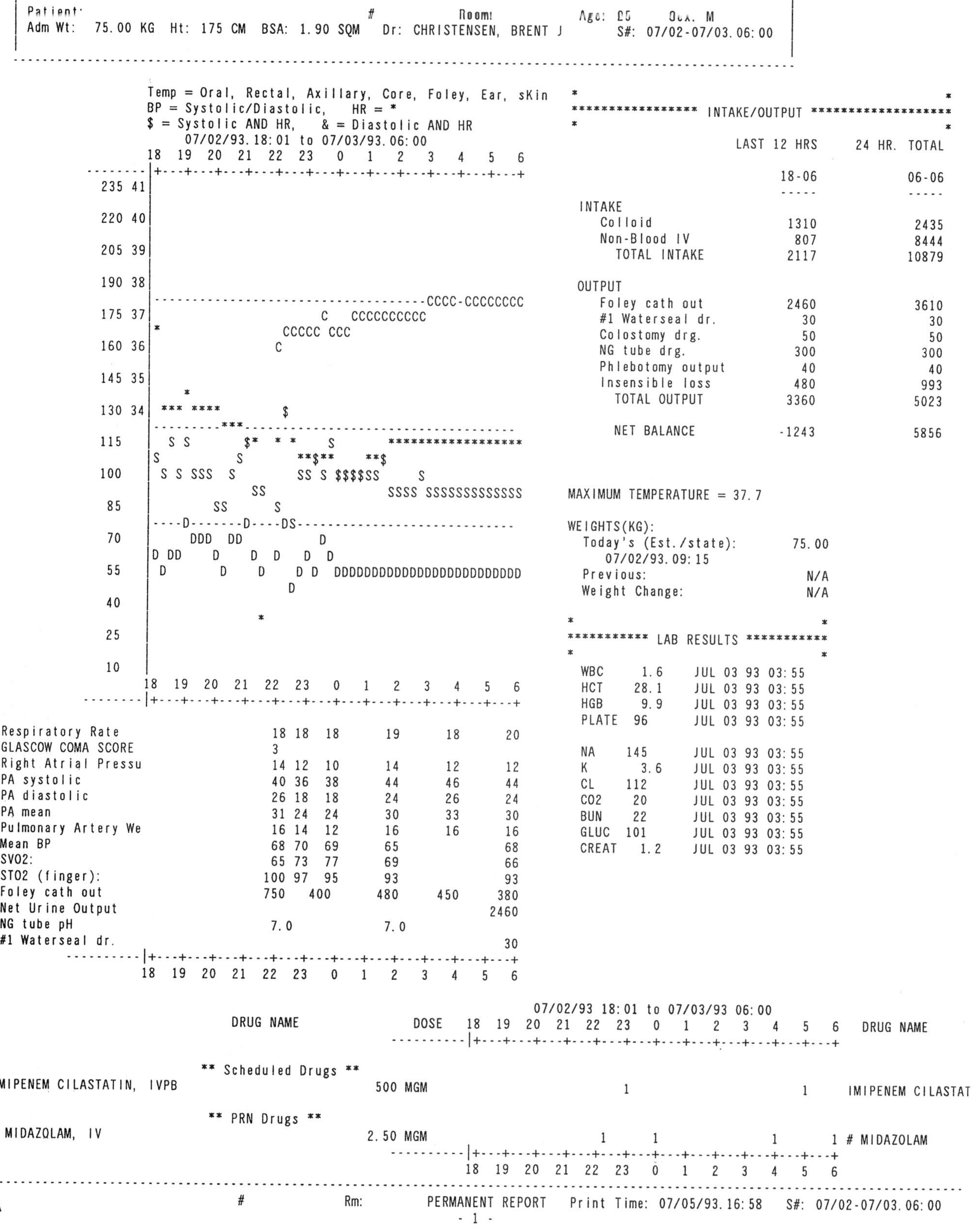

```
------------------------------------------- SHIFT REPORT ----------------------------------------
                          07/02/93. 18:01 to 07/03/93. 06:00

Patient:                                 #          Room:          Age: 55     Sex. M
Adm Wt:   75.00 KG  Ht: 175 CM  BSA: 1.90 SQM  Dr: CHRISTENSEN, BRENT J     S#: 07/02-07/03. 06:00
-------------------------------------------------------------------------------------------------

Temp = Oral, Rectal, Axillary, Core, Foley, Ear, sKin
BP = Systolic/Diastolic,     HR = *
$ = Systolic AND HR,     & = Diastolic AND HR
     07/02/93. 18:01 to 07/03/93. 06:00
        18  19  20  21  22  23   0   1   2   3   4   5   6
-------|+---+---+---+---+---+---+---+---+---+---+---+---+
235 41 |
220 40 |
205 39 |
190 38 |
       |-----------------------------------CCCC-CCCCCCCC
175 37 |                        C   CCCCCCCCCC
       |*                 CCCCC CCC
160 36 |                  C
145 35 |
       |    *
130 34 | *** ****           $
       |---------***-----------------------------------
115    | S S      $*  * *     S        ******************
       |S         S      **$**    **$
100    | S S SSS  S      SS S $$$$$SS     S
       |           SS               SSSS SSSSSSSSSSSSS
85     |       SS      S
       |----D-------D----DS---------------------------
70     |     DDD  DD          D
       |D DD    D     D  D    D  D
55     | D       D     D     D D  DDDDDDDDDDDDDDDDDDDDDDDDD
       |                      D
40     |
       |              *
25     |
10     |
        18  19  20  21  22  23   0   1   2   3   4   5   6
-------|+---+---+---+---+---+---+---+---+---+---+---+---+
```

	18	19	20	21	22	23	0	1	2	3	4	5	6
Respiratory Rate					18	18	18		19		18		20
GLASCOW COMA SCORE					3								
Right Atrial Pressu					14	12	10		14		12		12
PA systolic					40	36	38		44		46		44
PA diastolic					26	18	18		24		26		24
PA mean					31	24	24		30		33		30
Pulmonary Artery We					16	14	12		16		16		16
Mean BP					68	70	69		65				68
SVO2:					65	73	77		69				66
STO2 (finger):					100	97	95		93				93
Foley cath out					750		400		480		450		380
Net Urine Output													2460
NG tube pH					7.0				7.0				
#1 Waterseal dr.													30

```
*                                                        *
***************** INTAKE/OUTPUT ******************
*                                                        *
```

	LAST 12 HRS 18-06	24 HR. TOTAL 06-06
INTAKE		
Colloid	1310	2435
Non-Blood IV	807	8444
TOTAL INTAKE	2117	10879
OUTPUT		
Foley cath out	2460	3610
#1 Waterseal dr.	30	30
Colostomy drg.	50	50
NG tube drg.	300	300
Phlebotomy output	40	40
Insensible loss	480	993
TOTAL OUTPUT	3360	5023
NET BALANCE	-1243	5856

MAXIMUM TEMPERATURE = 37.7

WEIGHTS(KG):
Today's (Est./state): 75.00
07/02/93. 09:15
Previous: N/A
Weight Change: N/A

```
*                                   *
*********** LAB RESULTS ***********
*                                   *
```

WBC	1.6	JUL 03 93 03:55
HCT	28.1	JUL 03 93 03:55
HGB	9.9	JUL 03 93 03:55
PLATE	96	JUL 03 93 03:55
NA	145	JUL 03 93 03:55
K	3.6	JUL 03 93 03:55
CL	112	JUL 03 93 03:55
CO2	20	JUL 03 93 03:55
BUN	22	JUL 03 93 03:55
GLUC	101	JUL 03 93 03:55
CREAT	1.2	JUL 03 93 03:55

07/02/93 18:01 to 07/03/93 06:00

DRUG NAME	DOSE	18	19	20	21	22	23	0	1	2	3	4	5	6	DRUG NAME
** Scheduled Drugs **															
IMIPENEM CILASTATIN, IVPB	500 MGM						1						1		IMIPENEM CILASTAT
** PRN Drugs **															
# MIDAZOLAM, IV	2.50 MGM						1		1			1		1	# MIDAZOLAM

```
A              #        Rm:        PERMANENT REPORT  Print Time: 07/05/93. 16:58   S#: 07/02-07/03. 06:00
                                         - 1 -
```

Figure 196–15. *A and B,* Shift report for a 12-hour ICU nursing shift.

Illustration continued on following page

```
                                                                                18  19  20  21  22  23   0   1   2   3   4   5   6
                                                                      ----------|+---+---+---+---+---+---+---+---+---+---+---+---+
# MORPHINE, IV                                            5.00 MGM                                   1   2                      11 # MORPHINE

                                  ** Infusions **
DOPAMINE 400 MGM, IVD                                                           |                          111111111111111111111111 DOPAMINE
    <D5W 100 ML, INJ>                                                           |                   4478880000000000000000000000000
                                                 RATE      .100 MCG/KG/M        |                   4419999777777777777777777777777
--------------------------------------------------------------------------------|------------------------------------------------
LACTATED RINGERS 100 ML, IVD                                                    |                   22111                           LACTATED RINGERS
                                                                                |                   22000
                                                 RATE         1 ML/HOUR         |                   55000
--------------------------------------------------------------------------------|------------------------------------------------
NACL 0.45% 607 ML, IVD                                                          |                                                   NACL 0.45%
                                                 RATE       100 ML/HOUR         |                          11111111111111111111111
--------------------------------------------------------------------------------|------------------------------------------------
FRESH FROZEN PLASMA 230 ML, IVD                                                 |                              **                   FRESH FROZEN PLAS
    <O  POSITIVE, 0.>                                                           |
    <NO.    2089887>                                                            |
FRESH FROZEN PLASMA 230 ML, IVD                                                 |                               **                  FRESH FROZEN PLAS
    <O  POSITIVE, 1>                                                            |
    <NO.    1359868>                                                            |
FRESH FROZEN PLASMA 230 ML, IVD                                                 |                                *                  FRESH FROZEN PLAS
    <O  POSITIVE, 1>                                                            |
    <NO.    1359834>                                                            |
FRESH FROZEN PLASMA 180 ML, IVD                                                 |                                 **                FRESH FROZEN PLAS
    <O  POSITIVE, 1>                                                            |
    <NO.    133637>                                                             |
FRESH FROZEN PLASMA 230 ML, IVD                                                 |                                  **               FRESH FROZEN PLAS
    <O  POSITIVE, 1>                                                            |
    <NO.    1359888>                                                            |
FRESH FROZEN PLASMA 210 ML, IVD                                                 |                                  *                FRESH FROZEN PLAS
    <O  POSITIVE, 1>                                                            |
    <NO.    1836597>                                                            |
                                                                      ----------|+---+---+---+---+---+---+---+---+---+---+---+---+
                                                                                18  19  20  21  22  23   0   1   2   3   4   5   6

JUL 03 93     pH     PCO2     HCO3     BE    HB   CO/MT   PO2   SO2   O2CT   %O2  AVO2  VO2   C.O.   A-a  Qs/Qt  PK/ PL/PP  MR/SR
              --     ----                                 ---
NORMAL HI    7.45    39.3     25.1    2.5  17.7   2/ 1                                5.5  300   7.30   18    5
NORMAL LOW   7.35    25.9     15.0   -2.5  13.7   0/ 1     69    92   18.7            3.0  200   2.90         0

03 04:01 V   7.40    34.7     21.2   -2.4   9.8   2/ 1     32    67    9.3    40                                      /    / 5  18/
03 04:00 A   7.42    30.0     19.3   -3.6  10.0   2/ 1     87    96   13.5    40     4.05 308   7.60  116   13        /    / 5  18/
             SAMPLE # 11, TEMP 37.0, BREATHING STATUS : ASSIST/CONTROL
             NORMAL ARTERIAL ACID-BASE CHEMISTRY
             SEVERELY REDUCED O2 CONTENT (13.5) DUE TO ANEMIA (LOW HB)
             PULSE OXIMETER SO2  92.0
03 00:06 A   7.36    32.5     18.1   -5.9  12.0   2/ 1    128    97   16.5    80                        312            34/  29/ 5  18/
02 22:02 V   7.23    48.6     19.8   -7.5  11.3   2/ 1     33    63   10.0   100                                      /    / 5  18/
02 22:01 A   7.28    40.2     18.5   -7.5  11.2   2/ 1     82    94   14.9   100     4.98 254   5.10  471   29        /    / 5  18/
02 18:51 V   7.12    61.6     19.3  -10.1   9.4   2/ 1     46    71    9.4    93

------------------------------------------------------------ HEMODYMANICS -------------------------------------------------------

NORMAL HI        7.30  3.50  89 101  48 105  123 19  5.0  12  1.0  18  11.0  85
NORMAL LOW       2.90  2.80  49  47  38  70   80  9  1.0   4  0.5  12   8.0  48

TIME               CO    CI  HR  SV  SI  MP  MSP PA   RA  PW  PVR SVR   RWI LWI

JUL 03 04:00      7.6  4.00 116  66  34  64   77 33   12  16  2.2   7  12.7  29
          JUL 03 03:52  DOPAMINE (INTROPIN) 10.70 MCG/KG/MIN
          MODERATE LV DYSFUNCTION

JUL 02 22:10      5.1  2.68 114  45  24  66   77 31   14  16  2.9  10   6.7  19
          JUL 02 22:00  DOPAMINE (INTROPIN)  4.40 MCG/KG/MIN
          MODERATE LV DYSFUNCTION

                                                                                18  19  20  21  22  23   0   1   2   3   4   5   6
                                                                      ----------|+---+---+---+---+---+---+---+---+---+---+---+---+
  07/02/93.22:00  To 07/03/93.06:00                 CODY, RN                                *********************************



---------------------------------------------------------------------------------------------------------------------------------
B                                  #              Rm:          PERMANENT REPORT   Print Time: 07/05/93.16:58    S#: 07/02-07/03.06:00
                                                                     - 2 -
```

Figure 196–15 *Continued*

intervals that hemodynamic data are available, then arterial-to-venous oxygen content differences and oxygen consumption are calculated. Finally, the nurse or nurses who cared for the patient are shown, with the interval of care provision indicated by a row of asterisks.

THE FUTURE

The future of computers in the ICU is bright. With the improvement in performance of microprocessors and the continuous reduction in their cost, these devices will continue to become integral components of the ICU. The availability of adequate computer hardware will not be the limiting factor.

The use of computers to improve the speed and accuracy of communication of patient data is already well established. The use of computers to guide patient therapy is a new and exciting concept that, based on early experience, appears to be well accepted by medical professionals and that seems to provide improved outcomes. The limiting factors in the future use of computers in the ICU will be (1) human, cultural, and sociologic issues; (2) development of standards for sharing data and medical knowledge; (3) establishment of data acquisition methodologies that meet the competing demands of "What is enough data?" and "What can we afford?"; and finally, (4) societal views about the rationing of patient care.

SUMMARY: A MATCH MEANT TO BE!

Combining the computer and the modern ICU is certainly a match meant to be. Several advantages of computer systems in the ICU have been demonstrated. These systems can assist in data collection, provide computational capability, assist in data communications and integration of data, improve record keeping, enhance report generation, assist in medical decision making, and assist with protocol-directed care. As Dr. John J. Osborn, a pioneer in the field of computerized ICU, said so well 15 years ago,[56]

"The great mass of useful numbers we generate by computer has got to be tamed and controlled. We have learned how to make the measurements. Now we must learn how to handle the resulting data and present them in understandable terms. Used right, automation can integrate these data, simplify them, scan them and evaluate them. Automation is not a cold-blooded monster-machine between us and the patient. It is a tool to expand our medical power, to let us get closer to the patient, and take better care of him."

We who are now using the computer to assist with patient care and those who will be in the future should take confidence in Dr. Osborn's comments and make his dream our reality.

References

1. Medical Informatics: Computer Applications in Health Care. Shortliffe EH, Perreault LE (Eds). Reading, MA, Addison-Wesley Publishing Co, 1990.
2. Rennels GD, Shortliffe EH: Advanced computing for medicine. Sci Am 1987; 257:154–161.
3. Kroll DA: The automated record: Legal help or Pandora's box? J Clin Monit 1991; 7:77–78.
4. Brimm JE: Computers in critical care. Crit Care Q 1987; 9:53–63.
5. Gardner RM: Computerized data management and decision-making in critical care. Surg Clin North Am 1985; 65:1041.
6. Gardner RM: Computerized management of intensive care patients. MD Comput 1986; 3:36.
7. Tong HD, Gupta A: Personal computers. Sci Am 1982; 247:87.
8. Comerford R: Engineering workstations and PCs. IEEE Spectrum 1993; 30:37–76.
9. Barnett GO: The application of computer based medical records systems in ambulatory care. N Engl J Med 1984; 310:1643.
10. Dick RS, Steen EB (Eds): The computer-based patient record: An essential technology for health care. Washington, DC, National Academy Press, 1991.
11. Shortliffe EH, Tang PC, Detmer DE: Patient records and computers. Ann Intern Med 1991; 115:979–981.
12. McDonald CJ, Tierney WM: Computer-stored medical records: Their future role in medical practice. JAMA 1988; 259:3433–3440.
13. Whiting-O'Keefe QE, Simborg DW, Epstein WV, et al: A computerized summary medical record system can provide more information than the standard medical record. JAMA 1985; 254:1185.
14. Osheroff JA, Forsythe DE, Buchanan BG, et al: Physicians' information needs: Analysis of questions posed during clinical teaching. Ann Intern Med 1991; 114:476–481.
15. Hammond WE: Security, privacy, and confidentiality: A perspective. J Health Inf Manage Res 1992; 1:1–8.
16. Classen DC, Evans RS, Pestotnik SL, et al: The timing of prophylactic administration of antibiotics and the risk of surgical-wound infection. N Engl J Med 1992; 326:281–286.
17. Bradshaw KE, Gardner RM, Clemmer TP, et al: Physical decision-making: Evaluation of data used in a computerized ICU. Int J Clin Monit Comput 1984; 1:81.
18. Iglehart JK: The American health care system: Managed care. N Engl J Med 1992; 327:742–747.
19. Clinton W: The Clinton health care plan. N Engl J Med 1992; 327:804–807.
20. Reinhart UE: Politics and the health care system. N Engl J Med 1992; 327:809–811.
21. Tierney WM, Miller MM, Overhage JM, et al: Physician inpatient order writing on microcomputer workstations: Effects on resource utilization. JAMA 1993; 269:379–383.
22. Budd MC, Blaufuss J, Harada S: Nursing: A revenue center, not a cost center. Comp Healthcare, November 1988, pp 24–26.
23. Clemmer TP, Gardner RM: Medical Informatics in the Intensive Care Unit: State of the Art 1991. Int J Clin Monit Comput 1992; 8:237–250.
24. Bradshaw KE, Sittig DF, Gardner RM, et al: Computer-based data entry for nurses in the ICU. MD Comput 1989; 6:274–280.
25. Blaufuss J: Promoting the nursing process through computerization. Washington, DC, International Medical Informatics Association 86, 1986, pp 585–586.
26. Gardner RM, Bradshaw KE, Hollingsworth KW: Computerizing the intensive care unit: Current status and future directions. J Cardiovasc Nurs 1989; 4:68–78.
27. Shabot MM: Standardized acquisition of bedside data: The IEEE P1073 Medical Information Bus. Int J Clin Monit Comput 1989; 6:197–204.
28. IEEE P1073.3.1 Standard for Medical Device Communications, Transport Profile. Approved May 17, 1994.

28a. IEEE P1073.4.1 Standard for Medical Device Communications, Physical Layer–Cable Connection. Approved May 17, 1994.

29. IEEE 1073.1 (Proposed) Standard for Medicial Device Data Language (MDDL). Revision 0.10, January 24, 1994.
30. Gravenstein JS, deVries A Jr, Beneken JEW: Sampling intervals for monitoring of variables during anesthesia. J Clin Monit 1989; 5:17–21.
31. Gardner RM, Hawley WH, East TD, et al: Real time data acquisition: Recommendations for the medical information bus (MIB). Int J Clin Monit Comput 1992; 8:251–258.

31a. Oniki TA, Gardner RM: Computerized detection of arterial oxygen desaturations in an intensive care unit. Proc Annu Symp Comput Appl Med Care 1993; 17:356–360.

31b. Oniki TA, Clemmer TP, Gardner RM, et al: Computerized charting of vital signs in an intensive care unit. Proc Annu Symp Comput Appl Med Care 1994; 18:307–311.

32. McDonald CJ, Hammond WE: Standard formats for electronic record transfer of clinical data (Editorial). Ann Intern Med 1989; 110:333–335.
33. American Medical Informatics Association: Position Paper on Standards for Medical Identifiers, Codes and Messages Needed to Create an Efficient Computer-Stored Medical Record. J Am Med Informatics Assoc 1994; 1:1–7.
34. Rossing N: European Community research: Telematics for

health care and standardization. IEEE Trans Biomed Eng 1993; 12:70–74.
34a. Demming WE: Quality, Productivity, and Competitive Position. Cambridge, MA, Massachusetts Institute of Technology Center for Advanced Engineering Study, 1982.
35. Berwick DM: Continuous improvement as an ideal in health care. N Engl J Med 1989; 320:54–56.
36. Luce JM: Improving the quality and utilization of critical care. QRB Qual Rev Bull 1990; 16:398–403.
37. Weissman C, Mossel P, Haimet S, et al: Integration of quality assurance activities into a computerized patient management system in an intensive care unit. QRB Qual Rev Bull 1991; 17:42–47.
38. Sue DY: Development of an ICU patient care monitoring and evaluation system in a teaching hospital. QRB Qual Rev Bull 1991; 17:97–103.
39. Tate KE, Gardner RM, Weaver LK: A computerized laboratory alerting system. MD Comput 1990; 7:296–301.
39a. Tate KE, Gardner RM: Computers, quality and the clinical laboratory: A look at critical value reporting. Proc Annu Symp Comput Appl Med Care 1993; 17:193–197.
40. Elliott CG: Computer-assisted quality assurance: Development and performance of a respiratory care program. QRB Qual Rev Bull 1991; 17:85–89.
41. Classen DC, Pestotnik SL, Evans RS, et al: Computerized surveillance of adverse drug events in hospital patients. JAMA 1991; 266:2847–2851.
41a. Evans RS, Classen DC, Stevens LE, et al: Using a hospital information system to assess the effects of adverse drug events. Proc Annu Symp Comput Appl Med Care 1993; 17:161–165.
42. Fields MJ, Lohr KN (Eds): Guidelines for Clinical Practice: From Development to Use. Washington, DC, National Academy Press, 1992.
43. Eddy DM: Clinical decision making, from theory to practice: The challenge. JAMA 1990; 263:287–290.
44. Eddy DM: Clinical decision making, from theory to practice: Anatomy of a decision. JAMA 1990; 263:441–443.
45. Eddy DM: Clinical decision making, from theory to practice: Practice policies: Where do they come from? JAMA 1990; 263:1265–1275.
46. Gallagher TJ: Guidelines for care: The time has come. Crit Care Med 1991; 19:138.
47. Shabot MM, Gardner RM (Eds): Decision Support Systems for Critical Care. New York, Springer-Verlag 1994.
47a. Gardner RM, Shabot MM: The future of computerized decision support in critical care. *In*: Decision Support Systems for Critical Care. Shabot MM, Gardner RM (Eds). New York, Springer-Verlag, 1994, pp 396–409.
48. Gardner RM, West BJ, Pryor TA, et al: Computer-based ICU data acquisition as an aid to clinical decision-making. Crit Care Med 1982; 10:823.
49. Miller PL: Extending computer-based critiquing to a new domain: ATTENDING, ESSENTIAL-ATTENDING, and VQ-ATTENDING. Int J Clin Monit Comput 1986; 2:135.
50. Polaschek JX, Rutledge GW, Anderson SK, et al: Using belief networks to interpret qualitative data in the ICU. Respir Care 1993; 38:60–72.
51. Kuperman GJ, Gardner RM, Pryor TA: HELP: A Dynamic Hospital Information System. New York, Springer-Verlag, 1991.
52. Sittig DF, Pace NL, Gardner RM, et al: Implementation of a computerized patient advice system using the HELP clinical information system. Comp Biomed Res 1989; 22:474–487.
53. East TD, Morris AH, Wallace CJ, et al: A strategy for development of computerized critical care decision support systems. Int J Clin Monit Comput 1991; 8:263–269.
54. Henderson S, Crapo RO, Wallace CJ, et al: Performance of computerized protocols for management of arterial oxygenation in an intensive care unit. Int J Clin Monit Comput 1992; 8:271–280.
54a. Morris AH, Wallace C, Menlove R, et al: A computerized protocol-controlled randomized clinical trial of new therapy including PCIRV and extracorporeal CO_2 removal for ARDS. Am J Respir Crit Care Med 1994; 149:295–305.
55. Gardner RM, Huff SM: Computers in the ICU: Why? What? So What? (Editorial). Int J Clin Monit Comput 1992; 4:199–205.
56. Osborn JJ: Computers in critical care medicine: Promises and pitfalls. Crit Care Med 1982; 10:808–810.

CHAPTER 197

Computerization: Solutions to Problems in the Input, Manipulation, and Storage of Intensive Care Unit Data

Jeffrey S. Augenstein, MD, PhD

Nearly 15 years have passed since I first wrote on this topic for the first edition of this textbook. Over those 15 years, much progress has occurred in the intensive care unit and in the world of computers. The forces that drive computerization of the clinical world have increased.[1–2] They include demands for increased control of resources, decreased operational costs, and excellent quality care. The federal government, which is the United States' largest purchaser of healthcare, is expected to restructure the healthcare reimbursement system. In a similar fashion, employers are initiating major strategy changes to reduce their healthcare costs and are demanding that healthcare expenditures be carefully managed. The Institute of Medicine, an organization chartered by the National Academy of Sciences to advise the federal government on health policy, identified "the prompt development and implementation of computer-based patient records (CPRs)" as a key factor in the response to the present and future challenge of healthcare. The Institute of Medicine is referring to a totally computerized record-keeping environment in which clinicians perform all documentation duties at electronic workstations. The Institute of Medicine report, entitled "The Computer-Based Patient Record," specifies the following:

> *As its first step, the [Institute of Medicine] study committee examined why previous work had not resulted in widespread improvement of patient records and asked whether and how another effort might be successful. The committee identified five conditions in the current health care environment that increase the likelihood of success.*
>
> 1. The uses of and legitimate demands for patient data are growing. Part of this growth can be attributed to increased concern about the content and value of clinical therapies and a recent intense focus on health services research.
> 2. More powerful, affordable technologies to support computer-based patient records are now available.
> 3. Increasingly, computers are being accepted as a tool for enhancing efficiency in virtually all facets of everyday life.
> 4. Demographic factors such as aging population (which results in a growth in chronic diseases) and the continued mobility of Americans create greater pressures for patient records that can manage large amounts of information and are easily transferable among health care providers.
> 5. Pressures for reform in health care are growing, and automation of patient records is crucial to achievement of such reform.
>
> The combination of these factors led the committee to conclude that computerization can help to improve patient records and that improved patient records and information management of health care data are essential elements of the infrastructure of the nation's health care system."[3]

However, it is rare to find examples of CPRs in use in hospitals today. Component applications in which clinicians enter or review parts of the traditional paper and radiographic film record at computer workstations do exist.[4] The most common of these are laboratory results reporting systems.[5] Other applications are seen much less frequently; these include: intensive care flow sheet management, digital radiograph viewing via picture archiving computer systems (PACS), anesthesia record-keeping systems, and computer-based transcription of physician encounters.[6–11]

The increasing cost effectiveness of computer hardware and software is facilitating broad-based clinical computerization. Today, it is possible to build affordable, highly reliable, instantaneously responding systems.[12–15] Workstations can be located at all points where care is provided.[7, 16] Tools are available to develop and continually enhance software.[17, 18] The combination of the perceived need for clinical computer systems and the existence of affordable products may usher in an information revolution in hospital care. Computerized record keeping throughout the healthcare enterprise could soon be the norm.

A HEALTHCARE SCENARIO OF THE FUTURE

In this section, the care of a critically ill patient in a future healthcare scenario is described. The functionality of the CPR is emphasized. The information system components embody the perspective of the Institute of Medicine and others. Solutions to the system's challenges with respect to input, manipulation, and data storage are described in the section *The New Technology*.

While driving a new car, John Smith, a hypothetic patient, was involved in a severe head-on collision with a tree. The incident occurred at a remote location on the state turnpike. The transit times for police and rescue crews were optimally short because John's car was equipped with a crash alarming system. The system transmitted the exact location of the crash on the basis of global positioning coordinates.[19]

John was the sole occupant of the car and was found unconscious at the scene. Fortunately, he carried his healthcare record on a "smart card."[20] Using the rescue vehicle's card reader, an emergency medical technician was able to obtain critical information about John's history of arrhythmias and his current treatment regimen. All the information about observations and interventions was entered into a "pen-based" computer.[21] The computer functions like a clipboard; an electronic pen replaces the keyboard and the pointing device. The user interface includes a menu of choices whenever possible. Selections are made by pointing to the menu choices with the pen. This type of computer also recognizes handwritten letters and numbers. Diagrams can be drawn on the screen and stored as part of the record.[22] The locations of John's injuries were entered on anatomic diagrams that were brought up on the screen. The cardiac and blood pressure monitor provided direct input to the computer.[23] All data were simultaneously transmitted to the receiving trauma center by a radio transmission.[16]

The police used a similar computer to report the crash information. Electronic images of the scene and of the interior and exterior of the vehicle were obtained. Relevant views were transmitted to the trauma center, providing graphic documentation of the positioning of the occupant before extrication from the vehicle as well as data on the magnitude of the crash forces.[24] At the trauma center, all data from John's medical history, including recent radiographic images as well as the police and rescue crew information, were available. Monitored data and interventions, such as fluid infusions, were electronically entered into the computer system. In this future system, nurses chart observations and interventions, such as medication infusions, using radio-linked, pen-based computers. A coding system allows descriptions of diagnoses and procedures to be chosen from menus. These detailed descriptions form a problem list, which summarizes the care process.[25] The vocabulary in the menus is easy to understand yet is also detailed.[26, 27] Translations are made by the computer system to other standardized nomenclatures, such as the International Classification of Diseases, the Abbreviated Injury Score, and the Current Procedural Terminology.[28–31] Parenthetically, the standardized nomenclature is also used for performing searches of computerized literature.[32]

Unstructured comments are dictated. The system of this scenario makes possible electronic transcription of continuous speech.[33] Word recognition is almost 100% accurate, even with speakers who have pronounced accents. The system reviews all dictation for content. It informs the clinician who is dictating whenever codifiable diagnoses or procedures contained in the dictation are not included in the data base.[34] If appropriate, these elements are entered into the structured problem list.

All radiographs, scans, and ultrasound examinations are maintained in the computer system. High-resolution electronic "viewstations" throughout the trauma center allow multiple images to be reviewed simultaneously.[9] The data "superhighway" permits consultation on diagnostic images with geographically distant experts.[35–38]

Orders are entered into the computer system. Significant advantages accrue from the direct interface of the clinician with the system.[39] First, reference materials can be accessed on the same terminal. For example, the dosage of an ordered drug can be checked. Second, the system can provide "expert" review, using its artificial intelligence modules.[40–43] Complex software can evaluate orders for completeness, appropriateness, and cost effectiveness.

The distinct advantage of this CPR over traditional, manual record keeping is that patients can be included in research protocols much more easily. The system can review each patient's description to determine eligibility for various protocols. If inclusion opportunities exist, the system can inform the caregivers. Consent forms can be displayed on the pen-based computers. If the patient is to be included in a specific protocol, the relevant orders are added to the existing orders. In addition, appropriate investigators can be informed that a particular subject has been included through electronic mail or even electronic paging.

The accident victim, John, was taken to the operating room a short time after his arrival at the trauma center. Persistent hypotension was believed to be related to a hemoperitoneum. Ultrasonic evaluation had quickly confirmed the cause. In the operating room of the future, the anesthesiologist and nurse do all charting on the computer. The anesthesiologists' workstations permit mainly voice-entry of data so that these clinicians can keep their hands free for patient care. Again, all electronically recorded data, such as expired gas values, are entered directly. Nurses use a stationary central workstation. When a nurse documents the use of supplies, the inventory management system is updated. Replacement materials are automatically ordered as needed. Because of this computerized record keeping, the staffing needs in the central supply center are reduced compared with in today's hospitals, but the availability of supplies is excellent.

Another advantage of the CPR of the future is that the nurses', the surgeons', and the anesthesiologists' records of the operation identify the same times, diagnoses, procedures, and participating personnel. In comparison, today's separate nursing, anesthesiology, and surgical records of the same operation often differ significantly, even with respect to the time that the operation began.

The surgeon documented John Smith's operative procedure using a ceiling mounted camera and the laparoscopic camera. The procedure was a laparoscopic splenorrhaphy. Images of the injured organ before and after repair were included in the operative report. The healthcare system of the future requires extensive support documentation.

At the end of the case, the dictated (and electronically transcribed) operative report was supplemented by a description of the diagnoses and procedures that was based on the standardized nomenclature system. Any diagnoses that were previously entered could have been used. As mentioned earlier, John was believed to have a hemoperitoneum on resuscitation. The term *hemoperitoneum* was entered into the problem list at that time. The surgeon used that entry in his description for the justification for surgery.

In the intensive care unit, all of John's previously obtained data were available. In this case, it was very useful to have a complete record of fluid and medication interventions used during resuscitation and in the operating room.

In the intensive care unit of the future, the nurse uses a portable, radio-linked workstation for charting. It is incorporated into the bedside table; interaction is via a keyboard and mouse. Data are predominantly presented in a flow sheet format. All physician orders can be activated or deactivated through the workstation. A "kardex," the nursing task list, is a byproduct of this effort. The system informs the nurse of complex alarms; interventions and diagnostic procedures as they need to be performed; and newly available results from the laboratory.[8, 44, 45]

This system of the future allows clinicians to review the literature on problems stored in electronic libraries. These libraries are much more comprehensive than today's MEDLINE because they are able to provide complete electronic "reprints" on the screen. (As previously mentioned, the standardized nomenclature can be used to define search parameters.[32]) Moreover, the local as well as national experience with similar cases can be reviewed in the form of summaries or individual case histories.

Quality assurance and utilization review reports are a byproduct of the system's primary record-keeping functions. All professional and hospital bills emanate from the clinical data base. The various purchasers of the future refuse to pay for services when disparities exist in the descriptions of the care process as reported by the involved physicians and the hospital. The system eliminates discrepancies as well as many of the medicolegal initiatives that are based on poorly described care.

On the floor, a number of types of workstations are used. Desktop computers with large, high-resolution monitors are ubiquitous. They are identical to ones used during resuscitation, in the operating room, and in the intensive care unit. These workstations allow the review of images, text, flow sheets, and orders as well as voice- and keyboard-based data entry. They provide opportunities for multimedia education.[9, 46, 47] Lecture and other presentation packages that include still images, slides, voice, and moving images are available.[48, 49] Self-evaluations can be performed on the basis of clinical scenarios, and knowledge- and skill-based evaluations can be performed. Some of the presentations include surgery simulations in which lifelike anatomy and physiology are presented both initially and in response to intervention.

The data base can be reviewed by authorized personnel at these and other workstations. Graphic presentation of the information in the data base allows even a neophyte clinician to analyze the data flexibly. For example, a simple query would allow a clinician to review all recent cases of male patients who were involved in head-on car crashes and who received high-level, positive end-expiratory pressure ventilation. By connecting graphic images of the groups of data, the clinician can obtain the desired information.[50] These data can be transferred to a statistical program such as Statistical Package for Social Sciences (SPSS).[51]

The second type of workstation on the floor is a radio-linked, portable computer placed on nursing carts (e.g., the medication cart). Clinical observations and execution of orders are charted in this manner. The kardex, flow sheets, and assessments are available for entry or review from these devices. At all workstations electronic reference materials, such as the *Physician's Desk Reference,* are available.[52] In addition, an artificial intelligence system identifies the potential for drug interactions and allergic reactions.[5, 41, 53]

The physician uses a computer on a mobile cart that has telephone capabilities for dictation purposes. The computerized word recognition is excellent, even from these remote phones.

The CPR and associated computerization of police and rescue crew records described in the scenario could provide rapid and complete understanding of the healthcare system and the social structure within which it exists. It is hoped that they would facilitate improvements in the prevention, diagnosis, and treatment of health problems.

TECHNOLOGY IN TRANSITION

In the past, it would have been impossible to develop large-scale information systems with the complexity and scope described in the scenario. Impediments to building useful CPRs are quickly disappearing. In addition to high equipment costs, the insurmountable restrictions included the following:

- imperfect reliability
- inadequate speed of information presentation
- a small possible number of simultaneous users
- a limited data base size
- the inability to represent different information types on the same terminal with a coherent user interface
- the inability to support nontethered workstations

Software development limitations were equal to the hardware limitations. Traditional techniques of software creation required complex, error-prone, statement-by-statement programming. The traditional monolithic computer usually was limiting in some manner, typically in response time. To manage computer resources in the most efficient manner, programmers were required to use very rigid languages such as "assembler," "COBOL," or "C." The most efficient programs were written in languages that have close kinship to the commands the computer's central processor uses. However, these languages are extremely difficult to use. The productivity for even excellent programmers was 10 or 15 lines of program per day. The system of the future described earlier in the scenario would have thousands of lines of code. Traditional development strategies would not easily meet this challenge. Current system generation tools are up to the task of developing and maintaining large, complex systems. The maintenance alone of older, large-scale systems requires tremendous programming resources.

It is not clear as to what costs hospitals will incur to computerize medical record keeping. The present purchase price for the intensive care component of CPR systems is $20,000 to $30,000 per bed. To date, very few hospitals have bought systems. Even fewer have installed hospital-wide CPRs.[4] The economic equation is complex. One factor is the cost of purchasing, installing, and maintaining the hardware and software. Training personnel to use the system is included in this calculation. Another factor is the true cost of traditional record keeping. Hospitals spend a significant portion of their operational dollars on creating and maintaining the various components of the paper- and radiographic film–based medical record. The costs are influenced greatly by the time that clinicians, particularly nurses, spend writing the components of the record, interpreting unintelligible handwriting, and finding information.

The other significant "costs" associated with the paper- and film-based medical record include:

- storing and retrieving masses of paper and film objects that occupy a large amount of space
- inserting documents into the chart that are not available at the time of care, such as transcriptions
- copying records in response to patient, legal, and payer requests
- finding and organizing data in response to ever increasing reporting demands

Other costs are more difficult to calculate. These include adverse medicolegal judgments in cases of malpractice because the defense was forced to rely on incomplete or incomprehensible written documents.

The cost of computer systems relative to their performance is continually decreasing to the advantage of the purchaser. A full-page advertisement in a leading trade journal once boasted that if the automobile industry had made progress equal to that of the computer industry, a Rolls Royce would cost $1 and would get 1 million miles to the gallon. This is not a great exaggeration. Each year, consumers' purchasing power at least doubles with respect to disk storage capacity and processing speed.

THE NEW TECHNOLOGY

Technology is rapidly shifting from monolithic computers, called "mainframe" computers or "minicomputers," to "client server" networks.[54] The initial installation, maintenance, and growth of the former design were expensive, and the design itself was largely inflexible. The industry was dominated by a few vendors, and one of these dominated the market. Terminals presented limited displays of only words and numbers. Data bases were rarely accessible for research purposes.

Perhaps the most potent, enabling force on behalf of clinical computerization is the high-level processing, communication, and display performance offered by general-purpose, personal computers. They will be the clinical workstations of the future. Their ratio of price to performance will continue to improve. Computers, which provide high-quality, graphic user interfaces, are becoming essential business tools, as are multiline telephones. Medicine will benefit greatly as competition drives the prices of what will be general-purpose appliances down to the commodity price range. The current specialized workstation found in commercial intensive care information systems and which costs thousands of dollars will be replaced by an "off-the-shelf" personal computer that costs only a few hundred dollars. It is possible that the new bedside workstations will be general-purpose, portable computers that use wireless communication. Installation for an entire intensive care unit will take a few hours compared with the days and weeks that the setup of present systems requires.[16]

DATA SERVER TECHNOLOGY

In the new generation of technology, the data are maintained on optimized "servers." The data can be of multiple media (e.g., images and voice).[47, 55, 56] The common denominator is digitization. The success of commercial compact disks, on which music is stored digitally, demonstrates the acceptability of the numeric representation of data. In a similar fashion, radiographs, color pictures of histologic preparations, and even motion-based images such as ultrasound examinations and angiograms can be stored digitally.

As was stated, the costs of disk storage continually decrease relative to the amount of data that can be stored on them. The storage capacity of servers is typically 1 billion "bytes," or 1 "gigabyte."[12] A byte is basically equal to a single letter or number. Even small servers can hold the contents of a number of large city telephone directories. Because of the rapid computerization of data, new terms are entering everyday parlance. Many large corporations have disk-based records that are in the "terabyte," or trillion-byte, range,[12, 50] and some are in the "pedabyte," or 1 thousand–terabyte, range. It is said that 1 pedabyte of rain drops could float the largest of ships. Big hospitals that store multiple years' records, including images, will have data bases in the terabyte to pedabyte range.

A server capable of supporting hundreds of users simultaneously while managing gigabytes of data can be bought for a few thousand dollars. Server technology is optimized for data retrieval and storage. Servers can provide uninterrupted availability of data. Typically, the server responds to a command language. One of the most common languages is "structured query language."[56] The workstation sends a few commands to obtain any type or grouping of data.

"Relational" data bases are typically the containers for the servers' data. The data elements are maintained in coherent tables.[57, 58] The data structure looks much like a spreadsheet. Each column contains the same type of data, such as patients' names or ages. Rows contain unique instances of sets of data, such as the results of individual urine analyses. In a well-organized, relational data base, each table is a different type of record set. For example, individual tables may contain monitored cardiovascular data, such as heart rate and blood pressure; laboratory data, such as complete blood counts; or demographic information, such as name, address, and telephone number.

The unique identifier or "key" for each row of patient data in a table is typically a patient number as well as at least the date and the time of the encounter. The keys allow data tables to be combined. Thus, it is possible to generate a report on the name and age of each patient who had at least one heart rate of more than 150 beats per minute and who had a serum potassium level of less than 3 mmol/L, in temporal proximity to the tachycardia. This would involve connections among demographic, laboratory, and monitoring data.

Since servers have only to manage the data base and not address all the traditional monolithic computer's functions, they can be optimized for their tasks. They have a hardware and software configuration that facilitates the retrieval and storage of data. In addition, they can provide hardware and software "redundancy." This means that data will be available in the event of failure of a single component and even multiple components. Often, the data are maintained on duplicate disks and called "mirrored data," or they are spread across a number of disks and called "arrayed data."[59] Occasionally, the strategy involves utilizing paired servers. In this case, the programs and data are duplicated on each server. The failure of one server or its scheduled shutdown for maintenance barely affects the users. The protection of data availability provided by the software and hardware is referred to as "fault tolerance."[13] The critical nature of medical record data and the decreasing costs of even the best fault-tolerance strategies suggest that electronic record-keeping systems will be highly fault tolerant.

THE NETWORK LINK

The second part of the client-server technology is the network that links the hundreds of workstations and the data servers needed in even medium-sized hospitals. Present networks are based on "ethernet" or "token-ring" technologies.[60–62] They typically support data transmission rates of up to 10 megabytes per second (roughly equal to 1 million single letters or numbers). The technology of the future will likely employ the "asynchronous transmission mode," which will handle hundreds of millions of bytes of data per second.[63, 64] For example, many clinicians will need simultaneously to view their respective patients' radiographs at workstations throughout a hospital. Each image will be equivalent, minimally, to a 1 million–byte record. For all the images to appear instantaneously, the network capacity must be very high.

Traditional approaches use only wires or fiberoptic cables for transmission, whereas wireless communication typically employs radiofrequency technologies. Many of the terminals in a hospital could be movable and untethered, having nearly the functionality of desktop workstations. Communication strategies, previously found only in military applications (in particular, "spread spectrum"*), will provide high-speed communication among wireless workstations or other equipment with no interference.[16, 65]

Limitation of number of clients that can be serviced simultaneously and instantaneously has disappeared or will shortly disappear. There are commercial motivations, beyond medical applications, for the rapid increase in the capacity of networks to handle many users and vast amounts of data. One of the most potent market forces may be "interactive home television."[64] An example of this future level of home entertainment is access to movies "on demand." A viewer will purportedly be able to choose from thousands of titles and view a chosen movie whenever desired. Video objects, such as movies, will be digitized just as radiographs are today. The home television will become a multimedia workstation. The need to move the amount of data that movies comprise instantaneously to thousands of homes will increase the affordability of information technology used in hospitals.

The business potential of hundreds of millions of homes should motivate continuing improvement in not only the network components but also the server and workstation. Digital data, whether in the form of movies, radiographs, or the text of operative reports, will require similar technology for storage, transmission, and display. The proposed "high-definition television" of the home may be the basis of the workstation of the hospital. Thus, affordably managing digital radiograph images and other components of medical records should be achievable.

THE WORKSTATION

Present computer workstations, which cost several hundred dollars, can support the entry and review of the various components of the medical record. The ability to present multiple types of data and employ a graphic user interface are essential requirements. This form of display uses multiple "windows" of information and includes menus or choice lists.[66] A number of forms of "windowing" exist, such as Apple Computer's operating system (Apple Computer, Inc., Cupertino, CA) and Microsoft's "Windows" (Microsoft Corporation, Redmond, WA). In each case, multiple types of data can be presented, including traditional numbers and words, high-resolution images such as radiographs, and sound files such as dictations. The menus are used for navigating among applications as well as for making choices for data entry. A keyboard and a pointing device such as a mouse, trackball, pen, or even a finger are the tools of interaction. Windowing technology has made interaction with computers much more intuitive. Minimum training is necessary to accomplish complex tasks. This is largely because user interface rules exist and because most applications operate in a similar manner. The menus and included "Help" systems provide user direction and support. The user interface is standardized not only among applications but also among the various workstations. For example, the manner in which an order is written with a hand-held computer would be nearly identical with that of a large-screen desktop unit.

Strategies for entry and review of data must be optimized for these future information systems. Most clinical information systems merely emulate the paper-based processes. However, unprecedented amounts of data will be instantaneously available for decision making. Critical situations, such as progressive hypoxemia, should be clearly identified. With a complete electronic data base, much greater sophistication could exist in the processing and presentation of critical information than is possible with today's typically monitor-based alarms. Multiple parameters could be evaluated for patterns of change, whereas at present there is usually comparison of only one variable, such as heart rate, with a range of acceptable values. Fortunately, experience has been gained in the implementation of complex electronic alarming systems in critical environments. Since the late 1970s, electronic displays coupled with humanlike speech have been incorporated into commercial and military jet cockpits, replacing hundreds of gauges. These electronic presentations communicate information about a jet's moment-by-moment status and sound alarms in the event of dangerous conditions. The process of developing acceptable electronic communications in this critical environment is a model for the design of complex alerting systems.

Computerized systems should facilitate the process of understanding a patient's response to care. This often involves navigation through vast amounts of data. Currently, this process is relatively primitive. The facilitation of the process of asking and answering questions in an iterative fashion is a critical requirement of information systems. Let us imagine a situation in which an intensivist is reviewing a patient's response to care. The computer should ease the process of jumping from one set of information to another. If the clinician notes, for example, that a significant fever spike occurred each time a new antibiotic was administered, then he or she may want to review the literature concerning that constellation of events or review in-house patient experiences. The thought process should be greatly aided by the computer system's synthesizing of data.

Spreadsheets present the data to be analyzed in two-dimensional views. An analysis of fever response to an antibiotic requires a multidimensional navigation capability. This area of investigation and product development is called "on-line analytical processing."[50] Progress is being made on tools that could facilitate the complex review of clinical data during the process of care.

Some technologies for the components of workstations,

Spread spectrum: A radio transmission that continuously changes carrier frequency according to a unique pattern in both sending and receiving devices. It is used for security as well as to allow multiple wireless transmissions in the same space.

such as nomenclature standardization, voice recognition, handwriting recognition, and battery life for portable terminals, require maturation before the CPR can truly be developed.

A key to the organization of a medical record could be a concise problem list that outlines the care process.[26, 27] This would act as a table of contents or index of the many discrete components of the record. Ideally, the computer system should provide a nomenclature with which clinicians could define observations and therapeutic interventions. A menu-based system should facilitate the structured description of a patient's clinical course. In addition, the computer should search the contents of unstructured descriptions, such as operative dictations, in the search for components that may need to be added to the problem list. Translations from the clinician's description to other standardized nomenclatures, such as the International Classification of Diseases, should be accomplished in the background by the system.[28, 29, 34] For example, one descriptive effort by the clinician should prompt administrative functions, such as billing for hospital and professional services. There is optimism on the horizon for these systems to emerge. One of the most robust vocabularies with which to describe the spectrum of clinical medicine is the systematized nomenclature of medicine (SNOMED),[67] which was revised in 1993. Preliminary personal investigations suggest that it will provide an excellent basis for computerized descriptions. Included in its vast data base are translations to International Classification of Diseases codes. Menuing strategies must be developed if this excellent information source is to be accessed from workstations.

Voice recognition technology holds the promise of allowing clinicians to provide oral descriptions of complex events, such as surgeries or clinic visits. For the near future, dictation will be a significant component of medical record keeping. At the present time, the limitation has been the time and costs involved with manual transcription and document filing. Affordable electronic transcription systems are becoming commercially available. Some have meaningful clinical applications such as documentation of emergency room visits.[11, 33] Three factors have limited the clinical application of this technology. First, the systems' vocabularies have not been large enough to describe the spectrum of medical concepts adequately. Second, the systems have been unable to manage continuous speech satisfactorily. Thus, most applications require that users speak with unnatural separations between words. Third, most systems are reasonably speaker dependent; the speech of clinicians with pronounced accents often cannot be recognized. Certainly, these technologic limitations will soon be overcome. Even freeform text generated through dictation can be searched for key terms and concepts.[28, 34] Codifiable diagnoses and procedures can become integral components of the data base.

Handwriting recognition probably has a role in portable workstations.[68] Some presently available clinical workstations use a padlike user interface that is similar to the traditional clipboard. In the future, a clinician could carry a fully functional workstation that communicates with a network through a radiofrequency link.[21] In this scenario, traditionally typed data, such as clinician "sign-on" codes, would be entered by "writing" on the screen with a computer pen. Letters would be interpreted as if they were typed. The menu choices would be made by using the same pen.

The impetus for developing computers with handwriting recognition and operated by long-lasting, environmentally safe batteries is the vast market of business users who are demanding portable computers. A new commercial initiative is the "personal digital assistant."[69] This device is beginning to appear in the marketplace. It is a small, portable computer that typically is capable of handwriting recognition. Its primary function at this time is managing daily schedules and telephone directories. One of the most talked about of such products is Apple Computer's "Newton."[70] Its developers state that such devices will eventually incorporate cellular telephones, beepers, and wireless links to powerful data bases. Medical institutions will benefit from these technologies. Commercial opportunity in the general population will bring about necessary improvements in the affordability and functionality of these portable workstations. Improvements will be seen not only in handwriting recognition and battery life but also in the quality of displays and wireless data communication.

SOFTWARE DEVELOPMENT

The technology required to support clinical record keeping with window-based workstation displays, huge multimedia data networks, and vast server-based data bases is extremely complex. Previous programming techniques, with which past systems were developed line by line, will not meet this challenge. However, new technologies such as "fourth-generation languages" and "object-oriented programming" are reaching maturity.[8, 17, 71] These technologies minimize command level programming. Developers work on window-based workstations in which display screens, communication links, and data base functions are developed in part by manipulating objects on the screen. Within a few hours, a complex application can be developed that previously would have required months of conventional programming. The key is that the programs are largely "written" in the background by the development system itself. These tools will make clinical information projects manageable.

An impediment to CPR development is the lack of communication standards for computers. The ability to link many systems, some as small as a bedside cardiovascular monitor and others as large as a giant hospital information system, is mandatory if all relevant data are to appear on the CPR. Significant efforts are in progress to standardize the communication protocols among systems. Each system may store its data in a unique manner. If one computer requests data from another, the request would be formatted in a manner understandable to both computers. The data would be presented to the requesting computer in a standardized form. For example, if laboratory data are stored on one computer and a workstation in the operating room requests a flow sheet of the history of complete blood counts, the laboratory computer would package the data in an understandable manner. Such a transaction needs to occur instantaneously. Currently, several efforts to standardize and facilitate the exchange of health data are being made. Standards from the American Society for Testing and Materials (Philadelphia, PA) and Health Level Seven, Inc. (Chicago, IL) are representative of the current movement to develop data exchange standards.[72, 73] Both define formats for requesting data and for packaging data response.

A development strategy that may help address intercomputer data transmission is the object-oriented data base. In this strategy, the locations and methods of extracting the data from its parent computers are encoded in the data base. When the user at a workstation requests laboratory data, the server knows where to find it and what commands to employ to extract the data.

SUMMARY

American medicine may be about to embark on a journey into a new way of operating. In the future, the management of resources may be as critical as the care of patients. This chapter presented a scenario of the near future as a basis for describing the exciting potential of computerization. The hardware and software building blocks of the CPR, like wireless networks and data base servers, were described. Information will be much more accessible by caregivers. However, optimization of the system of care will occur only if educational and management strategies that take advantage of the potential are developed.

References

1. Lumsdon K: Holding networks together: Shared information will be glue for reformed health system. Hospitals 1993; 67:26–27.
2. Lumsdon K: Computerized patient records gain converts. Hospitals 1993; 67:44.
3. Richard SD, Elaine BS (Eds): The Computer-Based Patient Record: An Essential Technology for Health Care. Washington, DC, National Academy Press, 1991.
4. United Communications Group: National Report on Computers & Health. Presented in part at the Bedside Terminals: New Direction, Right Choices conference, Rockville, MD, July 27–28, 1992.
5. Bradshaw KE, Gardner RM, Pryor TA: Development of a computerized laboratory alerting system. Comput Biomed Res 1989; 22:575–587.
6. Hammond JE, Berger RG, Carey TS, et al: Making the transition from information systems of the 1970's to medical information systems of the 1990's: The role of the physician's workstation. J Med Syst 1991; 15:257–267.
7. Hard R: More hospitals move toward bedside systems. Hospitals 1992; 66:72.
8. Ball MJ, Hannah KJ, Jelger UG, et al (Eds): Nursing Informatics: Where Caring and Technology Meet. *In:* Computers in Health Care Series. New York, Springer-Verlag, 1988.
9. Englmeier KH, Fink U, Hilbertz T: Visualization of multimodal image information in medicine. American Medical Informatics Association. Presented at the Sixteenth Annual Symposium on Computer Applications in Medical Care Proceedings, Baltimore, MD, November 8–11, 1992, pp 25–29.
10. Gravenstein JS: The uses of the anesthesia record. J Clin Monit 1989; 5:256–265.
11. Linn NA, Rubenstein RM, Bowler AE, et al: Improving the quality of emergency department documentation using the voice-activated word processor: Interim results. American Medical Informatics Association. Presented in part at the Sixteenth Annual Symposium on Computer Applications in Medical Care Proceedings, Baltimore, MD, November 8–11, 1992, pp 772–778.
12. Ricciuti M. Terabytes of data: How to get at them? Datamation 1992; 38:38–44.
13. Gallie R: System fault tolerance. InfoWorld 1993; 15:65.
14. Gardner E: Internal medicine. LAN Magazine 1993; 8:129–135.
15. Snell N: Mainframe accounting moves down. Datamation 1992; 38:112.
16. Eisenberg A: PC's on the move. PC Sources 1993; 4:153–161.
17. Conway J: Case study: GE facilitates the transition to object-oriented programming. J Object-Oriented Programming 1993; 6:S4–S8.
18. Simpson D: Study predicts wider use of 4 GL's to handle large libraries, CASE. Digital News Rev 1992; 9:16.
19. User Service Plan for Emergency Notification and Personal Security: Program Plan for the Intelligent Vehicle Highway Systems (IVHS) Program (Draft). Washington, DC, US Department of Transportation, July 6, 1993.
20. Bulkeley W: "Get ready for smart cards in health care." Wall Street Journal, May 3, 1993, p 11B.
21. Lussier YA, Maksud M, Desruisseaux B, et al: A computerized patient record software for direct data entry by physicians using a keyboard-free pen-based portable computer. American Medical Informatics Association. Presented in part at the Sixteenth Annual Symposium on Computer Applications in Medical Care Proceedings, Baltimore, MD, November 8–11, 1992, pp 261–264.
22. Zimmerman MR: Separate but equal PDAs from Apple, Tandy/Casio. PC Week 1993; 10:25.
23. Gardner RM, West BJ, Pryor TA, et al: Computer-based ICU data acquisition as an aid to clinical decision-making. Crit Care Med 1982; 10:823.
24. Hunt RC, Brown RL, Cline KA, et al: Comparison of motor vehicle damage documentation in emergency medical services run reports compared with photographic documentation. Ann Emerg Med 1993; 22:651–656.
25. Osler T: Injury severity scoring: Perspectives in development and future directions. Am J Surg 1993; 165(Suppl 2A):43S–51S.
26. Mellner C, Selander H, Wolodarski J: The computerized problem-oriented medical record at Karolinska Hospital: Format and function, users acceptance and patient attitude. Methods Inf Med 1976; 15:11–20.
27. Weed LL. Medical records that guide and teach. N Engl J Med 1968; 278:593–600.
28. Stitt FW, Lu Y, Dickinson GM, et al: Automated severity classification of AIDS hospitalizations. Med Decis Making 1991; 11:S41–S45.
29. ICD-9 CM: International Classification of Diseases. Clinical Modification. 9th Revision. 3rd ed. Vol 1 and 2. Los Angeles, Product Management Information Corporation, 1991.
30. Association for the Advancement of Automotive Medicine: The abbreviated injury scale. 1990 revision. Des Plaines, IA, Association for Advancement of Automotive Medicine, 1990.
31. American Medical Association: Physicians' current procedural terminology. Chicago, American Medical Association, 1993.
32. Cimino JJ, Johnson SB, Aguirre A, et al: The Medline button. American Medical Informatics Association. Presented in part at the Sixteenth Annual Symposium on Computer Applications in Medical Care Proceedings, Baltimore, MD, November 8–11, 1992, pp 81–85.
33. Johnson K, Poon A, Shiffman S, et al: A history taking system that uses continuous speech recognition. American Medical Informatics Association. Presented in part at the Sixteenth Annual Symposium on Computer Applications in Medical Care Proceedings, Baltimore, MD, November 8–11, 1992, pp 757–761.
34. Gabrieli ER: Computer-assisted assessment of patient care in the hospital. J Med Systems 1988; 12:135–145.
35. Willett S: Construction of national data superhighway begins in Congress. InfoWorld 1993; 15:12.
36. Beatty P: Canada's bold new blueprint for a national electronic highway. Telecommunications 1993; 27:46.
37. Mace S: Clinton wants $14 million more to fund wide American network. InfoWorld 1993; 15:1.
38. McLachlan G: Rewiring America: Bill Clinton sees potential for an internet superhighway. LAN Comput 1993; 4:17.
39. Tierney WM, Miller ME, Overhage JM, et al: Physician inpatient order writing on microcomputer workstations: Effects on resource utilization. JAMA 1993; 269:379–383.
40. Miller PL, Black HR: Plan-analysis by computer: Critiquing the pharmacologic management of essential hypertension. Comput Biomed Res 1984; 17:38.
41. Shortliffe EH, Buchanan GB, Feigenbaum EA: Knowledge engineering for medical decision: A review of computer-based clinical decision aids. IEEE Proc 1979; 67:1207.
42. Miller PL, Black HR: HT-ATTENDING: Critiquing the pharmacological management of essential hypertension. J Med Syst 1984; 8:181.
43. Autio K, Kari A, Tikka H: Integration of knowledge-based system and database for identification of disturbances in fluid and electrolyte balance. Comput Methods Programs Biomed 1991; 34:201–209.
44. Cox HC, Harsanyi B, Dean LC: Computers and Nursing: Application to Practice, Education and Research. Norwalk, CT, Appleton & Lange, 1987.
45. Pluth JR, Smith HC, Schultz GL: The computerized intensive care unit: A comparative evaluation. Presented in part at the Second Henry Ford Hospital International Symposium on Cardiac Surgery, New York, NY, 1977, pp 152–156.

46. Yager T: Better than being there: Desktop video teleconferencing could change how you do business. Byte 1993; 18:129–134.
47. Adam JA: Interactive multimedia. Special report. IEEE Spectrum 1993; 30:22.
48. Altman M, Dev P, Nachbar M, et al: Gross anatomy and the missing link. The Journal (Technological Horizons in Education) 1993; 20:S4.
49. Perper EJ, Felciano R, Dev P: Real problems: A layered approach to constructing a patient simulation. American Medical Informatics Association. Presented in part at the Sixteenth Annual Symposium on Computer Applications in Medical Care Proceedings, Baltimore, MD, November 8–11, 1992, pp 707–711.
50. Codd EF, Codd SB, Salley CT: In depth: Beyond decision support. ComputerWorld 1993; 127:87–89.
51. Norusis MJ: Statistical Package for Social Sciences for Windows Professional Statistics. Release 5. Chicago, SPSS, Inc., 1992.
52. Physician's Desk Reference. 47th ed. Des Moines, IA, Medical Economics Data, 1993.
53. Held JP, Carlis JV: A shared conceptual schema for four medical expert systems. Presented in part at the Proceeding of the Sixth International Conference on Data Engineering, Los Angeles, CA, 1990, pp 410–419.
54. Ferguson CH, Morris CR: Computer Wars: How the West Can Win in a Post-IBM World. New York, Times Books, 1993.
55. Borsook P: Unix database servers are not for everyone. Byte 1993; 18:102.
56. Nath A: Guide to SQL Server. Reading, MA, Addison-Wesley Publishing, 1990.
57. Hutt ATF: A Relational Data Base: Management System. New York, John Wiley & Sons, 1979.
58. Maier D: The Theory of Relational Databases. Rockville, MD, Computer Science Press, 1983.
59. Nash KS: When it RAIDs, it pours. ComputerWorld 1993; 27:49.
60. Panettieri JC: Battle of the network stars. Inf Week 1993; No. 426, p 15.
61. Snyder J: The gestalt of ethernet. Digital News Rev 1992; 9:9–11.
62. Rymer JR: Ethernet vs. token-ring battles enter a new phase. Distributed Comput Monitor 1992; 7:31–33.
63. Musich P: ATM's power not yet tapped: Transport medium promises solution for high bandwidth. PC Week 1993; 10:43–45.
64. Leslie IM, McAuley DR, Tennenhouse DL: ATM everywhere? IEEE Network 1993; 7:40.
65. Loudermilk S: Spread-spectrum technology catches on. PC Week 1992; 9:45–47.
66. Microsoft Programming Series: The Windows Interface, An application Design Guide. Redmond, WA, Microsoft Corporation, 1992.
67. College of American Pathologists: SNOMED: Systematized nomenclature of medicine. Volume 1 Numeric Index. Northfield, IL, College of American Pathologists, 1993.
68. Lee Y: Handwriting recognition sputters: Low performance rate is an obstacle for pen computer development. InfoWorld 1992; 14:15–17.
69. Scheier RL: Took PDA's spell sea of change for the PC industry. PC Week 1992; 9:12.
70. Zimmerman M: Pen-based zoomer, newton phone services highlight consumer electronics show. PC Week 1993; 10:8.
71. Farber D: Charting a course for objects. PC Week 1993; 10:61–64.
72. American Society for Testing and Materials: A review of published standards and current projects committee. ASTM E-31. Philadelphia, PA, ASTM, 1992.
73. Health Level Seven: An application protocol for electronic data exchange in healthcare environments. Version 2.1. Chicago, Health Level Seven, Inc., 1990.

CHAPTER 198

Severity of Illness Indices and Outcome Prediction: Development and Evaluation

Michael G. Seneff, MD
Jack E. Zimmerman, MD, FACP, FCCP, FCCM
William A. Knaus, MD

Whether they are transferring an intensive care unit (ICU) patient to a regular ward or preparing a family for a loved one's death, physicians are acting on their expectations for a given patient. Thus, outcome prediction is routine in all ICUs. This kind of prediction is subjective and is largely based on published data or personal experience. Despite the development of increasingly accurate prognostic scoring systems for critically ill adults, physicians are generally unaware of the applicability of these systems, they consider them a research tool, or they shun their use on ill-defined ethical grounds.

Recent changes in the healthcare industry appear to mandate a change in attitude. Health care costs are spiraling upward, necessitating a change in the status quo. Visions of the future of medicine focus on cost containment through the broader use of managed care, health maintenance organizations, and umbrella health insurance. Medical treatment facilities and their specialized areas may thus have to compete for contracts with managed care organizations, whose consumers will demand increased value for their money. ICUs are likely to be one of the first areas affected by a new health policy because of their ever-increasing share of medical costs and perceived opportunities for improved cost efficiency. Intensivists attempting to improve the cost efficiency and overall effectiveness of intensive care are faced with realities that will make this task difficult. Even with spiraling costs, treatments for many severe illnesses are currently under-reimbursed,[1] and third-party payers will be reluctant to increase funding unless clear benefit is demonstrated. Unfortunately, for many ICU admissions, evidence for efficacy of treatment has been equivocal at best.[2] Third-party payers may also limit reimbursement for stable monitored-only patients, whose reimbursement surplus previously allowed some recoupment of costs invested in the care of the more severely ill.[3] Resolution of these conflicts will require that intensivists be not only excellent physicians but also excellent managers. Resources will need to be dedicated to patients who are likely to benefit, and cost containment will be a constant pressure. Through it all, any approach will have to maintain an unswerving respect for patient autonomy and for the primary importance of the doctor-patient relationship.[2a]

Accurate and objective outcome prediction is part of the solution to these daunting and formidable problems. To demonstrate cost efficiency while maintaining quality, hospitals will need to become fluent in analyzing, presenting, and maintaining utilization and outcome data. Demonstrating improved outcome for a given treatment will allow for financial and human resources to be allocated appropriately.[4] Accurate outcome data will result in better communication with patients and in treatment that is more likely to be consistent with the patient's value system.

In this chapter, we first define the term *outcome* and develop the rationale of outcome prediction as science by discussing concepts and limitations. We then describe the basic principles of outcome prediction and how predictive instruments are designed and validated. We then review two general prognostic scoring systems available for use in the ICU and discuss their implications for clinical practice. In Chapter 203, we review outcome data for selected diseases and include recommendations for their application in clinical practice. Our overall goal is to produce a better understanding of the science of outcome prediction to empower the intensivist with the tools needed to improve the quality and efficiency of intensive care.

WHAT IS OUTCOME?

A desirable outcome is often perceived differently by physicians, patients, and society. Modern clinical trials are designed to assess the impact of medical intervention on one or more traditional endpoints, typically survival or a quantifiable measure of disease activity, such as cardiac ejection fraction.[5] These endpoints, however, are not what concerns patients the most. Whereas physicians focus on chances for "disease-free" and "overall" survival, patients may be more concerned with the potential for returning to baseline function, for chronic disability, or for being a burden to their family. For many, some of these alternative outcomes are worse than death.[6-7]

Defining acceptable outcomes for individuals is particularly relevant for critical care because modern life-sustaining therapy often succeeds in postponing death but may be ineffective at restoring health. As the science of outcome prediction matures, qualitative outcomes, rather than mortality alone, will be increasingly measured. Efforts such as the SUPPORT (Study to Understand Prognosis and Preferences for Outcomes and Risks of Treatment) project[8] are ongoing and will provide data so that physicians can offer informed treatment options. Until better data are available, physicians learning to incorporate predictive models into their practice must bear in mind the limitations of using mortality as an endpoint.

IMPROVING ACCURACY OF MEDICAL DECISIONS

Medawar states "another property that sets the genuine sciences apart is . . . their predictive capability."[9] To comprehend how prognostic scoring systems can improve the accuracy of medical decision making and thus augment the predictive capability of medicine, one must first understand how decision making usually takes place. Medical decisions are made in an fashion that is analogous to the way individuals make everyday decisions and are based on a hypothetico-deductive model, heuristics, or rule-based behavior.[10-13] The reader is referred elsewhere for a full discussion of this topic[14] but is reminded that errors occurring with this type of decision making include allowing recall of recent (but not necessarily representative) experiences or for rare events (e.g., case reports) to disproportionately influence probability estimates. Inexperienced physicians in particular may be influenced by these factors. Probability estimates generated by predictive instruments help militate against errors introduced by standard clinical decision making[6, 14] by providing objective estimates based on a representative patient sample.

Another way to eliminate subjectivity and improve medical decision making is through the use of formal decision analysis.[15, 16] Most ICU patients require multiple diagnostic and therapeutic interventions, and construction of a basic decision tree using probability estimates derived from a predictive model provides a way to present outcomes for different treatment options scientifically rather than empirically (Fig. 198–1).[15] Use of this method can increase the precision of communication between physicians, patients, and families and can reduce physicians' reliance on emotional, poorly calibrated, or inaccurate, subjective estimates.[6]

Despite these considerations, most physicians are not yet ready to incorporate formal decision models or predictive instruments into everyday practice, and they remain skeptical of the accuracy of these instruments. Several comparisons of predictive instruments and clinical judgment have been made, with most of the studies focusing on predicting mortality for ICU patients.[14, 17-20] The predictive instruments have generally performed as well as or better than clinicians in discriminating outcome (i.e., predicting who will live or die) and have been better calibrated.[12] *Calibration* refers to how closely the predictions correlate with actual outcome across the entire range of risk. Clinicians are adept at selecting patients at high risk for mortality (frequently stated as >90% chance for death) but provide less accurate predictions for patients with moderate severity of illness. The importance of discrimination versus calibration depends on how a predictive instrument is to be used. For research or quality assurance, which usually involves groups of patients with varying risks of mortality, calibration is particularly important. For decisions about individual patients in whom measurement of an exact risk for mortality is desired, both discrimination and calibration are important.[10]

STATISTICS, PATIENT AUTONOMY, AND FUTILITY IN MEDICINE

Although probability estimates are generated using scientific principles, statistical considerations can introduce considerable uncertainty about their accuracy. A study of prognosis in patients with nontraumatic coma (see Chapter 203) is an excellent example of these uncertainties.[21] This 500-patient study used neurologic findings to predict outcome with excellent accuracy. However, opponents of using these data point out that even this relatively large study had a 5% false-positive rate in predicting chronic vegetative state, a condition that occurs in 1% of cases. This disparity implies that seven patients of the next 90 identified to have no chance of recovery or severe disability instead could have moderate disability or good recovery. This statistical consideration is virtually impossible to overcome. To achieve a 99% probability that a false-positive risk associated with a particular predictor of persistent vegetative state among survivors is no more than one in a 1000, a study would have to contain a subset of at least 4603 patients who meet that criterion, survive at least 3 months, and remain in a chronic vegetative state.[22]

Probability estimates will never approach 100% accuracy unless they are made so restrictive that they apply to very few patients and thus are rendered useless. Requiring prognostic tools to fulfill standards that virtually no other test in medicine can meet is unreasonable and counterproductive. Given those limitations, we must use the best data available and recognize that exceptions to the rule will always exist and that medicine cannot be practiced safely for the exceptions alone.

Even if a prognostic system were able to generate the kind of statistical accuracy noted earlier, many physicians would still be unable or reluctant to act on this information. Our society emphasizes the autonomy of each patient, and some patients want every intervention, no matter what the chances. Thus, for physicians who value life above all other considerations, even if outcome data were 100% accurate, life support would not be withdrawn or limited for the 99

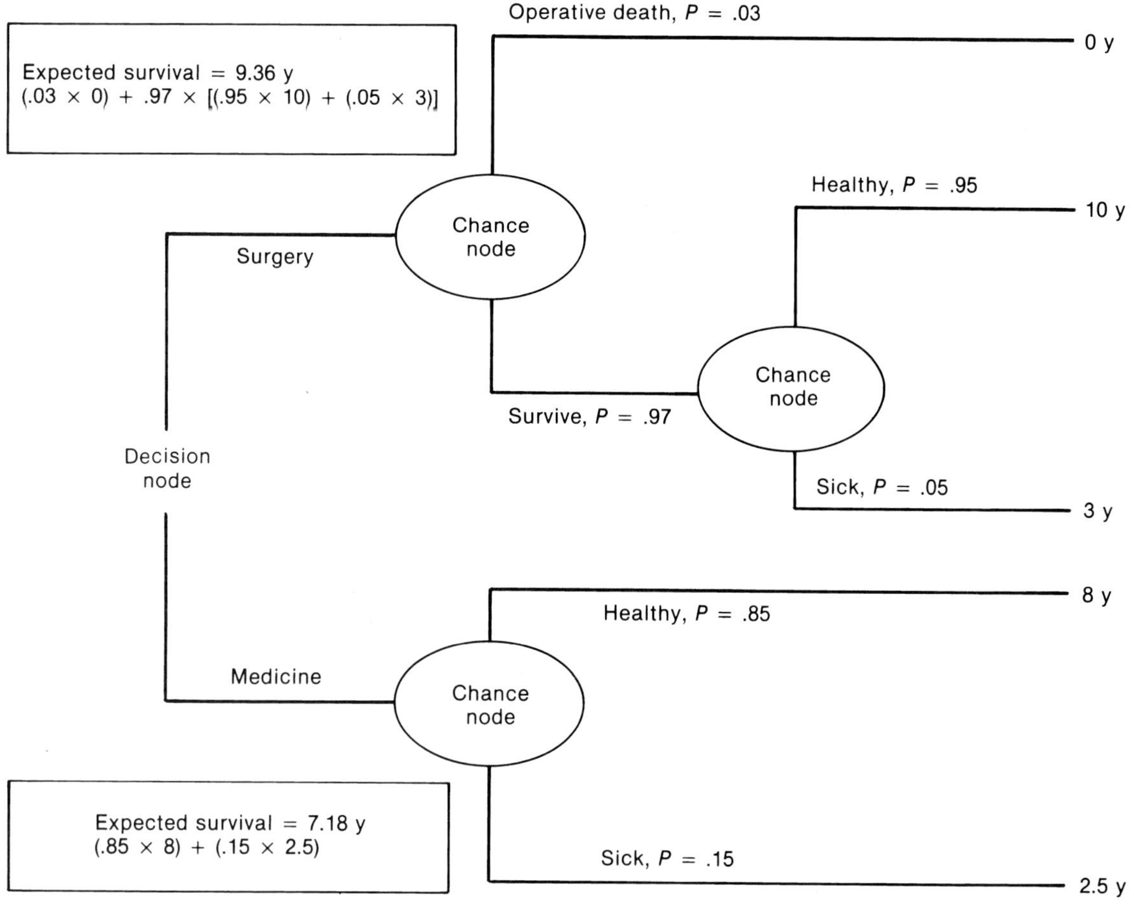

Figure 198–1. Example of formal decision tree analysis. (Adapted from Chalfin DB, Niederman MS, Fein AM: The application of decision analysis to critical care medicine. Intensive Care World 1992; 9:120–124.)

patients destined to die if the 100th patient is destined to survive. However, as already discussed, cost considerations are mandating a change in this paradigm, and although patient autonomy will always be respected, patients are unlikely to be able to insist on an intervention that is very unlikely to benefit them. Recent efforts to define futility in medicine are important indicators of the desire to provide guidelines to practitioners as to when they might consider continued treatment of a given case "futile."[23–26] One proposed definition of futility is treatment that has not benefited or has failed in the last 100 patients to whom it has been offered.[24] Defining a treatment as futile does not preclude the possibility that it could benefit a given patient, but it does provide a rationale for withholding the treatment. Although attempts to develop a numeric definition of futility oversimplifies a complex concept, objective estimates of outcome will be important in providing information that can be used for these difficult medical decisions. It will always be important to remember, however, that probability estimates are best used to support clinical decisions, not to make them.[27]

PRINCIPLES OF PROGNOSTIC SCORING AND OUTCOME PREDICTION

Several steps are necessary for devising an accurate and applicable outcome prediction model (Table 198–1).[28, 29] First, the outcome predicted must be defined and a model developed to relate how predictors influence outcome. Factors that influence outcome must be identified *(predictor variables)* and an accurate method for measuring and weighting each variable chosen. A data base is then collected that contains information about each predictor variable and the corresponding outcome. Next, statistical analysis is performed, a predictive instrument formulated, and predicted results compared with actual outcome. Finally, the instrument is validated, ideally by applying it to an independent patient data base. Because each of these steps is important in the development of a predictive instrument, they are reviewed in detail here.

Definition of Outcome

The outcome to be measured must be relevant to clinicians, easily recognized, and well defined so as to be free of ascer-

TABLE 198–1. Steps in the Development of a Prognostic Scoring System

- Establish a precise definition of the outcome being predicted.
- Develop a model of variables that directly influence outcome.
- Define each predictive variable with good measurement reliability.
- Collect data base with information on predictive variables and patient outcome.
- Formulate predictive instrument that anlayzes relationship of variables to the outcome.
- Validate the predictive instrument.

tainment bias. Hospital mortality is the outcome most commonly measured by currently available prognostic systems and meets all of these criteria. Hospital mortality is, and will remain, a highly relevant outcome for most physicians and patients. In the future, however, measuring other outcomes (e.g., quality of life) will also be important. Measuring quality of survival will be difficult and will be subject to ascertainment bias because it is difficult to define and is observer dependent. Fortunately, substantial progress has been made in the measurement of quality of life after hospitalization.[30] Because mortality remains the most relevant outcome for ICU physicians, the remainder of this discussion focuses on the designing of predictive models that use mortality as the measured outcome.

Model Development and Selection of Predictor Variables

Predictor variables include disease or other characteristics whose presence have an impact on mortality. Predictor variables may be as diverse as patient demographics, vital signs, or laboratory values. For a prognostic system to be consistent, predictor variables should be easily defined and reliably measured to ensure uniformity between institutions and to avoid acertainment bias.[31] To prevent circular reasoning, variables used in predicting an outcome must not be part of the outcome,[32] e.g., using a Glasgow Coma Scale of less than 7 to predict hepatic encephalopathy.

The variables that affect hospital mortality are shown in Table 198–2. The variables are divided into categories according to whether they can be measured before or after treatment. Although response to treatment is a powerful predictor of patient outcome, therapy varies greatly among institutions, and therefore bias is possible. One way in which Acute Physiology and Chronic Health Evaluation (APACHE) III differs from APACHE II is that serial measurements have been incorporated into the former, resulting in an improved and more dynamic predictive ability.

Two criticisms of current prognostic systems are that they can neither identify all variables that determine outcome nor account for unexpected or unpredictable events.[33] Because automated data collection, computer-bedside monitor links, and modern statistical analysis permit comprehensive evaluation of a wide variety of physiologic and laboratory variables, however, significant predictor variables are unlikely to be missed. Although predictive instruments will never have 100% accuracy, the use of serial measurements over time permits prognostic systems to better reflect the implications of treatment response and unexpected events on hospital outcome.

Pretreatment Predictor Variables

The ability to predict outcome before treatment can help decide whether or not therapy is effective or appropriate. Predicting that a patient is at low risk for requiring life support, for example, may allow triage to a step-down unit or to a regular floor rather than to an ICU. Similarly, predicting that a patient is at a greater than 95% risk of dying regardless of therapy can support allocation decisions when ICU resources are limited. Variables that determine outcome before treatment include type of disease; prior physiologic reserve, as reflected by age, chronic disease, and ability to perform activities of daily living; and severity of disease.

TABLE 198–2. Determinants of Outcome of Critical Illness

Information Availability	*Patient and Treatment Factors*
Before treatment	Type of disease
	Severity of Disease
	Physiologic reserve (age, comorbidity)
After treatment	Type and timing of therapy
	Response to therapy

TYPE OF DISEASE. This is an important determinant of patient outcome; for example, patients with septic shock have a higher risk of dying than do those with uncomplicated pneumonia. Disease labeling must be as precise as possible; inaccurate disease labeling introduces a potential error because patients are included in a prognostic system when they do not have the disease for which the system was designed. Not only must the disease be accurately labeled, but its cause may also be of equal importance. For example, acquired immunodeficiency syndrome patients who develop respiratory failure after bronchoscopy do not have the same prognosis as do those who develop respiratory failure from disease progression.[34] Accounting for different cause of the same disease is a major challenge to outcome prediction, especially for disease- or organ-specific systems.

Accurate disease labeling for critically ill patients is difficult because patients with serious preexisting diseases, or patients with two simultaneously occurring problems, are frequently admitted to ICUs. The outcome of a patient with leukemia and septic shock could be quite different from that of a previously normal person with sepsis. Outcome predictions can be made for either the short-term survival of the septic shock patient after treatment or for the long-term survival of the leukemic patient.

The more precisely a disease is identified, the more accurate is the final prediction. The value of this increased precision, however, must be balanced against the need to group patients into categories for analysis. Too limited a definition will mean too few patients are available for statistical analysis. Too broad a characterization will make analysis meaningless for clinical comparison.

PHYSIOLOGIC RESERVE. This term refers to the impact of a patient's prior health status on his or her ability to recover from acute illness. Clearly, a previously healthy 23-year-old patient is likelier to survive multiple traumatic injuries than is a chronically ill 75-year-old patient, but the difference is difficult to define and quantitate. Physiologic reserve is often assessed by use of such simple terminology as "appearing older than stated age," but more precise measurements are needed. Although age is an important factor, it is an imprecise indicator of physiologic reserve, and for some illnesses, it is a weak outcome predictor.[35, 36]

Chronic health problems accelerate the loss of physiologic reserve and decrease the probability of survival. Some diseases, such as cirrhosis of the liver, leukemia, lymphoma, and multiple myeloma, have a profound impact on outcome from critical illness and deserve special emphasis as predictor variables.[37] Other patients have diminished physiologic reserve but no well-defined comorbid process; other methods are required for their assessment. In some instances, tests such as serum albumin level determination provide insight about physiologic reserve and have prognostic significance.[38] The ability to perform activities of daily living is another way to quantify physiologic reserve. Until more reliable measures of physiologic reserve are developed, we must rely on the variables noted earlier to reflect baseline health.

SEVERITY OF DISEASE. This variable can be defined in different ways. One approach is to define severity by extent of injury, by using such instruments as the Burn Index[39] or the Injury Severity Scoring system for trauma.[40] Another approach is to assess the impact of disease or injury on organ function, by using such instruments as the Glasgow Coma Scale.[41] Each of these indices accurately stratifies patients into categories of risk for mortality, but they are limited in their application to specific diseases. The Therapeutic Intervention Scoring System (TISS)[42, 43] measures injury severity using the premise that the more therapy a patient receives, the greater the severity of illness. Various therapeutic, monitoring, and diagnostic tasks are assigned scores from 0 to 4, with higher scores given to the most invasive and labor-intensive tasks; for example, an intra-aortic balloon pump is assigned a score of 4, but hourly vital signs are given a score of 1. Although higher TISS points correlate with a higher probability of death, TISS has limited potential as a prognostic instrument because of its reliance on therapeutic intervention. This is because therapy for specific diseases varies greatly, not only between hospitals but also between physicians in the same hospital. A patient with bleeding esophageal varices may be treated with acute sclerotherapy in one hospital, transvenous intrahepatic portosystemic shunt in another, and balloon tamponade in a third.[44] The same patient with an identical severity of illness could thus have three different TISS scores, which would have an unpredictable effect on the estimation of prognosis. Because TISS directly measures the use of ICU technologic and personnel resources, it has proved useful for defining ICU resource use, nurse-patient ratios, and the need for additional ICU beds.[43]

We believe that physiologic measurements are the best way to measure severity of disease in the ICU. Physiologic variables, whether obtained from laboratory tests or from bedside observations, are readily available, objective, and well defined. The extent of physiologic abnormality is closely associated with subsequent hospital mortality rates in a wide variety of medical and surgical conditions.[45] If physiologic variables are used to measure disease severity, the issue then becomes which physiologic variables to use and how they should be weighted. For specific diseases, the choice of physiologic variables may be obvious, such as hemodynamic subsets in acute myocardial infarction.[46, 47] For a general classification system, however, choosing and weighting physiologic variables to reflect severity across a wide variety of diseases is more problematic. The selection and weighting of variables can be performed through two major methods, broadly defined as *objective* or *subjective*.[31]

The *subjective method* uses the literature or expert opinion to select physiologic variables and to assign relative weights or importance to each on the basis of clinical experience and available knowledge about their prognostic impact. The *objective method* requires some subjectivity in the initial choice of variables but then relies on computerized statistical procedures to determine their relative importance, based on the difference in values between survivors and nonsurvivors.[28] Although some controversy still exists regarding the most effective way to choose and weight physiologic variables, the availability of large data bases, on-line computerized data gathering, and sophisticated statistical analysis are encouraging more reliance on objective weighting of physiologic and other risk factors.

Posttreatment Predictor Variables

RESPONSE TO THERAPY. Currently, most triage decisions involving ICU treatment are relatively arbitrary, and few patients are denied ICU admission because of low acuity or because their illness is likely to lead to death, regardless of treatment. Many ICU admissions, however, fall in an intermediate range of severity, with a probability of death that ranges from 10% to 80%. After ICU admission and initiation of therapy, many patients respond to treatment and improve, some remain stable, and others deteriorate, despite full support. Responders are likelier to survive than nonresponders, and predictive models that include response to therapy in generating outcome estimates have improved accuracy.[48]

Quantitating improvement in critical illness, however, is a difficult task. For example, improvement might be defined as the movement of physiologic variables toward normal, but the issue is more complex. Among trauma, postoperative, and septic patients, studies have shown that individuals who respond to treatment by developing supranormal hemodynamic physiology, especially within the first 24 hours after the event, have improved survival.[49–52] Another study, however, showed that septic patients whose heart rate and cardiac index normalized at 24 hours had better survival.[53] Thus, even for a specific syndrome, defining improvement is difficult and is subject to conflicting results. For a general ICU population, the challenge is even greater and involves the accurate gauging of treatment response for a wide variety of illnesses. Although the exact pattern and consistency of physiologic responses for survivors versus nonsurvivors of ICU care is not yet totally clear, it is evident that refining prognostic probabilities to reflect response to therapy over time can improve prognostic precision.[54]

TYPE, TIMING, AND PROCESS OF THERAPY. Not all patients are treated in the same way or at the same time. A prognostic system developed to predict outcome from closed head trauma at an institution that employs early surgery and intracranial pressure monitoring might not be applicable for an institution that does not. Thus, variations in "standard" practice necessitate close examination of treatment variations when outcome from critical illness is evaluated.

The timing of therapy is a commonly overlooked but extremely important variable in the determination of outcome. A patient presenting to the emergency department with severe pneumonia has a better prognosis than does the patient admitted to a hospital ward 3 days earlier whose condition has deteriorated despite therapy. These two patients might have the same severity of illness on ICU admission, but one has already not responded to initial treatment. Likewise, some ICU patients are extensively treated and stabilized before ICU admission, whereas others are promptly admitted; differences in admission status may thus reflect variations in institutional practice rather than individual patient risk. Both of these forms of "lead-time bias" must be appropriately weighted if a prognostic system is to be applicable to all patients.[55, 56]

Data Base

Once variables are chosen, a data base that contains information on the variables and corresponding outcomes must be collected. The predictions derived from this patient data base provide risk assessments for future patients. The more patients in the data base with characteristics similiar to the new patients being evaluated, the more accurate and useful the risk assessments will be.[28] The data base must be carefully gathered and potential confounding variables identified to avoid selection bias. *Selection bias* refers to prediction errors caused by differences in current patients compared with the reference data base population. Collecting data in a large number of hospitals with different characteristics (size, teaching status, rural versus urban) avoids emphasizing practices that are unique to a single hospital type or region and minimizes the potential for selection bias.

Formulating the Predictive Instrument

After data collection is completed, an analysis of the relationship between predictor variables and outcome is necessary to formulate the predictive instrument and to generate probability estimates. Although predictor variables can be mathematically related to outcome in several ways, the commonest way is the use of univariate or multivariate regression techniques.[10, 57] Univariate regression analysis is generally used when there are a dichotomous dependent variable (e.g., death versus survival) and a continuous independent variable (e.g., the acute physiology score [APS] of APACHE). When multiple independent variables affect a dichotomous outcome, multivariate regression techniques provide a way to assess each predictor variable's relationship with the outcome independent of the other variables. For example, application of multivariate analysis to the APACHE III data base generated equations that predict the risk of hospital death from predictor variables that include APACHE III score (total points for age, chronic health evaluation, and APS); primary reason for ICU admission, location and length of stay before ICU admission; and surgical status.[58] Similarly, the mortality prediction model (MPM) used linear discriminant function and multiple logistic regression to predict mortality from 11 variables measured at ICU admission.[59]

Validation

Regardless of how predictive estimates are formulated, all prognostic systems must be validated. Validation is necessary for the detection of any bias that may have gone undetected in the original patient sample. Ideally, validation is performed using data from a "new" set of patients, but generating another data base from patients distinct from the test group is expensive and often impractical. Alternatively, the test group can be a sample of the original group from which the model was derived (referred to as cross-validation) or it can be a portion of the test group whose data were originally excluded when the model was formulated (split-sample technique). Whatever the methodology used, the accuracy of the predictive instrument is assessed by comparing predicted outcomes to the actual outcomes in the test group.

The statistical methods used to assess predictive accuracy include summary statistics, receiver-operator curves, goodness-of-fit tests, percent-correct classification, and R^2 analysis.[10, 57, 60, 61] Many physicians are unfamiliar with these statistical techniques and may even be suspicious that "number crunching" has caused data to appear more accurate than they really are. Reliance on a single summary number, such as R^2 or overall correct classification rate at a predefined risk level (conventionally 50%), reveals little about a prognostic system's overall performance or its utility in research or clinical applications.[28] We believe that it is more meaningful to examine the number of outcomes predicted to occur versus the actual number found (predictive value positive). This analysis can be displayed with bar graphs that plot observed versus predicted outcomes (Fig. 198–2). Such figures permit examination of the calibration of the system (how closely the predicted versus the observed outcomes match throughout the range of risks) and how well the system discriminates between individuals destined to live or die. Although the methods for assessing accuracy are complex and confusing, a working knowledge of statistical techniques is needed to evaluate and compare different predictive systems. The reader is referred elsewhere for a more complete discussion of all of these topics.[10, 57]

Outcome Prediction Models

Outcome prediction models can be broadly classified as disease specific or general. Prognostic indices for specific diseases include the Ranson criteria for acute pancreatitis,[62] the Child-Turcotte classification for cirrhosis,[63] the Burn Index,[39] the Injury Severity Score System,[40] the Glascow Coma Scale for assessing the neurologic function,[41] the Hunt-Hess scale for subarachnoid hemorrhage and the Sepsis Severity Scoring System.[64a] In addition, semistructured methods also exist for the stratification of patients with acute renal failure,[65] acute respiratory failure,[66] and multiple organ dysfunction syndrome.[67] Prognostic indices developed for specific disease have a conceptual advantage over general systems because they focus on predictors that are specific or peculiar to that entity. For example, patients with severe anoxic encephalopathy after cardiac arrest are unlikely to survive hospitalization even if otherwise physiologically stable.[68] Such a patient might have a relatively low APACHE score, which might otherwise portend a good outcome.

A general prediction model (e.g., APACHE III) is intended to estimate prognosis for a broad variety of diseases. Several considerations support the use of general over disease-specific systems. First, most ICUs admit patients with a broad range of diagnoses, and a general system that is accurate for all patients is more practical than is a different system for each patient. Second, for most diseases, physiologic abnormalities are not limited to a single organ system. For example, Ranson's criteria for assessing severity of acute

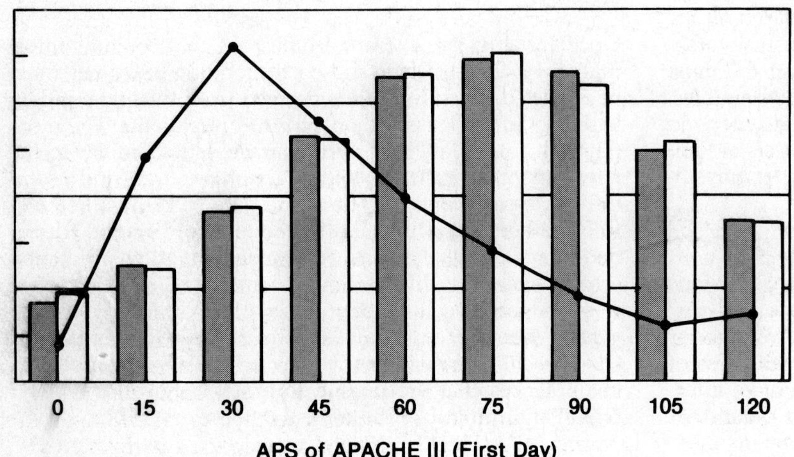

Figure 198–2. Example of a bar graph displaying predicted results *(white bars)* versus observed results *(gray bars)*. This example groups patients according to the first-day acute physiology score component of APACHE III. The number of cases *(solid line)* is displayed on the left scale, and the right scale could be calibrated to the outcome being predicted (e.g., mortality). Comparing predicted results with observed results within any single APS range (e.g., APS 60–70) demonstrates discrimination, whereas comparison across the entire range of scores refers to calibration. See the text for details.

pancreatitis include predominantly nonspecific variables, such as age, white blood cell count, blood urea nitrogen level, and PaO_2.[62] Because most of these variables are included in general prognostic systems, it is not surprising that systems such as APACHE II perform as well as do Ranson's criteria in predicting outcome from acute pancreatitis.[69–71] Finally, the large data bases and computer analyses used in developing general prognostic systems have permitted testing of multiple predictor variables and of their empirical importance by use of regression analysis. This methodology allows these systems to include a minimum number of variables, to simplify data collection, and yet to maintain prognostic accuracy. This approach has facilitated such discoveries as the importance of coma[72] and the impact of patient location before ICU admission[73] in predicting mortality for any disease category.

For these reasons, we believe that general prognostic systems have the widest applicability, and we encourage readers to familiarize themselves with these systems and their uses. Concerns regarding the applicability of these systems across disciplines (e.g., surgical patients)[74] or for specific entities, such as trauma,[75] have been addressed by the many examples of their accuracy and usefulness for these conditions. Reports of inaccurate prognostic estimates using general systems have also created considerable confusion.[76–79] We agree with others that many of these "negative" studies did not follow accepted methodology either in entering patients or in performing analysis and are not representative of the systems' abilities.[10, 80]

General Prognostic Scoring Systems

This section describes the two most widely used general severity and prognostic scoring systems, the MPM and the APACHE. The discussion focuses on their development and their uses for quality assessment, utilization review, risk stratification, and clinical decision support.

Mortality Prediction Model

The MPM[59, 81, 82] was designed to estimate the probability of hospital mortality at ICU admission, 24 and 48 hours after admission, and at other intervals during ICU stay. The methods used to develop the MPM differ substantially from those used for APACHE II.[82] Instead of using an expert panel to select and weight predictors according to perceived severity and impact on survival, the MPM is based on objective statistical modeling. Information was obtained on a large number of variables, followed by identification of a smaller subset of the strongest outcome predictors derived from statistical reduction techniques.

An admission model (MPM_0) estimates the probability of hospital mortality at the time of ICU admission. The MPM_0 contains 11 patient-specific variables: level of consciousness (coma or deep stupor), type of admission (elective, emergency), cardiopulmonary resuscitation performed immediately before ICU admission, cancer as part of the presenting problem, history of chronic renal failure, probable infection, age, ICU admission in previous 6 months, heart rate, surgical service, systolic blood pressure, and systolic blood pressure squared. A 14-variable, 24-hour model (MPM_{24}), and an 11-variable, 48-hour model (MPM_{48}) reflect patient status after treatment and develop hospital mortality predictions based on data collected during these time periods. In addition, a three-variable "over-time" model (MPM_{ot}) incorporates changes in probability of hospital mortality from previous evaluation points. The MPM was validated at 14 United States ICUs, and its performance was evaluated using goodness-of-fit testing.[82] The 24- and 48-hour models were evaluated on a subset of 948 patients who remained in the ICU for at least 48 hours.[83] The results of this study indicated that the MPM_0 did not fit when evaluated on this group; the MPM_{ot} had the highest sensitivity and the second highest specificity. Studies comparing the MPM, the Simplified APS, and the APACHE II suggest similar predictive accuracy based on first ICU day information.[83]

The MPM has been used to estimate probability of hospital mortality for ICU patient groups[83] and for identifying charts for ICU quality assessment review.[84] The MPM is not recommended for assessing prognosis for individual patients. Refinement is continuing, with the aim of improving the MPM's accuracy and usefulness.[85]

Acute Physiology and Chronic Health Evaluation

The original APACHE system was introduced in 1981[85] and consisted of two parts: (1) an APS that reflected the degree of physiologic derangement and (2) a chronic health evaluation that reflected the patient's status before the acute illness. The APS was developed by an expert panel of physicians who selected and weighted 34 laboratory and clinical measurements based on their perceived impact on mortality. APACHE provided a reliable and valid method for severity measurement and risk stratification[86–88] but was complex and required multihospital validation.

APACHE II was introduced in 1985 and incorporated major changes in the original APACHE system.[89] The number of physiologic variables was reduced from 34 to 12, and a higher score was assigned to acute renal failure and coma to better reflect their prognostic impact. Scoring for operative status, such as emergency surgery, was added, and chronic health evaluation was changed to reflect the impact of aging; immune deficiency; and chronic cardiac, pulmonary, renal, or liver disease. Finally, an equation was developed to estimate prognosis based on information collected during the first 24 hours in the ICU.

APACHE II consists of a numeric score (ranging from 0 to 71) derived from three components: (1) points for extent of abnormality of 12 physiologic parameters (APS), (2) points for increasing age, and (3) points for chronic health abnormalities. APACHE II scoring uses the worst values for the initial ICU day. An increasing APACHE II score reflects an increased severity of disease and a higher risk of hospital death. APACHE II can be used to predict the risk of death for multidiagnostic ICU patient groups based on aggregate individual estimates that account for the impact of disease, the risk imposed by emergency surgery, and first-day APACHE II score.[90] APACHE II has been used in over 300 published studies for outcome assessment, as a case-mix control in therapeutic trials, to evaluate ICU resource utilization, and as a quality assessment tool. The success and acceptance of APACHE II as a case-mix control and as a means for group risk stratification in clinical investigations is attributable to the system's statistical and clinical validity.

APACHE II's most important limitation is that the system was neither designed nor intended to predict mortality for individual patients, and it has an error rate of approximately 15% for the prediction of hospital mortality using a 0.50 decision point. Several investigators, however, have used APACHE II scoring over time to assess prognosis for individual patients.[48, 91, 92] Although these authors were able to place patients into ascending risk strata, their predictions were consistently high; for example all patients with a greater than 60% risk of death were predicted to die. APACHE II is also subject to selection and lead-time bias. Errors in prediction caused by differences in referral source[55, 93] and severity criteria relative to criteria used in creating APACHE II have led to inaccurate outcome estimates among patients with congestive heart failure[94] and MODS.[95] *Lead-time bias* refers to errors in prediction that result from variations in the timing of ICU admission. Unless the data from all admissions are entered at approximately the same time in the course of their illness, the resulting predictions may not calibrate well to new data bases.[55, 91]

APACHE III Prognostic System

APACHE III was introduced in 1991[54] to expand and improve the prognostic estimates provided by APACHE II. The APACHE III study[96] re-evaluated the selection and weighting of physiologic variables using objective statistical modeling; expanded the size and representativeness of the reference data base; examined how outcome is related to patient selection for, and timing of, ICU admission; and clearly distinguished the use of predictive estimates for patient groups from mortality estimates for individuals.

The APACHE III system consists of two parts: an APACHE III score, and a series of predictive equations linked to diagnosis and the APACHE III data base. The APACHE III score consists of points for (1) physiologic abnormalities, (2) age, and (3) chronic health status. Scoring is based on the degree of abnormality in 17 physiologic variables (APS), which reflects values for vital signs, laboratory tests, and neurologic status. In addition, points are added based on age and seven comorbid conditions shown to have a significant impact on short-term mortality. The sum of points for APACHE III's components yields a numeric score that theoretically ranges from 0 to 299; physiologic scoring contributes most (0–252) of the score, compared with age (0–24) and chronic health evaluation (0–23).

The APACHE III score can be used to measure severity of disease and to risk-stratify patients within a single diagnostic category or independently defined patient group. This is because an increasing score is associated with an increased risk of hospital death. APACHE III scores can also be used to compare patient outcomes but can only be used for ICU admissions meeting diagnostic and selection criteria similiar to those used in the APACHE III study.

APACHE III Predictive Equations

A series of APACHE III predictive equations estimate various outcomes by linking patient characteristics to a nationally representative data base of 17,440 United States ICU admissions. The risk of hospital death is based on the prognostic implications of first-day APACHE III score, disease classification, and patient selection for intensive care. The data base includes 212 potential diagnoses and provides weights for 66 specific diagnoses and 12 organ system–related residual categories. Patient selection is accounted for by variables that reflect whether or not ICU readmission or emergency surgery occurred and the patient's location and length of hospital stay before ICU admission. These variables are included to partly control for differences in patient selection and response to therapy, that is, selection and lead-time bias. In addition to predicting hospital mortality, equations using similiar, but not identical, variables are used to predict length of ICU stay, amount of therapy required, use of nursing resources, and risk for receiving active life-supporting therapy. Individual ICUs and institutions can thus compare outcome predictions based on their own patient and institutional characteristics with nationally derived figures, thereby providing a means for assessing ICU efficacy and efficiency.

Future Applications of Prognostic Systems

In the future, we expect that the use of prognostic systems for clinical research, quality improvement, and utilization review will become commoner and more sophisticated. We also believe that these systems will be used to assist in decision making about ICU admission and discharge, but we are uncertain about their exact role in individual patient care decisions. ICU clinicians could obtain and use probabilities at the patient's bedside in much the same way we currently use the results of laboratory tests. Unlike the results of a blood test, however, a risk probability is derived indirectly from patient characteristics and a reference data base.

Prognostic Systems in Clinical Research

A central problem in conducting clinical trials is the need to ensure that treatment and control groups are at equivalent baseline risk for death or other important outcome. Despite the use of categorical definitions, such as systemic inflammatory response syndrome,[97, 98] a large number of patient-related variations can lead to differences in pretreatment risk.[98, 99] Randomization is typically employed to spread risk factors evenly between experimental and control groups, and a comparison of mean values is used to ensure that risks are equally divided. Randomization, however, can ensure only that patients, not their risks, are randomly distributed, and mean values may not accurately define important variations in baseline risk.[100] In addition, exclusion criteria precisely define which patients are too well or too sick to benefit from the therapy being studied.

A prognostic scoring system that is capable of producing individual patient risk estimates can address these concerns by allowing investigators to risk-stratify patients before randomization to ensure proper patient selection and to ensure that risks are evenly distributed. Considering the expense required to enter patients into clinical experiments, any technique that can reduce the number of observations and improve the accuracy is valuable. Knaus and colleagues[101] demonstrated how estimating each patient's individual risk of death and using modern multivariate techniques can reduce the number of patients or observations needed to demonstrate statistical significance between the two treatment arms of a randomized trial. Individual risk estimates can also be used for an adjusted analysis of treatment results using a two-variable model, in which one variable is an indicator of treatment or control status and the second, a comprehensive measure of patient risk.[101] The same risk predictions could also be used to select patients and to monitor the effectiveness of new drugs once they are tested and approved.[101a]

Prognostic Systems and Quality Measurement

As health care costs have increased, outcome assessment has become a major priority for ICUs, hospitals, government, and third-party payers. Because an ICU in a rural, nonteaching hospital has a different patient population than does an urban teaching center, mortality and complication rates that are not adjusted for differences in patient mix are unlikely to reflect differences in quality of care.[102] A prognostic system that establishes a predicted mortality rate for each ICU based on a representative data base and a patient-by-patient measurement of risk allows ICUs to compare their observed versus their predicted outcomes. The difference between actual and predicted death rates provides an outcome-based measure of quality of care and provides insight into means for improving performance.

This approach was demonstrated by a 1986 evaluation of outcome from intensive care at 13 major United States medical centers.[90] When the actual mortality rate for each ICU was compared with its predicted rate, 11 of the 13 units performed within two standard deviations, but one ICU had significantly more deaths than predicted, and one had significantly fewer deaths. In a recently completed prospective study, unadjusted mortality rates at 42 ICUs ranged from 6.4% to 40%.[58] Analysis using the APACHE III prognostic scoring system revealed that 90% of this difference resulted from varying patient physiologic and demographic characteristics. The ratio of actual-to-predicted hospital death rates varied between 0.67 and 1.25, with risk adjusted mortality significantly better at five ICUs and worse at five ICUs ($P < .05$).[58]

In the future, ICUs will be able to monitor and compare their outcome performance using the methods discussed earlier. Through the use of an automated system to enter clinical and physiologic data, prognostic estimates can be generated that will allow ICUs to compare their observed outcomes with either a nationally representative sample or with ICUs with similar structural characteristics. For quality improvement activities, these methods will also facilitate analysis of group outcomes by specialty, diagnosis or severity of illness.

Prognostic Systems in Resource Allocation

Because cost containment is likely to dominate future health care policy, ICUs will find it increasingly important to improve the efficiency of patient selection and treatment. This goal can be achieved in three major ways: (1) limit ICU admission of patients at low risk for requiring life-supporting therapy, (2) limit admission or prolonged stays for patients who are unlikely to benefit from ICU therapy, and (3) monitor and seek to continuously improve the use of nursing, monitoring, and therapeutic resources.

Patients at less than a 10% risk for needing life-supporting therapy are commonly admitted to United States ICUs for monitoring and observation.[103–105] When all ICU beds are occupied, however, low-risk patients are frequently denied ICU admission, or their length of ICU treatment is shortened.[106–108] An objective method to identify these patients would be useful in supporting clinical judgment and in resolving competing demands regarding priorities for ICU admission when bed availability is limited. Studies using APACHE II have demonstrated the technical capability of accomplishing this goal, with modest cost savings and little effect on quality of care.[103, 104, 109] Although an estimate of risk for requiring unique ICU therapy is only one variable affecting the decision to admit a patient to an ICU, it can provide objective criteria for establishing priorities for admission and discharge. An automated system that incorporates a predictive equation can provide daily bedside estimates of risk for life-supporting treatment. These objective risk estimates could then be used to supplement clinical judgment regarding admission and discharge decisions.[109a]

Patients who are hopelessly ill and unlikely to benefit from ICU care are infrequently denied admission for reasons that range from prognostic uncertainty to denial of impending death on the part of patients, families, or physicians. Even commoner are patients who are already receiving ICU therapy but have either deteriorated or failed to respond to treatment. In the future, prognostic systems may be able to assist in identifying patients who are likely to die despite state-of-the-art medical support. When combined with clinical judgment these systems might be used to support decisions to withhold or withdraw treatment.[6, 110, 110a]

The applications of prognostic systems for resource allocation are not limited to evaluations of patient risk. ICU length of stay and aggregate treatment requirements can also be assessed as measures of unit performance.[58] Scientific methods to monitor performance and to define upper and lower control limits are the basis for modern quality management techniques.[111–114] Statistical controls also permit ICU clinicians to "manage by facts."[115] For example, length of ICU stay can be predicted based on individual patient characteristics referenced against a data base. An ICU medical director might discover that the length of stay in his or her ICU exceeds that of similiar units. Using this knowledge as a focus for problem diagnosis, potential causes can be identified and solutions designed and implemented. Continued monitoring would provide a means for confirming and maintaining improved performance.

Prognostic Systems and Individual Patient Decisions

For many clinicians, the most important question regarding prognostic scoring systems is how can they help with individual patient care decisions? Many physicians believe that group statistics do not apply to individuals. Although individual patients do have unique characteristics, they also share many common features with previous patients, and consideration of these similarities permits us to anticipate the patients' response and predict their outcome. If this kind of reasoning played no role in clinical decision making, then we would never be able to use past experience to guide future decisions. In fact, we do use past experiences every day when we choose one therapy over another, and we frequently base our decisions on the relative probability that a particular treatment will be successful in an individual patient.

Recent studies have explored the use of prognostic scores over time to update clinical predictions and thus better predict outcome.[48, 92, 110, 110a] It makes sense that a patient whose scores improve after the first 24 hours of ICU treatment is likelier to survive than is one whose scores worsen. Further investigation into the best way to assess scores over time, such as daily change in absolute scores or percentage change from baseline, is required before any specific approach can be recommended. Improvements in prognostic systems will also be related to expansion of the data bases used to generate their predictions. Every prognostic scoring system relies on data from previoiusly treated patients for the derivation of weights and the calibration of risk estimates. The larger and more representative the data base, the more accurate and useful the predictions will be for future patients.

Although the number of direct comparisons is still limited, statistical predictions of outcome produced by prognostic scoring systems are apparently at least as accurate as clinical predictions and are, in most circumstances, more reliable.[17, 19, 20, 116] These findings suggest that the predictions available from prognostic scoring systems could eventually be useful in aiding or supporting clinical judgment in decision making for individual patients.

CONCLUSIONS

Important social and financial considerations are changing American medicine. Physicians are, and should remain, uncomfortable with making treatment decisions based solely on financial factors, but the influence of these factors can no longer be avoided. In 1992, an estimated $809 billion was spent in the United States on health care, representing 13% of the gross national product.[117] Current practices will continue to escalate these expenditures, thus the mandate for change.

For financial, ethical, and medical reasons, intensive care is likely to be heavily scrutinized as part of any new health care delivery proposal. At high-cost facilities, the efficacy and cost efficiency of ICUs is already widely viewed as one important target for reduction. Policy analysts point at studies that suggest that 8% of ICU patients, "high-cost admissions," consumed as many resources as the remaining 92%.

Of the 8% designated as high-cost patients, 70% died in the hospital.[118, 119] Results of such studies, combined with a general societal concern over the amount of health care costs spent during the last year of life, are increasing concern that we are wasting substantial resources.

Cost control should never dictate withholding or withdrawal of care, and physicians must strive to maintain their role as the patient advocate. Physicians also need to recognize, however, that financial considerations are not necessarily at odds with their primary scientific and ethical obligations. When asked, most individuals do not desire invasive life-support measures if they will become dependent on them or if their lives will not be extended beyond 60 days. We need to engage our patients earlier and more frequently in discussions regarding their values and preferences for such interventions. Outcome predictions provide one source of support for such enhanced communication as well as a basis for discussions regarding the most appropriate allocation of resources. Predicting who will and who will not benefit from ICU care is an important new step in refining utilization of this very expensive therapy.

References

1. Butler PW, Bone RC, Field T: Technology under Medicare diagnosis-related groups prospective payment. Implications for medical intensive care. Chest 1985; 87:229–234.
2. National Institutes of Health Development Conference: NIH Consensus Development Conference Statement. JAMA 1983; 250:798.

2a. Siegler M: Falling off the pedestal: What is happening to the traditional doctor-patient relationship? Mayo Clin Proc 1993; 68:461–467.

3. Wagner DP, Wineland TD, Knaus WA: The hidden costs of treating severely ill patients: Charges and resource consumption in an intensive care unit. Health Care Fin Rev 1983; 5:81–86.
4. Outcomes and PORTs (Editorial): Lancet 1992; 340:1439.
5. Oye RK, Landefeld CS, Jayes RL: Outcomes in SUPPORT. J Clin Epidemiol 1990; 43:83S–87S.
6. Knaus WA, Wagner DP, Lynn J: Short-term mortality predictions for critically ill hospitalized adults: Science and ethics. Science 1991; 254:389–394.
7. Feinstein AR: An additional basic science for clinical medicine: 1. The constraining fundamental paradigms. Ann Intern Med 1983; 99:393–397.
8. Lynn J, Knaus WA: Background for SUPPORT. J Clin Epidemiol 1990; 43:1S–4S.
9. Medawar PB: The Limits of Science. New York, Harper & Row, 1984.
10. Schuster DP: Predicting outcome after ICU admission. The art and science of assessing risk. Chest 1992; 102:1861–1870.
11. Sox HC, Blatt MA, Higgens MC, et al: Medical Decision Making. Stoneham, MA, Butterworths, 1988.
12. Murphy DJ, Knaus WA: Outcome prediction in critical care medicine: The role of probability estimates in clinical decision-making and resource allocation. *In:* Critical Care: State of the Art Society of Critical Care Medicine. Vol. 11. Cerra FB, Shoemaker WC (Eds). Fullerton, CA, Society of Critical Care Medicine, 1990, pp 347–364.
13. Goldman GM: Judgmental error in intensive care practice. J Intensive Care Med 1990; 5:93–103.
14. Dawes RM, Faust D, Meehl PE: Clinical versus actuarial judgement. Science 1989; 245:1668–1674.
15. Chalfin DB, Niederman MS, Fein AM: The application of decision analysis to critical care medicine. Intensive Care World 1992; 9:120–124.
16. Greene HL, Johnson WP, Maricic MJ: Decision Making in Medicine. St. Louis, Mosby-Year Book, 1992.
17. Kruse JA, Thill-Baharozian MC, Carlson RW: Comparison of clinical assessment with APACHE II for predicting mortality risk in patients admitted to a medical intensive care unit. JAMA 1988; 260:1739–1742.
18. Schafer JH, Maurer A, Jochimsen F, et al: Outcome prediction models on admission in a medical intensive care unit: Do they predict individual outcome? Crit Care Med 1990; 18:1111–1117.
19. McClish DK, Powell SH: How well can physicians estimate mortality in a medical intensive care unit? Med Decis Making 1989; 9:125.
20. Brannen AL, Godfrey LJ, Goetter WE: Prediction of outcome from critical illness: A comparison of clinical judgment with a prediction role. Arch Intern Med 1989; 149:1083.
21. Levy DE, Bates D, Caronna JJ, et al: Prognosis in nontraumatic coma. Ann Intern Med 1981; 94:293–301.
22. Shewman DA, De Giorgio CM: Early prognosis in anoxic coma: Reliability and rationale. Neurol Clin 1989; 7:823–842.
23. Schneiderman LJ, Jecker N: Futility in practice. Arch Intern Med 1993; 153:437–441.
24. Schneiderman LJ, Jecker NS, Jonsen AR: Medical futility: Its meaning and ethical implications. Ann Intern Med 1990; 112:949–954.
25. Callahan D: Medical futility, medical necessity. The-problem-without-a-name. Hastings Cent Rep 1991; 21:30–35.
26. Loewy EH, Carlson RA: Futility and its wider implications: A concept in need of further examination. Arch Intern Med 1993; 153:429–431.
27. TPN and APACHE (Editorial): Lancet 1986; i:1478.
28. Seneff M, Knaus WA: Predicting patient outcome from intensive care: A guide to APACHE, MPM, SAPS, PRISM, and other prognostic scoring systems. J Intensive Care Med 1990; 5:33–52.
29. Seneff M, Knaus WA: APACHE: A prognostic scoring system. Probl Crit Care 1989; 3:563–577.
30. Katz S: The science of quality of life. J Chronic Dis 1987; 40:459–463.
31. Ruttiman UE: Severity of illness indices: Development and evaluation. *In:* Textbook of Critical Care. 2nd ed. Shoemaker WC, Thompson WL, Holbrook PH, et al. (Eds). Philadelphia, WB Saunders, 1988, pp 1442–1447.
32. Wasson JH, Sox HC, Neff RK, et al: Clinical prediction rules: Applications and methodological standards. N Engl J Med 1985; 313:793–799.
33. Civetta JM: The clinical limitations of ICU scoring systems. Probl Crit Care 1989; 3:681–695.
34. Luce JM, Wachter RM, Hopewell PC: Intensive care of patients with the acquired immunodeficiency syndrome: Time for a reassessment. Am Rev Respir Dis 1988; 137:1261–1263.
35. Pesau B, Falger S, Berger E, et al: Influence of age on outcome of mechanically ventilated patients in an intensive care unit. Crit Care Med 1992; 20:489–492.
36. Cox SC, Norwood SH, Duncan CA: Acute respiratory failure: Mortality associated with underlying disease. Crit Care Med 1985; 13:1005–1008.
37. Goldfarb G, Novel O, Poynard T, et al: Efficacy of respiratory assistance in cirrhotic patients with liver failure. Intensive Care Med 1983; 9:271.
38. Murray MJ, Marsh M, Wochos DN, et al: Nutritional assessment of intensive care unit patients. Mayo Clin Proc 1988; 63:1106–1114.
39. Feller I, Tholen D, Cornell RG: Improvements in burn care 1965 to 1979. JAMA 1980; 244:2074–2078.
40. Baker SP, O'Neal B, Haddun W, et al: The injury severity score: A method for describing patients with multiple injuries and evaluating emergency care. J Trauma 1974; 14:187.
41. Teasdale G, Jennet B: Assessment of coma and impaired consciousness. A practical scale. Lancet 1974; ii:81.
42. Keene AR, Cullen DJ: Therapeutic intervention scoring system: Update 1983. Crit Care Med 1983; 11:1–5.
43. Cullen DJ, Nemeskal AR: Therapeutic intervention scoring system (TISS). Probl Crit Care 1989; 3:545–562.
44. Ganger DR: Management of variceal bleeding. Intensive Crit Care Dig 1992; 11:42–45.
45. Wagner DP, Knaus WA, Draper EA: Physiologic abnormalities and outcome from acute disease. Evidence for a predictable relationship. Arch Intern Med 1986; 146:1389–1396.
46. Forrester JS, Diamost G, Chatterjee K, et al: Medical therapy of acute myocardial infarction by application of hemodynamic subsets (first of two parts). N Engl J Med 1976; 295:1356.

47. Forrester JS, Diamost G, Chatterjee K, et al: Medical therapy of acute myocardial infarction by application of hemodynamic subsets (Part 2). N Engl J Med 1976; 295:1404.
48. Chang RWS, Jacobs S, Lee B: Predicting outcome among intensive care unit patients using computerized trend analysis of daily APACHE II scores corrected for organ system failure. Intensive Care Med 1988; 14:558–566.
49. Bland RD, Shoemaker WC, Abraham E, et al: Hemodynamic and oxygen transport patterns in surviving and nonsurviving postoperative patients. Crit Care Med 1985; 13:85–90.
50. Shoemaker WC, Bland RD, Appel PL. Therapy of critically ill postoperative patients based on outcome prediction and prospective clinical trials. Surg Clin North Am 1985; 65:811–833.
51. Tuchsmidt J, Fried J, Swinney R, et al: Early hemodynamic correlates of survival in patients with septic shock. Crit Care Med 1989; 17:719–723.
52. Bishop MH, Shoemaker WC, Appel PL, et al: Relationship between supranormal circulatory values, time delays, and outcome in severely traumatized patients. Crit Care Med 1993; 21:56–63.
53. Parker MM, Shelhammer JH, Natanson C, et al: Serial cardiovascular variables in survivors and nonsurvivors of human septic shock: Heart rate as an early predictor of prognosis. Crit Care Med 1987; 15:923–929.
54. Knaus WA, Wagner DP, Draper EA, et al: The APACHE III prognostic system. Risk prediction of hospital mortality for critically ill hospitalized adults. Chest 1991; 100:1619–1636.
55. Feinstein AR, Horwitz RI: Double standards, scientific methods, and epidemiologic research. N Engl J Med 1981; 304:1292.
56. Dragsted L, Jorgenson J, Jensen NH, et al: Interhospital comparisons of patient outcome from intensive care: Importance of lead-time bias. Crit Care Med 1989; 17:418–422.
57. Kiefe C: Statistical methods used by ICU prognostic indices. Probl Crit Care 1989; 3:514–527.
58. Knaus WA, Wagner DP, Zimmerman JE, et al: Variation in mortality and length of stay in intensive care units. Ann Intern Med 1993; 118:753.
59. Lemeshow S, Teres D, Pastides H, et al: A method for predicting survival and mortality of ICU patients using objectively derived weights. Crit Care Med 1985; 13:519–525.
60. Metz CE: Basic principles of ROC analysis. Semin Nucl Med 1978; 8:283–294.
61. Lemeshow S, Hosner DW: A review of goodness-of-fit statistics for use in the development of logistic regression models. Am J Epidemiol 1982; 115:92–98.
62. Ranson JHC: Etiological and prognostic factors in human acute pancreatitis: A review. Am J Gastroenterol 1982; 77:633–638.
63. Christensen E, Schlichting P, Fauerholdt L, et al: Prognostic value of Child-Turcotte criteria in medically treated cirrhosis. Hepatology 1984; 4:420.
64. Hunt WE, Hess RM: Surgical risk as related to time of intervention in the repair of intracranial aneurysms. J Neurosurg 1968; 28:14–20.
64a. Knaus WA, Harrell FE, Fisher CJ, et al: The clinical evaluation of new drugs for sepsis: A prospective study design based on survival analysis. JAMA 1993; 270:12–33.
65. Bander SJ: The impact of acute renal failure on ICU patient survival. Probl Crit Care 1989; 3:631–638.
66. Crim C: The influence of respiratory failure on ICU patient outcome. Probl Crit Care 1989; 3:616–630.
67. Knaus WA, Draper EA, Wagner DP, et al: Prognosis in acute organ-system failure. Ann Surg 1985; 202:685–693.
68. Niskanen M, Kari A, Nikki P, et al: Acute physiology and chronic health evaluation (APACHE II) and Glascow Coma Scores as predictors of outcome from intensive care after cardiac arrest. Crit Care Med 1991; 19:1465–1473.
69. Agerwel N, Pitchumoni CS: Assessment of severity in acute pancreatitis. Am J Gastroenterol 1991; 66:1385–1391.
70. Demmy TL, Burch JM, Feliciano DV, et al: Comparison of multiple-parameter prognostic systems in acute pancreatitis. Am J Surg 1988; 156:452–456.
71. Wilson C, Heath DI, Imrie CW: Prediction of outcome in acute pancreatitis: A comparative study of APACHE II, clinical assessment and multiple factor scoring systems. Br J Surg 1990; 77:1260–1264.
72. Teres D, Brown RB, Lemeshow S: Predicting mortality of intensive care unit patients. The importance of coma. Crit Care Med 1982; 10:86–95.
73. Knaus WA, Wagner DP: Interpretation of hospital mortality rates: The current state of the art. Mayo Clin Proc 1990; 65:1627–1629.
74. Berger MM, Marazzi A, Freeman J, et al: Evaluation of the consistency of acute physiology and chronic health evaluation scoring in a surgical intensive care unit. Crit Care Med 1992; 20:1681–1687.
75. Rhee KJ, Baxt WG, Mackenzie JR, et al: APACHE II scoring in the injured patient. Crit Care Med 1990; 18:827–830.
76. Fedullo AJ, Swinburne AJ, Wahl GW, et al: APACHE II scoring and mortality in respiratory failure due to cardiogenic pulmonary edema. Crit Care Med 1988; 16:1218–1221.
77. Cerra FB, Negro F, Abrams J: APACHE II score does not predict multiple organ failure or mortality in postoperative surgical patients. Arch Surg 1990; 125:519–522.
78. Schein M, Gecelter G: APACHE II score in massive upper gastrointestinal hemorrhage from peptic ulcer: Prognostic value and potential clinical applications. Br J Surg 1989; 76:733–736.
79. Maher ER, Robinson KN, Scoble JE, et al: Prognosis of critically ill patients with acute renal failure: APACHE II score and other predictive factors. Q J Med 1989; 269:857–866.
80. Charlson ME, Ales KL, Simon R, et al: Why predictive indexes perform less well in validation studies. Arch Intern Med 1987; 147:2155–2161.
81. Lemeshow S, Teres D, Pastides H, et al: A method for predicting survival and mortality of ICU patients using objectively derived weights. Crit Care Med 1985; 13:519.
82. Teres D, Lemeshow S, Harris D, et al: Mortality prediction models (MPM) for ICU patients. Probl Crit Care 1989; 3:585.
83. Lemeshow S, Teres D, Avrunin JS, et al: A comparison of methods to predict mortality of intensive care unit patients. Crit Care Med 1987; 15:715.
84. Knaus WA, Zimmerman JE, Wagner DP, et al: APACHE—Acute physiology and chronic health evaluation: A physiologically based classification system. Crit Care Med 1981; 9:591.
85. Lemeshow S, Teres D, Klar J, et al: Mortality probability models (MPM_0 and MPM_{24}) based on 19,124 patients (Abstract). Crit Care Med 1993; 21:S175.
86. Durocher A, Saulnier F, Suescart R, et al: A comparison of three severity score indices in an evaluation of serious bacterial pneumonia. Intensive Care Med 1988; 14:39.
87. Dellinger EP, Wertz MJ, Meakins JL, et al: Surgical infection stratification system for intra-abdominal infection. A multicenter trial. Arch Surg 1985; 120:21.
88. Lavin M, McMahon MJ: APACHE II score for assessment and monitoring of acute pancreatitis. Lancet 1989; ii:201.
89. Knaus WA, Draper EA, Wagner DP, et al: APACHE II: A severity of disease classification system. Crit Care Med 1985; 13:818.
90. Knaus WA, Draper EA, Wagner DP, et al: An evaluation of outcome from intensive care in major medical centers. Ann Intern Med 1986; 104:410.
91. Bion JFD, Aitchison TC, Edlin SA, et al: Sickness scoring and response to treatment as predictors of outcome from critical illness. Intensive Care Med 1988; 14:167.
92. Chang RWS: Individual outcome predictions model for intensive care units. Lancet 1989; ii:143.
93. Escarce JJ, Kelley MA: Admission source to the medical intensive care unit predicts hospital death independent of APACHE II score. JAMA 1990; 264:2389.
94. Fedullo AJ, Swinburne AH, Wahl GW, et al: APACHE II scoring and mortality in respiratory failure due to cardiogenic pulmonary edema. Crit Care Med 1988; 16:1218.
95. Cerra FB, Negro F, Abrams J: APACHE II score does not predict multiple organ failure or mortality in postoperative surgical patients. Arch Surg 1990; 125:519.
96. Zimmerman JE (Ed): The Apache III study design: Analytic plan for evaluation of severity and outcome. Crit Care Med 1989; 17(Suppl):S169.
97. Bone RC, Fisher CJ, Clemmer TP, et al: Sepsis syndrome: A valid clinical entity. Crit Care Med 1989; 17:389.
98. Bone RC, Balk RA, Cerra FB, et al: Definitions for sepsis and

organ failure and guidelines for the use of innovative therapies in sepsis. Chest 1992; 101:1644.
99. Bone RC: Toward an epidemiology and natural history of SIRS. JAMA 1992; 268:3452.
100. Knaus WA, Wagner DP, Draper EA: The value of measuring severity of disease in clinical research on acutely ill patients. J Chron Dis 1984; 137:455.
101. Knaus WA, Sun X, Nystom PO, et al: Evaluation of definitions for sepsis. Chest 1992; 101:1656.
101a. Fisher CJ, Dhainaut JF, Opal SM, et al: Recombinant human interleukin 1 receptor antagonist in the treatment of patients with sepsis syndrome. JAMA 1994; 271:1836.
102. Ellwood PM: Outcomes management—A technology of patient experience. N Engl J Med 1988; 318:1549.
103. Henning RJ, McClish D, Daly B, et al: Clinical characteristics and resource utilization of ICU patients: Implications for organization of intensive care. Crit Care Med 1987; 15:264.
104. Oye RK, Bellamy PE: Patterns of resource consumption in medical intensive care. Chest 1991; 99:685.
105. Zimmerman JE, Knaus WA, Judson JA, et al: Patient selection for intensive care: A comparison of New Zealand and United States hospitals. Crit Care Med 1988; 16:318.
106. Strauss MJ, LoGerfo JP, Yeltatzie JA, et al: Rationing of intensive care unit services: An everyday occurrence. JAMA 1986; 255:1176.
107. Knaus WA: Rationing, justice, and the American physician (Editorial). JAMA 1986; 255:1176.
108. Singer DE, Carr PL, Mulley AG, et al: Rationing intensive care—Physician responses to a resource shortage. N Engl J Med 1983; 309:1155.
109. Wagner DP, Knaus WA, Draper EA: Identification of low risk monitor admissions to medical-surgical ICUs. Chest 1987; 92:423.
109a. Zimmerman JE, Wagner DP, Draper EA, et al: Improving intensive care unit discharge decisions: Supplementing physician judgment with predictions of next day risk for life support. Crit Care Med 1994; 23:1345.
110. Knaus WA, Rauss A, Alperovitch A, et al: Do objective estimates of chances for survival influence decisions to withhold or withdraw treatment? Med Decis Making 1990; 10:163.
110a. Wagner DP, Knaus WA, Harrell FE, et al: Daily prognostic estimates for critically ill adults in intensive care units. Crit Care Med 1994; 23:1354.
111. Berwick DM: Continuous improvement as an ideal in health care. N Engl J Med 1989; 320:53.
112. Laffel G, Blumenthal D: The case for using industrial management science in health care organizations. JAMA 1988; 162:809.
113. Walton M: The Deming Management Method. New York, Putnam, 1986.
114. Kritchevsky SB, Simmons BP: Continuous quality improvement: Concepts and applications for physician care. JAMA 1991; 266:1817.
115. Berwick DM, Godfrey AB, Roessner J: Curing Health Care: New Strategies for Quality Improvement. San Francisco, Josey-Bass, 1991.
116. Silverstein MD: Prediction instruments and clinical judgement in critical care (Editorial). JAMA 1988; 260:1758.
117. Sonnefield ST, Waldo DR, Lemieux JA, et al: Projections of national health expenditures through the year 2000. Health Care Fin Rev 1991; 13:1–27.
118. Schapira DV, Studnicki J, Bradham DD, et al: Intensive Care, survival, and expense of treating critically ill cancer patients. JAMA 1993; 269:783–786.
119. Clinical Outcomes, Costs, and Decision-Making. Washington DC: Office of Technology Assessment; 1984:3–51. Publication Y3. T22/2:2C82/2/Case 28.

CHAPTER 199

Evaluating Pediatric Intensive Care Units

Murray M. Pollack, MD

NATIONAL PERSPECTIVE

The 1980s were a time of rapid growth in pediatric intensive care. From 1980 to 1990, pediatric intensive care units (ICUs) increased from 211 to 335, a 59% increase, and the number of pediatric ICU beds increased from about 1600 to almost 2900, a 76% increase. During the same time period, the number of pediatric inpatient facilities decreased by 16%, from over 2800 facilities to fewer than 2400, and the number of pediatric inpatient beds decreased by 24%, from over 52,000 to fewer than 40,000. In 1990, approximately 14% of hospitals with pediatric inpatient facilities had pediatric ICUs, an 87% increase from 1980. In 1990, 7.2% of all pediatric inpatient beds were pediatric ICU beds, increased from only 3.1% in 1980, an increase of over 130%. Although this growth is substantial, little effort has been expended to evaluate the impact of this growth. A recent national survey of different types of ICUs indicated that despite this widespread growth, pediatric ICUs are still regional referral centers; compared with adult ICUs, a higher proportion of patients are referred to pediatric ICUs from other hospitals. However, evidence also suggested that pediatric ICUs have overexpanded. Pediatric ICUs had average occupancy rates of less than 80%, substantially lower than most other units.[1]

Coincident with this growth, the American Board of Pediatrics has instituted a certifying examination in pediatric intensive care. Other specialty boards have also instituted intensive care subspecialty boards that may be used to certify individuals to practice pediatric intensive care. By the year 2000, the number of certified intensivists available for the practice of intensive care will be approximately 800 if the number of fellowship positions remains stable.

The growth in pediatric intensive care is associated with a substantial diversity of size and organizational structure,[2] the importance of which is unknown. Nationally, almost half of all pediatric ICUs have six or fewer beds. Larger units are the exception: only 6% of all pediatric ICUs have more than 18 beds. For some diseases, an association exists between improved outcomes and increased patient volume.[3] If this volume-outcome relationship applies to pediatric intensive care diseases, the number of small pediatric ICUs will be very important because smaller units will suffer as a result of diminished experience. Fortunately, at this time, the available evidence indicates that severity-of-illness adjusted mortality rates for pediatric ICUs are not associated with volume of patients treated in them.[4]

The number of small pediatric ICUs nationally is also important for innovations in healthcare. Innovations that depend on sophisticated technologies will have a much smaller impact than those that can be delivered in the local communities. Technologies such as extracorporeal membrane oxygenation offer fewer opportunities for improving outcomes because they cannot be carried out in all pediatric ICUs.

Other significant differences among pediatric ICUs include the organization and structure of these units.[2] Only 80% of pediatric ICUs have full-time medical directors, and in only 64% is the medical director or designee automatically involved in the care of all patients. Seventy-five per cent of pediatric ICUs have a pediatric intensivist. Approximately half have in-house, dedicated physician coverage 24 hours a day. Some investigators have suggested that strong organization of units and integrated communication patterns are related to quality of care.[5] If organization and structure are important, then substantial numbers of pediatric ICUs do not have strong organizational structures or integrated communication patterns to foster improved outcomes.

Substantial diversity also exists in the way medicine is practiced in these pediatric ICUs. According to data acquired from university pediatric ICUs that had intensivists on staff during the 1980s, the incidence of the use of monitoring and care modalities varied substantially.[6] For example, the incidence of use of arterial catheters ranged from 18% to 71% in pediatric ICUs, the percentages of patients receiving cardiac output determinations varied from 1% to 9%, and the incidence of use of central venous pressure catheters ranged from 9% to 64%. Therapeutic interventions also differed substantially between pediatric ICUs. For example, the incidence of vasoactive agent infusions ranged from 2% to 36%, and incidence of nutritional support ranged from 6% to 45%. In some pediatric ICUs, antibiotics were used in fewer than half of patients, and in other ICUs, they were used in over 80% of patients.

Given the diversity and rapid growth in pediatric intensive care, it is important to assess if pediatric ICUs are improving the outcomes of children treated in these units. Only a single study has investigated this issue.[7] A prospective study in Oregon and southwestern Washington evaluated all critically ill children who had respiratory failure and head trauma over a 6-month period. Seventy-four of 76 hospitals participated; the two hospitals that did not participate were so small that they did not routinely care for children. After patient discharge, study nurses collected data on outcomes, Pediatric Risk of Mortality (PRISM) scores, and therapeutic and monitoring interventions. Tertiary hospitals all had separate ICUs for children and a core of important medical and surgical pediatric subspecialists. Overall, the mortality rate in tertiary care facilities was 23.4%, and in nontertiary care facilities, only 6.0%. However, when mortality rates were adjusted for the severity of illness of the children admitted to these units, the mortality rate for the tertiary units was appropriate, and that for the nontertiary care units was 39% higher than expected. For patients whose risk of dying was greater than 30%, the odds of dying in a nontertiary care center were over eight times those of dying in a tertiary care center. These outcome differences corresponded to the severity-of-illness adjusted rates for the use of monitoring and therapeutic care modalities. Nontertiary care units used personnel-intensive modalities, such as hourly vital sign measurements, more frequently than did tertiary care units, which used invasive monitoring modalities, such as arterial catheters, more frequently. Most important, tertiary care units used ICU therapies, including mechanical ventilation and vasoactive drug infusions, more frequently. If this geographic region is representative of the nation, then the number of children dying because they were hospitalized in the wrong location is approximately 1000 per year.

LOCAL PERSPECTIVE

Evaluating the Effectiveness of Individual Intensive Care Units

Evaluations of individual ICUs are evolving to meet at least two important national trends. The first trend is quality assessment and quality improvement. *Quality assessment* emphasizes local ICU performance assessment, often measured against national standards. *Quality improvement* is a modern management technique of improving quality through constant and continuous monitoring. The second trend is cost control, necessitated by the high cost of medical care. These efforts may have important implications both for the national need to reduce healthcare expenditures and for the local need to rely on competitive bidding for managed healthcare contracts. Because ICUs are expensive, directing utilization evaluations at this area is logical.

Measuring severity of illness is necessary for performance evaluations both of quality and of ICU costs. In the ICU, the concept of severity of illness follows closely from the observation that mortality rates increase as the number of organ system failures increases. For example, in pediatric ICUs, the mortality rates for one, two, three, and greater than four organ system failures are approximately 1%, 10%, 50%, and 75%, respectively.[8] Modern severity-of-illness assessment methods relevant to critically ill patients measure physiologic status and relate it to mortality risk. Measures of physiologic status provide a basic and important method for the assessment of many aspects of intensive care; they adjust data for the severity of illness of the population, enabling a standardization of the study population.

The pediatric mortality risk assessment method that is applicable to the wide variety of pediatric intensive care patients is the PRISM score.[9] PRISM is a revision of the Physiologic Stability Index (PSI).[10] The PSI was developed from the subjective input of experts. For the assessment tool, they chose 36 variables and 76 variables ranges. Each variable range was weighted to reflect the clinical significance of the abnormality. Of special importance to pediatrics, unmeasured variables are assumed to be normal; therefore, extra tests are not required. The PSI was prospectively validated by its relationship to mortality risk in eight pediatric ICUs. Although these eight pediatric ICUs had mortality rates ranging from 3.0% to 17.6%, the mortality rate differences could be explained by the distributions of patients with different degrees of severity of illness in each ICU. In all ICUs and in the total data base, both the numbers and the distribution of outcomes predicted by the PSI were not different from those expected.

The PSI was simplified using multivariate logistic regression techniques. The resulting PRISM score has only 14 variables and 23 ranges of these variables. The PRISM scoring system is shown in Table 199–1. The ranges of abnormality are weighted using a logistic scale according to their contribution to mortality risk. The most deviant recorded variable (found in the laboratory reports and in the bedside cardiovascular and neurologic vital sign sheets) for the admission day is used for scoring. As in the PSI, extra tests are not required or advised. If the patient dies during the admission day the preterminal period is not included in scoring. Mortality risks are calculated as indicated in Table 199–1.

The performance of PRISM is generally excellent. For example, in the original validation report, 105 deaths were observed, and 103.9 deaths were predicted. The corresponding mortality rates were 8.6% observed and 8.5% predicted. The agreement between the observed and the predicted outcomes, assessed with chi-squared goodness-of-fit tests, was excellent in each of the individual ICUs, in the major diagnostic categories, and in the patient classification groups of operative and nonoperative patients.

This performance is not unusual and has accounted for the widespread use of PRISM. The author has assessed the performance of approximately 10% of the pediatric ICUs in the United States. Approximately one third of all pediatric

TABLE 199–1. The Pediatric Risk of Mortality (PRISM) Score*

Variable	*Age Restrictions and Ranges*		*Scores*
	Infants	*Children All Ages*	
Systolic BP (mm Hg)	130–160	150–200	2
	55–65	65–75	2
	>160	>200	6
	40–54	50–64	6
	<40	<50	7
Diastolic BP (mm Hg)		>110	6
Heart Rate (beats/min)	>160	>150	4
	<90	<80	4
Respiratory Rate (breaths/min)	61–90	51–70	1
	>90	>70	5
	Apnea	Apnea	5
Pao_2/Fio_2†		200–300	2
		<200	3
$Paco_2$‡ (mm Hg)		51–65	1
		>65	5
Glasgow Coma Score§		<8	6
Pupillary Reactions		Unequal or dilated	4
		Fixed and dilated	10
PT/PTT		>1.5 × control	2
Total Bilirubin Level (mg/dL)		>3.5‖	6
Potassium Level (mEq/L)		3.0–3.5	1
		6.5–7.5	1
		<3.0	5
		>7.5	5
Calcium Level (mg/dL)		7.0–8.0	2
		12.0–15.0	2
		<7.0	6
		>15.0	6
Glucose Level (mg/dL)		40–60	4
		250–400	4
		<40	8
		>400	8
Bicarbonate Level¶ (mEq/L)		<16	3
		>32	3

*Score only 1 abnormality per variable. For the following equations, $PRISM_t$ = most recent PRISM score and $PRISM_a$ = admission-day PRISM score

$$P(\text{intensive care unit death}) = \exp(R)/(1 + \exp[R])$$

where

$$R = 0.207*PRISM_a - 0.005*\text{age (in months)} - 0.433*(\text{operative status}) - 4.782.$$

(operative status = 1 if postoperative, 0 if not postoperative)

Dynamic Objective Risk Assessment (DORA) score

$$P(\text{death within 24 hours}) = \exp(R)/(1 + \exp[R])$$

where

$$R = 0.160*PRISM_a - 6.427 \text{ if only } PRISM_a \text{ is available or}$$
$$R = 0.154*PRISM_t + 0.053*PRISM_a - 6.791 \text{ if more than 1 PRISM score is available.}$$

†Cannot be assessed in patients with intracardiac shunts or chronic respiratory insufficiency. Requires arterial blood sampling.

‡May be assessed with capillary blood gases.

§Assessed only if there is known or suspected central nervous system dysfunction. Cannot be assessed in patients during such conditions as iatrogenic sedation, paralysis, and anesthesia. Scores less than 8 correspond to deep stupor or coma. If sedation or paralysis continues throughout the first 24 hours, the latest pre-ICU coma assessment may be used.

‖Greater than 1 month.

¶Use measured values.

Abbreviations: BP = blood pressure; PT = prothrombin time; PTT = partial thromboplastin time.

ICUs in a recent survey of institutions that belong to the National Association of Children's Hospitals and Related Institutions use the PRISM score. Publications document its world-wide use.

Both the PSI and PRISM have also been validated in national pediatric trauma patient samples.[11] However, this result does not indicate that the score can be applied with equal accuracy to all diagnostic categories. Oncology disorders and acquired immunodeficiency syndrome are examples of diagnoses in which the general meaning of physiologic instability, which is relevant to most ICU patients, may be altered by the diagnosis.

The rigorous, multi-institutional validation of the PSI and PRISM scores is the backbone of their use in outcome-based, quantitative quality assurance. These same validation methods are available to individual hospitals and regions that have commonly available computer technology and appropriate software. The methods are not designed to replace other quality assurance tasks, such as evaluations of nosocomial infections and unplanned extubations. However, they are designed to provide objective, outcome-based quality assurance because they overcome the difficulties encountered in the use of crude mortality rates. They may also provide continuous severity-of-illness adjusted mortality rate monitoring, appropriate for quality improvement monitoring.

Studies demonstrate that quantitative quality assurance assessments that use objective predictors to compare observed and predicted numbers of outcomes can be successful. The prospective critical care quality study in Oregon and southwestern Washington referred to earlier illustrates the suitability of this type of methodology. In another study, severity-of-illness adjusted mortality rates compiled before a pediatric intensivist joined the hospital staff were compared with those compiled after the intensivist joined the staff. The ICU mortality rate improved after the intensivist was added to the staff.[12]

If an institution decides to use PRISM or PSI scores for quantitative quality assurance, the process follows the principles discussed earlier. First, a consecutive patient sample must be acquired. The power to detect a severity-of-illness outcomes difference from the predicted numbers will be related to the size of the sample and, especially, to the number of deaths. The more deaths that are accumulated during a study, the greater the power to detect statistically a deviation from the numbers expected. The estimated numbers of survivors and deaths are calculated by summing the individual patients' mortality risks. The comparison of the observed ICU survivors and ICU deaths with the estimated numbers of ICU survivors and ICU deaths is tested in two ways. First, the total number of observed outcomes is compared with the number of expected outcomes. Statistical tests, such as the z score as proposed by Flora, may be used.[13] This test is based on the z statistic and tests the total number of outcomes but not the distribution of outcomes. A second method is a goodness-of-fit test, which evaluates both the distribution of outcomes and the total numbers of outcomes.[14] This test follows the simple observation that a higher proportion of the very sick patients should be dying than should the healthiest patients. If the patients are divided into mortality risk groups on the basis of their estimated mortality risk, then both the total number of outcomes and the distribution of outcomes can be tested using a goodness-of-fit test that is based on the chi-squared statistic.

If the observed number and distribution of outcomes are similar to the predicted number and distribution of outcomes, then the performance of the institution is equivalent to those institutions that validated the predictor in the multi-institutional studies. If the performance of the institution is different than that expected, an explanation must be sought. As with any test, physicians using this quality assurance methodology need to understand its strengths and limitations and understand when false-positive and false-negative results, confounding variables, and peculiarities of the method can occur. If the goodness-of-fit methodology is used, a specific mortality risk interval can be targeted for in-depth chart reviews. The investigation of extra deaths detected by the mortality predictors may or may not indicate that unnecessary events have occurred. Legitimate explanations exist for extra ICU deaths. For example, if the ICU patient population is skewed toward diagnostic groups that have not been extensively tested (e.g., bone marrow transplant recipients, oncology patients), then the scores may not be applicable. Subjective chart reviews may determine that the deaths were expected. For example, a logical explanation for an underestimation of deaths in low–severity-of-illness strata might be that many physiologically stable patients with terminal conditions were admitted.

A smaller-than-expected number of deaths may also be detected. Of course, this result could indicate that the care delivered in the ICU is better than that delivered in the other institutions that validated the score. However, other explanations must also be sought. An important possibility is that resuscitative efforts before the patients' arrival in the ICU were less complete than those in other institutions. Therefore, some ICU admissions would have more treatable physiologic instability (and higher physiology scores) because of the less complete resuscitation used, compared with that used in the national sample to create and validate the PRISM score.[15] Improper use of the score may also explain the results. Data collectors who are also bedside caregivers might bias data by attempting to alter how sick the patient appears.

Because medicine is a dynamic specialty with a rapidly expanding knowledge base, the utility of any severity-of-illness assessment method will always reflect the data used to derive the score as well as the quality of the institutions that validate the score. To meet this constantly changing environment, all aspects of the PRISM score are currently being revised. The reader is encouraged to review the most recent publications on the PRISM methodology for such revisions.

Evaluating the Efficiency of Individual Intensive Care Units

Many ICUs are inefficiently utilized. Increased local pressures are likely to develop to improve efficiency in these units as managed health plans request information on the efficient utilization of ICUs before these plans contract with hospitals. Current methodology enables sophisticated evaluation of ICU bed use. As in the previous section, evaluations of ICU utilization equivalent to those discussed in this section can be performed with current, widely available computer technology and software. The time requirements are more extensive than quality assessments.

Evaluations of ICU utilization require a list of unique ICU therapies and a method of assessing severity of illness. Unique therapies are those that are best delivered in the ICU, such as mechanical ventilation and vasoactive agent infusions. Reasonable unique therapy lists exist for children.[16] In most studies, these therapies have been derived from the Therapeutic Intervention Scoring System score; however, individual ICUs can determine their own list of unique ICU therapies. Monitoring modalities generally carried out in the ICU (e.g., arterial catheters) should not be included as unique therapies, because monitoring philosophies differ widely.

The second requirement for evaluation of ICU utilization is a measure of severity of illness. Increasing physiologic instability correlates to increasing risk of requiring an active ICU therapy. The risk of requiring an active ICU therapy can be estimated by using the acute (<24-hour) mortality risk as measured with the Dynamic Objective Risk Assessment score.[17] Dynamic Objective Risk Assessment uses daily PRISM scores to reflect the changing nature of disease and recovery. The prediction equation for this score is given in Table 199–1. An acute mortality risk of less than 1% indicates a very low likelihood of requiring a unique therapy.

A new group of ICU efficiency terms has arisen from the concepts discussed in the previous paragraph. Low-risk monitor patients are those who do not receive a unique ICU therapy and have low daily risks of requiring an active ICU intervention (mortality risk < 1%) during every ICU day. Potential early-discharge patients are those who used a unique ICU therapy or had an acute mortality risk of greater than 1% during the early portion of their ICU stay but whose last consecutive days of ICU stay had the characteristics of the low-risk monitor patients (no unique therapy and low risk). Efficiency is defined using days of care as follows:

Efficiency = ([Total patient days of care]
− [days of low-risk monitor patients]
− [days of potential early discharge]) / (total patient days of care)

Using these concepts, studies indicate that a clear disparity exists among pediatric ICUs in the efficiency of their utilization.[16] In a study of eight pediatric ICUs, low-risk monitor patients constituted from 16% to 58% of the patients in individual ICUs, and they used from 5.4% to 34.5% of the total days of care. Potential early-discharge patients constituted from 12% to 29% of the patients, and their days of care ranged from 5.1% to 17.2% of the total days of care. Most important, efficiency ratings ranged from 0.89 to 0.55, with four ICUs having efficiency ratings greater than 0.8, and four having efficiency ratings of less than 0.8.[16]

These efficiency terms have not been designed to have direct clinical use. A physician's decision making must incorporate many facts about the patient's disease; the possibility of acute, life-threatening events; and the hospital's facilities and abilities outside of the ICU. However, efficiency evaluations will enable ICUs to compare their performances to those of other institutions. If institutions are functioning in a very inefficient manner, they may re-evaluate their admission-and-discharge criteria and other hospital services to enable more efficient utilization of the ICU. If these units have too many low-risk monitor patients, potential early-discharge patients, or low efficiency rates, creation of an intermediate care unit that provides the services for which these patients were admitted to the ICU may improve ICU utilization.

References

1. Groeger JS, Guntupalli KK, Strosberg M, et al: Descriptive analysis of critical care units in the United States: Patient characteristics and intensive care unit utilization. Crit Care Med 1993; 21:279–291.
2. Pollack MM, Cuerdon TC, Getson PR: Diversity of pediatric intensive care units: A national study. Crit Care Med 1993; 21:607–614.
3. Hannan El, O'Donnell JF, Bernard HR, et al: Investigation of the relationship between volume and mortality for surgical procedures performed in New York State hospitals. JAMA 1989; 262:503–510.
4. Ruttimann UE, Getson PR, Pollack MM: Response to letter. N Engl J Med 1992; 326:1162.
5. Knaus WA, Draper EA, Wagner DP, et al: An evaluation of outcome from intensive care in major medical centers. Ann Intern Med 1986; 104:410–418.
6. Pollack MM: Outcome analysis. *In:* Textbook of Pediatric Critical Care. Holbrook PR (Ed). Philadelphia, WB Saunders, 1993, pp 1151–1159.
7. Pollack MM, Alexander SR, Clarke N, et al: Improved outcomes from tertiary center, pediatric intensive care: A statewide comparison of tertiary and nontertiary care facilities. Crit Care Med 1991; 19:150–159.
8. Wilkinson JD, Pollack MM, Ruttimann UE, et al: Outcome of pediatric patients with multiple organ system failure. Crit Care Med 1986; 14:271–274.
9. Pollack MM, Ruttimann UE, Getson PR: The Pediatric Risk of Mortality (PRISM) Score. Crit Care Med 1988; 16:1110–1116.
10. Pollack MM, Ruttimann UE, Getson PR, et al: Accurate prediction of pediatric intensive care outcome: A new quantitative method. N Engl J Med 1987; 316:134–139.
11. Klem SA, Pollack MM, Glass NL, et al: Resource use, efficiency and outcome prediction in pediatric intensive care of trauma patients. J Trauma 1990; 30:32–36.
12. Pollack MM, Katz RW, Ruttimann UE, et al: Improving the outcome and efficiency of pediatric intensive care. The impact of an intensivist. Crit Care Med 1988; 16:11–17.
13. Flora JD: A method for comparing survival of burn patients to a standard survival curve. J Trauma 1978; 18:701–705.
14. Lemeshow S, Hosmer DW: A review of goodness-of-fit statistics for use in the development of logistic regression models. Am J Epidemiol 1982; 115:92–102.
15. Frank B, Pollack MM: Quantitative quality assurance in a community hospital pediatric intensive care unit. West J Med 1992; 157:149–151.
16. Pollack MM, Getson PR, Ruttimann UE, et al: Efficiency intensive care. A comparative analysis of eight pediatric intensive care units. JAMA 1987; 258:1481–1486.
17. Ruttimann UE, Pollack MM: Objective assessment of changing mortality risks in pediatric intensive care unit patients. Crit Care Med 1991; 19:474–483.

SECTION XVII

ETHICAL DECISION MAKING IN CRITICALLY ILL PATIENTS

Joann I. Lamb • Stephen M. Ayres

CHAPTER 200

Legal Issues Involved in the Delivery of Critical Care Medicine

Karen N. Swisher, MS, JD

With the advent of advanced and complex medical technology, and with the ever-increasing concern over patients' rights to make informed medical decisions, it is not surprising to see a concomitant increase in litigation over medical care decisions.

These are not, however, the traditional medical malpractice cases that most American courts are relatively familiar with. Rather, these cases now involve complex ethical, legal, and medical issues concerning a patient's "right to die" and right to demand or reject appropriate medical care. Moreover, it is unfortunate that the American legal and legislative systems have so much involvement in the making of what many would argue are medical decisions that are best left to the patient and to his or her attending physician.

Indeed, judicial cases in this area have become so numerous that the federal government recently enacted a new law, the Patient Self-Determination Act of 1991,[1] in an attempt to reduce the number of patient and medical provider controversies being resolved in the courts.

The Patient Self-Determination Act is significant new legislation. It requires all hospitals, skilled nursing facilities, home health agencies, hospice programs, and health maintenance organizations that receive Medicaid or Medicare funding to give written information to all incoming patients on a patient's right to create a "living will" or a medical power of attorney under applicable state laws.[2] The act does not require that a medical facility actually assist the patient in making these advance directives, but it does require that each medical facility have a written policy informing its patients of the assistance they can receive in adopting or rejecting these advance directives.

Because these advance directives are created by state law, the federal Patient Self-Determination Act has a secondary purpose of encouraging the state legislatures to reassess their own living will statutes—if they have them—and, it is hoped, revise prior state legislation in light of the newer empirical, ethical, and legal trends in medical decision making.

Although most states presently do have living will statutes, others do not, and even among the states with living will laws, the individual state statutes differ significantly. Moreover, despite the greater availability of state laws allowing more people to create a living will, sadly, few people choose to do so. In addition, because those who do have living wills seldom carry them on their person or make reference to them, hospital emergency rooms and intensive care units treating trauma patients usually do not have written documents to rely on. Finally, much confusion still surrounds living wills executed in one state if the patient is involved in an accident or a serious illness in another.

Accordingly, despite these important state and federal laws, which were largely created to avoid litigation, many of these medical-legal conflicts must still be resolved by the courts. And although these judicial controversies deal with medical, legal, and ethical issues, they can all be classified within general conceptual categories that assist the reader in understanding how the courts are attempting to resolve these troubling controversies. Each of these interrelated categories is discussed below.

WHO DECIDES WHEN LIFE-SUSTAINING TREATMENT SHALL BE PROVIDED, WITHHELD, OR WITHDRAWN?

The first general category of judicial cases involves the question of who decides when life-sustaining medical treatment shall be provided, withheld, or withdrawn. Where is the locus of appropriate decision making in this area? Is it with the patient, the patient's family members, the attending physician, a hospital committee, a court-appointed guardian for the patient, the court itself, or the state?

Medical Decisions Made by a Competent Adult Patient

A competent adult patient generally has the legal right in most states to refuse medical treatment and to be free of medical intervention, even at the risk of his or her death, and this legal right of a patient's self-determination normally outweighs the state's interest in preserving life or in safeguarding the integrity of the medical profession. Moreover, an incompetent patient may express this intent through a prior living will document or through the surrogate decision making of a relative.[3-5]

Medical treatment involving minors, however, is a very different matter, and numerous judicial cases have held that when medical treatment involves little risk to the child, but a failure to provide treatment would substantially endanger the child's life or health, then the state may step in, acting under its parens patriae power, and order such medical treatment over the objection of the child's parents.[6, 7]

Once an appropriate decision maker has been determined, another category of judicial opinions has dealt with what legal standards are involved in the making of the decision itself. As stated earlier, for competent patients with decision-making capacity, most courts respect patient autonomy and self-determination as long as the patient is given all the elements of informed consent. The elements normally include the risks and benefits of treatment, the alternatives to treatment, and the consequences of foregoing such treatment. In this situation, the medical decision is for the patient alone to make.

Indeed, even in the controversial *Cruzan* case, the United States Supreme Court reasserted the constitutional liberty right of a patient to consent to—or to refuse—any type of medical treatment, including life-sustaining medical care. Stated the Court:

> *The Fourteenth Amendment provides that no State shall "deprive any person of life, liberty, or property, without due process of law." The principle that a competent person has a constitutionally protected liberty interest in refusing unwanted medical treatment may be inferred from our prior opinions. . . . [F] or the purpose of this case, we assume that the United States Constitution would grant a competent person a constitutionally protected right to refuse lifesaving hydration and nutrition.*[8]

Likewise, in the case of *Bartling v Superior Court*,[9] a California appellate court held that a competent adult person with a serious illness that was probably incurable but not diagnosed as terminal had the legal right, over the objections of his physicians and the hospital, to have life-support equipment disconnected, despite the fact that the withdrawal of such medical devices would surely hasten his death.

Medical Decisions Made on Behalf of an Incompetent Adult Patient

Although a competent adult patient may choose to forgo medical treatment—even though that choice may result in the patient's death—making medical decisions for an incompetent patient is a different matter entirely. According to an article written by Roth and associates,[10] five tests for competency have been proposed in the literature or have been inferable from judicial commentary: (1) evidencing of a choice, (2) "reasonable" outcome of choice, (3) choice based on "rational" reasons, (4) ability to understand, and (5) actual understanding.

The *evidencing a choice test* for competency is set at a very low level and is the most respectful test for the autonomy of patient decision making. Under this test, the competent patient is one who evidences a preference for or against treatment. The test focuses not on the quality of the patient's decision, but on the presence or absence of a decision. This test of competency encompasses, at a minimum, the unconscious patient. In psychiatry, it encompasses the mute patient who cannot, or will not, express an opinion.

The *reasonable outcome of choice test* involves an evaluation of a patient's capacity to reach the "reasonable," "right," or "responsible" decision. The emphasis of this test is on the outcome rather than on the mere fact of the decision or on how it was reached. Thus, the patient who fails to make a decision that a reasonable person under like circumstances would make is viewed as incompetent.

The *choice based on rational reasons test* is a third test that is based on whether the reasons for the patient's decision are "rational"—that is, whether the patient's decision is a product of mental illness. As in the reasonable outcome test, if the patient decides in favor of appropriate medical treatment, then the issue of the patient's competency seldom arises because of the medical profession's bias toward consent to treatment and its countervailing bias against refusal of treatment. In this test, the quality of a patient's thinking is the salient feature.

A fourth test is called the *ability to understand test.* This test, which consists of ascertaining the ability of the patient to understand the risks, benefits, and alternatives to treatment (including refusal of treatment), is most consistent with the law of informed consent. Decision making need not be rational in either process or outcome, and unwise choices are permitted. Nevertheless, the patient at a minimum must manifest evidence of a sufficient ability to understand the information about medical treatment, even if the patient weighs this information differently from his or her attending physician.

The fifth and final test is the *actual understanding test.* Under this test, the physician has an obligation to educate the patient and to ascertain whether the patient has understood the risks and benefits of medical treatment or nontreatment. This test arguably requires a fairly high level of sophisticated understanding by the patient and a high level of competency that may be difficult to achieve.[10]

The 1980 President's Commission on Making Health Care Decisions, however, viewed the elements of patient capacity in this manner:

> *In the view of the Commission, any determination of the capacity to decide on a course of treatment must relate to the individual abilities of a patient, the requirements of the task at hand, and the consequences likely to flow from the decision. Decision-making capacity requires, to greater or lesser degree: (1) possession of a set of values and goals; (2) the ability to communicate and to understand information; and (3) the ability to reason and to deliberate about one's choices.*[11]

Although patient competency to make an informed medical decision thus appears to be an extremely complex and difficult issue to determine, it is actually not that complicated for many reasons. First, many states have enacted statutory definitions that cover patient competency and capacity, but these statutory definitions are generally broadly drafted to provide interpretive room for the person making the ultimate decision regarding patient capacity, and that person most frequently is the attending physician who is involved in providing his or her patient with the elements of informed consent.

Physicians likewise apply their own common sense test in determining patient competency and capacity to make medical decisions. The general rule seems to be that if the physician recommends an indicated medical treatment and the patient agrees, then capacity is presumed to exist. However, if the physician recommends a medical treatment and the patient disagrees, then the physician might question the patient's reasons and the patient's capacity for making this contrary choices.

Once a determination is made that the patient does not have the capacity to make medical decisions, the courts must then apply additional legal tests to determine who will make such medical decisions in lieu of, and on behalf of, the incompetent patient.

Choosing a Surrogate for Medical Decision Making

Determining who are appropriate surrogate decision makers has been the crux of many legal controversies and lawsuits. If the patient is now deemed incompetent but once did have the capacity for decision making, the surrogate assigned to make the medical decision on the patient's behalf is required to make his or her decision based on what the patient would have wanted. This legal standard for surrogate decision making is called the *substituted judgment test.*

For example, in the highly regarded and very influential case of *In re Conroy*,[12] the New Jersey Supreme Court held that life-sustaining medical treatment could be withheld or withdrawn from an incompetent patient when the particular patient would clearly have refused the treatment under the circumstances involved. The question in the *Conroy* case is not what a reasonable or average person would have chosen to do under the circumstances, but what choice the particular patient would have made if he or she were able.

The patient's intent can be ascertained in many ways. First, under a *limited-objective test*, life-sustaining treatment may be withheld or withdrawn from a patient when trustworthy evidence exists that the patient would have refused the treatment, and the decision maker is satisfied that the burdens of the patient's continued life with the treatment clearly outweigh the benefits of life to him or her.

This limited-objective standard thus permits the termination of treatment for a patient who had not unequivocally expressed his or her desires before becoming incompetent, when it is clear that the treatment in question would merely prolong the patient's suffering. This limited-objective test also requires trustworthy evidence that the patient would have wanted the medical treatment terminated.

In the absence of such trustworthy evidence, or in the absence of any evidence at all that the patient would have declined the treatment, life-saving medical treatment may still be withheld or withdrawn from a formerly competent person if a *pure-objective test* is satisfied. Under this test, the net burdens of the treatment should outweigh any benefits that the patient might receive from continued life. Further, the pain and suffering of continued treatment should be so severe that administering life-sustaining treatment would be inhumane.

The *Conroy* court expressly declined to authorize surrogate decision making based on assessments of the personal worth or social utility of another's life or on the value of that life to others. Moreover, the primary focus should be the patient's desires and experience of pain and enjoyment—not the type of treatment involved.[12]

Should incompetent patients in persistent vegetative states also be bound by this *Conroy* test? In two subsequent decisions,[13, 14] the New Jersey Supreme Court stated that by definition, patients in persistent vegetative states do not experience the benefits and burdens that the *Conroy* balancing tests were intended to appraise, and therefore these *Conroy* tests should not be applied to patients in persistent vegetative states. Moreover, if close and caring family members are willing to make this medical decision on behalf of the incompetent patient, a guardian need not be appointed.[15]

Thus, a surrogate decision maker attempts to establish, with as much accuracy as possible, what decision the patient would make if he or she were competent to do so. Employing this theory, the surrogate decision maker first tries to determine if the patient had expressed any explicit intent regarding the type of medical treatment preferred before he or she became incompetent. In cases in which no clear intent exists, the patient's personal value system must guide the surrogate decision maker. For example, in the *Brophy* case,[16] the Massachusetts Supreme Court held that food and hydration could be withheld from a comatose adult patient based on a substituted-judgment, surrogate decision-making test that included the following factors: (1) Brophy's expressed preferences, (2) his religious convictions and their relation to a refusal of medical treatment, (3) the impact on his family, (4) the probability of adverse side effects, and (5) the intrusiveness of the procedure, such as the need to use a feeding tube. Although Brophy never had discussed specifically whether the gastrostomy tube or the feeding tube should be withdrawn if he was diagnosed as being in a persistent vegetative state after his surgery, the surrogate decision maker inferred that if Brophy were presently competent, he would choose to forgo artificial nutrition and hydration by means of a gastrostomy tube.

Traditionally, physicians and the courts look to the patient's family as appropriate surrogate decision makers. The family usually is most knowledgeable about the patient and desires to do what is best for the patient. The President's Commission suggests five reasons for this deference to family members as surrogate decision makers: (1) the family is generally most concerned about the good of the patient; (2) the family is also usually most knowledgeable about the patient's goals, preferences, and values; (3) the family deserves recognition as an important social unit that ought to be treated, within limits, as a responsible decision maker in matters that intimately affect its members; (4) especially in a society in which many other traditional forms of community have eroded, participation in a family is often an important dimension of personal fulfillment; and (5) because a protected sphere of privacy and autonomy is required for the flourishing of this interpersonal union, institutions and the state should be reluctant to intrude, particularly regarding matters that are personal and on which a wide range of opinion in society exists.[17] Consulting with family members also neutralizes the possibility of subsequent medical malpractice claims, and this element also accounts for its current popularity.[18]

Family members have traditionally, legally, and morally made a vast number of important decisions concerning other family members in many related areas of family law.[19] It is very unfortunate, therefore, that the good intentions of the family were almost totally disregarded in the *Cruzan* case, which held that the individual states could establish tough evidentiary hurdles for surrogate decision makers to cross when the surrogates make medical choices on behalf of an incompetent patient.[20] It would have been more logical, more humane, and more in keeping with prior family law precedent for the court to have established a "rebuttable presumption" that family members are making the best choice for the patient. Therefore, from a legal standard, it is presumed the family is acting in the best interests of the patient. The burden to prove otherwise shifts to the person protesting the family's decision. Fortunately, however, the *Cruzan* case is legally binding in only a few states in addition to Missouri, where the original decision was handed down.[21]

Problems may still arise, however, when family members disagree as to what would constitute appropriate medical treatment for the incompetent patient, or when family members may not be acting in the best interests of the patient, or when a patient has never had the capacity to make medical decisions. Some patients, for example, because of mental illness, mental retardation, or infancy, have never had the capacity to make medical decisions relating to their own definition of "quality of life." For these patients, many courts are increasingly using a *best interests* test as enunciated in the *Saikewicz* case:[22]

> *The "best interests" of an incompetent person are not necessarily served by imposing on such persons results not mandated as to competent persons similarly situated. It does not advance the interest of the State or the incompetent patient to treat the incompetent patient as a person of lesser status or dignity than others. . . . If a competent person faced with death may choose to decline treatment which not only will not cure the person but which substantially may increase suffering in exchange for a possible yet brief prolongation of life, then it cannot be said that it is always in the "best interests" of the incompetent patient to require submission to such treatment.*

One major problem with this best interests test is that many courts apparently have a difficult time conceding to the reality of an impending death in the same manner that many Americans evidence a general denial of death. Thus, when court-appointed guardians are used to determine the best interests of the incompetent patient, they often choose to continue aggressive medical care, despite poor outcomes or despite additional suffering by the patient. The debatable logic behind this questionable approach is that any prolongation of life is a better "interest" than is death, and any act that can be performed to prolong life, despite the medical futility of such an act, and despite the suffering of the patient, is defined as being in the best interests of the patient. However, many horrible results place into question the proper application of this best interests test, at least as a per se rule.[23]

Like any other test, the best interests test should use a flexible approach, based on the facts surrounding each patient, the "totality of the circumstances," and not a small measure of basic common sense and human compassion. It is an approach best left to the family of an incompetent patient, as his or her surrogate decision maker, and to the patient's attending physician.[24]

As a concurring and dissenting judge in the Maryland appellate case of *Mack v Mack*[25] aptly observed:

> *The best interests test mandates that the decision to terminate life support be made relying on objective criteria rather than the family members' opinions as to what the patient would have chosen if the patient could choose. Perhaps the best interests test has applicability (1) where there is no available surrogate decision maker who is familiar with the patient; and (2) as a safeguard against bad faith or improper decisions by family members to terminate life support. Where a family's motives are suspect, a court could refuse to effectuate the family's decision to terminate life support if the court finds that decision is contrary to the patient's best interests.*
>
> *The best interests test may also be helpful where there are conflicting opinions by family members, as occurred in the instant case. Measuring contrasting opinions against the objective criteria of the best interests test may aid the court in resolving the conflict.*

Judicial Limitations on a Patient's Medical Choices

Ethical and legal decisions in patient right-to-die cases usually begin with a discussion of the foundations of patient autonomy because the right to accept or decline medical treatment is embedded in the common law right to self-determination. The right to accept or decline medical treatment is perhaps also a state and federal constitutional right, of both competent and incompetent patients, to refuse life-sustaining medical treatment.[26, 27] Therefore, a patient must decide whether he or she wants a particular medical treatment before a physician can treat the patient. However, a patient's right to decide whether he or she wants medical treatment is meaningless unless the patient has information regarding the risks and benefits of the proposed medical treatment. This is the concept of informed consent, and it constitutes the legal basis for the medical, legal, and ethical principle of patient autonomy.

Patient autonomy, however, is not an absolute principle, and complete patient autonomy is not always possible, because a patient cannot possess all of the medical knowledge held by his or her physician. Physicians have never been legally required to make a complete and total disclosure of every possible treatment, every possible risk, or every conceivable benefit. For example, a physician normally makes a threshold decision as to the relevance of a medical risk or a medical benefit to the decision a patient must make. By necessity, then, a patient's autonomy is largely shaped by the physician's prior medical judgment.[28]

Moreover, in assessing a patient's right to reject life-sustaining medical treatment, the state also has many countervailing interests in sustaining a person's life, including preserving life, preventing suicide, protecting innocent third parties, protecting the integrity of the medical profession, and encouraging charitable and humane care.[29]

Judicial Limits on Patient Autonomy

Various courts throughout the United States have affirmed a group of state interests that could supersede a patient's right to choose or to refuse medical treatments. These interests include preserving life; preventing suicide; protecting innocent third persons, such as children; preserving the integrity of the medical profession; and encouraging the charitable and humane care of afflicted persons. Although most courts recognize the same interests, the terms and philosophies used in defining them differ greatly. The varied and ambiguous nature of the judicial attempts to define such state interests is simply a reflection of diversified values in a pluralistic American society.

State's Interest in the Preservation of Life

The state's interest in preserving life is commonly considered the most significant state interest. It may be seen as embracing two separate but related concerns: an interest in preserving the life of the particular patient and an interest in preserving the sanctity of all life. One of the first cases in which a court had to weigh the state's interest in the preservation of life against a patient's right to choose was the case of Karen Quinlan, a 22-year-old woman who was diagnosed to be in a persistent vegetative state in 1975. The court held that

> *. . . the claimed interests of the state in this case are essentially the preservation and sanctity of human life. . . . Ultimately there comes a point at which the individual's rights overcome the State interest, it is for that reason that we believe Karen's choice if she were competent to make it, would be vindicated by law.*[30]

State's Interest in the Prevention of Suicide

Courts have struggled to distinguish between the affirmative act of taking one's life and the act of discontinuing artificial life support to let nature take its course. The case of *McKay v Bergstedt* illustrates this point. The patient, 31-year-old Kenneth Bergstedt, was a respirator-dependent quadriplegic. His parents had cared for him for 10 years at home. After the death of his mother, and faced with the imminent death of his father from cancer, Kenneth petitioned his local court for an order permitting the removal of his respirator by a medical person who could also administer a sedative to relieve pain. He sought an order of legal immunity for any person assisting him and a decree that his actions would not constitute suicide. Kenneth's father reluctantly approved of his son's actions. The State of Nevada contested the action as promoting "state-sponsored suicide."

The Supreme Court of Nevada finally held (posthumously) that Kenneth had a right to refuse treatment, even if the refusal would result in his death. The court used three factors to distinguish the action desired by Kenneth from suicide: attitude, physical condition, and prognosis. The court concluded that Kenneth did not wish to commit suicide. He simply wished to live only as long as his condition would permit without artificial support. Refusing medical intervention merely allows the disease or the effects of an injury to take a natural course. Death, therefore, would be the result of the underlying disease or injury, and not the result of self-inflicted injury.[31]

State's Interest in Protecting Innocent Third Parties

Courts have always taken a strong interest in the protection of children. Therefore, when parents refuse to consent for medical treatment deemed necessary to save the life of a child, courts often overrule the parents' desires, whether they be based on religious convictions or other reasons.

Another situation that moves courts to invoke this state interest is when parents cannot agree on a treatment decision for a terminally ill child. *In re Jane Doe, A Minor,* involved a 13-year-old terminally ill child in a nearly complete unconsciousness state. One parent consented to a do-not-resuscitate but the other parent refused to consent. Because the parents could not agree on the care to be provided, the hospital requested a hearing, and an independent guardian ad litem was appointed for the child.

The court found that if either parent made a decision to continue medical support, that decision must be respected. The integrity of the family was the issue that the court wished to protect, stating that

> *A court ruling authorizing termination against the wishes of one parent at the behest of another parent could be very detrimental to family harmony and create a serious precedent allowing courts to interfere in such major familial decision, all in violation of public policy.*[32]

Protecting the Integrity of the Medical Profession

Although it is always mentioned by state courts as an interest to be protected, no court has ever defined the state interest in protecting the integrity of the medical profession. A 1977 Massachusetts Supreme Court decision involving withdrawal of care from an incompetent mentally retarded patient stated

> *The state interest requiring discussion is that of the maintenance of the ethical integrity of the medical profession as well as allowing hospitals the full opportunity to care for people under their control. The force and impact of this interest is lessened by the prevailing medical ethical standards. Prevailing medical ethical practice does not, without exception, demand that all efforts toward life prolongation be made in all circumstances. Rather, the prevailing ethical practice seems to be to recognize that the dying are more often in need of comfort than treatment.*[33]

Encouragement of Charitable and Humane Care

The encouragement of charitable and humane care was introduced in the McKay case discussed earlier. The court recognized that state and national public policy dictated that efforts must be made to enhance the quality of life among those who are disabled. The court stated

> *It appeared to us that Kenneth needed some type of assurance that society would not cast him adrift in a sea of indifference. . . . Absent Kenneth's intervening death, it would have been necessary to fully inform him of the care alternatives that would have been available to him after his father's death or incapacity.*

CONCLUSIONS

Taking into account all of these countervailing interests (including patient autonomy versus appropriate medical treatment), current medical and ethical thought, buttressed by numerous influential judicial decisions, strongly suggests that physicians now have the moral and legal responsibility to respect the wishes of competent patients and the wishes of surrogate decision makers for incompetent patients, in the termination of life-sustaining medical treatment or futile medical care.

The troubling corollary to patient autonomy and right-to-die cases is the scenario of a patient's "right to demand medical care," even though the attending physician believes that such medical treatment would be futile. Here again, limits to patient autonomy exist, and patients have never had a generally recognized legal right to demand unlimited medical care.

However, as America moves toward a national health system that surely will place more limitations on the type and the amount of medical care that Americans will receive, more legal controversies in this area are very likely. When people do not get what they want, they increasingly resort to the courts. Health care rationing, or the process of making rational choices for medical care under new budgetary and personnel restrictions, will thus undoubtedly constitute the next horizon of judicial involvement in this medical-legal brave new world.

References

1. 42 USCA §1395.
2. 42 USCA §1395cc(a)(1)(f)(1)(A).
3. *In re Conroy,* 98 NJ 321, 486 A2d 1209 (1985).
4. *John F. Kennedy Memorial Hospital v Bludworth,* 452 So2d 921 (FLa 1984).
5. Childress, *Refusal of Lifesaving Treatment by Adults,* 23 J Fam L 191 (1984).
6. *Jehovah's Witnesses v King County Hospital,* 278 F Supp 488 (WD Wash 1967) affirmed 390 US 598 (1968).
7. *Custody of a Minor,* 375 Mass 733, 379 NE2d 1053 (1978).
8. *Cruzan v Director, Missouri Dept. of Health,* 110 SCt 2841 (1990).
9. *Bartling v Superior Court,* 163 Cal App3d 186, 209 Cal Rptr 220 (1984).
10. Roth LH, Meisel A, Lidz CW: Tests of competence to consent to treatment. Am J Psychiatry 1977; 134:279.
11. President's Commission for the Study of Ethical Problems in Medicine and Biomedical and Behavioral Research: Making Health Care Decisions. Washington, DC, US Government Printing Office, 1982, p 57.
12. 98 NJ 321, 486 A2d 1209 (1985).
13. *In re Jobes,* 108 NJ 394, 529 A2d 434 (1987).
14. *In re Peter,* 108 NJ 365, 529 A2d 419 (1987).
15. 529 A2d 447 (1987).
16. *Brophy v New England Sinai Hospital, Inc.,* 398 Mass 417, 497 NE2d 626 (1986).
17. President's Commission: Deciding to Forgo Life-Sustaining Treatment. Washington, DC, US Government Printing Office, 1983, p 127.
18. Furrow BR, Johnson SH, Jost TS, et al: Bioethics: Health Care Law and Ethics. St. Paul, West Publisher, 1991, p 280.
19. Gregory JD, Swisher PN, Scheible SL: Understanding Family Law. New York, Matthew Bender Publisher, 1993, pp 161–183.
20. *Cruzan v Director, Missouri Dept. of Health,* 110 SCt 2841 (1990).
21. Stewart, "Right to Die, But . . ." 76 ABAJ 40 (Sept 1990).
22. *Superintendent of Belchertown State School v Saikewicz,* 373 Mass 728, 370 NE2d 417 (1977).
23. *In re Storar,* 52 NY2d 363, 438 NYS2d 266 (1981).
24. Francis, *The roles of the Family in Making Health Care Decisions for Incompetent Patients,* Utah L Rev 861 (1992).
25. *Mack v Mack,* 329 Md 188, 618 A2d 744 (Md Ct App 1993).
26. *Brophy v New England Sinai Hospital,* 398 Mass 417, 497 NE2d 626 (1986).
27. *In re Conroy,* 98 NJ 321, 486 A2d 1209 (1985).
28. *Canterbury v Spence,* 464 F2d 772, 787 (1972).
29. Swisher K, Ayres S: Who decides when care is futile? Intensive Crit Care Digest 1992; 11(4):59–64.
30. *In re Quinlan,* 70 NJ 10, 355 A2d 266 (1976).
31. *McKay v Bergstedt,* 801 P2d 617 (Nev 1990).
32. *In re Jane Doe, A Minor Civil Action* No. D-93064, Super Ct of Fulton County, Georgia (Order, October 17, 1991).
33. *Superintendent of Belchertown State School v Saikewicz,* 373 Mass 728, 370 NE2d 417 at 425–427 (1977).

CHAPTER 201

Medical Futility

Stuart J. Youngner, MD

Over the past two decades, our society has established the primacy of informed consent to medical treatment. Implied in the doctrine of informed consent is that patients not only have a right to choose between alternative treatments, but they also may decide to have no treatment at all. Of course, decisions to refuse treatment are most weighty when the medical interventions being refused are life saving or life prolonging. After struggling with this issue over the past two decades, we have reached a broad consensus that competent adult patients may refuse any and all life-sustaining interventions, from dialysis and mechanical ventilation to the technical provision of fluids and nutrition. If physicians disagree with patients' treatment refusals and have explained their reasons to no avail, they have but two morally acceptable alternatives—either transfer care to another physician or follow the patient's wishes.

However, what is the physician's role when he or she determines that additional or continued life-sustaining measures are futile? Physicians are concerned that too often they are forced into giving futile end-of-life interventions, like cardiopulmonary resuscitation (CPR). Must such measures be offered to patients and their families? Must they be given when patients or families ask for or demand them? Can physicians simply say no? These questions, under the general rubric of *medical futility,* have been hotly debated in the medical literature over the past 10 years.

Increasingly, physicians, hospitals, professional organizations,[1–3] and even some state legislatures[4] have endorsed or adopted policies that recognize that limits exist as to what physicians are obligated to do at the end of a patient's life, regardless of the wishes of the patient or family. Many think that the pendulum has swung too far in the direction of consumerism and away from professional responsibility. They believe that physicians should shoulder more of the weight, relieving families of unnecessary guilt and protecting patients from "high-technology placebos."[5] Interest in medical futility has been greatly enhanced by growing concerns about efficiency and resource allocation in the health care system.

Nonetheless, many questions about futility remain unanswered. For instance, little agreement exists about the definition of futility. If a right to treatment does exist, how should we understand that right? Once physicians have determined that a given intervention is futile, how should they proceed? Should they inform the patient that the intervention will not be given, or should they wait for the patient to bring it up? Could do-not-resuscitate orders be written not only without patient or family permission, but without informing them as well? What is the difference between futility and rationing? Why would patients or families demand interventions that competent and compassionate health professionals have told them will do no good and may well cause considerable harm? How can we better communicate with patients and families to avoid confrontations about futility? The rest of this chapter attempts to answer some of these difficult questions.

HISTORICAL CONTEXT

The discussion of treatment limitation in the United States has largely taken place in the context of patient autonomy and the right to refuse treatment. Famous court cases, from Karen Quinlan in the 1970s to Nancy Cruzan in the 1990s, have centered around patients or families who sought to limit life-sustaining treatment in opposition to physicians who insisted it be continued. These court cases and dozens of others have established the right of patients or appropriate surrogates to refuse life-sustaining treatment. Patients' rights were elevated almost to the level of a movement. During this period, malpractice litigation (and with it, physicians' legal paranoia) grew dramatically.

At the same time, critical care physicians were learning from experience that patients at the end stage of chronic illness or those with multisystem organ failure rarely benefited from aggressive interventions such as CPR. And, although the famous cases involved patients and families who refused treatment when physicians wanted it to continue, more often patients, and, in particular, families demanded aggressive interventions when physicians had decided that sufficient treatment had been administered. Because of legal fears and a mistaken notion of patients' rights, we have established an unfortunate tradition of asking the question, "Do you want us to do everything?" and then following this direction when the answer comes back, "Yes."

POSITIVE VERSUS NEGATIVE RIGHTS AND THE INTEGRITY OF THE MEDICAL PROFESSION

It is a fallacy that because patients have a moral right to refuse life-sustaining treatment they have an unqualified right to demand it. The rights defined in the treatment refusal court cases were *negative* rights—the right that no treatment be given to the patient. *Positive* rights, conversely, "in the physician-patient context—the right that something *be* done—endorses the patient's right to select a particular intervention and implies a coexisting obligation of the physician to make that intervention available."[6] Claims to negative rights are generally considered to be more powerful than are those to positive rights and can be traced to different areas of moral theory and the law.

The right to refuse treatment is found in the constitutional rights of privacy and liberty or in the common law right against battery. The negative right to refuse treatment has been firmly established and rooted in our constitutional and common law heritage. Positive rights to have treatment may exist, but, if they do, they must be understood and justified separately from the right to refuse treatment. In fact, in a nation that is currently debating the appropriate level of access to beneficial health care, it seems a cruel irony that we feel obliged to give nonbeneficial care to persons in critical care environments simply because they demand that we do so.

The doctrine of informed consent specifies that patients have a right to an informed choice or a refusal of treatments offered to them within the standard of medical care; it does not say that they have a right to ask for any and all treatments in a physician's armamentarium. This observation is confirmed in everyday medical practice. A surgeon who has determined that a patient would not benefit from surgery does not feel obligated to ask: "Do you want me to do it anyway?" Nor must an internist prescribe antibiotics for a viral upper respiratory infection or give vitamin B_{12} injections because the patient wants them. As Brett and McCullough wrote, the patient's ability to exercise positive rights to treatment is limited by the physician's clinical judgment:

> *Because the physician is a necessary element in the dyad, his or her moral and medical values obviously are not extraneous factors in clinical decision making. . . . The foundation of the clinical encounter is a specified body of knowledge and expertise about what is beneficial for patients.*

When a patient seeks to exercise a positive right to an intervention, a necessary condition is that there is either an established or theoretical medical basis for this patient's request.[6]

Society has entrusted physicians with the responsibility for making clinical judgments. Physicians are held accountable for those judgments, and they are also given some authority to make them. In fact, these judgments form the basis of the medical profession. Physicians are more than technicians who follow the orders of patients, and medicine has goals that the physician must promote—above all, to benefit patients and do them no harm.

Furthermore, by offering desperately ill persons and their families futile treatments, we hardly promote the ideal of patient autonomy. The act of offering a futile intervention sends a mixed message that may actually undermine patient autonomy.[7] After all, why would a physician offer a treatment if it was not going to be successful?

DEFINING FUTILITY

Although the word *futility* has a categoric ring, it is difficult to define precisely. Some elements of the definition are clear, however. Futility must always be discussed in relation to an identified goal. Intervention A is futile if it is not successful in achieving goal B. Intervention A may not be futile in relation to goal C. Thus, the futility of an intervention is difficult to determine without identification of the goal. Numerous possible goals may be identified for any given intervention.[8] For example, we can understand an intervention purely in *physiologic* terms. By this standard, we would judge the administration of intravenous bicarbonate futile if it failed to correct an electrolyte disturbance. Other potential goals include postponing the moment of death, extending life for a specific period of time, and achieving an acceptable quality of life. We might also define futility by the *probability* of a given intervention's achieving a goal. Below a certain probability, an intervention would be considered futile.

Thus, communicating using the word futility, without first identifying goals, can be confusing and misleading. Moreover, the further we get away from physiologic futility (e.g., by defining it in terms of length or quality of life) and a zero probability of achieving a worthwhile goal, the more we begin to introduce value judgments about the worthiness of the goals we can achieve or the requisite probability that distinguishes an unacceptably low chance from a chance worth taking. But if value judgments inevitably come into play, whose values should be determinant, those of the patient and family or those of the physician?

Some authors have argued that physicians have a right, and indeed, an obligation to act on value judgments both about the probability of achieving certain goals and about whether the goals themselves are worthy. Tomlinson and Brody claim that "physicians must be able to restrict the alternatives made available to patients and must be able to employ value judgments in doing so."[9] Schneiderman and his colleagues distinguish between the effects of an intervention and its benefits: "We believe that the goal of medical treatment is not merely to cause an effect on some portion of the patient's anatomy, physiology, or chemistry, but to benefit the patient as a whole."[10] They argue that futility should be defined within the context of evolving standards of care and that the goal of medicine is to achieve a benefit above a certain minimum *qualitative* or *quantitative* threshold.[10] They have proposed very specific standards for determining futility in both of these dimensions.

They define as *qualitatively* futile "any treatment that merely preserves permanent unconsciousness or that fails to end total dependence on intensive medical care."[10] They consider both of these results to be of no benefit to the patient. *Quantitative* futility is "any effort to achieve a result that is possible but that reasoning or experience suggests is highly improbable and that cannot be systematically produced."[10] More specifically, they propose:

When physicians conclude (either through personal experience, experiences shared with colleagues, or consideration of reported empiric data) that in the last 100 cases a medical treatment has been useless, they should regard that treatment as futile.[10]

They justify this position by noting that although observing no successes in the last 100 trials does not mean that the treatment never works, such an observation would serve as a point estimate of the probability of success, and using statistical methods, a range of values that include the true success rate can be estimated with a specified probability. Thus, no successes have occurred in 100 consecutive cases, the clinician can be 95% confident that no more than three successes would occur in each of 100 comparable trials.[10]

Schneiderman and colleagues acknowledged that their proposals would be controversial and invited "examination and challenge" to them, a response that was quickly forthcoming. Truog and coworkers[11] challenged Schneiderman and colleagues' statistical approach. They pointed to the literature that documented problems with physicians' estimates of prognosis. Asking physicians to remember their last 100 similar cases is probably unrealistic, but even if empirical studies identify 100 consecutive patients who did not respond to a given treatment, the authors asked, "How similar must the patients be?" In assessing the efficacy of mechanical ventilation to treat pneumonia, for example, is it sufficient simply to recall the 100 most recent patients who received artificial ventilation for pneumonia, or must this group be stratified according to age, etiologic organism, or coexisting illness?[11] Callahan raised a more general concern.[12] He likened futility to other issues that have both factual and value elements, for example, abortion and the definition of death, noting that "no social 'ought' can be drawn from a scientific 'is.' " Lantos and his colleagues[13] made a similar point, saying that "Because futility determinations . . . combine technical considerations, patient values, and clinical judgments, the framework for these determinations should be one of shared decision-making."

Others have criticized Schneiderman and colleagues' notion of qualitative futility. Veatch and Spicer,[14] for example, argued that when a medical intervention will prolong life and physicians think continued life is not beneficial, the "situation must be resolved with a bias in favor of life." Addressing Schneiderman and colleagues' assignment of permanent unconsciousness to the realm of futility, they replied,

Life-prolonging care is fundamental, precisely because we can imagine ourselves in the minority desiring this care, and we would go to great lengths to assure that if we were in the minority, we would have some opportunity to gain access. . . . Even those not usually identified with pro-life positions would recognize how offensive it must be to a patient who believes in the ultimate value of biological life to be prohibited access to life-prolonging care by one's clinician.[14]

Schneiderman and colleagues' other example of nonbeneficial (and hence qualitatively futile) treatment is keeping someone alive who is totally dependent on intensive care. Sometimes, however, keeping such a patient alive allows time for good-byes and settling of unfinished business. It is hard to understand how these goals are not beneficial or how critical care physicians could turn off a ventilator or stop vasopressor administration for a patient who wanted to be kept alive for these purposes.

Clearly, although widespread sympathy with the notion of medical futility exists, little agreement exists about how to define it.

UNITED STATES COURTS AND MEDICAL FUTILITY

Few cases of futility have been tested in the courts. The best known case is that of Helga Wanglie, a woman in her nineties who was ventilator dependent and in a persistent vegetative state.[15] After several months, her physicians at Hennepin County Hospital recommended that mechanical ventilation be discontinued and that she be allowed to die.[16] Her husband objected and reported that she would have wanted to live as long as possible under the current circumstances. The hospital went to court to have an independent conservator appointed. The patient's husband objected, and the court appointed him as conservator.[17] Because the patient died shortly after this ruling, the right of the physicians to override the husband's wishes was never directly addressed by the court.

Some persons hailed the outcome of the Wanglie case as a victory for the rights of families.[17, 18] Others, sympathetic to the notion of futility, nonetheless thought a tactical error had been committed because this first major case hinged on such a subjective notion of futility, that is, a judgment that the patient's quality of life was unacceptable.

DANGERS OF APPLYING FUTILITY

Several other concerns have been raised about physicians using futility as a rationale for unilaterally limiting treatment. First, because determinations of futility are so value laden, until standards (such as those of Schneiderman and colleagues) are set for the profession as a whole, definitions of futility will likely vary from physician to physician. If all physicians unilaterally acted on their judgments about futility, similar cases would be treated differently,[18a] opening the way for accusations of abuse and prejudice.

Second, some argue that condoning unilateral decision making by physicians would set back shared decision making between patient, family, and physician, returning us to an earlier era of unbridled paternalism that our society has found unsatisfactory.[11, 13, 14] Even strong proponents of futility, like Schneiderman and colleagues[10] and Tomlinson and Brody,[9] agree that physicians should not *act* unilaterally until a much broader public discussion of the issues has occurred. Such a public discussion could be stimulated by several methods, including (1) formulation of institutional policies on futility after wide discussion within the hospital and the community of persons it serves, (2) publishing and dissemination of standards or guidelines by professional groups, (3) taking of selected cases to court, and (4) education of health professionals and the general public about these issues.

Third, concern exists that rationing and futility are becoming confused.[8, 11, 19] This issue is important because both futility and rationing have very different meanings, moral implications, and methods for resolution. Jecker and Schneiderman as well as Morreim described the common economic, historical, and demographic factors that have brought both concepts into the foreground,[19, 19a] including (1) a dramatic and continuing increase in healthcare costs and a concomitant call for measures to stop it, (2) the development of high-technology medicine and increased options for aggressive intervention, (3) an aging society that requires more and more medical care, and (4) a general recognition of the limits of individual autonomy as the needs of the greater society become more pressing—for example, allocation of scarce medical resources.

The differences between futility and rationing are important. A futile treatment is one that offers no benefit to the patient. Rationing implies denial of beneficial treatment to some persons because the treatment is not available in sufficient quantities to treat these persons. Limiting futile treatments may in fact help conserve resources and may make our health care system more efficient, but futile treatments could and should be limited, even in times of resource abundance.[19] "Circumstances of rationing always presuppose scarcity," Jecker notes, and "ethical rationing must meet standards articulated in theories of distributive justice."[19] Conversely, *futility* implies a cause-and-effect relationship between a medical intervention and its intended outcome in a specific patient. The distribution of scarce resources (rationing) is a matter for society, not individual physicians, to decide. Physicians owe their allegiance to their patients, who trust them to look after their interests, not the interests of others.[20] Rationing is an extremely sensitive topic; in our pluralistic society, little agreement exists about who should be excluded from treatment when insufficient quantities of the treatment exist. As Jecker and Schneiderman wisely caution, futility could become a "subterfuge for allocation decisions."[19]

MOTIVES FOR DEMANDING FUTILE TREATMENT

Most troubling, perhaps, is that rather than learning to understand the reasons why patients and their families demand futile interventions, physicians may use medical futility as a shortcut to decision making. Too often, the discussion of futility in the medical literature concerns cases in which extreme positions have already been taken—patients or their families demanding interventions that physicians have determined are useless.[21] However, these cases do not adequately portray the historical, social, and personal context in which these situations arise that motivate people to demand futile treatment. Better understanding of these motives will not resolve the futility debate, but it can prevent a confrontation about medical futility from occurring in many cases. Understanding what motivates people to ask for or demand futile therapy offers physicians an opportunity to provide optimal care for dying patients and their families and to promote shared decision making.

Failure to Set Timely Treatment Goals

In their discussions with patients, families, and each other, physicians too often focus on specific treatments rather than on the goals they may or may not achieve.[7, 8, 21]

CASE HISTORY

Mrs. Smith, a 95-year-old woman with severe dementia and a diagnosis of metastatic adenocarcinoma, was admitted to the hospital from a nursing home because of sepsis, renal failure, congestive heart failure, and gastrointestinal bleeding. Meeting the family for the first time, a house officer tells them the serious nature of patient's condition and then asks the question, "Do you want us to do everything?"

Mr. Jones, an otherwise healthy 70-year-old man, was admitted to a cardiac monitoring unit with chest pain. The house officer approached his wife with the question, "If your husband's heart stops, do you want us to try to start it again?" "Of course I want you to try," she replied. Later, she told her family physician about the incident. "What did that young man think? That I wanted my husband to die?"

The questions posed by the house officers in these two cases are meaningless or even misleading until the potential goals of treatment have been clarified and set. As we have seen, whatever one's definition of futility, it must be defined in relationship to a specific goal. Interventions like the use of ventilators, vasopressors, or CPR, are not ends in themselves but are means to ends that have been chosen through shared decision making.

Of course, patients and their families most often seek the goal of saving and restoring life. Sometimes, the highest priority is to help them realize that this goal is not achievable. Physicians often have difficulty with this task and postpone it until the last days or hours before the patient dies. Some physicians feel a sense of failure when they cannot save their patients' lives, whereas for others, the illusion of control brings a sense of power or narcissistic gratification. In both cases, to admit that the patient is going to die is to admit failure. Discussing death and dying is also emotionally difficult and time consuming, and many physicians avoid it. Effectively talking about these issues requires great interpersonal skills, self-awareness, and timing. It is little wonder, then, that families and patients demand treatment when they have understood neither the reality of the patient's overall condition nor the various goals individual treatments may or may not serve.

Worthwhile goals might include keeping the patient comfortable while allowing death to occur as quickly as possible, restoring the patient to a previous satisfactory quality of life, keeping the patient alive long enough to say goodbye to loved ones, and achieving a reduced, but still satisfactory, quality of life. Undesirable goals might include keeping the patient alive for a short while but with great pain, suffering, and indignity; restoring the patient to a quality of life that was, and remains, unacceptable to the patient; and achieving a reduced quality of life (e.g., bedridden, incontinent, dependent on others) that is unacceptable to the patient. Individual treatments may achieve some of these goals and not others. Of the goals that are achievable, some may be desired by the patient, others not.

Discussions with patients and their families are most effective if they identify goals first and the treatments that may or may not achieve them second.

Ignorance

Sometimes, people demand futile treatment when they simply do not understand the facts. When Mr. Jones' wife was outraged by the house officer's implication that she might not have wanted to "start up" her husband's heart if it stopped, she had little notion of what this process might involve or what the likely outcome would be if her husband were to receive full CPR.

In the report of a study of multiply impaired, elderly nursing home residents, Murphy found that only 10% had do-not-resuscitate orders written in their charts.[22] He changed the way the issue was approached by encouraging discussion and avoiding misleading language like, "Would you want us to do everything to save your life if your heart stopped beating?" When he spoke candidly to patients and families about their medical conditions, poor prognoses, and the unpleasant realities of dying in an intensive care unit, they uniformly (23 of 24 patients and all but one relative) rejected the use of CPR.[22] By acting proactively, Murphy empowered his patients and avoided a later confrontation over medical futility.

Confusion

People sometimes demand futile treatment because they are confused—often because they have been given inconsistent and contradictory information from health professionals.[21] Several causes exist for such confusion.

First, no evidence exists that practicing physicians agree on a single definition of futility. A patient will inevitably be confused after speaking with clinicians who have different thresholds for determining either qualitative or quantitative futility; such differences exist between different services, for example, the experimental oncology ward and the intensive care unit.[23] Oncologists have initiated treatments with patient and family consent and are less willing to call off aggressive interventions when the patient's condition deteriorates than are their critical care colleagues, who have not invested as much in the initial treatment and see more failures of cancer therapy than successes.

Second, the phenomenon of multiconsultants breeds confusion. Patients in critical care units in large tertiary medical centers may have many consultants, each of whom watches the progress of one problem. A steady stream of consultant teams passes by the patient's bedside, examining one part of the patient, one part of the chart, and one part of the lab results. Comments to the family similarly reflect a narrow focus—"the patient is no longer bleeding," "there is no sign of infection," "the heart is beating stronger today"—failing to convey an overall picture of the patient's deterioration. Such inadequate communication only exacerbates the patient and family's preoccupation with treatments or laboratory values as if they were ends in themselves, while the overall treatment plan is ignored.

Finally, confusion is aggravated by the fragmentation of care that results from monthly rotations of house officers and attending physicians and from shift changes for nurses. These characteristics of the health care system make it likely that patients and families will get different facts, different interpretations of similar facts, and different prognoses. Physicians should not unfairly give the futility justification when patients and families have been confused by multiple messages.

Mistrust

Another reason why patients may not accept physicians' pronouncements of futility is because they do not trust the physicians.[21] Some people are mistrusting by nature; others may have heard previous predictions of doom that did not materialize.

More important, perhaps, is how socioeconomic and cultural factors influence perceptions and attitudes. African Americans, for example, have many reasons to mistrust both the medical profession and the institutions where they receive their care. The Tuskegee medical experiments and the fact that until recently, most hospital wards were segregated provide historical reasons for mistrust. Unfortunately, subtler forms of racial and economic discrimination persist. Very few nurses and physicians are African American, and many poor and minority patients have inadequate access to health care unless they are critically ill.[24–26] Some data demonstrate that minority status and lower socioeconomic status are associated with preferences for more aggressive care.[27, 28]

By understanding the motives that lead to requests for futile treatment, physicians can take steps to prevent a confrontation near the end of a patient's life. By helping patients and families set treatment goals, physicians can avoid meaningless debates about the utility of specific interventions. By giving full disclosure about the invasiveness and poor outcomes (in most situations) of CPR, they can reduce unreasonable demands for this procedure. By providing continuity and consistency of care, they can minimize the confusion that too often results in unrealistic demands for treatment. Mistrust, however, is a more difficult problem that cannot be overcome until we have more minority health professionals and a more equitable health care system.

MEDICAL FUTILITY IN THE FUTURE

It is hoped that physicians will use what we have learned from the futility debate to communicate more effectively with patients and their families, thereby preventing unproductive and painful confrontation. Perhaps, as more institutions and professional societies develop medical futility policies, our society will recognize the difference between the negative right to refuse treatment and the positive right to demand it, letting physicians make more professional judgments about how to determine when end-of-life interventions offer little or no benefit.

Undoubtedly, the courts will hear more futility cases, and they are unlikely to give physicians the formal power to make unilateral futility judgments in any but the most narrow physiologic meanings of futility. At the same time, increasing pressure to conserve medical resources will make overt rationing (we covertly ration now, e.g., by ability to pay) an inevitability. In a society in which great inequity, racial division, and a pluralism of religious and cultural values exist, the confusion between futility and rationing will frequently manifest itself. Clinical studies will identify more situations in which outcomes are poor, and statistical models will better predict hopeless situations, but most dying patients will continue to fall into ambiguous categories. Physicians may have less, rather than more, time to optimally plan with their patients, who, because of the nature of our health care system, will often be strangers to them.

References

1. American Thoracic Society: Withholding and withdrawing life-sustaining therapy. Ann Intern Med 1991; 115:478–486.
2. Task Force on Ethics, Society of Critical Care Medicine: Consensus report on ethics of foregoing life-sustaining treatments in the critically ill. Crit Care Med 1990; 18:1435–1439.
3. Council on Ethical and Judicial Affairs, American Medical Association: Guidelines for the appropriate use of do-not-resuscitate orders. JAMA 1991; 265:1868–1871.
4. The Virginia Health Care Decisions Act of 1992. Virginia Code 8.§54.1-2990.
5. Blackhall LJ: Must we always use CPR? N Engl J Med 1987; 317:1281–1285.
6. Brett AS, McCullough LB: When patients request specific interventions: Defining the limits of the physician's obligation. N Engl J Med 1986; 315:1347–1351.
7. Tomlinson T, Brody H: Ethics and communication in do-not-resuscitate order. N Engl J Med 1988; 318:43–46.
8. Youngner SJ: Who defines futility? JAMA 1988; 260:2094–2095.
9. Tomlinson T, Brody H: Futility and the ethics of resuscitation. JAMA 1990; 264:1276–1280.
10. Schneiderman LJ, Jecker NS, Jonsen AR: Medical futility: Its meaning and ethical implications. Ann Intern Med 1990; 112:949–954.
11. Truog RD, Brett AS, Frader J: The problem of futility. N Engl J Med 1992; 326:1560–1564.
12. Callahan D: Medical futility, medical necessity: The-problem-without-a-name. Hastings Cent Rep 1991; 21:30–35.
13. Lantos JD, Singer PA, Walker RM, et al: The illusion of futility in clinical practice. Am J Med 1989; 87:81–84.
14. Veatch RM, Spicer CM: Medically futile care: The role of the physician in setting limits. Am J Law Med 1992; 18:15–36.
15. *In re Wanglie* No. PX-91-283, 4th JD, Hennepin County, Minn, July, 1991.
16. Miles SH: Informed demand for "non-beneficial" medical treatment. N Engl J Med 1991; 325:512–515.
17. Brennan TA: Physicians and futile care: Using ethics committees to slow the momentum. Law Med Health Care 1992; 20:336–339.
18. Angell M: The case of Helga Wanglie: A new kind of "right to die" case. N Engl J Med 1991; 325:511–512.

18a. McCrary SV, Swanson JW, Youngner SJ, et al: Physicians' qualitative assessment of medical futility. J Clin Ethics 1994; 5:100–105.

19. Jecker NS, Schneiderman LJ: Futility and rationing. Am J Med 1992; 92:189–196.

19a. Morreim EH: Profoundly diminished life: The casualties of coercion. Hastings Cent Rep 1994; 24:33–42.

20. Angel M: Cost containment and the physician. JAMA 1985; 254:1203–1207.
21. Youngner SJ: Applying futility: Saying no is not enough. J Am Geriatr Soc 1994; 42:887–889.
22. Murphy DJ: Do-not-resuscitate orders: Time for reappraisal in long-term-care institutions. JAMA 1988; 260:2098–2101.
23. Youngner SJ, Allen M, Montenegro H, et al: Resolving problems at the intensive care unit/oncology unit interface. Perspect Biol Med 1988; 31:299–308.
24. Wenneker MB, Weissman JS, Epstein AM: The association of payer with utilization of cardiac procedures in Massachusetts. JAMA 1990; 264:1255–1260.
25. Buckle JM, Horn SD, Oates VM, et al: Severity of illness and resource use differences among white and black hospitalized elderly. Arch Intern Med 1992; 152:1596–1603.
26. Braverman PA, Egerter A, Bennett R, et al: Differences in hospital resource allocation among sick newborns according to insurance coverage. JAMA 1991; 266:3300–3308.
27. Danis M, Patrick DL, Southerland LI, et al: Patients' and families' preferences for medical intensive care. JAMA 1988; 260:797–802.
28. Garrett JM, Harris RP, Norburn JK, et al: Life-sustaining treatment during terminal illness: Who wants it? J Gen Intern Med 1993; 8:361–368.

CHAPTER 202

Foregoing Life-Sustaining Therapy in Intensive Care

Michael A. DeVita, MD • Ake Grenvik, MD, PhD

In 1939, 37% of all deaths in the United States occurred in hospitals, but in 1989, as many as 85% did. Approximately 70%[1] of these deaths followed a decision to either withhold or withdraw some form of therapy. It is important for the intensivist to understand the rationale for such a decision, assist patients and surrogates in their decision making, and carry out therapeutic options in a way that preserves patient dignity and prevents suffering. This chapter reviews briefly the rationale for foregoing life-sustaining therapy and provides practical comments about making such decisions.

BRIEF HISTORY OF WITHHOLDING SUPPORT

The origins of withholding support are found in ancient times. In his *The Art,* Hippocrates stated that the role of medicine was "to do away with the sufferings of the sick, to lessen the violence of their diseases, and to refuse to treat those who are overmastered by their diseases, realizing that in such cases, medicine is powerless." Thus, the physician must try to cure those who may be cured, decrease morbidity of diseases where possible, and when unable to do so, he or she should ensure comfort for a patient. Finally, when a disease has "won" and a patient will die, the physician is obligated to recognize this, and ease the dying process. This characterization remains peculiarly pertinent to intensive care more than two millennia after Hippocrates.

During the long history of medicine, and until very recently, the physician has been accorded the responsibility of dictating therapy to be considered and then choosing the course for a patient to follow. The patient, in turn, was obligated to follow "doctor's orders."

Although the attempt to forestall death has been present in physicians' actions throughout time, it was not until the recent past that physicians could significantly impact upon the prevention of death without influencing the likelihood of recovery. That is, with the advent of techniques that support failed organs for a potentially indefinite period of time, physicians can now breathe, pump blood, excrete wastes, and provide nutrition for their patients. Thus, a new category of patient was created as a result of medical advancement: the "nearly dead," or one who is alive only because he or she is receiving life-support in the intensive care unit (ICU).

When ICUs were first created, they were filled not with the old, but with young patients who were more likely to benefit from the interventions provided in them.[2] As the benefits became more apparent, older and sicker patients were also treated in these ICUs. In the early 1960s, cardiopulmonary resuscitation and dialysis made a major impact on public and medical expectations and results. With these new interventions, death could be forestalled for long periods (e.g., in a patient with the previously fatal condition of renal failure) and lethal processes reversed. The decisions in the United States to provide dialysis for all patients and to widely train people in cardiopulmonary resuscitation created the expectation that all individuals had a right to all possible therapy.

With time, virtually all organs could be supported nearly indefinitely. Thus, cancers could be treated more aggressively, failed organs could be replaced with artificial or transplanted new ones, and infections could be cured because patients were alive longer and could receive more antibiotics. However, some survivors cannot recover and return to society. The new dilemma of how to deal with the incurable, life-supported ICU patient was recognized.

Physicians recognized that patients who had sustained a lethal brain injury and in fact had irreversibly absent brain function were kept "alive" on ventilators.[3, 4] Breathing was provided by a ventilator, and even the heart could be supported by a pacemaker. In this situation, it was realized that lack of cardiac function should not be an absolute criterion included in the definition of death. Several conventions of physicians and ethicists[5, 6] and legislative actions[7] forwarded the concept of *"brain death"* (see Chapters 171 and 173). This currently well-accepted term equates irreversible cessation of all brain function with death of the individual. The original purpose of such a concept and legislation was to allow physicians to ethically and legally terminate support and to enable these patients to donate viable organs for procurement and transplantation after death had been established.

The late 1960s thus brought the ability to terminate life support with an ethical justification that relied on the patient's already being dead. In the 1970s, it was further recognized that other individuals on support were not dead but clearly would not benefit from continued treatment. One such patient was Karen Ann Quinlan,[8] a young woman with severe anoxic encephalopathy following drug overdose. Her parents wished to have her life support terminated, stating that she would never have wanted such support in her current condition and would never have agreed to it. The resultant New Jersey Supreme Court ruling indicated that patients have the right to refuse even life-supporting therapy based on their autonomy and right to decide what should be allowed to happen to their bodies; essentially, this is the same legal and ethical basis of informed consent. It is also important to realize that physicians have no obligation to treat diseases when there is no hope of recovery. If they agree, physicians and patients are now widely accorded the ability and right to withdraw futile therapy in the face of terminal illness.

In 1991, the U.S. Congress passed and implemented the Patient Self-Determination Act, which further supports the right of patients to refuse therapy and recommends the use of advance directives to make their wishes known. Thus, at present, removal of life support for patients who are not expected to benefit from this therapy is widely accepted.

DISTINCTION BETWEEN WITHHOLDING AND WITHDRAWING SUPPORT

The discussion of terminating life-sustaining therapy in hopelessly ill patients has been an emotive one from its onset. Many healthcare professionals have been uncomfortable with removal of such support from these patients, believing that by doing so they become active agents of death. Some prefer to withhold support rather than withdraw it. *Withholding support* is defined as never providing the patient with the therapy in question. For example, a patient who develops irreversible renal failure would require dialysis for continued life. Physicians who prefer to withhold support would never start dialysis of patients unlikely to benefit. They feel that in this scenario the renal failure causes the patient to die.

Withdrawing support refers to discontinuing already instituted therapy. Proponents may feel more comfortable withdrawing support than withholding it because the therapy has already been shown not to benefit the patient. Those favoring this approach believe that withdrawing the therapy results in the patient's underlying disease being able to overwhelm the patient.

The phrase "foregoing therapy" refers both to the withdrawing and the withholding of therapy. Because both the withdrawing and the withholding of therapy result in the disease's unimpeded progression, the two focuses of foregoing therapy are considered ethically equivalent. However, it is important to note that many families, despite understanding the equivalence, may feel uncomfortable terminating support because of the temporal relationship between the removal of support and the patient's death, if it occurs. The involved physicians should be aware of the potential for this emotional response and try to understand and help families deal with their feelings.

Interventions *intended* to hasten death directly are considered *active euthanasia,* which is currently illegal in the United States. An example of active euthanasia is the delivery of a lethal intravenous dose of potassium chloride, which causes cardiac arrest.

Assisted suicide refers to the practice of helping a person to take his or her own life but not of directly performing the action that causes death. An example would be placement of an intravenous catheter into a patient, supplying the lethal medication, and instructing the patient in how to use it to commit suicide. Although assisted suicide is not equivalent to euthanasia per se, the two terms are often considered together because of the intention and active induction of death as their goals. In the United States, the practice is prohibited by law in most states; however, in recent years, statutes have been challenged in some areas.

WITHDRAWING MECHANICAL VENTILATORY ASSISTANCE

Foregoing life-sustaining support encompasses both withholding support and removal of unwanted support already being provided. However, not providing therapy may be easier to order than removal of therapy already started. In particular, removing respiratory support requires special attention because of its emotive nature and the significant distress that it can cause for the patient, his or her family, and the professional staff. Therefore, removal of ventilatory assistance is discussed separately from the withdrawal of other types of life support.

The major goal of the removal of ventilatory assistance is the withdrawal of unwanted therapy while maintaining a patient's comfort. Patients who have their ventilatory assistance withdrawn are likely to suffer respiratory distress unless their physicians anticipate this occurrence and act to prevent and treat it. Sedation in the form of narcotics administration (to suppress feelings of dyspnea) and the use of anxiolytics (to suppress anxiety) are almost always necessary. In dosing these medications, it is important to remember the therapeutic goals. It is crucial that comfort be maintained, even if providing the needed medication also hastens death. This has been referred to as the "double effect." For example, a hypotensive patient who has respiratory discomfort should still receive narcotics, even though his or her blood pressure may decrease further as a result, and death may occur sooner. The physician's *primary* intent—to relieve suffering—is crucial to legitimize giving medications that may also hasten death as a secondary effect.

Most physicians choose to give morphine or diazepam, or both, to relieve anxiety and to prevent dyspnea before they initiate therapy withdrawal. As withdrawal of mechanical ventilation progresses, more sedation is usually required. Physicians and nursing staff carefully watch for signs of distress and alleviate them immediately. It is important to recognize that respiratory drive is a potent force in the cause of this distress. Many ICU patients have developed some tolerance to opioids and sedatives. Therefore, very large doses of these medications may be required.[9] Some patients may need hundreds of milligrams of morphine if adequate control is to be achieved.[10] Experienced physicians are able to titrate the sedation to prevent rather than to relieve discomfort, and this is a laudable practice. As long as the patient remains comfortable, weaning from ventilatory support may proceed, but the rate of progression is dependent on patient tolerance.

Sample orders for sedation and comfort during terminal weaning are indicated in Table 202–1. These orders are directed at *preventing* distress through the continuous delivery of medication. An alternative approach directed at *alleviating* distress would use less (or no) continuous infusion sedative but rather would require giving sedation as needed in response to perceived mild distress. Both methods (prevention and alleviation) are clearly directed toward maintaining patient comfort and expeditious removal of the ventilator. The decision as to whether to extubate the patient must be considered by the medical team, the patient, and his or her family. The endotracheal tube may have symbolic value for the patient, family, or physician that may dictate whether the tube should remain in place or be removed. If it is removed, care must be taken to prevent acute airway obstruction, which can cause the patient significant distress. Use of an oral or nasal airway is usually sufficient for this purpose.

TABLE 202–1. Sample Orders for Withdrawal of Mechanical Ventilatory Assistance*

1. Patient to receive comfort measures only.
2. Morphine, 5 mg, and diazepam, 5 mg intravenously immediately.
3. Begin continuous morphine intravenous infusion at 5 mg/h.
4. Change ventilator mode to intermittent mandatory ventilation.
5. Decrease ventilator rate by four breaths every 5 minutes.
6. When rate decreased to zero, remove ventilator.
7. If patient's respiratory rate is greater than 20 breaths per minute, give morphine, 5 mg intravenously every 5 minutes, until respiratory rate is less than or equal to 20, and increase morphine infusion by 5 mg/h.
8. Do not withhold medications for treatment of low blood pressure.

*The doses of medication are not recommendations but are used for illustrative purposes only.

Most commonly, the physician remains at the bedside to titrate the medications. Careful documentation of dosage and of the rationale for the medication is warranted. Some nurses who are experienced in the withdrawal of support are able to enact terminal weaning orders as long as an experienced physician is readily available to oversee and assist this activity.

The goal of ventilator withdrawal is to remove the unwanted or nonbeneficial therapy while guaranteeing patient comfort and dignity. In the United States, it is unlawful to cause patient death, although death remains the expected outcome of removing ventilatory support. In some instances, physicians have discontinued withdrawal of mechanical ventilation because of patient intolerance and were reluctant to provide the large doses of narcotics and sedatives required because of fear of "killing" the patient. Other caregivers may place patient sedation and the hastening of death as priorities. This was exemplified in a study[11] reporting that 36% of physicians ordered and 39% of nurses delivered sedation with the hastening of death as their intent. Such intention remains illegal.

Solomon and coworkers[12] stated that physicians commonly provide care against their conscience to patients not expected to benefit from it. In their study, physicians also reported a reluctance to remove such patients from life support, even if the patients or their families had expressed a desire to forego such support. This dichotomy of understanding that continued therapy may not be in a patient's best interest points out the ethical and social ambiguity to which physicians are prey.

Vincent[13] surveyed European ICU physicians about similar issues. Thirty-one per cent of responding physicians indicated that they discuss do-not-resuscitate status with the patients, whereas 57% instead stated that they discuss this issue with the families. Do-not-resuscitate orders were frequently given but were usually oral and not written. Eighty-three per cent of the responding physicians included withholding of support as part of their practice, 63% withdrew initiated therapy, and 36% stated that they practice euthanasia. It is interesting that when considering the example of an irreversibly ill and comatose patient whose family wants "everything to be done," over 100 of the 242 respondents stated they would withhold support, and more than 30 would even withdraw therapy anyway.

Miller[14] has supported the physician's role in the dying process and further calls for recognition of the obligation the physician has to the dying. The physician must actively choose not to try to prevent death (when appropriate) and in fact must help facilitate it if the autonomy or dignity of the individual is threatened. Osler demonstrated this when caring for his patients and at the time of his own death. Hinohara[15] cites Osler's approval of the use of medications under certain circumstances when a patient is terminally ill. Osler, as his own death approached, turned from the use of medications for his chronic bronchitis to the use of opium, which made him comfortable. He recognized the importance of dying as a process, which must be psychologically and, if necessary, medically supported to eliminate pain—whether it be spiritual, physical, or mental.

It is possible that the nursing staff may be working with a different understanding and goal of therapy. For this reason, it is important to include the nursing staff in family discussions and the decision-making process. If not, once a decision is made, the physician must discuss the plan with the nursing staff. Without such a discussion, the ordered (intended) therapy may not be the same as the delivered therapy. The nursing staff may give less or more medication than required based on their own interpretation, which may be different from the physician's intent.

Patient preferences[16] for ICU care clearly support the desire of patients to live, if that outcome is reasonably likely. It is equally clear that if the outcome is likely to be poor, then most patients disagree with the continuation of life support. However, fully 25% of the patients in this study preferred life support even in the face of either a permanent vegetative state or terminal illness.

Although many clinicians may be concerned about the ethics and legality of foregoing life-sustaining therapy, the clinician in virtually all cases does not need a judge to permit such activity. Mishkin[17] has reported that no physician was ever found liable for terminating treatment at the request of a competent adult. This is because all interventions require consent, which reflects the voluntariness of the patient's participation. This effectively precludes the physician from liability. Still, physicians may fear litigation. In this situation, Mishkin argues that the courts and judges are not adequately trained to handle and lack the experience to confront such biomedical-ethical situations. It is the responsibility of hospitals to design policies regarding the management of such problems. On the other hand, by *not* complying with a request to terminate treatment, the physician does become vulnerable to a new type of legal action: The right to die suit. In fact, doctors of a patient in such a situation were found liable for pain and suffering caused by unwanted care.[17]

When we wean a patient from his or her ventilator, we usually order that intermittent mandatory ventilation be used. Assist-control ventilation cannot be used because all breathing attempts are supported by a full machine breath. Under such conditions, decreased support can only result from eradication of all respiratory drive. Pressure support, inspired oxygen concentration, and end-expiratory pressure can all be reduced gradually or rapidly.

Several groups have attempted to facilitate removal of life support from hopelessly ill patients. Some have focused on creating a comprehensive supportive care team[18] that provides an alternative to the ICU or ward environment by concentrating on the physical and psychosocial needs of the dying patients. Kwack and Grenvik have created a plan modeled after a practice observed in Korea.[19] It allows patients (or families) to make the decision whether to have life support withdrawn at home, with family members present, thereby lessening the intrusion of technology into an intensely personal and emotional event. Others have created futility policies, which restate the physician's duty to treat only when hope of benefit can be expected. With comfort measures always provided, these policies permit physicians to withdraw futile therapy from hopelessly ill patients even if the patients themselves or their families request continued treatment.[20–23] Although termination of life support is usually decided upon jointly by the physician, the patient, and the family (or surrogates), some reports describe involvement of third parties whose goal is to prevent withdrawal of therapy.[24–26]

WITHDRAWING NONVENTILATORY LIFE SUPPORT

In addition to mechanical ventilation, other forms of life-sustaining support can be foregone. Therapy with antibiotics, blood products, and antiarrhythmic agents is usually discontinued abruptly. There seldom is great controversy or difficulty in foregoing most of these forms of therapy. However, removal of other therapies may be more emotive because of some special symbolism or significance. Discontinuation of hydration and nutrition have been particularly difficult to rationalize for some,[27, 28] but the majority of physicians,[29–33] court opinions,[34, 35] and the public[36] equate all therapy. That is, all important therapy (with the exception of comfort measures) sustains life. The United States courts and most of the medical literature certainly agree on the equality in this regard of mechanical ventilation and assisted circulation, on the one side, and artificial feeding and fluid administration, on the other. However, the difference between such therapies as mechanical ventilation and nutrition is the immediacy of the effects of their deprivation on a patient.

As in discontinuation of mechanical ventilation, the withdrawal of other mechanical, hemodynamic, or homeostatic support requires ethical justification. Once the decision is made, the patient's comfort must be maintained as a primary goal. Most nonventilatory therapies do not have the same potential to stimulate distress as does withdrawal of ventilatory support. Discontinuation of antibiotics and blood products, for example, is not associated with pain or discomfort. For those therapies that may cause distress when removed, the physician must consider this possibility and treat or preferably prevent its occurrence. For example, hunger may be caused by the discontinuation of feedings. Another example is the potential anxiety that patients who understand that treatment is being discontinued may experience. However, these problems can be treated or prevented through the use of narcotics, sedatives, or anxiolytics, all of which are able to suppress those sensations. We always administer anxiolytics and narcotics to those patients who *possibly* may experience such sensations, even if they are not very likely to occur.

Examples of support whose withdrawal does not typically cause distress are cardiac bypass, dialysis, cardiac pacing, antibiotic use, and the administration of blood products. Examples of therapies whose discontinuation sometimes may be associated with discomfort are nutrition (hunger), hydration (thirst), use of pressor and inotropic agents (dyspnea from congestive failure), and dialysis in patients with volume overload (dyspnea).

Foregoing therapy always requires careful discussion with a patient's family and, if possible, with the patient. Early communication before any decisions are made builds trust and is effective in educating the involved persons about legal, medical, ethical, religious, and prognostic considerations. The discussions enable the physicians and patient or family to create a rational framework for agreeing on therapy that considers all of these considerations.

Families have demonstrated the ability to rationalize various combinations of therapy that are acceptable to them. For example, two recent patients had similar poor prognoses for recovery from pneumonia and persistent vegetative conditions. Both were intubated and mechanically ventilated. Careful discussion with one patient's family revealed the patient's desire not to be kept alive by machines if there was no hope of recovery but that the patient approved of all other therapies, such as the administration of antibiotics and bedsore prophylaxis. The second family reported that their loved one would not desire further therapy but did not want the ventilator disconnected because the patient believed that this was placing God's work into man's hands. The physicians discontinued the former patient's ventilator therapy only and the latter patient's medical and diagnostic therapy. In both cases, the families believed that the correct decision had been made, and the physicians were comfortable that nonbeneficial or unwanted therapy had been appropriately withdrawn.

EUTHANASIA

The rationale for foregoing therapy has been framed in terms of enhancing patient autonomy and avoiding futile (nonbeneficial) therapy, while allowing death to occur with dignity and quality at the end of the patient's life. Euthanasia arguments are virtually the same but differ in extent.

Euthanasia has received greatest acceptance when it is considered for patients who have terminal illness and are unresponsive to therapeutic interventions that are acceptable to the patient. These patients commonly suffer from pain or unremitting psychologic anguish. Miller[14] has stated that "the physicians, [patients,] and surrogates must be ready and willing to decide not to intervene in the dying process, indeed to hasten it when they see the autonomy and dignity of patients are threatened." However, hastening death remains an illegal action in the United States. Unfortunately, current legality depends on intentions and semantics. Cameron writes that "the difference between euthanasia and letting the patient die by omitting life-sustaining treatment is a moral quibble."[37]

Colloquially, *euthanasia* refers to active intervention to hasten the death of an individual. Foregoing support, by contrast, is the removal or avoidance of futile therapy that might temporarily postpone but not prevent death. Groups such as the Hemlock Society, which has more than 38,000 members,[38] have formed to support social acceptance of and foster legislation permitting euthanasia. They have been active in promoting the same goals for foregoing support as well.

Euthanasia has received considerable media attention. Jack Kevorkian, a retired pathologist, has become renowned because he has aided several patients to commit suicide. His actions have caught the attention of lay people, legislators, and ethicists, if not the entire world. States such as Michigan have passed statutes making assisting suicide a felony offense. However, the interest kindled may prove to set the stage for further debate and change.

In his book *Final Exit,* Derek Humphrey[39] argues that "when cure is no longer possible and the patient seeks relief through euthanasia, the help of physicians is most appropriate." In contrast, a trustee of the American Medical Association was quoted as saying that the assistance of suicide or euthanasia by physicians would destroy the therapeutic relationship of trust necessary for patients and physicians. Others contend that making these options widely available would raise the likelihood that individuals would inappropriately commit suicide or even permit murder. Humphrey's book is explicit with regard to step-by-step methods, dosages, and pitfalls in suicide and euthanasia. As a testament to the public's interest in this matter, in 1992 the book made the *New York Times* bestseller list.

Several states have contemplated legislation permitting so-called "rational suicide" or "assisted suicide." However, no state has passed such a statute to date.[40] In the Netherlands, many physicians have helped thousands of patients commit suicide and have also participated in euthanasia for patients. Although not legal, the practice is largely overlooked by legislators and prosecutors. The Dutch Parliament has recently passed a law that protects physicians from legal sanction if they participate in assisted suicide or euthanasia provided that accepted guidelines are followed.[41] Thus, even though the practice is not strictly legal, engaging in it does not result in prosecution.

The Dutch have created a set of practice guidelines that seek to ensure that only "appropriate" patients are considered for euthanasia. The request must be made voluntarily by the patient, who must be well informed about the procedure and alternatives; he or she must be suffering unbearably, without hope of recovery. Furthermore, the patient's decision must remain unchanged over time. The hope is to prevent depressed or impulsive individuals from acting upon a poorly grounded decision. The physician must consult with at least one colleague experienced in these matters, and adequate written documentation must demonstrate that the noted requirements have been met.

Although the practice is now approved by the Dutch Parliament, not all Dutch physicians are pleased with the decision. Eleven per cent state that they would refuse to participate,[40] and one has been quoted as saying, "Today, the Netherlands abolished the Hippocratic oath."[40]

HOSPITAL POLICY FORMATION

In the United States, legislation requiring hospitals to adopt policies regarding advance directives has given further impetus to the trend toward the development of policies concerning withdrawal of support. Since 1975, the University of Pittsburgh Medical Center has had a policy that provides guidelines for the withdrawal of support.[42] In 1992, those guidelines were revised for the third time. A summary of the policy is found in the Appendix of this chapter. The major changes from past practice are two. First, a specific mechanism for a decision-making process now exists for those individuals who are unable to speak for themselves, whose wishes are unknown, and for whom there are no surrogates. Before the policy revision, such cases were decided by the courts or by the clinicians based on a loose "best interest of the patient" premise, or they were left undecided. The new policy uses existing resources, especially the clinicians and the ethics committee, which represent both patient and clinician perspectives and viewpoints, to come to a decision without involving the judicial system. To date, the mechanism has been effective in making such difficult decisions and in providing an effective forum for all viewpoints to be considered.

The second major change in the policy involves level of care. The new policy has three levels in recognition of the fact that patients and their families place different values on various therapies. For instance, patients may decide on various components of resuscitation (e.g., include intubation, but exclude chest compressions) because of their likelihood of success and because of the values that these therapies may have for them. The policy allows patients and physicians to specify which therapies are to be provided and which are to be foregone.

It has been recognized[21, 43, 44] that situations in which families and physicians cannot reach an agreement regarding further provision of care are arising with increasing frequency. When patients or families want care to be provided and the physician believes that the therapy is not indicated, a stalemate of sorts may ensue. The University of Pittsburgh Medical Center policy, which is based on patient autonomy and cooperation, may be ill-suited in some circumstances to deal with this problem. This may occur even though a policy may explicitly state that patients and surrogates may not compel a physician to provide therapy that is against his judgment (as does the University of Pittsburgh Medical Center policy [see Appendix]). Therefore, some institutions have policies[21] or committees[43] that serve as a mechanism to withdraw care without family consent or over family refusal. They usually require third-party review by another physician and by an ethicist, as well as some sort of formal presentation of the problem for discussion. Stell cites the need to inform the surrogates of such a decision before its implementation, allowing the surrogates the opportunity to appeal or to transfer care to another physician or institution. The formalization of the process and the assurance that it seems to provide physicians appears to have resulted in lifting the burden of decision making from families unable to reach these decisions on their own. The policy seems to have resulted in increasing communication and diminishing conflict between surrogates and caregivers.[44] However, to date, no higher court decisions in the United States have supported or refuted the applicability of such intrainstitutional policies.

CONCLUSION

Foregoing therapy in the ICU is common in the United States and an accepted practice in most countries. However, the legality, practice, and societal acceptance of this option vary widely among and within countries. Because physicians are now empowered with newer and increasingly more effective therapies to prevent death, more and more people die only as a result of an active decision not to provide some form of therapy. Already, most hospitalized patients die following a decision to forego therapy. The physician must be aware of the rationale for foregoing support and be able to effectively prevent pain and distress as the end of life approaches. Physicians must be just as prepared to approach the making of such decisions as they are in approaching other medical dilemmas. Many resources available to caregivers can facilitate the decision-making process. Effective ICU care includes creating appropriate policies and utilizing a team approach to deal with decisions of an ethical nature. A team may variously include nurses, physicians, social workers, clergy, patient representatives, family members, or even the patients themselves.

References

1. Faber-Langendoen K, Bartels D: Process of forgoing life-sustaining treatment in a university hospital: An empirical study. Crit Care Med 1992; 20:570.
2. Rapin M: The ethics of intensive care (Editorial). Intensive Care Med 1987; 13:300.
3. Lofstedt S, von Reis G: Intracranial lesions with abolished passage of x-ray contrast through the internal carotid arteries. Opuscula Medica 1956; 8:199.
4. Mollaret P, Goulon M: Le coma dépassé. Rev Neurol (Par) 1959; 101:3.
5. Wolstenholme G, O'Connor M (Eds): 1966 Ciba Foundation Symposium: Ethics in Medical Progress with Special Reference to Transplantation. Boston, Little, Brown and Co, 1966.
6. Beecher H: A definition of irreversible coma: Special communication: Report of the Ad Hoc Committee of the Harvard Medical School to Examine the Definition of Brain Death. JAMA 1968; 205:337.
7. Wasmuth CE, Stewart BH: Medical and legal aspects of human organ transplantation. Cleveland-Marshall Law Review 1965; 14:464.
8. *In re Quinlan,* 355 A 2d647 (NJ 1976).
9. Carlson JP: Managing pain and suffering in the dying patient. Minn Med 1990; 73:35.
10. DeVita M, Grenvik A: Personal communication, June 1, 1993.
11. Wilson WC, Smedira NG, Fink C, et al: Ordering and administering of sedatives and analgesics during the withholding and withdrawal of life support from critically ill patients. JAMA 1992; 267:949.
12. Solomon MZ, O'Donnell LO, Jennings B: Decisions near the end of life: Professional views on life-sustaining treatments. Am J Public Health 1993; 83:14.
13. Vincent JL: European attitudes towards ethical problems in intensive care medicine: Results of an ethical questionnaire. Intensive Care Med 1990; 16:256–264.
14. Miller PJ: Death with dignity and the right to die: Sometimes doctors have a duty to hasten death. J Med Ethics 1987; 13:81.
15. Hinohara S: Sir William Osler's philosophy on death. Ann Intern Med 1993; 118:638.
16. Elpern EH, Patterson PA, Gloskey D, et al: Patients' preferences for intensive care. Crit Care Med 1992; 20:43.
17. Mishkin DB: You don't need a judge to terminate treatment. J Intensive Care Med 1990; 5:201–204.
18. Field BE, Devich LE, Carlson RW: Impact of a comprehensive supportive care team on management of hopelessly ill patients with multiple organ failure. Chest 1989; 96:353.
19. Kwack IY, Grenvik A: Personal communication, September 3, 1989.
20. Paris JJ, Crone RK, Reardon F: Physicians refusal of requested treatment. N Engl J Med 1990; 322:1012.
21. Stell LK: Stopping treatment on grounds of futility: A role for institutional policy. St. Louis University Public Law Review 1992; 11:481.
22. Hansen-Flaschen JH: When life support is futile (Editorial). Chest 1991; 100:1191.
23. Marsh FH, Staver A: Futile cardiopulmonary resuscitation and physician authority for unilateral do-not-resuscitate orders. J Crit Care 1991; 6:221.
24. McCormick RA: "Moral considerations" ill considered. America 1992; 166:210.
25. Swanson H: Murder and the right to die. Newsweek 1989; 113:33.
26. Burnell GM: My mother wants to die. A lawyer won't let her. Med Econ 1988; 65:57.
27. Ramsey P: The indignity of 'death with dignity.' *In:* Death Inside Out: The Hastings Center Report. Steinfels P, Veatch RM (Eds). New York, Harper & Row, 1974, pp 81–96.
28. Rosner F: Withholding therapy and anti-cruelty policies (Letter). Ann Intern Med 1986; 105:468.
29. Steinbrook R, Lo B: Artificial feeding: Solid ground, not a slippery slope. N Engl J Med 1988; 318:286.
30. Council on Ethical and Judicial Affairs of the American Medical Association: Guidelines for the appropriate use of do-not-resuscitate orders. JAMA 1991; 265:1868.
31. Orentlicher D: The right to die after Cruzan. JAMA 1990; 264:2444.
32. Lo B, Dornbrand L: The case of Claire Conroy: Will administrative review safeguard incompetent patients? Ann Intern Med 1986; 104:869.
33. O'Rourke K: The AMA statement on tube feeding: An ethical analysis. America 1986; 155:321.
34. *Cruzan v Director, Missouri Department of Health,* 110 S Ct 284 (1990).
35. *In re Conroy,* 98 NJ 321, 486 A 2d 1209 (1985).
36. Pinkney D: "N.Y. law allows home-bound patients to refuse resuscitation." American Medical News, August 12, 1991, p 3.
37. Cameron DCS: The Truth About Cancer. Englewood Cliffs, NJ, Prentice-Hall, 1956, p 116.
38. Henry WA III: Do-it-yourself death lessons. Time 1991; 138(7):55.
39. Humphrey D: Final Exit. Secaucus, NJ, Hemlock Society, 1991.
40. Steinfels P: "Help for the helping hands in death." New York Times, February 14, 1993, Section 4, p 1.
41. Simons M: Dutch parliament approves law permitting euthanasia. New York Times, February 10, 1993, p A5.
42. Meisel A, Grenvik A, Pinkus RL, et al: Hospital guidelines for deciding about life-sustaining treatment: Dealing with health "limbo." Crit Care Med 1986; 14:239.

43. Brennan TA: Do-not-resuscitate orders for the incompetent patient in the absence of family consent. Law Med Health Care 1986; 14:13.
44. Stell LK: Personal communication, May 4, 1993.

Appendix: Summary of University of Pittsburgh Medical Center Guidelines on Foregoing Life-Sustaining Treatment (1992 Revision of Previously Published Guidelines[42])

PURPOSE

The purpose of this summary is to provide access to information contained in the University of Pittsburgh Medical Center Guidelines on Forgoing Life-Sustaining Treatment. It is not to be used as a substitute for those guidelines, which should be referred to when specific medical-ethical dilemmas occur.

INTRODUCTION

No ethically relevant distinction exists between failing to institute new treatment and discontinuing treatment that has already been initiated. Therefore, the term "forego" is used to include stopping treatment already begun as well as not starting a new treatment. These guidelines are applicable to all kinds of life-sustaining treatment and are not limited to decisions to forego cardiopulmonary resuscitation.

STATEMENT OF GENERAL PRINCIPLES

General Principles Governing Decision Making

As a general rule, all adult patients who do not lack decision-making capacity may decline any treatment or procedure. Patients who lack decision-making capacity have the same ethical and legal rights as do patients who possess such capacity, but healthcare decisions must be made on their behalf by a surrogate decision maker. Provision is made for a process to make decisions for patients who do not have surrogates. This process includes ethics committee review. It is the ethical and legal right of an individual physician to decline to participate in the limitation or withdrawal of therapy, if he or she considers this action inappropriate. However, no physician may abandon his or her patient until care by another physician has been secured. Further, a patient or his surrogate may not compel the physician to provide any treatment which in the physician's professional judgment is unlikely to provide the patient with significant benefit, i.e., the treatment is not medically indicated. Procedures for assessing decision-making capacity, for selecting a surrogate decision maker, and for Ethics Committee consultation are outlined in this section.

ADVANCE DIRECTIVES

The definition of, weight to be given to, and procedures for handling advance directives (living wills) are outlined in this section.

Documentation of Decisions and Entry of Orders

When it has been determined that a particular life-sustaining procedure is to be foregone, the resulting order must be written into the patient's medical record and an appropriate progress note written, including information on diagnosis, prognosis, patient's or surrogate's wishes, the recommendations of the treating team, and a description of the patient's decision-making ability. It is the physician's responsibility to communicate this information to other members of the healthcare team.

Detailed orders are usually required. Three categories of care are outlined.

All Appropriate Therapy: These patients are treated vigorously, using indicated diagnostic and therapeutic interventions.

Limited Therapy: This category includes patients for whom the decision has been made to forego some therapy. Therapy already initiated will be limited by specific written order only. Patients, their families or surrogates, and their physicians will accord different values, risks, benefits, and burdens imposed by various therapies and diagnostics. Thus, it is reasonable to allow involved parties to choose the appropriate interventions for that particular group of individuals. For example, patients with similar problems and prognoses may choose with their doctors to have in one case mechanical ventilation, but not hemodynamic support, and in another, the reverse. It is important for the physician to document such decisions and their rationale in the patient medical record.

Comfort Measures Only: These patient will only receive nursing, hygienic care, and medications appropriate to maintain comfort as ordered. Therapy (e.g., administration of narcotics) which is necessary for comfort may be utilized even if it contributes to cardiorespiratory depression. Therapies already initiated will be reviewed by the physician and discontinued if not related to comfort or hygiene.

CHAPTER 203

Outcome Prediction for Specific Conditions

Michael G. Seneff, MD • *Jack E. Zimmerman, MD*
William A. Knaus, MD

Subtle differences in disease presentation can have profound impact on a patient's outcome. For example, treatment recommendations may vary greatly for two patients with fulminant hepatic failure and similar serum biochemical abnormalities treated at the same institution. Owing to the importance on outcome of age, the cause of liver failure, and differences in prothrombin time, one patient may be treated "conservatively," and the other transferred to a liver transplantation facility. This chapter summarizes current data for predicting outcome for conditions that, by their uniqueness and widely ranging medical and social impact, deserve special emphasis. They include nontraumatic coma, in-hospital cardiac arrest, metastatic and hematologic malignancy, acquired immunodeficiency syndrome (AIDS), cirrhosis, and multiple organ dysfunction syndrome. Readers interested in outcomes for syndromes or diseases other than those mentioned are referred to other chapters in this text that deal with the topic of interest or to those that review the general severity of disease prognostic systems.

COMA

Mental status changes are frequent in critical illness and have important prognostic implications.[1, 1a] Coma is particularly important because of its prevalence, negative impact on survival, and the possibility for severe chronic disability.[2] Many efforts have been made to predict outcome from coma, and some have engendered confusion and controversy because of imprecise definitions of diagnosis or outcome, poor study design, and the tendency for poor prognoses to be self-fulfilling.[3] This confusion has resulted in variations in approach that range from withdrawal of support when the probability of death or persistent vegetative state is high[4] to aggressive support as long as any chance for recovery exists. The latter approach was suggested in a review of prognosis in nontraumatic coma by Shewman and DiGiorgio.[3] They stated:

> *Given this inherent unreliability of early predictors for individual patients, given that decisions to continue life support are reversible, whereas decisions to withdraw it are usually not, and given that the death of a patient with potential for recovery is a more serious error than the (typically) transient prolongation of life of a patient destined soon to die anyway or (much less commonly) to remain in a vegetative state, it would seem prudent to continue life support for all patients during the first few weeks or months of coma or vegetative state, regardless of early indicators of poor outcome.*

Despite conflicting opinions, rational prognostication for coma patients is possible. Relevant considerations include the following:

1. Mortality is not the only important outcome measured. Poor quality of life, particularly persistent vegetative state, is considered even worse than death by most individuals. These potential outcomes (e.g., mild, moderate, or severe disability) should be defined precisely and measured prospectively to limit ascertainment bias.
2. Prognostic estimates should be attempted only after a reasonable amount of time to ensure exclusion of reversible conditions, such as the influence of drugs or metabolic disturbances. Drug elimination can be prolonged and unpredictable in critically ill patients, and encephalopathy due to reversible infectious, renal, and hepatic causes is frequent.
3. Poor prognoses must not become self-fulfilling prophecies, that is, the practice of withdrawing care from patients with poor prognoses can ensure death and a poor prognosis.

A wealth of literature deals with prognostication for both traumatic[5–13] and nontraumatic coma.[3, 14–30] The following discussion is limited to nontraumatic coma, but many of the prognostic factors identified for nontraumatic coma are also important for traumatic coma.

Despite extensive study conducted since the mid-1980s, the most useful prognostic estimates for nontraumatic coma were developed from multi-institutional studies by Levy and coworkers.[17] They prospectively studied 500 patients with nontraumatic coma that lasted at least 6 hours after admission. Serial neurologic examinations were performed and outcome analyzed with reference to findings on clinical examination. Investigators did not interfere with treatment decisions, and patients were treated by their own physicians, "most of whom continued with strong or maximal efforts until the patient died." Neurologic outcomes were defined, and patients were classified according to the best condition achieved, regardless of other outcome (even death). Causes of coma included subarachnoid hemorrhage, hypoxia-ischemia, other cerebrovascular disease, hepatic encephalopathy, infection, mass lesions, and metabolic disturbances. Overall mortality of the group was high, and approximately three fourths of the patients experienced no recovery or remained in a vegetative state.

The study's general findings included a lack of importance for age as a predictive variable, a tendency for almost all surviving coma patients to awaken after 2 to 1 weeks, and the importance of improvement on serial examinations in predicting final recovery, regardless of initial presentation. The presence of certain neurologic findings at 6 hours and at 1, 3, and 7 days predicts likely outcome (Fig. 203–1). For example, 120 of the 500 patients had zero or only one brain stem reflex (corneal, pupillary, or oculovestibular) present at 6 hours, and only 1 of these patients attained sufficient neurologic recovery to be classified as having moderate disability or good recovery (this patient later died in the hospital). Although physicians may not be willing to prognosticate as early as at 6 hours, the guidelines presented for 1, 3, and 7 days are similarly accurate and allow time to ensure the absence of reversible factors and to permit discussions with the family to take place.

The findings of Levy and coworkers have verified the accuracy of brain stem reflexes and best motor response in predicting outcome. Formal vestibulo-ocular reflex testing with cold water is a more potent stimulus than head movement and may improve assessment of coma,[24] but clinical features, such as seizure or myoclonus,[23] and additional tests, such as electroencephalography, or somatosensory evoked potentials,[25–28] have contributed little to overall prognostication.

As previously noted, many physicians have been reluctant to use these estimates for individual patients because of concern about overall accuracy and highly publicized case reports of emergence from prolonged persistent vegetative states.[31, 32] None of the patients in these two reports, however, would have been placed in a poor prognostic group if the data of Levy and coworkers were used. For physicians not comfortable with withdrawal of therapy, recognition that a patient has a poor prognosis still provides useful information regarding the benefits of continuing therapy. Levy and coworkers' study included patients from England as well as the United States. Patient demographics were similar, but a detailed analysis of the first 310 patients entered into the study revealed that three times as many laboratory tests (electroencephalography, angiography, computed tomography scans) were performed on the patients in the United States as in the United Kingdom.[33] Overall outcomes were similar, although a higher percentage of the total deaths occurred within the first 72 hours in the United Kingdom compared with the United States (mortality at 1 month was not different).

CARDIOPULMONARY RESUSCITATION IN HOSPITALIZED INDIVIDUALS

Cardiopulmonary resuscitation (CPR) has achieved the unique position of a treatment that *will* be administered unless there are specific orders to the contrary. These orders, known as *do-not-resuscitate* (DNR) *orders,* have become a subject of intense debate concerning patient autonomy versus a physician's right to withhold ineffective therapy.[34–36] In reality, CPR is a medical treatment with specific benefits and indications that was never intended to be utilized on all patients dying in a hospital.[37] In this section, studies of outcome from in-hospital CPR that can be used to assist in making DNR decisions are reviewed.

Multiple studies of outcome from in-hospital CPR have demonstrated remarkably consistent findings.[38–47a] Overall, 40% to 50% of patients have vital signs restored, but only 5% to 15% are eventually discharged alive from the hospital.

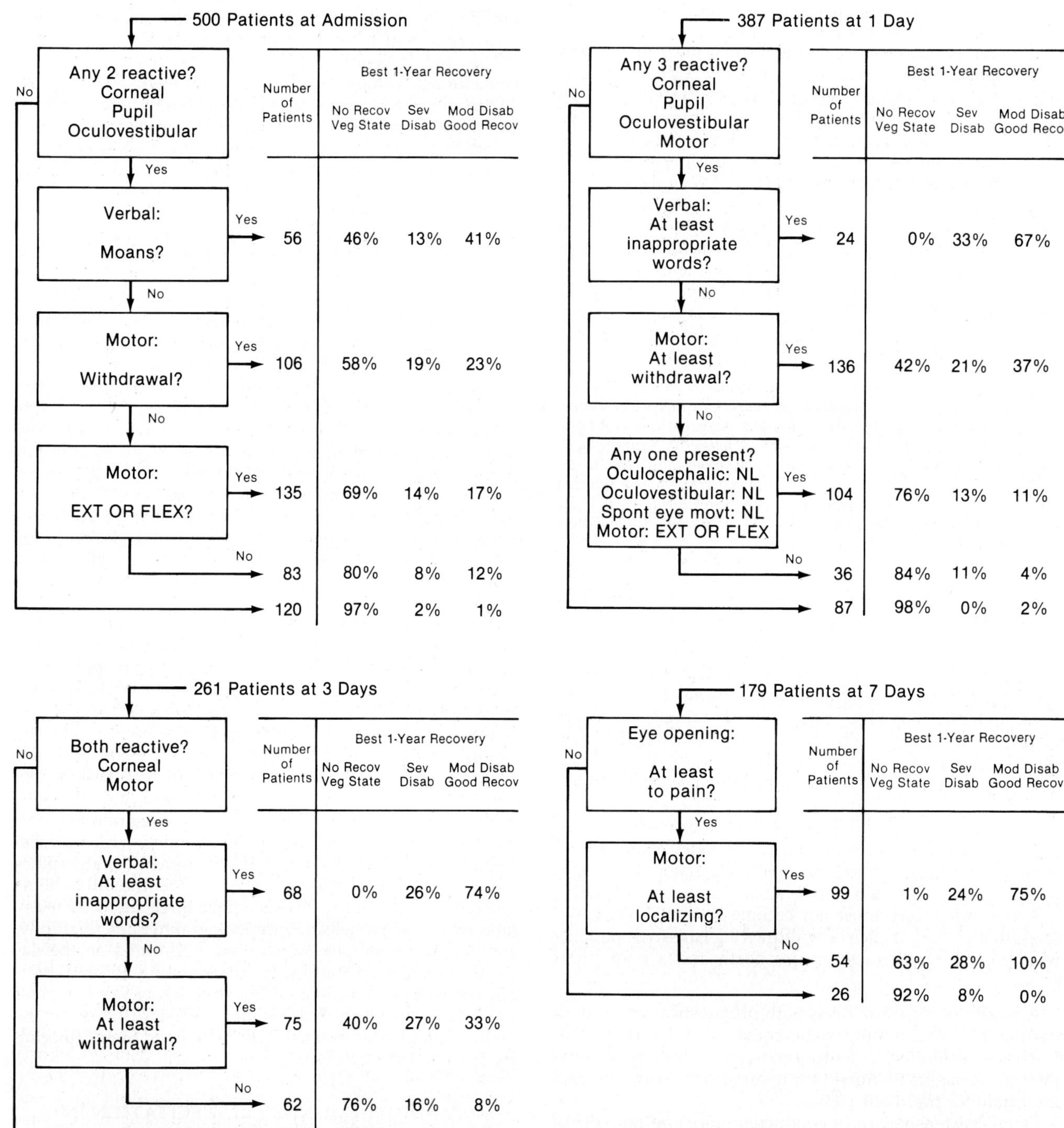

Figure 203–1. Relationship of clinical examination findings to outcome in patients admitted with coma. See text for details. (Reproduced with permission from Levy DE, Bates D, Caronna JJ, et al: Prognosis in nontraumatic coma. Ann Intern Med 1981; 94:293–301.)

Most deaths occur within the first week following CPR. Cardiovascular patients with ischemic heart disease or arrhythmias have the best outcome; success rates are higher for patients in coronary care units and lowest for those in ICUs and general medical or surgical wards.[42, 44, 46, 48] In large part, underlying disease, response times, and the number of witnessed versus unwitnessed arrests account for these differences. Patients with poor physiologic reserve because of age, chronic disease, and multiple organ dysfunction have a dismal prognosis, with a 0% to 5% survival rate at discharge. A substantial percentage of patients discharged alive remain functional at 1 year. This seems surprising but again emphasizes that good outcomes following CPR most commonly occur in patients with good baseline health and an acute reversible process such as myocardial infarction.[38, 43, 47]

Bedell and associates[38] prospectively identified predictor variables among 294 consecutive patients undergoing resuscitation in a university teaching hospital; 44% were successfully resuscitated, but only 41 (14%) were discharged alive, of whom 30 (10%) survived for 6 months. Multivariate logistic regression analysis identified predictors of mortality be-

TABLE 203–1. Predictors of Hospital Mortality After Cardiopulmonary Resuscitation

Characteristic	*Estimated Coefficient**
Before Arrest	
Hypotension (blood pressure < 100 mm Hg)	2.69
Pneumonia	2.85
Renal failure (blood urea nitrogen > 50 mg/dL)	2.75
Cancer	2.06
Homebound lifestyle	2.13
During Arrest	
Arrest duration > 15 min	2.51
Intubation	2.35
Hypotension (blood pressure < 100 mm Hg)	2.70
Pneumonia	2.48
Homebound lifestyle	2.24
After Resuscitation	
Coma	2.40
Need for pressors	2.16
Arrest duration > 15 min	1.87

(From Bedell SE, Delbanco TL, Cook EF, et al: Survival after cardiopulmonary resuscitation in the hospital. N Engl J Med 1983; 309:569–576. Reprinted by permission of *The New England Journal of Medicine*.)
*By multivariate logistic regression analysis.

fore, during, and after CPR (Table 203–1). Patients with one or more of these conditions at the time of arrest had a 95% mortality, whereas patients with none of these conditions had a 34% mortality. No patient with metastatic cancer or oliguria survived, and only 6 (4%) of 137 patients who were homebound before admission survived.

Other studies verify the uniformly dismal prognosis after CPR for patients with chronic disease, particularly those with malignancy, cerebral vascular accidents, chronic renal or hepatic failure, chronic obstructive pulmonary disease, and AIDS.[39, 46–48] In addition, patients with asystole, continued arrest after 15 minutes of CPR, or with a history of more than one cardiac arrest do not survive to be discharged from the hospital.[40, 47] In a prospective study of CPR in AIDS patients, only 1 of 43 patients was discharged from the hospital, and the survivor's arrest was iatrogenic in nature.[49] A retrospective review of CPR in medical and surgical ICUs demonstrated a 5% hospital discharge rate, and all survivors were dead or disabled at 1 year. A study of CPR in elderly patients revealed equally dismal results.[50]

Although studies reveal earlier and increased use of DNR orders in ICUs since the mid-1980s,[51, 52, 52a] prolonged, futile efforts are a continuing problem.[53] A frustrating but common scenario in the modern ICU is the admission of a terminally ill cancer patient following CPR for whom all agree that CPR was not indicated. Justification for CPR is usually stated as "that's what the patient wanted," but the real reasons are usually more complex and often center around poor communication and exchange of information. The reasons why CPR is attempted on patients who are unlikely to benefit include misunderstanding of ethical and legal guidelines, unwillingness to initiate DNR discussions, unrealistic patient expectations, and fear that DNR orders will cause appropriate care to be withheld. Many physicians are unaware of guidelines for the appropriate use of DNR orders presented by the Council on Ethical and Judicial Affairs of the American Medical Association.[54] These guidelines recommend DNR orders in several situations in which CPR, in our experience, is now widely used.

Some have argued for greater physician autonomy in the writing of DNR orders,[55, 56] but most physicians are uncomfortable with such orders that are unilaterally written. Hopefully, the public discussion and implementation of federally mandated notification regarding advance directives will improve opportunities for communication. Although better communication allows physicians to make decisions based on knowledge of a patient's preferences and values, accurate information about the likelihood of success of CPR is also essential to decision making.

AIDS

Few issues have received more attention than the medical, social, and financial impact of human immunodeficiency virus (HIV) infection. Early experience with respiratory failure in AIDS patients due to *Pneumocystis carinii* pneumonia (PCP) demonstrated an 84% to 100% hospital mortality rate, with many of the survivors dying within 6 months.[57–60] Subsequent articles and editorials discussed the futility of mechanical ventilation and ICU admission for these patients[61–65] but also emphasized that non-AIDS patients with a similar prognosis (e.g., metastatic cancer) were routinely offered ICU care. They also emphasized that it would be unethical to triage individuals with AIDS differently than patients with other disorders[64–66] and warned about promoting a self-fulfilling prophecy for AIDS patients by providing less aggressive care, thereby ensuring a continued high mortality rate. In the late 1980s, these concerns proved prophetic as hospital survival rates for patients with PCP and respiratory failure increased to 38% to 55%.[67–72] Improved survival was not due to differences in patient selection,[68, 69] and speculation about the reasons for improved prognosis included the impact of zidovudine (AZT), better nutrition, improved antibiotic treatment of PCP, and the use of steroids for patients with respiratory failure.[68, 71, 73, 73a] The improved outcome experience with AIDS patients demonstrates the pitfalls of using historical data to predict current outcome for a new disease that is the focus of dynamic research and new treatments.

Since the mid-1980s, our experience in an urban ICU that treats a large number of HIV-infected individuals mirrors the national experience.[74] We have been admitting fewer HIV patients with PCP and an increasing number of individuals with other infections, especially those with pneumococci and other gram-positive bacteria. Many of these patients have not yet developed AIDS and otherwise have excellent functional status. Their prognosis does not differ from that of similar patients who are not infected with HIV.[75, 76] With improved prophylaxis for PCP, an expanding patient population at risk, and the emergence of other infections such as multiple drug–resistant tuberculosis,[77] the increase in ICU admissions for HIV-infected individuals will continue.[73] Given the huge number of patients at risk and the substantial financial impact of providing them with critical care, accurate prognostication is essential.

Attempts to apply existing severity and prognostic systems for outcome prediction in AIDS patients have met with limited success. The Acute Physiology and Chronic Health Evaluation II (APACHE II) was developed before the AIDS epidemic and did not study patients with AIDS. APACHE II underpredicts mortality for patients with PCP and respiratory failure but has generally been accurate for non-PCP patients.[59] Attempts to modify APACHE II for AIDS patients with PCP by adding other variables, such as lactic dehydrogenase serum levels and organ failure scores, have improved accuracy.[78, 79] The APACHE III prognostic system does provide outcome estimates and includes independent predictor variables for parasitic pneumonia and AIDS as a definable chronic disease. We believe that APACHE III will be an accurate and effective means to predict outcome for HIV-infected individuals, but further information and independent validation is needed.

Until a validated general or disease-specific prognostic system for AIDS is available, intensivists need to subjectively estimate prognosis on a case-by-case basis. In general, HIV-infected patients without AIDS have a prognosis similar to non–HIV-infected individuals. Individuals with AIDS early in its course usually have adequate nutritional stores and organ function and frequently respond well to therapy. Even survival after prolonged mechanical ventilation for respiratory failure secondary to PCP is not uncommon.[72, 73] Patients with late-stage AIDS frequently have severe wasting and multiple organ dysfunction and do not respond well to critical care and life-support measures. These patients should be treated like any other patients with terminal disease and not viewed differently because they have AIDS; that is, futility is defined based on prognosis, and not on disease.[73, 80] In our experience, critical care is withheld more frequently from those with AIDS than from those with other terminal diseases. One reason for this is because an AIDS patient is more likely to request therapeutic limits, either through a living will or a surrogate.

Although HIV is a horrible contagion, it has taught us many important lessons. In general, homosexual activity is the most prevalent risk factor for patients at our hospital, and the gay community in Washington, D.C., is a politically active and united group that is extremely well informed about HIV, AIDS, and its treatment. Many of our patients have seen loved ones die from the disease and are knowledgable about and willing to discuss the effectiveness of medical intervention. This has resulted in an open, informed environment in which physicians, patients, and their representatives discuss therapeutic options and the advisability of life-support measures. A consensus regarding what represents "futile" therapy is common, and many terminally ill patients die without receiving artificial ventilation, CPR, or intensive care. Advance directives and power of attorney for healthcare decisions are frequently granted to others should the need arise.

We believe the AIDS experience should serve as a model for physicians and patients with other end-stage diseases. Terminal AIDS and metastatic cancer are not that different in terms of physiologic effects and prognosis, but physicians and the public view them as such. Physicians should bring the experience gained in discussing the prognosis and effectiveness of therapy with AIDS patients to other patients with equally poor prognoses so that limited ICU resources can be used more effectively.[66]

MULTIPLE ORGAN DYSFUNCTION SYNDROME

Multiple organ dysfunction syndrome (MODS) describes a dynamically changing continuum of organ dysfunction in which organ systems are not capable of maintaining homeostasis.[81] MODS is preferable to the term *multiple organ system failure,* which falsely implies a static, arbitrarily defined state that is either present or absent. A typical scenario is a septic or trauma patient admitted to the ICU who has severe physiologic abnormalities. Despite initial control of the inciting event and optimal support, the patient develops, over days or weeks, sequential dysfunction of multiple organ systems that frequently terminates with death. Although the syndrome has been recognized since the early 1970s,[82, 83] its cause remains uncertain. It is a source of extreme frustration for intensivists who sometimes view themselves as helpless engineers on a MODS freight train with a predetermined destination. In many ICUs, MODS is the most frequent cause of death; patients have protracted ICU stays, consume inordinate amounts of resources, and generate enormous costs. In one study, the average total hospital and rehabilitation charge per survivor was $385,000.[84]

Ongoing research is providing insight into potential causes and methods for prevention that may be the most effective way to improve outcome.[85–87] Until effective treatment is available, however, intensivists must be cognizant of the prognostic implications of MODS so that they can optimize resource allocation, counsel families, and act on advance directives. Studies of prognosis in MODS have demonstrated that death rate rises as the number of organ failures increases. Mortality increases from 5% to 30% for single-organ failure, 40% to 60% for double-organ failure, 60% to 80% for triple-organ failure, and from 95% to 100% for those with failure of four or more organs.[88–92] Patients with trauma generally fare better than do patients with other diseases. Unfortunately, the ability to compare outcomes in MODS has been confounded by variations in the timing and definition of organ failure. This accounts for much of the variation in the outcomes cited above and emphasizes the importance of daily severity scoring and risk stratification to describe the course and extent of organ dysfunction.[93]

Knaus and colleagues prospectively studied outcome for 2179 ICU admissions with one or more organ system failure (OSF).[94] This study defined five OSFs based on objective physiologic criteria that, with one exception, were independent of therapeutic intervention (the exception being dependence on mechanical ventilation for 72 hours or longer). The five definitions were applied to each 24-hour period for 7 days and ensured that maximal therapy was ongoing. This data was subsequently expanded to include 2405 ICU admissions at 27 French hospitals.[95] Findings were consistent regardless of hospital or country; prognosis worsened as the duration and number of OSFs increased. Mortality was greater than or equal to 93% for patients with three or more OSFs lasting 3 or more days, and virtually all survivors were younger than 40 years of age. Age was an important prognostic factor, with the mortality rate averaging 20% to 30% greater for patients older than 65 years. Only neurologic failure was associated with a higher mortality (40%) when compared with the approximately 30% rate for other organ systems. With the exception of neurologic failure, various OSF combinations did not result in substantially different outcomes, although data suggest that hepatic dysfunction may also be disproportionately important in predicting outcome for MODS.[96, 97]

A pilot study reported in 1990[98] demonstrated the potential value of prognostic data in MODS. In this study, daily estimates of risk for hospital mortality for patients with OSF were provided to ICU physicians practicing in selected French hospitals. The type, frequency, and reason for limiting or stopping therapy were then compared with the same for a control period when probability estimates were not available. Compared with the control period, a small but significant increase in decisions to stop active treatment and provide comfort care was limited to patients with three or more OSFs. Although the number of patients affected was small, this study demonstrated how probability estimates can be used to supplement clinical decision making in MODS.

ACUTE AND CHRONIC LIVER DISEASE

Cirrhosis

The scoring system developed by Child and Turcotte (the CTC, or Child's criteria)[99] and a subsequent modification by

Pugh and coworkers[100] are the most familiar and useful measures of severity and prognosis in liver disease. The CTC uses the extent of abnormality for 5 variables—serum bilirubin, albumin, ascites, neurologic dysfunction, and nutritional status—to classify patients into groups A, B, or C, which reflect increasing severity of disease. Pugh and coworkers assigned a score of 1 for CTC A variables, 2 for CTC B variables, and 3 for CTC C variables, and they used prothrombin time to replace the less reliably measured nutritional status. Child's criteria were developed to risk-stratify patients for portosystemic shunting. Mortality after shunting increases from 4% for group A patients to 43% for group C patients.[101] Child's criteria have also been used to risk-stratify cirrhotic patients undergoing other types of elective or emergency surgery, but there are significant limitations in using the criteria as a prognostic tool. The limitations include overlapping levels of severity among individual criteria, interobserver variation for subjective criteria (nutritional status), and a lack of prospective evaluation of predictive efficacy.

Several retrospective and longitudinal studies have evaluated the significance of variables other than the CTC in predicting outcome from liver disease.[102–106] Most of these studies were retrospective, did not include ICU patients, and attempted to identify variables that influenced 1- and 5-year mortality. Although these studies provide insight into measuring the severity of cirrhosis, they were primarily intended for group risk stratification rather than for individual prognostication.

Among the few studies that have specifically examined the prognosis of cirrhotic patients admitted for critical care, the most useful have focused on the efficacy of mechanical ventilation. Goldfarb and associates[107] evaluated outcome from intubation and mechanical ventilation among 100 ICU admissions with cirrhosis and severe complications. Overall mortality was 89%, but three variables—severe cirrhosis, septic shock, and hepatic coma due to superimposed acute hepatitis—were associated with 100% mortality. Severe cirrhosis was defined as jaundice, ascites, hepatic encephalopathy, or malnutrition (15% weight loss over the preceding 6 months). Shellman and coworkers[108] reported similar outcomes in a retrospective review of 100 ICU admissions with serious liver disease. Mortality was 91% among patients receiving assisted ventilation, 89% for Child's group C patients, and 93% for patients with creatinine values greater than 1.3 mg%. Patients with all three variables had a 2% survival rate. Variables such as sepsis, hyponatremia, oliguria, and low urine sodium levels were also associated with an increased mortality rate, but only three variables—assisted ventilation, Child's group C, and creatinine values greater than 1.3 mg%—were independently significant outcome predictors. Moreau and colleagues[109] also reported 100% mortality for Child's group C patients with septic shock treated in the ICU. Renal failure complicating severe cirrhosis has a similar dismal prognosis. Hospital mortality rates are as high as 95% among ICU admissions with the hepatorenal syndrome.[110,111] However, these data apply only when liver transplantation is not an option.

Together, these studies provide effective guidance in selecting cirrhotic patients for ICU care and for subsequent management decisions. Patients admitted with a problem isolated to a single organ system, such as upper gastrointestinal bleeding, deserve a trial of therapy because hospital and 2-month mortality for Child's group C patients with upper gastrointestinal bleeding ranges from 26% to 68%.[112] Patients who present with or subsequently develop MODS, require artificial ventilation, or both, have a poor prognosis, and decisions to limit or withdraw therapy are often appropriate.

Fulminant Hepatic Failure

Fulminant hepatic failure (FHF) is a syndrome due to acute massive liver necrosis and is characterized by progressive neurologic deterioration within 8 weeks of onset.[113] Average mortality for FHF is approximately 80%, despite the fact that it often afflicts previously healthy, young individuals. Identification of variables that predict outcome early in the syndrome is important because hepatic transplantation has resulted in improved survival for some patients. Onset of grade 4 hepatic encephalopathy and a prothrombin time greater than 100 seconds are independently associated with a mortality rate of greater than 95%. Other important prognostic factors include age, bilirubin level, and the cause of FHF (the outcomes of patients with acetaminophen overdose and hepatitis A are better than those of patients with other causes).[114]

O'Grady and coworkers[115] developed a prognostic model by performing univariate and multivariate analysis on data from 588 patients admitted to the hospital with FHF between 1973 and 1985. They then tested the model on 175 patients admitted between 1986 and 1987. Predicted mortality was 95% for patients with a prothrombin time greater than 100 seconds or the presence of any three of the following five variables: age under 10 or over 40 years; FHF caused by non-A, non-B hepatitis, halothane, or a drug other than acetaminophen; jaundice lasting longer than 7 days before encephalopathy is recognized; a prothrombin time greater than 50 seconds; and a serum bilirubin level greater than 17.7 mg%. Among patients not meeting these criteria, 82% survived with conventional treatment. Use of the above predictor variables identifies patients unlikely to survive conventional therapy and who might benefit from transfer to a hepatic transplantation center.

METASTATIC AND HEMATOLOGIC MALIGNANCIES

A real problem exists in determining the outcome of malignant disease treatment and the outcomes of individual ICU hospitalizations that are common in such patients. Most studies of cancer deal with disease-specific outcomes at 1 and 5 years. Staging, histologic subtyping, flow cytometry, and response to initial therapy guide the choice of therapy and influence outcome. There are studies of the outcomes of individual ICU admissions on overall cancer prognosis. Carlon (see Chapter 147) provides a list of acute problems in cancer patients who may require ICU admission but writes that "decisions must continue to be based on experience and conscience."

Overall mortality from ICU care for patients with malignancy ranges from 22% to 55%,[116–119] but overall mortality figures are not relevant because many of these ICU admissions are postoperative, for local or limited disease, or for a specific, acute, reversible problem such as hypercalcemia. In all the studies cited, mortality was markedly increased for patients with metastatic disease and multiorgan dysfunction, particularly those with respiratory disease requiring mechanical ventilation.

Several studies have demonstrated an extremely high mortality for cancer patients with respiratory failure. Snow and coworkers[120] reviewed outcomes for 180 patients with a variety of malignancies who required mechanical ventilation. Among the patients studied, 41% had hematologic, 15% lung, and 9% breast malignancies. Reasons for respiratory failure included atelectasis, upper airway obstruction, pleural effusion, and pneumonia; 26% of patients survived until extubation, and 13% and 7% were alive at 2 and 6 months, respectively. There were no 6-month survivors among patients with acute lymphocytic or myelogenous leukemia and adenocarcinoma of the lung, but breast cancer patients had a 24% 6-month survival. Patients who developed renal failure had a mortality of 91%. The most striking predictor of mortality was dysfunction of an increasing number of organ systems. Among patients with dysfunction of four or more systems, there were no 6-month survivors, and only one patient survived for 2 months.[120] Ewer and associates[121] analyzed outcome among 46 patients with inoperable lung cancer undergoing mechanical ventilation. Respiratory failure had a variety of causes, but the most common was progressive malignant disease. Ventilation was maintained for 1 to 145 days, with a median of 4 days for survivors and 6 days for nonsurvivors; 39 patients (85%) died while on the ventilator, and 7 were weaned on or before the 6th day. Three of these patients died before hospital discharge, and of the 4 patients who went home, 3 died within 4 months and only 1 was alive at 6 months.

Patients with hematologic malignancies and respiratory failure requiring mechanical ventilation have a hospital mortality of 80% to 95%.[122–127] This high mortality must be viewed in perspective, since long-term survival is sometimes possible if the primary disease responds to appropriate chemotherapy. However, persistent leukopenia, an increasing number of organ failures, and relapse or failure to respond to therapy increase the chance of dying while in the hospital. Patients with persistent leukopenia who require mechanical ventilation for 5 days or longer have a 95% to 100% chance of dying.

Until further information is available, how is a physician to interpret and use existing outcome data for patients with malignancies? Many patients develop reversible problems that can be treated with a high likelihood of success. These patients should be aggressively treated in the ICU. But what about the patient with metastatic cancer or hematologic malignancy in relapse who develops multiorgan dysfunction or respiratory failure? At many institutions, including our own, this type of patient often causes considerable friction and disagreement between critical care specialists and oncologists. This is understandable because the same patient is perceived differently.[128] Oncologists often see an individual with whom they have a long-standing relationship that developed under difficult circumstances. Treatment options were discussed, promises made, and expectations developed. The intensivist has no prior relationship with the patient but is aware that the need for life support, particularly mechanical ventilation, dramatically alters prognosis regardless of prior expectations. The intensivist perceives a chronic incurable illness with a low probability for survival and a high probability of prolonged dying. The potential for conflict is obvious.

Additional studies need to focus on identifying variables that accurately predict prognosis for cancer patients admitted to ICUs, but until more information is available, a solution to the above dilemma requires cooperation and mutual education. The intensivist must rely on the oncologist to provide an accurate prognostic estimate for the malignancy, concentrating on expected survival after ICU discharge. The oncologist must depend on the intensivist for an accurate prognostic estimate for the acute process and likelihood of ICU discharge. Only with accurate input from both parties can a reasonable and beneficial decision be reached.

CONCLUSION

In this and a previous chapter, we have attempted to present a dispassionate summary of the state of the art of outcome prediction. We have tried to show how a thorough knowledge of outcome prediction can not only facilitate communication with family and other professionals but also focus and improve the certainty of diagnostic and therapeutic maneuvers. In the past, many physicians who have attempted to incorporate outcome prediction into their practices have been frustrated by the sometimes conflicting nature of probability estimates and patient autonomy. However, the evolving societal healthcare debate will likely result in changes that will mandate more efficient healthcare and improved utilization of resources. A consensus on the concept of futility is also being developed, and such a consensus could have significant impact for the care of critically ill patients unlikely to survive their illness. These developments will only increase the importance of outcome prediction to critical care practice, and a thorough knowledge of both general and disease-specific outcome data will better prepare the intensivist for the future.

References

1. Sprung CL, Peduzzi PN, Shatney CH, et al: Veterans Administration Systemic Sepsis Cooperative Group: The impact of encephalopathy and physiologic derangements in the sepsis syndrome. Crit Care Med 1990; 18:801.

1a. Bastos PG, Sun X, Wagner DP, et al: Glasgow Coma Scale score in the evaluation of outcome in the intensive care unit: Findings from the Acute Physiology and Chronic Health Evaluation III Study. Crit Care Med 1993; 21:1459–1465.

2. Plum F, Posner JB: The Diagnosis of Stupor and Coma. 3rd ed. Philadelphia, FA Davis, 1982.
3. Shewman DA, DiGiorgio CM: Early prognosis in anoxic coma: Reliability and rationale. Neurol Clin 1989; 7:823–842.
4. Veatch R: The definition of death: Ethical, philosophical and policy confusion. Ann N Y Acad Sci 1978; 315:307.
5. Benzer A, Mitterschiffthaler G, Marosi M, et al: Prediction of non-survival after trauma: Innsbruck Coma Scale. Lancet 1991; 338:977–978.
6. Choi SC, Muizelaar JP, Barnes TY, et al: Prediction tree for severely head-injured patients. J Neurosurg 1991; 75:251–255.
7. Sazbon L, Groswasser Z: Outcome in 134 patients with prolonged posttraumatic unawareness. Part 1: Parameters determining late recovery of consciousness. J Neurosurg 1990; 72:75–80.
8. Groswasser Z, Sazbon L: Outcome in 134 patients with prolonged posttraumatic unawareness. Part 2: Functional outcome of 72 patients recovering consciousness. J Neurosurg 1990; 72:81–84.
9. Changaris DG, McGraw CP, Richardson JD, et al: Correlation of cerebral perfusion pressure and Glasgow Coma Scale to outcome. J Trauma 1987; 27:1007–1013.
10. Barelli A, Valente MR, Clemente A, et al: Serial multimodality-evoked potentials in severely head-injured patients: Diagnostic and prognostic implications. Crit Care Med 1991; 19:1374–1381.
11. Houlden DA, Li C, Schwartz ML, et al: Median nerve somatosensory evoked potentials and the Glasgow Coma Scale as predictors of outcome in comatose patients with head injuries. Neurosurgery 1990; 27:701–708.
12. Judson JA, Cant BR, Shaw NA: Early prediction of outcome from cerebral trauma by somatosensory evoked potentials. Crit Care Med 1990; 18:363–368.
13. Sazbon L, Fuchs C, Costeff H: Prognosis for recovery from prolonged post-traumatic unawareness: Logistic analysis. J Neurol Neurosurg Psychiatr 1991; 54:149–152.
14. Reinmuth OM, Vaagenes P, Abramson NS, et al: Predicting outcome after resuscitation from clinical death. Crit Care Med 1988; 16:1043–1052.
15. Maiese K, Caronna JJ: Coma following cardiac arrest: A review of the clinical features, management, and prognosis. J Intensive Care Med 1988; 3:153–163.
16. Bates D. Defining prognosis in medical coma. J Neurol Neurosurg Psychiatry 1991; 54:569–571.
17. Levy DE, Bates D, Caronna JJ, et al. Prognosis in nontraumatic coma. Ann Intern Med 1981; 94:293–301.

18. Bertini G, Margheri M, Giglioli C, et al: Prognostic significance of early clinical manifestations in postanoxic coma: A retrospective study of 58 patients resuscitated after prehospital cardiac arrest. Crit Care Med 1989; 17:627–633.
19. Longstreth WT, Inui TS, Cobb LA, et al: Neurologic recovery after out-of-hospital cardiac arrest. Ann Intern Med 1983; 98:588–592.
20. Longstreth WT, Diehr P, Inui TS: Prediction of awakening after out-of-hospital cardiac arrest. N Engl J Med 1983; 308:1378–1382.
21. Cerebral Resuscitation Study Group of the Belgian Society for Intensive Care: Predictive value of Glasgow coma score for awakening after out-of-hospital cardiac arrest. Lancet 1988; i:137–140.
22. Sacco RL, VanGool R, Mohr JP, et al: Nontraumatic coma: Glasgow coma score and coma etiology as predictors of 2-week outcome. Arch Neurol 1990; 47:1181–1184.
23. Krumholz A, Stern B, Weiss HD: Outcome from coma after cardiopulmonary resuscitation: Relation to seizures and myoclonus. Neurology 1988; 38:401–405.
24. Mueller-Jensen I, Neunzig HP, Emskotter T: Outcome prediction in comatose patients: Significance of reflex eye movements. J Neurol Neurosurg Psychiatry 1987; 50:389–392.
25. Austin EJ, Wilkus RJ, Longstreth WT: Etiology and prognosis of alpha coma. Neurology 1988; 38:773–777.
26. Alving J, Moller M, Sindrup E, et al: 'Alpha pattern coma' following cerebral anoxia. Electroencephalogr Clin Neurophysiol 1979; 47:95–101.
27. Ganes T, Lundar T: EEG and evoked potentials in comatose patients with severe brain damage. Electroencephalogr Clin Neurophysiol 1988; 69:6–13.
28. Rothstein TL, Thomas EM, Sumi SM: Predicting outcome in hypoxic-ischemic coma: A prospective clinical and electrophysiologic study. Electroencephalogr Clin Neurophysiol 1991; 79:101–107.
29. Falk RH: Physical and intellectual recovery following prolonged hypoxic coma. Postgrad Med J 1990; 66:384–386.
30. Brown J: The persistent vegetative state: Time for caution? Postgrad Med J 1990; 66:697–698.
31. Rosenberg GA, Johnson SF, Brenner RP: Recovery of cognition after prolonged vegetative state. Ann Neurol 1977; 2:167–168.
32. Shuttleworth E: Recovery to social and economic independence from prolonged postanoxic vegetative state. Neurology 1983; 33:372–374.
33. Bates D, Caronna JJ, Cartlidge NEF, et al: A prospective study of nontraumatic coma: Methods and results in 310 patients. Ann Neurol 1977; 2:211–220.
34. Paris JJ, Reardon FE: Moral, ethical, and legal issues in the intensive care unit. J Intensive Care Med 1991; 6:175–195.
35. Spenser SS: Code or no code: A non-legal opinion. N Engl J Med 1979; 300:138–141.
36. Lawler J: The ethical dilemma of resuscitation. The Lamp 1976; 33:27–28.
37. Emergency Cardiac Care Committee and Subcommitttees, American Heart Association: Guidelines for cardiopulmonary resuscitation and emergency cardiac care. JAMA 1992; 268:2282.
38. Bedell SE, Delbanco TL, Cook EF, et al: Survival after cardiopulmonary resuscitation in the hospital. N Engl J Med 1983; 309:569–576.
39. Roberts D, Landolfo K, Light RB, et al: Early predictors of mortality for hospitalized patients suffering cardiopulmonary arrest. Chest 1990; 97:413–419.
40. Kyff J, Puri VK, Raheja R, et al: Cardiopulmonary resuscitation in hospitalized patients: Continuing problems of decision-making. Crit Care Med 1987; 15:41–43.
41. Hollingsworth JH: The results of cardiopulmonary resuscitation: A 3-year university hospital experience. Ann Intern Med 1969; 71:459–466.
42. Scott RPF: Cardiopulmonary resuscitation in a teaching hospital: A survey of cardiac arrests occurring outside intensive care units and emergency rooms. Anaesthesia 1981; 36:526–530.
43. Peatfield RC, Taylor D, Sillett RW, et al: Survival after cardiac arrest in hospital. Lancet 1977; i:1223–1225.
44. Hershey CO, Fisher L: Why outcome of cardiopulmonary resuscitation in general wards is poor. Lancet 1982; i:31–34.
45. Tweed WA, Bristow G, Donen N, et al: Evaluation of hospital-based cardiac resuscitation, 1973–1977. Can Med Assoc J 1980; 122:301–304.
46. Castagna J, Weil MH, Shubin H: Factors determining survival in patients with cardiac arrest. Chest 1974; 65:527–529.
47. Suljaga-Pechtel K, Goldberg E, Strickon P, et al: Cardiopulmonary resuscitation in a hospitalized population: Prospective study of factors associated with outcome. Resuscitation 1984; 12:77–95.
47a. Schneider AP, Nelson DJ, Brown DD: In-hospital cardiopulmonary resuscitation: A 30-year review. J Am Board Fam Pract 1993; 6:91–101.
48. Landry FJ, Parker JM, Phillips, YY: Outcome of cardiopulmonary resuscitation in the intensive care setting. Arch Intern Med 1992; 152:2305–2308.
49. Raviglione MC, Battan R, Taranta A: Cardiopulmonary resuscitation in patients with the acquired immunodeficiency syndrome: A prospective study. Arch Intern Med 1988; 148:2602–2605.
50. Murphy DJ, Murray AM, Robinson BE, et al: Outcomes of cardiopulmonary resuscitation in the elderly. Ann Intern Med 1989; 111:199–205.
51. Zimmerman JE, Knaus WA, Sharpe SM, et al: The use and implications of do not resuscitate orders in intensive care units. JAMA 1986; 255:351–356.
52. Jayes RL, Zimmerman JE, Wagner DP, et al: Do not resuscitate order writing in intensive care units: Current practices and recent changes. JAMA 1993; 270:2213–2217.
52a. Parker JM, Landry FJ, Phillips YY: Use of do-not-resuscitate orders in an intensive care setting. Chest 1993; 104:1592–1596.
53. Stern SG, Orlowski JP: DNR or CPR: The choice is ours. Crit Care Med 1992; 20:1263.
54. Council on Ethical and Judicial Affairs: Guidelines for the appropriate use of Do-Not-Resuscitate orders. JAMA 1991; 265:1868–1871.
55. Blackhall LJ: Must we always use CPR? N Engl J Med 1987; 317:1281–1284.
56. Tomlinson T, Brody H: Ethics and communication in do-not-resuscitate orders. N Engl J Med 1988; 318:46.
57. Schein RMH, Fischl MA, Pitchenik AE, et al: ICU survival of patients with the acquired immunodeficiency syndrome. Crit Care Med 1986; 14:1026–1027.
58. Rosen MJ, Cucco RA, Teirstein AS: Outcome of intensive care in patients with the acquired immunodeficiency syndrome. J Intensive Care Med 1986; 1:55–60.
59. Smith RL, Levine SM, Lewis ML: Prognosis of patients with AIDS requiring intensive care. Chest 1989; 96:857–861.
60. Wachter RM, Luce JM, Turner J, et al: Intensive care of patients with the acquired immunodeficiency syndrome: Outcome and changing patterns of utilization. Am Rev Respir Dis 1986; 134:891–896.
61. Stover DE: Intensive care for AIDS victims: A new dilemma. J Intensive Care Med 1986; 1:4.
62. Luce JM, Wachter RM, Hopewell PC: Intensive care of patients with the acquired immunodeficiency syndrome: Time for a reassessment? Am Rev Respir Dis 1988; 137:1261–1263.
63. Lo B, Raffin TA, Cohen NH, et al: Ethical dilemmas about intensive care for patients with AIDS. Rev Infect Dis 1987; 9:1163–1167.
64. Sprung CL, Steinberg A: Acquired immunodeficiency syndrome and critical care. Crit Care Med 1990; 18:1300–1302.
65. Layon AJ, D'Amico R: Intensive care for patients with acquired immunodeficiency syndrome: Medicine versus ideology. Crit Care Med 1990; 18:1297–1299.
66. Wachter RM, Luce JM, Hearst N, et al: Decisions about resuscitation: Inequities among patients with different diseases but similar prognoses. Ann Intern Med 1989; 111:525–532.
67. Rogers PL, Lane C, Henderson DK, et al: Admission of AIDS patients to a medical intensive care unit: Causes and outcome. Crit Care Med 1989; 17:113–117.
68. Friedman Y, Franklin C, Rackow EC, et al: Improved survival in patients with AIDS, *Pneumocystis carinii* pneumonia, and severe respiratory failure. Chest 1989; 96:862–866.

69. Wachter RM, Russi MB, Bloch DA, et al: *Pneumocystis carinii* pneumonia and respiratory failure in AIDS: Improved outcomes and increased use of intensive care units. Am Rev Respir Dis 1991; 143:251–256.
70. El-Sadr W, Simberkoff MS: Survival and prognostic factors in severe *Pneumocystis carinii* pneumonia requiring mechanical ventilation. Am Rev Respir Dis 1988; 137:1264–1267.
71. Montaner JSG, Russell JA, Ruedy J, et al: Acute respiratory failure secondary to *Pneumocystis carinii* pneumonia in the acquired immunodeficiency syndrome: A potential role for systemic corticosteroids. Chest 1989; 95:881–884.
72. Efferen LS, Nadarajah D, Palat DS: Survival following mechanical ventilation for *Pneumocystis carinii* pneumonia in patients with the acquired immunodeficiency syndrome: A different perspective. Am J Med 1989; 87:401–404.
73. Wachter RM, Luce JM, Hopewell PC: Critical care of patients with AIDS. JAMA 1992; 267:541–547.
73a. Staikowsky F, Lafon B, Guidet B, et al: Mechanical ventilation for *Pneumocystis carinii* pneumonia in patients with the Acquired Immunodeficiency Syndrome: Is the prognosis really improved? Chest 1993; 104:756–762.
74. Gregg RW, Friedman BC, Williams JF, et al: Continuous positive airway pressure by face mask in *Pneumocystis carinii* pneumonia. Crit Care Med 1990; 18:21–24.
75. Janoff EN, Breiman RF, Daley CL, et al: Pneumococcal disease during HIV infection: Epidemiologic, clinical, and immunologic perspectives. Ann Intern Med 1992; 117:314–324.
76. Pesola GR, Charles A: Pneumococcal bacteremia with pneumonia: Mortality in acquired immunodeficiency syndrome. Chest 1992; 101:150.
77. Frieden TR, et al. The emergence of drug-resistant tuberculosis in New York City. N Engl J Med 1993; 328:521.
78. Benson CA, Spear J, Hines D, et al: Combined APACHE II score and serum lactate dehydrogenase as predictors of in-hospital mortality caused by first episode *Pneumocystis carinii* pneumonia in patients with acquired immunodeficiency syndrome. Am Rev Respir Dis 1991; 144:319–323.
79. Montaner JSG, Hawley PH, Ronco JJ, et al: Multisystem organ failure predicts mortality of ICU patients with acute respiratory failure secondary to AIDS-related PCP. Chest 1992; 102:1823–1828.
80. Rie MA: A further comment on acquired immunodeficiency syndrome. Crit Care Med 1992; 20:1361.
81. The ACCP/SCCM Consensus Conference Committee: Definitions for sepsis and organ failure and guidelines for the use of innovative therapies in sepsis. Chest 1992; 101:1644–1655.
82. Tilney NL, Bailey GL, Morgan AP: Sequential system failure after rupture of abdominal aortic aneurysms: An unsolved problem in postoperative care. Ann Surg 1973; 178:117.
83. Baue AE: Multiple, progressive, or sequential systems failure: A syndrome of the 1970s. Arch Surg 1973; 110:779.
84. Barton R, Cerra FB: The hypermetabolism multiple organ failure syndrome. Chest 1989; 96:1153.
85. Mainous MR, Deitch EA: Bacterial translocation and its potential role in the pathogenesis of multiple organ failure. J Intensive Care Med 1992; 7:101–108.
86. Fink MP: Why the GI tract is pivotal in trauma, sepsis, and MOF. J Crit Illness 1991; 6:253–276.
87. Bihari DJ, Tinker J: The therapeutic value of vasodilator prostaglandins in multiple organ failure associated with sepsis. Intensive Care Med 1988; 15:2–7.
88. Wilson GL: The impact of infection and multiple system organ failure syndrome on ICU outcome. Probl Crit Care 1989; 3:651–661.
89. Shen PF, Zhang S: Acute renal failure and multiple organ system failure. Arch Surg 1987; 122:1131.
90. Goris RJA, te Boekhorst TPA, Nuytinck JKS, et al: Multiple-organ failure: Generalized autodestructive inflammation? Arch Surg 1985; 120:1109.
91. Fry DE, Garrison RN, Williams HC: Patterns of morbidity and mortality in splenectomy for trauma. Ann Surg 1980; 46:28.
92. Fry DE, Pearlstein L, Fulton RL, et al: Multiple system organ failure: The role of uncontrolled infection. Arch Surg 1980; 115:136.
93. Knaus WA, Sun X, Nystrom PO, et al: Evaluation of definitions for sepsis. Chest 1992; 101:1656.
94. Knaus WA, Draper EA, Wagner DP, et al. Prognosis in acute organ-system failure. Ann Surg 1985; 202:685–693.
95. Knaus WA, Wagner DP: Multiple systems organ failure: Epidemiology and prognosis. Crit Care Clin 1989; 5:221–232.
96. Matuschak GM, Rinaldo JE: Organ interactions in the adult respiratory distress syndrome during sepsis: Role of the liver in host defense. Chest 1988; 94:400–406.
97. Pinsky MR, Matuschak GM: Multiple systems organ failure: Failure of host defense homeostasis. Crit Care Clin 1989; 5:199–220.
98. Knaus WA, Rauss A, Alperovitch A, et al: Do objective estimates of chances for survival influence decisions to withhold or withdraw treatment? Med Decis Making 1990; 10:163–171.
99. Child CG, Turcotte JG: Surgery and portal hypertension. *In:* The Liver and Portal Hypertension. Child CG (Ed). Philadelphia, WB Saunders, 1964, pp 50–64.
100. Pugh RNH, Murray-Lyon IM, Dawson JL, et al: Transection of the oesophagus in bleeding oesophageal varices. Br J Surg 1973; 60:648.
101. Conn HO: A peek at the Child-Turcotte classification. Hepatology 1981; 1:673.
102. Schlichting P, Christensen E, Anderson PK, et al: Prognostic factors in cirrhosis identified by Cox's regression model. Hepatology 1983; 3:889.
103. Christensen E, Schlichting P, Fauerholdt L, et al. Prognostic value of Child-Turcotte criteria in medically treated cirrhosis. Hepatology 1984; 4:430.
104. Saunders JB, Walters JRF, Davies P, et al: A 20-year prospective study of cirrhosis. Br Med J 1981; 282:263–266.
105. D'Amico G, Morabito A, Pagliaro L, et al: Survival and prognostic indicators in compensated and decompensated cirrhosis. Dig Dis Sci 1986; 31:468–475.
106. Orrego H, Blake JE, Blendis LM, et al: Prognosis of alcoholic cirrhosis in the presence and absence of alcoholic hepatitis. Gastroenterology 1987; 92:208–214.
107. Goldfarb G, Novel O, Poynard T, et al: Efficacy of respiratory assistance in cirrhotic patients with liver failure. Intensive Care Med 1983; 9:271.
108. Shellman RG, Fulkerson WJ, DeLong E, et al: Prognosis of patients with cirrhosis and chronic liver disease admitted to the medical intensive care unit. Crit Care Med 1988; 16:671–678.
109. Moreau R, Hadenague A, Soupison T, et al: Septic shock in patients with cirrhosis: Hemodynamic and metabolic characteristics and intensive care unit outcome. Crit Care Med 1992; 20:746–750.
110. Pinzani M, Zipser RD: The hepatorenal syndrome. Intensive Care Med 1987; 13:148.
111. Linas SL, Schaeffer JW, Moore EE, et al: Peritoneal venous shunt in the management of the hepatorenal syndrome. Kidney Int 1986; 30:736.
112. Murphy DJ, Knaus WA, Lynn J: Study population in SUPPORT: Patients (as defined by disease categories and mortality projections), surrogates, and physicians. J Clin Epidemiol 1990; 43:S11–S28.
113. Arora S, Kaplan MM: How to improve survival in fulminant hepatic failure. J Crit Illness 1991; 6:43–54.
114. O'Grady JG, Gimson AES, O'Brien CJ, et al: Controlled trials of charcoal hemoperfusion and prognostic factors in fulminant hepatic failure. Gastroenterology 1988; 94:1186–1192.
115. O'Grady JG, Graeme JMA, Hayaller K, et al: Early indicators of prognosis in fulminant hepatic failure. Gastroenterology 1989; 97:439–445.
116. Schapira DV, Studnicki J, Bradham DD, et al: Intensive care, survival, and expense of treating critically ill cancer patients. JAMA 1993; 269:783–786.
117. Turnbull A, Goldiner P, Silverman D, et al: The role of an intensive care unit in a cancer center: An analysis of 1035 critically ill patients treated for life-threatening complications. Cancer 1976; 37:82–84.
118. Hauser MJ, Tabak J, Baier H: Survival of patients with cancer in a medical critical care unit. Arch Intern Med 1982; 142:527–529.
119. Headley J, Theriault R, Smith TL: Independent validation of APACHE II severity of illness score for predicting mortality in

patients with breast cancer admitted to the intensive care unit. Cancer 1992; 70:497–503.
120. Snow RM, Miller WC, Rice DL, et al: Respiratory failure in cancer patients. JAMA 1979; 241:2039–2042.
121. Ewer MS, Ali MK, Atta MS, et al: Outcome of lung cancer patients requiring mechanical ventilation for pulmonary failure. JAMA 1986; 256:3364–3366.
122. Schuster DP, Marion JM: Precedents for meaningful recovery during treatment in a medical intensive care unit. Am J Med 1983; 75:402–408.
123. Peters SG, Meadows JA, Gracey DR: Outcome of respiratory failure in hematologic malignancy. Chest 1988; 94:99–102.
124. Estopa R, Marti AT, Kastanos N, et al: Acute respiratory failure in severe hematologic disorders. Crit Care Med 1984; 12:26–28.
125. Lloyd-Thomas AR, Wright I, Lister TA, et al: Prognosis of patients receiving intensive care for life-threatening medical complications of haematological malignancy. Br Med J 1988; 296:1025–1028.
126. Yau E, Rohatiner AZS, Lister TA, et al: Long-term prognosis and quality of life following intensive care for life-threatening complications of haematological malignancy. Br J Cancer 1991; 64:938–942.
127. Johnson MH, Gordon PW, Fitzgerald FT: Stratification of prognosis in granulocytopenic patients with hematologic malignancies using the APACHE II severity of illness score. Crit Care Med 1986; 14:693–697.
128. Poses RM, Bekes C, Copare FJ, et al: The answer to "What are my chances, Doctor?" depends on whom is asked: Prognostic disagreement and inaccuracy for critically ill patients. Crit Care Med 1989; 17:827–833.

CHAPTER 204

Critical Care Practice in the Era of Consumerism

Arthur H. Combs, MD, FCCM

The vocabulary of healthcare has become firmly centered around access, quality, and cost. *Access* clearly embraces supply and demand, whereas *quality* and *cost* are universally understood consumer concerns. We live and practice in the era of medical consumerism.[1]

Critical care has evolved rapidly into one of the ultimate consumer products: it is both high risk and high volume; it is extraordinarily expensive; every American is a potential and likely consumer; and it often involves literally life and death.

Nearly 6 million patients were treated in intensive care units (ICUs) in 1990 at a cost of 1% of the gross domestic product (GDP). Although accounting for only 8% of acute care hospital beds, ICUs generated 28% of acute care hospital costs, with 17% of all hospital patients spending some time in an ICU.[2] These data are not surprising because the principal causes of mortality in both adults and children are treated almost exclusively in a critical care setting.

The problem is not so simple as providing expensive care to a large number of patients while maintaining quality. The landmark cases of Karen Ann Quinlan and Nancy Cruzan have made it clear that life and death are not the only possibilities and that consumers desperately wish to control less desirable outcomes.[3] The paradox of contemporary critical care is that, although meaningful prolongation of life is not always possible, the postponement of death frequently is. Thus, "end-of-life" issues have moved increasingly to the forefront for both consumers and providers alike.

Control of the moments at the end of life is a pervasive issue in critical care—whether it be neonatal, pediatric, medical, surgical, or specialized; however, it is infrequently considered in advance by consumers. Numerous surveys concur that fewer than 20% of the elderly have completed an advance directive, despite the objective reality and imminent relevance of end-of-life issues for this population. People older than 65 years account for 58% of adult ICU admissions[4] but represent only 12.5% of the general population.

Although advance directives remain substantially underutilized, by law we have officially entered the age of patient self-determination. There are numerous obstacles to making this idealistic concept a practical reality. Some of the obstacles lie in the nature of the American consumer, who may run the full spectrum from "I want everything done" (even in hopeless cases) to "I never want to be kept alive on a machine" (even temporarily through a finite crisis). Other major impediments stem from the law's provision of mechanisms to make and enforce decisions without a program to educate the consumer—not about advance directives, but about the very issues and circumstances that they are trying to control.

To understand the elements that currently frustrate the optimization of access, cost, and quality in critical care, the nature of the product, the consumer, and the forces that govern their interaction must be examined.

THE PRODUCT

The many chapters of diverse content contained in this third edition of the *Textbook of Critical Care* define the science, sociology, and practice of critical care. The remarkable advances in critical care practice have brought with them a series of new issues as significant improvements in practice advance from capability to expectation and even to a perceived general "right." Cardiopulmonary resuscitation (CPR), introduced by Kouwenhoven and coworkers in 1960,[4a] soon became the only medical procedure that required a physician's order for it *not* to be performed. Although the merits of CPR in certain settings are well established (see Chapter 202), studies have shown that it is of no benefit, and may even be harmful, to some groups of patients. Nonetheless, in the state of New York, for example, a physician may only write a do-not-resuscitate order with the patient's or his or her surrogate's permission. In some situations, a concurring physician and witness may be required. It is easy to see how unrealistic consumer expectations, stimulated by the medical industry itself, are likely to grow and even evolve into a series of perceived civil rights.

Resources

Prior to 1992, little organized information about critical care resources in the United States was available. In 1984, Greenbaum provided important insight into the size, capability, and staffing of ICUs.[5] Because his study was published before subspecialty recognition and certification, it is likely that the shape of critical care has changed significantly in the years that followed. In 1992, Groeger and associates (see Chapter 1)[6] reported the results of a Task Force of the Society of Critical Care Medicine (SCCM) that conducted an extensive survey of all American Hospital Association hospitals with at least one ICU. Their description was based on 40% of such hospitals (4233), representing 32,850 ICU beds

TABLE 204–1. Desirable Characteristics of Critical Care Units and Unit Staff

Characteristic	%
Unit contains all potentially beneficial technology.	9.6
Unit has a full-time medical director.	39.0
Medical director is CCM certified.	44.1
Staff registered nurses are AACN certified.	20.1
Unit has an assigned respiratory therapist.	48.0
Admission and discharge and triage conflicts are resolved by the medical director or the CCM attending physician.	48.0

(Data from Groeger JS, Guntupalli KK, Strosberg MA, et al: Descriptive analysis of critical care units in the United States: Patient characteristics and intensive care unit utilization. Crit Care Med 1992; 20:846.)

Abbreviations: CCM = Critical Care Medicine; AACN = American Association of Critical Care Nurses.

and 25,871 patients from 2876 units in 1706 institutions. These data relate a great deal of information about the quantity and quality of the critical care resources available to American consumers.

Table 204–1, adapted from the study of Groeger and associates,[6] shows a wide disparity in the characteristics that most would agree describe an adequate ICU. The table suggests that less than half of ICUs meet relatively permissive criteria.[7] The unexpected occurrence of critical illness or injury finds individuals unprepared and unable to "shop" for the unit most appropriate to his or her needs. After admission, insufficient opportunity often exists for the individual and family to have a partnership role with physicians and nurses to exert their own autonomy.

Access, cost, and quality are inextricably woven together in an ICU. Inappropriate admissions imply poor quality. Unnecessary costs are experienced, and beds are denied to patients who might benefit from the specialized care available. Critical care professionals must work together to ensure the general availability of high quality care. The *Agenda for the 1990s* attempts to formalize the goals for such an undertaking.[2]

THE CONSUMER

The consumer of critical care has no specific identifying characteristics. Eighty per cent of all Americans experience the need for critical care at some time in their lives, either as a patient or as a family member. The experience is usually unanticipated and unplanned. The issues raised by life-threatening illness or injury cut squarely to the heart of an individual's personal values and rights. Because the issues are frequently matters of life and death, and because the decisions frequently involve loved ones, opinions and values are often vehemently expressed. The courts become involved because of the intensity and ambiguity of the issues, but, as with individuals, legal precedent is not consistent.

The United States and most other developed nations are societies of individuals governed by laws designed to empower and protect the rights of each member of those societies. Also, deliberate protection of dissenting minority opinions is provided for. The concept of informed consent is rooted in the patient's autonomy to accept or reject proposed treatments. One person's desire for critical care and life support may be quite different from that of another under remarkably similar circumstances.

Numerous surveys of public opinion and in various specific cohorts have tried to elucidate the desires of consumers. After a survey of more than 500 primary care outpatients and members of the general public, Emanuel and colleagues[8] concluded that about 70% of people would decide against life-sustaining treatments if they were incompetent and had a poor prognosis. These data have meaning as information about consumer preferences but have no potential to guide policy, since they imply that 30% of people would want critical care even under what others consider the worst of circumstances.

Frankl and coworkers[9] surveyed life-support preferences of 200 inpatients admitted to the general medical service of a major medical center. Their results indicate that the percentage of consumers who would want life support is 90% if they could be restored to health; 30% if they could not care for themselves; 16% if their condition were hopeless; and 6% if they would remain in a persistent vegetative state. The implications of these data would be profound if they were confirmed for the entire population. More than 6 million people are treated each year in ICUs. Thus, the 10% who do not desire critical care under the best conditions (restoration to health) would represent a loss of 600,000 productive lives each year. The 6% who would request critical care even though they were in a persistent vegetative state could represent 360,000 ICU beds occupied indefinitely on an annual basis. The reported cost of Nancy Cruzan's care for the period she was in a persistent vegetative state (tube feedings, no mechanical ventilation) was $112,000 per year.[10] The implications for access and cost are obvious.

The data from Groeger and associates and the SCCM Task Force[4] indicate that nationally, bed occupancy in ICUs averages 87% of available beds. Seventeen per cent of the patients have been in the ICUs for longer than 14 days, and 49% of all units report having at least one chronic (>14-day length of stay) patient. The number of chronic patients averages 2.2 in the smallest of hospitals and increases to 21 in hospitals with more than 500 beds. Unavailability of a lower acuity bed is the largest single reason for inability to transfer ICU patients appropriately, but between 8.6% and 20.3% of units, depending on type, cite "other" reasons that include patient, family, or physician unwillingness and medicolegal concerns.[4] These phenomena seem not to be the result of recent technologic advances nor of a major shift in consumer sentiment. A comparison of Medicare expenditures for the last year of life between 1976 and 1988 indicates that the per cent of the total budget spent on decedents fluctuated between 27.2% and 30.6%, and that payments for care in the last 60 days of life remained constant at 52% of the payments for the entire last year.[11] The authors concluded that persons in the last year of life do not account for a larger share of Medicare expenditures than in the past.

Frankl and coworkers[9] concluded that patients base their preferences for life support on perceived outcomes. What basic information forms the basis for consumer perceptions likely varies considerably from person to person, and what other influences affect these perceptions, especially in the absence of objective information, are unknown. A singular or small number of anecdotal experiences, which may not have been first-hand, often represent the consumer's only frame of reference. However, it is clear that if the consumer exercises his or her individual rights in the fashion and proportions indicated by published surveys, "consumer perception" is one of the most powerful forces shaping the issues of access, cost, and quality in critical care.

THE FOUNDATION FOR CRITICAL CARE

The Foundation for Critical Care was conceived and founded in the early 1980s by the leadership of SCCM. In collaboration with the American Association of Critical Care

Nurses, it focused in its early years on family support, the waiting room experience, and general heightening of public awareness of critical care. In recent years, the Foundation has sharpened its focus and redirected its mission toward consumer advocacy.

In 1992, the Foundation gathered preliminary data from elderly consumers regarding their knowledge base, experiences, and preferences with respect to critical care issues. The cohort of 224 respondents represented 70 elderly persons who were interviewed in person and 154 who returned surveys included in educational materials that they had requested from the Foundation. The data, although adequate only to serve as rationale for a much larger and statistically based effort, should be viewed in the context of three characteristics: respondents were all of retirement age (those who represent the largest group of critical care consumers); respondents were highly motivated consumers who had read an article about critical care, written to request educational materials, and received and completed a survey; and 85.4% of respondents had either been critical care patients or family members of one, validating the statistic that 80% of Americans experience critical care in their lifetimes.

Table 204–2 represents selected survey data grouped to emphasize the challenges to public education and consumer advocacy. The results also reveal the nature of American consumers who may desire treatment that they either know little about or believe to be infrequently successful. For example, 77% indicated that they knew what "CPR" means, whereas only 26% knew what "DNR" means. Thirty-five per cent believed that CPR is usually successful, whereas 84% wanted CPR for themselves at least under some circumstances. Similar apparent contradictions exist regarding attitudes toward respirator use and critical care in general.

When viewed as a consumer product, the individual's experience of critical care, either as a patient or as a family member, may well be as important in shaping consumer perception as pure outcome. The Foundation's survey found that 96% believe that the patient is not the only one who suffers, 44% believe that ICUs are frightening places, and fewer than 30% believe that being in a waiting room is a positive experience. Regardless of outcome, it is possible for the consumer to have a negative experience that then forms the basis for consumer perception and its ramifications.

THE PATIENT SELF-DETERMINATION ACT OF 1990

The Patient Self-Determination Act (PSDA) went into effect December 1, 1991.[12] The law was designed to increase patients' involvement in decisions regarding life-sustaining treatments, to ensure that advance directives would be available at the time such decisions were made, and to inform those who had not prepared such documents of their legal right to do so.[10] The law requires healthcare providers in hospitals and other settings to (1) ask all new patients whether they have prepared an advance directive and include this information in the chart, (2) give patients written information about the institution's policies concerning advance directives and about the patients' right to prepare them in accordance with the law, and (3) develop written policies and educational programs about advance directives for staff and the community. These stipulations of the PSDA are necessary conditions for Medicare and Medicaid reimbursement to care providers.

Before the effective date of the PSDA, between 4% and 17.5% of adults had prepared an advance directive.[13] At the same time, approximately 25% of Americans had prepared an ordinary will.[14] It has been observed that in the absence of a written will, applicable statutes ordinarily accomplish a decedent's wishes, distribute property and assets to his or her spouse and children, and at least are unlikely to do a great disservice to an individual's unstated wishes.[15] The same cannot be said regarding critical care decisions in the absence of an advance directive; thus, in the wake of the *Cruzan* decision, both impetus for increased use of advance directives[8, 10] and expectations for the impact of the PSDA have been heightened.

Even before the PSDA went into effect, its content and stipulations were extensively critiqued.[8, 13, 16] Anticipated limits of its effectiveness included (1) no mandate for physician involvement in the discussion of advance directives, leaving this task to others; (2) reliance on inpatient facilities; (3) no encouragement for advance directives to be prepared before decisions regarding hospitalization or long-term care arise (except for those enrolled in health maintenance organizations); (4) inability to discuss issues in a meaningful way because of illness (similar limitations may exist on admission to a nursing home); and (5) the absence of specific funding to implement the PSDA.[10] The SCCM has also filed suggestions for amendment to the final rule to enhance portability of advance directives, to prevent advance directive policies from creating "anti-dumping" conflicts, and to broaden the scope to include certain outpatient settings such as same-day surgery and ambulatory dialysis units, which serve particularly vulnerable patient populations.[17]

The number of people formalizing advance directives remains small, and many small studies have been undertaken to test strategies for increasing utilization. Numerous obsta-

TABLE 204–2. Foundation for Critical Care Survey of Elderly Consumers*

Consumer Beliefs or Desires	*Yes (%)*	*No (%)*	*Don't Know (%)*
Understand what critical care is	85	8	7
ICUs are frightening places	44	41	15
Being in a waiting room is a positive experience	30	40	30
Knew who was in charge of ICU	37	43	20
Never want to be in an ICU	9	81	10
Know the meaning of CPR	77	10	13
Know the meaning of do-not-resuscitate orders	26	53	21
Think CPR is usually successful in the hospital	35	21	45
Never want CPR	16	74	10
Know what a respirator is	95	1	4
Think there is a good chance of recovery on a respirator	38	30	32
Never want to be on a respirator	16	66	18
Have discussed wishes with family	69	28	4
Have discussed wishes with physician	25	69	6

*Results reported as a percentage of all respondents and grouped to illustrate inconsistencies in both knowledge and opinion.

cles have been identified; these fall under three general categories: (1) lack of knowledge about advance directives and the issues they embrace; (2) patient-related behavior; and (3) physician-related behavior. Although simple procrastination has been cited as a prevalent untoward patient behavior,[18, 19] the main behavioral obstacle has been reticence on the part of both patients and physicians to initiate discussions about end-of-life issues, life support, and advance directives.[20–22]

The PSDA encourages and empowers people to formulate advance directives. The decisions involved are nonetheless profound and likely to be difficult. Writing an advance directive should represent the culmination of a process that begins with the gathering of objective information, the formulation of reasonable expectations for certain scenarios, and the blending of those expectations with personal values. Although this hypothesis has not been tested directly, two studies examining interventions that provided only information about advance directives per se showed no increase in the number of advance directives written after the interventions.[18, 19] In another study, elderly persons were presented with outcome data pertaining to CPR that resulted in a change in expressed preferences in three of five hypothetical scenarios.[23]

Specific concerns have been raised over the implementation of the PSDA, focusing on how and by whom a person is informed of their rights. The impact of the law would likely be neutralized if an admissions clerk executed the procedure in a manner similar to recitation of the *Miranda* rights. Most authors advocate physician involvement, particularly in the primary care outpatient setting.

The most serious concern raised, however, is not related to failure to prepare advance directives but rather that they will not be honored in detail or even ignored. Danis and colleagues[24] prospectively studied 126 mentally competent nursing home residents and the surrogates of an additional 49 incompetent patients for a 2-year period. They observed 96 outcome events that in 24 cases were inconsistent with written advance directives in the patients' records. They concluded that advance directives may be ineffective as much as 25% of the time, and that some providers may give higher priority to other considerations than to patient autonomy. Careful reading of the study indicates that inconsistency between advance directives and the patients' care resulted at times because patients and family members changed their minds and because some physician interventions were made in a spirit of beneficence.

The PSDA is strongly supported by the SCCM, the Foundation for Critical Care, and critical care practitioners. The issues of life support, its appropriateness, and the rights and wishes of patients and their families are considered daily in every ICU in the land. Improved access, reduced cost, better quality, and improved provider-patient relationships could be achieved if more patients were able to consider life-support issues before their need was evident and if their expressed directive were regularly honored.

THE CONSUMER'S INFLUENCE ON CONSUMPTION OF SERVICES

McGinnis and Foege have reviewed actual causes of death in the United States.[25] They found that for 1990, half of all deaths could be attributed to factors that are external (nongenetic) and that owe largely to consumer behavior. The use of tobacco, alcohol, drugs and firearms; diet and activity patterns; motor vehicle safety; sexual behavior; and other factors are all potentially controllable consumer characteristics. The most common causes of death—cardiovascular disease, cancer, trauma, chronic obstructive pulmonary disease, pneumonia, acquired immunodeficiency syndrome, and others—are major critical care concerns potentially altered by changes in consumer behavior. The implications for coronary artery disease, chronic obstructive pulmonary disease, and trauma are obvious, whereas the impact of the 1 million unintentional teenage pregnancies annually is unknown with regard to the number of low-birth-weight infants, congenital anomalies, and other neonatal and pediatric critical care concerns.

Fries and coworkers[26] have suggested that healthcare costs can be substantially reduced by interventions that reduce the need and demand for services. They document many instances of cost savings accruing to both prevention and alteration in consumer behavior. Their review indicates that the programs that educate the consumer about self-management and appropriate use of services and that raise consumer confidence in healthcare decision making are the most effective. Such programs have the double benefit of reducing cost through reduction in demand, and of improved well-being for the individual.

Carlon and associates have shown that the majority of critical care services are consumed by the minority of patients who do not survive their hospitalization.[27] In this population of predominantly cancer patients, two thirds of all Therapeutic Intervention Scoring System (TISS) points accrued to the 46% of ICU patients who did not leave the hospital alive. In a community general hospital, a similar pattern was documented, with 50% of all TISS points accounted for by the 30% who died in the hospital.[28] These studies emphasize several points. First, although the TISS points represent interventions per se, they nonetheless extrapolate to the issues of access, cost, and quality. The interventions themselves imply time and effort, consumption of resources, bed occupancy, and the suffering of patients and families alike, all of which are then added to the effect of a negative outcome. Second, the degree to which these data are consumer driven is not yet known, but the many cases that enter litigation indicate that it may be substantial. Third, patients in ICUs need to be re-evaluated, and adjustments to their care made. As prognoses change, appropriate limitation of further interventions or even withdrawal of therapies, including life support, may be the most humane as well as the most cost-effective care plan. Finally, consumption of the majority of resources by the minority of patients who ultimately die must represent a system error for which the consumer, the physician, or the communication between them is responsible. Proper ICU management must take these data into account if the trend is to be reversed, resources appropriately allocated to potential survivors, and the consumer guided toward decisions that are not ultimately self-defeating.

THE INFLUENCE OF PROVIDERS

The benefits of trained critical care physicians serving as managers and practitioners have already been reviewed. It has also been noted that they are far from ubiquitous in currently operating ICUs. Moreover, more than 90% of units are "open," with physicians other than those with critical care training having the ability to admit and guide management for patients.[6]

Many studies have documented the reluctance of practitioners outside of the critical care environment to discuss advance directives, CPR, and "code status."[20] Additionally, physician attitudes regarding end-of-life issues in general and CPR in particular have been found to be influenced more by their personal feelings than by the results of published studies.[20] These personal responses and attitudes persist regardless of level of training or experience.[29, 30] It has also been shown that the value placed on critical care services by physicians bears no correlation with that of involved patients and families.[31] Greco and Eisenberg have recently reviewed the merits of various strategies for changing physicians' practices and their considerable resistance.[32]

Many reviews have offered information and guidance for all physicians dealing with end-of-life issues[1, 33] and specific critical care physician concerns.[34, 35] Formal guidelines have been formulated by the SCCM Ethics Task Force for the most difficult issue of foregoing life support.[35] The enhanced visibility and topicality of these issues in recent years are just beginning to have measurable effects. A review by Jayes and colleagues has shown both greater and earlier implementation of do-not-resuscitate orders in ICUs, which they attribute to greater knowledge of outcomes and greater dialogue about the issues among both families and physicians.[36]

The physician community is not homogeneous nor uniformly informed about the PSDA and related issues. Neither does it view its responsibilities for improving the delivery of critical care in a cohesive way. The position of some emergency physicians, for example, is that the emergency department is not the place for implementation of institutional obligations under the PSDA.[37] Such a position must be viewed in a context that considers that almost half of all ICU admissions enter the hospital through the emergency department and that virtually all patients who are resuscitated, intubated, or receiving vasopressors will be admitted to an ICU whether or not the intervention or critical care is desired by the patients. Such ICU admissions, regardless of appropriateness, have an immediate impact on access to and cost for the unit and present the more problematic issues of withdrawal of life support versus the humane withholding of such intervention in accordance with the patient's wishes.

THE INFLUENCE OF LAW

The nature of some state laws such as those of Missouri and New York ironically create precisely the kind of undesirable conditions for consumers—in the guise of protecting their autonomy—that most would avoid if their wishes were known.[38] Illinois has passed a healthcare surrogate law in the aftermath of the Samuel Linares incident, in which a father disconnected his 15-month-old son from a respirator at gunpoint. Others have advanced healthcare proxy laws to help overcome the limitations of the living will statutes that currently exist in more than 40 states.[39] These also have limitations, including that they represent yet another set of forms for the consumer to complete.

The PSDA has not been in effect long enough for its impact to be measured. However, there does not appear to be measurable change in either consumer behavior or in the utilization of advance directives.[40] Schneiderman and associates have also found no impact on medical treatment or costs in a randomized trial of the effects of applying advance directives.[41] In an indirect way, these disappointing observations support the hypothesis that the consumer will unlikely embrace his empowerment under the PSDA and that advance directives created at this time will not have the desired effects because fundamental information, such as outcome data, is not being provided to the consumer—information that either emphasizes the importance of the issues or that serves as a basis for realistic expectations and thus constructive advance directives.

The PSDA has the potential to fulfill its intention of protecting patient autonomy in healthcare decisions. The law is currently far from being optimally implemented and thus continues to have limited impact. The courts cannot determine the disposition of every patient in a persistent vegetative state, nor could consistency be expected if they did; and no federal or state law will have the salutary effect that an informed consumer, a well-trained critical care physician, and a properly managed ICU can have when operating in concert.

CONCLUSIONS AND RECOMMENDATIONS

The issues of access, cost, and quality are in sharp focus in critical care. In order that they be optimized, critical care physicians should be encouraged to do the following:

1. Support the SCCM paradigm of the well-trained critical care physician and encourage full-time, coordinated, collaborative unit management by credentialed medical and nursing directors.
2. Participate in healthcare reform to ensure that critical care is properly considered in basic benefits packages and that accountable health partnerships foster appropriate critical care management.
3. Support efforts to regionalize critical care for major trauma and the most intensive and expensive technologies (such as extracorporeal membrane oxygenation) while working to upgrade both the standard and the consistency of critical care in community hospitals.
4. Support the Foundation for Critical Care in its efforts to educate consumers about critical care and to help them plan effectively for an ICU experience.
5. Support the optimal implementation of the PSDA in their own institutions by taking part in consumer and professional education, developing hospital policies, and participating in the hospital's ethics committee.
6. Develop a unit environment that fosters humane caring for both patients and families, facilitates communication among all caregivers and consumers, and is founded on realism and patient advocacy.

Relman has defined good, cost-effective medical care as "the care provided by a competent and compassionate physician who has no incentive to do more or less than is judged appropriate in each case."[42] Critical care physicians can realistically approach this paradigm in the delivery of critical care. In the era of medical consumerism, it is required that they embrace their roles in political process, hospital policy, unit management, ethics committees, public and professional education, patient advocacy, and family support with the same passion that has achieved such substantial success at the bedside of the critically ill and injured.

ACKNOWLEDGMENT

Special acknowledgment and gratitude are extended to Louise Matthews, MD (anticipated 1995, Georgetown University School of Medicine), Kathryn McIntire, MD, and Debralynn Zickafoose, MD, for their scholarship, research assistance, and dedication to the mission of the Foundation for Critical Care.

References

1. Ruark JE, Raffin TA, et al: Initiating and withdrawing life support. N Engl J Med 1988; 318:25.
2. Coalition for Critical Care Excellence: Critical care blueprint for the future. Anaheim, CA, Society of Critical Care Medicine, 1992.

3. Pearlman RA, Cain KC, Patrick DL, et al: Insights pertaining to patient assessments of states worse than death. J Clin Ethics 1993; 4:33.
4. Groeger JS, Guntupalli KK, Strosberg MA, et al: Descriptive analysis of critical care units in the United States: Patient characteristics and intensive care unit utilization. Crit Care Med 1992; 20:846.
4a. Kouwenhoven WB, Jude JR, Knickerbocker GG: Closed chest cardiac massage. JAMA 1960; 173:1064.
5. Greenbaum DM: Availability of critical care personnel, facilities, and services in the United States. Crit Care Med 1984; 12:1073.
6. Groeger JS, Strosberg MA, Halpern NA, et al: Descriptive analysis of critical care units in the United States: Patient characteristics and intensive care unit utilization. Crit Care Med 1992; 20:846.
7. Ayres SM, Combs AH: A tale of two intensive care units? All intensive care units are not the same! Crit Care Med 1992; 20:727.
8. Emanuel LL, Barry MJ, Stoeckle JD, et al: Advance directives for medical care: A case for greater use. N Engl J Med 1991; 324:889.
9. Frankl D, Oye RK, Bellamy PE: Attitudes of hospitalized patients toward life support: A survey of 200 medical inpatients. Am J Med 1989; 86:645.
10. Greco PJ, Schulman KA, Lavizzo-Mourey R, et al: The patient self-determination act and the future of advance directives. Ann Intern Med 1991; 115:639.
11. Lubitz JD, Riley GF: Trends in Medicare payments in the last year of life. N Engl J Med 1993; 328:1092.
12. Omnibus Budget Reconciliation Act of 1990. Public Law No. 101–508.
13. La Puma J, Orentlicher D, Moss RJ: Advance directives on admission: Clinical implications and analysis of the Patient Self-Determination Act of 1990. JAMA 1991; 266:402.
14. Rowland M: "Tackling the dreaded w-word." The New York Times, November 11, 1990, Section 3, p 17.
15. Menikoff JA, Sachs GA, Siegler M: Beyond advance directives: Healthcare surrogate laws. N Engl J Med 1992; 327:1165.
16. Wolf SM, Boyle P, Callahan D, et al: Sources of concern about the patient self-determination act. N Engl J Med 1991; 325:1666.
17. Cerra FB, Hyman AI: BPD-718-IFC: Interim final rule on advance directives. Personal communication to the Honorable William Toby by the Society of Critical Care Medicine, May 1992.
18. Sachs GA, Stocking CB, Miles SH: Empowerment of the older patient? A randomized, controlled trial to increase discussion and use of advance directives. J Am Geriatr Soc 1992; 40:269.
19. High DM: Advance directives and the elderly: A study of intervention strategies to increase use. Gerontologist 1993; 33:342.
20. Brunetti LL, Carperos SD, Westlund RE: Physicians' attitudes towards living wills and cardiopulmonary resuscitation. J Gen Intern Med 1991; 6:323.
21. Kinsella TD, Stocking CB: Failed communication about life-support therapy: Silent physicians and mute patients. Am J Med 1989; 86:643.
22. Joos SK, Reuler JB, Powell JL, et al: Outpatients' attitudes and understanding regarding living wills. J Gen Intern Med 1993; 8:259.
23. Schonwetter RS, Walker RM, Kramer DR, et al: Resuscitation decision making in the elderly: The value of outcome data. J Gen Intern Med 1993; 8:295.
24. Danis M, Southerland LI, Garrett JM, et al: A prospective study of advance directives for life-sustaining care. N Engl J Med 1991; 324:882–888.
25. McGinnis JM, Foege WH: Actual causes of death in the United States. JAMA 1993; 270:2207.
26. Fries JF, Koop CE, Beadle CE, et al: Reducing health care costs by reducing the need and demand for medical services. N Engl J Med 1993; 329:321.
27. Carlon GC, Turnbull AD, Howland WS: Intensive care of the cancer patient. *In:* Textbook of Critical Care. 2nd ed. Shoemaker WC, Ayres SM, Grenvik A, et al (Eds). Philadelphia, WB Saunders, 1989, pp 944–945.
28. Ruona D, Combs AH: Prediction of outcome for patients with critical illness using the therapeutic intervention scoring system (Abstract). *In:* Critical Care Knows No Borders. American Association of Critical Care Nurses, 1988, p 211.
29. Varon J, Combs AH: Resuscitation desires of physicians at various levels of training (Abstract). Chest 1992; 102 (Suppl):S150.
30. Varon J, Fromm RE, Combs AH, et al: Discrepancy in resuscitation beliefs among physicians at various levels of training. Am J Emerg Med 1993; 11:290.
31. Danis M, Gerrity MS, Southerland LI, et al: A comparison of patient, family, and physician assessments of the value of medical intensive care. Crit Care Med 1988; 16:594.
32. Greco PJ, Eisenberg JM: Changing physicians' practices. N Engl J Med 1993; 329:1271.
33. Wanzer SH, Federman DD, Adelstein SJ, et al: The physicians responsibility toward hopelessly ill patients. N Engl J Med 1989; 320:844.
34. Troug RD: Triage in the ICU. Hastings Center Report, May–June 1992, pp 13–17.
35. Task Force on Ethics of the Society of Critical Care Medicine: Consensus report on the ethics of foregoing life-sustaining treatments in the critically ill. Crit Care Med 1990; 18:1435.
36. Jayes RL, Zimmerman JE, Wagner DP, et al: Do-not-resuscitate orders in intensive care units: Current practices and recent changes. JAMA 1993; 270:2213.
37. Rosen P: "Let the emergency department do it": A simple solution to a complex problem (Editorial). J Emerg Med 1991; 9:75.
38. Belkin L: "New York rule compounds dilemma over life support." New York Times, May 12, 1992, p A1.
39. Annas GJ: The health care proxy and the living will. N Engl J Med 1991; 324:1210.
40. Emanuel L: Advance directives: What have we learned so far? J Clin Ethics 1993; 4:8.
41. Schneiderman LJ, Kronick R, Kaplan RM, et al: Effects of offering advance directives on medical treatments and costs. Ann Intern Med 1992; 117:599.
42. Relman AS: Controlling costs by "managed competition": Would it work? (Editorial). N Engl J Med 1993; 328:133.

CHAPTER 205

The Ethics of Resource Allocation in the Intensive Care Unit

Stephen M. Ayres, MD • Karen N. Swisher, MS, JD

Many physicians, particularly intensivists, are intuitively compelled to ration scarce resources on a daily basis. The demand for well-staffed and well-equipped intensive care unit (ICU) beds frequently exceeds the local supply, and physicians must provide ICU care for some, knowing that they may in the process deny care to others who might benefit from that care. Using only their professional knowledge and a sense of equity, intensivists regularly decide whether to admit one more patient to a crowded ICU, transfer a patient to a less well-staffed unit in favor of one who shows greater promise of benefiting from ICU treatment, or transfer a patient who now shows little chance of benefit from ICU treatment.[1] Although ethicists, attorneys, and others worry about the legal and ethical bases for rationing care, intensivists practice rationing of ICU resources regularly. Since these patients are seriously ill, the reason for rationing is almost always based on the scarcity of resources rather than on the insurance status of the patients.

Strauss and coworkers,[2] in a 1986 study entitled "Rationing of Intensive Care Unit Services: An Every Day Occurrence," analyzed admission decision making in an 18-bed general ICU in a hospital associated with a medical school. Admission decisions were made by two specified physicians, the senior surgical resident and senior medical resident assigned to the unit. A statistically significant inverse correlation existed between bed availability and the age and severity of illness among those admitted to the unit. Patients admitted when beds were scarce were significantly sicker than those admitted when beds were plentiful! No significant differences were observed in the percentage of patients intubated, the ICU death rate, and the total length of stay in the hospital after ICU discharge. Discharges from the unit were 3.4 times more likely when no empty beds were available compared with when five empty beds were available. In economic terms, admission to the ICU was elastic in relation to bed availability.

Medical directors of special care units and other physicians are increasingly asked to make administrative decisions, such as determining the appropriateness of the admission of one patient over another to an ICU bed. Continuing pressures from regulators, administrators, and third-party payers will intensify the need for physicians as well as other clinical professionals to make decisions about the cost effectiveness of diagnostic and treatment procedures.[3] Many hospitals have decentralized their administrative and management functions, creating more opportunities for clinician-managers. Hospitals are placing greater responsibility upon clinicians in a number of ways: through reorganization, so that allocation decisions are delegated to front-line health professionals; in the creation of programs to provide cost information to physicians and other health professional decision-makers; and by changing physician behavior through utilization management programs that attempt to improve their efficiency and effectiveness.[4] Physicians assigned to these new roles are frequently poorly prepared for the ethical consequences of such resource allocation decisions. They are traditionally trained to be advocates for individual patients, and their frame of reference emphasizes patient and professional autonomy. Frequently, their insistence on individual patient needs comes into conflict with the financial needs of the institution.

Hiller[5] has provided a useful description of the physicians' dilemma by classifying the levels of their ethical conflicts. *Microlevel conflicts* are those that involve individual or professional values; *mesolevel conflicts* are those that involve institutional values; and *macrolevel conflicts* are those that involve community or cultural values. Physicians asked to make meso- or macrolevel decisions often feel that such considerations inevitably compromise the traditional doctor-patient relationship. Physicians perceive conflict between their role as clinicians and their role as advocates for the hospital. On a personal level, physician conflicts may include (1) expectations by hospital administration of actions that are incongruent with the orientations and values of the individual physician; (2) time overloading, if various role expectations exceed the available times and resources; and (3) role ambiguity, if information regarding the scope of responsibilities or the expectations of others are uncertain.[6] Administrators and clinicians must realize the potential role conflict experienced by those clinicians who now must make allocation choices. They can never hope to achieve a sound policy that purports to enhance quality of patient care in a time of resource limitation. Manager-physicians must broaden their ethical perspective and training to include the implications of their actions. Clinical ethical training has only a limited role to play here. In 1984, Hiller[5] noted that no comprehensive framework existed in the literature for the study of ethics in healthcare administration. Hospital administrators themselves are frequently poorly trained in business ethics and can offer little guidance to clinicians embarking upon a new career.

The demand for increased rationality in the matching of available resources to patients' need requires increased communication, understanding, and integration of clinical and business ethics among all healthcare professionals.

ALLOCATION, RATIONING, AND THE BUSINESS OF HEALTHCARE

Healthcare services have never been considered a basic American right. Instead, healthcare is considered to be a commodity that is, just like any other commodity, allocated and rationed through the marketplace. Services are available to those who can afford healthcare; those who cannot afford it frequently go without. The long-delayed move to healthcare reform has been fueled in large part by the belief held by many Americans that it is unfair and unjust to link access to healthcare to socioeconomic status.

Important distinctions between allocation and rationing can be made. *Allocation* decisions determine to what extent a society devotes its resources to a particular service. Funding levels for Medicare and Medicaid in the United States or those for national health systems in other countries are examples of "macro" allocation policies. Conversely, *rationing* is usually a "micro" level issue because decisions are made as to who receives resources for a particular purpose. Through rationing, a society decides who gets a particular heart transplant and who can go on dialysis. Obviously, allocation decisions affect rationing decisions; the almost universal availability of hemodialysis through Medicare reduces the need for rationing decisions. Federal and state allocation decisions, in turn, have a major impact on the strategic planning of hospitals and other healthcare organizations. The more resources allocated for a given clinical problem, the more profitable it is to provide such services. Hospitals attempt to increase their market share of reimbursed services by vigorously promoting their programs in transplantation or cardiac surgery but not for poorly reimbursed services such as treatments for multiple injury.

The implicitly accepted idea that the intensivist serves as the agent of rationing suggests that some agreed-upon definition of the word "rationing" itself exists. The definition espoused by the Catholic Health Association is "the withholding of potentially beneficial healthcare services because practices and policies establish limits on the resources available for healthcare."[7] A contrasting definition is "not all care expected to be beneficial is provided to all patients." The Catholic Health Association definition clearly indicates that it is the issue of "potential benefit" that determines whether the limitation of certain services is actually rationing. The patients discharged earlier from the intensive care unit studied by Strauss and coworkers[2] apparently did not experience rationing because there was no evidence of unfavorable outcome after they were transferred. Although ethicists may set rules for rationing, by this definition, only physicians can define the potential benefit of an intervention and know, therefore, whether rationing has actually occurred.

Henry J. Aaron, the Brookings Institution scholar who wrote *The Painful Prescription: Rationing Hospital Care* with William Schwartz in 1984, has an even more limiting definition of rationing. He believes that rationing can only be said to exist when the limited activity is known to be beneficial and is not available to individuals even if they could pay for it.[8]

A major emotional distinction exists between statistical and identifiable lives when rationing is under consideration.

Governments and insurers make decisions whether to pay for a specific procedure on the basis of population statistics and the number of lives that might be spared or lost as a result of these decisions. In contrast, when a particular child who requires organ transplantation dies while his or her family is trying to raise funds for the procedure, the child becomes a very identifiable individual. Furrow has pointed out that,

> *It is a commonplace that society will expend almost limitless resources to save the identifiable life, but is willing to sacrifice statistical lives at a much lower cost. The more overtly and explicitly a government is responsible, the more difficulty the government will face in saying no, in refusing to provide the resource necessary to save a life or to relieve suffering. This distinction is related to the preceding one, in that allocation decisions usually affect statistical lives—rationing, identifiable lives.*[9]

Healthcare reform is shifting rationing and allocation decisions from the marketplace to the political arena. Such a shift has great impact on the legal system. Once government makes eligibility for a specific procedure conditional, litigation inevitably increases as individuals are given the right to appeal conditional decisions. Healthcare reform will almost certainly create much more litigation in the healthcare industry than has been seen under the present system, in which most legal action is related to the allegation of medical malpractice.

THE IMPACT OF THE LEGAL SYSTEM ON ALLOCATION AND RATIONING

Physicians and hospitals are gravely concerned about the rising frequency and severity of medical malpractice claims. Physicians are held to a standard of care for all patients. How well the courts will consider and incorporate the realities of rationing and allocation into these decisions is not clear at this time. Physicians rightly fear that the limitation of ICU beds at any given moment will not be fully understood by the courts when a particular physician is forced to deny a particular patient access to one of these beds.

This issue was tested in the Maryland courts in 1993, when a 3-year-old child with a long history of complex seizure disorders that were often life threatening required urgent admission to a hospital. The protocol for the emergency medical service used by the family required that the child be transported to the nearest hospital, where he would be stabilized and then transferred to Johns Hopkins Hospital for further treatment. The doctors at Johns Hopkins Hospital, in cooperation with the child's parents, developed a new protocol that would allow the child to be transported directly to the hospital, even though the child was not stable. The physician treating the child wrote a letter in 1991 describing the procedure and stating that "it would be better to transport the child directly to the Hopkins Pediatric Emergency Room with advance warning by radio to the emergency room and pediatric neurology. There are always risks in transporting a seizing child, but I feel that they are in this case justified. These risks have been explained to the parents who understand and support this decision. . . ." In 1992, the child began seizing and was taken by ambulance to the designated helicopter for transportation. During transport, the ambulance called Johns Hopkins Hospital to inform physicians there of the child's impending arrival. The call was transferred directly to the staff of the pediatric ICU which replied that they could not admit the child because the unit was on "fly-by" status (i.e., new patients were not to be accepted because of staff and facilities shortages). Following hospital policy, the resident stated that the child should be taken to the nearest hospital or to Children's Hospital in Washington, D.C., only 6 minutes farther away. The father of the child refused and insisted that the child go to Johns Hopkins Hospital. The Johns Hopkins physicians then conferred briefly about the possibility of creating a place for the child. They agreed that the director of the pediatric ICU, who alone had the authority to suspend the fly-by status, should be called at her home. That physician reaffirmed that the child should be taken to Children's Hospital. Again the father demanded that the child be brought to Johns Hopkins. The unit director then stated, "Tell them to come on, I guess; I don't know what else to do; there's refusal to go to Children's Hospital." Immediately thereafter, that physician spoke to the charge nurse and determined which of the 11 children in the unit could be moved out of the unit with the least risk. One child was transferred out of the pediatric ICU, and the convulsing child was moved in. He was stabilized but suffered permanent brain damage in the course of his seizures. The parents sued the hospital, alleging that the 5- to 10-minute delay occasioned by the initial refusal to accept the child caused the damage. The court ruled on behalf of the hospital, stating that "a hospital is under no duty to accept a person with an emergency condition where there are no facilities available to treat the person properly. A hospital cannot be placed in the position where the admission of an additional patient will jeopardize the care of its existing patients." The hospital won its case, in large part owing to a well-established hospital policy regarding fly-by status and to an elaboration of the responsibility of the pediatric ICU director in making exceptions to the policy.[10]

In another legal case, H. Tristam Engelhardt, an ethicist, and Michael Rie, a physician,[1] discussed the ethical and legal consequences of inadvertent and perhaps inept rationing of scarce resources to a patient already in an ICU bed. They describe a $13 million court award to the survivors of Susan Von Stetina, a previously healthy 27-year-old woman who was accidently disconnected from a respirator. She had been injured in an automobile accident and suffered a fracture of the right femur and complete transsection of the pancreas. She developed the respiratory distress syndrome on the fourth day after trauma and was intubated, placed on a mechanical ventilator, and pharmacologically paralyzed to permit control of ventilation. She was successfully resuscitated after ventilation was restored but never regained consciousness because of chronic anoxic brain injury. She made a complete recovery from her traumatic injuries.

The court, in reaching its verdict, was influenced by evidence that only three nurses were available for the care of seven patients, even though the patient required the full attention of one nurse. Evidence presented at the trial indicated that one patient in the unit almost met the criteria for brain death and died 36 hours later. Two patients were to be electively discharged the next morning. In addition, three other hospitals in the community probably were better staffed at the moment and could have provided care for the patient. However, neither a medical director nor an administrative policy for dealing with census/staff relationships was available to address triage or transfer issues. If the facts in this case were those presented at trial, it certainly appeared that a breakdown occurred in the implicit or explicit rationing of scarce resources on the basis of expected benefit to be realized by ICU treatment.

These two cases, the outcome of one for and that of the other against the hospital, demonstrate the need for published policies that provide prescribed rules for making allocation and rationing decisions. Physicians can only be required to provide the standard of care that is appropriate under the circumstances, and sometimes under-staffing, fly-by status, or the need to triage patients for limited ICU beds requires physicians to refuse to admit patients to their unit. The development of criteria for admission is important but controversial. Most physicians would agree that the likelihood of potential benefit should guide such decision making, but issues of patient desire, sex, income, age, preexisting illness, and social worth frequently make it almost impossible for them to develop universally acceptable criteria.

THEORIES OF JUSTICE

Although physicians make clinical decisions based on the ethical concepts of patient autonomy, nonmaleficence, beneficence, and confidentiality, management decisions regarding allocation and rationing are heavily premised on theories of distributive justice. This principle states that benefits and burdens should be distributed equitably, that resources should be allocated fairly, and that one should act in such a manner that no one person or group bears a disproportionate share of benefits or burdens. Physicians frequently wonder whether it is morally right to prioritize patient admissions based on some criterion such as potential benefit. Ethicists Arras and Rhoden[11] point out that such judgments frequently lead to a win-lose framework and ignore the moral impact of the decision on each patient involved:

> *. . . Relativism, if taken seriously, has the odd implication that all moral reflection and deliberation are in fact quite irrelevant. Take the all-too-frequent medical dilemma concerning whether it would be wrong to terminate the life of a patient who is slowly and painfully dying. Ethical relativism would not have us search for a solution based upon consideration of mercy nor would it ask us what we would do if we were in the patient's place. Rather, it would seem that ethical relativism would have us consult a sociologist, for our dilemma could only be resolved by discovering the prevailing societal attitudes. In turn, this points to another difficulty with ethical relativism, namely, that often there is no prevailing attitude. . . . But we don't take this split as an indication that there is no right or wrong in these matters; rather we take it as an indication that, for the moment at least, we don't know what is right and what is wrong in these cases.*[11]

Many formulations of rationing draw heavily on the concept of justice put forth by John Rawls in his many writings and in his comprehensive work, *A Theory of Justice.*[12] Rawls begins by discussing "justice as fairness" and suggests that "society is well-ordered when it is not only designed to advance the good of its members but when it is also regulated by a public conception of justice." He points out that most people agree with the need for a general code of justice but frequently disagree over what principles should determine the assignment of "basic rights and duties" and "the proper distribution of the benefits and burdens of social cooperation." Since part of the disagreement over the distribution of societal goods is based on each individual's position in society, Rawls suggests that such decisions be made behind a "veil of ignorance," when one does not know whether he will become rich or poor, healthy or ill. This concept must be:

> *. . . understood as a purely hypothetical situation characterized so as to lead to a certain conception of justice. Among the essential features of this situation is that no one knows his place in society, his class position, or social status, nor does anyone know his fortune in the distribution of natural assets and abilities, his intelligence, strength, and the like. . . . The principles of justice are chosen behind a veil of ignorance. This insures that no one is advantaged or disadvantaged in the choice of principles by the outcome of natural chance or the contingency of social circumstances. Since all are similarly situated and no one is able to design principles to favor his particular condition, the principles of justice are the result of a fair agreement or bargain* (p 12).[12]

Rawls goes on to suggest that these principles of justice be embodied in a social contract between the body politic and the social institution or country. He rejects classic utilitarianism, which suggests that "society is rightly ordered and therefore just, when its major institutions are arranged so as to achieve the greatest net balance of satisfaction summed over all the individuals belonging to it." This suggests that some members of a group are forced to make sacrifices for others in order to maximize the success of the whole. Whereas this may be a useful concept in times of national struggle, it does not fit Rawls' idea of justice as fairness. He summarizes his views in two principles of justice:

> 1. Each person is to have an equal right to the most extensive basic liberty compatible with a similar liberty for others.
>
> 2. Social and economic inequalities are to be arranged so that they are both (a) reasonably expected to be to everyone's advantage and (b) attached to positions and offices open to all (p 60).[12]

Rawls repeatedly rejects the utilitarian views that disadvantages in power or income of one group may be tolerated if they are outweighed by the advantages of another. Instead, he insists that "social and economic inequalities, for example inequalities of wealth and authority, are just only if they result in compensating benefits for everyone, and in particular for the least advantaged members of society (p 14)."[12] Rawls' interpretation of justice as fairness is based on "Kant's notion of autonomy" and his "idea that moral principles are the objects of rational choice." It is little wonder, therefore, that Kantian ethical theories have achieved predominance in the field of bioethics.

APPLIED JUSTICE IN HEALTHCARE POLICY

Norman Daniels in his provocatively entitled book, *Just Health Care,*[13] suggests that Rawls' approach to justice as fairness may be applied to healthcare by claiming that such care, like education, is necessary to ensure equality of opportunity. One of us (SMA)[14] has argued that healthcare should be distributed on the basis of need and that its use be limited "to those who could benefit from it." In this view, either underutilization or overutilization is wrong. Daniels accepts this "functional" approach to the distribution of healthcare, but points out that the existence of significant "need" itself is not morally sufficient because it does not explain why the need for healthcare is different from any other human preference or need.

Daniels points out that each individual's genetic make-up provides him or her with a "normal opportunity range." It is considered "morally acceptable that there are winners and losers, even in races where the prize is a share of important social goods, provided the race is *fair* to all participants." Disease and disability reduce the range of available opportunities, and measures that reverse or moderate these disadvantages can be morally justified because they help provide a more "level playing field." However, society cannot provide every healthcare service that an individual might like; thus, agreement on what are *essential* healthcare services is necessary. He summarizes his view of the opportunity principle:

> *I urge the fair equality of opportunity principle as an appropriate principle to govern macro decisions about the design of our health care system. Such a principle defines, from the perspective of justice, what the moral* function *of the health care system must be—to help guarantee fair equality of opportunity.*[13]

THE PRESIDENT'S COMMISSION FOR THE STUDY OF ETHICAL PROBLEMS

As the United States and other countries embark on the road of major healthcare reform, a full national debate on access to such care and related issues is necessary. The federal government has regularly advanced such debates over a wide range of issues in healthcare by establishing national interdisciplinary commissions to marshall the facts and arguments that relate to each issue and often to make recommendations for governmental action. The ethical problems of unequal access to healthcare have concerned most of the nations of this world. A 1932 report of the national Committee on the Costs of Medical Care pointed out that "many persons do not receive service which is adequate either in quantity or quality, and the costs of service are inequably distributed. The result is a tremendous amount of preventable physical pain and mental anguish, needless deaths, economic inefficiency, and social waste."[15] A half century later, in 1974, the President's Commission for the Study of Ethical Problems in Medicine and Biomedical and Behavioral Research was created; the Commission completed its work in 1978.[16] In addition to making recommendations, the Commission concluded that equity in healthcare can only be realized by providing an adequate level of care for all Americans. It is not surprising for readers to see analogies between the President's Commission's requirement for adequate levels of care for all Americans as an example of John Rawls' interpretation of a social contract:

> *Understanding equitable access to health care to mean that everyone should be able to secure an adequate level of care has several strengths. Because an adequate level of care may be less than "all beneficial care" and because it does not require that all needs be satisfied, it acknowledges the need for setting priorities within health care and signals a clear recognition that society's resources are limited and that there are other goods besides health care. Thus, interpreting equity as access to adequate care does not generate an open-ended obligation. One of the chief dangers of interpretations of equity that require virtually unlimited resources is that they encourage the view that equitable access is an impossible ideal. Defining equity as an adequate level of care for all avoids an impossible commitment of resources without falling into the opposite error of abandoning the enterprise of seeking to ensure that health care is in fact available for everyone.*[16]

The Commission's letter to the President and to the leaders of Congress stated that "In examining the special nature of health care, we discern in our country's traditional commitment to fairness an ethical obligation on the part of society to ensure that all Americans have access to an adequate level of health care without the imposition of excessive burdens."

Thus, the President's Commission appears to support rationing (the withholding of potentially beneficial care) for certain individuals on the grounds that certain kinds of beneficial care do not need to be provided for everyone because they exceed the definition of what is adequate. There is a clear suggestion in the report that the kind of care that may be ethically denied is care that is too expensive and therefore cannot be provided from public resources for economic reasons.

The final paper in the appendix to the President's report is a fascinating discussion entitled, "Health care and the 'deserving poor' " by George Sher of the University of Vermont.[17] Because intensivists frequently care for injured drunken drivers and gunshot wound victims who are involved in criminal activity, Sher's discussion is quite relevant. He begins by recalling that "the idea that some poor persons deserve to be helped while others do not has long been influential in this country" and that "the blameworthy poor—the paupers were relegated to poorhouses," whereas the "blind, the deaf-mute and other blameless classes of the poor were helped in much less humiliating ways." The fact that some people are believed to be poor because of their own actions and that others become ill because of drinking, smoking, reckless driving, inappropriate sexual activity, or other risky behavior makes it attractive to create a class of "undeserving poor" or "undeserving ill" who might be excluded from governmentally funded healthcare services. Although people should expect their "desserts," he doubts whether American society is ready to withhold care from those who have squandered their ability to obtain health insurance because it seems "inhumane, and indeed indecent, to let someone suffer or die for lack of easily available care." Even the undeserving poor should have access to the "adequate" care proposed by the President's Commission.

Although many of these recommendations will surely be considered by the Clinton administration, the President's Commission of 1974 is not without its limitations. Daniel Callahan[18] criticized the Commission as limiting itself to a description of the rights and privileges of individuals exercising their individual autonomy but failed entirely to provide procedures or mechanisms for how such autonomous choices should be made. He states:

> *We have gone through an important era that has established many new rights and privileges in the face of the power and potency of biomedicine. We have been told that we are autonomous and can make free choices—that autonomy is a key ingredient in the thread of consensus that runs through the reports of the President's Commission. In the next stage, we must begin work on the content of that freedom. For it is here that consensus will most desperately be needed; otherwise, the newly gained freedoms will turn out to be either empty or dangerous.*[18]

State governments, perhaps, have made more significant progress toward consensus on bioethical issues, particularly those dealing with allocation of medical resources, than has the federal government. A year after the President's Commission completed its report, the state of New York developed its own Task Force on Law and Life. This task force has released several comprehensive reports. Although other states have followed New York's lead in developing interdisciplinary commissions, Oregon is perhaps best known for its attempt to actually implement rationing of care to its poorest citizens.

In the early 1990s, the state of Oregon decided to limit Medicaid costs by rank-ordering 709 diagnosis-treatment pairs out of the more than 10,000 diagnoses. The pairs were ranked by estimates of net benefit, but the cutoff was arbitrarily placed at the 587th pair based on the state's budgeted amount for Medicaid expenditures. No consideration was given to the intensity or appropriateness of care for each individual. This is what some—but not all—would consider rationing. State employees and other insured people could receive whatever their physicians believed to be necessary, whereas Medicaid recipients were limited to whatever the state could afford. Oregon leaders soon realized the important difference between statistical lives and individuals' lives as public outcry subjected the state government to what some might call "symbolic blackmail." The impetus for formal healthcare rationing arose from the shifting of funding from organ transplantation to comprehensive prenatal care. In 1987, one child—Coby Howard—was turned into a "national martyr" when attempts to collect donations for a needed bone marrow transplant failed and he died. In 1990, a chastened Oregon restored Medicaid funding for organ transplants. The Oregon plan to ration healthcare for the poor but not the affluent ran into considerable opposition on both political and moral grounds. It uses an arbitrary ranking system to redistribute healthcare resources among the poor. Current Medicaid recipients receive less care, the uninsured poor receive more care, and the insured continue to receive their same level of benefits. The Bush administration declined to support the Oregon plan on the basis of noncompliance with the Americans with Disabilities Act of 1990. Interestingly, it was the requirement for a treatment to return an individual to "asymptomatic" life that caused the greatest concern. An asymptomatic existence suggested a quality of life test, and the Clinton Administration insisted on its removal before it granted the necessary waiver.

Fox and Leichter, writing in the summer of 1993, concluded their report by suggesting that:

Three lessons emerge from the Oregon experience. The first is that citizen participation is a politically and legally flawed strategy to gain widespread acceptance for innovative reform. The second is that specificity (the infamous "List") can become a political albatross. No state has emulated the list or seems likely to do so soon. . . . The final lesson of Oregon is ironic. Oregon lawmakers backed into defining a minimum basic package of services. In so doing, they showed that it is possible to design and implement a plan that puts a floor of coverage under everyone in the state.[19]

In 1993, a federal court maintained that Medicaid had to fund all children in need of transplants, thus adding unanticipated millions into state Medicaid budgets. It is anticipated that litigation for patient rights of access to federal programs will only increase during healthcare reform.

In an article entitled, "Why a two-tier system is morally unavoidable," Engelhardt probably spoke for many others when he congratulated the authors of the Oregon plan and suggested that it

. . . provides a heuristic (philosophic jargon for "method") for resolving the public policy challenge. The creation of a basic adequate package through communal funds can be regarded as a prudent act of self-insurance, as a limited act of solidarity with others, or as a limited act of altruism. These and probably other reasons and goals will motivate citizens to create a basic package whose secular authority will be derived from a communal decision. The existence of a private luxury tier, supported through private insurance and direct out-of-pocket payments, represents a recognition of the limits of communal authority to define the proper ways in which justice and fairness ought to be achieved; the right of individuals to deploy their private resources and energies as they wish, once they have discharged their limited civic duties; and the diversity of human values with regard to health, disease, health care, and the avoidance of risks.[20]

THEORIES OF JUSTICE AND THE PRACTICE OF CRITICAL CARE MEDICINE

Theories of justice are most useful in making meso- and macro-ethical decisions but have limitations when clinician managers are faced with the decision as to whether to admit the individual with a myocardial infarction and unstable blood pressure or the gunshot victim to the last monitored bed in the ICU. These physicians are making distributive decisions, and such decisions are almost always based on the chances of clinical benefit to the patient. If survival rates appear to be similar, physicians usually start considering the patients' preexisting health status, their age, and the likelihood of full restoration of health.

In recent years, attempts have been made to measure health status in order to better understand the allocation of resources. Conceptions of good health vary from person to person, and Kaplan and Bush[21] at the University of California at San Diego have attempted to quantify levels of health or well-being. Their general health policy model includes mortality and quality of life and may be expressed as a continuum, using arbitrary values. The quality of life measure may then be modified by the likelihood of serious illness and its successful treatment and multiplied by the estimated years of remaining life to arrive at an estimate of "quality-adjusted life-years." Engelhardt and Rie,[1] in discussing the Von Stetina case, suggested using the potential benefit of a treatment (P), the quality of life expected (Q), and the remaining length of life (L) divided by the cost (C) to develop an "ICU treatment entitlement index (ICU-EI)":

$$\text{ICU-EI} = \frac{PQL}{C}$$

Preparing for the inevitable criticism over the use of such a mathematical analysis, Engelhardt and Rie concluded that "The point remains that some calculation of an index for treatment is better than no such calculation. Only through such an index, however informally drawn, will one be able to provide a basis for creating a society-endorsed and implementable policy regarding the use of scarce resources in general, and ICU resources in particular."[1] Consistent with their belief that a two-tier system is morally unavoidable, they also argue that the ICU-EI could be specified for government-guaranteed health policy contracts and that the affluent could be permitted to purchase a lower level of permissible ICU-EI.

JUSTICE AND COST

The concept of "health," to use the jargon of the economist, is clearly elastic. The Rand Health Insurance Study estimated that 80% of the general population has no dysfunction, but that 88% of the population will report symptoms at any time. Since the presence of symptoms leads to physician intervention, it is essential to distinguish between the "ill" and the "worried well." The total cost to the nation of all healthcare is dependent on how much care is given to those without serious illness as well as to the 20% of Americans who are ill. It could, for example, cost the nation far more to treat headaches with aspirin than to perform heart, kidney, lung, and bone marrow transplantations on relatively few patients. Thus, total cost is "elastic" to the perception of medical need and the cost of medical intervention, but the usual market expectation of demand driving down cost almost never occurs. The perverse incentives of fee-for-service practice, which have rewarded physicians for satisfying the desires of patients for increasing amounts of "magic," high-technology care, have prevented them from doing what is "right." Little has been written, in a market-organized economy, to emphasize how much the competition to perform expensive and presumably useful techniques has raised the cost of healthcare. If it is morally necessary to calculate the numerator of Engelhardt and Rie's equation[1] (PQL), is it not also morally necessary to define appropriate cost?

Analysis of the prevalence of coronary artery bypass surgery demonstrates how the proliferation of technology-rich tertiary care has increased the cost of medical care while probably decreasing its quality. In 1986, 702 hospitals performed bypass surgery; only one third of them performed more than 100 procedures. Both mortality rates and medical costs were substantially lower in those hospitals that performed more than 100 procedures. By 1993, 827 hospitals in the United States were performing bypass surgery. Los Angeles County alone had 37 "open heart centers," as they became called, but many of these only did a few operations. A survey of American hospitals revealed almost nine cardiac surgical units for every trauma unit, presumably because the payment system favors care for heart disease over trauma care. In the mid-1980s, Luft and associates[22] and Showstack and colleagues[23] began to study the results of certain surgical operations and discovered that the results of some operations depended on how often a surgeon actually performed surgery. Luft found substantially higher death rates for hospitals that performed fewer than 200 bypass operations compared with those that performed more. Whereas practice seems to make perfect, results also appeared to differ among surgeons. A careful study conducted by the Northern New England Cardiovascular Disease Study Group[24] showed that even when the severity of a patient's condition was taken into consideration, the mortality rates for individual surgeons ranged from about 2% to greater than 9%!

TOWARD AN ETHIC FOR RESOURCE ALLOCATION

The frustrations experienced by intensivists charged with the allocation of a fixed number of ICU beds are similar to those of many other clinician-managers. Lemieux-Charles[25] attempted to deal with these issues through a series of focus groups held at the University of Toronto. Twenty-eight clinician-managers were asked to discuss what they perceived to be the ethical issues affecting their daily practice. These issues were then classified by Hiller's taxonomy.[5] Microlevel issues dealt with the conflicts between their moral obligation to provide high-quality care and the interest of the institution in cost containment. They pointed to conflicts between physician payment incentives and institutional objectives, and to their own interpersonal conflicts regarding the various roles they were asked to assume. Macrolevel issues included determining priorities for care, conflicts between standards of individual health professions, conflict between clinicians and clinician-managers, relationship of unit activities to the hospital's mission, and the equitable allocation of resources throughout the hospital. They identified the needs of the community versus the needs of the hospital as their major macrolevel issue.

Lemieux-Charles' observations[25] have important implications for healthcare organizations and their professionals. She suggests that "(1) organizational approaches that aim to control expenditures and improve quality of care will be more successful if both roles and their obligations are treated as separate but related problems; (2) Ethical considerations should be acknowledged early in the development of any process of institutional change and considered regularly as part of a hospital's strategic planning, implementation, and evaluation of such changes; (3) Role expectations and the obligations they create should be the subject of both informal and formal hospital discussions within the institution; (4) Mechanisms for orientation and education should be developed at all hospitals to address conflicts experienced by individuals as well as those in working groups or treatment teams."

It is important for institutional interdisciplinary committees to create written policies regarding major rationing and allocation choices. Such policies should specify not only who makes such decisions but also the criteria on which these decisions are based. These policies should become part of the medical standard of care, thereby decreasing liability for physicians and hospitals that follow such policies. The role of hospital ethics committees should be extended from its traditional emphasis on individual patient care decisions to one that analyzes the way that institutions respond to the complex moral issues that they regularly encounter. The stakes in allocation ethics are high, and, to the most practical extent possible, such policies should be published and debated within the population served by the hospital. Objective information is critical to resource allocation and to decision making on the part of both health professionals and their patients. Only when accurate assessments of the outcomes of treatment on the duration and quality of subsequent life are available will it be possible to allow society to adopt the morally appealing principle of providing potentially beneficial care to all who require it.

The relationships among access to care, cost of such care, and appropriate levels of care for any given population should be freely debated by the public. Cost issues cannot be ignored, of course, and common sense would always dictate a less expensive approach if the same outcome could be achieved. Reducing cost and increasing the precision of medical decision making will permit society to adopt the morally appealing principle of providing potentially beneficial care to all who require it. Institutional ethics committees need to address the ethical dilemmas that they face as part of their business planning, as well as clinical ethical dilemmas. Finally, academic institutions training hospital administrators and clinicians must include training in allocation ethics into their curricula. The substantial benefits anticipated in the "brave new world" of healthcare reform will only be realized if structural change is accompanied by broad interdisciplinary training of the individuals who are expected to perform expanded roles that extend far beyond the traditional health professional–patient relationship.

References

1. Engelhardt HT, Rie MA: Intensive care units, scarce resources, and conflicting principles of justice. JAMA 1986; 255:1159–1164.
2. Strauss MJ, LoGerfo JP, Yeltazie JA, et al: Rationing of intensive care unit services: An every day occurrence. JAMA 1986; 255:1143–1146.
3. Begun JW, Lippincott RC: Strategic Adaptation in the Health Professions: Meeting the Challenges of Change. San Francisco, Jossey-Bass, 1993.
4. Leatt P, Vayda E, Williams JI: Medical Staff Organization in Canadian Hospitals. Unpublished research report prepared for the Social Sciences and Humanities Council of Canada, Toronto, 1987.
5. Hiller MD: Ethics and health care administration: Issues in education and practice. J Health Admin Educ 1984; 2:148–192.
6. Ruelas E, Leatt P: The roles of physician-executives in hospitals: A framework for management education. J Health Admin Educ 1985; 3:151–169.
7. With Justice For All? The Ethics of Healthcare Rationing. St. Louis, Catholic Health Association of the United States, 1991.
8. Aaron HJ: The Oregon experiment. *In*: Rationing America's Medical Care: The Oregon Plan and Beyond. Strosberg MA, Wiener JM, Baker R, et al (Eds.). Washington, DC, Brookings Institution, 1992, p 107.
9. Furrow BR, Johnson SH, Jost TS, et al: Bioethics: Health Care Law & Ethics. St. Paul, West, 1991.
10. *Davis v Johns Hopkins Hospital,* 622 A2d 128 (Md 1993).
11. Arras J, Rhoden N: Ethical Issues in Modern Medicine. 3rd ed. Mountain View, CA, Mayfield, 1989, pp 6–28.
12. Rawls J: A Theory of Justice. Cambridge, Belknap Press, 1971, pp 3–60.
13. Daniels N: Just Health Care. Cambridge, Cambridge University Press, 1985, pp 37–41.
14. Ayres S: Rationality, not rationing in health care. *In*: Rationing America's Medical Care: The Oregon Plan and Beyond. Strosberg MA, Wiener JM, Baker R, et al (Eds). Washington, DC, Brookings Institution, 1992, p 136.
15. Committee on the Costs of Medical Care: Medical Care for the American People. Washington, DC, Department of Health, Education, and Welfare, 1932, publication No. 28. New York, Arno Press, 1972 (reprinted).
16. President's Commission for the Study of Ethical Problems in Medicine and Biomedical and Behavioral Research: Securing Access to Health Care. Vol 1. Washington, DC, US Government Printing Office, publication No. 83-600501, 1983, p 20.
17. Sher G: Health care and the "deserving poor." *In*: Securing Access to Health Care. Vol 2. President's Commission for the Study of Ethical Problems in Medicine and Biomedical and

Behavioral Research. Washington, DC, US Government Printing Office, publication No. 82-600637, 1983, pp 293–301.
18. Callahan D: Morality and contemporary culture: The President's Commission and beyond. Cardozo Leg Rev 1984; 6:347.
19. Fox DM, Leichter HM: The ups and downs of Oregon's rationing plan. Health Aff (Millwood) 1993; 12:66–70.
20. Engelhardt R: Why a two-tier system of health care delivery is morally unavoidable. *In*: Rationing America's Medical Care: The Oregon Plan and Beyond. Strosberg MA, Wiener JM, Baker R, et al (Eds). Washington, DC, Brookings Institution, 1992, p 197.
21. Kaplan RM, Bush JW: Health-related quality of life measurement for evaluation research and policy analysis. Health Psychol 1982; 1:61–80.
22. Luft HS, Bunker J, Enthoven A: Should operations be regionalized? The empirical relationship between surgical volume and mortality. N Engl J Med 1979; 301:1364.
23. Showstack JA, Rosenfeld DW, Garnick DW, et al: Association of volume with outcomes of coronary artery bypass graft survival: Scheduled versus non-scheduled operations. JAMA 1987, 257:785.
24. O'Connor GT, Plume SK, Olmstead EM, et al: A regional prospective study of in-hospital mortality associated with coronary artery by-pass grafting. JAMA 1991; 266:803–809.
25. Lemieux-Charles L, Meslin EM, Aird C, et al: Ethical issues faced by clinician/managers in resource-allocation decisions. Hosp Health Serv Admin 1993; 38:267.

INDEX

Note: Page numbers in *italics* refer to illustrations; page numbers followed by t refer to tables.